Mandell, Douglas and Bennett's

Principles and Practice of
INFECTIOUS DISEASES

FOURTH EDITION

Edited by

GERALD L. MANDELL, M.D.

Professor of Medicine
Owen R. Cheatham Professor of the Sciences
Chief, Division of Infectious Diseases
University of Virginia Health Sciences Center
Charlottesville, Virginia

JOHN E. BENNETT, M.D.

Head, Clinical Mycology Section
Laboratory of Clinical Investigation
National Institute of Allergy and Infectious Diseases
National Institutes of Health
Bethesda, Maryland

RAPHAEL DOLIN, M.D.

Charles A. Dewey Professor of Medicine
Chair, Department of Medicine
University of Rochester School of Medicine and Dentistry
Rochester, New York

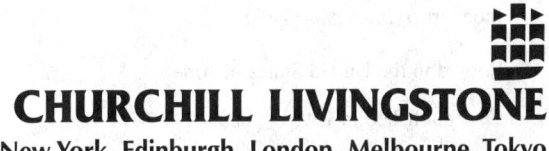

CHURCHILL LIVINGSTONE
New York, Edinburgh, London, Melbourne, Tokyo

Library of Congress Cataloging-in-Publication Data

Mandell, Douglas and Bennett's principles and practice of infectious
    diseases / edited by Gerald L. Mandell, John E. Bennett, Raphael
    Dolin. — 4th ed.
        p. cm.
        Rev. ed. of: Principles and practice of infectious diseases. 3rd
    ed. 1990.
        Includes bibliographical references and index.
        ISBN 0-443-08935-3
        1. Communicable diseases. I. Mandell, Gerald L. II. Douglas, R.
    Gordon (Robert Gordon), date. III. Bennett, John E. (John
    Eugene), date. IV. Principles and practice of infectious
    diseases.
        [DNLM: 1. Communicable Diseases. WC 100 M2713 1995]
    RC111.P78 1995
    616.9—dc20
    DNLM/DLC
    for Library of Congress   94-12792
                                                      CIP

Distributed in the United Kingdom by Churchill Livingstone, Robert Stevenson House, 1–3 Baxter's
Place, Leith Walk, Edinburgh EH1 3AF, and by associated companies, branches, and representatives
throughout the world.

Accurate indications, adverse reactions, and dosage schedules for drugs are provided in this book, but it
is possible that they may change. The reader is urged to review the package information data of the
manufacturers of the medications mentioned.

Acquisitions Editor: *Toni M. Tracy*
Editorial Assistant: *Laura Papach*
Copy Editor: *David Terry*
Production Supervisor: *Sharon Tuder*
Indexer: *Irving Conde Tullar*

Printed in the United States of America

First published in 1995   7 6 5 4 3 2

CONTRIBUTORS

N. FRANKLIN ADKINSON, Jr., M.D.
Professor, Department of Medicine, Johns Hopkins University School of Medicine; Co-Director, Division of Allergy and Clinical Immunology, Johns Hopkins Asthma and Allergy Center, Baltimore, Maryland

ROBERT H. ALFORD, M.D.
Clinical Professor, Department of Medicine, Vanderbilt University School of Medicine; Medical Director, Centennial Medical Center, Nashville, Tennessee

DAVID M. ALLEN, M.D.
Senior Fellow in Infectious Diseases, Department of Medicine, Cornell University Medical College; Assistant Attending Physician and Chief Medical Resident, Department of Medicine, The New York Hospital, New York, New York

GUY W. AMSDEN, PHARM.D.
Coordinator, Clinical Drug Research Service, St. Vincent Hospital, Worcester, Massachusetts

MICHAEL A. APICELLA, M.D.
Professor and Head, Department of Microbiology, University of Iowa College of Medicine, Iowa City, Iowa

GORDON L. ARCHER, M.D.
Professor, Departments of Medicine and Microbiology and Immunology, and Chairman, Division of Infectious Diseases, Virginia Commonwealth University Medical College of Virginia, Richmond, Virginia

DONALD ARMSTRONG, M.D.
Professor, Department of Medicine, Cornell University Medical College; Chief, Infectious Disease Service, and Director, Micro-biology Laboratory, Memorial Sloan-Kettering Cancer Center, New York, New York

CAROL J. BAKER, M.D.
Professor, Departments of Pediatrics and Microbiology and Immunology, and Head, Section of Infectious Diseases, Department of Pediatrics, Baylor College of Medicine, Houston, Texas

RONALD C. BALLARD, Ph.D.
Associate Professor, Department of Medical Microbiology, University of the Witwatersrand and South African Institute for Medical Research, Johannesburg, South Africa

KENNETH J. BART, M.D.
Associate Director for Child Health, Office of the Assistant Secretary for Health, Public Health Service, Department of Health and Human Services, Rockville, Maryland

MANUEL BATTEGAY, M.D.
Research Fellow, Liver Diseases Section, National Institute of Diabetes and Digestive and Kidney Diseases, National Institutes of Health, Bethesda, Maryland; Staff Physician, Department of Internal Medicine, Medizinische Universitats-Poliklinik, Basel, Switzerland

STEPHEN G. BAUM, M.D.
Professor, Department of Medicine, Albert Einstein College of Medicine of Yeshiva University; Director, Department of Medicine, Beth Israel Medical Center, New York, New York

MILES BEAMAN, M.D.
Senior Lecturer, University Department of Medicine, Fremantle Hospital, Fremantle, Western Australia, Australia

ROBERT BELSHE, M.D.
Professor, Department of Internal Medicine, St. Louis University School of Medicine; Director, Division of Infectious Diseases, Department of Internal Medicine, St. Louis University Hospital, St. Louis, Missouri

JOHN E. BENNETT, M.D.
Head, Clinical Mycology Section, Laboratory of Clinical Investigation, National Institut e of Allergy and Infectious Diseases, National Institutes of Health, Bethesda, Maryland

KENNETH W. BERNARD, M.D., D.T.M. & H.
Associate Director for Medical and Scientific Affairs, Office of International Health, Office of the Assistant Secretary for Health, Rockville, Maryland

ROBERT F. BETTS, M.D.
Professor, Department of Medicine, University of Rochester School of Medicine and Dentistry; Attending Physician, Department of Medicine, Strong Memorial Hospital, Rochester, New York

ALAN L. BISNO, M.D.
Professor, Department of Medicine, University of Miami School of Medicine; Chief, Medical Service, Miami Veterans Affairs Medical Center, Miami, Florida

MARTIN J. BLASER, M.D.
Addison B. Scoville Professor, Department of Medicine, Professor, Departments of Microbiology and Immunology, and Director, Division of Infectious Diseases, Vanderbilt University School of Medicine; Staff Physician, Department of Medicine, Veterans Affairs Medical Center, Nashville, Tennessee

THOMAS P. BLECK, M.D., F.C.C.M.

Associate Professor, Departments of Neurology and Neurological Surgery, and John T. and Louise Nerancy Associate Professor, Department of Neurology, University of Virginia School of Medicine; Director, Division of Critical Care, Department of Neurology, University of Virginia Health Sciences Center, Charlottesville, Virginia

DAVID A. BOBAK, M.D.

Assistant Professor, Departments of Medicine and Microbiology, University of Virginia School of Medicine, Charlottesville, Virginia

WILLIAM BONNEZ, M.D.

Assistant Professor, Department of Medicine, University of Rochester School of Medicine and Dentistry; Attending Physician, Department of Medicine, Strong Memorial Hospital, Rochester, New York

R.C. BOUCHER, M.D.

Professor, Department of Medicine, University of North Carolina at Chapel Hill School of Medicine, Chapel Hill, North Carolina

JOHN M. BOYCE, M.D.

Professor, Department of Medicine, Brown University School of Medicine; Associate Director, Infectious Diseases Section, Miriam Hospital, Providence, Rhode Island

BARRY D. BRAUSE, M.D.

Clinical Associate Professor, Department of Medicine, Cornell University Medical College; Associate Attending Physician, Department of Medicine, The New York Hospital and The Hospital for Special Surgery, New York, New York

ITZHAK BROOK, M.D.

Professor, Department of Pediatrics, Georgetown University School of Medicine, Washington, D.C.; Senior Investigator, Naval Medical Research Institute, Bethesda, Maryland

ARTHUR E. BROWN, M.D.

Professor of Clinical Medicine and Clinical Pediatrics, Departments of Medicine and Pediatrics, Cornell University Medical College; Attending Physician, Infectious Disease Service, Memorial Sloan-Kettering Cancer Center; Attending Pediatrician, Department of Pediatrics, The New York Hospital, New York, New York

EDWIN A. BROWN, M.D.

Assistant Professor, Division of Infectious Diseases, Department of Medicine, Medical University of South Carolina College of Medicine, Charleston, South Carolina

RALPH T. BRYAN, M.D.

Medical Epidemiologist, National Center for Infectious Diseases, Centers for Disease Control and Prevention, Atlanta, Georgia

RICHARD E. BRYANT, M.D.

Professor, Department of Medicine, and Director, Division of Infectious Disease, Oregon Health Sciences University School of Medicine, Portland, Oregon

WARD E. BULLOCK, M.D.

Professor, Department of Medicine, and Dean, University of Connecticut School of Medicine, Farmington, Connecticut

JAMES E. BURNS, M.D.

Division of Infectious Diseases, Department of Pediatrics, University of Virginia School of Medicine, Charlottesville, Virginia

LARRY M. BUSH, M.D., F.A.C.P.

Chairman, Department of Infectious Diseases, John F. Kennedy Medical Center, West Palm Beach, Florida; formerly Assistant Clinical Professor, Department of Medicine, Medical College of Pennsylvania, Philadelphia, Pennsylvania

THOMAS BUTLER, M.D.

Professor and Chief, Division of Infectious Diseases, Department of Internal Medicine, Texas Tech University Health Sciences Center School of Medicine; Consultant, Department of Internal Medicine, University Medical Center, Lubbock, Texas

JASON CALHOUN, M.D.

Professor, Department of Surgery, and Chief, Division of Orthopaedic Surgery, University of Texas Medical Branch, University of Texas Medical School at Galveston, Galveston, Texas

ELLIS S. CAPLAN, M.D., F.A.C.P.

Associate Professor, Division of Infectious Diseases, Department of Medicine, University of Maryland School of Medicine; Chief, Division of Infectious Diseases, Department of Medicine, R.A. Cowley Shock Trauma Center, Baltimore, Maryland

CHARLES C.J. CARPENTER, M.D.

Professor, Department of Medicine, Brown University School of Medicine; Physician-in-Chief, Miriam Hospital, Providence, Rhode Island

RICHARD E. CHAISSON, M.D.

Associate Professor, Departments of Medicine and Epidemiology, Johns Hopkins University School of Medicine; Director, AIDS Service, Johns Hopkins Hospital, Baltimore, Maryland

MARY E. CHAMBERLAND, M.D., M.P.H.

Chief, Epidemiologic Studies Activity, HIV Infections Branch, Hospital Infections Program, National Center for Infectious Diseases, Centers for Disease Control and Prevention, Atlanta, Georgia

HENRY F. CHAMBERS, M.D.

Associate Professor, Department of Medicine, University of California, San Francisco, School of Medicine; Chief, Division of Infectious Diseases, San Francisco General Hospital, San Francisco, California

STANLEY W. CHAPMAN, M.D.

Professor, Department of Medicine, Associate Professor, Department of Microbiology, and Director, Division of Infectious Diseases, University of Mississippi School of Medicine, Jackson, Mississippi

ANTHONY W. CHOW, M.D., F.R.C.P.(C)

Professor, Department of Medicine, and Head, Division of Infectious Diseases, University of British Columbia Faculty of Medicine; Head, Department of Medicine, Vancouver General Hospital, Vancouver, British Columbia, Canada

JEFFREY D. CHULAY, M.D., D.T.M.H.

Associate Director, Infectious Diseases and Immunology, Burroughs Wellcome Co., Research Triangle Park, North Carolina

H. FRED CLARK, M.D.

Adjunct Associate Professor, Department of Epidemiology, University of Pennsylvania School of Veterinary Medicine; Research Professor, Department of Pediatrics, Children's Hospital of Philadelphia, Philadelphia, Pennsylvania

ROBERT A. CLARK, M.D.

Professor, Chairman, and Dan F. Parman Distinguished Chair, Department of Medicine, University of Texas Medical School at San Antonio, San Antonio, Texas

C. GLENN COBBS, M.D.

Professor, Department of Medicine, University of Alabama School of Medicine; Chief, Medical Service, Birmingham Veterans Affairs Medical Center, Birmingham, Alabama

MYRON S. COHEN, M.D.

Professor, Departments of Medicine and Microbiology and Immunology, and Chief, Division of Infectious Diseases, University of North Carolina at Chapel Hill School of Medicine, Chapel Hill, North Carolina

LAWRENCE COREY, M.D.

Professor, Departments of Laboratory Medicine, Microbiology, and Medicine, University of Washington School of Medicine; Head, Division of Virology, Pacific Medical Center, Seattle, Washington

KENT B. CROSSLEY, M.D.

Professor, Department of Medicine, University of Minnesota Medical School, Minneapolis, Minnesota; Chief, Department of Medicine, St. Paul Ramsey Medical Center, St. Paul, Minnesota

JAMES W. CURRAN, M.D., M.P.H.

Director, AIDS Program, and Associate Director for AIDS, Center for Infectious Diseases, Centers for Disease Control and Prevention, Atlanta, Georgia

RABIH O. DAROUICHE, M.D.

Assistant Professor, Departments of Medicine and Physical Medicine and Rehabilitation, Baylor College of Medicine; Staff Physician, Infectious Disease Section and Spinal Cord Injury Service, Veterans Affairs Medical Center, Houston, Texas

LISA M. DEMETER, M.D.

Assistant Professor, Department of Medicine, University of Rochester School of Medicine and Dentistry; Attending Physician, Department of Medicine, Strong Memorial Hospital, Rochester, New York

PETER DENSEN, M.D.

Professor, Department of Internal Medicine, University of Iowa College of Medicine, Iowa City, Iowa

ROGER M. DES PREZ, M.D.

Professor, Department of Medicine, Vanderbilt University School of Medicine; Chief, Medical Service, Department of Medicine, Veterans Affairs Medical Center, Nashville, Tennessee

RICHARD D. DIAMOND, M.D.

Professor, Department of Medicine, and Research Professor, Department of Biochemistry, Boston University School of Medicine; Head, Section of Infectious Disease, Evans Memorial Department of Clinical Research, University Hospital, Boston, Massachusetts

CHARLES A. DINARELLO, M.D.

Professor, Departments of Medicine and Pediatrics, Tufts University School of Medicine; Staff Physician, Division of Geographic Medicine and Infectious Diseases, Department of Medicine, New England Medical Center, Boston, Massachusetts

WILLIAM E. DISMUKES, M.D.

Professor and Interim Chairman, Department of Medicine, and Director, Division of Infectious Diseases, University of Alabama School of Medicine; Director, Medical House Staff, University of Alabama Medical Center, Birmingham, Alabama

WILLIAM O. DOBBINS III, M.D.

Professor Emeritus, Department of Internal Medicine, University of Michigan Medical School, Ann Arbor, Michigan

BRADLEY N. DOEBBELING, M.D.

Assistant Professor, Department of Medicine, University of Iowa College of Medicine; Staff Physician, Department of Medicine, University of Iowa Hospitals and Clinics; Director, Section of Employee Health, Veterans Affairs Medical Center, Iowa City, Iowa

RAPHAEL DOLIN, M.D.

Charles A. Dewey Professor of Medicine and Chair, Department of Medicine, University of Rochester School of Medicine and Dentistry, Rochester, New York

GERALD R. DONOWITZ, M.D.

Professor, Department of Internal Medicine, and Associate Chairman for Education, Department of Medicine, University of Virginia School of Medicine; Associate Director, Hematology-Oncology Unit, Department of Medicine, University of Virginia Medical Center, Charlottesville, Virginia

GEORGE L. DRUSANO, M.D.

Professor of Medicine and Pharmacology and Director, Division of Clinical Pharmacology, Department of Medicine, Albany Medical College, Albany, New York

J. STEPHEN DUMLER, M.D.

Assistant Professor, Department of Pathology, University of Maryland School of Medicine; Associate Director, Clinical Microbiology Laboratories, and Staff Pathologist, Department of Pathology, University of Maryland Medical Systems, Baltimore, Maryland

J. STEPHEN DUMMER, M.D.

Associate Professor, Departments of Medicine and Surgery, Vanderbilt University School of Medicine, Nashville, Tennessee

HERBERT L. DuPONT, M.D.

Mary W. Kelsey Professor of the Medical Sciences, Division of Infectious Diseases, Department of Internal Medicine, University of Texas Medical School at Houston, Houston, Texas

DAVID T. DURACK, M.B., D.PHIL.

Chairman, Department of Medicine, and Chief, Division of Infectious Diseases, Health Care International, Clydebank, Scotland; Consulting Professor of Medicine, Duke University Medical Center, Durham, North Carolina

MICHAEL B. EDMOND, M.D., M.P.H.

Fellow Associate, Division of General Medicine, Clinical Epidemiology, and Health Services Research, Department of Internal Medicine, University of Iowa College of Medicine, Iowa City, Iowa

JOHN E. EDWARDS, Jr., M.D.

Professor, Division of Infectious Diseases, Department of Medicine, University of California, Los Angeles, UCLA School of Medicine, Los Angeles, California

MORVEN S. EDWARDS, M.D.

Associate Professor, Department of Pediatrics, Baylor College of Medicine, Houston, Texas

BARRY I. EISENSTEIN, M.D.

Professor, Department of Medicine, Indiana University School of Medicine; Vice President, Lilly Research Laboratories, Eli Lilly and Company, Indianapolis, Indiana

JERROLD J. ELLNER, M.D.

Professor, Department of Medicine, Case Western Reserve University School of Medicine; Director, Division of Infectious Diseases, Department of Medicine, University Hospitals, Cleveland, Ohio

STANLEY FALKOW, Ph.D.

Professor, Departments of Microbiology and Immunology and Medicine, Stanford University School of Medicine, Stanford, California

BARRY M. FARR, M.D.

Associate Professor, Department of Medicine, University of Virginia School of Medicine; Hospital Epidemiologist, Department of Internal Medicine, University of Virginia Health Sciences Center, Charlottesville, Virginia

W. EDMUND FARRAR, M.D.

Professor Emeritus, Department of Medicine, Medical University of South Carolina College of Medicine, Charleston, South Carolina

ANTHONY S. FAUCI, M.D.

Director, National Institute of Allergy and Infectious Diseases, National Institutes of Health, Bethesda, Maryland

STEPHEN M. FEINSTONE, M.D.

Chief, Laboratory of Hepatitis Research, Division of Virology, Center for Biologics Evaluation and Research, United States Food and Drug Administration, Bethesda, Maryland

ROBERT FEKETY, M.D.

Professor, Department of Internal Medicine, and Head, Division of Infectious Diseases, University of Michigan School of Medicine; Chief, Adult Infectious Diseases Service, University Hospital, Ann Arbor, Michigan

BERNARD N. FIELDS, M.D.

Adele Lehman Professor and Chairman, Department of Microbiology and Molecular Genetics, and Professor, Department of Medicine, Harvard Medical School; Member, Division of Infectious Disease, Department of Medicine, Brigham and Women's Hospital, Boston, Massachusetts

SYDNEY M. FINEGOLD, M.D.

Professor, Departments of Medicine and Microbiology and Immunology, University of California, Los Angeles, UCLA School of Medicine; Staff Physician, Medical Service, Wadsworth Veterans Administration Medical Center, Los Angeles, California

ANTHONY E. FIORE, M.D.

Fellow, Division of Infectious Diseases, Department of Medicine, University of Maryland School of Medicine, Baltimore, Maryland

GERALD W. FISCHER, M.D.

Professor, Department of Pediatrics, and Director, Pediatric Infectious Disease Fellowship Program, Uniformed Services University of the Health Sciences F. Edward Hébert School of Medicine; Attending Physician, Walter Reed Army Medical Center, Bethesda, Maryland

DANIEL B. FISHBEIN, M.D.

Coordinator, Scientific Studies International Branch, Division of Field Epidemiology, Epidemiology Program Office, Centers for Disease Control and Prevention, Atlanta, Georgia

MICHAEL O. FRANK, M.D.

Assistant Professor, Department of Medicine, Indiana University School of Medicine, Indianapolis, Indiana

JOHN I. GALLIN, M.D.

Chief, Laboratory of Host Defenses, National Institute of Allergy and Infectious Diseases, and Director, Clinical Center, National Institutes of Health, Bethesda, Maryland

ROBERT C. GALLO, M.D.

Chief, Laboratory of Tumor Cell Biology, National Cancer Institute, National Institutes of Health, Bethesda, Maryland

ROBERT H. GELBER, M.D.

Clinical Professor, Department of Epidemiology and Biostatistics, University of California, San Francisco, School of Medicine; Medical Director, San Francisco Regional Hansen's Disease Program, San Francisco, California

JEFFREY A. GELFAND, M.D.

Professor and Vice Chairman, Department of Medicine, Tufts University School of Medicine; Associate Physician-in-Chief, New England Medical Center, Boston, Massachusetts

ANNE A. GERSHON, M.D.

Professor, Department of Pediatrics, and Director, Division of Pediatric Infectious Diseases, Columbia University College of Physicians and Surgeons, New York, New York

DAVID N. GILBERT, M.D.

Professor, Department of Medicine, Oregon Health Sciences University School of Medicine; Director of Medical Education and Director, Earle A. Chiles Research Institute, Providence Medical Center, Portland, Oregon

VEE J. GILL, Ph.D.

Chief, Microbiology Service, Department of Clinical Pathology, National Institutes of Health, Bethesda, Maryland

P.H. GILLIGAN, Ph.D.

Associate Professor, Departments of Microbiology and Immunology and Pathology, University of North Carolina at Chapel Hill School of Medicine; Associate Director, Clinical Microbiology/Immunology Laboratories, University of North Carolina Hospitals, Chapel Hill, North Carolina

ELLIE J.C. GOLDSTEIN, M.D.

Clinical Professor, Department of Medicine, University of California, Los Angeles, UCLA School of Medicine, Los Angeles, California; Director, R.M. Alden Research Laboratory, Santa Monica Hospital Medical Center, Santa Monica, California

J. THOMAS GRAYSTON, M.D.

Professor, Department of Epidemiology, School of Public Health and Community Medicine, University of Washington, Seattle, Washington

W. RICHARD GREEN, M.D.

Odd Fellows Professor, Department of Ophthalmology, and Associate Professor, Department of Pathology, Johns Hopkins University School of Medicine; Chief, Eye Pathology Laboratory, Johns Hopkins Hospital, Baltimore, Maryland

JOHN E. GREENLEE, M.D.

Professor, Department of Neurology, University of Utah School of Medicine; Chief, Neurology Service, Veterans Affairs Medical Center, Salt Lake City, Utah

WILLIAM B. GREENOUGH III, M.D.

Professor, Department of Medicine, Johns Hopkins University School of Medicine, and Professor, Department of International Health, Johns Hopkins University School of Hygiene and Public Health, Baltimore, Maryland

DIANE E. GRIFFIN, M.D.

Professor, Departments of Medicine and Neurology, Johns Hopkins University School of Medicine; Active Staff, Johns Hopkins Hospital, Baltimore, Maryland

BARBARA M. GRIPSHOVER, M.D.

Assistant Professor, Division of Infectious Diseases, Department of Medicine, Case Western Reserve University School of Medicine; Attending Physician, Division of Infectious Diseases, Department of Medicine, University Hospitals of Cleveland, Cleveland, Ohio

DIETER H.M. GRÖSCHEL, M.D.

Professor, Departments of Pathology and Internal Medicine, and Director, Division of Microbiology, University of Virginia School of Medicine, Charlottesville, Virginia

DAVID I. GROVE, M.D.

Clinical Professor, Department of Medicine and Microbiology, University of Adelaide; Director of Clinical Microbiology and Infectious Diseases, The Queen Elizabeth Hospital, Adelaide, South Australia, Australia

RICHARD L. GUERRANT, M.D.

Professor, Department of Internal Medicine, and Head, Division of Geographic Medicine, University of Virginia School of Medicine; Attending Physician, Department of Medicine, University of Virginia Health Sciences Center, Charlottesville, Virginia

IAN D. GUST, M.D.

Professional Associate, University of Melbourne Faculty of Medicine, Dentistry and Health Sciences, Parkville, Victoria, Australia; Professor, Monash University Faculty of Medicine, Chadstone; Director, Research and Development, CSL Limited, Victoria, Australia

JACK M. GWALTNEY, Jr., M.D.

Professor, Department of Internal Medicine, and Head, Division of Epidemiology and Virology, University of Virginia School of Medicine, Charlottesville, Virginia

DAVID W. HAAS, M.D.

Assistant Professor, Department of Medicine, Vanderbilt University School of Medicine; Director, Inpatient Infectious Diseases Services, Department of Medicine, Vanderbilt University Hospital, Nashville, Tennessee

ASHLEY T. HAASE, M.D.

Professor and Head, Department of Microbiology, University of Minnesota Medical School, Minneapolis, Minnesota

STEPHEN C. HADLER, M.D.

Director, Division of Epidemiology and Surveillance, National Immunization Program, Centers for Disease Control and Prevention, Atlanta, Georgia

CAROLINE BREESE HALL, M.D.

Professor, Departments of Pediatrics and Medicine, University of Rochester School of Medicine and Dentistry; Attending Physician, Department of Medicine, University of Rochester Medical Center, Rochester, New York

WILLIAM J. HALL, M.D.

Professor of Medicine and Pediatrics, University of Rochester School of Medicine and Dentistry; Chief, General Medicine/Geriatrics Unit, Strong Memorial Hospital, Rochester, New York

W. LEE HAND, M.D.

Professor and Regional Chairman, Department of Internal Medicine, Texas Tech University Health Sciences Center School of Medicine, El Paso, Texas

H. HUNTER HANDSFIELD, M.D.

Professor, Department of Medicine, University of Washington School of Medicine; Director, Sexually Transmitted Disease Control Program, Seattle-King County Department of Public Health, Seattle, Washington

BARRY J. HARTMAN, M.D.

Associate Professor of Clinical Medicine, Department of Medicine, Cornell University Medical College; Associate Attending Physician, Department of Medicine, The New York Hospital, New York, New York

DIANE V. HAVLIR, M.D.

Assistant Professor, Division of Infectious Diseases, Department of Medicine, University of California, San Diego, School of Medicine, San Diego, California

RODERICK J. HAY, D.M.

Mary Dunhill Professor, Department of Cutaneous Medicine, St. John's Institute of Dermatology, Guy's Hospital, London, England

FREDERICK G. HAYDEN, M.D.

Professor, Departments of Internal Medicine and Pathology; Stuart S. Richardson Professor of Clinical Virology, Department of Internal Medicine; and Associate Director, Clinical Microbiology Laboratory (Virology), University of Virginia School of Medicine, Charlottesville, Virginia

CRAIG W. HEDBERG, Ph.D., M.S.

Epidemiologist, Acute Disease Epidemiology Section, Minnesota Department of Health, Minneapolis, Minnesota

FREDERICK P. HEINZEL, M.D.

Assistant Professor, Division of Geographic Medicine, Department of Medicine, Case Western Reserve University School of Medicine, Cleveland, Ohio

DAVID K. HENDERSON, M.D.

Associate Director for Quality Assurance and Hospital Epidemiology, and Hospital Epidemiologist, Warren G. Magnuson Clinical Center, National Institutes of Health, Bethesda, Maryland

J. OWEN HENDLEY, M.D.

Professor, Department of Pediatrics, and Head, Division of Pediatric Infectious Diseases, University of Virginia School of Medicine, Charlottesville, Virginia

KELLY J. HENRICKSON, M.D.

Assistant Professor, Division of Infectious Diseases, Departments of Pediatrics and Microbiology, Medical College of Wisconsin, Milwaukee, Wisconsin

ERIK L. HEWLETT, M.D.

Professor, Departments of Internal Medicine and Pharmacology, and Chief, Division of Clinical Pharmacology, University of Virginia School of Medicine, Charlottesville, Virginia

DAVID R. HILL, M.D.

Associate Professor, Department of Medicine, University of Connecticut School of Medicine; Director, International Traveler's Medical Service, Division of Infectious Diseases, Department of Medicine, University of Connecticut Health Center, Farmington, Connecticut

ALAN R. HINMAN, M.D., M.P.H.

Assistant Surgeon General, and Director, National Center for Prevention Services, Centers for Disease Control and Prevention, Atlanta, Georgia

MARTIN S. HIRSCH, M.D.

Professor, Department of Medicine, Harvard Medical School; Physician, Department of Medicine, Infectious Diseases Unit, Massachusetts General Hospital, Boston, Massachusetts

MONTO HO, M.D.

Professor and Chairman, Department of Infectious Diseases and Microbiology, and Professor, Department of Medicine, University of Pittsburgh School of Medicine; Physician, Department of Medicine, Presbyterian-University Hospital, Pittsburgh, Pennsylvania

GARY S. HOFFMAN, M.D.

Chairman, Department of Rheumatic and Immunologic Diseases, The Cleveland Clinic Foundation, Cleveland, Ohio

ELIZABETH L. HOHMANN, M.D.

Instructor, Department of Medicine, Harvard Medical School; Clinical Associate, Infectious Disease Unit, Massachusetts General Hospital, Boston, Massachusetts

STEVEN M. HOLLAND, M.D.

Assistant Professor of Medicine, Division of Infectious Diseases, Johns Hopkins University School of Medicine; NIAID Investigator, Laboratory of Host Defenses, National Institute of Allergy and Infectious Diseases, National Institutes of Health, Bethesda, Maryland

JAY H. HOOFNAGLE, M.D.

Director, Division of Digestive Diseases and Nutrition, and Senior Investigator, Liver Diseases Section, National Institutes of Diabetes and Digestive and Kidney Diseases, National Institutes of Health, Bethesda, Maryland

DAVID C. HOOPER, M.D.

Associate Professor, Department of Medicine, Harvard Medical School; Associate Physician, Department of Medicine, Infectious Disease Unit, Massachusetts General Hospital, Boston, Massachusetts

DAVID L. HOOVER, M.D.

Associate Professor, Department of Medicine, Uniformed Services University of the Health Sciences F. Edward Hébert School of Medicine, Bethesda, Maryland

EDWARD A. HOROWITZ, M.D.

Assistant Professor, Departments of Medicine and Medical Microbiology, Creighton University School of Medicine; Attending Physician, Department of Medicine, Omaha Veterans Affairs Medical Center, Omaha, Nebraska

HENRY H. HSU, M.D.

Clinical Instructor, Department of Medicine, Stanford University School of Medicine, Stanford, California; Senior Research Fellow, Department of Gastroenterology, Stanford University Medical Center, Palo Alto, California

JAMES M. HUGHES, M.D.

Director, National Center for Infectious Diseases, Centers for Disease Control and Prevention; Clinical Associate Professor, Department of Medicine, Emory University School of Medicine, Atlanta, Georgia

JOHN A. JERNIGAN, M.D.

Assistant Professor, Department of Medicine, Division of Infectious Diseases, Emory University School of Medicine, Atlanta, Georgia

CAROLINE C. JOHNSON, M.D.

Assistant Professor, Department of Medicine, Medical College of Pennsylvania; Staff Physician, Department of Medicine, Veterans Affairs Medical Center, Philadelphia, Pennsylvania

KARL M. JOHNSON, M.D.

Formerly, Chief, Special Pathogens Branch, Centers for Disease Control, Atlanta, Georgia

WARREN D. JOHNSON, JR., M.D.

Professor, Department of Medicine, and Chief, Division of International Medicine, Cornell University Medical College; Attending Physician, Department of Medicine, The New York Hospital, New York, New York

ROBERT B. JONES, M.D.

Professor, Departments of Medicine and Microbiology and Immunology, and Chief, Division of Infectious Diseases, Indiana University School of Medicine, Indianapolis, Indiana

MANJARI JOSHI, M.D.

Clinical Assistant Professor, Department of Medicine, University of Maryland School of Medicine; Attending Physician, Division of Infectious Diseases, Department of Medicine, R.A. Cowley Shock Trauma Center, Baltimore, Maryland

ALLEN B. KAISER, M.D.

Professor, Department of Medicine, Vanderbilt University School of Medicine; Vice Chairman, Department of Medicine, Vanderbilt University Medical Center, Nashville, Tennessee

ADOLF W. KARCHMER, M.D.

Professor, Department of Medicine, Harvard Medical School; Chief, Division of Infectious Diseases, Department of Medicine, New England Deaconess Hospital, Boston, Massachusetts

DONALD KAYE, M.D.

Professor and Chairman, Department of Medicine, Medical College of Pennsylvania; Chief, Department of Medicine, Hospital of the Medical College of Pennsylvania, Philadelphia, Pennsylvania

MICHAEL C. KEEFER, M.D.

Assistant Professor of Medicine, Infectious Diseases Unit, University of Rochester School of Medicine; Attending Physician, Strong Memorial Hospital, Rochester, New York

DOUGLAS S. KERNODLE, M.D.

Assistant Professor, Department of Medicine, Vanderbilt University School of Medicine; Chief, Infectious Diseases Section, Veterans Affairs Medical Center, Nashville, Tennessee

CHARLES H. KING, M.D.

Associate Professor, Section of International Health, Division of Geographic Medicine, Department of Medicine, Case Western Reserve University School of Medicine; Attending Physician, Department of Medicine, University Hospitals of Cleveland, Cleveland, Ohio

LOUIS V. KIRCHHOFF, M.D., M.P.H.

Associate Professor, Department of Internal Medicine, University of Iowa College of Medicine; Staff Physician, Department of Medicine, Veterans Affairs Medical Center, Iowa City, Iowa

JEROME O. KLEIN, M.D.

Professor, Department of Pediatrics, Boston University School of Medicine; Director, Division of Pediatric Infectious Diseases, Maxwell Finland Laboratory for Infectious Diseases, Boston City Hospital, Boston, Massachusetts

MARY E. KLOTMAN, M.D.

Senior Research Investigator, Laboratory of Tumor Cell Biology, National Cancer Institute, National Institutes of Health, Bethesda, Maryland

M.R. KNOWLES, M.D.

Associate Professor, Pulmonary Division, Department of Medicine, University of North Carolina at Chapel Hill School of Medicine, Chapel Hill, North Carolina

EDWARD L. KRAWITT, M.D.

Professor of Medicine, Department of Medicine, University of Vermont; Director, Department of Gastroenterology, Medical Center Hospital of Vermont, Burlington, Vermont

JOHN N. KRIEGER, M.D.

Professor, Department of Urology, University of Washington School of Medicine; Attending Surgeon, Department of Urology, University of Washington Medical Center, Seattle, Washington

DONALD J. KROGSTAD, M.D.

Henderson Professor and Chair, Department of Tropical Medicine, Tulane University School of Public Health and Tropical Medicine; Professor and Chair, Department of Parasitology, Tulane University Graduate School; Professor, Department of Medicine, Tulane University School of Medicine, New Orleans, Louisiana

STANLEY M. LEMON, M.D.

Professor, Departments of Medicine and Microbiology and Immunology, University of North Carolina at Chapel Hill School of Medicine, Chapel Hill, North Carolina

PHILLIP I. LERNER, M.D.

Professor, Department of Medicine, Case Western Reserve University School of Medicine; Chief, Division of Infectious Diseases, Mt. Sinai Medical Center, Cleveland, Ohio

D.P. LEVINE, M.D.

Associate Professor, Division of Infectious Diseases, Department of Internal Medicine, Wayne State University School of Medicine; Chief, Section of Infectious Diseases, Detroit Receiving Hospital, Detroit, Michigan

MATTHEW E. LEVISON, M.D.

Professor, Department of Medicine, and Chief, Division of Infectious Diseases, Medical College of Pennsylvania, Philadelphia, Pennsylvania

DANIEL LEW, M.D.

Professor, Department of Medicine, Geneva University Faculty of Medicine; Chief, Division of Infectious Diseases, Department of Medicine, Geneva University Hospital, Geneva, Switzerland

NATHAN LITMAN, M.D.

Associate Professor, Department of Pediatrics, Albert Einstein College of Medicine of Yeshiva University; Assistant Chief of Service and Associate Director, Department of Pediatrics, Montefiore Medical Center, Bronx, New York

RICHARD M. LOCKSLEY, M.D.

Professor, Departments of Medicine and Microbiology and Immunology, and Chief, Division of Infectious Diseases, University of California, San Francisco, School of Medicine, San Francisco, California

BENNETT LORBER, M.D.

Thomas M. Durant Professor, Department of Medicine, and Professor, Department of Microbiology and Immunology, Temple University School of Medicine; Chief, Section of Infectious Diseases, Department of Medicine, Temple University Hospital, Philadelphia, Pennsylvania

KRISTINE L. MacDONALD, M.D.

Adjunct Assistant Professor, Department of Epidemiology, University of Minnesota School of Public Health; Assistant State Epidemiologist and Assistant Chief, Acute Disease Epidemiology Section, Minnesota Department of Health, Minneapolis, Minnesota

ROB ROY MacGREGOR, M.D.

Professor, Department of Medicine, and Director, AIDS Clinical Trials Unit, Division of Infectious Diseases, University of Pennsylvania School of Medicine; Attending Physician, Department of Medicine, Hospital of the University of Pennsylvania, Philadelphia, Pennsylvania

JON T. MADER, M.D.

Professor, Department of Internal Medicine, University of Texas Medical Branch, University of Texas Medical School at Galveston; Chief, Department of Marine Medicine, Marine Biomedical Institute, University of Texas Medical Branch, University of Texas Medical School at Galveston, Galveston, Texas

EL SHEIKH MAHGOUB, M.D.

World Health Organization, Regional Office for the Eastern Mediterranean, Alexandria, Egypt

ADEL A.F. MAHMOUD, M.D., Ph.D.

John H. Hord Professor and Chairman, Department of Medicine, Case Western Reserve University School of Medicine; Physician-in-Chief, University Hospitals of Cleveland, Cleveland, Ohio

GERALD L. MANDELL, M.D.

Professor of Medicine, Owen R. Cheatham Professor of the Sciences, and Chief, Division of Infectious Diseases, University of Virginia Health Sciences Center, Charlottesville, Virginia

LIONEL A. MANDELL, M.D.

Professor, Department of Medicine, and Head, Division of Infectious Diseases, McMaster University School of Medicine, Hamilton, Ontario, Canada

BARBARA J. MANN, Ph.D.

Assistant Professor of Research, Division of Infectious Diseases, Department of Internal Medicine, University of Virginia School of Medicine, Charlottesville, Virginia

FRANCINE MARCIANO-CABRAL, Ph.D.

Associate Professor, Department of Microbiology and Immunobiology, Medical College of Virginia, Richmond, Virginia

LEWIS MARKOFF, M.D.

Chief, Laboratory of Vector-borne Virus Diseases, Division of Viral Products, Center for Biologics Evaluation and Research, United States Food and Drug Administration, Bethesda, Maryland

THOMAS J. MARRIE, M.D., F.R.C.P.(C)

Professor, Department of Medicine, Dalhousie University Faculty of Medicine, Halifax, Nova Scotia, Canada

MICHAEL A. MARTIN, M.D.

Associate Professor, Division of Infectious Diseases, Department of Medicine, Oregon Health Sciences University School of Medicine, Portland, Oregon

HENRY MASUR, M.D.

Clinical Professor, Department of Medicine, George Washington University School of Medicine, Washington, D.C.; Chief, Department of Critical Care Medicine, Clinical Center, National Institutes of Health, Bethesda, Maryland

GLENN E. MATHISEN, M.D.

Assistant Professor, Department of Medicine, University of California, Los Angeles, UCLA School of Medicine, Los Angeles, California; Physician Specialist and Chief, Infectious Diseases Service, Department of Medicine, Olive View Hospital, Sylmar, California

KENNETH H. MAYER, M.D.

Professor, Department of Medicine and Community Health, Brown University School of Medicine, Providence, Rhode Island; Chief, Division of Infectious Disease, Memorial Hospital of Rhode Island, Pawtucket, Rhode Island

ROBERT E. McCABE, M.D.

Assistant Professor, Department of Medicine University of California, Davis, School of Medicine, Davis, California

CAROL A. McCARTHY, M.D.

Assistant Professor, Department of Pediatrics, University of Chicago Division of the Biological Sciences Pritzker School of Medicine, Chicago, Illinois

WILLIAM M. McCORMACK, M.D.

Professor, Departments of Medicine, Obstetrics, and Gynecology, State University of New York Health Science Center at Brooklyn College of Medicine; Chief, Division of Infectious Diseases, Department of Medicine, State University of New York Health Science Center, Brooklyn, New York

JOHN E. McGOWAN, JR., M.D.

Professor, Departments of Medicine and Pathology and Laboratory Medicine, Emory University School of Medicine; Director, Clinical Microbiology Laboratory, Grady Memorial Hospital, Atlanta, Georgia

KENNETH McINTOSH, M.D.

Professor, Department of Pediatrics, Harvard Medical School; Chief, Division of Infectious Disease, Children's Hospital, Boston, Massachusetts

PHILIP B. MEAD, M.D.

Professor, Department of Obstetrics and Gynecology, University of Vermont College of Medicine; Attending Physician, Department of Obstetrics and Gynecology, Medical Center Hospital of Vermont, Burlington, Vermont

ANTONE A. MEDEIROS, M.D.

Professor, Department of Medicine, Brown University School of Medicine; Chief, Division of Infectious Disease, Miriam Hospital, Providence, Rhode Island

MICHAEL H. MERSON, M.D.

Executive Director, Global Programme on AIDS, World Health Organization, Geneva, Switzerland

FRANÇOISE MEUNIER, M.D., Ph.D.

Director, Central Office—Data Center, and Chairman, Invasive Fungal Infections Cooperative Group, European Organization for Research and Treatment of Cancer, Brussels, Belgium

SAMUEL I. MILLER, M.D.

Associate Professor, Department of Microbiology and Molecular Genetics, Harvard Medical School; Assistant Physician, Infectious Disease Unit, Massachusetts General Hospital, Boston, Massachusetts

JOHN F. MODLIN, M.D.

Professor, Departments of Pediatrics and Medicine, Dartmouth Medical School, Lebanon, New Hampshire

ROBERT C. MOELLERING, JR., M.D.

Shields Warren-Mallinckrodt Professor of Medical Research, Department of Medicine, Harvard Medical School; Chairman and Physician-in-Chief, New England Deaconess Hospital, Boston, Massachusetts

THOMAS P. MONATH, M.D.

Professor, Department of Tropical Public Health, Harvard School of Public Health, Boston, Massachusetts

E. RICHARD MOXON, M.D.

Professor, Department of Paediatrics, Oxford University Faculty of Medicine; Head, Department of Paediatrics, John Radcliffe Hospital, Headington, Oxford, England

ROBERT R. MUDER, M.D.

Assistant Professor, Department of Medicine, University of Pittsburgh School of Medicine; Chief, Infection Control, Veterans Affairs Medical Center, Pittsburgh, Pennsylvania

DANIEL M. MUSHER, M.D.

Professor, Departments of Medicine and Microbiology and Immunology, Baylor College of Medicine; Chief, Division of Infectious Disease, Medical Service Section, Veterans Affairs Medical Center, Houston, Texas

THEODORE H. NASH, M.D.

Medical Officer and Senior Scientist, Laboratory of Parasitic Diseases, National Institute of Allergy and Infectious Diseases, National Institutes of Health, Bethesda, Maryland

WILLIAM M. NAUSEEF, M.D.

Professor, Department of Internal Medicine, University of Iowa College of Medicine, Iowa City, Iowa

JOHN M. NEFF, M.D.

Professor, Department of Pediatrics, and Associate Dean, University of Washington School of Medicine; Medical Director, The Children's Hospital and Medical Center, Seattle, Washington

HAROLD C. NEU, M.D.

Professor, Departments of Medicine and Pharmacology, Columbia University College of Physicians and Surgeons; Hospital Epidemiologist, Department of Epidemiology, Presbyterian Hospital, New York, New York

THALIA I. NICAS, Ph.D.

Research Scientist, Infectious Disease Research Division, Lilly Research Laboratories, Eli Lilly and Company, Indianapolis, Indiana

TERRENCE P. O'BRIEN, M.D.

Assistant Professor, Department of Ophthalmology, Johns Hopkins University School of Medicine; Director, Department of Ocular Microbiology, Johns Hopkins Hospital, Baltimore, Maryland

PAUL A. OFFIT, M.D.

Associate Professor, Department of Pediatrics, University of Pennsylvania School of Medicine; Chief, Section of Infectious Diseases, Children's Hospital of Philadelphia, Philadelphia, Pennsylvania

STEVEN M. OPAL, M.D.

Assistant Professor, Department of Medicine, Brown University School of Medicine, Providence, Rhode Island; Staff Physician, Division of Infectious Disease, Memorial Hospital of Rhode Island, Pawtucket, Rhode Island

WALTER A. ORENSTEIN, M.D.

Director, National Immunization Program, Centers for Disease Control and Prevention, Atlanta, Georgia

MICHAEL T. OSTERHOLM, Ph.D.

Adjunct Associate Professor, Department of Epidemiology, University of Minnesota School of Public Health; State Epidemiologist, and Chief, Acute Disease Epidemiology Section, Minnesota Department of Health, Minneapolis, Minnesota

MICHAEL N. OXMAN, M.D.

Professor, Departments of Medicine and Pathology, University of California, San Diego, School of Medicine; Infectious Diseases Section, Department of Veterans Affairs Medical Center, San Diego, California

RICHARD D. PEARSON, M.D.

Professor, Departments of Internal Medicine and Pathology, University of Virginia School of Medicine, Charlottesville, Virginia; Attending Physician, Department of Internal Medicine, University of Virginia Hospital, Charlottesville, Virginia

DAVID A. PEGUES, M.D.

Research Fellow, Harvard Medical School; Research and Clinical Fellow in Medicine, Infectious Disease Unit, Massachusetts General Hospital, Boston, Massachusetts

ROBERT L. PENN, M.D.

Professor, Department of Medicine, Louisiana State University School of Medicine in Shreveport; Chief, Section of Infectious Diseases, Department of Medicine, Louisiana State University Medical Center-Shreveport, Shreveport, Louisiana

JAMES E. PENNINGTON, M.D.

Clinical Professor, Department of Medicine, University of California, San Francisco, School of Medicine, San Francisco, California; Director, Department of Medical Research, Miles Biological, Berkeley, California

CLARENCE J. PETERS, M.D.

Chief, Special Pathogens Branch, Division of Viral and Rickettsial Diseases, National Center for Infectious Diseases, Centers for Disease Control, Atlanta, Georgia

PHILLIP K. PETERSON, M.D.

Professor, Department of Medicine, University of Minnesota Medical School—Minneapolis; Director, Section of Infectious Diseases, Hennepin County Medical Center, Minneapolis, Minnesota

WILLIAM A. PETRI, Jr., M.D., Ph.D.

Associate Professor, Departments of Internal Medicine, Pathology, and Microbiology, University of Virginia School of Medicine; Attending Physician, Department of Internal Medicine, University of Virginia Hospital, Charlottesville, Virginia

ELIZABETH ANNE PIERCY, M.D.

Assistant Professor, Department of Internal Medicine, University of Texas Southwestern Medical Center at Dallas Southwestern Medical School, Dallas, Texas

PETER PIOT, M.D.

Director, Research and Intervention Development, Global Programme on AIDS, World Health Organization, Geneva, Switzerland

PHILIP A. PIZZO, M.D.

Head, Infectious Disease Section, and Chief, Pediatric Branch, National Cancer Institute, National Institutes of Health, Bethesda, Maryland

MICHAEL A. POLIS, M.D.

Senior Investigator, Laboratory of Immunoregulation, National Institute of Allergy and Infectious Diseases, National Institutes of Health, Bethesda, Maryland; Associate Clinical Professor, Department of Emergency Medicine, George Washington University Medical Center, Washington, D.C.

MATTHEW POLLACK, M.D.

Professor, Department of Medicine, Uniformed Services University of the Health Sciences F. Edward Hébert School of Medicine; Attending Physician and Infectious Diseases Consultant, Department of Internal Medicine, National Naval Medical Center, Bethesda, Maryland

AMY C. PORTMORE, M.D.

Assistant Professor of Medicine, University of Rochester School of Medicine and Dentistry; Medical Director, Adult AIDS Center, Strong Memorial Hospital, Rochester, New York

DIDIER RAOULT, M.D.

Rickettsia Unit, Bacteriology-Serology-Virology Laboratory, Groupe Hospitalier de la Timone; Director, National Rickettsia Reference Center, Marseilles, France

JONATHAN I. RAVDIN, M.D.

Professor and Vice Chairman, Department of Medicine, and Professor, Department of International Health, Case Western Reserve University School of Medicine; Chief, Medical Service, Veterans Affairs Medical Center, Cleveland, Ohio

RANJIT RAY, Ph.D.

Associate Professor, Division of Infectious Diseases, Department of Internal Medicine, St. Louis University School of Medicine, St. Louis, Missouri

ANNETTE C. REBOLI, M.D.

Assistant Professor, Department of Medicine, Hahnemann University School of Medicine, Philadelphia, Pennsylvania

RICHARD C. REICHMAN, M.D.

Professor, Departments of Medicine and Microbiology and Immunology, University of Rochester School of Medicine and Dentistry; Attending Physician, Department of Medicine, Strong Memorial Hospital, Rochester, New York

MICHAEL F. REIN, M.D.

Professor, Division of Infectious Diseases, Department of Internal Medicine, University of Virginia School of Medicine; Medical Director, Sexually Transmitted Disease Clinic, Thomas Jefferson Health Center, Charlottesville, Virginia

DAVID A. RELMAN, M.D.

Assistant Professor, Departments of Medicine and Microbiology and Immunology, Stanford University School of Medicine, Stanford, California; Staff Physician, Medical Service, Veterans Affairs Medical Center, Palo Alto, California

JACK S. REMINGTON, M.D.

Professor, Division of Infectious Diseases and Geographic Medicine, Department of Medicine, Stanford University School of Medicine, Stanford, California; Marcus A. Krupp Research Chair and Chairman, Department of Immunology and Infectious Diseases, Research Institute, Palo Alto Medical Foundation, Palo Alto, California

ANGELA RESTREPO M., Ph.D.

Head, Mycology Laboratory, and Investigator, Corporacion para Investigaciones Biológicas, Medellin, Colombia

JOHN H. REX, M.D.

Assistant Professor, Department of Medicine, University of Texas Medical School at Houston and School of Public Health, Houston, Texas

HERBERT Y. REYNOLDS, M.D.

J. Lloyd Huck Professor and Chairman, Department of Medicine, Pennsylvania State University College of Medicine, Hershey, Pennsylvania

NORBERT J. ROBERTS, JR., M.D.

Professor, Departments of Internal Medicine and Microbiology and Immunology, and Director, Division of Infectious Diseases, University of Texas Medical Branch, University of Texas Medical School at Galveston, Galveston, Texas

WILLIAM S. ROBINSON, M.D.

Professor, Department of Medicine, Stanford University School of Medicine; Attending Physician, Department of Medicine, Stanford University Hospital, Stanford, California

MARK E. RUPP, M.D.

Assistant Professor, Department of Medicine, University of Nebraska College of Medicine; Assistant Professor, Department of Medical Microbiology, Creighton University School of Medicine, Omaha, Nebraska

THOMAS A. RUSSO, M.D., C.M.

Assistant Professor, Division of Infectious Disease, Department of Medicine, State University of New York at Buffalo School of Medicine and Biomedical Sciences, Buffalo, New York

ALFRED J. SAAH, M.D., M.P.H.

Associate Professor, Department of Epidemiology, Johns Hopkins University School of Hygiene and Public Health; Associate Professor, Department of Medicine, Johns Hopkins University School of Medicine, Baltimore, Maryland

MERLE A. SANDE, M.D.

Professor and Vice Chairman, Department of Medicine, University of California, San Francisco, School of Medicine; Chief, Medical Service, San Francisco General Hospital, San Francisco, California

W. EUGENE SANDERS, JR., M.D.

Professor, Department of Medical Microbiology, Creighton University School of Medicine; Attending Physician, Department of Medicine, St. Joseph Hospital and Veterans Affairs Medical Center, Omaha, Nebraska

JAY P. SANFORD, M.D.

Professor, Department of Internal Medicine, University of Texas Southwestern Medical Center at Dallas Southwestern Medical School; Dean Emeritus, Uniformed Services University of the Health Sciences F. Edward Hébert School of Medicine, Bethesda, Maryland

FRANK T. SAULSBURY, M.D.

Professor and Head, Division of Immunology and Rheumatology, Department of Pediatrics, University of Virginia School of Medicine, Charlottesville, Virginia

MARIA C. SAVOIA, M.D.

Associate Professor of Clinical Medicine, Department of Medicine, University of California, San Diego, School of Medicine; Associate Dean for Curriculum and Student Affairs, University of California, San Diego, School of Medicine, San Diego, California

W. MICHAEL SCHELD, M.D.

Professor, Departments of Internal Medicine and Neurosurgery, University of Virginia School of Medicine, Charlottesville, Virginia

JEROME J. SCHENTAG, PHARM.D.

Professor, Departments of Pharmaceutics and Pharmacy, State University of New York at Buffalo School of Medicine and Biomedical Sciences; Director, Clinical Pharmacokinetics Laboratory, Millard Fillmore Hospital, Buffalo, New York

STEPHEN C. SCHIMPFF, M.D.

Professor, Departments of Medicine and Pharmacology, Program of Oncology, University of Maryland School of Medicine; Executive Vice President, University of Maryland Medical System, Baltimore, Maryland

CHARLES J. SCHLEUPNER, M.D.

Associate Professor, Department of Internal Medicine, University of Virginia School of Medicine, Charlottesville, Virginia; Chief, Infectious Diseases Section, Veterans Affairs Medical Center, Salem, Virginia

DAVID SCHLOSSBERG, M.D.

Professor, Department of Medicine, Medical College of Pennsylvania; Director, Department of Medicine, Episcopal Hospital, Philadelphia, Pennsylvania

ROBERT T. SCHOOLEY, M.D.

Professor, Department of Medicine, and Head, Division of Infectious Diseases, University of Colorado School of Medicine, Denver, Colorado

CYNTHIA L. SEARS, M.D.

Associate Professor, Divisions of Infectious Diseases and Gastroenterology, Department of Medicine, Johns Hopkins University School of Medicine, Baltimore, Maryland

RICHARD L. SIMMONS, M.D.

George Vance Foster Professor and Chairman, Department of Surgery, University of Pittsburgh School of Medicine; Chief, Department of Surgery, Presbyterian-University Hospital, Pittsburgh, Pennsylvania

LEONARD N. SLATER, M.D.

Associate Professor, Division of Infectious Diseases, Department of Medicine, University of Oklahoma College of Medicine; Staff Physician, Medical Service, Oklahoma City Veterans Affairs Medical Center; Attending Physician, Department of Medicine, The University Hospitals; Consultant, Oklahoma State Department of Health, Oklahoma City, Oklahoma

JAMES W. SMITH, M.D.

Professor, Department of Internal Medicine, University of Texas Health Science Center at Dallas Southwestern Medical School; Chief, Infectious Diseases Section, Veterans Affairs Medical Center, Dallas, Texas

JACK D. SOBEL, M.D.

Professor, Division of Infectious Diseases, Department of Internal Medicine, Wayne State University School of Medicine; Chief, Section of Infectious Diseases, Department of Internal Medicine, Detroit Medical Center, Detroit, Michigan

ANASTACIO DE QUEIROZ SOUSA, M.D.

Assistant Professor, Department of Medicine, Federal University of Ceara, Fortaleza, Brazil

P. FREDERICK SPARLING, M.D.

Professor and Chairman, Department of Medicine, University of North Carolina at Chapel Hill, Chapel Hill, North Carolina

CAROL A. SPIEGEL, Ph.D., A.B.M.M.

Associate Professor, Department of Pathology and Laboratory Medicine, University of Wisconsin Medical School; Director, Department of Clinical Microbiology, University of Wisconsin Hospital and Clinics, Madison, Wisconsin

HAROLD C. STANDIFORD, M.D.

Professor, Department of Medicine, University of Maryland School of Medicine; Chief, Infectious Diseases Section, Veterans Affairs Medical Center, Baltimore, Maryland

SHARILYN K. STANLEY, M.D.

Senior Clinical Investigator, Laboratory of Immunoregulation, National Institute of Allergy and Infectious Diseases, National Institutes of Health, Bethesda, Maryland

ALLEN C. STEERE, M.D.

Professor, Department of Medicine, and Chief, Division of Rheumatology and Immunology, Tufts University School of Medicine, Boston, Massachusetts

NEAL H. STEIGBIGEL, M.D.

Professor, Department of Medicine, Albert Einstein College of Medicine of Yeshiva University; Head, Division of Infectious Diseases, Montefiore Medical Center, Bronx, New York

JAMES P. STEINBERG, M.D.

Assistant Professor, Department of Medicine, Emory University School of Medicine; Associate Chief, Department of Medicine, Crawford Long Hospital of Emory University, Atlanta, Georgia

DAVID A. STEVENS, M.D.

Professor, Department of Medicine, Stanford University School of Medicine, Stanford, California; Chief, Division of Infectious Diseases, Department of Medicine, Santa Clara Valley Medical Center; Principal Investigator, Infectious Diseases Research Laboratory, California Institute for Medical Research, San Jose, California

MARK Y. STOECKLE, M.D.

Associate Professor, Department of Medicine, Cornell University Medical College; Associate Attending Physician, Department of Medicine, The New York Hospital, New York, New York

CHARLES W. STRATTON, M.D.

Associate Professor, Departments of Medicine and Pathology, Vanderbilt University School of Medicine; Director, Clinical Microbiology Laboratory, Vanderbilt University Medical Center, Nashville, Tennessee

STEPHEN E. STRAUS, M.D.

Chief, Laboratory of Clinical Investigation, National Institute of Allergy and Infectious Diseases, National Institutes of Health, Bethesda, Maryland

ALAN M. SUGAR, M.D.

Associate Professor, Department of Medicine, Boston University School of Medicine, Boston, Massachusetts

MORTON N. SWARTZ, M.D.

Professor, Department of Medicine, Harvard Medical School; Chief, James Jackson Medical Services, Massachusetts General Hospital, Boston, Massachusetts

ROBERT V. TAUXE, M.D.

Chief, Epidemiology Section, Enteric Diseases Branch, Division of Bacterial Diseases, Center for Infectious Diseases, Centers for Disease Control and Prevention, Atlanta, Georgia

DAVID TAYLOR-ROBINSON, M.D.

Professor, Departments of Genitourinary Microbiology and Medicine, St. Mary's Hospital Medical School, Paddington, London; Head, Division of Sexually Transmitted Diseases, Clinical Research Centre, Harrow, Middlesex; Research Director, Jefferies Research Wing of the Praed Street Clinic, St. Mary's Hospital, London, England

MICHAEL G. THRELKELD, M.D.

Clinical Instructor, Department of Family Medicine, University of Tennessee, Memphis, College of Medicine; Consultant, Division of Infectious Diseases; Epidemiologist; and Employee Health Physician, Hospital of St. Joseph, Memphis, Tennessee

EDMUND C. TRAMONT, M.D.

Professor, Department of Medicine, and Director, Medical Biotechnology Center, University of Maryland School of Medicine, Baltimore, Maryland

JOHN TREANOR, M.D.

Associate Professor, Infectious Disease Unit, Department of Medicine, University of Rochester School of Medicine and Dentistry, Rochester, New York

CARMELITA U. TUAZON, M.D.

Professor, Department of Medicine, and Director, Division of Infectious Disease, George Washington University School of Medicine, Washington, D.C.

ALLAN R. TUNKEL, M.D., Ph.D.

Associate Professor, Department of Medicine, Medical College of Pennsylvania; Attending Physician, Department of Medicine, Medical College Hospitals, Philadelphia, Pennsylvania

KENNETH L. TYLER, M.D.

Associate Professor, Departments of Neurology, Medicine, and Microbiology, University of Colorado School of Medicine, Denver, Colorado

BETH L.P. UNGAR, M.D.

Scientific Advisor, Division of AIDS, National Institute of Allergy and Infectious Diseases, National Institutes of Health, Bethesda, Maryland

IVO van de RIJN, Ph.D.

Professor, Department of Microbiology and Immunology, Bowman Gray School of Medicine of Wake Forest University; Associate in Infectious Diseases, Department of Medicine, Wake Forest University Medical Center, Winston-Salem, North Carolina

PAUL A. VOLBERDING, M.D.

Professor, Department of Medicine, and Chief, AIDS Activities Division, University of California, San Francisco, School of Medicine, San Francisco, California

KENNETH F. WAGNER, D.O.

Associate Professor, Department of Internal Medicine, Uniformed Services University of the Health Sciences F. Edward Hébert School of Medicine; Director, HIV Research Clinic; Senior Research Physician, Henry M. Jackson Foundation; and Attending Physician, Infectious Diseases Division, Department of Internal Medicine, National Naval Medical Center, Bethesda, Maryland

FRANCIS A. WALDVOGEL, M.D.

Professor, Department of Medicine, Faculty of Medicine, University of Geneva Medical School; Chairman and Physician-in-Chief, Department of Medicine, Medical Therapy Clinic, University Hospital, Geneva, Switzerland

DAVID H. WALKER, M.D.

Professor and Chairman, Department of Pathology, University of Texas Medical Branch, University of Texas Medical School at Galveston, Galveston, Texas

RICHARD J. WALLACE, JR., M.D.

Professor and Chairman, Department of Microbiology, and Professor, Department of Medicine, University of Texas Medical School at Tyler, Tyler, Texas

PETER D. WALZER, M.D.

Professor, Department of Internal Medicine, University of Cincinnati College of Medicine; Chief, Infectious Disease Section, Veterans Affairs Medical Center, Cincinnati, Ohio

CHRISTINE A. WANKE, M.D.

Assistant Professor, Department of Medicine, Harvard Medical School; Member, Division of Infectious Diseases, Department of Medicine, New England Deaconess Hospital, Boston, Massachusetts

JOHN W. WARD, M.D.

Chief, Surveillance Branch, Division of HIV/AIDS, National Center for Infectious Diseases, Centers for Disease Control and Prevention, Atlanta, Georgia

JOHN W. WARREN, M.D.

Professor, Department of Medicine, and Head, Division of Infectious Diseases, University of Maryland School of Medicine, Baltimore, Maryland

RONALD G. WASHBURN, M.D.

Associate Professor, Section of Infectious Diseases, Department of Medicine, Bowman Gray School of Medicine of Wake Forest University, Winston-Salem, North Carolina

JOHN A. WASHINGTON, M.D.

Professor, Department of Pathology, Ohio State University College of Medicine, Columbus, Ohio; Vice Chairman, Division of Pathology and Laboratory Medicine; Chairman, Department of Clinical Pathology; and Head, Section of Microbiology, The Cleveland Clinic Foundation, Cleveland, Ohio

BRYNMOR A. WATKINS, Ph.D.

Visiting Associate, Laboratory of Tumor Cell Biology, National Cancer Institute, National Institutes of Health, Bethesda, Maryland

DAVID J. WEBER, M.D., M.P.H.

Associate Professor, Departments of Medicine, Pediatrics, and Epidemiology, University of North Carolina at Chapel Hill School of Medicine; Medical Director of Hospital Epidemiology, University of North Carolina Hospitals, Chapel Hill, North Carolina

ARNOLD N. WEINBERG, M.D.

Professor, Department of Medicine, Harvard Medical School, Boston, Massachusetts; Medical Director, Massachusetts Institute of Technology, Cambridge, Massachusetts; Physician, Department of Medicine, Massachusetts General Hospital, Boston, Massachusetts

MICHAEL E. WEISS, M.D.

Assistant Clinical Professor, Department of Medicine, University of Washington School of Medicine, Seattle, Washington

DAVID F. WELCH, Ph.D.

Associate Professor, Division of Infectious Diseases, Department of Pediatrics, University of Oklahoma College of Medicine; Director, Clinical Microbiology Laboratories, Pathology Service, University Hospitals, Oklahoma City, Oklahoma

RICHARD P. WENZEL, M.D.

Professor, Department of Internal Medicine, and Director, Division of General Medicine, Clinical Epidemiology, and Health Services Research, University of Iowa College of Medicine; Hospital Epidemiologist, University of Iowa Hospitals and Clinics, Iowa City, Iowa

RICHARD J. WHITLEY, M.D.

Professor, Departments of Pediatrics, Microbiology, and Medicine, University of Alabama School of Medicine, Birmingham, Alabama

BARBARA BRAUNSTEIN WILSON, M.D.

Associate Professor, Department of Dermatology, University of Virginia School of Medicine, Charlottesville, Virginia

CHRISTOPHER B. WILSON, M.D.

Professor, Departments of Pediatrics and Immunology, and Head, Division of Pediatric Immunology and Rheumatology, University of Washington School of Medicine; Associate, Division of Infectious Diseases, Children's Hospital and Medical Center, Seattle, Washington

DREW J. WINSTON, M.D.

Associate Clinical Professor, Department of Medicine, University of California, Los Angeles, UCLA School of Medicine; Attending Physician, Department of Medicine, UCLA Medical Center, Los Angeles, California

BRIAN WISPELWEY, M.D.

Associate Professor, Department of Internal Medicine, University of Virginia School of Medicine; Director, Department of Medicine, Infectious Diseases/HIV Clinic, University of Virginia Medical Center, Charlottesville, Virginia

MARTIN S. WOLFE, M.D.

Clinical Professor, Department of Medicine, George Washington University School of Medicine and Health Science, and Clinical Associate Professor, Department of Medicine, Georgetown University School of Medicine; Director, Traveler's Medical Service of Washington, Washington, D.C.

SHELDON M. WOLFF, M.D.*

Endicott Professor and Chairman, Department of Medicine, Tufts University School of Medicine; Physician-in-Chief, New England Medical Center Hospital, Boston, Massachusetts

SIN-YEW WONG, M.D.

Senior Registrar, Singapore General Hospital, Singapore

GAIL L. WOODS, M.D.

Professor, Departments of Pathology and Microbiology, and Director, Division of Clinical Microbiology and Immunology, University of Texas Medical Branch, University of Texas Medical School at Galveston, Galveston, Texas

---

*Deceased.

EDWARD J. YOUNG, M.D.

Professor, Departments of Medicine and Microbiology and Immunology, Baylor College of Medicine; Chief of Staff, Veterans Affairs Medical Center, Houston, Texas

LOWELL S. YOUNG, M.D.

Clinical Professor, Department of Medicine, University of California, San Francisco, School of Medicine; Chief, Division of Infectious Diseases, California Pacific Medical Center, and Director, Kuzell Institute for Arthritis and Infectious Diseases, California Pacific Medical Center Research Institute, San Francisco, California

VICTOR L. YU, M.D.

Professor, Department of Medicine, University of Pittsburgh School of Medicine; Chief, Infectious Disease Section, Veterans Affairs Medical Center, Pittsburgh, Pennsylvania

ROGER W. YURT, M.D.

Professor and Vice-Chairman, Department of Surgery, Cornell University Medical College; Director, Trauma Center, The New York Hospital, New York, New York

STEPHEN H. ZINNER, M.D.

Professor, Department of Medicine, Brown University School of Medicine; Director, Infectious Diseases Section, Department of Medicine, Roger Williams General Hospital; Consultant in Infectious Disease, Rhode Island Hospital, Veterans Affairs Medical Center, Miriam Hospital, and Women and Infants Hospital, Providence, Rhode Island

PREFACE TO THE FOURTH EDITION

The first edition of this book was published in 1979 before the recognition of AIDS, Lyme disease, hepatitis C and E, resistant Enterococci, hantavirus pulmonary syndrome, and the discovery of the etiology of cat scratch disease, just to mention a few new developments. Therapeutic advances have been spectacular with new and potent antiviral, antifungal, and antimicrobial agents. We are witnessing the dawn of the era of immunomodulator therapy.

The fourth edition of *Principles and Practice of Infectious Diseases* reflects the rapid pace of developments in the broad field of infectious diseases. All these areas and many more new aspects are covered in depth.

All the chapters have been revised, many have been completely rewritten by new authors and a number of new chapters have been added.

We are grateful to the dedicated clinicians, scientists, microbiologists, and pharmacologists who have made this book possible.

Special thanks go to our wives, Judith, Shirley, and Kelly, for putting up with preoccupied husbands for the two-year incubation period of the fourth edition. We are also grateful to Toni Tracy and her dedicated staff at Churchill Livingstone, especially Laura Papach and David Terry, for their excellent work.

Gerald L. Mandell, M.D.
John E. Bennett, M.D.
Raphael Dolin, M.D.

PREFACE TO THE FIRST EDITION

Infectious diseases traverse the usual boundaries established by medical specialists. All organ systems may be involved, and all physicians caring for patients may have to deal with infected patients. The format of this book was chosen with the intent that it would contain the necessary information to aid the practitioner in the understanding, diagnosis, and treatment of infectious diseases. Thus, internists, family or general practitioners, pediatricians, surgeons, obstetrician-gynecologists, urologists, residents and fellows in training, medical students, hospital infection control personnel, and clinical microbiologists should find the book a valuable reference.

In planning this book the editors considered several different patterns of organization. The system adopted allows the reader to approach an infected patient three different ways: (a) by major clinical syndrome, (b) by specific etiologic organism, and (c) by host characteristics for patients who are compromised.

Principles and Practice of Infectious Diseases consists of four major parts. The book may be perused as whole, or individual chapters may be examined when the reader is concerned with a specific problem. Part I covers the basic principles necessary for a clear understanding of the concepts of diagnosis and management of infectious disease. Chapters dealing with microbial virulence factors, host defense mechanisms, the epidemiology of infectious diseases, and the clinician and microbiology laboratory are included. In addition, there is a comprehensive discussion of anti-infective chemotherapy.

Part II considers major clinical syndromes. The syndromes are described, followed by a discussion of the potential etiologic agents, evaluation of differential diagnostic possibilities, and an outline of presumptive therapy. All major infectious diseases are discussed in this part of the book.

Part III describes all important pathogenic microbes for man and the diseases they cause. The pathogen is classified and described, the epidemiology is discussed, clinical manifestations are listed, and specific information on therapy and prevention is presented. The most comprehensive discussion of a disease entity can be found by reading about both the etiologic agent and the clinical syndrome. Thus, a comprehensive treatment of pneumococcal pneumonia could be found in reading the appropriate sections of the chapters on acute pneumonia and *Streptococcus pneumoniae*. We attempted to make the chapters dealing with etiologic agents and those dealing with syndromes complete. Therefore some repetition was unavoidable.

The final section, Part IV, covers special problems in infectious diseases including nosocomial infections, infections in impaired hosts, immunizations, and protection of travelers.

The editors are grateful to our expert contributors. These physicians are the world's leaders in their fields, and they diligently prepared carefully written, well-referenced "state of the art" chapters. Our secretaries were skillful and meticulous in their attention to the complexities of assembling *Principles and Practice of Infectious Diseases*. John de Carville, executive editor of John Wiley & Sons, encouraged, cajoled, and advised us from the formative steps all the way through to completion. Lastly, and perhaps most important, we are grateful to our wives and children for putting up with interminable editorial work and meetings.

Gerald L. Mandell, M.D.
R. Gordon Douglas, Jr., M.D.
John E. Bennett, M.D.

CONTENTS

Volume 1

PART I. BASIC PRINCIPLES IN THE DIAGNOSIS AND MANAGEMENT OF INFECTIOUS DISEASES

SECTION A. MICROBIAL VIRULENCE FACTORS

1. Toxins and Other Virulence Factors 2
   Erik L. Hewlett

2. Microbial Adherence 11
   William A. Petri, Jr., and Barbara J. Mann

3. A Molecular Perspective of Microbial Pathogenicity 19
   David A. Relman and Stanley Falkow

SECTION B. HOST DEFENSE MECHANISMS

4. General or Nonspecific Host Defense Mechanisms 30
   Edmund C. Tramont and David L. Hoover

5. Antibodies 36
   Frederick P. Heinzel

6. Complement 58
   Peter Densen

7. Granulocytic Phagocytes 78
   Peter Densen, Robert A. Clark, and William M. Nauseef

8. Cell-Mediated Immunity and Its Role in Host Defense 102
   Richard M. Locksley and Christopher B. Wilson

9. Evaluation of the Patient with Suspected Immunodeficiency 149
   Steven M. Holland and John I. Gallin

SECTION C

10. Epidemiology of Infectious Diseases 158
    Michael T. Osterholm, Craig W. Hedberg, and Kristine L. MacDonald

SECTION D

11. The Clinician and the Microbiology Laboratory 169
    Gail L. Woods and John A. Washington

SECTION E. ANTI-INFECTIVE THERAPY

12. Principles of Anti-Infective Therapy 199
    Robert C. Moellering, Jr.

13. Mechanisms of Antibiotic Resistance 212
    Kenneth H. Mayer, Steven M. Opal, and Antone A. Medeiros

14. Pharmacology of Anti-Infective Agents 225
    George L. Drusano

15. Penicillins 233
    Henry F. Chambers and Harold C. Neu

16. Cephalosporins 247
    Adolf W. Karchmer

17. Other β-Lactam Antibiotics 264
    Henry F. Chambers and Harold C. Neu

18. β-Lactam Allergy 272
    Michael E. Weiss and N. Franklin Adkinson, Jr.

19. Fusidic Acid 278
    Lionel A. Mandell

20. Aminoglycosides 279
    David N. Gilbert

21. Tetracyclines and Chloramphenicol 306
    Harold C. Standiford

22. Rifamycins 317
    Barry M. Farr

23. Metronidazole 329
    Sydney M. Finegold and Glenn E. Mathisen

24. Macrolides and Clindamycin 334
    Neal H. Steigbigel

25. Vancomycin and Teicoplanin 346
    Robert Fekety

26. Sulfonamides and Trimethoprim 354
    Stephen H. Zinner and Kenneth H. Mayer

27. Quinolones 364
    David C. Hooper

28. Urinary Tract Agents: Nitrofurantoin and Methenamine 376
    David C. Hooper

29. Topical Antibacterials 381
    Allan R. Tunkel

30. Antimycobacterial Agents 389
    Robert H. Alford and Richard J. Wallace, Jr.

31. Antifungal Agents 401
    John E. Bennett

xxiii

32. Antiviral Agents   411
    Frederick G. Hayden

33. Immunomodulators   450
    Michael O. Frank and Gerald L. Mandell

34. Antiparasitic Agents   458
    John A. Jernigan and Richard D. Pearson

35. Tables of Antimicrobial Agent Pharmacology   492
    Guy W. Amsden and Jerome J. Schentag

PART II. MAJOR CLINICAL SYNDROMES

SECTION A. FEVER

36. Pathogenesis of Fever and the Acute Phase   Response
    530
    Charles A. Dinarello and Sheldon M. Wolff

37. Fever of Unknown Origin   536
    Jeffrey A. Gelfand and Sheldon M. Wolff

38. The Acutely Ill Patient with Fever and Rash   549
    David J. Weber and Myron S. Cohen

SECTION B. UPPER RESPIRATORY INFECTIONS

39. The Common Cold   561
    Jack M. Gwaltney, Jr.

40. Pharyngitis   566
    Jack M. Gwaltney, Jr.

41. Acute Laryngitis   572
    Jack M. Gwaltney, Jr.

42. Acute Laryngotracheobronchitis (Croup)   573
    Caroline Breese Hall

43. Otitis Externa, Otitis Media, Mastoiditis   579
    Jerome O. Klein

44. Sinusitis   585
    Jack M. Gwaltney, Jr.

45. Epiglottitis   590
    James E. Burns and J. Owen Hendley

46. Infections of the Oral Cavity, Neck, and Head   593
    Anthony W. Chow

SECTION C. PLEUROPULMONARY AND BRONCHIAL INFECTIONS

47. Acute Bronchitis   606
    Jack M. Gwaltney, Jr.

48. Chronic Bronchitis and Acute Infectious
    Exacerbations   608
    Herbert Y. Reynolds

49. Bronchiolitis   612
    Caroline Breese Hall and William J. Hall

50. Acute Pneumonia   619
    Gerald R. Donowitz and Gerald L. Mandell

51. Pleural Effusion and Empyema   637
    Richard E. Bryant

52. Lung Abscess   641
    Sydney M. Finegold

53. Chronic Pneumonia   646
    William E. Dismukes

54. Cystic Fibrosis   657
    M.R. Knowles, P.H. Gilligan, and R.C. Boucher

SECTION D

55. Urinary Tract Infections   662
    Jack D. Sobel and Donald Kaye

SECTION E

56. Sepsis Syndrome   690
    Lowell S. Young

SECTION F

57. Peritonitis and Other Intra-Abdominal Infections   705
    Matthew E. Levison and Larry M. Bush

SECTION G. CARDIOVASCULAR INFECTIONS

58. Endocarditis and Intravascular Infections   740
    W. Michael Scheld and Merle A. Sande

59. Infectious Disorders of Prosthetic Valves and Intravascular
    Devices   783
    Michael G. Threlkeld and C. Glenn Cobbs

60. Prophylaxis of Infective Endocarditis   793
    David T. Durack

61. Myocarditis and Pericarditis   799
    Maria C. Savoia and Michael N. Oxman

62. Mediastinitis   813
    Mark E. Rupp and Gordon L. Archer

SECTION H. CENTRAL NERVOUS SYSTEM INFECTIONS

63. Anatomic Considerations in Central Nervous System
    Infections   821
    John E. Greenlee

64. Acute Meningitis   831
    Allan R. Tunkel and W. Michael Scheld

65. Chronic Meningitis   865
    Barbara M. Gripshover and Jerrold J. Ellner

66. Encephalitis, Myelitis, and Neuritis   874
    Diane E. Griffin

67. Prion Diseases of the Central Nervous System
    (Transmissible Neurodegenerative Diseases)   881
    Kenneth L. Tyler

68. Brain Abscess   887
    Brian Wispelwey and W. Michael Scheld

69. Subdural Empyema   900
    John E. Greenlee

70. Epidural Abscess   903
    John E. Greenlee

71. Suppurative Intracranial Phlebitis   907
    John E. Greenlee

SECTION I. SKIN AND SOFT TISSUE INFECTIONS

72. Cellulitis and Subcutaneous Tissue Infections 909
Morton N. Swartz

73. Myositis 929
Morton N. Swartz

74. Lymphadenitis and Lymphangitis 936
Morton N. Swartz

SECTION J. GASTROINTESTINAL INFECTIONS AND FOOD POISONING

75. Principles and Syndromes of Enteric Infection 945
Richard L. Guerrant

76. Esophagitis 962
Michael A. Polis

77. Nausea, Vomiting, and Noninflammatory Diarrhea 965
Richard L. Guerrant and David A. Bobak

78. Antibiotic-Associated Colitis 978
Robert Fekety

79. Inflammatory Enteritides 987
Richard L. Guerrant

80. Enteric Fever and Other Causes of Abdominal Symptoms with Fever 998
Richard D. Pearson and Richard L. Guerrant

81. Food-Borne Disease 1012
Robert V. Tauxe and James M. Hughes

82. Tropical Sprue 1025
Christine A. Wanke and Richard L. Guerrant

83. Whipple's Disease 1030
William O. Dobbins III

SECTION K. BONE AND JOINT INFECTIONS

84. Infectious Arthritis 1032
James W. Smith and Elizabeth Anne Piercy

85. Osteomyelitis 1039
Jon T. Mader and Jason Calhoun

86. Infections with Prostheses in Bones and Joints 1051
Barry D. Brause

SECTION L. DISEASES OF THE REPRODUCTIVE ORGANS AND SEXUALLY TRANSMITTED DISEASES

87. Genital Skin and Mucous Membrane Lesions 1055
Michael F. Rein

88. Urethritis 1063
William M. McCormack and Michael F. Rein

89. Vulvovaginitis and Cervicitis 1074
Michael F. Rein

90. Infections of the Female Pelvis 1090
Philip B. Mead

91. Prostatitis, Epididymitis, and Orchitis 1098
John N. Krieger

SECTION M. EYE INFECTIONS

92. Conjunctivitis 1103
Terrence P. O'Brien and W. Richard Green

93. Keratitis 1110
Terrence P. O'Brien and W. Richard Green

94. Endophthalmitis 1120
Terrence P. O'Brien and W. Richard Green

95. Periocular Infections 1129
Terrence P. O'Brien and W. Richard Green

SECTION N. HEPATITIS

96. Acute Viral Hepatitis 1136
Henry H. Hsu, Stephen M. Feinstone, and Jay H. Hoofnagle

97. Chronic Hepatitis 1153
Edward L. Krawitt

98. Granulomatous Hepatitis 1159
Anthony S. Fauci and Gary S. Hoffman

SECTION O. ACQUIRED IMMUNODEFICIENCY SYNDROME (AIDS)

99. Global Perspectives on HIV Infection and AIDS 1164
Peter Piot and Michael H. Merson

100. Epidemiology and Prevention of AIDS and HIV Infection 1174
Mary E. Chamberland, John W. Ward, and James W. Curran

101. Immunology of AIDS and HIV Infection 1203
Sharilyn K. Stanley and Anthony S. Fauci

102. Clinical Manifestations of HIV Infection 1217
Richard E. Chaisson and Paul A. Volberding

103. Detection of HIV-1 Infection 1253
Charles J. Schleupner

104. Therapy of HIV Infection 1267
Lawrence Corey

105. Management of Opportunistic Infections Associated with HIV Infection 1280
Henry Masur

106. Vaccines for HIV-1 Infection 1294
Raphael Dolin and Michael C. Keefer

SECTION P. MISCELLANEOUS SYNDROMES

107. Chronic Fatigue Syndrome 1306
Robert T. Schooley

108. Cat Scratch Disease 1310
Gerald W. Fischer

Index

Volume 2

PART III. INFECTIOUS DISEASES AND THEIR ETIOLOGIC AGENTS

SECTION A. VIRAL DISEASES

109.   Introduction to Viruses and Viral Diseases   1314
Kenneth L. Tyler and Bernard N. Fields

DNA VIRUSES

Poxviridae

110.   Introduction   1325
John M. Neff

111.   Vaccinia Virus (Cowpox)   1325
John M. Neff

112.   Variola (Smallpox) and Monkeypox Viruses   1328
John M. Neff

113.   Parapoxviruses and Molluscum Contagiosum and Tanapox Viruses   1329
John M. Neff

Herpesviridae

114.   Introduction to Herpesviridae   1330
Stephen E. Straus

115.   Herpes Simplex Virus   1136
Martin S. Hirsch

116.   Varicella-Zoster Virus   1345
Richard J. Whitley

117.   Cytomegalovirus   1351
Monto Ho

118.   Epstein-Barr Virus (Infectious Mononucleosis)   1364
Robert T. Schooley

119.   Human Herpesvirus 6 and Human Herpesvirus 7   1377
Mark Y. Stoeckle

120.   Herpes B Virus   1379
Stephen E. Straus

Adenoviridae

121.   Adenovirus   1382
Stephen G. Baum

Papovaviridae

122.   Papillomaviruses   1387
William Bonnez and Richard C. Reichman

123.   JC, BK, and Other Polyomaviruses; Progressive Multifocal Leukoencephalopathy   1400
Lisa M. Demeter

Hepadnaviridae

124.   Hepatitis B Virus and Hepatitis D Virus   1406
William S. Robinson

Parvoviridae

125.   Parvoviruses (Erythema Infectiosum, Aplastic Crisis)   1439
Amy C. Portmore

RNA VIRUSES

Reoviridae

126.   Colorado Tick Fever   1446
Thomas P. Monath

127.   Reovirus and Orbivirus   1447
Thomas P. Monath

128.   Rotavirus   1448
Paul A. Offit and H. Fred Clark

Togaviridae

129.   Alphaviruses   1455
Lewis Markoff

130.   Rubella Virus (German Measles)   1459
Anne A. Gershon

Flaviviridae

131.   Flaviviruses (Yellow Fever, Dengue, Dengue Hemorrhagic Fever, Japanese Encephalitis, St. Louis Encephalitis, Tick-Borne Encephalitis)   1465
Thomas P. Monath

132.   Hepatitis C Virus   1474
Stanley M. Lemon and Edwin A. Brown

Coronaviridae

133.   Coronavirus   1486
Kenneth McIntosh

Paramyxoviridae

134.   Parainfluenza Viruses   1489
Kelly J. Henrickson, Ranjit Ray, and Robert Belshe

135.   Mumps Virus   1496
Stephen G. Baum and Nathan Litman

136.   Respiratory Syncytial Virus   1501
Caroline Breese Hall and Carol A. McCarthy

137.   Measles Virus (Rubeola)   1519
Anne A. Gershon

Rhabdoviridae

138.   Vesicular Stomatitis Virus and Related Viruses   1526
Mark Y. Stoeckle

139.   Rabies Virus   1527
Daniel B. Fishbein and Kenneth W. Bernard

Filoviridae

140.   Marburg and Ebola Virus Hemorrhagic Fevers   1543
        Clarence J. Peters

Orthomyxoviridae

141.   Influenza Virus   1546
        Robert F. Betts

Bunyaviridae

142.   California Encephalitis Viruses, Hantaviruses, and Other
        Bunyaviridae   1567
        Clarence J. Peters and Karl M. Johnson

Arenaviridae

143.   Lymphocytic Choriomeningitis Virus, Lassa Virus, and
        Other Arenaviruses   1572
        Clarence J. Peters and Karl M. Johnson

Retroviridae

144.   Introduction—Type C Oncoviruses Including
        Human T-Cell Lymphotropic Virus Types I
        and II   1579
        Mark Y. Stoeckle

145.   Lentiviruses: An Overview   1584
        Ashley T. Haase

146.   Human Immunodeficiency Viruses   1590
        *Brynmor A. Watkins, Mary E. Klotman, and
        Robert C. Gallo*

Picornaviridae

147.   Introduction   1606
        John F. Modlin

148.   Poliovirus   1613
        John F. Modlin

149.   Coxsackieviruses, Echoviruses, and Newer Enteroviruses
        1620
        John F. Modlin

150.   Hepatitis A Virus   1636
        *Manuel Battegay, Ian D. Gust,
        and Stephen M. Feinstone*

151.   Rhinovirus   1656
        Jack M. Gwaltney, Jr.

Unclassified Viruses

152.   Hepatitis E Virus   1663
        Stanley M. Lemon

Caliciviridae

153.   Norwalk Viruses and Other Caliciviruses   1666
        John Treanor and Raphael Dolin

Astroviridae

154.   Astroviruses   1672
        John Treanor and Raphael Dolin

SECTION B. PRIONS

155.   Prions   1674
        Kenneth L. Tyler

SECTION C. CHLAMYDIAL DISEASES

156.   Introduction   1676
        Robert B. Jones

157.   Chlamydia Trachomatis (Trachoma, Perinatal
        Infections, Lymphogranuloma Venereum, and   Other
        Genital Infections)   1679
        Robert B. Jones

158.   Chlamydia Psittaci (Psittacosis)   1693
        David Schlossberg

159.   Chlamydia Pneumoniae (TWAR)   1696
        J. Thomas Grayston

SECTION D. MYCOPLASMA DISEASES

160.   Introduction   1701
        Stephen G. Baum

161.   Mycoplasma Pneumoniae and Atypical
        Pneumonia   1704
        Stephen G. Baum

162.   Ureaplasma Urealyticum (T-Strain Mycoplasma)
        and Mycoplasma Hominis   1713
        David Taylor-Robinson

SECTION E. RICKETTSIOSIS

163.   Introduction   1719
        Alfred J. Saah

164.   Rickettsia Rickettsii and Other Spotted Fever Group
        Rickettsiae (Rocky Mountain Spotted Fever and
        Other Spotted Fevers)   1721
        David H. Walker and Didier Raoult

165.   Rickettsia Akari (Rickettsialpox)   1727
        Alfred J. Saah

166.   Coxiella Burnetii (Q Fever)   1727
        Thomas J. Marrie

167.   Rickettsia Prowazekii (Epidemic or Louse-Borne
        Typhus)   1735
        Alfred J. Saah

168.   Murine Typhus   1737
        J. Stephen Dumler and David H. Walker

169.   Rickettsia Tsutsugamushi (Scrub Typhus)   1740
        Alfred J. Saah

170.   Rochalimaea Species (Recently Renamed
        Bartonella)   1741
        Leonard N. Slater and David F. Welch

171.   Ehrlichia Chaffeensis (Human Ehrlichiosis) and
        Other Ehrlichiae   1747
        David H. Walker and J. Stephen Dumler

SECTION F. BACTERIAL DISEASES

172.   Introduction   1752
        Thalia I. Nicas and Barry I. Eisenstein

GRAM-POSITIVE COCCI

173. Staphylococcus Aureus (Including Toxic Shock Syndrome) 1754
      Francis A. Waldvogel

174. Staphylococcus Epidermidis and Other Coagulase-Negative Staphylococci 1777
      Gordon L. Archer

175. Classification of Streptococci 1784
      Alan L. Bisno and Ivo van de Rijn

176. Streptococcus Pyogenes 1786
      Alan L. Bisno

177. Nonsuppurative Poststreptococcal Sequelae: Rheumatic Fever and Glomerulonephritis 1799
      Alan L. Bisno

178. Streptococcus Pneumoniae 1811
      Daniel M. Musher

179. Enterococcus Species, Streptococcus Bovis, and Leuconostoc Species 1826
      Robert C. Moellering, Jr.

180. Streptococcus Agalactiae (Group B Streptococcus) 1835
      Morven S. Edwards and Carol J. Baker

181. Viridans Streptococci and Groups C and G Streptococci 1845
      Caroline C. Johnson and Allan R. Tunkel

182. Streptococcus Intermedius Group 1861
      Charles W. Stratton

GRAM-POSITIVE BACILLI

183. Corynebacterium Diphtheriae 1865
      Rob Roy MacGregor

184. Other Corynebacteria and Rhodococcus 1872
      Arthur E. Brown

185. Listeria Monocytogenes 1880
      Donald Armstrong

186. Bacillus Anthracis (Anthrax) 1885
      Daniel Lew

187. Other Bacillus Species 1890
      Carmelita U. Tuazon

188. Erysipelothrix Rhusiopathiae 1894
      Annette C. Reboli and W. Edmund Farrar

GRAM-NEGATIVE COCCI

189. Neisseria Meningitidis 1896
      Michael A. Apicella

190. Neisseria Gonorrhoeae 1909
      H. Hunter Handsfield and P. Frederick Sparling

191. Moraxella Catarrhalis and Other Gram-Negative Cocci 1926
      Dieter H.M. Gröschel

GRAM-NEGATIVE BACILLI

192. Vibrio Cholerae and Cholera 1934
      William B. Greenough III

193. Other Pathogenic Vibrios 1945
      Charles C.J. Carpenter

194. Campylobacter and Related Species 1948
      Martin J. Blaser

195. Helicobacter Pylori and Related Organisms 1956
      Martin J. Blaser

196. Enterobacteriaceae 1964
      Barry I. Eisenstein

197. Pseudomonas Aeruginosa 1980
      Matthew Pollack

198. Pseudomonas Species (Including Melioidosis and Glanders) 2003
      Jay P. Sanford

199. Acinetobacter Species 2009
      David M. Allen and Barry J. Hartman

200. Salmonella (Including Salmonella Typhi) 2013
      Samuel I. Miller, Elizabeth L. Hohmann, and David A. Pegues

201. Shigella Species (Bacillary Dysentery) 2033
      Herbert L. DuPont

202. Haemophilus Influenzae 2039
      E. Richard Moxon

203. Haemophilus Species (Including Chancroid) 2045
      W. Lee Hand

204. Gardnerella Vaginalis and Mobiluncus Species 2050
      Carol A. Spiegel

205. Brucella Species 2053
      Edward J. Young

206. Francisella Tularensis (Tularemia) 2060
      Robert L. Penn

207. Pasteurella Species 2068
      John M. Boyce

208. Yersinia Species (Including Plague) 2070
      Thomas Butler

209. Bordetella Species 2078
      Erik L. Hewlett

210. Streptobacillus Moniliformis (Rat-Bite Fever) 2084
      Ronald G. Washburn

211. Legionella Pneumophila (Legionnaires' Disease) 2087
      Victor L. Yu

212. Other Legionella Species 2097
      Robert R. Muder and Victor L. Yu

213. Capnocytophaga 2103
      Vee J. Gill

214. Other Gram-Negative Bacilli 2106
      John E. McGowan, Jr., and James P. Steinberg

SPIROCHETES

215. Treponema Pallidum (Syphilis)   2117
      Edmund C. Tramont

216. Treponema Species (Yaws, Pinta, Bejel)   2133
      Jeffrey D. Chulay

217. Leptospira Species (Leptospirosis)   2137
      W. Edmund Farrar

218. Borrelia Species (Relapsing Fever)   2141
      Warren D. Johnson, Jr.

219. Borrelia Burgdorferi (Lyme Disease, Lyme Borreliosis)   2143
      Allen C. Steere

220. Spirillum Minus (Rat-Bite Fever)   2155
      Ronald G. Washburn

ANAEROBIC BACTERIA

221. Anaerobic Bacteria: General Concepts   2156
      Sydney M. Finegold

222. Clostridium Tetani   2173
      Thomas P. Bleck

223. Clostridium Botulinum   2178
      Thomas P. Bleck

224. Gas Gangrene and Other Clostridium-Associated Diseases   2182
      Bennett Lorber

225. Bacteroides, Prevotella, and Fusobacterium Species (And Other Medically Important Anaerobic Gram-Negative Bacilli)   2195
      Bennett Lorber

226. Anaerobic Cocci   2204
      Itzhak Brook

227. Anaerobic Gram-Positive Nonsporulating Bacilli   2206
      Itzhak Brook

MISCELLANEOUS BACTERIA

228. Bartonella Bacilliformis (Bartonellosis)   2209
      Norbert J. Roberts, Jr.

229. Calymmatobacterium Granulomatis (Donovanosis, Granuloma Inguinale)   2210
      Ronald C. Ballard

MYCOBACTERIAL DISEASES

230. Mycobacterium Tuberculosis   2213
      David W. Haas and Roger M. Des Prez

231. Leprosy (Hansen's Disease)   2243
      Robert H. Gelber

232. Mycobacterium Avium Complex   2250
      Diane V. Havlir and Jerrold J. Ellner

233. Other Mycobacterium Species   2264
      Edward A. Horowitz and W. Eugene Sanders, Jr.

DISEASES DUE TO HIGHER BACTERIA

234. Nocardia Species   2273
      Phillip I. Lerner

235. Agents of Actinomycosis   2280
      Thomas A. Russo

SECTION G. MYCOSES

236. Introduction   2288
      John E. Bennett

237. Candida Species   2289
      John E. Edwards, Jr.

238. Aspergillus Species   2306
      John E. Bennett

239. Agents of Mucormycosis and Related Species   2311
      Alan M. Sugar

240. Sporothrix Schenckii   2321
      John H. Rex

241. Agents of Chromomycosis   2324
      Kenneth F. Wagner

242. Agents of Mycetoma   2327
      El Sheikh Mahgoub

243. Cryptococcus Neoformans   2331
      Richard D. Diamond

244. Histoplasma Capsulatum   2340
      Ward E. Bullock

245. Blastomyces Dermatitidis   2353
      Stanley W. Chapman

246. Coccidioides Immitis   2365
      David A. Stevens

247. Dermatophytosis and Other Superficial Mycoses   2375
      Roderick J. Hay

248. Paracoccidioides Brasiliensis   2386
      Angela Restrepo M.

249. Miscellaneous Fungi, and Prototheca   2389
      John E. Bennett

SECTION H. PROTOZOAL DISEASES

250. Introduction   2393
      Jonathan I. Ravdin

251. Entamoeba Histolytica (Amebiasis)   2395
      Jonathan I. Ravdin and William A. Petri, Jr.

252. Free-Living Amebae   2408
      Francine Marciano-Cabral and William A. Petri, Jr.

253. Plasmodium Species (Malaria)   2415
      Donald J. Krogstad

254. Leishmania Species: Visceral (Kala-Azar), Cutaneous, and Mucosal Leishmaniasis   2428
      Richard D. Pearson and Anastacio de Queiroz Sousa

255. Trypanosoma Species (American Trypanosomiasis, Chagas Disease): Biology of Trypanosomes 2442
Louis V. Kirchhoff

256. Agents of African Trypanosomiasis (Sleeping Sickness) 2450
Louis V. Kirchhoff

257. Toxoplasma Gondii 2455
Miles Beaman, Robert E. McCabe, Sin-Yew Wong, and Jack S. Remington

258. Pneumocystis Carinii 2475
Peter D. Walzer

259. Giardia Lamblia 2487
David R. Hill

260. Trichomonas Vaginalis 2493
Michael F. Rein

261. Babesia 2497
Jeffrey A. Gelfand

262. Cryptosporidium 2500
Beth L.P. Ungar

263. Isospora Belli, Sarcocystis Species, Balantidium Coli, Blastocystis Hominis, and Cyclospora 2510
Cynthia L. Sears

264. Microsporidia 2513
Ralph T. Bryan

SECTION I. DISEASES DUE TO HELMINTHS

265. Introduction 2525
Adel A.F. Mahmoud

266. Intestinal Nematodes (Roundworms) 2526
Adel A.F. Mahmoud

267. Tissue Nematodes (Trichinosis, Dracunculiasis, Filariasis) 2531
David I. Grove

268. Trematodes (Schistosomiasis) and Other Flukes 2538
Adel A.F. Mahmoud

269. Cestodes (Tapeworms) 2544
Charles H. King

270. Visceral Larva Migrans and Other Unusual Helminth Infections 2553
Theodore E. Nash

SECTION J. ECTOPARASITES

271. Introduction 2558
Barbara Braunstein Wilson

272. Lice (Pediculosis) 2558
Barbara Braunstein Wilson

273. Scabies 2560
Barbara Braunstein Wilson

274. Myiasis 2562
Barbara Braunstein Wilson

275. Mites (Including Chiggers) 2564
Barbara Braunstein Wilson

276. Ticks 2565
Barbara Braunstein Wilson

SECTION K. DISEASES OF UNKNOWN ETIOLOGY

277. Kawasaki Syndrome 2567
Frank T. Saulsbury

PART IV. SPECIAL PROBLEMS

SECTION A. NOSOCOMIAL INFECTIONS

278. Infection Control 2572
Michael B. Edmond and Richard P. Wenzel

279. Isolation 2575
Michael B. Edmond and Richard P. Wenzel

280. Sterilization, Disinfection, and Disposal of Infectious Waste 2579
Michael A. Martin and Richard P. Wenzel

281. Bacteremia Due to Percutaneous Intravascular Devices 2587
David K. Henderson

282. Nosocomial Respiratory Infections 2599
James E. Pennington

283. Nosocomial Urinary Tract Infections 2607
John W. Warren

284. Nosocomial Viral Hepatitis and Infections Transmitted by Blood and Blood Products 2616
Bradley N. Doebbeling and Richard P. Wenzel

285. HIV-1 in the Health Care Setting 2632
David K. Henderson

286. Nosocomial Herpesvirus Infections 2656
David K. Henderson

SECTION B. INFECTIONS IN SPECIAL HOSTS

287. Infections in the Cancer Patient—Diagnosis, Prevention, and Treatment 2666
Stephen C. Schimpff

288. Infections in Patients with Acute Leukemia and Lymphoma 2675
Françoise Meunier

289. Empirical Therapy and Prevention of Infection in the Immunocompromised Host 2686
Philip A. Pizzo

290. Infections in Intravenous Drug Abusers 2696
D.P. Levine and Jack D. Sobel

291. Infections in Transplant Recipients 2709
Monto Ho and J. Stephen Dummer

292. Infections in Bone Marrow Transplant Recipients 2717
Drew J. Winston

293. Infections in Solid Organ Transplant Recipients 2722
J. Stephen Dummer, Monto Ho, and Richard L. Simmons

294. Infections in Patients with Spinal Cord Injury 2732
Rabih O. Darouiche and Daniel M. Musher

295. Infections in the Elderly 2737
Kent B. Crossley and Phillip K. Peterson

SECTION C. SURGICAL AND TRAUMA-RELATED INFECTIONS

296. Postoperative Infections and Antimicrobial Prophylaxis 2742
Douglas S. Kernodle and Allen B. Kaiser

297. Approach to Infection in the Multiply Traumatized Patient 2756
Anthony E. Fiore, Manjari Joshi, and Ellis S. Caplan

298. Burns 2761
Roger W. Yurt

299. Bites 2765
Ellie J.C. Goldstein

SECTION D

300. Immunization 2770
Walter A. Orenstein, Alan R. Hinman, Kenneth J. Bart, and Stephen C. Hadler

SECTION E

301. Zoonoses 2790
Arnold N. Weinberg

SECTION F

302. Protection of Travelers 2796
Martin S. Wolfe

Index

BASIC PRINCIPLES
IN THE DIAGNOSIS
AND MANAGEMENT
OF INFECTIOUS DISEASES

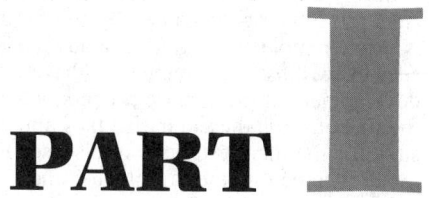

PART I

1. TOXINS AND OTHER VIRULENCE FACTORS

ERIK L. HEWLETT

Although humans are continually exposed to a vast array of microorganisms in the environment, only a small portion of those microbes are capable of interacting with the host in such a way that infection and disease result. The capacity to cause disease is determined by the production of a variety of virulence factors by the infecting organism. Although it was once thought that all microorganisms elicit their adverse effects on hosts by elaboration of toxins, it is now clear that the pathogenic process is complex and represents a well-orchestrated sequence of events in which many microbial components, such as enzymes and other biologically active molecules not technically considered toxins, are required.[1]

The first step in this process is the initial interaction of host and parasite. The adherence of microorganisms to host surfaces or tissues is now recognized to be highly specific and essential for subsequent events in the pathogenic process to occur. The specificity, mechanisms, and pathogenic significance of bacterial attachment are addressed in Chapter 2.

For some bacteria, the association with a mucosal surface represents the final destination. These bacteria, such as *Vibrio cholerae, Bordetella pertussis, Helicobacter pylori,* and some *Escherichia coli,* remain largely in the mucus layer or attached to the mucosa and exert their ill effects by cell contact and/or elaboration of toxins that interact with adjacent or distant cells. For many other organisms, however, the attachment process represents only the establishment of a beach-head from which tissue penetration and/or cell invasion can be launched. Organisms such as *Salmonella, Yersinia, Listeria,* and invasive *E. coli* penetrate the anatomic barriers of the host and either enter cells or pass through them to disseminate within the body. To survive under these conditions, all of these organisms have special virulence factors that enable them to avoid or disarm host defenses. Some are true toxins, in the classic sense, that kill, damage, or alter the function of host cells, but others, such as staphylococcal protein A, the polysaccharide capsule of a variety of bacteria, and a number of virulence factors that facilitate intracellular survival, provide protection without being directly harmful to individual cells.

Survival and continued proliferation of the infecting organisms are often accompanied by the production of toxins, that is, protein molecules capable of adversely affecting cells or tissues of the host. In some cases, these toxins only enhance the development of the disease process, whereas in others they are the sine qua non thereof in that they appear to be totally responsible for the manifestations of disease. Examples in this latter group include diphtheria, tetanus, and botulinum toxins.

Finally, one of the following three outcomes results: *(1)* The proliferation of organisms and production of toxic products impair the host to such an extent that the host dies. *(2)* A state of relative equilibrium is reached with the establishment of a chronic infection. *(3)* Host defense mechanisms, with or without the aid of exogenous factors such as antibiotics, supervene, and the infecting organism is cleared. It is of note that in some cases, elimination of the causative organism may not be sufficient to terminate the disease process because the toxic effects or immunologic reactions may persist in the absence of microbes. In addition, some bacterial products, such as staphylococcal superantigen, may precipitate responses in the host that are the principal cause of a clinical illness (toxic shock syndrome).

The remainder of this chapter is devoted to the role of bacterial toxins and other virulence factors in the development of human diseases. Recent data on the complex, integrated systems employed by pathogens to regulate virulence factor production will be discussed. Additional information on each example cited herein can be obtained from the chapters on specific causative organisms.

TOXINS

Classification and Structure of Toxins

The word *toxin* is derived from the Greek *toxikon,* bow poison, referring to the poisonous material placed on arrows by Greek warriors. The implication of this choice of terms is that the bacterium produces a molecule that it "releases" to affect host cells at a distance. The term was first used by Roux and Yersin[2] to describe the factor released into the culture medium by *Corynebacterium diphtheriae* that caused the death of recipient animals. Subsequently, many toxins have been identified, and confusion has arisen concerning the terminology used to describe and classify different toxins. *Exotoxin* was previously used to refer to toxins produced by and released from gram-positive bacteria during growth, whereas *endotoxin* was used for the intracellular and cell-associated toxic components of gram-negative organisms, including the lipopolysaccharide component that now bears the name *endotoxin.* Because gram-negative bacteria are now recognized to elaborate classic protein toxins, it seems prudent that the term *exotoxin* be used for bacterial products that are protein in nature, are released from the bacterium during exponential growth, and are toxic for target cells or experimental animals. As noted earlier, this definition excludes protein toxins that are intracellular and released only with lysis of the bacterial cells (intracellular or cell-associated toxins), gram-negative bacterial lipopolysaccharide, and bacterial virulence factors that may be involved in attachment, local or systemic dissemination, and acquisition of nutrients but that possess no capacity for direct toxicity to the host.

Although exotoxins occur in many forms, there is a general structural model to which a number of the important exotoxins conform (Table 1). According to the A–B model described by Gill,[20] each of these toxins is composed of a binding (B) domain, component, or subunit portion and an enzymatic (A) portion, which is responsible for the toxic effect once inside the cell. Isolated A subunits are enzymatically active but lack binding and cell entry capability and thus have no biologic activity (the ability to intoxicate intact cells). Isolated B subunits, on the other hand, may bind to target cells and even block the action of holotoxin, but they are, in most instances, nontoxic and biologically inactive.

Other criteria by which toxins may be classified are their cellular or tissue target of action (i.e., enterotoxins, neurotoxins, leukotoxins), their mechanisms of action (ADP-ribosylating toxins, adenylate cyclase toxins; Table 1), their major biologic effects (dermonecrotic toxin, edema-producing toxin, hemolytic toxin, lymphocytosis-promoting toxin), and their contribution to the pathogenicity of the disease process. Quite clearly the

TABLE 1. General Characteristics of Toxins

Toxin Family	Toxin	Organism	Subunit Structure[a]	Target Cell Receptor	Molecular Mechanism	Biologic Effects
ADP-ribosylating toxins	Cholera toxin	V. cholerae	A-5B[b]	Ganglioside (GM₁)	ADP-ribosylation of Gsα	Activation of enterocyte adenylate cyclase; secretory diarrhea
	Diphtheria toxin	C. diphtheriae	A/B	Heparin-binding, EGF-like growth factor precursor[c]	ADP-ribosylation of elongation factor II	Inhibition of protein synthesis; cell death
	Heat-labile enterotoxins[d]	E. coli	— Similar or identical to cholera toxin —			
	Exotoxin A	P. aeruginosa	A/B	α₂-Macroglobulin/ LDL receptor[e]	— Similar or identical to diphtheria toxin —	
	Pertussis toxin	B. pertussis	A-5B[f]	Different carbohydrate moeities in different cells[g]	ADP-ribosylation of several G proteins involved in signal transduction	Inhibition of signal transduction mediated by G protein target
	C2 toxin	C. botulinum	A + B[h]	Unknown	ADP-ribosylation of actin	Inhibition of actin polymerization; cell rounding; intestinal fluid accumulation
	Iota toxin	C. perfringens	— Similar or identical to C2 toxin —			
Adenylate cyclase toxins	Adenylate cyclase toxin	B. pertussis	A/B	None known	Calmodulin-activated adenylate cyclase; formation of ion-permeable pore	Increased target cell cAMP levels; hemolysis
	Edema factor (EF)[i]	B. anthracis	A + B	Unknown glycoprotein	— Similar or identical to AC toxin —	
RNA glycosidase toxins	Shiga toxin	S. dysenteriae	A-5B	Globotriaosylceramide (Gb₃)	N-glycosidase cleavage of rRNA	Inhibition of protein synthesis; cell death
	Shiga-like toxins	Shigella species, E. coli, others[j]	— Similar or identical to shiga toxin —			
Metallo protease toxins	Tetanus toxin	C. tetani	A/B	Probably ganglioside (GT₁ and/or GD₁ᵦ)	Zn²⁺-dependent protease cleavage of synaptobrevin[k]	Inhibition of neurotransmitter release; spastic paralysis
	Botulinum toxin	C. botulinum	A/B	Probably ganglioside	Zn²⁺-dependent protease, substrate: synaptobrevin[k]	Inhibition of neurotransmitter release; flaccid paralysis
	Lethal factor[i]	B. anthracis	A + B	Unknown	Zn²⁺-dependent protease, substrate unknown[k]	Induction of cytokine release; death of target cells and experimental animals

[a] A-5B or A-B indicates subunits synthesized separately and associated by noncovalent bonds; A/B denotes domains of a single protein that may be separated by proteolytic cleavage; A + B indicates two separate proteins that interact at target cell surface.
[b] Binding component composed of five identical B subunits; proteolytic cleavage and reduction of a disulfide bond within the A subunit yields two peptides, A₁ (possessing ADP ribosyltransferase activity) and A₂ (involved in association with B subunits) (3).
[c] Receptor recently identified as transmembrane EGF-like growth factor precursor (4).
[d] The heat-labile enterotoxins of E. coli are now recognized to be a family of related molecules with antigenic and receptor-binding differences, but identical mechanisms of action (5).
[e] Receptor recently identified as transmembrane, α₂-macroglobulin/LDL-receptor (6).
[f] Pentameric B subunit composition has stoichiometry of S₂·S₃·2S₄·S₅; noncovalent association with A subunit (S₁) (7).
[g] Binding to carbohydrates (glycoproteins/glycolipids), perhaps different receptors on different target cells (8–11).
[h] C2 is a binary toxin in which component II is responsible for binding and must undergo proteolytic activation, allowing component I to bind and enter (12). C3 is a separate ADP-ribosyltransferase produced by C. botulinum types C and D; it ADP-ribosylates several small molecular weight GTP-binding proteins (rho, etc.), but has no known toxic effects (13).
[i] Three component toxins in which PA (protective antigen) serves as binding subunit; as a result of proteolytic cleavage at target cell surface, PA is activated to bind either EF (edema factor) or LF (lethal factor) for internalization via receptor-mediated endocytosis (14–16).
[j] Shiga-like toxins are produced by a number of gram-negative organisms (17).
[k] Protease activity recently discovered and implicated as mechanism of toxin action (tetanus toxin [18]; botulinum toxin [18]; lethal factor, [19]).

difficulties associated with describing and classifying these bacterial products reflect limitations in our knowledge of their production, target cell interaction, mechanism of action, and clinical significance. The use of powerful investigative techniques provided by cellular and molecular biology has resulted in an explosion of information on bacterial toxins and other virulence factors, including discovery of new toxins, determination of the primary sequence and crystal structure of many toxins, recognition of molecular mechanism of action, and identification of family relationships among apparently disparate molecules.

Control of Synthesis and Release of Toxins

Molecular biologic approaches have revealed an unanticipated level of complexity in the regulation of toxin production and secretion.[21] Synthesis of many bacterial toxins and other virulence factors is tightly controlled by regulatory systems that are responsive to environmental conditions (see Chapter 3). For example, the production of diphtheria toxin is virtually eliminated by the presence of iron in the medium,[22] virulence gene expression in Yersinia is repressed by calcium,[23] and the expression of cholera toxin and associated virulence factors is con-

trolled by environmental osmolarity.[24] In many cases, two-component, environmental-sensing systems are responsible for coordinate control of the expression of a group of toxins and virulence factors associated in a regulon, allowing for their concurrent production in one phase of infection.[25] Recently, Mahan et al.[26] developed a genetic selection system to allow detection of bacterial genes activated in vivo, thus providing a powerful tool for evaluating putative virulence genes. In B. pertussis, induction of the synthesis of different virulence components is staggered, such that attachment factors are produced initially to establish the infection, and toxins are synthesized and released later to protect against the host response and promote survival.[27]

In addition to the regulatory elements within given toxin operon, there may be one or more structural genes encoding the toxin and other genes for proteins involved in activation and export of the toxin after synthesis.[21,28] Furthermore, the regulatory and structural genes may be chromosomal in location, as is the case for cholera toxin.[29] Production of the family of immunologically and functionally homologous heat-labile toxins of Escherichia coli is, on the other hand, plasmid mediated.[29] The structural gene for diphtheria toxin is located on a β-phase, but the inhibition of toxin synthesis by excess iron is mediated through a metalloregulatory protein, DtxR, which is of bacterial origin.[30] The structural gene for tetanus toxin is located on a large (75 kilobase [kb]) plasmid.[31] The pertussis toxin gene is chromosomal and is present in three *Bordetella* species but is expressed only in *B. pertussis* due to mutations in the promoter region of the gene in *B. parapertussis* and *B. bronchiseptica*.[32,33] Finally, the gene for staphylococcal enterotoxin may be either chromosomal or plasmid in location, but its production is regulated by genes on a plasmid.[34]

The processes by which large protein molecules, such as toxins, are exported from the bacterial cell have been further elucidated by analysis of the toxin operons. The mechanisms involved are thoroughly discussed in reviews by Randall et al.[35] and Pugsley.[36] Many of the classic exotoxins are synthesized with an NH-terminal signal or leader sequence consisting of a few (1–3) charged amino acids and a stretch (14–20) of hydrophobic amino acids. The signal sequence may bind and be inserted into the cytoplasmic membrane during translation such that the polypeptide is secreted while being synthesized. The signal peptide is then cleaved, which leaves the intact toxin molecule free in the periplasm. Alternatively, the protein may be synthesized intracytoplasmically. Subsequent binding via the leader sequence to the cytoplasmic membrane may cause a conformational change, allowing the protein to traverse the membrane with or without the help of pores or transport molecules. Frequently, chaperone proteins are required to guide this process. As is the case with many toxins, the synthesis and release of *E. coli* hemolysin,[28] *B. pertussis* adenylate cyclase toxin,[37] and pertussis toxin[38] clearly entail a process requiring the products of multiple genes involved in processing and/or transport. Some multicomponent toxins, such as cholera toxin, have their subunits secreted separately; they are then assembled in the periplasmic space with the assistance of disulfide isomerase-like enzymes.[39] In gram-negative organisms, however, the outer membrane provides an additional barrier to prevent escape of periplasmic protein molecules. Middeldorp and Witholt[40] have proposed that some toxins, such as *E. coli* heat-labile toxin, may not be released in soluble form, but rather delivered to target cells while contained in vesicles of the outer membrane. These vesicles would possess outer membrane-associated attachment factors, enabling them to act as "bombs" capable of interacting with and possibly entering target cells to release their contents of toxin.

Attachment and Entry of Toxins

Some toxins, such as the hemolytic phospholipases, are bacteria exoenzymes that appear to interact with the external surface of host cell membranes by catalyzing their specific reactions and thereby eliciting their specific toxic effects without cell entry.[41] A number of toxins, however, act on intracellular substrates and thus require cell entry to be effective. Most of these conform to the A–B model described earlier[20] and have binding components that interact with specific receptors on target cells, such as the sialoganglioside GM_1 for cholera toxin, GT_1 for tetanus toxin, and probably GD_{1b} for botulinum toxin.[42] The relatively wide distribution of GM_1 ganglioside among cell types accounts for the apparent lack of specificity of cholera toxin in vitro. The specificity of the effect of cholera toxin during infection (secretory diarrhea), however, is due to the localization of the organisms and the toxin to the intestinal tract. Pertussis toxin has been shown to interact with sialic acid–containing glycoproteins,[8–11] and most cells are sensitive to intoxication by pertussis toxin. Recent evidence suggests, however, that the toxin may be reacting with different carbohydrate-containing receptors on different cell types.[8–11] Diphtheria toxin and *Pseudomonas* exotoxin A catalyze the identical reaction intracellularly and are both distributed systemically, yet the resultant disease processes are quite distinct. The differences between the two appear to reside, at least in part, at the level of target cell specificities,[43] with diphtheria toxin binding to an epidermal growth factor (EGF) percursor molecule[4] and exotoxin A to the α_2-macroglobulin/low-density lipoprotein (LDL) receptor.[6]

There are several different mechanisms by which the A subunits of A/B toxins enter the target cell. In each case, however, a large protein molecule must insert into or cross the lipid bilayer.[20,44] This activity is reflected in the ability of a number of intact A/B toxins or their B subunits to insert into artificial lipid bilayers, creating ion-permeable pathways.[45–48] In some cases, such as diphtheria toxin, there appears to be binding to a surface receptor, uptake into an endocytotic vesicle, and acidification of that vesicle so as to result in a conformational change that enables a part of the toxin molecule to traverse the membrane.[49] The final step in diphtheria toxin translocation is energy requiring and dependent on membrane potential and a proton gradient.[50] *Pseudomonas* exotoxin A appears to be internalized somewhat differently, with endocytosis into coated pits and routing to the trans-Golgi where proteolytic activation occurs before entry into the cytosol.[51] Toxins with identical enzymatic mechanisms may enter cells by completely separate and distinct pathways. Adenylate cyclase toxins from *B. pertussis* and *Bacillus anthracis* both catalyze the production of cAMP from host intracellular ATP stores.[14,15,52] Anthrax toxin (edema factor plus protective antigen [EF + PA]) enters by receptor-mediated endocytosis, whereas pertussis adenylate cyclase toxin utilizes a different mechanism to traverse the cell membrane directly.[15] For many toxins, such as pertussis toxin and tetanus toxin, putative receptors have been identified, but the entry mechanisms remain a mystery.

Mechanism of Toxin Action and Role in Clinical Disease

As noted earlier, bacterial toxins do not operate in isolation to cause disease. With the exception of performed toxins responsible for food-borne illnesses, toxins are produced by organisms during the course of local or systemic infection of the host, and a complex array of virulence factors is generally involved. In the following sections, a number of toxins are described in terms of their mechanism of action and their apparent role in the clinical disease with which they are associated. This list is by no means complete, but rather includes examples of major toxins that are well-studied and for which the information is more complete. Many toxins that contribute importantly to infectious diseases are not discussed.[53]

Diphtheria Toxin.   One of the most extensively studied of all bacterial toxins is that produced by β-phage–infected *C. diphtheriae*.[49] Diphtheria toxin is the prototype ADP-ribosylating toxin, which inhibits cellular protein synthesis by catalyzing the transfer of ADP-ribose from nicotinamide adenine dinucleotide (NAD) to a novel amino acid (diphthamide) on transfer factor II, a host protein required for translocation of the ribosomal mRNA. Although other bacterial products are undoubtedly involved in establishment of the infection and production and dissemination of the toxin, the widespread control of diphtheria with the use of diphtheria toxoid attests to the dominant role of this toxin both in the local infection and in the systemic toxicity, morbidity, and mortality of clinical diphtheria. Diphtheria toxin has been crystallized and its structure resolved to 2.5 Å, allowing for intimate understanding of its functional domains.[54] Recently, the receptor for diphtheria toxin on eukaryotic cells was identified by Naglich et al.[4] The toxin appears to bind to the extracellular domain of a heparin-binding, EGF-like precursor molecule that also has transmembrane and cytosolic domains. An additional host cell component that may interact with the receptor has been identified by Iwamoto et al.[55] Bound diphtheria toxin then enters the cell by receptor-mediated endocytosis, with the A subunit being released into the cytosol.

As noted in Table 1, exotoxin A of *Pseudomonas aeruginosa* catalyzes the identical reaction to that of diphtheria toxin, but is associated with disease processes that are clearly distinct from diphtheria. The host cell receptor for exotoxin A has recently been identified as the α_2-macroglobulin/LDL receptor.[6] It is likely that the distinct differences between diphtheria and infection with an exotoxin A–producing *P. aeruginosa* are due to different receptors with different cellular distributions and to the fact that exotoxin A is only one of a number of virulence factors involved in *Pseudmonas*-induced disease.[56]

Hybrid toxin molecules using a portion of the diphtheria gene fused to ligand-binding moieties, such as a fragment of interleukin (IL)-2, have been prepared and are in clinical trial for treatment of IL-2-receptor-positive leukemias and other malignancies.[57] This construct is an example of a family of hybrid toxins being developed and tested for use as therapeutic agents.[57–59]

Tetanus Toxin.   In contrast to diphtheria, immunization with tetanus toxoid has no effect on the establishment of infection with *Clostridium tetani*. The resultant antibody response does, however, totally prevent the disease process of clinical tetanus, the major pathogenic role of tetanus toxin (tetanospasmin). Tetanus toxin exhibits striking selectivity for neural tissue and is believed to be taken up at myoneural junctions for retrograde axonal transport within α-motoneurons following binding to a receptor, which may be a ganglioside, GT_1 or GD_{1b}.[60,61] It ultimately crosses the synapses in a retrograde direction by an unknown mechanism to reach the axons of inhibitory γ-aminobutyric acid (GABA) neurons in the spinal cord. It is the toxin-induced inhibition of neurotransmitter release, specifically in the inhibitory neuron, that results in the spasms characteristic of the disease. At higher concentrations, however, tetanus toxin can cause inhibition of acetylcholine release at the myoneural junction and flaccid paralysis equivalent to that elicited by botulinum toxin.[62] These data and sequence homologies between the light chains (A subunits) of the two toxins suggested a common mechanism of action.[63] Very recently data from Schiavo et al.[18] revealed that tetanus toxin is a zinc-dependent metalloprotease that appears to act by selective cleavage of a protein component of synaptic vesicles, synaptobrevin II. Toxicity can be prevented by metalloprotease inhibitors, such as the angiotensin-converting enzyme inhibitor captopril, raising the possibility of specific therapeutic intervention, which has not been available heretofore. Although the data for botulinum toxin are less clear with regard to proteolytic substrate, it appears that it may act by a similar mechanism (see below). It remains to be determined whether the distinctiveness of the clinical syndromes produced by these two related toxins is solely the result of binding specificities and differential trafficking within the neurons or also to selectivity of the enzymatic activities of the molecules.

Botulinum Toxin.   Botulinum toxin is among the most potent toxins known, with a lethal dose (toxin type A) of approximately 1 ng/kg.[64] "Botulinum toxin" consists of a family of seven immunologically distinct molecules, most of which cause flaccid paralysis by inhibiting myoneural junction acetylcholine release.[65] The mechanism of this neurotoxic activity appears to be similar or identical to that of tetanus toxin, namely, proteolytic cleavage of synaptobrevin II.[18] The classical presentation of clinical botulism results from the ingestion of performed toxin in improperly prepared foods, but a subacute intoxication can occur in infants (infant botulism) and adults harboring *C. botulinum* in their gastrointestinal tracts.[66,67] In most cases, the low-level toxin absorption results in listlessness and hypotonia, but the course can be fulminant, and infant botulism has been proposed as a cause of sudden infant death syndrome.[66] The ability of botulinum toxin to block muscle contraction at the myoneural junction has led to its use therapeutically in disorders such as blepharospasm, spastic torticollis, and strabismus.[68]

Many strains of *C. botulinum* types C and D also produce a different molecule, C2 toxin, that ADP-ribosylates actin, inhibiting its polymerization, affecting the shape of target cells and resulting in enterotoxin activity in vivo.[12] This toxin is now known to represent a family of clostridial ADP-ribosylating toxins that modify actin.[12]

Cholera Toxin and E. coli Heat-Labile Toxin.   Cholera and *E. coli* heat-labile enterotoxin (LT) are discussed together because their structures are similar and their mechanisms of action appear to be identical.[69,70] It is now known, however, that the heat-labile enterotoxins of *E. coli* represent a more heterogeneous group, with some (type II) being nonimmunologically cross-reactive and interacting with a different receptor despite operating by an apparently identical mechanism of action.[5] Cholera toxin and the LTs promote isotonic intestinal secretion by catalyzing the ADP-ribosylation of the B subunit of the stimulatory guanine nucleotide protein G_s.[69,70] This covalent modification causes semipermanent activation of the cellular adenylate cyclase, increased cAMP accumulation, and enhancement of chloride and water secretion. In addition, there is evidence that the production of prostaglandins and other mediators may be involved in this process.[71] While these enterotoxins reproduce the secretory diarrhea when administered experimentally, it is clear that multiple other bacterial components, such as attachment factors and mucinase, are required for establishment of infection and perhaps toxin delivery in order for the disease process to occur.

Enterotoxin effects can be prevented by the addition of specific antibody in animal assay systems,[72] but the use of parenteral toxoid immunization has been largely unsuccessful in preventing clinical cholera. The combination of killed whole *Vibrio cholerae* organism and purified nontoxic B subunit administered orally has shown efficacy in vaccine trials.[73] Genetically engineered vaccines consisting of organisms that produce inactive toxin have also been shown to provide some protection.[74] The occurrence of diarrhea in patients receiving cholera strains with genetically inactivated cholera toxin has led to the recognition of other toxins, such as zonula occludens toxin (ZOT), that have an unknown role in clinical cholera.[75,76]

Enterotoxins related to cholera toxin and LT are produced by a variety of other gram-negative organisms, such as *Klebsiella*, *Salmonella*, *Aeromonas*, and *Plesiomonas*, but the relative frequency of diarrhea caused by these organisms and the roles of such toxins in that disease are unknown.

Escherichia coli Heat-Stable Toxin.   *Escherichia coli* organisms can cause diarrhea by a variety of mechanisms[77] and produce other than the heat-labile toxin discussed above. Heat-stable toxin, own as ST_a or ST-I, is synthesized as a peptide of 72 amino acids and is cleaved to an active species of 18 or 19 amino acids.[78] It causes diarrhea by binding to and activating the endogenous particulate guanylate cyclase, thus eliciting cGMP production.[79–81] Unlike cholera toxin and LT, ST_a exhibits striking target cell specificity with little activity in extraintestinal tissues,[82] except when the cells have been transfected with the gene for particulate guanylate cyclase.[83] The endogenous ligand for this receptor, called *guanylin*, has been identified in extracts of rat jejunum and shown to stimulate cGMP production and chloride secretion in intestinal cells.[84]

St_a is poorly immunogenic alone, but antitoxin antibody may be elicited against hybrid toxins in which ST_a is covalently linked to LT-B subunits.[85] Enteroaggregative *E. coli* have recently been found to produce a closely related heat-stable toxin that may be responsible for the diarrhea occurring in patients infected with those organisms.[86] Other bacterial species, such as *Yersinia enterocolitica*, non-01 *Vibrio cholerae*, and *Citrobacter freundii*, also produce toxins related to ST_a, but their role in diarrheal illnesses is unclear.[87]

Toxins of Bordetella pertussis. *Bordetella pertussis,* the causative agent of whooping cough, produces several toxins that have striking effects in experimental systems and are hypothesized to be major contributors to the pathogenesis of the clinical illness.[88] Pertussis toxin, also known as *lymphocytosis-promoting factor, histamine-sensitizing factor,* or *islet-activating protein,* is expressed only by *B. pertussis,* although a transcriptionally silent copy of the gene is present in *B. parapertussis* and *B. bronchiseptica.*[33] Pertussis toxin acts by ADP-ribosylation of several members of the family of guanine nucleotide–binding (G) proteins involved in signal transduction.[89,90] The result of this covalent modification is inhibition of G protein function and, consequently, interruption of the signal from a variety of receptors to effector systems, such as inhibition of adenylate cyclase, activation of phospholipases, and modulation of ion channels. Although pertussis toxin is clearly a virulence factor for *B. pertussis* and a protective antigen, its role in clinical pertussis remains unclear.[91–93] Unlike tetanus and diphtheria, however, pertussis is not a single toxin disease, as illustrated by the study in which pertussis toxin (1 µg/kg iv) was given to human volunteers who neither got whooping cough nor suffered adverse effects.[94]

Bordetella species also produce other toxins that are significant virulence factors; these include adenylate cyclase toxin[15,52,91] and tracheal cytotoxin.[95] Adenylate cyclase toxin enters host cells to catalyze the production of supraphysiologic levels of cAMP, which impair the normal activities of neutrophils and other immune effector cells.[52,96,97] Tracheal cytotoxin is a disaccharide-tetrapeptide that is derived from the bacterial peptidoglycan.[95] It is cytotoxic to respiratory epithelial cells, apparently by eliciting IL-1 release and nitric oxide production.[98]

Anthrax Toxins. *Bacillus anthracis* produces three toxin components that are novel in their interaction with cells.[14] None of the three components, edema factor (EF), lethal factor (LF), or protective antigen (PA), has toxin activity alone. PA is the binding moiety that interacts with target cells to promote the entry of EF or LF. PA binds to a glycoprotein receptor on target cells and is cleaved by a host protease that is furin or furin-like.[16] This process results in the release of a 20 kD fragment and activates the remaining portion of PA to allow EF or LF binding. The complex is internalized by receptor-mediated endocytosis.[99] PA has been shown to produce an ion-permeable pore in lipid bilayers,[46,47] an activity that is presumed to be involved in the delivery of EF or LF to the cell interior. When EF enters the cytosol, it is activated by calmodulin to produce supraphysiologic levels of cAMP.[14] LF appears to be toxic only for macrophages. Klimpel et al.[19] have recently shown that LF is a zinc-dependent protease that may be having its lethal effect by cleavage of some critical intracellular substrate in a manner analogous to the actions of tetanus and botulinum toxins. PA and LF together also elicit mediator (IL-1 and others) release, and that process may well be involved in or responsible for the rapid death that occurs in experimental animals given these components.[100]

Protective antigen is so named because it is a protective component in anthrax vaccine. The genes for all three toxin proteins are located on plasmids.[101]

Shiga and Shiga-like Toxins. Shiga toxin is the prototype of a family of toxins produced by *Shigella dysenteriae* (shiga toxin), *E. coli, C. freundii,* and other organisms (shiga-like toxins SLT-I and SLT-II, previously known as Vero toxins).[102,103] The SLT-I molecules react with antiserum to shiga toxin, whereas the SLT-IIs do not, despite possessing a common mechanism of action. The members of this family conform to the A/B model with subunit structure similar to that of cholera toxin (A-5B).[104] The binding pentamer interacts with the glycolipid globotriaosylceramide (Gb_3), and the toxin is internalized via receptor-mediated endocytosis through clathrin-coated pits trafficking eventually to the trans-Golgi apparatus.[102,105] Within the cytoplasm, the A subunit causes inhibition of protein synthesis by enzymatic inactivation of the 28S RNA within the 60S ribosomal subunit.[106,107] This occurs by enzymatic removal of adenine from a specific adenosine residue, the same process catalyzed by the plant toxin ricin.

Despite the cytotoxicity elicited in vitro, the role of these toxins in shigellosis and diarrhea associated with infection by SLT-positive, enterohemorrhagic *E. coli* and others remains controversial.[102] Shiga toxin, especially in combination with lipopolysaccharide, causes damage to vascular endothelial cells in a fashion that may explain the hemolytic-uremic syndrome known to be associated with infection by *S. dysenteriae* and enterohemorrhagic *E. coli.*[108,109] Even the enterotoxin activity (intestinal fluid accumulation) may represent toxin effects on the villus cells and on the vasculature of the intestinal mucosa. As with other toxins, the genetic regulation of toxin production is different for the variant toxins.[102]

Pyrogenic Exotoxins. *Staphylococcus aureus* and group A streptococci produce toxins that are now recognized to constitute a family of molecules with the ability to elicit massive activation of the immune system.[110] Included in this family are streptococcal scarlet fever toxins, toxic shock syndrome toxin 1 (TSST-1), staphylococcal enterotoxins, and, less closely related, streptococcal M protein and staphylococcal exfoliative toxin. These proteins share the ability to stimulate T-cell proliferation by interaction with the class II MHC complex on antigen-presenting cells and specific Vβ chains of the T-cell receptor and are thereby designated *superantigens.*[110,111] The important feature of this interaction is the resultant production of cytokines (IL-1, tumor necrosis factor, plus other monokines and lymphokines), which appear to be the principal mediators of the disease processes associated with these toxins. For example, toxic shock syndrome mimics endotoxic shock and, in experimental animal models, can be attenuated by treatment of the study subject with corticosteroids or cyclosporin to prevent the acute immunoactivation.[112] It is not clear, however, whether the superantigen activity is the sole mechanism of these illnesses or whether other actions of the toxins may contribute. For example, TSST-1 has been shown to be cytotoxic for aortic endothelial cells in vitro, a setting in which cytokines should not be present.[113] Thus, it is possible that the various clinical syndromes produced by the organisms that make these toxins reflect the activities of numerous bacterial components directly on the host cells, as well as the effects of the massive mediator release via their function and superantigens.

Other Toxins. The list of toxins discussed in the preceding sections is, by no means, all inclusive. It is, however, representative of those toxins that are most extensively characterized with regard to their role in pathogenesis. There are many other toxins that have been the subject of basic investigations concerning structure and molecular mechanisms of action, with little knowledge of their contribution to clinical disease. Some of these are mentioned below.

Clostridium difficile produces two toxins, A and B, that are implicated in antibiotic-associated pseudomembranous colitis.[114] The two toxins are structurally related and exhibit cytotoxic activity, but in vivo toxin A alone has enterotoxic activity, while toxin B is cytotoxic only following administration of toxin A. The cytotoxic effects appear to involve alterations of the target cell's cytoskeletal elements, but by unknown mechanisms.[114,115] *Helicobacter pylori,* the organism implicated in gastric ulcer disease, has been shown to produce an 87 kD toxin that causes vacuolation of cultured cells, but its role in gastric disease remains to be determined.[116] *Legionellae* also produce several potential toxins that exhibit cytotoxic and hemolytic activities in vitro, but there are insufficient data to establish a contribution by these products to clinical disease.[117]

A large number of toxins have the ability to lyse erythrocytes and are thus defined as "hemolysins." They act by a variety of mechanisms, including phospholipase C activity, resulting in membrane damage from the cell exterior[41] and pore formation leading to osmotic lysis.[118–120] Some of these hemolysins also have leukotoxic activity and have been found, on the basis of amino acid sequence, to contain a glycine-rich repeat region and thus belong to a family of toxins termed RTX (for *repeat in toxin*).[28] Others, such as listerolysin produced by *Listeria monocytogenes,* are essential for intracellular growth of the organism for reasons that are still to be elucidated.[121] Despite the thorough investigation of their biologic effects and strong evidence that they are relevant virulence factors, definitive determination of their actual contribution to the disease processes with which they are associated is lacking.

OTHER BACTERIAL VIRULENCE FACTORS

In contrast to toxins, "other virulence factors" are, by definition, not directly toxic to host cells. Although bacterial virulence is often quantitated by the number of organisms required to kill 50 percent of challenged experimental animals (LD_{50}) and toxin potency is measured similarly (by ED_{50} or by minimum lethal dose), single nontoxin virulence factors alone are unlikely to have any effect on a host animal. The infection process is a complex one, involving the concerted action of microbial products for attachment to the appropriate surfaces (see Chapter 2), entry into the host, and, in some instances, individual host cells, dissemination, acquisition of nutrients, proliferation, survival by avoidance or disarming of host defenses, and, frequently, production of tissue damage.[1] The loss of virulence in association with the elimination of a specific bacterial component that is not required for survival in vitro is suggestive of a role for that factor in the pathogenic process. Production of one or more putative virulence factors by an avirulent strain, however, does not mean that it is not a virulence factor; it may indicate that the pathophysiologic process cannot proceed without the full cast. Molecular biological approaches, such as transposon and site-directed mutagenesis, and gene cloning, transfer, and expression have facilitated the evaluation of individual and groups of candidate virulence components for their relevance to disease in experimental models. It has therefore been possible to test hypotheses that have long been beyond the reach of experimental approach. In addition, a number of "virulence genes" have been identified prior to any information about the proteins they encode, the regulatory systems they control, or their exact involvement in disease.

Although not considered directly "toxic," many virulence factors possess specific biologic activities that interfere with normal host function to the advantage of the microbe.[122,123] The discussion of these other virulence factors will focus on those responsible for circumventing the major host defenses: *(1)* anatomic barriers; *(2)* serum (humoral) factors; and *(3)* phagocytic cells (Table 2).

Virulence Factors for Overcoming Anatomic Barriers

The first line of host defense against microorganisms is the anatomic barrier of skin and mucous membranes. These "external" surfaces are colonized by the normal flora, which in itself provides an impediment to the uncontrolled proliferation of potentially pathogenic bacteria. Thus, in order for pathogens to survive and proliferate in sufficient numbers to cause disease, they must compete successfully with the other organisms present. Many bacteria secrete bacteriocins, toxins directed at other microbes, in order to defend their niche in the normal flora.[124] Not only do these products provide a protective advantage, but some even exhibit activity against host cells, such as mononuclear

TABLE 2. Other Virulence Mechanisms

Survival at and penetration of anatomic barriers
  Protection against normal flora
  Invasion of mucosal surfaces and cells
  Disruption of connective tissues
  Paralysis of ciliary activity
Disruption or avoidance of humoral factors
  Degradation of antibodies
  Disruption of other humoral factors
  Resistance to serum lysis
  Assimilation of host proteins on external surface
  Molecular mimicry of host factors
Avoidance or inactivation of phagocytic cells
  Inhibition of adherence to phagocytic cells
  Suppression of phagocytosis
  Impairment of oxidative burst
  Prevention of phagosome-lysosomal fusion
Resistance to lysosomal enzymes and other host factors

phagocytes.[125] Since antibiotics may dramatically alter the composition of the normal flora, enzymes that confer antibiotic resistance may aid the bacterium in maintaining itself in a position to take advantage of the void created when other organisms are killed.

Although many bacteria are able to enter the body through skin that has been disrupted by laceration, abrasion, puncture wound, or insect bite, there are no bacteria known to be capable of penetrating intact skin as are some parasites, such as *Schistosoma mansoni, Strongyloides stercoralis, Ancylostoma duodenale,* and *Necator americanus.* Noninvasive organisms can penetrate the mucosae of the respiratory, gastrointestinal, and genitourinary tracts through breaks created in conjunction with manipulations, such as tooth brushing, dental extraction, and instrumentation (endoscopy). Unless armed with other virulence components that allow evasion of other defenses (as discussed below), such organisms are quickly killed by complement or phagocytes. Other organisms, in contrast, have the ability to invade and traverse intact eukaryotic cells, allowing them to enter the body from mucosal surfaces. These invasive organisms, including members of the genera *Escherichia, Legionella, Listeria, Salmonella, Shigella,* and *Yersinia,* are now recognized to possess complex machinery for cellular invasion and intracellular survival.[21,28,126] These systems involve nontoxin virulence factors that are similar among the different organisms, and, in most cases, there is built-in redundancy to allow for differing growth conditions and to provide back-up protection for the bacteria. Several illustrative examples are described below, and there are excellent reviews on the invasive determinants of *Listeria*[121] and *Shigella* invasion.[121,127,128]

Legionella pneumophila enter mononuclear phagocytic cells by accumulation of the complement component C3bi on their surface and using that host protein to serve as the ligand for binding to the macrophage CR3 receptor.[129] They elicit specialized coiling phagocytosis[130] and remain within vacuoles that do not fuse with lysosomes, apparently due to the influence of other bacterial components (at least one possibly a toxin).[117,131] Little is known of the mechanisms involved in these processes, due in part to the difficulties of genetic manipulations of *Legionella.*

Salmonella possess at least two different genetic loci that regulate their entry into eukaryotic cells. The first is the *inv* operon (*invA* through *invH*) in which mutations yield organisms capable of adhering to target cells without being internalized.[132] These observations suggest that one or more protein encoded within the *inv* operon stimulates a signal transduction pathway within the host cell.[133] The second locus is present on a large DNA fragment that is different from *inv* and is able to confer invasive capabilities on recipient *E. coli.*[134] Even greater redundancy is present in *Yersinia,* which have three separate pathways for cell entry. The invasin (*inv*) gene encodes a 108 kD protein that not only promotes adhesion to β_1-integrins, but also activates the cytochalasin-dependent entry process.[135] Invasin can confer invasive capacity on noninvasive *E. coli* and even latex particles, further supporting the idea of these bacterial proteins stimulating an active process by the host cell.[136] The product of a separate invasion locus, *ail,* plays a role in adherence/invasion, but also makes *Y. enterocolitica* serum resistant.[137] Finally, a large plasmid, identified earlier by Portnoy and Falkow, in all pathogenic Yersinia isolates allows for less efficient entry in the absence of the *inv* and *ail* loci.[126] All of these invasive organisms must, however, also possess mechanisms for intracellular survival; these are discussed below.

In addition to these cell surface proteins involved in cell entry, a number of bacteria produce and release extracellular enzymes, such as hyaluronidase, neuraminidase, elastase, and collagenase, which are not considered "toxins." Hirakata et al.[138] have shown that output of these products from *Pseudomonas aeruginosa* may be suppressed by subinhibitory concentrations of erythromycin, reflecting a process by which nonlytic antibiotic levels provide an advantage to the host. While some of the exoenzymes may contribute to cellular invasion, they are more likely to be responsible for reducing intercelular tissue barriers to promote extracellular spread of the organisms.

Virulence Factors for Avoiding or Disrupting Humoral Defenses

A secondary line of defense against microbial infections is provided by humoral factors, such as antibody, complement, complement-induced mediators, and an assortment of other soluble host proteins including clotting factors, β-lysin, and transferrin. Although some organisms have the ability to interfere with antibody production by several different mechanisms,[139–141] including the massive, but disruptive, activation of the immune system by superantigens,[110] most bacteria protect themselves from the humoral factors by enzymes that degrade the antibodies or by modifications in their external surface to avoid hazardous interactions.

While there is little complement present at mucosal surfaces, antibodies such as secretory IgA may be active against microorganisms even before invasion. In response to this host defensive measure, some bacteria, such as *Neisseria gonorrheae, Haemophilus influenzae, Proteus mirabilis,* clostridial species, and *Streptococcus pneumoniae,* product IgA-specific proteases that cleave and inactivate the molecule.[139–144] Similarly, the ability of organisms to elaborate factors that modify or degrade serum components, such as fibrin and other clotting factors, is recognized to be associated with increased virulence. The binding of the Fc domain of host immunoglobulin molecules by staphylococcal protein A is postulated to represent a protective mechanism, but the presence of protein A in a range of virulent and avirulent strains has hampered the testing of this hypothesis.

Resistance to the lytic effects of complement is almost a universal requirement for pathogens that traverse mucosal or skin barriers but remain in the extracellular environment. It has long been recognized that blood stream isolates are serum resistant, explaining why disseminated *N. gonorrheae* are serum resistant, while those isolated from the genital tract are predominantly serum sensitive.[142,145,146] The serum lytic effect in gram-negative organisms is complement-mediated, but can be initiated by either the classical or alternative pathway.[147,148] Antibodies involved in either process have arisen from prior exposure to the organism or reflect cross-reactivity with antigens from common organisms in the environment. There are several mechanisms by which serum resistance occurs, including (1) failure to bind and activate complement; (2) shedding of the surface molecules that activate the system; (3) interruption of the complement cascade before the formation of C5b–C9; and enhancement of the formation of nonlytic complexes.[149] All of these involve alteration of the bacterial surface by endogenous or exogenous factors. For example, the change in *Y. enterocolitica* conferred by the product of the *ail* gene, which facilitates

invasion, also mediates serum resistance.[137] In addition, YadA, the product of another *Yersinia* virulence gene, enhances serum resistance by degrading C3b and inhibiting the generation of the membrane attack complex.[150] *Neisseria gonorrheae* organisms grown under anaerobic conditions become serum resistant by sialylating their lipooligosaccharide via a bacterial sialyl transferase,[151] perhaps with the help of a host factor.[152] The modification of the bacterial cell surface by sialylation, other surface components, or nonbactericidal blocking antibodies protect against the lytic effects of serum.[153–155] As noted above, *Legionellae* coat their surface with C3b to facilitate cell entry via the CR3 receptor,[129] but without being susceptible to complement-mediated lysis. Thus, a major host defense can be circumvented by creative pathogens in a variety of ways.

Nontoxin Virulence Factors Directed at Phagocytic Cells

As with humoral defenses, pathogenic bacteria have developed an array of mechanisms to stave off the attack of phagocytic cells, another main line of protection for the host consisting of polymorphonuclear leukocytes, monocytes, and macrophages. The phagocytosis and killing of microorganisms are part of a specific sequence of events consisting of (1) attraction of the phagocyte by a chemotactic gradient of bacterial products; (2) migration of the phagocyte to the site of infection; (3) contact between the organism and the phagocyte; (4) phagocytosis (ingestion) of the organism; (5) generation of oxidative and nonoxidative products directed at the organism; (6) fusion of the phagosome and lysosome with exposure of the organism to lysosomal contents; and (7) death and degradation of the ingested organism (see Ch. 7). In the evolution of virulence mechanisms, pathogens have developed methods to elude, inactivate, or ignore most of these steps.[1,156] Recent illustrative examples of some of these are provided below.

Phenotypic variation that results in periodic changes in the surface of a number of organisms is an important means of avoidance of host defenses. This topic is, however, covered in detail in Chapter 2 on microbial adherence. Some polysaccharide capsules constitute antibody-resistant, antiphagocytic surfaces that prevent productive interaction between phagocyte and microbe.[142,157–160]

A number of virulence genes have been identified that facilitate intracellular survival of bacteria, apparently by interference with some of the steps of phagocytosis and killing (see Ch. 3). For example, Miller[161] has described a series of "pags" that are genes activated by PhoP/PhoQ, a two-component regulatory system involved in *Salmonella* virulence. The pags encode for bacterial factors that confer resistance to defensins and other mediators of intracellular killing by unknown mechanisms. Other organisms are able to inhibit specifically the regulatory components of the oxidative burst. *Yersinia* produce a tyrosine phosphatase that dephosphorylates several substrates in macrophages and, apparently thereby, inhibits phagocytosis.[162] Similarly, *Legionella* possess a phosphatase that acts to block superoxide generation production, but the substrate proteins are unknown.[117] Finally, several organisms block phagosome-lysosome fusion,[117,163,164] but it is not clear that this activity is essential for virulence.[165]

In summary, pathogenic bacteria possess an almost endless collection of adaptations that allow them to overcome or avoid the defenses of the eukaryotic host. Recent advances using molecular genetic approaches have enriched understanding of the bacterial armamentarium, but it is also clear that many more genes are involved and waiting to be discovered and studied (see Ch. 3).

REFERENCES

1. Smith H. Pathogenicity and the microbe in vivo. The 1989 Fred Griffith Review Lecture. J Gen Microbiol. 1990;136:377–93.

2. Roux E, Yersin A. Contribution a l'etude de la diphtherie. Ann Inst Pasteur. 1888;2:629–61.
3. Gill DM. The arrangement of subunits of cholera toxin. Biochemistry. 1976; 15:1242–8.
4. Naglich JG, Metherall JE, Russel DW, et al. Expression cloning of a diphtheria toxin receptor: Identity with a heparin-binding EGF-binding growth factor precursor. Cell. 1992;69:1051–61.
5. Pickett CL, Twiddy EM, Coker C, et al. Cloning, nucleotide sequence, and hybridization studies of the type IIb heat-labile enterotoxin gene of Escherichia coli. J Bacteriol. 1989;171:4945–52.
6. Kounnas MZ, Morris RE, Thompson MR, et al. The α_2-macroglobulin receptor/low density lipoprotein receptor–related protein binds and internalizes Pseudomonas exotoxin A. J Biol Chem. 1992;267:12420–3.
7. Tamura M, Nogimori K, Murai S, et al. Subunit structure of islet-activating protein, pertussis toxin, in conformity with the A–B model. Biochemistry. 1982;21:516–22.
8. Brennan MJ, David JL, Kenimer JG, et al. Lectin-like binding of pertussis toxin to a 165-kilodalton Chinese hamster ovary cell glycoprotein. J Biol Chem. 1988;263:4895–9.
9. Saukkonen K, Burnette WN, Mar VL, et al. Pertussis toxin has eurkaryotic-like carbohydrate recognition domains. Proc Natl Acad Sci USA. 1992;89:118–22.
10. Clark CG, Armstrong GD. Lymphocyte receptors for pertussis toxin. Infect Immun. 1990;58:3840–6.
11. Sindt K, Redpath G, Hewlett E, et al. Inhibition of pertussis toxin-induced platelet activation by antibodies to platelet surface glycoproteins. Program of the 93rd Annual Meeting of the American Society for Microbiology, abstract B27, May 1993.
12. Aktories K, Mohr C, Koch G. Clostridial actin–ADP–ribosylating toxins. In: Aktories K, ed. Current Topics in Microbiology and Immunology. Berlin: Springer-Verlag; 1992:97–113.
13. Aktories K, Braun U. Botulinum ADP-ribosyltransferase C3. In: Moss J, Vaughn M, eds. ADP-Ribosylating Toxins and G Proteins. Washington, DC: American Society for Microbiology; 1990:79–95.
14. Leppla SH. Anthrax toxin edema factor: A bacterial adenylate cyclase that increases cyclic AMP concentrations in eukaryotic cells. Proc Natl Acad Sci USA. 1982;79:3162–6.
15. Gordon VM, Young WW, Lechler SM, et al. Adenylate cyclase toxins from Bacillus anthracis and Bordetella pertussis: Different processes for interaction with and entry into target cells. J Biol Chem. 1989;264:14792–6.
16. Klimpel KR, Molloy SS, Thomas G, et al. Anthrax toxin protective antigen is activated by a cell surface protease with the sequence specificity and catalytic properties of furin. Proc Natl Acad Sci USA. 1992;89:10277–81.
17. O'Brien AD, Tesh VL, Donohoe-Rolfe A, et al. Shiga toxin: Biochemistry, genetics, mode of action, and role in pathogenesis. Curr Top Microbiol Immunol. 1992;180:65–94.
18. Schiavo G, Benfenati F, Poulain B, et al. Tetanus and botulinum-B neurotoxins block neurotransmitter release by proteolytic cleavage of synaptobrevin. Nature. 1992;359:832–5.
19. Klimpel K, Arora N, Leppla SH. Anthrax toxin lethal factor has homology to the thermolysin-like proteases and displays proteolytic activity. Program of the 93rd Annual Meeting of the American Society for Microbiology, abstract B111, May 1993.
20. Gill DM. Seven toxic peptides that cross cell membranes. In: Jeljaszewicz J, Wadstrom T, eds. Bacterial Toxins and Cell Membranes. New York: Academic Press; 1978:291–332.
21. DiRita VJ, Mekalanos JJ. Genetic regulation of bacterial virulence. Annu Rev Genet. 1989;23:455–82.
22. Pappenheimer AM Jr. Diphtheria toxin. Annu Rev Biochem. 1977;46:69–94.
23. Straley SC, Plano GV, Skrzypek E, et al. Regulation by Ca^{2+} in the yersinia low-Ca^{2+} response. Mol Microbiol. 1993;8:1005–10.
24. Miller VL, Taylor RK, Mekalanos JJ. Cholera toxin transcriptional activator toxR is a transmembrane DNA binding protein. Cell. 1987;48:271–9.
25. Miller JF, Johnson SA, Black WJ, et al. Constitutive sensory transduction mutations in the Bordetella pertussis bvgS gene. J Bacteriol. 1992;174:970–9.
26. Mahan MJ, Slauch JM, Mekalanos JJ. Selection of bacterial virulence genes that are specifically induced in host tissues. Science. 1993;259:686–8.
27. Scarlato V, Arico B, Domenighini M, et al. Environmental regulation of virulence factors in Bordetella species. Bioessays. 1993;15:99–104.
28. Welch RA. Pore-forming cytolysins of gram-negative bacteria. Mol Microbiol. 1991;5:521–8.
29. Betley MJ, Miller VL, Mekalanos JJ. Genetics of bacterial enterotoxins. Annu Rev Microbiol. 1986;40:577–605.
30. Tao X, Murphy JR. Binding of the metalloregulatory protein DtxR to the diphtheria tox operator requires a divalent heavy metal ion and protects the palindromic sequence from DNase I digestion. J Biol Chem. 1992;267:21761–4.
31. Finn CW, Silver RP, Habig WH, et al. The structural gene for tetanus neurotoxin is on a plasmid. Science. 1984;224:881–4.
32. Locht C, Keith JM. Pertussis toxin gene: Nucleotide sequence and genetic organization. Science. 1986;232:1258–64.
33. Arico B, Rappuoli R. Bordetella parapertussis and Bordetella bronchiseptica contain transcriptionally silent pertussis toxin genes. J Bacteriol. 1987;169:2847–53.
34. Dyer DW, Iandolo JJ. Plasmid-chromosomal transition of genes important in staphylococcal enterotoxin B expression. Infect Immun. 1981;33:450–8.
35. Randall LL, Hardy SJS, Thom JR. Export of protein: A biochemical view. Annu Rev Microbiol. 1987;41:507–41.
36. Pugsley AP. The complete general secretory pathway in gram-negative bacteria. Microbiol Rev. 1993;57:50–108.
37. Bellalou J, Ladant D, Sakamoto H. Synthesis and secretion of Bordetella pertussis adenylate cyclase as a 200-kilodalton protein. Infect Immun. 1990; 58:1195–200.
38. Weiss AA, Johnson FD, Burns DL. Molecular characterization of an operon required for pertussis toxin secretion. Proc Natl Acad Sci USA. 1993;90:2970–4.
39. Yu J, McLaughlin S, Freedman RB, et al. Cloning and active site mutagenesis of Vibrio cholerae DsbA, a periplasmic enzyme that catalyzes disulfide bond formation. J Biol Chem. 1993;268:4326–30.
40. Middeldorp JM, Witholt B. K88-mediated binding of Escherichia coli outer membrane fragments to porcine intestinal epithelial cell brush borders. Infect Immun. 1981;31:42–51.
41. Mollby R. Bacterial phospholipases. In: Jeljaszewicz J, Wadstrom T, eds. Bacterial Toxins and Cell Membranes. New York: Academic Press; 1978; 367–424.
42. Eidels L, Proia RL, Hart DA. Membrane receptors for bacterial toxins. Microbiol Rev. 1983;47:596–620.
43. Middlebrook JL, Dorland RB. Response of cultured mammalian cells to the exotoxins of Pseudomonas aeruginosa and Corynebacterium diphtheriae: Differential cytotoxicity. Can J Microbiol. 1977;23:183–9.
44. Saelinger CB. Toxin structure and function. In: Saelinger CB, ed. Trafficking of Bacterial Toxins. Boca Raton, FL: CRC Press; 1990;2–13.
45. Kagan BL, Reich KA, Collier RJ. Orientation of the diphtheria toxin channel in lipid bilayers. Biophys J. 1984;45:102–4.
46. Blaustein RO, Koehler TM, Collier RJ, et al. Anthrax toxin: channel-forming activity of protective antigen in planar phospholipid bilayers. Proc Natl Acad Sci USA. 1989;86:2209–13.
47. Finkelstein A. Channels formed in phospholipid bilayer membranes by diphtheria, tetanus, botulinum and anthrax toxin. J Physiol Paris. 1990;84:188–90.
48. Hewlett W, Gray M, Weiss A, et al. Adenylate cyclase toxin produces an ion-permeable pore in a phospholipid bilayer. Program of the 93rd Annual Meeting of the American Society for Microbiology, abstract B30, May 1993.
49. Collier RJ. Diphtheria toxin: structure and function of a cytocidal protein. In: Moss J, Vaughan M, eds. ADP-Ribosylating Toxins and G Proteins. Washington, DC: American Society for Microbiology; 1990;3–19.
50. Hudson TH, Scharff J, Kimak MAG, et al. Energy requirements for diphtheria toxin translocation are coupled to the maintenance of a plasma membrane potential and a proton gradient. J Biol Chem. 1988;263:4773–81.
51. Morris RE. Interaction between pseudomonas exotoxin A and mouse LM fibroblast cells. In: Saelinger CB ed. Trafficking of Bacterial Toxins. Boca Raton, FL: CRC Press; 1990:50–70.
52. Hewlett EL, Gordon VM. Adenylate cyclase toxin of Bordetella pertussis. In: Wardlaw AC, Parton R, eds. Pathogenesis and Immunity in Pertussis. Chichester, England: John Wiley & Sons; 1988:193–209.
53. Alouf JE, Freer JH (eds). Sourcebook of Bacterial Protein Toxins. San Diego: Academic Press; 1991.
54. Choe S, Bennett MJ, Fujii G, et al. The crystal structure of diphtheria toxin. Nature. 1992;357:216–22.
55. Iwamoto R, Senoh H, Okada Y, et al. An antibody that inhibits the binding of diphtheria toxin to cells revealed the association of a 27-kDa membrane protein with diphtheria toxin receptor. J Biol Chem. 1991;266:20463–9.
56. Pollack M, Young LS. Protective activity of antibodies to exotoxin A and lipopolysaccharide at the onset of Pseudomonas aeruginosa septicemia in man. J Clin Invest. 1979;863:276–86.
57. Murphy JR, Lakkis FG, vanderSpek JC, et al. Protein engineering of diphtheria toxin. Development of receptor-specific cytotoxic agents for the treatment of human disease. Targ Diagn Ther. 1992;7:365–82.
58. Kreitman RJ, Fitzgerald D, Paston I. Targeting growth factor receptors with fusion toxins. Int J Immunopharm. 1992;14:465–72.
59. Meville DM, Jr, Scharff J, Srinivasachar K. In vivo T-cell ablation by a holo-immunotoxin directed at human CD3. Proc Natl Acad Sci USA. 1992;89:2585–9.
60. Mellanby J, Green J. How does tetanus toxin act? Neuroscience. 1981;6:281–300.
61. van Heyningen S. Tetanus toxin. In: Dorner F, Drews J, eds. Pharmacology of Bacterial Toxins. IEPT Section 199. Oxford: Pergamon Press; 1986; 549–70.
62. Habermann E, Dreyer F, Bigalke H. Tetanus toxin blocks the neuromuscular transmission in vitro like botulinum A toxin. Naunyn Schmiedbergs Arch Pharmacol. 1980;311:33–40.
63. Eisel U, Jaransch W, Goretzki K, et al. Tetanus toxin: primary structure, expression in E. coli and homology with botulinum toxins. EMBO J. 1986; 5:2495–502.
64. Gill DM, Bacterial toxins: a table of lethal amounts. Microbiol Rev. 1982; 46:86–94.
65. Simpson LL. Clostridial and related protein toxins: A short overview. In: Witholt B, Alouf JE, et al., eds. Bacterial Protein Toxins. Stuttgart: Gustav Fischer Verlag; 1992:20–30.
66. Arnon SS. Infant botulism. Annu Rev Med. 1980;31:541–60.
67. Chia JK, Clark JB, Ryan CA, et al. Botulism in an adult associated with food-borne intestinal infection with Clostridium botulinum. N England J Med. 1986;315:239–41.

68. Tim R, Massey JM. Botulinum toxin therapy for neurologic disorders. Post-grad Med. 1992;91:327–32.

69. Moss J, Vaughn M. Mechanisms of action of choleragen and *E. coli* heat-labile enterotoxin: Activation of adenylate cyclase by ADP-ribosylation. Mol Cell Biochem. 1981;37:75–90.

70. Holmgren J, Lonnorth I. Structure and function of enterotoxins and their receptors. In: Ouchterlony O, Holmgren J, eds. Cholera and Related Diarrheas. Basel: Karger, 1980:88–103.

71. Liang YF, Peterson JW, Reitmeyer JC. Inhibitory effect of aspirin on cholera toxin–induced phospholipase and cyclo-oxygenase activity. FEMS Microbiol Lett. 1990;60:137–41.

72. Pierce NF, Cray WC Jr, Sacci JB Jr. Oral immunization of dogs with purified cholera toxin, its B-subunit or a crude culture filtrate of *Vibrio cholera*: Evidence for synergistic protection by antitoxic and antibactericidal mechanisms. Infect Immun. 1982;37:687–94.

73. Holmgren J, Svennerholm AM, Jertborn M, et al. An oral B subunit: Whole cell vaccine against cholera. Vaccine. 1992;10:911–4.

74. Levine MM, Kaper JB. Live oral vaccines against cholera: An update. Vaccine. 1993;11:207–12.

75. Baudry B, Fasano A, Ketley J et al. Cloning of a gene (zot) encoding new toxin produced by *Vibrio cholerae*. Infect Immun. 1992;60:428–34.

76. Johnson JA, Morris JG, Kaper JB. Gene encoding zonula occludens toxin (zot) does not occur independently from cholera enterotoxin genes (ctx) in *Vibrio cholerae*. J Clin Microbiol. 1993;31:732–3.

77. Guerrant RL. Yet another pathogenic mechanism for *Escherichia coli* diarrhea? N Engl J Med. 1980;302:113–4.

78. Rasheed K, Guzman-Verduzco LM, Kupersztoch YM. Two precursors of the heat-stable enterotoxin of *Escherichia coli:* Evidence of extracellular processing. Mol Microbiol. 1989;4:941–8.

79. Field ML, Graf LH, Laird WJ, et al. Heat-stable enterotoxin of *Escherichia coli:* In vitro effects of guanylae cyclase activity, cGMP concentration, and ion transport in small intestine. Proc Natl Acad Sci USA. 1978;75:2800–4.

80. Hughes JM, Murad F, Chang B, et al. Role of cyclic GMP in the action of heat-stable enterotoxin of *Escherichia coli*. Nature. 1978;271:755–6.

81. Schulz S, Green CK, Yuen PST, et al. Guanylyl cyclase is a heat-stable enterotoxin receptor. Cell. 1990;63:941–8.

82. Guerrant RL, Hughes JM, Chang B, et al. Activation of intestinal guanylate cyclase by heat-stable enterotoxin of *Escherichia coli:* Studies of tissue specificity, potential receptors, and intermediates. J Infect Dis. 1980;142:97–120.

83. De Sauvage FJ, Camerato TR, Goeddel DV. Primary structure and functional expression of the human receptor for *Escherichia coli* heat-stable enterotoxin. J Biol Chem. 1991;17:912–8.

84. Forte LR, Eber SL, Turner JT, et al. Guanylin stimulation of C1-secretion in human intestinal T84 cells via cyclic guanosine monophosphate. J Clin Invest. 1993;91:2423–8.

85. Klipstein FA, Engert RF, Clemens JD, et al. Vaccine for enterotoxigenic *Escherichia coli* based on synthetic heat-stable toxin cross-linked to the B subunit of heat-labile toxin. J Infect Dis. 1983;147:318–26.

86. Savarino SJ, Fasano A, Watson J, et al. Enteroaggregative *Escherichia coli* heat-stable enterotoxin 1 represents another subfamily of *E. coli* heat-stable toxin. Proc Natl Acad Sci USA. 1993;90:3093–7.

87. Guarino A, Caparo G, Malamisura B, et al. Production of *Escherichia coli* ST$_a$ heat-stable enterotoxin by *Citrobacter freundii* isolated from humans. J Clin Microbiol. 1987;25:110–4.

88. Weiss AA, Hewlett EL. Virlence determinants of *Bordetella pertussis*. Annu Rev Microbiol. 1986;40:661–86.

89. Ui M. Pertussis toxin as a valuable probe for G-protein involvement in signal transduction. In: Moss J, Vaughan M, eds. ADP-Ribosylating Toxins and G proteins. Washington, DC: American Society for Microbiology; 1990:45–77.

90. Birnbaumer L, Mattera R, Yatani A, et al. Recent advances in the understanding of multiple roles of G proteins in coupling of receptors to ionic channels and other effectors. In: Moss J, Vaughan M, eds. ADP-Ribosylating Toxins and G Proteins. Washington, DC: American Society for Microbiology; 1990:225–66.

91. Weiss AA, Hewlett EL, Myers GA, et al. Pertussis toxin and extracytoplasmic adenylate cyclase as virulence factors of *Bordetella pertussis*. J Infect Dis. 1984;150:219–22.

92. Sato H, Sato Y. *Bordetella pertussis* infection in mice: Correlation of specific antibodies against two antigens, pertussis toxin, and filamentous hemagglutinin with mouse protectivity in an intracerebral or aerosol challenge system. Infect Immun. 1984;46:415–21.

93. Edwards KM. A cellular pertussis vaccines—A solution to the pertussis problem? J Infect Dis. 1993;168:15–20.

94. Toyota T, Kai Y, Kakizaki M, et al. Effect of islet-activating protein (IAP) on blood glucose and plasma insulin in health volunteers (phase I studies). Tohoku J Exp Med. 1980;130:105–20.

95. Cookson BT, Cho HL, Goldman WE. Biological activities and chemical composition of purified tracheal cytotoxin of *Bordetella pertussis*. Infect Immun. 1989;57:2223–9.

96. Confer DL, Eaton JW. Phagocyte impotence caused by an invasive bacterial adenylate cyclase. Science. 1982;217:948–50.

97. Pearson RD, Symes P, Conboy M, et al. Inhibition of monocyte oxidative responses by *Bordetella pertussis* adenylae cyclase toxin. J Immunol. 1987;139:2749–54.

98. Nixon-Heiss LJ, Lancaster JR, Corbett JA, et al. Nitric oxide mediates *Bordetella pertussis* tracheal cytotoxin damage to the respiratory epithelium.

Program of the 93rd Annual Meeting of the American Society for Microbiology, abstract B34, May 1993.

99. Gordon V, Leppla S, Hewlett E. Inhibitors of receptor-mediated endocytosis block entry of *Bacillus anthracis* adenylate cyclase toxin but not that of *Bordetella pertussis* adenylate cylcase toxin. Infect Immun. 1988;56:1066–9.

100. Hanna PC, Acosta D, Collier RJ. On the role of macrophages in anthrax. Proc Natl Acad Sci USA. 1993;90:1318–9.

101. Robertson DL, Leppla SH. Molecular cloning and expression in *Escherichia coli* of the lethal factor gene of *Bacillus anthracis*. Gene. 1986;4:71–8.

102. O'Brien AD, Tesh VL, Donohue-Rolfe A, et al. Shiga toxin: Biochemistry, genetics, mode of action, and role in pathogenesis. Curr Top Microbiol Immun. 1992;180:65–94.

103. Schmidt H, Montag M, Bockemuhl J, et al. Shiga-like toxin II-related cyto-toxins in *Citrobacter freundii* strains from humans and beef samples. Infect Immun. 1993;61:534–43.

104. Stein PE, Boodhoo A, Tyrrell GJ, et al. Crystal structure of the cell-binding B oligomer of verotoxin-1 from *E. coli*. Nature 1991;355:748–50.

105. Sandvig K, Garred O, Prydz K, et al. Retrograde transport of endocytosed Shiga toxin to the endoplasmic reticulum. Nature. 1992;358:510–2.

106. Reisbig R, Olsnes S, Eiklid K. The cytotoxin activity of *Shigella* toxin: Evidence for catalytic inactivation of the 60S ribosomal subunit. J Biol Chem. 1981;256:8739–41.

107. Obrig TG, Morgan TP, Colinas RJ. Ribonuclease activity associated with the 60S ribosome-inactivating proteins ricin A, phytolaccin and Shiga toxin. Biochem Biophys Res Commun. 1985;130:879–84.

108. Louise CB, Obrig TG. Shiga toxin-associated hemolytic uremic syndrome: Combine cytotoxic effects of shiga toxin and lipopolysacchardie (endotoxin) on human vascular endothelial cells in vitro. Infect Immun. 1992;60:1536–43.

109. Cohen MB, Giannella RA. Hemorrhagic colitis associated with *Escherichia coli*. Adv Intern Med. 1992;37:173–95.

110. Schlievert PM. Role of superantigens in human disease. J Infect Dis. 1993; 167:997–1002.

111. Marrack P, Kappler J. The staphylococcal enterotoxins and their relatives. Science. 1990;248:705–11.

112. Schwab JH, Brown RR, Anderle SK, et al. Superantigen can reactivate bacterial cell wall-induced arthritis. J Immun. 1993;150:4151–9.

113. Lee PK, Vercellotti GM, Deringer JR, et al. Effects of staphylococcal toxic shock syndrome toxin 1 on aortic endothelial cells. J Infect Dis. 1991;164: 711–9.

114. Bartlett JG. *Clostridium difficile:* Clinical considerations. Rev Infect Dis. 1990;12:243–51.

115. Muller H, von Eichel-Streiber C, Habermann E. Morphological changes of cultured endothelial cells after microinjection of toxins that act on the cytoskeleton. Infect Immun. 1992;60:3007–10.

116. Cover TL, Blaser MJ. Purification and characterization of the vacuolating toxin from *Helicobacter pylori*. J Biol Chem. 1992;267:10570–5.

117. Dowling JN, Saha AK, Glew RH. Virulence factors of the family *Legionellaceae*. Microbiol Rev. 1992;56:32–60.

118. Menestrina G, Belmonte G, Parisi V, et al. Structural features of the pore formed by *Staphylococcus aureus* alpha-toxin inferred from chemical modification and primary structure analysis. FEMS Microbiol Immun. 1992;5: 19–28.

119. Alouf JE. Streptococcal toxins (streptolysin O, streptolysin S, erythrogenic toxin). In: Dorner F, Drews J, eds. Pharmacology of Bacterial Toxins. IEPT Section 119. Oxford: Pergamon Press; 1986:635–92.

120. Supersac G, Prevost G, Piemont Y. Sequencing of leucocidin R from *Staphylococcus aureus P83* suggests that staphylococcal leucocidins and gamma-hemolysin are members of a single two-component family of toxins. Infect Immun. 1993;61:580–7.

121. Cossart P, Mengaud J. Listeria monocytogenes—A model system for the molecular study of intracellular parasitism. Mol Biol Med. 1989;6:463–74.

122. Brubaker RR. Mechanisms of bacterial virulence. Annu Rev Microbiol. 1985; 39:21–50.

123. Roth JA. Virulence Mechanisms of Bacterial Pathogens. Washignton, DC: American Society for Microbiology; 1988.

124. Smith HW, Huggins MB. Further observations on the association of the colicine V plasmic of *Escherichia coli* with pathogenicity and with survival in the alimentary tract. J Gen Microbiol. 1976;92:335–50.

125. Aguero ME, Cabelo FC. Relative contributions of Col V plasmid and K1 antigen to the pathogenicity of *Escherichia coli*. Infect Immun. 1983;40: 359–68.

126. Falkow S, Isberg RR, Portnoy DA. The interaction of bacteria with mammalian cells. Annu Rev Cell Biol. 1992;8:333–63.

127. Hale TL. Genetic basis of virulence in *Shigella* spcies. Microbiol Rev. 1991; 55:206–24.

128. Sansonetti PJ. Genetic and molecular basis of epithelial cell invasion by *Shigella* species. Rev Infect Dis. 1991;13:285–92.

129. Payne NR, Horwitz MA. Phagocytosis of *Legionella pneumophila* is mediated by human monocyte complement receptors. J Exp Med. 1987;166: 1377–89.

130. Horwitz MA. Phagocytosis of the Legionnaires' disease bacterium *(Legionella pneumophila)* occurs by a novel mechanism: Engulfment within a pseudopod coil. Cell. 1984;36:27–33.

131. Hacker J, Ott M, Ludwig B et al. Intracellular survival and expression of virulence determinants of *Legionella pneumophila*. Infection. 1991;19(Suppl 4):S198–201.

132. Galan JE, Curtiss R. Cloning and molecular characterization of genes whose

products allow *Salmonella typhimurium* to penetrate tissue culture cells. Proc Natl Acad Sci USA. 1989;86:6383–7.

133. Ginnochio C, Pace J, Galan JE. Identification and molecular characterization of a *Salmonella typhimurium* gene involved in triggering the internalizaton of salmonellae into cultured epithelial cells. Proc Natl Acad Sci USA. 1992; 89:5976–80.

134. Elingshorst EA, Baron LS, Kopecko DJ. Penetration of human intestinal epithelial cells by *Salmonella:* Molecular cloning and expression of *Salmonella typhi* invasion determinants in *Escherichia coli*. Proc Natl Acad Sci USA. 1989;86:5173–7.

135. Isberg RR. Pathways for the penetration of enteropathogenic *Yersinia* into mammalian cells. Mol Biol Med. 1990;7:73–82.

136. Young VB, Falkow S, Schoolnik GK, et al. The invasion protein of *Yersinia enterocolitica:* Internalization of invasin-bearing bacteria by eukaryotic cells is associated with reorganization of the cytoskeleton. J Cell Biol. 1992;116: 197–207.

137. Bliska JB, Falkow S. Bacterial resistance to complement killing mediated by the Ail protein of *Yersinia enterocolitica*. Proc Natl Acad Sci USA. 1992; 89:3561–5.

138. Hirakata Y, Kaku M, Mizukane R, et al. Potential effects of erythromycin on host defense systems and virulence of *Pseudomonas aeruginosa*. Antimicrob Agents Chemother. 1992;36:1922–7.

139. Kilian M. Bacterial enzymes degrading human IgA. In: Robbins JR, Hill JC, Sadoff JC, eds. Seminars in Infectious Disease. v. 4. Bactrial Vaccines. New York: Thieme-Stratton; 1982:213–8.

140. Munson RS Jr. *Haemophilus influenzae:* Surface antigens and aspects of virulence. Can J Vet Res. 1990;54:63–7.

141. Poulsen K, Brandt J, Hjorth JP, Thogersen HC, Kilian M. Cloning and sequencing of the immunoglobin A1 protease gene (iga) of *Haemophilus influenzae* serotype b. Infect Immun. 1989;57:3097–105.

142. Meyer TF. Pathogenic neisseriae—A model of bacterial virulence and genetic flexibility. Int J Med Microbiol. 1990;274:135–54.

143. Senior BW, Loomes LM, Kerr MA. The production and activity in vivo of *Proteus mirabilis* IgA protease in infections of the urinary tract. J Med Microbiol. 1991;35:203–7.

144. Hashim OH, Hassan H. Actions of three clostridial IgA proteases on distinct forms of immunoglobulin A molecules. Immunol. 1991;73:235–8.

145. Schoolnik GK, Buchanan TM, Holmes KK. Gonococci causing disseminated gonococcal infection are resistant to the bactericidal action of normal human sera. J Clin Invest. 1976;58:1163–73.

146. Sparling PF, Tsai J, Cornelissen CN. Gonococci are survivors. Scand J Infect Dis. 1990;69:125–36.

147. Frank M, Joiner K, Hammer C. The function of antibody and complement in the lysis of bacteria. Rev Infect Dis. 1987;9(Suppl 5):S537–45.

148. Fearon DT, Austen KF. The alternative pathway of complement: A system for host resistance to microbial infection. N Engl J Med. 1980;303:259–63.

149. Joiner KA. Complement evasion by bacteria and parasites. Annu Rev Microbiol. 1988;42:201–30.

150. Pilz D, Vocke T, Heesemann J, et al. Mechanism of YadA-mediated serum resistance of *Yersinia enterocolitica* serotype 0.3. Infect Immun. 1992;60: 189–95.

151. Frangipane JV, Rest RF. Anaerobic growth and cytidine 5′-monophospho-*N*-acetylneuraminic acid act synergistically to induce high-level serum resistance in *Neisseria gonorrheae*. Infect Immun. 1993;61:1657–66.

152. Constantinidou C, Beadle D, Zhou XH, et al. A high Mr factor in human blood which confers serum resistance on gonococci: Some properties and synergism with CMP-NANA. Microb Pathogen. 1992;12:421–32.

153. Howard CJ, Glynn AA. The virulence for mice of strains of *Escherichia coli* related to the effects of K antigens on their resistance of phagocytosis and killing by complement. Immunology. 1971;20:767–77.

154. McCutchan JS, Katzenstein D, Norquist D, et al. Role of blocking antibody in disseminated gonococcal infection. J Immunol. 1978;121:1884–8.

155. Parsons NJ, Curry A, Fox AJ, et al. The serum resistance of gonococci in the majority of urethral exudates is due to sialylated lipopolysaccharide seen as a suface coat. FEMS Microbiol Lett. 1992;69:295–9.

156. Cross AS, Kelly NM. Bacteria-phagocyte interactions: Emerging tactics in an ancient rivalry. FEMS Microbil Immun. 1990;2:245–58.

157. Podschun R, Penner I, Ullmann U. Interaction of *Klebsiella* capsule type 7 with human polymorphonuclear leucocytes. Microb Pathogen. 1992;13: 371–9.

158. Marques MB, Kasper DL, Pangburn MK, et al. Prevention of C3 deposition by capsular polysaccharide is a virulence mechanism of type III group B streptococci. Infect Immun. 1992;60:3986–93.

159. Martin TR, Ruzinski JT, Rubens CE, et al. The effect of type-specific polysaccharide capsule on the clearance of group B streptococci from the lungs of infant and adult rats. J Infect Dis. 1992;165:306–14.

160. Williams AE, Maskell DJ, Moxon ER. Relationship between intracellular survival in macrophages and virulence of *Haemophilus influenzae* type B. J Infect Dis. 1991;163:1366–9.

161. Miller SI. PhoP/PhoQ: Macrophage-specific modulators of *Salmonella* virulence? Mol Microbiol. 1991;5:2073–8.

162. Bliska JB, Clemens JC, Dixon JE, et al. The *Yersinia* tyrosine phosphatase: Specificity of a bacterial virulence determinant for phosphoproteins in the J774A.1 macrophage. J Exp Med. 1992;176:1625–30.

163. Buchmeier NA, Heffron F. Inhibition of macrophage phagosome–lysosome fusion by *Salmonella typhimurium*. Infect Immun. 1991;59:2232–8.

164. Ishibashi Y, Arai T. Specific inhibition of phagosome–lysosome fusion in murine macrophages mediated by *Salmonella typhimurium* infection. FEMS Microbiol Immun. 1990;2:35–43.

165. Ishibashi Y, Nobuta K, Arai T. Mutant of *Salmonella typhimurium* lacking the inhibitory function for phagosome–lysosome fusion in murine macrophages. Microb Pathogen. 1992;13:317–23.

2. MICROBIAL ADHERENCE

WILLIAM A. PETRI, Jr.
BARBARA J. MANN

Adherence is the initial interaction of a pathogenic microorganism with its host. Adherence is the route to cellular invasion by intracellular parasites and the first step in host cell killing and toxin delivery by microbial pathogens. Adhesins are microbial molecules that mediate adherence or binding of microbes to the host (Fig. 1). Receptors are the host molecules or ligands that microbial adhesins bind to initiate adherence. A single adhesin may have more than one receptor, and a single receptor may be recognized by many different adhesins.

EXPERIMENTAL IDENTIFICATION OF AN ADHESIN

Understanding a microbe's adherence mechanism begins with the development of an adherence assay (Table 1). Care must be

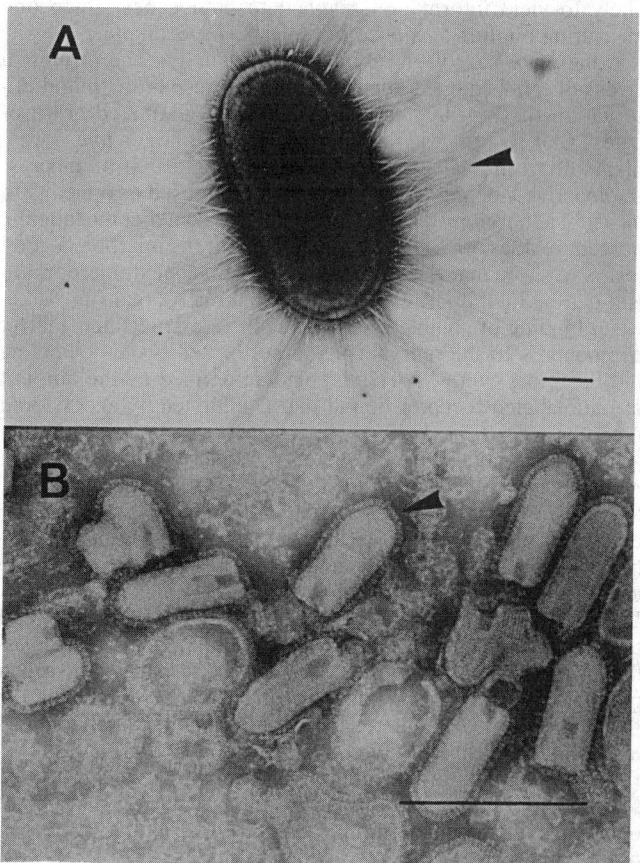

FIG. 1. Vesicular stomatitis virus and *E. coli* adhesins. Electron micrographs of **(A)** *E. coli* expressing P fimbriae (arrowhead) and **(B)** vesicular stomatitis virus, demonstrating the spikelike protrusions (arrowhead) of the viral adherence glycoprotein. Bar = 0.25 μm. (Fig. A from Klemm,[76] with permission.)

TABLE 1. Approaches to the Identification of Adhesins of Pathogenic Microorganisms

Develop assay that measures adherence to a physiologically relevant substrate.
Inhibit adherence with simple sugars or Fab fragments of monoclonal antibodies directed against the microorganism.
Demonstrate receptor binding activity of the purified putative adhesin and show that excess adhesin blocks adherence of intact organism.
Mutate the adhesin gene and demonstrate a change in the adhesive phenotype of the organism.

taken that the assay is designed to measure adherence and not motility or invasion. Experiments to measure adherence are often performed at 4°C, a temperature at which motility and invasion are inhibited. Juxtaposition of microbe and target cell can be accomplished by centrifugation, so that motility of the microbe is not required for adherence to take place. Bacterial adherence to cells may also be distinguished from invasion by adding aminoglycosides to the medium after adherence has occurred. Only extracellular bacteria should be killed, as the aminoglycosides do not penetrate into the cells in sufficient quantities to kill intracellular bacteria. Other approaches include mild fixation of the target cells to prevent intracellular invasion.

A physiologically relevant substrate can also be an important component of an adherence assay. Receptors for some microorganisms such as influenza or *Entamoeba histolytica* are ubiquitous, so that there is little if any observable species or tissue restriction to adherence in vitro. However, the adherence of many microorganisms, such as polioviruses and rhinoviruses, are species specific, and in the case of pathogens such as Epstein-Barr virus (EBV) and the human immunodeficiency virus, are species and cell type specific. An adherence assay that measures hepatitis B virus binding to human hepatocytes is more likely to yield information relevant to pathogenesis than one measuring binding to mouse fibroblasts, for example.

Adherence can often be measured visually. The influenza virus adhesin is named *hemagglutinin* because of the initial observation that purified influenza virions agglutinated erythrocytes. Cell rosetting assays performed with larger microorganisms are a modification of these hemagglutination assays. Radioactive labeling of the microbe is often used as a means to measure adherence to cells. Care must be taken that the labeling procedure does not kill or significantly alter the microbe; a good test is to show that the binding of the radiolabeled microorganism can be inhibited by excess unlabeled microorganism. Likewise, binding of soluble receptors such as extracellular matrix components to microorganisms is performed by radiolabeling the receptors, with "specific" binding defined as the amount of radiolabeled receptor bound that is inhibited by excess cold receptor.

Once an assay has been developed to measure the adherence of a pathogen to a cell or substrate, steps can be taken to identify the microbial components participating in adherence. As the binding of many microbes to host tissues is mediated by microbial lectins, an initial approach is to test whether adherence can be blocked with simple sugars or complex oligosaccharides. Definition of the carbohydrate specificity of adherence can lead to identification of the responsible adhesin via carbohydrate affinity chromatography. Another common approach is to screen monoclonal antibodies produced against the microorganism for their ability to block adherence; inhibitory monoclonal antibodies can be used to identify and purify the putative adhesin.

Antibody inhibition of adherence is most convincing if performed with Fab fragments of antibody, to reduce the likelihood of nonspecific effects of the antibodies from agglutination, steric hindrance or cross-linking on the microbial surface; or with monoclonal antibodies, where an epitope-specific inhibition of adherence can be demonstrated (monoclonal antibody to some but not all epitopes on an adhesin block its adhesive function, thereby making nonspecific effects of the monoclonal antibody less likely). The purified putative adhesin should be demon-

strated to bind to the microbe's receptor, and excess adhesin should be able to inhibit adherence of the intact microbe competitively by preventing binding to the host receptor.

EXPERIMENTAL IDENTIFICATION OF A HOST RECEPTOR

Identification of the receptor for an adhesin is important to the understanding of interactions of microbial pathogens with their hosts (Table 2). There are several examples where the species specificity, or tissue or cell tropism, of a microorganism can be explained by the presence or absence of a receptor for the microbial adhesin. Examples include the B-lymphocyte CR2 receptor for EBV,[1] the T-cell CD4 receptor for human immunodeficiency virus (HIV),[2,3] and the aminopeptidase N receptor for the pig coronavirus TGEV.[4,5] Species specificity of adherence of microbial pathogens has also been demonstrated for poliovirus[6,7] and the major group of rhinoviruses,[8–10] where viral receptors are present on human but not murine cells (Tables 3 and 4).

Species or tissue specificity for receptors for microbial adhesins suggests an obvious approach to their identification: transfection of DNA from a receptor (+) to a receptor (−) cell line, followed by identification and sequencing of the DNA segment that confers receptor positivity. This approach has been suc-

TABLE 2. Approaches to the Identification of Host Cell Receptors for Pathogenic Microorganisms

Transfect DNA from a permissive to a nonpermissive cell; identify the transfected DNA that confers permissiveness. This technique exploits the fact that many microorganisms have restricted host ranges (e.g., rhinovirus infects only human and chimpanzee cells) and tissue tropism (e.g., HIV and CD4 cells, Epstein-Barr virus, and B cells)
Produce monoclonal antibodies (mAb) against host cell-surface antigens; screen the mAb for inhibition of binding or infection. Characterize the antigen recognized by mAb.
Identify lectin (carbohydrate recognition) activity of microorganism's adhesin by blocking adherence and/or infectivity of permissive cell with simple or complex carbohydrates (e.g., sialic acid and influenza hemagglutinin; HIV and galactosyl cerebroside).
Affinity purify the host cell receptor using microbial adhesin (rarely successful, because of the generally low affinity of the adhesin for the solubilized receptor).

TABLE 3. Classes of Host Cell Receptors for Microbial Adhesins

Sugars: Sialic acid (ortho- and paramyxoviruses, polyomaviruses, galactose (*E. histolytica*), galactosylcerebroside (HIV)
Immunoglobulin superfamily: ICAM-1 (rhinoviruses, major group), CD4 (HIV), polioviruses receptor (polio)
Growth factors or growth factor receptors: EGF receptors (vaccinia), erythropoietin receptor (Friend leukemia virus), interleukin-6 (hepatitis B virus)
Integrins: VLA-2 (echovirus)
Extracellular matrix components: Laminin (*Toxoplasma gondii*), fibronectin (streptococci)
Transport proteins: Basic amino acid and phosphate transporter (certain retroviruses)
Complement receptors: CR2 (Epstein-Barr virus)
Antibody-dependent or complement-dependent enhancement of adherence: Antibody-coated Dengue virus entry into macrophages via Fcγ1 and IgA-coated Epstein-Barr virus entry via IgA receptor; HIV antibody-dependent enhancement via CR2

TABLE 4. Classes of Microbial Adhesins for Host Cell Receptors

Lectins: Sialic acid binding (hemagglutinin envelope glycoproteins of orthomyxoviruses), galactose binding (*Entamoeba histolytica* adherence lectin), galactosylcerebroside binding (HIV gp120/gp41), trans-sialidase (*Trypanosoma cruzi*)
Fimbriae (Pili): Filamentous bacterial adhesins of *E. coli* (P, S, type 1, K-88, K-99, CFA-1), *Neisseria gonorrhea* (type 4), *Salmonella* (type 1), *Vibrio cholerae* (Tcp)
Nonfimbrial bacterial adhesins: *Yersinia* (Inv and Ail proteins), *B. pertussis* (pertactin), *M. pneumoniae* (P1 cytoadhesin), *Treponema pallidum* (fibronectin-binding protein)
Lipid: *Streptococcus pyogenes* (lipoteichoic acid), *Leishmania* (lipophosphoglycan)
Glycosaminoglycan: *Chlamydia trachomatis* (heparin sulfate-like glycosaminoglycan)
Viral capsid proteins: Rhinovirus (VP1/VP3); aphthovirus (VP1)
Mechanical: *Giardia lamblia* (gripping disc)

cessfully used to identify ICAM-1 as the human receptor for the major group of rhinoviruses[9,10] and to identify the poliovirus receptor, a member of the immunoglobulin gene superfamily.[6,7] The advantage of this approach to receptor identification is that the receptor is cloned and sequenced at the same time that it is identified.

When a restricted host range or tissue tropism cannot be exploited, monoclonal antibodies produced against the host cell have been used to identify the receptor. Monoclonal antibodies that block adherence to, or infection of, host cells were used to identify ICAM-1 as the major group rhinovirus receptor,[8] CD4 as the HIV receptor,[2,3] aminopeptidase N as the TGEV coronavirus receptor,[4,5] and VLA-2 as the receptor for echovirus-1.[11]

If the microbial adhesin is a lectin, the carbohydrate structure recognized by the adhesin on host cells can be determined by the effect of different oligosaccharides on inhibition of adherence. In this manner, the detailed structure of the sialic acid–containing oligosaccharide recognized by influenza virus hemagglutinin has been obtained.[12]

If the adhesin itself is purified it can be used to affinity purify its receptor from the host cell. This approach is not likely to be successful if the interaction of adhesin with receptor is of low affinity, which may be a particular problem when adhesin and receptor have been solubilized in purification. However this approach successfully identified CR2 as the receptor for EBV.

CENTRAL CONCEPTS IN THE INTERACTIONS OF ADHESINS AND RECEPTORS

Many adhesins require post-translational processing, especially proteolytic fragmentation, to manifest full biologic activity (Table 5). The membrane fusion activity of the hemagglutinin (HA), which is required for viral infectivity, requires processing by a host protease of the intact hemagglutinin (HA$_0$) into HA$_1$ and HA$_2$. This proteolytic fragmentation exposes a highly conserved hydrophobic sequence at the amino terminus of HA$_2$ that, at acidic pH, is involved in viral entry into the cell by fusion of the viral membrane to the endocytic vacuole cell membrane (Fig. 2).[12] Similar processing events are required for the gp160 adhesin of HIV to have functional cell fusion activity, as will be described below. The requirement for host proteases to activate the fusion activity of adhesins may partly explain tissue tropisms of microbial pathogens, since proteases required to activate the adhesins may only be present in certain tissues.

A second important concept is the "canyon hypothesis," in which the active site of the adhesin may be inaccessible to antibody because of its location in a "canyon" or depression in the molecule. This shields the receptor site from antibody and enables the microbe to conserve the amino acids required for formation of the binding site in the face of antibody-driven variation in the rest of the adhesin sequence. For example, the sialic acid–binding site of the influenza HA is formed by the highly conserved amino acids tyr 98, trp 153, his 183, glu 190, and leu 194, which are found in an antibody-inaccessible depression at the distal end of the HA; while the surface-exposed residues are subject to antigenic variation.[12] In a similar manner,

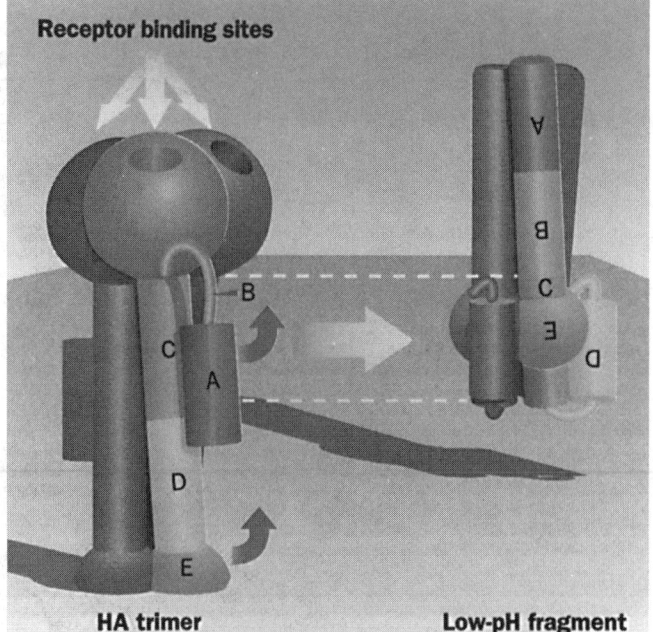

Receptor binding sites

HA trimer   **Low-pH fragment**

FIG. 2. Schematic representation of the conformation of the influenza hemagglutinin molecule at neutral and acidic pH. The HA trimer is shown protruding from a plane representing the surface of the viral membrane. The main structural units of the low pH structure (from about residues 40 to 155 of the HA$_2$ chain) are labeled A to E from the N-terminal end. The fusion peptide, N-terminal to unit A, would protrude well above the heads bearing the receptor binding sites, ideally placed to engage the membrane of the target cell. (From Stuart D, Nature 1994; 371:19–20, with permission.)

the binding site on the major group of rhinoviruses for the ICAM-1 receptor is located in a canyon formed by the capsid proteins that is only partially accessible to antibody (Fig. 3).[13]

Human adhesins such as LFA-1, CR3, and integrins require activation in addition to cell surface expression to mediate adherence,[14,15] and microbial adhesins also exist in active and inactive states. One example is the galactose-specific adhesin of *E. histolytica:* Antibodies against different epitopes on this adhesin either enhance or inhibit the galactose-binding activity of the adhesin, presumably by altering conformations from inactive to active configurations (see below).

Conformational changes in adhesin may also activate other functions of the adhesin, such as the fusion activities of enveloped virus glycoproteins. Some viral adherence glycoproteins, upon binding to a receptor, or upon exposure to low pH in endosomes, undergo conformational changes that expose the hydrophobic fusion domains of the envelope glycoproteins.[16,17]

Single adhesins can have multiple receptors. For example, gp120/41 of HIV binds to CD4 on T cells, galactosyl cerebroside on CD4− neural cell lines, and interacts with a membrane-bound serine proteinase prior to initiation of viral–host cell membrane fusion.

The immune response to an adhesin, in particular antiadhesin antibodies, may enhance adherence and/or infectivity by facilitating alternative routes of adherence and invasion. Examples of this phenomenon can be found in infections with HIV, *E. histolytica*, Dengue virus, and EBV. Enhancement of adherence and infection of Fc-receptor (+) monocytes and macrophages by subneutralizing antibodies has been demonstrated for some flaviviruses, including Dengue. However, the importance of antibody-dependent enhancement in the pathogenesis of Dengue hemorrhagic fever remains controversial.[18] Epstein-Barr virus entry into a human epithelial cell line was promoted by poly-

TABLE 5. Key Concepts in Microbial Adhesin-Host Cell Receptor Interactions

Proteolytic processing of the adhesin is often required for the full biologic activity of the adhesin to be manifest

Canyon hypothesis postulates that active sites of adhesins for receptor interaction will reside in antibody-inaccessible pockets in the adhesin

Activity of adhesins may be conformationally controlled, especially in the case of adhesins that also function as fusion proteins

Multiple receptors may bind to the same adhesin

Anti-adhesin antibodies may enhance infection by altering adhesin–receptor interactions

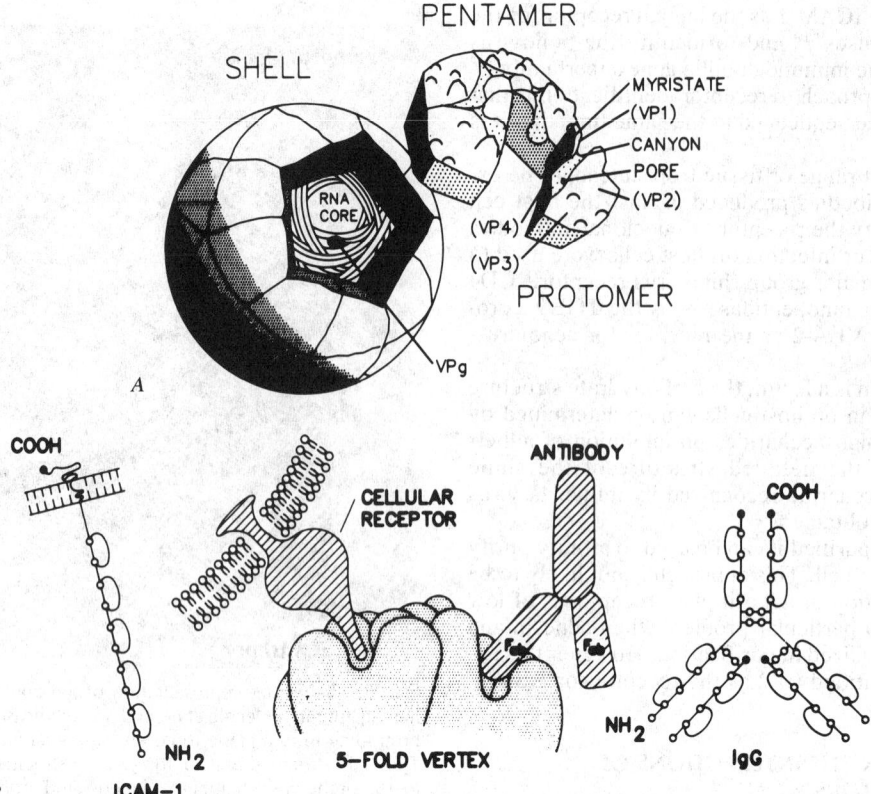

FIG. 3. Key features in the adherence function of a typical picornavirus. **(A)** Exploded diagram showing location of canyon in the middle of the center of the viral capsid protein VP4 pentamer. **(B)** Binding of cellular receptor to the floor of the canyon. Note that the binding site of the ICAM-1 molecule, identified as ICAM-1 for major group rhinoviruses, has a diameter roughly half that of an IgG antibody molecule. (From Rueckert,[78] with permission.)

meric IgA specific for EBV. The virus entered the cells via secretory component–mediated transport when bound to IgA instead of the usual route of entry via the CR2 receptor in B cells and other epithelial cell lines.[19]

The species, tissue, and/or cell tropism of a microbe is often determined by adhesin–receptor interactions. Examples include EBV and the CR2 receptor on B cells, polio virus and the polio virus receptor of human cells, and rhinoviruses and the human ICAM-1 receptor.

SPECIFIC ADHERENCE MECHANISMS AND THEIR ROLES IN PATHOGENESIS

HIV gp120/160

The development of an immune response to the adhesin of HIV, gp120/41, to block adherence and invasion by the virus, has been an important approach to the development of HIV vaccines, as discussed in Chapter 106.[20,21] Infection of cells with HIV and other enveloped viruses requires fusion of the viral and cell membranes. The fusion event releases the viral nucleocapsid into the cell cytoplasm, initiating the process of viral infection and replication.[22] This fusion event can occur at the cell surface between the plasma membrane and the viral membrane, as it does for paramyxoviruses, or it can occur between the endosome and viral membranes after phagocytosis of the virus, as in influenza virus infection. The adherence and fusion events are generally mediated by the same viral glycoprotein. In the case of HIV, it appears that the fusion event occurs at the plasma membrane, because neutralization of acidic endosomes with weak bases does not interfere with viral entry, and mutation of CD4 to a glycolipid-anchored form that is endocytosed poorly also has no effect on HIV entry.[23,24]

The HIV cell surface glycoprotein is synthesized as a 160 kDa

glycoprotein. Proteolytic cleavage of gp160 to gp120 and gp41 at a site containing several basic amino acids (arginine and lysine) is required for activation of the glycoprotein and production of infectious virions. gp160 cleavage is thought to occur in the trans-Golgi compartment and has been shown in vitro to be mediated by the endoproteinase furin, which cleaves at the consensus sequence arg-X-lys/arg-arg.[25] Furin also activates the hemagglutinin protein of the fowl plague influenza virus. In fact, the cleavage sites of the fusion proteins for orthomyxoviruses, paramyxoviruses, and retroviruses are all remarkably conserved. Inhibition of gp160 cleavage with peptide moieties containing the furin consensus sequence, or by the ionophore monensin, blocks HIV glycoprotein-induced syncytia formation and results in the production of virions with greatly reduced infectivity (25). Mutation of the carboxy-terminal amino acid 518 of gp120 from arginine to threonine abolishes both gp160 cleavage and syncytia formation (26).

Cleavage of gp160 results in the production of gp41 and gp120 and activates the fusion ability of the viral glycoprotein. gp41 contains the transmembrane carboxy terminus of gp160; gp120 remains attached to the virion via noncovalent interactions with gp41. The amino terminus created on gp41 by cleavage of gp160 is hydrophobic and contains the phe-X-gly sequence present in the amino termini of the activated fusion proteins of the paramyxoviruses. Mutations in gp160 that affect fusion activity map to the amino terminus of gp41. Thus the requirement for cleavage of gp160 to gp41 and gp120 is in large part because of the need to expose the fusion domain of gp41 for the virion to enter the cell via viral–cell plasma membrane fusion.[23–26]

Binding of HIV to CD4 and galactosylcerebroside is mediated by gp120.[2,3,27,28] Binding of CD4 by gp120 is a high-affinity interaction and results in the exposure of cryptic epitopes on gp120 and gp41 and shedding of gp120 from the virion, which indicates

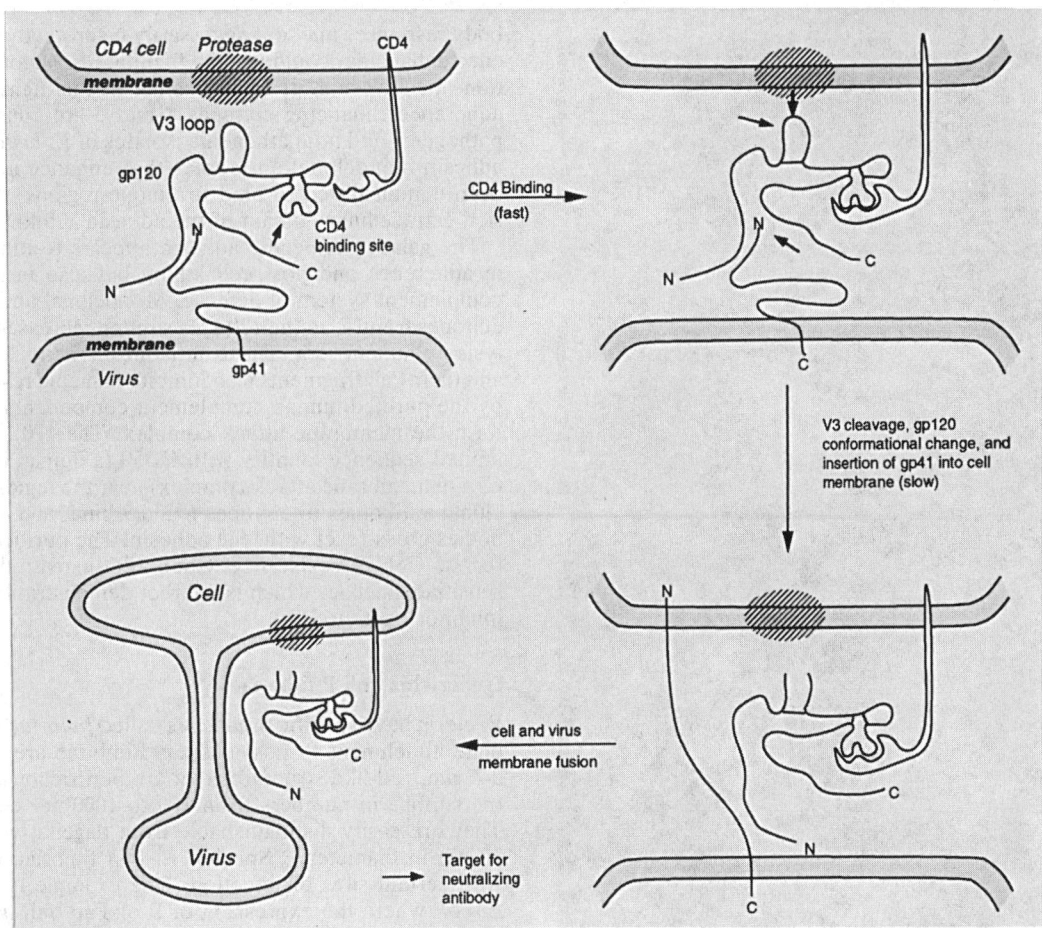

FIG. 4. Adherence and fusion mechanisms of HIV gp120/gp41. After gp120 binds to CD4, a cellular protease is proposed to cleave gp120 within the V3 loop and a conformational change in gp120 ensues. This change allows the amino terminus of gp41 to insert into the membrane of the CD4 cell and causes the membrane of the virus and cell to fuse. Membrane fusion thus allows the contents of the virus to enter the cell. (From Putney,[24] with permission.)

that CD4 binding has resulted in a conformational change in the virion glycoproteins.[29] Binding of HIV to CD4 is insufficient for fusion of viral and cell membranes, since cell surface expression of CD4 in murine cells enabled HIV to bind to, but not infect, the cells.[30]

Cell tropism (T4 cells vs. macrophages) of HIV-1 is determined in large part by the sequence of the third variable (V3) loop. Production of a chimeric gp120 containing the V3 loop of the macrophage-tropic BaL isolate of HIV-1 conferred macrophage tropism on the HTLV-IIIB strain, which is normally a T-cell tropic virus. The sensitivity of HIV isolates to inhibition by soluble CD4 is also determined by the sequence in the V3 loop.[31–34] Amino acid substitutions in the V3 loop block cell fusion and infectivity without affecting gp160 processing to gp120/gp41 or CD4 binding.[35] Recent evidence has demonstrated interaction of the V3 loop of gp120 with distinct membrane-bound serine proteinases from T-cell and promonocytic cell lines. These membrane-bound proteinases cleave gp120 at the V3 loop only upon prolonged (several hours) incubation in vitro, so it is not clear if the proteinase functions solely as a second receptor for gp120 or it protease-mediated cleavage of gp120 at the V3 loop is required for viral–cell membrane fusion (Fig. 4).[36]

Galactosyl cerebroside apparently acts as a receptor for gp120 on neural cells, which are infected by HIV but lack CD4. Galactosyl cerebroside is an abundant glycolipid in oligodendrocytes in the central nervous system in Schwann cells in the peripheral nervous system. Recombinant gp120 binds specifically to galactosyl ceramide, and antibodies against galactosyl ceramide in-

hibited HIV internalization and infection of two CD4 − cell lines derived from the nervous system.[27,28]

Enhancement of HIV infection of cells has also been observed in the presence of anti-gp120/gp41 antibodies. Most of the antibodies enhancing HIV infection have been mapped to the V3 loop; enhancement of infection appears to occur when anti-V3 loop antibodies derived from infection or immunization with gp120 from one strain cross-react with, but do not neutralize, the V3 region of another strain. Apparently V3 hypervariable loops from one isolate may elicit antibodies enhancing infection by another HIV isolate.[37] Antibody-mediated enhancement of HIV infection may be independent of complement or may be mediated by complement and the CR2 receptor; antibodies to the CR2 receptor blocked enhanced infectivity in one experimental system.[38]

Entamoeba histolytica Galactose Adhesin

Entamoeba histolytica trophozoites adhere to human colonic mucins and mammalian cells in culture via a surface lectin or adhesin that preferentially recognizes galactose in a β1–4 linkage to *N*-acetylglucosamine (Fig. 5).[39–41] Colonic mucins, by binding to and neutralizing the galactose-specific lectin, may serve as receptors for amebic colonization and also provide a nonimmune defense against amebic invasion, preventing adherence and contact-dependent killing of the intestinal epithelial cells.

Contact-dependent killing of host cells requires the activity of the galactose adhesin. Blockade of the galactose adhesin in

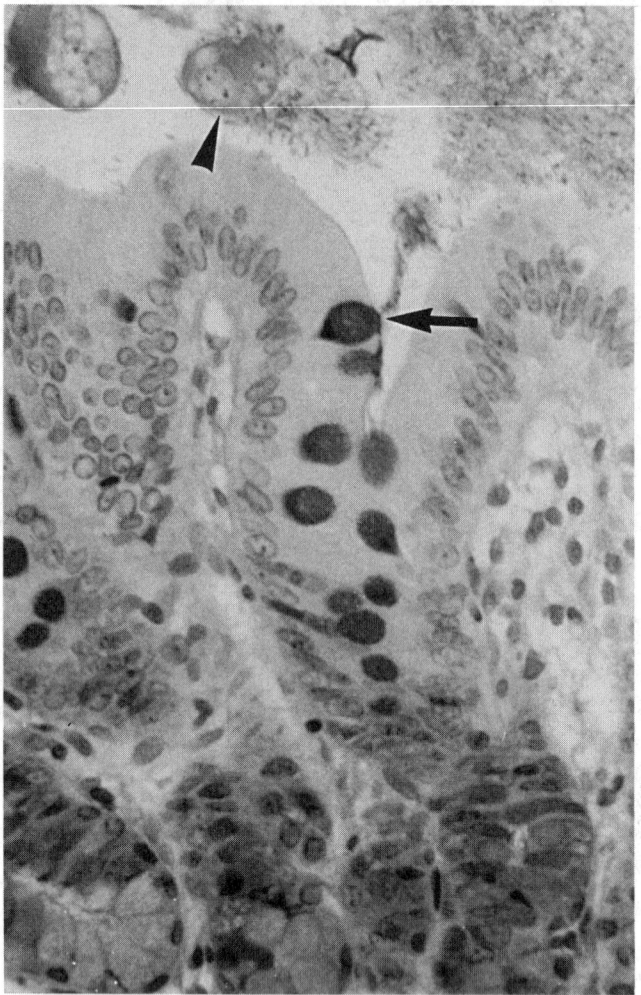

FIG. 5. *Entamoeba histolytica* trophozoites (arrowhead) adhering to colonic mucins in rat colon. Note the goblet cell with apical protrusion (arrow) in the interglandular epithelium. Bar = 0.06 mm. (HRE, ×312) (From Petri,[79] with permission.)

vitro with colonic mucins or galactose prevents amebic contact-dependent cytolysis of immune effector cells, including human macrophages and neutrophils.[39,40,42,43] The ability of antiadhesin monoclonal antibody to block cytolysis after adherence has occurred suggests that the adhesin either signals the initiation of cytolysis or directly participates in the cytolytic event.[44,45]

The role of the galactose lectin in adherence has been demonstrated in several ways. Inhibition of lectin activity with galactose or anti-lectin antibodies completely inhibited adherence to human colonic mucin glycoproteins and Chinese hamster ovary (CHO) cells.[39,40] The adhesin, purified by galactose-affinity chromatography, was shown to bind to CHO cells in a galactose-specific manner, and thereby competitively inhibit amebic adherence to CHO cells.[41,46] Chinese hamster ovary cells deficient in terminal *N*-acetyl-lactosamine (galactose β1–4 glucosamine) residues on their glycoproteins and glycolipids were resistant to amebic adherence and killing.[47,48]

The galactose lectin may resemble other eukaryotic adhesins such as LFA-1 and CR3 in requiring activation in addition to surface expression to mediate adherence. Monoclonal antibodies that bound to epitopes 1 and 2 on the 170 kD subunit increased the galactose-binding activity of the lectin, apparently by inducing a change to the active configuration of the lectin.[49] Activation and deactivation of the adhesin may explain the observed ability of amebae both to attach to and to detach from galactose-containing substrates. In addition, antiadhesin anti-

body responses may not necessarily be protective and, if adherence enhancing, could instead facilitate *E. histolytica* colonization and invasion. It is interesting in this light that only the adherence-enhancing epitopes 1 and 2 are conserved in both pathogenic and nonpathogenic isolates of *E. histolytica*.[50] Antiadhesin monoclonal antibodies that enhance adherence have been demonstrated to bind to unique regions of the cysteine-rich extracellular domain of the adhesin 170 kD subunit.[51]

The galactose-specific adhesin appears to function not only in adherence and host cell killing but also in evasion of the complement system of defense. Monoclonal antibodies against epitopes 6 and 7 on the 170 kDa subunit increased *E. histolytica* lysis by human sera. These antiadhesin monoclonal antibodies and their Fab fragments also inhibited amebic resistance to lysis by the purified human complement components C5b–9, which form the membrane attack complex. The 170 kD subunit has limited sequence identity with CD59 (a human inhibitor of the C5b–9 membrane attack complex) near the region where monoclonal antibodies to epitopes 6 and 7 bind, and anti-CD59 antibodies cross-react with, the adhesin. The purified adhesin conferred C5b–9 resistance when reconstituted into C5b–9-sensitive amebae, which is a direct demonstration of its C5b–9 inhibitory activity.[52]

Escherichia coli P fimbriae

Bacteria have specific organelles called *fimbriae* or *pili* that mediate attachment to host tissues. Fimbriae are proteinaceous, 2–7 nm, rod-like structures that are peritrichously arranged on the surface in numbers from 100 to 1000 per cell (Fig. 1).[53,54] They are easily distinguishable from flagella, which are about 20 nm in diameter.[55] Specific *E. coli* fimbriae are associated with certain sites of infection. One example is uropathogenic *E. coli* where the expression of P or Pap (*p*ili *a*ssociated with *p*yelonephritis) fimbriae[56–58] has been clearly established as a virulence factor that promotes urinary tract colonization and invasion.

The association of P fimbriae and uropathogenic *E. coli* has been demonstrated by comparing the frequency of P fimbriae expression on *E. coli* isolates from feces and the urinary tract system.[58] Isolates from all sources expressed type 1 fimbriae. P fimbriae were expressed on 100 percent of *E. coli* isolates from the urine of patients with pyelonephritis, but only on 17 percent of *E. coli* isolates from urine of patients with asymptomatic bacteriuria.

P fimbriae have been shown to bind specifically uroepithelial cells and P blood group antigens on human erythrocytes. The receptors for P fimbriae on these cells are globoseries glycolipids containing the disaccharide α-D-galactopyranosyl-(1,4)-β-D-galactopyranose (gal-gal).[57,59] Gal-gal, which is the minimal receptor moiety, can inhibit hemagglutination[60] and block the attachment of P fimbriated bacteria to uroepithelial cells.[61] The attachment and hemagglutination by P fimbriated strains of *E. coli* have been found to be completely dependent on the presence of P blood group antigens.[62]

Women with recurrent infections are two to three times more likely to be nonsecretors of P blood group substance. Uroepithelial cells from nonsecretors show more adherence of P fimbriated bacteria than do cells from secretors.[62] It has been speculated that the gal-gal receptors on nonsecretor cells may be more accessible because of the lack of fucosyltransferase-mediated synthesis of A, B, and H antigens and that the presence of these histo-blood group antigens on secretor cells may block or modify the essential gal-gal receptors.[62] Other investigators have reported the isolation of unique globoseries glycolipids present on nonsecretor uroepithelial cells and absent from secretor cells, which bind uropathogenic *E. coli*.[63] These results raise the possibility that the increased risk of urinary tract infections in nonsecretors may be due to the presence of a unique receptor for P fimbriated bacteria on their uroepithelial cells.

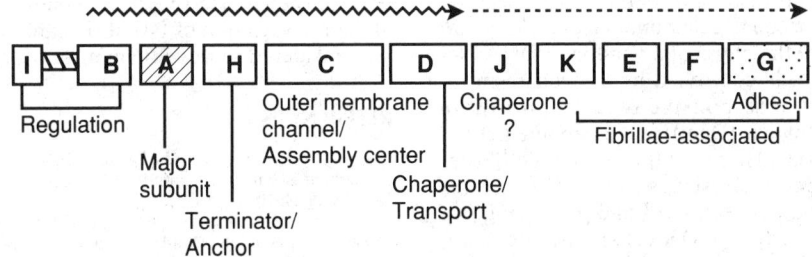

FIG. 6. Organization of the genes of the *pap* operon. Proposed functions for each gene are listed. The hatched bar represents the operator–promoter region of the DNA that binds the regulatory proteins described in text. Wavy lines represent mRNA transcripts. Polycistronic transcription has been shown to occur through *pap*D.[70] The dotted line indicates that transcription probably continues to *pap*G, but this has not been conclusively demonstrated.

P fimbriae biosynthesis, assembly, and regulation are encoded by the *pap* gene operon found on the *E. coli* chromosome (Fig. 6).[64,65] In *E. coli* many genes with related functions are often organized in operons. In the *pap* operon, a regulatory protein and RNA polymerase bind to DNA at specific sites, called *operator* and *promoter* sites, respectively, located just upstream of the structural genes. As RNA transcription proceeds, a single polycistronic mRNA transcript is made that encodes all of the structural genes. This type of system allows for the coordinate expression and regulation of all the genes that are essential for fimbriae production. One consequence of polycistronic transcription is that a mutation in a gene upstream that causes transcription or translation termination could produce what is called a *polar effect*, in that the expression of the genes located downstream from the mutation may be reduced or eliminated.

The functional roles of the genes in the *pap* operon have been elucidated by analyzing the phenotypes of nonpolar mutations in each gene.[64,65] *pap*I and *pap*B have been found to encode positive regulatory proteins that are necessary for the expression of the structural genes. *pap*A codes for the major fimbrial subunit that polymerizes to form the fimbrial rod. *pap*H mutants have unusually long fimbriae, and it has been proposed that PapH functions as an anchor or terminator of fimbrial polymerization. Mutations in *pap*C, *pap*D, *pap*K, or *pap*J failed to express fimbriae on the bacterial surface, indicating a role for these genes in surface assembly. The PapC protein has been found in the outer membrane and appears to function as a channel for translocation of the fimbrial subunits and also appears to function as an assembly center for fimbrial polymerization. A mutation in *pap*D resulted in rapid degradation of the other major and minor fimbrial subunits. PapD has been isolated as complexes with PapG and PapE. It has been suggested that PapD acts as a "chaperone" in fimbrial assembly. Chaperones stabilize other proteins and assist in maintaining or assuming the correct conformation that will allow the protein to be secreted across the cytoplasmic membrane or to assemble at the proper time. PapJ may also function as a chaperone. Bacterial strains with mutations in *pap*E, *pap*F, and *pap*G all produce fimbriae but do not bind gal-gal residues. They all also share some amino acid sequence homology with PapA. A model for fimbrial assembly and structure is depicted in Figure 7.[66] PapG has been identified as the actual gal-gal binding subunit by complementation studies[67] and localized to the tip of the fibrillae by immunoelectron microscopy (Fig. 8).

P fimbriae undergo a type of phase variation in which an individual bacteria can turn on or off the expression of the fimbrial genes. Consequently within a clonal population not all bacteria containing the P fimbrial genes will be expressing P fimbriae on their surface. The ability to control the expression of P fimbriae may be advantageous to the bacteria by enabling detachment and migration to different sites or by providing a mechanism of antigenic variation to avoid recognition by the immune system.

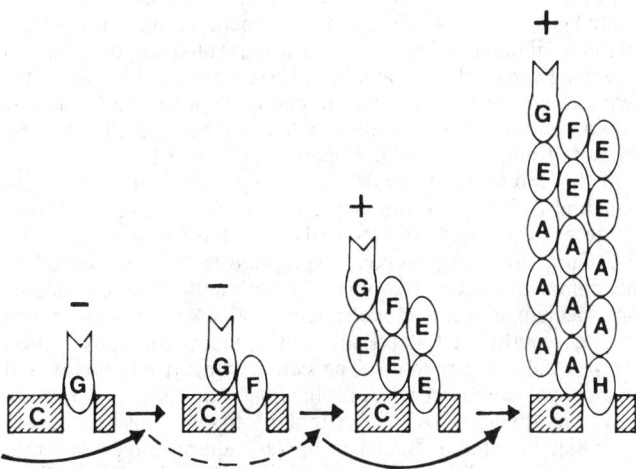

FIG. 7. Model for P fimbriae structure and assembly. Four successive stages of assembly are shown from left to right; +/− indicate the ability of the structure to bind gal-gal receptors. (From Lindberg et al.,[66] with permission.)

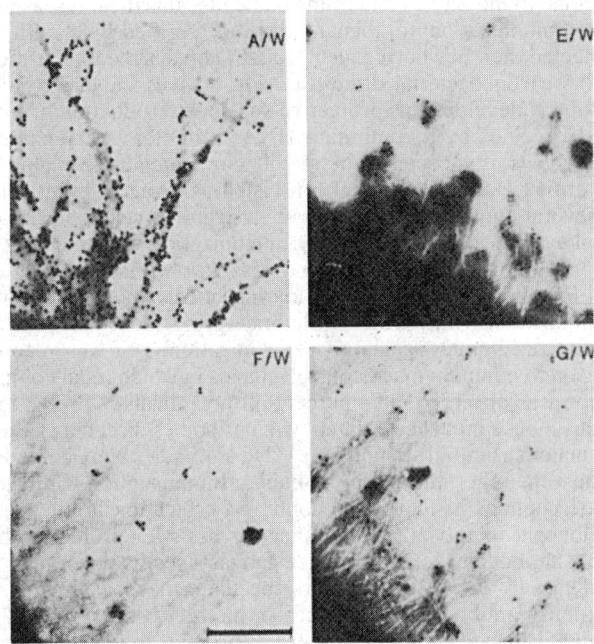

FIG. 8. Electron micrographs of P fimbriae reacted with sera specific for PapA in A/W, PapE in E/W, PapF in F/W, and PapG in G/W. Bound antibodies were visualized by the addition of colloidal gold–labeled protein A. Bar = 500 nm. (From Lindberg et al.,[66] with permission.)

P fimbrial phase variation is distinct from the phase variation systems of type 1 fimbriae or the flagellar antigen of *Salmonella typhimurium,* which involve the physical inversion of DNA element. P fimbriae expression is controlled by a mechanism involving PapB, PapI, leucine-responsive regulatory protein (Lrp), deoxyadenosine methylase (Dam), and catabolite activator protein (CAP).[69] P fimbrial phase variation involves differential methylation of the adenosine residues in two GATC sites located in the DNA situated between *pap*I and *pap*B (Fig. 6). In cells expressing P fimbriae (phase ON cells), one site is unmethylated ($GATC_{1028}$) and the other is methylated ($GATC_{1130}$). In phase OFF cells, the $GATC_{1028}$ site is methylated and the $GATC_{1130}$ site is nonmethylated. The methylation is regulated by the binding of Lrp and PapI to these sites. DNAse footprinting of Lrp/PapI to unmethylated *pap* regulatory region has demonstrated that Lrp binds to a region surrounding $GATC_{1130}$. PapI did not bind DNA in the absence of Lrp; however, when PapI and Lrp were added together, an additional footprint around $GATC_{1028}$ was observed. Dam methylation of these sites inhibited binding of Lrp/PapI.[70] These results support a model in which Dam methylase and PapI/Lrp compete for binding sites near the *pap* promoter. The binding of PapI/Lrp to $GATC_{1028}$ would facilitate the binding of RNA polymerase and thereby promote transcription of the operon.

In this model for ON/OFF switching, competition between Dam and Lrp/PapI for binding to the $GATC_{1028}$ controls P fimbriate expression.[69] In ON cells, Lrp/PapI is bound to the $GATC_{1028}$ site. For *pap* gene expression to be switched OFF, this complex must be removed, so that methylation can occur. One mechanism for removal might be DNA replication. Once the site is methylated, Lrp/PapI cannot bind, so the transcription of *pap* would be turned off. The switch from OFF to ON would require two rounds of DNA replication in order to reproduce a fully unmethylated $GATC_{1028}$ site. OFF to ON transition occurs on minimal media in about 1 in 10,000 bacteria, suggesting that competition conditions more often favor Dam binding and the methylated state.

Fimbriae are logical targets for antimicrobial therapy and vaccine development. Purified fimbriae have been effective, well-established vaccines for veterinary use for several years. One of the first effective fimbrial vaccines was based on K-88 antigen, a fimbriae found on *E. coli* strains that cause diarrheal disease in pigs. Immunization of pregnant pigs with purified K-88 antigen protected their newborn piglets from *E. coli* diarrhea.[71] Purified fimbriae from bacterial strains that infect calves and lambs have also been developed as protective vaccines. Production of fimbrial vaccines by recombinant DNA technology has enabled these types of vaccines to be readily commercially available.[72]

Purified P fimbriae have been tested as protective antigens in several animal models. Protection against pyelonephritis in monkeys has been achieved by immunization with purified P fimbriae. Protection was shown to correlate with a high titer of anti-P fimbrial antibodies.[73] In a murine model of pyelonephritis, immunization with purified P fimbriae protected 49 percent of immunized animals against renal colonization. This was in comparison to nonimmunized control animals in which renal colonization was observed in 94 percent of the animals.[74] Protection in this mouse model correlated with antibodies directed against the major structural subunit PapA. No antibodies were detected against the other minor pilus subunits. Immunization with synthetic peptides of PapA also conferred protection in a murine pyelonephritis model.[75] The molecular basis for protection by PapA antibodies is unclear, since gal-gal–specific adherence is mediated by PapG. The authors speculate that the binding of anti-PapA antibodies may directly or indirectly affect a conformational change in PapG or other Pap proteins that is unfavorable for gal-gal binding.[75] These reports suggest that P fimbrial proteins have potential as protective vaccine candidates. The application of DNA recombinant technology to express specific protective epitopes, possibly from more than one fimbrial protein, may increase the effectiveness of fimbrial vaccines. The antigenic variation of P fimbriae and other fimbriae will have to be considered in development of a broadly effective vaccine.

REFERENCES

1. Fingeroth JD, Weiss JJ, Tedder TF, et al. Epstein-Barr virus receptor of human B lymphocytes is the C3d receptor CR2. Proc Natl Acad Sci USA. 1984;81:4510–4.
2. Dagleish AG, Beverley PCL, Clapham PR, et al. The CD4 (T4) antigen is an essential component of the receptor for the AIDS retrovirus. Nature. 1984; 312:763–7.
3. Klatzmann D, Champagne E, Chamaret S, et al. T lymphocyte T4 molecule behaves as the receptor for human retrovirus LAV. Nature. 1984;312:767–8.
4. Delmas B, Gelfi J, L'Haridon R, et al. Aminopeptidase N is a major receptor for the enteropathogenic coronavirus TGEV. Nature. 1992;357:417–20.
5. Yeager CL, Ashmun RA, Williams RK, et al. Human aminopeptidase N is a receptor for human coronavirus 229E. Nature. 1992;357:420–2.
6. Mendelsohn CL, Wimmer E, Racaniello VR. Cellular receptor for poliovirus: Molecular cloning, nucleotide sequence, and expression of a new member of the immunoglobulin superfamily. Cell. 1989;56:855–65.
7. Koike S, Horie H, Ise I, et al. The poliovirus receptor protein is produced both as membrane-bound and secreted forms. EMBO J. 1990;9:3217–24.
8. Tomassini JE, Colonno RJ. Isolation of a receptor protein involved in attachment of human rhinoviruses. J Virol. 1986;58:290–95.
9. Greve JM, Davis G, Meyer AM, et al. The major human rhinovirus receptor is ICAM-1. Cell. 1989;56:839–47.
10. Staunton DE, Merluzzi VJ, Rothlein R, et al. A cell adhesion molecule, ICAM-1, is the major surface receptor for rhinoviruses. Cell. 1989;56:849–53.
11. Bergelson JM, Shepley MP, Chan BMC, et al. Identification of the integrin VLA-2 as a receptor for echovirus 1. Science. 1992;255:1718–20.
12. Wiley DC, Skehel JJ. The structure and function of the hemagglutinin membrane glycoprotein of influenza virus. Annu Rev Biochem. 1989;56:365.
13. Rossman MG, Arnold E, Erickson JW et al. The structure of a human common cold virus (rhinovirus 14) and its functional relations to other picornaviruses. Nature. 1985;317:145–53.
14. Altieri DC, Edginton TS. A monoclonal antibody reacting with distinct adhesion molecules defines a transition in the functional state of the receptor CD11b/CD18 (Mac-1). J Immunol. 1988;141:2656.
15. Dustin ML, Springer TA. T cell receptor cross-linking transiently stimulates adhesiveness through LFA-1. Nature. 1989;341:619.
16. Flynn DC, Meyer WJ, MacKenzie JM Jr, et al. A conformational change in Sindbis virus glycoprotein E1 and E2 is detected at the plasma membrane as a consequence of early virus–cell interaction. J Virol. 1990;64:3643–53.
17. Wahlberg JM, Garoff H. Membrane fusion process of Semliki forest virus I: Low pH-induced rearrangement in spike protein quaternary structure precedes virus penetration into cells. J Cell Biol. 1992;116:339–48.
18. Halstead SB. Pathogenesis of Dengue: Challenges to molecular biology. Science. 1988;239:476–81.
19. Sixbey JW, Yao QY. Immunoglobulin A induced shift of Epstein-Barr virus tissue tropism. Science. 1992;255:1578–80.
20. Emini EA, Schleif WA, Nunberg JH, et al. Prevention of HIV-1 infection in chimpanzees by gp120 V3 domain-specific monoclonal antibody. Nature. 1992;355:728–30.
21. Hu SL, Abrams K, Barber GN, et al. Protection of macaques against SIV infection by subunit vaccines of SIV envelope glycoprotein gp160. Science. 1992;255:456–9.
22. White J, Kielian M, Helenius A. Membrane fusion proteins of enveloped animal viruses. Q Rev Biophys. 1983;16:151–95.
23. Nara PL, Garrity RR, Goudsmit J. Neutralization of HIV-1: A paradox of humoral proportions. FASEB J. 1991;5:2437–55.
24. Putney S. How antibodies block HIV infection: Paths to an AIDS vaccine. Trends Biochem Sci. 1992;17:191–6.
25. Hallenberger S, Bosch V, Angliker H, et al. Inhibition of furin-mediated cleavage activation of HIV-1 glycoprotein gp160. Nature. 1992;360:358–61.
26. Freed EO, Myers DJ, Risser R. Mutational analysis of the cleavage sequence of the human immunodeficiency virus type 1 envelope glycoprotein precursor gp160. J Virol. 1989;63:4670–5.
27. Harouse JM, Bhat S, Spitalnik SL, et al. Inhibition of entry of HIV-1 in neural cells by antibodies against galactosyl ceramide. Science. 1991;253:320–3.
28. Bhat S, Spitalnik SL, Gonzalez-Scarano F, et al. Galactosyl ceramide or a derivative is an essential component of the neural receptor for human immunodeficiency virus type 1 envelope glycoprotein gp120. Proc Natl Acad Sci USA. 1991;88:7131–4.
29. Sattentau QJ, Moore JP. Conformational changes induced in the human immunodeficiency virus envelope glycoprotein by soluble CD4 binding. J Exp Med. 1991;174:407–15.
30. Maddon PJ, Dalgleish AG, McDougal JS, et al. The T4 gene encodes the AIDS virus receptor and is expressed in the immune system and brain. Cell. 1986;47:333.
31. Safrit JT, Fung MSC, Andrews CA, et al. hu-PBL-SCID mice can be protected from HIV-1 infection by passive transfer of monoclonal antibody to the principal neutralizing determinant of envelope gp120. AIDS. 1993;7:15–21.
32. Hwang SS, Boyle TJ, Lyerly HK, et al. Identification of the envelope V3 loop as the primary determinant of cell tropism in HIV-1. Science. 1991;253: 71–4.

33. Hwang SS, Boyle TJ, Lyerly HK, et al. Identification of the envelope V3 loop as the major determinant of CD4 neutralization sensitivity of HIV-1. Science. 1992;257:535–7.

34. Shioda T, Levy JA, Cheng-Mayer C. Macrophage and T cell tropisms of HIV-1 are determined by specific regions of the envelope gp120 gene. Nature. 1991; 349:167–9.

35. Page KA, Stearns SM, Littman DR. Analysis of mutations in the V3 domain of gp160 that affect fusion and infectivity. J Virol. 1992;66:524–33.

36. Avril LE, Martino-Ferrer MD, Barin F, et al. Interaction between a membrane-associated serine proteinase of U-937 monocytes and peptides from the V3 loop of the human immunodeficiency virus type 1 gp 120 envelope glycoprotein. FEBS Lett. 1993;317:167–72.

37. Jiang S, Lin K, Neurath AR. Enhancement of human immunodeficiency virus type 1 infection by antisera to peptides from the envelope glycoproteins gp120/gp41. J Exp Med. 1991;174:1557–63.

38. Tremblay M, Meloche S, Sekaly RP, et al. Complement receptor 2 mediates enhancement of human immunodeficiency virus 1 infection in Epstein-Barr virus carrying B cells. J Exp Med. 1990;171:1791–6.

39. Ravdin JI, Guerrant RL. Role of adherence in cytopathic mechanisms of *Entamoeba histolytica*. Study with mammalian tissue culture cells and human erythrocytes. J Clin Invest. 1981;68:1305–13.

40. Chadee K, Petri WA Jr, Innes DJ, et al. Rat and human colonic mucins bind to and inhibit the adherence lectin of *Entamoeba histolytica*. J Clin Invest. 1987;80:1245–54.

41. Saffer LD, Petri WA Jr. *Entamoeba histolytica*: recognition of α- and β-galactose by the 260 kDa adherence lectin. Exp Parasitol. 1991;72:106–8.

42. Guerrant RL, Brush J, Ravdin JI, et al. Interaction between *Entamoeba histolytica* and human polymorphonuclear neutrophils. J Infect Dis. 1981;143: 83–93.

43. Chadee K, Meerovitch E. *Entamoeba histolytica*: Early progressive pathology in the cecum of the gerbil *(Meriones unguiculatus)*. Am J Trop Med Hyg. 1985;34:283–91.

44. Ravdin JI, Croft BY, Guerrant RL. Cytopathogenic mechanisms of *Entamoeba histolytica*. J Exp Med. 1980;152:377–90.

45. Saffer LD, Petri WA Jr. Role of the galactose lectin of *Entamoeba histolytica* in adherence-dependent killing of mammalian cells. Infect Immun. 1991;59: 4681–3.

46. Petri WA Jr, Smith RD, Schlesinger PH, et al. Isolation of the galactose binding lectin of *Entamoeba histolytica*. J Clin Invest. 1987;80:1238–44.

47. Li E, Becker A, Stanley SL. Chinese hamster ovary cells deficient in *N*-acetylglucosaminyltransferase I activity are resistant to *Entamoeba histolytica*–mediated cytotoxicity. Infect Immun. 1989;57:8–12.

48. Ravdin JI, Stanley P, Murphy CF, et al. Characterization of cell surface carbohydrate receptors for *Entamoeba histolytica* adherence lectin. Infect Immun. 1989;57:2179–86.

49. Petri WA Jr, Snodgrass TL, Jackson TFHG, et al. Monoclonal antibodies directed against the galactose-binding lectin of *Entamoeba histolytica* enhance adherence. J Immunol. 1990;144:4803–9.

50. Petri WA Jr, Jackson TFHG, Gathiram V, et al. Pathogenic and nonpathogenic strains of *Entamoeba histolytica* can be differentiated by monoclonal antibodies to the galactose-specific adherence lectin. Infect Immun. 1990;58: 1802–6.

51. Mann BJ, Chung CY, Braga LL, et al. Neutralizing monoclonal antibody epitopes of the *Entamoeba histolytica* galactose adhesin map to the cysteine-rich extracellular domain of the 170 kDa subunit. Infect Immun. 1993;61: 1772–8. In press.

52. Braga LL, Ninomiya H, McCoy JJ, et al. Inhibition of the complement membrane attack complex by the galactose-specific adhesin of *Entamoeba histolytica*. J Clin Invest. 1992;90:1131–7.

53. Brinton CC Jr. The structure, function, synthesis and genetic control of bacterial pili and a molecular model for DNA and RNA transport in gram negative bacteria. Trans NY Acad Sci. 1965;27:1003–54.

54. Houwink AL, van Itersen W. Electron microscopic observations on bacterial cytology. II. A study on flagellation. Biochim Biophys Acta. 1950;5:10–44.

55. Silverman M, Simon MI. Bacterial flagella. Annu Rev Microbiol. 1977;31: 397–419.

56. Hull RA, Gill RE, Hsu P, et al. Construction and expression of recombinant plasmids encoding type 1 or D-mannose–resistant pili from a urinary tract infection *Escherichia coli* isolate. Infect Immun. 1981;33:933–8.

57. Kallenius G, Mollby R, Svenson SB, et al. The p^k antigen as receptor for the haemagglutinin of pyelonephritic *Escherichia coli* strains. FEMS Microbiol Lett. 1980;7:297–302.

58. O'Hanley P, Low D, Romero I, et al. Gal-gal binding and hemolysin phenotypes and genotypes associated with uropathogenic *Escherichia coli*. N Engl J Med. 1985;313:414–20.

59. Leffler H, Svanborg-Eden C. Chemical identificaton of glycosphingolipid receptor for *Escherichia coli* attaching to human urinary tract epithelial cells and agglutinating human erythrocytes. FEMS Microbiol Lett. 1980;8:127–34.

60. O'Hanley P, Lark D, Normark S, et al. Mannose-sensitive and gal-gal binding pili of *Escherichia coli* from recombinant strains. J Exp Med. 1983;158: 1713–19.

61. Svanborg-Eden C, Freter R, Hagberg L, et al. Inhibition of experimental ascending urinary tract infection by an epithelial cell-surface receptor analogue. Nature. 1982;298:560–2.

62. Lomberg H, Cedergren B, Leffler H, et al. Influence of blood group antigen on the availability of receptors for attachment of uropathogenic *Escherichia coli*. Infect Immun. 1986;51:919–26.

63. Stapleton A, Nudelman E, Clasuen H, et al. Binding of uropathogenic *Escherichia coli* R45 to glycolipids extracted from vaginal epithelial cells in dependent on histo-blood group secretor status. J Clin Invest. 1992;90:965–72.

64. Hultgren SJ, Normark S. Chaperone-assisted assembly and molecular architecture of adhesive pili. Annu Rev Microbiol. 1991;45:383–415.

65. Tennent JM, Hultgren S, Marklund B, et al. Genetics of adhesin expression in *Escherichia coli*. In: Iglewski BH, Clark VL, eds. The Bacteria. XI New York: Academic Press; 1990:79–110.

66. Lindberg F, Lund B, Johansson L, et al. Localization of the receptor-binding protein adhesin at the tip of the bacterial pilus. Nature. 1987;328:84–7.

67. Lund B, Lindberg F, Marklund BI, et al. The PapG protein is the α-D-galacto-pyranosyl-(1-4)-β-D-galactopyranose-binding adhesin of uropathogenic *Escherichia coli*. Proc Natl Acad Sci USA. 1987;84:5898–902.

68. Kuehn MJ, Heuser J, Normark S, et al. P pili in uropathogenic *E. coli* are composite fibres with distinct fibrillar adhesive tips. Nature. 1992;356:252–5.

69. Van der Woude MW, Braaten BA, Low DA. Evidence for global regulatory control of pilus expression in *Escherichia coli* by Lrp and DNA methylation: Model building based on analysis of *pap*. Mol Microbiol. 1992;6:2429–35.

70. Nou X, Skinner B, Braaten B, et al. Regulation of pyelonepritis-associated pili phae variation in *Escherichia coli*: Binding of the PapI and Lrp regulatory proteins is controlled by DNA methylation. Mol Microbiol. 1993;7:545–53.

71. Rutter JM, Jones GW. Protection against enteric disease caused by *Escherichia coli*—A model for vaccination with a virulence determinant? Nature. 1973;242:531–2.

72. Greenwood PE, Clark SJ, Cahill AD, et al. Development and protective efficacy of a recombinant-DNA derived fimbrial vaccine against enterotoxic colibacillosis in neonatal piglets. Vaccine. 1988;6:389–92.

73. Roberts J, Hardaway K, Kaack B, et al. Prevention of pyelonephritis by immunization with P-fimbriae. J Urol. 1984;131:602–7.

74. Pecha B, Low D, O'Hanley P. Gal-gal pili vaccines prevent pyeleonephritis by piliated *Escherichia coli* in a murine model. J Clin Invest. 1989;83:2102–8.

75. Schmidt MA, O'Hanley P, Lark D, et al. Synthetic peptides corresponding to protective epitopes of *Escherichia coli* digalactoside-binding pilin prevent infection in a murine pyelonephritis model. Proc Natl Acad Sci USA. 1988; 85:1247–51.

76. Klemm P. Fimbrial adhesins of *Escherichia coli*. Rev Infect Dis. 1985;7: 321–40.

77. Wiley DC, Skehel JJ. Viral membranes. In: Fields BN, Knipe DM, eds. Fields Virology. 5th ed. New York: Raven Press, 1990:63–85.

78. Rueckert RR. Picornaviridae and their replication. In: Fields BN, Knipe DM, eds. Fields Virology. 2nd ed. New York: Raven Press; 1990:507–48.

79. Petri WA Jr. Invasive amebiasis and the galactose lectin of *Entamoeba histolytica*. ASM News. 1991;57:299–306.

3. A MOLECULAR PERSPECTIVE OF MICROBIAL PATHOGENICITY

DAVID A. RELMAN
STANLEY FALKOW

The study of microbial pathogenicity at the molecular level has altered the way we view the host–parasite relationship and has forced the redefinition of some commonly used terms. *Infection, infectious disease,* and *virulence* have been defined and used in numerous and sometimes misleading ways. The essential feature of most infections, however, is the successful multiplication of a microbe on or within a host. This process is often of benefit to both participants. Thus, following birth, human exposure to a myriad of microorganisms leads to the establishment of a protective microbial flora, stimulates the immune system, and in addition provides small amounts of human accessory growth factors. The human participants in these infections are most often asymptomatic or exhibit subclinical signs but are generally better off for their encounter with the infecting organism(s). It is probably fair to say that this is the usual outcome of most infections.

The term *infectious disease* applies when signs and symptoms result from infection and its associated damage or altered physiology. A *pathogen* is usually defined as any microorganism that has the capacity to cause disease. Yet not all pathogens have an equal probability of causing disease in the same host population. *Virulence* provides a quantitative measure of pathogenicity, or the likelihood of causing disease. For example, encapsulated pneumococci are more virulent than are nonencapsulated pneumococci, and type b encapsulated *Haemophilus influenzae* organisms are more virulent than are other *H. influenzae* capsular types. *Virulence factors* refers to the properties (i.e., gene products) that enable a microorganism to establish itself on or within a host of a particular species and enhance its potential to cause disease.

If one is to examine microbial pathogenicity in detail, it is useful to distinguish ''principal'' pathogens, which *regularly* cause disease in some proportion of susceptible individuals with apparently *intact* specific and nonspecific defense systems from other potentially pathogenic microorganisms. Certain microorganisms do not meet this definition of a principal pathogen because they do not regularly cause disease in individuals with intact host defenses. *Pseudomonas aeruginosa* is a good example. This microorganism does not usually cause disease in people with intact host defense systems; yet it can clearly cause devastating disease in many hospitalized and immunocompromised patients. It is probable that virtually any microorganism with a capacity for sustained multiplication in humans can cause disease more readily in individuals with underlying chronic disease or who are otherwise compromised. The common term *opportunist* suits this category of pathogen well. One could extend this argument to say that, for most organisms classified as principal pathogens, for example, *Staphylococcus aureus* and the pneumococcus, there must be some impairment or local breakdown of the normal host defense mechanisms in order for these bacteria to cause disease. On the other hand, it seems clear that the capacity of certain microorganisms to cause disease in seemingly uncompromised human hosts on a regular basis reflects some fundamental difference in their virulence capabilities as compared with opportunists or nonpathogens.

THE ATTRIBUTES OF MICROBIAL PATHOGENS

To be successful, a pathogen must find an appropriate host niche and multiply there. Disease is arguably only an inadvertent outcome of microbial multiplication. To cause infection, a microorganism must possess an interactive group of complementary genetic properties, sometimes coregulated, that promote its interaction with a particular host. For a given microorganism these genetic traits define unique attributes[1] that enable it to follow a common sequence of steps used by organisms that are successful in establishing infection or subsequent disease.[2] These traits are reflected as phenotypes for which one or more genes and their gene products may be responsible. Elegant molecular techniques have permitted the identification, isolation, and characterization of many of these genes and their products. Precise manipulation of the pathogen's genome has led to the determination of the roles for some of these putative virulence factors.

An initial step required of a pathogen is for it to gain access to the host in sufficient numbers. Gaining access to a potential host requires that the microorganism not only make contact with an appropriate surface but also then reach its unique niche or microenvironment on or within the host. This requirement is not trivial. Some pathogens must survive for varying lengths of time in the external environment. Others have evolved an effective and suitable means of transmission. To accomplish this goal the infecting microbe may make use of motility, chemotactic properties, and adhesive structures, or adhesins, that mediate binding to specific eukaryotic cell receptors.[3] Preexisting microorganisms, the normal flora, provide competition against establishment of the newcomer; in addition, the latter must

adapt, at least temporarily, to the particular nutrient environment in which it now finds itself.

Normal host defense mechanisms pose the next and most difficult set of obstacles to the arriving pathogen. For any set of specific host defenses an individual pathogen may have devised a unique and distinctive counterstrategy. Some of the best known mechanisms for countering host defenses include the use of an antiphagocytic capsule and the elaboration of toxins and microbial enzymes that act on host immune cells and destroy anatomic barriers. In addition, microorganisms may employ subtle mechanisms to avoid or even subvert host defenses, including immunoglobulin-specific protease, iron sequestration mechanisms, or coating themselves with host proteins so as to confuse the immune surveillance system. Examples of these mechanisms include the production of IgA1 protease by *H. influenzae,* the use of receptors for iron-saturated human transferrin and lactoferrin by *Neisseria gonorrhoeae,* and the coating of *Treponema pallidum* with human soluble fibronectin. Antigenic variation and intracellular invasion are other common strategies used by successful pathogens to avoid immune detection.

The ability to multiply is a characteristic of all living organisms. Whether the pathogen's niche in the relevant host be intracellular or extracellular, mucosal or submucosal, within the blood stream or within a privileged anatomic site, the pathogen will have evolved a distinct set of biochemical tactics to achieve this goal. The success of a pathogen, indeed of any microorganism, is measured by the degree with which it can multiply upon reaching its specific niche and secure its potential transmission to a new susceptible host.

Thus, the outcome of the events just described is determined by the degree to which the pathogen has perpetuated itself and by the nature of the relationship it has established with its host. The result may be altered host physiology, tissue damage, and even clinical manifestations of disease. Death of the host is a rare event and one that must be viewed as most often detrimental to both parties involved! The more usual outcome is sufficient multiplication of the pathogen to ensure its establishment within the host (transient or long-term colonization) or its successful transmission to a new susceptible host.

Why do some pathogens cause disease more readily than others do? The strategy used for multiplication on or within the host often defines fundamental differences between pathogens that commonly cause disease and those that do not. If a microorganism succeeds by multiplying within deep fascial planes, it is far more likely to cause disease than is a nontoxinogenic microorganism that is content to grow on a mucosal surface. If a microorganism has evolved a means to nullify or destroy phagocytic cells in order to multiply successfully, it is more likely a disease-causing pathogen. Furthermore, an organism that can reach and multiply in privileged anatomic sites away from the competitive environment of skin and some mucosal surfaces is likely to disrupt homeostasis in the host and cause disease. Commensal organisms are content to multiply just enough, in the midst of competing microflora, to persist but not damage the host's self-preserving homeostatic mechanisms. It is important to emphasize that a microorganism exceptionally equipped to cause infection may be an unexceptional pathogen and only infrequently, if ever, cause clinically manifested disease.

Why are some organisms like *P. aeruginosa* only opportunists despite their impressive array of virulence factors? An organism has no presupposition about the state of the host defenses when it encounters a human host. For opportunistic pathogens that state is the main determinant of whether disease will be the outcome of their interaction with the host. This reflects the fact that these organisms may lack an effective means to overcome normal host defense mechanisms. Opportunists may be very adept at establishing an infection, but because of their preferred growth locale (e.g., the mucosal surface) and preferred growth conditions (e.g., a microaerophilic environment) they may have limited growth opportunities outside of their restricted niche in an unimpaired individual. As a result, disease may be only a rare consequence of the host–microbe encounter.

Pathogens were once viewed as organisms, largely unadapted to their hosts, that elaborated potent toxins or other powerful aggressive factors that caused the signs and symptoms of disease. The current view is that a microbial pathogen is a highly adapted organism that follows a strategy for survival requiring multiplication on or within another living organism. Occasionally this survival strategy produces overt damage to the host. Of course, some infectious diseases occur predominantly in dramatic epidemic form, arguing against the evolution of a balanced host–parasite relationship; however, in many such epidemics there are mitigating circumstances that involve herd immunity and other underlying social, economic, and political issues that impinge upon this relationship. Furthermore, some of the most serious infectious diseases occur when humans are infected by microorganisms that prefer and are better adapted to another mammalian host.

THE CLONAL NATURE OF BACTERIAL PATHOGENS

Pathogenicity is not a microbial trait that has appeared by chance. Instead, particular microbial strains and species have evolved to carry very specific arrays of virulence-associated genes. By examining the genetic organization of pathogens, opportunists, and nonpathogenic bacteria one can begin to understand the origins of pathogenicity.

Techniques used in the study of genetic relatedness include primary protein or nucleic acid sequence comparisons and DNA hybridization methods. Some genetic sequences, such as those of the small and large subunit ribosomal RNAs, have been used as reliable evolutionary clocks.[4] Comparative analysis of these sequences allows one to infer phylogenetic relationships among all known cellular life. Multilocus enzyme electrophoresis is a method by which chromosomal structure or genotype is deduced from the electrophoretic mobility variations in a number of common metabolic enzymes.[5] The grouping of strains according to electrophoretic type assumes the absence of selective pressure favoring any particular electrophoretic enzyme variant. On the other hand, it avoids comparisons of phenotypes (i.e., gross observable characteristics of a microbe, which can be unreliable). When these techniques are employed, a consistent finding emerges concerning the population structure of microorganisms.

Most natural populations of microorganisms consist of a number of discrete clonal lineages with preserved genotypes.[6] This finding implies that the rates of recombination of chromosomal genes between different strains of the same species and between different bacterial species are very low. Clonal organization has been substantiated by the concordance between evolutionary trees derived from unrelated chromosomal sequences. At first view, this may seem somewhat unexpected, since there exist well-established naturally occurring mechanisms for horizontal genetic exchange between and within species, including transformation, transduction, and conjugation. But bacteria are haploid creatures. If horizontal transfer of genetic material and subsequent recombination were frequent occurrences, one would expect to see homogenization of bacterial species and little specialization. In fact, the opposite is true. Bacterial species have remained discrete and distinct taxonomic entities.[7] This is because the bacterial chromosome is a highly integrated and coadapted entity that has resisted rearrangement.

Analysis of natural populations of *Escherichia coli*[6,8] as well as other species with pathogenic potential, including *Salmonella* spp.,[9] *Borrelia burgdorferi, Bordetella pertussis, H. influenzae, Legionella* spp., and *Streptococcus* spp.,[10] has revealed the prominent representation of a relatively few clones. In fact, most cases of serious disease may be caused by a small proportion of the total number of extant clones that constitute a patho-

TABLE 1. Proportion of Certain Infectious Diseases Caused by Common Bacterial Clonal Types

Species	Total Number of Clonal Types Identified	Number of Clonal Types Commonly Isolated from Cases of Disease	Percentage of Disease Due to Common Clonal Types
B. bronchiseptica	21	3	87
B. parapertussis	1	1	100
B. pertussis	2	2	100
H. influenzae type b			
North America	104	6	81
Europe	60	3	78
L. pneumophila			
Global	50	5	52
Wadsworth VA Hospital	10	1	86
S. sonnei	1	1	100

(Modified from Selander et al.,[11] with permission.)

genic bacterial species (Table 1). For example, from 182 distinct *H. influenzae* type b clones identified in natural populations worldwide, 9 account for approximately 80 percent of all invasive disease. Conversely, one *H. influenzae* clone, rarely associated with invasive disease, is frequently carried in the upper respiratory tract without associated symptoms.[12] The differences between pathogenic and nonpathogenic clones of the same species should provide considerable insight into the virulence mechanisms of these microorganisms. It has been noted that, in many instances, the proper unit of study in bacterial pathogenicity is not a phenotypic trait such as biotype or serotype but rather the clone. Phenotypic traits do not correlate directly with genotype and do not distinguish one clonal lineage from another. Indeed, in some extreme cases all members of a species such as *Shigella sonnei* or *B. pertussis* belong to the same electrophoretic type or small group of closely related types. Although it is true of most that have been studied, not all pathogenic bacterial species reveal this pattern of clonal organization. Two notable exceptions are *N. gonorrhoeae* and *P. aeruginosa,* which appear to use chromosomal recombination to increase their genetic diversity. The genetic variability among gonococcal isolates from discrete geographical locations suggests that this organism is essentially sexual. *Neisseria meningitidis* also demonstrates random chromosomal rearrangement; however, since single clones disseminate rapidly during an epidemic, the population structure of this species may falsely appear to be clonal.[13] In addition, while the population structure of most *Salmonella* serovars is clonal, there is evidence indicating that some diversity seen among members of other serovars can be best explained by horizontal genetic transmission.[9] *Salmonella* population analysis also suggests that serovars that are most adapted to a specific host species are less genetically diverse than are those that infect a wider range of hosts.

Clonal analysis using multilocus enzyme electrophoresis has generated other important conclusions concerning the evolution of bacterial species and pathogenic strains in particular. The study of *E. coli* populations in the human intestinal tract indicates that only a small number of clonal lineages persist while numerous unrelated cell lines appear and disappear.[6] The nonrandom association of particular versions of different genes within a distinct clone has led to speculation that this species has evolved, not by means of accumulated random recombinational events, but by "random sampling" of clonal populations from the environment with periodic selection and extinction. *Escherichia coli* urinary tract pathogens causing symptomatic disease in humans are even less genetically diverse than are *E. coli* strains found in the intestinal flora or those that cause asymptomatic urinary tract colonization.[6]

PLASMIDS, PHAGES, INSERTION ELEMENTS, AND PATHOGENICITY

The study of natural populations of bacteria suggests that the genetic potential for pathogenicity within a bacterial species has arisen among a small number of unrelated clones. It has arisen through means that do not compromise the genetic individuality of the organism or its unique place in nature but nonetheless in a fashion that provides the microbe with genetic and biochemical flexibility for a competitive environment. How might this have happened? Although periodic selection of mutant clones may play some role in the evolution of pathogenesis, it does not explain many of the differences seen between pathogenic and nonpathogenic clones of the same species.

A number of separate observations indicate that microbes frequently carry virulence-associated genes on mobile genetic elements.[1] Bacteriophages and extrachromosomal elements such as bacterial plasmids are supplements to the bacterial genome that allow a microbe to maintain the integrity of its chromosome and still increase its genetic diversity. Some of these mobile elements are able to enter a wide variety of host organisms and may facilitate the transfer of genes that have been selected for their ability to function in diverse genetic backgrounds.[14] Clinicians are painfully aware that genes encoding antibiotic resistance are efficiently disseminated among different microbial species in nature by such means. The presence of virulence factors in pathogenic bacteria is also associated with the presence of plasmids,[15,16] transposons, and bacteriophages to a striking degree, both in gram-positive and gram-negative species (Table 2).

Comparisons of pathogenic and nonpathogenic representatives of a single genus or species usually demonstrate the nonpathogens to be totally devoid of genetic sequences encoding the pathogenic trait(s). Inactive mutational variants or portions of virulence-associated genes infrequently occur in nonpathogenic strains of the same species. Not uncommonly, virulence-specific sequences are bounded by repeated DNA segments, some of which represent known insertion elements. This suggests that these virulence genes were once associated with a mobile genetic element or that these genes formerly occupied another chromosomal locale in either the same species or another microorganism all together. Thus, it often seems that microbes gain pathogenic potential through the inheritance of unique genetic information. Acquisition of an adhesin, toxin, or serum-resistance factor might lead a previously nonpathogenic organism to cause disease in a host that had previously been nonsusceptible. Some bacteria readily exchange random fragments of their chromosome with other members of their species through a process known as *transformation*. For some of these species, such as *N. gonorrhoeae*, tranformation in nature may provide an additional means of acquiring genes that are advantageous to their growth in the host.

Plasmids, transposons, and phages provide bacteria with the potential for relatively rapid adaptation to an unfavorable, changing, or new environment. Although these mobile genetic elements are often dispensable to the host bacterium, they are typically conserved over substantial periods of time within diverse cell lineages.[18] This is hardly surprising if the mobile element enables the organism to multiply successfully in a host. Often the mobile element carries multiple virulence-associated genes as a coadapted block. When such gene blocks are accompanied by a separate self-regulatory system that is responsive to a changing microbial environment, they influence the pathogenic potential even more.

THE REGULATION OF BACTERIAL PATHOGENICITY

All bacteria respond to environmental changes with metabolic alterations. A successful host–parasite relationship demands that a pathogen be capable of sensing its local host environment; it must distinguish between conditions favorable to rapid growth and those that are threatening and require a protective response. Consequently, regulating the expression of virulence factors is an additional, yet essential complication of a pathogenic microbe's life. When it first encounters a host, a pathogen must adapt dramatically to its changed environment. A study of the environmental regulation of microbes should recognize biases that arise from the peculiarities of laboratory culture conditions. These conditions may be inappropriate or irrelevant to the natural environments encountered by a microorganism. Given these limitations, some studies indicate that bacteria may be found in a "viable but nonculturable state" in their natural external environment.[19] *Vibrio cholerae*, for example, is thought to persist in this state in brackish estuaries and other saline aquatic environments, sometimes associated with the chitinous exoskeleton of various marine organisms.[20–22] Transition from this milieu to the contrasting environment of the human small intestinal lumen must be accompanied by substantial genetic regulatory events.

Less dramatic changes in the surrounding environment affect the expression of the determinants of virulence. Some pathogens (e.g., *B. pertussis*, *V. cholerae*, *E. coli*, *Shigella* spp., and *Yersinia* spp.) regulate their virulence determinants in response to changes in temperature, ionic conditions, oxygen concentra-

TABLE 2. Examples of Plasmid and Phage-Encoded Virulence Determinants

Organism	Virulence Factor	Biologic Function
Plasmid-encoded		
Enterotoxigenic *E. coli*	Heat-labile, heat-stable enterotoxins (LT, ST)	Activation of adenyl/guanylcyclase in the small bowel, which leads to diarrhea
	CFA/I and CFA/II	Adherence/colonization factors
Extraintestinal *E. coli*	Hemolysin	Cytotoxin
Shigella spp. and enteroinvasive *E. coli*	Gene products involved in invasion	Induces internalization by intestinal epithelial cells
Yersinia spp.	Adherence factors and gene products involved in invasion	Attachment/Invasion
B. anthracis	Edema factor, lethal factor, and protective antigen	Edema factor has adenylcyclase activity
S. aureus	Exfoliative toxin	Causes toxic epidermal necrolysis
C. tetani	Tetanus neurotoxin	Blocks the release of inhibitory neurotransmitter, which leads to muscle spasms
Phage-encoded		
C. diphtheriae	Diphtheria toxin	Inhibition of eukaryotic protein synthesis
S. pyogenes	Erythrogenic toxin	Rash of scarlet fever
C. botulinum	Neurotoxin	Blocks synaptic acetylcholine release, which leads to flaccid paralysis
Enterohemorrhagic *E. coli*	Shiga-like toxin	Inhibition of eukaryotic protein synthesis

(Data from Elwell et al.,[15] and Falkow et al.[17])

tion, pH, and calcium, iron, and other metal concentrations.[23] The environmental regulatory signals that prepare the microbe for its transition from an extra- to an intracellular state may include some of these parameters. Other microbial pathogens (e.g., *N. gonorrhoeae*, *Borrelia recurrentis*, and *Trypanosoma brucei*) periodically vary prominent antigenic components of their surface and, by so doing, may avoid the host immune response.

The number of well-characterized virulence regulatory systems is rapidly increasing. At the same time relatively little is known about both the specific environmental signals to which these systems respond and the rationale for these responses in the human host. The examples of regulation of bacterial virulence factors that are provided below illustrate two common themes for the response of prokaryotes to their environmental stimuli. First, the mechanism for transducing environmental signals typically involves a two-component regulatory system that acts on gene expression, usually at the transcriptional level.[24,25] Such systems make use of similar pairs of proteins; one protein of the pair spans the cytoplasmic membrane, contains a transmitter domain, and may act as a sensor of environmental stimuli, whereas the other is a cytoplasmic protein ("response regulator") with a receiver domain and regulates responsive genes or proteins. Sensor proteins are often kinases that phosphorylate themselves at a conserved histidine residue. These high-energy intermediates then transfer their phosphate groups to a conserved aspartate residue within the receiver domain of the response regulator proteins. Competing dephosphorylases determine an overall phosphorylation state of these response regulators and hence their level of activity. Many of these regulators are DNA-binding proteins that regulate transcription of multiple gene targets. Systems of this type control, for example, the permeability properties of the *E. coli* cell envelope in response to osmotic stimuli (EnvZ/OmpR), motor control involved in *E. coli* chemotaxis (CheA/CheY, CheB), the switch from vegetative growth to sporulation by *Bacillus subtilis* (KinA/SpoOF, SpoOA), and even the ability of the soil bacterium *Agrobacterium tumefaciens* to induce tumors in susceptible plant cells in response to phenols found within plant wound exudates (VirA/VirG). *V. cholerae* ToxR and the Bvg proteins of *B. pertussis* share several features common to these systems, but they also retain significant differences (discussed below).

The coordinated control of pathogenicity illustrates a second common feature of bacterial regulation, that is, the *regulon*. A regulon is a group of operons controlled by a common regulator, usually a protein activator or repressor. This regulator may, in some cases, also be a receiver protein in a two-component system as described above. A regulon provides a means by which many genes can respond in concert to a particular stimulus. At other times the same genes may respond independently to other signals. The concept of a regulon is integral to the study of bacterial physiology. However, only recently has it been appreciated that microbial virulence determinants can be under the control of such a global regulatory network (Table 3). The apparent complexity of virulence regulation in a single microbial

pathogen is magnified by the coexistence of multiple interacting ("cross-talking") two-component systems and by regulons within regulons.

Bordetella pertussis synthesizes a group of surface-associated or extracellular products that are responsible for the pathologic and clinical findings of pertussis. These products include pertussis toxin (Ptx), filamentous hemagglutinin (Fha), adenylate cyclase (Cya), dermonecrotic toxin (Dnt), fimbrial protein (Fim), and pertactin. Coordinate expression of these and other virulence factors is orchestrated by the two encoded products of the chromosomal *bvgAS* locus (formerly *vir*).[27,28] Trans-activation and trans-repression are features of the Bvg regulon in which at least 20 unlinked chromosomal *vir*-activated genes are expressed, and a group of other *vir*-repressed genes silenced, or vice versa, depending on the nature of the immediate environment (Fig. 1).

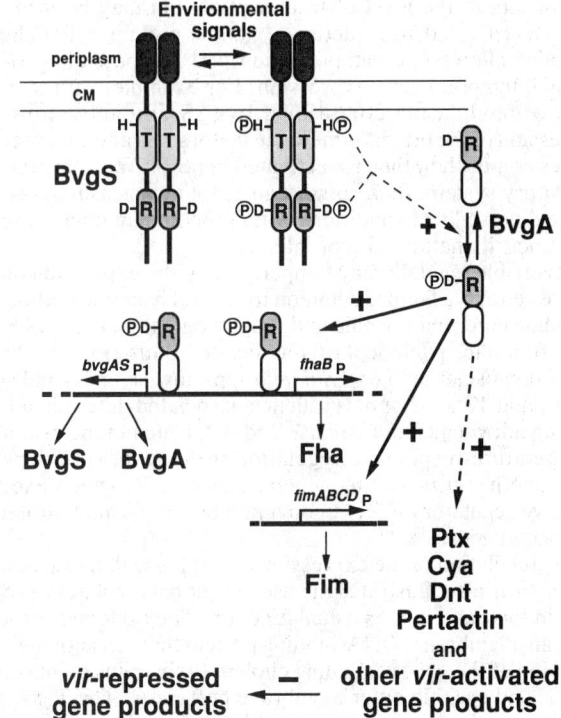

FIG. 1. Schematic model of the *B. pertussis* Bvg (*vir*) regulatory system, by which a variety of virulence-associated genes are either coordinately expressed or repressed in response to specific environmental signals (see text). This type of "two-component" regulatory system is found in a number of other microbial pathogens. CM, bacterial cytoplasmic membrane; T, transmitter protein domain; R, receiver protein domain; H, histidine; D, aspartic acid; P, phosphorylated residue; P subscript, transcriptional promoter; + and − indicate positive and negative regulatory signals, respectively; Ptx, pertussis toxin; Cya, adenylate cyclase; Dnt, dermonecrotic toxin; Fha, filamentous hemagglutinin; Fim, fimbrial protein.

TABLE 3. Examples of Bacterial Virulence Regulatory Systems

Organism	Regulatory Gene(s)	Environmental Stimuli	Regulated Functions
E. coli	drdX	Temperature	Pyelonephritis-associated pili
	fur	Iron concentration	Shiga-like toxin, siderophores
B. pertussis	bvgAS	Temperature, ionic conditions, nicotinic acid	Pertussis toxin, filamentous hemagglutinin, adenylate cyclase, others
V. cholerae	toxR	Temperature, osmolarity, pH, amino acids	Cholera toxin, pili, outer membrane proteins
Yersinia spp.	lcr loci	Temperature, calcium	Outer membrane proteins
	virF	Temperature	Adherence, invasiveness
Shigella spp.	virR	Temperature	Invasiveness
S. typhimurium	pag genes	pH	Virulence, macrophage survival
S. aureus	agr	pH	α-, β-hemolysins; toxic shock syndrome toxin 1, protein A

(Data from Miller et al.[26] and Mekalanos et al.[23])

BvgS is a member of the histidine kinase sensor class of bacterial regulatory proteins, but, unlike most other members of this class, it also contains a receiver communication module and a regulatory carboxy-terminal domain (Fig. 1). BvgS spans the cytoplasmic membrane and may exist as a multimer.[29] A periplasmic domain responds to temperature and ionic conditions, modulating BvgS activity. At 37°C, BvgS autophosphorylates its transmitter and receiver domains and subsequently donates a phosphate group to the receiver domain of BvgA, a member of the class of bacterial protein response regulators.[30] BvgA then binds to a DNA recognition sequence located upstream of both the *bvgAS* operon and the Fha structural gene and promotes transcription of these genes.[31] There is also a potential BvgA DNA recognition sequence upstream of a fimbrial gene cluster. Although BvgS and BvgA are also required for expression of the other *vir*-activated genes, the factor(s) that participate directly in the transcriptional activation of the latter have not yet been clearly identified. *vir*-Gene repression probably also occurs at the level of transcription and may be mediated by a *vir*-activated *trans*-acting regulator protein.[32] Regulatory cascades allow signal amplification and the possibility of sequential temporal gene expression. For example, with removal of downmodulating conditions, bvgAS autoactivation and expression of the crucial adherence factors Fha and Fim precede expression of the other *vir*-activated genes.[33] With this type of regulatory system, *B. pertussis* can adapt in a measured fashion to the diverse local conditions within the human upper respiratory tract, its natural site of infection.

Reversible regulation by temperature of the expression of virulence genes is a feature common to several bacterial pathogens, including enteropathogenic and uropathogenic *E. coli* (K-88 and K-99 fimbriae, pyelonephritis-associated pilus (Pap) fimbriae, and K-1 capsular antigen), *Shigella* spp. (invasiveness and shiga toxin), and *Yersinia* spp. (virulence-associated determinants including a low calcium response and outer membrane proteins). Temperature-responsive regulation in *Shigella* spp. depends upon another *trans*-acting genetic locus, *vir*R, which exerts a negative regulatory effect upon a number of plasmid virulence-associated genes.[34]

The regulation of the expression of virulence determinants by *V. cholerae* also illustrates the use of a global regulatory protein that, in this case, serves a dual function. The *tox*R gene product is a transmembrane, DNA-binding protein that can activate transcription of the genes encoding cholera toxin, pilus colonization factor, and specific outer membrane proteins.[35] The ToxR protein is also thought to sense a variety of other environmental regulatory signals, including osmolarity, amino acid concentration, temperature, and pH.[36] ToxR directs expression of these genes indirectly by activating transcription of ToxT, a member of the AraC family of trancriptional regulators.[37] At the level of amino acid sequence as well, the ToxR protein contains features of both sensor and regulator proteins from the two-component sensory transduction system. The combination of these features into one protein may lead to an increased specificity of action.

Antigenic variations in *S. typhimurium* and *N. gonorrhoeae* provide examples of alternative molecular mechanisms (i.e., DNA rearrangements) that mediate the regulation of the expression of virulence factors. *Salmonella typhimurium* varies an immunodominant antigen by alternating between the expression of two different flagellin genes, H1 and H2. The mechanism for this form of variation has been well characterized: Inversion of a 995 basepair (bp) chromosomal DNA sequence orients a promoter such that transcription of the H2 flagellin gene occurs together with that of a gene encoding a *trans*-acting repressor of the H1 gene.[38] The opposite orientation allows relief of H1 gene repression and prevents transcription of H2. Inversion is catalyzed by the *hin* gene product. It promotes site-specific recombination between the 14 bp inverted repeats that flank the invertible segment. In this manner, *S. typhimurium* avoids the host antibody response directed against it.

Pili are essential for virulence of the gonococcus in the human host, probably as a result of their role in adherence to the mucosal target surface.[39] They also elicit a specific local and systemic host antibody response.[40] Intermittent production of pili, as well as variation in the antigenic type of pilus, may be strategies used by the gonococcus to avoid the host immune response. The molecular mechanisms behind these strategies are complex. In general terms, phase and antigenic variation results from DNA rearrangements that move pilin-related sequences scattered around the gonococcal chromosome (in silent *pil*S loci) to the expression site (*pil*E locus).[41] Numerous different pilus types may be expressed by derivatives of a single *N. gonorrhoeae* strain. Gene conversion and other recombination mechanisms may be involved. Among other microbial pathogens DNA rearrangements account for the antigenic variation of variant surface glycoproteins of *T. brucei*[42] and the antigenic variation of variable major proteins in *Borrelia* spp.[43] A DNA rearrangement is also associated with the expression of type I pili in *E. coli*.

Proper presentation of certain virulence-associated gene products on the microbial surface is now recognized to be as important to pathogenicity as the initial expression of these genes. Presentation entails export pathways, association with other periplasmic or surface factors, and sometimes macromolecular assembly at the surface, and is also subject to regulation. Among bacterial pathogens, shared homology is apparent among families of proteins involved in these processes. One family of export and surface localization proteins that share homology is represented by *Shigella flexneri* Mxi/Spa and *Yersinia enterocolitica* Ysc proteins.[44] These proteins control localization of Ipa and Yop virulence factors, respectively. Another family consists of proteins that are known as *chaperones* and *ushers*, concepts first proposed in a model for the assembly of uroepithelium-adherent *E. coli* P pili.[45] Periplasmic chaperones, such as PapD, escort protein subunits from the cytoplasmic to outer membrane and assist in their proper folding. Outer membrane ushers, such as PapC, target these complexes to a surface assembly site. Folding, transport, and assembly enable a microorganism to present a specific array of surface molecules necessary for eukaryotic cell tropism, intoxication, or entry.[46] A precise configuration of microbial surface molecules might be viewed as an "attack complex," with properties not found in any of the individual components.

MICROBIAL PATHOGENS AS INTRACELLULAR PARASITES

Despite their capacity for an extracellular existence, a wide variety of bacterial and protozoal pathogens have evolved the means to enter, survive, and multiply within host eukaryotic cells. The advantages to the microorganism include avoidance of the host immune defenses and access to a variety of restricted nutrients.[47] These advantages impose a strong selective evolutionary pressure that is dramatically reflected in the refined strategies developed by microbial pathogens for life within a host cell. These strategies include molecular mimicry, coercion, and intimate adaption to eukaryotic cellular processes. Collaborative efforts of molecular microbiologists and cell biologists have begun to reveal some of the details of these strategies. Some common themes are described below.

To a large degree, the mechanisms used by a microorganism to adhere to a eukaryotic cell dictate whether and how it enters the cell and its subsequent intracellular fate. Most if not all intracellular pathogens have multiple means for attachment to a eukaryotic cell surface; the particular combination of microbial attachment factors and cognate host receptors selects one of several entry pathways and predetermines basic features of the intracellular vacuole. However, in a general sense, it is unclear to what extent microbial pathogens accept preprogrammed pathways dictated by phagocytic (e.g., complement and Fc receptors) and nonphagocytic receptors and to what extent they may be able to modify these pathways. *Toxoplasma gondii* invades and replicates within all types of nucleated mammalian cells. After entry, through unidentified receptors, *T. gondii* resides within a parasitophorous vacuole that is permanently incapable of fusion with other intracellular organelles, including lysosomes. Parasite survival within this vacuole depends on the accompanying lack of acidification, exclusion of lysosomal contents, and specific mechanisms for nutrient acquisition and environmental sensing.[48] However, when this organism is directed to enter eukaryotic cells by means of an alternative pathway (i.e., mediated by receptors for the constant region of immunoglobulin G, Fc) this vacuole fusion block is overcome.[49] Presumably, parasite-directed modifications of the surrounding vacuolar membrane and exclusion of certain host proteins during the earliest stages of entry help to create conditions necessary for growth and development of the pathogen.

Some pathogenic microorganisms seem to regulate when and where they enter host cells by utilizing preexistent host signaling pathways.[50] Enteropathogenic Yersinae bind to phagocytic and nonphagocytic cells by expressing invasin, YadA, and other adhesins, but these organisms select only certain types of host cells for entry. Bacterial internalization may result from a particularly high affinity interaction between invasin and multiple eukaryotic β1 integrin receptors,[51] whose more common functions include recognition of extracellular matrix proteins. Integrin ligation and clustering initiate an elaborate cascade of transmembrane signals, mediated in part by tyrosine phosphorylation. Subsequent cytoskeletal rearrangements are essential to the process by which *Yersinia* and many other intracellular pathogens enter and interact with host cells. It therefore would seem hardly accidental that *Yersinia* secrete a variety of environmentally regulated outer membrane proteins that can modify critical host cell processes and inactivate those host constitutive entry pathways that might lead to bacterial death.[52] Of these, YopH, for example, is a potent protein tyrosine phosphatase,[53] virulence factor, and antiphagocytic factor.

Microbial pathogens that have adapted to an intracellular environment possess diverse and specific strategies for survival and replication. Some pathogens remain within a vacuole (e.g., *Toxoplasma, Salmonella*) and some lyse the initial phagosomal membrane and replicate within the host cell cytoplasm *(Shigella, Listeria, Trypanosoma,* some *Rickettsia)*. Maintenance of specific and favorable vacuolar conditions may entail inhibition of phagolysosomal fusion and acidification *(Toxoplasma)*, association of eukaryotic organelles with bacteria-containing vacuoles *(Legionella, Salmonella)*, and regulation of pH *(Salmonella)*. Some of the details of the molecular mechanisms behind these phenomena are now available. For example, a single *Legionella pneumophila* gene appears to play a role in inhibition of phagolysosomal fusion as well as recruitment of vesicles, mitochondria, and ribosomes to the bacterial phagosome.[54] Furthermore, *S. typhimurium* delays and attenuates macrophage phagosomal acidification, during which various regulons (e.g., the PhoP/PhoQ two-component system) mediate bacterial adaptation to a radically changing environment.[55] Some of these regulated *Salmonella* gene products, such as the PhoP-activated PagC, are essential for survival within macrophages and recognize pH as a transcriptional signal.

Early escape from the vacuole is essential for growth and virulence of some intracellular pathogens. *Listeria monocytogenes* relies on several molecules for lysis of the early phagosome, including a pore-forming hemolysin (listeriolysin O) and two forms of phospholipase C.[56] Once in the cytoplasm, *Listeria* replicates and induces its own movement through a remarkable process of host cell actin polymerization and formation of microfilaments within a comet-like tail. *Shigella* also lyses the phagosomal vacuole and induces formation of similar structures for the purpose of intracytoplasmic movement and cell–cell spread. In both cases, bacterial factors involved in actin polymerization

have been identified.[57,58] In the same way that microbial pathogens fare differently in their interactions with phagocytic cells, the outcome of intracellular parasitism for the host cell also varies considerably, depending on the specific host cell and pathogen involved. In an interesting twist of fate, *Shigella flexneri* has been found to induce apoptosis, or programmed cell death, in cultured macrophage cell lines, an observation that is consistent with the colonic histopathology of the natural disease.[59]

THE IDENTIFICATION AND CHARACTERIZATION OF VIRULENCE GENES

The characterization of microbial pathogenicity at the molecular level begins with the identification of a virulence-associated phenotype. This may come from clinical observation, epidemiologic investigation, or the use of a model system that reliably reproduces the microbial phenotype in a manner similar to that seen in the natural infection. Traditionally, a virulent strain was compared with a naturally occurring avirulent variant. Such variants, however, may have complex genotypic alterations involving multiple genetic loci. The comparison of strains of naturally occurring virulent and nonvirulent organisms may be even more confounding since we now understand that they may represent entirely different clones.

Analysis using mutant strains of identical genetic background is a more desirable approach to the definition of virulence phenotypes. The goal is to define a single, well-defined genetic lesion that alters a recognizable phenotype and then test the effect of this alteration on the pathogenicity or virulence of the organism in an appropriate model system. The use of insertional elements (e.g., antibiotic-resistant transposons) as mutational agents is an attractive means of accomplishing this aim. Transposons are pieces of DNA that are able to translocate from one genomic site to another. Insertion into a gene usually disrupts its function. Transposons have the advantage of marking the mutagenized genetic locus with a new selectable phenotype, typically antibiotic resistance. The development of broad host range plasmid vectors carrying well-defined transposons has extended this method of analysis to a number of pathogenic species for which a method of genetic manipulation was not previously available.[60] Consequently, the comparison of organisms with identical genetic backgrounds, differing only in a single, defined mutation, is employed widely to identify putative virulence genes. Once identified, more precise characterization of such genes and the identification of the gene products usually follow.

Molecular cloning has been the method preferred by many investigators in recent years to isolate specific virulence genes and to modify them in a precise way.[61] A description of the methodologies available for the isolation and characterization of virulence genes is outside the scope of this discussion; however, it may be useful to point out several basic approaches.

Single genes are usually isolated by screening a "library" of overlapping pieces of a fragmented microbial genome that have been inserted into an appropriate plasmid or bacteriophage vector, which is then introduced into a carrier microorganism, typically *E. coli* K-12. In some instances only a few hundred carrier organisms bearing such recombinant molecules need to be examined to screen effectively an entire, average-sized bacterial genome.[62] Typical strategies for screening a genomic library may or may not depend on expression of the cloned gene of interest by the carrier organisms.

Genes encoding putative virulence determinants may not express their gene products in the *E. coli* carrier strain, either because the product is lethal to the cell or because the appropriate mechanisms for transcription or translation are not available. Screening techniques based on hybridization with DNA probes avoid the need for expression of the cloned gene, although not the possible lethal effects of expression. These probes may derive from previously isolated genes known to be homologous to the gene of interest,[63] from an oligonucleotide corresponding to the amino-terminal amino acid sequence of the gene product[64] or from DNA flanking an insertion element that has been used to mutagenize the gene in the original host.[60] In the case of the last method, DNA flanking a transposon-marked gene can be easily isolated by screening an initial genomic library for a clone with the appropriate antibiotic resistance phenotype.[65]

Screening recombinant clones for the presence of a cloned gene whose product is stable and expressed at adequate levels is often accomplished by using labeled antibodies directed against the gene product. Although transcription and translation of the cloned gene and stability of the gene product may be enhanced by special expression vectors,[66] appropriate antibodies are not always available. It some cases a recombinant host expressing the cloned gene will display a corresponding phenotype that can be exploited for screening purposes: Expression of the cloned *inv* locus from *Yersinia pseudotuberculosis* confers on the *E. coli* host an ability to invade certain types of cultured eukaryotic cells in vitro.[67] The carrier organisms bearing the recombinant clones, once intracellular, are uniquely resistant to the killing effect of gentamicin, which acts only on extracellular bacteria.

A number of powerful methods have been developed for the identification of virulence-associated genes based on the recognition that these genetic loci are regulated by the transitions between external and internal host and cellular environments. For example, one can select for mutations that cause a defect in the intracellular growth of certain bacterial pathogens, by studying auxotrophic strains that die upon replication in conditions that mimic those found within the host cell. One then imposes a requirement upon a pool of mutagenized auxotrophs that they survive serial passage within host cells under these limiting conditions. This type of method has revealed a *Legionella* gene that is necessary for intracellular growth.[54] In addition, one can select for genes and promoters that are preferentially expressed by a microbial pathogen within a host cell or within a host organ by cloning them in specially designed vectors such that when these genes are expressed they complement a preselected growth-attenuating defect in the pathogen. Initial results suggest that some genes identified with this strategy may be required for virulence.[68]

Subtractive hybridization techniques permit detection of subtle differences between two populations of DNA or RNA. A recent modification of these techniques incorporates the polymerase chain reaction to enrich for molecules present in one population and not in the other.[69] The result is a method known as *representational difference analysis* that may be suited for identifying only those genes that are expressed by a microbial pathogen in selected environments.

To isolate the cloned gene on a DNA fragment of minimal size the boundaries of the gene must be mapped on the initial recombinant vector insert. Transposon mutagenesis may be used for this purpose. The smallest restriction endonuclease fragment that carries the virulence-associated gene is then subcloned. Further characterization at this point includes introducing specific mutations in the gene and defining their effect on a function of its protein product. Site-directed mutagenesis,[70] rapid DNA sequencing,[71] and in vitro coupled transcription–translation of plasmid-encoded proteins[72,73] are techniques that facilitate such analyses. Final proof, however, that the cloned and characterized gene is associated with pathogenicity requires its return to the strain of origin and that certain criteria be met.

ASSOCIATION OF GENES WITH VIRULENCE: PROOF BY A MOLECULAR FORM OF KOCH'S POSTULATES

Technical advances have brought about a proliferation of reports describing the cloning and sequencing of genes thought to be involved in microbial pathogenicity. At the same time these advances have dramatized the need for defined criteria by which genes may be assigned a role in pathogenesis. In a manner analogous to Koch's original postulates, these criteria must include the return of the putative causal agent (the cloned virulence-associated gene mutated or intact) to the host of origin. Unless one can demonstrate an effect on pathogenicity by this kind of controlled genetic manipulation, causality with respect to virulence has not been proved. Just as the original Henle-Koch postulates have provided a reference point for later revised criteria of microbial causality,[74] the criteria outlined below best serve as guidelines, in this case, for an experimental approach to the molecular genetic basis of pathogenicity.

A molecular form of Koch's postulates[75] can be stated as follows: *(1)* The phenotype or property under investigation should be associated significantly more often with pathogenic members of a genus or pathogenic strains of a species than with nonpathogenic members or strains. *(2)* Specific inactivation of the gene or genes associated with the suspected virulence trait should lead to a measurable decrease in virulence. If inactivation of the gene has taken place in a cloned copy carried by a recombinant host, then this mutated gene must be exchanged for the wild-type copy of the gene in the host of origin; the latter must suffer a loss of virulence following the exchange. *(3)* Restoration of full pathogenicity should accompany replacement of the mutated version of the gene with the wild-type version in the strain of origin.

Technical limitations often face the investigator who wishes to apply these postulates to an organism poorly characterized from a genetic standpoint. The ability to exchange alleles in the organism under investigation is crucial because it allows a virulence-associated gene to be studied in an isogenic background. Until 1986 this was an impossible task with the respiratory tract pathogen *B. pertussis*. Although the complementation of chromosomal mutations was possible by using recombinant multiple-copy plasmids, there was no easy means of replacing a chromosomal gene with a cloned copy, thereby avoiding a multiple gene dose effect. The construction of a suicide vector, pRTP1,[76] provided a solution to this problem and illustrates some of the principles by which this kind of problem can be approached in other organisms.

Homologous recombination is the process by which a segment of DNA replaces an equivalent segment elsewhere that has identical or nearly identical nucleotide sequences. Enzymes that catalyze DNA repair and synthesis mediate this process. Cloned genes, carried into the strain of origin on plasmid vectors, are exchanged for the analogous chromosomal version of the same genes by means of homologous recombination. A suicide plasmid cloning vector can be used for this purpose. Such vectors carry DNA sequences responsible for transfer of the plasmid to a broad range of hosts so that the plasmid can be mated, by conjugation, into a variety of gram-negative organisms. A suicide plasmid also carries *E. coli* DNA sequences that allow it to replicate in this gram-negative organism but not many others. pRTP1 is such a plasmid vector that can be transferred to *B. pertussis* but cannot replicate there. When conjugation is performed in the presence of an antibiotic that selects for the presence of the suicide plasmid, the plasmid becomes recombined into the recipient organism's chromosome because of the homology with the cloned gene copy in the plasmid. Subsequent antibiotic selection against the presence of the suicide plasmid causes a second recombinational event to occur that results in excision of the plasmid and replacement of the original *B. pertussis* chromosomal gene copy with that carried by the plasmid. In this way, chromosomal virulence genes can be modified in a directed fashion.

Another difficulty in the application of a molecular form of Koch's postulates is similar to a problem that faced Koch in his own day: finding an appropriate animal model system. This is a problem that limits the study of microbial pathogenesis as much as any other. It does little good to return a carefully constructed virulence gene mutation to the original strain if there is no way to evaluate its effect on a particular virulence phenotype. A model must duplicate relevant pathology commonly observed in the normal host. The animal host must become consistently infected by using a natural route. Clearly, a model of this sort does not exist for many pathogens. At the same time, it should be remembered that exposure to a known human pathogen does not uniformly lead to disease in all humans.

The postulates just outlined are meant to provide principles by which one may study the genes and gene products associated with microbial pathogenesis. This kind of approach can also be used to analyze the internal structure of these genes and the corresponding functional domains of the encoded proteins.

UNDERSTANDING VIRULENCE: CLINICAL CORRELATIONS AND APPLICATIONS

Do these concepts of microbial pathogenicity have a practical impact on the practice of clinical infectious diseases? It is already apparent that studies of microbial pathogenicity at the molecular level have made substantial contributions to our understanding of the epidemiology, clinical manifestations, diagnosis, and immunoprophylaxis of infectious diseases.

Infectious disease epidemiology hinges on clear definition of the clinical problem under study and, moreover, precise identification of the etiologic agent. Molecular techniques, including multilocus enzyme electrophoresis and diagnostic DNA probe hybridization, provide for both sensitive and specific detection of putative pathogens and a means for establishing relationships among multiple isolates of the same species. As a result, seemingly unrelated cases occurring during an outbreak have been connected; similarly, geographically or temporally distinct outbreaks have been linked to the same pathogenic clone. Molecular techniques have been employed in other epidemiologic investigations to study transmission mechanisms and the role of avirulent microbial variants in the spread of disease.

Multilocus enzyme electrophoresis has been used in epidemiologic investigations to define clonal relationships among pathogens in numerous outbreaks. These include *E. coli* O157:H7 strains associated with hemorrhagic colitis and hemolytic uremic syndrome,[77] *Streptococcus pyogenes* strains causing toxic shock-like syndrome,[78] and *Bordetella* spp. isolated from diverse hosts at different times and locations[79]; all demonstrate the prevalence of a relatively few distinct clonal lineages. Other molecular techniques commonly used in infectious disease epidemiology include plasmid analysis and restriction endonuclease genomic fingerprinting.[80] Investigations into the spread of chloramphenicol-resistant *Salmonella newport* in the food chain[81] and an outbreak of *Legionella* spp. prosthetic valve endocarditis[82] illustrate the usefulness of these methods.

One of the most exciting and profound technical advances in the past decade has been the development of nucleic acid amplification techniques and their application to the study of microbial pathogenesis. The polymerase chain reaction (PCR), originally described by Mullis et al.[83] is currently the most widely used of these techniques.[84,85] When using this technique it is possible to detect the presence of a single target DNA or RNA sequence in a sample of 10^5 cells. This degree of sensitivity is far greater than that achieved by Southern hybridization with a specific DNA probe. Specific PCR assays and DNA probes are now available for a long and rapidly growing list of microbial pathogens.[86,87] The more informative of these assays target microbial genetic sequences that encode specific virulence determinants or antimicrobial resistance factors. Probes linked to nonradioactive detection systems are readily applied to field investigations and are widely used in laboratory diagnosis, both with cultivated microbial pathogens and directly with clinical samples. On the other hand, the extraordinary sensitivity of the PCR and potential problems with cross-contamination have thus far restricted its use to reference and research laboratories. Other nucleic acid and probe amplification methods include self-sustaining sequence replication (3SR), strand displacement amplification (SDA), ligase chain reaction (LCR), and Qβ replicase-based probe amplification.[87]

Southern hybridization-DNA probe technology has had widespread application to infectious disease outbreak investigations and field surveillance. One of the first applications of the former technique was the detection of enterotoxigenic *E. coli* by colony hybridization with a probe for the LT gene.[88] With specific DNA probes *Yersinia pestis* can be detected in situ in its normal host vector, the rat flea.[89] In addition, DNA probes have been used for strain identification in epidemiologic investigations: Analysis of Swedish *C. diphtheriae* isolates from recent years by using a probe against a specific multicopy transposable DNA insertion element has linked most epidemic diphtheria cases to a single clonal strain and provided important information about the epidemiology of this disease.[90]

The epidemiology of tuberculosis, a rapidly emerging public health concern, has also been addressed with similar techniques. DNA insertion elements (IS) are randomly scattered throughout the *Mycobacterium tuberculosis* chromosome. The polymorphisms created by hybridizing chromosomal restriction fragments with an IS probe define a unique "fingerprint" for independent strains.[91] Fingerprint patterns have been used to track isolates and to incriminate one strain in multiple cases of disease.[92]

PCR-based methods may supplant Southern hybridization techniques in many of these sorts of investigations. For example, a variety of arthropod-borne microbial pathogens (such as *Y. pestis*, *Rickettsia rickettsii*, *Babesia microti*, and some arboviruses) are readily detected in their natural vectors with the PCR. *Borrelia burgdorferi* sequences have been amplified from archival tick samples and used to clarify the geographic and temporal origins of Lyme disease in the United States.[93] Arbitrarily primed (AP)-PCR is a variant form of this amplification technique in which random oligonucleotides serve as primers under conditions of low stringency. AP-PCR generates strain-specific chromosomal fingerprints that can be used to trace bacterial isolates during an epidemic outbreak.[94]

The clinical manifestations of numerous infectious diseases are more readily understood as a result of the molecular analysis of microbial virulence factors. Methods by which genes encoding virulence determinants can be isolated, modified, and returned to the original strain have been described earlier. Further techniques are available to create specific internal mutations within these genes, e.g., site-directed mutagenesis.[70] In this manner, not only can virulence factors be correlated with specific manifestations of disease, but particular protein domains can be correlated with specific biologic activities. This kind of analysis has revealed the amino acid residues that are crucial for ADP-ribosyltransferase activity of the pertussis toxin S1 subunit.[95,96]

Improvements in the diagnosis of infectious diseases have followed in step with many of the advances in epidemiologic investigation. In particular, DNA probe technology and PCR amplification techniques seem destined to have major impacts on diagnosis. The list of pathogens for which there are diagnostic DNA probes and specific PCR-based assays are already quite impressive.[86,87] PCR assays for detection of the human immunodeficiency virus are now available in many clinical microbiology laboratories.[97] In situ PCR is confined to the research laboratory at the present time but may soon permit ready anatomic localization of PCR-amplified signals within clinical samples.[98,99] As these two technologies become simplified and more widely used, it will be increasingly important to distinguish target sequences that are virulence associated from those that are not.

Current methods for the identification of microbial pathogens rely heavily on cultivation or propagation in the laboratory. A number of bacteria that are resistant to cultivation have now been identified with nonculture-based methods. One of these methods utilizes highly conserved small subunit rRNA gene sequences[100,101] as PCR primer binding sites in order to amplify rDNA sequences directly from digested, infected human tissue.[102] The evolutionary relationships of the previously unidentified pathogens are then established from analysis of the amplified rDNA sequences. With this approach, the bacterial agents of bacillary angiomatosis (see Ch. 170) and Whipple's disease (see Ch. 84) have been identified.[102–104] Findings from similar investigations of environmental microbial communities suggest that this kind of approach has the potential to reveal for the first time the true diversity of human microbial pathogens and commensal microorganisms.[105]

The application of molecular techniques and theory to infectious disease therapeutics and prophylaxis is in its infancy. As virulence factors for essential steps in pathogenesis are identified in individual pathogens, it should be possible to interfere with their function. For example, one might design competitive inhibitors of microbial adherence factors or invasion-promoting proteins.[106] As they become better characterized, manipulation of global virulence regulatory systems may have therapeutic value. New acellular or recombinant live attenuated vaccines will likely result from the identification of immunoprotective antigens with molecular approaches.[96] A growing understanding of microbial pathogenesis at the molecular level will foster these kinds of practical developments. The result should be a more informed and effective approach to the detection and treatment of infectious diseases.

REFERENCES

1. Falkow S, Small P, Isberg R, et al. A molecular strategy for the study of bacterial invasion. Rev Infect Dis. 1987;9:450–5.
2. Finlay BB, Falkow S. Common themes in microbial pathogenicity. Microbiol Rev. 1989;53:210–30.
3. Jones GW, Isaacson RE. Proteinaceous bacterial adhesins and their receptors. CRC Crit Rev Microbiol. 1983;10:229–60.
4. Woese CR. Bacterial evolution. Microbiol Rev. 1987;51:221–71.
5. Selander RK, Caugant DA, Ochman H, et al. Methods of multilocus enzyme electrophoresis for bacterial population genetics and systematics. Appl Environ Microbiol. 1986;51:873–84.
6. Selander RK, Caugant DA, Whittam TS. Genetic structure and variation in natural populations of Escherichia coli. In: Neidhardt FC, ed. Escherichia coli and Salmonella typhimurium. Washington, DC: American Society for Microbiology; 1987:1625–48.
7. Ochman H, Wilson AC. Evolutionary history of enteric bacteria. In: Neidhardt FC, ed. Escherichia coli and Salmonella typhimurium. Washington, DC: American Society for Microbiology; 1987:1649–54.
8. Ochman H, Selander RK. Evidence for clonal population structure in Escherichia coli. Proc Natl Acad Sci USA. 1984;81:198–201.
9. Selander RK, et al. Evolutionary genetic relationships of clones of Salmonella serovars that cause human typhoid and other enteric fevers. Infect Immun. 1990;58:2262–75.
10. Selander RK, Musser JM, Caugant DA, et al. Population genetics of pathogenic bacteria. Microbial Pathogen. 1987;3:1–7.
11. Selander RK, Muser JM. The population genetics of bacterial pathogenesis. In: Iglewski BH, Clark VL, eds. Molecular Basis of Bacterial Pathogenesis. Orlando, FL: Academic Press; 1990:11–36.
12. Musser JM, et al. Global genetic structure and molecular epidemiology of encapsulated Haemophilus influenzae. Rev Infect Dis. 1990;12:75–111.
13. Maynard Smith J, Smith NH, O'Rourke M, Spratt BG. How clonal are bacteria? Proc Natl Acad Sci USA. 1993;90:4384–8.
14. Campbell A. Evolutionary significance of accessory DNA elements in bacteria. Annu Rev Microbiol. 1981;35:55–83.
15. Elwell LP, Shipley PL. Plasmid-mediated factors associated with virulence of bacteria to animals. Annu Rev Microbiol. 1980;34:465–96.
16. Kopecko DJ, Formal SB. Plasmids and the virulence of enteric and other bacterial pathogens (Editorial). Ann Intern Med. 1984;101:260–2.
17. Falkow S, Portnoy DA. Bacterial plasmids—An overview. Clin Invest Med. 1983;6:207–12.
18. Mercer AA, Morelli G, Heuzenroeder M, et al. Conservation of plasmids among Escherichia coli K1 isolates of diverse origins. Infect Immun. 1984; 46:649–57.
19. Roszak DB, Colwell RR. Survival strategies of bacteria in the natural environment. Microbiol Rev. 1987;51:365–79.
20. Huq A, Small EB, West PA, et al. Ecological relationships between Vibrio cholerae and planktonic crustacean copepods. Appl Environ Microbiol. 1983;45:275–83.
21. Tamplin ML, Colwell RR. Effects of microcosm salinity and organic substrate concentration on production of Vibrio cholerae enterotoxin. Appl Environ Microbiol. 1986;52:297–301.
22. Perez-Rosas N, Hazen TC. In situ survival of Vibrio cholerae and Escherichia coli in tropical coral reefs. Appl Environ Microbiol. 1988;54:1–9.
23. Mekalanos JJ. Environmental signals controlling the expression of virulence determinants in bacteria. J Bacteriol. 1992;174:1–7.
24. Stock JB, Stock AM, Mottonen JM. Signal transduction in bacteria. Nature. 1990;344:395–400.
25. Parkinson JS. Signal transduction schemes of bacteria. Cell. 1993;73:857–71.
26. Miller JF, Mekalanos JJ, Falkow S. Coordinate regulation and sensory transduction in the control of bacterial virulence. Science. 1989;243:916–22.
27. Weiss AA, Falkow S. Genetic analysis of phase change in Bordetella pertussis. Infect Immun. 1984;43:263–9.
28. Arico B, et al. Sequences required for expression of Bordetella pertussis virulence factors share homology with prokaryotic signal transduction proteins. Proc Natl Acad Sci USA. 1989;86:6671–5.
29. Stibitz S, Yang MS. Subcellular localization and immunological detection of proteins encoded by the vir locus of Bordetella pertussis. J Bacteriol. 1991; 173:4288–96.
30. Uhl MA, Miller JF. Autophosphorylation and phosphotransfer in the Bordetella pertussis BvgAS signal transduction cascade. Proc Natl Acad Sci USA. 1994; 91;1163–7.
31. Roy CR, Falkow S. Identification of Bordetella pertussis regulatory sequences required for transcriptional activation of the fhaB gene and autoregulation of the bvgAS operon. J Bacteriol. 1991;173:2385–92.
32. Beattie DT, Mahan MJ, Mekalanos JJ. Repressor binding to a regulatory site in the DNA coding sequence is sufficient to confer transcriptional regulation of the vir-repressed genes (vrg genes) in Bordetella pertussis. J Bacteriol. 1993;175:519–27.
33. Scarlato V, Arico B, Prugnola A, Rappuoli R. Sequential activation and environmental regulation of virulence genes in Bordetella pertussis. EMBO J. 1991;10:3971–5.
34. Maurelli AT, Sansonetti PJ. Identification of a chromosomal gene controlling temperature-regulated expression of Shigella virulence. Proc Natl Acad Sci USA. 1988;85:2820–4.
35. Miller VL, Taylor RK, Mekalanos JJ. Cholera toxin transcriptional activator toxR is a transmembrane DNA binding protein. Cell 1987;48:271–9.
36. Miller VL, Mekalanos JJ. A novel suicide vector and its use in construction of insertion mutations: Osmoregulation of outer membrane proteins and virulence determinants in Vibrio cholerae requires toxR. J Bacteriol. 1988;170: 2575–83.
37. DiRita VJ, Parsot C, Jander G, et al. Regulatory cascade controls virulence in Vibrio cholerae. Proc Natl Acad Sci USA. 1991;88:5403–7.
38. Simon M, Zieg J, Silverman M, et al. Phase variation: Evolution of a controlling element. Science. 1980;209:1370–4.
39. McGee ZA, Johnson AP, Taylor-Robinson D. Pathogenic mechanisms of Neisseria gonorrhoeae: Observations on damage to human fallopian tubes in organ culture by gonococci of colony type 1 or type 4. J Infect Dis. 1981; 143:413–22.
40. McChesney D, Tramont EC, Boslego JW, et al. Genital antibody response to a parenteral gonococcal pilus vaccine. Infect Immun. 1982;36:1006–12.
41. Seifert HS, So M. Genetic mechanisms of bacterial antigenic variation. Microbiol Rev. 1988;52:327–36.
42. Borst P. Discontinuous transcription and antigenic variation in trypanosomes. Anu Rev Biochem. 1986;55:701–32.
43. Meier JT, Simon MI, Barbour AG. Antigenic variation is associated with DNA rearrangements in a relapsing fever borrelia. Cell. 1985;41:403–9.
44. Andrews GP, Maurelli AT. mxiA of Shigella flexneri 2a, which facilitates export of invasion plasmid antigens, encodes a homolog of the low-calcium response protein, LcrD, of Yersinia pestis. Infect Immun. 1992;60:3287–95.
45. Jones CH, et al. Adhesin presentation in bacteria requires molecular chaperones and ushers. Infect Immun. 1992;60:4445–51.
46. Hultgren SJ, et al. Pilus and nonpilus bacterial adhesins: assembly and function in cell recognition. Cell. 1993;73:887–901.
47. Falkow S. Bacterial entry into eukaryotic cells. Cell. 1991;65:1099–102.
48. Joiner KA, Dubremetz JF. Toxoplasma gondii: A protozoan for the nineties. Infect Immun. 1993;61:1169–72.
49. Joiner KA, et al. Toxoplasma gondii: Fusion competence of parasitophorous vacuoles in Fc receptor-transfected fibroblasts. Science. 1990;249:641–6.
50. Bliska JB, Galan JE, Falkow S. Signal transduction in the mammalian cell during bacterial attachment and entry. Cell. 1993;73:903–20.
51. Isberg RI. Discrimination between intracellular uptake and surface adhesion of bacterial pathogens. Science. 1991;252:934–8.
52. Straley SC, et al. Yops of Yersinia. spp. pathogenic for humans. Infect Immun. 1993;61:3105–10.
53. Clemens JC, et al. Microbial pathogenesis and tyrosine dephosphorylation: Surprising "bedfellows." Mol Microbiol. 1991;5:2617–20.
54. Berger K, Isberg RR. Two distinct defects in intracellular growth complemented by a single genetic locus in Legionella pneumophila. Mol Microbiol. 1993;7:7–19.
55. Aranda CMA, et al. Salmonella typhimurium activates virulence gene transcription within acidified macrophage lysosomes. Proc Natl Acad Sci USA. 1992;89:10079–83.
56. Camilli A, Tilney LG, Portnoy DA. Dual roles of plcA in Listeria monocytogenes pathogenesis. Mol Microbiol. 1993;8:143–57.
57. Goldberg MB, Barzu O, Parsot C, Sansonetti PJ. Unipolar localization and ATPase activity of IcsA, a Shigella flexneri protein involved in intracellular movement. J Bacteriol. 1993;175:2189–96.

58. Kocks C, et al. *L. monocytogenes*–induced actin assembly requires the *actA* gene product, a surface protein. Cell. 1992;68:521–31.
59. Zychlinsky A, Prevost MC, Sansonetti PJ. *Shigella flexneri* induces apoptosis in infected macrophages. Nature. 1992;358:167–9.
60. Weiss AA, Hewlett EL, Myers GA, et al. Tn5-induced mutations affecting virulence factors of *Bordetella pertussis*. Infect Immun. 1983;42:33–41.
61. Macrina FL. Molecular cloning of bacterial antigens and virulence determinants. Annu Rev Microbiol. 1984;38:193–219.
62. Collins J. *Escherichia coli* plasmids packageable in vitro in lambda bacteriophage particles. Methods Enzymol. 1979;68:309–26.
63. Pearson GDN, Mekalanos JJ. Molecular cloning of *Vibrio cholerae* enterotoxin genes in *Escherichia coli* K-12. Proc Natl Acad Sci USA. 1982;79:2976–80.
64. Livey I, Duggleby CJ, Robinson A. Cloning and nucleotide sequence analysis of the serotype 2 fimbrial subunit gene of *Bordetella pertussis*. Mol Microbiol. 1987;1:203–9.
65. Stibitz S, Weiss AA, Falkow S. Genetic analysis of a region of the *Bordetella pertussis* chromosome encoding filamentous hemagglutinin and the pleiotropic regulatory locus *vir*. J Bacteriol. 1988;170:2904–13.
66. Shatzman AR, Rosenberg M. Expression, identification, and characterization of recombinant gene products in *Escherichia coli*. Methods Enzymol. 1987;152:661–73.
67. Isberg RR, Falkow S. A single genetic locus encoded by *Yersinia pseudotuberculosis* permits invasion of cultured animal cells by *Escherichia coli* K-12. Nature. 1985;317:262–4.
68. Mahan MJ, Slauch JM, Mekalanos JJ. Selection of bacterial virulence genes that are specifically induced in host tissues. Science. 1993;259:686–8.
69. Lisitsyn N, Lisitsyn N, Wigler M. Cloning the differences between two complex genomes. Science. 1993;259:946–51.
70. Botstein D, Shortle D. Strategies and applications of in vitro mutagenesis. Science. 1985;229:1193–201.
71. Sanger F, Nicklen S, Coulson AR. DNA sequencing with chain-terminating inhibitors. Proc Natl Acad Sci USA. 1977;74:5463–7.
72. Frazer AC, Curtiss R. Production, properties and utility of bacterial minicells. Curr Top Microbiol Immunol. 1975;69:1–84.
73. Sancar A, Hack AM, Rupp WD. Simple method for identification of plasmid-coded proteins. J Bacteriol. 1979;137:692–3.
74. Evans AS. Causation and disease: The Henle-Koch postulates revisited. Yale J Biol Med. 1976;49:175–95.
75. Falkow S. Molecular Koch's postulates applied to microbial pathogenicity. Rev Infect Dis. 1988;10(Suppl):274:6.
76. Stibitz S, Black W, Falkow S. The construction of a cloning vector designed for gene replacement in *Bordetella pertussis*. Gene. 1986;50:133–40.
77. Whittam TS, Wachsmuth IK, Wilson RA. Genetic evidence of clonal descent of *Escherichia coli* 0157:H7 associated with hemorrhagic colitis and hemolytic uremic syndrome. J Infect Dis. 1988;157:1124–33.
78. Musser JM, et al. *Streptococcus pyogenes* causing toxic-shock-like syndrome and other invasive diseases: Clonal diversity and pyrogenic exotoxin expression. Proc Natl Acad Sci USA. 1991;88:2668–72.
79. Musser JM, Hewlett EL, Peppler MS, et al. Genetic diversity and relationships in populations of *Bordetella* spp. J. Bacteriol. 1986;166:230–7.
80. Tompkins LS. The use of molecular methods in infectious diseases. N Engl J Med. 1992;327:1290–7.
81. Spika JS, Waterman SH, Hoo GW, et al. Chloramphenicol resistant *Salmonella newport* traced through hamburger to dairy farms. N Engl J Med. 1987;316:565–70.
82. Tompkins LS, Roessler BJ, Redd SC, et al. *Legionella* prosthetic-valve endocarditis. N Engl J Med. 1988;318:530–5.
83. Saiki RK, Gelfand DH, Stoffel S, et al. Primer-directed enzymatic amplifica-
tion of DNA with a thermostable DNA polymerase. Science. 1988;239:487–91.
84. Eisenstein BI. The polymerase chain reaction: A new method of using molecular genetics for medical diagnosis. N Engl J Med. 1990;322:178–83.
85. Erlich HA, Gelfand D, Sninsky JJ. Recent advances in the polymerase chain reaction. Science. 1991;252:1643–51.
86. Tenover FC. Diagnostic deoxyribonucleic acid probes for infectious diseases. Clin Microbiol Rev. 1988;1:82–101.
87. Persing DH, Smith TF, Tenover FC, White TJ, eds. Diagnostic Molecular Microbiology: Principles and Applications. Washington, DC: American Society for Microbiology, 1993.
88. Moseley SL, Huq I, Alim AR, et al. Detection of enterotoxigenic *Escherichia coli* by DNA colony hybridization. J Infect Dis. 1980;142:892–8.
89. McDonough KA, Schwan TG, Thomas RE, et al. Identification of a *Yersinia pestis*–specific DNA probe with potential for use in plague surveillance. J Clin Microbiol. 1988;26:2515–9.
90. Rappuoli R, Perugini M, Falsen E. Molecular epidemiology of the 1984–1986 outbreak of diphtheria in Sweden. N Engl J Med. 1988;318:12–4.
91. Hermans PWM, et al. Insertion element IS986 from *Mycobacterium tuberculosis*: A useful tool for diagnosis and epidemiology of tuberculosis. J Clin Microbiol. 1990;28:2051–8.
92. Daley CL, et al. An outbreak of tuberculosis with accelerated progression among persons infected with the human immunodeficiency virus: An analysis using restriction-fragment-length polymorphisms. N Engl J Med. 1992;326:231–5.
93. Persing DH, et al. Detection of *Borrelia burgdorferi* DNA in museum specimens of *Ixodes dammini* ticks. Science. 1990;249:1420–3.
94. Welsh J, McClelland M. Fingerprinting genomes using PCR with arbitrary primers. Nucleic Acids Res. 1990;18:7213–8.
95. Black WJ, Munoz JJ, Peacock MG, et al. ADP-ribosyltransferase activity of pertussis toxin and immunomodulation by *Bordetella pertussis*. Science. 1988;240:656–9.
96. Pizza M, et al. Mutants of pertussis toxin suitable for vaccine development. Science. 1989;246:497–500.
97. Ou CY, Kwok S, Mitchell SW, et al. DNA amplification for direct detection of HIV-1 in DNA of peripheral blood mononuclear cells. Science. 1988;239:295–7.
98. Haase AT, Retzel EF, Staskus KA. Amplification and detection of lentiviral DNA inside cells. Proc Natl Acad Sci USA. 1990;87:4971–5.
99. Bagasra O, et al. Detection of human immunodeficiency virus type 1 provirus in mononuclear cells by in situ polymerase chain reaction. N Engl J Med. 1992;326:1385–91.
100. Lane DJ, et al. Rapid determination of 16S ribosomal RNA sequences for phylogenetic analyses. Proc Natl Acad Sci USA. 1985;82:6955–9.
101. Chen K, Neimark H, Rumore P, et al. Broad range DNA probes for detecting and amplifying eubacterial nucleic acids. FEMS Microbiol Lett. 1989;48:19–24.
102. Relman DA, Loutit JS, Schmidt TM, et al. The agent of bacillary angiomatosis: An approach to the identification of uncultured pathogens. N Engl J Med. 1990;323:1573–80.
103. Wilson KH, Blitchington R, Frothingham R, et al. Phylogeny of the Whipple's-disease–associated bacterium. Lancet. 1991;338:474–5.
104. Relman DA, Schmidt TM, MacDermott RP, et al. Identification of the uncultured bacillus of Whipple's disease. N Engl J Med. 1992;327:293–301.
105. Relman DA. The identification of uncultured microbial pathogens. J Infect Dis. 1993;168:1–8.
106. Isberg RR, Voorhis DL, Falkow S. Identification of invasin: A protein that allows enteric bacteria to penetrate cultured mammalian cells. Cell. 1987;50:769–78.

SECTION B. HOST DEFENSE MECHANISMS

4. GENERAL OR NONSPECIFIC HOST DEFENSE MECHANISMS

EDMUND C. TRAMONT
DAVID L. HOOVER

General or nonspecific host defense mechanisms refer to a formidable array of host resistance factors that interfere with and provide defense against microbes. The protective effects are due to innate steady-state resistance (e.g., intact skin, lysozyme, complement) or as a consequence of the presence or invasion of any foreign substance (e.g., cytokines, natural killer cells). These mechanisms are a critical first encounter for any microorganism. Because of their general nature, the nonspecific host defense mechanisms are difficult to quantitate, and because they are so efficient, they are often taken for granted (Table 1). Taken as a whole, the effect of this first line of defense is impressive; taken individually, each mechanism or factor is less effective than are responses that confer resistance to specific infectious agents (i.e., antibodies, cytotoxic lymphocytes).

NORMAL INDIGENOUS MICROBIAL FLORA

A microorganism must gain access into or onto the host in order to develop a particular relationship with that host (a preformed toxin such as that produced by *Clostridium botulinum* would be an exception). This host-parasite relationship may be *symbiotic*, *commensal*, or *parasitic*, depending upon the particular situation that is encountered. For example, *Escherichia coli* is a commensal organism in the gastrointestinal tract, but it is a parasite in the lung. Certain organisms always behave in a predictable fashion. For example, in humans, the rabies virus is always considered a pathogen, whereas the lactobacillus seldom is. From the point of view of the microorganism, the better adapted it becomes to exist in a symbiotic or commensal relationship with its host, the better its chances for survival.

The normal commensal flora plays an important role in protecting the host from microbial invasion by "pathogenic" organisms.[1] Mechanisms of this protection include the following: *(1)* competition for the same nutrients (interference); *(2)* competition for the same receptors on host cells (tropism); *(3)* production of bacteriocins, that is, bacterial products that are toxic to other organisms, usually of the same species; *(4)* production of volatile fatty acids[2] or other metabolites; *(5)* continual stimulation of the immune system to maintain low but constant levels of class II histocompatibility (DR) molecule expression on macrophages and other antigen presenting cells[3]; and *(6)* stimulation of cross-protective immune factors such as the so-called natural antibodies.

The ultimate effect of the first three protective mechanisms is to limit the quantity or dominance of any one species or organism. For example, broad-spectrum antibiotic therapy decreases the numbers of bacteria in the gut. This results in an increased proportion of normally commensal fungal species and resistant bacterial strains. When the antibiotic therapy is stopped, a rebound results and the gut is repopulated, but to the advantage of the faster-growing aerobic Enterobacteriaceae over the slower-metabolizing anaerobes.[4]

The microbial flora harbored by the host can be divided into two groups: *(1)* normal resident flora that is regularly found and, if perturbed, promptly reestablishes itself and *(2)* a transient flora that may colonize the host for periods ranging from hours to weeks but does not permanently establish itself.

Certain organisms characteristically colonize certain body sites (tropism). This is obviously taken into consideration when deciding whether a particular organism is behaving in a pathogenic fashion. Bacteria and fungi make up the great majority of commensal and symbiotic organisms. Protozoa are less ubiquitous, almost always reside in the gastrointestinal tract, and are more prevalent in underdeveloped countries. Mycoplasmas and viruses are much less prevalent.

The species that make up the normal commensal flora are obviously influenced by environmental factors such as diet, san-

TABLE 1. Factors Contributing to Host Nonspecific Resistance to Infection

Normal indigenous microflora
Genetic factors
Natural antibodies
Morphologic integrity
Normal excretory secretions and flow
Phagocytosis
Natural killer cells
Nutrition
Non-antigen-specific immune response
Fibronectin
Hormonal factors

TABLE 2. Cytokines and PAF in the Acute Phase Response

Cytokine	Actions	Main Sources
IL-1, TNF-α	Induces fever; augments leukocyte production, expression of adhesion molecules, phagocyte antimicrobial activity, catabolic effects; promotes IL-8 release	M, K, E, NK
IL-6	Induces fever; augments production of acute phase reactants by liver; inhibits IL-1 and TNF production	M, E
IL-8	Enhances adherence and chemotaxis of PMN; induces PMN granule release	M, E
IFN-α	Induces fever; increases expression of adhesion molecules; augments production of IFN-γ by NK cells	M, F, NK
IFN-γ	Enhances production of IL-1, TNF, IL-6; augments phagocyte microbicidal activity	NK, T
IL-2	Enhances phagocyte microbicidal activity	T
IL-3, GM-CSF, G-CSF, SCF	Augments production and function of leukocytes	T, M
IL-12	Augments production of IFN-γ by NK cells	B, M
TGF-β	Inhibits production of TNF, IL-1	M, F, E, P
IL-4, IL-10, IL-13	Inhibits production of TNF, IL-1; inhibits phagocyte microbicidal activity	T (TH2)
Lipid mediator		
PAF	Augments adhesion molecules; induces vasodilatation, increased vascular permeability	P, E, M, PMN

Abbreviations: IL, interleukin; CSF, colony-stimulating factor; GM-GSF, granulocyte-macrophage CSF; G-CSF, granulocyte CSF; IFN, interferon; PAF, platelet activating factor; SCF, stem cell factor; TGF, tissue growth factor; B, B lymphocytes; E, endothelial cell; K, keratinocyte; M, monocyte–macrophage; NK, natural killer cell; P, platelet; PMN, polymorphonuclear leukocyte; T, T lymphocyte.

itary conditions, air pollution, and hygienic habits.[4] For example, lactobacilli are common intestinal commensals whenever dairy products make up a significant proportion of the dietary intake; protozoa are common intestinal inhabitants of those living where sanitation is poor; and a patient with underlying chronic bronchitis is more likely to harbor *Haemophilus influenzae* in the tracheobronchial tree.

The normal flora is also influenced by hormones. Premenarchal and postmenopausal vaginal flora differ significantly from that present during the childbearing period.

An important effect of the normal flora on the immune system is to keep it "primed" and thus more rapid and efficient in its response to invading microorganisms. Antigens must be presented to the immune system in an ordered and specified way. For example, helper (CD4) T cells recognize antigens only after they are displayed on the surface of a macrophage (or other antigen-presenting cells) in physical association with a class II histocompatibility (DR) molecule. Normally, 75–85 percent of circulating monocytes in adults maintain relatively high levels of DR molecule expression. DR expression is much lower on monocytes of human newborns,[3] neonatal mice, and germ-free animals. Thus, the constant stimulation by the host's indigenous microbial flora maintains the high level of DR molecule expression on macrophages and perhaps other antigen-presenting cells, and this serves to keep the immune system primed. This modulation is due, at least in part, to low-level production of interferon-γ, interleukin-4 (IL-4), and other cytokines by activated T cells (see below under "Cytokines") (Table 2). This process can also be detrimental by stimulation of blocking antibodies, cross-reactive responses to host tissues, or inappropriate T-cell responses.

TISSUE TROPISMS AND HEREDITARY FACTORS

Receptors exist on tissues that permit the attachment of microorganisms. The attachment of a microorganism to a receptor is dependent upon the presence of a complementary ligand or adhesin on that microorganism[5] (see Ch. two). The ligand and the receptor vary independently as to their specificity—a receptor binding to one or many different organisms (ligands), a ligand binding one or many different receptors. Thus, most organisms preferentially colonize certain tissues and spare others. This phenomenon is referred to as *tissue tropism*. For example, influenza virus and mycoplasmas preferentially adhere to respiratory epithelial cells, *E. coli* and *Vibrio cholerae* to intestinal cells, and *Streptococcus mutans* to tooth enamel; also, gram-positive organisms more readily attach to heart valves than do gram-negative organisms. *Treponema pallidum,* on the other hand, binds to many different tissue receptors, and untreated late syphilis may involve any organ.

Receptors on host cells may change. For example, there is evidence to suggest that viral illness may affect tissue tropisms of the oropharynx to allow easier colonization by gram-negative organisms.[6] Also, urinary epithelial cells from people prone to develop urinary tract infections support the attachment of urinary pathogens over urinary epithelial cells from healthy people.[7] The genetics of tissue tropisms are unknown, but the role of these factors in determining susceptibilities of a host to a particular infection is obviously important.

The relationship of genetic factors to susceptibilities to infectious agents has been appreciated for many years.[8,9] Infections have been one of the strongest selective pressures in human evolution. Tuberculosis, measles, and smallpox had devastating effects on the native American populations. Conversely, the protective effects of sickle cell trait on the outcome of falciparum malaria have benefitted inhabitants living in falciparum malarious areas.

Histocompatibility antigens have been linked to a predisposition to some infectious complications. The HLA-B27 and reactive arthropathy or Reiter syndrome and the predisposition of individuals with blood group O to cholera, presumably linked to the expression of glycosphingolipids in the small bowel mucosa, were the earliest associations recognized. There is evidence of HLA-linked determinants in tuberculoid leprosy,[10] acute glomerulonephritis,[11] paralytic poliomyelitis,[12] HIV,[12a] and responsiveness to antigenic stimuli.[13] The list is destined to grow.

Natural Antibodies

Natural antibodies are antibodies specific to a microbe found in healthy people without a previous history of infection by the microbe. These antibodies are of great importance in the immunity to many bacteria, especially encapsulated bacteria such as *Neisseria meningitidis* and *H. influenzae* type b.

They are stimulated by colonization in the oropharynx, gut, or elsewhere of organisms sharing cross-reactive (cross-protective) antigens.[13] However, these antibodies are not always beneficial. For example, specific serum IgA antibodies to *N. meningitidis* may predispose an otherwise immune person to become susceptible by preferentially attaching to the organism, thus blocking the beneficial bactericidal effect of the protective IgG and IgM antibodies.[14] The blood group antibodies are a consequence of colonization in the gut of microorganisms bearing cross-reactive antigens.

NATURAL BARRIERS TO THE ENTRY OF MICROORGANISMS INTO THE BODY

The morphologic integrity of the body surface is an important and effective first line of defense.

Skin and Mucous Membranes

The intact skin forms a very effective mechanical barrier to invasion by microorganisms. Since very few organisms have the innate ability to penetrate the skin, they must gain access by some physical means such as by an arthropod vector, trauma, surgical incision, or intravenous catheter.

The specific antimicrobial properties of skin have not been exhaustively studied. However, the relative dryness or desiccating effect of skin, the mild acidity (acid mantle, pH 5–6), and the normal skin flora act in concert to form an effective prohibitive environment. Inflamed skin is more permeable to water and therefore leads to greater colonization. It has been speculated that oily skin may retard evaporation of water, resulting in increased numbers of colonizing organisms. The acidity of the skin results from the breakdown of lipids into fatty acids. Sebum contains few esterified fatty acids, but the normal skin flora partially hydrolyzes the triglycerides, thereby liberating fatty acids. Desquamation of skin scales also aids in the elimination of microorganisms.

The mucous membranes support a larger number of microorganisms. They are bathed in secretions with antimicrobial properties. For example, cervical mucus, prostatic fluid, and tears have been shown to be toxic to a variety of microorganisms. One of the more potent antimicrobial substances is lysozyme, which is found in every mucosal secretion. It is an enzyme that lyses bacteria by splitting the muramic acid B-(1–4)-N-acetyl-glucosamine linkage in the bacterial cell wall and is especially effective against gram-positive organisms. Local secretions also contain specific immunoglobulins, principally IgG and secretory IgA (which act primarily to block the attachment of organisms to host cells and significant amounts of iron-binding proteins. The importance of iron for microorganisms is well recognized, and all fluids that are potentially exposed to microbes are enriched with iron-binding proteins, which act to keep this important factor from the microorganisms.[15] Body iron stores that have been chelated to deferioxamine can be utilized as an iron source for some organisms. This may account for the susceptibility to mucormycosis and yersiniosis in patients treated with deferioxamine.

Respiratory Tract

The respiratory tract has formidable antimicrobial defense mechanisms.[16] First, the inhaled particles must survive and penetrate the aerodynamic filtration system of the upper airway and tracheobronchial tree. The airflow in these areas in quite turbulent, causing large particles to impact on the mucosal surfaces. Humidification also causes hydroscopic organisms to increase in size, thus aiding phagocytosis.

Once deposited, the mucociliary blanket transports the invading offender away from the lung. Coughing obviously aids this expulsion. This system is amazingly efficient: 90 percent of deposited material is cleared in less than 1 hour. In addition, the bronchial secretions contain various antimicrobial substances (e.g., lysozyme).

Once a particle reaches the alveoli, physical expulsion becomes much less effective, and the alveolar macrophage and tissue histiocytes play a more prominent role in protecting the host. When the lungs become inflamed, they are aided by the influx of polymorphonuclear leukocytes and monocytes, which become even more efficient when specific immune mechanisms such as opsonins are present.

Like all defense mechanisms, these nonspecific mechanisms can be overcome by the introduction of large numbers of invading organisms (e.g., contaminated respirator), particularly when the host is exposed over an extended period of time. Furthermore, their effectiveness is decreased by air pollutants (e.g., cigarette smoke), mechanical respirators, tracheostomy, concomitant infection, and allergenic agents.

Intestinal Tract

The acid pH of the stomach, the antibacterial effect of the various pancreatic enzymes, and bile and intestinal secretions are effective antimicrobial factors. Peristalsis and the normal loss of epithelial cells also act to purge the intestinal tract of harmful microorganisms. Alteration of these parameters can lead to increased susceptibility of the host to infection. For example, *Salmonella* and tuberculosis infections are more common in achlorhydric patients, and slowing peristalsis with belladonna or opium alkaloids prolongs symptomatic shigellosis. Intubated patients treated with inhibitors of gastric acid secretion have a higher incidence of aspiration pneumonia.

Normal bowel flora competition (10^{12} organisms per gram of feces) plays an extremely important protective role. Altering this flora with broad-spectrum antibiotics can lead to overgrowth with inherently pathogenic organisms (e.g., *Salmonella typhimurium*) or suprainfection with ordinarily commensal organisms (e.g., *Candida albicans*). The interfering competitive capacity of the normal flora can be overcome by large numbers of virulent organisms. For example, the rate of development of salmonellosis has been directly related to the number of *Salmonella* organisms ingested.

Genitourinary Tract

Urine is normally sterile. The factors that contribute to the ability of the urinary tract to resist infection are quite complex. Urine is bactericidal for some strains of bacteria. This is mostly due to the pH of the urine, but factors such as urea and other solutes play a role.

The lower urinary tract is flushed with urine four to eight times each day, eliminating potential pathogenic organisms unless they are capable of firmly attaching to epithelial cells of the urinary tract, such as *Neisseria gonorrhoeae* and certain strains of *E. coli*. The length of the male urethra (20 cm in the adult) also provides protection, and bacteria seldom gain access to the bladder in men unless introduced by instrumentation. The female urethra is much shorter (5 cm in the adult) and more readily traversed by microorganisms, which may be one reason

why urinary tract infections are 14 times more common in women than in men. The hypertonic state of the kidney medulla presents an unfavorable milieu for most microorganisms. Tamm-Horsfall protein is a glycoprotein produced by the kidneys and excreted in large amounts in urine (approximately 50 mg/L). Certain bacteria avidly bind to it, suggesting that it prevents them from gaining a foothold in the urinary tract, thereby acting as a natural host defense mechanism against colonization and subsequent infection.[17]

The vagina has a unique mechanism of protection. Under hormonal influence, especially estrogens, the vaginal epithelium contains increased amounts of glycogen that Döderlein's bacilli and other commensals metabolize into lactic acid. *Döderlein's bacilli* is an all-encompassing term used to describe acidogenic gram-positive rods residing in the vagina. Normal vaginal secretions contain up to 10^8 of such bacteria per milliliter. Thus an acid environment is established that is unfavorable to most pathogenic bacteria. The vaginal secretions of women with nonspecific vaginitis, a pertubation of the normal vaginal ecology, is usually characterized by an elevated pH.

The Eye

Constant bathing of the eyes by tears is an effective means of protection. Foreign substances are continually diluted and washed away via the tear ducts into the nasal cavity. Tears also contain large amounts of lysozyme and other antimicrobial substances.

STEADY-STATE COMPONENTS OF NONSPECIFIC IMMUNITY

After microbes breach the integumentary barriers, they encounter additional host defenses mediated by either soluble factors or cells. The level and localization of these humoral and cellular components are regulated by cytokines and other products of the immune system.

Complement

Complement refers to a group of upwards of 20 serum proteins that interact with each other in an orderly fashion that is referred to as the *complement cascade*. Although most often activated in conjunction with specific immunity through the classical pathway, complement can also be activated by the surface of some microorganisms via the alternative pathway. Complement activation can lead to microbial lysis, but also plays important roles in phagocytosis, cytokine production, and attraction of leukocytes to infected sites. The lytic action of complement is very effective: the overwhelming majority of intestinal bacteria are susceptible to complement-mediated lysis. In contrast, strains of enteric bacteria that cause invasive disease typically resist complement-mediated serum bactericidal activity. Most complement components are synthesized by macrophages, with increased production in response to infection[18] (see Ch. 6).

Fibronectin

Fibronectin is a high-molecular-weight glycoprotein found in plasma and on cell surfaces that plays a central role in cell adhesion. It covers the receptors of surface cells, blocking the attachment of many organisms, such as *Pseudomonas aeruginosa*, but enhances the binding of other organisms, such as *S. aureus*, to host cells.[19]

Phagocytosis

Microorganisms that enter the lymphatics, lung, or blood stream are engulfed and killed by a variety of phagocytic cells. Polymorphonuclear leukocytes and monocytes, which circulate in blood and migrate through the tissues, are attracted to sites of inflammation. Opsonin-independent phagocytosis by polymorphonuclear cells is related to contact angle between microorganism and the surface on which it rests. As a consequence of this relationship, phagocytosis is most efficient when organisms are trapped in small tissue spaces (e.g., alveoli) than residing on smooth, open surfaces (e.g., synovium).[20]

Mononuclear phagocytes in blood, lymph nodes, spleen, liver, bone marrow, and lung constitute the reticuloendothelial system. This system removes particulate matter, including microbes and damaged or senescent host cells, from the lymph and blood. Particles are recognized via receptors on the macrophage surface. Fibronectin, for example, coats fragments of damaged cells, collagen debris, altered platelets, and fibrinogen-fibrin complexes and enhances their clearance by macrophages. Host-derived ligands such as complement and fibronectin may also adhere to microorganisms to permit recognition.[21] Alternatively, macrophages recognize microbial surface components such as lipopolysaccharide. Mannose-binding protein on macrophage membranes may bind surface mannans of fungi and mediate attachment to phagocytes. Persons whose spleens have been surgically or functionally eliminated dramatically demonstrate the importance of the reticuloendothelial system: encapsulated bacteria such as pneumococci can replicate freely in the blood, leading to overwhelming infection.

Ingested microorganisms are killed by the action of toxic oxygen metabolites (e.g., hydrogen peroxide, superoxide, hydroxyl radical) or by granule-bound antibacterial molecules. These molecules, including defensins, azurocidin, cathepsin G, and bactericidal/permeability-increasing (BPI) protein, kill microbes and some enveloped viruses by permeabilizing their membranes.[22,23]

ACUTE PHASE RESPONSE

When an invader sufficiently perturbs the baseline defensive capabilities of humoral components and phagocytes, a generalized, coordinated, but nonspecific reaction termed the *acute phase response* ensues. This response augments the concentration of humoral defensive components, increases the number and function of phagocytic cells, facilitates delivery of humoral and cellular components to sites of inflammation, and initiates antigen-specific responses. These components of the acute phase response are mediated by reactions of pre-existing humoral defenses and by de novo production of active regulatory molecules (e.g., cytokines, prostaglandins and other eicosanoids, hormones) by phagocytes, lymphocytes, and endothelial cells.

Cytokines

Production of cytokines, hormonelike peptides that regulate numerous cellular responses, is triggered by phagocytosis, adherence of microbes or their products to cell surfaces, complement fragments, host cell stress proteins, and altered cell surface adhesion molecules (Fig. 1, Table 2). The intricacy, pleomorphism, and redundancy of the cytokine network has become increasingly apparent (see Ch. 8). Most cytokines are secreted by more than one cell type; most cells that secrete one cytokine secrete many cytokines. In addition, cytokines may enhance or diminish the release of themselves, other cytokines, or other components of the regulatory network.

Four major cell types contribute most heavily to the acute phase cytokine response: mononuclear phagocytes, natural killer (NK) cells, T lymphocytes that bear the γ- and δ-chains

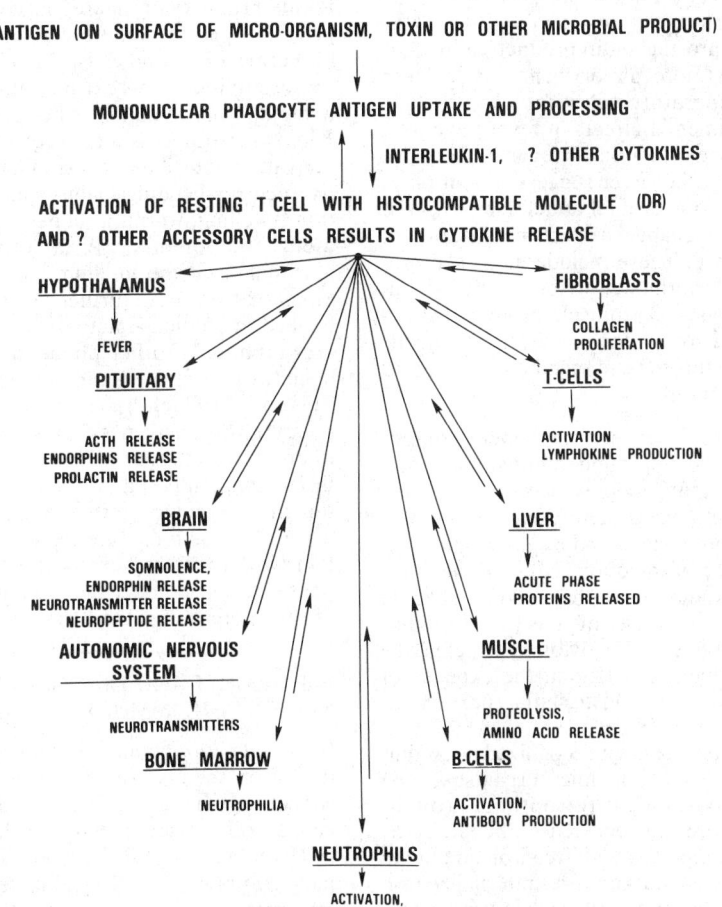

FIG. 1. The cytokine cascade.

of the T-cell receptor (γδ-T cells), and endothelial cells. Mononuclear phagocytes, the most broadly reactive cells of this group, are an important source of the pro-inflammatory cytokines IL-1, tumor necrosis factor (TNF)-α, and IL-6 and of interferon α (IFN-α), an important nonspecific antiviral molecule and enhancer of T-cell-mediated immune responses. Moreover, macrophages produce prostaglandins and other arachidonic acid metabolites that play a prominent role in inflammation and generally provide feedback inhibition on pro-inflammatory cytokine release.

Endothelial cells also secrete IL-1, TNF-α, and IL-6, particularly in response to TNF-α, IL-1, and gram-negative bacterial lipopolysaccharide. Endothelial cells may be important sources of cytokines because of their numbers and their location at the blood-tissue interface. In addition, they produce large amounts of IL-8, an important mediator of polymorphonuclear localization.[24]

Both NK cells and γδ-T cells recognize a 70-kD stress (heat shock) protein expressed by macrophages after ingestion of microbes. Also, microbes themselves express heat shock proteins that may trigger NK cell responses. The most important product of both NK cells and γδ-T cells is IFN-γ augmented by cytokines IL-2 and IL-12.[25,26] IFN-γ profoundly enhances IL-1, TNF-α, and IL-6 produced by macrophages. These stimulatory activities are regulated by negative feedback circuits, in which cytokines such as IL-4 and IL-10 released by the TH2 subset of helper T lymphocytes, participate.[26a] Macrophages and platelets release TGF-β and soluble receptors for stimulatory cytokines, which also downregulate the acute phase response.[27] Cytokines also induce release of adrenocorticotropic hormone, endorphins, prolactin, neurotransmitters, and growth hormone, which further regulate nonspecific and specific immune responses.[28]

Metabolic Changes. Fever is the most obvious sign of the acute phase response. Numerous cytokines, notably IL-1, TNF-α, IL-6, and IFN-α, increase prostaglandin production by cells in or near the hypothalamic thermoregulatory center.[29,29a] These prostaglandins raise the temperature set point and result in fever. The beneficial vs. detrimental effects of fever have long been debated. The consistent expression of fever in response to moderate to severe infection, however suggests that it plays a beneficial role in resistance to microbial attack (see Ch. 37).

A number of other metabolic changes reflect mobilization of the host's resources for defense. These include increased production of thyroid-stimulating hormone, vasopressin, insulin, and glucagon. Profound catabolism of muscle protein also occurs, as amino acids are used for synthesis of defensive cells and proteins and increased resting muscle metabolic activity or shivering to raise body temperature.

Soluble Defensive Molecules. Serum complement components, fibronectin, mannose-binding protein, haptoglobin, amyloid A protein, C-reactive protein, lipopolysaccharide-binding protein (LPS-BP), a number of glycoproteins, and certain protease inhibitors including α₁-antitrypsin and α₂-macroglobulin, also increase as a consequence of infection. LPS-BP mediates binding of LPS to monocytes and macrophages via a specific receptor (CD14) and increases sensitivity of cells to LPS stimulation.[30] Increased hepatic synthesis of many of these defensive proteins occurs under the influence of IL-6 at the expense of serum albumin synthesis, as host metabolism shifts from homeostasis to defense.[31]

A decrease in serum iron has long been recognized as a component of the acute phase response. Many microorganisms must scavenge iron from their environment for optimal growth. Transferrin, an iron-binding protein secreted by hepatocytes under the influence of IL-6, complexes with free iron and limits its availability to microorganisms. Macrophages internalize iron transferrin complexes, retain the iron, and recycle transferrin, further reducing both free and total serum iron.[32]

Increased Phagocyte Number and Function. Numbers and functions of phagocytes also increase as an immediate consequence of infection (see Ch. 7). Production of IL-1, TNF-α, IL-3, and stem cell factor by macrophages and/or lymphocytes enhances replication of bone marrow stem cells. Replication and differentiation of bone marrow cells toward mature phagocytes are further augmented by granulocyte-macrophage colony-stimulating factor (GM-CSF) and granulocyte colony-stimulating factor (G-CSF).[33]

In addition to providing increased numbers of phagocytes available for defense, cytokines play an important role in enhancing microbicidal activity. TNF-α, IL-1, GM-CSF, IFN-γ and IL-2, alone or in various combinations, lead to increased destruction of microbes by increasing production of toxic oxygen products and release of granule-bound antimicrobial molecules. TNF-α and IL-1 also promote expression of complement receptor 3 (CR3), the receptor of iC3b, and thereby enhance ingestion of organisms opsonized by complement.[34]

Inflammation. As part of the acute phase response, phagocyte and soluble antimicrobial substances are directed to sites of microbial invasion. Cytokines, especially TNF-α and IL-1, increase expression of adhesion molecules on endothelial cells, polymorphonuclear leukocytes (PMN), and monocytes.[36] Production of IL-8 by endothelial cells, monocytes, and PMN in response to cytokines or microbial products further modulates expression of adhesion molecules and provides a chemotactic signal that promotes emigration of PMN from the blood to the inflammatory site. Moreover, IL-8 directly induces release of granule contents from PMN.[24] Chemotaxis and release of granule contents in response to complement components (e.g., C5a) or microbial products (e.g., lipopolysaccharide, formylmethionine-leucine-phenylalanine) is also enhanced by IFN-α. These granule contents increase vascular permeability. Other, noncytokine products of macrophages, such as the arachidonic acid products, prostaglandins, and leukotrienes, also increase vascular permeability and cause vasodilatation. As a consequence of these activities, local extravasation of soluble defensive components and plasma and further emigration of phagocytes occur. Kinins generated as a consequence of the coagulation cascade activation contribute to vasodilatation and stimulate pain-sensitive neuronal endings. Thus, the classic hallmarks of inflammation (swelling, warmth, redness, pain) appear. As more complement components, fibronectin, PMN, and macrophages accumulate at the inflammatory site, they release more cytokines that promote further chemotaxis, inflammation, and enhanced microbicidal activity.

A number of other phenemona, of uncertain import, also occur as part of the acute phase reaction. Zinc levels decrease. This metal, which has no known tissue stores, enhances lymphocyte responsiveness, aids wound healing, and participates in protein synthesis.[37] Zinc plays a crucial role in regulation of DNA transcription and RNA translation. Its decrease in infection may reflect its increased use by actively metabolizing cells.

Ceruloplasmin, a superoxide scavenging, copper-binding protein synthesized by hepatocytes, also increases during the acute phase response under the influence of IL-6. The consequences of this increase for the host are not known.

IMPAIRMENT AND EXAGGERATION OF NONSPECIFIC IMMUNITY

Impaired natural immunity, most conveniently detected by testing for cutaneous delayed hypersensitivity, can occur as a consequence of numerous illnesses. In the United States, end-stage cancer, renal disease, end-stage human immunodeficiency virus (HIV) infection (AIDS), liver disease, and alcoholism are the most common underlying illnesses resulting in diminished cellular immune responsiveness. Worldwide, malnutrition is the leading cause of increased susceptibility to and severity of several infections. These include life-threatening bacterial infections of the middle ear, pervasive dental caries, and common childhood infections, especially measles and HIV.[38,38a]

Aging

Although the data regarding aging are confusing and sometimes conflicting, this process has many important effects on the immune system that can be best summarized as immunosenescence. Superimposed and interrelated with this generalized impairment are social isolation and age-related decrements in organ structure and function. Regardless of the setting, there is a higher incidence of pneumonias, cholangitis, diverticulitis, bacteremia, asymptomatic bacteriuria, urinary tract infections, reactivation of varicella-zoster virus and tuberculosis, and even bacterial endocarditis.[39] In general, cellular immunity is decremented most severely with aging[40] and includes both functional and quantitative cell counts.[41,42]

Stress

A growing body of evidence demonstrates a relationship between stress and immune function.[43,44]

Hormones

Increased adrenocorticotropic hormone production occurs during the acute phase response and appears to augment the host's survival potential. The depressive effect of excess corticosteroids on inflammation are well known. Estrogen affects the lining of the vagina, resulting in increased nonspecific resistance. Cellular immunity declines during pregnancy, which may account for the severity of certain infections, such as poliomyelitis, group A β-hemolytic streptococci, and N. gonorrhoeae particularly in the third trimester.[45]

Dysregulation

The initial nonspecific response is usually quite effective in controlling microbial invasion. With overwhelming infection and release of large amounts of microbial products, however, failure of feedback control may lead to the catastrophic syndrome of septic shock. In addition, if infections are not controlled and become chronic, some acute derangements (e.g., decreased serum albumin, iron sequestration) become profound. Prolonged infection also results in muscle wasting, which may be clearly evident within days.

REFERENCES

1. Mackowiak PA. The normal microbial flora. N Engl J Med. 1982;307:83–6.
2. Tazume S, Ozawa A, Yamamoto T, et al. Ecological study on the intestinal bacterial flora of patients with diarrhea. Clin Infect Dis 1993;16(2):S77–82.
3. Stiehm ER, Sztein MB, Steeg PS, et al. Deficient antigen expression on human cord blood monocytes. Reversal with lymphokines. Clin Immunol Immunopathol. 1984;30:430–6.
4. Moore WEC, Burmeister JA, Brooke CW, et al. Investigation of the influences on puberty, genetics and environment on the composition of subgingival periodontal flora. Infect Immun. 1993;61:2891–8.
5. Beachey EH. Bacterial adherence: Adhesion–receptor interactions mediating the attachment of bacteria to mucosal surfaces. J Infect Dis. 1981;143:325.
6. Ramirez-Ronda CH, Fuxench-Lopez Z, Nevarez M. Increased pharyngeal bacterial colonization during viral illness. Arch Intern Med. 1981;141:1599.
7. Svanburg-Eden C, Jodal V. Attachment of E. coli to urinary sediment epithelial cells from urinary tract infection prone to healthy children. Infect Immun. 1979;26:837.
8. Kaslow RA, Shaw S. The role of histocompatibility antigens (HLA) in infection. Epidemiol Rev. 1981;3:90.
9. Whisnant JK, Rogentine N, Gradmick MA, et al. Host factors and antibody response to Haemophilus influenzae type b meningitidis and epiglottitis. J Infect Dis. 1976;133:488.
10. Van Eden W, de Vries RRP, Mehra NK, et al. HLA segregation of tuberculoid leprosy: Confirmation of the DR2 marker. J Infect Dis. 1980;141:693.
11. Sasazuki I, Hayose R, Wanto I, et al. HLA and acute poststreptococcal glomerulonephritis. N Engl J Med. 1979;301:1184.
12. Zander H, Gross-Wilde H, Kuntz B, et al. HLA-A, -B, and -D antigens in paralytic poliomyelitis. Tissue Antigens. 1979;13:310.
12a. Kaslow RA, Duquesnox R, VanRaden M, et al. A1, Cw7, B8, DR3 HLA antigen combination associated with rapid decline of T-helper lymphocytes in HIV-1 infection. Lancet. 1990;335:927–30.
13. Schneerson R, Robbins JB. Induction of serum Haemophilus influenzae type b capsular antibodies in adult volunteers fed cross reacting Escherichia coli 075:K100:H5. N Engl J Med. 1975;292:1093.
14. Griffiss JM. Bactericidal activity by IgA of lytic antibody in human convalescent sera. J Immunol. 1975;114:1779.
15. Weinberg ED. Iron withholdings: A defense against infection and neoplasia. Physiol Rev. 1984;64:65–102.
16. Green GM. In defense of the lung. Am Rev Respir Dis. 1970;102:691.
17. Israde V, Darabi A, McCracken GH. The role of bacterial virulence factors and Tamm-Horsfall protein in the pathogenesis of E. coli urinary tract infections in infants. Am J Dis Child. 1993;147:1230–4.
18. Colten HR. Tissue-specific regulation of inflammation. J Appl Physiol. 1992;72:1–7.
19. Vandaux P, Didier P, Haeberli A, et al. Fibronectin is more active than fibrin or fibrinogen in promoting S. aureus adherence to inserted intravascular catheters. J Infect Dis. 1993;167:633–41.
20. Van Oss CJ, Gillman CF. Phagocytosis as a surface phenomenon. I. Contact angles and phagocytosis of nonopsonized bacteria. J Reticuloendothel Soc. 1972;12:283.
21. Proctor RA. Fibronectin: A brief overview of its structure, function, and physiology. Rev Infect Dis. 1984;9:S317–21.
22. Boman HG. Antibacterial peptides: Key components needed in immunity. Cell 1991;65:205–7.
23. Vaara M. Agents that increase the permeability of the outer membrane. Microbiol Rev. 1992;56:395–411.
24. Huber AR, Kunkel SL, Todd RFI, Weiss SJ. Regulation of transendothelial neutrophil migration by endogenous IL-8. 1991;254:99–102.
25. Romagnani S. Induction of TH1 and TH2 responses: A key role for the "natural" immune response? Immunol Today. 1992;13:379–81.
26. Scott P. IL-12: Initiation cytokine for cell-mediated immunity. 1993;260:196–7.
26a. Minty A, Chalon P, Derocq JM, et al. Interleukin-13 is a new human lymphokine regulating inflammatory and immune responses. Nature. 1993;362:248–50.
27. Sher A, Gazzinelli RT, Oswald IP, et al. Role of T-cell derived cytokines in the downregulation of immune responses in parasitic and retroviral infection. Immunol Rev. 1992;127:183–204.
28. Sullivan GW, Mandell GL. The role of cytokines in infection. Curr Opin Infect Dis. 1991;4:344–9.
29. Dinarello CA, Endogenous pyrogens: The role of cytokines in the pathogenesis of fever. In: Mackowiak P, ed. Fever: Basic Mechanisms and Management. New York: Raven Press, 1991:23–47.
29a. Dinarello CA, Wolff SM. The role of interleukin-1 in disease. N Engl J Med. 1993;328:106–113.
30. Wright SD, Ramos RA, Tobias PT, et al. CD14, a receptor for complexes of lipopolysaccharide (LPS) and LPS binding protein. Science. 1990;249:1431–3.
31. Heinrich PC, Castell JV, and Andus T. Interleukin-6 and the acute phase response. Biochem J. 1990;265:621–36.
32. Ward CG. Influence of iron on infection. Am J Surg. 1986;151:291–5.
33. Hamilton JA. Colony stimulating factors, cytokines and monocyte-macrophages—Some controversies. Immunol Today. 1993;14:18–24.
34. Thompson HL, Matsushima K. Human polymorphonuclear leucocytes stimulated by tumour necrosis factor alpha show increased adherence to extracellular matrix proteins which is mediated via the CD11b/18 complex. Clin Exp Immunol. 1992;90:280–5.
35. Thiery JP, Boyer B. The junction between cytokines and cell adhesion. Curr Opin Cell Biol. 1992;4:782–92.
36. Bevilacqua MP, Nelson RM. Selectins. J Clin Invest. 1993;91:379–87.
37. Keen CL, Gershwin ME. Zinc deficiency and immune function. Annu Rev Nutr. 1990;10:415–31.
38. Corman LC. The relationship between nutrition, infection, and immunity. Med Clin North Am. 1985;69:519–31.
38a. Semba RD, Graham NMH, Caiatta WT, et al. Increased mortality associated with vitamin A deficiency during HIV type 1 infection. Arch Int Med. 1993;153:2149–54.
39. Yoshikawa TT, Norman DC: Aging and Clinical Practice; Infectious Diseases, Diagnosis, and Treatment. Igaku-Shoin: New York, 1987.
40. Saltzman RL, Peterson PK. Immunodeficiency of the elderly. Rev Infect Dis. 1987;1127–39.
41. Bender BS, Nagel JE, Adler WH, et al: Absolute peripheral blood lymphocyte count and subsequent morality in elderly men: The Baltimore longitudinal study of aging. J Am Geriatr Soc. 1986;34:649–54.
42. Powers DC, Belshe RB. Effects of age in cytotoxic lymphocyte memory as well as serum and local antibody responses elicited by inactivated influenza virus vaccine. J Infect Dis. 1993;167:584–92.
43. Cohen S, Tyrrell DAJ, Smith AP. Psychological stress and susceptibility to the common cold. N Engl J Med. 1991;325:606–12.
44. Peterson PK, Chao CC, Moliter T, et al. Stress and pathogenesis of infectious disease. Rev Infect Dis. 1991;13:710–12.
45. Weinberg ED. Pregnancy-associated depression of cell-mediated immunity. Rev Infect Dis. 1984;6:814–31.

5. ANTIBODIES

FREDERICK P. HEINZEL

Antibodies are complex glycoprotein immunoglobulins that can bind specifically to a wide variety of protein or polysaccharide antigens. Once bound to antigen, the antibody can elicit focused cellular and molecular responses important in antimicrobial immunity. In conjunction with the complement system, antibodies are the major effector molecules of humoral immunity, and their presence in the circulation or on mucosal surfaces defines acquired resistance against many infectious agents. Two critical functions are encoded within the structure of the immunoglobulin molecule. The amino-terminal end of the molecule contains the variable (or V) region that defines the antigen recognition site and that is provided from a repertoire of up to 10^8 possible amino acid sequences with distinct antigen-binding specificities. The relatively conserved carboxy-terminal portion of the molecule belongs to one of nine structural classes and subclasses that define the *isotype* of the immunoglobulin (i.e., IgD, IgM, IgG$_{1-4}$, IgA$_{1-2}$, or IgE). Each immunoglobulin isotype possesses distinct functional attributes that are specialized for coping with various biologic tasks. In particular, the class-specific structure of the immunoglobulin determines the efficiency with which it can activate complement and leukocyte responses or distribute throughout different anatomic compartments.

Antibodies are produced by B lymphocytes (or B cells) that express surface-bound immunoglobulins of a single specificity. When these antigen receptors are engaged by the appropriate ligand, the B cell proliferates and begins to secrete soluble antibodies directed against the target molecule. B cells additionally function as antigen-presenting cells that can assist in T-lymphocyte-mediated immune responses (further defined in Ch. 8). Antibody responses are essential for the cure and prevention of many bacteria and viral infections. However, antibodies also may contribute to the immunopathology of infectious diseases when they manifest as immune complexes or autoantibodies. Inherited or acquired defects in any of these B lymphocyte functions can be associated with clinically significant immunodeficiencies that predispose to frequent severe infections as a result of antibody underproduction. The significant benefit for these patients that follows transfusion with immunoglobulin preparations further illustrates the clinical importance of the antibody system.

IMMUNOGLOBULINS

Structure and Chemistry

All classes of immunoglobulin have the same basic molecular structure, consisting of two identical peptide heterodimers

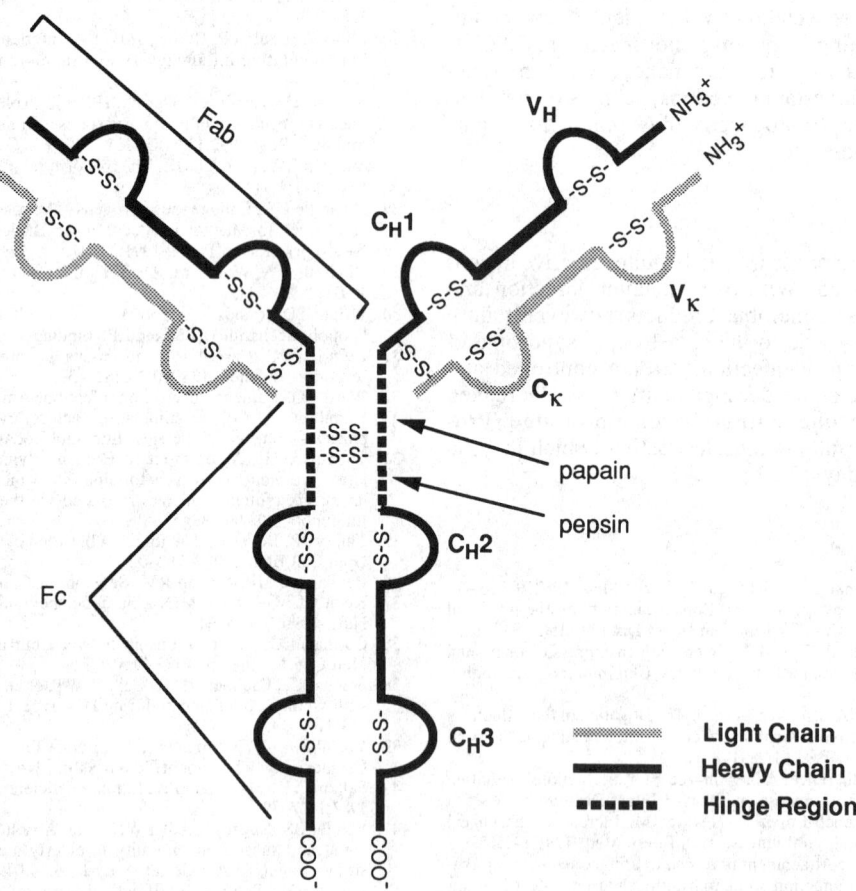

FIG. 1. Schematic illustration demonstrating the structure of an IgG molecule. Two γ heavy chains and two κ light chains (shown as black or gray lines) are linked together by disulfide bonds (−S−S−). Individual domains are designated as V$_H$ and V$_\kappa$ for variable domains, and C$_H$1−3 and C$_\kappa$ for the three constant domains of the heavy chain and one constant domain of the light chain. The antigen-binding site is defined by the combination of V$_H$ and V$_\kappa$ sequences and is contained within the Fab fragment released upon digestion by papain (indicated by the arrow). Also shown is the Fc portion of the molecule involved in activation of both the complement cascade and leukocyte Fc receptors. The heavy chain hinge region is shown as cross-hatched line. IgE and IgM each contain an additional C$_H$4 domain.

linked by disulfide bonds. Each heterodimer consists of a *heavy chain* and a *light chain*, also joined by disulfide bridges (Fig. 1). Both chains are further subdivided into two to five structurally related peptide *domains* of approximately 110 amino acids, each domain containing one intrachain disulfide bond. The domain closest to the amino terminus of both heavy and light chains consists of framework peptide sequences interspersed with three hypervariable regions, stretches of 10–12 amino acid residues with markedly variant sequences. Light and heavy chain variable domains (V_L and V_H, respectively) jointly form a quaternary structure that defines the antigen-binding site of the fully assembled antibody.[1] Since the basic immunoglobulin molecule is composed of two H + L heterodimers, antibodies are bivalent for antigen binding.

In addition to the one variable domain, heavy chains possess a *constant region* composed of three to four constant domains (C_H1, C_H2, C_H3, and C_H4). Within the constant region are peptide segments that determine the ability of the intact antibody to mediate important biologic functions following antigen binding.[2] Each H-chain constant region is the product of distinct genes that define the class of immunoglobulin produced and that are identified by Greek letters (i.e., δ, μ, γ, α, ϵ). The number and location of inter-heavy chain disulfide bridges vary in different immunoglobulin class. However, disulfide linkages between heavy chains at the IgG C_H1 or IgM C_H2 site define a region with varying degrees of molecular flexibility called the immunoglobulin *hinge*. This structure determines rotation and flexion, or the variable reach of the antigen-binding regions around the heavy chain stem. Immunoglobulin isotypes differ markedly in hinge region length and flexibility, suggesting that this may correlate with their disparate abilities to activate effector functions.[3]

Enzymatic cleavage of immunoglobulins has provided insights into the functional organization of the immunoglobulin molecule. Papain cleaves immunoglobulins proximal to the inter-heavy chain disulfide bond(s), generating three fragments. Two, referred to as *Fab* fragments, are identical, bind to antigen, but cannot activate complement or leukocyte Fc receptors (Fig. 1). A third crystallizable, or *Fc*, fragment does not bind antigen, but retains the ability to activate effector functions. Fab fragments are heterodimers composed of intact light chains covalently joined via disulfide bond to the variable (V_H) and first constant (C_H1) domains of the adjacent heavy chain. Each Fab fragment contains one antigen-binding site for a single antigenic determinant. The portion of the antigen recognized by the Fab fragment is referred to as the antigenic *epitope*; the complementary structure of the Fab binding site is called the antibody *para-*

tope. Structural analysis of Fab–antigen complexes have revealed much about the mechanism by which antibody binds antigen. Both heavy and light chains generate a polypeptide pocket bounded by V_H and V_L hypervariable loops into which the antigenic epitope fits by virtue of complementary molecular charge, size, and conformation. Rather than being a strictly "lock and key" fit, conformational changes can occur also during binding to provide an "induced fit."[4] The enzyme pepsin cleaves immunoglobulins on the carboxy-terminal side of the inter-H-chain disulfide bridge to generate a single large F(ab')$_2$ fragment consisting of two Fab fragments linked together by their H-chains. As with monovalent Fab fragments, F(ab')$_2$ molecules also bind antigens with affinities similar to the parent molecule, but lack the constant region domains required for activation of effector functions.

The Fc portion release by enzymatic cleavage is a homodimer composed of disulfide-linked heavy chains, truncated to include only the two to three domains closest to the carboxy terminus of the protein (Fig. 1). It is this region of the molecule that interacts with C1q to activate the complement system or that binds to defined immunoglobulin receptors on the surface of immune effector cells (referred to as Fc receptors). Amino acid sequences within the IgG C_H2 and C_H3 domains define the C1q and Fc receptor-binding sites; immunoglobulin isotypes that are poor activators of these effector systems do not possess these sequences or contain steric impediments that block access to these sites.[5,6] Membrane-spanning domains may be added to the carboxy terminus of the heavy chain by alternative splicing of precursor RNA, thus providing a mechanism for producing immunoglobulin that is either anchored to the surface of the B cell to act as an antigen receptor or released as a soluble antibody.[7] IgM and IgA also contain additional carboxy-terminal sequences that are recognition sites for J-chain cross-linking and polymerization.

Immunoglobulin Classes

Five immunoglobulin classes, defined by their heavy chain composition, have been identified that share the basic structure discussed above.[8–11] Molecular differences include disparities in size, charge, and association into antibody multimers (Table 1). IgG and IgA classes are further divided into subclasses that are derived from distinct heavy chain genes. Each heavy chain gene product gives rise to a different immunoglobulin isotype. Allelic differences within each heavy chain locus also result in serologically recognizable *allotypes*. There are two classes of light chains, the κ and λ proteins, encoded by a single

TABLE 1. Selected Molecular and Functional Properties of Human Immunoglobulins

	IgG	IgA	IgM	IgD	IgE
Basic structure	Monomer	Monomer/dimer	Pentamer	Monomer	Monomer
Molecular weight	150,000	160,000/400,000	900,000	180,000	190,000
Molecular formula	γ_2L_2	$\alpha_2L_2/(\alpha_2L_2)2$, SC, J	$(\mu_2L_2)_5$J	δ_2L_2	ϵ_2L_2
Mean serum concentration in mg/dL (range)	989 (600–1,600)	200 (60–330)	120 (45–150)	Trace	Trace
	IgG$_1$ 670–1,050				
	IgG$_2$ 250–420				
	IgG$_3$ 54–100				
	IgG$_4$ 38–67				
Serum T$_{1/2}$ (days)	23	6	5	3	2
Complement activation					
Classical pathway (C1q binding)	+ +	0	+ + + +	0	0
Alternative pathway	+	+	+	+	+
Opsonic activity (FcR binding)	+ + + +	+ +	0	0	0
Reaginic activity	0	0	0	0	+ + + +
Functions as antigen receptor on B-cell surface	+	±	+ + + +	+ + + +	±

Abbreviations: L, light chain (either λ or κ); SC, secretory component; J, J chain.

(Adapted from Stites et al.,[270] with permission.)

Cκ locus and four distinct Cλ genes. Only a single class of light chain is expressed during the life span of each B-cell clone. Although all the heavy chain classes can associate with either κ or λ peptides, the ratio of actual useage of κ to λ is about 7 to 3.

IgM. IgM is present in the serum as a 950-kD pentameric immunoglobulin. IgM can also be expressed as a transmembrane monomer on the surface of B cells, where it functions as an antigen receptor capable of transducing activating signals when bound to antigen. The IgM heavy chain consists of four constant domains, and the C_H4 domain at the carboxy-terminus contains an 18 amino acid extension required for polymerization. Each IgM member of the pentamer is covalently linked to the others, either by direct intermolecular disulfide bonds or by indirect attachments through a 15-kD polypeptide called the J-chain (Fig. 2).[12] The J-chain is cosynthesized by the IgM-secreting B cell

and is necessary for IgM polymerization, a process catalyzed by a sulfhydryl oxidase on the surface of these cells.[13]

IgM is the first class of immunoglobulin synthesized by infants and is also the first isotype to appear following an immune response to new antigen.[14] Although the affinity of each IgM monomer for antigen is usually less than that of IgG, the pentameric structure of IgM may compensate for this deficiency by increasing the total number of antigen–antibody interactions. Pentavalent binding also assists in complement activation and in the aggregation of antigen or microbes. These virtues of the IgM molecule make it an important first response to microbial infection until IgG with higher affinity and more specialized function can be generated.

IgM usually constitutes only 10 percent of serum immunoglobulins. Much of the circulating IgM consists of low-affinity antibody against common environmental determinants, including phosphocholine, dextrans, and other polysaccharide deter-

IgM Pentamer

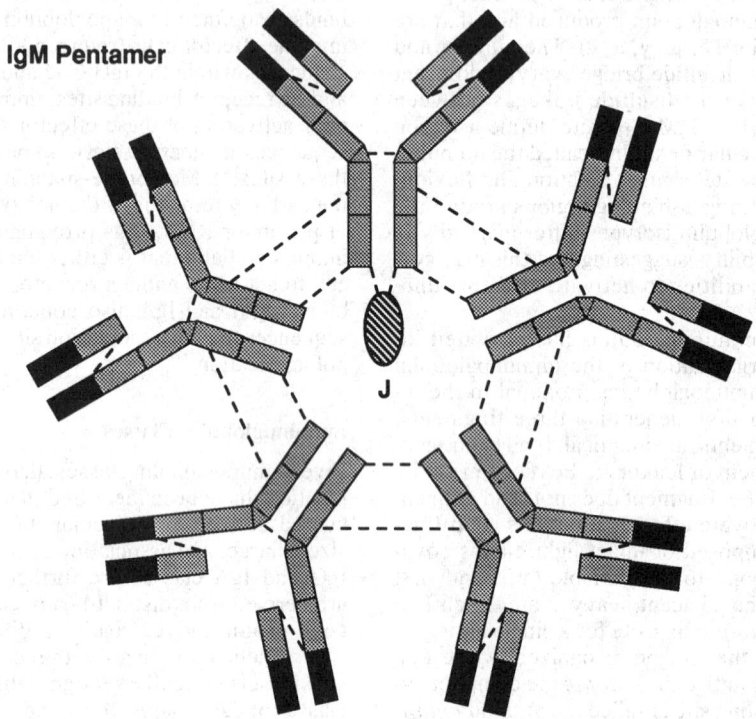

IgA Dimer

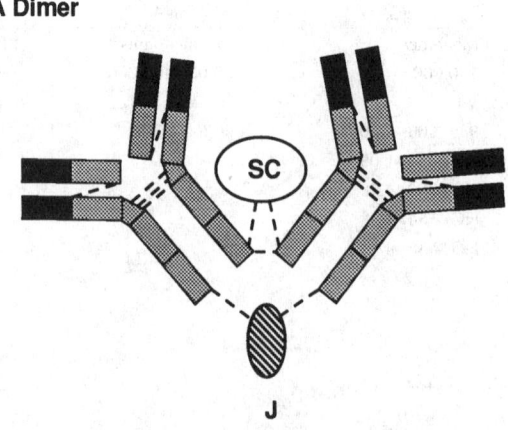

FIG. 2.   Schematic illustration of the molecular structure of an IgM pentamer and an IgA dimer. Individual immunoglobulins are joined to each other through intermolecular disulfide bonds, as shown by dashed lines. Similar disulfide linkages attach the J chain (J) or the secretory component (SC) to the antibody multimers. Constant domains are shown in gray and variable domains in black.

minants.[15] These include blood type—specific isohemagglutin antibodies, probably generated in response to cross-reactive carbohydrate determinants provided by exposure to common environmental proteins or gastrointestinal bacteria.

IgD. IgD is a 175-kD protein produced as a monomer. The greater size of the IgD molecule compared with IgG reflects the possession of an especially long hinge region. IgD is not abundant in the serum, constituting less than 0.2 percent of serum immunoglobulins. Instead, most of the IgD synthesized is expressed as surface-bound antigen receptor on B cells. Membrane IgD can be anchored to the cell surface either via a hydrophobic transmembrane peptide domain or via a glycosophosphoinositol linkage synthesized after peptide translation.[16]

IgG. IgG is the most abundant immunoglobulin in the serum of normal adults, providing 75 percent of the total immunoglobulin mass, and is more broadly distributed through tissues than are other isotypes. IgG crosses the placenta and provides much of the maternal antibody present during the first 6 months of life. IgG is also prevalent in the lower respiratory tract and appears at mucosal sites during exudative responses.[17] The four subclasses of IgG are each encoded by a different $C\gamma$ heavy chain gene consisting of three C_H domains. The different IgG isotypes vary in abundance ($IgG_1 > IgG_2 > IgG_3 > IgG_4$) and possess distinct functional capabilities. IgG_3 and IgG_1 both fix complement well, although several IgG molecules are required to provide the multivalent binding required for activation of C1q. IgG_1 and IgG_3, but not IgG_2 and IgG_4, can bind and activate leukocyte Fc receptors for IgG. Despite the relative inability of IgG_2 to activate Fc receptor–mediated functions, IgG_2 may activate complement if bound on microbial surfaces in high concentration.[18] In adults, IgG_2 is the predominant isotype generated with specificity for dense polysaccharide determinants on encapsulated bacteria.[19] Genetic or cellular deficiencies leading to defective IgG_2 production are sometimes associated with an increased frequency and severity of infections caused by *Streptococcus pneumoniae* and *Haemophilus influenzae*.[20–22] IgG_4 is the least abundant isotype in the serum and has the least functional capability. Specifically, the short, inflexible hinge region of IgG_4 may result in steric hindrance by the Fab arms of the complement-fixing motif in C_H2.[6] IgG_4 is often produced in concert with IgE, leading to speculation that IgG_4 can block IgE interactions with antigen and the IgE Fc receptor.[23]

IgA. IgA is present as either a 160-kD monomer or a 400-kD dimer, with heavy chains provided by either the IgA_1 or IgA_2 genes.[24–26] Each heavy chain consists of three constant domains; the C_H3 domain contains the peptide sequence necessary for polymerization via J-chain (Fig. 2). Although IgA constitutes only about 15 percent of total serum immunoglobulins, its serum half-life is shortened relative to IgG, and IgA production actually exceeds that of IgG (66 vs. 30 mg/kg/day).[27] Generally, IgA_1 is produced in the bone marrow and provides most of the IgA present in the serum, 80 percent of which is monomeric. In contrast, both IgA_1 and IgA_2 are produced in the gut-associated lymphoid tissue as homodimeric molecules that can be secreted onto the mucosal surfaces.[28] Some IgA is polymerized beyond the dimer stage.

Transport of dimeric IgA from the intestinal submucosa to the lumen of the gut is mediated by a unique receptor-linked mechanism. A 100-kD peptide, called the *secretory component*, is expressed as an integral membrane protein on the basolateral surface of epithelial cells and serves as a receptor for dimeric IgA.[27,29] Engagement of the secretory component receptor by IgA induces endocytosis, transcytoplasmic transport, and release of the immunoglobulin from the apical cellular surface into the mucosal lumen. During this process, the secretory component receptor is cleaved, and the IgA retains a piece of this covalently linked peptide. IgM can be transported similarly and constitutes a minor population of secretory antibodies.[25,30] Recently, secretory component–mediated IgA transport was identified as responsible for a shift in the cellular tropism of Epstein-Barr virus from B lymphocytes to the nasopharyngeal epithelium following extensive coating of the virus with IgA.[31] IgA bound to antigen can also be transported through epithelial tissues by secretory component, and this may be a mechanism for disposal of submucosal antigen and viral particles.[32]

Secretory IgA is the predominant immunoglobulin present in the gastrointestinal fluids, nasal secretions, saliva, tears, and other mucous secretions of the body, where it provides an important host defense against infection entering via enteric or respiratory routes.[24] Colostrum is an especially abundant source of IgA, and the passive contribution of this maternal antibody to breast-fed infants may be responsible for their lower incidence of infection compared with formula-fed children.[33] Although secretory IgA does not activate complement well (nor are complement proteins abundant on mucosal surfaces), IgA can neutralize toxin activity and disrupt adherence of pathogens to mucosal cellular receptors. Passive protection mediated by IgA has been described in models of viral, bacterial, and protozoan infection.[34–36] Fc receptors capable of initiating phagocytosis of IgA-coated microorganisms have been recognized on neutrophils and monocytes derived from the pulmonary mucosa.[37] This suggests a broader role for mucosal IgA in mediating opsonophagocytosis. Although IgA is resistant to digestion by gastrointestinal proteases, some bacteria have evolved IgA-specific proteases that may confer a survival advantage to the pathogen.[38]

Another important function of IgA may be to mask commonly encountered dietary or environmental peptides and thereby avoid undesirable inflammatory responses mediated by T-cell responses or by other antibody isotypes.[39] The relative inability of IgA to activate proinflammatory effector mechanisms would allow these antigens to be sequestered without deleterious consequences.[40] This form of "antigenic exclusion" of dietary proteins may account for the increased frequency of autoimmune or allergic diseases in patients with IgA deficiencies.[41,42]

IgE. IgE is a 190-kD immunoglobulin composed of ϵ heavy chains containing four constant domains. Although present in low abundance in the serum, IgE can be expressed on the cell surface of mast cells and basophils through noncovalent binding to high-affinity IgE Fc receptors.[43] Immediate-type hypersensitivity, or reaginic, responses are triggered when cytophilic IgE encounters antigen and activates cellular degranulation and the synthesis of eicosanoid and peptide mediators of hypersensitivity (see discussion under IgE Fc Receptors, below). These potentially deleterious reactions presumably subserve some host defense role that remains poorly defined. The expulsion of gastrointestinal nematodes mediated by the peristaltic and exudative effects of mast cell degranulation has been suggested as one protective role for IgE. Consistent with this, elevated IgE serum levels and tissue mastocytosis develop during intestinal infection with worms.[44,45] Epidemiologic evidence has also pointed to a direct correlation between elevated IgE levels and decreased reinfection rates with *Schistosoma haematobium*. Increased levels of IgG_4, IgG_2, and IgM that may block IgE interaction with antigen were associated with more frequent reinfection.[46] The protective effects of IgE in this disease may be mediated in part by IgE-directed antibody-dependent cellular cytotoxicity (ADCC; reviewed by Capron and Dessaint[47]). Putative effector cells in this response include monocytes, eosinophils, and platelets bearing the low-affinity IgE Fc receptor (FcεRII). However, this may not be true for all helminthic infections, as in vivo neutralization of IgE does not prevent recovery from experimental infection with worms that dwell in the gut lumen.[48]

Distribution and Catabolism of Antibodies

Concentrations of different immunoglobulin isotypes in the serum reflect disparate rates of synthesis and catabolism unique to each class of antibody (Table 1). Human immunoglobulins are synthesized at estimated rates of 66 mg/kg/day for IgA, 30 mg/kg/day for IgG, and 2 mg/kg/day for IgM. IgE and IgD are produced at even lower rates. Due to differing rates of catabolism, immunoglobulin half-lives do not correlate strictly with these rates of synthesis; half-lives are 21 days for IgG, 6 days for IgA, 5 days for IgM, and 3 days for IgE and IgD.[49] Diseases that affect catabolic and/or synthetic rates of these proteins can sometimes lead to detectable immunoglobulin deficiencies (discussed under Immunoglobulin and Antibody Deficiency States, below). The catabolic rate of IgG seems to be directly proportional to its own concentration within the serum, perhaps accounting for the increased clearance of nonmalignant antibodies in patients with paraproteinemias. Possession of an intact Fc portion protects against degradation, Fab fragments of antibody being rapidly cleared. It has been proposed that saturable receptors for immunoglobulin are present in the body that act to prevent degradation or that high concentrations of antibody promote the formation of IgG aggregates that are then cleared from the circulation.[50]

IgG and IgA are the most widely distributed of the immunoglobulins throughout different anatomic compartments. Only 50 percent of total IgG and IgA are present in the circulation, whereas 75 percent of IgM and IgD remain serum associated. IgG is the only class of immunoglobulin capable of crossing placental barriers and thus provides much of the maternal antibodies present during neonatal life. Although IgA is the major immunoglobulin present at mucosal sites, IgG is actually present in greater concentrations in the lower respiratory tract and, in the presence of IgA deficiency, secretory IgM may replace IgA on mucosal surfaces.[17,30]

Immunoglobulin Fc Receptor

Cellular Fc receptors are transmembrane protein complexes that bind to the Fc portion of immunoglobulin and activate cell-specific functions (Table 2).[51] Fc receptors are specific for individual immunoglobulin classes; those that bind to IgA, IgE, and IgG are designated as FcαR, FcεR, and FcγR, respectively. The receptor subunits responsible for recognition and binding of different immunoglobulin Fc regions are related members of a gene family with highly conserved extracellular immunoglobulin binding domains and richly diverse cytoplasmic sequences capable of mediating a wide variety of cellular functions.[52] Accessory molecules necessary for receptor complex assembly and signal transduction are often shared between different Fc receptors. These may include ζ homodimers normally present in the T-cell receptor complex.[53] In contrast, the low-affinity receptor for IgE (FcεRII) is genetically distinct, being related to animal lectin receptors.[54] Whatever their specificity, Fc receptors may mediate similar types of cell responses, including degranulation, phagocytosis, uptake of immune complexes, cytokine generation, and synthesis of eicosanoid and amine inflammatory mediators. However, the variety of Fc receptors expressed suggests a degree of specialization providing for distinct antibody-mediated effector responses in different cells.

IgG Fc Receptors. IgG$_1$ and IgG$_3$ induce phagocytosis of coated particles by neutrophils, monocytes, and macrophages, either by interacting as monomers with high-affinity FcγRI receptors or as multivalent complexes with low-affinity FcγRII and FcγRIII receptors (reviewed by Ravetch and Kinet[52]). IgG$_2$ and IgG$_4$ do not participate significantly in FcγR engagement. Phagocytosis mediated by FcγR triggers important microbicidal responses in granulocytes and macrophages, including activation of the oxidative burst[55] and generation of proinflammatory monokines.[56] Although FcγRII is also present on B lymphocytes, the cytoplasmic portion of this receptor is truncated and cannot mediate phagocytosis.[52] The B-cell receptor isoform may instead inhibit cellular responses when engaged by immune complexes, presumably providing a form of feedback inhibition during states of antibody excess.[57] Transmembrane FcγRIII on natural killer (NK) cells and macrophages can trigger ADCC; cross-linking of FcγRIII on NK cells additionally elicits γ-interferon (γ-IFN) production that may assist in control of infection.[58,59] Granulocyte FcγRIII is attached to the cell surface by phosphoinositolglycan anchors. Since this may disrupt the usual mechanisms for signal transduction, the function of this receptor is not well understood.[60]

IgE Fc Receptors. The high-affinity receptor for IgE (FcεRI) is expressed on mast cells and basophils (for review, see Metzger et al.[43]). As with other FC receptors, FcεRI is a transmembrane protein multimer consisting of an IgE-binding α-chain associated with β- and γ-chains essential for assembly and signal transduction.[61] Because of the high affinity for its ligand, receptors capture and stably display monomeric IgE. Cellular functions are activated when this cytophilic IgE is cross-linked by antigen. Activated mast cells discharge granule contents containing preformed vasoactive amine and eicosanoid mediators that mediate the clinical manifestations of urticaria, anaphylaxis, and asthma—or *reaginic* responses. Mast cells and basophils activated by IgE receptor cross-linking also generate cytokines, such as interleukin (IL)-4, IL-3, IL-5, and granulocyte macrophage colony-stimulating factor (GM-CSF) that may influence T-cell and B-cell responses developing at the time of mast cell activation.[62]

Low-affinity IgE receptors (FcεRII) are expressed on IL-4–stimulated B cells and many other leukocytic cells. Binding of IgE–antigen complexes to the receptor results in endocytosis and may lead to antigen processing with presentation of peptides

TABLE 2. Immunoglobulin Fc Receptors: Distribution and Function

Type	Cellular Distribution	Function
IgG Fc receptors		
FcγRI (high affinity) CD64	Monocytes, activated neutrophils	Antibody-dependent cytotoxicity (ADCC), phagocytosis, cell degranulation
FcγRII (low affinity) CD32	Monocytes, neutrophils, eosinophils, B lymphocytes, platelets	Endocytosis of immune complexes, ADCC, phagocytosis, cell degranulation, superoxide anion generation; the B-cell isoform inhibits immunoglobulin production
FcγRIII (low affinity) CD16	Macrophages, neutrophils, NK cells	Phagocytosis, removal of immune complexes, ADCC, cytokine generation
IgE Fc receptors		
FcεRI (high affinity)	Mast cells, basophils	Degranulation, leukotriene production, cytokine production
FcεRII (low affinity) CD23	Eosinophils, T and B lymphocytes, macrophages, platelets	Antigen uptake, phagocytosis, ADCC
IgA Fc receptors		
FcαR	Macrophages, granulocytes	Phagocytosis, superoxide anion production

to T cells.[63] Alternatively, spliced variants of FcεRII are expressed on macrophages, platelets, and eosinophils and can trigger phagocytosis, degranulation, and ADCC. This response has been suggested to protect against reinfection by *Schistosoma haematobium*.[47]

IgA Fc Receptor.   Part of the protective effect of IgA at mucosal surfaces may be mediated by enhanced phagocytosis of IgA-coated microbial pathogens. Mucosal macrophages and granulocytes, particularly in the lung, express a receptor for monomeric and dimeric IgA that was cloned and identified as a relative of IgG Fc receptors.[64] Engagement of this receptor triggers both phagocytosis and generation of superoxide.[65]

ANTIMICROBIAL FUNCTIONS OF ANTIBODIES

Complement Activation

The classical pathway of complement is activated when multiple sites on the hexameric C1q initiator molecule are engaged by the Fc regions of IgG and IgM. Defined peptide sequences within the C_H2 domains of IgG_1 and IgG_3 or the C_H3 domain of IgM are required for this noncovalent association.[2] Aggregation of IgG on a microbial surface is a prerequisite for complement fixation by this pathway, as immobilized IgG binds C1q with 10,000-fold increased affinity compared with soluble IgG.[66] Although pentameric IgM more readily activates complement when present at lower densities than does monomeric IgG, binding of IgM to substrate also is required for complement activation. This apparently reflects structural changes in the Fc region that interact with C1q, thereby preventing inappropriate activation by soluble antibody.[67] IgG_2 is less capable of C1q binding, although it may be effective when presented in high local concentrations, as would be expected when it binds to densely clustered polysaccharide determinants on encapsulated bacteria.[18] In contrast, IgG_4, IgE, and IgA do not have significant C1q-binding activities.

Activation of complement on bacterial cell surfaces mediates both lytic and opsonizing activities important in the resolution of infection.[68] Opsonizing antibodies of this sort have been identified during infection with pneumonococcus, *Streptococcus pyogenes*, *H. influenzae*, and *Staphylococcus aureus*.[69-72] Further discussion of the complement cascade and the role of complement products in inflammation is given in Chapter 6. Although the alternative pathway of complement activation is typically defined by its antibody-independent nature, aggregates of immunoglobulin may facilitate the generation of C3 convertase by providing a favorable glycosylated substrate.[73,74]

Phagocytosis

All three classes of IgG Fc receptors can efficiently mediate phagocytosis of antibody-coated particles by neutrophils, macrophages, and monocytes.[55,75,76] This process is generally limited to organisms coated with IgG_1 and/or IgG_3, although IgA opsonizes microbes for ingestion via FcαR-mediated uptake by mucosal phagocytes.[65] Although FcR interactions alone are sufficient to mediate phagocytosis, in most cases efficient ingestion of encapsulated bacteria will require coating with both antibody and complement.[72,77] The respective roles of Fc receptors and complement receptors in opsonophagocytosis are addressed in Chapters 6 and 7. Cross-linking of FcγR and FcαR may also trigger an oxidative burst and the release of proinflammatory mediators, such as IL-1, tumor necrosis factor (TNF), and eicosanoids, as part of a coordinated microbicidal response.

Antibody-Dependent Cellular Cytotoxicity

Engagement of Fc receptors on leukocytes can induce contact-dependent killing of antibody-coated microbes or parasitized host cells.[78] Antibody provides both the target specificity and the activating stimulus for these responses. NK cells expressing the low-affinity FcγRIII receptor can thus lyse cells infected with virus when they express viral antigens on their surface.[79] When the density of bound antibody is sufficient to cross-link the Fc receptor, degranulation occurs with release of cytolytic perforin molecules and the synthesis of cytotoxic cytokines, such as IFN-γ and TNF.[80] ADCC is also mediated by the FcγRII receptor on macrophages and neutrophils.[81] IgE-coated parasites can be targeted and killed in vitro by FcεRII-bearing eosinophils that release toxic molecules, such as major basic protein (MBP), onto the parasite surface in response to receptor cross-linking.[47]

Neutralization of Microbial Toxins

The ability of antibodies to neutralize disease-causing microbial toxins was among the earliest recognized forms of protective immunity and directly led to the clinical use of horse antiserum to treat diphtheria.[82] The mechanism of neutralization presumably reflects steric disruption of toxin uptake and action through specific cellular receptors (see Ch. 1). The role of passive and active immunization in the prevention of toxin-mediated diseases, such as tetanus,[83] botulism,[84] and pertussis[85] are further discussed in the appropriate chapters of this text.

More recently, the use of antiendotoxin antibodies as therapy for gram-negative septic shock has been aggressively studied. Antibodies directed against outer carbohydrate determinants on bacterial endotoxins are capable of detoxifying this normally proinflammatory substance and markedly reducing lethality in animal models.[86] However, the extreme diversity of serogroups expressed by pathogenic bacteria has confounded the formulation of broadly reactive immunoglobulins. Instead, monoclonal antibodies generated against common determinants of the invariant core region of lipopolysaccharide (provided by *Escherichia coli* J5 lipopolysaccharide) have been used in an attempt to generate a single immunologic agent active against a variety of pathogenic gram-negative bacteria. Despite the successful use of polyclonal antisera against J5 lipopolysaccharide in the prevention of bacteremic death,[87] recent clinical trials with two different monoclonal antibody preparations have not shown consistent benefit.[88-90]

Neutralization of Viruses

Antibodies of the IgG, IgM, or IgA class inhibit the ability of extracellular viruses to infect host cells.[91,92] This is best illustrated by the neutralizing antibody response to influenza, where attachment, fusion with cell membrane, and subsequent uncoating are all inhibited by immunoglobulin A present on the mucosal surface.[93] Antibodies directed to determinants remote from the viral binding site may prevent infection by inducing deleterious conformations or altering important charge characteristics of the pathogen. A single antibody may thus neutralize infectivity despite the presence of as many as 60 separate binding sites on picornaviruses.[94] Antibodies may also coat and inactivate viral ribonucleoproteins required for transcription of viral genes.[95] The protective role of neutralizing antibodies in infections caused by viruses, especially hepatitis, polio, and rabies viruses, are reviewed in their respective chapters in this textbook and in Chapter 300.

Antibody responses are probably less effective against viruses that spread largely by direct cell–cell transfer, including herpesviruses and the human immunodeficiency virus (HIV). However, antibodies recognizing cell-associated viral antigen may direct ADCC responses involved in viral clearance.[79] Furthermore, in epithelial cells possessing the polymeric IgA receptor, antibody may inhibit intracellular virus replication when virus and immunoglobulin are colocalized within the cytoplasm during IgA transport.[96] This may constitute an important barrier defense against viral pathogens that initiate infection within the mucosal tissues.

Antiadhesion Antibodies

Most pathogenic microbes adhere to host tissues as a prelude to tissue invasion or local proliferation. Since this requires interactions between distinct bacterial ligands and host cell receptors,[97] antibodies generated against microbial surface molecules have the capacity to disrupt adherence and thereby abort infection.[26,98] The antiadhesion effects of IgA in the gut may depend on poorly defined interactions with the mucous layer, as demonstrated in studies of the anti-*Campylobacter* IgA responses.[99]

Agglutination

Polyvalent immunoglobulins have the ability to cross-link microbes and/or microbial antigens extensively. These IgM, IgG, or IgA antigenic complexes can then effect removal of the offending substance when complement is activated by classical or alternative pathways. Agglutination of microbes by IgA may assist in mucociliary clearance of the subsequent particulate material within the respiratory tract.

IMMUNOPATHOLOGY CAUSED BY ANTIBODIES

Hypergammaglobulinemia

Chronic infection and inflammation can be associated with exaggerated antibody responses resulting in abnormally high serum levels of immunoglobulin. This is commonly observed during infective endocarditis, secondary syphilis, infectious mononucleosis, AIDS, parasitic infection, and cystic fibrosis.[100–103] Polyclonal responses are thought to represent "bystander" activation of B cells producing antibody specificities unrelated to the infecting agent. Because Epstein-Barr viruses transiently infect and activate B cells, a variety of irrelevant antibody responses may occur during infectious mononucleosis as a result of polyclonal stimulation. These are frequently observed as antibody responses to nuclear antigens, leukocytes, and ampicillin.[104] Otherwise, polyclonal gammopathies resulting from infection are usually not linked to any definable pathology unless they are accompanied by formation of immune complexes or cryoglobulins.

Immune Complexes

Under favorable stoichiometric conditions, antigen and antibody can combine into immune complexes that may result in overt tissue damage during infectious diseases. The pathologic potential of immune complexes depends on size, valency, charge characteristics, and the site at which the complex is generated.[105] Damage is mediated through activation of leukocyte Fc receptors, causing release of proteases and the production of reactive oxygen intermediates. Local complement activation by immune complexes further contributes to pathology.[106] The classic manifestation of immune complex–related pathology is seen in the immune glomerulopathies resulting from infection with hepatitis B, hepatitis C, and *Strep. pyogenes*.[107] Any source of chronic microbial antigen release into the circulation, such as occurs during endocarditis and venticuloatrial shunt infections ("shunt nephritis"), may lead to these complications.[108] Because of their undesirable effects, normal hosts maintain mechanisms for the clearance of these immune complexes. Prominent among these are removal by low-affinity Fc receptors on phagocytic cells and, when the immune complex activates the classical pathway of complement activation, by complement receptors on erythrocytes. Complement proteins may also help to solubilize aggregated IgG by disrupting noncovalent attractions between IgG Fc regions.[109]

Rheumatoid Factor

Rheumatoid factors (RF) are IgM or IgG antibodies that are directed specifically against autologous IgG.[15,110] Although originally characterized as a pathologic concomitant of rheumatoid arthritis, it has become obvious that IgM RF factor is a frequent product of normal B-cell responses. This reflects the preferential expression of a small number of V_H and V_L genes that naturally encode RF activity in their germline sequence.[111,112] Perhaps because of their low affinity for antigen, RF-positive B cells are not normally deleted during early development. In fact, B cells bearing surface antibody with this specificity are surprisingly abundant in healthy individuals, especially within the CD5+ B cell population. Similarly, 10 percent of IgM paraproteinemias are composed of RF antibody. The conservation of such a strong bias in specificity suggests that RF-positive B cells and their immunoglobulin products serve an important immunologic or host defense role. In this regard, it has been speculated that RF enhances opsonization of pathogens when IgG reactive with microbes is insufficiently concentrated on the target or of the wrong IgG subclass to permit efficient complement activation.[15] The normally weak affinity of natural RF for soluble IgG is overcome when the IgG is immobilized on solid surfaces, permitting multivalent binding. Rheumatoid factor may similarly accelerate the clearance of immune complexes containing IgG-coated antigen. An intriguing hypothesis has been advanced that RF+-positive B cells fulfill important accessory cell functions by efficiently capturing IgG complexed to antigen, this amplifying T-cell activation in response to low levels of antigen.[15,113] Rheumatoid factor responses become pathogenic when the autoantibody response increases in titer, the RF isotype switches to IgG, and higher affinity RF variants appear as a result of somatic mutation or altered germline sequence usage.[112]

Cryoglobulinemia

Type II or mixed cryoglobulinemia is a vasculitis associated with purpura, arthralgias, and glomerulonephritis caused by cryoprecipitable immune complexes generated in the presence of IgM RF and elevated serum levels of polyclonal IgG. Infections with hepatitis C or hepatitis B virus are frequently associated with this syndrome.[114,115]

Autoantibodies

The formation of antibodies against host tissue determinants is surprisingly frequent during infectious diseases. Most commonly, this represents the stimulation of RF or other low-affinity IgM molecules with broad reactivity toward polysaccharide and phospholipid determinants. These may be sufficiently predictable to permit indirect serodiagnosis of infection, as illustrated by the cold hemagglutinin response associated with *Mycoplasma* infections. Similarly, antibodies that are cross-reactive with cardiolipin are generated during syphilis. Cross-reactivity between microbes and humans may also reflect similarities in peptide sequence—so-called molecular mimicry.[116] For instance, autoimmunity against neural tissue during Chagas' disease has been linked to a cross-reactive 12-amino acid antigenic peptide common to both *Trypanosoma cruzi* and mammalian neurons.[117] Highly conserved sequences within the heat shock proteins of humans and various microbial pathogens similarly induce autoimmune responses that may present as rheumatologic disease.[118] Cross-reactive epitopes shared by the M protein of *Strep. pyogenes* and proteins within the myocardial sarcolemma may contribute to the pathogenesis of rheumatic heart disease.[119]

CELLULAR MECHANISMS IN ANTIBODY PRODUCTION

Antibody responses are clinically manifest by the appearance of protective or diagnostic antibodies following antigenic exposure. Antibodies produced during the *primary antibody response* following an encounter with a new antigen are typically of the IgM isotype, appear at 5–10 days after antigenic exposure, and express relatively low affinities for antigen. *Secondary antibody responses* result in the more rapid appearance of antibodies (within 1–3 days) that are more abundant and that are more likely to consist of IgG, IgA, or IgE. During the secondary response, the affinity of the antibody is also increased for its respective antigen, a process referred to as *affinity maturation*. The more rapid onset and greater amplitude of the secondary antibody response reflects the increased number of antigen-specific B cells generated previously during the primary response. These *memory cells* also are more likely to produce mature antibody isotypes, and this process of *isotypic switching* is closely controlled by T cells and their cytokine products. Secondary antibody responses to protein antigens are quantitatively and qualitatively distinct from those elicited by polymeric polysaccharide antigens. This reflects different T-cell–dependent and –independent mechanisms of B-cell activation, as will be discussed in more detail below.

The ability of an individual to produce antibodies against a broad range of exogenous antigens introduced by infection or immunization, while minimizing wasteful or autoreactive immune reactions, testifies to the complex and highly regulated biology of the B cell. The following discussion will highlight important functions of B cells with regard to antibody production and immunologic specialization

The Generation of Antigen-Binding Diversity

The immunoglobulin antigen-binding repertoire is created during early B-lymphocyte development through the linear assembly of DNA segments derived from large families of related, but sequence-disparate variable region genes.[120–122] An estimated 10^8 possible antigen-binding specificities (idiotypes) result from this process. Similar mechanisms generate diversity in T-cell receptor genes. Although heavy chain genes rearrange first during B-cell ontogeny, the light chain complexes are of simpler design and will be discussed first.

Gene complexes encoding the constant and variable region genes of the κ light chain are located on chromosome 2, and the genes for λ constant and variable regions are on chromosome 22. The variable region sequence of each light chain gene is generated by the fusion of a single member of nearly 200 separate V segment genes with one of 5–10 short joining (J) segment genes (Fig. 3). Although these gene segments are separated by as much as 1 million base pairs, these loci are juxtaposed when the intervening DNA is deleted by recombinase activity.[123] A role for the RAG-1 and RAG-2 gene products in this process has been identified recently.[124] The κ light chain complex contains one Cκ gene adjacent to the site of Vκ/Jκ joining, so that a single recombination forms a linear array of genes that can be transcribed to generate mature light chain mRNA. The λ complex is differently constructed, having six or more Cλ genes, each adjacent to a distinct Jλ gene segment. Excision of inter-

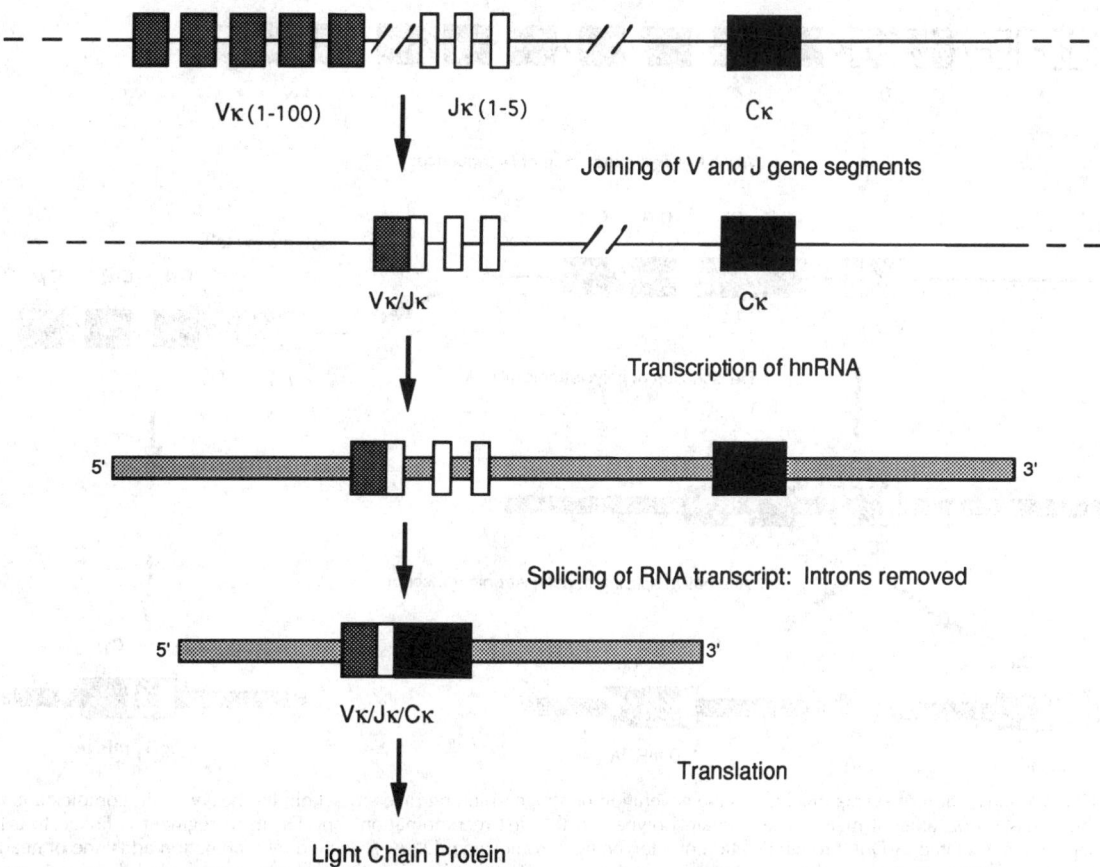

FIG. 3. Illustration of events involved in the generation of antigen binding diversity within the κ light chain gene complex. Recombination results in one of nearly a hundred Vκ gene segments being brought into proximity with one of the indicated Jκ segments through deletion of the intervening chromosomal DNA. Continuity with the rest of the chromosome is indicated by the dashed lines at either end of the gene complex. Transcription of the recombined gene complex leads to heterogeneous nuclear RNA (hnRNA) containing introns and irrelevant exons that are subsequently deleted during RNA processing to produce the mature messenger RNA.

vening DNA associates one of several hundred Vλ sequences with any one of these Jλ/Cλ pairs to produce a complete transcriptional unit. In either case, diversity of the light chain variable region is generated through the great number of possible V and J joinings. The relative inaccuracy of the joining process contributes an additional source of diversity by introducing one or two randomly selected amino acids at the VJ splice site. Only one successful variable region rearrangement is allowed per cell; the first rearranged gene product suppresses recombination at the other three light chain loci so that each mature B cell expresses only a single light chain isotype (κ or λ).

The genes of the heavy chain complex on chromosome 14 rearrange in a similar fashion (Fig. 4). About 500 V_H genes and 4 J_H segments are available for fusion, providing 2,000 possible VJ combinations. In addition, there are 10 or more short, diversity-generating (D_H) segment genes available for insertion between the V and J segments during variable region assembly, increasing the number of possible V-region gene combinations to 20,000. One or two amino acid codons, called N sequences, are added to the VDJ splice sites by the enzyme terminal doxy-

nucleotidyltransferase.[125] The successfully rearranged VDJ gene can be expressed in conjunction with any of nine heavy chain constant region genes that, when translated, define the isotype of the final immunoglobulin. These C_H genes are arranged in linear fashion near to the VDJ recombination site in the following order: Cμ, Cδ, Cγ3, Cγl, Cα1, Cγ2, Cγ4, Cε, and Cα2. At first, transcription initiated within the VDJ assembly extends only through the two proximal C_H genes, creating a polycistronic message that can be selectively spliced to produce either μ or δ heavy chains without further rearrangement of DNA. Heavy chain switching can occur under the control of extrinsic immunologic signals, whereby antigen-binding specificity is maintained but antibody class is altered. Isotypic switching is accomplished through the excision of intervening DNA and the juxtaposition of the intact variable region sequence with a new distal C_H gene. Excision occurs at defined "switch" regions and is preceded by the appearance of a long RNA molecule spanning the future deletion site. This transcript is not translated and has been proposed to function as a template to guide the excisional and splicing process.[126]

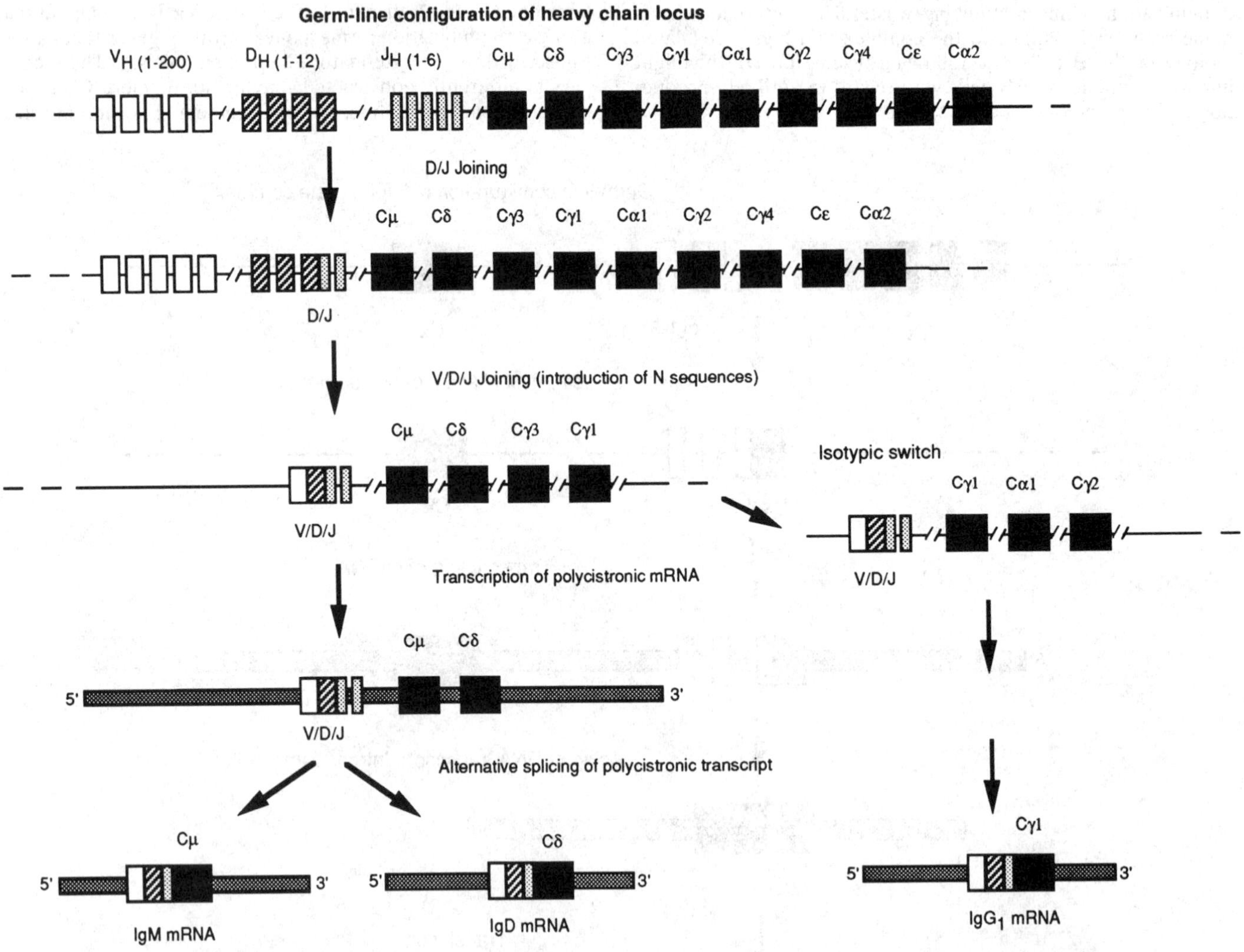

FIG. 4. Illustration of events involved in the generation of antigen-binding diversity within the heavy chain complex and in the formation of different mature heavy chain isotypes. In the first recombination, one D_H gene segment is linked to a J_H segment (designated as D/J) through deletion of intervening chromosomal DNA. A second recombination adds one of nearly 200 V_H segments to the nascent variable region gene (V/D/J). At this time, junctional diversity is created through inexact joining of these segments and through addition of N-sequence amino acid codons. Transcription through the V/D/J gene and through the adjacent μ and δ heavy chain constant genes generates a polycistronic nuclear RNA (hnRNA) that can be spliced to provide mature mRNA encoding either IgM or IgD. Other types of alternative splicing may lead to the deletion or addition of a region within the tail of the heavy chain that determines if the final immunoglobulin product is expressed on the surface of the B cell or is released as soluble antibody (not shown). Alternatively, deletion of intervening DNA can lead to the association and expression of the unaltered variable region sequences with a distal heavy chain gene.

Because C_H genes proximal to the new splice site are deleted from the genome, isotypic switches to IgG, IgE, or IgA phenotype are irreversible. Therefore, the order of C_H genes in the genome crudely approximates the order of appearance of isotypes during advanced B-cell differentiation, IgM and IgD being the first immunoglobulins produced and IgG, IgE, or IgA appearing during later differentiation. The antigen-binding specificity is preserved during isotypic switches, as heavy and light chain variable regions are not affected by this process. The switch to IgE and IgG4 production or to IgA expression in response to appropriate regulatory signals has been well studied, and it is apparent now that each switch occurs as a single excisional deletion of intervening C_H genes and not in multiple, transient recombinations.[127] The control of immunoglobulin isotype switching by T cells and T-cell–derived cytokines is further discussed below. Whatever the isotype, heavy chain genes can generate either membrane-bound or soluble immunoglobulins, depending on the inclusion or deletion of two exons encoding a 40 amino acid hydrophobic transmembrane domain.

In summary, antigen-binding diversity is generated through the *recombination* of V, D, and J sequences, *junctional diversity* introduced by the inexact joining of these segments and the addition of N sequences and the *quaternary association* of both V_H and V_L into a complete antigen-binding site during immunoglobulin assembly. A fourth nonrecombinatorial mechanism further increases idiotype diversity following primary exposure to antigen. Specifically, comparisons of immunoglobulin gene sequences before and after secondary or tertiary antigenic challenges demonstrate increasing numbers of single-base mutations in the hypervariable regions of light and heavy chains[128] (for review, see French et al.[129]). These mutations are restricted to select areas within the hypervariable regions and are usually point mutations. It is thought that this process of *somatic mutation* underlies the phenomenon of affinity maturation, where repeated antigenic challenges result in production of antibodies with incrementally increased affinity for the eliciting epitope.

Surface Molecules of the B Cell

Mature B lymphocytes are defined by their expression of surface immunoglobulin. Initially B cells are surface IgM and IgD positive, but with isotypic switching IgG, IgA, and IgE can be expressed as well. Further differentiation into antibody-secreting plasma cells results in the loss of surface immunoglobulin expression. Other molecules expressed on the B-cell surface have defined functions in B-cell activation and differentiation (Table 3), but are too numerous for all but the most important to

be reviewed here (see Banchereau and Rousset[130] for complete review).

The B-Cell Receptor Complex

Surface immunoglobulin functions as the antigen receptor of the B cell, and cross-linking of this molecule by the appropriate ligand induces activating signals that are conducted via associated surface proteins into the B-cell cytoplasm.[130-132] Parallels between the multimeric T-cell receptor complex and the B-cell receptor complex are apparent in these functional and structural details[133] (Fig. 5). Accessory molecules of the B-cell receptor complex include nonimmunoglobulin transmembrane proteins (Igα and Igβ) that form a disulfide-linked heterodimer noncovalently associated with surface immunoglobulin. Cross-linking of surface immunoglobulin by antigen probably causes conformational changes resulting in the activation of Src family tyrosine kinases (Fyn, Lyn, and Blk) by signals mediated through the cytoplasmic domains of Igα and Igβ.[134] Other transmembrane molecules are associated noncovalently with the B-cell receptor complex and probably contribute to B-cell activation as well. One of these is CD21, the complement receptor 2 (CR2) molecule capable of binding to the C3d, C3dg, and C3g degradation products of activated complement.[135] CD21 is also the cellular ligand for the B-cell specific Epstein-Barr virus. Because CD21 is closely associated with the transmembrane protein CD19 and because CD19 can lower the activation threshold of B lymphocytes nearly 100-fold when cross-linked to surface immunoglobulin, CD21 and CD19 may have a physiologic role in B-cell activation when coaggregated by complement-coated complexes of antigen and antibody. This could result in a valuable increase in B-cell sensitivity in response to monomeric protein antigens that normally would not be able to cross-link surface immunoglobulin extensively. Another member of the B-cell receptor complex, CD22, is a surface-associated tyrosine kinase that may help to initiate cytoplasmic signals following antigen binding.[136]

The first intracellular event resulting from cross-linking of the B-cell receptor complex by antigen is the phosphorylation of transmembrane and cytoplasmic proteins by several tyrosine kinases. These include the aforementioned CD22 protein and the Src family of kinases that interact with cytoplasmic domains of Igα and Igβ.[134] Phosphorylation activates phospholipase Cγ2 that hydrolyzes plasma membrane phosphoinositides to release the active intermediate molecules inositol triphosphate (IP$_3$) and diacylglycerol (DAG). Diacylglycerol activates protein kinase C (PKC), and IP$_3$ mobilizes intracellular calcium ions that then activate calcium-dependent calcium channels within the cell

TABLE 3. Important B-Cell Surface Molecules

Molecules	Function
IgM, IgD	Antigen-specific receptor on B-cells; triggers cell activation and endocytosis of bound antigen
Igα, Igβ	Accessory molecules of the B-cell receptor complex. Associates with IgM and IgD and transduces activating signals via cytoplasmic domains
B7	Marker of activated B cells; induced by cross-linking of surface immunoglobulin or MHC II; adhesion receptor for T-cell CD28; provides critical costimulus for T-cell activation
CD5	Ligand for CD72; expressed by the B1 subset of B cells; may modulate activation signals
CD19	Associates with surface immunoglobulin and CD21; lowers threshold for activation during Ig cross-linking
CD21 (CR2)	Binds the C3dg fragment(s) of C3 and is the receptor for Epstein-Barr virus; coassociates with CD19
CD22	Transmembrane molecule with tyrosine kinase activity; involved in signal transduction; adhesion receptor for T-cell CD45RO and other uncharacterized ligands
CD40	Ligand for T-cell membrane molecule gp39 and the receptor for T-cell help; transduces signals necessary for growth and differentiation of activated B cells; genetic deficiency in gp39 function is the cause of hyper-IgM syndrome
CD45	Protein phosphatase required for activation; expressed throughout B-cell ontogeny
CD72	Ligand for CD5 expressed on T-cells and the B1 subset of B-cells
Fc receptors	See Table 2
MHC II	Involved in presentation of antigenic peptides to complementary T-cell receptor heterodimer
Cytokine receptors	Transduce signals required for proliferation, activation, and differentiation

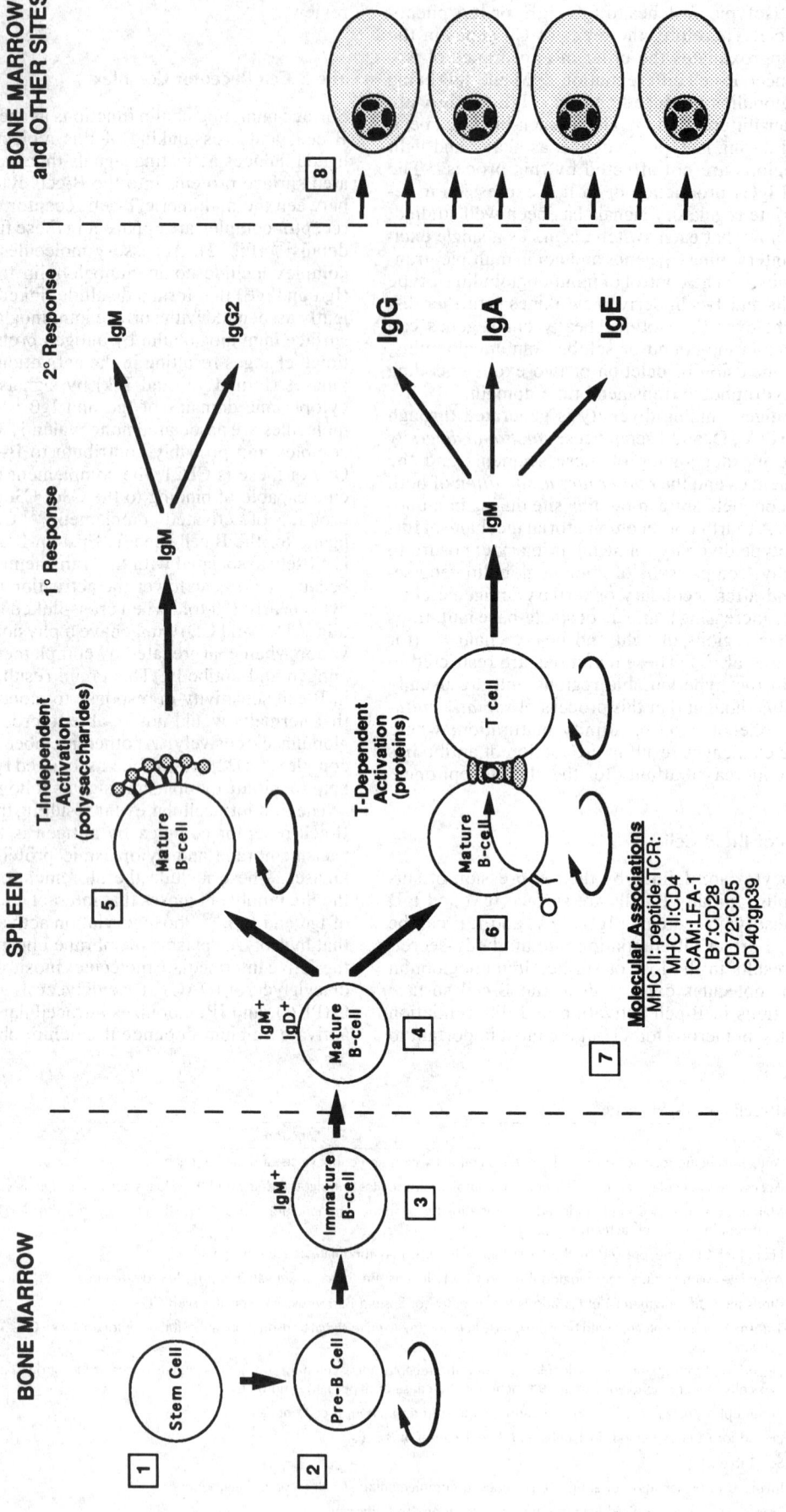

BONE MARROW and OTHER SITES

Plasma Cells

8

2° Response

IgM

IgG2

1° Response

IgM

T-Independent Activation (polysaccharides)

SPLEEN

Mature B-cell

5

IgM⁺ IgD⁺

Mature B-cell

4

T-Dependent Activation (proteins)

T cell

Mature B-cell

6

IgM

IgG

IgA

IgE

Molecular Associations
MHC II: peptide:TCR:
MHC II:CD4
ICAM:LFA-1
B7:CD28
CD72:CD5
CD40:gp39

7

BONE MARROW

Stem Cell

1

Pre-B Cell

2

IgM⁺ Immature B-cell

3

membrane and contribute to PKC activity. The combination of activities mediated by tyrosine kinases, PKC, and fluctuating levels of intracellular calcium eventually leads to the transcription of cellular genes required for cell division, differentiation, and antibody production.

However, recognition of antigen alone is rarely sufficient for the full expression of B-cell function. Depending on the nature of the eliciting antigen, B cells may require further signals provided by physical interaction with activated T "helper" cells—so-called *T-cell–dependent (TD) B-cell activation.* This requires that the B-cell function as an antigen-presenting cell by internalizing and processing antigen to be provided as peptides complexed on major histocompatibility complex (MHC) II for recognition by the appropriate T-cell partner.[137] The joint recognition of the same antigen by both B cells and T cells constitutes the phenomenon previously identified as hapten-carrier cooperation.[138] The B-cell receptor generally binds to native, unprocessed protein determinants, whereas the T-cell receptor is limited to the recognition of linear peptide determinants previously processed by the B cell. A very different type of B-cell activation takes place in response to highly polymerized antigens, characteristically bacterial polysaccharides, that cause extensive cross-linking of the B-cell receptor complex and generate activation signals of sufficient intensity to drive B-cell proliferation and antibody production in the absence of cognate T-cell interactions. This is referred to as *T-independent (TI) B-cell activation.*

T-Cell–Dependent B-Cell Activation

Both the B-cell receptor and its bound ligand are internalized and delivered to a protease-rich lysosomal compartment where antigen is processed into component peptides that are complexed with nascent MHC II molecules.[139] B cells constitutively express large amounts of MHC II on their surface in support of their accessory cell functions. In contrast to other antigen-presenting cells, such as macrophages and dendritic cells, that process antigens from proteins obtained by bulk endocytosis, the high affinity of B-cell antigen receptors for their ligand means that B cells can activate T cells when specific antigen is present in concentrations nearly 10,000-fold less than that required for macrophage antigen-presenting cell function.[140] This ability to present antigens efficiently during secondary immune responses is markedly increased when the previous encounter has increased the available number of antigen-specific B cells in the lymphoid tissues.

The formation of a T- and B-cell cognate pair is a highly orchestrated event dependent on multiple noncovalent interactions between complementary adhesion molecules expressed on the surface of each cell.[137] Many of these molecules also transduce functionally important signals through their cytoplasmic domain or through associated transmembrane molecules. This results in a bidirectional, antigen-specific activation of the engaged lymphocytes during the transient intercellular adhesion process. Antigen specificity is provided by the recognition of MHC II–peptide complexes by the appropriate T-cell receptors. The usually weak interactions involved in the coupling of MHC II, peptide, and T-cell receptors are stabilized by specific and inducible interactions between CD4, CD28, CD5, and LFA-1 on T cells and their complementary B-cell ligands MHC II, B7, CD72, and ICAM.[141,142,143] This process is reviewed in detail in Chapter 8. Some of these receptor–ligand pairings generate signals important in B-cell function. Specifically, binding of B-cell CD40 to its respective T-cell ligand, called *gp39* or *CD40 ligand,* is essential for continued B-cell proliferation and viability following activation by antigen.[141,144] Because signals provided by CD40 ligation are necessary for B-cell differentiation into IgG-, IgA-, and IgE-producing cells, disabling mutations within the CD40-ligand gene cause a severe immunodeficiency characterized by deficient production of these isotypes. Instead, antibody responses are dominated by IgM and are inadequate to defend against bacterial and viral pathogens.[145] The hyper-IgM immunodeficiency syndrome is further discussed below (see Immunoglobulin and Antibody Deficiency States). Similarly, patients who lack LFA-1 (the leukocyte adheson deficiency syndrome) are less able to generate antibodies against protein antigens, but their production of antipolysaccharide antibodies is unimpaired.[146]

T-Cell–Independent B-Cell Activation

Certain polymeric antigens, especially bacterial polysaccharides containing repetitive carbohydrate determinants, can activate B cells without requiring cognate signals from T cells. The polymeric structure of these antigens suggests that extensive cross-linking of surface immunoglobulin is an important feature of T-

---

FIG. 5. Important stages in the development of B cells from primitive bone marrow stem cells to antibody secreting plasma cells. **(1)** Antigen-independent proliferation of bone marrow stem cells leads to large numbers of pre-B cells. Proliferative stages are indicated by the semicircular arrow. **(2)** Recombination of heavy and light chain gene complexes occurs during the pre-B cell stage and generates the antigen-binding diversity of the future B-cell repertoire. **(3)** Approximately 10 percent of cells achieve a functional recombination and thereupon express surface IgM. These surface IgM-positive cells are defined as immature B cells until they are capable of activation by antigen exposure. At this stage autoreactive B cells are removed by programmed cell death (apoptosis) should they recognize a self-antigen. **(4)** Survivors of this process of negative selection evolve into mature B cells (surface IgM- and IgD-positive cells) that can be activated to proliferate and produce antibodies following recognition of their respective antigen. Activation by two distinct pathways is shown at this stage. **(5)** In the T-cell–independent pathway, B cells are activated when surface immunoglobulins are extensively cross-linked by polymeric antigens—such as the repetitive carbohydrate structure of bacterial polysaccharides, leading to antigen-specific B-cell proliferation and IgM production during the primary antibody response (1° Response). T-cell–independent activation results in poor memory cell formation; therefore the amount of antibody produced during the secondary response (2° Response) is low. Little differentiation of isotype occurs, the secondary response is composed largely of IgM with some production of IgG (often IgG2). **(6)** In the T-cell–dependent pathway, specific immunoglobulin receptors identify and internalize low concentrations of monomeric antigens that are processed and incorporated as peptide fragments bound to surface MHC II. T cells recognize and bind to the MHC II–peptide complex, thereby activating multiple intercellular molecular interactions as listed **(7)**. This results in mutual activation of T and B cells. Activated B cells proliferate and produce IgM as part of the primary antibody response. Compared with T-cell–independent responses, T-cell–dependent responses result in more efficient memory cell formation and a consequently larger secondary antibody response (indicated by the larger type). Affinity maturation of antibody takes place in the germinal center at this time. Isotypic switching results in the appearance of IgG, IgA, and IgE isotypes during the secondary response. The type of immunoglobulin made is controlled by T cells through their ligation of B-cell CD40 and through the generation of soluble cytokines such as IL-4, which promotes IgE formation, and IL-5/TGF-β, which induce IgA production. **(8)** With repeated stimulation, short-lived plasma cells producing large amounts of antibody production appear in the bone marrow and in other tissues.

independent B-cell responses. Antibody responses generated by T-independent activation are distinct from that induced by T-dependent B-cell activation, and this has important clinical ramifications. First, immunoglobulin isotypes produced in response to T-independent antigens, typified by *Strep. pneumonia* or *H. influenzae* polysaccharide vaccines, consist largely of IgM and IgG2.[19] Second, memory cell formation is inefficient during T-independent B-cell activation, and repeated antigenic challenges generate low-level antibody responses compared with T-dependent antigens. This poses a practical problem for vaccine design when the immunogen is a bacterial polysaccharide that elicits only low titers of antibody that may be nonprotective. Fortunately, coupling the desired determinants with a protein antigen can convert a T-independent response into a T-cell–driven immune reaction and result in strong IgG recall responses. This is well illustrated by the greater vaccine efficacy of *H. influenza* type b capsular polysaccharide antigen when it is coupled to diphtheria or tetanus toxoid.[147]

B-Cell Ontogeny and Differentiation

Nearly a billion B cells are produced in the adult bone marrow daily. These arise continuously from stem cells and proceed through a series of highly programmed maturational stages before emerging into the peripheral lymphoid system as fully competent B cells defined by their expression of surface immunoglobulin.[148] Following initial differentiation into spontaneously proliferating, surface immunoglobulin-negative B-cell precursors (referred to as *pre-B cells*), the future antigenic specificity of these cells is generated by immunoglobulin gene rearrangements that, if successful, lead to the synthesis of a μ heavy chain and a λ or κ light chain, as previously discussed. Gene rearrangement occurs first in the heavy chain gene complex, starting in one parental chromosome and progressing to the other if the first does not provide a functional rearrangement. Cytoplasmic μ heavy chain appears when this is complete. It has been recently appreciated that a temporary membrane-bound receptor is generated through assembly with a surrogate light chain that is not used in mature B cells; the functional significance of this pre-B-cell receptor is undefined.[149] One of the four κ or λ light chain gene complexes is next to rearrange, with sequential activation of the remaining gene complexes if the initial rearrangements are dysfunctional. Due to frame shift errors and mutations during VJ or VDJ joining, a great majority of immunoglobulin gene rearrangements are nonfunctional. Nearly 90 percent of pre-B cells encounter such difficulty and are removed through a process of programmed cell death or apoptosis.[150] With successful light and heavy chain recombination, IgM is synthesized and expressed on the surface of the B cell. Only one functional light chain or heavy chain rearrangement is observed per cell, as production of intact immunoglobulin suppresses further gene recombination. When an immunoglobulin chain suppresses activation of the analogous gene locus on the other parental chromosome, this process is termed *allelic exclusion*. Concurrent suppression of κ-chain rearrangement by successful λ-chain recombination (or vice versa) is referred to as *isotypic exclusion*.

Antigen-independent proliferation ceases with attainment of the B-cell phenotype. During a brief *immature B-cell stage*, the newly emerged IgM-positive B cells are subjected to a process of negative selection to remove or suppress autoreactive specificities. Exposure to self-antigen within the bone marrow or in the periphery removes nascent self-reactive clones. Apparently surface immunoglobulin-mediated signals are transiently programmed to induce cell death by apoptosis,[151,152] whereas failure to detect self-antigen during this critical period allows further maturation into an antigen-responsive or *mature* B cell.[152] Intermediate degrees of self-reactivity may instead result in *tolerance*, where the autoreactive B-cell clone does not die but is rendered unresponsive to future activating stimuli.[153] However,

the mere presence of tolerized B-cell specificities in the body introduces the potential for future autoimmune responses.[154]

Whereas immature B cells express only surface IgM, mature B cells surviving negative selection are both surface IgM and IgD positive. The reason for maintaining two different isotypes of B-cell receptor is not well defined. Signaling through either IgM or IgD receptors does not provide for distinct tolerizing or activating responses,[155] and IgD-deficient mice suffer only a delay in the onset of affinity maturation following B-cell activation.[156] These mature B cells leave the bone marrow and next appear in the periarteriolar sheath of the spleen and peripheral lymph node tissues. When activated by exposure to antigen, through mechanisms described previously, the B cells are triggered to proliferate and differentiate into antibody-secreting cells and/or memory cells. The proliferative phase that follows primary or secondary sensitization by antigen is associated with a translocation of the activated B-cell from the periarteriolar sheath into the germinal center, where the cells enlarge into "centroblasts" as defined by morphologic criteria. Affinity maturation occurs during this phase, reflecting a process of somatic hypermutation within the hypervariable regions of the immunoglobulin and subsequent selection by antigen-expressing follicular dendritic cells (FDC).[157,158] High-affinity or kinetically favorable receptor–antigen interactions are preserved for further clonal amplification, whereas low-affinity somatic mutants are removed by apoptotic death.[159] Responses engendered by a single antigen may result in each germinal center being occupied by only a few amplified clones derived from a single antigen-response precursor cell.[158] Follicular dendritic cells are critically involved in this selection process through their presentation to B cells of antigenic complexes. These antigens are displayed on the cell surface of the FDC for prolonged periods of time and are capable of supporting B-cell proliferation and affinity maturation long after circulating antigen has disappeared.[160]

B-Cell Differentiation

Following primary antigenic exposure, the activated B cells may undergo isotypic switching, wherein the expressed immunoglobulin isotype is changed to IgG, IgA, or IgE with preserved variable regions and antigenic specificity.[127] Although the bulk of B cells previously exposed to antigen and capable of priming the secondary response (memory B cells) remain surface IgM positive, they are capable of rapid production of IgG isotype following restimulation.[161] This process of isotypic switching is regulated by exposure to T-cell cytokines and T-cell cognate interactions. Heavy chain switching to produce IgE requires that the responding B cells receive differentiating stimuli provided by the T-cell lymphokine IL-4 and the engagement of the B-cell CD40 molecule by its respective T-cell ligand.[144] Similarly, CD40 ligation in the presence of transforming growth factor-β and IL-5 results in switching to the IgA isotype. A variety of cytokine combinations promote IgG production. Thus the expression of IgG, IgA, and IgE by B cells will tend to reflect the dominant cytokine milieu provided by antigen-responsive CD4+ T cells. As discussed in greater detail in the chapter on T-cell immunity, this may explain the propensity for B cells to evolve into IgA-secreting cells within the gut-associated lymphatics, where the local T-cell environment is strongly biased in favor of T-helper type 2 cytokine responses that would support IgA isotypic switches.

With continued stimulation, some B cells leave the lymphoid tissues and evolve into surface immunoglobulin-negative, non-proliferating plasma cells that are characterized by markedly expanded endoplasmic reticulum and Golgi structures committed to the sole function of producing large quantities of antibody.[130] Plasma cells are present mostly in the bone marrow and in the lamina propria of the gut and are an important source of circulating IgG and IgA. Infiltration of nonlymphoid tissues by plasma cells may characterize many chronic infectious diseases associated with hypergammaglobulinemia.

B1 Cells

A subpopulation of B lymphocytes with distinct immunologic functions is characterized by expression of surface protein CD5, normally a surface antigen of T cells. CD5+ B1 cells are distributed within peritoneal and other serosal cavities, but are rare within the lymph nodes and spleen, where the more numerous CD5− B2 cells reside.[162,163] B1 cells appear to replicate autonomously at these sites, leading to some speculation that they arise from distinct precursor cells and constitute a separate lymphocyte lineage altogether. Of clinical significance, B1 cells produce IgM with polyreactive specificities to phosphocholine, DNA, and polysaccharide-related determinants. A role for these constitutively expressed antibodies as a type of early-acting "natural" humoral immunity against infectious agents bearing determinants cross-reactive with these common moieties has been suggested.[164,165] The B1 cell repertoire is also biased to include more autoreactive idiotypes than observed in CD5− B2 cells. Low-affinity RF is prominent within the B1 population and may provide these cells with special functions in antigen presentation and nonspecific immunity (see above discussion of rheumatoid factor).

The Regulation of B-Cell Activity

A variety of regulatory mechanisms have evolved to avoid development of autoreactive B cells and to select simultaneously for high-affinity antibodies directed against foreign antigens. As discussed, the antibody repertoire is actively shaped at different times in the B-cell life span. Negative selection during the immature B-cell stage removes autoreactive specificities through programmed cell death. B-cell tolerance to less intensely activating self-epitopes occurs both in the bone marrow and in the peripheral tissues and provides another layer of control over potentially autodestructive specificities. During the secondary response, both positive and negative selection results in the emergence of a few high-affinity B-cell clones within the germinal center. In addition, suppressor CD8+ T cells may inhibit antibody production in response to some antigens, although the mechanisms involved are still not well understood.[166] Antibody overproduction may be regulated as well, either by feedback inhibition through downregulatory B-cell Fc receptors or via anti-idiotypic antibody networks where inhibitory antibodies are generated against the overexpressed idiotype.[167]

IMMUNOGLOBULIN AND ANTIBODY DEFICIENCY STATES

These immunodeficiencies embrace a wide range of genetic and acquired disorders characterized at the extremes by either the absence of circulating antibodies resulting in repeated, potentially fatal infections or by the selective loss of a single class or subclass that may be wholly asymptomatic. Several of the more significant humoral immunodeficiencies are single-gene defects within the X chromosome and are thus diseases of young boys.[168] Because severe forms of antibody deficiency can be usefully treated with intravenous immunoglobulins, children or adults presenting with unusually frequent bacterial infections should be evaluated for immunoglobulin deficiencies. Delayed diagnosis is associated with worsened prognosis.[169]

The severe manifestations of agammaglobulinemia are most obviously related to the loss of IgG- and IgM-mediated serum opsonic, lytic, and neutralizing activities that critically defend against infection with encapsulated bacteria and many types of virus. The cause of susceptibility to infection in partial immunoglobulin deficiencies, such as IgG subclass disorders, may be driven as much by dysfunctional primary antibody responses

as by quantitative changes in serum immunoglobulin levels. This can be measured in the patient's inability to generate antibody against defined bacterial polysaccharide or protein antigens. Several genetic diseases result in combined humoral and cellular immune deficiencies and are discussed in further depth in Chapter 8.[171] Immunoglobulin deficiencies or functional abnormalities can be secondary manifestations of preexisting diseases that alter production or clearance of antibody. In these cases, the underlying disease may separately contribute to the enhanced susceptibility to infection.

Common Clinical Features of Antibody Deficiencies

The most severe antibody deficiencies, such as X-linked agammaglobulinemia, common variable immunodeficiency, and X-linked hyper-IgM syndrome, usually manifest in children or young adults as recurrent infections involving many different organ systems.[169–173] Unusually severe or recurrent pulmonary infections with *Strep. pneumoniae, H. influenzae, Mycoplasma* spp., and meningococci are especially characteristic. The persistent or repetitive nature of the infections can lead to chronic morbidity from bronchiectasis and related pulmonary disease. Chronic sinusitis and otitis are also frequent problems. Gastrointestinal infections are increased in severity and incidence and are caused by common pathogens, such as *Salmonella, Shigella, Campylobacter,* and rotavirus.[169,174] Intestinal giardiasis may be prolonged in patients with hypergammaglobulinemia, reflecting a key role for secretory antibody in the control of this parasite.[175] Chronic giardiasis can result in prolonged malabsorption associated with nodular submucosal hyperplasia of lymphoid tissues in the small intestine.[176] However, gluten-sensitive enteropathies or Crohn's disease are suspected to be more common in these patients.[169,177]

Rheumatologic disease occurs in about 10–30 percent of patients with humoral immunodeficiency.[178] This includes septic arthritis caused by the usual bacterial agents, but also embraces joint infections caused by *Mycoplasma* and *Ureaplasma* spp. that may pose unusual diagnostic and therapeutic problems. *Mycoplasma* spp. are associated with a destructive arthritis with a subacute onset in these patients that is usually, but not always, associated with intra-articular purulence.[169,178,179] Diagnosis requires specialized culture procedures adapted for *Mycoplasma,* and empiric therapy with doxycycline should be considered whenever these patients develop arthritis that is culture negative using conventional microbiologic techniques. Rheumatoid-like, polyarticular synovitis also occurs in the absence of a definable infectious etiology. Infusion with intravenous immunoglobulins may lead to clinical improvement. A syndrome that closely resembles polymyositis or dermatomyositis is caused by enteroviral infection of the skeletal muscle.[180] Finally, the incidence of autoimmune disorders, such as systemic lupus erythematosus, Sjögren's syndrome, and autoimmune hematologic disorders is increased to as much as 20 percent in patients with common variable immunodeficiency and IgA deficiency. These complications are notably lacking in patients with X-linked agammaglobulinemia.[172,173]

Other unique infectious disease manifestations of hypogammaglobulinemia are noteworthy. Enterovirus can cause chronic meningitis that is often fatal despite the institution of combined intrathecal and intravenous immunoglobulin therapies.[169,173,181] Although the humoral immune deficiencies do not generally predispose to fungal or parasitic infections, the occurrence of *Pneumocystis carinii* pneumonia in several agammaglobulinemic patients has been described.[182] This may reflect the frequent occurrence of neutropenia in these disorders[183] or relate to defects in T-cell function resulting from disrupted intracellular signaling between B cells and T cells.[145,184] Similarly, viral infections normally controlled by cell-mediated immunity, such as herpes simplex, can become recurrent or severe in these patients.[185]

Other immunologic functions unrelated to control of infection are affected by the loss of immunoglobulins. Serum and mucosal IgA is thought to play an important role in sequestering frequently encountered antigens derived from the diet or from the environment. Failure to mask these potential allergens may result in undesirable IgE-mediated responses. Indeed, a high rate of atopic disorders is observed in patients with isolated IgA deficiency.

Diagnosis of Antibody Deficiencies

Although frequent infections can also result from complement deficiencies, cystic fibrosis, dysmotile cilia syndrome, and the acquired immunodeficiency syndrome (AIDS); the availability of accurate laboratory assays of serum IgM, IgG, and IgA levels or of IgG subclass concentrations make the diagnosis of immunoglobulin deficiency relatively straightforward.[186] The biggest impediment to the diagnosis of agammaglobulinemia is usually a failure to suspect the disorder. However, the clinician should be aware of important caveats in the interpretation of serum immunoglobulin levels.[171] The laboratory threshold defining the lower limits of normal are based on statistical, not functional, criteria. As such, most patients found to have low levels of immunoglobulin—5 percent of the population by definition—will not be truly immunodeficient. A more useful rule of thumb is that susceptibility to recurrent infection more typically occurs in patients with levels of IgG that are 50 percent or less of the lower limit of normal—typically less than 200 mg/dl. Those antibody deficiencies most likely to require intravenous immunoglobulin (IVIG) will have no detectable IgM or IgG in the serum. Additionally, normal immunoglobulin levels vary with age, and the laboratory should provide appropriate age-adjusted normal levels upon request.

Low levels of immunoglobulin do not always correlate with the patients' ability to generate specific antibody responses against new antigens.[171] In fact, the majority of patients with demonstrably low IgG subclass levels will have clinically adequate antibody responses to defined antigens. In situations in which a strong history of recurrent infection is associated with isolated subclass deficiencies or modestly depressed immunoglobulin levels, a useful functional test of humoral adequacy is to evaluate antibody responses to tetanus toxoid, pneumococcal vaccine, *H. influenzae* type B toxoid conjugate vaccine, or hepatitis B vaccine. ELISA determinations of these antibodies are available through commercial laboratories. A relatively normal antibody response either before or after immunization implies functional normalcy and argues strongly against a need for immunoglobulin replacement therapy. Similar tests may also be useful in the evaluation of diseases associated with dysfunctional antibody responses and only modestly abnormal immunoglobulin levels, including ataxia telangiectasia, and Wiskott-Aldrich syndrome.[187]

In situations in which diagnostic ambiguity exists or when resources are easily available, circulating B-lymphocyte numbers can be quantitated using fluorescent monoclonal antibodies and fluorescence activated flow cytometry (FACS). X-linked agammaglobulinemia, but not common variable immunodeficiency, will be associated with an absence of peripheral B cells.[171,186] Measurement of in vitro immunoglobulin production in response to B-cell mitogens is a research tool in selected institutions. The coordinated use of these tests in conjunction with assays of complement, phagocyte, T-lymphocyte function, and ciliary function, as well as tests for cystic fibrosis and AIDS, are described in further detail in Chapter 9.

Treatment of IgG Deficiency

The goals of therapy in these patients are threefold: *(1)* to treat acute infection effectively, *(2)* to prevent repeated infections through infusion of IVIG, and *(3)* to prevent or treat pulmonary disease resulting from repeated pneumonias and bronchitis.[171,188] Because agammaglobulinemia leads to a failure of serum opsonization, acute infections require aggressive therapy with antibiotics. Antimicrobials should be given intravenously and for longer periods of time than is the usual practice. Empiric therapy should always include antibiotics active against typical encapsulated bacterial pathogens, notably *Strep. pneumoniae* and *H. influenzae*. Since infection may consume the small amounts of serum immunoglobulin available, IVIG administration during acute infection is probably indicated if serum immunoglobulin levels are considered subtherapeutic.

Prophylaxis against infection is based on the administration of preparations of human immunoglobulins specially formulated for intravenous delivery.[188-190] Historically, IgG replacement had been attempted using intramuscular gammaglobulin, but the limited volume tolerable by this route of delivery made normalization of serum IgG levels unrealistic. Immunoglobulin preparations for intravenous injection are now available that can be administered in quantities sufficient to normalize serum IgG levels. These preparations are 95–99 percent IgG, with trace quantities of IgA, IgM, IgD, and IgE; the half-life of the delivered IgG is variable, but averages about 20 days.[188] The efficacy of IVIG in improving symptoms and preventing infection among patients with severe hypogammaglobulinemias has been well documented. The average patient with complete immunoglobulin deficiency may require doses of anywhere from 300 to 600 mg/kg delivered every 3–4 weeks to achieve protection. A comparative study showed that higher dose regimens resulted in decreased incidence of pneumonia and meningitis and fewer days in the hospital and may prevent long-term sequelae, such as bronchiectasis or other chronic pulmonary disease.[191] Monitoring of trough immunoglobulin levels may assist in defining the optimal duration between doses, as IgG clearance may vary considerably among patients. It has been recommended that trough levels be maintained at 400–500 mg/dl during therapy of humoral immunodeficiencies.[188] The efficacy of therapy can be followed also by obtaining yearly pulmonary function tests and through the maintenance of patient diaries to document frequency of infections.

Intravenous immunoglobulin is typically well tolerated, although rate-related side effects can be common. About 3–12 percent of patients experience fever, chills, headache, myalgia, and nausea with infusion. When symptoms are severe enough, the rate of infusion should be slowed (to less than 5 mg/kg/min) and the patient pretreated with acetaminophen, antihistamines, and hydrocortisone to reduce these side effects.[171,188,190] Tolerance to these effects develops after several doses, and the rate of infusion can be increased to minimize inconvenience. Home administration of IVIG has been advocated as a convenient and cost-conserving measure,[192] although the potential for complications needs to be considered.[188] Special precautions are necessary when treating isolated IgA deficiency with IVIG, as anti-IgE antibodies may develop against the exogenous IgA contained in the infusate and cause anaphylactic reactions.[193] The process used to prepare human immunoglobulins for infusion inactivates most viral pathogens, and HIV has never been reported to be passaged by IVIG.[188] However, hepatitis C virus contaminating several lots of infusate caused an outbreak of non-A, non-B hepatitis before screening could be instituted to remove this infectious threat.[194]

Treatment of the chronic pulmonary disease resulting from repeated infection is also required, as structural lesions within the lung further predispose to infection and cor pulmonale. Pulmonary disease is an important cause of death in patients with agammaglobulinemia. Postural drainage or other physiotherapy may be required to clear pooled respiratory secretions. The role of prophylactic antibiotics or antibiotic "clean-outs" akin to that used in patients with lung disease resulting from cystic fibrosis have not been studied in cases of humoral immunodeficiency.

The ultimate treatment for genetic humoral immunodeficiencies is to provide the affected individual with normal bone marrow stem cells. This can be achieved with bone marrow transplants in cases of severe combined immunodeficiency, X-linked agammaglobulinemia, and Wiskott-Aldrich syndromes, although the risks of allogeneic transplant in the absence of suitable related donors may contraindicate this approach. However, the recent identification of the genetic lesions responsible for X-linked agammaglobulinemia and X-linked hyper-IgM syndrome has given rise to interest in adoptive gene therapy.[195]

Primary Disorders: Pure Antibody Deficiency

X-Linked Agammaglobulinemia (XLA). Originally described by Bruton[196] in 1952, XLA represents the first immunodeficiency disorder to be described. This disorder was recently mapped to a previously uncharacterized protein-tyrosine kinase that contained inactivating mutations in all the affected individuals studied.[197] The XLA genotype in males results in abortive B-cell development at the pre-B-cell stage. As a consequence, B cells and plasma cells are markedly diminished (less than 1 percent of normal) in blood, lymph node, and bone marrow.[198] Although VDJ rearrangement occurs in nascent B cells, heavy chain transcripts do not contain variable region sequences.[199] IgG, IgM, and IgA are reduced to undetectable or extremely low levels in the serum. Affected infants are usually asymptomatic until 5–6 months of age, at which time maternal antibodies are reduced to levels ineffective against infection. The hypogammaglobulinemia will then usually manifest as recurrent middle ear, sinopulmonary, and gastrointestinal tract infections with or without complicating bacteremia, meningitis, and cellulitis.[198] Less commonly, recurrent infections are clinically unappreciated until progressive pulmonary disease and bronchiectasis are identified. The presence of pulmonary disease at the time of diagnosis is considered a poor prognostic factor as mortality, usually in the second or third decade of life, is caused by progressive respiratory failure. Vaccination with inactivated antigen is usually futile, and live virus vaccinations are strictly contraindicated because of the risk of opportunistic infection. Poliomyelitis has occurred in several patients with agammaglobulinemia.[171]

Diagnosis rests on the characteristic family history of severe illnesses in young males and the failure to detect IgM, IgG, and IgA in the serum. IgG levels in particular are usually less than 100 mg/dl, a level below which antibody-dependent serum opsonization is severely affected. When appropriate laboratory resources are available, the absence of B cells in the peripheral blood and lymphatic tissues can be documented.[200] Antibody deficiency can also be identified by the absence of IgM isohemagglutinins against ABO incompatibilities and an inability to generate antibodies against vaccine antigens following routine immunization. Although rarely indicated for diagnosis of X-linked agammaglobulinemia, biopsy specimens from appropriate tissues demonstrate a complete absence of plasma cells in the germinal centers of lymph nodes and the lamina propria of the gut. Cellular immunity is completely intact. Many patients may have an associated cyclic or transient neuropenia that further aggravates their predisposition to infection. Related syndromes include X-linked hypogammaglobulinemia with isolated growth hormone deficiency and autosomal recessive hypogammaglobulinemia.[201]

Transient Hypogammaglobulinemia of Infancy. Transient hypogammaglobulinemia of infancy represents a delay in production of endogenous IgM and IgG, leading to an exaggerated form of the normal reduction in serum IgG levels that occurs at 5–6 months.[202] Serum IgG levels may drop as low as 350 mg/dl, and the infant may be subject to the same type of infections as children with X-linked hypogammaglobulinemia. In contrast to XLA, these infants are able to generate normal antibody responses to diptheria, tetanus, and pertussis vaccines.[203] Because of their transient immunodeficiency, these children should not be immunized with live virus vaccine until recovery of serum immunoglobulins is established. Treatment with IVIG is only rarely required for severe infections. Indeed, infusion of immunoglobulin may be detrimental if it suppresses production of endogenous immunoglobulins.

Common Variable Immunodeficiency (CVI). The CVI antibody deficiencies probably embrace several different disorders that have in common a later onset (15–25 years of age), hypogammaglobulinemia, and recurrent bacterial infections.[172,204] Because disease becomes manifest in adulthood, this disorder is often referred to as "acquired" hypogammaglobulinemia, although the strong familial occurrence suggests a genetic etiology. The possession of rare alleles of complement genes within the MHC III complex on chromosome 6 is strongly associated with the development of CVI and/or IgA-deficiency.[205] The estimated prevalence of CVI is anywhere from $1:50,000$ to $1:200,000$.[172]

The underlying etiology of CVI-related antibody deficiency remains poorly defined. Early B-cell maturation is intact, and normal numbers of B cells are evident in the circulation and in lymph nodes, although their ability to secrete antibody is clearly lacking.[206] At least part of the defect may be intrinsic to the B cell, although T cells from these patients are poor producers of IL-2, suggesting that the lesion of CVI perturbs activation of both lymphocytes.[207,208] A separate T-cell defect would also explain the increased risk of neoplasm and autoimmunity encountered in these patients. As described earlier, genetic linkages to the MHC III complex and the intrafamilial concurrence of both CVI and IgA deficiency suggest that these two disorders may be mechanistically related. Indeed, some patients with IgA deficiency later develop CVI.[205]

Common variable immunodeficiency is distinct in its manifestation compared with XLA.[204] While IgG levels are invariably below 250 mg/dl in symptomatic patients, with comparable decreases in the levels of other immunoglobulins, this pattern is less pronounced or consistent when compared with that of patients with X-linked hypogammaglobulinemia. Mature B cells expressing surface immunoglobulin are apparent in near-normal numbers in the circulation. Common variable immunodeficiency affects men and women equally, and the infections are often less severe than that of X-linked hypogammaglobulinemia. Some patients may merely experience an increased number or severity of sinopulmonary infections. Patients are predisposed to sprue-like malabsorption or regional enteritis and are also especially prone to autoimmune illnesses. In contrast to XLA, generalized lymphoid hyperplasia with or without splenomegaly is a common finding. Patients with CVI are highly predisposed to malignancy and have an estimated 57-fold increased risk of gastric cancer and a 438-fold increased risk of developing lymphomas later in life.[172,209]

The treatment of patients with the acquired form is similar to that of those with X-linked hypogammaglobulinemia and relies on the use of aggressive antibiotic therapy for acute infection combined with monthly infusions of IVIG to prevent future infections. Affected patients may require therapy for associated autoimmune disorders, and screening for malignancies should be aggressively pursued.

X-linked Hyper-IgM Syndrome (XHM). Affected males have elevated serum IgM levels and diminished or absent IgG levels and suffer from recurrent pyogenic infections.[210–212] This humoral immunodeficiency is also uniquely associated with an increased incidence of *Pneumocystis* pneumonia. Although initial B-cell maturation is intact, appropriate activating stimuli do not result in differentiation into IgG- or IgA-producing cells. Consequently, there is a characteristic increase in serum IgM concentrations in association with low-to-absent levels of IgA and IgG and a paucity of circulating B cells expressing IgG or IgA. It had been appreciated for some time that this may be traced to a defect in T-cell function normally required to support IgG production.[213] Recently, families with XHM were discovered to have a variety of mutations in a gene on the X chromosome that encoded the T-cell ligand for B-cell CD40.[145] In previous studies, activation of B cells via CD40 had been identified as a prerequisite for the appearance of IgG- and IgA-producing cells. The described genetic defect therefore provides a satisfactory explanation for the observed B-cell dysfunction.[144] Treatment is similar to that of the other hypogammaglobulinemic disorders outlined above. As in CVI, lymphoid hyperplasia is characteristic and may result in diagnostic misdirection.

Selective IgA Deficiency. Selective IgA deficiency is the most common disorder of antibody production with an incidence of about 1:300–600 in the normal population.[42,214] Whereas the majority of people with IgA deficiency are clinically normal, it is clear that this defect predisposes to a variety of diseases similar to those seen in CVI, including (1) recurrent sinopulmonary infections, (2) atopy, (3) gastrointestinal tract disease, (4) autoimmune disorders (e.g., systemic lupus erythematosus, rheumatoid arthritis, pernicious anemia), and (5) malignancy (diffuse histiocytic lymphoma or gastrointestinal carcinoma). These clinical manifestations are probably due to the absence of protective IgA on mucosal surfaces[26] and the loss of serum IgA blocking antibody directed against environmental antigens. Affected patients have markedly reduced levels of IgA in both serum (<50 mg/dl) and secretions, generally without abnormalities within the other major immunoglobulin classes.[42,214] Usually both IgA subclasses are affected, although selected deficiencies in IgA_2 have been described.[215] Some patients with IgA deficiency may have decreased levels of IgG subclasses, notably IgG_2 and IgG_4 with or without an absence of serum IgE.

The variability in the predisposition of IgA-deficient individuals to infection is still largely unexplained; it has been speculated that associated IgG_2 subclass deficiencies account for such susceptibility.[20] However, cases of combined IgA–IgG_2 deficiency caused by deletions of heavy chain genes have been identified by screening of blood donors without any history of increased susceptibility to infection.[216,217] Secretory IgM directed against microbial antigens is present in greater concentrations in these subjects and may provide adequate compensation for deficient dimeric IgA at mucosal sites.[30] There is little evidence that IVIG therapy is required in patients with IgA deficiency. Patients may require frequent follow-up for the management of atopic or autoimmune disease and are at increased risk of malignancy. Occasional IgA-deficient patients develop common variable immunodeficiency.

Allergies in these patients are often directed to common dietary antigens, such as bovine albumin contained in milk products.[218] As a consequence, patients who are totally IgA deficient are at risk of developing IgE-mediated anaphylactic reactions directed against exogenous IgA neoantigens.[193] When identified, these subjects should not receive immunoglobulin preparations containing IgA and should only receive extensively washed red cell transfusions.

IgG Subclass Deficiency. Isolated deficiency of IgG_1 is rare and, since this subtype accounts for approximately 70 percent of the IgG class, results in recognizable reductions in total IgG levels.[21] The clinical presentation with increased bacterial infections is very much like that of hypogammaglobulinemia patients. Replacement gammaglobulin therapy is usually effective in reducing the incidence of infections.

IgG_2 subclass deficiencies have been identified that are usually combined with parallel decreases in IgG_4, IgE, and IgA. Total levels of IgG are often in the normal range, reflecting the small contribution of IgG_2 to total IgG concentration. A subset of these patients may be at risk for recurrent bacterial infec-

tions.[20,22] However, most individuals with IgG_2 deficiency do not have an increased susceptibility to infectious disease.[219] It is likely that the predisposition to pulmonary infection instead reflects functional defects in the ability to generate specific anticapsular antibodies by a subset of patients with subclass deficiency.[220,221] Because the majority of IgG subclass-deficient patients may not be at risk for infection, IVIG therapy should be reserved for those patients who have clear-cut evidence of increased susceptibility to infectious diseases and who have demonstrated an inability to respond to capsular polysaccharide vaccines.

Combined T-Cell and Antibody Deficiencies

Severe Combined Immunodeficiency Disorders. A number of primary immunodeficiency disorders have been described in which both antibody production and cellular immunity are impaired. The most prominent include the severe combined immunodeficiency disorders (SCID), which result from a common inability to generate either mature B or T cells.[170,171] These infants are subject to a complex variety of infectious diseases and rarely survive past their second year of life. The etiology and variant types of this immunodeficiency are discussed in greater detail in Chapters 8 and 9. Due to extremely low immunoglobulin levels, these individuals are at increased risk of bacterial pneumonia, otitis, and septicemia. However, the clinical picture is mostly dominated by opportunistic infections resulting from deficient cellular immunity. Treatment consists of bone marrow transplantation or enzyme replacement (when the deficiency is due to loss of adenosine deaminase).

Wiskott-Aldrich Syndrome. Wiskott-Aldrich syndrome is a rare X-linked recessive disorder characterized by a triad of thrombocytopenia, severe eczematoid dermatitis, and deficient T-cell– and B-cell–mediated immune responses.[222,223] Young boys with this genotype usually present at a very early age with gastrointestinal bleeding or with severe eczema. The immunodeficiency is associated not only with an increased risk of infection but also with an approximately 10 percent lifetime risk of cancer.[224] Because of the great risk of premature death from bleeding, sepsis, or malignancy in these young patients, bone marrow transplantation is often considered as a curative measure. The precise genetic defect leading to the complex pathophysiology of Wiskott-Aldrich syndrome is not yet characterized, although abnormalities in O-glycosylation are well defined and associated with decreased expression of adhesion-mediating proteins, such as lymphocyte surface protein CD43.[225] Although affected patients have normal numbers of B and T cells, IgM and IgG levels are low, IgE and IgA levels are high, and de novo synthesis of antibodies to T-independent antigens—such as bacterial polysaccharides—are subnormal.[226] B-cell signal transduction following surface immunoglobulin ligation is significantly perturbed and may contribute to humoral immunodeficiency.[227] Not surprisingly, severe infections with pneumococci and *H. influenzae* are common and may necessitate frequent antibiotic and IVIG prophylaxis.[222] The recent isolation of the genetic lesion to the short arm of the X chromosome has provided a mechanism for prenatal and carrier detection.

Ataxia-Telangiectasia. Ataxia-telangiectasia is a rare genetic disorder linked to chromosome 11 and is associated with heterogenous defects in immunoglobulin levels and antigen-specific B-cell and T-cell responses.[228] The clinical picture is dominated by the progressive and disabling neurologic manifestations of the syndrome. Ocular telangiectasias are also present in nearly all affected individuals. Markedly perturbed DNA repair mechanisms are characteristic of ataxia-telangiectasia syndrome; chromosomal damage near the T-cell receptor and immunoglobulin genes have been suggested as reasons for the observed defects in immunity. Because immunoglobulin levels are not usually critically diminished, the use of IVIG should be restricted to patients with recurring infection who are unable to generate antibodies against *H. influenzae* B toxoid conjugate or other childhood vaccines.[171,188]

Secondary Antibody Deficiencies

Malignancy. Lymphoreticular or hematopoietic malignancies, especially lymphoma, lymphosarcoma, and thymoma, can be accompanied by profound deficiencies in one or more classes of immunoglobulins.[229,230] Chronic lymphocytic leukemia is even more commonly associated with clinically significant antibody deficiency.[231,232] The etiology of the hypogammaglobulinemia is not certain, but low levels of IgG and decreased antipneumococcal antibody titers in these patients are correlated with more frequent infectious morbidity. Such patients may benefit modestly from regular administration of intravenous immunoglobulin,[233] although the cost-effectiveness of this approach has been questioned.[234]

Antibody dyscrasias, such as multiple myeloma and Waldenstrom's macroglobulinemia, are associated with suppressed antibody responses by nonmalignant B cells.[235] This is related both to decreased numbers of normal B cells and to functional disorders that might be due to triggering of immune feedback mechanisms in response to monoclonal hypergammaglobulinemia.[236] Increased catabolism of immunoglobulins may also contribute to decreased levels of nonmalignant types of IgG. Infections with encapsulated and gram-negative bacteria are prominent in these patients.[237,238] Immunoglobulin supplementation is thought to be of little help, given that the clearance of antibodies is increased.[239]

Protein Wasting States. Immunoglobulin catabolism is increased in some patients with severe burns, protein-losing enteropathies, and the nephrotic syndrome. Immunoglobulins can be lost excessively in burned tissues,[240] whereas gastrointestinal or urinary tract losses of IgG are responsible for hypogammaglobulinemia in the other disorders. Treatment of the primary disease process will bring about a reversal of these conditions.

Splenectomy and Sickle Cell Anemia. The spleen provides a multitude of important host defense functions.[241] It serves as a phagocytic filter that can nonspecifically remove circulating antigenic complexes, microbes, and parasitized erythrocytes. The spleen is especially efficient at removing poorly opsonized pathogens.[242] Antigen-presenting cells within the spleen are available for processing the captured antigens and presenting them to T cells contained in this organ. The spleen is also an important site of IgM production and memory B-cell differentiation during primary humoral responses.[243] Consequently, removal of the spleen by surgery or by disease results in a heightened predisposition to sepsis syndrome caused by pneumococci, other streptococci, *H. influenzae,* meningococci, and a variety of other encapsulated bacteria, such as *Capnocytophaga canimorsus* (DF2).[244,245] Splenic hypofunction also predisposes to severe infection with intraerythrocytic parasites such as *Babesia microti.* Splenectomy during childhood is most associated with enhanced susceptibility to infection, although adult splenectomy is also accompanied by similar risks. The immune defect is probably related to decreased phagocytic removal of poorly opsonized bacteria from the blood stream.[242,246]

Although the titer of antibody produced in response to pneumococcal vaccine is less than that of eusplenic patients, the protective efficacy had been reported as being at least 85 percent.[247] Since antipneumococcal antibody responses decline over 2–5 years in asplenic hosts, revaccination 2 years after primary immunization has become accepted practice.[248,249] *Haemophilus influenzae* type B conjugate vaccine administered to children undergoing splenectomy generates antibody responses deemed adequate for prophylaxis against infection.[250]

Therefore, it is recommended that asplenic patients be vaccinated with *H. influenzae* type B conjugate and pneumococcal vaccines twice over a period of 2–3 years. Although these patients are also at risk for meningococcemia and respond well to meningococcal vaccine, the currently available preparations do not provide protection against the group B serotype common in the United States.[251] Daily oral penicillin is still considered a mainstay therapy to prevent infection in the splenectomized child or adult.[252] In contrast to these studies of patients splenectomized because of trauma, the removal of the spleen as part of the staging study for Hodgkin's disease results in diminished responsiveness to pneumococcal vaccine after splenectomy, probably reflecting the deleterious effect of cytotoxic or lymphoid irradiation therapies on B-cell responses.[253] However, the ability to generate antibody to polysaccharide vaccines remains intact prior to splenectomy, and vaccination is recommended 2 weeks before the spleen is scheduled to be removed.

Sickle cell patients, who are functionally asplenic following infarction of that organ, also suffer from a 30 to 100-fold increased incidence of pneumococcal, *Haemophilus,* and meningococcal infections, including both pneumonia and septicemia.[254,255] The increased susceptibility to infection in these patients has been variously ascribed to the loss of splenic clearance mechanisms, to poor anticapsular antibody responses, and to deficient serum opsonizing activity. In contrast to splenectomy, sickle cell disease is more clearly associated with a deficient response to available pneumococcal vaccines.[255] However, *H. influenzae* type b polysaccharide–tetanus protein conjugate vaccine stimulates antibody levels comparable to those of normal children.[256] Antibiotic prophylaxis and aggressive vaccination are advised to prevent infection with pneumococcus or *H. influenzae* in young sickle cell patients.[255,257]

Bone Marrow Transplantation. The preparative regimen used prior to bone marrow transplant effectively removes bone marrow precursor B cells and memory B-cell populations in the lymphoid organs. Despite the prolonged half-life of serum immunoglobulin, the long time required for full engraftment of donor bone marrow usually results in a dramatic decrease in serum immunoglobulin levels that slowly return to normal over 3–4 months.[258] In some respects this process recapitulates the transient hypogammaglobulinemia of infancy in that IgM recovery precedes IgG and IgA. After normalization of serum immunoglobulin levels, some patients remain functionally antibody deficient in the face of bacterial and viral infections. In this regard, combinations of IVIG and ganciclovir have proven of benefit to some bone marrow transplant patients with clinically overt cytomegalovirus infection.[259] Intravenous immunoglobulin is also used after allogeneic transplantation to prevent acute graft-vs.-host disease and interstitial pneumonitis.[260] The ability of IVIG to reduce bacterial infections significantly in these patients remains controversial.[261]

HIV-Related Antibody Deficiency. Infection with HIV is associated with aberrant immunoglobulin production and B-cell function. Although adult patients may have normal to increased immunoglobulin levels, their ability to generate or maintain specific antibody responses to bacterial antigens is severely impaired even before CD4+ T-lymphocyte counts begin to decline. This commonly manifests as poor antibody responses to polysaccharide and protein vaccines[262,263] and an increasing inability to seroconvert during primary infections. Children typically have a much more severe humoral deficiency, probably because they have not formed sufficient memory B cells before CD4+ helper T-cell functions are lost. Both children and adults have markedly increased rates of pneumococcal and *H. influenzae* pneumonia and bacteremia.[264] Although immunization with pneumococcal vaccine does not reliably provoke strong antibody responses in AIDS patients, *H. influenzae* capsular antigens linked to diphtheria toxoid were markedly more effective than capsular polysaccharide alone in inducing adequate humoral responses.[265] Therefore, HIV-positive patients should receive pneumococcal, *H. influenzae*–toxoid conjugate and influenza vaccines as early in the course of disease as possible. Therapy with intravenous immunoglobulin was recently demonstrated to reduce the incidence of bacterial infections in HIV-infected children with CD4+ counts of greater than 200 cells/mm^3 and may be indicated for severe repeated bacterial infections.[266,267] There were no differences in the rate of opportunistic infections.

In contrast, production of IgE may actually be increased during HIV infection. This is associated with an increased frequency (30–68 percent) of allergic rhinitis and sinusitus, leading to frequent bacterial sinusitis as a complication. Patients in the later stages of disease develop new allergies documentable by skin testing and maintain serum levels of IgE that are three- to five-fold increased over normal values.[268] This spontaneous shift in immunoglobulin isotype during AIDS may reflect alterations in the balance of T-helper types 1 and 2 CD4+ activities during the evolution of AIDS.[269]

REFERENCES

1. Capra JD, Kehoe JM. Hypervariable regions, idiotypy, and the antibody-combining site. Adv Immunol. 1975;20:1–33.
2. Burton DR, Woof JM. Human antibody effector function. Adv Immunol. 1992;51:1–84.
3. Nezlin R. Internal movements in immunoglobulin molecules. Adv Immunol. 1990;48:1–40.
4. Rini J, Schulze-Gahmen U, Wilson IA. Structural evidence for an induced fit as a mechanism for antibody–antigen recognition. Science. 1992;255:959–65.
5. Canfield SM, Morrison SL. The binding affinity of human IgG for its high affinity Fc receptor is determined by multiple amino acids in the C_H2 domain and is modulated by the hinge region. J Exp Med. 1991;173:1483–91.
6. Tao MH, Canfield SM, and Morrison SL. The differential ability of human IgG1 and IgG4 to activate complement is determined by the COOH-terminal sequence of the C_H2 domain. J Exp Med. 1991;173:1025–8.
7. Kehry M. The immunoglobulin μ chains of membrane-bound and secreted IgM molecules differ in their C-terminal segments. Cell. 1980;21:393.
8. Natvig J, Kunkel H. Immunoglobulins: Classes, subclasses, genetic variants, and idiotypes. Adv Immunol. 1973;16:1–26.
9. Goodman JW. Immunoglobulin structure and function. In: Stites D, Terr AI (eds): Basic Clinical Immunology. 7th ed. San Mateo, CA: Appleton & Lange; 1991:109–21.
10. Porter RR. Structural studies of immunoglobulins. Science. 1973;180:713–6.
11. Spiegelberg HL. Biological activities of immunoglobulins of different classes and subclasses. Adv Immunol. 1974;19:259–94.
12. Koshland ME. The coming of age of the immunoglobulin J chain. Annu Rev Immunol. 1985;3:425–53.
13. Roth RA, Koshland ME. Identification of a lymphocyte enzyme that catalyzes pentamer immunoglobulin M assembly. J Biol Chem. 1981;256:4633–9.
14. Buckley RH, Dees SC, and O'Fallon WM. Serum immunoglobulins. I. Levels in normal children and in uncomplicated childhood allergy. Pediatrics. 1968;41:600–11.
15. Carson DA, Chen PP, Kipps TJ. New roles for rheumatoid factor. J Clin Invest 1991;87:379–83.
16. Wienands J, Reth M. Glycosyl-phosphatidylinositol linkage as a mechanism for cell-surface expression of immunoglobulin D. Nature. 1992;356:246–9.
17. Reynolds HY. Immunoglobulin G and its function in the human respiratory tract. Mayo Clin Proc. 1988;63:161–74.
18. Michaelsen TE, Garred P, Aase A. Human IgG subclass pattern of inducing complement-mediated cytolysis depends on antigen concentration and to a lesser extent on epitope patchiness, antibody affinity and complement concentration. Eur J Immunol. 1991;21:11–6.
19. Siber GR, Schur PH, Aisenberg AC, et al. Correlation between serum IgG2 concentrations and the antibody response to bacterial polysaccharide antigens. N Engl J Med. 1980;303:178–81.
20. Oxelius VA, Laurell AB, Lindquist B, et al. IgG subclasses in selective IgA deficiency. Importance of IgG2–IgA deficiency. N Engl J Med. 1981;304:1476–7.
21. Schur P, Borel H, Gelfand G, et al. Selective gamma-G globulin deficiencies in patients with recurrent pyogenic infections. N Engl J Med. 1970;283:631–5.
22. Bjorkander J, Bake B, Oxelius V, et al. Impaired lung function in patients with IgA deficiency and low levels of IgG2 or IgG3. N Engl J Med. 1985;313:720–4.
23. Stanworth DR, Smith AK. Inhibition of reagin-mediated PCA reactions in baboons by the human IgG4 suB class. Clin Allergy. 1973;3:37–41.
24. Underdown B, Schiff M. Immunoglobulin A: Strategic defense initiative at the mucosal surface. Ann Rev Immunol. 1986;389–417.
25. Tomsai TB, Plaut AG. Humoral aspects of mucosal immunity. In: Gallin J, Fauci A, eds. Advances in Host Defense Mechanisms. New York: Raven Press; 1985:31–62.
26. Childers NK, Bruce MG, McGhee JR. Molecular mechanisms of immunoglobulin A defense. Annu Rev Microbiol. 1989;43:503–36.
27. Mestecky J, McGhee JR. Immunoglobulin A (IgA): Molecular and cellular interaction involved in IgA biosynthesis and immune response. Adv Immunol. 1987;40:153–89.
28. Lamm ME. Cellular aspects of immunoglobulin A. Adv Immunol. 1976;22:223–90.
29. Mostov KE, Deitcher DL. Polymeric immunoglobulin receptor expressed in MDCK cells transcytoses IgA. Cell. 1986;46:613–21.
30. Mellander L, Bjorkander J, Carlsson B, et al. Secretory antibodies in IgA-deficient and immunosuppressed individuals. J Clin Immunol. 1986;6:284–90.
31. Sixbey JW, Yao QY. Immunoglobulin A–induced shift of epstein-Barr virus tissue tropism. Science. 1992;255:1578–80.
32. Kaetzel CS, Robinson JK, Chintalacharuvu KR, et al. The polymeric immunoglobulin receptor (secretory component) mediates transport of immune complexes across epithelial cells: A local defense function for IgA. Proc Natl Acad Sci USA. 1991;88:8796–800.
33. Welsh JK, May JT. Antiinfective properties of breast milk. J Pediatr. 1979;94:1–9.
34. Ogra PL, Karzon DT, Righthand F, et al. Immunoglobulin response in serum and secretions after immunization with live and inactivated poliovaccine and natural infection. N Engl J Med. 1968;279:894–902.
35. Heyworth MF. Immunology of *Giardia* and *Cryptosporidium* infections. J Infect Dis. 1992;166:465–72.
36. Bessen D, Fischetti VA. Passive acquired mucosal immunity to group A streptococci by secretory immunoglobulin A. J Exp Med. 1988;167:1945–50.
37. Hostoffer RW, Krukovets I, Berger M. Increased FcαR expression and IgA-mediated function on neutrophils induced by chemoattractants. J Immunol. 1993;150:4532–40.
38. Kilian M, Mestecky J, Russell MW. Defense mechanisms involving Fc-dependent functions of immunoglobulin A and their subversion by bacterial immunoglobulin A proteases. Microbiol Rev. 1988;52:296–303.
39. Brandtzaeg P. Humoral immune response patterns of human mucosae: Induction and relation to bacterial respiratory tract infections. J Infect Dis 1992;165(Suppl 1):S167–76.
40. Stokes CR, Soothill JR, Turner MW. Immune exclusion is a function of IgA. Nature. 1975;255:745–6.
41. Walker W, Isselbacher KJ, Block K. Intestinal uptake of macromolecules: Effect of oral immunization. Science. 1972;177:608–10.
42. Burks A, Steele RW. Selective IgA deficiency. Ann Allergy. 1986;57:3–8.
43. Metzger H, Alcaraz G, Hohman R, et al. The receptor with high affinity for immunoglobulin E. Annu Rev Immunol. 1986;4:419–70.
44. Jarrett EE, Miller H. Production and activities of IgE in helminth infection. Prog Allergy. 1982;31:178–84.
45. Miller H. The protective mucosal response against gastrointestinal nematodes in ruminants and laboratory animals. Vet Immunol. 1984;6:167–74.
46. Hagan P, Blumentahl U, Dunn D, et al. Human IgE, IgG4 and resistance to reinfection with *Schistosoma haematobium*. Nature. 1991;349:243–6.
47. Capron A, Dessaint JP. Immunologic aspects of schistosomiasis. Annu Rev Med. 1992;43:209–18.
48. Urban JF, Madden KB, Svetic A, et al. The importance of Th2 cytokines in protective immunity to nematodes. Immunol Rev. 1992;127:205–20.
49. Zuckier LS, Rodriquez LD, Scharff MD. Immunological and pharmacological concepts of monoclonal antibodies. Semin Nucl Med. 1989;19:166–86.
50. Waldmann TA, Strober W. Metabolism of immunoglobulins. Prog Allergy. 1969;13:1–110.
51. Fridman WH. Fc receptors and immunoglobulin binding factors. FASEB J. 1991;5:2684–90.
52. Ravetch JV, Kinet JP. Fc receptors. Annu Rev Immunol. 1991;9:457–92.
53. Kinet JP. The γ–ζ dimers of Fc receptors as connectors to signal transduction. Curr Opin Immunol. 1992;4:43–8.
54. Conrad DH. FcεRII/CD23: The low affinity receptor for IgE. Annu Rev Immunol. 1990;8:623–45.
55. Huizinga T, van Kemenade F, Koenderman L, et al. The 40-kDa Fcγ receptor (FcRII) on human neutrophils is essential for the IgG-induced respiratory burst and IgG-induced phagocytosis. J Immunol. 1989;142:2365–9.
56. Debets JM, Van der Linden CJ, Dieteren IEM, et al. Fc-receptor cross-linking induces rapid secretion of tumor necrosis factor (cachectin) by human peripheral blood monocytes. J Immunol. 1988;141:1197–201.
57. Bich LT, Revillard JP. Selective suppression of human B lymphocyte differentiation into IgG-producing cells by soluble Fc receptors. J Immunol. 1982;129:150–9.
58. Cassatella M, Anegon I, Cuturi MC, et al. FcγR (CD16) interaction with ligand induces Ca^{2+} mobilization and phosphoinositide turnover in human natural killer cells: Role in transcription and expression of lymphokine genes. J Exp Med. 1989;169:549–67.
59. Azzoni L, Kamoun M, Salcedo TW, et al. Stimulation of FcγRIIIA results in phospholipase C-γ1 tyrosine phosphorylation and p56[lck] activation. J Exp Med. 1992;176:1745–50.
60. Hibbs ML, Selvaraj P, Carpen O, et al. Mechanisms for regulating expression of membrane isoforms of FcγRIII (CD16). 1989;246:1608–11.
61. Blank U, Ra C, Miller L, et al. Complete structure and expression in transfected cells of high affinity IgE receptor. Nature. 1989;337:187–9.

62. Paul WE, Seder RA, Plaut M. Lymphokine and cytokine production by FceRI⁺ cells. Adv Immunol. 1993;53:1–29.
63. Kehry MR, Yamashita LC. Role of the low-affinity Fce receptor in B lymphocyte antigen presentation. Res Immunol. 1990;141:77–81.
64. Maliszewski CR, March CJ, Schoenborn MA, et al. Expression cloning of a human Fc receptor for IgA. J Exp Med. 1990;172:1665–72.
65. Shen L, Lasser R, Fanger MW. My43, a monoclonal antibody that reacts with human myeloid cells, inhibits monocyte IgA binding and triggers function. J Immunol. 1989;143:4117–21.
66. Burton DR. Immunoglobulin G: Functional sites. Mol Immunol. 1985;22: 161–206.
67. Borsos T, Rapp HJ. Complement fixation on cell surfaces by 19S and 7S antibodies. Science. 1965;150:505–6.
68. Frank M, Joiner K, Hammer C. The function of antibody and complement in the lysis of bacteria. Rev Infect Dis. 1987;9:S537–45.
69. Giebink GS, Verhoef J, Peterson P. Opsonic requirements for phagocytosis of *Streptococcus pneumoniae* types VI, XVIII, XXIII, and XXV. Infect Immunol. 1977;18:291–7.
70. Anderson P, Johnston R. Human serum activities against *Hemophilus influenzae,* type B. J Clin Invest. 1972;51:31–8.
71. Peterson P, Wilkinson B, Kim Y, et al. The key role of peptidoglycan in the opsonization of *Staphylococcus aureus.* J Clin Invest. 1978;61:597–609.
72. Horowitz MA. Phagocytosis of microorganisms. Rev Infect Dis. 1982;4: 104–18.
73. Schneiderman RD, Lint TL, Knight KL. Activation of the alternative pathway of complement by 12 different rabbit-mouse chimeric transfectoma IgA isotypes. J Immunol. 1990;145:233–7.
74. Pfaffenbach G, Lamm ME, Gigli I. Activation of the guinea pig alternative complement pathway by mouse IgA immune complexes. J Exp Med. 1982; 155:231–47.
75. Fanger MW, Erbe DV. Fc gamma receptors in cancer and infectious disease. Immunol Res. 1992;11:203–16.
76. Anderson CL, Shen L, Eicher DM. Phagocytosis mediated by three distinct Fcγ receptor classes on human leukocytes. J Exp Med. 1990;171:1333–45.
77. Johnston R, Anderson P, Rosen F, et al. Characterization of human antibody to polyribose phosphate, the capsular antigen of *Haemophilus influenzae* type b. Clin Immunol Immunopathol. 1973;1:234–40.
78. Clark RA, Klebanoff SJ. Studies on the mechanism of antibody-dependent polymorphonuclear leukocyte-mediated cytotoxicity. J Immunol. 1977;119: 1413–8.
79. Sissons J, Oldstone M. Killing of virus infected cells by cytotoxic lymphocytes. J Infect Dis. 1980;142:114–9.
80. Trinchieri G. Biology of natural killer cells. Adv Immunol. 1989;47:187–376.
81. Fanger MW, Shen L, Graziano RF, et al. Cytotoxicity mediated by human Fc receptors for IgG. Immunol Today. 1989;10:92–9.
82. Ehrlich P. Die Wertbemessung des Diphtherieserums und deren theoretische Grundlagen. Klin Jahrbuch. 1897;6:299–312.
83. Blake PA, Feldman RA, Buchanan TM, et al. Serologic therapy of tetanus in the United States, 1965–1971. JAMA. 1976;235:42–4.
84. Metzer JF, Lewis GE. Human-derived immune globulins for the treatment of botulism. Rev Infect Dis. 1979;1:689–94.
85. English PC. Diphtheria and theories of infectious disease: Centennial appreciation of the critical role of diphtheria in the history of medicine. Pediatrics 1985;71:1–9.
86. Johns M, Skehill A, McCabe WR. Immunization with rough mutants of *Salmonella minnesota.* IV. Protection by antisera to O and rough antigens of endotoxin. J Infect Dis. 1983;147:57–63.
87. Ziegler E, McCutchan J, Fierer J, et al. Treatment of gram-negative bacteremia and shock with human antiserum to a mutant *Escherichia coli.* N Engl J Med. 1982;307:1225–30.
88. Ziegler E, Fisher C, Sprung C, et al. Treatment of gram-negative bacteremia and septic shock with HA-1A human monoclonal antibody against endotoxin: A randomized, double-blind, placebo-controlled trial. N Engl J Med. 1991; 324:429–36.
89. Greenman R, Schein R, Martin M, et al. A controlled clinical trial of E5 murine monoclonal IgM antibody to endotoxin in the treatment of gram-negative sepsis. JAMA. 1991;266:1097–102.
90. Warren HS, Danner RL, Munford RS. Anti-endotoxin monoclonal antibodies (Editorial). N Engl J Med. 1992;326:1153–7.
91. Mandel B. Neutralization of animal viruses. Adv Virus Res. 1974;23:205–69.
92. Dimmock NJ. Mechanisms of neutralization of animal viruses. Gen Virol. 1984;65:1015–22.
93. Taylor HP, Dimmock NJ. Mechanism of neutralization of influenza virus by secretory IgA is different from that of monomeric IgA or IgG. J Exp Med. 1985;161:198–209.
94. Rossman MG. Neutralization of small RNA viruses by antibodies and antiviral agents. FASEB J. 1989;3:2335–43.
95. Armstrong SJ, Dimmock NJ. Neutralization of influenza virus by low concentrations of hemagglutinin-specific polymeric immunoglobulin A inhibits viral fusion activity, but activation of the ribonucleoprotein is also inhibited. J Virol. 1992;66:3823–32.
96. Mazanec MB, Kaetzel CS, Lamm ME, et al. Intracellular neutralization of virus by immunoglobulin A antibodies. Proc Natl Acad Sci USA. 1992;89: 6901–5.
97. Finlay BB, and Falkow S. Common themes in microbial pathogenicity. Microbiol Rev. 1989;53:210–30.
98. Williams RC, Gibbons RJ. Inhibition of bacterial adherence by secretory immunoglobulin A: A mechanism of antigen disposal. Science. 1972;697–9.
99. McSweegan E, Burr DH, Walker RI. Intestinal mucus gel and secretory antibody are barriers to *Campylobacter jejui* adherence to INT 407 cells. Infect Immun. 1987;55:1431–5.
100. Moss RB. Hypergammaglobulinemia in cystic fibrosis. Chest 1987;91:523–6.
101. Phair J, Clarke J. Immunology of infective endocarditis. Prog Cardiovasc Dis. 1979;22:137–44.
102. Kobayakawa T, Louis J, Izui S, et al. Autoimmune response to DNA, red blood cells and thymocyte antigens in association with polyclonal antibody synthesis during experimental African trypanosomiasis. J Immunol. 1979; 122:296–301.
103. Rosen A, Gergely P, Jondal M, et al. Polyclonal Ig production after Epstein-Barr virus infection of human lymphocytes in vitro. Nature. 1977;267:53–6.
104. Carter RL. Antibody formation in infectious mononucleosis. II. Other 19S antibodies and false positive serology. Br J Haematol. 1966;12:268–72.
105. Theofilopoulous AN, Dixon FJ. The biology and detection of immune complexes. Adv Immunol. 1979;28:89–199.
106. Hoiby N, During G, Schiotz K. The role of immune complexes in the pathogenesis of bacterial infections. Annu Rev Microbiol. 1986;40:29–53.
107. Couser WG. Mechanisms of glomerular injury in immune-complex disease. Kidney Int. 1985;28:569–83.
108. Strickler GB, Shin M, Bureke E. Diffuse glomerulonephritis associated with infected ventriculoatrial shunt. N Engl J Med. 1968;279:1077–82.
109. Schifferli J, Ng YC, Peters DK. The role of complement and its receptor in the elimination of immune complexes. N Engl J Med. 1986;315:488–95.
110. Carson DA, Chen PP, Fox RI, et al. Rheumatoid factor and immune networks. Annu Rev Immunol. 1987;5:109–26.
111. Radoux V, Chen PP, Sorge JA, et al. A conserved human germline Vκ gene directly encodes rheumatoid factor light chains. J Exp Med. 1986;164: 2119–24.
112. Pascual V, Randen I, Thompson K, et al. The complete nucleotide sequences of the heavy chain varible regions of six monospecific rheumatoid factors deived from Epstein-Barr virus-transformed B cells isolated from the synovial tissue of patients with rheumatoid arthritis. J Clin Invest. 1990;86: 1320–8.
113. Roosnek E, Lanzavecchia A. Efficient and selective presentation of antigen–antibody complexes by rheumatoid factor B cells. J Exp Med. 1991; 173:487–89.
114. Agnello V, Chung RT, Kaplan LM. A role for hepatitis C virus infection in type II cryoglobulinemia. N Engl J Med. 1992;327:1490–5.
115. Misiani R, Bellavita P, Fenili D, et al. Hepatitis C virus infection in patients with essential mixed cryoglobulinemia. Ann Intern Med. 1992;117:573–77.
116. Fritzler MJ, Salazar M. Diversity and origin of rheumatologic autoantibodies. Clin Microbiol Rev. 1991;4:256–69.
117. Van Voorhis WC, Schlekewy L, Trong HL. Molecular mimicry by *Trypanosoma cruzi:* The Fl-160 epitope that mimics mammalian nerve can be mapped to a 12-amino acid peptide. Proc Natl Acad Sci USA. 1991;8:5993–7.
118. Cohen IR, Young DB. Autoimmunity, microbial immunity and the immunological humunculus. Immunol Today. 1991;12:105–7.
119. Dale JB, Beachey EH. Epitopes of streptococcal M proteins shared with cardiac myosins. J Exp Med. 1985;162:583–91.
120. Tonegawa S. Somatic generation of antibody diversity. Nature. 1983;302: 575–81.
121. Alt FW, Blackwell TK, Yancopoulos G. Development of the primary antibody repertoire. Science. 1987;238:1079–87.
122. Yancopoulos GD, Alt FW. Regulation of the assembly and expression of variable-region genes. Annu Rev Immunol. 1986;4:339–68.
123. Schatz DG, Oettinger MA, Schlissel MS. V(D)J recombination: Molecular biology and regulation. Annu Rev Immunol. 1992;10:359–83.
124. Shinkai Y, Rathbun G, Lam K, et al. RAG-2 deficient mice lack mature lymphocytes owing to inability to initiate V(D)J rearrangement. Cell. 1991; 68:855–67.
125. Landau NR, Schatz DG, Rosa M, et al. Increased frequency of N-regional insertion in a murine pre-B cell line infected with a terminal deoxynucleotidyl transferase retroviral expression vector. Mol Cell Biol. 1987;7:3237–43.
126. Harriman W, Volk H, Defranoux N, et al. Immunoglobulin class switch recombination. Annu Rev Immunol. 1993;11:361–84.
127. Coffman RL, Lebman DA, Rothman P. Mechanism and regulation of immunoglobulin isotype switching. Adv Immunol. 1993;54:229–70.
128. Siekevitz M, Kocks C, Rajewsky K, et al. Analysis of somatic mutation and class switching in naive and memory B cells generating adoptive primary and secondary responses. Cell. 1987;48:757–70.
129. French DL, Laskov R, Scharff M. The role of somatic hypermutation in the generation of antibody diversity. Science. 1989;244:1152–7.
130. Banchereau J, Rousset F. Human B lymphocytes: Phenotype, proliferation, and differentiation. Adv Immunol. 1992;52:125–251.
131. Clark EA, Lane PJ. Regulation of human B cell activation and adhesion. Annu Rev Immunol. 1991;9:97–127.
132. Reth M. Antigen receptors on B lymphocytes. Annu Rev Immunol. 1992; 10:97–121.
133. Malissen B, Schmitt-Verhulst AM. Transmembrane signalling through the T cell receptor-CD3 complex. Curr Opin Immunol. 1993;5:324–3.
134. Clark M, Campbell K, Kazlauskas A, et al. The B cell antigen receptor complex: Association of Ig-α and Ig-β with distinct cytoplasmic effectors. Science. 1992;258:123–6.
135. Cooper NR, Moore MD, Nemerow GR. Immunobiology of CR2, the B lym-

phocyte receptor for Epstein-Barr virus and the C3d complement fragment. Annu Rev Immunol. 1988.

136. Clark EA. CD22, a B cell-specific receptor, mediates adhesion and signal transduction. J Immunol. 1993;150:4715–8.

137. Parker DC. T cell-dependent B cell activation. Annu Rev Immunol. 1993; 11:331–60.

138. Mitchinson NA. The carrier effect in the secondary response to hapten-carrier conjugates. II. Cellular cooperation. Eur J Immunol. 1971;1:18–26.

139. Germain RN, Margulies DH. The biochemistry and cell biology of antigen processing and presentation. Annu Rev Immunol. 1993;11:403–50.

140. Chestnut RW, Grey HM. Antigen presentation by B cells and its significance in T–B interactions. Adv Immunol. 1986;39:51–95.

141. Lederman S, Yellin JJ, Covey LR, et al. Non-antigen signals for B cell growth and differentiation to antibody secretion. Curr Opin Immunol. 1993;5: 439–44.

142. Van de Velde H, von Hoegen I, Luo W, et al. The B cell surface protein CD72/LyB 2 is the ligand for CD5. Nature. 1991;351:662–5.

143. Linsley PS, Ledbetter JA. The role of the CD28 receptor during T cell responses to antigen. Annu Rev Immunol. 1993;11:191–212.

144. Banchereau J, Rousset F. Growing human B lymphocytes in the CD40 system. Nature. 1991;353:678–9.

145. Aruffo A, Farrington M, Hollenbaugh D, et al. The CD40 ligand, gp39, is defective in activated T cells from patients with X-linked hyper-IgM syndrome. Cell. 1993;72:291–300.

146. Fischer A, Durandy A, Sterkers G. Role of the LFA-1 molecule in cellular interactions required for antibody production in humans. J Immunol. 1986; 136:3198–203.

147. Santosham M, Wolff M, Reid R, et al. The efficacy in Navajo infants of a conjugate vaccine consisting of *Haemophilus influenzae* type b polysaccharide and *Neisseria meningitidis* outer-membrane protein complex. N Engl J Med. 1991;324:1767–72.

148. Cooper MD. B lymphocytes: Normal development and function. N Engl J Med. 1987;317:1452–6.

149. Nishimoto N, Kubagawa H, Ohno T, et al. Normal pre-B cells express a receptor complex of μ heavy chains and surrogate light-chain proteins. Proc Natl Acad Sci USA. 1991;88:6284–8.

150. Motyka B, Reynolds JD. Apoptosis is associated with the extensive B cell death in the sheep ileal Peyer's patch and the chicken bursa of fabricus: A possible role in B cell selection. Eur J Immunol. 1991;21:1951–8.

151. Cohen J, Duke RC, Fadoik VA, et al. Apoptosis and programmed cell death in immunity. Annu Rev Immunol. 1992;10:267–94.

152. Hartley S, Crosbie J, Brink R, et al. Elimination from peripheral lymphoid tissues of self-reactive B lymphocytes recognizing membrane-bound antigens. Nature. 1991;353:765–9.

153. Goodnow CC. B cell tolerance. Curr Opin Immunol. 1992;4:703–10.

154. Goodnow CC, Brink R, Adams E. Breakdown of self-tolerance in anergic B lymphocytes. Nature. 1991;352:532–6.

155. Brink R, Goodnow CC, Crosbie J, et al. Immunoglobulin M and D antigen receptors are both capable of mediating B lymphocyte activation, deletion, or angergy after interaction with specific antigen. J Exp Med. 1992;176: 991–1005.

156. Roes J, Rajewsky K. Immunoglobulin D (IgD)-deficient mice reveal an auxiliary receptor function for IgD in antigen-mediated recruitment of B cells. J Exp Med. 1993;177:43–55.

157. Kelsoe G, Zheng B. Sites of B cell activation in vivo. Curr Opin Immunol. 1993;5:418–22.

158. Jacob J, Kelsoe G, Rajewsky K, et al. Intraclonal generation of antibody mutants in germinal centers. Nature. 1991;354:389–92.

159. Foote J, Milstein C. Kinetic maturation of an immune response. Nature. 1991;352:530–2.

160. Schriever F, Nadler LM. The central role of follicular dendritic cells in lymphoid tissue. Adv Immunol. 1992;51:243–84.

161. Gray D. Immunological memory. Annu Rev Immunol. 1993;11:49–77.

162. Kearney JF. CD5 + B cell networks. Curr Opin Immunol. 1993;5:223–6.

163. Kantor AB, Herzenberg LA. Origin of murine B cell lineages. Annu Rev Immunol. 1993;11:501–38.

164. Briles DE, Nahm M, Schroer K, et al. Antiphosphorylcholine antibodies found in normal mouse serum are protective against intravenous infections with type 3 *S. pneumoniae*. J Exp Med. 1981;153:694–705.

165. Goni F, Frangione B. Amino acid sequence of the Fv region of a human monoclonal IgM (protein WEA) with antibody activity against 3,4-pyruvylated galactose in *Klebsiella* polysaccharides K30 and K33. Proc Natl Acad Sci USA. 1983;80:4837–41.

166. Murphy DB. T cell mediated immunosuppression. Curr Opin Immunol. 1993; 5:411–7.

167. Nisonoff A. Idiotypes: Concepts and applications. J Immunol. 1991;147: 2429–38.

168. Conley ME. Molecular approaches to analysis of X-linked immunodeficiencies. Annu Rev Immunol. 1992;10:215–38.

169. Hermaszewski RA, Webster AD. Primary hypogammaglobulinaemia: A survey of clinical manifestations and complications. Q J Med. 1993;86:31–42.

170. Rosen FSJ, Cooper MD, Wedgwood RJP. The primary immunodeficiencies. N Engl J Med. 1984;311:235–42.

171. Buckley RH. Immunodeficiency diseases. JAMA. 1992;268:2797–806.

172. Sneller MC, Strober W, Eisenstein E, et al. New insights into common variable immundeficiency. Ann Intern Med. 1993;118:720–30.

173. Spickett GP, Misbah SA, Chapel HM. Primary antibody deficiency in adults. Lancet. 1991;337:281–4.

174. Saulsbury FT, Winkelstein JA, Yolken RH. Chronic rotavirus infection in immunodeficiency. J Pediatr. 1980;97:61–5.

175. Roberts-Thomson IC. Genetic studies of human and murine giardiasis. Clin Infect Dis. 1993;16(Suppl 2):S98–104.

176. Ochs HD, Ament ME, Davis SD. Giardiasis with malabsorption in X-linked agammaglobulinemia. N Engl J Med. 1972;287:341–3.

177. Abramowsky CR, Sorensen RU. Regional enteritis-like enteropathy in a patient with agammaglobulinemia: Histologic and immunocytologic studies. Hum Pathol. 1988;19:483–90.

178. Lee AH, Levinson AI, Schumacher HR. Hypogammaglobulinemia and rheumatic disease. Semin Arthritis Rheum. 1993;22:252–64.

179. Forgacs P, Kundsin RB, Margles SW, et al. A case of *Ureaplasma urealyticum* septic arthritis in a patient with hypogammaglobulinemia. Clin Infect Dis. 1993;16:293–4.

180. Crennan JM, Van Scoy RE, McKenna CH, et al. Echovirus polymyositits in patients with hypogammaglobulinemia. Failure of high-dose intravenous gammaglobulin therapy and review of the literature. Am J Med. 1986;81: 35–42.

181. McKinney RE, Katz SE, Wilfert CM. Chronic enteroviral meningoencephalitis in agammaglobulinemic patients. Rev Infect Dis. 1987;9:334–56.

182. Saulsbury FT, Bernstein MT, Winkelstein JA. *Pneumocystis carinii* pneumonia as the presenting infection in congenital hypogammaglobulinemia. J Pediatr. 1979;95:559–61.

183. Webster A, Platts-Mills T, Jannossy G, et al. Autoimmune blood dyscrasias in five patients with hypogammaglobulinemia: Response of neutropenia to vincristine. J Clin Immunol. 1981;1:113–8.

184. Farrington ML, Grosmaire LS, Nonoyama S, et al. CD40 ligand expression in patients with primary immunodeficiency (Abstract). J Immunol. 1993;150: 102A.

185. Straus SE, Seidlin M, Takiff H, et al. Oral acyclovir to suppress recurring herpes simplex virus infections in immunodeficient patients. Ann Intern Med. 1984;100:522–4.

186. Lopez M, Fleisher T, deShazo RD. Use and interpretation of diagnostic immunologic laboratory tests. JAMA. 1992;268:2970–90.

187. Gross S, Blaiss MS, Herrod HG. Role of immunoglobulin subclasses and specific antibody determinations in the evaluation of recurrent infection in children. J Pediatr. 1992;121:516–22.

188. Buckley RH, Schiff RI. The use of intravenous immune globulin in immunodeficiency diseases. N Engl J Med. 1991;325:110–7.

189. Stiehm ER, Ashida E, Kim KS, et al. Intravenous immunoglobulins as therapeutic agents. Ann Intern Med. 1987;107:367–82.

190. Berkman SA, Lee ML, Gale RP. Clinical uses of intravenous immunoglobulins. Ann Intern Med. 1990;112:278–92.

191. Liese JG, Wintergerst U, Tympner KD, et al. High- vs low-dose immunoglobulin therapy in the long-term treatment of X-linked agammaglobulinemia. Am J Dis Child 1992;146:335–9.

192. Kobayashi RH, Dobayashi AD, Lee N, et al. Home self-administration of intravenous immunoglobulin therapy in children. Pediatrics. 1990;85:705–9.

193. Burks AW, Sampson HA, Buckley RH. Anaphylactic reactions after gamma globulin administration in patients with hypogammaglobulinemia: Detection of IgE antibodies to IgA. N Engl J Med. 1986;314:560–4.

194. Weiland O, Mattsson L, Glaumann H. Non-A, non-B hepatitis after intravenous gammaglobulin. Lancet 1986;1:976–7.

195. Cournoyer D, Caskey CT. Gene therapy of the immune system. Annu Rev Immunol. 1993;11:297–329.

196. Bruton OC. Agammaglobulinemia. Pediatrics. 1952;9:722–8.

197. Vetrie D, Vorechovsky I, Sideras P, et al. The gene involved in X-linked agammaglobulinaemia is a member of the *src* family of protein-tyrosine kinases. Nature. 1993;361:226–233.

198. Lederman HM, Winkelstein JA. X-linked agammaglobulinemia: An analysis of 96 patients. Medicine. 1985;64:145–56.

199. Anker R, Conley ME, Pollok BA. Clonal diversity in the B cell repertoire of patients with X-linked agammaglobulinemia. J Exp Med. 1989;169:2109–19.

200. Pezacalsakak G, Lim J, Good R. B lymphocytes in primary and secondary deficiencies of humoral immunity. Birth Defects. 1975;11:33–8.

201. Fleisher T, White R, Broder S, et al. X-linked hypogammaglobulinemia and isolated growth hormone deficiency. N Engl J Med. 1980;302:1429–34.

202. Tiller TL, Buckley R. Transient hypogammaglobulinemia of infancy: Review of the literature, clinical and immunologic features of 11 new cases, and long-term follow up. J Pediatr. 1978;92:347–53.

203. McGready SJ. Transient hypogammaglobulinemia of infancy: Need to reconsider name and definition. J Pediatr. 1987;110:47–50.

204. Hermans P, Diaz-Buxo J, Stobo J. Idiopathic late onset immunoglobulin deficiency. Clinical observations in 50 patients. Am J Med. 1976;61:221–32.

205. Volanakis J, Zhu Z, Schaffer F, et al. Major histocompatibility complex III genes and susceptibility to immunoglobulin A deficiency and common variable immunodeficiency. J Clin Invest. 1992;89:1914–22.

206. Spickett GP, Webster A, Farrant J. Cellular abnormalities in common variable immunodeficiency. Immunodeficiency Rev. 1990;2:199–219.

207. Sneller MC, Strober W. Abnormalities of lymphokine gene expression in patients with common variable immunodeficiency. J Immunol. 1990;144: 3762–9.

208. Eisenstein EM, Jaffe J, Sneller MC, et al. Impaired and intact differentiation pathways in CD4 lymphocytes of patients with common variable immunodeficiency. J Allergy Clin Immunol. 1992;89:167.

209. Kinlen LJ, Webseter A, Bird A, et al. Prospective study of cancer in patients with hypogammaglobulinaemia. Lancet. 1985;1:263–5.

210. Levitt D, Haber P, Rich K, et al. Hyper IgM immunodeficiency. J Clin Invest. 1983;72:1650–7.

211. Stiehm ER, Fudenberg HH. Clinical and immunologic features of dysgammaglobulinemia type I. Am J Med. 1966;40:805–15.

212. Geha RS, Hyslop N, Alami S, et al. Hyper immunoglobulin M immunodeficiency (dysgammaglobulinemia). J Clin Invest. 1979;64:385–91.

213. Mayer L, Kwan SP, Thompson C, et al. Evidence for a defect in ''switch'' T cells in patients with immunodeficiency and hyperimmunoglobulinemia M. N Engl J Med. 1986;314:409–13.

214. Ammann AJ, Hong R. Selective IgA deficiency: Presentation of 30 cases and a review of the literature. Medicine. 1971;50:223–36.

215. Van Loghem E, Zegers BJM, Bast EJEG, et al. Selective deficiency of immunoglobulin A2. J Clin Invest. 1983;72:1918–23.

216. Migane N, Oliviero S, DeLange G, et al. Multiple-gene deletions within the human immunoglobulin heavy chain cluster. Proc Natl Acad Sci USA. 1984;5811–5.

217. Carbonara A, Demarchi M. Genetics and techniques: Ig isotype deficiency caused by gene deletions. Monogr Allergy. 1986;20:13–7.

218. Cunningham-Rundles C, Brandeis W, Good R, et al. Milk precipitins, circulating immune complexes and IgA deficiency. Proc Natl Acad Sci USA. 1978;75:3387–92.

219. Lefranc MP, Hammarstrom L, Smith C. Gene deletions in the human immunoglobulin heavy chain constant region locus: Molecular and immunological analysis. Immunol Rev. 1991;2:265–81.

220. Insel RA, Anderson PW. Response to oligosaccharide–protein conjugate vaccine against Hemophilus influenzae b in two patients with IgG2 deficiency unresponsive to capsular polysaccharide vaccine. N Engl J Med. 1986;315:499–503.

221. Umetsu DT, Ambrosino DM, Geha RS. Children with selective IgG subclass deficiency and recurrent sinopulmonary infection: Impaired response to bacterial capsular polysaccharide antigens. Mongr Allergy. 1986;20:57–61.

222. Standen GR. Wiskott-Aldrich syndrome: A multidisciplinary disease. J Clin Pathol. 1991;44:979–82.

223. Peacocke M, Siminovitch K. Wiskott-Aldrich syndrome: New molecular and biochemical insights. J Am Acad Dermatol. 1992;27:507–19.

224. Perry GS, Spector B, Schuman L, et al. The Wiskott-Aldrich syndrome in the United States and Canada (1892–1979). J Pediatr. 1980;97:72–8.

225. Park J, Rosenstein Y, Remold-O'Donnell E, et al. Enhancement of T-cell activation by the CD43 molecule whose expression is defective in Wiskott-Aldrich syndrome. Nature. 1991;350:706–9.

226. Spitler LE, Levein AS, Stites DP, et al. The Wiskott-Aldrich syndrome. Immunologic studies in nine patients and selected family members. Cell Immunol. 1975;19:201–18.

227. Simon HU, Mills GB, Hashimoto S, et al. Evidence for defective transmembrane signaling in B cells from patients with Wiskott-Aldrich syndrome. J Clin Invest. 1992;90:1396–405.

228. Woods CG, Taylor AM. Ataxia telangiectasia in the British Isles: The clinical and laboratory features of 70 affected individuals. Q J Med. 1992;82:169–79.

229. Miller DG. Patterns of immunologic deficiency in lymphomas and leukemias. Ann Intern Med. 1972;57:703–6.

230. Weitzman SA, Aisenberg AC, Siber GR. Impaired humoral immunity in treated Hodgkin's disease. N Engl J Med. 1977;297:245–8.

231. Ultmann J, Winthrop F, Osserman E, et al. The clinical implications of hypogammaglobulinemia in patients with chronic lymphocytic leukemia and lymphocytic lymphosarcoma. Ann Intern Med. 1959;51:501–16.

232. Chapel HM, Bunch C. Mechanisms of infection in chronic lymphocytic leukemia. Semin Hematol. 1987;24:291–6.

233. Cooperative Group for the Study of Immunoglobulin in Chronic Lymphocytic Leukemia. Intravenous immunoglobulin for the prevention of infection in chronic lymphocytic leukemia: A randomized, controlled clinical trial. N Engl J Med. 1988;319:902–7.

234. Weeks JC, Tierney MR, Weinstein MC. Cost effectiveness of prophylactic intravenous immune globulin in chronic lymphocytic leukemia. N Engl J Med. 1991;325:81–6.

235. Birgens H, Esperson F, Hertz J, et al. Antibody response to pneumococcal vaccination in patients with myelomatosis. Scand J Haematol. 1982;30:324–30.

236. Pilarksi LM, Andrews E, Mant MJ, et al. Humoral immune deficiency in multiple myeloma patients due to compromised B cell function. J Clin Immunol. 1986;6:491–501.

237. Meyers BR, Hirschman SZ, Axelrod J. Current patterns of infection in multiple myeloma. Am J Med. 1972;52:87–92.

238. Savage DG, Lindenbaum J, Garrett T. Biphasic pattern of bacterial infection in multiple myeloma. Ann Intern Med. 1982;96:47–50.

239. Gordon DS, Hearn EB, Spira TJ, et al. Phase I study of intravenous gamma globulin in multiple myeloma. Am J Med. 1984;76:111–6.

240. Hansbrough J, Miller L, Field T, et al. High dose intravenous immunoglobulin therapy in burn patients. Pharmacokinetics and effects on microbial opsonization and phagocytosis. Pediatr Infect Dis J. 1988;7:S49–56.

241. Bohnsack JF, Brown EJ. The role of the spleen in resistance to infection. Annu Rev Med. 1986;37:49–59.

242. Hosea S, Brown E, Hamburger M, et al. Opsonic requirements for intravascular clearance after splenectomy. N Engl J Med. 1981;304:245–50.

243. Lockwood CM. Immunological functions of the spleen. Clin Haematol. 1983;12:449–65.

244. Brigden ML. Overwhelming postsplenectomy infections still a problem. West J Med. 1992;157:440–3.

245. Styrt B. Infection associated with asplenia: Risks, mechanisms, and prevention. Am J Med. 1990;88:33N–42N.

246. Brown E, Hosea SW, Frank MM. The role of the spleen in experimental pneumococcal bacteremia. J Clin Invest. 1981;67:975–82.

247. Bolan G, Broome CV, Facklam RR, et al. Pneumococcal vaccine efficacy in selected populations in the United States. Ann Intern Med. 1986;104:1–6.

248. Konradsen HB, Pedersen F, Henrichsen J. Pneumococcal revaccination of splenectomized children. Pediatr Infect Dis J. 1990;9:258–63.

249. Grimfors G, Soderqvist M, Holm G, et al. A longitudinal study of class and subclass antibody responses to pneumococcal vaccination in splenectomized individuals with special reference to patients with Hodgkin's disease. Eur J Haematol. 1990;45:101–8.

250. Ambrosino D, Lee M, Chen D, et al. Response to *Haemophilus influenzae* type B conjugate vaccine in children undergoing splenectomy. J Pediatr Surg 1992;27:1045–7.

251. Ruben F, Hankins WA, Zeigler Z, et al. Antibody response to meningococcal polysaccharide vaccine in adults without a spleen. Am J Med. 1984;76:115–21.

252. Murdoch IA, Dos Anjos R. Continued need for pneumococcal prophylaxis after splenectomy. Arch Dis Child. 1990;65:1268–9.

253. Siber GR, Goman C, Martin P, et al. Antibody response to pretreatment immunization and post treatment boosting with bacterial polysaccharide vaccines in patients with Hodgkin's disease. Ann Intern Med. 1986;104:467–75.

254. Wong WY, Powars DR, Chan L, et al. Polysaccharide encapsulated bacterial infection in sickle cell anemia: A thirty year epidemiologic experience. Am J Hematol. 1992;39:176–82.

255. Wong WY, Overturf GD, Powars DR. Infection caused by *Streptococcus pneumoniae* in children with sickle cell disease: Epidemiology, immunologic mechanisms, prophylaxis and vaccination. Clin Infect Dis. 1992;14:1124–36.

256. Kaplan SL, Duckett T, Mahoney DH, et al. Immunogenicity of *Haemophilus influenzae* type b polysaccharide-tetanus protein conjugate vaccine in children with sickle hemoglobinopathy or malignancies, and after systemic *Haemophilus influenzae* type b infection. J Pediatrics. 1992;120:367–70.

257. Gaston MH, Verter JI, Woods G, et al. Prophylaxis with oral penicillin in children with sickle cell anemia: A randomized trial. N Engl J Med. 1986;314:1593–9.

258. Witherspoon RP, Storb R, Ochs HD. Recovery of antibody production in human allogeneic marrow graft recipients: Influence of time posttransplantation, the presence or absence of chronic graft-versus-host disease and antithymocyte globulin treatment. Blood. 1981;58:360–8.

259. Morgan M, Gale RP, Winston D. Intravenous immunoglobulin in bone marrow transplantation. Cancer. 1991;68(Suppl 6):1451–3.

260. Sacher RA. Intravenous gammaglobulin therapy: Current role in bone marrow transplant, malignancy, and autoimmune hematologic disorders. Semin Hematol. 1992;29(Suppl 2):1–5.

261. Wolff S, Fay JW, Herzig R, et al. High-dose weekly intravenous immunoglobulin to prevent infections in patients undergoing autologous bone marrow transplantation or severe myelosuppressive therapy. Ann Intern Med. 1993;118:937–42.

262. Huang KL, Ruben FL, Rinaldo CR, et al. Antibody response after influenza and pneumococcal immunization in HIV-infected homosexual men. JAMA. 1987;257:2047–50.

263. Collier AC, Corey L, Murphy VL, et al. Antibody to human immunodeficiency virus (HIV) and suboptimal response to hepatitis B vaccination. Ann Intern Med. 1988;109:101–5.

264. Janoff EN, Breiman RF, Daley CL, et al. Pneumococcal disease during HIV infection. Epidemiologic, clinical and immunologic perspectives. Ann Intern Med. 1992;117:314–24.

265. Steinhoff MC, Auerbach BS, Nelson KE, et al. Antibody responses to *Haemophilus influenzae* type b vaccines in men with human immunodeficiency virus infection. N Engl J Med. 1991;325:1837–42.

266. Mofenson L, Moye J, Bethel J, et al. Prophylactic intravenous immunoglobulin in HIV-infected children with CD4+ counts of 0.20 × 10⁹/L or more. Effect on viral, opportunistic and bacterial infections. JAMA. 1992;268:483–4.

267. The National Institute of Child Health and Human Development Intravenous Immunoglobulin Study Group. Intravenous immune globulin for the prevention of bacterial infections in children with symptomatic human immunodeficiency virus infection. N Engl J Med. 1991;325:73–80.

268. Small C, Kaufman A, Armenaka M, et al. Sinusitis and atopy in human immunodeficiency virus infection. J Infect Dis. 1993;167:283–90.

269. Salk J, Bretscher PA, Salk PL, et al. A strategy for prophylactic vaccination against HIV. Science. 1993;260:1270–2.

270. Stites DP, Stobo JD, Wells JV, eds. Basic and Clinical Immunology. 7th ed. Los Altos, CA: Appleton & Lange; 1991.

6. COMPLEMENT

PETER DENSEN

Functional activity attributable to the complement system was first described in the period between 1888 and 1894.[1] These experiments demonstrated that fresh serum contained a heat-labile bactericidal factor termed *alexin*. Subsequently it was shown that a heat-stable factor present in convalescent serum also contributed to bactericidal activity. At the turn of the century Paul Erlich employed the terms *complement* to describe the heat-labile factor and *ambocepto* (antibody) to describe the heat-stable factor. With the nineteenth century came the recognition that complement was composed of more than one component. However, it was not until 1941 that Louis Pillemer was able to separate functionally distinct components of the classical pathway from various serum fractions. In the early 1950s Pillemer and coworkers also described and characterized an antibody-independent mechanism for complement activation that they termed the *properdin pathway*.[1-3] However, the protein purification techniques of the time were unable to provide complement components of sufficient purity to convince others of the existence of this pathway. With the 1960 and 1970s came the development of a mathematical model capable of describing the sequential activation of complement as well as new techniques for the purification of the individual complement components. The latter development led to the rediscovery of Pillemer's work, the characterization of these proteins, and the delineation

of mechanisms controlling their activity. The 1980s brought the recognition that the complement system consists not only of plasma proteins but also of membrane proteins that protect host cells from the detrimental effects of complement activation. In addition, the explosion in molecular biology has led to the cloning and structural chacterization of all the complement proteins as well as an understanding of the molecular basis for their deficiency states.

At the present time the complement system is comprised of more than 30 proteins (Table 1). Their activation results in the sequential triggering of the various proteins and in this regard exhibits many similarities to the clotting cascade. The beneficial effects of complement activation for the host include the development of an inflammatory response and the elimination of microbial pathogens and immune complexes.

The antibody and complement systems are grouped together because of their historical and functional association and because they are soluble serum proteins.[4] However, antibody-mediated events are characterized by a high degree of specificity dictated by a given antibody for a given antigenic epitope. Consequently, after initial exposure to antigen there is a significant delay while protective antibody is synthesized to influence the course of the disease. In contrast, the complement system is activated by a wide variety of chemically diverse substances even in the absence of antibody. Consequently, the multiplicity of its physiologic effects is felt early in the course of infection. In many instances antibody and complement are synergistic in providing effective host defense. The presence of specific antibody leads to more rapid and efficient complement activation and serves to direct complement deposition to appropriate sites

TABLE 1. Complement Plasma Proteins

Component	Approximate Serum Concentration (μg/ml)	Molecular Weight	Chain Structure[a]	Number of Genetic Loci	Chromosomal Assignment[b]
Classical pathway					
C1q	70	410,000	(A, B, C) × 6	3 (A, B, C)	1p
C1r	34	170,000	Dimer of 2 identical chains	1	12p
C1s	31	85,000	Dimer of 2 identical chains	1	12p
C4	600	206,000	$\beta-\alpha-\gamma$	2 (C4A, C4B)	6p
C2	25	117,000	1 chain	1	6p
Alternative pathway					
D (adipsin)	1	24,000	1 chain	1	ND
C3	1300	195,000	$\beta-\alpha$	1	19q
B	200	95,000	1 chain	1	6p
Membrane attack complex					
C5	80	180,000	$\beta-\alpha$	1	9q
C6	60	128,000	1 chain	1	5q
C7	55	120,000	1 chain	1	5q
C8	65	150,000	3 nonidentical chains $\alpha---\gamma, \beta$	3 (A, B, G)	α, β 1p γ 9q
C9	60	79,000	1 chain	1	5p
Control proteins					
Positive regulation					
Properdin	25	220,000	Cyclic polymers of a single 57 kD chain	1	Xp
Negative regulation					
C1 INH	200	105,000	1 chain	1	11q
C4 bp	250	550,000	7 idential chains	1	1q
Factor H	500	150,000	1 chain	1	1q
Factor I	34	90,000	$\beta-\gamma$	1	4q
Anaphylatoxin inactivator (carboxypeptidase B)	35	280,000	Dimer of 2 nonidentical chains (H, L) × 2	ND	ND
S protein (vitronectin)	500	80,000	1 chain	1	ND
SP-40, 40 (clusterin)	50	80,000	$\alpha-\beta$	1	8p

Abbreviations: ND, not determined; C1-INH, C1 inhibitor.

[a] For multichain components parentheses are used to indicate subunit structure; commas indicate noncovalent linkage of chains arising from separate genes; solid lines indicate covalent linkage of chains arising from post-translational cleavage of a proenzyme molecule, chains being listed in order beginning at the amino terminus of the proenzyme molecule; dashed line indicates covalent linkage of chains arising from separate genes.

[b] p indicates the short arm and q the long arm of the chromosome.

on the surface of invading pathogens. Opsonization of infectious agents with both antibody and complement leads to more efficient ingestion and killing of these microbes than does opsonization with either substance alone. Similarly, the presence of receptors on lymphocytes for immunoglobulin and complement suggest a cooperative role for these substances in both the affector and effector pathways of the immune response. "In such a way a highly specific response mediated by the tertiary structure of an antibody molecule can be coupled with the more general cellular or humoral responses of the phagocytic and complement system to eradicate attacking organisms."[4]

COMPLEMENT SYNTHESIS, CATABOLISM, AND DISTRIBUTION

Studies employing cultured hepatocytes coupled with an examination of complement component polymorphisms in patients before and after orthotopic liver transplantation have established that the liver is responsible for the synthesis of at least 90 percent of the complement proteins in plasma.[5-7] The normal concentration of many individual complement components fluctuates over time. In part this fluctuation reflects the fact that many of the components are acute-phase reactants, and their synthesis can be modulated by a variety of immune modulators. These substances, including the interleukins (IL-1 and IL-6), tumor necrosis factor, and dexamethasone, increase hepatic synthesis two- to fivefold.[8,9]

Complement synthesis also occurs in a variety of other cells, most notably monocytes and macrophages.[10] Synthesis varies with the site of isolation of the cell. For example, bronchoalveolar fluid, breast milk, and monocyte-derived macrophages differ with respect to the proportion of the cells secreting C2, average rate of C2 production per cell, and amount of C2-specific RNA.[11] Complement synthesis by monocytes can be modulated by interferon-γ, endotoxin,[12,13] IL-1, and tumor necrosis factor. In most cases enhanced synthesis is mediated at the transcriptional level.

Synthesis of the early components of both activating pathways of complement by mononuclear phagocyte cells is believed to be an important aspect of complement-mediated host defense in tissues. In vitro studies have demonstrated that these cells can synthesize sufficient amounts of these components to promote opsonization, ingestion, and killing of bacteria or other target cells with which they have been coincubated.[14]

A detailed examination of the metabolic fate of all complement components has not been carried out. However, studies have demonstrated fractional catabolic rates for C3, C4, C5, and factor B that range from 1 to 2 percent per hour, indicating that they are among the most rapidly metabolized of all plasma proteins. Catabolic rates of C3 and C4 are independent of serum levels, whereas their synthetic rates correlate with serum levels, indicating that the rate of synthesis is the major determinant of plasma concentration.[15]

In healthy individuals the vast majority of complement is found in blood. Concentrations of complement proteins in normal mucosal secretions are approximately 5–10 percent of serum levels and in normal spinal fluid even lower, perhaps 1 percent or less. In the presence of local inflammation complement concentrations in mucosal secretions and in cerebrospinal fluid increase, most likely as a result of altered vascular permeability barriers but also as a consequence of enhanced synthesis and secretion by local mononuclear cells.

Serum complement activity is reduced in preterm infants in proportion to the magnitude of their immaturity.[16] In contrast, complement levels in healthy term infants range from 60 to 100 percent of those in healthy adults. Despite these nearly normal levels, defective complement activation via either the classical or alternative pathway has been noted in as many as 40 percent of such infants.[17-19]

COMPLEMENT ACTIVATION

Generation of the Classical Pathway C3 Convertase

Activation of the classical pathway most commonly occurs as a consequence of antigen–antibody recognition. Only IgM and certain IgG subclasses (3 > 1 > 2) are capable of initiating complement activation.[20] The CH3 region of IgM, especially glycosylation at Asn 402, and the CH2 and CH3 regions of IgG play particularly important roles in the association of C1 with antibody.[21,22] Amino acid sequence differences in the CH2 region may account for the different complement-activating potential among the IgG subclasses.[23]

C1 is a trimolecular complex containing one molecule of C1q and two molecules each of C1r and C1s. C1q consists of a central core with six radiating collagenlike fibrillar strands that terminate in globular heads, which contain the antibody-binding sites.[20,24] In the case of IgM, functionally important C1q binding occurs following the change in configuration that accompanies binding of a single IgM molecule to multiple sites on the target particle. In contrast, for IgG, functionally effective C1q binding requires that two IgG molecules be cross-linked via the globular heads on C1q. This topographic stipulation dictates that many IgG molecules be bound to a target particle to ensure sufficient density for doublet formation. At a functional level this requirement means that complement activation by IgG is less efficient than that by IgM, since the latter requires only that a single molecule be bound in the correct configuration.[20,24]

Although antibody–antigen interactions are the most common means of initiating classical pathway activation, C1q can bind directly to anionic structures, for example, lipid A keto-deoxy-octonoate (KDO) complexes exposed on the surface of rough gram-negative bacteria. Binding in this manner initiates the full range of classical pathway–mediated activities. In addition, mannan-binding protein (MBP), pulmonary surfactant proteins A (SP-A) and D, the macrophage scavenger receptor, and bovine conglutinin are structurally homologous with C1q in terms of having both collagenlike and globular domains. These proteins bind to polyanionic molecules through their collagenlike domains, and several can mediate opsonization via the C1q receptor.[25,26] Moreover, particle-bound MBP, but not SP-A,[27] appears able to substitute for C1q in activating the classical pathway, although there is debate regarding the mechanism by which activation occurs.[28-30]

C1 binding by antibody results in a change in the structural configuration of the C1q molecule such that the C1r and C1s tetramer contained within the cagelike structure formed by the radiating pods of C1q becomes autocatalytically active. This structural alteration may involve the release of C1 inhibitor, which binds reversibly to proenzyme C1. C1r and C1s are structurally related molecules consisting of a head bearing the serine esterase enzymatic site and a tail bearing the binding site. The subunits are aligned linearly such that the central portion of the tetramer is formed by two C1r subunits linked through their catalytic domains. Each C1r molecule is joined to a C1s molecule via the binding site in the tail region of the respective subunits. This linear arrangement allows the tetramer to assume a figure eight configuration such that all four catalytic domains are in close proximity. In this configuration each C1r molecule is believed to activate the other C1r molecule, which in turn activates C1s.[20,31,32]

Expression of enzymatic activity by C1r and C1s represents the initial activation and amplification step in the classical pathway. Thus many molecules of substrate are cleaved by a given enzyme complex, resulting in the fixation of subsequent complement components in the cascade in close proximity to the antibody-binding site on the surface of the target particle. Hence antibody serves not only to activate complement in a kinetically efficient manner but also to direct complement deposition to specific sites on the target surface.

Activated C1s cleaves a 9 kD fragment, C4a, from the amino

terminus of the α-chain of C4. This results in the exposure of an internal thiolester bond linking the SH group of a cysteine residue with the terminal COOH group of glutamic acid. This bond is subject to nucleophilic attack by hydroxyl or amino groups, leading to the formation of covalent ester or amide linkages.[20,33,34] Through this reaction and the analogous one involving C3 (see Fig. 2), the complement system acquires a chemically stable association with the target surface. Of interest with regard to the formation of these covalent bonds is that due to gene duplication there are two slightly different C4 genes, C4A and C4B. The product of the C4A gene preferentially forms amide bonds with target surfaces and is hemolytically less active than the product of the C4B gene, which preferentially forms ester bonds.[36–38] Consequently, C4A binds more effectively to proteins, for example, antigen–antibody complexes, than does C4B.[37,39,40] The molecular basis for this difference in binding efficiency appears to be the presence of an aspartic acid residue in the C4A molecule and a histidine residue in the C4B molecule at a site distant from the thiolester. Although distant from the thiolester in the primary structure of C4, the tertiary configuration of the molecule probably brings these charged amino acids into close proximity with the thiolester such that they influence the nucleophilic attack of the thiolester bond by amino or hydroxyl groups on the target surface. The difference in reactivity of the C4A and C4B molecules may play a role in determining the clinical picture observed in patients with inherited deficiencies of these respective genes.[41]

Activated C1s also cleaves C2 to produce a small fragment, C2b, which is released into the environment, and a larger fragment, C2a, which binds to C4b on the surface of the target particle. This complex, C4b2a, is the classical pathway C3 convertase (Fig. 1). It is inherently labile, but after its dissociation C4b can bind newly generated C2a derived from further cleavage of C2 by C1s.[20,30]

Generation of the Alternative-Pathway C3 Convertase

Activation of complement by the alternative pathway displays several unique features. First, antibody is not required, although it can facilitate the activation process. Second, activation proceeds both in the fluid phase and on cell surfaces. Fluid-phase activation occurs continuously at a low rate that is controlled by plasma regulatory proteins. Spillover from the fluid phase results in complement deposition on cells of the host as well as intruding microorganisms. Thus host cells must possess a mechanism to limit the effects of complement fixation (i.e., they are "nonactivators"), whereas intruding microorganisms must provide a surface that allows complement activation to proceed further (i.e., they are "activators").[30,42,43] Third, a component of the activation process, C3b, is also a product of the reaction, thereby generating a positive-feedback loop that amplifies the activation process. Consequently, C3b deposition resulting from C3 cleavage by either the alternative- or the classical-pathway C3 convertase can initiate the alternative-pathway amplifi-

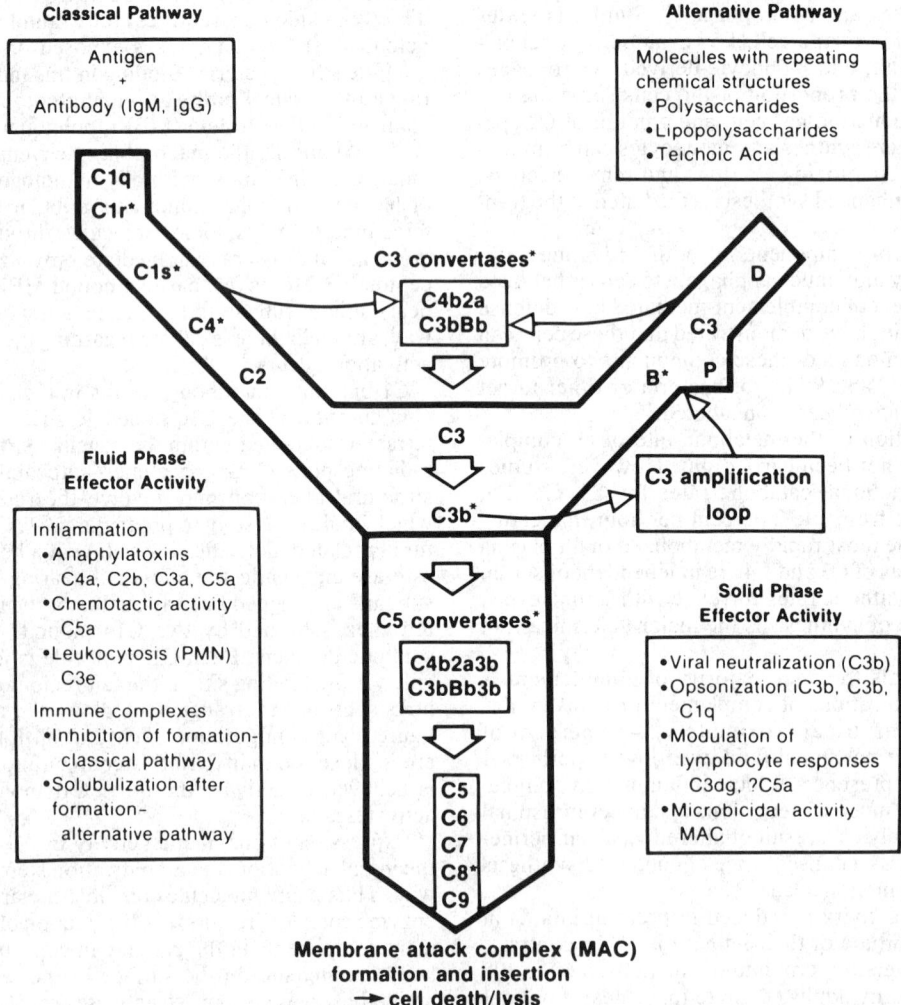

FIG. 1. The complement cascade. Within each pathway the components are arranged in order of their activation and aligned opposite their functional and structural analog in the opposite pathway. Asterisks indicate sites of downregulation of complement activity (see Table 2).

cation loop (Fig. 1).[30,42,43] The time required until amplification occurs makes complement activation via the alternative pathway three to five times kinetically less efficient than via the classical pathway on the same target.[44] This delay in activation is characteristic for a given target and differs among different target particles.[42,43] Fourth, in contrast to the classical pathway in which antibody directs covalent C4b binding in clusters about the antibody-binding site, covalent C3b binding mediated by the alternative pathway occurs randomly over the surface of the target particle.[42,43] The random nature of this process contributes in part to the delay in complement activation via this pathway.

C3 is the critical reactant of the alternative pathway. It is structurally and functionally analogous to C4 (Fig. 1) and contains the same internal thiolester bond within its α-chain. This internal thiolester bond undergoes spontaneous low-rate hydrolysis to form $C3(H_2O)$, as shown in Figure 2. For a brief moment before its inactivation by the control proteins factors H and I, $C3(H_2O)$ can form a complex with factor B. Once bound to C3, factor B can be cleaved by factor D to yield $C3(H_2O)Bb$—the fluid phase C3 convertase. $C3(H_2O)Bb$ reacts with intact C3 to cleave a 9 kD peptide fragment, C3a, from the amino terminus of the α-chain.[42,43] Analogous to the situation with C4, this process results in the exposure of the internal thiolester in the α-chain. The resulting metastable C3b can form covalent ester or amide linkages with appropriate chemical constituents on the surface of nearby cells. Surface-bound C3b can bind additional factor B, which in turn can be cleaved by factor D to produce C3bBb. This complex is the alternative-pathway C3 convertase, which is capable of cleaving additional C3, thereby initiating the amplification phase of the alternative pathway. Like its classical-pathway analog, this convertase is inherently labile and has a half-

life of approximately 90 seconds. Properdin binding to C3bBb stabilizes the complex and prolongs its half-life by 5- to 10-fold,[45,46] thereby providing reaction conditions sufficient for further C3 cleavage and signaling the initiation of the amplification phase of alternative-pathway activation.

From these considerations it is apparent that any substance that stabilizes the alternative-pathway convertase will also promote C3 consumption. This situation arises in patients who develop autoantibodies to C3bBb that stabilize the convertase.[47] In addition, cobra venom contains a C3b-like factor that forms an extremely stable complex with factor B that functions as a C3 convertase except that it is resistant to the action of the control proteins. Thus, the addition of cobra venom factor to serum leads to the dramatic consumption of C3.[42,48–50] Consequently, infusion of this factor can be used in experimental animals to delineate the role of the complement cascade in host defense or other disease processes.

Although antibody is not required for activation of the alternative pathway, it acts synergistically with properdin to facilitate the activation process.[51,52] Facilitation is dependent on the Fab portion of the antibody molecule rather than the Fc fragment responsible for classical-pathway activation.[52–56] Not all antibodies can enhance activation, for example, guinea pig IgG1 but not IgG2 can augment alternative-pathway activation.[57] The molecular basis for facilitation is uncertain but probably requires carbohydrate moieties present on IgG.[58] Antibody deposited on target surfaces can serve as a potential binding site for the covalent linkage of C3.[53] Moreover, the alternative-pathway C3 convertase C3bBb that is formed on IgG is relatively resistant to the action of the regulatory proteins.[59,60] This property may contribute to the ability of antibody to facilitate alternative-pathway activation.

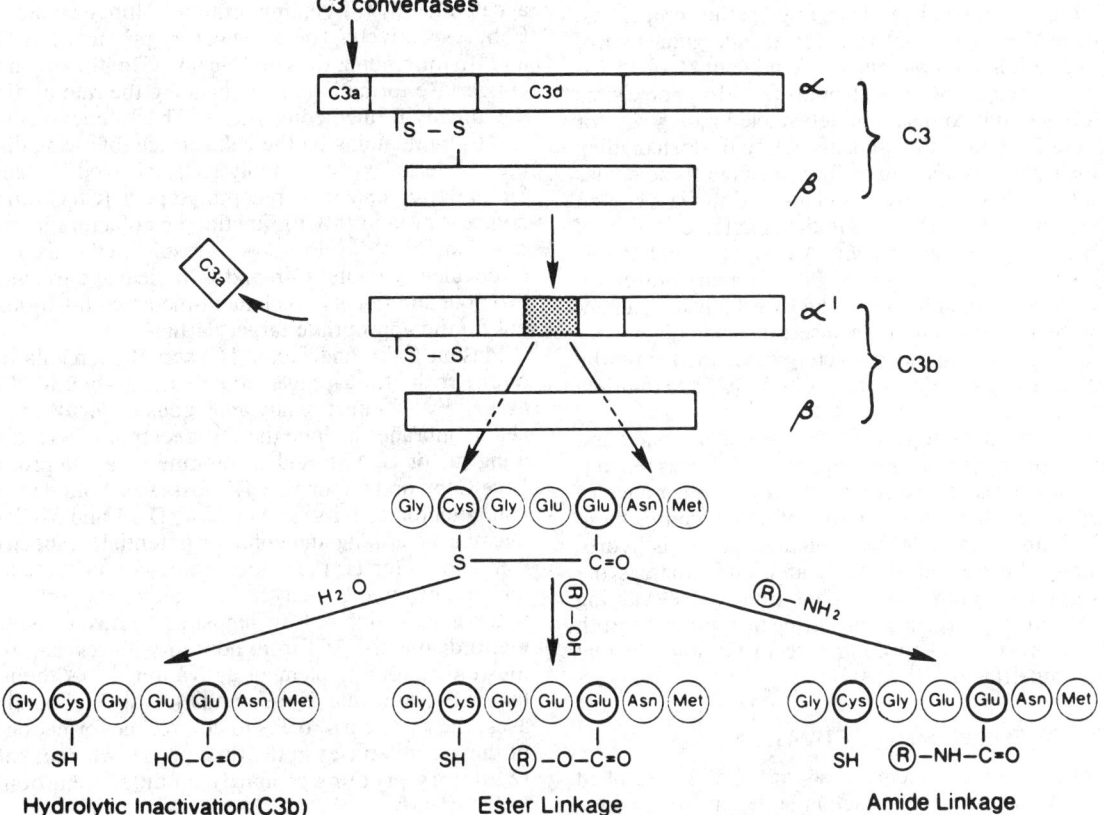

FIG. 2. C3 activation and fate of the internal thiolester bond. During activation C3a is released from the amino terminus of the α-chain of C3. The exposed internal thiolester bond becomes accessible to nucleophilic attack and can react with water or available hydroxyl or amine groups on cell surfaces. Analogous reactions occur with C4. Together these reactions involving C3 and C4 are responsible for covalently linking complement deposition to the cell surface. (From Gordon et al.,[35] with permission.)

C3—The Linchpin of the Complement System

The critical importance of C3 in the complement cascade is evident from its position at the convergence of the classical and alternative pathways, its role in activating and amplifying alternative-pathway activation, the multidue of functional activities associated with its various cleavage products, the fact that it is a major point of regulation of complement activity (Fig. 1), and the fact that its concentration in plasma (1.6 mg/ml) exceeds by 2- to 10-fold the concentration of all other complement components (Table 1).[61] The α-chain of C3b is subject to proteolytic cleavage by factor I to yield iC3b and by less well-defined proteases to C3dg and C3d. Each of these progressively smaller C3 fragments remains linked to the cell surface via the original covalent bond, and each can react with specific receptors on phagocytic and lymphocytic cells. However, only C3b can perpetuate complement activation. C3b binding to the C3 convertases generates new complexes, C4bC2aC3b and C3bBbC3b, the C5 convertases, which are responsible for cleaving C5 and initiating assembly of the membrane attack complex (MAC).

Assembly of the Membrane Attack Complex

C5 is the structural homolog of C4 and C3 except that its α-chain does not contain an internal thiolester bond. Instead, the amino acids cysteine and glutamine, which form the internal thiolester in C4 and C3, have been replaced by serine and alanine.[62,63] Analogous to C4 and C3, activation of C5 proceeds via cleavage of an 11.2 kD fragment, C5a, from the amino terminus of its α-chain. The resulting C5b binds noncovalently to the surface of the target particle.[64] The remaining terminal complement components C6, C7, C8β, C8α-γ, and C9, share a high level of structural organization at both the DNA and protein levels.[65–67] Unlike the early components of the classical and alternative pathways, these proteins lack enzymatic activity but as a group are characterized by their amphipathic properties. They circulate in plasma in hydrophilic form, undergoing hydrophobic transformation upon binding to the nascent MAC.[64] Assembly of the MAC begins when C5b binds to hydrophobic sites on the cell surface and expresses a metastable binding site for C6. Both C6 and C7 bind to the α-chains of C5b through binding domains in their carboxy termini to form a stable trimolecular complex, C5b67.[64] Subsequently, C8 binds to C5b via a site on its β-chain.[68,69] In the final step, C8 initiates polymerization of C9 through a binding site on C8α-γ.[70] A current model of this process suggests that the function of C5b8 is to create a discontinuity in the membrane lipid bilayer, thereby establishing an environment for the stepwise unfolding, insertion, and polymerization of monomeric C9.[71] In its completely assembled state the MAC consists of a single molecule each of C5b–C8 and multiple (1–18) molecules of C9.[64]

Fully inserted and polymerized C9 has a tubular shape and the properties of an integral membrane protein.[64,71] It is responsible for the characteristic electron microscopic appearance of the membrane holes that appear during effective complement activation. The inner aspect of this tubular structure is hydrophilic and allows the passage of water and ions, whereas the outer surface of the structure is hydrophobic and causes varying degrees of membrane disorganization during insertion.[64,71] Both of these effects are thought to contribute to the microbicidal and cytolytic properties of the MAC.

REGULATION OF COMPLEMENT ACTIVATION

A major feature of the complement cascade is the controlled production of an inflammatory reaction sufficient to enhance host defense and the immune response yet not lead to host injury. Amplificatory regulation of this process is achieved via the inherent property of enzymes to turn over multiple substrate molecules rapidly and by stabilization of enzyme complexes (e.g., by properdin). Downregulation is achieved in a temporal fashion by the short half-lives of the enzymatic complexes and the anaphylatoxins and in a spacial manner by directing complement activation to the target surface (e.g., by antibody). Modulation of the potential injurious effects of indiscriminant complement activation is achieved by specific regulatory proteins acting at three major levels: activation (C1), effector initiation (C3), and cytolysis (MAC). Unique disease entities resulting from a deficiency of these control proteins are testimony to the importance of complement regulation.

Regulation of C1 Activation

As described earlier, C1 esterase inhibitor (C1-INH) binds reversibly to pro-C1, thereby preventing its spontaneous activation.[24] Binding of C1q to antibody subverts this control by causing dissociation of C1-INH from pro-C1 and allowing autocatalytic cleavage to proceed. At some point after C1 activation C1-INH binds to the serine esterase sites on C1r and C1s, inactivating their catalytic function and dissociating them from C1q. Complete inactivation requires the binding of four molecules of C1-INH, one per catalytic site. In contrast to its binding to pro-C1, C1-INH binding to C1r and C1s is irreversible, thereby preventing cleavage of C4 and controlling the initial amplification step of classical-pathway activation.[24,72]

Regulation of the C3 Convertases

As indicated in Figure 1, the classical- and alternative-pathway C3 convertases are functionally analogous molecules. Control of their activity occurs by three basic mechanisms and uses functionally identical or shared regulator proteins (Table 2).[30,42,43,47] First, both of the convertases are inherently labile and undergo spontaneous decay with the loss of C2a or Bb from the complex. Second, the rate of spontaneous decay can be accelerated by C4-binding protein (C4bp) or factor H to C4b or C3b, respectively. These regulatory proteins compete with C2a and Bb for binding sites on C4b and C3b, thereby inhibiting new convertase formation and enhancing the rate of dissociation of the already formed convertases. Third, functionally active C3b and C4b remaining on the cell surface following dissociation of the convertases are proteolytically cleaved by factor I. C4bp, factor H, complement receptor type 1 (CR1), and membrane cofactor protein (MCP) function as cofactors in mediating this reaction.[30,42,43,47,73] Proteolysis results in the display of an array of covalently bound C4b and C3b cleavage fragments that can promote additional complement-mediated functions when present on the appropriate target particle.

Plasma C4bp and factor H exert their regulatory influence over both fluid-phase and surface-bound C3 convertases.[30,42,73,74] Functionally analogous molecules present in host cell membranes include the C3b receptor (CR1), decay accelerating factor (DAF), and membrane cofactor protein (MCP).[75] Like C4bp and factor H, CR1 possesses both decay acclerating and cofactor activity. In contrast, DAF and MCP exhibit only decay accelerating and cofactor potential, respectively. Unlike C4b and factor H, these membrane-bound proteins do not exhibit pathway specificity.[73,74] Together they play a major role in the inactivation of C3b deposited on host cells, thereby serving to distinguish self from nonself with respect to the deleterious effects of complement activation.[73,74] Although C4bp and factor H contribute to the regulation of cell-bound C3 convertases, their principal role is to control the formation and activity of these convertases in the fluid phase, whereas the membrane regulatory proteins primarily modulate cell-bound C3b and C4b.[73,74]

The assembly and insertion of the MAC has also been shown to inhibit C3 convertase formation and to accelerate the decay of the alternative-pathway convertase. Feedback inhibition of this sort may serve to protect the host from the detrimental effects of continued complement activation.[76,77]

TABLE 2. Plasma and Membrane Proteins that Regulate or Mediate Complement Activity

Location, Protein	Specifity	Function
Plasma		
C1-INH	C1r, C1s	Binds to and removes C1r and C1s from C1 complex
C4bp	C4b	Inhibits assembly and accelerates decay of C4b2a Cofactor for C4b cleavage by factor I
Factor H	C3b	Inhibits assembly and accelerates decay of C3bBb Cofactor for C3b cleavage by factor I
Factor I	C4b, C3b	Proteolytic inactivation of C4b and C3b
S protein (vitronectin), SP-40/40 (clusterin)	C5b-7	Bind fluid-phase C5b-7; prevent attachment of C5b-7 and C5b-9 to membranes
Carboxypeptidase B	C4a, C3a, C5a	Inactivates these anaphylatoxins by removal of carboxy-terminal arginine
Cell membranes		
CR1 (CD35)	C3b, C4b, iC3b	Inhibit assembly and accelerates decay of C3 convertases
MCP (CD46)	C3b, C4b	Cofactor for cleavage of C4b/C3b by factor I
DAF (CD55)	C4b2a, C3bBb	
CR1 (CD35)	C3b, C4b, iC3b	Binds immune complexes to erythrocytes; phagocytosis
CR2 (CD21)	C3d, C3dg iC3b, C3b	Phagocytosis Modulates B-cell responses Epstein-Barr virus receptor
CR3 (CD11b/CD18)	iC3b	Phagocytosis
CR4 (CD11c/CD18)	C3dg, C3d	Phagocytosis
HRF; CD59 (MACIF, MIRL)	C8 in C5b-8	Bind to C8 Inhibit polymerization of C9
C3a/C4aR	C3a, C4a	Vasodilation
C5aR	C5a, C5a des arg	Chemotaxis
C1qR	C1q	Phagocytosis

Regulation of the Membrane Attack Complex

Control of the assembly of the MAC is exerted at two levels. First, plasma clusterin and S protein (vitronectin) bind to the amino-terminal cysteine-rich domains of C6, C7, C8, and C9 through its heparin-binding domain to inhibit the association of C5b67 with membranes and prevent assembly of the MAC on host cells.[78,79] Second, CD59 and homologous restriction protein (HRP) present on many types of peripheral blood cells bind C8 and prevent C9 polymerization.[80,81]

Nucleated eukaryotic cells are quite resistant to complement-mediated cytolysis even in the face of a nonhomologous complement source. Resistance is associated with the capacity of the cell to maintain high synthetic rates of membrane lipids and the ability to shed MAC from the cell surface.[82–84] Insertion of the MAC in eukaryotic cell membranes is accompanied by a rapid influx of calcium, generation of multiple signals, and stimulation of arachidonic acid metabolism.[85–91] These events probably promote normal physiologic functions as well as contribute to host cell injury.

The Basis for Discriminating between Host and Microbial Cell Surfaces

The capacity of C4 and C3 to form covalent bonds with reactive groups on cell surfaces, thereby establishing the nidus for C3 convertase formation, is inherently incapable of distinguishing between host and microbial cells. Consequently, in order for the beneficial effects of complement activation to be expressed as an effective host defense mechanism, additional factors must allow the discrimination between self and nonself:[74] inhibiting activation of complement amplification on host cells ("nonactivators") yet permitting amplification on the surface of microbial organisms ("activators"). One element of this discriminatory process is the presence of the complement regulatory proteins in the membranes of host cells but not on the cells of microbial organisms.[74] The other important determinant of complement activation is the chemical composition of the cell surface. Moreover, since covalent bond formation is nondiscriminatory, the basis for discrimination must lie in the capacity for chemical differences to affect the outcome of the competition between

factor B and factor H for the binding site on C3b, which in turn determines C3 convertase formation or decay and whether a particular cell surface will activate the alternative pathway. For example, C3b bound to the surface of a nonactivating particle binds factor H with about a 100-fold greater affinity than C3b bound to an activator particle. Consequently, factor B binding and subsequent amplification of complement activation is favored on the latter particle.[30,42,43,47]

Chemical constituents that influence the competition between factor B and factor H for C3b include sialic acid and sulfated acid mucopolysaccharides (e.g., heparin sulfate). These chemical molecules are present on most human cells and enhance the affinity of factor H for C3b, thereby contributing to the nonactivator status of host cells.[92–94] From the standpoint of infectious diseases it is interesting that sialic acid is a prominent chemical constituent of the capsular polysaccharides present on type 3 group B streptococci, K1 Escherichia coli, and groups B and C meningococci.[47] Consequently, the capsules of these organisms are nonactivators of the alternative pathway and, since sialic acid is a constituent of host cells, constitute a poor stimulus for antibody production. In this context it is noteworthy that K1 E. coli, group B streptococci, and group B meningococci are prominent causes of neonatal and infant sepsis and meningitis. Moreover, the frequent absence in these individuals of specific antibody to activate the classical pathway coupled with bacterial sialic acid–mediated inhibition of alternative-pathway activity may provide the ideal clinical setting for infection with these organisms.

Chemical constituents other than sialic acid must also affect the outcome of the competition between factors B and H for C3b. For example, sheep and human erythrocytes contain an extensive amount of sialic acid on their surface and are normally nonactivators of the alternative pathway.[92,95] Enzymatic removal of sialic acid from these cells converts sheep but not human erythrocytes into activating particles. Moreover, the chemical introduction of lipopolysaccharide molecules capable of activating the alternative pathway into the membrane of sheep erythrocytes converts them from a nonactivating to an activating particle despite the presence of sialic acid.[95]

In summary, the C3 convertases represent the major site of

both complement amplification and regulation. The membranes of host cells contain specific proteins that act to downregulate the C3 convertases as well as other chemical constituents that enhance the affinity of fluid-phase factor H for surface-bound C3b and promote its regulatory activity. In contrast, most microbial surfaces lack specific factors capable of downregulating complement activation and possess a chemical composition that decreases the affinity of factor H for cell-bound C3b. Thus, factor B binding to C3b and alternative-pathway activation and amplification are favored on most microbial surfaces.

COMPLEMENT RECEPTORS

Complement receptors have been described primarily on peripheral blood cells, including erythrocytes, neutrophils, monocytes, B and T lymphocytes, and platelets. They fall into two broad categories: those that bind complement components deposited on cell surfaces such that the component serves as a bifunctional ligand linking the target cell to the receptor and those that bind diffusible complement fragments released during activation of the complement cascade. The latter are responsible for many of the manifestations of the inflammatory response.

The former category of receptors includes C1qR, CR1, CR2, CR3, and CR4. The C1qR is a carbohydrate-rich protein expressed on phagocytic cells and lymphocytes that modulates phagocytosis, cytokine release, cytotoxicity, and interactions with endothelial cells. Functional ligands in addition to C1q that are recognized by C1qR include MBP, Sp-A, and conglutinin, all of which exhibit structural homology with C1q.[25]

Receptors for the cleavage products of C3 and C4 (CR1, CR2, CR3, and CR4) have been studied more extensively. Although they recognize closely related ligands, each of these receptors is structurally distinct and exhibits a unique pattern of distribution on peripheral blood cells.[96,97] A portion of these receptors is linked to the cellular cytoskeleton, an association that is probably important in signal transduction.[98]

CR1, the C3b/C4b receptor, is present on erythrocytes, neutrophils, monocytes, B cells, subpopulations of T cells, follicular dendritic cells, and glomerular podocytes. It mediates immune complex binding and clearance, ingestion of C3b/C4b-bearing particles, modulates certain lymphocyte functions,[96,97] and carries certain blood group antigens.[99] There are four polymorphic variants that range in size (190–280 kD) and number of C3b/C4b-binding sites.[100]

CR3 and CR4 are members of the integrin family of heterodimeric proteins.[101] They recognize C3bi as their major binding ligand. However, CR3 also binds to C3b and C3dg and bears a lectinlike domain that recognizes specific carbohydrates on microbial surfaces.[102] The three amino acid sequence arg-gly-asp, which is present in C3 and other ligands, represents an important binding motif for CR3.[103,104] Together CR3 and CR4, particularly the former, recognize the various combinations of C3b, C3bi, and C3dg present on the surface of microbial cells and play a major role in their elimination by phagocytic cells. In addition, CR3 plays an important role in the adherence-related functions of neutrophils (see Ch. 7).

CR2 is present on B lymphocytes and follicular dendritic cells and serves to recognize C3dg.[105] The association of CR2 and CD19 in the B-cell membrane constitutes an important mechanism for B-cell activation.[106] CR2 acts to localize C3dg-bearing particles or immune complexes to lymphocyte-rich areas in the spleen and lymph nodes, thereby driving antigen activation of these cells.

Receptors for complement-derived mediators of the inflammatory response, including C4a, C3a, and C5a, have also been described. Of these the high-affinity C5a receptor has been best studied. It is present on neutrophils and monocytes, and its perturbation causes directed migration (chemotaxis) of these cells in the direction of increasing C5a concentration. Experimental evidence suggests the presence of receptors for C3a on guinea pig ileum, vascular endothelium, and mast cells.[107]

FAMILIES OF COMPLEMENT PROTEINS

The preceding material and the representation of the complement cascade presented in Figure 1 emphasize features shared by both pathways with respect to their activation and regulation. It is apparent from these similarities that a number of complement components belong to several different protein families. These include the serine protease family (C1r, C1s, C2, factor D, factor B, and factor I); disulfide-linked, multichained molecules with homology to an ancestral protein that contained an internal thiolester bond (C4, C3, and C5); proteins that are the products of class 3 major histocompatibility complex (MHC) genes located on chromosome 6 (C2, factor B, C4A, and C4B); proteins that bind C3 and C4 fragments and belong to a closely clustered supergene family located on the long arm of chromosome 1 (C4bp, factor H, DAF, MCP, CR1, and CR2); and proteins sharing homology with the low-density lipoprotein (LDL) receptors (C6, C7, C8α, C8β, and C9).[108]

Among these families current interest has focused on those components that are the products of the class 3 MHC genes, the regulatory protein supergene family on chromosome 1, and the proteins with homology to the LDL receptor. Class 3 MHC genes are located between the class 1 and class 2 loci on the short arm of chromosome 6.[109] The genetic material in this region appears to have undergone two duplication events resulting on the one hand in the structurally and functionally related proteins C2 and factor B and on the other the C4 and 21-hydroxylase A and B variants.[108–110] Recombinant events in this region of the chromosome tend to be suppressed, thereby leading to the usual inheritance of the entire region intact from each parent.[111] The polymorphic variants of the complement components encoded by these genes in a given individual are referred to as *complotypes*.[112] The association of specific complotypes with specific products of the class 1 and class 2 MHC genes probably contributes to the association of specific complotypes with certain disease states (e.g., systemic lupus erythematosus).[113]

Proteins encoded by the complement regulatory protein loci on the long arm of chromosome 1 share a common organization with each other, with other proteins capable of binding to C3 and C4 (e.g., C2 and factor B), and with some complement and noncomplement proteins that do not bind these two components.[114,115] These proteins contain tandem repeats of approximately 60 amino acids that share a consensus sequence. Each is encoded within a separate exon, the number of repeats varying from as few as 2 in C1r to as many as 30 in CR1. The functional significance of these repeats, in addition to their C3- and C4-binding properties, remains to be clearly delineated.[115]

The LDL receptor-related complement proteins are cysteine-rich molecules. Each molecule contains an even number of cysteine residues that are clustered at the amino and carboxy ends of the protein and participate in disulfide bond formation. Those clustered at the amino terminus of the molecule share homology with the LDL receptor, while those at the carboxy terminus share homology with epidermal growth factor. The large number of disulfide bonds in these molecules is thought to convey a tertiary structure that facilitates the hydrophilic–hydrophobic transition that occurs upon their interaction with lipid membranes during the assembly of the MAC.[65,66,107]

COMPLEMENT-MEDIATED FUNCTIONS

Complement plays a major role in initiating the inflammatory response, clearing immune complexes, modulating immunoglobulin production, opsonizing microbial pathogens, and killing certain gram-negative bacteria (Fig. 1). Small, diffusable peptide fragments released from C4, C3, C5, and probably C2 during their activation help to mediate the inflammatory response.[107]

Collectively C4a, C3a, and C5a are referred to as *anaphylatoxins*, and together they stimulate histamine release from mast cells (C3a), promote vascular dilation (C3a, C4a), increase endothelial permeability (C3a), and stimulate neutrophil responses (C5a). Carboxypeptidase B-mediated removal of the carboxy terminal arginine from these molecules abrogates their functional activity by preventing their interaction with specific receptors.[107] In the case of C5a des arg (the inactivated form of C5a), chemotactic activity is restored by association with vitamin D–binding protein.[116,117] The activity of this complex is inhibited by free Bb, which is found in the sera of some patients with SLE.[118]

The incorporation of complement in immune complexes enhances their clearance and helps to minimize their potential for causing tissue damage.[119,120] This process includes the inhibition of immune complex precipitation from solution, the solubilization of immune complexes, and the clearance of C3b-bearing immune complexes via the CR1 receptor. Under conditions of antibody excess or antibody–antigen equivalence, the attachment of both antigen-binding sites on a single antibody to epitopes on a single antigen and the binding of multiple antibody molecules to a given molecule of antigen provide an opportunity for antibody–antibody interactions via their Fc fragments, a condition that leads to immune complex precipitation.[119] C1q binding inhibits these Fc–Fc interactions and leads to complement activation with covalent binding of C3b to the immune complex. Subsequent recruitment of the alternative pathway via the C3b amplification loop promotes further C3b deposition within the immune complex lattice, thereby reducing the forces holding the lattice together and causing separation (solubilization) of smaller complexes from the lattice network. Thus the classical pathway functions to inhibit immune complex precipitation, whereas the alternative pathway promotes solubilization of the immune complex.[119,120]

Small immune complexes bearing C3b are bound to cells bearing C3b receptors (CR1). The number of these receptors per cell varies from a low of 950 for erythrocytes to a high of 57,000 for neutrophils.[121] However, since red cells outnumber white cells by a thousandfold, 95 percent of the total CR1 receptors in the peripheral circulation are located on red cells. Consequently, immune complexes bearing C3b are 500–1000 times more likely to be cleared from the circulation via red cells than white cells.[121] These complexes are removed from the red cell during passage through the liver by an as yet undefined mechanism.[122]

Substantial data indicate that C3 modulates the immune response.[123] This evidence includes (1) the absolute requirement for C3 in antigen localization within splenic germinal centers; (2) the presence of CR1, CR2, and CR3 on B and T lymphocytes, follicular dendritic cells, and other antigen-presenting cells; (3) impaired antibody responses in animals or humans lacking one of the complement components (C1, C2, C4, C3) required for classical pathway C3 convertase formation and the restoration of the immune response by replacement of the missing component; and (4) the association of these deficiencies in man with significantly depressed concentrations of IgG4 and IgG2.[124–128] In general, these studies demonstrate that soluble C3 fragments inhibit immune responses, whereas the same products covalently linked to target particles enhance these reactions by reducing the concentration of antigen required to initiate an optimal response.[123] For example, the association of ligand bearing CR2 with CD19 in B cell membranes is an important signal for the activation of these cells.[106] In addition to enhancing responses to primary antigenic exposure, C3 fragments facilitate isotype switching and anamnestic responses following secondary antigenic exposure.[123] An intriguing observation in this regard is the apparent inverse correlation between the extent of C3b degradation on a given pneumococcal polysaccharide and the ability of that polysaccharide to elicit an immune response when administered as part of the polyvalent vaccine.[129] Thus,

although an absolute complement requirement does not exist for the generation of the humoral immune response, C3 clearly helps to promote an optimal response by facilitating antigen localization and presentation, by participating directly in the activation of B cells, and by promoting cytokine synthesis indirectly.

Cell-bound fragments of C3, particularly C3b and iC3b, serve as bifunctional ligands linking target particles with cells bearing receptors for these fragments. In the case of bacteria, opsonization with C3b or iC3b, especially in conjunction with IgG, promotes ingestion of the organism and triggers the microbicidal mechanisms of phagocytic cells (see Ch. 7). Ingestion appears to be more efficient when the organism is opsonized with iC3b than with C3b.[35,130] A small fragment, C3e, derived from the α-chain of C3, promotes the development of leukocytosis. This observation may account for the failure of some C3-deficient patients to develop leukocytosis in response to infection.[30]

The complete activation of the complement cascade with the assembly of the MAC and its effective insertion into cell membranes results in the death and eventual lysis of the cell. Death and lysis are independent events, and in the case of prokaryotes evidence suggests that a metabolic response is required by the organism before the lethal effects of the MAC can be expressed.[131] For some organisms the assembly of the MAC through C8 is sufficient for killing[132]; however, in all cases the incorporation of C9 accelerates this process. Complement-mediated virucidal activity has also been well described and in some cases seems to require deposition of only the early components of the classical pathway.[133]

MICROBIAL INTERACTIONS WITH THE COMPLEMENT SYSTEM

A common theme encountered in the pathogenesis of infection is the evolution of microbial strategies to elude host defense mechanisms. In the case of complement, these strategies parallel those employed by host cells to circumvent injury during the inflammatory response. That is, they are focused on decreasing complement activation and accelerating the decay or blocking the effect of activated components.[134,135] Indeed, in many instances the microbial proteins responsible for these effects share molecular, structural, immunologic, and functional homology with their human counterparts. In addition, a number of intracellular pathogens take advantage of various complement receptors to gain access to the interior of the cell.

Elegant experiments correlating virulence with lipopolysaccharide composition and complement activation in three isogenic *Salmonella typhimurium* variants have demonstrated the importance to bacteria of limiting complement deposition on their surface. These variants differ only in the chemical structure of their lipopolysaccharide side chains, yet their relative in vivo virulence is inversely proportional to their ability to activate complement via the alternative pathway. The rate of C3 consumption and extent of C3b deposition on the surface of these bacteria parallel one another, the greatest consumption and deposition occurring on the least virulent strains. Additional studies demonstrated that the magnitude of C3b binding is a function of the fine structure of the lipopolysaccharide O antigen and that while this structure affects C3 binding it has no effect on the subsequent cleavage and breakdown of the bound C3b. The effect of O antigen structure is expressed at the level of alternative-pathway amplification rather than degradation as shown by a greater affinity of factor B for C3b on the surface of the least virulent as compared with the most virulent strains, whereas the affinity of factor H for C3b is the same on all strains.[136–141]

Other examples of microbial surface structures that decrease complement activation include the sialic acid capsular polysaccharides found on serogroup B and Y meningococci and type III group B streptococci. In general, capsules also block the interaction group between C3 deposited on subcapsular structures and complement receptors on phagocytic cells. This phenomenon accounts in large measure for the antiphagocytic property of these structures. The ability of capsular-specific antibody to reverse this effect is testimony to the importance of antibody to redirect complement deposition to a relevant site on the organism surface.[142] Capsular polysaccharides and outer membrane blebs are shed during organism growth and complement attack. Shedding serves to abort complement attack at the organism surface. In addition, surface molecules released into the environment may act to decoy complement activation away from the intact organism.[134]

To date, molecules analogous to the complement regulatory proteins that accelerate the decay of the C3 convertases have not been identified in bacteria, although they are well described in multicellular parasites and viruses. The striking metamorphosis that protozoans undergo during transformation from insect to human infective forms is often accompanied by the acquisition of resistance to complement-dependent killing. This phenomenon has been studied most extensively in *Trypanosoma cruzi* for which two surface proteins, gp72 and gp160, have been identified that block the assembly and promote the decay of the alternative pathway C3 convertase.[134,135,143] Thus, they function in a manner identical to human CR1 and DAF (see Table 2). In the case of gp160, structural homology to DAF appears to be the underlying basis for the functional homology. Functionally analogous proteins are present on Epstein-Barr virus. In addition, vaccinia virus bears a C4bp structural and functional homolog that accelerates the decay of the classical pathway convertase.[135,144,145]

There is some evidence that parasites may adsorb human proteins onto their surface that then serve to downregulate complement activity. A variation of this theme occurs in serum-sensitive gonococci isolated from individuals with symptomatic local genital disease. These organisms possess a sialyl transferase but lack the ability to synthesize cytidine monophospho-*N*-acetyl neuraminic acid (CMP-NANA). Consequently they are incapable of endogenous sialylation of their lipopolysaccharide; rather they appropriate host CMP-NANA for this purpose. Exogenous sialylation confers serum resistance to these gonococci by reducing the binding of bactericidal antibody.[146] It also reduces phagocytic uptake and may alter C3 cleavage and intracellular survival. *T. cruzi* accomplishes the same effect via a *trans*-sialidase that removes terminal sialic acid residues from host glycoconjugates and transfers them to acceptor molecules on the parasite surface.[143]

The demonstration by Roantree and Rantz[147] that gram-negative bacteria isolated from blood cultures were almost always resistant to complement-mediated killing while two-thirds of those isolated from mucosal surfaces were serum sensitive was one of the first to suggest an important role for complement bactericidal activity. Enteric gram-negative bacilli like *Salmonella* owe their serum resistance to the long O-antigen side chains on their lipopolysaccharides. These chains lead to complement activation at sites distant from the outer membrane and hinder access of C5b-9 complexes to it. The failure of these complexes to localize to hydrophobic domains in the outer membrane results in their shedding and the survival of the organism.[134,148]

Gram-negative bacteria possessing truncated lipopolysaccharide molecules, for example, *Haemophilus influenzae*, meningococci, and gonococci, are not innately resistant to the bactericidal effects of the complement system but require antibody for effective sensitization and complement deposition. The absence of bactericidal antibody renders these organisms serum resistant and contributes to the greater frequency of *H. influenzae* and meningococcal disease during the first several years of life.

Gonococci isolated from individuals with disseminated gonococcal infection are resistant to the bactericidal activity of normal human serum.[149] The serum resistance of these strains is multifactorial. In the absence of bactericidal antibody the MAC is assembled on the organism surface but fails to insert properly into the outer membrane.[150,151] MAC insertion and killing occur normally in the presence of antilipopolysaccharide IgG found in the convalescent serum of some individuals with this infection.[152,153] However, some sera also contain IgG specific for gonococcal outer membrane protein 3.[154,155] This antibody competes with bactericidal antibody for binding sites on the surface of the organism, thereby blocking its bactericidal effect. Although the blocking antibody promotes complement deposition on the organism, it apparently does so at sites that do not lead to the killing of the organism.[156] Blocking antibody also appears to account for the resistance of meningococci to killing by the serum of many adults who acquire this infection.[157,158] These findings illustrate the interplay between the composition of the outer membrane of gram-negative bacteria in determining sensitivity to complement-mediated killing and the importance to the host of specific antibody in overcoming the resistance of these organisms to killing.[159]

Other organisms owe their serum resistance to functional homologs of CD59, the protein that interferes with MAC assembly on host cell membranes. For example, the galactose-specific adhesion of *Entamoeba histolytica* not only functions in this manner but also shares DNA sequence homology and antigenic cross reactivity with CD59.[160] Plasmids in *Salmonella typhimurium* and *Yersinia enterocolitica* contain the rck and Ail genes, respectively, which encode products of a family of virulence-associated outer membrane proteins. By preventing C9 polymerization these proteins mediate serum resistance and thus function similarly to CD59.[161,162]

Recently there has been a growing appreciation for the number of intracellular pathogens that utilize complement receptors to gain entry into cells. Entry in this fashion varies as to whether it initiates an appropriate signal transduction response and whether it is sufficient to establish effective intracellular infection. For example, Epstein-Barr and human immunodeficiency type 1 (HIV-1) viruses utilize CR2 to gain entry to B cells. The resulting cellular transformation may contribute to the polyclonal gammopathy observed early in the course of disease caused by these pathogens.[163–165] In contrast, *Leishmania* species, *Legionella pneumophila*, and various *Mycobacteria* spp. and *Babesia* spp. utilize CR1 and CR3, alone or in combination, to gain intracellular access. The effect of this mode of entry on cellular activation processes has not been as well elucidated as that for Epstein-Barr virus. In most instances the microbial ligand interacting with complement receptors has not been identified. Exceptions are the gp350 and gp63 molecules on Epstein-Barr virus and *Leishmania major*, respectively.[135]

Finally, several groups have reported that *Candida albicans* bears a surface protein that binds iC3b and reacts with antibodies to CR3.[166,167] Expression of this integrin-like molecule is upregulated by glucose and associated with increased association of *Candida* with endothelial cells, presumably through an interaction with an intercellular adhesion molecule (ICAM-1) on the endothelial surface.[168]

COMPLEMENT DEFICIENCY STATES

Frequency

Complement deficiency states may be either acquired or inherited. Acquired deficiency states can occur acutely, as part of an abrupt insult such as infection, or in conjunction with more chronic diseases such as rheumatologic or autoimmune processes. The frequency of inherited complement deficiencies in the general population is about 0.03 percent. Since these states are rare, the utility of screening tests is greatest in populations that contain the clinical correlates of abnormal complement inheritance, that is, persons with rheumatologic diseases and/or recurrent bacterial infections.[169,170] The frequency of complement deficiencies reported in these disorders is affected by both methodologic and biologic factors.[171] The most important methodologic variables are the sample size and degree of ascertainment. The most important biologic considerations are the ethnic makeup of the population and the incidence of the target disease in that population.

In one such study, a single individual with homozygous C2 deficiency was detected among 545 patients with rheumatologic diseases.[172] This frequency (0.2 percent) is approximately 10-fold greater than that in the general population. In addition, 19 individuals with a definite, probable, or possible heterozygous C2 deficiency state were detected among the 545 rheumatologic patients as compared with only 6 possible heterozygotes among 509 individuals without these diseases. Thus, this study provides clear support for the association of complement deficiency states with certain rheumatologic disorders, in particular, systemic lupus erythematosus (SLE).[172]

Reports of an association between systemic meningococcal and gonococcal infections and an inherited deficiency of C5, C6, C7, or C8 have led to several studies of the frequency of these deficiencies among patients with these infections. Such studies have uncovered as few as 0 of 47 (<2 percent) to as many a 8 of 16 (50 percent) complement-deficient individuals presenting with a first episode of documented meningococcal disease.[170,171] Analysis of these studies reveals an inverse relationship between the prevalence of complement deficiency in persons with meningococcal disease and the incidence of the disease in the general population (Fig. 3). This relationship suggests that the overall prevalence of complement deficiencies is relatively constant (0.03–0.11 percent), but that, among populations in which the level of immunity is low and meningococcal disease is epidemic, more normal than complement-deficient persons will be infected because there are significantly more of the former than the latter. As the level of immunity in the population increases, the incidence of meningococcal disease falls. However, because the prevalence of complement deficiency in the general population is relatively stable, the frequencies of these states among individuals with meningococcal disease increase, that is, complement deficiency becomes a greater determinant of the risk of infection.[171] Thus, the best estimate of inherited complement deficiency states among patients with

endemic neisserial disease is about 5–10 percent, although the likelihood of a complement deficiency is increased dramatically (31 percent) among patients who have had more than one episode of meningococcal infection.

Classical-Pathway Deficiencies

The association of immune disorders, in particular SLE, with complement deficiency states is most evident in individuals lacking C1, C4, C2, or C3 (Table 3). The clinical presentation of SLE in individuals with a deficiency of one of these components differs from that in the general population in that males are commonly affected, renal disease is less severe, antinuclear antibody titers are low or absent, and there is an increased prevalence of Ro antibodies.[173–175]

In contrast to the relationship with infection in which an association is apparent only in homozygous deficient individuals, an increased frequency of collagen vascular diseases is apparent in individuals with either homozygous or heterozygous deficiency. The basis for this phenomenon has not been precisely delineated, although impaired immune complex handling and tight genetic linkage of the C2 and C4 loci to the class I and class II MHC genes appear to contribute to the association.[176] Of these variables, impaired immune complex clearance probably exerts a greater impact since the association is apparent for all four of these complement proteins, whereas only C4 and C2 are MHC linked. The role of the early components of the classical pathway in inhibiting immune complex precipitation has been confirmed in the sera from patients with these deficiencies.[177,178] Moreover, abnormal humoral immune system regulation and the presence of autoantibodies, including rheumatoid factors, have been demonstrated in C2- and C4-deficient guinea pigs.[179]

The low frequency of infection (20 percent) in individuals with a deficiency of C1, C4, or C2 as compared with other component deficiencies (Table 3) is attributed to the presence of an intact alternative pathway in these patients. When it occurs, bacterial infection is usually caused by encapsulated bacteria, especially *Streptococcus pneumoniae*, and may be recurrent. The most common sites of infection are the sinopulmonary tree, meninges, and blood.[169,170]

Consequent to the linkage disequilibrium with other MHC

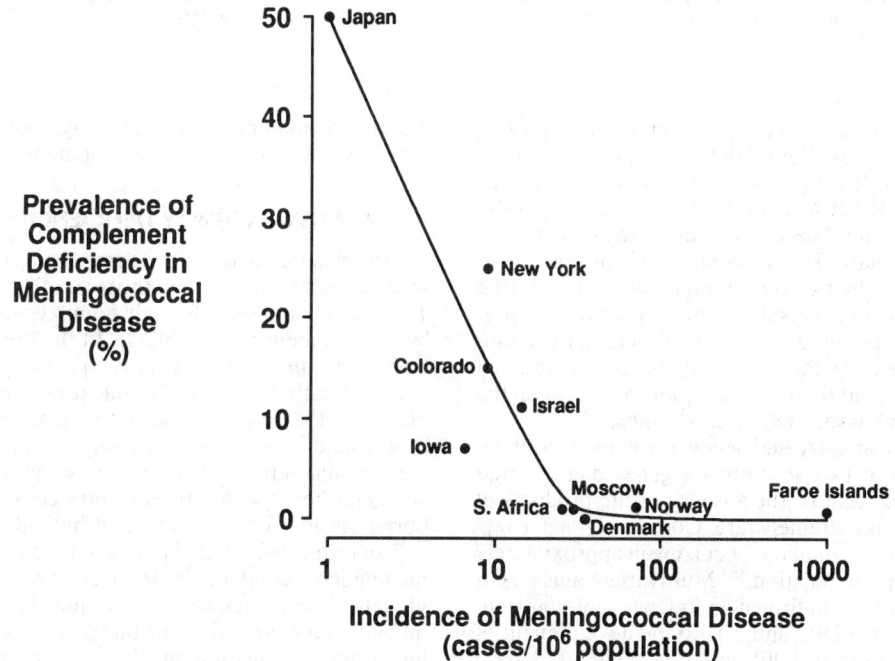

FIG. 3.   Relationship between the prevalence of complement deficiency and the incidence of meningococcal disease. (From Figueroa and Densen,[171] with permission.)

TABLE 3. Complement Deficiency States

Component	No. of Reported Patients	Mode of Inheritance	Functional Defects	Disease Associations
Classical pathway				
C1qrs	31	ACD	Impaired IC handling, delayed C' activation, impaired immune response	CVD, 48%; infection (encaps bact), 22%; both, 18%; healthy, 12%
C4	21	ACD		
C2	109	ACD		
Alternative pathway				
D	3	ACD	Impaired C' activation in absence of specific antibody	Infection (meningococcal), 74%; healthy, 26%
P	70	XL		
Junction of classical and alternative pathways				
C3	19	ACD	Impaired IC handling, opson/phag; granulocytosis, CTX, immune response and absent SBA	CVD, 79% recurrent infection (encaps bact), 71%
Terminal components				
C5	27	ACD	Impaired CTX; absent SBA	Infection (Neisseria, primarily meningococcal), 58%; CVD, 4%
C6	77	ACD		Both, 1%
C7	73	ACD	Absent SBA	Healthy, 25%
C8	73	ACD		
C9	165	ACD	Impaired SBA	Healthy, 91%; infection, 9%
Plasma proteins regulating C' activation				
C1-INH	many	AD / Acq	Uncontrolled generation of an inflammatory mediator upon C' activation	Hereditary angioedema
H	13	ACD	Uncontrolled AP activation → low C3	CVD, 40% / CVD + infection (encaps bact), 40%; healthy, 20%
I	14	ACD	Uncontrolled AP activation → low C3	Infection (encaps bact), 100%
Membrane proteins regulating C' activation				
DAF HRF CD59	Many	Acq	Impaired regulation of C3b and C8 deposited on host RBC; PMN, platelets → cell lysis	Paroxysmal nocturnal hemoglobinuria
CR3	>20	ACD	Impaired PMN adhesive functions, i.e., margination, CTX, iC3b-mediated opson/phag	Infection (S. aureus, Pseudomonas spp.), 100%
Autoantibodies, C3 nephritic factors	>59	Acq	Stabilize AP, convertase → low C3	MPGN, 41%; PLD, 25%; infection (encaps bact), 16% / MPGN + PLD, 10%; PLD + infection, 5%; MPGN + PLD + infection, 3%; MPGN + infection, 2%
C4 nephritic factor		Acq	Stabilize CP, C3 convertase → low C3	Glomerulonephritis, 50%; CVD, 50%

Abbreviations: ACD, autosomal codominant; XL, X-linked; AD, autosomal dominant; Acq, acquired; IC, immune complex; C', complement; opson/phag, opsonophagocytosis; CTX, chemotaxis; SBA, serum bactericidal activity; AP, alternative pathway; RBC, red blood cells; PMN, polymorphonuclear neutrophils; CVD, collagen vascular disease; encaps bact, encapsulated bacteria; MPGN, membrano-proliferative glomerulonephritis; PLD, partial lymphadystrophy.

(Data from refs. 169, 170.)

loci, the C2 and C4 null genes occur predominantly as part of distinct extended haplotypes. For C2 deficiency, this haplotype is DR2;C2Q0;BfS;C4A-4;C4B-2;B18;A25,[180] and for C4 deficiency it is DR3;C2C;BfS;C4AQ0;C4B-1;B8.[181] The specific haplotype associated with C2 deficiency occurs in about 93 percent of affected individuals. The molecular basis of this defect is a 28 bp gene deletion that causes skipping of exon 6 during mRNA splicing, which in turn results in the generation of a premature stop codon and synthesis of a nonfunctional protein. The bases of the deficiency in the remaining 7 percent of affected individuals is unknown, but there is no relationship between the basis for the defect and associated disease states.[182,183]

The molecular basis of C4A deficiency involves gene deletion.[181] The existence of two separate C4 genes dictates that complete C4 deficiency, that is, the absence of the products of all four C4 genetic loci, is extremely rare. Conversely, heterozygous C4 deficiency is very common, occurring in approximately 25 percent of the general population.[184] Multivariate analysis of DR and C4 gene types has confirmed an independent contribution of the C4AQ0 and the DR2 antigens to the development of SLE. The C4B null gene (C4Q0) was not associated with SLE.[185] The chemical preference of the internal thiolester in C4A to form amide bonds during complement activation and to

react with immune complexes may contribute to the effect of the C4A null gene on the development of SLE.[37,39,40]

ALTERNATIVE-PATHWAY DEFICIENCIES

Inherited deficiencies of the components of the alternative pathway are less common than those of other complement proteins. To date, no individuals with homozygous factor B deficiency have been identified (Table 3). In the presence of specific antibody, persons with alternative-pathway defects activate the classical pathway normally, but the absence of antibody, coupled with the defect in alternative-pathway activation, leads to a profound abnormality in complement activation and serum bactericidal activity. Consequently, infection in such individuals might be expected to have dire consequences, a prediction borne out in properdin-deficient individuals (Table 4).

Properdin deficiency is an X-linked trait that predisposes to meningococcal infections in three-quarters of the affected individuals. These infections are frequently characterized by a fulminant course and high mortality rate. Consequently, recurrent infections are uncommon.[186,187] Three properdin-deficient variants have been described: type 1, characterized by extremely low concentrations (<0.1 μg/ml) and absent properdin func-

TABLE 4. Comparison of Meningococcal Disease in Normal and Late Complement Component– and Properdin-Deficient Individuals

Characteristics	Normal	C5–C8	C9	Properdin Deficient[a]
No. of homozygotes	—	250	165	54–70
No. with meningococcal disease	—	146	15	25–37
Frequency of infection (%)	0.0072	58	9.1	46–53
Median age (year), first episode	3	17	16	14–11.5
Recurrence rate (%)	0.34	44	0	2–1.4
Relapse rate (%)	0.6	7.9	0	0
Mortality/100 episodes (%)	19	1.5	0	12–51.4
Infecting serogroup				
No. of isolates	3,184	67	2	16
B (%)	50	19.4	50	18.7
Y (%)	4.4	32.8	0	37.5

[a] Where a range is given the first number refers to documented cases and the second number refers to documented plus probable and possible cases.

(From Densen,[171] with permission.)

tions[186,187]; type 2 characterized by a low concentration (~2 μg/ml) of antigenically detectable but functionally altered properdin; and type 3, characterized by a normal concentration of antigenically detectable properdin (~25 μg/ml) but absent function.[188,189]

C3 Deficiency

C3 deficiency is uncommon (Table 3). As expected from its position and function as the linchpin of the complement cascade, virtually all individuals with this defect are seriously ill.[169,170] Approximately three-quarters develop SLE or a related rheumatologic syndrome. Moreover, the inability to use either the classical or alternative pathway results in a multitude of severe defects in host defense, including impairments in opsonization, immune response, neutrophil chemotaxis, and the ability to generate serum bactericidal activity. Consequently, severe and recurrent pneumococcal, *H. influenzae,* and meningococcal infections involving the sinopulmonary tree, meninges, and blood stream are common, occurring in about 70 percent of such patients.[169,170] The molecular basis for primary C3 deficiency has been characterized in two patients. In one individual, an 800 bp genomic deletion affecting exons 22 and 23 was responsible for the defect,[190] whereas, in the second patient, the defect was due to a splicing abnormality resulting in partial deletion of exon 19.[191]

A comparable clinical picture is observed in individuals with an inherited deficiency of either factor H or factor I and in individuals who develop autoantibody to C3 (C3 nephritic factor).[169,170] The similar clinical picture results from uncontrolled alternative-pathway activation and resultant low levels of C3 (less than 10 percent) in serum. Recurrent infection and collagen vascular disorders occur less commonly in individuals with C3 nephritic factor, presumably due to the somewhat higher levels of C3 in these patients. Patients with autoantibody to C3 have an increased incidence of membranoproliferative glomerulonephritis and/or partial lipodystrody (Table 3).[192,193] Recently, complement factor D and adipsin, a secretory product of adipocytes that is deficient in several animal models of obesity, have been shown to be the same protein.[194,195] This finding has led to the recognition that adipose tissue is a significant site of synthesis for alternative-pathway components.[196] The subsequent demonstration that C3 nephritic factor can promote adipocyte lysis suggests a potential explanation for the association of this antibody with partial lipodystrophy.[197]

LATE COMPLEMENT COMPONENT DEFICIENCIES

Individuals with a deficiency of one of the terminal complement components exhibit a striking susceptibility to systemic neisserial infections, especially meningococcal disease. Despite the chemotactic defect associated with C5 deficiency, the clinical manifestations of meningococcal disease in persons with this defect and those with other terminal component deficiencies is remarkably similar.[171] Thus the basis for the association of meningococcal disease in these persons appears due to their inability to assemble the membrane attack complex and express complement-dependent bactericidal activity. This conclusion is supported by detailed population-based epidemiologic studies demonstrating an approximate 5000-fold increase in risk of meningococcal disease in C7-deficient compared with complement-sufficient Japanese. In contrast, C9-deficient Japanese experienced an approximate 700-fold increase in risk.[198] The increased risk of meningococcal disease in C5–C8-deficient persons relative to C9-deficient individuals is consistent with in vitro studies demonstrating that C9-deficient sera can kill meningococci, albeit at a slower rate.[132] This dose-response relationship coupled with the fact that the structural genes encoding these proteins are located on multiple chromosomes provides strong evidence for a cause and effect relationship between the absence of complement-dependent bactericidal activity and the increased susceptibility of these individuals to meningococcal disease.

The molecular bases for these deficiency states remain largely undefined, although a single C → T exchange in exon 9 of C8β, which produces a premature stop codon, appears to be the most common cause of this defect.[199] As with other genetic deficiencies, heterogeneous mechanisms are likely. For example, the structural genes for C6 and C7 are tightly located on chromosome 9, yet both combined and individual deficiencies of these proteins have been described.[170]

MENINGOCOCCAL INFECTION IN COMPLEMENT DEFICIENCY STATES

Meningococcal disease is the single most common infection sustained by complement-deficient individuals, accounting for 75–85 percent of etiologically identified infections.[169,170] Although meningococcal disease has been reported in individuals with a deficiency of any of the plasma complement proteins, it is most common in properdin-, C5-, C6-, C7-, or C8-deficient individuals, of whom 50–60 percent experience at least one episode during their lifetime. This striking association confirms the importance of the complement system in host defense against meningococci.

Meningococcal disease in these complement deficiencies exhibits several unique features that help to distinguish it from that in complement-sufficient persons (Table 4). These features provide valuable clinical clues suggesting the need to screen for a complement deficiency state. These features are unlikely to result solely from ascertainment bias for the following reasons. First, they have been confirmed in multiple studies in different populations around the world. Second, each feature has been borne out by investigations of complement-deficient families following exclusion of the proband from the analysis. Third, at least in the case of the late complement component deficiencies, family studies fail to reveal undiagnosed infections and unexplained or premature deaths.

Data compiled from the literature as well as a detailed population-based study suggest that these complement deficiency states increase the risk of meningococcal disease 5,000–10,000-fold. In contrast to persons in the general population in whom the median age of meningococcal infection is 3 years and 56 percent of the infections occur before 5 years of age, the median age of first infection in complement-deficient individuals is 17 years and only 10 percent of the infections occur before age 5 years. Thus, most deficient persons pass through the age of life when the deficiency might be expected to increase maximally their susceptibility to meningococcal disease without evincing evidence of that susceptibility. The basis for this observation is unknown, but it suggests that unidentified factors may modulate the susceptibility of deficient individuals to infection later in life.

Meningococcal disease in complement-deficient individuals is caused by uncommon serogroups, particularly groups Y, W135, and X, more often than in normal individuals.[169,170] Conversely, the prevalence of these deficiencies is increased among individuals with meningococcal disease caused by these serogroups.[200] The physiologic basis for this observation is not known with certainty, but factors that may be important include (1) the critical requirement for anticapsular antibody for prevention of disease in deficient compared with normal individuals; (2) the more ready elimination of group B isolates by phagocytic cells in the absence of capsular antibody[201]; and (3) the propensity for uncommon meningococcal serogroup organisms to cause disease in older individuals.[202] Nevertheless, meningococci and gonococci isolated from complement-deficient individuals with systemic neisserial infection do not differ significantly in their biologic properties compared with the same organisms isolated from complement-sufficient individuals.[203] Thus, the absence of complement-dependent bactericidal activity does not automatically provide access to the blood stream by less virulent serum-sensitive organisms.

Recurrent meningococcal disease, defined as a new infection occurring more than 1 month following a previous episode, occurs in about 40–45 percent of C5–C8-deficient individuals. This recurrence rate is approximately 100–150 times greater than that in the general population. Statistical analysis of the number of individuals with a specified number of episodes of meningococcal disease is consistent with the interpretation that the risk of meningococcal disease in complement-deficient individuals is independent of prior infection.[170] That is, prior disease does not reduce the risk of subsequent meningococcal infection in these individuals. In that study, the estimated probability of each infection was 0.39.[170] A similar analysis, utilizing a slightly different statistical approach, arrived at an identical conclusion and resulted in an estimate of the probability of infection of 0.6.[204,205] The latter analysis also demonstrated that the interval between infections (4–5 years) did not differ, again suggesting that prior disease does not reduce the risk of subsequent meningococcal infection. The explanation for the failure of prior infection to reduce the risk of subsequent episodes of meningococcal disease in these complement-deficient persons appears to lie in their critical dependence on capsular antibodies for protection and the fact that infection constitutes a relatively poor stimulus for production of these antibodies. These antibodies are highly efficient in promoting opsonophagocytic elimination of meningococci. In contrast, antibodies to subcapsular antigens, although bactericidal and protective in the normal host, are poor opsonins and thus afford little protection in complement-deficient individuals who lack the effector proteins necessary for the expression of bactericidal activity.[206]

Relapse of meningococcal disease, defined as infection with the same serogroup occurring less than 1 month following the initial infection, occurs in 7.6 percent of the C5–C8-deficient individuals with meningococcal disease reported in the literature. This frequency is approximately 10 times greater than that in the general population and suggests that meningococci may be sequestered intracellularly where they may be relatively protected from antibiotics.

One of the most striking aspects of meningococcal disease in late complement component-deficient individuals is that, despite a several-thousand-fold increase in the risk of infection, they experience a 5- to 10-fold reduction in the chance of dying from the disease compared with normal persons. Thus, the identical defect that predisposes to infection appears to provide protection from the lethal consequences of the disease. This re-

markable observation suggests that the host's exuberant response to the organism is as much responsible for the clinical manifestations and outcome as the organism itself. This deduction is supported by the report of Brandzaeg et al.[207] of a close correlation between the extent of complement activation and mortality in meningococcal disease and suggests that the latter is in part dependent on the assembly of the membrane attack complex.

The basis for the lower mortality from meningococcal disease in late complement-deficient persons is unknown, but variables that may be relevant include milder disease[204]; the possibility that fewer organisms are required to initiate infection; an ability to tolerate better a given endotoxin load[208]; and less host cell injury.

The possibility that fewer organisms may be required to establish systemic meningococcal disease in deficient than normal individuals is attractive, although data addressing this point are conspicuously absent in the literature. Such an effect would account for the increased number of infections as well as milder disease and the decreased case fatality rate since mortality is directly related to the number of organisms in the blood stream.[209,210] A reduction in the organism load might translate into a lower concentration of circulating endotoxin and less systemic inflammation. Alternatively, since insertion of the MAC into the outer membrane of gram-negative organisms results in the release of free endotoxin, the inability of late complement component-deficient persons to assembly the MAC may be associated with a reduction in the quantity of circulating endotoxin for a given load of organisms. This reduction in turn might lessen ongoing complement activation and decrease secretion of various cytokines linked to the development of septic shock in meningococcal disease.[207,211–215] Finally, insertion of the MAC into host cell membranes might occur in vivo as a consequence of exuberant complement activation in the vicinity of innocent bystander cells or as a consequence of endotoxin binding to these cells and subsequent complement activation on their surfaces. Insertion of the MAC into the membrane of host cells, while not lethal, has been associated with profound effects,[216,217] for example, leukocyte activation with the resultant release of a plethora of potentially noxious mediators[218] and the increased expression of procoagulant molecules on the surface of endothelial cells.[219] Interruption of these processes in the late complement component-deficient individual would result in an improved ability to tolerate a given load of organisms and endotoxin.

Other Complement Deficiency States

Hereditary Angioedema–C1 Inhibitor Deficiency. Individuals lacking C1-INH present with a distinctive clinical picture historically referred to as hereditary angioneurotic edema (HANE or HAE).[220] The hereditary form of this disease was recognized over 100 years ago, whereas an acquired variant has been identified as a distinct entity only within the last 25 years. The genetic form of the disease is inherited as an autosomal dominant trait and exhibits two variants. Type 1 HAE is more common and accounts for 75–85 percent of cases and is characterized by the presence of low (5–30 percent) levels of normally functioning C1-INH protein. In contrast, type 2 HAE is characterized by the presence of normal to elevated levels of antigenic C1-INH that is functionally abnormal.[72,220,221] The acquired forms of this disorder occur considerably less commonly, and two variants are recognized. One, occurring in association with B-lymphocyte disorders, is due to a reaction of circulating anti-idiotype antibodies, with the monoclonal immunoglobulin expressed on the surface of the abnormal B cells.[222] The resulting immune complex leads to C1-INH consumption and secondarily to the clinical picture of angioedema. The second type derives from the presence of autoantibody to C1-INH. In this situation, angioedema develops as a consequence of inhibition of C1-INH activity.[223]

Since the hereditary form of this disorder is inherited as an autosomal dominant trait, the serum from all of these individuals contains some normally functioning C1-INH.[72] In contrast, individuals with the acquired variants have markedly reduced or absent functional C1-INH activity in their serum. As a consequence of this basic difference, the serum from individuals with the hereditary form of this disorder contains normal amounts of C1 and C1q but reduced levels of C4 and C2, whereas the serum from individuals with the acquired variants contains strikingly reduced amounts of C1, C1q, C4, and C2.[72,220,221]

The health of individuals with this disorder is punctuated by attacks of nonpitting, nonpruritic, and nonpainful edema of the extremities, face, or larynx. Angioedema of the larynx is the most severe complication of the disorder and is a common cause of death in these individuals. The gastrointestinal tract may also be affected, and such attacks present as episodes of acute, crampy abdominal pain frequently associated with nausea, vomiting, and occasionally diarrhea. In the inherited form of the disorder, attacks generally begin in childhood, increase in frequency and worsen in severity during adolescence, increase during menstruation, are markedly reduced during pregnancy, and diminish gradually in the fifth and sixth decades of life. A typical attack lasts 2–3 days. Impeded androgens increase the biosynthesis of C1-INH in vitro and have been employed successfully to treat individuals with the hereditary form of the disease.[72,220]

Although C1-INH is the only recognized inhibitor of C1 esterase activity, it also participates in regulating the plasma kinin system and some of the enzymes in the coagulation and fibrinolytic cascades.[72,220] Plasma from these patients exhibits an impaired ability to inactivate kallikrein, and it has been suggested that this impairment is responsible for the manifestations of HAE. However, subcutaneous injection of bradykinin produces pain and swelling, and intravenous infusion induces hypotension, none of which are characteristic of HAE.[72] In contrast, intradermal injection of activated C1s leads to nonpainful, nonpruritic swelling in both humans and guinea pigs. This response does not occur if activated C1 is injected into C2-deficient individuals or guinea pigs, but is observed following injection into a C3-deficient patient.[224] Consequently, these data favor the hypothesis that the clinical manifestations of this disorder are due to the release of an anaphylatoxic-like peptide from the C2b fragment of the C2 molecule. It is also possible that symptoms result from the interaction of several factors from these cascade systems.[72]

As expected from the different C1-INH protein phenotypes, the genetic basis for HAE is heterogeneous. A substantial proportion of the type I HAE defects are associated with mutations within Alu clusters. These mutations cause a variety of rearrangements leading to deletions or duplications within the gene, impaired transcription, and reduced levels of specific mRNA and plasma concentrations of C1-INH. In contrast, type II HAE, which is generally associated with normal concentrations of a dysfunctional protein, is typically caused by point mutations. These mutations usually affect the arginine at the reactive center of the molecule or amino acids in its immediate vicinity. Occasionally mutations affect C1-INH glycosylation. In all instances the mutation leads to the synthesis of a protein with an altered ability to react with its substrates. The resulting altered catabolism is responsible for the normal or elevated concentration of plasma C1-INH.[225,226]

Paroxysmal Nocturnal Hemoglobinuria. Another syndrome in which the function of complement regulatory proteins is deranged is paroxysmal nocturnal hemoglobinuria (PNH).[227,228] The basic problem in such individuals is an increased susceptibility of their red blood cells to hemolysis. The disease is uncommon but usually presents in young adults during the third to fifth decades. Occasionally it may be observed in association with drug-induced aplastic anemia, but in most instances there is no apparent inciting event. Classically, individuals present with bouts of hemolysis that are worse at night and last for several days to weeks. The precipitating events responsible for these bouts of hemolysis are usually inapparent, although occasionally they are associated with infection. The basis for the increased hemolysis at nighttime is not clear but may relate to a lower pH in the small vessels of the peripheral venous circulation. Although this is the classic picture of the disease, the more common presentation, occurring in about half of the patients, is one of chronic hemolysis. Patients may have back pain, crampy abdominal pain, and headaches. Some of these individuals are prone to venous thrombosis, especially after surgery, while others may have slightly more frequent infections. Thrombocytopenia and/or leukopenia develop in most individuals at some point during their illness.[227,228]

The peripheral blood of individuals with PNH contains varying proportions of three populations of red blood cells. PNH type 1 cells are normal, whereas type 2 and type 3 PNH cells exhibit 3- to 6- and 15- to 25-fold increases in sensitivity to complement-mediated lysis, respectively. The severity of the clinical picture correlates best with the proportion of type 3 cells present in the peripheral circulation.[229]

Identification of cell surface proteins that modulate the effects of complement deposition on host cells led to the discovery that PNH cells lack the complement regulatory proteins DAF and CD59.[230,231] Moreover, if normal erythrocytes are treated with antibody to DAF, they behave like PNH type 2 cells, and if DAF is inserted in the membrane of type 2 cells, they behave like normal (type 1) cells. However, insertion of DAF into the membrane of PNH type 3 cells, while circumventing increased C3b uptake, has no effect on their increased susceptibility to complement-mediated lysis.[232] Thus, although both PNH type 2 and 3 cells lack DAF, the greatly increased sensitivity to complement-mediated lysis, which is the physiologic basis for the clinical manifestations of the disorder, appears to be due to the absence of CD59.[231–233] This conclusion is further buttressed by the observation that individuals with an inherited defect affecting expression of just DAF on their red cell membranes do not exhibit the PNH phenotype, whereas individuals lacking solely CD59 do manifest this phenotype.[234,235] The absence of DAF and CD59 from platelets and neutrophils from patients with DNH may help to explain the increased susceptibility of these individuals to episodes of venous thrombosis and infection.[236] The fact that these molecules are present in normal amounts on endothelial cells in individuals with PNH supports the clonal origin of this disorder within bone marrow precursor cells.

PNH cells are also missing a number of other surface proteins, including acetylcholinesterase, alkaline phosphatase, lymphocyte-function-associated antigen 3 (LFA-3), and FcγRIII receptors.[237] The feature shared by these proteins is that they are all bound to the cell membrane through a carboxy-terminal glycolipid linkage. Thus, although the physiologic basis for the clinical symptomatology in this disorder is the absence of DAF and CD59 from PNH cells, the molecular basis lies in an abnormality in the synthetic pathway by which these proteins are anchored to the cell membrane through glycolipid linkages. Genetic complementation studies indicate that this defect affects the first step in the synthesis of the glycosylphosphatidylinositol anchor itself, in which an enzyme catalyzes the transfer of activated N-acetyl glucose to a phosphatidylinositol acceptor in the endoplasmic reticulum.[238,239] The gene encoding this transferase presumably bears a mutation that affects its function.

COMPLEMENT IN DISEASE STATES

Complement activation has been demonstrated in a wide variety of diseases, which suggests that products of this activation may play a role in the development of symptoms or in the outcome of these disorders. Evidence supporting this suggestion includes the fact that the extent of complement activation parallels disease activity, that complement deposition can be demonstrated at the site of tissue injury, the finding of altered complement metabolism in various disease states, and the demonstration that complement activation modulates the course of disease in animal models of these disorders. In this context, the role of complement has been most extensively studied in infectious diseases, rheumatologic conditions, renal diseases, and hemolytic states. The demonstration of the MAC in ischemic myocardium,[240–244] renal tissue in various immune and nonimmunologic renal diseases,[245–252] the skin of individuals with immunologically mediated dermatitis,[253] the cerebrospinal fluid of individuals with central nervous system lupus erythematosus,[254] and the serum and peripheral nerves of individuals with Guillain-Barré syndrome as well as other demyelinating diseases[255–257] implicates this complex in tissue damage in these disorders. Hyperacute graft rejection of xenogeneic transplants is complement dependent and can be prevented by complement depletion or infusion of proteins that regulate complement activation such as soluble CR1 and CD46.[258–261] Similarly CR1 infusion reduces inflammation and the extent of myocardial infarction in an animal model of reperfusion injury.[262]

Infectious Diseases

Complement activation probably occurs during most infections but can be particularly impressive in diseases like dengue fever, bacterial endocarditis, and bacteremia in which the organisms or their products react with antibodies to form circulating immune complexes and initiate complement consumption. Complement consumption is particularly striking in meningococcal disease and other forms of gram-negative bacteremia. Complement activation via the alternative pathway has been well documented in gram-negative sepsis, with the greatest degree of activation occurring in patients with shock.[263] Whether complement activation contributes to shock or is a consequence of the development of shock itself has been a matter of debate. Circulating C5a has been associated with the development of the acute respiratory distress syndrome in humans[264,265] and in a monkey model of gram-negative shock.[266] In the latter, mortality could be prevented and morbidity attenuated by the administration of antibody to C5a.[266] The observation that individuals with inherited C5, C6, C7, or C8 deficiency have a 6000-fold greater frequency of meningococcal disease but 10-fold less mortality than do persons with a normal complement system (Table 4) suggests that the ability to assemble the MAC may increase mortality (see above).[169]

Complement, in conjunction with the organs of the reticuloendothelial system, plays a critical role in the removal of encapsulated bacteria from the blood stream.[267] Delineation of the contribution of these variables to the clearance process has been accomplished in an animal model of pneumococcal bacteremia and has demonstrated that the more virulent the organism, the greater the role of the spleen in performing this clearance function.[268,269] Complement depletion of the animals led to a significant decrease in the number of pneumococci needed to kill 50 percent of the animals, thus demonstrating an important role for complement in the clearance function. In addition, clearance of pneumococci was similar in healthy and C4-deficient animals, thus indicating that complement activation and fixation to the bacteria via the alternative pathway was particularly relevant in this process. Last, the presence of immune antibody shifted the burden of clearance from the spleen to the liver, but this effect was absolutely dependent on a functional alternative complement pathway.[270]

An increased susceptibility to infection is observed in both individuals undergoing splenectomy and individuals with intact but nonfunctioning spleens, for example, patients with sickle cell anemia.[271,272] The incidence of infection varies from a low of approximately 1 percent in individuals undergoing incidental

splenectomy to a high of approximately 25 percent in individuals undergoing splenectomy as treatment for thalassemia.[272] The mortality rate in these individuals varies between 40 and 80 percent, depending on the underlying condition prompting splenectomy. A wide variety of organisms have been reported to cause overwhelming sepsis in splenectomized individuals, but the pneumococcus accounts for 50–70 percent of such infections, with the bulk of the remainder being accounted for by the meningococcus, *H. influenzae,* and to a lesser extent *E. coli.*[272] The typical presentation of such individuals is that of septic shock, disseminated intravascular coagulopathy, and the adult respiratory distress syndrome occurring in the absence of a primary site of infection.[273]

Rheumatologic Disorders

Substantial clinical and experimental evidence links complement deficiency syndromes and complement activation to a variety of rheumatologic diseases, most notably SLE.[274] Additional support for this relationship is the finding that pharmacologic agents, for example, hydralazine and isoniazid, associated with the drug-induced form of SLE inactivate C4 by nucleophilic attack on its internal thiolester and formation of amide bonds.[275] Evidence that complement activation may be associated with the manifestations of the disease and tissue injury includes the demonstration of C3 and immune complex deposition at the dermal–epidermal junction in the cutaneous lesions from patients with both SLE and discoid lupus erthematosus. Similar immunohistochemical alterations have been demonstrated in biopsy specimens of healthy skin from the same individuals. However, the recent finding of MACs in areas of affected but not unaffected skin from these individuals strengthens the hypothesis that complement activation may partly mediate tissue injury in these disorders.[253]

In addition to these effects in the tissues, the sera from about 40 percent of patients with SLE contain an inhibitor of C5a-derived chemotactic activity.[276–278] Its presence correlates with disease activity and the resultant chemotactic defect with the enhanced susceptibility of these patients to infection. The inhibitor has been identified as the Bb fragment of factor B, and it exerts its effect by blocking the interaction of C5a des arg with its cochemotaxin in serum.[118] The presence of free Bb in the serum of these individuals reflects alternative-pathway activation and substantiates the utility of complement component quantitation in assessing disease activity.

Incorporation of C3 into immune complexes promotes their binding to C3b receptors (CR1) on erythrocytes, and the number of these receptors is reduced in individuals with disorders like SLE that are characterized by circulating immune complexes.[275,279] The degree of CR1 reduction correlates well with disease activity and the extent of complement activation. These and other data indicate that erythrocyte CR1 is removed along with immune complexes during passage through the liver and spleen. The decrease in CR1 coupled with the inability of circulating red cells to resynthesize them further exacerbates the defect in immune complex clearance, thereby promoting their deposition in the tissues, with resultant damage to the host.

Renal Disorders

Complement deposition in renal disease associated with immune disorders is related to the deposition of immune complexes within the kidney.[245–248,250–252] whereas complement deposition in the absence of immune complexes is postulated to occur by activation of the alternative pathway.[249] Recently, a rat model of chronic tubulointerstitial disease has been used to investigate the mode of complement deposition and its role in producing injury.[246] In the diseased rats, the loss of renal mass and function was correlated with increased ammonia production and systemic acidosis. Under these conditions, peritubular deposition of C3 and the MAC was readily demonstrated. However, deposition of these components and evidence of tubulointerstitial inflammation were markedly decreased in diseased animals treated with sodium bicarbonate. These and other results suggest that ammonia attacks the C3 internal thiolester to form amidated C3. Amidated C3 serves to activate the alternative complement pathway in the fluid phase, leads to C3 and C5b-9 deposition in the tissue, and elicits an inflammatory response and tissue injury.[249,280] The resulting intrarenal complement depletion may also contribute to the development of chronic bacterial pyelonephritis.[281]

Local ammonia production may also play a role in complement deposition in ischemic tissue. The mechanisms of ammonia formation in such tissues involves the release of adenosine from affected cells and its deamination to ammonia by the adenosine deaminase present in circulating erythrocytes.[282–283]

The use of C6-sufficient and -deficient rabbits and the infusion of C8-deficient serum into rats has clearly demonstrated that the development of proteinuria in membranous glomerulonephritis is dependent on the assembly and deposition of a complete MAC on the glomerular epithelial cells.[247,251] A substantial portion of this injury results from MAC-mediated stimulation of prostaglandin and thromboxane synthesis, since the proteinuria could be inhibited by treatment with indomethacin, an inhibitor of cyclo-oxygenase.[284]

Many patients with chronic renal disease ultimately require hemodialysis. Exposure of plasma to first-use filter membranes during dialysis results in complement activation.[285] Anaphylatoxins released during this process, for example, C5a, have been associated in a concentration-dependent and temporal fashion with the onset of respiratory distress in some dialysis patients.[265,285,286] This association is believed to relate in part to C5a-dependent neutrophil aggregation and stimulation and the formation of microemboli and their deposition in the lung (see Ch. 7).[265]

EVALUATION AND TREATMENT OF COMPLEMENT DISORDERS

Evaluation

Evaluation of the complement system is indicated when the diagnosis of a complement deficiency state is being considered or when specific measures of complement proteins are being used to assess disease activity or response to therapy. As pointed out earlier, several clinical clues should lead the clinician to suspect a complement deficiency state.[169,170] Foremost among these is a medical or family history of recurrent systemic infection caused by encapsulated bacteria, especially meningococci. A family history of fulminant meningococcal disease occurring in males in skipped generations should suggest the possibility of X-linked properdin deficiency. Meningococcal disease occurring in individuals over 10 years of age, especially when caused by non-group B meningococci, warrants evaluation of the complement system since 5–10 percent of these individuals will have a complement deficiency state, even in the absence of recurrent disease. Likewise, a history of SLE in family members or the occurrence of atypical features of SLE should also suggest the need to evaluate the complement system. Specific syndromes including partial lipodystrophy, angioedema, and PNH are other indications for the specific measurement of complement function or related activities.

Since any of a number of specific complement deficiencies can produce one of the typical clinical syndromes associated with these disorders, it is important to use a test that measures the function of the entire complement cascade during the initial evaluation of such patients. The most common of these tests is the CH_{50}, which measures the functions of the classical and terminal complement pathways. When defects in the alternative pathway are being considered, an analogous test evaluating al-

ternative-pathway function should be requested. Many hospital laboratories do not perform the latter test, so it may be necessary to contact a research or commercial laboratory with specific expertise in this area. A negative or extremely low result in either of these two assays warrants further diagnostic evaluation. The combined results of the tests of classical- and alternative-pathway functions should suggest which additional tests need to be performed. If both the classical- and alternative-pathway CH_{50} values are extremely low, the defect must lie in one of the components shared by both pathways, i.e., C3 through C9 (Fig. 1). If the alternative pathway is normal but the classical pathway is not, the deficient component must be C1, C2, or C4. Conversely, a normal classical but defective alternative pathway suggests a defect in factors D or B or in properdin. The diagnosis of these specific defects can frequently be accomplished by using immunochemical methods to demonstrate an absence of the relevant antigen. However, several complement deficiency states involve absent function in the presence of normal amounts of antigenic protein. Hence confirmation of the diagnosis of a specific component deficiency should be documented using specific functional assays for the protein under consideration and by demonstrating that replacement of the missing component restores both specific as well as total complement activity. Such assays usually require the expertise of a complement laboratory.

Treatment

There are two aspects of the treatment of complement deficiency states: replacement of the missing protein and prevention of infection. Although advances in our knowledge of the molecular basis for the various complement deficiency states may provide an alternative means of therapy in the future, replacement of a deficient component at the present time generally requires the infusion of fresh frozen plasma. This approach has been successfully employed in therapy for acute attacks of angioedema[72,220] in restoring C3 levels toward normal in individuals with C3 deficiency and in the successful treatment of a C2-deficient individual with SLE unresponsive to conventional therapy.[287] This approach suffers from several drawbacks. First, the half-life of most complement proteins in vivo is short,[15] although a notable exception occurs in patients with low C3 levels secondary to factor I deficiency. In these patients, replacement therapy restores factor I activity, thereby markedly reducing the accelerated breakdown of C3 that is observed in this disorder.[288] Second, replacement of a genetically absent protein may stimulate the production of antibody to the missing component, thereby limiting the value of subsequent therapy. This consideration is of limited concern in individuals with autosomally inherited disorders such as hereditary angioedema whose sera contain some normal protein or in individuals with other complement deficiency disorders characterized by the presence of antigenically normal amounts of a dysfunctional protein. Third, the relative infrequency of infection in most of these individuals must be balanced against the potential risk of acquiring a variety of blood-borne infections during plasma infusion, especially since alternative modes of therapy are available. Whether the acute infusion of fresh frozen plasma might be beneficial in the treatment of life-threatening infections,[289] especially in properdin-deficient patients, remains an untested possibility. The use of impeded androgens to enhance the in vivo biosynthesis of C1-INH provides a long-term alternative approach to the replacement of this protein.[72,220,290]

Prevention of infection in complement-deficient patients is best achieved through vaccination. All deficient individuals should be vaccinated with the tetravalent meningococcal vaccine. Individuals with classical pathway deficiencies should also receive the polyvalent pneumococcal and conjugated *H. influenzae* vaccines. Successful vaccination leads to the production of anticapsular antibodies that promote utilization of the classical pathway in individuals with an alternative-pathway defect and facilitate alternative-pathway utilization in individuals lacking one of the classical-pathway components.[51,187] In such individuals, these antibodies may promote bactericidal activity as well as microbial elimination by enhancing opsonophagocytosis. Although anticapsular antibody cannot enhance serum bactericidal activity in individuals with a deficiency of one of the terminal complement proteins, it promotes opsonization and killing of these organisms by phagocytic cells.[201] In view of experimental evidence indicating a suboptimal response to protein and polysaccharide antigens in C1-, C2-, C4-, and C3-deficient humans and animals, documentation of the patient's response to vaccination with these antigens seems prudent.

An alternative strategy for the prevention of meningococcal disease is the use of prophylactic antibiotics.[291] This approach significantly reduces the frequency of infection in C6-deficient individuals and has its greatest utility in populations in whom group B disease is highly prevalent.[292] It is unclear whether prophylaxis should be lifelong or whether the development of antibiotic resistance will limit the efficacy of this approach.

REFERENCES

 1. Ross GD. Introduction and history of complement research. In: Ross GD, ed. Immunobiology of the Complement System. Orlando, FL: Academic Press; 1986:1–20.
 2. Ratnoff WD. A war with the molecules: Louis Pillemer and the history of properdin. Perspect Biol Med. 1980;23:638–57.
 3. Lepow IH. Louis Pillemer, properdin, and scientific controversy. J Immunol. 1980;125:471–8.
 4. Root RK, Ryan JL. Humoral immunity and complement. In: Mandell GL, Douglas RG Jr, Bennett JE, eds. Principles and Practice of Infectious Diseases. 2nd ed. New York: Churchill Livingstone; 1985:31–56.
 5. Morris KM, Aden DP, Knowles BB, et al. Complement biosynthesis by the human hepatoma-derived cell line HepG2. J Clin Invest. 1982;70:906–13.
 6. Perlmutter DH, Colten HR. Molecular immunobiology of complement biosynthesis: A model of single-cell control of effector–inhibitor balance. Annu Rev Immunol. 1986;4:231–51.
 7. Alper CA, Raum D, Awdeh ZL, et al. Studies of hepatic synthesis in vivo of plasma proteins, including orosomucoid, transferrin, α_1-antitrypsin, C8, and factor B. Clin Immunol Immunopathol. 1980;16:84–9.
 8. Mier JW, Dinarello CA, Atkins MB, et al. Regulation of hepatic acute phase protein synthesis by products of interleukin 2 (IL-2)-stimulated human peripheral blood mononuclear cells. J Immunol. 1987;139:1268–72.
 9. Baumann H, Richards C, Gauldie J. Interaction among hepatocyte-stimulating factors, interleukin 1, and glucocorticoids for regulation of acute phase plasma proteins in human hepatoma (HepG2) cells. J Immunol. 1987;139:4122–8.
10. Beatty DW, Davis AE III, Cole FS, et al. Biosynthesis of complement by human monocytes. Clin Immunol Immunopathol. 1981;18:334–43.
11. Cole FS, Auerbach HS, Goldberger G, et al. Tissue-specific pretranslational regulation of complement production in human mononuclear phagocytes. J Immunol. 1985;134:2610–6.
12. Strunk RC, Cole FS, Perlmutter DH, et al. γ-Interferon increases expression of class III complement genes C2 and factor B in human monocytes and in murine fibroblasts transfected with human C2 and factor B genes. J Biol Chem. 1985;260:15280–5.
13. Strunk RC, Whitehead AS, Cole FS. Pretranslational regulation of the synthesis of the third component of complement in human mononuclear phagocytes by the lipid A portion of lipopolysaccharide. J Clin Invest. 1985;76:985–90.
14. Hetland G, Eskeland T. Formation of the functional alternative pathway of complement by human monocytes in vitro as demonstrated by phagocytosis of agarose beads. Scand J Immunol. 1986;23:301–8.
15. Ruddy S, Carpenter CB, Chin KW, et al. Human complement metabolism: An analysis of 144 studies. Medicine (Baltimore). 1975;54:165–78.
16. Notarangelo LD, Chirico G, Chiara A, et al. Activity of classical and alternative pathways of complement in preterm and small for gestational age infants. Pediatr Res. 1984;18:281–5.
17. Johnston RB Jr, Altenburger KM, Atkinson AW Jr, et al. Complement in the newborn infant. Pediatrics. 1979;64(Pt 2, Suppl):781–6.
18. Mills EL, Björksten B, Quie PG. Deficient alternative complement pathway activity in newborn sera. Pediatr Res. 1979;13:1341–4.
19. Edwards MS, Buffone GJ, Fuselier PA, et al. Deficient classical complement pathway activity in newborn sera. Pediatr Res. 1983;17:685–8.
20. Lachmann PJ, Hughes-Jones NC. Initiation of complement activation. Springer Semin Immunopathol. 1984;7:143–62.
21. Muraoka S, Shulman MJ. Structural requirements for IgM assembly and cytolytic activity. Effects of mutations in the oligosaccharide acceptor site at Asn402. J Immunol. 1989;142:695–701.
22. Wright JF, Shulman MJ, Isenman DE, et al. C1 binding by mouse IgM. The

23. Tao M-H, Canfield SM, Morrison SL. The differential ability of human IgG1 and IgG4 to activate complement is determined by the COOH-terminal sequence of the C_H2 domain. J Exp Med. 1991;173:1025–8.
24. Cooper NR. The classical complement pathway: Activation and regulation of the first complement component. Adv Immunol. 1985;37:151–216.
25. Malhotra R, Sim RB, Reid KBM. Interaction of C1q, and other proteins containing collagen-like domains, with the C1q receptor. Biochem Soc Trans. 1990;18:1145–8.
26. Acton S, Resnick D, Freeman M, et al. The collagenous domains of macrophage scavenger receptors and complement component C1q mediate their similar, but not identical, binding specificities for polyanionic ligands. J Biol Chem. 1993;268:3530–7.
27. Tenner AJ, Robinson SL, Borchelt J, et al. Human pulmonary surfactant protein (SP-A), a protein structurally homologous to C1q, can enhance FcR- and CR1-mediated phagocytosis. J Biol Chem. 1989;264:13923–8.
28. Schweinie JE, Ezekowitz RAB, Tenner AJ, et al. Human mannose-binding protein activates the alternative complement pathway and enhances serum bactericidal activity on a mannose-rich isolate of Salmonella. J Clin Invest. 1989;84:1821–9.
29. Lu J, Thiel S, Wiedemann H, et al. Binding of the pentamer/hexamer forms of mannan-binding protein to zymosan activates the proenzyme $C1r_2C1s_2$ complex, of the classical pathway of complement, without involvement of C1q. J Immunol. 1990;144:2287–94.
30. Matsushita M, Fujita T. Activation of the classical complement pathway by mannose-binding protein in association with a novel C1s-like serine protease. J Exp Med. 1992;176:1497–502.
31. Arlaud GJ, Colomb MG, Gagnon J. A functional model of the human C1 complex. Immunol Today. 1987;8:106–11.
32. Schumaker VN, Zavodszky P, Poon RH. Activation of the first component of complement. Annu Rev Immunol. 1987;5:21–42.
33. Fearon DT. Complement. J Allergy Clin Immunol. 1983;71:520–9.
34. Müller-Eberhard HJ. Molecular organization and function of the complement system. Annu Rev Biochem. 1988;57:321–47.
35. Gordon DL, Hostetter MK. Complement and host defense against microorganisms. Pathology. 1986;18:365–75.
36. Isenman DE, Young JR. The molecular basis for the difference in immune hemolysis activity of the Chido and Rodgers isotypes of human complement component C4. J Immunol. 1984;132:3019–27.
37. Law SKA, Dodds AW, Porter RR. A comparison of the properties of two classes, C4A and C4B, of the human complement component C4. EMBO J. 1984;3:1819–23.
38. Dodds AW, Law SK, Porter RR. The origin of the very variable haemolytic activities of the common human complement component C4 allotypes including C4-A6. EMBO J. 1985;4:2239–44.
39. Schifferli JA, Steiger G, Paccaud J-P, et al. Difference in the biological properties of the two forms of the fourth component of human complement (C4). Clin Exp Immunol. 1986;63:473–7.
40. Schifferli JA, Hauptmann G, Paccaud J-P. Complement-mediated adherence of immune complexes to human erythrocytes. FEBS Lett. 1987;213:415–8.
41. Naama JK, Niven IP, Zoma A, et al. Complement, antigen–antibody complexes and immune complex disease. J Clin Lab Immunol. 1985;17:59–67.
42. Pangburn MK, Müller-Eberhard HJ. The alternative pathway of complement. Springer Semin Immunopathol. 1984;7:163–92.
43. Pangburn MK. The alternative pathway. In: Ross GD, ed. Immunobiology of the Complement System. Orlando, FL: Academic Press; 1986:45–62.
44. Densen P, McRill C, Ross SC. The contribution of the alternative and classical complement pathways to gonococcal killing and C3 fixation. In: Poolman JT, Zanen HC, Meyer TF, et al, eds. Gonococci and Meningococci. Dordrecht: Kluwer Academic Publishers; 1988:693–7.
45. Fearon DT, Austen KF. Properdin: Initiation of alternative complement pathway. Immunology. 1975;72:3220–4.
46. Fearon DT, Austen KF. Properdin: Binding to C3b and stabilization of the C3b-dependent C3 convertase. J Exp Med. 1975;142:856–63.
47. Fearon DT, Austen KF. The alternative pathway of complement—a system for host resistance to microbial infection. N Engl J Med. 1980;303:259–63.
48. Hunsicker LG, Ruddy S, Austen KF. Alternate complement pathway: Factors involved in cobra venom factor (CoVF) activation of the third component of complement (C3). J Immunol. 1973;110:128–38.
49. Müller-Eberhard HJ, Schreiber RD. Molecular biology and chemistry of the alternative pathway of complement. Adv Immunol. 1980;29:1–53.
50. Vogel C-W, Smith CA, Müller-Eberhard HJ. Cobra venom factor: Structural homology with the third component of human complement. J Immunol. 1984;133:3235–41.
51. Söderström C, Braconier JH, Danielsson D, et al. Bactericidal activity for Neisseria meningitidis in properdin-deficient sera. J Infect Dis. 1987;156:107–12.
52. Schenkein HA, Ruddy S. The role of immunoglobulins in alternative complement pathway activation by zymosan. II. the effect of IgG on the kinetics of the alternative pathway. J Immunol. 1981;126:11–5.
53. Ratnoff WD, Fearon DT, Austen KF. The role of antibody in the activation of the alternative complement pathway. Springer Semin Immunopathol. 1983;6:361–71.
54. Winkelstein JA, Shin HS. The role of immunoglobulin in the interaction of pneumococci and the properdin pathway: Evidence for its specificity and

lack of requirement for the Fc portion of the molecule. J Immunol. 1974; 112:1635–42.

55. Nelson B, Ruddy S. Enhancing role of IgG in lysis of rabbit erythrocytes by the alternative pathway of human complement. J Immunol. 1979;122: 1994–9.

56. Schenkein HA, Ruddy S. The role of immunoglobulins in alternative complement pathway activation by zymosan. I. Human IgG with specificity for zymosan enhances alternative pathway activation by zymosan. J Immunol. 1981;126:7–10.

57. Nicholson-Weller A, Daha MR, Austen KF. Different functions for specific guinea pig IgG1 and IgG2 in the lysis of sheep erythrocytes by C4-deficient guinea pig serum. J Immunol. 1981;126:1800–4.

58. Capel PJA, Groeneboer O, Grosveld G, et al. The binding of activated C3 to polysaccharides and immunoglobulins. J Immunol. 1978;121:2566–72.

59. Fries LF, Gaither TA, Hammer CH, et al. C3b covalently bound to IgG demonstrates a reduced rate of inactivation by factors H and I. J Exp Med. 1984;160:1640–55.

60. Joiner KA, Fries LF, Schmetz MA, et al. IgG bearing covalently bound C3b has enhanced bactericidal activity for *Escherichia coli* 0111. J Exp Med. 1985;162:877–89.

61. Lambris JD, Müller-Eberhard HJ. The multifunctional role of C3: Structural analysis of its interactions with physiological ligands. Mol Immunol. 1986; 23:1237–42.

62. Wetsel RA, Lemons RS, Le Beau MM, et al. Molecular analysis of human complement component C5: Localization of the structural gene to chromosome 9. Biochemistry. 1988;27:1474–82.

63. Lundwall AB, Wetsel RA, Kristenson T, et al. Isolation and sequence analysis of a cDNA clone encoding the fifth complement component. J Biol Chem. 1985;260:2108–12.

64. Müller-Eberhard HJ. The membrane attack complex of complement. Annu Rev Immunol. 1986;4:503–28.

65. Stanley K, Luzio P. A family of killer proteins. Nature. 1988;334:475–6.

66. Tschopp J, Mollnes T-E. Antigenic crossreactivity of the α subunit of complement component C8 with the cysteine-rich domain shared by complement component C9 and low density lipoprotein receptor. Proc Natl Acad Sci USA. 1986;83:4223–7.

67. Haefliger J-A, Tschopp J, Nardelli D, et al. Complementary DNA cloning of complement C8β and its sequence homology to C9. Biochemistry. 1987; 26:3551–6.

68. Monahan JB, Sodetz JM. Binding of the eighth component of human complement to the soluble cytolytic complex is mediated by its β subunit. J Biol Chem. 1980;255:10579–82.

69. Stewart JL, Kolb WP, Sodetz JM. Evidence that C5b recognizes and mediates C8 incorporation into the cytolytic complex of complement. J Immunol. 1987;139:1960–4.

70. Stewart JL, Sodetz JM. Analysis of the specific association of the eighth and ninth components of human complement: identification of a direct role for the α subunit of C8. Biochemistry 1985;24:4598–602.

71. Stanley KK, Page M, Campbell AK, et al. A mechanism for the insertion of complement component C9 into target membranes. Mol Immunol. 1986; 23:451–8.

72. Davis AE III. C1 inhibitor and hereditary angioneurotic edema. Annu Rev Immunol 1988;6:595–628.

73. Holers VM, Cole JL, Lublin DM, et al. Human C3b- and C4b-regulatory proteins: A new multi-gene family. Immunol Today. 1985;6:188–92.

74. Atkinson JP, Farries T. Separation of self from non-self in the complement system. Immunol Today. 1987;8:212–5.

75. Nicholson-Weller A, Burge J, Fearon DT, et al. Isolation of a human erythrocyte membrane glycoprotein with decay-accelerating activity for C3 convertases of the complement system. J Immunol. 1982;129:184–9.

76. Bhakdi S, Maillet F, Muhly M, et al. The cytolytic C5b-9 complement complex: Feedback inhibition of complement activation. Proc Natl Acad Sci USA. 1988;85:1912–6.

77. Densen P, McRill CM, Ross SC. Assembly of the membrane attack complex promotes decay of the alternative pathway C3 convertase on *Neisseria gonorrhoeae*. J. Immunol. 1988;141:3902–9.

78. Tschopp J, Masson D, Schafer S, et al. The heparin binding domain of S-protein/vitronectin binds to complement components C7, C8, and C9 and perforin from cytolytic T-cells and inhibits their lytic activities. Biochemistry. 1988;27:4103–9.

79. Fritz IB, Murphy B. Clusterin. Insights into a multifunctional protein. TEM. 1993;4:41–5.

80. Shin ML, Hänsch G, Hu VW, et al. Membrane factors responsible for homologous species restriction of complement-mediated lysis: Evidence for a factor other than DAF operating at the stage of C8 and C9. J Immunol. 1986; 136:1777–82.

81. Rollins SA, Zhao J, Ninomiya H, et al. Inhibition of homologous complement by CD59 is mediated by a species-selective recognition conferred through binding to C8 within C5b-8 or C9 within C5b-9. J Immunol. 1991;146:2345–51.

82. Carney DF, Koski CL, Shin ML. Elimination of terminal complement intermediates from the plasma membrane of nucleated cells: The rate of disappearance differs for cells carying C5b-7 or C5b-8 or a mixture of C5b-8 with a limited number of C5b-9. J Immunol 1985;134:1804–9.

83. Ramm LE, Whitlow MB, Koski CL, et al. Elimination of complement channels from the plasma membranes of U937, a nucleated mammalian cell line: Temperature dependence of the elimination rate. J Immunol. 1983;131: 1411–5.

84. Schlager SI, Ohanian SH, Borsos T. Correlations between the ability of tumor cells to resist humoral immune attack and their ability to synthesize lipid. J Immunol. 1978;120:463–71.

85. Campbell AK, Luzio JP. Intracellular free calcium as a pathogen in cell damage initiated by the immune system. Experientia. 1981;37:1110–2.

86. Imagawa DK, Osifchin NE, Paznekas WA, et al. Consequences of cell membrane attack by complement: Release of arachidonate and formation of inflammatory derivatives. Proc Natl Acad Sci USA. 1983;80:6647–51.

87. Betz M, Hansch GM. Release of arachidonic acid: A new function of the late complement components. Immunobiology. 1984;166:473–83.

88. Hänsch GM, Seitz M, Martinotti G, et al. Macrophages release arachidonic acid, prostaglandin E₂, and thromboxane in response to late complement components. J Immunol. 1984;133:2145–50.

89. Suttorp N, Seeger W, Zinsky S, et al. Complement complex C5b-8 induces PGI₂ formation in cultured endothelial cells. Am J Physiol. 1987;253:13–32.

90. Carney DF, Lang TJ, Shin ML. Multiple signal messengers generated by terminal complement complexes and their role in terminal complement complex elimination. J Immunol. 1990;145:623–9.

91. Halperin JA, Taratuska A, Nicholson-Weller A. Terminal complement complex C5b-9 stimulates mitogenesis in 3T3 cells. J Clin Invest. 1993;91:1974–8.

92. Fearon DT, Austen KF. Activation of the alternative complement pathway with rabbit erythrocytes by circumvention of the regulatory action of endogenous control proteins. J Exp Med. 1977;146:22–33.

93. Fearon DT. Regulation by membrane sialic acid of β1H-dependent decay-dissociation of amplification C3 convertase of the alternative complement pathway. Proc Natl Acad Sci USA. 1978;75:1971–5.

94. Kazatchkine MD, Fearon DT, Austen KF. Human alternative complement pathway: Membrane-associated sialic acid regulates the competition between B and β1H for cell-bound C3b. J Immunol. 1979;122:75–81.

95. Pangburn MK, Morrison DC, Schreiber RD, et al. Activation of the alternative complement pathway: Recognition of surface structures on activators by bound C3b. J Immunol. 1980;124:977–82.

96. Ross GD, Medof ME. Membrane complement receptors specific for bound fragments of C3. Adv Immunol. 1985;37:217–67.

97. Wilson JG, Andriopoulos NA, Fearon DT. CR1 and the cell membrane proteins that bind C3 and C4. A basic and clinical review. Immunol Res. 1987; 6:192–209.

98. Jack RM, Ezzell RM, Hartwig J, et al. Differential interaction of the C3b/C4b receptor and MHC class I with the cytoskeleton of human neutrophils. J Immunol. 1986;137:3996–4003.

99. Moulds JM, Nickells MW, Moulds JJ, et al. The C3b/C4b receptor is recognized by the Knops, McCoy, Swain-Langley, and York blood group antisera. J Exp Med. 1991;173:1159–63.

100. Krych M, Hourcade D, Atkinson JP. Sites within the complement C3b/C4b receptor important for the specificity of ligand binding. Proc Natl Acad Sci USA. 1991;88:4353–7.

101. Hynes RO. Integrins: A family of cell surface receptors. Cell. 1987;48: 549–54.

102. Wright SD, Levin SM, Jong MTC, et al. CR3 (CD11b/CD18) expresses one binding site for arg-gly-asp-containing peptides and a second site for bacterial lipopolysaccharide. J Exp Med. 1989;169:175–83.

103. Wright SD, Reddy A, Jong MTC, et al. C3bi receptor (complement receptor type 3) recognizes a region of complement protein C3 containing the sequence arg-gly-asp. Proc Natl Acad Sci USA. 1987;84:1965–8.

104. Ruoslahti E, Pierschbacher MD. Arg-gly-asp: A versatile cell recognition signal. Cell. 1986;44:517–8.

105. Myones BL, Dalzell JG, Hogg N, et al. Neutrophil and monocyte cell surface p150,95 has iC3b-receptor (CR4) activity resembling CR3. J Clin Invest. 1988; 81:64–51.

106. Matsumoto AK, Kopicky-Burd J, Carter RH, et al. Intersection of the complement and immune systems: A signal transduction complex of the B lymphocyte–containing complement receptor type 2 and CD19. J Exp Med. 1991; 173:55–64.

107. Hugli TE. Biological activities of fragments derived from human complement components. Prog Immunol. 1983:419–26.

108. Perlmutter DH, Colten HR. Complement molecular genetics. In: Gallin JI, Goldstein IM, Snyderman R, eds. Inflammation: Basic Principles and Clinical Correlates. New York: Raven Press; 1988:75–88.

109. Campbell RD. The molecular genetics and polymorphism of C2 and factor B. Br Med Bull. 1987;43:37–49.

110. Campbell RD, Law SKA, Reid KBM, et al. Structure, organization, and regulation of the complement genes. Annu Rev Immunol. 1988;6:161–95.

111. Awdeh ZL, Raum D, Yunis EJ, et al. Extended HLA/complement allele haplotypes: Evidence for T/t-like complex in man. Proc Natl Acad Sci USA. 1983;80:259–63.

112. Alper CA, Raum D, Karp S, et al. Serum complement "supergenes" of the major histocompatibility complex in man (complotypes). Vox Sang. 1983; 45:62–7.

113. Porter RR. Complement polymorphism, the major histocompatibility complex and associated diseases: A speculation. Mol Biol Med. 1983;1:161–8.

114. Kristensen T, D'Eustachio P, Ogata RT, et al. The superfamily of C3b/C4b-binding proteins. Fed Proc. 1987;46:2463–9.

115. Reid KBM, Bentley DR, Campbell RD, et al. Complement system proteins which interact with C3b or C4b. A superfamily of structurally related proteins. Immunol Today. 1986;7:230–4.

116. Perez HD, Kelly E, Chenoweth D, et al. Identification of the C5a des arg

cochemotaxin. Homology with vitamin D–binding protein (group-specific component globulin). J Clin Invest. 1988;82:360–3.

117. Kew RR, Webster RO. Ge-globulin (vitamin D–binding protein) enhances the neutrophil chemotactic activity of C5a and C5a des arg. J Clin Invest. 1988;82:364–9.

118. Perez HD, Hooper C, Volanakis J, et al. Specific inhibitor of complement (C5)-derived chemotactic activity in systemic lupus erythematosus related antigenically to the Bb fragment of human factor B. J Immunol. 1987;139: 484–9.

119. Miller GW, Nusenzweig V. A new complement function: Solubilization of antigen–antibody aggregates. Proc Natl Acad Sci USA. 1975;72:418–22.

120. Schifferli JA, Ng YC, Peters DK. The role of complement and its receptor in the elimination of immune complexes. N Engl J Med 1986;315:488–95.

121. Siegel I, Liu TL, Gleicher N. The red-cell immune system. Lancet. 1981;2: 556–9.

122. Cornacoff JB, Hebert LA, Smead WL, et al. Primate erythrocyte-immune complex-clearing mechanism. J Clin Invest. 1983;71:236–47.

123. Erdei A, Fust G, Gergely J. The role of C3 in the immune response. Immunol Today. 1991;12:332–7.

124. Bird P, Lachmann PJ. The regulation of IgG subclass production in man: Low serum IgG4 in inherited deficiencies of the classical pathway of C3 activation. J Immunol. 1988;18:1217–22.

125. Papamichail M, Gutierrez C, Embling P, et al. Complement dependence of localisation of aggregated IgG in germinal centres. Scand J Immunol. 1975; 4:343–7.

126. Ochs HD, Wedgwood RJ, Frank MM, et al. The role of complement in the induction of antibody responses. Clin Exp Immunol. 1983;53:208–16.

127. Böttger EC, Bitter-Suermann D. Complement and the regulation of humoral immune responses. Immunol Today. 1987;8:261–4.

128. Ochs HD, Wedgwood RJ, Heller SR, et al. Complement, membrane glyco-proteins, and complement receptors: Their role in regulation of the immune response. Clin Immunol Immunopathol. 1986;40:94–104.

129. Hostetter MK. Serotypic variations among virulent pneumococci in deposi-tion and degradation of covalently bound C3b: Implications for phagocytosis and antibody production. J Infect Dis. 1986;153:682–93.

130. Hostetter MK, Krueger RA, Schmeling DJ. The biochemistry of opsoniza-tion: Central role of the reactive thiolester of the third component of comple-ment. J Infect Dis. 1984;150:653–61.

131. Taylor PW. Bactericidal and bacteriolytic activity of serum against gram-negative bacteria. Microbiol Rev. 1983;47:46–83.

132. Harriman GR, Esser AF, Podack ER, et al. The role of C9 in complement-mediated killing of Neisseria. J Immunol. 1981;127:2386–90.

133. Cooper NR, Nemerow GR. Complement-dependent mechanisms of virus neutralization. In: Ross GD, ed. Immunobiology of the Complement System. Orlando, FL: Academic Press; 1986:139–62.

134. Joiner K. Comlement evasion by bacteria and parasites. Annu Rev Micro-biol. 1988;42:201–30.

135. Cooper NR. Complement evasion strategies of microorganisms. Immunol Today. 1991;12:327–32.

136. Leive LL, Jimenez-Lucho VE. Lipopolysaccharide O-antigen structure con-trols alternative pathway activation of complement: Effects on phagocytosis and virulence of Salmonella. In: Leive L, ed. Microbiology. Washington, DC: American Society for Microbiology; 1986:14–7.

137. Liang-Takasaki C-J, Mäkelä PH, Leive L. Phagocytosis of bacteria by macrophages: Changing the carbohydrate of lipopolysaccharide alters inter-action with complement and macrophages. J Immunol. 1982;128:1229–35.

138. Liang-Takasaki C-J, Saxén H, Mäkelä PH, et al. Complement activation by polysaccharide of lipopolysaccharide: An important virulence determinant of Salmonella. Infect Immun. 1983;41:563–9.

139. Grossman N, Leive L. Complement activation via the alternative pathway by purified Salmonella lipopolysaccharide is affected by its structure but not its O-antigen length. J Immunol. 1984;132:376–85.

140. Grossman N, Joiner KA, Frank MM, et al. C3b binding, but not its break-down, is affected by the structure of the O-antigen polysaccharide in lipopoly-saccharide from Salmonella. J Immunol. 1986;136:2208–15.

141. Jimenez-Lucho VE, Joiner KA, Foulds J, et al. C3b generation is affected by the structure of the O-antigen polysaccharide in lipopolysaccharide from Salmonella. J Immunol. 1987;139:1253–9.

142. Brown EJ. Interaction of gram-positive microorganisms with complement. Curr Top Microbiol Immunol. 1985;121:159–97.

143. Hall BF, Joiner KA. Developmentally regulated virulence factors of Trypa-nosoma cruzi and their relationship to evasion of host defences. J Euk Micro-biol. 1993;40:207–13.

144. Kotwal GJ, Moss B. Vaccinia virus encodes a secretory polypeptide structur-ally related to complement control proteins. Nature. 1988;335:176–8.

145. Kotwal GJ, Isaacs SN, McKenzie R, et al. Inhibition of the complement cascade by the major secretory protein of vaccinia virus. Science. 1990;250: 827–30.

146. Smith H, Cole JA, Parsons NJ. The sialylation of gonococcal lipopolysaccha-ride by host factors: A major impact on pathogenicity. FEMS Microbiol Lett 1992;100:287–92.

147. Roantree RJ, Rantz LA. A study of the relationship of the normal bactericidal activity of human serum to bacterial infection. J Clin Invest. 1960;39:72–81.

148. Joiner KA, Grossman N, Schmetz M, et al. C3 binds preferentially to long-chain lipopolysaccharide during alternative pathway activation by Salmo-nella montevideo. J Immunol. 1986;136:710–5.

149. Schoolnik GK, Buchman TM, Holmes KK. Gonococci causing disseminated

150. Joiner KA, Warren KA, Brown EJ, et al. Studies on the mechanism of bacte-rial resistance to complement-mediated killing. IV. C4b-9 forms high molecu-lar weight complexes with bacterial outer membrane constituents on serum-resistant but not on serum-sensitve Neisseria gonorrhoeae. J Immunol. 1983; 131:1443–51.

151. Harriman GR, Podack ER, Braude AI, et al. Activation of complement by serum-resistant Neisseria gonorrhoeae. J Exp Med. 1982;156:1235–49.

152. Rice PA, Kasper DL. Characterization of gonococcal antigens responsible for induction of bactericidal antibody in disseminated infection. J Clin Invest. 1977;60:1149–58.

153. Densen P, Gulati S, Rice PA. Specificity of antibodies against Neisseria gonorrhoeae that stimulate neutrophil chemotaxis. Role of antibodies di-rected against lipooligosaccharides. J Clin Invest. 1987;80:78–87.

154. Rice PA, Kasper KL. Characterization of serum resistance of Neisseria gonorrhoeae that disseminate. Roles of blocking antibody and gonococcal outer membrane proteins. J Clin Invest. 1982;70:157–67.

155. Rice PA, Vayo HE, Tam MR, et al. Immunoglobulin G antibodies directed against protein III block killing of serum-resistant Neisseria gonorrhoeae by immune serum. J Exp Med. 1986;164:1735–48.

156. Joiner KA, Scales R, Warren KA, et al. Mechanism of action of blocking immunoglobulin G for Neisseria gonorrhoeae. J Clin Invest. 1985;76: 1765–72.

157. Griffiss MJ, Bertram MA. Immunoepidemiology of meningococcal disease in military recruits. II. Blocking of serum bactericidal activity by circulating IgA early in the course of invasive disease. J Infect Dis. 1977;136:733–9.

158. Griffiss JM. Epidemic meningococcal disease: Synthesis of a hypothetical immunoepidemiologic model. Rev Infect Dis. 1982;4:159–72.

159. Frank MM, Joiner K, Hammer C. The function of antibody and complement in the lysis of bacteria. Rev Infect Dis. 1987;9(Suppl 5):537–45.

160. Braga LL, Ninomiya H, McCoy JJ, et al. Inhibition of the complement mem-brane attack complex by the galactose-specific adhesin of Entamoeba histo-lytica. J Clin Invest 1992;90:1131–7.

161. Heffernan EJ, Reed S, Hackett J, et al. Mechanism of resistance to comple-ment-mediated killing of bacteria encoded by the Salmonella typhimurium virulence plasmid gene rck. J Clin Invest. 1992;90:953–64.

162. Bliska JB, Falkow S. Bacterial resistance to complement killing mediated by the Ail protein of Yersinia enterocolitica. Proc Natl Acad Sci USA. 1992; 89:3561–5.

163. Cooper NR, Moore MD, Nemerow GR. Immunobiology of CR2, the B lym-phocyte receptor for Epstein-Barr virus and the C3d complement fragment. Annu Rev Immunol. 1988;6:85–113.

164. Fingeroth JD, Weis JJ, Tedder TF, et al. Epstein-Barr virus receptor of human B lymphocytes is the C3d receptor CR2. Proc Natl Acad Sci USA. 1984;81:4510–4.

165. Montefiori DC, Stewart K, Ahearn JM, et al. Complement-mediated binding of naturally glycosylated and glycosylation-modified human immunodefi-ciency virus type 1 to human CR2 (CD21). J Virol. 1993;67:2699–2706.

166. Edwards JE Jr, Gaither TA, O'Shea JJ, et al. Expression of specific binding sites on candida with functional and antigenic characteristics of human com-plement receptors. J Immunol. 1986;137:3577–83.

167. Gilmore BJ, Retsinas EM, Lorenz JS, et al. An iC3b receptor on Candida albicans: Structure, function, and correlates for pathogenicity. J Infect Dis. 1988;157:38–46.

168. Gustafson KS, Vercellotti GM, Bendel CM, et al. Molecular mimicry in Candida albicans. Role of an integrin analogue in adhesin of the yeast to human endothelium. J Clin Invest. 1991;87:1896–1902.

169. Ross SC, Densen P. Complement deficiency states and infection: Epidemiol-ogy, pathogenesis and consequences of neisserial and other infections in an immune deficiency. Medicine (Baltimore). 1984;63:243–73.

170. Figueroa JE, Densen P. Infectious diseases associated with complement defi-ciencies. Clin Microbiol Rev. 1991;4:359–95.

171. Densen P. Human complement deficiency states and infection. In: Whaley K, Loos M, Weiler JM, editors. Complement in Health and Diseae. Dor-drecht, The Netherlands: Kluwer Academic Publishers; 1993:173–97.

172. Glass D, Raum D, Gibson D, et al. Inherited deficiency of the second compo-nent of complement. J Clin Invest. 1976;58:853–61.

173. Agnello V. Complement deficiency states. Medicine (Baltimore). 1978;57: 1–23.

174. Agnello V. Lupus diseases associated with hereditary and acquired deficien-cies of complement. Springer Semin Immunopathol. 1986;9:161–78.

175. Provost TT, Arnett FC, Reichlin M. Homozygous C2 deficiency, lupus ery-thematosus, and anti-Ro (SSA) antibodies. Arthritis Rheum. 1983;26: 1279–82.

176. Davis AE III. The efficiency of complement activation in MHC-linked dis-eases. Immunol Today. 1983;4:250–2.

177. Schifferli JA, Peters DK. Complement, the immune-complex lattice, and the pathophysiology of complement-deficiency syndromes. Lancet. 1983;2: 957–9.

178. Schifferli JA, Steiger G, Hauptmann G, et al. Formation of soluble immune complexes by complement in sera of patients with various hypocomplemen-temic states. J Clin Invest. 1985;76:2127–33.

179. Böttger EC, Hoffmann T, Hadding U, et al. Guinea pigs with inherited defi-ciencies of complement components C2 or C4 have characteristics of immune complex disease. J Clin Invest. 1986;78:689–95.

180. Awdeh ZL, Raum DD, Glass D, et al. Complement-human histocompatibility antigen haplotypes in C2 deficiency. J Clin Invest. 1981;67:581–3.
181. Kemp ME, Atkinson JP, Skanes VM, et al. Deletion of C4A genes in patients with systemic lupus erythematosus. Arthritis Rheum. 1987;30:1015–22.
182. Johnson C, Densen P, Cole FS, et al. Molecular heterogeneity of human C2 deficiency. N Engl J Med. 1992;326:871–4.
183. Johnson CA, Densen P, Hurford R, et al. Type I human complement C2 deficiency: A 28-base pair gene deletion causes skipping of exon 6 during RNA splicing. J Biol Chem. 1992;267:9347–53.
184. Hauptmann G, Goetz J, Uring-Lambert B, et al. Component deficiencies. 2. The fourth component. Progr Allergy. 1986;39:1232–49.
185. Howard PF, Hochberg MC, Bias WB, et al. Relationship between C4 null genes, HLA-D region antigens, and genetic susceptibility to systemic lupus erythematosus in Caucasian and Black Americans. Am J Med. 1986;81:187–93.
186. Sjöholm AG, Braconier J-H, Söderström C. Properdin deficiency in a family with fulminant meningococcal infections. Clin Exp Immunol. 1982;50:291–7.
187. Densen P, Weiler JM, Griffiss JM, et al. Familial properdin deficiency and fatal meningococcemia. Correction of the bactericidal defect by vaccination. N Engl J Med. 1987;316:922–6.
188. Sjöholm AG, Söderström C, Nilsson L-A. A second variant of properdin deficiency: The detection of properdin at low concentration in affected males. Complement. 1988;5:130–40.
189. Sjöholm AG, Kuijper EJ, Tijssen CC, et al. Dysfunctional properdin in a Dutch family with meningococcal disease. N Engl J Med. 1988;319:33–7.
190. Botto M, Fong KY, So AK, et al. Homozygous hereditary C3 deficiency due to a partial gene deletion. Proc Natl Acad Sci USA. 1992;89:4957–61.
191. Botto M, Fong KY, So AE, et al. Molecular basis of hereditary C3 deficiency. J Clin Invest. 1990;86:1158–63.
192. Sissons JGP, West RJ, Fallow J, et al. The complement abnormalities of lipodystrophy. N Engl J Med. 1976;294:461–5.
193. Ipp MM, Minta JO, Gelfand EW. Disorders of the complement system in lipodystrophy. Clin Immunol Immunopathol. 1977;7:281–7.
194. Rosen BS, Cook KS, Yaglom J, et al. Adipsin and complement factor D activity: An immune-related defect in obesity. Science. 1989;244:1483–7.
195. White RT, Damm D, Hancock N, et al. Human adipsin is identical to complement factor D and is expressed at high levels in adipose tissue. J Biol Chem. 1992;267:9210–3.
196. Choy LN, Rosen BS, Spiegelman BM. Adipsin and an endogenous pathway of complement from adipose cells. J Biol Chem. 1992;267:12736–41.
197. Mathieson PW, Wurzner R, Oliveira DBG, et al. Complement-mediated adipocyte lysis by nephritic factor sera. J Exp Med. 1993;177:1827–31.
198. Nagata M, Hara T, Aoki T, et al. Inherited deficiency of ninth component of complement: An increased risk of meningococcal meningitis. J Pediatr. 1989;114:260–4.
199. Kaufmann T, Hänsch G, Rittner C, et al. Genetic basis of human complement C8β deficiency. J Immunol. 1993;150:4943–7.
200. Fijen CA, Kuijper EJ, Hannema AJ, et al. Complement deficiencies in patients over ten years old with meningococcal disease due to uncommon serogroups. Lancet. 1989;2:585–8.
201. Ross SC, Rosenthal PJ, Berberich HM, et al. Killing of Neisseria meningitidis by human neutrophils: Implications for normal and complement-deficient individuals. J Infect Dis. 1987;155:1266–75.
202. Anonymous. Analysis of endemic meningococcal disease by serogroup and evaluation of chemoprophylaxis. J Infect Dis. 1976;134:201–4.
203. Ross SC, Berberich HM, Densen P. Natural serum bactericidal activity against Neisseria meningitidis isolates from disseminated infections in normal and complement-deficient hosts. J Infect Dis. 1985;152:1332–5.
204. Beloborodov VB, Platonov AE. Meningococcal disease in the USSR in patients with deficiencies in late complement components. In: Achtman M, Kohl P, Marchal C, et al. Neisseriae 1990. Berlin: Walter de Gruyter; 1991:659–63.
205. Platonov AE, Beloborodov VB. Vershinina IV. Meningococcal disease in patients with late complement deficiency: Studies in the U.S.S.R. Medicine. 1993;72:374–92.
206. Andreoni J, Käyhty H, Densen P. Vaccination and the role of capsular polysaccharide antibody in prevention of recurrent meningococcal disease in late complement component-deficient individuals. J Infect Dis. 1993;168:227–31.
207. Brandtzaeg P, Mollnes TE, Kierulf P. Complement activation and endotoxin levels in systemic meningococcal disease. J Infect Dis. 1989;160:58–65.
208. Brown DL, Lachmann PJ. The behaviour of complement and platelets in lethal endotoxin shock in rabbits. Int Arch Allergy. 1973;45:193–205.
209. Zwahlen A, Waldvogel FA. Magnitude of bacteremia and complement activation during Neisseria meningitidis infection. Study of two co-primary cases with different clinical presentations. Eur J Clin Microbiol. 1984;3:439–41.
210. Sullivan TD, LaScolea LJ Jr. Neisseria meningitidis bacteremia in children: Quantitation of bacteremia and spontaneous clinical recovery without antibiotic therapy. Pediatrics. 1987;80:63–7.
211. Brandtzaeg P, Kierulf P, Gaustad P, et al. Plasma endotoxin as a predictor of multiple organ failure and death in systemic meningococcal disease. J Infect Dis. 1989;159:195–204.
212. Waage A, Brandtzaeg P, Halstensen A, et al. The complex pattern of cytokines in serum from patients with meningococcal septic shock. Association between interleukin 6, interleukin 1, and fatal outcome. J Exp Med. 1989;169:333–8.
213. Girardin E, Grau GE, Dayer JM, et al. Tumor necrosis factor and interleukin-1 in the serum of children with severe infectious purpura. N Engl J Med. 1988;319:397–400.
214. Waage A, Halstensen A, Espevik T. Association between tumour necrosis factor in serum and fatal outcome in patients with meningococcal disease. Lancet. 1987;1:355–7.
215. Waage A, Halstensen A, Shalaby R, et al. Local production of tumor necrosis factor α, interleukin 1, and interleukin 6 in meningococcal meningitis: Relation to the inflammatory response. J Exp Med. 1989;170:1859–67.
216. Morgan BP. Mechanisms of tissue damage by the membrane attack complex of complement. Complement Inflamm. 1989;6:104–11.
217. Sims PJ, Wiedmer T. The response of human platelets to activated components of the complement system. Immunol Today. 1991;12:338–42.
218. Platonov AE, Gracheva AM. Effects of lipopolysaccharide on human granulocyte lysis and chemiluminescence. In: Achtman M, Kohl P, Marchal C, et al., eds. Neisseriae 1990. Berlin, FRG: Walter de Gruyter; 1991:627–31.
219. Hamilton KK, Hattori R, Esmon CT, et al. Complement proteins C5b–9 induce vesiculation of the endothelial plasma membrane and expose catalytic surface for assembly of the prothrombinase enzyme complex. J Biol Chem. 1990;265:3809–14.
220. Frank MM, Gelfand JA, Atkinson JP. Hereditary angioedema: The clinical syndrome and its management. Ann Intern Med. 1976;84:580–93.
221. Frank MM. C1 esterase inhibitor: Clinical clues to the pathophysiology of angioedema. J Allergy Clin Immunol. 1986;78:848–50.
222. Geha RS, Quinti I, Austen KF, et al. Acquired C1-inhibitor deficiency associated with antiidiotypic antibody to monoclonal immunoglobulins. N Engl J Med. 1985;312:534–40.
223. Alsenz J, Bork K, Loos M. Autoantibody-mediated acquired deficiency of C1 inhibitor. N Engl J Med. 1987;316:1360–6.
224. Strang CJ, Auerbach HS, Rosen FS. C1s-induced vascular permeability in C2-deficient guinea pigs. J Immunol. 1986;137:631–5.
225. Agostini A, Cicardi M. Hereditary and acquired C1-inhibitor deficiency: Biological and clinical characteristics in 235 patients. Medicine. 1992;71:206–15.
226. Donaldson VH, Bissler JJ. C1 inhibitors and their genes: An update. J Lab Clin Med. 1993;119:330–3.
227. Rosse WF. Paroxysmal nocturnal hemoglobinuria. In: Williams WJ, Beutler E, Erslev AJ, et al., eds. Hematology. New York: McGraw-Hill; 1972:460–74.
228. Rosse WF, Parker CJ. Paroxysmal nocturnal haemoglobinuria. Clin Haematol. 1985;14:105–25.
229. Rosse WF. The control of complement activation by the blood cells in paroxysmal nocturnal hemoglobinuria. Blood. 1986;67:268–9.
230. Nicholson-Weller A, March JP, Rosenfeld SI, et al. Affected erythrocytes of patients with paroxysmal nocturnal hemoglobinuria are deficient in the complement regulatory protein, decay accelerating factor. Proc Natl Acad Sci USA. 1983;80:5066–70.
231. Holguin MH, Fredrick LR, Bernshaw NJ, et al. Isolation and characterization of a membrane protein from normal human erythrocytes that inhibits reactive lysis of the erythrocytes of paroxysmal nocturnal hemoglobinuria. J Clin Invest. 1989;84:7–17.
232. Medof ME, Gottlieb A, Kinoshita T, et al. Relationship between decay accelerating factor deficiency, diminished acetylcholinesterase activity, and defective terminal complement pathway restriction in paroxysmal nocturnal hemoglobinuria erythrocytes. J Clin Invest. 1987;80:165–74.
233. Holguin MH, Wilcox LA, Bernshaw NJ, et al. Relationship between the membrane inhibitor of reactive lysis and the erythrocyte phenotypes of paroxysmal nocturnal hemoglobinuria. J Clin Invest. 1989;84:1387–94.
234. Merry AH, Rawlinson VI, Uchikawa M, et al. Studies on the sensitivity to complement-mediated lysis of erythrocytes (Inab phenotype) with a deficiency of DAF (decay accelerating factor). Br J Haematol. 1989;73:248–53.
235. Yamashina M, Ueda E, Kinoshita T, et al. Inherited complete deficiency of 20-kilodalton homologous restriction factor (CD59) as a cause of paroxysmal nocturnal hemoglobinuria. N Engl J Med. 1990;323:1184–9.
236. Nicholson-Weller A, Spicer DB, Austen KF. Deficiency of the complement regulatory protein, "decay-accelerating factor," on membranes of granulocytes, monocytes, and platelets in paroxysmal nocturnal hemoglobinuria. N Engl J Med. 312:1091–7.
237. Rosse WF. Phosphatidylinositol-linked proteins and paroxysmal nocturnal hemoglobinuria. Blood. 1990;75:1595–601.
238. Armstrong C, Schubert J, Ueda E, et al. Affected paroxysmal nocturnal hemoglobinuria T lymphocytes harbor a common defect in assembly of N-acetyl-D-glucosamine inositol phospholipid corresponding to that in class A thy-1-murine lymphoma mutants. J Biol Chem. 1992;267:25347–51.
239. Takeda J, Miyata T, Kawagoe K, et al. PIG-A is the responsible gene for paroxysmal nocturnal hemoglobinuria (PNH). FASEB J. 1993;7:A1049.
240. Schafer H, Mathey D, Bhakdi HF. Deposition of the terminal C5b–9 complement complex in infarcted areas of human myocardium. J Immunol. 1986;137:1945–9.
241. Rus HG, Niculescu F, Vlaicu R. Presence of C5b–9 complement complex and S-protein in human myocardial areas with necrosis and sclerosis. Immunol Lett. 1987;16:15–20.
242. Rus HG, Niculescu F, Constantinescu E, et al. Immunoelectron-microscopic localization of the terminal C5b–9 complement complex in human atherosclerotic fibrous plaque. Atherosclerosis. 1986;61:35–42.
243. Maroko PR, Carpenter CB, Chiariello M, et al. Reduction by cobra venom factor of myocardial necrosis after coronary artery occlusion. J Clin Invest. 1978;61:661–70.

244. Pinckard RN, O'Rourke RA, Crawford MH, et al. Complement localization and mediation of ischemic injury in baboon myocardium. J Clin Invest. 1980; 66:1050–6.

245. Biesecker G, Katz S, Koffler D. Renal localization of the membrane attack complex in systemic lupus erythematosus nephritis. J Exp Med. 1981;151: 1790–1.

246. Falk RJ, Dalmasso AP, Kim Y, et al. Neoantigen of the polymerized ninth component of complement. Characterization of a monoclonal antibody and immunohistochemical localization in renal disease. J Clin Invest. 1983;72: 560–73.

247. Groggel GC, Adler S, Rennke HG, et al. Role of the terminal complement pathway in experimental membranous nephropathy in the rabbit. J Clin Invest. 1983;72:1948–57.

248. Adler S, Baker PJ, Pritzl P, et al. Detection of terminal complement components in experimental immune glomerular injury. Kidney Int. 1984;26:830–7.

249. Nath KA, Hostetter MK, Hostetter TH. Pathophysiology of chronic tubulointerstitial disease in rats. Interactions of dietary acid load, ammonia, and complement component C3. J Clin Invest. 1985;76:667–75.

250. Cybulsky AV, Rennke HG, Feintzeig ID, et al. Complement-induced glomerular epithelial cell injury. Role of the membrane attack complex in rat membranous nephropathy. J Clin Invest. 1986;77:1096–107.

251. Cybulsky AV, Quigg RJ, Salant DJ. The membrane attack complex in complement-mediated glomerular epithelial cell injury: Formation and stability of C5b-9 and C5b-7 in rat membranous nephropathy. J Immunol. 1986;137: 1511–6.

252. Rus HG, Niculescu F, Nanulescu M, et al. Immunohistochemical detection of the terminal C5b-9 complement complex in children with glomerular diseases. Clin Exp Immunol. 1986;65:66–72.

253. Biesecker G, Lavin L, Ziskind M, et al. Cutaneous localization of the membrane attack complex in discoid and systemic lupus erythematosus. N Engl J Med. 1982;306:264–70.

254. Sanders ME, Alexander EL, Koski CL, et al. Detection of activated terminal complement (C5b-9) in cerebrospinal fluid from patients with central nervous system involvement of primary Sjögren's syndrome or systemic lupus erythematosus. J Immunol. 1987;138:2095–9.

255. Koski CL, Sanders ME, Swoveland PT, et al. Activation of terminal components of complement in patients with Guillain-Barré syndrome and other demyelinating neuropathies. J Clin Invest. 1987;80:1492–7.

256. Cammer W, Brosnan CF, Basile C, et al. Complement potentiates the degradation of myelin proteins by plasmin: Implications for a mechanism of inflammatory demyelination. Brain Res. 1986;364:91–101.

257. Mollnes TE, Vandvik B, Lea T, et al. Intrathecal complement activation in neurological diseases evaluated by analysis of the terminal complement complex. J Neurol Sci. 1987;78:17–28.

258. Platt JL, Vercellotti GM, Dalmasso AP, et al. Transplantation of discordant xenografts: A review of progress. Immunol Today. 1990;11:450–5.

259. Dalmasso AP, Vercellotti GM, Fischel RJ, et al. Mechanism of complement activation in the hyperacute rejection of porcine organs transplanted into primate recipients. Am J Pathol. 1992;140:1157–66.

260. Xia W, Fearon DT, Kirkman RL. Effect of repetitive doses of soluble human complement receptor type 1 on survival of discordant cardiac xenografts. Transplant Proc. 1993;25:410–1.

261. Loveland BE, Johnstone RW, Russell SM, et al. CD46 (MCP) confers protection from lysis by xenogeneic antibodies. Transplant Proc. 1993;25:396–7.

262. Weisman HF, Bartow T, Leppo MK, et al. Soluble human complement receptor type 1: in vivo inhibitor of complement suppressing post-ischemic myocardial inflammation and necrosis. Science. 1990;249:146–51.

263. Fearon DT, Ruddy S, Schur PH, et al. Activation of the properdin pathway of complement in patients with gram-negative bacteremia. N Engl J Med. 1975;292:937–40.

264. Weaver LJ, Craddock PR, Jacob HS. Association of complement activation and elevated plasma-C5a with adult respiratory distress syndrome. Pathophysiological relevance and possible prognostic value. Lancet. 1980;1:947–9.

265. Jacob HS, Craddock PR, Hammerschmidt DE, et al. Complement-induced granulocyte aggregation. An unsuspected mechanism of disease. N Engl J Med. 1980;302:789–94.

266. Stevens JH, O'Hanley P, Shapiro JM, et al. Effect of anti-C5a antibodies on the adult respiratory distress syndrome in septic primates. J Clin Invest. 1986;77:1812–6.

267. Hosea SW, Brown EJ, Frank MM. The critical role of complement in experimental pneumococcal sepsis. J Infect Dis. 1980;142:903–9.

268. Brown EJ, Hosea SW, Frank MM. The role of the spleen in experimental pneumococcal bacteremia. J Clin Invest. 1981;67:975–82.

269. Bohnsack JF, Brown EJ. The role of the spleen in resistance to infection. Annu Rev Med. 1986;37:49–59.

270. Brown EJ, Hosea SW, Frank MM. The role of antibody and complement in the reticuloendothelial clearance of pneumococci from the bloodstream. Rev Infect Dis. 1985;5(Suppl):797–805.

271. Singer DB. Postsplenectomy sepsis. Perspect Pediatr Pathol. 1973;1: 285–311.

272. Winkelstein JA, Drachman RH. Deficiency of pneumococcal serum opsonizing activity in sickle-cell disease. N Engl J Med. 1968;279:459–66.

273. Bisno AL, Freeman JC. The syndrome of asplenia, pneumococcal sepsis, and disseminated intravascular coagulation. Ann Intern Med. 1970;72:389–93.

274. Atkinson JP. Complement activation and complement receptors in systemic lupus erythematosus. Springer Semin Immunopathol. 1986;9:179–94.

275. Sim E, Gill EW, Sim RB. Drugs that induce systemic lupus erythematosus inhibit complement component C4. Lancet. 1984;2:422–4.

276. Clark RA, Kimball HR, Decker JL. Neutrophil chemotaxis in systemic lupus erythematosus. Ann Rheum Dis. 1974;33:167–72.

277. Perez HD, Lipton M, Goldstein IM. A specific inhibitor of complement (C5)-derived chemotactic activity in serum from patients with systemic lupus erythematosus. J Clin Invest. 1978;62:29–38.

278. Perez HD, Goldstein IM. Polymorphonuclear leukocyte chemotaxis in systemic lupus erythematosus. J Rheumatol. 1987;14:53–8.

279. Ross GD, Yount WJ, Walport MJ, et al. Disease-associated loss of erythrocyte complement receptors (CR1, C3b receptors) in patients with systemic lupus erythematosus and other diseases involving autoantibodies and/or complement activation. J Immunol. 1985;135:2005–14.

280. Gordon DL, Krueger RA, Quie PG, et al. Amidation of C3 at the thiolester site: Stimulation of chemiluminescence and phagocytosis by a new inflammatory mediator. J Immunol. 1985;134:3339–45.

281. Beeson PB, Rowley D. The anticomplementary effect of kidney tissue. Its association with ammonia production. J Exp Med. 1959;110:685–98.

282. Hostetter MK, Gordon DL. Biochemistry of C3 and related thiolester proteins in infection and inflammation. Rev Infect Dis. 1987;9:97–109.

283. Rubio R, Berne RM, Katori M. Release of adenosine in reactive hyperemia of the dog. Am J Physiol. 1969;216:56–62.

284. Cybulsky AV, Lieberthal W, Quigg RJ, et al. A role for thromboxane in complement-mediated glomerular injury. Am J Pathol. 1987;128:45–51.

285. Hakim RM, Breillatt J, Lazarus MJ, et al. Complement activation and hypersensitivity reactions to dialysis membranes. N Engl J Med. 1984;311:878–82.

286. Craddock PR. Complement and granulocyte activation and deactivation during hemodialysis. In: Lysaght MJ, Gurland JG, eds. Plasma Separation and Plasma Fractionation. Basel: S Karger AG; 1983:14–21.

287. Steinsson K, Erlendsson K, Valdimarsson H. Successful treatment with plasma infusions in a patient with deficiency of the second component of complement and systemic lupus erythematosus. Clinical experience over a 45 month period. Arthritis Rheum. 1989;32:906.

288. Barrett DJ, Boyle MDP. Restoration of complement function in vivo by plasma infusion in factor I (C3b inactivator) deficiency. J Pediatr. 1984;104: 76–81.

289. Rao CP, Minta JO, Laski B, et al. Inherited C8β subunit deficiency in a patient with recurrent meningococcal infections: In vivo functional kinetic analysis of C8. Clin Exp Immunol. 1985;60:183–90.

290. Pitts JS, Donaldson VH, Forristal J, et al. Remissions induced in hereditary angioneurotic edema with an attenuated androgen (danazol): Correlation between concentrations of C1-inhibitor and the fourth and second components of complement. J Lab Clin Med. 1978;92:501–7.

291. Densen P, Brown EJ, O'Neill GJ. Inherited deficiency of C8 in a patient with recurrent meningococcal infections: Further evidence for a dysfunctional C8 molecule and nonlinkage to the HLA system. J Clin Immunol. 1983;3:90–9.

292. Potter PC, Frasch CE, van der Sande WJ, et al. Prophylaxis against *Neisseria meningitidis* infections and antibody reseponses in patients with deficiency of the sixth component of complement. J Infect Dis. 1990;161:932–7.

7. GRANULOCYTIC PHAGOCYTES

PETER DENSEN
ROBERT A. CLARK
WILLIAM M. NAUSEEF

Granulocytes are the most numerous leukocytes in the peripheral circulation. The granulocytic cell series consists of basophils, eosinophils, and neutrophils. These cells share in common a multilobed nucleus, the presence of numerous membrane-bound, characteristically staining cytoplasmic granules, as well as a primary site of action in the tissues. Functionally, however, their differences are greater than are their similarities.

White cells were first recognized in blood in the 1760s by William Hewson in England. A century later, Elya Metchnikoff reported his observations on phagocytosis and formulated his theory of cellular immunity. In 1903–1904, Wright and Douglas demonstrated the importance of serum factors in phagocytosis and coined the term *opsonins* for these factors. Their work provided the impetus for the experimental resolution of the conflict between the theories of cellular and humoral immunity.[1,2] The past 20 years have seen the progressive understanding of neutrophil function in biochemical terms. Central to this understanding has been the clinical recognition of qualitative defects in neutrophil function and the experimental elucidation of the basis for these defects.

NEUTROPHILS

Development

Neutrophils are derived from pluripotential stem cells located in the bone marrow. Several low-molecular-weight proteins have been identified as colony-stimulating factors (CSF) for myeloid cells.[3] These molecules influence the survival and direct the maturation and proliferation of myeloid cells. Each factor is named for the colony produced under its influence: GM-CSF, for granulocytes and macrophages; G-CSF, for neutrophils; M-CSF, for monocytes and macrophages; and multi-CSF (or interleukin [IL]-3), for a variety of colonies including neutrophils, macrophages, eosinophils, megakaryocytes, and erythroid cells. IL-1 and stem cell factor act very early in myelopoiesis and are synergistic with the other CSF.[4,5] Recent studies indicate that cytokines, including GM-CSF and G-CSF, may prolong neutrophil survival by preventing the apoptosis these cells usually undergo.[6]

Granulocyte development and maturation in the bone marrow occurs in two phases, a mitotic phase and a nonmitotic phase. Each phase lasts approximately 1 week. During the mitotic phase, cells mature sequentially from myeloblasts into promyelocytes and myelocytes.[7] Maturation is associated with the appearance of the characteristic granules in the cytoplasm of neutrophils, basophils, and eosinophils. The nonmitotic phase of development includes metamyelocytes, band (or immature) neutrophils, and mature neutrophils.

Morphologic development is accompanied by changes in the physical properties of the cell, the appearance of specific cell surface antigens, and maturation of cell function.[8] Thus, Fc receptors appear as the cells develop into promyelocytes; phagocytic ingestion in the early myelocyte stage; complement receptors in the late myelocyte and metamyelocyte stage; oxygen-dependent microbicidal activity in the early metamyelocyte stage; oxidative activity and oxygen-dependent microbicidal activity at the metamyelocyte stage; and increased adhesiveness, cell motility, and chemotactic responses in the late metamyelocyte-band stage.[8,9] In addition, there is a coordinated expression of genes encoding the granule proteins that is synchronized with early stages of meyloid development. Morphologically mature neutrophils in the bone marrow exhibit lower stimulated oxidative responses than do mature neutrophils in the peripheral circulation.[9] A reduction in net surface charge, due primarily to the loss of sialic acid, occurs during maturation and has been implicated in the release of cells from the bone marrow.[10]

Morphologic and Structural Characteristics

Based on histochemical staining, there are two classes of neutrophil granules, those that stain for peroxidase activity and those that are peroxidase negative. The peroxidase-positive granules represent one of the major populations of neutrophil granules, the primary or azurophilic granules.[11] Those that are perioxidase negative include the secondary or specific granules as well as additional granule types.[11–15] Sophisticated subcellular fractionation and analysis of neutrophil organelles have suggested that at least two additional compartments exist, a gelatinase-rich tertiary granule and a labile, alkaline, phosphatase-containing secretory vesicle.[14–16]

Features of the best characterized granule types, the primary

TABLE 1. Characteristics of Neutrophil Granules

Characteristics	Primary (Azurophil)	Specific (Secondary)
Contents	Acid hydrolases	Lactoferrin
	β-Glucuronidase	Lysozyme
	α-Mannosidase	Vitamin B_{12}-binding protein
	Arylsulfatase	Collagenase (?)
	5′-Nucleotidase	Monocyte chemotactic factor
	Acid protease (cathepsin)	C3 and C5 cleaving proteases
	Neutral proteases	Membrane-bound receptors
	Cathepsin G	CR-3
	Elastase	CR-4
	Collagenase (?)	C5a
	Myeloperoxidase	FMLP
	Cationic proteins	Laminin
	Defensins	Membrane-bound
	Lysozyme	components of NADPH
	Acid mucopolysaccharide	oxidase system
		Cytochrome b_{558}
pH optimum	5.5–6.5	7.0–7.5
Degranulation	Degranulation delayed >50% Into phagosome	Degranulates first >90% Exocytosis
Function	Microbial killing Digestion	Inflammatory process

Abbreviation: FMLF: formylmethyl-leucyl-phenylaline.

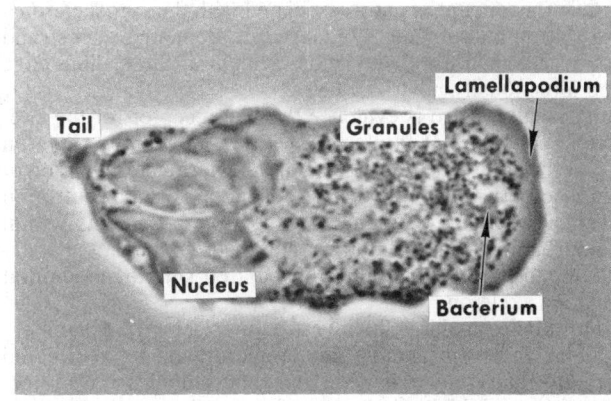

FIG. 1. Phase-contrast photomicrograph of a human neutrophil.

and the specific granules, are summarized in Table 1. Primary granules appear first, stain blue, and are subject to reduction in number during mitosis. Specific granules arise during the nonmitotic stage of development and thus do not undergo numerical reduction. Consequently in the mature neutrophil, specific granules outnumber primary granules 2–3 : 1.[7,11] Primary granules are true lysosomes since they contain acid hydrolases in addition to neutral proteases, myeloperoxidase, cationic proteins, defensins, lysozyme, and acid mucopolysaccharide. Specific granules contain lactoferrin, lysozyme, and vitamin B_{12}-binding protein. Importantly, the membranes of specific granules contain CD11b/CD18, the formyl-methionyl-leucyl-phenylalanine (FMLP) receptor, and cytochrome b_{558}, thereby serving as a recruitable reservoir of functionally important membrane proteins for the plasma membrane.

During maturation, the nucleus becomes segmented and cytoskeletal elements—microfilaments and microtubules—appear in the cytoplasm. A meshwork of microfilaments makes up the clear cortical veil that surrounds the cell and forms the lamellipodium of an advancing cell (Fig. 1). These structures are polymers of actin, a protein representing 5–10 percent of the total cellular protein. Actin, together with a number of other interacting proteins, constitutes the contractile machinery of the cell that generates locomotion.[17–19] Actin monomers (G-actin), in the presence of actin-binding protein, polymerize to form cross-linked actin filaments (F-actin). Regulation of the length of the filaments and the degree of cross-linking provide for the physicochemical fluctuation of actin between the gel and sol states. Filament length is controlled by several different proteins. Profilin serves to sequester G-actin and may provide a mechanism for rapid transport of actin to sites of polymerization. Acumentin, by initiating multiple sites of filament formation (nucleation) and preferentially inhibiting actin monomer exchange from the "slow growing" end of elongating filaments, maintains actin in short filaments. Gelsolin, a calcium-modulated protein that initiates filament nucleation, binds to the "fast growing" end of the filaments and can split preformed actin filaments. In the presence of ATP, myosin repetitively dissociates and binds to cross-linked actin. Myosin binding changes the cross-linking angle between actin filaments from 90 to 45 degrees, which results in movement of the filaments. Thus myosin serves to harness the changes in the physicochemical state of actin to give directionality to cell movement. Changes in calcium concentration that occur with membrane perturbation, directly and in concert with calmodulin, exert control over the contractile process by regulating myosin kinase and gelsolin. As a result, intracellular calcium gradients provide for an increase in polymerized actin in regions of high calcium concentrations.[17–19]

Actin filaments are associated with the cytoskeleton or with the plasma membrane via membrane skeletal proteins.[20] Stimulation of the cell with chemotactic factors causes an abrupt increase in the amount of actin associated with the cytoskeleton[21] and a shift in microfilament organization from a parallel strand to a crosshatched meshwork most evident at the leading edge of the directionally polarized cell.[22]

Additionally, there is evidence that the receptor for the chemotactic peptide FMLP interacts with the membrane skeleton and that this interaction contributes to the normal termination of oxidase activity.[23,24] Thus, signal transduction during neutrophil activation results in reorganization of protein domains within the neutrophil plasma membrane, and this reorganization is dependent, in part, on the actin-associated subplasmalemmal membrane skeleton.[25,26]

Microtubules are large, hollow structures composed of dimers of tubulin. In contrast to the role of microfilaments in directed locomotion and changes in cell shape, microtubules appear necessary for the initial orientation of the cell in a chemotactic gradient as well as the spatial organization of structures within the cell during locomotion. They also may be involved in degranulation and in the regulation of cell surface microviscosity during phagocytosis.[27,28]

Mature neutrophils (Figs. 1 and 2) are characterized by a pau-

city of ribosomal material and mitochondria, which reflects the relative lack of synthetic processes in these cells. Glycogen granules fill the cytoplasm and serve as a source of energy for neutrophil function.

Receptors with specificity for a number of humoral substances, including IgG, IgA, C3b, iC3b, and several chemotactic factors, most notably the FMLP receptor family, have been identified and characterized both functionally and structurally.[29–32] These receptors are homogeneously distributed over the surface of the resting cell. Upon polarization of the cell in response to a chemotactic stimulus, receptors for IgG and concanavalin A undergo an asymmetric clustering at the front of the cell. It is now clear that the distribution of receptors with different ligand specificity can be independently regulated even though stimulation via these receptors may result in similar functional effects.[33–35] Moreover, the various neutrophil functional responses exhibit differential requirements for receptor occupancy. Thus, maximal degranulation requires brief receptor occupancy whereas sustained oxidative responses are dependent on continuous ligand binding to the receptor.[36]

Neutrophil Kinetics

The daily production of mature neutrophils (PMN) is on the order of 10^{11} cells. This granulocyte reserve contains up to 10 times the normal daily neutrophil requirement. During acute infection or other inflammatory stresses, neutrophils are mobilized from the marrow. In the face of a continuing stimulus this reserve may be depleted, thus necessiating additional means for increasing delivery to meet demands. Increased stem cell input, increased mitoses during the mitotic stage of development, use of a store of cells whose maturation had been inhibited (so-called hiatal cells), and shortening of the maturation time within the marrow may all occur.[37] Multiplication and differentiation of stem cells is stimulated by the CSF produced by peripheral blood monocytes, tissue macrophages, and stimulated lymphocytes.[37,38] Lithium carbonate, a drug used primarily for the treatment of manic-depressive disorders, accelerates neutrophil production by stimulating clonal proliferation and leading to an increase in the total circulating neutrophil mass.[39]

Approximately 5 percent ($\sim 4 \times 10^8$ cells/kg body weight) of the granulocyte pool is located in similar-sized, intravascular circulating and marginating compartments. The intravascular half-life of these cells is 6–8 hours, whereas their persistence in extravascular sites ranges from 7 hours to 14 days. Granulocytosis, the hallmark of acute inflammation, is a consequence of certain physiologic and pharmacologic stimuli. These stimuli typically alter the distribution of neutrophils among the various granulocyte pools rather than increasing cell production. For example, the acute administration of corticosteroids or endotoxin, perhaps mimicking pathophysiologic events that occur in severe infection, promotes granulocyte release from the marrow reserve. In contrast, chronic steroid administration produces granulocytosis by decreasing neutrophil adherence and shifting cells from the marginating to the circulating pool. Similarly, exercise, stress, epinephrine, hypoxia, aspirin, and alcohol cause granulocytosis by mobilizing marginating cells.

Delivery to the Inflammatory Site

Intravascular neutrophils are heterogeneous, being composed of a large population (80 percent) with IgG rosetting properties and a smaller population lacking this characteristic.[41] This heterogeneity probably reflects maturational differences within a single cell line, but its functional significance is uncertain. Differences in the distributions of these cells may contribute to the development of "impaired" neutrophil function in certain disease states.[42] In contrast, tissue neutrophils are homogeneous, greater than 96 percent being capable of IgG rosette formation.[41] They contain fewer lysosomal granules and more glycogen than

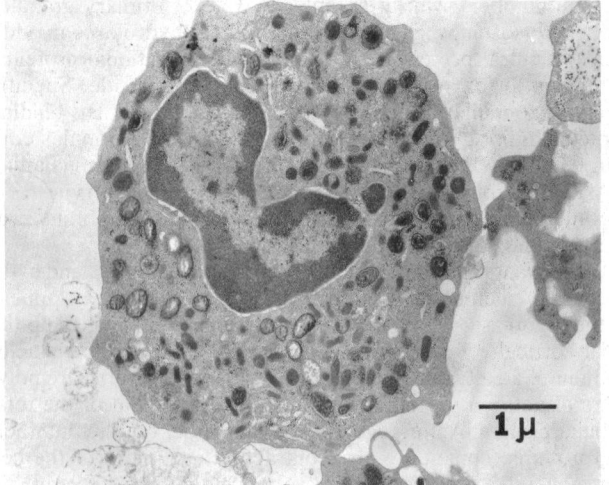

FIG. 2. Electron micrograph of a human neutrophil. Note the granules (large oval structures), glycogen particles (small dark particles), but few other visible organelles.

1 μ

their circulating counterparts.[43] Anaerobic glycolysis of these glycogen stores provides the energy for cell movement through the tissues.

The recent delineation of the basis for distinct neutrophil adhesion defects has contributed greatly to our understanding of the molecular events underlying the directed process by which neutrophils leave the vascular space and home in on sites of microbial invasion. This process involves at least three discrete steps: rolling adhesion, firm adhesion, and transmigration (Fig. 3).[43,44] A broad array of inflammatory mediators, including microbial products, cytokines, activated complement components, and arachidonic acid metabolites, act on both neutrophils and endothelial cells to initiate these events. Modulation of these events occurs through the activation of autocrine and paracrine feedback loops as well as the continued generation of phlogistic mediators at the site of inflammation.

Normally, neutrophils arriving in the postcapillary venules enter either the circulating or the marginating granulocyte pool (Fig. 3). Through a process of repetitive ligand–receptor binding and release, marginating granulocytes become lightly adherent to endothelial cells and, under the influence of the physiologic shear forces of blood flow, tumble or roll slowly along the vessel wall. The molecules mediating rolling adhesion are called selectins "to highlight the amino terminal lectin domain and to indicate [their] selective function and cellular expression."[44] These

molecules are homologous to C-type lectins and thus require calcium for expression of binding activity. Individual members of this family are named for the cell type on which they were originally identified (E, endothelia; L, lymphocytes; P, platelets). Although recent attention has focused on binding to sialylated Lewis x and a (sLe^x, sLe^a) oligosaccharides, selectins also interact with sulfated and phosphated polysaccharides such as heparin and mannose-6-phosphate. Individual selectins exhibit different but overlapping binding specificities, the basis for which largely remains to be determined.[45-47] However, L-selectin predominantly binds to a 50-kD mucin-like glycoprotein, which has been named Gly CAM-1 (glycosylation-dependent cell adhesion molecule-1).[48]

The presence of unique selectins on endothelial cells and neutrophils means that rolling adhesion can be modulated bidirectionally. For example, L-selectin is constitutively expressed on neutrophils and appears to be shed after cell activation. In contrast, little or no E-selectin is present on resting endothelial cells both *in vitro* and *in vivo*. Stimulation of these cells leads to inducible and transient E-selectin expression, which peaks about 4 hours following stimulation and dissipates over 24 hours.[44]

When neutrophils tumbling along the venule wall encounter inflammatory mediators and stimulated endothelial cells, adhesion between the two cell types rapidly shifts to a high-affinity

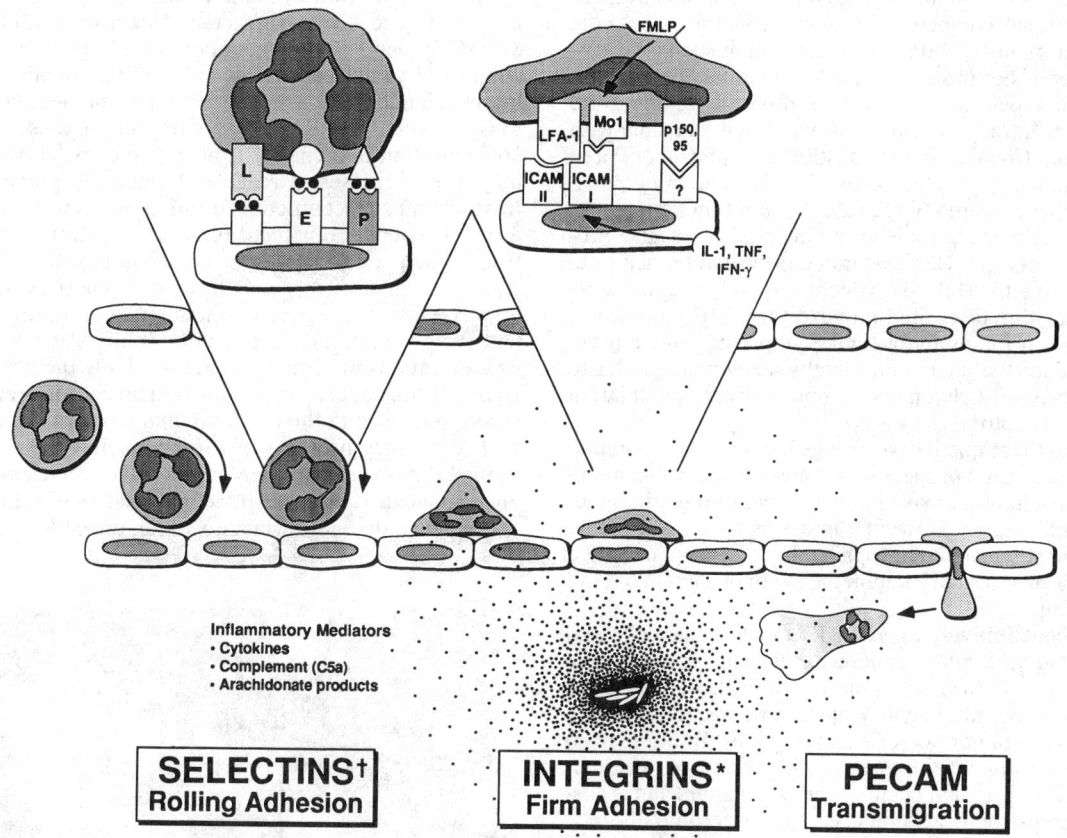

FIG. 3. Steps in the emigration of neutrophils from the vascular space. Neutrophils are depicted entering the marginating pool in a postcapillary venule. Initial adhesion is mediated by neutrophil (L) and endothelial (E, P) selectins and by their respective carbohydrate ligands on the opposing cell surface. Blood flow shear forces propel the lightly adherent neutrophils forward with a rolling or tumbling motion. Inflammatory mediators diffusing into the blood stream from sites of microbial invasion in the tissues bind to specific receptors and upregulate the functional expression of β_2-integrins (LFA-1; Mo-1; p150,95) on neutrophils as well as intercellular adhesion molecules (ICAM) on endothelial cells. These alterations promote a change in neutrophil shape and the firm adhesion of these cells to the vessel wall. Platelet/endothelial cell adhesion molecules (PECAM) localized to interendothelial cell junctions interact with PECAM on the neutrophil surface to permit neutrophil migration between endothelial cells. Once in the tissues, the polarized neutrophils move up the mediator concentration gradient to reach the site of microbial invasion. Type 2 leukocyte adhesion deficiency (†) is caused by the absence on neutrophil glycoproteins of the primary carbohydrate ligand (small dots in diagram), sLe^x, for E-selectin. Type 1 leukocyte adhesion deficiency (*) is caused by the lack of β_2-integrin expression on the neutrophil surface.

state. Neutrophils change from spherical granulocytes with relatively little surface area involved in cell–cell contact to flattened cells with a broad surface area for cellular interactions (Fig. 3). Blood flow shear forces are no longer able to propel them forward along the vessel wall. This type of firm adhesion is mediated through interactions between β_2-integrins on neutrophils and intercellular adhesion molecules, ICAM-1 and -2, on endothelial cells.[43,44,49]

The β_2 or leukocyte integrins are members of a large family of heterodimeric molecules that mediate cell–cell and cell–matrix interactions. This family is subdivided on the basis of eight different β-chains, any one of which can associate with multiple α-chains to form a unique α, β pair. Both the α- and β-chains are transmembrane molecules with short cytoplasmic tails and large extracellular globular heads that interact to form the ligand-binding site. The three neutrophil integrins have a common 95-kD β-chain, which is identical to CD18, and distinct α-chains. These molecular complexes are also referred to as LFA-1 (αLβ_2, CD11a/CD18), Mo-1 or Mac-1 (αMβ_2, CD11b/CD18), and p150,95 (αXβ_2, CD11c/CD18).[50] Mo-1 and p150,95 also function as receptors (CR3 and CR4, respectively) for the opsonic C3 fragments iC3b and C3d. Endothelial counterreceptors for the β_2-integrins include ICAM-1 and ICAM-2. LFA-1 binds to both ICAM-1 and -2, whereas Mo-1 binds only to ICAM-1 (on a different site from that for LFA-1). The cellular ligand for p150,95 is unknown.[44,50]

Integrin regulation exhibits both qualitative and quantitative features. Functional competence requires calcium, a specific membrane environment, and appropriate stimuli such as chemoattractant peptides or protein kinase C activators. These stimuli appear to modulate integrin binding affinity by altering the interaction of the intracytoplasmic tails with each other and with the cytoskeleton. Changes in the constitutively phosphorylated α-chain are inhibitory, whereas changes in the inducibly phosphorylated β-chain positively regulate integrin function. These mediators also regulate intracellular phospholipases and promote the release of a 340-Da unsaturated fatty acid termed integrin-modulating factor (IMF-1), which positively regulates receptor function. Smyth et al.[50] propose that IMF-1 promotes the dissociation of the inhibitory intracytoplasmic α-chain tail from the stimulatory β-chain tail, thereby allowing the latter to interact with the cytoskeleton and complete affinity modulation of the integrin receptor.

In addition to these qualitative changes, granulocyte stimulation promotes the fusion of specific granule and neutrophil membranes and a resultant increase in the number of integrin molecules on the cell surface. However, integrins are constitutively expressed on unstimulated neutrophils; thus, these quantitative changes appear of secondary importance with respect to overall integrin function.

ICAM-2 is constitutively expressed on endothelial cells and thus may provide the initial endothelial ligand underlying the rapid development of firm adhesion. In contrast, ICAM-1, like E-selectin, undergoes marked upregulation when endothelia are exposed to IL-1 or tumor necrosis factor (TNF). It differs from E-selectin in that low-level expression is present on unstimulated cells, peak expression occurs over 12–24 hours and is sustained, and expression is also induced by interferon (IFN)-γ.[44] The ability of corticosteroids to inhibit E-selectin and ICAM-1 upregulation in the face of endotoxin, a potent stimulus for their expression, attests to the feasibility of anti-inflammatory strategies directed at adhesion molecules.[51]

Endothelial cells play an active role in upregulating adherence events. Not only do they secrete a number of cytokines, for example, IL-8, a neutrophil chemoattractant, but their stimulation promotes surface expression of platelet-activating factor.[44,52] Interaction of this factor with its receptor on neutrophils does not result directly in adherence, but does constitute a potent stimulus for integrin-mediated adherence. Lastly, experimental data suggest that the interaction between E-selectin and

its ligands on the neutrophil surface promotes the functional competency of the β_2-integrins. This effect may be due to the fact that β_2-integrins bear sLe^x, a known E-selectin ligand, within their carbohydrate moieties.[44]

Transmigration is the final step in neutrophil emigration into the tissues (Fig. 3). Platelet/endothelial cell adhesion molecule-1 (PECAM-1; CD31), a 130-kD glycoprotein selectively localized to the intercellular junctions betweeen endothelial cells, is crucial for this step. PECAM-1 is also expressed on platelets and a wide array of leukocytes. Homophilic interactions between PECAM molecules on endothelial and neutrophil membranes as well as heterophilic interactions with an as yet unknown ligand provide the molecular basis for this critical event.[53]

Neutrophil emigration from the vascular space and migration through the tissues is the consequence of a carefully regulated process involving the sequential release and compartmentalization of a wide variety of inflammatory mediators. Early (0–5 hour) neutrophil influx into an area of induced injury appears predominantly to reflect the effects of IFN-γ, C5a, and leukotriene B4 (LTB4). IL-8 and IL-6 appear in a second wave of mediator activity (5–24 hours); IL-1β, GM-CSF, and TNF-α in a third wave of activity (8–24 hours); whereas IL-1α, IL-2, and IL-4 concentrations remain unchanged.[54] C5a, LTB4, and IL-8, as well as hydroxyeicosatetraenoic acids (HETE) and microbial oligopeptides analogous to FMLP, are potent neutrophil chemoattractants.

Chematactic stimuli bind to high-affinity receptors on the leukocyte surface. Chemoattractant receptors (e.g., those for IL-8, FMLP, and C5a) are members of a large family of proteins comprised of an external ligand-binding domain, seven membrane-spanning segments, and cytoplasmic regions that couple to G proteins.[55–57] When the neutrophil is exposed to a uniform concentration of a chemoattractant, the speed or frequency of migration increases, a reaction termed *chemokinesis*. In contrast, chemoattractant concentration differences across the cell as small as 0.1–1.0 percent (e.g., as the attractant diffuses out from a focus of infection) cause ligand-linked receptors to distribute asymmetrically and lead to a polarized response that imparts a directional component to locomotion (chemotaxis) and the net accumulation of neutrophils at sites of increasing concentrations of attractant (Fig. 4). How the chemoattractant signal is transduced to cell movement is not precisely understood, but calcium fluxes, actin, and a number of actin-binding and regulatory proteins of the cyoskeleton are centrally involved.[28] Also critical are interactions between leukocyte adherence molecules and the extracellular matrix, since migration can take place only on a surface to which the cells can attach. For-

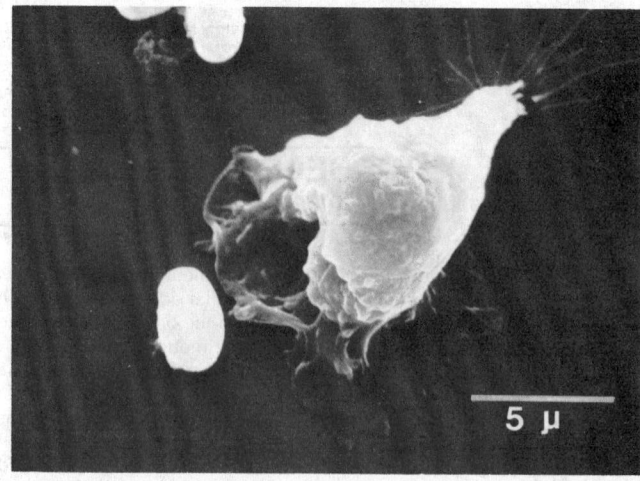

FIG. 4. Scanning electron micrograph of a neutrophil extending a pseudopod toward *Candida albicans*.

ward progress appears to be made either by gliding along a surface with caudad displacement of dorsal folds or cycles of partial release of the lamellipodium from the substrate with anterior advance followed by lamellipodial reassociation with the substrate.[58]

The binding of chemoattractants to their receptors also initiates elements of the microbicidal response, namely, degranulation and the respiratory burst, although these responses generally require higher concentrations of the stimulus than does chemotaxis. Thus, the activation of these distal events may be delayed until the cell is in close proximity to the infected tissue site. Fusion of granule and cell membranes during limited degranulation increases the number of chemotactic receptors.[59] As the cell moves in an increasing chemotactic gradient, these receptors become occupied and are rapidly internalized. The resultant decrease in receptor number and perhaps a decrease in affinity of the remaining receptors may control chemotactic responsiveness. The oxidative and degranulation responses induced in the neutrophil by increasing concentrations of mediators promote the inactivation of unbound chemotactic mediators.[60,61] In addition, lysozyme release dampens both the chemotactic and oxidative responsiveness of the cell.[62] In concert, this multitude of effects serves to attract and retain neutrophils at the site of bacterial invasion.

Phagocytosis

Phagocytosis is a two-step process involving attachment and engulfment of the phagocytic particle. Ingestion, but not attachment, is an active process requiring energy from anaerobic glycolysis. Optimal ingestion requires the presence of calcium and magnesium ions. Some microorganisms may be ingested by neutrophils in the absence of serum factors. This type of ingestion is frequently mediated by surface proteins on one or both cells recognizing specific sugars on the other cell. This process has been called *lectinophagocytosis*.[63] However, most bacteria must be coated with opsonins (humoral substances that enhance microbial ingestion) for attachment to and ingestion by neutrophils to occur.

Specific IgG and complement are the major opsonic factors promoting recognition and ingestion of most microorganisms by neutrophils. Antibody promotes phagocytic uptake by neutralizing antiphagocytic molecules on the bacterial surface, e.g., capsular polysaccharide; efficiently activating the classical pathway of complement and promoting deposition of opsonic fragments of C3 on the bacterial surface; physically linking the organism to the neutrophils; and activating the neutrophil ingestion mechanism through interaction of IgG with its receptor in the neutrophil membrane. Activation of complement via either the alternative or classical pathway lead to C3b and iC3b deposition on the microbial surface (see Ch. 6). In addition, C1q deposition enhances Fc receptor–dependent ingestion.[64]

Receptors for IgG (FcγRI–III), but not other immunoglobulins, and for C3b (CR-1) and iC3b (CR-3) are present in the neutrophil membrane.[29,30] These receptors are biochemically, topographically, and functionally distinct. In addition to its iC3b-binding site, CR3 also bears a carbohydrate recognition domain that may play a role in lectinophagocytosis. Data suggest that Fcγ receptors mediate phagocytosis via calcium-dependent pathways, whereas CR-1 and -3 use calcium-independent pathways.[65] FcγRII and III are low to moderate affinity receptors that are constitutively expressed, whereas the high-affinity FcγRI is present only after cell stimulation, for example, by IFN-γ.[66] Intracellular pools of Fc receptors have not been identified. In contrast, such pools have been described for both CR-1 and CR-3, the latter clearly being associated with the specific granules.[67] These receptor pools are rapidly mobilized to the surface after stimulation of the cell by a variety of inflammatory mediators. It is likely that C3 receptors enjoy only low-level expression on circulating neutrophils and that differences

in resting expression levels are attributable to the presence of miniscule amounts of mediators (e.g., endotoxin) in the isolation procedures used during neutrophil purification.

In contrast to upregulation, which occurs primarily through an increase in receptor numbers, downregulation of receptor-mediated processes occurs principally via diminished receptor function. Receptor oxidation as a consequence of the normal stimulation of the neutrophil oxidative burst contributes to decreased receptor function. Consequently, neutrophil receptor half-life and function are enhanced in individuals with impaired oxidase activity (e.g., chronic granulomatous disease) or in whom the generation of certain oxidative reactants is depressed (e.g., myeloperoxidase deficiency).[68,69] The balance between these regulating events is probably an important modulating factor in the inflammatory response and in limiting tissue damage.

Both IgG and C3 binding increase the rate of phagocytosis of appropriately sensitized erythrocytes, but in the unprimed cell only interactions via the Fc receptor initiate microfilament polymerization and ingestion of this target.[70–72] However, complement deposition alone is sufficient to promote ingestion of a number of bacteria, a finding that emphasizes the heterogeneity among opsonic requirements for different particles. In most cases phagocytosis is most efficient when organisms are coated with both IgG and C3, thereby allowing cooperative interaction of the two types of receptors.

Ingestion is the result of the sequential interaction between opsonic ligands distributed homogeneously over the particle surface and their receptors on the phagocyte membrane. The sequential interaction of these opsonic ligands with their receptors in the phagocytic membrane initiates polymerization of actin microfilaments in the cytoplasm underlying the site of a particle attachment and results in the circumferential flow of the cell membrane about the opsonized particle and its enclosure within a phagosome (Figs. 4 and 5).[17,73,74]

In addition to acting as ligands between the phagocytic particle and the phagocyte, complement and specific immunoglobulin alter the surface characteristics of the phagocytic particle. The surface of bacteria, which has antiphagocytic properties, is hydrophilic relative to the surface of the neutrophil. Upon opsonization the surfaces of these bacteria become relatively more hydrophobic than that of the neutrophil, and they are readily engulfed. Alterations in surface properties may also promote ingestion by reducing charge repulsion between the particle and the phagocyte.[75] Different bacterial species, as well as mutants

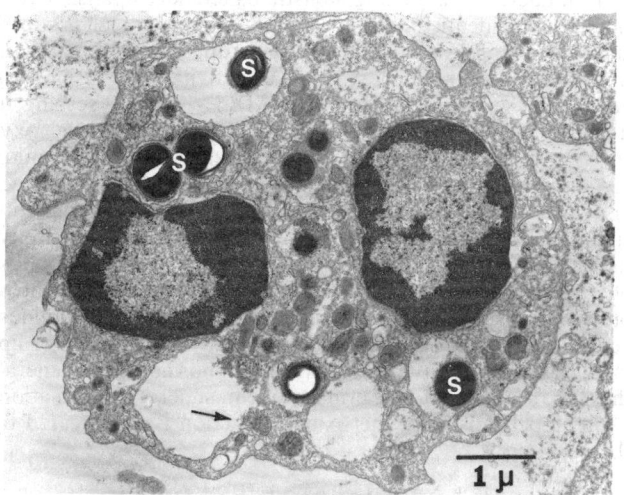

FIG. 5. Electron micrograph of a neutrophil that has ingested *Staphylococcus aureus* (S). Bacteria are in phagocytic vacuoles formed by invagination of external cell membrane. Degranulation into a phagocytic vacuole can be seen at the lower left (arrow).

within the same species, may vary in their opsonic requirements for optimal phagocytosis.

Increased attention has been paid to the important role that nonspecific factors play in the phagocytic process, especially in soft tissues where the functional impact of the neutrophil is most critical. Chief among these factors are fibronectin and laminin, proteins that constitute part of the extracellular matrix secreted by endothelial cells. These proteins contain the arg-gly-asp amino acid recognition sequence through which they bind to specific but separate membrane receptors.[76] Since the different receptors recognize the same binding sequence, specificity must be conferred by other aspects of the structure of these matrix proteins.[76] In the fluid phase or by themselves these proteins fail to promote ingestion of target particles. However, when neutrophils adherent to surfaces coated with these proteins are stimulated with a variety of chemotactic factors, their capacity to ingest either IgG- or C3-coated particles, in particular, the latter, is substantially enhanced. This effect requires neutrophil adherence to the matrix protein but not the interaction of the matrix protein with the target particles or an increase in FcγR or C3 receptor number. Hence these proteins are not opsonins. Rather, they enhance phagocytosis primarily by promoting the conversion of C3 receptors from a binding to an ingesting function. Thus chemotactic mediators and extracellular matrix proteins cooperate to prepare neutrophils for their primary phagocytic function as they migrate from the circulation to sites of infection.[77,78]

Postphagocytic Events

During the internalization of microorganisms within a phagocytic vacuole a coordinated sequence of events leading to the activation of microbicidal systems is initiated. The critical elements are a burst of oxidative metabolism that generates toxic products of oxygen and the delivery to the phagocytic vacuole of antimicrobial granule proteins by the process of degranulation. Both of these processes are triggered by the interaction of neutrophil membrane receptors with either ligands bound to the microbial surface (e.g., opsonins) or soluble mediators such as C5a, formylmethionyl peptides, or LTB4.

Oxidative Burst.   The oxidative or respiratory burst is mediated by a multicomponent system present as an enzymatically active complex in the plasma membrane and phagocytic vacuole membrane of activated neutrophils.[79–84] Such enzymatic activity is not detected in resting, nonstimulated neutrophils. A very similar, if not identical, enzyme system is found as well in stimulated eosinophils, monocytes, and macrophages, although neutrophils express the highest levels of activity. The respiratory burst enzyme is functionally an NADPH oxidase, serving to transport electrons from cytosolic NADPH to molecular oxygen. The immediate product of the reaction is superoxide anion (O_2^-), the one-electron reduction product of oxygen. A number of other events accompany the oxidative burst, including consumption of oxygen, formation of hydrogen peroxide, hydroxyl radical and singlet oxygen, enhancement of hexose monophosphate shunt activity, membrane depolarization, movement of protons across the membrane, emission of light (chemiluminescence), iodination of protein, and increased metabolism of lipids, proteins, carbohydrates, and certain hormones. In general, these are secondary to the primary event, superoxide formation.

The biochemistry of the oxidase reaction is represented by the equation:

$$2O_2 + NADPH \rightarrow 2O_2^- + H^+ + NADP^+$$

Important features of the reaction include the 1:1 stoichiometry between oxygen consumption and superoxide formation, the two-electron oxidation of the pyridine nucleotide compared with the one-electron reduction of oxygen, the formation of protons,

and the generation of $NADP^+$, which must be reduced back to NADPH in order to sustain the reaction.

Most of the superoxide formed readily undergoes dismutation to hydrogen peroxide and oxygen:

$$2O_2^- + 2H^+ \rightarrow H_2O_2 + O_2$$

This reaction occurs spontaneously with rapid kinetics at acidic pH where a significant portion of the superoxide exists in its protonated form, the perhydroxy radical (HO_2^-). This is due to the very high rate constant for the reaction between O_2^- and HO_2^-. Thus, in the acidic environment of the phagocytic vacuole superoxide is converted quantitatively to hydrogen peroxide. Since one mole of oxygen is regenerated for each mole of hydrogen peroxide formed, there is a net 1:1 stoichiometry between oxygen consumption and hydrogen peroxide formation, but a 2:1 relationship between O_2^- and H_2O_2.

Detoxification of O_2^- and H_2O_2 is carried out by cellular enzyme systems. At neutral pH superoxide dismutase markedly accelerates the dismutation reaction. H_2O_2 is metabolized either by catalase or through the glutathione system:

Catalase: $2H_2O_2 \rightarrow 2H_2O + O_2$
Glutathine peroxidase: $H_2O_2 + 2GSH \rightarrow 2H_2O + GSSG$
Glutathione reductase: $GSSG + H^+ + NADPH \rightarrow 2GSH + NADP^+$

Catalase converts H_2O_2 directly to water and oxygen, whereas glutathione peroxidase utilizes reduced glutathione (GSH) to reduce H_2O_2 to water. NADPH provides the reducing equivalents for the glutathione reductase-catalyzed regeneration of GSH from glutathione (GSSG).

NADPH levels must be maintained in order to support both the superoxide-forming oxidase and the glutathione cycle. The reduced pyridine nucleotide is regenerated by the activity of the hexose monophosphate shunt, which is enhanced 15- to 30-fold during phagocytosis.[85] The first two enzymes in the shunt pathway, glucose-6-phosphate dehydrogenase and 6-phosphogluconate dehydrogenase, utilize $NADP^+$, which is reduced to NADPH.

The dormant respiratory burst oxidase of the resting neutrophil is activated as the cell is stimulated, for example, via engagement of receptors for opsonins during phagocytosis. The lag period between stimulus exposure and expression of NADPH oxidase activity varies from 10 or 20 seconds up to a minute or two, depending on the stimulus. It appears that the lag time reflects the period required for the assembly of the multiple components of the oxidase at the cytoplasmic face of the plasma membrane or phagocytic vacuole membrane. On the basis of studies in both intact neutrophils and *in vitro* cell-free systems, the components of the NADPH oxidase comprise integral membrane proteins as well as soluble cytosolic proteins (Fig. 6).

Within the membrane is cytochrome b_{558}, so designated because of a characteristic 558-nm peak in its redox difference spectrum.[86–94] It is a heterodimer composed of large and small subunits, gp91*phox* and p22*phox* (*phox* stands for *ph*agocyte *ox*idase), respectively, which are firmly, though noncovalently associated. This protein has two different types of redox centers, a flavin adenine dinucleotide (FAD) domain and two (or possibly more) heme prosthetic groups.[95–97] There is evidence that cytochrome b_{558} is the sole catalytic subunit of the oxidase, although this is not yet unequivocally established. According to this view the substrate, NADPH, binds to a domain within the flavoprotein portion of the molecule and is oxidized by the transfer of two electrons to FAD. Then follow two single-electron reductions of the heme groups ($Fe^{3+} \rightarrow Fe^{2+}$). The very low midpoint potential of the reduced hemes allows them to react directly with molecular oxygen, reoxidizing the iron moieties and forming two molecules of superoxide, O_2^-.

Although cytochrome b_{558} appears to mediate the catalytic functions of the respiratory burst oxidase, other proteins are required for enzyme activation and activity. Two necessary pro-

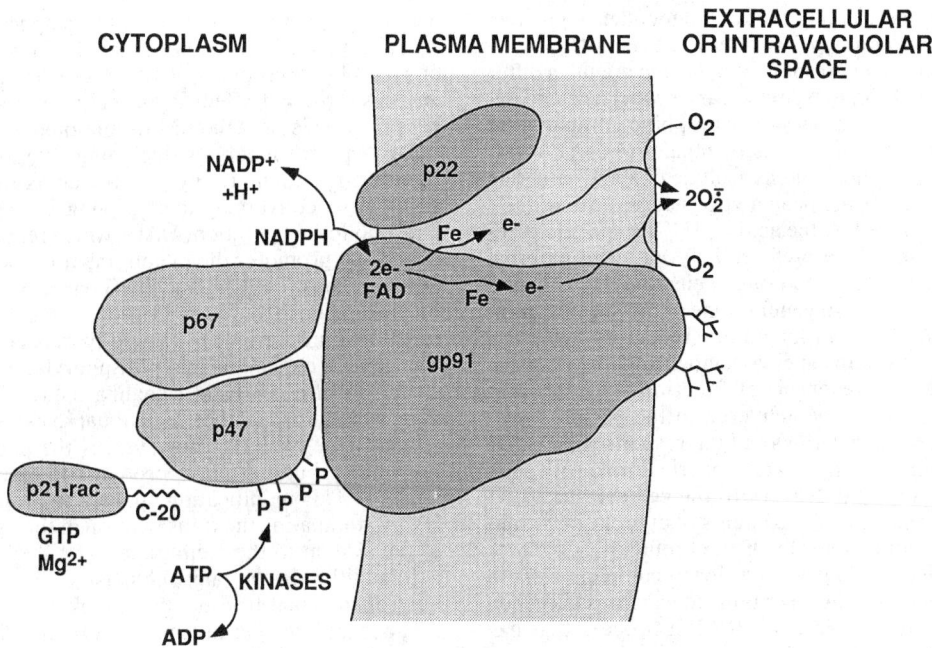

FIG. 6. Model of the assembled neutrophil respiratory burst oxidase. (See text for details.)

teins, p47*phox* and p67*phox*, are present in neutrophil cytosol,[99-103] existing, at least in part, as a complex with one another.[82,104] The complex may well include other as yet unidentified proteins. The primary structure of p47*phox* includes a very cationic carboxy-terminal domain containing several serine residues that serve as substrates for phosphorylation by protein kinase C (PKC) or related enzymes.[84,102] In the stimulated neutrophil p47*phox* is, in fact, phosphorylated by a PKC-like enzyme and the partially phosphorylated protein then translocates to the plasma membrane where additional sites are phosphorylated.[105-109] There is also evidence for phosphorylation-independent determinants of p47*phox* translocation.[110] Cytochrome b_{558} appears to be the membrane docking site for p47*phox*, and a specific cytoplasmic domain of the gp91*phox* subunit has been implicated in this function.[111,112] Neutrophil stimulation also results in the membrane translocation of p67*phox*, likely due to its association with p47*phox* since p67*phox* fails to translocate in the absence of p47*phox*, although p47*phox* is competent for translocation by itself.[108].

Both p47*phox* and p67*phox* contain two copies of a 50 amino acid domain related to a region of the *src* oncoprotein designated SH3 (*src* homology region 3).[101,103] Proline-rich motifs similar to those that bind to SH3 domains in other proteins[113,114] are present in p47*phox*, p67*phox*, and p22*phox*. In general, SH3 domains are thought to mediate binding to cytoskeletal and membrane elements. It seems likely that both SH3 and proline-rich segments of the oxidase proteins are involved in the protein–protein interactions required for oxidase activation and function. The net effect of phosphorylation and translocation of cytosolic components is the assembly on the membrane of the active oxidase complex, comprised of the cytochrome b_{558} subunits, p47*phox*, p67*phox*, and perhaps other constituents.

In cell-free model systems requirements for additional proteins have been demonstrated. In keeping with the enhancement of oxidase activation in these systems by GTP or nonhydrolyzable GTP analogs,[99,115-117] proteins related to the p21 *ras* family of low-molecular-weight GTP-binding proteins have been found to be necessary. One of two closely related proteins, *rac*1 or *rac*2, has been implicated, depending on species and type of phagocytic cell.[118-121] The *rac* proteins are isolated together with another protein, *rho*GDI (the GDP dissociation inhibitor of p21*rho*), which may also be involved in the oxidase system.

Modification of the carboxyterminus of *rac* by isoprenylation with a 20-carbon (geranyl geranyl) fatty acid, and carboxymethylation promotes association with *rho*GDI and with membranes and is required for optimal activity.[122,123] It is not yet known what role the *rac* proteins play or whether they associate directly with other oxidase components. Another small GTP-binding protein, *Rap*1A, is closely associated with cytochrome b_{558}, but whether it is involved in NADPH oxidase assembly or function is unknown.[124-126]

The active respiratory burst oxidase is topographically oriented in the membrane to promote the delivery of toxic products of oxygen reduction to the ingested microorganism. The binding site for NADPH is on the cytoplasmic face of the membrane, whereas the reaction product superoxide is formed at the vacuolar side of the membrane. Oxidase activation on the external plasma membrane results in extracellular release of superoxide, a process important in the oxidative attack on attached but uningested organisms such as protozoa and on adjacent host cells. The respiratory burst is sustained through an ongoing cycle of activation and inactivation. The inactivation is mediated in part by negative feedback inhibition. The products of the respiratory burst, particularly those generated through the catalytic activity of myeloperoxidase, oxidatively inactivate components of the neutrophil, including the oxidase itself.[127]

Degranulation.   Occurring in parallel with the oxidative burst is the process of degranulation. The cytoplasmic granules of the neutrophil approach the membrane of the developing phagocytic vacuole and the plasma membrane. The granule membrane fuses with either the vacuolar membrane delivering granule contents to the phagocytic vacuole or with plasma membrane resulting in the extracellular secretion of granule proteins. There is only limited understanding of the mechanisms involved in degranulation. Energy requirements are met by ATP formed largely through the glycolytic pathway. Cytoskeletal elements are intimately involved. Microtubules appear to mediate granule translocation, whereas remodeling of the actin microfilaments is essential in permitting the juxtaposition of granule and plasma membranes.[128] Cyclic nucleotides and calcium participate in the regulation of these processes.[129,130]. Membrane fusion is likely mediated by certain fusogenic proteins, prominent candidates including the annexins, a family of Ca^{2+}-dependent cytosolic proteins capable of promoting *in vitro* fusion events.[131-133]

The different classes of neutrophil cytoplasmic granules differ substantially in lumenal contents, membrane properties, and degranulating behavior. The primary or azurophilic granules fuse predominantly with the membranes of phagocytic vacuoles. Their contents of microbicidal and hydrolytic enzymes are thus delivered to the interior of the phagocytic vacuole, where their enzymatic action is favored by the acidic pH. The specific granules, on the other hand, fuse preferentially with the external plasma membranes, thereby secreting their contents into the extracellular milieu. The limiting membrane of the specific granules contains a number of transmembrane receptors, adhesion molecules, and other proteins such as cytochrome b_{558}. These granules thus serve as a reservoir of functionally important membrane proteins that can be delivered to the plasma membrane to reinforce or sustain various cellular responses.[134] Other classes of labile secretory vesicles are similarly armed with such membrane proteins for rapid delivery to the cell surface.

The extracellular release of the contents of cytoplasmic granules occurs by two morphologically distinct routes.[135] Granules can fuse with the nascent phagosome prior to complete closure of the phagocytic vacuole. The degranulated enzymes may then be free to leak into the extracellular fluid, a process that has been termed regurgitation during feeding. Alternatively, granule membranes can fuse directly with the external plasma membrane in the process of exocytosis. This occurs when the cell is activated by the binding of soluble stimuli to surface receptors or when it encounters ligands attached to a nonphagocytosable surface, for example, a basement membrane with deposits of immune complexes. The latter phenomenon has been referred to as *reverse endocytosis* or *frustrated phagocytosis*.

Signal Transduction

Exposure of the neutrophil to various stimuli is linked to functional responses through receptor-dependent generation of intracellular second messengers. The biochemical nature of the stimulus and the physical form of its presentation are primary determinants of the response. For example, opsonic factors (e.g., iC3b) fixed to a particle such as a microorganism elicit a focal response resulting in phagocytosis. Soluble stimuli lead to a generalized response as receptors are activated in all portions of the plasma membrane. Stimuli such as C5a that induce locomotion may trigger a nondirectional enhancement of migratory activity (chemokinesis) if present in a uniform concentration or directed migration (chemotaxis) if present in a concentration gradient. Chemoattractants are capable of stimulating locomotion at very low concentrations, generally in the nanomolar range, but must be present at substantially higher concentrations in order to induce a respiratory burst and degranulation.

Once a receptor on the neutrophil surface binds its specific ligand a series of reactions takes place at the membrane level as well as in the cytoplasm. A key initial feature is the activation of a phospholipase that cleaves specific membrane phospholipids to generate active products. Phospholipase C is a prototype in neutrophils as well as in a wide variety of other cells. The link between an occupied receptor and the phospholipase is provided by a G protein. Dissociation of the active α-subunit, the GTP-binding component, leads to activation of the phospholipase. In the case of phospholipase Cγ, phosphatidylinositol 4,5-bisphosphate is then cleaved to form inositol 1,4,5-trisphosphate (IP_3) and diacylglycerol (DAG).[136] The water-soluble IP_3 diffuses into the cytoplasm where it binds to high-affinity receptors in the membranes of intracellular Ca^{2+} storage organelles. The IP_3 receptor functions as a ligand-gated Ca^{2+} channel permitting the rapid release into the cytosol of a large amount of Ca^{2+} from high-capacity, low-affinity Ca^{2+} storage proteins.[137] The resulting initial spike in cytoplasmic Ca^{2+} concentration may then be supplemented by an influx of Ca^{2+} through plasma

membrane channels. These channels appear to be opened by a signal generated via emptying of the intracellular Ca^{2+} stores or possibly by products of IP_3 metabolism, including IP_4.[138] In any case, the net effect is an increase in cytosolic Ca^{2+} from baseline levels of <100 nM to micromolar concentrations.

Ca^{2+} has many targets, including cytoskeletal proteins and a number of enzymatic systems such as the Ca^{2+}-dependent PKC. Also converging at this point is the second product of phospholipase Cγ action, DAG, which remains membrane associated and promotes the membrane translocation and activation of PKC. Thus, both IP_3 and DAG participate in PKC activation. PKC then phosphorylates a variety of regulatory proteins whose functional properties are altered by this covalent modification. The general concept is that phosphorylation acts as a molecular switch to turn on distal signaling pathways, although specific PKC substrates and their functional roles remain poorly characterized. One example, however, is the phosphorylation of the respiratory burst oxidase protein p47*phox* by a PKC-like enzyme.[109] This modification appears to promote oxidase assembly by stimulating the translocation of the cytosolic components of the system to the membrane.

In addition to the phospholipase C pathway, mechanisms of neutrophil signal transduction involving phospholipases D and A2 appear to be operative under certain conditions.[138] Phospholipase D cleaves phosphatidylcholine to form phosphatidic acid. This product may trigger distal activation pathways either directly or via its conversion by a phosphohydrolase enzyme to DAG, which then activates PKC. Phospholipase A2 acts on phospholipids or phosphatidic acid to form lyso-phospholipds or lyso-phosphatidic acid, respectively, plus free arachidonic acid. Both the lyso compounds and arachidonate may go on to signal cellular activation, although the mechanisms remain poorly understood. It is known, however, that in cell-free systems the respiratory burst oxidase can be activated by arachidonate, phosphatidic acid, or lyso-phosphatidic acid.

Various pharmacologic agents can either block intracellular signaling at various points or bypass proximal signaling elements to activate distal pathways. Specific inhibition can be mediated at the G protein level by pertussis toxin, which catalyzes ADP-ribosylation of certain $G_α$-subunits. The IP_3–Ca^{2+} pathway is disrupted by heparin, which binds to the IP_3 receptor and inhibits its function. PKC is blocked by a number of inhibitors such as staurosporine. The phorbol ester tumor promotors serve as direct activators of PKC and can thus bypass the receptor, phospholipase, and IP_3–Ca^{2+} steps. Certain compounds known as ionophores insert into the cell membrane and promote the entry of Ca^{2+}, thereby activating some cell functions in a phospholipase and IP_3-independent manner. These various pharmacologic agents have served as useful probes for understanding signal transduction, but have not been adapted as therapeutic agents.

Priming of Neutrophil Responses

Concentrations of mediators sufficiently low enough not to stimulate neutrophils directly nevertheless prepare the cell for an enhanced response to a second unrelated stimulus.[140] This phenomenon is referred to as priming and is likely to be important in vivo since it appears to be cell specific. That is, bacterial infection primes neutrophils, whereas parasitic infection or allergic responses prime eosinophils.[141] A broad array of inflammatory mediators, including chemotactic factors, endotoxin, cytokines, and certain lipids, can prime the neutrophil, and the primed state exists with respect to each of the major aspects of neutrophil function. This state of enhanced responsiveness persists for an extended period of time (>20 minutes) relative to the response elicited by direct stimulation of the cell. Presentation of the same agonist in both the priming and stimulating steps results in decreased cellular responses, indicating the existence of chemical pathways for desensitization in addition to those for priming. The chemical basis for these different pathways is uncertain. Current evidence suggests that, in contrast to directly stimulated responses, primed responses are independent of PKC activation and translocation. Changes in the physicochemical properties of the lipid bilayer have been invoked as the physiologic basis for this phenomenon.[141]

Microbicidal Mechanisms

The postphagocytic events described above are designed to deliver the products of degranulation and the respiratory burst to the phagocytic vacuole. The phagosome plays an important role in this process because it provides a closed space in which an ingested microbe is exposed to high concentrations of toxic substances, and the exposure of the phagocyte and other cells to these metabolites is minimized (Fig. 5).[142]

Oxygen-dependent bactericidal mechanisms can be divided into myeloperoxidase-dependent and -independent reactions.[143] The essential requirements for the myeloperoxidase-mediated bactericidal mechanisms as first described by Klebanoff are myeloperoxidase, released from the primary granule; hydrogen peroxide, generated by the respiratory burst; and a halide ion. In addition, the low pH present in the phagocytic vacuole enhances myeloperoxidase activity. Hydrogen peroxide by itself has bactericidal properties, but in the presence of myeloperoxidase the potency of this system for bacteria is enhanced 50-fold. The halide used in the myeloperoxidase–hydrogen peroxide reaction also has an effect on potency: iodide > bromide > chloride. However, on the basis of concentration, chloride appears to be the physiologic cofactor for this reaction in the cell.[143]

Hypochlorous acid, formed by the neutrophil when chloride is the relevant halide, is a potent oxidizing and microbicidal agent.[143] The precise event responsible for the microbicidal activity of this system is incompletely characterized.[144] Candidate sites in bacteria include components of the electron transport chain, iron-sulfur centers, penicillin-binding proteins, and sites in bacterial membranes necessary for initiation of chromosomal replication.[145–149] Oxidation of some of these molecules may lead to the release of free iron, which can then participate in the formation of the highly reactive hydroxyl radical.[150,151] In addition to these effects, the myeloperoxidase–hydrogen peroxide–halide system promotes the formation of singlet oxygen, decarboxylation of amino acids to form toxic aldehydes, and generation of chloramines.[152] These agents may contribute to neutrophil microbicidal activity.[153]

Metabolites of oxygen for which a role in neutrophil bactericidal activity has been suggested include hydrogen peroxide, superoxide, singlet oxygen, and hydroxyl radical. The fact that catalase, which destroys hydrogen peroxide, protects bacteria from the bactericidal effects of neutrophils[154] and that the bactericidal activity of myeloperoxidase-deficient neutrophils remains high are strong pieces of evidence supporting a direct germicidal effect of hydrogen peroxide. Superoxide, by itself, is thought to play little role in the killing of microorganisms. This conclusion is based on the demonstration that bacteria incubated in a cell-free, superoxide-generating system survive normally. However, under appropriate conditions superoxide can react with other products of oxygen to gnerate hydroxyl radical and singlet oxygen. The bactericidal effect of these oxygen-derived free radicals may be due to the initiation of a chain of oxidizing events in the bacterial cell wall.[143,153] Hydroxyl radical is a potent bactericidal agent that can be formed by the direct reaction of superoxide with hydrogen peroxide. This reaction occurs too slowly to be of biologic importance, but it can be catalyzed by ferric salts.[155,156]

Because hydroxyl radical is highly reactive and therefore short lived, detection methods such as electron spin resonance using spin traps are necessary for identifying such reactive species in biologic systems.[156,157] Using such detection systems, the evidence indicates that activated neutrophils can produce hydroxyl radical by two different mechanisms. One mechanism

is dependent on the catalytic activity of myeloperoxidase,[157] whereas the other requires participation of transition metals in the Haber-Weiss reaction.[158–161] The relative contribution of each mechanism to the overall production of hydroxyl radical *in vivo* depends on the availability of exogenous transition metals, usually iron. In the presence of supplemental iron, hydroxyl radical generation occurs through the Haber-Weiss reaction. However, *in vivo* lactoferrin and transferrin bind iron in a form that cannot catalyze this reaction. Thus under most physiologic conditions, the small amount of hydroxyl radical generated by stimulated neutrophils is derived from the myeloperoxidase-dependent pathway.

The presence of oxygen-independent microbicidal mechanisms in neutrophils is clearly demonstrated by the ability of these cells to kill some organisms under anaerobic conditions.[162] Substances contributing to oxygen-independent microbicidal activity include acid, defensins, bactericidal permeability increasing protein (BPI), lactoferrin, lysozyme, and a variety of cationic proteins. In human neutrophils, the pH in the phagosome decreases to about 6.0.[163] Although pneumococci are readily killed by the effect of acid alone, most bacteria are little affected by the acid environment. The main effect of the low pH in the phagocytic vacuole is to enhance the activity of the granule enzymes important in the killing and digestion of ingested microorganisms.

Defensins are potent antimicrobial peptides in the primary granules of neutrophils[164,165] as well as in intestinal mucosal epithelial cells.[166,167] Defensins and closely related proteins are widely distributed in nature (e.g., the hemolymph of insects[168]) and likely represent an ancient mechanism for host defense. In general, defensins are small (3–4 kD), rich in arginine, and contain a characteristic disulfide motif. Elegant studies have defined many of the physical properties of purified defensins[169–171] and may provide insight into their mechanism of action. The spectrum of organisms against which defensins are active is extremely broad, including gram-positive and gram-negative bacteria, fungi, and enveloped viruses.

BPI is a 59-kD protein located in the primary granule of neutrophils. Its antimicrobial activity resides in a 25-kD amino-terminal fragment.[172–174] In addition, BPI binds to lipopolysaccharide (LPS)[175] and blocks the release of TNF elicited by bacteria,[174] properties that portend a potential clinical use of recombinant BPI, or a fragment thereof, in the therapy or prevention of LPS-dependent sequelae of acute bacterial infection.

Lactoferrin is an iron-binding protein found in secretions bathing mucosal membranes as well as in neutrophils.[176] Its presence in the specific granules of neutrophils suggests that the primary site of its action lies extracellularly. Lactoferrin's bacteriostatic effect is related to its ability to deprive bacteria of the iron required for growth, and this effect is eliminated by saturation of both iron-binding sites.[176] Lactoferrin plays a role in the alteration of the physicochemical properties of the neutrophil membrane that occurs during degranulation,[177] the modulation of hydroxyl radical production,[156] the regulation of granulopoiesis,[178] and the modulation of complement function.[179]

Lysozyme is found mainly in the specific granules but is also present in the primary granules. This enzyme hydrolyzes the glycoside bond between *N*-acetylmuramic acid and *N*-acetylglucosamine, a component of the peptidoglycan in bacterial cell walls. The bactericidal properties of lysozyme are due to this reaction. However, in most bacteria, peptide substitutions on the *N*-acetylmuramic acid residue make this bond inaccessible to lysozyme. The bacteriolytic properties of lysozyme are correspondingly limited. The action of lysozyme is enhanced by the presence of other substances, for example, complement, which damages the bacterial cell wall, thereby allowing access of lysozyme to its site of action.[143]

A number of additional cationic proteins have been isolated from neutrophil primary granules.[172,180] The reactions of these proteins with acidic groups on the bacterial surface are associated with inhibition of bacterial growth. Some of these proteins preferentially inhibit specific bacterial species.[181] These proteins include a 37-kD cationic antimicrobial protein, the activity of which is favored by the intraphagosomal acid pH[180,182,183] p15s,[184] azuricidin,[185,186] indolicin,[187] and bactenectins.[188–190] The exact mode of action of these various proteins is incompletely understood. In some cases it involves temperature-independent binding to the organism via ionic interactions followed by temperature dependent insertion into the outer membrane via hydrophobic interactions.[172,180] These events result in increased permeability of the bacterial outer membrane which in turn is associated with death of the organism. Intracellular killing of bacteria may also be enhanced by antibody and complement independently of the role of these ligands in opsonization and triggering the respiratory burst.[191,192]

Microbial Defenses Against Phagocytes

A basic principle of microbial pathogenesis, illustrated in the chapter on complement (see Ch. 6) and reiterated here for neutrophils, is that organisms have evolved molecular strategies for neutralizing one or more of the discrete steps in host defense.[193] In general, acute bacterial infections are caused by organisms that have developed tactics to avoid ingestion by phagocytic cells. In contrast, chronic infections are more typically caused by organisms that are readily ingested but have evolved strategies to elude intracellular killing mechanisms. The form category includes organisms like *Neisseria gonorrhoeae* that fail to generate complement-derived chemotactic factors and cause disseminated gonococcal infection. Capsular polysaccharides present on *Pneumococcus, Meningococcus,* and *Haemophilus influenzae* inhibit opsonization and phagocytosis. The latter category includes organisms like *Legionella pneumophila, Mycobacterium tuberculosis,* and *Toxoplasmia gondii,* which inhibit degranulation, and *Legionella micdadei* and *Salmonella typhi,* which limit the respiratory burst.[195] Alternatively, these processes may take place normally, but the microorganisms are relatively resistant to granule protein (e.g., mycobacteria, salmonella), or reactive oxygen derivatives (e.g., *S. aureus, Listeria*). Some species produce cytolytic toxins that damage phagocytes directly (e.g., *Pseudomonas, S. aureus, S. pyogenes*).[193]

The genetic basis for these strategies and their regulation is increasingly being understood in molecular terms. A fundamental principle emerging from these studies is the bidirectional nature of the process: that is, organisms both send and receive chemical signals that modify their environment and their responses, respectively. Host cells presumably utilize a similar process.[195,196] In the case of bacterial responses, this process involves a mechanism for sensing environmental changes and another leading to the coordinate expression of a number of gene products, some of which are virulence factors.[195,197] For example, during infection in mice, *Salmonella tyhpimurium* reside within a "safe site" in splenic neutrophils.[198] *Salmonella* resistance to neutrophil (and gut) defensins and oxidative products appears to involve the *phoQ–phoP* regulon in which the former gene encodes a membrane protein that senses environmental signals and undergoes a change that activates a carboxy-terminal kinase in the intracellular portion of the protein. Kinase activation leads to phosphorylation of the *phoP* product, a transciptional regulatory protein that binds to DNA and coordinates the expression of a multitude of genes. Most of these gene products remain to be identified, but presumably some mediate *Salmonella* resistance to neutrophil microbicidal mechanisms.[199–201] Candidate gene products mediating microbial resistance to neutrophil oxidative products include superoxide dismutase and catalase, which catalyze the ultimate reduction of these products to water.[201]

Tissue Injury—The Dark Side of Neutrophil Function

Ordinarily, degranulation and the oxidative burst are restricted to the points of contact between an opsonized organism and the developing phagolysosome.[203] Downregulation of receptor-mediated events during continuous exposure to homologous stimuli (desensitization) and during exposure to products of the oxidative burst,[69] oxidative inactivation of inflammatory mediators[60] and the oxidase itself,[127] and the release of lactoferrin to bind environmental iron in a form in which it is not available to catalyze hydroxyl radical formation[204] further limit neutrophil activation and confine the toxic effects of oxygen-dependent and -independent microbicidal systems to the vicinity of the organism. However, the toxic potential of these microbicidal systems can be unleashed and cause damage to host tissues in diseases associated with autoantibody formation, immune complex deposition, the intravascular release of excessive quantities of inflammatory mediators, or chronic low-grade inflammation. Thus various granule proteins and products of the neutrophil oxidative burst have been implicated in the pathogenesis of immune- and nonimmune-mediated arthropathies and nephropathies as well as pulmonary and cardiac injury.[205] Inflammatory cytokines such as TNF and IL-1 activate neutrophils and may contribute to tissue damage.

The intravascular activation of complement and generation of circulating C5a that can occur during the initiation of hemodialysis, cardiopulmonary bypass, or septic shock has been shown to stimulate neutrophil aggregation, oxidative activity, and degranulation. Aggregation of neutrophils leads to the formation of microemboli that lodge in the lung and accounts for the neutropenia observed in these situations. The release of toxic products of oxygen metabolism, coupled with the discharge of granule contents from aggregated neutrophils in the pulmonary circulation, leads to endothelial damage and has been implicated in the development of the adult respiratory distress syndrome both in vitro and in vivo.[206,207] However, the occurrence of the adult respiratory distress syndrome in neutropenic patients indicates that factors other than intravascular neutrophil aggregates also contribute to the development of this syndrome.[208] Substantial evidence implicates neutrophil products in the development of pulmonary emphysema. In this scenario neutrophils infiltrate the lung and are activated consequent to inflammation-provoking substances in cigarette smoke. Cigarette smoke and products of activated neutrophils inactivate α_1-antitrypsin, the major inhibitor of neutrophil elastase. Neutrophil elastase released during cellular stimulation then promotes proteolytic destruction of the lung architecture.[209,210]

Defects in Neutrophil Function

Defects in neutrophil function can result from decreased numbers of mature neutrophils or abnormalities in chemotaxis, ingestion, or bactericidal mechanisms.[211] Table 2 summarizes these defects. Infections resulting from quantitative or qualitative defects in neutrophil function share in common a tendency to be prolonged, to respond slowly to antibiotics, and to be recurrent. Staphylococci, gram-negative organisms, and fungi are the usual organisms responsible for these infections. Patients with defective opsonic activity suffer from infections due to encapsulated bacteria.

Qualitative defects may be intrinsic or extrinsic to the neutrophil. In general, the intrinsic defects of qualitative neutrophil function are more severe than are the extrinsic defects. Chemotactic defects are frequently expressed as cutaneous infections with associated adenitis. Unlike quantitative defects or defects in phagocytosis or intracellular killing, they rarely result in bacteremia or metastatic spread of infection. This is probably due to the fact that, although neutrophil accumulation is delayed, phagocytosis and bactericidal activity frequently proceed normally once neutrophils encounter the microorganism.

NEUTROPENIA

The most common granulocyte defect encountered is the absolute reduction of circulating neutrophils. The lower limit of nor-

TABLE 2. Defects in Neutrophil Function

Neutropenia
  Acquired
    Drug induced
    Autoimmune
    Cancer related
  Hereditary
    Infantile genetic agranulocytosis
    Familial neutropenia
    Cyclic neutropenia
Qualitative defects
  Adhesion defects
    Leukocyte adhesion deficiency
      Type 1, integrin deficiency
      Type 2, E-selectin ligand deficiency
  Chemotactic defects
    Humoral
      Complement deficiency
      Inhibitors
      Immune complexes
      Hyperimmunoglobulinemia E (Job's) syndrome
    Cellular
      Chédiak-Higashi syndrome
      Hypophosphatemia
      Lazy leukocyte syndrome
  Opsonic defects
    Complement deficiency
    Antibody deficiency
  Defects in intracellular killing
    Abnormal respiratory burst
      Chronic granulomatous disease
      G6PD deficiency
    Granule abnormalities
      Myeloperoxidase deficiency
      Specific granule deficiency
      Chédiak-Higashi syndrome

Abbreviation: G6PD: glucose-6-phosphate dehydrogenase.

mal for circulating neutrophils is 1500–2000/mm³. The risk of acquiring an infection increases progressively with both the duration and the magnitude of the granulocytopenia below 1500 cells/mm³. Below 500 neutrophils/mm³, there is a dramatic increase in the incidence of infection.[212]

The acquired neutropenias are most often related to drug therapy and may be a predictable result of therapy or an idiosyncratic reaction. The former are frequently encountered during chemotherapy for various neoplastic and immunologic disorders. Neutropenia as a result of an idiosyncratic drug reaction is observed with phenothiazines, sulfonamides, penicillins, cephalosporins, and vancomycin. Chloramphenicol can cause both a predictable and an idiosyncratic neutropenia. The latter is uncommon but is frequently fatal. Increased granulocyte destruction may occur as a result of splenic sequestration. Splenic sequestration of neutrophils may be immunologically mediated by antibody[213] or secondary to any of the causes of hypersplenism. Splenectomy may be beneficial in restoring neutrophil counts toward normal.

The availability of recombinant CSF has afforded clinicians a therapeutic option for acquired cytopenias (see Ch. 33). Most clinical experience has been with G-CSF and GM-CSF, and use has been primarily during the granulocytopenia associated with cancer chemotherapy and bone marrow transplantation.[214] For example, use of G-CSF increases circulating neutrophils by stimulating release from storage pools and by shortening the maturation time in bone marrow. These agents have been used to stimulate hematopoiesis in myelodysplastic syndromes, aplastic anemia, and cytopenias secondary to chemotherapy. Likewise, GM-CSF has been used to overcome HIV-mediated leukopenias and, in some cases, to permit use of myelosuppressive antiviral agents. Not only is the number of circulating cells increased but the biologic function and bactericidal activity of the recruited cells are normal.[215–217] However, current data do not support their use as an adjunct to antibiotics in infected patients with normal neutrophil production.

Hereditary neutropenia is observed either as a solitary defect or in association with other defects, for example, orotic aciduria. The neutropenia may be severe as in infantile genetic agranulocytosis, moderate as in familial (benign) neutropenia, or cyclic. Infantile genetic agranulocytosis is an autosomal recessive disorder characterized by granulocyte maturation arrest and severe infection with death in infancy. Some hereditary neutropenias are accompanied by an apparent compensatory monocytosis. Cyclic neutropenia is a rare autosomal dominant defect of myelopoiesis that is characterized by the periodic disappearance of neutrophils and other blood elements from the circulation. Early granulocyte precursors are present in the marrow during the neutropenia, which suggests a transient maturation arrest. The duration of neutropenia ranges from 5 to 8 days, followed by a 2- to 5-week period with normal numbers of circulating neutrophils. In a given patient, the periodic oscillations are constant. During the neutropenic state, the patients suffer from aphthous stomatitis, fever, malaise, and cutaneous infections. The disease is usually recognized during childhood, and there is no amelioration with age. Treatment with either recombinant G-CSF (3–10 μg/kg/day)[218] or alternate-day prednisolone (25 mg qod)[219] attenuates the oscillation in neutrophil maturation.

LEUKOCYTE ADHESION DEFICIENCY SYNDROMES

The hallmark of the leukocyte adhesion deficiency (LAD) syndromes is severe, prolonged, and recurrent infection in the face of a marked granulocytosis, cell counts often being 2–20 times normal even in the absence of infection. Despite this impressive granulocytosis, pus formation (the accumulation of neutrophils in tissues) is poor, and patients develop "cold" abscesses. This abnormality reflects impaired adhesion of affected cells within the vasculature and their inability to emigrate into the tissue. Two types of LAD have been described: type 1, in which integrin expression is abnormal, and type 2, in which expression of the primary selectin ligand sLe^x on granulocytes is essentially absent (Fig. 3). *In vivo*, cells from type 2–deficient individuals fail to adhere to stimulated venules exposed to normal shear forces, and they do not exhibit rolling adhesion. Because integrin function is intact, these cells can adhere to the vessel wall and can emigrate into the tissues if shear forces are absent. In contrast, cells from type 1–deficient individuals display normal rolling adhesion *in vivo* but are unable to adhere firmly to the venule walls and to emigrate from the vasculature.[220]

Type 2 LAD is an autosomal recessive disorder that has been described in two unrelated Arab families. These individuals have a distinct facial appearance, short stature, microcephaly, and mental retardation. In addition, they possess the rare Bombay blood phenotype and are both secretor negative and Lewis antigen negative. They develop recurrent bacterial infections, primarily pneumonia, beginning early in life. Periodontal infections, otitis media, and focal cellulitis have also been reported, but infection caused by a predominant organism has not been striking.[221]

In vivo assessment of neutrophil function reveals a marked impairment of both random motility and directed migration. Oxidative response to a particulate stimulus is within the normal range, although lower than that from simultaneously evaluated normal cells. Phorbol myristate acetate, a soluble stimulus, also evokes a normal although somewhat greater than average oxidative response from these cells. Lymphocyte number, subset distribution, and mitogenic responses are normal, as is natural killer cell activity.[222]

The basis for type 2 LAD has not been fully established. However, the Bombay phenotype is caused by an inability to form fucose-1,2-galactose linkages. Similarly, Lewis blood group antigen and sLe^x expression as well as secretor status are fucose dependent. Despite this similarity, the specific fucose linkages present in these antigens are formed by unique fucosyltransferases. Hence, a more general defect in fucose metabolism, perhaps involving a universal fucose donor, may be the cause of this syndrome.[222] At present the tissue specificity of this defect requires further clarification. A global deficiency would impact on both neutrophils and endothelial cells, whereas a cell-specific defect might affect only leukocytes or granulocytes.

Type I LAD is inherited in an autosomal recessive manner, and there is frequently a history of consanguinity. Severe and moderate phenotypes are recognized. Patients with this syndrome typically present with prolonged and/or recurrent staphylococcal and *Pseudomonas* infections beginning in infancy, often in the perinatal period. Patients with the severe phenotype exhibit poor wound healing. As a consequence they often have delayed separation of the umbilical cord and may develop omphalitis. Infections involving the soft tissues, mucosal surfaces, and the intestinal tract are common. Cutaneous infections frequently become necrotic. Initially they may resemble ecthyma gangrenosum, whereas later they may assume a pyoderma gangrenosum appearance. Individuals surviving infancy universally develop acute gingivitis with eruption of primary dentition. The ginivitis persists and results in progressive gingival hypertrophy and alveolar bone loss. Although survival into adulthood is well described, particularly in patients with the moderate phenotype, 41 percent of affected individuals die before the age of 2 years.[223,224]

Evaluation of neutrophil function demonstrates impaired adherence to artificial substrates, impaired chemotaxis *in vivo* and *in vitro,* and impaired respiratory burst in response to the ingestion of particles coated with iC3b but not IgG.[211,223] Affected neutrophils exhibit an above- or below-normal burst in oxidative metabolism after stimulation with soluble stimuli, depending on which stimulus is used and the nature of the association between its receptor and the cytoskeleton.[225]

Leukocytes from individuals with the severe phenotypic expression of this disorder bear less than 0.3 percent of the normal quantity of all three β_2-integrins, whereas integrin expression on cells from moderately affected individuals is 2.5–6 percent of that in healthy people.[224] In affected individuals the surface expression of both the α- and β-chains is abnormal. However, the α-chain is present in normal amounts within the cell. The predominant basis for this syndrome is abnormal β-chain synthesis and the requirement for intracellular assembly of the $\alpha\beta$-heterodimer for transport of the molecular complex to the cell surface.[226] Molecular analysis has demonstrated a spectrum of β-gene mutations that cause abnormalities ranging from the failure to produce mRNA in some individuals with the severe disease phenotype, to the production of an abnormally sized precursor β-protein, to the absence of a readily apparent defect.[227]

CHEMOTACTIC DEFECTS

Extrinsic Abnormalities

Neutrophil chemotactic defects due to factors extrinsic to the cell may be secondary to abnormalities involving the complement cascade. These include genetic deficiencies (C3, C5), as well as decreased synthesis (cirrhosis, kwashiorkor, premature infants), hypercatabolism, and increased loss (severe burns) of serum proteins. Some investigators have noted a depression in neutrophil chemotactic responses in patients with diabetes mellitus that is independent of serum osmolality. The defect is mild and is most readily demonstrated in juvenile-onset diabetics. Chemotactic responsiveness of diabetic neutrophils can be restored in vitro by incubation with insulin.[228]

Chemotactic inhibitors may express their effect directly or indirectly by neutralizing the chemotactic effect of complement. Polymeric IgA is cytophilic for neutrophils and can markedly depress chemotaxis.[229] Defective chemotaxis has been described in a number of diseases characterized by circulating immune complexes. These include rheumatoid arthritis, sys-

temic lupus erythematosus, and subacute bacterial endocarditis. Neutrophils exposed to immune complexes have high rates of oxidative metabolism and granule release in the resting state as well as an abnormal response to chemotactic stimuli. The sera from about 40 percent of patients with systemic lupus erythematosus contain an inhibitor that is specific for C5-derived chemotactic activity. This inhibitory factor does not interfere with the expression of other C5-mediated functions. Its presence correlates with disease activity and the resultant chemotactic defect with the enhanced susceptibility of these patients to infection.[230] The inhibitor has been identified as the Bb fragment of complement factor B, and it exerts its effect by inhibiting the interaction of C5a des-arg with cochemotaxin in serum.[231]

A chemotactic defect has been described in patients with juvenile periodontitis, a familial disorder characterized by periodontitis occurring in the absence of severe dental disease. Serum from some of these patients contains an inhibitor of chemotaxis, and the resultant defect in chemotaxis has been postulated to play a role in the pathogenesis of this disease.[232] In addition, neutrophils from some of these patients bear fewer chemotactic receptors than do cells from unaffected individuals, and an apparent structural abnormality of certain isoforms of the formyl peptide chemoattractant receptor has been reported.[333,334] Of particular note in this regard is the report of an acquired neutrophil chemotactic defect in two adults with gingival infection due to *Capnocytophaga* (*Bacteroides ochraceus*). Eradication of infection resulted in a return to normal of neutrophil function. Sonicates of *Capnocytophaga* and filtrates of broth in which the organism had been grown inhibited the chemotactic response of normal neutrophils. These findings suggest that the chemotactic defect associated with some forms of periodontal disease may be due to the presence of bacterial products in the circulation.[235]

Chemotactic inhibitors whose mode of action appears to be the inactivation of chemotactic substances have been described in Hodgkin's diesase, sarcoidosis, leprosy, and cirrhosis. These inhibitors are usually present in low concentration in normal serum and affect chemotaxis only when present in high concentrations. Recurrent skin infections and abnormal neutrophil chemotaxis have also been associated with an IgG antineutrophil antibody.[236]

A number of pharmacologic agents including alcohol, steroids, tetracyclines, and amphotericin B inhibit chemotaxis in vitro. Alcohol may exert its effect by elevating cyclic AMP levels. The inhibitory effect of tetracyclines may be related to their ability to chelate calcium.

Intrinsic Abnormalities

Chédiak-Higashi Syndrome. The Chédiak-Higashi syndrome is a rare autosomal recessive trait involving a generalized dysfunction of granule-containing cells. Giant granules have been found in melanocytes, Schwann cells, renal tubular cells, thyroid cells, and all types of leukocytes (Fig. 7). These abnormal granules account for many of the physical findings including partial oculocutaneous albinism, rotatory nystagmus, peripheral neuropathy (both sensory and motor), and recurrent infection. In neutrophils, they are formed during cell maturation by fusion of the two granule types.[237] Laboratory abnormalities include anemia, leukopenia, thrombocytopenia, and evidence of intramedullary destruction of all blood elements with an associated elevation in serum lysozyme levels and deficiencies in iron and folate concentrations. Abnormal natural killer (NK) cell function has also been reported.[238] In a number of patients with the Chédiak-Higashi syndrome, the disease undergoes a transformation to an accelerated phase. This phase is characterized by hepatosplenomegaly, lymphadenopathy, and lymphocytic organ infiltration. Unexplained febrile episodes occur, and patients frequently die of infection or less commonly of hemorrhage at an early age.[239]

Neutrophils from patients with the Chédiak-Higashi syn-

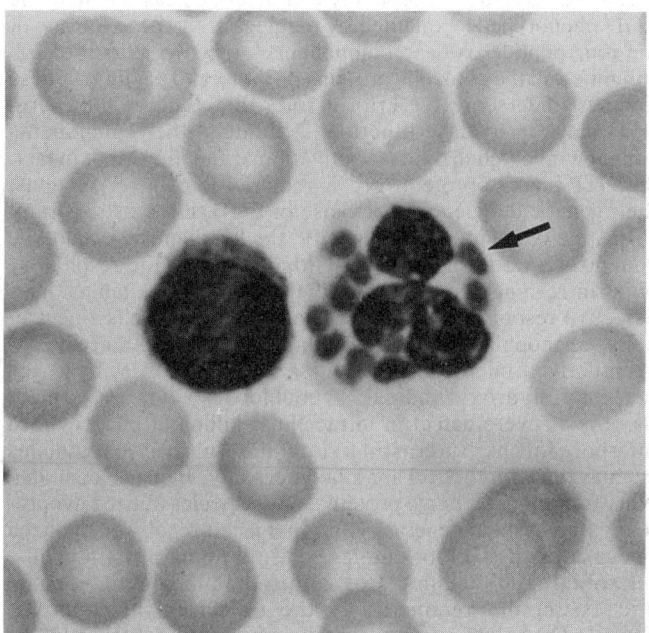

FIG. 7. Neutrophil and lymphocyte from a patient with Chédiak-Higashi syndrome. Note the large abnormal granules (arrow).

drome exhibit a defective chemotactic response, but ingestion occurs normally.[240] Many bacteria, including both catalase-positive and catalase-negative species, exhibit prolonged survival within these neutrophils. Bacterial killing rates are most abnormal during the first 20 minutes of contact in vitro but approach normal levels at 2 hours. The faulty release of the large neutrophil granules is associated with the delayed appearance of myeloperoxidase within phagocytic vacuoles. The metabolic burst is normal.[241] The intracellular killing defect thus appears primarily due to delayed delivery of granule enzymes to the phagosome.

The biochemical abnormality underlying the neutrophil dysfunction in the Chédiak-Higashi syndrome is unknown. Abnormal function of a diverse number of cell types suggests that the defect involves some basic aspect of cell function. The bulk of current evidence suggests that the defect involves the microtubule apparatus: cell ultrastructure studies confirm a decreased number of centriole-associated microtubules in some patients; membrane fluidity is enhanced and has been suggested as a possible explanation for the abnormal fusion of the azurophil and specific granules; the level of tyrosylated tubulin is abnormally high; and pharmacologic agents, such as ascorbic acid, that affect microtubule assembly may improve cell function in occasional patients. In addition, agents that decrease the cyclic AMP/GMP ratio have been reported to improve neutrophil function. Many of these agents also affect microtubule assembly, and changes in cyclic nucleotide metabolism now appear to be a consequence of these alterations.[228,242]

Hyperimmunoglobulinemia E with Impaired Chemotaxis (Job Syndrome). Job syndrome, as originally described, is an affliction of fair-skinned, red-haired females that is characterized by eczema, recurrent "cold" staphylococcal skin abscesses, sinusitis, and otitis media.[243,244] However, the disorder occurs in blacks and males as well. Many of the patients have coarse facial features and a broad nasal bridge. In addition to cutaneous staphylococcal infection, recurrent pneumonia and mucocutaneous candidiasis are common. Patients may have mild eosinophilia, and, although variable, the neutrophils of most patients exhibit a chemotactic abnormality. The chemotactic defect appears to correlate best with the severity of the eczema, and

patients have been reported in whom a chemotactic defect could be demonstrated only during relapses of their dermatitis. Mononuclear cells from these patients but not from individuals either with or without atopy spontaneously produce a factor that inhibits the chemotactic responses of normal neutrophils and monocytes.[245] All patients have markedly elevated (>10 times normal) serum levels of IgE due to a decreased fractional catabolic rate of this immunoglobulin.[246] Antistaphylococcal and anti-*Candida* IgE antibodies have been demonstrated in the sera from patients with Job syndrome but not from healthy people, from patients with hyperimmunoglobulinemia E due to atopic disease or parasitic infection, or from patients with chronic staphylococcal infections. Antistaphylococcal antibody of the IgM class is also elevated in the sera from these patients, whereas specific IgA is low and IgG no different from that in healthy people. Infection is inversely related to the levels of specific IgE, IgA, and IgM, thus suggesting that these antibodies normally exert a protective rather than a permissive effect against staphylococci.[247] Thus it appears that Job syndrome does not represent an intrinsic defect of neutrophil function but rather is the result of aberrant immune regulation.

A well-controlled clinical trial established that levamisol, which had been reported to improve neutrophil function in patients with Job syndrome, failed to reduce and was actually associated with an increase in the number of infections.[248] Thus, management should be directed toward early detection of infection, prolonged treatment with antibiotics, and early surgical drainage of "cold" abscesses.[244]

Other Disorders. A mild and variable chemotactic defect has been described in patients with Kartagener (immotile cilia) syndrome in which there is an abnormality in the linkage between microtubules and cilia.[224] An acquired but reversible defect in neutrophil function has been documented with severe hypophosphatemia (less than 1 mg/dl) secondary to phosphate-free hyperalimentation. The defect in these cells is thought to be due to an inability to generate ATP from anaerobic glycolysis.[249]

Abnormal Phagocytosis

Defective opsonization occurs with inherited or acquired deficiencies of the early complement components (especially C3) or immunoglobulin. Similar derangements accompany the paraproteinemias as well as a number of other neoplastic and nonneoplastic disorders characterized by hypoglobulinemia and/or hypocomplementemia. Patients with these types of opsonic disorders frequently have recurrent infections with encapsulated bacteria, particularly pneumococci and *Haemophilus influenzae*. Infection with these organisms in the splenectomized person can present as fulminant bacteremia or meningitis accompanied by disseminated intravascular coagulation.[250]

In 1968, Miller et al.[251] reported that sera from 5–7 percent of the population were defective in opsonizing baker's yeast. A number of these individuals suffered recurrent upper respiratory tract infections, and some had diarrhea with associated failure to thrive.[251] The basis for this defect remained obscure until Turner and coworkers[252] discovered that the concentration of mannan-binding protein (MBP) was low in these persons. MBP acts to enhance complement activation and deposition on mannose-rich surfaces.[253,254] The usual molecular basis for this defect is a point mutation resulting in the replacement in exon 1 of a glycine residue with aspartic acid. This change is postulated to interfere with MBP triple helix formation with consequent retention of the protein and intracellular degradation.[255]

Defects in Intracellular Killing

Impaired neutrophil intracellular microbicidal activity may be a consequence of either an abnormal respiratory burst oxidase or the absence or failure of delivery of granule enzymes. Those diseases in which microbicidal defects have been well-characterized represent inherited disorders. Although functional decreases in microbial killing have been described in patients with certain acquired inflammatory, metabolic, and malignant diseases, these observations have been neither widely confirmed nor characterized at a biochemical level.

Abnormal Respiratory Burst. CHRONIC GRANULOMATOUS DISEASE. Patients with the hereditary disorder chronic granulomatous disease (CGD) characteristically experience recurrent and often severe pyogenic infections, a granulomatous tissue response, and impaired phagocyte microbicidal activity due to the absence of respiratory burst oxidase activity.[256–263] Classically, CGD was described as an X-linked disorder in males whose mothers and some sisters are heterozygous carriers. However, the inheritance of CGD follows an autosomal recessive pattern in some kindreds. Since the respiratory burst oxidase is now known to comprise both membrane and cytosolic components, the various forms of CGD (Table 3) can be partially characterized by analysis of subcellular neutrophil fractions in the broken cell oxidase system. All patients with X-linked CGD, which includes about 55 to 60 percent of the total, have a membrane-associated functional abnormality, whereas in most patients with autosomally transmitted CGD the subcellular defect is localized to the cytosol.

The membrane component of the NADPH oxidase is the heterodimeric cytochrome b_{558}. The gene for the large subunit (gp91phox) is located on the X chromosome and is the site of mutation in all patients with X-linked CGD.[87,264] Rarely (in < 5 percent of CGD patients) mutations occur in the gene for the small subunit (p22phox),[265] which is on chromosome 16. In most cases deletion or frameshift mutations result in a failure to synthesize the affected subunit of the cytochrome. When one subunit is absent neither is inserted into the membrane, and the characteristic heme spectrum featuring a 558-nm peak is not present.[266] In rare kindreds single point missense mutations are present in either the large[267] or small[268] subunit. In these cases the cytochrome with a single amino acid substitution is present and has a normal heme spectrum but absent redox function. In certain instances the specific site of the altered amino acid maps to a critical functional domain such as the binding site for NADPH.[96]

In most patients with autosomally inherited CGD the neutrophils lack the cytosolic oxidase component p47phox.[260,261] Mutations in the p47phox gene account for approximately one-third of all cases of CGD. Unlike the cytochrome b mutations, which comprise many different lesions, one particular mutation seems to account for most examples of p47phox deficiency.[82,269,270] This is a two-base deletion at an exon splice site that results in a frameshift and early termination of translation. Most of the patients studied to date appear to be homozygous for this deletion, although examples have been described of patients who are compound heterozygotes for this mutation and either a single-base frameshift deletion at another site or missense mutations.[82,270] Mutations in the gene for p67phox are less common, accounting for perhaps 5 percent of CGD cases.[261] The p67phox protein is absent, but specific mutations have not yet been defined.

Importantly, in all thoroughly characterized cases to date the CGD phenotype is explained by a defect in the gene for one of the four peptide oxidase components—the two cytochrome b subunits and the cytosolic proteins p47phox and p67phox. These findings underscore the critical roles that each of these proteins plays in oxidase function. Although other components could be involved in oxidase activation or function, and, in fact, the GTP-binding protein rac2 is required in cell-free systems, their genetic deficiency as a cause of CGD, if it exists, is rare.

In spite of genetic heterogeneity, the biochemical phenotype common to all forms of CGD is the failure of the respiratory burst in response to any phagocytic or soluble stimulus. This defective response is observed in all phagocytic cells—neutrophils, eosinophils, monocytes, anhd macrophages. Since no oxygen-derived microbicidal agents (e.g., superoxide, hydrogen peroxide, hydroxyl radical, hypochlorous acid) are formed, there is a severe defect in intracellular killing of phagocytized microorganisms. Interestingly, catalase-negative organisms such as the streptococci are killed normally. Because of an inability to synthesize heme proteins, these species utilize flavoprotein pathways that generate H_2O_2 that is not readily catabolized because of the lack of catalase, also a heme protein. Thus, microbial H_2O_2 accumulates within the phagocytic vacuole and essentially reconstitutes the defective myeloperoxidase–H_2O_2–halide system, thereby leading to bacterial killing in spite of the failure of the neutrophil itself to produce H_2O_2. The preservation of microbicidal activity of CGD cells against catalase-negative microorganisms translates into an absence of major clinical infections caused by these species in patients with CGD.

In general the clinical manifestations of the different genetic forms of CGD are quite similar, notwithstanding some evidence for a more severe course in X-linked vs. autosomally inherited disease. Infectious complications often begin in infancy and recur throughout childhood and adolescence. In those patients who survive into adulthood, there may be a lessening of clinical severity. Occasionally, there is a relatively mild clinical course during childhood, and some patients may not come to medical attention until they are adolescents or even adults.[271,272] Infections may involve virtually any organ system, but the most common manifestations are suppurative lymphadenitis, subcutaneous abscesses, pneumonia, lung abscess, liver abscess, and osteomyelitis. Stomatitis, blepharitis, and pyogenic dermatitis are often seen as recurring problems. The most characteristic pathogens are *S. aureus, Serratia marcescens, Pseudomonas cepacia,* and *Aspergillus* spp., although a wide variety of other catalase-positive bacteria and fungi may cause disease as well. *Serratia marcescens* osteomyelitis is particularly suggestive of the diagnosis of CGD. Infections can follow an acute course, but more often there is a subacute or chronic progression with poor wound healing, a mixed acute and chronic inflammatory response, and granuloma formation. The basis for the granulomatous inflammation is not clear, though it is thought to relate to the persistence of viable intracellular microorganisms. In certain tissue sites obstructive lesions may develop as in xanthogranulomatous urinary tract disease[273] or granulomatous bowel involvement that resembles Crohn's disease.[274] Perirectal involvement with fissures or inflammatory masses is a rather common mani-

TABLE 3. Genetic Types of Chronic Granulomatous Disease

Defective Component	Relative Frequency (%)[a]	Gene Locus	Mutations	Biochemical Features	
				Membranes	Cytosol
gp91phox	55–60	Xp21.1	Large deletions, deletion/frameshift, missense	Cytochrome b absent in most, but present in missense mutations	Normal
p22phox	<5	16q24	Deletion/frameshift missense	Same as for gp91phox	Normal
p47phox	30–35	7q11.23	Deletion/frameshift missense	Normal	p47phox absent
p67phox	<5	1q25	Unknown	Normal	p67phox absent

[a] Percent of all CGD patients.[260,261]

festation. In patients with X-linked CGD, gene deletions may involve the nearby Xp21.1 loci for Duchene's muscular dystrophy and retinitis pigmentosa. Also in this region is the gene for the Kell-related blood group antigen K_X, the absence of which results in the McLeod red cell phenotype, hemolytic anemia, and difficulty in transfusion cross-matching.

The physical examination often shows dermatitis, lymphadenitis, enlargement of liver and spleen, and retardation of normal rates of growth and development. Routine laboratory studies may indicate anemia of chronic disease, leukocytosis to a moderate level (generally less than 15,000–20,000 per mm^3), hyperglobulinemia, and an elevated erythrocyte sedimentation rate. Pathologic examination of infected tissues usually demonstrates inflammatory masses with granulomas that may progress to areas of frank necrosis, sometimes with well-defined abscesses. Lipid-filled histiocytes are found in liver, spleen, lymph nodes, gut, and other tissues of some CGD patients.

The diagnosis of CGD can be made using assays for any of the products of the neutrophil respiratory burst. The most useful method is the nitroblue tetrazolium (NBT) slide test.[275] Neutrophils adherent to a microscope coverslip are stimulated in the presence of NBT, a soluble yellow dye that is reduced by superoxide to formazan, an insoluble precipitate that stains the cells dark blue or black. In normal control subjects essentially 100 percent of the neutrophils stain with NBT. In contrast, neutrophils from CGD patients are uniformly NBT negative, whereas female carriers of X-linked CGD exhibit a mixture of NBT-positive and -negative cells due to the expression of only one of the X chromosomes in any somatic female cell (lyonization). Although the average distribution of the two cell types is 50/50, skewing toward a higher proportion of either defective (i.e., CGD) or normal cells occurs. Most female carriers of CGD maintain good health and normal host defenses, but some develop either a cutaneous syndrome similar to discoid lupus or systemic lupus erythematosus.[276,277] Rarely, these carriers may experience recurrent infections. In general, the severity of the clinical problems in X-linked carriers is related directly to the proportion of their neutrophils that express the CGD phenotype.

The management of patients with CGD is based largely on the early recognition and aggressive treatment of infections. Specific microbiologic diagnosis should be established whenever possible. If empiric therapy is necessary it should be based on the characteristic pathogens encountered (i.e., *S. aureus* and certain gram-negative bacilli). Surgical incision and drainage are often required, although the surgeon may encounter an inflammatory granulomatous mass rather than a discrete abscess. Since the utility of granulocyte transfusions has not been established, they are not generally recommended, although their use in severe infections unresponsive to standard treatment may be worth considering. Prophylactic use of antimicrobial agents is of well-established benefit in patients with CGD.[278] Effective agents include trimethoprim–sulfamethoxazole, antistaphylococcal penicillins, clindamycin, and perhaps rifampin if combined with another agent to retard the emergence of resistant staphylococci. In patients who continue to experience morbidity from infections in spite of prophylactic antimicrobial agents, the use of recombinant IFN-γ should be considered. This agent given in a dose of 50 μg/m^2 three times weekly by the subcutaneous route was shown to result in an overall 72 percent reduction in the incidence of serious infections.[279] Efficacy was demonstrated in both X-linked and autosomal forms of the disease, and relatively few side effects were noted. Notwithstanding the effects of IFN-γ on oxidative metabolism and microbicidal activity of CGD phagocytes,[280–282] the mechanism of action in patients is not clear.[283] In a rare kindred with a defect in the regulatory domain of the gp91*phox* subunit of cytochrome b$_{558}$, the cytokine appears to upregulate gene expression and restore cytochrome synthesis and function to normal.[284] Clearly this is not the mechanism of action in the large majority of patients having mutations affecting the coding regions of the genes. In

the IFN-γ study there was also a trend toward improvement in obstructive disease of the gastrointestinal and urinary tracts, although this was not statistically significant. Anecdotal experience has raised the issue of corticosteroid therapy for these obstructive lesions, but the efficacy of this approach remains questionable.

Long-term reconstitution of normal phagocyte function in CGD patients might be achieved by bone marrow transplantation. However, the morbidity and mortality of this mode of treatment are quite high, and results in a few CGD patients have been variable. Gene transfer may ultimately prove to be the preferred means of definitive treatment. At this point *in vitro* reconstitution of oxidase function in CGD cells has been achieved in several systems,[270,285–287] but gene therapy has not yet been attempted in patients. The prognosis in CGD patients has improved considerably over the last 20 years based on increased recognition, aggressive treatment of infections, and prophylactic approaches to preventing infectious complications. Whereas most patients were previously reported to die during childhood, the majority can now expect to survive into adulthood.

GLUCOSE-6-PHOSPHATE DEHYDROGENASE DEFICIENCY. Although erythrocyte and leukocyte glucose-6-phosphate dehydrogenase (G6PD) are products of the same gene, the common form of G6PD deficiency that presents as a hemolytic anemia in blacks is not associated with neutrophil dysfunction. This discrepancy is explained by the fact that this deficiency is due to an unstable enzyme, the activity of which diminishes over a period of time that exceeds the life expectancy of the neutrophil. Neutrophil dysfunction does occur in rare cases of G6PD deficiency in whites missing or having less than 5 percent of the normal levels of G6PD. The basis for neutrophil dysfunction in this disorder is that in the absence of G6PD glucose cannot be metabolized via the hexose monophosphate shunt. As a consequence, NADPH, used by the oxidase, cannot be regenerated from NADP. Aside from the presence of a hemolytic anemia, the clinical, laboratory, and genetic (X-linked) presentation is very similar to CGD. The NBT test is negative or low, as are other parameters of the respiratory burst. The failure of methylene blue to stimulate hexose monophosphate shunt activity and low levels of G6PD distinguish this defect from CGD.[288]

Granule Abnormalities. Once thought to be a rare disorder, neutrophil myeloperoxidase (MPO) deficiency is now recognized as the most common of all neutrophil functional disorders, with a frequency of 1 per 2000–4000 people for whom leukocyte counts are performed. This discrepancy is accounted for by the fact that the overwhelming majority of such individuals are healthy and that detection of this condition has been greatly facilitated by the widespread use of flow cytometry techniques that use peroxidase staining for leukocyte differential counts.[289] Eosinophil peroxidase is not affected in this disorder. An autosomal recessive manner of inheritance has been reported, but the heterogeneous expression of the defect has led to the suggestion that inheritance may be under polygenic control. Of all the patients recognized with this disorder, only six have had serious infections. Systemic candidiasis occurred in four of these patients, three of whom had diabetes mellitus.[290]

Since the cell is devoid of MPO-dependent but not other oxidative killing mechanisms, there is delayed but not absent intracellular killing in MPO-deficient neutrophils. Delayed killing is more pronounced for fungi than for bacteria,[291] which suggests an explanation for the clinical findings in this disorder. Chemotaxis, phagocytosis, and degranulation are normal, but the respiratory burst is enhanced. The supranormal oxidative metabolism may be due to absent MPO-dependent inactivation of the oxidase system[127] and may help explain the lack of clinical expression of this defect in most patients.

Normal MPO is the product of a single gene on chromosome

17. Post-translational processing of a glycosylated (89 kD) primary gene product results in a mature molecule containing heavy α (59-kD) and light β (13.5-kD) chains.[290,292, 293] The current structural model suggests that the chain content of mature MPO is $\alpha_2\beta_2$ and that processing and lysosomal targeting are independent of the mannose-6-phosphate receptor system.[294] Granule extracts from normal neutrophils contain an 80- to 90-kD MPO-related peptide in addition to the mature α- and β-chains, whereas similar extracts from completely deficient MPO neutrophils contain only the 80- to 90-kD peptide.[292] This finding strongly suggests that MPO deficiency is due to a defect in the post-translational modification of the 89-kD precursor protein, although there is a case reported that is consistent with a pre-translational defect.[295] Restriction endonuclease DNA mapping and analysis of MPO-specific mRNA obtained from the bone marrow of deficient individuals indicates that a number of heterogenous molecular defects are responsible for the phenotypic deficit in processing.[290] Recently a single missense mutation of arginine to tryptophan at codon 569 has been identified as one of the genotypes responsible for inherited MPO deficiency.[296] MPO deficiency has also been recognized as an acquired defect accompanying some myeloproliferative disorders, particularly acute myelogenous leukemia (AML). In the leukemic but not the preleukemic state this deficiency is associated with an increased risk of infection.[290] This finding coupled with analogous observations in the inherited form of the disorder indicates that the occurrence of MPO deficiency by itself does not alter the host's susceptibility to infection but, in conjunction with an additional insult (e.g., diabetes mellitus, AML), may tip the balance in favor of infection.

Specific Granule Deficiency. The absence of specific granules has been recognized in five patients with recurrent infection.[297] The peripheral white blood cell count in such individuals is normal when they are uninfected, and the diagnosis is established by the apparent absence of intracellular granules on routine Wright stain (primary granules do not take up Wright stain). Close examination reveals a bilobed nuclear morphology with nuclear blocks and clefts. In addition, eosinophils are affected in this disorder.[298] Specific granule contents (e.g., lactoferrin, vitamin B$_{12}$–binding protein) are absent, as is membrane alkaline phosphatase.[297] Unexpectedly, the neutrophils of affected patients are nearly completely devoid of defensins, proteins that normally constitute one-third of the azurophilic granule contents.[299] These findings coupled with the presence of apparently empty granule vesicles in one of these patients and the abnormal nuclear morphology suggests that the responsible defect may be a more general disorder involving membrane assembly rather than a defect unique to specific granules.[297]

Specific granules are a rich source of substances that modulate the inflammatory response, and their membranes contain receptors for a number of opsonic ligands and inflammatory mediators. Hence, it is not surprising that in vitro upregulation of these receptors is impaired and that there are associated impairments in chemotaxis, phagocytosis, and oxidase activity with certain stimuli. Of particular note, however, is the demonstration of an in vivo chemotactic defect for both neutrophils and monocytes from patients with this disorder, whereas only neutrophils exhibit a chemotactic defect in vitro. This finding supports a role for defective chemotaxis in the genesis of infection in these patients and further suggests that a constituent of specific granules may normally modulate monocyte infiltration to sites of inflammation. Neutrophils from severely burned patients and from neonates share some of the characteristics of specific granule-deficient cells.[297]

Therapy for Neutrophil Defects

Antimicrobial Therapy. The recurrent and severe infections that occur in many patients with abnormal neutrophil function

have made the administration of prophylactic antibiotics common despite concerns about colonization and infection with resistant microorganisms. The low prevalence of these disorders has made controlled trials of prophylactic antibiotics nearly impossible, although one study evaluating cloxacillin prophylaxis in the Chédiak-Higashi syndrome did not show any benefit.[300] The administration of lipid-soluble antibiotics such as rifampin and trimethoprim–sulfamethoxazole that penetrate phagocytic cells[301,302] has been advocated for patients with impaired neutrophil bactericidal activity. In this regard, the broad antimicrobial spectrum of trimethoprim–sulfamethoxazole against both gram-positive and gram-negative bacteria, coupled with its penetration and concentration within neutrophils, probably explains its apparent effectiveness in reducing infections in patients with CGD.[303] Prophylactic antibiotic therapy in patients with CGD has been associated with an increase in the infection-free interval from 9.6 to 40 months.[278] The effect of antibiotics on the intracellular killing mechanisms has received attention with the demonstration that staphylococci exposed to sublethal concentrations of cell wall active antibiotics for a short time were more readily killed by neutrophils than were staphylococci grown in the absence of antibiotics. Improved killing was due to an enhancement in nonoxidative bactericidal mechanisms and was both organism and antibiotic specific.[304] The significance of these findings for patient management is unknown.

Cytokine Therapy. Incubation of IFN-γ with granulocytic cells from patients with CGD enhances superoxide production, restores killing of S. aureus, and increases cytochrome b$_{558}$ content. In total, cells from 15 of 18 patients with cytochrome b–positive (primarily autosomal) CGD but only 7 of 21 individuals with cytochrome b–negative (primarily X-linked) CGD responded to IFN-γ. In vitro testing appeared predictive of a response in vivo in five patients who received subcutaneous injections of recombinant human IFN-γ. Moreover in vivo responses persisted for 3–5 weeks following cessation of therapy.[280–282] A controlled international cooperative study has demonstrated clinical benefits in treating patients with IFN-γ,[279] although the biochemical basis for the clinical improvement is not known.[283] In addition, a number of laboratories are developing techniques for gene therapy directed at the specific molecular defect in CGD.[283] In contrast, administration of recombinant IFN-γ to a patient with type 1 LAD failed to increase neutrophil β$_2$-integrin expression and did not affect the outcome of the disorder.[305]

Granulocyte Transfusion. Granulocyte transfusions have been used therapeutically in febrile granulocytopenic patients. To achieve a theoretic blood neutrophil count of 1000 cells/mm^3 after transfusion, approximately 1×10^{10} neutrophils (all the neutrophils in 2–3 liters of blood) are required for the average adult per day. However, many patients will show no significant rise in the peripheral white cell count after transfusion of this number of cells.[306] Two basic methods of procurement have been devised: centrifugation and filtration leukopheresis. The former method uses differences in density among blood cells to achieve separation. Filtration uses the ability of neutrophils to adhere to nylon wool to achieve separation from other cells. Cells obtained by both procedures are functional both in vitro and in vivo, but those obtained by filtration leukopheresis exhibit cytoplasmic vacuolization and surface distortion as well as a loss of granule contents and reduced bactericidal capacity.[306,307] In addition, up to 75 percent of the recipients of cells obtained by leukopheresis will have transfusion reactions, predominantly fever and chills, as compared with 15 percent of the recipients of cells obtained by centrifugation.[308] Despite these differences, administration of cells obtained by either method to granulocytopenic patients with infection has been beneficial in some but not all controlled trials.[309,310] Granulocytopenic patients with proven bacterial infection who received daily granulocyte transfusions for the duration of their infection survived longer than did infected nontranfused control patients. Both groups received therapy appropriate for their infection.[308,311] Leukocyte transfusions have also been therapeutically successful when administered to a limited number of patients with neutrophil bactericidal defects and progressive infection. By using a positive NBT test as a marker, delivery to and persistence of transfused normal leukocytes at the site of infection has been documented in a patient with CGD.[312]

Although leukocyte transfusion may be beneficial for certain infected granulocytopenic patients, associated complications have limited their use. These complications include *(1)* transfusion-associated cytomegalovirus infection, *(2)* allosensitization to HLA antigens, *(3)* difficulties in locating adequate numbers of suitable donors, *(4)* risks to the donor, *(5)* extreme cost of the procedure, and *(6)* an increased incidence of acute pulmonary reactions when transfusions are given in conjunction with amphotericin B.[313,314] This latter complication is a major concern since one accepted indication for the use of leukocyte transfusions is the treatment of unrelenting fungal infection in the neutropenic host. This reaction most commonly occurs when amphotericin B treatment is initiated simultaneously with or after transfusion. It is characterized by the acute onset of respiratory decompensation, pulmonary infiltrates, and intra-alveolar hemorrhage.[314] A potentially serious complication of red cell or white cell transfusions in patients with CGD is related to the Kell-related antigen K_x. This antigen is present on the surface of red and white cells from healthy people and patients with autosomally transmitted CGD. K_x is absent from the neutrophils of most patients with the X-linked form of the disease due to the close linkage of the CGD and X_k genes on the X chromosome.[315–317] Failure to recognize this antigenic abnormality can result in severe transfusion reactions.[318] As a consequence of these complicating aspects, leukocyte transfusion seems best reserved for the patient with severe granulocytopenia or functionally defective neutrophils who has a serious bacterial or fungal infection that has not responded to appropriate antimicrobial therapy. Donors should preferably be seronegative for cytomegalovirus.

Bone Marrow Transplanation. Several patients, one with LAD and three with CGD,[319] have undergone successful bone marrow engraftment and clinical improvement. Two of the latter patients ultimately rejected their transplant but continued to enjoy clinical improvement. This result illustrates the difficulty in the meaningful evaluation of this procedure in these types of patients. Moreover, given the increased infection-free interval and survival observed with the use of prophylactic antibiotics in CGD,[278] it seems reasonable to reserve such aggressive therapy for unusual situations.

Evaluating Phagocyte Function

The most important step in the evaluation of possible abnormalities of neutrophil function is to obtain a good clinical history and white blood cell count with a differential count. Serum immunoglobulin and complement levels should be determined. An NBT test, requiring only a drop or two of blood, is simple and can be performed quickly. Further evaluation depends on the results of these simple screening tests (Table 4).[319,320]

TABLE 4. Evaluation of Neutrophil Function

White blood cell count and differential count
Adherence
Migration to site[321]
Chemotaxis[322]
Phagocytosis and bactericidal activity[323]
Postphagocytic activity
    Oxygen consumption[324]
    Hexose monophosphate shunt[325]
    Iodination[326]
    NBT reduction[275,327]
    Degranulation[328]
    Chemiluminescence[329]

EOSINOPHILS

Eosinophils are primarily tissue-based granulocytes located subjacent to the skin and mucosal lining of the respiratory and gastrointestinal tracts. In these locations they play a role in host defense against helminthic infection; hypersensitivity diseases, especially bronchial asthmia; and certain dermatologic conditions.[330,331]

Eosinophils develop from marrow stem cells over a 5–6 day period.[332] Eosinophilopoiesis in humans appears uniquely dependent on IL-5. IL-3 and GM-CSF also mediate an increase in the number of eosinophils. However, the concentrations of IL-3 and GM-CSF required for this effect are an order of magnitude greater than that for their effect on neutrophil and macrophage production, and the absolute increase in eosinophils is small in comparison with the increase in neutrophils and macrophages. More importantly, IL-5 concentrations coincide temporally with the appearance and magnitude of eosinophilia *in vivo*.[331,333]

Eosinophil maturation is accompanied by the appearance of three characteristic granule populations: primary, secondary, and small granules (Fig. 8). Primary granules are electron dense and appear during the promyelocyte stage of development. Secondary granules are recognized by their size, electron-dense crystalloid core containing major basic protein, and electron lucent matrix containing eosinophil cationic protein, eosinophil-derived neurotoxin, and eosinophil peroxidase. Small granules contain acid phosphatase and arylsulfatase B. Mature eosinophils also possess secretory IgA receptors as well as low-affinity IgG (FcγRII) and IgE receptors. Receptors for complement (CR1, CR3, C1qR, C5a), cytokines (IL-5, IL-3, GM-CSF, IFN-γ, TNF), platelet-activating factor, and LTB4 have also been reported.[331] The number and functional competence of these receptors are presumably regulated in a manner analogous to that documented for neutrophils.

Circulating eosinophils can be separated into two populations based on their buoyant density. Most of the eosinophils in normal individuals are characterized as dense or normodense. Hypodense eosinophils are cells that have been activated: they express a greater number of functionally competent receptors, exhibit a higher resting level of oxidative metabolism, and predominate in the blood and tissues of persons with eosinophilia.[331] As with eosinophilopoiesis, IL-5 appears to play a major role in initiating this activated state.[331,333]

The intravascular half-life of eosinophils is about 2 hours. Eosinophil migration from the vasculature has not been as well clarified as for neutrophils. Basal adherence to endothelial cells is high and involves divalent cations. It is inhibited at 4°C, sug-

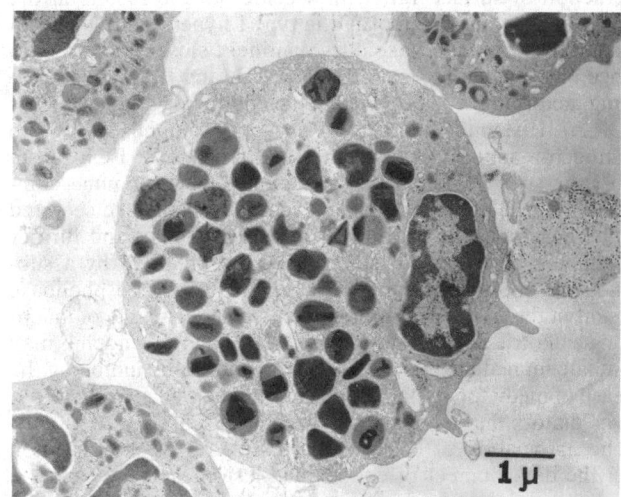

FIG. 8. Electron micrograph of a human eosinophil. Note the prominent granules with crystalloid cores.

gesting that selectin-dependent attachment, which is temperature independent, may not play a role in this process. Moreover, E-selectin is clearly not involved in eosinophil–endothelial cell interactions. β_2-Integrin–ICAM-1 interactions play a significant role in eosinophil adherence, but the observation that eosinophil transmigration is normal in type 1 LAD provides evidence for an added level of specificity in this process. This specificity appears to be mediated by IL-5–dependent upregulation of very late activation antigen-4 (VLA-4) on eosinophils and its counterreceptor, vascular cell adhesion molecule-1 (VCAM-1), on endothelial cells.[334]

In murine models of helminthic infection the major source of IL-5 is the T-helper cell subset, TH-2. The outcome of the infection appears to depend on whether TH-1 or TH-2 cell responses predominate as well as on the identity of the parasites. Since IL-5 is intimately involved in eosinophil production, activation, and transmigration in humans, its modulation is an attractive therapeutic strategy for affecting this type of eosinophil-dependent event.[331,333]

Substantial evidence supports a role for eosinophils in immunity to helminthic parasites as demonstrated by the greater worm burden and tissue damage in animals treated with antieosinophil serum and by the finding that the transfer of passive immunity requires the presence of these cells. This conclusion is buttressed by the demonstration of eosinophils on and around degenerating parasites *in vivo* and by the ability of eosinophils to kill these organisms *in vitro*.[335,336]

Killing of parasites is related to exocytosis of eosinophil granule contents onto the parasite surface while it is in close apposition to the eosinophils.[337,338] The eosinophil peroxidase, hydrogen peroxide, halide oxidation system plays a minor role in anthelminthic activity.[330,339] Rather, the cationic granule proteins are responsible for the bulk of this activity. These proteins appear to have different sites of action as inferred from different morphologic alterations in the parasite surface and internal tissues that are observed upon incubation of the organism with purified preparations of the various proteins. Synergistic activity among proteins with different loci of action may occur. On a molar basis eosinophil cationic protein exerts a more potent antihelminthic effect than does major basic protein, but the greater quantity of the latter in the eosinophil makes its contribution more significant.[331] The effect of these proteins is also specific for different stages in the life cycle of the parasite.[331,340]

Recognition that eosinophil granules contain a number of substances capable of inactivating the chemical mediators of anaphylaxis has led to the suggestion that the eosinophil may modulate the severity of type I hypersensitivity reactions.[341,342] In this scenario, stimulation of basophils and mast cells by the interaction of surface IgE with specific antigen results in the release of substances important in type I hypersensitivity reactions. These include vasoactive amines, slow-reacting substance of anaphylaxis (leukotrienes C, D, and E), platelet-activating factor, and eosinophil chemotactic factor of anaphylaxis (ECF-A). Histamine and ECF-A attract eosinophils to the site of antigen reaction with basophils and mast cells. ECF-A can also stimulate eosinophil degranulation, as can immune complexes that the eosinophil phagocytizes. Histaminase secreted by the eosinophil may inactivate local histamine, and further histamine secretion by basophils may be inhibited by a substance present in eosinophils. Arylsulfatase and phospholipase present in the smaller eosinophil granules are capable of inactivating leukotrienes C, D, and E and PAF. Thus, eosinophils may modulate immediate hypersensitivity reactions by inhibiting the release of mediators of the type I reaction as well as by destroying mediators that have already been released.[330, 342]

The association of eosinophilia of several weeks' duration with the development of endocardial lesions and the isolation of an eosinophil-derived neurotoxin capable of reproducing the neurologic picture observed in patients with cerebrospinal fluid eosinophilia strongly supports a role for the eosinophil in the

pathogenesis of tissue injury in certain disorders. Most prominent among these disorders is bronchial asthma. Here substantial evidence indicates that eosinophil major basic protein (MBP) is an important mediator of tissue injury. For example, increased quantities of MBP are detectable in the bronchial washings from patients with asthma but not other pulmonary disorders. Nanomolar concentrations of MBP but not other cationic proteins cause exfoliation of epithelial cells, impaired ciliary function, net chloride secretion, and bronchial hyperreactivity. Immunofluorescent staining of bronchial epithelium in autopsy specimens from patients dying of asthma reveals extensive deposition of MBP in the peribronchial areas and overlying regions of bronchial epithelial denudation. These findings were not observed in autopsy material obtained from patients whose deaths were related to other pulmonary diseases. The importance of epithelial denudation lies in the resultant enhanced responsiveness of the underlying bronchial smooth muscle to contractile agonists, including acetylcholine, and histamine, as well as leukotriene C_4 produced by eosinophils.[331]

REFERENCES

1. Silverstein AM. Cellular versus humoral immunity: Determinants and consequences of an epic 19th century battle. Cell Immunol. 1979;48:208.
2. Hirsch JG. Host resistance to infectious diseases—A centennial. Adv Host Defense Mech. 1982;1:1.
3. Starnes HF Jr. Biological effects and possible clinical applications of interleukin 1. Semin Hematol. 1991;28(Suppl 2):34–41.
4. Bagby GC. Interleukin-1 and hematopoiesis. Blood. 1989;3:152–61.
5. Heyworth CM, Whetton AD, Nicholls S, et al. Stem cell factor directly stimulates the development of enriched granulocyte-macrophage colony-forming cells and promotes the effects of other colony-stimulating factors. Blood. 1992;80:2230–6.
6. Colotta F, Re F, Polentarutti N, et al. Modulation of granulocyte survival and programmed cell death by cytokines and bacterial products. Blood. 1992; 80:2012–20.
7. Bainton DF. Differentiation of human neutrophilic granulocytes: Normal and abnormal. Prog Clin Biol Res. 1977;13:1.
8. Glasser L, Fiederlein RL. Functional differentiation of normal human neutrophils. Blood. 1987;69:937–44.
9. Zakhireh B, Root RK. Development of oxidase activity by human bone marrow granulocytes. Blood. 1979;54:429.
10. Lichtman MA, Chamberlain JK, Weed RI, et al. The regulation of the release of granulocytes from normal marrow. Prog Clin Biol Res. 1977;13:53.
11. Bainton DF, Farquhar MG. Origin of granules in polymorphonuclear leukocytes. J Cell Biol. 1966;28:277.
12. Bretz U, Baggiolini M. Biochemical and morphological characterization of azurophil and specific granules of human neutrophilic polymorphonuclear leukocytes. J Cell Biol. 1974;63:251.
13. West BC, Rosenthal AS, Gelb NA, et al. Separation and characterization of human neutrophil granules. Am J Pathol. 1974;77:41.
14. Dewald B, Bretz U, Baggiolini M. Release of gelatinase from a novel secretory compartment of human neutrophils. J Clin Invest. 1982;70:518–25.
15. Brederoo P, van der Meulen J, Mommaas-Kienhuis AM. Development of the granule population in neutrophil granulocytes from human bone marrow. Cell Tissue Res. 1983;234:469–96.
16. Calafat J, Kuijpers TW, Janssen H, et al. Evidence for small intracellular vesicles in human blood phagocytes containing cytochrome b558 and the adhesion molecule CD11b/CD18. Blood. 1993;81:3122–9.
17. Southwick FS, Stossel TP. Contractile proteins in leukocyte function. Semin Hematol. 1983;20:305.
18. Stossel TP, Hartwig JH, Yin HL, et al. The motor of leukocytes. Fed Proc. 1984;43:2760–3.
19. Stossel TP. On the crawling of animal cells. Science. 1993;260:1086–94.
20. Stevenson KB, Clark RA, Nauseef WM. Fodrin and band 4.1 in a plasma membrane-associated fraction of human neutrophils. Blood. 1989;74: 2136–43.
21. White JR, Naccache PH, Sha'afi RI. Stimulation by chemotactic factor of actin association with the cytoskeleton in rabbit neutrophils. J Biol Chem. 1983;258:14041–7.
22. Ryder MI, Weinreb RN, Niederman R. The organization of actin filaments in human polymorphonuclear leukocytes. Anat Rec. 1984;209:7–20.
23. Jesaitis AJ, Tolley JO, Painter RG, et al. Membrane-cytoskeleton interactions and the regulation of chemotactic peptide-induced activation of human granulocytes: The effects of dihydrocytochalasin B. J Cell Biochem. 1985; 27:241–53.
24. Jesaitis AJ, Tolley JO, Allen RA. Receptor-cytoskeleton interactions and membrane traffic may regulate chemoattractant-induced superoxide production in human granulocytes. J Biol Chem. 1986;261:13662–9.
25. Quinn MT, Parkos CA, Jesaitis AJ. The lateral organization of components of the membrane skeleton and superoxide generation in the plasma mem-

brane of stimulated human neutrophils. Biochim Biophys Acta. 1989;987: 83–94.

26. Jesaitis AJ. Signal transduction in neutrophil membrane domains. Comments Mol Cell Biophys. 1992;8:97–114.
27. Berlin RD, Fera JP. Changes in membrane microviscosity associated with phagocytosis: Effects of colchicine. Proc Natl Acad Sci USA. 1977;74:1072.
28. Snyderman R, Goetzl EJ. Molecular and cellular mechanisms of leukocyte chemotaxis. Science. 1981;213:830.
29. Messner RP, Jelinek J. Receptors for human gamma-globulin on human neutrophils. J Clin Invest. 1970;49:2165.
30. Lay WH, Nussenzweig V. Receptors for complement on leukocytes. J Exp Med. 1968;129:991.
31. Williams LT, Snyderman R, Pike MC, et al. Specific receptor sites for chemotactic peptides on human polymorphonuclear leukocytes. Proc Natl Acad Sci USA. 1977;74:1204.
32. Chenoweth DE, Hughli TE. Demonstration of specific C5a receptor on intact human polymorphonuclear leukocytes. Proc Natl Acad Sci USA. 1978;75: 3943.
33. Walter RJ, Berlin RD, Oliver JM. Asymmetric Fc receptor distribution on human PMN oriented in a chemotactic gradient. Nature. 1980;286:724.
34. Weinbaum DL, Sullivan JA, Mandell GL. Receptors for concanavalin A cluster at the front of polarized neutrophils. Nature. 1980;286:725.
35. Bender JG, Van Epps DE, Chenoweth DE. Independent regulation of human neutrophil chemotactic receptors after activation. J Immunol. 1987;139: 3028–33.
36. Korchak HM, Wildenfeld C, Rich AM, et al. Stimulus response coupling in the human neutrophil. J Biol Chem. 1984;259:7439–45.
37. Walker RI, Willemze R. Neutrophil kinetics and regulation of granulopoiesis. Rev Infect Dis. 1980;2:282–92.
38. Sachs L. The molecular control of blood cell development. Science. 1987; 238:1374–9.
39. Rothstein G, Clarkson DR, Larsen W, et al. Effect of lithium on neutrophil mass and production. N Engl J Med. 1978;298:178.
40. Klempner MS, Gallin JI. Separation and functional characterization of human neutrophil subpopulations. Blood. 1978;51:659.
41. Gallin JI. Human neutrophil heterogeneity exists, but is it meaningful? Blood. 1984;63:977–83.
42. Robinson JM, Karnovsky ML, Karnovsky MJ. Glycogen accumulation in polymorphonuclear leukocytes, and other intracellular alterations that occur during inflammation. J Cell Biol. 1982;95:933.
43. Butcher EC. Leukocyte-endothelial cell recognition: Three (or more) steps to specificity and diversity. Cell. 1991;67:1033–6.
44. Bevilacqua MP. Endothelial-leukocyte adhesion molecules. Annu Rev Immunol. 1993;11:767–804.
45. Lasky LA. Selections: Interpretors of cell-specific carbohydrate information during inflammation. Science. 1992;258:964–9.
46. Polley MJ, Phillips ML, Wayner E, et al. CD62 and endothelial cell-leukocyte adhesion molecule 1 (ELAM-1) recognize the same carbohydrate ligand, sialyl-Lewis x. Proc Natl Acad Sci USA. 1991;88:6224–8.
47. Larsen GR, Sako D, Ahern TJ, et al. P-selectin and E-selectin. Distinct but overlapping leukocyte ligand specificities. J Biol Chem. 1992;267:11104–10.
48. Lasky LA, Singer MS, Dowbenko D, et al. An endothelial ligand for L-selectin is a novel mucin-like molecule. Cell. 1992;69:927–38.
49. Lawrence MB, Springer TA. Leukocytes roll on a selectin at physiologic flow rates: Distinction from and prerequisite for adhesion through integrins. Cell. 1991;65:859–73.
50. Smyth SS, Joneckis CC, Parise LV. Regulation of vascular integrins. Blood. 1993;81:2827–43.
51. Cronstein BN, Kimmel SC, Levin RI, et al. A mechanism for the antiinflammatory effects of corticosteroids: The glucocorticoid receptor regulates leukocyte adhesion to endothelial cells and expression of endothelial-leukocyte adhesion molecule 1 and intercellular adhesion molecule 1. Proc Natl Acad Sci USA. 1992;89:9991–5.
52. Huber AR, Kunkel SL, Todd RF, III, et al. Regulation of transendothelial neutrophil migration by endogenous interleukin-8. Science. 1991;254:99–102.
53. Muller WA, Weigl SA, Deng X, et al. PECAM-1 is required for transendothelial migration of leukocytes. J Exp Med. 1993;178:449–60.
54. Kuhns DB, DeCarlo E, Hawk DM, et al. Dynamics of the cellular and humoral components of the inflammatory response elicited in skin blisters in humans. J Clin Invest. 1992;1734–40.
55. Gerard NP, Gerard C. The chemotactic receptor for human C5a anaphylatoxin. Nature. 1991;349:614–7.
56. Boulay F, Mery L, Tardif M, et al. Expression cloning of a receptor for C5a anaphylatoxin on differentiated HL-60 cells. Biochemistry. 1991;30:2993–9.
57. Murphy PM, Tiffany HL. Cloning of complementary DNA encoding a functional human interleukin-8 receptor. Science. 1991;253:1280–3.
58. Sullivan JA, Mandell GL. Motility of human polymorphonuclear neutrophils. J Reticuloendothel Soc. 1983;3:11.
59. Fletcher MP, Gallin JI. Degranulating stimuli increase the availability of human neutrophils for the chemoattractant f-met-leu-phe. J Immunol. 1980; 124:1585.
60. Clark RA. Chemotactic factors trigger their own oxidative inactivation by human neutrophils. J Immunol. 1982;129:2725.
61. Lee CW, Lewis RA, Corey EJ, et al. Oxidative inactivation of leukotriene C4 by stimulated human polymorphonuclear leukocytes. Proc Natl Acad Sci USA. 1982;79:4166.

62. Gordon LI, Douglas SD, Kay NE, et al. Modulation of neutrophil function by lysozyme. J Clin Invest. 1979;64:226.
63. Ofek I, Sharon N. Lectinophagocytosis: A molecular mechanism of recognition between cell surface sugars and lectins in the phagocytosis of bacteria. Infect Immun. 1988;556:539–47.
64. Bobak DA, Gaither TA, Frank MM, et al. Modulation of FcR function by complement: Subcomponent C1q enhances the phagocytosis of IgG-opsonized targets by human monocytes and culture-derived macrophages. J Immunol. 1987;138:1150–6.
65. Lew DP, Andersson T, Hed J, et al. Ca^{2+}-dependent and Ca^{2+}-independent phagocytosis in human neutrophils. Nature. 1985;315:509–11.
66. Petroni KC, Shen L, Guyre PM. Modulation of human polymorphonuclear leukocyte IgG Fc receptor and Fc receptor-mediated functions by IFN-γ and glucocorticoids. J Immunol. 1988;140:3467–72.
67. Berger M, O'Shea J, Cross AS, et al. Human neutrophils increase expression of C3bi as well as C3b receptors upon activation. J Clin Invest. 1984;74: 1566–71.
68. Stendahl O, Coble B-I, Dahlgren C, et al. Myeloperoxidase modulates the phagocytic activity of polymorphonuclear neutrophil leukocytes. Studies with cells from a myeloperoxidase-deficient patient. J Clin Invest. 1984;73: 366–73.
69. Gaither TA, Medley SR, Gallin JI, et al. Studies of phagocytosis in chronic granulomatous disease. Inflammation. 1987;11:211–27.
70. Lawrence WD, Packman CH, Rowe JM, et al. Attachment of particle bound IgG and complement to human neutrophils. Blood. 1981;58:772.
71. Stossel TP. Phagocytosis recognition and ingestion. Semin Hematol. 1975; 12:83.
72. Newman S, Johnston RB Jr. Role of binding through C3b and IgG in polymorphonuclear neutrophil function: Studies with trypsin generated C3b. J Immunol. 1979;123:1839.
73. Griffin FM, Griffin JH, Leider JE, et al. Studies on the mechanism of phagocytosis. I. Requirements for circumferential attachment of particle bound ligands to specific receptors on the macrophage plasma membrane. J Exp Med. 1975;142:1263.
74. Griffin FM, Griffin JA, Silverstein SC. Studies on the mechanism of phagocytosis. II. The interaction of macrophages with anti-immunoglobulin IgG-coated bone marrow derived lymphocytes. J Exp Med. 1976;144:788.
75. van Oss CJ. Phagocytosis as a surface phenomenon. Annu Rev Microbiol. 1978;32:19.
76. Ruoslahti E, Pierschbacher MD. Arg-Gly-Asp: A versatile cell recognition signal. Cell. 1986;44:517–8.
77. Wright SD, Griffin FM. Activation of phagocytic cells' C3 receptors for phagocytosis. J Leukocyte Biol. 1985;38:327–39.
78. Brown EJ. The role of extracellular matrix proteins in the control of phagocytosis. J Leukocyte Biol. 1986;39:579–91.
79. Clark RA. The human neutrophil respiratory burst oxidase. J Infect dis. 1990; 161:1140–7.
80. Babior BM. The respiratory burst oxidase and the molecular basis of chronic granulomatous disease. Am J Hematol. 1991;37:263–6.
81. Segal AW, Abo A: The biochemical basis of the NADPH oxidase of phagocytes. Trends Biochem Sci. 1993;18:43–7.
82. Heyworth PG, Peveri P, Curnutte JT: Cytosolic components of NADPH oxidase: Identity, function, and role in regulation of oxidase activity. In: Cochrane CG, Gimbrone MA, eds. Cellular and Molecular Mechanisms of Inflammation. New York: Academic Press; 1992;43–81.
83. Rossi F. The O_2-forming NADPH oxidase of the phagocytes: Nature, mechanisms of activation and function. Biochim Biophys Acta. 1986;853:65–89.
84. Bellavite P: The superoxide-forming enzymatic system of phagocytes. Free Radic Biol Med. 1988;4:225–61.
85. Eggleston LV, Krebs AA. Regulation of the pentose phosphate cycle. Biochem J. 1974;138:424.
86. Segal AW. Absence of both cytochrome b-245 subunits from neutrophils in X-linked chronic granulomatous disease. Nature. 1987;326:88–91.
87. Teahan C, Rowe P, Parker P, et al. The X-linked chronic granulomatous disease gene codes for the b-chain of cytochrome b-245. Nature. 1987;327: 720–1.
88. Segal AW, Jones OTG. Novel cytochrome b system in phagocytic vacuoles of human granulocytes. Nature. 1978;276:515–7.
89. Segal AW, Jones OTG, Webster D, et al. Absence of a newly described cytochrome b from neutrophils of patients with chronic granulomatous disease. Lancet. 1978;2:446–9.
90. Segal AW, Cross AR, Garcia RC, et al. Absence of cytochrome b-245 in chronic granulomatous disease. A multicenter European evaluation of its incidence and relevance. N Engl J Med. 1983;308:245–51.
91. Borregaard N, Simons ER, Clark RA. Involvement of cytochrome b-245 in the respiratory burst of human neutrophils. Infect Immun. 1982;38:1301–3.
92. Gabig TG, Schervish EW, Santinga JT. Functional relationship of the cytochrome b to the superoxide-generating oxidase of human neutrophils. J Biol Chem. 1982;257:4114–9.
93. Parkos CA, Allen RA, Cochrane CG, et al. Purified cytochrome b from human granulocyte plasma membrane is comprised of two polypeptides with relative molecular weights of 91,000 and 22,000. J Clin Invest. 1987;80: 732–42.
94. Dinauer MC, Orkin SH, Brown R, et al. The glycoprotein encoded by the X-linked chronic granulomatous disease locus is a component of the neutrophil cytochrome b complex. Nature. 1987;327:717–20.
95. Quinn MT, Mullen ML, Jesaitis AJ. Human neutrophil cytochrome *b* con-

tains multiple hemes. Evidence for heme associated with both subunits. J Biol Chem. 1992;267:7303–9.

96. Rotrosen D, Yeung CL, Leto TL, et al. Cytochrome b_{558}: The flavin-binding component of the phagocyte NADPH oxidase. Science. 1992;256:1459–62.

97. Segal AW, West I, Wientjes F, et al. Cytochrome b_{-245} is a flavocytochrome containing FAD and the NADPH-binding site of the microbicidal oxidase of phagocytes. Biochem J. 1992;284:781–8.

98. Sumimoto H, Sakamoto N, Nozaki M, et al. Cytochrome b_{558}, a component of the phagocyte NADPH oxidase, is a flavoprotein. Biochem Biophys Res Commun. 1992;186:1368–75.

99. Volpp BD, Nauseef WM, Clark RA. Two cytosolic neutrophil oxidase components absent in autosomal chronic granulomatous disease. Science. 1988; 242:1295–7.

100. Nunoi H, Rotrosen D, Gallin JI, et al. Two forms of autosomal chronic granulomatous disease lack distinct neutrophil cytosol factors. Science. 1988; 242:1298–301.

101. Volpp BD, Nauseef WM, Donelson JE, et al. Cloning of the cDNA and functional expression of the 47 kilodalton cytosolic component of the human neutrophil respiratory burst oxidase. Proc Natl Acad Sci USA. 1989;86:7195–9.

102. Lomax KJ, Leto TL, Nunoi H, et al. Recombinant 47-kilodalton cytosol factor restores NADPH oxidase in chronic granulomatous disease. Science. 1989;245:409–12.

103. Leto TL, Lomax KJ, Volpp BD, et al. Cloning of a 67-kD neutrophil oxidase factor with similarity to a noncatalytic region of p60^{c-src}. Science. 1990;248:727–30.

104. Park J-W, Ma M, Ruedi JM, et al. The cytosolic components of the respiratory burst oxidase exist as a M_r (approx.) 240,00 complex that acquires a membrane-binding site during activation of the oxidase in a cell-free system. J Biol Chem. 1992;267:17327–32.

105. Heyworth PG, Shrimpton CF, Segal AW. Localization of the 47 kDa phosphoprotein involved in the respiratory-burst NADPH oxidase of phagocytic cells. Biochem J. 1989;260:243–8.

106. Rotrosen D, Leto TL. Phosphorylation of neutrophil 47-kDa cytosolic oxidase factor. Translocation to membrane is associated with distinct phosphorylation events. J Biol Chem. 1990;265:19910–5.

107. Clark RA, Volpp BD, Leidal KG, et al. Two cytosolic components of the human neutrophil respiratory burst oxidase translocate to the plasma membrane during cell activation. J Clin Invest. 1990;85:714–21.

108. Heyworth PG, Curnutte JT, Nauseef WM, et al. Neutrophil nicotinamide adenine dinucleotide phosphate oxidase assembly. Translocation of p47-*phox* and p67-*phox* requires interaction between p47-*phox* and cytochrome b_{558}. J Clin Invest. 1991;87:352–6.

109. Nauseef WM, Volpp BD, McCormick S, et al. Assembly of the neutrophil respiratory burst oxidase. Protein kinase C promotes cytoskeletal and membrane association of cytosolic oxidase components. J Biol Chem. 1991;266:5911–7.

110. Nauseef WM, McCormick S, Renee J, et al. Functional domain in an arginine-rich carboxyl-terminal region of p47phox. J Biol Chem. 1993;268:23646–51.

111. Rotrosen D, Kleinberg ME, Nunoi H, et al. Evidence for a functional cytoplasmic domain of phagocyte oxidase cytochrome b558. J Biol Chem. 1990;265:8745–50.

112. Kleinberg ME, Mital D, Rotrosen D, et al. Characterization of a phagocyte cytochrome b_{558} 91-kilodalton subunit functional domain: Identification of peptide sequence and amino acids essential for activity. Biochemistry. 1992;31:2686–90.

113. Ren R, Mayer BJ, Cicchetti P, et al. Identification of a ten-amino acid proline-rich SH3 binding site. Science. 1993;259:1157–61.

114. Pawson T, Schlessinger J. SH2 and SH3 domains. Curr Biol. 1993;3:434–42.

115. Seifert R, Schultz G. Fatty-acid–induced activation of NADPH oxidase in plasma membranes of human neutrophils depends on neutrophil cytosol and is potentiated by stable guanine nucleotides. Eur J Biochem. 1987;162:563–9.

116. Gabig TG, English D, Akard LP, et al. Regulation of neutrophil NADPH oxidase activation in a cell-free system by guanine nucleotides and fluoride. J Biol Chem. 1987;262:1685–90.

117. Ligeti E, Doussiere J, Vignais PV. Activation of the O₂-generating oxidase in plasma membrane from bovine polymorphonuclear neutrophils by arachidonic acid, a cytosolic factor of protein nature, nonhydrolyzable analogues of GTP. Biochemistry. 1988;27:193–200.

118. Abo A, Pick E, Hall A, et al. Activation of the NADPH oxidase involves the small GTP-binding protein p21^{rac1}. Nature. 1991;353:668–70.

119. Abo A, Pick E. Purification and characterization of a third cytosolic component of the superoxide-generating NADPH oxidase of macrophages. J Biol Chem. 1991;266:23577–85.

120. Knaus UG, Heyworth PG, Evans T, et al. Regulation of phagocyte oxygen radical production by the GTP-binding protein Rac 2. Science. 1991;254:1512–5.

121. Knaus UG, Heyworth PG, Kinsella BT, et al. Purification and characterization of Rac 2. A cytosolic GTP-binding protein that regulates human neutrophil NADPH oxidase. J Biol Chem. 1992;267:23575–82.

122. Philips MR, Pillinger MH, Staud R, et al. Carboxyl methylation of Ras-related proteins during signal transduction in neutrophils. Science. 1993;259:977–80.

123. Ando S, Kaibuchi K, Sasaki T, et al. Post-translational processing of *rac* p21s is important both for their interaction with the GDP/GTP exchange proteins and for their activation of NADPH oxidase. J Biol Chem. 1992;267:25709–13.

124. Quinn MT, Parkos CA, Walker L, et al. Association of a Ras-related protein with cytochrome b of human neutrophils. Nature. 1989;342:198–200.

125. Bokoch GM, Quilliam LA, Bohl BP, et al. Inhibition of Rap1A binding to cytochrome b_{558} of NADPH oxidase by phosphorylation of Rap1A. Science. 1991;254:1794–6.

126. Quinn MT, Mullen ML, Jesaitis AJ, et al. Subcellular distribution of the Rap1A protein in human neutrophils: Colocalization and cotranslocation with cytochrome b_{559}. Blood. 1992;79:1563–73.

127. Jandl RC, Andre-Schwartz J, Borges-Dubois L, et al. Termination of the respiratory burst in human neutrophils. J Clin Invest. 1978;61:1176.

128. Moore PL, Bank HL, Brissie NT, et al. Association of microfilament bundles with lysosomes in PMN leukocytes. J Cell Biol. 1976;71:659.

129. Smolen JE, Sandborg RR. Ca²⁺-induced secretion by electropermeabilized human neutrophils. The roles of Ca²⁺, nucleotides and protein kinase C. Biochim Biophys Acta Mol Cell Res. 1990;1052:133–42.

130. Smolen JE. Neutrophil signal transduction: Calcium, kinases, and fusion. J Lab Clin Med. 1992;120:527–32.

131. Ernst JD, Hoye E, Blackwood RA, et al. Purification and characterization of an abundant cytosolic protein from human neutrophils that promotes Ca²⁺-dependent aggregation of isolated specific granules. J Clin Invest. 1990;85:1065–71.

132. Ernst JD. Annexin III translocates to the periphagosomal region when neutrophils ingest opsonized yeast. J Immunol. 1991;146:3110–4.

133. Francis JW, Balazovich KJ, Smolen JE, et al. Human neutrophil annexin I promotes granule aggregation and modulates Ca²⁺-dependent membrane fusion. J Clin Invest. 1992;90:537–44.

134. Borregaard N, Heiple JM, Simons ER, et al. Subcellular localization of the b-cytochrome component of the human neutrophil microbicidal oxidase. Translocation during activation. J Cell Biol. 1983;97:52–61.

135. Goldstein IM. Polymorphonuclear leukocyte lysosomes and immune tissue injury. Prog Allergy. 1976;20:301.

136. Berridge MJ. Inositol trisphosphate and calcium signalling. Nature. 1993;361:315–25.

137. Mikoshiba K. Inositol 1,4,5-trisphosphate receptor. Trends Pharmacol Sci. 1993;14:86–9.

138. Putney JW Jr, Bird GSJ. The signal for capacitative calcium entry. Cell. 1993;75:199–201.

139. Baggiolini M, Boulay F, Badwey JA, et al. Activation of neutrophil leukocytes: Chemoattractant receptors and respiratory burst. FASEB J. 1993;7:1004–10.

140. Bender JG, McPhail LC, Van Epps DE. Exposure of human neutrophils to chemotactic factors potentiates activation of the respiratory burst enzyme. J Immunol. 1983;130:2316–23.

141. Bass DA, Gerard C, Olbrantz P, et al. Priming of the respiratory burst of neutrophils by diacylglycerol. J Biol Chem. 1987;262:6643–9.

142. Densen P, Mandell GL. Gonococcal interactions with polymorphonuclear neutrophils. Importance of the phagosome for bactericidal activity. J Clin Invest. 1978;62:1161.

143. Klebanoff SJ. Antimicrobial mechanisms in neutrophilic PMN leukocytes. Semin Henatol. 1975;12:117.

144. Klebanoff SJ. Myeloperoxidase: Occurrence and biological function. In: Everse J, Everse K, Grisham M, eds. Peroxidases in Chemistry and Biology. Boca Raton, FL: CRC Press; 1991:1–36.

145. Rakita RM, Michel BR, Rosen H. Differential inactivation of *Escherichia coli* membrane dehydrogenases by a myeloperoxidase-mediated antimicrobial system. Biochemistry. 1990;29:1075–80.

146. Rosen H, Orman J, Rakita RM, et al. Loss of DNA-membrane interactions and cessation of DNA synthesis in myeloperoxidase-treated *Escherichia coli*. Proc Natl Acad Sci USA. 1990;87:10048–52.

147. Rakita RM, Rosen H. Penicillin-binding protein inactivation by human neutrophil myeloperoxidase. J Clin Invest. 1991;88:750–4.

148. Rakita RM, Michel BR, Rosen H. Myeloperoxidase-mediated inhibition of microbial respiration: Damage to *Escherichia coli* ubiquinol oxidase. Biochemistry. 1989;28:3031–6.

149. Hurst JK, Barrette WC Jr, Michel BR, et al. Hypochlorous acid and myeloperoxidase-catalyzed oxidation of iron-sulfur clusters in bacterial respiratory dehydrogenases. Eur J Biochem. 1991;202:1275–82.

150. Rosen H, Klebanoff SJ. Oxidation of *Escherichia coli* iron centers by the myeloperoxidase-mediated microbicidal system. J Biol Chem. 1982;257:13731–5.

151. Rosen H, Klebanoff SJ. Oxidation of microbial iron-sulfur centers by the myeloperoxidase–H₂O₂–halide antimicrobial system. Infect Immun. 1985;47:613–8.

152. Thomas EL, Jefferson MM, Grisham MB. Myeloperoxidase-catalyzed incorporation of amines into proteins: Role of hypochlorous acid and dichloramines. Biochemistry. 1982;24:6299–308.

153. Klebanoff SJ. Oxygen-dependent cytotoxic mechanisms of phagocytes. Adv Host Defense Mech. 1982;1:111.

154. Mandell GL. Catalase, superoxide dismutase, and virulence of *S. aureus*. J Clin Invest. 1975;55:561.

155. Klebanoff SJ. The iron–H₂O₂–iodide cytotoxic system. J Exp Med. 1982;156:1262–7.

156. Cohen MS, Britigan BE, Hassett DJ, et al. Phagocytes, O₂ reduction, and hydroxyl radical. Rev Infect Dis. 1988;10:1088.

157. Ramos CL, Pou S, Britigan BE, et al. Spin trapping evidence for myelopero-

xidase-dependent hydroxyl radical formation by human neutrophils and monocytes. J Biol Chem. 1992;267:8307–12.

158. Britigan BE, Rosen GM, Chai Y, et al. Do human neutrophils make hydroxyl radical? Detection of free radicals generated by human neutrophils activated with a soluble or particulate stimulus using electron paramagnetic resonance spectrometry. J Biol Chem. 1986;261:4426–31.

159. Britigan BE, Coffman TJ, Adelberg DR, et al. Mononuclear phagocytes have the potential for sustained hydroxyl radical production: Use of spin trapping techniques to investigate mononuclear phagocyte free radical production. J Exp Med. 1988;168:2367–72.

160. Rosen GM, Britigan BE, Cohen MS, et al. Detection of phagocyte-derived free radicals with spin-trapping techniques: Effects of temperature and cell metabolism. Biochim Biophys Acta. 1988;969:238–41.

161. Pou S, Cohen MS, Britigan BE, et al. Spin trapping and human neutrophils: Limits of detection of hydroxyl radical. J Biol Chem. 1989;264:12299–302.

162. Mandell GL. Bactericidal activity of aerobic and anaerobic polymorphonuclear neutrophils. Infect Immun. 1974;9:337.

163. Mandell GL. Intraphagosomal pH of human polymorphonuclear neutrophils. Proc Soc Exp Biol Med. 1970;134:447.

164. Lehrer RI, Ganz T, Selsted ME. Defensins: Endogenous antibiotic peptides of animal cells. Cell. 1991;64:229–30.

165. Lehrer RI, Lichtenstein AK, Ganz T. Defensins: Antimicrobial and cytotoxic peptides of mammalian cells. Annu Rev Immunol. 1993;11:105–28.

166. Ouellette AJ, Miller SI, Henschen AH, et al. Purification and primary structure of murine cryptdin-1, a Paneth cell defensin. FEBS Lett. 1992;304:146–8.

167. Selsted ME, Miller SI, Henschen AH, et al. Enteric defensins: Antibiotic peptide components of intestinal host defense. J Cell Biol. 1992;118:929–36.

168. Hoffmann JA, Hetru C. Insect defensins: Inducible antibacterial peptides. Immunol Today. 1992;13:411–5.

169. Hill CP, Yee J, Selsted ME, et al. Crystal structure of defensin HNP-3, an amphiphilic dimer: Mechanisms of membrane permeabilization. Science. 1991;251:1481–5.

170. Zhang X-L, Selsted ME, Pardi A. NMR studies of defensin antimicrobial peptides. 1. Resonance assignment and secondary structure determination of rabbit NP-2 and human HNP-1. Biochemistry. 1992;31:11348–56.

171. Pardi A, Zhang X-L, Selsted ME, et al. NMR studies of defensin antimicrobial peptides. 2. Three-dimensional structures of rabbit NP-2 and human HNP-1. Biochemistry. 1992;31:11357–64.

172. Elsbach P, Weiss J. Oxygen-independent bactericidal systems of polymorphonuclear leukocytes. In: Weissmann G, ed. Advances in Inflammation Research v. 2. New York: Raven Press; 1981:95.

173. Ooi CE, Weiss J, Elsbach P, et al. A 25-kD NH₂-terminal fragment carries all the antibacterial activities of the human neutrophil 60-kD bactericidal/permeability-increasing protein. J Biol Chem. 1987;262:14891.

174. Weiss J, Elsbach P, Shu C, et al. Human bactericidal/permeability-increasing protein and a recombinant NH-terminal fragment cause killing of serum-resistant Gram-negative bacteria in whole blood and inhibit tumor necrosis factor release induced by the bacteria. J Clin Invest. 1992;90:1122–30.

175. Weersink AJL, Van Kessel KPM, van den Tol ME, et al. Human granulocytes express a 55-kDa lipopolysaccharide-binding protein on the cell surface that is identical to the bactericidal/permeability-increasing protein. J Immunol. 1993;150:253–63.

176. Oram JD, Reiter B. Inhibition of bacteria by lactoferrin and other iron-chelating agents. Biochim Biophys Acta. 1968;170:351.

177. Boxer LA, Coates TD, Haak RA, et al. Lactoferrin deficiency associated with altered granulocyte function. N Engl J Med. 1982;387:404.

178. Broxmeyer HE, Smithyman A, Eger RR, et al. Identification of lactoferrin as the granulocyte-derived inhibitor of colony-stimulating activity production. J Exp Med. 1978;148:1052.

179. Kijlstra A, Jeurissen HM. Modulation of classical C3 convertase of complement by tear lactoferrin. Immunology. 1982;47:263.

180. Sptiznagel JK, Shafer WM. Neutrophil killing of bacteria by oxygen-independent mechanisms: A historical summary. Rev Infect Dis 1985;7:398.

181. Zeya AT, Spitznagel JK. Arginine-rich proteins of PMN leukocyte lysosomes. J Exp Med. 1968;127:927.

182. Shafer WM, Martin LE, Spitznagel JK. Cationic antimicrobial proteins isolated from human neutrophil granulocytes in the presence of diisopropyl flurophosphate. Infect Immun. 1984;45:29.

183. Shafer WM, Martin LE, Spitznagel JK. Late intraphagosomal hydrogen ion concentration favors the in vitro antimicrobial capacity of a 37-kilodalton cationic granule protein of human neutrophil granulocytes. Infect Immun. 1986;53:651.

184. Levy O, Weiss J, Zarember K, et al. Antibacterial 15-kDa protein isoforms (p15s) are members of a novel family of leukocyte proteins. J Biol Chem. 1993;268:6058–63.

185. Campanelli D, Detmers PA, Nathan CF, et al. Azurocidin and a homologous serine protease from neutrophils. Differential antimicrobial and proteolytic properties. J Clin Invest. 1990;85:904–15.

186. Almeida RP, Melchior M, Campanelli D, et al. Complementary DNA sequence of human neutrophil azurocidin, an antibiotic with extensive homology to serine proteases. Biochem Biophys Res Commun. 1991;177:688–95.

187. Selsted ME, Novotny MJ, Morris WL, et al. Indolicidin, a novel bactericidal tridecapeptide amide from neutrophils. J Biol Chem. 1992;267:4292–5.

188. Zanetti M, Litteri L, Gennaro R, et al. Bactenecins, defense polypeptides of bovine neutrophils, are generated from precursor molecules sorted into the large granules. J Cell Biol. 1990;111:1363–71.

189. Del Sal G, Storici P, Schneider C, et al. cDNA Cloning of the neutrophil bactericidal peptide indolicidin. Biochem Biophys Res Commun. 1992;187:467–72.

190. Zanetti M, Del Sal G, Storici P, et al. The cDNA of the neutrophil antibiotic Bac5 predicts a pro-sequence homologous to a cysteine proteinase inhibitor that is common to other neutrophil antibiotics. J Biol Chem. 1993;268:522–6.

191. Leijh PCJ, van den Barselaar MTh, van Zwet TL, et al. Requirement of extracellular complement and immunoglobulin for intracellular killing of microorganisms by human monocytes. J Clin Invest. 1979;63:772.

192. Tedesco F, Rottini G, Patriarca P. Modulating effect of the late acting components of the complement system on the bactericidal activity of human polymorphonuclear leukocytes on E. coli 0111:34. J Immunol. 1981;127:1910.

193. Densen P, Mandell GL. Phagocyte strategy vs. microbial tactics. Rev Infect Dis. 1980;2:817.

194. Donowitz GR, Reardon I, Dowling J, et al. Ingestion of Legionella micdadei inhibits human neutrophil function. Infect Immun. 1990;58:3307–11.

195. Miller JF, Mekalonas JJ, Falkow S. Coordinate regulation and sensory transduction in the control of bacterial virulence. Science. 1989;243:916–22.

196. Finlay BB, Heffron F, Falkow S. Epithelial cell surfaces induce Salmonella proteins required for bacterial adherence and invasion. Science. 1989;243:940–3.

197. Groisman EA, Saier Jr MH. Salmonella virulence: New clues to intramacrophage survival. TIBS. 1990;15:30–3.

198. Dunlap NE, Benjamin Jr WH, Berry AK, et al. A "safe-site" for Salmonella typhimurium is within splenic polymorphonuclear cells. Microbial Pathogenesis. 1992;13:181–90.

199. Buchmeier NA, Heffron F. Intracellular survival of wild-type Salmonella typhimurium and macrophage-sensitive mutants in diverse populations of macrophages. Infect Immun. 1989;57:1–7.

200. Fields PI, Groisman EA, Heffron F. A Salmonella locus that controls resistance to microbicidal proteins from phagocytic cells. Science. 1989;143:1059–62.

201. Miller SI, Pulkkinen WS, Selsted ME, et al. Characterization of defensin resistance phenotypes associated with mutations in the phoP virulence regulon of Salmonella typhimuriuim. Infect Immun. 1990;58:3706–10.

202. Hassett DJ, Cohen MS. Bacterial adaptation to oxidative stress: Implications for pathogenesis and interaction with phagocytic cells. FASEB J. 1989;3:2574–82.

203. Ohno YI, Hirai KI, Kanoh T, et al. Subcellular localization of H₂O₂ production in human neutrophils stimulated with particles and an effect of cytochalasin-B on the cells. Blood. 1982;60:253.

204. Britigan BE, Hassett DJ, Rosen GM, et al. Neutrophil degranulation inhibits potential hydroxyl radical formation: Differential impact of myeloperoxidase and lactoferrin release on hydroxyl radical production by iron supplemented neutrophils assessed by spin trapping techniques. Biochem J. 1989;264:447–465.

205. Cross CE, Halliwell B, Borish ET, et al. Oxygen radicals and human disease. Ann Intern Med. 1987;107:526.

206. Hammerschmidt DE. Activation of the complement system and of granulocytes in lung injury: The adult respiratory distress syndrome. In: Weissmann G, ed. Advances in Inflammation Research. v. 5. New York: Raven Press; 1983:147.

207. Smedley LA, Tonnesen MG, Sandhaus RA, et al. Neutrophil-mediated injury to endothelial cells: Enhancement by endotoxin and essential role of neutrophil elastase. J Clin Invest. 1968;77:1233.

208. Ognibene FP, Martin SE, Parker MM, et al. Adult respiratory distress syndrome in patients with severe neutropenia. N Engl J Med. 1986;315:547.

209. Wewers MD, Gadek JE. The protease theory of emphysems. Ann Intern Med. 1987;107:761.

210. Carrell RW. α₁-Antitrypsin: Molecular pathology, leukocytes and tissue damage. J Clin Invest. 1986;78:1427.

211. Malech HL, Gallin JI. Neutrophils in human diseases. N Engl J Med. 1987;317:687.

212. Bodey GP, Buckley M, Sathe YS, et al. Quantitative relationship between circulating leukocytes and infection in patients with acute leukemia. Ann Intern Med. 1966;64:328.

213. Wright DG. Autoimmune leukopenia. In Lichtenstein LM, Fauci AS, eds: Current Therapy in Allergy and Immunology. Toronto: BC Decker; 1983:277.

214. Peters WP. The myeloid colony-stimulating factors: Introduction and overview. Semin Hematol. 1991;28(Suppl 2):1–5.

215. Scadden DT. The clinical applications of colony-stimulating factors in acquired immunodeficiency syndrome. Semin Hematol. 1992;29(Suppl 3):33–57.

216. Baldwin GC, Gasson JC, Quan SG, et al. GM-CSF enhances neutrophil function in AIDS patients. Proc Natl Acad Sci USA. 1988;85:2763–6.

217. Groopman JE, Mitsuyasu RT, DeLeo MJ, et al. Effect of recombinant granulocyte-macrophage colony stimulating factor on myelopoiesis in the acquired immunodeficiency syndrome. N Engl J Med. 1987;317:593–8.

218. Hammond WP, Price TH, Souza LM, et al. Treatment of cyclic neutropenia with granulocyte colony-stimulating factor. N Engl J Med. 1989;320:1306–11.

219. Wright DG, Fauci AS, Dale DC, et al. Correction of human cyclic neutropenia with prednisolone. N Engl J Med. 1978;298:295.

220. von Andrian UH, Berger EM, Ramezani L, et al. In vivo behavior of neutrophils from two patients with distinct inherited leukocyte adhesion deficiency syndromes. J Clin Invest. 1993;91:2893–7.

221. Frydman M, Etzioni A, Eidlitz-Markus T, et al. Rambam-Hasharon syn-

drome of psychomotor retardation, short stature, defective neutrophil motility and Bombay phenotype. Am J Med Genet. 1992;44:297–302.

222. Etzioni A, Frydman M, Pollack S, et al. Recurrent severe infections caused by a novel leukocyte adhesion deficiency. N Engl J Med. 1992;327:1789–92.

223. Anderson DC, Springer TA. Leukocyte adhesion deficiency: An inherited defect in the Mac-1, LFA-1, and p169,95 glycoproteins. Annu Rev Med. 1987;38:1975–94.

224. Anderson DC, Schmalsteig FC, Finegold MJ, et al. The severe and moderate phenotypes of heritable Mac-1, LFA-1 deficiency: Their quantitative definition and relation to leukocyte dysfunction and clinical features. J Infect Dis. 1985;152:668.

225. Nauseef WM, de Alarcon P, Bale JF, et al. Aberrant activation and regulation of the oxidative burst in neutrophils with Mo-l glycoprotein deficiency. J Immunol. 1986;137:636.

226. Springer TA, Thompson WS, Miller LJ, et al. Inherited deficiency of the Mac-1, LFA-1, p150,95 glycoprotein family and its molecular basis. J Exp Med. 1984;160:1901.

227. Kishimoto TK, Hollander N, Roberts TM, et al. Heterogeneous mutations in the β subunit common to the LFA-1, Mac-1, and p150,95 glycoproteins cause leukocyte adhesion deficiency. Cell. 1987;50:193.

228. Gallin JI. Abnormal phagocyte chemotaxis: Pathophysiology, clinical manifestations, and management of patients. Rev Infect Dis. 1981;3:1196.

229. Van Epps DE, Williams RC. Suppression of leukocyte chemotaxis by human IgA myeloma components. J Exp Med. 1976;144:1227.

230. Perez HD, Lipton M, Goldstein IM. A specific inhibitor of complement (C5)–derived chemotactic activity in serum from patients with systemic lupus erythematosus. J Clin Invest. 1978;62:29.

231. Perez HD, Hooper C, Volanakis J, et al. Specific inhibitor of complement derived chemotactic activity in systemic lupus erythematosus related antigenically to the Bb fragment of human factor B. J Immunol. 1987;139:484.

232. Clark RA, Page RC, Wilde G. Defective neutrophil chemotaxis in juvenile periodontis. Infect Immun. 1977;18:694.

233. Van Dyke TE. Role of the neutrophil in oral disease: Receptor deficiency in leukocytes from patients with juvenile periodontitis. Rev Infect Dis. 1985;7:419.

234. Perez HD, Kelly E, Elfman F, et al. Defective polymorphonuclear leukocyte formyl peptide receptor(s) in juvenile periodontitis. J Clin Invest. 1991;87:971–6.

235. Shurin SB, Socransky SS, Sweeney E, et al. A neutrophil disorder induced by capnocytophaga. A dental micro-organism. N Engl J Med. 1979;301:849.

236. Kramer N, Perez HD, Goldstein IM. An immunoglobulin (IgG) inhibitor of polymorphonuclear leukocyte motility in a patient with recurrent infection. N Engl J Med. 1980;303:1253.

237. Rausch PG, Pryzwansky KB, Spitznagel JK. Immunochemical characterization of Chédiak-Higashi neutrophils. N Engl J Med. 1978;298:693.

238. Haliotis T, Roder J, Klein M, et al. Chédiak-Higashi gene in humans. I. Impairment of natural killer function. J Exp Med. 1980;151:1039.

239. Blume RS, Wolff SM. The Chédiak-Higashi syndrome: Studies in four patients and a review of the literature. Medicine (Baltimore). 1972;51:247.

240. Clark RA, Kimball HR. Defective granulocyte chemotaxis in the Chédiak-Higashi syndrome. J Clin Invest. 1971;50:2645.

241. Root RK, Rosenthal AS, Balestra DJ. Abnormal bactericidal, metabolic, and lysosomal functions of Chédiak-Higashi syndrome leukocytes. J Clin Invest. 1972;51:649.

242. Pryzwansky KB, Schliwa M, Boxer LA. Microtubule organization of unstimulated and stimulated adherent human neutrophils in Chédiak-Higashi syndrome. Blood. 1985;66:1398.

243. Davis SD, Schaller J, Wedgwood RJ. Job's syndrome. Recurrent "cold" staphylococcal abscesses. Lancet. 1966;1:1013.

244. Donabedian H, Gallin JI. The hyperimmunoglobulinemia E recurrent-infection (Job's) syndrome Medicine (Baltimore). 1983;62:195.

245. Donabedian H, Gallin JI. Mononuclear cells from patients with the hyperimmunoglobulinemia E recurrent infection syndrome produce an inhibitor of leukocyte chemotaxis. J Clin Invest. 1982;69:1155.

246. Dreskin SC, Goldsmith PK, Strober W, et al. Metabolism of immunoglobulin E in patients with markedly elevated serum immunoglobulin E levels. J Clin Invest. 1987;79:1764.

247. Dreskin SC, Goldsmith PK, Gallin JI. Immunoglobulins in the hyperimmunoglobulin E and recurrent infection (Job's) syndrome. J Clin Invest. 1985;75:26.

248. Donabedian H, Alling DW, Gallin JI. Levamisole is inferior to placebo in the hyperimmunoglobulin E recurrent-infection (Job's) syndrome. N Engl J Med. 1982;307:290.

249. Craddock PR, Yawata P, Van Santen L, et al. Acquired phagocyte dysfunction. A complication of the hypophosphatemia of parenteral hyperalimentation. N Engl J Med. 1974;290:1403.

250. Bisno AL, Freeman JC. The syndrome of asplenia, pneumococcal sepsis, and disseminated intravascular coagulation. Ann Intern Med. 1970;72:389.

251. Miller ME, Seals J, Kaye R, et al. A familial, plasma associated defect of phagocytosis: A new cause of recurrent bacterial infections. Lancet. 1968;2:60–3.

252. Super M, Thiel S, Lu J, et al. Association of low levels of mannan-binding protein with a common defect of opsonisation. Lancet. 1989;1236–9.

253. Turner MW, Seymour ND, Kazatchkine MD, et al. Suboptimal C3b/C3bi deposition and defective yeast opsonization. I. Evidence for the absence of essential co-factor activity. Clin Exp Immunol. 1985;62:427–34.

254. Super M, Levinsky RJ, Turner MW. The level of mannan-binding protein regulates the binding of complement-derived opsonins to mannan and zymosan at low serum concentrations. Clin Exp Immunol. 1990;79:144–50.

255. Garred P, Thiel S, Madsen HO, et al. Gene frequency and partial protein characterization of an allelic variant of mannan binding protein associated with low serum concentrations. Clin Exp Immunol. 1992;90:517–21.

256. Tauber AI, Borregaard N, Simons ER, et al. Phagocyte oxidase deficiency syndrome (PODS): A revised nosology of chronic granulomatous disease and related acquired disorders. Medicine (Baltimore). 1983;62:286–309.

257. Smith RM, Curnutte JT. Molecular basis of chronic granulomatous disease. Blood. 1991;77:673–86.

258. Curnutte JT. Chronic granulomatous disease: The solving of a clinical riddle at the molecular level. Clin Immunol Immunopathol. 1993;67:S2–15.

259. Babior BM, Woodman RC. Chronic granulomatous disease. Semin Hematol. 1990;27:247–59.

260. Casimir C, Chetty M, Bohler M-C, et al. Identification of the defective NADPH-oxidase component in chronic granulomatous disease: A study of 57 European families. Eur J Clin Invest. 1992;22:403–6.

261. Clark RA, Malech HL, Gallin JI, et al. Genetic variants of chronic granulomatous disease: Prevalence of deficiencies of two cytosolic components of the NADPH oxidase system. N Engl J Med. 1989;321:647–52.

262. Ezekowitz RAB. Chronic granulomatous disease: An update and a paradigm for the use of interferon-gamma as adjunct immunotherapy in infectious diseases. Curr Top Microbiol Immunol. 1992;181:283–92.

263. Dinauer MC, Orkin SH. Chronic granulomatous disease. Annu Rev Med 1992;43:117–24.

264. Royer-Pokora B, Kunkel LM, Monaco AP, et al. Cloning the gene for an inherited human disorder—chronic granulomatous disease—on the basis of its chromosomal location. Nature. 1986;322:32–8.

265. Parkos CA, Dinauer MC, Walker LE, et al. Primary structure and unique expression of the 22-kilodalton light chain of human neutrophil cytochrome b. Proc Natl Acad Sci USA. 1988;85:3319–23.

266. Parkos CA, Dinauer MC, Jesaitis AJ, et al. Absence of both the 91 kD and 22 kD subunits of human neutrophil cytochrome b in two genetic forms of chronic granulomatous disease. Blood. 1989;73:1416–20.

267. Dinauer MC, Curnutte JT, Rosen H, et al. A missense mutation in the cytochrome b heavy chain in cytochrome-positive X-linked chronic granulomatous disease. J Clin Invest. 1989;84:2012–16.

268. Dinauer MC, Pierce EA, Erickson RW, et al. Point mutation in the cytoplasmic domain of the neutrophil p22-*phox* cytochrome *b* subunit is associated with a nonfunctional NADPH oxidase and chronic granulomatous disease. Proc Natl Acad Sci USA. 1991;88:11231–5.

269. Casimir CM, Bu-Ghanim HN, Rodaway ARF, et al. Autosomal recessive chronic granulomatous disease caused by deletion at a dinucleotide repeat. Proc Natl Acad Sci USA. 1991;88:2753–7.

270. Volpp BD, Lin Y. In vitro molecular reconstitution of the respiratory burst in B lymphoblasts from p47-*phox*–deficient chronic granulomatous disease. J Clin Invest. 1993;91:201–7.

271. Clark RA, Klebanoff SJ. Chronic granulomatous disease: Studies of a family with impaired neutrophil chemotactic, metabolic and bactericidal function. Am J Med. 1978;65:941–8.

272. Schapiro BL, Newburger PE, Klempner MS, et al. Chronic granulomatous disease presenting in a 69-year-old man. N Engl J Med. 1991;325:1786–90.

273. Aliabadi H, Gonzalez R, Quie PG. Urinary tract disorders in patients with chronic granulomatous disease. N Engl J Med. 1989;321:706–8.

274. Ament ME, Ochs HD. Gastrointestinal manifestations of chronic granulomatous disease. N Engl J Med. 1973;288:382–7.

275. Ochs HD, Igo RP. The nitroblue tetrazolium slide test: A simple screening method for detecting chronic granulomatous disease and female carriers. J Pediatr. 1973;83:77–82.

276. Sillevis Smitt JH, Weening RS, Krieg SR, et al. Discoid lupus erythematosus-like lesions in carriers of X-linked chronic granulomatous disease. Br J Dermatol. 1990;122:643–50.

277. Hafner J, Enderlin A, Seger RA, et al. Discoid lupus erythematosus-like lesions in carriers of X-linked chronic granulomatous disease. Br J Dermatol. 1992;127:446–7.

278. Gallin JI, Buescher ES, Seligmann BE, et al. Recent advances in chronic granulomatous disease. Ann Intern Med. 1983;99:657–74.

279. International Chronic Granulomatous Disease Study Group. A controlled trial of interferon gamma to prevent infection in chronic granulomatous disease. N Engl J Med. 1991;324:509–16.

280. Sechler JMG, Malech HL, White CJ, et al. Recombinant human interferon-γ reconstitutes defective phagocyte function in patients with chronic granulomatous disease of childhood. Proc Natl Acad Sci USA. 1988;85:4874–8.

281. Ezekowitz RAB, Orkin SH, Newburger PE. Recombinant interferon gamma augments phagocyte superoxide production and X-chronic granulomatous disease gene expression in X-linked variant chronic granulomatous disease. J Clin Invest. 1987;80:1009–16.

282. Ezekowitz RAB, Dinauer MC, Jaffee HS, et al. Partial correction of the phagocyte defect in patients with X-linked chronic granulomatous disease by subcutantous interferon gamma. N Engl J Med. 1988;319:146–51.

283. Woodman RC, Erickson RW, Rae J, et al. Prolonged recombinant interferon-gamma therapy in chronic granulomatous disease: Evidence against enhanced neutrophil oxidase activity. Blood. 1992;79:1558–62.

284. Newburger PE, Ezekowitz RAB. Cellular and molecular effects of recombinant interferon gamma in chronic granulomatous disease. Hematol Oncol Clin North Am. 1988;2:267–76.

285. Sekhsaria S, Gallin JI, Linton GF, et al. Peripheral blood progenitors as

a target for genetic correction of p47^{phox}-deficient chronic granulomatous disease. Proc Natl Acad Sci USA. 1993;90:7446–50.

286. Chanock SJ, Faust LRP, Barrett D, et al. O$^-_2$ production by B lymphocytes lacking the respiratory burst oxidase subunit p47^{phox} after transfection with an expression vector containing a p47^{phox} cDNA. Proc Natl Acad Sci USA. 1992;89:10174–7.

287. Thrasher A, Chetty M, Casimir C, et al. Restoration of superoxide generation to a chronic granulomatous disease–derived B-cell line by retrovirus mediated gene transfer. Blood. 1992;80:1125–9.

288. Babior GL, Crowley CA. Chronic granulomatous disease and other disorders of killing by phagocytes. In: Steinbury JB, Wyngaarden JB, Frederickson DS, et al. eds. The Metabolic Basis of Inherited Disease. 5th ed. New York: McGraw-Hill; 1983:1969.

289. Parry MF, Root RK, Metcalf JA, et al. Myeloperoxidase deficiency. Prevalance and clinical significance. Ann Intern Med. 1981;95:293.

290. Nauseef WM. Myeloperoxidase deficiency. Hematol Oncol Clin North Am. 1988;2:135.

291. Lehrer RJ, Cline MJ. Leukocyte myeloperoxidase deficiency and disseminated candidiasis: The role of myeloperoxidase in resistance to candida infection. J Clin Invest. 1969;48:1478.

292. Nauseef WM, Root RK, Malech HL. Biochemical and immunologic analysis of hereditary myeloperoxidase deficiency. J Clin Invest. 1983;71:1297.

293. Koeffler HP, Ranyard J, Pertcheck M. Myeloperoxidase: Its structure and expression during myeloid differentiation. Blood. 1985;65:484.

294. Nauseef WM, McCormick S, Yi H. Roles of heme insertion and the mannose-6-phosphate receptor in processing of the human myeloid lysosomal enzyme, myeloperoxidase. Blood. 1992;80:2622–33.

295. Tobler A, Selsted ME, Miller CW, et al. Evidence for a pretranslational defect in hereditary and acquired myeloperoxidase deficiency. Blood. 1989; 73:1980–6.

296. Nauseef WM, Brigham S, Cogley M. Hereditary myeloperoxidase deficiency due to a missense mutation of arginine to tryptophan. J Biol Chem. 1994; 369:1212–6.

297. Gallin JI. Neutrophil specific granule deficiency. Annu Rev Med. 1985;36: 263.

298. Rosenberg HF, Gallin JI. Neutrophil-specific granule deficiency includes eosinophils. Blood. 1993;82:268–73.

299. Ganz T, Metcalf JA, Gallin JI, et al. Microbicidal/cytotoxic proteins of neutrophils are deficient in two disorders: Chediak-Higashi syndrome and ''specific'' granule deficiency. J Clin Invest. 1988;82:552–6.

300. Wolff SM, Dale DC, Clark RA, et al. The Chédiak-Higashi syndrome: Studies of host defenses. Ann Intern Med. 1972;76:293.

301. Ezer G, Soothill JF. Intracellular bactericidal effects of rifampicin in both normal and chronic granulomatous disease polymorphs. Arch Dis Child. 1974;49:463.

302. Mandell GL. Interaction of intraleukocytic bacteria and antibiotics. J Clin Invest. 1973;52:1673.

303. Gmümder RK, Seger RA. Chronic granulomatous disease: Mode of action of sulfamethoxazole/trimethoprim. Pediatr Res. 1981;15:1533.

304. Yourtee EL, Root RK. Antibiotic-neutrophil interactions in microbial killing. Adv Host Defense Mech. 1982;1:187.

305. Weening RS, Bredius RGM, Vomberg PP, et al. Recombinant human interferon-gamma treatment in severe leucocyte adhesion deficiency. Eur J Pediatr. 1992;151:103–7.

306. Herzig GP, Graw RG. Granulocyte transfusion for bacterial infections. Prog Hematol. 1975;9:207.

307. Klock JC, Bainton DF. Degranulation and abnormal bactericidal function of granulocytes procured by reversible adhesion to nylon wool. Blood. 1976; 48:149.

308. Herzig RH, Herzig GP, Grano RG, et al. Successful granulocyte transfusion therapy for gram-negative septicemia. N Engl J Med. 1977;296:701.

309. Strauss RG, Connett JE, Gale RP, et al. A controlled trial of prophylactic granulocyte transfusions during initial induction chemotherapy for acute myelogenous leukemia. N Engl J Med. 1981;305:597.

310. Winston DJ, Winston GH, Gale RP. Therapeutic granulocyte transfusions for documented infections. Ann Intern Med. 1982;97:509.

311. Alavi JB, Root RK, Djerassi I, et al. A randomized clinical trial of granulocyte transfusions for infections in acute leukemia. N Engl J Med. 1977;296: 706.

312. Buescher ES, Gallin JI. Leukocyte transfusion in chronic granulomatous disease. N Engl J Med. 1982;307:800.

313. Young LS. Prophylactic granulocytes in the neutropenic host. Ann Intern Med. 1982;96:240.

314. Wright DG, Robichaud KJ, Pizzo PA, et al. Lethal pulmonary reactions associated with the combined use of amphotericin B and leukocyte transfusions. N Engl J Med. 1981;304:1185.

315. Marsh WL, Oyen R, Nichols ME. K$_x$ antigen, the McLeod phenotype, and chronic granulomatous disease: Further studies. Vox Sang. 1976;31:356.

316. Densen P, Wilkinson-Kroovand S, Mandell GL, et al. K$_x$: Its relationship to chronic granulomatous disease and genetic linkage with Xg. Blood. 1981; 58:34.

317. Frey D, Machler M, Seger R, et al. Gene deletion in a patient with chronic granulomatous disease and McLeod syndrome: Fine mapping of the Xk gene locus. Blood. 1988;71:252.

318. Giblett ER, Klebanoff SJ, Pincus SH, et al. Kell phenotypes in chronic granulomatous disease: A potential transfusion hazard. Lancet. 1971;1:1235.

319. van der Meer JWM, van den Broek PJ. Present status of the management of patients with defective phagocyte function. Rev Infect Dis. 1984;6:107.

320. Metcalf JA, Gallin JI, Nauseef WM, et al. Laboratory of Neutrophil Function. New York: Raven Press; 1985.

321. Rebuck JW, Crowley JH. A method of studying leukocyte functions in vivo. Ann NY Acad Sci. 1955;59:757.

322. Nelson RB, Quie PG, Simmons RL. Chemotaxis under agarose: A new and simple method for measuring chemotaxis and spontaneous migration of human polymorphonuclear leukocytes and monocytes. J Immunol. 1975;155: 1650.

323. Mandell GL, Hook EW. Leukocyte function in chronic granulomatous disease of childhood. Studies on a 17 year old boy. Am J Med. 1969;57:473.

324. Holmes B, Page A, Good R. Studies of the metabolic activity of leukocytes from patients with genetic abnormality of phagocytic function. J Clin Invest. 1967;46:1422.

325. Root RK, Rosenthal AS, Balestra DJ. Abnormal bactericidal metabolic and lysosomal functions of Chédiak-Higashi syndrome leukocyte. J Clin Invest. 1972;51:649.

326. Klebanoff SJ, Clark RA. Iodination of human polymorphonuclear leukocytes: A re-evaluation. J Lab Clin Med. 1977;89:675.

327. Baehner RL, Nathan DG. Quantitative nitroblue tetrazolium dye test in chronic granulomatous disease. N Engl J Med. 1968;278:971.

328. Stossel TP, Root RK, Vaughan M. Phagocytosis in chronic granulomatous disease and the Chédiak-Higashi syndrome. N Engl J Med. 1972;286:120.

329. Allen RC, Loose LD. Phagocytic activation of a luminol-dependent chemiluminescence in rabbit alveolar and peritoneal macrophages. Biochem Biophys Res Commun. 1976;69:245.

330. Weller PF, Goetzl EJ. The human eosinophil. Roles in host defense and tissue injury. Am J Pathol. 1980;100:790.

331. Gleich GJ, Adolphson CR, Leiferman KM. The biology of eosinophilic leukocyte. Annu Rev Med. 1993;44:85–101.

332. Spry CJE. Mechanisms of eosinophilia. V. Kinetics of normal and accelerated eosinopoiesis. Cell Tissue Kinet. 1971;4:351.

333. Sanderson CJ. Interleukin-5, eosinophils, and disease. Blood. 1993;12: 3101–9.

334. Dobrina A, Menegazzi R, Carlos TM, et al. Mechanisms of eosinophil adherence to cultured vascular endothelial cells. Eosinophils bind to the cytokine-induced endothelial ligand vascular cell adhesion molecule-1 via the very late activation antigen-4 integrin receptor. J Clin Invest. 1991;88:20–6.

335. David JR, Vadas MA, Butterworth AE, et al. Enhanced helminthotoxic capacity of eosinophils from patients with eosinophilia. N Engl J Med. 1980; 303:1147.

336. Mahmoud AAF, Warren KS, Peters PA. A role for the eosinophil in acquired resistance to *Schistosoma mansoni* infection as determined by antieosinophil serum. J Exp Med. 1975;142:805.

337. McLaren DJ, MacKenzie CD, Ramalho-Pinto FJ. Ultrastructural observations on the in vitro interaction between rat eosinophils and some parasitic helminths (*Schistosoma mansoni, Trichinella spiralis* and *Nippostrongylus brasiliensis*). Clin Exp Immunol. 1977;30:105.

338. Densen P, Mahmoud AAF, Sullivan J, et al. Demonstration of eosinophil degranulation on the surface of opsonized schistosomules by phase-contrast cinemicrography. Infect Immun. 1978;22:282.

339. Bass DA. Eosinophil behavior during host defense reactions. Adv Host Defense Mech. 1982;1:211.

340. Grove DI, Mahmoud AAF, Warren KS. Eosinophils and resistance to *Trichinella spiralis*. J Exp Med. 1977;145:755.

341. Butterworth AE, David JR. Eosinophil function. N Engl J Med. 1981;304: 154.

342. Goetzl EJ, Wasserman SI, Austen KF. Eosinophil polymorphonuclear leukocyte function in immediate hypersensitivity. Arch Pathol. 1975;99:1.

BIBLIOGRAPHY

Klebanoff SJ, Clark RA. The Neutrophil. Function and Clinical Disorders. Amsterdam: North Holland; 1978.

8. CELL-MEDIATED IMMUNITY AND ITS ROLE IN HOST DEFENSE

RICHARD M. LOCKSLEY
CHRISTOPHER B. WILSON

Cell-mediated immunity (CMI) is generally considered to include those aspects of the immune response that are mediated or modulated by T lymphocytes, natural killer (NK) cells and mononuclear phagocytes. Although CMI is commonly viewed as being important in the control of infections due to microbes that survive and replicate intracellularly, it is now clear that these cells and their products play a pivotal role in regulating all aspects of the immune response. This occurs in an orchestrated manner. Thus, NK cells and macrophages, components of the phylogenetically more primitive, innate immune system, are important not only in the early phase of the cell-mediated immune response prior to development of antigen-specific, T-cell–mediated immunity, but also influence the nature of the subsequent T-cell response. The central importance of T cells, particularly the CD4 subset of T cells, in all aspects of the immune response has been clearly illustrated by the devastating effect on immune function that occurs in the acquired immunodeficiency syndrome (AIDS), in which these cells are preferentially affected. Thus, although not part of CMI in a classic sense, the optimal function of B lymphocytes and the nature of the humoral immune response are dependent on and governed by T cells and the cellular immune response.

Historically, CMI was recognized by the delayed-type hypersensitivity (DTH) response. Delayed-type hypersensitivity is manifested by the development of induration and erythema at the site of intradermal injection of antigen, which is generally maximal at about 48 hours. This is associated with the influx of lymphocytes and macrophages into the site and can be passively transferred with T cells but not with serum. Resistance to intracellular pathogens can be transferred in a similar fashion.[1,2] The understanding of these processes is progressing rapidly, reflecting advances in cellular, molecular, and structural biology. Nonetheless, our current knowledge remains incomplete.

In this chapter, the essential components of CMI are presented first. Thereafter, their integrated function in host defense is discussed. Finally, conditions in which CMI is impaired and potential strategies for augmenting CMI are presented.

MAJOR HISTOCOMPATIBILITY COMPLEX MOLECULES RESTRICT AND DETERMINE THE CAPACITY FOR THE IMMUNE RESPONSE TO ANTIGENS

Major Histocompatibility Genes and Molecules

The major histocompatibility complex (MHC) is a cluster of genetic loci, located in humans on the short arm of chromosome 6, that encode genetically polymorphic cell membrane molecules involved in binding peptides for T-cell recognition; these molecules are known in humans as human leukocyte antigens (HLA). The MHC locus encodes two structurally different types of molecules, referred to as class I and class II molecules.[3–5] Both are members of the immunoglobulin superfamily. There are three MHC class I genes in humans, designated HLA-A, -B, and -C, that encode polymorphic proteins involved in classic immune responses, including reactivity to virus-infected cells, tissue grafts, and tumors. There are three known additional nonclassic MHC class I genes (class Ib genes), designated HLA-E, -F, and -G, whose functions remain incompletely defined. In general, class Ib molecules are less polymorphic and are ex-

pressed in a tissue-restricted fashion (see below). The major human class II molecules are denoted HLA-DR, -DQ, and -DP; additional class II molecules of uncertain function have also been demonstrated. A cluster of genes that encode components of the cell cytosolic proteolytic complex, termed the *proteosome*, and transmembrane transporter genes are also in the class II gene cluster. These proteins are thought to be involved in the processing and transport of peptides to class I molecules (see below). The genes for class I and class II molecules are in separate clusters on chromosome 6 and are separated by the class III region, containing at least 36 genes, including those for complement factors C2, C4, and Bf, the cytokines tumor necrosis factor (TNF) and lymphotoxins α and β, and the heat-shock protein (Hsp) 70 genes.

Additional HLA genetic elements are also present, but those studied to date appear not to be functional genes. Each chromosome contains a complete set of these molecules. Accordingly, two alleles each of HLA-A, -B, and -C and HLA-DR, -DP, and -DQ, are simultaneously expressed on the cells of each individual. The number of alleles for each HLA molecule varies: 40 B but only about 10 C and 20 A alleles are expressed at significant frequencies in human populations; the number of D region alleles is less well known, but DR appears to be the most diverse. The diversity provided by two alleles of each HLA antigen has evolved to permit immune recognition by most individuals of the array of microbes and antigens that they encounter. Populations in which the MHC alleles are less polymorphic, such as Native Americans, may be at greater risk for some infections due to limitations in the capacity to present antigenic peptides.[6]

Structure and Assembly

The function of MHC molecules as peptide receptors is intimately tied to their assembly within the cell.[7,7a] In each case, bound peptides are involved in stabilization of the completed multimeric MHC complexes for transport and expression on the cell surface. As a rule, MHC class I molecules present peptides derived from the protein pool synthesized within the cell, whereas MHC class II molecules present peptides derived from the endocytic/lysosomal pathway (Fig. 1). The mechanisms for assembly of MHC class I and class II molecules ensure their capacities to acquire peptides from the appropriate cellular compartment. Alternative pathways by which exogenous peptides are presented with class I and cytosolic peptides with class II have been noted[8–10]; the former may be particularly adapted by macrophages.[8,11]

MHC Class I.   The heterodimeric MHC class I molecule is composed of a polymorphic heavy chain of about 350 amino acids linked noncovalently to an invariant light chain, β_2-microglobulin, of about 100 amino acids.[12] β_2-Microglobulin is required to generate stable MHC class I complexes; mice made deficient in β_2-microglobulin through gene disruption are unable to express stable MHC class I molecules on the cell surface.[13] Both are synthesized in the endoplasmic reticulum (ER). The complex is stabilized by association with a Ca^{2+}-binding protein, calnexin,[14] and perhaps other associated components that ensure proper folding. As revealed by x-ray crystallographic studies, the extracellular domains of the heavy chain, designated α_1, α_2, and α_3, are structured such that the α_1- and α_2-domains form a groove consisting of a platform of β-pleated sheets bordered by two α-helices.[15] Amino acid substitutions that generate the polymorphisms in MHC class I alleles are mostly located in the α_1- and α_2-peptide–binding domains. Peptides within the ER compete for binding within the groove in accordance with their affinities and abundance.

Peptides for MHC class I binding are generally derived from proteins within the nucleus or cytoplasm, although origin from proteins from mitochondria and from particulate antigens phagocytosed by macrophages into vacuolar compartments[8] has also been detected. Most cellular proteins targeted for degradation are processed by a large, multimeric, complex termed the

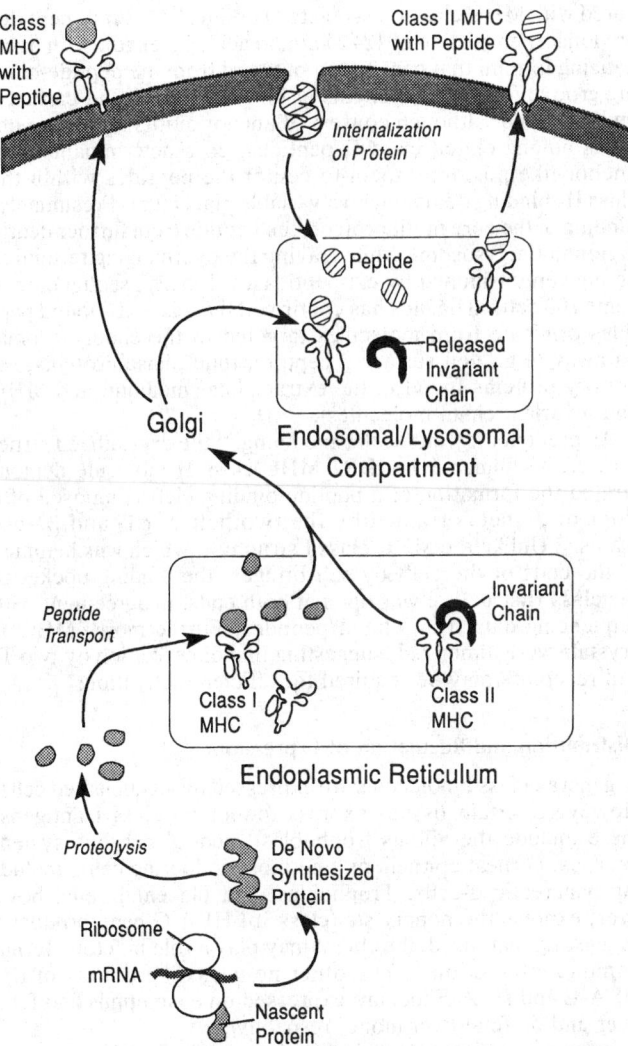

FIG. 1. Intracellular pathways of antigen presentation. Peptides that bind to class I MHC molecules are derived predominantly from cytoplasmic proteins synthesized de novo within the cell; binding takes place within the endoplasmic reticulum and is facilitated by peptide transporters (*TAP*1 and *TAP*2). The invariant chain binds to class II MHC molecules and prevents them from binding peptides until they reach an endosomal/lysosomal compartment. In this compartment, the invariant chain is released and peptides derived from internalized proteins may now bind to class II MHC. (From Lewis and Wilson,[484] with permission.)

proteasome.[16] The barrel-shaped proteasome is composed of 13–15 distinct subunits as well as 10–20 larger polypeptides and comprises up to 1 percent of the protein in mammalian cells. In conjunction with ATP hydrolysis, proteins are degraded to peptides. Although direct experimental proof that the proteasome is responsible for the production of the peptide pool available for binding by MHC class I molecules remains lacking, circumstantial evidence suggests that this occurs.[17,18] First, two genes, *Lmp*2 and *Lmp*7, are encoded within the MHC class II loci and are homologous to proteasome subunits. Second, antisera that precipitate Lmp proteins or proteasomes precipitate similar polypeptides, and both have proteolytic activity. Third, the catalytic activity of the proteasome includes an endopeptidase specific for the carboxylic side of hydrophobic amino acids, a structural motif common to peptides sequenced directly from MHC class I molecules. Despite these data, mutant cell lines lacking the *Lmp* genes were capable of presenting antigens with MHC class I.[19,20] Flanking sequences in the protein do influence the capacity to process efficiently and present peptides,[21,22] indicating that some constraints on the peptide-generating system do occur.

Following their generation in the cytosol and nucleus, peptides are thought to be transported across the ER membrane by ATP-dependent membrane transport proteins. The genes for two such proteins, *Tap*1 and *Tap*2, have been localized to the MHC class II loci. Mutant cell lines deficient in these transport proteins are markedly deficient in their surface expression of MHC class I molecules, whereas transfection of the *Tap*1/*Tap*2 cDNA restores expression to normal.[23–25] Mice with disruption of the *Tap*1 gene are deficient in MHC class I expression.[26] In the rat, polymorphisms in one of these transporters has been demonstrated to alter the spectrum of bound peptides,[27] suggesting a potential additional mechanism for generating peptide diversity, although similar polymorphisms have not been identified in humans. Although most peptides are thought to be transported to the ER, several instances in which signal sequences used normally to direct synthesized proteins into the ER have been found bound to MHC class I molecules, demonstrating that this alternate pathway also occurs.[28,29] Most biochemical and immunohistochemical studies suggest that loading of peptides onto MHC class I molecules occurs in the ER and *cis*-Golgi.[30]

Evidence suggests that the MHC class I complex in the ER participates actively in the selection of peptides for presentation, possibly by protecting the bound peptide from further proteolytic degradation. Thus the same peptides are presented by the H-2K class I molecule whether it is expressed in mouse or human cells, indicating that the proteolytic and transport pathways are conserved across species. Bound peptides in turn serve to stabilize the heavy chain–β_2-microglobulin complex, which is otherwise unstable at physiologic temperatures (31). The peptide-stabilized complexes are exported from the ER and post-translationally assembled into tetramers that are transported through the Golgi to the cell surface.[32]

Elution and sequencing of peptides bound to MHC class I complexes have begun to clarify the rules governing binding of peptides to discrete MHC molecules. Initial studies with the murine class I MHC molecules H-2K^b and H-2K^d, isolated from cells infected with viruses, identified immunodominant peptides of eight or nine amino acids.[33,34] Comparison with other known H-2K^d peptides revealed a conserved motif consisting of tyrosine in position 2 and the aliphatic residues leucine or isoleucine in position 9. Direct sequencing of pools of peptides bound to immunoprecipitated MHC class I molecules in normal cells confirmed the physical restraints to MHC-bound self-peptides that have subsequently been extended to additional mouse and human MHC class I alleles.[35,36] First, the length constraints are such that most MHC molecules preferentially bind nonamers, with some exceptions; murine H-2K^b preferentially accepts octamers, and peptides of one or two additional amino acids can be accommodated if the peptide is allowed to bulge up from the MHC groove. Second, conserved positions, called *anchor residues*, occur most frequently at position 2 and at the carboxy termini. The knowledge of length constraints and the positions of unique anchor residues for different MHC alleles allows the prediction of allele-specific peptide motifs that have been used to forecast predicted immunodominant class I–binding peptides. Third, the sequences of naturally occurring class I peptides frequently align with innate cytosolic proteins, including histones, ribosomal proteins, and heat-shock proteins or, less frequently, with signal sequences derived from normal proteins transported to the ER.

Direct x-ray crystallographic studies of discrete MHC class I–peptide complexes have demonstrated that the peptide lies within the groove of the MHC molecule in an extended linear conformation.[37–40] Over 75 percent of the peptide is buried within the groove, largely due to interactions with the ends of the peptide in pockets that accommodate the conserved anchor residues. Extensive hydrogen bonding to the peptide backbone and the positioning of minor pockets along the floor of the β-sheet allows tremendous promiscuity for the intervening peptide sequence while maintaining the high affinity required to stabilize the structure. The flexibility of the parallel α-helices allows accommodation of diverse amino acid side chains in minor pockets or through interactions with water molecules.[41] The amino acids from the middle of the peptide can variably bulge from the center of the groove, thus contributing the recognition site for the T-cell antigen receptor. These important findings explain the capacity of relatively few MHC class I alleles to bind a diverse set of peptides with high affinity.

Interest in the function of the nonpolymorphic class Ib alleles has been stimulated by the demonstration that a murine allele, H-2M3, preferentially presents peptides containing a formylated amino-terminal methionine, as occurs in prokaryotic organisms, and can present bacterial-derived peptides to cytotoxic T cells during infection with *Listeria*.[42] Direct sequencing of peptides derived from Qa-2, another murine class Ib molecule, has confirmed similar length restrictions and anchor positions as classic class I molecules, but substantially more ligand stringency, presumably reflecting the lack of significant polymorphisms.[43] As with H-2M3 ligands, screening data banks for predicted binding motifs yielded an unusually large number of matches with infectious organisms. Some γ/δ T cells have been identified that recognize antigen in conjunction with MHC CD1b molecules.[44]

MHC Class II.   MHC class II molecules are composed of noncovalently associated heterodimeric α and β transmembrane glycoproteins that are synthesized in the ER with a third component, termed *invariant chain*. Dimerization of the α- and β-chains is mediated by structural motifs in the transmembrane domains.[45] Despite its name, invariant chain exists in several distinct forms, reflecting variable translation initiation and alternative splicing forms of the molecule. A trimeric variant chain core complex associates with three α/β-dimers to form a stable nine-member subunit.[46] The associated invariant chains prevent stable peptide binding to the MHC class II molecules and facilitate export from the ER by preventing interaction with resident retention proteins. After passage through the Golgi, sorting sequences in the cytoplasmic tail of the invariant chains target the complex to an early endosomal compartment.[47,48]

Transit of the MHC class II complex from early endosomes occurs relatively rapidly, but diminished rate of transport into late endosomal and prelysosomal compartments is also mediated by sequences within the cytoplasmic tail of invariant chain.[49] This slow progression toward lysosomal compartments coincides with degradation of the associated invariant chains by proteases and restoration of the peptide-binding capacity of the MHC class II molecules. Presumably, these changes may lengthen the time for endosomal vesicle fusion to occur, thus enhancing exposure of endocytosed antigens to MHC class II molecules.

Peptides for interaction with MHC class II molecules are generally derived from proteins that are directed to the endosomal/lysosomal protein degradation pathway, whether internalized after interaction with cell surface ligands (immunoglobulin receptor, Fc receptors), by fluid phase pinocytosis, or by the targeting of endogenous cellular proteins to this compartment (transferrin receptor or invariant chain or MHC class II molecules themselves).[50] Proteases in the lysosomal pathway, particularly members of the cathepsin family, degrade proteins to expose linear sequences capable of binding to the peptide-binding regions of the MHC class II molecules. Peptides bind to MHC molecules in this low pH environment, resulting in stabilization of the complex in a more compact conformational state and enhancing their transit to and expression on the cell surface.[51] The less stable empty MHC class II molecules can be detected on the cell surface, raising the possibility that recycling into endolysosomal compartments for reloading by peptides may occur.

Direct sequencing of naturally occurring MHC class II–associated peptides has demonstrated several differences as compared with MHC class I–associated peptides.[52,53] First, peptides are longer, consisting of 12–24 amino acids in length, with overhanging termini that can extend outward from the peptide-binding groove for varying lengths at both the amino and carboxyl ends. Second, although conserved anchor motifs are not as obvious among eluted class II peptides, core determinants with anchor-like positions seem to center the peptides within the class II–binding domain with a variable placement. Presumably, binding of the core motif protects the peptide from further degradation in the lysosome while leaving the overhanging termini to be unevenly trimmed by exopeptidases. Finally, sequencing of some 200 natural ligands has confirmed that class II–bound peptides originate from molecules targeted to the endolysosomal pathway (e.g., cell surface receptors, fluid phase proteins, secretory proteins found in the extracellular medium, and MHC and invariant chain molecules).

As predicted by molecular modeling,[54] the crystallized structure of the human HLA-DR1 MHC class II molecule demonstrated the formation of a peptide-binding cleft composed of a floor of β-sheets framed by the two helical α1- and β1-domains.[55] Unlike the MHC class I structure, which was hemmed at the ends of the cleft by salt bridges, the binding pocket of the class II structure was open at both ends, in agreement with sequencing data from eluted peptides. Furthermore, MHC II crystals were dimerized, suggesting that dimerization by two T-cell receptors may be required for efficient activation.

Distribution and Regulation of Expression

In general, class I molecules are expressed by all nucleated cells. However, certain tissues express few or no class I antigens; these include the villous trophoblast, central nervous system neurons, corneal epithelium, and most endocrine cells, including pancreatic β-cells. Trophoblast and placental cells, however, express the nonclassic (class Ib) HLA-G gene products, suggesting that this determinant may play a role in fetomaternal immune interaction.[56] The other nonclassic products of the HLA-E and HLA-F loci are expressed on eosinophils and fetal liver and on fetal liver alone, respectively.[4]

Expression of class II molecules is normally restricted to antigen-presenting cells (APC). Dendritic cells and Langerhans cells in the skin constitutively express large amounts of MHC class II molecules and serve a major role in trapping and presenting antigens to the immune system.[57] Mature B cells constitutively express lower levels of class II, and circulating monocytes and tissue macrophages each express proportionately still lower amounts.

Cytokines modulate the levels of MHC expression on a variety of cell types, thus serving to focus antigen recognition at sites of cell activation. This is particularly true for MHC class II expression, which is normally more restricted in distribution. Interferon-γ (IFN-γ) enhances class II expression on Langerhans cells and mononuclear phagocytes and induces class II expression on endothelial and epithelial cells. Expression can also be induced on endocrine and stromal cells by high levels of IFN-γ, whereas neuronal cells are not affected. Class II induction allows these cells to function as APC when necessary but to be negative normally. Aberrant expression of class II molecules by such cells may lead to autoimmune injury, as demonstrated in murine models of autoimmune diabetes. Class II molecules are induced on resting B cells, and, less well, on mononuclear phagocytes, by interleukin-4 (IL-4). In various systems, induction of class II can be antagonized by bacterial lipopolysaccharides, prostaglandins, and glucocorticoids, emphasizing the important role of regulation in the expression of class II molecules. Class I expression is also increased by IFN-γ, and additional cytokines, including IFN-α and -β, and TNF. Control of MHC expression by IFN-γ is medicated at the transcriptional level and is coordinatedly regulated with associated molecules such as invariant chain, β$_2$-microglobulin, and the proteosome and peptide transporter genes located within the class II MHC loci.

T LYMPHOCYTES

The T-Cell Antigen Receptor Complex

T cells are lymphocytes that bear specific cell surface receptors for protein-derived antigen. Antigen-specific T-cell receptors (TCR) are heterodimeric molecules composed either of α- and β-chains (Fig. 2) or of γ- and δ-chains. The amino-terminal portion of each of the TCR chains is variable and involved in antigenic peptide recognition.[58,59] As discussed below, the highly variable nature of this portion of the TCR is due, in large part, to the process of TCR gene rearrangement. In contrast, the carboxy-terminal region of each of the four TCR chains is monomorphic or constant. Although the crystal structure of the TCR is not yet known, considerable insights have been gained through molecular modeling and mutagenesis studies, as well as the development of transgenic mice expressing cloned TCR of defined specificities. By comparison to immunoglobulin molecules, the TCR α/β-chains have been predicted to form analogous domains, designated CDR1, CDR2, and CDR3 (complementarity-determining regions).[58] The CDR1 and CDR2 domains are encoded within the variable regions of the TCR genes, whereas the CDR3 domain is encoded by the hypervariable region formed by the junction of the V and J regions in the TCR α- and γ-chains or V, D, and J regions in the TCR β- or δ-chains. This structure predicts that the CDR1 and CDR2 regions of Vα and Vβ sit atop the α-helices bordering the cleft of the MHC molecule, and the variable CDR3 domain sits above the peptide within the cleft itself (Fig. 2). Thus the part of the TCR that encodes variability due to the rearrangement of the TCR genes is positioned above variable peptides, whereas the relatively constant regions of the V genes are used to maintain the interaction with MHC. Studies using mice transgenic for either a TCR α- or β-chain specific for a single peptide have confirmed that reciprocal amino acid changes within the CDR3 regions can alone account for changes in specificity of the TCR.[60] Although other studies have demonstrated strong conservation of V region gene products with variable CDR3 domains for some peptides, the bulk of data suggest that the V regions are important in the generation of the structure that positions the CDR3 domain over the peptide in the MHC cleft. Thus transfer of the CDR3 region alone was incapable of conferring peptide–MHC specificity.[61] Examples for orientation of the TCR in either direction relative to the amino terminus of the peptide have been reported.[61,62] In contrast to the role of the CDR3 domain in peptide-MHC recognition by α/β TCR, peptide may not be involved in the recognition of MHC by γ/δ TCR.[62a]

The TCR dimer on the cell surface is invariably associated with the CD3 complex, a group of at least five different proteins (Fig. 2). The CD3 complex is involved in transducing a signal to the interior of the cell after the TCR has been engaged by antigenic peptide. The typical TCR complex begins assembly in the ER as dimers consisting of the α/β-heterodimer, two noncovalently associated dimers containing ε, ε/γ and ε/δ, and the ζ-homodimer (or ζ complexed to one of the other two members of the ζ family). The association between TCRαβ and CD3γδε complexes requires the presence of oppositely charged amino acids within their transmembrane domains. Basic residues in the cytoplasmic domains of the γ- and δ-chains mediate ER retention that may be required for efficient assembly.[63] Export from the ER through the Golgi complex requires the assembly of all the components except ζ, but this partial complex is degraded in lysosomes. The ζ-homodimer is required for rescue of the heptameric TCRαβ–CD3γδε2 complex for expression at the cell surface.[64] Chemical cross-linking and studies using transgenic mice expressing human CD3ε suggest that the minimal final complex consists of a TCRαβ complex in close association with the ζ-homodimer, with a CD3δε dimer flanking the TCRα chain and a CD3γε dimer flanking the TCRβ chain.[65]

α/β T cells, which bear αβ-TCR, predominate in lymphoid organs, including the thymus, lymph nodes, and spleen, as well as in the circulation. In humans, γ/δ T cells, which bear γδ-TCR, are found in only small numbers at these sites and are more abundant in certain mucosal tissues, such as the intestinal epithelium.[66] The differentiation and immunologic function of γ/δ T cells is less clear and will be discussed separately from that for α/β T cells.

Thymocyte Development and the Generation of T-Cell Receptor Diversity

Differentiation within the thymus is an obligatory step for most α/β T cells, although in mice small populations of α/β T cells found in the gut epithelium and liver may develop by a thymus-independent pathway.[67–69] It is in the thymus that, as a consequence of a rigorous selection process, recognition of antigenic peptide–MHC complexes by the αβ-TCR on mature T cells is assured of being MHC restricted (i.e., there is preferential recognition of peptides bound to self-MHC class I or class II as opposed to non-self MHC alleles).

Our current working concepts of T-cell development in the thymus are based on data derived largely from the mouse, in which normal T-cell ontogeny can be manipulated in a variety of ways, and on the phenotype of human lymphoid leukemia cell lines. Based on these data, thymocyte progenitors of the α/β-lineage of T cells can be divided into three major populations (types I–III) that reflect progressively more mature stages of development. Type I thymocytes, the least mature population, lack αβ-TCR–CD3 complexes on their surface. Since most, but not all, of these cells also lack CD4 and CD8 (accessory cell surface molecules present on nearly all mature α/β T cells), they are often referred to as double-negative (CD4−CD8−) or triple-negative (CD4−CD8−CD3−) cells. It is at this stage that rearrangement of TCR genes occurs. Type II thymocytes, a more mature population, are found mainly in the thymic cortex. These cells express low to moderate amounts of αβ-TCR–CD3 complexes on their surface along with high amounts of CD4 and CD8 (double-positive cells). It is primarily during this stage that a rigorous selection process based on TCR specificity occurs. Type III thymocytes are the most mature thymocyte population,

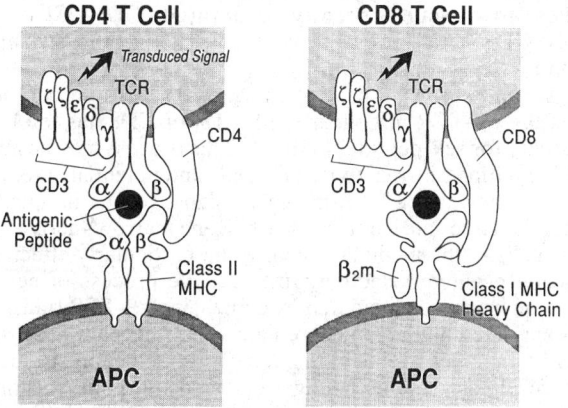

FIG. 2. T-cell recognition of antigen and activation. The α/β-T-cell receptor (TCR) recognizes antigen presented by the antigen presenting cell (APC) in the form of antigenic peptide bound to MHC molecules on the APC surface. Most CD4+ T cells recognize peptides bound to class II MHC, while most CD8+ T cells recognize peptides bound to class I MHC. This MHC restriction is determined, in part, by the affinity of the CD4 and CD8 molecules for the class II and class I MHC molecules, respectively. Once antigen is recognized, the CD3 complex of proteins, which is invariably associated with the α/β-TCR, transduces an intracellular signal that leads to T cell activation. (From Lewis and Wilson,[484] with permission.)

found mainly in the thymic medulla. They express high levels of αβ-TCR–CD3 complexes with either CD4 or CD8 in a mutually exclusive fashion (single-positive cells).

Thymocyte differentiation begins when the prothymocyte, an immature lymphoid bone marrow–derived cell in which the TCR genes have been neither rearranged nor expressed, enters into the nonlymphoid thymic rudiment. Recently, human thymocyte development has been reconstituted by transplantation of bone marrow and human fetal thymic stromal tissue into an immuno-deficient mouse (the severe combined immunodeficiency dis-ease [SCID]–human chimera system). This system indicates that human prothymocytes in the adult bone marrow are con-tained within a cell population that expresses the CD34 molecule but lacks markers for other mature cell lineages.[70] Human pro-thymocytes also may express the CD7 molecule, a protein found on thymocytes, mature T cells, and NK cells.[71] In experimental systems, a single prothymocyte appears sufficient to initiate the entire sequence of thymocyte development.[72] The thymus prob-ably does not have a population of self-replenishing stem cells and therefore requires a continual input of prothymocytes to maintain thymocytopoiesis.[73]

Their microenvironment somehow triggers type I α/β-lineage thymocytes to rearrange highly dispersed V, D, and J segments encoding the TCR β-chain gene. Subsequently, V and J seg-ments encoding the TCR α-chain are rearranged. This permits the TCR β- and α-chain genes to be transcribed and expressed as an intact protein (Fig. 2).[74] RAG-1 and RAG-2, two proteins uniquely expressed in T (and B) lymphoid progenitor cells, are required for rearrangement of TCR genes. These proteins pre-sumably form a recombinase enzyme complex that recognizes conserved recombination sequences flanking each V, D, and J segment.[75–77] Since TCR and immunoglobulin rearrangement is also abnormal in SCID mice, but the SCID mutation is located on a chromosome different than the RAG-1 or RAG-2 genes, at least one additional gene is required for effective rear-rangement.[78]

In its unrearranged, germ-line configuration, the human TCR β-chain gene consists of at least 57 V (variable) gene segments. There are two C (constant) regions, each associated with one D (diversity) and six J (joining) segments. These segments are spread over more than 600 kb of DNA on chromosome 7.[79,80] V_β segments can be divided into at least 24 families based on their sequence homology[81]; family members are typically not clustered together but, rather, widely dispersed.[79] The human TCR α-gene locus is less well characterized, but contains ap-proximately 100 V segments and 50–100 J segments. The rear-rangement of the TCR β-chain gene occurs prior to the TCR α-chain gene. Initially, the D segment rearranges to a J segment located downstream with the deletion of intervening DNA. This is followed by rearrangement of a V segment to the DJ segment. The transient expression of a complete TCR β-chain protein on the cell surface in the absence of TCR α-chain may somehow direct the development of type I thymocytes into type II thymo-cytes[82–84]; a pre-TCR complex of β-chain associated with a de-velopmentally regulated protein, gp33, may transduce signals through the CD3 complex.[84a] Rearrangement of the TCR α-chain is similar to that for the TCR β-chain gene, except that V segments are directly joined to J segments without intervening D segments.[85]

In cases in which rearrangement of the TCR β-chain gene on one of the chromosomes encoding it is does not result in a functional protein, rearrangement may proceed at the other al-lele. However, a functional VDJ TCR β-chain gene rearrange-ment appears to block rearrangement at the other allele, a pro-cess known as *allelic exclusion*. The mechanism for allelic exclusion of the TCR β-chain is poorly understood. Allelic ex-clusion is usually observed for the TCR α-chain gene as well. Once the type II thymocyte expresses a complete αβ-TCR on the cell surface, engagement of the TCR during the thymic selec-tion process may terminate RAG-1 and RAG-2 expression[86] and

prevent further gene rearrangement. The end result of the allelic exclusion is that the thymocyte normally synthesizes a single αβ-TCR protein, although the cell has the genetic information to produce two different TCR α- and β-chains.

T-cell receptors diversity is generated in part by the largely random use of V, (D), and J segments in assembling individual TCR α- and β-chain genes. In addition to this combinatorial diversity, several other mechanisms increase potential diversity at the junctions between V, D, and J. First, the recombinase is imprecise in cleaving the ends of the segments for recombination so that variable numbers of nucleotides are lost.[87] Second, TdT, an enzyme expressed at high levels in TCR gene-rearranging thymocytes, can add nucleotides (called *N-nucleotides*), appar-ently at random, to the ends of segments undergoing rearrange-ment.[87] Finally, one or two nucleotides (called *P-nucleotides*) encoded at the join region may be duplicated and added to it.[88] Together, these mechanisms for generating diversity can theo-retically result in as many as 10^{15} types of αβ-TCR.[74]

Thymocytes Are Selected Via Their Surface αβ-T-Cell Receptors

Type II thymocytes in which the rearrangement of both TCR α- and TCR β-gene are functional express moderate amounts of αβ-TCR with the CD3 complex proteins, as well as high levels of both CD4 and CD8.[89] Cells at this stage must pass a selective process that tests the appropriateness of their TCR receptor specificity, known as *positive selection*. Positive selection ap-pears to require that the αβ-TCR recognize self-peptides bound to MHC molecules.[84a,90] Type II thymocytes appear destined to self-destruct (apoptose) unless appropriate TCR-mediated in-tracellular signals from positive selection supervene. Apoptosis is due, at least in part, to activation of a nuclear DNase that destroys the genome.[91] The precise identity of peptides and their cellular sources involved in positive selection remain controver-sial. The peptides appear to be presented by class I and class II MHC molecules found on epithelial cells of the thymic cor-tex.[92–94] Recognition by the αβ-TCR of a class II MHC–associ-ated peptide may instruct the thymocyte to stop expressing CD8 and retain expression of CD4,[95,96] while recognition by the αβ-TCR of a class I–associated peptide is proposed to instruct the thymocyte to cease expression of CD4 while maintaining CD8 expression (the instructional model).[96–98] However, other evi-dence favors a random loss of CD4 or CD8 expression by CD4 + CD8 + thymocytes and that positive selection merely serves to rescue recently generated CD4 + CD8 − or CD4 − CD8 + thymocytes from cell death (the stochastic model).[99–101]

A second selective process, negative selection, can occur when the αβ-TCR in concert with CD4 or CD8 has too high a reactivity for self-peptide–MHC.[102] This process may be impor-tant in limiting self-reactivity of T cells and potential autoimmu-nity. In this case, a TCR-mediated signal results in apoptosis rather than a rescue from cell death. Bone marrow–derived den-dritic cells in the medulla appear to be particularly effective in inducing negative selection. In mice, the process of negative selection has been elucidated by expressing αβ-TCR transgenes for experimentally administered antigens[103] or natural self-anti-gens.[104] In many strains of mice, negative selection also occurs as a result of proteins (v-sags) encoded by mouse mammary tumor virus, an endogenous retroviruses.[105,106] Unlike most peptide antigens, v-sags bind to the variable portion of the TCR β-chain outside of the usual groove for antigenic peptide.[107] As a result, T cells expressing a particular V_β reactive with the v-sag may be eliminated during thymic development and not ap-pear in the periphery. Although endogenous retroviral se-quences are also common in humans, there is, as yet, no evi-dence that an analogous form of V_β-specific negative selection occurs during human thymocyte development.[108]

How positive selection and negative selection, both of which involve the interaction of TCR with peptide–MHC complexes, are independently controlled during thymic development remains unsolved.[84a,109] Positive versus negative selection might depend on whether the avidity of the αβ-TCR for peptide–MHC is low or high, respectively. Alternatively, distinct APC in positive versus negative selection might provide different signals, independently of the TCR–peptide/MHC interaction, which impact on outcome. Neither of these models excludes the possibility that thymocytes at different stages of maturation are differentially susceptible to signals involved in positive versus negative selection. As a net result of either the failure to rearrange productively an α and β TCR gene, the lack of positive selection or the occurrence of negative selection, the majority (~95 percent) of thymic precursors die rather than become mature single-positive thymocytes.[110]

Postselection Maturation in the Thymus

TCR αβ-bearing CD4+CD8− and CD4−CD8+ thymocytes are the most mature T-cell population in the thymus and predominate in the thymic medulla. Many of the phenotypic and functional differences between peripheral CD4+ and CD8+ T cells appear to be established during the later stages of thymic maturation, presumably as a result of differentiation induced by positive selection: CD4+CD8− thymocytes, like peripheral CD4+ T cells, are enriched in cells that can secrete certain cytokines, such as IL-2, and provide help for B cells in producing immunoglobulin. CD4−CD8+ thymocytes, like peripheral CD8+ T cells, are relatively limited in their ability to produce IL-2, but, once primed by antigen, are effective in mediating cytotoxic activity.[111,112] CD4+CD8− and CD4−CD8+ thymocytes enter into the circulation where they colonize peripheral lymphoid tissue. It is also during this stage of thymocyte development that thymocytes in the human cease to express the RO isoform of the leukocyte common antigen CD45 and express the RA isoform, a marker generally associated with virgin (naive) peripheral T cells (see below).

Thymocyte Growth and Differentiation Factors

The cell–cell interactions and factors secreted within the thymic microenvironment that are essential for thymocyte development are only partly understood. Studies in mice using specific gene targeting have shown that the expressions of the TCR–CD3 complex,[113] CD4,[114] CD8,[115] the *lck* tyrosine kinase (which associates with CD4 and CD8),[116] and class I[117] and class II[118] MHC are essential for normal thymic development. In contrast, other surface molecules, such as CD2,[119] and certain cytokines, such as IL-2 and IL-4,[120,121] are not essential for this process in the mouse, even though these are normally expressed within the thymus. Although IL-2 is not necessary for normal development of T cells in the thymus of mice, T-cell development in the thymus is blocked at an early stage in humans with X-linked SCID associated with mutations in the γ-chain of the IL-2 receptor.[122] This reflects sharing of the IL-2 receptor γ-chain for signalling by most T-cell growth factors, including IL-2, IL-4, and IL-7, and probably IL-9, IL-13, and IL-15 as well.[122a] TNF-α, which is normally produced intrathymically, appears to have an important role in thymocyte development.[123] IL-1 and IL-7, which are expressed by nonlymphoid cells in the thymus and can augment the growth of human fetal or postnatal thymocytes, may also support thymocyte growth and differentiation.[124–126] The subsequent steps in T-cell development and function are critically linked to their recognition of foreign antigen.

T Cells Scan Surface MHC Molecules for Foreign Peptides

As summarized above, MHC molecules constantly present peptides from the two major cellular compartments that degrade antigens—the proteosome via the incorporation into newly formed MHC class I molecules and the endolysosomal degradation system via newly formed MHC class II molecules. Under normal conditions, self-peptides do not elicit recognition by circulating T cells, since, as noted above, self-reactive T cells are deleted in the thymus or are peripherally silenced by deletion or anergy (see below). Viral infection of cells results in production of a number of new peptides within the cytosol, some of which meet the defined requirements for binding to one or more of the various MHC class I molecules expressed by an individual and become expressed on the surface of the infected cell. Since all nucleated cells express MHC class I, all such cells could present viral peptides to signal intracellular infection. At the same time, circulating viral antigens can be complexed with antibodies. The immune complexes are cleared by cells bearing Fc immunoglobulin receptors, such as macrophages. Internalization of complexes leads to degradation in the endolysosomal compartment and the potential for complexing to MHC class II antigens expressed on these cells. It is these foreign peptides, presented with host MHC molecules, that serve as the ligand for the T-cell antigen receptor. Experimental data using MHC class II–bound peptides suggest that 100–200 MHC molecules on the cell surface are sufficient to active T cells when bound to the appropriate peptide.

There are several major differences between the ways in which the T-cell and B-cell antigen receptors interact with ligands. B cells, through the surface immunoglobulin receptor, recognize intact antigens and thus the conformational determinants provided by the secondary and tertiary structures assumed by molecules in solution. T cells, in contrast, recognize peptides that assume extended linear positions within MHC molecules, an energetically unfavorable conformation for antigens in solution. Thus T cells must see antigens presented on the surface of cells expressing the appropriate MHC molecules. Second, immunoglobulins generally interact with high affinity with ligand due to their capacity to undergo affinity maturation by somatic mutation during the primary immune response. A typical antibody receptor may have a $K_d = 10^{-8}–10^{-10}$ M based on the affinity for the antibody in solution. Direct measurements of the affinity of the TCR for the MHC–antigen complex have become possible using genetically engineered soluble TCR and MHC complexes. Both indirect competition assay and direct measurements have suggested a markedly lower affinity, with K_d in the range of $4–6 \times 10^{-5}$ M.[127,128] These data have suggested that T cells survey the surface of APC through interactions with cell surface adhesion molecules prior to the cognate interaction with peptide–MHC.[129] Recognition of the latter complex in numbers sufficient to cross-link surface TCR subsequently leads to affinity upregulation of expressed adhesion molecules and lowering of the threshold for activation through the TCR.

Adhesion Receptor–Ligand Pairs Guide Antigen-Nonspecific Interactions for T-Cell Surveillance and Costimulation

A number of low-affinity receptor–ligand interactions enable T cells to survey the surface of APC, allowing reversible attachment and detachment as MHC–peptide complexes are scanned.[130,131] Resting T cells express the glycoprotein ICAM-3, a member of the immunoglobulin superfamily of receptor molecules, which forms a ligand–receptor pair with LFA-1 expressed on APC.[132] LFA-1 is a member of the β2-integrin family of adhesion receptors and is expressed as a heterodimer consisting of a unique chain (CD11α) paired with a conserved chain, CD18, shared by other members of the β2-integrin family. The reciprocal interaction between ICAM-3 expressed on monocytes and B cells, and LFA-1 expressed on T cells, also occurs. The critical role of LFA-1 in cell adhesion has been demonstrated by the capacity of blocking antibodies to inhibit T-cell adhesion to target cells and to inhibit T-cell proliferation. Importantly, stimulation through the T-cell receptor results in enhancement in the adhesiveness of LFA-1 that peaks within 5–10 minutes and returns to the low avidity state within 1–2 hours, depending on the degree of TCR cross-linking, thus allowing for de-adhesion. This regulation of LFA-1:ICAM avidity has been termed inside-out signaling.[133] Activation of the T cell results in expression of another, inducible, member of the ICAM family, ICAM-1 (CD54), that further promotes adhesion through binding to LFA-1.

A second important receptor–ligand pair involved in antigen-independent adhesion occurs between CD2, a member of the immunoglobulin superfamily expressed on T cells and some NK cells, and at least three ligands: LFA-3 (CD58), a glycoprotein member of the immunoglobulin superfamily, that is widely expressed on most cells, including APC; CD59, a glycoprotein expressed on red cells and leukocytes that inhibits complement-mediated lysis in serum; and CD48, a glycosyl phosphatidylinositol (GPI)–anchored glycoprotein member of the immunoglobulin superfamily that is structurally homologous to LFA-3 and is expressed on activated B cells, T cells, monocytes, and endothelial cells.[134,135] The genes for CD48, CD2, and LFA-3 each lie on chromosome 1 in humans, suggesting that these ligands arose through gene duplication. A role for CD2–LFA-3 conjugate formation between T cells and APC is suggested by the inhibitory effects of blocking monoclonal antibodies to these proteins, which inhibition is further enhanced by the addition of anti-LFA-1–blocking antibodies. The nuclear magnetic resonance (NMR) spectra-deduced structure of CD2 together with mutagenesis and proteolysis studies have demonstrated that binding occurs via the amino-terminal, most external of the two immunoglobulin-like domains.[136] As compared with LFA-3, binding to CD59 appears to occur at a distinct but overlapping binding site within the CD2 molecule.

T-Cell–APC Ligand Pairs: Costimuli for T-Cell Activation

The CD2 family of ligands is involved not only in cell adhesion but also in costimulation with signals through the TCR.[137] Signaling occurs both through CD2 to the T cell and through its ligands to the APC, resulting in a lowering of the threshold stimulation through the CD3–TCR complex required for activation of the T cell. Such interactions are thought to lower the energy required for cell activation through the recruitment of tyrosine kinases involved in phosphorylation of critical signal-transducing molecules, as addressed below.

Although the CD2 system is perhaps best studied, a number of other receptor–ligand interactions have been shown to contribute to what is called the *alternative pathway of T-cell activation*. Such pathways, however, require coexpression of the CD3–TCR complex and probably serve to lower the stimulation requirements by recruiting kinases and enhancing Ca^{2+} fluxes required for activation. Like CD48, a number of such molecules exist as GPI-anchored forms in the membrane, such as Thy-1 and CD59, or as transmembrane molecules, such as CD5, a member of the scavenger receptor cysteine-rich glycoproteins. The ligand for CD5 has been shown to be CD72, a B-cell surface homodimeric glycoprotein.[138] Other less well-understood ligands that seem to initiate or augment T-cell activation include CD23, CD26, CD27, CD44, and CD73.

CD4 and CD8. T cells can be divided functionally into cells that provide help for other cells of the immune system, such as B-cell antibody production, and cells that mediate cytotoxicity, such as against virally infected targets. Helper T cells express the cell surface glycoprotein CD4, whereas cytotoxic T cells express CD8. This dichotomy reflects the ability of the external domains of CD4 or CD8 to bind monomorphic determinants on MHC class II or class I molecules, respectively. Mice with disruption of the MHC class I[117] or MHC class II[95,118] genes

are unable to develop mature CD8 or CD4 cells, respectively, emphasizing the critical co-receptor roles for these two glycoproteins in T-cell development. Conversely, mice with disruption of the CD4[114] or CD8[115] genes have markedly abrogated T helper or cytotoxic function, respectively. CD4 and CD8 function not only as adhesion molecules but also as costimulatory molecules important in amplifying stimulation through the TCR.[139–141] Both are members of the immunoglobulin superfamily.

CD4 is a single polypeptide with four immunoglobulin-like domains, a transmembrane domain, and a cytoplasmic domain. The molecule extends as a rigid rod from the cell surface, enabling the distal two immunoglobulin domains to interact with a site on the β2-domain of MHC class II,[142,143] perhaps stabilized by interaction with the α2-domains formed by the dimeric class II structure.[55] The binding site for human immunodeficiency virus (HIV) seems to localize to the CDR2-like region of domain 1.[144]

CD8 consist of either α-chain homodimers or of α/β-heterodimers. The α- and β-chains consist of highly conserved transmembrane and cytoplasmic domains. Each CD8 molecule consists of a single immunoglobulin-like domain at the end of an extended glycosylated rod-like region.[145] Mutational analysis has demonstrated that CD8 binds MHC class I using the CDR-like domains 1 and 2 to interact with the α3-domain of the MHC molecule.[146] One CD8 dimer has the capacity to interact with two MHC class I molecules. Most peripheral CD8 cells express the α/β-heterodimer, which may be more efficient than α/α-homodimers in augmenting cytokine production by virtue of sequences in the external domain of the β-chain.[147] An alternatively spliced soluble form of the CD8 α-chain has also been demonstrated.[148]

T-cell activation can be markedly enhanced by coaggregation of the TCR–CD3 complex with CD4 or CD8. This costimulation is maximal when the same MHC molecule presenting antigen to the TCR is bound by CD4 or CD8.[149,150] Stimulation through the TCR seems to result in changes in the avidity with which CD4 or CD8 interacts with MHC class II or class I, respectively, perhaps by induced changes in conformation, thus enhancing cell adhesion. Furthermore, cysteine motifs within the cytoplasmic tails of CD4 and CD8 allow association with a tyrosine kinase, *lck*, that is critically involved in enhancing signaling generated through TCR activation.[151]

CD28 and B7/BB1. Optimal activation of the T cell requires stimulation not only of the TCR complex but also of a costimulatory signal delivered by the APC. This is particularly true for the initial response of T cells to a novel antigen (i.e., the primary response by virgin T cells; see below). Stimulation using monoclonal antibodies or fixed ligands without this second signal typically result in anergy, a state of unresponsiveness to subsequent stimulation, even when subsequent stimulation provides the second signal.[152] More recent studies suggest that the critical costimulatory signal necessary for effective T-cell activation is the engagement of CD28 on T cells by its ligands, members of the B7/BB1 family on APC.[153] Costimulation of the homodimeric CD28 antigen on T cells during TCR activation results in a 30-fold enhancement of IL-2 production, due both to enhanced IL-2 transcription[154] and to stabilization of the mRNA for IL-2 (and for other cytokines).[155]

The three B7/BB1 antigens are transmembrane glycoproteins and members of the immunoglobulin superfamily. Importantly, expression of B7/BB1 correlates with the capacity of various APC to activate naive T cells.[153,155a,155b] Dendritic cells are the most potent APC in humans, and perhaps the only APC capable of activating naive T cells, defined as mature peripheral T cells that have not been previously activated through the TCR. Besides MHC class I and class II molecules, dendritic cells constitutively express B7/BB1 as well as other adhesion ligands, including ICAM-1 (CD54), LFA-3 (CD58), and LFA-1 (CD11α/

CD18),[156] the ligands for LFA-1, CD2, and ICAM-3 and -1, respectively, on T cells. In contrast, B7/BB1 is not expressed on resting B cells and monocytes, but is induced with activation, including stimulation of B cells through the immunoglobulin receptor or IL-4 or of monocyte/macrophages with IFN-γ. Stimulation of B-cell lines by cross-linking of MHC class II molecules has been shown to upregulate B7/BB1 expression through signals mediated by the short cytoplasmic domain of MHC class II.[157] Additionally, gp39 (CD40 ligand), which is expressed primarily on activated CD4 T cells, can induce B-cell B7/BB1 expression following binding to CD40.[158] Thus B cells and monocytes become recruited into the pool of effective APC with activation, serving to enhance and amplify the initial stimulation of naive T cells by dendritic cells. Activated T lymphocytes and NK cells have been demonstrated to express functional B7/BB1 late after activation,[159] raising the possibility of autocrine or paracrine costimulation.

Activation of T cells leads to the appearance of a related molecule, CTLA-4, that binds B7/BB1 with higher avidity, although expression of CTLA-4 is only 3 percent of that for CD28.[160] These two antigens, which likely arose from a gene duplication event, may cooperate to activate T-cell proliferation maximally. Blockade of CD28/CTLA-4 at the time of T-cell activation results in anergy.[161] Interest in induction of anergy has increased with the demonstration that such blockade can prolong the survival of allografts[162,163] and that tranfection of B7 into malignant cells prior to challenging animals allows their recognition and rejection by host CD8+ T cells.[164,165]

T-Cell Activation Occurs through Engagement of the TCR Complex

These nonantigen-specific ligand pair interactions may transiently stabilize adhesion between the T cell and the APC, and some of the costimulatory pathways may poise the cell to receive a final activation signal through the T-cell receptor. Subsequent engagement of the TCR receptor results in rapid (5-second) tyrosine phosphorylation of a number of intracellular substrates, and inhibition of tyrosine phosphorylation results in failure of T-cell activation. These observations have focused intense interest on tyrosine kinases that are coupled to the TCR and mediate early biochemical events in the cell.[166–168] The use of molecularly engineered chimeric receptors, in which the outer ligand-binding domain consists of a convenient marker antigen and the cytoplasmic, signaling domain consists of various components of the CD3 complex, has allowed the identification of cytoplasmic domains of this complex that can mediate downstream signaling events.[169] Such analyses have identified reiterated sequence motifs within the CD3 complex, which have been designated antigen recognition activation motifs, or ARAM. ARAM are 17-amino acid sequences identified by properly spaced tyrosine and leucine or isoleucine residues. One ARAM is present in the cytoplasmic domains of both the CD3 γ- and ε-chains, and three copies occur in tandem in the ζ-chain.[170–172] Related cytoplasmic sequences occur in the immunoglobulin-associated proteins that mediate signaling in B cells and the β- and γ-chains of the FcεR on basophils and mast cells. The tyrosines within the ARAM sequence become phosphorylated following ligation of the TCR, an event required for the functional activity of the sequence. Because the patterns of cellular tyrosine phosphorylation are overlapping but not identical following stimulation of individual chimeric molecules, it is possible that the different signaling components of the TCR interact with distinct tyrosine kinases and signal transduction substrates.

The major tyrosine kinases implicated in TCR signaling include *lck*, *fyn*, and ZAP-70; the first two are members of the *src* family of tyrosine kinases. Typical *src* family kinases contain, from the amino terminus, a myristoylation site that may allow anchoring in lipid membranes, an adjoining cysteine-rich motif where CD4 and CD8 have been shown to bind, two "*src* homology domains," designated SH3 and SH2, that contain substrate interactive sites, and a kinase domain that contains critical tyrosines whose phosphorylation regulates the intrinsic kinase activity.

Lck is expressed primarily in T cells and is noncovalently associated with the cytoplasmic domains of CD4 and CD8 through cysteine residues within the *lck* amino-terminal domain. Thus CD4 and CD8 coreceptors may function not only to enhance avidity of the T cell with the MHC–peptide complex but also to bring *lck* close to the cytoplasmic domains of the TCR to mediate tyrosine phosphorylation of the ARAM sequences.[173] Mutant cells deficient in *lck* have defective signal transduction through the TCR,[174] and mice with disruption of the *lck* gene have abnormal T-cell development.[116] Sequestration of *lck* away from the TCR complex by cross-linking CD4 prior to antigen stimulation also markedly impairs TCR-mediated signal transduction.[175] The stoichiometric association of cellular *lck* is greater with CD4 (75–95 percent) than with CD8 (5–10 percent), suggesting differences in activation pathways between the two subsets.[176]

One of the two alternatively spliced forms of *fyn* is restricted to hematopoietic cells. *fyn* kinase activity has been immunoprecipitated with the TCR complex,[177] a rapid increase in *fyn* kinase activity can be measured following TCR activation, and overexpression of *fyn* in transgenic mice resulted in enhanced TCR responses.[178] *fyn* may be associated with CD3 as opposed to *lck,* which is associated with the CD4 and CD8 coreceptors. Mice with disruption of the *fyn* gene, however, had abnormalities of signal transduction predominantly in isolated single-positive thymocytes, whereas signaling in peripheral T cells was reduced minimally, suggesting that additional unknown kinases may also play a role in TCR signaling.[179,180]

ZAP-70 (zeta-associated protein, 70 kD) is expressed in T cells and NK cells and is most homologous to the *syk* tyrosine kinase expressed in B cells. ZAP-70 rapidly associates with phosphorylated ζ-chains.[181] This suggests that CD3 and ζ-phosphorylation at ARAM sequences by *lck* or *fyn* may precede binding of ZAP-70 to phosphorylated ζ. Both ζ and ZAP-70 become tyrosine phosphorylated during TCR activation. ZAP-70 binds to ζ through its own SH2 domains; this presumably serves to activate the kinase activity of ZAP-70 itself.

A final requisite component of the tyrosine activation pathway involves CD45, a transmembrane phosphatase expressed on T cells in multiple isoforms, reflecting the differential use of exons 3 through 7 during transcription.[182] Some 10 percent of the lymphocyte surface is covered by CD45, a carbohydrate-rich glycoprotein expressed only by nucleated hematopoietic cells. The external amino-terminal part of the molecule is a heavily glycosylated (at both *O*-linked and *N*-linked sites), elongated structure, and it is in this domain that the alternative splicing creates differences in sequence and overall length between the various isoforms. The transmembrane and long (705-amino acid) cytoplasmic domains are conserved among isoforms and substantially conserved across species, suggesting that preservation of signaling function is critical. Duplicated phosphatase domains are present in this cytoplasmic sequence. Mature thymocytes express the low-molecular-weight isoform CD45RO, whereas peripheral blood T cells express a variety of isoforms. Although monoclonal antibodies to distinct isoforms of CD45 have been used to distinguish subpopulations of human cells involved in inducer suppressor (CD4+2H4+) and helper (CD4+UCHL-1+) populations, it is clear that the expression of CD4+ isoforms can change with TCR activation[183] and that, in the mouse, interconversion of these phenotypes can be observed in vivo.[184] Differences in the extracellular domains of CD45 suggest that distinct ligands exist on different cells or as different soluble ligands. Binding of one isoform to the CD22 B-cell adhesion molecule has been demonstrated.[185] Coimmunoprecipitation and capping studies have demonstrated that CD45 can physically associate with a number of stimulatory antigens on the T-cell surface, including CD3, CD2, CD4, CD8, and Thy-

1, suggesting that CD45 is required for activation of the T cell. Indeed, mutant T cells lacking CD45 are deficient in TCR-mediated signaling through CD3 (or CD2) and reconstitution of CD45 by transfection restored signaling.[186,187] Furthermore, CD45 is itself phosphorylated on tyrosine following TCR stimulation.

The critical role of the CD45 phosphatase may be to dephosphorylate the carboxy-terminal tyrosine that maintains *src* family kinases in an inactive conformation. As best studied using *lck*, phosphorylation of the carboxy-terminal tyrosine Y505 may allow intramolecular binding of Y505 to its own SH2 domain, thus rendering the kinase domain inactive. Dephosphorylation by CD45 would expose the kinase domain, allowing binding of the exposed SH2 domains to tyrosine-phosphorylated substrates, such as the ARAM in CD3. CD45 has been coprecipitated with *lck*, suggesting physical association between these proteins. Evidence has been presented that *fyn* may also serve as a substrate for CD45, although the possibility that the phosphorylation state of *fyn* is mediated by other phosphatases has been suggested. Importantly, the cytoplasmic domain of CD45 was alone sufficient to restore functional TCR signal transduction in CD45-deficient mutant cell lines.[188,189] The use of chimeric ligands with an extracellular epidermal growth factor receptor domain demonstrated that dimerization of CD45 by external ligands negatively regulated TCR signal transduction, suggesting that ligation of CD45 functionally inactivates its phosphatase activity in situ.[190] Thus, CD45 may be constitutively active in vivo and may be brought into the TCR complex at the time of T-cell activation in order to activate critical tyrosine kinases by dephosphorylation. Engagement of the ligand for CD45 would then shut off further signaling by dimerization of the phosphatase, an event potentially mediated by autodephosphorylation of CD45 itself.

A number of other proteins besides CD45 are phosphorylated on tyrosine following TCR engagement. One important early substrate is a phospholipase C, PLC-γ1, whose enzymatic function becomes activated following tyrosine phosphorylation by TCR-mediated activation of tyrosine kinases.[191,192] PLC-γ1 is largely cytosolic, but translocates to the membrane to bind activated, phosphorylated receptors via its own SH2 domain. Phosphorylation results in enzymatic activation, and the proximity to the membrane allows the enzymatic hydrolysis of the lipid phosphatidylinositol 4,5-biphosphate (PIP$_2$) to the intracellular second messengers, diacylglycerol (DAG) and inositol 1,4,5-triphosphate (IP$_3$).[193] These two molecules are respectively responsible for activation of protein kinase C (PKC), a serine and threonine kinase, and the immediate mobilization of Ca^{2+} from both intracellular, sequestered stores within the ER and the sustained flow of Ca^{2+} from the extracellular medium, perhaps through activation of transmembrane Ca^{2+} channels. An IP$_3$ receptor has been localized to the plasma membrane in proximity to the activated TCR antigen receptor.[194] PKC is responsible for phosphorylation of CD3 γ- and δ-chains. The critical role for these second-messenger pathways is suggested by the capacity of PKC activation using phorbol esters to stimulate T-cell activation in the presence of Ca^{2+} ionophore. Activation of PKC has been closely linked to expression of CD69, a dimer expressed on the T-cell surface within 2–4 hours following stimulation. CD69 may play a role in mediating the Ca^{2+} influx, since some anti-CD69 monoclonal antibodies induce Ca^{2+} influx following PKC activation.[195] Another important target for PKC is a myristoylated, alanine-rich C-kinase substrate (MARCKS).[196] MARCKS binds to calmodulin and actin and has been implicated in cell motility, secretion, and membrane trafficking. A related protein, MacMARCKS, is highly enriched in macrophages. Additional second messengers in T cells include *vav*, a protein expressed only in hematopoietic cells that is tyrosine phosphorylated after stimulation, perhaps by *lck*, which functions as a guanine nucleotide-releasing protein. Activated *vav* and inhibition of *ras*-GAP allow the activation of ras, small GTP-

binding proteins implicated in mediating cell proliferation.[197,198] Downstream of this in the signaling pathway are other kinases, including MAP and ribosomal S6 kinases, both of which are activated following phosphorylation by more proximal kinases (e.g., *c-raf* and PKC). This may lead to the activation of preformed transcriptional regulatory proteins (e.g., the release of *elf*-1 from an inhibitory interaction with the retinoblastoma protein[199]) or induce de novo synthesis of transcription factors that regulate genes induced in response to T-cell activation (e.g., a newly synthesized subunit of the nuclear factor of activated T cells, NF-AT[200]). Elevated Ca^{2+} levels activate the calmodulin-dependent phosphatase calcineurin, which allows translocation of the cytoplasmic component of NF-AT to the nucleus, where it combines with the newly synthesized nuclear component to contribute to the transcriptional activation of the IL-2 gene and certain other lymphokine genes. The critical role for calcineurin in T-cell activation was defined by the demonstration that immunosuppressants like cyclosporin and FK506 interact with cellular binding proteins, termed *immunophilins,* to form a complex that binds and inhibits calcineurin. Sequestration of calcineurin inhibits IL-2 production by activated T cells, thus accounting for the immunosuppression mediated by these compounds.[200]

In summary, a cascade of biochemical events, many regulated through phosphorylation and dephosphorylation of constitutive cellular substrates, occurs following TCR stimulation, culminating in production of IL-2 and progression of the cell into the cell cycle. The ultimate result is proliferation and clonal expansion, a process accompanied by differentiation of the cell, thus generating effector cells required to deal efficiently with the origin of the foreign peptides. Markers of the generation of effector T cells include the expression of unique adhesion antigens and the capacity to produce cytokines, soluble molecules that are critical in amplifying the immune response.

Activation by Microbial Superantigens

A number of microbial pathogens secrete intermediate-sized proteins that share the capacity to bind to monomorphic determinants on both discrete families of the V$_\beta$ region of the TCR and MHC class II molecules.[201] The best studied are the staphylococcal toxins, including the enterotoxins (SEA, SEB, etc.) and toxic shock syndrome toxin (TSST), although other organisms contain related toxins, including streptococcal pyrogenic exotoxins, M proteins, and the nucleocapsid of rabies virus. In mice, murine mammary tumor viruses express a similar molecule. When the virus becomes integrated and infectious particles are no longer formed, the endogenous antigen, encoded in the proviral 3′ long terminal repeat, may be expressed and mediate cellular activation in a manner similar to the bacterial antigens.[202,203] Some of these proviruses encode the endogenous genetic elements underlying the minor lymphocyte stimulation, or Mls, antigens in mice.[204]

The capacity of these antigens to stimulate both T cells and APC through their ability to establish tight adhesion between the TCR–MHC class II complex has characterized these molecules as "superantigens." Superantigens do not require processing and associate with MHC class II molecules outside of the peptide-binding groove.[205] In general, toxins bind best to HLA-DR, and less well to -DQ, and the association with different families of V$_\beta$ are different for each. TSST binds to V$_{\beta 2}$, thus resulting in activation of approximately 10 percent of all peripheral T cells, as contrasted with about 1 in 10^5 T cells that are activated by conventional peptide antigens. The crystal structure of SEB together with mutational analysis suggest that each molecule of SEB may cross-link two MHC class II molecules with V$_\beta$ chains.[206] The resulting activation of both T cells and APC results in massive release of cytokines, such as TNF-α, which mediate many of the systemic manifestations of shock.[207] Patients studied during an episode of toxic shock syndrome demonstrate tremendous expansion of V$_{\beta 2}$-bearing T cells, from a normal level of about 9 percent to as high as 50 percent.[208]

Although evidence for the existence of endogenous superantigens in humans, such as the Mls system in mice, has not been established, many human peripheral blood γ/δ T cells can be stimulated to proliferate by a small number of ligands, including mycobacterial antigens, staphylococcal superantigens, and surface molecules on tumor cell lines.[209,210] The reactive cells use the $V_{\gamma}9$ TCR product and express junctional region diversity in the TCR,[211] and proliferation is not restricted by classic MHC molecules. These properties are consistent with selection by a superantigen[212] and perhaps represent a primitive defense system to microbial pathogens.

Initial Activation of Memory T Cells Results in Long-Lasting Phenotypical and Functional Changes

After mature T cells have first responded to an antigen (the primary response) and ceased to proliferate, their phenotype and function remain significantly altered. Previously activated or "primed" cells are larger with increased RNA content compared with antigenically naive, virgin T cells and express increased levels of molecules involved in adhesion to the APC and to endothelium.[213,214] Primed T cells also do not require all of the costimulatory signals from the APC necessary for activation of antigenically naive T cells. These and other alterations may account for the ability of the host upon rechallenge with antigen to mount a more rapid and greater T-cell response in terms of T-cell proliferation, cytokine production, and cytotoxicity (the secondary response). Enhanced secondary responses by T cells can be observed months to decades after an initial single exposure to antigen, indicating that the initial response has generated a population of memory T cells. Whether the maintenance of memory T cells in vivo requires continual or intermittent exposure of T cells to the original antigen or a cross-reactive one remains controversial.

In humans, CD4+ α/β T cells with memory-like function (defined by proliferation to previously administered antigens) are contained predominantly within a subset that comprises about 40 percent of CD4+ α/β T cells in the adult circulation.[213–215] A reciprocal population, which comprises about 60 percent of adult peripheral blood T cells, appears to contain virgin CD4+ T cells that have not previously encountered their cognate antigen.[214–216] Putative memory CD4+ T cells mostly express on their surface the low-molecular-weight isoform of the CD45 protein CD45RO and relatively high levels of CD29,[214,215] while virgin CD4+ T cells express the high-molecular-weight isoforms of CD45, CD45RA but not CD45RO, and have lower amounts of CD29.[213,217] For CD8+ T cells, it is controversial whether selective expression of CD45RA and CD45RO as clearly demarcate the virgin and memory populations.[217,218] A number of other proteins are differentially expressed by memory versus naive CD4+ and CD8+ T cells.[214]

Putative memory T cells differ from virgin cells in their increased capacity to produce certain cytokines (e.g., IL-4 and IFN-γ) but not others (IL-2), to adhere more tightly to and to migrate across endothelium in nonlymphoid tissues, and to provide help for antibody production by B cells. Unlike virgin T cells, which appear to migrate preferentially from the blood to peripheral lymphoid tissue, memory cells in the circulation preferentially adhere to and migrate across the endothelium of inflamed tissues.[219,220] Memory T cells are also more readily activated to proliferate than virgin T cells with a variety of stimuli, such as anti-CD2 or -CD3 monoclonal antibodies,[221–223] a feature that may contribute to the more rapid and vigorous secondary response they mediate in vivo. It is hypothesized that CD45RA + CD29lo virgin T cells are the precursors of CD45RO + CD29hi memory cells.[213–216] Activation of virgin T cells in vitro, which may mimic the generation of memory T cells in vivo, converts the virgin T-cell phenotype in many respects to a memory T-cell phenotype: these cells acquire an enhanced capacity to produce IL-4 and IFN-γ but not IL-2, to provide

help for antibody production,[224] and to proliferate vigorously in response to anti-CD3 monoclonal antibody.[225] In addition, they become predominantly CD45RO + CD29hi.[214,215] This pathway of differentiation, if correct, may not be unidirectional, since some CD45RO+ T cells appear to become CD45RA+ in vivo.[226]

Lymphocyte Adhesion Molecules in Trafficking and Recirculation

In addition to expression of CD45RA, newly derived virgin (naive) T cells characteristically express high levels of the L-selectin adhesin and low levels of many other adhesins, including CD44 (Pgp-1), CD2, LFA-1, LFA-3, and ICAM-1. L-selectin is a homing receptor for peripheral lymph node high endothelial venules (HEV) and contributes to the primary emigration of naive T cells from blood, across HEV into the lymph nodes, and then back to blood via the efferent lymphatics and thoracic duct.[227,227a] L-selectin functions as a Ca^{2+}-dependent lectin that binds to a mucin-like, sulfated glycoprotein, GlyCAM-1 (glycosylation-dependent cell adhesion molecule-1), expressed on HEV.[228,229] The low levels of most adhesion molecules expressed on naive T cells are consistent with their more stringent activation requirements by APC, such as dendritic cells, that express high levels of these ligands together with B7/BB1.

As noted above, compared with virgin T cells, memory T cells have the capacity to respond to TCR stimulation with more rapid generation and diversity of cytokines, the soluble mediators of the immune response (see below). Similarly, in addition to the rapid alteration in adhesion receptor–ligands that occurs with T-cell activation and lasts for minutes to days, permanent alterations in adhesin expression accompany the transition to the memory phenotype. This appears to account for the fact that memory T cells follow a different recirculation pattern than naive T cells. They leave the blood across endothelium at distinct tissue sites and enter the regional lymph nodes through afferent lymphatics, before returning to the blood via efferent lymphatics and the thoracic duct. As previously noted, memory T cells frequently express the CD45RO isoform, but also express two- to four-fold higher levels of CD3, LFA-1, LFA-3, and CD44 while downregulating expression of L-selectin, the peripheral lymph node receptor. CD44 is a member of the cartilage link and proteoglycan core family of proteins and has been implicated in lymphocyte binding to HEV in lymph nodes associated with mucosal sites and in the synovium.[230] CD44 exists in at least 10 alternatively spliced forms, one of which, containing exon 6, is expressed following lymphocyte activation in lymph nodes and by tumor cells with metastatic potential[231]; expression of the CD44 splice variant may be required for lymphocyte entry into lymphoid and certain other tissues. Additional adhesion markers expressed only on subsets of activated or memory cells allow these cells to home to areas of inflammation or to restricted areas of the body, such as epithelial sites or Peyer's patches in the gut. Prominent among these are members of the very late antigens (VLA), a subfamily of β_1-integrins, so named because of the expression of VLA-1 ($\alpha 1/\beta 1$) and VLA-2 ($\alpha 2/\beta 1$) 2–4 weeks after stimulation with antigen. Both VLA-1 and -2 bind to laminin and collagen and may be important in the interaction of activated T cells with the extracellular matrix. Additional members of the integrin family expressed on T cells include VLA-4 (α_4/β_1), VLA-5 (α_5/β_1), VLA-6 (α_6/β_1), and an α_4/β_7-integrin.[232] These integrins also bind to extracellular matrix components, including fibronectin and laminin. VLA-4 also binds to VCAM-1, an immunoglobulin superfamily member expressed on endothelium that has been activated with inflammatory mediators, including cytokines. Unlike VLA-1 and -2, VLA-4, -5, and -6 are expressed on resting T cells, but assume a high avidity binding state rapidly after T cell activation,[233] thus enhancing primary activation and allowing activated cells to interact with the extracellular matrix or traverse inflamed endothelium. As with other adhesion molecules, expression of these VLA molecules is enhanced three- to four-fold on memory T cells. Augmented expression of adhesion molecules on memory cells contributes to their more rapid response to stimulation and their less stringent requirements during activation of APC. Thus B cells and macrophages present antigens much more efficiently to memory T cells than to naive cells.

The combinatorial expression of members of the integrin family confers specificity and diversity to the T-cell memory population. Distinct homing receptors are thought to be acquired within unique microenvironments at the time of initial T-cell priming whose expression ensures the recirculation of the T cell back through the tissue where antigen was initially encountered.[227a] Circulation out of the endothelium in different tissues is thought to be mediated by vascular "addressins," specific ligands for different T-cell homing molecules. Memory T cells from cutaneous sites express a novel homing receptor, CLA, that binds to E-selectin on endothelium and is involved in the targeted recirculation of a skin-associated subpopulation of memory T cells.[234,235] Memory T cells from Peyer's patch and gut tissues express the $\alpha_4\beta_7$ integrin that binds to a mucosal and gut endothelial addressin, MAdCAM-1 (mucosal addressin cell adhesion molecule-1),[236] and α^E/β_7- and $\alpha HML\beta_7$-integrins that bind to intestinal epithelial cells.[237] An additional endothelial molecule that mediates lymphocyte adhesion in peripheral lymph nodes, tonsil, and synovium, named *vascular adhesion protein-1* (VAP-1) has also been identified.[238] Expression of the α_4-integrins on CD4+ T cells has been shown to be required for entry into brain parenchyma.[239] Such a system ensures that pathogens encountered at individual sites, such as skin or gut epithelia, will be met the next time with memory T cells capable of more rapid responses in effecting control of infection.

T Cells in the Mucosal Immune System

The mucosal immune system denotes lymphocytes in the intestine, oral, nasal, and genitourinary tracts, and the mammary gland. Of these, the intestinal system has been most studied. In the mouse, a substantial number of the total peripheral T-cell population is comprised of the intestinal-associated lymphocyte population designated *intraepithelial lymphocytes* (IEL). The major lymphocyte phenotypes that comprise IEL consist of CD8+ cells that use CD8α/β-heterodimers, an $\alpha\beta$-TCR, and express Thy-1, and CD8+ cells that use CD8α/α-homodimers, express $\alpha\beta$- or $\gamma\delta$-TCR, and do not express Thy-1.[67] A small population of CD4+, $\alpha\beta$-TCR+ cells is also present. The unique α/α CD8+ population is thymus independent, as demonstrated by its normal presence in T-cell–deficient animals and by the support of T-cell development by fetal intestinal grafts.[69] Furthermore, IEL, in contrast to peripheral T cells, contain mRNA for the RAG genes required for rearrangement of TCR genes into functional surface receptors. Intermediate, CD4+CD8+ populations of IEL are reminiscent of T-cell differentiation that occurs in the thymus. Up to 40 percent of the peripheral T-cell compartment in mice may differentiate using this extrathymic pathway and remain in the intestine.

A substantial number of CD8+ IEL, in contrast to peripheral CD8+ cells, contain cytoplasmic granules, perforin, and granzyme transcripts typical of activated peripheral CD8 cytotoxic cells. These cells mediate cytotoxicity in redirected lysis assays.[240] IEL producing IFN-γ and IL-5 have been described[241]; IL-5 with TGF-β, produced by epithelial cells, can direct B-cell immunoglobulin switching to IgA, the predominant immunoglobulin secreted into the intestinal lumen. Unlike the mouse, in which 50–75 percent of the IEL population is comprised of a restricted population of γ/δ T cells using the $V_{\gamma5}/V_{\delta4}$ or $V_{\delta6}$ TCR, human IEL are comprised predominantly of α/β T cells. Similar to the mouse, human IEL are also oligoclonal, suggesting that these cells arise following clonal expansion in response to a restricted set of antigens derived from the gut.[242,243] Poised

at the basolateral surface of epithelial cells, IEL are capable of responding rapidly to gut-derived antigens presented on epithelial cells. A jejunal-derived human IEL cell line was restricted by the nonclassic MHC class I molecule, CD1c, consistent with selection of these oligoclonal cells by monomorphic MHC determinants.[244] Nonclassic MHC class I molecules, including members of the CD1 and TLa families, have been localized to intestinal epithelial cells. Members of the CD1 family have been demonstrated to present peptides derived from pathogenic microbes.[44] Perhaps contributing to their localization, over 95 percent of IEL express the α^E/β_7- and $\alpha HML\beta_7$-integrins, which are expressed by less than 2 percent of peripheral blood T cells.[245] TGF-β1 markedly enhances expression of this unique integrin, which may be important in mediating homing and cell–cell adhesion between IEL and epithelial cells.[246]

LYMPHOKINES AND CYTOKINES

Definitions and Overview

Lymphokines are proteins or glycoproteins secreted by lymphocytes that act as molecular signals for communication between cells of the immune system and as systemic mediators of the host response to infection; as such, their function is analogous to that of neurotransmitters and hormones, respectively. It is now clear that a number of other cell types, particularly mononuclear phagocytes, release and/or respond to such substances. In recognition of this, *cytokines,* a more general term that includes lymphokines, monokines (cytokines produced by mononuclear phagocytes), and other such mediators, is most commonly used.[247] The two terms are often used interchangeably.

Cytokines were originally detected in experimental systems that defined them by a specific biologic effect. Modern molecular biologic techniques have enabled the use of cloned recombinant materials. For a number of cytokines, it has become apparent that more than one cytokine can mediate biologic effects previously ascribed to a specific molecule and that pairs of cytokines can synergize with or antagonize one another, depending on the experimental system. Thus, definitions based solely on biologic effects can be misleading. Until it is cloned and molecularly characterized, a cytokine is generally referred to as a *factor* and is named according to its biologic effect(s), recognizing that this may or may not represent a single molecule. Once the amino acid sequence of the human form has been determined, however, it may be assigned an interleukin (IL) number. However, some cytokines, including interferons, TNF, and most of the colony-stimulating factors, have retained their original names even though cloned and molecularly characterized. For purposes of clarity and because many of the important cytokines originally described as factors have been cloned, this chapter focuses on those that have been molecularly characterized. The reader should recognize that this necessarily oversimplifies the true complexity of the system; many factors that are not molecularly characterized and not fully discussed are likely to play a role in the processes that will be discussed.

Cytokines Act to Amplify or Attenuate Immune Responses Coordinately

The actions of cytokines are not antigen specific. However, their effects in many cases serve to transduce antigen-specific signals. Such is the case for the T-cell–derived cytokines, since their production follows stimulation of the TCR by foreign peptides bound to MHC molecules. Similarly, certain microbial antigens, such as lipopolysaccharide from gram-negative bacteria or components of *Listeria,* can directly stimulate cytokine production by macrophages. Activation of cells by microbial products results in the release of cytokines in the same location, thus focusing the inflammatory response where it is needed. In general, cytokines coordinately regulate the clonal expansion of effector T- and B-cell populations, recruit additional effector cells to sites of inflammation through effects on adhesion molecules on both endothelial cells and leukocytes, activate effector cells to more potent microbicidal states, and deactivate the response in order to minimize tissue damage and coordinate the healing response after the pathogen has been killed. These responses tend to be localized; indeed, systemic circulation of high levels of cytokines can be detrimental, as in septic shock. Systemic effects mediated by cytokines include early regulation of the nonspecific immune response, including fever and the acute phase reaction, and stimulation of the bone marrow to replace cells required in the inflammatory response. Thus, multiple cytokines, pleiotropic in their activities, mediate the complex regulatory network between lymphoid cells, hematopoietic cells, and endothelial cells.

Table 1 lists the principal cytokines that have been molecularly characterized and describes their basic characteristics, the major cell sources and stimuli triggering their secretion, and their major biologic effects. Progress in this field remains rapid. In many cases, specific receptors for these molecules are much more widely distributed on cells than are the known biologic effects. Thus, it is to be anticipated that additional effects of importance will be discovered with time.

General Biochemical Properties of Cytokines

With the possible exception of mast cells,[248,249] cytokines are not stored preformed within cells. Their production requires new protein synthesis and in most cases new mRNA synthesis. Many contain a conserved series of repeated sequences in the 3′ untranslated sequence of the mRNA that directs rapid degradation of the message[250,251]; activation stimuli frequently result not only in new gene transcription but also in enhanced mRNA stability with a prolongation of the mRNA half-life. Conversely, glucocorticoids tend to enhance the mechanism mediating the inherent message instability of the cytokines. Most cytokines are encoded as propeptides and (with the notable exceptions of IL-1 and TNF) have an amino-terminal sequence directing their transport to the Golgi apparatus, where they are glycosylated (for those that are glycoproteins) and promptly secreted. The cleavage of the signal peptide yields the mature protein of a lower molecular mass. Each cytokine is encoded by a unique mRNA, and most are encoded by a single gene. However, alternatively spliced forms that generate different proteins, including soluble and transmembrane forms, exist for several cytokines, and IL-12 is composed of a heterodimer that is the product of two different genes.[252,253]

Structural Considerations

Cytokines can exist a monomers (e.g., granulocyte colony-stimulating factors [G-CSF], IFN-β), dimers (e.g., macrophage colony-stimulating factors [M-CSF], IL-5, IL-8, IL-10, IFN-γ, TGF-β), and even trimers (TNF) in their native state. Crystallographic and NMR studies have delineated common folding patterns within groups of cytokines that allow their assignment to families based on tertiary structures. A frequent structure is the "four-α-helix bundle" topology identified in studies of IL-2,[254] IL-4,[255] IL-5,[256] M-CSF,[257] G-CSF,[258] and GM-CSF[259] as well as growth hormone. These cytokines also share common exon–intron organization. The secondary structures of IL-6, IL-7, IL-10, IL-11, stem cell factor, and erythropoietin have been predicted to assume a similar structure. The occurrence of these conserved structures despite the absence of any significant sequence similarity suggests important evolutionary constraints in interactions with cytokine receptors on cells and/or other physicochemical constants. Human IFN-γ has a compact, largely α-helical, structure that has folding topology similar to IFN-β, despite their dissimilar sequences.[260] TNF forms a compact, conical trimer, with remarkable structural similarity to the

"jelly-role" motif of viral capsid proteins.[261] IL-1β and fibroblast growth factor form all-β-sheet structures with a threefold axis of symmetry.[262] Again, constraints on binding to specific receptors may underlie these topologic findings.

Cytokine Receptors

Cytokine receptor molecules have also been assigned to families based on conserved motifs within their primary and secondary structures.[122a,263] The largest, termed the *hematopoietic cytokine receptor superfamily,* defines a group of receptors that share four conserved cysteine residues in the amino-terminal half of the molecule and a repeated tryptophan-serine (WSXWS) motif at the carboxy-terminus close to the external side of the membrane. Members of this superfamily include IL-2-R (β- and γ-chains), IL-3-R, IL-4-R, IL-5-R, IL-6-R, IL-7-R, IL-9-R, EPO-R, G-CSF-R, GM-CSF-R, and LIF-R (leukemia inhibitory factor receptor). The IFN-α/β-R and the IFN-γ-R are also related by homologous domains that are more distantly related to the hematopoietic cytokine receptor superfamily.

A family of TNF/nerve growth factor (NGF) receptors has been identified based on the presence of four extracellular cysteine-rich domains, each with six conserved cysteines. Members of this family include the two TNF receptors, designated p55 and p75, CD40 on B cells, CD27 on T cells, and the low-affinity NGF-R (nerve growth factor receptor).[264] The Fas antigen was recently cloned and demonstrated to be another member of this family.[265] Since some antibodies to Fas can mediate apoptosis, or programmed cell death, it may be that several of these receptors either abrogate or induce programmed cell death under the appropriate conditions. Additional cytokine receptor families include the TGF-β-R[266] and the chemokine family of receptors[267,268]; the latter are members of an even larger family of the "serpentine" G-protein–coupled receptors that cross the membrane seven times. The two IL-1-R, designated type 1 on T cells, fibroblasts, and endothelial cells and type 2 on B cells, macrophages, and neutrophils, are members of the immunoglobulin superfamily.

A number of cytokine receptors are multichain receptors. Combinatorial arrangements of different chains result in receptors with differing affinities for the cytokine or differential ability to transduce a competent signal. Regulation of expression of the different chains allows another level of control in modulating cytokine activity. The IL-2-R consists of three chains: the IL-2 α-, β-, and γ-chains; the latter two are members of the WSXWS hematopoietic cytokine receptor superfamily.[269] Although both the α- and β-chains bind IL-2 with low affinity ($K_d = 10^{-7}$–10^{-8} M), coexpression with the γ-chain is required to produce a high-affinity ($K_d = 10^{-11}$ M) receptor that transduces an IL-2–dependent signal. An intermediate-affinity, signal-transducing receptor can be formed by a β/γ-heterodimer. The Il-2-R γ-chain is shared by components of the IL-4 and IL-7 (and probably IL-9, IL-13, and IL-15).[122a]

The GM-CSF, IL-3, and IL-5 high-affinity receptors are composed of α-chains that uniquely bind each distinct cytokine but a shared β-chain.[270] The heterodimer is required for both high-affinity binding and signal transduction, which is characterized by activation of a tyrosine phosphorylation cascade involving the p92c-*fes* (c-*fps/fes*) protooncogene.[271] Use of a common component may underlie some of the shared properties of these hematopoietic growth factors, whereas the unique α-chains may contribute to the lineage- and cytokine-specific effects. Interestingly, the unique extracellular domains of the α-chains seems to confer specificity to the patterns of intracellular tyrosine kinase activation.[272]

The complexities of combinatorial arrangements have been further delineated using the IL-6-R.[122a,273] Although the IL-6-R binds IL-6 with low affinity, coexpression of another molecule, termed gp130, is required both to form a high-affinity receptor and to transduce an effective signal. Two other molecules, LIF

TABLE 1. Cytokines

Name	Physicochemical Characteristics (Human)	Principal Cell Sources	Major Biologic Effects
Interleukin-1	Two proteins; α and β; both Mr ~17.5 kD	Many cell types; mononuclear phagocytes are a major source	Fever, acute phase response, ACTH release; cofactor for B-cell proliferation, T-cell activation, bone marrow stem cell proliferation; endothelial cell activation; enhances or induces TNF, IL-1, IFN, and CSF production
Interleukin-1 receptor antagonist (IL-1ra)	Protein ~18 kD and glycoprotein ~22 kD	Mononuclear phagocytes contain secreted form; epithelial cells and keratinocytes contain intracellular form	Binds to IL-1-R (type 1 > type 2); fails to transduce IL-1 signal, thus competing with active IL-1
Interleukin-2	Glycoprotein ~15 kD	T cells	Major mediator of T-cell proliferation; promotes production of other cytokines; enhances CTL and NK function; cofactor for B-cell proliferation and immunoglobulin secretion
Interleukin-3	Glycoprotein ~14–28 kD	T cells, mast cells	Promotes proliferation of pluripotent marrow stem cells
Interleukin-4	Glycoprotein ~20 kD	T cells, mast cells, basophils	Promotes proliferation of B and T cells; induces IgE isotype synthesis; enhances MHC class II and CD23 expression on B cells and macrophages; inhibits macrophage activation; enhances LAK activity
Interleukin-5	Glycoprotein ~18 kD	T cells, (eosinophils, mast cells)	Enhances eosinophil production and function; synergistic induction of IgA and IgM in the mouse
Interleukin-6	Glycoprotein ~21–29 kD	Many cell types; mononuclear phagocytes are a major source; T cells, endothelial cells	Mediates the acute phase response; enhances B-cell proliferation and differentiation to immunoglobulin-secreting plasma cell; cofactor for T-cell proliferation; enhances megakaryocyte growth
Interleukin-7	Glycoprotein ~25 kD	Bone marrow stromal cells	Growth of B-cell precursors; thymocyte development; cofactor for T-cell growth; macrophage activation
Chemokine α family (C-X-C): IL-8, PF-4, GRO/MGSA, βTG, IP-10, NAP 2, ENA-78, MIP-2 (murine)	Glycoproteins ~8–10 kD	Many cell types; mononuclear phagocytes are a major source; endothelial cells, epithelial cells, T cells	Neutrophil chemoattractants
Chemokine β family (C-C): MCP-1, RANTES, MIP-1α, MIP-1β	Proteins ~8–10 kD	Many cells types; mononuclear phagocytes are a major source; endothelial cells, epithelial cells, T cells	Lymphocyte and monocyte chemoattractants; eosinophil and basophil chemoattractants and activators
Interleukin-9	Glycoprotein ~32–39 kD	CD4+ T cells	Cofactor for some CD4+ T-cell clones; mast cell growth
Interleukin-10	Glycoprotein ~19 kD	Mononuclear phagocytes, CD4+ T cells, B cells, keratinocytes	Inhibits cytokine synthesis by macrophages, T cells, NK cells; downregulates MHC class II on macrophages; enhances B-cell growth and secretion of immunoglobulin; cofactor for mast cell growth
Interleukin-11	Protein ~23 kD	Bone marrow stromal cells	Mediates acute phase protein synthesis; enhances B-cell growth and differentiation to plasma cells; enhances megakaryocyte production
Interleukin-12	Heterodimer composed of two glycoproteins of ~35 and 40 kD	Mononuclear phagocytes; B cells	Induces IFN-γ production from T, NK cells; enhances T, NK cytotoxicity; growth factor for activated T cells; induces TH1 development
Interleukin-13	Protein ~10 kD; glycoprotein ~17 kD	T cells	Induces MHC class II and CD23 expression on mononuclear phagocytes, B cells; B-cell proliferation and immunoglobulin production; enhances IgE, IgG4 isotype switching; downregulates expression of macrophage inflammatory cytokines; synergistic enhancement of IFN-γ from NK cells
Interferon-α	Family of peptides 18–20 kD	Mononulcear phagocytes; lymphocytes	Interferes with viral replication; increases MHC class I; enhances IgG2a and IgG3 and inhibits IgE isotype production in the mouse; enhances NK function
Interferon-β	Glycoprotein 23 kD	Fibroblasts; epithelial cells	Interferes with viral replication; enhances NK function; induces MHC class I
Interferon-γ	Glycoprotein 20–25 kD	T cells, NK cells	Same as IFN-α and -β; increases MHC class II; macrophage activation; inhibits IgE production; inhibits proliferation of TH2 cells
TNF-α	Secreted protein 17 kD; membrane form 26 kD	Mononuclear phagocytes; T cells; NK cells; mast cells; eosinophils	Fever; endothelial cell activation and angiogenesis; cofactor for macrophage activation; enhances expression of adhesion molecules on leukocytes; induces catabolic state; cofactor for B-, T-cell proliferation; membrane form may mediate cytotoxicity
Lymphotoxin-α	Glycoprotein ~25 kD	Lymphocytes	Same as TNF-α, although generally less potent

(Continued)

TABLE 1. (*Continued*)

Name	Physicochemical Characteristics (Human)	Principal Cell Sources	Major Biologic Effects
Lymphotoxin-β	Membrane glycoprotein ~33 kD; forms heterotrimers with lymphotoxin α	Lymphocytes	Role in cytotoxicity postulated
GM-CSF	Glycoprotein ~14–35 kD	T cells, endothelial cells, mononuclear phagocytes; fibroblasts; mast cells	Growth of granulocyte macrophage precursors; enhances granulocyte, macrophage function
M-CSF	Glycoprotein ~20–25 kD and 35–45 kD forms	Monocytes; endothelial cells; fibroblasts	Growth of mononuclear phagocytes; enhances macrophage function
G-CSF	Glycoprotein 19 kD	Mononuclear phagocytes; epithelial cells; fibroblasts	Promotes granulocyte production; enhances granulocyte function
Steel Factor	Glycoprotein 31–36 kD	Bone marrow stromal cells	Promotes hematopoietic precursors (synergy with IL-7, GM-CSF); mast cell growth and activation

(leukemia inhibitory factor) and OM (oncostatin M), are less well-characterized cytokines that share many structural and functional properties with IL-6; each of these cytokines also uses gp130 in the formation of high-affinity signaling receptors. IL-11, which also shares a number of activities with IL-6, may also utilize this signal transduction pathway through association with its own unique binding molecule. Similarly, the p35 and p40 components of IL-12 share homologies with IL-6 and the IL-6-R, respectively, suggesting that a gp130-like signal-transducing molecule may exist for this cytokine as well.[274] Such associations may underlie some of the overlapping and pleiotropic effects of a number of the cytokines.

A number of cytokine receptors, including IL-1-R, IL-2-R α and β, IL-4-R, IL-6-R, IL-7-R, IL-9-R, G-CSF-R, gp130, IFN-γ-R, and TNF-R, can also exist in soluble forms.[275] Such soluble receptors may modulate the activity of cytokines by competing with binding to membrane-associated receptors. Gene capture of several of these soluble receptors by a number of viruses[276] suggests that modulation of the inflammatory response in this manner may play a role in viral pathogenicity.

Specific Cytokines Produced by Mononuclear Phagocytes

Monocytes and macrophages are important sources of IL-1α and -1β, IL-1 receptor antagonist protein (IL-1ra), IL-6, IL-8 and other members of the chemokine family, IL-10, IL-12, IFN-α, TNF-α, GM-CSF, G-CSF, and M-CSF. Studies performed primarily in vitro indicate that each of these cytokines is also produced by other human cells; human endothelial cells and fibroblasts are probably important sources of CSF, IL-1, and IL-6; B lymphocytes of IL-1, IL-10, and IL-12; T lymphocytes of TNF-α, IL-6, and IL-10; and NK cells of TNF-α. IFN-β, which is related to IFN-α and shares similar biologic activity, is produced by fibroblasts and epithelial cells. Other cell types may produce one or more of these cytokines; this may be of physiologic importance in specific anatomic sites. Most of the cytokines produced by mononuclear phagocytes have potent and diverse systemic effects in addition to their effects on immune function.

In general, stimulation of mononuclear phagocytes induces transcription of specific cytokine mRNA and translation into proteins, followed by prompt extracellular secretion. Adherence of freshly isolated monocytes induces mRNA expression for IL-1β, IL-6, TNF-α, and M-CSF, although translation and secretion appear to require a second signal.[277,278] Such "primed" cells may be important in allowing the more rapid production of cytokine protein by mononuclear phagocytes in response to infectious or inflammatory stimuli in vivo than would be possible if all protein was derived from newly synthesized mRNA.

A common set of stimuli lead to the production of cytokines by mononuclear phagocytes. Bacteria and their products, such as lipopolysaccharide and microbial superantigens, are potent inducers of TNF-α, IL-1, IL-6, IL-8 and other members of the chemokine family, IL-10, IL-12, IFN-α, and the CSFs by mononuclear phagocytes. Viruses also induce IFN-α and perhaps IL-1. An important property of these cytokines is their capacity to induce or enhance their own or each other's production. Thus, TNF-α and IL-1 directly induce production of IL-1, TNF-α, IL-6, and CSF by human mononuclear cells, endothelial cells, and fibroblasts. Cytokines can also enhance production induced by other stimuli. GM-CSF and IFN-γ enhance production of TNF-α and IL-1 and of M-CSF and G-CSF. Activated complement components and immune complexes also stimulate cytokine production by human mononuclear phagocytes through distinct receptors. Other cell surface ligands implicated in cytokine generation include LFA-3, CD44, and CD45 in inducing TNF-α and IL-1 release[279] and CD14 in mediating the number of cytokines released in response to lipopolysaccharide bound to serum lipopolysaccharide-binding protein (see below).

Stimulation of macrophage cytokine production by microbial products with amplification by other cytokines allows a rapid response to minimize microbial invasion but has the potential for overproduction in response to overwhelming infection; this may contribute to deleterious effects such as septic shock, as discussed below. Importantly, the host has mechanisms for focusing production at the site of infection by downregulating production of cytokines and limiting their systemic release.

One mechanism for focusing the effects of the cytokines would be to limit their production to the local site. Resting tissue macrophages appear to have a more limited capacity to release TNF-α, and particularly IL-1, than do inflammatory macrophages and monocytes, and may release greater amounts of inhibitory cytokines, such as IL-1ra.[280] Thus, the intrinsic tissue macrophages may have limited capacities to promote inflammation through cytokine release, consistent with their role in remodeling tissue in a manner that preserves tissue integrity. In contrast, the higher capacity of macrophages in inflammatory sites to promote an inflammatory response may relate in part to their more recent derivation from monocytes and to their exposure to high local concentrations of microbial products, chemotactic complement components, and cytokines. Such recently recruited macrophages release a number of cytokines, such as the chemokines, which serve to attract additional inflammatory cells[281]; TNF-α and IL-1, which induce adhesion molecules on endothelial cells and inflammatory cells to promote egress from the vasculature[282]; IL-12, which enhances IFN-γ production from NK and T cells[283]; and CSF and TNF-α, which potentiate the microbicidal systems of recruited cells. As organisms are killed and the stimulus abates, a number of deactivating molecules are produced that downregulate the response in order that homeostasis can be achieved. These include IL-10, which inhibits the release of a number of macrophage proinflammatory cytokines in an autocrine manner[284]; IL-ra, a member of the IL-1 gene family that competes with active IL-

1 for available receptors but does not transduce a signal[285]; and TGF-β, important in both deactivation of macrophages and induction of tissue repair through remodeling of the extracellular matrix.[286,287] Both TNF-α and IL-1 induce production of prostaglandins (PG), particularly PGE$_2$, which downregulate their own production and certain effects of IL-1. IL-1 appears to be unique in its ability to enhance production of certain pituitary hormones, including ACTH and α-MSH. ACTH, by enhancing glucocorticoid production, can negatively regulate production of itself, TNF, and other cytokines, including the CSF, interferons, and IL-2 to IL-6. In addition to inhibiting cytokine production, glucocorticoids and α-MSH inhibit the effects of IL-1 on many cell types. The effects of excessive amounts of a number of cytokines are also attenuated by their ability to downregulate their own receptors. Thus inflammation is controlled; tissue repair, including angiogenesis, mediated by such cytokines as TNF-α, TGF-β, and IL-8, ensues; and homeostasis is restored. The macrophage plays a central role in this process through the elaboration of this wide array of cytokines.

Cytokines Produced by T Cells

With the exception of certain tumors, T lymphocytes are the sole source of IL-2 and IL-9 (and possibly IL-13) and are a major source of lymphotoxin α and β (with B cells and lymphokine-activated killer cells), IL-3 and IL-4 (with mast cells and basophils, IL-5 (with eosinophils), and IFN-γ (with NK cells). T cells also produce IL-6, IL-10, GM-CSF, and TNF-α. Unlike macrophages, which produce and secrete cytokines in response to a number of stimuli, T cells secrete lymphokines in response to activation by antigen in the context of HLA molecules. Following activation through the signaling systems discussed above, the genes encoding these cytokines are transcribed within a few hours, followed rapidly by their production and prompt secretion. Production continues to increase over the first 24–72 hours after stimulation, depending on the conditions, and then declines. TNF-α and lymphotoxin are unique in their ability to be expressed as transmembrane molecules (in addition to secreted forms) on the surface of activated T cells.[288,289] Such forms may be important in focusing the effects of these cytokines locally and avoiding their potential for systemic adverse effects. Membrane lymphotoxin occurs as a trimer, with the lymphotoxin β-molecule tethering the secreted lymphotoxin α-chains to the membrane.

Activation of a mixed population of T lymphocytes and APC, such as blood, tonsillar, or splenic mononuclear cells, usually leads to coordinate production of each of these cytokines, although the rate and time to maximal production of each vary slightly. This reflects the aggregate production of lymphokines by all cells in the population. However, evidence suggests that the production of individual cytokines may be differentially regulated.

CD4 cells of humans and mice produce each of these cytokines. However, the capacity to secrete specific cytokines appears to be restricted to subsets of CD4 cells.[290] Naive CD4 cells, exemplified by newborn umbilical cord blood cells, secrete relatively large amounts of IL-2 but small amounts of other cytokines. These cells, designated THp (T-helper precursors) in the mouse, require priming by potent APC, such as dendritic cells, but subsequently acquire the ability to secrete a broader array of additional cytokines, including IL-2, IL-4, IL-5, IL-10, and IFN-γ, upon restimulation a second time. Such restimulation can be achieved by a broader range of APC, including B cells and macrophages. These cells, designated TH0 cells,[291] generate the large number of cytokines required to orchestrate the cognate immune response through the supply of T- and B-cell growth factors and macrophage-activating factors. Under still incompletely defined conditions, CD4 cells can be strongly primed and restimulated such that the subsequent cytokine profiles further differentiate into highly polarized populations, des-

ignated TH1 and TH2 cells.[292] In the mouse, TH1 cells produce IL-2, IFN-γ, and lymphotoxin, whereas TH2 cells produce IL-4, IL-5, IL-6, IL-9, IL-10, and IL-13. Other cytokines, such as IL-3 and GM-CSF, are produced by both TH1 and TH2 subsets. In the human, IL-6 and IL-10, and occasionally IL-2, are less restricted in their distribution between subsets, and responses more commonly are characterized by populations with mixed cytokine profiles (neither distinctly TH1 or TH2) than in the mouse. The presence of each of these subsets has been demonstrated both in vitro and in vivo in both mice and humans.[290,293]

Very different immune responses are mediated by TH1 and TH2 cells, as predicted by the different cytokines produced. Importantly, the collection of cytokines produced by each of these subsets coordinately regulates different cell types in order to focus discrete immunologic responses. TH1 cells release macrophage-activating factors (principally IFN-γ), mediate DTH, and promote immunoglobulin switching to isotypes that mediate complement fixation and antibody-dependent cellular cytotoxicity (ADCC). Some TH1 cells also acquire a cytotoxic phenotype.[294] Such responses are optimally focused against intracellular organisms, such as viruses and intracellular parasites, by promoting immunoglobulin isotypes that neutralize pathogens or enhance their interaction with fixed phagocytic cells, coupled with activation of those cells to a microbicidal state. Clearly, such responses require close regulation and, in a number of mouse models and some human diseases, TH1 cells have been associated with autoimmune disease.[295,296] In contrast, TH2 cells release cytokines that favor B-cell growth and differentiation (particularly IL-4, IL-6, and, in humans, IL-13), isotype switching to IgE antibody (IL-4 and, in humans, IL-13), upregulation of low-affinity Fc receptors for IgE (CD23) on B cells and macrophages (IL-4, IL-13), eosinophil differentiation and activation (IL-5), and mast cell differentiation and activation (IL-4, IL-9, and IL-10). Such responses have been demonstrated in animal models to be protective in establishing gut immunity against parasitic nematodes.[297] Again, close regulation is required. Not unexpectedly, based on the activation of the above cell types, TH2 cells have been implicated in human allergic and hypersensitivity states.[298,299]

The mechanisms for the development of CD8 T cell effector functions have been less clearly defined. Although both CD4 and CD8 T cells produce IL-2 and IFN-γ when stimulated with nonspecific mitogens or in response to allogeneic cells, production of IL-2 in response to antigens appears to be restricted primarily to CD4 cells. Production of other cytokines by CD8 T cells in response to antigens appears to be almost completely dependent on IL-2 production by CD4 cells. These findings highlight the critical importance of CD4 helper T cells in lymphokine production and provide an explanation for the devastating effects that result from the ablation of CD4 cells in AIDS.

As with macrophages, important regulatory mechanisms act to attenuate the secretion of T-cell–derived cytokines. First, IL-2 does not stimulate its own production. In addition, with mouse T-cell clones, the capacity of IL-2 to enhance lymphokine production is maximum within the first 24–48 hours after T cells have been activated by antigen and is virtually absent 7 days later. Reciprocally, exposure of T cells to high concentrations of IL-2 impairs their activation through the antigen receptor and may induce apoptosis.[300] In addition, activated T cells produce TGF-β that inhibits IL-2–induced T-cell proliferation and inhibits IFN-γ production. Mice with disruption of the TGF-β gene die shortly after birth with massive lymphocyte and macrophage infiltration of internal organs,[301] consistent with failure to restrict expansion of potentially autoreactive T cells, or production of proinflammatory cytokines by macrophages. Furthermore, monocytes exposed to IFN-γ produce PGE$_2$ and 1,25-dihydroxyvitamin D$_3$ (calcitriol), which inhibit IL-2 and IFN-γ production. Thus, like the production of cytokines by macrophages, both positive and negative regulatory signals act to modulate the strength and duration of T-cell cytokine production.

Cytokine Production by NK Cells and B Cells

The repertoire of cytokines produced by NK and B cells is more limited. NK cells are a major source of IFN-γ, which is largely dependent on the inducing capacity of IL-12. Maximal secretion of IFN-γ occurs with stimulation by the combination of IL-12, IL-2, and TNF-α[302]; IFN-α may also play a role. IL-13 may contribute synergistically to IFN-γ production by human NK cells.[303] NK cells may also release low levels of TNF-α and IL-1. B cells can also release low levels of IL-1, but are important sources of IL-10 and IL-12 and may also produce IL-6 and TNF. In the mouse, B cells that express the surface antigen CD5 are the major source of IL-10.[304] Thus, like macrophages, B cells acting as APC can influence the differentiation of activated T cells through the elaboration of these cytokines.

Important Immunologic Response Pathways Are Regulated by Cytokines

To provide a conceptual framework for understanding the function of cytokines in the immune response, several examples of cytokine-regulated responses are discussed below. These discussions are necessarily oversimplified, and additional complexities are likely.

Fever.   Fever is associated with an elevation of the normal temperature set point for an individual; although the mean body temperature is increased, the normal diurnal fluctuation of temperature is not altered (see Ch. 37). Fever may play a beneficial role in host resistance to infection both by inhibiting the growth of certain microorganisms directly and by enhancing certain aspects of the immune response. The elevation of temperature is mediated primarily by endogenous pyrogens. Studies to define pyrogenic molecules have, by necessity, been done largely in experimental animals. Recombinant IL-1 (α and β), TNF (α and β), and MIP-1α (a member of the chemokine family)[305] are directly pyrogenic in rabbits. IL-1 and TNF appear to act directly on vascular endothelial cells in the hypothalamic area to cause local production of PGE_2, which then acts on cells within the anterior hypothalamus to cause fever. The antipyretics, such as aspirin and acetaminophen, act by blocking the production of PGE_2 in the brain. MIP-1α acts independently of PGE_2. Bacterial lipopolysaccharide (LPS) can induce each of these mediators; LPS can also act directly on the hypothalamus to induce fever, accounting for the biphasic fever seen in response to this substance. Other cytokines, including interferons and IL-6, cause fever in experimental animals, but these are less potent and may act indirectly through induction of the major endogenous cytokine mediators.

The Acute Phase Response in Infection.   *Acute phase response* is a term describing collectively the range of metabolic changes occurring during systemic infection and inflammation (see Ch. 4). Striking effects include those on hepatic protein synthesis, lipid metabolism, and tissue catabolism. The liver undergoes a characteristic response to stress by downregulating albumin synthesis while upregulating the synthesis of a number of acute phase proteins that reach very high levels in serum. The acute phase proteins are thought to play a role in nonspecific host defense, in part by enhancing phagocytosis and assisting in complement activation. The two classes of acute phase proteins, designated class 1 and class 2, are regulated predominantly by IL-1 and TNF, or combinations of IL-1/TNF with IL-6 or combinations of IL-6 with glucocorticoids, respectively. Class 1 proteins include C-reactive protein, serum amyloid A, complement C3, haptoglobin and α₁-glycoprotein. Class 2 proteins include fibrinogen, α₁-anti-

trypsin, and α₁-antichymotrypsin. Studies in animals suggest that IL-6 is the primary mediator in the transcriptional control of the acute phase protein response and that TNF and IL-1 mediate their effects through the indirect induction of IL-6. The promoter region of the IL-6 gene contains a unique DNA sequence that binds a protein designated NF-IL-6 (possibly as a heterodimer with a related protein, NF-IL-6β[306]), that is induced by IL-1, TNF, lipopolysaccharide, and IL-6 itself.[307] Importantly, the same NF-IL-6–binding site exists in the promoter of the acute phase proteins, thus accounting for the coordinated regulation of this systemic response to stress. The IL-6-R is expressed on circulating human monocytes, but is rapidly downregulated after stimulation with LPS or IL-1. Conversely, IL-6 expression and secretion is induced by these stimuli, and IL-6-R are induced on human hepatocytes. This serves effectively to transfer signaling by IL-6 from the monocytes to the liver to coordinate the acute phase response.[308]

Both TNF and IL-1 inhibit lipoprotein lipase and stimulate hepatic lipogenesis, thereby causing lipemia, which is characteristic of certain chronic infections. The role of TNF-α in cachexia related to infection or malignancy has been postulated based on its effects on food intake and catabolism. Transgenic mice bearing tumors constitutively secreting TNF-α develop progressive anorexia and wasting,[309] and recombinant TNF-α–induced tissue catabolism, lipolysis, and lipemia occur when administered to humans. It is likely that IL-1, and possibly additional cytokines, contributes to the wasting seen in chronic inflammatory conditions. Under physiologic conditions in humans, excess production of multiple cytokines (e.g., TNF-α and IFN-α) in patients with AIDS and superimposed secondary infections[310] is required to induce wasting.

Septic Shock.   Septic shock is a complex systemic response to products of microbial organisms that is characterized by high levels of circulating cytokines (see Ch. 56). Infusion of endotoxin into experimental animals and humans causes the sequential release of TNF-α, peaking after 2 hours, followed within hours by IL-1, IL-6, and IL-8 and later by IFN-γ and CSF.[311–315] Circulating LPS is rapidly bound by a plasma protein, lipopolysaccharide-binding protein (LBP), which in humans is present in considerable concentrations at steady state; LBP is also an acute phase protein, and hepatic synthesis and secretion are induced with inflammatory stimuli, resulting in 100-fold increases in serum levels.[316] LBP binds LPS, forming a complex that binds to a monocyte/macrophage surface antigen termed CD14.[317] Engagement of CD14 by LPS complexed with LBP, in turn, results in TNF-α, IL-1, IL-6, and IL-8 synthesis and secretion by monocytes and macrophages.[318] CD14 also exists in a soluble form, can bind to LPS–LBP complexes, and subsequently be bound by an unidentified receptor on endothelial and epithelial cells, thus contributing to the LPS sensitivity of these cells.[319] Consistent with its role as an LPS receptor, transgenic mice expressing human CD14 become hypersensitive to LPS.[320] Although additional molecules on mononuclear phagocytes, such as the CR3 receptor,[321] may be involved in binding LPS, physiologically CD14 may be the major LPS receptor relevant to its agonist effects.

The primary role of TNF-α in mediating the downstream events in the sepsis syndrome is suggested by the ability of recombinant TNF-α to induce this syndrome,[322] by the capacity of treatment with neutralizing antibodies to TNF to protect against a subsequently administered lethal dose of LPS in experimental animals,[323,324] and by the resistance of mice with disruption of the p55 TNF-R gene to lethal doses of LPS.[325] Furthermore, serum TNF-α levels are markedly elevated in human sepsis, and higher levels are associated with a morbid outcome.[326–328] It is likely that TNF-α initiates a cytokine and second-messenger cascade, including arachidonic acid metabolites, platelet-activating factor (PAF), and kinins, with wide-ranging effects on endothelial cells and circulating neutrophils.[329] Many of these effects of TNF are augmented synergistically by other cytokines, particularly IL-1[329a]. The induction by these cytokines of endothelial cell adhesion molecules, including ICAM-1, VCAM-1, and E-selectin, together with the induction of the integrins LFA-1 and CR3 on neutrophils, contributes to margination of leukocytes and prolonged secretion of reactive oxygen products with the capacity of substantial endothelial cell damage.[330] These cytokines and LPS can also induce the release of IL-1 and IL-6 from endothelial cells, thus contributing to a positive feedback cycle. TNF and IL-1 also inhibit the antithrombotic properties of endothelium through thromboplastin synthesis and suppression of the thrombomodulin/protein C anticoagulation pathway and through synthesis of PAF. These cytokines also induce plasminogen activator inhibitor-1 and induce prostacyclin synthesis, both of which activate the fibrinolytic system. Vascular tone is reduced through induction of prostacyclin, generation of nitric oxide (NO), a potent vasodilator, and production of endothelin. These responses are thought to contribute to the decrease in systemic vascular resistance, capillary leakage, disseminated intravascular coagulation, vessel thrombosis, and hemorrhagic necrosis, particularly in the bowel, which occur in experimental and human septic shock. Inhibition of the synthesis of pulmonary surfactant proteins SP-A and SP-B by TNF-α may contribute to the high incidence of adult respiratory distress syndrome (ARDS).[331] The appreciation of the role of cytokine dysregulation in septic shock has spawned a number of therapeutic interventions, mostly in animal systems, including the use of neutralizing monoclonal antibodies or antagonistic soluble receptors that bind TNF or IL-1, the use of IL-1ra, the use of IL-4 and IL-10 (which downregulate macrophage inflammatory cytokine production and stimulate IL-1ra release), and the use of drugs that interfere with the synthesis or secretion of TNF. Further study will be required before the therapeutic efficacy of such interventions can be fully assessed. This is discussed more fully below (see Immunoattenuation to Decrease Immunologically Mediated Injury).

HEMATOPOIESIS

Hematopoietic cells are derived in the bone marrow from pluripotent stem cells found in association with a complex stromal cell network of diverse cell types.[332] Constitutive hematopoiesis occurs in the absence of immunologic stimuli, suggesting that a combination of adhesion molecules and cytokines produced by stromal cells are alone sufficient to mediate stem cell renewal and hematopoiesis. Many of these factors remain incompletely characterized, although M-CSF, IL-7, IL-11, and stem cell factor (steel factor or kit ligand) are produced constitutively by stromal cells, and GM-CSF may be produced constitutively by bone marrow microvascular endothelium. Spontaneous mutations in mice in stem cell factor or its ligand, the transmembrane tyrosine kinase c-kit, result in severe deficiencies in erythroid and mast cell lineages and in lesser effects on the myeloid and lymphoid lineages.[333] Similarly, mutations in the murine M-CSF receptor result in a paucity of osteoclasts, which is manifested as osteopetrosis and diminished numbers of macrophages,[334] and immunologically induced G-CSF deficiency causes granulocytopenia in dogs.[335] Thus, at minimum, these three cytokines play a role in constitutive hematopoiesis.

Cytokines derived from activated macrophages and CD4+ T cells play a major role in inducible hematopoiesis, an inflammatory response that represents an important component of host defense against microorganisms. IL-1 and TNF derived from stimulated macrophages amplify the response by inducing IL-1, IL-6, and CSF from fibroblasts, endothelial cells, and marrow stromal cells. IL-1α, IL-3, and IL-6 stimulate proliferation of early pluripotent stem cells; IL-3 and GM-CSF stimulate proliferation of cells capable of forming granulocytes, erythrocytes, macrophages, and megakaryocytes; GM-CSF stimulates granulocytes and macrophage precursors to proliferate; M-CSF and G-CSF stimulate proliferation of their respective committed precursors; IL-5 stimulates eosinophil production; and IL-3, IL-9, and IL-10 enhance mast cell cell production. TNF, interferons, and MIP-1α may act as negative feedback signals to downregulate marrow expansion. Note that the factors acting on the most mature precursors of phagocytes (M-CSF and G-CSF) are rapidly produced by macrophages and other nonhematopoietic cells in response to microbial or inflammatory stimuli. This may be important in allowing rapid mobilization of marrow reserves in response to infection. In contrast, the T-cell–derived products act either to augment production of cells at earlier stages of differentiation (IL-3, GM-CSF) or to stimulate production of eosinophils (IL-5) or mast cells (IL-3, IL-9, IL-10).

THE ROLE OF CYTOKINES IN T-CELL PROLIFERATION AND MATURATION

IL-2 is the major lymphokine required for T-cell proliferation under most conditions. As discussed above, the capacity to respond optimally to IL-2 is determined by the expression of the trimeric, high-affinity IL-2-R.[269] Lymphoid cells constitutively express the IL-2-R γ-chain, whereas the β-chain is expressed constitutively on CD8+ T cells but not on CD4+ T cells, and is induced by activation. The α-chain is induced only with T-cell activation, as is the IL-2 ligand itself. Expression of the γ-chain is required for signal transduction, probably via the capacity of the cytoplasmic domain to associate physically and functionally with the *src* family of kinases, p56*lck*, and p59*fyn*. Rapid tyrosine phosphorylation of cellular proteins occurs following stimulation of cells by IL-2. The demonstration that mutations in the IL-2-R γ-chain are associated with cases of human X-linked SCID and absence of mature T cells[122] would seem to implicate signaling through this receptor in normal T-cell development, consistent with the use of the IL-2-R γ-chain with multiple T-cell growth factors.[122a]

Expression of both IL-2 and the high-affinity receptor are coordinately regulated by signaling through the T-cell antigen receptor in the presence of appropriate costimulation; coexpression of receptor and ligands ensures that activated T cells are capable of responding to IL-2 in both an autocrine and paracrine fashion. Although cognate interactions of T cells with antigen-presenting macrophages induce IL-1 production in macrophages,[336] the inability of the IL-1 antagonist IL-1ra to block human T-cell responses to mitogens, antigens, or alloantigens[285] suggests that IL-1 may not be a required accessory molecule for T-cell activation.

The most important IL-2–independent cytokine capable of supporting T-cell proliferation is IL-4. Competence to respond to IL-4 also requires cognate activation by APC and appropriate costimulation through the CD28/B7 pathway. Signaling pathways mediated in T cells through the IL-4-R remain less completely characterized, but involve tyrosine phosphorylation of phosphatidylinositol 3-kinase, an interaction associated with cell proliferative pathways mediated by insulin. Indeed, common elements between signaling pathways mediated by IL-4 and insulin have been identified.[337]

Several other cytokines have been demonstrated to enhance T-cell activation or proliferation synergistically. IL-6 and IL-7 can activate T-cell proliferation in an IL-2–independent fashion under certain conditions, IL-9 can support the growth of certain murine and human T-cell lines, IL-12 can synergize with IL-2 in supporting resting T-cell proliferation and can support the proliferation of activated T cells, and TNF-α can synergize in the proliferation of IL-2–stimulated T cells.

The mechanisms by which effector TH1 and TH2 populations become established have not been fully elucidated. Contributions by different populations of APC and different MHC molecules have been suggested by animal studies.[338,339] Several cytokines, however, have been implicated in mediating this developmental regulation of CD4 T cells. IL-12 has been identified as an important cytokine that mediates the maturation of TH1 cells in vitro in both human and mouse[340,341] and in vivo in the mouse.[342] Some of the effects of IL-12, such as suppression of IL-4–induced IgE production, may be independent of its capacity to induce IFN-γ.[343] IFN-α and TGF-β may contribute to TH1 development in certain instances. IL-4 has proven to be the strongest inducer of TH2 maturation in both human and mouse studies in vitro and in mouse studies in vivo.[344–347] Mice with disruption of the IL-4 gene are impaired in their capacity to generate TH2 cells.[348] The best evidence, as derived from studies in transgenic mice expressing a single TCR, suggests that all naive T cells have the capacity to differentiate into TH0, TH1, or TH2 cells, presumably dependent on the cytokine milieu at the time of stimulation through the TCR.[349,350]

Highly established TH1 or TH2 cell responses occur in part due to the capacity of each of the subsets to regulate the other negatively through the cytokines they produce. TH1 cells inhibit proliferation of TH2 cells, isotype switching to IgE, and eosinophil recruitment through elaboration of IFN-γ.[351–353] Conversely, TH2 cells inhibit macrophage activation by IFN-γ and the release of macrophage-derived proinflammatory cytokines through the actions of IL-4, IL-10, and IL-13,[354–356] and inhibit the use of IL-2 as a T-cell growth factor by downregulating IL-2-R expression through IL-4.[357] The latter forces T cells to use IL-4 as a primary growth factor. Such cross-regulation may occur during normal immune responses to ensure balanced cellular and humoral responses and to prevent the outgrowth of autoimmune reactive cells. Importantly, the elucidation of TH1 and TH2 subsets has explained early observations in experimental immunology, demonstrating that cellular and humoral responses could be dissociated at different doses of antigen, so-called split tolerance or low-zone tolerance.

Recent evidence suggests that CD8 + T lymphocytes may also differentiate into TH1-like (type 1) and TH2-like (type 2) phenotypes. In human leprosy, CD8 + clones from patients with immunologically reactive tuberculoid disease secreted IFN-γ and mediated cytotoxicity in vitro. In contrast, CD8 + clones from patients with the nonreactive lepromatous form of disease secreted IL-4 and IL-5 and mediated suppression of lymphocyte proliferation in vitro.[358] Studies with mouse CD8 + T cells demonstrated the capacity of IL-4 to mediate the outgrowth of T cells that have lost CD8 expression and cytolytic activity but acquired the capacity to secrete IL-4, IL-5, and IL-10 and provide B-cell help, each activities of TH2 CD4 + T cells.[359] Further study will be required to establish whether such activities occur in vivo in the CD8 + population.

An important maturation step for T cells is the development of memory cells that can respond to secondary challenge with more rapid secretion of effector cytokines. The surface phenotype and trafficking patterns of these cells have been discussed above. Conditions promoting memory T-cell development remain poorly defined. Whether persistence of antigen may be required to maintain a stable memory cell population beyond a finite interval is controversial.[360] TGF-β may play a role in the establishment of the memory phenotype.[361]

ROLE OF CYTOKINES AND T CELLS IN B CELL ACTIVATION, DIFFERENTIATION, AND IMMUNOGLOBULIN ISOTYPE SWITCHING

B cells are activated by specific antigens through surface immunoglobulin that acts as an antigen receptor. Once activated, they replicate and then differentiate into immunoglobulin-secreting B cells and subsequently into memory B cells or plasma cells. This process is controlled by T cells, macrophages, and the cytokines secreted from these cells. This appears to be a sequential process involving first antigen-induced activation and then DNA synthesis and proliferation, followed by differentiation into immunoglobulin-secreting cells.

Antibody responses to antigens consisting of proteins or of protein-derived peptides are T-cell dependent. This dependence results from the need for direct T cell–B cell interaction. This occurs when the interaction is cognate (i.e., when CD4 T cells engage antigenic peptides presented in association with class II MHC on the B cell). The specific binding of the CD4 molecule on helper T cells to class II MHC molecules, which are expressed constitutively on B cells, facilitates this cognate interaction. Signals derived from this T–B interaction, and from engagement of surface immunoglobulin on the B-cell by the antigen from which the peptides were derived, results in B-cell activation. The important role that the CD4 molecule plays in this cognate interaction is consistent with the function of CD4 T cells as helper T cells—they provide help for B-cell proliferation and immunoglobulin production. Other ligand pairs appear to play an important role in this interaction, thereby facilitating both T- and B-cell activation. Two critical interactions appear to be those between CD40 and the CD40 ligand and between CD28 and its ligand B7/BB1.[361a]

The CD40 molecule is expressed on all B cells, whereas the CD40 ligand is expressed transiently by CD4 T cells following activation.[362,363] The CD40 ligand is a membrane-bound molecule with homology to the cytokine TNF. In the presence of accessory signals provided by lymphokines (e.g., IL-4 or IL-10), engagement of CD40 on the B cell by its ligand on activated CD4 T cells enhances B-cell proliferation and immunoglobulin class switch (e.g., from IgM to IgE). The CD40–CD40 ligand interaction appears to be permissive for class switching and development of memory B cells, whereas the nature of the cytokines and other interactions determine the isotype of the immunoglobulin(s) produced and whether memory B cells or plasma cells are produced. The expression of the CD40 ligand in humans is consistent with this role. Although not present on resting blood T cells, it is present on blood T cells that have been activated in vitro. CD40 ligand is expressed by CD4 T cells in the secondary lymphoid follicles and the periarteriolar lymphoid sheath in vivo, where CD4 T cells provide contact-dependent help for B cells.[364] In earlier studies it was found that the CD45RO + memory subset of human CD4 T cells efficiently provides B-cell help.[365,366] This difference in capacity for B-cell help may reflect the broader capacity of memory as compared with naive CD4 T cells to express lymphokines (e.g., IL-4) that facilitate B-cell proliferation; poor expression of the CD40 ligand may also be a contributing factor to the inability of naive T cells to provide B-cell help, since naive CD4 T cells from human neonates express minimal amounts of the CD40 ligand after activation (unpublished observations). The critical importance of this form of T-cell help is illustrated by a form of genetic immunodeficiency, the X-linked hyperimmunoglobulin M syndrome. In this disorder mutations in the CD40 ligand gene, which prevent expression of a functional protein, are associated with a marked deficiency in production of specific antibody and in switching from IgM to other immunoglobulin classes.[367]

The CD28 molecule is expressed constitutively on CD4 and most CD8 T cells. It binds to B7 molecules, which are expressed on dendritic cells and on activated B cells and macrophages (see above). The engagement of CD28 on T cells provides a critical costimulus for TCR-dependent activation of T cells, as shown by the profound inhibition of antigen-dependent T-cell activation by antagonists of CD28–B7 interaction.[161–163] For example, CD28 plays an important role in the induction of the CD40 ligand. Other pairs of ligands that contribute to the bidirectional interaction between T and B cells include LFA-1/CD54 and CD5/CD72.[132,138]

The initial activation of B cells and T cells through cognate signaling plays a critical role in the initiation of B-cell proliferation and antibody production. Such interactions are often mimicked in the laboratory by the use of mitogens, for example, by cross-linking surface antigen receptors or by staphylococcal protein A. These stimuli, like soluble antigen, provide the first signals in B-cell activation, but full activation requires secreted lymphokines. Thus, although cross-linking of CD40 and the surface immunoglobulin receptor supports the long-term proliferation of human B cells in vitro, only low levels of IgM, IgG, and IgA are produced.[368] In vitro studies in murine and human systems have demonstrated that a number of cytokines, including IL-2, IL-4, IL-5, IL-6, IL-10, IL-11, TNF-α, IFN-α, and IFN-γ, can modulate B-cell activation, proliferation, and/or differentiation. Studies in the mouse have critically implicated IL-2, IL-4, and IL-6 in driving activated B cells to immunoglobulin production.[369] A role for IL-5 in promoting B-cell differentiation has been clearly established only in the mouse. IL-6 may be important in terminal differentiation and growth of plasma cells. Studies in the CD40 in vitro system with human B cells demonstrated that IL-4 markedly potentiates B-cell proliferation and growth and enhances secretion of IgM, IgG, and IgE. The addition of IL-10 results in synergistic B-cell growth, and, in cooperation with TGF-β, IgA is also produced. Thus B-cell expansion and recovery of all of the major classes of immunoglobulin can be mimicked in this in vitro system.

Experiments in mice in which the IL-2, IL-4, or IFN-γ genes or their receptors have been disrupted by homologous recombination suggest that these predominantly T-cell–derived cytokines are not essential for B-cell development, but are important for regulation of the isotype of immunoglobulin produced.[120,370,371] Cytokines have been implicated in immunoglobulin isotype switching using both in vitro and in vivo systems.[372] Cytokines act as switch factors by altering the chromatin near the 5′ ends of the IgH loci to which switching is directed and induce the accumulation of germ line transcripts for the appropriate heavy chain.[373] IL-4 appears to be the major switch factor in the mouse for IgE and also influences the capacity to produce IgG1. Mice with disruption of the IL-4 gene do not make IgE and have blunted IgG1 responses.[120] IFN-γ is capable of counterregulating the effects of IL-4 in the mouse and promotes IgG2a and IgG3 production. Mice with disruption of the IFN-γ-R gene had blunted IgG2a and IgG3 responses.[371] IFN-α has similar effects as IFN-γ in the mouse, although somewhat less potent.[374] The murine isotypes induced by IFN-γ fix complement and bind efficiently to IgG Fc receptors on phagocytes, whereas IgE induced by IL-4 binds to IgE Fc receptors on mast cells and basophils. This has led to the suggestion that IFN-γ plays an important role in defense against viral and other intracellular pathogens that induce IFN production[375,376] and that IL-4 contributes to defense against metazoan parasites that induce its production.[377] In humans, IL-4 has been implicated in IgE and IgG4 production. In contrast to the mouse, human IL-13 can also promote isotype switching to IgE and IgG4 that is independent of IL-4.[378] CD23, the low-affinity IgE receptor, can also promote IL-4–induced IgE production through binding to an alternative ligand, the cell surface protein CD21.[379] IL-8 inhibits IgE production by IL-4–stimulated human B cells.[380] IFN-γ, as well as IFN-α and PGE₂, can impair IL-4–mediated IgE production by human B cells.[381] In both human and mouse, TGF-β promotes the production of IgA under various costimulatory conditions and, in the mouse, production of IgG2b by activated B cells.[382] IL-5 may boost IgA production in the mouse.[383]

Antigens other than proteins are not presented by MHC and thus are not capable of mediating cognate T cell–B cell interaction. It is unclear if naturally occurring, fully T-cell–independent (type 1) antigens exist in humans; in the mouse such antigens are usually large, multivalent, synthetic molecules. Partially T-cell–independent (type II) antigens are oligovalent antigens with repetitive sites, such as the polysaccharide antigens of encapsulated bacteria. Such antigens may be rendered T dependent through natural association with proteins. In these cases the protein component of the antigen would be presented to T cells, while the multivalent lipid or polysaccharide components may serve to mediate cognate interaction of the B cell with helper T cells. This is the strategy used to convert capsular polysaccharides, which themselves are poor immunogens, to better immu-

nogens (e.g., *Haemophilus influenzae* conjugate vaccines). In the absence of such an association, these nonprotein antigens poorly induce the development of memory B cells and the production of immunoglobulin isotypes other than IgM. The production of isotypes other than IgM directed to nonprotein antigens may result from antigen nonspecific T-cell help for B cells, which is derived from T cells activated by other APC in the B cell's local environment. This is mediated in part by lymphokines secreted by the T cells. It is possible that a recently activated T cell expressing CD40 ligand and with upregulated expression of other ligands/adhesins for B-cell surface molecules may provide direct, albeit noncognate, help for B cells. It is not clear at present whether such interactions occur under physiologic conditions.

COUNTERIMMUNOMODULATORY FUNCTIONS OF T CELLS: SUPPRESSION

The most critical function of the immune system is self/nonself discrimination, which effects the removal of invading microbes while minimizing host injury. As noted above, there are multiple mechanisms that act to retain T cells potentially reactive with nonself, while deleting or rendering unresponsive those reactive to self. The mature T cells that are retained modulate the immune response both through the production of soluble lymphokines and through cell–cell interactions. Both mechanisms participate in T-cell help for B-cell proliferation, differentiation, and immunoglobulin class switching. There is also a body of experimental evidence indicating that T cells may inhibit the function of B cells, T cells, and macrophages. This inhibition may be an active or dominant process, commonly referred to as *suppression*. The lack of firm experimental evidence for the existence of a distinct subset of cells and a definable molecular mechanism by which these cells mediate antigen-specific suppression has engendered considerable skepticism regarding the relevance of these phenomena.[384]

Such cells have been invoked as the cause for the anergy associated with polar lepromatous leprosy. In this disease[384] and in experimental forms of autoimmune disease,[385] induction of suppression is antigen specific but the effector phase is nonspecific and mediated by cytokines. As part of the antigen-specific inductive phase, direct cell–cell interaction by CD8 T cells directed against TCR peptides recognized as nominal antigen (possibly in association with class I MHC molecules on the T cell expressing that specific receptor) is proposed to lead to the production of soluble antigen-specific suppressor factors. The molecular composition of such factors has not been clarified, raising doubt as to their existence. One group suggests that TCR α-chain, in association with other unidentified components not including the β-chain of the TCR, is one component of such a factor.[386] These findings require confirmation. More compelling evidence indicates that inhibition of CD4 T-cell responses by CD8 or other CD4 T cells occurs in these disease states through an antigen nonspecific, nocytotoxic mechanism by release of regulatory cytokines. These include TGF-β,[386–388] IL-4, and IL-10.[384,386]

This work addresses phenomena of considerable potential importance to our understanding of self/nonself discrimination and host defense. Clarification of these phenomena in molecular detail is required before their role in proper regulation of the immune response can be established.

EFFECTOR CELLS AND CYTOKINES MEDIATE AND MODULATE THE ANTIMICROBIAL ACTIVITY OF THE CELLULAR IMMUNE SYSTEM

The preceding sections focused on the role of CMI in the induction of the immune response and regulation of the humoral immune response. CMI also plays a direct and often primary role in controlling infection. This is particularly true for infections

TABLE 2. Cytokine and T-Cell Subsets Implicated in Resistance or Susceptibility to Infection *In Vivo*[a]

	Protection	Susceptibility/Injury
Bacteria		
Mycobacterium tuberculosis/BCG	IFN-γ, TNF-α, TH1, CD8	
Mycobacterium avium-intracellulare	TNF-α, IFN-γ(±)	
Mycobacterium leprae	IFN-γ, TH1	IL-4, TH2
Legionella pneumophila	IFN-γ, TNF-α	
Listeria monocytogenes	IFN-γ, TNF-α, IL-12, TH1	IL-10
Salmonella typhimurium	IFN-γ, TNG-α	
Franciscella tularensis	IFN-γ, TNF-α	IL-4
Chlamydia trachomatis	IFN-γ	
Fungi		
Histoplasma capsulatum	IFN-γ	
Candida albicans	IFN-γ, NK cells, CD4, CD8	IL-4
Candida neoformans	IFN-γ, CD4	
Protozoa		
Toxoplasma gondii	IFN-γ, IL-12, TNF-α(±), CD8, TH1	IL-6, IL-10, IL-4
Leishmania major	IFN-γ, IL-12, TNF-α, TH1	TH2, IL-4, IL-10
Leishmania donovani	IFN-γ, TH1, CD8	IL-10
Trypanosoma cruzi	IFN-γ, TNF-α, CD8	
Plasmodia	CD8, TH1, TNF-α, IFN-γ	Excess CD8, TH1, TNF-α, IFN-γ, cerebral injury
Cryptosporidium	IFN-γ	
Metazoa		
Heligmosomoides polygyrus (murine intestinal pathogen)	IL-4	
Schistosoma mansoni	IFN-γ	IL-2, TH2
Trichinella spiralis	TH1	TH2
Representative viruses		
Cytomegalovirus	IFN-γ, CD8, TH1	
Herpes simplex virus	IFN-γ, CD8, TH1	
Vaccinia virus	IFN-γ, TNF-α, TH1	
Influenza virus	IFN-γ, CD8, TH1	
Measles virus	TH1	

Abbreviations: IFN-γ: interferon-γ; TNF-α: tumor necrosis factor α; TH1: type 1 helper (CD4) T cells; TH2: type 2 helper (CD4) T cells.
[a] Data are from studies in mice with the exception of *M. leprae, L. major,* and *L. donovani,* for which there are preliminary treatment or correlative data in man; see text for details.

(Modified from Scott and Kaufman,[456] with permission.)

with microbes that survive and replicate within host cells (Table 2). Immunity to these facultative and obligate intracellular pathogens is mediated by effector cells, including antigen-specific cytotoxic T cells, NK cells and activated macrophages, and cytokines. CMI also appears to play an important, direct role in defense against multicellular metazoan pathogens (Table 2). In addition to their role as direct mediators of cellular immunity, T cells and cytokines can also enhance or attenuate the cell-mediated effector response, paralleling their role as modulators of the humoral immune response. CMI also modulates the host response against pyogenic bacterial pathogens, although some evidence suggests that T cells may play a more direct role in defense against certain of these microbes (e.g., *Pseudomonas aeruginosa, Bacteroides fragilis*).[389,390]

Cytotoxic T Cells

Most cytotoxic T cells express CD8 and mediate antigen-specific, class I MHC-restricted cytolytic activity. This may be functionally desirable since antigens that are presented by class I MHC molecules are generally derived from proteins synthe-

sized within the cell, thus focusing the cytotoxic activity toward cells in which microbes (e.g., viruses) are replicating rather than cells that may have acquired antigen by endocytosis from the extracellular environment. Cytotoxic CD8 T cells are thought to play a particularly important role in defense against viral pathogens,[2] although they also contribute to resistance against other intracellular pathogens (e.g., *Listeria;* see below). The role of these cells in specific infectious diseases is discussed more completely below. CD4 T cells may exhibit cytotoxicity in vitro in response to some agents. That CD4 T cells may be functionally cytotoxic in vivo is supported in part by the ability of mice that lack class I MHC and CD8 T cells to clear many viral infections normally,[2] although it is not clear that CD4 T-cell–dependent viral clearance in these mice is mediated by cytotoxicity or that such mice correctly reflect the role played by CD4 T cells in normal animals or in man.

In the absence of recent stimulation by infection or immunization, CD8 T cells that are isolated from the blood or tissues are not cytolytic, with the exception of HIV infection. However, subsequent exposure to antigen through infection or immunization stimulates the development of CD8 T cells with antigen-specific and MHC class I–restricted cytolytic activity. The activation of CD8 T cells through the TCR is augmented by the interaction of CD2 and LFA-1 with their respective ligands: LFA-3 and ICAM-1, -2, and -3 (and between CD28 and B7 if the latter is present on the target cells). CD4 T cells facilitate development of cytotoxic T lymphocytes (CTL) by production of multiple cytokines. The most important of these appears to be IL-2, which appears to be required for efficient CTL generation in vitro and in vivo[391,392]; most definitive in this regard is the defect in development of CTL in mice in which the IL-2 gene has been ablated.[370,393] Other cytokines that appear to facilitate CTL development in vitro include IL-4, IL-7, IL-10, IL-12, and IFN-γ.[253,394–398] However, the importance of most of these for CTL generation has not been tested rigorously in vivo, with the exception of IFN-γ. In mice in which either the IFN-γ or the IFN-γ receptor genes have been ablated, development of CTL was found to be normal or at most minimally diminished,[371,398] suggesting that IFN-γ does not play an obligatory role in CTL development. The ability of cytokines to facilitate CTL development is governed in part by the expression of their respective receptors. In this regard the critical role of IL-2 in CTL development and the restriction of high-affinity IL-2 receptor expression to T cells that have recently been activated by recognition of specific antigen in association with MHC appropriately constrains cytotoxicity to those cells recently activated by specific antigen.

The biochemical changes associated with the acquisition of cytotoxic capacity have been explored in considerable depth. Nevertheless, the mechanisms by which cytotoxic T cells kill their targets remain controversial, perhaps reflecting multiple, in part redundant, mechanisms. The best characterized changes are the synthesis of perforin and of a family of proteases (granzymes) that are stored within the granules of differentiated CTL. Perforin, like the membrane attack complex of complement, can form pores in the plasma membrane of target cells and organisms.[399] The granzymes are serine proteases.[391,400,401] Development of cytotoxic function in murine T cells in vitro is associated with acquisition of perforin and granzymes. Recent experiments suggest that one of the granzymes plays an important role in the cytolytic function of these cells in vitro.[401] Other studies suggest that under some conditions cytolysis is not mediated by these granule components.[402,403] Alternative mediators of cytotoxicity include cytokines produced by CD8 T cells, such as TNF-α and lymphotoxin,[404] or perhaps cell-associated forms of these mediators, including the recently described lymphotoxin α/β-heterotrimer.[289] The relative role of each of these in killing remains to be resolved and may vary depending on the target cell. Furthermore, the overall importance of cytotoxicity in the function of CD8 T cells has been questioned by some, who suggest that local and focused production of cytokines like TNF-α, lymphotoxin, and IFN-γ by CD8 T cells may be more important.[405] Since CD4 T cells are also efficient producers of these cytokines, it is possible that the relative preservation of resistance to viral infection in mice lacking CD8 T cells[2] is due to this mechanism rather than to cytotoxicity.

NK CELLS

Natural killer cells are a lymphocyte subset, originally identified by their morphologic appearance as large granular lymphocytes. In humans they can be identified by the expression of the CD16 and/or CD56 surface antigens and the absence of surface expression of the CD3 complex.[406,407] Most NK cells in the adult express CD57, and many express CD2. The latter is a marker expressed on all T lymphocytes. Other evidence suggests that NK cells are most closely related to T lymphocytes. Multiple components of the CD3 complex are expressed in human fetal NK cells and are transiently expressed in activated NK cells from adults. One component of the CD3 complex, the ζ-chain, is important in the function of mature NK cells. CD3 ζ-chain and the immunoglobulin Fc receptor CD16 are expressed as a complex on NK cells, the ζ-chain being required for cell surface expression of CD16. Unlike T cells, NK cells develop normally in the absence of a thymus, do not exhibit rearrangement of TCR or immunoglobulin genes, and are present in normal or increased numbers in mice and many humans with SCID, which lack mature T and B cells.[407,408]

NK cells were originally defined by their ability to lyse target cells in a manner not restricted by MHC antigens and not requiring presensitization. Recent evidence suggests that this involves a novel and more phylogenetically and ontogenetically primitive system for self/nonself discrimination. NK cells appear to recognize the absence of self-MHC expression[408,409] in contrast to T cells, which recognize foreign antigen in the context of self-MHC or the presence of foreign MHC. This property endows NK cells with the capacity to reject bone marrow grafts from individuals lacking recipient MHC even if they do not express foreign MHC (a phenomenon referred to as *hybrid resistance* and important in bone marrow transplantation). In addition, in certain tumors and in certain viral-infected cells, self-MHC expression is inhibited or perhaps masked by the presence of foreign peptides, leading to recognition by NK cells. The receptors that endow NK cells with the capacity to recognize lack of self are not completely defined, but are likely to exhibit only limited polymorphism.[409,410] The existing data suggest that certain of these putative NK receptors associate with the CD3 ζ-chain, as does the NK cell Fc receptor CD16. The cytotoxic activity of NK cells is triggered by engagement of antigen–IgG complexes through the CD16 Fc receptor (a process referred to as *antibody-dependent cell-mediated cytotoxicity* [ADCC]) or by binding of NK cells to targets recognized as lacking self (referred to as *natural cytotoxicity*).

NK cells may play an important role in defense against intracellular infectious pathogens, particularly against infection with the herpes group viruses. Most of the data are derived from studies in mice challenged with herpes simplex virus,[411] cytomegalovirus,[412] *Toxoplasma gondii*,[413] or *Listeria monocytogenes*.[1,414] However, rare patients who have few or no detectable NK cells experience severe initial infection with multiple herpes group viruses, suggesting that this is also true in humans (unpublished observation).[415]

NK cells proliferate in response to IL-2, which is augmented by IL-12, IL-7, and IFN-γ.[416,417] Their cytotoxic activity is enhanced by IL-2, IL-12, IFN-γ, and IFN-α/β. In addition to their cytolytic activity, NK cells are important producers of IFN-γ and TNF-α in the early phases of the immune and inflammatory response; NK cells also produce GM-CSF.[417] Cytokine production is induced by engagement of Fc receptors by IgG or by exposure to IL-2 or IL-12. NK cells may influence the development of CD4+ T cells through production of IFN-γ, which biases CD4 T cells preferentially to produce the TH1 cytokines, IFN-γ, IL-2, and other cytokines favorable to defense against infection.[418] NK cells also play a role in dampening the immune response through inhibition of T- and B-cell hematopoietic precursor cell proliferation.

MONONUCLEAR PHAGOCYTES

The mononuclear phagocyte system includes bone marrow progenitors, circulating monocytes, and tissue macrophages. In the adult, the promonocyte is the first recognizable precursor cell, although it is presumably derived from a common myeloid stem cell precursor. Promonocytes are actively dividing cells that mature into monocytes, which are generally nonreplicating. Monocytes are released from the marrow within 24 hours and circulate in the blood for 1–3 days before moving to the tissues under steady-state conditions. Their growth and maturation in the marrow and function are regulated by specific CSF and other cytokines.

Once leaving the blood, unlike lymphocytes, monocytes do not recirculate, but differentiate into macrophages, which are present in all tissues. The estimated life-span of tissue macrophages is 4–12 weeks. Under steady-state conditions, more than 95 percent of mononuclear phagocytes are mature tissue macrophages and less than 2 percent are monocytes. Data from bone marrow transplants indicate that tissue macrophages are derived from blood monocyte precursors, although tissue macrophages are capable of self-renewal to some degree. Differentiation of monocytes into macrophages is associated with some common maturational changes and others that are unique to the specific tissues.

Resting tissue macrophage play an important role in clearing small numbers of microbes that gain access to tissues and the removal of damaged or effete cells or extracellular matrix. These cells express on their plasma membrane three forms of the receptor for the Fc portion of IgG, which differ in regard to their affinity for different IgG isotypes and the receptor for the Fc portion of IgA.[419] They also express the CR1 and CR3 receptors for complement C3b and C3bi,[420] receptors for lipopolysaccharide,[421] and receptors for high mannose and fucose.[422,4243] The latter allows these cells to recognize, in an antigen nonspecific manner, unencapsulated bacteria, yeast, influenza virus, and effete host cells, since these but not normal host cells express high mannose containing carbohydrates on their surface. These receptors allow high-affinity binding. Cross-linking of receptors through multivalent interactions with their respective ligand triggers phagocytosis, which encloses the microbe in vacuoles into which the macrophage secretes a variety of potentially microbicidal compounds. These include reactive oxygen products, such as superoxide anion, hydrogen peroxide, or their reactive derivative, hydroxyl radical. This oxygen-dependent mechanism is of particular importance in the killing of catalase-containing pyogenic microbes.[424] Microbicidal granule proteins, including the cationic proteins cathepsin G, BPI, lysozyme, and phagosomal acidification, constitute the principal oxygen-independent mechanisms of resident human tissue macrophages; human macrophages do not appear to contain defensins, which are important components of the oxygen-independent mechanisms of human neutrophils and macrophages from some species.[425] Whether killing and/or degradation of phagocytosed organisms is effective depends at least in part on the characteristics of the organism, the receptors involved in phagocytosis, and the functional state of the mononuclear phagocyte. In contrast to circulating neutrophils and monocytes and to activated macrophages (see below), the microbicidal activity of macrophages resident in most tissues is relatively modest. This may be important in allowing macrophages to remove small numbers of microbes and tissue debris, without excessively damaging tissues through the release of potentially toxic compounds. However, the capacity of such cells may be overwhelmed by infection with numerous or highly virulent pathogens. An effective response in these situations may require the recruitment of other leukocytes from the blood and the activation of macrophages to a state of enhanced antimicrobial activity.

Recruitment of Monocytes and Activation of Macrophages in Response to Infection

In the process of phagocytosis, in response to lipopolysaccharide or other microbial components or in response to mediators derived from the humoral immune system (e.g., complement components), tissue macrophages release mediators that lead to the recruitment of leukocytes from the blood. Other tissue cells also contribute. The nature of the mediators produced may vary with the type of infection and over the course of an infection and thereby determine the nature of the inflammatory response that develops. Lipid-derived mediators, such as leukotriene B4 and PAF are produced rapidly from preformed precursors, whereas IL-1, TNF-α, and the chemotactic cytokines (chemokines) are produced somewhat later by synthesis. In response to acute pyogenic infection or injury, these mediators act in a concerted fashion to direct an initial recruitment of neutrophils. If infection is effectively controlled, this is followed within 6–12 hours by the influx of monocytes and lymphocytes. The determinants of this sequential influx of leukocyte types may relate to the slower migration of monocytes and lymphocytes, the preferential expression late in the reaction of lymphokines (chemokines) and vascular endothelial adhesion molecules that favor the influx of mononuclear cells, or both.[227a]

The adhesion molecules, which are known to play a central role in leukocyte adhesion to endothelium, the first step in leukocyte emigration into tissues, are members of one of three families of cell surface glycoproteins: the selectins, the integrins, and certain members of the immunoglobulin gene superfamily.[130,426–428]

The selectins are named by the cell types in which they are primarily expressed: L-selectin by leukocytes, E-selectin by endothelial cells, and P-selectin by platelets and endothelial cells. Selectins are named for their ability to bind to specific types of carbohydrates that are selectively expressed on different tissues; binding is mediated through a lectin-like domain found in all family members. The integrins are dimeric proteins composed of an α- and a β-chain. There are multiple integrins differing in chain composition.

Mononuclear phagocytes express L-selectin and each of the three β2-integrins. L-selectin is expressed on naive T cells. All lymphocytes express the LFA-1 (CD11α/CD18) and some express the Mac-1/CR3 (CD11β/CD18) integrin. Monocytes and memory T cells also express the $\alpha_4\beta_1$-integrin VLA-4 (very late antigen-4).[232,428] ICAM-2 is constitutively expressed on endothelium, whereas ICAM-1 expression is increased markedly by exposure to inflammatory mediators, including IL-1, TNF-α, and lipopolysaccharide. ICAM-3 is expressed primarily on other myeloid and lymphoid cells and is important for interactions between these cells, but not between these cells and endothelium.[132] VCAM, also a member of the immunoglobulin gene superfamily, is expressed only on endothelium activated by exposure to cytokines or bacterial products such as lipopolysaccharide. In response to activation of monocytes and T cells, L-selectin expression diminishes. This effect persists, such that memory T cells generally express lower amounts of L-selectin. Activation also results in an increase in the abundance and avidity of the β1- and β2-integrins for their endothelial ligands. The upregulation of the avidity of the β1- and β2-integrins mediates leukocyte adhesion to and migration through the endothelium.[429] Since VLA-4 is present on mononuclear but not neutrophilic leukocytes, it may be a contributing factor in the ability of monocytes and memory T cells to enter tissues in states not

associated with neutrophilic inflammatory responses, such as DTH. The expression of VLA-4 may also account for the capacity of monocytes but not neutrophils to enter tissues in the leukocyte adhesion deficiency syndrome, which is due to the lack of expression of β2-integrins.[430]

Many of the factors that are chemotactic for neutrophils also induce monocyte chemotaxis. These include bacterial products such as FMLP, activated complement components such as C5a, and lipid products including leukotriene B4 and PAF. However, those chemokines (Table 1) that are chemotactic for neutrophils are not generally chemotactic for monocytes and vice versa. For example, IL-8 and other type I chemokines are chemotactic for neutrophils but not for monocytes, whereas type II chemokines, including MCP-1, MIP-1α, and -1β, and RANTES selectively activate and attract monocytes.[431] The coordinate influx of monocytes and lymphocytes may be related to the ability of the MIP-1α to attract CD8 T cells and MIP-1β and RANTES to attract CD4 T cells.[432]

Unlike the acute inflammatory response, DTH responses are characterized by an influx of mononuclear phagocytes and lymphocytes, with minimal or no neutrophilic influx. This response reaches a maximum at 24–72 hours after antigen infiltration. Recent experimental evidence in mice and humans undergoing DTH reactions suggests that this process is governed, at least in part, by cytokines. These include IL-1 and TNF-α, produced by epidermal Langerhans cells (which are marrow-derived dendritic cells) and by epithelial cells, and IL-2 and IFN-γ, produced by T cells infiltrating the subcutaneous tissues.[433,434] The expression of these cytokines and the induction by IFN-γ of class II MHC antigen reaches its maximum before the peak influx of cells and induration, consistent with a role in causation.

Regulation of the Immune and Inflammatory Responses by Monokines

Monocytes and macrophages play important roles in regulation of the afferent and efferent phases of the immune response. As noted above, mononuclear phagocytes and the related dendritic cells are important APC. The production by macrophages of cytokines facilitates this process and modulates the efferent immune and inflammatory responses (Table 1). Monocytes and macrophages, particularly primed and activated macrophages, produce IL-1, chemokines (e.g., IL-8), TNF-α, IFN-α, and G-CSF, and M-CSF; macrophages also produce IL-10 and IL-6. Whether macrophages or other cells (e.g., endothelial cells) are the major source of these cytokines varies depending on the inciting stimulus for their production and the tissue. Most cytokines produced by mononuclear phagocytes have potent and diverse systemic effects in addition to their effects on functions of other cells of the immune system (see above).

In general, phagocytosis, lipopolysaccharide or cognate interaction with T cells (to which antigen is being presented) stimulate macrophages to synthesize specific cytokine mRNA and proteins, followed by cytokine secretion. In some cases, low-level expression of the mRNA encoding certain of these cytokines has been observed in normal tissues, but protein is not known to be produced in the absence of stimulation. Many of these cytokines induce or modulate each other's production: TNF-α and IL-1 directly induce production of IL-1, TNF-α, IL-6, and G-, M-, and GM-CSF by mononuclear phagocytes and other cells such as endothelial cells. Compared with TNF-α and IL-1, IL-6 and IL-10 are expressed later after activation, and they inhibit production of TNF-α and IL-1.[435] Similarly, mononuclear phagocytes produce an antagonist of IL-1, the IL-1 receptor antagonist (IL-1ra), the production of which also occurs later after stimulation.[285,436] The late production of these counterregulatory cytokines may dampen the response and attenuate immune-mediated injury. Reciprocally, activation of macrophages by T-cell–derived products, particularly IFN-γ, leads to enhanced production of proinflammatory cytokines and attenuates production of IL-10.[437] Thus, production of cytokines by mononuclear phagocytes is normally temporally restricted to those cells in contact with agonistic stimuli at sites of infection or inflammation and is under positive and negative control. Excess production of TNF-α, IL-1, IFN-γ, and other proinflammatory cytokines plays a deleterious role in septic shock and related syndromes (ARDS), underscoring the importance of closely regulated and anatomically restricted production of these cytokines.[329,438]

Macrophage Activation: A Cytokine-Regulated Process

Along with the recruitment of monocytes and T cells into sites of infection and inflammation, enhancement of the antimicrobial and proinflammatory functions of macrophages contributes to host defense. This process is commonly referred to as *macrophage activation*. It was first described by Mackaness[439] in the 1960s. In these and related studies, resistance to intracellular pathogens, such as *Mycobacterium* spp., *Listeria*, and *Toxoplasma*, could be transferred adoptively from immune to naive animals by T lymphocytes and did not develop in T-cell–deficient nude mice. As the infection was brought under control macrophages at sites of infection were found to have enhanced microbicidal activity not only against the specific pathogen but also against a wide range of microbes. Dissection of this process in vitro indicated that the T cells activated in response to specific antigens secreted lymphokines that primed macrophages for enhanced microbicidal activity. The predominant lymphokine that activates macrophages appears to be IFN-γ.[394,413,440–442] Subsequent exposure to microbes or to their products and host factors derived from cells of the innate immune system (NK cells and phagocytes) further enhances their activity, in part by inducing TNF-α production. The increased microbicidal activity is associated with increased expression of type I Fc receptors for IgG[443,444] and enhanced chemotactic and phagocytic capacity.

The efficiency with which activated macrophages kill varies between organisms. For example, activated human macrophages are microbicidal for *Toxoplasma gondii* and *Leishmania donovani*, inhibit but do not kill *Chlamydia psittaci*, and have variable activity against mycobacteria. This reflects in part an increased capacity to generate reactive oxygen metabolites.[440] In mice, the de novo induction of the inducible nitric oxide synthase enables activated macrophages to generate nitric oxide and other reactive nitrogen metabolites. These compounds appear to be the predominant mediators of murine macrophage activity against many intracellular protozoan and bacterial pathogens and Cryptococci.[445–447] However, the available evidence suggests that activated human macrophages do not express the inducible nitric oxide synthase, suggesting that nitric oxide may not play a parallel role in the human.[448] Other antimicrobial mechanisms are induced in activated macrophages. These include the degradation of tryptophan and scavenging of iron, which may impede the intracellular replication of *Chlamydia psittaci* and *Toxoplasma*[449–451] and of *Legionella pneumonophila*,[452] respectively. The variety of mechanisms contributing to the enhanced antimicrobial activity of activated macrophages likely reflects both a useful redundancy and the coevolution of host defenses and microbes, each seeking to counter the newest or most efficient gambits of the other. The mechanisms by which pathogens have evolved to evade various components of these defenses are discussed below.

More recent data[413,440,453–455] indicate that activated macrophages are not only an essential element of defense against nonviral intracellular pathogens but play a more general role in host defense. This may reflect (1) their enhanced capacity for antigen processing and presentation due to increased expression of MHC class I and II and of MHC class I–linked peptide transporters and (2) their important role in the production of cytokines that regulate the inflammatory and acute phase responses to infection.

Macrophage activation is only one component of the T-cell–dependent and lymphokine-mediated immunity originally identified through the studies of adoptive protection noted above. Effector CD4 and CD8 T cells acquire enhanced capacity to release lymphokines that impede replication of intracellular pathogens not only in macrophages but also in other host cells. Cytotoxic T cells lyse cells infected with viruses and nonviral intracellular pathogens.[1,2] Several types of information indicate the importance of lymphokines, particularly IFN-γ, in this overall process (Table 3). One is the capacity of lymphokines when given before or soon after experimental infection to provide protection; a second is the impairment of immunity in experimental animals that are treated either with antibodies that neutralize the activity of a specific lymphokine or in which a specific lymphokine gene has been ablated genetically by homologous recombination; finally, a wide variety of microbes express proteins that function as antagonists of specific cytokines and that in some cases can be shown by genetic means to be important for the pathogenesis of infection with these agents. This information is summarized in Table 3 and discussed below in the context of specific pathogens.

ROLE OF CMI IN DEFENSE AGAINST SPECIFIC TYPES OF INFECTIOUS PATHOGENS

CMI appears to be the central mechanism by which infection with intracellular pathogens is controlled. This includes virtually all viral pathogens. In addition, CMI plays a critical role in defense against nonviral, nonpyogenic microbes: the facultative or obligate intracellular pathogens, which are capable of or are restricted to replication within host cells, respectively, and extracellular metazoan pathogens. CMI also contributes to protection against some fungi, in concert with neutrophils, antibody, and complement. In Table 2, the role of specific T-cell subsets and cytokines is given for those organisms in which there are sufficient data, either in experimental animal models or in some infections of humans, to support their role in protection from or susceptibility to infection or infection-associated injury. The list is representative rather than exhaustive, particularly for the viral pathogens. For some agents the information is more detailed than for others; the absence of information regarding the role for a specific T-cell subset or cytokine does not indicate that they play no role in that infection, merely that the information is not available. In many cases in vitro studies suggest that similar mechanisms are at least in part applicable to other related pathogens. This section discusses general paradigms, using illustrative pathogens as examples. Specific details about other pathogens may be sought in the chapters on those agents. Immunomodulatory therapy is discussed at the end of this section.

Nonviral Pathogens: Intracellular

Each of the bacterial and protozoan pathogens, which are listed in Table 2, and the fungus *Histoplasma capsulatum* are facultative or obligate intracellular pathogens. Other agents in this class include species of *Brucella*, *Yersinia*, *Nocardia*, and *Rickettsia*. For these organisms entry into macrophages (and for some agents, e.g., *Toxoplasma*, *Plasmodia*, *Chlamydia*, other host cells as well) plays an important role in their pathogenesis, in contrast to extracellular, pyogenic microbes for which ingestion by phagocytes usually results in death.

Based to a large extent on experiments performed in rodent models, the principal mechanisms of host defense against these pathogens appear to be mediated by the conserted and sequential action of the innate and then antigen-specific components of the immune system: NK cells and macrophages, and later

TABLE 3. Virus Proteins Known or Predicted To Effect Immune and Inflammatory Responses

Virus Family	Virus	Product	Host Target	Role In Vivo	Reference
Adenoviruses		VA RNA	IFN (α/β)	Unknown	Mathews and Shenk (1991)[649]
		E3-gp 19K	Class I MHC		Wold and Gooding (1991)[650]
		E3-14.7K	TNF	No effect on replication; diminish injury	Wold and Gooding (1991)[650]
		E-3-10, 4/14.5K	TNF		Wold and Gooding (1991)[650]
		E1B-19K	TNF		Wold and Gooding (1991)[650]
					Wold and Gooding (1991)[650]
Poxviruses	Shope fibroma/myxoma	T2	TNF		Smith et al. (1991)[651]
	Vaccinia	VCP	Complement	Increase viral replication; impede inflammatory response	Kotwal et al., (1990),[652]
	Vaccinia/cowpox	B15R	IL-1		Spriggs et al., (1992),[653] Alcami and Smith (1992)[655]
	Cowpox	crmA	IL-1		Ray et al. (1992)[655]
	Myxoma	MT7	IFN-γ		Upton (1992)[656]
Herpesviruses	Epstein-Barr virus	EBER RNA	IFN (α/β)	Unknown	Bhat and Thimmappaya (1983)[657]
	Epstein-Barr virus	BCRF1	Cytokine synthesis	Unknown	Hsu et al. (1990)[658]
	Cytomegalovirus	UL18	Class I MHC	Unknown	Browne et al. (1990)[659]
	Cytomegalovirus	US28	MIP-1αR	Unknown	Gao et al. (1993)[660]
	Herpes simplex I/II	gC-1	Complement	Unknown	Harris et al. (1990)[661]
	Herpes simplex I/II	gE-g1	Antibody	Unknown	Bell et al. (1990)[662]
	Herpes saimiri	CCPH	Complement	Unknown	Albrecht and Fleckenstine (1992)[663]
	Herpesvirus saimiri	ECRF3	IL-8 R, type B	Unknown	Gao et al. (1993)[660]

Abbreviations: IFN: interferons; CTL: cytotoxic T lymphocytes; TNF: Tumor necrosis factor; IL: interleukin.
(Modified from Gooding,[276] with permission.)

in infection, antigen-specific T lymphocytes and the cytokines produced by these cells. In the early phase of the immune response (the first 5–7 days) the efficiency of the pathogen nonspecific, innate immune response determines whether infection is limited or disseminates widely. This phase of the immune response is independent of classic αβ-TCR–bearing T cells and B cells and is generally not curative. In the later phase of the immune response, antigen-specific immunity serves to eliminate active infection, resulting either in eradication of the organism or the cessation of active infection and the establishment of latency.

In the first days of infection, recruitment of monocytes to the loci of infection and the activation of NK cells to produce IFN-γ appear to be important factors in host resistance; this has been most completely explored in infections with *Listeria*, *Leishmania*, and *Toxoplasma*.[283,413,414,456,457] The importance of monocyte recruitment may relate to the greater capacity of these cells than resident tissue macrophages to kill these organisms[413,457] and with their greater capacity to produce cytokines that help control infection, such as TNF-α. The production of IFN-γ is detectable in infected mice before antigen-specific T cells are detectable, suggesting that it is derived from NK cells. This process has been best elucidated in nude mice or mice with SCID, which lack or have few T cells but which have NK cell numbers and function that are equal to or exceed those of normal mice. Microbial products appear to induce TNF-α and IL-12 production from mononuclear phagocytes, and these in concert stimulate NK cells to produce IFN-γ. Recent data strongly suggest that IL-12, also called *NK-stimulating factor*, is the essential cytokine produced by macrophages in response to these microbes, which stimulates the production of IFN-γ from NK cells.[283,341,342] The role of TNF-α in IFN-γ induction appears to result primarily from its enhancement of IL-12 production. Conversely the deleterious effects of IL-10 and IL-4 in these infections may result, at least in part, from their inhibition of IL-12 production. Together IFN-γ and TNF-α enhance the capacity of macrophages to kill these organisms (see description of macrophage activation, above). T cells expressing γδ-TCR also appear to contribute to resistance in the early phase of infection with *Listeria*, *Salmonella*, and *Mycobacterium*.[1,458] Whether these cells are responding to microbial components or

host components induced in the stress response to infection is not clear.

Recent evidence strongly suggests that an autosomal recessive gene linked to a locus on chromosome 1 in the mouse, is of critical importance in resistance to *Leish. donovanii*, *Salmonella typhimurium*, and mycobacteria (BCG strain of *Mycobacterium bovis*, *M. avium*, and *M. lepraemurium* [the murine lepra bacillus]). This locus is commonly referred to as the *Bcg/Ity/Lsh* locus.[459] This locus also appears to correlate with resistance to primary infection resulting from ingestion of *Toxoplasma* oocysts.[460] Macrophages from resistant strains of mice are able to restrict the intracellular replication of these microbes, whereas these microbes replicate much more readily in macrophages from sensitive strains. A candidate gene from this locus has recently been cloned and encodes a novel protein *(Nramp)* with homology to a bacterial nitrate transport protein from a prokaryote.[461] This has led to the suggestion that the enhanced ability of macrophages from resistant strains of mice to kill these microbes may be related to a greater ability to deliver microbicidal nitric oxide metabolites into the phagosome. A nonconservative amino acid difference is present in the coding sequence of the gene in susceptible vs. resistant strains. Formal proof that this is the basis for the difference in resistance is still needed. This gene may be a major factor in human disease susceptibility as well.

There are clear differences in susceptibility of humans to infection with these or related organisms. For leprosy, the ability of the bacterium to establish infection is genetically inherited in an autosomal recessive manner, but the locus is not known.[384] A region on chromosome 2q in the human is syntenic with the murine *Bcg/Ity/Lsh* locus. Although it is not known whether resistance to leprosy in humans is genetically linked to this region, this locus is a strong candidate. Similarly, susceptibility to infection with *M. tuberculosis* is genetically determined in humans, although the genetic locus (or loci) has not been mapped.[462] Once infection with the lepra bacillus is established, risk for progression to multibacillary lepromatous disease is associated with genes in the MHC complex. Linkage of subsequent disease course to the MHC is consistent with the critical role that antigen-specific T cells play in eradication of infection. For example, mice lacking mature T cells ultimately succumb from infection even though NK function and the efficiency of the early containment phase of infection is more robust in such animals. It also appears that the nature of the response in the early containment phase plays a critical role in determining the qualitative nature of the subsequent T-cell–mediated response.

The importance of the functional qualities of antigen-specific T cells is most clearly illustrated by one well-characterized murine disease model, infection with *Leishmania major,* and by one human disease, leprosy. The development of antigen-specific immunity during primary infection results from the presentation of microbial antigens in association with class II MHC molecules on APC. Engagement of receptors on CD4 T cells for antigen–MHC in association with relevant accessory molecules (e.g., B7) on the APC leads to activation of these cells. In certain inbred strains of mice the nature of the CD4 T cells that develop appear to play a critical role in the subsequent outcome of infection. In strains (e.g., BALB/c) that develop progressive cutaneous and then disseminated infection, the CD4 T cells exhibit a distinct TH2 profile, producing IL-4 but little IFN-γ, whereas strains that are resistant to infection develop CD4 T cells with a TH1 profile, with abundant production of IFN-γ and little or no IL-4.[377] It appears that robust generation of TH1 T cells is the proximate cause of the susceptibility of the BALB/c strain. This can be blocked by partial depletion or inhibition of proliferation of CD4 T cells or by administration of antibodies to IL-4, conditions that favor the development of TH2 T cells. Reciprocally, resistant strains of mice can be rendered susceptible by excess IL-4.[463] Results similar to these have been obtained in humans infected with *Leishmania braziliensis.*[464] Recent data suggest that a major factor determining whether TH1 or TH2 T cells develop is the extent to which macrophages or B cells of the mice produce IL-12 or IL-10 (which may act by blocking IL-12 production) in response to infection.[283,342,456] As noted above, IL-12 acts to stimulate IFN-γ production by T cells and NK cells and to inhibit IL-4 production by T cells, thereby biasing CD4 development into TH1 effector cells. These cytokines exert opposite effects on the ability of macrophages to kill *Leishmania:* IFN-γ in concert with TNF-α activates macrophages to kill the parasite, whereas IL-4 and IL-10 inhibit macrophage activation.[435,446,465–467] In this infection, in which the organism infects almost exclusively macrophages and resides within a phagocytic vacuole, it is likely that the difference in macrophage activation by cytokines is the principal determinant of outcome. Mechanisms of defense against the causative agent of visceral leishmaniasis in man, *Leish. donovani,* appear to be similar, at least as regards resistance to primary infection.[468,469]

The polar nature of *Leish. major* infection in inbred mice parallels in many ways the spectrum of disease observed in leprosy.[384] Patients with the tuberculoid form have a strong cellular immune response dominated by the presence of CD8 and CD4 T cells with a TH1 profile (good producers of IL-2, IFN-γ, and TNF-α), few lesions, and very small numbers of viable *Mycobacterium leprae.*[470,471] In contrast, patients with the lepromatous form have a TH2-like response associated with greater amounts of antibody than patients with the tuberculoid form and an extraordinarily high body burden of leprosy bacilli. These differences have been observed both by examination of the abundance and profile of cells in the lesions of patients by immunohistochemistry and in situ hybridization and by examination of the capacity of lymphocytes isolated from patients to produce cytokines in vitro[472]; however, by the latter technique some investigators have failed to observe a clear association between TH2 cytokines and lepromatous disease.[473] Whether the polar variations in disease pattern and T-cell responses in leprosy result from genetic differences in the nature of the innate immune response, as suggested for *Leish. major* infection in mice, is not known.

Although the spectrum of responses observed in these two infections is not so clearly evident in those due to other intracellular pathogens, it appears that many of the basic principles

are similar. Some differences in mechanisms of protection may result from the wide variety of strategies by which intracellular pathogens evade killing by resident macrophages.[1,474] For example, *Toxoplasma* evades killing since it is both relatively resistant to and fails to trigger an effective production of microbicidal oxygen metabolites or phagolysosome fusion.[475–477] *Trypanosoma cruzi* evades oxygen metabolites and lysosomal proteins by escaping from the cytoplasmic vacuole into the cytoplasm. Other intracellular pathogens use one or more of these strategies to survive in macrophages and other cells. Although there are variations, there is considerable evidence that the production of IFN-γ, and other cytokines produced efficiently by TH1 CD4 T cells and CD8 T cells, is a central feature of effective host defense for each.

In *Toxoplasma* infection, the production of IFN-γ by T cells appears to be the single most important factor in resolution of acute infection, in the prevention of recrudescence of chronic, latent infection, and in protection from secondary infection.[413,478,479] This is suggested (1) by the quantitative correlation between the amount of IFN-γ produced and resistance to infection, (2) by the protection afforded by administration of IFN-γ, and (3) by the ability of antibodies to IFN-γ to accelerate the development of lethal acute infection or cause recrudescence of dormant central nervous system infection. IFN-γ activates macrophages to kill this organism and inhibits its growth in other cells. The importance of T cells as producers of IFN-γ in *Toxoplasma* infection is indicated (1) by the development of CD4 T cells that produce a TH1 pattern of cytokines and of CD8 T cells that produce IFN-γ in mice resolving infection, (2) by the ability of such cells to transfer resistance adoptively, and (3) by the abrogation of resistance to acute and latent infection by depletion of these cells. Both CD4 and CD8 T cells appear to play an important role in this process, since depletion of both subsets is required to abrogate immunity; CD8 T cells may be the most important. It is interesting to note that *Toxoplasma,* a pathogen that replicates solely within cytoplasmic vacuoles, is nevertheless a target for recognition by CD8 T cells, which see antigen in the context of class I MHC. Since antigenic peptides that associate with class I MHC generally do so in the ER or in the cytosol, these data suggest that proteins or peptides derived from this organism gain access to this compartment. The importance of CD8 T cells in defense against *Toxoplasma* may reflect the fact that this parasite, unlike *Leishmania,* infects virtually all nucleated cells, not just macrophages, so that activation of the macrophages' ability to kill ingested parasites would not be sufficient to control infection. Although IFN-γ is required for CD8 T cells to provide protection against *Toxoplasma,* it is possible that CD8 T cells also act in part by lysing infected cells.[413,480] *Toxoplasma* infection is particularly problematic in adults with AIDS in whom the principal deficiency is the functional and numerical loss of CD4 T cells; however, in advanced HIV infection CD8 T cells are also affected. Among the other cytokines, TNF-α and IL-1 appear to act with IFN-γ to enhance resistance in vivo. In contrast, IL-6 and IL-10, which may be produced by macrophages and TH2 CD4 T cells, antagonize the enhancement of macrophage anti-*Toxoplasma* activity induced by IFN-γ in vitro.

Mechanisms of resistance to *Listeria, Mycobacterium,* and other bacteria (Table 2) that are facultative intracellular pathogens parallels to a large extent those for *Toxoplasma* with some exceptions. Infection with these bacteria differs in that (1) they infect macrophages readily but other cells poorly, (2) they may either replicate within a vacuole (e.g., *M. tuberculosis, Yersinia*) or within the cytoplasm of the cell (e.g., *Listeria*) rather than in an intracellular vacuole, and (3) infection is usually eradicated by protective immunity, whereas in *Toxoplasma* infection protective immunity maintains the infection in a latent state but is not usually curative.[1,478,481,482]

In rodent models, the production of IFN-γ by NK cells and by CD4 T cells appears to play an important role in protection from *Toxoplasma* infection. However, IFN-γ is unable by itself to endow macrophages with the capacity to kill *Listeria* or mycobacteria. Rather, IFN-γ in concert with TNF-α (or microbial products that induce TNF-α) are needed.[1,413,414] Together, these cytokines activate rodent macrophages to produce reactive nitrogen intermediates that are toxic to *Listeria*. Neutralization of endogenous IFN-γ, TNF-α, and/or IL-1 abrogates the immune response to *Listeria* in mice.[1,414] Mice that are unable to produce or respond to IFN-γ or TNF-α, due to genetic ablation of the IFN-γ gene, the IFN-γ receptor gene, or the type I TNF-α receptor gene, are more susceptible to *Listeria, M. tuberculosis,* and BCG.[325,371,398] CD8 T cells are much more efficient than CD4 T cells at transferring immunity.[1,482,483] The protection by CD8 T cells, unlike CD4 T cells, is not dependent on production of IFN-γ, but rather may reflect their capacity to lyse infected cells.[482] Finally, recent data suggest that T cells other than those of the CD4 or CD8 subset (perhaps γδ-TCR–expressing T cells) may contribute to endogenous resistance to primary or secondary *Listeria* infection.[1,481,483a] Both *Listeria* and *Toxoplasma* infections are unduly severe in human neonates, which parallels the markedly diminished capacity of their T cells to produce IFN-γ and perhaps the modest reduction in TNF-α production by their macrophages.[484]

Cytotoxic T cells and NK cell-mediated cytotoxicity may play a role in control of infections other than *Listeria*. Murine macrophages infected with *M. tuberculosis* and *M. leprae* are also lysed by cytotoxic T cells in an antigen–MHC-restricted manner.[1] *Nocardia asteroides* is also susceptible to killing by cytotoxic T cells.[495] NK cells may contribute to resistance to cryptococci, *Leishmania, Plasmodia,* and *Trypanosoma* in animal models.[486]

CMI appears to be the sole mechanism of resistance to *Listeria* and mycobacteria. Antibody appears to play no beneficial role.[1] Based on studies in animal models and with human cells in vitro, antibody may play only a limited role in protection against *Salmonella* and *Legionella*.[487,488] Antibody does provide some protection against *Toxoplasma* in animal models. Mice that have been depleted of B cells and cannot mount an antibody response are slightly more susceptible to late death from *Toxoplasma*.[489] However, it was not proved in these studies that B cells acted solely through antibody production. Antibody and complement do lyse the tachyzoite form, and antibody-coated tachyzoites are killed even by resident tissue macrophages.[476] Passively derived antibody alone provides minimal protection in adult and newborn mice, but does enhance protection mediated by activated macrophages.[490] Nevertheless, T-cell–deficient mice are much more susceptible than are antibody-deficient mice and are not protected by antibody. Antibody may contribute to protection against *Leishmania* amastigotes by inhibiting their uptake into resident macrophages in which they replicate.[491]

Extracellular Pathogens: Pneumocystis, Metazoans, and Bacteria

There is no infection in which the importance of CMI is more clearly evident than that due to *Pneumocystis*. This has been most clearly demonstrated by the extraordinary susceptibility of patients with AIDS to this organism, which often heralds the onset of their immunologic impairment. The majority of infections in adults appear to result from recrudescence of dormant infection, which is held in check by CMI and occurs when the numbers of CD4 lymphocytes fall (see Chs. 103 and 261). In children with perinatal AIDS, infection may develop at times when the numbers of CD4 T cells are normal.[492] This may reflect the functional immaturity of T cells in the neonate and infant, different requirements for protection from the initial infection than from recrudescent infection, or both. *Pneumocystis* is also common in individuals with iatrogenic immunosuppression by a variety of agents, most commonly corticosteroids or

cyclosporin, or with depressed CMI associated with malnutrition. These effects can be modeled in experimental animals in which treatment with corticosteroids or cyclosporin is used to induce active infection and disease. Also nude mice that have a genetic immunodeficiency of the T-cell system or SCID mice readily develop *Pneumocystis* pneumonia.[493,494] In these immunodeficient mice resistance can be conferred by transfer of CD4 but not CD8 T cells. Similarly, depletion of CD4 but not CD8 T cells in otherwise immunocompetent mice leads to the development of active infection.[493,495,496] It appears that TNF-α[497,498] and IL-1[499] may play important roles in the CD4 T-cell–mediated clearance of *Pneumocystis*, although exogenous administration of IFN-γ did facilitate clearance of the organism.[500] A possible role for γδ-TCR–expressing T cells has also been suggested.[498] The exact mechanism by which clearance of *Pneumocystis* is mediated has not been demonstrated. Ingestion and degradation of *Pneumocystis* by alveolar macrophages is observed during resolution. This may be mediated through ingestion of the organism by the macrophage mannose receptor.[501] Since this receptor is downregulated by IFN-γ, this may explain the lack of importance of endogenous IFN-γ in resistance.[497] It has been suggested that nitric oxide produced by murine and human alveolar macrophages during ingestion of *Pneumocystis* contributes to killing of the parasite.[502] TNF-α might act by enhancing production of nitric oxide in this setting, but this requires experimental confirmation. Overall, the animal data parallel the observed risk in humans and clearly identify the CD4 T cell as the critical mediator of resistance. In the absence of an effective CD4 T-cell–mediated response, an ineffective and potentially injurious inflammatory response may be observed. This may account for the apparent benefit of corticosteroid therapy in reducing disease severity, when used as an adjunct to effective antimicrobial therapy in human disease.[503]

The role of CMI in defense against helminths is complex and appears to be controlled by CD4 T cells, with the outcome depending in part on the relative balance between production of lymphokines typically produced by TH1 or TH2 CD4 T cells. The best characterized is infection with *Schistosoma mansoni*. The response to this parasite includes components of typical cell-mediated immune responses, with T cells, macrophages, and granulomas, and in addition eosinophils and IgE antibodies.[297,377,504] Previous observations suggested that each contributed to a protective immune response. However, more recent data in animal models suggest that the IgE- and eosinophil-mediated response, which is associated with TH2 cytokine-producing CD4 T cells producing IL-4 and IL-5, does not facilitate protective immunity to infection with the adult worms. In contrast, inhibition of IFN-γ does impair protective immunity to the adult worm. The eggs, deposited in the portal vasculature by the adults, release the antigens that stimulate the TH2-type response that contributes to the injury by inducing a robust granulomatous response to the eggs. In individuals with high egg burdens and a robust granulomatous response, production of IFN-γ and killing of schistosomules by macrophages are impaired. These data suggest that the TH2 response in this disease may be deleterious.

Similarly, protection from infection with nematodes that enter through the gut and migrate to and produce pathology in the tissues may be more dependent on TH1 than TH2 responses. This is suggested in *Trichinella spiralis* infection in which strains of mice that efficiently expel the adult worms are high IFN-γ, low IL-5 producers (TH1 profile); conversely, those that have delayed worm expulsion have the opposite (TH2) profile. It is important to note that these data report an association only and that more definitive experiments in which T-cell subsets or lymphokines are blocked are needed to substantiate the relative importance of these findings. These results contrast in part with data regarding two murine models of intestinal nematode infection. Infection with *Heligmosomoides polygyrus* is restricted to the intestinal lumen. In this infection CD4 T cells and IL-4 appear to play an important role in protective immunity.[297] In infection with another nematode, *Nippostrongylus brasiliensis,* CD4 T cells are required for worm expulsion but no single lymphokine is required for this process. In contrast, a combination of exogenous IL-3 and IL-4 (cytokines produced efficiently by TH2 CD4 T cells) markedly reduces intestinal parasites in T-cell–deficient mice; this suggests that TH2 cytokines may contribute to protection, even though they may not be required. These differences suggest that control of infection and the pathology of infection with these (and probably other) metazoan pathogens is modulated in complex ways by CD4 T cells and their products. The most clear example of a protective role of T cells against intestinal nematodes is illustrated in humans by the *Strongyloides* hyperinfection syndrome, which occurs in immunodepressed individuals (see Ch. 269).

CMI may also contribute to resistance with certain extracellular pathogens that more typically produce disease in individuals with defective phagocyte number or function. *Candida* spp. are a common cause of systemic infection in such patients, but evidence suggests that depressed CMI may play a contributing role in many such cases. Mucocutaneous infection with *Candida* is common in individuals with selective defects in CMI, including patients with primary immunodeficiency, AIDS, or iatrogenic immunosuppression. Studies in experimental animals suggest that a deficit in NK-cell or T-cell function, and particularly both, increases the risk not only of superficial infection but also of invasive infection and that IFN-γ may be an important mediator of resistance.[505,506] Similar mechanisms may contribute to resistance to other fungal pathogens, but the data are less complete.[507]

The role of the innate component of CMI in regulating the inflammatory and acute phase is now known to be an important determinant of outcome in many infections. However, the role of antigen-specific, T-cell–mediated cellular immunity in control of pyogenic bacterial infection is less clear. The regulation of the development of intraperitoneal abscesses caused by *Bacteroides fragilis*[389,508] likely reflects the role of T cells in modulation of inflammation. However, in mice with peritoneal infection due to *Pseudomonas aeruginosa,*[390] immune T cells are protective in the absence of antibody and neutrophils.[390,509] This appears to be mediated by T-cell–derived lymphokines, and, as predicted by this, induction of resistance but not protection is antigen specific. In a broader sense, the regulation by T cells of antibody production and of antibody isotype plays an important role in protection against pyogenic pathogens.

Viruses

Since nonviral intracellular pathogens are obligate intracellular pathogens, many of the concepts discussed for them are applicable to host defenses against viruses: mechanisms that act to restrict replication within cells or to block cell–cell spread of virus are critical for effective host defense. Clinical experience indicates that deficits in CMI that accompany the physiologic immune deficiencies of the fetus, neonate, and aged, primary immune deficiency and AIDS, and iatrogenic immunosuppression of transplant recipients are major factors predisposing to a variety of viral infections. Antibody may play a role in protection when provided actively or passively prior to exposure. However, with the exception of enteroviruses, which have a predilection for causing severe and potentially fatal chronic infection in individuals with isolated antibody deficiency,[510] antibody does not appear to be the critical mediator in elimination of active viral infection.

Because they are particularly problematic in individuals with impaired CMI, the herpes group viruses are useful prototypes for discussion. These viruses produce an acute infection of varying acuity and then establish a latent infection with periodic reactivation thereafter. In response to the initial infection, the antiviral immune response can generally be divided into an early

antigen-nonspecific phase (the first 5–7 days) and a later phase.[411] In the early phase, infection may either be contained or disseminate widely, whereas in the later phase antigen-specific immunity acts to eliminate active infection, resulting in the establishment of latency. The antigen-specific immune system, and particularly T cells, appears to play an important role in the maintenance of viral latency, as indicated by the frequency of recurrent and severe infections with herpes simplex virus and cytomegalovirus in patients with congenital or acquired immune deficiency. In the case of herpes simplex virus infection, the tempo of the disease is initially acute, so that the early containment phase of the response may be relatively more important than it is in the less rapidly progressive infection with cytomegalovirus.

The important mediators of resistance in the early containment phase of infection appear to be mononuclear phagocytes and NK cells and the interferons produced by these cells. Mononuclear phagocytes may adsorb or phagocytose viruses. Herpes simplex virus infection of monocytes usually results in abortive infection.[511] In contrast, infection of tissue macrophages may result in productive infection, depending on the tissue from which the cells were derived and, as suggested by murine studies, perhaps the host from which they were obtained.[512,513] Infection of macrophages induces the production of IFN-α,[514] which restricts the ability of these viruses to replicate in the macrophages and a wide variety of other cell types. Other cytokines, such as TNF-α, may impede viral replication in some cases[515,516] or enhance replication, for example of HIV.[517] The relevance of mononuclear phagocytes in protection against herpes simplex virus is indicated by studies in mice, in which the severity of infection is greater following the administration of agents that deplete macrophages, although their relative importance may vary depending on the mode of acquisition of infection.[518,519]

The other cell that appears to play an important role in resistance is the NK cell. As indicated above, NK cells are capable of lysing virus-infected cells directly and also are important producers of cytokines, particularly IFN-γ and TNF-α, which impede viral replication and augment other aspects of antiviral immune responses. The relevance of NK cells in defense against infection with herpes group viruses is demonstrated by the unusual severity of infections with herpes simplex virus, cytomegalovirus, and varicella in the rare patients with a selective deficiency of NK cells (unpublished observations).[415] Consistent with this, innate resistance to CMV in mice maps to a region in which multiple genes linked to NK cell function are located.[412] Data in mice indicate that early containment of infection is critically dependent on the production of IFN-α and -β and on the presence of functional NK cells.[520–522] The role of NK cells is apparent only during the early phase of herpes simplex virus infection: depletion of NK cells 5 days after infection has no effect.[522] IFN-γ derived from NK cells in the early phase of the infection and IFN-α produced largely by macrophages may influence the development of CD4 T cells into the TH1 type that are effective mediators of antiviral defense (see above). IFN-α and -β also act by inducing resistance to viral infection in cells, by enhancing NK cytolytic activity, and by increasing class I MHC expression on cells, which augments presentation of viral antigens on infected cells and thereby recognition by CD8 T cells.

The late containment phase of the immune response to viral infection is antigen specific and mediated by T and B cells.[411,523] Antigen-specific responses are detectable near the end of the first week of HSV infection and peak at 2–3 weeks after onset. The CD4 subset of T cells, acting through cell–cell interactions and the production of lymphokines, facilitates the development of antibody-producing B cells and MHC class I–restricted antigen-specific cytotoxic CD8 T cells. CD4 T cells may also directly participate in cytolysis of class II MHC–expressing, viral-infected cells. Because antibody production by B cells in response to viral protein and glycoprotein antigens is T-cell dependent, it is often difficult to assess independently the specific role of B and T cells in viral resistance. In some cases of severe and at least partially selective T-cell immunodeficiency, a predilection for severe infection with herpes group viruses is seen (nucleoside phosphorylase deficiency, AIDS), but this is not the case in others (DiGeorge syndrome).[492,524,525] This may reflect in part the greater degree of T-cell impairment in the former disorders. Nude mice, which are markedly deficient in mature T cells but have normal or increased NK activity, develop severe herpes simplex virus infection that is only manifested in the late phase of infection.[522,526] These mice are protected by adoptive transfer of T cells, whereas passive administration of antibody limits viral spread initially but does not confer ultimate protection. Infections with herpes simplex virus (and other herpes group viruses) are most severe in those forms of immunodeficiency in which both T- and B-cell immunity are impaired,[527,528] and are usually not impaired in pure B-cell immunodeficiency. Collectively these data suggest that T-cell–mediated immunity is most important but antibody may facilitate containment of infection. Whether antibody acts primarily to neutralize extracellular virus or to allow enhanced killing by NK cells and phagocytes through ADCC is not clear.

The mechanisms by which T cells mediate defense against herpes simplex virus are likely to be multiple, but include cytolysis of virus-infected cells and the production of cytokines. Cytolytic T cells of both the CD4 and CD8 subsets can be derived from infected humans.[523,529] However, the overall importance of cytoxicity compared with other functions, such as lymphokine secretion, in the action of CD8 T cells is not clear. Of the T-cell–derived cytokines, IFN-γ may play a particularly important role. In mice, T cells, IFN-γ, and IL-2 appear to contribute to the inflammatory response to herpes simplex virus infection that results in the containment of infection in tissues, but may contribute to injury in the cornea.[530] Furthermore, studies in experimental models of herpes simplex virus infection suggest that IFN-γ is an important factor in protection from severe primary infection and from recurrent infection.[531,532] A delay in the development of antigen-specific T cells that produce IFN-γ correlates with the markedly increased severity of disease due to herpes simplex virus in human neonates,[533] although other factors including diminished NK cell function are likely factors in the neonate's predisposition.[484]

Mechanisms protecting against other herpes group viruses appear to be similar to those acting in herpes simplex virus infection. CD8 cytotoxic T cell (CTL) function has been implicated strongly in control of infection with cytomegalovirus in humans,[534] and adoptive transfer of cloned cytomegalovirus specific CTL appears to diminish the risk of cytomegalovirus pneumonia in bone marrow transplant recipients.[535] CD8 CTL also transfer protection in mice. IFN-γ appears to contribute to protection against cytomegalovirus, although the evidence is not as clear as for herpes simplex virus.[536] The pathology in acute Epstein-Barr virus (EBV) infection is largely derived from a brisk CD8-mediated host immune response to infected B cells.[537] Conversely, inhibition of T-cell–mediated immunity with cyclosporin or antilymphocyte globulin or transfer of lymphocytes from infected humans into mice with combined immunodeficiency is associated with the development of polyclonal B-cell lymphomas. Variants of EBV that may allow the virus to avoid recognition by CD8 T cells through alteration of a critical peptide recognized by these cells in association with specific class II MHC molecules (HLA-A11) were observed in a population in which HLA-A11 was highly prevalent, suggesting that CD8 T cells had driven evolution of the virus[538]; similar mechanisms have been postulated to drive evolution of HIV within infected individuals. This suggests that T-cell–mediated immunity plays a critical role in maintaining viral latency.[539] A unique form of human immunodeficiency, the X-linked immunodeficiency syndrome, is associated with aberrations in control of

infection with EBV.[540] Although thought to reflect a T-cell abnormality, this has not been proved.

The importance of the cell-mediated immune response and of cytokines in host defense against viruses is strongly supported by the multitude of recently discovered viral genes that may allow the virus to evade or modulate the immune and inflammatory responses.[276,541,542] As shown in Table 3, among the herpes group viruses, EBV produces an analog of IL-10, BCRF1. Like IL-10, BCRF1 inhibits production of cytokines, including IFN-γ, that facilitate the host immune response. Both proteins also enhance growth of B cells in which the virus replicates. A chemokine receptor homolog is present in the cytomegalovirus genome, which could act to block recruitment of macrophages and T cells, although this has yet to be tested experimentally. Other proteins produced by herpes group viruses impede MHC class I expression and thereby perhaps CD8 T-cell recognition or may engage and impede the actions of IgG antibody and complement. However, the role of these proteins has not been tested formally in vivo.

In contrast to the lack of data regarding the role of viral derived modulators of the immune response in infection with herpes group viruses, such proteins have been shown to affect infection due to vaccinia and other pox viruses and adenoviruses in animal models.[276] Members of the family of poxviruses produce homologs of TNF, IL-1, and IFN-γ receptors and a protein that blocks the processing of the biologically inactive IL-1β precursor into biologically active IL-1β. Genetic mutants in which any one of these proteins has been deleted have diminished virulence. This is associated with an increased recruitment of inflammatory cells to the site of infection. IFN-γ is important in defense against vaccinia virus, since mice in which the IFN-γ receptor has been deleted are much more susceptible to this infection.[371] One member of this family is known to produce a homolog of the IFN-γ receptor, which binds and inhibits the action of IFN-γ in vitro. Thus, poxviruses appear to have incorporated antagonists of proinflammatory cytokines (and also complement) into their complex genomes as a means to enhance their virulence. Adenoviruses, which produce a less acute infection, appear to have done the opposite. These viruses express proteins that impede transport of class I MHC proteins to their cell surface and that block the intracellular signal induced by TNF. Viruses in which these genes have been deleted replicate equally well in vivo but induce greater injury since the inflammatory response is more robust. The advantage to this virus of impeding the inflammatory response is not clear, but could relate to improved viral persistence. These and other immunomodulatory viral genes are likely to represent only a fraction of those that exist. They strongly suggest that viruses have evolved in parallel with the host immune response. Analysis of the role of these genes in viral pathogenesis along with studies that perturb specific aspects of the host immune system offer the promise for a much more detailed understanding of the protective or deleterious aspects of the host immune response.

CMI contributes both to protection and to injury with pathogens that infect the respiratory tree. The best studied is influenza virus infection. Results from murine models of influenza, parainfluenza, or respiratory syncytial virus infection suggest that resolution of both the primary infection and the illness associated with primary infection are T-cell mediated. Antibody plays little role in the primary response but does contribute to resistance to secondary infection.[2,543,544] The initial nonantigen-specific phase of primary infection is associated with an influx of macrophages, neutrophils, and NK cells in the lungs. Resistance to influenza appears to be related to the actions of type I IFNs (α and β), since induction by these IFN of the Mx gene correlates with resistance.[545] Subsequently, by days 6–7 in experimental models, antigen-specific CD8 and CD4 T cells are detected in the regional lymph nodes and soon thereafter in the airways. The response in the airways is progressively dominated by CD8 T cells. Mice that are depleted of or lack either CD4 or CD8 T cells clear influenza virus normally; depletion of both T-cell subsets results in progressive infection and death. Both subsets appear to contribute to the inflammatory response and pneumonia that accompany primary infection. Conversely, both protect if transferred adoptively into naive recipients and protect against secondary infection. CD4 T cells contribute to resistance by enhancing B-cell antibody production, and perhaps through cytotoxicity and lymphokine production. The lymphokines found in mice with resolving influenza virus infection are consistent with a dual T- and B-cell response. CD4 T cells expressing IL-4 and IL-10, lymphokines that facilitate B-cell responses, and CD8 T cells expressing IFN-γ and lymphotoxin, lymphokines acting to impede intracellular viral replication and enhance the inflammatory response, are both observed.[546] Similarly, both CD4 and CD8 T cells appear to contribute to viral clearance in respiratory syncytial virus infection.[543] When both T-cell subsets are depleted, virus is not cleared, but no disease results. It is not certain that complete depletion was achieved so that the small number of residual T cells or γ/δ T cells not depleted by this mechanism may contribute to protection. Infection with the Sendai strain of parainfluenza virus is more severe in mice lacking CD8 T cells and lethal in those deficient in both CD4 and CD8 T cells.[544] Overall, the data suggest that, as in infection with herpes group and vaccinia viruses, resolution of infection with these respiratory viruses is dependent on a T-cell–mediated, antigen-specific immune response. However, unlike the more lytic infections due to the former viruses, most of the injury associated with these viral infections appears to be a consequence of the immune response. Results in humans are generally consistent with the experimental studies in mice. Individuals with primary or acquired immunodeficiency, including AIDS, experience prolonged viral excretion and increased morbidity with influenza, respiratory synctial, parainfluenza, and measles viruses.[547–549]

PROSPECTS FOR IMMUNOLOGIC INTERVENTION

Exogenous Cytokines or Effector Cells as Treatment Adjuncts in Infectious Diseases

A better definition of host defense mechanisms offers the promise that more effective prevention or treatment regimens can be developed, particularly cytokine-based therapies (see Ch. 33). Interferon-α has been licensed for the treatment of condyloma acuminatum and chronic hepatitis B and hepatitis C (non-A/non-B) infections. It is being studied for use in other viral infections, such as laryngeal papillomatosis. Rather than acting to modulate the immune response, the primary action of IFN-α in these diseases is more likely mediated by direct inhibition of viral replication. It is also licensed for the treatment of noninfectious processes in which it probably acts through its antiproliferative, not immunomodulatory, properties.

There are several important considerations regarding possible use of cytokines as adjunct treatment of established infections: *(1)* Although cytokines such as IFN-α or TNF-α have shown efficacy in various animal models, treatment generally is effective in established infections only in those diseases (e.g., leishmaniasis, mycobacterial infection) of a chronic or slowly progressive nature. In more rapidly progressive infection (e.g., listeriosis) IFN-γ appears to be most critical in the early phase of infection and may be a less useful adjunct once infection is established. *(2)* Cytokines are secreted by lymphocytes locally and in a vectorial fashion so that they are preferentially secreted in the direction of the APC or, in the case of CD8 T cells, the infected cell. Exogenous administration of cytokines fails to reproduce the local, focused effect. Thus, concentrations at the site of infection may be too low to achieve the desired effect without resulting in unacceptable systemic toxicity. *(3)* Systemic administration that delivers cytokines to sites distant from the focus of infection may actually lead to alterations in effector

cell migration away from the focus of infection by inducing vascular adhesins at other sites. *(4)* Finally, in the natural situation, multiple complementary and counterregulatory cytokines are produced that are not reproduced by exogenous administration. Nevertheless, preliminary data suggest that in certain situations exogenous, systemically administered cytokines may have a therapeutic role.

Infections due to nonviral intracellular pathogens have been investigated to the greatest extent. In patients with lepromatous leprosy, both recombinant IL-2 and IFN-γ have been associated with improvement when administered in open trials and in conjunction with conventional multidrug therapy. Short courses of intradermal IL-2 were associated with increased infiltration by CD4 T cells and with increased class II MHC expression in the skin.[471] This was most marked at the sites of injection, but an overall total body reduction in bacilli was estimated to be about fivefold. The effects of IL-2 were believed to result indirectly from induction of IFN-γ.[550] Similar histologic changes and reductions in bacillary load were observed in certain patients with short courses of intradermal IFN-γ. In patients who receive more prolonged courses of intermittent intradermal IFN-γ in doses of 100 μg every 2–4 weeks for 6–11 months, a sustained approximate 10-fold reduction in bacillary load and an increased incidence of erythema nodosum leprosum was observed (6 of 10 vs. historical rates of 15 percent).[551] Although monocytes isolated from treated patients have enhanced function consistent with exposure to IFN-γ, there was no reversal of the underlying phenotype—lepromatous patients remained anergic to *M. leprae*. The apparent clinical improvement needs to be corroborated in randomized trials in larger groups of patients.

Similar studies have been done in patients with visceral *Leish. donovani* infection. Conventional therapy with pentavalent antimony generally results in an approximate 85 percent cure rate. Initial studies assessed the use of IFN-γ in doses of 100–400 μg/m^2, as an adjunct.[552] In eight patients who had previously failed antimony therapy, six were successfully treated with combination therapy; two responded but relapsed when therapy was discontinued. An additional nine patients were treated with the combination initially, and eight of these were successfully treated. Comparison of these patients with historical controls suggested that the rate of improvement was accelerated and that combination therapy may be successful in some of those who are refractory to conventional therapy. Subsequent treatment of 14 more antimony-treatment failures has been less successful: only 6 of 14 were successfully treated with the first course of therapy, although 9 of 14 were ultimately treated successfully.[553] Relapses have occurred in some who appeared to be parasite negative during therapy. Therapy with these doses of IFN-γ, which are considerably higher than those used in leprosy, was associated with fever in most patients, but this was tolerable and did not limit therapy. Other side effects were uncommon. The relative role and optimal dose and duration of combined IFN-γ/antimony for treatment are not yet known. Randomized treatment trials will be needed before this can be considered standard therapy.

Diffuse cutaneous leishmaniasis is rare and is associated with large numbers of organisms and a poor immune response to the organism, resembling lepromatous leprosy. It is generally resistant to chemotherapy, but preliminary trials in six patients suggest that combined therapy with IFN-γ and antimony may be useful.[553] In one patient therapy was associated with a clinical remission of longer than 1 year and the development of skin test reactivity to leishmania antigen, suggesting that development of efficient immunity may have occurred.

Ongoing trials of IFN-γ are continuing in these diseases and in patients with AIDS. Low-dose intermittent IFN-γ in combination with TNF-α (both at 10 μg/m^2) does not appear efficacious in treatment of HIV infection, since neither indices of viral burden nor of immunologic status were affected.[554] Treatment trials in which IFN-γ is being tested as an adjunct to therapy for infection with *M. avium* and *Toxoplasma* in AIDS patients are in progress. However, patients with AIDS have developed cryptococcal meningitis and *Pneumocystis* pneumonia during treatment with IFN-γ, and IFN-γ therapy did not affect established cytomegalovirus infection.[555,556] The failure of IFN-γ in these cases may reflect onset of infection early during IFN-γ therapy, failure of systemic administration to focus delivery at sites of infection, or a lack of activity of IFN-γ–activated effector cells in these infections.

Therapy with low-dose soluble IL-2 or a longer acting preparation in which IL-2 is fused to polyethylene glycol (PEG IL-2) have been used in combination with zidovudine in preliminary trials in AIDS patients.[557–559] In these studies no change in indices of viral burden were observed. However, modest increases in CD4 T-cell numbers, improved DTH skin test response, and some improvement in lymphocyte responses tested in vitro were observed. It remains to be seen whether these changes will be associated with long-term benefit. In the lower dose studies ($<2 \times 10^5$ units)[558] no toxicity or increased rate of systemic bacterial infections were observed, both of which have occurred in cancer patients treated in high-dose intravenous IL-2 protocols.[560,561]

Adoptive transfer of antigenic-specific T cells is an alternative to exogenous cytokine therapy, which offers the potential for regulated and focused delivery of the effector response at sites of infection. Such an approach parallels the successful use of adoptive transfer in the protection of experimental animals against viral and nonviral intracellular pathogens. Recently, in vitro activated and propagated effector T cells entered preliminary trials as immunotherapeutic agents for persistent and refractory infection with cytomegalovirus or HIV.[535] Preliminary data indicate that such cells persist in individuals and retain their effector functions. However, their ability to provide protection is as yet unknown.

Cytokines as Vaccine Adjuvants

Promising studies suggest that cytokines, particularly IL-2, may be useful as components of recombinant vaccines. This was first shown with vaccinia virus recombinants in which IL-2, IFN-γ, or TNF-α were expressed as secreted products by the recombinant virus.[405] Such vaccines result in local production of cytokine at sites of live viral vaccine replication. In the case of the IL-2–producing virus, local host immune cells were recruited efficiently to sites of infection with this virus and acted through NK cells to effect viral clearance in an IFN-γ–dependent manner. Such vaccines appear to be safe even in immunodeficient mice lacking functional T cells, which normally succumb to vaccinia virus infection. Focused production of the lymphokine appeared to be important—injection of recombinant IL-2 along with a vaccinia vector not producing cytokines was lethal rather than protective. Vaccinia vectors that express TNF-α and IFN-γ have been produced and also are safe in immunodeficient mice.[405] In contrast to these favorable results, vaccinia virus vectors expressing influenza virus antigens and IL-2 resulted in greater antibody production to the influenza virus antigens compared with those achieved with vectors not producing IL-2, but protection against subsequent influenza challenge was not different. Similarly, incorporation of IL-2 into vaccinia virus vectors expressing herpes simplex virus antigens did not result in greater protection against subsequent herpes simplex virus challenge than did vectors without IL-2.

In some cases coadministration of cytokines may facilitate the development of protective immunity. Recombinant IFN-γ given with inactivated influenza virus vaccine provided significantly greater protection against subsequent viral challenge and early antibody production in mice than did vaccine alone.[562] Coadministration of IL-2 and TNF-α in these studies did not improve vaccine-induced protection. The data in humans are limited. Exogenous IL-2 did not enhance the antibody response

to hepatitis B vaccine in one randomized trial in normal individuals[563] but did in a smaller nonrandomized study of renal dialysis patients, in whom the response is usually poor.[564] A larger controlled trial of IFN-γ given with hepatitis B vaccine in hemodialysis patients did not show a significant advantage for the IFN-γ group, although the rate of response in this and in a second smaller study were greater in the IFN-γ group.[565]

Based on animal data, it is possible that cytokines may be used in the future to effect not simply the magnitude but the nature of immune response. For example, administration of IFN-γ or IL-12 has the potential to favor the development of an immune response weighted toward a cell-mediated immune response.[283,565,565a] This may be desirable for vaccines against viral or nonviral intracellular pathogens. Reciprocally, coadministration of cytokines, such as IL-4 or IL-10, might be anticipated to favor the development of antibody responses. Although appealing, there are no data to date to indicate whether such an approach is likely to be productive in humans.

Immunoattenuation to Decrease Immunologically Mediated Injury

In certain disease states, an excessive immune or inflammatory response results in tissue damage. As described above, in septic shock and the often coexistent condition of ARDS there is considerable evidence that proinflammatory cytokines, including TNF-α, IL-1, and IFN-γ, play an injurious role. When the production and action of these cytokines is anatomically and temporally restricted to sites of infection or inflammation, they facilitate clearance of microbes and development of the specific immune response at those sites. In septic shock, the normal counterregulatory mechanisms that act to attenuate this response and to restrict the locus of action of these cytokines are overwhelmed. Contemporary approaches seek to modulate these responses in a manner that allows the development of protective immunity while ameliorating injury.

The most thoroughly studied agents are corticosteroids. In experimental animals, early administration of corticosteroids before septic shock is fully established ameliorates the process and decreases mortality; later administration is less effective. This may reflect the ability of corticosteroids to inhibit production of proinflammatory cytokines if added before or concomitantly with agonists (e.g., LPS), but not after.[566] In humans corticosteroids are not effective in the management of septic shock,[503] perhaps reflecting the necessary delay in administration, relative to experimental models. The one exception to this is shock associated with severe typhoid fever[503] in which corticosteroids appear to be effective. Whether the greatest efficacy in this infection reflects a different tempo of disease or the nature of the pathogen (i.e., an intracellular pathogen) is not clear. Corticosteroids do appear to be useful in certain other inflammatory conditions (tuberculous pericarditis and *Pneumocystis* pneumonia) and are possibly effective in certain others.[503] Comparative trials indicate that children with meningitis due to *H. influenzae* who receive dexamethasone at the time antibiotic therapy is initiated have fewer long-term sequelae, primarily hearing loss.[567] The beneficial effect has been suggested to result in part from inhibition of the production of TNF-α and other cytokines, which are increased in concentration in the cerebrospinal fluid in this disease. Caveats regarding the evidence preclude definitive conclusions regarding efficacy at this time.

At the present time there is an intensive effort to develop agents that more selectively antagonize the actions or production of proinflammatory cytokines, particularly TNF-α and IL-1. The most extensively studied is the natural antagonist of IL-1, IL-1ra. In animal models this antagonist diminishes LPS-induced local inflammation and markedly improves survival in endotoxin-induced septic shock.[285,436,568] However, none of these studies tested efficacy once severe septic or shock was established. A preliminary report of a placebo-controlled, randomized human trial indicated diminished survival in the group treated with a continuous infusion of IL-1ra.[569] These results suggest caution regarding extrapolation of the results of animal trials to humans. Antagonists of TNF have also been developed, and cytokines that block the release of TNF-α and other proinflammatory cytokines, such as IL-10, are candidates for therapeutic use in sepsis.[570,571] Studies in animals show that both TNF antagonists and IL-10 protect against endotoxin-induced shock, but neither were tested after shock was established.[572] It seems likely that these and related antagonists may be more useful in the modulation of local inflammation or cell-mediated immunity than in the management of established sepsis. For example, parallels between the murine models of *Leish. major* infection and the nonhealing variants of *Leishmania* and mycobacterial infection in humans suggest that intervention to impede counterproductive immune responses associated with excess production of IL-4, IL-10, or other TH2 cytokines may be useful in these human diseases.[573]

DEFECTS IN CELLULAR IMMUNITY

Physiologically Diminished CMI in the Fetus and Neonate

Immune function in the fetus and neonate and its relationship to infection at this stage of life has been reviewed recently.[484] The human fetus and neonate are unduly susceptible to infection with a variety of pathogens, including infections due to those against which CMI is the major mechanism of host defense. These include the herpes group viruses, herpes simplex virus and cytomegalovirus (and, although uncommon, varicella-zoster virus), *Toxoplasma gondii, Listeria monocytogenes,* and *Treponema pallidum.* It is noteworthy that for cytomegalovirus and *Toxoplasma,* congenital infection that results from primary maternal infection in the first half of gestation is associated with the most severe sequelae, whereas sequelae are milder and less common when fetal infection occurs near or at term. This is also true for congenital infection with rubella virus. In contrast, infection with herpes simplex virus, varicella-zoster virus, and *Listeria* may be severe even when infection is acquired in the latter part of gestation or at term. These observations suggest that important host defenses for cytomegalovirus and for *Toxoplasma* may mature before those acting to protect from infection with herpes simplex virus and *Listeria.*

Infections that occur in the first 10 weeks of human gestation do so at a time when the fetus has few detectable T or B cells, and, if infection begins before the sixth week of gestation, NK cells also will be absent. Furthermore, the numbers and repertoire for antigen recognition of T cells, B cells, and antibody-secreting plasma cells are limited in the first half of gestation. It is reasonable to suggest that the extraordinary susceptibility to severe injury from infection with each of these agents in the first half of gestation reflects quantitative deficits in these cells. In contrast, when infection occurs at later stages of gestation, the immune system is more fully developed. By midgestation the numbers of NK, T, and B cells are equal to or exceed those in adults, and the potential for the generation of a diverse repertoire of antigen-specific TCR and immunoglobulin appears not to be limiting. Functional rather than numerical differences between the fetal and neonatal immune systems and that of mature hosts are likely to account for the predisposition at this age. Differences in function exist both in cells of the innate immune system and in T cells.

For protection against herpes simplex virus, deficits in the early antigen-nonspecific phase of viral resistance may be a critical factor in neonates, given the rapid progression of disease to involve vital organs. The cytotoxic activity of blood mononuclear cells, monocytes, and purified NK cells from neonates is impaired in the neonate against a variety of targets, including cells infected with herpes simplex virus and in assays measuring

natural cytotoxicity and ADCC. The deficit in NK-cell function is likely related to the poor cytolytic function of neonatal NK cells, which is approximately 50 percent of that mediated by cells from adults.[406,574] This is consistent with the observation that only about 50 percent of neonatal NK cells are CD56+. Nearly all adult NK cells are CD56+, and it is this subset that is cytolytic. Furthermore, unlike NK cells from adults, the cytolytic activity of neonatal NK cells is poorly augmented by interferons, whereas IL-2 augments the cytolytic activity of both.[406,574,575] The ability of neonatal NK cells to produce IFN-γ in response to the combination of live herpes simplex virus and IL-2, although modest, appeared not to differ from cells from adults in one study.[576] This may be mediated in part through IL-12, although this has not been tested directly. However, indirect evidence for a deficit in the production of IFN-γ by human neonatal NK cells under such conditions comes from the failure of IL-2 and human neonatal blood mononuclear cells to mediate adoptive protection against herpes simplex virus in neonatal mice, in contrast to adult blood mononuclear cells. This protection is dependent on IL-2–facilitated IFN-γ production by the transferred mononuclear cells.[577] Although human adult mononuclear cells will protect neonatal mice from herpes simplex virus in combination with antibody, IFN-α, IFN-γ, or IL-2, human neonatal mononuclear cells protect only in combination with IFN-γ, but not under any other conditions tested to date.[532]

The failure of neonatal cells to confer protection unless exogenous IFN-γ is provided is consistent with the marked deficit in production of IFN-γ by neonatal T cells.[578,579] The deficit in production of IFN-γ by neonatal T cells appears to derive in large part from the lack of previous exposure to exogenous antigens. As described above, in the mature host, CD4 T cells that respond to antigens to which the individual has been previously exposed (often referred to as *memory* or *memory effector* CD4 T cells) differ in the expression of certain cell surface molecules and express a broader range of lymphokines than do cells that have not been primed by previous exposure to antigens (naive T cells). Consistent with residence in a protected environment, the T cells of the fetus and neonate appear almost solely to have the characteristics of naive T cells. Like adult naive T cells, neonatal T cells express IL-2 well, but produce many other cytokines either slightly (TNF-α, GM-CSF) or markedly less (IL-3, IL-4, IL-5, IFN-γ) well than do memory T cells from adults.[484] Neonatal T cells that have been propagated in vitro in a manner that mimics exposure to antigen acquire the surface phenotype and capacity to produce lymphokines that parallels that of adult memory T cells. Nevertheless, studies performed ex vivo suggest that the acquisition of antigen-specific T cell–mediated immune responses is commonly diminished and/or delayed in their development in human neonates compared with adults. Multiple studies have shown a delay in development of antigen-specific responses as detected by lymphocyte proliferation in neonates as compared with adults with primary herpes simplex virus infection.[533,580,581] We recently found in a longitudinal analysis that there was a 3-week delay in the development of herpes simplex virus antigen-specific lymphocyte proliferation in neonates compared with adults with primary herpes simplex virus infection, and this was paralleled by a delay in antigen-specific production of IFN-γ.[553] The basis for this delay is not completely clear. It is interesting that once human infants who were infected as neonates subsequently develop herpes simplex virus antigen-specific T cells, as indicated by a detectable proliferative response, antigen-specific IFN-γ production was usually detectable as well.[533] This is consistent with the notion that the lack of antigen-specific memory T cells is the major cause of the deficit in production of IFN-γ (and certain other cytokines) by neonatal T cells.

The delay in the acquisition of antigen-specific T cells and cytokine production may be an important factor in the neonate's greater susceptibility to infection with herpes simplex virus. It is unknown if this is accompanied by a similar delay or deficit in T-cell–mediated, antigen-specific cytotoxicity. However, antiviral cytotoxicity is likely to be impaired since cytotoxicity to other targets has generally been found to be diminished. Together, the diminished and delayed T-cell–mediated responses to herpes simplex virus along with deficits in NK function are likely to be important factors in the predisposition of the neonate to infection with this virus.

Like herpes simplex virus, severe infection with *Listeria* and untoward sequelae secondary to *Toxoplasma* infection commonly results from fetal infection in the latter part of gestation, although for *Toxoplasma* the outcome is not as devastating as when infection occurs early in gestation. Immaturity in the early antigen-nonspecific phase of immunity, particularly in NK function and in mononuclear phagocyte recruitment, is likely to contribute to more severe disease. The deficits in NK function have been alluded to above. Production of monokines that facilitate recruitment of monocytes and activation of NK cells (i.e., TNF-α and IL-1) are generally normal in term infants,[484] but TNF-α production by monocytes from preterm infants is about 75 percent less than by cells from term infants and adults. Production of TNF-α by monocyte-derived and tissue (placental) macrophages from term neonates is reduced to a greater extent than that by blood monocytes and appears to be upregulated less by IFN-γ than in cells from adults. Similarly, in neonatal rats challenged with LPS or *Lis. monocytogenes* at less than 8 days of age, TNF-α production is not detectable in vivo and reaches adult levels in response to these agonists only after 16 days of age.[582,583] IFN-γ does not enhance TNF-α production in the less mature rats. Deficient production of IFN-γ by neonatal T cells may further compound the deficit in TNF-α production in humans (see above), and decreased production of IFN-γ by NK cells and T cells in neonatal rats may be a contributing factor to the decreased production of TNF-α and diminished resistance to *Lis. monocytogenes*. Although the maturity of the neonatal rodent immune system is less than that of human neonates, these results appear to parallel those in human neonates.

Results in infants with congenital *Toxoplasma* infection suggest that infection of the fetus in utero may in some cases further impede the development of memory T cells and that in such cases cells capable of producing protective TH1 cytokines may not always develop in parallel with antigen-specific T-cell proliferation. In the first months of life proliferative responses of T cells from neonates to *Toxoplasma* antigen are often not detectable above background, although most develop a detectable response thereafter.[584] In the study by McLeod et al.[585] none of eight congenitally infected infants studied in the first 15 months of life had blood mononuclear cells that produced IFN-γ or IL-2, even though antigen-specific proliferative responses were detectable in some. More detailed analysis is needed to determine the basis for the protracted impairment in the development of effective T-cell–mediated responses in these infants. Impairment in the development of antigen-specific T-cell responses has also been observed in infants with congenital infection due to cytomegalovirus and rubella (see above). These findings contrast with the less persistent delay in development of antigen-specific T-cell responses in children infected with herpes simplex virus at term and raise the possibility that infection occurring at a time of greater immunologic immaturity may lead to a state of relative anergy, as observed in rodents.

CMI in Aging

In the aged both an increased incidence of infection with viral and nonviral intracellular pathogens and of autoimmunity are observed.[586] This is commonly ascribed to deficits in T-cell–mediated defenses and regulation of the B-cell response, although a direct cause and effect relationship has not been proved. Aging related changes in T-cell phenotype and function are well described.[587,588] These include thymic involution, diminished DTH responses, diminished responses to certain vaccines (e.g., influenza), and phenotypic and functional changes in T-cell responses as assayed in vitro. For many of these differences similar and more consistent differences are observed in aged animals. However, there appear to be a variety of factors that affect immunosenescence, including genetic factors and other associated diseases. Most consistently observed has been a diminished proliferative response to mitogens and antigens, which appears to be related in large part to a diminished production of IL-2. This is associated with an increase with age of T cells expressing the low-molecular-weight isoform of CD45 and other markers of memory T cells. Changes in relative or absolute numbers of other T-cell subsets have been inconsistent, as have results regarding production of other lymphokines. It has been suggested that aging is associated with a relative imbalance in favor of TH2-mediated and humoral immune responses over TH1 and cellular responses, based on the diminution in production of IFN-γ, a lymphokine commonly produced by memory and TH1 T cells. However, conflicting results have been obtained in some studies.

Primary Immunodeficiency

Primary immunodeficiencies are genetically determined or linked disorders in which the immune system is the sole or major system affected by the genetic defect. They have been recently reviewed.[589,590] These disorders occur with a frequently of about 1 : 10,000. The most common forms, common variable immunodeficiency and X-linked agammaglobulinemia, are manifested primarily or solely as defects in B cell/humoral immunity. Less common are those forms of primary immunodeficiency in which the cellular immunity is impaired. Those disorders that affect cellular immunity generally result from deficits in the numbers and/or the function of T lymphocytes with or without a concomitant defect directly affecting the B-cell lineage. Given the central role of T cells, particularly of CD4 T cells, in regulating all aspects of the immune response, profound deficits in T-cell function will lead to secondary deficits in B-cell function and humoral immunity as well. Accordingly, T-cell deficits generally result in combined (cellular and humoral) immune deficiency. These disorders most commonly manifest as *(1)* an increased severity or frequency of infection with pathogenic microbes and *(2)* opportunistic infections with microbes of low virulence. It may be less obvious that disorders that result in incomplete loss of cell-mediated immunity often are associated with autoimmune disorders. These may reflect either deficits in the capacity for self/nonself discrimination (a central function of T cells) or from the induction by chronic or undetected microbial infection of aberrant, self-cross-reactive immune responses.

When deficits are profound, SCID occurs (Table 4). SCID can be inherited in an autosomal recessive or X-linked fashion. The X-linked disorder affects T cells most severely and their NK cells; B-cell numbers are generally normal. This disorder has recently been shown to result from mutations in the γ-chain of the IL-2 receptor.[122] The autosomal recessive form most commonly is associated with diminution in B-cell numbers as well as T-cell numbers, whereas numbers of NK cells are generally normal. These patients almost always present in the first year of life with severe and/or recurrent infections due to opportunistic organisms, such as cytomegalovirus and *Pneumocystis carinii*, often in association with sinopulmonary infections caused by conventional capsulated bacterial pathogens. Chronic diarrhea and chronic mucocutaneous candidiasis are common, as is eczema, which may become superinfected. Most infants fail to grow normally. The defect in SCID may vary somewhat in severity: T cells may be decreased in number and/or abnormal in phenotype rather than absent, and some function (e.g., weak proliferative responses to nonspecific mitogens) may be present. However, antigen-specific responses are minimal or absent.

TABLE 4. Primary Immunodeficiencies Affecting Cellular Immunity

Designation	Serum Immunoglobulin	Circulating B Cells	Circulating T Cells	Presumed Pathogenesis	Inheritance	Associated Features
Severe combined immunodeficiency (SCID)						
X-linked	Decreased	Normal or increased	Markedly decreased	IL-2-R γ-chain defect	XL	
Autosomal recessive	Decreased	Markedly decreased or normal	Markedly decreased	Maturation defect of both T and B cells; possible DNA repair defect	AR	Variants with normal numbers of T cells occur
Adenosine deaminase (ADA) deficiency	Decreased	Progressive decrease	Progressive decrease	T-cell and B-cell defects from toxic metabolites due to enzyme deficiency	AR	Cartilage abnormalities
Purine nucleoside phosphorylase (PNP) deficiency	Normal or decreased	Normal	Progressive decrease	T-cell defect from toxic metabolites due to enzyme deficiency	AR	Autoimmune hemolytic anemia, neurologic symptoms
MHC deficiency (bare lymphocyte syndrome)	Normal or decreased	Normal	Normal	Defect of regulatory gene for transcription of MHC class II molecules	AR	Class II deficiency ± class I deficiency
Reticular dysgenesis	Decreased (maternal)	Markedly decreased	Markedly decreased	Defective maturation of T and B cells and myeloid cells (stem cell defect)	AR	Granulocytopenia, thrombocytopenia
Omenn syndrome	Increased IgE, others variable	Decreased	Oligoclonal	Maturation defect T and B cells	AR	Variant of SCID, oligoclonal T-cell proliferation, graft-vs.-host–like disease, eosinophila
Short-limbed dwarfism, cartilage-hair hypoplasia	Normal or decreased	Normal	Variably decreased	Unknown	AR	
CD3γ or CD3ε deficiency	Normal	Normal	Normal	Defective transcription of CD3γ or CD3ε chain	AR	Phenotype variable
CD8 deficiency	Normal	Normal	Decreased	Mutation in ZAP-70	AR	T-cell signaling is abnormal
CD4 deficiency	Decreased	Normal	Decreased	Defect of DC4 expression or maturation	?	
T-cell signaling defect	Normal	Normal	Normal	Defect in proximal T-cell signal transduction	?	Recurrent sinopulmonary infection, autoimmune hemolytic anemia
Hyper-IgM syndrome	Increased IgM; decreased IgG, IgA	Normal	Normal	CD40L mutation / Unknown	XL / AR	Recurrent sinopulmonary, gastrointestinal infections; granulocytopenia
Lymphokine production deficit						
IL-2 selective	Decreased	Normal	Mildly decreased	IL-2 gene or regulatory factor defect	?	One case of selective IL-2 deficiency had intact B-cell, decreased T-cell function; others presented as SCID
Multiple	Decreased	Normal	Normal or decreased	Abnormal gene regulation factor(s)	?	
Wiskott-Aldrich syndrome	Decreased IgM; antibody to polysaccharides particularly decreased	Normal	Progressive decrease	Cell membrane defect affecting hematopoietic stem cell derivatives	XL	Thrombocytopenia; small defective platelets; eczema; lymphoreticular malignancies; autoimmune disease
Ataxia-telangiectasia	Often decreased IgA, IgE, and IgG subclasses; increased IgM monomers; antibodies variably decreased	Normal	Decreased	Chromosomal instability	AR	Ataxia-telangiectasia; increased α-fetoprotein lymphoreticular malignancies
DiGeorge anomaly	Normal or decreased	Normal	Decreased or normal	Embryopathy of thymic development	Unknown	Cardiac outflow tract malformation abnormal facies; hypoparathyroidism; partial monosomy of 22q11.pter or 10 p in some patients
NK cell deficiency	Normal	Normal	Normal		Unknown	Absent NK cells; severe initial infection with herpes group viruses

(Modified from ref. 589, with permission.)

SCID patients who have normal numbers of NK cells may have a degree of resistance but fail to develop protective immunity.

The clinical presentation of SCID is similar to that of perinatally acquired AIDS. Differentiation can best be accomplished by serologic testing of the mother and infant or by assays to detect HIV virus in the infant. Unlike patients with perinatal HIV infection who commonly have diffuse lymphadenopathy, patients with SCID usually lack detectable lymphoid tissue. One variant of autosomal recessive SCID, Omenn syndrome, may initially suggest perinatal AIDS. Omenn syndrome often presents with enlargement of lymph nodes, liver, and spleen, diffuse erythroderma, eosinophilia, and increased IgE.[591] However, in Omenn syndrome the T-cell lymphoproliferative process is usually oligoclonal, often resulting in a markedly abnormal distribution of T cells expressing the α/β or γ/δ receptor or CD4 or CD8. It is associated with an imbalance of lymphokine production in which IL-4 production is increased relative to production of IFN-γ and IL-2.[579,591] Omenn syndrome resembles graft-vs.-host disease, but the T cells that proliferate and invade normal tissues are of host origin. SCID and Omenn syndrome are usually fatal in the first year of life without specific treatment.

Combined immunodeficiency results from a deficiency in the adenosine deaminase enzyme in approximately 20 percent of cases. This results in progressive depletion of T cells and B cells due to the accumulation of toxic purine metabolites. A less severe disorder in which B-cell number and function are better preserved results from a defect in purine nucleoside phosphorylase. *Bare lymphocyte syndrome* refers to combined immunodeficiency that results from the markedly diminished MHC expression, particularly class II MHC expression, that results from defects in expression of proteins that regulate the expression of MHC proteins. In these patients the T-cell numbers and subsets are commonly normal, but T-cell and antibody responses to specific antigens are markedly impaired. Reticular dysgenesis appear to result from a defect in hematopoietic maturation, since lymphocytes, granulocytes, and often platelets are markedly diminished or absent. Each of these disorders is autosomal recessive.

In Table 4, several other variants of primary combined or cellular immunodeficiency are noted. It is evident that their phenotypes vary considerably. In some, numbers of T and B cells and concentrations of serum immunoglobulins are normal. However, one or more functions of T cells is deficient, particularly antigen-specific responses, including DTH responses. The genetic basis for most is not yet clear, although deficiencies in specific proteins that function as components of the TCR–CD3 complex or that act to regulate lymphokine production have been identified in some. The clinical presentation of these more heterogeneous disorders varies as well. Some present as SCID, whereas others present with less life-threatening infections with opportunistic pathogens, recurrent sinopulmonary infections with capsulated pathogens, or autoimmune conditions (e.g., hemolytic anemia).[592-596]

The DiGeorge syndrome, which results from a defect in thymic development due to an abnormality in embryogenesis of the third and fourth branchial clefts, is highly variable. Most patients have little or no immunologic defect, but the more severely affected patients, who have T-cell numbers of less than 10–20 percent of normal, are immunodeficient. This is manifested in markedly diminished numbers of T cells with a resultant secondary defect in B-cell function. Risk for infection parallels the immunologic defect. The Wiskott-Aldrich syndrome affects a variety of cell types and is associated with abnormalities in several cell surface glycoproteins expressed on hematopoietic cells. There is a resultant defect in T-cell and B-cell functions and thrombocytopenia. Patients with ataxia-telangiectasia have a DNA repair defect that appears to affect adversely TCR and immunoglobulin gene rearrangement and class switching. The immunologic defect is most commonly manifested as diminished production of immunoglobulin classes requiring the most distal switch and recurrent sinopulmonary infections, although defects in T-cell numbers and function occur. Lymphoid malignancies are common in ataxia-telangiectasia and the Wiskott-Aldrich syndrome.

Two more circumscribed immunodeficiency disorders are worth noting. Biron et al.[415] described a patient with absent NK cells and severe initial infections with herpes group viruses, including varicella, cytomegalovirus, and herpes simplex virus. Once the initial infection was resolved, recurrences were not common. This differs from T-cell disorders in which failure to resolve the initial infection and frequent or severe recurrences are characteristic. The clinical picture is compatible with the primary role of NK cells in the initial containment of these infections. We have also seen a patient with a similar disorder (unpublished observation). The X-linked lymphoproliferative syndrome appears to represent a lacunar defect in the control of infection with EBV. These patients present either with severe and often fatal infectious mononucleosis or acquired hypogammaglobulinemia, apparently reflecting an unmodulated attack of CD8 T cells against EBV-infected cells, or with B-cell lymphoma.[540]

Chronic mucocutaneous candidiasis is a condition of unknown etiology in which the principal manifestation is that suggested by the name. The age of onset, severity of disease, and association with other clinical features vary. One variant is associated with autoimmune endocrinopathy. There are no diagnostic laboratory findings. Numbers and functions of T cells are generally normal. However, most fail to manifest DTH responses to *Candida* and often fail to respond to *Candida* antigen in vitro.

Immunodeficiency Secondary to Drug or Radiation Therapy

Immunodeficiency in clinical practice is commonly secondary to drug or radiation therapy. In the management of patients undergoing transplantation or as part of cancer therapy protocols multiple drugs and radiation therapy are commonly combined. Combinations, which act to inhibit the immune response in multiple ways, are associated with more severe impairment of CMI (and often other aspects of the host response) and with a greater risk for infection. The nature of the underlying disease may dictate the nature and intensity of the immunosuppressive regimen and also may directly affect the immune response independently of therapy. The insult provided by the chemotherapy is then superimposed on the underlying immune abnormality. With modern combination immunosuppressive therapies it is often not possible to differentiate the specific contribution of individual drugs or the disease.[597]

Several general principles have emerged. In patients receiving organ transplants and combined immunosuppressive therapy with corticosteroids, azathioprine, and cyclosporin, there is a clearly increased risk of infection with a variety of opportunistic pathogens, including those listed in Table 2, particularly the herpes group viruses. Infections with the latter are particularly severe when primary cytomegalovirus[598] or varicella[599] infection occurs during this period. This may reflect the greater ability of certain classes of drugs to inhibit a primary response rather than an established or secondary immune response. In addition to typical infectious disease processes, such patients are at markedly increased risk for the development of EBV-related B-cell lymphoproliferative disorders.[539,600] These are often polyclonal initially but with time progress to become oligo- or monoclonal lymphomas.

In general, single-drug regimens are less likely to result in opportunistic infection. This may be related to the fact that such regimens are commonly employed in the treatment of diseases that themselves are not associated (or are less likely associated with abnormal cellular immunity. For example, the incidence of EBV-related lymphomas in patients with rheumatoid arthritis and other autoimmune diseases who were treated with cyclosporin is much less (2 of 2,600) than observed in transplant patients.[601] In contrast, EBV-associated lymphomas, *P. carinii* pneumonia, and disseminated herpes zoster have been reported in patients with rheumatoid arthritis receiving relatively low doses of methotrexate with or without concomitant corticosteroids.[602] The conditions generally improved when immunosuppressive therapy was stopped. It has been argued that patients with rheumatoid arthritis and other autoimmune conditions are at greater risk than those with conditions not clearly associated with aberrant, systemic immune responses (e.g., psoriasis and asthma). Nevertheless, patients who receive moderate doses of corticosteroids for asthma are at increased risk of lethal primary infection with varicella.[603] Overall, it is prudent to assume that patients receiving therapeutic doses of one or more agents that interfere with T-cell and/or mononuclear phagocyte function may have an impaired ability to respond to primary infection with an effective CMI response. Patients receiving therapy with more intense and prolonged multidrug regimens may also exhibit increased risk of recrudescent infection with opportunistic pathogens.

Corticosteroids. The most commonly used drugs that impede the function of the cellular immune system are corticosteroids. Although humans are less sensitive to depletion of T cells by corticosteroids than are rodents, potent effects on CMI are observed. Corticosteroids inhibit the immune system through multiple direct effects on lymphocytes and macrophages and also impede other aspects of the inflammatory response relevant to CMI.[604] In vivo administration of a single therapeutic dose of corticosteroids results in redistribution of lymphocytes and monocytes from the peripheral circulation, resulting in an approximate 70 and 90 percent reduction, respectively, at 4–6 hours with a return to normal by 24 hours. This effect recurs with repeated dosing. Continued administration will result in an alteration in the availability of these cells for recruitment into sites of infection or DTH skin tests. The effects on monocytes and macrophages also include a diminution in clearance of particles, including those opsonized by IgG or complement. Antigen-specific immune responses are inhibited by pharmacologic doses, with the effects on T-cell–mediated immune response being most apparent. Synthesis of specific antibodies in response to immunization with most common antigens and serum immunoglobulin concentrations are not affected by conventional doses. However, pulses of high-dose methylprednisolone are associated with inhibition of specific antibody production and a diminution of immunoglobulins of all classes that reaches a nadir at 2–4 weeks.

The effects of glucocorticoids are mediated in part by their ability to block activation of lymphocytes and macrophages. The early events induced by antigen-specific stimulation of T cells are not inhibited, but subsequent events that lead to the transcription and production of lymphokines are blocked. The inhibition of IL-2 production[605,606] is likely central to the inhibition of T-cell proliferation and the generation of cytotoxic T cells. Glucocorticosteroids also inhibit the production by macrophages of lipid mediators of inflammation, including the leukotrienes and prostaglandins. Macrophage production of cytokines, including TNF-α, IL-1, and chemokines, and microbicidal activity, including production of nitric oxide, are also inhibited. These effects on macrophages are the probable cause for the inhibition of fever by corticosteroids.

Cyclosporin and FK506. Cyclosporin, a fungal product, has been in clinical use for some time; FK506 is a macrolide antibiotic under investigation.[607] Although dissimilar in chemical structure, these compounds act as immunosuppressants to block calcium-dependent events in lymphocyte signaling by forming a ternary complex with one or more specific binding proteins and the calcium-dependent phosphatase calcineurin B.[608] The result is a blockade in T-cell activation, inhibition of production of IL-2 and other lymphokines including IFN-γ, and, as a result, inhibition of proliferation. Generation of cytotoxic T cells is blocked, and the killing of targets by existing CTL is inhibited. Effects on B-cell activation and proliferation are more variable. Production of specific antibodies in vivo is inhibited, which likely reflects effects on T-cell help and to some extent direct effects on B cells. The major clinical effects of cyclosporin are exhibited as inhibition of CMI and the resultant increased risk of infection with intracellular pathogens.[609] The profound and relatively selective effects of these drugs on T-cell function may account for the frequency of B-cell lymphoproliferative disorders, including polyclonal or frank malignant lymphoma, associated with EBV.[539,600,610]

Azathioprine, Cyclophosphamide, Chlorambucil, and Related Drugs. Azathioprine is related to 6-mercaptopurine and acts to inhibit proliferation of cells of all types. The immune suppression is directly related to this effect. Thus, prolonged therapy is generally associated with some degree of lymphopenia. These and related compounds appear to inhibit the development of primary responses by diminishing antigen-driven lymphocyte proliferation at the step of DNA synthesis.[611] They have little effect on an established immune response other than by diminishing the numbers of monocytes and lymphocytes available for recruitment into loci of ongoing immune responses. There are some variations in the relative impact of these agents on different subsets of cells. For example, azathioprine generally results in a greater relative diminution of T cells and NK cells than of B cells, whereas the akylating agents chlorambucil and cyclophosphamide may have a greater impact on B cells and primary antibody responses.[597,612] These compounds have little or no effect on the inflammatory response.

Methotrexate. Methotrexate, like azathioprine, blocks proliferation of cycling cells. It inhibits the development of primary immune responses more efficiently than secondary immune responses. Its mechanism of action as an immunopressant is not as well characterized as the drugs noted above. It was initially developed for cancer therapy, but has recently been employed extensively for the treatment of psoriasis, rheumatoid arthritis, and other autoimmune diseases. As noted in the introductory portion of this section, it appears to impede CMI sufficiently that patients receiving this drug for autoimmune disease alone or in combination with corticosteroids have developed infections with opportunistic pathogens, including *Pneumocystis* and herpes zoster.[613]

Antithymocyte Globulin and Anti-T-Cell Monoclonal Antibodies. Antithymocyte globulin acts primarily by depleting T cells and secondarily by inhibiting T-cell activation. These preparations of polyclonal antibodies vary in their potency and selectivity for T cells. OKT3 is the only licensed monoclonal antibody for use as an immunosuppressive agent. It produces a T-cell lymphopenia but also impairs T-cell function in part by down-regulation of the TCR–CD3 complex. With initial administration it activates T cells, which commonly results in fever, chills, and other cytokine-mediated side effects. Subsequently T cells are rendered anergic to subsequent activation by specific antigen. Accordingly, it is a potent suppressor of T-cell–mediated immunity. It is generally only used for short periods, but during this time patients are at considerably increased risk of infection with opportunistic pathogens, particularly cytomegalovirus.[597]

Total Lymphoid Irradiation. Total lymphoid irradiation was initially used as a form of immunosuppressive therapy for Hodgkin's disease, but more recently has been used to manage rejection episodes in patients with solid organ transplants. Total lymphoid irradiation inhibits the development of primary antigen-specific immune responses, advantageous in transplantation since a state of partial tolerance may be induced.[614] It results in about 50 percent reduction in circulating T and B cells[615,616] and a similar reduction in lymphocyte proliferative responses in vitro; these reduced values persist for the first 6–12 months and return to baseline in 2–3 years. There are also marked effects on the thymus and lymphoid organs. In mice an imbalance in CD4 T-cell function is induced. Cells secreting the TH2 cytokines IL-4 and IL-5 recover more quickly than those secreting IL-2 and IFN-γ,[617] which could impede defenses against intracellular pathogens. Clinically, total lymphoid irradiation has been associated with an increased risk of disease due to cytomegalovirus and varicella-zoster virus.[614]

Immunodeficiency Secondary to Tumors

Most malignancies do not directly impair CMI. CMI may become impaired due to the effects of chemotherapy or malnutrition that may accompany the tumor. However, certain tumors involving the lymphoid system appear to have a direct effect on CMI.

Thymomas are associated with marked aberrations of the immune response, most severely affecting humoral immunity.[618] Patients are most commonly between 40 and 70 years of age. They may present with antibody-mediated autoimmune diseases, such as myasthenia gravis, or with recurrent infections, most commonly sinopulmonary infections due to capsulated bacteria. This parallels a profound depletion of B cells and of serum immunoglobulins. However, defective CMI, as indicated by absent DTH responses and reduced CD4 T cells, occurs in many. These patients may develop opportunistic infections with herpes group viruses and *Pneumocystis* and chronic mucocutaneous candidiasis.

Hodgkin's disease is commonly associated with defective CMI. Even in untreated patients with minimal or no symptoms, DTH responses are often reduced or absent. Various abnormalities of T- and NK-cell functions as assayed in vitro have been reported.[619,620] The degree to which other forms of lymphoid malignancies result in altered CMI independent of treatment varies. Patients with hairy cell leukemia are commonly pancytopenic and exhibit increased susceptibility to bacterial and invasive fungal pathogens. However, they also have a very high incidence of infection with *M. avium*-intracellulare, herpes group viruses, *Toxoplasma*, and *Pneumocystis*, consistent with defective CMI. There are moderate alterations in T-cell subsets in the disease, but these do not appear to be sufficient to account for the overall degree of impairment.[621] Other lymphoid malignancies occasionally present with opportunistic infections suggestive of altered CMI.[622]

Immunodeficiency Secondary to Malnutrition

With HIV infection, protein energy malnutrition is the most frequent cause of impaired cell-mediated immunity on a global scale.[623] It frequently complicates other diseases and may play a major role (e.g., in cancer) or a contributing role (e.g., in HIV infection) in immunologic impairment in such disorders. Malnutrition results in involution of the thymus and a parallel reduction in T-cell–dependent areas in the lymph nodes and spleen. Circulating numbers of T cells are diminished, with a greater decrease in CD4 T cells than in CD8 T cells. Antigen-specific responses are diminished in vivo and in vitro, as detected by DTH skin tests, proliferation assays, and lymphokine production. B-cell numbers and antibody production are better preserved, although T-cell–dependent antibody responses may be impaired. The clinical impact of these changes on resistance to infection are multiple: fatal measles virus infection is a major problem related to malnutrition, risk of progressive or severe tuberculosis and herpes virus infections is greater, and the origi-

nal descriptions of *Pneumocystis* pneumonia were in malnourished children (see Ch. 258). The impairment in CMI and T-lymphocyte numbers is reversible over weeks to months with restoration of nutrition.

Selective deficiency of nutrients may also impair cell-mediated immunity. The most clear evidence for impairment of T-cell function is in zinc deficiency,[624] but severe deficiency of iron has also been associated with impaired CMI. However, the evidence that these specific nutrient deficiencies impair CMI sufficiently that they result in increased predisposition to infection is not compelling. Deficiencies of specific vitamins or cofactors resulting from a genetic defects in transcobalamin II, carboxylase, and other enzymes result in abnormalities in multiple organs, including impairment of the immune response.[589]

Immunodeficiency Secondary to Infectious Processes

Infectious diseases have been noted to impair host defenses since the original observation that measles was associated with a transient loss of tuberculin reactivity almost a century ago.[625] Viral infections in particular are commonly associated with impaired CMI. These include, most notably, HIV infection, the immunopathology of which is discussed in more detail in Chapter 101. Mechanisms by which viruses impair CMI are multiple.[625,626] These include direct infection of lymphocytes and/or mononuclear phagocytes, which may either lead to depletion of the cell type or affect function. Measles virus, each of the herpes group viruses (cytomegalovirus, EBV, and HHV6, in particular), influenza virus, and the respiratory syncytial virus are some examples. In addition, viruses can directly produce proteins that impair the function of components of the cellular immune system, as discussed above and shown in Table 3. Alternatively, viruses may induce host cells that directly or through the production of soluble mediators downregulate CMI. Direct inhibition of responses by CD8 T cells against the infecting virus has been shown best with lymphocytic choriomeningitis virus in mice.[626] As regards soluble mediators, viral infection is a potent inducer of interferons, and interferons by inhibiting cell proliferation may dampen lymphocyte responses.[398,625,627] Respiratory syncytial virus induces the production by human blood mononuclear cells of IL-1 receptor antagonist in excess over IL-1,[628] and this in part accounts for the inhibition of lymphocyte proliferation caused by respiratory syncytial virus in vitro. Finally, some viruses may alter the balance of T-cell lymphokine production toward the production of cytokines that impede effective anti-viral CMI (i.e., TH2-like cytokines).[629] This has been most clearly shown for murine AIDS, which is not retrovirally induced.[629] Recent data suggest that a similar pattern may occur in humans with AIDS as disease progresses.[630,631]

In AIDS, the effects on the immune system are progressive and profound and clearly result in increased susceptibility to opportunistic infections against which CMI is critical. In the other infections, the alteration in CMI is transient. In many of these infections lymphopenia or alterations in T-cell subsets, often an absolute or relative decrease in CD4 T cells with an accompanying relative or absolute increase in CD8 T cells, occur. This is common in individuals with infectious mononucleosis due to EBV or in those with similar acute infectious syndromes caused by HIV, cytomegalovirus, or *Toxoplasma* infection. In the acute infection these effects may reflect an actual increase in total numbers of CD8 T cells responding to the acute intracellular infection and alterations in T-cell homing.

Unlike AIDS, in most of the other infections evidence that the initial viral infection results in clinically significant increased risk of opportunistic infections is lacking. One exception is measles, which appears to be associated with an increased risk of tuberculosis. In other cases, subsequent infections with another agent may reflect the underlying immunologic cause for the initial infection rather than impairment of the immune response to one infection by another.[633] The most common secondary infections are pyogenic in nature (e.g., bacterial pneumonia complicating influenza) rather than other opportunistic infections with intracellular pathogens.[633,634] This suggests that tissue injury or impairment of the inflammatory response may be the more clinically important effect of the primary viral infection. However, there are some circumstances in which clinically significant impairment of CMI occurs. For example, cytomegalovirus infection has been reported in humans and in experimental animals to increase the risk of secondary infections, for example, with *Pneumocystis* or *Toxoplasma*.[635,636] Influenza is associated with clear inhibition of general cell-mediated immunity, whereas an effective influenza-specific immune response develops. This has been argued to reflect the appropriate focusing of host defenses to control the initial infection rather than a true state of immunodeficiency.[637] At present, an independent role of viral-induced impairment of CMI in predisposition to infection is not established for most agents.

Impairment of CMI is also evident in certain protozoan infection, infection with intracellular bacterial pathogens, and in severe infection with pyogenic infections. In these infections it seems likely that alterations in T-cell subsets and the lymphokines they produce, or changes in lymphocyte traffic associated with systemic cytokine production, play an important role in the impairment of CMI. Strong evidence supports a role for infection-induced abnormalities in CMI in the pathogenesis of progressive *Leishmania* infection and in lepromatous leprosy (see above). In the former disease a predominant TH2 response of CD4 T cells and in the latter a CD8 subset that atypically and preferentially produces IL-4 have been implicated in antigen-specific impairment of CMI. In malaria and in infections due to African trypanosomes and *Trypanosoma cruzi*, CD8 T cells that inhibit IL-2 production have been invoked to explain the more general inhibition of CMI that occurs.[377,638] It is not clear if mechanisms similar to these account for the impairment of CMI in other diseases with intracellular pathogens such as typhoid fever, brucellosis, and tuberculosis, in which the clinical significance of the impairment in CMI resulting from the infection is not readily separated from other events (e.g., impairment in nutrition) that commonly accompany these infections.

A variety of other disease processes are associated with impaired CMI. These include uremia, burns, major surgery, sarcoidosis, and graft-vs.-host disease. More details of these and other secondary immunodeficiencies may be found in review by Shearer and Anderson[639] and by Lachman et al.[640]

Cytokines Therapy in Immunodeficiency States

To date, specific recombinant cytokines have found their greatest established utility in the management of conditions predisposing to infection rather than in the treatment of specific infections. With the exception of recombinant CSF, only IFN-γ has been licensed for clinical use, to prevent or ameliorate infection in patients with chronic granulomatous disease. This condition results from a genetic defect in one of the proteins that compose the phagocyte oxidase (see Ch. 7). These patients develop infections with catalase-positive microbes, most commonly pyogenic bacteria and fungi. A multicenter collaborative study of recombinant IFN-γ administered three times per week resulted in a diminution in numbers of serious infections in all groups of patients when used alone or in concert with prophylactic trimethoprim-sulfamethoxazole.[641,642] Anecdotal reports also suggest that IFN-γ may improve the ability of these patients to control infection with filamentous fungi.[643,644] The mechanism of action is uncertain but may be related to the enhancement by IFN-γ of phagocyte antimicrobial mechanisms, which help to compensate for the lack of effective oxygen-radical–dependent killing. A patient with combined immunodeficiency related to a deficiency in the production of IL-2 has been treated with recombinant IL-2 with apparent benefit.[592] However, the efficacy of this form of therapy in other patients with primary immunodefi-

ciency and defective IL-2 production is not known. In preliminary trials of a longer acting IL-2 preparation, PEG IL-2 administration to a small group of patients with common variable immunodeficiency was associated with improved antibody production and T-cell help for antibody production in vitro[645]; no effects were observed in vivo, but the study was not designed to test in vivo efficacy.

Clinical Evaluation of Individuals with Suspect Cellular Immunodeficiency

In general, clinical suspicion of an abnormality of cellular immunity is most often raised by an increased frequency or severity of infections with opportunistic viral or nonviral intracellular pathogens (Table 2), certain fungal pathogens (e.g., mucocutaneous *Candida* infection, disseminated coccidiodomycosis), intestinal protozoan, and occasionally metazoans (e.g., *Cryptosporidium parvum, Strongyloides stercoralis*). Disordered CMI is also commonly associated with impaired antibody production, autoimmune conditions (e.g., autoimmune hemolytic anemia, thrombocytopenia), and malignancies, particularly lymphoid malignancies. Most often more than one of these manifestations will develop over time, but the presenting feature may be any one of the above, depending to some extent on the age of onset and exposure of individuals to specific agents. Accordingly, a careful history is often the most important feature that directs the initial evaluation. Although most forms of genetic immunodeficiency are autosomal recessive, a detailed family history is often revealing in cases of X-linked immunodeficiency or in cases of consanguinity. Most forms of primary cellular immune deficiency (Table 4) produce obvious disease in the first months of life. Milder defects, which are now more commonly appreciated, may not present as early or with the multiplicity of problems usually observed with classic SCID. Secondary immunodeficiencies will be suspected based on an appropriate history, including risk factors for HIV infection.

Physical examination is useful in identifying associated clinical features and manifestations of secondary infections. For example, patients with short-limbed dwarfism/cartilage hair hypoplasia have characteristic skeletal features, and patients with DiGeorge syndrome have characteristic facies (hypertelorism, antimongoloid slant to eyes, low-set ears, and micrognathia) and associated abnormalities of the cardiovascular system. Severe, recalcitrant eczema is a common manifestation in many forms of immunodeficiency, particular Omenn and Wiskott-Aldrich syndromes. In patients with classic SCID, lymphoid and thymic tissue is absent or markedly reduced. In contrast, in Omenn syndrome (a variant of autosomal recessive SCID) and in HIV infection lymphadenopathy is common. Radiographic abnormalities of cartilage are present in adenosine deaminase deficiency and in short-limbed dwarfism.

DTH skin tests may be useful for a screening evaluation. DTH is reduced or absent in most individuals with substantive defects of cellular immunity. Intact DTH, with induration at 48–72 hours of at least 5 mm to one or more common recall antigens indicates that severe impairment of CMI is absent. Conversely, particularly in individuals with acquired immune deficiencies, considerable depletion of T cells or alterations in T-cell functional profiles may occur before complete anergy to recall antigens is observed. In early infancy, DTH skin test reactivity is not detectable, and reactivity is unreliable as a measure of CMI up to 2 years of age. This reflects both a lack of exposure to the test antigens and the physiologic impairment in several components of the immune response necessary to manifest normal DTH reactivity. Finally, despite recent attempts to improve standardization of skin test antigens and procedures,[589,646] there are many technical pitfalls in their use for evaluation of CMI.

For these reasons, laboratory evaluation is generally indicated when there is more than minimal clinical suspicion of a defect in CMI. A complete blood count and flow cytometric evaluation of lymphocyte subsets are the two most important methods for laboratory evaluation of CMI. Proper standardization of procedures and the use of appropriate antibody reagents is important in obtaining valid results by flow cytometry.[647] It is important that results for absolute and relative numbers of T cells, B cells, NK cells, and their subsets be compared with age-specific norms. For example, absolute and relative numbers of CD4 T cells are higher in infants and young children than in adults, and the percentage of CD56+ NK cells is about 50 percent less in infants than in adults, although the percentage of CD16+ NK cells is similar.[484] In patients with many forms of SCID, flow cytometry will confirm a paucity of T cells or NK cells or show abnormalities in T-cell subsets or in expression of components of the TCR complex. In such cases evaluation of lymphocyte proliferative responses to mitogens usually suffices to provide confirmation of markedly diminished T-cell function and confirm a diagnosis of SCID (see Table 4). In cases with less complete forms of cellular immunodeficiency, flow cytometry and evaluation of proliferative responses to mitogens or autologous mononuclear cells (mixed leukocyte reaction) may provide an incomplete picture of the degree to which function is impaired. In those cases, evaluation of responses to specific antigens or the production of specific lymphokines or cell surface molecules important for cell–cell interaction in the immune system are important. Such testing is generally best performed by individuals familiar with clinical evaluation of the immune response. It may include proliferation and production of specific lymphokines in response to mitogens and recall antigens, evaluation of the capacity to produce specific antibody, the ability to develop a recall response on secondary immunization, and to switch from IgM to IgG production as part of the recall response; such tests provide a particularly stringent test of combined T-cell and B-cell function.[589,648]

If diagnosis of primary cellular immunodeficiency is established, testing to determine if SCID has resulted from adenosine deaminase deficiency is important, since enzyme replacement therapy or gene therapy may be considered as an alternate to bone marrow transplantation. Other specific causes (e.g., IL-2-R γ-chain deficiency, bare lymphocyte syndrome) can be identified by appropriate testing. In combined immunodeficiency due to lymphokine production defects, proliferative responses can usually be restored by addition of IL-2 production to the cultures. The identification of specific gene defects in other forms of genetic immunodeficiency and further development of specific gene therapy can be anticipated in the upcoming years.

The findings in secondary immunodeficiency are highly variable, reflecting the differences in mechanism. Most commonly abnormal are tests of antigen-specific responses, particularly the development of responses to neoantigens rather than to recall antigens. Such abnormalities can be found when other tests of CMI yield normal results. This is particularly true in children with HIV infection, who frequently present with opportunistic infections at times when the number of CD4 T cells is normal. Thus, a routine part of all evaluations for defects in CMI should include testing to detect HIV infection. In children in the first 15 months of life it is not possible to establish a diagnosis by serologic testing alone. However, seropositivity in the mother and/or child strongly suggests the diagnosis in the face of clinical immunodeficiency; however, tests that directly detect the virus or its products are needed for confirmation of the diagnosis in infancy.

ACKNOWLEDGMENTS

This work was supported in part by grants from the National Institutes of Health to R.M.L. and C.B.W.

REFERENCES

1. Kaufmann SHE. Immunity to intracellular bacteria. Annu Rev Immunol. 1993;11:129–64.
2. Doherty PC, Allan W, Eichelberger M, et al. Roles of αβ and γδ T cell subsets in viral immunity. Annu Rev Immunol. 1992;10:123–52.
3. Bjorkman PJ, Parham P. Structure, function and diversity of class I major histocompatibility complex molecules. Annu Rev Biochem. 1990;59:253–88.
4. Geraghty DE. Structure of the HLA class I region and expression of its resident genes. Curr Opin Immunol. 1993;5:3–7.
5. Monaco JJ. Structure and function of genes in the MHC class II region. Curr Opin Immunol. 1993;5:17–20.
6. Black FL. Why did they die? Science. 1992;258:1739–40.
7. Rammensee H-G, Falk K, Rotzschke O. MHC molecules as peptide receptors. Curr Opin Immunol. 1993;5:35–44.
7a. Germain RN. MHC-dependent antigen processing and peptide presentation: providing ligands for T lymphocyte activation. Cell. 1994;76:287–99.
8. Pfeifer JD, Wick MJ, Roberts RL, et al. Phagocytic processing of bacterial antigens for class I MHC presentation to T cells. Nature. 1993;361:359–62.
9. Nuchtern JB, Biddison WE, Klausner RD. Class II MHC molecules can use the endogenous pathway of antigen presentation. Nature. 1990;343:74–6.
10. Malnati MS, Marti M, LaVaute T, et al. Processing pathways for presentation of cytosolic antigen to MHC class II-restricted T cells. Nature. 1992;357:702–4.
11. Kovacsovics-Bankowski M, Clark K, Benacerraf B, et al. Efficient major histocompatibility complex class I presentation of exogenous antigen upon phagocytosis by macrophages. Proc Natl Acad Sci USA. 1993;90:4942–46.
12. Bijlmakers M-J, Ploegh HL. Putting together an MHC class molecule. Curr Opin Immunol. 1993;5:21–6.
13. Zijlstra M, Bix M, Simister NE, et al. β2-Microglobulin deficient mice lack CD4−8+ cytolytic T cells. Nature. 1990;344:742–6.
14. Ahluwalia N, Bergeron JJM, Wada I, et al. The p88 molecular chaperone is identical to the endoplasmic reticulum protein, calnexin. J Biol Chem. 1992;267:10914–18.
15. Bjorkman PJ, Saper MA, Samaoui B, et al. Structure of the human class I histocompatibility antigen HLA-A2. Nature. 1987;329:506–12.
16. Goldberg AL, Rock KL. Proteolysis, proteasomes and antigen presentation. Nature. 1992;357:375–9.
17. Brown MG, Driscoll J, Monaco JJ. Structural and serological similarity of MHC-linked LMP and proteasome (multicatalytic proteinase) complexes. Nature. 1991;353:355–7.
18. Glynne R, Powis SH, Beck S, et al. A proteasome-related gene between the two ABC transporter loci in the class II region of the human MHC. Nature. 1991;353:357–60.
19. Arnold D, Driscoll J, Androlewicz M, et al. Proteasome subunits encoded in the MHC are not generally required for the processing of peptides bound by MHC class I molecules. Nature. 1992;360:171–4.
20. Momburg F, Ortiz-Navarrete V, Neefjes J, et al. Proteasome subunits encoded by the major histocompatibility complex are not essential for antigen presentation. Nature. 1992;360:174–7.
21. Del Val M, Schlicht H-J, Ruppert T, et al. Efficient processing of an antigenic sequence for presentation by MHC class I molecules depends on its neighboring residues in the protein. Cell. 1991;66:1145–53.
22. Eisenlohr LC, Yewdell JW, Bennink JR. Flanking sequences influence the presentation of an endogenously synthesized peptide to cytotoxic T lymphocyes. J Exp Med. 1992;175:481–7.
23. Powis SJ, Townsend ARM, Deverson EV, et al. Restoration of antigen presentation to the mutant cell line RMA-S by an MHC-linked transporter. Nature. 1991;354:528–31.
24. Kelly A, Powis SH, Kerr L-A, et al. Assembly and function of the two ABC transporter proteins encoded in the human major histocompatibility complex. Nature. 1992;355:641–4.
25. Attaya M, Jameson S, Martinez CK, et al. Ham-2 corrects the class I antigen-processing defect in RMA-S cells. Nature. 1992;355:647–9.
26. Van Kaer L, Ashton-Rickardt PG, Ploegh HL, et al. TAP1 mutant mice are deficient in antigen presentation, surface class I molecules, and CD4−8+ T cells. Cell. 1992;71:1205–14.
27. Powis SJ, Deverson EV, Coadwell WJ, et al. Effect of polymorphism of an MHC-linked transporter on the peptides assembled in a class molecule. Nature. 1992;357:211–5.
28. Wei ML, Cresswell P. HLA-A2 molecules in an antigen-processing mutant cell contain signal sequence-derived peptides. Nature. 1992;356:443–6.
29. Henderson RA, Michel H, Sakaguchi K, et al. HLA-A2.1–associated peptides from a mutant cell line: a second pathway of antigen presentation. Science. 1992;255:1264–6.
30. Kleijmeer MJ, Kelly A, Geuze HJ, et al. Location of MHC-encoded transporters in the endoplasmic reticulum and cis-Golgi. Nature. 1992;357:342–4.
31. Elliot T, Cerundolo V, Elvin J, et al. Peptide-induced conformational change of the class I heavy chain. Nature. 1991;351:402–6.
32. Krishna S, Benaroch P, Pillai S. Tetrameric cell-surface MHC class I molecules. Nature. 1992;357:164–7.
33. Rotzschke O, Falk K, Deres K, et al. Isolation and analysis of naturally processed viral peptides as recognized by cytotoxic T cells. Nature. 1990;348:252–4.
34. Van Bleek GM, Nathenson SG. Isolation of an endogenously processed immunodominant viral peptide from the class I H-2Kb molecule. Nature. 1990;348:213–6.
35. Falk K, Rotzschke O, Stevanovic S, et al. Allele-specific motifs revealed by sequencing of self-peptides eluted from MHC molecules. Nature. 1991;351:290–6.
36. Jardetzky TS, Lane WS, Robinson RA, et al. Identification of self peptides bound to purified HLA-B27. Nature. 1991;353:326–9.
37. Madden DR, Gorga JC, Strominger JL, et al. The structure of HLA-B27 reveals nonamer self-peptides bound in an extended conformation. Nature. 1991;353:321–5.
38. Fremont DH, Matsumura M, Stura EA, et al. Crystal structures of two viral

peptides in complex with murine MHC class I H-2Kb. Science. 1992;257: 919–27.

39. Zhang W, Young ACM, Imarai M, et al. Crystal structure of the major histocompatibility complex class I H-2Kb molecule containing a single viral peptide: Implications for peptide binding and T cell receptor recognition. Proc Natl Acad Sci USA. 1992;89:8403–7.

40. Silver ML, Guo H-C, Strominger JL, et al. Atomic structure of a human MHC molecule presenting an influenza virus protein. Nature. 1992;360: 367–9.

41. Matsumura M, Fremont DH, Peterson PA, et al. Emerging principles for the recognition of peptide antigens by MHC class I molecules. Science. 1992; 257:927–34.

42. Pamer EG, Wang C-R, Flaherty L, et al. H-2M3 presents a *Listeria monocytogenes* peptide to cytotoxic T lymphocytes. Cell. 1992;70:215–23.

43. Rotzschke O, Falk K, Stevanovic S, et al. Qa-2 molecules are peptide receptors of higher stringency than ordinary class I molecules. Nature. 1993;361: 642–4.

44. Porcelli S, Morita CT, Brenner MB. CD1b restricts the response of human CD4−8− T lymphocytes to a microbial antigen. Nature. 1992;360:593–7.

45. Cosson P, Bonifacino JS. Role of transmembrane domain interactions in the assembly of class II MHC molecules. Science. 1992;258:659–62.

46. Roche PA, Marks MS, Cresswell P. Formation of a nine-subunit complex by HLA class II glycoproteins and the invariant chain. Nature. 1991;354: 392–4.

47. Lotteau V, Teyton L, Peleraux A, et al. Intracellular transport of class II MHC molecules directed by invariant chain. Nature. 1990;348:600–1.

48. Bakke O, Dobberstein B. MHC class II-associated invariant chain contains a sorting signal for endosomal compartments. Cell. 1990;63:707–16.

49. Romagnoli P, Layet C, Yewdell J, et al. Relationship between invariant chain expression and major histocompatibility complex class II transport into early and late endocytic compartments. J Exp Med. 1993;177:583–96.

50. Chicz RM, Urban RG, Corga JC, et al. Specificity and promiscuity among naturally processed peptides bound to HLA-DR alleles. J Exp Med. 1993; 178:27–47.

51. Germain RN, Hendrix LR. MHC class II structure, occupancy and surface expression determined by post-endoplasmic reticulum antigen binding. Nature. 1991;353:134–9.

52. Rudensky AY, Preston-Hurlburt P, Hong S-C, et al. Sequence analysis of peptides bound to MHC class II molecules. Nature. 1991;353:622–7.

53. Hunt DF, Michel H, Dickinson TA, et al. Peptides presented to the immune system by the murine class II major histocompatibility complex molecule I-Ad. Science. 1992;256:1817–20.

54. Brown JH, Jardetzky T, Saper MA, et al. A hypothetical model of the foreign antigen binding sites of class II histocompatibility molecules. Nature. 1988; 332:845–50.

55. Brown JH, Jardetzky TS, Gorga JC, et al. Three dimensional structure of the human class II histocompatibility antigen HLA-DRI. Nature. 1993;364: 33–9.

56. Hunt JS, Orr HT. HLA and maternal-fetal recognition. FASEB J. 1992;6: 2344–8.

57. Steinman RM. The dendritic cell system and its role in immunogenicity. Annu Rev Immunol. 1991;9:271–96.

58. Davis MM, Bjorkman PJ. T cell antigen recpetor genes and T cell recognition. Nature. 1988;334:395–401.

59. Weiss A. Structure and function fo the T cell antigen receptor. J Clin Invest. 1990;86:1015–22.

60. Jorgensen JL, Esser U, Fazekas de St. Groth B, et al. Mapping T cell receptor–peptide contacts by variant peptide immunization of single-chain transgenics. Nature. 1992;355:224–30.

61. Patten PA, Rock EP, Sonoda T, et al. Transfer of putative complementarity-determining region loops of T cell receptor V domains confers toxin reactivity but not peptide/MHC specificity. J Immunol. 1993;150:2281–94.

62. Hong SC, Cheloche A, Lin RH, et al. An MHC interaction site maps to the amino-terminal half of the T cell receptor alpha chain variable domain. Cell. 1992;69:999–1009.

62a. Schild H, Mavaddat N, Litzenberger C, et al. The nature of major histocompatibility complex recognition by γδ T cels. Cells. 1994;76:29–37.

63. Letourneur F, Klausner RD. A novel di-leucine motif and a tyrosine-based motif independently mediate lysosomal targeting and endocytosis of CD3 chains. Cell. 1992;69:1143–57.

64. Geisler C, Kuhlmann J, Rubin B. Assembly, intracellular processing, and expression at the cell surface of the human ab T cell receptor/CD3 complex. J Immunol. 1989;143:4069–77.

65. de la Hera A, Muller U, Olsson C, et al. Structure of the T cell antigen receptor (TCR): Two CD3ε subunits in a functional TCR/CD3 complex. J Exp Med. 1991;173:7–17.

66. Bucy RP, Chan C-LH, Cooper MD. Tissue localization and CD 8 accessory molecule expression of Tγδ cells in humans. J Immunol. 1989;142:3045–9.

67. Guy-Grand D, Cerf-Bensussan N, Malissen B, et al. Two gut intraepithelial CD8+ lymphocyte populations with different T cell receptors: A role for the gut epithelium in T cell differentiation. J Exp Med. 1991;173:471–81.

68. Ohteki T, Okuayama R, Seki S, et al. Age-dependent increase of extrathymic T cells in the liver and their appearance in the periphery of older mice. J Immunol. 1992;149:1562–70.

69. Mosley RL, Klein JR. Peripheral engraftment of fetal intestine into athymic mice sponsors T cell development: Direct evidence for thymopoietic function of murine small intestine. J Exp Med. 1992;176:1365–73.

70. Peault B, Weissman IL, Baum C, et al. Lymphoid reconstitution of the human fetal thymus in SCID mice with CD34+ precursor cells. J Exp Med. 1991;174:1283–6.

71. Haynes BF, Martin ME, Kay HH, Kurtzberg J. Early events in human T cell ontogeny. Phenotypic characterization and immunohistologic localization of T cell precursors in early human fetal tissues. J Exp Med. 1988;168:1061–80.

72. Williams GT, Kingston R, Owen MJ, et al. A single micromanipulated stem cell gives rise to multiple B-cell receptor gene rearrangements in the thymus in vitro. Nature. 1986;324:63–4.

73. Donskoy E, Goldschneider I. Thymocytopoiesis is maintained by bloodborne precursors throughout postnatal life. A study of parabiotic mice. J Immunol. 1992;148:1604–12.

74. Davis MM, Bjorkman PJ. T-cell antigen receptor genes and T-cell recognition. Nature. 1988;334:395–402.

75. Oettinger MA, Schatz DG, Gorka C, et al. RAG-1 and RAG-2, adjacent genes that synergistically activate V(D)J recombination. Science. 1990;248: 1517–23.

76. Mombaerts P, Iacomini J, Johnson RS, et al. RAG-1-deficient mice have no mature B and T lymphocytes. Cell. 1992;68:869–77.

77. Shinkai Y, Rathbun G, Lam K-P, et al. RAG-2-deficient mice lack mature lymphocytes owing to inability to initiate V(D)J rearrangement. Cell. 1992; 68:855–67.

78. Schatz DG, Oettinger MA, Baltimore D. The V(D)J recombination activating gene, RAG-1. Cell. 1989;59:1035–48.

79. Wilson RK, Lai E, Concannon P, et al. Structure, organization and polymorphism of murine and human T-cell receptors α and β chain gene families. Immunol. Rev. 1988;101:149–72.

80. Royer H-D, Acuto O, Reinhertz EL. Chromosomal location of human T-cell receptor gene Tiβ. Science. 1984;226:348–9.

81. Robinson MA. The human T cell receptor β-chain gene complex contains at least 57 variable gene segments. Identification of six Vβ genes in four new gene families. J Immunol. 1991;146:4392–7.

82. Kishi H, Borgulya P, Scott B, et al. Surface expression of the β T cell receptor (TCR) chain in the absence of other TCR or CD3 proteins on immature T cells. EMBO J. 1991;10:93–100.

83. Mombaerts P, Clarke AR, Rudnicki MA, et al. Mutations in T-cell antigen receptor genes α and β block thymocyte development at different stages. Nature. 1992;360:225–31.

84. Shinkai Y, Koyasu S, Nakayama K-I, et al. Restoration of T cell development in RAG-2-deficient mice by functional TCR transgenes. Science. 1993; 259:822–5.

84a. Von Boehmer H. Positive selection of lymphocytes. Cell. 1994;76:219–28.

85. Klein MH, Concannon P, Everett M, et al. Diversity and structure of human T-cell receptor α-chain variable region genes. Proc Natl Acad Sci USA. 1987; 84:6884–8.

86. Turka LA, Schatz DG, Oettinger MA, et al. Thymocyte expression of RAG-1 and RAG-2: Termination of T cell receptor cross-linking. Science. 1991; 253:778–81.

87. Siu G, Kronenberg M, Strauss E, et al. The structure, rearrangement and expression of Dβ gene segments of the murine T-cell antigen receptor. Nature. 1984;311:344–50.

88. Ferguson SE, Thompson CB. A new break in V(D)J recombination. Curr Biol. 1993;3:51–3.

89. Lanier LL, Allison JP, Phillips JH. Correlation of cell surface antigen expression on human thymocytes by multi-color flow cytometric analysis: Implications for differentiation. J Immunol. 196:137:3501–7.

90. Nikolic-Zugic J, Bevan MJ. Role of self-peptides in positively selecting the T-cell repertoire. Nature. 1990;344:65–7.

91. Peitsch MC, Polzar B, Stephan H, et al. Characterization of the endogenous deoxyribonuclease involved in nuclear DNA degradation during apoptosis (programmed cell death). EMBO J. 1993;12:3710–7.

92. Bill J, Palmer E. Positive selection of CD4+ T cells mediated by MHC class II-bearing stromal cell in the thymic cortex. Nature. 19898;341:649–51.

93. Benoist C, Mathis D. Positive selection of the T cell repertoire: Where and when does it occur? Cell. 1989;58:1027–33.

94. von Boehmer H, Kisielow P. Self-nonself discrimination by T cells. Science. 1990;248:1369–72.

95. Cosgrove D, Gray D, Dierich A, et al. Mice lacking MHC class II molecules. Cell. 1991;66:1051–66.

96. Borgulya P, Kishi H, Müller U, et al. Development of the CD4 and CD8 lineage of T cells: Instruction versus selection. EMBO J. 1991;10:913–18.

97. Robey EA, Fowlkes BJ, Gordon JW, et al. Thymic selection in CD8 transgenic mice supports an instructive model for commitment to a CD4 or CD8 lineage. Cell. 1991;64:99–107.

98. Seong RH, Chamberlain JW, Parnes JR. Signal for T-cell differentiation to a CD4 cell lineage is delivered by CD4 transmembrane region and/or cytoplasmic tail. Nature. 1992;356:718–20.

99. Teh HS, Garvin AM, Forbush KA, et al. Participation of CD4 coreceptor molecules in T-cell repertoire selection. Nature. 1991;349:241–3.

100. Davis CB, Killeen N, Casey Crooks ME, et al. Evidence for a stochastic mechanism in the differentiation of mature subsets of T lymphocytes. Cell. 1993;73:237–247.

101. von Boehmer H, Kisielow P. Lymphocyte lineage commitment: Instruction versus selection. Cell. 1993;73:207–8.

102. Robey EA, Ramsdell F, Kioussis D, et al. The level of CD8 expression can determine the outcome of thymic selection. Cell. 1992;69:1089–96.

103. Murphy KM, Heimberger AB, Loh DY. Induction by antigen of intrathymic apoptosis of CD4+ CD8+ TCRlo thymocytes in vivo. Science. 1990;250: 1720–3.

104. Kisielow P, Blüthmann H, Staerz UD, et al. Tolerance in T-cell–receptor transgenic mice involves deletion of nonmature CD4+CD8+ thymocytes. Nature. 1988;333:742–6.

105. Kappler JW, Staerz U, White J, et al. Self-tolerance eliminates T cell specific or Mls-modified products of the major histocompatibility complex. Nature. 1988;332:35–45.

106. Korman AJ, Bourgarel P, Tommaso M, et al. The mouse mammary tumour virus long terminal repeat encodes a type II transmembrane glycoprotein. EMBO J. 1992;11:1901–5.

107. Pullen AM, Bill J, Kubo RT, et al. Analysis of the interaction site for the self superantigen M1s-1ᵃ on T cell receptor Vβ. J Exp Med. 1991;173:1183–92.

108. Baccala R, Kono DH, Walker S, et al. Genomically imposed and somatically modified human thymocyte Vβ gene repertoires. Proc Natl Acad Sci USA. 1991;88:2908–12.

109. Nossal GJV. Negative selection of lymphocytes. Cell. 1994;76:229–39.

110. von Boehmer H, Teh HS, Kisielow P. The thymus selects the useful, neglects the useless and destroys the harmful. Immunol Today. 1989;10:57–61.

111. Ceredig R, Glasebrook AL, MacDonald HR. Phenotypic and functional properties of murine thymocytes. I. Precursors of cytolytic T lymphocytes and interleukin 2-producing cells are all contained within a subpopulation of "mature" thymocytes as analyzed by monoclonal antibodies and flow microfluorometry. J Exp Med. 1982;155:358–79.

112. Ceredig R, Dialynas DP, Fitch FW, et al. Precursors of T cell growth factor producing cells in the thymus: Ontogeny, frequency, and quantitative recovery in a subpopulation of phenotypically mature thymocytes defined by monoclonal antibody GK-1.5. J Exp Med. 1983;158:1654–70.

113. Philpott KL, Viney JL, Kay G, et al. Lymphoid development in mice congenitally lacking T cell receptor αβ-expressing cells. Science 1992;256:1448–52.

114. Rahemtulla A, Fung-Leung WP, Schilham MW, et al. Normal development and function of CD8⁺ cells but markedly decreased helper cell activity in mice lacking CD4. Nature. 1991;353:180–4.

115. Fung-Leung W-P, Schilham MW, Rahemtulla A, et al. CD8 is needed for development of cytotoxic T cells but not helper T cells. Cell. 1991;65:443–9.

116. Molina TJ, Kishihara K, Siderovski DP, et al. Profound block in thymocyte development in mice lacking p56ˡᶜᵏ. Nature. 1992;357:161–4.

117. Zijlstra M, Bix M, Simister NE, et al. β₂-Microglobulin deficient mice lack CD4⁻8⁺ cytolytic T cells. Nature. 1990;344:742–6.

118. Grusby MJ, Johnson RS, Papaioannou VE, et al. Depletion of CD4⁺ T cells in major histocompatibility complex class II–deficient mice. Science. 1991; 253:1417–20.

119. Killeen N, Stuart SG, Littman DR. Development and function of T cells in mice with a disrupted CD2 gene. EMBO J. 1992;11:4329–36.

120. Kühn R, Rajewsky K, Müller W. Generation and analysis of interleukin-4 deficiency mice. Science. 1991;254:707–10.

121. Schorle H, Holtschke T, Hünig T, et al. Development and function of T cells in mice rendered interleukin-2 deficient by gene targeting. Nature. 1991;352: 621–4.

122. Noguchi M, Yi H, Rosenblatt HW, et al. Interleukin-2 receptor γ chain mutation results in X-linked severe combined immunodeficiency in humans. Cell. 1993;73:147–57.

122a.Kishimoto T, Taga T, Akira S. Cytokine signal transduction. Cell. 1994;76: 253–62.

123. de Kossodo S, Grau GE, Daneva T, et al. Tumor necrosis factor α is involved in mouse growth and lymphoid tissue development. J Exp Med. 1992;176: 1259–64.

124. Fabbi M, Groh V, Strominger JL. IL-7 induces proliferation of CD3-/low CD4⁻ CD8⁻ human thymocyte precursors by an IL-2 independent pathway. Int Immunol. 1992;4:1–5.

125. Uckun FM, Tuel-Ahlgren L, Obuz V, et al. Interleukin 7 receptor engagement stimulates tyrosine phosphorylation, inositol phospholipid turnover, proliferation, and selective differentiation to the CD4 lineage by human fetal thymocytes. Proc Natl Acad Sci USA. 1991;88:6323–27.

126. Dalloul AH, Fourcade C, Debré P, et al. Thymic epithelial cell-derived supernatants sustain the maturation of human prothymocytes: Involvement of interleukin 1 and CD23. Eur J Immunol. 1991;21:2633–6.

127. Weber S, et al. Specific low-affinity recognition of major histocompatibility complex plus peptide by soluble T cell receptor. Nature. 1992;356:793–5.

128. Matsui K, et al. Low affinity interaction of peptide-MHC complexes with T cell receptors. Science. 1991;254:1788–91.

129. Davis MM, Chien Y-H. Topology and affinity of T cell receptor mediated recognition of peptide-MHC complexes. Curr Opin Immunol. 1993;5:45–9.

130. Springer TA. Adhesion receptors of the immune system. Nature. 1990;346: 425–34.

131. Dustin ML, Springer TA. Role of lymphocyte adhesion receptors in transient interactions and cell locomotion. Annu Rev Immunol 1991;9:27–66.

132. Fawcett J, Holness CLL, Needham LA, et al. Molecular cloning of ICAM-3, a third ligand for LFA-1, constitutively expressed on resting leukocytes. Nature. 1992;360:481–4.

133. Dustin ML, Springer TA. T cell receptor cross-linking transiently stimulates adhesiveness through LFA-1. Nature. 1989;341:619–24.

134. Hahn WC, et al. Overlapping but nonidentical binding sites on CD2 for CD58 and a second ligand CD59. Science. 1992;256:1805–7.

135. Kato K, et al. CD48 is a counter-receptor for mouse CD2 and is involved in T cell activation. J Exp Med. 1992;176:1241–9.

136. Driscoll PC, Cyster JG, Campbell ID, Williams AF. Structure of domain 1 of rat T lymphocyte CD2 antigen. Nature. 1991;353:762–5.

137. Brown MH, et al. The CD2 antigen associates with the T cell antigen receptor CD3 antigen complex on the surface of human T lymphocytes. Nature. 1989; 339:551–3.

138. Van de Velde H, von Hoegen I, Luo W, et al. The B cell surface protein CD72/Lyb-2 is the ligand for CD5. Nature. 1991;351:662–5.

139. Miceli MC, von Hoegen P, Parnes JR. Adhesion versus coreceptor function of CD4 and CD8: Role of the cytoplasmic tail in coreceptor activity. Proc Natl Acad Sci USA. 1991;88:2623–7.

140. Norment AM, et al. Cell-cell adhesion mediated by CD8 and MHC class I molecules. Nature. 1988;336:79–81.

141. O'Rourke AM, Rogers J, Mescher MF. Activated CD8 binding to class I protein mediated by the T cell receptor results in signalling. Nature. 1990; 346:187–9.

142. Cammarota G, Scheirle A, Takacs B, et al. Identification of a CD4 binding site on the β₂ domain of HLA-DR molecules. Nature. 1992;356:799–801.

143. Konig R, Huang L-Y, Germain RN. MHC class II interaction with CD4

144. Ryu S-E, et al. Crystal structure of an HIV-binding recombinant fragment of human CD4. Nature. 1990;348:419–26.

145. Parham P. CD8 and CD4: The box and the rod. Nature. 1992;357:538–9.

146. Salter RD, et al. A binding site for the T cell receptor CD8 on the α3 domain of HLA-A2. Nature. 1990;345:41–6.

147. Wheeler CJ, von Hoegen P, Parnes JR. An immunological role for the CD8 β-chain. Nature. 1992;357:247–9.

148. Norment AM, Lonberg N, Lacy E, et al. Alternatively spliced mRNA encodes a secreted form of human CD8a. J Immunol. 1989;142:3312–19.

149. Connolly JM, Hansen TH, Ingold AL, et al. Recognition by CD8 on cytotoxic T lymphocytes is ablated by several substitutions in the class I α3 domain: CD8 and the T cell receptor recognize the same class I molecule. Proc Natl Acad Sci USA. 1990;87:2137–41.

150. Kupfer A, Singer SJ, Janeway CA, et al. Coclustering of CD4 molecule with the T cell receptor is induced by specific direct interaction of helper T cells and antigen-presenting cells. Proc Natl Acad Sci USA. 1987;84:5888–92.

151. Turner JM, et al. Interaction of the unique N-terminal region of tyrosine kinase p56ˡᶜᵏ with cytoplasmic domains of CD4 and CD8 is mediated by cysteine motifs. Cell. 1990;60:755–65.

152. Jenkins MK, Miller RA. Memory and anergy: Challenges to traditional models of T lymphocyte differentiation. FASEB J. 1992;6:2428–33.

153. Schwartz RH. Costimulation of T lymphocytes: The role of CD28, CTLA-4, and B7/BB1 in interleukin-2 production and immunotherapy. Cell. 1992; 71:1065–8.

154. Fraser JD, Irving BA, Crabtree GR, et al. Regulation of interleukin-2 gene enhancer activity by the T cell accessory molecule CD28. Science. 1991;251: 313–6.

155. Lindsten T, June CH, Ledbetter JA, et al. Regulation of lymphokine messenger mRNA stability by a surface-mediated T cell activation pathway. Science. 1989;244:339–43.

155a. Azuma M, Ito D, Yagita H, et al. B70 antigen is a second ligand for CTLA-4 and CD28. Nature. 1993;366:76–9.

155b. Boussiotis V, Freeman G, Gribben J, et al. Activated human B lymphocytes express three CTLA-4 counterreceptors that costimulate T cell activation. Proc Natl Acad Sci USA. 1993;90:11059–63.

156. Young JW, Koulova L, Soergel SA, et al. The B7/BB1 antigen provides one of several costimulatory signals for the activation of CD4 + T lymphocytes by human blood dendritic cells in vitro. J Clin Invest. 1992;90:229–37.

157. Nabavi N, Freeman GJ, Gault A, et al. Signalling through the MHC class II cytoplasmic domain is required for antigen presentation and induces B7 expression. Nature. 1992;360:266–8.

158. Ranheim EA, Kipps TJ. Activated T cells induce expression of B7/BB1 on normal or leukemic B cells through a CD40-dependent signal. J Exp Med. 1993;177:925–35.

159. Azuma M, Yssel H, Phillips JH, et al. Functional expression of B7/BB1 on activated T lymphocytes. J Exp Med. 1993;177:845–50.

160. Linsley PS, Greene JL, Tan P, et al. Coexpression and functional cooperation of CTLA-4 and CD28 on activated T lymphocytes. J Exp Med. 1992; 176:1595–604.

161. Tan P, Anasetti C, Hansen JA, et al. Induction of alloantigen-specific hyporesponsiveness in human T lymphocytes by blocking interaction of CD28 with its natural ligand B7/BB1. J Exp Med. 1993;177:165–73.

162. Lenschow DJ, Zeng Y, Thistlethwaite JR, et al. Long-term survival of xenogeneic pancreatic islet grafts induced by CTLA-4. Science. 1992;257:789–92.

163. Turka LA, Linsley PS, Lin H, et al. T-cell activation by the CD28 ligand B7 is required for cardiac allograft rejection in vivo. Proc Natl Acad Sci USA. 1992;89:11102–5.

164. Townsend SE, Allison JP. Tumor rejection after direct costimulation of CD8+ T cells by B7-transfected melanoma cells. Science. 1993;259:368–70.

165. Chen L, Ashe S, Brady WA, et al. Costimulation of antitumor immunity by the B7 counterreceptor for the T lymphocyte molecules CD28 and CTLA-4. Cell. 1992;71:1093–1102.

166. Klausner RD, Samelson LE. T cell antigen receptor activation pathways: The tyrosine kinase connection. Cell. 1991;64:875–8.

167. Perlmutter RM. Molecular dissection of lymphocyte signal transduction pathways. Pediatr Res. 1993;33:S9–15.

168. Malissen B, Schmitt-Verhulst A-M. Transmembrane signalling through the T cell receptor-CD3 complex. Curr Opin Immunol. 1993;5:324–33.

169. Weiss A. T cell antigen receptor signal transduction: A tale of tails and cytoplasmic protein-tyrosine kinases. Cell. 1993;73:209–12.

170. Irving BA, Weiss A. The cytoplasmic domain of the T cell receptor Z chain is sufficient to couple the receptor-associated signal transduction pathways. Cell. 1991;64:891–901.

171. Letourneur F, Klausner RD. Activation of T cells by a tyrosine kinase activation domain in the cytoplasmic tail of CD3ε. Science. 1992;255:79–82.

172. Wegener A-M, Letourneur F, Hoeveler A, et al. The T cell receptor/CD3 complex is composed of at least two autonomous transduction modules. Cell. 1992;68:83–95.

173. Barber EK, Dasgupta JD, Schlossman SF, et al. The CD4 and CD8 antigens are coupled to a protein-tyrosine kinase (p56lck) that phosphorylates the CD3 complex. Proc Natl Acad Sci USA. 1989;86:3277–81.

174. Strauss DB, Weiss A. Genetic evidence for the involvement of the Lck tyrosine kinase in signal transduction through the T cell antigen receptor. Cell. 1992;70:585–93.

175. Haughn L, Gratton S, Caron L, et al. Association of tyrosine kinase p56lck with CD4 inhibits the induction of growth through the αβ T cell receptor. Nature. 1992;358:328–31.

176. Julius M, Maroun CR, Haughn L. Distinct roles for CD4 and CD8 as coreceptors in antigen receptor signalling. Immunol Today. 1993;14:177–83.

177. Samelson LE, Phillips AF, Luong ET, et al. Association of the fyn protein-

tyrosine kinase with the T cell antigen receptor. Proc Natl Acad Sci USA. 1990;87:4358–62.

178. Cooke MP, Abraham KM, Forbush KA, et al. Regulation of T cell receptor signaling by a *src* family protein-tyrosine kinase (p59*fyn*). Cell. 1991;65:281–91.

179. Stein PL, Lee H-M, Rich S, et al. p59*fyn* mutant mice display differential signaling in thymocytes and peripheral T cells. Cell. 1992;70:741–50.

180. Appleby MW, Gross JA, Cooke MP, et al. Defective T cell receptor signaling in mice lacking the thymic isoform of p59*fyn*. Cell. 1992;70:751–63.

181. Chan AC, Iwashima M, Turck CW, et al. ZAP-70: A 70 kd protein-tyrosine kinase that associates with the TCR Z chain. Cell. 1992;71:649–62.

182. Koretzky GA. Role of the CD45 tyrosine phosphatase in signal transduction in the immune system. FASEB J. 1993;7:420–6.

183. Rothstein D, Yamada A, Schlossman SF, et al. Cyclic regulation of CD45 isoform expression in a long term human CD4+CD45RA+ T cell line. J Immunol. 1991;146:1175–83.

184. Bell EB, Sparshott SM. Interconversion of CD54R subsets of CD4 T cells in vivo. Nature. 1990;348:163–6.

185. Stamenkovic I, Sgroi D, Aruffo A, et al. The B lymphocyte adhesion molecule CD22 interacts with leukocyte common antigen CD45RO on T cells and α2–6 sialyltransferase, CD75, on B cells. Cell. 1991;66:1133–44.

186. Koretzky GA, Picus J, Schultz T, et al. Tyrosine phosphatase CD45 is required for T cell antigen receptor and CD2-mediated activation of a protein tyrosine kinase and interleukin 2 production. Proc Natl Acad Sci USA. 1991; 88:2037–41.

187. Koretzky GA, Kohmetscher MA, Kadleck T, et al. Restoration of T cell receptor-mediated signal transduction by transfection of CD45 cDNA into a CD45-deficient variant of the Jurkat T cell line. J Immunol. 1992;149:1138–42.

188. Hovis RR, Donovan JA, Musci MA, et al. Rescue of signaling by a chimeric protein containing the cytoplasmic domain of CD45. Science. 1993;260:544–6.

189. Volarevic S, Niklinska BB, Burns CM, et al. Regulation of TCR signaling by CD45 lacking transmembrane and extracellular domains. Science. 1993;260:541–4.

190. Desai DM, Sap J, Schlessinger, et al. Ligand-mediated negative regulation of a chimeric transmembrane receptor tyrosine phosphatase. Cell. 1993;73:542–54.

191. Mustelin T, Coggeshall KM, Isakov N, et al. T cell antigen receptor-mediated activation of phospholipase C requires tyrosine phosphorylation. Science. 1990;247:1584–7.

192. Weiss A, Koretzky G, Schatzman RC, et al. Functional activation of the T cell antigen receptor induces tyrosine phosphorylation of phospholipase C-γ1. Proc Natl Acad Sci USA. 1991;88:5484–58.

193. Berridge MJ. Inositol trisphosphate and calcium signalling. Nature. 1993;361:315–25.

194. Khan AA, Steiner JP, Klein MG, et al. IP3 receptor: Localization to plasma membrane of T cells and cocapping with the T cell receptor. Science. 1992;257:815–8.

195. Testi R, Phillips JH, Lanier LL. T cell activation via Leu-23 (CD69). J Immunol. 1989;143:1123–30.

196. Aderem A. The MARCKS brothers: A family of protein kinase C substrates. Cell. 1992;71:713–6.

197. Gulbins E, Coggeshall KM, Baier G, et al. Tyrosine kinase-stimulated guanine nucleotide exchange activity of *Vav* in T cell activation. Science. 1993;260:822–5.

198. Downward J, Graves JD, Warne PH, et al. Stimulation of p21^ras upon T-cell activation. Nature. 1990;346:719–23.

199. Wang C-Y, Petryniak B, Thompson CB, et al. Regulation of the *Ets*-related transcription factor *Elf*-1 by binding to the retinoblastoma protein. Science. 1993;260:1330–5.

200. Schreiber S, Crabtree GR. The mechanism of action of cyclosporin A and FK506. Immunol Today. 1992;13:136–42.

201. Marrack P, Kappler J. The staphylococcal enterotoxins and their relatives. Science. 1990;248:705–11.

202. Choi Y, Kappler JW, Marrack P. A superantigen encoded in the open reading frame of the 3′ long terminal repeat of mouse mammary tumor virus. Nature. 1991;350:203–7.

203. Woodland DL, Lund FE, Happ MP, et al. Endogenous superantigen expression is controlled by mouse mammary tumor proviral loci. J Exp Med. 1991;174:1255–8.

204. Frankel WN, Rudy C, Coffin JM, et al. Linkage of *Mls* genes to endogenous mammary tumor viruses of inbred mice. Nature. 1991;349:526–8.

205. Dellabona P, Peccoud J, Kappler JW, et al. Superantigens interact with MHC class II molecules outside of the antigen groove. Cell. 1990;62:1115–21.

206. Swaminathan S, Furey W, Pletcher J, et al. Crystal structure of staphylococcal enterotoxin B, a superantigen. Nature. 1992;359:801–6.

207. Miethke T, Wahl C, Heeg K, et al. T cell-mediated lethal shock triggered in mice by the superantigen staphylococcal enterotoxin B: Critical role of tumor necrosis factor. J Exp Med. 1992;175:91–8.

208. Choi Y, Lafferty JA, Clements JR, et al. Selective expansion of T cells expressing Vβ2 in toxic shock syndrome. J Exp Med. 1990;172:981–4.

209. De Libero G, Lanzavecchia A. Selection by two powerful antigens may account for the presence of the major population of human peripheral γδ+ T-cells. J Exp Med. 1991;173:1311–22.

210. Kabelitz D, Bender A, Prospero T, et al. The primary response of human γδ+ T-cells to mycobacterium tuberculosis is restricted to Vγ9-bearing cells. J Exp Med. 1991;173:1331–8.

211. Ohmen JD, Barnes PF, Uyemura K, et al. The T cell receptors of human

212. γδ T cells reactive to *Mycobacterium* tuberculosis are encoded by specific V genes but diverse V-J junctions. J Immunol. 1991;147:3353–9.

212. Pfeffer K, Schoel B, Plesnila N, et al. A lectin-binding, protease-resistant mycobacterial ligand specifically activates Vγ9+ human γδ T cells. J Immunol. 1992;148:575–83.

213. Sanders ME, Makgoba MW, Shaw S. Human naive and memory T cells: Reinterpretation of helper-inducer and suppressor-inducer subsets. Immunol Today. 1988;9:195–9.

214. Sanders ME, Makgoba MW, Sharrow SO, et al. Human memory T lymphocytes express increased levels of three cell adhesion molecules (LFA-3, CD2, and LFA-1) and three other molecules (UCHL1, CD29, and Pgp-1) and have enhanced IFN-γ production. J Immunol. 1988;141a:1401–7.

215. Akbar AN, Terry L, Timms A, et al. Loss of CD45R and gain of UCHL1 reactivity is a feature of primed T cells. J Immunol. 1988;140:2171–8.

216. Teder TF, Clement LT, Cooper MD. Human lymphocyte differentiation antigens HB-10 and HB-11. I. Ontogeny of antigen expression. J Immunol. 1985;134:2983–8.

217. de Jong R, Brouwer M, Miedema F, et al. Human CD8+ T lymphocytes can be divided into CF45RA+ and CD45RO+ cells with different requirements for activation and differentiation. J Immunol. 1991;146:2088–94.

218. Okumura M, Fujii Y, Inada K, et al. Both CD45RA+ and CD45RA− subpopulations of CD8+ T cells contain cells with high levels of lymphocyte function-associated antigen-1 expression, a phenotype of primed T cells. J Immunol. 1993;150:429–37.

219. Damle NK, Doyle LV. Ability of human T lymphocytes to adhere to vascular endothelial cells and to augment endothelial permeability to macromolecules is linked to their state of post-thymic maturation. J Immunol. 1990;144:1233–40.

220. Pitzalis C, Kingsley GH, Covelli M, et al. Selective migration of the human helper-inducer memory T cell subset: Confirmation by in vivo cellular kinetic studies. Eur J Immunol. 1991;21:369–76.

221. Byrne JA, Butler JL, Reinherz EL, et al. Virgin and memory T cells have different requirements for activation via the CD2 molecule. Int Immunol. 1989;1:29–35.

222. Byrne JA, Butler JL, Cooper MD. Differential activation requirements for virgin and memory T cells. J Immunol. 1988;141:3249–57.

223. Sanders ME, Makgoba A, June CH, et al. Enhanced responsiveness of human memory T cells to CD2 and CD3 receptor-mediated activation. Eur J Immunol. 1989;19:803–8.

224. Clement LT, Yamishita N, Martin AM. The functionally distinct subpopulations of human CD4+ helper/inducer T lymphocytes defined by anti-CD45R antibodies derive sequentially from a differentiation pathway that is regulated by activation-dependent post-thymic differentiation. J Immunol. 1988;141:1464–70.

225. Koulova L, Yang SY, Dupont B. Identification of the anti-CD3-unresponsive subpopulation of CD4+, CD45RA+ peripheral T lymphocytes. J Immunol. 1990;145:2035–43.

226. Michie CA, McLean A, Alcock C, et al. Lifespan of human lymphocyte subsets defined by CD45 isoforms. Nature. 1992;360:264–5.

227. Mackay CR. Homing of naive, memory and effector lymphocytes. Curr Opin Immunol. 1993;5:423–7.

227a.Springer TA. Traffic signals for lymphocyte recirculation and leukocyte emigration: The multistep paradigm. Cell. 1994;76:301–14.

228. Lasky LA, Singer MS, Dowbenko D, et al. An endothelial ligand for L-selectin is a novel mucin-like molecule. Cell. 1992;69:927–38.

229. Imai Y, Lasky LA, Rosen SD. Sulphation requirement for GlyCAM-1, an endothelial ligand for L-selectin. Science. 1993;361:555–7.

230. Haynes BF, Telen MJ, Hale LP, et al. CD44—A molecule involved in leukocyte adherence and T cell activation. Immunol Today. 1989;10:423–8.

231. Arch R, Wirth K, Hofmann M, et al. Participation in normal immune responses of a metastasis-inducing splice variant of CD44. Science. 1992;257:682–4.

232. Hemler ME. VLA proteins in the integrin family: Structure, functions, and their role on leukocytes. Annu Rev Immunol. 1990;8:365–400.

233. Shimuzu Y, Van Seventer GA, Horgan KJ, et al. Regulated expression and binding of three VLA (β1) integrin receptors on T cells. Nature. 1990;345:250–3.

234. Picker LJ, Kishimoto TK, Smith CW, et al. ELAM-1 is an adhesion molecule for skin-homing T cells. Nature. 1991:349:796–9.

235. Picker LJ, Treer JR, Ferguson-Darnell B, et al. Control of lymphocyte recirculation in man. II. Differential regulation of the cutaneous lymphocyte-associated antigen, a tissue-selective homing receptor for skin-homing T cells. J Immunol. 1993;150:1122–36.

236. Briskin MJ, McEvoy LM, Butcher EC. MAdCAM-1 has homology to immunoglobulin and mucin-like adhesion receptors and to IgA1. Nature. 1993;363:461–4.

237. Parker CM, Cepek KL, Russel GJ, et al. A family of β7 integrins on human mucosal lymphocytes. Proc Natl Acad Sci USA. 1992;89:1924–8.

238. Salmi M, Jalkanen S. A 90-kilodalton endothelial molecule mediating lymphocyte binding in humans. Science. 1992;257:1407–9.

239. Braon JL, Madri JA, Ruddle NH, et al. Surface expression of α4 integrin by CD4 T cells is required for their entry into brain parenchyma. J Exp Med. 1993;177:57–68.

240. Guy-Grand D, Malassis-Seris M, Briottet C, et al. Cytotoxic differentiation of mouse gut thymodependent and independent intraepithelial T lymphocytes is induced locally. J Exp Med. 1991;173:1549–52.

241. Yamamoto M, Fujihashi K, Beagley KW, et al. Cytokine synthesis by intestinal intraepithelial lymphocytes. J Immunol. 1993;150:106–14.

242. Van Kerckhove C, Russel GJ, Deusch K, et al. Oligoclonality of human intestinal intraepithelial T cells. J Exp Med. 1992;175:57–63.

243. Blumberg RS, Yockey CE, Gross GG, et al. Human intestinal intraepithelial lymphocytes are derived from a limited number of T cell clones that utilize multiple Vβ T cell receptor genes. J Immunol. 1993;150:5144–53.

244. Balk SP, Ebert EC, Blumenthal RL, et al. Oligoclonal expansion and CD1 recognition by human intestinal intraepithelial lymphocytes. Science. 1991; 253:1411–5.

245. Cerf-Bensussan N, Jarry A, Brousse N, et al. A monoclonal antibody (HML-1) defining a novel membrane molecule present on human intestinal lymphocytes. Eur J Immunol. 1987;17:1279–86.

246. Cepek KL, Parker CM, Madara JL, et al. Integrin αEβ7 mediates adhesion of T lymphocytes to epithelial cells. J Immunol. 1993;150:3459–70.

247. Arai K-I, Lee F, Miyajima A, et al. Cytokines: Coordinators of immune and inflammatory responses. Annu Rev Biochem. 1990;59:783–836.

248. Gordon JR, Galli SJ. Mast cells as a source of both preformed and immunologically inducible TNF-α/cachectin. Nature. 1990;346:274–6.

249. Bradding P, Feather IH, Howarth PH, et al. Interleukin 4 is localized to and released by human mast cells. J Exp Med. 1992;176:1381–6.

250. Shaw G, Kamen R. A conserved AU sequence from the 3′ untranslated region of GM-CSF mRNA mediates selective mRNA degradation. Cell. 1986; 46:659–7.

251. Caput D, Beutler B, Hartog K, et al. Identification of a common nucleotide sequence in the 3′-untranslated region of mRNA molecules specifying inflammatory mediators. Proc Natl Acad Sci USA. 1986;83:1670–4.

252. Wolf SF, Temple PA, Kobayashi M, et al. Cloning of cCNA for natural killer cell stimulatory factor, a heterodimeric cytokine with multiple biologic effects on T and natural killer cells. J Immunol. 1991;146:3074–81.

253. Gubler U, Chua AO, Schoenhaut DS, et al. Coexpression of two distinct genes is required to generate secreted bioactive cytotoxic lymphocyte maturation factor. Proc Natl Acad Sci USA. 1991;88:4143–7.

254. Brandhuber BJ, Boone T, Kenney WC, et al. Three-dimensional structure of interleukin-2. Science. 1987;238:1707–9.

255. Powers R, Garrett DS, March CJ, et al. Three-dimensional solution structure of human interleukin-4 by multidimensional heteronuclear magnetic resonance spectroscopy. Science. 1992;256:1673–7.

256. Milburn MV, Hassel AM, Lambert MH, et al. A novel dimer configuration revealed by the crystal structure at 2.4 A resolution of human interleukin-5. Nature. 1993;363:172–6.

257. Pandit J, Bohm A, Jancarik J, et al. Three-dimensional structure of dimeric human recombinant macrophage colony-stimulating factor. Science. 1992; 258:1358–62.

258. Hill CP, Osslund TD, Eisenberg D. The structure of granulocyte-colony-stimulating factor and its relationship to other growth factors. Proc Natl Acad Sci USA. 1993;90:5167–71.

259. Diederichs K, Boone T, Karplus PA. Novel fold and putative receptor binding site of granulocyte-macrophage colony-stimulating factor. Science. 1991; 254:1779–82.

260. Ealick SE, Cook WJ, Vijay-Kumar S, et al. Three-dimensional structure of recombinant human interferon-γ. Science. 1991;252:698–702.

261. Jones EY, Stuart DI, Walker NPC. Structure of tumor necrosis factor. Nature. 1989;338:225–8.

262. Habazetti J, Gondol D, Wiltscheck R, et al. Structure of hisactophilin is similar to interleukin-1β and fibroblast growth factor. Nature. 1992;359: 855–8.

263. Taga T, Kishimoto T. Cytokine receptors and signal transduction. FASEB J. 1993;7:3387–96.

264. Smith CA, Davis T, Anderson D, et al. A receptor for tumor necrosis factor defines an unusual family of cellular and viral proteins. Science. 1990;248: 1019–23.

265. Itoh N, Yonehara S, Ishii A, et al. The polypeptide encoded by the cDNA for human cell surface antigen Fas can mediate apoptosis. Cell. 1991;66: 233–43.

266. Massague J. Receptors for the TGF-β family. Cell. 1992;69:1067–70.

267. Holmes WE, Lee J, Kuang W-J, et al. Structure and functional expression of a human interleukin-8 receptor. Science. 1991;253:1278–80.

268. Murphy PM, Tiffany HL. Cloning of complementary DNA encoding a functional human interleukin-8 receptor. Science. 1991;253:1280–3.

269. Taniguchi T, Minami Y. The IL-2/IL-2 receptor system: An overview. Cell. 1993;73:5–8.

270. Nicola NA, Metcalf D. Subunit promiscuity among hemopoietic growth factor receptors. Cell. 1991;67:1–4.

271. Hanazono Y, Chiba S, Sasaki K, et al. c-fps/fes protein-tyrosine kinase is implicated in a signaling pathway triggered by granulocyte-macrophage colony-stimulating factor and interleukin-3. EMBO J. 1993;12:1641–6.

272. Chiba T, Nagata Y, Machide M, et al. Tyrosine kinase activation through the extracellular domains of cytokine receptors. Nature. 1993;362:646–8.

273. Kishimoto T, Akira S, Taga T. Interleukin-6 and its receptor: a paradigm for cytokines. Science. 1992;258:593–7.

274. Gearing DP, Cosman D. Homology of the p40 subunit of natural killer cell stimulatory factor (NKSF) with the extracellular domain of the interleukin-6 receptor. Cell. 1991;66:9–10.

275. Fernandez-Botran R. Soluble cytokine receptors: Their role in immunoregulation. FASEB J. 1991;5:2567–74.

276. Gooding LR. Virus proteins that counteract host immune defenses. Cell. 1992;71:5–7.

277. Haskill S, Johnson C, Eierman D, et al. Adherence induces selective mRNA expression of monocyte mediators and proto-oncogenes. J Immunol. 1988; 140:1690–4.

278. Navarro S, Debili N, Bernaudin J-F, et al. Regulation of the expression of IL-6 in human monocytes. J Immunol. 1989;142:4339–45.

279. Webb DSA, Shimizu Y, Van Seventer GAV, et al. LFA-3, CD44 and CD45: Physiologic triggers of human monocyte TNF and IL-1 release. Science. 1990;249:1295–7.

280. Janson RW, Hance KR, Arend WP. Production of IL-1 receptor antagonist by human in vitro–derived macrophages. Effects of lipopolysaccharide and granulocyte-macrophage colony stimulating factor. J Immunol. 1991;147: 4218–23.

281. Oppenheim JJ, Zachariae COC, Mukaida N, et al. Properties of the novel proinflammatory supergene "intercrine" cytokine family. Annu Rev Immunol. 1991;9:617–48.

282. Mantovani A, Bussolino F, Dejana E. Cytokine regulation of endothelial cell function. FASEB J. 1992;6:2591–9.

283. Locksley RM. Interleukin 12 in host defense against microbial pathogens. Proc Natl Acad Sci USA. 1993;90:5879–80.

284. Howard M, O'Garra A. Biological properties of interleukin 10. Immunol Today. 1992;13:198–200.

285. Arend WP. Interleukin 1 receptor antagonist. A new member of the interleukin 1 family. J Clin Invest. 1991;88:1445–51.

286. Tsunawaki S, Sporn M, Ding A, et al. Deactivation of macrophages by transforming growth factor-β. Nature. 1988;334:260–2.

287. Rappolee DA, Mark D, Banda MJ, et al. Wound macrophages express TGF-β and other growth factors in vivo: Analysis by mRNA phenotyping. Science. 1988;241:708–12.

288. Kinkhabwala M, Sehajpal P, Skolnik E, et al. A novel addition to the T cell repertoire. Cell surface expression of tumor necrosis factor/cachectin by activated normal human T cells. J Exp Med. 1990;171:941–6.

289. Browning JL, Ngam-ek A, Lawton P, et al. Lymphotoxin β, a novel member of the TNF family that forms a heteromeric complex with lymphotoxin on the cell surface. Cell. 1993;72:847–56.

290. Mosmann TR, Coffman RL. TH1 and TH2 cells: Different patterns of lymphokine secretion lead to different functional properties. Annu Rev Immunol. 1989;7:145–73.

291. Firestein GS, Roeder WD, Laxer JA, et al. A new murine CD4+ T cell subset with an unrestricted cytokine profile. J Immunol. 1989;143:518–25.

292. Scott P. Selective differentiation of CD4+ T helper cell subsets. Curr Opin Immunol. 1993;5:391–7.

293. Romagnani S. Human TH1 and TH2 subsets: Doubt no more. Immunol Today. 1991;12:256–9.

294. Del Prete GF, De Carli M, Ricci M, et al. Helper activity for immunoglobulin synthesis of T helper type 1 (TH1) and TH2 human T cell clones: The help of TH1 clones is limited by their cytolytic capacity. J Exp Med. 1991;174: 809–13.

295. Merrill JE, Kong DH, Clayton J, et al. Inflammatory leukocytes and cytokines in the peptide-induced disease of experimental allergic encephalomyelitis in SJL and B10.PL mice. Proc Natl Acad Sci USA. 1992;89:574–8.

296. Olsson T, Wei Zhi W, Hojeberg B, et al. Autoreactive T lymphocytes in multiple sclerosis determined by antigen-induced secretion of interferon-γ. J Clin Invest. 1990;86:981–5.

297. Finkelman FD, Urban JF. Cytokines: Making the right choice. Parasitol Today. 1992;8:311–4.

298. Parronchi P, Macchia D, Piccinni M-P, et al. Allergen- and bacterial antigen-specific T cell clones established from atopic donors show a different profile of cytokine production. Proc Natl Acad Sci USA. 1991;88:4538–42.

299. Robinson DS, Hamid Q, Ying S, et al. Predominant TH2-like bronchoalveolar T-lymphocyte population in atopic asthma. N Engl J Med. 1992;326: 298–304.

300. Lenardo M. Interleukin-2 programs mouse αβ T lymphocytes for apoptosis. Nature. 1991;353:858–61.

301. Shull MM, Ormsby I, Kier AB, et al. Targeted disruption of the mouse transforming growth factor-β1 gene results in multifocal inflammatory disease. Nature. 1992;359:693–9.

302. Tripp CS, Wolf SF, Unanue ER. Interleukin 12 and tumor necrosis factor α are costimulators of interferon-γ production by natural killer cells in severe combined immunodeficiency mice with listeriosis, and interleukin 10 is a physiologic antagonist. Proc Natl Acad Sci USA. 1993;90:3725–9.

303. Minty A, Chalon P, Derocq J-M, et al. Interleukin-13 is a new human lymphokine regulating inflammatory and immune responses. Nature. 1993;362: 248–51.

304. O'Garra A, Chang R, Go N, et al. Ly-1 B (B-1) cells are the main source of B cell–derived interleukin 10. Eur J Immunol. 1992;22:711–6.

305. Davatelis G, Wolpe SD, Sherry B, et al. Macrophage inflammatory protein-1: A prostaglandin-independent endogenous pyrogen. Science. 1989;243: 1066–8.

306. Kinoshita S, Akira S, Kishimoto T. A member of the C/EBP family, NF-IL-6b, forms a heterodimer and transcriptionally synergizes with NF-IL-6. Proc Natl Acad Sci USA. 1992;89:1473–6.

307. Chen-Kiang S, Hsu W, Natkunam Y, et al. Nuclear signaling by interleukin 6. Curr Opin Immunol. 1993;5:124–8.

308. Bauer J, Bauer TM, Kalb T, et al. Regulation of interleukin 6 receptor expres-

sion in human monocytes and monocyte-derived macrophages. Comparison with the expression in human hepatocytes. J Exp Med. 1989;170:1537–49.

309. Oliff A, Defeo-Jones D, Boyer M, et al. Tumors secreting human TNF/cachectin induce cachexia in mice. Cell. 1987;50:555–63.

310. Grunfel C, Feingold KR. Metabolic disturbances and wasting in the acquired immunodeficiency syndrome. N Engl J Med. 1992;327:329–37.

311. Michie HR, Manogue KR, Spriggs DR, et al. Detection of circulating tumor necrosis factor after endotoxin administration. N Engl J Med. 1988;318:1481–6.

312. Cannon JG, Thompkins RG, Gelfand JA, et al. Circulating interleukin-1 and tumor necrosis factor in septic shock and experimental endotoxin fever. J Infect Dis. 1990;161:79–84.

313. Martich GD, Danner RL, Ceska M, et al. Detection of interleukin 8 and tumor necrosis factor in normal humans after intravenous endotoxin: The effect of antiinflammatory drugs. J Exp Med. 1991;173:1021–4.

314. Van Zee KJ, DeForge LE, Fischer E, et al. IL-8 in septic shock, endotoxemia and after IL-1 administration. J Immunol. 1991;146:3478–82.

315. Cross AS, Opal SM, Sadoff JC, et al. Choice of bacteria in animal models of sepsis. Infect Immun. 1993;61:2741–7.

316. Schumann RR, Leong SR, Flaggs GW, et al. Structure and function of lipopolysaccharide binding protein. Science. 1990;249:1429–31.

317. Wright SD, Ramos RA, Tobias PS, et al. CD14, a receptor for complexes of lipopolysaccharide (LPS) and LPS binding protein. Science. 1990;249:1431–3.

318. Dentener MA, Bazil V, Von Asmuth EJU, et al. Involvement of CD14 in lipopolysaccharide-induced tumor necrosis factor-α, IL-6 and IL-8 release by human monocytes and alveolar macrophages. J Immunol. 1993;150:2885–91.

319. Pugin J, Schurer-Maly C-G, Leturcq D, et al. Lipopolysaccharide activation of human endothelial and epithelial cells is mediated by lipopolysaccharide-binding protein and soluble CD14. Proc Natl Acad Sci USA. 1993;90:2744–8.

320. Ferrero E, Jiao D, Tsuberi BZ, et al. Transgenic mice expressing human CD14 are hypersensitive to lipopolysaccharide. Proc Natl Acad Sci USA. 1993;90:2380–4.

321. Wright SD, Levin SM, Jong MTC, et al. CR3 (CD11b/CD18) expresses one binding site for Arg-Gly-Asp-containing peptides and a second site for bacterial lipopolysaccharide. J Exp Med. 1989;169:175–83.

322. Tracey KJ, Beutler B, Lowry SF, et al. Shock and tissue injury induced by recombinant human cachectin. Science. 1986;234:470–4.

323. Tracey KJ, Fong Y, Hesse DG, et al. Anti-cachectin/TNF monoclonal antibodies prevent septic shock during lethal bacteremia. Nature. 1987;330:662–4.

324. Fong Y, Tracey KJ, Moldawer LL, et al. Antibodies to cachectin/tumor necrosis factor reduce interleukin 1β and interleukin 6 appearance during lethal bacteremia. J Exp Med. 1989;170:1627–33.

325. Pfeffer K, Matsuyama T, Kundig TM, et al. Mice deficient for the 55 kd tumor necrosis factor receptor are resistant to endotoxic shock, yet succumb to L. monocytogenes infection. Cell. 1993;73:457–67.

326. Girardin E, Grau GE, Dayer J-M, et al. Tumor necrosis factor and interleukin-1 in the serum of children with severe infectious purpura. N Engl J Med. 1988;319:397–400.

327. Waage A, Brandtzaeg P, Halstensen A, et al. The complex pattern of cytokines in serum from patients with meningococcal septic shock. J Exp Med. 1989;169:333–8.

328. Taveira da Silva AM, Kaulback HC, Chuidian FS, et al. Shock and multiple-organ dysfunction after self-administration of Salmonella endotoxin. N Engl J Med. 1993;328:1457–60.

329. Glauser MP, Zanetti G, Baumbartner J-D, et al. Septic shock: Pathogenesis. Lancet. 1991;338:732–6.

329a. Casey LC, Balk RA, Bone RC. Plasma cytokine and endotoxin levels correlate with survival in patients with the sepsis syndrome. Ann Intern Med. 1993;119:771–8.

330. Nathan CF. Neutrophil activation on biological surfaces. J Clin Invest. 1987;80:1550–60.

331. Wispe JR, Clark JC, Warner BB, et al. Tumor necrosis factor-α inhibits expression of pulmonary surfactant protein. J Clin Invest. 1990;86:1954–60.

332. Zipori D. The renewal and differentiation of hemopoietic stem cells. FASEB J. 1992;6:2691–7.

333. Witte ON. Steel locus defines new multipotent growth factor. Cell. 1990;63:5–6.

334. Wiktor-Jedrzejczak W, Bartocci A, Ferrante AW Jr, et al. Total absence of colony-stimulating factor 1 in the macrophage-deficient osteopetrotic (op/op) mouse. Proc Natl Acad Sci USA. 1990;87:4828–32.

335. Hammond WP, Csiba E, Canin A, et al. Chronic neutropenia: A new canine model induced by human granulocyte colony-stimulating factor. J Clin Invest. 1991;87:704–10.

336. Koide S, Steinman RM. Induction of interleukin 1a mRNA during the antigen-dependent interaction of sensitized T lymphoblasts with macrophages. J Exp Med. 1988;168:409–41.

337. Wang L-M, Keegan AD, Li W, et al. Common elements in interleukin 4 and insulin signaling pathways in factor-dependent hematopoietic cells. Proc Natl Acad Sci USA. 1993;90:4032–36.

338. Gajewski TF, Pinnas M, Wong T, et al. Murine TH1 and TH2 clones proliferate optimally in response to distinct antigen-presenting cell populations. J Immunol. 1991;146:1750–8.

339. Murray JS, Madri J, Pasqualini T, et al. Functional CD4 T cell subset interplay in an intact immune system. J Immunol. 1993;150:4270–6.

340. Manetti R, Parronchi P, Giudizi G, et al. Natural kiler cell stimulatory factor

341. (interleukin 12) induces T helper type 1 (TH1)-specific immune responses and inhibits the development of IL-4-producing TH cells. J Exp Med. 1993;177:1199–204.

341. Hsieh C-S, Macatonia SE, Tripp CS, et al. Development of TH1 CD4+ T cells through IL-12 produced by Listeria-induced macrophages. Science. 1993;260:547–9.

342. Heinzel FP, Schoenhaut DS, Rerko RM, et al. Recombinant IL-12 cures mice infected with Leishmania major. J Exp Med. 1993;177:1505–9.

343. Kiniwa M, Gately M, Gubler U, et al. Recombinant interleukin-12 suppresses the synthesis of immunoglobulin E by interleukin-4 stimulated human lymphocytes. J Clin Invest. 1992;90:262–6.

344. Swain SL, Weinberg AD, English M, et al. IL-4 directs the development of TH2-like helper effectors. J Immunol. 1990;145:3796–806.

345. Abehsira-Amar O, Gibert M, Joliy M, et al. IL-4 plays a dominant role in the differential development of TH0 into TH1 and TH2 cells. J Immunol. 1992;148:3820–9.

346. Maggi E, Parronchi P, Manetti R, et al. Reciprocal regulatory effects of IFN-γ and IL-4 on the in vitro development of human TH1 and TH2 clones. J Immunol. 1992;148:2142–7.

347. Sadick MD, Heinzel FP, Holaday BJ, et al. Cure of murine leishmaniasis with anti-IL-4 monoclonal antibody. J Exp Med. 1990;171:115–27.

348. Kopf M, LeGros G, Bachmann M, et al. Disruption of the murine IL-4 gene blocks Th2 cytokine responses. Nature. 1993;363:245–8.

349. Hsieh C-S, Heimberger AB, Gold JS, et al. Differential regulation of T helper phenotype development by interleukins 4 and 10 in an αβ T-cell-receptor transgenic system. Proc Natl Acad Sci USA. 1992;89:6065–9.

350. Seder RA, Paul WE, Davis MM, et al. The presence of interleukin 4 during in vitro priming determines the lymphokine-producing potential of CD4+ T cells from T cell receptor transgenic mice. J Exp Med. 1992;176:1091–8.

351. Gajewski TF, Fitch FW. Antiproliferative effect of IFN-γ in immune regulation. I. IFN-γ inhibits the proliferation of TH2 but not TH1 murine helper T lymphocyte clones. J Immunol. 1988;140:4245–51.

352. Snapper CM, Paul WE. Interferon-γ and B cell stimulatory factor-1 reciprocally regulate Ig isotype production. Science. 1987;236:944–7.

353. Iwamoto I, Nakajima H, Endo H, et al. Interferon γ regulates antigen-induced eosinophil recruitment into the mouse airways by inhibiting the infiltration of CD4+ T cells. J Exp Med. 1993;177:573–6.

354. Essner R, Rhoades K, McBride WH, et al. IL-4 down-regulates IL-1 and TNF gene expression in human monocytes. J Immunol. 1989;142:3857–61.

355. Vannier E, Miller LC, Dinarello CA. Coordinated antiinflammatory effects of interleukin 4: Interleukin 4 suppresses interleukin 1 production but up-regulates gene expression and synthesis of interleukin 1 receptor antagonist. Proc Natl Acad Sci USA. 1992;89:4076–80.

356. de Waal Malefyt R, Abrams J, Bennett B. Interleukin 10 (IL-10) inhibits cytokine synthesis by human monocytes: An autoregulatory role of IL-10 produced by monocytes. J Exp Med. 1991;174:1209–20.

357. Martinez AM, Gibbons RS, Garovoy MR, et al. IL-4 inhibits IL-2 receptor expression and IL-2-dependent proliferation of human T cells. J Immunol. 1990;144:2211–5.

358. Salgame P, Abrams JS, Clayberger C, et al. Differing lymphokine profiles of functional subsets of human CD4 and CD8 T cell clones. Science. 1991;254:279–82.

359. Erard F, Wild M-T, Garcia-Sanz JA, et al. Switch of CD8 T cells to noncytolytic CD8−CD4− cells that make TH2 cytokines and help B cells. Science. 1993;260:1802–5.

360. Gray D. Immunological memory. Annu Rev Immunol. 1993;11:49–77.

361. Swain SL. Polarized patterns of cytokine secretion. Curr Biol. 1993;3:115–7.

361a. Clark EA, Ledbetter JA. How B and T cells talk to each other. Nature. 1994;367:425–8.

362. Noelle RJ, Ledbetter JA, Aruffo A. CD40 and its ligand, an essential ligand–receptor pair for thymus-dependent B-cell activation. Immunol Today. 1992;13:431–3.

363. Spriggs MK, Armitage RJ, Strockbine L, et al. Recombinant human CD40 ligand stimulates B cell proliferation and immunoglobulin E secretion. J Exp Med. 1992;176:1543–50.

364. Lederman S, Yellin MJ, Inghirami G, et al. Molecular interactions mediating T–B lymphocyte collaboration in human lymphoid follicles. Roles of T cell–B cell-activating molecule (5c8 antigen) and CD40 in contact-dependent help. J Immunol. 1992;149:3817–26.

365. Rudd CE, Morimoto C, Wong LL, et al. The subdivision of the T4 (CD4) subset on the basis of the differential expression of L-C/T200 antigens. J Exp Med. 1987;166:1758–73.

366. Mosmann TR, Cherwinski H, Bon MW, et al. Two types of murine helper T cell clone. I. Definition according to profiles of lymphokine activities and secreted proteins. J Immunol. 1986;136:2348–57.

367. Aruffo A, Farrington M, Hollenbaugh D, et al. The CD40 ligand, gp39, is defective in activated T cells from patients with X-linked hyper-IgM syndrome. Cell. 1993;72:291–300.

368. Bancherau J, Rousset F. Growing human B lymphocytes in the CD40 system. Nature. 1991;353:678–9.

369. Croft M, Swain SL. B cell response to fresh and effector T helper cells. Role of cognate T–B interaction and the cytokines IL-2, IL-4 and IL-6. J Immunol. 1991;146:4055–64.

370. Schimpl A, Schorle H, Holschke T, et al. Development and function of T cells in mice rendered IL-2 deficient by targeted disruption of the IL-2 locus (Abstract). Cytokine. 1992;3:515.

371. Huang S, Hendriks W, Althage A, et al. Immune response in mice that lack the interferon-γ receptor. Science. 1993;259:1742–5.

372. Finkelman Fd, Holmes J, Katona IM, et al. Lymphokine control of in vivo immunoglobulin isotype selection. Annu Rev Immunol. 1990;8:303–33.

373. Purkerson J, Isakson P. A two-signal model for regulation of immunoglobulin isotype switching. FASEB J. 1992;6:3245–52.

374. Finkelman FD, Svetic A, Gresser I, et al. Regulation by interferon α of immunoglobulin isotype selection and lymphokine production in mice. J Exp Med. 1991;174:1179–88.

375. Coutelier J-P, van der Logt JTM, Heessen FWA, et al. IgG2a restriction of murine antibodies elicited by viral infections. J Exp Med. 1987;165:64–9.

376. Coutelier J-P, van der Logt JTM, Heessen FWA, et al. Virally induced modulation of murine IgG antibody subclasses. J Exp Med. 1988;168:2373–8.

377. Sher A, Coffman RL. Regulation of immunity to parasites by T cells and T cell-derived cytokines. Annu Rev Immunol. 1992;10:385.

378. Punnonen J, Aversa G, Cocks BG, et al. Interleukin 13 induces interleukin 4–independent IgG4 and IgE synthesis and CD23 expression by human B cells. Proc Natl Acad Sci USA. 1993;90:3730–4.

379. Aubry J-P, Pochon S, Graber P, et al. CD21 is a ligand for CD23 and regulates IgE production. Nature. 1992;358:505–7.

380. Kimata H, Yoshida A, Ishioka C, et al. Interleukin 8 (IL-8) selective inhibits immunoglobulin E production induced by IL-4 in human B cells. J Exp Med. 1992;176:1227–31.

381. Pène J, Rousset F, Brière F, et al. IgE production by normal human lymphocytes is induced by interleukin 4 and suppressed by interferons γ and α and prostaglandin E₂. Proc Natl Acad Sci USA. 1988;85:6880–4.

382. McIntyre TM, Klinman DR, Rothman P, et al. Transforming growth factor β1 selectively stimulates immunoglobulin G2b secretion by lipopolysaccharide-activated murine B cells. J Exp Med. 1993;177:1031–7.

383. Sonoda E, Matsumoto R, Hitoshi Y, et al. Transforming growth factor β induces IgA production and acts additively with interleukin 5 for IgA production. J Exp Med. 1989;170:1415–20.

384. Bloom BR, Modlin RL, Salgame P. Stigma variations: Observations on suppressor T cells and leprosy. Annu Rev Immunol. 1992;10:453–88.

385. Miller A, Lider O, Weiner H. Antigen-driven bystander suppression after oral administration of antigens. J Exp Med. 1991;174:791–8.

386. Dorf ME, Kuchroo VK, Collins M. Suppressor T cells: Some answers but more questions. Immunol Today. 1992;13:241–3.

387. Espevik T, Figari IS, Shalaby MR, et al. Inhibition of cytokine production by cyclosporin A and transforming growth factor β. J Exp Med. 1987;166:571–6.

388. Lee G, Ellingsworth LR, Gillis S, et al. β Transforming growth factors are potential regulators of B lymphopoiesis. J Exp Med. 1987;166:1290–9.

289. Onderdonk AB, Markahm RB, Zeleznik DF, et al. Evidence for T cell–dependent immunity to *Bacteroides fragilis* in an intraabdominal abscess model. J Clin Invest. 1982;69:9–16.

390. Powderly WG, Schreiber JR, Pier GB, et al. T cells recognizing polysaccharide-specific B cells function as contrasuppressor cells in the generation of T cell immunity to *Pseudomonas aeruginosa*. J Immunol. 1988;140:2746–52.

391. Gromo G, Geller RL, Inverardi L, et al. Signal requirements in the stepwise functional maturation of cytotoxic T lymphocytes. Nature. 1987;327:424–6.

392. Gately MK, Wilson DE, Wong HL. Synergy between recombinant interleukin (rIL2) and IL 2-depleted lymphokine-containing supernatants in facilitating allogeneic human cytolytic T lymphocyte responses in vitro. J Immunol. 1986;136:1274–82.

393. Balkwill F. Cytokines in health and disease. Immunol Today. 1993;14:149–50.

394. Farrar MA, Schreiber RD. The molecular cell biology of interferon-γ and its receptor. Annu Rev Immunol. 1993;11:571–611.

395. Widmer MB, Acres RB, Sassenfeld HM, et al. Regulation of cytolytic cell populations form human peripheral blood by B cell stimulatory factor 1 (interleukin 4). J Exp Med. 1987;166:1447–55.

396. Chen W-F, Zlotnik A. IL-10: A novel cytotoxic T cell differentiation factor. J Immunol. 1991;147:528–34.

397. Hickman CJ, Crim JA, Mostowski HS, Siegel JP. Regulation of human cytotoxic T lymphocyte development by IL-7. J Immunol. 1990;145:2415–20.

398. Dalton DK, Pitts-Meek S, Keshav S, et al. Multiple defects of immune cell function in mice with disrupted interferon-γ genes. Science. 1993;259:1739–42.

399. Podack ER, Hengartner H, Lichtenheld MG. A central role of perforin in cytolysis. Annu Rev Immunol. 1991;9:129–57.

400. Masson D, Tschopp J. A family of serine esterases in lytic granules of cytolytic T lymphocytes. Cell. 1987;49:679–85.

401. Talento A, Nguyen M, Law S, et al. Transfection of mouse cytotoxic T lymphocyte with an antisense granzyme A vector reduces lytic activity. J Immunol. 1992;149:4009–15.

402. Helgason CD, Prendergast JA, Berke G, Bleackley RC. Peritoneal exudate lymphocyte and mixed lymphocyte culture hybridomas are cytolytic in the absence of cytotoxic cell proteinases and perforin. Eur J Immunol. 1992;22:3187–90.

403. Dennert G, Anderson CG, Prochazka G. High activity of *N*-benzyloxycarbonyl-L-lysine thiobenzyl enter serine esterase and cytolytic perforin in cloned cell lines is not demonstrable in in vivo–induced cytotoxic effector cells. Proc Natl Acad Sci USA. 1987;84:5004–8.

404. Young JD-E, Liu C-C. How do cytotoxic T lymphocytes avoid self-lysis? Immunol Today. 1988;9:14–5.

405. Ramsay AJ, Ruby J, Ramshaw IA. A case for cytokines as effector molecules in the resolution of virus infection. Immunol Today. 1993;14:155–7.

406. Phillips JH, Hori T, Nagler A, et al. Ontogeny of human natural killer (NK) cell: Fetal NK cells mediate cytolytic function and express cytoplasmic CD3ε,δ proteins. J Exp Med. 1992;175:1055–66.

407. Lanier LL, Spits H, Phillips JH. The relationship between NK and T cells. Immunol Today. 1992;13:392–5.

408. Versteeg R. NK cells and T cells: Mirror images? Immunol Today. 1992;13:244–7.

409. Raulet DH. A sense of something missing. Nature. 1992;358:21–22.

410. Moretta L, Ciccone E, Moretta A, et al. Allorecognition by NK cells: Nonself or no self? Immunol Today. 1992;13:300–6.

411. Kohl S. The neonatal human's immune response to herpes simplex virus infection: A critical review. Pediatr Infect Dis J. 1989;8:67–74.

412. Scalzo AA, Fitzgerald NA, Wallace CR, et al. The effect of *Cmv*-1 resistance gene, which is linked to the natural killer cell gene complex, is mediated by natural killer cells. J Immunol. 1992;149:581–9.

413. Beaman MH, Wong S-Y, Remington JS. Cytokines, *Toxoplasma* and intracellular parasitism. Immunol Rev. 1992;127:97–117.

414. Bancroft GJ, Schreiber RD, Unanue ER. Natural immunity: A T-cell-independent pathway of macrophage activation, defined in the *scid* mouse. Immunol Rev. 1991;124:5–24.

415. Biron CA, Byron KS, Sullivan JL. Severe herpesvirus infections in an adolescent without natural killer cells. N Engl J Med. 1989;320:1731–5.

416. Naume B, Gately M, Espevik T. A comparative study of IL-12 (cytotoxic lymphocyte maturation factor)–, IL-2–, and IL-7–induced effects on immunomagnetically purified CD56⁺ NK cells. J Immunol. 1992;148:2429–36.

417. Perussia B. Lymphokine-activated killer cells, natural killer cells and cytokines. Curr Opin Immunol. 1991;3:49–55.

418. Romagnani S. Induction of TH1 and TH2 responses: A key role for the ''natural'' immune response? Immunol Today. 1992;13:379–81.

419. Maliszewski CR, March CJ, Schoenborn MA, et al. Expression cloning of a human Fc receptor for IgA. J Exp Med. 1990;172:1665–72.

420. Colten HR, Rosen FS. Complement deficiencies. Annu Rev Immunol. 1992;10:809–34.

421. Wright SD. Multiple receptors for endotoxin. Curr Opin Immunol. 1991;3:83–90.

422. Kuhlman M, Joiner K, Ezekowitz RAB. The human mannose-binding protein functions as an opsonin. J Exp Med. 1989;169:1733–45.

423. Ezekowitz RAB, Sastry K, Bailley P, et al. Molecular characterization of the human macrophage mannose receptor: Demonstration of multiple carbohydrate recognition-like domains and phagocytosis of yeasts in Cos-1 cells. J Exp Med. 1990;172:1785–94.

424. Smith RM, Curnutte JT. Molecular basis of chronic granulomatous disease. Blood. 1991;77:673–86.

425. Lehrer RI, Lichenstein AK, Ganz T. Defensins: Antimicrobial and cytotoxic peptides of mammalian cells. Annu Rev Immunol. 1993;11:105–28.

426. Lasky LA. Selectins: Interpreters of cell-specific carbohydrate information during inflammation. Science. 1992;258:964–9.

247. Bevilacqua MP, Nelson RM. Selectins. J Clin Invest. 1993;91:379–87.

428. Butcher EC. Leukocyte-endothelial cell recognition: Three (or more) steps to specificity and diversity. Cell. 1991;67:1033–6.

429. Hynes RO. Integrins: Versatility, modulation, and signaling in cell adhesion. Cell. 1992;69:11–25.

430. Yang KD, Hill HR. Neutrophil function disorders: Pathophysiology, prevention, and therapy. J Pediatr. 1991;119:343–54.

431. Miller MD, Krangel MS. Biology and biochemistry of chemokines: A family of chemotactic and inflammatory cytokines. Crit Rev Immunol. 1992;12:17–46.

432. Taub DD, Conlon K, Lloyd AR, et al. Preferential migration of activated CD4⁺ and CD8⁺ T cells in response to MIP-1α and MIP-1β. Science. 1993;260:355–8.

433. Enk AH, Katz SI. Early molecular events in the induction phase of contact sensitivity. Proc Natl Acad Sci USA. 1992;89:1398–402.

434. Tsicopoulos A, Hamid Q, Varney V, et al. Preferential messenger RNA expression of Th1-type cells (IFN-γ⁺, IL-2⁺) in classical delayed-type (tuberculin) hypersensitivity reactions in human skin. J Immunol. 1992;148:2058–61.

435. Moore KW, O'Garra A, de Waal Malefyt R, et al. Interleukin-10. Annu Rev Immunol. 1993;11:165–90.

436. Dinarello CA. Interleukin-1 and interleukin-1 antagonism. Blood. 1991;77:1627–52.

437. Chomarat P, Rissoan M-C, Banchereau J, et al. Interferon γ inhibits interleukin 10 production by monocytes. J Exp Med. 1993;177:523–7.

438. Pollack M. New therapeutic strategies in gram-negative sepsis and septic shock based on molecular mechanisms of pathogenesis. In Mandell GL, Douglas RG, Bennett JE (eds): Principles and Practice of Infectious Diseases. New York: Churchill Livingstone; Update 8, 1990:3–18.

439. Mackaness GB. The immunological basis of acquired cellular immunity. J Exp Med. 1964;120:105–20.

440. Murray HW. The interferons, macrophage activation, and host defense against nonviral pathogens. J Interferon Res. 1992;12:319–22.

441. Drapier J-C, Wietzerbin J, Hibbs JB Jr. Interferon-γ and tumor necrosis factor induce the L-arginine-dependent cytotoxic effector mechanism in murine macrophages. Eur J Immunol. 1988;18:1587–92.

442. Ding AH, Nathan CF, Stuehr DJ. Release of reactive nitrogen intermediates

and reactive oxygen intermediates from mouse peritoneal macrophages. J Immunol. 1988;141:2407–12.

443. Ravetch JV, Kinet J-P. Fc Receptors. Annu Rev Immunol. 1991;9:457–92.

444. van de Winkel JGJ, Anderson CL. Biology of human immunoglobulin G Fc receptors. J Leukocyte Biol. 1991;49:511–24.

445. Nathan CF, Hibbs JB Jr. Role of nitric oxide synthesis in macrophage antimicrobial activity. Curr Opin Immunol. 1991;3:65–70.

446. Gazzinelli Rt, Oswald IP, James SL, et al. IL-10 inhibits parasite killing and nitrogen oxide production by IFN-γ–activated macrophages. J Immunol. 1992;148;1792–6.

447. Green SJ, Crawford RM, Hockmeyer JT, et al. *Leishmania major* amastigotes initiate the L-arginine–dependent killing mechanism in IFN-γ stimulated macrophages by induction of tumor necrosis factor-α. J Immunol. 1990; 145:4290–7.

448. Schneemann M, Schoedon G, Hofer S, et al. Nitric oxide synthase is not a constituent of the antimicrobial armature of human mononuclear phagocytes. J Infect Dis. 1993;167:1358–63.

449. Pfefferkorn ER. Interferon-γ blocks the growth of *Toxoplasma gondii* in human fibroblasts by inducing the host cells to degrade tryptophan. Proc Natl Acad Sci USA. 1984;81:908–12.

450. Byrne GI, Lehamnn LK, Landry GJ. Induction of tryptophan catabolism is the mechanism for gamma-interferon–mediated inhibition of intracellular *Chlamydia psittaci* replication in T24 cells. Infect Immun. 1986;53:347–51.

451. Niesel DW, Hews CB, Cho YJ, et al. Natural and recombinant interferons inhibit epithelial cell invasion by *Shigella* spp. Infect Immun. 1986;52:838–3.

452. Byrd TF, Horwitz MA. Interferon gamma-activated human monocytes downregulate transferrin receptors and inhibit the intracellular multiplication of *Legionella pneumophila* by limiting the availability of iron. J Clin Invest. 1989;83:1457–65.

453. Johnston RB Jr. Monocytes and macrophages. N Engl J Med. 1988;318: 747–52.

454. Adams DO, Koerner TJ. Gene regulation in macrophage development and activation. In Cruse JM, Lewis RE Jr (eds): The Year in Immunology 1988: Cellular, Molecular, and Clinical Aspects. v. 5. Basel: Karger;1989:159–80.

455. Rutherford MS, Witsell A, Schook LB. Mechanisms generating functionally heterogeneous macrophages: Chaos revisisted. J Leukocyte Biol. 1993;53: 602–18.

456. Scott P, Kaufmann SHE. The role of T-cell subsets and cytokines in the regulation of infection. Immunol Today. 1991;12:346–8.

457. Steigbiegel RT, Lambert LH Jr, Remington JS. Phagocytic and bactericidal properties of normal human monocytes. J Clin Invest. 1974;53:131–42.

458. Emoto M, Naito T, Nakamura R, et al. Different appearance of γδ T cells during salmonellosis between Ity^r and Ity^s mice. J Immunol. 1993;150: 3411–20.

459. Skamene E, Pietrangeli CE. Genetics of the immune response to infectious pathogens. Curr Opin Immunol. 1991;3:511–7.

460. McLeod R, Skamene E, Brown CR, et al. Genetic regulation of early survival and cyst number after peroral *Toxoplasma gondii* infection of AxB/BxA recombinant inbred and B10 congenic mice. J Immunol. 1989;143:3031–4.

461. Vidal SM, Malo D, Vogan K, et al. Natural resistance to infection with intracellular parasites: Isolation of a candidate for *Bcg*. Cell. 1993;73:469–85.

462. Stead WW. Genetics and resistance to tuberculosis. Could resistance be enhanced by genetic engineering? Ann Intern Med. 1992;116:937–41.

463. Leal LMCC, Moss DW, Kuhn R, et al. Interleukin-4 transgenic mice of resistant background are susceptible to *Leishmania major* infection. Eur J Immunol. 1993;23:566–9.

464. Pirmez C, Yamamura M, Uyemura K, et al. Cytokine patterns in the pathogenesis of human Leishmaniasis. J Clin Invest. 1993;91:1390–5.

465. te Velde AA, Huijbens RJF, de Vries JE, et al. IL-4 decreases FCγR membrane expression and FcγR-mediated cytotoxic activity of human monocytes. J Immunol. 1990;144:3046–51.

466. Fenton MJ, Buras JA, Donnelly RP. IL-4 reciprocally regulates IL-1 and IL-1 receptor antagonist expression in human monocytes. J Immunol. 1992; 149:1283–8.

467. Larner AC, Petricoin EF, Nakagawa Y, et al. IL-4 attenuates the transcriptional activation of both IFN-α– and IFN-γ–induced cellular gene expression in monocytes and monocytic cell lines. J Immunol. 1993;150:1944–50.

468. Holaday BJ, de Lima Pompeu MM, Evans T, et al. Correlates of Leishmania-specific immunity in the clinical spectrum of infection with *Leishmania chagasi*. J Infect Dis. 1993;167:411–7.

469. Carvalho EM, Barral A, Pedral-Sampaio D, et al. Immunologic markers of clinical evolution in children recently infected with *Leishmania donovani chagasi*. J Infect Dis. 1992;165:535–40.

470. Modlin RL, Melancon-Kaplan J, Young SMM, et al. Learning from lesions: Patterns of tissue inflammation in leprosy. Proc Natl Acad Sci USA. 1988; 85:1213–7.

471. Kaplan G. Recent advances in cytokine therapy in leprosy. J Infect Dis. 1993;167(Suppl 1):S18–22.

472. Cooper CL, Mueller C, Sinchaisri T-A, et al. Analysis of naturally occurring delayed-type hypersensitivity reactions in leprosy by in situ hybridization. J Exp Med. 1989;169:1565–81.

473. Mutis T, Kraakman EM, Cornelisse YE, et al. Analysis of cytokine production by *Mycobacterium*-reactive T cells. J Immunol. 1993;150:4641–551.

474. Moulder JW. Comparative biology of intracellular parasitism. Microbiol Rev. 1985;49:298–337.

475. Murray HW. How protozoa evade intracellular killing. Ann Intern Med. 1983;98:1016–8.

476. Wilson CB, Tsai V, Remington JS. Failure to trigger the oxidative metabolic burst by normal macrophages. J Exp Med. 1980;151:328–46.

477. Wilson CB, Haas JE. Cellular defenses against *Toxoplasma gondii* in newborns. J Clin Invest. 1984;73:1606–16.

478. Gazzinelli RT, Hakim FT, Hieny S, et al. Synergistic role of CD4$^+$ and CD8$^+$ T lymphocytes in IFN-γ production and protective immunity induced by an attenuated *Toxoplasma gondii* vaccine. J Immunol. 1991;146:286–92.

479. Gazzinelli R, Xu Y, Hieny S, et al. Simultaneous depletion of CD4$^+$ and CD8$^+$ T lymphocytes is required to reactivate chronic infection with *Toxoplasma gondii*. J Immunol. 1992;149:175–80.

480. Hakim FT, Gazzinelli RT, Denkers E et al. CD8$^+$ T cells from mice vaccinated against *Toxoplasma gondii* are cytotoxic for parasite-infected or antigen-pulsed host cells. J Immunol. 1991;147:2310–6.

481. Dunn PL, North RJ. Limitations of the adoptive immunity assay for analyzing anti-*Listeria* immunity. J Infect Dis. 1991;164:878–82.

482. Harty JT, Schreiber RD, Bevan MJ. CD8 T cells can protect against an intracellular bacterium in an interferon γ-independent fashion. Proc Natl Acad Sci USA. 1992;89:11612–6.

483. Orme I, Anderson P, Boom WH. T cell response to *Mycobacterium tuberculosis*. J Infect Dis. 1993;167:1481–97.

483a.Mombaerts P, Arnoldi J, Russ F, et al. Different roles of αβ and γδ T cells in immunity against an intracellular bacterial pathogen. Nature. 1993;365: 53–6.

484. Lewis DB, Wilson CB. Developmental immunology and the role of host defense in neonatal susceptibility to infection. In Remington JS, JO Klein (eds): Infectious Diseases of the Fetus and Newborn Infant. 4th ed. Philadelphia: WB Saunders; 1993. In press.

485. Deem RL, Doughty FA, Beaman BL. Immunologically specific direct T lymphocyte–mediated killing of *Nocardia asteroides*. J Immunol. 1983;130: 2401–6.

486. Albright JW, Munger WE, Henkart PA, et al. The toxicity of rat large granular lymphocyte tumor cells and their cytoplasmic for rodent and African trypanosomes. J Immunol. 1988;140:2774–8.

487. Joiner KA, Hammer CH, Brown EJ, et al. Studies on the mechanism of bacterial resistance to complement-mediated killing. J Exp Med. 1982;155: 797–808.

488. Horwitz MA, Silverstein SC. Interaction of the Legionnaire's disease bacterium (*Legionella pneumophila*) with human phagocytes. J Exp Med. 1980; 153:386–97.

489. Frenkel JK, Taylor DW. Toxoplasmosis in immunoglobulin M–suppressed mice. Infect Immun. 1982;38:360.

490. Eisenhauer P, Mack DG, McLeod R. Prevention of peroral and congenital acquisition of *Toxoplasma gondii* by antibody and activated macrophages. Infect Immun. 1988;56:83–7.

491. Chang K-P. Antibody-mediated inhibition of phagocytosis in *Leishmania donovani*–human phagocyte interactions in vitro. Am J Trop Med Hyg. 1981; 30:344–9.

492. Koup RA, Wilson CB. The clinical immunology of HIV infected children. In Pizzo P, Wilfert CM (eds): Pediatric AIDS. 2nd ed. Baltimore. Williams and Wilkins. 1993. In press.

493. Harmsen AG, Stankiewicz M. Requirement for CD4$^+$ cells in resistance to *Pneumocystis carinii* pneumonia in mice. J Exp Med. 1990;172:937–45.

494. Roths JB, Sidman CL. Both immunity and hyperresponsiveness to *Pneumocystis carinii* result from transfer of CD4$^+$ but not CD8$^+$ T cells into severe combined immunodeficiency mice. J Clin Invest. 1992;90:673–8.

495. Beck JM, Warnock ML, Curtis JL, et al. Inflammatory responses to *Pneumocystis carinii* in mice selectively depleted of helper T lymphocytes. Am J Respir Cell Mol Biol. 1991;5:186–97.

496. Chellito J, Suzara VV, Blumenfeld W, et al. A new model of *Pneumocystis carinii* infection in mice selectively depleted of helper T lymphocytes. J Clin Invest. 1990;85:1686–93.

497. Chen W, Havell EA, Harmsen AG. Importance of endogenous tumor necrosis factor alpha and gamma interferon in host resistance against *Pneumocystis carinii* infection. Infect Immun. 1992;60:1279–84.

498. Harmsen AG, Chen W. Resolution of *Pneumocystis carinii* pneumonia in CD4$^+$ lymphocyte-depleted mice given aerosols of heat-treated *Escherichia coli*. J Exp Med. 1992;176:881–6.

499. Chen W, Havel EA, Moldawer LL, et al. Interleukin 1: An important mediator of host resistance against *Pneumocystis carinii*. J Exp Med. 1992;176: 713–8.

500. Beck JM, Liggitt HD, Brunette EN, et al. Reduction in intensity of *Pneumocystis carinii* pneumonia in mice by aerosol administration of gamma interferon. Infect Immun. 1991;59:3859–62.

501. Ezekowitz RAB, Williams DJ, Koziel H, et al. Uptake of *Pneumocystis carinii* mediated by the macrophage mannose receptor. Nature. 1991;351: 155–8.

502. Sherman MP, Lorom L, Wong VZ, et al. Cytokine- and *Pneumocystis carinii*–induced L-arginine oxidation by murine and human alveolar macrophages. J Protozol. 1991;38:234–65.

503. McGowan JE Jr, Chesney PJ, Brossley KB, et al. Guidelines for the use of systemic glucocorticosteroids in the management of selected infections. J Infect Dis. 1992;165:1–13.

504. Cox FEG, Liew FY. T-cell subsets and cytokines in parasitic infections. Immunol Today. 1992;13:445–8.

505. Cenci E, Romani L, Vecchiarelli A, et al. T cell subsets and IFN-γ productcion in resistance to systemic candidosis in immunized mice. J Immunol. 1990;144:4333–9.

506. Mahanty S, Greenfield RA, Joyce WA, et al. Inoculation candidiasis in a murine model of severe combined immunodeficiency syndrome. Infect Immun. 1988;56:3162–6.

507. Levitz SM. Overview of host defenses in fungal infections. Clin Infect Dis. 1992;14(Suppl 1):S37–42.

508. Shapiro ME, Kasper DL, Zaleznik DF, et al. Cellular control of abscess formation: Role of T cells in the regulation of abscesses formed in response to *Bacteriodes fragilis*. J Immunol. 1986;137:341–6.

509. Markham RB, Powderly WG. Exposure of mice to live *Pseudomonas aeruginosa* generates protective cell-mediated immunity in the absence of an antibody response. J Immunol. 1988;140:2039–45.

510. McKinney RE Jr, Katz SL, Wilfert CM. Chronic enteroviral meningoencephalitis in agammaglobulinemic patients. Rev Infect Dis. 1987;9:334–56.

511. Daniels CA, Kleinerman ES, Snyderman R. Abortive and productive infections in human mononuclear phagocyte by type 1 herpes simplex virus. Am J Pathol. 1978;91:118–29.

512. Drew WL, et al. Growth of herpes simplex and cytomegalovirus in cultured human alveolar macrophages. Am Rev Respir Dis. 1979;119:287.

513. Mims CA, Gould J. The role of macrophages in mice infected with murine cytomegalovirus. J Gen Virol. 1978;41:143–53.

514. Stanwick TL, Campbell DE, Nahmias AJ. Cells infected with herpes simplex virus induce human monocyte-macrophages to produce interferon. Immunobiology. 1981;158:207–12.

515. Wong GHW, Goeddel DV. Tumour necrosis factors α and β inhibit virus replication and synergize with interferons. Nature. 1986;323:819–22.

516. Paya CV, Denmotsu N, Schoon RA, et al. Tumor necrosis factor and lymphotoxin secretion by human natural killer cells leads to antiviral cytotoxicity. J Immunol. 1988;141:1989–95.

517. Fauci AS, Schnittman SM, Poli G, et al. Immunopathogenic mechanisms in human immunodeficiency virus (HIV) infection. Ann Intern Med. 1991;114:678–93.

518. Zisman B, Hirsch MS, Allison AC. Selective effects of anti-macrophage serum, silica and anti-lymphocyte serum on pathogenesis of herpes virus infection of young adult mice. J Immunol. 1970;104:1155–9.

519. McGeorge MB, Morahan PS. Comparison of various macrophage-inhibitory agents on vaginal and systemic herpes simplex virus type 2 infections. Infect Immun. 1978;22:623–6.

520. Gresser I, Tovey MG, Maury C, et al. Role of interferon in the pathogenesis of virus diseases in mice as demonstrated by the use of antiinterferon serum. I. Rapid evolution of encephalomyocarditis virus infection. J Exp Med. 1976;144:1316–23.

521. Engler H, Zawatzky R, Kirchner H, et al. Experimental infection of inbred mice with herpes simplex virus. IV. Comparison of interferon production and natural killer cell activity in susceptible and resistant adult mice. Arch Virol. 1982;74:239–47.

522. Habu S, Akamatsu K-I, Tamaoki N, et al. In vivo significance of NK cell on resistance against virus (HSV-1) infections in mice. J Immunol. 1984;133:2743–7.

523. Schmid DS, Rouse BT. The role of T cell immunity in control of herpes simplex virus. Curr Top Microbiol Immunl. 1992;179:57–74.

524. Nahmias AJ, Coleman RM. The significance of herpes simple virus infections in humans. In Rouse BT, Lopez C (eds): Immunobiology of Herpes Simplex Virus Infection. Boca Raton, FL: CRC Press, 1984:1–8.

525. Rijksen G, et al. A new case of purine nucleoside phosphorylase deficiency: Enzymologic, clinical and immunologic characteristics. Pediatr Res. 1987;21:13.

526. Nagaguchi S, Oda H, Mori R, et al. Mechanism of acquired resistance to herpes simplex virus infection as studied in nude mice. J Gen Virol. 1979;44:715–23.

527. Ammann AJ, Hong R. Disorders of the T-cell system. In Stiehm ER (ed): Immunologic Disorders in Infants and Children. Philadelphia: WB Saunders, 1989:257–315.

528. St. Geme JW Jr, Prince JT, Burke B, et al. Impaired cellular resistance to herpes-simplex virus in Wiskott-Aldrich syndrome. N Engl J Med. 1965;273:229–34.

529. Koelle DM, Tigges MA, Burke RL, et al. Herpes simplex virus infection of human fibroblasts and keratinocytes inhibits recognition by cloned CD8+ cytotoxic T lymphocytes. J Clin Invest. 1993;91:961–8.

530. Hendricks RL, Tumpey TM, Finnegan A. IFN-γ and IL-2 are protective in the skin but pathologic in the corneas of HSV-1-infected mice. J Immunol. 1992;149:3023–8.

531. Weinberg A, Konrad M, Merigan TC. Regulation of interleukin-2 of protective immunity against recurrent herpes simplex virus type 2 genital infection in guinea pigs. J Virol. 1987;61:2120–7.

532. Kohl S. Protection against murine neonatal herpes simplex virus infection by lymphokine-treated human leukocytes. J Immunol. 1990;144:307–12.

533. Burchett SK, Corey L, Mohan KM, et al. Diminished interferon-γ and lymphocyte proliferation in neonatal and postpartum primary herpes simplex virus infection. J Infect Dis. 1992;165:813–8.

534. Quinnan GV Jr, Kirmani N, Rook AH, et al. Cytotoxic T cells in cytomegalovirus infection. HLA-restricted T-lymphocyte and non-T-lymphocyte cytotoxic responses correlate with recovery from cytomegalovirus infection in bone-marrow-transplant recipients. N Engl J Med. 1982;307:7–13.

535. Riddell SR, Watanabe KS, Goodrich JM, et al. Restoration of viral immunity in immunodeficient humans by the adoptive transfer of T cell clones. Science. 1992;257:238–41.

536. Fennie EH, Lie YS, Low M-AL, et al. Reduced mortality in murine cytomeg-

alovirus infected mice following prophylactic murine interferon-γ treatment. Antiviral Res. 1988;10:27–39.

537. Finberg R, Hom R. The role of T cell immunity in infection with the herpes group viruses. Year Immunol. 1986;2:267–8.

538. de Campos-Lima P-O, Avioli R, Zhang Q-J, et al. HLA-A11 epitope loss isolates of Epstein-Barr virus from a highly A11+ population. Science. 1993;260:98–100.

539. Cohen JI. Epstein-Barr virus lymphoproliferative disease associated with acquired immunodeficiency. Medicine. 1991;70:137–60.

540. Grierson H, Purtilo DT. Epstein-Barr virus infections in males with the X-linked lymphoproliferative syndrome. Ann Intern Med. 1987;106:538–45.

541. Upton C, Mossman K, McFadden G. Encoding of a homolog of the IFN-γ receptor by myxoma virus. Science. 1992;258:1369–72.

542. Murphy PM. Molecular mimicry and the generation of host defense protein diversity. Cell. 1993;72:823–6.

543. Graham BS, Bunton LA, Wright PF, et al. Role of T lymphocyte subsets in the pathogenesis of primary infection and rechallenge with respiratory syncytial virus in mice. J Clin Invest. 1991;88:1026–33.

544. Hou S, Doherty PC, Zijlstra M, et al. Delayed clearance of Sendai virus in mice lacking class I MHC-restricted CD8+ T cells. J Immunol. 1992;149:1319–25.

545. Ronni T, Melen M, Malygin A, Julkunen I. Control of IFN-inducible MxA gene expression in human cells. J Immunol. 1993;150:1715–26.

546. Carding SR, Allan W, McMickle A, et al. Activation of cytokine genes in T cells during primary and secondary murine influenza pneumonia. J Exp Med. 1993;177:475–82.

547. Hall CB, Powell KR, MacDonald NE, et al. Respiratory synctial viral infection in children with compromised immune function. N Engl J Med. 1986;315:77–81.

548. Fishaut M, Tubergen D, McIntosh K. Cellular response to respiratory viruses with particular reference to children with disorders of cell-mediated immunity. J Pediatr. 1980;96:179–86.

549. Jarvis Wr, Middleton PJ, Gelfand EW. Significance of viral infections in severe combined immunodeficiency disease. Pediatr Infect Dis. 1983;2:187–92.

550. Nathan C, Squires K, Griffo W, et al. Widespread intradermal accumulation of mononuclear leukocytes in lepromatous leprosy patients treated systemically with recombinant interferon γ. J Exp Med. 1990;172:1509–12.

551. Sampaio EP, Moreira SL, Sarno EN, et al. Prolonged treatment with recombinant interferon γ induces erythema nodosum leprosum in lepromatous leprosy patients. J Exp Med. 1992;175:1729–37.

552. Badaro R, Falcoff E, Badaro FS, et al. Treatment of visceral leishmaniasis with pentavalent antimony and interferon gamma. N Engl J Med. 1990;322:16–21.

553. Badaro R, Johnson WD Jr. The role of interferon-gamma in the treatment of visceral and diffuse cutaneous leishmaniasis. J Infect Dis. 1993;167(Suppl 1):S13–7.

554. Agosti JM, Coombs RW, Collier AC, et al. A randomized, double-blind, phase I/II trial of tumor necrosis factor and interferon-gamma for treatment of AIDS-related complex (Protocol 025 from the AIDS Clinical Trials Group). AIDS Res Hum Retroviruses. 1992;8:581–7.

555. Murray HW, Scavuzzo D, Jacobs JL, et al. In vitro and in vivo activation of human mononuclear phagocytes by gamma interferon: Studies with normal and AIDS monocytes. J Immunol. 1987;138:2457–62.

556. Parkin JM, Eales LJ, Moshtael O, et al. A preliminary report of the use of interferon-gamma in patients with the acquired immunodeficiency syndrome. In Staquet MJ, Hemmer R, Baert AE (eds): Clinical Aspects of AIDS and AIDS-Related Complex. Oxford: Oxford University Press; 1986:167–74.

557. Teppler H, Kaplan G, Smith K, et al. Prolonged immunostimulatory effect of low-dose polyethylene glycol interleukin 2 in patients with human immunodeficiency virus type 1 infection. J Exp Med. 1993;177:483–92.

558. Tappler H, Kaplan G, Smith K, et al. Efficacy of low doses of the polyethylene glycol derivative of interleukin-2 in modulating the immune response of patients with human immunodeficiency virus type 1 infection. J Infect Dis. 1993;167:291–8.

559. Wood R, Montoya JG, Kundu SK, et al. Safety and efficacy of polyethylene glycol-modified interleukin-2 and zidovudine in human immunodeficiency virus type I infection: A phase II/II study. J Infect Dis. 1993;167:519–25.

560. Maoleekoonpairoj S, Mittelman A, Savona S, et al. Lack of protection against bacterial infections in patients with advanced cancer treated by biologic response modifiers. J Clin Microbiol. 1989;27:2305–8.

561. Pockaj BA, Topalian SL, Steinberg SM, et al. Infectious complications associated with interleukin-2 administration: A retrospective review of 935 treatment courses. J Clin Oncol. 1993;11:136–47.

562. Cao M, Sasaki O, Yamada A, Imanishi J. Enhancement of the protective effect of inactivated influenza virus vaccine by cytokines. Vaccine. 1992;10:238–42.

563. Rose RM, Rey-Martinez J, Croteau C, et al. Failure of recombinant interleukin-2 to augment the primary humoral response to a recombinant hepatitis B vaccine in healthy adults. J Infect Dis. 1992;165:775–7.

564. Meuer SC, Dumann H, zum Büschenfelde K-HM, Köhler H. Low-dose interleukin-2 induces systemic immune responses against HBsAg in immunodeficient nonresponders to hepatitis B vaccination. Lancet. 1989;1:15–7.

565. Heath AW, Playfair JHL. Cytokines as immunological adjuvants. Vaccine. 1992;10:427–34.

565a.Afonso L, Scharton T, Vieira L, et al. The adjuvant effect of interleukin-12 in a vaccine against *Leishmania major*. Science. 1994;263:235–7.

566. Vassali P. The pathophysiology of tumor necrosis factors. Annu Rev Immunol. 1992;10:411–52.

567. Odio CM, Faingezicht I, Paris M, et al. The beneficial effects of early dexamethasone administration in infants and children with bacterial meningitis. N Engl J Med. 1991;324:1525–31.

568. Dinarello CA, Wolff SM. The role of interleukin-1 in disease. N Engl J Med. 1993;328:106–13.

569. Fisher CJJ, Slotman GJ, Opal S, et al. Interleukin-1 receptor antagonist reduces mortality in patients with sepsis syndrome (Abstract). Presented at the Annual meeting of the American College of Chest Physicians, San Francisco, November 7, 1991.

570. Gérard C, Bruyns C, Marchant A, et al. Interleukin 10 reduces the release of tumor necrosis factor and prevents lethality in experimental endotoxemia. J Exp Med. 1993;177:547–50.

571. Howard M, Muchamuel T, Andrade S, et al. Interleukin 10 protects mice from lethal endotoxemia. J Exp Med. 1993;1205–8.

572. Ashkenazi A, Marsters SA, Capon SJ, et al. Protection against endotoxic shock by a tumor necrosis factor receptor immunoadhesin. Proc Natl Acad Sci USA. 1991;88:10535–9.

573. Bloom BR. The power of negative thinking. J Clin Invest. 1993;91:1265–6.

574. Sancho L, de la Hera A, Casas J, et al. Two different maturational stages of natural killer lymphocytes in human newborn infants. J Pediatr. 1991;119:446–54.

575. Seki H, Ueno Y, Taga K, et al. Mode of in vitro augmentation of natural killer cell activity by recombinant human interleukin 2: A comparative study of Leu-11$^+$ and Leu-11$^-$ cell populations in cord blood and adult peripheral blood. J Immunol. 1985;134:2351–6.

576. Hayward AR, Herberger M, Saunders D. Herpes simplex virus-stimulated γ-interferon production by newborn mononuclear cells. Pediatr Res. 1986;20:398–401.

577. Kohl S, Loo LS, Drath DB, et al. Interleukin-2 protects neonatal mice from lethal herpes simplex virus infection: A macrophage-mediated, γ interferon-induced mechanism. J Infect Dis. 1989;159:239–47.

578. Wilson CB, Westall J, Johnston L, et al. Decreased production of interferon-gamma by human neonatal cells: Intrinsic and regulatory deficiencies. J Clin Invest. 1986;77:860–7.

579. Wilson CB, Penix L, Melvin A, et al. Lymphokine regulation and the role of abnormal regulation in immunodeficiency. Clin Immunol Immunopathol. 1993;67:S25–32.

580. Yeager AS, Arvin AM, Urbani LJ, et al. Relationship of antibody to outcome in neonatal herpes simplex virus infections. Infect Immun. 1980;29:532–8.

581. Sullender WM, Miller JL, Yasukawa LL, et al. Humoral and cell-mediated immunity in neonates with herpes simplex virus infection. J Infect Dis. 1987;155:28–37.

582. Bortolussi R, Rajaraman K, Serushago B. Role of tumor necrosis factor-α and interferon-γ in newborn host defense against *Listeria monocytogenes* infection. Pediatr Res. 1992;32:460–4.

583. Chen Y, Nakane A, Minagawa T. Recombinant murine gamma interferon induces enhanced resistance to *Listeria monocytogenes* infection in neonatal mice. Infect Immun. 1989;57:2345–9.

584. Wilson CB, Desmonts G, Couvreur J, et al. Lymphocyte transformation in the diagnosis of congenital toxoplasma infection. N Engl J Med. 1980;302:785–8.

585. McLeod R, Mack DG, Boyer K, et al. Phenotypes and functions of lymphocytes in congenital toxoplasmosis. J Lab Clin Med. 1990;116:623–35.

586. Gardner ID. The effect of aging on susceptibility to infection. Rev Infect Dis. 1980;2:801–10.

587. Murasko DM, Goonewardene IM. T-cell funtion in aging: Mechanisms of decline. Annu Rev Gerontol Geriatri. 1990;10:71–96.

588. Thoman ML, Weigle WO. The cellular and subcellular bases in immunosenescence. Adv Immunol. 1989;46:221.

589. Report of a WHO Scientific Group. Primary immunodeficiency diseases. Immunodeficiency Rev. 1992;33:195–236.

590. Fischer A. Severe combined immunodeficiencies. Immunodeficiency Rev. 1992;3:83–100.

591. Schandene L, Ferster A, Mascart-Lemone F, et al. T helper type 2-like cells and therapeutic effects of interferon-γ in combined immunodeficiency with hypereosinophilia (Omenn's syndrome). Eur J Immunol. 1993;23:56–60.

592. Pahwa R, Chatila T, Pahwa S, et al. Recombinant interleukin 2 therapy in severe combined immunodeficiency disease. Proc Natl Acad Sci USA. 1989;86:5069–73.

593. Weinberg K, Parkman R. Severe combined immunodeficiency due to a specific defect in the production of interleukin-2. N Engl J Med. 1990;322:1718–23.

594. Le Deist F, Thoenes G, Corado J, et al. Immunodeficiency with low expression of the T cell receptor/CD3 complex. Effect on T lymphocyte activation. Eur J Immunol. 1991;21:1641–7.

595. Sorenson RU, Boehm K, Kaplan D, et al. Cryptococcal osteomyelitis and cellular immunodeficiency associated with interleukin-2 deficiency. J Pediatr. 1992;121:873–9.

596. Arnaiz-Villena A, Timon M, Rodriguez-Gallego C, et al. Human T-cell activation deficiencies. Immunol Today. 1992;13:259–65.

597. Rees AJ, Lockwood CM. Immunosuppressive drugs in clinical practice. In Lackham PJ, Peters K, Rosen FS, et al. (eds): Clinical Aspects of Immunology. 5th ed. v. 2. London: Blackwell Scientific; 1993:929–69.

598. Cytomegalovirus infections: Epidemiology, diagnosis, and treatment strategies. Rev Infect Dis. 1990;12(Suppl 7):S691–849.

599. Lynfield R, Herrin JT, Rubin RH. Varicella in pediatric renal transplant recipients. Pediatrics. 1992;90:216–20.

600. Malatack JJ, Gartner JC, Urbach AH, et al. Orthotopic liver transplantation, Epstein-Barr virus, cyclosporine, and lymphoproliferative disease: A growing concern. J Pediatr. 1991;118:667–75.

601. Sany J. Immunological treatment of rheumatoid arthritis. Clin Exp Rheum. 1990;8(Suppl 5):81–8.

602. Kamel OW, van de Rijn M, Weiss LM, et al. Reversible lymphomas associated with Epstein-Barr virus occurring during methotrexate therapy for rheumatoid arthritis and dermatomyositis. N Engl J Med. 1993;328:1317–21.

603. Dowell SF, Bresee JS. Severe varicella associated with steroid use. Pediatrics. 1993;92:223–8.

604. Boumpas DT, Paliogianni F, Anastassiou ED, et al. Glucocorticosteroid action on the immune system: Molecular and cellular aspects. Clin Exp Rheumatol. 1991;9:413–23.

605. Northrop JP, Crabtree GR, Mattila PS. Negative regulation of interleukin 2 transcription by the glucocorticoid receptor. J Exp Med. 1992;175:1235–45.

606. Paliogianni F, Raptis A, Ahuja SS, et al. Negative transcriptional regulation of human interleukin 2 (IL-2) gene by glucocorticoids through interference with nuclear transcription factors AP-1 and NF-AT. J Clin Invest. 1993;91:1481–9.

607. Sigal NH, Dumont FJ. Cyclosporin A, FK-506, and rapamycin: Pharmacologic probes of lymphocyte signal transduction. Annu Rev Immunol. 1992;10:519–60.

608. Clipstone NA, Crabtree GR. Identification of calcineurin as a key signalling enzyme in T-lymphocyte activation. Nature. 1992;357:695–7.

609. Kim JH, Perfect JR. Infection and cyclosporine. Rev Infect Dis. 1989;11:677–90.

610. Randhawa PS, Jaffe R, Demetris AJ, et al. Expression of Epstein-Barr virus–encoded small RNA (by the EBER-1 gene) in liver specimens from transplant recipients with post-transplantation lymphoproliferative disease. N Engl J Med. 1992;327:1710–4.

611. Dayton JS, Turka LA, Thompson CB, et al. Comparison of the effects of mizoribine with those of azathioprine, 6-mercaptopurine, and mycophenolic acid on T lymphocyte proliferation and purine ribonucleotide metabolism. Mol Pharmacol. 1992;41:671–6.

612. Chiappelli F, Myers LW, Ellison GW, et al. Preferential reductions in lymphocyte sub-populations induced by monthly pulses of chlorambucil: Studies in patients with chronic progressive multiple sclerosis. Int J Immunopharmacol. 1991;13:455–61.

613. Shiroky JB, Frost A, Skelton JD, et al. Complications of immunosuppression associated with weekly low dose methotrexate. J Rheumatol. 1991;18:1172–5.

614. Strober S, Dhillon M, Schubert M, et al. Acquired immune tolerance to cadaveric renal allografts. N Engl J Med. 1989;321:28–33.

615. Evans MA, Schomberg PJ, Rodeheffer RJ, et al. Total lymphoid irradiation: A novel and successful therapy for resistant cardiac allograft rejection. Mayo Clin Proc. 1992;67:785–90.

616. Stober S, Farinas MC, Field EH, et al. Treatment of lupus nephritis with total lymphoid irradiation: Observations during a 12–79-month followup. Arthritis Rheum. 19988;31:850–7.

617. Bass H, Adkins B, Strober S. Thymic irradiation inhibits the rapid recovery of TL1-like functions of CD4$^+$ T cells after total lymphoid irradiation. Cell Immunol. 1991;137:316–28.

618. Ochs HD, Wedgwood RJ. Disorders of the B cell system. In Stiehm ER (ed): Immunologic Disorders in Infants and Children. 3rd ed. Philadelphia: WB Saunders, 1989:226–56.

619. Caldera LH, Leon-Ponte M, Acquatell G, et al. Bone marrow and peripheral blood natural killer cell activity in lymphomas. Its response to IL-2. Clin Exp Immunol. 1992;88:143–8.

620. Mangge H, Beaufort F, Neubauer M, et al. Peripheral blood lymphocytes of nonleukemic lymphoma patients exhibit aberrant expression of T-cell activation markers after polyclonal stimulation in vitro. Cancer. 1990;66:677–83.

621. van der Horst FAL, van der Marel A, den Ottolander GJ, et al. Decrease of memory T helper cells (CD4$^+$ CD45RO$^+$) in hairy cell leukemia. Leukemia. 1993;7:46–50.

622. Furukawa Y, Nakamura H, Sakamoto S, et al. Cytomegalovirus gastritis as an initial manifestation of a patient with adult T-cell leukemia. Acta Haematol. 1988;80:216–8.

623. Chandra RK. Nutrition and immunity. In Lackham PJ, Peters K, Rosen FS, et al. (eds): Clinical Aspects of Immunology. 5th ed. v. 2. London: Blackwell Scientific; 1993:1325–38.

624. Allen JI, Kay NE, McClain CJ. Severe zinc deficiency in humans: Association with a reversible T-lymphocyte dysfunction. Ann Intern Med. 1981;95:154–7.

625. Rouse BT, Horohov DW. Immunosuppression in viral infections. Rev Infect Dis. 1986;8:850–73.

626. Zinkernagal RM, Hengartner H. Virally induced immunosuppression. Curr Opin Immunol. 1992;4:408–12.

627. Peska S, Lagen LA, Zoon KC, et al. Interferons and their actions. Annu Rev Biochem. 1987;56:757–80.

628. Salkind AR, McCarthy DO, Nichols JE, et al. Interleukin-1–inhibitor activity induced by respiratory synctytial virus: Abrogation of virus-specific and alternate human lymphocyte proliferative responses. J Infect Dis. 1991;163:71–7.

629. Sher A, Gazzinelli RT, Oswald IP, et al. Role of T-cell derived cytokines in

the downregulation of immune responses in parasitic and retroviral infection. Immunol Rev. 1992;127:183–204.

630. Maggi E, Macchia D, Parronchi P, et al. Reduced production of interleukin 2 and interferon-gamma and enhanced helper activity for IgG synthesis by cloned C4⁺ T cells from patients with AIDS. Eur J Immunol. 1987;17:1685–90.

631. Salk J, Bretscher PA, Salk PL, et al. A strategy for prophylactic vaccination against HIV. Science. 1993;260:1270–2.

632. Gorensek MJ, Stewart RW, Keys TF, et al. Symptomatic cytomegalovirus infection as a significant risk factor for major infections after cardiac transplanation. J Infec tDis. 1988;158:884–7.

633. Couch RB. The effects of influenza on host defenses. J Infect Dis. 1981;144:284–91.

634. Gardner ID. Suppression of antibacterial immunity by infection with influenza virus. J Infect Dis. 1981;144:225–31.

635. Rand KH, Pollard RB, Merigan TC. Increased pulmonary superinfection in cardiac transplant patients undergoing primary cytomegalovirus infection. N Engl J Med. 1978;298:951–3.

636. Pomeroy C, Filice GA, Hitt J, Jordan MC. Cytomegalovirus-induced reactivation of *Toxoplasma gondii* pneumonia in mice: Lung lymphocyte phenotypes and suppressor function. J Infect Dis. 1992;166:677–81.

637. Roberts NJ Jr. The concept of immunofocusing illustrated by influenza virus infection. Rev Infect Dis. 1988;10:1071–4.

638. Tarleton RL. Regulation of immunity in *Trypanosoma cruzi* infection. Exp Parasitol. 1991;73:106–9.

639. Shearer WT, Anderson DC. The secondary immunodeficiencies. In Stiehm ER (ed): Immunologic Disorders in Infants and Children. 3rd ed. Philadelphia: WB Saunders; 1989:400–38.

640. Lachman PJ, Peters K, Rosen FS, et al. Clinical Aspects of Immunology. 5th ed. London: Blackwell Scientific; 1993.

641. The International Chronic Granulomatous Disease Cooperative Study Group. A controlled trial of interferon gamma to prevent infection in chronic granulomatous disease. N Engl J Med. 1991;324:509–16.

642. Curnutte JT. Conventional versus interferon-γ therapy in chronic granulomatous disease. J Infect Dis. 1993;167:S8–12.

643. Bernhisel-Broadbent J, Camargo EE, Jaffe HS, et al. Recombinant human interferon-γ as adjunct therapy for *Aspergillus* infection in a patient with chronic granulomatous disease. J Infect Dis. 1991;163:908–11.

644. Williamson PR, Kwon-Chung KJ, Gallin JI. Successful treatment of *Paecilomyces varioti* infection in a patient with chronic granulomatous disease and a review of *Paecilomyces* species infections. Clin Infect Dis. 1992;14:1023–6.

645. Cunningham-Rundles C, Mayer L, Sapira E, et al. Restoration of immunoglobulin secretion in vitro in common variable immunodeficiency by in vivo treatment with polyethylene glycol-conjugated human recombinant interleukin-2. Clin Immunol Immunopath. 1992;64:46–56.

646. Centers for Disease Control and Prevention. Purified protein derivative (PPD)-tuberculin anergy and HIV infection: Guidelines for anergy testing and management of anergic persons at risk of tuberculosis. MMWR. 1991;40:27–32.

647. Centers for Disease Control and Prevention. Guidelines for the performance of CD4⁺ T-cell determinations in persons with human immunodeficiency virus infection. MMWR. 1992;41:1–17.

648. Pyun KH, Ochs HD, Wedgwood RJ, et al. Human antibody responses to bacteriophage φX174. Sequential induction of IgM and IgG subclass antibody. Clin Immunol Immunopathol. 1989;51:252–63.

649. Mathews MB, Shenk T. Adenovirus virus-associated RNA and translation control. J Virol 1991;65:5657–62.

650. Wold WSM, Gooding LR. Region E3 of adenovirus: A cassette of genes involved in immunosurveillance and virus-cell interaction. Virology. 1991;184:1–8.

651. Smith CA, Davis T, Wignall JM, et al. T2 open reading frame from the Shope fibroma virus encodes a soluble form of the TNF receptor. Biochem Biophys Res Commun. 1991;176:335–42.

652. Kotwal GJ, Isaacs SN, McKenzie R, et al. Inhibition of the complement cascade by the major secretory protein of vaccinia virus. Science. 1990;250:827–30.

653. Spriggs MK, Hruby DE, Maliszewski CR et al. Vaccinia and cowpox viruses encode a novel secreted interleukin-1-binding protein. Cell. 1992;71:145–52.

654. Alcami A, Smith GL: Cell. A soluble receptor for interleukin-1β encoded by vaccinia virus. Cell. 1992;71:153–67.

655. Ray CA, Black RA, Kronheim SR, et al. Viral inhibition of inflammation: Cowpox virus encodes an inhibitor of the interleukin-1β converting enzyme. Cell. 1992;69:597–604.

656. Upton C, Macen JL, Schreiber M, McFadden G: Myxoma virus expresses a secreted protein with homology to the tumor necrosis factor receptor gene family that contributes to viral virulence. Virology. 1991;184:370–82.

657. Bhat RA, Thimmappaya B. Two small RNAs encoded by Epstein-Barr virus can functionally substitute for the virus-associated RNAs on the lytic growth of adenovirus. Proc Natl Acad Sci USA. 1983;80:4789–93.

658. Hsu D-H, de Waal Malefyt R, Florentino DF, et al. Expression of interleukin-10 activity by Epstein-Barr virus protein BCRF1. Science. 1990;250:830–32.

659. Browne H, Smith G, Beck S, Minson T. A complex between the MHC class I homologue encoded by human cytomegalovirus and β2 microglobin. Nature. 1990;347:770–72.

660. Gao J, Kuhns DB, Tiffany HL, et al. Structure and functional expression of the human macrophage inflammatory protein 1α/RANTES receptor. J Exp Med. 1993;177:1421–7.

661. Harris SL, Frank I, Yee A, et al. Glycoprotein C of herpes simplex virus type I prevents complement-mediated cell lysis and virus neutralization. J Infect Dis. 1990;162:331–37.

662. Bell S, Cranage M, Borysiewicz L, Minson T. Induction of immunoglobulin C fc receptors by recombinant vaccinia viruses expressing glycoproteins E and I of herpes simplex virus type I. J Virol. 1990;64:2181–86.

663. Albrecht J-C, Fleckenstein B. New member of the multigene family of complement control proteins in Herpesvirus saimiri. J Virol. 192;66:3937–80.

9. EVALUATION OF THE PATIENT WITH SUSPECTED IMMUNODEFICIENCY

STEVEN M. HOLLAND
JOHN I. GALLIN

The most common causes of immunodeficiency are iatrogenic, with the widespread use of therapies that modulate the immune system either by design or incidentally. With the expanding recognition, characterization, and, in an increasing number of cases, correction of immune abnormalities, making the correct diagnosis is no longer of only academic interest. The identification and cloning of disease-related genes has now made precise antenatal diagnosis and genetic counseling a reality. The promise of the emerging field of gene transfer technology makes a sensible, problem-oriented approach to the patient in whom these issues are raised essential. Following are some general principles involved in the consideration of whether a patient may have an immunodeficiency and how to proceed with a diagnostic evaluation before or as an adjunct to referral or discussion with a specialist.

THE INDEX OF SUSPICION

Concern about the immune status of a patient is usually raised on the basis of the frequency, severity, distribution, or the infectious agent of one or more episodes that are, or are thought to be, infectious. Table 1 lists some infectious organisms and the affected limb of host defense implied by their isolation. Obviously not every isolation of a herpesvirus or a *Staphylococcus* implies an immunodeficiency in a specific patient. However, in the setting of abnormally frequent infections or failure to thrive, isolation of these organisms from patient samples should make one consider possible underlying diagnoses. In contrast, isolation of *Pseumocystis carinii, Pseudomonas cepacia, Aspergillus,* or *Nocardia* from a patient without a known immunodeficiency is sufficient grounds for pursuing the probability of an underlying defect.

Recurrent hematogenous neisserial infections indicate deficiencies in the late components of complement.[1] *Pn. carinii* pneumonia indicates T-cell abnormalities.[2] *Ps. cepacia* bacteremia strongly suggests chronic granulomatous disease.[3] Some specific immunodeficiencies are listed in Table 2, along with the gene defect, if known, and some pertinent findings. Recognition and appreciation of the genetic basis of these disorders has been critical to development of treatments for them and is fundamental to the curative approaches that are now underway.

INITIAL EVALUATION

The screening approach to the patient with suspected immunodeficiency is listed in Table 3. Careful attention to historical detail is critical. Age of onset of illness is helpful; Job syndrome often has onset within the first days to weeks of life, whereas

TABLE 1. Selected Disease-Associated Pathogens

Pathogen	History	Host Defense Affected	Clinical Examples
Pneumocystis carinii, Cryptococcus neoformans, herpesviruses	Disseminated infections, opportunistic infections, persistent viral infections	T cells	Severe combined immunodeficiency, acquired immunodeficiency syndrome
Haemophilus influenzae, Streptococcus pneumoniae, Giardia lamblia, Campylobacter spp., enteroviruses	Recurrent respiratory infections with encapsulated organisms, chronic diarrhea, aseptic meningitis	B cells	Common variable immunodeficiency, X-linked agammaglobulinemia
Staphylococcus aureus, Pseudomonas cepacia, Serratia marsescens, Aspergillus spp., Nocardia spp.	Gingivitis, aphthous ulcers, recurrent pyogenic infections, delayed umbilical stump separation	Phagocytes	Chronic granulomatous disease, Chédiak-Higashi syndrome, leukocyte adhesion deficiency
Neisseria spp.	Recurrent bacteremia, recurrent meningitis	Complement	Late complement component deficiency
Staphylococcus aureus, Haemophilus influenzae, Streptococcus pneumoniae, Candida albicans	Eczema, kyphoscoliosis, bony deformities and fractures, pulmonary and cutaneous infections, mucocutaneous candidiasis	T cells, phagocytes	Hyper immunoglobulin E and recurrent infections (Job syndrome)

antibody deficiency states only appear after several months of life when maternal immunoglobulin levels have fallen.[4] Failure to thrive and diarrhea are important points in favor of a substantial problem but are not specific in terms of etiology. Birth history should include the condition and time of separation of the umbilical stump, as this is abnormally delayed in leukocyte adhesion deficiency.[5] The past medical history should note the administration of vaccines, especially for measles, mumps, rubella, vaccinia, and Calmette-Guérin bacillus (BCG), difficulties with which are suggestive of dysfunctional T-cell immunity. A dental history can be quite informative, as patients with abnormalities of phagocytic defense often have gingivitis with periodontal disease.[6] Specific questioning regarding parental consanguinity is critical.

The physical examination can yield findings diagnostic or highly suggestive of lesions in specific arms of the immune system. Facial anomalies, including hypertelorism, a shortened philtrum, and downslanting palpebral fissures, are encountered in DiGeorge syndrome,[2] while hypertelorism, coarse facies, and a triangular mandible are seen in the syndrome of extremely elevated IgE and recurrent infections (Job syndrome).[7] Hair with a silvery sheen and irregular melanization is seen in Chédiak-Higashi syndrome.[8] In general, poor dentition, gingivitis, aphthous ulcers, and tooth loss are seen in phagocytic defects such as chronic granulomatous disease and leukocyte adhesion deficiency, whereas supernumerary teeth are encountered in Job syndrome.[6] Cutaneous signs of immune defects include telangiectases over the bulbar conjunctivae and skin in ataxia telangiectasia, severe eczema that accompanies Job syndrome, or dystrophic scarring seen in leukocyte adhesion deficiency.

The initial laboratory examination should consist of a complete blood count with differential, platelet count, review of the peripheral smear, and erythrocyte sedimentation rate. Chédiak-Higashi syndrome and neutrophil specific granule deficiency can be detected on peripheral smear, whereas Kostmann syndrome (congenital agranulocytosis) and Wiskott-Aldrich syndrome can be excluded by normal neutrophil or platelet counts, respectively. An immunoglobulin profile with total levels of IgA, IgM, and IgG will help detect cases of IgA deficiency as well as hypogammaglobulinemia. In cases in which eczema is a prominent feature or Job syndrome is suspected, measures of IgE levels are indicated. A functional challenge of the humoral immune system, such as pre- and postimmunization antibody levels, may be informative. Testing of total hemolytic complement (CH_{50}) gives a quick assessment of the functional integrity of the classical component of the complement cascade from C1 through the membrane attack complex (C5–C9). Plain radiographs of the chest can demonstrate pulmonary scarring, pneumatoceles, and destruction, often encountered in phagocyte defects and Job syndrome. Kyphoscoliosis, osteoporosis, rib, and long bone fractures and their sequelae are seen frequently in Job syndrome.[7]

LYMPHOCYTE IMMUNE DEFECTS

T Cells and Cell-Mediated Immunity

The initial presentation of congenital T-cell defects is usually, but not always, within the first few months of life and includes severe mucocutaneous candidiasis, recurrent, persistent respiratory infections, diarrhea, and failure to thrive. There is a broad spectrum of onset and severity. Reticular dysgenesis presents within the first weeks of life, with pancytopenia, infection, and early demise.[9,10] The lymphocyte enzymopathies (adenosine deaminase deficiency and purine nucleoside phosphorylase deficiency) tend to present after several months of life when lymphocyte counts begin to fall due to the accumulation of the toxic metabolites dATP and dGTP, respectively.[11,12] The occurrence of *Pn. carinii* pneumonia, disseminated BCG infection following vaccination, persistent polio virus infection after oral polio vaccination, or persistent respiratory virus infection should initiate a consideration of a defect in lymphocyte function.[13] Graft versus host disease, either acquired from in utero transfer of maternal lymphocytes or through transfusion of unirradiated blood, may be the underlying cause of cutaneous eruptions, transaminase elevations, or malabsorption and diarrhea and is a strong indicator of defective T-cell immunity.[13]

In many forms of T-cell abnormality, B-cell function is also compromised, leading to both cell-mediated and humoral deficiencies, a state referred to as *severe combined immunodeficiency* (SCID).[13] This syndrome tends to be recognized after maternal antibody levels wane and recurrent bacterial infections begin. The finding of low immunoglobulin levels in association with marked lymphopenia in the appropriate setting should lead to the consideration of SCID.[2]

The most direct and simplest assessment of T-cell immune status is the determination of the lymphocyte number, which is obtained in the screening differential count. Circulating lymphocyte number ranges from about 7000 cells/μl in the infant to 4000 cells/μl in children and about 2000 cells/μl in adolescents and adults through old age.[14] Of these lymphocytes, roughly half are T cells, with the remainder split between B cells and natural killer cells. Severe quantitative abnormalities of lymphocytes are relatively uncommon; low absolute lymphocyte numbers are encountered in the great majority of cases of SCID, as well as in several other congenital immunodeficiencies (Table 2). The acquired immunodeficiency syndrome (AIDS), high plasma corticosteroids (iatrogenic or endogenous), obstructed lymphatic circulation (e.g., intestinal lymphangiectasia), severe systemic illness (e.g., carcinomatosis, miliary tuberculosis), systemic lupus erythematosus, sarcoid, cytotoxic, or immunosuppressive therapy, and severe right-sided congestive heart failure can also cause lymphocytopenia.

T-lymphocyte function is initially and most easily assayed in vivo by testing of type IV cell-mediated immunity, delayed-type hypersensitivity (DTH) (Table 4). DTH is elicited by the intra-

TABLE 2. Congenital Immunodeficiencies

Clinical Disease	Affected Gene Product[a]	Chromosomal Location	Inheritance	Functional Defect	Important Findings	References
T cells						
Severe Combined Immunodeficiency (SCID)						13
X-linked SCID	Interleukin-2 receptor γ-chain	Xq13–21.1	X	T-cell proliferation, antibody production	Lymphopenia, hypogammaglobulinemia	71
Adenosine deaminase deficiency (ADA)	Adenosine deaminase	20q13–ter	AR	T-cell functions, antibody production	Absent ADA activity, lymphopenia, hypogammaglobulinemia	11, 72, 73
Purine nucleoside phosphorylase deficiency (PNP)	Purine nucleoside phosphorylase	14q13.1	AR	T-cell functions	Absent PNP activity, low CD3 + cells, increased NK cells, low uric acid	12, 72, 74
Defective MHC molecules	MHC classes I and II, RF-X	19q13	AR	Cell-mediated immunity	B cells normal, Ig normal or low, absent MHC molecules	21, 75
IL-2 deficiency	Nuclear factor activated T cells (NFAT)	?	AR	Cell-mediated immunity, antibody production	Lymphopenia, hypogammaglobulinemia	18–20
Reticular dysgenesis	?	?	AR	Pancytopenia	Pancytopenia	9, 10
DiGeorge syndrome	?hox 1.5	22q11.21–q11.23	AD	Anomalous development 3rd and 4th pharyngeal pouches	Thymic aplasia, parathyroid aplasia, cardiac anomalies, abnormal facies	23, 24
Ataxia-telangiectasia	?	11q22.3	AR	DNA repair, T cells	Low IgA, Low CD3 and CD4 cells	25, 76, 77
Wiskott-Aldrich	CD43, sialophorin	Xq11–11.3	X	T cells and platelets	Thrombocytopenia, Low IgM, high IgA	26–28
B cells						
X-linked agammaglobulinemia	B-cell progenitor kinase (BPK)	Xq22	X	B cells	Very low antibody levels	78, 79
X-linked immunodeficiency with hyper IgM	CD40 ligand (gp39)	Xq26	X	B cells	High IgM, Low IgG, IgA	80, 81
X-linked lymphoproliferative syndrome (Duncan syndrome)	?	Xq26–27	X	EBV response	Low EBNA antibody	31, 82
Common variable immunodeficiency	?	?	?	Antibody synthesis	Low IgG, poor antibody response, low IgA common	32
IgA deficiency	IgA	?6p21.3	AR	IgA	Associated with other immunodeficiencies	32
Phagocytes						
Chronic Granulomatous Disease (CGD)						
X-linked CGD	gp91[phox]	Xp21.1	X	Bacterial and fungal killing defective in all forms of CGD	Infections with catalase + microbes, granulomas, and absent NBT reduction and superoxide generation 60% of CGD	47, 83, 84, 85
Autosomal recessive CGD	p22[phox]	16q24	AR		5% of CGD	86, 87
	p47[phox]	7q11.23	AR		30% of CGD	87, 88
	p67[phox]	1q25	AR		5% of CGD	87, 89
Cyclic neutropenia	?G-CSF	?5q	AR	Neutropenia	Cyclic hematopoiesis, cycle about 21 days	34
Chédiak-Higashi syndrome	?	?1q43	AR	Chemotactic defect, neutropenia	Giant granules in neutrophils, oculocutaneous albinism	8, 36, 37
Leukocyte adhesion deficiency type 1	CD18	21q22.3	AR	Absent integrins	Chronic leukocytosis, delayed umbilical cord separation, recurrent infections	5, 90, 91
Leukocyte adhesion deficiency type 2	Sialyl-Lewis X	?19q	AR	E-selectin ligand, ?fucose metabolism	Short stature, mental retardation	39
Neutrophil specific granule deficiency	?	?	AR	Neutrophil granule products	Absent neutrophil-specific granules	42, 43
Myeloperoxidase deficiency	Myeloperoxidase	17q21–q23	AR	Conversion superoxide to hydrogen peroxide	Absent myeloperoxidase, usually unassociated with infections	45
Hyper IgE recurrent infection syndrome (Job syndrome)	?	?	AD	Intermittently poor chemotaxis, ?CD8 T-cell dysfunction	Extremely high IgE, eczema, facial and bony abnormalities, pneumatocele formations	4, 7, 60

(Continued)

TABLE 2. (Continued)

Clinical Disease	Affected Gene Product[a]	Chromosomal Location	Inheritance	Functional Defect	Important Findings	References
Complement						
Classical pathway				Antibody-dependent complement lysis is depressed in all forms of classical complement component deficiencies	Low CH₅₀ is seen with all forms of classical complement component deficiency. Individual components are very low or absent. Autoimmune disease common in early component deficiencies (C1–C4). Bacteremia and meningitis are common in all types of complement deficiency	1
C1q deficiency	C1q	1p	AR			
C1r deficiency	C1r	12p13	AR			
C1s deficiency	C1s	12p13	AR			
C2 deficiency	C2	6p21.3	AR			
C3 deficiency	C3	19p13.2–p13.11	AR			
C4A deficiency	C4A	6p21.3	AR			
C4B deficiency	C4B	6p21.3	AR			
C5 deficiency	C5	9q22–q34	AR			
C6 deficiency	C6	5	AR			
C7 deficiency	C7	1p22	AR			
C8 deficiency	C8	1p36.2–p22.1	AR			
C9 deficiency	C9	5p14–p12	AR			
Alternative pathway				Antibody-independent complement lysis is depressed in alternative complement component deficiencies	More severe susceptibility to infection than classical component deficiencies.	
Properdin deficiency	Properdin	Xp21–p11	X			
Factor H deficiency	Factor H	1q32	AR			
Factor I deficiency	Factor I	4q25	AR			

Abbreviations: X, X-linked inheritance; AR, autosomal recessive; AD, autosomal dominant.
[a] The affected gene product is not always the gene in which the lesion has occurred. The genetic lesion may disable a regulatory gene required for expression or function of the affected gene product.

TABLE 3. Screening Evaluations for Immune Defects

History
  Medications and treatments
  Relatedness of parents, umbilical stump separation, age of onset
  Frequency, severity, distribution, type of infections
  Vaccination history, especially live vaccines
  Causative infectious agents

Physical
  Weight and height
  Hair: sheen, pigmentation
  Abdomen: organomegaly
  Skin: dystrophic scars, telangiectases, eczema
  Oropharynx: thrush, ulcers, gingivitis
  Facies: hypertelorism, eye slant, philtrum
  Skeleton: kyphoscoliosis, fractures

Routine Laboratory
  Complete blood count
    Differential: lymphopenia, neutropenia, eosinophilia
    Peripheral smear: giant granules, specific (secondary) granules
    Platelet count: thrombocytopenia
    Erythrocyte sedimentation rate: usually elevated in infection
  Chemistries
    Serum calcium
    Serum uric acid
    Liver functions
  Immunoglobulins
    IgA, IgM, IgG, IgE
    Isohemagglutinins
    Antibody titers (tetanus, pneumococcus, etc.)
  Complement
    Total hemolytic complement (CH₅₀)

Radiographs
  Plain chest films: kyphoscoliosis, pneumatoceles, scarring

TABLE 4. Directed Tests of Immune Function

T cells
  Fluorescence-activated cell sorting (FACS)
  Delayed-type hypersensitivity: mumps, Candida, tetanus, trichophyton
  Lymphocyte enzymes (adenosine deaminase and purine nucleoside phosphorylase)
  Cytokine production and response
  In vitro proliferation: stimulation with antigen, lectin, antibody, allogeneic cells phosphokinase C stimulants and calcium ionophores

B cells
  Fluorescence activated cell sorting (FACS)
  Antigen challenge, recall or new
  In vitro antibody production

Phagocytes
  Fluorescence activated cell sorting (FACS) for leukocyte adhesion molecules
  Nitroblue tetrazolium reduction
  Superoxide generation, hydrogen peroxide generation
  Adherence
  Staphylococcidal activity
  Chemotaxis
  Phagocytosis

Complement
  Assay of individual complement components, functional or quantitative

dermal injection of an antigen to which the patient has been exposed. Antigen-specific CD4+ T cells are recruited that in turn recruit macrophages with resulting interstitial fibrin deposition and induration. Erythema and edema are seen early after the injection but are not indicative of DTH. Frank induration is appreciated best between 24 and 48 hours and then gradually falls off. Effective DTH is indicated by induration. In the screening evaluation for immune defects, it is important to consider the patient's antigenic experience, such as immunizations, previous infections, and regional exposures in the selection of antigens. It is critical to test several different antigens simultaneously for the determination of T-cell responsiveness, such as mumps, can-

dida, trichophyton, streptococcal antigens, and tetanus. The demonstration of intact DTH confirms the presence of functional CD4+ T cells and excludes most of the congenital defects in cell-mediated immunity. Importantly, DTH can be preserved until relatively late into human immunodeficiency (HIV) infection. Therefore, the presence of DTH should not be considered evidence against HIV infection per se. Selective anergy to the antigens of the offending organism has been observed in active visceral leishmaniasis and lepromatous leprosy. These specific defects have reversed following successful treatment of the underlying infection.[15] Complete anergy to a battery of antigens is a relatively nonspecific finding in terms of etiology, insofar as the differential diagnosis includes all the entities that cause lymphopenia. However, anergy makes further evaluation of the cell-mediated immune system reasonable.

Fluorescence-activated cell sorting (FACS) analysis now allows rapid enumeration and characterization of lymphocyte subsets.[16] Access to FACS analysis is widely available. Lymphocyte subset determination, specifically for CD4+ T cells, is standard in the management of HIV infection in order to provide guideposts for initiation of antiviral and prophylactic therapies. With the recent identification and cloning of certain immunodeficiency-related genes, FACS may be able to confirm or exclude specific diagnoses.

Evaluation of T-cell function in vitro requires laboratory personnel skilled in the isolation, preparation, and stimulation of peripheral blood mononuclear cells. Stimulation is typically done on unseparated peripheral blood mononuclear cells and therefore represents the product of both lymphocyte and monocyte contributions. Proliferation is usually measured as ^{3}H-thymidine incorporation into the DNA of dividing lymphocytes following stimulation with cell membrane binding lectins (phytohemagglutinin, concanavalin A, pokeweed mitogen), direct stimulants of cellular signalling pathways that bypass the need for membrane components (phorbol myristate acetate and calcium ionophore), antigens (PPD, candida, tetanus), cytokines (interleukin-2 [IL-2], or allogeneic cells (mixed lymphocyte reaction).[16] Significantly low proliferation in vitro can result from absent cell surface receptors, such as the CD3 complex,[17] antigen-specific anergy as in leishmaniasis,[15] IL-2 deficiencies,[18-20] or major histocompatibility complex abnormalities.[21] Recently two important CD4+ T-cell subsets were recognized. Th1 cells produce interferon-γ and IL-2 and are the predominant cells in the DTH response. Th2 cells produce interleukins 4, 5, and 10 and can regulate the differentiation of B cells and eosinophils. Both of these cell types regulate each other and therefore open new areas for the likely discovery of immune defects and new therapeutic manipulations of their relationship.[22] Cytokine levels in the supernatants of stimulated and unstimulated cells can be readily determined and may demonstrate states of either deficiency[18-20] or excess.

DiGeorge syndrome is caused by anomalous development of the third and fourth pharyngeal pouches with agenesis of the thymus and parathyroids and subsequent immunodeficiency and hypocalcemia. Neonatal tetany is an expected presentation.[23] The recent duplication of some of the cardinal features of DiGeorge syndrome in mice with disruption in one of the homeobox genes (hox 1.5) has raised the possibility of a defect in a homeobox-controlling gene in humans.[24] Ataxia-telangiectasia is associated with low IgA, CD3+ and CD4+ T-cell levels, progressive ataxia, and oculocutaneous telangiectases. These patients usually experience recurrent bacterial respiratory infections and are at increased risk of malignancy due to abnormalities in DNA repair.[2,25] Wiskott-Aldrich syndrome is characterized by eczema, thrombocytopenia, and recurrent opportunistic infections.[26] Recently, a gene product defective in Wiskott-Aldrich syndrome was identified as sialophorin, CD43.[27,28]

B Cells and Humoral Immunity

It is little over 40 years since the first description of an immunodeficiency syndrome, X-linked agammaglobulinemia (XLA), by Colonel Bruton.[29] The clinical presentation of immunoglobulin defects is distinct from that of T-cell or combined defects. The age of onset for congenital deficiencies is between 6 months and 2 years, and the presenting infections are predominantly with encapsulated bacteria. The thymus gland is present and apparently normal in XLA, but peripheral lymphoid tissues such as tonsils and lymph nodes are essentially absent.[30] B cells and plasma cells in the circulation and the periphery are rare despite normal numbers of pre-B cells in the bone marrow. These patients have elevated T-cell numbers, normal T-cell subsets, and intact T-cell functions. Although they have significant problems with bacterial infections, XLA patients also have severe difficulty with persistent, disseminated echoviral infections, especially in the central nervous system. Immunoglobulins G, A, and M levels are extremely low, as are those of isohemagglutinins. There is no antibody detectable to either new or previously administered antigens. In contrast, patients with another X-linked B-cell defect, immunoglobulin deficiency with elevated IgM, may have preserved lymphoid tissue mass, hepatosplenomegaly, normal numbers of B cells and T cells, and variable neutropenia. Autoimmune phenomena such as Coombs positive hemolytic anemia and thrombocytopenia are common. IgM is elevated, and IgG and IgA are usually quite low; isohemagglutinins may be elevated.[30] The X-linked lymphoproliferative disease Duncan syndrome occurs in males only after infection with Epstein-Barr virus and results in a full blown immunodeficiency syndrome that can be fatal.[31] Some abnormality in response to Epstein-Barr virus is thought to underlie this disorder, which can lead to malignancy.

The initial test for the integrity of the humoral arm of immunity is the determination of levels of isohemagglutinins (see below) and levels of IgG, IgA, and IgM. Normal immunoglobulin levels are relatively low in infancy and childhood and increase with age. If immunoglobulin levels are appropriate, both XLA and immunoglobulin deficiency with elevated IgM can be excluded. Low immunoglobulin levels may be seen within the first year of life in the transient hypogammaglobulinemia of infancy.[2,30] However, these infants usually have detectable isohemagglutinins and can mount antibody responses to new antigenic challenges. Despite family histories notable for relatives with immunodeficiencies, patients with transient hypogammaglobulinemia of infancy tend to normalize their immunoglobulin levels over the first 2 years of life. The finding of depressed levels of immunoglobulin, especially in an adult with recurrent bacterial sinopulmonary infections, raises the possibility of common variable immunodeficiency.[32] Common variable immunodeficiency is a heterogeneous group of diseases that share the features of hypogammaglobulinemia and an increased susceptibility to chronic enteric infections with *Giardia lamblia, Campylobacter,* and disseminated echoviral infections in addition to sinopulmonary bacterial infections. Patients with common variable immunodeficiency often have low isohemagglutinins and abnormal DTH and fail to make antibody to new antigens. IgG subclass analysis may show selective defects in IgG 1 and 3 or 2 and 4 in addition to IgA.[32]

Isohemagglutinins are IgM antibodies directed against blood groups A and B antigens, which occur in all healthy people except those with blood group AB. By the age of 3, 98 percent of blood groups A, B, or O patients have isohemagglutinins with a titer of at least 1:16.[32] Isohemagglutinin levels are determined in blood banks as a prerequisite to transfusion. Challenge with antigen is probably the most effective method for determining the functional integrity of the humoral immune system. Use of a recall antigen allows for testing of anamnestic responses. Novel antigens such as bacteriophage ΦX174 or keyhole limpet hemocyanin make possible the testing of antibody responses during immunoglobulin administration. Pneumococcal vaccination examines the response to polysaccharide antigen, whereas tetanus challenge is more specific for peptide responses. Serum titers should be checked before and 2 weeks after immunization.

PHAGOCYTE IMMUNE DEFECTS: NEUTROPHILS

The clinical presentations of patients with neutrophil disorders often share common features: gingivitis, periodontal disease, and oral ulceration.[6] Cutaneous infections with *Staphylococcus aureus* are recurrent and can be severe. In neutrophil disorders characterized by inadequate inflammation (neutropenia, leukocyte adhesion deficiency, Chédiak-Higashi syndrome, neutrophil-specific granule deficiency), infections can extend locally and subcutaneously with little reaction until marked destruction has taken place. Visceral and especially sinopulmonary involvement are features that help distinguish neutrophil defects from other syndromes in the differential diagnosis. Hepatic abscess is a frequent manifestation of chronic granulomatous disease and is most often due to *S. aureus,* an organism rarely encountered at that anatomic site in patients with normal neutrophils.

Neutropenia

A neutrophil count below 500 cells/μl carries a profound risk of bacterial and fungal infection.[33] Although this principle was first extensively documented and is still most frequently displayed in cancer and leukemia patients undergoing combination chemotherapy, its importance has been confirmed in patients with genetic disorders that affect neutrophil number. Cyclic neutropenia or cyclic hematopoiesis is a rare disease occurring in autosomal dominant, spontaneous, and acquired forms characterized by regular 21-day oscillations in the levels of blood neutrophils, monocytes, eosinophils, lymphocytes, platelets, and reticulocytes.[34] The defect is at the level of the hematopoietic stem cell and is associated with abnormal colony-stimulating factor responses in bone marrow precursor cells. It is postulated that cyclic neutropenia may represent dysregulated feedback from the circulating cell pool to the marrow. Patients usually present in childhood and have recurrent episodes of fever, malaise, mucosal ulcers, and, occasionally, life-threatening infections associated with periods of profound neutropenia (<200/μl).[34] Adult onset cases have been described with an associated clonal proliferation of large granular lymphocytes as well. Neutrophil number is transiently impaired, but function is normal. The diagnosis is suspected in children with recurrent stomatitis, gingivitis, cutaneous infections, lymphadenopathy, and fever. The diagnosis can only be established after repeated white blood cell counts with differentials at least three times per week for at least 6 weeks. In congenital agranulocytosis (Kostmann syndrome[35]), neutrophil counts are consistently low from birth and show no periodicity. Both syndromes are successfully treated with recombinant granulocyte colony-stimulating factor.

Chédiak-Higashi Syndrome

Chédiak-Higashi syndrome is a rare autosomal recessive disorder characterized by recurrent bacterial infections, partial oculocutaneous albinism, photophobia, nystagmus, and peripheral neuropathy. Many patients die in childhood from infection. About half of the patients who survive into adolescence develop an aggressive "lymphoproliferative" phase with diffuse organ infiltration and death. Several patients have lived into adulthood at which time an aggressive, severe, debilitating peripheral neuropathy is a common feature.[8] Pathologically, giant abnormal granules are found in neutrophils, melanocytes, hair, Schwann cells, the central nervous system, peripheral ganglia, capillary epithelium, renal tubular epithelium, erythroid precursors, fibroblasts, and other granule containing cells.[8] In neutrophils the granules are formed mainly by fusion of azurophilic or primary granules to each other and to a lesser extent to specific or secondary granules.[36]

Features of Chédiak-Higashi syndrome include central and peripheral nervous system involvement with peripheral neuropathy, myopathy, autonomic dysfunction, and leptomeningeal involvement.[8] Lymphohistiocytic infiltration of axons and myelin sheaths occurs in patients with peripheral neuropathy and in ganglia in patients with autonomic neuropathy. Melanin granules seen in the neurons of the substantia nigra are large, irregular, and clumped. These aggregates of melanosomes seem to increase in size and number with age. Low intelligence has been noted in some series.[8] The diagnosis of Chédiak-Higashi syndrome is easily made by inspection of the peripheral smear for giant lysosomes or microscopic examination of hair for characteristic melanin clumps. Although no candidate genes have been proposed so far, the defect probably maps to chromosome 1q43.[37]

Leukocyte Adhesion Deficiency

Leukocyte adhesion to endothelium and other leukocytes is mediated by several sets of molecules, among which are the integrins and the selectins. It is now recognized that defects in either of these two intercellular adhesion pathways can lead to overlapping clinical phenotypes. Leukocyte adhesion deficiency type 1 (LAD 1) is a rare autosomal recessive disorder involving one set of the leukocyte integrins, the molecules required for leukocyte adherence to endothelium, other leukocytes, and bacteria.[38] Deficiency of the integrin component CD18 leads to a corresponding deficiency of the complexes LFA-1, Mac-1, and p150,95 and resulting abnormalities of cellular adhesion. These abnormalities are predictable from the basic defect. The absence of a marginated pool of neutrophils leads to chronic leukocytosis, while the poor inflammatory response leads to recurrent infections.

LAD1 falls into two broad categories, severe and moderate, depending on the degree of CD18 deficiency.[5] Patients with severe deficiency (<0.5 percent) of normal protein expression are characterized by delayed umbilical stump separation, umbilical stump infection, persistent leukocytosis in the absence of active infection(>15,000/μl), and severe, destructive periodontitis with associated loss of dentition and alveolar bone. Recurrent infections of the skin, upper and lower airways, bowel and perirectal area and septicemia are common and usually due to *S. aureus* or gram-negative rods, most notably *Pseudomonas* spp. Infections tend to be necrotizing and may progress to ulceration, but demonstrate an almost complete absence of neutrophil invasion on histopathology. Patients with the moderate form of disease (3–10 percent of normal expression) tend to have normal umbilical stump separation, be diagnosed later in life, and less commonly have life-threatening infections. Leukocytosis is still the rule, as is delayed wound healing and periodontal disease. Although the patients with the moderate form of the disease are less ill and tend to live past childhood, deaths from infection have been reported in young adults.[5]

Laboratory findings in general reflect the clinical differences between severe and moderate phenotypes of the disease, with the severe form showing more profound deficiencies than the moderate form. Abnormalities include grossly defective granulocyte and mononuclear cell mobilization into Rebuck skin windows in vivo and diminished neutrophil migration in response to the bacterial chemoattractant f-met-leu-phe in vitro, despite normal numbers of receptors.[5] These laboratory abnormalities are demonstrated in vivo in histologic sections of infected tissues, showing the presence of some mononuclear cells but very low numbers of neutrophils. Patient granulocyte adherence to glass, plastic, nylon wool, and to other LAD granulocytes is greatly reduced and is not stimulated by exposure to f-met-leu-phe or phorbol myristate acetate (PMA). The absence of CD18 leads to the absence of Mac-1 and the iC3b receptor CR3. Therefore, complement-mediated phagocytosis is severely impaired whereas IgG-mediated phagocytosis is normal. Although viral infections are not usually special problems in LAD, antibody-dependent cellular cytotoxicity by patient cells is also diminished. Oxidative metabolism in response to PMA or calcium ionophore is normal in patient granulocytes as measured by nitroblue tetrazolium reduction or chemiluminescence. Neutrophil primary and secondary granule release in response to PMA or chemoattractants are normal in LAD cells, whereas the response after zymosan particle ingestion is depressed.

Diagnosis is established through a thorough history with special attention to depressed inflammation in the neonatal period with delayed umbilical stump separation and recurrent infections. A dental history is helpful, as most of these patients have severe problems with gingivitis, periodontal disease, tooth loss, and alveolar bone erosion. Wounds often heal abnormally, leaving dystrophic, paper thin scars. The diagnosis is confirmed by FACS, which shows reduction or absence of the components of the leukocyte adhesion molecules CD18, CD11a, CD11b, and CD11c.

In leukocyte adhesion deficiency type 2 (LAD 2), neutrophil adherence to endothelial cells is defective, presumably on the basis of the absence of the sialyl-Lewis X antigen on the neutrophil surface, which is the binding site for E-selectin.[39–41] The patients reported are the products of consanguineous marriages. They have had neutrophilia, recurrent pulmonary, periodontal, and cutaneous infections, abnormal chemotaxis, mental retardation, short stature, distinctive facies, and the Bombay (hh) blood phenotype. The underlying defect is probably autosomal recessive and appears to be in fucose metabolism.[39]

Neutrophil-Specific Granule Deficiency

Neutrophil-specific (secondary) granule deficiency is a rare (five cases reported), heterogeneous, probably autosomal recessive disease characterized by the profound reduction or absence of neutrophil-specific granules and their contents.[42] Associated abnormalities in the few patients reported include bi- or tri-lobed neutrophil nuclei, absence of some neutrophil primary (azurophil) granule proteins, mononuclear eosinophils without eosinophil granules, and dysfunction of platelet α-granules. The neutrophil-specific granule protein lactoferrin has been shown to be diminished or absent in these patients' neutrophils, and the defective production of lactoferrin is relatively tissue specific with normal production by lacrimal glands.[42,43] Sibling deaths at early ages, consanguineous marriages in parents of patients, and occurrence of the syndrome in females lead to the assumption of an autosomal recessive pattern of inheritance for neutrophil-specific granule deficiency.

Myeloperoxidase Deficiency

Myeloperoxidase (MPO; also called *verdoperoxidase*), the heme-binding protein that makes pus green, catalyses the conversion of hydrogen peroxide to hypochlorous acid (bleach). MPO deficiency is the most common neutrophil disorder, affecting about 1 in 2000 persons, but is quite silent in most cases. Neutrophil function is affected by MPO deficiency in a variety of ways. The respiratory burst in MPO-deficient neutrophils is prolonged, resulting in exaggerated amounts of hydrogen peroxide produced.[45] The increased hydrogen peroxide production probably compensates functionally for the defect in hypochlorous acid production. Phagocytosis is normal to increased in MPO-deficient neutrophils, whereas bactericidal activity is somewhat slower than normal. Killing of *Aspergillus* conidia by MPO-deficient neutrophils is retarded, whereas the combination of MPO-deficient neutrophils with chronic granulomatous disease neutrophils (see below), which are unable to generate hydrogen peroxide but do produce MPO, results in normal killing of *Aspergillus* conidia.[46] Pathologic sequelae of MPO deficiency are only brought out in the presence of other impairments of host defense such as diabetes mellitus. A very few MPO-deficient diabetic patients have had severe yeast infections.

Chronic Granulomatous Disease

Chronic granulomatous disease (CGD) is a genetically heterogeneous group of disorders of phagocytic cell oxidative metabolism characterized by recurrent life-threatening infections with bacteria and fungi and dysregulated granuloma formation. The estimated frequency is 1 in 1 million persons, but may well be higher. CGD is caused by a defect in the NADPH oxidase that is responsible for the respiratory burst and the generation of hydrogen peroxide. Clinically, CGD is quite variable, ranging in time of presentation from infancy to late adulthood, with the majority of patients diagnosed as toddlers and young children. However, a significant number of patients are diagnosed later in life.[47,48] Children with CGD tend to be short and small for their age but tend eventually to achieve the height predicted by their parents' heights.[49]

The frequent infections are pulmonary, cutaneous, lymphatic, and hepatic. Osteomyelitis, perianal abscess, and gingivitis are also common.[48] The microbiology of the infections of CGD is remarkable for its relative specificity. As in other neutrophil abnormalities, the most common offender in CGD is *S. aureus*. Whereas the typical case of liver abscess in the immunologically normal patient involves enteric organisms and is liquid and easily drainable, the liver abscesses encountered in CGD are dense, caseous, and staphylococcal. Likewise lung, skin, and bone infections are usually staphylococcal. However, *Aspergillus* spp. and some of the rarer fungi such as *Exophiala dermatitidis*[50] and *Paecelomyces* spp.[51] are encountered in CGD. *Nocardia* sp., *Chromobacterium violaceum*, *Serratia marcescens*, and *Ps. cepacia* are other infections that are seen with unusual frequency in CGD and should suggest the diagnosis.[3,48,52] Bony involvement can occur by direct extension in the case of *Aspergillus* or hematogenously as in the case of *Staphylococcus* and *Nocardia*.[53] The advent of antibiotic prophylaxis has altered the frequency of infections in CGD and reduced the frequency of staphylococcal infections in particular.[3,52] The rate of fungal infections in CGD is lower than that for bacterial infections and has apparently not changed in the setting of prophylactic antibiotics.[54]

The granulomata that occur in CGD are presumed to originate from the inflammatory response to infectious or irritative foci (e.g., sutures) that fails to eradicate the infection or irritation. This persistent inflammatory reaction leads to exuberant and often obstructive granulomatous lesions. The gastrointestinal and genitourinary tracts are frequently involved by granulomatous lesions in CGD, sometimes as the site of the presenting complaint, sometimes asymptomatically. Ament and Ochs[55] noted frequent malabsorption, intrinsic factor unresponsive vitamin B$_{12}$ deficiency, abundant lipid-pigmented histiocytes in small bowel biopsy specimens, and pigmented histiocytes and granulomata in rectal biopsy material. These findings were present in both autosomal and X-linked patients. Esophageal, jejunal, ileal, cecal, rectal, and perirectal involvement with granulomata, often mimicking Crohn's disease, have been described. Gastric outlet obstruction is an especially common manifestation and may be the initial presentation of CGD. In a comprehensive review of genitourinary manifestations, Walther et al.[56] found that 38 percent of CGD patients had some kind of urologic event, including bladder granulomata, ureteral obstruction, and urinary tract infection.

Diagnosis of CGD is made by assays of superoxide or hydrogen peroxide production, such as nitroblue tetrazolium reduction or chemiluminescence. Mothers of boys with the X-linked form of CGD are obligate carriers of a defective X chromosome. Therefore, by lyonization, a certain proportion of the mother's cells will fail to reduce nitroblue tetrazolium, giving a characteristic mosaic pattern. By performing a nitroblue tetrazolium test on the mother's blood, one can comfortably determine the broad lines of inheritance of CGD in a given male.

An important adjunct to therapy is interferon γ, a cytokine with neutrophil and monocyte–macrophage stimulating properties that has reduced the frequency and severity of infections in CGD.[57] Although granulocyte transfusions supply only a small portion of the body's normal neutrophil output in a day, we believe they maybe effective in helping to clear severe infections. Transfused granulocytes produce superoxide, which can be used by the intact MPO system in CGD neutrophils, bypassing their biochemical defect.[58] The granulomatous complications of CGD pose a special problem in management. Although these patients are already somewhat immunocompromised, the judicious use of corticosteroids in conjunction with antibiotics has been successful in opening and maintaining patency of hollow visci in CGD patients.[59]

Hyper Immunoglobulin E-Recurrent Infection Syndrome (Job Syndrome)

Job syndrome is a rare disorder characterized by recurrent infections, typically of the lower respiratory system and skin, eczema, extremely elevated levels of IgE, and eosinophilia. The majority of patients have facial abnormalities, including ocular hypertelorism, a prominent, protruding, triangular mandible, and a broad, somewhat bulbous nose.[4,7,60] Supranumerary teeth are not infrequent. Most patients develop moderate to severe kyphoscoliosis. Many also have abnormalities of bone formation and metabolism, including *osteogenesis imperfecta tarda*, which may result in fractures and short stature, and craniosynostosis.[60-62] Job syndrome appears to occur spontaneously in all racial and ethnic groups, and in some cases it is apparently transmitted as an autosomal dominant trait.[4,63]

Patients usually present within the first days to months of life with severe eczema, mucocutaneous candidiasis, and cutaneous, sinus, or pulmonary infections predominantly with *S. aureus* or *Haemophilus influenzae*. Pneumatoceles are often noted early in life. Otitis media and externa are relatively common, as are intertriginous infections and breast abscesses. Infections occur less frequently in bone and joints, and very infrequently in liver, kidneys, and the gastrointestinal tract. Documented sepsis is rare. Deep tissue infections are frequently extensions of paronychia or apical abscesses. Recurrent "cold" abscesses of the skin are commonly due to staphylococci. These are a cutaneous manifestation of the impaired inflammatory response in these patients, insofar as substantial infection may elicit only modest reaction and is often unassociated with a sense of illness on the part of the patient. Pathogens that have been recovered from patients with Job syndrome include *S. aureus*, *H. influenzae*, *Aspergillus* spp., *P. aeruginosa*, *Streptococcus pneumoniae*, group A streptococci, *Cryptococcus neoformans*, and *Candida albicans*.[4,7,60]

The syndrome is defined by marked elevations of IgE (>2000 IU/ml), with levels of more than 50,000 IU/ml reported.[4] Levels may start out elevated in cord blood and then climb through infancy and childhood.[63] Therefore, although a high IgE level is part of the diagnostic criteria for Job syndrome, authentic cases do at times lack this particular feature. The catabolism of IgE is abnormally reduced in both Job syndrome and atopic dermatitis, contributing further to the elevated levels of IgE seen in these syndromes.[64] A high proportion of the IgE in Job syndrome binds to *S. aureus* and *C. albicans*.[65] That this is specific was shown by the absence of binding to *Escherichia coli* and *S. pneumoniae*. The lack of similar binding activity in other patients infected frequently with *S. aureus* indicates that this abnormality is host, and not organism, driven. The presence of elevated anti-*S. aureus* IgE is specific for Job syndrome and can help in the discrimination of this syndrome from severe atopic dermatitis with high IgE levels.[65] White blood cell counts are typically normal, but have been reported to range from 60,000 to 1700/μl.[4,7] Chronic leukopenia with borderline neutropenia has been observed in several patients.[7] Mild to moderate eosinophilia is the rule, although there are exceptions. There is no correlation between IgE levels and degree of eosinophilia or clinical disease. Chemotaxis is abnormal in this syndrome at least some of the time in most of the patients.

Complement-Mediated Immunity

Expectedly, deficiencies in complement components present clinically as recurrent systemic bacterial infections. Bacteremia and meningitis are common in all the complement deficiencies.[1] Pneumonia is common in the early classical pathway (C1, C4, C2) and alternative pathway (factors I, H, properdin, C3) defects. The late component defects (C5–C9) are associated with recurrent *Neisseria* spp. bacteremia and meningitis. Surprisingly, the bacteremias associated with late component defects occur at a much later age (average 17 years) than meningococcal bacteremia in the healthy population. Although these patients also have much higher rates of relapse and reinfection than healthy people, their mortality from the infection is lower than normal. Patients with deficiencies of the early components of complement, C1, C4, C2, and C3 tend to have considerably higher rates of collagen-vascular diseases such as systemic and discoid lupus erythematosus than either the healthy population or patients with late component defects.

Except for properdin deficiency, which is X-linked, the complement deficiency states are inherited as autosomal recessive disorders. Heterozygotes have 50 percent of normal levels while homozygous defective persons tend to have very low levels, if any, of the affected component. Screening for the presence of complement deficiencies is best accomplished by use of the test for total hemolytic complement (CH_{50} assay). This test examines the integrity of the classical pathway of the complement system by determining the ability of complement in patient serum to lyse antibody-coated sheep erythrocytes in vitro. Cell lysis leads to the release of hemoglobin, which can be determined spectrophotometrically. Specific classic complement component defects can be detected by a modified CH_{50} assay that uses purified proteins and selectively omits the one to be assayed, allowing patient serum to supply the missing factor.[16] Direct determinations of immunologically reactive protein, including members of the alternative pathway, can be performed using enzyme-linked immunosorbent assays or diffusion assays. These types of assay systems do not offer functional data, but can help to quantify apparent functional defects.

Acquired Immune Deficiencies

The most common forms of immunodeficiency encountered are acquired after birth and are not clearly traceable to an immune genetic basis. Like other immunodeficiencies, they are best approached by a thorough history and physical examination to search for associated findings and to guide diagnostic testing. Special attention to the infecting organisms can point to underlying abnormalities in host defense. AIDS[66] is caused by human immunodeficiency virus (HIV), which induces progressive CD4+ T-cell depletion. A recently described syndrome that presents like AIDS with opportunistic infections but is unassociated with HIV infection is idiopathic CD4+ lymphopenia.[67] The diagnosis is made by excluding all other known causes of immunodeficiency, including HIV, and determining that the CD4+ T-cell count is ≤300/μl. Certain malignancies, particularly hematopoietic and lymphoid, cause immune dysfunction by causing deficiency of the immune effector cells or dysregulation of such things as antibody synthesis and are associated with severe or opportunistic infections. Drug therapy can be complicated by rare or idiosyncratic reactions such as the aplastic anemia with chloramphenicol or drug-induced neutropenia.[68] Iron overload and chelation therapy with desferroximine provide a hospitable environment for certain bacteria, notably *Yersinia enterocolitica*.[69,92,93] Splenectomy, especially post-traumatic, predisposes to overwhelming infection with encapsulated organisms such as *St. pneumoniae* and *Capnocytophaga canimorsus* (DF-2) and parasites such as *Babesia microti* and malaria.[94] Severe thermal injury is associated with selective degranulation of neutrophil-specific granules, decreased chemotaxis, and profound susceptibility to infections.[95]

REFERENCES

1. Ross SC, Denson P. Complement deficiency states and infection: Epidemiology, pathogenesis and consequences of neisserial and other infections in an immune deficiency. Medicine. 1984;63:243–73.
2. Buckley RH. Immunodeficiency diseases. JAMA. 1992;268:2797–806.
3. O'Neil KM, Herman JH, Modlin JF, et al. *Pseudomonas cepacia:* An emerging pathogen in chronic granulomatous disease. J Pediatr. 1986;108:940–2.
4. Buckley RH, Becker WG. Abnormalities in the regulation of human IgE synthesis. Immunol Rev. 1978;41:288–314.
5. Anderson DC, Schmalsteig FC, Finegold MJ, et al. The severe and moderate phenotypes of heritable Mac-1, LFA-1 deficiency: Their quantitative definition and relation to leukocyte dysfunction and clinical features. J Infect Dis. 1985;152:668–89.

6. Charon JA, Mergenhagen SE, Gallin JI. Gingivitis and oral ulceration in patients with neutrophil dysfunction. J Oral Pathol 1985;14:150–5.
7. Donabedian H, Gallin JI. The hyperimmunoglobulin E recurrent infection (Job's) syndrome: A review of the NIH experience and the literature. Medicine. 1983;62:195–208.
8. Blume RS, Wolff SM. The Chediak-Higashi syndrome: Studies in four patients and a review of the literature. Medicine. 1972;51:247–80.
9. Ownby DR, Pizzo SV, Blackmon L, et al. Severe combined immunodeficiency with leukopenia (reticular dysgenesis) in siblings: Immunologic and histopathologic findings. J Pediatr. 1976;89:382–7.
10. Roper M, Parmley RT, Crist WM, et al. Severe congenital leukopenia (reticular dysgenesis): Immunologic and morphologic characterizations of leukocytes. Am J Dis Child. 1985;139:832–5.
11. Hirschhorn R. Adenosine deaminase deficiency. Immunodef Rev. 1990;2:175–98.
12. Markert ML. Purine nucleoside phosphorylase deficiency. Immunodef Rev. 1991;3:45–81.
13. Fisher A. Severe combined immunodeficiencies. Immunodef Rev. 1992;3:83–100.
14. Williams WJ, Nelson DA, Morris MW. Examination of the blood. In: Williams WA, Beutler E, Erslev AJ, Lichtman MA, eds. Hematology. 4th eds. New York: McGraw-Hill; 1990:9–24.
15. Carvalho EM, Bacellaro O, Barral A, et al. Antigen specific immunosuppression in visceral leishmaniasis is cell mediated. J Clin Invest. 1989;83:860–4.
16. Lopez M, Fleisher T, deShazo RD. Use and interpretation of diagnostic immunologic laboratory tests. JAMA. 1992;268:2970–90.
17. Alarcon B, Regueiro JR, Arnaiz-Villena A, Terhorst C. Familial defect in the surface expression of the T cell receptor–CD3 complex. N Engl J Med. 1988;319:1203–8.
18. Pahwa R, Chatila T, Pahwa S, et al. Recombinant interleukin 2 therapy in severe combined immunodeficiency disease. Proc Natl Acad Sci USA. 1989;86:5069–73.
19. Weinberg K, Parkman R. Severe combined immunodeficiency due to a specific defect in the production of interleukin 2. N Engl J Med. 1990;322:1718–23.
20. Chatila T, Castigli E, Pahwa R, et al. Primary combined immunodeficiency resulting from defective transcription of multiple T-cell lymphokine genes. Proc Natl Acad Sci USA. 1990;87:10033–7.
21. Griscelli C, Lisowska-Grospierre B, Mach B. Combined immunodeficiency with defective expression in MHC class II genes. Immunodef Rev. 1989;1:135–53.
22. Mossmann TR, Moore KW. The role of IL10 in cross regulation of Th1 and Th2 responses. Immunol Today. 1991;12:A48–53.
23. Muller W, Peter HH, Wilken M, et al. The DiGeorge syndrome: I. Clinical evaluation and course of partial and complete forms of the syndrome. Eur J Pediatr. 1988;147:496–502.
24. Chisaka O, Capecchi MR. Regionally restricted developmental defects resulting from targeted disruption of the mouse homeobox gene hox 1.5. Nature 1991;350:473–9.
25. Gatti RA, Boder E, Vinters HV, et al. Ataxia-telangiectasia: An interdisciplinary approach to pathogenesis. Medicine. 1991;70:99–117.
26. Aldrich RA, Steinberg AG, Campbell DC. Pedigree demonstrating a sex-linked recessive condition characterized by draining ears, eczematoid dermatitis, and bloody diarrhea. Pediatrics. 1954;13:133–9.
27. Park JK, Rosenstein YJ, Remold-O'Donnell E, et al. Enhancement of T-cell activation by the CD43 molecule whose expression is defective in Wiskott-Aldrich syndrome. Nature. 1991;350:706–9.
28. Rosenstein Y, Park JK, Hahn WC, et al. CD43, a molecule defective in Wiskott-Aldrich syndrome, binds ICAM-1. Nature. 1991;354:233–5.
29. Bruton OC. Agammaglobulinemia. Pediatrics. 1952;9:722–8.
30. Waldmann TA. Immunodeficiency diseases: Primary and acquired. In: Samter M, ed. Immunological Diseases. 4th ed. New York: Little Brown; 1988:411–65.
31. Sullivan JL, Woda BA. X-linked lymphoproliferative syndrome. Immunodef Rev. 1989;1:325–47.
32. Sneller MC, Strober W, Eisenstein E, et al. New insights into common variable immunodeficiency. Ann Intern Med. 1993;118:720–30.
33. Bodey GP, Buckley M, Sathe YS, Freireich EJ. Quantitative relationships between circulating leukocytes and infection in patients with acute leukemia. Ann Intern Med. 1966;64:328–40.
34. Wright DG, Dale DC, Fauci AS, Wolff SM. Human cyclic neutropenia: Clinical review and long term follow up of patients. Medicine. 1981;60:1–13.
35. Bonilla MA, Gillio AP, Ruggiero M, et al. Effects of recombinant human granulocyte colony-stimulating factor on neutropenia in patients with congenital agranulocytosis. N Engl J Med. 1989;320:1574–80.
36. Rausch PG, Pryzwansky KB, Spitznagel JK. Immunocytochemical identification of azurophilic and specific granule markers in the giant granules of Chediak-Higashi neutrophils. N Engl J Med. 1978;298:693–8.
37. Jenkins NA, Justice MJ, Gilbert DJ, et al. Nidogen/entactin (Nid) maps to the proximal end of mouse chromosome 13 linked to beige (bg) and identifies a new region of homology between mouse and human chromosomes. Genomics. 1991;9:401–3.
38. Kishimoto TK, Larson RS, Corbi AL, et al. The leukocyte integrins. Adv Immunol. 1989;46:149–82.
39. Etzioni A, Frydman M, Pollack S, et al. Brief report: Recurrent severe infections caused by a novel leukocyte adhesion deficiency. N Engl J Med. 1992;327:1789–92.
40. Springer TA. Adhesion receptors of the immune system. Nature. 1990;346:425–34.
41. Butcher EC. Leukocyte-endothelial cell recognition: 3 (or more) steps to specificity and diversity. Cell. 1991;67:1033–6.
42. Gallin JI, Fletcher MP, Seligmann BE, et al. Human neutrophil specific granule deficiency: A model to assess the role of the neutrophil specific granules in the evolution of the inflammatory response. Blood. 1982;59:1317–29.
43. Lomax KJ, Gallin JI, Rotrosen D, et al. Selective defect in myeloid cell lactoferrin gene expression in neutrophil specific granule deficiency. J Clin Invest. 1989;83:514–9.
44. Rosenberg HF, Gallin JI. Neutrophil specific granule deficiency includes eosinophils. Blood. 1993;82:268–73.
45. Nauseef WM. Myeloperoxidase deficiency. Hematol Oncol Clin North Am. 1988;2:135–58.
46. Rex JH, Bennett JE, Gallin JI, et al. Normal and deficient neutrophils can cooperate to damage Aspergillus fumigatus hyphae. J Infect Dis. 1990;162:523–8.
47. Gallin JI, Malech HL. Update on chronic granulomatous disease of childhood: immunotherapy and potential for gene therapy. JAMA. 1990;263:1533–7.
48. Muoy R, Fisher A, Vilmer E, et al. Incidence, severity and prevention of infections in chronic granulomatous disease. J Pediatr. 1989;114:555–60.
49. Buescher ES, Gallin JI. Stature and weight in chronic granulomatous disease. J Pediatr. 1984;104:911–3.
50. Kenney RT, Kwon-Chung KJ, Waytes AT, et al. Successful treatment of systemic Exophiala dermatitidis infection in a patient with chronic granulomatous disease. Clin Infect Dis. 1992;1:235–42.
51. Williamson PR, Kwon-Chung KJ, Gallin JI. Successful treatment of Paecilomyces varioti infection in a patient with chronic granulomatous disease and a review of Paecilomyces species infections. Clin Infect Dis. 1992;5:1023–6.
52. Gallin JI, Buescher ES, Seligmann BE, et al. Recent advances in chronic granulomatous disease. Ann Intern Med. 1983;99:657–74.
53. Sponseller PD, Malech HL, McCarthy EF, et al. Skeletal involvement in chronic granulomatous disease of childhood. J Bone Joint Surg. 1991;73A:37–51.
54. Margolis DM, Melnick DA, Alling DW, Gallin JI. Trimethoprim-sulfamethoxazole prophylaxis in the management of chronic granulomatous disease. J Infect Dis. 1990;162:723–6.
55. Ament ME, Ochs HD. Gastrointestinal manifestations of chronic granulomatous disease. N Engl J Med. 1973;288:382–7.
56. Walther MM, Malech H, Berman A, et al. The urologic manifestations of chronic granulomatous disease. J Urol. 1992;147:1314–8.
57. Gallin JI, Malech HL, Weening JT, et al. A controlled trial of interferon gamma to prevent infection in chronic granulomatous disease. International Chronic Granulomatous Disease Cooperative Study. N Engl J Med. 1991;324:509–16.
58. Buescher ES, Gallin JI. Leukocyte transfusions in chronic granulomatous disease: Persistence of transfused leukocytes in sputum. N Engl J Med. 1982;307:800–3.
59. Chin TW, Steihm ER, Falloon J, Gallin JI. Corticosteroids in treatment of obstructive lesions of chronic granulomatous disease. J Pediatr. 1987;111:349–52.
60. Geha RS, Leung DYM. Hyper immunoglobulin E syndrome. Immunodef Rev. 1989;1:155–72.
61. Lallemand D, Kalifa G, Buriot D, et al. Constitutional bone anomalies in congenital immune deficiencies. Ann Radiol. 1978;22:108–18.
62. Leung DYM, Key L, Steinberg JJ, et al. Increased in vitro bone resorption by monocytes in the hyperimmunoglobulin E syndrome. J Immunol. 1988;140:84–8.
63. Dreskin SC, Gallin JI. Evolution of the hyper immunoglobulin E and infection (HIE, Job's) syndrome in a young girl. J Allergy Clin Immunol. 1987;80:746–51.
64. Dreskin SC, Goldsmith PK, Strober W, et al. Metabolism of immunoglobulin E in patients with markedly elevated serum immunoglobulin E levels. J Clin Invest 1987;79:1764–72.
65. Berger M, Kirkpartrick CH, Goldsmith PK, Gallin JI. IgE antibodies to Staphylococcus aureus and Candida albicans in patients with the syndrome of hyperimmunoglobulin E and recurrent infections. J Immunol. 1980;125:2437–43.
66. Pantaleo G, Graziosi C, Fauci AS. The immunopathogenesis of human immunodeficiency virus infection. N Engl J Med. 1993;328:327–35.
67. Smith DK, Neal JJ, Holmberg SD, Centers for Disease Control Idiopathic CD4+ T-lymphocytopenia task force. Unexplained opportunistic infections and CD4+ T-lymphocytopenia without HIV infection—An investigation of cases in the United States. N Engl J Med. 1993;328:373–9.
68. Singh N, Yu VL, Mielles LA, Wagener MM. Beta-lactam antibiotic induced leukopenia in severe hepatic dysfunction: Risk factors and implications for dosing in patients with liver disease. Am J Med. 1993;94:251–6.
69. Leighton PM, MacSween HM. Yersinia hepatic abscesses subsequent to long term iron therapy. JAMA. 1987;257:964–5.
70. Tacket CO, Brenner F, Blake PA. Clinical features and an epidemiologic study of Vibrio vulnificus infections. J Infect Dis. 1984;149:558.
71. Noguchi M, Yi H, Rosenblatt HM, et al. Interleukin-2 receptor gamma chain mutation results in X-linked severe combined immunodeficiency in humans. Cell. 1993;73:147–58.
72. Markert ML, Hershfield MS, Schiff RI, Buckley R. Adenosine deaminase and purine nucleoside phosphorylase deficiencies: Evaluation of therapeutic interventions in eight patients. J Clin Immun. 1987;7:389–99.

73. Parkman R, Gelfand EW, Rosen FS, et al. Severe combined immunodeficiency and adenosine deaminase deficiency. N Engl J Med. 1975;292:714–9.

74. Rich KC, Mejias E, Fox IH. Purine nucleoside phosphorylase deficiency: improved metabolic and immunologic function with erythrocyte transfusions. N Engl J Med. 1980;303:973–7.

75. de Preval C, Lisowska-Grospierre B, et al. The lack of expression of HLA class II antigens in severe immunodeficiency reveals the existence of a trans-acting class II regulatory gene, unlinked to the MHC. Nature. 1985;318:291–3.

76. McFarlin DE, Strober W, Waldmann TA. Ataxia-telangiectasia. Medicine. 1972;51:281–314.

77. Gatti RA, Berkel I, Boder E, et al. Localization of an ataxia-telangiectasia gene to chromosome 11q22–23. Nature. 1988;336:577–580.

78. Tsukada S, Saffran DC, Rawlings DJ, et al. Deficient expression of a B cell cytoplasmic tyrosine kinase in human X-linked agammaglobulinemia. Cell. 1993;72:279–90.

79. Vetrie D, Vorechovsky I, Sideras P, et al. The gene involved in X-linked agammaglobulinaemia is a member of the *src* family of protein-tyrosine kinases. Nature. 1993;361:226–33.

80. Allen RC, Armitage RJ, Conley ME, et al. CD40 ligand gene defects responsible for X-linked hyper-IgM syndrome. Science. 1993;259:990–3.

81. Aruffo A, Farrington M, Hollenbaugh D, et al. The CD40 ligand, gp39, is defective in activated T cells from patients with X-linked hyper-IgM syndrome. Cell. 1993;72:291–300.

82. Sullivan JL, Byron KS, Brewster FE, et al. X-linked lymphoproliferative syndrome: Natural history of the immunodeficiency. J Clin Invest. 1983;71:1765–78.

82a. Grierson H, Purtilo DT. Epstein-Barr virus infections in males with the x-linked lymphoproliferative syndrome. Ann Intern Med. 1987;106:538–45.

83. Royer-Pokora B, Kunkel LM, Monaco P, et al. Cloning the gene for an inherited human disorder—chronic granulomatous disease—on the basis of its chromosomal location. Nature. 1986;322:32–8.

84. Bolsher BGJM, deBoer M, de Klein A, et al. Point mutations in the B-subunit of cytochrome b558 leading to X-linked chronic granulomatous disease. Blood 1991;77:2482–7.

85. Shapiro BL, Newburger PE, Klempner MS, Dinauer MC. Chronic granulomatous disease presenting in a 69-year-old man. N Engl J Med. 1991;325:1786–90.

86. Dinauer MC, Pierce EA, Bruns GA, et al. Human neutrophil cytochrome b light chain (p22-phox). Gene structure, chromosomal location, and mutations in cytochrome negative autosomal recessive chronic granulomatous disease. J Clin Invest. 1990;86:1729–37.

87. Clark RC, Malech HL, Gallin JI, et al. Genetic variants of chronic granulomatous disease: Prevalence of deficiencies of two cytosolic components of the NADPH oxidase system. N Engl J Med. 1989;321:647–52.

88. Casimir CM, Bu-Ganim HN, Rodaway ARF, et al. Autosomal recessive chronic granulomatous disease caused by deletion at a dinucleotide repeat. Proc Natl Acad Sci USA. 1991;88:2753–2757.

89. Kenney RT, Malech HL, Leto TL. Structural characterization of the p67phox gene. Clin Res. 1992;40:261A.

90. Kishimoto TK, Hollander N, Roberts TM, et al. Heterogeneous mutations in the β subunit common to the LFA-1, Mac-1, and P150,95 glycoproteins cause leukocyte adhesion deficiency. Cell. 1987;50:193–202.

91. Corbi AL, Larson RS, Kishimoto TK, et al. Chromosomal location of the genes encoding the leukocyte adhesion receptors LFA-1, Mac-1, and P150,95: Identification of a gene cluster involved in cell adhesion. J Exp Med 1988; 167:1597–607.

92. Gallant T, Freedman MH, Vellend H, Francombe WH. *Yersinia* sepsis in patients with iron overload treated with desferroxamine (Letter). N Engl J Med. 1986;314:1643.

93. Mofenson HC, Caraccio TR, Sharieff N. Iron sepsis: *Yersinia* enterocolitica septicemia possibly caused by an overdose of iron (Letter). N Engl J Med. 1987;316:1092–3.

94. Case 29-1986: DF-2 sepsis in a splenectomized patient. N Engl J Med. 1986; 315:241–9.

95. Davis JM, Dineen P, Galin JI. Neutrophil degranulation and abnormal chemotaxis after thermal injury. J Immunol. 1990;124:1467–71.

SECTION C

10. EPIDEMIOLOGY OF INFECTIOUS DISEASES

MICHAEL T. OSTERHOLM
CRAIG W. HEDBERG
KRISTINE L. MacDONALD

Epidemiology is the study of the distribution of health-related conditions or events and factors associated with the occurrence of these conditions or events in defined populations. The science of epidemiology was originally derived from the study of epidemics and now has been broadened to encompass all phenomena related to health in populations.[1] Simply stated, epidemiology involves the careful description of events within populations and the comparison of rates at which these events occur between groups within those populations. Similar concepts and methods of epidemiology apply to both infectious and noninfectious diseases.[2] The strength and adaptability of epidemiologic methods comes from their underlying simplicity. For example, John Snow's application of epidemiologic study methods resulted in the classic investigation of the Broad Street pump outbreak of cholera in London in 1851. His work was based on a careful description of his observations and his quantitative approach in analyzing the occurrence of cholera among the citizens of London. The influence of his work led to legislation mandating that all of the water companies in London filter their water. Of note, it was not until 1883 that Robert Koch discovered *Vibrio cholerae*.[3]

GOALS OF EPIDEMIOLOGIC ANALYSIS

As applied to infectious diseases, there are at least 10 primary goals of epidemiologic analysis. These are to (1) describe patterns of infection and disease occurrence in populations; (2) identify outbreaks or unusual rates of disease occurrence; (3) facilitate laboratory-based efforts to identify infectious agents; (4) describe the occurrence of asymptomatic infection and the spectrum of disease associated with specific agents; (5) provide population-based descriptions of clinical illness to improve the specificity of diagnosis for individual diseases; (6) assist in the understanding of disease pathogenesis; (7) identify and characterize factors in the chain of infection that contribute to agent transmission and development of disease; (8) develop and evaluate treatment protocols through clinical trials; (9) develop and evaluate primary, secondary, and tertiary prevention and control measures for individuals; and (10) describe and assess the use of prevention measures on a community-wide basis. These comprehensive goals far exceed the often considered goal of epidemiologic analysis to investigate and control epidemics or outbreaks.

These goals can be illustrated by a historical review of the unfolding of the human immunodeficiency virus (HIV) epidemic. After the acquired immunodeficiency syndrome (AIDS) was initially described in 1981, a national epidemiologic surveillance case definition was developed. Subsequent disease surveillance was initiated to characterize the cases by standard measures of time, place, and person and to identify population groups at risk. Based on these efforts, an infectious etiology was hypothesized early in the epidemic, before the first laboratory evidence of an etiologic agent was presented. Combined clinical, epidemiologic, and laboratory studies led to identification of

HIV as the cause of AIDS and development of sensitive and specific serologic tests for infection. This in turn led to studies that have characterized the spectrum of illness associated with HIV infection. Epidemiologic studies of persons infected with HIV (with or without AIDS) have characterized the routes of HIV transmission, have shown that the occurrence of other sexually transmitted diseases can increase the risk of HIV transmission, and have demonstrated that HIV infection can enhance the transmission of other agents such as *Mycobacterium tuberculosis*. Clinical trials have been conducted (or are ongoing) to assess the efficacy of certain antiretroviral agents. Multiple other trials have also been conducted to assess the efficacy of a range of antimicrobial agents aimed at preventing a variety of opportunistic infections. Finally, community-based programs developed on the basis of epidemiologic data have been developed to promote behavior change aimed at reducing the risk of HIV transmission. Epidemiologic methods have also been applied to evaluation of these community-based programs. These examples illustrate the broad role that epidemiologic methods have played in understanding and controlling the HIV epidemic.

DEFINING INFECTIONS, DISEASES, AND POPULATIONS

An essential aspect of any epidemiologic study is the careful definition of the infection, disease, condition, or factor that is being studied. The ability to detect meaningful and valid statistical associations between health status and risk factors is frequently dependent on the precision and reliability with which the study variables can be defined. For example, the occurrence of toxic shock syndrome (TSS) in menstruating women was initially associated with the use of a single brand of tampons.[4] However, that brand had a disproportionately increased share of the high absorbency tampon sales compared with all other brands. Another epidemiologic study that controlled for the absorbency of tampons demonstrated that the use of all tampon brands was associated with TSS.[5]

Specificity and sensitivity are concepts that are frequently used in reference to laboratory test performance, particularly tests that are used for screening purposes.[1] However, with the epidemiologic study of infectious diseases, it is important to also apply the concepts of specificity and sensitivity more broadly in terms of diagnosis of infection and disease. For example, the diagnosis of smallpox infection and disease was both highly specific and sensitive. Few other diseases could be confused with smallpox (i.e., the diagnosis was specific) and most people who became infected with smallpox virus developed clinical disease (i.e., the diagnosis was sensitive). These qualities, in addition to the fact that humans were the only important reservoir for the smallpox virus and the development of highly immunogenic vaccines, led to the successful eradication of smallpox.[6] In contrast, the diagnosis of infection and disease with *Borrelia burgdorferi* (i.e., Lyme disease), is neither highly specific nor sensitive. This has led to widespread controversy regarding the diagnosis and clinical spectrum of Lyme disease.[7] Without a specific and sensitive case definition for *B. burgdorferi* infection, surveillance efforts have been hampered, and, thus, an accurate description of the epidemiology of this disease in the community has been limited.

Some clinical conditions or syndromes may be caused by more than one etiologic agent (e.g., meningitis or hemolytic uremic syndrome). In such situations, for epidemiologic methods to be successful, the case definition needs to be kept as specific as possible. Conversely, some agents may lead to a broad spectrum of clinical illnesses. Depending on the goals of a particular study, investigators may choose a case definition that casts a wide net or may choose a more narrow case definition. The type of definition can impact substantially on study results and

should be considered carefully before a specific study is undertaken.

Epidemiologic studies may be designed to evaluate outcome variables other than infection or disease occurrence. In these situations, how the outcome variables are defined and measured can affect the interpretation of the results and the validity of the conclusions. For example, in the development of recombinant vaccines for hepatitis B virus (HBV), two vaccine formulations that differed primarily in the amount of hepatitis B surface antigen (HBsAg) in each dose were evaluated.[8] Although subjects who were administered the vaccine with 20 μg HBsAg per dose developed higher antibody titers than did those who were provided the vaccine with 10 μg HBsAg per dose, similar proportions of both groups developed sufficient levels of antibody to be considered protected against infection. Based on similar qualitative responses in clinical trials, both vaccines were licensed by the Food and Drug Administration (FDA). However, among Minnesota hospital employees, those persons who received the vaccine with 20 μg HBsAg per dose were more likely than persons given the other vaccine to have detectable antibody when tested within 6 months after completing the three-dose series.[9] Results of this investigation suggested that sociodemographic factors of the population studied, such as age, gender, weight, and smoking, affected the outcome of vaccination programs.

Establishing specific enrollment criteria for cases of infection or disease in epidemiologic studies is critical to obtaining valid and biologically meaningful results. For example, a large multistate outbreak of salmonellosis was recently identified through recognition of the increased isolation of an uncommon *Salmonella* serotype from clinical specimens evaluated in public health laboratories.[9] The unexpected number and temporal clustering of these infections suggested a common source in the community. However, further biologic characterization of these *Salmonella* isolates revealed both a common outbreak-associated strain and unrelated, sporadic isolates of the same serotype. Including these cases of sporadic infection, due to an unrelated strain of the same serotype, in the outbreak investigation would have weakened the observed associations between illness and specific risk factors, thus diminishing the likelihood of finding the cause of the outbreak.

A similar issue regarding the definition of cases and the population in which they occur confronts public health officials when they must consider intervention activities due to a possible outbreak of some selected infectious disease. It is a common practice to define outbreaks as the occurrence of cases of disease at a frequency greater than expected.[1] It is important to determine if the reported illnesses (i.e., the numerator) are caused by a single outbreak-associated strain or by the coincidental occurrence of several unrelated strains of the etiologic agent (i.e., no outbreak). Similarly, it is necessary to define the population at risk (i.e., the denominator) if an accurate measure of the rate of disease is to be calculated. For example, it is not unusual to recognize a cluster of cases of *Neisseria meningitidis* disease in the community. Because outbreaks of invasive *N. meningitidis* disease are known to occur in closed populations, such as dormitories and barracks, and because a vaccine and antibiotic chemoprophylaxis are available to prevent or control these outbreaks, the occurrence of multiple cases of meningococcal disease inevitably prompts a rapid public health assessment. Since cases of meningococcal disease tend to occur during well-described seasonal-peak periods, there is the likelihood of a cluster of unrelated cases occurring in a defined population. The need for public health intervention is quite different for a cluster of cases related to a single outbreak-associated strain vs. a cluster of cases where each is caused by a different group or strain of *N. meningitidis*. However, in many situations, strains are not available for further subtyping as laboratory capacity to distinguish strains is limited.

A companion problem to defining the cases is the definition of the population at risk. To determine if the occurrence of cases of disease is at a frequency greater than expected, it is necessary to consider baseline incidence rates of disease. For example, in the United States, *N. meningitidis* invasive disease occurs at a rate of approximately one to two cases per 100,000 persons per year.[10] However, many of these cases occur seasonally (i.e., winter months) and among young children. Thus, expected temporal clustering in the winter months could make a short-term observed rate of occurrence appear excessive when compared with the annual rate of disease. A similar issue is the fact that cases often occur in one or more identified populations (i.e., school, work-place, church-group) that are of limited size; therefore, rate comparisons may be meaningless. For example, one case of meningococcal disease in a school of 1000 students could be represented as a rate of 100 per 100,000 persons per year. Although this is 50 times the expected annual population rate, it cannot reasonably be interpreted as defining an outbreak. Thus, timely decisions regarding major community-based interventions due to the observation of a cluster of meningococcal cases will often be made without adequate information regarding the status of a possible outbreak. Similar situations also occur with other pathogens.

Two common measures of the occurrence of disease in populations are incidence and prevalence.[1] *Incidence* represents the occurrence of new cases of infection or disease per unit of population per time period. It is common to express incidence rates in terms of person-years of exposure. *Prevalence* describes the number of current cases of disease per population unit at the time of observation. The relationship between incidence and prevalence depends on the duration of infection or disease. For example, the incidence of measles over the period of a year will always be greater than its prevalence at a given point in time because the disease has a very short duration. In contrast, the prevalence of HIV infection will always be greater than its incidence because the infection is chronic and infected persons may live for years after the initial infection.

BIOLOGY AND STATISTICS

The results of epidemiologic studies to compare risk between infection or disease and the presence or absence of specific risk factors are presented in terms of relative risks and odds ratios. A *relative risk* is the ratio of the rate of illness or infection among persons who were exposed and the rate of illness or infection in persons who were not exposed (Fig. 1). Relative risks may also be called *rate ratios* and are the products of cohort studies. In case-control studies, *odds ratios* are determined and approximate the relative risk. The odds ratio provides a valid estimate of the relative risk under conditions that prevail in most case-control studies; these include that the cases of disease are newly diagnosed, that prevalent cases are not included in the control group, and that the selection of cases and controls is not based on exposure status.[11]

An increased relative risk or odds ratio (i.e., >1.0) for an exposure variable indicates that the exposure is related to an increased risk of disease. Similarly, a decreased relative risk or odds ratio (i.e., <1.0) indicates that the exposure variable is related to a decreased risk of disease. For example, the consumption of undercooked eggs has been associated with an increased risk of *Salmonella enteritidis* infection in outbreak settings and for sporadic *S. enteritidis* infections in the community.[12] While relative risks and odds ratios do provide a measure of the risk of disease associated with a specific factor, they do not directly describe how much disease in the community can be attributed to that factor. Rather, the *attributable risk* or *fraction* considers both the relative risk for an exposure variable and the proportion of the population exposed to that variable. In Minnesota, persons who consumed undercooked eggs had approximately a four times greater risk of *S. enteritidis* infection than those who did not eat undercooked eggs. Based on an estimate for the frequency of eating undercooked eggs

A   The relative risk is calculated as: $\dfrac{[a/(a+b)]}{[c/(c+d)]}$

The odds ratio is calculated as: $\dfrac{a/c}{b/d}$

B   Calculation of population-attributable risk percent:

$$\frac{(\text{Prevalence of exposure})(\text{relative risk}-1)}{1 + [(\text{Prevalence of exposure})(\text{relative risk}-1)]}$$

FIG. 1. **(A)** The calculation of and relationship between relative risks and odds ratios. **(B)** Calculation of population-attributable risk percentage. Prevalence of exposure and relative risk are usually not known precisely in a population, but can be estimated from case-control studies. Prevalence of exposure of controls—b/(b + d)—in the study population is assumed to be the prevalence of exposure in the entire population. The odds ratio determined in the study is assumed to be the relative risk of persons exposed in the whole population. The validity of this approach is limited by how representative controls are of the population and how well the odds ratio estimates the relative risk.

among the general population, investigators estimated that 37 percent of sporadic *S. enteritidis* infections in Minnesota adults could be attributed to consumption of undercooked eggs.[13] Thus, both relative risk and the attributable risk are important measures for describing the epidemiology of infectious diseases and determining public health priorities.

In the process of studying the epidemiology of infectious diseases, many factors are evaluated to determine their relationship or association with a specific disease. Statistical associations, both positive and negative, may represent a true causal relationship, a confounding relationship with another factor, or a chance occurrence. When more than one factor is statistically associated with infection or disease status in univariate or single variable analyses, the relationship between individual factors and infection or disease status can be evaluated using multivariate regression analysis.[14] These procedures allow the investigator to control simultaneously for a combination of factors in the analysis and to determine whether any of the risk factors are associated with infection or disease status independently of other factors. Another critical way of distinguishing between causation, confounding, and chance is by assessing the biologic plausibility of the association. An unexpected statistical association found in conjunction with an epidemiologic study may result in a new understanding of how agent transmission or disease occurs. The temptation to stretch the plausibility of biology to provide meaning to statistical results is a constant danger. However, such results may be a useful guide to evaluate new hypotheses in future studies.

Furthermore, "statistically significant results" may be unimportant from a disease control or a practical perspective. Statistical significance, which has historically been considered to be an event that happens less than once every 20 times by chance alone (i.e., $p < 0.05$), is a combination of both the sample size and the strength or degree of the association. Studies with a large number of persons enrolled can produce statistically significant results of weak associations (i.e., relative risks or odds ratios of greater than one but less than two), whereas studies with a limited number of persons enrolled may not be able to produce statistically significant results even with moderately strong or increased associations (i.e., relative risks or odds ratios greater than five).

DETERMINING EPIDEMIOLOGIC METHODS APPROPRIATE TO THE STUDY SETTING

The clinical trial is cited as the gold standard of epidemiologic research. However, many epidemiologic studies cannot take place under such rigorously controlled conditions. Taking advantage of opportunities to study diseases in clinical and community settings is one of the strengths of epidemiology. In the setting of a clinical practice, epidemiology may involve studying a series of patients, participating in multicenter trials, or being a reporting source for cases of disease to public health officials. This last aspect of epidemiologic study may be a legal obligation, but should also be viewed as an opportunity for all practicing clinicians to participate in the practice of community-based epidemiology. Academic-based research centers are often settings for clinical trials, studies requiring newly developed laboratory methods, or studies derived from referrals to clinical specialty groups. Public health departments typically do not have direct access to or contact with patients for clinical trials, but are responsible for surveillance of reportable diseases and the investigation of outbreaks. Each of these settings provides opportunities for epidemiologic studies that have made major contributions to the understanding, prevention, and control of infectious diseases.

There are several major constraints confronted in the design of epidemiologic studies of infectious diseases. Time is frequently a problem in the investigation of outbreaks. The need to design and conduct outbreak investigations quickly limits the investigator's ability to explore the outbreak setting fully and can result in the loss of information. In any study involving the retrospective collection of data, information may be lost because of the difficulty in recalling exposures or in verifying information about the exposure.

For many infectious diseases, it may also be difficult to identify sufficient numbers of cases in clinical settings to conduct meaningful epidemiologic studies. For example, in Minnesota, 117 cases of hemolytic uremic syndrome occurred in residents less than 18 years of age from 1979 through 1988.[15] Thus, describing the epidemiology and clinical aspects of such a disease in Minnesota and its possible relationship to *Escherichia coli* O157:H7 infection required a statewide approach coordinated through the state health department.

TYPES OF EPIDEMIOLOGIC STUDIES

There are several schemes for classifying or defining types of epidemiologic studies (Table 1). Studies can be classified as *descriptive* or *analytic* and *observational* or *experimental*. A descriptive study is designed only to describe the existing distribution of case characteristics without regard to causal or other hypotheses.[16] For example, results of community-based surveillance for *Campylobacter* infections may include a summary of all cases reported in a given year by the date of onset, county

of residence, age, sex, and race. An analytic study is one designed to examine associations, particularly hypothesized causal relationships.[16] A case-control study could be designed to examine whether consumption of unpasteurized milk is a risk factor for cases with *Campylobacter* infections identified through surveillance activities. In addition to case-control studies, cohort studies, clinical trials, and cross-sectional surveys are common types of analytic studies. In practice, most epidemiologic studies involve both descriptive and analytic elements.

A more relevant distinction can be made between observational and experimental studies. Observational studies are conducted in natural settings where changes in one characteristic are studied in relation to others without the intervention of the investigator.[17] Observational studies comprise the bulk of epidemiologic research because they focus on events, exposures, and diseases occurring in the population during the course of routine living conditions. In contrast, experimental studies are ones in which the study conditions are under the direct control of the investigator.[17] Such studies may include randomization of subjects to treatment or placebo groups and blinding of subject and investigator to the placement status. Clinical trials are the prototypical experimental study. On a broader scale, community intervention trials can also be conducted.

OBSERVATIONAL STUDIES

Disease Surveillance

Disease surveillance is an ongoing process that involves the systematic collection, analysis, and distribution of information regarding the occurrence of diseases in defined populations.[18] Surveillance can be conducted in the community and in institutional settings, where it may form the basis for an infection control program. For most infectious diseases, community-based surveillance is the domain of public health departments at the local or state level. All jurisdictions require licensed physicians to report the occurrence of selected diseases to the health department.[19] Typically, these include sexually transmitted diseases, vaccine-preventable diseases, blood-borne pathogens, tuberculosis, and enteric infections caused by *Salmonella, Shigella,* and *Campylobacter.* In addition to categorical reporting, most states require reporting of disease outbreaks, regardless of the cause, and have some provision to solicit reports of new and emerging diseases.

Surveillance can be conducted in an active or passive manner. *Active surveillance* involves a regular, systematic effort to contact reporting sources or to review records within an institution to ascertain information on the occurrence of newly diagnosed diseases or infections. An example of a community-based active surveillance system is the federally supported active surveillance for AIDS cases conducted by state and some local health departments. *Passive surveillance* relies on the individual clinician or laboratory to initiate the report.

Two key qualities of community-based surveillance for infectious diseases that must be considered in interpreting surveillance data are representativeness and timeliness. These will vary by disease and depend on multiple factors. The first factor of importance is that the patient must seek medical attention. It is not common for persons with mild or limited illnesses to seek medical attention. Second, the physician must seek laboratory testing of appropriate clinical specimens to confirm the diagnosis. Third, the laboratory must have the capability to identify the agent when a laboratory diagnostic test is available. Fourth, the physician and laboratory must report the clinical and laboratory findings to public health officials in a timely manner. Even in states where laboratory-based infectious disease reporting is required, there may be confusion between the physician and the laboratory officials over who has responsibility for reporting. Finally, public health agencies must have the resources to conduct timely and routine follow-up of such reports to ascer-

TABLE 1. Classification of Epidemiologic Studies

	Observational	Experimental
Descriptive	Surveillance	
	Case series	
Analytic	Outbreak investigations	Clinical trials
	Cross-sectional surveys	Community interventions
	Seroprevalence surveys	
	Case-control studies	
	Cohort studies	
	Seroincidence studies	

tain basic case demographic and other relevant data. A failure at any step of this process will result in loss of information to the community-based surveillance system.

The efficiency of community-based surveillance systems varies greatly depending on the disease and how the diagnosis is made and the resources targeted toward the surveillance effort.[18] Diseases that require a diagnosis based on clinical presentation, such as Lyme disease, present difficulties because many patients may not be seen when the typical clinical manifestations of the disease are present and laboratory testing is not adequate to establish the diagnosis. In contrast, the diagnosis of measles can be confirmed by specific serologic testing whether or not the physician sees the patient when the pathognomonic clinical features of the disease are present. Surveillance for invasive bacterial diseases, such as those caused by *H. influenzae* type b and *N. meningitidis,* is facilitated by the need for medical treatment due to the relative severity of the disease and the laboratory-supported diagnosis. For diseases such as these, active case-ascertainment can greatly enhance the effectiveness of surveillance activities. However, active surveillance requires the commitment of personnel and other resources that are limited for many reportable diseases. Typically, active surveillance may be conducted for a limited time period when complete data are most critical. Examples include the characterization of emerging diseases such as AIDS or special surveillance projects aimed at assessing an intervention, such as evaluating the efficacy of *H. influenzae* type b vaccine in a defined population.[20]

Most infectious disease surveillance conducted by public health departments in the United States is passive in that it relies on the physician or the laboratory to initiate the report. Passive surveillance systems are subject to selection bias because disease reports are likely to come from a nonrepresentative sample of practicing physicians who may report specific diseases because of personal interest.[18] In addition, some data (i.e., age and gender vs. clinical and pathologic information) may be more readily reported because of ease of ascertainment.[18]

Active surveillance is relatively more common in the hospital setting. For example, surveillance of nosocomial infections is an important hospital infection control activity.[21] This highly specialized surveillance system has the operational advantage of a defined population, routine clinical observation of the patient population, and direct access to the laboratory. Hospital-based surveillance has been a primary epidemiologic tool in the study of drug-resistant organisms.[22]

Case Series

A common type of descriptive study that is conducted in clinical settings is the case series. A case series describes the clinical features of a disease and the demographic profiles and other interesting features of patients with the disease. They are typically the domain of practicing clinicians and serve as a way of communicating significant clinical observations. For example, a review of eight patients referred to Arkansas Children's Hospital suggested that ceftriaxone is not effective in treating infections with *Franciscella tularensis.*[23]

Case-Control Studies

In case-control studies, persons with infection or disease are compared to controls (i.e., persons without the infection or disease under study) with respect to prior exposures likely to be related to agent transmission.[1] Case-control studies by nature are retrospective because the outcome (i.e., case status) is known at the outset of the study. Case-control studies are the most widely conducted type of epidemiologic study because they are relatively cheap, powerful, and adaptable to many settings.[14] For example, in a multi-state outbreak of *Salmonella javiana* and *Salmonella oranienburg* infections, the results of a case-control study identified mozzarella cheese and shredded

cheese as the source of the outbreak, even though regulatory officials were not able to isolate the outbreak-associated strains of *Salmonella* from several hundred cheese samples from the implicated source.[9] When the outbreak-associated *Salmonella* was eventually isolated from cheese, it was shown to be present at levels of 2–16 cells per pound of cheese, levels which rendered microbiologic surveillance of cheese insensitive.

The primary considerations in designing case-control studies are defining cases, establishing enrollment criteria, identifying suitable controls, and developing interview or other data collection processes that do not systematically result in different standards of data collection for cases compared with controls. In the community setting, it is customary to select controls from the same area of residence as the case. It is desirable for controls to resemble cases with respect to variables that are not being studied. Controls may also be matched on age, gender, or any other factor that the investigator wishes to consider. For example, in studying risk factors for TSS in menstruating women, it was important to select or match controls based on gender. The use of male controls could have produced spurious associations between illness and any menses-related event. However, overmatching, such as requiring controls to have the same birthday as the case may make it difficult to identify and recruit controls. Also, once a variable is used as a matching criterion it is no longer available for evaluation. Thus, in the studies of TSS in menstruating women, requiring controls to use the same catemenial products (i.e., tampons) as the case would have eliminated the possibility of studying this factor. In hospital settings, controls are frequently selected from patients with unrelated diagnoses who might otherwise be comparable to the cases.

Analysis of case-control studies involves comparing exposure differences between cases and controls. This allows for associations between exposure and disease to be studied even when the disease is a rare outcome of the exposure. For example, a case-control study of Guillen-Barré syndrome (GBS) demonstrated an association between *Campylobacter* infection and GBS.[24] This association could not have been easily evaluated in a prospective cohort study due to the required population size necessary to identify a similar number of GBS cases. The power of the case-control methodology comes from the fact that although illnesses may be uncommon outcomes of a given exposure, the common history of exposure among cases may stand in stark contrast to the exposure history of controls.

Cohort Studies

In cohort studies, the development of infection or disease is observed in groups who are either exposed or not exposed to the previously defined risk factors.[1] Cohort studies are traditionally considered prospective studies. However, this nomenclature is misleading because in reality cohort studies can be prospective or retrospective, depending on how the exposed and comparison groups were identified and followed. Cohort studies provide the advantage of a direct measurement of illness rates by exposure status; this allows the direct measurement of relative risks. Furthermore, when conducted prospectively, cohort studies allow the investigator better control over data collection and identification of potential confounding variables. The use of cohort studies is limited to groups in which exposures can be defined and measured.

Cohort studies of homosexual men have helped to evaluate risk factors for transmission of HIV, HBV, and hepatitis C virus (HCV).[25,26] These studies are also examples of *seroincidence surveys* in which the appearance of antibody to an agent in the second of two sequentially collected specimens indicates infection with that agent somewhere between the two times of collection.[27] Seroincidence surveys allow the investigator to (1) define total infection rates, (2) relate infection rates to prior antibody levels, and (3) identify risk factors for infection.[27] Prospective cohort studies are limited because of the enrollment size and observation period requirements for diseases of low incidence. Retrospective cohort studies, in which previous exposures can be identified, offer the advantage of not requiring additional observation periods. However, they may be limited by recall of study subjects or the adequacy of available medical records.

Cross-Sectional Surveys

Cross-sectional surveys provide a point-in-time assessment of the population or study group. These surveys may be conducted to determine the prevalence of a disease in the community, but a more common use is to establish the prevalence of risk factors or serologic markers of infection.[11] For example, a cross-sectional survey of patients attending a sexually transmitted disease (STD) clinic demonstrated that HCV infection occurred infrequently; however, patients with a history of intravenous drug use had a significantly higher rate of serologic markers for HCV infection.[28]

An important type of cross-sectional survey is the *seroprevalence survey*. Serologic prevalence data reflect total infection rates, representing both clinical and subclinical (or asymptomatic) infections. Thus, seroprevalence surveys can provide information on patterns of infection or immunity to agents that could not be obtained by ordinary surveillance methods based on the reporting of clinical cases.[27] For example, the federally funded survey of newborn infants for antibody to HIV conducted by state and local health departments has provided population-based HIV infection rates for childbearing women throughout the United States.[29]

Outbreak Investigations

A final category of observational study that integrates multiple epidemiologic methods is the outbreak investigation. A special feature of outbreak investigations is that they are frequently conducted with a sense of urgency because of the ongoing occurrence of cases, the need to implement control measures rapidly, and the potential for intense public and media interest in the outbreak. The investigation of the first documented outbreak of legionnaire's disease and the 1993 outbreak of hantavirus-associated respiratory illness in the southwestern United States, were lead stories for national news media. Standard methods for conducting outbreak investigations have been published.[17]

Specific surveillance systems have been established for outbreaks of food-borne and water-borne diseases, influenza, and a range of infections in institutional settings. At the local or state level, outbreaks may be reported because a physician or the public is aware of the health department's existence and desires some intervention. Once an outbreak has been recognized it is necessary to determine its extent in terms of person, place, and time. For example, an outbreak of shigellosis among members of a professional football team served to index a larger outbreak involving consumption of food served on an international airline.[30] Furthermore, an outbreak of a food-borne disease among patrons of a single fast-food restaurant may actually index a contaminated food product that is being distributed to other restaurants in multiple states. Determining the source of the outbreak is frequently a two-stage process. For example, in the first stage of a community-wide food-borne outbreak investigation, cases may need to be compared to well persons in the community to confirm that the outbreak is associated with a particular eating establishment. In the second stage, cases can be compared to well persons who also patronized the establishment to confirm that the outbreak is associated with a particular food item. At both stages, appropriate controls are required to confirm the source of the outbreak.

EXPERIMENTAL STUDIES

Clinical Trials

Clinical trials are research activities that involve the administration of a test regimen to humans to evaluate its safety and efficacy.[1] In general, these involve comparing the clinical outcomes in patients receiving treatment with the outcomes of a comparable control group. Most clinical trials of interest in infectious disease epidemiology involve trials of antimicrobial agents and vaccines. An early forerunner to the modern clinical trial was a U.S.-based smallpox trial conducted in 1800.[31] During the 1950s, several multicenter trials were developed to evaluate chemotherapy in the treatment of tuberculosis.[32] In 1953, the U.S. poliomyelitis vaccine trials were conducted in collaboration with the U.S. Public Health Service and state health departments.[33]

There are many considerations in designing a clinical trial. First, should the trial be conducted at all? This requires some knowledge of the immunogenicity of candidate vaccines or the in vitro activity of an antibiotic against specific pathogens. Second, would patients be harmed by withholding either the treatment or the vaccine? These issues have gained particular attention regarding trials of drugs for the treatment of HIV infection. Concern expressed by AIDS activists and some clinicians about withholding potentially life-extending treatments has forced the FDA to sanction the use of a secondary and less rigorous treatment and evaluation protocol in designated AIDS clinics.[34]

Other considerations include the specification of both test and control treatments, an outcome measure for evaluating the treatments, a bias-free method for assigning patients to treatment groups, and calculation of the necessary sample size.[35] Sample size calculations are affected by the number of treatment groups to be studied, the desired significance level for rejecting the null hypothesis, the statistical power to detect a difference, and the desired detectable treatment difference.

Community Intervention Trials

Community intervention trials are related to the clinical trial, but are carried out on a larger scale. These are experiments in which large groups or communities are selected to receive a therapeutic or preventive regimen.[35] For example, the efficacy of normal human immunoglobulin prophylaxis to control outbreaks of hepatitis A virus (HAV) in child-care facilities was demonstrated in a community trial in Phoenix.[36] Community trials are particularly well suited to interventions targeted for public utilities or community services.

THE HOST-AGENT RELATIONSHIP

Although advances in medical science have made us less vulnerable to some infectious disease epidemics and pandemics, they continue to occur as they have throughout human history. As recently as the late 1960s, it was suggested by leading medical authorities in this country, including the Surgeon General, that it was time "to close the book on infectious diseases."[37] However, infectious diseases remain the leading cause of death worldwide. The world's human and animal populations continue to struggle against an increasingly recognized number of viral, bacterial, protozoal, helminthic, and fungal agents.

For the study of infectious disease epidemiology, it is important to consider both infection and disease, for these may be different. *Infection* results from an encounter with a potentially pathogenic agent with a susceptible human host in conjunction with a suitable portal of entry. The source of most human infections occurs outside the individual human host; thus, exposure to the environment or other infected hosts is a key factor. *Disease* is one of the possible outcomes of infection, and its development is related to factors of both the host and the agent.

While the clinician is primarily concerned with disease, the epidemiologist is interested in both infection and disease. Since infection without disease occurs frequently for many agents, a study of only clinical illness may provide a misleading understanding of the epidemiology of a specific infectious disease in the community. For example, adults infected with HAV frequently experience clinical hepatitis, while infants and toddlers with HAV infection are usually asymptomatic.[38] Thus, to determine the incidence of hepatitis A infection associated with child-care facilities and subsequent transmission to family members and child-care providers, investigators need to determine both the diagnosis of asymptomatic HAV infection and the level of HAV-related disease.

If the balance between agent and host favors the agent, infection (and in some instances disease) will occur. This relationship between the agent, the route or mechanism of transmission, and the host is referred to as the *chain of infection*. The control and prevention of infections depends on sufficient understanding of the dynamics of these interrelating factors.

Frequently, characteristics of the agent or host are seen as independent factors. However, it is necessary to consider both the host and the agent together in any discussion of the relationship resulting in infection and disease causation. For example, smallpox was a disease of dramatic human suffering; historically, it has been one of the most feared of all infectious diseases. Yet, the ability of the smallpox virus (variola virus) to infect and cause disease only in humans and subhuman primates was an important consideration in approaches to control and prevention (i.e., vaccination of the human population).[39] Consideration of the smallpox virus as highly virulent must be tempered by the fact that inoculation studies of this virus into many animal species did not result in infection. In contrast, most *Salmonella* serotypes may cause mild to severe infections in man and a variety of animal species. A notable exception is *S. typhi*, which causes infections only in humans. Thus, any description of the characteristics of either the agent or the host must be understood in the context of their interrelationship.

Agent

Any agent or microorganism is of epidemiologic importance if it can be transmitted through the environment, causes infection in a host (either human or animal), and produces clinical disease. These agents, regardless of their classification as bacterial, viral, protozoal, helminthic, or fungal, are considered the first necessary component of the chain of infection. Three characteristics of agents must be considered in terms of their epidemiologic importance.[40] These are *(1)* those characteristics of agents that are involved in their spread or transport through the environment, *(2)* the agent characteristics that are involved in the production of infection, and *(3)* those characteristics that are involved in the production of disease.

The characteristics of agents involved in spread through the environment vary depending on the method of transmission. However, regardless of the method of transmission, it is necessary for a minimum number of organisms to survive transport through the environment to reach and enter a susceptible host. For agents that are transmitted by direct person-to-person contact, their ability to survive stressful environmental conditions (such as changes in temperature, humidity, or pH) tend to be minimal. In contrast, agents that are capable of actual multiplication within the environment (i.e., in food products, water, soil, and plants) have a unique advantage for survival. Some agents such as *Legionella pneumophila* or *Bacillus anthracis* do not necessarily multiply within the environment; however, they can survive for months in relatively hostile conditions including distilled water or soil.[41,42] For those agents for which humans are the only known reservoir, the longer the time between likelihood of contact between two susceptible hosts, the greater the resistance that the agent must have to environmental conditions such as heat, drying, ultraviolet light, or dilution due to airflow.

Finally, some agents have the capacity to infect a nonhuman host, such as animals, birds, or an insect vector. Such nonhuman hosts may play an important role in the maintenance of the agent in the environment.

The ability of an agent to cause infection or disease has to be considered in the context of host characteristics. For example, an agent is considered to *colonize* a host when its presence in that host does not cause a specific immune response to infection. However, should the relationship between the agent and the host change, such as the introduction of *E. coli* from the gastrointestinal tract into the blood stream, infection can result. These types of infection are known as *endogenous*. If the agent is transported from an external source to the host (*exogenous infection*) and the balance between the agent and host favors the agent, infection usually develops.

There are several aspects of the host-agent relationship that can be related to the agent. Other aspects must be considered only in the context of both agent and host characteristics. For example, *infectiousness* is a characteristic of an agent that is concerned with the relative ease with which it is transmitted to appropriate hosts. A droplet-spread infection, such as that caused by a respiratory virus, tends to be more infectious than an infection transmitted by direct contact, such as an STD. Characteristics of the portals of exit and entry are thus determinants of infectiousness, as are the agent's characteristics of ability to survive away from the host. Some factors that are often ascribed to an agent are actually the result of both agent and host characteristics. They include infectivity, pathogenicity, virulence, and antigenicity or immunogenicity.

Infectivity typically is defined as the characteristic of the infectious agent that embodies its capability to enter, survive, and multiply in the host. A measure of infectivity is the *secondary attack rate*. Infectivity is often expressed as the number infected per the number susceptible and exposed. A population with an increased number of individuals with compromised specific or nonspecific immune responses may result in a higher proportion of exposed individuals actually becoming infected. For example, individuals who have decreased gastric acidity due to antacid use are at a higher risk of developing salmonellosis at a lower infectious dose than those with normal gastric pH.[43]

Pathogenicity is the property of an agent that determines the extent to which overt disease is produced in an infected population.[1] The pathogenicity of an agent is measured by the ratio of the number of persons developing clinical disease to the number of persons becoming infected. Again, this is frequently considered a sole property of the agent; however, host characteristics play an important role in defining pathogenicity. For example, as noted above, the ratio of disease to total infections related to HAV varies widely by host age.[38] In general, those agents with the highest levels of pathogenicity possess characteristics that protect them against nonspecific host defenses. In addition, they may elaborate a number of enzymes or toxins or induce host-mediated disease associated with immune response to the infection.

The *gradient of infection* or *biologic gradient* is the range of manifestations of illness in the host as a result of infection with an agent. It extends from death at one extreme to inapparent or subclinical illness at the other. In this regard, *virulence* is frequently used as a quantitative expression of the disease-producing potential of a pathogenic agent. It is defined as the ratio of the number of cases of serious or disability-producing infections among the total number of people infected.[1] When death is the only criterion in determining severity, it is referred to as the *case fatality rate*.

From the epidemiologic perspective, the virulence of an organism must be viewed in light of the host. For example, the clinical outcome of HBV infection, ranging from limited, subclinical infection to the development of acute fulminant hepatitis, is related to immune-mediated disease and important genetic factors of the host.[44] Similarly, the severity of tuberculosis is increased among African-Americans given similar host characteristics of cases in other races.[45] The development of drug resistance among organisms (regardless of mechanism) is an important consideration related to virulence. Infection that is caused by agents sensitive to a variety of antimicrobial drugs is less likely to cause serious disease if treated in a timely and appropriate manner than infection caused by a highly resistant organism. With rapidly increasing drug resistance among all groups of infectious agents, this virulence characteristic will become even more important in the future.[46,47]

Finally, the last characteristic usually ascribed to an agent is *antigenicity* or *immunogenicity*. It is defined as the ability of an agent to produce a systemic or local immunologic reaction in the host.[1] However, this characteristic also must be considered in the context of both agent and host. The antigenicity of an agent is important from a clinical perspective because it is a primary determinant in the host's ability to mount an initial immune response to infection, thus affecting both pathogenicity and virulence. It also determines the host's development of long-term immunity to a specific agent.

A number of factors affect host immune responses, including genetic, age, metabolic, environmental, anatomic, and physiologic factors. An example of the complex nature of the interaction between an agent and host can be demonstrated by the relationship between *H. influenzae* type b and age of the host. Children younger than 2 years of age do not mount an effective immune response to agents with capsular polysaccharide (i.e., *H. influenzae* type b, *N. meningitidis, Streptococcus pneumoniae*).[48] Polysaccharide antigens are T-cell-independent antigens, in contrast to protein antigens, which induce a T-cell effect. T-cell-independent antigens are poorly immunogenic in children younger than 2 years of age due to the lack of maturation of their immune system. Thus, recent efforts to develop vaccines for *H. influenzae* in younger children required that the *H. influenzae* type b polysaccharide be conjugated to various carrier proteins.[20,48] This combination of polysaccharide and protein has resulted in vaccines with enhanced immunogenicity by inducing a T-cell response in infants. The use of the second-generation *H. influenzae* conjugate vaccines in infants in the United States has resulted in a dramatic decrease in the occurrence of invasive *H. influenzae* type b disease in children in that age group.[49] Since the use of vaccines has proved to be one of the most cost-effective methods of preventing infectious diseases, the need to understand antigenicity in terms of both the agent and the host is a high priority.

Host

As noted in the previous section regarding agent, characteristics of the host also play an important role in the eventual outcome of an agent-host interaction. Host factors that influence exposure, infection, and disease are summarized in Table 2. Factors can be divided into two categories: those that influence exposure and those that influence the likelihood of infection and occurrence and severity of disease.

All of the factors that influence human exposure to an infectious agent depend on contact with sources of infection within the environment or promotion of person-to-person transmission.[40] The importance of the factors that influence exposure tend to change by host age, culture, geographic residence, season, and family status.

While most of the factors that influence infection and occurrence and severity of disease are related to the host, the characteristics of both agent and host, as described by pathogenicity, virulence, and antigenicity, are important. Also, agent infectious dose, mechanisms of disease production, antibiotic resistance of the infecting agent, and portal of entry contribute to infection and disease status.[40] For most infections, two host factors play a key role in determining the likelihood of developing clinical illness and the severity of that illness; they are the

TABLE 2. Host Factors That Influence Exposure, Infection, and Disease

Factors that influence exposure	
Animal exposure, including pets	Hospitalization or outpatient medical care
Behavioral factors related to age, drug usage, alcohol consumption	Hygienic practices, including toilet training and handwashing
Blood or blood product receipt	Occupation
Child day care attendance	Recreational activities, including sports
Closed living quarters: military barracks, dormitories, homeless shelters, facilities for the elderly and mentally handicapped, prisons	Sexual activity: hetero- and homosexual, type and number of partners
	School attendance
	Socioeconomic status
Food and water consumption	Trauma that damages skin or membrane integrity
Familial exposure	Travel, especially to developing countries
Gender	Vector exposure

Factors that influence infection, occurrence, and severity of disease	
Age at the time of infection	Gender
Alcoholism	Genetic makeup, especially influences on the immune response
Anatomic defect	
Antibiotic resistance (agent)	Immune state at time of infection, including immunization status
Antibiotic use (host)	
Coexisting noninfectious diseases, especially chronic	Immunodeficiency (specific or nonspecific): natural, drug-induced, or viral (HIV)
Coexisting infections	
Dosage: amount and virulence of organism to which host is exposed	Mechanism of disease production: inflammatory, immunopathologic, or toxic
Duration of exposure to organism	Nutritional status
	Receptors for organism on cells needed for attachment or entry of organism
Entry portal of organism and presence of trauma at site of entry	

(Adapted from Evans and Brachman,[40] with permission.)

immune status of the host and the age at the time of infection. The highest level of pathogenicity and virulence associated with the agent-host relationship tends to occur very early in life, when immune disease mechanisms are immature, or during old age, when they may be deteriorating. Finally, genetic factors tend to influence both susceptibility and disease outcome, although they are primarily related to the host immune response to infection.

ROUTES OF TRANSMISSION

The transmission of infectious agents is defined as any mechanism by which an infectious agent is spread through the environment or to another person.[1,50] These mechanisms can be classified as either direct or indirect.

There are three different modes of direct agent transmission. The most common mode is associated with a direct and immediate transfer of an infectious agent to a receptive portal of entry through which the human infection is established. This type of direct contact transmission occurs in association with touching, kissing, or sexual intercourse, or by the direct projection (droplet spread) of droplet spray from an infected host onto the conjunctiva or onto the mucous membranes of the nose or mouth. Typically, droplet spread is usually limited to a distance of approximately 1 m. The second type of direct transmission occurs when host-susceptible tissue is exposed to the agent such as by the bite of a rabid animal or when it comes in contact with soil or decaying matter in which the agent usually leads a saprophytic existence (e.g., the systemic mycosis). Finally, transplacental transmission is another form of direct transmission.

There are three primary mechanisms of indirect agent transmission that occur; they include vehicle-borne, vector-borne, and air-borne. Vehicle-borne transmission occurs when any material serves as an intermediate means by which an infectious agent is transported or introduced into the susceptible host through a suitable portal of entry. These materials may include water, food, biologic products including blood, serum, plasma, tissues, organs, and objects (fomites) such as toys, soiled clothing, bedding, or surgical instruments. It is not necessary that the agent multiply or develop in or on the vehicle before it is transmitted.

The second method of indirect transmission is vector borne. There are two different types of vector-borne transmission: mechanical or biologic. Mechanical transmission occurs when an insect through the soiling of its feet or proboscis or through carriage in its gastrointestinal tract spreads an infectious agent. Mechanical transmission does not require multiplication or development of the organism. In contrast, biologic vector-borne transmission occurs when the propagation (multiplication), cyclic development, or a combination of these (cyclopropagative) is required before the arthropod can transmit the infected form of the agent to humans.

The third type of indirect transmission is air-borne. This involves a dissemination of aerosols with infectious agents to a suitable portal of entry in a host, usually the respiratory tract. These aerosols are suspensions in the air of particles consisting partially or wholly of infectious agents. The particles are in the range of 1–5 μm. (Note, air-borne transmission does not include droplets and other large particles that promptly settle out. As noted above, these are included under direct transmission.) Some infections transmitted by the air-borne route may be carried great distances from their sources, as documented by outbreaks of legionnaire's disease or Q fever.

DISEASE PREVENTION AND CONTROL

Individual, Institutional, and Community-Based Strategies

Disease prevention and control activities for infectious agents occur at three levels. The first level is targeted to the individual and is predominantly the domain of the clinician. A variety of prevention activities can be targeted to individuals through their primary care provider. Use of chemoprophylaxis to prevent surgical wound infections is an example of a control measure targeted to the individual. The second level is that of the institution; this is predominately the domain of the infection control practitioner or the school health official. This level includes health-care facilities, nursing homes, correctional facilities, other residential facilities, and schools. Programs to prevent the spread of blood-borne pathogens or tuberculosis to health care workers in hospitals are examples of control strategies targeted at the institutional level. The third level is targeted to the community in general. This is predominantly the domain of public health agencies (at the local, state, and national levels). The removal of a contaminated food product from the market is an example of a control measure targeted to the community.

While some control measures are specific to these different levels, a substantial amount of overlap can also occur. For example, immunization programs operate at all three levels. Clinicians play an important role in the health maintenance of their individual patients by providing immunizations against a variety of pathogens. Immunization programs are also an important activity at the institutional level, such as routine annual immunization against influenza in nursing homes and immunization of health care workers against HBV. Finally, public health agencies monitor vaccination levels in the community and provide vaccination clinics open to the public.

When assessing or developing disease prevention and control activities targeted to infectious diseases, the weakest link in the chain of infection (agent, transmission, host) also needs to be considered for each specific pathogen. In some situations, control of the agent in a specific reservoir may be the best way to reduce disease occurrence. Chlorination of water is an example of destroying the agent in its reservoir or eliminating a possible mode of transmission.

Strategies aimed at the level of transmission need to be tailored to the type of transmission involved. For example, the use of condoms in the prevention of STDs is a control strategy targeted to preventing contact transmission. Transmission through common vehicles frequently involves food and water and may also involve other vehicles such as blood in the case of transfusions. Irradiation of food or screening blood for infectious agents are control activities targeted to a common vehicle. An example of a control activity targeted to air-borne transmission is use of masks and respirators to prevent transmission of tuberculosis in the health care setting. Finally, control of vector-borne transmission can be targeted toward destroying the vector or use of protective clothing and repellents.

In some instances, the best mechanism to prevent disease occurrence is through modification of the host, such as developing or boosting immunity through active or passive immunization. Other examples of control activities targeted to the host include improving nutritional status or providing chemoprophylaxis against a variety of agents.

Assessment of Risk, Feasibility, Cost, and Effectiveness

When developing disease prevention and control strategies several issues needed to be considered. These include risk, feasibility, cost, and effectiveness. Risk can be defined by the potential for exposure. Epidemiologic studies or analysis of surveillance data can serve to define persons or populations at risk and can also quantify risks within different populations. At the individual level, risk can be evaluated by assessing host characteristics, such as the need for prophylaxis against *Pneumocystis carinii* pneumonia for persons with HIV infection and T-cell depletion.[51] An example of evaluating risk at the institutional level is assessing occupational exposure to infectious agents such as blood-borne pathogens. At the community level, groups at risk for a variety of conditions can be defined by demographic features (such as age, race, country of origin, socioeconomic status, and geographic location). For example, persons born outside the United States are at increased risk of developing infectious diseases such as tuberculosis or of being chronic carriers of infections such as HBV. Screening programs targeted to these populations with subsequent interventions (such as isoniazid prophylaxis for persons with *M. tuberculosis* infection or immunization of susceptible household contacts of HBV carriers) can serve as important community-based strategies to prevent infectious disease occurrence.[52,53] Another example of defining risk at the community level is assessing behaviors that increase risk for specific diseases, such as intravenous drug use as a risk behavior for acquiring HIV infection. Education and drug treatment programs targeted to this population can serve as an important HIV prevention and control strategy.

In developing control programs, the feasibility of a strategy also needs to be assessed. Feasibility is dependent on the sociodemographic factors of the population involved. For example, high immunization rates can clearly prevent the occurrence of certain infectious diseases. In the United States, immunizations should be readily available; however, in the late 1980s numerous large outbreaks of measles occurred in U.S. inner-city populations because of low immunization rates.[54] A variety of sociodemographic factors contributed to these low rates, such as inadequate access to medical care and other barriers to immunizations. Until such barriers are removed and control strategies are developed to target such populations specifically, adequate control of vaccine-preventable diseases in the United States cannot be accomplished.[55]

Cost and availability of resources also need to be considered when developing control strategies. Adequate water treatment facilities and distribution systems in developing countries would do much to eliminate the spread of cholera. However, in many countries, resources to build and develop such facilities are not available. Consequently, control strategies need to be focused on simpler, less expensive methods, such as boiling water or improving water storage in the home.

Finally, control strategies need to be evaluated for their effectiveness. For example, this is a critical issue in evaluating ways to curb the HIV epidemic in the absence of effective treatment or vaccination. Evaluation of HIV prevention educational programs or HIV counseling and testing programs is essential in assessing the effectiveness of currently available strategies.

Primary, Secondary, or Tertiary Prevention

Prevention strategies can be characterized as primary, secondary, or tertiary.[1] *Primary prevention* is defined as the protection of health by personal and community-wide efforts. *Secondary prevention* includes measures available to individuals and populations for early detection and effective intervention. *Tertiary prevention* consists of measures available to reduce or eliminate long-term impairments and disabilities and to minimize suffering caused by existing departures from good health.

Primary Prevention. A key example of primary prevention is immunoprophylaxis, which can be active or passive (see Ch. 300). Active immunoprophylaxis involves administration of all or part of a microorganism (live or inactivated) or a product of that microorganism (such as a toxoid) to alter the host by stimulating an immunologic response aimed at protecting against infection.[50] There are currently at least four types of active immunization programs. First is routine childhood immunization. Current practices include routine childhood immunization against measles, mumps, rubella, tetanus, diphtheria, pertussis, *H. influenzae* type b, and HBV.[56] In many parts of the world, Bacille Calmette-Guérin (BCG) vaccine is also given routinely in early childhood. Additional childhood immunizations may be recommended for routine use in the near future, including vaccines against hepatitis A virus and varicella-zoster virus.[57] As the routine childhood immunization schedule becomes increasingly complex, new methods of vaccine delivery need to be developed. Of particular interest is the development of new multiple-antigen vaccines to simplify the routine schedule and maximize efficiency of vaccine delivery. The goals of routine childhood immunization are twofold: first to protect the individual and second to provide herd immunity, which can be effective in controlling certain diseases at the population level (such as measles, mumps, rubella, and *H. influenzae*).[58] Ongoing adequate surveillance for these diseases is essential to monitor the effectiveness of population-based immunization programs so that strategies can be adapted as needed. The expansion of measles immunization to a two-dose schedule in the United States in 1989 is an example of using surveillance data to revise immunization practices.[59]

A second type of immunization program is travel-related immunization (see Ch. 302). Examples include administration of typhoid, yellow fever, Japanese encephalitis, and meningococcal vaccines for travel to areas endemic for these conditions. The third type of program is immunization of selected at-risk populations. For example, influenza vaccine is currently recommend in the United States annually for persons over age 65 years, residents of nursing homes, adults with certain chronic diseases, and children who are receiving long-term aspirin therapy and may be at risk for Reye syndrome (see Ch. 141). Pneumococcal vaccine is also recommended to selected high-risk populations, including persons over age 65 years, persons with certain chronic diseases, and persons with certain immunosuppressive conditions. The final type of program is immunization based on occupational exposure. Examples include immunization of laboratory workers against anthrax and rabies in settings where occupational exposure may occur and immunization of health case workers against HBV based on exposure to bloodborne pathogens. Active immunization is also used after exposure to certain agents unrelated to an occupational setting, such as following exposure to *N. meningitidis*, HBV, measles, pertussis, and rabies. Some of these vaccines are given in conjunc-

tion with various types of immunoglobulin in the postexposure setting.

Passive immunization involves the administration of preformed antibodies, often to specified agents (see Chs. 33 and 300). The broadest form of passive immunization is use of normal human immune globulin (also referred to as γ-globulin). It is most often used following exposure to HAV and may be effective if given within 14 days after exposure.[53] Normal human immune globulin is also recommended prior to travel to countries endemic for hepatitis A. It may also be effective in reducing clinical disease in persons exposed to measles if provided within 6 days after exposure.[59] There are also multiple specific types of immune globulin that are used in postexposure settings to prevent infection or reduce the severity of disease if infection occurs. Examples include immune globulin specific to HBV, cytomegalovirus, rabies, varicella-zoster virus, and tetanus.

A second type of primary prevention is antibiotic prophylaxis, often referred to as *chemoprophylaxis*. Use of effective chemoprophylaxis requires that the infectious agent be susceptible to the antimicrobial used. As a primary prevention strategy, it may be employed before or after exposure to prevent infection. Examples of chemoprophylaxis in the postexposure setting include exposure to pertussis (i.e., erythromycin), *N. meningitidis*, influenza virus (e.g., amantadine or rimantadine), and *H. influenzae* type b (e.g., rifampin). Prophylaxis against surgical wound infections prior to surgery (see Ch. 296) and prophylaxis of neonates against ophthalmia neonatorum are examples of chemoprophylaxis used in the hospital setting. In such situations, chemoprophylaxis is used because a likelihood of exposure to pathogenic organisms is present, even though exposure is not clearly documented. Chemoprophylaxis is also used in anticipation of exposure during travel (such as prevention of malaria through the use of chloroquine or mefloquine) or the use of antimicrobials against enteric pathogens to prevent traveler's diarrhea (see Ch. 302).

In addition to immuno- and chemoprophylaxis, there are other important primary prevention activities at the individual, institutional, and community levels. Examples of these have been discussed in earlier sections of this chapter.

Secondary Prevention. Secondary prevention activities traditionally employ chemoprophylaxis and involve identifying early or asymptomatic infection with subsequent treatment so that such infections are eradicated and sequelae are prevented. Although most secondary prevention programs involve intervention at the individual level through the use of chemoprophylaxis, such programs often operate within the context of a population-based or institutional-based screening effort. Routine screening programs for sexually transmitted agents, such as *Chlamydia*, are examples of secondary prevention strategies.[60,61] Contact investigations for partners of persons with STDs are also part of a secondary prevention strategy focused at those at highest risk of infection (i.e., those with known exposure).[60] Another example of a secondary prevention program using chemoprophylaxis is screening of high-risk populations for tuberculosis infection and subsequent therapy with an antimicrobial such as isoniazid (INH) to prevent active disease.

Although most secondary prevention strategies involve chemoprophylaxis (and, rarely, immunoprophylaxis), the concept can be broadened to other prevention efforts aimed at intervention and correction of a recognized specific health hazard. Most such efforts occur at the community level. Examples of community-based secondary prevention efforts include the early identification of contaminated products through outbreak investigations and subsequent removal of such products from the market to prevent additional illnesses and restore ''the community's health.'' A ''boil water order'' for a water-borne disease outbreak of cryptosporidiosis is another example of a secondary prevention strategy aimed at correcting an existing community-wide problem.

Tertiary Prevention Tertiary prevention efforts are measures to eliminate long-term impairments and disabilities from an existing condition. Since most infectious diseases are treatable, tertiary prevention activities are less common than those found with chronic diseases such as hypertension, diabetes, and coronary artery disease. However, this concept is still applicable in the control of infectious diseases, since some viral infections are chronic and cannot be eradicated. Current treatment of HIV infection, including prophylaxis against other opportunistic agents, is an example of a tertiary prevention activity. Treatment of chronic active hepatitis due to HBV or HCV infection is an additional example of tertiary prevention aimed at minimizing the consequences of a chronic infection.

REFERENCES

1. Last JM, ed. A Dictionary of Epidemiology. 2nd ed. New York: Oxford University Press; 1988.
2. Barrett-Connor E. Infectious and chronic disease epidemiology: Separate and unequal? Am J Epidemiol. 1979;109:245–9.
3. Snow J. On the Mode of Communication of Cholera. London, 1855. Reprinted in: Frost WH, ed. Snow on Cholera. New York: Commonwealth Fund; 1936.
4. Centers for Disease Control and Prevention. Follow-up on toxic shock syndrome. MMWR. 1980;29:297–9.
5. Osterholm MT, Davis JP, Gibson RW, et al. Tri-state toxic-shock syndrome study. I. Epidemiologic findings. J Infect Dis. 1982;145:431–40.
6. World Health Organization. Global eradication of smallpox. Bull WHO. 1980; 58:161–3.
7. Steere AC, Taylor E, McHugh GL, et al. The overdiagnosis of Lyme disease. JAMA. 1993;269:1812–6.
8. Wood RC, MacDonald KL, White KE, et al. Risk factors for lack of detectable antibody following hepatitis B vaccination of Minnesota health care workers. JAMA. 1993;270:2935–9.
9. Hedberg CW, Korlath JA, D'Aoust J-Y, et al. A multi-state outbreak of *Salmonella javiana* and *Salmonella oranienberg* infections due to consumption of contaminated cheese. JAMA. 1992;268:3203–7.
10. Centers for Disease Control and Prevention. Summary of notifiable diseases, United States, 1992. MMWR. 1992;41:41.
11. Hennekens CH, Burning JE. Epidemiology in Medicine. Boston: Little, Brown, and Company; 1987.
12. St. Louis ME, Morse DL, Potter ME, et al. The emergence of grade A eggs as a major source of *Salmonella enteritidis* infections. New implications of the control of salmonellosis. JAMA. 1988;259:2103–7.
13. Hedberg CW, David MJ, White KE, et al. Role of egg consumption in sporadic *Salmonella enteritidis* and *Salmonella typhimurium* infections in Minnesota. J Infect Dis. 1993;167:107–11.
14. Schlesselman JJ, Stolley PD. Case-Control Studies. Design, Conduct, Analysis. New York: Oxford University Press; 1982.
15. Martin DL, MacDonald KL, White KE, et al. The epidemiology and clinical aspects of the hemolytic uremic syndrome in Minnesoa. N Engl J Med. 1990; 323:1161–7.
16. Lilienfeld AM, Lilienfeld DE. Foundations of Epidemiology. 2nd ed. New York: Oxford University Press; 1980.
17. Kelsey JL, Thompson WD, Evans AS. Methods in Observational Epidemiology: Monographs in Epidemiology and Biostatistics. v. 10. New York: Oxford University Press; 1986.
18. Thacker SB, Berkelman RL. Public health surveillance in the United States. Epidemiol Rev. 1988;10:164–90.
19. Chorba TL, Berkelman RL, Saffor SK, et al. Mandatory reporting of infectious diseases by clinicians. JAMA. 1989;262:3018–26.
20. Osterholm MT, Rambeck JH, White KE, et al. Lack of efficacy of *Haemophilus* b polysaccharide vaccine in Minnesota. JAMA. 1988;260:1423–8.
21. Centers for Disease Control and Prevention. Public health: Surveillance, prevention and control of nosocomial infections. MMWR. 1992;41:783–7.
22. Williams REO. Changing perspectives in hospital infection. In: Proceedings of the International Conference on Nosocomial Infections. Atlanta: Centers for Disease Control; 1970:1–10.
23. Cross JT, Jacobs RF. Tularemia: Treatment failures with outpatient use of ceftriaxone. Clin Infect Dis. 1993;17:976–80.
24. Mishu B, Blaser MJ. Role of infection due to *Campylobacter jejuni* in the initiation of Guillain-Barré syndrome. Clin Infect Dis. 1993;17:104–8.
25. Moss AR, Osmond D, Bacchetti P, et al. Risk factors for AIDS and HIV seropositivity in homosexual men. Am J Epidemiol. 1987;125:1035–47.
26. Osmond DH, Charlebois E, Sheppard HW, et al. Comparison of risk factors for hepatitis C and hepatitis B infection in homosexual men. J Infect Dis. 1993;167:66–71.
27. Evans AS, ed. Viral Infections of Humans. Epidemiology and Control. 3rd ed. New York: Plenum Medical Book Company; 1991.
28. Weinstock HS, Bolar G, Reingold AL, et al. Hepatitis C virus infection among patients attending a clinic for sexually transmitted diseases. JAMA. 1993;269: 392–4.
29. Gwinn M, Pappaioanou M, George JR, et al. Prevalence of HIV infection in childbearing women in the United States. Surveillance using newborn blood samples. JAMA. 1991;265:1764–14.
30. Hedberg CW, Levine WC, White KE, et al. An international foodborne outbreak of shigellosis associated with a commercial airline. JAMA. 1992;268: 3208–12.
31. Waterhouse B. A Prospect for Exterminating the Smallpox. Cambridge, England: Cambridge Press; 1800.
32. Tucker WB. The evolution of the cooperative studies in the chemotherapy of tuberculosis of the Veteran's Administration and Armed Forces of the USA: An account of the evolving education of the physician in clinical pharmacology. Adv Tuber Res. 1960;10:1–68.
33. Francis T, Karns RF, Voight RB, et al. An evaluation of the 1954 poliomyelitis vaccine trial: Summary report. Am J Public Health. 1955;45 (part II, May Suppl):1–51.
34. Austin SC, Stolley PD, Lasky T. The history of malariotherapy for neurosyphilis. Modern parallels. JAMA. 1992;268:516–9.
35. Meinert CL. Clinical Trials. Design, Conduct and Analysis. Monographs in Epidemiology and Biostatistics. v. 8. New York: Oxford University Press; 1986.
36. Hadler SC, Erben JJ, Matthews D, et al. Effect of immunoglobulin on hepatitis A in day-care centers. JAMA. 1983;249:48–53.
37. Berkelman RL, Hughes JM. The conquest of infectious diseases: Who are we kidding? Ann Intern Med. 1993;119:426–8.
38. Hadler SC, Webster HM, Erben JJ, et al. Hepatitis A in day care centers—A community-wide assessment. N Engl J Med. 1980;302:1222–7.
39. Benenson AS. Smallpox. In: Evans AS, ed. Viral Infections of Humans: Epidemiology and Control. New York: Plenum Medical Book Company; 1991: 633–57.
40. Evans AS, Brachman PS, eds. Bacterial Infections of Humans: Epidemiology and Control. 2nd ed. New York: Plenum Medical Book Company; 1991.
41. Fox M, Kaufmann AF, Zendel SA, et al. Anthrax in Louisiana, 1971: Epizootiologic study. J Am Vet Med Assoc. 1973;163:446–51.
42. Skaliy P, McEachern HV. Survival of the Legionnaires' disease bacterium in water. Ann Intern Med. 1979;90:577–80.
43. Black PH, Swartz MN. Salmonellosis—A review of some unusual aspects. N Engl J Med. 1960;262:811–16, 846–70, 921–7.
44. Lau JYN, Wright TL. Molecular virology and pathogenesis of hepatitis B. Lancet. 1993;342:1335–9.
45. Stead WW, Senner JW, Reddick WT, et al. Racial differences in susceptibility to infection by *Mycobacterium tuberculosis*. N Engl J Med. 1990;322:422–7.
46. Cohen ML. Epidemiology of drug resistance: Implications for a post-antimicrobial era. Science. 1992;257:1050–5.
47. Levy SB. Confronting multidrug resistance: A role for each of us. JAMA. 1993;269:1840–2.
48. Granoff DM, Munson RS Jr. Prospects for prevention of *Haemophilus influenzae* type b disease by immunization. J Infect Dis. 1986;153:448–61.
49. Murphy TV, White KE, Pastor P, et al. Declining incidence of *Haemophilus influenzae* type b since introduction of vaccination. JAMA. 1993;269:246–8.
50. Benenson AS, ed. Control of Communicable Diseases in Man. 15th ed. Washington, DC: American Public Health Association; 1990.
51. Centers for Disease Control and Prevention. Recommendations for prophylaxis against *Pneumocystis carinii* pneumonia for adults and adolescents infected with human immunodeficiency virus. MMWR. 1992;41(No. RR-4);1–11.
52. American Thoracic Society. Control of tuberculosis in the United States. Am Rev Respir Dis. 1992;146:1623–33.
53. Centers for Disease Control and Prevention. Protection against viral hepatitis: Recommendations of the Immunization Practices Advisory Committee. MMWR. 1990;39(No. RR-2):1–26.
54. The National Vaccine Advisory Committee. The measles epidemic: The problems, barriers, and recommendations. JAMA. 1991;266:1547–52.
55. Shalala DE. Giving pediatric immunizations the priority they deserve. JAMA. 1993;269:1844–5.
56. Peter G, Lepow ML, McCracken GH Jr, et al, eds. Report of the Committee of Infectious Diseases. 22nd ed. Elk Grove Village, IL: American Academy of Pediatrics: 1991.
57. Katz SL. Prospects for childhood immunization in the next decade. Pediatr Ann. 1993;22:733–8.
58. Fine PE. Herd immunity: History, theory, practice. Epidemiol Rev. Epidemiol Rev. 1993;15:265–302.
59. Centers for Disease Control and Prevention. Measles prevention: Recommendations of the Immunization Practices Advisory Committee. MMWR. 1989; 38(No. S-9):1–13.
60. Centers for Disease Control and Prevention. 1993 sexually transmitted diseases treatment guidelines. MMWR. 1993;42(No. RR-14):1–102.
61. Centers for Disease Control and Prevention. Recommendations for the prevention and management of *Chlamydia trachomatis* infections, 1993. MMWR. 1993;42(No. RR-12):1–39.

SECTION D

11. THE CLINICIAN AND THE MICROBIOLOGY LABORATORY

GAIL L. WOODS
JOHN A. WASHINGTON

The purpose of the microbiology laboratory is to isolate and identify microorganisms that cause disease and to determine their susceptibility to antimicrobial agents that assist in their eradication. There is, however, no other area of the clinical laboratory in which specimen sources and types are so diverse, in which specimen selection and collection are so important, and in which close communication with the clinician is so vital.

SPECIMEN COLLECTION AND PROCESSING

There are several general guidelines on selection and collection of the specimen that bear emphasis. First of all, the specimen selected should be representative of the disease process. Material swabbed from the orifice of a sinus tract is, for example, more apt to yield harmless saprophytic microorganisms present on the skin than would material obtained by curettage or biopsy of the base of the tract. Second, an adequate quantity of material should be obtained for complete examination. All too frequently, a small or even invisible amount of material is obtained with a swab, which makes it nearly impossible for the laboratory to make appropriate smears and adequate cultures. Characteristically, chronic lesions contain few organisms. These may be missed readily in smears, cultures, and histopathologic sections. Third, scrupulous attention must be given to avoiding contamination of the specimen by the many varieties of organisms indigenous to the skin and mucous membranes (see Ch. 4), culture of which may often be more confusing and misleading than helpful. Sterile equipment and aseptic technique should be used for collecting specimens, particularly those from normally sterile sites. Fourth, material should be forwarded promptly to the laboratory. Fastidious organisms may not survive prolonged storage or may be overgrown by less fastidious organisms before cultures can be made. Last, specimens should be obtained before antimicrobial agents have been administered and, in the case of viral infections, early in the acute phase of illness to enhance recovery of the virus.

Hospital procedure guides should contain reasonably precise guidelines for the collection and transport of specimens from various sites (Table 1). There are numerous kinds of devices and containers available for this purpose. Swabs of every description and composition are available. If a swab is used to collect a sample for virus culture, calcium alginate should be avoided because it could inactivate herpes simplex virus. For culture of *Chlamydia trachomatis*, swabs with wooden shafts should not be used. Many commercially manufactured swab tubes contain a transport medium that is designed to preserve a variety of organisms and to prevent the multiplication of rapidly growing organisms. The swab, however, should be limited in its use to collecting material from the skin and mucous membranes, principally because the amount of material that can be collected with it is limited and is often negligible in practice. For recovery of most bacteria, myobacteria, and fungi, a swab should never

be submitted in lieu of curettings, biopsy material, pus, or fluid or tissue removed surgically. All too frequently, biopsy specimens or excised materials are placed in their entirety into formalin for histopathologic examination, and the microbiology laboratory receives one swab for a variety of smears and cultures.

Because of the frequency with which anaerobic bacteria play a role in causing infectious diseases, fluids or pus from the brain, thoracic and abdominal cavities, transtracheal and suprapubic aspirations, the pelvis, and the musculoskeletal system should be placed into a transport vial or tube in which anaerobes can survive for several hours. Alternatively, the syringe used to aspirate such materials may be used for their transport to the laboratory, provided the transport time is short. Anaerobe transport vials or tubes are available commercially. Vials should contain a transport medium with an indicator, for example, resazurin, which in its colorless state shows that the interior of the vial is anaerobic at the time a specimen is introduced. Anaerobic swab devices are also commercially available; however, their use is inadvisable because of the limited amount of material generally collected on swabs. Specimen containers should be sterile; they should not contain nonviable but stainable organisms that may provide misleading results.

SPECIFIC GUIDELINES FOR SPECIMEN COLLECTION AND PROCESSING

Respiratory Tract

Many types of specimens originate from the respiratory tract. The means of their collection and transport are outlined in Table 1, whereas the procedures recommended for their microscopic examination and culture are listed in Table 2.

Nasopharynx. Cultures of the nose are occasionally made to detect carriers of *Staphylococcus aureus;* however, the results of such cultures are seldom of any epidemiologic value and are not indicated except when serious focal outbreaks of nosocomially acquired staphylococcal infections occur. The results of cultures of the nose have been shown by Evans et al.[1] to correlate poorly with those of sinus aspirates and are, therefore, of little value in establishing the microbial etiology of sinusitis. Since aerobic, anaerobic, and facultatively anaerobic bacteria as well as fungi and viruses have been shown to cause sinusitis, it is necessary to take appropriate precautions with sinus aspirates to ensure the recovery of such a variety of organisms. There is similarly little value in making cultures of nose material to establish the microbial cause of otitis media. Although seldom necessary in acute cases because of the rather predictable findings of *Haemophilus influenzae, Streptococcus pneumoniae,* and *Streptococcus pyogenes,* tympanocentesis is probably warranted in cases with chronic otitis media due to this condition's variable bacteriologic etiology.

Cultures of the nasopharynx may be used to detect carriers of *Strep. pyogenes* (i.e., group A streptococci), *Neisseria meningitidis, Corynebacterium diphtheriae,* and *Bordetella pertussis.* Some have advocated their use in determining the cause of pneumonia in infants and children; however, nasotracheal aspiration is likely to provide material that is more representative of the disease process. Nasopharyngeal suction, as described by Auger,[2] is preferred for establishing the bacteriologic diagnosis of pertussis. A no. 8 French 16-in suction catheter with a safety valve is satisfactory in most cases. It is important to remember that cultures for *N. meningitidis, C. diphtheriae,*

TABLE 1. Guidelines for Microbiologic Specimen Collection and Transport

Specimen	Container or Transport Device	Volume (ml)	Other Considerations
Respiratory tract			
Nasopharynx	Flexible wire calcium alginate tipped swab or aspiration with a no. 8 French 16″ suction catheter into a sterile jar	NA	Used to detect carrier states of *Streptococcus pyogenes*, *Neisseria meningitidis*, *Corynebacterium diphtheriae*, and *Bordetella pertussis*; and *Chlamydia trachomatis* pneumonia in infants. Aspirates are useful in the diagnosis of pertussis and washings for viral infections.
Sinus aspirate	Anaerobic transport vial	NA	
Tympanocentesis	Anaerobic transport vial	NA	
Oral cavity	Swab	NA	
Throat	Swab		Swab tonsils, tonsillar areas, posterior pharynx, and areas of inflammation, exudation, ulceration, or capsule formation. Notify laboratory when *Mycoplasma pneumoniae* pneumonia, diphtheria, pertussis, or gonococcal pharyngitis is suspected clinically. Also useful for detection of enteroviruses, adenovirus, herpes simplex virus, and cytomegalovirus.
Tracheal aspirate	Sterile, screw-capped tube or jar	NA	Specimen unsuitable for anaerobic culture.
Bronchial washings	Sterile, screw-capped tube or jar	NA	Specimen unsuitable for anaerobic culture unless obtained with double-lumen, distally occluded catheter.
Transtracheal aspirate	Anaerobic transport vial	3–5	
Sputum			
Bacteria	Sterile, screw-capped jar	NA	Collect fresh specimen resulting from deep cough. Instruct patient not to expectorate saliva or postnasal discharge into container. Specimen unsuitable for anaerobic culture.
Mycobacteria	Sterile, screw-capped jar	5–10 ⎫	Collect three early morning, fresh specimens resulting from deep cough or induced by heated aerosol of 10% glycerin and 15% NaCl. Send to laboratory promptly or store under refrigeration. DO NOT COLLECT 24-HOUR SPECIMENS.
Fungi	Sterile screw-capped jar	3–5 ⎬	
Lung abscess, empyema fluid	Anaerobic transport vial	NA	
Urinary tract			
Clean-voided midstream urine or urine obtained by catheterization or cystoscopy for	Sterile, screw-capped tube or jar		
Viruses		1–10 ⎫	Send to laboratory promptly or store under refrigeration. DO NOT COLLECT 24-HOUR SPECIMENS. Specimen unsuitable for anaerobic cultures. Urine culture for *C. trachomatis* is suitable only for men.
C. trachomatis		1–10	
Bacteria		1–10 ⎬	
Mycobacteria		>20	
Fungi		>20 ⎭	
Suprapubic aspirate	Anaerobic transport vial	(As above)	Only valid means of establishing diagnosis of anaerobic bacteriuria.
Voided urine for parasites	Clean, screw-capped container	24-hour collection	Primarily collected to detect eggs of *Schistosoma haematobium*.
Blood			
Cultures for			
Viruses	Heparinized or clot tube	5–10; 30–50 for HIV	
Bacteria	Blood culture bottles containing broth or lysis–centrifugation tube	20–30 from adults, 1–3 from infants and children	Collect three separate blood samples during a 24-hour period; intervals between cultures are determined by urgency of clinical situation. More than three cultures per 24 hours are rarely necessary.
Brucellae and fungi	Lysis–centrifugation tube or biphasic blood culture bottle	(As for bacteria)	(As for bacteria)
Leptospires	Sterile, heparinized tube	1	(As for bacteria)
Examination for			
Borreliae	Peripheral smear	NA	Examine wet mount by darkfield microscopy or smear stained with aniline dyes
Malaria	Thick and thin films on clean glass slide	NA	
Filaria	Sterile tube containing anticoagulant (citrate, oxalate, heparin)	5	Wet mount of drop of blood or concentrated hemolyzed blood preferable to stained thick and thin films.
Trypanosomes			

(Continued)

TABLE 1. (Continued)

Specimen	Container or Transport Device	Volume (ml)	Other Considerations
Fluids			
Exudates, transudates, drainage, pus	Anaerobic transport vial	1–5	
Abdomen, chest	Anaerobic transport vial	1–5 for bacteria, >10 for mycobacteria or fungi	
Synovial	Anaerobic transport vial	1–5 for bacteria, >10 for mycobacteria or fungi	Inoculate modified Thayer-Martin medium in cases of suspected gonococcal arthritis.
Cerebrospinal	Sterile, screw-capped tube	1–2 for bacteria or viruses, >2 for mycobacteria or fungi	Send to laboratory immediately.
Catheters			
Intravascular	Sterile, screw-capped tube; Culturette (with swab removed)	NA	Disinfect skin entry site, remove catheter, clip off end into tube.
Suction, drainage	Sterile, screw-capped tube	NA	
Skin and soft tissues			
Cultures	Swab; anaerobic transport vial	NA NA	
Scrapings for dermatophytes	Sterile Petri dish	NA	
Gastrointestinal tract			
Stool culture or examination for			
Bacteria	Sterile, screw-capped jar; transport medium swab	NA	Freshly collected specimen mandatory; transport medium less desirable. Request cultures for vibrios, *Yersinia*, *E. coli* O157:H7, or enteric adenoviruses when suspected clinically.
Viruses	(As for bacteria)		
Ova and parasites	Stool carton sealed in plastic bag with polyvinyl alcohol preservative	NA	
Anal swab for pinworm	Sterile plastic swab in tube (SWUBE)	NA	Swab perianal area, preferably on arising in morning and before bathing or defecation.
Sexually transmitted diseases			
Neisseria gonorrhoeae	Swab; modified Thayer-Martin medium (Transgrow, JEMBEC)	NA	Women Cervix—moisten speculum with water; insert swab into cervical canal. Anal canal—insert swab approximately 1 in. to sample anal crypts. Urethral or vaginal—culture if cervix not accessible. Men Urethral—obtain material for smear and culture with swab or a sterile bacteriologic loop, which is used to inoculate medium directly and for preparing smears of exudates from men.
Haemophilus ducreyi	Swab	NA	
Treponema pallidum	Serous exudate on clean glass slide or in capillary pipet	NA	Abrade lesion with clean dry sponge. Examine preparation by darkfield microscopy *immediately*.
Chlamydia trachomatis	Sucrose-phosphate solution (2 SP)	NA	Extract urethral or cervical material on swab in solution and refrigerate during storage.
Ureaplasma urealyticum	(As for *Chlamydia*)	(As for *Chlamydia*)	(As for *Chlamydia*)
Candida albicans	Swab	NA	
Trichomonas vaginalis	Swab	NA	
Herpes simplex virus	Swab	NA	Avoid calcium alginate, refrigerate during storage.
Genitourinary tract excluding sexually transmitted diseases			
Cervical, vaginal discharge	Swab	NA	Specimen unsuitable for anaerobic culture.
Culdocentesis fluid	Anaerobic transport vial	NA	
Abscess			
Pelvic, tubal, ovarian	Anaerobic transport vial	NA	
Prostatic secretion	Sterile, screw-capped bottle	NA	
Eye			
Corneal lesion or scraping	Material should be inoculated directly onto appropriate media and applied directly to clean microscope slides for staining and microscopic examination.		
Conjunctiva examination for			
Bacteria, fungi, viruses	Swab		
Neisseria gonorrhoeae	Modified Thayer-Martin medium (Transgrow, JEMBEC)	NA	Inoculate swab directly onto medium.
Chlamydia trachomatis	Sucrose-phosphate solution (2 SP); swab for direct smear	NA	Extract material on swab in solution and refrigerate during storage.
Tissue	Sterile, screw-capped bottle	Representative samples	Specimen must be of sufficient size to ensure recovery of small numbers of organisms.

TABLE 2. Microscopic Examination for Respiratory Tract Pathogens

Source	Organism Sought or Disease Suspected	Gram Stain	FA[a]	Acid-Fast	KOH or Calcofluor	Toluidine Blue	Methenamine Silver
Nasopharynx	Streptococcus pyogenes		+				
	Bordetella pertussis		+				
	Viruses		+				
Paranasal sinus (aspirate)	Sinusitis	+					
Ear (aspirate)	Otitis media	+					
Mouth	Acute necrotizing ulcerative gingivitis (Vincent's)	+					
	Thrush					+	
Throat	S. pyogenes		+				
Sputum	Bacteria	+					
	Legionella		+				
	Mycobacteria			+			
	Nocardia			+[b]			
	Fungi				+		
	Pneumocystis carinii		+				
Bronchial lavage or brush	Bacteria	+					
	Legionella		+				
	Mycobacteria			+			
	Nocardia			+[b]			
	Fungi				+		
	Pneumocystis carinii		+			+	+
	Viruses		+				
Pleural fluid	Empyema						
	Nonsurgical	+		+			
	Surgical	+					
Lung tissue	Bacteria	+					
	Legionella		+				
	Mycobacteria			+			
	Nocardia			+[b]			
	Fungi				+		
	Pneumocystis carinii		+			+	+
	Viruses		+				

[a] Immunofluorescence performed on smear for respiratory syncytial virus, influenza A and B, parainfluenza viruses, adenovirus and *Pneumocystis carinii, S. pyogenes* is best detected when FA is done on centrifuged sediment of a 2–4-hour broth culture of a throat swab. Immunofluorescence testing for *Legionella* is not routinely recommended.
[b] Modified acid fast stain.

TABLE 3. Viruses Detectable in Nasopharyngeal Specimens and the Diseases They Cause

Disease	Viruses[a]
Common cold	Rhinoviruses, PIV, RSV, influenza viruses
Croup	PIV, RSV, influenza viruses
Acute bronchiolitis	RSV, PIV, influenza viruses, rhinoviruses
Pneumonia	Influenza viruses, RSV, PIV, adenovirus
Measles	Rubeola virus[b]

Abbreviations: PIV: parainfluenza viruses; RSV: respiratory syncytial virus
[a] Listed in order of most commonly to least commonly associated virus. Frequency of association of viruses with specific disease varies with age.
[b] Usually diagnosed serologically.

(Modified from Woods and Gutierrez,[19] with permission).

and *B. pertussis* must be requested specifically since these organisms either will not grow or will fail to be recognized on conventional bacteriologic media. Pertussis may be presumptively diagnosed by staining a smear of nasopharyngeal aspirate with anti-*B. pertussis* fluorescein-labeled conjugate, although the reported sensitivities and specificities of this test vary widely.

Nasopharyngeal specimens—aspirates, washings, and swabs—are recommended for diagnosis of many viral respiratory infections (Table 3), and they are useful in the diagnosis of measles and pneumonia caused by *Chlamydia trachomatis* in infants. Naso- or oropharyngeal specimens may be tested by direct fluorescent antibody methods to detect influenza A and B viruses; parainfluenza viruses, types 1, 2, and 3; respiratory syncytial virus; and adenoviruses. The sensitivity of direct fluorescent antibody testing is directly related to the quality of the specimen and the number of columnar epithelial cells (as opposed to squamous epithelial cells) that are present in the specimen. For this reason, nasopharyngeal aspirates or washes are superior to nasopharyngeal swabs. Enzyme immunoassay (EIA) can also be used for direct specimen testing for respiratory viruses; however, the procedure takes longer to perform than direct fluorescent antibody testing and is most economical when batches of specimens are tested. Nasopharyngeal aspirates and washings are superior to swabs for detection of viruses, but swabs are more convenient and, therefore, often are submitted. An aspirate is collected as described above, and a wash is obtained from the nose using a rubber suction bulb by instilling and withdrawing 3–7 ml of sterile phosphate-buffered saline. To collect nasopharyngeal secretions and cells with a swab, all mucus is removed from the nasal cavity first, after which a small, flexible nasopharyngeal swab is inserted along the nasal septum to the posterior pharynx and rotated several times against the mucosa. For detection of viruses, these specimens are placed into 2–4 ml of transport medium, such as veal infusion broth with 0.5% gelatin or Hanks' balanced salt solution with or without antibiotics, and to detect *C. trachomatis* the swab is placed in 2-sucrose phosphate transport medium. Specimens should be transported promptly to the laboratory or stored briefly in the refrigerator.

Oral Cavity. Cultures of the oral cavity are seldom helpful because of the millions of microorganisms normally resident in it. Direct examination of potassium hydroxide (KOH) preparations may, however, be helpful in confirming the diagnosis of oral thrush, and a Gram- or methylene blue-stained smear may be helpful in the diagnosis of acute necrotizing ulcerative gingivitis (Vincent's angina or fusospirochetal disease).

Throat. Most cultures of the throat are made to diagnose streptococcal pharyngitis since its clinical presentation is highly variable and is often indistinguishable from that of viral pharyngitis. Moreover, it is not at all uncommon for there to be concurrent viral and group A streptococcal infections of the throat. Sampling errors in swabbing the throat are frequent, and the patient's interests are best served by vigorous rather than gentle application of the swab to the posterior portion of the pharynx, tonsillar areas, and areas of ulceration, exudation, and membrane formation. Gram-stained smears are of little use or reliability since streptococci of all kinds occur normally and in large numbers in the mouth, and there is little that is distinctive about the microscopic appearance of group A streptococci.

A large number of rapid group A streptococcal antigen detection kits are commercially available for direct testing of throat swabs. Although these tests are highly specific, their sensitivity ranges from 45 to 100 percent, depending on the population studied, culture method used for comparison purposes, experience of the person doing the test, and the criteria (i.e., number of colonies) used to define a positive culture.[3,4] Since the sensitivity of antigen detection kits is directly correlated with the number of group A streptococci present in the specimen, kit sensitivity is lowest with specimens yielding few colonies of group A streptococci in cultures. Manufacturers have tended to discount false-negative kit test results under these circumstances as clinically unimportant; however, since the seroconversion (antistreptolysin O [ASO] and/or anti-DNase B) rate in children with both positive antigen test and culture results is virtually identical to that in children with negative antigen test results and positive cultures,[5] the number of group A streptococci in the specimen often reflect sampling variation and are seldom helpful in distinguishing between infection and colonization or the carrier state. Thus, although antigen tests have a high positive predictive value (100 percent), their negative predictive value may be substantially lower. Antigen tests may, therefore, not be acceptable as a culture substitute, particularly in areas where there has been a resurgence of acute rheumatic fever. Although it has been shown that the treatment rate is markedly higher for cases detected by antigen tests than for those detected by culture,[6] it is likely that inappropriate treatment rates are also markedly higher when a screening test is known to have a sensitivity of only 45 percent.

A throat swab is the specimen of choice for culture of *Mycoplasma pneumoniae;* however, pneumonia caused by *M. pneumoniae* often is diagnosed on the basis of clinical manifestations alone or on serologic tests. Culture of *M. pneumoniae* must be requested specifically, because a special culture medium is required for its recovery.

In expert hands, a Loeffler's alkaline methylene blue smear of material collected from the margin of a membrane may suggest the diagnosis of diphtheria; however, such expertise is rare in the United States today, and culture remains the principal means of establishing this diagnosis.

It must also be remembered that acute pharyngitis may be caused by *Neisseria gonorrhoeae,* which will not grow on media usually used for throat cultures. If gonococcal pharyngitis is suspected on clinical or epidemiologic grounds, the laboratory should be notified accordingly; however, it is preferable to inoculate modified Thayer-Martin or other selective media directly at the time the swab is taken.

Viral pharyngitis usually is a component of one of the syndromes listed in Table 3, and for optimal detection of the causative agent a nasopharyngeal specimen should be collected. Adenoviruses or, occasionally, enteroviruses also may cause pharyngitis, and a throat specimen—washings obtained by gargling with 5 ml of viral transport medium containing antibiotics or by a swab—is recommended for detection of these agents. Both of these viruses, however, may be shed in the pharynx months after resolution of an illness; therefore, a stool specimen should be cultured concurrently. Detection of the virus in both throat and stool suggests that it is likely to be responsible for current symptoms.

A throat specimen also is useful for diagnosis of congenital infection with herpes simplex virus (HSV) or cytomegalovirus (CMV) and for diagnosis of primary HSV stomatitis. In immunocompromised patients, such as organ transplant recipients, culture of throat specimens has been used to detect shedding of CMV, but the presence of CMV in the throat cannot be equated with CMV disease. Similarly, detection of HSV in the throat, except in newborns and seronegative persons with primary stomatitis, does not necessarily indicate that the virus is causing disease. Epstein-Barr virus (EBV) may be recovered from the throat of persons with infectious mononucleosis or healthy seropositive persons, but culture is not done in most clinical laboratories. Infectious mononucleosis is diagnosed serologically.

Sputum. The microbiologic examination of sputum is fraught with numerous problems. The patient is usually poorly instructed as to the type of specimen required; supervision is generally lacking during specimen collection; and the specimen often remains on the patient's night table for hours before being delivered to the laboratory, during which time it becomes overgrown with bacteria normally present in saliva. Ideally, patients should be instructed to rinse out their mouths with water and to provide only material resulting from a deep cough. Several attempts may be necessary before a suitable specimen of sputum is obtained. The specimen should then be transported to the laboratory promptly. If bacterial infection is suspected clinically, examination under low power ($\times 100$) of a Gram-stained smear of a carefully selected aliquot of the specimen, as described by Chodosh,[7] is a rapid means of determining its suitability for culture (Fig. 1). The presence of many squamous epithelial cells (>25 per low-power field[lpf]) indicates that the specimen consists substantially of saliva and contains an abundance of oropharyngeal microflora.[8,9] It is advisable not to culture this specimen but to reject it and request another one. If few squamous epithelial cells (<25/lpf) are present, the smear should be examined carefully under oil immersion ($\times 1000$) to determine whether bacteria morphologically typical of certain species (e.g., pneumococci, staphylococci) are present and the specimen should be cultured. In cases of suspected legionellosis, sputum should be cultured on buffered charcoal yeast extract medium containing antibiotics (BMPA medium). The most important consideration, however, in the laboratory diagnosis of pneumococcal and other bacterial pneumonias is the attention given to proper specimen collection.[10]

Although the degree of oropharyngeal contamination is not as critical in sputum specimens submitted for mycobacterial or fungal examination, every effort should still be made to collect material resulting from a deep cough and to minimize the specimen's contamination since the overgrowth by aerobic and facultatively anaerobic bacteria of mycobacterial and fungal cultures may severely limit the laboratory's ability to recover these pathogens. Twenty-four-hour specimens should not be collected for mycobacterial or fungal cultures. In some cases collection of sputum induced by a heated aqueous aerosol of 10% glycerin and 15% sodium chloride is useful for recovering mycobacteria and fungi. Specimens that cannot be processed within 1–2 hours after collection should be refrigerated during their storage and transport; failure to do so may result in a decreased yield of mycobacteria or fungi.

In suspected mycobacterial or fungal disease, appropriately prepared smears should be examined. A fluorochrome stain provides the most rapid means of examining a smear for mycobacteria. Phase-contrast microscopy, a KOH preparation or a smear stained with calcofluor white represent the best means of looking for fungi (Fig. 2).[11] It is important to remember that *Nocardia,* which may be seen in Gram-stained smears or KOH preparations of respiratory tract specimens, may not be seen in carbol fuchsin (Ziehl-Neelsen or Kinyoun) acid-fast–stained smears unless decolorized with 0.5–1% sulfuric acid without alcohol.

Bronchoscopy. Bronchoscopy is a relatively safe technique that provides secretions directly from bronchial drainage sites of infection. Examination of bronchoscopy specimens should

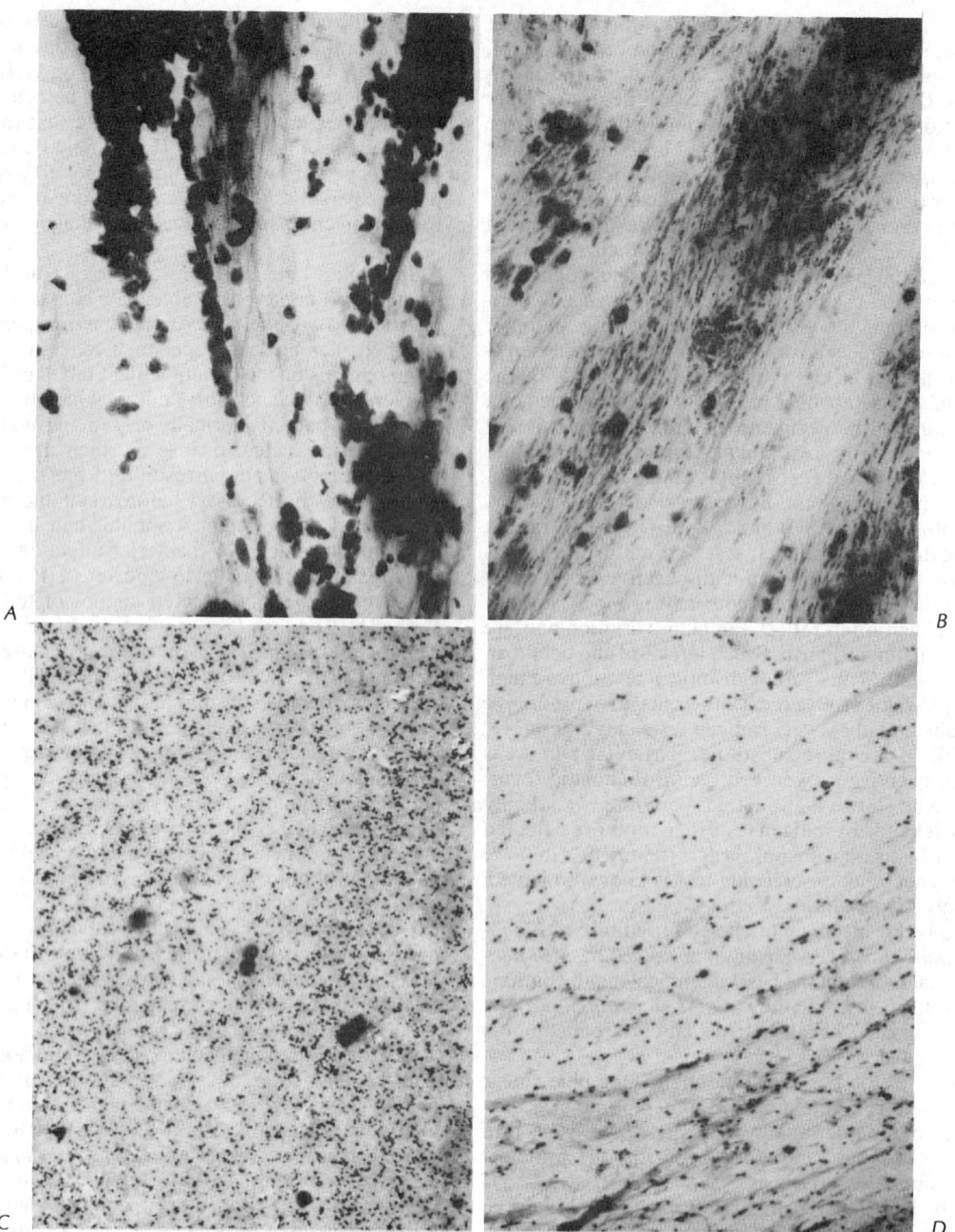

FIG. 1. Smears of representative sputum specimens. (Gram stain, ×100) **(A)** Group 1: leukocytes, <10; epithelial cells, >25. **(B)** Group 3: leukocytes, >25; epithelial cells, >25. **(C)** Group 4: leukocytes, >25; epithelial cells, 10–25. **(D)** Group 5: leukocytes, >25; epithelial cells, <10. (From Murray and Washington,[8] with permission.)

be considered in two categories: *(1)* studies to detect microorganisms (e.g., *Legionella, Mycobacterium tuberculosis, Pneumocystis carinii, Rhodococcus equi,* and *Cryptococcus neoformans*) that pose no problem in interpretation even in the presence of upper respiratory contamination and *(2)* studies for bacteria that may comprise upper respiratory flora but in which differentiation between upper and lower respiratory origin is necessary.[12] Bronchoscopy, including washings, biopsy, or lavage procedures, is suitable for the first category of examination, whereas bronchoscopy with a protected specimen brush has been advocated for the second category, particularly when accompanied by quantitative cultures for aerobic and anaerobic bacteria.[12] Quantitative cultures of fluid collected by bronchoalveolar lavage also may be useful for diagnosis of bacterial pneumonia.[13]

Pleural Fluid.   Pleural or empyema fluid is of particular value in the diagnosis of anaerobic pleuropulmonary infections and legionnaires' disease. In such cases, a Gram-stained smear can be very helpful, although it is necessary to prolong the period of counterstaining with safranin for several minutes to detect *Legionella.* A more specific approach to the diagnosis of this disease is by direct immunofluorescent staining of a smear of pleural fluid. Obviously, pleural or empyema fluid can be examined and cultured for other etiologic agents of pulmonary disease.

Lung Tissue.   Obtained at substantial cost and some risk to the patient, lung tissue specimens warrant special attention by all concerned.[12] The microbiologist needs to know the suspected clinical diagnosis and what the histopathologic studies show. It

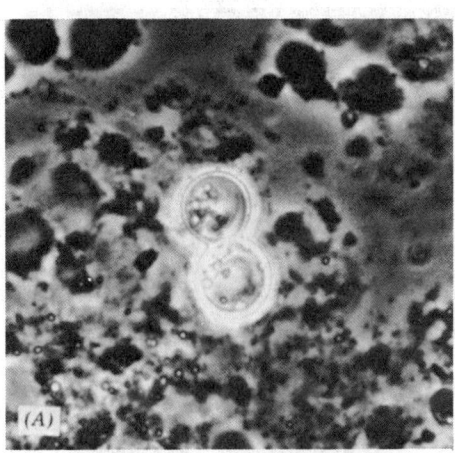

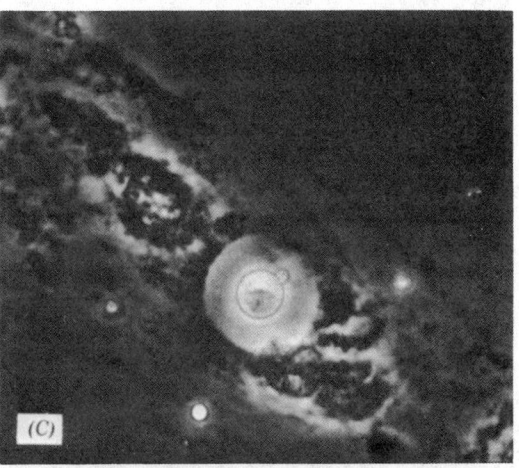

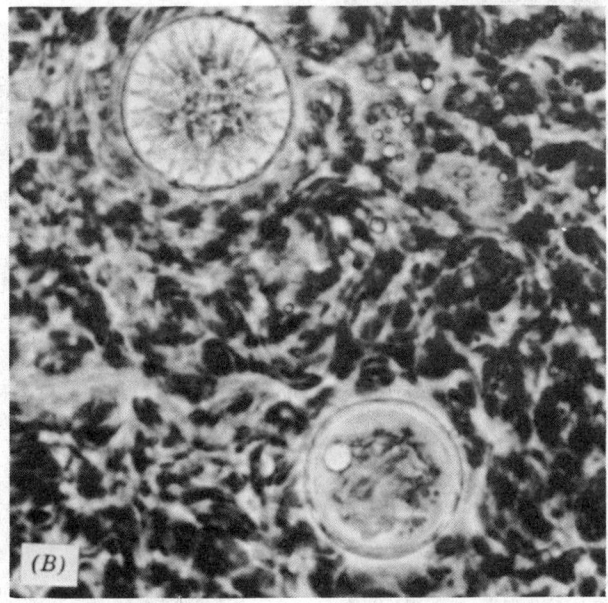

FIG. 2. Phase-contrast microscopy of clinical specimens. (× 2000) **(A)** *Blastomyces dermatitidis* in sputum. The characteristic yeast form has a budding cell attached by a broad base. Also note the "double contoured" appearance of the cell wall. **(B)** *Coccidioides immitis* in sputum. Large thick-walled spherules with few endospores are scattered within the interior of the spherule (lower) or cleavage furrows developing along the periphery to form endospores (upper). **(C)** *Cryptococcus neoformans* in sputum. Spherical yeast is surrounded by a large capsule with a small bud arising from the parent cell. *(Figure continues)*

should be stressed that few organisms may be present in a chronic inflammatory lesion and that an adequate quantity of the lesion should be submitted for examination and cultures. Impression smears of tissue are especially useful in the diagnosis of *Pneumocystis carinii* infections and legionnaires' disease. *Pneumocystis carinii* is readily seen in smears stained with Gomori methenamine silver, toluidine blue 0, or Giemsa. Also, monoclonal antibodies for immunofluorescence staining are commercially available and are likely the most sensitive technique for visualizing *P. carinii*.[14,15] Impression smears for *Legionella* are fixed with 10% formalin for 10 minutes and are stained with specific fluorescein-labeled conjugate.

Gram stain, an acid-fast stain, and Gomori methenamine silver stain are satisfactory for screening tissue sections for microorganisms.[12] Dieterle silver-impregnation stain will demonstrate *Legionella* in paraffinized tissue sections, but the stain is not specific for *Legionella*.[12]

Tissue for culture is finely minced with sterile scissors and is then ground in a tissue grinder or with a small amount of sterile abrasive (alundum) in a sterile mortar with a pestle. A 10–20 percent suspension is prepared with nutrient broth and is used to inoculate cultures. Alternatively, tissue may be macerated in a stomaching device and the extract used for microbiologic examination. Such suspensions are saved, most conveniently in a sterile 60-ml dropper bottle, until after the tissue sections and special stains have been reviewed in case additional cultures are indicated.

Urinary Tract

Clean-voided midstream urine is preferred for bacterial, mycobacterial, and fungal cultures. Twenty-four-hour collections are suitable only for parasitologic study (Table 1). Catheterization is not recommended for obtaining urine unless the procedure fulfills a diagnostic or therapeutic purpose. Suprapubic aspiration is recommended for establishing the diagnosis of bacteriuria in infants and small children, for determining the significance of borderline counts of bacteria in repeated clean-voided midstream specimens, and for determining the presence of anaerobic bacteriuria.

Because the distal urethra of both men and women is normally colonized with large numbers of aerobic, facultatively anaero-

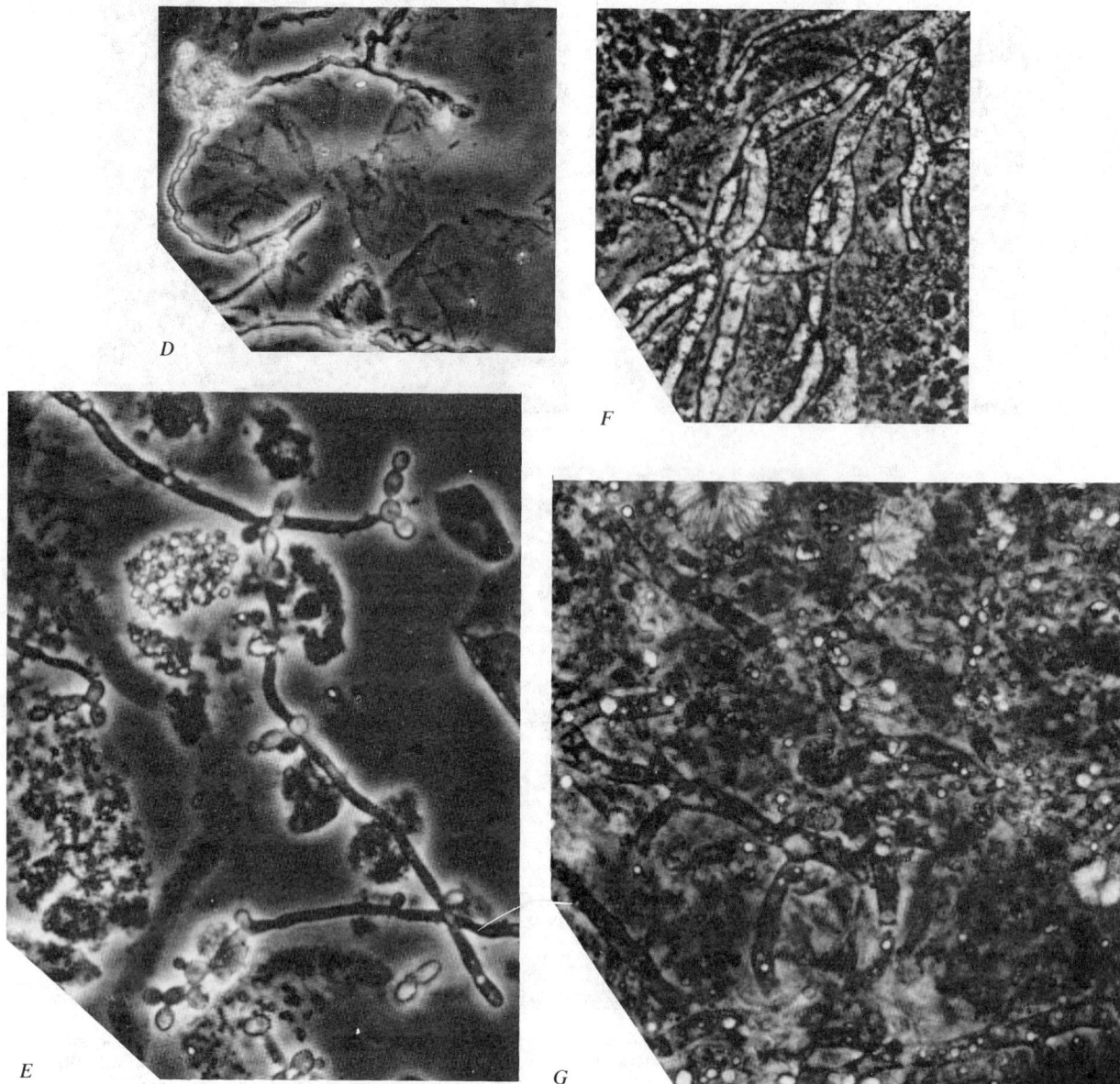

FIG. 2. *(Continued).* **(D)** Dermatophyte in a skin scraping. Septate hyphae intertwine among squamous cells. **(E)** *Candida albicans* in urine. Hyphae and budding yeasts appear among epithelial cells. **(F)** *Mucor* sp. in pus from a skin lesion. The large, branching, ribbonlike aseptate hyphae are indicative of a zygomycete. **(G)** *Aspergillus fumigatus* in sputum. The septate hyphae show dichotomous branching. (Courtesy of Dr. Glenn D. Roberts, Rochester, MN.)

bic, and anaerobic bacteria, the diagnosis of clinically significant bacteriuria in a clean-voided, midstream specimen requires quantitative cultures. Moreover, a Gram stain of a drop (allow to dry without spreading) of well-mixed urine will provide a means of determining the adequacy of its collection and the diagnosis of significant bacteriuria ($\geq$100,000 cfu/ml) when at least two bacteria per oil immersion ($\times$1000) field are found. The correlation of the results of this test in expert hands with those of quantitative cultures should be at least 90 percent. Essential to the validity of these results is proper specimen collection and transport to the laboratory. Unless refrigerated during storage and transport, no urine arriving in the laboratory more than 2 hours after its collection should be cultured. The presence of many squamous epithelial cells on microscopic examination of the urine is indicative of poor technique in its collection, and another specimen should be requested.

Quantitation of bacteriuria in cultures can be most conveniently accomplished by streaking a measured volume (e.g., 0.01 or 0.001 ml) of well-mixed urine onto the surface of culture media with a calibrated milk dilution platinum loop. A general-purpose medium (e.g., blood agar) and a gram-negative differential medium (e.g., eosin-methylene blue [EMB] or Mac-Conkey) should be used. Broth cultures of clean-voided urine are meaningless and should not be made since the growth of even a few bacteria of urethral origin will render the broth turbid and will provide misleading results. Precision in reporting the number of colonies isolated on solid media is unnecessary, and the results can be reported as approximate colony counts (e.g., $<10^3$, 10^4–10^5, $>10^5$ cfu/ml). Provided the specimen has been properly collected, colony counts of $\geq$10^4 ml are usually significant; however, as few as 100 cfu/ml may be significant in women with the acute dysuric syndrome, and as few as 1000 cfu/ml may be significant in males. Unless specimens are very carefully collected and transported to the laboratory, such low numbers of cfu/ml may be highly nonspecific.

Commercially available screening tests for significant bacteriuria include bioluminescence, miniaturized culture systems, dipstick method for nitrite and leukocyte esterase (Chemstrip

L-N), and staining of bacteria and leukocytes on filter paper (Bac-T-Screen, Filtra Check-UTI).[16] Regardless of the principle involved in the test, sensitivity is maximal with at least 10^5 cfu/ml, although it may vary with the populations of patients studied. The sensitivity of the L-N test may be enhanced by using the additional tests for blood and protein that are available on the Chemstrip 9.[17]

Cultures of the urine for other microorganisms (e.g., brucellae, leptospires, mycobacteria, fungi, mycoplasmas, and viruses) entail selective processes for their isolation, but the same requirements for careful specimen collection and transport apply because selective procedures are not uniformly successful in eliminating any bacterial contamination that may be present and that may overgrow cultures or otherwise interfere with the isolation of these other microorganisms. Decontamination and selective isolation procedures for these other organisms are described in detail elsewhere.[18,19] *Chlamydia trachomatis* urethritis in men may be diagnosed by detecting the organism in urine by enzyme immunoassay.[20]

Septicemia

The successful isolation of microorganisms from blood requires an understanding of the intermittency and low order of magnitude of most bacteremias, the great variety of organisms capable of causing septicemia, and a broad range of microbiologic considerations involved in the isolation of microorganisms from blood. Each of these factors is reviewed in detail elsewhere.[21,22] There are two major variables that warrant emphasis here: timing of blood collections and volume of blood collected for culture. Most bacteremias are intermittent, so blood collections for culture should be made intermittently during a 24-hour period. Studies have shown that the sensitivity of two to three separately collected blood cultures within a 24-hour period in establishing the cause of clinically significant bacteremias is nearly 100 percent and that the sensitivity of a single blood culture within this same time period is approximately 80–90 percent. The bacteremia associated with subacute bacterial endocarditis is usually continuous, so only two cultures will yield the etiologic agent in nearly all cases. It is apparent, therefore, that two separate blood cultures should be collected within a 24-hour period and that it is seldom necessary to perform more than two blood cultures within this same time period, especially if the anticipated pathogen is different from organisms that are normally present on the skin. When the anticipated pathogen might be one ordinarily considered to be a contaminant (e.g., coagulase-negative *Staphylococcus* in a patient with a prosthetic valve), it is advisable to obtain three or four separate cultures. A single culture in either instance should never be considered adequate.

Most bacteremias, with the exception of those occurring in infants, are of a very low order of magnitude; therefore, an adequate volume of blood should be collected for each set of cultures. It is suggested that 20 ml be obtained from adults and that 1–5 ml be obtained from infants and small children. It is important to consider the volume of blood cultured and the number of blood cultures obtained as independent variables; therefore, we should avoid the obvious temptation to use one venipuncture to obtain an unusually large volume of blood that is then inoculated into several sets of cultures. Although the rate of recovery of bacteria from blood is directly related to the volume of blood cultured, the yield from several separate sets of blood cultures is related, in turn, to the usual intermittency of bacteremia. Both factors, therefore, must be kept in mind when making blood cultures.

The proposed venipuncture site requires careful disinfection since bacteria normally resident in the skin include species that frequently are associated with infections of implanted prosthetic material. Their isolation from blood cultures can cause considerable confusion unless the skin has been carefully prepared for venipuncture with a suitable antiseptic agent and multiple sets of blood cultures have been inoculated with blood obtained from separate venipunctures.

Proper selection of blood culture bottles, although important, is difficult because of the many currently available conventional, semiautomated, automated, and specialized (e.g., Isolator, Wampole Laboratories, Cranbury, NJ) systems.

Generally, blood is inoculated into two blood culture bottles on a 10% vol/vol basis, which provides optimal neutralization of the serum bactericidal activity. Exceptions are the high-blood-volume bottles used with the BACTEC nonradiometric system (Becton Dickinson, Sparks, MD), for which the optimal ratio of blood to broth is 1:3.5 rather than 1:10. In the past, leaving one of the inoculated bottles unvented (relatively anaerobic) was recommended. Since that practice was suggested, the frequency of anaerobic bacteremia in some centers has decreased and that of fungemia has increased.[23] Given this trend, considering a blood culture protocol composed of two aerobic bottles or one aerobic bottle and one fungal medium and only selective use of anaerobic blood cultures has been recommended.[24] Depending on the type of system used, cultures are examined at least once per day for macroscopic, infrared spectrophotometric, or colorimetric evidence of growth for 5–7 days; longer periods of incubation may be indicated in cases of suspected endocarditis.[25] If a conventional broth system is used, subcultures may be made from aerobic bottles without macroscopic evidence of growth, optimally between 6 and 24 hours after initial inoculation. Subcultures of bottles yielding growth are made onto media that will allow recovery of aerobic, facultative, and anaerobic bacteria and differentiation of mixtures of different species of bacteria, because polymicrobial bacteremia occurs in about 10 percent of cases. Turbid broth or colonies from bottles yielding growth may be used for direct antimicrobial susceptibility testing after a short incubation period and adjustment of the inoculum size to that used in standardized methodology.

In cases of suspected meningococcemia or gonococcemia, media without sodium polyanetholsulfonate (SPS) should be inoculated because of this polyanion's inhibitory effects on some strains of pathogenic neisseriae. Otherwise, SPS, which has antiphagocytic, anticomplement, and anticoagulant activity, should be incorporated at concentrations of 0.025–0.05 percent into all blood culture media. The value of penicillinase in media inoculated with blood from patients receiving penicillins is uncertain, but its addition is probably advisable provided it is tested concurrently for its sterility. The value of resins in blood culture systems remains controversial with specific regard to the enhanced recovery of bacteria from blood cultures of patients receiving antimicrobial therapy.

Nutritionally deficient streptococci (*Streptococcus defectivus* and *Streptococcus adjacens*), which require pyridoxal (vitamin B6) for growth, are easily isolated in broth blood culture systems. Growth in the broth medium is recognized, a smear stained with the Gram stain shows gram-positive cocci in chains, but subcultures to solid media are sterile. Organisms are recovered by performing a "Staph streak": a lawn of the organism from the blood culture broth is spread over the surface of a blood agar plate and streaked with an isolate of *Staphylococcus aureus*, which provides the necessary pyridoxal. Laboratories that use only the Isolator system for blood cultures, however, will not detect nutritionally deficient streptococci unless the inoculated agar plate is supplemented with pyridoxal. Therefore, in the latter case the physician must inform the laboratory personnel when infection with nutritionally deficient streptococci is suspected (e.g., a patient with endocarditis and negative routine blood cultures) so the appropriate measures can be taken to allow its recovery.

Brucellae are most likely to be recovered from blood that is cultured early in the course of the disease and that has been processed by the Isolator tube and inoculated onto suitable culture media. Leptospires can be recovered only in some cases during the first week of illness and from essentially none thereafter. Cultures should be made by inoculating a few drops of fresh or anticoagulated blood into each of several tubes containing a leptospiral semisolid culture medium such as Fletcher's or Ellinghausen, McCullough, Johnson and Harris (EMJH) medium. Cultures should be incubated at 30°C for 2 or 3 weeks and should be examined with darkfield or immunofluorescent microscopy twice weekly. Direct darkfield microscopic examination of blood or blood cultures should be interpreted very cautiously because of the formation of motile "pseudospirochetes" from blood components.

Bartonella (Rochalimaea) henselae recently has been identified as a cause of persistent fever and bacteremia, as well as bacillary angiomatosis, bacillary peliosis hepatis, and catscratch disease. The organism is most likely to be recovered from blood that has been processed by the Isolator system and inoculated onto enriched media supplemented with blood or charcoal-yeast extract agar. Given these special requirements, the clinician must communicate with the laboratory personnel when *B. henselae* is in the differential diagnosis. Most currently available blood culture systems provide effective recovery of yeasts causing fungemia; however, lysis-centrifugation (Isolator) is the only system available today for the recovery of dimorphic fungi causing deep mycotic infections (e.g., *Histoplasma capsulatum*).[25]

Malassezia furfur, which causes fungemia primarily in patients receiving intravenous lipids, grows well in broth blood culture systems. If the microbiology laboratory uses only the Isolator system, the clinician must inform the laboratory personnel when fungemia with *M. furfur* is suspected so appropriate measures can be taken to ensure its recovery. *Malassezia furfur* requires lipid for growth; therefore, the agar medium inoculated with the sediment from an Isolator tube must be covered with a thin layer of sterile olive oil, coconut oil, or another lipid source.

Intra-Abdominal Infections

According to Finegold,[26] the incidence of infections involving anaerobic bacteria in this site generally is 86 percent. Anaerobes are involved in pyogenic abscesses of the liver in 50–100 percent of the cases and in at least 90 percent of tubo-ovarian and pelvic abscesses. Appropriate measures must, therefore, be taken to ensure the survival of anaerobes during the specimen's transport to the laboratory. Fluid or pus should be aspirated into a syringe, and air bubbles expelled, and its contents should be injected into an anaerobic vial for transport to the laboratory. Swabs are generally not suitable for this purpose.

Granulomatous lesions of the liver, spleen, or lymph nodes should be cultured for mycobacteria and fungi, as well as for aerobic and facultatively anaerobic bacteria. Complete microbiologic examination of material removed surgically is essential in patients undergoing abdominal exploration for fever of unexplained origin. Because the distribution of organisms in tissue may not be uniform, generous portions of tissue should be removed for histologic and microbiologic examination.

Amebic abscesses of the liver are rarely confused histologically with pyogenic abscesses and are mainly composed of necrotic granular and eosinophilic material with considerable nuclear debris and few or no cells. The amebae are usually found near the capsule and not in the central necrotic material. Microscopic examination of the pus may be facilitated by its enzymatic digestion with streptodornase and the preparation of wet mounts from centrifuged sediment. Serologic tests often are useful for diagnosis of extraintestinal amebiasis.

Central Nervous System Infections

The cerebrospinal fluid from a patient suspected of having meningitis demands immediate attention from the microbiologist.

This urgency is dictated by the lethality of acute bacterial meningitis if untreated, its morbidity if inadequately treated, and its curability if treated early with appropriate antimicrobial agents. The prompt detection, isolation, and identification of the etiologic agent and determination of its antimicrobial susceptibility play a crucial role in the management of meningitis.

Cerebrospinal fluid must be collected aseptically, both to prevent the inadvertent introduction of organisms into the central nervous system and to avoid contamination with organisms indigenous to the skin or other body surfaces, culture of which may delay or confuse the diagnosis. Aspirations of cerebrospinal fluid shunts must be made very carefully since bacteria associated with infections of such shunts frequently belong to species that are ordinarily indigenous to the skin. Careful preparation of the skin must be carried out with a suitable antiseptic such as chlorhexidine or an iodophor; aqueous benzalkonium chloride should be avoided for skin antisepsis.

Specimen containers in lumbar puncture trays, whether prepared in-house or commercially, should be tested occasionally by the microbiology laboratory for sterility, absence of stainable but nonviable bacteria, and effectiveness of closure to prevent leakage during transport. Many hospitals use pneumatic tube systems to transport medically urgent specimens to the laboratory, and it is not uncommon for leakage from certain kinds of tubes to occur under these conditions. Cerebrospinal fluid should not be stored or refrigerated, and it should be transported to the laboratory for examination as rapidly as possible.

Although the number of bacteria per milliliter of cerebrospinal fluid in cases with meningitis usually exceeds 10^5 cfu/ml, numbers significantly below this level do occur. Moreover, if present, the numbers of mycobacteria and fungi in cerebrospinal fluid are often few. It is, therefore, important for a sufficient volume (Table 1) of fluid to be sent to the laboratory to ensure its proper examination. Additional fluid is, of course, required for cell counts and biochemical analyses. Ideally, fluid for microbiologic studies should be placed in separate containers from that needed for other studies to expedite processing and to minimize contamination.

Fluid should be examined microscopically in the laboratory (Table 4). Centrifuged sediment is generally examined microscopically; however, it is important to realize that some bacteria usually require a force of at least $10,000 \times g$ for 10 minutes to sediment and that 60 minutes may be required to accomplish the same purpose with the conventional bench-top laboratory

TABLE 4. Microbiologic Examination of Cerebrospinal Fluid

Suspected Cause	Essential	Supplemental	Culture
Bacterial	Gram-stained smear	Quellung reaction, latex agglutination	Blood agar, chocolate blood agar, ± automated system
Viral		Serologic tests for measles, HTLV-1, HIV, rabies virus, or viral encephalitis	Cell culture for mumps, enterovirus, HSV, VZV, HIV, or CMV
Syphilis	VDRL		
Mycobacterial	Acid-fast smear		Bactec TB, Septi-Check AFB, Lowenstein Jensen, 7H11
Fungal	Latex agglutination or EIA for Cryptococcus	India ink smear for Cryptococcus	Brain–heart infusion, Sabouraud's agar
Amebae	Phase-contrast microscopy		1.5% agar in distilled water or cocultivation with E. coli

centrifuge, which develops a maximum force of only 1000 × g. In most cases, the presence of inflammatory cells will hasten the sedimentation process; however, there may only be a few polymorphonuclear leukocytes in the cerebrospinal fluid early in the course of acute bacterial meningitis. Published reports of the sensitivity of the Gram-stained smear of cerebrospinal fluid sediment from patients with acute bacterial meningitis vary but approximate 70 percent. For this reason as well as because of possible misinterpretation of findings in the smear, other methods of bacterial detection in cerebrospinal fluid have been developed, the most rapid and specific of which are immunologic. The first such test was counterimmunoelectrophoresis, which has been replaced in almost all clinical laboratories by the more rapid and more sensitive latex particle agglutination (LPA) and coagglutination (CoA) tests.

Latex particle agglutination and coagglutination tests have been positive upon initial evaluation of cerebrospinal fluid in 95 (range, 78–100) and 94 (range, 83–100) percent, respectively, of patients with *Haemophilus influenzae* meningitis.[27] The corresponding figures for LPA and CoA in meningococcal meningitis are 78 (range, 20–100) and 39 (range, 33–50) percent, respectively, and for pneumococcal meningitis are 67 (range, 50–100) and 82 (range, 60–100) percent, respectively.[27] The sensitivities of LPA and CoA are much less in cases in which the Gram-stained smear of cerebrospinal fluid was negative than in those in which the smear was positive.[27] False-positive immunologic test results (i.e., positive for antigen and a negative culture) on cerebrospinal fluid are uncommon. Whether such false-positive results actually represent false-negative cultures, technical errors, cross-reactions, or, in the case of tests of urine in which false-positives occur more frequently, antigenuria in asymptomatic carriers or recently immunized children remains uncertain.[27,28]

The major question regarding rapid antigen tests of cerebrospinal fluid is how the information they provide is used clinically. In one study of this question, appropriate therapy for *H. influenzae* type b meningitis was initiated before the results of latex particle agglutination were known, and in no case did the results of the test alter therapy.[28] Granoff et al.[28] concluded that physicians believed that the risks of error in the test were not acceptable in the management of an infection that is potentially fatal without appropriate antimicrobial therapy and that culture results rather than antigen test results were being used for management decisions. Antigen tests of cerebrospinal fluid may be helpful in partially treated patients.

In suspected fungal meningitis, an India ink wet mount preparation of cerebrospinal fluid sediment can be examined for the presence of encapsulated, budding yeasts resembling cryptococci. Care must be taken not to confuse red blood cells, white blood cells, or starch granules with the characteristically encapsulated cryptococci. The sensitivity of this procedure is less than the latex agglutination or enzyme immunoassay tests for cryptococcal antigen. Properly controlled, the sensitivity of an antigen test approximates that of culture. Because false-positive antigen tests occur, diagnosis must be confirmed by culture. Wet mount preparations are not usually useful in establishing the diagnosis of coccidioidal meningitis. Cultures should be made but are infrequently positive for *C. immitis*. Most patients develop complement-fixing antibodies to *Coccidioides* in their spinal fluid.

Darkfield microscopy of cerebrospinal fluid may be helpful in establishing the diagnosis of leptospirosis; however, the presence of leptospires in cerebrospinal fluid closely parallels that in blood. Darkfield examinations and cultures should therefore be made during the first week of illness.

The motile amebae (*Naegleria, Acanthamoeba* group) may be seen with phase microscopy. They may be cultured on plain agar by placing a drop of cerebrospinal fluid onto a loopful of *E. coli* spread in a 1-cm² area in the center of the plate.

Brain abscesses contain anaerobic bacteria in nearly 90 per-

cent of cases.[26] Often their presence is suggested in Gram-stained smears made directly with pus from the abscess. Appropriate precautions must be taken to ensure the survival of anaerobes during the specimen's transport to the laboratory, and anaerobic cultures should be prepared.

Media to be inoculated with cerebrospinal fluid are listed in Table 4 according to the etiologic agent suspected. It is important to concentrate the specimen before its inoculation either by centrifugation or by membrane filtration. In the latter case, fluid is forced through a 0.45-μm disposable membrane filter device (e.g., Swinnex, Millipore Corporation), and the filter is cultured by placing it "upstream" side down on the agar surface. After 24–48 hours of incubation, the filter is moved to determine whether colonies may have arisen at its site of application.

Processing cerebrospinal fluid for diagnosis of viral infections involves conventional culture or, for some viruses, serologic tests. Of the viruses that could be detected in cerebrospinal fluid, enteroviruses are recovered most frequently in the clinical laboratory. HSV, varicella-zoster virus (VZV), and CMV are isolated infrequently from cerebrospinal fluid, but brain tissue is preferred for detection of these viruses. Mumps virus is easily cultured in the clinical laboratory, but this must be specifically requested. Rabies virus, lymphocytic choriomeningitis virus, human T-cell leukemia virus type I (HTLV-I), and human immunodeficiency virus (HIV) may be isolated from the cerebrospinal fluid, but these tests usually are available only in reference laboratories. Polymerase chain reaction (PCR) of cerebrospinal fluid is available in some research laboratories for detection of CMV.

Detection of antibodies in cerebrospinal fluid is useful for diagnosis of subacute sclerosing panencephalitis and neurologic disease caused by HTLV-I or HIV. Tests for specific immunoglobulin M, which generally are performed only in special reference laboratories, are useful in diagnosing several viral encephalitides: western equine, eastern equine, Venezuelan equine, St. Louis, Japanese, and LaCrosse.

Musculoskeletal Infections

Most musculoskeletal infections are due to bacteria (aerobic, facultatively anaerobic, anaerobic, and mycobacterial) and less frequently to fungi. Microorganisms are usually recovered from previously unopened and undrained abscesses, provided the pus has been properly collected and transported to the laboratory. "Sterile" pus is usually due to carelessness on the part of the person collecting the specimen or to the ineptness of the laboratory personnel examining it. In chronic lesions the number of organisms is often small, so an adequate quantity of specimen should be obtained. Swabs are usually unsatisfactory for this purpose, and material should be collected with a sterile syringe and needle. If necessary, irrigation of the lesion with bacteriostat-free saline or Ringer lactate solution is satisfactory. Sinus tracts often originate in bone or lymph nodes, and their microbial cause is seldom elucidated by swabbing the tract's orifice.[29] The orifice should be cleansed with an antiseptic, and curettings should be taken of the tract as close to its base as possible. A deep biopsy specimen is preferable. Cultures of swabs of ulcers may also be misleading, and it is suggested that curetting or biopsy specimens be taken from the base or undermined edge of such lesions. Cultures of previously opened abscesses usually yield a great variety of microorganisms, identification of which taxes the technologist and defies rational antimicrobial therapy. Again, a carefully collected specimen does much to minimize confusion.

Wounds, both traumatic and nosocomial in origin, are increasingly found to be infected with gram-negative bacilli and anaerobic bacteria. Media appropriate for the isolation and identification of these bacteria should be used for cultures of wound material. Quantitative bacteriology of biopsy specimens from acute and chronic wounds has been shown to provide valuable prognostic information on the risk of sepsis at the time of closure.[30] In addition, quantitative bacteriology of biopsy specimens of burn wounds has been found to reflect infection more accurately than have surface culture techniques.[31] As a general rule, the risk of wound sepsis increases significantly if there are more than 10^5 cfu/g of tissue, whereas wounds with fewer than 10^5 cfu/g have little risk of developing sepsis when closed primarily.[32] Gram-stained smears of biopsy material may be made to provide quantitative results within 30 minutes after receipt of the specimen in the laboratory.[30]

Post-traumatic mycobacterial infections are often due to the *Mycobacterium fortuitum-chelonae* complex and to *Mycobacterium marinum*.[32] Sources of the former group of mycobacteria have included soil, lower animals, dirty skin, foreign bodies, contaminated needles or syringes, and contaminated injectable material, whereas those of *M. marinum* have included tropical fish aquariums, swimming pools, and tributaries. When granulomas are suspected of being due to *M. marinum*, the laboratory should be notified so cultures are incubated at 25°–30°C; *M. marinum* grows slowly if at all at 37°C. On solid media, colonies of *M. marinum* require 2 weeks or longer to develop, whereas those of the *M. fortuitum-chelonae* complex will usually appear within 7 days of incubation. Mycobacterial infections of the bones and joints may also be due to several species including *M. tuberculosis, M. bovis,* and *M. kansasii*.[32] Their growth requires at least 2 weeks on solid media, but growth may be detected earlier in broth media.

The significance of mycobacteria other than tubercle bacilli that are isolated from the musculoskeletal system and wounds must be interpreted cautiously because of their occurrence in nature as well as in clinically asymptomatic humans, especially in superficial lesions. Their significance is increased if isolated from an abscess or closed lesion, when present in large numbers, and if isolated in repeated cultures. Acid-fast bacteria may not be seen in as many as half of the tissues from which tubercle bacilli are isolated, so acid-fast stains are helpful only when positive.

Osseous lesions may occur in disseminated forms of brucellosis, cryptococcosis, coccidioidomycosis, blastomycosis, and sporotrichosis. The presence of granulomas in frozen sections of bone should therefore prompt a request for cultures for mycobacteria, brucellae, and fungi (see Table 4 for suitable media).

Gastritis

Helicobacter pylori is commonly associated with gastritis. Definitive diagnosis is made by staining gastric biopsies with hematoxylin and eosin (H&E) or silver impregnation stain and observing the characteristic curved bacteria on the gastric epithelium. Cultures of gastric biopsies may also be diagnostic; however, incubation in a microaerophilic atmosphere for up to 5 days may be necessary for recovery of the organism. A presumptive diagnosis of *H. pylori* infection may also be made by placing a biopsy specimen in a urea broth and observing the medium for a pH change as a result of the organism's ability to rapidly hydrolyze urea. The presence of IgA, IgM, and IgG antibodies in serum may also be used diagnostically, and a decline in IgG antibody titers over a period of several months is indicative of a therapeutic response.

Acute-Onset Diarrhea

Acute-onset diarrhea may be caused by a variety of bacterial, parasitic, and viral agents. Included among bacterial etiologic agents are *Bacillus cereus, Campylobacter jejuni, Clostridium difficile, Clostridium perfringens,* enterotoxigenic, enterohemorrhagic, and enteroinvasive *E. coli,* salmonellae, shigellae, *Vibrio cholerae* and halophilic vibrios, and *Yersinia enterocolitica*. Among parasitic agents, those most frequently encountered in the United States are *Giardia lamblia* and *Entamoeba histolyt-*

ica; however, cryptosporidiosis has become a serious problem in patients with acquired immunodeficiency syndrome (AIDS) and can cause diarrhea in previously healthy persons. Other parasites more recently recognized as human pathogens are microsporidia (*Enterocytozoon bienusi*) and *Cyclospora* spp. (previously called *Cyanobacterium*-like bodies), both of which cause chronic diarrhea. Microsporidiosis has been diagnosed almost exclusively in persons with AIDS. *Cyclospora* has been detected in a few persons with AIDS and also has been responsible for three outbreaks of diarrhea (one in Chicago and two in Kathmandu, Nepal) in immunocompetent persons. Viral causes of acute-onset diarrhea are rotavirus, Norwalk and similar agents, calicivirus, and adenovirus.

Unexplained renal failure in children with diarrhea or bloody diarrhea should raise the possibility of *E. coli* O157:H7. This agent is easily missed on culture for routine enteric pathogens and is best detected on sorbitol MacConkey agar. Commercially available antiserum to O157 can be used to test the colorless colonies from this medium.

The diagnosis of *Clostridium difficile*–associated diarrhea requires toxin detection, for which the reference method is cell culture assay to detect the cytotoxic activity of toxin B. Drawbacks to the cell culture assay are lack of standardization, which makes comparison of data from different studies difficult, long turn-around time (24–48 hours), sensitivity of less than 100%, and the requirement that personnel performing the test be familiar with cell culture.[33] For these reasons, alternative methods for toxin detection have been developed. A commercially available latex agglutination test is technically simple to do and provides results in 30 minutes or less. The test, however, detects glutamate dehydrogenase, not toxin A as initially believed, and gives positive reactions with nontoxigenic strains of *C. difficile* and other anaerobes that might be present in stool.[34,35] Moreover, the sensitivity of the latex test in some studies has been as low as 75–80 percent compared with the cell culture assay.[36] Commercially available enzyme immunoassays that detect toxin A or both toxins A and B are relatively simple to perform, have a turn-around time of 2.5–4 hours, are highly specific and more sensitive than the latex test.[37] Isolation of the organism from stool is nonspecific and, therefore, is not recommended for diagnosis of *C. difficile*–associated disease.

To examine stool for the more conventional pathogenic bacteria, the laboratory should receive a freshly passed stool or freshly collected rectal swab. The specimen should be inoculated onto blood agar, a gram-negative differential medium (EMB or MacConkey agar), a selective medium for *Salmonella* and *Shigella* (xylose-lysine-deoxycholate [XLD] or Hektoen enteric [HE] agar), and enrichment broth (gram-negative [GN] or selenite), and selective media for *Campylobacter jejuni* and, when specifically requested, *Y. enterocolitica* or sorbitol MacConkey for enterohemorrhagic *E. coli* (O157:H7). Should infection with vibrios be suspected on the basis of recent travel in an endemic area (*V. cholerae*) or recent ingestion of raw seafood or shellfish (*V. cholerae* or *V. parahaemolyticus*), the laboratory should be so notified so that thiosulfate-citrate-bile salts (TCBS) agar can also be inoculated, although these organisms grow well on blood agar and many grow on gram-negative differential and selective media. *Bacillus cereus* food poisoning has been only infrequently recognized in the United States but becomes manifested either by upper gastrointestinal tract symptoms, similar to those seen in staphylococcal food poisoning, or by lower intestinal tract symptoms, similar to those seen in clostridial food poisoning. Diagnosis of the former syndrome can only be established by the isolation of large numbers of *B. cereus* in incriminated food; however, diagnosis of the latter syndrome is limited to isolation of the organism from stool and determining whether it is enterotoxigenic.

In suspected parasitic infections, loose watery stools should be promptly submitted to the laboratory since protozoan trophozoites may degenerate rapidly, especially at room or incubation temperatures. If the stools are formed, it is preferable to obtain a saline-purged stool on each of 3 consecutive days after having the patient ingest 15 ml of magnesium sulfate (Epsom salt) early in the day. Specimens that are mailed or in which delivery is delayed should be placed in 10% formalin or polyvinyl alcohol (PVA) fixative in a small, plastic, screw-capped container. For brief periods of storage (≤2 hours), refrigeration is advisable. Studies have shown that in most cases examination of a single specimen is all that is required.[38] Moreover, in patients developing diarrhea after being hospitalized for over 3 days, examination of stool for parasites rarely is productive.[39] Specimens are examined grossly for the presence of proglottids or adult worms and for areas of blood or mucus that should be examined microscopically in direct and concentrated wet mounts and in permanently stained smears. Concentration procedures by formalin-ether sedimentation or zinc sulfate flotation techniques increase the likelihood of detection of protozoan cysts and helminthic eggs and larvae. Trichrome and iron hematoxylin are commonly used for preparing permanent stains.

Detection of cryptosporidia, microsporidia, and *Cyclospora* spp. requires special procedures; therefore, in most clinical microbiology laboratories, these tests must be specifically requested. Oocysts of cryptosporidia are detected by staining a smear of a fixed stool specimen or a routine stool concentrate with a modified acid-fast stain or a commercially available monoclonal antibody. Concentration of stool using Sheather's sugar flotation is an excellent procedure for recovery and identification of *Cryptosporidium* oocysts, but it is not necessary for diagnosis. Microsporidiosis is diagnosed by histologic examination of biopsies of the small intestine, most optimally the duodenum, followed by the jejunum. These organisms also can be detected by light microscopic examination of smears of stool samples or duodenal aspirates stained with a modified trichrome stain. This stain, however, is not available in many laboratories, in which case sending the specimen to a laboratory with experienced personnel is recommended. *Cyclospora* species may be visualized in wet-mount preparations of fresh, unpreserved stool, in smears stained with the modified acid-fast stain, and in smears examined under ultraviolet light.

Norwalk-like agents are important causes of epidemic gastroenteritis but require special immune electron microscopy or radioimmunoassay or enzyme immunoassay techniques for their detection. Rotavirus causes a syndrome characterized by diarrhea, fever, and vomiting but may also be shed asymptomatically; thus, detection of rotavirus in feces may have little utility in distinguishing between those who are infected (as evidenced by antibody titer rise) and those who are carriers. Nonetheless, detection of rotavirus has epidemiologic utility since viral shedding is the major means of transmission of the virus. The major diagnostic tests available commercially for detection of rotavirus in feces are enzyme immunoassay and latex agglutination. Latex agglutination is comparable to enzyme immunoassay in the acute phase of rotaviral infection since large amounts of antigen are excreted during the first days of illness; however, latex agglutination has less sensitivity than does enzyme immunoassay later in the course of disease or in the detection of asymptomatic carriers.[40] Enteric adenoviruses may be detected in the clinical laboratory. Detection may be made by enzyme immunoassay, or it may require inoculation of a special cell line; therefore, laboratory personnel must be informed in advance that infection with this virus is suspected.

Despite the many advances that have been made in determining the etiology of diarrheal disease, the diagnostic capabilities of the clinical laboratory remain limited to cultures for *Salmonella, Shigella, Campylobacter, Yersinia, Vibrio,* and the enteric adenoviruses; examination for ova and parasites; detection of *C. difficile* toxin and rotavirus antigen; and culture plus serotyping or toxin detection for the enterohemorrhagic *E. coli.* Detection of enterotoxigenic, enteroinvasive, and enteropatho-genic strains of *E. coli,* Norwalk-like agents, caliciviruses, and astroviruses await further technologic developments.

Genital Infections

Syphilis. Although usually diagnosed serologically, syphilis can in its primary and secondary stages be diagnosed by darkfield or direct fluorescent antibody microscopic examination of serous exudate from infectious lesions. Lesions should be abraded with a dry sponge to provoke exudation; however, it is important to minimize bleeding since the presence of red cells will make the examination more difficult. The exudate is applied directly to a clean coverslip that is inverted on a glass slide. The edges of the coverslip can be sealed to minimize evaporation since *Treponema pallidum* is very sensitive to desiccation. The slide should, at any rate, be examined as soon as possible. Spirochetes of *T. pallidum* are motile, 6–15 μm in length, and have 5–20 rigid and regular spirals. Because of the normal presence of nonpathogenic treponemes in the mouth, darkfield microscopic examinations of material from this source should not be performed.

Serologic tests for syphilis are divided into nontreponemal tests, including the Venereal Disease Research Laboratory (VDRL) test, and treponemal tests, including the fluorescent treponemal antibody absorption (FTA-ABS) test and microhemagglutination tests such as MHA-TP. The sensitivity of the VDRL test is high in secondary syphilis and early latent syphilis and less sensitive in primary syphilis. Its specificity is high (99.5–100 percent) in healthy persons but reduced (75–85 percent) in sick persons.[41] The VDRL test is the preferred test for screening asymptomatic persons and, when positive, should be confirmed by a hemagglutination test. The VDRL should then be followed at 3, 6, and 12 months to determine the adequacy of treatment. Although the CSF-VDRL test is a highly specific indicator of neurosyphilis, it is positive in only 22–69 percent of patients with active neurosyphilis. Because of its lack of specificity, the CSF-FTA-ABS is not recommended for use in this country.

Gonorrhea. The diagnosis of gonorrhea in men can be established presumptively by the findings of gram-negative intracellular diplococci in stained smears of urethral discharge (Fig. 3). Gram-stained smears of cervical drainage lack sensitivity and specificity,[42] and it is probably advisable for laboratories other than those in sexually transmitted disease clinics not to make them at all. Nonpathogenic neisseriae, anaerobic cocci, overdecolorized gram-positive cocci, and short forms of gram-negative

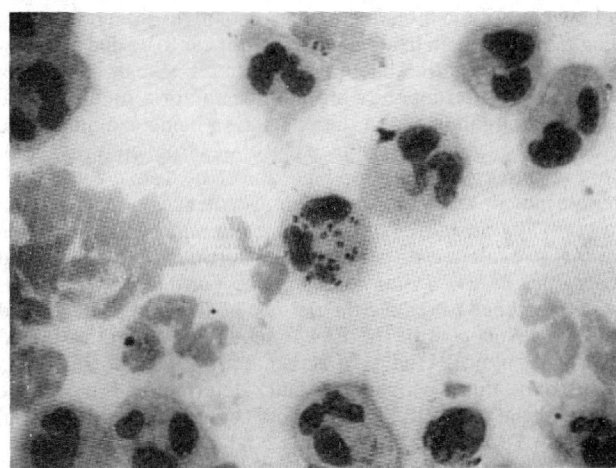

FIG. 3. Intracellular diplococci in a smear of urethral exudate from a male with gonorrhea. (Gram stain, ×1000) (From Washington,[42] with permission.)

bacilli that may normally be found in the vagina and may appear to be within or adherent to leukocytes render interpretation of Gram-stained smears of this area especially difficult and are subject to potentially serious error. To confirm the diagnosis in men and to establish it in women, it is necessary to make cultures for *N. gonorrhoeae*. In the absence of a urethral discharge, which may sometimes be obtained by "milking" the urethra, material should be obtained either by inserting a thin calcium alginate swab or small-diameter, smooth bacteriologic loop into the urethra. Cervical material should be obtained by direct visualization with the aid of a speculum. In all women and in homosexual men suspected of having gonorrhea it is also recommended that the anal crypts be swabbed for culture since this may be the only site from which gonococci may be recovered. In cases of suspected gonococcal pharyngitis, the posterior portion of the pharynx and tonsillar areas should be vigorously swabbed for any throat culture. In cases of suspected gonococcemia, blood should be inoculated into media without SPS, as has already been described.

Specimens from sites normally inhabited by fungi or other bacteria should be inoculated promptly onto selective media such as modified Thayer-Martin medium (MTM) containing vancomycin (3 µg/ml), colistin (7.5 µg/ml), and nystatin (12.5 units/ml) or, preferably, anisomycin (10 µg/ml). The addition of trimethoprim (5 µg/ml) to MTM is desirable to prevent swarming by *Proteus*. Concurrent inoculation of chocolate blood agar without antibiotics might be considered to allow growth of vancomycin-susceptible gonococci, another cause of false-positive smears. Incubation in an atmosphere of at least 70 percent humidity and 3–7 percent carbon dioxide should be done as quickly as possible. Gonococci are sensitive to drying and wide fluctuations in temperature.

Several devices are available commercially that permit the physician to inoculate MTM directly with clinical material. The necessary carbon dioxide is either already provided in the device by its manufacturer (e.g., Transgrow) or a carbon dioxide–generating effervescent tablet is placed in a chamber at the time the MTM is inoculated (e.g., JEMBEC). Such devices may then be transported to a laboratory for examination; however, it is important that they be incubated at 35°C overnight before mailing, and failure to do so will significantly decrease recovery of *N. gonorrhoeae*.

An enzyme immunoassay (EIA) for the detection of gonococcal antigen is commercially available and has been found to be as sensitive as Gram-stained smears of male urethral specimens and more sensitive than are Gram-stained smears of cervical specimens for the detection of *N. gonorrhoeae*. Compared with culture of endocervical specimens, the sensitivity of EIA has varied between 75 and 100 percent, whereas specificity has varied between 95 and 99 percent. False-positives in endocervical specimens have been troublesome and appear to be due to cross-reactive gram-negative bacteria. Whether EIA can serve as a culture substitute depends on multiple factors, including the prevalence of gonorrhea in the population being examined, the incidence of antibiotic resistance of isolates from cultures, laboratory resources, turn-around time, and cost. A small false-positive rate may be acceptable in a high-prevalence population seen in a sexually transmitted disease clinic but may be unacceptable in a low-prevalence private practice setting. The turnaround time of the EIA is 4 hours but may be considerably longer if tests are batched to reduce the per-test cost. Even on a batched basis, however, cost of the EIA exceeds that of Gram-stained smear and culture. Finally, if screening for *N. gonorrhoeae* is by EIA only, this obviously precludes determining β-lactamase activity or the susceptibility of gonococci to other antimicrobial agents.

Recently, an acridinium-ester–labeled nucleic acid probe for detection of *N. gonorrhoeae* became commercially available. The probe is highly specific and sensitive when used for culture confirmation, and it appears to be similarly reliable when used

for direct detection of *N. gonorrhoeae* in clinical specimens.[43,44] In a preliminary evaluation, the ligase chain reaction for direct detection of *N. gonorrhoeae* in endocervical secretions had a sensitivity and specificity nearly equal to those of culture.[45] However, as is true of EIA, use of either the probe or nucleic acid amplification for direct detection precludes determining antimicrobial susceptibility of the infecting strain.

Chlamydia. From men, a urine sample is acceptable if an approved EIA or perhaps PCR is used to detect the organism. Dacron-, rayon-, or cotton-tipped swabs are acceptable; however, swabs with wooden shafts should be avoided because wood is toxic to the organism. To collect a specimen from the urethra, any discharge is removed, a swab is inserted 3–4 cm into the anterior urethra and gently rotated for 10–15 seconds, and placed in the appropriate transport medium, which depends on the detection method used in the laboratory. If direct fluorescence using monoclonal antibodies (DFA) is done, the swab is rolled over the surface of a glass microscope slide and the material is immediately fixed (the slide and fixative are provided in the specimen collection kit). Endocervical specimens are collected after the cervix is visualized with the aid of a speculum moistened only with warm water. The cervix first is cleaned with a swab; then a second swab is inserted a few millimeters into the cervical canal, rotated firmly for 15–30 seconds, removed without touching the walls of the vagina, and either rolled on the surface of a glass slide or placed in the appropriate transport medium, depending on what test is performed in the laboratory.

Chlamydia trachomatis may be detected in genitourinary specimens by cell culture, DFA, enzyme immunoassay, nucleic acid hybridization, or nucleic acid amplification. Currently, cell culture is considered the reference method and must be used when the diagnosis is disputed or in criminal cases such as sexual assault and abuse investigations. Specimens for culture are placed in transport medium (2-sucrose phosphate [2 SP]) and delivered promptly to the laboratory. If a delay is unavoidable, the specimen in 2 SP is stored in the refrigerator or at −70°C if for longer than 72 hours. To culture the sample, shell vials or 24-well plates containing coverslips seeded with McCoy or Buffalo green monkey kidney cells are inoculated; and cultures are centrifuged, incubated for 48 hours, and stained with fluorescein-conjugated monoclonal antibodies. Disadvantages of cell culture are its cost, delay in turn-around time (results are not available for 48–96 hours), and its sensitivity, which for culture of a single endocervical specimen is estimated to be 70–80 percent. For these reasons, the nonculture methods mentioned above were developed.

Detection of *C. trachomatis* by DFA involves direct visualization of elementary bodies in smears stained with fluorescein-conjugated monoclonal antibodies specific for its major outer membrane protein or lipopolysaccharide. The sensitivity of DFA in women ranges from 70 to 100 percent, depending on the prevalence of disease in the population being evaluated; for urethral specimens from men, the sensitivity is about 70 percent.[46] In general, the sensitivity is greater in populations with a high prevalence of disease. The specificity of DFA is greater than 95 percent. With DFA, specimen adequacy can be assessed and results could be available within 1 hour of receiving the specimen; however, a high-performance fluorescent microscope is essential, interpretation is subjective, and operator fatigue limits the number of specimens that can be processed in a day.

EIA kits provide objective results in 30 minutes (for membrane-based systems) to a few hours. Sensitivities and specificities are similar to those of DFA.[47] False-positive results can be reduced by improving the specimen collection technique and by using blocking antibodies.[48,49] An acridinium-ester–labeled DNA probe complementary to *C. trachomatis* ribosomal RNA provides results within a few hours and for endocervical specimens has a sensitivity and specificity comparable with those of cell culture.[50] The PCR for detection of *C. trachomatis* in endocervical specimens or in urine specimens from men with urethritis appears to be more sensitive than culture and just as specific.[51]

Mycoplasma and Ureaplasma. The role of the genital mycoplasmas and ureaplasmas in producing urethritis and pelvic inflammatory disease remains unclear, although there are circumstantial data implicating *Ureaplasma urealyticum* (T-strain mycoplasmas) in nongonococcal urethritis. Swabs transported in 2-SP are suitable for culture of genital mycoplasmas; however, the results of cultures should be interpreted cautiously because of the frequency of isolation of mycoplasmas from genital areas of asymptomatic patients.

Gardnerella vaginalis. The role of *Gardnerella vaginalis* in causing bacterial vaginosis remains uncertain since it is found in the vaginal flora of many asymptomatic women and since the entity of bacterial vaginosis appears to be associated with the isolation of *G. vaginalis,* anaerobic curved rods (*Mobiluncus* spp.), and anaerobic gram-negative bacilli. Amsel et al.[52] have proposed three of the four following criteria adequate for a diagnosis of bacterial vaginosis: *(1)* vaginal pH greater than 4.5; *(2)* thin, homogeneous, milklike discharge; *(3)* release of fishy amine odor on addition of a drop of KOH (10% solution) to a a drop of vaginal discharge; and/or *(4)* the presence microscopically of clue cells in a saline wet mount of the vaginal discharge. Culture is not recommended for diagnostic purposes.

Pelvic Inflammatory Disease. The cause of pelvic inflammatory disease is difficult to determine and varies according to the population of patients studied, the types of specimens examined, and the investigator bias as to the types of microorganisms being studied. Pelvic inflammatory disease may be classified as gonococcal and nongonococcal or as sexually transmitted and nonsexually transmitted.[53] The major causes of the sexually transmitted disease are *Neisseria gonorrhoeae* and *Chlamydia trachomatis.* The possible roles of *Mycoplasma hominis* and *Ureaplasma urealyticum* remain controversial.[53] The major causes of nonsexually transmitted pelvic inflammatory disease are aerobic and anaerobic bacteria, often in mixed culture.[53] Diagnosis of gonococcal disease is facilitated by the isolation of *N. gonorrhoeae* from the endocervix, while the preferred method of diagnosis of disease due to aerobic and anaerobic bacteria is by aspiration with a needle and syringe or surgical incision and drainage or excision.[26] Anaerobic cultures should be routinely performed with such specimens as well as with material obtained by culdocentesis. Cultures of material aspirated from the uterine cavity should be limited to those obtained with a double-lumen, distally occluded catheter, which will minimize contamination of the specimen by normal vaginal and cervical flora.

Both *Chlamydia trachomatis* and genital tract mycoplasmas have been implicated as causes of acute salpingitis after their recovery from material obtained by laparoscopy.[54] Tests of endocervical or tubal material for *C. trachomatis* are therefore of value in elucidating the cause of salpingitis. The interpretation of endocervical cultures yielding mycoplasmas, however, remains problematic because of the frequency of isolation of this group of organisms from asymptomatic women.

Herpes Simplex Virus. Sexually transmitted disease caused by HSV may be diagnosed by direct observation of characteristic uninucleate or multinucleate cells with intranuclear inclusions in smears of cells stained with the Wright stain (Tzanck

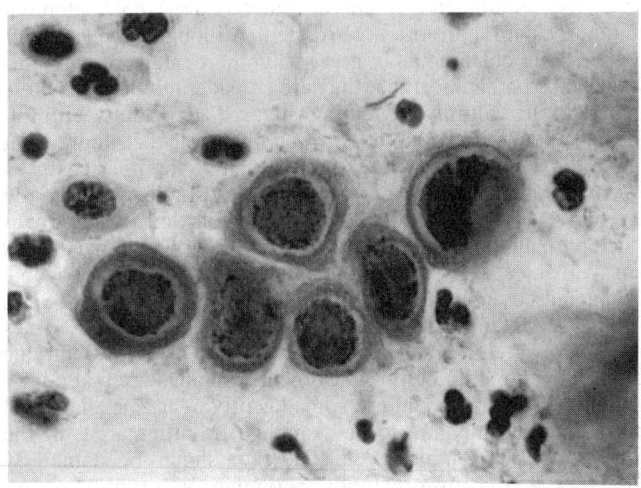

FIG. 4. Typical inclusions of herpes simplex virus in smear of endocervical cells. (Papanicolau stain, ×256)

preparation) or Papanicolau stain (Fig. 4), by detection of HSV antigens in smears stained with monoclonal antibodies or in swab specimens tested by EIA, or by isolating the virus in cell culture. The sensitivity of detecting typical inclusions in stained smears is about 50–70 percent for a vesicle and much lower if the vesicle has crusted or if there is no visible lesion.[55] Moreover, cytologic changes caused by HSV and VZV are identical and cannot be distinguished. Staining smears with monoclonal antibodies provides an identification, but the sensitivity is only 70–80 percent. The sensitivity of EIA for direct detection of HSV has ranged from 100 percent for vesicular lesions to 75 percent for nonvesicular ones.[56] Conventional cell culture is the reference method (and the most sensitive technique) for detection of HSV, and in most cases typical cytopathic changes in the inoculated cells are visible within 1–3 days.

Specimens useful for detection of HSV are urethral or endocervical swab specimens, collected as described earlier for *Chlamydia trachomatis* (but avoiding calcium alginate swabs). If a vesicle is present, the fluid may be aspirated with a 27-gauge needle on a tuberculin syringe, or the vesicle may be unroofed and the base firmly scraped with a swab. Likewise for ulcers, the base is firmly scraped with a swab. Both vesicle fluid and swab specimens should be placed in an appropriate viral transport medium and promptly taken to the laboratory or refrigerated if a delay in transport cannot be avoided. If examination of a smear is desired, the swab specimen should be rolled on the surface of a glass slide, and a second swab specimen should be collected for culture.

Trichomonas. *Trichomonas vaginalis* accounts for about one-fourth of clinically significant vaginal infections in the United States.[57] Typically, the infection is diagnosed by visualizing motile trichomonads in wet mount preparations of vaginal discharge. Organisms also may be seen in wet mount preparations of urethral discharge from symptomatic males. *Trichomonas vaginalis* may be isolated from vaginal or urethral discharge, but culture is not available in most clinical laboratories.

Ocular Infections

The difficulties of determining the cause of conjunctivitis on the basis of Gram-stained smears and bacteriologic cultures have been emphasized by Leibowitz et al.,[58] who found a poor correlation between the initial clinical impression and the results of microbiologic studies and between the findings in Gram-stained smears and in cultures. Although bacteriologic studies of conjunctivitis are useful primarily in gonococcal conjunctivitis, microbiologic studies for chlamydiae and viruses (e.g., adenovirus, herpesvirus) are often warranted. Although Giemsa stains demonstrate chlamydiae in a very high percentage of neonates with inclusion blennorrhea, they are considerably less sensitive than is tissue culture in detecting chlamydiae in adults with follicular conjunctivitis due to *C. trachomatis*. Direct fluorescent antibody-stained smears are highly sensitive in either case.

Corneal ulcers require careful laboratory studies as described elsewhere by Jones et al.[59] and by François and Rysselaere.[60] The ophthalmologist should ensure that the following materials are available: sterile swabs, spatula, clean glass microscopic slides and coverslips, proparacaine hydrochloride (Ophthaine, 0.5%), alcohol lamp, and media suitable for cultivation of bacteria, mycobacteria, and fungi. The swabs are used for obtaining conjunctival and lid cultures. Corneal scrapings are taken with the aid of a slit lamp and are spread gently over a small area of each slide and medium to be examined. Multiple areas of the ulcer should be sampled. One slide each should be stained by the Gram and Giemsa methods. Scrapings on a third slide are examined under a coverslip in a potassium hydroxide preparation. If indicated, the remaining slides may be stained with a fluorochrome or carbol fuchsin technique for mycobacteria and by a silver impregnation method for fungi. In cases with corneal ulcers in contact lens wearers, corneal scrapings should be cultured for *Acanthamoeba*.

Intraocular infections, including those related to surgery, may be due to a variety of microorganisms. Material obtained by ocular paracentesis requires scrupulous attention with appropriate smears and cultures for bacteria (including anaerobic), mycobacteria, fungi, and viruses.

IDENTIFICATION OF ORGANISMS

The laboratory can provide preliminary or definitive identification of etiologic agents based on: *(1)* microscopic examination of specimens, of growth occurring in cultures of those specimens, or of indirect evidence of growth in tissue culture (e.g., cytopathic effects); *(2)* immunologic techniques that detect microbial antigens or antibodies in body fluids or in cultures of those fluids; *(3)* DNA probes to detect microorganisms or genetically encoded characteristics of microorganisms in specimens or cultures; and *(4)* growth or biochemical characteristics of organisms isolated in cultures.

Microscopy

Unstained. Wet mount preparations of specimens can be examined with an ordinary light microscope for evidence of fungi or parasites. The substage condenser should be raised and lowered during examination to achieve optimal illumination and contrast. Practical applications include direct examination for fungi in sputum and other body fluids, bronchial aspirates, skin and hair scrapings, and urinary sediments mixed with 10% potassium hydroxide on a clean glass microscopic slide. A coverslip is placed over the mixture, and the slide is gently heated by passing it through a flame. Wet mounts are also used for examining fecal material for the presence of protozoan trophozoites and helminth larvae. Contrast can be increased in examining cerebrospinal fluid for cryptococci by mixing centrifuged sediment with India ink or Nigrosin. Contrast can also be enhanced with phase microscopy (Fig. 2) or with darkfield microscopy, the latter being the procedure of choice for the detection of spirochetes in skin or mucosal lesions in early cases of syphilis or in the cerebrospinal fluid or urine in early cases of leptospirosis.

Wet mounts of urinary sediment, with or without methylene blue, will provide reliable evidence of the presence of significant bacteriuria when at least 20 bacteria per high dry objective field ($\times 430$) are seen.

In each of these cases microscopy can provide rapid and de-

TABLE 5. Stains Commonly Used for Detection of Microorganisms

Stain	Organisms detected
Gram	Bacteria, *Candida*
Auramine-rhodamine[a]	Mycobacteria
Ziehl-Neelsen	Mycobacteria
Kinyoun	Mycobacteria
Modified Kinyoun	*Nocardia*, cryptosporidia, *Isospora, Cyclospora*
Giemsa	Plasmodia, trypanosomes, leishmania, *Toxoplasma gondii, Histoplasma capsulatum, Pneumocystis carinii* (trophozoites), *Borrelia* spp. (causing relapsing fever)
Gomori's methenamine silver (GMS)	*P. carinii* (cysts), fungi
Toluidine blue	*P. carinii* (cysts)
Dieterle	*Legionella* spp., spirochetes, *Bartonella (Rochalimaea)*
Trichrome[a]	Parasites (cysts and trophozoites)
Calcofluor white	Fungi
Mucicarmine	*Cryptococcus neoformans*

[a] More sensitive and easier to read than Ziehl-Neelsen and Kinyoun stains.

finitive identification of an etiologic agent in a specimen, assuming, of course, that organisms display typical morphologic characteristics. All these procedures are limited by the occurrence of small or rare numbers of organisms in the specimen, by the findings of artifacts that may resemble organisms, and by the presence of atypical forms of organisms that are not readily identifiable. Training and experience are required to prevent over- or underinterpretation of findings.

Stains. Innumerable stains have been described for the examination of specimens or organisms. The one most frequently used in the clinical laboratory—for direct examination of smears prepared from clinical material, from positive blood cultures, or from isolated colonies—is the Gram stain, performed as follows:

1. Drop or roll the material to be examined onto the surface of a clean glass slide. Allow it to dry or heat it on a slide warmer or by passing it through a flame.
2. Flood the slide with crystal violet and let it stand without drying for 30 seconds. Rinse with tap water.
3. Flood the slide with iodine and let it stand without drying for 60 seconds. Rinse with tap water.
4. Decolorize with acetone-alcohol (95% ethanol) until no violet color washes off (about 10 seconds), and rinse with tap water.
5. Flood the slide with safranin and let it stand without drying for 30–60 seconds. Rinse with tap water and allow the smear to dry.
6. Examine under oil immersion.
7. To ensure proper procedure, control slides should be stained and examined at least weekly.

Other commonly used stains and their main purposes are listed in Table 5.[61,62] The interested reader is referred to standard references for details about reagents and procedures for other stains.

Immunoassays and DNA Probe Hybridization Techniques

New technologies that provide rapid detection or identification of specified microorganisms or specific characteristics of microorganisms are exciting developments that are likely to alter the practice of medical microbiology substantially. The number of commercially available nucleic acid hybridization methods is expanding too rapidly to permit a complete list, but among the most useful are the chemiluminescent (nonradioactive) probes (Gen-Probe, San Diego, CA), some of which detect the target organism directly in clinical specimens (*Chlamydia trachomatis, Neisseria gonorrhoeae*, and group A streptococci), whereas others (*Coccidioides immitis, Histoplasma capsulatum, Blastomyces dermatitidis, Mycobacterium tuberculosis* complex, *Mycobacterium avium* complex, *Mycobacterium gordonae*, *Mycobacterium kansasii,* and several other bacteria) identify the organism once growth is apparent (culture confirmation). Nucleic acid hybridization tests, in general, are based on the ability of complementary nucleic acid strands to align specifically and associate to form stable double-stranded complexes. The Gen-Probe system uses chemiluminescent (acridinium-ester)-labeled, single-stranded DNA probes that are complementary to ribosomal RNA (rRNA) of the target organism. To do the test, the specimen or colony is agitated and heated to release the rRNA from the organism, and the labeled probe is added. If the probe is complementary to the target organism's rRNA, a stable DNA–RNA hybrid is formed. This hybrid is separated from the nonhybridized probe, and chemiluminescence is measured in a luminometer. These relatively simple tests have shortened identification of several molds and mycobacteria (listed above) to hours what would once have required weeks and specialized expertise to accomplish.

Amplification techniques, such as the polymerase chain reaction (PCR), provide added sensitivity and are becoming available for clinical laboratory use. This methodology is, however, technically complex and requires extreme care to prevent false-positive reactions due to contamination. PCR is replacing culture for the rapid detection of the human immunodeficiency virus (HIV-1). Numerous other applications of amplification techniques are anticipated, particularly for the detection of non-cultivatable, slow growing, or fastidious organisms.

Other Immunologic Techniques

Direct Immunofluorescence. Direct immunofluorescence technique involves the attachment of antigen or antibody labeled with fluorescein isothiocyanate (FITC) to its antibody or antigen, respectively, and detection of the labeled product with fluorescence microscopy. Practical applications of direct staining include the identification of *S. pyogenes* (group A) in throat swabs or cultures; *B. pertussis* in nasopharyngeal swabs, aspirates, or cultures; *Cryptosporidium* in stool specimens; *Brucella, Francisella tularensis,* and *Yersinia pestis* in clinical specimens; *Legionella* in lung tissue or respiratory secretions; *C. trachomatis* in ocular, nasopharyngeal, and genital specimens; *Pneumocystic carinii* in respiratory tract secretions; and several viruses (see Table 2) in nasopharyngeal specimens.

Direct immunofluorescence is a rapid and sensitive method of staining organisms in specimens or cultures. Fluorescent antibody procedures for screening clinical material and cultures for fungi have been described by Kaufman and Reiss at the Centers for Disease Control and Prevention[63]; however, labeled reagents are not available from commercial sources. The accuracy of immunofluorescence depends on many factors, including technical expertise, properly functioning equipment, the sensitivity of the reagents and their specificity, and the source of the specimen being examined. Immunofluorescence is not necessarily a substitute for culture since it does not yield a viable organism for antimicrobial susceptibility testing or other specific studies. Nonetheless, it can provide rapid detection and often at least presumptive identification of many microorganisms, and it has become an indispensable tool for many laboratories.

Agglutination. Agglutination tests to identify etiologic agents in specimens are limited in number. The most important one in use today is the latex agglutination test for *Cryptococcus neoformans* antigen in cerebrospinal fluid and serum. The sensitivity of this test exceeds that of the India ink preparation for examination of cerebrospinal fluid. Specificity of the cryptococcal latex agglutination test may be reduced by the presence of rheumatoid factor or other interfering proteins; however, treatment of the specimen with a protease (pronase) will eliminate false-positive results due to interfering proteins.[64]

As discussed earlier, latex and coagglutination may be useful in the diagnosis of bacterial meningitis of partially treated children or in those children in whom the inflammatory response and various biochemical indices in the cerebrospinal fluid do not clearly distinguish between bacterial and viral meningitis.

Latex agglutination, coagglutination, the quellung reaction and counterimmunoelectrophoresis have been used to detect pneumococcal antigen in sputum from patients with suspected pneumococcal pneumonia. The sensitivity of each of these tests relative to documented pneumococcal pneumonia is approximately 80 percent and is therefore higher than that of a Gram-stained smear (approximately 50 percent) in which a positive result is defined by a predominance of lancet-shaped diplococci in each of several oil immersion fields ($\times 1000$). Specificities of the antigen tests may, however, be only about 70 percent since false-positive results occur, particularly in patients with chronic bronchitis and pneumococci in their sputum. Latex agglutination tests for group A streptococci are widely available commercially. Although highly specific, these tests are only relatively sensitive, so antigen-negative tests should be backed up by cultures, particularly in areas in which there is a high prevalence of acute rheumatic fever or in which there has been a resurgence of acute rheumatic fever.

Latex agglutination has also been used to detect *Candida* antigenemia; however, the test lacks sufficient sensitivity and specificity to be clinically useful.

Enzyme Immunoassays. EIA systems useful for diagnosis of infectious diseases are those for detection of HSV, respiratory syncytial virus, influenza A virus, rotavirus, p24 antigen of HIV *Chlamydia trachomatis, Streptococcus pyogenes, Clostridium difficile* toxin(s), *Neisseria gonorrhoeae* (primarily used in sexually transmitted disease clinics), *Cryptococcus neoformans, Giardia lamblia,* and cryptosporidia.

Growth or Biochemical Characteristics

The presence of growth can usually be readily recognized by the development of colonies on solid media, colonies or turbidity in liquid media, or cytopathic changes in cell culture. The rate of growth, however, is a function of the original inoculum size and the group of organisms involved. Most pathogenic bacteria, for example, require only a few hours to produce visible growth, whereas it may take many weeks for colonies of mycobacteria to become evident. It is important for the clinician to know what are reasonable reporting times for various kinds of cultures. It is equally important for the laboratory to establish a system for reporting important preliminary results by telephone and in writing.

The initial identity of an organism may be suggested by the source of the material cultured, its pattern of growth on nutrient and selective media, its colonial morphology on the various media inoculated, its hemolytic or fermentative properties, and its microscopic appearance. This process requires careful training and experience and provides information that is essential for all further procedures required to identify the organism. The experienced microbiologist can often provide a reasonably accurate preliminary identification of an organism at this point.

Bacteria. Most clinically important bacteria grow under both aerobic and anaerobic conditions and are called *facultatively anaerobic.* Certain bacteria, such as *Streptococcus pneumoniae, Haemophilus influenzae,* and *Neisseria* spp. require an atmosphere of increased CO_2 for optimal growth. Some, such as *Pseudomonas aeruginosa,* are strict aerobes. For practical purposes, anaerobic bacteria are those that grow only in an atmosphere of reduced oxygen tension and do not grow on solid media in an atmosphere with 10% CO_2 in air.[26] The term *microaerophilic* has no standard meaning but is commonly applied to bacteria preferring an incubation atmosphere of 10% CO_2 in air to aerobic or anaerobic atmospheres of incubation. The term, more accurately, applies to organisms that grow only in an atmosphere containing reduced oxygen (e.g., *Campylobacter, Helicobacter*). General schemes for differentiating the major groups of gram-positive and gram-negative bacteria are shown in Figures 5 and 6.

AEROBIC AND FACULTATIVELY ANAEROBIC BACTERIA. *Gram-Positive Cocci.* The gram-positive cocci usually grow satisfactorily on blood agar and are inhibited in their growth on gram-negative differential media such as EMB and MacConkey agar. Staphylococci possess catalase that produces oxygen bubbles when a drop of hydrogen peroxide (H_2O_2) is placed on a colony on a glass microscope slide or on a medium without red blood cells; streptococci are catalase negative. Staphylococci may or may not exhibit hemolytic properties. Streptococci may display β-hemolytic (complete), α-hemolytic (partial), or nonhemolytic (called γ) properties on blood agar. This method of classifying streptococci is complicated by other schema that place them into pyogenes, viridans, and enterococcal groups based on their biologic properties and into serologic (Lancefield) groups based on group-specific carbohydrate precipitin patterns (Fig. 5) (Fig. 6). Although many β-hemolytic strains are pyogenic and belong to a specific Lancefield group, Lancefield's group D includes α-, β-, and nonhemolytic strains. Both α- and nonhemolytic strains (other than those belonging to group D) are frequently classified as viridans streptococci.

More recent changes in streptococcal taxonomy include the reclassification of what were formerly salt-tolerant group D streptococci into the genus *Enterococcus*, including the species *E. faecalis, E. faecium,* and *E. durans*, and the reclassification, by some workers, of "*S. milleri*," *S. intermedius, S. constellatus*, and minute or small colony-forming β-hemolytic streptococci that are nongroupable or possess the group A, C, F, or G antigens into the species *S. anginosus*.

Vancomycin-resistant α- and γ-hemolytic gram-positive cocci belong to the genera *Leuconostoc, Pediococcus*, and *Lactococcus*. Moreover, in many areas of the United States, vancomycin-resistant enterococci have become a problem.

Most clinical laboratories perform the coagulase test by a tube test or slide agglutination with catalase-positive cocci resembling staphylococci and report *Staphylococcus aureus* or coagulase-negative *Staphylococcus* accordingly. Although *S. epidermidis* constitutes the predominant coagulase-negative staphylococcal species of clinical importance, *S. saprophyticus* is an important cause of the acute dysuric syndrome. Other coagulase-negative species of *Staphylococcus* are infrequently pathogenic. The novobiocin test for presumptive identification of *S. saprophyticus*, which is novobiocin resistant, can be limited to urinary isolates of coagulase-negative staphylococci from young female outpatients in the sexually active age group. Otherwise, speciation of coagulase-negative staphylococci is seldom indicated.

The bile solubility test, performed by observing lysis of colonies of α-hemolytic streptococci when a solution of 10% deoxycholate is applied to the agar surface, is useful for presumptive identification of *Streptococcus pneumoniae*. Pneumococci are also inhibited by low concentrations of ethyl hydrocuprein hydrochloride or optochin (P disk). Presumptive identification of group A streptococci can be made on the basis of their inhibition by low amounts of bacitracin contained in a paper disk (A disk) that is applied to the surface of agar to which the organism has been subcultured. Although it is rare for a group A *Streptococcus* to be resistant to bacitracin, between 5 and 10 percent of nongroup A β-hemolytic streptococci (generally belonging to groups B, C, and G) are inhibited. Group B β-hemolytic streptococci can be identified on the basis of their ability to hydrolyze hippurate. Group D streptococci tolerate 40% bile and hydrolyze esculin; those growing in the presence of 6.5% sodium chloride or hydrolyzing L-pyrrolidonyl-β-naphthalamide (PYR) represent enterococcal species. Group A streptococci also hydrolyze PYR, and in many laboratories this test has replaced bacitracin for identification of *S. pyogenes*. Viridans streptococci represent a group of at least nine species, including *Streptococcus pneumoniae*. Most so-called microaerophilic strains belong to these species. In practice, however, it is sufficient to call them viridans streptococci.

Immunofluorescence, latex agglutination, or coagglutination can be used for the rapid identification of groups A, B, C, and G β-hemolytic streptococci. Lancefield grouping is otherwise performed by capillary precipitin techniques. Typing of group A streptococci, based on their M or T proteins, may be useful for epidemiologic purposes.

Gram-Negative Cocci. Presumptive identification of the pathogenic neisseriae is based on the growth of gram-negative cocci on modified Thayer-Martin medium and a positive oxidase reaction. Definitive identification and differentiation of *N. gonorrhoeae* and *N. meningitidis* require carbohydrate utilization tests. Immunofluorescence, coagglutination, or nucleic acid hybridization can be used to identify colonies of *N. gonorrhoeae;* however, anti-*N. meningitidis* fluorescein-labeled conjugates tend to cross-react with *N. gonorrhoeae*. Another species, *Neisseria lactamica*, also grows on Thayer-Martin agar and closely resembles *N. meningitidis* in its carbohydrate utilization properties; however, it utilizes lactose, which *N. meningitidis* does not. *Neisseria lactamica* is rarely pathogenic. *Moraxella catarrhalis* has assumed increasing importance in otitis media and as an opportunistic lower respiratory pathogen; it frequently produces β-lactamase.

Gram-Negative Bacilli. The identification of gram-negative bacilli is complex and is based on the interpretation of numerous biochemical tests. The number of tests required for speciation of the various groups in Figure 6 depends on technical expertise, interest, economics, epidemiologic necessity, and clinical relevance. Commercially prepared devices containing multiple tests for identifying the Enterobacteriaceae have become widely used and have generally proved to be convenient and accurate. In most kits individual test results are reduced to profile or code numbers. It should be emphasized that the reproducibility of these numbers reflects the reproducibility of individual test reactions and that some of these reactions are sufficiently variable to render unreliable the use of the numbers ("biotypes") for epidemiologic purposes. Devices are also available for the identification of nonfermenters; however, the identification of these organisms remains rather complex, and the tests provided in the devices often need to be supplemented with other tests to obtain a definitive identification.

There are, in addition, gram-negative bacilli that require enriched media and, in many cases, added carbon dioxide during incubation for their growth. Included in this group are *Campylobacter, Haemophilus, Cardiobacterium, Actinobacillus, Capnocytophaga, Bordetella, Brucella,* and *Francisella*.

Species of *Haemophilus* of clinical importance are *H. influenzae, H. parainfluenzae, H. aphrophilus, H. paraphrophylus*, and *H. ducreyi*. Although *H. influenzae* is readily identifiable on the basis of its colonial morphology, characteristic odor, oxidase activity, requirements for hemin (X factor) and nicotinamide adenine dinucleotide (V factor), and antigenic characteristics, the other species are not and require a more complex series of tests for their differentiation. These species are being recognized increasingly, along with *Actinobacillus, Cardiobacterium, Kingella*, and *Eikenella*, for their role in causing endocarditis. The identification of *Brucella* and *Francisella* can be expedited with direct immunofluorescent staining.

Gram-Positive Bacilli. Gram-positive bacilli are either sporulating or nonsporulating. The most commonly isolated nonsporulating bacilli are the corynebacteria ("diphtheroids") that normally inhabit the skin but may cause infections of implanted prosthetic material, a possibility that is strongly suggested by their repeated isolation from normally sterile fluids or sites. When isolated from blood or cerebrospinal fluid, it is important

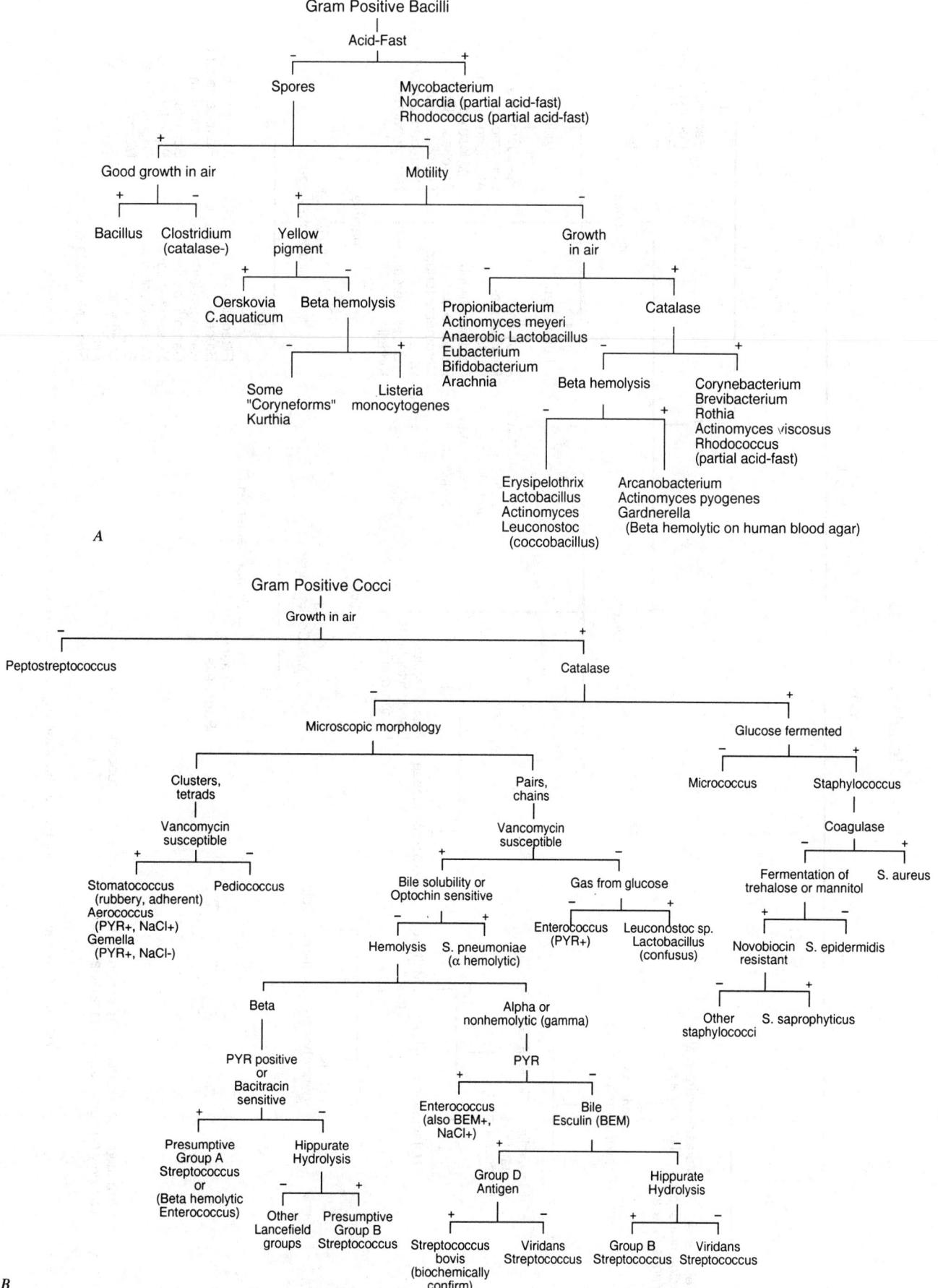

FIG. 5. Schematic outline for the identification of **(A)** gram-positive bacilli; **(B)** gram-positive cocci. (Adapted from Washington,[18] with permission.)

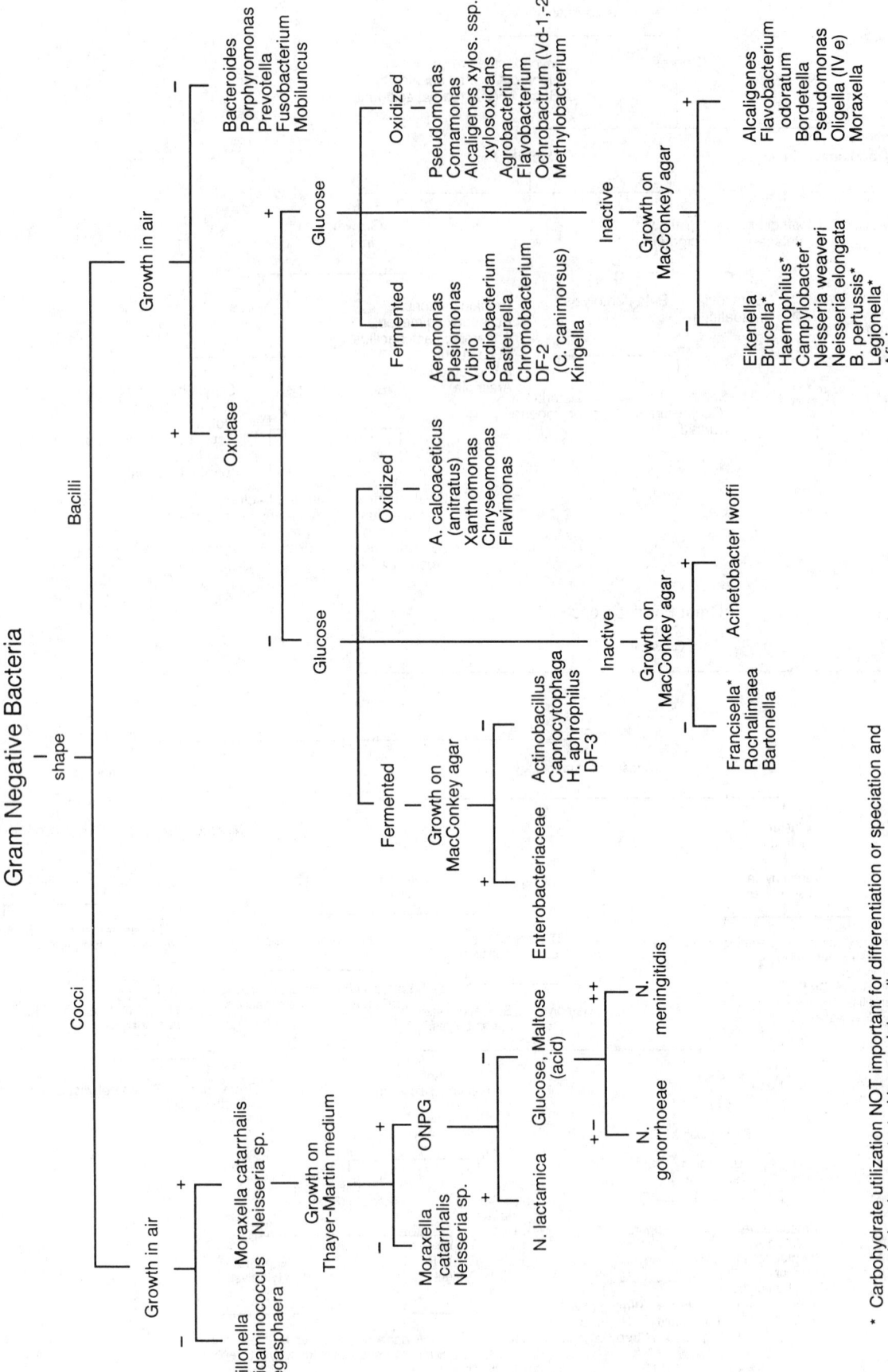

FIG. 6. Schematic outline for the identification of gram-negative bacteria. (From Washington,[22] with permission.)

* Carbohydrate utilization NOT important for differentiation or speciation and can only be demonstrated in special media.

to distinguish corynebacteria, which produce catalase and are usually not motile, from another nonsporulating gram-positive bacillus, *L. monocytogenes,* which is motile at room temperature and may cause meningitis in newborn infants and in immunosuppressed hosts.

The isolation of *C. diphtheriae,* a nonsporulating rod, or *Bacillus anthracis,* a large sporulating rod, requires that the laboratory be notified so appropriate media are inoculated and toxigenicity tests performed. Otherwise, these organisms, if isolated, are apt to be discarded as contaminants.

ANAEROBIC BACTERIA. Most infections occurring in proximity to a mucosal surface, particularly those in the abdomen and the pelvis, are due to a combination of facultatively anaerobic (e.g., *E. coli* and *Enterococcus*) and anaerobic bacteria, including *Bacteroides* spp., fusobacteria, anaerobic cocci, clostridia, and nonsporulating gram-positive bacilli. The presence of anaerobic bacteria is often suspected on the basis of their pleomorphism in Gram-stained smears of appropriately collected specimens and is subsequently confirmed in cultures on selective and nonselective media. Since cultures are often mixed and since definitive identification of anaerobic bacteria is time-consuming and expensive, the extent of identification provided must first reflect clinical need and then laboratory resources. When several different groups of anaerobic bacteria are present in a culture, it may be sufficient to characterize them superficially according to their Gram-stained morphology and to determine whether any anaerobic gram-negative bacilli that may be present produce β-lactamase. Although not necessarily predictive of β-lactam activity, a positive β-lactamase test (nitrocefin) finding is generally indicative of the presence of the *Bacteroides fragilis* group in the culture, although some species of *Prevotella* and *Porphyromonas* and some fusobacteria also produce β-lactamase. In the case of perirectal lesions and sacral decubiti, it may be sufficient to report the presence of mixed fecal flora. Definitive identification may be reserved for isolates in pure culture and those from blood, brain abscesses, and other critical areas and may be carried out with one of several commercially available rapid identification kits.

Because of continuing debate about the relevance of in vitro susceptibility test results to clinical response, the variability of results provided by the different methods that are available for susceptibility testing of anaerobic bacteria, disagreement over break points for defining susceptibility, and the relatively slow turnaround time for isolating and performing susceptibility test of individual isolates of anaerobic bacteria, testing should be limited to those isolates from brain abscesses, bone and joint infections, infections of implanted prosthetic materials or devices, endocarditis, and persistent or recurrent bacteremia. Otherwise, susceptibility testing should be done to monitor susceptibility patterns on a regional or local basis and to evaluate the activity of new antimicrobial agents.

Mycobacteria

Traditionally, culture of mycobacteria has involved inoculation of at least one egg-based and one agar-based medium (Lowenstein-Jensen and Middlebrook 7H11, respectively, frequently are used), which are incubated for 6–8 weeks. Isolates then are identified on the basis of growth rate, colony morphology, pigmentation with and without exposure to light, and results of biochemical tests.[65] These tests identify almost all species of mycobacteria, but results usually are not available for several weeks to months after growth is apparent.

The isolation on a solid medium after 2 or more weeks of incubation of slowly growing, nonpigmented, and rough colonies is strongly suggestive of *M. tuberculosis,* confirmation of which is obtained with a positive niacin test result. Calmette-Guérin bacillus (BCG) mutants of *M. bovis* have been isolated from patients receiving immunotherapy for cancer and are distinguishable from *M. tuberculosis* in that they are inhibited by

thiophene-2-carboxylic acid hydrazide (TCH). *Mycobacterium kansasii,* which causes lesions resembling tuberculosis, grows slowly (2–3 weeks) on solid media and produces raised, rough, colorless, or buff-colored colonies that become yellow to orange when exposed to light (photochromogenic). Similar characteristics are displayed by *M. marinum,* which, however, grows best at 30°C and is usually isolated from superficial lesions. Also photochromogenic at 25°C is *Mycobacterium szulgai,* which produces lesions resembling tuberculosis; this organism grows slowly and produces pale yellow colonies (scotochromogenic) whether exposed to light or not when incubated at 37°C. *Mycobacterium scrofulaceum* is a slowly growing (1–3 weeks) scotochromogen that is widely distributed in nature and may cause cervical adenitis in children.

Mycobacterium xenopi is a slowly growing (3–4 weeks) organism that grows best at 42°–45°C, is found in water, and has been associated with pulmonary lesions. It resembles *Mycobacterium intracellulare,* which is closely related to *M. avium,* hence the term *M. avium-intracellulare* complex ("Battey bacillus"). Although members of the *M. avium-intracellulare* complex are highly resistant to most antimicrobial agents, *M. xenopi* is not.

Mycobacterium fortuitum is a rapidly growing (1–3 days) soil mycobacterium that is closely related to *Mycobacterium chelonae* and for which the term *M. fortuitum-chelonae* complex has been proposed. Rarely the cause of pulmonary disease, this group of organisms has caused wound infections, postinjection abscesses, and contamination of porcine valves used for heart valve replacement in humans.

Mycobacterium malmoense, which produces visible colonies on solid medium in 2–3 weeks, is uncommonly encountered in the United States. It is predominantly a pulmonary pathogen, typically causing chronic lung disease in middle-aged men who have a pneumoconiosis. *Mycobacterium haemophilum* is unique among the mycobacteria in its growth requirement for hemoglobin, iron, or hemin. Human infections caused by this organism are uncommon. Disease usually is manifested as multiple cutaneous nodules, ulcers, or painful swellings, most frequently involving the extremities, that increase in size and occasionally develop into abscesses and open fistulas that drain purulent material. Most infected persons have an underlying immunodeficiency, such as lymphoma, exogenous immunosuppression after organ transplantation, or AIDS.

Mycobacterium genavense is a recently described species that has been reported to cause disseminated infections in AIDS patients. Most isolates have been recovered from blood. The organism grows optimally in broth media; growth on solid media has required supplementation with mycobactin J. For identification, nucleic acid analysis has been necessary; conventional biochemical tests and chromatographic methods have not been adequate.

Mycobacterium ulcerans grows slowly (3–4 weeks) at 30°C but not at 37°C, is nonphotochromogenic, and produces chronic skin ulcers ("Buruli ulcer") on the extremities of patients living in the tropics. *Mycobacterium leprae* causes leprosy in humans but cannot be cultured on artificial media. It is identified in tissue sections and smears by the arrangement of acid-fast bacilli in intracellular bundles called "globi." Bacilli may be abundant in lepromatous leprosy but are rare in tuberculoid lesions.

Given the resurgence of tuberculosis in this country and the increasing number of other mycobacterial infections, especially in persons with AIDS, more rapid methods of mycobacterial detection and identification are important. The radiometric BACTEC TB system utilizes broth media (13A for direct inoculation of blood samples and 12B for all other specimen types) that contain labeled substrate. If mycobacteria are present, they utilize the labeled substrate, releasing $^{14}CO_2$ into the head space above the broth. The amount of $^{14}CO_2$ is measured by an instrument (the BACTEC 460), and a growth index is calculated. Advantages of the BACTEC TB are rapid detection of mycobacterial growth and detection of more positive cultures, although for optimal detection of mycobacteria in specimens other than blood, inoculating one solid medium in addition to the BACTEC TB vial is recommended. The BACTEC TB system, however, is more costly than conventional culture, it entails more technologist time, and disposal of the radioactive media may require special attention.

Other uses of the BACTEC TB system include distinguishing isolates of *Mycobacterium tuberculosis* complex (MTBC) from nontuberculous mycobacteria with NAP (*p*-nitro-α-acetylamino-β-hydroxy-propiophenone) and susceptibility testing. NAP, an intermediate compound in the synthesis of chloramphenicol, inhibits growth of mycobacteria belonging to MTBC almost completely, whereas growth of other mycobacteria are inhibited only slightly or not at all. Results of the NAP test are available 3–5 days after acid-fast bacilli are detected in a BACTEC TB vial, which is much more rapid than can be accomplished with conventional biochemical tests. Likewise, using the BACTEC TB system to test susceptibility of MTBC to primary antimycobacterial drugs provides results more rapidly than is possible with the standard proportion method of susceptibility testing (5–7 days with BACTEC TB vs. 21 days with the proportion method).

The Septi-Chek AFB system consists of a broth medium and a paddle with three types of agar media enclosed in a plastic chamber. The broth is inoculated with the specimen, the paddle is secured to the bottle, and the assembly is inverted, allowing the broth to flow over the agar surfaces. Rates of detection of mycobacteria with this system and the BACTEC TB are comparable. The time to detection of growth with Septi-Chek AFB, in general, is longer than with the BACTEC TB, but more rapid than conventional solid media.

Rapid methods currently available for identification of mycobacteria include chemiluminescent DNA probes and high-performance liquid chromatography (HPLC). With probes, sediment from a positive BACTEC TB vial or isolated colonies may be tested, and results are available in 1–2 hours. Their major limitation is the number of species that can be identified: *Mycobacterium tuberculosis, M. avium* complex (separate probes for *M. avium* and *M. intracellulare* also are available), *Mycobacterium gordonae,* and *M. kansasii.* HPLC will identify virtually all species of mycobacteria in 2–4 hours, but colonies must be tested for reliable, reproducible results. HPLC also requires expensive equipment and technical expertise that personnel in a clinical mycobacteriology laboratory typically do not have; therefore, the test is done primarily in reference and research laboratories. Nucleic acid amplification methods, such as PCR, that will allow direct detection of MTBC in clinical specimens within at least 24 hours of specimen receipt are being developed and should be commercially available soon.

Fungi. The diagnosis of fungal infection can often be made by mixing a portion of the specimen with a drop of 10% potassium hydroxide on a clean glass microscope slide, applying a coverslip, gently flaming the slide, and examining the material microscopically (Fig. 2). The fluorescent calcofluor stain is more sensitive and requires less expertise to read. Fungal cultures most often yield yeasts, the most frequently isolated species of which is *Candida albicans,* followed by *Torulopsis glabrata, C. tropicalis, C. parapsilosis, C. krusei,* and *Saccharomyces.* The interpretation of these results is complicated by the normal occurrence of these yeasts in the oropharynx, gastrointestinal tract, and vagina. However we decide to identify isolates from these sources, a minimal requirement is that all clinical laboratories should be able to isolate and identify *Cryptococcus neoformans* and *C. albicans* from normally sterile body fluids and tissues. Yeasts isolated from these sources should be screened for urease production. The production of urease should strongly suggest *C. neoformans,* the identification of which should be confirmed with carbohydrate and nitrate assimilation tests or Niger seed agar.[18] *Candida albicans* is identified by inoculating

a colony into 0.5 ml of normal human serum, incubating the test at 37°C for 3 hours, and examining the suspension microscopically for germ tube formation. A variety of kits and devices are available commercially for identifying other species of *Candida.*

The identification of the filamentous fungi is more complex and time-consuming. Their colonial morphology is seldom characteristic and is highly medium dependent. Rates of growth vary widely. *Coccidiodes immitis* colonies may appear after only a day's incubation, whereas colonies of *Blastomyces dermatitidis* and *Histoplasma capsulatum* may take as long as 1 month to appear. Definitive identification is based therefore on microscopic examination of the hyphae and the arrangement and appearance of the spores. Demonstration of the saprobic and parasitic forms of the thermal dimorphic fungi is usually required. In some cases animals, most often mice, must be inoculated to convert the dimorphic fungi to the parasitic or yeast form. Recognition of the morphology characteristic of the various species requires experience, and it is suggested that photographs and other illustrative material be used as reference material with which to compare the morphology of isolates. An excellent six-volume *Atlas of Clinical Mycology* may be obtained for this purpose from the American Society of Clinical Pathologists. Moreover, exoantigen tests and nucleic acid probes allow more rapid identification of colonies of *Histoplasma capsulatum, Blastomyces dermatitidis,* and *Coccidioides immitis.*[66]

Viruses. Growth of viruses is detected in the clinical laboratory by visualization of cytopathic changes in cell cultures. Three types of cultured cells may be used to recover viruses from clinical specimens: *(1)* Primary cell cultures, such as primary monkey kidney cells, are established from tissue taken freshly from animals. They are capable of limited growth in vitro. *(2)* Diploid cell cultures, such as MRC-5 cells, consist of a single cell type that always retains a diploid chromosome number. These cell lines can undergo up to 50 divisions in vitro before dying. *(3)* Continuous cell cultures, such as HEp-2 and A-549 cells, are composed of a single cell type that is capable of indefinite propogation in vitro. After multiple passages, however, diploid and continuous cell lines frequently become less permissive to viral infection, viral replication, or both. Cell lines commonly used in the clinical virology laboratory may be obtained from the American Type Culture Collection (ATCC) and passaged in the laboratory, or tissue culture tubes seeded with these cells may be purchased from various manufacturers. In general, different cell lines are used in the clinical laboratory to allow detection of the broadest variety of clinically significant viruses. For example, MRC-5 is a general purpose cell line that provides a high level of sensitivity for growth of a wide spectrum of viruses, such as the herpes viruses, cytomegalovirus, varicella zoster virus, and enteroviruses. The HEp-2 cell line has a high level of sensitivity for respiratory syncytial virus and adenoviruses. Finally, the primary monkey kidney cell line is especially useful for the isolation of influenza and parainfluenza viruses.

Several viruses encountered in the clinical laboratory are named presumptively, based on the light microscopic appearance of the cytopathic effect (CPE) induced in the cell monolayer, its rate of progression, and the cell lines in which it occurred (Fig. 7). The identification can be confirmed by staining the infected cells with virus-specific monoclonal antibodies. Some isolates of influenza A and B viruses and most parainfluenza and mumps virus isolates do not induce a distinctive CPE. They do, however, possess hemagglutinins that have an affinity for erythrocytes and, therefore, can be detected by hemadsorption. Once the presence of a hemadsorbing virus is known, the specific virus is identified by staining the infected cells with monoclonal antibodies.

A drawback to conventional cell culture is the prolonged time (as long as 4 weeks for CMV) often required for the development of CPE. Because effective antiviral therapy is available for sev-

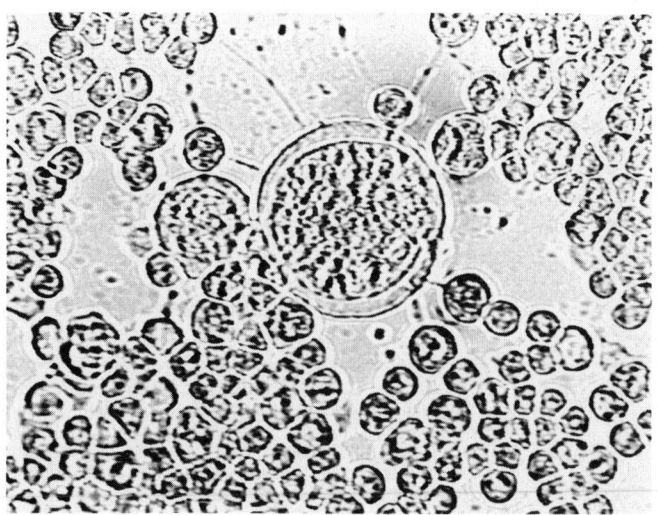

FIG. 7. Cytopathic effect produced by herpes simplex virus in A-549 cells. (× 40) (From Woods and Gutierrez,[19] with permission.)

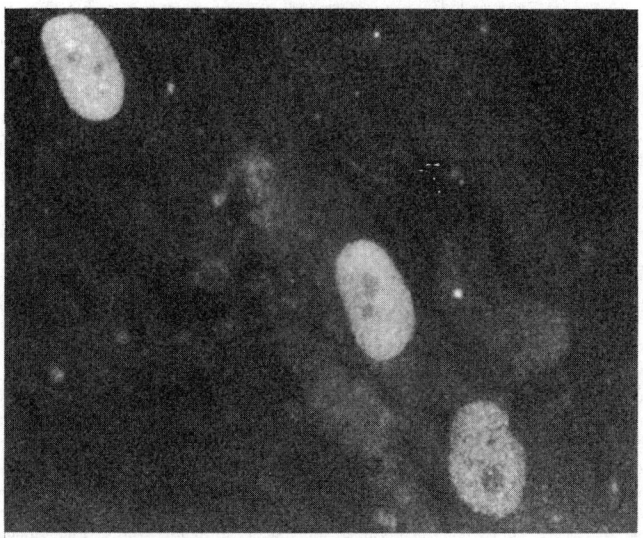

FIG. 8. Centrifugation culture shows the typical intranuclear inclusions associated with the early nuclear antigen of cytomegalovirus. (× 256) (From Woods and Gutierrez,[19] with permission.)

eral viruses, more rapid detection methods are essential. Centrifugation culture (also called the *shell vial assay*) significantly shortens the time to detection of CMV and may be used to detect other viruses such as HSV, VZV, adenoviruses, influenza and parainfluenza viruses, and RSV.[67–72] Sterile circular glass coverslips in shell vials or individual wells of a 24-well plate are seeded with cells permissive to the suspected virus and inoculated with the clinical specimen. Vials or plates are centrifuged and incubated overnight (or longer, depending on the virus). The cell monolayer is fixed and stained with monoclonal antibodies directed against the suspected virus. Coverslips are mounted on microscope slides and viewed with a fluorescent microscope; fluorescent inclusions indicate that the virus is present (Fig. 8).

DETECTION OF ANTIBODIES

Cultures of certain bacteria, fungi, parasites, and viruses may be unavailable because the methodology remains undeveloped (e.g., *T. pallidum,* hepatitis B virus), is unsafe (e.g., rickettsiae), or is impractical for all but a few research and reference labora-

tories (e.g., HIV, EBV). Moreover, cultures may be negative because of prior antimicrobial therapy or because of the chronic state of the disease. Under these circumstances, the detection of nonspecific (Table 6) or specific (Tables 7 and 8) antibodies may be of considerable diagnostic and epidemiologic use. Antibody response to infection is, however, quite variable, so serologic tests may vary considerably in sensitivity and specificity. An elevated single antibody titer usually does not permit a distinction to be made between active and past infection, and the absence of a measurable antibody titer may reflect a lack of immunogenicity of the etiologic agent, the use of an inappropriate test for detecting the antibody, or insufficient time from the onset of infection for an antibody response to have occurred. For these reasons, test selection and timing of the collection of specimens are essential to the proper use and interpretation of serologic tests. As a general rule, therefore, unless the test is being done to determine immune status only, a specimen taken during the acute phase of the disease and a specimen (convalescent) taken 1 or more weeks thereafter should be tested concurrently. A fourfold or greater rise in antibody titer usually provides unequivocal evidence of recent infection. Serologic testing is for this reason often of confirmatory or epidemiologic value.

Antibodies may be detected by agglutination, immunodiffusion, immunofluorescence, immunoassay, and many other techniques. No single technique is universally applicable for measuring antibody responses to all microorganisms. Techniques are selected on the basis of their sensitivity, specificity, ease and speed of performance, and cost-effectiveness.

The commonly available bacterial antibody tests are described in Table 7. Antibodies to the 0 antigens of *Proteus vulgaris, Brucella, Francisella,* and *Salmonella* have commonly been included in a "febrile agglutinin" test battery, which, either because of the infrequency of the diseases involved or the lack of specificity of the tests involved, is not recommended.

Infections caused by several viruses typically are diagnosed serologically: EBV, HHV-6, parvovirus B19; hepatitis A, B, C, D, and E viruses; mumps, measles, and rubella viruses; Colorado tick fever virus; Eastern, Western, and Venezuelan equine encephalitis viruses; dengue virus; yellow fever virus; St. Louis, Japanese, and California encephalitis viruses; Rift Valley fever virus; Hantaan virus; Crimean-Congo hemorrhagic fever virus; lymphocytic choriomeningitis virus; Lassa virus; Junin and Machupo viruses; filoviruses; HTLV-I and -II; and HIV-1 and -2.

DETERMINATIONS OF ANTIMICROBIAL ACTIVITY

Susceptibility Tests

General indications for performing susceptibility tests are *(1)* the isolation of organisms with unpredictable susceptibility to antimicrobial agents (e.g., staphylococci, Enterobacteriaceae, and pseudomonads) and *(2)* the isolation of organisms of clinical significance (e.g., isolates from normally sterile sources, wounds and abscesses, and urine if present in significant numbers). Susceptibility tests are usually performed with organisms that grow rapidly and well on artificial media, so variables such as inoculum size, medium, atmosphere and duration of incubation, and interpretative criteria can be standardized. Standards, therefore, have been established for testing the rapidly growing aerobic and facultatively anaerobic bacteria and anaerobes.[73,75] Standards are under development for testing mycobacteria and yeasts, although procedures have been described in the literature for testing these organisms, as well as viruses.

Susceptibility testing of anaerobic bacteria should be limited to isolates from more serious or persistent infections (e.g., bacteremia); brain abscess; and bone, joint, or intraocular infections. Periodic testing of large numbers of anaerobes should be carried out by large reference laboratories to determine whether any alterations in susceptibility have occurred.

Given the resurgence of tuberculosis in the United States and

TABLE 6. Nonspecific Antibody Tests

Disease	Test	Antigen or Hapten	Comments
Infectious mononucleosis due to EBV	Heterophile agglutination	Sheep erythrocytes	Test is negative in about 10% of cases.
Inflammation disorder, acute infection	C-reactive protein	C-reactive protein	Nonspecific indicator of active tissue-damaging process.
Mycoplasma pneumoniae	Cold agglutinins	Human O erythrocytes	Titers rise in only about 50% of cases and may rise in cases with hemolytic anemias and liver disease.
Syphilis	Nontreponemal (VDRL, RPR, ART)	Cardiolipin	If reactive, test should be confirmed with specific treponemal antigen test.

Abbreviations: EBV: Epstein-Barr virus; RPR: rapid plasma reagin; ART: automated reagin test.

TABLE 7. Commonly Available Bacterial Serologic Tests

Disease	Antigen(s)	Test(s)	Interpretation
Brucellosis	Brucella abortus	Agglutination	Titers of more than 1:80 are suggestive of past infection, whereas titers of more than 1:160 are highly suggestive of active infection. Titers of less than 1:80 occur occasionally in cases of active infection. Cross-reactions occur in patients with Francisella, Yersinia, or Vibrio infections or immunizations.
Tularemia	Francisella tularensis	Agglutination	Titers of 1:40 or more are indicative of past infection; titers usually rise to more than 1:160 during active infection. Minor cross-reactions occur in patients with Brucella infection or immunization.
Legionellosis	Legionella pneumophila and other species	Immunofluorescence	Fourfold titer rise to 1:128 is indicative of recent infection. Titers of 1:256 or more may occur in asymptomatic population.
Leptospirosis	Multiple Leptospira serovars	Agglutination	Titers of 1:100 or more are indicative of recent or past infection.
Rickettsioses	Group specific	Immunofluorescence	Fourfold titer rise, single titer of 1:128 or more, or any IgM titer is indicative of infection.
		Complement fixation	Fourfold titer rise is significant; however, CF test is less sensitive and specific than is the immunofluorescent antibody test.
Streptococcal infection (group A)	Streptolysin O DNase B	Neutralization (ASO) Neutralization (anti-DNase B)	Approximately 45% of children with pharyngitis and positive throat cultures for group A streptococci have a fourfold rise in ASO and/or anti-DNase B titers. Approximately 10% of such children will have a fourfold rise in ASO but not in anti-DNase B titer or vice versa. ASO titers usually do not rise in cases of streptococcal pyoderma.
	"Extracellular products"	Agglutination (streptozyme)	Sensitivity is equivalent to but the specificity is less than either ASO or anti-DNase B. False-positives may be due to non-group A β-hemolytic streptococci.
Syphilis	Treponema pallidum	Immunofluorescence (FTA-ABS) Hemagglutination (MHA-TP)	These tests are used to confirm positive nontreponemal or reagin test.
Psittacosis	Chlamydia psittaci	Immunofluorescence (Micro-IF)	Fourfold titer rise (IgG) for presence of IgM antibody is indicative of recent chlamydial infection. LGV-1 antigen cannot distinguish between infection by C. trachomatis and C. psittaci.
Other Chlamydia	Chlamydia trachomatis (LGV-1)	Immunofluorescence (Micro-IF)	There is a high incidence of seroreactors among venereal disease populations. IgM antibody (>1:32) and IgG antibody (≥1:2000) titers occur in patients with active lymphogranuloma venereum. IgM antibody titers of 1:128 or more occur in infants with C. trachomatis pneumonitis.
	Chlamydia pneumoniae	Immunofluorescence (Micro-IF)	Fourfold rise in IgG titer, single IgG titer ≥1:512, or an IgM titer ≥1:16 is consistent with acute infection
Mycoplasma	Mycoplasma pneumoniae	Complement fixation	Fourfold titer rise is indicative of recent infection. High IgG titers may persist for more than 1 year. A positive IgM titer is consistent with acute infection.

the recent outbreaks of drug-resistant tuberculosis, susceptibility testing of Mycobacterium tuberculosis from previously untreated patients is recommended. Moreover, susceptibility testing is indicated for M. tuberculosis isolated from previously treated patients who have relapsed after a course of chemotherapy, from patients whose sputum smears continue to show acid-fast bacilli after 2–3 months of treatment or whose cultures are persistently positive after 5–6 months of treatment, and from patients who acquired their disease outside the United States or from possible contacts with drug-resistant tuberculosis. Because they are often resistant to the commonly recommended antimycobacterial agents, clinically significant mycobacteria other than M. tuberculosis probably should be tested. Susceptibility testing of M. tuberculosis is based on the principle that when more than 1 percent of tubercle bacilli are drug resistant in vitro therapy with that agent is not likely to be effective. Inocula of mycobacteria are therefore adjusted with the standard agar proportion method so that colony-forming units can

be enumerated, and the percentage or proportion surviving in the presence of various agents is calculated.[65] Direct drug susceptibility studies of specimens may be performed if the initial smear demonstrates that sufficient numbers of acid-fast bacilli are present. The radiometric BACTEC TB system is a suitable alternative for testing M. tuberculosis[65] and is recommended because results are available in 5–7 days rather than 21 days with the agar proportion method. Agents to be tested against mycobacteria include the primary antituberculous drugs isoniazid, streptomycin, rifampin, pyrazinamide, and ethambutol. The secondary drugs include ethionamide, amikacin, capreomycin, cycloserine, and paraaminosalicylic acid and are usually only given in cases with infections due to mycobacteria that are resistant to the primary drugs. As has already been discussed, susceptibility testing of mycobacteria should be limited to laboratories expert in this area.

The indications for performing susceptibility tests of fungi are quite limited, probably reflecting the small number of antifungal

TABLE 8. Commonly Available Fungal Serologic Tests

Infection	Antigen(s)	Test(s)	Interpretation
Aspergillosis	*Aspergillus fumigatus* *Aspergillus niger* *Aspergillus flavus*	Immunodif-fusion	Preciptins can be found in 95% of the fungus ball cases and 50% of the allergic bronchopulmonary cases
Blatomycosis	*Blastomyces dermatitidis* Yeast form	Complement fixation	Titers of 1:8 to 1:16 are highly suggestive of active infection; titers of 1:32 or greater are indicative. Cross-reactions occur in patients having coccidioidomycosis or histoplasmosis; however, titers are usually lower. A decreasing titer is indicative of regression. Most patients (75%) having blastomycosis have negative test findings.
	Yeast culture filtrate	Immunodiffusion	An A precipitin band may occur in as many as 80% of proven cases of blastomycosis.
Candidiasis	*Candida albicans*	Immunodiffusion, CIE	The test is difficult to interpret because precipitins are found in 20–30% of the normal population, and reports in the literature are conflicting. Clinical correlation must exist for the test to be useful.
Coccidioidomycosis	Coccidioidin	Complement fixation	Titers of 1:2 to 1:4 have been seen in active infection. Low titers should be followed by repeat testing at 2–3 wk intervals. Titers of greater than 1:16 are usually indicative of active infection. Cross-reactions occur in patients having histoplasmosis, and false-negative results occur in patients with solitary pulmonary lesions. Titer parallels the severity of infection.
	Coccidioidin	Immunodiffusion	Results correlate with complement fixation test and can be used as a screening test—should be confirmed by performing complement fixation test. A concentration (8- to 10-fold) of specimen enhances antibody detection
	Coccidioidin	Latex agglutination	Precipitins occur during first 3 wk of infection and are diagnostic but not prognostic—useful as a screening test for precipitins in early infection. False-positive tests are frequent when diluted serum or cerebrospinal fluid specimens are used.
Cryptococcosis	No antigen—latex particles coated with hyperimmune anticryptococcal globulin	Latex agglutination or EIAS for cryptococcal antigen	The presence of cryptococcal polysaccharide in body fluids is indicative of cryptococcosis. Rheumatoid factor presents false-positive reactions, and an RA test must be performed as a control. A decrease in antigen titer indicates regression. Positive tests (in CSF) have been seen in 95% of cryptococcal meningitis cases and 30% of nonmeningitis cases. Serum is less frequently positive than CSF. Disseminated infections usually present positive results in serum. The test may be performed by using serum and CSF, and is more sensitive than the India ink preparation.
Histoplasmosis	Histoplasmin and yeast form of *Histoplasma capsulatum*	Complement fixation	Titers of 1:8 to 1:16 are highly suspicious of infection; however, titers of 1:32 or greater are usually indicative of active infection. Cross-reactions occur in patients having aspergillosis, blastomycosis, and coccidioidomycosis, but titers are usually lower. Several follow-up serum samples should be tested—drawn at 2–3 week intervals. Some disseminated infections are nonreactive to the complement fixation test. Recent skin tests in persons who have had prior exposure to *H. capsulatum* will cause an elevation in the complement fixation titer. This occurs in 17–20% of persons tested. The yeast antigen gives positive reactions in 75–80% of cases, and the histoplasmin gives positive reactions in 10–15% of cases. In 10% of cases both are positive simultaneously.
	Histoplasmin	Immunodiffusion	H and M bands appearing simultaneously are indicative of active infection. M band may appear alone and can indicate early infection or chronic infection. Also the M band may appear after a recent skin test. The H band appears later than the M band does and disappears earlier, but is infrequently positive.
	Histoplasmin	Latex agglutination	The test is unreliable. Many false-positive and negative test results may be observed. Any positive test result should be confirmed by the complement fixation test.
Sporotrichosis	Yeast of *Sporothrix schenckii*	Agglutination	Titers of 1:80 or greater are usually indicative of active infection. Some cutaneous infections present negative test findings; however, extracutaneous infections present positive test results.

(From Koneman et al.,[86] with permission.)

agents available, the limited number of people expert in their administration, the technical difficulties involved in testing yeasts and, especially, filamentous fungi reproducibly, and problems correlating clinical response with in vitro activity. Amphotericin B has a broad range of activity in vitro against fungi, including the yeasts, dimorphic fungi, and strictly filamentous fungi; therefore, determination of its antifungal activity is rarely indicated in clinical practice. Although most clinically significant yeasts are initially susceptible to flucytosine, resistance is acquired during therapy in a substantial number of cases. For this reason, the drug is seldom administered alone, and it is usually used in conjunction with amphotericin B, with which it acts synergistically unless the organism is resistant to it. It is therefore probably important to determine the susceptibility to flucytosine of yeasts isolated from serious infections so that its use with amphotericin B can be considered. A standard method for both flucytosine and ketoconazole has been adopted by the National Committee for Clinical Laboratory Standards (NCCLS) but is too time-consuming for routine use.

Currently, antiviral susceptibility testing is available only in a few reference or research laboratories, and standards for such testing are much further from development than are those for testing mycobacteria or fungi. The need for susceptibility testing of a viral isolate depends on the frequency with which resistant viruses occur, whether resistant strains are associated with clini-

cally significant disease, whether in vitro resistance predicts lack of clinical response, and whether results of in vitro susceptibility testing will affect patient management. In immunocompromised patients, primarily patients with AIDS and organ transplant recipients, who previously were treated with antiviral agents, clinically significant disease due to acyclovir-resistant HSV, acyclovir-resistant VZV, or ganciclovir-resistant CMV has occurred, and alternative drugs effective against these viruses are available. Therefore, in such a patient, failure to respond to first-line therapy or disease progression after an apparent response may be an indication for susceptibility testing.

Selection of Antimicrobial Agents

Suggested guidelines for selecting agents to be tested are listed in Table 9. Additions to and perhaps deletions from this list can be anticipated as new agents are introduced and older ones become infrequently used. Additional guidelines are provided by the NCCLS.[73,74] Close coordination between the laboratory and the hospital formulary committee is of utmost importance for the final selection of antimicrobial agents to be tested. Sulfonamides, except in combination with trimethoprim, are not included in this list because their principal use is in the treatment of uncomplicated lower urinary tract infections that are usually due to susceptible strains of *E. coli*, the most accurate suscepti-

TABLE 9. Guidelines for Selection of Antibacterial Agents for Susceptibility Testing

Agent	Staphylococci	Enterococci	Nonenterococcal Streptococci	Pseudomonads	Enterobacteriaceae
Amikacin				S	P
Ampicillin	S	P			P
Ampicillin/sulbactam (or amoxicillin/clavulanate)	S				S
Azlocillin (or mezlocillin, piperacillin or ticarcillin)				P	
Aztreonam				S	S
Cefamandole (or cefonicid or cefuroxime)					S
Cefotaxime (or cefoperazone, ceftazidime, ceftizoxime, or ceftriaxone)					P
Cefoxitin (or cefotetan)					S
Ceftazidime (or cefoperazone)				P	
Cephalothin	P[a]		P		P[b]
Chloramphenicol	S			S	S
Ciprofloxacin or ofloxacin	S			S	S
Clindamycin	P		P		
Erythromycin	P		P		
Gentamicin (or tobramycin)	S	S[c]		P	P
Imipenem				S	S
Mezlocillin (or piperacillin or ticarcillin)					P
Netilmicin				S	S
Oxacillin (or methicillin or nafcillin)	P[b]				
Penicillin G	P		P		
Tetracycline	S				S, U
Ticarcillin/clavulanate					S
Trimethoprim/sulfamethoxazole	S			S[d]	P
Vancomycin	P	S			
Cinoxacin (or nalidixic acid)					U
Nitrofurantoin	U	U	U		U
Norfloxacin	U	U	U	U	U
Trimethoprim	U				U

Abbreviations: P: primary agents to be tested routinely; S: secondary agents to be tested under special circumstances such as in institutions harboring endemic or epidemic resistance to one or more of the primary agents, for therapy for patients allergic to a primary agent, or as an epidemiologic aid; U: urinary tract–specific agent to be tested against urinary isolates only.

[a] Oxacillin (or methicillin- or nafcillin)-resistant staphylococci should be considered resistant to cephalosporins, penicillins (including combinations with β-lactamase inhibitors), and imipenem.

[b] Although cephalothin can be used to predict the in vitro activity of other first-generation cephalosporins, cefazolin should not be used for the same purpose because cefazolin is more active than are other first-generation cephalosporins vs. *E. coli.*

[c] Gentamicin should be tested at concentration of 500 or 2000 μg/ml to detect high-level resistant strains that are not synergistically affected by the combination of a penicillin and gentamicin.

[d] Applies only to species other than *P. aeruginosa.*

(Data modified from National Committee for Clinical Laboratory Standards.[73,74])

bility test of which is their eradication within the first 48–72 hours of therapy. Oxacillin or nafcillin is preferable to methicillin because of its greater stability in disks or solution. Demonstration of resistance of staphylococci to the penicillinase-resistant penicillins often requires the addition of NaCl (2% in broth, 4% in agar) to Mueller-Hinton medium and incubation at temperatures not exceeding 35°C for 24 hours. Cephalosporins, imipenem, and some β-lactam/β-lactamase inhibitor combinations may appear to be active against methicillin-resistant staphylococci in vitro; however, there is clinical evidence that these compounds are not effective in treating serious infections due to methicillin-resistant staphylococci. Thus, staphylococci that are resistant in vitro to oxacillin, nafcillin, or methicillin should be considered resistant to other β-lactams and reported as such. Because of this characteristic, cephalosporins are not tested in some laboratories against staphylococci, and all oxacillin-, nafcillin-, or methicillin-susceptible staphylococci are considered to be susceptible to cephalosporins.

Of the currently available aminoglycosides, only three—gentamicin, tobramycin, and amikacin—generally appear in hospital formularies. Testing of any one or all of these should depend on which one or ones are in the formulary, which might, in turn, reflect the local prevalence of resistance to gentamicin or tobramycin and local bias regarding the relative toxicity of each aminoglycoside. Since resistance of enterococci to the synergistic activity of penicillin or ampicillin plus streptomycin or gentamicin can be predicted from their resistance to 2000 μg strepto-

mycin/ml or 500 or 1000 μg gentamicin/ml, it is recommended that susceptibility testing of enterococci from blood, tissue, and normally sterile body fluid cultures be tested at these high concentrations of streptomycin and gentamicin. Enterococci should also be tested for vancomycin susceptibility.

The most complex issue facing formulary committees and microbiologists is the proliferation of expanded-spectrum β-lactams. Selection of a few from among the many for the hospital formulary and for laboratory testing requires familiarity with their similarities and dissimilarities in vitro and in vivo and a substantial amount of commitment and fortitude. Aztreonam and all third-generation cephalosporins are equally active in vitro against the Enterobacteriaceae; therefore, aztreonam, cefotaxime, ceftazidime, ceftizoxime, or ceftriaxone, could be selected for testing. It would be advisable to test either cefoperazone or ceftazidime against *Pseudomonas.* Whether to test aztreonam against *Pseudomonas* in this instance might reflect its position in the formulary. Although neither aztreonam nor all third-generation cephalosporins are listed as primary antibiotics in Table 9, there are probably few settings in which one or more of these compounds are not included in the formulary and are not being tested. The *Pseudomonas*-active penicillins are usually administered with an aminoglycoside, and have equivalent efficacy. Thus, selection of the one for the formulary and for testing should not be based solely on in vitro activity and could be based on competitive bidding.

Resistance among microorganisms such as *Haemophilus in-*

fluenzae, Neisseria gonorrhoeae, and *Streptococcus pneumoniae* that were previously considered to be uniformly susceptible to penicillins and some other commonly recommended agents has created a need for determining their susceptibility on a more routine basis. Initially, it was sufficient to test isolates of *H. influenzae* and *N. gonorrhoeae* to detect plasmid-mediated β-lactamases; however, chromosomally mediated resistance to penicillins, which is not related to β-lactamase production and is, therefore, not detectable by β-lactamase testing, has occurred in both species so that susceptibility testing of β-lactamase–negative isolates to penicillins is becoming necessary. Resistance of *N. gonorrhoeae* to ceftriaxone, which is currently recommended for its treatment, has not yet been reported. Although isolates of pneumococci with penicillin minimal inhibitory concentrations (MICs) between 0.12 and 1.0 have been recognized for many years, strains with penicillin MICs of ≥ 2 μg/ml are being increasingly recognized. Resistance to ceftriaxone is also emerging. Since pneumococci with MICs of 0.12–1.0 μg/ml may not respond to penicillin therapy in cases of meningitis and since infections due to penicillin-resistant pneumococci fail to respond to therapy with penicillin and antibiotics other than vancomycin, it is imperative for the laboratory to test clinically significant isolates of pneumococci against penicillin and ceftriaxone. A useful screening technique for penicillin resistance is to use a 1-μg oxacillin disc in the Kirby-Bauer test.

Methods

Dilution. The principle of dilution tests is to determine the lowest or minimal concentration of the antimicrobial agent that is required to inhibit the growth of a microorganism. The MIC is usually expressed in micrograms per milliliter. Approved standards describing the methods to be used for dilution testing have been published by the NCCLS.[74] Dilution tests may be performed in agar or in broth, the latter of which can be readily adapted to microdilution, which is currently in widespread use in clinical and research laboratories. Dilution tests are often preferred because they are incorrectly perceived as being more accurate than disk diffusion tests and because laboratory personnel incorrectly assume that MICs are preferred by clinicians. In fact, dilution and diffusion tests are directly correlated, and most clinicians other than those with subspecialty interest in infectious diseases require interpretation of MICs. Thus, the indications for dilution testing are *(1)* investigations of new antimicrobial agents, *(2)* testing of microorganisms that grow slowly or have special growth requirements, *(3)* determination of precise susceptibility when the preferred therapy is with a relatively nontoxic but not highly active β-lactam, and *(4)* as an alternative to disk diffusion testing when inocula replica plating is deemed cost-effective. Replicate inoculation of a single microorganism into microwells containing biochemical substrates for microbial identification and antimicrobial agents for susceptibility testing is a common feature of many commercially available devices today.

Disk Diffusion. The principle of the disk diffusion technique is that the diameter of a zone of inhibition about an antimicrobial-impregnated paper disk relates approximately linearly to the antimicrobial's $\log_2$ MIC. Zone diameters are interpreted as signifying susceptibility, intermediate susceptibility, or resistance to each antimicrobial agent tested according to published criteria.[73] Obviously, these criteria retain their validity only as long as standard procedures are followed.[73] It should be equally obvious that the interpretative criteria apply only to organisms that grow rapidly on Mueller-Hinton agar, with or without whole or chocolatized blood, when incubated at 35°C for 16–18 hours in room air, that is, staphylococci, Enterobacteriaceae, and pseudomonads. The disk diffusion test may also be used reliably to determine whether *H. influenzae* is susceptible to ampicillin.

No disk diffusion method is uniformly reliable for determining the susceptibility of anaerobic bacteria.

E-Test. The E-test is a relatively new in vitro method of susceptibility testing developed to determine the MIC (in μg/ml) of individual antimicrobial agents on an agar medium. The test consists of an impenetrable, inert, thin reagent carrier strip that is placed on an agar plate that has been inoculated with a standardized inoculum of test bacterium. On one side of the strip is a predefined continuous concentration gradient of dried and stabilized drug. The plate is incubated under appropriate conditions (atmosphere, temperature) for the required time, after which inhibitory concentrations are seen as an elliptical zone of inhibited growth. The intersection between the value printed on the strip edge and the zone of inhibition is the MIC. This test is most useful for testing fastidious bacteria, such as *Streptococcus pneumoniae, H. influenzae, N. gonorrhoeae,* fastidious streptococci, and anaerobes. Currently, its major drawback is cost.

Disk Elution. Elution of antimicrobial agents into liquid or solid media occurs rapidly and completely. The concept has been applied to automated rapid susceptibility testing, including the Organon Teknika Autobac and the Abbott MS-2. Formerly used for testing of anaerobes, disk elution has been shown to be inaccurate and is no longer recommended for this purpose.

Anaerobic Bacteria. Standard methods have been developed for both agar and broth microdilution,[75] but testing is rarely indicated. Resistance to β-lactam/β-lactamase inhibitor combinations, chloramphenicol, and carbapenems remains rare. With the exception of certain nonsporeforming gram-positive bacilli, metronidazole resistance is also rare.

Bactericidal Tests

Broth. The principle of the broth test is to determine the lowest or minimal concentration of antimicrobial agent that kills at least 99.9 percent of the inoculum used for the test. The minimal bactericidal concentration (MBC) or minimal lethal concentration (MLC) is obtained by subculturing measured aliquots from broth in tubes containing no visible growth (inhibitory phase) to antimicrobial-free media. Although the inhibitory phase of this test has been standardized, the volume of the aliquot subcultured, the subculture medium, the subculture method (pour vs. streak plates), and the duration of incubation have not. There have been consequently numerous technical variations of this test in the literature. Most investigators agree on the need to quantify the original inoculum to determine the lowest concentration of antimicrobial agent that destroys at least 99.9 percent of it. Recommended procedures for performing bactericidal tests have been described by Pearson et al.[76] and in a tentative guideline published by the NCCLS.[77] Critical components of the methodology include an inoculum of at least 5×10^5 cfu/ml and a subculture volume of 0.01 ml to allow accurate estimation of at least 99.9 percent killing.[76,77]

There are very few indications for bactericidal testing. Although the MBC is an accepted parameter in the evaluation of a new antimicrobial agent, its clinical value is debatable, especially since the test is very method dependent and interpretation of the results is not well defined. A related issue is that of tolerance, about which much has been written but about which there are substantial definitional problems.[78,79] Among the technical problems involved are *(1)* the fact that stationary-phase cultures result in diminished killing rates, *(2)* bacteria may escape exposure to the antibiotic by adhering to the side of the tube above the meniscus, *(3)* sufficient antibiotic may be transferred in subcultures to inhibit surviving organisms, and *(4)* the rate of bactericidal activity may vary according to duration of incubation, medium content, and pH.[78,79] For all of these reasons it appears that the most reliable method for determining tolerance, defined as a reduced rate of killing, is by timed killing curve studies in which an exponential phase of growth of the organism is adjusted to provide an inoculum of approximately 5×10^5 cfu/ml that is exposed to a concentration of the antibiotic that is eight times its MIC and the number of survivors after 4–6 hours of incubation is compared with those at 2 hours or 0 time. Determination of the number of persisters can be made by quantitative subculture after 24 hours of incubation.[79]

Combination Studies. Studies of combinations of antimicrobial agents are performed when there is multiple resistance to antimicrobials singly, when there are contraindications to the use of preferred antimicrobials, when therapeutic failure has occurred with a current antimicrobial regimen, and when the potential for toxicity exists during a prolonged therapeutic regimen.

There are two major approaches to performing combination studies.[80]

METHODS WITH SOLID MEDIUM. Antimicrobials can be combined in a single disk to determine whether their activity is greater (or less) than that of either agent singly. A frequently used example of this approach is the trimethoprim-sulfamethoxazole disk. The synergistic interaction of this combination can be seen if its components are tested separately by placing disks containing each proximately on the seeded agar surface. A modification of this technique is to place two filter paper strips, each containing a different antimicrobial, at right angles to one another on the seeded agar surface. Bacteriostatic synergism is indicated by inhibition of growth within the angle formed by the two strips. Bactericidal interactions between two antimicrobial agents may be determined by the cellophane transfer technique wherein a cellophane tambour inoculated on the inside with the test organism is applied to an agar surface into which antimicrobials have prediffused from filter paper strips placed at right angles.[80] The antimicrobials and nutrients from the agar diffuse through the cellophane. After overnight incubation, the tambour is removed from the agar surface, transferred to an antimicrobial-free medium, and incubated for an additional 24 hours. Synergism is indicated when growth is absent within the area formerly encompassed by the angle formed by the two antimicrobial-containing strips.

METHODS WITH LIQUID MEDIUM. There are two techniques for combination studies in liquid medium.[80] In the two-dimensional ("checkerboard") method serial, twofold dilutions of two agents, alone and in combination, are inoculated with the test organism. After incubation for 16–18 hours, those tubes containing broth without visible growth are subcultured, as for the MBC, to antimicrobial-free media. The results are then depicted according to isobologram criteria as demonstrating synergy, antagonism, or indifference (Fig. 9). In the timed killing curve two or more fixed concentrations of two or more antimicrobials, singly and in combination, are inoculated with the test organism and subcultured quantitatively over time to compare the rate of killing by the combinations with that of either antimicrobial by itself (Fig. 10).[81]

Synergism is usually defined by the significantly greater activity of the combination than would be expected from the sum of the separate effects of the antimicrobials being tested.[80] In the checkerboard method, synergism is defined when the fractional inhibitory concentration (FIC) or fractional bactericidal concentration (FBC) index is 0.5 or less, whereas in killing curve studies synergy is defined as a 2 $\log_{10}$ cfu/ml or greater decrease between the combination and its most active component after 24 hours of incubation, assuming that at least one of the antimicrobials in the combination does not produce inhibitory or killing activity by itself (Fig. 10). Antagonism is defined in the checkerboard method by an FIC or FBC index of greater than 4.0 and in the killing curve method by a 2 $\log_{10}$ or less decrease in killing by the combination at 24 hours as compared with the

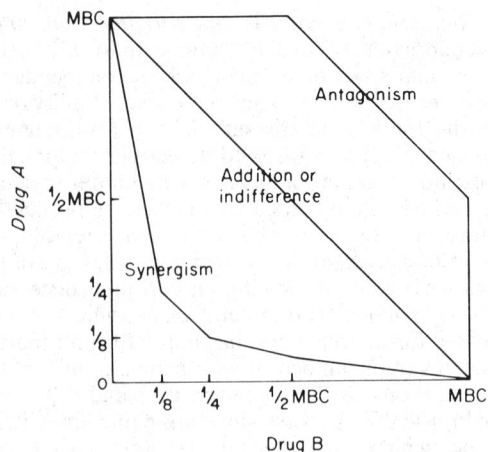

FIG. 9. Isobologram depicting three possible interactions between two antimicrobial agents when tested in combination by the two-dimensional ("checkerboard") technique. (From Washington,[18] with permission.)

most active antimicrobial by itself. Between synergy and antagonism are additive and indifferent effects.

Although the interpretative results of both the checkerboard and timed killing curve methods often agree, differences do occur, often reflecting differences between methods in inoculum size and growth phase as well as in sampling times.[82] Because of the extremely laborious nature of these methods and because of difficulties in applying the results in clinical practice, their use should probably be restricted to investigational studies.

Serum Bactericidal Test. The dilution of serum that is inhibitory or bactericidal to an organism isolated from a patient receiving antimicrobial therapy has been used for years as an indirect method of monitoring the antimicrobial dosage. First described by Schlichter et al.[83] as a test of the serum's bacteriostatic activity at the anticipated trough level of antibiotics, the test has undergone innumerable modifications as regards the timing of blood collection, inoculum size, serum diluent, subculture volume and medium, and endpoints. Tentative guidelines for performing the test have been published by the NCCLS[84]; however, the interpretative guidelines provided are limited by several factors. First, exclusive of infections associated with implanted prosthetic materials, most cases of endocarditis and osteomyelitis are successfully treated with currently recommended antibiotic regimens, so the correlation between treatment failure and any range of titers is based on a very small sample. Accordingly, although the predictive value of a titer, for example, 1:64 or greater, for cure may be high, that for failure with a lesser titer is not, particularly when confidence limits are applied to any published predictive values for failure related to titers below 1:64. Second, although the serum bactericidal test is considered an indirect assay of antimicrobial activity in vitro, the test is subject to all of the methodological variables that have been described for the MBC. Third, there is an inherent risk in promoting a particular minimal acceptable titer in that efforts to increase a low titer might result in an inappropriate increase in the dosage of a potentially toxic antibiotic. In conclusion, although the determination of serum bactericidal titers may provide another piece of information about the antimicrobial properties in vivo of a new investigational antimicrobial agent, there are few clinical indications for its use.

Assays

Assays of antimicrobial concentrations in serum should be made when there is dysfunction of excretory or metabolic organs or systems, when there is an in vivo response that is inconsistent

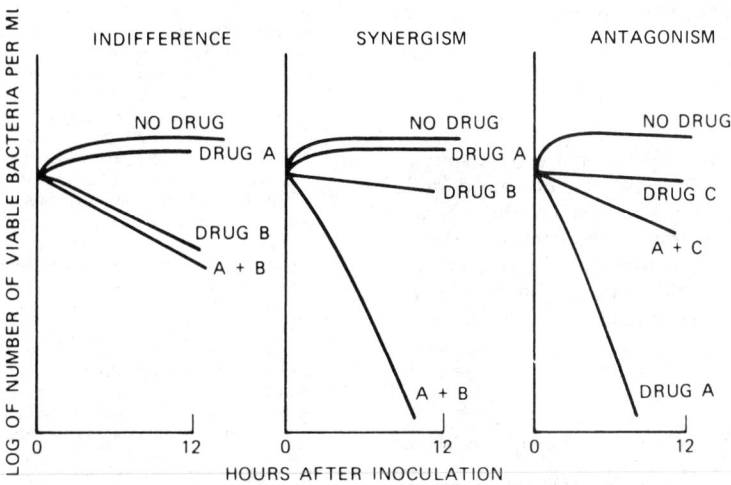

FIG. 10. Schematic representation of bactericidal action in vitro shows the possible types of results seen when one drug or two drugs act on a homogeneous population of bacteria under conditions permitting growth. (From Jawetz,[81] with permission.)

with in vitro susceptibility test results, when there is variability in the pharmacokinetics of an antimicrobial agent, and when potentially toxic antimicrobial agents are being administered. Assays are particularly useful when therapeutic concentrations of an agent approximate its potentially toxic concentrations. For example, therapeutic concentrations of gentamicin are in the range of 4–8 μg/ml, whereas potentially toxic concentrations are 12 μg/ml or greater. Assays in this case assist in adjusting the antibiotic dosage to achieve therapeutic concentrations in serum and, at the same time, provide a means of monitoring the dosage to ensure that potentially toxic levels are not being attained. Although many formulas have been published to assist in adjusting antibiotic dosage, changing renal status often renders these calculations invalid, and assays should be made to monitor antimicrobial therapy.

There are many methods for performing antimicrobial assays, but the methods most frequently used in clinical laboratories are microbiologic assay or bioassay, radioimmunoassay (RIA), chromatography, and nonisotopic immunoassays (e.g., fluorescence polarization).

Bioassay. Bioassays compare the responses of a highly susceptible test organism to known concentrations of an antimicrobial with the response of the same organism under identical test conditions to an unknown concentration of the same antimicrobial. Bioassays may be made by serial dilution methods; however, the accuracy of such methods is ±1 $\log_2$ dilutions, and they are generally not suitable for assays of agents with narrow toxic:therapeutic ratios.

Many bioassays are performed by the more accurate agar diffusion method. In the diffusion assay a standard curve is constructed from the inhibitory zone diameters produced by standards with varying concentrations of antimicrobial. The zone diameter of inhibition produced by an unknown sample is extrapolated from the standard curve to a concentration (μg/ml). Standards and unknown materials to be assayed are placed into a cylinder or onto a paper disk applied to the seeded agar surface (Fig. 11). Alternatively, samples can be placed into wells punched out of the seeded agar. By increasing the inoculum size, it is often possible to shorten the incubation time of the bioassay. Most aminoglycosides, for example, can be assayed within a 4-hour period.

Fluids to be assayed often contain more than one antimicrobial agent. In the bioassay this problem is circumvented by selecting a test organism that is very susceptible to the agent to be assayed and resistant to other agents, by inactivating interfering antimicrobials, or by diluting the fluid to eliminate detectable

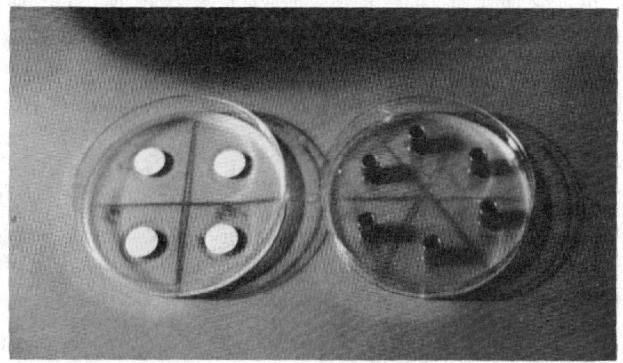

FIG. 11. Agar diffusion assays using stainless steel cylinders (right) and paper disks (left) to contain the standards and samples to be tested.

activity of any agents present in low concentrations to assay one that is present in high concentrations. In practice, the first two approaches are commonly used. Organisms with the desired susceptibility patterns can be obtained from reference laboratories or can be selected from isolates encountered in the laboratory. These organisms should be tested at regular intervals to ensure that they have retained their original susceptibility patterns. Penicillins and cephalosporins can be inactivated with β-lactamases, whereas aminoglycosides can be inactivated with calcium hydroxide or sodium polyanetholsulfonate.

It is essential for physicians ordering assays to provide the laboratory with information on the dosage and time interval since the last dose of the antimicrobial to be assayed as well as what other antimicrobials are being administered concurrently. Failure to do so may not only delay completion of the assay but can also lead to spurious results.

Immunoassay. Today, assays for aminoglycosides and glycopeptides are performed almost exclusively with rapid, commercially available enzyme immunoassay systems. These assays are sensitive and specific and can be performed with equipment that is commonly available in clinical chemistry laboratories, thereby allowing optimal utilization of equipment and purchase of reagents.[85]

High-Pressure Liquid Chromatography. Generally available only in research laboratories, HPLC assays provide sensitive and specific techniques for the assay of the great majority of available antimicrobial agents today. The technology is, however, complex and not readily amenable to testing large numbers of specimens.

Chemical Tests for β-Lactamase

The determination of production of β-lactamase by staphylococci, *H. influenzae,* and *N. gonorrhoeae* is of considerable clinical value in the treatment of diseases caused by these organisms. There are both rapid acidimetric and iodometric methods, as well as a rapid chromogenic cephalosporin test, available for this purpose. These can be used with isolated colonies of bacteria and provide results within a few minutes.

REFERENCES

1. Evans FO, Sydnor JB, Moore WEC, et al. Sinusitis of the maxillary antrum. N Engl J Med. 1975;293:735–9.
2. Auger WJ. An original method of obtaining sputum from infants and children with reference to the incidence of pneumococci in the nasopharynx. J Pediatr. 1939;15:640–5.
3. Facklam RR. Specificity study of kits for detection of group A streptococci directly from throat swabs. J Clin Microbiol. 1987;25:504–6.
4. Radetsky M, Solomon JA, Todd JK. Identification of streptococcal pharyngitis in the office laboratory: Reassessment of new technology. Pediatr Infect Dis J. 1987;6:556–63.
5. Gerber MA. Rapid diagnosis of group A beta-hemolytic streptococcal pharyngitis. Use of antigen detection tests. Diagn Microbiol Infect Dis. 1986; 4(Suppl):5–15.
6. Lieu TA, Fleisher GR, Schwartz JS. Clinical performance and effect on treatment rates of latex agglutination testing for streptococcal pharyngitis in an emergency department. Pediatr Infect Dis. 1986;5:655–9.
7. Chodosh S. Examination of sputum cells. N Engl J Med. 1970;282:854–7.
8. Murray PR, Washington JA II. Microscopic and bacteriologic analysis of sputum. Mayo Clin Proc. 1975;50:339–44.
9. Geckler RW, Gremillion DH, McAllister CK, et al. Microscopic and bacteriological comparison of paired sputa and transtracheal aspirates. J Clin Microbiol. 1977;6:396–9.
10. Thorsteinsson SB, Musher DM, Fagan T. The diagnostic value of sputum culture in acute pneumonia. JAMA. 1975;233:894–5.
11. Harrington BJ, Hageage GJ. Calcofluor white: Tips for improving its use. Clin Microbiol Newslett. 1991;13:3–5.
12. Bartlett JG. Invasive diagnostic techniques in pulmonary infections. In: Pennington JE, ed. Respiratory Infections: Diagnosis and Management. New York: Raven Press; 1989:69–96.
13. Kahn FW, Jones JM. Diagnosing bacterial respiratory infection by bronchoalveolar lavage. J Infect Dis. 1987;155:862–9.
14. Chalvardjian AM, Grawe LA: A new procedure for the identification of *Pneumocystis carinii* cysts in tissue sections and smears. J Clin Pathol. 1963;16: 383–4.
15. Cregan P, Yamamoto A, Lum A, et al. Comparison of four methods for rapid detection of *Pneumocystis carinii* in respiratory specimens. J Clin Microbiol. 1990;28:2432–6.
16. Pezzlo M. Detection of urinary tract infections by rapid methods. Clin Microbiol Rev. 1988;1:268–80.
17. Jones RN. Contemporary perspectives on clinical laboratory diagnosis of urinary tract infections: Two protocols that function in a cost-containment outpatient medical practice. In: Smith JW, ed. The Role of Clinical Microbiology in Cost-Effective Health Care. Skokie, IL: College of American Pathologists; 1985:427–36.
18. Washington JA II (ed): Laboratory Procedures in Clinical Microbiology. 2nd ed. New York: Springer-Verlag; 1985.
19. Woods GL, Gutierrez Y. Diagnostic Pathology of Infectious Diseases. Philadelphia: Lea & Febiger; 1993.
20. Chernesky M, Castriciano S, Sellors J, et al. Detection of *Chlamydia trachomatis* antigens in urine as an alternative to swabs and cultures. J Infect Dis. 1990;161:124–6.
21. Wilson ML (ed). Blood cultures. Clin Lab Med. 1994;14:102.
22. Washington JA II. Blood cultures: Issues and controversies. Rev Infect Dis. 1986;8:792–802.
23. Dorsher CW, Rosenblatt JE, Wilson WR, et al. Anaerobic bacteremia: Decreasing rate over a 15-year period. Rev Infect Dis. 1990;13:633–6.
24. Murray PR, Traynor P, Hopson D. Critical assessment of blood culture techniques: Analysis of recovery of obligate and facultative anaerobes, strict aerobic bacteria, and fungi in aerobic and anaerobic blood culture bottles. J Clin Microbiol. 1992;30:1462–8.
25. Masterson KC, McGowan JE Jr. Detection of positive blood cultures by the Bactec NR660. Am J Clin Pathol. 1988;90:91–4.
26. Finegold SM: Anaerobic bacteria in Human Disease. New York: Academic Press; 1977.
27. Wilson CB, Smith AL. Rapid tests for the diagnosis of bacterial meningitis. In: Remington JS, Swartz MN, eds. Current clinical topics in infectious diseases 7. New York: McGraw Hill; 1986:134–56.
28. Granoff DM, Murphy TV, Ingram DL, et al. Use of rapidly generated results in patient management. Diagn Microbiol Infect Dis. 1986;4(Suppl):157–66.
29. Mackowiak PA, Jones SR, Smith JW. Diagnostic value of sinus-tract cultures in chronic osteomyelitis. JAMA. 1978;239:2772–5.
30. Krizek TJ, Robson MC: Evolution of quantitative bacteriology in wound management. Am J Surg. 1975;130:579–84.
31. Loebel EC, Marvin JA, Heck EL, et al. The method of quantitative burn-wound biopsy cultures and its routine use in the care of the burned patient. Am J Clin Pathol. 1974;61:20–4.
32. Woods GL, Washington JA II. Mycobacteria other than *Mycobacterium tuberculosis:* Review of microbiologic and clinical aspects. Rev Infect Dis 1987; 9:275–94.
33. Gerding DN. Disease associated with *Clostridium difficile* infection. Ann Intern Med. 1989;110:255–7.
34. Lyverly DM, Krivan HC, Wilkins TD. *Clostridium difficile:* Its disease and toxins. Clin Microbiol Rev. 1988;1:1–18.
35. Lyverly DM, Barroso LA, Wilkins TD. Identification of the latex reactive protein of *Clostridium difficile* as glutamate dehydrogenase. J Clin Microbiol. 1991;29:2639–42.
36. Woods GL, Iwen PC. Comparison of a dot immunobinding assay, latex agglutination and cytotoxin assay for laboratory diagnosis of *Clostridium difficile*–associated diarrhea. J Clin Microbiol. 1990;28:855–7.
37. DeGirolami PC, et al: Multicenter evaluation of a new enzyme immunoassay for detection of *Clostridium difficile* enterotoxin A. J Clin Microbiol. 1992; 30:1085–8.
38. Morris AJ, Wilson ML, Reller LB. Application of rejection criteria for stool ovum and parasite examinations. J Clin Microbiol. 30:3213–6.
39. Siegel DL, Edelstein PH, Nachamkin I. Inappropriate testing for diarrheal diseases in the hospital. JAMA. 1990;263:979–82.
40. Yolken RH, Miotti P, Viscidi R. Immunoassays for the diagnosis and study of viral gastroenteritis. Pediatr Infect Dis. 1986;5(Suppl):46–52.
41. Hart G. Syphilis tests in diagnostic and therapeutic decision making. Ann Intern Med. 1986;104:368–76.
42. Washington JA II. What can you reasonably ask and expect of the microbiology laboratory? Med Times. 1977;105:20–7.
43. Panke ES, Yang LI, Leist PA, et al. Comparison of Gen-Probe DNA test and culture for the detection of *Neisseria gonorrhoeae* in endocervical specimens. J Clin Microbiol. 1991;29:883–8.
44. Hale YM, Melton ME, Lewis JS, et al. Evaluation of the PACE 2 *Neisseria gonorrhoeae* assay by three public health laboratories. J Clin Microbiol. 1993; 31:458–9.
45. Birkenmeyer L, Armstrong AS. Preliminary evaluation of the ligase chain reaction for specific detection of *Neisseria gonorrhoeae.* J Clin Microbiol. 1992;30:3089–94.
46. Tilton RC, Judson FN, Barnes RC, et al. Multicenter comparative evaluation of two microscopic methods and culture for detection of *Chlamydia trachomatis* in patient specimens. J Clin Microbiol. 1988;26:167–70.
47. Barnes RC. Laboratory diagnosis of human chlamydial infections. Clin Microbiol Rev. 1989;2:119–36.
48. Kellogg JA, Sieple JW, Murray CL, et al. Effect of endocervical specimen quality on detection of *Chlamydia trachomatis* and on the incidence of false-positive results with the Chlamydiazyme method. J Clin Microbiol. 1990;28: 1108–13.
49. Mills RD, Young A, Cain K, et al. Chlamydiazyme plus blocking assay to detect *Chlamydia trachomatis* in endocervical specimens. Am J Clin Pathol. 1992;97:209–12.
50. Iwen PC, Blair TMH, Woods GL. Comparison of the Gen-Probe PACE 2 system, direct fluorescent-antibody and cell culture for detecting *Chlamydia trachomatis* in cervical specimens. Am J Clin Pathol. 1991;95:578–82.
51. Loeffelholz MJ, Lewinski CA, Silver SR, et al. Detection of *Chlamydia trachomatis* in endocervical specimens by polymerase chain reaction. J Clin Microbiol. 1992;30:2847–51.
52. Amsel R, Totten PA, Spiegel CA, et al. Nonspecific vaginitis: Diagnostic criteria and microbial and epidemiologic associations. Am J Med. 1983;74: 14–22.
53. Burnakis TG, Hildebrandt NB. Pelvic inflammatory disease: A review with emphasis on antimicrobial therapy. Rev Infect Dis. 1986;8:86–116.
54. Mardh P-A. An overview of infectious agents of salpingitis, their biology, and recent advances in methods of detection. Am J Obstet Gynecol. 1980;138: 933–51.
55. Nahass GT, Goldstein BA, Zhu WY, et al. Comparison of Tzanck smear, viral culture, and DNA diagnostic methods in detection of herpes simplex and varicella-zoster infection. JAMA. 1992;268:2541–4.
56. Dorian KJ, Beatty E, Atterbury KE. Detection of herpes simplex virus by the Kodak SureCell herpes test. J Clin Microbiol. 1990;28:2117–9.
57. Osborne NF, Grubin L, Pratson L. Vaginitis in sexually active women: Relationship to nine sexually transmitted organisms. Am J Obstet Gynecol. 1982; 142:962–7.
58. Leibowitz HM, Pratt MV, Flagstad IJ, et al. Human conjunctivitis. I. Diagnostic evaluation. Arch Ophthalmol. 1976;94:1747–9.
59. Jones DB, Liesegang TJ, Robinson NM. Cumitech 13. In: Washington JA II, ed. Laboratory Diagnosis of Ocular Infections. Washington: American Society for Microbiology; 1981.
60. François J, Rysselaere M: Oculomycoses. Springfield, IL: Charles C Thomas; 1972.
61. Gosey LL, Howard RM, Witebsky FG, et al. Advantages of a modified tolu-

idine blue O stain and bronchoalveolar lavage for the diagnosis of *Pneumocystis carinii* pneumonia. J Clin Microbiol. 1985;22:803–7.

62. Shimono LH, Hartman B. A simple and reliable rapid methenamine silver stain for *Pneumocystis carinii* and fungi. Arch Pathol Lab Med. 1986;110: 855–6.

63. Kaufman L, Reiss E. Serodiagnosis of fungal diseases. In: Rose NR, Friedman H, Fahey JL, et al., eds. Manual of Clinical Laboratory Immunology. 4th ed. Washington, DC: American Society for Microbiology; 1992;506–528.

64. Roberts GD, Koneman EW, Kim YK. Specificity of latex test for cryptococcal antigen: A rapid, simple method for eliminating interference factors. J Clin Microbiol. 1982;16:965–7.

65. Roberts GD, Koneman EW, Kim YK. *Mycobacterium*. In Balows A, Hausler WJ Jr, Herrmann KL, et al, eds. Manual of Clinical Microbiology. 5th ed. Washington, DC: American Society for Microbiology; 1991;304–39.

66. Hall GS, Pratt-Rippin K, Washington JA. Evaluation of a chemiluminescent probe assay for identification of *Histoplasma capsulatum* isolates. J Clin Microbiol. 1992;30:3003–4.

67. Gleaves CA, Smith TF, Shuster EA, et al. Rapid detection of cytomegalovirus in MRC-5 cells inoculated with urine specimens by using low-speed centrifugation and monoclonal antibody to an early antigen. J Clin Microbiol. 1984;19: 917–9.

68. Paya CV, Wold AD, Smith TF. Detection of cytomegalovirus infections in specimens other than urine by shell vial assay and conventional tube cell cultures. J Clin Microbiol. 1987;25:755–7.

69. Woods GL, Young A, Johnson A, et al. Detection of cytomegalovirus by 24-well plate centrifugation assay using a monoclonal antibody to an early nuclear antigen and by conventional cell culture. J Virol Methods. 1987;18:207–14.

70. Woods GL, Mills RD. Conventional tube cell culture compared with centrifugal inoculation of MRC-5 cells and staining with monoclonal antibodies for detection of herpes simplex virus in clinical specimens. J Clin Microbiol. 1988; 26:570–2.

71. Woods GL, Yamamoto M, Young A. Detection of adenovirus by rapid 24-well plate centrifugation and conventional cell culture with dexamethasone. J Virol Methods. 1988;20:109–14.

72. Mills RD, Cain KJ, Woods GL. Detection of influenza virus by centrifugal inoculation of MDCK cells and staining with monoclonal antibodies. J Clin Microbiol. 1989;27:2505–8.

73. National Committee for Clinical Laboratory Standards. Performance Standards for Antimicrobial Disk Susceptibility Tests. Approved Standard NCCLS Publication M2A5. Villanova, PA: NCCLS; 1993.

74. National Committee for Clinical Laboratory Standards. Dilution Procedures for Susceptibility Testing of Aerobic Bacteria. Approved Standard NCCLS Publication M7-A3. Villanova, PA: NCCLS; 1993.

75. National Committee for Clinical Laboratory Standards. Methods for Antimicrobial Susceptibility Testing of Anaerobic Bacteria. Approved Standard. NCCLS Document M11-A3. Villanova, PA: NCCLS; 1993.

76. Pearson RD, Steigbigel RT, Davis HT, et al. Method for reliable determination of minimal lethal concentrations. Antimicrob Agents Chemother. 1980;18: 699–708.

77. National Committee for Clinical Laboratory Standards. Methods for Determining Bactericidal Activity of Antimicrobial Agents. Tentative Guideline. NCCLS Document M26-T. Villanova, PA: NCCLS; 1992.

78. Handwerger S, Tomasz A. Antibiotic tolerance among clinical isolates of bacteria. Rev Infect Dis. 1985;7:368–86.

79. Sherris JC. Problems in vitro determination of antibiotic tolerance in clinical isolates. Antimicrob Agents Chemother. 1986;30:633–7.

80. Eliopoulos GM, Moellering RC Jr. Antimicrobial combinations. In Lorian V, ed. Antibiotics in Laboratory Medicine. 3rd ed. Baltimore: Williams & Wilkins; 1991;432–492.

81. Jawetz E. Combined antibiotic action. Some definitions and correlations between laboratory and clinical results. Antimicrob Agents Chemother. 1967: 203–9.

82. Bayer AS, Morrison JO. Disparity between timed-kill and checkerboard methods for determination of in vitro bactericidal interactions of vancomycin plus rifampin versus methicillin-susceptible and -resistant *Staphylococcus aureus*. Antimicrob Agents Chemother. 1984;26:220–3.

83. Schlichter JG, Maclean H, Milzer A. Effective penicillin therapy in subacute bacterial endocarditis and other chronic infections. Am J Med Sci. 1949;217: 600–8.

84. National Committee for Clinical Laboratory Standards. Methodology on the Serum Bactericidal Test. Tentative Guideline. NCCLS Document M21-T. Villanova, PA: NCCLS; 1992.

85. Chapin-Robertson K, Edberg SC. Measurement of antibiotics in human body fluids: Techniques and significance. In Lorian V, ed. Antibiotics in Laboratory Medicine. 3rd ed. Baltimore: Williams & Wilkins; 1991;295–366.

86. Koneman EW, Roberts GD. Clinical and laboratory diagnosis of mycotic disease. In: Henry JB, ed. Clinical Diagnosis and Management by Laboratory Methods. 17th ed. Philadelphia: WB Saunders; 1984;1205.

SECTION E. ANTI-INFECTIVE THERAPY

---

12. PRINCIPLES OF ANTI-INFECTIVE THERAPY

ROBERT C. MOELLERING, Jr.

Although the discovery of effective agents to prevent and treat infection caused by bacteria and other pathogenic microorganisms is one of the most important developments of modern medicine, the use of such agents has not been limited to the present era. Substances with anti-infective potential have been applied medically for thousands of years. Indeed, more than 2500 years ago the Chinese were aware of the therapeutic properties of moldy soybean curd applied to carbuncles, boils, and other infections,[1] and the ancient Greek physicians, including Hypocrates, routinely used substances with antimicrobial activity including wine, myrrh, and inorganic salts in their treatment of wounds.[2] Until the discovery of the microbiologic basis of infections in the nineteenth century, however, the therapy for infections remained strictly empirical. Heavy metals such as arsenic and bismuth were found to be useful against a number of infections, including syphilis in the early 1900s; but the modern era of chemotherapy did not really begin until the discovery and initial clinical use of the sulfonamides in 1936.[1] This was followed in the 1940s by the discovery of the therapeutic value of penicillin and streptomycin, and by 1950 the "golden age" of antimicrobial chemotherapy was well underway.

It is the result of the relatively recent work in this area since 1936 that forms the basis for this and each of the succeeding chapters on anti-infective therapy. The major emphasis in this chapter is on antibacterial agents, because there are more data available on these drugs. However, many of the principles to be discussed can also be applied to the use of antifungal, antiviral, and, to some extent, antiparasitic drugs.

CHOICE OF THE PROPER ANTIMICROBIAL AGENT

In choosing the appropriate antimicrobial agent for therapy for a given infection, a number of important factors must be considered. First, the identity of the infecting organism must be known, or at the very least it must be possible to arrive at a reasonable statistical guess as to its identity on the basis of clinical information. Second, we must have as accurate information as possible about the antimicrobial susceptibility (or potential susceptibility) of the infecting organism. Finally, a series of so-called host factors must be taken into consideration to arrive at the optimal choice of antimicrobial agent. Each of these items will be considered in this section.

Identification of the Infecting Organism

Several methods for the rapid identification of pathogenic bacteria in clinical specimens are available. A Gram stain preparation is perhaps the simplest, least expensive, and most useful of all the "rapid methods" of identification of bacterial (and some fungal) pathogens. This technique can be used to identify the presence and morphologic features of microorganisms in body fluids that are normally sterile (cerebrospinal fluid, pleural fluid, synovial fluid, peritoneal fluid, urine). On occasion, Gram staining of a buffy coat preparation of blood will reveal phagocytosed organisms in the polymorphonuclear leukocytes of patients with bacteremia or fungemia. Similar preparations of sputum will also be helpful in revealing the nature of the infecting organism in patients with bacterial bronchitis or pneumonia. Gram stain of a stool specimen may also produce useful information. In patients with staphylococcal enterocolitis, the Gram stain reveals sheets of gram-positive cocci replacing the normal stool flora. The presence of polymorphonuclear leukocytes in the stool also provides a helpful clue to the cause of certain cases of diarrhea. Polymorphonuclear leukocytes are not found in normal stools. When present, they suggest the possibility of a bacterial gastroenteritis such as shigellosis, salmonellosis, or campylobacteriosis or invasive *Escherichia coli* gastroenteritis. Polymorphonuclear leukocytes are not found in the stools of patients with viral gastroenteritis, food poisoning, cholera, and diarrhea due to noninvasive taxigenic *E. coli*.[3] *Campylobacter* may be identified in the stools of patients by its characteristic gull-wing appearance on smears of stool.[4]

Immunologic methods for antigen detection (such as enzyme-linked immunoabsorbent assay [ELISA] or latex agglutination) may also provide clues for the rapid identification of the infecting pathogens. New molecular techniques are also being applied to the detection and identification of antimicrobial agents. The polymerase chain reaction (PCR) has been used to identify DNA of viruses, bacteria, and other microorganisms in the blood of patients,[5,6] and this technique and others including the use of DNA probes have proven helpful in rapid identification of organisms that have been cultured in the laboratory.[7] At present, however, these techniques are not widely available. Final and definitive identification of pathogenic organisms therefore usually requires cultural techniques. It is thus imperative that appropriate specimens be obtained for culture before beginning antimicrobial therapy. Once anti-infective therapy has been started, cultures often are rendered sterile, even though viable organisms remain in the host.

In most cases, it may be impossible to determine the exact nature of the infecting organisms before the institution of antimicrobial therapy. In these cases the use of bacteriologic statistics may be particularly helpful.[8,9] The term *bacteriologic statistics* refers to the application of knowledge of the organisms most likely to cause infection in a given clinical setting. For example, a person with normal host defense mechanisms who develops cellulitis of the arm after a minor abrasion most likely has an infection due to *Staphylococcus aureus* or group A streptococci, and antimicrobial therapy should be tailored accordingly, even though there is no material available for examination with Gram stain. Similarly, a young child with acute otitis media almost certainly has an infection due either to a virus or to one of four major bacterial pathogens: *Haemophilus influenzae, Streptococcus pneumoniae, Moraxella (Branhamella) catarrhalis,* or a group A streptococcus.

Determination of Antimicrobial Susceptibility of Infecting Organisms

Since different organisms vary in their susceptibility to antimicrobial agents, it is imperative that we have some means for determining the antimicrobial susceptibility of the actual (or presumed) infecting organism(s). If the pathogen is isolated from a culture, it can be subjected to direct susceptibility testing as described in Chapter 11. A number of methods for determining antimicrobial susceptibility are available. The commonly used disk-diffusion method is simple to perform and is relatively inexpensive, but it provides at best only semiquantitative or qualitative data about the susceptibility of a given organism to a given agent. It is not useful for many slow-growing or fastidious organisms and has not been standardized for anaerobes. Nonetheless, if the test is carefully done, it provides data that are clinically useful. A recently described variant of the diffusion test, the E test, uses diffusion of a continuous concentration gradient of an antimicrobial agent from a plastic strip into an agar medium to yield quantitative measurement of antimicrobial susceptibility.[10]

Quantitative data are also provided by methods that incorporate serial dilutions of antimicrobials in agar-containing or broth culture media. The lowest concentration of the antimicrobial agent that prevents visible growth after an 18- to 24-hour incubation period is the minimal inhibitory concentration (MIC). The minimal bacterial concentration (MBC) or minimal lethal concentration (MLC) may be determined in broth dilution tests by subculturing the containers that show no growth onto antibiotic-free agar-containing media. The lowest concentration of antimicrobial that totally suppresses growth on antibiotic-free media (or results in a 99.9 percent or greater decline in colony count) after overnight incubation is known as the MBC (or MLC). The aforementioned techniques are based on an 18- to 24-hour incubation period. A variety of "rapid methods" are now available as well.[11] These are based on a determination of changes in bacterial growth rates caused by antimicrobial agents and can provide susceptibility in 4–8 hours.

Susceptibility testing is particularly important for certain organisms such as *S. aureus* and the various facultative and aerobic gram-negative bacilli. The widespread clinical and agricultural use of antibiotics since the 1930s and 1940s has resulted in the emergence of many strains of bacteria resistant to one or more antimicrobial agents.[12] In most cases in which adequate studies have been done, it appears that the role of antimicrobial agents is to exert selective pressure that results in the emergence of resistant organisms. In some cases the organisms are naturally resistant to the antibiotic used. Examples of this include gram-positive organisms such as staphylococci and streptococci, which are naturally resistant to the polymyxins. Many gram-negative bacilli are naturally resistant to penicillin G, erythromycin, and clindamycin. In other cases the resistant bacterial strains have acquired genes encoded on transposons or plasmids that enable them to resist antimicrobial inhibition. These genes may provide the organisms with the ability to synthesize enzymes that modify or inactivate the antimicrobial agent; they may result in changes in the bacterial cell's ability to accumulate the antimicrobial agent or may permit the cell to produce metabolic enzymes resistant to inhibition by the antimicrobial agent.[12] Examples of each of these mechanisms of resistance are well known. Most strains of *S. aureus* that are resistant to penicillin contain plasmids that enable them to produce an extracellular β-lactamase that hydrolyzes and inactivates penicillin G.[12] Many gram-negative bacilli that are resistant to aminoglycosidic aminocyclitol antibiotics such as streptomycin, kanamycin, tobramycin, gentamicin, and amikacin contain genes on plasmids that code for the production of periplasmic enzymes that catalyze a modification of the aminoglycosidic aminocyclitols by phosphorylation, acetylation, or adenylylation.[12] Efflux mechanisms (which may be plasmid or transposon mediated) can cause resistance to tetracycline and other agents in *S. aureus* and gram-negative bacilli.[13] *Escherichia coli* resistant to trimethoprim have been found to contain R factors that enable them to synthesize a new dihydrofolate reductase (the enzyme specifically inhibited by trimethoprim) that is 10,000 times less susceptible to the in vitro effects of trimethoprim than is the host bacteria's own chromosomal enzyme.[12]

The aforementioned developments provide the rationale for

performing tests of antimicrobial susceptibility whenever there is reasonable doubt about the susceptibility of a given organism. There are certain cases in which routine susceptibility testing need not be done, but they make up an ever-diminishing list. All group A streptococci remain susceptible to the penicillins and cephalosporins; meningococci likewise are universally susceptible to chloramphenicol; virtually all anaerobes except *Bacteroides* spp. are susceptible to penicillin G. Thus, testing these organisms against the agents listed need not be routinely carried out at the present time. Even a statement such as this is fraught with a certain amount of danger. The discoveries of penicillin-resistant meningococci and pneumococci in South Africa, the emergence of penicillin-resistant gonococci in Asia and Africa, the rapid spread of ampicillin-resistant (and even chloramphenicol-resistant) strains of *H. influenzae* in the United States and Europe and the proliferation of vancomycin-resistant enterococci and staphylococci make us realize that, in time, strains of virtually any organism may be found that are resistant to antimicrobial agents that previously had been effective against them.[14]

It is important to consider geographic differences in patterns of susceptibility of organisms when choosing antimicrobial agents. In many cases, there may be variations in susceptibility patterns between hospitals and the community or among hospitals themselves. The emergence of gram-negative bacilli that are resistant to gentamicin is a good example of this. Most of the aminoglycoside-resistant organisms are found in hospitals, whereas most isolates from nonhospitalized patients remain susceptible to gentamicin.[12,15] The possibility of significant geographic variations in antimicrobial susceptibility must be remembered as we examine Table 1, which is a compendium of antimicrobial agents of choice for various commonly encountered infectious agents. The data in Table 1 are based on material accumulated primarily in the United States and are similar in many aspects to data published periodically in the *Medical Letter on Drugs and Therapeutics*.[16]

Host Factors

It is obviously important to determine the identity and antimicrobial susceptibility of the organism(s) causing a given infection. However, optimal therapy is impossible unless we also consider a number of host factors that may influence the efficacy and toxicity of antimicrobial agents.[17]

History of Previous Adverse Reactions to Antimicrobial Agents. Simply obtaining an adequate history of previous adverse reactions to drugs may prevent the inadvertent administration of an antimicrobial agent to which the patient is allergic. A failure to do so can have serious (and sometimes fatal) consequences.

Age. The age of the patient is a major factor to consider in the choice of antimicrobial agents. Gastric acidity varies with age. The pH of gastric secretions is higher in young children and does not reach adult levels of acidity until approximately the age of 3 years. At the other end of the age spectrum, there is also a decline in gastric acidity such that gastric achlorhydria is found in 5.3 percent of people 20–29 years of age, in 16 percent of those 40–49, and in 35.4 percent of those over 60.[17] The absorption of a number of antimicrobials via the oral route depends on their acid stability and the pH of gastric secretions. Penicillin G is an excellent example of this phenomenon. The oral absorption of penicillin G is markedly reduced by gastric acid. However, in young children and in older achlorhydric patients, the absorption of the drug is markedly enhanced. As a result, various orally administered penicillins will produce high serum levels in young children and in elderly patients who have achlorhydria. It makes no sense to give such a patient the more expensive acid-resistant forms of penicillin such as phenox-

ymethyl penicillin (penicillin V), since these drugs will not be absorbed any better than the less expensive penicillin G. The absorption of other orally administered β-lactam antibiotics is probably also enhanced in achlorhydric patients; however, evidence is convincing only in the case of the penicillins.[18] Gastric acidity does not always have a negative influence on the absorption of antimicrobials. Drugs that are weak acids such as ketoconazole may be better absorbed at a low pH. Thus, absorption of ketoconazole is impaired by the administration of antacids, cimetidine, or even food.[19]

Renal function, likewise, varies with age. It is relatively diminished in premature and newborn children and reaches "adult levels" between 2 and 12 months of age.[17] Thus, the serum half-lives of drugs that are primarily excreted by the kidneys may be considerably increased in neonates. As a result, doses of antimicrobial agents such as penicillin G and its various semisynthetic derivatives as well as the aminoglycosides must be altered in neonates.

Aging results in the decline of a number of physiologic processes, including renal function.[18] It is especially important to realize that creatinine clearance may be significantly reduced in elderly patients even though they have normal blood urea nitrogen (BUN) or serum creatinine concentrations. In view of this, high doses of the penicillins or cephalosporins must be given with caution to elderly patients to prevent the development of excessively high serum levels that may produce severe neurotoxic reactions such as myoclonus, seizures, and coma.[17,18] It is likewise possible that other adverse reactions to the penicillins such as reversible neutropenia may be dose related and may occur with increased frequency when high doses of such drugs are given to elderly patients with physiologic renal impairment.[18] This, however, has not been proved. Impaired renal excretion of the aminoglycoside antibiotics may result in elevated serum concentrations, which in turn may be associated with an increasing incidence of ototoxicity in elderly patients.[20]

In addition to the toxicity that may result from impaired renal excretion in neonates and elderly patients, other adverse effects of antimicrobial agents may also be age related.[18,21] Hepatic function in the neonate is underdeveloped by adult standards. This can result in difficulties if such patients are administered drugs that are normally excreted or inactivated by the liver. Chloramphenicol is inactivated by conjugation to the glucuronide form in the liver. However, in the neonate, hepatic levels of glucuronyl transferase are relatively insufficient. Thus, when neonates are given large doses of chloramphenicol, high serum levels of unconjugated chloramphenicol result. Such high concentrations of unconjugated chloramphenicol are toxic and can result in shock, cardiovascular collapse, and death (the so-called gray syndrome).[17,22] For this reason, chloramphenicol should be avoided if possible in the neonate. If it is necessary to use the drug, however, it may be safely administered if given in a dosage that has been reduced appropriately for the patient's age.[22,23]

The sulfonamides compete with bilirubin for binding sites on serum albumin. When given to neonates, they produce increased serum levels of unbound bilirubin that predispose the child to kernicterus.[22,23] For this reason, these agents should not be administered to neonates. Hyperbilirubinemia per se may be associated with the administration of novobiocin to neonates.[22] This is due to the ability of this drug to inhibit hepatic glucuronyl transferase, which in turn diminishes the ability of the liver to conjugate and excrete bilirubin. Hence, novobiocin should be avoided in newborn infants.

The tetracyclines are avidly bound to developing bone and tooth structures. As they bind to developing teeth, tetracyclines may cause a number of adverse effects, ranging from purplish to brownish discoloration of the teeth to actual enamel hypoplasia.[17,22] The tetracyclines readily cross the placenta.[24] Thus, when administered during the latter half of pregnancy or from birth to the age of 6 months, they may cause these effects on

TABLE 1. Antimicrobial Agents of Choice

Organism	Antimicrobial of Choice	Alternative Agents
Gram-positive cocci		
Staphylococcus aureus		
Non-penicillinase producing	Penicillin	A cephalosporin,[a] vancomycin, clindamycin, imipenem, erythromycin, fluoroquinolone[b]
Penicillinase producing	A penicillinase-resistant penicillin[c]	A cephalosporin,[a] vancomycin, clindamycin, imipenem, erythromycin, fluoroquinolone[b]
β-Streptococci (groups A, B, C, and G)	Penicillin	A cephalosporin,[a] erythromycin, vancomycin
α-Streptococci (viridans streptococci)	Penicillin	A cephalosporin,[a] vancomycin, erythromycin
Streptoccus bovis	Penicillin	A cephalosporin,[a] vancomycin, erythromycin
Enterococci		
Endocarditis or other serious infection	Penicillin (or ampicillin) plus gentamicin or streptomycin	Vancomycin plus gentamicin or streptomycin
Uncomplicated urinary tract infection	Ampicillin or amoxicillin	Nitrofurantoin, fluoroquinolone[b]
Streptococcus pneumoniae	Penicillin	A cephalosporin,[a] erythromycin, chloramphenicol, vancomycin, cefotaxime or ceftriaxone (penicillin-resistant strains)
Gram-negative cocci		
Neisseria meningitidis	Penicillin	Ceftizoxime, ceftriaxone, cefotaxime, chloramphenicol, cefuroxime, a sulfonamide
Neisseria gonorrhoeae		
Non-β-lactamase producing	Penicillin	Spectinomycin, ampicillin, amoxicillin, cefoxitin, ceftriaxone, cefuroxime, cefotaxime, trimethoprim-sulfamethoxazole, cefpodoxime, cefixime, fluoroquinolone[b]
β-Lactamase producing	Ceftriaxone	Cefoxitin, cefuroxime, amoxicillin-clavulanate, spectinomycin, chloramphenicol, cefotaxime, trimethoprim-sulfamethoxazole, cefpodoxime, cefixime, fluroquinolone[b]
Gram-negative bacilli		
Acinetobacter spp. *(mima, herellea)*	Imipenem	Tobramycin, gentamicin, or amikacin, sulfisoxazole, trimethoprim-sulfamethoxazole, ticarcillin, mezlocillin, piperacillin, doxycycline
Brucella spp.	Tetracycline (± streptomycin)	Chloramphenicol (± streptomycin)
Campylobacter jejuni	Erythromycin	Fluoroquinolone[b,d] tetracycline, gentamicin
Enterobacter spp.	Gentamicin or tobramycin or imipenem	Carbenicillin, ticarcillin, mezlocillin, piperacillin, aztreonam, netilmicin, amikacin, third-generation cephalosporin,[e] cefoperazone, tetracycline, chloramphenicol, trimethoprim-sulfamethoxazole, fluoroquinolone[b]
Escherichia coli		
Uncomplicated urinary tract infection	Trimethoprim-sulfamethoxazole or amoxicillin-clavulanate	Fluoroquinolone,[b] a cephalosporin,[a] a tetracycline, ampicillin, amoxicillin
Systemic infection	Third-generation cephalosporin,[e] cefoperazone	A cephalosporin,[a] carbenicillin, mezlocillin, piperacillin, gentamicin, tobramycin, kanamycin, amikacin, netilmicin, fluoroquinolone,[b] imipenem, aztreonam, ampicillin, amoxicillin, ampicillin-sulbactam, ticarcillin-clavulanate, piperacillin-tazobactam
Francisella tularensis	Streptomycin	Tetracycline, chloramphenicol
Haemophilus influenzae		
Meningitis	Third-generation cephalosporin[e]	Ampicillin (if β-lactamase–negative), chloramphenicol
Other infections	Ampicillin or amoxicillin,[f] amoxicillin-clavulanate or ampicillin-sulbactam	Trimethoprim-sulfmethoxazole, cefuroxime cefaclor, cefprozil, cefpodoxime, cefixime, cefamandole, sulfisoxazole, fluoroquinolone[b]
Klebsiella pneumonia	A cephalosporin[a] (for serious infections, third-generation cepholosporin[e])	Imipenem, aztreonam, trimethoprim-sulfamethoxazole, cefuroxime, cefamandole, amikacin, netilmicin, gentamicin, tobramycin, fluoroquinolone,[b] chloramphenicol, tetracycline
Legionella spp.	Erythromycin ± rifampin	Trimethoprim-sulfamethoxazole, fluoroquinolone[b,d]
Proteus mirabilis	Ampicillin	Gentamicin or tobramycin, a cephalosporin,[a] imipenem, aztreonam, ticarcillin, mezlocillin, piperacillin
Other *Proteus* spp. *(P. rettgeri, M. morganii, P. vulgaris)*	Gentamicin or tobramycin or third-generation cephalosporin[e]	Carbenicillin, ticarcillin, mezlocillin, piperacillin, amikacin, kanamycin, netilmicin, imipenem, aztreonam, trimethoprim-sulfamethoxazole, chloramphenicol, fluoroquinolone[b]
Providencia spp.	Gentamicin or tobramycin or third-generation cephalosporin[e]	Amikacin, kanamycin, netilmicin, carbenicillin, ticarcillin, mezlocillin, piperacillin, imipenem, aztreonam, trimethoprim-sulfamethoxazole, chloramphenicol, fluoroquinolone[b]
Pseudomonas aeruginosa	Tobramycin or gentamicin plus ticarcillin, carbenicillin, azlocillin, mezlocillin, or piperacillin	Fluoroquinolone,[b] amikacin, netilmicin, imipenem, aztreonam, ceftazidime
Salmonella spp.	Fluoroquinolone,[b] ceftriaxone	Chloramphenicol, ampicillin or amoxicillin, trimethoprim-sulfamethoxazole[d]
Serratia marcescens	Gentamicin or amikacin or third-generation cephalosporin[e]	Carbenicillin, ticarcillin, mezlocillin, piperacillin, imipenem, aztreonam, tobramycin, netilmicin, chloramphenicol
Shigella spp.	A fluoroquinolone[b]	Trimethoprim-sulfamethoxazole, ampicillin, chloramphenicol, nalidixic acid
Yersinia pestis	Streptomycin	Tetracycline, chloramphenicol, gentamicin

(Continued)

TABLE 1. (Continued)

Organism	Antimicrobial of Choice	Alternative Agents
Anaerobes		
Anaerobic streptococci	Penicillin	Clindamycin, erythromycin, chloramphenicol, a cephalosporin,[a] tetracycline
Bacteroides spp.		
Oropharyngeal stains	Penicillin	Clindamycin, tetracycline, chloramphenicol, metronidazole, cefoxitin, cefotetan
Gastrointestinal strains	Clindaymicin or metronidazole	Chloramphenicol, cefoxitin, cefotetan, carbenicillin, ticarcillin, piperacillin, mezlocillin, imipenam, ticarcillin cavulanate, ampicillin-sulbactam, piperacillin-tazobactam
Clostridium spp.	Penicillin	Chloramphenicol, clindamycin, metronidazole

[a] The term *cephalosporin* refers to the first-generation cephalosporins cephalothin, cefazolin, cephapirin, cephradine, cephalexin, cefaclor, and cefadroxil.
[b] Ciprafloxacin or ofloxacin (or, for urinary tract infections, norfloxacin, lomefloxacin, or enoxacin)
[c] Methicillin, nafcillin, oxacillin, or dicloxacillin.
[d] Not approved for this indication by the U.S. Food and Drug Administration.
[e] The term *third-generation cephalosporin* refers to ceftriaxone, cefotaxime, ceftizoxime, and ceftazidime.
[f] For strains that do not produce β-lactamase.

the deciduous teeth of the infant. From the age of 6 months to 6–8 years, similar damage to the permanent teeth may occur. In view of this, tetracycline should be avoided, if possible, in young children.

The quinolone antimicrobials including the newer agents such as ciprofloxacin, norfloxacin, ofloxacin, pefloxacin, and others have been shown to cause cartilage damage and arthropathy in young animals. As a result, they are not recommended for use in prepubertal children.[25]

Adverse effects due to a number of antimicrobial agents have been noted to occur with increased incidence in the elderly.[18] In some cases (and perhaps in all if adequately studied), this relationship may be shown to be due to specific disease states or to impairment of physiologic processes associated with aging, as noted earlier. However, in certain cases no specific factors other than age can be identified. The hepatotoxicity associated with isoniazid administration is a good example of this. A small percentage of patients receiving isoniazid develop toxic hepatitis that may be fatal if not recognized in time.[26] Liver damage from isoniazid almost never occurs in patients under 20 years of age. In patients 20–34 years of age, the incidence of isoniazid hepatotoxicity is 0.3 percent and rises steadily with age to reach 2.3 percent in patients 50 years of age or more. Because of this, it is currently recommended that routine prophylactic use of isoniazid for patients discovered to have positive tuberculin test reactions be limited to people under the age of 35, but the risk-benefit of these recommendations is not universally accepted.[27]

Nephrotoxic reactions to certain antimicrobial agents likewise appear to be more frequent or to occur with lower doses of drugs among the elderly. This has been demonstrated to occur with cephaloridine[28] and colistin[17,29] and may be true for other nephrotoxic antimicrobials as well.

Finally, hypersensitivity reactions to antimicrobial agents also appear to be more common in elderly than in younger patients.[17] This appears to be due to the fact that older patients are more likely to have been previously exposed and, thus, sensitized to these agents. In addition, prior exposure to drugs such as the aminoglycosidic aminocyclitols, which produce irreversible cochlear damage, can result in cumulative toxicity on repeat exposure.[18]

Genetic or Metabolic Abnormalities. The presence of genetic or metabolic abnormalities may also have a significant effect on the use or toxicity of a given antimicrobial agent. The rate at which isoniazid is conjugated and biologically inactivated by acetylation in the liver is genetically determined.[17] Rapid acetylators are more commonly found among Oriental populations, whereas 45–65 percent of U.S. and North European populations are slow acetylators. Several studies have suggested that polyneuritis is seen more frequently as a complication of isoniazid therapy in slow than in rapid acetylators.[17] It was once thought that hepatotoxicity due to isoniazid is related to the

conversion of isoniazid to acetylhydrazine and other related hepatoxic derivatives and is more common among rapid acetylators,[30] but this does not appear to be true.

A number of antimicrobial agents have been shown to be capable of provoking hemolysis in patients with glucose-6-phosphate dehydrogenase (G6PD) deficiency, including the sulfonamides, nitrofurantin, furazolidone, diaminodiphenylsulfone, and chloramphenicol.[17] Sulfonamides may likewise cause hemolytic reactions in the presence of certain hemoglobinopathies, including hemoglobin Zurich and hemoglobin H.[17]

The presence of metabolic disorders such as diabetes mellitus may also pose problems in antimicrobial therapy. Certain agents such as the sulfonamides (especially the long-acting types) and chloramphenicol can potentiate the hypoglycemic activity of sulfonylurea hypoglycemic agents such as tolbutamide and chlorpropamide.[18] In the case of the sulfonamides, this action may be related to their structural similarity to the sulfonylurea drugs. Chloramphenicol inhibits microsomal enzyme activity in the liver, and this impairs the metabolism of the sulfonylurea hypoglycemic agents. The dextrose load infused with intravenous antibiotics dissolved in dextrose-containing vehicles may be sufficient to produce hyperglycemia and glucosuria in diabetic patients. Another kind of ''glucosuria'' can occur in patients receiving antimicrobial agents. The cephalosporins, chloramphenicol, isoniazid, nalidixic acid, nitrofurantoin, penicillin, streptomycin, sulfanilimide, and the tetracyclines can all cause false-positive test results when urine sugar levels are determined by a method (such as the Benedict test or Clinitest) that measures reducing substances in the urine.[18] Tests that are specific for glucose (i.e., that use glucose oxidase) such as Dextrostix or Labstix are not affected by antimicrobial agents.

The absorption of intramuscularly administered antibiotics may be impaired in diabetic patients. Diabetics with bacterial endocarditis who failed to respond to intramuscular penicillin have been described.[17] Administration of the same dose of penicillin by the intravenous route, however, resulted in bacterial eradication.[17] Because of the potential impaired absorption of intramuscularly administered antimicrobial agents, it is probably prudent to initiate therapy by the intravenous route when using drugs such as the aminoglycosides to treat diabetic patients with gram-negative bacteremia (especially if accompanied by hypotension) or other serious infections.

The concomitant administration of chloramphenicol has been noted to delay the reticulocyte response to vitamin B₁₂ or iron therapy in patients with pernicious anemia or iron deficiency anemia.[17] As noted previously, patients with pernicious anemia and gastric achlorhydria may exhibit enhanced serum levels of antimicrobials such as penicillin G when given by the oral route.

Rifampin may increase the hepatic metabolism and therefore decrease the effect of oral anticoagulants, oral contraceptives, and barbiturates. See Rizack and Hilman[32] for a comprehensive list of drug interactions.

Pregnancy. Patients who are pregnant and nursing mothers also pose certain problems in the selection of appropriate antimicrobial agents. All antimicrobial agents cross the placenta in varying degrees.[33,34] Thus, the use of such agents in pregnant women provides direct exposure of the fetus to the adverse effects of the drug. Although there are few solid data on the teratogenic potential of most antimicrobial agents in humans, experience suggests that certain drugs such as the penicillins (with the possible exception of ticarcillin[35]), the cephalosporins, and erythromycin are unlikely to be teratogenic and are safe for pregnant women to use.[22,33,34] Metronidazole and ticarcillin have been shown to be teratogenic in rodents and thus should be avoided in pregnancy.[35,36] The teratogenic potential of many other drugs in humans, including the fluoroquinolones, rifampin, and trimethoprim, is simply unknown.

A number of antimicrobials have been shown to be deleterious in pregnancy. Tetracycline heads the list. The possible adverse effects of this drug on fetal dentition have already been noted. In addition, pregnant women receiving tetracycline are particularly vulnerable to certain toxic effects including acute fatty necrosis of the liver, pancreatitis, and probably renal damage.[17] The liver damage may be severe and can result in death. When administered to patients with impaired renal function, these effects may be magnified, particularly if the agent is one of the tetracyclines that is primarily excreted by the kidneys. These adverse effects are dose related and may be more frequent after intravenous administration. Although it has been suggested that tetracyclines may be given to pregnant women by the oral route in doses of 1 g or less per 24 hours, it is probably safer to avoid these agents entirely in pregnancy.[17,22]

The aminoglycosidic aminocyclitol antibiotics cross the placenta. Thus far fetal toxicity has been reported only for streptomycin when used to treat tuberculosis in pregnant women. Even in that setting, the toxicity has been mild, detectable only by formal vestibular testing or by an audiogram.[37] Psychomotor retardation, myoclonus, and convulsions have been reported in a small uncontrolled series of children whose mothers received isoniazid for tuberculosis during pregnancy.[38] This observation has not been confirmed to date.

Another aspect of drug therapy in pregnancy has been examined. It has been found that serum levels after a given dose of ampicillin are lower in pregnant than in nonpregnant women.[39] This is related to more rapid clearance of the drug and to a greater volume of distribution (probably due to increased plasma volume) in pregnancy. Thus, higher doses of ampicillin are required to achieve therapeutic blood levels in pregnancy. It is likely that these observations will also apply to other antimicrobial agents, but data on this are not presently available.

Virtually all antimicrobial agents appear in measurable concentrations in breast milk when administered in therapeutic doses to nursing women.[40] The amount of drug excreted into breast milk depends on its degree of ionization, its molecular weight, and its solubility in fat and water. Under usual circumstances, the concentrations of antibiotics found in breast milk are quite low. However, even these small amounts may cause significant adverse reactions in the nursing infant. Nalidixic acid and the sulfonamides in breast milk have been shown to cause hemolysis in infants with G6PD deficiency. Sulfonamides in breast milk may be dangerous to premature babies, because even small doses of ingested sulfonamides may produce increased levels of unbound bilirubin by displacing bilirubin from its albumin-binding sites. As noted previously, this predisposes the child to kernicterus.[40] The possibility that antimicrobial agents in breast milk can sensitize newborn children is a theoretic one, but it has not been convincingly demonstrated. Although tetracycline is excreted in breast milk, it is unlikely to produce damage to the nursing child's bones or teeth because the calcium in the milk forms an insoluble chelate with tetracyclines, which is not absorbable by the oral route.[40]

Renal and Hepatic Function. The ability of the patient to metabolize or excrete antimicrobial agents is one of the most important host factors to consider, especially when high serum or tissue concentrations of the administered drugs are potentially toxic. From a practical point of view, this means that one must carefully assess the patient's renal and hepatic function, since these organs serve as the major (and in most cases the *only*) routes of excretion and/or inactivation of antimicrobials. Renal excretion is the most important route of elimination for most antimicrobial agents.[41–46] Table 2 lists those drugs that must be used with particular care in patients with decreased renal function. Doses for these drugs may be found in the chapters dealing with the individual agents and in Chapter 35. In general those agents that require no dosage change in impaired renal function are excreted effectively by extrarenal routes (usually the hepatobiliary system) in patients with renal failure. Their use in normal doses does not result in the appearance of toxic serum levels in this situation, although the urine levels of a number of these agents such as doxycycline and chloramphenicol may be significantly diminished.

Toxic serum levels of the remaining agents may develop if they are used without dosage modification in patients with impaired renal function. Excessive serum levels of penicillin G, carbenicillin, or imipenem may be associated with neuromuscular hyperexcitability, myoclonus, seizures, or coma.[17] Excessive serum levels of semisynthetic penicillins such as carbenicillin and ticarcillin or of cephalothin or moxalactam may cause hemostatic defects in patients with impaired renal failure because of interference with platelet function.[47,48] Elevated serum levels of aminoglycosidic aminocyclitol antibiotics or vancomycin may result in eighth nerve damage.[20,46] Neurotoxic reactions including respiratory arrest and death may occur in patients with excessive serum levels of certain aminoglycosidic aminocyclitols or the polymyxins.[17,29] Bone marrow suppression may occur in patients with renal failure who receive inappropriately high doses of 5-fluorocytosine.[49] In all the above situations, the possibility of toxic reactions can be significantly lessened or eliminated if the doses of the antimicrobial agents are appropriately reduced in the presence of renal insufficiency.

The tetracyclines (except doxycycline and possibly minocycline) are contraindicated in patients with impaired renal function because the elevated serum levels that result may produce a significant worsening of the uremic state due to their antianabolic effect. Moreover, they may cause enhanced hepatotoxicity in this situation.[17] Cephaloridine and the long-acting sulfonamides should be avoided in this situation because they are potentially nephrotoxic.

Certain antimicrobial agents, including erythromycin, chloramphenicol, lincomycin, and clindamycin, should be used with caution in patients with impaired hepatic function.[50] These drugs

---

TABLE 2. Antimicrobial Use in Patients with Varying Degrees of Impaired Renal Function

Antimicrobial agents requiring no dosage change regardless of renal function
  Erythromycin, clindamycin, chloramphenicol, doxycycline, cefoperazone, oxacillin, cloxacillin, dicloxacillin, nafcillin, rifampin, amphotericin B,[a] cefaclor, ceftriaxone, metronidazole
Antimicrobial agents requiring dosage change only with severe renal failure
  Penicillin G, amoxicillin, ampicillin, methicillin, cephalothin, cephalexin, cefamandole, cefoxitin, cefotaxime, ceftizoxime, piperacillin, isoniazid, ethambutol, trimethoprim-sulfamethoxazole, cefotetan, ceftazidime, cefuroxime, cefonicid, mezlocillin, nalidixic acid, ciprofloxacin, norfloxacin
Antimicrobial agents requiring dosage change with impaired renal function
  Carbenicillin, ticarcillin, cefazolin, moxalactam, streptomycin, kanamycin, gentamicin, tobramycin, amikacin, netilmicin, polymyxin B, colistin, vancomycin, flucytosine, imipenem, ofloxacin
Antimicrobial agents contraindicated in renal failure
  Tetracyclines (except doxycycline and possibly minocycline), nitrofurantoin, cephaloridine, long-acting sulfonamides, methenamine, para-aminosalicyclic acid

[a] Even though amphotericin B is excreted primarily by nonrenal means, this drug must be used with caution in patients with impaired renal function because of its nephrotoxicity.

are primarily excreted or detoxified in the liver. Bone marrow suppression due to chloramphenicol is much more likely to occur in patients with impaired hepatic function; because of this, it has been suggested that the dose of chloramphenicol be cut at least in half in patients with cirrhosis and other severe liver disease.[51] The serum half-life of clindamycin is increased in patients with severe liver disease; because of this, the dose should be decreased in this situation. The tetracyclines may produce elevations in serum transaminase levels in patients recovering from viral hepatitis.[17] They should be avoided or used with extreme caution in patients with underlying liver disease. The serum half-lives of both rifampin and isoniazid are prolonged in patients with cirrhosis.[52] Other drugs that should be used with caution or for which serum levels should be monitored in patients with severe liver disease include metronidazole, ketoconazole, miconazole, fluconazole, itraconazole, nitrofurantoin, fusidic acid, and pyrazinamide.[50] It has recently been suggested that β-lactam antibiotic-induced leukopenia occurs more frequently in patients with impaired hepatic function.[53] Hepatobiliary disease influences antimicrobic therapy in still another way. The biliary concentrations of many antimicrobial agents, including ampicillin and nafcillin, that are normally excreted in high concentration in the bile may be significantly reduced in patients with liver disease or biliary obstruction.[17]

Site of Infection. Of all the host factors to be considered in the choice of an antimicrobial agent, none is more important than the site of infection. The locus of the infectious process determines not only the choice of the agent but also its dose and the route by which it should be administered. For antimicrobial therapy to be effective, an adequate concentration of the drug must be delivered to the site of infection. In most cases, this means that the local concentration of the antimicrobial agent should at least equal the MIC of the infecting organism. Concentrations representing multiples of the MIC are generally felt more likely to be efficacious, but in many cases such local concentrations may be difficult or impossible to achieve. A failure to achieve local concentrations of antibiotics higher than the MIC of the infecting organism may not always be disastrous, however, because there is evidence that subinhibitory concentrations of drugs may produce antimicrobial effects that aid the host defenses against infections. It has been clearly demonstrated that subinhibitory concentrations of antibiotics can alter bacterial morphology,[54] adherence properties,[55] and opsonic requirements[56]; can enhance phagocytosis[57]; and can even aid intracellular killing of bacteria by polymorphonuclear leukocytes.[58] This may explain the clinical observation that, on occasion, doses of antimicrobials that produce seemingly inadequate serum levels may still result in clinical cure. In spite of such observations, most infectious disease clinicians feel that optimal therapy requires concentrations of antimicrobials that are above the MIC.

Serum concentrations of antimicrobial agents are relatively easy to determine and therefore are often used as a guide in the therapy. However, except in cases of bacteremia, antimicrobial efficacy is more likely determined by the tissue concentration than by blood level, as noted earlier. Moreover, there are some agents such as spiromycin and certain macrolides such as azithromycin that are effective in vivo despite an inability to achieve serum levels above the MIC of certain organisms.[59] This may be explained by the ability to achieve intracellular and tissue concentrations that far exceed those obtained in serum.[60,61] Binding to serum proteins may affect both the tissue distribution and the activity of antimicrobial agents in the blood. Although much careful investigation has been done on protein binding, the precise clinical significance of this phenomenon remains to be determined. For example, it has been shown that only the unbound form of a given antimicrobial agent is active in vitro (and presumably also in vivo) against infecting organisms.[62] However, since protein binding is rapidly reversible,[63] the activity of even highly protein-bound agents may not be absolutely limited by protein binding. The penetration of antimicrobial agents into interstitial fluid and lymph is related to protein binding, since only the free form of the agent is able to pass through the capillary wall.[62] Penetration of antibiotics into fibrin clots (which may be analogous to the penetration of the drugs to reach the site of infection in patients with bacterial endocarditis) is likewise related to the amount of unbound antibiotic in the surrounding fluid.[64] Nevertheless, it is often difficult to correlate therapeutic outcome with in vitro susceptibility and protein binding unless several variables are carefully controlled.[65,66] The reason for this is simply that it is the concentration of antibiotic at the site of infection that is the major determinant in the successful therapy. Such concentrations are often difficult to assess because they are the result of a complex interaction between local factors that may bind, inactivate, or enhance the activity of a given antimicrobial agent. The ability of an antibiotic to pass through membranes by nonionic diffusion is related to its lipid solubility. Thus, lipid-soluble agents such as chloramphenicol, rifampin, trimethoprim, and isoniazid are all more adept at penetrating membranes than are the more highly ionized compounds.[62] These agents rapidly cross the blood-brain barrier and produce better cerebrospinal fluid levels than do more highly ionized compounds such as the aminoglycosidic aminocyclitols. Except in neonates, none of the aminoglycosides produces effective cerebrospinal fluid levels when given parenterally. To be effective for the treatment of meningitis, they must be given via the intrathecal or intraventricular route in adults.[67] This is an excellent example of the importance of the site of infection in determining the most efficacious antimicrobial therapy. For the treatment of bacterial meningitis in adults, we either must choose agents such as chloramphenicol or the third-generation cephalosporins (e.g., cefotaxime, ceftriaxone, or ceftazidime) that cross the blood-brain barrier reasonably well, or we must use high concentrations of parenteral doses of drugs such as penicillin G, ampicillin, or nafcillin that penetrate into the cerebrospinal fluid only with difficulty. Agents such as the aminoglycosidic aminocyclitols and first-generation cephalosporins that produce inadequate cerebrospinal fluid levels even after high-dose parenteral therapy must be administered directly into the cerebrospinal fluid or must be avoided entirely.

The vegetations of bacterial endocarditis, bones, and devitalized tissue represent examples of other areas in which the penetration of antimicrobial agents to the site of infection may be borderline or inadequate. Because of this, high-dose and prolonged parenteral therapy is usually required for the effective treatment of bacterial endocarditis and osteomyelitis. In some cases, we may take advantage of the physiologic handling of antimicrobials to achieve therapeutic success. Agents that are excreted by the liver and are concentrated in the bile such as ampicillin or doxycycline may be more effective in treating cholangitis than are agents such as the first-generation cephalosporins or aminoglycosidic aminocyclitols that are not greatly concentrated in bile. The new fluoroquinolones may owe some of their effectiveness in the treatment of osteomyelitis to their ability to achieve superior concentrations in bone.[68] Likewise, these agents penetrate far more effectively into the prostate than the β-lactams or aminoglycosides, and this undoubtedly accounts for their superior therapeutic efficacy in prostatitis.[69]

Even the achievement of "therapeutic concentrations" of antimicrobial agents at the site of infection may not be sufficient for cure. The reason for this is that a number of local factors may influence the activity of antimicrobial agents. These, too, must be considered in designing an appropriate therapeutic regimen. Aminoglycosidic aminocyclitols and the polymyxins are bound to and inactivated by purulent material.[70] This is one of many reasons why surgical drainage is imperative when treating abscesses with agents such as these. Interestingly, carbenicillin does not lose activity in pus.[70] Although carbenicillin (and other penicillins) may be more active in purulent material, clinical experience strongly suggests that appropriate drainage procedures greatly enhance the efficacy of these agents as well. While penicillin G, like carbenicillin, is not inactivated by purulent material per se,[62] recent studies suggest that the presence of β-lactamase–producing organisms such as *Bacteroides fragilis* in abscesses may result in local inactivation of penicillin G and other β-lactam antibiotics.[71]

Pencillins and tetracyclines are also bound by hemoglobin and thus may be less effective in the presence of significant hematoma formation.[62] In vitro *Pseudomonas aeruginosa* is protected from the action of the aminoglycosidic aminocyclitols and polymyxins by high concentrations of calcium or magnesium in the culture medium.[72] The clinical significance of this observation, if any, remains to be determined. Local decreases in oxygen tension such as occur in abscesses and intraperitoneal infections may also have an effect on the activity of certain antimicrobial agents. The aminoglycosidic aminocyclitols, for example, are inactive against anaerobes and may also be less effective against facultative organisms under anaerobic conditions because oxygen is required for the transport of these agents into the bacterial cell.[73]

Local alterations in pH such as occur in abscesses and especially in the urine may have an important effect on the activity of a number of antimicrobial agents. Methenamine, nitrofurantoin, novobiocin, and chlortetracycline are more active at an acid pH, whereas alkalinization enhances the activity of erythromycin, lincomycin, clindamycin, and the aminoglycosidic aminocyclitol antibiotics. Indeed, the aminoglycosidic aminocyclitols show a marked loss of activity at a low pH. These observations have been used in treating patients with urinary tract infections, a situation in which the local pH can be altered by the addition of acidifying or alkalinizing agents.[74,75]

The presence of foreign bodies also has a profound effect on the activity of antimicrobial agents. Thus, it is often necessary to remove the foreign material to cure an infection in the vicinity of a prosthetic heart valve or joint implant.[76] The mechanism by which foreign bodies potentiate infection is not clear, but they probably cause localized impairment of host defense mechanisms.[77] In addition, the foreign body often serves as a nidus on which organisms can adhere and produce extracellular substances such as glycocalyx or slime that may interfere with phagocytosis and impair the penetration of antibiotics to the underlying organisms.[78] It has also been demonstrated that antimicrobial agents themselves may cause alterations in host defenses. Clinically achievable concentrations of many different agents have been shown to have adverse effects on leukocyte chemotaxis, lymphocyte transformation, monocyte transformation, delayed hypersensitivity, antibody production, phagocytosis, and the microbicidal action of polymorphonuclear leukocytes.[79–85] It is not clear, however, whether any of these effects (largely demonstrated by in vitro studies) are of clinical significance.[85] Nonetheless, the possibility that antimicrobial agents can cause immunosuppression exists, and this fact should discourage the indiscriminate use of antibiotics, especially in patients who are already immunosuppressed because of their underlying disease or because of their concomitant drug therapy.[83] Finally, antimicrobial agents such as the β-lactams that cause rapid lysis of bacteria may also release endotoxins or cell wall components that have potentially deleterious local and/or systemic effects in the host. The local inflammatory consequences of such activity have been clearly defined in experimental models of bacterial meningitis,[86] but their significance in other settings such as gram-negative sepsis remains to be determined.[87]

ANTIMICROBIAL COMBINATIONS

Most infections in humans with normal host defenses can be treated with a single antimicrobial agent, but there are clear-cut

(as well as borderline) indications for the use of combinations (usually two) of antimicrobials. Because combinations may provide more broad-spectrum coverage than single agents can, the physician is often tempted to use combinations for the sense of security they provide, even in situations in which they are not indicated. Such inappropriate use of antimicrobial combinations may have significantly deleterious effects. In this section, we will examine indications for the use of combinations and the potential disadvantages of this approach to therapy. Although we will consider briefly the use of combination therapy in neutropenic patients, this discussion will not attempt to deal with combination therapy in severely immunocompromised patients such as those undergoing organ transplantation or with severe immunodeficiency states such as occur in patients with HIV infections. In these settings, under specialized circumstances, clinicians are often forced to use broad-spectrum combinations of antibacterial, antiviral, antifungal, and even, at times, antiparasitic agents.

In Vitro Results of Combination Therapy

When two antimicrobial agents are combined, they may have one of three types of activity against a given organism in vitro: *(1)* an additive effect (sometimes called an *indifferent effect*), *(2)* synergism, and *(3)* antagonism.[88] Two drugs are said to be additive when the activity of the drugs in combination is equal to the sum (or a partial sum) of their independent activities when studied separately. The combined effect of a synergistic pair of antimicrobials is greater than the sum of their independent activities when measured separately. If two drugs are antagonistic, the activity of the combination is less than the sum of their independent effects when measured alone. These concepts are illustrated by "time-kill curves" in Figure 1. The various methods used to determine the in vitro effects of antibiotic combinations are beyond the scope of this chapter but have been reviewed in detail.[89]

Indications for the Clinical Use of Antimicrobial Combinations

Five reasons have been advanced to justify the use of antimicrobial combinations. The first three of these are discussed in detail in other chapters and, therefore, will be given only brief mention here.

Prevention of the Emergence of Resistant Organisms. Although the use of antimicrobial agents to prevent the emergence of resistant organisms would seem to be a major indication for the use of such therapy, combination therapy has been clearly documented as effective in preventing resistance only during the treatment of tuberculosis (see Chs. 30 and 230). There is somewhat less epidemiologic evidence in support of this concept as it applies to the use of rifampin for the treatment of nonmycobacterial infections, but it nonetheless appears that one of the major benefits of using rifampin in combination with a second agent for treating staphylococcal infections, for example, is that the combination prevents the rapid emergence of resistance to rifampin, which is evident when this drug is used alone.[90,91]

Polymicrobial Infections. In most infections, even those due to more than one organism, a single effective agent can be found. For example, cellulitis due to *S. aureus* and group A streptococci can be treated with a penicillinase-resistant penicillin alone. However, there are certain types of infections due to such a broad variety of organisms that more than one antimicrobial agent may be required to provide adequate coverage. Examples of such infections include intraperitoneal and pelvic infections due to mixed aerobic and anaerobic organisms. However, many of the newer carbapenems and β-lactam–β-lactamase inhibitor combinations have such broad spectra of activity that

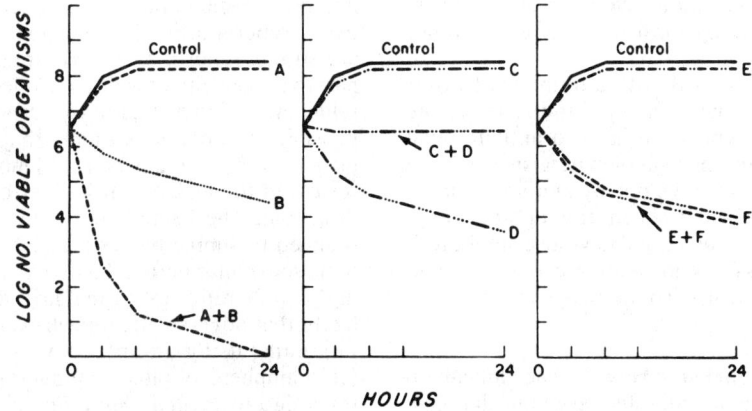

FIG. 1. Antibacterial effects of antibiotic combinations. *Left* (A and B): synergism; *center* (C and D): antagonism; *right* (E and F): indifference (additive). (From Moellering,[94] with permission.)

they can be effectively employed as "monotherapy" for intraabdominal and pelvic sepsis.[92,93]

Initial Therapy. In neutropenic patients or other patients with presumed infection in whom the nature of the infection is not clear, it may be reasonable to begin broad-spectrum coverage, usually with two agents such as ticarcillin plus gentamicin or tobramycin while awaiting the results of cultures. In this setting, it is often possible to switch to a single drug after the results of cultures are available (see Chs. 288 and 289). The development of new drugs with broad spectra of activity makes it possible to use a single agent for most cases of initial therapy, but it would be premature to advocate a general application of this concept at present.

Decreased Toxicity. Many of the drugs used in therapy for infections are potentially toxic (e.g., aminoglycosidic aminocyclitols). Therefore, a major goal of combination therapy has been to reduce the amount of drug required for treatment and, thus, to reduce dose-related toxicity. Unfortunately, at present there are no data from clinical trials that establish beyond doubt that combination therapy with different agents permits a reduction of the drug dose sufficient to reduce dose-related toxicity.

Synergism. The use of synergistic combinations of antimicrobial agents to treat infections due to resistant or relatively resistant organisms represents one of the most appealing ways to use these agents. There are numerous examples of in vitro synergism, but thus far synergistic antimicrobial combinations have proved more effective than are single agents in only a limited number of clinical settings.[94,95]

Perhaps the best known application of synergistic combinations of antimicrobial agents is for the treatment of enterococcal endocarditis. Treatment of this disease with penicillin alone results in an unacceptable relapse rate because enterococci are relatively resistant to penicillin.[96] Indeed, penicillin alone seems to act as a bacteriostatic and not a bactericidal agent.[97] The addition of an aminoglycoside such as streptomycin or gentamicin results in both in vitro and in vivo synergism and yields clinical cure rates comparable to those achieved for endocarditis caused by less resistant streptococci.[96,97] Penicillin enhances the uptake of aminoglycosides by enterococci; the result of this interaction is the synergistic killing of the organisms.[98] In recent years some enterococci have been found to be resistant to penicillin-streptomycin, penicillin-kanamycin, and penicillin-amikacin synergism due to high-level resistance (MIC > 2000 μg/ml) to streptomycin and/or to kanamycin.[99] Strains may resist synergism if they are ribosomally resistant to streptomycin[100] or if they contain plasmid-mediated enzymes that inactivate streptomycin, kanamycin, or amikacin.[101] The prevalence of en-

terococci with high-level resistance to gentamicin appears to be increasing rapidly.[102,103] Moreover, the use of penicillin-gentamicin therapy in such patients may result in a failure to eradicate the infecting organisms.[104] Therefore, it is important to test for high-level resistance to streptomycin and gentamicin before embarking on a therapeutic regimen for enterococcal endocarditis or meningitis.

Penicillin-streptomycin combinations are also synergistic against viridans streptococci and have been used for the treatment of endocarditis due to these organisms.[95] However, viridans streptococci are usually very susceptible to penicillin, and penicillin alone has been used successfully for treatment of this kind of endocarditis.[105,106]

A similar type of synergism occurs when semisynthetic penicillinase-resistant penicillins such as nafcillin or oxacillin are combined with gentamicin against *S. aureus*.[107] Thus far there are no data to document that the use of combination therapy for *S. aureus* infections in humans has any advantage over therapy with a penicillin or cephalosporin alone.[108]

Combinations of carbenicillin, ticarcillin, mezlocillin, azlocillin, or piperacillin with gentamicin, tobramycin, or amikacin exhibit synergism against many strains of *P. aeruginosa*.[109,110] The mechanism of synergism in this setting is similar to that described for enterococci (i.e., enhanced uptake of the aminoglycoside in the presence of the antipseudomonal penicillin). Studies with experimental animals convincingly demonstrate the superiority of such combinations for the treatment of serious *Pseudomonas* infections.[111] Although the information available from limited human trials to date is also consistent with enhanced activity of these combinations for *Pseudomonas* infections, this form of therapy has not been subjected to definitive controlled study.[89] A recent large prospective (but uncontrolled) study of patients with *Pseudomonas* bacteremia documented an increased survival in patients receiving antimicrobial combinations as compared with single-drug therapy. Interestingly, the presence or absence of synergism seemed less important than administration of combination therapy in this population.[112]

Synergism occurs by a different mechanism when sulfonamides are combined with trimethoprim. In this case, the two agents are synergistic because they act to inhibit sequential steps in the microbial pathway of folic acid metabolism.[113] As a result, combinations of sulfonamides with trimethoprim are often useful for the treatment of infections due to organisms that may be resistant to sulfonamides alone. A fixed combination of sulfamethoxazole and trimethoprim is available for clinical use and has been shown effective for the treatment and prevention of chronic urinary tract infections, even when due to sulfonamide-resistant organisms.[114] The combination has also been shown to be useful for the treatment of typhoid fever and shigellosis caused by organisms resistant to ampicillin and/or chloramphenicol, for the treatment of infections due to ampicillin-resistant *H. influenzae* and for therapy for a wide variety of other infections as well.[89,115-117]

Combinations of amphotericin B with a number of other agents including 5-fluorocytosine, rifampin, and tetracycline have been shown to result in enhanced in vitro antimicrobial activity against fungi.[118] The mechanism of synergism seems to involve damage to the fungal cell envelope by amphotericin B, with resultant enhanced intracellular penetration of 5-fluorocytosine and other agents.[118] Flucytosine and low-dose amphotericin B have been used successfully in treating candidiasis and cryptococcosis when the patient's isolate was susceptible to both drugs.[119,120]

Synergism and Infections in Impaired Hosts.   The clinical applications of antimicrobial combinations discussed thus far have all represented attempts to use a synergistic interaction for enhanced efficacy in the treatment of infections due to relatively resistant organisms. Another use of such therapy is to obtain enhanced antimicrobial activity in the treatment of infections due to susceptible organisms occurring in patients with abnormalities of host defense systems. Several groups have conducted randomized trials of various combinations of two agents chosen from among carbenicillin, ticarcillin, piperacillin, the cephalosporins, gentamicin, tobramycin, and amikacin for the treatment of severe infections in patients with impaired host defense mechanisms. Both Lau et al.[121] and Klastersky et al.[122] have demonstrated improved survival rates in such patients treated with combinations that were synergistic against the infecting organisms as compared with patients receiving nonsynergistic combinations. These studies add strong support to the concept that synergistic combinations of antimicrobials may be an important determinant of success in the treatment of serious infections, especially when due to gram-negative organisms in patients with impaired host defenses. However, there is no absolute proof that synergistic combinations are more effective in this setting than are single agents that have a sufficiently broad spectrum and that produce sufficiently high serum bactericidal titers against the infecting organisms.[123]

Disadvantages of the Inappropriate Use of Antimicrobial Combinations

Whereas the clinical use of synergistic combinations of antimicrobial agents may have beneficial results as noted above, the inappropriate use of antimicrobial combinations may have important adverse effects, three of which are discussed below.

Antagonism.   The medical literature contains a large number of reports of in vitro antagonism between antimicrobial agents.[94,95] In view of this, it is surprising that there are only a few well-documented clinical examples of antagonism. Perhaps the most impressive is the study of Lepper and Dowling,[124] who demonstrated conclusively in 1951 that penicillin is more effective than is the combination of penicillin with chlortetracycline for the treatment of pneumococcal meningitis. The fatality among patients treated with penicillin alone was 21 percent, whereas that among patients treated with penicillin plus chlortetracycline was 79 percent. A study of childhood meningitis has also demonstrated the superiority of single-drug therapy. Mathies et al.[125] treated a group of children suffering from bacterial meningitis with either ampicillin alone or a combination of ampicillin, chloramphenicol, and streptomycin. The mortality among 140 children treated with ampicillin alone was 4.3 percent, whereas the mortality among 124 children receiving the antibiotic combination was 10.5 percent, a difference that reached statistical significance. There are several other reports of the influence of antagonism on the treatment of urinary tract infections and streptococcal pharyngitis, but none are particularly impressive.[94] Considering the extensive clinical use of anti-

microbial combinations and especially in view of the large number of reports of in vitro antagonism, it is surprising that there are so few reports of in vivo antagonism. This may be due in part to the paucity of well-controlled studies in this area or to the reluctance of investigators to report adverse results. Another possible explanation is simply that clinically significant antagonism is not a common event. In most cases, in vitro antagonism results in the loss or partial loss of activity of the most active drug (e.g., the bactericidal activity of such an agent may be reduced to simple bacteriostasis), but the combination still retains some antimicrobial activity. As long as the patient receiving such therapy has normal host defense mechanisms, it is unlikely that adverse effects will be seen. This has been the case in studies using an antagonistic combination of antibiotics (chloramphenicol plus gentamicin) to treat experimental infections due to *Proteus mirabilis* in mice.[126] In healthy mice, in vivo antagonism could not be demonstrated, but after irradiation to render the animals neutropenic, gentamicin alone was more effective than gentamicin plus chloramphenicol was. This combination has also been shown to be antagonistic in experimentally produced meningitis due to *P. mirabilis* in rabbits.[127] Thus, it seems that clinically important antagonism is most likely to be manifested in patients with generalized impairment of host defense mechanisms (such as seen in leukemia, cancer patients who are neutropenic, and so forth) or in patients with infections such as meningitis or endocarditis in whom localized host defenses may be inadequate.

The observation of in vivo antagonism in the treatment of bacterial meningitis raises some questions about the recommendations of the use of ampicillin plus chloramphenicol in the initial treatment of childhood meningitis (see Ch. 64) because of the emergence of ampicillin-resistant strains of *H. influenzae*.[12] Combinations of penicillin plus chloramphenicol have been shown to exhibit in vitro antagonism against pneumococci and other organisms.[95] However, this antagonism takes the form of lessened bactericidal activity of penicillin in the presence of chloramphenicol. Since chloramphenicol alone is quite active against the organisms likely to cause childhood meningitis. (*H. influenzae, S. pneumoniae, Neisseria meningitidis*) and since there is no evidence that penicillin or ampicillin antagonizes the activity of chloramphenicol, it seems unlikely that the use of ampicillin-chloramphenicol therapy for pediatric meningitis will result in in vivo antagonism when used to treat the organisms listed above.[95]

Studies documenting the effectiveness of cephalosporins such as cefotaxime and ceftriaxone[128,129] for childhood meningitis make it unnecessary to continue to use combination therapy in this setting.

There has been a recent upsurge of interest in the use of the newer broad-spectrum β-lactams in combination with each other to obtain broad-spectrum coverage without exposing the patient to the possible toxicity of an agent such as chloramphenicol or an aminoglycosidic aminocyclitol.[130] For the most part, this seems reasonable. However, there is in vitro and in vivo evidence that some β-lactam–β-lactam combinations may be antagonistic against certain organisms such as *Enterobacter, Serratia,* or *Pseudomonas*. This antagonism seems to be the result of the induction or derepression of chromosomally mediated β-lactamases by one of the agents, leading to inactivation of the second.[131] The exact clinical significance of this phenomenon is not presently clear, but it must be kept in mind when one considers the clinical use of such combinations.

Most of the examples of in vitro antagonism are the result of interactions of the antimicrobial agents as they act at a subcellular level on a given microorganism. However, another type of antagonism should also be included in this discussion. This may result from the direct interaction of drugs before they reach the microorganism. If chloramphenicol and erythromycin are inadvertently mixed together in the same parenteral infusion solution, they form insoluble precipitates and hence lose activity. In recent years, it has become clear that the mixing of penicillins (especially carbenicillin or ticarcillin) with aminoglycosides results in the inactivation of the aminoglycoside.[132] Because the reaction occurs slowly, this is usually not a problem in vivo, provided the drugs are given by separate routes of administration. However, in uremic patients in whom the serum half-life of aminoglycosides is greatly prolonged, in vivo inactivation can occur.[133] The clinical significance of this observation, however, has not yet been elucidated.

Cost. With the possible exception of penicillin G, ampicillin, and certain of the tetracyclines and sulfonamides, antimicrobials are expensive drugs. Thus the inappropriate use of antimicrobial combinations (when a single agent would be adequate) can add greatly to the cost of the patient's illness.

Adverse Effects. It has been estimated that approximately 5 percent of the patients receiving a given antibiotic in the hospital will experience some sort of adverse reaction.[19,134] Obviously the possibility of such adverse reactions (including hypersensitivity reactions and direct toxic effects) is increased without any enhanced therapeutic benefit when one inappropriately uses combinations of antimicrobial agents. Moreover, when an adverse reaction occurs in a patient receiving more than one drug, it is often difficult to be certain of the agent that caused the reaction. This may mean that treatment with several or all drugs must be stopped. If combination drug therapy is to be used in such a patient, each drug must be tested carefully before use to make certain that it was not the cause of the original adverse reaction. This is time consuming and expensive and may needlessly deprive the patient of the benefits of a useful agent.

CHOICE OF APPROPRIATE ROUTE OF ADMINISTRATION OF ANTIMICROBIAL AGENTS AND EVALUATION OF EFFICACY

Route of Administration

Once the physician has determined the most appropriate drug or drugs with which to treat a given infection, he or she must decide which route of administration to use to obtain maximum benefits from the therapy. In most cases this is a choice between oral and parenteral routes. In general, the oral route of administration is chosen for those infections that are mild and can be treated on an outpatient basis. Not all antibiotics can be administered in this way. Drugs such as vancomycin, the polymyxins, the aminoglycosidic aminocyclitols, and amphotericin B are absorbed so poorly from the gastrointestinal tract that they cannot be administered orally to treat systemic infections. When drugs are administered by the oral route, the physician must ascertain that the patient will reliably take them as ordered. The absorption of certain agents such as penicillin G is markedly impaired if taken with meals, whereas the absorption of acid-stable penicillins such as penicillin V is not affected by food or gastric acidity. The concomitant administration of antacids or iron-containing preparations may severely impair the absorption of tetracycline, since this drug forms insoluble chelates in the presence of Mg^{2+}, Ca^{2+}, or Fe^{2+} ions. Antacids and histamine antagonists may also interfere with the absorption of the fluoroquinolones such as ciprofloxacin and norfloxacin.[135] More detailed information on the oral absorption of antimicrobial agents may be found in the chapters on the individual drugs.

The parenteral route of administration is used for agents that are inefficiently absorbed from the gastrointestinal tract and for the treatment of patients with serious infections in whom high serum concentrations of antimicrobial agents are required. The aminoglycosidic aminocyclitols and polymyxins may be given by intramuscular injection and are well tolerated when given this way. For most infections, adequate serum concentrations are achieved after the intramuscular administration of these

drugs. However, in life-threatening infections, especially in the presence of shock (or in diabetic patients as discussed earlier), intravenous administration is preferred. Intravenous administration allows large doses of drugs to be given with a minimum of discomfort to the patient when high serum concentrations are required for the effective treatment of disease processes such as meningitis, endocarditis, and osteomyelitis. Whether intravenously administered drugs should be given by continuous infusion or by intermittent bolus infusion remains a matter of controversy. The former method has the advantage of simplicity; because pulses containing very high concentrations of drugs are avoided, it may result in less venous irritation and phlebitis. Studies in animal models suggest that the concentration of drugs such as penicillins and cephalosporins in fibrin clots is related to the peak serum levels achieved. Thus, greater concentrations of drugs are achieved in the clots in the face of intermittent bolus therapy.[136] It has been suggested that these data may be applicable to therapy for infective endocarditis and other infections in which high tissue concentrations of antibiotics are required. More recent evidence, however, strongly suggests that the clinical effectiveness of β-lactam antibiotics is optimal when the concentration of the antimicrobial agent at the site of infection exceeds the MIC of the infecting organism for a prolonged period of time. Since it is easier to maintain such concentrations persistently above the MIC by continuous infusion, these studies lend support to the concept of administering β-lactam antibiotics by continuous infusion for serious systemic infections.[137] On the other hand, antimicrobial agents such as the aminoglycosides exhibit concentration-dependent killing (which is not seen with the β-lactams), and, for this reason, giving these drugs by once-a-day bolus infusion is attractive from a pharmacodynamic point of view.[138] Thus, the high peak levels obtained after bolus dosing cause more rapid killing of the infecting pathogen. Once-a-day dosing of aminoglycosides also leads to lower (or absent) trough levels, which may be advantageous in terms of potential toxicity.[138] Definitive clinical studies providing unequivocal support for these concepts, however, remain to be carried out.

As discussed earlier, the intrathecal or intraventricular route of administration may be necessary for the treatment of meningeal infections with drugs such as the aminoglycosidic aminocyclitols, polymyxins, bacitracin, and possibly vancomycin, all of which cross the blood-brain barrier with considerable difficulty. The parenteral administration of antimicrobial agents results in adequate concentrations in pleural, peritoneal, pericardial, and synovial fluids.[139,140] Thus, direct instillation of antibiotics into these areas is not necessary.

Monitoring the Response of the Patient to Antimicrobial Therapy

Although several laboratory tests are available to assist in the monitoring of antimicrobial therapy, clinical assessment remains the most important method for determining the efficacy of treatment. It is not uncommon to see patients fail to respond in the face of laboratory studies that suggest adequate therapy and vice versa. The reasons for this may usually be found among the many host factors that affect therapy as described earlier.

Nonetheless, the measurement of serum concentrations of antimicrobial agents and a determination of serum bactericidal titers are often of considerable use. The details concerning these tests are given in Chapter 11 and will not be repeated here. The major value of the direct determination of serum concentrations of antimicrobial agents is to avoid toxicity from excessive levels of agents such as the aminoglycosidic aminocyclitols, especially in patients with impaired renal or hepatic function. These tests are also useful for determining inadequate serum levels due to insufficient dosing or unusually rapid clearance.

Another method used to monitor the effectiveness of antimicrobial therapy is the serum bactericidal titer (sometimes called the *serum antimicrobial dilution titer*). This test was originally described by Schlichter and MacLean[141] as a guide for effective therapy for subacute bacterial endocarditis. Subsequently this test has been used to monitor therapy in patients with infective endocarditis, osteomyelitis, septic arthritis, empyema, and bacteremia.[122,142] In this test, serial dilutions of the patient's serum are incubated with an inoculum of the infecting organism; after incubation, the highest dilution that inhibits and/or kills the organism is determined. Most investigators feel that a serum bactericidal titer of at least 1:8 can be correlated with a successful therapeutic outcome.[122,141,143,144] A more recent multicenter study has suggested that peak and trough titers of at least 1:64 and 1:32, respectively, are good predictors of a successful therapeutic outcome in patients with infective endocarditis.[145] However, a lack of standardization and a lack of consistency in specifying the point (peak, trough, or midpoint serum levels) at which the test should be done have hindered attempts at more widespread application and evaluation of this test.[146–149]

CONCLUSION

Optimal use of antimicrobial agents demands consideration of a large number of important factors that may influence the choice of an appropriate agent and that determine the most effective dose and route of administration of a drug. A number of these factors have been outlined in this chapter. In the final analysis, sound clinical judgment remains the most important determinant of a successful outcome.

REFERENCES

1. Weinstein L. General considerations. In: Goodman LS, Gilman A, eds. The Pharmacological Basis of Therapeutics. New York. Macmillan; 1970:1154.
2. Majno G. The Healing Hand: Man and Wound in the Ancient World. Cambridge, MA: Harvard University Press; 1975:154, 215.
3. Harris JC, Dupont HL, Hornick RB. Fecal leukocytes in diarrheal illness. Ann Intern Med. 1972;76:697.
4. Ho D, Ault MJ, Ault MA, et al. Campylobacter enteritis. Early diagnosis with Gram's stain. Arch Intern Med. 1982;142:1858.
5. Zipeto D, Revello MG, Silini E, et al. Development and clinical significance of a diagnostic assay based on the polymerase chain reaction for detection of human cytomegalovirus DNA in blood samples from immunocompromised patients. J Clin Microbiol. 1992;30:527.
6. Peter J. The polymerase chain reaction: Amplifying our options. Rev Infect Dis. 1991;13:166.
7. Desmond EP. Molecular approaches to the identification of mycobacteria. Clin Microbiol Newslett. 1992;14:145.
8. Weinstein L. Common sense (clinical judgment) in the diagnosis and antibiotic therapy of etiologically undefined infections. Pediatr Clin North Am. 1968;15:141.
9. Moellering RC Jr. A rational approach to the choice of antimicrobial agents in bacterial infections. In: Seminar on Gram-Negative Infections. St Louis: CV Mosby;1974:5.
10. Huang MB, Baker CN, Bannerjee S, Tenover FC. Accuracy of the E test for determining antimicrobial susceptibility of staphylococci, enterococci, Campylobacter jejuni, and gram-negative bacteria resistant to antimicrobial agents. J Clin Microbiol. 1992;30:3243.
11. Jorgensen JH. Antibacterial susceptibility tests: Automated or instrument-based methods. In: Balows A, Hausler WJ Jr, Herrmann KL, et al., eds. Manual of Clinical Microbiology. Washington, DC. American Society for Microbiology;1991:1166.
12. Murray BE, Moellering RC Jr. Patterns and mechanisms of antibiotic resistance. Med Clin North Am. 1978;62:899.
13. Levy SB. Active efflux mechanisms for antimicrobial resistance. Antimicrob Agents Chemother. 1992;36:695.
14. Puoff KL. Gram-positive vancomycin-resistant clinical isolates. Clin Microbiol Newslett. 1989;11:1.
15. Moellering RC Jr, Kunz LJ, Poitras JW, et al. Microbiologic basis for the rational use of antibiotics. South Med J. 1977;70(Suppl):8.
16. Abramowicz M, ed. The choice of antibacterial drugs. Med Lett. 1992;34:49.
17. Weinstein L, Dalton AC. Host determinants of response to antimicrobial agents. N Engl J Med. 1968;279:467.
18. Moellering RC Jr. Factors influencing the clinical use of antimicrobial agents in elderly patients. Geriatrics. 1978;33:83.
19. Mannisto PT, Mantyla R, Nykanen S, et al. Impairing effect of food on ketoconazole absorption. Antimicrob Agents Chemother. 1982;21:730.
20. Jackson GG, Arcieri G. Ototoxicity of gentamicin in man: A survey and controlled analysis of clinical experience in the United States. J Infect Dis. 1969;119:432.
21. Calderwood S, Moellering RC Jr. Common adverse effects of antibacterial agents on major organ systems. Surg Clin North Am. 1980;60:65.
22. Moellering RC Jr. Antimicrobial agents in pregnancy and the postpartum period. Clin Obstet Gynecol. 1989;22:277.
23. McCracken GH Jr. Pharmacologic basis for antimicrobial therapy in newborn infants. Am J Dis Child. 1974;128:407.
24. Kline AH, Blattner RJ, Lunin M. Transplacental effect of tetracyclines on teeth. JAMA. 1964;118:178.
25. Hoyer D, Wolfson J. Adverse effects of quinolone antibiotics. In: Hooper D, Wolfson J, eds. Quinolone Antimicrobial Agents. Washington, DC: American Society for Microbiology; 1989:249–271.
26. Garibaldi RA, Drusin RE, Ferebee SH, et al. Isoniazid-associated hepatitis. Am Rev Respir Dis. 1972;106:357.
27. Rose DN, Schechter CB, Silver AL. The age threshold for isoniazid chemoproplylaxis. JAMA. 1986;256:2709.
28. Foord RD. Cephaloridine, cephalothin and the kidney. J Antimicrob Chemother. 1975;1(Suppl):119.
29. Koch-Weser J, Sidel VW, Federman EB, et al. Adverse effects of sodium colistimethate. Ann Intern Med. 1970;72:857.
30. Van Scoy RE. Antituberculous agents. Mayo Clin Proc. 1977;52:694.
31. Young DS, Thomas DW, Friedman RB, et al. Effects of drugs on clinical laboratory tests. Clin Chem. 1972;18:1041.
32. Rizack MA, Hilman CDM. The Medical Letter Handbook of Drug Interactions. New Rochelle, NY: The Medical Letter; 1983.
33. Hamod KA, Khouzami VA. Antibiotics in pregnancy. In: Nietyl JR, (ed). Drug Use in Pregnancy. Philadelphia: Lea & Febiger; 1982:31.
34. Philipson A. The use of antibiotics in pregnancy. J Antimicrob Chemother. 1983;12:101.
35. Anonymous. Ticarcillin. Med Lett. 1977;19:17.
36. Anonymous. Is Flagyl dangerous? Med Lett. 1975;17:53.
37. Conway N, Birt BD. Streptomycin in pregnancy: Effect in foetal ear. Br Med J. 1965:2:260.
38. Monnet P, Kalb JC, Pujol M. Toxic influence of isoniazid on fetus. Lyon Med. 1967;218:431.
39. Philipson A. Pharmakokinetics of ampicillin during pregnancy. J Infect Dis. 1977;136:370.
40. Vorherr H. Drug excretion in breast milk. Postgrad Med. 1974;56:97.
41. Reeves DS. The effect of renal failure on the pharmacokinetics of antibiotics. J Antimicrob Chemother. 1988;21:5.
42. Jackson EA, McLeod DC. Pharmacokinetics and dosing of antimicrobial agents in renal impairment, part i. Am J Hosp Pharm. 1974;31:36.
43. Jackson EA, McLeod DC. Pharmacokinetics and dosing of antimicrobial agents in renal impairment, part ii. Am J Hosp Pharm. 1974;31:137.
44. Moellering RC Jr., Eliopoulos GM. Principles of anti-infective therapy. In: Stein JH ed. Internal Medicine. St. Louis: CV Mosby, 1994:1800.
45. Bennett WM, Aronoff GR, Morrison G, et al. Drug prescribing in renal failure: Dosing guidelines for adults. Am J Kidney Dis. 1983;3:155.
46. Cooper K, Bennett WM. Nephrotoxicity of common drugs used in clinical practice. Arch Intern Med. 1987;147:1213.
47. Natelson EA, Brown CH III, Bradshaw MW, et al. Influence of cephalosporin antibiotics on blood coagulation and platelet function. Antimicrob Agents Chemother. 1976;9:91.
48. Neu HC. Adverse effects of new cephalosporins. Ann Intern Med. 1983;98:415.
49. Kaufman CA, Frame PT. Bone marrow toxicity associated with 5-fluorocytosine therapy. Antimicrob Agents Chemother. 1977;11:244.
50. Davey PG. Pharmacokinetics in liver disease. J Antimicrob Chemother. 1988;21:1.
51. Suhrland LG, Weisberger AS. Chloramphenicol toxicity in liver and renal disease. Arch Intern Med. 1963;112:747.
52. Pessayre D, Allemand H, Benhamou J-P. Effets des maladies du foie et des voies biliaires sur le métabolisme des médicaments. Nouv Presse Med. 1977; 35:3209.
53. Singh N, Yu VL, Mieles LA, et al. β-Lactam-antibiotic-induced leukopenia in severe hepatic dysfunction: Risk factors and implications for dosing in patients with liver disease. Am J Med. 1993;94:251.
54. Lorian V, Atkinson B. Killing of oxacillin-exposed staphylococci in human polymorphonuclear leukocytes. Antimicrob Agents Chemother. 1980;18:807.
55. Ofek IE, Beachey H, Eisenstein BI, et al. Suppression of bacterial adherence by subminimal inhibitory concentration of β-lactam and aminoglycoside antibiotics. Rev Infect Dis. 1979;1:832.
56. Gemmell CG, Peterson PK, Schmeling DJ, et al. Potentiation of opsonization and phagocytosis of Streptococcus pyogenes following growth in the presence of clindamycin. J Clin Invest. 1981;67:1249.
57. Friedman HH, Warren GH. Enhanced susceptibility of penicillin-resistant staphylococci to phagocytosis after in vitro incubation with low dose of nafcillin. Proc Soc Exp Biol Med. 1974;146:707.
58. Elliott GR, Peterson PK, Verbrugh HA, et al. Influence of subinhibitory concentrations of penicillin, cephalothin, and clindamycin on Staphylococcus aureus growth in human phagocytic cells. Antimicrob Agents Chemother. 1982;22:781.
59. Moellering RC Jr. Revolutionary changes in the macrolide and azalide antibiotics. Am J Med. 1991;91:1S.
60. Smith CR. The spiramycin paradox. J Antimicrob Chemother. 1988;22(Suppl B):141.
61. Foulds G, Johnson RB. Selection of dose regimens of azithromycin. J Antimicrob Chemother 1993;31(Suppl E):39.
62. Craig WA, Kunin CM. Significance of serum protein and tissue binding of antimicrobial agents. Annu Rev Med. 1976;27:287.
63. Peterson LR, Gerding DN. Interaction of cephalosporins with human and canine serum proteins. J Infect Dis. 1978;137:452.
64. Barza M, Samuelson T, Weinstein L. Penetration of antibiotics into fibrin

loci in vivo. II. Comparison of nine antibiotics: Effect of dose and degree of protein binding. J Infect Dis. 1974;129:66.

65. Kunst MW, Mattie H. Cefazolin and cephradine. Relationship between antibacterial activity in vitro and in mice experimentally infected with *Escherichia coli*. J Infect Dis. 1978;137:391.

66. Merrikin DJ, Briant J, Rolinson GN. Effect of protein binding on antibiotic activity in vivo. J Antimicrob Chemother. 1983;11:233.

67. Kaiser AB, McGee ZA. Aminoglycoside therapy of gram-negative bacillary meningitis. N Engl J Med. 1975;293:1215.

68. Waldvogel FW. Treatment of osteomyelitis and septic arthritis with quinolone antimicrobial agents. In: Hooper D, Wolfson J, eds. Quinolone antimicrobial Agents. Washington DC: American Society for Microbiology; 1989: 177–86.

69. Naber KG. The role of quinolones in the treatment of chronic bacterial prostatitis. In: Hooper D, Wolfson J, eds. *Quinolone Antimicrobial Agents*. 2nd ed. Washington, DC: American Society for Microbiology; 1993;285.

70. Bryant RE, Howard D. Interaction of purulent material with antibiotics used to treat *Pseudomonas* infections. Antimicrob Agents Chemother. 1974;6:702.

71. O'Keefe JP, Tally FP, Barza M, et al. Inactivation of penicillin G during experimental infection with *Bacteroides fragilis*. J Infect Dis. 1978;137:437.

72. Zimelis VM, Jackson GG. Activity of aminoglycoside antibiotics against *Pseudomonas aeruginosa*. Specificity and site of calcium and magnesium antagonism. J Infect Dis. 1973;127:663.

73. Bryan LE, Van Den Elzen HM. Streptomycin accumulation in susceptible and resistant strains of *Escherichia coli* and *Pseudomonas aeruginosa*. Antimicrob Agents Chemother. 1976;9:928.

74. Zinner SH, Sabath LD, Casey JI, et al. Erythromycin and alkalinization of the urine in the treatment of urinary tract infections due to gram-negative bacilli. Lancet. 1971;1:1267.

75. Sabath LD, Gerstein DA, Leaf CD, et al. Increasing the usefulness of antibiotics: Treatment of infections caused by gram-negative bacilli. Clin Pharmacol Ther. 1970;11:161.

76. Karchmer AW, Dismukes WE, Buckley MJ, et al. Late prosthetic valve endocarditis. Am J Med. 1978;64:99.

77. Zimmerli W, Waldvogel FA, Vaudaux P, et al. Pathogenesis of foreign body infection: Description and characteristics of an animal model. J Infect Dis. 1982;146:487.

78. Dickinson GM, Bisno AL. Infections associated with indwelling medical devices. Antimicrob Agents Chemother. 1989;33:597.

79. Forsgren A, Schmeling D, Quie PG. Effect of tetracycline on the phagocytic function of human leukocytes. J Infect Dis. 1974;130:412.

80. Seklecki MM, Quintiliani R, Maderazo EG. Aminoglycoside antibiotics moderately impair granulocyte function. Antimicrob Agents Chemother. 1978; 13:552.

81. Chaperon EA, Sanders WE Jr. Suppression of lymphocyte responses by cephalosporins. Infect Immun. 1978;19:378.

82. Mandell LA. Effects of antimicrobial and antineoplastic drugs on the phagocytic and microbicidal function of the polymorphonuclear leukocyte. Rev Infect Dis. 1982;4:683.

83. Hauser WE, Remington JS. Effect of antibiotics on the immune response. Am J Med. 1982;72:711.

84. Manzella JP, Clark JK. Effects of moxalactam and cefuroxime on mitogen-stimulated human mononuclear leukocytes. Antimicrob Agents Chemother. 1983;23:360.

85. Daschner FD. Antibiotics and host defense with special reference to phagocytosis by human polymorphonuclear leukocyte function in vivo. Antimicrob Agents Chemother. 1985;27:712.

86. Wispelway B, Lesse AJ, Hansen EJ, et al. *Haemophilus influenzae* lipopolysaccharide-induced blood-brain barrier permeability during experimental meningitis in the rat. J Clin Invest. 1988;82:1339.

87. Evins ME, Pollack M. Effect of antibiotic class and concentration on the release of lipopolysaccharide from *Escherichia coli*. J Infect Dis. 1993;167: 1336.

88. Jawetz E. Combined antibiotic action: Some definitions and correlations between laboratory and clinical results. Antimicrob Agents Chemother. 1967,1968;203.

89. Eligondos GM, Moellering RC Jr. Antimicrobial combinations. In: Lorian V, ed. Antibiotics in Laboratory Medicine. 3rd ed. Baltimore: Williams & Wilkins; 1991:432–92.

90. VanderAuwera P, Meunier-Carpentier F, Klastersky J. Clinical study of combination therapy with oxacillin and rifampin for staphylococcal infections. Rev Infect Dis. 1983;5(Suppl 3):515.

91. Karchmer AW, Archer GL, Dimukes WE. Rifampin treatment of prosthetic valve endocarditis due to *Staphylococcus epidermidis*. Rev Infect Dis. 1983; 5(Suppl 3):543.

92. Solomkin JS, Dellinger EP, Christou NV, et al. Results of a multicenter trial comparing imipenem/cilastatin to tobramycin/clindamycin for intra-abdominal infections. Ann Surg. 1990;212:581.

93. Brismar B, Malmborg AS. Tunevall G, et al. Piperacillin-tazobactam versus imipenem-cilastatin for treatment of intra-abdominal infections. Antimicrob Agents Chemother. 1992;36:2766.

94. Moellering RC Jr. Use and abuse of antibiotic combinations. RI Med J. 1972; 55:341.

95. Rahal JJ Jr. Antibiotic combinations: The clinical relevance of synergy and antagonism. Medicine (Baltimore). 1978;57:179.

96. Mandell GL, Kaye D, Levison ME, et al. Enterococcal endocarditis. An

analysis of 38 patients observed at the New York Hospital–Cornell Medical Center. Arch Intern Med. 1970;125:258.

97. Moellering RC Jr, Wennersten C, Weinberg AN. Studies on antibiotic synergism against enterococci: I. Bacteriologic studies. J Lab Clin Med. 1971;77: 821.

98. Moellering RC Jr, Weinberg AN. Studies on antibiotic synergism against enterococci: II. Effect of various antibiotics on the uptake of ^{14}C-labelled streptomycin by enterococci. J Clin Invest. 1971;50:2580.

99. Moellering RC Jr, Wennersten CBG, Medrek T, et al. Prevalence of high-level resistance to aminoglycosides in clinical isolates of enterococci. Antimicrob Agents Chemother. 1970, 1971;335.

100. Zimmermann RA, Moellering RC Jr, Weinberg AN. Mechanism of resistance to antibiotic synergism in enterococci. J Bacteriol. 1971;105:873.

101. Krogstad DJ, Korfhagen TR, Moellering RC Jr, et al. Aminoglycoside-inactivating enzymes: An explanation for resistance to penicillin-aminoglycoside synergism in enterococci. J Clin Invest. 1978;62:480.

102. Mederski-Samoraj BD, Murray BE. High-level resistance to gentamicin in clinical isolates of enterococci. J Infect Dis. 1983;147:751.

103. Moellering RC Jr. The enterococcus: High-level resistance to gentamicin and production of beta-lactamase. Clin Microbiol Newslett. 1988;10:129.

104. Fernandez-Guerrero ML, Barros C, Tudela JLR, et al. Aortic endocarditis caused by gentamicin-resistant *Enterococcus*. Eur J Clin Microbiol. 1988;7: 525.

105. Wolfe JC, Johnson WD Jr. Penicillin-sensitive streptococcal endocarditis. Ann Intern Med. 1974;81:178.

106. Karchmer AW, Moellering RC Jr, Maki D, et al. Single antibiotic therapy of streptococcal endocarditis. JAMA. 1979;241:1801.

107. Watanakunakorn C, Glotzbecker C. Enhancement of the effects of antistaphylococcal antibiotics by aminoglycosides. Antimicrob Agents Chemother. 1974;6:802.

108. Korzeniowski O, Sande MA. The National Collaborative Endocarditis Study Group: Combination antimicrobial therapy for *Staphylococcus aureus* endocarditis in patients addicted to parenteral drugs and in nonaddicts. Ann Intern Med. 1982;97:496.

109. Smith CB, Dans PE, Wilfert JN, et al. Use of gentamicin in combination with other antibiotics. J Infect Dis. 1969;119:370.

110. Eliopoulos GM, Moellering RC Jr. Azlocillin, mezlocillin and piperacillin: New broad-spectrum penicillins. Ann Intern Med. 1982;97:755.

111. Adriole VT. Antibiotic synergy in experimental infection with *Pseudomonas*: II. The effect of carbenicillin, cephalothin or cephanone combined with tobramycin or gentamicin. J Infect Dis. 1974;129:124.

112. Hilf M, Yu VL, Sharp JA, et al. Antibiotic therapy for *Pseudomonas aeruginosa* bacteremia: Outcome correlations in a prospective study of 200 patients. Am J Med. 1989;87:540.

113. Then R. Synergism between trimethoprim and sulfonamides. Science. 1977; 197:1301.

114. Harding GKM, Ronald AR. A controlled study of antimicrobial prophylaxis of recurrent urinary tract infections in women. N Engl J Med. 1974;291:597.

115. Gilman RN, Terminel M, Levine MM, et al. Comparison of trimethoprim-sulfamethoxazole and amoxicillin in therapy of chloramphenicol-resistant and chloramphenicol-sensitive typhoid fever. J Infect Dis. 1975;132:630.

116. Chang MJ, Dunkle LM, Van Reken D, et al. Trimethoprim-sulfamethoxazole compared to ampicillin in the treatment of shigellosis. Pediatrics. 1977;59: 726.

117. Quintiliani R, Levite RE, Nightingale CH. Potential role of trimethoprim-sulfamethoxazole in the treatment of serious hospital-acquired infections. Rev Infect Dis. 1987;9(Suppl 2):160.

118. Kwan CN, Medoff G, Kobayashi G, et al. Potentiation of the anti-fungal effects of antibiotics by amphotericin B. Antimicrob Agents Chemother. 1972;2:61.

119. Titsworth E, Grunberg E. Chemotherapeutic activity of 5-fluorocytosine and amphotericin B against *Candida albicans* in mice. Antimicrob Agents Chemother. 1973;4:306.

120. Bennett J, Dismukes W, Duma R, et al. A comparison of amphotericin B alone with amphotericin B plus flucytosine in the treatment of cryptoccal meningitis. N Engl J Med. 1979;301:126.

121. Lau WK, Young LS, Block RE, et al. Comparative efficacy and toxicity of amikacin/carbenicillin versus gentamicin/carbenicillin in leukopenic patients. Am J Med. 1977;62:959.

122. Klastersky J, Hensgens C, Meunier-Carpentier F. Comparative effectiveness of combinations of amikacin with penicillin G and amikacin with carbenicillin in gram-negative septicemia: Double-blind clinical trial. J Infect Dis. 1976; 134(Suppl):433.

123. Moellering RC Jr. Monotherapy with expanded-spectrum cephalosporins for empiric treatment of serious infections diseases. In: Hoepelman IM, Moellering RC Jr, eds. New Directions in Cephalosporin Therapy: The Expanded Spectrum Cephalosporins. Winchester, UK: Theracom; 1988:49.

124. Lepper MH, Dowling HF. Treatment of pneumococcic meningitis with penicillin compared with penicillin plus aureomycin. Arch Intern Med. 1951;88: 489.

125. Mathies AW Jr, Leedom JM, Ivier D, et al. Antibiotic antagonism in bacterial meningitis. Antimicrob Agents Chemother. 1967;7:218.

126. Sande MA, Overton JW. In vivo antagonism between gentamicin and chloramphenicol in neutropenic mice. J Infect Dis. 1973;128:247.

127. Strausbaugh LJ, Sande MA. Factors influencing the therapy of experimental *Proteus mirabilis* meningitis in rabbits. J Infect Dis. 1978;137:251.

128. Schaad UB, Suter S, Gianella-Borradori A, et al. A comparison of ceftriaxone and cefuroxime for the treatment of bacterial meningitis in children. N Engl J Med. 1990;322:141.

129. Del Rio MDL, Chrane D, Shelton S, et al. Ceftriaxone versus ampicillin and chloramphenicol for treatment of bacterial meningitis in children. Lancet. 1983;1:1241.

130. Moellering RC Jr. Rationale for the use of antibiotic combinations. Am J Med. 1983;75(2A):4.

131. Sanders CC. Novel resistance selected by the new expanded spectrum cephalosporins: A concern. J Infect Dis. 1983;147:585.

132. McLaughlin JE, Reeves DS. Clinical and laboratory evidence for inactivation of gentamicin by carbenicillin. Lancet. 1971;1:261.

133. Riff LJ, Jackson GG. Laboratory and clinical conditions for gentamicin inactivation by carbenicillin. Arch Intern Med. 1972;130:887.

134. Seidl LG, Thornton GF, Smith SW, et al. Studies on epidemiology of adverse drug reactions. III. Reactions in patients on general medical service. Bull Johns Hopkins Hosp. 1966;119:299.

135. Drusano GL. Pharmacokinetics of quinolone antimicrobial agents. In: Hooper D, Wolfson J, eds. Quinolone Antimicrobial Agents. Washington, DC: American Society for Microbiology; 1989:71–105.

136. Barza M, Brusch J, Bergeron M, et al. Penetration of antibiotics into fibrin loci in vivo. III. Intermittent versus continuous infusion and the effect of probenicid. J Infect Dis. 1974;129:73.

137. Craig WA, Ebert SC. Continuous infusion of β-lactam antibiotics. Antimicrob Agents Chemother. 1992;36:2577.

138. Gilbert DN. Once-daily aminoglycoside therapy. Antimicrob Agents Chemother. 1991;35:399.

139. Nelson JD. Antibiotic concentrations in septic joint effusions. N Engl J Med. 1971;284:349.

140. Gerding DN, Hall WH. The penetration of antibiotics into peritoneal fluid. Bull NY Acad Med. 1975;51:1016.

141. Schlichter JG, MacLean H. A method of determining the effective therapeutic level in the treatment of subacute bacterial endocarditis with penicillin. Am Heart J. 1947;34:209.

142. Reller LB, Stratton CW. Serum dilution test for bactericidal activity. II. Standardization and correlation with antimicrobial assays and susceptibility tests. J Infect Dis. 1977;136:196.

143. Carrizosa J, Kaye D. Antibiotic concentrations in serum, serum bactericidal activity, and results of therapy of streptococcal endocarditis in rabbits. Antimicrob Agents Chemother. 1977;12:479.

144. Levy J, Klastersky J. Serum bactericidal test: A review with emphasis on its role in the evaluation of antibiotic combination. In: Klastersky J, Staquet MJ, eds. Combination Antibiotic Therapy in the Compromised Host. New York: Raven Press; 1982:43.

145. Weinstein MP, Stratton CW, Ackley A, et al. Multicenter collaborative evaluation of a standardized serum bactericidal test as a prognostic indicator in infective endocarditis. Am J Med 1985;78:262.

146. Pien FD, Vosti KL. Variation in performance of the serum bactericidal test. Antimicrob Agents Chemother. 1974;6:330.

147. Stratton CW, Reller LB. Serum dilution test for bactericidal activity. I. Selection of a physiologic diluent. J Infect Dis. 1977;136:187.

148. Mellors JW, Colman DL, Andriole VT. Value of the serum bactericidal test in management of patients with bacterial endocarditis. Eur J Clin Microbiol. 1986;5:67.

149. Reller LB. The serum bactericidal test. Rev Infect Dis. 1986;8:803.

13. MECHANISMS OF ANTIBIOTIC RESISTANCE

KENNETH H. MAYER
STEVEN M. OPAL
ANTONE A. MEDEIROS

MOLECULAR GENETICS OF ANTIBIOTIC RESISTANCE

Genetic variability is essential in order for microbial evolution to occur. Antimicrobial agents exert strong selective pressures upon bacterial populations favoring those organisms that are capable of resisting them.[1,2] Genetic variability may occur by a variety of mechanisms. Point mutations may occur in a nucleotide base pair, which is referred to as *microevolutionary change*. These mutations may alter the target site of an antimicrobial agent, interfering with its activity.

A second level of genomic variability in bacteria is referred to as a *macroevolutionary change* and results in whole-scale rearrangements of large segments of DNA as a single event. Such rearrangements may include inversions, duplications, insertions, deletions, or transposition of large sequences of DNA from one location of the bacterial chromosome to another. These whole-scale rearrangements of large segments of the bacterial chromosome are frequently created by specialized genetic elements known as *transposons* or *insertion sequences,* which have the capacity to move independently from the rest of the bacterial chromosome.[2]

A third level of genetic variability in bacteria is created by the acquisition of foreign DNA carried by plasmids, bacteriophages, or transposable genetic elements. Inheritance of these extrachromosomal elements further contributes to the organism's ability to cope with selection pressures imposed by antimicrobial agents.[3] These mechanisms endow bacteria with the seemingly unlimited capacity to develop resistance to any antimicrobial agent. Once an antibiotic resistance gene evolves, this resistance determinant may spread to other bacteria by transformation, transduction, conjugation, or transposition. Favored clones of bacteria may then proliferate in the flora of patients who receive antibiotics.

Plasmids

Extrachromosomal elements were present in bacteria prior to the advent of antibiotics.[4] However, the introduction of antibiotics into clinical medicine over the past five decades has created selection pressures that favored the dissemination of antibiotic resistance genes via mobile genetic elements (e.g., plasmids, transposons, and other mobile genes). Rapid increases in the spread of antibiotic resistance within and between species often correlate with the dissemination of specific resistance (R) genes. Plasmids are particularly well-adapted to serve as agents of genetic evolution and resistance gene dissemination.[5] Plasmids are extrachromosomal genetic elements that are made of circular double-stranded DNA molecules that range in size from less than 10 to greater than 400 kilobase pairs and are extremely common in bacteria.[6] While multiple copies of a specific plasmid and/or multiple different plasmids may be found in a single bacterial cell, closely related plasmids often cannot coexist in the same cell. This observation has led to a classification scheme of plasmids based upon incompatibility groups.[7]

Plasmids may determine a wide range of functions, besides antibiotic resistance, including virulence and metabolic capacities. Plasmids are autonomous, self-reproducing genetic elements that require an origin for replication and regions that facilitate its stable maintenance in host bacteria.[7] Conjugative plasmids require additional genes that can initiate self-transfer.[8]

The transfer of plasmid DNA between bacterial species is a complex process, and thus conjugative plasmids tend to be larger than nonconjugative ones. Some small plasmids may be able to utilize the conjugation apparatus of a coresident conjugative plasmid. Many plasmid-encoded functions enable bacterial strains to persist in the environment by resisting noxious agents, such as heavy metals. For example, mercury released from dental fillings may increase the number of antibiotic-resistant bacteria in the oral flora.[9] Compounds such as hexachlorophene are used as topical bacteriostatic agents, and plasmid-mediated resistance to these agents has increased significantly.[10]

Plasmids may be involved in the dissemination of antibiotic resistance in several ways (Fig. 1). A single clone of a specific organism may become resistant by mutation or by the inheritance of a resistance plasmid. The resultant resistant organism may have genes that are particularly well adapted to a specific niche and thus be able to disseminate widely. The single clone

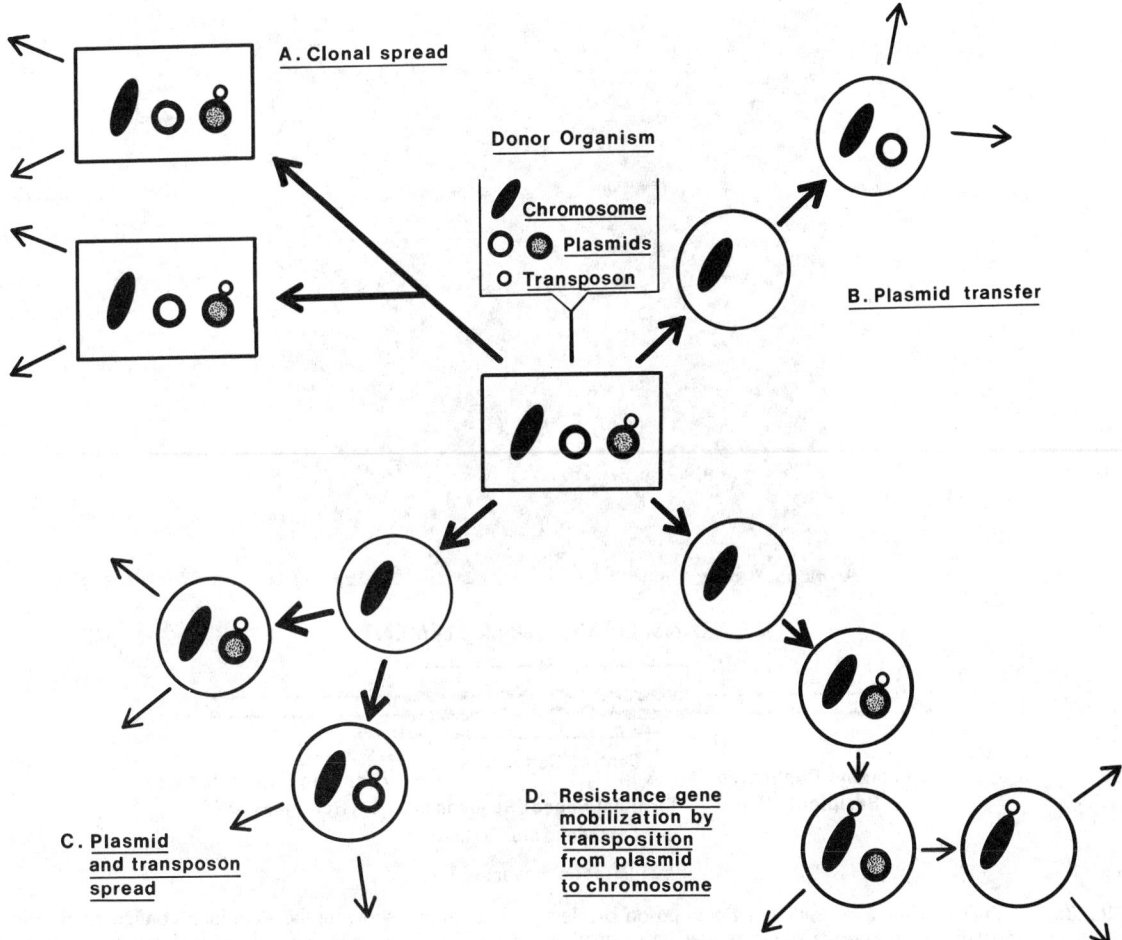

FIG. 1. Examples of the molecular spread of antibiotic resistance. The donor organism has a chromosome, two plasmids, and a transposon. **(A)** If it is well adapted to a particular niche, it may remain stable in the environment and continue to replicate itself and thus disseminate through clonal spread. **(B)** If the organism comes into close physical contact with another bacterium that may not possess extrachromosomal DNA, attachment between the two cells from different bacterial species may allow for the introduction of one of the plasmids by conjugation. **(C)** The donor organism may be able to spread resistance genes through several mechanisms, including the spread of transposons, as well as plasmids. Transposons may be able to hop between plasmids, as shown in Fig. C, or **(D)** they may be able to allow for the mobilization of resistance genes by being transferred on a conjugative plasmid into new bacterial species and then hopping from the plasmid to the chromosome. Some transposons may subsequently become integrated into the host chromosome and be spread as a stable genetic element in the chromosome without any subsequent transfer via plasmid DNA.

may be responsible for multiple and/or recurrent outbreaks of antibiotic resistance. Conjugative plasmids may be transferred from one species to another and result in new outbreaks of antibiotic resistance in previously susceptible species.[11] Transposons create the potential for even wider dissemination of antibiotic resistance genes.[12]

Transposable Genetic Elements

Transposons can translocate from one area of the bacterial chromosome to another or between the chromosome and plasmid or bacteriophage DNA. Transposable genetic elements possess a specialized system of recombination that is independent of the generalized recombination system that classically permits recombination of largely homologous sequences of DNA by crossover events (the recA system of bacteria). The recA-independent recombination system of transposable elements usually occurs in a random fashion between nonhomologous sequences of DNA resulting in whole-scale modifications of large sequences of DNA as a single event (Fig. 2).[1,3]

There are two types of transposable genetic elements, referred to as *transposons* and *insertion sequences*, which have

similar characteristics. Transposons (Tn) differ from insertion sequences (IS elements) in that they mediate a recognizable phenotypic characteristic such as an antibiotic resistance marker. Either element can translocate as an independent unit. Both elements are flanked on either end by short identical sequences of DNA in reverse order ("inverted repeats"). These inverted repeat DNA termini are essential to the transposition process. Transposons and insertion sequences are incapable of autonomous self-replication and therefore must exist on a replicon such as the chromosome, bacteriophage, or plasmid in order to be replicated and maintained in a bacterial population. A new class of transposable elements has been described that has the capability to move from the chromosome of one bacterium to another without becoming incorporated into a plasmid or bacteriophage. These elements are referred to as *conjugative* transposons and have been found primarily in aerobic and anaerobic gram-positive organisms.[13,14]

Transposition usually results in localized replication of the transposable element from the original donor sequence of DNA as well as the insertion of a copy of the transposable element into the recipient sequence of DNA (replicative transposition).[1–3] Transposition is a continuous and ongoing process in bacterial

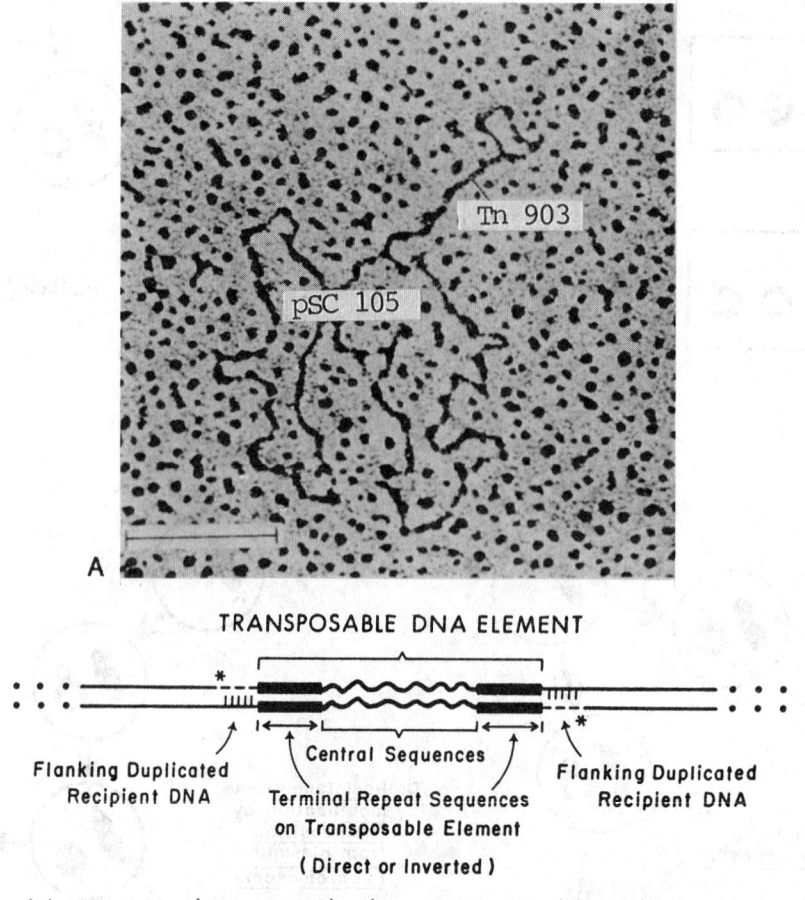

FIG. 2. **(A)** Characteristic appearance of a transposon by electron microscopy showing the stem-loop configuration. The kanamycin resistance transposon Tn903 is inserted into a small plasmid (pSC105). Following denaturation, intrastrand annealing of the complementary 1000 base pair, inverted repeat, terminal sequences of the transposon form the stem structure. The kanamycin resistance gene and the genes necessary for transposition are located in the central loop structure. **(B)** Structure of a transposable element inserted into a recipient DNA sequence. The transposon (depicted by the rectangles and wavy lines) consists of a central sequence containing the phenotypic marker gene(s) (antibiotic resistance gene) and the "transposase" genes. The terminal repeat sequences of the transposon flank the central sequences on both sides. Insertion of the transposon results in single-strand, staggered cuts in the recipient DNA (marked by asterisks). Subsequent gap-filling DNA synthesis and ligation results in duplication of a short sequence of recipient DNA at either end of the transposon.

populations. An example of this phenomenon is the spread of a tetracycline resistance transposon among *Neisseria gonorrhoeae, Mycoplasma hominis,* and *Ureaplasma urealyticum.*[15,16] Transposons are also essential in the evolution of R plasmids that contain multiple antibiotic resistance determinants.[12] Single transposons may encode multiple antibiotic resistance determinants within their inverted repeat termini as well.[3]

Our recognition of the extent of genetic exchange of antibiotic resistance determinants between bacteria of different genera and species is expanding.[17,18] Identical erythromycin resistance genes occur in streptococci and *Campylobacter,*[19] and enterococci have apparently acquired aminoglycoside[20] and β-lactam[21] resistance from staphylococci. Thus, given the appropriate environmental selection pressures, the ongoing evolution of multiresistant species is inevitable, and prevention will be difficult.[22–24]

DNA INTEGRATION ELEMENTS

The structural genes that mediate antibiotic resistance are often closely linked and may exist in tandem along the bacterial chromosome or plasmid. Genetic analysis of sequences of DNA adjacent to antibiotic resistance genes has revealed that unique integration units often exist near promoter sites.

These integration elements, known as *integrons,*[25] function as recombinational "hot spots" for site-specific recombination

events between largely nonhomologous sequences of DNA. The integron provides an integrase function to facilitate this recA-independent recombination and a common integration site consisting of a 59 base pair sequence of highly conserved DNA. This 59 base pair sequence is preserved at the 3′ end of inserted antibiotic resistance genes.[26]

While these integration elements differ structurally and functionally from transposons, they appear to be widespread in bacterial populations and play an important role in the dissemination of antibiotic resistance genes. They provide a convenient site for insertion of resistance genes from foreign DNA sources. Integrons also serve as expression cassettes for resistance genes in that an efficient promotor site is provided in close proximity to the 5′ end of the newly inserted DNA sequence. Numerous clusters of different antibiotic resistance genes have been identified that have evolved through specific insertions into common integrons.[27]

MECHANISMS OF ANTIBIOTIC RESISTANCE

At least eight distinctive mechanisms of antibiotic resistance have been described in bacteria[28] (Table 1).

Enzymatic Inhibition

β-Lactamases.   Resistance to β-lactam antibiotics is due mainly to the production of β-lactamases, enzymes that inacti-

TABLE 1. Major Mechanisms of Antibiotic Resistance

Resistance Mechanism	β-Lactams	Amino-glycosides	Chloram-phenicol	Macro-lides	Lincos-amides	Sulfon-amides	Trimeth-oprim	Tetra-cyclines	Quino-lones	Van-comycin	Rifampin	Polymyxin
Enzymatic inhibition	B	B	P	P	—	—	—	—	—	—	—	—
Membrane impermeability	C	C	P	—	—	C	C	B	—	C	—	C
Active pumping out of antibiotic (efflux)	—	—	—	C	C	—	—	B	C	—	—	—
Alteration of ribosomal target	—	C	C	B	B	—	—	B	—	—	—	—
Alteration of cell wall precursor target	—	—	—	—	—	—	—	—	—	B	—	—
Alteration of target enzymes	C	—	—	—	—	B	B	—	C	—	C	—
Overproduction of target enzyme	—	—	—	—	—	C	C	—	—	—	—	—
Auxotrophs that bypass inhibited steps	—	—	—	—	—	B	B	—	—	—	—	—

Abbreviations: P, plasmid mediated; C, chromosomally mediated; B, both; —, not yet described.

vate these antibiotics by splitting the amide bond of the β-lactam ring. Numerous β-lactamases exist, encoded either by chromosomal genes or by transferable genes located on plasmids or transposons.[29]

Three evolutionarily distinct classes of β-lactamases have been defined on the basis of amino acid and nucleotide sequence studies. Class A β-lactamases have molecular weights around 29,000, possess a serine residue at their active site, and preferentially hydrolyze penicillins. An example is the TEM-1 β-lactamase, which is widely prevalent in gram-negative bacilli. Class B are metalloenzymes that have a zinc-binding thiol group required for β-lactamase activity. Class C includes the β-lactamase determined by the chromosomal *ampC* gene of *Escherichia coli* K-12, which shares extensive sequence homology with chromosomally mediated β-lactamases of *Shigella* and *Klebsiella* species. These enzymes are large proteins of molecular weight about 39,000 with mainly cephalosporinase activity. They also have serine at their active site, but share little homology with the class A β-lactamases.[30] However, the tertiary structures of class A and class C β-lactamases show striking similarities to penicillin-binding proteins (PBPs), from which both class A and class C enzymes may have evolved.[31–34] Class D β-lactamases are oxacillin-hydrolyzing enzymes.

GRAM-POSITIVE BACTERIA. Among the gram-positive bacteria staphylococci are the major pathogens that produce β-lactamase. Staphylococcal β-lactamases preferentially hydrolyze penicillins. Most are inducible and are excreted extracellularly.[29] The genes that determine staphylococcal β-lactamases are usually carried on small plasmids or transposons. Larger plasmids encoding β-lactamase and other resistances also exist and can transfer by conjugation, not only between strains of *Staphylococcus aureus* but also between *S. aureus* and *Staphylococcus epidermidis*.[35]

Enterococci produce a plasmid-determined β-lactamase that appears to be of staphylococcal origin.[36] Since the appearance of the first strain in Texas in 1981, β-lactamase-producing enterococci have been found throughout the United States and in South America.[37] The genes often coexist with genes that determine high-level resistance to gentamicin and may occur on transposons as well as on plasmids. Interestingly, these transposons are similar to staphylococcal β-lactamase transposons and may be derived from them.[38]

GRAM-NEGATIVE BACTERIA. Gram-negative bacteria produce a much greater variety of β-lactamases than do gram-positive bacteria. This diversity has led to several classification schemes. A recent classification by Bush[39,40] groups β-lactamases according to substrate profiles and inhibition by clavulanic acid (Table 2).

Many β-lactamases are determined by plasmids.[41] All are produced constitutively and can be grouped into six broad classes:

TABLE 2. Bush Classification of β-Lactamases

Group	Characteristics	Typical Enzymes
1	Cephalosporin-hydrolyzing β-lactamases not inhibited by clavulanic acid	P99, *E. cloacae* (C); ampC, *E. coli* (C); S&A, *P. aeruginosa* (C)
2a	Penicillin-hydrolyzing β-lactamases inhibited by clavulanic acid	PC1, *S. aureus* (P); *B. cereus* 569 (C); NPS-1 (P)
2b	Broad spectrum β-lactamases inhibited by clavulanic acid	TEM-1 (P), SHV-1 (B), ROB-1 (P)
2b'	Extended-broad-spectrum β-lactamases inhibited by clavulanic acid	TEM-3 (P); SHV-2 (P); K1, *K. oxytoca* (C)
2c	Carbenicillin-hydrolyzing β-lactamases inhibited by clavulanic acid	PSE-1 (P), CARB-3 (P), BRO-1 (P), AER-1 (P)
2d	Cloxacillin-hydrolyzing β-lactamases inhibited by clavulanic acid	OXA-1 (P), PSE-2 (P)
2e	Cephalosporin-hydrolyzing β-lactamases inhibited by clavulanic acid	L2, *X. maltophilia* (?C); *P. vulgaris* SC10950 (?C)
3	Metallo-β-lactamases	L1, *X. maltophilia* (?C); CcrA, *B. fragilis* (C)
4	Penicillin-hydrolyzing β-lactamases not inhibited by clavulanic acid	*P. cepacia* 249 (C), *B. fragilis* G-237 (C), LCR-1 (P)

Abbreviations: P, plasmid determined; C, chromosomally determined; B, both.

(1) those that hydrolyze benzylpenicillin and cephaloridine at similar rates (broad-spectrum enzymes); *(2)* those that hydrolyze oxacillin and related penicillins rapidly (oxacillinases); *(3)* those that break down carbenicillin readily (carbenicillinases); *(4)* enzymes that inactivate oxyimino β-lactams such as cefotaxime, ceftazidime, or aztreonam (extended-spectrum β-lactamases; point mutations and recombination have resulted in 24 variants of the widely prevalent TEM and in 4 variants of the SHV β-lactamases;[42] *(5)* enzymes that break down oxyimino-β-lactams and are resistant to clavulanate (cephalosporinases; the genes that encode these enzymes are similar in nucleotide sequence to chromosomal β-lactamase genes of *Enterobacter*, *Citrobacter*, or *Klebsiella oxytoca* and have similar biochemical characteristics[43–46]); and *(6)* an unusual β-lactamase found in *Pseudomonas aeruginosa* that hydrolyzes imipenem (carbapenemase).[47] Properties of the plasmid-determined β-lactamases are summarized in Table 3.

ANAEROBIC BACTERIA. The resistance of anaerobic bacteria to β-lactam antibiotics also involves production of β-lactamases.[48,49] The β-lactamases of *Fusobacteria* and *Clostridia* are principally penicillinases.[50] Those produced by *Bacteroides fragilis* are predominantly cephalosporinases, some of which have been found to hydrolyze cefoxitin and imipenem and may be transferable.[51–54] Most of the cephalosporinases are inhibited by clavulanate, sulbactam, or tazobactam. The carbapene-

TABLE 3. Properties of Plasmid-Determined β-Lactamases

β-Lactamase	pI	Prevalence	Host Bacteria	Specific Features
Broad Spectrum				
HMS-1	5.2	Rare	Enterobacteriaceae	
TRI (Sal & Guer)	5.2	Rare	E. Coli	TEM derivatives resistance to clavulanate
TRC-1	5.25	Rare	E. coli	A TEM derivative resistant to calvulanate
TEM-1	5.4	Very common	Enterobacteriacease P. aeruginosa H. influenzae N. gonorrhoeae Vibrio cholerae	Most common type in nearly all bacterial species
TLE-1	5.55	Rare	E. coli	Closely related to TEM-1
TEM-2	5.6	Common	Enterobacteriaceae	Differs from TEM-1 by one amino acid
LCR-1	5.85	Rare	P. aeruginosa	Not inhibited by clavulanic acid
NPS-1	6.5	Rare	P. aeruginosa	Cefsulodin induces conformational change
TLE-2	6.5	Rare	K. pneumoniae	High affinity for cefsulodin and cefotetan
LXA-1	6.7	Uncommon	Enterobacteriaceae	Very low affinity for benzylpenicillin, confers low-level β-lactam resistance
OHIO-1	7.0	Uncommon	Enterobacteriaceae	Only found in isolates from Ohio
SHV-1 (PIT-2)	7.6	Common	Enterobacteriaceae	Often encoded by chromosomal genes in K. pneumoniae
ROB-1	8.1	Uncommon	H. influenzae H. pleuropneumoniae P. multocida	Found in both human and animal isolates
Oxacillinase				
OXA-9	?	Rare	K. pneumoniae	Encoded by transposon Tn 1331
Unnamed (GN11499)	6.9	Rare	B. fragilis	
OXA-3	7.1	Uncommon	Enterobacteriaceae P. aeruginosa	
OXA-1	7.4	Common	Enterobacteriaceae P. aeruginosa	Second most common type in E. coli
OXA-4	7.45	Rare	Enterobacteriaceae	Closely related to OXA-1
OXA-8	7.6?	Rare	?	Encoded by p40Tn2
OXA-5	7.62	Rare	P. aeruginosa	
OXA-7	7.65	Rare	E. coli	
OXA-6	7.68	Rare	P. aeruginosa	
OXA-2	7.7	Common	Enterobacteriaceae P. aeruginosa	Second most common type in salmonellae
Carbenicillinase				
CARB-4	4.3	Rare	P. aeruginosa	Confers resistance to cefsulodin
SAR-1	4.9	Rare	V. cholerae	
PSE-4 (CARB-1)	5.3	Uncommon	P. aeruginosa Enterobacteriaceae	
BRO-1, -2, -3	Multiple bands (5.3–7.7)	Common	Branhamella	Confers resistance to ampicillin and cefaclor; found in M. catarrhalis; plasmid location uncertain; may be on a conjugative transposon
PSE-1 (CARB-2)	5.7	Common	P. aeruginosa Enterobacteriaceae	Most common type in P. aeruginosa
CARB-3	5.75	Rare	P. aeruginosa	
AER-1	5.9	Rare	A. hydrophila	
Unnamed (N-3)	6.0 (5.73)	Rare	P. mirabilis	Similar to PSE-1
PSE-2	6.1	Uncommon	P. aeruginosa Enterobacteriaceae	Hydrolyzes oxacillin rapidly
CARB-5	6.3	Rare	A. calcoaceticus	Susceptible to ticarcillin combined with clavulanate
PSE-3	6.9	Uncommon	P. aeruginosa Enterobacteriaceae	
Unnamed (N-29)	6.9 (6.93)	Rare	P. mirabilis	
Extended-Spectrum (Oxyimino-β-Lactamases)				
TEM-3 to TEM-26	5.2–6.3	Nosocomial outbreaks worldwide	K. pneumoniae, less common in other Enterobacteriaceae	One to five amino acid substitutions in the TEM-1 or TEM-2 structure; confer resistance mainly to ceftazidime or aztreonam; susceptible to clavulanate
SHV-3 to SHV-5	7.0–7.8	Nosocomial outbreaks worldwide	K. pneumoniae, less common in other Enterobacteriaceae	One to three amino acid substitutions in the SHV-1 structure; more resistant to cefotaxime than TEM derivatives
Cephalosporinase				
CEP-1	8.0	Rare	P. mirabilis	
CEP-2	8.1	Rare	Achromobacter	
CMY-2	8.1	Rare	K. pneumoniae	Similar to Citrobacter chromosomal β-lactamase
′R-1	8.4	Nosocomial outbreak	K. pneumoniae	Similar to E. cloacae chromosomal β-lactamase
1	8.4	Rare	E. coli	Similar to K. oxytoca chromosomal β-lactamase
	8.8	Rare	E. coli	Similar to Citrobacter chromosomal β-lactamase
ase				
	9.0	Rare	P. aeruginosa	A metalloenzyme that hydrolyzes imipenem; resistant to clavulanate

mases, however, are metalloenzymes inhibited by EDTA but not clavulanate or sulbactam.

DISTRIBUTION IN CLINICAL ISOLATES. The existence of β-lactamase genes on plasmids and transposons ensures that a β-lactamase originally confined to one group of bacteria sooner or later may appear in other groups. Widespread use of antibiotics fosters selection of the resistant organisms that rise in prevalence locally, then spread worldwide. A prime example of this process occurred with the TEM-1 β-lactamase, which has spread from the Enterobacteriaceae to *Haemophilus-influenzae*[55] and *N. gonorrhoeae*.[56] Clinical isolates may produce two, and even three, plasmid-determined β-lactamases. In nearly all cases TEM-1 is one of the β-lactamases produced. A large number of strains from South America and the Far East have had novel and/or multiple plasmid β-lactamases.[41]

The success of the pharmaceutical industry in developing new β-lactams resistant to hydrolysis by β-lactamases led to the introduction into clinical use of the third-generation β-lactam antibiotics around 1978 in Europe and 1981 in the United States. These antibiotics were very resistant to hydrolysis by the known plasmid-determined β-lactamases. Then, in 1983 in Germany, isolates of *Klebsiella pneumoniae* and then other enterobacteriaceae were discovered that produced a plasmid-determined β-lactamase that hydrolyzed cefotaxime, as well as to other newer cephalosporins. This new β-lactamase, called SHV-2, derived from a mutation in the well-known SHV-1 β-lactamase commonly found in *Klebsiella*. The mutation resulted in an enhanced affinity of the SHV-1 β-lactamase for cefotaxime.[57] Subsequently, ceftazidime-resistant strains of *K. pneumoniae* producing a novel plasmid-encoded ceftazidime-hydrolyzing β-lactamase, designated CTX-1, were isolated in several French hospitals.[58] Nucleotide sequencing studies showed that this enzyme differed from TEM-2 by only two amino acids. Since then there has been a rapid increase in the number and variety of extended-spectrum β-lactamases.[42] The numbers of derivatives of the TEM and SHV β-lactamases proven to be unique by sequencing or oligotyping have now reached 24 and 4, respectively.[42,59] Several occur in many countries (SHV-2, SHV-4, SHV-5, TEM-6), whereas others seem to occur more commonly in one or two countries. For example, TEM-3 is prevalent in France and TEM-10 and TEM-12 in the United States and England.[42,60] The varying national patterns of antibiotic use in hospitals probably account for the differences in distribution of these enzymes. Most of the clinical isolates that produce extended-spectrum β-lactamases have come from hospitalized patients and have frequently caused nosocomial outbreaks, mostly due to *K. pneumoniae*. Recent surveys of hospital isolates of *Klebsiella pneumoniae* in England,[61] France,[62] and Portugal[63] show that 14–16 percent produce extended-spectrum β-lactamases. In France the prevalence rose from less than 1 percent in 1985 to the current level by 1988. Extended-spectrum β-lactamases are also found in nearly all other species of Enterobacteriaceae, but they occur infrequently. In a recent French survey 2–3 percent of *Enterobacter* species and *K. oxytoca* but only 0.1 percent of *E. coli* produced extended-spectrum β-lactamases.[62] Surveys of strains isolated since 1988 in England and Portugal also document a low frequency in *E. coli*.[61,64] Curiously, reports of extended-spectrum β-lactamases in *Proteus mirabilis* have been rare.[65–67] In this species, spread of extended-spectrum β-lactamases may be limited by a low frequency of plasmid conjugation.[68]

Sporadic nosocomial outbreaks due to strains producing extended-spectrum β-lactamases seem to have led to an endemic problem in some hospitals. Sometimes patients from nursing homes and other long-term care institutions bring such strains into the hospital.[69] Then selection pressure from widespread hospital use of a β-lactam apparently enhances colonization of the digestive or respiratory tracts of other patients, and infection follows.[59,70] Not surprisingly, outbreaks have often been associated with prolonged hospital stay, surgery, or the presence of urinary or arterial catheters, especially in patients in intensive care units.[70]

Failure to control outbreaks has resulted in the appearance of new mutant type extended-spectrum β-lactamases in the same institution and, sometimes, in the same patient. For example, in Clermont-Ferrand hospital, eight different extended-spectrum β-lactamases (TEM-3, TEM-5, CAZ-2, CAZ-3, CAZ-6, CAZ-7, SHV-4, and SHV-5) have appeared since the first surfaced in 1984.[71] Both plasmid and strain dissemination has occurred. Furthermore, the finding of CAZ-7 producing *K. pneumoniae* and *E. coli* in the same patient led to the discovery that the CAZ-7 and amikacin genes were on a fragment that could translocate to different plasmids. Other extended-spectrum β-lactamase genes (i.e., TEM-3 and TEM-12) are known to reside on transposons.[72–74] TEM-12 arose as the result of a single point mutation in a TEM-1-bearing plasmid that had been seen 12 years earlier in one hospital.[75] Apparently, single point mutations and recombinations between different β-lactamase genes are yielding new extended-spectrum β-lactamases in the "hot house" environments where these genes are endemic.[75,76]

Other genetic events may also be contributing to the resistance mediated by extended-spectrum β-lactamases. IS1-like elements that insert into the promoter of the gene for TEM-6 and increase its strength have been found in many strains producing TEM-6 and other TEM variants, causing high-level production of these extended-spectrum β-lactamases.[77] Indeed, even high-level production of the parent β-lactamase SHV-1 confers resistance to ceftazidime and aztreonam.[78]

Isolates of *E. coli* that produce a new class of TEM-derived plasmid-borne β-lactamase have been found recently in France, Scotland, and Spain.[79–81] These so-called TRI β-lactamases confer resistance to β-lactamase inhibitors (clavulanate, sulbactam) but not to the oxyimino-β-lactams such as cefotaxime, aztreonam, and ceftazidime.

β-LACTAMASES DETERMINED BY CHROMOSOMAL GENES. Virtually all gram-negative bacteria produce some chromosomally determined β-lactamase. Furthermore, the types of β-lactamase produced are often specific for species and sometimes for subspecies. β-Lactamase activity is frequently very low, particularly in ampicillin-susceptible isolates, but may increase due to either induction or alteration in the number of β-lactamase genes on the chromosome.[82] Also, mutation of genes that regulate induction may lead to constitutive hyperproduction of inducible β-lactamases.[83] Selection of hyperproducer mutants caused emergence of resistance to third-generation cephalosporins in 19 percent of patients receiving third-generation cephalosporins for *Enterobacter* bacteremia.[84] Most of the clinically relevant chromosomally determined β-lactamases belonging to Bush group 1 preferentially hydrolyze cephalosporins and are resistant to inhibition by clavulanic acid. They inactivate many of the third-generation β-lactams that are resistant to hydrolysis by most of the plasmid-determined β-lactamases. The metallo-β-lactamases (Bush group 3) that hydrolyze carbapenems are a growing threat of great concern.[85]

Chromosomally determined β-lactamases nearly always differ in their biochemical properties from the plasmid-determined enzymes. The exception is a chromosomal β-lactamase found in many isolates of *K. pneumoniae* that is indistinguishable from the SHV-1 β-lactamase. It may be that the SHV-1 β-lactamase gene evolved as a chromosomal gene in *Klebsiella* and was later incorporated into a plasmid.[86] As yet no such ancestral chromosomal gene has been found for the much more common TEM-1 β-lactamase or for any of the other plasmid-determined β-lactamases.

Chromosomal genes have incorporated into plasmids, a long-feared threat. In Providence, RI, nosocomial isolates of *K. pneumoniae* and *E. coli* were found to produce the MIR-1 β-lactamase, a plasmid-determined *ampC*-type β-lactamase derived from *Enterobacter cloacae*.[43] Besides resistance to oxyimino-β-lactams, the strains were also highly resistant to the 7α-methoxy-β-lactams and the clavam and sulfone β-lactamase inhibitors. Recently, plasmid-borne genes determining *ampC*-type β-lactamases from *Citrobacter freundii* (CMY-2, BIL-1)[44,45] and *K. oxytoca* (MEN-1)[46] have also been found. The plasmids were in strains of *K. pneumoniae* and *E. coli* from France, Greece, and Pakistan, demonstrating that the formidable threat posed by them is already worldwide. The discovery in Japan of a strain of *P. aeruginosa* producing a plasmid-mediated β-lactamase that confers resistance to imipenem and all other β-lactams presents an even greater threat.[47]

CONTRIBUTION OF β-LACTAMASES TO β-LACTAM ANTIBIOTIC RESISTANCE. The level of antibiotic resistance mediated by a particular β-lactamase in a population of bacteria is determined by several variables. The efficiency of the β-lactamase in hydrolyzing an antibiotic depends on both its rate of hydrolysis (V_{max}) and its affinity for the antibiotic (K_m). Other variables are the amount of β-lactamase produced by the bacterial cell, the susceptibility of the target protein (PBP) to the antibiotic, and the rate of diffusion of the antibiotic into the periplasm of the cell.

Within the bacterial cell, β-lactamases contribute to antibiotic resistance in several ways. The simplest model is that of penicillinase-producing staphylococci in which the bacteria, upon exposure to penicillin, begin to produce β-lactamase, which they excrete extracellularly. Two events then take place concurrently: *(1)* penicillin lyses bacteria, and *(2)* β-lactamase hydrolyses penicillin. If viable bacterial cells remain after the level of penicillin has fallen below the minimal inhibitory concentration, regrowth of bacteria occurs.[30]

Another model is exemplified by gram-negative bacilli, which *(1)* produce a β-lactamase that remains trapped in the periplasmic space and *(2)* have no barrier to antibiotic penetration. An example is *H. influenzae* strains that produce the TEM-1 β-lactamase.[87] In both this model and the first one discussed, a marked inoculum effect occurs in that the minimal inhibitory concentration for a large inoculum (10^6 organisms/ml) may be a thousandfold greater than with a small inoculum (10^2 organisms/ml). The low level of resistance of single cells has made it possible for ampicillin to cure some infections caused by β-lactamase-producing strains of *H. influenzae* when the inoculum of infecting bacteria was low.

Another model is exemplified by ampicillin resistance of *E. coli* strains that produce the TEM-1 β-lactamase. These bacteria have a barrier to entry of β-lactam molecules (the outer membrane), and they produce a β-lactamase that remains localized to the periplasmic space. In this model, the kinetics are more complicated. The enzyme is strategically situated between the barrier to antibiotic penetration (outer membrane) and the antibiotic targets (PBPs on the cytoplasmic membrane). In this position the enzyme can sequentially destroy antibiotic molecules as they make their way through the barrier, analogous to a sharpshooter with abundant ammunition who aims at targets passing through a single entry point. As a consequence, high levels of resistance occur with single bacterial cells, unlike the previous example.[30]

Variations on this model occur when the amount of β-lactamase produced increases with exposure to a β-lactam (induction), as occurs in *Enterobacter* and *Pseudomonas* species. High levels of β-lactamase are produced only after a period of exposure to the inducing antibiotic, and hence resistance may be expressed late. When *Enterobacter* strains are exposed to two β-lactam antibiotics, one of which is a potent inducer (e.g., cefamandole), antagonism between the two antibiotics may result.[88]

Aminoglycoside Resistance-Modifying Enzymes. Among aerobic bacteria, aminoglycoside resistance is most commonly due to modifying enzymes that are coded by genes on plasmids or the chromosome.[89] Several of the aminoglycoside-modifying enzymes have been shown to be carried on transposons.[12]

More than two dozen aminoglycoside-modifying enzymes that have been identified are capable of three general reactions: *N*-acetylation, *O*-nucleotidylation, and *O*-phosphorylation. For each of these general reactions there are several different enzymes that attack a specific amino or hydroxyl group. The nomenclature for these enzymes lists the molecular site where the modification occurs after the type of enzymatic activity. For example, an aminoglycoside acetyltransferase (AAC) that acts at the 3' site is designated AAC(3') (Table 4).[35] However, there may be more than one enzyme that will catalyze the same reaction, and thus roman numerals may be necessary (e.g., AAC[3']-IV).

Enzymatic aminoglycoside resistance is achieved by modification of the antibiotic in the process of transport across the cytoplasmic membrane.[89] Resistance to a particular aminoglycoside is a function of two different rates, that of drug uptake versus that of drug inactivation. An important factor in determining the level of resistance is the affinity of the modifying enzyme for the antibiotic. If an enzyme has a high affinity for the specific aminoglyoside, then drug inactivation can occur at very low concentrations.

The differences in the worldwide distribution of aminoglycoside-modifying enzymes may partially be a function of antibiotic selection pressures and have had profound implications on the choice of antibiotics used at specific medical centers.[90] APH(3') and APH(3″) are widely distributed among gram-positive and gram-negative species worldwide and thus have led to decreased utilization of kanamycin and streptomycin. The ANT(2″) gene has been associated with multiple nosocomial outbreaks over the past decade across the United States. The AAC(6')-I gene has been found to be more prevalent in East Asia.[91] The AAC(3) group of enzymes have been responsible for outbreaks of antibiotic resistance in South America, Western Europe, and the United States. Although each outbreak of aminoglycoside-resistant Enterobacteriaceae has its own pattern, the most typical manner of spread has been the appearance of a plasmid-carrying aminoglycoside-resistant strain of *K. pneumoniae* usually carrying the ANT(2″) gene, with subsequent dissemination to other strains of the species and further spread later to other species and genera of Enterobacteriaceae.[92]

In recent years, major increases in plasmid-mediated aminoglycoside resistance have been noted among enterococci,[20,93,94] initially in the developing world[95] but increasingly in the United States and Europe.[96,97] The plasmids that carry the aminoglycoside-modifying genes in enterococcal outbreaks are heterogeneous.[98] Their clinical impact is exacerbated by the frequent cotransmission of β-lactamases, resulting in loss of synergy when combination therapy is employed for serious enterococcal infections. *S. aureus* and *S. epidermidis* have become increasingly resistant to aminoglycosides because of the inter- and intraspecies dissemination of plasmid-mediated aminoglycoside-modifying enzymes.[99]

Chloramphenicol Acetyltransferase. Resistance to chloramphenicol in gram-positive and gram-negative organisms is pri-

TABLE 4. Aminoglycoside-Modifying Enzymes

Enzymes	Usual Antibiotics Modified	Common Genera
Phosphorylation		
APH(2″)	K, T, G	SA, SR
PH(3')-I	K	E, PS, SA, SR
APH(3')-III	K, ±A	E, PS, SA, SR
Acetylation		
AAC(2')	G	PR
AAC(3)-I	±T, G	E, PS
AAC(3)-III, -IV, or -V	K, T, G	E, PS
AAC(6')	K, T, ±A	E, PS, SA
Adenylation		
ANT(2″)	K, T, G	E, PS
ANT(4')	K, T, A	SA

Abbreviations: K, kanamycin; A, amikacin; SR, streptococci; T, tobamycin; E, Enterobacteriaceae; PS, pseudomonads; G, gentamicin; SA, staphylococci; PR, *Providencia/Proteus*.

marily mediated by an inactivating enzyme known as *Chloramphenicol acetyltransferase*. This is an intracellular enzyme that inactivates the drug by 3-*O*-acetylation[100] and is encoded by plasmid borne or chromosomal genes. Despite homology at the active site of this enzyme, there is considerable diversity between chloramphenicol acetyltransferase enzymes isolated from gram-positive and gram-negative organisms.[101]

Erythromycin Esterase. While resistance to erythromycin and other macrolides is frequently the result of alteration in the ribosomal target site, several substrate-inactivating enzymes have recently been characterized.[102] Erythromycin esterases have been isolated from *E. coli*, which hydrolyze the lactone ring of the antibiotic, resulting in its inactivation.[103] This is a plasmid-mediated resistance determinant that is constitutively produced and results in high-level resistance to erythromycin (minimum inhibitory concentration [MIC] > 2000 μg/ml).[104] Other plasmid-mediated macrolide, lincosamide, streptogramin (MLS) inactivating enzymes have been described in *Streptococcus hemolyticus* and *S. aureus* that adenylate,[105] acetylate,[106] or hydrolyze[107] substrate. These resistance determinants may limit the utility of oral erythromycin in reducing the aerobic gram-negative flora of the intestinal tract prior to gastrointestinal surgical procedures.

Alterations of Bacterial Membranes

Outer Membrane Permeability. It was recognized early in the history of antibiotic development that penicillin was effective against gram-positive bacteria but not against gram-negative bacteria.[108] This difference in susceptibility to penicillin is due in large part to the outer membrane, a lipid bilayer that acts as a barrier to the penetration of antibiotics into the cell.[109] Situated outside the peptidoglycan cell wall of gram-negative bacteria, this outer membrane is absent in gram-positive bacteria. The outer portion of this lipid bilayer is composed principally of lipopolysaccharide made up of tightly bound hydrocarbon molecules that impede entry of hydrophobic antibiotics, such as nafcillin or erythromycin.[110,111] Agents that disrupt the integrity of the lipopolysaccharide layer such as polymixin, or mutations that lead to production of defective lipopolysaccharides, result in increased permeability of hydrophobic antibiotics.[112]

The passage of hydrophilic antibiotics through this outer membrane is facilitated by the presence of porins, proteins that are arranged so as to form water-filled diffusion channels through which antibiotics may traverse.[113] Bacteria usually produce a large number of porins; approximately 10^5 porin molecules are present in a single cell of *E. coli*. Bacteria are able to regulate the relative number of different porins in response to the osmolarity of the surrounding media. Thus, in hyperosmolar media *E. coli* may repress production of the larger porins (OmpF) while continuing to express smaller ones (OmpC).[114]

The rate of diffusion of antibiotics through this outer membrane is a function not only of the numbers and properties of the porin channels but also of the physicochemical characteristics of the antibiotic. Generally, the larger the antibiotic molecule, the more negative charges, and the greater the degree of hydrophobicity, the less likely it is to penetrate through the outer membrane.[109,115] Small, hydrophilic molecules with a zwitterionic charge, such as imipenem, are highly permeable. Conversely, larger highly charged molecules such as carbenicillin are much less permeable.

Mutations resulting in the loss of specific porins can occur in clinical isolates and determine increased resistance to β-lactam antibiotics. For example, a strain of *Salmonella typhimurium* obtained from a perirenal abscess became resistant to multiple cephalosporins during therapy with cephalexin.[116] The parent strain produced both OmpF and OmpC proteins, but the mutant produced only OmpF. The mutant was resistant to β-lactam antibiotics only when tested in media of high osmolarity, compa-

rable to that in the patient's tissues. Under these conditions the production of the OmpF protein was repressed completely, leaving the microorganism devoid of either species of porin and impermeable to the cephalosporins. Resistance to aminoglycosides and carbapenems emerging during therapy has also been associated with lack of production of outer membrane proteins.[117,118] In *P. aeruginosa* resistance to imipenem appears to be due to interplay between chromosomal β-lactamase activity and loss of a specific entry channel, the D2 porin.[119]

Resistance to nalidixic acid and other quinolones has been associated with alterations of outer membrane proteins in *Serratia marcescens*[120] as well as *P. aeruginosa*. However, single-step high-level mutational resistance to nalidixic acid by aerobic gram-negative bacilli occurs with a 10^{-7} frequency, whereas only low-level resistance to the newer quinolones ($<10 \times$ MIC) is usually obtained with a single-step selection of $<10^{-9}$.[121] Plasmid-mediated chloramphenicol resistance due to decreased permeability has been demonstrated in *E. coli*.[122]

Inner Membrane Permeability. The rate of entry of aminoglycoside molecules into bacterial cells is a function of them binding to a usually nonsaturable anionic transporter, whereupon they retain their positive charge and are subsequently "pulled" across the cytoplasmic membrane by the internal negative charge of the cell.[123] This process requires energy and a threshold minimal level of internal negative charge of the cell that has to be present before significant transport occurs ("proton motive force").[124] The level of the internal charge that is required may depend on the actual aminoglycoside concentration at a given time. The energy generation or the proton motive force that is required for substrate transport into the cell may be altered in mutants resistant to aminoglycosides.

These aminoglycoside-resistant isolates with altered proton motive force occur rarely, but develop in the course of long-term aminoglycoside therapy.[125] These isolates usually have a "small colony" phenotype due to their reduced rate of growth. They may be unstable and revert back to a sensitive phenotype in the absence of selective aminoglycoside pressure. The clinical significance of these isolates is not clear. They may retain some virulence[126] and may cause fatal bacteremia rarely.[127] Because oxidative metabolism is essential for aminoglycoside uptake action, as well as cell growth and development, *Pseudomonas* mutants have been found that have been deficient in specific cytochromes.[123] Resistant mutants with defective electron transport systems have been described in *E. coli*, *S. aureus*, and *Salmonella* spp. Facultative organisms grown anaerobically are resistant to aminoglycosides because of a marked reduction of the uptake of the antibiotic.[89]

Promotion of Antibiotic Efflux

The major mechanism of resistance to tetracycline found in enteric gram-negative organisms results from the decreased accumulation of tetracycline. This reduced uptake is an energy-dependent process that is related to the generation of an inner membrane protein produced by the tetracycline resistance determinant. The primary mechanism for decreased accumulation of tetracycline is due mainly to active efflux of the antibiotic across the cell membrane.[128,129] Decreased uptake of tetracycline from the extracellular environment also accounts for decreased accumulation of tetracycline inside resistant cells. These resistance determinants may be found on the chromosome or plasmids and are frequently found on transposable genetic elements. Tetracycline resistance genes are generally inducible by subinhibitory concentrations of tetracycline. An active efflux system for removal of norfloxacin has been demonstrated in *E. coli*.[130] This system may represent a potential mechanism for resistance to the newer quinolones, but has not been found to be common among quinolone-resistant clinical isolates. Active efflux of 14-member ring macrolides, azalides, and streptogramins has been detected in *S. epidermidis* via an inducible ATP-binding protein that functions as a drug efflux pump. Plasmid-associated erythromycin resistance in *S. epidermidis* has also been demonstrated in conjunction with a similar protein, but its clinical significance is not yet known.

Alteration of Ribosomal Target Sites

Resistance to a wide variety of antimicrobial agents, including tetracyclines, macrolides, lincosamides, and the aminoglycosides, may result from alteration of ribosomal binding sites. Failure of the antibiotic to bind to its target site(s) on the ribosome disrupts its ability to inhibit protein synthesis and cell growth. For the MLS, this is the principal mechanism of multiple-agent resistance among aerobic and anaerobic gram-positive organisms.[131] Resistance occurs as the result of at least eight classes of methylase enzymes that dimethylate adenine residues on the 23S ribosomal RNA of the 50S subunit of the prokaryotic ribosome, disrupting the binding of MLS to the ribosome. Different classes of this resistance determinant may be located on plasmids or on the bacterial chromosome.[132] MLS resistance due to ribosomal methylation has been described in *S. aureus*, *Streptococcus sanguis*, *B. fragilis*, and *Clostridium perfringens*. MLS resistance may be constitutive or inducible by either older macrolides (e.g., erythromycin) or newer azalides. Tetracycline resistance may also occur by a mechanism that interferes with the ability of tetracycline to bind to the ribosome. The ubiquitous *tetM* resistance gene protects the ribosome from tetracycline action. The precise mechanism of action of this resistance gene is unclear at present.[133] The *tetM* determinant is widely dispersed in gram-positive organisms[133] in addition to *Mycoplasma*,[134] *Ureaplasma*,[16] *Campylobacter*,[135] and *Neisseria* spp.[15]

Resistance to aminoglycosides may also be mediated at the ribosomal level. Mutations of the S12 protein of the 30S subunit has been shown to interfere with binding streptomycin to the ribosome. Ribosomal resistance to streptomycin may be a significant cause of streptomycin resistance among enterococcal isolates.[136] Ribosomal resistance to the 2-deoxystreptamine aminoglycosides (gentamicin, tobramycin, amikacin) appears to be uncommon and may require multiple mutations in that these aminoglycosides appear to bind to several sites on the 30 and 50S subunits of the prokaryotic ribosome. Ribosomal resistance is often associated with decreased intracellular accumulation of the drug.[137]

Alteration of Cell Wall Precursor Targets

Vancomycin and other glycopeptide antibiotics such as teicoplanin bind to D-alanine–D-alanine, which is present at the termini of peptidoglycan precursors. The large glycopeptide molecules prevent the incorporation of the precursors into the cell wall. Resistance of enterococci to vancomycin has been classified as A, B, or C based on levels of resistance to vancomycin and susceptibility or resistance to teicoplanin.[138] Strains of *Enterococcus faecium* and *Enterococcus faecalis* with high-level resistance to both vancomycin and teicoplanin have class A resistance. Either vancomycin or teicoplanin can induce resistance in these strains. Class A resistance to glycopeptides transfers by conjugation from *E. faecium* to other gram-positive bacteria,[139] including *E. faecalis*,[140] *Streptococcus pyogenes* and *S. sanguis*, as well as *Listeria monocytogenes*. The *vanA* gene on the plasmid encodes an inducible protein that is related to the D-alanine–D-alanine ligases involved in cell wall synthesis in *E. coli*.[141] This protein synthesizes peptidoglycan precursors that have a depsipeptide terminus (D-alanine–D-lactate) instead of the usual D-alanine–D-alanine. The modified peptidoglycan binds glycopeptide antibiotics with reduced affinity, thus conferring resistance to vancomycin and teicoplanin.[142,143]

Strains of *E. faecium* and *E. faecalis* with class B resistance have levels of resistance to vancomycin that range from high (MIC 1024 µg/ml) to low (MIC 4 µg/ml) and are susceptible to teicoplanin. Vancomycin, but not teicoplanin, can induce resistance to both vancomycin and teicoplanin in these strains. The genes determining the *vanB* phenotype are self-transferrable by conjugation to other *Enterococcus* strains.[144]

All isolates of *Enterococcus gallinarum* and *Enterococcus casseliflavus* possess low-level resistance to vancomycin and are susceptible to teicoplanin (class C phenotype). The resistance is thought to be mediated by a chromosomal gene.[145]

Alteration of Target Enzymes

β-Lactams. β-Lactam antibiotics inhibit bacteria by binding covalently to PBPs in the cytoplasmic membrane. These target proteins catalyze the synthesis of the peptidoglycan that forms the cell wall of bacteria.[146] Alterations of PBPs can lead to β-lactam antibiotic resistance.[147]

In gram-positive bacteria resistance to β-lactam antibiotics may be associated either with a decrease in the affinity of the PBP for the antibiotic[148] or with a change in the amount of PBP produced by the bacterium.[149] Multiple mechanisms appear to be present in some clinical isolates. For example, penicillin-resistant strains of *S. pneumoniae* isolated in South Africa have shown several changes in their PBPs (i.e., decreased affinity of some PBPs, loss of others, and appearance of PBPs not present in the more susceptible cells).[150] The genes that encode these PBPs are mosaics, made up of segments from susceptible pneumococci and segments from resistant commensal streptococci.[151] In *S. aureus*[152–154] and *E. faecium*[154,155] additional PBPs may be inducible (i.e., their production is stimulated by exposure of the microorganism to the β-lactam antibiotic). These inducible PBPs have a lower affinity for β-lactam antibiotics, making them less susceptible to inhibition by low concentrations of drug. Changes in the types of PBPs observed in susceptible and resistant strains have also been seen with viridans streptococcal species *Streptococcus mitis*.[156]

Factors that regulate the induction of PBPs are poorly understood. The induction of a low-affinity PBP in methicillin-resistant *S. aureus* (MRSA) occurs to a larger extent when the microorganisms are grown at 32°C rather than at 37°C, conditions known to favor the expression of methicillin resistance.[157] There is evidence that the production of this inducible PBP is under the control of plasmid-borne genes that regulate staphylococcal penicillinase production. The structural gene (*mecA*) that determines the low-affinity PBP of MRSA shares extensive sequence homology with a PBP of *E. coli*, and the genes that regulate the production of the low-affinity PBP have considerable sequence homology with the genes that regulate the production of staphylococcal penicillinase.[158] Thus, the production of this low-affinity penicillin-binding protein in MRSA may be mediated by a fusion of gene segments from *E. coli* and *S. aureus*. Another gene (*femA*) also influences expression of methicillin resistance by mechanisms unknown.[159]

The PBPs of β-lactamase-negative penicillin-resistant strains of *N. gonorrhoeae*, *Neisseria meningitidis*, and *H. influenzae* have shown reduced penicillin-binding affinity.[160–163] Their PBPs appear to be encoded by hybrid genes containing segments of DNA scavenged from resistant strains of related species, similar to penicillin-resistant pneumococci.[164] Mutations leading to loss of outer membrane proteins may also be associated with acquisition of penicillin resistance in non-penicillinase-producing strains of *N. gonorrhoeae*, suggesting that altered permeability may also contribute to the resistance.[165] Permeability changes and decreased affinity of PBPs are mechanisms jointly found in clinical isolates of *P. aeruginosa*[166] and in non-β-lactamase-producing strains of *H. influenzae* as well.[167] Thus, multiple mutations may be necessary in order to effect this type of resistance.

Sulfonamides and Trimethoprim. Sulfonamides compete with para-aminobenzoic acid to bind the enzyme dihydropteroate synthetase, thereby halting the generation of pteridines and nucleic acids. Sulfonamide resistance may be mediated by the production of a dihydropteroate synthetase that is resistant to binding by sulfonamides.[168] The high prevalence of resistance to sulfonamides among gram-negative bacteria may be attributed to the spread of R plasmids that contain genes that elaborate resistant enzymes. The most common mechanism of transferable trimethoprim resistance occurs in a similar fashion, by making a drug-resistant dihydrofolate reductase (DHFR).[169] Trimethoprim-resistant DHFRs have been found on the chromosome, and multiple forms have been found to be plasmid mediated.[170]

Quinolones. DNA gyrase is necessary for the supercoiling of chromosomal DNA in bacteria in order to have efficient cell division.[171] This enzyme consists of two A subunits encoded by the *gyrA* gene and two B subunits encoded by the *gyrB* gene. Although spontaneous mutations in the *gyrA* locus have resulted in resistance to multiple fluoroquinolones, B subunit alterations may also affect resistance to these drugs. Mutations in a variety of chromosomal loci have been described, resulting in altered DNA gyrases that are resistant to nalidixic acid and the newer fluroquinolones in Enterobacteriaceae and *P. aeruginosa*.[172,173] Many of these mutations involve the substitution of single amino acids at key enzymatic sites that are involved in the generation of the DNA gyrase–bacterial complex.[174,175] Clinical isolates of *C. freundii* in Japan have been found to be highly resistant to the newer quinolones via alterations in the DNA gyrase.[176] Alterations in the DNA gyrases of clinical isolates of other enterobacteriaceae, particularly *E. coli*, have been described[177,178] and are thought to involve a mechanism that is similar to that found in quinolone-resistant *S. aureus* and other gram-positive species.

Bypass of Antibiotic Inhibition

Another mechanism for acquiring resistance to specific antibiotics is by the development of auxotrophs, which have growth factor requirements different from those of the wild strain. These mutants require substrates that normally are synthesized by the target enzymes, and thus, if the substrates are present in the environment, the organisms are able to grow despite inhibition of the synthetic enzyme. For example, bacteria that lose the enzyme thymidilate synthetase are "thymine dependent" and cannot synthesize thymidilate in the usual way. They therefore require exogenous supplies of thymidine to synthesize thymidilate via salvage pathways and are thus highly resistant to trimethoprim.[179]

CONTROL OF ANTIBIOTIC RESISTANCE

Although the emergence of antibiotic-resistant bacteria has generally been correlated with the rise and fall of specific antibiotic use in clinical practice, the chain of causality is not always clear cut.[180] Bacterial strains contain complex aggregations of genes that may be linked together. Thus the use of one antibiotic may select for the emergence of resistance to another. Although the development of antibiotic resistance may be inevitable, the rate at which it develops may be diminished by the rational use of antibiotics.[181]

The wider accessibility to computers, and the ability to track antibiotic resistance genes with molecular techniques have enhanced the ability to track the spread of antibiotic resistance. With the appropriate computerized surveillance, a hospital laboratory may be able to rapidly detect the emergence of a new type of resistance or the presence of a new microbial strain within a specific unit or patient population. Techniques such as restriction endonuclease digestion analyses of bacterial

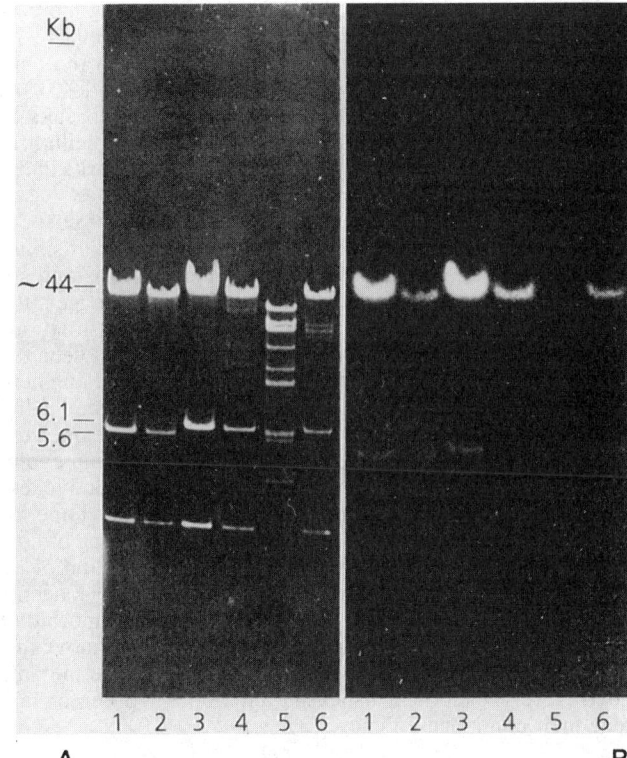

FIG. 3. **(A)** Agarose gel of *Eco*RI-digested plasmids derived from four isolates that contain a nosocomial trimethoprim resistance plasmid (known as pBWH10) from a Boston hospital (lanes 1–4). Another nosocomial plasmid from the same hospital that does not contain trimethoprim resistance genes (lane 5), and one in which both the trimethoprim-resistant and -sensitive plasmids are present in the same isolate (lane 6). **(B)** To show that the "fingerprints" from the trimethoprim-resistant plasmids in lanes 1–4 and 6 contain the same gene, DNA-DNA hybridization of the same six plasmids was performed using a type II DHFR probe. The probe and the restriction endonuclease analyses helped pinpoint the location and genetic homology of this trimethoprim resistance gene.

plasmids and chromosomes and genetic probes of resistance genes make it possible to confirm the presence of new genes in the environment. This information may then be correlated with the phenotypic measures determined by the clinical microbiology surveillance system (Fig. 3).[182] Utilization of molecular techniques greatly augments surveillance data, since large data sets may obscure subtle changes ("mini epidemics") that may be more amenable to the institution of stringent infection control measures.

The study of the genetics of antibiotic resistance, particularly the awareness of the great mobility of plasmids and transposons, leads one to the conclusion that ultimately each antibiotic used may inexorably alter its microenvironment, creating selective advantages for resistant organisms. Since prokaryotic organisms all contribute to a common "gene pool," favorable genes mediating antibiotic resistance may disseminate among bacterial populations. In less than a decade, newly utilized inexpensive drugs such as trimethoprim have gone from being highly effective in the treatment of dysentery in developing countries to becoming unusable in several of these areas.[183] Other recent examples of the emergence of polyresistant organisms have had clinical significance in the management of out-patient, as well as nosocomial, infections. The increased use of erythromycin for the management of streptococcal pharyngitis in Finland in the 1980s has been paralleled by a dramatic increase in the prevalence of multiresistant streptococci isolated from pharyngeal, as well as blood, cultures.[184] The clinical importance of this finding is that in β-lactam-intolerant or allergic patients, the range of effective antistreptococcal drugs is becoming increasingly limited. Even more worrisome is the specter of multiresistant enterococci as nosocomial pathogens,[185] given their increasing resistance to β-lactams,[186] and aminoglycosides,[187] as well as vancomycin[188] and other glycopeptides. Outbreaks of vancomycin-resistant *E. faecalis* and vancomycin/ampicillin-resistant *E. faecium* have occurred in London, New York, Philadelphia, and Providence, RI.[189–193]

Similar concerns exist regarding the management of nosocomial staphylococcal infections, given the rapid spread of simultaneous β-lactam, aminoglycoside, and quinolone-resistant isolates.[194–196] Rational antibiotic usage policies would suggest the curtailment of the unnecessary use of antibiotics in situations such as animal husbandry, although the causal link between the use of antibiotic for animal growth promotion and their augmentation of the resistance in human pathogens has been disputed.[197] New drug discoveries have allowed us to be one step ahead of the bacterial pathogens. Nonetheless, the rapid evolution of resistance has limited the duration of the effectiveness of specific agents against certain pathogens. The best hope for the future is the development of a greater understanding of how antimicrobial resistance spreads and the implementation of effective infection control strategies. Newer antimicrobial agents have had a substantial impact in decreasing human morbidity and mortality rates over the past half century. It behooves us to expand our surveillance of antibiotic resistance determinants and to exercise caution in dispensing antibiotics in order to maximize their continued efficacy.

REFERENCES

1. Kopecko D. Specialized genetic recombination systems in bacteria: Their involvement in gene expression and evolution. Prog Mol Subcell Biol. 1980;7:135–243.
2. Kopecko DJ. Involvement of specialized recombination in the evolution and expression of bacterial genes. In: Stutgart C, Rozel KR, eds. Plasmids and Transposons. New York: Academic Press; 1980:165–206.
3. Lupski JR. Molecular mechanisms for transposition of drug-resistance genes and other movable genetic elements. Rev Infect Dis. 1987;9:357–68.
4. Datta N. Plasmids as organisms. In: Helinski DR, Cohen SN, Clevwell DB, et al., eds. Plasmids in Bacteria. New York: Plenum Press; 1985;383–95.
5. O'Brien T, del Pilar Pla M, Mayer KH, et al. Intercontinental spread of a new antibiotic resistance gene on an epidemic plasmid. Science. 1985;230:87–8.
6. Timmis KN, Gonalez-Carrero MI, Sekizaki T, Rojo F. Biological activities specified by antibiotic resistance plasmids. J Antimicrob Chemother. 1986;18:1–12.
7. Nordstrom K. Replication, incompatibility and partition. In: Helinski DR, Cohen SN, Clewell DB, et al., eds. Plasmids in Bacteria. New York: Plenum Press; 1985:119–23.
8. Thompson R. R plasmid transfer. J Antimicrob Chemother. 1986;18:13–23.
9. Summers AO, Wireman J, Vimy MJ, et al. Mercury released from dental silver fillings provokes an increase in mercury-resistant and antibiotic-resistant bacteria in oral and intestinal floras of primates. Antimicrob Agents Chemother. 1993;37:825–34.
10. Foster TJ. Plasmid-determined resistance to antimicrobial drugs and toxic metal ions in bacteria. Microbiol Rev. 1983;43:361–409.
11. Mayer KH, Hopkins JD, Gilleece ES, et al. Molecular evolution, species distribution and clinical consequences of an endemic aminoglycoside resistance plasmid. Antimicrob Agents Chemother. 1986;29:628–33.
12. Rubens CE, McNeill WF, Farrar WE Jr. Evolution of multiple-antibiotic-resistance plasmids mediated by transposable plasmid deoxyribonucleic acid sequences. J Bacteriol. 1979;140:713–9.
13. Franke AE, Clewell DB. Evidence for a chromosome-borne resistance transposon (Tn916) in *Streptococcus faecalis* that is capable of "conjugal" transfer in the absence of a conjugative plasmid. J Bacteriol. 1981;145:494–502.
14. Solh NE, Allignet J, Bismuth R, et al. Conjugative transfer of staphylococcal antibiotic resistance markers in the absence of detectable plasmid DNA. Antimicrob Agents Chemother. 1986;30:161–9.
15. Morse SA, Johnson SR, Biddle JW, Roberts MC. High-level tetracycline resistance in *Neisseria gonorrhoeae* is the result of acquisition of streptococcal tetM determinant. Antimicrob Agents Chemother. 1986;30:664–70.
16. Roberts MC, Kenny GE. Dissemination of the tetM tetracycline resistance determinant to *Ureaplasma urealyticum*. Antimicrob Agents Chemother. 1986;29:350–2.
17. DeFlaun MF, Levy SB: Genes and their various hosts. In: Levy SB, Miller RV (eds). Gene Transfer in the Environment. New York: McGraw Hill; 1989:1–32.

18. Brisson-Noel A, Arthur M, Courvalin P: Evidence for natural gene transfer from gram positive cocci to *Escherichia coli*. J Bacteriol. 1988;170:1739–45.
19. Papadopoulou B, Courvalin P: Dispersal in *Campylobacter spp.* of aphA-3, a kanamycin resistance determinant from gram positive cocci. Antimicrob Agents Chemother. 1988;32:945–8.
20. Courvalin P, Carlier C, Collatz E: Plasmid-mediated resistance to aminocyclitol antibiotics in group D streptocci. J Bacteriol. 1980;143:541–51.
21. Zscheck KK, Hull R, Murray BE: Restriction mapping and hybridization studies of a β-lactamase-encoding fragment from *Streptococcus* (Enterococcus) *faecalis*. Antimicrob Agents Chemother. 1988;32:768–69.
22. Courvalin P: Resistance of enterococci to glycopeptides. Antimicrob Agents Chemother. 1990;34:2291–6.
23. Neu HC: The crisis in antibiotic resistance. Science. 1992;257:1064–73.
24. Cohen ML: Epidemiology of drug resistance: Implications for a post-antimicrobial era. Science. 1992;257:1050–5.
25. Stokes HW, Hall RM. A novel family of potentially mobile DNA elements encoding site-specific gene-integration functions: Integrons. Mol Microbiol. 1989;3:1669–83.
26. Cameron FH, Groot Obbink DJ, Ackerman VP, Hall RM. Nucleotide sequence of the AD (2″) aminoglycoside adenylyl transferase determinant *aadB*. Evolutionary relationship of this region with those surrounding *aadA* in R538-1 and *dhFrII* in R388. Nucleic Acids Res. 1986;14:8625–35.
27. Ouellette M, Bissonnette L, Roy P. Precise insertion of antibiotic resistance determinants into Tn21-like transposons: Nucleotide sequence of the OXA-1 beta-lactamase gene. Proc Natl Acad Sci USA. 1987;84:7378–82.
28. Jacoby GA, Archer GL. New mechanisms of bacterial resistance to antimicrobial agents. N Engl J Med. 1991;324:601–12.
29. Medeiros AA. Beta-lactamases. Br Med Bull. 1984;40:18–27.
30. Sykes RB, Matthew M. The beta-lactamases of gram-negative bacteria and their role in resistance to beta-lactam antibiotics. J Antimicrob Chemother. 1976;2:115–57.
31. Joris B, Ghuysen J-M, Dive G, et al. The active-site-serine penicillin-recognizing enzymes as members of the *Streptomyces* R61 DD-peptidase family. Biochem J. 1988;250:313–24.
32. Moews PC, Knox JR, Dideberg O, et al. Beta-lactamase of *Bacillus licheniformis* 749/C at 2 Å resolution. Proteins. 1990;7:156–71.
33. Herzberg O. Refined crystal structure of β-lactamase from *Staphylococcus aureus* PC1 at 2 Å resolution. J Mol Biol. 1991;217:701–19.
34. Kelly JA, Dideberg O, Charlier P, et al. On the origin of bacterial resistance to penicillin: Comparison of a beta-lactamase and a penicillin target. Science. 1986;231:1429–31.
35. McDonnell RW, Sweendy HM, Cohen S. Conjugational transfer of gentamicin resistance plasmids intra- and interspecifically in *Staphylococcus aureus* and *Staphylococcus epidermidis*. Antimicrob Agents Chemother. 1983;23:151–60.
36. Murray BE, Mederski-Samoraj B, Foster SK, et al. In-vitro studies of plasmid-mediated penicillinase from *Streptococcus faecalis* suggest a staphylococcal origin. J Clin Invest. 1986;77:289–93.
37. Murray BE. Beta-lactamase-producing enterococci. Antimicrob Agents Chemother. 1992;36:2355–9.
38. Rice LB, Marshall SH. Evidence of incorporation of the chromosomal beta-lactamase gene of enterococcus-faecalis-CH19 into a transposon derived from staphylococci. Antimicrob Agents Chemother. 1992;36:1843–6.
39. Bush K. Classfication of beta-lactamases: Groups 2c, 2d, 2e, 3, and 4. Antimicrob Agents Chemother. 1989;33:271–6.
40. Bush K. Classification of beta-lactamases: Groups 1, 2a, 2b, and 2b′. Antimicrob Agents Chemother. 1989;33:264–70.
41. Medeiros AA. Plasmid-determined beta-lactamases. In: Bryan LE, ed. Handbook of Experimental Pharmacology. v. 91. Heidelberg: Springer-Verlag; 1989:101–28.
42. Jacoby GA, Medeiros AA. More extended-spectrum beta-lactamases. Antimicrob Agents Chemother. 1991;35:1697–704.
43. Papanicolaou GA, Medeiros AA, Jacoby GA. Novel plasmid-mediated beta-lactamase (MIR-1) conferring resistance to oxyimino- and alphamethoxy-beta-lactams in clinical isolates of *Klebsiella pneumoniae*. Antimicrob Agents Chemother. 1990;34:2200–9.
44. Bauernfeind A, Mangold P, Schweighart S, et al. Molecular analysis of a transferable cephamycinase in *Klebsiella pneumoniae* (Abstract). In: Program Abstr 32nd Intersci Conf Antimicrobial Agents and Chemotherapy. 1992:322.
45. Payne DJ, Woodford N, Amyes SGB. Characterization of the plasmid mediated beta-lactamase BIL-1. J Antimicrob Chemother. 1992;30:119–27.
46. Barthelemy M, Peduzzi J, Bernard H, et al. Close amino acid sequence relationship between the new plasmid-mediated extended-spectrum beta-lactamase MEN-1 and chromosomally encoded enzymes of *Klebsiella oxytoca*. Biochim Biophys Acta. 1992;1122:15–22.
47. Watanabe M, Iyobe S, Inoue M, Mitsuhashi S. Transferable imipenem resistance in *Pseudomonas aeruginosa*. Antimicrob Agents Chemother. 1991;35:147–51.
48. Nord CE. Mechanisms of beta-lactam resistance in anaerobic bacteria. Rev Infect Dis. 1986;8(Suppl 5):S543–8.
49. Appelbaum PC. Patterns of resistance and resistance mechanisms in anaerobes. Clin Microbiol Newslet. 1992;14:49–53.
50. Tuner K, Lindqvist L, Nord CE. Purification and properties of a novel beta-lactamase from *Fusobacterium nucleatum*. Antimicrob Agent Chemother. 1985;27:943–7.
51. Cuchural GJ Jr, Tally FP, Storey JR, Malamy MH. Transfer of beta-lactam-

ase-associated cefoxitin resistance in *Bacteroides fragilis*. Antimicrob Agents Chemother. 1986;29:918–20.

52. Cuchural GJ Jr, Mulamy MH, Tally FP. Beta-lactamase-mediated imipenem resistance in *Bacteroides fragilis*. Antimicrob Agents Chemother. 1986;30: 645–8.

53. Hedberg M, Edlund C, Lindqvist L, et al. Purification and characterization of an imipenem hydrolysing metallo-beta-lactamase from *Bacteroides fragilis*. J Antimicrob Chemother. 1992;29:105–13.

54. Yotsuji A, Minami S, Inoue M, Mitsuhashi S. Properties of novel beta-lactamase produced by *Bacteroides fragilis*. Antimicrob Agents Chemother. 1983; 24:925–9.

55. Medeiros AA, O'Brien TF. Ampicillin-resistant *Haemophilus influenzae* type B possessing a TEM-type beta-lactamase but little permeability barrier to ampicillin. Lancet. 1975;1:716.

56. Elwell LP, Roberts M, Mayer LW, Falkow S. Plasmid-mediated beta-lactamase production in *Neisseria gonorrhoeae*. Antimicrob Agents Chemother. 1977;11:528–33.

57. Kliebe C, Nies BA, Meyer JF, et al. Evolution of plasmid-coded resistance to broad-spectrum cephalosporins. Antimicrob Agents Chemother. 1985;28: 302–7.

58. Brun-Buisson C, Legrand P, Philippon A, et al. Transferable enzymatic resistance to third-generation cephalosporins during nosocomial outbreak of multiresistant *Klebsiella pneumoniae*. Lancet. 1987;1:302–6.

59. Naumovski L, Quinn JP, Miyashiro D, et al. Outbreak of ceftazidime resistance due to a novel extended-spectrum beta-lactamase in isolates from cancer patients. Antimicrob Agents Chemother. 1992;36:1991–6.

60. Sanders CC, Sanders WE. Beta-lactam resistance in gram-negative bacteria—Global trends and clinical impact. Clin Infect Dis. 1992;15:824–39.

61. Liu PYF, Gur D, Hall LMC, Livermore DM. Survey of the prevalence of beta-lactamases amongst 1000 gram-negative bacilli isolated consecutively at the Royal London Hospital. J Antimicrob Chemother. 1992;30:429–47.

62. Sirot DL, Goldstein FW, Soussy CJ, et al. Resistance to cefotaxime and seven other beta-lactams in members of the family *Enterobacteriaceae*: A 3-year survey in France. Antimicrob Agents Chemother. 1992;36:1677–81.

63. Ferreira HMN, Sousa JC, Peixe LM. [Characterization of the beta-lactamases responsible for the resistance of hospital strains of *Klebsiella pneumoniae* to beta-lactam antibiotics.] Rev Portuguesa Doencas Infecciosas. 1992;15:207–9.

64. Sousa JC, Carneiro G, Peixe ML, et al. Characterization of beta-lactamases encoded by pathogenic strains of *Escherichia coli* from Portugal. J Antimicrob Chemother. 1991;27:437–40.

65. Watanabe Y, Yokota T, Higashi Y, et al. In vitro and in vivo transferable beta-lactam resistance due to a new plasmid-mediated oxyminocephalosporinase from a clinical isolate of *Proteus mirabilis*. Microbiol Immunol. 1991; 35:87–97.

66. Espinasse F, Mariotte S, Labia R, Nicolas MH. Each epidemic cefotaxime (CTX) resistant strain of *Proteus mirabilis* is related to an extended spectum beta-lactamase (Abstract). In: Program Abstr 32nd Intersci Conf Antimicrobial Agents and Chemotherapy. 1992:323.

67. Rossi MA, Gutkind G, Quinteros M, et al. A *Proteus mirabilis* with a novel extended spectrum beta-lactamase and 6 different aminoglycoside (AG) resistance genes (Abstract). In: Program Abstr 31st Intersci Conf Antimicrobial Agents and Chemotherapy 1991:255.

68. Mariotte S, Nordmann P, Nicolas MH. Spread of extended-spectrum beta-lactamases (ES Bla) in *Proteus mirabilis* (P.m.) may be limited by low frequency of plasmid conjugation (Abstract). In: Program Abstr 31st Intersci Conf Antimicrobial Agents and Chemotherapy. 1991:255.

69. Wiener J, Quinn J, Kowalczyk M, et al. Production of TEM-10 beta-lactamase in ceftazidime-resistant (CFZ-R) enterobacteriaceae from multiple nursing homes (NHs) (Abstract). In: Program Abstr 32nd Intersci Conf Antimicrobial Agents and Chemotherapy. 1992:217.

70. Lucet JC, Chevret S, Vanjak D, et al. Risk factors for acquiring extended-spectrum beta-lactamases enterobacteriaceae (ESBLE) in ICU patients (Abstract). In: Program Abstr 32nd Intersci Conf Antimicrobial Agents and Chemotherapy. 1992:217.

71. Sirot D, deChamps C, Chanal C, et al. Translocation of antibiotic resistance determinants including an extended-spectrum beta-lactamase between conjugative plasmids of *Klebsiella pneumoniae* and *Escherichia coli*. Antimicrob Agents Chemother. 1991;35:1576–81.

72. Jiang H, Hopkins JD, Zieg J, et al. Origin and transposition of a gene encoding a TEM12 beta-lactamase on pBWH102 and pBWH501 in ceftazidime resistant (CAZ-R) isolates of *Klebsiella pneumoniae* at one U.S. Medical Center (Abstract). In: Program Abstr 30th Intersci Conf Antimicrobial Agents and Chemotherapy. 1990:117.

73. Heritage J, Hawkey PM, Todd N, Lewis IJ. Transposition of the gene encoding a TEM-12 extended-spectrum beta-lactamase. Antimicrob Agents Chemother. 1992;36:1981–6.

74. Mabilat C, Lourencaovital J, Goussard S, Courvalin P. A new example of physical linkage between tn1 and tn21—The antibiotic multiple-resistance region of plasmid pCFF04 encoding extended-spectrum beta-lactamase TEM-3. Mol Gen Genet. 1992;235:113–21.

75. Jiang H, Zieg J, O'Brien TF. Observation of the acquisition of an amikacin resistance gene by an endemic nosocomial plasmid encoding a ceftazidime resistance gene (Abstract). In: Program Abstr 32nd Intersci Conf Antimicrobial Agents and Chemotherapy. 1992:184.

76. Chanal C, Poupart MC, Sirot D, et al. Nucleotide sequences of CAZ-2, CAZ-6, and CAZ-7 beta-lactamase genes. Antimicrob Agents Chemother. 1992; 36:1817–20.

77. Goussard S, Sougakoff W, Mabilat C, et al. An IS1-like element is responsible for high-level synthesis of extended-spectrum beta-lactamase TEM-6 in enterobacteriaceae. J Gen Microbiol. 1991;137:2681–7.

78. Petit A, Ben Yaghlane-Bouslama H, Sofer L, Labia R. Does high level production of SHV-type penicillinase confer resistance to ceftazidime in enterobacteriaceae? FEMS Microbiol Lett. 1992;92:89–94.

79. Thomson CJ, Amyes SGB. TRC-1—Emergence of a clavulanic acid-resistant TEM beta-lactamase in a clinical strain. FEMS Microbiol Lett. 1992;91: 113–7.

80. Vedel G, Belaaouaj A, Gilly L, et al. Clinical isolates of *Escherichia coli* producing TRI beta-lactamases: Novel TEM-enzymes conferring resistance to beta-lactamase inhibitors. J Antimicrob Chemother. 1992;30:449–62.

81. Alos JI, Blazquez J, Baquero F. A new plasmid mediated TEM-1 type beta-lactamase resistant to clavulanic acid, sulbactam and tazobactam detected in a clinical *Escherichia coli* isolate (Abstract). In Program Abstr 32nd Intersci Conf Antimicrobial Agents and Chemotherapy. 1992:207.

82. Sanders CC. Chromosomal cephalosporinases responsible for multiple resistance to newer beta-lactam antibiotics. Annu Rev Microbiol. 1987;41:573–93.

83. Korgmann G, Sanders CC, Moland ES. Altered phenotypes associates with ampD mutations in *Enterobacter cloacae*. Antimicrob Agents Chemother. 1991;35:358–64.

84. Chow JW, Fine MJ, Shlaes DM, et al. Enterobacter bacteremia—Clinical features and emergence of antibiotic resistance during therapy. Ann Intern Med. 1991;115:585–90.

85. Livermore DM. Carbapenemases. J Antimicrob Chemother. 1992;29:609–12.

86. Nugent ME, Hedges RW. The nature of the genetic determinant for the SHV-1 beta-lactamase. Mol Gen Genet. 1979;175:239–43.

87. Moxon ER, Medeiros AA, O'Brien TF. Beta-lactamase effect on ampicillin treatment of *Haemophilus influenzae* bacteremia and meningitis in infant rats. Antimicrob Agents Chemother. 1977;12:461–4.

88. Sanders CC, Sanders WE, Goering RV. In vitro antagonism of beta-lactam antibiotics by cefoxitin. Antimicrob Agents Chemother. 1982;21:968–75.

89. Bryan LE. Aminoglycoside resistance. In: Bryan LE, ed. Antimicrobial Drug Resistance. Orlando, FL: Academic Press; 1984:241–77.

90. Mayer KH. Review of epidemic aminoglycoside resistance world-wide. Am J Med. 1986;80(Suppl 6B):56–64.

91. Shimizu K, Kumada T, Hsieh W, et al. Comparison of aminoglycoside resistance patterns in Japan, Formosa, and Korea, Chile, and the United States. Antimicrob Agents Chemother. 1985;28:282–8.

92. John JF Jr, Twitty JA. Plasmids as epidemiologic markers in nosocomial gram-negative bacilli: Experience at a university and review of the literature. Rev Infect Dis. 1986;8:693–704.

93. Horodniceanu T, Bougueleret G, El-Sohi N, et al. High level plasmid-borne resistance to gentamicin in *Streptococcus faecalis* subsp. *zymogenes*. Antimicrob Agents Chemother. 1979;16:686–9.

94. Mederski-Samoraj B, Murray BE: High level resistance to gentamicin in clinical isolates of enterococci. J Infect Dis. 1983;147:751–7.

95. Murray BE, Tsao J, Panida J: Enterococci from Bangkok, Thailand, with high level resistance to currently available aminoglycosides. Antimicrob Agents Chemother. 1983;23:799–802.

96. Zervos MJ, Kauffman CA, Therasse PM, et al. Nosocomial infection by gentamicin-resistant *Streptococcus faecalis:* an epidemiological study. Ann Intern Med. 1987;106:687–91.

97. Hoffman SA, Moellering RC: The enterococcus: "Putting the bug in our ears." Ann Intern Med. 1987;106:757–61.

98. Zervos MJ: Gentamicin resistance plasmids of enterococci from diverse geographic areas are heterogeneous. J Infect Dis. 1988;158:212–6.

99. Lyon BR, Skurray R: Antimicrobial resistance of *Staphylococcus aureus:* Genetic basis. Microbiol Rev. 1987;51:88–134.

100. Gaffney DF, Foster TJ, Shaw WV. Chloramphenicol acetyl transferases determined by R-plasmids from gram (−) bacteria. J Gen Microbiol. 1978;109: 351–8.

101. Davies J. General mechanisms of antimicrobial resistance. Rev Infect Dis. 1979;1:23–7.

102. Leclercq R, Courvalin P: Resistance to macrolides, azalides, and streptogramins. In: HC Neu, LS Young, SH Zinner, eds. The New Macrolides, Azalides, and Streptogramins. New York: Marcel Dekker; 1993:33–40.

103. Barthelemy P, Autissier D, Gerbaud G, Courvalin P. Enzymatic hydrolysis of erthromycin by a strain of *Escherichia coli*: A new mechanism of resistance. J Antibiot. 1984;37:1692–6.

104. Andremont A, Gerbaud G, Courvalin P. Plasmid-mediated high-level resistance to erythromycin in *Escherichia coli*. Antimicrob Agents Chemother. 1986;29:515–8.

105. Brisson-Noel A, et al. Inactivation of lincosaminide antibiotics in *Staphylococcus*. J Biol Chem. 1988;263:15880–7.

106. Le G'offic F, et al. Plasmid-mediated pristinamycin resistance; PH1A, a pristinamycin 1A hydrolase. Ann Microbiol (Inst Pasteur). 1977;128:471–4.

107. Allignet J, et al: Nucleotide sequence of a staphylococcal plasmid gene, vgb, encoding a hydrolase inactivating the B components of virginiamycin-like antibiotics. Plasmid 1988;20:271–5.

108. Fleming A. On the antibacterial action of cultures of a *Penicillium*, with special reference to their use in the isolation of *B. influenzae*. Br J Exp Pathol. 1929;10:226–36.

109. Nikaido H. Role of permeability barriers in resistance to beta-lactam antibiotics. Pharmacol Therapeut. 1985;27:197–231.

110. Labischinski H, Barnickel G, Bradaczek H, et al. High state of order of isolated bacterial lipopolysaccharide and its possible contribution to the permeation barrier property of the outer membrane. J Bacteriol. 1985;162:9–20.

111. Takeuchi Y, Nikaido H. Physical interaction between lipid A and phospholipids: A study with spin-labeled phospholipids. Rev Infect Dis. 1984;6:488–92.

112. Vaara M. Polymyxin B nonapeptide complexes with lipopolysaccharide (Letter). FEMS Microbiol. 1983;18:117–21.

113. Nikaido H, Vaara M. Molecular basis of the permeability of outer membrane permeability. Microbiol Rev. 1985;49:1–32.

114. Hasegawa Y, Yamada H, Mizushima S. Interactions of outer membrane proteins 0-8 and 0-9 with peptidoglycan sacculus of Escherichia coli K-12. J Biochem. 1976;80:1401–9.

115. Yoshimura F, Nikaido H. Diffusion of beta-lactam antibiotics through the porin channels of Escherichia coli K-12. Antimicrob Agents Chemother. 1985;27:84–92.

116. Medeiros AA, O'Brien TF, Rosenberg EY, Nikaido H. Loss of OmpC porin in a strain of Salmonella typhimurium causes increased resistance to cephalosporins during therapy. J Infect Dis. 1987;156:751–7.

117. Goldstein FW, Gutmann L, Williamson R, et al. In vivo and in vitro emergence of simultaneous resistance to both beta-lactam and aminoglycoside antibiotics in a strain of Serratia marcescens. Ann Microbiol (Inst Pasteur). 1983;134A:329–37.

118. Quinn JP, Dudek EJ, DiVincenzo CA, et al. Emergence of resistance to imipenem during therapy for Pseudomonas aeruginosa infections. J Infect Dis. 1986;154:289–94.

119. Livermore DM. Interplay of impermeability and chromosomal beta-lactamase activity in imipenem-resistant Pseudomonas aeruginosa. Antimicrob Agents Chemother. 1992;36:2046–8.

120. Sanders CC, Sanders WE Jr, Goering RV, Werner V. Selection of multiple antibiotic resistance by quinolones, beta-lactams, and aminoglycosides with special reference to cross-resistance between unrelated drug classes. Antimicrob Agents Chemother. 1984;26:797–801.

121. Hooper DC, Wolfson JS, Ng EY, Swartz MN: Mechanisms of action and resistance to ciprofloxacin. Am J Med. 1987;82:2–11.

122. Gaffney DF, Cundiffe E, Foster TJ. Chloramphenicol resistance that does not involve chloramphenicol acetyltransferase encoded by plasmids from gram (−) bacteria. J Gen Microbiol. 1981;125:113–21.

123. Bryan LE, Kwan S. Roles of ribosomal binding membrane potential and electron transport in bacterial uptake of streptomycin and gentamicin. Antimicrob Agents Chemother. 1983;23:835–45.

124. Mates SM, Esenberg ES, Mandel LF, et al. Membrane potential and gentamicin uptake in Staphylococcus aureus. Proc Natl Acad Sci USA. 1982;79:6693–7.

125. Rusthoven JJ, Davies A, Lerner SA. Clinical isolation and characterization of aminoglycoside-resistant small colony varients of Enterobacter aerogenes. Am J Med. 1979;67:702–6.

126. Musher DN, Baughan RE, Merrell GL. Selection of small-colony variants of Enterobacteriaceae by in vitro exposure to aminoglycosides: Pathogenicity for experimental animals. J Infect Dis. 1979;140:209–14.

127. Funada H, Hattori K, Kosaki N. Catalase-negative Escherichia coli isolated from the blood. J Clin Microbiol. 1978;7:474–8.

128. McMurry L, Petrucci RE, Levy SB. Active efflux of tetracycline encoded by four genetically different tetracycline resistance determinants in Escherichia coli. Proc Natl Acad Sci USA. 1980;71:3974–7.

129. McMurry LM, Park BH, Burdette V, Levy SB. Energy-dependent efflux mediated by class L (tetL) tetracycline resistance determinant from streptococci. Antimicrob Agents Chemother. 1987;31:1648–50.

130. Cohen SP, Hooper DC, Wolfson JS, et al. Endogenous active efflux of norfloxacin in susceptible Escherichia coli. Antimicrob Agents Chemother. 1988;32:1187–90.

131. Engel HWB, Soedirman N, Rost JA, et al. Transferability of macrolide, lincomycin, and streptogramin resistances between group A, B, and D streptococci, Streptococcus pneumoniae, and Staphylococcus aureus. J Bacteriol. 1980;142:407–13.

132. Weisblum B. Inducible resistance to macrolides, lincosamides and streptogramin type B antibiotics: The resistance phenotype, its biological diversity, and structural elements that regulate expression—A review. J Antimicrob Chemother. 1985;16(Suppl A):63–90.

133. Burdette V. Streptococcal tetracycline resistance mediated at the level of protein synthesis. J Bacteriol. 1986;165:564–9.

134. Roberts MC, Koutsy LA, Holmes KK, et al. Tetracycline-resistant Mycoplasma hominis strains contain streptococcal tetM sequences. Antimicrob Agents Chemother. 1985;28:141–3.

135. Taylor DE, Kiratsuka K, Ray H, Manavathu EK. Characterization and expression of a cloned tetracycline resistance determinant from Campylobacter jejuni plasmid pUA466. J Bacteriol. 1987;169:2984–9.

136. Eliopoulos GM, Farber BF, Murray BE, et al. Ribosomal resistance of clinical enterococcal isolates to streptomycin. Antimicrob Agents Chemother. 1984;25:398–9.

137. Ahmad MH, Rechenmacher A, Boch A. Interaction between aminoglycoside uptake and ribosomal resistance mutations. Antimicrob Agents Chemother. 1980;18:798–806.

138. Dutka-Malen S, LeClercq R, Coutant V, eᵗ al. Phenotypic and genotypic

139. Leclercq R, Derlot E, Weber M, et al. Transferable vancomycin and teicoplanin resistance in Enterococcus faecium. N Engl J Med. 1988;319:157–61.

140. Shlaes DM, Bouvet A, Devine C, et al. Inducible, tranferable resistance to vancomycin in Enterococcus faecalis A256. Antimicrob Agents Chemother. 1989;33:198–203.

141. Nicas TI, Cole CT, Preston DA, et al. Activity of glycopeptides against vancomycin-resistant gram-positive bacteria. Antimicrob Agents Chemother. 1989;33:1477–81.

142. Bugg TD, Wright GD, Dutka-Malen S, et al. Molecular basis for vancomycin resistance in Enterococcus faecium BM4147: Biosynthesis of a depsipeptide peptidoglycan precursor by vancomycin resistance proteins VanH and VanA. Biochemistry. 1991;30:10408–15.

143. LeClercq R, Dutkamalen S, Brissonnoel A, et al. Resistance of enterococci to aminoglycosides and glycopeptides. Clin Infect Dis. 1992;15:495–501.

144. Quintiliani R, Jr., Evers S, Courvalin P. The vanB gene confers various levels of self-transferable resistance to vancomycin in enterococci. J Infect Dis. 1993;167:1220–3.

145. LeClercq R, Dutkamalen S, Duval J, Courvalin P. Vancomycin resistance gene vanC is specific to Enterococcus gallinarum. Antimicrob Agents Chemother. 1992;36:2005–8.

146. Waxman DJ, Strominger JL. Penicillin-binding proteins and the mechanism of action of beta-lactam antibiotics. Annu Rev Biochem 1983;52:825–69.

147. Malouin F, Bryan LE. Modification of penicillin-binding proteins as mechanisms of beta-lactam resistance. Antimicrob Agents Chemother. 1986;30:1–5.

148. Williamson R. Resistance of Clostridium perfringens to beta-lactam antibiotics mediated by a decreased affinity of a single essential penicillin-binding protein. J Gen Microbiol. 1983;129:2339–42.

149. Giles AF, Reynolds PE. Bacillus megaterium resistance to cloxacillin accompanied by a compensatory change in penicillin binding proteins. Nature. 1979;280:167–8.

150. Hakenbeck R, Tarpay M, Tomasz A. Multiple changes of penicillin-binding proteins in penicillin-resistant clinical isolates of Streptococcus pneumoniae. Antimicrob Agents Chemother. 1980;17:364–71.

151. Spratt BG, Dowson CG, Zhang Q-Y, et al. Mosaic genes, hybrid penicillin-binding proteins, and the origins of penicillin resistance in Neisseria meningitidis and Streptococcus pneumoniae. In: Campisi J, Cunningham DD, Inouye M, et al., eds. Perspectives on Cellular Regulation: From Bacteria to Cancer. New York: Wiley-Liss; 1991:73–83.

152. Hartman BJ, Tomasz A. Low-affinity penicillin-binding protein associated with beta-lactam resistance in Staphylococcus aureus. J Bacteriol. 1984;158:513–6.

153. Ubukata K, Yamashita N, Konno M. Occurrence of a beta-lactam-inducible penicillin-binding protein in methicillin-resistant staphylococci. Antimicrob Agents Chemother. 1985;27:851–7.

154. Fontana R. Penicillin-binding proteins and the intrinsic resistance to beta-lactams in gram positive cocci. J Antimicrob Chemother. 1985;16:412–6.

155. Fontana R, Grossato A, Rossi L, et al. Transition from resistance to hypersusceptibility to beta-lactam antibiotics associated with loss of low-affinity penicillin-binding protein in a Streptococcus faecium mutant highly resistant to penicillin. Antimicrob Agents Chemother. 1985;28:678–83.

156. Farber BF, Eliopoulos GM, Ward JI, et al. Multiply resistant viridans streptococci: Susceptibility to beta-lactam antibiotics and comparison of penicillin-binding protein patterns. Antimicrob Agents Chemother. 1983;24:702–5.

157. Sabath LD. Chemical and physical factors influencing methicillin resistance of Staphylococcus aureus and Staphylococcus epidermidis. J Antimicrob Chemother. 1977;3(Suppl C):47–51.

158. Song MD, Wachi M, Doi M, et al. Evolution of an inducible penicillin target protein in methicillin-resistant Staphylococcus aureus by gene fusion. FEBS Lett. 1987;226:167–71.

159. Berger-Bachi B, Barberis-Maino L, Strassle A, Kayser FH. FemA, a host-mediated factor essential for methicillin resistance in Staphylococcus aureus: Molecular cloning and characterization. Mol Gen Genet. 1989;219:263–9.

160. Dougherty TJ, Koller AE, Tomasz A. Penicillin binding proteins of penicillin-susceptible and intrinsically resistant Neisseria gonorrhoeae. Antimicrob Agents Chemother. 1980;18:730–7.

161. Mendelman PM, Chaffin DO, Kalaitzoglou G. Penicillin-binding proteins and ampicillin reistance in Haemophilus influenzae. J Antimicrob Chemother. 1990;25:525–34.

162. Dougherty TJ. Genetic analysis and penicillin-binding protein alterations in Neisseria gonorrhoeae with chromosomally mediated resistance. Antimicrob Agents Chemother. 1986;30:649–52.

163. Mendelman PM, Campos J, Chaffin DO, et al. Relative penicillin G resistance in Neisseria meningitidis and reduced affinity of penicillin-binding protein 3. Antimicrob Agents Chemother. 1988;32:706–9.

164. Spratt BG, Zhang Q-Y, Jones DM, et al. Recruitment of a penicillin-binding protein gene from Neisseria flavescens during the emergence of penicillin resistance in Neisseria meningitidis. Proc Natl Acad Sci USA. 1989;86:8988–92.

165. Faruki H, Kohmescher RN, McKinney WP, Sparling PF. A community based outbreak of infection with penicillin-resistant Neisseria gonorrhoeae

not producing penicillinase (chromosomally mediated resistance). N Engl J Med. 1985;313:607–11.

166. Mirelman D, Nuchamowitz Y, Rubinstein E. Insensitivity of peptidoglycan biosynthetic reactions to beta-lactam antibiotics in a clinical isolate of *Pseudomonas aeruginosa*. Antimicrob Agents Chemother. 1981;19:687–95.

167. Parr TR, Bryan LE. Mechanism of resistance of an ampicillin-resistant beta-lactamase-negative clinical isolate of *Haemophilus influenzae* type b to beta-lactam antibiotics. Antimicrob Agents Chemother. 1984;25:747–53.

168. Hamilton-Miller JMT. Resistance to antibacterial agents acting on antifolate metabolism. In: Bryan LE, ed. Antimicrobial Drug Resistance. Orlando, FL: Academic Press; 1984;173–88.

169. Huovinen P. Trimethoprim resistance. Antimicrob Agents Chemother. 1987; 31:1451–6.

170. Steen R, Skold O. Plasmid-borne or chromosomally mediated resistance by Tn7 is the most common response to ubiquitous use of trimethoprim. Antimicrob Agents Chemother. 1985;27:933–7.

171. Wolfson JS, Hooper DC. The fluoroquinolones: Structures, mechanisms of action and resistance, and spectra of activity in vitro. Antimicrob Agents Chemother. 1985;28:581–6.

172. Hane MW, Wood TH. *Escherichia coli* K-12 mutants resistant to nalidixic acid: Genetic mapping and dominance studies. J Bacteriol. 1969;99:238–41.

173. Robillard NJ, Scarpa AL. Genetic and physiological characterization of ciprofloxacin resistance in *Pseudomonas aeruginosa* PAO. Antimicrob Agents Chemother. 1988;32:535–9.

174. Wolfson JS, Hooper DC: The fluoroquinolones: Structures, mechanisms of action resistance, and spectra of activity in vitro. Antimicrob Agents Chemother. 1985;28:581–6.

175. Fisher LM, Hopewell R, Oram M, Sreedharan S: The molecular basis of quinolone action and resistance. In: Neu HC, ed. New Antibacterial Strategies. New York: Churchill Livingstone; 1990:177–190.

176. Aoyama H, Fujimaki K, Sato K, et al. Clinical isolate of *Citrobacter freundii* highly resistant to new quinolones. Antimicrob Agents Chemother. 1988;32: 922–4.

177. Nakamura S, Nakamura M, Kojima T, Yoshida H: gyrA and gyrB mutations in quinolone-resistant strains of *Escherichia coli*. Antimicrob Agents Chemother. 1989;33:128–30.

178. Sullen ME, Wyke AW, Kuroda R, Fisher LH: Cloning and characterization of a DNA gyrase A gene from *Escherichia coli* that confers clinical resistance to 4-quinolones. Antimicrob Agents Chemother. 1989;33:886–94.

179. Maskell R, Okubagejo OA, Payne RH. Human infections with thymine-requiring bacteria. J Med Microbiol. 1978;33–42.

180. McGowan JE. Antimicrobial resistance in hospital organisms and its relation to antimicrobial use. Rev Infect Dis. 1983;5:1033–48.

181. Levy SB. Resistance to th tetracyclines. In: Bryan LE, ed. Antimicrobial Drug Resistance. Orlando, FL: Academic Press; 1984:192–234.

182. Mayer KH, Hopkins JD, Gilleece ES, et al. Computer-assisted correlations between antibiotypes of clinical isolates and the endonuclease restriction fragment of types of their plasmids. In: Mitsuhasi S, Rosival L, Kromery V, eds. Transferrable Antibiotic Resistance: Plasmids and Gene Manipulation. Prague: Czechoslovak Press; 1984:163–9.

183. Murray BE, Alvarado T, Kim K-H. Increasing resistance to trimethoprim-sulfamethoxazole among isolates of *Escherichia coli* in developing countries. J Infect Dis. 1985;152:1107–13.

184. Seppala H, Nissinen A, Jarvinen H, et al. Resistance to erythromycin in group A streptococci. N Engl J Med. 1992;326:292–7.

185. Moellering RC: Emergence of *Enterococcus* as a significant pathogen. Clin Infect Dis. 1992;14:1173–78.

186. Grayson ML, Eliopoulos GM, Wennersten CB, et al. Increasing resistance to beta-lactam antibiotics among clinical isolates of *E. faecium*: A 22-year review at one institution. Antimicrob Agents Chemother. 1991;35:2180–4.

187. Rhinehart E, Smith NE, Wennersten C, et al: Rapid dissemination of beta-lactamase-producing, aminoglycoside-resistant *Enterococcus faecalis* among patients and staff on an infant-toddler surgical ward. N Engl J Med. 1990;323:1814–8.

188. Bugg TDH, Dutka-Malen S, Arthur M, et al. Identification of vancomycin resistance protein VanA as a D-alanine:D-alanine ligase of altered substrate specificity. Biochemistry. 1991;30:2017–21.

189. Rubin LG, Tucci V, Cercenado E, et al. Vancomycin-resistant *Enterococcus faecium* in hospitalized children. Infect Control Hosp Epidemiol. 1992;13: 700–5.

190. Karanfil LV, Murphy M, Josephson A, et al. A cluster of vancomycin-resistant *Enterococcus faecium* in an intensive care unit. Infect Control Hosp Epidemiol. 1992;13:195–200.

191. Livornese LL, Dias S, Samel C, et al. Hospital-acquired infection with vancomycin-resistant *Enterococcus faecium* transmitted by electronic thermometers. Ann Intern Med. 1992;117:112–6.

192. Uttley AHC, Collins CH, Naidoo J, George RC. Vancomycin-resistant enterococci. Lancet. 1988;1:57–8.

193. Boyce JM, Opal SM, Chow JW, et al. Outbreak of multidrug-resistant *Enterococcus faecium* with transferable *vanB* class vancomycin resistance. J Clin Microbiol. 1994;32:1148–53.

194. Schaefler S: Methicillin-resistant strains of *Staphylococcus aureus* resistant to quinolones. J Clin Microbiol. 1989;27:335–6.

195. Shalit I, Berger SA, Gorea A, Frimerman H: Widespread quinolone resis-

tance among methicillin-resistant *Staphylococcus aureus* isolates in a general hospital. Antimicrob Agents Chemother. 1989;33:593–4.

196. Banerjee SN, Emori TG, Culver DH, et al: Secular trends in nosocomial primary bloodstream infections in the United States, 1980–1989. Am J Med. 1991;3B-86S–9S.

197. Holmberg SD, Solmon SL, Blake PA. Health and economic impacts of antimicrobial resistance. Rev Infect Dis. 1987;6:1065–78.

14. PHARMACOLOGY OF ANTI-INFECTIVE AGENTS

GEORGE L. DRUSANO

Administration of an antimicrobial agent should inhibit or kill the microorganism causing the infection. An assumption underlying the necessity for determination of a drug's pharmacologic profile is that there is a relationship between drug exposure in the patient—in the blood, in certain cells, or at the specific site of infection (e.g., central nervous system, prostate)—and the therapeutic effects that are then observed.

DRUG EXPOSURE AND RESPONSE

When an anti-infective agent is administered, it develops a plasma concentration-time profile that can be characterized in a number of ways. Furthermore, this concentration-time profile must be seen relative to an index of the potency of the drug for the microorganism in question (e.g., minimum inhibitory concentration [MIC], minimum bactericidal concentration [MBC], minimum fungicidal concentration [MFC], or effective concentration for 50% (95%) of strains [EC_{50}, EC_{95}]). Consequently, one can then attempt to link aspects of the concentration-time profile to the therapeutic and toxic outcomes observed. On a theoretical basis, one would expect different aspects of the pharmacologic profile to be linked to therapeutic outcome (e.g., peak/MIC, area under the concentration-time curve (AUC)/MIC, and time plasma concentrations above the MIC), depending on the microbiologic properties of the drug in question.

For clarity, we examine the case of a cidal antibacterial agent and gram-negative bacilli, but the principles may be applied to other microbes. The drug in question can be characterized as being relatively concentration dependent in kill rate or as being relatively concentration-independent in kill rate. This simple dichotomous characterization of one of the drug's properties has important implications for dosing the agent so as to obtain an optimal outcome (Fig. 1).

The number of organisms killed after drug administration is linked to the manner in which it kills (concentration dependently vs. independently). In the case of a relatively concentration-independent killer (e.g., β-lactam antibiotics,[1] it is immediately apparent that peak cannot be directly linked to outcome, as the kill rate engendered at high concentrations is virtually identical to kill rates engendered by concentrations near the middle of the curve or even down near the MIC (i.e., a high peak concentration does not measurably improve kill rate). Consequently, an approximation of the total number of organisms killed after a dose of drug is merely the kill rate (nearly a constant) times the time that plasma concentrations exceed the MIC (or MBC, if greatly different). If therapeutic success is linked to the ability to eradicate the causative microbe, then increasing success (up to a maximum value) will be had with increasing the duration that drug concentrations exceed the MIC for drugs that are relatively concentration independent in the kill rate engendered.

Drugs that are highly concentration-dependent in kill rate,

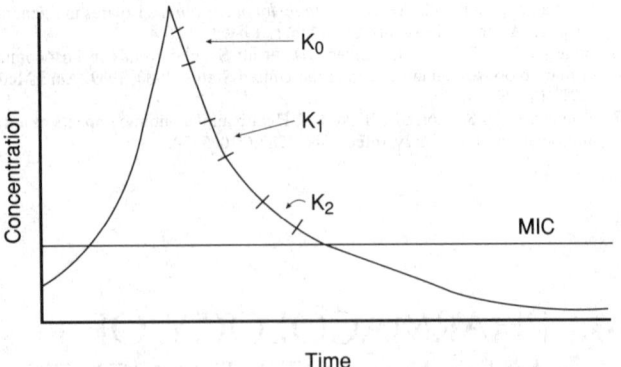

FIG. 1. Schematic diagram showing relationship between antibiotic concentration, MIC, and rates of kill at three different times after infusion (k_0, k_1, k_2). For drugs that kill in a concentration-independent manner, $k_0 \cong k_1 \cong k_2$, and the total number of organisms killed is the nearly constant kill rate times the time drug concentrations exceed the MIC (or MBC). An example is the β-lactam class of drugs. For drugs that are concentration dependent in kill rate, $k_0 > k_1 > k_2$, and the total organism kill is a path integral, which can be related to the AUC, itself an integral of the concentration-time curve. Examples are aminoglycoside and fluoroquinolone classes of anti-infectives.

such as aminoglycosides and fluoroquinolones,[1,2] should, on a theoretical basis, have a different aspect of their pharmacologic profile linked to therapeutic outcome. Here, the kill rate engendered by concentrations near the peak is greater than that engendered by concentrations near the middle of the curve, which, in turn, is greater than that engendered by concentrations near the MIC (Fig. 1). The kill rate continuously changes with concentration (time in the patient), and the total number of organisms killed is an integral of the concentration-dependent kill rate with respect to time. Drugs of this type should have the therapeutic outcome linked to the AUC, which is, itself, an integral of the concentration-time curve.

The importance of obtaining high peak concentrations can only be demonstrated by introducing an additional concept. It is therapeutically advantageous to prevent the emergence of resistance. It is here that peak concentration may be important. Large total populations of the microorganisms lead to an increasing probability that a subpopulation of the organisms will have acquired a mutation that renders them less susceptible to the anti-infective agent being employed. The probability increases as a function of two factors, the absolute population size (as opposed to density) and the frequency of mutation to a less susceptible state. The obvious clinical example is seen with *Mycobacterium tuberculosis*,[3] but others have been clearly demonstrated, such as fluoroquinolone resistance among bacteria[4] and, less well documented but highly likely, alteration of EC_{50} of nucleoside analogs for HIV-1.[5] Less clear is whether obtaining high peak concentrations allows the suppression of both parent organism and the more resistant mutants. It is likely that, when resistant mutants are limited in the increase in MIC relative to the parent strain and the kill rate is concentration dependent (e.g., fluoroquinolones and the gyrA mutation), obtaining high peak concentrations can suppress the parent strain and mutant organisms as well.

An exception to the above may occur when an antimicrobial agent is highly ion trapped within cells. This may violate the above scenarios in a number of different ways. If the pathogen being treated is intracellular and the amount of active antibiotic in the infected cell is linked to the amount of ion trapped and if the residence time of the trapped molecule in the cell is much longer than the plasma half life, then, on a theoretical basis, one would expect to see AUC linked to outcome. This is because the amount of drug entering the cell and then becoming trapped will be linked to AUC. Likewise, if the cell is only a carrier for

the drug and disgorges it at the primary infection site (e.g., the azalide azithromycin), one would expect to see the same thing.

Optimal Modes of Administration for Different Drug Classes

For β-lactams, aminoglycosides, fluoroquinolones, and antiretrovirals, data will be presented supporting an optimal mode of administration. In general, these data will be organized as coming from in vitro model systems, animal model systems, and human trials.

One must exercise caution in the interpretation of findings from in vitro models. As Haag and colleagues[6] have pointed out, physical factors such as adherence of *Pseudomonas* to the walls of the reaction vessel can dramatically alter the findings of the model. Nonetheless, these in vitro experiments can provide valuable insights into the process of the therapy of infections.

β-Lactams

In Vitro Models. However, even with the caveat provided above, the in vitro model system evaluated by Blaser et al.[7] seems to correlate well with clinical outcome. Zinner and colleagues[8] used this system to evaluate the dosing of 4 g per day of cefoperazone, with the experiments differing by fractionation schedule (4 g qid vs. 2 g q12h). They found that as long as plasma concentrations of drug exceeded the MIC of the pathogen for the full 24 hours (as was the case with *Escherichia coli* and *Klebsiella pneumoniae*), both regimens were equivalent. However, with more resistant pathogens with higher MICs, the more frequent schedule provided a full 24 hours with concentrations in excess of the MIC, but the once daily regimen did not. This translated into significantly greater bacterial growth with the once daily regimen as compared with the more frequently administered regimen. It should be pointed out that this system did not evaluate the effect of protein binding and that clinical results may be altered by this factor.[9]

Animal Models. There is a wealth of data in the literature examining the relationship of plasma concentrations to outcome (organism kill) for β-lactam antibiotics. Gerber and colleagues[10] examined the influence of dosing schedule on the ability of ticarcillin to kill *Pseudomonas aeruginosa* at the primary infection site in a neutropenic mouse though infection model. The more frequent regimen provided significantly better control of the infection at the primary site in this neutropenic animal model. This is consistent with theory in that the higher peak plasma concentrations seen with less frequently administered regimens should not provide greater organism kill, as kill rate is relatively insensitive to concentration for β-lactam drugs.

Roosendaal et al.[11,12] examined ceftazidime administered as either a continuous or intermittently in a rat pneumonia model with *K. pneumoniae*. Cohorts of animals were made neutropenic or had normal host defenses. Whether animals were normal or neutropenic, continuous administration was significantly better in preventing mortality than intermittent administration. The differences are magnified by alteration of host defenses, with neutropenic animals requiring 15 times more drug to salvage a cohort completely by intermittent administration than by continuous infusion.

Vogelman et al.[13] and Leggett et al.[14] examined multiple β-lactams against several different organisms, both gram-positive as well as gram-negative. The animal models employed were neutropenic and had primary infections in the mouse thigh and pneumonia. These investigators examined a great many schedules and performed regression analysis so as to determine which variable (peak/MIC, AUC/MIC, time above the MIC) was most strongly linked to outcome. For each β-lactam examined, the time above the MIC was always most strongly linked to the kill of organisms at the primary infection site. This held true for cephalosporins as well as penicillins.

Animal model data are often denigrated because small animal pharmacokinetics differs dramatically from the kinetic profile in humans. Flückiger et al.[15] attacked this drawback by developing the man-adapted mouse model. In this model, doses are given in a highly fractionated fashion so that the resultant plasma concentration-time profile observed is nearly identical to that seen in humans. They then used imipenem as a probe in their system, with *Pseudomonas* serving as the challenge organism. Once again, the time that plasma concentrations remained above the MIC correlated best with the ability of this β-lactam to kill organisms at the primary infection site.

Clearly, then, several investigators, employing many different β-lactams, models, and challenge strains come to concordant findings. In vitro data and animal model data support the concept that the time that plasma concentrations (and hence concentrations at primary infection sites) spend above the MIC of the causative pathogen determines the ability of the regimen to kill that pathogen.

Clinical Trial Data. Some of the earliest clinical data were generated in a neutropenic cancer patient by Bodey and colleagues.[16] In that investigation, febrile neutropenic patients were randomized to one of three therapies: *(1)* cefamandole by continuous infusion (12 g per day) plus carbenicillin by intermittent infusion; *(2)* cefamandole (3 g every 6 hours) plus carbenicillin, both by intermittent administration; or *(3)* cefamandole (3 g every 6 hours) plus tobramycin, both by intermittent administration. One weakness of the study design is that multiple agents were used (at the time, a necessity in the patient population under study), and the continuous infusion therapy arm, which maximizes time above the MIC, is adulterated by an intermittent administration schedule for carbenicillin. These weaknesses are mitigated by the actual schedule of administration for carbenicillin, which was every 4 hours, with each dose being given as a 2-hour infusion. In reality then, the double β-lactam arms can be effectively thought of as more nearly (arm 1) continuous infusion and less nearly (arm 2) continuous infusion. Any differences observed are likely to be clinically significant. Patients with profound, persistent neutropenia benefitted significantly from continuous infusion of cefamandole. These conclusions are softened by the combination nature of the therapeutic intervention. Nonetheless, the outcome recapitulates the lessons learned from in vitro and animal model systems.

In another study[17] in which cefoperazone and cefamandole/tobramycin were compared for the empiric therapy of gram-negative sepsis, 120 patients were randomized, with 60 receiving cefoperazone. Ten of these patients had a single-organism, gram-negative bacteremia documented. With the hypothesis that coverage of the entire dosing interval with free drug at a concentration above the MIC would maximize success, our group predicted that there would be six successes and four failures. The matched observations revealed five successes and five failures. The mispredicted patient was a physiologic and not a pharmacologic failure. Of possible further import is the fact that it was important to correct for protein binding in this evaluation. Given the relatively small number of patients evaluated, these results need to be viewed with caution. Nonetheless, this is certainly consistent with the lessons learned in animal models of infection.

One very controversial point is the importance of protein binding. Certainly, in the data cited above, it would appear that protein binding plays a determinative role. However, certain very highly bound agents such as ceftriaxone produce clinically acceptable outcomes against pathogens such as *E. coli* and *K. pneumoniae,* even at less than maximal doses, where free drug concentrations decline to levels below the MIC. This becomes understandable when one takes into account the relatively low molecular weight serum factor discovered by Leggett and

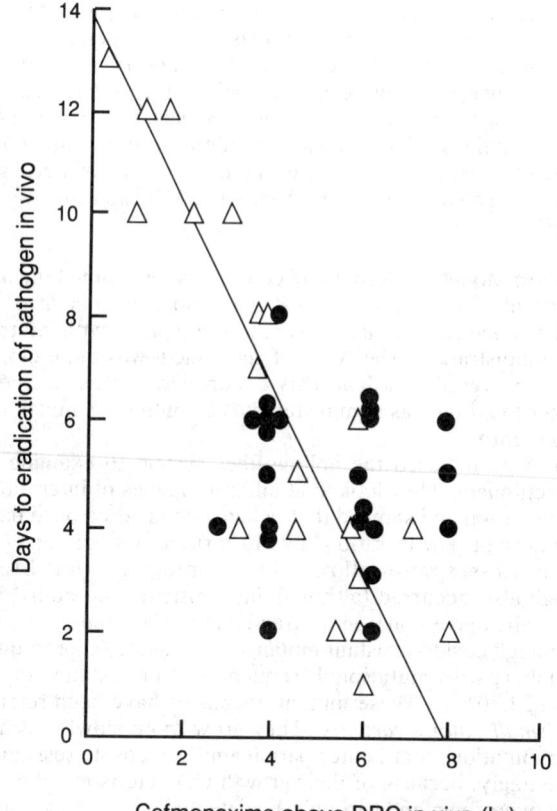

FIG. 2. Relationship between the time cefmenoxime serum concentrations exceeded the dynamic response concentration (DRC; this approximates the MIC) for retrospectively (△) and prospectively (●) treated patients and the days to bacterial eradication in vivo. Each data point represents one pathogen. The regression line describing the retrospective data took the form of the equation: days to eradication = 13.86 − 1.78 × (time > DRC), r = 0.89, p < 0.001. This correlation was not seen for the prospectively treated patients. (From Schentag et al.,[19] with permission.)

Craig.[18] This factor improves the activity of highly bound β-lactams against the Enterobacteriaceae, resulting in a functional lowering of the MIC. Interestingly, this factor does not affect either *Staphylococcus aureus* or *P. aeruginosa.* The good clinical outcomes that one sees with such agents that would not be predicted on a priori principles then become understandable.

Further clinical data were provided by Schentag and colleagues.[19] In their trial, a different end point was evaluated. They examined the time to eradication of pathogens identified in the lower respiratory tract. The relationship between increasing time above the MIC and the number of days to eradication was then determined by regression analysis. These results are displayed in Figure 2. It is clear that an increasing time above the MIC is associated with a linear decrease in the time to eradication of a gram-negative pathogen from the lower respiratory tract of intubated patients in the intensive care unit.

For β-lactams, then, in vitro models, animal models, and clinical trial data provide concordant findings. The best microbiologic and clinical outcomes are obtained by increasing the amount of time drug concentrations and perhaps, more conservatively, free drug concentrations remain above the MIC of the infecting pathogen.

Aminoglycosides

With aminoglycoside antibiotics, as will also be seen with the fluoroquinolones, there is some disagreement regarding which aspect of the concentration-time curve is most closely linked to some measure of outcome. As with the fluoroquinolones, it is likely that resistant mutants that exist in dense populations of organisms account for a great deal of the observed discrepancies. Variance in study design, as well as the covariance that exists among the pharmacodynamic variables, also explains the different findings. That is, on a fixed administration schedule, it is difficult, if not impossible, to examine the impact of increasing dose on peak/MIC separately from AUC/MIC and time above the MIC.

In Vitro Models.   Gerber and colleagues[20] examined the aminoglycoside gentamicin against *P. aeruginosa* in an in vitro system. Dynamic continuous infusion was compared with intermittent administration. The AUC of gentamicin was quite closely linked to organism kill in this experiment, irrespective of whether the drug was administered as a continuous infusion or intermittently.

Blaser et al.[7] used the hollow fiber system to examine the drug netilmicin. They looked at different modes of intermittent administration and showed that, when administered once daily, obtaining a peak/MIC ratio above 10 ensured sterilization of the system. Lesser ratios allowed breakthrough growth. Breakthrough also occurred (although intermittently) at equivalent AUCs when given on a more fractionated schedule.

Aminoglycoside-resistant mutants are actually quite frequent in number, with mutational frequencies to resistance on the order of $1/10^{6-7}$.[21] These mutant organisms have been referred to as *small colony variants*. They grow quite slowly because of the mutations that confer partial aminoglycoside resistance. Interestingly, because of their growth characteristics, they are easily overgrown and can only be detected when grown under selective pressure.[22]

Aminoglycosides gain entry into gram-negative cells as a function of the transmembrane $\Delta\Psi$.[23] Mutations in one or more of the electron transport chain enzymes causes less aminoglycoside entry, functionally increasing the MIC (usually two- to fourfold).[24] It is likely that obtaining a high enough peak/MIC ratio (≥ 10) allows these slow-growing mutants to be suppressed along with the parent strain. Otherwise, at lower ratios, or with fewer mutants in the population, the AUC becomes the controlling variable.

Animal Models.   Once again, as with β-lactams, there is a considerable amount of animal model data relating to the optimal mode of administration of aminoglycosides. Also, as with the in-vitro data, there is disagreement as to which pharmacodynamic variable is most closely linked to outcome.

Gerber and Feller-Segessenmann[25] examined kill patterns of *P. aeruginosa* in a granulocytopenic mouse thigh infection model with the aminoglycoside gentamicin. They were able to demonstrate that one large administration of gentamicin effected greater kill of the organism in vivo than the same dose administered on a more fractionated schedule. They then concluded that peak was important, as the AUC was the same for both regimens and the time above the MIC was greater for the more fractionated schedule. Neither regimen, however, was able to shut off regrowth through continued drug administration.

This regrowth was almost assuredly regrowth of the small colony variant resistant mutants. This was shown elegantly in a different investigation by Gerber et al.[26] These variants are selected quite quickly in the setting of granulocytopenia. The coadministration of a β-lactam prevents the emergence of these resistant mutants.

Other investigators, however, have concluded that AUC might be most closely linked to cell kill with aminoglycosides. Vogelman et al.[13] demonstrated in a mouse thigh infection model that, when different doses and schedules are employed, multivariate analysis chooses AUC as the variable most closely linked to outcome if the dosing intervals considered are limited to 12 hours. At longer intervals, the analysis also adds time

above the MIC. As the authors point out, this is likely because the longer dosing intervals range longer than the time above the MIC plus the postantibiotic effect (PAE).[27]

This was again well demonstrated by Leggett et al.,[14] who explicitly modeled the effect of dose on organism kill. They showed the lack of effect of interval on the dose mediating 50% reduction in bacterial population (P_{50}) for intervals up to these lengths, in contrast to the markedly increasing P_{50}s seen with β-lactams with increasing intervals. These studies were performed in a neutropenic model. This is important, as it helps to explain the findings of Kapusnik et al.,[28] who studied neutropenic guinea pigs with *Pseudomonas* pneumonia. In this investigation, once-daily aminoglycoside administration was less efficacious than the same total dose administered on a 4-hour schedule. This was not seen with non-neutropenic animals, and the likely explanation is that the interval in the neutropenic animals exceeded the time above the MIC plus the PAE. In the normal animals granulocyte-mediated killing plus, perhaps, the postantibiotic leukocyte enhancement effect blocks this breakthrough growth.[29] In a non-neutropenic setting, once again, Wood et al.[30] found that AUC was most closely linked to bacteriologic outcome when studying aminoglycosides.

Clinical Trial Data.   Some of the first data examining outcome as a function of achieved plasma concentration were provided by Noone et al.[31] These investigators measured peak concentrations of gentamicin (defined as 15 minutes after the end of the infusion) in 68 patients with serious gram-negative infection. These patients included 29 individuals with pneumonia and 15 patients with gram-negative bacteremia. A factor ameliorating the impact of this study was the use of a concomitant β-lactam in 22 patients. Nonetheless, patients with measured concentrations greater than 5 µg/ml obtained in the first 3 days of therapy (except for pneumonia, when a concentration greater than 8 µg/ml was required) had a significantly better outcome.

Once-daily tobramycin therapy was compared with the continuous infusion of tobramycin in patients with cystic fibrosis by Powell and colleagues.[32] Thirty-one patients were randomized, 16 receiving continuous infusion, 15 receiving once-daily therapy. Mean symptom scores at therapy initiation and at end of therapy did not show differences by analysis of variance. This study clearly indicates that AUC was linked to outcome; if it were time above the MIC, the continuous infusion group would have had the better resolution, while if peak concentration controlled outcome, the once-daily group would have been superior. It must be pointed out that this study did not examine any microbiologic end points and did not look for emergence of resistance.

Finally, Moore et al.[33–35] published a series of studies using logistic regression analysis or discriminant function analysis to link plasma concentrations of aminoglycosides (or their ratio to the MIC) to the observed outcomes. These investigators analyzed data collected in three randomized, double-blind clinical trials involving gentamicin, tobramycin, and amikacin. In all of the various examinations of all or some of the data, peak concentration was shown to be strongly linked to the ultimate outcome. However, sampling of plasma concentrations in this study was sparse (peaks and troughs only) and, perhaps more importantly, the dosing interval was fixed at every 8 hours, irrespective of renal function. This last factor absolutely guarantees maximal covariance among peak/MIC, AUC/MIC, and time above the MIC. Nonetheless, in all the studies of the in vitro model, animal model, and clinical trial data presented, it is clear that, for aminoglycosides, when the kill rate is highly concentration dependent it is either the peak/MIC ratio or the AUC/MIC ratio that is linked to outcome.

Fluoroquinolones

Fluoroquinolones share many of the microbiologic properties of aminoglycosides, such as concentration-dependent killing, great potency, and the existence of spontaneously resistant mutants at relatively high frequency, but with a relatively small MIC increase.[36,37] It should come as no surprise, therefore, that fluoroquinolones share the pharmacodynamic linkages seen with aminoglycosides.

In Vitro Models.   Blaser and colleagues[7] published early studies of the in vitro dynamic properties of fluoroquinolones. These authors studied the quinolone enoxacin. They examined both *K. pneumoniae* and *P. aeruginosa* as the challenge organisms. They examined the kill of *Klebsiella* after exposure to two regimens of enoxacin, one administering the whole dose every 24 hours and the other administering half the dose every 12 hours. Each experiment was replicated three times. In one of the q12h replications, but in none of the once-daily experiments, there was breakthrough growth by the *Klebsiella*. Clearly, administering the whole dose once daily allowed for the best outcome. These authors also examined other doses. Reference to Figure 3 displays that, identically to aminoglycosides, the attainment of a peak/MIC ratio of greater than 10/1 results in complete sterilization of the system in every instance. This is almost assuredly due to the suppression of resistant mutants. Resistance to fluoroquinolones among gram-negative persons can often be mediated by a gyrA mutation, which usually confers an eightfold increase in MIC (but may increase it by as much as 32-fold) or by a transport mutation, in which MIC can increase by two- to fourfold. Consequently, it is understandable that peak/MIC ratios above 10/1 can often suppress not only the parent strain, but the mutant organisms as well.

Dudley and colleagues[38] examined the effect of ciprofloxacin on *P. aeruginosa* in the same system. They characterized the susceptibility of the population to ciprofloxacin at baseline, at 12 hours and at 24 hours. They documented the emergence of resistant organisms between the baseline determination and the 12-hour point (the first dosing interval), with a further increase in population resistance over the next interval. This model system demonstrates the superiority of single, high-dose administration (implying that peak may be linked to outcome) and also shows that the regrowth phenomenon is linked to emergence of resistant mutants.

Animal Models.   Leggett et al.[39] examined ciprofloxacin against *P. aeruginosa* in a neutropenic mouse thigh infection model and against *K. pneumoniae* in both neutropenic mouse thigh infections and neutropenic mouse pneumonia studies. In both instances the authors noted a minimal effect of increasing dosing interval on the P_{50} (dose mediating a 50 percent reduction in bacterial population) for both *Pseudomonas* and *Klebsiella*, out to a maximum value (6–8 hours for *Pseudomonas*, 12 hours for *Klebsiella*). This indicates that AUC/MIC may be the dynamically linked variable for quinolones.

Drusano and colleagues[40] examined lomefloxacin in a neutropenic rat model of *Pseudomonas* sepsis. A dose of 80 mg/kg was administered to cohorts of 50 animals as a single daily dose, as 40 mg/kg every 12 hours or as 20 mg/kg every 6 hours. Plasma concentration-time profiles were determined to document the peak/MIC ratios, the AUC/MIC ratios, and the time that plasma concentrations exceeded the MIC for each regimen. The once daily regimen is shown in Figure 4, with the highest peak/MIC ratio having a significantly better survivorship compared with the more fractionated regimens (74 vs. 32 vs. 36 percent). Both fractionated regimens had approximately the same survivorship curves. Decreasing the dose to 40 mg/kg/day and administering this as a once daily dose vs. 20 mg/kg every 12 hours provides virtually identical survivorship curves.

The size of the challenge used may explain the difference in findings between the two studies above. In Leggett's study, the inoculum was on the order of 10^6 organisms. With a mutational frequency to resistance usually cited as being between $1/10^7$ and $1/10^8$, it is far less likely that the inoculum would contain resistant mutants in Leggett's study. In Drusano's study, the challenge inoculum was 10^9. It is much more likely, therefore, that

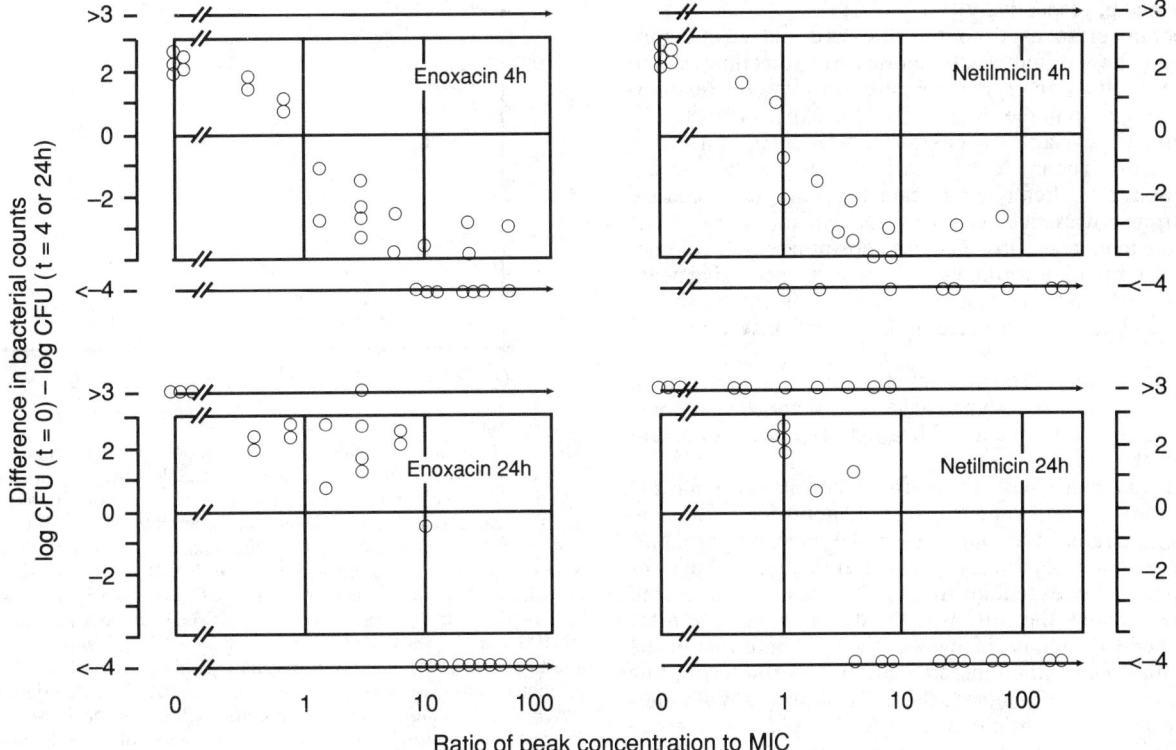

FIG. 3.   Antibacterial effect of multiple-dose regimens of enoxacin and netilmicin against five organisms. Changes in bacterial numbers during treatment periods of 4 and 24 hours are plotted against the ratios of peak concentration to MIC. t = time. (From Blaser et al.,[7] with permission.)

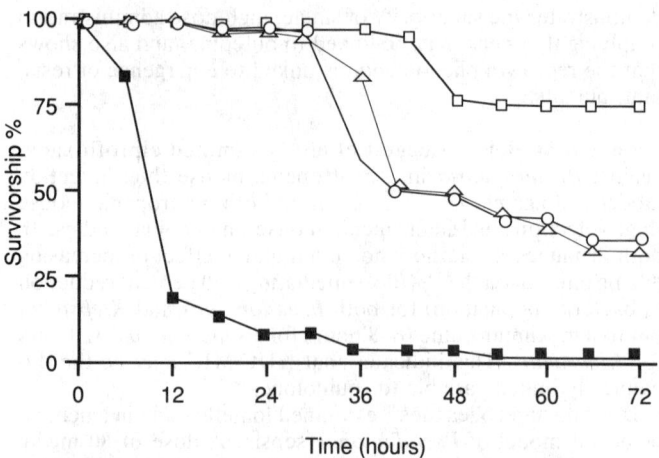

FIG. 4. Dose fractionation experiment. The MIC of lomefloxacin for the challenge organism was 1 µg/ml. Regimens of 80 mg/kg every 24 hours (□), 40 mg/kg every 12 hours (△), and 20 mg/kg every 6 hours (○) were evaluated. Control animals received a saline placebo injection (■). There were 50 animals evaluated per group. (From Drusano et al.,[40] with permission.)

there were resistant mutants in the challenge population. The large once-daily dose (80 mg/kg once daily) obtained peak/MIC ratios on the order of 20/1. The more fractionated schedules were less than 10/1 and would have a much greater chance of allowing breakthrough growth with a resistant mutant.

Further experiments in Drusano's study examined the influence of changing MIC (MIC of 1, 2, and 8 µg/ml) on survivorship. As one would expect, altering the MIC in an isogenic background alters the survivorship when the treatment does not change (survivorships of 65, 15, and 0 percent). However, producing the same peak/MIC ratio by changing dose instead of MIC produces essentially an identical survivorship curve (a comparison of challenge organisms of 1 and 4 µg/ml treated with 20 and 80 mg/kg, respectively).

The other important aspect of this study is displayed in Figure 5. It explains how different laboratories can sometimes come to differing results. Each panel of Figure 5 displays the relationship of survivorship in the single daily dose experiments to different dynamic variables (peak/MIC, AUC/MIC, and time above the MIC). The model with each variable displays an extremely good, statistically significant fit to the data because there is strong covariance between these dynamic variables. It is impossible to increase dose in a fixed dosing interval, volume, and clearance situation without simultaneously increasing peak/MIC, AUC/MIC and time above the MIC. This will be shown to have considerable importance in the following section.

Clinical Trial Data. The amount of clinical trial information regarding which pharmacodynamic variable optimizes outcome is limited. The two relevant publications represent different analyses of the same data set.

Peloquin and colleagues[41] analyzed 50 patients receiving 200 mg of ciprofloxacin intravenously every 12 hours for gram-negative lower respiratory tract infection in the intensive care unit. The study design was virtually identical to that cited above for cefmenoxime. After examining the data, these authors indicated that the time above the MIC was the dynamic variable most closely linked to outcome. However, they did note that in the patients with *Pseudomonas* infection, from whom uniformly low peak/MIC ratios were obtained, there was a high rate of emergence of resistance to ciprofloxacin. Indeed, resistance emerged in 10 of 13 of these patients.

Three years later, after adding 24 new patients, Forrest and colleagues[42] reanalyzed these data. Among the new patients, 6 infected with *Pseudomonas* also received azlocillin in combina-

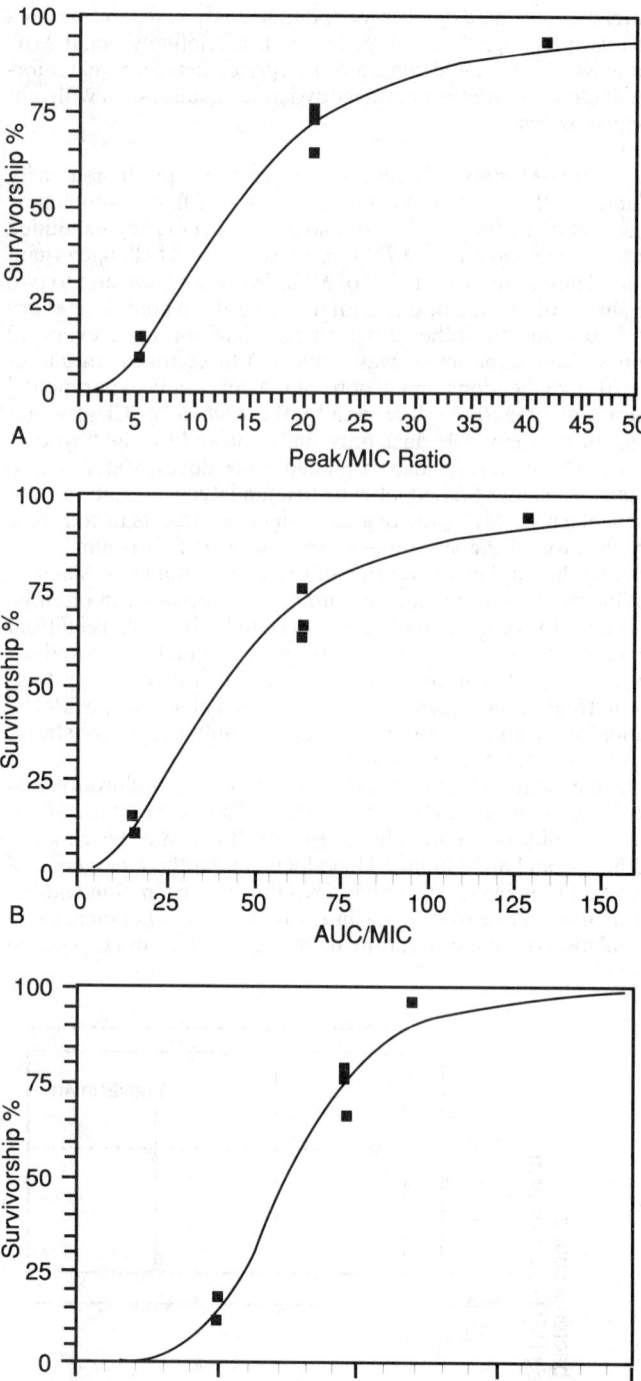

FIG. 5. Modified Hill's (sigmoid E_{max}) model evaluating survivorship as a function of three different independent variables: **(A)** the peak/MIC ratio; **(B)** the AUC/MIC ratio; and **(C)** the time that the concentration in the plasma was above the MIC. In Fig. A, % Survivorship = 100 × (peak/MIC ratio)$^{2.18}$/[(13.3)$^{2.18}$ + (peak/MIC ratio)$^{2.18}$]. r^2 = 0.989; weighted sum of squares = 6.1314; $p < 0.001$. In Fig. B, % Survivorship = 100 × (AUC/MIC ratio)$^{2.18}$/[(41.1)$^{2.18}$ + (AUC/MIC ratio)$^{2.18}$]. r^2 = 0.989; weighted sum of squares = 6.1314; $p < 0.001$. In Fig. C, % Survivorship = 100 × (t > MIC)$^{4.71}$/[(7.75$^{4.71}$ + (t > MIC)$^{4.71}$], where t > MIC is the time that concentration in plasma was above the MIC. r^2 = 0.985; weighted sum of squares = 8.3915; $p < 0.001$. This demonstrates that when administration schedule is a constant, there is maximal covariance between the pharmacodynamic variables and outcome (survivorship). (From Drusano et al.,[40] with permission.)

tion with ciprofloxacin. Another 11 patients had serious staphylococcal infections, with 5 receiving the combination of rifampin plus ciprofloxacin. Data were analyzed for both microbiologic outcome and clinical outcome. In this reanalysis, AUC/MIC was the variable most closely linked to outcome in a multivariate analysis by logistic regression. The time for the lower respiratory tract to be cleared of the pathogen was also highly significantly related to the AUC/MIC achieved. The relationships are displayed in Table 1. The probabilities of obtaining a clinical or microbiologic cure rise with increasing AUC/MIC ratio, and the time to bacterial eradication decreases.

This analysis found AUC/MIC and not peak/MIC to be most significant for a clear reason. Twenty-five patients had *P. aeruginosa* as their pathogen. Another 11 had *Staphylococcus aureus*. There were a number of *Enterobacter* spp. recovered that also achieved low (<10/1) peak/MIC ratios. Greater than half the study population had a peak/MIC ratio less than 10. The finding of AUC/MIC as the pharmacodynamically linked variable is then perfectly consistent with the animal model data cited above. Furthermore, the emergence of resistance in *Pseudomonas* commented on by Peloquin et al.[41] in this setting of low peak/MIC ratio (10 of 13 patients with *P. aeruginosa* as their pathogen had emergence of resistance to ciprofloxacin during therapy) is once again consistent with both the in vitro and animal model data. The suppression of this emergence of resistance by higher ratios has been cited above as a possible explanation for the better survivorship in the animal model system with the once daily dosing regimen.

For fluoroquinolones, as for both β-lactams and aminoglycosides, the in vitro, animal model and clinical data come to concordant results. Here, the importance of obtaining high peak concentrations (to suppress resistant mutants) is most clearly seen and the ultimate outcome (microbial kill) is seen most clearly to be linked to AUC/MIC. If one does not obtain a high enough peak/MIC ratio, the mutant subpopulation may emerge, as is seen in the in vitro model system. This can lead to significantly greater rates of failure of therapy, as was seen in the animal model data of Drusano et al.[40] This emergence of resistance in situations of low peak/MIC was well demonstrated clinically by Peloquin and colleagues.[41]

For aminoglycosides and fluoroquinolones, both concentration dependent in kill rate, attainment of high peak/MIC ratios and large AUC/MIC ratios is important. Both of these aims can be attained by the administration of single daily doses. For aminoglycosides, this chain of logic has already led to the institution of once-daily therapy at two institutions, although general adaptation of this strategy must await more clinical data.[43,44] β-Lactams, on the other hand, being relatively concentration independent in kill rate, need to be administered on a more frequent basis, keeping trough concentrations (probably of free drug) above the MIC of the infecting pathogen. Because there is a slight concentration dependency of kill rate for β-lactams up to two to four times the MIC, and because penetration to some specialized sites of infection results in lower concentrations than observed in plasma, it may be wise to attempt to obtain two to

four times the MIC of free drug at trough for β-lactams as a clinical goal.

Schentag and colleagues[45] have published a paper in which they indicate that AUC/MIC is the pharmacodynamically linked variable for β-lactams and fluoroquinolones. They come to this conclusion on the basis of the same AUC/MIC ratio (of 125–250) being predictive of a good outcome for both β-lactams and fluoroquinolones. However, the preponderance of evidence (see above) indicates that time above the MIC is the most important variable linked to outcome of β-lactam therapy. This raises the question as to why the Schentag et al.[45] analysis was able to find both drug classes having the same AUC/MIC breakpoint for a good clinical outcome. The answer can be found in the fact that there was a fixed dosing interval in both trials. There was an increase in the covariance seen between peak/MIC, AUC, MIC, and time above the MIC. That is, one cannot increase the AUC/MIC on a fixed schedule without simultaneously increasing the peak/MIC as well as the time above the MIC. Indeed, this can be seen in the animal model data presented in Figure 5. All these data are from fixed interval experiments (once daily). Each pharmacodynamic variable precisely and statistically significantly describes the outcome. This is because of covariance. However, as the data of Drusano et al.[40] demonstrate, peak/MIC or AUC/MIC are the causally linked pharmacodynamic variables. This explains why two different analyses of essentially the same data set[41,42] could arrive at different pharmacodynamically linked variables (time above the MIC vs. AUC/MIC).

However, one can use this AUC/MIC ratio breakpoint to advantage, as long as the clinician already has the patient on an optimal schedule. The daily AUC/MIC can then be measured and drug dosage adjusted to ensure the best probability of a good outcome.

Antiretroviral Agents

In Vitro and Animal Models. Therapy with antiretroviral agents is still in its infancy. Bilello et al.[46] have adapted the in vitro model system of Blaser et al.[7] to examine the growth of HIV and to determine the impact of different antiretroviral agents on the replication of HIV. They demonstrated that there was no difference in the impact on viral replication when 2',3'-dideoxy-didehydroxythymidine (D4T) was administered as a continuous infusion or an every 12 hour dose with matching AUC. They further demonstrated that D4T started to lose its viral inhibitory effect on the HIV-1 MN strain examined as doses of less than 0.5 mg/kg/day, a value in excellent agreement with that seen in clinical trials.[47,48]

The use of animal models for HIV-related research has not focused to any great degree on the pharmcodynamics of effect. However, two groups have demonstrated that continuous administration of zidovudine was more effective than intermittent administration in suppression of two different murine leukemia viruses in a mouse model.[49,50] However, one needs to exercise caution regarding the interpretation of animal data in this instance, as murine cells anabolize zidovudine much differently than do human cells.[51]

Clinical Trial Data. Pizzo et al.[52] and Balis et al.[53] examined the continuous infusion of zidovudine in HIV-positive children. However, while showing good effect, this study did not examine intermittently administered zidovudine.

The nucleoside analog ddI has had two demonstrations of linkage of effect to a measured dynamic variable. Drusano and colleagues[54] analyzed the phase I clinical trial data reported by Lambert et al.[55] They examined two different surrogate markers, CD4 count change and suppression of p24 from baseline, and attempted to link these variables to measured exposure to ddI as indexed to area under the concentration-time curve. CD4 counts were found to change mainly as a function of the baseline

TABLE 1. AUC/MIC Vs. Percentage of Clinical and Microbiologic Cures

AUC/MIC Range	Total No. of Patients	Clinical No. of Patients	%	Microbiologic No. of Patients	%
0–62.5	9	4	44	2	22
62.5–125	10	4	40	3	30
125–250	16	14	88	13	81
250–500	7	5	71	6	86
500–5541	22	17	77	18	82

(From Forrest et al.,[42] with permission.)

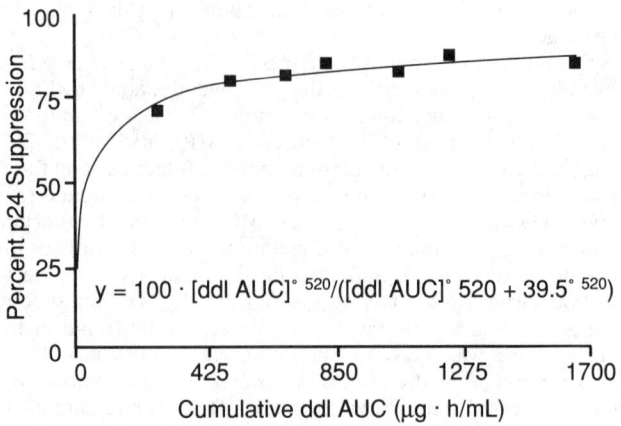

FIG. 6. Relation between the suppression of p24 antigen and the cumulative area under the plasma concentration-time curve of dideoxyinosine (ddI) in a typical patient. This figure shows the relation between ddI exposure by cumulative ddI area under the curve (AUC) and suppression of p24 antigen from the baseline value as analyzed by a sigmoid E_{max} model ($r^2 = 0.84$, $p < 0.001$). (From Drusano et al.,[54] with permission.)

count of CD4 cells and was not importantly influenced by the amount of ddI exposure. However, suppression of p24 was found to be directly linked to the cumulative AUC of exposure of the patient to ddI. This can be seen for a typical patient in Figure 6.

Drusano et al.[54] used the relationship detailed above in conjunction with the findings of Yarchoan et al.,[56] who showed that the ability to stay on ddI therapy decreased dramatically at doses higher than 10 mg/kg/day, to predict that lower doses of ddI (in the range of 200 mg bid) would be at least as good as higher doses of ddI. This prediction was supported by the results of ACTG trial 116B/117,[57] in which 250 mg bid was at least as good as 375 mg of ddI bid.

Pizzo, Balis, and coworkers also demonstrated in a study of ddI use in HIV-infected children that the AUC of ddI was significantly associated with change in IQ score.[58] In some studies, outcome of ddI therapy could be linked to measured exposure to the drug. This underlines the need to continue to develop these relationships for other drugs used for antiretroviral chemotherapy.

For antiretrovirals, as for antibacterials, relationships can be demonstrated between measures of drug exposure and the outcome of the patient's infection. Not addressed in this chapter, but of critical importance, is the fact that many anti-ineffective agents have concentration-related adverse effects. These relationships also need delineation, and the best results for seriously ill patient populations can be achieved when the treating physician employs a dose and schedule of drug (whether antibacterial, antifungal, or antiviral) that develops the best clinical outcome for the smallest cost in attendant toxicity.

REFERENCES

1. Craig WA, Ebert SC. Killing and regrowth of bacteria in vitro: A review. Pediatr Infect Dis J. 1991;S74:63–70.
2. Smith JT. Awakening the slumbering potential of the 4-quinolone antibacterials. Pharmacol J. 1984;233:299–305.
3. David HL, Newman CM. Some observations on the genetics of isoniazid resistance in the tubercle bacilli. Am Rev Respir Dis. 1971;104:508–15.
4. Peterson LR. Quinolone resistance in clinical practice: Occurrence and importance. In: Hooper DC, Wolfson JS, eds. Quinolone Antimicrobial Agents. 2nd Ed. Washington DC: American Society for Microbiology; 1993:119–37.
5. St. Clair MH, Hartigan PM, Andrews JC, et al. Zidovudine resistance, syncytium-inducing phenotype, and HIV disease preogression in a case-control study. J AIDS. 1993;6:891–7.
6. Haag R, Lexa P, Werkhauser I. Artifacts in dilution pharmacokinetic models caused by adherent bacteria. Antimicrob Agents Chemother. 1986;29:765–768.
7. Blaser J, Stone BB, Groner MC, et al. Comparative study with enoxacin and
netilmicin in a pharmacodynamic model to determine importance of ratio of antibiotic peak concentration to mic for bacterial activity and emergency of resistance. Antimicrob Agents Chemother. 1987;31:1054–70.
8. Zinner ZH, Dudley MN, Gilbert D, et al. Effect of dose and schedule on cefoperazone pharmacoynamics in an in vitro model of infection in a neutropenic host. Am J Med. 1988;85(Suppl 1A):56–8.
9. Merrikin DJ, Briant J, Rolinson GN. Effect of protein binding on antibiotic activity in vivo. J Antimicrob Chemother. 1983;11:233–8.
10. Gerber AU, Craig WA, Brugger HP, et al. Impact of dosing intervals on activity of gentamicin and ticarcillin against *Pseudomonas aeruginosa* in granulocytopenic mice. J Infect Dis. 1983;147:910–7.
11. Roosendaal R, Bakker-Woudenber IA, van den Berg JC, et al. Therapeutic efficacy of continuous versus intermittent administration of ceftazidime in an experimental *Klebsiella pneumoniae*. J Infect Dis. 1985;152:373–8.
12. Roosendaal R, Bakker-Woudenberg IA, Berghe-Van Raffe M, et al. Continuous versus intermittent administration of ceftazidime in experimental *Klebsiella pneumoniae* pneumonia in normal and leukopenic rats. Antimicrob Agents Chemother. 1986;30:403–8.
13. Vogelman B, Gudmundsson S, Leggett J, et al. Correlation of antimicrobial pharmacokinetic parameters with therapeutic efficacy in an animal model. J Infect Dis. 1988;158:831–47.
14. Leggett JE, Fantin B, Ebert S, et al. Comparative antibiotic dose-effect relations at several dosing intervals in murine pneumonitis and thigh-infection models. J Infect Dis. 1989;159:281–92.
15. Flückiger U, Segessenmann C, Gerber AU. Integration of pharmacokinetics and pharmacodynamics of imipenem in an human-adapted mouse model. Antimicrob Agents Chemother. 1991;35:1905–1910.
16. Bodey GP, Ketchel SJ, Rodriguez V. A randomized study of carbenicillin plus cefamandole or tobramycin in the treatment of febrile episodes in cancer patients. Am J Med. 1979;67:608–16.
17. Drusano GL. Role of pharmacokinetics in the outcome of infections. Antimicrob Agents Chemother. 1988;32:289–97.
18. Leggett JE, Craig WA. Enhancing effect of serum ultrafiltrate on the activity of cephalosporins against gram-negative bacilli. Antimicrob Agents Chemother. 1989;33:35–40.
19. Schentag JJ, Smith IL, Swanson DJ, et al. Role for dual individualization with cefmenoxime. Am J Med. 1984;77(Suppl 6a):43–50.
20. Gerber AU, Wiprachtiger P, Stettler-Spichiger U, et al. Constant infusion vs. intermittent doses of gentamicin against *Pseudomonas aeruginosa* in vitro. J Infect Dis. 1982;145:554–60.
21. Nilsson LT, Soren L. Selective growth of resistant variants during incubation of Enterobacteriaceae with four aminoglycosides. J Antimicrob Chemother. 1986;18:317–24.
22. Gerber AU, Craig WA. Aminoglycoside-selected subpopulations of *Pseudomonas aeruginosa*: Characterization and virulence in normal and neutropenic mice. J Lab Clin Med. 1981;100:671–681.
23. Bryan LE, Kwan S. Roles of ribosomal binding, membrane potential, and electron transport in bacterial uptake of streptomycin and gentamicin. Antimicrob Agents Chemother. 1983;23:835–45.
24. Bryan LE, Kwan S. Aminoglycoside-resistant mutants of *Pseudomonas aeruginosa* deficient in cytochrome d, nitrite reductase, and aerobic transport. Antimicrob Agents Chemother. 1981;19:958–64.
25. Gerber AU, Feller-Segessenmann C. In-vivo assessment of in-vitro killing patterns of *Pseudomonas aeruginosa*. J Antimicrob Chemother. 1985;15(Suppl A):201–6.
26. Gerber AU, Vastola AP, Brandel J, Craig WA. Selection of aminoglycoside-resistant variants of *Pseudomonas aeruginosa* in an in vivo model. J Infect Dis. 1982;146:691–7.
27. Bundtzen RW, Gerber AU, Cohn DL, et al. Postantibiotic suppression of bacterial growth. Rev Infect Dis. 1981;3:28–37.
28. Kapusnik JE, Hackbarth CJ, Chambers HF, et al. Single, large, daily dosing versus intermittent dosing of tobramycin for treating experimental *Pseudomonas* pneumonia. J Infect Dis. 1988;158:7–12.
29. Pruul H, McDonald PJ. Enhancement of leukocyte activity against *Escherichia coli* after brief exposure to chloramphenicol. J Antimicrob Chemother. 1979;16:695–700.
30. Wood CA, Norton DR, Kohlhepp SJ, et al. The influence of tobramycin dosage regiments on nephrotoxicity, ototoxicity, and antibacterial efficacy in a rat model of subcutaneous abscess. J Infect Dis. 1988;158:13–22.
31. Noone PT, Parsons MC, Pattison JR, et al. Experience in monitoring gentamicin therapy during treatment of serious gram-negative sepsis. Br Med J 1974;1:477–81.
32. Powell SH, Thompson WL, Luthe MA, et al. Once-daily vs. continuous aminoglycoside dosing: Efficacy and toxicity in animal and clinical studies of gentamicin, netilmicin, and tobramycin. J Infect Dis. 1983;14:918–32.
33. Moore RD, Lietman PS, Smith CR. Clinical response to aminoglycoside therapy: Importance of the ratio of peak concentration to minimal inhibitory concentration. J Infect Dis. 1987;155:93–9.
34. Moore RD, Smith CR, Lietman PS. The association of aminoglycoside plasma levels with mortality in patients with gram-negative bacteremia. J Infect Dis. 1984;149:443–8.
35. Moore RD, Smith CR, Lietman PS. Association of aminoglycoside plasma levels with therapeutic outcome in gram-negative pneumonia. Am J Med. 1984;77:657–62.
36. Hooper DC, Wolfson JS, Ng EY, et al. Mechanism of action of and resistant to ciprofloxacin. Am J Med 1987;82(Suppl. 4A):12–20.

37. Dudley MN. Pharmacodynamics and pharmacokinetics of antibiotics with special reference to the fluoroquinolones. Am J Med. 1991;91:45S–50S.
38. Dudley MN, Mandler HD, Gilbert D, et al. Pharmacokinetics and pharmacodynamics of intravenous ciprofloxacin. Am J Med. 1987;82:363–8.
39. Leggett JE, Ebert S, Fantin B, et al. Comparative dose-effect relations at several dosing intervals for beta-lactam, aminoglycoside and quinolone antibiotics against gram-negative bacilli in murine thigh-infection and pneumonitis models. Scand J Infect Dis. 1991;74:179–84.
40. Drusano GL, Johnson DE, Rosen M, Standiford HC. Pharmacodynamics of a fluoroquinolone antimicrobial agent in a neutropenic rat model of *Pseudomonas* sepsis. Antimicrob Agents Chemother. 1993;37:483–90.
41. Peloquin CA, Cumbo TJ, Nix DE, et al. Evaluation of intravenous ciprofloxacin in patients with nosocomial lower respiratory tract infections. Arch Intern Med. 1989;149:2269–73.
42. Forrest A, Nix DE, Ballow CH, et al. Pharmacodynamics of intravenous ciprofloxacin in seriously ill patients. Antimicrob Agents Chemother. 1993; 37:1073–81.
43. Gilbert DN. Once-daily aminoglycoside therapy. Antimicrob Agents Chemother. 1991;35:399–405.
44. Nicolau DP, Belliveau PP, Freeman CH, et al. Once daily aminoglycosides: Experience with 500 patients in a hospital-wide program (Abstract 85). Program and Abstracts of the 33rd Interscience Conference on Antimicrobial Agents and Chemotherapy. New Orleans, Louisiana, October 17–20, 1993.
45. Schentag JJ, Nix DE, Adelman MH. Mathematical examination of dual individualization principles (i): Relationships between AUC above MIC and area under the inhibitory curve for cefmenoxime, ciprofloxacin, and tobramycin. Ann Pharmacother. 1991;25:1050–7.
46. Bilello JA, Bauer G, Dudley MN, et al. The effect of 2′,3′-dideoxy-2′,3′-didehydrothymidine (D4T) in an in vivo hollow fiber pharmacodynamic model system correlates with results of dose ranging clinical studies. 1993. In Press.
47. Anderson R, Myer W, Balch F, et al. Antiviral effects of stavudine (d4T) therapy. Abstract WeB1010. VIIIth International Conference on AIDS. Amsterdam, The Netherlands, 1992.
48. Browne MJ, Mayer KH, Chafee SB, et al. 2′,3′-Didehydro-3′-deoxythymidine (d4T) in patients with AIDS or AIDS-related complex: A phase I trial. J Infect Dis. 1993;167:21–9.
49. Sinet M, Harcouet L, Desforges B, et al. Efficacy of continuous zidovudine infusion at early stages of retroviral infection in mice. J AIDS. 1992;5:557–82.
50. Bilello JA, Eiseman JL, Standiford HC, et al. Impact of dosing schedule upon suppression of a retrovirus in a murine model of AIDS encephalopathy. Antimicrob Agents Chemother. 1994;38:628–31.
51. Ho H, Hitchcock MJM. Cellular pharmacology of 2′,3′-dideoxy-2′,3′-didehydrothymidine, a nucleoside analogue active against human immunodeficiency virus. Antimicrob Agents Chemother. 1989;33:844–9.
52. Pizzo PA, Eddy J, Falloon J, et al. Effect of continuous intravenous infusion of zidovudine (AZT) in children with symptomatic HIV infection. N Engl J Med. 1988;319:889–96.
53. Balis FM, Pizzo PA, Murphy RF, et al. The pharmacokinetics of zidovudine administered by continuous infusion in children. Ann Intern Med. 1989;110: 279–85.
54. Drusano GL, Yuen GJ, Lambert JS, et al. Relationship between dideoxyinosine expose, CD4 counts, and p24 antigen levels in human immunodeficiency virus infection. A phase 1 trial. Ann Intern Med. 1992;116;562–6.
55. Lambert JS, Seidlin M, Reichman RC, et al. 2′,3′-Dideoxyinosine (ddi) in patients with the acquired immunodeficiency syndrome or AIDS-related complex. A phase 1 trial. N Engl J Med. 1990;322:1333–40.
56. Yarchoan R, Pluda JM, Thomas RV, et al. Long-term toxicity/activity profile of 2′,3′-dideoxyinosine in aids or aids-related complex. Lancet. 1990;336: 526–529.
57. Kahn JO, Lagakos SW, Richman DD, et al. A controlled trial comparing continued zidovudine with didanosine in human immunodeficiency virus infection. N Engl J Med. 1992;327:581–7.
58. Butler KM, Husson RN, Balis FM, et al. Dideoxyinosine in children with symptomatic human immunodeficiency virus infection. N Engl J Med. 1991; 324:137–44.

15. PENICILLINS

HENRY F. CHAMBERS
HAROLD C. NEU

Penicillin was discovered by Fleming[1] in 1928. He isolated penicillin from *Penicillium notatum* in 1929 but was unsuccessful in attempts to obtain significant amounts of the agent. The work of Florey, Chain, and associates in 1941 made possible the commercial production of penicillin G. In 1939 Florey at the Sir William Dunn School of Pathology began to work out the isolation, structure, and properties of the compound. In 1940 his group showed that penicillin protected mice experimentally infected with streptococci, and by 1941 they had produced enough penicillin to treat a few patients, the first of whom was a British policeman infected with both staphylococci and streptococci. As a result of World War II, production of penicillin was undertaken in the United States. Initial clinical trials at Yale and the Mayo Clinic were so successful that the U.S. Army began to use the material to treat streptococcal, gonococcal, and treponemal infections. As fermentation techniques improved, production of large amounts of pure drug became possible, and by the end of the 1940s penicillin G was available for general use in the United States.

CHEMISTRY

The basic structure of the majority of commercially available penicillins is a nucleus that consists of a thiazolidine ring, the β-lactam ring, and a side chain (Fig. 1). The penicillin nucleus is a condensation of alanine and β-dimethylcysteine. Penicillins currently in use are dextrorotatory and usually exist as salts combined with alkaline earth metals such as sodium or potassium. The β-lactam ring is essential for antibacterial activity. The side chain determines in large part the antibacterial spectrum and pharmacologic properties of a particular penicillin. Although biosynthesis of penicillin has been achieved, it has not proved to be a useful technique, and fermentation remains the method of production of penicillin G.

The appearance of β-lactamase-producing organisms, particularly *Staphylococcus aureus,* prompted studies to develop compounds with resistance to hydrolysis by β-lactamases and also to find agents more active than penicillin G against gram-negative species. In 1959, Batchelor et al.[2] isolated the penicillin nucleus 6-amino-penicillanic acid from a precursor-depleted fermentation of *Penicillium chrysogenum.* This made possible the production and testing of numerous semisynthetic penicillins, the first of which was methicillin, active against β-lactamase-producing *S. aureus;* followed by ampicillin, active against selected gram-negative bacilli; and carbenicillin, which had activity against *Pseudomonas aeruginosa.* Since then scores of agents with different pharmacologic and antimicrobial properties have been developed.

MECHANISM OF ACTION

We do not know precisely how penicillins kill bacterial cells. Study of the action of penicillins has elucidated many aspects of bacterial physiology, but recent advances suggest that the

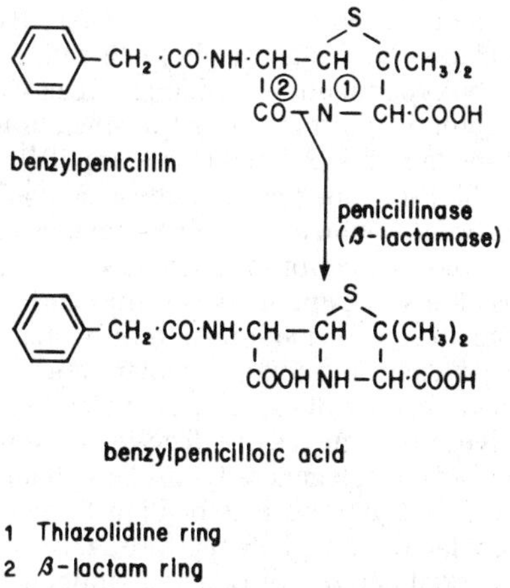

FIG. 1. Structure of penicillin and site of β-lactamase attack.

concept that penicillin kills simply by blocking the last step in cell wall synthesis is a simplistic one. The cell wall of bacteria is assembled in a series of enzymatic steps that involve at least 30 enzymes.

Bacterial Cell Walls

The cell walls of both gram-positive and gram-negative bacteria are held in a rigid manner, protecting against osmotic rupture by the peptidoglycan, also called *murein sacculus*.[3,4] The cell wall of gram-positive bacteria is a large, 50–100 molecular layer, whereas the peptidoglycan component of gram-negative bacteria is only one or two molecules thick. An outer lipopolysaccharide layer, which is not found in gram-positive bacteria, is present on top of the peptidoglycan in gram-negative species.

Peptidoglycans are long polysaccharide chains in which N-acetylglucosamine (NAG) and N-acetylmuramic (NAM) acid alternate in a linear form. Individual chains are cross-linked by short peptides linked in amide linkage to the penultimate D-alanyl group of the N-acetylmuramic acid. In gram-negative species the 6-amino group of diaminopimelic acid is linked to the carboxyalanine terminus of another chain.[4] Interestingly, percent cross-linking is less in *Escherichia coli* (25 percent) than in *S. aureus* (90 percent).[5]

Peptidoglycan synthesis has been divided into three stages. The first is the synthesis of UDP-NAM-pentapeptide and UDP-NAG. These two compounds are transported across the cytoplasmic membrane by a lipid-soluble carrier that is a C_{55} isoprenyl alcohol phosphate. Transglycosylation of disaccharide monomer into peptidoglycan polymer occurs at this stage. The final reaction is cross-linking the new peptidoglycan into the existing peptidoglycan. In this final reaction a free amino group on the third amino acid (or on the terminal residue of a short peptide chain attached to the third amino acid) of the NAM-pentapeptide of one strand displaces the terminal D-alanine from a pentapeptide of a second strand in a transpeptidation reaction. This transpeptidation reaction is sensitive to inhibition by penicillin. There appear to be distinct transpeptidases that provide for anchoring of new peptidoglycan to old that cross-link special structures and that make the cell wall septum. Although there are other penicillin-sensitive reactions, such as the effects on carboxypeptidase, these reactions do not seem to be critical in gram-negative species. The most telling argument that penicillin inactivates transpeptidases was the stereochemistry modeling performed by Strominger's group,[6] which supports an acylenzyme intermediate because of the structural similarity of penicillin and the acyl-D-alanyl-D-alanine.

Penicillin-Binding Proteins

Bacteria produce four types of penicillin-binding proteins (PBPs), which structurally resemble and probably are derived from serine proteases.[7] High-molecular-weight PBPs (i.e., more than 50 kD) and low-molecular-weight PBPs catalyze transpeptidation and carboxypeptidation reactions of cell wall assembly. Penicillin receptor PBPs transmit a transmembrane signal for induction of β-lactamases. β-Lactamases are PBPs that catalyze hydrolysis of the β-lactam ring, thereby inactivating the drug. PBPs are membrane bound except for β-lactamases, which may be either secreted or membrane associated. Transpeptidases form the cross-links in peptidoglycan, and carboxypeptidases possibly are important for modification of peptidoglycan. Both high-molecular-weight and low-molecular-weight PBPs are inhibited by β-lactam antibiotics, which covalently bind by acylation of the active site serine residue. The critical functions essential for survival of the cell generally reside with high-molecular-weight PBPs. Consequently, it is binding to and inhibition of the high-molecular-weight PBPs that probably are responsible for the antibacterial activity of β-lactam antibiotics.

PBPs of a given organism are numbered according to molecular weight, with the highest molecular weight protein being designated PBP 1, the next highest, PBP 2, and so on. If what initially seemed to be one PBP (e.g., PBP 2) is subsequently found to be two or more distinct proteins, rather than renumbering all the PBPs, letters are used to differentiate the individual PBPs of similar molecular weight (e.g., PBP 2a, PBP 2b, and PBP 2x), or the newly identified PBP may be designated with a prime sign (e.g., PBP 2'). PBPs assigned the same number but produced by different species are not necessarily related or of similar function, and the numbering of PBPs for gram-positive bacteria bears no relation to the numbering for gram-negative bacteria.

PBPs account for approximately 1 percent of membrane proteins. PBPs vary both in amounts present and in the physiologic functions they serve during cell wall assembly. They also differ in their affinities for binding β-lactam antibiotics, which explains at least in part why the β-lactam antibiotics differ in their antibacterial properties and spectrum of activity. Spratt's studies[8,9] in *E. coli* were the first to elucidate the different functions of PBPs. Inhibition of PBP 1b or a substitute enzyme 1a results in cell lysis. PBP 1 is speculated to be important for cell elongation. Inhibition of PBP 2 results in formation of round cells that eventually lyse, suggesting that PBP 2 has a role in an initial step in cell elongation and in determining the rod shape of *E. coli*. Inhibition of PBP 3 produces long, filamentous cells, indicating that it is important for the ordered process of cross wall formation and cell division. The functions performed by PBPs in other species have not been well defined, but presumably also are distinct.

No single PBP species is the target of β-lactam antibiotics, which produce their lethal effect on bacteria by inactivation of multiple PBPs simultaneously.[10] The lethal effect in both gram-positive and gram-negative organisms appears to be cell cycle dependent with inhibition of PBPs leading to disruption of a critical event probably at the time of cell division.[11,12] Unopposed action of autolysins when PBPs are inhibited by β-lactam antibiotics may also contribute to the antibacterial effect in some organisms.

BACTERIAL RESISTANCE

Three mechanisms account for clinically significant bacterial resistance to β-lactam antibiotics: destruction of antibiotic by β-lactamase, failure of antibiotic to penetrate to PBP targets, and low-affinity binding of antibiotic to PBPs. Of these three mechanisms, β-lactamase destruction of antibiotic is the most important.[13] β-Lactamases, which are a type of PBP, covalently react with the β-lactam bond to form an acyl-enzyme intermediate, which undergoes rapid hydrolysis, thereby destroying the activity of the drug. β-Lactamases are classified on the basis of their affinity for β-lactam compounds and amino acid composition (Fig. 2). β-Lactamase of staphylococci is plasmid encoded and inducible by β-lactam antibiotics. Although it may be membrane bound, staphylococcal β-lactamase, which acts primarily as a penicillinase, is an exoenzyme that is liberated into the surrounding medium in which it destroys penicillin before it can reach the target PBPs. The activities of methicillin and the isoxazolyl penicillins are due to their stability to staphylococcal β-lactamase.

β-Lactamases of gram-negative bacteria are cell-associated enzymes located in the periplasmic space that lies between the inner (cytoplasmic) membrane and outer lipopolysaccharide membrane. Thus, gram-negative β-lactamases are concentrated and strategically located to protect the target PBPs from exposure to active β-lactam antibiotics. Gram-negative β-lactamases may be encoded either on the chromosome or on plasmids, produced constitutively or as inducible enzymes, with affinity for penicillins or cephalosporins or both types of compounds. All gram-negative species probably contain at least small amounts of β-lactamase. Differences among β-lactam compounds in

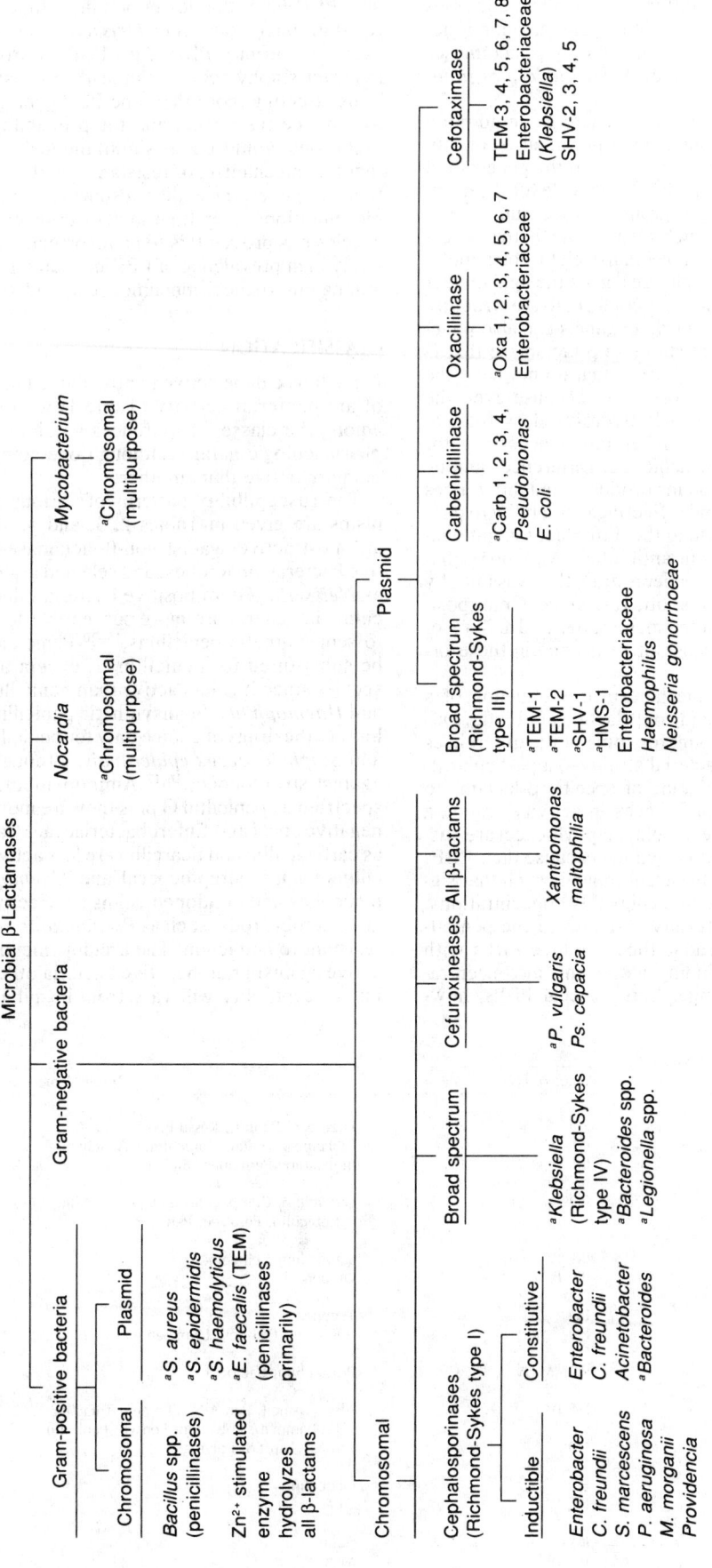

FIG. 2. Diagrammatic representation of β-lactamases.

binding affinity and susceptibility to hydrolysis by gram-negative β-lactactamases and the type of β-lactamase that is produced account for some of the differences in their activities against gram-negative bacteria. For example, carbenicillin is destroyed at a much slower rate than ampicillin by β-lactamases produced by *Enterobacter cloacae* or *Morganella morganii;* consequently, it is more active.

The outer membrane of gram-negative bacteria, in addition to concentrating β-lactamase within the periplasm, also contributes to resistance because it acts as a barrier to the penetration of β-lactam compounds to target PBPs. To provide for the entry of essential nutrients into the cell, gram-negative outer membrane contains porin proteins, which form channels that selectively permit penetration of low-molecular-weight polar molecules of appropriate structure and charge across the lipid bilayer into the cell. β-Lactam compounds that conform to the structure and charge requirements of these porin channels can also penetrate into the cell and, if they are stable to β-lactamase that is present, bind to target PBPs. Compounds that do not have the appropriate structure penetrate poorly and, because even the most stable compounds can be slowly hydrolyzed by β-lactamase, the minimum intracellular concentration necessary for binding to target PBPs cannot be achieved. Differences among bacteria with respect to porin proteins produced and differences in structure of β-lactam compounds affecting their ability to pass through porin channels contribute to the differences in antibacterial activity among the β-lactam antibiotics. Mutations that alter porin protein structure may render a strain that was initially susceptible to a given β-lactam antibiotic resistance. Gram-positive bacteria do not have an outer membrane, and failure of antibiotic penetration is not a cause of resistance in these organisms.

The third type of resistance mechanism is production of a PBP that has low affinity for binding of β-lactam antibiotic. Differences in binding of PBPs account for some of the differences in susceptibility of individual bacterial strains to a particular β-lactam antibiotic. Differential binding of specific β-lactams to target PBPs also accounts for differences in activity against a single organism or species. For example, staphylococci are susceptible to penicillinase-resistant penicillins because their PBPs have relatively high affinity for these compounds such that significant binding occurs at clinically achievable concentrations. Enterococci, however, are naturally resistant to the penicillinase-resistant penicillins because they produce PBPs with lower affinity, and significant binding occurs only at concentrations above the therapeutic range. Enterococcal PBPs, however, generally have high affinity for penicillin and ampicillin, and thus they are susceptible to these drugs. Mutations in resident PBP genes that lower binding affinity (e.g., as in penicillin-resistant pneumococci or *Neisseria* spp.) or the presence of an extra low affinity PBP (e.g., PBP 2a produced by methicillin-resistant staphylococci) can lead to resistance. Multiple mutations affecting more than one PBP gene generally are required to produce resistance, and the probability that several unique mutations would occur simultaneously is remote, suggesting that this mechanism of resistance might not be clinically important. However, the ability of some bacteria to accumulate multiple mutations over time and to transfer mutant genes across species has proven this to be incorrect, as evidence by the relatively high prevalence of PBP-mediated resistance to penicillins among enterococci, pneumococci, and staphylococci.[14]

CLASSIFICATION

Penicillins can be conveniently divided into classes on the basis of antibacterial activity (Table 1) with considerable overlap among the classes. Differences within a class usually are of a pharmacologic nature, although one compound in a class may be more active than another.

The susceptibility patterns of various species of microorganisms are given in Tables 2, 3, and 4. The natural penicillins are most active against non-β-lactamase-producing gram-positive bacteria, anaerobes, and selected gram-negative cocci, such as *Neisseria.* Gram-positive bacteria inhibited by natural penicillins in general are more susceptible to these penicillins than to semisynthetic penicillins.[15–20] Penicillin V (used orally) can be substituted for penicillin G, except against gram-negative species since it is less active than penicillin G against *Neisseria* and *Haemophilus.* Semisynthetic penicillinase-resistant penicillins are the drugs of choice only for penicillin-resistant *S. aureus* and *Staphylococcus epidermidis,* although they also are active against streptococci.[16,17] Aminopenicillins possess the same spectrum as penicillin G plus they are more active against gram-negative cocci and Enterobacteriaceae. Carboxypenicillins such as carbenicillin and ticarcillin are less active than the ureidopenicillins against streptococcal and *Haemophilus* spp. Carboxypenicillins and ureidopenicillins have activity against gram-negative aerobic rods, such as *Pseudomonas aeruginosa,* which are resistant to ampicillin. The ureidopenicillins generally are more active against gram-negative bacteria other than *Pseudomonas,* but susceptibility will vary from hospital to hospital and from

TABLE 1. Classification of Penicillins

	Routes of Use	Trade Names
Natural penicillins		
Penicillin G	PO	Pfizerpen, Pentids, Kesso-Pen
	IM	Procaine-Wycillin, Duracillin, Crysticillin
	IM	Benzathine-Permapen, Bicillin
Penicillin G potassium or sodium	IV	
Penicillin V	PO	Ledercillin, Compocillin, Betapen, V-cillin, Veetids, Uticillin, S-K penicillin, Robicillin, Pen-Vee, Penapar
Penicillinase-resistant penicillins		
Methicillin	IM, IV	Staphcillin, Celbenin
Nafcillin	IM, IV	Unipen
Isoxazolyl penicillins		
Cloxacillin	PO	Tegopen
Dicloxacillin	PO	Veracillin, Pathocil, Dynapen
Flucloxacillin	PO	
Oxacillin	PO, IM, IV	Prostaphlin, Bactocill
Aminopenicillins		
Ampicillin	IM, IV	Alpen, Amcil, Pen A/N, Omipen, Totacillin, Super, S-K ampicillin, Principen, Probampcin, Polycillin, Pensyn, Penbritin
Amoxicillin	PO	Amoxil, Larotid, Polymax
Carboxy and indanyl penicillins		
Indanylcarbenicillin	PO	Geocillin
Ticarcillin	IM, IV	Ticar
Extended-spectrum ureidopenicillins		
Azlocillin	IM IV	Azlin
Mezlocillin	IM, IV	Mezlin
Piperacillin	IM, IV	Pipral, Pipracil

TABLE 2. Usual Minimal Inhibitory Concentrations (MIC) of Penicillins Against Cocci

	Mean Minimun Inhibitory Concentration (μg/ml)							
	Penicillin G	Penicillin V	Ampicillin, Amoxicillin	Methicillin	Oxacillin, Cloxacillin Dicloxacillin	Nafcillin	Ticarcillin	Azlocillin Mezlocillin Piperacillin
Streptococcus pneumoniae	0.01[a]	0.02[a]	0.02[a]	0.1[a]	0.04	0.02	0.4	0.02
Streptococcus pyogenes	0.005	0.01	0.02	0.2	0.04	0.02	0.2	0.02
Streptococcus agalactiae	0.005	0.01	0.02	0.2	0.06	0.02	0.2	0.15
Viridans streptococci	0.01	0.01	0.05	0.1	0.1	0.06	0.2	0.12
Enterococcus faecalis	3.0	6.0	1.5[c]	>25	>25	>25	50	1.5
Peptostreptococcus	0.2	0.5	0.2	2.0	0.6	0.5	0.4	0.8
Staphylococcus aureus Penase-negative	0.02	0.02	0.05	1.0	0.3	0.25	1.2	0.8
Penase-positive	>25	>25	>25	2.0	0.4	0.25	25	25
Staphylococcus epidermidis	0.02[b]	0.02[b]	0.05[b]	0.8[b]	0.2[b]	0.2[b]	0.8[b]	1.6[b]
Neisseria gonorrhoeae[d]	0.01[b]	0.1	0.3[b]	12.0	12.0	12.0	0.3[b]	0.05[b]
Neisseria meningitidis	0.05	0.25	0.05	6.0	6.0	6.0	0.1	0.05

[a] Rare isolates resistant to penicillins have been found MIC >5 μg/ml.
[b] Many isolates resistant.
[c] Amoxicillin has a mean MIC of 0.4.
[d] Can range from 0.005 to 100.

TABLE 3. Activity of Penicillins Against Selected Bacilli and Anaerobic Organisms

	Mean Minimum Inhibitory Level (μg/ml)				
Organism	Penicillin G	Ampicillin, Amoxicillin[12]	Oxacillin[b]	Ticarcillin[a]	Azlocillin, Mezlocillin, Piperacillin[a]
Clostridium perfringens	0.5	0.05	> 0.5	0.5	0.05
Corynebacterium diphtheriae	0.1	0.02	> 0.1	0.1	1.0
Listeria monocytogenes	0.5	0.5	> 4.0	4	0.5
Haemophilus influenzae[c]	0.8	0.5	> 25	0.5	0.1
Prevotella melaninogenica	0.5	0.5	> 25	0.5	0.2
Fusobacterium nucleatum	0.5	0.1	>100	0.5	0.5
Bacteroides fragilis	32	32	>500	64	32

[a] Minor differences do occur.
[b] Oxacillin is used as representative of isoxazoyl penicillins.
[c] β-Lactamase-producing strains occur and are resistant to the penicillins.

TABLE 4. Activity of Penicillins Against Enterobacteriaceae and *Pseudomonas*

	Mean Minimum Inhibitory Levels (μg/ml)				
	Penicillin G	Ampicillin, Amoxicillin	Oxacillin[b]	Ticarcillin	Azlocillin,[a] Mezlocillin, Piperacillin
Escherichia coli[c]	100	3	>1000	6	8
Proteus mirabilis	50	3	>1000	1.5	1
Klebsiella spp.	>400	200	>1000	>400	16
Enterobacter spp.	>500	>500	>1000	50	16
Citrobacter diversus	>500	>100	>1000	12	8
Citrobacter freundii	>500	50	>1000	12	32
Serratia	>500	>500	>1000	100	32
Salmonella[c]	10	1.5	>1000	3	4
Shigella[c]	20	1.5	>1000	3	8
Proteus vulgaris	>500	>500	>1000	12	16
Providencia	>500	>500	>1000	12	8
Morganella	>500	200	>1000	25	8
Pseudomonas, other	>500	>500	>500	100	>100
Acinetobacter	>500	250	>1000	25	32
Pseudomonas aeruginosa	>500	>500	>1000	50	16[b]

[a] Some isolates, particularly *Klebsiella*, are resistant to azlocillin but susceptible to mezlocillin and piperacillin.
[b] Used as representative antistaphylococcal penicillin.
[c] Amoxicillin is twofold more active against *Salmonella* and twofold less active against *Shigella*. Strains containing the TEM plasmid β-lactamase are resistant except to temocillin.

community to community. Most of the anaerobic gram-positive bacteria are susceptible to all the penicillins. Gram-negative anaerobic bacteria are susceptible to most penicillins, with the exception of isolates of *Bacteroides fragilis,* and are inhibited by high levels of penicillin G or the semisynthetic anti-*Pseudomonas* agents—azlocillin, carbenicillin, mezlocillin, piperacillin, and ticarcillin.[19] Strains of *Fusobacterium varium* often are resistant to all penicillins.

PHARMACOLOGIC PROPERTIES

Penicillins differ markedly in their oral absorption (Table 5). Penicillin G is not stable in acid and has a half-life of less than 20 minutes at pH 2. In contrast, at pH 4 it has a half-life of 1 hour. Methicillin and all the anti-*Pseudomonas* penicillins are acid labile. However, acid stability is not a guarantee of oral absorption, and there can be major differences in oral absorption

TABLE 5. Pharmacokinetic Properties of Penicillins

Antibiotic	Oral Adsorption (%)	Food Decreases Adsorption	Protein Binding (%)	Percentage of Dose Metabolized (%)	Serum Level[a] Total Drug (μg/ml)	Serum Level[a] Free Drug (μg/ml)	Serum $T_{1/2}$ (hr)[b] Normal ($C_{cr} > 90$ ml/min)	Serum $T_{1/2}$ (hr)[b] Renal Failure ($C_{cr} < 10$ ml/min)	Liver Impairment Increases (T_i)	Na$^+$ Content[c] (mEq/g)
Penicillin G	20	Yes	55	20	2	0.9	0.5	10	+	2.7
Penicillin V	60	No	80	55	4	0.8	1	4		
Methicillin	Nil		35	10			0.5	4		3.1
Oxacillin	30	Yes	93	45	6	0.4	0.5	1		
Cloxacillin	50	Yes	94	20	10	0.6	0.5	1	+ +	
Dicloxacillin	50	Yes	97	10	15	0.45	0.5	1.5	+ +	
Nafcillin	Erratic	Yes	87				0.5	1.5	+ + +	
Ampicillin[c]	40	Yes	17	10	3.5	2.9	1	8	+ +	3.4
Amoxicillin	75	No	17	10	7.5	6.2	1	8	+	
Indanyl carbenicillin	30	No	50		15	7.5	1.1	15	+ +	
Ticarcillin	Nil		50	15			1.2	15	+ +, 18–20 hr	4.7
Mezlocillin	Nil		50				1.1	4	+ +	1.8
Piperacillin	Nil		50				1.3	4	+ +	1.8
Azlocillin	Nil		20				0.8	4	+ +	2.2
Temocillin	Nil		85	10			4	17	+ +	

[a] After 500 mg dose taken fasting.
[b] Values have been rounded of to approximate values.
[c] Na$^+$ content based on IV preparations.

of compounds from within the same class. Penicillin V is well absorbed even when ingested with food, and the greatest absorption of penicillin V is with the potassium salt.[21] The semisynthetic penicillins except nafcillin are well absorbed. Ampicillin is only partially absorbed, 30–60 percent,[16] whereas amoxicillin is almost totally absorbed.[20] Although carbenicillin is not absorbed, esters of the compound such as indanyl carbenicillin are adequately absorbed to provide urinary concentration to treat urinary tract infections.[22]

The majority of penicillins are absorbed so they yield peak levels 1–2 hours after ingestion. Absorption is delayed to yield peak serum levels 2–3 hours after ingestion with food, and peak levels are lower, except for amoxicillin.

Repository forms of penicillin G are available. These are procaine penicillin G and benzathine penicillin G. These are absorbed more slowly from intramuscular sites than are the crystalline salts. Procaine or lidocaine can also be used as a diluent for intramuscular injection of anti-*Pseudomonas* penicillins, but the half-life of these drugs is not prolonged by this maneuver.

Penicillins are bound to protein in varying degrees from 17 percent for the aminopenicillins to 97 percent for dicloxacillin (Table 5). The major protein to which they bind is albumin.[16] Only unbound drug exerts antibacterial activity, since the bound drug is not free to interact with PBPs. However, protein binding is a reversible process, and it is possible for bound penicillin to be released and to kill bacteria in tissue or in the blood stream. The major mechanism by which they are removed from the body is by excretion as intact molecules via the kidney.[23] Penicillins are metabolized to a minor degree.[24] Even minor differences in metabolism can result in clinically significant differences among half-lives in the presence of renal failure. Biliary excretion of penicillins does occur, but it probably is important only for nafcillin and the anti-*Pseudomonas* penicillins.[25]

The mechanism of excretion of penicillins is via renal tubular cells. Penicillins are rapidly excreted into urine, and hence they have a short half-life, ranging from less than 30 minutes for penicillin to 72 minutes for carbenicillin. The ability of the renal tubular cells to excrete penicillin varies with the agents, but up to 4 g/hr of penicillin G can be excreted. This excretion can be blocked by probenecid, which prolongs the serum half-life of all the penicillins.[26] Probenecid also competes for binding sites on albumin; hence, there is more free drug in the presence of probenecid. Renal excretion of all penicillins by the newborn is

TABLE 6. Antibiotic Dosage Change in Renal Disease and after Dialysis

Agent	Dosage Change in Renal Failure[a] Creatinine Clearance (30–50 ml/min)	Dosage Change in Renal Failure[a] Creatinine Clearance (<10 ml/min)	Dosage after Hemodialysis
Penicillin G	NC	1.6×10^6 units/6 hr	Yes (1.6×10^6 units)
Penicillin V	NC	250 mg/6 hr	Yes (250 mg)
Methicillin	NC	2 g/8 hr	Slight (2 g)
Oxacillin	NC	NC	Slight (as in uremia)
Cloxacillin	NC	NC	Slight (as in uremia)
Dicloxacillin	NC	NC	Slight (as in uremia)
Nafcillin	NC	NC	Slight (as in uremia)
Ampicillin	NC	0.5–1 g/8 hr	Yes (500 mg)
Amoxicillin	NC	500 mg/12 hr	Yes (250 mg)
Ticarcillin[b]	2 g/4 hr	2 g/12 hr	Yes (2 g)
Indanyl carbenicillin	NC	Avoid	
Azlocillin	NC	3 g/8–12 hr	Yes (2 g)
Mezlocillin	NC	3 g/8–12 hr	Yes (2 g)
Piperacillin	NC	3 g/8–12 hr	Yes (2 g)
Temocillin	1 g/24 hr	1 g/48 hr	Yes (1 g)
Amdinocillin	NC	1 g/8 hr	Yes (1 g)

Abbreviations: NC: no change.
[a] Refers to maximum dose used.
[b] Only carbenicillin and ticarcillin need adjustment of dosage after peritoneal dialysis.

markedly less than in older children since tubular function is not fully developed. Hence, the dosage programs for penicillins must be modified when given to newborns or low-birth-weight infants.

Reduction in renal function is an important consideration in the administration of certain penicillins (e.g., ticarcillin). If the creatinine clearance is greater than 10 ml/min, it is necessary to make only minor adjustments in the dosage of other penicillins. In the presence of anuria, reduction in total daily dose of the natural penicillins, of many of the penicillinase-resistant penicillins, and of the aminopenicillins is necessary[27] (Table 6).

Peritoneal dialysis removes variable amounts of the penicillins. In general, after peritoneal dialysis only the dosage programs of ticarcillin need to be adjusted. After hemodialysis it is necessary to replace the dialyzed penicillin G, ampicillin, amoxicillin, ticarcillin, azlocillin, mezlocillin, and piperacillin, but not nafcillin or the isoxazolyl penicillins.[27]

Penicillins are well distributed to most areas of the body such as lung, liver, kidney, muscle, bone, and placenta. The levels of penicillins in abscesses, middle ear, and pleural, peritoneal, and synovial fluids are sufficient in the presence of inflammation to inhibit most susceptible bacteria.[28-32] Most penicillins are relatively insoluble in lipid and penetrate cells relatively poorly. Distribution of all the penicillins to eye, brain, cerebrospinal fluid, or prostate is nil in the absence of inflammation.[33] Inflammation alters normal barriers, permitting entry of penicillins, but more importantly it interferes with the anion pump that removes penicillins from areas such as cerebrospinal fluid. Low protein-bound penicillins reach levels in fetal serum equivalent to levels in maternal serum 30–60 minutes after injection. In contrast, the highly protein-bound semisynthetic penicillins achieve low concentrations in both amniotic fluid and fetal serum.[34]

Urinary concentrations of all penicillins are high, even in the presence of moderately reduced renal function, but in people with creatinine clearances below 10 ml/min the urinary levels may not exceed those in the blood. Cortical and medullary concentrations of penicillins during normal hydration and in hydropenia exceed serum levels.[35]

Most penicillins are actively secreted into the bile, yielding biliary concentrations well in excess of those in serum. The levels of penicillin G, ampicillin, and amoxicillin are at least 10 times those in the serum, and the levels of nafcillin and mezlocillin are as high as 100 times the simultaneous serum level. In the presence of common duct obstruction, the levels of all penicillins in bile are markedly reduced. Since the biliary transport system is a saturable one, at very high serum levels the biliary levels are not significantly increased over those obtained at lower serum levels.

UNTOWARD REACTIONS

The major adverse effects of the penicillins are hypersensitivity reactions, which range in severity from rash to immediate anaphylaxis (Table 7) (see Ch. 18).[36,37] Penicillins are capable of acting as haptens to combine with proteins contaminating the solution or with human protein after the penicillin has been administered to humans. Penicilloyl and penicillanic derivatives are the major determinants of penicillin allergy. The penicilloyl determinant, which is produced through opening of the β-lactam ring, thereby allowing amide linkage to body proteins (Fig. 3), is the most important antigenic component. Penicillanic acid and derivatives of penicillanic acid are produced when reconstituted penicillins break down in solution due to acidity or temperature elevation. Minor determinants of allergy are benzyl penicillin itself or sodium benzyl penicilloate, which can act either as sensitizing agents or on their own elicit an allergic reaction.[36,37] Both major and minor determinants may be involved in anaphylactic reactions, as well as in urticarial reactions. These reactions are mediated by IgE antibody. Minor determinants are the major cause of anaphylactic reactions. When a person has been sensitized by the hapten-carrier complex, he or she can have a reaction to penicillin alone or to penicillin that has formed dimers or polymers in solution. Anaphylactic reactions to penicillins are uncommon, occurring in only 0.2 percent of 10,000 courses of treatment, with 0.001 percent out of 100,000 courses resulting in fatality.[38] People with atopic dermatitis or allergic rhinitis appear not to be at increased risk of a penicillin reaction.[39]

Serum sickness does occur with penicillins, but it is very uncommon today. It probably is due to IgG antibodies to the benzyl penicilloyl hapten. The illness is characterized by fever, urticaria, joint pains, and angioneurotic edema. Exfoliative dermatitis and Stevens-Johnson syndrome are rare forms of allergic reactions to penicillins. The morbilliform eruptions that

TABLE 7. Adverse Reactions to Penicillins[a]

Type of Reaction	Frequency (%)	Occurs Most Frequently with[a]
Allergic		
IgE antibody	0.004–0.4	Penicillin G
Anaphylaxis		
Early urticaria (<72 hr)		
Cytotoxic antibody	Rare	Penicillin G
Hemolytic anemia		
Ag-Ab complex disease	Rare	Penicillin G
Serum sickness		
Delayed hypersensitivity	4–8	Ampicillin
Contact dermatitis		
Idiopathic	4–8	Ampicillin
Skin rash		
Fever		
Late onset urticaria		
Gastrointestinal	2–5	
Diarrhea	2–5	Ampicillin
Enterocolitis	<1	Ampicillin
Hematologic		
Hemolytic anemia	Rare	Penicillin G
Neutropenia	1–4	Penicillin G Nafcillin Oxacillin Piperacillin
Platelet dysfunction	3	Carbenicillin ticarcillin
Hepatic		
Elevated SGOT level	1–4	Oxacillin Nafcillin Carbenicillin
Electrolyte disturbance		
Sodium overload	Variable	Ticarcillin
Hypokalemia	Variable	Ticarcillin
Hyperkalemia—acute	Rare	Penicillin G
Neurologic		
Seizures	Rare	Penicillin G
Bizarre sensations		Procaine Penicillin
Renal		
Interstitial nephritis	1–2	Methicillin
Hemorrhagic cystitis	Rare	Methicillin

[a] All the reactions can occur with any of the penicillins.

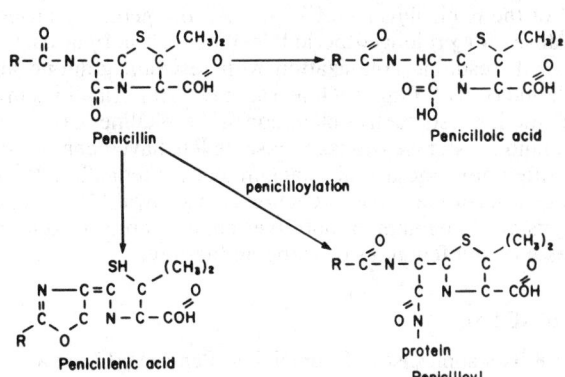

FIG. 3. Mechanisms for formation of antigens from penicillins.

develop after penicillin therapy probably are due to IgM antibody to the benzyl penicilloyl hapten and to the minor determinants. In many patients these rashes will disappear, even if the penicillin is continued, due to the production of IgG blocking antibody. There is a risk, however, that the rash could progress to generalized desquamation. If an allergic reaction does occur, epinephrine given intramuscularly or intravenously will usually abort the reaction. Antihistamines and corticosteroids have not been shown to be of benefit.

Another allergic reaction to penicillins is that of allergic vasculitis with development of cutaneous and visceral lesions similar to that found with periarteritis nodosa. This reaction is extremely rare.

Hematologic toxicity is rare, although neutropenia has been

encountered with the use of all types of penicillins, particularly when large doses are used.[40] The mechanism of the neutropenia is unknown, and white blood cell counts return to normal rapidly if the offending agent is discontinued. Sometimes a lower dose of drug can be used without production of neutropenia. Coombs-positive hemolytic anemia occurs rarely.[41] All penicillins at high concentrations, but particularly carbenicillin and ticarcillin, bind to the adenosine diphosphate receptor site in platelets, preventing normal platelet aggregation. Clinically significant bleeding occurs relatively infrequently.[42]

Renal toxicity from penicillins has varied from allergic angiitis to interstitial nephritis.[43,44] Interstitial nephritis occurs most commonly with methicillin, but is seen with all penicillins. The clinical syndrome is one of fever, macular rash, eosinophilia, proteinuria, eosinophiluria, and hematuria. Initially the reaction is one of nonoliguric renal failure with a decrease in creatinine clearance and a rise in serum urea nitrogen and serum creatinine concentrations. This reaction can progress to anuria and renal failure. Biopsy specimens of the kidney show an interstitial infiltrate of mononuclear and eosinophilic cells with tubular damage but no glomerular lesions. Discontinuation of the penicillin will result in the return of renal function to normal in most cases.[45]

Administration of massive doses of any penicillin, but most often carbenicillin and ticarcillin, may result in hypokalemia due to the large dose of nonreabsorbable anion presented to the distal renal tubules, which alters $[H^+]$ excretion and secondarily results in K^+ loss.[43]

Central nervous system toxicity in the form of myoclonic seizures can follow administration of massive doses of penicillin G, ampicillin, or methicillin. If there is reduced renal function, the drugs accumulate, and this toxicity is more likely.[46] Direct instillation of small doses of methicillin, oxacillin, or nafcillin into the ventricles at the time of surgery for placement of atrioventricular shunts has not resulted in seizures. Direct application of penicillin to the cortex will provoke seizure activity.

Gastrointestinal disturbances have followed the use of any of the oral forms but have been most pronounced with ampicillin. Enterocolitis due to *Clostridium difficile* has followed the use of all of the penicillins (see Ch. 78). All the penicillins used at high doses for prolonged periods will abolish normal bacterial flora with resulting colonization with resistant gram-negative bacilli and/or with fungi such as *Candida*. Abnormalities in hepatic function tests such as elevation of the alkaline phosphatase and aminotransferase (transaminase) levels have been reported most often after the use of oxacillin and carbenicillin.[40,47] The pathogenesis of the hepatic reaction is unknown. Major hepatic injury is very uncommon, and liver enzymes return to normal values within a few days of stopping therapy.

CLINICAL USE

Table 8 lists some uses of penicillins. Penicillin G remains the primary agent for treatment of *Streptococcus pyogenes, S. pneumoniae,* and enterococcal infections. None of the newer penicillins or agents in other classes has been shown to be more effective. *Streptococcus pneumoniae* resistant to penicillin have been isolated in many countries, including United States. In the U.S. *S. pneumoniae* of relative resistance to penicillin, minimum inhibitory concentration (MIC) values of 0.1–1 μg/ml are increasingly common with prevalences up to 22 percent in some areas. Much higher doses of penicillin are required to kill these organisms. Nearly all *Neisseria meningitidis* strains are susceptible to penicillin G. *Neisseria gonorrhoeae* vary in susceptibility to penicillin G. Strains can be resistant due to β-lactamase production, to altered PBPs, or to membrane changes (see Ch. 13). Penicillin G is the drug of choice for treponemal infection in all its forms. Puerperal infections due to anaerobic streptococci or group B streptococci *(Streptococcus agalactiae),* as well as genital clostridial infections, are treated with penicillin G. Infections produced by anaerobic mouth flora including

gram-positive and gram-negative cocci and the *Actinomyces* can be treated with penicillin G, although *Prevotella melaninogenica* that produce a β-lactamase and are resistant to penicillin are being encountered.

PROPHYLACTIC USE

Penicillins have been used in a number of situations for prevention of infection. Oral administration of 200,000 units of penicillin G or penicillin V every 12 hours has resulted in a significant reduction in recurrences of rheumatic fever. Because of the problems with compliance with oral therapy, intramuscular injections of 1.2 or 2.4 million units of benzathine penicillin given once each month have also been used with excellent results.

Outbreaks of streptococcal infection due to *S. pyogenes* have been aborted by the use of oral penicillin G or V given twice a day for 5 days, by single injections of procaine penicillin daily, or by administration of benzathine penicillin. One of the most important prophylactic uses of penicillin is for prevention of bacterial endocarditis (see Ch. 60).

Antistaphylococcal penicillins may be used prophylactically at the time of implantation of an artificial joint or heart valve. These agents should be given just before the surgery, during the procedure, and in the immediate postoperative period. There are no studies that delineate the best penicillin agent for such procedures, and many physicians prefer to use a cephalosporin (see Ch. 296).

Ampicillin or amoxicillin has been administered orally to asplenic children or to children with agammaglobulinemia to prevent infections caused by *H. influenzae* and *S. pneumoniae.* Penicillin prophylaxis has not been of benefit in prevention of meningococcal infection, bacterial infection after viral respiratory infection, or pneumonia after coma, shock, or congestive heart failure.

PROPERTIES OF INDIVIDUAL PENICILLINS

Dosages of penicillins are given in Tables 9 and 10.

Natural Penicillins

Penicillin G. Penicillin G or benzylpenicillin G (Fig. 4) is available in oral, parenteral, and repository salts for intramuscular injection. Oral salts are either the sodium or potassium forms, which are available as suspensions for pediatric use or as tablets in doses of 50,000 to 1 million units (200,000 units equals 125 mg). Because of its instability in acid there is no reason to use oral penicillin G, and penicillin V or amoxicillin should be used instead.

Crystalline penicillin G in aqueous solution has been used intramuscularly, subcutaneously, intravenously, and intrathecally. It is available either as the potassium or sodium salt. The sodium salt is much more expensive than the potassium salt, and it rarely needs to be used since the amount of potassium present in 6 million units, an amount a patient with reduced renal function would receive, is less than 10 mEq. Given intramuscularly as an aqueous solution, penicillin G is very rapidly cleared from the body, and it is preferable to use a repository form. It is available as sterile dry powder in ampules or vials containing 200,000 to 20 million units per vial. Each million units of penicillin G contains 1.7 mEq of sodium or potassium.

Repository penicillins provide tissue depots from which the drug is absorbed over hours in the case of procaine penicillin or over days in the case of benzathine penicillin. Repository penicillins are only for intramuscular use and cannot be used intravenously or subcutaneously or to irrigate wounds. Procaine penicillin is a mixture of equal molar parts of procaine and penicillin. Thus 300,000 units contains 120 mg of procaine. Use of this suspension delays the peak of activity but provides serum and tissue levels for at least 12 hours. Doubling the dose of

TABLE 8. Antimicrobial Spectrum of Penicillin[a]

Organisms	Penicillin of Choice	Alternative Acceptable Penicillin	Frequency of Resistance to Penicillins (%)
Gram-positive cocci			
Streptpcoccus pneumoniae	G	V	Uncommon
Streptococcus pyogenes (A)	G	V	None
Steptococcus agalactiae (B)	G	Ampicillin	None
Viridans streptococci	G		None
Streptococcus bovis (D)	G		None
Enterococcus faecalis	Ampicillin	Mezlocillin	Rare, <1
Staphylococcus aureus (nonpenicillinase)	G	Penase-resistant	80
Staphylococcus aureus (penicillinase)	Penase-resistant		100
Staphylococcus aureus (methicillin-resistant)	None	None	100
Staphylococcus epidermidis	Penase-resistant		80
Staphylococcus epidermidis (methicillin-resistant)	None	None	100
Gram-negative cocci			
Neisseria meningitidis	G	Ampicillin	Very rare
Neisseria gonorrhoeae	G	Ampicillin	1–40
Gram-positive bacilli			
Bacillus anthracis	G		None
Corynebacterium diphtheriae	G		None
Listeria monocytogenes	Ampicillin	G	None
Anaerobic species			
Peptostreptoccoccus	G	Ampicillin	None
Actinomyces israeli	G	V	None
Bacteroides melaninogenicus	G	C, T	10
Fusobacterium	G	Ampicillin	1–10
Bacteroides fragilis	M, PA		75
Clostridium	G	Ampicillin	<1
Gram-negative bacilli			
Haemophilus	Ampicillin	G	5–30
Escherichia coli	Ampicillin		30
Proteus mirabilis	Ampicillin	G	<5
Salmonella typhi	Ampicillin		20
Salmonella other spp.	Ampicillin		20
Klebsiella	None	95	
Enterobacter spp.	M, P, T		70
Citrobacter freundii	M, P, T		80
Proteus, indole-positive	M, P, T		20
Serratia	M, P, T		90
Pseudomonas aeruginosa	A, P, T		20–30
Pseudomonas, other	None		95
Acinetobacter	T	A, G, P	50
Providencia	M, P, T		20–30
Xanthomonas	None		95
Other organisms infrequently encountered			
Erysipelothrix	G	Ampicillin	None
Pasteurella multocida	G		Rare, <1
Streptobacillus moniliformis	G		None
Spirillum minus	G		None
Treponema pallidum	G		None

Abbreviations: A: azlocillin; M: mezlocillin, P: piperacillin; T: ticarcillin.
[a] In each case it is assumed that a route of administration would be used that would achieve levels in serum and tissue to eradicate the organism. If there is no entry in the alternate column, it means that an antibiotic in another class would be a more appropriate choice. Amoxicillin can be used in place of ampicillin in all situations except with *Shigella*.

TABLE 9. Dosage of Penicillins

Compound	Oral	Intramuscular	Intravenous
Penicillin G			25,000–500,000 units/kg/day, 6 doses
Procaine		300,000–600,000 units every 12 hr	
Benzathine		1.2–2.4 mega units every 15–20 days	
Pencillin V	Infant: 50 mg/kg/day, 3 doses 125–500, 4 doses		
Ampicillin	25–200 mg/kg/day, 4 doses	100–200 mg/kg/day, 4 doses	100–300 mg/kg/day, 6 doses
Amoxicillin	25–50 mg/kg/day, 3 doses		
Methicillin			
Oxacillin		100 mg/kg/day, 4 doses	100–300 mg/kg/day, 6 doses
Nafcillin			
Cloxacillin	25–100 mg/kg/day, 4 doses		
Dicloxacillin	12–25 mg/kg/day, 4 doses		
Ticarcillin		50–100 mg/kg/day, 4 doses	50–300 mg/kg/day, 6 doses
Indanylcarbenicillin	50–65 mg/kg/day, 4 doses		
Azlocillin		50–100 mg/kg/day, 4 doses	200–300 mg/kg/day, 4 doses
Mezlocillin		50–100 mg/kg/day, 4 doses	200–300 mg/kg/day, 4 doses
Piperacillin		50–100 mg/kg/day, 4 doses	200–300 mg/kg/day, 4 doses

TABLE 10. Dosage of Antibiotics in Newborn Infants

Compound	Infants Less than 1 Week Old		Infants 1 Week–1 Month Old	
	Dose (per kg/day)	Interval between Doses (in hours)	Dose (per kg/day)	Interval between Doses (in hours)
Penicillin G	50,000–100,000 units	12	100,000 units	8
Ampicillin	100 mg	12	200 mg	6
Oxacillin	100 mg	12	200 mg	6
Methicillin	100 mg	12	300 mg	6
Nafcillin	100 mg	12	200 mg	6
Ticarcillin	150 mg	8	300 mg	6
Mezlocillin	75 mg	12	300 mg	6
Azlocillin	75–100 mg	12	300 mg	6

$$R-NH\cdot CH-CH \quad \overset{S}{\underset{}{C(CH_3)_2}}$$
$$CO-N-CH\cdot COOH$$

Structure of side chain R

Penicillin G
benzylpenicillin — ⬡–CH₂·CO–

Penicillin V
phenoxymethylpenicillin — ⬡–O·CH₂·CO–

Phenethicillin
DL–α–phenoxyethylpenicillin — ⬡–O·CH·CO– / CH₃

FIG. 4.   Structures of penicillin G and penicillin V.

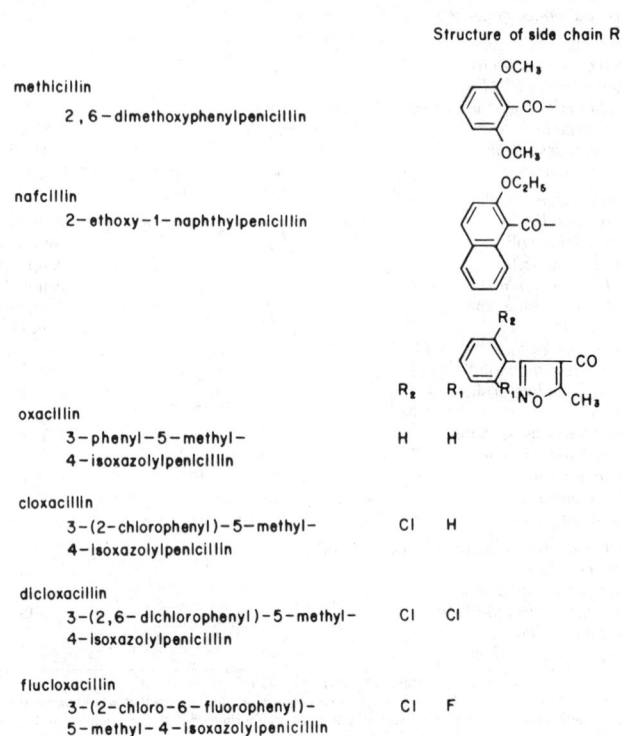

$$R-NH\cdot CH-CH \quad \overset{S}{\underset{}{C(CH_3)_2}}$$
$$CO-N-CH\cdot COOH$$

Structure of side chain R

methicillin
2,6–dimethoxyphenylpenicillin

nafcillin
2–ethoxy–1–naphthylpenicillin

oxacillin
3–phenyl–5–methyl–
4–isoxazolylpenicillin — R₂ H   R₁ H

cloxacillin
3–(2–chlorophenyl)–5–methyl–
4–isoxazolylpenicillin — Cl   H

dicloxacillin
3–(2,6–dichlorophenyl)–5–methyl–
4–isoxazolylpenicillin — Cl   Cl

flucloxacillin
3–(2–chloro–6–fluorophenyl)–
5–methyl–4–isoxazolylpenicillin — Cl   F

FIG. 5.   Antistaphylococcal penicillins.

procaine penicillin given at a single injection site does not double the serum level. To increase the peak level it is necessary to use two body sites, as was done in the treatment of gonorrhea, for example, with 2.4 million units of procaine penicillin given in each buttock. Marketed procaine penicillin preparations are of two types: one is an aqueous solution of the crystalline salt, and the other contains 2% aluminum monosterate as a dispensing agent. The preparations are marketed in cartridges and vials in doses of 300,000, 500,000, and 600,000 units in 1–4 ml and as 2.4 million units/4 ml.

Benzathine penicillin is a repository form of penicillin, which is a combination of 1 mol of penicillin and 2 mol of an ammonium base. It is available for intramuscular injection in 10-ml vials containing 300,000 units/ml and as prefilled syringes containing 600,000 units/ml in 1-, 2-, and 4-ml sizes. It provides detectable serum levels for 15–30 days, depending on the size of the dose. Concentrations of penicillin G in the spinal fluid after use of benzathine penicillin probably are inadequate to treat treponemal infections of the nervous system.

Penicillin V.   Phenoxymethyl penicillin (Fig. 4) is available only for oral use as sodium or potassium salts in suspension or tablets in doses of 125, 250, and 500 mg. The potassium salt produces higher blood levels than the other salts. Serum levels are from two to five times those obtained with penicillin G. Absorbed penicillin V is handled in the body similarly to penicillin G. Penicillin V can be substituted for penicillin G in most situations in which it is reasonable to treat an infection by the oral route. However, penicillin V is less active than penicillin G against *Haemophilus, Neisseria,* and enteric organisms. Blood levels after 500 mg given to an adult are equivalent to the levels achieved with 600,000 units of procaine penicillin given intramuscularly. The usual dosage for children is 25–50 mg/kg/day and for adults, 1–4 g/day. The interval between dosages is 6–8 hours.

Penicillinase-Resistant Penicillins (Fig. 5)

Methicillin.   Methicillin (2,6-dimethoxyphenylpenicillin) is a penicillin resistant to staphylococcal β-lactamase.[31] Susceptible strains of staphylococci are inhibited by 2–4 μg/ml. Methicillin-resistant *S. aureus* and coagulase-negative staphylococci are resistant not because of β-lactamase activity but by virtue of a unique, low-affinity penicillin-binding protein, PBP 2a. These organisms have become a serious problem in some parts of the United States. Methicillin inhibits *S. pyogenes* and *S. pneumoniae* at levels of 0.2 μg/ml, but it has no useful activity against *Enterococcus fecalis* and gram-negative bacilli. Methicillin is acid-unstable and must be given parenterally. Absorption after an intramuscular injection is rapid, as is excretion, with peak levels after 1 g of 17 μg/ml but subinhibitory levels by 4 hours. Methicillin is less protein bound than the other antistaphylococcal penicillins, and, although its intrinsic activity is less than the other antistaphylococcal penicillins, it is as active in the presence of serum as are the more intrinsically active oxacillin and nafcillin. Methicillin is available as a sodium salt, but since it is unstable in acidic media, it is used as a buffered solution. It is packaged as 1-, 4-, and 6-g vials and can be diluted with sodium chloride or dextrose in water. When diluted, buffered solutions are stable at room temperature for 8 hours. It is preferable to administer the drug every 4 hours if used intravenously. Methicillin should be used only for the treatment of penicillin G–resistant staphylococcal infections. Toxicity is that seen with an penicillin, although interstitial nephritis may be more common. The usual dosage is 6–12 g/day for adults and 200–300 mg/kg/day for children given in four or six doses.

Nafcillin. Nafcillin (2-ethoxy-1-naphthylpenicillin) has more intrinsic activity than methicillin against both staphylococci and streptococci and is also not active against gram-negative bacteria. Nafcillin is highly protein bound, and in the presence of serum its activity is similar to methicillin. Although nafcillin is absorbed when taken by mouth, absorption is erratic whether the drug is taken fasting or with food, and hence serum levels are low.[31] Levels after intramuscular injection are low, and the preferred route of administration is intravenously. The antibiotic is primarily excreted by the liver and to a lesser extent by the kidney. Serum levels are elevated and the half-life is prolonged by probenecid. Although nafcillin is available as capsules (250 mg) and a suspension, cloxacillin or dicloxacillin should be used for oral administration. Sterile vials of 500 mg/1, 2, or 4 g of the sodium salt can be reconstituted in most solutions and are stable for up to 4 hours at room temperature. The usual dosage of nafcillin is 6–9 g/day, depending on the severity of the infection, and 100–200 mg/kg/day for children.

Isoxazolyl Penicillins. All these agents are stable to staphylococcal β-lactamase and inhibit both penicillin-sensitive and penicillin-resistant staphylococci at mean concentrations of 0.2–0.4 μg ml. Methicillin-resistant staphylococci are resistant to these penicillins. Isoxazolyl penicillins inhibit streptococci and pneumococci but are virtually inactive against gram-negative bacilli. All are absorbed after oral administration, but absorption is adversely affected by food. There are differences in serum levels among the drugs after oral ingestion, with the serum level of cloxacillin twice that of oxacillin and the levels of dicloxacillin twice that of cloxacillin; all the drugs are highly bound to serum proteins; oxacillin and cloxacillin are equally bound, but dicloxacillin is bound to a greater extent. Thus, actual free serum concentrations of the drugs are greater for cloxacillin and dicloxacillin than oxacillin (Table 5). After intravenous infusion of 1 g over 15 minutes, peak serum levels are 70–100 μg/ml, with levels of 25 μg/ml at 1 hour and less than 1 μg/ml at 6 hours. The isoxazoyl penicillins undergo some metabolism but are excreted primarily by the kidney with slight biliary excretion. Oxacillin undergoes more rapid degradation in the body than does cloxacillin or dicloxacillin.

OXACILLIN. Oxacillin is available as a sodium salt for oral use in 250- and 500-mg capsules and as a powder for suspension at 250 mg/5 ml. It should be taken 1–2 hours before meals. The daily dosage for adults is 1–4 g taken in four parts. The dosage for children is 50–100 mg/kg/day taken in four parts. Oxacillin sodium for injection may be given intramuscularly or intravenously. It is available in 500-mg and 1-, 2-, or 4-g vials and is stable in most saline and dextrose solutions for 6 hours at room temperature. Adult dosage is 2–12 g/day and for children, 100–300 mg/kg/day given every 4–6 hours.

CLOXACILLIN. Cloxacillin sodium is available in the United States only as an oral solution (125 mg/5 ml) or capsules of 250 and 500 mg. Dosage for children is 50–100 mg/kg/day given as four equal doses. Dosage for adults is 1–4 g/day given as four equal doses. In Europe cloxacillin is available parenterally for intramuscular or intravenous administration in 250-mg vials. It yields serum levels similar to those achieved with oxacillin.

DICLOXACILLIN. Dicloxacillin sodium is available as a suspension (62.5 mg/5 ml) and as capsules of 125 and 250 mg. The dosage for children less than 40 kg is 25 mg/kg/day given as four doses. Some authorities recommend doses as above for cloxacillin. For adults, a dosage of 250 mg to 1 g every 6 hours can be given, depending on the severity of the infection.

Aminopenicillins

The antibacterial activities of all aminopenicillins are similar (Fig. 6).[48] They are not stable to β-lactamases of either gram-positive or gram-negative bacteria. The aminopenicillins are only slightly less active than penicillin G against *S. pyogenes, S. pneumoniae,* and *S. agalactiae.* They are slightly more active against enterococci. Activity of the compounds against clostridial species, *Actinomyces,* corynebacteria, and *N. meningitidis* is equal to that of penicillin G. They are more active than penicillin G against *Listeria monocytogenes.* Sensitivity of *N. gonorrhoeae* (see Ch. 191) varies from highly sensitive to completely resistant in strains that bear a plasmid-mediating production of a β-lactamase. *Haemophilus influenzae* (both typeable and nontypeable strains) and *Haemophilus parainfluenzae* are usually susceptible, except for the isolates that produce β-lactamases (see Chs. 203, 204). Although many domiciliary *E. coli* are sensitive to aminopenicillins, plasmid resistance is common in hospital isolates. *Shigella sonnei,* many salmonellae, including many *Salmonella typhi,* are resistant because of β-lactamases. Most *Klebsiella, Serratia, Acinetobacter,* indole-positive *Proteus, Pseudomonas,* and *Bacteroides fragilis* are resistant to the penicillins of this class.

Ampicillin. Ampicillin is moderately well absorbed after oral administration, but peak levels are delayed and lowered if it is ingested with food. Peak blood levels of 3 μg/ml occur 1–2 hours after ingestion of 0.5 g. Peak blood levels occur later in diabetic patients with neurologic disease and in patients with renal failure. Drug can be detected in the serum for 4–6 hours. After intramuscular injection of 0.5 g peak levels of 10 μg are achieved in 1 hour and persist for 4 hours. Probenecid increases the height of peak levels and prolongs the period in which the drug can be detected in serum. Ampicillin is well distributed to body compartments and achieves therapeutic concentrations in cerebrospinal fluid and in pleural, joint, and peritoneal fluids in the presence of inflammation after parenteral administration. Urinary levels are high even in the presence of markedly reduced renal function. Peritoneal dialysis is ineffective in removing the drug, but hemodialysis removes approximately 40 percent in a 6-hour period.

Ampicillin is available for oral use as the sodium salt or as the trihydrate in capsules of 125, 250, and 500 mg, as a suspension of 125 and 250 mg/5 ml, as drops of 100 mg/ml, and as 125 mg chewable tablets. It is also prepared as a suspension, which contains 3.5 g of ampicillin trihydrate and 1 g of probenecid. It is available as ampicillin trihydrate in 2.5-g vials only for intra-

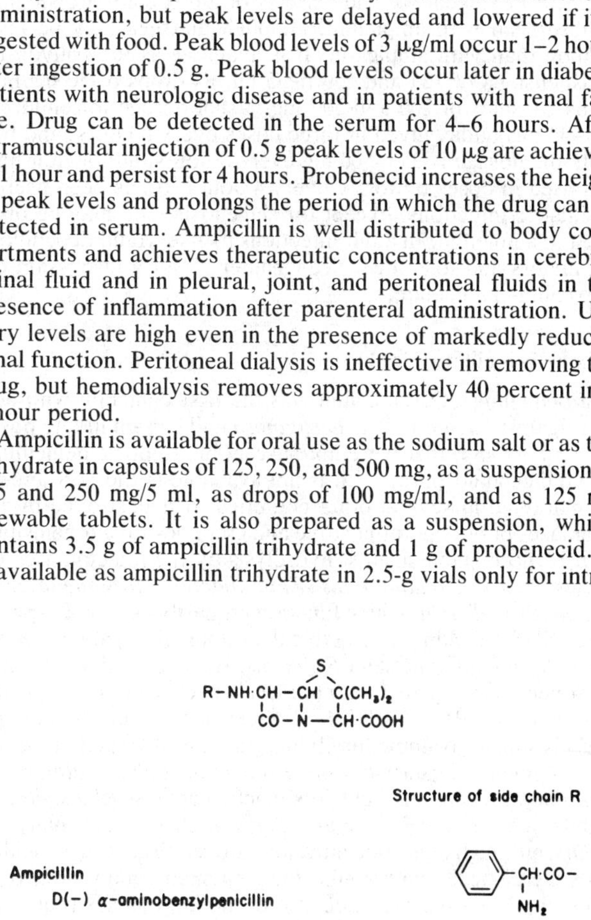

$$R-NH\cdot CH - CH \begin{array}{c} S \\ | \quad | \end{array} C(CH_3)_2$$
$$CO - N - CH\cdot COOH$$

Structure of side chain R

Ampicillin
  D(−) α-aminobenzylpenicillin

Amoxicillin
  D(−) α-amino-p-hydroxybenzylpenicillin

FIG. 6. Aminopenicillins.

muscular use. As a sodium salt in vials of 0.125, 0.5, 2, and 4 g it can be used either intramuscularly or intravenously. It is stable in sodium chloride for 8 hours at concentrations up to 30 mg/ml, but for intravenous use at concentrations greater than 2 mg/ml it is stable at room temperature for less than 4 hours and hence would preferably be administered by "piggy back" within 0.5–1 hour. Dosage varies with the age of the patients, the status of renal function, and the severity of the disease. For children above 1 month of age the oral dosage is 50–100 mg/kg/day in four doses; the intramuscular or intravenous dosage is 100–300 mg/kg/day in four or six doses. For adults the oral dosage is 2–4 g/day given in a dose every 6 hours. For severe infection the parenteral dosage is 6–12 g/day given in divided doses every 4 hours. See Chapter 17 for a discussion of ampicillin–sulbactam.

Amoxicillin. Amoxicillin differs from ampicillin only in the presence of a hydroxyl group in the para position of the benzene side chain. It has in vitro activity similar to ampicillin. It is significantly better absorbed when given by mouth than is ampicillin.[20] Peak blood levels are from two to two and a half times those achieved with a similar dose of ampicillin, and food does not decrease absorption. Oral amoxicillin produces blood levels similar to those produced by intramuscularly administered sodium ampicillin or ampicillin trihydrate. Urinary excretion of amoxicillin is greater than that of ampicillin. Tissue distribution is similar to that of ampicillin. Clinical studies with amoxicillin have been extensive, and it has been used in the treatment of otitis media, bronchitis, pneumonia, typhoid, gonorrhea, and urinary tract infections.[49] It has been used as a single 3-g dose for therapy for bacterial cystitis in women.[50] It is not useful as treatment of shigellosis. Side effects of amoxicillin are similar to those seen with ampicillin, although diarrhea may be less common than with ampicillin. It is available as the trihydrate in suspensions of 125 and 250 mg/5 ml, as drops of 50 mg/ml, and as capsules of 250 and 500 mg. Usual dosage for children is 20–40 mg/kg/day given in three doses every 8 hours, and for adults the dosage is 250–500 mg every 8 hours, although it has been used in doses up to 1 g every 4 hours. It has been useful in pediatric infections, except for shigellosis, and may be preferred to ampicillin. In adult infections its use would depend on cost factors and tolerance. See Chapter 17 for a discussion of amoxicillin-clavulanate.

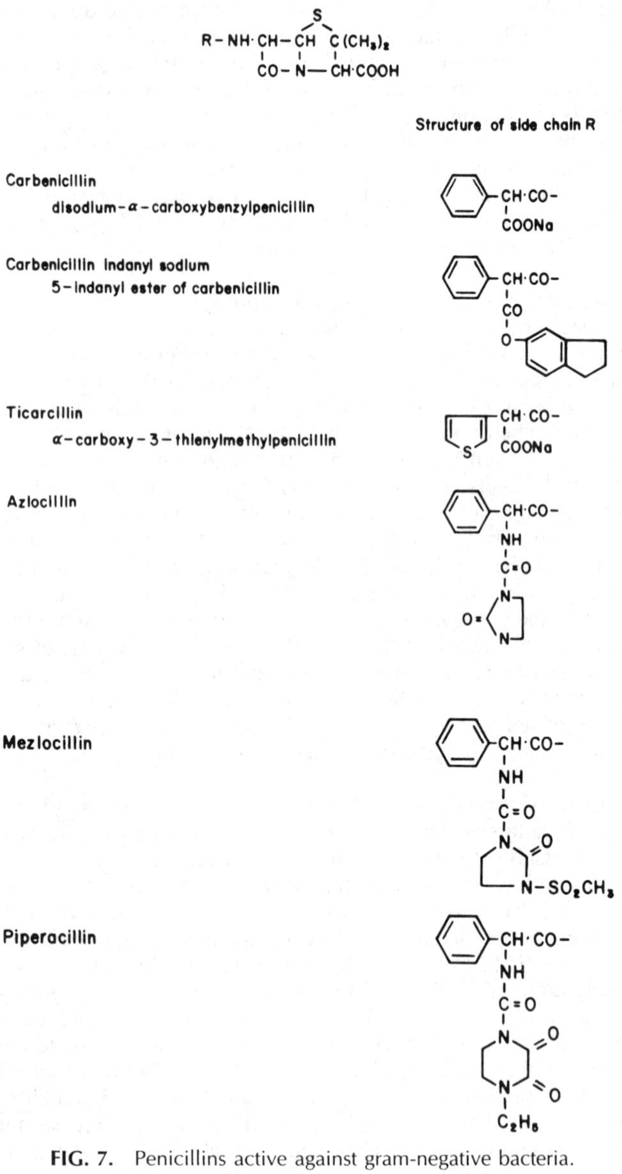

Carboxy Penicillins (Fig. 7)

Carbenicillin. Carbenicillin was the first penicillin with activity against *Pseudomonas aeruginosa* and certain indole-positive *Proteus* spp. that were not susceptible to other penicillins or to the cephalosporins.[32] It is not available in the U.S. but is still marketed in several other countries. It is destroyed by β-lactamases of both gram-positive and gram-negative organisms, but it is more stable against hydrolysis by the β-lactamases of species such as *Pseudomonas, Enterobacter, Morganella,* and *Proteus-Providencia,* which function primarily as cephalosprorinases. Carbenicillin is less active than ampicillin against *S. pyogenes, S. pneumoniae,* and *E. fecalis.* It is less active than the ureidopenicillins against streptococcal species and *Listeria.* Its activity against *Haemophilus, N. gonorrhoeae,* and *N. meningitidis* is similar to ampicillin. It has gram-negative activity similar to ampicillin against *E. coli, Proteus mirabilis, Salmonella* spp., and *Shigella* spp., but it is inactive against *Klebsiella.* It inhibits some *Enterobacter* and *Serratia* strains and many *B. fragilis,* although high concentrations are required. Carbenicillin acts synergistically with amikacin, gentamicin, and tobramycin to inhibit *P. aeruginosa.* Because of the large doses required, greater potential for toxicity, and the availability or more potent alternatives, it should no longer be used.

Ticarcillin. The antibacterial spectrum of ticarcillin is identical to that of carbenicillin, except that it is from two to four times

FIG. 7.   Penicillins active against gram-negative bacteria.

more active against *P. aeruginosa.*[51] The pharmacokinetics of ticarcillin and carbenicillin are virtually identical, as are the side effects.[53] Ticarcillin is not absorbed by mouth but can be given by intramuscular or intravenous administration. After an intramuscular dose of 1 g, peak serum levels of 20 μg/ml are reached in 1 hour. Serum levels of 150–200 μg/ml will be maintained when it is given at dosages of 70–100 mg/kg over 1–2 hours. Ticarcillin is excreted by renal tubules, but since less is converted to penicilloic acid, its half-life (72 minutes) is longer than that of penicillin G, and it accumulates in the presence of renal failure.[32,52] Greater accumulation occurs if there is combined hepatic and renal dysfunction. Hemodialysis reduces plasma concentrations. Probenecid delays renal excretion and increases serum concentrations. Tissue distribution is similar to ampicillin, but concentrations in the cerebrospinal fluid are not adequate for *Pseudomonas.* Side effects are similar to those seen with penicillins. Ticarcillin binds to the adenosine diphosphate (ADP) receptor site on platelets and prevents normal contraction; hence, bleeding occurs on occasion in the presence of high serum levels such as in the presence of renal failure. Ticarcillin can be used at dosages of 200–300 mg/kg/day. It is available in 1-, 3-, and 6-g vials. The advantage of ticarcillin over carbenicillin is that it is more active against *Pseudomonas.*[54] Another advantage is a reduced dose of ticarcillin (with the same therapeutic efficacy) resulting in less platelet dysfunction and less hypokalemia. See Chapter 17 for a discussion of ticarcillin-clavulanate.

Indanyl Carbenicillin

Indanyl carbenicillin (carindacillin) is an α-carboxy ester of carbenicillin. It has no intrinsic activity of its own, but as a sodium ester it is highly acid stable and relatively well absorbed from the gastrointestinal tract. Ingestion with food may actually enhance absorption. The ester is immediately hydrolyzed to free carbenicillin, and only trace amounts of ester are found in serum or urine. Peak serum levels after 1 g taken orally are 10 μg at 1–2 hours. Urine levels are 300–1000 μg/ml with 30 percent of a dose recovered in the first 6 hours. The compound does not provide adequate serum or tissue levels for systemic infections, and it is useful only for the treatment of urinary tract infections. In the presence of decreased renal function, urine levels are lower and may be inadequate to treat *Pseudomonas* infections. Side effects are those of all the penicillins, but gastrointestinal irritation has been a problem in some people. It is available as 500-mg capsules (containing 382 mg of carbenicillin). The usual dosage is 1 g every 6 hours for adults. Quinolones should replace this agent for treatment of urinary tract infections and prostatitis.

Ureidopenicillins

Azlocillin. Azlocillin is an acylureido penicillin that is 8–16 times more active than carbenicillin against *Pseudomonas aeruginosa* and is less active against indole-positive *Proteus* spp. It has the same activity as ampicillin against streptococcal species.[55] It is destroyed by β-lactamases of both gram-positive and gram-negative bacteria. It is not orally absorbed and must be given by the intravenous route to provide adequate serum levels to treat *Pseudomonas* infection. The half-life is approximately 50 minutes, and administration of 4 g yields peak levels of 285 μg/ml.

Azlocillin shows nonlinear pharmacokinetics. The peak serum concentrations and the area under the drug curve are not proportional; that is, a 4- or 5-g dose produces serum levels that are greater than four or five times the 1-g dose.[56] The drug thus could be administered in larger doses at intervals of 6 hours. Azlocillin also does not accumulate in renal failure to the same degree as do carbenicillin and ticarcillin, since its half-life rises only to 4 hours with creatinine clearances below 7 ml/min.[57–59] Azlocillin enters the cerebrospinal fluid in the presence of meningeal inflammation, but levels are only 10 percent of the serum level. Azlocillin also causes less increase in bleeding time than does carbenicillin, since it apparently has less affinity for the ADP receptor site. Azlocillin is used primarily to treat *Pseudomonas* infections. It has proved to be a useful drug in a variety of clinical situations.[58] It is available in 1-, 2-, 3-, and 4-g vials, which contain 2.17 mEq sodium per gram of drug.

Mezlocillin. Mezlocillin is an acylureido penicillin similar in antibacterial spectrum to carbenicillin and ticarcillin but with some significant differences.[55] It is more active in vitro against *E. faecalis* than either of the above-mentioned agents. It inhibits about 75 percent of *Klebsiella* species at a concentration of 25 μg/ml, whereas less than 5 percent would be inhibited by 100 μg/ml of carbenicillin.[60] It is also more active than carbenicillin or ticarcillin against *H. influenzae* and is more active than carbenicillin against *B. fragilis*. It is, however, not more stable to β-lactamase hydrolysis than is carbenicillin; hence its greater intrinsic activity is due to other factors such as greater affinity for PBPs and better entry into the bacterial periplasmic space. It acts synergistically against gram-negative bacteria when combined with aminoglycosides. The drug must be given parenterally. Like azlocillin and piperacillin, mezlocillin shows dose-

related nonlinear kinetics. Peak serum levels, half-life, and area under the time curve are greater with larger doses. Administration of 4 g produces peak levels of 300 μg/ml.[61] Its half-life increases only to 4 hours in patients in renal failure. Mezlocillin is the least likely of the broad-spectrum penicillins to alter bleeding times. Clinical studies in the United States and Europe have shown that it is effective therapy for respiratory, urinary, gynecologic, and surgical infections.[58,62–67] It causes less increase in bleeding time than does carbenicillin. Usual doses have been 12–18 g/day for adults. It is available in 1-, 2-, 3-, and 5-g vials, which contain 1.85 mEq of sodium per gram.

Piperacillin. Piperacillin is an acylueido penicillin derivative that is similar in activity to ampicillin against gram-positive species.[68] It has excellent activity against streptococcal species and against *Neisseria* and *Haemophilus* and many Enterobacteriaceae. It also has excellent activity against both cocci and bacilli anaerobic species. It inhibits 60 percent of *Pseudomonas* species at 3 μg/ml and 90 percent at 12μg/ml.[68,69] It is hydrolyzed by plasmid-mediated β-lactamases of gram-positive and gram-negative bacteria. Its acts synergistically against *Pseudomonas* and against some of the Enterobacteriaceae when combined with aminoglycosides.[68] The human pharmacology of piperacillin is similar to that of azlocillin and mezlocillin.[70–73] Administration of 4 g by the intravenous route produces peak serum levels of 300 μg/ml. It shows kinetics that are dose dependent. It accumulates in renal failure to a lesser degree than does carbenicillin, and its half-life is only 4 hours in renal failure.[74] It is removed by hemodialysis. Piperacillin has shown adverse reactions similar to those of the other penicillins noted earlier. After prolonged administration at high doses neutropenia has been reported. Alteration of bleeding time and hypokalemia occur but less frequently than with carbenicillin. Clinical studies have shown that it is a useful agent in treatment of a variety of infections.[58,75–81] It is administered in daily doses to adults of 12–18 g. It is available in vials of 2, 3, and 4 g, which contain 1.85 mEq of sodium per gram of drug. Piperacillin-tazobactam is discussed in Chapter 17.

REFERENCES

1. Fleming A. On the antibacterial action of cultures of a penicillium, with special reference to their use in the isolation of *B. influenzae*. Br J Exp Pathol. 1929; 10:226.
2. Batchelor FR, Doyle FP, Naylor JHC, et al. Synthesis of penicillin: 6-Aminopenicillanic acid in penicillin fermentations. Nature. 1959;183:257.
3. Tipper DJ, Wright A. The structure and biosynthesis of bacterial cell walls. In: Sokatch JR, Ornstein LA, eds. The Bacteria. v 7. New York: Academic Press, 1979:291.
4. Strominger JL. Penicillin-sensitive enzymatic reactions in bacterial cell wall synthesis. Harvey Lect. 1970;64:179.
5. Mirelman D. Biosynthesis and assembly of cell wall peptidoglycan. In: Inouye M, ed. Bacterial Outer Membranes. New York: John Wiley & Sons; 1980: 166.
6. Waxman DL, Yocum RR, Stominger JL. Penicillins and cephalosporins are active site-directed acylating agents: Evidence in support of the substrate analogue hypothesis. Philos Trans R Soc Lond [Biol]. 1980;289:257.
7. Ghuysen JM. Serine beta-lactamases and penicillin-binding proteins. Annu Rev Microbiol. 1991;45:37.
8. Spratt BG. Distinct penicillin binding proteins involved in the division, elongation and shape of *Escherichia coli*, K 12. Proc Natl Acad Sci USA. 1975;72: 2999.
9. Spratt BG. Biochemical and genetical approaches to the mechanism of action of penicillin. Philos Trans R Soc Lond [Biol]. 1980;289:273.
10. Georgopapadakou NH, Liu FY. Binding of β-lactam antibiotics to penicillin-binding proteins of *Staphylococcus aureus* and *Streptococcus faecalis* in relation to antibacterial activity. Antimicrob Agents Chemother. 1980;18:834.
11. Spratt BG, Bowler LB, Edelman A, et al. Membrane topology of PBPs 1B and 3 of *E. coli* and the production of water-soluble forms of high molecular weight PBPs. In: Shockman GD, ed. Antibiotic Inhibition of Bacterial Cell Surface Assembly and Function. Washington, DC: American Society for Microbiology; 1988:292.
12. Maidhof H, Johannssen L, Labischinski H, et al. Onset of penicillin induced bacteriolysis in staphylococci is cell cycle dependent. J Bacteriol. 1989;171: 2252.

13. Sykes RB, Matthew M. The β-lactamases of gram-negative bacteria and their role in resistance to β-lactam antibiotics. J Antimicrob Agents Chemother. 1976;2:115.
14. Smith JM, Dowson CG, Spratt BG. Localized sex in bacteria. Nature. 1991; 349:29.
15. Barber M, Waterworth PM. Antibacterial activity of the penicillins. Br Med J. 1962;1:1159.
16. Rolinson GN, Sutherland R. Semisynthetic penicillins. Adv Pharmacol Chemother. 1973;11:152.
17. Marcy SM, Klein JO. The isoxazolyl penicillins: Oxacillin, cloxacillin and dicloxacillin. Med Clin North Am. 1970;54:1127.
18. Finland M, Garner C, Wolcox C, et al. Susceptibility of pneumococci and *Haemophilus influenzae* to antibacterial agents. Antimicrob Agents Chemother. 1976;9:274.
19. Sutter VL, Finegold SM. Susceptibility of anaerobic bacteria to 23 antimicrobial agents. Antimicrob Agents Chemother. 1976;10:736.
20. Neu HC. Antimicrobial activity and human pharmacology of amoxicillin. J Infect Dis. 1974;129 (Suppl):123.
21. McCarthy CG, Finland M. Absorption and excretion of four penicillins: penicillin G, penicillin V, phenethicillin and phenylmercaptomethyl penicillin. N Engl J Med. 1960;263:315.
22. Butler K, English AR, Briggs B, et al. Indanyl carbenicillin: chemistry and laboratory studies with a new semisynthetic penicillin. J Infect Dis. 1973; 127(Suppl):97.
23. Eagle H, Newman E. Renal clearance of penicillin. F, G, K, and X in rabbits and man. J Clin Invest. 1947;26:903.
24. Cole M, Kening MD, Hewitt VA. Metabolism of penicillins to penicilloic acidosis and 6-aminopenicillanic acid in man and its significance in assessing penicillin absorption. Antimicrob Agents Chemother. 1973;3:463.
25. Acocella G, Mattiussi R, Nichols FB, et al. Biliary excretion of antibiotics in man. Gut. 1968;9:536.
26. Gilbaldi M, Swartz MA. Apparent effect of probenecid on the distribution of penicillins in man. Clin Pharmacol Ther. 1968;9:345.
27. Appel GB, Neu HC. Infections and antibiotic usage in patients with renal diseases. In: Martinez-Maldonado M, ed. Handbook of Renal Therpeutics. New York: Plenum; 1983:227.
28. Parker RH, Schmid FR. Antibacterial activity of synovial fluid during therapy of septic arthritis. Arthritis Rheum. 1971;14:96.
29. Barza M, Weinstein L. Penetration of antibiotics into fibrin loci in vivo. I. Comparison of penetration of ampicillin into fibrin clots, abscesses and interstitial fluid. J Infect Dis. 1974;129:59.
30. Pancoast SJ, Neu HC. Antibiotic levels in human bone and synovial fluid. Orthop Rev. 1980;9:49.
31. Neu HC. Antistaphylococcal penicillins. Med Clin North Am. 1982;66:51.
32. Neu HC. Carbenicillin and ticarcillin. Med Clin North Am. 1982;66:61.
33. Fishman RA. Blood-brain and CSF barriers to penicillin and related organic acids. Arch Neurol. 1966;15:13.
34. Depp R, Kind AC, Kirby WMM, et al. Transplacental passage of methicillin and dicloxacillin into the fetus and amniotic fluid. Am J Obstet Gynecol. 1970; 197:1054.
35. Whelton A, Carter GG, Bryant HH, et al. Carbenicillin concentrations in normal and diseased kidneys. A therapeutic consideration. Ann Intern Med. 1973;78:659.
36. Levine BB, Redmond AP, Feller MF, et al. Penicillin allergy and the heterogeneous immune response of man to benzylpenicillin. J Clin Invest. 1966;45: 1895.
37. Saxon A. Immediate hypersensitivity reactions to β-lactam antibiotics. Rev Infect Dis. 1983;5(Suppl 2):368.
38. Idsoe O, Gothe T, Wilcox RR, et al. Nature and extent of penicillin side reactions with particular reference to fatalities from anaphylactic shock. Bull WHO. 1968;38:159.
39. Green GR, Rosenblum A. Report of the penicillin study group, American Academy of Allergy. J Allergy Clin Immunol. 1971;48:331.
40. Parry MF, Neu HC. The safety and tolerance of mezlocillin. J Antimicrob Chemother. 1982;9(Suppl A):273.
41. Kerr RO, Cardamone J, Dalmasso AP, et al. Two mechanisms of erthrocyte destruction in penicillin-induced hemolytic anemia. N Engl J Med. 1972;287: 1322.
42. Brown CH, Natelson EA, Bradshaw W, et al. The hemostatic defect produced by carbenicillin. N Engl J Med. 1974;291:265.
43. Appel GB, Neu HC. The nephrotoxicity of antimicrobial agents. N Engl J Med. 1977;296:63.
44. Appel GB, Neu HC. Acute interstitial nephritis induced by β-lactam antibiotics. In: Fillastre JP, ed. Nephrotoxicity-Ototoxicity of Drugs. Rouen: Inserum Publ de l'Université de Rouen; 1981:195.
45. Baldwin DS, Levine BB, McCluskey RT, et al. Renal failure and interstitial nephritis due to penicillin and methicillin. N Engl J Med. 1968;279:1245.
46. Bloomer HA, Barton LJ, Maddock RJ Jr. Penicillin-induced encephalopathy in uremic patients. JAMA. 1967;200:121.
47. Wilson FM, Belamavic J, Lauter CB, et al. Anicteric carbenicillin hepatitis. Eight episodes in four patients. JAMA. 1967;232:818.
48. New HC. Aminopenicillins: Clinical pharmacology and use in disease states. Int J Clin Pharmacol Biopharm. 1975;11:132.

49. Prince AS, Neu HC. New penicillins and their use in pediatrics. Pediatr Clin North Am. 1983;30:3.
50. Fang LST, Tolokoff-Rubin NE, Rubin RH. Efficacy of single-dose and conventional amoxicillin therapy in urinary tract infection localized by antibody-coated bacteria technique. N Engl J Med. 1978;298:413.
51. Fuchs PC, Thornsberry C, Barry AL, et al. Ticarcillin: A collaborative in vitro comparison with carbenicillin against 9,000 clinical bacterial isolates. Am J Med Sci. 1977;274:255.
52. Hoffman TA, Cestero R, Bullock WE. Pharmacodynamics of carbenicillin in patients with hepatic and renal failure. Ann Intern Med. 1970;73:173.
53. Neu HC, Garvey GG. Comparative in vitro activity and clinical pharmacology of ticarcillin and carbenicillin. Antimicrob Agents Chemother. 1975;8:457.
54. Parry MF, Neu HC. Ticarcillin for treatment of serious infections with gram-negative bacteria. J Infect Dis. 1976;134:476.
55. Fu KP, Neu HC. Azlocillin and mezlocillin: New ureido penicillins. Antimicrob Agents Chemother. 1978;13:930.
56. Bergen T. Review of the pharmacokinetics and dose dependency of azlocillin in normal subjects and patients with renal insufficiency. J Antimicrob Agents. 1983;11(Suppl B):101.
57. Whelton A, Stout RL, Delgado FA. Azlocillin kinetics during extracorporeal haemodialysis and peritoneal dialysis. J Antimicrob Chemother. 1983; 11(Suppl B):89.
58. Drusano GL, Schimpff SC, Hewitt WL. The acylampicillins: Mezlocillin, piperacillin, and azlocillin. Rev Infect Dis. 1984;6:13.
59. Lowenbraun S, Fox N, Cunitz D. Azlocillin, cephalothin and tobramycin therapy in solid tumor patients with chemotherapy-induced leukopenia. Cancer. 1987;60:14.
60. Parry MF, Folta D. The in vitro activity of mezlocillin against community hospital isolates in comparison to other penicillins and cephalosporins. J Antimicrob Chemother. 1983;11(Suppl C):97.
61. Meyers BR, Mendelson MH, Srulevitch-Chin E, et al. Pharmacokinetic properties of mezlocillin in ambulatory elderly subjects. J Clin Pharmacol. 1987; 27:678.
62. Pancoast SJ, Jahre JA, Neu HC. Mezlocillin in the therapy of serious infections. Am J Med. 1979;67:747.
63. Issell BF, Bodey GP. Mezlocillin for treatment of infections in cancer patients. Antimicrob Agents Chemother. 1980;17:1008.
64. Melikian V, Wise R, Allum WH, et al. Mezlocillin and gentamicin in the treatment of infections in seriously ill and immunosuppressed patients. J Antimicrob Chemother. 1981;7:657.
65. Ramirez-Ronda CH, Gotierrez J, Bermudez RH. Comparative effectiveness, safety and tolerance of mezlocillin and ticarcillin: A prospective randomized trial. J Antimicrob Chemother. 1982;9(Suppl A):125.
66. Faro S, Phillips LE, Baker JL, et al. Comparative efficacy and safety of mezlocillin, cefoxitin, and clindamycin plus gentamycin in post-partum endometritis. Obstet Gynecol. 1987;69:760.
67. Alvarez RD, Kilgore LC, Huddlestone JF. A comparison of mezlocillin versus clindamycin/gentamicin for the treatment of post-caesarean endomyometritis. Am J Obst Gynecol. 1988;158:425.
68. Fu KP, Neu HC. Piperacillin, a new penicillin active against many bacteria resistant to other penicillins. Antimicrob Agents Chemother. 1978;13:358.
69. Verbist L. Comparison of the activities of the new ureido-penicillins—piperacillin, mezlocillin, azlocillin and Bay K4999—against gram-negative organisms. Antimicrob Agents Chemother. 1979;16:115.
70. Bergen T. Overview of acylureidopenicillin pharmacokinetics. Scand J Infect Dis. 1981;29:33.
71. Tjandramaga TB, Mollie A, Verbesselt R, et al. Piperacillin pharmacokinetics after intravenous and intramuscular administration. Antimicrob Agents Chemother. 1978;14:829.
72. Martens MG, Faro S, Feldman S, et al. Pharmacokinetics of the acylureidopenicillins piperacillin and mezlocillin in the post-partum patient. Antimicrob Agents Chemother. 1987;31:2015.
73. Brattstrom C, Malmborg AS, Tyden G. Penetration of clindamycin, cefoxitin, and piperacillin into pancreatic juice in man. Surgery. 1988;103:563.
74. Francke EL, Appel GB, New HC. Pharmacokinetics of intravenous piperacillin in patients undergoing chronic hemodialysis. Antimicrob Agents Chemother. 1979;16:788.
75. Winston DJ, Murphy W, Young LS, et al. Piperacillin therapy for serious bacterial infections. Am J Med. 1980;69:255.
76. Wade JC, Schimpff SC, Newman KA, et al. Piperacillin or ticarcillin plus amikacin: a double blind prospective comparison of empiric antibiotic therapy for febrile granulocytopenic cancer patients. Am J Med. 1981;71:983.
77. Pancoast SJ, Prince AS, Francke EL, et al. Clinical evaluation of piperacillin for therapy of infection. Arch Intern Med. 1981;141:1447.
78. Prince AS, Neu HC. Use of piperacillin, a semisynthetic penicillin, in the therapy of acute exacerbations of pulmonary disease in patients with cystic fibrosis. J Pediatr. 1980;97:148.
79. Hemsell DL, Hemsell PG, Heard MC. Piperacillin and a combination of clindamycin and gentamicin for the treatment of hospital and community-acquired acute pelvic infections including pelvic abscess. Surg Gynecol Obstet. 1987; 165:223.
80. Menichetti F, Del Favero A, Guerciolini R, et al. Empiric antimicrobial therapy in febrile granulocytopenic patients. Randomized prospective comparison of amikacin plus piperacillin with or without parenteral trimethoprim/sulfamethoxazole. Infection. 1986;14:61.
81. Holmes B, Richard DM, Brodgen RN, et al. Piperacillin: A review of its antibacterial activity, pharmacokinetic properties, and their therapeutic use. Drugs. 1984;28:375.

16. CEPHALOSPORINS

ADOLF W. KARCHMER

The cephalosporins, among the most widely prescribed antimicrobials, take origin from the work of Giuseppe Brotzu, a Professor of the University of Cagliari, in the mid-1940s. Brotzu hypothesized that the apparent periodic clearing of microorganisms from the water in the vicinity of a sewage outlet in the harbor at Cagliari, Sardinia, might result from the inhibitory effects of substances produced by another microbe. His search for a microbe producing such a substance in the seawater at the harbor sewage outlet ultimately led to the isolation of a fungus, *Cephalosporium acremonium* (now called *Acremonium chrysogenum*), the first microbial source of a cephalosporin.[1] Brotzu found that the growth of certain gram-positive and gram-negative bacteria was inhibited by this organism. Furthermore, filtrates from cultures of *C. acremonium* seem to produce antibacterial effects on infections in animals and patients. In fact, Brotzu injected this material into boils and other skin infections with some apparent success and subsequently administered it parenterally to local patients with typhoid fever and brucellosis.[2] In 1948, unable to proceed further with his work on the antimicrobial substance produced by *C. acremonium,* he sent a culture of the organism to Sir Howard Florey at Oxford. There workers, led by Professor Edward P. Abraham, proceeded to identify several fermentation products of *C. acremonium* that possessed antimicrobial activity.

Three antimicrobial substances were ultimately isolated from cultures of *C. acremonium* by workers at Oxford; one of these gave rise to the cephalosporins. Initially they identified a steroid, called cephalosporin P, with activity against only gram-positive bacteria. Later they found cephalosporin N, a compound with antibacterial activity against gram-negative bacteria. This material was subsequently shown to be a penicillin with an aminocarboxybutyl side chain and it was renamed penicillin N. Ultimately, a third substance, cephalosporin C, was identified. This material, which was less active against *Salmonella typhi* and staphylococci than penicillin N, was of interest because it was not destroyed by the penicillinase of staphylococci and *Bacillus cereus* and was relatively acid stable.[2] Ultimately cephalosporin C became the foundation upon which our current cephalosporin antimicrobials are constructed.

CHEMISTRY

Cephalosporin C (Fig. 1) is a β-lactam compound in which the β-lactam ring is fused to a six-membered dihydrothiazine ring (yielding the cephem nucleus; Fig. 2) in contrast to penicillins

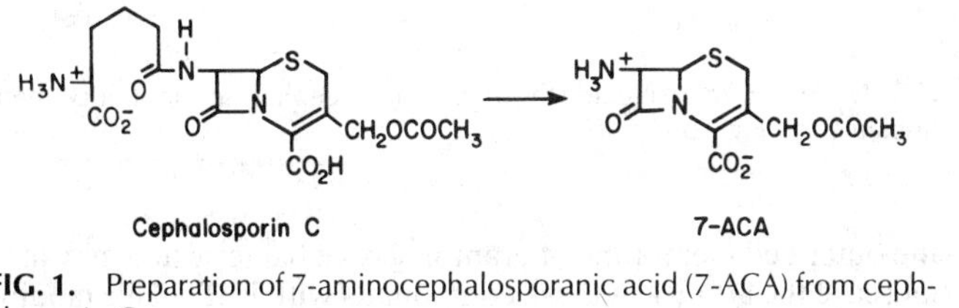

FIG. 1. Preparation of 7-aminocephalosporanic acid (7-ACA) from cephalosporin C.

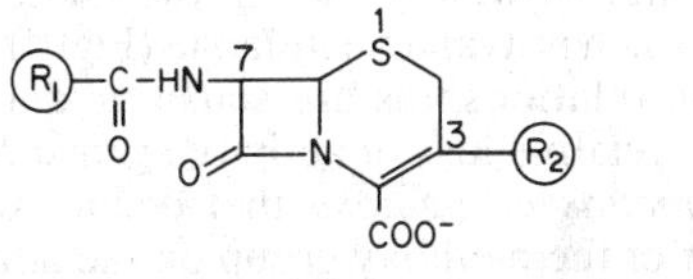

FIG. 2. Basic structure of a cephalosporin (cephem nucleus).

wherein the comparable unit is a five-membered thiazolidine ring. The knowledge that substitution of different side chains at the 6-acylamino site of the 6-aminopenicillanic acid nucleus resulted in semisynthetic penicillins of increased potency set the stage for attempts to modify cephalosporin C and thus enhance its potency.[3] Acid hydrolysis of cephalosporin C resulted in a 7-aminocephalosporanic acid (7-ACA; Fig. 1) and the basic structure for future development of the cephalosporins.[4] The basic molecule of the cephalosporins (the fused β-lactam and dihydrothiazine rings) is numbered beginning in the dihydrothiazine ring with the sulfur moiety at position 1 (Fig. 2). There is an unsaturated bond between positions 3 and 4. The modification of this basic structure by substitutions at position 1, by the addition of substituents at position 3 or 7, or by the addition of different acyl side chains from position 7 has given rise to the family of cephalosporin antibiotics. Modifications at position 7 alter antimicrobial activity while substituents added at position 3 predominantly effect changes in metabolic and pharmacokinetic parameters.[5–7]

The factors involved in the net antibacterial activity of β-lactam antibiotics, as well as the resistance of bacteria to these agents, include the ability of the antibiotic to reach its sites of action, the resistance of the antibiotic to destruction by inactivating enzymes (β-lactamases), and the affinity of the agent for its targets. The targets of β-lactam antibiotics are enzymes situated in the bacterial cytoplasmic membrane called *penicillin-binding proteins* (PBP) that are essential for cell division and survival. Modifications of the cephalosporin nucleus that impact on one or more of these factors may alter antimicrobial activity.

Cephalothin and cephaloridine were the initial clinically useful cephalosporins; they were active against gram-positive cocci (except enterococci and methicillin-resistant staphylococci), *Escherichia coli, Klebsiella pneumoniae,* and *Proteus mirabilis.* Cephaloridine, which differs from cephalothin only at position 3, where cephaloridine has a pyridine group (Fig. 3), has greater bactericidal activity relative to cephalothin for bacteria that lack β-lactamases. This property is attributable to an increased affinity of cephaloridine for essential PBP.[6]

The enhanced activity of early cephalosporins against gram-negative bacilli resulted from the presence of a methoxy group at position 7, replacing a hydrogen.[8,9] Cefoxitin, the initial antibiotic with this structure, was isolated from a culture of *Streptomyces lactamdurans* and is technically a cephamycin.[8] The clinically available cephamycins, which now are synthesized from 7-ACA and include cefoxitin, cefotetan, and cefmetazole, are nevertheless considered among the cephalosporins (Fig. 3). The addition of the methoxy at position 7, replacing a hydrogen, results in enhanced stability of these compounds to β-lactamases of many gram-negative rods, especially those of *Bacteroides fragilis,* and hence increased antibacterial activity against these organisms.[6–9] However, the substitution for the hydrogen at position 7 results in poor binding of these agents to the PBP of gram-positive cocci.[9] As a consequence of this, the cephamycins have reduced activity against staphylococci and streptococci. Cefuroxime, a true cephalosporin, contains a furyl group on the acyl side and an iminomethoxy at the α-position on this chain. Compared with early cephalosporins, it has increased β-lactamase stability as well as retained activity against streptococci and to a lesser degree against methicillin-susceptible staphylococci.[10,11]

Further modifications of the acyl side chain at position 7 by the addition of an aminothiazole group resulted in markedly enhanced activity of cephalosporins against many Enterobacteriaceae.[12,13] The addition of an iminomethoxy group to the α-site of this side chain results in an aminothiazolylmethoxy side chain that confers stability to many of the β-lactamases of gram-negative bacteria while retaining high activity against streptococci and to a lesser degree against methicillin-susceptible *Staphylococcus aureus.*[12–14] The addition of this side chain appears to enhance the penetration of the cephalosporin through

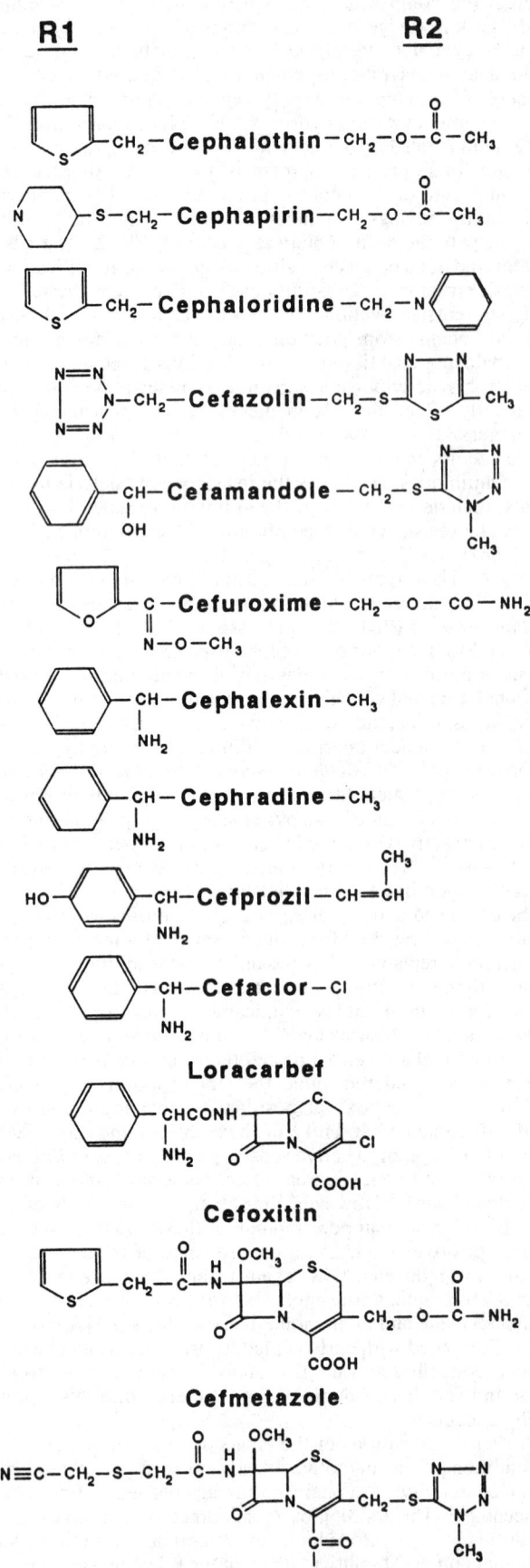

FIG. 3.   Structure of selected first- and second-generation cephalosporins (for cephem nucleus, see Fig. 2).

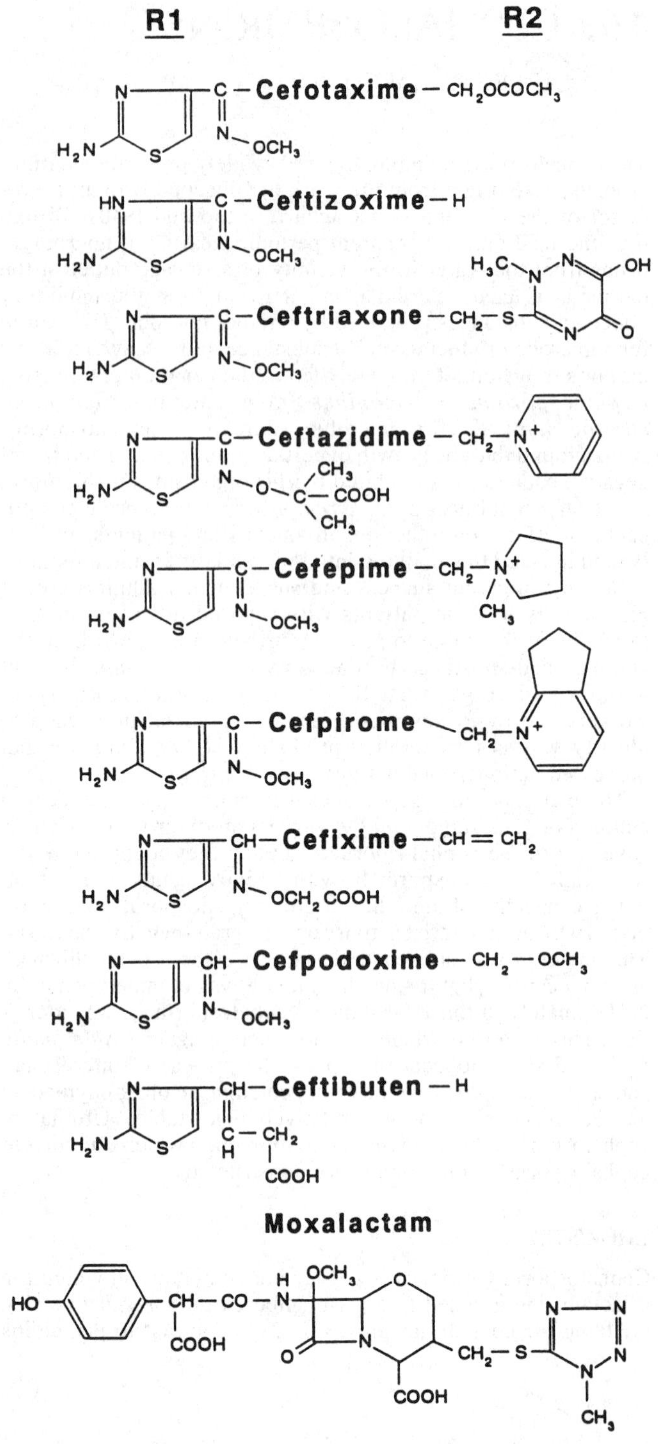

FIG. 4.   Structure of selected third-generation cephalosporins (for cephem nucleus, see Fig. 2).

the outer cell membrane of gram-negative bacteria and may also increase the affinity of these compounds with PBP.[7] This modification, in conjunction with various substituents at the 3 position of the dihydrothiazine ring, results in cefotaxime, ceftizoxime, and ceftriaxone, all widely used in the United States, and cefmenoxime, which is available in Japan (Fig. 4). That these structure-function relationships are sensitive and specific is illustrated by the relative loss of activity against *S. aureus, E. coli*, and *Pseudomonas aeruginosa* that occurs with a shift in the stereoisomer of the methoxy group on the aminothiazolylmethoxy side chain of cefotaxime and ceftizoxime. This change in antimicrobial activity is a consequence of a decrease in affinity for PBP rather than a reduction in β-lactamase stability or penetration through the outer cell membrane.[13,15]

The addition of an acidic moiety to the acyl side chain at position 7 enhances activity against *P. aeruginosa*.[7] A propylcarboxy addition to the aminothiazolyl side chain plus a pyridine at position 3 characterizes ceftazidime (Fig. 4), the clinically used cephalosporin most active against *P. aeruginosa*.[6,16–18] Ceftazidime, to a significant degree, retains the antistreptococcal activity of the other aminothiazolyl cephalosporins (cefotaxime, ceftizoxime, ceftriaxone) but has lost its activity against methicillin-susceptible *S. aureus*.[18] This loss of activity is a consequence of reduced binding to staphylococcal PBP.[19] Cefoperazone, with a ureido(—NH—C—H—)2,3 dioxopiperazine on the acyl side chain and a methylthiotetrazole (MTT) moiety at position 3, achieves modest activity against *P. aeruginosa*. Attempts to maintain good activity against streptococci and *S. aureus*, while achieving increased activity against β-lactamase–producing gram-negative rods including *P. aeruginosa* and the Enterobacteriaceae with inducible chromosomal β-lactamases (*Enterobacter* spp., *Citrobacter freundii*, and *Serratia* spp.) have involved substitutions at positions 3 in aminothiazolylmethoxy cephalosporins. Two such compounds, cefepime and cefpirome, with a pyrolidine and a cyclopentopyridinium moiety at position 3, respectively (Fig. 4), have been evaluated extensively. These dipolar ionic cephalosporins penetrate the gram-negative bacteria outer cell membrane faster than other aminothiazolyl cephalosporins, have good affinity for essential PBP, and low affinity for many β-lactamases, including the inducible β-lactamases of the Enterobacteriaceae (the latter feature correlates with increased β-lactamase stability).[20]

Moxalactam, although considered with the cephalosporins, is an oxacephem since the sulfur at position 1 has been replaced by an oxygen (Fig. 4). Because this shift not only enhanced antibacterial activity against gram-negative bacteria without β-lactamases but also decreased β-lactamase stability, a methoxy group was inserted at position 7 to replace a hydrogen (as seen in the cephamycin). A carboxyl group is present on the acyl side chain, further improving β-lactamase stability, and there is an MTT moiety at position 3. Of note, as in the cephamycins, the replacement of hydrogen at position 7 results in reduced binding to the PBP of gram-positive cocci with significant loss of activity against methicillin-susceptible *S. aureus* and streptococci.[6,20]

Major modifications of the cephem nucleus at position 3 have been initiated in the search for useful cephalosporins resulting from alterations of pharmacokinetic features. Cephalexin, the initial cephalosporin absorbed from the gastrointestinal tract, contains an aminobenzyl substituent on the acyl side chain and, importantly for gastrointestinal absorption, a methyl group at position 3 (Fig. 3). Cephradine, which has a cyclohexadine group replacing the phenol group of cephalexin, and cefadroxyl, with a hydroxy aminobenzyl on the acyl side chain, both have a methyl moiety at position 3 (Fig. 3). They are also absorbed from the gastrointestinal tract, suggesting that the simple moiety at position 3, in contrast to the bulky substituents in this position on cephalothin, cephapirin, and cefazolin, has a major impact on bioavailability after ingestion. Cefaclor, which has a chlorine replacing the methyl group at position 3 of cephalexin, and cefprozil, which has a vinyl methyl replacing this methyl group in cefadroxil, are also well absorbed after ingestion. Loracarbef resembles cefaclor; however, it is a carbacephem in which a carbon has replaced the sulfur of the dihydrothiazine ring (Fig. 3). Cefixime, an aminothiazolyl cephalosporin with anticipated activity against a broad group of gram-negative bacteria, has a vinyl group at position 3. The bioavailability after ingestion of all of these compounds is adversely impacted by the polarity of the carboxyl group at position 4, a group required for the activity of the β-lactam ring. Esterification of this carboxyl group results in an inactive prodrug that can be cleaved by intestinal mucosal esterases during absorption to liberate an active cephalosporin into the circulation. Cefuroxime axetil and cefpodoxime proxetil are compounds in which esterification of this carboxyl has facilitated gastrointestinal absorption of cephalosporins with an iminomethoxy group as the furyl and aminothiazolyl, respectively.[7,21,22] Alteration of the substitution at position 3 may have other pharmacokinetic effects. Markedly enhanced protein binding and a prolonged serum half-life are noted in cefonicid when a sulfamethyl group replaces the methyl group on the MTT moiety at position 3 in cefamandole.[7]

Modifications of the cephalosporin basic unit to achieve a given pharmacokinetic effect may have unanticipated and undesirable consequences. The MTT substituent at position 3 of some cephalosporins and cephamycins (cefamandole, cefmenoxime, cefoperazone, moxalactam, cefmetazole, cefotetan) has been associated with prolongation of the prothrombin time and, in association with alcohol consumption, a disulfiramlike reaction.

CLASSIFICATION

Several complex classifications of the cephalosporins using microbiologic, pharmacokinetic, and β-lactamase stability have been proposed. No classification has been entirely suitable; nevertheless, the somewhat arbitrary system that is most widely used combines the parenteral and oral cephalosporins into generations based on their spectrum of microbiologic activity (Tables 1 and 2). The first-generation compounds have a relatively narrow spectrum of activity focused primarily on the gram-positive cocci. The second-generation cephalosporins have variable activity against gram-positive cocci but have increased activity against gram-negative bacteria. In spite of relatively increased potency against gram-negative aerobic and anaerobic bacilli, the cephamycins are included in the second generation. Those cephalosporins with very marked activity against the gram-negative bacteria are grouped in a third generation; some of these compounds have limited activity against gram-positive cocci, particularly methicillin-susceptible *S. aureus*. Cefsulodin and cefmenoxime, parenterally administered cephalosporins not listed in Table 1, are grouped with the third-generation cephalosporins even though the clinically relevant activity of cefsulodin is directed only at *P. aeruginosa*. Recently, several compounds have been considered possibly to merit classification as a fourth generation. These cephalosporins, which include cefepime and cefpirome, have activity against gram-positive cocci and a broad array of gram-negative bacteria, including *P. aeruginosa* and many of the Enterobacteriaceae with inducible chromosomal β-lactamases.

MECHANISM OF ACTION

The antimicrobial activity of the cephalosporins, like that of other β-lactam antibiotics, results at least in part from their ability to interfere with the synthesis of the peptidoglycan component of the bacterial cell wall. The peptidoglycan of the gram-positive bacteria forms an outermost thick permeable structure immediately overlying the cell's cytoplasmic membrane. The analogous component overlying the cytoplasmic membrane of the gram-negative bacteria is relatively thin in comparison. External to the peptidoglycan of gram-negative bacteria and separated from it by the periplasmic space is a complex lipopolysaccharide membrane with interspersed proteins. The peptidoglycans are long polysaccharide chains in which *N*-acetylglucosamine (NAG) and *N*-acetylmuramic acid (NAM) residues alternate in a linear form. Using the pentapeptide side chain of NAM residues, these polysaccharide strands are cross-linked into a netlike structure. The NAG and NAM-pentapeptide components of peptidoglycan are synthesized in the cytoplasm and transported across the cytoplasmic membrane. Thereafter these residues are inserted into the existing cross-linked peptidogly-

TABLE 1. Selected Parenteral Cephalosporins by Generation and Dosing Range

Generic Name (Proprietary Name)	Formulation	Dosing Range		Children[a]
		Adults		
		Dose/Interval	Daily Dose, Severe Infection	Dose (mg/kg/day)/Interval
First generation				
Cephalothin (Keflin, Seffin)	IV	0.5–2 g q4–6h	6–12 g	75–125/q4–6h
Cefazolin (Ancef, Kefzol)	IV/IM	0.5–1.5 g q6–8h	3–6 g	50–100/q6–8h
Cephapirin (Cefadyl)	IV/IM	0.5–2 g q4–6h	6–12 g	40–80/q4–6h
Cephradine (Velosef)	IV/IM	0.5–2 g q4–6h	4–12 g	50–100/q6h
Second generation				
Cefamandole (Mandol)	IV/IM	0.5–2 g q4–6h	6–12 g	100–150/q4–8h
Cefonocid (Monocid)	IV/IM	0.5–2 g q24h	2 g	40/q24h[b]
Cefuroxime (Kefurox, Zenacef) (Cephamycins)	IV/IM	0.75–1.5 g q6–8h	4.5–6 g	100–240/q6–8h
Cefoxitin (Mefoxin)	IV/IM	1–2 g q4–6h	6–12 g	80–160/q4–6h
Cefotetan (Cefotan)	IV/IM	1–3 g q12h	4–6 g	40–80/q12h[b]
Cefmetazole (Zefazone)	IV	2 g q6–12h	8 g	—[b]
Third generation				
Cefotaxime (Claforan)	IV/IM	1–2 g q4–8h	6–12 g	100–180/q4–6h
Ceftizoxime (Cefizox)	IV/IM	1–4 g q8–12h	6–12 g	150–200/q6–8h
Ceftriaxone (Rocephin)	IV/IM	0.5–2 g q12–24h	2–4 g	50–100/q12–24h
Cefoperazone (Cefobid)	IV/IM	2–4 g q8–12h	6–12 g	100–150/q8–12h[b]
Ceftazidine (Fortaz, Tazidime, Tazicef)	IV/IM	0.5–2 g q8–12h	6 g	90–150/q8h
Cefpirome (investigational)	IV/IM	1–2 g q12h		
Cefpiramide (investigational)	IV	1–4 g q24h		

[a] Dose for infants in first month of life (neonates) may differ; consult specific reference.
[b] Pediatric experience limited; not approved for pediatric use.

TABLE 2. Selected Oral Cephalosporins by Generation: Formulation and Dosing Range

Generic Name (Proprietary Name)	Formulation	Dosing Range	
		Adults Dose/Interval	Children mg/kg/d Interval
First generation			
Cephalexin (Keflex, Keftab, Biocef)	0.25, 0.5 g tabs/caps 125, 250 mg/5 ml susp	0.25–1 g q 6h	25–100/q6h
Cephradine (Velosef, Anspor)	0.25–0.5 g caps 125, 250 mg/5 ml susp	0.25–1 g q6h	25–50/q6h
Cefadroxil (Duricef, Ultracef)	0.5, 1.0 g tabs 125, 250, 500 mg/5 ml susp	0.5–1 g q12–24h	30/q12–24h
Second generation			
Cefaclor (Ceclor)	0.25, 5 g caps 125, 187, 250, 375 mg/5 ml susp	0.25–.5 g q8h	40/q8h
Cefuroxime axetil (Ceftin)	0.125, 0.25, 0.5 tabs	0.25–.5 g q12h	30–40g/q12h[a]
Cefprozil (Cefzil)	0.25, 0.5 caps 125, 250 mg/5 ml susp	0.25–.5g q12–24h	30/q12h
Loracarbef (Lorabid)	0.20 g tabs 100, 200 mg/5 ml susp	0.2–.4 q12h	15–30/q12h[a]
Third generation			
Cefixime (Suprax)	0.2, .5 g caps 100 mg/5 ml susp[b]	0.2 g q12h 0.4 g q24h[c]	8/q12 or 24h
Cefpodoxime proxetil (Vantin)	0.1, 0.2 g tabs 50, 100 mg/5 ml susp	0.2–0.4 q12h[c]	10/q12h
Ceftibuten (investigational)		0.2–0.4 q12h	9/q24h

[a] Higher listed dose recommended for otitis media.
[b] Higher serum concentrations with suspension.
[c] Lower urinary tract infection: cefuroxime axetil, 0.125–0.25 g q12h; loracarbcef, 0.20 g qd; cefpodoxime, 0.1 g q12h.

can as part of cell growth and division by transpeptidases, carboxypeptidases, and endopeptidases. These enzymes, located in the cytoplasmic membrane, are the site of action for β-lactam antibiotics and are called *penicillin-binding proteins* (PBP). Because the amide component of the β-lactam antibiotic is structurally similar to the D-alanyl–D-alanine natural substrate of these enzymes, the antibiotic may bind to the PBP. As a result of its long-lived covalent bond with the β-lactam antibiotic, the PBP is rendered inactive.[23,24] The PBP of cells vary structurally, quantitatively, functionally, and in their affinity for β-lactam antibiotics. The effect of a given β-lactam antibiotic on a cell is related to which PBP are inactivated and to the role of those PBP in peptidoglycan synthesis and cell survival.[25–29] How cephalosporins and other β-lactam antibiotics exert bactericidal

or lytic effects through the inhibition of PBP is not completely understood.

MECHANISMS OF RESISTANCE

Microbial resistance to cephalosporins, as well as to other β-lactam antibiotics, can be mediated through three mechanisms: alteration of a PBP target that is essential for cell survival, production of β-lactamases that inactivate the cephalosporin, or decreased ability of the antibiotic to reach its PBP target. Often multiple mechanisms may work in concert to render a cell resistant.

While gram-negative bacteria can utilize the reduced ability of some cephalosporins to penetrate to the PBP target site in order to enhance resistance, this option is not available to gram-positive bacteria. In gram-positive bacteria the cytoplasmic membrane resides immediately beneath the relatively porous outermost peptidoglycan structure. The peptidoglycan does not exclude molecules the size of cephalosporins; hence these antibiotics easily reach the PBP. In contrast, the gram-negative bacteria have a complex outer membrane composed of lipids, polysaccharides, and proteins; this membrane constitutes a significant barrier to cephalosporins and other molecules.[30] Cephalosporins penetrate this outer cell membrane primarily through water-filled channels, called *porins*, that are formed by various outer membrane proteins. The movement of antibiotics through porins is selective based on their size, shape, charge, and hydrophilic properties.[31,32] Although the relative permeability of this outer membrane for a specific β-lactam antibiotic is an intrinsic feature of the organism, changes in porins as a consequence of exposure to an antimicrobial may reduce penetration further and thus enhance resistance.[33] It is unlikely that porin permeability barriers alone will result in the resistance of gram-negative bacteria to cephalosporins.[34] Nevertheless, the rate of a β-lactam antibiotic's penetration through the outer membrane is intrinsically linked to resistance mediated by β-lactamases.[35–37]

Reduced affinity of PBP for β-lactam antibiotics is a mechanism by which some *Neisseria gonorrhea* and *Streptococcus pneumoniae* have become relatively resistant to penicillins. Methicillin-resistant *S. aureus* produce PBP2′ (also called PBP2a), which has markedly reduced affinity for penicillinase-resistant penicillins and cephalosporins.[32,39] The ability of this novel PBP to functionally replace essential PBP that have higher affinity for these antibiotics ultimately mediates the resistance of methicillin-resistant *S. aureus* to all cephalosporins.

Production of β-lactamase is the mechanism by which clinically relevant gram-negative bacteria are most frequently resistant to cephalosporins. These inactivating enzymes are encoded chromosomally or extrachromosomally through plasmids or transposons and may be produced constitutively or induced. β-Lactamases are widely distributed in gram-negative bacteria and are present in some gram-positive bacteria, most notably staphylococci. These enzymes, like the PBP themselves, belong to a family of serine proteases. The binding of β-lactamase to an antibiotic catalyzes a rapid reaction resulting in hydrolysis at the critical amide bond of the β-lactam ring and antibiotic inactivation. In contrast, upon the binding of a β-lactam antibiotic to a PBP, the reaction proceeds slowly or not at all, resulting in effective inactivation of the PBP. The net ability of a β-lactamase to protect a cell from an antibiotic results from a complex interaction of antibiotic concentration, stability of the antibiotic to the β-lactamase, affinity of the antibiotic for the β-lactamase, and concentration of the β-lactamase in the cell environment.[40] Gram-positive bacteria release β-lactamase directly into their immediate environs. In the presence of a cephalosporin, the survival of otherwise susceptible gram-positive bacteria depends on the collective ability of the cells to inactivate the cephalosporin enzymatically. In fact, most cephalosporins, with the exception of cephaloridine, are poorly hydrolyzed by staphylococcal β-lactamase. The antistaphylococcal effect, therefore, is largely related to the cephalosporin's affinity for essential staphylococcal PBP. The cephamycins and ceftazidime, which are relatively β-lactamase stable, have reduced antistaphylococcal activity as a consequence of poor affinity for the PBP of *S. aureus*.[6]

β-Lactamase–mediated resistance to cephalosporins among gram-negative bacteria is more complex. In these organisms, β-lactamase is confined to the periplasmic space. Entry of cephalosporins into this space, as noted above, is regulated by porins. Given suitable affinity for the cephalosporins, both β-lactamase unstable cephalosporins and ones that are relatively β-lactamase stable can be effectively inactivated by β-lactamases within the confines of the periplasmic space. Reduced penetration of ceph-

alosporins into the periplasmic space will enhance the efficiency with which the β-lactamase protects the cell while the converse will occur with increased penetration.[40] Increased production of β-lactamase or production of a new β-lactamase with enhanced affinity may result in resistance to cephalosporins among gram-negative bacilli. High-level production of TEM-1 or SHV-1 β-lactamases, two of the most commonly encountered plasmid-mediated β-lactamases among Enterobacteriaceae, due to increases in the number of gene copies per cell has been associated with not only resistance to penicillin/β-lactamase inhibitor combinations but also to cephalothin, cefamandole, and cefoperazone.[40,41] *Enterobacter* spp., *Citrobacter freundii, Morganella, Serratia, Providencia,* and *Pseudomonas aeruginosa* have an inducible chromosomally encoded cephalosporinase (a Bush group 1 β-lactamase) with sufficient affinity for currently available cephamycins and cephalosporins, including those of the third generation, that it can inactivate these antibiotics in the periplasmic space. The induction or stable derepression of this chromosomal β-lactamase during prior exposure to cephamycins and third-generation cephalosporins results in resistance to all of the currently available cephalosporins.[40,41] Emergence of this form of resistance is frequent when infection due to these organisms, particularly *Enterobacter cloacae* and *P. aeruginosa,* are treated with broad-spectrum cephalosporins. Furthermore, this resistance often translates to failure of the β-lactam antibiotic therapy.[42] New plasmid-mediated extended-spectrum β-lactamases (ESBL) have been discovered. These derived from a point mutation of TEM-1, TEM-2, or SHV-1 that results in a single amino acid substitution at the enzyme's active site. At least 26 TEM-related and 5 SHV-related distinct EBSL have been described.[43,44] Although occasionally found in other Enterobacteriaceae, ESBL have been noted predominantly in *Klebsiella pneumoniae.* The ESBL mediate high-level resistance to ceftazidime and aztreonam but also confer reduced susceptibility to other third-generation cephalosporins. Bacteria containing an ESBL do not appear notably resistant to third-generation cephalosporins other than ceftazidime. Consequently, clinical laboratories not testing for ceftazidime may overlook strains with ESBL. Nosocomial outbreaks of infection caused by strains with ESBL appear to result from both strain and plasmid dissemination. Barring the presence of concurrent mechanisms of resistance, TEM- and SHV-related ESBL strains remain susceptible to cephamycins and imipenem.[43] The potential for expanded cephalosporin resistance mediated by β-lactamase is foretold by the detection of *K. pneumoniae* and *E. coli* resistant to all β-lactams except imipenem. This resistance was mediated by an *E. cloacae* chromosomal gene that had become incorporated into a plasmid.[44]

PHARMACOLOGY

The pharmacologic properties of selected cephalosporins are presented in Table 3.[21,22,45–48] Absorption from the gastrointestinal tract occurs for cephalexin, cephradine, and cefadroxil among the first-generation agents, for cefaclor, cefuroxime axetil, cefprozil, and the carbapenem loracarbef among the second-generation compounds, and for cefixime and cefpodoxime proxetil among the third-generation agents. The absorption of cefuroxime and cefpodoxime is facilitated by their formulation as esters; the compounds are cleaved to active drug by intestinal mucosal esterases during absorption. Cefetamef and cefteram, which are investigational aminothiazolyl cephalosporins, have also been esterified to facilitate oral administration. Absorption of esterified cephalosporins is enhanced by administration with food as an apparent consequence of the more prolonged contact with the gastric mucosa that results from a food-associated delay in gastric emptying.[21] Bioavailability of cefpodoxime is decreased by H2 antagonist and nonabsorbable antacids, presumably due to incomplete dissolution of drug.[21] Cefixime and cefpodoxime are slowly absorbed and reach lower maximum serum

TABLE 3. Pharmacologic Properties of the Cephalosporins

Generic Name	Adult Dose for Serious Infection[a]	Peak Serum Concentration[b] (μg/ml)	Half-life (hour)	Effect of Food on Peak Serum Concentration	Cerebrospinal Fluid Conc (range, μg/ml)	Serum Protein Binding (%)	Route of Excretion
First generation							
Cefazolin	1 g q8h	80 (1)	1.8			80	Renal
Cephalothin	1–2 g q4–6h	30 (1)	0.6			71	Renal
Cefadroxil	0.5 g q12h po	16 (0.5)	1.2	None		20	Renal
Cephalexin	0.5–1 g q6h po	18 (0.5)	0.9	None		10	Renal
Cephradine	0.5 g q6h po	18 (0.5)	0.7	None		10	Renal
Second generation							
Cefamandole	1–2 g q4–6h	150 (2)	0.8			75	Renal
Cefonicid	1–2 g q24h	260 (2)	4.5			98	Renal
Cefotetan	2–3 g q12h	230 (2)	3.5			90	Renal
Cefoxitin	2 g q4–6h	150 (2)	0.8			70	Renal
Cefmetazole	2 g q6h	140 (2)	1.1			65	Renal
Cefuroxime	1.5 g q8h	100 (1.5)	1.3		1.1–17	35	Renal
Cefaclor	0.25–0.5 g q8h po	13 (0.5)	0.8	Decreased		25	Renal
Cefuroxime axetil	0.25–0.5 g q12h po	8–9 (0.5)	1.3	Increased[c]		35	Renal
Loracarbef	0.4 g q12h po	15 (0.4)	1.1	Decreased		35	Renal
Cefprozil	0.5 g q12h po	10 (0.5)	1.2	None		42	Renal
Third generation							
Cefixime	0.4 g q24h po	3.9 (0.4)	3.7	None		67	Renal 50%; ? other
Cefpodoxime proxetil	0.4 g q12h po	4 (0.4)	2.2	Increased[c]		40	Renal
Ceftibuten	0.2 g q12h po	11 (0.2)	2.5			63	Renal
Cefotaxime	2 g q6–8h	130 (2)	1.0		5.6–44	35	Renal
Ceftizoxime	2 g q8–12h	130 (2)	1.7		0.5–29	30	Renal
Ceftriaxone	1–2 g q12h	250 (2)	8.0		1.2–39	83–96	Renal 50%; biliary 40%
Moxalactam	1–2 g q8h	200 (2)	2.2		0.8–33	50	Renal
Cefmenoxime	2 g q6–8h	100 (2)	1.0			77	Renal
Third-generation cephalosporins with anti-pseudomonas activity							
Cefoperazone	2 g q8–12h	250 (2)	2.0			87–93	Biliary 70%; renal 25%
Cefepime	1–2 g q12h	130 (2)	2.1			20	Renal
Cefpiramide[d]	1–4 g q12–24h	166 (1)	5.4			94–98	Biliary 80%; renal 20%
Cefpirome[d]	1–2 g q12h	100 (1)	2.0		1.3–7.5	10	Renal
Ceftazidime	2 g q8h	160 (2)	1.8		0.5–30	17	Renal

[a] All doses are parenteral unless otherwise stated.
[b] Level after noted gram amount (in parentheses) of drug given intravenously or, where noted in column 2, orally. Peak serum concentrations reported in the literature vary, depending on the time over which a drug is given and time of serum sampling. Representative values are noted.
[c] H₂ antagonist and nonabsorbable antacids decrease absorption.
[d] Investigational.

concentrations relative to the other orally administered cephalosporins. The oral administration of ceftibuten, an investigational third-generation agent, rapidly generates high peak serum concentrations and is comparable to the absorption of cephalexin.[21,22] It is recommended that cephalothin and cephapirin, which cause pain when administered intramuscularly, be limited to the intravenous route. The other parenteral cephalosporins can be administered intravenously or intramuscularly, although the volumes required for administration often limit dosing. The modest discomfort of intramuscular cephalosporin administration has been reduced by adding 1% lidocaine solution to the diluent (see specific package insert). Peak serum concentrations after parenteral administration of cephalosporins are similar; they range between 100 and 150 μg/ml after doses of 2 g.

With a few exceptions, the cephalosporins achieve excellent penetration into tissues and fluid compartments, including lung, female genital tissues, kidney, and synovial, pericardial, peritoneal, and pleural fluids. Cefpiramide, cefoperazone, and ceftriaxone, all of which have significant biliary routes of excretion, achieve high concentration in bile.[49,50] Penetration of cephalosporins into the aqueous humor of the eye may be sufficient with high-dose parenteral therapy to allow effective treatment of anterior chamber infection caused by susceptible gram-positive and gram-negative bacteria. Cephalosporins do not achieve significant concentration in the posterior chamber of vitreous humor. For therapeutic purposes, significant penetration into the cerebrospinal fluid occurs only with cefuroxime, cefotax-

ime, ceftriaxone, ceftizoxime, cefmenoxime, moxalactam, and ceftazidime. Penetration is less satisfactory with cefoperazone.[50,51]

Most cephalosporins are excreted through the kidney and hence achieve exceptionally high urine concentrations. The excess urine concentration relative to the minimum inhibitory concentration (MIC) of the usual urinary tract pathogen often allows effective treatment of urinary tract infection with reduced doses. Alternatively, dose adjustments are required with modest to severe renal dysfunction (Table 4). Cefoperazone, ceftriaxone, and cefpiramide, with significant biliary excretion, do not require dose adjustment in azotemic patients. The half-life of cefotaxime is not significantly increased with renal failure; however, its desacetyl and other metabolites accumulate significantly. Consequently, reduced cefotaxime dosing is warranted with severe azotemia. Cefoperazone and ceftriaxone are not removed by hemodialysis and do not require additional dosing after dialysis. Severe hepatic disease, even in the absence of ascites and its effect on volume of distribution, can alter the pharmacokinetics of cefperazone, cefpiramide, and cefotaxime; there is little impact on ceftriaxone.[50,53] Reduced desacetylation as a result of liver disease may increase the half-life of cefotaxime slightly. In contrast, the half-life of cefoperazone and cefpiramide may increase significantly because of liver disease. In the setting of liver disease, compensatory renal excretion generally occurs. Accumulation of cefoperazone, cefpiramide, ceftriaxone, and cefotaxime is likely to occur in the setting of combined

TABLE 4. Dosing of Selected Cephalosporins in Patients with Renal Insufficiency[a]

Agent	Usual Adult Dose in Serious Infection (Parenteral Unless Indicated)	Maintenance Dose (g)/Dosing Interval (h) GFR (ml/min)			Dosing During Dialysis	
		90–50	50–10	<10	Hemodialysis[b]	CAPD
Cefazolin	1 g q8h	Usual	0.5–1/8–12	0.5–1/24	0.5–1 g	0.5 g q12h
Cephapirin	2 g q6h	Usual	2/8	2/12	2 g	2 q12h
Cephalexin	0.5 g q6h po	Usual	0.5/8–12	0.5/12	0.25 g	0.25 g q8h
Cephradine	0.5 g q6h po	Usual	0.5/8	0.25/12	0.5 g	0.25 g q6h
Cefadroxil	0.5 g q12h po	Usual	0.5/24	0.5/36	0.5 g	0.5 g q24h
Cefamandole	2 g q6h	Usual	2/8	1/12	1 g	1 g q12h
Cefonicid	2 g q24h	Usual	1/24	1/72	None	1 g q72h
Cefotetan	2 g q12h	Usual	2/24	2/48	1 g	1 g q24h
Cefoxitin	2 g q6h	2/8	2/12	1/12	2 g	1 g q24h
Cefuroxime	1.5 g q8h	Usual	1.5/12	0.75/24	1.5 g	0.75 g q24h
Cefuroxime axetil	0.5 g q12h po	Usual	Usual	0.5/24	0.5 g	0.5 g q24h
Cefprozil	0.5 g q12h po	Usual	0.5/24	0.25/24	0.5 g	0.25 g q12h
Cefaclor	0.5 g q8h po	Usual	Usual	0.5/12	0.5 g	0.5 g q8h
Loracarbef	0.4 g q12h po	Usual	0.4/24	0.4/72	0.4 g	0.4 g q24h
Cefixime	0.4 g q24h po	Usual	0.2/24	0.2/24	0.2 g	0.2 g q24h
Cefpodoxime	0.4 g q12h po	Usual	0.4/24	0.2/24	0.4 g	0.2 g q24h
Ceftizoxime	2 g q8h	Usual	1/12	0.5/12	1 g	0.5 g q24h
Cefotaxime	2 g q6–8h	Usual	2/12	2/24	1 g	1.0 g q24h
Ceftazidime	2 g q8h	Usual	1/12	1/24	1 g	0.5 g q24h

[a] Ceftriaxone, cefoperazone: no change in dosing required.
[b] Supplement given after hemodialysis during maintenance therapy.

hepatic and renal failure, and dose adjustment is likely to be required.[50,52]

Cephalosporins with an acetyl group at position 3 on the dihydrothiazine ring (cephalothin, cephapirin, and cefotaxime) undergo in vivo metabolism to a desacetyl form. While the desacetyl form is a less potent antimicrobial, desacetyl cefotaxime may be synergistic with the parent compound and contribute to cefotaxime's net antibacterial effect.[53]

The interplay of cephalosporin pharmacokinetics in the eradication of bacteria merits consideration. Cephalosporins do not, in contrast to quinolones and aminoglycosides, exhibit concentration-dependent killing of bacteria. Bactericidal effect of cephalosporins reaches a maximum at four to five times the MIC of the organism. Furthermore, regrowth of bacteria after exposure to cephalosporins occurs promptly; there is a nonexistent or very brief postantibiotic effect for gram-negative bacteria and an abbreviated effect for streptococci and staphylococci. These considerations suggest that the amount of time a cephalosporin is above the MIC of the pathogen at the site of infection is the important pharmacokinetic parameter for enhanced efficacy. A brief time with a high peak concentration followed by a significant period with concentrations below the MIC is not ideal. Studies using animal models as well as those correlating pharmacokinetic, microbiologic, and clinical observations in patients support this concept.[57–59] Continuous infusion therapy, shorter dose to dose intervals, or strategies to delay excretion may warrant additional attention in cephalosporin therapy.

ADVERSE REACTIONS

The cephalosporins have a highly favorable toxicity profile compared with other antimicrobials. With a few unique exceptions, the adverse events caused by cephalosporins are similar across the group (Table 5).

Local Reactions

Thrombophlebitis, a common complication with intravenously administered medications, occurs in 1–5 percent of cephalosporin recipients and is not uniquely associated with a specific

TABLE 5. Adverse Events Associated with Cephalosporins

	Frequency (%)
Hypersensitivity reactions	
Maculopapular rash	1–3
Urticaria	
Pruritis	
Anaphylaxis/angioedema	Rare
Serum sickness (↑ with cefaclor)	
Eosinophilia	1–7
Hematologic reactions	
Reversible neutropenia	<1
Thrombocytosis	2–5
Coombs test positive (hemolysis is rare)	1–5
Coagulation abnormalities	
Hypoprothrombinemia (related to MTT group)	
Reduced platelet aggregation (moxalactam)	
Gastrointestinal reactions	
Abnormal liver function tests (mild)	1–7
Diarrhea, nonspecific; Clostridium difficile related	
Biliary sludge (ceftriaxone-dose related)	20
Nephrotoxicity	
Interstitial nephritis	Rare
Phlebitis	

agent. Pain at the site of intramuscular injection is not uncommon and can be ameliorated by adding lidocaine to the diluent.

Hypersensitivity Reactions

Hypersensitivity reactions are the most common systemic adverse events encountered with cephalosporin treatment. Nevertheless, immediate (30–60 minutes after administration) and accelerated (1–72 hours after administration) IgE-mediated anaphylactic or urticarial reactions are rare (especially with second- and third-generation compounds) relative to the frequency of 0.01 percent associated with penicillin.[60,61] Skin rash with or without fever and eosinophilia occurs in 1–3 percent of patients after variable periods of cephalosporin therapy.[61–64] With the exception of an apparent increased incidence of a serum sickness syndrome in children receiving cefaclor, there are no data to indicate that hypersensitivity reactions are more common with any individual cephalosporin.

The cross-reactivity among cephalosporins and between

cephalosporins and penicillins has been examined in laboratory and clinical settings; nevertheless, this complex issue remains unresolved.[60,61] The specific haptens involved in cephalosporin hypersensitivity are not known. The number of potential haptens is quite large, since both side chain and nuclear components of the cephalosporins may participate in the hypersensitivity reaction.[60] Laboratory test systems suggest that cephalosporin derivatives show less cross-reactivity among themselves than do penicillin derivatives but that the cross-reactivity between cephalosporins is greater than between cephalosporins and penicillins.[60] In the absence of information detailing cephalosporin haptenic determinants, these assessments, however, are severely limited. At a clinical level early studies suggested that cephalosporin reactions occurred in 5–15 percent of persons with a history of penicillin allergy as compared with 1–2.5 percent of those having no history of penicillin allergy.[65] Those data have been challenged, and the rates for cephalosporin reactions among patients with a history of penicillin allergy were reestimated at 3–7 percent.[60] Even these estimates may be high. Among ceftazidime recipients, for example, 2.7 percent of patients with a history of penicillin reactions experienced a reaction as contrasted with 1.6 percent of those with no prior history of penicillin allergy, yielding a relative risk of 1.66 for ceftazidime reactions in persons with a history of penicillin allergy.[61] This is significantly less than the relative risk of 4 estimated from earlier cephalosporin cross-reaction data.[66] Additionally, of 99 patients with a history of penicillin allergy and a positive skin test with the major and minor penicillin determinants who received a cephalosporin, only 1 had a reaction.[60] This rate is lower than the 22 percent reaction rate noted when a similarly defined population was challenged with penicillin.[67] Although the frequency of primary hypersensitivity reactions to cephalosporins is less than for penicillin, they do occur. Similarly, among patients with a history of penicillin allergy or proven allergy, the risk of reactions upon challenge with a cephalosporin is relatively low, and lower than noted on penicillin rechallenge. However, there is no test system with which to predict who is at risk for these reactions. Skin testing with cephalosporin compounds is unreliable and not recommended. Selection of antibiotic therapy in patients with a history of a reaction to a cephalosporin or penicillin must be guided by the severity of the reaction and the availability of suitable non-β-lactam therapy. Therapy with non-β-lactam antibiotics should be used if severe β-lactam reactions, especially those mediated by IgE, have occurred.[68,69] If cephalosporin therapy is highly desirable and the allergy history is imprecise, skin test reactivity with penicilloyl polylysine and a minor determinant mixture can be assessed. Reactivity to both reagents may reflect an increased risk of a cephalosporin reaction and may warrant alternative therapy.[69] Although patients with a history of non-IgE–mediated penicillin allergy, even with negative skin tests, are at increased risk of a reaction on receiving a cephalosporin, these reactions are rarely severe, and a cephalosporin can be used, if necessary.[70]

Hematologic Reactions

Eosinophilia occurs in 1 to 7 percent of cephalosporin recipients and may be noted as an isolated finding. Neutropenia that reverses promptly after discontinuation of a cephalosporin is seen during prolonged high-dose therapy; the frequency of neutropenia is less than 1 percent. Approximately 5 percent of cephalosporin recipients have thrombocytosis. Although a positive reaction to the Coomb's test occurs in 3 percent of patients receiving earlier cephalosporins, hemolytic anemia is very uncommon.[71] Cephalosporins can alter hemostasis mechanisms.[72,73] Although antibiotic therapy may inhibit the synthesis and absorption of vitamin K by inhibition of gut flora, hypoprothrombinemia has been associated with the competitive inhibition by the MTT group of the vitamin K-dependent carboxylase that is responsible for converting clotting factors II, VII, IX, and

X to their active forms.[74–78] The MTT group, which occupies position 3 in cefamandole, cefoperazone, cefotetan, moxalactam, cefmetazole, and cefmenoxime, may also inhibit, like coumadin, vitamin K 2,3-epoxide reductase, which converts inactive vitamin K to its active form.[76] The frequency of hypoprothrombinemia in recipients of these compounds is variable (range 4–68 percent) and is markedly enhanced by poor nutritional status, debilitation, recent gastrointestinal surgery, and renal failure.[72,79,80] Bleeding occurs less frequently and has been associated primarily with moxalactam, cefoperazone, and cefotetan.[79,81] Vitamin K treatment will over 24–36 hours restore the prothrombin time to normal. Weekly prophylaxis with vitamin K has been recommended when MTT-bearing cephalosporins are administered to patients at high risk for hypothrombinemia. Moxalactam, in addition, reversibly suppresses ADP-induced platelet aggregation with consequent prolongation of the bleeding time.[82] Other cephalosporins do not significantly impair platelet function. Use of moxalactam has been curtailed because it was associated with relatively frequent and severe bleeding complications.[72,83]

Gastrointestinal Tract Toxicity

Mild elevations in transaminases and alkaline phosphatase have been noted during cephalosporin therapy but rarely necessitate discontinuation of therapy.[64,70] The frequency of nonspecific antibiotic-associated diarrhea is 2–5 percent in cephalosporin recipients. It is postulated that diarrhea is more frequent with cefoperazone and ceftriaxone as a consequence of biliary excretion and subsequent impact on gastrointestinal flora. Cephalosporin therapy is associated with pseudomembranous or *Clostridium difficile* toxin-related colitis; the risk, however, is not increased for specific cephalosporins or for cephalosporins compared with penicillins or clindamycin. Ceftriaxone has been associated with the formation of sonographically identifiable sludge in the gallbladder and common bile duct. While commonly asymptomatic, the biliary tract sludge may be associated with symptoms of cholecystitis.[84,85] Risk factors for ceftriaxone-associated sludge formation, also called *pseudolithiasis,* include childhood, prolonged or high dose (greater than 2 g/day), and biliary stasis (receipt of total parenteral nutrition).[84–86] If the ceftriaxone excreted into the bile and concentrated there exceeds its solubility product it precipitates as crystals of a ceftriaxone-calcium salt.[86] The sludge, which may form in 20–45 percent of patients receiving ceftriaxone 2 g daily, clears between 10 and 60 days after therapy.[84,141] Occasionally ceftriaxone-calcium crystals may coalesce to form cholelithiasis and precipitate symptomatic disease.[85]

Nephrotoxicity

Cephaloridine was associated with dose-dependent nephrotoxicity; however, this agent is no longer used.[68] Nephrotoxicity due to currently available cephalosporins, when used in recommended doses, is generally rare. Acute tubular necrosis has occasionally been attributed to extremely high doses of cephalothin or to standard high-dose therapy in the elderly.[87,88] Furthermore, cephalothin may enhance the nephrotoxicity of aminoglycosides.[89,90] Ceftazidime, which shares a pyridine substituent at position 3 with cephaloridine, may cause some decrease in glomerular and tubular function[91]; however, clinically significant nephrotoxicity has not been noted.[63] Interstitial nephritis occurs as an apparent hypersensitivity response to cephalosporins.

Disulfiranlike Reactions

Ingestion of alcohol by patients receiving cephalosporins with the MTT group at position 3 (see Hematologic Toxicity, above) has been associated with difulfiramlike reactions.[92,93] These are characterized, depending on severity, by rapid onset of flushing, tachycardia, headache, sweating, thirst, nausea, vomiting, hypotension, confusion, and blurred vision. The MTT group, the standard configuration of which is similar to that of disulfiram, appears to block alcohol metabolism at the acetaldehyde step. The accumulation of acetaldehyde is associated with these symptoms.

FIRST-GENERATION CEPHALOSPORINS

The first-generation cephalosporins (Tables 1 and 2) are very active against gram-positive cocci and have moderate activity against community-acquired *Moraxella catarrhalis*, *E. coli*, *Proteus mirabilis* (indole-negative), and *K. pneumoniae* (Tables 6 and 7).[23,68–70,109–113] The antibacterial activity of these agents for other Enterobacteriaceae is unpredictable and should not be

assumed. While active against most of the penicillin-susceptible oral cavity anaerobes, the *Bacteroides fragilis* group are resistant. These agents have poor activity against *H. influenzae* and are not active against methicillin-resistant staphylococci, penicillin-resistant pneumococci, and *Enterococcus* spp. Even when in vitro susceptibility tests suggest cephalosporins are likely to be effective against methicillin-resistant staphylococci, these agents are not effective therapeutically.[114] With the exception of cefazolin, which has slightly enhanced activity for some Enterobacteriaceae, the antibacterial activity of both the oral and parenteral first-generation cephalosporins is similar.[22,109–113]

Drugs

Cephalothin (Keflin) is a parenteral agent that distributes throughout body tissues and fluids with the exception of the

TABLE 6. In Vitro Antibacterial Activity of Selected Oral Cephalosporins

Organism					MIC$_{90}$					
	Cephalexin	Cephradine	Cefadroxil	Cefaclor	Cefprozil	Loracarbef	Cefuroxime	Cefpodoxime	Cefixime	Ceftibuten
S. pneumoniae[a]	2	2	2	0.5	0.12	0.5	≤0.06	≤0.06	0.25	4
S. agalactiae	2	2	2	2	0.25	0.5	<0.12	0.12	0.25	16
B. fragilis	>32	>32	>32	>32	>32	>32	>32	>32	>32	>32
P. aeruginosa	>32	>32	>32	>32	>32	>32	>32	>32	>32	>32
S. pyogenes	2	2	2	0.5	0.12	0.5	≤0.06	0.06	0.25	2
S. aureus[b]	4	4	4	4	2	4	4	4	>32	>32
H. influenzae[b]	8	16	32	8	8	2	0.5	0.06	0.06	0.06
N. gonorrhoeae[b]	2	4	4	1	1	0.12	0.25	0.06	0.06	0.004
M. catarrhalis[b]	4	4	4	1	2	1	0.5	0.25	0.06	2
E. coli[a]	>16	>16	>16	>16	2	>16	8	0.5	0.25	0.12
C. diversus	4	4	4	0.5	1	0.5	4	0.5	0.06	0.06
Klebsiella spp.[b]	>16	>16	>16	>16	>16	>16	2	0.12	0.06	0.03
P. mirabilis	16	16	16	1	1	2	2	0.06	0.06	≤0.015
Salmonella spp.[b]	>16	>16	>16	16	0	8	4	0.12	0.06	0.06
Shigella spp.[b]	>16	>16	>16	16	8	8	2	0.12	≤0.06	≤0.06
C. freundii	>32	>32	>32	>32	>32	>32	>32	>32	>32	>32
E. aerogenes	>32	>32	>32	>32	>32	>32	>32	0.5	2	1
E. cloacae	>32	>32	>32	>32	>32	>32	>32	>32	>32	>32
M. morganii	>32	>32	>32	>32	>32	>32	>32	8	8	2
P. vulgaris	>32	>32	32	>32	>32	>32	>32	0.12	0.25	0.03
P. rettgeri	>32	>32	>32	>32	>32	>32	16	0.03	0.06	0.06
P. stuartii	>32	>32	>32	>32	>32	>32	>32	0.5	0.06	0.06
Serratia spp.	>32	>32	>32	>32	>32	>32	>32	>32	>32	4

[a] Penicillin-sensitive isolates.
[b] β-Lactamase-producing isolates.

(Modified from Neu,[22] with permission.)

TABLE 7. In Vitro Antibacterial Activity of Selected Parenteral Cephalosporins[a]: MIC$_{50}$/MIC$_{90}$ (μg/ml)[b]

Antibiotic	S. pyogenes	S. pneumoniae[a]	S. aureus[d]	H. influenzae[e]	E. coli	P. mirabilis	K. pneumoniae	E. cloacae	E. aerogenes	C. freundii	M. morganii	P. aeruginosa	B. fragilis
Cefazolin	0.1/0.1	0.12/0.12	1/1	4/8	<2/16	>2/<2	<2/4	>32/>32	>32/>32	>32/>32	>32/>32	>32/>32	64/>64
Cefamandole	0.06/0.06	0.12/0.12	<0.25/1	16/32	2/16	0.5/1	1/8	32/>64	2>64	32/64	>32/>32	>32/>32	64/>64
Cefuroxime	<0.03/0.06	0.06/0.06	0.8/4	0.5/2	4/8	<2/<2	2/8	>32/>64	8/>32	4/>32	32/>32	32/>32	64/>64
Cefoxitin	0.5/1	1/2	2/4	1/4	2/8	2/8	2/8	>32/>32	>32/>32	>32/>32	8/8	>32/>32	4/32
Cefotetan	2/4	8/>32	<4/16	4/4	0.12/.48	0.25/0.25	0.12/0.25	8/64	>8/>64	2/64	4/4	>32/>32	8/>64
Cefmetazole	0.5/0.5	1/8	2/4	1/4	1/4	2/4	1/2	>32/>32	4/32	>32/>32	4/8	>32/>32	8/16
Cefotaxime	0.06/0.06	0.06/0.06	2/4	0.06/0.06	0.12/0.12	0.12/0.12	0.12/0.12	0.5/>32	0.12/32	0.25/0.5	0.5/8	16/32	32/>64
Ceftizoxime	0.01/0.01	0.01/0.02	4/16	0.01/0.01	0.25/0.25	0.25/0.25	0.25/0.25	0.25/32	0.25/32	0.25/>32	0.25/2	>32/>32	16/>64
Ceftriaxone	0.01/0.03	0.25/0.5	2/4	0.01/0.01	0.25/0.25	0.25/0.25	0.25/0.25	0.26/>64	0.25/16	0.25/>64	0.25/1	16/>32	32/>64
Ceftazidime	0.12/0.25	0.25/0.25	8/16	0.06/0.12	0.12/0.12	0.12/0.25	0.12/0.5	0.25/>16	0.25/>32	0.05/>16	0.12/4	2/>16	>32/>2
Cefepime	0.02/0.04	0.04/0.25	2/4	0.06/0.12	0.04/0.06	0.04/0.1	0.12/0.25	0.06/2	0.06/0.5	0.05/8	0.03/0.05	<4/16	32/256
Cefpirome	0.02/0.05	0.08/0.12	0.5/1	0.06/0.12	0.12/0.12	0.12/0.12	0.12/0.25	0.12/0.5	0.03/0.12	0.03/0.06	0.12/0.5	4/>16	32/256

[a] Values are approximations from references 18, 20, 94–108.
[b] MICs for 50 and 90 percent of strains in μg/ml.
[c] Penicillin susceptible (MIC < 0.1 μg/ml).
[d] Methicillin susceptible S. aureus.
[e] β-lactamase producing.

cerebrospinal fluid. The acetoxy substituent at position 3 is cleaved from 20–30 percent of the parent compound to form a desacetyl metabolite. Both the desacetyl product and unmetabolized cephalothin are excreted in the urine. The elimination half-life is short (30–40 minutes). Among the cephalosporins, cephalothin is the least hydrolyzed by staphylococcal β-lactamase; hence it is considered the optimal cephalosporin for treatment for staphylococcal endocarditis and other severe nonmeningeal staphylococcal infections.[115]

Cefazolin (Ancef, Kefzol) is well tolerated when given intramuscularly or intravenously. Serum concentrations of cefazolin are higher than those achieved with comparable doses of cephalothin, in part because cefazolin has a smaller volume of distribution. The serum half-life is 1.8 hours. Cefazolin is not metabolized; with normal renal function 80 percent of the administered dose is excreted through the kidney by glomerular filtration.[116] The antimicrobial spectrum of cefazolin is similar to that of cephalothin, although cefazolin is slightly more potent against *E. coli* and *Klebsiella* spp.[113] Cefazolin is more readily hydrolyzed by staphylococcal β-lactamase than cephalothin.[117,118] Although this relatively increased β-lactamase vulnerability has not been clearly demonstrated to be clinical significance, some experts prefer cephalothin for the treatment of life-threatening *S. aureus* infections.[115] Because its pharmacokinetics allow 8 hourly dosing, cefazolin has become the most widely utilized parenteral first-generation cephalosporin.

Cephapirin (Cefadyl), a parenterally administered cephalosporin, is very similar to cephalothin in terms of its pharmacokinetics, metabolism, antimicrobial activity, and clinical utility.[111]

Cephalexin (Keflex, Keftab, Biocef) is exceptionally well absorbed from the gastrointestinal tract; maximum serum concentrations of 15–18 μg/ml are attained in 1 hour after a 0.5 g oral dose. Ninety percent of the oral dose is excreted in the urine as native drug. The serum half-life is approximately 50–55 minutes.[22,109,119]

Cephradine (Anspor, oral; Velosef, oral and parenteral) is similar to cephalexin structurally except that it has a cyclohexidine ring on its acyl side chain where cephalexin has a phenol group. The compound is rapidly absorbed from the intestinal tract, it is not metabolized, and it is rapidly excreted in the urine (half-life, 30–40 minutes). Because cephradine is fully bioavailable after oral administration, peak serum concentrations (15–18 μg/ml) and area under the curve after either a 0.5 g oral or intramuscular dose, are similar.[120]

Cefadroxil (Duricef, Ultracef), the parahydroxy analog of cephalexin, is almost 100 percent absorbed after oral administration and has a slightly longer half life than cephalexin and cephradine (1.1 hour). The more sustained serum and urine concentrations of cefadroxil allow treatment of less severe infections (skin, pharyngeal, urinary tract) with once or twice daily dosing schedules.[22,109]

Clinical Use

The first-generation cephalosporins are appropriate treatment for *S. aureus* and nonenterococcal streptococcal infections when it is desirable to avoid penicillins. Most commonly, these include skin and soft tissue infection, streptococcal pharyngitis, and community-acquired pneumonia caused by *Streptococcus pneumoniae*. These antibiotics are not ideal for treatment of infections that are likely to be caused by *Haemophilus influenzae* or *Moraxella catarrhalis* (sinusitis, otitis media, and some lower respiratory tract infections). They may be used for treatment of community-acquired, uncomplicated urinary tract infection; however, trimethoprim-sulfamethoxazole is more effective and less costly. First-generation cephalosporins are not used to treat infections of the central nervous system and because of their limited activity against gram-negative bacilli are not appropriate choices for empiric therapy of nosocomial infections. Oral first-generation cephalosporins are not effective

treatment for infections caused by *Pasturella multocida* (animal bites and scratches).[121] Because of its spectrum of action, favorable toxicity profile, relatively long half-life, modest cost, and proven efficacy, cefazolin is the prophylactic antibiotic of choice for surgical procedures involving foreign body implantation and many clean and clean-contaminated procedures wherein there is a relatively high risk for infection.[122,123] These include cardiac surgery, arterial reconstruction, insertion of orthopedic devices, head and neck surgery that crosses the oropharyngeal mucosa, high-risk gastroduodenal and biliary tract procedures, vaginal and abdominal hysterectomy, high-risk cesarian sections, and procedures on fresh trauma wounds. These agents are not recommended as prophylaxis for colorectal surgery, appendectomy, or when methicillin-resistant *S. aureus* is a particular threat.

SECOND-GENERATION CEPHALOSPORINS

The second-generation cephalosporins should be considered in two groups: The true cephalosporins and the cephamycins (cefoxitin, cefotetan, and cefmetazole; Tables 1 and 2). The true cephalosporins in this group include a range of parenteral and oral antibiotics that provide, in comparison with the first-generation agents and comparable to enhanced activity against staphylococci and nonenterococcal streptococci, significantly improved activity against *H. influenzae*, *Moraxella catarrhalis*, *Neisseria meningitidis*, and *Neisseria gonorrhoeae* and in selected instances increased in vitro activity against some Enterobacteriaceae (Tables 6 and 7).[10,11,22,124–130] In comparison with first-generation compounds and the second-generation true cephalosporins, the cephamycins have inferior activity against staphylococci and streptococci, but they, particularly cefotetan, have an enhanced antibacterial effect against selected Enterobacteriaceae. Their activity against *Neisseria* spp. is good. They are noteworthy as the cephems most active against *Bacteroides* spp., particularly *B. fragilis*.[95–98,131–136]

Drugs

Cefamandole (Mandol), a parenteral cephalosporin, is excreted in the urine and has a serum half-life of 50 minutes. Bearing an MTT group at position 3, cefamandole has manifested the toxicities associated with that moiety. Cefamandole has excellent activity against gram-positive cocci, appearing superior to cefazolin against selected *S. aureus* and coagulase-negative staphylococci. Although cefamandole has improved activity against β-lactamase–negative *H. influenzae*, significant inactivation by β-lactamase renders cefamandole unreliable against TEM-1 plasmid-bearing strains of *H. influenzae*.[124,126]

Ceforanide (Precef), similar in structure to cefamandole including a modified MTT group at position 3, produces peak serum concentration comparable to cefazolin, has a half-life of 2.6 hours, and is excreted unmetabolized in the urine. Except for having reduced activity against *H. influenzae*, its spectrum of antibacterial activity is similar to that of cefamandole. Ceforanide can be administered every 12 hours.

Cefonocid (Monocid), which is structurally and biologically similar to cefamandole, is unique because it is 98 percent serum protein bound and has a serum half-life of 4.4 hours.[130] Although it has been used effectively as once daily dosing for infection caused by susceptible organisms, failures have been noted in more serious infection, including *S. aureus* bacteremia.[137] A single preoperative dose of cefonocid reduced the incidence of wound infection in patients undergoing breast surgery or herniorraphy.[138]

Cefuroxime (Kefurox, Zenacef), because of an iminomethoxy group on the acyl side chain, has significantly enhanced stability to the β-lactamases of *H. influenzae* and *N. gonorrhoeae* (TEM-1) and some Enterobacteriaceae, relative to the first-generation cephalosporins and cefamandole. Accordingly, it has notably improved activity against both β-lactamase positive and negative *H. influenzae, N. gonorrhoeae,* and *Moraxella catarrhalis* and significantly increased activity against *E. coli, Proteus mirabilis, Klebsiella* spp., *Citrobacter* spp., and *Morganella.* It does not have good activity against *Proteus vulgaris, Serratia* spp., and *Providencia* (Tables 6 and 7).[10,11,22] Although somewhat less potent against *S. aureus,* it is significantly more active against *Streptococcus pneumoniae* and *Streptococcus pyogenes* than the first-generation cephalosporins.[10,11,22] Cefuroxime has a serum half-life of 1.3–1.5 hours and thus can be administered intramuscularly or intravenously at 8-hour intervals. As the only second-generation cephalosporin to demonstrate significant penetration into the cerebrospinal fluid, cefuroxime has provided effective treatment for bacterial meningitis caused by *N. meningitidis, Streptococcus pneumoniae,* and *H. influenzae.*[139,140] However, in a direct randomized comparison to ceftriaxone in the treatment of meningitis in children, cefuroxime was associated with delayed sterilization of the cerebrospinal fluid and a greater frequency of moderate to prolonged hearing loss.[141]

Cefprozil (Cefzil) is structurally similar to cefadroxil except that cefprozil contains a vinyl-methyl group at position 3 of the cephem nucleus instead of a methyl group. Because of this difference, cefprozil is more active than the first-generation oral cephalosporins against *Streptococcus pneumoniae, Streptococcus pyogenes,* and other streptococci; *Neisseria* spp., and, to a lesser degree, against *S. aureus.* Its activity against *H. influenzae,* both β-lactamase negative and positive strains, is only modestly increased beyond that of cephalexin and cefadroxil; it is comparable to that noted with cefaclor and less than that of cefuroxime. Cefprozil is more active than first-generation cephalosporins against *E. coli, Proteus mirabilis, Klebsiella* spp. and *Citrobacter* spp., it is not active against the indole-positive *Proteus, Providencia,* and *Enterobacter* spp. (Tables 6 and 7).[22,120] The 90 percent bioavailability of orally administered cefprozil is not affected by feeding or simultaneous administration of nonabsorbable antacids. A 0.5-g dose yields a peak serum concentration of 10 μg/ml. Cefprozil has a serum half-life of 1.2–1.4 hours. It is excreted primarily in the urine; consequently the half-life increases significantly (to >5 hours) when creatinine clearance is less than 30 ml/min. It is effectively removed by hemodialysis. The pharmacokinetics of cefprozil support twice daily dosing for mild to moderate infections.[21,142]

Cefuroxime axetil (Ceftin), the acetoxyethyl ester of cefuroxime that is hydrolyzed to the parent compound during absorption, has a bioavailability to 30–50 percent after oral administration; absorption is increased by food and diminished by antacids or H$_2$ receptor antagonists. The serum half-life allows twice daily dosing for mild to moderate infections. Cefuroxime axetil is not available in suspension, and crushed tablets have an unacceptably bitter taste.[143,144]

Cefaclor (Ceclor), an orally administered cephalosporin, has pharmacokinetic and biologic activities similar to those of cephalexin. Relative to cephalexin, it has moderately increased activity against *H. influenzae, Moraxella catarrhalis, E. coli* and *Proteus mirabilis.* It is, however, significantly destroyed by the TEM-1 and Bro-1 β-lactamases of some *H. influenzae* and *Moraxella catarrhalis,* respectively.[22,101] Cefaclor is not stable in human plasma, has a half-life of 0.8 hours, and should be administered at 8-hour intervals.

Loracarbef (Lorabid) is an orally administered carbacephem antibiotic, having a carbon at position 1 of the cephem nucleus instead of a sulfur; otherwise, the molecule is structurally similar to cefaclor. Relative to cefaclor, loracarbef has comparable activity against *S. aureus, Streptococcus pneumoniae,* and streptococci but has modestly increased activity against *H. influenzae* and *Moraxella catarrhalis* (particularly those strains of each that are β-lactamase producing) and some Enterobacteriaceae. It is not active in vitro against *Citrobacter, Enterobacter,* indole-positive *Proteus, Providencia,* and *Serratia* spp.

Loracarbef is destroyed by the ESBL.[22,101,128] Virtually all of the orally administered dose is absorbed and excreted in the urine. Absorption is more rapidly and peak serum concentrations are significantly higher with the suspension formulation than with capsules; food decreases absorption. After a 400-mg dose, peak serum concentrations are 14–18 μg/ml. Loracarbef is excreted in the urine and has a serum half-life of 1.1 hours; azotemia (creatinine clearance < 30 ml/min) increases the half-life to 5 hours, thus warranting dose adjustments. The compound is effectively removed by hemodialysis.[21,22,145] Loracarbef is stable in human plasma at body temperature for greater than 100 hours as compared with the rapid deterioration of cefaclor.[22,146]

Cefoxitin (Mefoxin), a cephamycin, is notably resistant to the β-lactamases produced by gram-negative bacilli and is a highly effective inducer of β-lactamase production by some Enterobacteriaceae.[42] Cefoxitin is more active against *E. coli, Klebsiella,* and the indole-negative *Proteus* spp. than first-generation cephalosporins; less active against *H. influenzae* than the second-generation true cephalosporins; and has significantly reduced antibacterial activity against gram-positive cocci compared with first- and second-generation cephalosporins.[131] Cefoxitin is the most potent of the cephalosporins against the *Bacteroides fragilis* group. Among *B. fragilis,* resistance to cefoxitin (MIC breakpoint ≥ 32 μg/ml) ranges from 4 to 31 percent, whereas resistance among *B. thetaiotaomicron, B. distasonis,* and *B. ovatus* is significantly greater, ranging from 24 to 56 percent.[96,98] Cefoxitin has good activity against *N. gonorrhoeae,* including those that produce β-lactamase. After parenteral administration, cefoxitin is rapidly excreted in the urine. The serum half-life is 40–45 minutes; thus dosing at 4–6 hour intervals is required.

Cefotetan (Cefotan), another cephamycin, has antibacterial activity similar to cefoxitin. It is similar to cefoxitin in potency against *B. fragilis* but less active against the non-*B. fragilis* members of the *B. fragilis* group.[96,98] Its activity against facultative gram-negative bacilli is greater than that of the second-generation cephalosporins and approaches that of the third-generation agents.[147] It is not active against *Pseudomonas* spp. but is highly effective against *N. gonorrhoeae,* including those that produce β-lactamase. The serum half-life of 3.5 hours allows cefotetan to be administered at 12-hour intervals and in perioperative prophylaxis as a single dose. Cefotetan has an MTT group and has been associated with hypoprothrombinemia and bleeding.

Cefmetazole (Zefazone) is the most recently available cephamycin; compared with cefoxitin, it is slightly less active against the *B. fragilis* group and moderately more active against some Enterobacteriaceae. Cefmetazole is not as potent against gram-negative bacilli as cefotetan, and none of the cephamycins are highly active against the *Enterobacter, Providencia,* indole-positive *Proteus, C. freundii,* or *Serratia* spp.[136] Cefmetazole is administered parenterally, achieves peak serum concentrations of 140 μg/ml 30 minutes after a 2g infusion, has a serum half-life of 1.1 hours, and is excreted unchanged in the urine by tubular secretion. The molecule has an MTT chain at position 3; however, the frequency with which it causes the known associated adverse reactions has not been established. It does not impair platelet aggregation, as is noted with moxalactam.[148]

Clinical Use

The activity of cefuroxime against *Streptococcus pneumoniae, H. influenzae,* and *Moraxella catarrhalis,* including β-lactamase–producing strains of the latter two, has prompted use of cefuroxime in the treatment of patients hospitalized for community-acquired, presumed bacterial (sputum not diagnostic) pneumonia.[149,150] Other serious infections caused by susceptible bacteria, including epiglotitis, complicated sinusitis, bacteremia, soft tissue infection, and uncomplicated urinary tract infection, can also be treated with cefuroxime. Cefuroxime is effective therapy for meningitis due to *H. influenzae, N. meningitidis,* and *Streptococcus pneumoniae*. However, as a result of the increased potency of third-generation cephalosporins against these organisms, the more favorable penetration of these cephalosporins into the cerebrospinal fluid, and the outcome of a direct clinical comparison, third-generation cephalosporins have become the agents of choice for empiric therapy of meningitis or therapy of meningitis caused by *H. influenzae*.[51,139-141] Although its spectrum of activity is similar to that of cefuroxime, cefamandole, with less favorable pharmacokinetics, inferior in vitro activity against *H. influenzae*, potential toxicity due to an MTT substituent, and lack of penetration into the central nervous system, is less widely used. Neither cefamandole nor cefuroxime should be considered for empiric treatment of nosocomial pneumonia or other nosocomial infections that are potentially caused by *Enterobacter*, *Citrobacter*, indole-positive *Proteus*, *Providencia*, *Morganella*, *Serratia*, or *P. aeruginosa*. These organisms are likely to be intrinsically resistant or to become resistant through induction (or derepression) of chromosomal β-lactamases.[40-42]

The oral second-generation cephalosporins, including cefuroxime axetil, cefprozil, cefaclor, and loracarbef, are agents that can be used to treat effectively a spectrum of mild to moderate community-acquired uncomplicated infections.[151-163] Such infections include skin and soft tissue infection, urinary tract infection, pneumonia, acute bronchitis, acute exacerbation of chronic bronchitis, streptococcal pharyngitis, sinusitis, and otitis media. In some of these settings more cost-effective or narrow-spectrum therapy is desirable (e.g., a penicillinase-resistant oral penicillin or cephalexin for skin infection or trimethoprim-sulfamethoxazole for uncomplicated urinary tract infections). Given these considerations, the oral second-generation agents should be used primarily for the treatment of infections of the respiratory tract and its appendages. Trials comparing these agents among themselves, to amoxicillin-clavulanate and to amoxicillin have not demonstrated a superior agent in a given infection. The studies examining the efficacy of these agents for respiratory tract infections have not contained large numbers of β-lactamase–producing pathogens, a situation that might obscure differences in efficacy between the agents. It may be prudent to consider the relatively enhanced potency of cefuroxime axetil and loracarbef against *H. influenzae* and *Moraxella catarrhalis* when selecting from among these agents to treat respiratory tract infections. For example, limited data suggest that among children with otitis media, the recovery of *H. influenzae* during therapy is increased in those treated with cefprozil or cefaclor as opposed to cefuroxime axetil or amoxicillin-clavulanate.[164] Cefuroxime axetil is an effective alternative to doxycycline and penicillins for the treatment of early (erythema migrans-associated) Lyme disease.[165]

Cefoxitin, cefotetan, and cefmetazole have been demonstrated efficacious in the treatment of intra-abdominal infections, pelvic and gynecologic infections, infected decubitus ulcers, foot infections in diabetics, and mixed aerobic-anaerobic soft tissue infections.[132,166-170] All of these infections represent entities wherein facultative gram-negative bacilli and anaerobic organisms, especially *B. fragilis*, are likely to play a prominent role. Although the experience is most extensive with cefoxitin, available comparative trials suggest similar efficacy for each agent. The clinical significance of the reduced in vitro activity of cefotetan and cefmetazol against the non-*B. fragilis* species in the *B. fragilis* group is not clear. Furthermore, as many as 15 percent of *B. fragilis* may be resistant to the cephamycin antibiotics. Accordingly, these agents should not be used, in the absence of susceptibility information, to treat life-threatening *B. fragilis* infection. Metronidazole, chloramphenicol, a β-lactam/β-lactamase combination or imipenem, which are active against virtually all *B. fragilis*, would be preferred in this setting.[95] These cephalosporins are not highly active against *S. aureus* and are often inactive in the setting of induced (or derepressed) chromosomal β-lactamases in Enterobacteriaceae both

of which might be encountered in nosocomial infections.[40-42] Accordingly, these agents should not be considered optimal single-drug therapy when the above infections occur in patients who have been hospitalized and received antibiotic therapy. Cefoxitin and cefotetan have been demonstrated to be effective therapy for urogenital gonorrhea but for financial and logistical reasons are not recommended as a therapy of choice.[172,173] Cefoxitin and cefotetan are recommended, in combination with doxycycline, as a therapy of choice for treatment of pelvic inflammatory disease.[173,174] Cefoxitin, cefotetan, and cefmetazole have been shown effective and comparable as systemic prophylaxis for surgery performed at various levels of the gastrointestinal tract, for appendectomy, and for selected gynecologic procedures.[122,171,175-177] These agents have not been proven superior to cefazolin other than in the setting of colorectal surgery and appendectomy and hence are recommended only in these settings.[122,123,177] Although in elective colorectal surgery the benefits of systemic prophylaxis in addition to an oral erythromycin-neomycin preoperative bowel preparation have not been fully established, it is common practice to use one of these agents in this setting.[177]

THIRD-GENERATION CEPHALOSPORINS

The third-generation cephalosporins are commonly viewed as the most potent cephalosporins against facultative gram-negative bacilli (Tables 6 and 7).[69] In addition, however, they have superior antimicrobial activity against *Streptococcus pneumoniae* (including those with relative penicillin resistance) *Streptococcus pyogenes*, other streptococci, and, with the exception of ceftazidime, have modest activity against *S. aureus*. They also have excellent activity against *H. influenzae*, *N. meningitidis*, *N. gonorrhoeae*, and *Moraxella catarrhalis*. In spite of wide use, these agents have retained an unusually high degree of activity against *E. coli*, *Klebsiella*, *Proteus mirabilis*, indole-positive *Proteus*, *Providencia*, and *Serratia*.[69,94,99,100,178] Third-generation cephalosporins may be subdivided based on their activity against *Pseudomonas aeruginosa*; cefotaxime, ceftizoxime, ceftriaxone, moxalactam (an oxacephem), cefixime, cefpodoxime proxetil, and the investigational agents cefmenoxime, cefodizime, ceftibuten, cefetamet, cefteram, and cefdinir lack activity against *P. aeruginosa*. In contrast, antipseudomonal activity is found in cefoperazone, ceftazidime, and the investigational agents cefsulodin, cefepime, cefpirome, and cefpiramide. The third-generation cephalosporins, like all of the compounds based on the cephem nucleus, lack activity against *Enterococcus* spp. methicillin-resistant staphylococci, highly penicillin-resistant *Streptococcus pneumoniae*, *Listeria*, and *Xanthomonas*. They are variably active against *Acinetobacter*.

The superior broad activity of these agents against the Enterobacteriaceae has recently been challenged by β-lactamase–mediated resistance (see Mechanisms of Resistance, above, and Ch. 13). Chromosomally encoded β-lactamases (Bush group 1; see Ch. 13) that are inducible or that can be stably derepressed and that mediate resistance to all cephalosporins have resulted in an increasing number of infections due to *Enterobacter* spp. and *Citrobacter freundii*. Although less frequently encountered as causes of infection, *Serratia*, *Morganella*, *Proteus vulgaris* and *Aeromonas* may express resistance to these agents through inducible β-lactamases.[20,40-42] Additionally, the plasmid-mediated ESBL, which mediate resistance to third-generation cephalosporins as a consequence of point mutations in the TEM or SHV genes, represent a widening threat to the utility of these agents.[43,44]

Drugs

Cefotaxime (Claforan) has superior activity against *Streptococcus pneumonia*, *Streptococcus pyogenes*, and other streptococci, *H. influenzae*, and *Neisseria*; it has modest activity against *S. aureus*. It remains highly potent against *E. coli, Proteus mirabilis, Klebsiella*, and other Enterobacteriaceae that do not express Bush 1 β-lactamases or contain ESBL.[18,94] Cefotaxime is not active against *Pseudomonae aeruginosa, Xanthomonas*, and non-*aeruginosa* pseudomonads. Cefotaxime's activity against *B. fragilis* is less than that of the cephamycins; nevertheless, 47–66 percent of strains have an MIC below the susceptibility break point.[95,178] Cefotaxime is metabolized to desacetyl cefotaxime, which, while less potent than the parent compound, has a longer half-life and may act synergistically with cefotaxime to allow effective dosing at 8-hour intervals in patients with moderate infections.[179] Cefotaxime reliably enters the cerebrospinal fluid when dosed at 2 g every 4 hours.[51,140]

Ceftizoxime (Cefizox) shares the pattern of antibacterial activity seen with cefotaxime except that it inhibits a larger percentage of *B. fragilis* (66–80 percent).[18,95,99,100,180] The serum half-life of ceftizoxime is 1.7 hours, allowing dosing at 8-hour intervals. Ceftizoxime is excreted in the urine, and doses must be adjusted in azotemic patients. Clinically effective cerebrospinal fluid concentrations are achieved with doses of 3 g every 8 hours.[51,140]

Ceftriaxone (Rocephin) possess antibacterial activity similar to that of cefotaxime and ceftizoxime.[18,99,100,181] Against several organisms (e.g., *N. gonnorrhoeae, N. meningitidis*, and *H. influenzae*) it is the most potent third-generation cephalosporin.[18] Ceftriaxone, however, has truly unique pharmacokinetics; it is 90 percent protein bound, excreted through both the biliary and urinary tracts, and has a serum half-life of 8 hours. As a consequence, most serious infections can be treated with once daily dosing (meningitis: adults, 1–2 g every 12 hours; children, 50 mg/kg every 12 hours). Isolated renal or hepatic dysfunction does not require dose adjustment; however, with failure of both organs dose adjustment is necessary.[50]

Moxalactam (Moxam), an oxacephem with a methoxy group at position 7 similar to the cephamycins, has activity against gram-negative bacteria similar to other third-generation cephalosoporins; it, however, is less active against gram-positive cocci than cefotaxime.[50] It inhibits 75–85 percent of *B. fragilis*.[95] Moxalactam has been associated with hypoprothrombinemia related to the MTT group at position 3 and with a platelet-aggregating defect also.[50] The associated coagulopathy has resulted in significant bleeding complications and recommendations that moxalactam not be used.

Cefmenoxime (investigational) is a parenterally administered aminothiazolyl-iminomethoxy cephalosporin with an antibacterial spectrum very similar to those of cefotaxime, ceftizoxime, and ceftriaxone.[6,18] Its pharmacokinetics are similar to those of cefotaxime except that it is not metabolized. Cefmenoxime has an MTT group. It is not active against *P. aeruginosa* or *Acinetobacter* and is effective against only 50 percent of *B. fragilis*.[18]

Cefodizime (investigational), an aminothiazolyl cephalosporin, is administered parenterally, achieving serum concentrations of 100 μg/ml 30 minutes after intravenous administration of 1 g. It is excreted unchanged in the urine and has a serum half-life of 2.5–3.5 hours. The antibacterial activity of cefodizime is similar to that of cefotaxime.[182] Cefodizine enhances the bactericidal activity of neutrophils against both opsonized and nonopsonized bacteria.[183]

Cefixime (Suprax), an orally administered third-generation cephalosporin with a prolonged serum half-life, can be administered once daily and is highly effective against *Streptococcus pyogenes, Streptococcus pneumoniae, H. influenzae, Neisseria*, and many of the Enterobacteriaceae. It has poor activity against methicillin-susceptible *S. aureus*.[21,22,184,185]

Cefpodoxime proxetil (Vantin), an esterified third-generation cephalosporin, is absorbed after oral administration (absorption increased by food), is excreted unchanged in the urine, and has a serum half-life of 2.2 hours.[21,22] The microbiologic activity of cefpodoxime is similar to that of cefixime, except cefpodoxime retains moderate antistaphylococcal activity.[22]

Ceftibuten (investigational), an orally administered third-generation cephalosporin, is rapidly and nearly completely absorbed, is excreted in the urine, and has a half-life of 2.5 hours.[21,22] Ceftibuten is not active against *S. aureus* and has moderate activity against *Streptococcus pneumoniae* similar to that seen with first-generation cephalosporins. It is highly active against the Enterobacteriaceae (except those with derepressed Bush 1 β-lactamase), *H. influenzae, Neisseria*, and *Moraxella catarrhalis*. Of note, ceftibuten is not hydrolyzed by some of the ESBL and remains active against organisms bearing these β-lactamase genes.[22]

Cefdinir (investigational) is an orally administered aminothiazolyl hydroximino cephalosporin with antibacterial activity against the Enterobacteriaceae that is two- to fourfold less than that of cefixime. Its antistaphylococcal and antistreptococcal activities are similar to those of cefpodoxime.[22,186,187] Cefdinir is hydrolyzed by the ESBL.[22]

Specific Agents With Anti-*Pseudomonas* Activity

Cefoperazone (Cefobid) has moderate anti-*Pseudomonas* activity; at least 50 percent of *P. aeruginosa* are susceptible (MIC ≤ 16 μg/ml). However, cefoperazone is less active than cefotaxime against gram-negative bacteria and gram-positive cocci.[18,99,100] Cefoperazone is highly protein bound, has a relatively small volume of distribution, and, although it achieves very high serum concentrations after parenteral administration, does not reliably penetrate into the cerebrospinal fluid.[50,51] It is excreted primarily in the bile. The half-life of 2.0 hours allows dosing every 12 hours in moderate infections. Disulfiramlike reactions and hypoprothrombinemia with bleeding, both consequences of the MTT group at position 3, have been noted in some cefoperazone recipients.[50,188]

Ceftazidime (Fortaz, Tazidime, Tazicef) is a unique third-generation cephalosporin. It has a low affinity for many inducible β-lactamases and is a weak inducer of β-lactamase itself.[6] It has excellent activity against gram-negative bacteria, including *P. aeruginosa*. In many series the MIC$_{50}$ for *P. aeruginosa* is 2 μg/ml.[18,69,99,100] Among the third-generation cephalosporins, ceftazidime has little activity against *B. fragilis* and has poor (only 15–25 percent are susceptible) antistaphylococcal activity.[18,69,95,100] Ceftazidime penetrates into the cerebrospinal fluid and is the treatment of choice for meningitis due to *P. aeruginosa*.[51]

Cefpirome (investigational), a parenterally administered cephalosporin, has been called a fourth-generation agent and has superior activity against streptococci, *S. aureus, Neisseria, H. influenzae*, and the Enterobacteriaceae.[18,20,190] Although 50 percent of *P. aeruginosa* isolates are inhibited by cefpirome at 6.0 μg/ml, it is less active against these strains than ceftazidime.[190,200] Cefpirome appears stable to some Bush 1 and extended spectrum β-lactamases (20). Cefpirome is excreted in the urine and has a half-life of 2.0 hours. It is cleared by hemodialysis.[191] Limited studies indicated penetration into the cerebrospinal fluid when the meninges are inflamed.[192]

Cefepime (maxipime) has been, like cefpirome, proposed as a fourth-generation cephalosporin because of its exceptionally broad spectrum of antibacterial activity. It has superior activity against *Streptococcus pneumoniae, Streptococcus pyogenes, S. aureus, H. influenzae, Neisseria*, and the Enterobacteriaceae.[106–108] Fifty percent of *P. aeruginosa* are inhibited by cefepime at concentrations less than 8 μg/ml.[20] Cefepime is resistant to hydrolysis by Bush 1 β-lactamases and by many ESBL.[20] Cefepime is excreted in the urine, has a half-life of 2.1 hours in patients with normal renal function, and will be removed by hemodialysis.

Cefpiramide (investigational) has antipseudomonal activity similar to that of cefoperazone but is less active than other third-generation cephalosporins against Enterobacteriaceae.[193,194] Like cefoperazone, it is primarily excreted into the biliary tract; renal excretion increases in the presence of liver disease.[49,52]

Clinical Use

The third-generation cephalosporins have become important agents in clinical medicine. Exceptional antimicrobial potency and spectrum of activity, a very acceptable toxicity profile, and, in selected instances, beneficial pharmacokinetics have allowed these compounds to assume a major role in antimicrobial therapy. The unique aspect of the antimicrobial activity of these agents is their superior activity against gram-negative bacilli that are resistant to other β-lactam antibiotics. Because these relatively resistant bacilli are rarely the cause of community-acquired infection, physicians are urged not to use third-generation cephalosporins routinely for community-acquired infections but rather to use less potent or more specifically targeted alternatives. Third-generation cephalosporins, however, may be beneficial in the treatment of severe community-acquired infections due to less resistant gram-negative bacilli (e.g., *E. coli*, *Proteus mirabilis*, and *K. pneumoniae*).

Cefotaxime, ceftizoxime, and ceftriaxone have provided effective treatment for a variety of nosocomial infections caused by susceptible gram-negative bacilli, including pneumonia, wound infection, and complicated urinary tract infection.[195–198] When treatment is instituted empirically in this setting, the potential for infecting pathogens that are resistant to these agents (e.g., *P. aeruginosa*, methicillin-resistant *S. aureus*, and enterococci) must be considered and combination antimicrobial therapy (usually with an aminoglycoside) used until microbiologic data allow the design of specific therapy. With the widespread use of potent β-lactam antibiotics capable of inducing or precipitating derepression of chromosomal β-lactamase in *Enterobacter* spp., *Citrobacter freundii*, *Serratia*, and other gram-negative bacilli, it is increasingly likely that nosocomial infections caused by highly β-lactam antibiotic resistant Enterobacteriaceae will be encountered.[42,199] In particular, *Enterobacter cloacae* causing infection in this setting may be resistant to these agents. Third-generation cephalosporins must be used cautiously in this setting, and severely ill patients may benefit from combination therapy.[199]

Cefotaxime, ceftriaxone, and, to a lesser degree, ceftizoxime have been demonstrated to be effective therapy for meningitis caused by *H. influenzae*, *Streptococcus pneumoniae*, and *N. meningitidis* and in children are at least as effective as previously used regimens (ampicillin plus chloramphenicol, ampicillin plus gentamicin).[201–204] Cefotaxime or ceftriaxone is now recommended for treatment of *H. influenzae* meningitis and as part of the regimen for empiric therapy for meningitis in children and adults greater than 50 years of age.[140] These agents have also been proven uniquely effective in the treatment of meningitis due to gram-negative bacilli other than *P. aeruginosa* and *Enterobacter* spp.[205,206] Ceftazidime is the agent of choice for meningitis due to *P. aeruginosa*.[207] Meningitis caused by *Enterobacter* spp. that does not respond to a third-generation cephalosporin may be treated with trimethoprim-sulfamethoxazole.[208] Finally, ceftriaxone has been effective therapy for meningitis caused by pneumococci that are relatively resistant to penicillin (penicillin MIC, 0.1–1.0 μg/ml).[209]

Ceftazidime, because of its unique antipseudomonal activity, should be reserved for treatment of infections in which the role of *P. aeruginosa* is established or highly likely. Third-generation cephalosporins have been used as part of empiric combination antimicrobial therapy for the febrile neutropenic patient. Because of its antipseudomonal efficacy ceftazidime is often used in combination with an aminoglycoside for empiric treatment of neutropenic patients.[210] Similarly, combination therapy has also been used in the nonneutropenic patient with severe *P. aeruginosa* infection. Ceftazidime, often as single-drug therapy, has been effective for treatment of acute exacerbations of chronic pulmonary infection in patients with cystic fibrosis.[210] Cefoperazone, in spite of moderate antipseudomonal activity, does not have an important role in the treatment of serious infections caused by *P. aeruginosa*.

As a consequence of the unique antibacterial activity of the third-generation cephalosporins or the combination of antimicrobial activity and unique pharmacokinetics, third-generation cephalosporins have become established therapy in specific settings. Because of increasing chromosomal and β-lactamase–mediated resistance among *N. gonorrhoeae* isolated in the United States, ceftriaxone, which remains highly active against both resistant and susceptible strains, has become recommended for therapy of all forms of gonococcal infection and pelvic inflammatory disease.[173] Cefixime has been proven effective for uncomplicated anogenital gonorrhea, including that caused by penicillinase-producing strains, and is recommended for single-dose oral therapy.[173–211] Additionally, single-dose ceftriaxone is recommended therapy for chancroid.[173–212] Ceftriaxone has been shown effective treatment of Lyme disease and is recommended for treatment of stages of disease with neurologic findings (except isolated Bell's palsy), carditis, arthritis, and refractory late constitutional symptoms.[213,214] Cefotaxime appears to provide therapy comparable to that with ceftriaxone for late Lyme neuroborreliosis. The potent antistreptococcal activity of ceftriaxone and pharmacokinetics allowing once daily dosing have created a role for ceftriaxone in the outpatient therapy of nonenterococcal streptococcal endocarditis.[215,216] When treatment with trimethoprim-sulfamethoxazole or a fluoroquinolone is not feasible, acute uncomplicated cystitis or mild uncomplicated pyelonephritis in women can be treated with cefpodoxime proxetil for 7–14 days.

Prompted by unusual antibiotic activity against difficult gram-negative pathogens causing complex infections, third-generation cephalosporins have been evaluated and additional therapeutic niches established. Ceftazidime in combination with trimethoprim-sulfamethoxazole has been demonstrated more effective than the previous standard therapy for severe infections caused by *Pseudomonas pseudomallei*.[217] Ceftriaxone is an effective therapy for typhoid fever.[218] Third-generation cephalosporins have provided effective therapy for brain abscess caused by gram-negative bacilli, focal salmonella infection, and endocarditis caused by fastidious gram-negative coccobacilli.[219]

The major clinical successes of the third-generation cephalosporins have led to spectacularly increased utilization of these agents. Frequently when these agents are administered, the therapeutic indications are not appropriate and less-broad-spectrum therapy would be equally effective.[220] Furthermore, these agents and cephamycins are often used for prophylaxis when a less-broad-spectrum antimicrobial would be equally efficacious. Overutilization has revealed the Achilles' heel of the available third-generation cephalosporins. The relentless pressure of β-lactam antibiotics on the Enterobacteriaceae flora has yielded a prominent array of β-lactamase–producing organisms that are resistant to many of the most potent and previously reliable antimicrobials.[41,42,44,189,199,220] Additionally, these newly resistant gram-negative rods play increasing roles as nosocomial pathogens and agents of secondary infection. Similarly, organisms intrinsically resistant to cephalosporins are emerging as major causes of nosocomial infection. Thus, in a case-control study, nosocomial enterococcal bacteremia was significantly associated with prior treatment using a second- or third-generation cephalosporin.[221] Enhanced infection control efforts and enforced guidelines for utilization of antibiotics may be necessary if the clinical efficacy of potent antimicrobials, such as the cephalosporins, is to be maintained.[220]

REFERENCES

1. Abraham EP. Cephalosporins 1945–1986. In: Williams JD, ed. The Cephalosporin Antibiotics. Auckland: Adis Press; 1987:1–14.
2. Abraham EP, Loder PB. Cephalosporin C. In: Flynn EH, ed. Cephalosporins and Penicillins: Chemistry and Biology. New York: Academic Press; 1972: 2–26.

3. Rolinson GN. The influence of 6-aminopenicillanic acid on antibiotic development. J Antimicrob Chemother. 1988;22:5–14.

4. Huber FM, Chauvette RR, Jackson BG. Preparative methods for 7-aminocephalosporanic acid and 6-aminopenicillanic acid. In: Flynn EH, ed. Cephalosporins and Penicillins. New York: Academic Press; 1972:27.

5. Neu HC. Structure-activity relations of new beta-lactam compounds and in vitro activity against common bacteria. Rev Infect Dis. 1983;5(Suppl):S319–37.

6. Neu HC. Relation of structural properties of beta-lactam antibiotics to antibacterial activity. Am J Med. 1985;79(Suppl 2A):2–13.

7. Allan JD, Eliopoulos GM, Moellering RC Jr. Antibiotics: Future directions by understanding structure-function relationships. In: Root RK, Trunkey DD, Sande MA, eds. Contemporary Issues in Infectious Diseases. v. 6. New York: Churchill Livingstone; 1987:263–84.

8. Onishi HR, Daoust DR, Zimmerman SB, et al. Cefoxitin, a semisynthetic cephamycin antibiotic: Resistance to β-lactamase inactivation. Antimicrob Agents Chemother. 1974;5:38–48.

9. Stapley EO, Birnbaum J. Chemistry and microbiological properties of the cephamycins. In: Salton MRJ, Shockman GD, eds. Beta-lactam antibiotics. New York: Academic Press; 1981:327–51.

10. O'Callaghan CH, Sykes RB, Griffith A, et al. Cefuroxime, a new cephalosporin antibiotic: Activity in vitro. Antimicrob Agents Chemother. 1976;9:511–9.

11. Neu HC, Fu KP. Cefuroxime, a β-lactamase–resistant cephalosporin with a broad spectrum of gram-positive and negative activity. Antimicrob Agents Chemother. 1978;13:657–64.

12. Dunn GL. Ceftizoxime and other third generation cephalosporins: Structure-activity relationships. J Antimicrob Chemother. 1982;10(Suppl C):1.

13. Boucourt R, Bormann D, Heymes R, et al. Chemistry of cefotaxime. J Antimicrob Chemother. 1980;6(Suppl A):63–7.

14. Neu HC. β-Lactam antibiotics: Structural relationships affecting in vitro activity and pharmacologic properties. Rev Infect Dis. 1986;8(Suppl 3):S237–59.

15. Shigi Y, Kojo H, Waksugi M, et al. Differences between ceftizoxime and its stereoisomer in antibacterial activity and affinity for penicillin-binding proteins. Antimicrob Agents Chemother. 1981;19:393–6.

16. Neu HC, Labthavikul P. Antimicrobial activity and beta-lactamase stability of ceftazidime, an aminothiazolyl cephalosporin potentially active against *Pseudomonas aeruginosa*. Antimicrob Agents Chemother. 1982;4:11–8.

17. Phillips I, Warren C, Shannon K, et al. Ceftazidime: In vitro antibacterial activity and susceptibility to beta-lactamases compared with that of cefotaxime, moxalactam, and other beta-lactam antibiotics. J Antimicrob Chemother. 1981;8(Suppl B):13–31.

18. Thornsberry C. Review of in vitro activity of third-generation cephalosporins and other newer beta-lactam antibiotics against clinically important bacteria. Am J Med 1985;79(Suppl 2A):14–20.

19. Neuman M. Mechanisms of action of beta-lactam antibiotics: Relationship between PBP (penicillin-binding proteins) and autolysis. Drugs Exp Clin Res. 1981;7:363–7.

20. Sanders CC. Cefepime. Clin Infect Dis. 1993;17:369–79.

21. Fassbender M, Lode H, Schaberg T, et al. Pharmacokinetics of new oral cephalosporins, including a new carbacephem. Clin Infect Dis. 1993;16:646–53.

22. Neu HC. Oral β-lactam antibiotics from 1960 to 1993. Infect Dis Clin Pract. 1993;6:394–404.

23. Waxman DJ, Yocum RR, Stominger JL. Penicillins and cephalosporins are active site-directed acylating agents: Evidence in support of the substrate analogue hypothesis. Philos Trans R Soc Lond (Biol). 1980;289:257–71.

24. Yocum RR, Rasmussin JR, Strominger SL. Mechanism of action of penicillin: Penicillin activates the active site of *Bacillus stearothermophilus* D-alanine carboxypeptidase. J Biol Chem. 1980;255:3977–86.

25. Spratt BG. Properties of the penicillin-binding proteins of *Escherichia coli* K12. Eur J Biochem. 1977;72:341–52.

26. Neu HC. Penicillin-binding proteins and role of amdinocillin in causing bacterial cell death. Am J Med. 1983;75(Suppl 2A):9–20.

27. Matsuhashi S, Kamiryo T, Blumberg PM, et al. Mechanism of action and development of resistance to a new amdino penicillin. J Bacteriol. 1974;117:578–87.

28. Waxman DJ, Strominger JL. Penicillin-binding proteins and the mechanism of action of β-lactam antibiotics. Annu Rev Biochem. 1983;52:825–69.

29. Tomasz A. Penicillin-binding proteins and the antibacterial effectiveness of β-lactam antibiotics. Rev Infect Dis. 1986;8(Suppl 3):S260–78.

30. Nikaido H, Nakae T. The outer membrane of gram-negative bacteria. Adv Microb Physiol. 1979;20:163–250.

31. Yoshimura F, Nikaido H. Diffusion of β-lactam antibiotics through the porin channels of *Escherichia coli* K12. Antimicrob Agents Chemother. 1985;27:84–92.

32. Gutmann L, Williamson R, Collatz E. The possible role of porins in antibiotic resistance. Ann Intern Med. 1984;101:554–7.

33. Hopkins JM, Towner KJ. Enhanced resistance to cefotaxime and imipenem associated with outer membrane protein alterations in *Enterobacter aerogenes*. J Antimicrob Chemother. 1990;25:49–55.

34. Nikaido H. Outer membrane barrier as a mechanism of antimicrobial resistance. Antimicrob Agents Chemother. 1989;33:1831–6.

35. Richmond MH. Factors influencing the antibacterial action of β-lactam antibiotics. J Antimicrob Chemother. 1978;4(Suppl B):1–14.

36. Bush K, Sykes RB. Interaction of β-lactam antibiotics with β-lactamases as a cause for resistance. In: Bryan LE, ed. Antimicrobial Drug Resistance. Orlando: Academic Press; 1984:1–31.

37. Sawai T, Yamaguchi A, Hiruma R. Effect of interaction between outer membrane permeability and β-lactamase production on resistance to β-lactam agents in gram-negative bacteria. Rev Infect Dis. 1988;10:761–4.

38. Hartman BJ, Tomasz A. Low affinity penicillin binding proteins associated with β-lactam resistance in *Staphylococcus aureus*. J Bacteriol. 1984;158:513–6.

39. Utsui Y, Yokota T. Role of an altered penicillin-binding protein in methicillin and cephem-resistant *Staphylococcus aureus*. Antimicrob Agents Chemother. 1985;28:397–403.

40. Sanders CC. β-Lactamases of gram-negative bacteria: New challenges for new drugs. Clin Infect Dis. 1992;14:1089–99.

41. Sanders CC, Sanders E Jr. β-Lactam resistance in gram-negative bacteria: Global trends and clinical impact. Clin Infect Dis. 1992;15:824–39.

42. Sanders WE Jr, Sanders CC. Inducible β-lactamases: Clinical and epidemiologic implications for use of newer cephalosporins. Rev Infect Dis. 1988;10:830–8.

43. Jacoby GA, Medeiros AA. More extended-spectrum β-lactamases. Antimicrob Agents Chemother. 1991;35:1697–704.

44. Medeiros AA. Nosocomal outbreaks of multiresistant bacteria: Extended-spectrum beta-lactamases have arrived in North America. Ann Intern Med. 1993;119:429–9.

45. Brogard JM, Conte F. Pharmacokinetics of the new cephalosporins. Antibiot Chemother. 1982;31:145–210.

46. Bergan T. Pharmacokinetic properties of the cephalosporins. In: Williams JD, ed. The Cephalosporin Antibiotics. Auckland: Adis Press; 1987:89–104.

47. Patel IH, Kaplan SA. Pharmacokinetic profile of ceftriazone in man. Am J Med. 1984;77(Suppl 4G):17–25.

48. Wise R. The pharmacokinetics of the oral cephalosporins—A review. J Antimicrob Chemother. 1990;26(Suppl E):13–20.

49. Brogard JM, Jehl F, Aldoff M, et al. High hepatic excretion in humans of cefpiramide, a new cephalosporin. Antimicrob Agents Chemother. 1988;32:1360–4.

50. Barriere SL, Flaherty JF. Third generation cephalosporins: A critical evaluation. Clin Pharm. 1984;3:351–73.

51. Cherubin CE, Eng RHK, Norrby R, et al. Penetration of newer cephalosporins into cerebrospinal fluid. Rev Infect Dis. 1989;11:526–48.

52. Demotes-Mainard F, Vincon G, Amouretti M, et al. Pharmacokinetics and protein binding of cefpiramide in patients with alcoholic cirrhosis. Clin Pharmacol Ther. 1991;49:263–9.

53. Chin NX, Neu HC. Cefotaxime and desacetyl cefotaxime: An example of advantageous antimicrobial metabolism. Diagn Microbiol Infect Dis. 1984;2:215.

54. Craig WA, Ebert SC. Killing and regrowth of bacteria in vitro. A review. Scand J Infect Dis. 1991;74(Suppl):63–70.

55. Bundtzen R, Gerber AU, Cohn D, et al. Post-antibiotic suppression of bacterial growth. Rev Infect Dis. 1981;3:28–37.

56. Vogelman B, Gudmundssun S, Turnidge J, et al. In vivo post-antibiotic effect in thigh infection in neutropenic mice. J Infect Dis. 1988;157:287–9.

57. Vogelman B, Gundmundsson S, Leggett J, et al. Correlation of antimicrobial pharmacokinetic parameters with therapeutic efficacy in an animal model. J Infect Dis 1988;158:831–47.

58. Leggett J, Fantin B, Ebert S, et al. Comparative antibiotic dose-effect relations at several dosing intervals in murine pneumonitis and thigh infection models. J Infect Dis. 1989;159:281–92.

59. Schentag JJ, Smith IL, Swanson DJ, et al. Role for dual individualization with cefmenoxime. Am J Med. 1984;77(Suppl 6A):43–50.

60. Saxon A, Beall GN, Rohr AS, et al. Immediate hypersensitivity reactions to beta-lactam antibiotics. Ann Intern Med. 1987;107:204–15.

61. Lin R. A perspective on penicillin allergy. Arch Intern Med. 1992;152:930–7.

62. Platt R. Adverse effects of third-generation cephalosporins. J Antimicrob Chemother. 1982;10(Suppl C):135–40.

63. Meyers BR. Comparative toxicities of third-generation cephalosporins. Am J Med. 1985;79(Suppl 2A):96–103.

64. Norrby SR. Side effects of cephalosporins. Drugs. 1987;34(Suppl 2):105–20.

65. Petz LD. Immunologic reactions of humans to cephalosporins. Postgrad Med J. 1971;Feb(Suppl):64–9.

66. Petz LD. Immunologic cross-reactivity between penicillins and cephalosporins: A review. J Infect Dis. 1978;137:S74–9.

67. Sogn DD, Evans R III, Shepherd GM, et al. Results of the national institute of allergy and infectious diseases collaborative trial to test the predictive value of skin testing with major and minor penicillin derivatives in hospitalized adults. Arch Intern Med. 1992;152:1025–32.

68. Moellering RC, Jr, Swartz MN. The newer cephalosporins. N Engl J Med. 1976;294:24.

69. Donowitz GR, Mandell GL. Beta-lactam antibiotics. N Engl J Med. 1988;313:490–500.

70. Gustaferro CA, Steckelberg JM. Cephalosporin antimicrobial agents and related compounds. Mayo Clin Proc. 1991;66:1064–73.

71. Bang N, Kammer RB. Hematologic complications associated with beta-lactam antibiotics. Rev Infect Dis. 1983;5(Suppl 2):S380–93.

72. Sattler FR, Weitekamp MR, Ballard JO. Potential for bleeding with the new beta-lactam antibiotics. Ann Intern Med. 1986;105:924–31.

73. Nichols RL, Wikler MA, McDevitt JT, et al. Coagulopathy associated with extended-spectrum cephalosporins in patients with serious infections. Antimicrob Agents Chemother. 1987;31:231–5.

74. Conly JM, Ramotar K, Chubb H, et al. Hypoprothrombinemia in febrile, neutropenic patients with cancer: Association with antimicrobial suppression of intestinal microflora. J Infect Dis. 1984;150:202–12.

75. Lipsky JJ, Lewis JC, Novick WJ Jr. Production of hypoprothrombinemia by moxalactam and 1-methyl-5-thiotetrazole in rats. Antimicrob Agents Chemother. 1984;25:380–1.

76. Bechtold H, Andrassy K, Jahnchen E, et al. Evidence for impaired hepatic vitamin K₁ metabolism in patients treated with N-methyl-thiotetrazole cephalosporins. Thromb Haemost. 1984;51:358–61.

77. Barza M, Furie B, Brown AE, et al. Defects in vitamin K–dependent carboxylation associated with moxalactam treatment. J Infect Dis. 1986;153:1166–9.

78. Agnelli G, Del Favero A, Parise P, et al. Cephalosporin-induced hypoprothrombinemia: Is the N-methylthiotetrazole side chain the culprit? Antimicrob Agents Chemother. 1986;29:1108–9.

79. Sattler FR, Colao DJ, Caputo GM, et al. Cefoperazone for empiric therapy in patients with impaired renal function. Am J Med. 1986;81:229–36.

80. Baxter JG, Marble DA, Whitfield LR, et al. Clinical risk factors for prolonged PT/PTT in abdominal sepsis patients treated with moxalactam or tobramycin plus clindamycin. Ann Surg. 1985;201:96–102.

81. Conjura A, Bell W, Lipsky JJ. Cefotetan and hypoprothrombinemia. Ann Intern Med. 1988;108:643.

82. Weitekamp MR, Caputo GM, Al-Mondhiry HA, et al. The effect of latamoxef, cefotaxime, and cefoperazone on platelet function and coagulation in normal volunteers. J Antimicrob Chemother. 1985;16:95–101.

83. Pakter RL, Russel TR, Mielke H, et al. Coagulopathy associated with the use of moxalactam. JAMA. 1982;248:1100.

84. Heim-Duthoy KL, Caperton EM, Pollock R, et al. Apparent biliary pseudolithiasis during ceftriaxone therapy. Antimicrob Agents Chemother. 1990;34:1146–9.

85. Lopez AJ, O'Keefe P, Morrissey M, et al. Ceftriaxone-induced cholelithiasis. Ann Intern Med. 1991;115:712–4.

86. Park HZ, Lee SP, Schy AL. Ceftiraxone-associated gallbladder sludge: Identification of calcium-ceftriaxone salt as a major component of gallbladder precipitate. Gastroenterology. 1991;100:1665–70.

87. Pasternack DP, Stephen BG. Reversible nephrotoxicity associated with cephalothin therapy. Arch Intern Med. 1975;135:599–602.

88. Barza M. Nephrotoxicity of cephalosporins: An overview. J Infect Dis. 1978;137(Suppl):S60–73.

89. Wade JC, Petty BG, Conrad G, et al. Cephalothin plus an aminoglycoside is more nephrotoxic than methicillin plus an aminoglycoside. Lancet. 1978;2:604–6.

90. Lutt FC. Cephalosporin and aminoglycoside interactions: Clinical and toxicologic implications. In: Whelton A, Neu HC, eds. The Aminoglycosides: Microbiology, Clinical Use and Toxicology. New York: Marcel Dekker; 1982:387–96.

91. Alestig K, Trollfors B, Anderson R, et al. Ceftazidime and renal function. J Antimicrob Chemother. 1984;13:177–81.

92. Foster RS, Raehl CL, Wilson HD. Disulfiram-like reactions associated with a parenteral cephalosporin. Am J Hosp Pharm. 1980;37:858–9.

93. Buening MK, Wold JS, Israel KS, et al. Disulfiram-like reactions to β-lactams. JAMA. 1981;245:2027.

94. Neu HC. Cephalosporins—Cefotaxime 10 years later, a major drug with continued use. Infection. 1991;19(Suppl 6):S309–15.

95. Cuchural GH Jr, Tally FP, Jacobus NV, et al. Comparative activities of newer β-lactam agents against members of the Bacteroides fragilis group. Antimicrob Agents Chemother. 1990;34:479–80.

96. Appleman MD, Heseltine PNR, Cherubin CE. Epidemiology, antimicrobial susceptibility, pathogenicity, and significance of Bacteroides fragilis group organisms isolated at Los Angeles County—University of Southern California Medical Center. Rev Infect Dis. 1991;13:12–8.

97. Jones RN. Microbiologic observations of cefmetazole and other cephamycins. Hosp Ther. 1990;15(Suppl 4):3–15.

98. Lee K, Jang IH, Kim YJ, et al. In vitro susceptibilities of the Bacteroides fragilis group to 14 antimicrobial agents in Korea. Antimicrob Agents Chemother. 1992;36:195–7.

99. Jones RN, Pfaller MA, Allen SD, et al. Antimicrobial activity of cefpirome: An update compared to five third-generation cephalosporins against nearly 6000 recent clinical isolates from five medical centers. Diagn Microbiol Infect Dis. 1991;14:361–4.

100. Murray RP, Jones RN, Allen SD, et al. Multilaboratory evaluation of the in vitro activity of 13 β-lactam antibiotics against 1474 clinical isolates of aerobic and anaerobic bacteria. Diagn Microbiol Infect Dis. 1993;16:191–203.

101. Jorgensen JH, Doern GV, Maher LA, et al. Antimicrobial resistance among respiratory isolates of Haemophilus influenzae, Moraxella catarrhalis, and Strepcococcus pneumoniae in the United States. Antimicrob Agents Chemother. 1990;34:2075–80.

102. Neu HC, Chin NX, et al. The in vitro activity and beta lactamase stability of cefpirome (HR 810), a pyridine cephalosporin agent active against staphylococci, enterobacteriaceae, and Pseudomonas aeruginosa. Infection. 1985;13:146–55.

103. King A, Boothman C, Phillips I. Comparative in vitro activity of cefpirome and cefepime, two new cephalosporins. J Clin Micro Infect Dis. 1990;9:677–85.

104. Chin NX, Gu Jin, et al. In vitro activity and β-lactamase stability of GR69153, a new long acting cephalosporin. Antimicrob Agents Chemother. 1991;35:259–66.

105. Neu HC, Chin NX, Jules K, et al. The activity of BMY 28142, a new broad spectrum β-lactamase stable cephalosporin. J Antimicrob Chemother. 1986;17:441–52.

106. Steele HCH, Edwards, Rissing JP. In-vitro activity of BMY 28142, a new aminothiazolyl cephalosporin. J Antimicrob Chemother. 1985;16:463–8.

107. Norden CW, Neiderriter K. In vitro activity of BMY-28142, a new cephalosporin. Chemotherapy. 1987;33:15–7.

108. Masuyoshi S, Hiraoka M, Inoue M, et al. Comparison of the in vitro and in vivo antibacterial activities of cefepime (BMY-28142) with ceftazidime, cefuzonam, cefotaxime and cefmonoxime. Drugs Exp Clin Res. 989;15:1–10.

109. Hartstein AI, Patrick KE, Jones SR, et al. Comparison of pharmacologic antimicrobial properties of cephadroxil and cephalexin. Antimicrob Agents Chemother. 1977;12:93–7.

110. Silver MS, Counts GW, Zeleznik D, et al. Comparison of in vitro antibacterial activity of three oral cephalosporins: Cefaclor, cephalexin and cephadrine. Antimicrob Agents Chemother. 1977;12:591–6.

111. Renzini G, Ravagnan G, Oliva B. In vitro and in vivo microbiological evaluation of cephapirin, a new antibiotic. Chemotherapy. 1975;21:289–96.

112. Klein JO, Eickhoff TC, Tilles JG, et al. Cephalothin: Activity in vitro, absorption and excretion in normal subjects and clinical observations in 40 patients. Am J Med Sci. 1964;248:640–56.

113. Sabath LD, Wilcox C, Garner C, et al. In vitro activity of cefazolin against recent clinical bacterial isolates. J Infect Dis. 1973;128(Suppl):S320–6.

114. Myers JP, Linneman CC Jr. Bacteremia due to methicillin-resistant Staphylococcus aureus. J Infect Dis. 1982;145:532–6.

115. Quinn EL, Pohlod D, Madhavan T, et al. Clinical experience with cefazolin and other cephalosporins in bacterial endocarditis. J Infect Dis. 1983;128(Suppl):S386–91.

116. Bergeron MG, Brusch JL, Barza M, et al. Bactericidal activity and pharmacology of cefazolin. Antimicrob Agents Chemother. 1973;4:396–401.

117. Regamey C, Libke RD, Engelking ER, et al. Inactivation of cefazolin, cephaloridine, and cephalothin by methicillin-sensitive and methicillin-resistant strains of Staphylococcus aureus. J Infect Dis. 1975;131:291–4.

118. Fong IW, Engelking ER, Kirby WMM. Relative inactivation by Staphylococcus aureus of eight cephalosporin antibiotics. Antimicrob Agents Chemother. 1976;9:939–44.

119. Meyers BR, Kaplan K, Weinstein L. Cephalexin microbiological effects and pharmacologic parameters in man. Clin Pharmacol Ther. 1969;10:810–6.

120. Neiss E. Cephradine: Summary of preclinical studies and clinical pharmacology. J Irish Med Assoc. 1973;66(Suppl):1–12.

121. Weber DJ, Wolfson JS, Swartz MN, et al. Pasteurella multocida infections: Report of 34 cases and review of the literature. Medicine. 1984;63:133–54.

122. Kaiser AB. Antimicrobial prophylaxis in surgery. N Engl J Med. 1986;315:1129–38.

123. Antimicrobial prophylaxis in surgery. Medical Letter. 1993;35:91–4.

124. Sanders CV, Greenberg RN, Marier RL. Cefamandole and cefoxiton. Ann Intern Med. 1985;103:70–8.

125. Fraser DG. Drug therapy reviews: Antimicrobial spectrum, pharmacology and therapeutic use of cefamandole and cefoxitin. Am J Hosp Pharm. 1979;36:1503–8.

126. Delgado DG, Crau CJ, Cobbs CG, et al. Clinical and laboratory evaluation of cefamandole in therapy of Haemophilus sp. Bronchopulmonary infections. Antimicrob Agents Chemother. 1979;15:807–12.

127. Meyers BR, Hirschman SZ. Antibacterial activity of cefamandole in vitro. J Infect Dis. 1978;137(Suppl):S25–31.

128. Doern G. In vitro activity of loracarbef and effects of susceptibility test methods. Am J Med. 1992;92(Suppl 6A):75–155.

129. Thornsberry C. Review of the in vitro antibacterial activity of cefprozil, a new oral cephalosporin. Clin Infect Dis. 1992;14(Suppl 2):S189–94.

130. Actor P. In vitro experience with cefonicid. Rev Infect Dis. 1984;6(Suppl 4):S783–90.

131. Birnbaum J, Stapley EO, Miller AK, et al. Cefoxitin, a semi-synthetic cephamycin: A microbiologic overview. J Antimicrob Chemother. 1978;4:15–32.

132. Ward A, Richards DM. Cefotetan: A review. Drugs. 1985;30:382–426.

133. Ayres LW, Jones RN, Barry AL, et al. Cefotetan, a new cephamycin. Antimicrob Agents Chemother. 1982;22:859–77.

134. Aldridge KE, Sanders CC, Janney A, et al. Comparison of the activities of penicillin G and new β-lactam antibiotics against clinical isolates of Bacteroides species. Antimicrob Agents Chemother. 1984;26:410–3.

135. Goldstein EJC, Citron DM. Annual incidence, epidemiology and comparative in vitro susceptibilities to cefoxitin, cefotetan, cefmetazole and ceftizoxime of recent community-acquired isolates of the Bacteroides fragilis group. J Antimicrob Chemother. 1988;26:2361–6.

136. Jones RN. Review of the in-vitro spectrum and characteristics of cefmetazole (CS = 1170). J Antimicrob Chemother. 1989;12(Suppl D):1–12.

137. Jacob LS, Layne P. Cefonicid: An overview of clinical studies in the United States. Rev Infect Dis. 1984;6(Suppl 4):S791.

138. Platt R, Zaleznik DF, Hopkins CC, et al. Perioperative antibiotic prophylaxis for herniorrhaphy and breast surgery. N Engl J Med. 1990;322:153–60.

139. Marks WA, Stutman HR, Marks MI, et al. Cefuroxime versus ampicillin plus chloramphenicol in childhood bacterial meningitis: A multicenter randomized controlled trial. J Pediatr. 1986;109:123–30.

140. Tunkel AR, Wispelway B, Scheld WM. Bacterial meningitis: Recent advances in pathophysiology and treatment. Ann Intern Med. 1990;112:610–23.

141. Schaad UB, Suter S, Gianella-Borradori A, et al. A comparison of ceftiraxone and cefuroxime for the treatment of bacterial meningitis in children. N Engl J Med. 1990;322:141–7.

142. Barriere SL. Pharmacology and pharmacokinetics of cefprozil. Clin Infect Dis. 1992;14(Suppl 2):S184–8.

143. Harding SM, Williams PEO, Ayrton J. Pharmacology of cefuroxime as the 1-acetoxyethyl ester in volunteers. Antimicrob Agents Chemother. 1984;25:78–82.

144. Sommers D, Wan Wyk M, Williams PEO, et al. Pharmacokinetics and tolerance of cefuroxime axetil in volunteers during repeated dosing. Antimicrob Agents Chemother. 1984;25:344–7.

145. DeSante KA, Zeckel ML: Pharmacokinetic profile of loracarbef. Am J Med. 1992;92(Suppl 6A)16S–25S.

146. Cooper RDG. The carbacephems: A new beta-lactam antibiotic glass. Am J Med. 1992;92(Suppl 6A):2S–6S.

147. Morel C, Vergnaud M, Langeard MM, et al. Cefotetan: Comparative study in vitro against 266 gram-negative clinical isolates. J Antimicrob Chemother. 1983;11(Suppl A):31–6.

148. Peters GR, Metzler CM. The effects of cefmetazole and latamoxef on platelet function in healthy human volunteers. J Antimicrob Chemother. 1989;23(Suppl D):119–23.

149. Pines A, Raafat HH, Khorasani M, et al. Cefuroxime and ampicillin compared in a double-blind study in the treatment of lower respiratory tract infections. Chemotherapy. 1981;27:459–65.

150. Mehtar S, Parr JH, Morgan DJR. A comparison of cefuroxime and cortimoxazole in severe respiratory tract infections. J Antimicrob Chemother. 1982;9:479–84.

151. Schleupner CJ, Anthony WC, Tan J, et al. Blinded comparison of cefuroxime to cefaclor for lower respiratory tract infections. Arch Intern Med. 1988;148:343–8.

152. Dere WH. Acute bronchitis: Results of U.S. and European trials of antibiotic therapy. Am J Med. 1992;92(Suppl 6A):53S–57S.

153. Zeckel ML. Loracarbef (LY163892) in the treatment of actue exacerbations of chronic bronchitis: Results of U.S. and European comparative clinical trials. Amer J Med 1992;92(Suppl 6A):58S–64S.

154. Hyslop DL. Efficacy and safety of loracarbef in the treatment of pneumonia. Am J Med. 1992;92(Suppl 6A):65S–9S.

155. McCarty J. Loracarbef versus penicillin VK in the treatment of streptococcal pharyngitis and tonsillitis in an adult population. Am J Med. 1992;92(Suppl 6A):74S–9S.

156. McCarty J, Ruoff GE, Jacobson KD. Loracarbef (LY163892) versus cefaclor in the treatment of bacterial skin and skin-structure infections in an adult population. Am J Med. 1992;92(Suppl 6A):80S–5S.

157. Hyslop DL, Bischoff W. Loracarbef (LY163892) versus cefaclor and norfloxacin in the treatment of uncomplicated pyelonephritis. Am J Med. 1992;92(Suppl 6A):86S–93S.

158. Stutman HR, Arguedas AG. Comparison of cefprozil with other antibiotic regimens in the treatment of children with acute otitis media. Clin Infect Dis. 1992;14(Suppl 2):S204–8.

159. McCarty JM, Renteria A. Treatment of pharyngitis and tonsillitis with cefprozil: Review of three multicenter trials. Clin Infect Dis. 1992;14(Suppl 2):S224–30.

160. Pelletier LL Jr. Review of the experience with cefprozil for the treatment of lower respiratory tract infections. Clin Infect Dis. 1992;14(Suppl 2):S238–43.

161. Iravani A. Multicenter comparison of safety and efficacy of cefprozil vs. cefaclor in the treatment of acute uncomplicated urinary tract infections. Clin Infect Dis. 1992;14(Suppl 2):S252.

162. Nolen TM. Clinical trials of cefprozil for treatment of skin and skin-structure infections: Review. Clin Infect Dis. 1992;14(Suppl 2):S255–63.

163. Davies BL, Maesen FDV, Teengs JP. Cefuroxime axetil in acute purulent exacerbations of chronic bronchitis infections. Infection. 1987;15:253–6.

164. Klein JO. Microbiologic efficacy of antibacterial drugs for acute otitis media. Pediatr Infect Dis J. 1993;12:973–5.

165. Nadelman RB, Luger SW, Frank E, et al. Comparison of cefuroxime axetil and doxycycline in the treatment of early Lyme disease. Ann Intern Med. 1992;117:273–80.

166. Poindexter AN III, Sweet R, Ritter M. Cefotetan in the treatment of obstetric and gynecologic infections. Am J Obstet Gynecol. 1986;154:946–50.

167. Lefrock JL, Blais F, Schell RD, et al. Cefoxitin in the treatment of diabetic patients with lower extremity infections. Infect Surg. 1983;2:361–74.

168. Drusano GL, Warren W, Saah AJ, et al. A prospective randomized controlled trial of cefoxitin versus clindamycin-aminoglycoside in mixed anaerobic-aerobic infections. Surg Gynecol Obstet. 1982;154:715–20.

169. Wilson SE, Boswick JA, Duma RJ, et al. Cephalosporin therapy in intra-abdominal infections: A multicenter randomized, comparative study of cefotetan, moxalactam and cefoxitin. Am J Surg. 1988;155(Suppl 5A):61–6.

170. Sweet R, Gall SA, Gobbs RS, et al. Multicenter clinical trial comparing cefotetan with moxalactam or cefoxitin as therapy for obstetric gynecologic infections. Am J Surg. 1988;155(Suppl 5A):56–60.

171. Griffith DL, Novak E, Greenwald CA, et al. Clinical experience with cefmetazole sodium in the United States: An overview. J Antimicrob Chemother. 1989;23(Suppl D):21–33.

172. Moran JS, Zenilman JM. Therapy for gonococcal infections: Options in 1989. Rev Infect Dis. 1990;12(Suppl 6):S633–44.

173. Centers for Disease Control and Prevention. 1993 Sexually transmitted diseases treatment guidelines. MMWR. 1993;42(No. RR-14):20, 56–66, 75–81.

174. Peterson HB, Galaid EI, Zenilman JM. Pelvic inflammatory disease: Review of treatment options. Rev Infect Dis. 1990;12(Suppl 6):S656–64.

175. Orr JW, Varner RE, Kilgore LC, et al. Cefotetan versus cefoxitin as prophylaxis in hysterectomy. Am J Obstet Gynecol. 1986;154:960–3.

176. McGregor JA, French JI, Makowski E. Single dose cefotetan versus multi-dose cefoxitin for prophylaxis in cesarean section in high risk patients. Am J Obstet Gynecol. 1986;154:955–60.

177. Gorbach SL. The role of cephalosporins in surgical prophylaxis. J Antimicrob Chemother. 1989;23(Suppl D):61–70.

178. Neu HC. Pathophysiologic basis for the use of third-generation cephalosporins. Amer J Med. 1990;88(Suppl 4A):3S–11S.

179. Trenholme GM, Schmitt BA, Nelson JA, et al. Comparative study of three different dosing regimens of cefotaxime for gram-negative bacteremia. Diagn Microbiol Infect Dis. 1989;12:107–12.

180. Fu KP, Neu HC. Antibacterial activity of ceftizoxime, a β-lactamase stable cephalosporin. Antimicrob Agents Chemother. 1980;17:583–90.

181. Cleeland R, Squires E. Antimicrobial activity of ceftriaxone, a review. Am J Med. 1984;77:3–11.

182. Jones RN, Barry Al, et al. In vitro activity of evaluation of cefodizime (HR221), a new semisynthetic cephalosporin. Antimicrob Agents Chemother. 1981;20:760–8.

183. Labro MT, Amit N, et al. Cefodizime (HR221) potentiation of human neutrophil oxygen-dependent bactericidal activity. J Antimicrob Chemother. 1987;19:331–41.

184. Neu HC, Chin NX, Labthavikul P. Comparative in vitro activity and β-lactamase stability of FR 17027, a new orally active cephalosporin. Antimicrob Agents Chemother. 1984;26:174–80.

185. Jones RN. Antimicrobial activity spectrum and pharmacokinetics of old and new orally administered cephems. Antimicrob Newslett. 1988;5:1–8.

186. Neu HC, Saha G, Chin NX. Comparative in vitro activity and β-lactamase stability of FK482, a new oral cephalosporin. Antimicrob Agents Chemother. 1989;33:1795–1800.

187. Briggs BN, Jones RN, Erwin ME, et al. In vitro activity evaluations of cefdinir (FK482, CI-983, and PD134393): A novel orally administered cephalosporin. Diagn Microbiol Infect Dis. 1991;14:425–34.

188. Brogen RN, Carmine A, Heel RC, et al. Cefoperazone, a review of its in vitro antimicrobial activity, pharmacological properties and therapeutic efficacy. Drugs. 1981;22:423–60.

189. Rice LB, Willey SH, Papanicolaou GA, et al. Outbreak of ceftazidime resistance caused by extended-spectrum β-lactamases at a Massachusetts chronic care facility. Antimicrob Agents Chemother. 1990;34:2193–9.

190. Schafer V, Shah PM, Doerr HW, et al. In vitro activity of cefpirome against isolates from patients with urinary tract, lower respiratory tract and wound infections. J Antimicrob Chemother. 1992;29(Suppl A):7–12.

191. Meyer BH, Muller FO, Luus HG, et al. Safety, tolerance and pharmacokinetics of cefpirome administered intramuscularly to healthy subjects. J Antimicrob Chemother. 1992;29(Suppl A):63–70.

192. Wolff M, Chavanet P, Kazmierczak A, et al. Diffusion of cefpirome into the cerebrospinal fluid of patients with purulent meningitis. J Antimicrob Chemother. 1992;29(Suppl A):59–62.

193. Pfaller MA, Niles AC, Murray PR. In vitro antibacterial activity of cefpiramide. Antimicrog Agents Chemother. 1984;25:368–72.

194. Fukasawa M, Noguchi H, Okuda T, et al. In vitro antibacterial activity of SM-1652 a new broad-spectrum cephalosporin with anti-pseudomonal activity. Antimicrob Agents Chemother. 1983;3:195–200.

195. Young JPW, Husson JM, Bruch K, et al. The evaluation of efficacy and safety of cefotaxime: A review of 2500 cases. J Antimicrob Chemother. 1980;6(Suppl A):293–300.

196. Daikos GK, Kosmidis J, Giamarellou H, et al. Evaluation of cefotaxime in a hospital with high antibiotic resistance rates. J Antimicrob Chemother. 1980;6(Suppl A):255–61.

197. Scully BE, Neu HC. The use of ceftizoxime in the treatment of critically ill patients infected with multiply antibiotic resistant bacteria. J Antimicrob Chemother. 1982;10(Suppl C):141–50.

198. Eron LJ, Park CH, Goldenberg RI, et al. Ceftriaxone therapy of serious bacterial infections. J Antimicrob Chemother. 1983;12:65–78.

199. Chow JW, Fine MJ, Shlaes DM, et al. *Enterobacter* bacteremia: Clinical features and emergence of antibiotic resistance during therapy. Ann Intern Med. 1991;115:585–90.

200. Norrby SR. Role of cephalosporins in the treatment of bacterial meningitis in adults: Overview with special emphasis on ceftazidime. Am J Med. 1985; Suppl 2A:56–61.

201. Jacobs RJ, Wells TG, Steele RW, et al. A prospective randomized comparison of cefotaxime vs ampicillin and chloramphenicol for bacterial meningitis in children. Pediatr Infect Dis. 1986;4:362–8.

202. Barson WJ, Miller MA, Brady MT, et al. Prospective comparative trial of ceftriaxone vs conventional therapy for treatment of bacterial meningitis in children. Pediatr Infect Dis. 1986;4:362–8.

203. Congeni BL. Comparison of ceftriaxone and traditional therapy of bacterial meningitis. Antimicrob Agents Chemother. 1984;25:40–4.

204. Bryan JP, Rocha H, daSilva HR, et al. Comparison of ceftriaxone and ampicillin plus chloramphenicol for therapy of acute bacterial meningitis. Antimicrob Agents Chemother. 1985;28:361–8.

205. Lecour H, Seara A, Miranda A, et al. Treatment of 160 cases of acute bacterial meningitis with cefotaxime. J Antimicrob Chemother. 1984;14(Suppl B):195–202.

206. Mullaney DT, John JF. Cefotaxime therapy: Evaluation of its effects on bacterial meningitis, CSF drug levels, and bactericidal activity. Arch Intern Med. 1983;143:1705–8.

207. Fong IW, Tompkins KB. Review of *Pseudomonas aeruginosa* meningitis with special emphasis on treatment with ceftazidime. Rev Infect Dis. 1985; 7:604–12.

208. Wolff MA, Young CL, Ramphal R. Antibiotic therapy for enterobacter meningitis: A retrospective review of 13 episodes and review of the literature. Clin Infect Dis. 1983;16:772–7.

209. Viladrich PF, Gudiol F, Linares J, et al. Characteristics and antibiotic therapy of adult meningitis due to penicillin-resistant pneumococci. Am J Med. 1988;84:839–46.

210. Hughes WT, Armstrong D, Bodey GP, et al. Guidelines for the use of antimicrobial agents in neutropenic patients with unexplained fever. J Infect Dis. 1990;161:381–96.

211. Handsfield HH, McCormack WM, Hook EW, et al. A comparison of single-dose cefixime with ceftriaxone as treatment for uncomplicated gonorrhea. N Engl J Med. 1991;325:1337–41.

212. Schmid GP. Treatment of chancroid, 1989. Rev Infect Dis. 1990;12(Suppl 6):S580–9.

213. Dattwyler RJ, Halperin JJ, Pass H, et al. Ceftiraxone as effective therapy in refractory Lyme disease. J Infect Dis. 1987;155:1322–5.

214. Dattwyler RJ, Halperin JJ, Volkman DJ, et al. Treatment of late Lyme borreliosis—randomized comparison of ceftriaxone and penicillin. Lancet. 1988; 1:1191–4.

215. Francioli P, Etienne J, Hoigne R, et al. Treatment of streptococcal endocarditis with a single daily dose of ceftriaxone sodium for 4 weeks. JAMA. 1992; 267:264–7.

216. Stamboulian D, Bonvehi P, Arevalo C, et al. Antibiotic management of outpatients with endocarditis due to penicillin-susceptible streptococci. Rev Infect Dis. 1991;13(Suppl 2):S160–3.

217. Sookpranee M, Boonma P, Susaengrat W, et al. Multicenter prospective randomized trial comparing ceftazidime plus co-trimoxazole with chloramphenicol plus doxycycline and co-trimoxazole for treatment of severe melioidosis. Antimicrob Agents Chemother. 1992;158–62.

218. Islam A, Butler T, Nath SK, et al. Randomized treatment of patients with typhoid fever by using ceftriaxone or chloramphenicol. J Infect Dis. 1988; 158:742–7.

219. Finch RG. Third-generation cephalosporins in the treatment of rare infections. Am J Med. 1990;88(Suppl 4A):25S–31S.

220. Bamberger DM, Dahl SL. Impact of voluntary vs enforced compliance of third-generation cephalosporin use in a teaching hospital. Arch Intern Med. 1992;152:554–7.

221. Pallares R, Pujol M, Pena C, et al. Cephalosporins as risk factors for nosocomial *Enterococcus faecalis* bacteremia. A matched case-control study. Arch Intern Med. 1993;153:1581–6.

17. OTHER β-LACTAM ANTIBIOTICS

HENRY F. CHAMBERS
HAROLD C. NEU

CARBAPENEMS

Carbapenems are differentiated from penicillins and cephalosporins by a methylene replacement for sulfur in the five-membered α-ring structure, which, like the cephalosporins, also contains a double bond. They are derivatives of thienamycin, a compound produced by *Streptomyces cattleya*.[1]

Imipenem

Chemistry. In addition to those features noted above, imipenem differs from the conventional β-lactams in the nature and conformation of its side chain. All conventional penicillins and cephalosporins contain an acylamino side chain, whereas imipenem has a hydroxyethyl side chain. Furthermore, the side chain in the conventional β-lactams is in a cis configuration, whereas the hydroxyethyl side chain of imipenem is in a trans configuration. It is this trans conformation that is responsible

FIG. 1.   Imipenem.

for the β-lactamase stability of imipenem. This has been demonstrated by the discovery of other carbapenems, the epithienamycins, whose side chains are in a cis conformation and are not β-lactamase–stable.

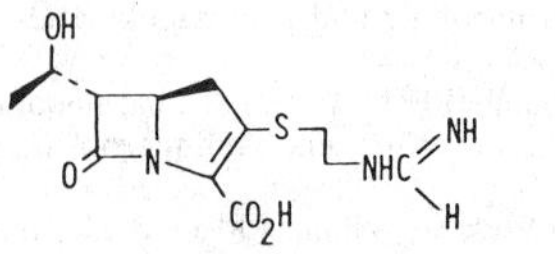

Antibacterial Activity. Imipenem is the *N*-formimidoyl derivative of thienamycin (Fig. 1). Imipenem has excellent in vitro activity against aerobic gram-positive species such as the hemolytic streptococci of the Lancefield classifications A, B, C, and G, with minimal inhibitory (MIC) values of 0.2 μg/ml or less (Table 1).[2,3] *Streptococcus pneumoniae* organisms are inhibited by less than 0.1 μg/ml, and many, but not all, penicillin-resistant strains of *S. pneumoniae* (MIC values >4 μg/ml) are inhibited by 1 μg/ml or less. Penicillin-susceptible strains of *Enterococcus faecalis* are inhibited by less than 1.5 μg/ml; however, like penicillin, imipenem is bacteriostatic, not bactericidal, against sus-

TABLE 1. Comparative Activity of Imipenem and Meropenem against Aerobic and Anaerobic Bacteria

Organism	MIC₉₀ (μg/ml)	
	Imipenem	Meropenem
Staphylococcus aureus[a,b]	0.03	0.3
Coagulase-negative staphylococci[a,b]	0.1	1
Streptococcus pyogenes	0.03	0.1
S. agalactiae	0.03	0.1
S. pneumoniae	0.02	0.03
Enterococcus faecalis	2	8
Haemophilus influenzae	2	0.1
Neisseria gonorrhoeae	0.1	0.03
N. meningitidis	0.1	0.01
Listeria monocytogenes	0.3	0.3
Klebsiella pneumoniae[a]	0.3	0.1
Enterobacter cloacae[a]	1	0.1
E. aerogenes[a]	1	0.1
Escherichia coli[a]	0.1	0.03
Klebsiella oxytoca[a]	1	0.03
Aeromonas hydrophila[a]	8	0.3
Citrobacter freundii[a]	1	0.1
C. diversus[a]	0.5	0.02
Serratia marcescens[a]	4	0.1
Proteus marabilis[a]	4	0.1
Morganella morganii[a]	4	0.2
P. vulgaris[a]	4	0.1
Acinetobacter anitratus	0.5	1
Pseudomonas aeruginosa[a]	4	2
P. maltophilis	>50	>50
P. cepacia	16	32
Bacteroides fragilis	2	1
Bacteroides melaninogenicus[c]	0.1	0.1
Clostridium difficile	4	2
Clostridium perfringens	0.1	0.02
Anaerobic gram-positive cocci	0.5	0.3
Campylobacter jejuni	0.03	0.02

[a] Both β-lactamase- and non-β-lactamase-containing strains.
[b] Methicillin-susceptible strains; methicillin-resistant strains are also resistant to imipenem and meropenem.
[c] Now called *Prevotella melaninogenica*.

(Data from Edwards et al.[2] and Sentochnik et al.[3])

ceptible enterococci. Non-β-lactamase–producing penicillin-resistant strains of enterococci and *E. faecium* are resistant to imipenem. *Staphylococcus aureus* and *Staphylococcus epidermidis* are inhibited by less than 0.2 and 1.5 μg/ml, respectively. Methicillin-resistant staphylococci also are resistant to imipenem. *Listeria* and *Bacillus* spp. are inhibited by less than 1 μg/ml.[4]

Most of the Enterobacteriaceae are inhibited by concentrations of imipenem less than or equal to 1 μg/ml. Some *Proteus* strains have MIC values of 2–4 μg/ml. *Haemophilus infuenzae* and *Neisseria gonorrhoeae*, including their β-lactamase–producing isolates, are inhibited by less than 0.5 μg/ml.

Pseudomonas aeruginosa, including strains resistant to antipseudomonal penicillins and cephalosporins, are inhibited by 1–6 μg/ml.[5] *Xanthomonas maltophilia* is resistant, as are many strains of *Pseudomonas cepacia*. Most *Acinetobacter* organisms are inhibited by less than 1 μg/ml.

Imipenem inhibits most anaerobic species, including *Bacteroides fragilis*.[6,7] Most *Clostridium* spp. are inhibited by 1 μg/ml or less, with the exception of *Clostridium difficile*, which is resistant. *Fusobacterium, Actinomyces, Campylobacter,* and *Yersinia* are inhibited by imipenem, and many *Nocardia asteroides* strains are inhibited by 1 μg/ml. It also inhibits *Mycobacterium avium-intracellulare* and some *Legionella* spp.

Mechanism of Action.   Imipenem binds with high affinity to high-molecular-weight penicillin-binding proteins (PBPs) of both gram-positive and gram-negative bacteria, binding initially to PBP2 and subsequently to 1a, causing lysis of cells of gram-positive and gram-negative bacteria. It is not hydrolyzed by most β-lactamases, penicillinases, cephalosporinases, plasmid or chromosomally mediated, of *S. aureus, Escherichia coli, Enterobacter cloacae, Citrobacter freundii, Proteus rettgeri, Serratia marcescens, Proteus vulgaris, Klebsiella oxytoca, Pseudomonas aeruginosa, Pseudomonas cepacia,* and *B. fragilis*. It is hydrolyzed by a *X. maltophilia* β-lactamase, some *Bacillus,* and *Bacteroides* enzymes.

Carbapenems show a postantibiotic effect (PAE) against gram-negative organisms, in contrast to penicillins and cephalosporins and similar to aminoglycosides and fluoroquinolones. The PAE varies by organism and species. It is best seen with *P. aeruginosa* and allows the drug to be administered less frequently than one normally would suspect on the basis of the activity present in serum. This PAE is noted in the presence of nutrient broth, urine, and serum.

Resistance.   In *X. maltophilia* there is production of a β-lactamase that will hydrolyze imipenem and other carbapenems. A similar enzyme exists in some *P. cepacia* as well. However, most of the resistance is due to loss of an outer membrane protein, referred to as D2, which is in contrast to outer membrane proteins F and C, through which cephalosporins and penicillins traverse the outer membrane of gram-negative organisms. This has been primarily a problem in *P. aeruginosa*. Recently some hyperproducers of chromosomal β-lactamase in *E. cloacae* have been isolated that are also deficient in outer membrane protein and hence can destroy imipenem, since imipenem will induce a large amount of β-lactamase in the periplasmic space.

Pharmacology.   Imipenem cannot be absorbed after oral ingestion due to its instability in gastric acid. Imipenem is removed from the circulation by glomerular filtration and secretion. It is hydrolyzed by the renal peptidase dehydropeptidase-1, located on the brush border of the proximal renal tubules. To overcome the problem of the destruction of imipenem in urine, a dehydropeptidase inhibitor was synthesized. This molecule, called *cilastatin,* is administered in equal amounts to imipenem. Cilastatin has no antibacterial activity, nor does it alter the antibacterial activity of imipenem. Cilastatin does not affect zinc metalloenzyme peptidases or angiotensin-converting en-

zymes. Metabolites of imipenem in the absence of cilastatin are nephrotoxic.

Imipenem is not destroyed in the general circulation and is widely distributed to various body compartments.[8,9] There is minimal biliary secretion of imipenem, and there is minimal change in bowel flora. In the absence of meningeal inflammation only minor amounts of imipenem enter the cerebrospinal fluid (CSF). In the presence of meningeal inflammation CSF levels of 1–5 μg/ml have been recorded. Imipenem has a high affinity for brain cells.

After 20–30 minutes of infusion of 250 mg imipenem plus 250 mg cilastatin, mean peak serum levels of imipenem are 13 μg/ml. After 500 mg, mean peak serum levels are 33 μg/ml; 1000 mg produces a peak concentration of 52 μg/ml.[10,11] The half-life of imipenem is 1 hour in healthy people. The serum half-life is 4 hours in patients whose creatinine clearance is less than 10 ml/min. The half-life of cilastatin increases to a much greater extent than does that of imipenem and reaches 16 hours in anuria.[12] Imipenem and cilastatin are removed from the body by hemodialysis, with dialysis half-lives of 2.5 hours and 3.8 hours, respectively. In the presence of cilastatin, urinary recovery of imipenem is 70 percent, with a 25–29 percent recovery of the metabolites. Fecal elimination of imipenem is less than 1 percent.[13]

Adverse Reactions.   Imipenem has generally been well tolerated.[14] It causes minimal phlebitis when used IV. It can cause immediate hypersensitivity,[15] and cross-reactions with penicillins have occurred. No major adverse effects such as diarrhea, pseudomembranous colitis, coagulation abnormalities, nephrotoxicity, or hepatotoxicity have been reported. Rapid infusion of imipenem has produced nausea and emesis in about 1 percent of patients. About 2–4 percent of imipenem-treated patients will have from a one- to twofold elevation of serum glutamic-oxaloacetic transaminase and/or serum glutamic-pyruvic transaminase (SGOT, SGPT) values. Leukopenia has occurred, but infrequently. No drug interactions have been reported. The most serious toxicity is seizures, an infrequent side effect that occurs most often in patients with underlying central nervous system pathology and in individuals with decreased renal function in whom dose adjustment has not been made. In some series seizures have been reported in up to 1.5 percent of patients, although the manufacturer reports an incidence of 0.4 percent.

Clinical Use.   Animal infection studies have demonstrated the utility of imipenem in therapy for staphylococcal endocarditis (but not enterococcal endocarditis where high relapse rates were noted),[16,17] bacteremia due to *P. aeruginosa* in neutropenic rats,[18] and pyelonephritis in rats. Some of these observations have been extended to humans, in whom imipenem has been found to be useful in the treatment of bone and soft tissue infections, obstetric and gynecologic infections, complicated urinary tract infections, intra-abdominal sepsis, pneumonia, and endocarditis due to *S. aureus*.[19-25] Imipenem has been found to be effective as a single agent in the treatment of febrile neutropenic patients, although the number of patients treated to date has been small.[26] Imipenem has activity against *Nocardia asteroides* in vitro and in a murine model of cerebral infection.[27] Clinical experience is limited.[28]

In cystic fibrosis patients receiving imipenem as a single agent for the treatment of pulmonary exacerbations, a significant number of *P. aeruginosa* isolates resistant to imipenem have been encountered.[29] In addition, the treatment of pneumonia due to *P. aeruginosa* in noncystic fibrosis patients with imipenem as a single agent has had a disappointingly low success rate.[30] These observations suggest that imipenem not be used alone in therapy for serious pseudomonal infections, particularly those involving the respiratory tract.

The use of imipenem is most appropriate in the treatment of infections due to cephalosporin-resistant Enterobacteriaceae, particularly those due to *Citrobacter freundii* and *Enterobacter* spp.; as empiric therapy in the treatment of serious infections in patients previously treated with multiple antibiotics because the likelihood of encountering organisms resistant to more conventional β-lactams is high; possibly as a single agent in the treatment of the febrile, neutropenic patient, although this still is not clearly established; and in the treatment of polymicrobial infections where otherwise multiple-drug regimens of higher cost and potentially more adverse side effects would be necessary. The recommended dose of imipenem for serious infections is 0.5–1 g administered intravenously every 6–8 hours for patients with normal renal function. The pediatric dose is 15–25 mg/kg every 6 hours. Dosage adjustment is required for creatinine clearance below 50 ml/min.

Meropenem

Chemistry. Meropenem's acyl side chain is in a cis position rather than a trans position as seen in penicillin and cephalosporins. However, it has a dimethylcarbanoyl pyrolidiolidyn derivative on position 2 of the ring in contrast to the *N* formidyl group present in imipenem. This makes it stable to dihydropeptidase 1.

Mechanism of Action. Excellent penetration into bacteria, high affinity for PBPs, and stability to β-lactamases account for its activity. Studies with *K. pneumoniae, E. coli* and *Salmonella* spp. using liposomal membranes reconstituted from purified protein porins of outer membranes of *P. aeruginosa* show that meropenem penetrates these gram-negative organisms more readily than does imipenem, accounting for its greater activity against these organisms.[31]

Antibacterial Activity. Meropenem is slightly more active than imipenem against gram-negative organisms. It inhibits *P. aeruginosa* resistant to imipenem by virtue of more rapid entry into these organisms. There is no cross resistance to ceftazidime or other cephalosporins nor with the antipseudomonas ureidopenicillins such as piperacillin. Meropenem shows a PAE against *P. aeruginosa* similar to that of imipenem and LJ 10627, another dihydropeptidase 1 compound previously referred to as CS 533 and referred to now as biapenem; biopenem has completed preregistration studies in Japan. It is also stable to dihydropeptidase 1.

Resistance. Similar to imipenem, meropenem is hydrolyzed, albeit slowly, by β-lactamases such as the zinc-dependent β-lactamase that exists in *X. maltophila*. It also does not bind to PBPs of *E. faecium*, which utilizes PBP5 and 6 to make cell wall. Because it is more rapidly transported through the D2 porin of gram-negative organisms than is imipenem, resistance due to permeability is uncommon.

Pharmacology. Meropenem is a dimethylcarbamoyl pyrolidinyl derivative of thienamycin (Fig. 2). Its spectrum of antibacterial activity is very similar to that of imipenem (Table 1), with potent activity against a variety of gram-positive species, gram-negative aerobes, and anaerobic species. It is slightly less active than imipenem against gram-positive bacteria, but more active

against gram-negative organisms, including some imipenem-resistant strains of *Pseudomonas aeruginosa*.[2,3]

Meropenem, unlike imipenem, is not significantly degraded by renal tubular dehydropeptidase-1 and therefore it does not require coadministration of an inhibitor, such as cilistatin. Its pharmacology is otherwise very similar to that of imipenem. The mean peak serum concentration with intravenous administration of a single 500 mg dose over 30 minutes is approximately 30 µg/ml in healthy individuals and 50 µg/ml in those with end-stage renal disease, and half-lives are 1 hour and 10 hours, respectively. Clearance is linerally proportional to glomerular filtration rate.[32] Metabolites may have markedly prolonged half-lives, up to 35 hours. Meropenem is removed by hemodialysis and should be administered after each dialysis session. It penetrates inflamed meninges, into bile, bone, synovial fluid, and most tissues. Cerebrospinal fluid concentrations are approximately 1–5 µg/ml.[33]

The toxicity profile of meropenem is similar to that of imipenem except that data from animals suggest that meropenem may be less epileptitogenic and less nephrotoxic. The relative lack of nephrotoxicity is due to its lack of susceptibility to degradation by renal peptidases.

Clinical experience with meropenem is limited. Because of its similarity to imipenem, it would be expected to be therapeutically equivalent and to have similar indications for use. Meropenem has been shown to be effective in several animal models.[34] It has been used successfully to treat pneumonia, meningitis, intra-abdominal infections, bacteremia, urinary tract infections, and febrile episodes in neutropenic patients.[35,36] Single-drug therapy of serious *Pseudomonas aeruginosa* infections has been accompanied by emergence of resistance to meropenem, and combination therapy should be used if possible.[37] The recommended adult dose for patients with a creatinine clearance greater than 50 ml/min is 500–1000 mg IV every 6–8 hours. The pediatric dose is 10 to 20 mg/kg every 6 to 8 hours.

MONOBACTAMS

The development of new methods by Sykes and colleagues[38] to screen large numbers of organisms for the production of β-lactam antibiotics showed that a number of bacteria, par-ticularly *Gluconobacter* and *Acinetobacter,* produced mono-cyclic β-lactam antibiotics with antibacterial activity. From *Chromobacterium violaceum* a monocyclic compound was isolated and the structure confirmed. This compound was sub-sequently modified to yield a highly active therapeutic agent, aztreonam.

AZTREONAM

Aztreonam is a monocyclic β-lactam (Fig. 3). Aztreonam has no appreciable antibacterial activity against gram-positive or anaerobic bacteria. This is because it does not bind to PBPs in these species. Aztreonam binds primarily to PBP 3 in Enterobacteriaceae, *Pseudomonas,* and other gram-negative aerobic organisms. It produces long filamentous structures that are not viable. Aztreonam readily passes through the outer membrane of gram-negative species. It is not hydrolyzed by most plasmid and chromosomal β-lactamases but is hydrolyzed by *K. oxytoca* and *Pseudomonas cepacia* and by the cefotaxime-hydrolyzing plasmid enzymes.

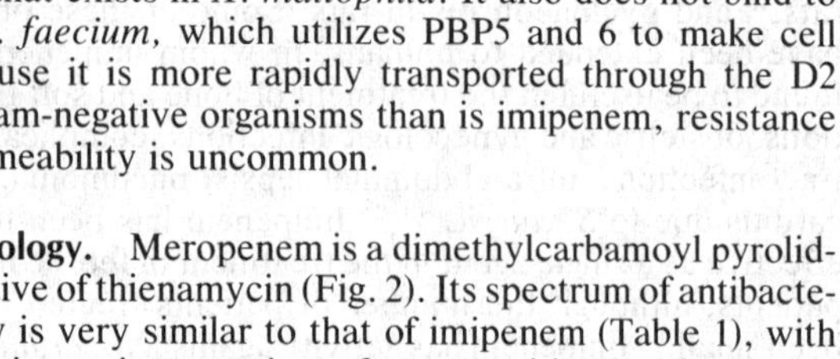

FIG. 2. Meropenem.

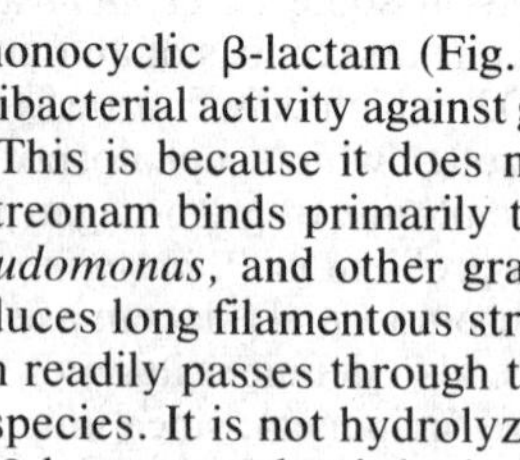

FIG. 3. Aztreonam.

TABLE 2. In Vitro Activity of Aztreonam

Organism	MIC$_{90}$ (μg/ml)
Escherichia coli	0.25
Klebsiella pneumoniae	1
K. oxytoca	1
Enterobacter cloacae	16
E. aerogenes	8
E. agglomerans	1
Citrobacter freundii	8
C. diversus	0.25
Serratia marcescens	4
Proteus mirabilis	0.01
P. vulgaris	0.12
P. rettgeri	0.12
Morganella morganii	0.25
Providencia	0.025
Salmonella enteritidis	0.25
Shigella	0.12
Arizona hinshawii	0.12
Aeromonas hydrophila	0.12
A. shigelloides	0.12
Yersinia enterocolitica	2
Pasteurella multocida	0.12
Salmonella typhi	0.12
Haemophilus influenzae	0.12
Neisseria gonorrhoeae	0.25
N. meningitidis	0.025
Pseudomonas aeruginosa	16
P. maltophilia	>128
Pseudomonas, other (*P. cepacia, P. diminuta, P. stutzeri, P. fluorescens*)	>128
S. pyogenes	16
S. pneumoniae	16
Enterococci	>128
Clostridium	>128
Bacteroides spp.	>128

Antibacterial Activity

Aztreonam inhibits most Enterobacteriaceae at concentrations below 0.5 μg/ml (Table 2); some *P. aeruginosa, E. cloacae,* and *C. freundii* strains are resistant. Most *P. aeruginosa* organisms are inhibited by less than 16 μg/ml. Most *P. cepacia* and *X. maltophilia* are resistant, as are many *Acinetobacter* spp.; *Haemophilus* and *Neisseria,* including β-lactamase–producing isolates, are inhibited by less than 0.2 μg/ml. *Yersinia* and *Aeromonas* are inhibited by less than 0.5 μg/ml. In general, the antibacterial activity is minimally affected by inoculum size except for *P. aeruginosa,* and there is no major difference between MIC and minimum bactericidal concentration (MBC) values.[39–41] Aztreonam acts synergistically with aminoglycosides against *P. aeruginosa* and some Enterobacteriaceae. Enterobacteriaceae and *P. aeruginosa* can be resistant due to a failure to penetrate the outer membrane, destruction by β-lactamases (i.e., *X. maltophilia*), and a failure to bind to PBPs.

Pharmacokinetics

Aztreonam is not absorbed from the gastrointestinal tract.[42] It is rapidly and completely absorbed after IM administration, with peak serum concentrations attained within 1 hour.[43–46] A 500 mg IM aztreonam dose produces serum concentrations of 21–27 μg/ml at 1 hour, 3.8–5.9 μg/ml at 6 hours, and 1.5–3.3 μg/ml at 8 hours. After IV infusion of a single 0.5, 1, or 2 g dose of aztreonam in healthy adults over a period of 30 minutes, peak serum concentrations of the drug immediately after completion of the infusion average 55–65, 90–160, or 200–255 μg/ml, respectively. Aztreonam serum concentrations 1 hour after an IM dose are the same as after an IV dose.

Aztreonam is widely distributed into body tissues and fluids.[43] Therapeutic levels are present in adipose tissue, bone, gallbladder, liver, lungs, kidney, heart, intestinal tissue, and prostatic tissue. It is also present in saliva, sputum, bronchial secretions, bile, and pericardial, pleural, peritoneal, and synovial fluids.

Aztreonam enters the CSF after IV administration, with CSF concentrations at 1 and 4 hours after a 2 g dose of 2 and 3.2 μg/ml, respectively.[47] In neonates and children 3 months to 2 years of age with bacterial meningitis who received a 30 mg/kg dose of aztreonam by IV injection over a period of 3 minutes, CSF aztreonam concentrations ranged from 2.1 to 20.8 μg/ml at 0.8–4.3 hours after the dose.[48]

Aztreonam is primarily removed from the body by renal mechanisms of both glomerular filtration and tubular secretion. No active metabolites have been found in serum or urine. In adults with normal renal and hepatic function, the distribution half-life of aztreonam averages 0.2–0.7 hours, and the elimination half-life averages 1.3–2.2 hours. The half-life of aztreonam averages 1.7 hours in children 2 months to 12 years of age.[48] In neonates 7 days old, the half-life of aztreonam averages 5.5–9.9 hours in neonates weighing less than 2.5 kg.[48]

Serum concentrations of aztreonam are higher and the serum half-life prolonged in patients with renal impairment.[48,49] In adults with renal impairment, the half-life of aztreonam averages 3.5, 5.6, 7.8, and 8.5 hours in adults with creatinine clearances of 30–80, 10–30, 10 or less, and 2 ml/min, respectively. The half-life of aztreonam is only slightly prolonged in patients with hepatic impairment.

Aztreonam is excreted as unchanged drug by both glomeruler filtration and tubular secretion. Approximately 58–74 percent of the dose is excreted unchanged and 1–7 percent as open ring metabolites.[43] In adults with normal renal function, urinary concentrations of aztreonam after a single 0.5 or 1 g IV dose average 250–330 and 710–720 μg/ml, respectively, 4–6 hours after the dose.[46]

Aztreonam and its renal metabolite are removed by hemodialysis.[49,50] The serum half-life of aztreonam averages 2.7 hours during hemodialysis and 6–8 hours between dialysis sessions. A 4-hour period of hemodialysis removes 25–50 percent of a dose. Aztreonam is removed to a lesser extent by peritoneal dialysis. With a 6-hour dwell time, about 10 percent of a single 1 g IV dose of aztreonam is removed.[51]

Adverse Reactions

No major adverse reactions to aztreonam have been reported.[52] Skin rashes have occurred. Neither anaphylaxis nor rashes have followed its use in patients with positive skin test reactions to penicillins (see Ch. 18). About 2–4 percent of patients will have increases in serum transaminase values two times above normal when receiving aztreonam. No hematologic, gastrointestinal, nephrotoxic, or neurotoxic reactions have been noted with this agent.

Clinical Use

Aztreonam has been used for the treatment of a variety of infections such as cystitis, pyelonephritis, lower respiratory tract infections including pneumonia and bronchitis, septicemia, skin and skin structure infections, infections of postoperative wounds or ulcers and burns, intra-abdominal infection including peritonitis, and gynecologic infections including endometritis and pelvic cellulitis due to gram-negative aerobic bacteria.[52–62] Because of its lack of cross-reactivity with other β-lactam antibiotics, aztreonam can be safely used in patients with serious allergy to penicillins or cephalosporins. The usual dose is 1–2 g q6–8h IV or IM with a daily dose for serious infection of 6 g. The drug is not approved for pediatric use but has been given 18.75–37.5 mg/kg q6h IV or IM.

Because aztreonam has a spectrum of activity limited to aerobic gram-negative bacteria, the drug should not be used singly for empiric therapy in seriously ill patients if there is any possibility that the infection may be caused by gram-positive aerobic bacteria or if a mixed aerobic-anaerobic bacterial infection is suspected. An anti-infective agent effective against the suspected organism(s) should be used concomitantly. Aztreonam has been used safely and effectively in conjunction with clinda-mycin, erythromycin, metronidazole, penicillins, and vanco-mycin.

β-LACTAMASE INHIBITORS

β-Lactamase inhibitors are clavulanic acid and penicillanic acid sulfone derivatives. These compounds, which have weak anti-bacterial activity, are potent inhibitors of many plasmid-encoded and some chromosomal β-lactamases. Thus, these com-pounds can restore antibacterial activity of amoxicillin, ampicil-lin, piperacillin, mezlocillin, and cefoperazone, all of which can be destroyed by β-lactamases commonly produced by gram-positive and gram-negative bacteria (Table 3). Al-though competitive inhibition is seen, β-lactamase inhibitor pri-marily acts as a suicide substrate that forms a stable acyl-enzyme intermediate, that renders the enzyme inactive.

Three β-lactamase inhibitors are in clinical use: clavulanic acid, sulbactam, and tazobactam. Each inhibitor is available only as a fixed combination preparation that includes an active β-lactam antibiotic as the companion agent. There are minor differences in potency, activity, and pharmacology among the β-lactamase inhibitors, but clinically they can be considered therapeutically equivalent except for some *Klebsiella* spp. where clavulanate inhibits isolates resistant to sulbactam and tazobactam. The antibacterial activity of inhibitor-antibiotic combination is determined by the spectrum of the companion β-lactam antibiotic.

β-Lactamase inhibitors are most effective against β-lacta-mases produced by *S. aureus, H. influenzae, B. catarrhalis, Bacteroides* spp., and some Enterobacteriaceae. *Serratia* spp., *Citrobacter freundii, Enterobacter* spp., *P. aeruginosa*, and some Enterobacteriaceae produce chromosomal β-lactamases that are inhibited poorly by β-lactamase inhibitors.

β-Lactamase inhibitors are most active against plasmid-encoded β-lactamases. The most common is TEM-1, so-called for the initials of the original patient from whom the *E. coli* β-lactamase containing isolate was derived. There are also TEM-2; oxacillin-hydrolyzing enzymes OXA-1, -2, and -3; sulfhydro-inhibited enzymes SHV-1 and HMS; and PSE-1, PSE-2, PSE-3, and PSE-4, originally thought to be enzymes found only in *Pseudomonas* but now found occasionally in *E. coli*. All of these plasmid enzymes are inhibited, as are the new cefotaxime–cef-tazidime hydrolyzing enzymes TEM-3, -4, -5, -6, -7, up to 27; and SHV-2, -3, -4, and -5, -7, -8 (Table 4).

Inhibition of chromosomal β-lactamases by β-lactamase in-hibitors is variable. The most important chromosomal β-lacta-mases, which generally fall into the Richmond-Sykes class I type of chromosomal β-lactamases (see Fig. 2 in Ch. 15) are present in *Acinetobacter, Citrobacter, Enterobacter, Proteus,*

TABLE 3. Activity of Amoxicillin–Clavulanate against Amoxicillin-Resistant Organisms

Organism	Amoxicillin	Augmentin[a]
Staphylococcus aureus	256	1.0
Staphylococcus epidermidis	256	2.0
Staphylococcus aureus (MRSA)	256	16.0
Haemophilus influenzae	64	0.5
Branhamella catarrhalis	16	0.25
Neisseria gonorrhoeae	128	1.0
Escherichia coli	>256	8.0
Klebsiella pneumoniae	128	4.0
Proteus mirabilis	>256	4.0
Proteus vulgaris	>256	2.0
Bacteroides fragilis	32	0.5
Enterobacter, Citrobacter, Serratia spp. and *Pseudomonas aeruginosa*	>128	>128

[a] Contains amoxicillin and clavulanate in a 2:1 ratio.

TABLE 4. Inhibition of β-Lactamases by β-Lactam Inhibitors

β-Lactamase	Name	Organisms	Inhibited by Clavulanate, Sulbactam, and Tazobactam
Plasmid		*S. aureus*	Yes
Plasmid	TEM-1	*E. coli*	Yes
		Haemophilus	
		N. gonorrhoeae	
		Salmonella	
		Shigella	
Plasmid	TEM-2	*E. coli*	Yes
Plasmid	TEM-3 to -8	*Klebsiella*	Yes
Plasmid	SHV-1	*Klebsiella*	Yes
Plasmid	SHV-2 to -5	Enterobacteriaceae	Yes
Plasmid	OXA-1, 2, 3	*E. coli*	Variable
Plasmid	PSE-1, 2, 3	*Pseudomonas*	Variable
Chromosomal	Type 1a[a]	*Enterobacter*	No
		Morganella	
		Citrobacter	
		Serratia	
Chromosomal	Type Id[a]	*Pseudomonas*	No
Chromosomal	Type IV, K1[a]	*Klebsiella*	Yes
Chromosomal		*Bacteroides*	Yes
Chromosomal		*Legionella*	Yes
Chromosomal		*Branhamella*	Yes

[a] Richmond and Sykes[63] classification.

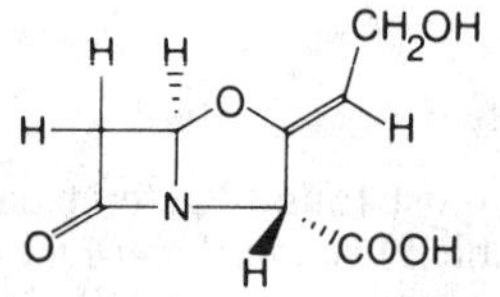

FIG. 4. Clavulanate.

Pseudomonas, and *Serratia*.[63] These are inducible enzymes that are not inhibited by β-lactamase inhibitors except at very high concentrations, which are only possible in test tube conditions. β-Lactamases are produced constitutively by some *Enterobac-ter, Citrobacter freundii*, and *Aeromonas* spp., and these are not inhibited. However, chromosomal β-lactamases of *Legio-nella* and *Bacteroides* are inhibited by β-lactamase inhibitors, as are some other chromosomally mediated β-lactamases, such as the class IV enzymes produced by *Klebsiella*.[64–67]

Clavulanate

The β-lactamase inhibitor clavulanate (Fig. 4) was found in cul-tures of *Streptomyces clavuligerus*. It showed only a low level of antibacterial action, but, when the compound was combined with penicillin G, inhibition of a *Klebsiella* isolate normally re-sistant to penicillin was noted. Clavulanate has subsequently been shown to inhibit certain types of β-lactamases from a num-ber of clinically important gram-positive and gram-negative or-ganisms.[68,69] Clavulanate in combination with amoxicillin is available for oral administration, and a parenteral preparation is available in many countries, but not the United States. Clavu-lanate in combination with ticarcillin is available for intravenous administration in the United States.

Pharmacology. Clavulanate is moderately well absorbed from the gastrointestinal tract, with peak serum levels occurring 40–120 minutes after ingestion. Mean peak serum levels for 62.5 mg are 1 μg/ml; for 125 mg, 4 μg/ml; and for 250 mg, 6 μg/ml.[70,71] Combining clavulanate with amoxicillin does not signifi-cantly alter the pharmacologic parameters of either drug. The pharmacokinetics of orally administered clavulanate in children in terms of peak serum levels and plasma half-lives of the drug are similar to those in adults.[72,73]

The absorption of clavulanate is unaffected by the simultaneous administration of food, milk, or aluminum hydroxide-containing antacids. After IV infusion of clavulanate combined with either amoxicillin or ticarcillin, the drug is rapidly distributed. Peak serum concentrations are approximately 11 μg/ml after a 200 mg IV dose, with drug detectable to levels of 0.2 μg/ml at 6 hours.[74,75] Peak serum concentrations of clavulanate in children receiving 5 mg/kg have been 19 μg/ml with less than 1 μg/ml present at 3 hours.[73]

The serum half-life of clavulanate is slightly less than that of amoxicillin, 0.76–1.4 hours. No accumulation of clavulanate occurs until creatinine clearances fall below 10 ml/min.[70] Dose adjustment is made by adjustment for amoxicillin or ticarcillin. Clavulanate has been shown to be degraded in vivo in animals, with metabolites being excreted via lung, feces, and urine and only 20–60 percent appearing unchanged in urine 6 hours after an oral dose. After a dose of 125 mg of clavulanate, urine levels are 115–508 μg/ml for 0–2 hours and 45–74 μg/ml for 4–6 hours.[76]

Concentrations less than 1 μg/ml of clavulanate are achieved in sputum after the oral administration of amoxicillin-clavulanate, but pleural fluid levels are 46–91 percent of peak serum levels. There is rapid penetration of clavulanate into peritoneal fluid, with mean peritoneal fluid levels of clavulanate 66 percent of serum levels.[74,77] After 200 mg of clavulanate, peritoneal fluid levels fall below 5 μg/ml after about 0.5 hours and below 1 μg/ml after about 3 hours. Clavulanate does not penetrate noninflamed meninges, but after large IV doses in patients with meningitis CSF levels of clavulanate have been in the range of 1 μg/ml. Clavulanate produces therapeutic levels in bile, middle ear fluid, and tonsil tissue.[77] Clavulanate crosses the placenta and may be found in the cord blood of newborns and in the amniotic fluid, but no clavulanate can be detected in breast milk.

Adverse Reactions. No new or major adverse reactions to the use of clavulanate combined with either amoxicillin or ticarcillin have been reported. The incidence of skin reactions has been similar to that with penicillin used alone. Diarrhea has followed the use of 250 mg clavulanate given three times daily, and some nausea has occurred with this dose program. Parenteral use of amoxicillin-clavulanate and ticarcillin–clavulanate has not caused undue diarrhea.

Amoxicillin-Clavulanate

Amoxicillin-clavulanate (Augmentin) has been used in a number of different clinical settings. The combination has proved useful as therapy for acute otitis media in children that is caused by β-lactamase–producing *Haemophilus influenzae* and *Branhamella catarrhalis*.[78] It has also been used to treat sinusitis and, rarely, pharyngitis in individuals whose large tonsillar tissue contains β-lactamase-producing *Prevotella melaninogenica* (*Bacteroides melaninogenicus*).[78] Amoxicillin-clavulanate has proved useful in lower respiratory tract infections such as exacerbations of bacterial bronchitis or pneumonitis due to β-lactamase-producing bacteria. It has proved particularly useful to treat bite wounds of human or animal origin. Skin structure infections due to streptococci and staphylococci have responded to amoxicillin-clavulanate with results comparable to oral antistaphylococcal agents and oral cephalosporins.[79] Amoxicillin-clavulanate has been used to treat diabetic foot infections since it has activity against staphylococci, anaerobes, and aerobic gram-negative bacteria. The agent is formulated as 250–500 mg of amoxicillin to 125 mg of clavulanate, and dosing is as for the amoxicillin component. The usual dose is 0.25–0.50 g (of amoxicillin) q8h by mouth. In children the dose is 6.6–13.3 mg/kg q8h by mouth.

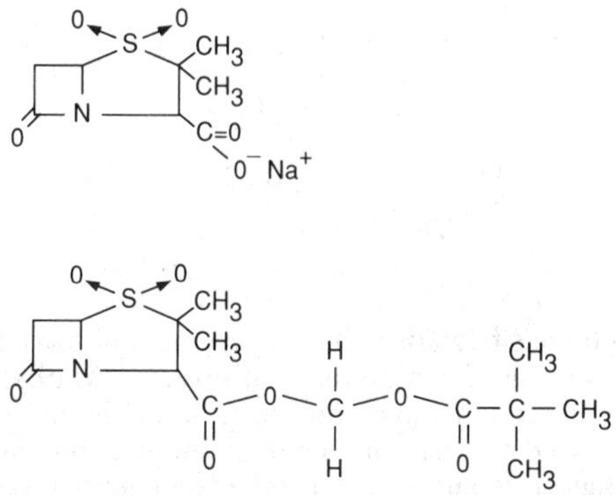

FIG. 5. Sulbactam (top) and sulbactam oral ester (bottom).

Ticarcillin-Clavulanate

Ticarcillin-clavulanate has been used as treatment of community- and hospital-acquired pneumonia, particularly where there has been aspiration of oral secretions and aerobic gram-negative bacilli.[80] Intra-abdominal infections and gynecologic infections have been treated successfully, as have skin structure infections and osteomyelitis.[81,82] When ticarcillin–clavulanate has been used to treat febrile neutropenic patients, it has been necessary to combine it with an aminoglycoside. The usual doses are 3.1 g administered every 4–6 hours. The dose should be reduced in patients with creatinine clearance of less than 30 ml/min (see Ch. 35).

Sulbactam

Sulbactam (Fig. 5) is a 6-desaminopenicillin sulfone. Sulbactam is a broader spectrum β-lactamase-inhibitor than clavulanic acid, but less potent. Sulbactam does not induce chromosomal β-lactamases, nor does it select for derepressed β-lactamase-producing bacteria. Sulbactam is available in the United States only in combination with ampicillin (Unasyn) in a ratio of 0.5 g of sulbactam per 1 g of ampicillin as a parenteral formulation primarily for intravenous administration.

Pharmacology. Sulbactam has pharmacokinetics in humans similar to those of ampicillin.[83,84] Peak serum levels after im injections of 0.250 and 0.5 g are 7 and 13 μg/ml, respectively, with a serum half-life of 1.1–1.3 hours. After the IV infusion of 0.5 g, peak serum levels of 30 μg/ml are achieved, and after 1 g, 68 μg/ml are achieved. The serum half-life is 1 hour. Sulbactam is excreted by the kidney and has a urinary recovery rate of 70–80 percent of a dose. Biliary excretion is minimal, and metabolism is less than 25 percent. Renal excretion is blocked by probenecid. The half-life is not significantly altered until creatinine clearance falls below 30 ml/min. With clearances between 15 and 30, the half-life is 5.1 hours; with clearances of 5–15, the half-life is 9.2 hours, and the half-life of anuric patients is 20 hours. It can be removed by hemodialysis. Concentrations of sulbactam in interstitial fluid and peritoneal secretions are comparable to levels in serum. Penetration of sulbactam into inflamed meninges is low, with levels of 0.1–10 μg/ml found in the CSF after a 1 g infusion.

Adverse Reactions. The clinical studies of the combination of sulbactam plus ampicillin have reported no major hematologic, renal, hepatic, or central nervous system reactions.[85–87] Diarrhea has not been a major problem after IV use. Skin reactions are similar to those found for ampicillin, and there is occasional elevation of transaminase levels.

Clinical Use. Sulbactam–ampicillin and amoxicillin–clavulanate have the same spectrum of antibacterial activity. Sulbact-

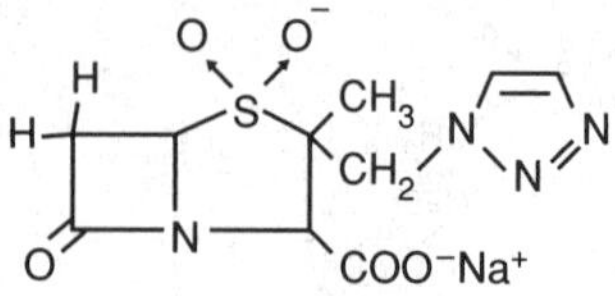

FIG. 6.   Tazobactam.

am-ampicillin has been used in the treatment of mixed bacterial infections such as intra-abdominal infections, obstetric and gynecologic infections, and soft tissue and bone infections.[88,89] It has been used to treat meningitis in infants and children and to treat epiglottitis and selected other pediatric infections.[90,91] However, the pediatric experience is limited, and it would seem that third-generation cephalosporins would be preferred in such infections.

Tazobactam

Tazobactam is a penicillanic acid sulfone β-lactamase inhibitor with a structure similar to that of sulbactam (Fig. 6). Its spectrum of β-lactamase inhibition is like that of sulbactam, but its potency is more like that of clavulanic acid. It does not induce chromosomal β-lactamases.[92–94] It is available for parenteral administration only in combination with piperacillin (Zosyn) in an 8:1 ratio of piperacillin to tazobactam by weight.

Pharmacology.   Mean peak serum concentration after a 30-minute IV infusion of 500 mg of tazobactam is 25 μg/ml in healthy subjects.[95] The clearance of tazobactam is primarily renal, and dosage should be adjusted for creatinine clearances less than 40 ml/min. Combining tazobactam with piperacillin reduces clearance of tazobactam, but the clearance of piperacillin is not affected. Clearance of piperacillin and tazobactam are similar in subjects with normal renal function. Peak serum concentrations are approximately 50 percent higher in those with end-stage renal disease.[95] The half-life of tazobactam is 1 hour in subjects with normal renal function, increasing to 3.6 hours (vs. 2 hours for piperacillin) in those with a creatinine clearance less than 20 ml/min. The half-life of tazobactam is approximately 7 hours in patients with end-stage renal disease. Hemodialysis removes 31 and 39 percent of the administered dose of piperacillin and tazobactam, respectively. These differences in pharmacokinetics of piperacillin and tazobactam do not require adjusting the dose of tazobactam independent of piperacillin. The dose is adjusted based on the pharmacokinetics of piperacillin. Patients undergoing hemodialysis should have the dose of piperacillin-tazobactam administered after dialysis. Negligible amounts of either drug are removed by peritoneal dialysis.

Tissue levels of tazobactam reflect a percent penetration that is similar to that of piperacillin for each tissue type.[96] Tazobactam penetrates inflamed meninges. CSF concentrations of piperacillin and tazobactam were 16 and 32 percent of simultaneous serum concentrations, respectively, in a rabbit menegitis model.[97]

Adverse Reactions.   Limited clinical data do not indicate any new or unusual toxicity unique to tazobactam.

Clinical Use.   Published clinical studies with the piperacillin-tazobactam combination are limited and have been conducted mainly in adults. The indications for use of this combination in the treatment of pediatric infections have not been defined, and other agents would be preferred. The combination of piperacillin-tazobactam is equivalent in vitro to the combination of ticarcillin-clavulanate for most organisms. Slightly greater activity with the pipercillin-tazobactam combination vs. ticarcillin-clavulanate has been observed for some strains, presumably due to the greater intrinsic activity of piperacillin.[92,94] Thus, the types of infections that have been successfully treated with ticarcillin-clavulanate would also be expected to respond to therapy with piperacillin-tazobactam. Piperacillin-tazobactam has been effective in the treatment of intra-abdominal infections, skin and soft tissue infections, pneumonia, and febrile episodes in neutropenic patients.[98–103] The adult dose is 12–16 g/day of piperacillin (with 1.5–2 g/day of tazobactam) administered in divided doses every 6–8 hours for creatinine clearance greater than 40 ml/min.

REFERENCES

1. Kahan JS, Kahan FM, Goegleman R, et al. Thienamycin, a new beta-lactam antibiotic. 1. Discovery, isolation and physical properties. J Antibiot. 1979; 32:1–12.
2. Edwards JR, Turner PJ, Wannop C, et al. In vitro antibacterial activity of SM-7338, a carbapenem anatibiotic with stability to dehydropeptidase I. Antimicrob Agents Chemother. 1989;33:215–222.
3. Sentochnik DE, Eliopoulos GM, Ferraro MJ, et al. Comparative in vitro activity of SM7338, a new carbapenem antimicrobial agent. Antimicrob Agents Chemother. 1989;33:1232–1236.
4. Jones RN. Review of the in vitro spectrum of activity of imipenem. Am J Med. 1985;78:22–32.
5. Prince AS, Neu HC. Activities of new beta-lactam antibiotics against isolates of *Pseudomonas aeruginosa* from patients with cystic fibrosis. Antimicrob Agents Chemother. 1981;20:545–546.
6. Brown JE, Del Benes VE, Collins CD. In vitro activity of *N*-formimidoyl thienamycin, moxalactam and other new beta-lactam agents against *Bacteroides fragilis:* Contribution of beta-lactamase to resistance. Antimicrob Agents Chemother. 1981;19:248–252.
7. Kesado T, Hashizume T, Ashi Y, et al. Susceptibilities of anaerobic bacteria to *N*-formimidoyl thienamycin (MK0787) and to other antibiotics. Antimicrob Agents Chemother. 1982;21:1016–1022.
8. Norrby SR, Alestig K, Bjauorngard B, et al. Urinary recovery of *N*-formimidoyl thienamycin (MK0787) as affected by coadministration of *N*-formimidoyl thienamycin dehydropeptidase inhibitors. Antimicrob Agents Chemother. 1983;23:300–307.
9. Norrby SR, Alestig K, Ferber F, et al. Pharmacokinetics and tolerance of *N*-formimidoyl thienamycin (MK0787) in humans. Antimicrob Agents Chemother. 1983;23:293–299.
10. Drusano GL, Standiford HC, Ruslamante C, et al. Multiple dose kinetics of imipenem/cilastatin. Antimicrob Agents Chemother. 1984;26:715–721.
11. Drusano GL, Standiford HC. Pharmacokinetic profile of imipenem/cilastatin in normal volunteers. Am J Med. 1985;78:47–53.
12. Berman SJ, Sugihara JG, Nakumara JM, et al. Multiple dose study of imipenem/cilastatin in patients with end-stage renal disease undergoing long-term hemodialysis. Am J Med. 1985;78:105–108.
13. Norrby SR, Rogers JD, Ferber F, et al. Disposition of radio labeled imipenem and cilastatin in normal human volunteers. Antimicrob Agents Chemother. 1985;26:707–714.
14. Calandra GB, Ricci FM, Wang C, et al. Safety and tolerance comparison of imipenem-cilastatin to cephalothin and cefazolin. J Antimicrob Chemother. 1983;12(Suppl D):125–131.
15. Sadon A, Gilden BN, Rohr AS, et al. Immediate hypersensitivity reactions to beta-lactam antibiotics. Ann Intern Med. 1987;127:204–215.
16. Baumgardner JD, Galuser MP. Comparative imipenem treatment of *Staphylococcus aureus* endocarditis in the rat. J Antimicrob Chemother. 1983; 12(Suppl D):79–87.
17. Scheld WM, Keely J. Imipenem therapy of experimental *Staphylococcus aureus* and *Streptococcus faecalis* endocarditis. J Antimicrob Chemother. 1983;12(Suppl D):69–78.
18. Johnson De, Calia IM, Snyder MJ, et al. Imipenem therapy of *Pseudomonas aeruginosa* bacteremia in neutropenic rats. J Antimicrob Chemother. 1983; 12(Suppl D):89–96.
19. MacGregor RR, Gentry LO. Imipenem/cilastatin in the treatment of osteomyelitis. Am J Med. 1985;78:92–95.
20. Marier RL. Role of imipenem in the treatment of soft tissue infections. Am J Med. 1985;78:132–136.
21. Berkeley AS, Freedman K, Hirsch J, et al. Imipenem/cilastatin in the treatment of obstetric and gynecologic infections. Am J Med. 1985;78:71–76.
22. Cox CE, Corrado ML. Safety and efficacy of imipenem/cilastatin in treatment of complicated urinary tract infections. Am J Med. 1985;78:84–91.
23. Kager L, Nord CE. Imipenem/cilastatin in the treatment of intraabdominal infections: A review of worldwide experience. Rev Infect Dis. 1985;7(Suppl 3):518–521.
24. Salata RA, Gebhart RC, Palmer DL, et al. Pneumonia treated with imipenem/cilastatin. Am J Med. 1985;78:96–101.
25. Dickson G, Rodriguez K, Arcey S, et al. Efficacy of imipenem/cilastatin in endocarditis. Am J Med. 1985;78:109–118.
26. Bodey GP, Alvarez ME, Jones PG, et al. Imipenem/cilastatin as initial therapy for febrile cancer patients. Antimicrob Agents Chemother. 1986;30: 211–214.
27. Gombert ME, Aulicino TM, duBouchet L, et al. Therapy of experimental cerebral nocardiosis with imipenum, amikacin, trimethoprim-sulfamethoxazole, and minocycline. Antimicrob Agents Chemother. 1986;30:270–3.
28. Ertl G, Schall K, Kochsiek K. Nocardial endocarditis of an aortic valve prosthesis. Br Heart J. 1987;57:384–6.

29. Krilov LR, Blumer JL, Stern RC, et al. Imipenem/cilastatin in acute pulmonary exacerbations of cystic fibrosis. Rev Infect Dis. 1985;7(Suppl 3): 482–489.

30. Acar JF. Therapy for lower respiratory tract infections with imipenem/cilastatin: A review of worldwide experience. Rev Infect Dis. 1985;7:S513–S517.

31. Satake S, Yoshihara E, Nakae T. Diffusion of beta-lactam antibiotics through liposome membranes reconstituted from purified outer membranes of *Pseudomonas aeruginosa*. Antimicrob Agents Chemother. 1990;34:685–90.

32. Leroy A, Fillastre JP, Borsa-Lebas F, et al. Pharmacokinetics of meropenem (ICI 194,660) and its metabolite (ICI 213,689) in healthy subjects and in patients with renal impairment. Antimicrob Agents Chemother. 1992;36: 2794–2798.

33. Fujii R, Yoshioka H, Fujita K, et al. Pharmacokinetic and clinical studies in the pediatric field. Pediatric study group of meropenem. Jpn J Antibiotics. 1992;45:697–717.

34. Edwards JR, Williams S, Nairn K. Therapeutic activity of meropenem in experimental infections. J Antimicrob Agents 1989;24(Suppl A):279–285.

35. Sugiyama H, Horiuchi A, Hasegawa H, et al. Therapeutic effects of meropenem against severe infections in patients with hematopoietic disorders. Hanshin Study Group of Hematopoietic Disorders and Infection. Jpn J Antibiotics. 1992;45:687–696.

36. Kanellakopoulou K, Giamarellou H, Papadothomakos P, et al. Meropenem versus imipenem/cilastatin in the treatment of intraabdominal infections requiring surgery. Eur J Clin Microbiol Infect Dis. 1993;12:449–453.

37. Margaret BS, Drusano GL, Standiford HC. Emergence of resistance to carbapenem antibiotics in *Pseudomonas aeruginosa*. J Antimicrob Chemother 1989;24(Suppl A):161–167.

38. Sykes RB, Cimarausti CM, Bonner DP, et al. Monocyclic beta-lactam antibiotics produced by bacteria. Nature. 1981;291:489–491.

39. Neu HC, Labthavikul P. Antibacterial activity of a monocyclic beta-lactam SQ 26,776. J Antimicrob Chemother. 1981;9(Suppl E):111–112.

40. Barry AL, Thornsberry C, Jones RN, et al. Aztreonam: Antibacterial activity, beta-lactamase stability, and interpretive standards and quality control guidelines for disk-diffusion susceptibility tests. Rev Infect Dis. 1985;7(Suppl 4):594–604.

41. Sykes RB, Bonner DP, Bush K, et al. Aztreonam (SQ 26,776), a synthetic monobactam specifically active against aerobic gram-negative bacteria. Antimicrob Agents Chemother. 1982;21:85–92.

42. Swabb EA, Sugerman AA, Stern M. Oral bioavailability of the monobactam aztreonam (SQ 26,776) in healthy subjects. Antimicrob Agents Chemother. 1983;23:548–550.

43. Swabb EA. Review of the clinical pharmacology of the monobactam antibiotic aztreonam. Am J Med. 1985;78(Suppl 2A):11–18.

44. Jones PG, Bodey GP, Swabb EA, et al. Clinical pharmacokinetics of aztreonam in cancer patients. Antimicrob Agents Chemother. 1984;26:455–461.

45. Janicke DM, Cafarell RF, Parker SW, et al. Pharmacokinetics of aztreonam in patients with gram-negative infections. Antimicrob Agents Chemother. 1985;27:16–20.

46. Scully BE, Swabb EA, Neu HC. Pharmacology of aztreonam after intravenous infusion. Antimicrob Agents Chemother. 1983;24:18–22.

47. Duma RJ, Berry AJ, Smith SM, et al. Penetration of aztreonam into cerebrospinal fluid of patients with and without inflamed meninges. Antimicrob Agents Chemother. 1984;26:730–733.

48. Stutman HR, Marks MI, Swabb EA. Single-dose pharmacokinetics of aztreonam in pediatric patients. Antimicrob Agents Chemother. 1984;26:196–199.

49. Fillastre JP, Leroy A, Baudoin C, et al. Pharmacokinetics of aztreonam in patients with chronic renal failure. Clin Pharmacokinet. 1985;10:91–100.

50. Mihindu JC, Scheld WM, Bolton ND, et al. Pharmacokinetics of aztreonam in patients with various degrees of renal dysfunction. Antimicrob Agents Chemother. 1983;24:252–261.

51. Gerig JS, Bolton ND, Swabb EA, et al. Effect of hemodialysis and peritoneal dialysis on aztreonam pharmacokinetics. Kidney Int. 1984;26:308–318.

52. Henry SA, Bendush CB. Aztreonam: Worldwide overview of the treatment of patients with gram-negative infections. Am J Med. 1985;78(Suppl 2A): 57–64.

53. Daikos GK. Clinical experience with aztreonam in four Mediterranean countries. Rev Infect Dis. 1985;7(Suppl 4):831–839.

54. Giamarellou H, Galanakis N, Douzinas E, et al. Evaluation of aztreonam in difficult-to-treat infections with prolonged post-treatment follow-up. Antimicrob Agents Chemother. 1984;26:245–249.

55. Gibbs RS, Blanco JD, Bernstein S. Role of aerobic gram-negative bacilli in endometritis after cesarean section. Rev Infect Dis. 1985;7(Suppl E): 690–695.

56. Rodriguez JR, Ramirez-Ronda CH. Efficacy and safety of aztreonam versus tobramycin for aerobic gram-negative bacilli lower respiratory tract infections. Am J Med. 1985;78(Suppl 2A):42–43.

57. Romero-Vivas J, Rodriguez-Creixems M, Bouza E, et al. Evaluation of aztreonam in the treatment of severe bacterial infections. Antimicrob Agents Chemother. 1985;28:222–226.

58. Scully BE, Henry SA. Clinical experience with aztreonam in the treatment of gram-negative bacteremia. Rev Infect Dis. 1985;7(Suppl 4):789–793.

59. Scully BE, Neu HC. Use of aztreonam in the treatment of serious infections due to multiresistant gram-negative organisms, including *Pseudomonas aeruginosa*. Am J Med. 1985;78:251–261.

60. Scully BE, Ores CN, Prince AS, et al. Treatment of lower respiratory tract infections due to *Pseudomonas aeruginosa* in patients with cystic fibrosis. Rev Infect Dis. 1985;7(Suppl):669–674.

61. Simons WJ, Lee TJ. Aztreonam in the treatment of bone and joint infections caused by gram-negative bacilli. Rev Infect Dis. 1985;7(Suppl 4):783–788.

62. Gudiol F, Pallares R, Ariza X, et al. Comparative clinical evaluation of aztreonam versus aminoglycosides in gram-negative septicaemia. J Antimicrob Chemother. 1986;17:661–671.

63. Richmond MM, Sykes RB. The beta-lactamases of gram-negative bacteria and their possible physiological role. Adv Microb Physiol. 1973;9:31–88.

64. Neu HC. The contribution of beta-lactamases to bacterial resistance and mechanisms to inhibit beta-lactamases. Am J Med. 1986;79(Suppl 5B):2–12.

65. Neu HC. The role of beta-lactamase inhibitors in chemotherapy. In: Tipper PJ, ed. Antibiotic Inhibitors of Bacterial Cell Wall Biosynthesis. Oxford: Pergamon Press; 1987:241–258.

66. Neu HC. Penicillin-binding proteins and beta-lactamases: Their effects on the use of cephalosporins and other new beta-lactams. In: Remington JS, Swartz MN, eds. Current Clinical Topics in Infectious Diseases. New York: McGraw-Hill; 1987:37–83.

67. Bush K: Recent developments in beta-lactamase research and their implications for the future. Rev Infect Dis. 1988;10:681–690.

68. Reading C, Cole M. Clavulanic acid: A beta-lactamase inhibiting beta-lactam from *Streptomyces clavuligerus*. Antimicrob Agents Chemother. 1977;11: 852–857.

69. Neu HC, Fu KP. Clavulanic acid: A beta-lactamase–inhibiting beta-lactamase. Antimicrob Agents Chemother. 1978;14:650–655.

70. Munch P, Luthy R, Blaser J, et al. Human pharmacokinetics and CSF penetration of clavulanic acid. J Antimicrob Chemother. 1981;8:29–37.

71. Adam D, Visser I, Koeppe P. Pharmacokinetics of amoxicillin and clavulanic acid administered alone and in combination. Antimicrob Agents Chemother. 1982;22:353–357.

72. Nelson JD, Kusmiesz H, Shelton S. Pharmacokinetics of potassium clavulanate in combination with amoxicillin in pediatric patients. Antimicrob Agents Chemother. 1982;21:681–682.

73. Schaad UB, Casey PA, Copper DL. Single-dose pharmacokinetics of intravenous clavulanic acid with amoxicillin in pediatric patients. Antimicrob Agents Chemother. 1983;23:252–255.

74. Bennett S, Wise R, Weston D, et al. Pharmacokinetics and tissue penetration of ticarcillin combined with clavulanic acid. Antimicrob Agents Chemother. 1983;23:831–834.

75. Scully BE, Chin NX, Neu HC. Pharmacology of ticarcillin combined with clavulanic acid in humans. Am J Med. 1985;79(Suppl 5B):39–43.

76. Jackson D, Cockburn A, Cooper DL, et al. Clinical pharmacology and safety evaluation of Timentin. Am J Med. 1985;79(Suppl 5B):44–55.

77. Walsted RA, Hellum KB, Thurmann-Nielson E, et al. Pharmacokinetics and tissue penetration of Timentin: A simultaneous study of serum, urine, lymph, suction blister, and subcutaneous treatment fluid. J Antimicrob Chemother. 1986;17(Suppl C):71–80.

78. Kaleida PH, Bluestone DC, Rockette HE, et al. Amoxicillin–clavulanate potassium compared with cefaclor for acute otitis media in infants and children. Pediatr Infect Dis. 1987;6:265–271.

79. Neu HC, ed. Progress and perspectives on beta-lactamase inhibition: A review of Augmentin. Postgrad Med. 1984;3–295.

80. Neu HC, ed. Beta-lactamase inhibition: Therapeutic advances. Am J Med. 1985;79(Suppl 5B):1–196.

81. Gentry LO, Macko V, Lind R, et al. Ticarcillin plus clavulanic acid (Timentin) therapy for osteomyelitis. Am J Med. 1985;79(Suppl 5B):116–121.

82. Leigh DA, Phillips I, Wise R, eds. Timentin–ticarcillin plus clavulanic acid, a laboratory and clinical perspective. J Antimicrob Chemother. 1986; 17(Suppl C):1–244.

83. Foulds G, Stankewich JP, Marshall DC, et al. Pharmacokinetics of sulbactam in humans. Antimicrob Agents Chemother. 1983;23:692–699.

84. Hampel B, Lode H, Bruchnor G, et al. Comparative pharmacokinetics of sulbactam/ampicillin and clavulanic acid/amoxicillin in human volunteers. Drugs. 1988;35(Suppl 7):29–33.

85. Guneren MF. Clinical experience with intramuscular sulbactam/ampicillin in the out-patient treatment of various infections: A multicenter trial. Drugs. 1988;35(Suppl 7):57–68.

86. Dajani AS. Sulbactam/ampicillin in pediatric infections. Drugs. 1988; 35(Suppl 7):35–38.

87. Kass EH, Lode H, eds. Enzyme-mediated resistance to beta-lactam antibiotics: A symposium on sulbactam/ampicillin. Rev Infect Dis. 1986;8(Suppl 5): 465–650.

88. Reinhardt JF, Johnston L, Ruane P, et al. A randomized, double-blind comparison of sulbactam/ampicillin and clindamycin for the treatment of aerobic and aerobic-anaerobic infections. Rev Infect Dis. 1986;8(Suppl 5):569–575.

89. Hemsell DL, Heard MC, Hemsell PG, et al. Sulbactam/ampicillin versus cefoxitin for uncomplicated and complicated acute pelvic inflammatory disease. Drugs. 1988;35(Suppl 7):39–42.

90. Rodriguez WJ, Kahn WN, Puig N, et al. Sulbactam/ampicillin vs. chloramphenicol/ampicillin for the treatment of meningitis in infants and children. Rev Infect Dis. 1986;8(Suppl 5):620–629.

91. Wald E, Reilly JS, Bluestone CD, et al. Sulbactam/ampicillin in the treatment of acute epiglottis in children. Rev Infect Dis. 1986;8(Suppl 5):617–619.

92. Fass RJ, Prior RB. Comparative in vitro activity of piperacillin-tazobactam and ticarcillin-clavulanate. Antimicrob Agents Chemother. 1989;33: 1268–1274.

93. Aronoff SC, Jacobs MR, Johenning S, Yamabe S. Comparative activities of the β-lactamase inhibitors YTR 830, sodium clavulanate, and sulbactam combined with amoxicillin or ampicillin. Antimicrob Agents Chemother. 1984;26:580–582.

94. Kuck NA, Jacobus NV, Petersen, et al. Comparative in vitro and in vivo activities of piperacillin combined with the β-lactamase inhibitors tazobactam, clavulanic acid, and sulbactam. Antimicrob Agents Chemother. 1989; 33:1964–1969.

95. Johnson CA, Halstenson CE, Kelloway JS, et al. Single-dose pharmacoki-

netics of piperacillin and tazobactam in patients with renal disease. Clin Pharmacol Ther. 1992;51:32–41.

96. Kinzig M, Sörgel F, Brismar B, Nord CE. Pharmacokinetics and tissue penetration of tazobactam and piperacillin in patients undergoing colorectal surgery. Antimicrob Agents Chemother. 1992;36:1997–2004.

97. Kern W, Kennedy S, Sachdeva M, et al. Evaluation of piperacillin-tazobactam in experimental meningitis caused by a beta-lactamase producing strain of K1-positive Escherichia coli. Antimicrob Agents Chemother. 1990;34:697–701.

98. Brismar B, Malmborg AS, Tunevall G, et al. Piperacillin–tazobactam versus imipenem–cilastatin for treatment of intra-abdominal infections. Antimicrob Agents Chemother. 1992;36:2766–2727.

99. Micozzi A, Nucci M, Venditti M, et al. Piperacillin/tazobactam/amikacin versus piperacillin/tazobactam/amikacin/teicoplanin in empirical therapy of neutropenic patients. Eur J Clin Microbiol Infect Dis. 1993;12:1–8.

100. Mouton Y, Leroy D, Beuscart C, et al. Efficacy, safety and tolerance of parenteral piperacillin/tazobactam in the treatment of patients with lower respiratory tract infections. J Antimicrob Chemother. 1993;31(Suppl A):87–95.

101. Tassler H, Cullman W, Elhardt D. Therapy of soft tissue infections with piperacillin/tazobactam. J Antimicrob Chemother 1993;31(Suppl A):105–112.

102. Eklund RE, Nord CE. A randomized multicenter trial of piperacillin/tazobactam versus imipenem/cilastatin in the treatment of severe intra-abdominal infections. Swedish Study Group. J Antimicrob Chemother. 1993;31(Suppl A):79–85.

103. Niinikoski J, Havia T, Alhava E, et al. Piperacillin/tazobactam versus imipenem/cilastatin in the treatment of intra-abdominal infections. Surg Gynecol Obstet. 1993;176:255–261.

18. β-LACTAM ALLERGY

MICHAEL E. WEISS
N. FRANKLIN ADKINSON, Jr.

CLASSIFICATION OF β-LACTAM REACTIONS

Since the introduction of penicillin by Fleming in the mid-1940s the number of β-lactam antibiotics developed has grown dramatically. Currently there are 46 β-lactam antibiotics licensed for use in the United States. Other than allergy, these drugs have remarkably low toxicity when used in moderate doses. In fact, the principal toxicity of β-lactam antibiotics is allergic reactions. The first case of anaphylaxis due to penicillin was reported in 1946,[1] and the first reported death due to an allergic reaction was in 1949.[2] Allergic reactions occur in 7–40/1000 penicillin treatment courses.[3,4] Studies have indicated that as much as half of all allergic drug reactions occurring in hospitalized patients are attributable to β-lactam antibiotics.[5] A wide range of different allergic reactions have been caused by β-lactam antibiotics. It is possible to classify allergic reactions to β-lactam antibiotics using the Gell and Coombs[6] immunopathologic classification system, using Levine's classification system,[7] which is based on time of onset of the reaction, or by classifying the reaction based on the predominate clinical manifestation.

Gell and Coombs Classification

Gell and Coombs classified four different types of immunopathologic reactions, all of which have been seen with β-lactam antibiotics (Table 1):

Type I—Immediate Hypersensitivity. These reactions result from the interaction of β-lactam antigens with performed β-lactam–specific IgE antibodies that are bound to tissue mast cells and/or circulating basophils via high-affinity IgE receptors. Cross-linking two or more IgE receptors by β-lactam antigens leads to the release of both preformed mediators (histamine, proteases, and chemotactic factors) and newly formed mediators (prostaglandins, leukotrienes, and platelet activating factor), which are generated by the metabolism of arachidonic acid.[8] Release of these mediators can lead to urticaria, laryngeal edema, and bronchospasm with or without cardiovascular collapse. Anaphylactic reactions occur in 4–15/100,000 penicillin treatment courses.[4–9] Fatality from β-lactam anaphylaxis has been reported to occur once in every 32,000–100,000 treatment courses.[4,9] The use of β-adrenergic antagonists may increase the risk of death if anaphylaxis occurs, as treatment of an anaphylactic reaction is made more difficult.[10] IgE type I acute allergic reactions cause the greatest clinical concern because of the risk of life-threatening anaphylaxis.

Type II—Cytotoxic Antibodies (Usually IgG and/or IgM). These reactions result when β-lactam– specific IgG or IgM antibodies become attached to circulating blood cells or renal interstitial cells which have β-lactam antigens bound to their cell surface. This antigen–antibody interaction activates the complement system, resulting in cell lysis. Type II reactions may also be complement independent. IgG or IgM antibody may bind to beta-lactam antigens on cell membranes, resulting in neutrophil or macrophage attachment and activation via IgG or IgM Fc receptors. This opsonization can result in injury to the antigen-laden cell. Examples include hemolytic anemia, leukopenia, thrombocytopenia, or drug-induced nephritis. Long-term, high-dose β-lactam treatment is usually required for this form of allergic reaction.

Type III—Immune Complexes (Arthus Reaction). β-Lactam–specific IgG or IgM antibodies may form circulating complexes with β-lactam antigens. These circulating complexes can fix complement and then lodge in tissue sites, causing serum sickness-like reactions and possibly drug fever. In children, serum sickness is 15 times more likely to occur secondary to administration of cefaclor than with amoxicillin.[11] These reactions typically occur 7–14 days after the initiation of β-lactam therapy. The syndrome can occur even after the termination of therapy. Preliminary data, using sera from a small number of patients, suggests that cefaclor serum sickness may be predicted using a microsome metabolite lymphotoxic assay.[12]

Type IV—Cell-Mediated Hypersensitivity. These reactions are not mediated by an antibody, but rather by T lymphocytes. A T lymphocyte recognizes the β-lactam antigen through an antigen-specific T-cell receptor. This triggers the T cell to release cytokines that orchestrate an immune response by recruiting and stimulating proliferation of other lymphocytes and mononuclear cells that ultimately cause tissue inflammation and injury. Contact dermatitis is a clinical manifestation of a Type IV reaction. The high rate of penicillin related contact dermatitis (5–10%) in the 1940s led to the discontinuation of its use as a topical antibiotic.

Idiopathic Reactions

Some reactions to β-lactam antibiotics have an obscure pathogenesis and are not included in the Gell and Coombs classification system. These reactions include pruritus, maculopapular (morbilliform) exanthems, erythema multiforme, erythema nodosum, photosensitivity reactions, fixed drug reactions, and exfoliative dermatitis. The very common maculopapular rash appears late in the treatment course in 2–3 percent of penicillin treatments. Ampicillin (and amoxicillin)–induced rashes occur with much greater frequency (5.2–9.5 percent of treatment courses) in uncomplicated cases.[5,13,14] When ampicillin or amoxicillin is given during infections with Epstein-Barr virus or cytomegalovirus, or to patients with acute lymphocytic leukemia, a much higher incidence of rash (69–100 percent) occurs.[15] Other reactions caused by unknown mechanisms include the Stevens-Johnson syndrome involving rash (usually erythema multiforme) plus involvement of two or more mucous membranes and Lyell syndrome, also known as toxic epidermal ne-

TABLE 1. Classification of Immunopathologic Reactions According to the Scheme of Gell and Coombs

Type of Reactions	Description	Antibody	Cells	Other	Clinical Reactions
I	Anaphylactic, (reagenic), immediate hypersensitivity	IgE	Basophils, mast cells		Anaphylaxis, urticaria
II	Cytotoxic or cytolytic	IgG, IgM	Any cell with isoantigen	C', RES	Hemolytic anemia cytopenias; nephritis
III	Immune complex disease	Soluble immune complexes (Ag–Ab)	None directly	C'	Serum sickness; drug fever;
IV	"Delayed" or cell-mediated hypersensitivity	None known	Sensitized T lymphocytes		Contact dermatitis
V	Idiopathic		?	?	Maculopapular eruptions
			?	?	Eosinophilia
			?	?	Stevens-Johnson syndrome
			?	?	Exfoliative dermatitis

Abbreviations: C': complement; RES: reticuloendothelial system; Ag–Ab: antigen–antibody; ?: immunopathologic mechanism is in doubt.

(Modified from Weiss and Adkinson,[33] with permission.)

TABLE 2. Classification of Allergic Reactions to β-Lactam Antibiotics Based on Their Time of Onset

Reaction Type	Onset (Hours)	Clinical Reactions
Immediate	0–1	Anaphylaxis Hypotension Laryngeal edema Urticaria/angioedema Wheezing
Accelerated	1–72	Urticaria/angioedema Laryngeal/edema Wheezing
Late	>72	Morbilliform rash Interstitial nephritis Hemolytic anemia Neutropenia Thrombocytopenia Serum sickness Drug fever Stevens-Johnson syndrome Exfoliative dermatitis

(Adapted from Levine,[7] with permission.)

crolysis. Patients who have had Stevens-Johnson or Lyell syndrome associated with β-lactam antibiotics should not receive β-lactam drugs in the future. Attempts to desensitize individuals to β-lactam antibiotics that have caused these syndromes is also not recommended. Pseudoanaphylactic reactions have been observed after im or inadvertent iv injection of procaine penicillin. These reactions are most likely due to a combination of a toxic and embolic phenomena from procaine.[16]

Levine Classification

Levine[7] classified reactions to penicillin according to their time of onset (Table 2). Immediate reactions occur within the first hour after β-lactam administration, and they are almost IgE mediated (anaphylaxis and urticaria). Accelerated reactions occur 1–72 hours after initial treatment with β-lactams; they most commonly involve urticaria. Late reactions occur more than 72 hours after onset of therapy. Anaphylaxis does not occur later in the course of continuous β-lactam therapy; maculopapular reactions are most common, but types II to IV reactions also occur during this time frame. Allergic reactions may also be classified according to their predominate clinical manifestations, as listed in Table 3.

IMMUNOCHEMISTRY OF β-LACTAM ANTIBIOTICS

Penicillins consist of a β-lactam ring, on which antimicrobial activity depends, and a five-membered thiazolidine ring (Fig. 1). Since penicillin is a low-molecular-weight compound (356 Da) it must first covalently combine with tissue macromolecules (presumably proteins) to produce multivalent hapten–protein complexes, which are required for both the induction of an immune response and the later elicitation of an allergic reaction (Fig. 2).[17] The most common form of haptenization by penicillin is in the penicilloyl configuration. Since the penicilloyl determinant is the most abundant derivative of penicillin in vivo it has been labeled the *major determinant*. While the formation of the penicilloyl group has been shown to occur spontaneously under physiologic conditions, recent evidence suggests that penicillin haptenization may be facilitated by serum molecules.[18,19] This reaction occurs with the prototype benzylpenicillin and virtually all semisynthetic penicillins. Penicillin can also be degraded by other metabolic pathways to form additional antigenic determinants.[20] These derivatives are formed in small quantities and stimulate a variable immune response; hence they have been termed the *minor determinants*. Known precursors of minor determinants of penicillin include benzylpenicillin, its alkaline hydrolysis product (benzylpenicilloate), and an acid hydrolysis product (benzylpenilloate), collectively called the *minor determinant mixture* (MDM).

Therefore, for penicillin and other β-lactam antibiotics IgE antibodies can be produced against a number of haptenic determinants labeled major and minor determinants. Anaphylactic reactions to penicillin are usually mediated by IgE antibodies directed against minor determinants, although some anaphylac-

TABLE 3. Classification of Reactions to β-Lactam Antibiotics According to their Predominant Clinical Manifestations

Reaction	Manifestation
Anaphylaxis	Laryngeal edema Hypotension Bronchospasm
Cutaneous reactions	Urticaria/angioedema Vasculitis Stevens-Johnson syndrome Exfoliative dermatitis Contact sensitivity Fixed drug eruption Toxic epidermal necrolysis Pruritus Maculopapular (morbilliform) rash Erythema multiforme Erythema nodosum Photosensitivity reactions
Destruction of formed elements of blood	Hemolytic anemia Neutropenia Thrombocytopenia
Renal reactions	Interstitial nephritis Glomerulonephritis Nephrotic syndrome
Serum sickness	
Drug fever	
Systemic vasculitis	
Lymphadenopathy	

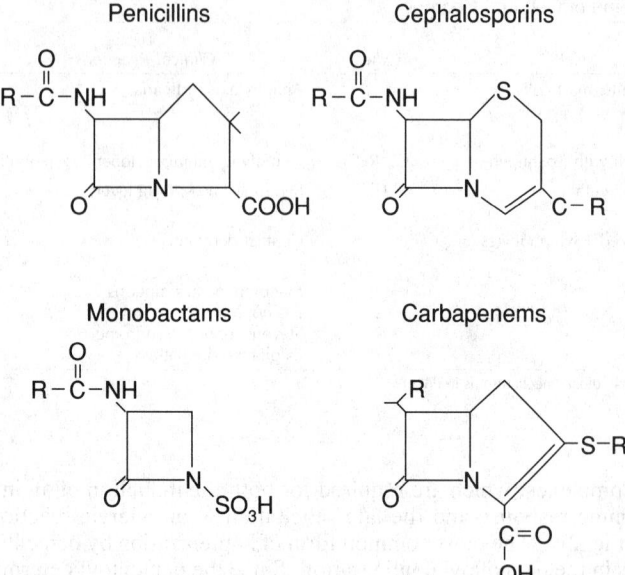

FIG. 1. Structure of four classes of β-lactam antibiotics in use in the United States.

in part by the genetic makeup of that individual.[22] The half-life of β-lactam IgE antibodies has been shown to range from as short as 10 days to an indeterminately long interval (more than 1000 days).[23] Obviously an individual whose β-lactam–specific IgE antibody response persists is at greater cumulative risk for allergic reactions to β-lactam antibiotics than one whose IgE antibody quickly disappears.

Parenteral administration of β-lactam antibiotics produces more allergic reactions than orally administered β-lactam antibiotics.[24] However, recent evidence suggests that this may be more related to dose than route of administration. When higher oral doses are given, as in the treatment of gonorrhea, the incidence of allergic reactions is no different from that of im procaine penicillin at a comparable dose.[25]

A history of atopy (allergic rhinitis, asthma, and/or atopic dermatitis) does not seem to be an independent risk factor for the development of β-lactam allergy,[23,26] although atopic individuals, especially those with asthma, seem to be predisposed to severe and fatal reactions should anaphylaxis occur.[9]

Individuals with a history of prior penicillin reactions have a four- to sixfold increased risk of subsequent reactions to β-lactam antibiotics compared with those without previous reaction histories.[26] The risk is particularly pronounced if the previous reaction was anaphylaxis or urticaria.[23] However, since most serious and fatal allergic reactions to β-lactam antibiotics occur in individuals who have never had a prior allergic reaction, a negative history of β-lactam allergy should not leave one with

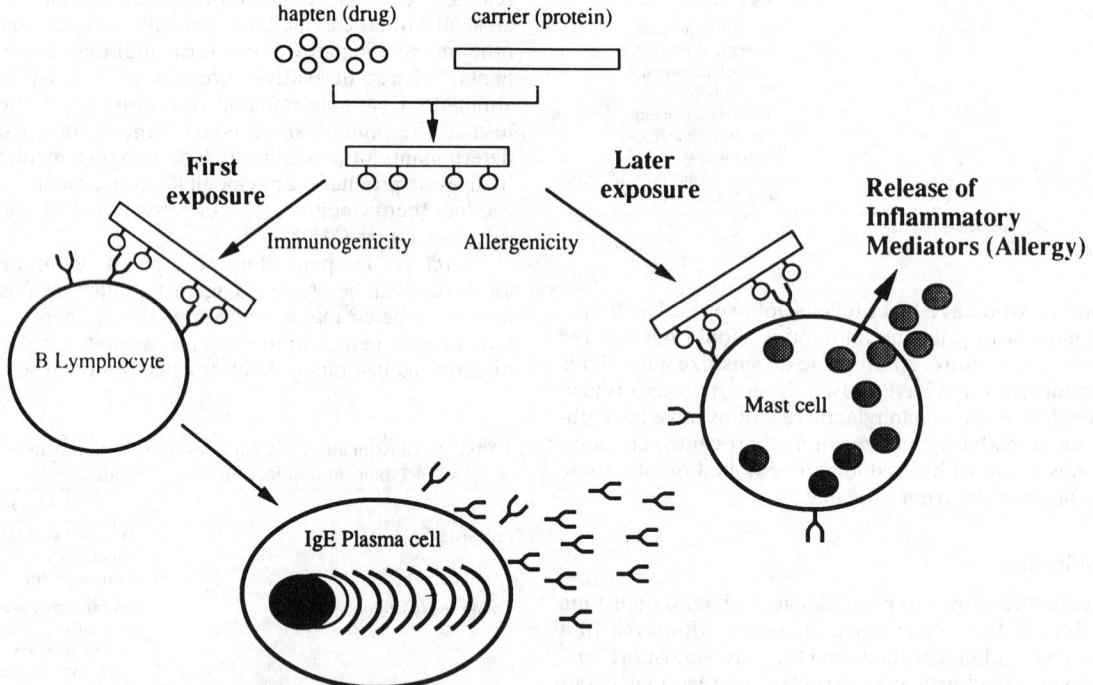

FIG. 2. Illustration of drug hapten combining with carrier molecule to induce IgE antibody production against drug (sensitization). On subsequent exposure, drug combines with IgE antibody on mast cell surface, leading to anaphylactic reaction (immune response).

tic reactions have occurred in patients with only penicilloyl-specific IgE antibodies.[7,20,21] Accelerated and late urticarial reactions are usually mediated by penicilloyl-specific IgE antibodies (major determinant).[7]

RISK FACTORS FOR β-LACTAM REACTIONS

Immune responses to β-lactam antibiotics occur in only a small percentage of exposed patients, and clinical expression of β-lactam allergy occurs in only a fraction of the patients demonstrating an immune responses. The generation of a sustained immune response to a β-lactam antibiotic is probably controlled

a false sense of security. Sensitization in these individuals probably occurred from their last therapeutic course of penicillin. A randomized, controlled trial of routine penicillin skin testing in history-negative patients was shown not to be cost effective, and therefore skin testing at this time is only recommended for patients with prior of history of β-lactam allergy.[27]

In general, the likelihood of sustaining IgE-specific β-lactam antibodies declines with increasing time from the previous reaction. Sullivan and collaborators[28] reported that skin tests done within the first 1 or 2 months after an acute allergic reaction were positive 80–90 percent of the time. Thereafter, there was a time-dependent decline in the rate of positive skin tests to less than 20 percent by 10 years.[28] Patients who have had serum sickness-like reactions to β-lactam antibiotics often persist with an intense antibody response and may remain at high risk for allergic reactions for many years.

Despite sparse evidence, it is generally thought that penicillin reactions occur less frequently in both children and the elderly than in nonelderly adults.[26,29] Although the frequency of anaphylactic reactions may be less in the elderly, fatal outcomes are more commonly due to compromised cardiopulmonary reserve.

DIAGNOSING β-LACTAM ALLERGY

An important question facing clinicians is how to assess patients with histories of prior β-lactam reactions who have a current clinical need for β-lactam antibiotics. Approximately 5–20 percent of patients give a history of prior reactions to β-lactam antibiotics. By current medical standards, all of these subjects would be denied therapy with β-lactam antibiotics the rest of their lives unless further evaluation is undertaken. The most useful single piece of information in assessing an individual's risk for a type I, IgE-mediated reaction (anaphylaxis and urticaria) is the skin test response to major and minor penicillin determinants.

The major (penicilloyl) determinant of penicillin can be assessed by skin testing with penicilloyl-polylysine (PPL). This commercially available skin test reagent (PRE-PEN, Swartz-Pharma, Milwaukee, WI) contains multiple penicilloyl molecules synthetically coupled to a weakly immunogenic polylysine carrier. Unfortunately, minor determinants of penicillin are not commercially available in the United States at present. It is hoped that this will change in the near future. In the meantime, benzylpenicillin alone (10,000 U/ml) can be substituted as a less efficient minor determinant reagent in patients without histories of anaphylactic sensitivity.

Skin testing should first proceed with an epicutaneous (prick-puncture) test for safety. If there is no induration (or systemic symptoms) after 15 minutes, intradermal injections are placed, raising 3–4-mm blebs in duplicate on the forearm. Testing should be done with PPL, MDM, a positive control (histamine), and a negative diluent control. The diameter of induration at 15–20 minutes is read; if it is greater than 5 mm, the test is considered positive.[30] Antihistamines, tricyclic antidepressants, and adrenergic drugs, all of which may inhibit skin test results, should be discontinued at least 48 hours prior to skin testing. Antihistamines with long half-lives need to be discontinued for appropriate intervals.

When properly performed with due consideration for preliminary epicutaneous tests and appropriate dilutions, skin testing with penicillin reagents can almost always be safely accomplished. Systemic reactions occur in about 1 percent of those tested[31,32]; there are usually mild but can be serious. Therefore skin tests should be done in the presence of a physician and with immediate access to medications needed to treat anaphylaxis.

In numerous studies in which both PPL and minor determinant skin tests were performed, only 7–35 percent of patients who gave histories of penicillin allergy were skin test positive to either reagent,[33] although one study found a positive skin test rate of 63 percent.[28] In general, with increasing time from the allergic reaction, the prevalence of positive skin tests to penicillin determinants decreases, although some patients have penicillin antibodies indefinitely.[28,34] Therefore, in patients who give a history of penicillin allergy, skin tests confirm that 65–93 percent can safely be given a β-lactam antibiotic. With negative histories of penicillin allergy, the rate of positive skin tests is about 2 percent.[27]

Extensive worldwide experience involving over 20,000 patients has shown that individuals with prior histories of penicillin reactions can be safely retreated with penicillin or related antibiotics if intradermal skin tests with PPL and a suitable MDM are shown to be negative.[35] When therapeutic doses of penicillin

are given to patients with histories of penicillin allergy but with negative skin tests to PPL and MDM, IgE-mediated reactions occur in 2–15 percent of patients, depending on clinical history; such reactions are almost always mild and self-limited. Penicillin anaphylaxis has not been reported in skin test–negative patients in the United States. When penicillin is given after negative skin tests, about 1–3 percent of patients will develop urticarial or other mild cutaneous reactions.[33] If the major determinant penicillin is used alone as a skin test reagent, approximately 10–25 percent of all potential positive reactions would be missed.[28] If one uses benzylpenicillin G, diluted to a concentration of 10,000 units/ml (10^{-2} M) as the sole minor determinant, about 5–10 percent of skin test–positive patients will be missed.[28] Since readministration of β-lactam antibiotics may resensitize a patient, retesting the patient with a history of IgE-mediated reactions is recommended before each new course of β-lactam antibiotics.

A limited number of skin test–positive patients have been treated with therapeutic doses of penicillin. The risk of an acute immediate or accelerated allergic reaction ranges from about 10 percent in history-negative to 50–70 percent in history-positive subjects.[33] Therefore, if skin tests are positive, an equally effective, noncross-reacting antibiotic should be substituted when available. Patients with a history of exfoliative dermatitis or Stevens-Johnson or Lyell syndrome, reactions that constitute absolute contraindications for penicillin administration, should not be evaluated by skin testing. Skin tests have no predictive value in non-IgE–mediated reactions, such as drug fever, serum sickness, cytopenias, interstitial nephritis, contact dermatitis, or maculopapular exanthems. Penicillin skin tests are indeterminate (usually erythema without wheal or discordant duplicates) in about 0.6–3 percent of patients with histories of penicillin allergy.[32,35] The meaning of such results is presently unclear.

Type II reactions, such as hemolytic anemias, cytopenias, and interstitial nephritis, usually follow high-dose, long-term β-lactam therapy. Anecdotal experience suggests that short courses of β-lactam therapy in moderate doses can be tolerated by most, if not all, patients with these histories. Penicillin skin testing is important to rule out concomitant type I sensitivity but would not be predictive of type II or III type reactions. If skin tests are negative in these patients and β-lactam antibiotics are strongly indicated, gradual dose escalation under careful medical observation can be prudently attempted. If cytopenia, hemolytic anemia, hematuria, or proteinuria develop, therapy should be promptly stopped and high-dose glucocorticoids administered. Most subjects can be retreated, however, without recurrence, especially if the prior history of reaction is remote.

Solid-phase immunoassays such as the radioallergosorbent test (RAST) have been developed to detect serum IgE antibodies directed against the penicilloyl determinant. At present there is no in vitro RAST for minor determinant antibodies.[30] Because it is more time consuming, more expensive, less sensitive for detection of the major determinant IgE antibodies than skin testing, and is presently unavailable for minor determinant antibody detection, the RAST and other in vitro analogs have limited clinical utility at this time.

SEMISYNTHETIC PENICILLINS WITH SPECIAL REFERENCE TO AMPICILLIN/AMOXICILLIN

Semisynthetic penicillins contain the same nuclear structure as benzylpenicillin with differing side chains. Since allergic reactions are thought to be due to neoantigens formed by the β-lactam nucleus interacting with native proteins, it has generally been considered unnecessary to skin test with specific derivatives of semisynthetic penicillins. Hapten inhibition theory would predict that antibodies directed against the unmodified side chain would not cause allergic reactions because of overwhelming hapten inhibition from unconjugated univalent drug.[36,37] Earlier studies showed that skin testing with derivatives of semisynthetic penicillins in addition to benzylpenicillin derivatives were not needed.[38] Recently Blanca and associated[39,40] in Spain questioned this dogma and suggested that skin testing with major and minor determinants of benzylpenicillin may not predict all individuals with ampicillin/amoxicillin specific allergy. Silviu-Dan et al.[41] subsequently reported that skin testing with derivatives of ampicillin/amoxicillin detected nine patients who otherwise were skin test negative to benzylpenicillin reagents.[41] These nine represented nearly half of all skin test–positive individuals. Unfortunately, this study does not provide information about benzylpenicillin skin test–negative and ampicillin/amoxicillin skin test–positive individuals challenged with a β-lactam. Mendelson et al. (personal communication) studied 443 patients with a history of penicillin allergy who were skin test negative to PPL and an MDM of benzylpenicillin. The 443 patients tolerated a 10-day penicillin challenge, but, when given 10 days of amoxicillin, 18.7 percent developed cutaneous reactions. Thus, amoxicillin/ampicillin seems to have a greater propensity for causing cutaneous allergic reactions. It has been postulated that the diamino acyl side chain contained in ampicillin/amoxicillin more readily allows for the formation of linear polymers of varying lengths, which may explain the higher cutaneous reaction rate seen with ampicillin/amoxicillin.[42] Except for that of Blanca et al.,[40] there have been no reports of any patient with negative skin tests to PPL and an MDM of benzylpenicillin and then treated with amoxicillin/ampicillin having had anything more than a cutaneous reaction. Studies in the 1960s showed that patients with late-occurring maculopapular rashes from ampicillin/amoxicillin could safely be retreated with the antibiotics without any increased risk for acute allergic reactions. In these individuals, skin testing with PPL and MDM may be useful to rule out concomitant type I, IgE-mediated sensitivity.

β-LACTAM DESENSITIZATION

Effective, non-cross-reacting alternative antibiotics are usually available for patients with positive skin tests to penicillin. If alternative drugs fail, induce unacceptable side effects, or are clearly less effective, then the administration of a β-lactam antibiotic using a desensitization protocol may be justified. Infections in which this may be considered include subacute endocarditis due to enterococci, brain abscess, bacterial meningitis, or overwhelming infections with Staphylococcus or Pseudomonas organisms such as osteomyelitis or sepsis, Listeria infections, neurosyphilis, or syphilis during pregnancy. Use of a desensitization protocol for penicillin skin test-positive patients markedly reduces the risk of anaphylaxis.

β-Lactam desensitization should only be performed in an intensive care setting. Any medical risk factor for anaphylaxis should be corrected. All β-adrenergic antagonists including ophthalmologic drops should be discontinued. Asthmatic patients should be under optimal control. An intravenous line should be established, and baseline electrocardiogram and spirometry should be performed. Continuous electrocardiogram monitoring should be instituted.

Protocols have been developed for beta-lactam desensitization using both the oral and parenteral route (Tables 4 and 5).[43] If an oral preparation is available and the patient has a functional gastrointestinal tract, then the oral route may be preferable for desensitization. Results from oral desensitization have shown that approximately one-third of patients will develop a transient allergic reaction during desensitization and two-thirds will develop one during penicillin treatment after desensitization. These reactions are usually mild and self-limited in nature, but may be serious.[24]

During desensitization any dose that causes mild systemic reactions such as pruritus, fleeting urticaria, rhinitis, or mild wheezing should be repeated until the patient tolerates the dose without systemic symptoms or signs. More serious reactions

TABLE 4. Protocol for Oral Desensitization of β-Lactam Antibiotic-Allergic Patients

Step	β-Lactam Drug (mg/ml)	Amount[a] (ml)	Dose Given[a,b] (mg)	Cumulative Dose (mg)
1	0.5	0.1	0.05	0.05
2	0.5	0.2	0.10	0.15
3	0.5	0.4	0.20	0.35
4	0.5	0.8	0.40	0.75
5	0.5	1.6	0.80	1.55
6	0.5	3.2	1.60	3.15
7	0.5	6.4	3.20	6.35
8	5.0	1.2	6.00	12.35
9	5.0	2.4	12.00	24.35
10	5.0	4.8	24.00	48.35
11	50.0	1.0	50.00	98.35
12	50.0	2.0	100.00	198.35
13	50.0	4.0	200.00	398.35
14	50.0	8.0	400.00	798.35

Note: Observe patient for 30 minutes. Administer 1 g of same agent intravenously.

[a] Drug suspension diluted in 30 ml of water for ingestion.
[b] Interval between doses, 15 minutes.

(From Sullivan,[43] with permission.)

TABLE 5. Protocol for Parenteral Desensitization of β-Lactam Antibiotic-Allergic Patients

Step	β-Lactam Drug (mg/ml)	Amount[a] (ml)	Dose Given[a,b] (mg)	Cumulative Dose (mg)
1	0.1	0.1	0.01	0.01
2	0.1	0.2	0.02	0.03
3	0.1	0.4	0.04	0.07
4	0.1	0.8	0.08	0.15
5	1.0	0.16	0.16	0.31
6	1.0	0.32	0.32	0.63
7	1.0	0.64	0.64	1.27
8	10	0.12	1.20	2.47
9	10	0.24	2.40	4.87
10	10	0.48	4.80	10
11	100	0.10	10	20
12	100	0.20	20	40
13	100	0.40	40	80
14	100	0.80	80	160
15	1000	0.16	160	320
16	1000	0.32	320	640
17	1000	0.64	640	1280

Note: Observe patient for 30 minutes. Administer 1 g of same agent intravenously.

[a] Doses administered subcutaneously (or intramuscularly or intravenously).
[b] Interval between doses, 15 minutes.

(From Sullivan,[43] with permission.)

such as hypotension, laryngeal edema, or asthma require appropriate treatment, and if desensitization is continued, the dose should be decreased by at least 10-fold and withheld until the patient is stable.[44]

Once desensitized, the patient's treatment with penicillin must not lapse or the risk of an allergic reaction increases. If the patient requires a β-lactam antibiotic in the future and still remains skin test positive to penicillin reagents, desensitization would be required again. Patients have been maintained on long-term, low-dose oral penicillin therapy (usually bid or tid) to sustain a chronic state of desensitization.[45]

CROSS-REACTIVITY AMONG β-LACTAM ANTIBIOTICS

Cephalosporins

Like penicillins, cephalosporins possess a β-lactam ring but the five-membered thiazolidine ring is replaced by the six-membered dihydrothiazine ring (Fig. 1). Shortly after cephalosporins came into clinical use allergic reactions were reported in penicillin allergic patients, and the question of cross-reactivity between cephalosporins and penicillins was raised.[46] To date, the degree of cross-reactivity between penicillins and cephalosporins remains a matter of considerable uncertainty. Complicating matters, the early cephalosporins were contaminated with trace amounts of penicillin,[47] potentially leading to overestimates of the degree of cross-reactivity. Nevertheless, studies in both animals and humans clearly demonstrated cross-reactivity between penicillins and first-generation cephalosporins using immuno- and bioassays to evaluate IgE, IgM, and IgG antibodies.[48–50] In general the degree of clinical cross-reactivity is much lower than the in vitro cross-reactivity between penicillins and cephalosporins. Small numbers of penicillin skin test–positive patients have been treated with cephalosporin antibiotics without allergic reactions.[51,52] Very few cephalosporin skin test–positive individuals have been challenged with cephalosporins to allow estimation of the predictive value of a positive skin test. Unfortunately major determinant analogs of cephalosporins are not currently available as skin test reagents, therefore limiting the utility of skin testing for cephalosporin allergy.

The incidence of clinically relevant cross-reactivity between the penicillins and cephalosporins is probably small, but rare cases of life-threatening anaphylactic cross-reactivity have occurred. The risk of administering a first-generation cephalosporin to a penicillin skin test–positive patient is lower than administering a penicillin antibiotic, but is not negligible. Antibodies to the second- and third-generation cephalosporins are often directed against the side chains rather than the ring structures, and therefore cross-reactivity with penicillins is less than first generation cephalosporins.[43] Patients with positive skin tests to any penicillin reagent probably should not receive cephalosporin antibiotics unless alternative drugs are clearly less desirable. If cephalosporin drugs are to be used, they should be administered with caution and with adequate precautions.

Carbapenems

These are a third class of β-lactam antibiotics of which imipenem is the prototype (Fig. 1). Recent studies have shown that approximately 50 percent of penicillin skin test–positive patients have positive skin reactions to analogous imipenem determinants,[53] suggesting appreciable cross-reactivity and indicating that these β-lactam antibiotics are relatively contraindicated in patients with positive penicillin skin tests.

Monobactams

The monobactams are a new class of β-lactam antibiotics that contain a monocyclic ring structure rather than the bicyclic structure of the penicillins, cephalosporins, and carbapenems (Fig. 1). The prototype monobactam licensed in the United States is aztreonam. In preclinical studies, negligible cross-reactivity in rabbits and in human subjects between aztreonam and penicillins or cephalosporins was found.[54] When subjects with positive penicillin skin tests were skin tested with analogous aztreonam reagents, appreciable cross-reactivity was not found.[55] In a subsequent trial, 20 patients with positive penicillin skin test were treated with therapeutic doses of aztreonam, and none had IgE-mediated reactions.[56] Taken together, these data suggest weak cross-reactivity between aztreonam and other β-lactam antibiotics and indicate that aztreonam may be safely administered to most if not all penicillin-allergic subjects.

UNANSWERED QUESTIONS

Important clinical questions remain for future research in β-lactam allergy. These include (1) the further elucidation of when side chain–specific allergies may be the cause of β-lactam reac-

tions, (2) the possible identification of genetic factors that predispose individuals to have β-lactam allergy, (3) the validation of testing procedures to evaluate clinical cross-reactivity between cephalosporin and penicillin antibiotics, and (4) the potential relationship of penicillin allergy to other medication reactions of structurally unrelated drugs.

REFERENCES

1. Gorevic PD. Drug-induced autoimmune disease. In: Kaplan A, ed. Allergy. New York: Churchill Livingstone; 1985:480.
2. Schwartz HJ, Sher TH. Anaphylaxis to penicillin in a frozen dinner. Ann Allergy. 1984;52:342–3.
3. Parker CW. Drug therapy (first of three parts). N Engl J Med. 1975;292:511–4.
4. International Rheumatic Fever Study Group. Allergic reactions to long-term benzathine penicillin prophylaxis for rheumatic fever. Lancet 1993;337:1308–10.
5. Arndt KA, Jick H. Rates of cutaneous reactions to drugs. A report from the Boston Collaborative Drug Surveillance Program. JAMA. 1976;235:918–22.
6. Gell PGH, Coombs RRA. Classification of allergic reactions responsible for clinical hypersensitivity and disease. In: Gell PGH, Coombs RRA, Hachmann PJ, eds. Clinical Aspects of Immunology. Oxford: Blackwell Scientific Publications; 1975:761–81.
7. Levine BB. Immunologic mechanisms of penicillin allergy. A haptenic model system for the study of allergic diseases of man. N Engl J Med. 1966;275:1115–25.
8. Ishizaka T. Mechanisms of IgE-mediated hypersensitivity. In: Middleton E Jr, Reed CE, Ellis EF, et al., eds. Allergy: Principles and Practice. St. Louis: CV Mosby; 1988:71–93.
9. Idsoe O, Guthe T, Willcox RR, et al. Nature and extent of penicillin side-reactions, with particular reference to fatalities from anaphylactic shock. Bull WHO 1968;38:159–88.
10. Jacobs RL, Geoffrey WR Jr, Fournier DC, et al. Potentiated anaphylaxis in patients with drug-induced beta-adrenergic blockade. J Allergy Clin Immunol. 1981;68:125–7.
11. Heckbert SR, Stryker WS, Coltin KL, et al. Serum sickness in children after antibiotic exposure: Estimates of occurrence and morbidity in a health maintenance organization population. Am J Epidemiol 1990;132:336–42.
12. Wheeler JG, Childress SH, Kearns GL. Cefaclor serum sickness: In vitro identification using microsome cytotoxicity and flow cytometry (Abstract). J Allergy Clin Immunol. 1993;91:363.
13. Levine B. Skin rashes with penicillin therapy: Current management. N Engl J Med. 1972;286:42–3.
14. Shapiro S, Siskin V, Slone D, et al. Drug rash with ampicillin and other penicillins. Lancet. 1969;2:7628.
15. Kerns DL, Shira JE, Go S, et al. Ampicillin rash in children. Relationship to penicillin allergy and infectious mononucleosis. Am J Dis Child. 1973;125:187–90.
16. Galpin JE, Chow AW, Yoshikawa TT, et al. "Pseudoanaphylactic" reactions from inadvertent infusion of procaine penicillin G. Ann Intern Med. 1974;81:358.
17. Eisen HN. Hypersensitivity to simple chemicals. In: Lawrence HS, ed. Cellular and Humoral Aspects of the Hypersensitive States. New York: PB Hoeber; 1959:111–6.
18. DiPiro JT, Hamilton RG, Adkinson NF Jr. Facilitation of penicilloation of proteins by serum cofactors (Abstract). J Allergy Clin Immunol. 1990;85:192.
19. Sullivan TJ. Facilitated haptenation of human proteins by penicillin (Abstract). J Allergy Clin Immunol. 1989;83:255.
20. Levine BB, Redmond AP. Minor haptenic determinant-specific reagins of penicillin hypersensitivity in man. Int Arch Allergy. 1969;35:445–55.
21. Levine BB, Redmond AP, Fellner MJ, et al. Penicillin allergy and the heterogeneous immune responses of man to benzylpenicillin. J Clin Invest. 1966;45:1895–1906.
22. Levine BB. Effect of combinations of inbred strain, antigen, and antigen dose on immune responsiveness and reagin production in the mouse. A potential mouse model for immune aspects of human atopic allergy. Int Arch Allergy Appl Immunol. 1970;39:156–71.
23. Adkinson NF Jr. Risk factors for drug allergy. J Allergy Clin Immunol. 1984;74:567–72.
24. Sullivan TJ, Yecies LD, Shatz GS, et al. Desensitization of patients allergic to penicillin using orally administered beta-lactam antibiotics. J Allergy Clin Immunol. 1982;69:275–82.
25. Adkinson NF Jr, Wheeler B. Risk factors for IgE-dependent reactions to penicillin. In: Kerr JW, Ganderton MA, eds. XI International Congress of Allergology and Clinical Immunology. London: MacMillan Press Ltd.; 1983:55–9.
26. Sogn DD. Prevention of allergic reactions to penicillin. J Allergy Clin Immunol. 1987;78:1051–2.
27. Adkinson NF Jr, Spence M, Wheeler B. Randomized clinical trial of routine penicillin skin testing. J Allergy Clin Immunol. 1984;73:163.
28. Sullivan TJ, Wedner HJ, Shatz GS, et al. Skin testing to detect penicillin allergy. J Allergy Clin Immunol. 1981;68:171–80.
29. Sogn DD. Penicillin allergy. J Allergy Clin Immunol. 1984;74:589–93.
30. Adkinson NF Jr. Tests for immunological drug reactions. In: Rose NF, Friedman H, eds. Manual of Clinical Immunology. Washington, DC: American Society for Microbiology; 1986:692–7.
31. Sullivan TJ. Penicillin allergy. In: Lichtenstein LM, Fauci A, eds. Current Therapy in Allergy. St. Louis: CV Mosby; 1985:57–61.

32. Gadde J, Spence M, Wheeler B, et al. Clinical experience with penicillin skin testing in a large inner city STD clinic. JAMA. 1993;270:2456–63.
33. Weiss ME, Adkinson NF Jr. Immediate hypersensitivity reactions to penicillin and related antibiotics. Clin Allergy. 1988;18:515–40.
34. Chandra RK, Joglekar SA, Tomas E. Penicillin allergy: Anti-penicillin IgE antibodies and immediate hypersensitivity skin reactions employing major and minor determinants of penicillin. Arch Dis Child. 1980;55:857–60.
35. Sogn DD, Casale TB, Condemi JJ, et al. Results of the NIAID collaborative clinical trial to test the predictive value of skin testing with major and minor penicillin derivatives in hospitalized adults. Arch Intern Med. 1992;152:1025–32.
36. De Weck AL, Schneider CH. Specific inhibition of allergic reactions to penicillin in man by a monovalent hapten. II. Clinical studies. Int Arch Allergy. 1972;42:798–815.
37. De Weck AL, Schneider CH. Specific inhibition of allergic reactions to penicillin in man by a monovalent hapten. Int Arch Allergy. 1972;42:782–97.
38. Warrington RJ, Simons FER, Ho HW, et al. Diagnosis of penicillin allergy by skin testing: The Manitoba experience. CMA J. 1978;11:787.
39. Blanca M, Vega JM, Garcia J, et al. Allergy to penicillin with good tolerance to other penicillins: Study of the incidence in subjects allergic to betalactams. Clin Exp Allergy. 1990;20:475–81.
40. Blanca M, Perez E, Garcia J, et al. Anaphylaxis to amoxycillin but good tolerance for benzylpenicillin. Allergy. 1988;43:508–10.
41. Silviu-Dan F, Mcphillips S, Warrington R. The frequency of skin test reactions to side-chain penicillin determinants. J Allergy Clin Immunol. 1993;91:694–701.
42. Adkinson Jr NF. Side-chain specific beta-lactam allergy. Clin Exp Allergy. 1990;20:445–7.
43. Sullivan TJ. Drug allergy. In: Middleton E, Reed C, Ellis E, et al., eds. Allergy: Principles and Practice. 4th ed. St. Louis: CV Mosby; 1993:1523–34.
44. Adkinson NF Jr. Penicillin allergy. In: Lichtenstein LM, Fauci A, eds. Current Therapy in Allergy, Immunology and Rheumatology. Ontario, Canada: BS Decker; 1983:57–62.
45. Naclerio R, Mizrahi EA, Adkinson NF Jr. Immunologic observations during desensitization and maintenance of clinical tolerance to penicillin. J Allergy Clin Immunol. 1983;71:294–301.
46. Grieco MH. Cross-allergenicity of the penicillins and the cephalosporins. Arch Intern Med. 1967;119:141–6.
47. Pedersen-Bjergaard J. Cephalothin in the treatment of penicillin sensitive patients. Act Allergol. 1967;XXII:299–306.
48. Petz L. Immunologic cross-reactivity between penicillins and cephalosporins: A review. J Infect Dis. 1978;137:S74–9.
49. Shibata K, Atsumi T, Itorivchi Y, et al. Immunological cross-reactivities of cephalothin and its related compounds with benzylpenicillin (penicillin G). Nature. 1966;212:419–20.
50. Abraham GN, Petz LD, Fudenberg HH. Immunohaematological cross-allergenicity between penicillin and cephalothin in humans. Clin Exp Immunol. 1968;3:343–57.
51. Solley GO, Gleich GJ, Van Dellen RG. Penicillin allergy: Clinical experience with a battery of skin-test reagents. J Allergy Clin Immunol. 1982;69:238–244.
52. Saxon A, Beall GN, Rohr AS, et al. Immediate hypersensitivity reactions to beta-lactam antibiotics. Ann Intern Med. 1987;107:204–15.
53. Saxon A. Immediate hypersensitivity reactions to beta-lactam antibiotics. Rev Infect Dis. 1983;5:S368.
54. Adkinson NF Jr, Swabb EA, Sugerman AA. Immunology of the monobactam aztreonam. Antimicrob Agents Chemother. 1984;25:93–7.
55. Saxon A, Hassner A, Swabb EA, et al. Lack of cross-reactivity between aztreonam, a monobactam antibiotic, and penicillin in penicillin-allergic subjects. J Infect Dis. 1984;149:16–22.
56. Adkinson NF Jr, Wheeler B, Swabb EA. Clinical tolerance of the monobactam aztreonam in penicillin allergic subjects (Abstract WS-26-4). Presented at the 14th International Congress of Chemotherapy, June 23–28, 1985. Kyoto, Japan.

19. FUSIDIC ACID

LIONEL A. MANDELL

STRUCTURE

Fusidic acid, a member of the fusidane class, is derived from the fungus *Fusidium coccineum* and is chemically related to the antibiotics helvolic acid and cephalosporin P1.[1] Despite its steroidlike structure, fusidic acid does not have steroid activity. The sodium salt of fusidic acid, termed *fucidin*, was developed by Leo Laboratories in Denmark and was first introduced into clinical practice in 1962.

MECHANISM OF ACTION

Fusidic acid is usually bacteriostatic but at higher concentrations may be bactericidal. It exerts its antibacterial effect by inhibiting protein synthesis but the exact mechanisms by which this inhibition occurs have not been fully elucidated.

Bacterial protein synthesis depends upon the translocation of peptidyl-tRNA from the ribosomal acceptor site to the peptidyl site. This requires protein elongation factor G and hydrolysis of GTP. At least part of fusidic acid's action reflects its ability to stabilize ribosome–elongation factor–GDP + inorganic phosphate complexes, thereby inhibiting GTP hydrolysis and blocking elongation of the nascent polypeptide chain.[2]

Resistance to fusidic acid may occur through a variety of mechanisms. Strains of *Staphylococcus aureus* may exhibit chromosome or plasmid-mediated resistance. Chromosomal mutations occur at a frequency of 1 in 10^{6-7} and result in alteration at the target site (i.e., elongation factor G). Plasmid-mediated resistance may be due to reduced permeability to the antibiotic.[3]

ANTIMICROBIAL ACTIVITY

Fusidic acid has an unusual and somewhat unique spectrum of antimicrobial activity. Susceptible organisms include selected aerobes and anaerobes. Although there are no official National Committee for Clinical Laboratory Standards guidelines for in vitro susceptibility testing, the usual accepted breakpoint is 2 mg/liter.

Fusidic acid is most active against *S. aureus* and *Staphylococcus epidermidis*, including strains that are methicillin resistant. Such organisms are generally sensitive to fusidic acid, as there is no cross-resistance between this agent and β-lactam antimicrobials. Minimum inhibitory concentrations (MICs) for methicillin-resistant *S. aureus* range from 0.03 to 0.8 mg/liter, but in one study of bacteremic isolates the MIC_{90} was 0.2 mg/liter.[4] However, fusidic acid is considerably less active against *Staphylococcus saprophyticus* strains and streptococci.

Corynebacteria are generally sensitive, as are *Neisseria gonorrhoeae* and *Meningococcus*. Aerobic gram-negative bacilli appear to be resistant.[5]

With the exception of *Fusobacterium necrophorum*, anaerobic organisms are generally quite sensitive to fusidic acid. Gram-positive anaerobes generally are very susceptible, with MIC_{90}s ranging from 0.25 to 1.0 mg/liter.[6] MIC_{90}s for *Clostridium difficile* are somewhat higher at 2.0 mg/liter. Gram-negative anaerobes are a little more variable in their susceptibility. The *Bacteroides* species *distasonis*, *ovatus*, *thetaiotaomicron*, and *fragilis* exhibit MIC_{90}s ranging from 2.0 to 16.0 mg/liter, whereas for the *Prevotella* species *buccae*, *oralis*, and *melaninogenica* and the *Bacteroides* species *ureolyticus* and *vulgatus*, MIC_{90}s range from only 0.25 to 1.0 mg/liter.

MICs are markedly increased in the presence of serum, and antimicrobial activity is also reduced in alkaline media. Reports of the effects of antimicrobial combinations containing fusidic acid have been somewhat inconsistent. In one study of drug combinations involving fusidic acid with either vancomycin or rifampin against isolates of methicillin-resistant *S. aureus*, neither synergy nor antagonism was demonstrated, while another study of fusidic acid with rifampin against methicillin resistant coagulase-positive and coagulase-negative staphylococci suggested some synergistic effect.[7,8]

PHARMACOLOGY

Fusidic acid may be used parenterally as an intravenous formulation, or it may be given orally or applied topically. Various formulations, dosages, and frequencies of administration are

TABLE 1. Dosage and Administration of Fusidic Acid

Route of Administration	Formulation	Dosage	Frequency of Administration
iv	Sodium fusidate	>50 kg BW, 500 mg[a]	tid
		<50 kg BW, 7 mg/kg	tid
po (film-coated tables)	Sodium fusidate	500 mg	tid
po (suspension)	Hemihydrate	0–1 year, 0.3 ml/kg BW	tid
		1–5 years, 5 ml	tid
		6–12 years, 10 ml	tid
		Adults, 15 ml	tid
Topical			
Cream (2%)	Fusidic acid		bid
Ointment (2%)	Sodium fusidate		bid
Gel (2%)	Sodium fusidate		bid
Ophthalmic			
Viscous eyedrops (1%)	Fusidic acid		bid

[a] 500 mg sodium fusidate is equivalent to 480 mg of fusidic acid.

given in Table 1. The new sodium salt iv formulation may be administered over 2–4 hours.

The drug is virtually completely absorbed after oral administration, achieving levels up to 71 mg/liter with repeated tid dosing. With repeated iv infusions, peak plasma concentrations of 123 mg/liter have been recorded. The drug is highly protein bound (95–97 percent), exhibits nonlinear kinetics, and has a half-life of approximately 14 hours. Fusidic acid is widely distributed to such tissues as synovial fluid, bone, subcutaneous fat, kidney, bronchial secretions, cardiac tissue, and aqueous humor.[9] The drug also crosses the placenta.

It is metabolized by the liver and is eliminated primarily by biliary excretion. About 2 percent of the drug can be recovered unchanged in the stool, but very little is recovered in urine. Dosage modification is not necessary for patients with renal failure or for those patients on hemodialysis. Little is known about the use of fusidic acid in patients with hepatic impairment, and the drug is probably best avoided in such circumstances.

ADVERSE REACTIONS

The adverse reactions depend upon the route of administration. With the iv formulation, thrombophlebitis and reversible jaundice have been noted. Reversible jaundice is also seen with the oral preparation, but to a lesser extent (6 vs. 17 percent).[10]

As the drug is avidly bound to albumin, it competes with bilirubin for binding sites. It should therefore be used with caution, if at all, in newborns, particularly if they are icteric, acidotic, or premature.[11] Oral use is generally well tolerated but has been associated with mild gastrointestinal upset. The ophthalmic preparations may occasionally cause mild to moderate local symptoms such as itching or stinging.

CLINICAL USE

Fusidic acid has been used in systemic (iv, po) and topical (ophthalmic, skin preparations) formulations primarily for treatment of staphylococcal infections. It is not available in the United States, although it may be obtained through compassionate release. The foci of infection, with and without associated bacteremia, have included acute and chronic osteomyelitis, septic arthritis, endocarditis, soft tissue infections including burns, and lower respiratory tract infections in patients with cystic fibrosis.[12–14]

Endocarditis has been treated with some success using fusidic acid in combination with a second drug. Fusidic acid has been given with a penicillinase-resistant semisynthetic penicillin such as flucloxacillin for staphylococcal endocarditis and with erythromycin for cases caused by diphtheroids.[15,16]

Given the increased incidence of methicillin-resistant *S. au-*

reus and methicillin-resistant *Staphylococcus epidermidis* infections, this drug may offer advantages over currently available agents. Topical use has been limited to external eye infections and superficial skin infections, including erythrasma caused by *Corynebacterium minutissimum.*

Initial concerns about emergence of resistant strains during therapy lead to the practice of combining fusidic acid with a second drug. Resistance may be more likely to occur in the setting of chronic infections if the drug is used alone.[3,17] However, experience over the past few decades has shown that even when used alone for the treatment of acute infections, resistance is seen in only 0–2 percent of cases, whereas resistance occurs in less than 1 percent of cases treated with combination therapy.

REFERENCES

1. Godtfredsen W, Roholt K, Tybring L. Fusidin. A new orally active antibiotic. Lancet. 1962;1:928–31.
2. von Daehne W, Godtfredsen WO, Rasmussen PR. Structure-activity relationships in fusidic acid-type antibiotics. Adv Appl Microbiol. 1979;25:95–146.
3. Shanson DC. Clinical relevance of resistance to fusidic acid in *Staphylococcus aureus*. J Antimicrob Chemother. 1990;25(Suppl B):15–21.
4. Van der Auwera P, Godard C, Denis C, et al. In vitro activities of new antimicrobial agents against multiresistant *Staphylococcus aureus* isolated from septicemic patients during a Belgian national survey from 1983 to 1985. Antimicrob Agents Chemother. 1990;34:2260–2.
5. Verbist L. The antimicrobial activity of fusidic acid. J Antimicrob Chemother. 1990;25(Suppl B):1–5.
6. Steinkraus GE, McCarthy LR. In vitro activity of sodium fusidate against anaerobic bacteria. Antimicrob Agents Chemother. 1979;16:120–2.
7. Foldes M, Munro R, Sorrell TC, et al. In-vitro effects of vancomycin, rifampicin, and fusidic acid, alone and in combination, against methicillin-resistant *Staphylococcus aureus*. J Antimicrob Chemother. 1983;11:21–6.
8. Farber BF, Yee YC, Karchmer AW. Interaction between rifampin and fusidic acid against methicillin-resistant coagulase-positive and -negative staphylococci. Antimicrob Agents Chemother. 1986;30:174–5.
9. Reeves DS. The pharmacokinetics of fusidic acid. J Antimicrob Chemother. 1987;20:467–76.
10. Eykyn SJ. Staphylococcal bacteremia and endocarditis and fusidic acid. J Antimicrob Chemother. 1990;25(Suppl B):33–8.
11. Brodersen R. Fusidic acid binding to serum albumin and interaction with binding of bilirubin. Acta Paediatr Scand. 1985;74:874–80.
12. O'Brien T, McManus F, MacAuley PH, Ennis JT. Acute haematogenous osteomyelitis. J Bone Joint Surg. 1982;64-B:450–3.
13. Gransden WR, Eykyn SJ, Phillips I. *Staphylococcus aureus* bacteraemia: 400 episodes in St. Thomas's Hospital. Br Med J. 1984;288:300–3.
14. Wright GLT, Harper J. Fusidic acid and lincomycin therapy in staphylococcal infections in cystic fibrosis. Lancet. 1970;1:9–14.
15. Moy RJD, George RH, de Giovanni JV, Silove ED. Improving survival in bacterial endocarditis. Arch Dis Child. 1986;61:394–9.
16. Jackson G, Saunders K. Prosthetic valve diphtheroid endocarditis treated with sodium fusidate and erythromycin. Br Heart J. 1973;35:931–6.
17. Faber M, Rosdahl VT. Susceptibility to fusidic acid among Danish *Staphylococcus aureus* strains and fusidic acid consumption. J Antimicrob Chemother. 1990;25(Suppl B):7–14.

20. AMINOGLYCOSIDES

DAVID N. GILBERT

Aminoglycoside antibiotics have been an important part of the antibacterial drug arsenal since the 1940s. They demonstrate concentration-dependent bactericidal activity against susceptible organisms. Several members of the aminoglycoside family have predictable in vitro activity against *Pseudomonas aeruginosa* and the vast majority of other aerobic gram-negative bacilli. Some aminoglycosides have useful activity against mycobacteria; one (paromomycin) has been used to treat selected colonic protozoan pathogens; and a related antibiotic, spectinomycin, has been used to treat infections due to *Neisseria gonorr-*

hoeae. The aminoglycoside antimicrobial activity may be additive or synergistic with penicillin or cephalosporins against infection due to aerobic gram-negative bacilli or aerobic gram-positive cocci. The prevalence of aminoglycoside resistance has remained low and emergence of bacterial resistance during therapy rare.

The aminoglycoside family shares the potential for nephrotoxicity, ototoxicity, and, rarely, neuromuscular blockade. Risk of toxicity may be decreasing as mechanisms are understood, new dosage strategies introduced, concomitant risk factors avoided, and shorter duration of treatment employed. Allergic reactions are rare. With patent expirations, the cost of many aminoglycosides is low. Although new β-lactams and fluoroquinolones share the same antibacterial spectrum, the efficacy of the aminoglycosides and resistance problems with the newer drugs presage a continued need.

NAMES AND SOURCES: INTRODUCTION TO CHEMISTRY

In the 1940s, soil actinomycetes (bacteria) were screened systematically for the elaboration of antimicrobial substances. Streptomycin was the first aminoglycoside found (Table 1).[1] Streptomycin was produced by a *Streptomyces* sp., and subsequent drugs were derived from either other *Streptomyces* spp. or *Micromonospora* spp.[2–5] The suffix indicates the source: that is, aminoglycosides with names ending in *mycin* derive directly or indirectly from *Streptomyces,* while aminoglycosides with names ending in *micin* derive directly or indirectly from *Micromonospora.*

Neomycin, kanamycin, and gentamicin are fermentation products with two or three chemical constituents. Amikacin, netilmicin, dibekacin, and isepamicin are semisynthetic derivatives of the natural product. Nine aminoglycosides (including spectinomycin) are available commercially at this time in the United States, sisomicin, dibekacin, and isepamicin are approved for human use in Japan, Europe, and elsewhere.

CHEMISTRY

Structure

All aminoglycosides have an essential six-membered ring with amino-group substituents and hence the name *aminocyclitol.*[2–5] The descriptor *aminoglycoside* results from the glycosidic bonds between the aminocyclitol and two or more amino-containing or non-amino-containing sugars. Spectinomycin differs

in that there is an aminocyclitol ring but no aminosugars and no glycosidic bonds.

The central aminocyclitol for streptomycin is streptidine, while for all other current aminoglycosides it is 2-deoxystreptamine (Fig. 1). The standard numbering convention is illustrated in Figure 1. Note the counterclockwise numbering of the aminocyclitol ring and the clockwise numbering of linked sugar molecules. Figure 1 also illustrates the structural basis of the aminoglycoside subgroups. Neomycin and paromomycin are derived from *Streptomyces* spp. and link to cyclic sugars at positions 4 and 5 of 2-deoxystreptamine. Both drugs contain a distinctive pentose linkage as well as linkage to two hexose sugars. Note that of the commonly used aminoglycosides neomycin contains the largest number, six, of free amino groups.

Kanamycin, tobramycin, amikacin, and dibekacin constitute the kanamycin family (Table 2).[3–10] All derive from *Streptomyces* spp. and link to cyclic sugars at positions 4 and 6 of 2-deoxystreptamine. Tobramycin is 3'-deoxykanamycin B. Amikacin is kanamycin A with the semisynthetic addition of 2-hydroxy-4-aminobutyric acid to the amino group at position 1 of the aminocyclitol.

Gentamicin is a mixture of three closely related constituents, C_1, C_{1a}, and C_2, elaborated by *Micromonospora* spp. with glycosidic linkages at positions 4 and 6. Sisomicin is the dehydro analog of gentamicin C_{1a}; netilmicin is derived from sisomicin by the addition of an ethyl group to the amino group at position 1 of the aminocyclitol.

There is an incomplete understanding of the aminoglycoside structure–activity relationships. Removal of amino and/or hydroxyl groups results in a concomitant loss of both antibacterial activity and toxic potential.[5–7]

Chemical Characteristics

The aminoglycosides are highly soluble in water and insoluble in organic solvents.[11,12] The latter correlates with the limited ability of aminoglycosides to cross lipid-containing cellular membranes.

The aminoglycosides have a molecular weight in the range of 445–600 Da.[11] The molecular structure is unchanged by freezing, heating to 100°C for up to 4 hours, or changes in solution pH ranging from 3.0 to 12 over several hours.[13–16] The ionization constants for individual amino groups are difficult to determine. The overall pK_a for gentamicin is about pH 8.4.[11] Hence, at pH 7.4, the aminoglycosides have a very high positive charge and are cationic.

TABLE 1. The Family of Aminoglycosides in Clinical Use[a]

Names				
Generic	Proprietary	Source	Year Reported	Chemistry
Streptomycin	None	*Streptomyces griseus*	1944	Unique central aminocyclitrol ring
Neomycin	Mycifradin, neobiotic	*Streptomyces fradiae*	1949	Roughly equal proportion of neomycin B and C
Kanamycin	Kantrex	*Streptomyces kanamyceticus*	1957	Mixture of 95% kanamycin A and 5% kanamycin B
Paromomycin	Humatin	*Streptomyces fradiae*	1959	Part of "neomycin" family
Gentamicin	Garamycin	*Micromonospora purpurea* and *Micromonospora echinospora*	1963	Roughly equal proportion of gentamicin C_1, C_{1a}, C_2
Tobramycin	Nebcin	*Streptomyces tenebrarius*	1968	Natural 3'-deoxy derivative of kanamycin B
Amikacin[b]	Amikin	*Streptomyces kanamyceticus*	1972	Semisynthetic derivative of kanamycin A
Netilmicin[b]	Netromycin	*Micromonospora inyoensis*	1975	N-ethyl derivative of sisomicin
Spectinomycin	Trobicin	*Streptomyces spectabilis*	1962	Chemically distinct but closely related to aminoglycosides
Sisomicin[c]	Siseptin	*Micromonospora inyoensis*	1970	Dehydro-analog of gentamicin C_{1a}
Dibekacin[b,c]	—	*Streptomyces kanamyceticus*	1971	Dideoxy derivative of kanamycin B
Isepamicin[b,c]	—	*Micromonospora purpurea*	1978	I-N-S-alpha hydroxy-B-aminopropionyl derivative of gentamicin B

[a] The drugs are listed by the year they were described with comments on their chemistry.[1–8]
[b] Semisynthetic aminoglycosides.
[c] Approved for human use in countries other than the United States.

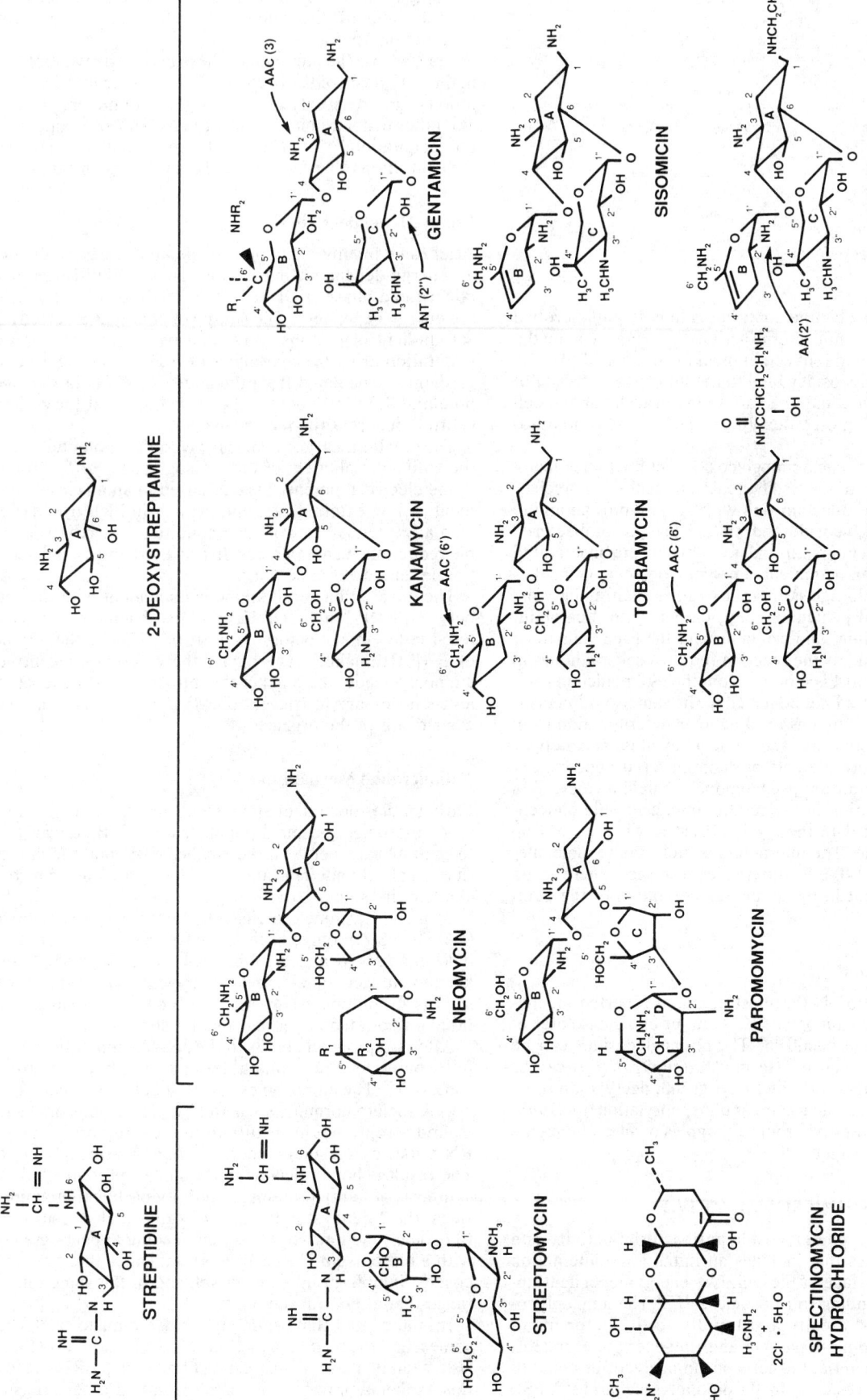

FIG. 1. Chemical structure of the aminoglycosides and spectinomycin. Neomycin contains approximately equal amounts of neomycin B ($R_1 = H$; $R_2 = CH_2NH_2$) and neomycin C ($R_1 = CH_2NH_2$; R_2-H). Kanamycin is principally kanamycin A, as shown. Gentamicin is gentamicin C complex with roughly equal amounts of C_1 ($R_1 = R_2 = CH_3$), C_{1a} ($R_1 = R_2 = H$), and C_2 ($R_1 = CH_3$; $R_2 = H$). The sites of action of four inactivating enzymes are shown; three acetyltransferases (AAC [3], AAC [2'], and AAC [6']) and one adenyltransferase (ANT [2'']).

TABLE 2. Chemical Families of Aminoglycoside Antibiotics

Family	Member
Streptomycin	Streptomycin
Kanamycin	Kanamycin A
	Kanamycin B
	Amikacin
	Tobramycin
	Dibekacin
Gentamicin	Gentamicin C_1, C_{1a}, C_2
	Sisomicin
	Netilmicin
	Isepamicin
Neomycin	Neomycin
	Paromomycin
Spectinomycin[a]	

[a] An aminocyclitol, no glycosidic bonds.

The overall positive charge contributes to both antimicrobial activity and toxicity. Antibacterial activity is enhanced in media with an alkaline pH and reduced in media with an acid pH.[15,16] The cationic aminoglycosides bind to the lipopolysaccharide of the cell wall of bacteria and to a variety of intracellular and cell membrane anionic molecules (e.g., DNA and phospholipids).[17–22]

Of interest, the cationic aminoglycosides interact chemically with β-lactam antibiotics.[23–29] The reaction results in a nucleophilic opening of the β-lactam ring with acylation of an amino group of the aminoglycoside and mutual loss of antibacterial activity. In vitro, gentamicin and tobramycin are inactivated with greater ease than netilmicin, amikacin, or isepamicin. Perhaps because their dosage is in grams rather than milligrams, the antipseudomonal penicillins (e.g., carbenicillin, ticarcillin, piperacillin, mezlocillin, and azlocillin) are the β-lactams most prone to the reaction. As the reaction requires several hours in vitro, the clinical import is limited. Nonetheless, penicillins and aminoglycosides should not be mixed in the same solution prior to infusion. Serum specimens for drug level determination from patients receiving both drugs should be assayed immediately or frozen. If renal failure patients are administered concomitant aminoglycoside and an antipseudomonal penicillin, there is a 10–20 percent reduction in the serum aminoglycoside concentration as compared with the levels observed when each drug is administered alone. The interaction is molecule to molecule, and, because of the 40-fold difference in dosage, there is no discernible decrement in the serum concentration of the penicillin.

Enzymatic Inactivation

Enzymatic inactivation is the most common reported mechanism of resistance to aminoglycosides among clinical isolates of aerobic gram-negative bacilli.[5,30] The aminoglycosides can be inactivated by adenylation (termed *adenyltransferases* or *nucleotidyltransferases*) of a hydroxyl group, acetylation *(acetyltransferase)* of an amino group, or phosphorylation *(phosphotransferases)* of a hydroxyl group. Examples of sites of enzyme activity are shown in Figure 1.

MECHANISM OF ANTIMICROBIAL ACTIVITY

The mechanism of aminoglycoside antibacterial activity is a multifactorial process that includes an initial ionic interaction with the external surface of the cell, two energy-dependent uptake phases, and binding to ribosomes.[5,31–33] The aminoglycosides bind electrostatically and rapidly to the outer membrane.[34–36] The binding is passive and non-energy-dependent. In gram-negative bacteria, the cationic aminoglycosides bind to negatively charged residues in the lipopolysaccharide (LPS), polar heads of phospholipids, and anionic outer membrane proteins.[17,18,32] The aminoglycosides displace competitively cell wall Mg^{2+} and Ca^{2+} that normally link adjacent LPS mole-

cules.[37,38] The result is a rearrangement of LPS with subsequent bleeding of the outer membrane, formation of transient holes in the cell wall, and disruption of the cell wall's normal permeability function.[39]

Once across the membrane, the drugs are irreversibly trapped in the cytoplasm of the bacteria. The trapping may be a manifestation of the reactivity of the charged cationic drugs with DNA and other cellular anionic constituents with subsequent internal coprecipitation.[33,40,41] The result is intracellular aminoglycoside concentrations that far exceed external concentrations.

Energy-Dependent Phase

After ionic binding, aminoglycoside uptake can be divided into an energy-dependent initial slow phase (EDP-I) and a subsequent rapid phase, EDP-II.[5,31–33,42–44] Both EDP-I and EDP-II are energy dependent. The source of energy is an electrochemical gradient of protons, generated by proton extrusion during respiration or by the hydrolysis of ATP.[31] The electrochemical gradient is calculated from the additive effects of the electrical potential difference across the membrane and the proton concentration across the membrane.

The greater the transmembrane electrical potential the greater the antibacterial effect of the aminoglycosides. The transmembrane electrical potential is decreased in an anaerobic environment, a low external pH, and growth in high osmolar culture media.[45,56] Under each of these conditions, there is a demonstrable reduction in aminoglycoside transport and associated reduction in antibacterial activity.

The onset of bacterial killing is coincident with the transient between EDP-I and EDP-II.[42,43] Most bacterial cells have suffered lethal injury before completion of more than 25 percent of EDP-II uptake.[43] The higher the external concentration of aminoglycoside, the quicker the intracellular drug level reaches levels necessary to trigger EDP-II uptake, which in turn forecasts death of the organism.[47]

Antimicrobial Mechanism

Early studies document aminoglycoside interaction with one or more microbial ribosomal-binding sites.[48,49] Binding is localized to the interface between the smaller (30S) and the larger (50S) ribosomal subunit. This area includes several proteins from the smaller ribosomal structure (proteins designated S3, S4, S5, S12) and at least one protein from the larger ribosomal structure (L6).[50–53] Streptomycin binding requires the presence of S12, but binding is localized to the region of S3 and S5. Neomycin, kanamycin, gentamicin, and tobramycin do not bind at the same sites as streptomycin (54). Multiple binding sites have been identified on both the larger and smaller subunits of the ribosomes.

After streptomycin binds to the 30S portion of the ribosomes, polysomes become unstable and break down to monosomes.[55–57] The monosomes can neither initiate chain formation nor dissociate normally so as to free active ribosomal subunits. Bound streptomycin results in misreading of the messenger RNA code as a result of incorrect codon–anticodon interaction. The result is both a decline in the rate of protein synthesis and synthesis of faulty proteins.[58] Activity of the other aminoglycosides, the 2-deoxystreptamine derivatives, also results in faulty ribosome function. However, misreading appears greater than with streptomycin.[59] Recent work indicates that the aminoglycosides inhibit group I intron splicing in the same micromolar range that alters translation.[60]

It is accepted that aminoglycosides bind to bacterial ribosomes, and the result is a measurable decrease in protein synthesis and an increase in misreading of messenger RNA. However, this explanation may be incomplete in that other drugs that inhibit protein synthesis (e.g., chloramphenicol) are only bacteriostatic and not bactericidal.[43,59,61] Bacterial death may be multifactorial.[5,31,33,62] Aminoglycoside binding to, and alteration of, the cell envelope plus ribosomal dysfunction and perhaps other yet unrecognized effects could act in concert to produce a rapid cidal result.[62]

AMINOGLYCOSIDE RESISTANCE

Bacteria defend themselves against aminoglycosides by some combination of three mechanisms: alteration in uptake, synthesis of modifying enzymes, or a change in ribosomal binding sites.[63–65] Enzymatic modification is the most common mechanism.

Enzymatic Modification

Aerobic gram-negative bacteria can alter the aminoglycoside molecule by acetylation of an amino group with acetyltransferases (AAC), adenylation of a hydroxyl group with nucleotidyltransferases (also known as *adenyltransferases*) (ANT), or phosphorylation of a hydroxyl group with phosphotransferases (APH).[5,24] The modified aminoglycoside binds poorly to ribosomes, and the EDP-II of accelerated drug uptake fails to occur; high-level resistance results.[66] An analysis of the enzymatic resistance mechanisms of 4228 clinical isolates collected worldwide between 1987 and 1991 demonstrate a diverse pattern of enzyme production.[30] Of the ACC group, a family of AAC (6′) enzymes is of particular import due to their ability to modify tobramycin, gentamicin, netilmicin, and amikacin (Fig. 1). Eight or more genes encode this enzymatic activity. ANT (2′′) enzymes result in gentamicin, tobramycin, and dibekacin resistance. At least three encoding genes are involved. APH enzymes produce resistance to neomycin, paromomycin, and kanamycin. Overall, the data suggest that most enzyme-mediated aminoglycoside resistance in gram-negative bacilli is due to more than one gene. There may be more homogeneity in the genetic resistance of gram-positive cocci. Aminoglycoside resistance surveys on strains collected prior to 1983 demonstrate a single resistant mechanism (i.e., one aminoglycoside-modifying enzyme).[30] In recent surveys, the majority of resistance strains manifest a combination of several resistance mechanisms. The presence of multiple resistance genes in a single integron is postulated.

Many of the resistance genes are associated with transposable genetic elements. Transposon 21 (Tr 21) is of particular interest in that it contains a region, termed the *integron,* in which many different resistance genes are located.[30] Susceptible bacteria also acquire aminoglycoside-resistance-encoding genes via conjugative or nonconjugative plasmids. The plasmids may encode resistance to other classes of antibiotics as well. The presence of resistance genes as part of movable genetic elements contributes to the rapid dissemination of these genes.

There are two theories as to the origin of aminoglycoside-modifying enzymes.[30] The enzymes may have been derived from the antinomycetes that synthesize the aminoglycosides. The enzymes would provide self-protection against the antibiotic synthesized. Alternatively, the aminoglycoside resistance genes may derive from mutation of genes that encode enzymes involved in normal cellular respiration.

The intracellular location of aminoglycoside-modifying enzymes is debatable. Available data are consistent with localization to the periplasmic space.

There is no evidence of regulation of the aminoglycoside resistance genes; gene transcription, with few exceptions, is constitutive. The enzymes are produced whether or not antibiotic is present. There is no evidence that the antibiotic is needed to induce resistance.

Altered Ribosome-Binding Sites

Although a single mutation of one protein (S12) of the 30S ribosome of a laboratory strain of *Escherichia coli* results in high levels of resistance to streptomycin, it is rare in clinical isolates of gram-negative bacilli.[50] This type of streptomycin resistance is found in clinical isolates of *N. gonorrhoeae* (also spectinomycin resistant) and in enterococci. In contrast to streptomycin, ribosomal resistance is rare as a mechanism of resistance of the deoxystreptamine group of aminoglycosides.

Altered Aminoglycoside Uptake

Mutant aerobic gram-negative bacilli and staphylococci with reduced uptake of aminoglycosides have been identified.[67] There is cross-resistance to all aminoglycosides, but the level of resistance is often less than that resulting from enzymatic modification.[67] In vitro, aminoglycoside concentrations 10 times the minimum inhibitory concentration (MIC) prevents emergence of mutant populations.[68]

Bacterial chromosomal mutations may result in defect(s) that influence any part of the binding and electrochemical gradient that leads to aminoglycoside uptake.[55,67,69,70] Emergence of resistant *Staphylococcus aureus* during aminoglycoside monotherapy is well recognized. The resistant organisms have alterations in their transmembrane electrical potential and/or electron transport chain. The organisms appear as small colonies on culture plates. Although the small colony variants are often less virulent, they are a mechanism of bacterial persistence during aminoglycoside therapy; after cessation of aminoglycoside treatment, the organism can revert to the original virulent phenotype and cause clinical relapse.[71] Concomitant β-lactam therapy should prevent the problem.[67]

A transient resistance to aminoglycosides is observed after the rapid, early concentration-dependent killing of susceptible bacteria.[36,72] The refractory state lasts beyond the postantibiotic effective period into the time of regrowth. This phenomenon is termed *adaptive resistance* rather than *emergence of unstable mutants*. It is believed to result from a temporary disruption of the EDP of aminoglycoside uptake.

The non-energy-dependent phases of uptake may lead to resistance based on altered permeability.[47] Alterations in cell wall lipopolysaccharide have been described for *P. aeruginosa*.

Laboratory isolates of *E. coli* resistant to amikacin have been reported that have both impaired aminoglycoside uptake and aminoglycoside phosphorylation.[73] Combined resistance mechanisms have not yet been reported in clinical isolates.

Aminoglycoside-Resistant Enterococci

There are well-documented cases of infective endocarditis due to enterococci with a high level of resistance to aminoglycosides.[74,75] Resistance results from disruption of the synergistic bactericidal interaction between cell wall active antimicrobials and aminoglycosides that requires enhanced intracellular penetration of the latter in the presence of cell wall active drug. Resistance based on β-lactamase activity or glycopeptide resistance is discussed elsewhere (see Chs. 13 and 179).

Enterococci are intrinsically resistant to low concentrations of aminoglycoside (e.g., 4–250 µg/ml) because of their anaerobic metabolism.[76] Since aminoglycoside uptake requires aerobic oxidative metabolism, enterococcal low-level resistance is believed to reflect a low level of cell membrane oxidative energization that results in poor active transport of drug.[33,77] Transport is also influenced by composition of the cell wall of enterococci.[78]

Resistance of enterococci to aminoglycosides can result from one or more of three mechanisms: alteration of the target site, interference with drug permeability, or enzymatic inactivation of drug. The first two types result from chromosome changes, and the third is usually mediated by plasmids.

There are increasing reports of isolation of enterococci with aminoglycoside MICs of 2000 µg/ml or more; strains with an MIC of 2000 µg/ml or more are arbitrarily defined as showing high-level resistance (HLR) to aminoglycosides.[74,75] The HLR is mediated by modifying enzymes, and, with the exception of a chromosomally encoded AAC (6′) of *Enterococcus faecium,* the responsible genes are found on plasmids.[79-83] Of concern, transposons encoding HLR to gentamicin are recognized.[84]

The modifying enzymes appear to represent a subset of those found in aminoglycoside-resistant staphylococci.[85] There are differences and similarities between the enzymes from gram-positive and gram-negative organisms.[79,86] Regardless of substrate profile differences, all enzymes are synthesized constitutively.[85] Overall, aminoglycoside resistance is determined by the result of the balance between rate of uptake and rate of detoxification of the antibiotic.

Based on the current knowledge of the substrate ranges of aminoglycoside-modifying enzymes from enterococci, some general suggestions include the following[85]: *(1)* In patients with severe enterococcal infection (e.g., endocarditis), the etiologic organism should be tested for HLR to aminoglycosides. *(2)* If there is HLR to streptomycin, streptomycin should not be used in combination with a β-lactam drug. If the HLR is to kanamycin, neither kanamycin nor amikacin should be combined with a β-lactam antibiotic. If the HLR is to gentamicin, then gentamicin, tobramycin, netilmicin, kanamycin, and amikacin should not be used with a beta-lactam. One report describes HLR to gentamicin but susceptibility to streptomycin.[87] *(3)* Results with tobramycin can be extrapolated to dibekacin. *(4)* Gentamicin and sisomicin HLR results are equivalent with the exception of a chromosomally encoded AAC (6′) that confers resistance to sisomicin but not gentamicin. In short, for endocarditis patients, whatever aminoglycoside is employed should be tested against the *Enterococcus* isolated from the patient for HLR.

There are a few clinical isolates of enterococci with HLR to streptomycin apparently on the basis of altered ribosomal affinity.[88] To date, HLR on the basis of impaired cell wall permeability has not been recognized.

Clinical Epidemiology of Aminoglycoside Resistance

In vitro resistance of clinical isolates of aerobic gram-negative bacilli to aminoglycosides varies with the specific drug, the target organism, the nature of the patient population and their underlying disease(s), and local/regional patterns of physician use of specific aminoglycosides. In 1992, at the Oregon Health Sciences University, the overall in vitro resistance of aerobic gram-negative bacilli to gentamicin, tobramycin, and amikacin varied from 0 to 5 percent (Table 3).[89] An exception was the in vitro resistance of 44 percent of *Enterobacter aerogenes* strains to amikacin despite the predominant clinical use of gentamicin. Of the *P. aeruginosa* isolates, 29 percent were resistant to gentamicin, 12 percent to amikacin, and 5 percent to tobramycin.

Selective use of one aminoglycoside, or one family of aminoglycosides, appears to alter subsequent susceptibility patterns. Over a 10 year period, the Minneapolis Veterans Affairs Medical Center monitored aminoglycoside resistance in 25,000 clinical

isolates of gram-negative bacilli while simultaneously controlling aminoglycoside usage.[90] On two occasions, amikacin was made available and became the most frequently prescribed aminoglycoside. On both occasions, there was a significant reduction in resistance of aerobic gram-negative bacilli to gentamicin and tobramycin. With the exception of *P. aeruginosa,* resistance to aminoglycosides remained under 5 percent of clinical isolates at the end of the 10 year period. Similar results were obtained at a university hospital in Louisiana.[91] Prior to the use of amikacin as the dominant aminoglycoside, the rates of resistance among aerobic and facultative gram-negative isolates were 13, 11, and 6 percent for gentamicin, tobramycin, and amikacin, respectively. After 30 months of sole usage of amikacin, the rates of resistance were 6, 4, and 3 percent for gentamicin, tobramycin, and amikacin, respectively. In addition, a decrease in the frequency of bacteremia due to gram-negative bacilli and a decrease in death associated with such bacteremia was observed. In a South African general hospital pediatric service with a high rate of tobramycin, gentamicin, and netilmicin resistance, amikacin was prescribed as the sole aminoglycoside over 18 months.[92] No appreciable amikacin resistance developed, and the resistance to tobramycin, netilmicin, and gentamicin decreased significantly.[92] Exclusive use of one aminoglycoside may eventually lead to resistant organisms. Exclusive amikacin use in a neonatal unit in Johannesburg pediatric unit was followed by an outbreak of *Serratia* spp. resistant to amikacin and an increase in amikacin resistance to other gram-negative pathogens from 8 to 28 percent.[93] Lastly, in Japan, the most commonly prescribed aminoglycosides have been members of the kanamycin family (i.e., kanamycin, amikacin, and dibekacin). Of the aminoglycoside-resistant strains from East Asia, 88 percent were found to have some type of 6′-AAC activity against the kanamycin family of aminoglycosides.[94] Hence, there is at least a strong association between the family of aminoglycoside prescribed and the frequency of aminoglycoside resistance for drugs of that family. Furthermore, the frequency of aminoglycoside resistance for a specific drug correlates with the frequency of usage of that drug or of a closely related aminoglycoside.

In distinction to β-lactams with activity against aerobic gram-negative bacilli, resistance rarely emerges during the course of aminoglycoside therapy. In a study of *Enterobacter* bacteremia in 129 adults, emergence of antimicrobial resistance during 4–18 days of therapy occurred in 6 of 31 patients administered a third-generation cephalosporin (19 percent) and in 1 of 89 patients administered an aminoglycoside (1 percent), $p = 0.001$.[95] Concomitant administration of an aminoglycoside did not decrease the emergence of resistance to the third-generation cephalosporin. This and other studies document the emergence of cephalosporin-resistant aerobic gram-negative bacilli during therapy; in contrast, the evolution of aminoglycoside resistance appears to require either long periods of exposure or a very large inocula of organisms, as is found in patients with burns or cystic fibrosis.

IN VITRO ANTIMICROBIAL ACTIVITY

Clinical Microbiology

The in vitro spectrum of activity of the aminoglycosides is compared with selected β-lactams and fluoroquinolones in Table 4.[96] The aminoglycosides demonstrate concentration-dependent bactericidal activity against a broad spectrum of aerobic and facultative gram-negative bacilli.[15,16,97-101] The spectrum of activity ranges from Enterobacteriaceae to *Pseudomonas* spp. to *Haemophilus* spp. Methicillin-susceptible, but not methicillin-resistant *S. aureus* are inhibited.[101] Streptomycin has the greatest activity in vitro against *Mycobacterium tuberculosis* while amikacin is more active against *Mycobacterium avium-intracellulare* and other atypical mycobacteria.[102-104] Streptomycin is the drug of choice for *Yersinia pestis* infection, and success

TABLE 3. In Vitro Susceptibility of Clinical Isolates of Aerobic Gram-Negative Bacilli at the Oregon Health Sciences University During 1992

Organisms	No. of Isolates	Percent susceptible to		
		Gentamicin	Tobramycin	Amikacin
Enterobacter aerogenes	56	98	100	56
Enterobacter cloacae	284	96	97	100
Escherichia coli	1101	98	99	100
Klebsiella pneumoniae	319	99	99	100
Proteus mirabilis	88	95	98	98
Proteus vulgaris	27	100	100	100
Serratia marcescens	92	100	99	92
Pseudomonas aeruginosa	730	71	95	88

(Data from Oregon Health Sciences University.[89])

TABLE 4. Comparison of the "Usual" In Vitro Spectrum of Activity of Aminoglycosides to Other Classes of Antimicrobial Agents against Selected Microorganisms

Organism	Aminoglycosides							ESP						Monobactam	ESC		Carbapenems		FQ		TMP/SMX
	Strepto-mycin	Kana-mycin	Genta-micin	Tobra-mycin	Ami-kacin	Netil-micin	Spectino-mycin	Ticar-cillin	Mezlo-cillin	Pipera-cillin	Amp/Sulb	Ticar/Clav	Piper/Tazo	Aztreo-nam	Ceftri-axone	Ceftazi-dime	Imi-penem	Mero-penem	Oflox-acin	Cipro-floxacin	
Gram-negative																					
Escherichia coli	+	+	+	+	+	+	0	+	+	+	+	+	+	+	+	+	+	+	+	+	+
Proteus mirabilis	+	+	+	+	+	+	0	+	+	+	+	+	+	+	+	+	+	+	+	+	+
Klebsiella sp.	+	+	+	+	+	+	0	0	+	+	+	+	+	+	+	+	+	+	+	+	+
Enterobacter sp.		0	+	+	+	+	0	+	+	+	+	+	+	+	+	+	+	+	+	0	+
Morganella sp.	+	+	+	+	+	+	0	+	+	+	+	+	+	+	+	+	+	+	+	0	+
Citrobacter sp.			+	+	+	+	0	+	+	+	+	+	+	+	+	+	+	+	+	+	+
Serratia sp.	+	+	+	+	+	+	0	+	+	0	+	+	0	+	+	+	+	+	+	+	+
Salmonella sp.				+		+	0	+	+	+	+	+	+	+	+	+	+		+	+	+
Providencia sp.			+	+	+	+	0	+	+	+	+	+	+	+	+	+	+		+	+	
Aeromonas sp.			+	+	+	+	0	+	+	+	+	+	+	+	+	+	+	+	+	+	+
Acinetobacter sp.		0	0	+	0	+		0	0	0	±	+	+	0	±	+	+		+	+	0
Pseudomonas aeruginosa	0	0	+	+	+	+	0	+	+	+	0	+	+	+	0	+	+		+	+	0
Pseudomonas cepacia	0	0	0	0	0	0	0	0		+	0	+	+	0	+	0	+		0	0	+
Xanthomonas maltophilia	0	0	0	0	0	0	0		±	±	0	+	0	0	0	0	0		0	0	+
Neisseria gonorrhoeae		±	0	0	0	0	+	+	+	+	+	+	+	+	+	+	+		+	+	±
Haemophilus influenzae		+	+	+	+	+	0	±	±	±	+		+	+	+	+	+		+	+	±
Yersinia pestis			+																		
Francisella tularensis	+	+	+																		
Gram-positive																					
Streptococcus pneumoniae	0	0	0	0	0	0	0	+	+	+	+	+	+	0	+	+	+		±	±	+
Staphylococcus aureus (MSSA)	+	+	+	+	+	+	0	0	0	0	+	+	+	0	+	+	+	+	+	+	+
Staphylococcus aureus (MRSA)	0	0	0	0	0	0	0	0	0	0	0	0	0	0	0	0	0		0	0	0
Miscellaneous																					
Mycobacterium tuberculosis	+	0	0	0	+	0	0	0	0	0	0	0	0	0	0	0	0		+	0	0
Mycobacterium avium-intracellulare	0	0	0	0	+	0	0	0	0	0	0	0	0	0	0	0	+		+	0	0
Bacteroides fragilis	0	0	0	0	0	0	0	0	0	0	+	+	+	0	0	0	+		0	0	0

Abbreviations: sensitive (relative degrees of sensitivity are not indicated); +: sensitive; ±: variable; 0: resistant; blank: data not available; ESP: representative extended spectrum penicillins; ESC: representative extended spectrum cephalosporins; FQ: fluoroquinolones; Amp/Sulb: ampicillin sulbactam; Ticar/clav: ticarcillin clavulanate; Piper/Tazo: piperacillin tazobactam; MSSA: methicillin sensitive S. aureus; MRSA: methicillin resistant S. aureus; TMP/SMX: trimethoprim-sulfamethoxazole.

(Adapted from Sanford,[96] with permission.)

with both streptomycin and gentamicin have been reported for *Francisella tularensis* infections.[16] Compared with the other 2-deoxystreptamine aminoglycoside(s), the spectrum of kanamycin is limited by the absence of predictable activity against *P. aeruginosa* and development of resistant Enterobacteriaceae. Equally important are the other bacteria against which the aminoglycosides have no predictable in vitro activity, such as *Streptococcus pneumoniae, Xanthomonas maltophilia, Pseudomonas cepacia, Bacteroides* spp., *Clostridium* spp., and other anaerobic organisms.[15,16,96] Resistance to aminoglycosides is one characteristic used to identify *X. maltophilia* and *P. cepacia* in clinical specimens. There is no clinically significant activity against rickettsia, fungi, *Mycoplasma,* and viruses.

While the spectrum of activity of streptomycin and kanamycin are limited, the spectrum of gentamicin, tobramycin, amikacin, and netilmicin are virtually identical. Table 4 defines *sensitive* as an in vitro MIC/minimum bactericidal concentration (MBC) that is within the range of blood concentrations achieved clinically with traditional twice- or thrice-a-day dosing.[105,106] Table 4 does not indicate relative degrees of in vitro potency. The MIC/MBC of gentamicin against *Serratia* spp. is consistently twofold lower than the other aminoglycosides; the MIC/MBC of tobramycin vs. *P. aeruginosa* is consistently twofold lower than the other aminoglycosides.[15,16,93–97] Although tobramycin is more active in animal models of pneumonia, to date there has been no clinical efficacy data that parallel these in vitro differences.

Aminoglycosides have in vitro activity against *Haemophilus* spp. and *Legionella* spp. but are not employed clinically for infections due to these organisms. *Legionella* are intracellular pathogens, and the intracellular penetration of aminoglycosides is low.[107] Nonetheless, aminoglycosides are used successfully in the treatment of intracellular infections such as brucellosis, tuberculosis, tularemia, and yersiniosis.[16] In vitro, streptomycin, gentamicin, and, to a lesser degree, netilmicin at "therapeutic" concentrations demonstrated cidal activity against intracellular *E. coli*.[108]

Only spectinomycin has been employed clinically for infections due to *N. gonorrhoeae*.[15] Aminoglycosides in combination with other drugs have been used successfully to treat infections due to staphylococci, streptococci, enterococci, *Listeria*, and mycobacteria.

Not shown in Table 4 is the activity of the aminoglycoside paromomycin against intestinal parasites. Paromomycin is too toxic for parenteral administration. Since the drug is not absorbed from the intestinal tract, it can be used safely as an alternative therapy for infections due to *Entamoeba histolytica*.[109] Recent anecdotal reports describe success clinically in acquired immunodeficiency syndrome (AIDS) patients infected with the protozoa *Cryptosporidium parvum*.[110]

As Table 4 indicates, many extended-spectrum penicillins (with and without a β-lactamase inhibitor), the monobactam aztreonam, the carbapenems, extended-spectrum cephalosporins, and the fluoroquinolones share with aminoglycosides the virtue of in vitro activity against a wide spectrum of fermentative and nonfermentative aerobic gram-negative bacilli. Some differences are apparent when other facets of in vitro antimicrobial sensitivity testing are considered.

Aminoglycosides are little influenced by the size of the test inoculum of bacteria; the MIC for 90 percent (MIC_{90}) of test strains is unchanged whether the initial inoculum is 10^5 bacteria/ml or 10^7 bacteria/ml.[15,16,97–101] In contrast, an increase in test inoculum often results in a substantive increase in the MIC_{90} of extended-spectrum penicillins or cephalosporins. Depending on the method employed, the reported percentage of aminoglycoside that is protein bound ranges between 0 and 30 percent and is considered inconsequential.[111] The higher the cation content of test media, the higher the MIC/MBC results vs. *P. aeruginosa* and, to a lesser degree, other gram-negative bacilli. Early in the evaluation of gentamicin, it was recognized that the Ca^{2+} and

Mg^{2+} and, to lesser extent, sodium concentrations of standard agar culture media varied widely from lot to lot.[112] Broth medium has very low concentrations of Ca^{2+} and Mg^{2+}. Subsequently, test culture media have been standardized as Mueller-Hinton broth supplemented with physiologic concentrations of calcium (50 mg/l) and magnesium (25 mg/liter).[113] Since netilmicin activity vs. *P. aeruginosa* is more influenced by the medium cation concentration than are other aminoglycosides, some authors recommend separate media with lower cation supplementation for netilmicin MIC testing.[114] There are no similar standards for cation content of test agar.[115] Some laboratories incorporate P-nitrophenylglycerol (PNPG) into agar susceptibility test media to prevent swarming of *Proteus* spp. PNPG is reported to increase the MIC of aminoglycosides against strains of *P. aeruginosa*.[116] An alkaline medium will yield an erroneously low MIC; an acid medium will yield an erroneously high MIC.[15,16]

Urine is known to inhibit the activity of aminoglycosides against urinary tract pathogens. Inhibition is believed to result from the low pH and high osmolality resulting from high salt and glucose concentrations. In addition, present data support the hypothesis that betaines, normally found in urine, permit expression of increased aminoglycoside resistance.[117] To date, there is no standardization of betaine concentrations in test media.

The other drugs listed in Table 4 were selected because their spectrum includes activity against aerobic gram-negative bacilli. Note the absence of activity of ampicillin/sulbactam, ceftriaxone, ofloxacin, and trimethoprim-sulfamethoxazole against *P. aeruginosa*.

Time Course of In Vitro Antimicrobial Activity

"Time-kill" curves are not practical for routine susceptibility testing but do illustrate three facets of aminoglycosides antibacterial activity: concentration-dependent killing, the presence of a postantibiotic effect (PAE), and synergism with other drugs.[118]

Aminoglycosides are rapidly bactericidal, and their rate of bacterial killing increases as the antibiotic concentration is increased regardless of the inoculum.[119–121] Standard in vitro test systems have a static drug concentration. In vitro kinetic models allow fluctuations of drug concentration that mimic in vivo pharmacokinetics. For netilmicin and amikacin in the latter model, exposure of test bacteria to the 24 hour aminoglycoside dose as a single bolus with the associated high peak drug concentration resulted in faster killing and a larger magnitude of cidal activity as opposed to the same total dose administered in smaller increments at regular intervals.[122,123] In years past, high concentrations were avoided for fear of toxicity. Now, transient high concentrations are considered a virtue and serve as a part of the rationale for once-daily dosing of aminoglycosides. Of interest, β-lactams do not exhibit concentration-dependent killing; bactericidal activity depends on maintaining drug concentrations at or above the target organism's MIC.[124,125]

Postantibiotic Effect

The PAE is the persistent suppression of bacterial growth after short antimicrobial exposure.[126] The PAE can be measured in vitro or in animal models of infection. In vitro, the aminoglycosides consistently demonstrate a PAE that varies from 1 to 3 hours in broth and serum for *P. aeruginosa* and from 0.9 to 2.0 hours for other Enterobacteriaceae.[127] An aminoglycoside PAE can be demonstrated after incubation with *S. aureus* but not after contact with *Strep. pneumoniae*.[125] The higher the initial aminoglycoside concentration, the longer the presence of the aminoglycoside in the culture medium; the smaller the inoculum and the higher the oxygen tension, the longer the PAE.[126–128] The lower the pH of the test medium, the shorter the PAE.[126] For those aerobic or facultative gram-negative rods tested, the combination of a β-lactam and an aminoglycoside results in the PAE of the aminoglycoside.[126] An exception is imipenem; imipenem plus tobramycin or gentamicin enhanced the PAE of the aminoglycoside alone.[129–130] Rifampin had a synergistic enhancement of the PAE induced in *P. aeruginosa* by tobramycin.[127]

An aminoglycoside-induced PAE is the second part of the rationale for once daily dosing of aminoglycosides. The last part is an attenuated risk of toxicity, as discussed below. In contrast, the β-lactam antibiotics, other than the carbapenems, have not demonstrated a PAE against aerobic and facultative gram-negative bacilli.[124–128]

Antimicrobial Synergy

Synergy between an aminoglycoside and a cell wall active antimicrobial (e.g., penicillin, cephalosporin, monobactam, carbapenem, glycopeptide) is a positive interaction.[118,131,132] The effect of the drugs in combination is greater than the anticipated results based on the effect of each individual drug. In short, there is more than an additive influence.

Several laboratory procedures are employed to study drug combinations for evidence of synergism. Although cumbersome and labor intensive, only the time-kill (or killing curve) method detects and quantitates bactericidal activity. The following comments and the data summarized in Table 5 are based on results from time-kill curves.[118] A great many additional studies describe synergism utilizing "checkerboard" or other techniques that indicate bacteriostatic activity as an endpoint and hence are excluded from the table.

The mechanism of aminoglycoside synergistic activity may not be the same for all target organisms. Study of the enterococcus indicates that intracellular accumulation of labeled streptomycin is enhanced significantly in the presence of penicillin or other cell wall active drugs (e.g., bacitracin, vancomycin).[78] Similar enhanced aminoglycoside uptake in the presence of an active cell-wall active drug has been demonstrated with viridans streptococci, *S. aureus,* and *P. aeruginosa*.[118]

The enterococci have been studied extensively since the original description of penicillin-streptomycin synergy in 1947.[133] Subsequently, the concept was extended to viridans streptococci and group B streptococci. Note that no aminoglycoside/cell wall drug combination is indicated as effective for methicillin-resistant *S. aureus.* There are laboratory reports of synergy between cephalothin plus kanamycin and for high concentrations of either oxacillin or cephalothin plus gentamicin.[118] Un-

fortunately, the latter regimens have not proven useful clinically.

There are many time-kill curve studies documenting synergism against *P. aeruginosa* and Enterobacteriaceae.[118,131,132] Because of the rapid bactericidal activity of high aminoglycoside concentrations, low to moderate aminoglycoside concentrations are employed to detect synergistic activity. The clinical inference might be that lower doses of aminoglycoside could be combined effectively with the cell wall active drug; from the opposite perspective, higher doses are desirable to maximize the concentration-dependent bactericidal activity of aminoglycosides.

Of equal import, the bactericidal activity of aminoglycosides can be antagonized by bacteriostatic agents such as chloramphenicol and tetracycline.[118] The mechanism is unclear. Postulates include inhibition of the energy-dependent uptake of aminoglycosides or interference with movement of the ribosome along messenger RNA.

ANTIBACTERIAL EFFICACY IN ANIMAL MODELS OF INFECTION

Historical Perspective

An idealistic goal is an animal model that mimics human infection so that the efficacy of aminoglycoside therapy, alone or in combination, can be maximized while simultaneously minimizing the risk of toxicity.[134] In a critical review of literature published through 1980, the use of aminoglycosides alone was not found very effective in animal models of pyelonephritis, osteomyelitis, endocarditis, peritonitis, and meningitis.[135] Aminoglycosides were more effective in experimental models of pneumonia.[135] In retrospect, the studies reviewed did not consider the influence of dosing regimens, the pretreatment interval, and other variables now recognized to influence therapeutic efficacy. The theoretic value of combined therapy with drugs with different targets of activity was well known, especially with respect to infections with the enterococci; however, cell wall active drugs with a spectrum of activity that included aerobic gram-negative bacilli have only become available in recent years. The bulk of animal model studies since 1980 have focused on pharmacokinetics or combination aminoglycoside/β-lactam therapy.

Aminoglycosides Alone

Several infection models have been used to study the influence of aminoglycoside pharmacokinetics on drug efficacy.[124,126] In

TABLE 5. Selected Examples of In Vitro Synergism of an Aminoglycoside Combined with a Cell Wall Active Antimicrobial[a]

Organism	Aminoglycoside(s)	Cell Wall Active Drug(s)
Enterococci	Streptomycin, kanamycin, gentamicin, tobramycin, netilmicin, sisomicin, amikacin	Penicillin, ampicillin, carbenicillin, nafcillin, vancomycin
Viridans streptococci	Streptomycin	Penicillin
Streptococcus pyogenes	Gentamicin	Penicillin, ampicillin
Staphylococcus aureus, MSSA	Kanamycin, gentamicin, tobramycin, netilmicin, sisomicin	Nafcillin, oxacillin, cephalothin, vancomycin
Staphylococcus aureus, MRSA		Teicoplanin (+ rifampin)
Staphylococcus epidermidis, MSSE	Gentamicin, tobramycin	Vancomycin (+ rifampin)
Staphylococcus epidermidis, MRSE		
Enterobacteriaceae	Gentamicin, tobramycin, amikacin	Piperacillin, cephalothin, cefoxitin, cefotaxime
Pseudomonas aeruginosa	Gentamicin, tobramycin, amikacin, netilmicin, sisomicin	Antipseudomonal penicillins,[b] aztreonam, ceftazidime, imipenem
Listeria monocytogenes	Streptomycin, gentamicin	Penicillin, ampicillin, imipenem
Corynebacteria JK	Gentamicin, tobramycin	Vancomycin, teicoplanin

Abbreviations: MSSA: methicillin-sensitive *S. aureus;* MRSA: methicillin-resistant *S. aureus;* MSSE: methicillin-sensitive *S. epidermidis;* MRSE: methicillin resistant *S. epidermidis.*
[a] Inclusion required killing curve data demonstrating bactericidal activity.
[b] Includes carbenicillin, ticarcillin, mezlocillin, azlocillin, piperacillin.

(Modified from Eliopoulos and Moellering,[118] with permission.)

the infected mouse thigh model, successful outcome of treatment of aerobic gram-negative rod infection correlated with the presence of granulocytes and with the peak serum aminoglycoside concentration.[124,126,127]

The growth of *P. aeruginosa* in thigh muscle increases rapidly in neutropenic mice as opposed to a plateau number of organisms in non-neutropenic animals.[136] Gentamicin therapy results in a rapid and continuing response in normal mice, while neutropenic mice display an initial response followed by, despite continued gentamicin therapy, regrowth with organisms resistant to gentamicin. The overgrowth of these small colony-resistant mutants is prevented by concomitant administration of an active antipseudomonal penicillin (e.g., ticarcillin).

In the neutropenic thigh model, the therapeutic efficacy of aminoglycosides correlated with the peak serum concentration and the area under the concentration curve over time (AUC).[137] Because the half-life of aminoglycosides in small animals is short (less than 1 hour), it is possible to separate the influence of the peak serum concentration from the area under the curve.[124] The short drug half-life also predicts a long time interval of sub-MIC serum levels implying an in vivo postantibiotic effect.

The in vivo PAE of aminoglycosides has been studied in at least five animal models.[126,138,139] Using the neutropenic mouse thigh infected with 15 clinical isolates of Enterobacteriaceae, the in vivo PAE after gentamicin therapy varied from 1.4 to 6.9 hours. In the same model infected with *P. aeruginosa*, increasing the dose of tobramycin fivefold increased the PAE from 2.2 to 7.3 hours.[138] The in vivo PAE is prolonged further in non-neutropenic animals. In experimental thigh infections with *Klebsiella pneumoniae* treated with an aminoglycoside, the PAE ranged from 2.6 hours in granulocytopenic animals to 12.8 hours in non-neutropenic mice.[139] The PAE is prolonged in renal-impaired neutropenic animals as compared with neutropenic mice with normal renal function.[139] Guinea pigs with *P. aeurginosa* pneumonia were treated with once-daily tobramycin.[120] Although drug levels were not directly measured, based on assumed serum levels and quantitation of lung bacteria, the PAE is estimated at 12 or more hours.

Animal models are influenced by other factors as well. In a model of *K. pneumoniae* empyema in rabbits, gentamicin alone effected a cure rate of 60 percent.[140] The cure rate increased to 100 percent in a shorter time when animals were maintained in a hyperbaric oxygen chamber.[140] The age of the experimental infection has a major influence. In both normal and granulocytopenic mice, a pretreatment interval of 6 or more hours abolished the bactericidal activity of gentamicin against *P. aeruginosa* in the thigh.[141]

In short, current animal data on the efficacy of aminoglycosides alone support the administration of large appropriately spaced doses rather than frequent small doses. In neutropenic animals, concomitant administration of an active β-lactam antibiotic was necessary to avoid selection of resistant mutants.

Combination Therapy

The organisms with demonstrable in vitro synergy between an aminoglycoside and a cell wall active antimicrobial are summarized in Table 5.[118,131,135,142–147] Many of the same combinations have been evaluated in animal models of endocarditis, meningitis, pneumonia, peritonitis/bacteremia, pyelonephritis, osteomyelitis, myositis (mouse thigh), subcutaneous infection with and without foreign body, and more. The results can be reviewed by the organ or tissue infected[135] (e.g., endocarditis) or by the etiologic organism.[142] The latter approach is summarized in Table 6. In general, when the etiologic organism is susceptible to both the aminoglycoside and the companion drug, an enhancement of antibacterial activity results. Note the lack of synergy of amikacin plus pefloxacin (a fluorinated quinolone) in a mouse peritonitis model. Although active against different targets, both classes of drugs have an intracellular target; virtually

all studies showing effectiveness of combined therapy utilized a cell wall active drug (β-lactam or glycopeptide) with the aminoglycoside.

Import of Dosing Regimen

For drug–organism combinations without a PAE, there is increasing evidence in support of β-lactam dosage regimens that maintain serum levels above the MIC of the infecting organism for the entire dosage interval.[124,125] In contrast, the optimal dosing regimen for aminoglycosides depends on the specific microbial target. For experimental enterococcal endocarditis, antimicrobial activity was best with frequent doses of aminoglycoside.[142] Presumably, both the penicillin and the aminoglycoside must be present at the same time to facilitate aminoglycoside uptake. In contrast, for penicillin-susceptible streptococcal endocarditis, combinations of penicillin and tobramycin are reported equally effective regardless of total daily dose or dosing regimen.[148] The bactericidal activity of penicillin alone is a likely explanation.

For experimental infections due to aerobic gram-negative bacilli, a single daily dose of aminoglycoside is reported as efficacious as the same total dose divided into multiple administrations.[120,150] The results are consistent with the known concentration-dependent killing and the long in vivo PAE of aminoglycosides. In neutropenic animals, the aminoglycoside PAE is much shorter. In contrast, an effective blood level of a β-lactam must be continuously present to ensure efficacy.[125] Of interest, in the neutropenic murine thigh model, the in vivo PAE was prolonged in animals given combination therapy for infections due to *S. aureus*, *E. coli*, *K. pneumoniae*, and *P. aeruginosa*, providing both the aminoglycoside and the companion drug demonstrated a PAE when used alone.[151]

Prevention of Emergence of Drug Resistance

Aminoglycoside as part of combination therapy may prevent or delay emergence of bacteria resistant to either the aminoglycoside or the comparison drug. In a series of studies, aminoglycosides were shown to reduce, but not fully prevent, the emergence of quinolone-resistant Enterobacteriaceae or *P. aeruginosa* in a murine model of peritonitis.[152–154] Of interest, β-lactams were more effective than the aminoglycosides.

As described above, the concomitant use of an active β-lactam appears to prevent the emergence of gentamicin-resistant subpopulations in neutropenic animals.[136] Another example is the treatment of *P. aeruginosa* soft tissue infection in the neutropenic mouse with carbenicillin or gentamicin plus carbenicillin.[155] In vivo "synergism" was believed to result from suppression by carbenicillin of the emergence of gentamicin-resistant subpopulations.

INTRA-ABDOMINAL PERITONITIS/ABSCESS

Experimental models of intraperitoneal infection differ in that the bacterial inocula is purposefully a polymicrobic mixture of the aerobic and anaerobic flora of the colon. Human or rat pooled colonic content are placed intraperitoneally, and shortly thereafter therapy is initiated.[156,157] In untreated animals, a two-stage disease develops: in the first few days 37 percent of the rats die of acute peritonitis and associated bacteremia; all the survivors developed intra-abdominal abscesses.[158] The early stage is primarily due to aerobic or facultative gram-negative bacilli; the late stage requires both the aerobic gram-negative bacilli and anaerobic gram-negative bacilli. The former includes Enterobacteriaceae and *P. aeruginosa*, while the latter is usually due to *Bacteroides fragilis*, especially heavily encapsulated strains.[159]

Treatment of infected animals with gentamicin markedly reduced mortality but had virtually no influence on the incidence

TABLE 6. Use of Aminoglycosides as part of Combination Therapy against Selected Bacteria in Animal Models of Infection

Organism	Infection (Animal)	Aminoglycoside	Drug(s) Combined with Aminoglycoside	Results
Enterococcus faecalis	Endocarditis (rat, rabbit)			
Penicillin susceptible		S, G	Penicillin/ampicillin	Combination synergistic
Penicillin resistant		S, G	Vancomycin	Combination synergistic
HLR streptomycin, kanamycin		G	Penicillin/ampicillin	Combination synergistic
HLR gentamicin		S (?)	Penicillin/ampicillin	
Enterococcus faecium				
Penicillin susceptible		G	Penicillin	Combination synergistic
Penicillin resistant		G	Penicillin or vancomycin	Penicillin combination failed; vanco effective
Vancomycin resistant, high level		G	Teicoplanin	Combination more effective
Viridans streptococci	Endocarditis (rabbit)	S	Penicillin	Combination synergistic
Staphylococcus aureus MSSA	Endocarditis (rabbit)			
		G	Nafcillin	Combination synergistic
MRSA		None	Vancomyinc + rifampin	Combination effective
Staphylococcus epidermidis MRSE	Endocarditis (rabbit)			
		G	Vancomycin + rifampin	Triple combination more effective
MGRSE		N, A	Amoxicillin/clavulanic acid	Triple combination effective
Enterobacteriaceae Variety of organisms	Peritonitis (mouse)	G, T	Ticarcillin, carbenicillin	Enhanced activity of combination
Escherichia coli	Endocarditis (rabbit)	G	Ceftriaxone + sulbactam	Combination effective
Klebsiella pneumoniae, Pseudomonas aeruginosa, Serratia marcescens	Peritonitis (rats)	A	Imipenem	Enhanced survival with combination
Klebsiella pneumoniae	Pneumonia (neutropenic mice)	G	Ceftazidime	Modest enhanced efficacy
Pseudomonas aeruginosa	Peritonitis (rat, mouse; neutropenic and non-neutropenic)	G, T	Ticarcillin, carbenicillin	Enhanced activity of combination
	Peritonitis (mouse)	A	Pefloxacin	No benefit of combination
	SQ chamber (rabbit)	A	Azlocillin	Combination more effective
	Infected thigh (neutropenic mice)	N	Azlocillin	Combination more effective
	Osteomyelitis (rabbit)	Sis	Carbenicillin	Combination synergistic
	Pneumonia (guinea pig)	T	Ceftazidime	Enhanced activity of combination
Listeria monocytogenes	Meningitis (rabbit)	G	Ampicillin	Enhanced activity of combination

Abbreviations: HLR: high level resistance; MSSA: methicillin-susceptible *S. aureus*; MRSA: methicillin-resistant *S. aureus*; MRSE: methicillin-resistant *S. epidermidis*; MGRSE: methicillin/gentamicin-resistant *S. epidermidis*; S: streptomycin; G: gentamicin; N: netilmicin; A: amikacin; Sis: sisomicin.
(Data from refs. 118, 131, 135, 142–147.)

of abscess formation.[156–159] Treatment with clindamycin or metronidazole reduced the incidence of abscess formation but had no effect on peritonitis/bacteremia or lethality.[160] Combination therapy reduced both acute mortality and late abscess formation.

The role of enterococci in intra-abdominal infections has been controversial. In the rat model, intraperitoneal implantation of only enterococci and *B. fragilis* resulted in abscess formation.[161] The clinical implications are discussed below.

The efficacy of the aminoglycosides has been surprising. Their activity is reduced significantly at low pH, low oxygen tension, and in the presence of drug-binding purulent debris.[15–21] The latter conditions characterize the murine intra-abdominal infection model, and yet beneficial aminoglycoside activity is demonstrable.

PHARMACOLOGY

Administration

Aminoglycosides are administered intravenously over 15–30 minutes. If large single daily doses are prescribed, it is reasonable to extend the infusion to 30–60 minutes to diminish the theoretic risk of a rapid rise in serum concentration that might precipitate neuromuscular blockade. Aminoglycoside administered

intramuscularly is absorbed completely, with maximal serum levels achieved between 30 and 90 minutes.[162] Absorption may be delayed in patients with hypotension and impaired tissue perfusion.

There is minimal absorption of aminoglycosides from the gastrointestinal tract.[163] Nonetheless, instances of deafness have occurred from oral neomycin administered to patients with hepatic encephalopathy and impaired renal function.[164,165] Also, there is theoretical concern of increased absorption in the presence of concomitant inflammatory bowel disease. In contrast, patients with AIDS and severe cryptosporidiosis have ingested large amounts of paromomycin over protracted periods without evidence of toxicity.[110] Other exposures may lead to systemic toxicity. Topical application of aminoglycoside on inflamed skin leads to no or minimal absorption. However, patients with extensive burns or other severe dermal injury may absorb drug and be at risk of toxicity.[166,167] Aminoglycosides can be instilled into either the pleural space or peritoneal cavity. Absorption is rapid, with resultant serum concentrations proportionate to concentration of drug instilled. Use of aminoglycosides in solutions used for abdominal irrigation is not recommended, as rapid absorption with subsequent neuromuscular blockade has been reported.[168] In contrast, aminoglycosides have been administered as a bladder irrigant, an aerosol, and by direct instillation into the lumbar sac or lateral ventricles without evidence of detectable concentrations in the blood.[169–171]

Distribution

As anticipated for drugs with a low level of protein binding of approximately 10 percent and a high level of solubility in water, the aminoglycosides are distributed freely in the vascular space and relatively freely in the interstitial spaces of most tissues.[111] The mean aminoglycoside concentration of interstitial fluids approximates the mean plasma concentration as achieved at steady state after repetitive dosing. The interstitial peak concentrations are lower, the oscillations between peak and trough levels are less, and the rate of elimination slower.[172] In the absence of disease and/or infection, the volume of distribution (V_D) is 0.2–0.3 liter/kg.[173] The V_D increases in edematous states to include ascites, in patients with burns, and in some severe infections. The V_D decreases in obese individuals.[174] Because of their size, polycationic charge, and lipid insolubility, aminoglycosides cross biologic membranes poorly with the exception of renal tubular cells and perhaps inner ear cells that have an inherent transport mechanism. The cells of renal proximal convoluted tubule can concentrate aminoglycosides to levels that exceed those of plasma or interstitial fluid.[175]

Parenteral aminoglycoside administration results in low concentrations of active drug in bronchial secretions.[171] Much higher concentrations can be achieved by administration via aerosol.[176] For success, it is necessary to use an aerosol generator that produces droplets of 1–3 μm in diameter.

Aminoglycosides traverse the blood–cerebrospinal fluid and blood–brain barriers poorly.[177] Penetration is somewhat better in newborns. Lumbar sac administration yields high local cerebrospinal fluid levels but poor intraventricular levels, whereas intraventricular administration results in high concentrations in both ventricular and spinal fluid.[178,179] Hence, the intraventricular route is recommended for meningitis due to aerobic gramnegative bacilli in adults in those rare cases where this therapy is necessary. In the newborn, intraventricular aminoglycoside is no more effective and perhaps more toxic than intravenous administration.[180]

Urine concentrations of aminoglycosides exceed peak plasma levels 25–100-fold within 1 hour of drug administration.[181,182] Due to renal tubular cell absorption and subsequent release, the urine concentrations remain above therapeutic levels for several days after a single dose. After termination of multiple dose regimen, the urine levels remain above therapeutic levels for days with a terminal half-life of 48–200 hours.[182–184]

The aminoglycosides enter synovial fluid easily with subsequent levels only slightly less than simultaneous serum concentrations.[185] The biliary tract is poorly penetrated by aminoglycosides, with bile drug levels only 30 percent of concomitant serum concentrations.[186,187] Aminoglycoside penetration into the tissues of the eye has been studied intensively.[188] Mean vitreous levels are only about 40 percent of serum levels over a 12 hour period.[189] In humans, subconjunctival injections yield high aqueous human levels,[190] but neither systemic nor subconjunctival administration in single doses produces reliable levels in vitreous humor of humans.[191] Direct intravitreal injection is recommended for the treatment of endophthalmitis.[188]

Metabolism

There is no evidence of in vivo metabolism of the aminoglycosides.

Excretion

Of a parenteral dose of aminoglycosides, 99 percent is excreted unchanged by the kidney. Less than 1 percent is eliminated in the feces and 1 percent in saliva.[192] Aminoglycosides undergo glomerular filtration. In animals, approximately 5 percent binds to the brush border of renal proximal tubular cells and is reabsorbed.[175,193–195] The tubular cell handling of the drug is discussed below under Toxicity. Reabsorbed drug is returned to tubular lumen and excreted. With normal renal function in adults, more than 90 percent of an administered dose is recovered in urine unchanged during the first 24 hours.[192,196] The remainder is slowly recycled to the tubular lumen with a tissue half-life of 30–700 hours.[196,197] Drug can be detected in urine for 20 days or longer after discontinuation of therapy.

Pharmacokinetics

All the aminoglycosides have similar pharmcokinetics. The pharmacokinetics occur in three interrelated phases.[198] The first (or alpha or distributive) phase is the result of drug distribution from the vascular to the extravascular space. This occurs with a half life, $T_{1/2}$, of 15–30 minutes.[198] It is suggested that "peak" aminoglycoside serum levels be drawn 30 minutes after the end of an intravenous infusion. As the infusion is often over 15–30 minutes, it is convenient to request that the serum be collected 1 hour after the start of the drug administration.

The second (or beta) phase of elimination results from excretion of drug from plasma and extravascular space. The second phase is determined by the glomerular filtration rate and hence is of greatest import in clinical dosage regimens. In adults and infants older than 6 months with normal renal function, the $T_{1/2}$ of all the aminoglycosides are similar and range from 1.5 to 3.5 hours.[173,199–202] The $T_{1/2}$ in infants less than 1 week old or in low-birth-weight prematures can be 8–11 hours.[203] The $T_{1/2}$ in neonates who weight over 2 kg is roughly 5 hours.[203] The $T_{1/2}$ is shortened in febrile illnesses and progressively prolonged with any process that decreases renal function. Prolongation of $T_{1/2}$ in the elderly is the result of age-related decrements in renal function.[204]

The third (or gamma) phase is the prolonged and slow elimination of drug that has accumulated in the kidney. The third phase is not considered in dosage calculations. Clinical dosing procedures are presented below.

TOXICITY

General

With the exception of the aminocyclitol spectinomycin, the aminoglycoside antibiotics share the potential for causing injury to the renal proximal convoluted tubules, damage to the cochlea and/or vestibular apparatus, and neuromuscular blockade (Table 7).[168,205,206] The inherent toxicity and relative toxic potential of the aminoglycosides correlates with their positive electrical charge at physiologic pH.[11] At intracellular sites, the pH is lower and the drugs more cationic.

Also important are those untoward effects that are encountered rarely. Hypersensitivity reactions are uncommon. The aminoglycosides do not provoke inflammation; hence, phlebitis at iv infusion sites is rare; im injection sites do not become painful; instillation into the pleural space, abdominal cavity, and cerebrospinal fluid is free of irritation; and incorporation into methylmethacrylate prosthetic joint cement is well tolerated over protracted periods. The aminoglycosides are not hepato-

TABLE 7. Estimated Frequency of Serious Adverse Reactions after Administration of Aminoglycoside Antibiotics[a]

Adverse Reaction	Estimated Frequency (%)
Nephrotoxicity	0–50 (205, 280–287)
Ototoxicity	
Cochlear	0–62 (206, 308, 309, 330, 332)
Vestibular	0–19 (206, 327, 328, 330, 332)
Neuromuscular blockade	Exceedingly rare (335)

[a] See text for explanation of large range. Numbers in parentheses are references.

toxic, do not induce photosensitivity, and have no identified adverse influence on hematopoiesis or the coagulation cascade.

Nephrotoxicity

Experimental Nephrotoxicity. PATHOGENESIS. Attempts to elucidate the mechanism(s) of aminoglycoside-induced injury of renal proximal tubular cells have utilized isolated enzyme systems, cell membrane vesicles, tissue culture of tubular cells, isolated perfused kidneys, and animal models—with and without active infection. A role for a genetic predisposition is suggested by differences in susceptibility between rats, rabbit, and other animals, and between inbred strains of a specific animal.[207] Furthermore, recent preliminary data indicate that a lymphocyte-mediated inflammatory response is necessary for the expression of tubular injury.[208]

Based on the accumulated current knowledge, a postulate of the pathophysiology of renal tubular damage can be constructed (Fig. 2) and thereby summarize a large body of research.[20,175,193,194,209–224] It has been suggested that the aminoglycosides bind to specific receptors and then undergo endocytosis via the same mechanism used to "scavenge" amino acids, small peptides, and perhaps polyamines from the glomerular filtrate.[225,226] Interaction of drug with the cells lining the S_1 and S_2 portions of the proximal convoluted tubules is manifest by an increase in the excretion of brush border enzymes; this enzymuria occurs after a single dose of drug and hence is too sensitive and does not serve as a useful clinical marker of toxicity.[212,213] Also, there is rapid increase in calcium and, to a lesser extent, magnesium

excretion.[214,215] The phosphatidylinositol (PI) membrane cascade serves a messenger function. In vitro and in vivo evidence indicates aminoglycoside disruption of agonist activation of the PI cascade, perhaps by binding between the polycationic drug and the polyanionic phosphatidylinositol 4,5-biphosphate.[20,216,217,227]

What is known about the intracellular pathways of aminoglycosides is consistent with knowledge of other ligands that undergo receptor-mediated endocytosis.[220] Delineation of movement of aminoglycosides within the cell has been technically difficult. Autoradiograph studies are by nature discontinuous but do document rapid uptake and localization in lysosomes within 1 hour.[175,193–195] The technique of videomicroscopy with fluoresceinated aminoglycoside allows continuous observation of drug movement in living cells. With the latter technique, aminoglycosides localize as early as 15 minutes in the perinuclear region, suggesting interaction with the Golgi apparatus and/or endoplasmic reticulum.[221] After an hour or more, localization to lysosomes is observed.[175,193–195] Lysosome interaction results in deposition of osmiophilic-membrane-appearing material in a layered whorl-like pattern that vaguely resembles myelin by electron microscopy and hence the term *myeloid body* (also called *cytosegresomes*).[20] In intact animals, myeloid bodies can be found in voided urine presumably as a result of lysosomal excretion. Myeloid bodies may result from inhibition of lysosomal enzymes by aminoglycosides.[20] Cell injury due to lysosome "phospholipidosis" is one postulated mechanism of drug-induced toxicity.[20,227] Myeloid bodies are

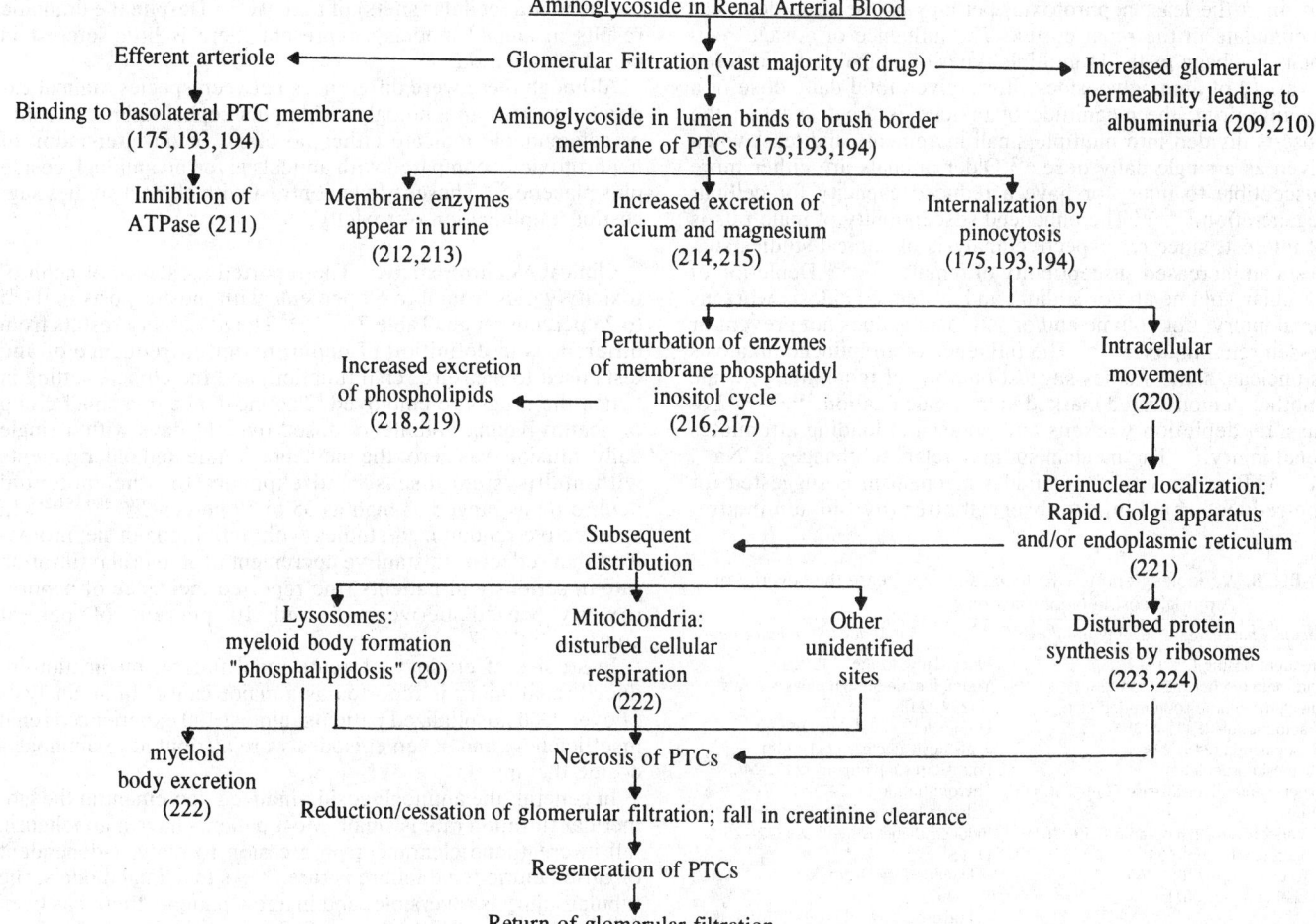

FIG. 2. A proposed pathway of the handling of aminoglycosides by the renal proximal tubular cells (PTCs). (Numbers in parentheses are references.)

not unique to aminoglycosides; they occur after administration of a wide variety of other cationic amphiphilic drugs.[227]

The aminoglycosides cause dysfunction of a variety of other cellular organelles and enzymes. It is unclear whether these toxicities represent primary sites of injury or reflect secondary dysfunction in a damaged or injured cell. Ribosomes, mitochondria, membrane Na^+, K^+-ATPase functional abnormalities are reported.[211,222–224] It is not yet clear which mechanism is primary and which are epiphenomena resulting from cell damage. Irreversible cell death is associated with changes in the intracellular compartmentalization of calcium.[227]

There is no agreement as to how injury and/or death of proximal tubular cells results in a fall in the glomerular filtration rate. Theories include (1) a release of vasoconstrictive hormones effecting the afferent arterioles; (2) backleak of waste products across damaged epithelium; (3) cellular debris obstructing individual nephrons; (4) or a change in glomerular fenestrae, with a decrease in the glomerular ultrafiltration coefficient.[205] One or a combination of these mechanisms may be operative.

Whatever the mechanism(s), the cell is relatively resistant. In intact animals given purposefully toxic doses, several days of drug administration are necessary before functional or anatomic evidence of toxicity occurs. Furthermore, aminoglycoside-induced renal tubular necrosis is reversible. Remarkably, the tubular cells can regenerate despite continued administration of the aminoglycoside.[228]

VARIABLES. Animal models, particularly with the rat, have been studied to delineate variables that may have clinical import or elucidate pathophysiology. Selected examples are summarized in Table 8. There is a hierarchy of nephrotoxic potential among the aminoglycosides.[229–231] Neomycin is the most toxic aminoglycoside precluding parenteral administration. Streptomycin is the least nephrotoxic, perhaps as the drug does not accumulate in the renal cortex. The influence of dosage regimens has been tested in multiple types of animals administered a variety of aminoglycosides. For a given total daily dose of a specific drug, the magnitude of toxicity is greatest when the dose is divided into multiple small increments and least when given as a single daily dose.[232] Older animals are either more susceptible to injury or have a reduced capacity for cellular regeneration.[234–237] The enhanced susceptibility of male rats is of interest, since retrospective analysis of clinical studies suggests an increased susceptibility of females.[238–240] Depletion of vascular volume and/or sodium and systemic acidosis worsens renal injury, but volume and/or salt loading does not prevent or lessen renal injury.[241,242] The influence of an induced alkalosis is unclear; some studies suggest blunting of renal injury, while another demonstrated marked kidney calcification.[241,243,244] Potassium depletion worsens and potassium loading attenuates renal injury.[245] The mechanism may relate to changes in Na^+, K^+-ATPase activity.[246] A similar mechanism is suggested for the reduced renal injury observed after thyroid administra-

tion.[247] Loop diuretics may amplify toxicity via volume depletion, hypokalemia, or acceleration of drug uptake by renal cells.[248,249]

Dietary calcium loading ameliorates gentamicin-induced acute renal failure and the associated decline in mitochondrial function.[250–252] The mechanism of protection remains unclear.[215,253]

The influence of experimental liver disease on aminoglycoside nephrotoxicity is unclear. One report describes amplification of drug-induced renal injury by experimental extrahepatic cholestasis.[254] A second study found no influence of experimental cirrhosis on the severity of aminoglycoside nephrotoxicity.[255] The accumulated clinical data indicate that concomitant liver disease is a risk factor for nephrotoxicity.

Animals with streptozotocin-induced experimental diabetes are reported to have attenuated aminoglycoside nephrotoxicity.[257,258] The mechanism and clinical relevance of this observation are unclear.

Various drugs influence the severity of experimental aminoglycoside nephrotoxicity. Vancomycin and the related drug teicoplanin amplify experimental aminoglycoside nephrotoxicity.[259,260] Neither drug alone exhibits a toxic potential. Of interest, vancomycin interacts with the kidney at sites other than the proximal tubular cell.[261] The extended-spectrum penicillins lower the risk of kidney injury.[262] Some data suggest that the protection is the result of the high sodium content of the penicillin salts.[263]

Polymers of aspartic acid dramatically reduce renal tubular injury despite accumulation of very high renal concentrations of aminoglycoside.[268–278] It is postulated that the anionic polyaspartic acid complexes the cationic aminoglycoside in cytoplasmic vacuoles and thereby precludes movement of aminoglycoside to intracellular site(s) of toxicity.[277] Despite the dramatic results in animal models, at present there is little interest in clinical evaluation.

Although there were differences between species, animal experiments with an aminoglycoside plus cephalothin, cefazolin, or cefamandole indicate either no effect or an attenuation of nephrotoxicity compared with animals given an aminoglycoside plus placebo.[279] These results contrast with clinical studies suggesting amplification of toxicity.

Clinical Nephrotoxicity. The reported incidence of nephrotoxicity varies from 0 to 50 percent, with most reports in the 5 to 25 percent range (Table 7).[279–287] The variability results from differences in definition of nephrotoxicity, frequence of and tests used to measure renal function, and the clinical setting in which the drugs are employed. The incidence in a small group of healthy young volunteers dosed over 11 days with a single daily infusion was zero; the incidence in infected older patients with multisystem disease and exposure to other potential nephrotoxins ranged as high as 35 to 50 percent.[205,280,281,288] In prospective randomized studies with definitions of nephrotoxicity that reflect a substantive decrement in glomerular filtration rate in seriously ill patients, the reported incidence of nephrotoxicity varied between 5 and 10 percent of patient courses.[282–287]

In studies of etiology of acute renal failure, medication-induced renal injury is reported as a major cause. In an analysis of over 2000 hospitalized patients, almost 100 experienced renal insufficiency, and seven episodes were attributed to aminoglycoside therapy.[289]

In general, the aminoglycoside-induced decrement in the glomerular filtration rate is small. Most patients have a nonoliguric fall in creatinine clearance; progression to dialysis-dependent oliguric–anuric renal failure is rare.[205] As in animal models, the tubular injury is reversible, and in a few patients there has been documented recovery of renal function despite continued administration of the aminoglycoside.[290]

Reported risk factors for aminoglycoside nephrotoxicity are

TABLE 8. Variables Reported To Increase or Decrease the Severity of Aminoglycoside Nephrotoxicity[a]

Factors That Increase Severity of Injury	Factors That Reduce Severity of Injury
Frequent dosing (232)	Once-daily dosing (232, 233)
Old male Fischer rats (234–238)	Young female Sprague-Dawley rats (234–238)
Infected, volume sodium-depleted, acidotic rats (241, 242)	Uninfected, euvolemic, role of alkalosis unclear (241–244)
Hypokalemia (245, 246)	Potassium supplements (245, 246)
Magnesium depletion	Thyroid hormone (247)
Experimental liver disease (254–256)	Calcium loading (250–253)
Drugs	Induced diabetes mellitus (257–258)
Vancomycin, teicoplanin (259–261)	Drugs
Methoxyflurane (264)	Extended-spectrum penicillins[b] (262, 263)
Cyclosporine (265, 266)	Polyaspartic acid (268–278)
cis-Platinum (267)	? Cephalothin (279)

[a] Numbers in parentheses are references.
[b] For example, carbenicillin, ticarcillin, mezlocillin, piperacillin.

TABLE 9. Risk Factors for Aminoglycoside Nephrotoxicity

Factors That Increase Risk of Toxicity	Factors That Decrease Risk of Toxicity
Patient factors	Patient factors
Older patients[a]	Younger patients[a]
Preexisting renal disease	Normal renal function
Female gender[b] (239); male gender (285)	
Volume depletion, hypotension[a]	Normotensive[a]
Hepatic dysfunction[b] (256, 291)	No hepatic dysfunction[b]
Aminoglycoside factors	Aminoglycoside factors
Recent aminoglycoside therapy[b]	No recent aminoglycoside therapy[b]
With larger doses[a]	With smaller doses[a]
Treatment of 3 or more days[a]	Treatment less than 3 days[a]
Drug choice, e.g., gentamicin[a] (283)	Drug choice, e.g., tobramycin[a] (283)
Frequent dosing interval[a] (150, 292–294)	Once-daily dosing[a] (150, 292–294)
Concomitant drugs	Concomitant drugs
Vancomycin[a] (295–297)	Extended spectrum penicillins[a,c] (298)
Amphotericin B	
Furosemide	
Clindamycin	
Piperacillin	
Cephalosporins (299–301)	
Methoxyflurane (302)	
Foscarnet[d]	
Intravenous radiocontrast agents[d]	

[a] In concurrence with experimental nephrotoxocity data.
[b] Contrary to experimental nephrotoxicity data.
[c] Extended-spectrum penicillins, e.g., carbenicillin, ticarcillin.
[d] Additive risk postulated.

(Data are from refs. 239, 240, 281, 285, and from those references given in parentheses.)

summarized in Table 9.[239,240,280,281,285] The factors listed can be grouped as relating to the patient, to the aminoglycoside, and to the influence of the selected concomitant drug. Many of the factors identified in clinical trials concur with data from animal models of nephrotoxicity. Female gender was identified as a risk factor in one study but not confirmed in others.[239,280,286,287] In a retrospective analysis, male gender was a risk factor.[285] Reported clinical studies with cephalosporins do not include an aminoglycoside-only group of patients, and hence it is not possible to ascertain if the cephalosporins had no influence, increased the risk, or decreased the risk of nephrotoxicity.

The correlation of increased risk of toxicity with age and/or preexisting renal disease may be misleading. It is unclear whether a risk exists when the dosing regimen is adjusted for preexisting decrease in glomerular filtration rate.

Hypotensive patients, especially those with septic shock or sepsis syndrome, have an increased incidence of renal insufficiency. The role of aminoglycosides is unclear in that infection-related low perfusion, consumptive coagulopathy, cytokine-mediated endothelial damage and other factors may be etiologic in the fall in glomerular filtration rate.

Liver disease was identified as a risk factor in the retrospective analysis of two large clinical trials and then was validated in two additional prospective trials.[256] Further support derives from a retrospective review of aminoglycoside-treated patients with biliary obstruction and/or cholangitis.[291]

The significance of recent aminoglycoside therapy is hard to define. In animals, the pattern of injury is cyclical. Administration of more aminoglycoside during the renal saturation phase may increase risk, while risk may be decreased if more drug is given when the tubular cells are in a regenerative phase.

Clinical trial data support the notion of a need for several days of therapy to cause nephrotoxicity of clinical consequence. In contrast, accidental massive overdosage of 1 day or less has not resulted in acute tubular necrosis.[303,304]

In the rat model of nephrotoxicity, tobramycin was found less nephrotoxic than gentamicin.[230] This hypothesis was tested in a randomized prospective clinical trial. The results indicated a lower incidence of nephrotoxicity in tobramycin recipients, but controversy surrounds the study methods and data interpreta-

tion.[283] The results of subsequent trials were mixed. Amikacin and gentamicin were found equivalent with respect to risk of nephrotoxicity.[282] One study reported a lower incidence of renal injury in netilmicin recipients than in patients administered tobramycin.[286]

Several international trials have compared traditional two-to-three-times-a-day dosing with a single daily administration.[150] In small groups of patients, no difference in efficacy or risk of toxicity was found. In recent larger studies, both delay in onset and reduction in incidence of nephrotoxicity are reported in adult and pediatric populations.[292–294] Details of dosing are described below.

The influence of concomitant drugs is difficult to interpret in patients with serious and/or complex disease states who are receiving multiple pharmaceuticals. Nonetheless, the majority of studies suggest an increased risk of fall in glomerular filtration rate when patients are administered the drugs listed in Table 9 concomitant with aminoglycosides.[239,240,280,281,285] The data are not always conclusive in that many studies suffer from the absence of a matched patient population given only an aminoglycoside. Three prospective studies, one of which was double blind, found the combination of cephalothin plus aminoglycoside more nephrotoxic than a penicillin derivative plus an aminoglycoside.[299–301] Subsequent multiple logistic regression risk factor analysis identified a variety of cephalosporins as risk factors. Two studies evaluated concomitant vancomycin; one analysis included a control group that received only an aminoglycoside.[295,296] Both studies indicated vancomycin was a risk factor. In children, vancomycin was not found to be a risk factor.[297]

In febrile neutropenic patients administered gentamicin or tobramycin plus carbenicillin or ticarcillin, the reported incidence of nephrotoxicity is 2–6 percent as compared with 10–15 percent or higher when the aminoglycoside is combined with other β-lactam antibiotics.[299,300] Of interest, a recent risk factor analysis found an increased risk with concomitant piperacillin but not carbenicillin or ticarcillin.[285] The authors speculated that the lower sodium content of piperacillin may explain the difference.[263]

Some concomitant drugs identified as risk factors intuitively made sense because the drug has its own inherent potential kidney toxicity (e.g., amphotericin B); some drugs may act indirectly by altering intravascular volume or electrolyte concentrations (e.g., furosemide); some are of theoretic concern because of their own inherent toxicity potential (e.g., foscarnet, iv radiocontrast agents); and some statistically identified risk factors defy explanation at present (e.g., clindamycin). Lastly, note that two drugs that amplify aminoglycoside experimental nephrotoxicity, cyclosporin and cis-platinum, do not appear to increase the risk of clinical nephrotoxicity in their clinical application.[265–267,305,306]

If deterioration of renal function occurs, it is advisable to discontinue aminoglycoside therapy. Spontaneous recovery occurs within a few days in the absence of other nephrotoxins, hypotension, renal cortical necrosis of another etiology, or other clinical factors. Progression to anuric renal failure is uncommon. In those patients in whom it is inadvisable to discontinue therapy (e.g., those with *P. aeruginosa* endocarditis), the aminoglycoside dosage is adjusted and therapy continued. Recovery of renal function concomitant with continued aminoglycoside therapy has been reported.[290]

Serum Levels and Nephrotoxicity. Note that serum levels are not included as a risk factor, although they are frequently identified as such.[239,240,285] In experimental animals and presumably in patients, the higher the dose of aminoglycoside, the higher the serum levels, the greater the area under the time-concentration curve, and the greater the risk of toxicity. Measurement of peak serum concentration is indicated to ensure that enough drug was given for antibacterial efficacy and to avoid a large overdosage. Trough levels are obtained to ensure the adequacy of renal clearance of drug. A high trough concentration is a reflection of impaired renal clearance of drug and indicates the need to adjust the dosage regimen as discussed below.

Ototoxicity

The aminoglycoside antibiotics may cause cochlear and vestibular damage in both experimental animals and humans. Streptomycin-induced hearing loss and dizziness were included in the first clinical report of the drug's efficacy.[307] Ototoxicity is of particular concern because it is usually irreversible and can appear after the end of treatment, and repeated exposures engender cumulative risk.[206] Because the target sites of injury are small and buried in bone, studies dealing with pathophysiology are fewer in number than those addressing nephrotoxicity. A given patient may suffer just cochlear damage, just vestibular damage, or rarely both organs are injured.

Cochlear Toxicity. INCIDENCE. Few recipients of aminoglycoside therapy complain of hearing loss, and yet the reported incidence is as high as 62 percent when asymptomatic high-frequency audiograms are performed repeatedly.[308] An overall incidence is quoted as 3–14 percent.[309]

Normal sound perception extends to frequencies of 20 kHz. The outer hair cells in the basal turn of the cochlea are most susceptible to aminoglycoside damage; the basal turn is the site of detection of high-frequency sound.[206] Perception of human speech requires sound detection in the 0.3–3 kHz range. Even in the speech frequency range, a loss of hearing threshold of 25–30 dB is necessary before the patient is aware of the deficit. Hence, considerable cochlear damage can occur without patient recognition. Further detection is difficult in ill patients with impaired cognition. Lastly, many audiometers do not test frequencies above 8 kHz.

Another problem in ascertaining incidence is the absence of a universally accepted definition for drug-induced ototoxicity. A commonly used definition is an increase in auditory threshold of 15 dB or greater at any of two or more frequencies.[206]

Controlled data on cochlear toxicity are sparse. In healthy adult male volunteers administered kanamycin sulfate, cochlear toxicity developed in 17 percent.[310] In contrast, ototoxicity was reported in 7.4 percent of infected patients treated with cefotaxime.[281] Also as a comparison, hearing deficits developed in 15 of 27 patients admitted to the hospital without exposure to antimicrobials or other known ototoxins.[311] In a series of prospective clinical studies that compared the efficacy and toxicity of gentamicin, tobramycin, or amikacin in combination with β-lactam antibiotics, 22 percent of the aminoglycoside recipients had documented audiometric toxicity; all but one patient had hearing loss at 4 or 8 kHz (312). Frequencies over 8 kHz were not tested. In a different study of 53 subjects administered gentamicin, tobramycin, or amikacin for at least 4 days tested at frequencies up to 20 kHz, 33 of the 53 patients suffered either a 20 dB or greater loss at one frequency, or a 10 dB or greater loss at two consecutive frequencies, or loss of response at three consecutive frequencies.[308] Of the ears with damage, 62 percent demonstrated hearing loss initially at or above 9 kHz.[308] Loss was unilateral in 55 percent and bilateral in 45 percent of patients. Treatment ranged from 4 to 32 days, and hearing loss was initially detected after a mean of 9 days of therapy.

Recent reports have suggested a molecular basis for human hypersensitivity to aminoglycoside antibiotics. Individuals with a specific mitochondrial DNA polymorphism were associated with aminoglycoside-induced deafness in two Japanese pedigrees.[312a] The same nucleotide mutation was found, rarely, in sporadic cases of aminiglycoside-induced deafness.[312b]

PATHOPHYSIOLOGY. Aminoglycosides are accumulated in the cochlear hair cells from drug in the bathing perilymph.[313] In the rat, hair cell uptake is rapid, dose dependent, and demonstrates both early saturation and an increasing tissue half-life

with prolonged dosing.[313] Phosphatidylinositol has been suggested as the aminoglycoside receptor.[314] In contrast to the cells of the renal proximal tubule, drug concentrations in inner ear tissue do not exceed plasma concentrations.[313] Binding of aminoglycoside to the plasma membrane of hair cells creates acute electrophysiologic changes that are antagonized by calcium.[315] Drug uptake by hair cells is energy dependent.[316]

Immunocytochemical studies demonstrate localization of gentamicin to the inner and outer hair cells of the organ of Corti.[317] Overall evidence suggests a cell traffic pattern similar to the kidney cells: endocytosis followed by transfer to the endoplasmic reticulum, Golgi complex and lysosomes.[317] Although originally considered irreversible, clinical reports and laboratory experiments document at least some potential for regeneration of hair cells.[318–320]

RISK FACTORS. Risk factors have been assessed in animal models of cochlear injury. Many of the results parallel those observed in the rat model of nephrotoxicity. To whit, toxicity is related to the dose and duration of aminoglycoside.[321] There is a hierarchy of toxic potential with neomycin the most toxic, followed in descending order by gentamicin, tobramycin, amikacin, and netilmicin.[321] Concomitant "loop" diuretics, vancomycin, and loud ambient noise increase the risk.[322–324] Once-daily dosing decreases the risk compared with the same total daily dose administered at frequent intervals or by continuous infusion.[325,326]

Risk factor analysis of human trials is difficult to assess in that patients were not studied for high-frequency hearing loss, and baseline data cannot be obtained with confidence in ill, febrile patients. Nonetheless, retrospective stepwise discriminant analysis of 135 patients enrolled in prospective double-blind clinical trials of aminoglycosides identified treatment duration, associated bacteremia, hypovolemia, degree of temperature elevation, and liver dysfunction as risk factors.[327] Another group employed multivariate analysis and identified only age as a risk factor.[328] With the currently available data, it is difficult to ascertain measurable differences in risk of cochlear toxicity between gentamicin, tobramycin, amikacin, and netilmicin.[309,329] In one study, netilmicin was found less cochleotoxic than tobramycin.[286] The development of renal impairment for whatever reason and a failure to lower the aminoglycoside daily dose, or to discontinue the aminoglycoside, results in higher serum levels, greater perilymph drug concentrations, and an increased risk of toxicity.[330]

CLINICAL FEATURES. Cochlear toxicity may be unilateral or bilateral.[330–333] Injury may occur days to weeks after termination of drug administration. Cochlear injury may be independent of nephrotoxicity. The cumulative dose and duration of therapy are more important than serum concentrations.

The risk of either cochlear or vestibular toxicity is greater in patients with renal impairment.[330] The use of neomycin, regardless of the route of administration (e.g., oral, intraperitoneal, topical on open wounds, or bladder irrigation), is particularly hazardous.[330]

High-frequency hearing loss can occur with no symptoms. Conversational hearing loss can occur without warning. Some patients complain of tinnitus or a sensation of "fullness in the ears," which may represent early injury.

Vestibular Toxicity. The target of drug toxicity is the type I hair cell of the summit of the ampullar cristae.[334] The true incidence of vestibular toxicity in ill patients is virtually impossible to determine.[331,332] Since vestibular injury can be compensated by visual and proprioceptive cues, patients can suffer considerable injury prior to the appearance of symptoms or clinical findings. Suspicion is raised at the bedside by complaints of nausea, vomiting, and vertigo. Symptoms are exacerbated in the dark, when the eyes are closed, or in other situations that block compensatory pathways. Nystagmus may be evident. Systematic surveillance of patients with electronystagmography (EMG) is seldom performed; in one clinical study utilizing EMG surveillance, abnormalities were found in 4–6 percent of patients receiving gentamicin or amikacin.[286,287,333]

Prevention. When aminoglycoside therapy is indicated, the risk of ototoxicity can be minimized by as short a duration of therapy as is clinically appropriate and by periodic assessments of renal function to avoid rising serum concentrations. If high-frequency audiometric testing is available and the patient's mental state allows valid responses to auditory stimuli, and a treatment duration of more than 4 days is likely, it seems reasonable to monitor serially the ability of the patient to hear high-frequency sound.

Neuromuscular Blockade

Neuromuscular blockade after aminoglycoside administration is a rare, but serious and potentially lethal, adverse effect. Neuromuscular blockade has been described in patients administered neomycin, streptomycin, kanamycin, tobramycin, gentamicin, amikacin, and netilmicin.[335] In general, blockade has occurred in clinical situations in which a disease state and/or a concomitant drug interferes with neuromuscular transmission.[335] A rapid rise in serum drug concentrations is also a risk factor.

Clinical manifestations of blockade may include weakness of respiratory musculature, flaccid paralysis, and dilated pupils.[335] Deep tendon reflexes may be absent, hypoactive, or present. Drug exposure may have been a result of intraperitoneal, intravenous, intramuscular, intrapleural, oral, topical, or retroperitoneal administration.[335] Both in vitro and in vivo, the greater the positive charge, the greater the propensity to cause blockade; hence, neomycin is the most potent of the aminoglycosides.[336]

The risk of blockade is amplified in patients also administered D-tubocuare, succinylcholine, or similar agents.[335] Hypomagnesemia, hypocalcemia, and perhaps calcium channel blockers amplify the risk.[337] Patients with infant botulism are at risk.[338] There are conflicting reports as to risk in patients with myasthenia gravis.[339,340]

Blockade results from inhibition of the presynaptic release of acetylcholine and blockage of postsynaptic receptor sites of acetylcholine. The aminoglycosides can prevent internalization of calcium into the presynaptic region of the axon.[341] Calcium internalization must occur prior to acetylcholine release. The drugs also blunt the response of the postsynaptic receptors for acetylcholine. Neomycin is more apt to inhibit presynaptic release while streptomycin and netilmicin are the most active drugs at the postsynaptic site.[342,343] The neuromuscular blockade is reversed rapidly by administering iv calcium gluconate.[344] The response to the neostigmine has been variable.

Blockade is preventable by infusing iv aminoglycoside over 20–30 minutes or more, especially in patients administered large doses once a day. There is no clear indication for instillation of high concentrations of aminoglycoside into the peritoneal cavity or pleural space.

CLINICAL INDICATIONS

The clinical indications for aminoglycosides are divided into empiric, specific, and prophylactic categories. The empiric and specific use are summarized respectively in Tables 10 and 11. In each table, other pertinent, textbook chapters are listed.

Empiric Therapy

The aminoglycosides are indicated when there is the clinical possibility of infection due to aerobic gram-negative bacilli. This is particularly true if *P. aeruginosa* infection is under considera-

TABLE 11. The Specific Indications for Aminoglycosides and Spectinomycin

Selected Pathogens	Aminoglycoside	Drugs Used in Combination
Aerobic gram-negative bacillus		
Klebsiella spp. (373)	A, G, N, T	APP, ESC
Enterobacter aerogenes (95, 374, 375)	A, G, N, T	APP, ESC
Serratia marcescens (376)	G	APP, ESC
Pseudomonas aeruginosa (377–379)	T	APP, APC
Francisella tularensis	St, G	No
Brucella abortus (380)	G or St	Doxycycline
Yersinia pestis	St, G	No
Aerobic gram-positive cocci		
Viridans streptococci	G	Penicillin G
Enterococcus faecalis	G	Penicillin G
Staphylococcus aureus	G	Nafcillin
Staphylococcus epidermidis	G	Vancomycin ± rifampin
Neisseria gonorrhoeae (383, 384)	Sp	No
Mycobacterium avium-intracellulare (385, 386)	A	Multiple
Mycobacterium tuberculosis (387, 388)	St	Multiple
Entamoeba histolytica (389)	P	No
Cryptosporidium parvum (110)	P	No

Abbreviations: A: amikacin; G: gentamicin; N: netilmicin; P: paromomycin; Sp: spectinomycin; St: streptomycin; T: tobramycin; ESC: extended-spectrum cephalosporin; APP: antipseudomonal penicillin; APC: antipseudomonal cephalosporin.

(Data are from refs. 109, 345, 358, and from those references given in parentheses.)

TABLE 10. Examples of Empiric Indications for Aminoglycosides

Type of Infection	Example(s)	Initial Use in Combination with Other Antimicrobials
Bacteremia possible (281–287)	Fever without obvious source	Yes
Burn wound (348)	Burn wound infection	Yes
Endocarditis, infective (349)	Streptococcal, enterococcal, staphylococcal	Yes
Intra-abdominal (160, 350, 351)	Appendicitis, diverticulitis, cholecystitis, peritonitis	Yes
Meningitis (177, 178, 180)	Post-trauma, postoperative	Yes
Neutropenia and fever (352, 353)	Postchemotherapy	Yes
Ocular (188, 191)	Endophthalmitis	Yes
Osteomyelitis/septic arthritis (346, 347, 354, 355)	Postoperative or post-trauma	Yes
Otitis (356, 357)	Malignant, external in a diabetic	Yes
Pneumonia (358, 359)	Respirator-associated pneumonia	Yes
Pyelonephritis (346, 347)	Patients with chronic Foley catheter	Yes
Sexually transmitted disease (360, 361)	Pelvic inflammatory disease	Yes
Skin-subcutaneous tissue (362, 363)	Infected diabetic foot	Yes

(Data are from refs. 118, 131, 132, 281, 329, 345–347, and from those references given in parentheses.)

tion because of the limited number of treatment options for this pathogen. In empiric therapy, the aminoglycosides are usually used in combination. Clinically it is often not possible, with confidence, to be sure that the infectious process is due to aerobic gram-negative bacilli as opposed to *S. aureus* or *Enterococcus* spp. Also, the empiric therapy may be directed at a mixed aerobic–anaerobic flora. Empiric combination therapy may be designed to take advantage of a synergistic or additive effect of an antimicrobial with a cell wall site of action as compared with the ribosome target of the aminoglycosides.

Other classes of antimicrobials, alone or in combination, may be equally efficacious in the empiric therapy of the infections listed in Table 10. Examples include the antipseudomonal penicillins (e.g., piperacillin), a penicillin combined with a β-lactamase inhibitor (e.g., ampicillin-sulbactam, ticarcillin-clavulanic acid, piperacillin-tazobactam), the extended-spectrum cephalosporins (e.g., ceftriaxone, ceftazidime), a carbapenem (e.g., imipenem-cilastatin), or the fluorinated quinolones (e.g., ciprofloxacin and ofloxacin).

The efficacy of empiric aminoglycoside therapy is documented in published symposia that describe the results of clinical trials that served as the basis for licensure, as well as in subsequent trials that compared one aminoglycoside with another or with a β-lactam.[281–287,329,345,364–369]. In febrile neutropenic patients, a high failure rate was experienced with monotherapy with an aminoglycoside, and, hence, the aminoglycosides are administered in combination with a β-lactam antibiotic active against aerobic gram-negative bacilli.[352,353]

The need for inclusion of an aminoglycoside in the empiric treatment of intra-abdominal infections may be decreasing.[350,351] Clinical trials indicate that extended-spectrum penicillins and cephalosporins, β-lactams in combination with a β-lactamase inhibitor, and fluoroquinolones can substitute for the activity of the aminoglycosides against aerobic gram-negative bacilli.[350,351] In some studies, the failure rate of the aminoglycoside combination regimen was statistically higher than monotherapy or a combination that did not include an aminoglycoside.[370–372] Aminoglycoside failures were theorized as due to the relative resistance of gram-negative organisms functioning as facultative anaerobes and/or the failure to achieve "therapeutic" peak serum levels rapidly. There is concern that the aminoglycosides may be more efficacious in the 5–18 percent of patients whose initial cultures yield *P. aeruginosa* or *Enterobacter* spp.[350] The weight of evidence suggests that the virulence of the *Enterococcus* is insufficient to warrant inclusion of the aminoglycoside in empiric therapy.[351] An exception may be the patient with underlying valvular heart disease.

Specific Therapy

After 1 or 2 days, when the patient is stabilized, the disease process is better understood, and the results of culture(s) obtained on admission are available, it may be possible, to increase the specificity of the patient's antimicrobial therapy (Table 11). If *P. aeruginosa* is isolated, an aminoglycoside is often continued with an antipseudomonal penicillin (e.g., ticarcillin) or an antipseudomonal cephalosporin (e.g., ceftazidime).[109,345,358] Occasionally, rifampin may be added to combination therapy.[379] In the non-neutropenic patient with infection of mild severity, monotherapy with an aminoglycoside may suffice. Because of greater activity in vitro and in animal models, tobramycin is the preferred aminoglycoside for *P. aeruginosa* infections.[16,118,131] Because gentamicin displays greater in vitro activity against *Serratia* spp., gentamicin is preferred when *Serratia* is the pathogen. For other aerobic gram-negative bacilli, the efficacy of amikacin, gentamicin, netilmicin, and tobramycin appears equivalent.

Streptomycin and gentamicin have proven efficacious in the treatment of plague and tularemia, as has gentamicin plus doxycycline in the treatment of brucellosis.[109,345,380] Other aminoglycosides may be effective, but there is no reported experience with them.

The aminoglycosides are often used in combination therapy as indicated in Table 11. With an increasing armamentarium of drugs of different classes with predictable activity against aerobic gram-negative bacilli, it is now possible and often advisable to discontinue the aminoglycoside after 2 or 3 days. Such a strategy takes advantage of the efficacy of aminoglycosides and, because of the short duration of therapy, minimizes the risk of aminoglycoside toxicity. Initiating empiric therapy with one of the nonaminoglycoside drugs is another treatment strategy. The emergence of resistant Enterobacteriaceae during the first few days of therapy with extended-spectrum cephalosporins is a concern.[95] It is theorized that this problem is inoculum dependent and hence less likely to occur after a few days of aminoglycoside or combined therapy including an aminoglycoside.

Prophylaxis

Genitourinary and gastrointestinal surgical procedures place the patient at risk of bacteremia due to enterococci. If the patient has underlying valvular heart disease, antimicrobial prophylaxis with the combination of ampicillin and gentamicin is recommended.[390] Vancomycin is substituted for ampicillin in the penicillin-allergic patient.

The risk of infection after elective colectomy is reduced by mechanical cleansing of the bowel plus the oral administration of neomycin and erythromycin.[391] One gram of each is given three times during the 18–24 hours prior to surgery.

DOSING OF AMINOGLYCOSIDES

The aminoglycosides are licensed for multiple administrations per day to patients with normal renal function; that is, twice a day for streptomycin and amikacin and three times a day for gentamicin, tobramycin, and amikacin. Based on laboratory and clinical investigation, there is a current interest in once-daily aminoglycoside therapy. Both methods will be described as they apply to adults. Dosing in the pediatric population and in other selected circumstances are reviewed separately.

Multiple Daily Dosing

Loading Dose. The treatment regimen is divided into an initial (loading) dose and maintenance doses. The purpose of the initial dose is to achieve rapidly a "therapeutic" peak plasma concentration. The targeted range of peak levels represents a compromise between the efficacy that correlates with higher concentrations and the desirability of excreting potentially toxic drug prior to the next dose. The indicated trough levels reflect the intention to maintain the trough concentrations at or above the MIC of the majority of susceptible aerobic gram-negative bacilli.

The loading dose is calculated based on ideal body weight in kilograms as derived from the following formulae:

Females: 45 kg + 2.3 kg/inch of height over 5 ft

Males: 50 kg + 2.3 kg/inch of height over 5 ft

The loading dose is independent of renal function. The peak serum level obtained is dependent on the volume of distribution. Since the volume of distribution is less in adipose tissue than in lean body mass, the initial dose is adjusted in patients with an actual body weight that is more than 30 percent above ideal weight. The ideal body weight is added to 40 percent of the excess weight and the total used as a basis for calculating the loading dose: ideal body weight + 0.4 (total body weight − ideal body weight).[174] Adjustment for excess adiposity is of particular import in the "morbidity" obese.[392]

Volume of distribution is increased in patients with severe

TABLE 12. Suggested Loading Doses, Maintenance Doses, and Desirable Serum Concentrations of Aminoglycosides in Adult Patients with an Estimated Creatinine Clearance above 90 ml/min

Drug[a]	Loading Dose (mg/kg)	Daily Maintenance Dose Total mg/kg	Daily Maintenance Dose Divided as mg/kg	Desired Serum Concentrations (µg/ml) Peak	Desired Serum Concentrations (µg/ml) Trough
Gentamicin	2	5.1	1.7 q8h	4–10	1–2
Tobramycin	2	5.1	1.7 q8h	4–10	1–2
Netilmicin	2	6	2 q8h	4–10	1–2
Amikacin	7.5	15	7.5 q12h	15–30	5–10
Streptomycin[b]	7.5	15	7.5 q12h	15–30	5–10

[a] All drugs, including streptomycin, can be given im or iv.
[b] Maximum daily dose, 2.0 g. Can administer 1.0 g im (or iv) daily for tuberculosis.

(Data from refs. 173, 397.)

burns, ascites, other edematous states, and, at least in theory, any disease process that results in a capillary "leak" syndrome. Conversely, dehydration or muscle wasting decreases the apparent volume of distribution. The latter conditions vary widely from patient to patient and hour to hour in critically ill patients.[393] Hence, it is recommended that after either the initial dose or the first maintenance dose a "peak" serum drug level be obtained.

The definition of a peak level varies from author to author.[394,395] For the clinician, a precise definition is not necessary. For patients treated with iv drug, the loading dose is infused over 15–30 minutes, as there is a theoretic risk of neuromuscular blockade with more rapid administration. Ideally, peak serum levels are obtained 30 minutes after the end of the infusion. Such careful timing is often not feasible or practical, and it is acceptable, and easier, to time the serum collection as 1 hour from the start of the 15–30 minute infusion. After im administration, serum is collected 1 hour later. Anticipated peak and trough concentrations are summarized in Table 12 and Chapter 35.

Maintenance Dose. Calculation of the maintenance dosage regimen requires an estimation of renal function, as aminoglycoside excretion correlates directly with glomerular filtration. Glomerular filtration falls normally with aging and with the result of disease status. The glomerular filtration rate is reflected by the endogenous creatinine clearance. The endogenous creatinine clearance (C_{cr}) is estimated by the equation of Cockcroft and Gault[396]:

$$C_{cr} = \frac{(140 - age)(wgt\ in\ kgs^*)}{Serum\ creatinine \times 72}$$

To adjust for females, multiply calculated C_{cr} by 0.85.

NORMAL RENAL FUNCTION. The suggested loading doses, maintenance doses, and desirable serum concentrations in patients with an estimated creatinine clearance above 90 ml/min are summarized in Table 12.[173,397] It is desirable to measure peak and trough serum aminoglycoside levels after the first or second maintenance dose and to adjust the maintenance dosage accordingly. Subsequently, the serum creatinine should be measured every 3–5 days. If the creatinine is stable, there is no reason to repeat serum aminoglycoside measurements. If renal function changes, dosage is recalculated, and serum levels are repeated after initiation of the new regimen.

Peak serum aminoglycoside levels are obtained to ensure that enough drug was administered for therapeutic efficacy. Data

from infected animals and analysis of clinical trial data support the correlation between high peak levels and antibacterial efficacy.[120,150,359,398,399] The clinical trial data are subject to some criticism.[394]

Among other risk factors, the larger the total daily dose and the longer the duration of therapy, the greater the risk of renal and/or ototoxicity.[239,281,285,327,328] Trough levels are a measure of renal function, as is the serum creatinine. Trough levels do not predict nephrotoxicity per se. If the dosage calculation is in error and the dosage administered exceeds the renal excretory capacity, the overdosage is reflected by a high trough concentration. Individualized pharmacokinetic dosing has been employed in some medical centers. There is no convincing evidence that customized dosing has reduced the incidence of nephrotoxicity.[285,400–402]

IMPAIRED RENAL FUNCTION. Various guidelines have been published to assist in aminoglycoside dosage calculation for patients with reduced glomerular filtration rates. Published reference tables allow the physician the option of reducing the individual dose while maintaining the standard 8–12 hour dosage interval or maintaining a larger maintenance dose and extending the dosage interval. The latter method has theoretic and practical advantages. The larger the individual dose, the higher the serum level, the greater concentration-dependent bactericidal activity, and the longer the postantibiotic effect. There is less patient and hospital staff inconvenience and some economy from reduced frequency of administration.

Sarubbi and Hull[403] provide a dosage chart that allows the physician to calculate a maintenance dose based on a percentage of the loading dose for incremental decrease in creatinine clearance; percentages for three dosing intervals are provided. Bennett et al.[173] group patients as having mild, moderate, or severe renal impairment and suggest dosage regimens either as dosage reduction or interval prolongation (Table 13). Maderazo et al.[404] suggest a percentage system based on the decrement in creatinine clearance. If normal creatinine clearance (Cl_{cr}) is defined as 100 ml/min, reduction in *dose* without change in interval is calculated as $Cl_{cr}/100 \times$ normal maintenance dose. Adjustment of the *dosage interval* is calculated as $100/Cl_{cr} \times$ normal dosage interval. In addition, some hospitals provide clinical pharmacy services to assist in selection of an initial empiric dosage regimen.[285] Regardless of how the maintenance regimen is calculated or who calculates it, it is highly desirable to validate the regimen with serum drug level measurements. Serum aminoglycoside levels and sequential serum creatinine concentrations are of particular import in the critically ill patient with a rapidly evolving disease process.

A rough estimate of predicted serum level (ug/ml) can be calculated from the equation

$$\frac{Dose\ (mg/kg) \times kg\ body\ weight}{Volume\ distribution\ (liter/kg) \times kg\ body\ weight}$$

The volume of distribution (V_D) of aminoglycoside is reported as 0.2–0.3 liter/kg.[173] Larger V_D values are reported for burn patients and edematous states.

DOSING OF DIALYSIS PATIENTS. Because aminoglycosides are dialyzable, it is necessary to give a supplemental dose of aminoglycoside after each hemodialysis.[173] The dosage suggested in Table 13 reflects the clearance of roughly two-thirds of serum aminoglycoside per dialysis. However, individual patients, especially septic and/or hemodynamically unstable patients, may vary widely in the effectiveness of a given dialysis. Hence, in critical patients it is mandatory to measure peak serum concentrations after administration of the postdialysis dose of aminoglycoside.

Continuous arteriovenous hemofiltration is employed with increasing frequency in the management of critically ill patients with acute renal failure.[405–407] Depending on variables that relate to both the patient and the filter, continuous hemofiltration results in the equivalence of a creatinine clearance of between 10

* Same weight as used for the loading dose. The most recent serum creatinine should be used. In disease states, the serum creatinine may change rapidly, up or down, and necessitate recalculation of the estimated creatinine clearance and the resulting dosage regimen.

TABLE 13. Adjustment of Dosage of Aminoglycoside Antibiotics in Patients with Variable Degrees of Impaired Renal Function Using the Method of Prolongation of the Dosage Interval[a]

| Drug | Maintenance Dose for Normal Renal function (mg/kg) | Estimated Creatinine Clearance (ml/min) | | | | Supplement after Hemodialysis[b] (mg/kg) | Supplement after CAVH[b] (mg/kg/day) | Supplement after CAPD-Peritonitis (mg/liter) | |
		80–90	50–80	10–50	<10			Continuous[c]	Intermittent[d]
Gentamicin	1.7 q8h	q12h	q12–24h	q24–48h	q48–72h	1–2	2.5	4–8	20
Tobramycin	1.7 q8h	q12h	q12–24h	q24–48h	q48–72h	1–2	2.5	4–8	20
Netilmicin	2 q8h	q12h	q12–24h	q24–48h	q48–72h	2	2.5	4–8	20
Amikacin	7.5 q12h	q12h	q12–24h	q24–48h	q48–72h	5–7	4.0	6–12	60

[a] Also shown are suggested doses of aminoglycoside for patients requiring hemodialysis, continuous arteriovenous hemofiltration (CAVH), and dosages to treat peritonitis in patients maintained by continuous ambulatory peritoneal dialysis (CAP).
[b] Rate and absolute amount of drug removed influenced by a variety of host disease and dialysis-related factors. In critically ill patients, serum aminoglycoside levels should be monitored.
[c] Aminoglycoside added to each exchange; usually four exchanges per day of 2 liters each with 6 hours dwell time.
[d] Aminoglycoside added in larger dosage to only one of four daily exchanges.

(Data from refs. 173, 405–408.)

and 50 ml/min. The filtered fluid is replaced continuously by parenteral fluid administration. It is suggested that gentamicin be given as a separate infusion, once daily in a dosage of 2.5 mg/kg body weight. With this dosage, the peak serum concentration should be in the range of 8–12 µ/ml and the trough level (at the end of 24 hours) between 1 and 2 µg/ml. Because of individual variability, serum levels should be measured. Suggested doses for tobramycin, netilmicin, and amikacin are summarized in Table 13.

Aminoglycosides are often employed in peritoneal dialysis fluid to treat peritoneal-dialysis-associated peritonitis due to aminoglycoside-susceptible organisms.[408] This method of drug administration is not recommended for patients with systemic infection. The aminoglycoside is added to the peritoneal dialysis fluid. It may be added in "therapeutic" concentration to each bag of dialysis fluid, or the aminoglycoside may be added in higher concentration to only one of the usual four exchanges of peritoneal dialysis fluid (Table 13). The once-a-day regimen is analogous to the once-daily parenteral aminoglycoside therapy.

Once-Daily Administration

It should be emphasized that data are currently not adequate to support an unqualified endorsement for once-daily dosing. Careful comparison of efficacy in a variety of infections will be required before one can conclude that efficacy is not reduced by extending dosing intervals.

Premise. The concept of once-daily aminoglycoside therapy evolved from three separate but related observations.[150] First, experimental nephrotoxicity and ototoxicity were less severe in animals administered a daily dose of drug as a single injection as opposed to the same daily dosage administered in two or three divided doses. Animals given a single daily dose accumulated less drug in the renal cortex. The same result was observed in patients who agreed to receive an aminoglycoside prior to elective nephrectomy. Patients given standard q8h doses had lower renal tissue concentrations of tobramycin, netilmicin, and amikacin as opposed to recipients given an equivalent amount of drug by continuous iv infusion.[409,410] Second, the aminoglycosides demonstrate a PAE against aerobic gram-negative bacilli both in vitro and in vivo.[126–128,138,139] The duration of the PAE is greater the higher the peak aminoglycoside concentration. In animals, the duration of PAE is much longer in intact animals as opposed to animals rendered neutropenic. Hence, the serum level of aminoglycoside can fall below the MIC of the pathogenic bacteria without loss of efficacy. Third, antibacterial efficacy of the aminoglycosides is enhanced with high peak drug concentrations.[119,126] Hence, once-a-day dosing offers the potential of both reducing the risk of oto- and nephrotoxicities while not sacrificing antibacterial efficacy.

Once-daily therapy proved safe and efficacious in infected animal models. Nephrotoxicity was delayed in onset and was

less severe in rats with subcutaneous abscesses dosed once daily as compared with rats given multiple daily doses.[411] In guinea pigs with pneumonia due to *P. aeruginosa*, once-daily dosing was as efficacious as multiple daily doses.[120] In neutropenic animals, once-daily aminoglycoside therapy was less efficacious unless combined with a β-lactam active against *P. aeruginosa*.[120]

Two small groups of healthy volunteers received single-dose aminoglycoside. No evidence of nephrotoxicity or ototoxicity was detected.[288,412,413]

Clinical Trials. Only one U.S. study has compared once-daily aminoglycoside therapy with standard multidose treatment. Young adults with cystic fibrosis were administered tobramycin as 11 mg/kg/day by continuous infusion or 11 mg/kg/day as a single dose.[233] No difference in efficacy or toxicity was seen in the 31 enrolled patients.

The international interest in once-daily dosing is evident by the increasing frequency of publication of clinical trials that include moderate to large numbers of patients.[150,292–294] Two of the reported trials include children.[294,414] Only one trial focused on febrile neutropenic patients.[415]

The initial reports are characterized by small numbers of patients and no demonstrable differences in efficacy or toxicity between once-daily or multiple-daily dose aminoglycoside.[150] Ter Braak et al.[292] reported that the laboratory abnormalities of nephrotoxicity took longer to appear after once-daily netilmicin as opposed to the group receiving two or three daily doses. Tulkens[416] found reduced urinary levels of PI in patients with pelvic inflammatory disease who received once-daily netilmicin or amikacin as opposed to thrice- or twice-daily dosage regimens of the same drugs. Prins et al.[293] reported equal efficacy but reduced nephrotoxicity in adults with serious infections who were administered once-daily gentamicin as opposed to the equivalent daily dose given three times a day. Marik et al.[294] randomized critically ill children and adults to once- versus twice-daily amikacin. The once-daily recipients experienced a significantly higher clinical cure rate as well as a significant reduction in nephrotoxicity. The pediatric once-daily subgroup had a significantly greater bacteriologic cure rate.

Clinical Practice. With once-daily therapy, each dose is a loading dose. Using the Cockcroft and Gault formula,[396] an estimated creatinine clearance is calculated using ideal body weight. Suggested dosage regimens for gentamicin and tobramycin by estimated creatinine clearance are presented in Table 14.[417] Similar suggestions for netilmicin, amikacin, kanamycin, and streptomycin are available elsewhere.[417] Note that as the creatinine clearance falls and the serum $T_{1/2}$ increases, the period of time at the end of each dose interval with serum levels under 1 µg/ml decreases. As the creatinine clearance falls to 20 ml/min or less, a 24 hour dosage interval results in modest peak concentrations and progressively higher trough serum levels. Because of

TABLE 14. Suggested Once Daily Dosage Regimens of Gentamicin and Tobramycin in Patients with Estimated Creatinine Clearance (Est Cr Cl) between 20 and 100 ml/min[a]

Est Cr Cl (ml/min)	Dosage Interval (h)	Dose (mg/kg)	T₁/₂ (h)	Times for Estimated Mean Serum Level (µg/ml)			
				1 h	12 h	18 h	24 h
100	24	5	2.5	20[b]	1.0	<1	<1
90	24	5	3.1	20	2.0	<1	<1
80	24	5	3.4	20	2.5	<1	<1
70	24	4	3.9	16	2.0	<1	<1
60	24	4	4.5	16	3.0	1.5	<1
50	24	3.5	5.3	14	3.5	1.0	<1
40	24	2.5	6.5	10	3.0	1.5	<1
30	24	2.5	8.4	10	4.0	2.5	1.5
				1 h	24 h	36 h	48 h
20	48	4.0	11.9	16	4.0	2.0	1.0
10	48	3.0	20.4	12	5.0	3.0	2.0
0[c]	48	1–2	69.3	8	7.0	6.0	5.0

[a] Every other day regimens for creatinine clearance below 20 ml/min. Predicted peak and trough serum levels are shown. Peak levels are calculated as

$$\frac{\text{mg admin: mg/kg} \times \text{kg body wt}}{V_D \text{ (liter/kg)} \times \text{kg body weight}}$$

Trough levels are calculated from peak concentration and published T₁/₂, at varying levels of renal function.
[b] Mean ± 2 SD yields range of 16–24 µg/ml.
[c] Example values for patient receiving every other day hemodialysis. Actual peak depends on efficiency of dialysis. Dose given postdialysis.

(From Gilbert and Bennett,[417] with permission.)

TABLE 15. Aminoglycoside Dosage Regimens for Neonates, Infants, and Children

Age	Drug and Dosage (mg/kg per day)[a]			
	Gentamicin	Tobramycin	Netilmicin	Amikacin
0–7 days[b]	5	4	5	15–20
Infants	5–7.5	5	7.5	20–30
Children	6–7.5	6–7.5	7.5	15

[a] Given in two or three divided doses.
[b] Assumes birth weight of 2000–2500 g or greater. Dose reduction necessary for neonates of lower weight.

(Data from refs. 96, 203, 418, 419.)

the theoretical reduction in antibacterial efficacy as the peak level falls, and to avoid an odd number of hours in the dosage interval, an every-48-hour dosage is suggested if the creatinine clearance is 20 ml/min or less. It is emphasized that the efficacy of once-daily therapy in patients with severe degrees of renal impairment has not been evaluated in depth. In patients with serious infections and until more data are available, it is desirable to administer a concomitant β-lactam antibiotic. Note that there is no difference in suggested treatment regimens for patients on hemodialysis.

For patients given 4–5 mg/kg of gentamicin or tobramycin as a single dose, the aminoglycoside is infused over 60 minutes rather than the customary 15–30 minutes as a precaution against potential neuromuscular blockade. Peak serum levels are measured only for academic interest unless there is clinical reason to suspect an unusually large volume of distribution or the patient has clinical evidence of a failure to respond. For patients with estimated creatinine clearance values of 60 ml/min or more, serum levels at 18 hours are suggested to ensure adequate renal clearance and to document that there is an end-of-dose time interval with serum levels below 1 µg/ml so as to take advantage of the PAE of aminoglycosides.

Special Circumstances

Children. The pharmacokinetics of aminoglycosides in newborns and infants differ from adults in at least two ways.[203,418,419] The renal clearance of aminoglycosides is reduced in newborns with a resultant prolongation of the T₁/₂ and need for a reduction in aminoglycoside dosage (Table 15).[96,203,418,419] The T₁/₂ is even

further prolonged in low-birth-weight infants. By 7 days in newborns with normal birth weight, the serum T₁/₂ is approaching adult values.

Furthermore, the volume of distribution of aminoglycosides is larger, as a percentage of body weight, in newborns than in adults. The larger volume of distribution compensates, but only in a modest way, for the reduction in renal clearance. Because of the unpredictable pharmacokinetics, particularly in low-birth-weight newborns, it is necessary to obtain peak and trough serum levels.

Note that neither kanamycin nor streptomycin are listed in Table 15, the former because of the frequency of resistance among Enterobacteriaceae and the latter because of risk of ototoxicity. Nonetheless, streptomycin therapy may prove necessary in patients with multidrug-resistant tuberculosis.

Cystic Fibrosis. The pharmacokinetics of aminoglycosides are altered in patients with cystic fibrosis. Although the mechanism is debated, cystic fibrosis patients demonstrate some combination of increased glomerular clearance, shortened T₁/₂, and an increased volume of distribution.[420] The result is low serum and sputum concentrations of aminoglycoside if standard doses are administered. In young adult cystic fibrosis patients with an acute exacerbation of airway infection, a continuous infusion of tobramycin, 11 mg/kg/day, was necessary to maintain a serum concentration of 5.2 µg/ml.[233] If the 11 mg/kg was given as a single injection, the mean peak serum level was 62 µg/ml. There was no observed difference in either efficacy or toxicity when comparing the continuous infusion and once-daily groups over a 10 day period. However, chronic parenteral therapy results in a high incidence of cochlear damage.[421]

The risk of cochlear toxicity is minimized by aerosol administration of tobramycin.[422] Compared with placebo, 600 mg of tobramycin in saline, delivered three times daily by a ultrasonic nebulizer, improved pulmonary function and reduced the sputum density of *P. aeruginosa* over a 28 day study period.[423]

Infective Endocarditis. There are no reported clinical trials that compare aminoglycoside dosage frequency in patients with infective endocarditis. Based on in vitro studies and animal models of endocarditis, some tentative generalizations are possible. The antibacterial effect of aminoglycosides against *Enterococcus* spp. requires the continuous presence of both an active cell wall β-lactam antibiotic (e.g., ampicillin) and an aminoglycoside. Hence, once-daily dosing does not seem justified. Assuming in vitro susceptibility and evidence of clinical response, the current consensus recommendation of an American Heart Association sponsored expert committee is penicillin G plus gentamicin, 3 mg/kg/day (assuming normal renal function), divided into a q8h dosage schedule, for viridans streptococcal and enterococcal endocarditis.[349]

Endocarditis due to aerobic gram-negative bacilli is exceedingly rare. Some success is reported with the combination of an aminoglycoside and an active β-lactam antibiotic.[424]

Spectinomycin and Gonorrhea. Spectinomycin is used exclusively to treat gonococcal infections.[425] It is not effective in the treatment of infections due to *Treponema pallidum* or *Chlamydia trachomatis*. The drug does not achieve therapeutic concentrations in saliva and hence does not eliminate pharyngeal gonococci. The drug is neither nephrotoxic or ototoxic. Spectinomycin is effective in the treatment of uncomplicated urethral or cervical or disseminated gonorrhea. It is an alternative therapy in patients allergic to penicillin or in patients infected with penicillinase-producing strains of gonococci. For infection of the cervix or urethra, the dose is 2 g as a single im injection. For gonococcemia, the suggested dose is 2 g im every 12 hours for 3 days. There is no iv form of the drug.

TABLE 16. Pharmaceutical Preparations of Aminoglycoside Antibiotics

| Drug | im/iv | Available Pharmaceutical Preparations | | | |
		Intrathecal	po	Ophthalmic	Topical
Streptomycin	im only				
Kanamycin	im/iv				
Gentamicin	im/iv	Yes		Yes	Yes
Tobramycin	im/iv			Yes	
Amikacin	im/iv				
Netilmicin	im/iv				
Neomycin	No		Yes[a]	Yes	Yes
Paromomycin			Yes		
Spectinomycin	im only				

[a] For bowel prep and hepatic coma.

(Data from Drug Facts and Comparisons.[426])

Pharmaceutical Preparations

A variety of approved aminoglycoside pharmaceutical preparations are available (Table 16).[426] Note that neomycin and paromomycin are not administered parenterally. Ophthalmic and topical preparations are often combined with other antimicrobials or glucocorticoids.

FUTURE USE

Coincident with the availability of other antimicrobial agents with antimicrobial activity against aerobic gram-negative bacilli, there has been a steady decline in the empiric use, specific therapy, and duration of therapy with aminoglycosides. Alternative agents include the extended-spectrum penicillins, penicillin–β-lactamase inhibitor combinations, extended-spectrum cephalosporins, the monobactam aztreonam, the carbapenems, and the fluorinated quinolones. Nonetheless, several factors suggest a continued place for aminoglycosides. There are disturbing reports of increased frequency of resistance of aerobic gram-negative bacilli to β-lactams and quinolones.[427] The emergence of resistance during therapy with extended-spectrum cephalosporins is particularly worrisome.[95] Aminoglycosides may be necessary as part of combination therapy for multidrug resistance *Mycobacterium tuberculosis*.[428]

The incorporation of aminoglycosides into liposomes may enhance drug delivery to intracellular sites.[429] Substances such as polyaspartic acid may provide protection against toxicity without loss of antibacterial activity.[268–278]

REFERENCES

1. Waksman SA, Schatz AI. Present status of streptomycin therapy. Lancet. 1946;66:77–78.
2. Rinehart KL Jr. Comparative chemistry of the aminoglycoside and aminocyclitol antibiotics. J Infect Dis. 1969;119:345–50.
3. Daniels PJL. Antibiotics (aminoglycosides). In: Grayson M, ed. Kirk-Othmer: Encyclopedia of Chemical Technology. 3rd ed, v. 5. New York: John Wiley & Sons; 1978:819.
4. Hooper IR. The naturally occurring aminoglycoside antibiotics. In: Umezawa H, Hooper IR, eds. Aminoglycoside Antibiotics. New York: Springer-Verlag; 1982:1.
5. Davies JE. Aminoglycoside-aminocyclitol antibiotics and their modifying enzymes. In: Lorian V, ed. Antibiotics in Laboratory Medicine. 3rd ed. Baltimore: Williams & Wilkins; 1991:691–713.
6. Umezawa S, Tsuchiya T. Total synthesis and chemical modification of the aminoglycoside antibiotics. In: Umezawa H, Hooper IR, eds. Aminoglycoside Antibiotics. New York: Springer-Verlag; 1982:37.
7. Price KE, Godfrey JC. Effect of structural modifications on the biological properties of aminoglycoside antibiotics containing 2-deoxystreptamine. Adv Appl Microbiol. 1974;18:191–307.
8. Price KE. Aminoglycoside research 1975–1985: Prospects for development of improved agents. Antimicrob Agents Chemother. 1986;29:543–8.
9. Nagabhushan TL, Miller GH, Weinstein MJ. Structure–activity relationships in aminoglycoside-aminocyclitol antibiotics. In: Whelton A, Neu HC, eds. The Aminoglycosides. New York: Marcel Dekker; 1982:3–27.
10. Leitner F, Price KE. Aminoglycosides under development. In: Whelton A, Neu HC, eds. The Aminoglycosides. New York: Marcel Dekker; 1982: 29–64.
11. Berdy J, Aszalos A, Bostian M, et al. CRC Handbook of Antibiotic Compounds. v I. Carbohydrate Antibiotics. Boca Raton, FL. CRC Press Inc.; 1980.
12. Weiss PJ, Andrew ML, Wright WW. Solubility of antibiotics in 24 solvents: Use in analysis. Antibiot Chemother. 1957;7:374–7.
13. Weinstein MJ, Wagman GH, Oden EM, et al. Biological activity of the antibiotic components of the gentamicin complex. J Bacteriol. 1967;94:789–90.
14. Gilbert DN, Kohlhepp SJ. New sodium hydroxide digestion method for measurement of renal tobramycin concentrations. Antimicrob Agents Chemother. 1986;30:361–5.
15. Moellering RC Jr. In vitro antibacterial activity of the aminoglycoside antibiotics. Rev Infect Dis. 1983;5(Suppl):S212–32.
16. Moellering RC Jr. Clinical microbiology and the in vitro activity of aminoglycosides. In: Whelton A, Neu HC, eds. The Aminoglycosides: Microbiology, Clinical Use and Toxicology. New York: Marcel Dekker; 1982:65–95.
17. Moore RA, Bates NC, Hancock REW. Interaction of polycationic antibiotics with *Pseudomonas aeruginosa* lipopolysaccharide and lipid A studied by using dansyl-polymyxin. Antimicrob Agents Chemother. 1986;29:496–500.
18. Rocque WJ, Fesik SW, Haug A, et al. Polycation binding to isolated lipopolysaccharide from antibiotic-hypersusceptible mutant strains of *Escherichia coli*. Antimicrob Agents Chemother. 1988;32:308–13.
19. Vandaux P, Waldvogel FA. Gentamicin inactivation in purulent exudates: role of cell lysis. J Infect Dis. 1980;142:586–93.
20. Laurent G, Kishore BK, Tulkens PM. Aminoglycoside-induced renal phospholipidosis and nephrotoxicity. Biochem Pharmacol. 1990;40:2383–92.
21. Ramphal R, Lhermitte M, Filliat M, et al. The binding of antipseudomonas antibiotics to macromolecules from cystic fibrosis sputum. J Antimicrob Chemother. 1988;22:483–90.
22. Bataillon V, Lhermitte M, Lafitte J-JH, et al. The binding of amikacin to macromolecules from the sputum of patients suffering from respiratory diseases. J Antimicrob Chemother. 1992;29:499–508.
23. McLaughlin JE, Reeves DS. Clinical and laboratory evidence for inactivation of gentamicin by carbenicillin. Lancet. 1971;1:261–264.
24. Waitz JA, Drube CG, Moss EL Jr, et al. Biological aspects of the interaction between gentamicin and carbenicillin. J Antibiot. 1972;25:219–225.
25. Pickering LK, Rutherford I. Effect of concentration and time upon inactivation of tobramycin, gentamicin, netilmicin, mezlocillin, and piperacillin. J Pharmacol Exp Ther 1981;217:345–9.
26. Glew RH, Pavuk RA. Stability of gentamicin, tobramycin, and amikacin in combination with four β-lactam antibiotics. Antimicrob Agents Chemother. 1983;24:474.
27. Wallace SM, Chan L-Y. In vitro interaction of aminoglycosides with β-lactam penicillins. Antimicrob Agents Chemother. 1985;28:274–81.
28. Walterspiel JN, Feldman S, Van R, et al. Comparative inactivation of isepamicin, amikacin, and gentamicin by nine β-lactams and two β-lactamase inhibitors, cilastatin and heparin. Antimicrob Agents Chemother. 1991;35: 1875–8.
29. Halstenson CE, Wong MU, Herman CS, et al. Effect of concomitant administration of piperacillin on the dispositions of isepamicin and gentamicin in patients with end-stage renal disease. Antimicrob Agents Chemother. 1992; 36:1832–6.
30. Shaw KJ, Rather PN, Hare RS, et al. Molecular genetics of aminoglycoside resistance genes and familial relationships of the aminoglycoside-modifying enzymes. Microbiol Rev. 1993;57:138–63.
31. Bryan LE, Kawan S. Roles of ribosomal binding, membrane potential, and electron transport in bacterial uptake of streptomycin and gentamicin. Antimicrob Agents Chemother. 1983;23:835–45.
32. Taber HW, Muller JP, Arrow AS. Bacterial uptake of aminoglycoside antibiotics. Microbiol Rev. 1987;51:439–57.
33. Hancock RE, Bellido F. Antibiotic uptake: unusual results for unusual molecules. J Antimicrob Chemother. 1992;29:235–9.
34. Bryan LE, Van Den Elzen HM. Effects of membrane-energy mutations and cations on streptomycin and gentamicin accumulation by bacteria: A model for entry of streptomycin and gentamicin in susceptible and resistance bacteria. Antimicrob Agents Chemother. 1977;12:163–77.
35. Hurwitz C, Rosano CL, Landau JV. Kinetics of loss of viability of *Escherichia coli* exposed to streptomycin. J Bacteriol. 1962;83:1210–6.
36. Jackson GE, Lolans VT, Daikos GL. The inductive role of ionic binding in the bactericidal and postexposure effects of aminoglycoside antibiotics with implications for dosing. J Infect Dis. 1990;162:408–13.
37. Hancock REW. Alterations in outer membrane permeability. Annu Rev Microbiol. 1984;38:237–64.
38. Peterson AA, Hancock REW, McGroarty EJ. Binding of polycationic antibiotics and polyamines to lipopolysaccharides of *Pseudomonas aeruginosa*. J Bacteriol. 1985;164:1256–61.
39. Martin NL, Beveridge TJ. Gentamicin interaction with *Pseudomonas aeruginosa*. Antimicrob Agents Chemother. 1986;29:1079–87.
40. Moskowitz M. Differences in precipitability of nucleic acids with streptomycin and dihydrostreptomycin. Nature. 1963;200:335–7.
41. Nichols WW, Young SN. Respiration-dependent uptake of dihydrostreptomycin by *Escherichia coli*. Its reversible nature and lack of evidence for a uniport process. Biochem J. 1985;228:505–12.
42. Hancock REW. Aminoglycoside uptake and mode of action—with special reference to streptomycin and gentamicin. I. Antagonists and mutants. J Antimicrob Chemother. 1981;8:249–76.
43. Hancock REW. Aminoglycoside uptake and mode of action—with special reference to streptomycin and gentamicin. II. Effects of aminoglycosides on cells. J Antimicrob Chemother. 1981;8:429–45.
44. Bryan LE. Mechanisms of action of aminoglycoside antibiotics. In: Root RK, Sande MA, eds. Contemporary Issues in Infectious Diseases. v. 1. New

Dimensions in Antimicrobial Therapy. New York: Churchill Livingstone; 1984:17–36.

45. Damper PD, Epstein W. Role of the membrane potential in bacterial resistance to aminoglycoside antibiotics. Antimicrob Agents Chemother. 1981; 20:803–8.

46. Mates SM, Patel L, Kaback HR, et al. Membrane potential in anaerobically growing *Staphylococcus aureus* and its relationship to gentamicin uptake. Antimicrob Agents Chemother. 1983;23:526–30.

47. Nicas TI, Hancock REW. Outer membrane protein H1 of *Pseudomonas aeruginosa*: involvement in adaptive and mutational resistance to ethylenediamine tetraacetate, polymyxin B, and gentamicin. J Bacteriol. 1980;143: 872–8.

48. Spots CR, Stainier RY. Mechanism of streptomycin action on bacteria: A unitary hypothesis. Nature. 1961;192:663.

49. Weisblum B, Davies J. Antibiotic inhibitors of the bacterial ribosome. Bacteriol Rev. 1968;32(Suppl):493–528.

50. Ozaki M, Mizushima S, Nomura M. Identification and functional characterization of the protein controlled by the streptomycin-resistant locus in *E. coli*. Nature 1969;222:333–9.

51. Schreiner G, Nierhaus KH. Protein involved in the binding of dihydrostreptomycin to ribosomes of *Escherichia coli*. J Mol Biol. 1973;81:71–82.

52. Kuhberger R, Piepersberg W, Petzet A, et al. Alteration of ribosomal protein L6 in gentamicin-resistant strains of *Escherichia coli*. Effects on fidelity of protein synthesis. Biochemistry 1979;18:187–93.

53. Hummel H, Piepersberg W, Bock A. 30S subunit mutations relieving restriction of ribosomal misreading caused by L6 mutations. Mol Gen Genet 1980; 179:147–53.

54. Chang FN, Flaks JG. Binding of dihydrostreptomycin to *Escherichia coli* ribosomes: Characteristics and equilibrium of the reaction. Antimicrob Agents Chemother. 1972;2:294–307.

55. Modolell J, Davis BD. Mechanism of inhibition of ribosomes by streptomycin. Nature. 1969;224:345–8.

56. Wallace BJ, Davis BD. Cyclic blockade of initiation sites by streptomycin-damaged ribosomes in *Escherichia coli*: an explanation for dominance of sensitivity. J Mol Biol 1973;75:377–90.

57. Wallace BJ, Tai PC, Davis BD. Effect of streptomycin on the response of *Escherichia coli* ribosomes to the dissociation factor. J Mol Biol. 1973;75: 391–400.

58. Davies J, Gorini L, Davis BD. Misreading of RNA code words induced by aminoglycoside antibiotics. Mol Pharmacol. 1965;1:93–106.

59. Pestka S. Inhibitors of protein synthesis. In: Weissback H, Pestka S, eds. Molecular Mechanisms of Protein Synthesis. New York: Academic Press; 1977:467.

60. vonAksen U, Noller HF. Footprinting the sites of interaction of antibiotics with catalytic group I intron RNA. Science. 1993;260:1500–3.

61. Davis BB. The lethal action of aminoglycosides. J Antimicrob Chemother. 1988;22:1–3.

62. Kodurugamuwa JL, Lam JS, Beveridge TJ. Interaction of gentamicin with the A band and B band lipopolysaccharides of *Pseudomonas aeruginosa* and its possible lethal effect. Antimicrob Agents Chemother. 1993;37:715–21.

63. Bryan LE. General mechanisms of resistance to antibiotics. J Antimicrob Chemother. 1988;22(Suppl A):1–15.

64. Mitsuhashi S, Kawabe H. Aminoglycoside antibiotic resistance in bacteria. In: Whelton A, Neu HC, eds. The Aminoglycosides. New York; Marcel Dekker; 1983;97–122.

65. Davies JE. Resistance to aminoglycosides: mechanism and frequency. Rev Infect Dis. 1983;5(Suppl):S261–7.

66. Dickie P, Bryan LE, Pickard MA. Effect of enzymatic adenylation on dihydrostreptomycin accumulation in *Escherichia coli* carrying an R-factor: Model explaining aminoglycoside resistance by inactivating mechanisms. Antimicrob Agents Chemother. 1978;14:569–80.

67. Bryan LE. Aminoglycoside resistance. In: Bryan LE, ed. Antimicrobial Drug Resistance. Orlando, FL. Academic Press; 1984:241–77.

68. Blaser J. Efficacy of once- and thrice-daily dosing of aminoglycosides in in vitro models of infection. J Antimicrob Chemother. 1991;27(Suppl C):21–8.

69. Ahmad MH, Rechenmacher A, Bock A. Interaction between aminoglycoside uptake and ribosomal resistant mutations. Antimicrob Agents Chemother. 1980;18:798–806.

70. Bryan LE, Kwan S. Mechanisms of aminoglycoside resistance of anaerobic bacteria and facultative bacteria grown anaerobically. J Antimicrob Chemother. 1981;8(Suppl D):1–8.

71. Rusthoven JJ, Davies TA, Lerner SA. Clinical isolation and characterization of aminoglycoside-resistance small colony variants of *Enterobacter aerogenes*. Am J Med. 1979;67:702–706.

72. Daikos GL, Jackson GG, Lolans VT, et al. Adaptive resistance to aminoglycoside antibiotics from first-exposure down-regulation. J Infect Dis. 1990; 162:414–20.

73. Perlin MH, Lerner SA. High-level amikacin resistance in *Escherichia coli* due to phosphorylation and impaired aminoglycoside uptake. Antimicrob Agents Chemother. 1986;29:216–24.

74. Murray BE. New aspects of antimicrobial resistance and the resulting therapeutic dilemmas. J Infect Dis. 1991;163:1185–94.

75. Moellering RC. The *Enterococcus*: A classic example of the impact of antimicrobial resistance on therapeutic options. J Antimicrob Chemother. 1991;28: 1–12.

76. Toala P, McDonald A, Wilcox C, et al. Susceptibility of group D *Streptococcus (Enterococcus)* to 21 antibiotics in vitro, with special reference to species differences. Am J Med Sci. 1969;258:416–30.

77. Bryan LE, Kowand SK, Van Den Elzen HM. Mechanism of aminoglycoside

antibiotic resistance in anaerobic bacteria. *Clostridium perfringens* and *Bacteroides fragilis*. Antimicrob Agents Chemother. 1979;15:7–13.

78. Moellering RC Jr, Weinberg AN. Studies on antibiotic synergism against enterococci. II. Effect of various antibiotics on the uptake of ^{14}C-labeled streptomycin by enterococci. J Clin Invest. 1971;50:2580–4.

79. Courvalin P, Carlier C, Collatz E. Plasmid-mediated resistance to aminocyclitol antibiotics in group D streptococci. J Bacteriol. 1980;143:541–51.

80. Courvalin P, Shaw WV, Jacob AE. Plasmid-mediated mechanisms of resistance to aminoglycoside-aminocyclitol antibiotics and to chloramphenicol in group D streptococci. Antimicrob Agents Chemother. 1978;13:716–25.

81. Kono M, Hamashima H, O'Harar K. Modification of aminoglycoside antibiotics by clinical isolates of *Streptococcus faecalis*. J Antibiot (Tokyo). 1981; 34:224–30.

82. Krogstad DJ, Korfhagen TR, Mollering RC Jr, et al. Aminoglycoside-inactivating enzymes in clinical isolates of *Streptococcus faecalis*. J Clin Invest. 1978;62:480–6.

83. Moellering RC Jr, Korzeniowski OM, Sande MA, et al. Species-specific resistance to antimicrobial synergism in *Streptococcus faecium* and *Streptococcus faecalis* J Infect Dis. 1979;140:203–8.

84. Hodel-Christian SL, Murray BE. Comparison of the gentamicin resistance transposon Tn 5281 with regions encoding gentamicin resistance in *Enterococcus faecalis* isolates from diverse geographic locations. Antimicrob Agents Chemother. 1992;36:2259–64.

85. Leclercq R, Dutka-Malen S, Brisson-Noel A, et al. Resistance of enterococci to aminoglycosides and glycopeptides. Clin Infect Dis. 1992;15:495–501.

86. Courvalin P, Carlier C, Collatz E. Structural and functional relationships between aminoglycoside-modifying enzymes from streptococci and staphylococci. In: Mitsuhashi S, Rosival S, Kremery V, eds. Medical and Biological Aspects of Resistant Strains. Berlin: Springer-Verlag; 1980;309–20.

87. Bhattacharya M, Warren JR. Treatment of infections due to enterococci with high level gentamicin resistance and streptomycin susceptibility. Clin Infect Dis. 1993;16:330–1.

88. Eliopoulos GM, Farber BF, Murray BE, et al. Ribosomal resistance of clinical enterococcal (isolates) to streptomycin. Antimicrob Agents Chemother. 1984;245:398–9.

89. Data supplied by Microbiology Section, Dept of Clinical Pathology, Oregon Health Sciences University, February 15, 1993.

90. Gerding DN, Larson TA, Hughes RA, et al. Aminoglycoside resistance and aminoglycoside usage: Ten years experience in one hospital. Antimicrob Agents Chemother. 1991;35:1284–90.

91. King JW, White MC, Todd JR, et al. Alterations in the microbial flora and in the incidence of bacteremia at a university hospital after adoption of amikacin as the sole formulary aminoglycoside..Clin Infect Dis. 1992;14:908–15.

92. Hesseling PB, Mouton WL, Henning PA, et al. A prospective study of long-term use of amikacin in a pediatrics department. S Afr Med J. 1990;768: 192–5.

93. Friedland IR, Funk E, Khoosal M, et al. Increased resistance to amikacin in a neonatal unit following intensive amikacin usage. Antimicrob Agents Chemother. 1992;36:1596–600.

94. Shimizu K, Jumada T, Hseih W-C, et al. Comparison of aminoglycoside resistance patterns in Japna, Formosa, Korea, Chile, and the U.S. Antimicrob Agents Chemother. 1985;28:282–8.

95. Chow JW, Fine MJ, Shlaes DM, et al. Enterobacter bacteremia: Clinical features and emergence of antibiotic resistance during therapy. Ann Intern Med. 1991;115:585–90.

96. Sanford JP. Guide to Antimicrobial Therapy 1993. Dallas: Antimicrobial Therapy Inc., 1994.

97. Briedis DJ, Robson HG. Comparative activity of netilmicin, gentamicin, amikacin, and tobramycin against *Pseudomonas aeruginosa* and Enterobacteriaceae. Antimicrob Agents Chemother. 1976;10:592–7.

98. Fu KP, Neu HC. In vitro study of netilmicin compared with other aminoglycosides. Antimicrob Agents Chemother. 1976;10:526–34.

99. Kabins SA, Nathan C, Cohen S. In vitro comparison of netilmicin, a semisynthetic derivative of sisomicin, and four other aminoglycoside antibiotics. Antimicrob Agents Chemother. 1976;10:139–45.

100. Dhawan V, Marso E, Martin WJ, et al. In vitro studies with netilmicin compared with amikacin, gentamicin, and tobramycin. Antimicrob Agents Chemother. 1977;11:64–73.

101. Young LS, Hewitt WL. Activity of five aminoglycoside antibiotics in vitro against gram-negative bacilli and *Staphylococcus aureus*. Antimicrob Agents Chemother. 1973;4:617–25.

102. Garcia-Rodriquez JA, Martin LF, Saenz GMC. Activity of amikacin against *Mycobacterium tuberculosis*. J Antimicrob Chemother. 1978;4:293–4.

103. Dalovisio JR, Pankey GA. In vitro susceptibility of *Mycobacterium fortuitum* and *Mycobacterium chelonei* to amikacin. J Infect Dis. 1978;137:318–21.

104. Chiu J, Nussbaum J, Bozzette S, et al., California Collaborative Treatment Group. Treatment of disseminated *Mycobacterium avium* complex infection in AIDS with amikacin, ethambutol, rifampin, and ciprofloxacin. Ann Intern Med. 1990;113:358–61.

105. National Committee for Clinical Laboratory Standards. Approved Standard M7-A: Methods for Dilution Antimicrobial Susceptibility Tests for Bacteria That Grow Aerobically. Villanova PA: National Committee for Clinical Laboratory Standards; 1985.

106. National Committee for Clinical Laboratory Standards. Approved Standard M2-A3: Performance Standards for Antimicrobic Disc Susceptibility Tests. Villanova, PA: National Committee for Clinical Laboratory Standards; 1984.

107. Hand WL, King-Thompson NL. Contrasts between phagocyte antibiotic uptake and subsequent intracellular bactericidal activity. Antimicrob Agents Chemother. 1986;29:135–40.

108. Utili R, Adinolfi LE, Dillilo M, et al. Activity of aminoglycosides against phagocytosed bacteria. J Antimicrob Chemother. 1991;28:897–904.

109. Drugs for parasitic infections. Med Lett. 1992;34:17–24.

110. Ficktenbaum CJ, Ritchie DJ, Powderly WG. Use of paromomycin for treatment of cryptosporidiosis in patients with AIDS. Clin Infect Dis. 1993;16:298–300.

111. Craig WA, Suh B. Protein binding and the antimicrobial effects: Methods for the determination of protein binding. In: Lorian V, ed. Antibiotics in Medicine, 3rd ed. Baltimore: Williams & Wilkins; 1991;367–402.

112. Gilbert DN, Kutscher E, Ireland P, et al. Effect of the concentrations of magnesium and calcium on the in vitro susceptibility of Pseudomonas aeruginosa to gentamicin. J Infect Dis. 1971;124:537–44.

113. Reller LB, Schoenknecht FD, Kenny MA, et al. Antibiotic susceptibility testing of Pseudomonas aeruginosa: selection of a control strain and criteria for magnesium and calcium content in media. J Infect Dis. 19794;130:454–63.

114. Barry AL, Miller GH, Thornsberry C, et al. Influence of cation supplements on activity of netilmicin against Pseudomonas aeruginosa in vitro and in vivo. Antimicrob Agents Chemother. 1987;31:1514–8.

115. Barry AL. Procedures and theoretical considerations for testing antimicrobial agents in agar media. In: Lorian V, ed. Antibiotics in Laboratory Medicine. 3rd ed. Baltimore: Williams & Wilkins; 1991;3–8.

116. Ward PB, Palladino S, Looker JC, et al. P-nitrophenylglycerol in susceptibility testing media alters the MICs of antimicrobials for Pseudomonas aeruginosa. J Antimicrob Chemother. 1993;31:489–96.

117. Peddie BA, Chambers ST. Effects of betaines and urine on the antibacterial activity of aminoglycosides. J Antimicrob Chemother. 1993;31:481–8.

118. Eliopoulos GM, Moellering RC. Antimicrobial combinations. In: Lorian V, ed. Antibiotics in Laboratory Medicine. 3rd ed. Baltimore: Williams & Wilkins; 1991;432–92.

119. Vogelman B, Craig WA. Kinetics of antimicrobial activity. J Pediatr. 1986;108(5 Pt 2):835–40.

120. Kapusnik JE, Hackbarth CJ, Chambers HF, et al. Single, large daily dosing vs intermittent dosing of tobramycin for treating experimental Pseudomonas pneumonia. J Infect Dis. 1988;158:7–12.

121. Gerber AU, Fellder-Segessenmann C. In vivo assessment of in vitro killing patterns of Pseudomonas aeruginosa. J Antimicrob Chemother. 1985;15(Suppl A):201–6.

122. Blaser JB, Stone B, Zinner SH. Efficacy of intermittent versus continuous administration of netilmicin in a two-compartment in vitro model. Antimicrob Agents Chemother. 1985;27:343–9.

123. Dudley MN, Zinner SH. Single daily dosing of amikacin in an in vitro model. J Antimicrob Chemother. 1991;27(Suppl C):15–9.

124. Drusano GL. Role of pharmacokinetics in the outcome of infections. Antimicrob Agents Chemother. 1988;32:289–97.

125. Craig WA, Ebert SC. Continuous infusion of beta-lactams. Antimicrob Agents Chemother. 1992;36:2577–83.

126. Craig WA, Gudmundsson S. Postantibiotic effect. In Lorain V, ed. Antibiotics in the Laboratory. 3rd ed. Baltimore: Williams & Wilkins; 1991;403–31.

127. Fantin B, Ebert S, Leggett J, et al. Factors influencing the duration of in vivo postantibiotic effect for aminoglycosides against gram-negative bacilli. J Antimicrob Chemother. 1990;27:829–36.

128. Craig WA, Ebert SC. Killing and regrowth of bacteria in vitro: A review. Scand J Infect Dis. 1991;74(Suppl):63–70.

129. Gudmundsson S, Erlendsdottir H. The impact of drug combinations on the postantibiotic effect (PAE). In: Programs and Abstracts of the 28th Interscience Conference on Antimicrobial Agents and Chemotherapy. Abstract 773. Washington, DC: American Society for Microbiology; 1988:246.

130. Hessen MT, Pitsakis PG, Levison ME. Absence of a postantibiotic effect in experimental Pseudomonas endocarditis treated with imipenem, with or without gentamicin. J Infect Dis. 1988;158:542–8.

131. Allan JD, Moellering RC Jr. Management of infections caused by gram-negative bacilli: The role of antimicrobial combinations. Rev Infect Dis. 1985;7(Suppl 4):S559–71.

132. Holm SE. Interaction between β-lactam and other antibiotics. Rev Infect Dis. 1986;8(Suppl 3):S305–14.

133. Hunter TH. Use of streptomycin in the treatment of bacterial endocarditis. Am J Med. 1947;2:436–42.

134. Zak O, O'Reilly T. Animal models in the evaluation of antimicrobial agents. Antimicrob Agents Chemother. 1991;35:1527–31.

135. Andriole VT. Aminoglycoside antibiotics: Antibacterial efficacy in animal models of infection. J Infect Dis. 1983;5(Suppl 2):S233–49.

136. Vastola AP, Brandel J, Craig WA. Selection of aminoglycoside-resistant variants of Pseudomonas aeruginosa in an in vivo model. J Infect Dis. 1982;146:691–7.

137. Gerber AU, Feller-Segessenmann C. In vivo assessment of in vitro killing patterns of Pseudomonas aeruginosa. J Antimicrob Chemother. 1985;15:201–6.

138. Vogelman B, Gudmundsson S, Turnidge J, et al. In vivo postantibiotic effect in a thigh infection in neutropenic mice. J Infect Dis. 1988;157:287–98.

139. Craig WA. Post-antibiotic effects in experimental infection models: Relationship to in vitro phenomena and to treatment of infections in man. J Antimicrob Chemother. 1993;31(Suppl D):149–58.

140. Sohet I, Yellin A, Meyerovitch J, et al. Pharmacokinetics and therapeutic efficacy of gentamicin in an experimental pleural empyema rabbit model. Antimicrob Agents Chemother. 1987;31:982–5.

141. Gerber AU, Grestes U, Segesseman C, et al. The impact of the pre-treatment interval on antimicrobial efficacy in a biological model. J Antimicrob Chemother. 1993;31(Suppl D):29–39.

142. Fantin B, Carbon C. In vivo antibiotic synergism. Contribution of animal models. Antimicrob Agents Chemother. 1992;36:907–12.

143. Chavanet P, Colin F, Muggeo E, et al. The in vivo activity of co-amoxiclav with netilmicin against experimental methicillin and gentamicin resistant Staphylococcus epidermidis infection in rabbits. J Antimicrob Chemother. 1993;31:129–38.

144. Trautman M, Bruckner O, Marre R, et al. Comparative efficacy of ciprofloxacin, ceftazidime and gentamicin, given alone or in combination, in a model of experimental septicemia due to Klebsiella pneumoniae in neutropenic mice. Infection. 1988;16:49–53.

145. Gerber AU. Impact of the antibiotic dosage schedule on efficacy in experimental soft tissue infections. Scand J Infect Dis. 1991;74(Suppl):147–54.

146. Chadwick EK, Shulman ST, Yogev R. Correlation of antibiotic synergy in vitro and in vivo: Use of an animal model of neutropenic gram-negative sepsis. J Infect Dis. 1986;154:670–5.

147. Gordin FM, Riusnak MG, Sande MA. Evaluation of combination chemotherapy in a lightly anesthetized animal model of Pseudomonas pneumonia. Antimicrob Agents Chemother. 1987;31:398–403.

148. Fantin B, Pangon B, Potel G, et al. Ceftriaxone-netilmicin combination in single-daily-dose treatment of experimental Escherichia coli endocarditis. Antimicrob Agents Chemother. 1989;33:767–70.

149. Herscovici L, Grise G, Thauvin C, et al. Efficacy and safety of once daily versus intermittent dosing of tobramycin in rabbits with acute pyelonephritis. Scand J Infect Dis. 1988;20:205–12.

150. Gilbert DN. Once daily aminoglycoside therapy. Antimicrob Agents Chemother. 1991;35:339–405.

151. Gudmundsson S, Einarsson S, Erlendstotter H, et al. The postantibiotic effect of antimicrobial combinations in a neutropenic murine thigh infection model. J Antimicrob Chemother. 1993;31(Suppl D):177–91.

152. Michea Hamzehpour M, Auckenthaler R, Regamey P, et al. Resistance occurring after fluoroquinolone therapy of experimental Pseudomonas aeruginosa peritonitis. Antimicrob Agents Chemother. 1987;31:1803–8.

153. Michea-Hamzehpour M, Pechere JC, Marchou B, et al. Combination therapy: A way to limit emergence of resistance? Am J Med. 1986;80(Suppl 6B):138–42.

154. Pechere JC, Marchou B, Michea-Hamzehpour M, et al. Emergence of resistance after therapy with antibiotics used alone or combined in a murine model. J Antimicrob Chemother. 1986;17(Suppl A):11–18.

155. Gerber AU, VaStola AP, Brandel J, Craig WA. Selection of aminoglycoside-resistant variants of Pseudomonas aeruginosa in an in vivo model. J Infect Dis. 1982;146:691–7.

156. Weinstein WM, Onderdonk AB, Bartlett JG, et al. Antimicrobial therapy of experimental intra-abdominal sepsis. J Infect Dis. 1975;131:282–6.

157. Nichols RL, Smith JW, Fossedal EN, et al. Efficacy of parenteral antibiotics in the treatment of experimentally induced intra-abdominal sepsis. Rev Infect Dis. 1979;1:302–12.

158. Weinstein WM, Onderdonk AB, Bartlett JG, et al. Experimental intra-abdominal abscesses in rats: development of an experimental model. Infect Immun. 1974;10:1250–5.

159. Onderdonk AB, Kasper DL, Cisneros RL, et al. The capsular polysaccharide of Bacteroides fragilis as a virulence factor: Comparison of the pathogenic potential of encapsulated and unencapsulated strains. J Infect Dis. 1977;136:82–9.

160. Nichols RL, Smith JW. Wound and intra-abdominal infections: Microbiological considerations and approaches to treatment. Clin Infect Dis. 1993;16(Suppl 4):S266–77.

161. Onderdonk AB, Bartlett JG, Louie T, et al. Microbial synergy in experimental intra-abdominal abscess. Infect Immun. 1976;13:22–6.

162. Barza M, Lauermann M. Why monitor serum levels of gentamicin? Clin Pharmacokinet. 1978;3:202–15.

163. Kunin CM, Chalmers TC, Leevy CM, et al. Absorption of orally administered neomycin and kanamycin. N Engl J Med. 1960;262:380–5.

164. Last PM, Sherlock S. Systemic absorption of oral administered neomycin in liver disease. N Engl J Med. 1960;262:385–9.

165. Breen KJ, Bryant RE, Levinson JD, et al. Neomycin absorption in man. Ann Intern Med. 1972;76:211–8.

166. Little PJ, Lynn KL. Neomycin toxicity. NZ Med J. 1975;81:445.

167. Bamford MFM, Jones LF. Deafness and biochemical imbalance after burns treatment with topical antibiotics in young children. Arch Dis Child. 1978;53:326–9.

168. Pittinger CB, Adamson R. Antibiotic blockade of neuromuscular function. Annu Rev Pharmacol. 1972;12:169–84.

169. Chamberlain G, Needham P. The absorption of antibiotics from the bladder. J Urol. 1976;116:172–3.

170. Lifschitz MI, Denning CR. Safety of kanamycin aerosol. Clin Pharmacol Ther. 1971;12:91–5.

171. Odio W, VanLeier E, Klastersky J. Concentrations of gentamicin in bronchial secretions after intramuscular and endotracheal administration. J Clin Pharmacol. 1975;15:518–24.

172. Van Etta LL, Kravitz GR, Russ TE, et al. Effect of method of administration on extravascular penetration of four antibiotics. Antimicrob Agents Chemother. 1982;21:873–80.

173. Bennett WM, Aronoff GR, Golper TA, et al. Drug Prescribing in Renal Failure. 2nd ed. Philadelphia, PA: American College of Physicians; 1991.

174. Schwartz SN, Pazin GJ, Lyon JA, et al. A controlled investigation of the pharmacokinetics of gentamicin and tobramycin in obese subjects. J Infect Dis. 1978;138:499–505.

175. Kunar MJ, Mak LL, Lietman PS. Localization of ^{3}H-gentamicin in the proximal renal tubule of the mouse. Antimicrob Agents Chemother. 1979;15: 131–3.
176. Ramsey BW, Dorkin HL, Eisenberg JD, et al. Efficacy of aerosolized tobramycin in patients with cystic fibrosis. N Engl J Med. 1993;328:1740–6.
177. Rahal JJ Jr, Hyams PJ, Simberkoff MS, et al. Combined intrathecal and intramuscular gentamicin for gram-negative meningitis. N Engl J Med. 1974; 290:1394–8.
178. Kaiser AB, McGee ZA. Aminoglycoside therapy of gram-negative bacillary meningitis. N Engl J Med. 1975;293:1215–20.
179. Wirt TC, McGee ZA, Oldfield EH, et al. Intraventricular administration of amikacin for complicated gram-negative meningitis and ventriculitis. J Neurosurg. 1979;50:95–9.
180. McCracken GH Jr, Mize S, Threlkeld N. Intraventricular gentamicin therapy in gram-negative bacillary meningitis of infancy. Lancet. 1980;1:787–91.
181. Wood MJ, Farrell W. Comparison of urinary excretion of tobramycin and gentamicin in adults. J Infect Dis. 1976;134(Suppl):S133–6.
182. Kahlmeter G, Kamme G. Prolonged excretion of gentamicin in a patient with unimpaired renal function. Lancet. 1975;1:286.
183. Kahlmeter G. Netilmicin: clinical pharmacokinetics and aspects on dosage schedules. An overview. Scand J Infect Dis. 1980;23:74–81.
184. Laskin OL, Longstreth JA, Smith CR, et al. Netilmicin and gentamicin multidose kinetics in normal subjects. Clin Pharmacol Ther. 1983;34:644–50.
185. Dee TH, Kozin F. Gentamicin and tobramycin penetration into synovial fluid. Antimicrob Agents Chemother. 1977;12:548–9.
186. Pitt HA, Roberts RB, Johnson WD Jr. Gentamicin levels in the human biliary tract. J Infect Dis. 1973;127:299–302.
187. Mendelson J, Portnoy J, Sigman H. Pharmacology of gentamicin in the biliary tract of humans. Antimicrob Agents Chemother. 1973;4:538–41.
188. Pflugfelder SC, Flynn HW. Infectious endophthalmitis. Infect Dis Clin North Am. 1992;6:859–73.
189. Barza M, Kane A, Baum J. Comparison of the effects of continuous and intermittent systemic administration on the penetration of gentamicin into infected rabbit eyes. J Infect Dis. 1983;147:144–8.
190. Gorden TB, Cunningham RD. Tobramycin levels in aqueous humor after subconjunctival injection in humans. Am J Ophthalmol. 1982;93:107–10.
191. Rubenstein E, Goldfarb J, Keren G, et al. The penetration of gentamicin into the vitreous humor in man. Invest Ophthalmol Vis Sci. 1983;24:637–9.
192. Wilson TW, Mahon WA, Inaba T, et al. Elimination of tritiated gentamicin in normal human subjects and in patients with severely impaired renal function. Clin Pharmacol Ther. 1973;14:815–22.
193. Collier VU, Lietman PS, Mitch WE. Evidence for luminal uptake of gentamicin in perfused rat kidney. J Pharmacol Exp. Ther. 1979;210:247–51.
194. Silberblatt FJ, Kuehn C. Autoradiography of gentamicin uptake by the rat proximal tubular cell. Kidney Int. 1979;15:335–45.
195. Beauchamp D, Gourde P, Bergeron MG. Subcellular distribution of gentamicin in proximal tubular cells, determined by immunogold labeling. Antimicrob Agents Chemother. 1991;35:2173–9.
196. Fabre J, Rudhardt M, Blanchard P, et al. Persistence of sisomicin and gentamicin in renal cortex and medulla compared with other organs and serum of rats. Kidney Int. 1976;10:444–9.
197. Schentag JJ, Jusko WJ: Renal clearance and tissue accumulation of gentamicin. Clin Pharmacol Ther. 1977;22:364–70.
198. Laskin OL, Longstreth JA, Smith CR, Leitman PS. Netilmicin and gentamicin multidose kinetics in normal subjects. Clin Pharmacol Ther. 1983;34: 644–50.
199. Gyselynck A-M, Forrey A, Cutler R. Pharmacokinetics of gentamicin: distribution and plasma and renal clearance. J Infect Dis. 1971;124(Suppl):S70–6.
200. Plantier J, Forrey AW, O'Neill MA, et al. Pharmacokinetics of amikacin in patients with normal or impaired renal function: radioenzymatic acetylation assay. J Infect Dis. 1976;134(Suppl):S323–30.
201. Barza M, Brown RB, Shen D, et al. Predictability of blood levels of gentamicin in man. J Infect Dis. 1975;132:165–74.
202. Clarke JT, Libke RD, Regamey C, Kirby WM. Comparative pharmacokinetics of amikacin and kanamycin. Clin Pharmacol Ther. 1974;15:610–6.
203. McCracken GH, Freij BJ. Clinical pharmacology of antimicrobial agents. In: Remington JS, Klein JO, eds. Infectious Diseases of the Fetus and Newborn Infant. 3rd ed. Philadelphia: WB Saunders; 1990;1020–76.
204. Welling PG, Baumueller A, Lau CC, et al. Netilmicin pharmacokinetics after single intravenous doses to elderly male patients. Antimicrob Agents Chemother. 1977;12:328–34.
205. Appel GB. Aminoglycoside nephrotoxicity. Am J Med. 1990;88(Suppl C): 16S–20S.
206. Brummett RE, Fox KE. Aminoglycoside-induced hearing loss in humans. Antimicrob Agents Chemother. 1989;33:797–800.
207. Reinhard MK, Hottendorf GH, Powell FD. Differences in the sensitivity of Fischer and Sprague-Dawley rats to aminoglycoside nephrotoxicity. Toxicol Pathol. 1991;19:66–71.
208. Vaamonde CA, Pardo V, Fajardo C, et al. The nude rat is protected against gentamicin nephrotoxicity (Abstract). Role of T cells. 12th Int Cong Nephrol. 1993;12:273.
209. Baylis C, Rennke HR, Brenner RM. Mechanisms of the defect in glomerular ultrafiltration associated with gentamicin administration. Kidney Int. 1977; 12:344–8.
210. De-Barrow-E-Silva ML, Varanda WA, Lachat JJ, et al. Glomerular permeability to macromolecules in gentamicin-treated rats. Brazel J Med Biol Res. 1992;25:409–17.
211. Lipsky JJ, Lietman PS. Neomycin inhibition of adenosine triphosphate: Evidence for a neomycin-phospholipid interaction. Antimicrob Agents Chemother. 1980;18:532–5.
212. Mondorf AQW, Breier J, Hendus J, et al. Effect of aminoglycosides on proximal tubular membranes of the human kidney. Eur J Clin Pharmacol. 1978;13:133–42.
213. Beck PR, Thompson RB, Chaudhuri AKR. Aminoglycoside antibiotics and renal function: Changes in urinary γ-glutamyltransferase excretion. J Clin Pathol. 1977;30:432–7.
214. Foster JE, Harpur ES, Garland HO. An investigation of the acute effect of gentamicin on the renal handling of electrolytes in the rat. J Pharmacol Exp Ther. 1992;281:38–43.
215. Elliott WB, Patchin DS. Aminoglycoside-mediated calcinosis. J Pharmacol Exp Ther. 1992;262:151–6.
216. Feldman S, Wang M-Y, Kaloyamides GJ. Aminoglycosides induce a phospholipidosis in the renal cortex of the rat: An early manifestation of nephrotoxicity. J Pharmacol Exp Ther. 1982;220:514–20.
217. Marche P, Koutouzov S, Girard A. Impairment of membrane phosphoinositide metabolism by aminoglycoside antibiotics. Streptomycin, amikacin, kanamycin, dibekacin, gentamicin, and neomycin. J Pharmacol Exp Ther. 1983; 227:415–20.
218. Josepovitz C, Levine R, Farrugella T, Kaloyanides G. Comparative effects of aminoglycosides on renal cortical and urinary phospholipids in the rat. Proc Soc Exp Biol Med. 1986;182:1–5.
219. Ibrahim S, Van der Auwera P, Meunier F, et al. Effect of netilmicin and amikacin on urinary phospholipid excretion in humans. Arch Toxicol Suppl. 1989;13:413–6.
220. Shepherd VL. Intracellular pathways and mechanisms of sorting in receptor-mediated endocytosis. TIPS. 1989;10:458–62.
221. Kohlhepp S, Bennett J, Leggett J, et al. Computerized fluorescent videomicroscopy demonstration of the renal cell handling of tobramycin in vitro. In: Programs and Abstracts of the 29th Interscience Conference on Antimicrobial Agents and Chemotherapy. Abstract 293. Washington, DC: American Society for Microbiology; 1989:385.
222. Sastrasink M, Weinberg JM, Humes HD. The effect of gentamicin on calcium uptake by renal mitochondria. Life Sci. 1982;30:2309–15.
223. Bennett WM, Mela-Riker L, Houghton DC, et al. Microsomal protein synthesis inhibition: An early manifestation of gentamicin nephrotoxicity. Am J Physiol. 1988;2255:F265–9.
224. Loveless MO, Kohlhepp SJ, Gilbert DN. The influence of aminoglycoside antibiotics on the in vitro function of rat liver ribosomes. J Lab Clin Med. 1984;103:294–303.
225. Kirschbaum BB. Interactions between renal brush border membranes and "polyamines." J Pharmacol Exp Ther. 1984;229:409–16.
226. Kaloyanides GJ, Ramsammy LS. Possible role of altered polyamine metabolism in gentamicin toxicity in OK cells. Contrib Nephrol. 1993;101:199–205.
227. Gilbert DN, Bennett WM. Progress in the elucidation of aminoglycoside nephrotoxicity. Contemp Iss Infect Dis. 1984;1:121–52.
228. Gilbert DN, Houghton DC, Bennett WM, et al. Reversibility of gentamicin nephrotoxicity in rats: Recovery during continuous drug administration. Proc Soc Exp Biol Med. 1979;160:99–103.
229. Luft FC, Bennett WM, Gilbert DN. Experimental aminoglycoside nephrotoxicity: accomplishments and future potential. Rev Infect Dis. 1983;5(Suppl 2):S268–93.
230. Gilbert DN, Plamp C, Starr P, et al. Comparative nephrotoxicity of gentamicin and tobramycin in rats. Antimicrob Agents Chemother. 1979;13:34–40.
231. Luft FC, Bloch R, Sloan RS, et al. Comparative nephrotoxicity of aminoglycoside antibiotics in rats. J Infect Dis. 1978;138:541–5.
232. Bennett WM, Plamp CE, Gilbert DN, et al. The influence of dosage regimen on experimental gentamicin nephrotoxicity: Dissociation of peak serum levels from renal failure. J Infect Dis. 1979;140:576–80.
233. Powell SH, Thompson WL, Luthe MA, et al. Once daily vs continuous aminoglycoside dosing: Efficacy and toxicity in animal and clinical studies of gentamicin, netilmicin, and tobramycin. J Infect Dis. 1983;147:918–23.
234. Beauchamp D, Gourde P, Thereault G, Bergeron MG. Age-dependent gentamicin experimental nephrotoxicity. J Pharmacol Exp. Ther. 1992;260:444–9.
235. Provoost A, Adeljuyigbe O, Wolfe ED. Nephrotoxicity of aminoglycosides in young and adult rats. Pediatr Res. 1985;19:1191–6.
236. Marre R, Tarara N, Louton T, Sack K. Age-dependent nephrotoxicity and the pharmacokinetics of gentamicin in rats. Eur J Pediatr. 1980;133:25–9.
237. McMartin DN, Engel SG. Effect of aging on gentamicin nephrotoxicity in rats. Res Commun Chem Pathol Pharmacol. 1982;38:193–207.
238. Bennett WM, Parker RA, Elliott WB, et al. Sex: A determinant of susceptibility to gentamicin nephrotoxicity in the rat. J Infect Dis. 1982;145:370–3.
239. Moore RD, Smith CR, Lipsky JJ, et al. Risk factors for nephrotoxicity in patients treated with aminoglycosides. Ann Intern Med. 1984;100:352–7.
240. Sawyers CL, Moore RD, Lerner SA, et al. A model for predicting nephrotoxicity in patients treated with aminoglycosides. J Infect Dis. 1985;153:1062–8.
241. Elliott WB, Parker RA, Houghton DC, et al. Effect of sodium bicarbonate and ammonium chloride ingestion in experimental gentamicin nephrotoxicity in rats. Res Commun Pathol Pharmacol. 1980;28:483–96.
242. Bennett WM, Hartnett MN, Gilbert D, et al. Effect of sodium intake on gentamicin nephrotoxicity in the rat. Proc Soc Exp Biol Med. 1976;151: 736–8.
243. Peterson LN, Borzecki JS. Inhibition of tobramycin reabsorption in nephron segments by metabolic alkalosis. Kidney Int. 1990;37:1492–9.
244. Chiu PJS, Miller GH, Long JF, et al. Renal uptake and nephrotoxicity of

gentamicin during urinary alkalinization in rats. Clin Exp Pharmacol Physiol. 1979;6:317–26.

245. Thompson JR, Simonsen R, Spindler MA, et al. Protective effect of KCl loading in gentamicin nephrotoxicity. Am J Kidney Dis. 1990;15:583–91.

246. Rodriquez HJ, Hogan WC, Hellman RN, et al. Mechanism of activation of renal Na$^+$-K$^+$-ATPase in the rat: Effects of potassium loading. Am J Physiol 1980;238:F315–23.

247. Cronin RE, Newman JA. Protective effect of thyroxine but not parathyroidectomy on gentamicin nephrotoxicity. Am J Physiol. 1985;248:F332–9.

248. Adelman RD, Spangler WL, Beasom F, et al. Furosemide enhancement of experimental gentamicin nephrotoxicity: Comparison of functional and morphological changes with activities of urinary enzymes. J Infect Dis. 1979; 140:342–52.

249. Nakahama H, Fukuhara Y, Osita Y, et al. Furosemide accelerates gentamicin accumulation in cultured renal cells (LLC-PK1 cells). Nephron. 1989;53: 138–41.

250. Bennett WM, Elliott WC, Houghton DC, et al. Reduction of experimental gentamicin nephrotoxicity in rats by dietary calcium loading. Antimicrob Agents Chemother. 1982;22:508–12.

251. Quarum ML, Houghton DC, Gilbert DN, et al. Increasing dietary calcium moderates experimental gentamicin nephrotoxicity. J Lab Clin Med. 1984; 103:104–14.

252. Humes HD, Sastrasinh M, Weinberg JM. Calcium is a competitive inhibitor of gentamicin–renal membrane binding interactions and dietary calcium supplementation protects against gentamicin nephrotoxicity. J Clin Invest. 1984; 73:134–47.

253. Ernst S. Model of gentamicin-induced nephrotoxicity and its amelioration by calcium and thyroxine. Med Hypoth. 1989;30:195–202.

254. Vakil N, Abu-Alfa A, Mujais SK. Gentamicin nephrotoxicity in extrahepatic cholestasis: Modulation by dietary calcium. Hepatology. 1989;9:519–24.

255. Camps J, Sola X, Rimola A, et al. Comparative study of aminoglycoside nephrotoxicity in normal rats and rats with experimental cirrhosis. Hepatology. 1988;8:837–44.

256. Lietman PS. Liver disease, aminoglycoside antibiotics, and renal dysfunction. Hepatology. 1988;4:966–8.

257. Teixeira RB, Kelley J, Alpert H, et al. Complete protection from gentamicin-induced acute renal failure in the diabetes mellitus rat. Kidney Int. 1982;21: 600–12.

258. Elliott WB, Houghton DC, Gilbert DN, et al. Experimental gentamicin nephrotoxicity: Effect of streptozotocin-induced diabetes. J Pharmacol Exp Ther. 1985;233:264–70.

259. Wood CA, Kohlhepp SJ, Kohnen PW, et al. Vancomycin enhancement of experimental tobramycin nephrotoxicity. Antimicrob Agents Chemother. 1985;30:20–4.

260. Kohlhepp SJ, Gilbert DN, Kohnen PW, et al. Teicoplanin enhancement of experimental tobramycin nephrotoxicity (Abstract). 31st Interscience Conference on Antimicrobial Agents Chemotherapy. Washington, DC: American Society for Microbiology; 1991.

261. Golper TA, Noonan HM, Elzinga L, et al. Vancomycin pharmacokinetics, renal handling and non-renal clearance in normal human subjects. Clin Pharmacol Ther. 1988;43:565–70.

262. English J, Gilbert DN, Kohlhepp SJ, et al. Attenuation of experimental tobramycin nephrotoxicity by ticarcillin. Antimicrob Agents Chemother. 1985; 276:897–902.

263. Sabra R, Branch RA. Role of sodium in protection by extended spectrum penicillins against tobramycin-induced nephrotoxicity. Antimicrob Agents Chemother. 1990;340:1020–5.

264. Barr GA, Mazze RI, Cousins MJ, et al. An animal model for combined methoxyflurane and gentamicin nephrotoxicity. Br J Anesthesiol. 1973;45: 306–31.

265. Whiting PH, Simpson JG. The enhancement of cyclosporin-A induced nephrotoxicity by gentamicin. Biochem Pharmacol. 1983;32:2025–8.

266. Ryffel B, Muller AM, Mihatsch MJ. Experimental cyclosporine nephrotoxicity: Risk of concomitant chemotherapy. Clin Nephrol 1988;25(Suppl 1): S121–5.

267. Jongejan HTM, Provoost AP, Molenaar JC. Potentiated nephrotoxicity of cisplatin when combined with amikacin comparing young and adult rats. Pediatr Nephrol. 198;31:290–5.

268. Williams PD, Hottdenford GH. Inhibition of renal membrane binding and nephrotoxicity of gentamicin by polyasparagine and polyaspartic acid in the rat. Res Commun Chem Pathol Pharmacol. 1985;47:317–20.

269. Gilbert DN, Wood CA, Kohlhepp SJ, et al. Polyaspartic acid prevents experimental aminoglycoside nephrotoxicity. J Infect Dis. 1989;159:945–53.

270. Swan SK, Kohlhepp SJ, Kohnen PW, et al. Long-term protection of poly-aspartic acid in experimental gentamicin nephrotoxicity. Antimicrob Agents Chemother. 1991;35:2591–5.

271. Gilbert DN, Kohlhepp SJ, Swan SK, et al. Pharmacologic limits of polyaspartic acid's protective effect on experimental gentamicin nephrotoxicity. Submitted for publication.

272. Swan SK, Gilbert DN, Kohlhepp SJ, Leggett JE, Kohnen PW, Bennett WM. Duration of the protective effect of polyaspartic acid on experimental gentamicin nephrotoxicity. Antimicrob Agents Chemother. 1992;36:2556–8.

273. Ramsammy LS, Josepovitz C, Lane BP, et al. Polyaspartic acid protects against gentamicin nephrotoxicity in the rat. J Pharmacol Exp Ther. 1989; 250:149–53.

274. Beauchamp D, Laurent G, Maldague P, et al. Reduction of gentamicin nephrotoxicity by the concomitant administration of poly-L-aspartic acid and poly-L-asparagine in rats. Arch Toxicol. 1986;9(Suppl):306–9.

275. Beauchamp D, Laurent G, Maldague P, et al. Protection against gentamicin-induced early renal alterations (phospholipidosis and increased DNA synthe-

276. Kishore BK, Ibrahim S, Lambrict P, et al. Comparative assessment of poly-L-aspartic and poly-L-glutamic acids as protectants against gentamicin-induced renal lysosomal phospholipidosis, phospholipiduria and cell proliferation in rats. J Pharmacol Exp. Ther. 1992;262:424–32.

277. Kohlhepp SJ, McGregor D, Gilbert DN. Determinants of the in vitro interaction of polyaspartic acid and aminoglycoside antibiotics. J Pharmacol Exp. Ther. 1992;263:1464–70.

278. Ramsammy L, Josepovitz C, Lane B, et al. Polyaspartic acid inhibits gentamicin-induced perturbations of phospholipid metabolism. Am J Physiol. 1990;258:C1141–9.

279. Luft FC. Cephalosporin and aminoglycoside interactions: Clinical and toxicologic implications. In: Whelton A, Neu HC, eds. The Aminoglycosides. New York: Marcel Dekker; 1982;387–99.

280. Kahlmeter G, Dahlager JI. Aminoglycoside toxicity—A review of clincal studies published between 1975 and 1982. J Antimicrob Chemother. 1984; 13(Suppl A):9–22.

281. Lietman PS, Smith CR. Aminoglycoside nephrotoxicity in humans. Rev Infect Dis. 1983;5(Suppl 2):284–92.

282. Smith CR, Baughman KL, Edwards CQ, et al. Controlled comparison of amikacin and gentamicin. N Engl J Med. 1977;296:349–53.

283. Smith CR, Lipsky JJ, Laskin OL, et al. Double-blind comparison of the nephrotoxicity and auditory toxicity of gentamicin and tobramycin. N Engl J Med. 1980;302:1106–9.

284. Smith CR, Ambinder R, Lipsky JJ, et al. Cefotaxime compared with nafcillin plus tobramycin for serious bacterial infections. Ann Intern Med. 1984;101: 469–77.

285. Bertino JS, Booker LA, Franck PA, et al. Incidence of and significant risk factors for aminoglycoside-associated nephrotoxicity in patients dosed by using individualized pharmacokinetic monitoring. J Infect Dis. 1993;167: 173–9.

286. Lerner AM, Cone LA, Jansen W, et al. Randomized, controlled trial of the comparative efficacy, auditory toxicity and nephrotoxicity of tobramycin and netilmicin. Lancet. 1983;1:1123–6.

287. Lerner SA, Schmitt BA, Seligsohn R, et al. Comparative study of ototoxicity and nephrotoxicity in patients randomly assigned treatment with amikacin and gentamicin. Am J Med. 1986;80(Suppl 5B):98–104.

288. Petty BG, Baumgardner JY, Leitman PS. Comparison of the renal effects of single vs. thrice daily dosing in healthy volunteers (Abstract). 26th Interscience Conference on Antimicrobial Agents and Chemotherapy. Washington DC: American Society of Microbiology; 1986.

289. Hou SH, Bushinsky DA, Wish JB, et al. Hospital-acquired renal insufficiency: A prospective study. Am J Med. 1983;74:243–8.

290. Trollfors B. Gentamicin-associated changes in renal function reversible during continued treatment. J Antimicrob Chemother. 1983;12:285–7.

291. Desai TK, Tsang T-K. Aminoglycoside nephrotoxicity in obstructive jaundice. Am J Med. 1988;85:47–50.

292. Ter Braak EW, DeVries PJ, Bouter KP, et al. Once daily dosing regimen for aminoglycoside plus β-lactam combination therapy of serious bacterial infections: Comparative trial with netilmicin plus ceftriaxone. Am J Med. 1990;89:58–66.

293. Prins JM, Buller HR, Kuijper EJ, et al. Once versus thrice daily gentamicin in patients with serious infections. Lancet. 1993;341:335–9.

294. Marik PE, Kipman J, Obilski S, et al. A prospective randomized study comparing once versus twice daily amikacin dosing in critically ill adult and pediatric patients. J Antimicrob Chemother. 1991;28:753–64.

295. Farber BF, Moellering RC. Retrospective study of the toxicity of preparations of vancomycin from 1974–1981. Antimicrob Agents Chemother. 1983; 23:138–41.

296. Rybak MJ, Albrecht LM, Boike SC, et al. Nephrotoxicity of vancomycin alone and with an aminoglycoside. J Antimicrob Chemother. 1990;25:679–87.

297. Nahata MC. Lack of nephrotoxicity in pediatric patients receiving vancomycin and aminoglycoside therapy. Chemotherapy. 1987;33:302–4.

298. Bennett WM, Wood CA, Houghton DC, et al. Modification of experimental aminoglycoside nephrotoxicity. Am J Kidney Dis. 1986;8:292–6.

299. The EORTC International Antimicrobial Therapy Project Group. Three antibiotic regimens in the treatment of infection in febrile granulocytopenic patients with cancer. J Infect Dis. 1978;137:14–29.

300. Klastersky J, Hensgens C, Debussscher I. Empiric therapy for cancer patients: Comparative study of ticarcillin-tobramycin, ticarcillin-cephalothin, and cephalothin-tobramycin. Antimicrob Agents Chemother. 1975;7:640–5.

301. Wade JC, Smith CR, Petty BG, et al. Cephalothin plus an aminoglycoside is more nephrotoxic than methicillin plus an aminoglycoside. Lancet. 1978; 3:604–6.

302. Mazze RI, Cousins MJ. Combined nephrotoxicity of gentamicin and methoxyflurane in man. Br J Anaesthes. 1973;45:394–8.

303. Green FJ, Lavelle KJ, Aronoff GR, et al. Management of amikacin overdose. Am J Kidney Dis. 1981;1:110–2.

304. Ho PW, Pien FD, Kominami N. Massive amikacin "overdose." Ann Intern Med. 1979;91:227–8.

305. Cooper B, Creger RJ, Soegiarso W, et al. Renal dysfunction during high-dose cisplatin therapy and autologous hematopoietic stein cell transplantation: Effect of aminoglycoside therapy Am J Med. 1993;94:497–504.

306. Leach CT, Kuhls TL, Brill JE, et al. Use of aminoglycosides during cyclosporine A immunosuppression after liver transplantation in children. Pediatr Infect Dis J. 1989;8:354–7.

307. Hinshaw HC, Feldman WH. Streptomycin in treatment of clinical tuberculosis: A preliminary report. Proc Staff Meet Mayo Clin. 1945;20:313–8.

308. Fausti SA, Henry JA, Schaffer HI, et al. High-frequency audiometric moni-

toring for early detection of aminoglycoside ototoxicity. J Infect Dis. 1992; 165:1026–32.

309. Govaerts PJ, Claes PH, DeHeyring PHV, et al. Aminoglycoside-induced ototoxicity. Toxicol Lett. 1990;52:227–51.
310. Sataloff J, Wagner S, Menduke H. Kanamycin ototoxicity in healthy men. Arch Otolaryngol. 1964;80:413–7.
311. Davey PG, Jabeen F, Harpur ES, et al. The use of pure-tone audiometry in the assessment of gentamicin auditory toxicity. Br J Audiol. 1982;16:151–4.
312. Moore RD, Smith CR, Lietman PS. Risk factors for the development of auditory toxicity in patients receiving aminoglycosides. J Infect Dis. 1984; 149:23–30.
312a. Hutchin T, Haworth I, Higashi K, et al. A molecular basis for human hypersensitivity to aminoglycoside antibiotics. Nucleic Acids Research. 1993;21: 4174–79.
312b. Fischel-Ghodsian N, Prezant TR, Bu X, et al. Mitochondrial ribosomal RNA gene mutation in a patient with sporadic aminoglycoside ototoxicity. Am J Otolaryngol. 1993;14:399–403.
313. Tran Ba Huy P, Bernard P, Schacht J. Kinetics of gentamicin uptake and release in the rat. Comparison of inner ear tissues and fluids with other organs. J Clin Invest. 1986;77:1492–500.
314. Schacht J. Isolation of an aminoglycoside receptor from guinea pig inner ear tissues and kidney. Arch Otorhinolaryngol. 1979;224:129–34.
315. Dulon D, Zajic G, Aran JM, Schacht J. Aminoglycoside antibiotics impair calcium entry but not viability and motility in isolated cochlear outer hair cells. J Neurosci Res. 1989;24:338–46.
316. Schact J. Molecular mechanisms of drug-induced hearing loss. Hear Res. 1986;22:297–304.
317. de Groot JCMJ, Meeuwsen F, Ruizendaal WE, et al. Ultrastructural localization of gentamicin in the cochlear. Hear Res. 1990;50:35–42.
318. Hashino E, Tanaka Y, Salvi RJ, et al. Hair cell regeneration in the adult budgerigar after kanamycin ototoxicity. Hear Res. 1992;59:46–58.
319. Lombarte A, Yan HY, Popper AN, et al. Damage and regeneration of hair cell ciliary bundles in a fish ear following treatment with gentamicin. Hear Res. 1993;64:166–74.
320. Forge A, Li L, Corwin JT, et al. Ultrastructural evidence for hair cel regeneration in the mammalian inner ear. Science. 1993;259:1616–21.
321. Brummett RE, Fox KE. Studies of aminoglycoside ototoxicity in animal models. In: Whetton A, Neu HC, eds. The Aminoglycosides: Microbiology, Clinical Use and Toxicology. New York: Marcel Dekker; 1982:419–51.
322. Brummett RE, Bendrick T, Himes D. Comparative ototoxicity of bumetanide and furosemide when used in combination with kanamycin. J Clin Pharmacol. 1981;21:628–36.
323. Brummett RE, Fox KE. Vancomycin- and erythromycin-induced hearing loss in humans. Antimicrob Agents Chemother. 1989;33:791–6.
324. Brummett RE, Fox KE, Kempton JB. Quantitative relationships of the interaction between sound and kanamycin. Arch Otolaryngol Head Neck Surg. 1992;118:498–500.
325. Tran Ba Huy PT, Deffrennes D. Aminoglycoside ototoxicity: Influence of dosage regimen on drug uptake and correlation between membrane binding and some clinical features. Acta Otolaryngol. 1988;105:511–5.
326. Pettarossi VE, Ferraresi A, Errico P, et al. The impact of different dosing regimens of the aminoglycosides netilmicin and amikacin on vestibulotoxicity in the guinea pig. Eur Arch Otorhinolaryngol. 1990;247:277–82.
327. Moore RD, Smith CR, Lietman PS. Risk factors for the development of auditory toxicity in patients receiving aminoglycosides. J Infect Dis. 1984; 149:23–30.
328. Gatell JM, Ferran F, Araujo V, et al. Univariate and multivariate analyses of risk factors predisposing to auditory toxicity in patients receiving aminoglycosides. Antimicrob Agents Chemother. 1987;31:1383–7.
329. Buring JE, Evans DA, Mayrent SL, et al. Randomized trials of aminoglycoside antibiotics: Quantitative overview. Rev Infect Dis. 1988;10:951–7.
330. Manian FA, Stone WJ, Alford R: Adverse antibiotic effects associatd with renal insufficiency. Rev Infect Dis. 1990;12:236–49.
331. Bendush CL. Ototoxicity: Clinical considerations and comparative information. In: Whelton A, Neu HC, eds. The Aminoglycosides. New York: Marcel Dekker; 1982;452–486.
332. DeOliveira JAA. Audiovestibular Toxicity of Drugs. vols I, II. Boca Raton: CRC Press; 1989.
333. Lerner SA, Martz GJ, Hawkins JE, eds. Aminoglycoside Ototoxicity. Boston: Little, Brown; 1981.
334. Amiko M, Bagger-Sjoback D, Wersall J, et al. Gentamicin binding to the isolated crista ampullaris of the guinea pig. Res Commun Chem Pathol Pharmacol. 1982;37:333–42.
335. Snavely SR, Hodges GR. The neurotoxicity of antibacterial agents. Ann Intern Med. 1984;101:92–104.
336. Talbot PA. Potentiation of aminoglycoside-induced neuromuscular blockade by protons in vitro and in vivo. J Pharmacol Exp Ther. 1987;241:686–94.
337. Del-Pozo E, Baezem, JM. Effects of calcium channel blockers on neuromuscular blockade induced by aminoglycoside antibiotics. Eur J Pharmacol. 1986;128:49–54.
338. Gay CT, Marks WA, Riley HD Jr, et al. Infantile botulism. South Med J. 1988;81:457–60.
339. Sanders DB, Kim YI, Howard JR Jr, et al. Intercostal muscle biopsy studies in myasthenia gravis: Clinical correlations and the direct effects of drugs and myasthenic serum. Ann NY Acad Sci. 1981;377:544–66.
340. Hokkanen E. The aggravating effect of some antibiotics on the neuromuscular blockade in myasthenia gravis. Acta Neurol Scand. 1964;40:346–52.
341. Wright JM, Collier B. The effects of neomycin upon transmitter release and action. J Pharmacol Exp Ther. 1977;200:576–87.
342. Lee C, DeSilva AJ. Acute and subchronic neuromuscular blocking characteristics of streptomycin: a comparison with neomycin. Br J Anaesth. 1979;51: 431–4.
343. Caputy AJ, Kim YI, Sanders DB. The neuromuscular blocking effects of therapeutic concentrations of various antibiotics on normal rat skeletal muscle: A quantitative comparison. J Pharmacol Exp Ther. 1981;217:369–78.
344. Antibiotic-induced paralysis of the mouse phrenic nerve-hemidiaphragm preparation, and reversibility by calcium and by neostigmine. Anesthesiology. 1978;48:418–24.
345. Neu HC. Clinical use of aminoglycosides. In: Whelton A, Neu HC, eds. The Aminoglycosides. New York: Marcel Dekker; 1982;611–28.
346. Sanford JP. Guide to Antimicrobial Therapy—1993. Dallas: Antimicrobial Therapy; 1993:2–38.
347. Choice of antimicrobials. Med Lett. 1992;34:49–60.
348. Warren S, Burke JF. Infection and burn wounds: Evaluation and management. Current Clin Top Infect Dis. 1991;11:206–17.
349. Bisno AL, Dismukes WE, Durack DT, et al. Antimicrobial treatment of infective endocarditis due to viridans streptococci, enterococci, and staphylococci. JAMA. 1989;261:1471–7.
350. Ho JL, Barza M. Role of aminoglycoside antibiotics in the treatment of intra-abdominal infection. Antimicrob Agents Chemother. 1987;31:485–91.
351. Gorbach SL. Treatment of intra-abdominal infections. J Antimicrob Chemother. 1993;31(Suppl A):67–78.
352. Hughes WT, Armstrong D, Bodey GP, et al. Guidelines for the use of antimicrobial agents in neutropenic patients with unexplained fever. J Infect Dis. 1990;161:381–96.
353. Pizzo PA. Management of fever in patients with cancer and treatment-induced neutropenia. N Engl J Med. 328:1323–32.
354. Ho G Jr. Bacterial arthritis. Curr Opin Rheumatol. 1992;4:509–15.
355. Gentry LO. Antibiotic therapy for osteomyelitis. Infect Dis Clin North Am. 1990;4:485–99.
356. Giamarellou H. Malignant otitis externa: The therapeutic evolution of a lethal infection. J Antimicrob Chemother. 1992;30:745–51.
357. Johnson MP, Ramphal R. Malignant external otitis: Report on therapy with ceftazidime and review of therapy and prognosis. Rev Infect Dis. 1900;12: 173–80.
358. Collins T, Garding DN. Aminoglycosides versus beta-lactams in gram-negative pneumonia. Semin Respir Infect. 1991;6:136–46.
359. Moore RD, Smith CR, Lietman PS. Association of aminoglycoside plasma levels with therapeutic outcome in gram-negative pneumonia. Am J Med. 1984;77:657–62.
360. Peterson HB, Galaid EI, Zenilman JM. Pelvic inflammatory disease: Review of treatment options. Rev Infect Dis. 1990;12(Suppl 6):S656–64.
361. Wolner-Hanssen P. Pelvic inflammatory disease. Curr Opin Obstet Gynecol 1991;3:687–91.
362. Lipsky BA. Diabetic foot infections: Pathophysiology, diagnosis, and treatment. Int J Dermatol. 1991;30:560–2.
363. Lipsky BA, Pecoraro RE, Wheat LJ. The diabetic foot: Soft tissue and bone infection. Infect Dis Clin North Am. 1990;4:409–32.
364. Jackson GG, Finland M, eds. International Symposium on Gentamicin. J Infect Dis. 1969;119:341–540.
365. Finland M, Hewitt WL, eds. Second International Symposium on Gentamicin. J Infect Dis. 1971;124:S1–S300.
366. Finland M, Neu HC, eds. Tobramycin. J Infect Dis. 1976;134(Suppl):S1–234.
367. Hewitt WL, Young LS. Symposium perspective. Am J Med 1977;62:863–7.
368. Netilmicin. Based on a symposium, Vienna, Austria, 28 August 1983. J Antimicrob Chemother. 1984;13(Suppl A):1–83.
369. Gruenwaldt G, Marget W, Weuta H. New aspects of aminoglycoside therapy: Sisomicin extended summarizes of papers presented at a symposium May 6–7, 1977, Geneva, Switzerland. Infection. 1979;7(Suppl 3):241–304.
370. Solomkin JS, Dellinger EP, Christou NV, Busuttil RW. Results of a prospective and double-blind trial of new beta-lactams in the treatment of appendicitis. Antimicrob Agents Chemother. 1990;28:639–42.
371. Williams RR, Hotchkin D. Aztreonam plus clindamycin versus tobramycin plus clindamycin in the treatment of intra-abdominal infections. Rev Infect Dis. 1991;13(Suppl 7):S629–33.
372. Bubrick MP, Heim-Duthoy KL, Yellin AE, et al. Ceftazidime/clindamycin versus tobramycin/clindamycin in the treatment of intra-abdominal infections. Am Surgeon. 1990;56:613–7.
373. Korvick JA, Bryan CS, Farber B, et al. Prospective observational study of Klebsiella bacteremia in 230 patients: outcome for antibiotic combinations versus monotherapy. Antimicrob Agents Chemother. 1992;36:2639–44.
374. Tunkel AR, Fisch MJ, Schlein A, Scheld WM. Enterobacter endocarditis. Scand J Infect Dis. 1992;24:233–40.
375. Bodey GP, Elting LS, Rodriquez S. Bacteremia caused by Enterobacter: 15 years of experience in a cancer hospital. Rev Infect Dis. 1991;13:550–8.
376. Saito H, Elting L, Bodey GP, et al. Serratia bacteremia: Review of 118 cases. Rev Infect Dis. 1989;11:912–20.
377. Rolston KV, Bodey GP. Pseudomonas aeruginosa infection in cancer patients. Cancer Invest. 1992;10:43–59.
378. Saha V, Stansfield R, Masterton R, et al. The treatment of Pseudomonas aeruginosa meningitis—Old regime or newer drugs? Scand J Infect Dis. 1993; 25:81–3.
379. Korvick JA, Peacock JE, Muder RR, et al. Addition of rifampin to combination antibiotic therapy for Pseudomonas aeruginosa bacteremia: Prospective trial using the Zelen protocol. Antimicrob Agents Chemother. 1992;36:620–5.
380. Montejo JM, Alberok I, Glez-Zarate P, et al. Open randomized trial of six antimicrobial regimens in the treatment of human brucellosis. Clin Infect Dis. 1993;16:671–6.
381. Chuang YC, Yuan CY, Liu CY, et al. Vibrio vulnificus infection in Taiwan:

Report of 28 cases and review of clinical manifestations and treatment. Clin Infect Dis. 1992;15:271–6.

382. Murphey DK, Septimus EJ, Waagner DC. Catfish-related injury and infection: Report of two cases and review of the literature. Clin Infect Dis. 1992; 14:689–93.

383. Moran JS, Zenilman JM. Therapy for gonococcal infections: Options in 1989. Rev Infect Dis. 1990;12(Suppl 6):S633–44.

384. 1989 sexually transmitted diseases treatment guidelines. A symposium. Atlanta, Georgia, 28–29 March 1989. Rev Infect Dis. 1990;12(Suppl 6): S577–690.

385. Jorup-Ronstrom C, Julander I, Petrini B. Efficacy of triple drug regimen of amikacin, ethambutol and rifabutin in AIDS patients with symptomatic *Mycobacterium avium* complex infection. J Infect. 1993;26:67–70.

386. de Lalla F, Maserati R, Scarpellini P, et al. Clarithromycin-ciprofloxacin-amikacin for therapy of *Mycobacterium avium intracellulare* bacteremia in patients with AIDS. Antimicrob Agents Chemother. 1992;36:1567–9.

387. Edlin BR, Tokars JI, Grieco MH, et al. An outbreak of multidrug-resistant tuberculosis among hospitalized patients with the acquired immunodeficiency syndrome. N Engl J Med. 1992;326:1514–21.

388. Riley LW, Arathoon E, Loverde VD. The epidemiologic patterns of drug-resistance *Mycobacterium tuberculosis* infections: A community-based study. Am Rev Respir Dis. 1989;139:1282–5.

389. Drugs for parasitic infections. Med. Lett. 1992;34:17–24.

390. Dajani AS, Bisno AL, Chung KJ, et al. Prevention of bacterial endocarditis. Recommendations by the American Heart Association. JAMA. 1990;264: 2919–22.

391. Gorbach SL. Antimicrobial prophylaxis for appendectomy and colorectal surgery. Rev Infect Dis. 1991;13(Suppl 10):S815–20.

392. Voytovich RM, Massaro MJ, Titus DL, et al. An aminoglycoside dosing regimen in a morbidly obese patient (Letter). DICP. 1990;24:100–2.

393. Hickling KG, Begg EJ, Perry RE, et al. Serum aminoglycoside clearance is predicted as poorly by renal aminoglycoside clearance as by creatinine clearance in critically ill patients. Crit Care Med. 1991;19:1041–7.

394. McCormack JP, Jewesson PJ. A critical reevaluation of the "therapeutic range" of aminoglycoside. Clin Infect Dis. 1992;14:320–9.

395. Edwards C, Bent AJ, Venables CW, et al. Sampling time for serum gentamicin levels. J Antimicrob Chemother. 1992;29:575–8.

396. Cockcroft DW, Gault MH. Prediction of creatinine clearance from serum creatinine. Nephron. 1976;16:31–41.

397. Physician's Desk Reference. 47th ed. Montvale, NJ: Medical Economics Data; 1993.

398. Moore RD, Lietman PS, Smith CR. Clinical response to aminoglycoside therapy: Importance of the ratio of peak concentration to minimal inhibitory concentrations. J Infect Dis. 1987;155:93–9.

399. Noone P, Rogers BT. Pneumonia caused by coliforms and *Pseudomonas aeruginosa*. J Clin Pathol. 1976;29:652–6.

400. Spector R, Park GD, Johnson GF, et al. Therapeutic drug monitoring. Clin Pharmacol Ther. 1988;43:345–53.

401. McInnes GT. The value of therapeutic drug monitoring to the practicing physician—An hypothesis in need of testing. Br J Clin Pharmacol. 1989;278: 281–4.

402. Matzke GR, Lucarotti RL, Shapiro HS. Controlled comparison of gentamicin and tobramycin nephrotoxicity. Am J Nephrol. 1983;3:11–7.

403. Sarubbi FA, Hull H. Amikacin serum concentrations: Prediction of levels and dosage guidelines. Ann Intern Med. 1978;89:612–8.

404. Maderazo EG, Sun H, Jay GT. Simplification of antibiotic dose adjustments in renal insufficiency: The DREM system. Lancet. 1992;340:767–70.

405. Golper TA, Wedel SK, Kaplan AA, et al. Drug removal during continuous arteriovenous hemofiltration: theory and clinical observations. Int J Artif Organs. 1985;2:307–12.

406. Bickley SK. Drug dosing during continuous hemofiltration. Clin Pharmacol. 1988;7:198–206.

407. Reetze-Bonorden P, Bohler J, Keller E. Drug dosage in patients during continuous renal replacement therapy. Clin Pharmacokinet. 1993;24:362–79.

408. Keane WF, Everett ED, Golper TA, et al. Peritoneal dialysis-related peritonitis treatment recommendations. 1993 update. Periton Dialysis Int. 1993; 13:14–28.

409. Verpooten GA, Giuliano RA, Verbist L, et al. Once-daily dosing decreases renal accumulation of gentamicin and netilmicin. Clin Pharmacol Ther. 1989; 45:22–7.

410. De Broe ME, Verbist L, Verpooten GA. Influence of dosage schedule on renal cortical accumulation of amikacin and tobramycin in man. J Antimicrob Chemother. 1991;27(Suppl C):41–7.

411. Wood CA, Norton DR, Kohlhepp SJ, et al. The influence of tobramycin dosage regimen on nephrotoxicity, ototoxicity and antibacterial efficacy in a rat model of subcutaneous abscess. J Infect Dis. 1988;158:13–22.

412. Pierre C, Blanchet F, Seta N, et al. Tolerance of once daily dosing of netilmicin and teicoplanin alone or in combination in healthy volunteers. Clin Pharmacol Ther. 1988;44:458–66.

413. Proctor L, Petty B, Lietman P, et al. Study of potential vestibulotoxic effects of one daily versus thrice daily administrations of tobramycin. Laryngoscope. 1987;97:1443–9.

414. Vigano A, Principi N, Brivio L, et al. Comparison of 5 mg of netilmicin per kilogram of body weight once daily versus 2 mg per kilogram thrice daily for treatment of gram-negative pyelonephritis in children. Antimicrob Agents Chemother. 1992;36:1499–503.

415. Rozdzinski E, Kern WV, Reichle A, et al. Once-daily versus thrice-daily dosing of netilmicin in combination with beta-lactam antibiotics as empiric therapy for febrile neutropenic patients. J Antimicrob Chemother. 1993;31: 585–98.

416. Tulkens PM. Efficacy and safety of aminoglycosides once-a-day: Experimental and clinical data. Scand J Infect Dis. 1991;74(Suppl):249–57.

417. Gilbert DN, Bennett WM. Use of antimicrobial agents in renal failure. Infect Dis Clin North Am. 1989;3:517–31.

418. Prober CG, Stevenson DK, Benitz WSE. The use of antibiotics in neonates weighing less than 1200 gm. Pediatr Infect Dis. 1990;9:111–21.

419. Klein JO. Antimicrobial agents. In: Feign RD, Cherry JD, eds. Textbook of Pediatric Infectious Diseases. 3rd ed. Philadelphia: WB Saunders; 1992; 2179–98.

420. Zebner R, Quinn JP. Antimicrobials in cystic fibrosis: Emergence of resistance and implications for treatment. Semin Respir Infect. 1992;7:210–7.

421. Mulherin D, Fahy J, Grant W, et al. Aminoglycoside induced ototoxicity in patients with cystic fibrosis. Ir J Med Sci. 1991;160:173–5.

422. Mukhopadkyay S, Baer S, Blanshard J, et al. Assessment of potential ototoxicity following high-dose nebulized tobramycin in patients with cystic fibrosis. J Antimicrob Chemother. 1993;31:429–36.

423. Ramsey BW, Dorkin HL, Eisenberg JD, et al. Efficacy of aerosolized tobramycin in patients with cystic fibrosis. N Engl J Med. 1993;328:1740–6.

424. Levine DP, Crane LR, Zervos MJ. Bacteremia in narcotic addicts at the Detroit Medical Center: II. Infectious endocarditis: A prospective comparative study. Rev Infect Dis. 1986;8:374.

425. Holloway WJ. Spectinomycin. Med Clin North Am. 1982;656:169.

426. Drug Facts and Comparisons. 1992 ed. St. Louis, MO: Facts and Comparisons, 1992.

427. Neu HC. The crisis of antibiotic resistance. Science. 1992;257:1064–73.

428. Dooley SW, Jarvis WR, Martone W, et al. Multidrug-resistant tuberculosis. Ann Intern Med. 1992;117:257–9.

429. Kawlowsky JA, Zhanel GG. Concepts of the use of liposomal antimicrobial agents: Applications for aminoglycosides. Clin Infect Dis. 1992;15:654–67.

21. TETRACYCLINES AND CHLORAMPHENICOL

HAROLD C. STANDIFORD

THE TETRACYCLINES

All the tetracyclines are primarily bacteriostatic at therapeutic concentrations and have a broad spectrum that includes gram-positive, gram-negative, aerobic, and anaerobic bacteria, spirochetes, mycoplasmas, rickettsia, chlamydiae, and some protozoa. The analogs can be divided into three groups based on differences in their pharmacology: *(1)* the short-acting compounds chlortetracycline, oxytetracycline, and tetracycline; *(2)* an intermediate group consisting of demeclocycline and methacycline; and *(3)* the more recently discovered, longer-acting compounds doxycycline and minocycline.

Structure, Derivation, Nomenclature, and Brand Names

Unlike the fortuitous discovery of penicillin by Fleming, the first tetracycline, chlortetracycline, was discovered by screening organisms obtained from the soil for their antimicrobial properties. Benjamin M. Duggar, a meticulous mycologist in his 70s, noted unusual antimicrobial activity from organisms that formed a golden yellow colony.[1] He designated the organism *Streptomyces aureofaciens* (L. *aurum*, golden) and named the product *aureomycin*. Oxytetracycline was derived from *Streptomyces rimosus* in 1950, and tetracycline was produced by the catalytic dehalogenation of chlortetracycline in 1953. The two long-acting compounds were derived semisynthetically: doxycycline in 1966 and minocycline in 1967. The generic names of the analogs are determined by the substitutions on the basic structure of tetracycline, which consists of a hydronaphthacene nucleus containing four fused rings (Fig. 1). The compounds currently available in the United States and their major brand names, doses, and costs are listed in Table 1. Of these, tetracycline HCl and doxycycline have emerged as the most useful clinically. Chlortetracycline (aureomycin), the first member of the family, is no longer available except for topical use, and methacycline (Rondomycin) has recently been withdrawn from the market.

Mechanism of Action

The tetracyclines enter bacteria by diffusion as a protonated form and are probably accumulated by a ΔpH-dependent process as a membrane-impermeable magnesium–tetracycline chelate complex.[2] Once within the cell, they reversibly bind primarily to the 30S ribosomal subunit at a position that blocks the binding of the aminoacyl-tRNA to the acceptor site on the mRNA–ribosome complex.[3] This prevents the addition of new amino acids into the growing peptide chain. The tetracyclines also inhibit protein synthesis in mammalian cells, particularly in mitochondrial ribosomes, but apparently are not in sufficient concentration in these structures to produce severe toxicity.[4]

In Vitro Activity

The antimicrobial spectra of all the tetracyclines are almost identical. Some differences, however, in the degree of activity against these organisms do exist among the analogs. In general, the lipophilic congeners are more active than are those that are more hydrophilic. It follows, therefore, that minocycline is the

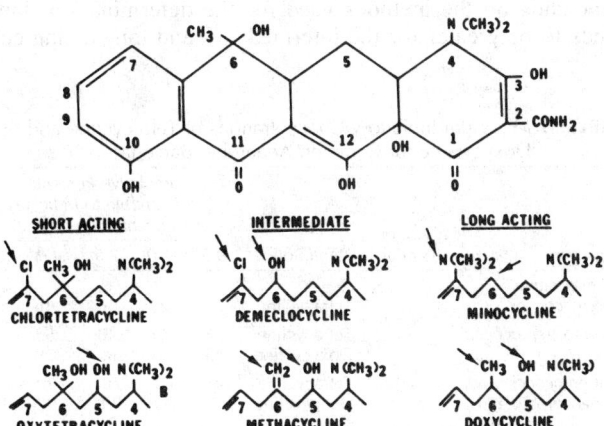

FIG. 1. Chemical structure of the tetracyclines. The analogs differ from tetracycline at the fifth, sixth, or seventh position, as indicated by the arrows.

most active of the analogs, closely followed by doxycycline. The minimum inhibitory concentration (MIC) of the more hydrophilic congeners oxytetracycline and tetracycline are two- to fourfold higher against many bacteria and are the least-active analogs. Despite these differences, for cost reasons it is recommended that tetracycline be used in the clinical microbiology laboratory to evaluate susceptibility for all the analogs.[5] MICs of tetracycline and doxycycline for many aerobic bacteria are given in Table 2. For the activities of the other analogs, the reader is referred to the extensive work from the laboratory of Finland et al.[7–9]

Although many of the aerobic and facultative anaerobic organisms are within the spectrum of the tetracyclines, more effective agents are available for the treatment of infections caused by most of these bacteria. The pneumococci and *Haemophilus influenzae* can be inhibited by concentrations of tetracyclines achieved in the serum, and this provides a rationale for their use in sinusitis and acute exacerbations of chronic bronchitis.[13] Gonococci and meningococci are extremely susceptible; unfortunately, gonococci resistant to penicillin G also tend to be resistant to tetracycline.[6,14] Most *Escherichia coli* acquired outside the hospital setting can be inhibited by concentrations achieved in the urine, if not the serum. Tetracyclines, therefore, are useful agents for the treatment of acute, uncomplicated, urinary tract infections and the acute urethral syndrome. *Pseudomonas pseudomallei* organisms are generally sensitive, and this has therapeutic importance, as does the high degree of susceptibility of *Brucella* spp.[10,15] *Vibrio cholerae*, *Vibrio vulnificus*, and other vibrios are generally susceptible, and the tetracyclines are important for therapy for diseases caused by this group of organisms.[16] Although *Campylobacter* spp. are generally susceptible, a high percentage of resistant isolates has been noted in some countries.[11,17,18] Therefore, it is not the drug of choice for infections caused by these bacteria. *Shigella* organisms have become increasingly resistant.[12] *Mycobacterium marinum* is susceptible and appears to respond clinically.[19]

The tetracyclines have activity against many anaerobic organisms (Table 3).[20] Their activity against *Actinomyces* is particularly relevant clinically. Doxycycline is more active against *Bacteroides fragilis* than tetracycline is, but clindamycin or metronidazole are the preferred agents for infections caused by this organism. The activity of the tetracyclines against anaerobic bacteria, however, may be partially responsible for the effectiveness of the neomycin–tetracycline combination and doxycycline alone as oral presurgical bowel preparations.[21,22] Many pathogenic spirochetes are susceptible, including *Borrelia burgdorferi*, the agent of Lyme disease.[23] Other organisms generally inhibited by this group of antibiotics include rickettsia, chlamydiae, mycoplasmas, and to a limited degree protozoa (malariae and *Entamoeba histotytica*).[24]

Bacteria develop resistance to the tetracyclines predomi-

TABLE 1. The Names, Preparations, and Usual Adult Oral Dosages for the Tetracyclines Currently Available in the United States

Generic Name (Major Brand Name[a])	Oral Preparations	Usual Adult Oral Dosage
Short-acting[b]		
Oxytetracycline (Terramycin, Pfizer)	Capsules: 125, 250 mg	500 mg q6h
Tetracycline HCl[c] (Achromycin V, Lederle)	Capsules: 100, 250, 500 mg	500 mg q6h
	Syrup: 125 mg/5 ml	
Intermediate		
Demeclocycline HCl (Declomycin, Lederle)	Capsules: 150 mg	300 mg q12h
	Tablets: 150, 300 mg	
Long-acting[d]		
Doxycycline (Vibramycin, Pfizer)	Capsules (hyclate): 50, 100 mg	200 mg (or 100 q12h for first day), then 100 mg q24h[e]
	Syrup (calcium): 50 mg/5 ml	
Minocycline (Minocin, Lederle)	Capsules and tablets: 50, 100 mg	200 mg, then 100 mg q12h
	Suspension: 50 mg/5 ml	

[a] Many other brands are available for some of the analogs.
[b] The short-acting tetracyclines are also available for intravenous administration at usual doses of 500 mg every 6–12 hours not to exceed 2 g daily. However, most prefer doxycycline for this route of administration. Preparation combined with a local anesthetic agent can be given intramuscularly, but these are not recommended.
[c] Tetracycline is also available as a tetracycline phosphate complex (Tetrex, Bristol) intended to enhance absorption, but its superiority has not been established.
[d] The longer-acting agents can be given intravenously in the same doses that are recommended for oral therapy. Doxycycline is available at 100 or 200 mg per vial and minocycline at 100 mg per vial.
[e] The treatment schedules for sexually transmitted diseases and for Lyme disease use 100 mg twice daily.

TABLE 2. Minimum Inhibitory Concentration of Tetracycline and Doxycycline for Common Aerobic and Facultative Anaerobic Bacteria

Organism	No. of Strains	Antibiotic	0.4	0.8	1.6	3.1	6.3
Gram-positive							
S. aureus	56	Tetracycline	0	2	20	65	67
		Doxycycline	2	25	63	65	68
S. pyogenes[a]	63	Tetracycline	10	50	80	87	90
		Doxycycline	56	90	90	95	95
S. pneumoniae[b]	35	Tetracycline	70	96	96	100	
		Doxycycline	100				
Streptococcus (group B)	12	Tetracycline	0	0	50	50	50
		Doxycycline	0	50	50	50	50
Enterococcus	36	Tetracycline	0	0	0	0	10
		Doxycycline	0	0	0	0	10
Gram-negative[c]							
N. gonorrhoeae[d]	25	Tetracycline	5	60	85	88	100
		Doxycycline	60	75	80	92	100
N. meningitidis[e]	10	Tetracycline	0	50		100	
		Doxycycline	0		50		100
H. influenzae	15	Tetracycline	0	0	0	33	87
		Doxycycline	0	0	60	93	100
E. coli	48	Tetracycline	0	0	0	5	35
		Doxycycline	0	0	0	5	35
K. pneumoniae	17	Tetracycline	0	0	0	0	5
		Doxycycline	0	0	0	0	12
Enterobacter spp.	10	Tetracycline	0	10	30	50	70
		Doxycycline	0	0	0	0	10
Pseudomonas pseudomallei	10	Tetracycline	0	0	60	100	
Campylobacter jejuni	172	Tetracycline	44	62	74	81	84
	107	Doxycycline	68	74	79	80	86
Shigella spp.	213	Tetracycline	0	10	12	50	50

[a] More recent series indicate that 20–40 percent of S. pyogenes have become resistant to the tetracyclines.
[b] Tetracycline-resistant S. pneumoniae strains are more common in some areas.
[c] Proteus mirabilis, indole-positive Proteus spp., and P. aeruginosa are generally resistant to 25 μg/ml.
[d] Gonococci resistant to penicillin G also tend to be resistant to tetracycline.[6,14]
[e] The medium inhibitory concentration of minocycline for meningococci is 1.6 μg/ml (range, 0.8–1.6 μg/ml).

(Data from refs. 7–12.) Organisms should be considered susceptible if the MICs are 4 μg/ml or less. A moderate susceptibility range of up to 8 μg/ml may be useful for the treatment of urinary tract infections.[5]

nantly by preventing the accumulation of tetracycline within the cell. This is accomplished by decreasing the influx or increasing the ability of the cell to export the antibiotic.[2] Rarely if ever are the tetracyclines inactivated biologically or altered chemically by resistant bacteria.[25–28] Resistance to one tetracycline usually implies resistance to all, although there are marked differences in the degree of resistance among species. The resistance among bacteria can be mediated by transferable resistance plasmids. The tetracyclines have been widely used in feeds to promote growth in animals. This may be a major factor in providing selective antibiotic pressure for the spread of plasmid-mediated resistance to these and other antibiotics.[29–31]

Pharmacology

Serum levels achieved by usual oral doses in adults are given in Figure 2. Absorption occurs primarily in the proximal small bowel and produces peak serum concentrations 1–3 hours after administration. The commonly used 500-mg therapeutic dose of tetracycline gives a serum level of 4 μg/ml, highest of all the short-acting analogs.[32] Doxycycline and minocycline (200 mg) achieve serum levels of about 2.5 μg/ml, slightly higher than levels attained by the larger therapeutic doses of the intermediate agents.[33–37]

After the intravenous administration of 500 mg, serum levels of the short-acting agents (not shown) are approximately 8 μg/

ml at 30 minutes and decrease to 2–3 μg/ml by 5 hours.[38] Intravenous injection of the usual 200-mg loading dose of the long-acting agents doxycycline and minocycline produces serum levels of approximately 4 μg/ml at 30 minutes. Once tissue distribution occurs for the long-acting analogs, levels are almost identical to concentrations achieved orally.[33,39] Thrombophlebitis is a frequent complication of the intravenous preparations. Intramuscular preparations are available for the short-acting compounds but are not recommended because of the severe pain produced on injection, even when they are mixed with local anesthetics.

Some of the pharmacokinetic properties of the tetracyclines are compared in Table 4. The high levels obtained orally with tetracycline as compared with other short-acting agents are due primarily to better absorption from the gastrointestinal tract. The long-acting analogs doxycycline and minocycline are absorbed almost completely; thus, high serum levels are achieved with relatively small doses.[33,34] The tetracyclines can be differentiated into three groups on the basis of their different half-lives. Doxycycline has the longest of all and allows therapeutic levels to be maintained with a single daily dose.[33] The 8-hour half-life of tetracycline[38] suggests that the dosage interval could be 8 hours for this antibiotic when it is used to treat minor infections. The half-lives of the compounds are determined mainly by the rate of excretion by the kidneys. Chlortetracycline is an exception: it has a short half-life despite a slow rate of clearance as a result of the marked instability of the compound in vitro as well as in vivo.[38] With the possible exception of chlortetracycline and minocycline, adequate therapeutic concentrations of all the tetracyclines are achieved in the urine for treatment of urinary tract infections caused by sensitive organisms. The degree of protein binding of the analogs is variable, depending on the methods used for the determination, but it tends to be greater for the intermediate- and long-acting com-

TABLE 3. Minimum Inhibitory Concentrations of Tetracycline and Doxycycline for Common Anaerobic Bacteria[a]

Organism	No. of Strains	Antibiotic	0.5	1.0	2.0	4.0	8.0
Gram-positive							
Peptococcus	59	Tetracycline	25	29	36	36	37
Peptostreptococcus	29	Tetracycline	38	41	48	52	72
		Doxycycline	45	45	66	79	97
Streptococci, anaerobic and microaerophilic	10	Tetracycline	50	60	70	90	90
		Doxycycline	70	90	90	90	100
Eubacterium	17	Tetracycline	24	59	65	65	77
		Doxycycline	59	65	77	82	88
Propionibacterium	12	Tetracycline	58	75	83	83	83
		Doxycycline	75	83	83	92	92
Clostridium perfringens	9	Tetracycline	22	22	56	67	67
		Doxycycline	67	67	67	78	89
Other clostridia	33	Tetracycline	36	46	49	52	61
		Doxycycline	49	52	61	68	82
Actinomyces	16	Tetracycline	56	69	94	94	94
		Doxycycline	63	69	94	100	
Gram-negative							
Gram-negative cocci	26	Tetracycline	54	69	73	73	73
		Doxycycline	58	69	73	81	96
Fusobacterium	34	Tetracycline	94	97	97	97	97
		Doxycycline	94	94	94	94	100
Bacteroides fragilis	76	Tetracycline	25	40	40	42	46
		Doxycycline	41	42	50	75	88
Prevotella melaninogenica	67	Tetracycline	75	76	79	87	94
		Doxycycline	75	78	90	96	97
Other Bacteroides	72	Tetracycline	33	35	43	50	60
Selenomonas		Doxycycline	40	43	53	68	79

[a] An organism with a MIC of 4 μg/ml or less should be considered susceptible.

(Modified from Sutter and Finegold,[20] with permission.)

pounds.[39–41] This may be one of the factors that determines their slow rate of renal excretion. The apparent volume of distribution for most of the tetracyclines is greater than that of extracellular body water, thus indicating sequestration in tissues, presumably the liver.[38] Minocycline and doxycycline have the smallest volume of distribution, another factor that tends to enhance their serum levels.[39]

Tissue Distribution. The tetracyclines can be found in small amounts in many tissues and fluids, including the lung, liver, kidney, brain, sputum, and mucosal fluid. For tetracycline, the levels in the cerebral spinal fluid are approximately 10–26 percent of the serum levels,[42,43] whereas concentrations in synovial fluid and the maxillary sinus mucosa approach serum levels.[44,45] All the tetracyclines are concentrated in unobstructed bile and produce levels in this fluid 5–20 times those obtained in the serum. It has been suggested that lipid solubility is a primary determinant for the diffusion in many tissues. Minocycline, followed by doxycycline, is more lipophilic at a physiologic pH than are the other drugs. This may explain why minocycline reaches sufficient concentrations in saliva and tears to eradicate the meningococcal carrier state, whereas the other tetracyclines do not.[46,47] The tetracyclines cross the placenta, and accumulate in fetal bone and teeth and therefore should not be given during pregnancy.[48] Because they are excreted in breast milk, caution is advised in the postpartum period.

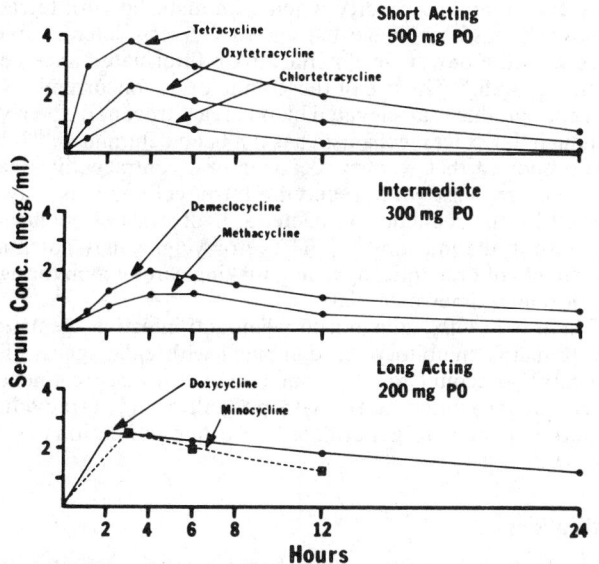

FIG. 2. Serum levels achieved with the usually recommended oral doses of the tetracyclines. Chlortetracycline and methacycline are no longer available for oral or parenteral administration. (Data from refs. 32–36.)

Renal and Hepatic Insufficiency. The tetracyclines should not be used in patients with renal failure. Doxycycline, the only exception, is excreted in the gastrointestinal tract under these circumstances. Neither the half-life nor the therapeutic dose of this antibiotic varies with alterations in renal function.[49] The tetracyclines are slowly removed by hemodialysis but not effectively by peritoneal dialysis. Hepatic disease is not known to cause elevated serum levels of the tetracyclines. However, they should be used very cautiously in such situations, because they have been noted to cause hepatic toxicity.

Assay

The tetracyclines can be measured by a number of different techniques. These include bioassay using *Bacillus cereus* as the test organism or by high-performance liquid chromatographic procedures,[50,51] but monitoring of serum levels during therapy is rarely indicated.

Toxicity

Skin and Allergy. Hypersensitivity reactions including anaphylaxis, urticuria, periorbital edema, fixed drug eruptions, and morbilliform rashes occur with tetracyclines but are not common.[52–54] When a patient is allergic to one analog, he should be considered to be allergic to all. Photosensitivity reactions consisting of a red rash on areas exposed to sunlight that is frequently associated with onycholysis are most common in patients receiving demeclocycline but occur with all analogs.[55,56] They appear to be a toxic rather than an allergic reaction. Prolonged administration of minocycline has been noted rarely to cause nail, skin, and scleral pigmentation, which is usually reversible, as well as an asymptomatic black pigmentation of the thyroid.[57,58]

Teeth and Bones. A gray-brown to yellow discoloration of the teeth has been noted in some communities in 80 percent of the children taking tetracyclines.[59] This side effect is permanent and may be associated with hypoplasia of the enamel[55,60] and depression of skeletal growth in premature infants.[61] The darkening effect of tetracyclines on permanent teeth appears to be related to the total dose of the antibiotic administered. In a retrospective study, cosmetically noticeable but mild darkening of the permanent teeth occurred in 3 of 14 children receiving five courses of tetracycline, whereas 4 of 6 children receiving eight courses had moderate darkening of the enamel.[62] Primary teeth generally show more darkening than do the larger, thicker, and more opaque permanent teeth. Since there is some variability in staining with similar tetracycline exposure, it is prudent not to administer these agents to pregnant women and to children up to the age of 8 years, the period when tooth enamel is being formed. For this reason, the Food and Drug Administration

TABLE 4. Pharmacokinetic Features of the Tetracyclines[a]

Antibiotic	GI Absorption (%)	Half-Life (hr)	Renal Clearance[b] (ml/min/1.73 m²)	Urinary Recovery (%)	Apparent Volume of Distribution[b] (Liters)	Protein Binding[c] (%)
Short acting						
Oxytetracycline	58	9	99	70	128	35
Tetracycline	77	8	74	60	108	65
Intermediate						
Demeclocycline	66	12	35	39	121	91
Methacycline	58	14	31	60	79	90
Long acting						
Doxycycline	93	18	20	42	50	93
Minocycline	95	16	9	6	60	76

[a] The pharmacokinetic values vary considerably from laboratory to laboratory. These values were selected in most instances because comparative data were available from reliable investigators.
[b] After single-dose intravenous administration
[c] Ultrafiltration technique.

(Data from refs. 33–35 and 38–41.)

(FDA) has withdrawn from the market the concentrated liquid dosage forms (drops) specifically intended for pediatric use.[63] It is not unreasonable, however, to administer a single course of tetracycline therapy to young children for specifically defined indications where the alternative regime may produce more severe toxicity. Thus, the tetracyclines may be indicated for children suspected of having Rocky Mountain spotted fever who can tolerate oral medications. Doxycycline binds less with calcium than do other tetracyclines and may cause dental changes less frequently in children.[64]

Gastrointestinal Symptoms. The tetracyclines are irritative substances and frequently produce gastrointestinal symptoms after oral administration. Esophageal ulcerations that are manifested as retrosternal pain exacerbated by swallowing have been clearly documented after tetracycline and doxycycline administration. In most cases, the patients were taking the capsules with little or no fluid just before going to bed. A word of caution to the patient is indicated in order to prevent this toxicity. The complication may also occur in patients with esophageal obstruction or motility disorders.[65,66] Nausea, vomiting, and epigastric distress are dose related and limit the dose of most of the analogs. The administration of food with doxycycline, minocycline, or oxytetracycline may ameliorate some of these symptoms, but food seriously decreases the absorption of the other tetracyclines. Diarrhea is most often associated with analogs that are poorly absorbed and appears to be related to alterations in the enteric flora. Doxycycline produces less of an effect on bowel flora than does tetracycline.[67] The diarrhea usually subsides when treatment with the antibiotic is stopped, but prolonged symptoms due to pseudomembranous colitis have been reported.[68] Tetracycline also has been noted, rarely, to cause pancreatitis with or without overt liver disease.[69]

Liver. The hepatoxicity of the tetracyclines, first described in patients receiving intravenous chlortetracycline but now described with other analogs, appears pathologically as a fine droplet fatty metamorphosis and results in a high mortality.[70,71] The administration of less than 2 g/day intravenously is not associated with liver dysfunction or injury except in pregnant women, who are particularly at risk,[72] and in patients with an excessive serum level due to renal failure.[73]

Renal Function. The tetracyclines aggravate pre-exisitng renal failure by inhibiting protein synthesis, which increases the azotemia from amino acid metabolism.[74] Nephrogenic diabetes insipidus is produced by demeclocycline, a side effect that has been used therapeutically to reverse chronic inappropriate antidiuretic hormone secretion[75]; renal failure has complicated its use for this purpose in patients with cirrhosis.[76] Outdated tetracycline has produced a reversible Fanconi-like syndrome with renal tubular acidosis, but tetracycline formulations producing this syndrome have been modified. It is unlikely that this complication will recur.[49]

Nervous and Sensory Systems. Vertigo is a side effect unique to minocycline. Symptoms of light-headedness, loss of balance, dizziness, and tinnitus usually begin on the second and third days of therapy and have been noted more frequently in women (70 percent) than in men (28 percent). The symptoms are reversible within several days after discontinuation of therapy with the antibiotic, but this side effect has seriously limited the use of minocycline.[77] Benign intracranial hypertension (pseudotumor cerebri) has been described in infants and adults with many of the analogs.[78,79]

Superinfection. Colonization by tetracycline-resistant organisms is a frequent occurrence during tetracycline therapy and is generally of little clinical significance. Rarely, a fulminating diarrhea resulting from clostridium difficile pseudomembranous colitis or staphylococcal enteritis may occur after oral or parenteral therapy.[80,81] More often and less serious, oral or vaginal monaliasis complicates treatment, a complication that may require specific therapy.

Significant Drug Interactions

Food adversely affects the absorption of tetracycline, chlortetracycline, methacycline, and demeclocycline. All the tetracyclines form complexes with divalent or trivalent cations. Therefore, absorption is markedly decreased when these drugs are administered simultaneously with calcium, magnesium, and aluminum in antacids, milk, or iron and iron-containing tonics.[82] Sodium bicarbonate also has an adverse effect on absorption and should not be administered simultaneously.[83] Cimetidine has been shown to decrease the absorption of tetracycline, but this is unlikely to be significant in the clinical situation.[84] Carbamazepine (Tegretol), diphenylhydantoin, and barbiturates decrease the normal half-life of doxycycline to almost one-half by increasing the hepatic metabolism of the antibiotic.[85,86] Chronic ethanol ingestion has also resulted in a shorter half-life of doxycycline but not tetracycline, presumably also through induction of hepatic microsomal enzymes.[87] Methoxyflurane anesthesia may cause nephrotoxicity when administered with tetracyclines.[88] It has been suggested that this adverse interaction occurs with the newer, less nephrotoxic fluorinated anesthetic agents as well.[89] The use of these antibiotics concurrently with diuretics produces an elevated blood urea nitrogen (BUN) level, although the exact mechanism has not been determined.[90] It has been reported that women receiving oral contraceptives have become pregnant while receiving tetracycline. This may be caused by the reduction in bacterial hydrolysis of conjugated estrogen in the intestine.[91,92] The tetracyclines may potentiate the effects of oral anticoagulants, making careful monitoring of prothrombin times essential.

There is in vitro antagonism when anti-infective agents that are primarily inhibitory are combined with cidal agents. This appears to account for the poor outcome in the treatment of pneumococcal meningitis with penicillin and tetracycline. Whether it can be generalized to other indications is not known.[93]

Indications

The tetracyclines are the drugs of choice or effective alternative therapy for a wide variety of bacterial, chlamydial, mycoplasma, and rickettsial infections (Table 5). The reader is referred to the pertinent chapters in this volume for details. The tetracyclines have no role in the treatment of viral or fungal diseases. Tetracycline or doxycycline can be used interchangeably for most of these indications. However, compliance may be better with doxycycline since it can be taken twice daily without regard to meals and cost is no longer an important factor. Doxycycline is preferred by most when intravenous administration is required.

CHLORAMPHENICOL

Soon after chloramphenicol was released in the United States in 1949, reports linked this highly effective agent with aplastic anemia, and it quickly fell into disfavor. The increased awareness of the pathogenicity of anaerobic organisms and the development of ampicillin-resistant *H. influenzae* accounted for an increase in the use of the compound. However, the availability of other agents for anaerobic infections has reduced the need for chloramphenicol for this indication, and its use for ampicillin-resistant *H. influenzae* also has been replaced by other agents.

TABLE 5. Major Therapeutic Indications for the Tetracyclines[a]

Major Indications	Effective Alternative Therapy
Borrelia burgdorferi (Lyme disease, early)	Acne, severe
Borrelia recurrentis (relapsing fever)	*Actinomyces israeli* (actinomycosis)
Brucellosis (with gentamicin in seriously ill patients)	Anthrax
Calymmatobacterium granulomatis (granuloma inguinale)	*Campylobacter fetus, jejuni*
Chlamydial infections	Chronic bronchitis (acute exacerbation)
Chlamydia pneumoniae (Twar strain)	*Clostridium tetani*
Epididymitis, acute (sexually transmitted form)	*Eikenella corrodens*
Inclusion conjunctivitis (adult)	*Francisella tularensis* (tularemia)
Lymphogranuloma venereum	*Leptospira* (Leptospirosis)
Ornithosis, psittacosis	*Mycobacterium marinum* (Minocycline)
Trachoma	
Urethral, endocervical, or rectal infections in adults	*Nocardia* (minocycline)
Helicobacter pylori (plus metronidazole plus bismuth subsalicylate)	
Pelvic inflammatory disease (acute, in combination with other antibiotics)	*Pasteurella multocida*
(doxycycline)	*Pseudomonas pseudomallei* (melioidosis) (doxycycline with TMP/SMX and
	chloramphenicol)
	Rat-bite fever (*Spirillum minus, Streptococcus moniliformis*)
Pseudomonas mallei (glanders) (streptomycin with a tetracycline)	*Rochalimaea henselae* (Bacillary angiomatosis)
	Treponema pallidum (syphillis)
Rickettsial infections (some prefer chloramphenicol for severe infections)	
Ehrlichiosis	*Treponema pertenue* (Yaws, nasopalatal)
Q fever	*Ureaplasma urealyticum*
Rickettsial pox	*Yersinina pestis* (plague)
Rocky Mountain spotted fever	*Xanthomonas maltophilia* (minocycline)
Typhus fever	
Urethritis, nonspecific	
Urethral syndrome, acute	*Alternative Prophylaxis*
Vibrio cholera (cholera)	Oral bowel preparation for intestinal surgery (tetracycline in combination with
Vibrio parahemolyticus	neomycin or doxycycline alone)
Vibrio vulnificus	Meningococcal disease prophylaxis (minocycline)

[a] Unless specified, tetracycline and doxycycline can be considered interchangeable.

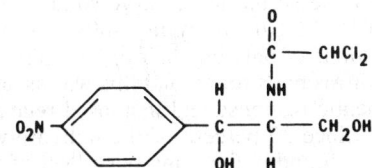

FIG. 3. Chemical structure of chloramphenicol.

Chloramphenicol remains a useful antibiotic, but only as alternative therapy in seriously ill patients.

Structure, Derivation, Brand Names, and Preparations

Like the early tetracyclines, chloramphenicol was discovered by screening organisms for their antimicrobial activity. Isolated independently by Burkholder from a mulched field near Caracas, Venezuela[94] and by workers at the University of Illinois from compost,[95] the organism producing the active compound was named *Streptomyces venezuelae*.[96] The structure of chloramphenicol is shown in Figure 3. It was the first antibiotic whose chemical synthesis was economically and technically practical for large-scale production.[97] It is available in 250-mg capsules (chloromycetin, Parke-Davis), suspension 150 mg/5 ml (chloromycetin palmitate), and as a parenteral formulation (chloromycetin sodium succinate, 1-g powder). Generic formulations are also available.

Thiamphenical, not available in the United States, is an analog in which the *p*-nitro group on the benzene ring is replaced by a methylsulfonyl group. Its spectrum of activity is similar to that of chloramphenicol, but it has not been reported to cause aplastic anemia.

Mechanism of Action

Chloramphenicol appears to enter the cell by an energy-dependent process.[98] Once within the cell it inhibits protein synthesis. This is accomplished by reversibly binding to the larger 50S subunit of the 70S ribosome at a locus that prevents the attachment of the amino acid-containing end of the aminoacyl-tRNA to its binding region. Without this attachment, the association of the amino acid substrate with peptidyltransferase does not occur, and peptide bond formation is prevented.[2] This block in protein synthesis produces a static effect against most sensitive microorganisms. However, chloramphenicol is bactericidal against some meningeal pathogens such as *H. influenzae, Streptococcus pneumoniae*, and *Neisseria meningitidis* but not group B streptococci or enteric gram-negative bacilli at concentrations that can be achieved therapeutically.[99–101] Although mammalian cells contain primarily 80S ribosomes that are unaffected by chloramphenicol, the mitochondria do contain 70S particles. The effect of chloramphenicol on these has been suggested as a cause for the dose-related bone marrow suppression of the compound but not the idiosyncratic aplastic anemia.[102]

In Vitro Activity

Chloramphenicol is extremely active against a variety of organisms, including bacteria, spirochetes, rickettsia, chlamydiae, and mycoplasmas. The MICs required for bacteria are listed in Table 6. Most of the gram-positive and gram-negative aerobic bacteria are inhibited by concentrations easily achieved in the serum of patients, but more active or less toxic therapeutic agents are available for most of these pathogens.[8–10,20,97,103–107] Salmonellae including *Salmonella typhi* are generally susceptible.[105] In the United States, resistant strains occasionally occur,[108] but imported strains may be highly resistant. The three most common organisms causing meningitis in childhood (*H. influenzae, S. pneumoniae*, and *N. meningitidis*) are highly susceptible,[9,109,110] although rare resistant strains of each species have been reported. The overall rate of *H. influenzae* resistance among clinical strains in the United States is approximately 0.6 percent.[111] Indeed, strains of *H. influenzae* that cause clinical infections and are resistant to both chloramphenicol and ampicillin have been isolated in several parts of the world.[112–114] These resistant isolates are rare in the United States and Canada but rather frequent in Spain.[115–117] Chloramphenicol is one of the most active antibiotics against anaerobic bacteria including *B. fragilis*, but clindamycin, metronidazole, and imipenem have

TABLE 6. Activity of Chloramphenicol Against Selected Bacteria[a]

Bacteria	No. of Strains	Cumulative Percentage Inhibited at Indicated Concentration (μg/ml)				
		0.4	0.8	1.6	3.1	6.3
Aerobic bacteria						
Gram-positive						
S. aureus	291	0	0	0	5	55
S. aureus (methicillin-resistant)	22	0	0	0	0	20
S. pyogenes	303	0	0	20	92	99
Streptococci, group B	146	0	0	0	85	99
Viridans streptococci	193	0	0	0	60	90
Enterococci	382	0	0	0	0	0
S. pneumoniae	78				50	100
Gram-negative						
H. influenzae	17			50	100	
N. meningitidis	7		50		100	
N. gonorrhoeae	106	5	52	97	100	
E. coli	71	0	0	5	30	75
K. pneumoniae	35	0	0	6	70	75
Enterobacter	10	0	0	0	10	20
Serratia marcescens	111	0	0	0	5	
P. mirabilis	209	0	0	0	20	60
Proteus (indole-positive)	32	0	0	0	10	40
Salmonella typhi	81	0	0	0	50	95
S. paratyphi A	31				28	97
Shigella spp.	44		20	30	75	90
Vibrio cholera	64					84
Brucella spp.	25	0	0	28	92	100
P. aeurginosa	11	0	0	0	0	0
P. pseudomallei	10	0	0	0	0	50
Bordetella pertussia	31	20	45	85	97	99
Anaerobic bacteria						
Gram-positive						
Peptococcus spp.	145	8	25	67	97	98
Peptostreptococcus spp.	72	11	37	63	96	100
Propionibacterium acnes	16	12	31	94	100	
Eubacterium lentum	14	14	14	28	71	100
Clostridium perfringens	34	0	0	15	100	
Clostridium spp.	17	12	12	53	88	100
Gram-negative						
Veilonella spp.	13	23	46	85	100	
B. fragilis	195	0	1	2	23	98
Prevotella melaninogenica	29	14	31	93	96	100
Fusobacterium spp.	18	39	44	56	89	100

[a] The National Committee for Clinical Laboratory Standards suggests that 4 μg/ml or less be considered susceptible when testing *H. influenzae* and 12 μg/ml or less be considered susceptible when testing other organisms.[5]

(Data from refs. 8–10, 12, 20, 97, and 103–118.)

become more important clinically to treat infections caused by these bacteria.[20,118–120]

Bacteria develop resistance to chloramphenicol by becoming impermeable to the drug or by producing an enzyme, acetyltransferase, that acetylates the antibiotic to an inactive diacetyl derivative.[121,122] This latter mechanism has been R factor–mediated and has been responsible for widespread epidemics of chloramphenicol-resistant typhoid fever and *Shigella* dysentery in Central and South America, Vietnam, India, and other countries.[123–126] It has been suggested that the unrestricted over-the-counter sales of chloramphenicol in the countries involved may be an important factor that provides antibiotic pressure for the development of these resistant strains.[125,126] In the United States, chloramphenicol resistance in *Salmonella* has been traced to the use of chloramphenicol on dairy farms.[31]

Pharmacology

Chloramphenicol serum levels achieved by different routes of administration and with different product forms are listed in Figure 4. Chloramphenicol in the encapsulated form is well absorbed from the gastrointestinal tract and results in peak serum levels of 12 μg/ml of active antibiotic after a 1-g dose.[127,128] Since it is a very bitter substance, aqueous solutions may not be accepted by children. A tasteless suspension in the form of chloramphenicol palmitate is available. This preparation must be hydrolyzed in the intestine to produce active chloramphenicol. Although earlier formulations sometimes produced erratic serum levels, the bioavailability of chloramphenicol palmitate in the current formulation is the same as in the capsules and is effective for children with *H. influenzae* meningitis (A. J. Glazko, Warner-Lambert/Parke-Davis Pharmaceutical Research Division, Ann Arbor, Michigan, personal communication).[129,130]

The intravenous preparation of the drug is the soluble but inactive chloramphenicol succinate ester that is rapidly hydrolized within the body to biologically active chloramphenicol.[131] This preparation produces active chloramphenicol levels in the serum that are 70 percent of those obtained after oral administration due to incomplete hydrolysis.[127] Bhutta et al. found consistently lower serum levels when treating typhoid fever compared to other diseases with intravenous chloramphenicol in children and suggested a dose of 75 mg/kg/day instead of 50 mg/kg/day to compensate.[132] Intramuscular injection is well tolerated and in most studies produces peak serum levels and areas under the serum level curve similar to intravenous administration.[133–136] One study in adults, however, showed peak concentrations of only one-half to two-thirds of those obtained by the intravenous route, and this was associated with a delayed therapeutic response and increased relapse rate of typhoid fever.[137] Since 30 percent of the unhydrolyzed inactive succinate ester is found in the urine regardless of which parenteral route is used, the lower serum levels produced by intramuscular injection appear to be due to delayed absorption of the ester from the site of injection rather than to decreased hydrolysis.[127] The intramuscular route should be used cautiously.

Chloramphenicol is metabolized primarily by the liver, where it is conjugated with glucuronic acid, and is excreted in this inactive form by the kidney. Only about 5–10 percent of the administered dose is recovered in the urine as biologically active chloramphenicol. Nevertheless, in the absence of renal disease, concentrations of 150–200 μg/ml of active drug are achieved, which is sufficient to treat urinary tract infections if necessary. Urinary concentrations are markedly diminished, however, in patients with renal failure.[138]

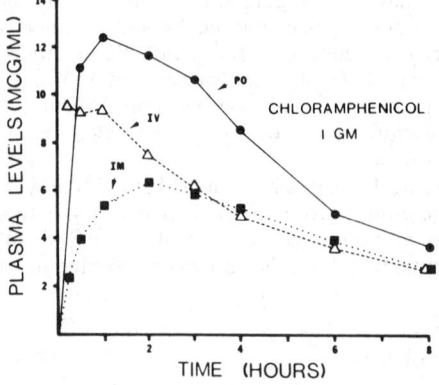

FIG. 4. Plasma levels of active chloramphenicol achieved with 1 g of chloramphenicol administered orally (Chloromycetin Kapseals) and with chloramphenicol sodium succcinate intravenously (iv) and intramuscularly (im). (Modified from Glazko,[127] with permission.)

The use of chloramphenicol in children has led to a better understanding of its pharmacokinetics. It is clear that there is a wide variation in the metabolism and excretion in that age group. Dosage requirements may vary threefold in children of the same age, with even greater variation noted in newborn and young infants. Because newborns metabolize the antibiotic at a slow rate, the initial dose for those less than 1 week old should be 25 mg/kg every 24 hours and for infants from 1–4 weeks old, 25 mg/kg every 12 hours instead of the usual 50 mg/kg/ day divided into 6-hour dosing intervals for older children and adults. However, the wide variation makes monitoring serum levels imperative.[136,139,140]

Chloramphenicol has a half-life in adults of 4.1 hours after single intravenous injections, is not highly bound to protein (25–50 percent), and has an apparent volume of distribution of 100 liters.[97,127,141] The antibiotic diffuses well into many tissues and body fluids. Kramer et al.[142] have shown levels in the brain to be 36 µg/ml, whereas corresponding serum levels were 4 µg/ ml. These high levels may reflect the antibiotic's high degree of lipid solubility in conjunction with low protein binding and small molecular size.[143] Levels in the cerebrospinal fluid even without inflamed meninges are generally 30–50 percent of serum concentrations, much higher than those of most other antibiotics.[97] Therapeutic levels are obtained in pleural, ascitic, and synovial fluids.[97,144] In the aqueous humor, levels are approximately 50 percent of those in the serum,[145] but studies in rabbits and humans suggest that topical administration may be more efficient in providing high aqueous concentrations.[146,147] Subconjuctival injections are not satisfactory.[148] The antibiotic crosses the placenta to the fetal circulation but produces negligible amounts in the amniotic fluid. Only small amounts of active chloramphenicol are recovered in the bile (0.14 percent of a 1-g dose).[97]

Renal and Hepatic Insufficiency.   The half-life of biologically active chloramphenicol in patients with renal disease differs only slightly from healthy subjects, whereas its metabolites increase markedly. The dose, however, should not be modified if therapeutic levels of the active drug are to be maintained. Fortunately, the metabolites do not appear to be as toxic as the active compound. Neither peritoneal nor hemodialysis alters serum levels sufficiently to require dose alterations.[141,149]

Patients with hepatic failure, as evidenced by jaundice or ascites, conjugate chloramphenicol at a slower rate. Serum levels of active chloramphenicol increase to levels capable of bone marrow suppression.[150] The regimen suggested for adults with hepatic insufficiency is an initial 1-g loading dose followed by 500 mg every 6 hours. The course of therapy should be limited when possible to 10–14 days.

Assay

Because of the narrow therapeutic-to-toxic ratio, it is important to monitor serum levels of this antibiotic, particularly in newborn and premature infants, in patients with hepatic disease, and in those patients taking interacting drugs. There are a number of very effective assays that can be used, including bioassays, radioenzymatic assays, competitive enzyme-linked immunoassays, and high-performance chromotography.[151–158] Serum levels in most cases should be maintained between 10 and 30 µg/ ml.

Toxicity

Hematologic.   The most important toxic effects of chloramphenicol occur in the bone marrow. The effects can be divided into two types. The first is a reversible bone marrow depression due to a direct pharmacologic effect of the antibiotic as a result of inhibition of mitochondrial protein synthesis. It is manifested by reticulocytopenia, anemia, leukopenia, thrombocytopenia, or any combination thereof. There is an increase in serum iron

in association with a reduced uptake of radioactive iron by the red blood cells, thus indicating diminished hemoglobin synthesis. The bone marrow reveals vacuolization of the erythyroid and myeloid precursors, but these changes are not specific for chloramphenicol. This type of toxicity is extremely common, occurs during the course of therapy, and is dose related.[159] It is more likely to occur in patients receiving 4 g or more per day or in patients in whom serum levels are above 25 µg/ml, a level that may occur in patients with severe liver disease who are receiving usual doses. It is reversible when treatment with the antibiotic is discontinued.[160]

The second type of toxicity is a rare but generally fatal "idiosyncratic" response that is most frequently manifested as aplastic anemia.[161] Indeed, chloramphenicol is the most common cause of this syndrome. According to the best epidemiologic studies in the United States, aplastic anemia occurs once in 24,500–40,800 patients who receive the antibiotic, a risk about 13 times greater than that for aplastic anemia in the general population.[162] The aplastic anemia most commonly occurs weeks to months after completion of therapy and is not necessarily dose related. It appears that this toxic effect is caused by a mechanism different from the direct bone marrow suppression previously described. Although the pathogenesis of this idiosyncratic response is not known, there have been several observations and theories that suggest the toxicity is very complex, involving interactions of the host and toxic intermediates of the antibiotic. This type of toxicity has occurred in identical twins, which suggests a genetic predisposition.[163] Morley et al.[164] have observed that mice given chloramphenicol after treatment with busulfan had a progressive decrease in the number of pluripotential stem cells, whereas control mice did not, suggesting that the aplastic anemia might result in patients with unrecognized pre-existing residual marrow damage either genetic or acquired. In 1967, Holt[165] observed that the aplastic anemia occurred only after oral administration of the antibiotic. He postulates that the fatal reaction may be caused by the absorption of toxic products produced by enzymatic degradation of chloramphenicol, perhaps as a result of specific types of bacteria colonizing the gut of affected people. Supporting this hypothesis, Jimenez and colleagues[166] have shown that one of chloramphenicol's metabolites, dehydrochloramphenicol, is 10- to 20-fold more cytotoxic than chloramphenicol yet is only one-third as effective in inhibiting protein synthesis, thus suggesting that this metabolite and perhaps others may play a significant role in this toxicity. These toxic metabolites may undergo further metabolic transformation in the bone marrow with on-site production of toxic intermediates.[167,168] Although the number of cases reported is greater after oral therapy, a number of cases of aplastic anemia from parenteral chloramphenicol even after the administration of eyedrops have also been reported.[169,170]

Although most cases of aplastic anemia from chloramphenicol become apparent after the completion of therapy, it should be emphasized that 22 percent of the cases occur concurrently with antibiotic administration.[161,170] Whether some of these episodes can be prevented by checking the blood counts of patients is not known. Until the pathogenesis of the toxicity is clearly understood, it is recommended that a complete blood count be obtained on a twice-a-week basis from all patients receiving chloramphenicol. If the white blood cell count decreases below 2500/mm³, it is desirable to discontinue treatment with the antibiotic if the clinical condition allows. It should be recognized, however, that low numbers of white blood cells may occur in illnesses for which chloramphenicol is used, such as typhoid fever.

Also of concern are the reports of childhood leukemia after the use of chloramphenicol. Although these cases generally follow the aplastic anemia, a population-based case-control interview study of 309 childhood leukemia cases and 618 age- and sex-matched controls showed a significant dose-response relation between chloramphenicol and the risk of both acute lymphocytic and nonlymphocytic leukemia, particularly after treatment for greater than 10 days in children without prior aplastic anemia. Until this is more clearly defined, it seems prudent to change therapy as quickly as possible to alternate agents when organisms prove susceptible to other equally effective and less toxic antibiotics.[171]

Chloramphenicol may also produce a hemolytic anemia in patients with the Mediterranean form of glucose-6-phosphate dehydrogenase (G6PD) deficiency. This apparently does not occur with the milder A type G6PD deficiency, which is the most common form in blacks.[172]

Gray Baby Syndrome.   The gray baby syndrome of neonates is characterized by abdominal distension, vomiting, flaccidity, cynosis, circulatory collapse, and death. The side effect results from a diminished ability of neonates to conjugate chloramphenicol and to excrete the active form in the urine.[173] If chloramphenicol is necessary in premature infants and neonates, the dose should be reduced to 25 mg/kg/day, and the antibiotic levels should be monitored. This syndrome has also been recognized in toddlers and after accidental overdoses in adults.[174,175] It is generally associated with serum concentrations of chloramphenicol of greater than 50 μg/ml and may present with unexplained metabolic acidosis.[176] Large-volume exchange transfusions or charcoal hemoperfusion have been used to accelerate drug removal. It is due in part to impaired myocardial contractility related to direct interference of myocardial tissue respiration and oxidative phosphorylatation.[177–180]

Optic Neuritis.   Optic neuritis resulting in decreased visual acuity has been described in patients receiving prolonged chloramphenicol therapy.[181] The symptoms are generally reversible, but loss of vision has occurred. Other neurologic sequelae such as peripheral neuritis, headache, depression, ophthalmoplegia, and mental confusion have also been described.

Other Types.   Hypersensitivity reactions (including rashes and drug fevers) and anaphylaxis are rare. Herxheimer-like responses during therapy for syphilis, brucellosis, and typhoid fever have been observed. Symptoms involving the gastrointestinal tract, including nausea, vomiting and diarrhea, glossitis, and stomatitis, occur but have not been a major problem. Bleeding due to decreased vitamin K synthesis has resulted from prolonged administration.

Significant Drug Interactions

Chloramphenicol prolongs the half-life of tolbutamide, chlorpropamide, phenytoin, cyclophosphamide, and warfarin (Coumadin), apparently by inhibiting hepatic microsomal enzymes.[182–185] Severe toxicity and death have occurred. Phenytoin, rifampin, and phenobarbital have been observed to decrease the serum concentration and increase the total body clearance of chloramphenicol, perhaps by inducing hepatic microsomal enzymes. Serum concentrations should be monitored when these drugs are administered concurrently.[186,187] The physician should be on the alert for toxicity from other agents that are metabolized by the liver when administering this agent and should monitor serum levels when these drugs are administered concurrently. Chloramphenicol may delay the response of anemias to iron, folic acid, and vitamin B$_{12}$.[188]

Chloramphenicol is primarily a bacteriostatic agent and will antagonize in vitro the bactericidal activity of the penicillins, cephalosporins, and aminoglycoside antibiotics. This has doubtful clinical significance in most instances. However, care should be exercised in the use of such combinations for infections that require bactericidal activity for efficacy such as for infections in the granulocytopenic host or in the treatment of endocarditis.[189] In the treatment of meningitis, the bacteriostatic activity of chloramphenicol against group B streptococci and its in vitro

TABLE 7. Indications for Chloramphenicol[a]

Indications	Comments
Therapy of choice	
None[b]	
Effective alternative therapy	
Bacterial meningitis	For penicillin-allergic patients. Also used
H. influenzae	for S. pneumoniae relatively resistant to
S. pneumoniae	penicillin
N. meningitidis	
Brain abscess	
Chlamydia psittaci (Psittacosis)	
Clostridium perfringens	
Ehrlichiosis	
Rickettsial infections	Preferred by many when patients require
Rocky Mountain spotted fever	parenteral therapy, during pregnancy,
Typhus (murine)	and for young children
Scrub typhus	
Tick-bite fever	
Q fever	
Pseudomonas mallei	Used with streptomycin
Pseudomonas pseudomallei	Used with doxycycline
(Melioidosis, acute)	
Typhoid fever and invasive	Strains in some areas may be
salmonellosis	chloramphenicol resistant; not used for
	gastroenteritis or carrier state.
Vibrio vulnificus cellulitis and/	
or sepsis	

[a] The usual recommended adult dose is 50 mg/day/day. Some prefer 75 mg/kg/day for the treatment of typhoid fever. For infections of the central nervous system, 100 mg/kg/day is suggested. See text for pediatric doses.
[b] In some countries, chloramphenicol remains the standard for the therapy of typhoid fever.

antagonism with ampicillin against this organism are of concern and should be considered in selecting therapy when this organism is likely to be a pathogen.[101]

Indications

The clinical indications for the use of chloramphenicol are listed in Table 7. With the possible exception of typhoid fever in areas where cost and availability make it the primary therapy, it is no longer the drug of choice for any specific infection. The third-generation cephalosporins have superseded chloramphenicol for the treatment of bacterial meningitis in infants and children, though chloramphenical is still used for the treatment of meningitis in the penicillin-allergic patients, for meningitis cases by relatively penicillin-resistant pneumococci, and as an oral alternative when the use of parenteral therapy is impossible.[190] Occasionally, the antibiotic is useful when the differential diagnosis includes both meningococcemia and Rocky Mountain spotted fever, diseases that may be difficult to distinguish on clinical characteristics.

Chloramphenicol is a valuable antimicrobial agent. Like many other agents, it is toxic and its use should be restricted to clearly defined situations in seriously ill patients.

REFERENCES

1. Finland M. Twenty-fifth anniversary of the discovery of Aureomycin: The place of the tetracyclines in antimicrobial therapy. Clin Pharmacol Ther. 1974;15:3.
2. Yamaguchi A, Onmori H, Kaneko-Ohdera M, et al. ΔpH-dependent accumulation of tetracycline in Escherichia coli. Antimicrob Agents Chemother. 1991;35:53.
3. Craven GR, Gavin R, Fanning T. The transfer RNA binding site of the 30 S ribosome and the site of tetracycline inhibition. Symp Quant Biol. 1969; 34:129.
4. Bread NS, Armentrout SA, Weisberger AS. Inhibition of mammalian protein synthesis by antibiotics. Pharmacol Rev. 1969;21:213.
5. National Committee for Clinical Laboratory Standards. Methods for dilution antimicrobial susceptibility tests for bacteria that grow aerobically: Approved standard. NCCLS Publication M7-A. Villanova, PA: NCCLS; 1985.
6. Centers for Disease Control. Antibiotic-resistant strains of Neisseria gonorrhoeae. MMWR. 1987;36(Suppl 55)1–18.
7. Steigbigel NH, Reed CR, Finland M. Susceptibility of common pathogenic bacteria to seven tetracycline antibiotics in vitro. Am J Med Sci. 1968;255: 179.
8. Finland M. Changing patterns of susceptibility of common bacterial pathogens to antimicrobial agents. Ann Intern Med. 1972;76:1009.

9. Sabath LD, Stumpf LL, Wallace SJ, et al. Susceptibility of *Diplococcus pneumoniae, Haemophilus influenzae*, and *Neisseria meningitidis* to 23 antibiotics. Antimicrob Agents Chemother. 1970;10:53–56.

10. Eickhoff TC, Bennett JV, Hayes PS, et al. *Pseudomonas pseudomallei* susceptibility to chemotherapeutic agents. J Infect Dis. 1970;121:95.

11. Karmali MA, DeGrandis S, Fleming PC. Antimicrobial susceptibility of *Campylobacter jejuni* with special reference to resistance patterns of Canadian isolates. Antimicrob Agents Chemother. 1981;19:593.

12. Gordon RC, Thompson TR, Carlson W, et al. Antimicrobial resistance of shigellae isolated in Michigan. JAMA. 1975;231:1159.

13. Neu HC. A symposium on the tetracyclines: A major appraisal. Introduction. Bull NY Acad Med. 1978;54:141.

14. Sparling PF. Antibiotic resistance in *Neisseria gonorrhoeae*. Med Clin North Am. 1972;56:1133.

15. Farrell ID, Hinchliffe PM, Robertson L. Susceptibility of *Brucella* spp. to tetracycline and its analogues. J Clin Pathol. 1976;29:1097.

16. Morris JG Jr., Black RE. Cholera and other vibrioses in the United States. N Engl J Med. 1985;312:343–50.

17. Chow AW, Patten V, Dominick B. Susceptibility of *Campylobacter fetus* to twenty-two antimicrobial agents. Antimicrob Agents Chemother. 1978;13:416.

18. Michel J, Rogol M, Dickman D. Susceptibility of clinical isolates of *Campylobacter jejuni* to sixteen antimicrobial agents. Antimicrob Agents Chemother. 1983;23:796.

19. Wallace RJ, Wiss K. Susceptibility of *Mycobacterium marinum* to tetracyclines and aminoglycosides. Antimicrob Agents Chemother. 1981;20:610.

20. Sutter VL, Finegold SM. Susceptibility of anaerobic bacteria to 23 antimicrobial agents. Antimicrob Agents Chemother. 1976;10:736.

21. Washington JA, Dearing WH, Judd ES, et al. Effect of preoperative antibiotic regimen on development of infection after intestinal surgery: Prospective, randomized, double-blind study. Ann Surg. 1974;180:567.

22. Hojer H, Wetterfors J. Systemic prophylaxis with doxycycline in surgery of the colon and rectum. Ann Surg. 1978;187:362.

23. Johnson SE, Klein GP, Schmid GP, et al. Susceptibility of the Lyme disease spirochete to seven antimicrobial agents. Yale J Biol Med. 1984;57:549–53.

24. Pang LW, Limsomwong N, Boudreau EF, et al. Doxycycline prophylaxis for *Falciparum malaria*: Lancet. 1987;1:1161–4.

25. Benveniste R, Davies J. Mechanisms of antibiotic resistance in bacteria. Annu Rev Biochem. 1973;42:471.

26. Sompolinsky D, Zemira S. Plasmid-determined resistance to tetracycline. Microbios. 1981;30:109.

27. Park BH, Hendricks M, Malamy MH, et al. Cryptic tetracycline resistance determinant (class F) isolated from *Bacteroides fragilis* mediates resistance in *Escherichia coli* by actively reducing tetracycline accumulation. Antimicrob Agents Chemother. 1987;31:1739–43.

28. Roberts MC, Kenny GE, Tet M. Tetracycline resistance determinants in *Ureaplasma urealyticum*. Antimicrob Agents Chemother. 1986;29:350–2.

29. Rapoport MI, Calia FM. The use of antibiotics in animal feeds. JAMA. 1974;229:1212.

30. VanLeeuwen WJ, VanEmbden J, Guinee PAM, et al. Decrease in drug resistance in *Salmonella* in the Netherlands. Antimicrob Agents Chemother. 1979;16:237.

31. Spika JS, Waterman SH, Soo Hoo GW, et al. Chloramphenicol-resistant *Salmonella newport* traced through hamburger to dairy farms. N Engl J Med. 1987;316:565–70.

32. Finland M, Garrod LP. Demethylchlortetracycline. Br Med J. 1960;2:959.

33. Fabre J, Milek E, Kalfopoulos P, et al. The kinetics of tetracyclines in man: Digestive absorption and serum concentrations. In: Doxycycline (Vibramycin): A Compendium of Clinical Evaluation. New York: Pfizer Laboratories; 1973;13–18.

34. Lederle Laboratories. Minocin: Minocycline. Pearl River, NY: Lederle Laboratories; 1975.

35. Rosenblatt JE, Barrett JE, Brodie JL, et al. Comparison of in vitro activity and clinical pharmacology of doxycycline with other tetracyclines. Antimicrob Agents Chemother. 1966;6:134–141.

36. Kirby WMM, Roberts CE, Burdick RE. Comparison of two new tetracyclines with tetracycline and demethylchlortetracycline. Antimicrob Agents Chemother. 1961;286–292.

37. Fabre J, Pitton JS, Junz JP, et al. Distribution and excretion of doxycycline in man. Chemotherapia. 1966;11:73.

38. Kunin CM, Dornbush AC, Finland M. Distribution and excretion of four tetracycline analogues in normal young men. J Clin Invest. 1959;38:1950.

39. MacDonald H, Kelley RG, Allen ES, et al. Pharmacokinetic studies on minocycline in man. Clin Pharmacol Ther. 1973;14:852.

40. Kunin CM. Comparative serum binding distribution and excretion of tetracycline and a new analogue methacycline. Proc Soc Exp Biol Med. 1962;110:311.

41. Bennett JV, Mickewait JS, Barrett JE, et al. Comparative serum binding of four tetracyclines under simulated in vivo conditions. Antimicrob Agents Chemother. 1965;5:180–2.

42. Wood WS, Kipnis GP. The concentrations of tetracycline, chlortetracycline and oxytetracycline in the cerebrospinal fluid after intravenous administration. In: Welch H, Marti-Ibanez F, eds. Antibiotics Annual, 1953–1954. New York: Medical Encyclopedia; 1953;98–101.

43. Yim CW, Flynn NM, Fitzgerald FT. Penetration of oral doxycycline into the cerebrospinal fluid of patients with latent or neurosyphilis. Antimicrob Agents Chemother. 1985;28:347.

44. Parker RH, Schmid F. Antimicrobial activity of synovial fluid during therapy of septic arthritis. Arthritis Rheum. 1971;14:96.

45. Lundberg C, Malmburg A, Ivemark BI. Antibiotic concentrations in relation to structural changes in maxillary sinus mucosa folowing intramuscular or peroral treatment. Scand J Infect Dis. 1974;6:187.

46. Fabre J, Milek E, Kalopoulos P, et al. The kinetics of tetracyclines in man. II. Excretion, penetration in normal and inflammatory tissues, behavior in renal insufficiency and hemodialysis. In: Doxycycline (Vibramycin): A Compendium of Clinical Evaluations. New York: Pfizer Laboratories; 1973; 19–28.

47. Hoeprich PD, Warshauer DM. Entry of four tetracyclines into saliva and tears. Antimicrob Agents Chemother. 1974;5:330.

48. LeBlanc AL, Perry JE. Transfer of tetracycline across the human placenta. Texas Rep Biol Med. 1967;25:541.

49. Whelton A. Tetracyclines in renal insufficiency: Resolution of a therapeutic dilemma. Bull NY Acad Med. 1978;54:223.

50. Bennett JV, Brodie JL, Benner EJ, et al. Simplified accurate method for antibiotic assay of clinical specimens. Appl Microbiol. 1966;14:170.

51. Ray A, Newton V. Use of high-performance liquid chromatography to monitor for stability of tetracycline and chlortetracycline in susceptibility determination. Antimicrob Agents Chemother. 1991;35:1264–6.

52. Csonka GW, Rosedale N, Walkden L. Balanitis due to fixed drug eruption associated with tetracycline therapy. Br J Vener Dis. 1970;47:42.

53. Fellner MJ, Baer RL. Anaphylactic reaction to tetracycline in a penicillin-allergic patient: Immunologic studies. JAMA. 1965;192:997.

54. Furey WW, Tan C. Anaphylactic shock due to oral demethylchlortetracycline. Ann Intern Med. 1969;70:357.

55. Carey BW. Photodynamic response of a new tetracycline. JAMA. 1960;172:1196.

56. Frost P, Weinstein GD, Gomez EC. Phototoxic potential of minocycline and doxycycline. Arch Dermatol. 1972;105:681.

57. Angeloni VL, Salasche SJ, Ortiz R. Nail, skin and scleral pigmentation induced by minocycline. Cutis. 1987;40:229–33.

58. Atwood HD, Dennet X. A black thyroid and minocycline treatment. Br Med J. 1976;2:1109.

59. Brearley LJ, Storey E. Tetracycline-induced tooth changes: Part 2. Prevalence, localization and nature of staining in extracted deciduous teeth. Med J Aust. 1968;2:714.

60. Witkop CJ, Wolf RO. Hypoplasia and intrinsic staining of enamel following tetracycline therapy. JAMA. 1963;185:1008.

61. Cohan S, Bevelander G, Tiamsic T. Growth inhibition of prematures receiving tetracycline. Am J Dis Child. 1963;105:453.

62. Grossman ER, Walcheck A, Freedman H. Tetracycline and permanent teeth: The relationship between doses and tooth color. Pediatrics. 1971;47:567.

63. Department of Health Education and Welfare. Tetracycline pediatric drops to be withdrawn from the market. FDA Drug Bull. 1978;8:23.

64. Forti G, Benincori C. Doxycycline and the teeth. Lancet. 1969;1:782.

65. Schneider R. Doxycycline esophageal ulcers. Am J Dig Dis. 1977;22:805.

66. Winckler K. Tetracycline ulcers of the oesophagus: Endoscopy, histology, and reoentgenology in two cases, and review of the literature. Endoscopy. 1981;13:225.

67. Hinton NA. The effect of oral tetracycline HCl and doxycycline on the intestinal flora. Curr Ther Res. 1970;12:341.

68. Gorbach SL, Bartlett JG. Anaerobic infections. N Engl J Med. 1974;290:1289.

69. Elmore MF, Rogge JD. Tetracycline induced pancreatitis. Gastroenterology. 1981;81:1134.

70. Lepper MH, Wolfe CK, Zimmerman HJ, et al. Effect of large doses of Aureomycin on human liver. Arch Intern Med. 1951;88:271.

71. Schultz JC, Adamson JS Jr, Workman WW, et al. Fatal liver disease after intravenous administration of tetracycline in high doses. N Engl J Med. 1963; 269:999.

72. Whalley PJ, Adams RH, Combes B. Tetracycline toxicity in pregnancy: Liver and pancreatic dysfunction. JAMA. 1964;189:357.

73. Damjanov I, Arnold R, Faour M. Tetracycline toxicity in a non-pregnant woman. JAMA. 1968;204:934.

74. Shils ME. Renal disease and the metabolic effects of tetracycline. Ann Intern Med. 1963;58:389.

75. Forrest JN, Cox M, Hong C, et al. Superiority of demeclocycline over lithium in the treatment of chronic syndrome of inappropriate secretion of antidiuretic hormone. N Engl J Med. 1978;298:173.

76. Carrilho F, Bosch J, Arroyo V, et al. Renal failure associated with demeclocycline in cirrhosis. Ann Intern Med. 1977;87:195.

77. Fanning WL, Gump DW, Sofferman RA. Side effects of minocycline: A double blind study. Antimicrob Agents Chemother. 1977;11:712.

78. Koch-Weser J, Gilmore EB. Benign intracranial hypertension in an adult after tetracycline therapy. JAMA. 1967;200:345.

79. Walters BNJ, Gubbay SS. Tetracycline and benign intracranial hypertension: Report of five cases. Br Med J. 1981;282:19.

80. Jackson GG, Haight TH, Kass EH, et al. Tetramycin therapy of pneumonia: Clinical and bacteriologic studies in 91 cases. Ann Intern Med. 1951;35:1175.

81. Lundsgaard-Hansen P, Senn A, Roos B, et al. Staphylococcal enteritis: Report of six cases with two fatalities after intravenous administration of *N*-(pyrrolidinomethyl) tetracycline. JAMA. 1960;173:1008.

82. Neuvonen PJ, Gothoni G, Hackman R, et al. Interference of iron with the absorption of tetracyclines in man. Br Med J. 1970;4:532.

83. Bar WH, Adir J, Garrettson L. Decrease of tetracycline in man by sodium bicarbonate. Clin Pharmacol Ther. 1971;12:779.

84. Fisher P, House F, Inns P, et al. Effect of cimetidine on the absorption of orally administered tetracycline. Br J Clin Pharmacol. 1980;9:153.

85. Neuvonen PJ, Pentitila O. Interaction between doxycycline and barbiturates. Br Med J. 1974;1:535.

86. Pentitla O, Neuvonen PJ, Lehtovaara R. Interaction between doxcycline and some antiepileptic drugs. Br Med J. 1974;2:470.

87. Neuvonen PJ, Penttila O, Roos M. Effect of long-term alcohol consumption on the half-life of tetracycline and doxycycline in man. Int J Clin Pharmacol. 1976;14:303.

88. Kuzucu EY. Methoxyflurane, tetracycline and renal failure. JAMA. 1970; 211:1162.

89. Semel JD. Renal failure and multiple organ toxicity associated with tetracycline operative prophylaxis. Infect Surg. 1988;June:405–8.

90. Boston Collaborative Drug Surveillance Program. Tetracycline and drug-attributed rises in blood urea nitrogen. JAMA. 1972;220:377.

91. Bacon JF, Chenfield GM. Pregnancy attributable to interaction between tetracycline and oral contraceptives. Br Med J. 1980;280:293.

92. Hansen PD. Drug Interactions. 5th ed. Philadelphia: Lea & Febiger; 1985: 239.

93. Lepper MH, Dowling HF. Treatment of pneumococcol meningitis with penicillin compared with penicillin plus aureomycin. Arch Intern Med. 1951;88: 489.

94. Ehrlich J, Bartz QR, Smith RM, et al. Chloromycetin, a new antibiotic from a soil actinomycete. Science. 1947;106:417.

95. Carter HE, Gottliebb D, Anderson HW. Comments and communications. Science. 107;113:947.

96. Ehrlich J, Gottlieb D, Burkholder PR, et al. *Streptomyces venezuelae*, N. sp., the source of Chloromycetin. J Bacteriol. 1948;56:467.

97. Woodward TE, Wisseman CL. Chloromycetin (Chloramphenicol). New York: Medical Encyclopedia; 1958.

98. Abdel-Sayed S. Transport of chloramphenicol into sensitive strains of *Escherichia coli* and *Pseudomonas aeruginosa*. J Antimicrob Chemother. 1987; 19:7–20.

99. Turk DC. A comparison of chloramphenicol and ampicillin as bactericidal agents for *Haemophilus influenzae* type B. J Med Microbiol. 1977;10:127.

100. Rahal JJ, Simberkoff MS. Bactericidal and bacteriostatic action of chloramphenicol against meningeal pathogens. Antimicrob Agents Chemother. 1979; 16:13.

101. Weeks JL, Mason EO Jr, Baker CJ. Antagonism of ampicillin and chloramphenicol for meningeal isolates of group B streptococci. Antimicrob Agents Chemother. 1981;20:281.

102. Roodyn DB, Wilkie D. The Biogenesis of Mitochondria. London: Methuen; 1968.

103. McGowan JE, Garner C, Wilcox C, et al. Antibiotic susceptibility of gram negative bacilli isolated from blood cultures: Results of tests with 35 agents and strains from 169 patients at Boston City Hospital during 1972. Am J Med. 1974;57:225.

104. Yow EM, Spink WW. Experimental studies on the action of streptomycin, Aureomycin and Chloromycetin on *Brucella*. J Clin Invest. 1949;28:871.

105. Robertson RP, Wahab MFA, Raasch FO. Evaluation of chloramphenicol and ampicillin in *Salmonella* enteric fever. N Engl J Med. 1968;278:171.

106. Rubinstein E, Shainberg B. In vitro activity of cinoxacin, ampicillin, and chloramphenicol against *Shigella* and non-typhoid *Salmonella*. Antimicrob Agents Chemother. 1977;11:577.

107. Wells EB, Chang SM, Jackson GG, et al. Antibiotic spectrum of *Hemophilus pertussis*. J Pediatr. 1950;36:752.

108. Cherubin CE, Neu HC, Rahal JJ, et al. Emergence of resistance to chloramphenicol in *Salmonella*. J Infect Dis. 1977;135:807.

109. Long SS, Phillips SE. Chloramphenicol-resistant *Hemophilus influenzae*. J Pediatr. 1976;90:1030.

110. Mathies AW Jr. Penicillins in the treatment of bacterial meningitis. *J R Coll Physicians Lond.* 1972;6:139.

111. Doern GV, Jorgensen JH, Thornsberry C, et al. Prevalance of antimicrobial resistance among clinical isolates of *Haemophilus influenzae*: A collaborative study. Diagn Microbiol Infect Dis. 1986;4:95–107.

112. MacMahon P, Sills J, Hall E, et al. *Haemophilus influenzae* type b resistant to both chloramphenicol and ampicillin in Britain. Br Med J. 1982;24:1229.

113. Bergeron MC, Claveau S, Simard P. Limited in vitro activity of cefamandole against 100 beta-lactamase and non–beta-lactamase-producing *Haemophilus influenzae* strains: Comparison of moxalactam, chloramphenicol and ampicillin. Antimicrob Agents Chemother. 1981;19:101.

114. Kenny JF, Isburg CD, Michaels RH. Meningitis due to *Haemophilus influenzae* type b resistant to both ampicillin and chloramphenicol. Pediatrics. 1980; 66:14.

115. Campos J, Garcia-Tornel S, San Feliu I. Susceptibility studies of multiply resistant *Haemophilus influenzae* isolated from pediatric patients and contacts. Antimicrob Agents Chemother. 1984;25:706.

116. Williams JD, Mossdeen F. Antibiotic resistance in *Haemophilus influenzae*. Epidemiology, mechanisms, and therapeutic possibilities. Rev Infect Dis. 1986;8(Suppl 5):555–61.

117. Kabani A, Joffe A, Jadavji T. Haemophilus Influenzae Type B resistant to Ampicillin and chloramphenicol. Pediatric Infectious Disease Journal 1991; 9:681.

118. Martin WJ, Gardner M, Washington JA II. In vitro antimicrobial susceptibility of anaerobic bacteria isolated from clinical specimens. Antimicrob Agents Chemother. 1972;1:148.

119. Cuchural GJ Jr, Talley FP, Jacobus NV, et al. Susceptibility of the *Bacteroides fragilis* group in the United States: Analysis by site of isolation. Antimicrob Agents Chemother. 1988;32:717–22.

120. Finegold SM, Wexler HM. Therapeutic implications of bacteriologic findings in mixed aerobic-anaerobic infections. Antimicrob Agents Chemother. 1988; 32:611–6.

121. Okamoto S, Mizuno D. Mechanism of chloramphenicol and tetracycline resistance in *Escherichia coli*. J Gen Microbiol. 1964;35:125.

122. Okamoto S, Suzuki Y. Chloramphenicol-, dihydrostreptomycin-, and kanamycin-inactivating enzymes from multiple drug-resistant *Escherichia coli* carrying episome "R." Nature. 1965;208:1301.

123. Gangarosa EJ, Bennett JV, Wyatt C, et al. An epidemic-associated episome? J Infect Dis. 1972;126:215.

124. Butler T, Linh NN, Arnold K, et al. Chloramphenicol-resistant typhoid fever in Vietnam associated with R-factor. Lancet. 1973;2:983.

125. Editorial: Drug resistance in salmonellas. Lancet. 1982;1:1391.

126. Halder KK, Dalal BS, Ghose E, Samyal S. Chloramphenicol resistant *Salmonella typhi*: The cause of recent outbreak of enteric fever in Calcutta. Indian J Pathol Microbiol. 1992;35:11–17.

127. Glazko AJ, Dill WA, Kinkel AW, et al. Absorption and excretion of parenteral doses of chloramphenicol sodium succinate in comparison with peroral doses of chloramphenicol (Abstract). Clin Pharmacol Ther. 1977;21:104.

128. Bartelloni PJ, Calia FM, Minchew BH, et al. Absorption and excretion of two chloramphenicol products in humans after oral administration. Am J Med Sci. 1969;258:203.

129. Pickering LK, Hoecker JL, Kramer WG, et al. Clinical pharmacology of two chloramphenicol preparations in children: Sodium succinate (IV) and palmitate (oral) esters. J Pediatr. 1980;96:757.

130. Tuomen EI, Powell KR, Marks MI, et al. Oral chloramphenicol in the treatment of *Haemophilus influzenae* meningitis. J Pediatr. 1981;99:968.

131. McCrumb FR, Snyder MJ, Hicken WJ. The use of chloramphenicol acid succinate in the treatment of acute infections. In Welch H, Marti-Ibanez F, eds.: Antibiotics Annual, 1957–1958. New York: Medical Encyclopedia; 1958:837–841.

132. Bhutta ZA, Niazi SK, Suria A. Chloramphenicol clearance in typhoid fever. Implications for therapy. Indian J Pediatr. 1992;59:213–9.

133. Ross S, Puig JR, Zarembra EA. Chloramphenicol acid succinate (sodium salt); some preliminary clinical and laboratory observations in infants and children. In Welch H, Marti-Ibanez F, eds.: Antibiotics Annual, 1957–1958. New York: Medical Encyclopedia; 1958:803–20.

134. McCrumb FR Jr, Snyder MJ, Hicken WJ. The use of chloramphenicol acid succinate in the treatment of acute infections. In Welch H, Marti-Ibanez F, eds.: Antibiotics Annual, 1957–1958. New York: Medical Encyclopedia; 1958:837.

135. Shann F, Linnenmann V, MacKenzie A, et al. Absorption of chloramphenicol sodium succinate after intramuscular administration in children. N Engl J Med. 1985;313:410–4.

136. Smith AL, Weber A. Pharmacology of chloramphenicol. Pediatr Clin North Am. 1983;30:209–36.

137. DuPont HL, Hornick RB, Weiss CF, et al. Evaluation of chloramphenicol acid succinate therapy of induced typhoid fever and Rocky Mountain spotted fever. N Engl J Med. 1970;282:53.

138. Lindberg AA, Nilsson LH, Bucht H, et al. Concentration of chloramphenicol in the urine and blood in relation to renal function. Br Med J. 1966;2:724.

139. Kauffman RE, Miceti JN, Strebel L, et al. Pharmacokinetics of chloramphenicol and chloramphenicol succinate in infants and children. J Pediatr. 1981; 98:315.

140. Kauffman RE, Thirumoorthi MC, Buckley JA, et al. Relative bioavailability of intravenous chloramphenicol succinate and oral chloramphenicol palmitate in infants and children. J Pediatr. 1981;99:363.

141. Kunin CM. A guide to use of antibiotics in patients with renal disease. Ann Intern Med. 1967;67:151.

142. Kramer PW, Griffith RS, Campbell RL, et al. Antibiotic penetration of the brain: A comparative study. J Neurosurg. 1969;31:295.

143. Braude AI: Antimicrobial Drug Therapy. Philadelphia: WB Saunders; 1976: 82.

144. Rapp GF, Griffith RS, Hebble WM. The permeability of traumatically inflamed synovial membrane to commonly used antibiotics. J Bone Joint Surg. 1966;48:1534.

145. Abraham RK, Burnett HH. Tetracycline and chloramphenicol studies on rabbit and human eyes. Arch Ophthalmol. 1955;54:641.

146. Beasley H, Boltralik JJ, Baldwin HA. Chloramphenicol in aqueous humor after topical application. Arch Ophthalmol. 1975;93:184.

147. George FJ, Hanna C. Ocular penetration of chloramphenicol. Arch Ophthalmol. 1977;95:879.

148. McPherson SD Jr, Presley GD, Crawford JR. Aqueous humor assays of subconjunctival antibiotics. Am J Ophthalmol. 1968;66:430.

149. Kunin CM, Glazko AJ, Finland M. Persistence of antibiotics in blood of patients with acute renal failure. II. Chloramphenicol and its metabolic products in the blood of patients with severe renal disease or hepatic cirrhosis. J Clin Invest. 1959;38:1498.

150. Suhrland LG, Weisberger AS. Chloramphenicol toxicity in liver and renal disease. Arch Intern Med. 1963;112:161.

151. Louie TJ, Tally FP, Bartlett JG, et al. Rapid microbiological assay for chloramphenicol and tetracyclines. Antimicrob Agents Chemother. 1976;9:874.

152. Jorgensen JH, Alexander GA. Rapid bioassay for chloramphenicol in the presence of other antibiotics. Am J Clin Pathol. 1981;76:474.

153. Lietman PS, White TJ, Shaw WV. Chloramphenicol: An enzymological microassay. Antimicrob Agents Chemother. 1976;10:347.
154. Smith AL, Smith DH. Improved enzymatic analysis of chloramphenicol. Clin Chem. 1978;24:1452.
155. Aravind MK, Miceli JN, Kauffman RE, et al. Simultaneous measurements of chloramphenicol and chloramphenicol succinate in body fluids utilizing HPLC. J Chromatogr. 1980;221:176.
156. Nahata MC, Powell DA. Simultaneous determination of chloramphenicol and its succinate ester by high-performance liquid chromatography. J Chromatogr. 1981;223:247.
157. Cambell GS, Mageau RP, Schwab B, et al. Detection and quantitation of chloramphenicol by competitive enzyme-linked immunoassay. Antimicrob Agents Chemother. 1984;25:205–11.
158. Abou-Khalil S, Abou-Khalil WH, Masoud AM, et al. High-performance liquid chromatographic determination of chloramphenicol and four analogues using reductive and oxidative electrochemical and ultraviolet detection. J Chromatogr. 1987;417:111–9.
159. Yunis AA. Chloramphenicol-induced bone marrow suppression. Semin Hematol. 1973;10:225.
160. Scott JL, Finegold SM, Belkin GA, et al. A controlled double-blind study of the hematologic toxicity of chloramphenicol. N Engl J Med. 1965;272:1137.
161. Best WR. Chloramphenicol-associated blood dyscrasias. A review of cases submitted to the American Medical Association Registry. JAMA. 1967;201:181.
162. Wallerstein RO, Condit PK, Kasper CK, et al. Statewide study of chloramphenicol therapy and fatal aplastic anemia. JAMA. 1969;208:2045.
163. Nagao T, Mauer AM. Concordance for drug-induced aplastic anemia in identical twins. N Engl J Med. 1969;281:7.
164. Morley A, Trainor K, Remes J. Residual marrow damage: Possible explanation for idiosyncrasy to chloramphenicol. Br J Haematol. 1976;32:525.
165. Holt R. The bacterial degradation of chloramphenicol. Lancet. 1967;1:1259.
166. Jimenez JJ, Arimura GK, Abou-Khalil WH, et al. Chloramphenicol-induced bone marrow injury: Possible role of bacterial metabolites of chloramphenicol. Blood. 1987;70:1180–5.
167. Jimenez JJ, Jimenez JG, Daghistani D, Yunis AA. Interaction of chloramphenicol and metabolites with colony stimulating factors: Possible role in chloramphenicol-induced bone marrow injury. Am J Med Sci. 1990;300:350–3.
168. Yunis AA. Chloramphenicol toxicity: 25 years of research. Am J Med. 1989;87 (3N):44N–8N.
169. Plaut ME, Best WR. Aplastic anemia after parenteral chloramphenicol: Warning renewal (Letter). N Engl J Med. 1982;306:1486.
170. Daum RS, Cohen DL, Smith AL. Fatal aplastic anemia following apparent "dose-related" chloramphenicol toxicity. J Pediatr. 1979;94:403.
171. Shu XO, Linet MS, Gao RN, et al. Chloramphenicol use and childhood leukaemia in Shanghai. Lancet. 1987;2:934–7.
172. Beutler E. Glucose 6-phosphate dehydrogenase deficiency. In: Williams WJ, Beutler E, Erslev AJ, et al., eds. Hematology. New York: McGraw-Hill; 1977:466.
173. Burns LE, Hodgman JE, Cass AB. Fatal circulatory collapse in premature infants receiving chloramphenicol. N Engl J Med. 1959;261:1318.
174. Craft AW, Brocklebank JT, Hey EN, et al. The "grey toddler": Chloramphenicol toxicity. Arch Dis Child. 1974;49:235.
175. Thompson WL, Anderson SE, Lipsky JJ, et al. Overdoses of chloramphenicol. JAMA. 1975;234:149.
176. Evans LS, Kleiman MB. Acidosis as a presenting feature of chloramphenicol toxicity. J Pediatr. 1986;108:475–7.
177. Fripp RR, Carter MC, Werner JC, et al. Cardiac function and acute chloramphenicol toxicity. J Pediatr. 1983;103:487–90.
178. Suarez CR, Ow EP. Chloramphenicol toxicity associated with severe cardiac dysfunction. Pediatr Cardiol. 1992;13:48–51.
179. Stevens DC, Kleinman MB, Lietman PS, et al. Exchange transfusion in acute chloramphenicol toxicity. J Pediatr. 1981;99:651.
180. Freundlick M, Cynamon H, Tamer A, et al. Management of chloramphenicol intoxication in infancy by charcoal hemoperfusion. J Pediatr. 1983;103:485.
181. Chloramphenicol blindness (Editorial). Br Med J. 1965;1:1511.
182. Christensen LK, Skovsted L. Inhibition of drug metabolism by chloramphenicol. Lancet. 1969;2:1397.
183. Petitpierre B, Fabre J. Chlorpropamide and chloramphenicol. Lancet. 1970;1:789.
184. Rose JQ, Choi HK, Schentag JJ. Intoxication caused by interaction of chloramphenicol and phenytoin. JAMA. 1977;237:2630.
185. Faber OK, Mouridsen HT, Skovsted L, et al. The effect of chloramphenicol and sulphaphenazole on the biotransformation of cyclophosphamide in man. Br J Clin Pharmacol. 1975;2:281.
186. Powell DA, Nahata MC, Durrell DC, et al. Interactions among chloramphenicol, phenytoin and phenobarbital in a pediatric patient. J Pediatr. 1981;98:1001.
187. Prober CG. Effect of rifampin on chloramphenicol levels. N Engl J Med. 1985;312:788–9.
188. JiJi RM, Gangarosa EJ, de la Macorra F. Chloramphenicol and its sulfamoyl analogue. Report of reversible erythropoietic toxicity in healthy volunteers. Arch Intern Med. 1963;11:70.
189. Sande MA, Overton JW. In vivo antagonism between gentamicin and chloramphenicol in neutropenic mice. J Infect Dis. 1973;128:247.
190. Klass PE, Klein JO. Therapy of bacterial sepsis, meningitis and otitis media in infants and children: 1992 poll of directors of programs in pediatric infectious diseases. Pediatr Infect Dis J. 1992;11:702–5.

22. RIFAMYCINS

BARRY M. FARR

Rifampin is a semisynthetic derivative of rifamycin B, a macrocyclic antibiotic compound produced by the mold *Streptomyces mediterranei*. First isolated from fermentation culture of a soil isolate in 1957, rifamycins were named for a then-current French movie, *Le Riffi*.[1] Rifampin, which is the 3-4-methyl-piperazinyl-iminomethyl derivative of rifamycin SV, is more soluble and active in vitro than is its parent compound (Fig. 1).[2] Rifampin is a zwitterion (inner salt) that is soluble in acidic aqueous solution, is even more soluble in organic solvents, and displays remarkable diffusion through lipids.[3]

MECHANISM OF ACTION

The rifamycins exert a bactericidal effect by inhibition of DNA-dependent RNA polymerase at the β-subunit, which prevents chain initiation but not elongation.[4] Mammalian mitochondrial RNA synthesis is not impaired at clinically achievable concentrations.

PHARMACOLOGY

Rifampin is available in the United States as a capsule of orange-red powder and as a solution for intravenous infusion. The oral preparation is almost completely absorbed from the gastrointestinal tract to yield peak plasma concentrations of approximately 7–10 µg/ml (range, 4–32) within 1–4 hours after ingestion of 600 mg in adults or 10 mg/kg of body weight in children. Higher doses such as 1200 mg in adults result in a similar, more-than-proportional increase in the peak ($\geq$30 µg/ml) serum concentration, because such doses exceed the biliary Tm for excretion of rifampin.[5] The area under the curve (AUC) shows a similar, more-than-proportional increase after saturation of the biliary Tm. For this reason, a single daily dose of 1200 mg results in higher AUC values for rifampin than do divided doses totaling 1200 mg.

The recommended dosage is usually 10–20 mg/kg (600 mg maximum) in a single daily administration. A 1% weight/volume oral suspension containing 10 mg/ml may be prepared by mixing the contents of four 300-mg capsules with 120 ml of any of sev-

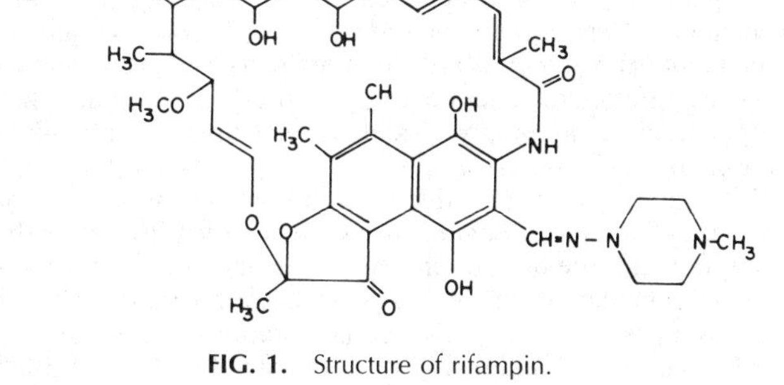

FIG. 1. Structure of rifampin.

eral commercially available syrups according to the directions in the package insert of the *Physician's Desk Reference*.[6] It should not be cosuspended with other antituberculosis agents such as isoniazid or pyrazinamide, or with ascorbic acid, because such cosuspensions are associated with a significant decline in detectable concentrations of the drugs.[7]

Dosage adjustment is unnecessary in renal failure, but rifampin should be avoided or used with caution (perhaps at a lower dosage) in patients with hepatic dysfunction. Food with a high fat concentration interferes with absorption by lowering and delaying peak blood levels.[8] Para-aminosalicylic acid also interferes with absorption.

The drug is 80 percent protein bound in serum and distributes into a volume calculated to be 160 percent of body weight. Plasma clearance is through hepatic uptake, deacetylation to an active metabolite, and biliary excretion. Deacetylation diminishes reabsorption and increases fecal excretion, but there is significant enterohepatic circulation. The half-life is initially 2–5 hours, but it decreases by 40 percent during the first 2 weeks of therapy due to enhanced biliary excretion. Slow acetylators of isoniazid have an accelerated clearance of rifampin. From 6 to 30 percent of a dose is excreted in the urine. Probenecid does not consistently affect rifampin serum levels. Renal excretion is reduced in the elderly, but serum levels remain similar to those in young adults because of hepatic clearance.[9] Pharmacokinetics in pediatric patients are similar to those in adults.[10] The intravenous preparation yields higher peak concentrations of about 27 μg/ml but otherwise similar pharmocokinetics.[11]

Rifampin penetrates well into almost all body tissues. It achieves concentrations in lung, liver, bile, cholecystic wall, and urine that exceed peak blood levels.[12] Peak concentrations average 300–350 μg/ml in urine.[5] The concentration in tears is similar to that in serum, and salivary concentrations are about 20 percent of those in serum. It achieves therapeutic levels in pleural exudate, sputum,[5] ascites, cavity fluid, milk, urinary bladder wall, skin blister fluid,[13] and soft tissues. It penetrates bone, with higher levels being reached in the presence of osteomyelitis.[12] Aqueous humor concentrations ranged from 0.2 to 1.3 μg/ml after a single oral dose of 600 mg in patients undergoing cataract removal.[14] In a rabbit model mean concentrations in the vitreous were approximately half those measured in the aqueous humor.[15] Levels in cerebrospinal fluid of 0–0.5 μg/ml have been achieved in healthy people, and higher levels (up to 1.3 μg/ml) have been observed during meningitis after a standard oral dosage of 600 mg/day. Rifampin has also been shown to penetrate and sterilize abscess fluid more readily than do most other antibiotics with similar antibacterial activity.[16,17] This may relate both to the drug's high lipid solubility and to its relatively unusual ability to enter living phagocytes and kill intracellular bacteria.[3,13,17]

ANTIMICROBIAL ACTIVITY

Rifampin exhibits bactericidal activity against a wide range of organisms (Table 1).[19,20] It is extremely active against staphylococci (both coagulase-positive and coagulase-negative strains) and is also effective against other gram-positive cocci, although somewhat less so than penicillin. It is active against the pulmonary pathogen *Rhodococcus equi*, which is usually resistant to penicillin.[21] *Neisseria meningitidis*, *Neisseria gonorrhoeae*, and *Haemophilus influenzae* are the most sensitive gram-negative species. Rifampin has less activity than do tetracycline, chloramphenicol, or aminoglycosides against most gram-negative aerobic bacilli.

Rifampin is the most active agent known against the various species and strains of *Legionella*, being clearly more active than erythromycin, the drug of choice for legionellosis.[20] It is as active as vancomycin in vitro against *Clostridium difficile*, the organism associated with pseudomembranous colitis.

Mycobacterium tuberculosis has remained quite sensitive to

TABLE 1. Susceptibility of Various Bacteria to Rifampin

Species (n)	MICs (μg/ml)		
	Range (Mode)	MIC$_{50}$	MIC$_{90}$
Gram-positive bacteria			
Staphylococcus aureus (26)	0.008–0.015 (0.015)	0.015	0.015
Staphylococcus epidermidis (25)	0.004–0.015 (0.015)	0.015	0.015
Group A streptococci (25)	0.03–0.12 (0.12)	0.12	0.12
Group B streptococci (25)	0.25–1 (1)	1.0	1.0
Streptococcus pneumoniae (28)	0.06–32 (0.06)	0.12	4.0
Viridans group			
Streptococci (34)	0.03–8 (0.06)	0.06	0.12
Enterococcus faecalis (16)	1.0–8 (2)	2.0	8.0
Haemophilus influenzae (26)	0.5–64 (1)	1.0	1.0
Neisseria gonorrhoeae (29)	0.06–2 (0.25)	0.25	0.5
Neisseria meningitidis (26)	0.015–1 (0.03)	0.03	0.5
Listeria monocytogenes (40)	≤0.12–0.25 (≤0.12)	≤0.12	0.25
Mycobacterium fortuitum (18)	16.0–>64 (>64)	>64	>64
Mycobacterium chelonae (15)	>64 (>64)	>64	>64
Gram-negative bacteria			
Escherichia coli (15)	8–16 (8)	8	16
Klebsiella pneumoniae (14)	16–32 (32)	32	32
Enterobacter agglomerans (14)	8–64 (32)	32	64
Enterobacter cloacae (13)	16–64 (32)	64	64
Enterobacter aerogenes (15)	16–64 (32)	32	64
Citrobacter freundii (4)	32 (32)	32	32
Citrobacter diversus (4)	32 (32)	32	32
Proteus mirabilis (15)	4–8 (4)	4	8
Proteus vulgaris (17)	8–32 (32)	16	32
Morganella morganii (15)	8–32 (32)	16	32
Providencia rettgeri (15)	8–64 (8, 16)	16	32
Providencia stuartii (15)	4–16 (8)	8	16
Serratia marcescens (15)	32–64 (64)	64	64
Acinetobacter species (15)	4–16 (8)	8	8
Pseudomonas aeruginosa (17)	32–>64 (32)	32	64
Pseudomonas species (12)	4–>64 (8)	8	32

Abbreviation: MIC: minimal inhibitory concentration.

(From Thornsberry et al.,[20] with permission.)

rifampin, with most epidemiologic surveys finding less than 4 percent initial resistance to the drug.[22–24] *Mycobacterium ulcerans* is equally sensitive. A spiropiperidyl rifamycin called *rifabutin* (ansamycin) has potent in vitro activity against many mycobacteria, including the *Mycobacterium avium-intracellulare* complex and *Mycobacterium fortuitum*,[25] as do the new derivatives, the benzoxazinorifamycins.[26]

The rifamycins possess antiviral and possible antitumor activity, but have not proved clinically useful at usual therapeutic levels. Rifampin is among the most active agents against *Chlamydia*, including *Chlamydia trachomatis* (lymphogranuloma venereum [LGV] and non-LGV strains) and *Chlamydia psittaci*.[27] *Ureaplasma urealyticum* and *Treponema pallidum* are usually resistant. Rifampin has shown synergy with amphotericin B in vitro and in animal models of infection with fungal species such as *Histoplasma capsulatum*, *Aspergillus* spp.,[28] and *Fusarium proliferatum*[29] and also with itraconazole against *Cryptococcus neoformans*.[30] The clinical significance of this, if any, is unclear.

Bacteria rapidly develop resistance to rifampin in vitro or in vivo due to mutations altering the β-subunit of the DNA-dependent RNA polymerase. These mutations may occur at many different sites in the RNA polymerase and lead to various degrees of resistance to rifampin.[31] Approximately 1 out of every 10^{11} tubercule bacilli is a resistant mutant. A national survey of 3313 isolates in the first quarter of 1991 found the incidence of rifampin resistance among previously untreated tuberculous patients to be 3.5 percent as compared with 9.0 percent of patients previously treated for tuberculosis. The rates of isoniazid resistance in this same survey were much higher, 8.2 and 21.5 percent for untreated and previously treated patients, respectively.[24]

The mutation rate to rifampin resistance among other bacteria is higher than that for *M. tuberculosis* (e.g., *Staphylococcus aureus*, 10^{-7}; *Streptococcus* spp., 10^{-7}; *H. influenzae* type B, 10^{-7}; *Meningococcus*, 10^{-7}; and *Escherichia coli*, 10^{-8}).[19,32] Except for short-term meningitis prophylaxis, rifampin should not be used alone because of this rapid development of resistance during monotherapy.

ADVERSE EFFECTS

Short-term meningitis prophylaxis with rifampin has been associated with mild, reversible symptoms in 20–25 percent of recipients as compared with about 10 percent of placebo recipients.[33,34] The symptoms reported most frequently have been dizziness, drowsiness, abdominal pain, diarrhea, nausea, vomiting, headache, visual change, pruritus, and rash. Each of these symptoms usually occurs in less than 5–10 percent of recipients.[34] An orange-red discoloration of urine and permanent staining of soft contact lenses may also occur with such brief regimens.

Chronic daily therapy is associated with a mild, usually self-limited maculopapular rash in up to 5 percent of patients. More severe rashes such as exfoliative dermatitis and toxic epidermal necrolysis have been rarely reported as being associated with rifampin.[35,36] Fixed drug eruptions have also been rarely reported.[37] Gastrointestinal complaints are noted by 1–2 percent of patients. Rantitidine, 150 mg twice daily, was shown in a randomized trial to reduce the frequency of gastrointestinal complaints with rifampin therapy without altering rifampin serum concentrations.[38] Asymptomatic elevation of serum enzyme levels is observed in up to 14 percent of adults patients,[19] and overt hepatitis in 1 percent of patients receiving rifampin with combination antituberculous therapy excluding isoniazid and in 2.6 percent of patients receiving both rifampin and isoniazid.[39] The addition of isoniazid to rifampin increases the risk of hepatitis, but the combination is usually considered acceptably safe in the absence of prior liver disease.[40] Hepatotoxicity is more common with alcoholism and with malnutrition.[41] Of 430 children treated with rifampin and isoniazid for tuberculosis, 14 (3.3 percent) were reported to have hepatotoxic reactions in a recent national survey.[42] In a study of rifampin (15 mg/kg/day) and higher dose isoniazid (15–20 mg/kg/day) therapy for children with severe tuberculosis, 36 of 44 developed an elevation of hepatic enzyme levels during therapy, and one child died of hepatitis.[43] A meta-analysis of seven pediatric studies showed that the combination of isoniazid with rifampin resulted in a significantly higher rate of clinical hepatitis (6.9 percent) than did isoniazid alone (0.2 percent).[39] Some patients develop cholestatic jaundice with rifampin therapy.[44] Rifampin causes an increase in serum bile acid levels and can cause slight elevations of serum bilirubin concentrations that return to normal during the first week of therapy in the absence of hepatitis. This increase in bilirubin appears to be due to a competitive inhibition of hepatic bilirubin metabolism.[39]

Acute renal failure has been reported during daily therapy and has occasionally required dialysis.[45] The renal failure has been related to a variety of different mechanisms, including interstitial nephritis, glomerulonephritis, and massive hemolysis.[46,47] Light-chain proteinuria has been reported to occur in a majority of patients receiving rifampin without apparent ill effect, but in the setting of dehydration these proteins may contribute to development of a cast nephropathy and acute renal failure on this basis.[48,49]

Intermittent administration (less than twice per week) and high individual dosages (greater than or equal to 1200 mg) have been associated with an increased incidence of side effects. A flulike syndrome with fever, chills, and myalgias may develop in up to 20 percent of patients after several months of intermittent therapy and correlates with the presence of antirifampin antibodies.[50] These patients may develop eosinophilia, interstitial nephritis, acute tubular necrosis, thrombocytopenia, hemolytic anemia, and even shock.[51–53] Acute massive hemolysis is rarely associated with such flulike reactions after intermittent therapy, in which case nausea, vomiting, flank pain, and brown turbid urine may be observed; most patients with massive hemolysis develop acute renal failure.[54–57] Anaphylaxis has been rarely reported.[58]

Various effects of rifampin on the central nervous system have been reported, including rare cases of organic brain syndrome. Pseudomembranous colitis has been observed in animal models after rifampin administration to animals colonized with a rifampin-resistant strain of *C. difficile*. One patient has also been reported with pseudomembranous colitis that developed with a rifampin-resistant *C. difficile* during rifampin therapy. This appears to be a very rare side effect with only a few reports of such an association despite widespread chronic use of rifampin in antituberculous chemotherapy.[59,60] Pancreatitis has been reported in rare cases. One case of hemorrhagic gastritis has been reported that responded to cessation of rifampin and recurred with readministration.[61] Patients have survived overdoses of up to 12 g, turning "lobster red" for several days; facial or periorbital edema, pruritus of the head, and vomiting each occur in a majority of cases of the "red man syndrome" after an overdose.[62,63]

Rifampin causes a reduction in 25-hydroxycholecalciferol levels without changing the levels of 1,25-dihydroxycholecalciferol or parathyroid hormone, and osteomalacia has been mentioned as a possible side effect with long-term treatment. It causes increased deiodination and biliary clearance of thyroxine and lowers the serum concentration of thyroxine. The serum concentration of triiodothyronine remains normal.

Immunosuppression has been an alleged side effect of rifampin therapy. Contradictory studies have found diminished or normal antibody responses to various antigens such as sheep red blood cells, pneumococcal vaccine, and tetanus toxoid. Some workers have suggested blunted cell-mediated immunity with a diminished response to phytohemagglutinin in vitro, whereas others have shown no change in response to phytohemagglutinin, concanavalin A, pokeweed mitogen, or purified protein derivative (PPD). Skin tests with PPD have not been consistently altered by rifampin therapy, and no ill effect from this possible immunosuppression in the form of opportunistic infection or an inability to heal tuberculosis has been reported.[64] Rifampin readily crosses the placenta and has caused teratogenic effects in rodents treated with high doses; such effects have not been observed in humans, except in patients with severe tuberculosis, but rifampin should only be used for severe tuberculous infections during pregnancy.[65]

DRUG INTERACTIONS

Rifampin competitively inhibits the hepatic uptake of several compounds such as cholecystografin and sulfobromophthalein. Rifampin is one of the most potent inducing agents for intestinal and hepatic microsomal enzymes,[66,67] leading to reduced oral bioavailability and to a decreased serum half-life for a number of compounds including prednisone, norethisterone, digitoxin,

TABLE 2. Medications for Which Serum Concentrations Are Decreased through Enhancement of Hepatic or Intestinal Metabolism by Rifampin[a]

Barbiturates	Doxycycline	Phenytoin
Chloramphenicol	Estrogens	Propafenone
Cimetidine	Fluconazole	Propranolol
Clofibrate	Haloperidol	Quinidine
Contraceptive, oral	Itraconazole	Sulfonylureas
Cyclosporine	Ketoconazole	Tertalol
Dapsone	Lorcainide	Tocainide
Digitoxin	Metaprolol	Theophylline
Digoxin	Methadone	Thyroxine
Diltiazem	Nifedipine	Verapamil
Diazepam	Nitrazepam	Warfarin
Disopyramide	Novobiocin	

[a] See Rizak and Hillman[273] for a complete list.

quinidine, ketoconazole, and the sulfonylureas (Table 2).[68–72] These effects have been reported to cause decreased efficacy of oral contraceptive agents, relapse of arrhythmias during quinidine therapy, decompensation of heart failure during digoxin or digitoxin therapy, and exacerbation of diabetes during oral hypoglycemic therapy. Rifampin also reduces the efficacy of warfarin, causing a reduction in prothrombin time in patients anticoagulated with this drug. Patients receiving glucocorticoid therapy for Addison's disease or asthma have relapsed, and transplant patients receiving cyclosporine therapy have developed acute rejection when given rifampin. Hypothyroid patients receiving replacement L-thyroxine may require an increased dosage.[71]

Aluminum hydroxide–containing antacids were associated with significantly lower rifampin peak concentrations in one randomized trial.[73] Rifampin significantly decreases the serum concentrations of ketoconazole, which in turn may decrease rifampin concentrations[74]; the U.S. Food and Drug Administration (FDA) has advised against using this drug combination.[75] Trimethoprim-sulfamethoxazole administration results in increased rifampin levels.[76,77]

THERAPEUTIC USES

Mycobacterial Infections

The unique pharmacology and bactericidal activity of rifampin have revolutionized chemotherapy for pulmonary tuberculosis, with rifampin-containing treatment courses of 6–9 months yielding cure rates equal to those achieved with 18 months of regimens without rifampin.[78] The regimen of choice for uncomplicated pulmonary or extrapulmonary tuberculosis (e.g., involving lymph nodes, pleura, or meninges) is now 6 months of daily rifampin (15 mg/kg/day; maximum, 600 mg) and isoniazid (10 mg/kg/day; maximum, 300 mg), with daily pyrazinamide being added for the first 2 months.[79–86] In most areas, a fourth drug, ethambutol or streptomycin, is recommended until susceptibility to isoniazid (INH) and rifampin is documented.[87] Combinations excluding rifampin have resulted in relapse rates exceeding 20 percent with such short courses.[88,89] Almost half of patients with pulmonary tuberculosis resistant to rifampin and isoniazid remain sputum culture positive despite multidrug therapy for years.[90] Tuberculous meningitis was successfully treated in a patient with hepatic failure using combination therapy including intraventricular administration of rifampin to avoid hepatic side effects.[91] Twice-weekly supervised administration after daily therapy for 2–8 weeks has been successful in noncompliant patients.[92,93] It should be emphasized that rifampin monotherapy is contraindicated in mycobacterial disease, as illustrated by one study in which 5 of 11 tuberculous patients developed rifampin-resistant isolates within 3 months when receiving rifampin alone.[94] The American Thoracic Society has recommended the use of rifampin (with or without ethambutol) as prophylactic therapy for infected contacts of persons with

known isoniazid-resistant tuberculosis.[79] Data regarding the efficacy of such prophylaxis are not available, however, and one failure of rifampin monoprophylaxis in such an instance has been reported in an alcoholic with questionable compliance.[95] For rifampin-resistant organisms pyrazinamide (PZA) plus either ciprofloxacin or ofloxacin has been suggested.

Rifampin-containing regimens have proved useful in therapy for *M. avium-intracellulare*,[96–99] *Mycobacterium kansasii*,[100,101] *Mycobacterium xenopi*,[102] *Mycobacterium marinum*,[103] and Calmette-Guerin bacillus (BCG) infections.[104,105]

Rifampin kills *Mycobacterium leprae* faster than do the sulfones. If used in patients with lepromatous leprosy, however, it should be combined with dapsone to prevent the development of resistance. The multidrug regimens recommended by the World Health Organization for adults are as follows: *(1)* for multibacillary leprosy, rifampin, 600 mg monthly (supervised); dapsone, 100 mg daily; and clofazimine, 300 mg monthly (supervised) and 50 mg daily for at least 2 years and until skin smear negativity if possible; and *(2)* for paucibacillary leprosy, rifampin, 600 mg monthly (supervised); and dapsone, 100 mg daily.[106] Monthly rifampin doses may be given without producing the flulike side effects seen more frequently with weekly rifampin administration.[107,108]

Meningitis Prophylaxis

Rifampin has been approved by the FDA as prophylaxis for close contact of patients with meningococcal meningitis at a daily dose of 10 mg/kg (600 mg maximum) for 4 days. As an alternative dose, the Centers for Disease Control and Prevention (CDC) recommends 600 mg every 12 hours for 2 days for adults and 10 mg/kg every 12 hours for 2 days for children. Rifampin has been shown to eradicate meningococci from the nasopharynx in approximately 90 percent of carriers.[109–112] Sulfadiazine was formerly recommended for meningococcal prophylaxis, but up to 70 percent of recent meningococcal isolates are resistant to sulfa. Minocycline is also an effective prophylactic agent, but it is associated with a higher incidence of side effects, especially vestibular symptoms.[113] Recent studies have suggested the efficacy of oral ciprofloxacin (4–10 doses) and also of a single intramuscular injection of ceftriaxone (250 mg for adults, 125 mg for children less than 15 years old).[114,115]

Epidemiologic studies of *H. influenzae* type B meningitis have shown a high incidence of secondary disease among preschool contacts.[116] Secondary disease attack rates for this group have been approximately 1 percent, which yields a relative risk approximately 600 times that of the general population.[117] Rifampin at a single daily dose of 20 mg/kg (up to a maximum dose of 600 mg) for 4 days has been shown to eradicate *H. influenzae* from the nasopharynx in over 90 percent of carriers and to reduce significantly the risk of secondary infection.[33] It has been recommended that families with young children exposed to another member of the household with invasive *H. influenzae* type B disease (e.g., meningitis, epiglottitis, or pneumonia) take rifampin prophylaxis.[117,119] The age below which child household contacts and their families should receive prophylaxis has been debated. All agree that prophylaxis should be given when there are children younger than 2 years, and some recommend prophylaxis when there are children under 4 years (see Ch. 202).[117–120] Pregnant family members should not take rifampin prophylaxis. Day care center staff (excluding pregnant women) and day care classmates of a child with such disease have also been advised to take rifampin prophylaxis if any of the exposed classmates are younger than 2 years old. Some authorities recommend prophylaxis after a single case in a day care center, while others have advocated instituting prophylaxis only if a second case occurs within 60 days.[119,121] Failure to provide simultaneous rifampin prophylaxis to all day care center contacts including those who have received *Haemophilus* B polysaccharide vaccine has been associated with persistent colonization of children in the center and subsequent cases of disease.[122] The prophylaxis should be given as rapidly as possible after identification of the index case, since a majority of secondary cases appear to occur in the week after the onset of the index case. Index cases with invasive *H. influenzae* disease should also be given the same rifampin regimen before hospital discharge because of the 1 per-rate of recurrent systemic disease in index cases after therapy and also the risk of exposing other children to the organism.[123] Attempts to eradicate nasopharyngeal carriage with other drugs active against *H. influenzae*, including ampicillin and trimethoprim-sulfamethoxazole, have been less successful; data regarding the efficacy of quinolones and third-generation cephalosporins for this indication are not yet available.

Endocarditis

The use of rifampin in the treatment of staphylococcal endocarditis remains an unsettled and controversial issue.[124] Rifampin was shown to be superior to therapy with vancomycin, gentamicin, or β-lactams in an experimental model of *Staphylococcus epidermidis* endocarditis in rabbits.[125] In another rabbit model of *S. epidermidis* endocarditis, rifampin plus teicoplanin proved more effective therapy than either agent alone.[126] A retrospective series of 75 cases of prosthetic valve endocarditis due to *S. epidermidis*, the most common cause of prosthetic valve endocarditis, suggested a trend toward higher survival ($p = 0.10$) in patients receiving rifampin (900–1200 mg/day) or an aminoglycoside plus vancomycin as opposed to vancomycin alone.[127] The only randomized trial of rifampin therapy in endocarditis compared patients with prosthetic valve endocarditis due to methicillin-resistant *S. epidermidis* who were treated with vancomycin (30 mg/kg/day) and rifampin (300 mg q8h) or with vancomycin and rifampin (same doses) plus gentamicin (3 mg/kg/day). The cure rate was 77 percent with the two-drug regimen and 85 percent with the three-drug regimen. Rifampin resistance developed in six patients receiving the two-drug regimen as compared with none receiving the three-drug regimen.[128] A separate study identified three patients in whom rifampin resistance developed during therapy for prosthetic valve *S. epidermidis* endocarditis with rifampin plus vancomycin.[129]

Several patients with endocarditis due to *Staphylococcus aureus* have been reported to respond only after the addition of rifampin to nafcillin or vancomycin.[19,130,131] Some in vitro studies with *S. aureus*, however, have suggested that rifampin frequently results in antagonism when added to oxacillin or ciprofloxacin.[132,133] Rifampin therapy for experimental endocarditis due to *S. aureus* in rabbits has been examined by Sande and Johnson[16] and Zak et al.[134] In one study, the combination of rifampin with penicillin was antagonistic in vitro against a strain of *S. aureus*, and there was a trend toward slower sterilization of vegetations with the rifampin combination than with penicillin alone. Sterilization of renal abscesses, however, occurred faster in the group receiving the rifampin combination than in the group receiving penicillin alone despite in vitro antagonism. It was suggested that this was due to rifampin's unique ability to penetrate and sterilize abscess fluid and living polymorphonuclear neutrophil (PMN) leukocytes.

In a subsequent study using the same animal model and a methicillin-sensitive strain of *S. aureus* it was found that rifampin plus cloxacillin was additive or synergistic in four of five different regimens studied; the only regimen showing antagonism combined a high dose of cloxacillin (100 mg/kg) with a low dose of rifampin (2 mg/kg).[134]

A combination of oral rifampin with ciprofloxacin (intravenous for 1 week and oral thereafter) was studied for 4-week therapy of right-sided endocarditis with a cure of all 10 patients who completed therapy.[135] A study of this combination in a rabbit model of *S. aureus* endocarditis found it to be as effective as vancomycin and to result in a lower rate of resistance to

ciprofloxacin developing during combination therapy than with monotherapy, but also noted that the combination was less effective than ciprofloxacin alone in reducing vegetation counts with one of the two strains tested.[136] An in vitro study also raised concern about antagonism between ciprofloxacin and rifampin when combined for *S. aureus*.[132] Early development of resistance has been reported during therapy of right-sided *S. aureus* endocarditis with this combination from one hospital.[137]

Kapusnik et al.[138] have concluded that rational treatment of staphylococcal endocarditis might involve initial therapy with a β-lactam or vancomycin alone or in combination with an aminoglycoside, which should result in rapid elimination of organisms from vegetations. They suggest the addition of rifampin for cases in which myocardial or metastatic abscesses are detected, while emphasizing the necessity of surgical drainage of abscesses.[138] Adding rifampin after several days of effective therapy with nafcillin or vancomycin plus gentamicin might be less likely to result in the development of rifampin resistance because the titer of organisms exposed to rifampin should then be lower.

The problem of methicillin-resistant *S. aureus* (MRSA) endocarditis has been studied in a rabbit model by Bayer and Lam,[139] who found that a combination of rifampin (20 mg/kg/day) plus vancomycin (30 mg/kg/day) was significantly more effective than was either drug alone in eliminating organisms from the valve and curing the animal. Rifampin resistance developed in two of four animals that were sacrificed after treatment with rifampin alone but was not found in any of the 21 animals given the combination.[139] One retrospective study of treatment of MRSA endocarditis in drug addicts did not demonstrate a higher cure rate for rifampin-containing regimens than for vancomycin alone, but such studies are likely to be biased, with only the more severely ill patients receiving rifampin. Randomized trials are needed to assess accurately the efficacy of rifampin for endocarditis due to MRSA.

The problem of rifampin resistance developing during therapy for endocarditis that has been noted with methicillin-resistant *S. epidermidis* has also been observed with MRSA during treatment with rifampin and vancomycin.[140,141] Acar and colleagues[131] reported that two of three patients with *S. aureus* endocarditis who had failed therapy with another regimen developed rifampin resistance when rifampin was added to either vancomycin or pristinamycin. It has been suggested by the results of one study that, although rifampin resistance may develop in the presence of a β-lactam such as nafcillin in vitro, the rate of developing such resistance is lower with this combination than with rifampin alone; in contrast, this study found that vancomycin did not suppress the emergence of rifampin resistance when incubated with rifampin in vitro.[142] The results of other studies, however, have suggested that incubation of vancomycin with rifampin in vitro can suppress the emergence of rifampin resistance.[143,144]

The efficacy of rifampin in *S. aureus* endocarditis will have to be demonstrated by randomized controlled trials. One small randomized trial of vancomycin compared with vancomycin plus rifampin for endocarditis due to MRSA showed slow clearance of bacteremia in both groups and no trend toward benefit for the combination.[145] It would appear reasonable to consider using rifampin in cases with renal, myocardial, splenic, or cerebral abscess formation or because of failure of conventional therapy. If rifampin were to be added, an optimal regimen would probably include at least two other drugs such as gentamicin and either nafcillin or vancomycin to minimize the probability of developing rifampin resistance during therapy.

The value of serum bactericidal titers and of in vitro synergy studies of antibiotic combinations including rifampin are of unclear value. Serum bactericidal titers have not been clearly demonstrated to predict the clinical outcome in patients with endocarditis,[146] and in vitro studies of rifampin and vancomycin or nafcillin with large batteries of staphylococcal isolates have produced inconsistent results in different laboratories, with most studies finding indifference for a majority of isolates.[147–154] Synergy studies performed with the same strain of *S. aureus* and the same concentrations of antibiotics have yielded directly contradictory results using checkerboard and time-kill methods.[147,150,155] Faster sterilization of renal abscesses has been shown in one animal model when a combination of rifampin and penicillin was administered despite in vitro evidence of antagonism.

One theme that has emerged from several synergy studies is that lower ratios of the concentration of rifampin to the concentration of oxacillin appear to be less bactericidal in vitro. Since highest peak concentrations and AUC values are achieved by administering a single large daily dose of rifampin (e.g., ≥600 mg for an adult),[5] this approach may be more effective than smaller divided doses would be.

Rifampin (300 mg PO BID) has also been recommended in combination with vancomycin and gentamicin for the treatment of endocarditis due to *Corynebacterium* spp.[156] One case of endocarditis due to psittacosis was refractory to several other antibiotics but subsequently responsive to rifampin.[157] Rifampin has activity against *Coxiella burnetii,* the cause of Q fever endocarditis, and has been used in combination with doxycycline or with fluoroquinolones. Although randomized trials have not been done, the currently favored regimen is doxycycline plus a fluoroquinolone for at least 3 years.[158,159]

Tolerant Staphylococci

Staphylococci with an antibiotic minimal bactericidal concentration (MBC) much greater than the minimal inhibitory concentration (MIC) (MBC equal to or greater than 32 × MIC) are said to be tolerant to the antibiotic in question. Tolerance to nafcillin and/or vancomycin has been described in several cases of persistent staphylococcal infection. The addition of rifampin has led to improved serum bactericidal levels and the successful treatment of such infections in several cases.[160,161] No randomized trials of such therapy for this indication are available.

Staphylococcal Carriage and Furunculosis

Rifampin has been shown to reduce the rate of staphylococcal nasal colonization markedly,[162–164] whereas systemic penicillinase-resistant penicillins or intranasal gentamicin cream has not eradicated nasal carriage.[165] Mandell and Sande (unpublished data) have used cloxacillin plus rifampin to eradicate nasal carriage and interrupt the course of recurrent furunculosis. Its role in preventing staphylococcal infections in dialysis patients continues to be studied.[166] Methicillin-resistant staphylococcal nasal carriage in nosocomial epidemics has been successfully eradicated by using a combination of rifampin plus vancomycin, trimethoprim-sulfamethoxazole, minocycline, novobiocin, or nasal mupirocin ointment.[165,167–171]

Methicillin-Resistant Staphylococcal Infection

Methicillin-resistant infections should be treated with vancomycin, to which they are uniformly sensitive. There are no data to support the routine addition of rifampin to vancomycin, but if there is inadequate response to vancomycin alone, then the addition of gentamicin, rifampin, or both should be considered. The development of rifampin resistance has been reported during therapy for MRSA infections with vancomycin plus rifampin,[131,141] and the addition of gentamicin to the regimen may help to prevent the development of rifampin resistance.[128]

Streptococcal Carriage

Chronic pharyngeal carriage of *Streptococcus pyogenes* in children has sometimes resulted in multiple courses of antibiotic therapy for apparent streptococcal pharyngitis with each new cold because of continuing positive cultures after completion of each course of therapy, and even in tonsillectomy. Eradication of carriage is not usually medically indicated for chronic carriers, but, when carriage eradication is desired, rifampin, 10 mg PO BID for 4 days, plus benzathine penicillin has been shown to eradicate *Streptococcus pyogenes* in 93 percent of cases.[172] Such therapy for the eradication of *Streptococcus pyogenes* was tried in patients with psoriasis, with apparent benefit to their skin disease,[173] but a randomized trial including 20 patients showed no benefit.[174]

Group B streptococci are the leading cause of sepsis and menigitis in neonates, and efforts to eradicate colonization are now being studied. A recent study of the treatment of experimentally exposed infant rats showed that rifampin plus penicillin eradicated group B streptococci for 80 percent of the animals, a significantly higher rate than for either drug alone.[175] Clinical data are not available.

Osteomyelitis and Septic Arthritis

Experimental animal data suggest that rifampin combined with another antistaphylococcal drug such as nafcillin or vancomycin provides better results than does single-drug therapy for chronic staphylococcal osteomyelitis, even when the drug combination is antagonistic in vitro.[176,177] In a rat model, azithromycin plus rifampin showed synergy against *Staphylococcus aureus* osteomyelitis, being slightly more active than a clindamycin-rifampin combination even though azithromycin alone was ineffective.[177] Controlled trials are necessary to confirm these data in human infection, however. The only randomized trial evaluating a rifampin-containing regimen in chronic staphylococcal osteomyelitis was halted after the enrollment of 18 patients: there was a trend toward a higher rate of favorable response in the group receiving rifampin and nafcillin (8 of 10) as compared with the group receiving nafcillin alone (4 of 8). The difference was not statistically significant ($p = 0.2$), but the statistical power was only 40 percent for detecting significance in the 30 percent higher rate of response that was observed because of the small sample size.[179]

An uncontrolled trial of rifampin combined with ciprofloxacin or a β-lactam antibiotic for therapy of streptococcal or staphylococcal orthopedic implant infection reported a success rate of 82 percent.[180]

Rifampin is not part of the usual regimen for staphylococcal arthritis, but it has been added with success in occasional patients initially refractory to nafcillin alone[181]; however, rifampin resistance has developed in one patient due to MRSA treated with vancomycin and rifampin.[142]

Legionella

Both *Legionella pneumophila* and *Legionella micdadei* are sensitive to rifampin. It has been suggested that rifampin be added to erythromycin for patients with legionnaires' disease when the illness does not respond to erythromycin alone, but data from randomized trials are lacking. In vitro studies show that combination of erythromycin with rifampin or pefloxacin is more active than erythromycin alone.[182]

Brucellosis

Rifampin has been shown to be superior to tetracycline in therapy for experimental brucellosis in rodents, and there have been several case reports of successful therapy for human infections.[183] In one uncontrolled study, relapses occurred after rifampin monotherapy, thus suggesting the need for combination therapy if rifampin is used.[184] Another case series identified 2 relapses in 10 cases treated with rifampin alone, 1 relapse after tetracycline and streptomycin therapy in 56 cases, and no relapses after tetracycline and rifampin therapy in 40 cases.[185] Four randomized trials comparing tetracycline (or doxycycline) regimens containing either rifampin or streptomycin consistently found that a significantly higher proportion of the rifampin recipients failed therapy or relapsed as compared with streptomycin recipients.[186–189] A more recent randomized trial with 61 patients compared doxycycline and rifampin with ofloxacin plus rifampin; only one failure (in the ofloxacin group) and one relapse in each group were found.[190] Rifampin resistance has also developed during such therapy and has been documented during clinical relapse. Several studies of rifampin and doxycycline therapy for patients with neurobrucellosis have suggested a high rate of efficacy, with relapse rates between 0 and 10 percent.[191]

Rickettsia: Mediterranean Spotted Fever

Rifampin has activity against *Rickettsia conorii,* the agent of Mediterrean spotted fever, and was shown to be effective clinically although with slower resolution of symptoms than with doxycycline, the drug of choice.[192] *Coxiella burnetii* (Q fever) has been treated successfully with rifampin, but doxycycline and fluoroquinolones are the preferred treatment at this time.[159]

Infection Occurring in Patients with Chronic Granulomatous Disease of Childhood

Rifampin has been shown to kill living intracellular staphylococci in neutrophils from healthy people and from patients with chronic granulomatous disease.[193] One patient with an axillary staphylococcal abscess responded dramatically to the addition of rifampin after months of unsuccessful therapy with vancomycin, nafcillin, and gentamicin.[194]

Infected Cerebrospinal Fluid Shunts, Vascular Grafts, and Implants

Cerebrospinal fluid shunt infections have responded to the addition of rifampin in several cases after an initial failure with multiple-drug therapy excluding rifampin.[195–198] Data from controlled trials of therapy are lacking, but a randomized trial of rifampin-trimethoprim prophylaxis at the time of shunt placement showed a trend favoring this approach (12 percent infection rate vs. 19 percent among placebo recipients). The trial was stopped early because of the high overall rate of infection and before statistical significance was achieved, so no recommendation can be made for routine prophylaxis until more trials are done.[199]

Three patients with *Staphylococcus epidermidis* infections of a penile prosthesis were successfully treated by removal of the prosthesis and 72 hours of continuous irrigation of the corpora cavernosa with rifampin before insertion of a new prosthesis.[200] Therapy with rifampin plus clindamycin for aortic Dacron grafts experimentally infected with *S. aureus* was found to cure the infection in seven of seven dogs as compared with five of seven dogs cured with cefazolin therapy.[201] Data from clinical trials are not available.

A rat model of chronic *S. aureus* foreign body infection using subcutaneous tissue cages showed that a combination of vancomycin with fleroxacin and rifampin was superior to regimens with fewer drugs.[202] An in vitro model of *S. epidermidis* biofilm on a foreign body showed that rifampin was the only drug of 35 tested with significant activity against organisms in a biofilm and that adding an agent with cell wall activity (e.g., vancomycin or a β-lactam) resulted in synergistic activity against the biofilm.[203]

Prevention of vascular graft infections using rifampin-impregnated grafts has been investigated recently.[204–209] In a sheep model 2 of 10 rifampin-impregnated Dacron grafts became infected as compared with 6 of 8 regular grafts.[210] Some high-risk patients have had rifampin-impregnated grafts implanted without complications.[211]

Cutaneous Leishmaniasis

When a patient with *Leishmania mexicana amazonensis* refractory to previous antileishmanial therapy was treated with rifampin and isoniazid for intercurrent mycobacterial infection, the cutaneous leishmaniasis improved.[212] Several uncontrolled case series have suggested that rifampin may be effective in 80 percent of patients with this disease,[213,214] but controlled trials are lacking.[215]

Urinary Tract Infection

A number of studies have been conducted that show the efficacy of rifampin in the treatment of urinary tract infections. Rifampin resistance has arisen with monotherapy, but combination therapy with trimethoprim has resulted in cure rates that are comparable to those of trimethoprim-sulfamethoxazole.[216] Rifampin combined with trimethoprim has been used with success in eradicating persistent, relapsing infections of the kidney or prostate.[216] Rifampin combinations are not the drug of choice for infections of the urinary tract but may be considered when conventional therapy fails.

Urethritis

Although not a first-line drug for gonococcal urethritis, rifampin (900 mg) plus erythromycin (1 g) as a single oral dose has been shown to cure 95 percent of patients with gonorrhea, with equivalent efficacy against penicillinase-producing *Neisseria gonorrhoeae* (PPNG) strains.[217,218] Despite excellent activity against chlamydia in vitro, a single dose of rifampin in combination with erythromycin showed poor efficacy in the treatment of chlamydial urethritis.[218]

Rhodococcus

Rhodococcus equi is a common equine pathogen that has recently been described as a rare cause of human pneumonia with cavity formation in 69 percent. Almost all cases have occurred in immunocompromised patients, including AIDS patients.[219] Optimal therapy in foals has been with rifampin combined with erythromycin. This regimen has been used successfully in patients as has vancomycin and vancomycin combined with rifampin. Therapy is recommended for 2–6 months.[220]

Chancroid

Rifampin has good activity against *Haemophilus ducreyi,* the causative agent of chancroid, and has been shown effective in treatment.[221] However, intramuscular ceftriaxone and oral erythromycin are the treatments of choice.[222]

Infections Due to Pseudomonas aeruginosa and Other Aerobic Gram-Negative Bacilli

Most isolates of *Pseudomonas aeruginosa* are relatively resistant to rifampin, with MICs ranging from 32 to 64 µg/ml. Occasional isolates of *P. aeruginosa,* however, are also resistant to available β-lactams, aminoglycosides, or both. In vitro data have suggested synergy of rifampin with ticarcillin and tobramycin, with imepenem and ciprofloxacin, and with ceftazidime or cefpirome and an aminoglycoside against such resistant strains even when some strains were resistant to all three individual drugs.[223,224] There are case reports of patients refractory to conventional therapy who have responded dramatically after the addition of rifampin to their regimen, suggesting that rifampin may be of value in combination therapy for such infections.[225] Rifampin combined with imipenem has also shown in vitro synergy against *P. aeruginosa* and *Enterobacter* spp. and an additive effect against *Serratia marcescens;* in vitro synergy was also shown for the combination of rifampin, imipenem, and ciprofloxacin against each of these three species.[226] Data from clinical trials are needed regarding the use of rifampin in such combination therapy. One randomized trial of rifampin added to β-lactam and aminoglycoside therapy for *Pseudomonas* bacteremia showed a lower rate of breakthrough bacteremia and of relapse in the rifampin group, but there was no significant difference in the survival rate.[227] An uncontrolled series of rifampin combined with ciprofloxacin for 6–12 weeks of therapy for malignant external otitis found that 10 of 11 were cured.[228]

Rhinoscleroma, a granulomatous disease of the nose due to *Klebsiella rhinosleromatis,* can be effectively treated with rifampin administered orally or as a topical ointment.[229] Brazilian purpuric fever, a life-threatening infection preceded by conjunctivitis, is caused by *Haemophilus influenzae* biogroup *aegyptius,* which was eradicated from the conjunctiva by oral rifampin (20 mg/kg/d for 4 days) in 100 percent of patients in one study.[230]

Anaerobic Infections

Data from experimental animal models suggest that rifampin is as effective as metronidazole in the prevention of abscess formation and eradication of *Bacteroides fragilis* after intraperitoneal injection of the organism. Clinical data are not available.[231,232]

Rifampin is highly active against *C. difficile* and has been used in combination with vancomycin to interrupt relapsing pseudomembranous colitis successfully in one series.[233] Rifampin plus bacitracin showed synergy against 85 percent of 55 strains in one study.[234]

Meningitis

Rifampin has been used successfully in the therapy of several cases of meningitis refractory to other available antibiotics. *Flavobacterium meningosepticum* is a rare cause of meningitis and occurs primarily in neonates but sometimes in adults after surgery. Most strains are susceptible to trimethoprim-sulfamethoxazole, imipenem, vancomycin, and rifampin. Rifampin has been used successfully as part of combination therapy with one or more of these other agents in curing such patients.[213,235] Randomized trials of such therapy are not available.

Rifampin was also added to the regimen of a patient with *H. influenzae* meningitis who had not responded clinically to therapy with chloramphenicol or subsequently with ampicillin and trimethoprim-sulfamethoxazole. The patient responded dramatically after the addition of rifampin.[236] A similar success was reported with rifampin and vancomycin therapy of previously unresponsive enterococcal meningitis.[237]

Rabies

A study of experimental rabies infection in mice suggested that rifampin might have some activity, but these findings require confirmation.[238]

OTHER RIFAMYCINS

Rifapentine

Rifapentine is a cyclopentyl rifamycin with antibacterial[239,240] and antimycobacterial[241,242] activity similar to that of rifampin but has a longer half-life of approximately 14–18 hours in animals (rat, mouse, and rabbit).[243] Sixty-five percent of an oral dose of 10 mg/kg is absorbed by such animals; its hepatic metabolism, biliary excretion, and wide distribution throughout body tissues are each similar to that of rifampin, as is its marked induction of hepatic microsomal oxidase activity.[244,245] This drug appears to be several times more active against *M. tuberculosis* and *M. leprae* than rifampin is, and its longer half-life may facilitate therapy by allowing less frequent administration. It was more active against *M. avium* in vitro and in a murine model than was rifampin.[246,247] Data from clinical trials are not yet available.

Rifabutin

Rifabutin (ansamycin, LM 427) is a semisynthetic spiropiperidyl derivative of rifamycin S that shows good activity against most species of mycobacteria, including all rifampin-sensitive *M. tuberculosis* strains and about one-third of rifampin-resistant strains; strains highly resistant to rifampin are usually resistant to rifabutin. Rifabutin shows better activity against the *M. avium-intracellulare* complex of organisms than rifampin; it inhibits 81 percent of these strains at a concentration of 1.0 μg/ml as compared with only 6 percent being inhibited by rifampin at this concentration.[248]

Rifabutin is absorbed from the gastrointestinal tract, with a peak level of 0.49 μg/ml about 4 hours after ingestion of 300 mg in an adult. The serum half-life is 16 hours, and protein binding is 20 percent. The drug is taken up by all tissues and especially concentrated in the lungs, where levels may be 10-fold higher than in serum. Both hepatic and renal clearances occur as with other rifamycins, and, although animal models suggest less of an effect on hepatic microsomal enzyme activity than rifampin has, several reports have suggested that rifabutin may increase corticosteroid metabolism in patients. The rates and types of side effects from rifabutin appear to be comparable to rifampin from initial reports, but better quantification of these reactions is needed from controlled clinical trials.[248]

Nine of 10 patients with AIDS-related complex developed arthralgia or arthritis when treated with more than 1050 mg per day. Two of these developed uveitis and mouth ulcers at a dose of 1800 mg per day.[249]

Rifabutin was ineffective as monotherapy in open trials for the treatment of *M. avium-intracellulare* disease in patients with acquired immunodeficiency syndrome,[250,251] but it has proven effective in preventing *M. avium* complex disease in AIDS patients with CD4 counts below 200 per cubic millimeter and is now recommended as routine prophylaxis for AIDS patients with CD4 counts below 100 by a Public Health Service Task Force.[252]

Rifabutin therapy for patients with newly diagnosed cavitary pulmonary tuberculosis had significantly less effect on bacilli in cavities than did rifampin in one randomized trial.[253] Rifabutin has been somewhat effective in combination therapy of various mycobacteria resistant to rifampin.[254,255]

Bezoxazinorifamycins

The benzoxazinorifamycins, a group of newly synthesized rifamycin derivatives, exhibited MICs more than 64-fold lower than those of rifampin against *M. tuberculosis, M. kansasii, M. scrofulaceum, M. avium,* and *M. intracellulare.*[256] Rifampin-resistant *M. tuberculosis* showed MICs eightfold lower than those for rifampin, and *M. fortuitum* and *M. chelonae* had MICs equal to those for rifampin.[256] One bezoxazinorifmaycin (KRM-1648) had MICs for *M. avium-intracellulare* ranging from 0.004 to 0.0625, lower than rifampin, rifabutin, and eight other antituberculous agents tested.[26] KRM-1648 administered in a nude mouse leprosy model was significantly more active than rifampin at equivalent oral doses of 1 mg/kg or 3 mg/kg twice weekly.[257] Against *M. avium* KRM-1648 MIC values were 32–128 times lower than for rifampin.[258]

Rifaximin

Rifaximin is a new rifamycin derivative that has only negligible oral absorption. After administration of 1600 mg to 13 subjects biliary concentrations could be detected in only 6, and concentrations were more than fivefold lower than those expected for a similar dose of rifampin.[259] The drug has been used primarily in Italy, with studies suggesting efficacy in uncomplicated diverticulitis, small bowel overgrowth syndrome, and hepatic encephalopathy.[260-263] In a randomized trial rifaximin was as effective as neomycin in lowering blood ammonia levels in patients with hepatic encephalopathy.[264]

NONINFECTIOUS DISEASES

Rifampin has been used successfully to decrease pruritus in patients with primary biliary cirrhosis.[265-267] The drug also has immunodulatory effects and has been studied for use in a number of conditions. Oral rifampin was given to eight rheumatoid arthritis patients without clear response.[268] Rifampin has been injected into the peripheral joints of patients with ankylosing spondylitis with reported decreases in erythrocyte sedimentation rate and Schober's test measurements, but no randomized trial has been done.[269]

Rifabutin and ethambutol were given to 10 patients with recurrent Crohn's disease without clinical or pathologic improvement.[270]

Antitumor activity has also been reported. One study showed additive effects of rifampin and tamoxifen against biliary tract carcinoma cell lines in vitro.[271] Another study reported prolonged remission in patients with acute myelogenous leukemia receiving rifampin.[272]

REFERENCES

1. Sensi P. History of the development of rifampin. Rev Infect Dis. 1983; 5(Suppl):402.
2. Sensi P, Maggi N, Furesz S, et al. Chemical modifications and biological properties of rifamycins. Antimicrob Agents Chemother. 1966;6:699.
3. Mandell GL. Interaction of intraleukocytic bacteria and antibiotics. J Clin Invest. 1973;52:1673.
4. Wehrli W, Knusel F, Schmid K, et al. Interaction of rifamycin with bacterial RNA polymerase. Proc Natl Acad Sci USA. 1968;61:667.
5. Acocella G. Pharmacokinetics and metabolism of rifampin in humans. Rev Infect Dis. 1983;5(Suppl):428.
6. Krukenberg CC, Mischler PG, Massad N, et al. Stability of 196 rifampin suspensions prepared in five syrups. Am J Hosp Pharm. 1986;43:2225–8.
7. Stewart HI, Perkin DP, Donald PR. Stability of isoniazid, rifampin and pyrazinamide in suspensions used for the treatment of tuberculosis in children. Pediatr Infect Dis J. 1991;10:827–31.
8. Purohit SD, Gupta ML, Gupta PR. Dietary constituents and rifampicin absorption. Tubercle. 1987;68:151.
9. Advenier C, Gobert C, Houin G, et al. Pharmacokinetic studies of rifampicin in the elderly. Ther Drug Monit. 1983;5:61–5.
10. Koup JR, Williams-Warren J, Viswanathan CT, et al. Pharmacokinetics of rifampin in children II. Oral bioavailability. Ther Drug Monit. 1986;8:17–22.
11. Roup JR, Williams-Warren J, Weber A, et al. Pharmacokinetics of rifampin in children I. Multiple dose intravenous infusion. Ther Drug Monit. 1986;8:11–6.
12. Furesz S. Chemical and biological properties of rifampicin. Antibiot Chemother. 1970;16:316.
13. Solberg CO, Halstensen A, Digranes A, et al. Penetration of antibiotics into human leukocytes and dermal suction blisters. Rev Infect Dis. 5:S468, 1983.
14. Outman WR, Levitz RE, Hill DA, et al. Intraocular penetration of rifampin in humans. Antimicrob Agents Chemother. 1992;36:1575–6.
15. Wong KW, D'Amico DJ, Oum BS, et al. Intraocular penetration of rifampin after oral administration. Graefes Arch Clin Exp Ophthalmol. 1990;228:40–3.
16. Sande MA, Johnson ML. Antimicrobial therapy of experimental endocarditis caused by Staphylococcus aureus. J Infect Dis. 1975;131:367.
17. Mandell GL, Vest TK. Killing of intraleukocytic Staphylococcus aureus by rifampin: In vitro and in vivo studies. J Infect Dis. 1972;125:486.
18. Mandell GL. The antimicrobial activity of rifampin: Emphasis on the relation to phagocytes. Rev Infect Dis. 1983;5(Suppl):463.
19. Farr BM, Mandell GL. Rifampin. Med Clin North Am. 1982;66:157.
20. Thornsberry C, Hill BC, Swenson JM, et al. Rifampin: Spectrum of antibacterial activity. Rev Infect Dis. 1983;5(Suppl):412.
21. Prescott JF. Rhodococcus equi: An animal and human pathogen. Clin Microb Rev. 1991;4:20–34.
22. Collins CH, Yates MD. Low incidence of rifampin resistant tubercle bacilli. Thorax. 1982;37:526.
23. Cauthen GM, Kilburn JO, Kelly GD, et al. Resistance to anti-tuberculosis drugs in patients with and without prior treatment: Survey of 31 state and large city laboratories, 1982–1986. Am Rev Respir Dis. 1988;137:260.
24. Alan Bloch. Personal communication regarding unpublished CDC data from a 1991 national survey, November 24, 1993.
25. Woodley CL, Kilburn JO. In vitro susceptibility of Mycobacterium avium complex and Mycobacterium tuberculosis strains to a spiro-piperidyl rifamycin. Am Rev Respir Dis. 1982;126:586.
26. Tomioka H, Saito H, Fujii K, et al. In vitro antimicrobial activity of benzoxazinorifamycin, KRM-1648, against Mycobacterium avium complex, determined by the radiometric method. Antimicrob Agents Chemother. 1993;37:67–70.
27. Schachter J. Rifampin in chalmydial infections. Rev Infect Dis. 1983; 5(Suppl):562.
28. Medoff G. Antifungal action of rifampin. Rev Infect Dis. 1983;5(Suppl):614.
29. Barrios NJ, Kirkpatrick DV, Murciano A, et al. Successful treatment of disseminated Fusarium infection in an immunocompromised child. Am J Pediatr Hematol Oncol. 1990;12:319–24.
30. Tucker RM, Denning DW, Hanson LH, et al. Interaction of azoles with rifampin, phenytoin, and carbamazepine: In vitro and clinical observations. Clin Infect Dis. 1992;14:165–74.
31. Wehrli W. Rifampin: Mechanisms of action and resistance. Rev Infect Dis. 1983;5(Suppl):407.
32. Yogev R, Melick C, Glogowski W. In vitro development of rifampin resistance in clinical isolates of Haemophilus influenzae type B. Antimicrob Agents Chemother. 1982;21:387.
33. Band JD, Fraser DW, Ajello G, et al. Prevention of Hemophilus influenzae type b disease. JAMA. 1984;251:2381–6.
34. Band JD, Fraser DW. Adverse effects of two rifampicin dosage regimens for the prevention of meningococcal infection. Lancet. 1984;1:101.
35. Goldin HM, Schweitzer WJ, Bronson DM. Rifampin and exfoliative dermatitis. Ann Intern Med. 1987;107:789.
36. Okano M, Kitano Y, Igarashi T. Toxic epidermal necrolysis due to rifampicin. J Am Acad Dermatol. 1987;17:303.
37. Mimouni A, Hodak E, Mimouni M. Fixed drug eruption following rifampicin treatment. DICP 1990;24:947–8.
38. Purohit SD, Johri SC, Gupta PR, et al. Ranitidine-rifampicin interaction. J Assoc Physicians India 1992;40:308–10.
39. Steele MA, Burk RF, DesPrez RM. Toxic hepatitis with isoniazid and rifampin. A meta-analysis. Chest. 1991;99:456–71.
40. Mandell GL, Sande MA. Drugs used in the chemotherapy of tuberculosis and leprosy. In: Goodman AG, Goodman LS, Gilman A, eds. The Pharmacological Basis of Therapeutics. 6th ed. New York: Macmillan; 1980:1203–6.
41. Gendrel D, Nardou M, Mouba JF, et al. Hepatotoxicity of the combination of isoniazid rifampicin in African children. Role of malnutrition and HB virus. Arch Fr Pediatrie. 1989;46:645–8.
42. O'Brien RJ, Long MW, Cross FS, et al. Hepatotoxicity from isoniazid and rifampin among children treated for tuberculosis. Pediatrics. 1983;72:491–9.
43. Tsagaropoulou-Stinga H, Mataki-Emmanouilidou T, Karida-Kavalioti S, et al. Hepatotoxic reactions in children with severe tuberculosis treated with isomazid-rifampin. Pediatr Infect Dis. 1985;4:270–3.
44. Taillan B, Chichmanian RM, Fuzibet JG, et al. Jaundice caused by rifampicin: 3 cases. Rev Med Int. 1989;10:409–11.
45. Qunibi WY, Godwin J, Eknoyan G. Toxic nephropathy during continuous rifampin therapy. South Med J. 1980;73:791.
46. Grosset J, Leventis S. Adverse effects of rifampin. Rev Infect Dis. 1983; 5(Suppl):440.
47. Murray AN, Cassidy MJD, Templecamp C. Rapidly progressive glomerulonephritis associated with rifampicin therapy for pulmonary tuberculosis. Nephron. 1987;46:373.
48. Soffer O, Nassar VH, Campbell WG Jr. Light chain cast nephropathy and acute renal failure associated with rifampin therapy. Am J Med. 1987;82:1052.
49. Winter RJD, Banks RA, Collins CMP, et al. Rifampicin induced light chain proteinuria and renal failure. Thorax. 1984;39:952.
50. Poole G, Stradling P, Worlledge S. Potentially serious side-effects of high dose twice weekly rifampicin. Postgrad Med J. 1971;47:742–7.
51. Girling DJ, Hitze HL. Adverse reactions to rifampicin. Bull WHO. 1979;57:45.
52. Fahal IH, Williams PS, Clark RE, et al. Thrombotic thrombocytopenic purpura due to rifampicin. BMJ 1992;304:882.
53. Lee CH, Lee CJ. Thrombocytopenia—A rare but potentially serious side effect of initial daily and interrupted use of rifampicin. Chest. 1989;96:202–3.
54. Tahan SR, Diamond JR, Blank JM, et al. Acute hemolysis and renal failure with rifampicin-dependent antibodies after discontinuous administration. Transfusion. 1985;25:124–7.
55. Pereira A, Sanz C, Cervantes F, et al. Immune hemolytic anemia and renal failure associated with rifampicin-dependent antibodies with anti-I specificity. Ann Hematol. 1991;63:56–8.
56. Levine M, Collin K, Kassen BO. Acute hemolysis and renal failure following discontinuous use of rifampin. DICP 1991;25:743–4.
57. Gupta A, Sakhuja V, Gupta KL, et al. Intravascular hemolysis and acute renal failure following intermittent rifampin therapy. Int J Leprosy Other Mycobacterial Dis. 1992;60:185–8.
58. Harland RW, Lindblom SS, Munnell MO. Anaphylaxis from rifampin. Am J Med. 1992;92:581–2.
59. Fekety R, O'Connor R, Silva J. Rifampin and pseudomembranous colitis. Rev Infect Dis. 1983;5(Suppl):524–7.
60. Miller DL, Sedlack JD, Holt RW. Perforation complicating rifampin-associated pseudomembranous enteritis. Arch Surg. 1989;124:1082.
61. Zargar SA, Thapa BR, Sahni A, et al. Rifampicin-induced upper gastrointestinal bleeding. Postgrad Med J. 1990;66:310–1.

62. Bolan G, Laurie RE, Broome CV. Red man syndrome: Inadvertent administration of an excessive dose of rifampin to children in a day-care center. Pediatrics. 77:633,1986.

63. Holdiness RM. A review of the redman syndrome and rifampicin overdosage. Med Toxicol Adverse Drug Exp. 1989;4:444–51.

64. Humber DP, Nsanzumuhire H, Aluoch HA, et al. Controlled double-blind study of the effect of rifampin on humoral and cellular immune responses in patients with pulmonary tuberculosis and in tuberculosis contacts. Am Rev Respir Dis. 1980;122:425.

65. Snider DE Jr, Layde PM, Johnson MW, et al. Treatment of tuberculosis during pregnancy. Am Rev Respir Dis. 1980;122:65.

66. Ohnhaus EE, Kirchhof B, Peheim E. Effect of enzyme induction on plasma lipids using antipyrine, phenobarbital, and rifampicin. Clin Pharmacol Ther. 1979;25:591.

67. Kolars JC, Schmiedlin-Ren P, Schuetz JD, et al. Identification of rifampin-inducible P450IIIA4 (CYP3A4) in human small bowel enterocytes. J Clin Invest. 1992;90:1871–8.

68. Twum-Barima Y, Carruthers SG. Quinidine-rifampin interaction. N Engl J Med. 1981;304:1466.

69. Brass C, Galgiani JN, Blaschke TF, et al. Disposition of ketoconazole, an oral antifungal, in humans. Antimicrob Agents Chemother. 1982;21:151.

70. Baciewicz AM, Self TH, Bekemeyer WB. Update on rifampin drug interactions. Arch Intern Med. 1987;147:565.

71. Baciewicz AM, Self TH. Rifampin drug interactions. Arch Intern Med. 1984; 144:1667–71.

72. Isley WL. Effect of rifampin therapy on thyroid function tests in a hypothyroid patient on replacement L-thyroxine. Ann Intern Med. 1987;107:517.

73. Gupta PR, Mehta YR, Gupta ML, et al. Rifampin-aluminum antacid interaction. J Assoc Physicians India 1988;36:363–4.

74. Pilheu JA, Galati MR, Yunis AS, et al. Pharmacokinetic interaction of ketoconazole, isoniazid and rifampicin. Med Buenos Aires 1989;49:43–7.

75. Borcherding SM, Baciewicz AM, Self TH. Update of rifampin drug interactions II. Arch Intern Med 1992;152:711–6.

76. Malhi R, Uppal R, Sharma PL. Drug interaction between rifampicin, isoniazid and cotrimoxazole in rabbits. Hum Exp Toxicol 1992;11:105–7.

77. Bhatia RS, Uppal R, Malhi R, et al. Drug interaction between rifampicin and cotrimoxazole in patients with tuberculosis. Hum Exp Toxicol 1991;10: 419–21.

78. British Thoracic Association: A controlled trial of six months chemotherapy in pulmonary tuberculosis. Second report: Results during the 24 months after the end of chemotherapy. Am Rev Respir Dis. 1982;126:460.

79. American Thoracic Society/CDC. Treatment of tuberculosis and tuberculous infection in adults and children. Am Rev Respir Dis. 1986;134:355–63.

80. McCarthy OR, Rudd RM. Six months' chemotherapy for lymph node tuberculosis. Respir Med. 1989;83:425–7.

81. Reis FJ, Bedran MB, Moura JA, et al. Six-month isoniazid-rifampin treatment for pulmonary tuberculosis in children. Am Rev Respir Dis. 1990;142: 996–9.

82. Ormerod LP, McCarthy OR, Rudd RM, et al. Short course chemotherapy for pulmonary tuberculosis. Respir Med. 1991;85:291–4.

83. Agounitestane D, Chiheb M, Khaled S, et al. A therapeutic trial of a combination of 3 essential drugs in a short course of chemotherapy in tuberculosis. Results 6 months after the end of treatment. Rev Des Mal Respir. 1990;7: 209–13.

84. Chatterjee G, Kaur S, Sharma VK, et al. Bacillemia in leprosy and effect of multidrug therapy. Leprosy Rev. 1989;60:197–201.

85. Alarcon F, Escalante L, Perez Y, et al. Tuberculous meningitis. Short course of chemotherapy. Arch Neurol. 1990;47:1313–7.

86. Dutt AK, Moers D, Stead WW. Tuberculous pleural effusion: 6-Month therapy with isoniazid and rifampin. Am Rev Respir Dis. 1992;145:1429–32.

87. Initial therapy for tuberculosis in the era of multidrug resistance. MMWR. 1993;42:1–8.

88. Felten MK. Importance of rifampicin in combined daily/intermittent chemotherapy for tuberculosis. S Afr Med J. 1989;75:524–6.

89. Balasubramanian R, Sivasubramanian S, Vijayan VK, et al. Five year results of a 3-month and two 5-month regimens for the treatment of sputum-positive pulmonary tuberculosis in south India. Tubercle. 1990;71:253–8.

90. Goble M, Iseman MD, Madsen LD, et al. Treatment of 171 patients with pulmonary tuberculosis resistant to isoniazid and rifampin. N Engl J Med. 1993;328:527–32.

91. Vincken W, Meysman M, Verbeelen D, et al. Intraventricular rifampicin in severe tuberculous meningo-encephalitis. Eur Respir J. 1992;5:891–3.

92. Castelo A, Jardim JR, Goihman S, et al. Comparison of daily and twice-weekly regimens to treat pulmonary tuberculosis. Lancet. 1989;2:1173–6.

93. Cohn DL, Catlin BJ, Peterson KL, et al. A 62-dose, 6 month therapy for pulmonary and extrapulmonary tuberculosis: A twice-weekly, directly observed, and cost-effective regimen. Ann Intern Med. 1990;112:407–14.

94. Baronti A, Lukinovich N. A pilot trial of rifampicin in tuberculosis. Tubercle. 1968;49:180.

95. Livengood JR, Sigler TG, Foster LR, et al. Isoniazid resistant tuberculosis: A community outbreak and report of a rifampin prophylaxis failure. JAMA. 1985;253:2847–9.

96. Hunter AM, Campbell IA, Jenkins PA, et al. Treatment of pulmonary infections caused by mycobacteria of the *Mycobacterium avium-intracellular* complex. Thorax. 1981;36:326.

97. Baron EJ, Young LS. Amikacin, ethambutol, and rifampin for treatment of disseminated *Mycobacterium avium-intracellular* infections in patients with acquired immune deficiency syndrome. Diagn Microbiol Infect Dis. 1986;5: 215–20.

98. Chiu J, Nussbaum J, Bozzette S, et al. Treatment of disseminated *Mycobacterium avium* complex infection in AIDS with amikacin, ethambutol, rifampin, and ciprofloxacin. California Collaborative Treatment Group. Ann Intern Med. 1990;113:358–61.

99. Dautzenberg B, Tuffot C, Mignon A, et al. Rifabutin in combination with clofazimine, isoniazid and ethambutol in treatment of AIDS patients with infections due to opportunistic mycobacteria. Tubercle. 1991;72:168–75.

100. Ahn CH, Lowell JR, Ahn SS, et al. Chemotherapy for pulmonary disease due to *Mycobacterium kansasii:* Efficacies of some individual drugs. Rev Infect Dis. 1981;3:1028.

101. Helm U, Kaustova J, Kubin M, et al. Susceptibility of *Mycobacterium kansasii* to ethambutol and its combination with rifamycins, ciprofloxacin and isoniazid. Eur J Clin Microbiol Infect Dis. 1992;11:51–4.

102. Bogaerts Y, Elinck W, van Renterghem D, et al. Pulmonary disease due to *Mycobacterium xenopi:* Report of two cases. Eur J Respir Dis. 1982;63:298.

103. Donta ST, Smith PW, Levitz RE, et al. Therapy of *Mycobacterium marinum* infections. Arch Intern Med. 1986;146:902–4.

104. Kallenius G, Moller E, Ringden O, et al. The first infant to survive a generalized BCG infection. Acta Paediatr Scand. 1982;71:161.

105. Izumi AK, Matsunaga J. BCG vaccine-induced lupus vulgaris. Arch Dermatol. 1982;118:171.

106. Gilbody JS. Impact of multidrug therapy on the treatment and control of leprosy. Int J Leprosy 1991;59:458–78.

107. Yawalkar SJ, McDougall AC, Longuillon J, et al. Once monthly rifampicin plus daily dapsone in initial treatment of lepromatous leprosy. Lancet. 1982; 1:1119.

108. Bullock WE. Rifampin in the treatment of leprosy. Rev Infect Dis. 1983; 5(Suppl):606–13.

109. Deal WB, Sanders E. Efficacy of rifampin in treatment of meningococcal carriers. N Engl J Med. 1969;281:641–5.

110. Devine LF, Rhode SL, Pierce WE. Rifampin: Effect of two-day treatment on the meningococcal carrier state and the relationship to the levels of drug in sera and saliva. Am J Med Sci. 1971;261:79–83.

111. Weidmer CE, Dunkel TB, Pettyjohn FS, et al. Effectiveness of rifampin in eradicating the meningococcal carrier state in a relatively closed population: Emergence of resistant strains. J Infect Dis. 1971;124:172–8.

112. Beaty HN. Rifampin and minocycline in meningococcal disease. Rev Infect Dis. 1983;5(Suppl):451–8.

113. Jacobson JA, Daniel B. Vestibular reactions associated with minocycline. Antimicrob Agents Chemother. 1975;8:453–6.

114. Schwartz B, Al-Ruwais A, A'Ashi J, et al. Comparative efficacy of ceftriaxone and rifampicin in eradicating pharyngeal carriage of group A *Neisseria meningitidis.* Lancet. 1988;1:1239–42.

115. Pugsley MP, Dworzack DL, Horowitz EA, et al. Efficacy of ciprofloxacin in the treatment of nasopharyngeal carriers of *Neisseria meningitidis.* J Infect Dis. 1987;156:211–3.

116. Broome CV, Mortimer EA, Katz SL, et al. Use of chemoprophylaxis to prevent the spread of *Hemophilus enfluenzae* B in day-care facilities. N Engl J Med. 1987;316:1226–8.

117. Anonymous. Update: Prevention of *Haemophilus influenzae* type b disease. MMWR. 1986;35:170–80.

118. Respiratory and Special Pathogens Epidemiology Branch (CDC): Prevention of secondary cases of *Haemophilus influenzae* type B disease. MMWR. 1982; 31:672.

119. Brunnel PA, Bass JW, Daum RS, et al. Revision of recommendation for use of rifampin prophylaxis of contact of patients with *Haemophilus influenzae* infection. Pediatrics. 1984;74:301–2.

120. American Academy of Pediatrics. Report of the Committee on Infectious Diseases. 22nd Ed. Elk Grove Village, IL: American Academy of Pediatrics; 1991:220–9.

121. Dashefsky B, Wald E, Li K. Management of contacts of children in day care with invasive *Haemophilus influenzae* type b disease. Pediatrics. 1986;78: 939–40.

122. Wilde J, Adler SP. Molecular epidemiology of *Haemophilus influenzae* type B: Failure of rifampin prophylaxis in a day care center. Pediatr Infect Dis. 1986;5:505–8.

123. Cates KL, Krause PJ, Murphy TV, et al. Second episodes of *Haemophilus influenzae* type b disease following rifampin prophylaxis of the index patients. Pediatr Infect Dis J. 1987;6:512–5.

124. Sande MA. The use of rifampin in treatment of nontuberculous infections. Rev Infect Dis. 1983;5(Suppl):399.

125. Vazquez GJ, Archer GL. Antibiotic therapy of experimental *Staphylococcus epidermidis* endocarditis. Antimicrob Agents Chemother. 1980;17:280–5.

126. Tuazon CU, Washburn D. Teicoplanin and rifampicin singly and in combination in the treatment of experimental *Staphylococcus epidermidis* endocarditis in the rabbit model. J Antimicrob Chemother. 1987;20:233–7.

127. Karchmer AW, Archer GL, Dismukes WE. *Staphylococcus epidermis* causing prosthetic valve endocarditis: Microbiological and clinical observations as guides to therapy. Ann Intern Med. 1983;48:447.

128. Karchmer AW, Archer GA. Methicillin-resistant *Staphylococcus epidermidis* (SE) prosthetic valve (PV) endocarditis (E): A therapeutic trial (Abstract 476). Program and Abstracts of the Twenty-fourth Interscience Conference on Antimicrobial Agents and Chemotherapy. October 8–10, 1984.

129. Chamovitz B, Bryant RE, Gilbert D, et al. Prosthetic valve endocarditis caused by *Staphylococcus epidermidis.* JAMA. 1985;253:2867–8.

130. Swanberg L, Tuazon CU. Rifampin in the treatment of serious staphylococcal infections. Am J Med Sci. 1984;287:49–54.

131. Acar JF, Goldstein EW, Duval J. Use of rifampin for the treatment of serious staphylococcal and gram-negative bacillary infections. Rev Infect Dis. 1983; 5(Suppl)502–6.

132. Roder BL, Gutschik E. In-vitro activity of ciprofloxacin combined with either fusidic acid or rifampicin against *Staphylococcus aureus*. J Antimicrob Chemother. 1989;23:347–52.

133. Moretti MV, Fiorio M, Pasticci MB, et al. Killing rate and serum bactericidal activity of oxacillin, rifampin and ciprofloxacin against *Staphylococcus aureus*. Microbiologica. 1989;12:297–306.

134. Zak O, Scheld M, Sande M. Rifampin in experimental endocarditis due to *Staphylococcus aureus* in rabbits. Rev Infect Dis. 1983;5(Suppl):481–90.

135. Dworkin RJ, Lee BL, Sande MA, et al. Treatment of right-sided *Staphylococcus aureus* endocarditis in intravenous drug users with ciprofloxacin and rifampicin. Lancet. 1989;2:1071–3.

136. Kaatz GW, Seo SM, Barriere SL, et al. Ciprofloxacin and rifampin, alone and in combination, for therapy of experimental *Staphylococcus aureus* endocarditis. Antimicrob Agents Chemother. 1989;33:1184–7.

137. Tebas P, Martinez Ruiz R, Roman F, et al. Early resistance to rifampin and ciprofloxacin in the treatment of right-sided *Staphylococcus aureus* endocarditis. J Infect Dis. 1991;163:204–5.

138. Kapusnik JE, Parenti F, Sande M. The use of rifampicin in staphylococcal infections—A review. J Antimicrob Chemother. 1984;13:61–6.

139. Bayer AS, Lam K. Efficacy of vancomycin plus rifampin in experimental aortic-valve endocarditis due to methicillin-resistant *Staphyloccus aureus:* In vitro–in vivo correlations. J Infect Dis. 1985;151:157–65.

140. Eng RHK, Smith SM, Tillem M, et al. Rifampin resistance. Development during the therapy of methicillin-resistant *Staphylococcus aureus* infection. Arch Intern Med. 1985;145:146–8.

141. Simon GL, Smith RH, Sande MA. Emergence of rifampin-resistant strains of *Staphylococcus aureus* during combination therapy with vancomycin and rifampin: A report of two cases. Rev Infect Dis. 1983;5(Suppl):507–8.

142. Eng RHK, Smith SM, Buccini FJ, et al. Differences in ability of cell-wall antibiotics to suppress emergence of rifampicin resistance in *Staphylococcus aureus*. J Antimicrob Chemother. 1985;15:201–7.

143. Hackbarth CJ, Chambers HF, Sande MA. Serum bactericidal activity of rifampin in combination with other antimicrobial agents against *Staphylococcus aureus*. Antimicrob Agents Chemother. 1986;29:611–3.

144. Foldes M, Munro R, Sorrell TC, et al. In-vitro effects of vancomycin, rifampicin, and fusidic acid, alone and in combination, against methicillin-resistant *Staphylococcus aureus*. J Antimicrob Chemother. 1983;11:21–6.

145. Levine DP, Fromm BS, Reddy BR. Slow response to vancomycin or vancomycin plus rifampin in methicillin-resistant *Staphylococcus aureus* endocarditis. Ann Intern Med. 1991;115:674–80.

146. Coleman DL, Horwitz RI, Andriole VT. Association between serum inhibitory and bactericidal concentrations and therapeutic outcome in bacterial endocarditis. Am J Med. 1982;73:260–7.

147. Traczewski MM, Goldmann DA, Murphy P. In vitro activity of rifampin in combination with oxacillin against *Staphylococcus aureus*. Antimicrob Agents Chemother. 1983;23:571.

148. Watanakunakorn C, Guerriero JC. Interaction between vancomycin and rifampin against *Staphylococcus aureus*. Antimicrob Agents Chemother. 1981; 19:1089.

149. Walsh TJ, Auger P, Tatem BA, et al. Novobiocin and rifampin in combination against methicillin-resistant *Staphylococcus aureus:* An in-vitro comparison with vancomycin plus rifampin. J Antimicrob Chemother. 1986;17: 75–82.

150. Varaldo PE, Debbia E, Schito GC. In vitro activity of teichomycin and vancomycin alone and in combination with rifampin. Antimicrob Agents Chemother. 1983;23:402–6.

151. Zinner SH, Lagast H, Klastersky J. Antistaphylococcal activity of rifampin with other antibiotics. J Infect Dis. 1981;144:365–71.

152. Van der Auwera P, Klastersky J. In vitro study of the combination of rifampin with oxacillin against *Staphylococcus aureus*. Rev Infect Dis. 1983;5(Suppl): 509–14.

153. Van der Auwera P, Klastersky J. Bactericidal activity and killing rate of serum in volunteers receiving teicoplanin alone or in combination with oral or intravenous rifampin. Antimicrob Agents Chemother. 1987;31:1002–5.

154. Ho JL, Klempner MS. In vitro evaluation of clindamycin in combination with oxacillin rifampin or vancomycin against *Staphylococcus aureus*. Diun Microbiol Infect Dis. 1986;4:133.

155. Bayer AS, Morrison JO. Disparity between timed-kill and checkerboard methods for determination of in vitro bactericidal interactions of vancomycin plus rifampin versus methicillin-susceptible and resistant *Staphylococcus aureus*. Antimicrob Agents Chemother. 1984;26:220–3.

156. Sande MA, Scheld WM. Combination antibiotic therapy of bacterial endocarditis. Ann Intern Med. 1980;92:390.

157. Jariwalla AG, Davies BH, White J. Infective endocarditis complicating psittacosis: Response to rifampin. Br Med J. 1980;280:155.

158. Raoult D. Treatment of Q fever. Antimicrob Agents Chemother. 1993;37: 1733–36.

159. Levy PY, Drancourt M, Etienne J, et al. Comparison of different antibiotic regimens for therapy of 32 cases of Q fever endocarditis. Antimicrob Agents Chemother. 1991;35:533–7.

160. Faville RJ, Zaske DE, Kaplan EL, et al. *Staphylococcus aureus* endocarditis: Combined therapy with vancomycin and rifampin. JAMA. 1978;240:1963.

161. Simmons NA. Synergy and rifampicin. J Antimcirob Chemother. 1977;3:109.

162. Wheat LJ, Kohler RB, White AL, et al. Effect of rifampin on nasal carriers of coagulase-positive staphylococci. J Infect Dis. 1981;144:177.

163. Wheat LJ, Kohler RB, Luft PC, et al. Long term studies of the effect of rifampin on nasal carriage of coagulase-positive staphylococci. Rev Infect Dis. 1983;5(Suppl):459–62.

164. McNally TP, Lewis MR, Brown DR. Effect of rifampin and bacitracin on nasal carriers of *Staphylococcus aureus*. Antimicrob Agents Chemother. 1984;25:422–6.

165. Locksley RM, Cohen ML, Quinn TC, et al. Multiply antibiotic-resistant *Staphylococcus aureus:* Introduction, transmission, and evolution of nosocomial infection. Ann Intern Med. 1982;97:317.

166. Zimmerman SW, Johnson CA. Rifampin use in peritoneal dialysis. Peritoneal Dialysis Int. 1989;9:241–3.

167. Ward TT, Winn RE, Hartstein AL, et al. Observations relating to an interhospital outbreak of methicillin resistant *Staphylococcus aureus:* Role of antimicrobial therapy in infection control. Infect Control. 1981;2:453.

168. Ellison H, Judson PN, Peterson LC. Oral rifampin trimethoprim-sulfamethoxazole therapy in symptomatic carriers of methicillin-resistant *Staphylococcus aureus* infections. West J Med. 1984;140:735–40.

169. Pearson JW, Christiansen KJ, Annear DI, et al. Control of methicillin-resistant *Staphylococcus aureus* (MRSA) in an Australian metropolitan teaching hospital complex. Med J Aust. 1985;142:103–8.

170. Darouiche R, Wright C, Hamill R, et al. Eradication of colonization by methicillin-resistant *Staphylococcus aureus* by using oral minocycline-rifampin and topical mupirocin. Antimicrob Agents Chemother. 1991;35:1612–5.

171. Arathoon EG, Hamilton JR, Hench CE, et al. Efficacy of short courses of oral novobiocin-rifampin in eradicating carrier state of methicillin-resistant Staphylococcus aureus and in vitro killing studies of clinical isolates. Antimicrob Agents Chemother. 1990;34:1655–9.

172. Tanz RR, Shulman ST, Barthel MJ, et al. Penicillin plus rifampin eradicates pharyngeal carriage of group A streptococci. J Pediatr. 1985;106:876–80.

173. Rosenberg EW, Noah PW, Zanolli MD, et al. Use of rifampin with penicillin and erythromycin in the treatment of psoriasis. J Am Acad Dermatol. 1986; 14:761–4.

174. Vincent F, Ross JB, Dalton M, et al. A therapeutic trial of the use of penicillin V or erythromycin with or without rifampin in the treatment of soriasis. J Am Acad Dermatol. 1992;26:458–61.

175. Millard DD, Shulman ST, Yogev R. Rifampin and penicillin for the elimination of group B streptococci in nasally colonized infant rats. Pediatr Res. 1985;19:1183–6.

176. Norden CW, Shaffer M. Treatment of experimental chronic osteomyelitis, due to *Staphylococcus aureus* with vancomycin and rifampin. J Infect Dis. 1983;147:352.

177. Dworkin R, Modin G, Kunz S, et al. Comparative efficacies of ciprofloxacin, pefloxacin, and vancomycin in combination with rifampin in a rat model of methicillin-resistant *Staphylococcus aureus* chronic osteomyelitis. Antimicrob Agents Chemother. 1990;34:1014–6.

178. O'Reilly T, Kunz S, Sande E, et al. Relationship between antibiotic concentration in bone and efficacy of treatment of staphylococcal osteomyelitis in rats: Azithromycin compared with clindamycin and rifampin. Antimicrob Agents Chemother. 1992;36:2693–7.

179. Norden CW, Bryant R, Palmer D, et al. Chronic osteomyelitis caused by *Staphylococcus aureus:* Controlled clinical trial of nafcillin therapy and nafcillin-rifampin therapy. South Med J. 1986;79:947–51.

180. Widmer AF, Gaechter A, Ochsner PE, et al. Antimicrobial treatment of orthopedic implant-related infections with rifampin combinations. Clin Infect Dis. 1992;14:1251–3.

181. Beam TR. Sequestration of *Staphylococcus aureus* at an inaccessible focus. Lancet. 1979;2:227.

182. Dournon E, Mayaud C, Wolff M, et al. Comparison of the activity of three antibiotic regimens in severe Legionnaires' disease. J Antimicrob Chemother. 1990;26(Suppl B):129–39.

183. Jacobs F, Abramowicz D, Vereerstraeten P, et al. *Brucella* endocarditis: The role of combined medical and surgical treatment. Rev Infect Dis. 1990; 12:740–4.

184. LLoren-Terol J, Busquets RM. Brucellosis treated with rifampicin. Arch Dis Child. 1980;55:486.

185. Shehabi A, Shakir K, el-Khateeb M, et al. Diagnosis and treatment of 106 cases of human brucellosis. J Infect. 1990;20:5–10.

186. Ariza J, Gudiol P, Pallares R, et al. Comparative trial of rifampin-doxycycline versus tetracycline-streptomycin in the therapy of human brucellosis. Antimicrob Agent Chemother. 1985;28:548–51.

187. Colmenero Castillo JD, Hernandez Marquez S, Reguera Iglesias JM, et al. Comparative trial of doxycycline plus streptomycin versus doxycycline plus rifampin for the therapy of human brucellosis. Chemotherapy. 1989;35: 146–52.

188. Solera J, Medrano F, Rodriguez M, et al. A comparative therapeutic and multicenter trial of rifampin and doxycycline versus streptomycin and doxycycline in human brucellosis. Med Clin. 1991;96:649–53.

189. Ariza J, Guidol F, Pallares R, et al. Treatment of human brucellosis with doxycycline plus rifampin or doxycycline plus streptomycin. A randomized, double-blind study. Ann Intern Med. 1992;117:25–30.

190. Akova M, Uzun O, Akalin HE, et al. Quinolones in treatment of human brucellosis: Comparative trial of ofloxacin-rifampin versus doxycycline-rifampin. Antimicrob Agents Chemother. 1993;37:1831–34.

191. Perez MAH, Rodriguez BA, Garcia AP, et al. Treatment of nervous system

brucellosis with rifampin and doxcycline (Letter). Neurology. 1986;36: 1408–9.

192. Bella F, Espejo E, Uriz S, et al. Randomized trial of 5-day rifampin versus 1-day doxycycline therapy for Mediterranean spotted fever. J Infect Dis. 1991;164:433–4.

193. Ezer G, Soothill JF. Intracellular bactericidal effect of rifampicin in both normal and chronic granulomatous disease polymorphs. Arch Dis Child. 1974;49:463.

194. Lorber B. Rifampin in chronic granulomatous disease. N Engl J Med. 1980; 303:111.

195. Archer G, Tenenbaum JM, Haywood HB. Rifampun therapy of S. epidermidis: Use in infections from indwelling artificial devices. JAMA. 1978;240: 751.

196. Bolton WK, Sande MA, Normansell DE, et al. Ventriculojugular shunt nephritis with Corynebacterium bovis. Am J Med. 1975;59:417.

197. Ring JC, Cates KL, Belani KK, et al. Rifampin for CSF shunt infection caused by coagulase-negative staphylocci. J Pediatr. 1979;95:317.

198. O'Keefe PT, Bayston R. Pneumococcal meningitis in child with ventriculoperitoneal shunt. J Infect. 1991;22:77–9.

199. Walters BC, Goumnerova L, Hoffman HJ, et al. A randomized controlled trial of perioperative rifampin/trimethoprim in cerebrospinal fluid shunt surgery. Childs Nervous Sys. 1992;8:253–7.

200. Teloken C, Souto JC, Da Ros C, et al. Prosthetic penile infection: "Rescue procedure" with rifamycin. J Urol. 1992;148:1905–6.

201. Wakefield TW, Schaberg DR, Pierson CL, et al. Treatment of established prosthetic vascular graft infection with antibiotics preferentially concentrated in leukocytes. Surgery. 1987;102:8–14.

202. Chuard C, Herrmann M, Vaudaux P, et al. Successful therapy of experimental chronic foreign-body infection due to methicillin-resistant Staphylococcus aureus by antimicrobial combinations. Antimicrob Agents Chemother. 1991; 35:2611–6.

203. Gagnon RF, Richards GK, Wisenfeld L. Staphylococcus epidermidis biofilms: Unexpected outcome of double and triple antibiotic combinations with rifampin. ASAIO Transactions. 1991;37:M158–60.

204. Colburn MD, Moore WS, Chvapil M, et al. Use of an antibiotic-bonded graft for in situ reconstruction after prosthetic graft infections. J Vasc Surg. 1992; 16:651–60.

205. Freyrie A, Curti T, Rodio M, et al. Interaction between vascular prostheses and rifampicin in the prevention of the grafts infection. An experimental study. Int Angiol. 1992;11:113–6.

206. Lundell A, Bergqvist D, Lindblad B, et al. The acute thrombogenicity of an infection-resistant rifampicin-soaked Dacron graft: An experimental study in sheep. 1992;6:403–7.

207. Goeau-Brissonniere O, Leport C, Bacourt F, et al. Prevention of vascular graft infection by rifampin bonding to a gelatin-sealed Dacron graft. Ann Vasc Surg. 1991;5:408–12.

208. Chervu A, Moore WS, Gelabert HA, et al. Prevention of graft infection by use of prostheses bonded with a rifampin/collagen release system. J Vasc Surg. 1991;14:521–5.

209. Avramovic Jr, Fletcher JP. Rifampicin impregnation of a protein-sealed Dacron graft: An infection-resistant prosthetic vascular graft. Aust NZ J Surg. 1991;61:436–40.

210. Avramovic J, Fletcher JP. Prevention of prosthetic vascular graft infection by rifampicin impregnation of a protein-sealed Dacron graft in combination with parenteral cephalosporin. J Cardiovasc Surg. 1992;33:70–4.

211. Strachan CJ, Newsom SW, Ashton TR. The clinical use of an antibiotic-bonded graft. Eur J Vasc Surg 1991;5:627–32.

212. Peters W, Shaw JJ, Lainson R, et al. Potentiating action of rifampicin and isomazid against Leishmania mexicana amazonensis. Lancet. 1981;1:1122.

213. Even-Paz Z, Weinrauch L, Livshin R, et al. Rifampicin treatment of cutaneous leishmaniasis. Int J Dermatol. 1982;21:110.

214. Joshi RK, Nambiar PM. Dermal leishmaniasis and rifampicin. Int J Dermatol. 1989;28:612–4.

215. Conti R, Parenti P. Rifampin therapy for brucellosis, Flavobacterium meningitis, and cutaneous leishmammasis. Rev Infect Dis. 1983;5(Suppl):600–5.

216. Brumfitt W, Dixson S, Hamilton-Miller JMT. Use of rifampin for the treatment of urinary tract infections. Rev Infect Dis. 1983;5(Suppl):573–82.

217. Desudchit P, Nunthapisud P, Rukjutitum S, et al. Rifampicin-erythromycin combination for the treatment of gonococcal urethritis in men. Southeast Asian J Trop Med Public Health. 1984;15:360–3.

218. Oriel JD, Ridway GL, Goldmeir D, et al. Treatment of gonococcal urethritis in men with a rifampicin-erythromycin combination. Sex Transm Dis. 1982; 9:208–11.

219. Lasky J, Pulkingham N, Powers M, et al. Rhodococcus equi causing human pulmonary infection: Review of 29 cases. South Med J. 1991;84:1217–20.

220. Gray B. Case report: Rhodococcus equi pneumonia in a patient infected by the human immunodeficiency virus. Am J Med Sci. 1992;303:180–3.

221. Plummer PA, Nsanze H, D'Costa LJ, et al. Short-course and single-dose antimicrobial therapy for chancroid in Kenya: Studies with rifampin alone and in combination with trimethoprim. Rev Infect Dis. 1983;5(Suppl):565–72.

222. Treatment of sexually transmitted diseases. Med Lett. 1988;30:5–10.

223. Kumar A, Wofford-McQueen R, Gordon RC. Ciprofloxacin, imipenem and rifampicin: iv-vitro synergy of two and three drug combinations against Pseudomonas cepacia. J Antimicrob Chemother. 1989;23:831–5.

224. Zuravleff JJ, Yu VL, Yee RB. Ticarcillin-tobramycin-rifampin: In vitro synergy of the triplet combination against Pseudomonas aeruginosa. J Lab Clin Med. 1983;101:896–902.

225. Yu VL, Zuravleff JJ, Peacock JE, et al. Addition of rifampin to carboxypenicillin-aminoglycoside combination for the treatment of Pseudomonas aerugionosa infection: Clinical experience with four patients. Antimicrob Agents Chemother. 1984;26:575–7.

226. Chin NX, Heu HC. Synergy of imipenen, a novel carbapenem, and rifampin and ciprofloxacin against Pseudomonas aeruginosa, Serratis marcescens and Enterobacter species. Chemotherapy. 1987;33:183–8.

227. Korvick JA, Peacock JE Jr., Muder RR, et al. Addition of rifampin to combination antibiotic therapy for Pseudomonas aeruginosa bacteremia: Prospective trial using the Zelen protocol. Antimicrob Agents Chemother. 1992;36: 620–5.

228. Rubin J, Stoehr G, Yu VL, et al. Efficacy of oral ciprofloxacin plus rifampin for treatment of malignant external otitis. Arch Otolaryngol Head Neck Surg. 1989;115:1063–9.

229. Gamea AM, el-Tatawi FA. The effect of rifampicin on rhinoscleroma: An electron microscopic study. J Laryngol Otol. 1990;104:772–7.

230. Perking BA, Tondella ML, Bortolotto IM, et al. Comparative efficacy of oral rifampin and topical chloramphenicol in eradicating conjunctival carriage of Haemophilus influenzae biogroup aegyptius. Pediatr Infect Dis J. 1992; 11:717–21.

231. Fu KP, Lasinski ER, Zoganas HC, et al. Therapeutic efficacy and pharmacokinetic properties of rifampicin in m a Bacteroides fragilis intra-abdominal abscess. J Antimicrob Chemother. 1984;14:633–40.

232. Fu KP, Lasinski ER, Zoganas HC, et al. Efficacy of rifampicin in experimental Bacteroides fragilis and Pseudomonas aeruginosa mixed infections. J Antimicrob Chemother. 1985;15:579–85.

233. Buggy BP, Fekety R, Silva J Jr. Therapy of relapsing Clostridium difficile associated diarrhea and colitis with the combination of vancomycin and rifampin. J Clin Gastroenterol. 1987;9:155–9.

234. Bacon AE, McGrath S, Fekety R, et al. In vitro synergy studies with Clostridium difficile. Antimicrob Agents Chemother. 1991;35:582–3.

235. Hirsh BE, Wong B, Kiehn TE, et al. A case of Flavobacterium meningosepticum bacteremia in an adult with acute leukemia. Use of rifampin to clear persistent infection. Diagn Microbiol Infect Dis. 1986;4:65–9.

236. Lewis MA, Priestley BL. Addition of rifampicin in persistent Haemophilus influenzae type B meningitis. 1986;292:448–9.

237. Ryan JL, Pachner A, Andriole VT, et al. Enterococcal meningitis: Combined vancomycin and rifampin therapy. Am J Med. 1980;68:449–451.

238. Zubovich IK, Votyakov VI, Mishaeva NP. Rifampicin protective action in experimental rabies infection of albino mice. Antibiot Khimioter. 1989;34: 123–5.

239. Varaldo PE, Debbia E, Schito GC. In vitro activities of rifapentine and rifampin, alone and in combination with six other antibiotics, against methicillin-susceptible and methicillin-resistant staphylococci of different species. Antimicrob Agents Chemother. 1985;27:615–8.

240. Korvic J, Yu VL, Sharp JA. Interaction of rifampicin or rifapentine with other agents against Pseudomonas aerugionosa. J Antimicrob Chemother. 1987;19:847–8.

241. Dickinson JM, Mitchison DA. In vitro properties of rifapentine (MDL473) relevant to its use in intermittent chemotherapy of tuberculosis. Tubercle. 1987;68:113–8.

242. Bermudez LEM, Wu M, Young LS. Intracellular killing of Mycobacterium avium complex by rifapentine and liposome-encapsulated amikacin. J Infect Dis. 1987;156:510–3.

243. Assandri A, Ratti B, Cristina T. Pharmacokinetics of rifapentine, a new long lasting rifamycin, in the rat, the mouse and the rabbit. J Antibiot (Tokyo). 1984;37:1066–73.

244. Durand DV, Hampden C, Boobis AR, et al. Induction of mixed function oxidase activity in man by rifapentine (MDL473), a long-acting rifamycin derivative. Br J Clin Pharmacol. 1986;21:1–7.

245. Liw DY, Wang YS. Inductive effects of rifapentine on mice hepatic mixed function oxidase system. Methods Findings Exp Clin Pharmacol. 1990;12: 109–13.

246. Klemens SP, Cynamon MH. Activity of rifapentine against Mycobacterium avium infection in beige mice. J Antimicrob Chemother. 1992;29:555–61.

247. Heifets LB, Lindholm-Levy PJ, Flory MA. Bactericidal activity in vitro of various rifamycins against Mycobacterium avium and Mycobacterium tuberculosis. Am Rev Respir Dis. 1990;141:626–30.

248. O'Brien RJ, Lyle MA, Snider DE. Rifabutin (ansamycin LM 427): A new rifamycin-S derivative for the treatment of mycobacterial diseases. Rev Infect Dis. 1987;9:519–30.

249. Siefal FP, Eilbott D, Burger H, et al. Dose-limiting toxicity of rifabutin in AIDS-related complex: syndrome of arthralgia/arthritis. AIDS. 1990;4: 433–41.

250. Hawkins CC, Gold JWM, Whimbey E, et al. Mycobacterium avium complex infections in patients with the acquired immunodeficiency syndrome. Ann Intern Med. 1986;105:184–8.

251. Masur H, Tuazon C, Gill V, et al. Effect of combined clofazimine and ansamycin therapy on Mycobacterium avium-Mycobacterium intracellulare bacteremia in patients with AIDS. J Infect Dis. 1987;155:126–9.

252. Masur H and the Public Health Service Task force on Prophylaxis and Therapy for Mycobacterium avium Complex. Recommendation on prophylaxis and therapy for disseminated Mycobacterium avium complex disease in patients infected with human immunodeficiency virus. N Engl J Med. 1993; 329:898–904.

253. Chan SL, Yew WW, Ma WK, et al. The early bactericidal activity of rifabutin

measured by sputum viable counts in Hong Kong patients with pulmonary tuberculosis. Tubercle Lung Dis. 1992;73:33–8.

254. Pretet S, Lebeaut A, Parrot R, et al. Combined chemotherapy including rifabutin for rifampicin and isoniazid resistant pulmonary tuberculosis. Eur Respir J. 1992;5:680–4.

255. Anonymous. Rifabutine in the treatment of mycobacterial infections resistant to rifampicin. Preliminary results. Rev Mal Repir. 1989;6:335–42.

256. Saito H, Tomioka H, Sato K, et al. In vitro antimycobacterial activities of newly synthesized benzoxazinorifamycins. Antimicrob Agents Chemother. 1991;35:542–7.

257. Gidoh M, Tsutsumi S, Yamane T, et al. Bactericidalaction at low doses of a new rifamycin derivative, 3'-hydroxy-5'-(4-isobutyl-1-piperazinyl) benzo-xazinorifamycin (KRM01648) on *Mycobacterium leprae* inoculated into foot-pads of nude mice. Leprosy Rev. 1992;63:319–28.

258. Yamamoto Y, Saito H, Tomioka KH, et al. In vitro and in vivo activities of KRM-1648, a newly synthesized benzoxazinorifamycin, against Mycobacterium marinum. Int J Med Microbiol Virol Parasitol Infect Dis. 1992;277:204–9.

259. Verardi S, Verardi V. Bile rifaximin concentration after oral administration in patients undergoing cholecystectomy. Farmaco. 1990;45:131–5.

260. Iosca N, Ferrieri A. The rifaximin therapy and prophylaxis of episodes of acute diverticulitis. Recent Prog Med. 1993;84:49–53.

261. Corazza GR, Sorge M, Strocchi A, et al. Non-absorbable antibiotics and small bowel bacterial overgrowth. Italian J Gastrol. 1992;24:4–9.

262. Papi C, Camarri E. Non-absorbable antibiotics in the treatment of divercu-lar disease of the colon. Italian J Gastrol. 1992;24:19–22.

263. Di Febo G, Claabrese C, Matassoni F. New trends in non-absorbable antibi-otics in gastrointestinal disease. Italian J Gastrol. 1992;24:10–3.

264. Pedretti G, Calzetti C, Missale, et al. Rifaximin versus neomycin on hyper-ammoniemia in chronic portal system encephalophathy of cirrhotics. A dou-ble-blind, randomized trial. Italian J Gastrol. 1991;23:175–8.

265. Bachs L, Pares A, Elena M, et al. Effects of long-term rifampicin administra-tion in primary biliary cirrhosis. Gastrology 1992;102:2077–80.

266. Podesta A, Lopez P, Terg R, et al. Treatment of pruritus of primary biliary cirrhosis with rifampin. Dig Dis Sci. 1991;36:216–20.

267. Cynamon HA, Andres JM, Iafrate RP. Rifampin relieves pruritus in children with cholestatic liver disease. Gastroenterology. 1990;98:1013–16.

268. Gabriel SE, Conn DL, Luthra H. Rifampin therapy in rheumatoid arthritis. J Rheumatol. 1990;17:163–6.

269. Caruso I, Cazzola M, Santandrea S. Clinical improvement in ankylosing spondylitis with rifamycin SV infiltrations of peripheral joints. J Int Med Res. 1992;20:171–81.

270. Rutgeerts P, Geboes K, Vantrappen G, et al. Rifabutin and ethambutol do not help recurrent Crohn's disease in the neoterminal ileum. J Clin Gastroenterol. 1992;15:24–8.

271. West CM, Reeves SJ, Brough W. Additive interaction between tamoxifen and rifampicin in human biliary tract carcinoma cells. Cancer Lett. 1990;55:159–63.

272. Burghouts J, Haanen C. A possible role of rifampicin in prolonging remission duration in acute myelogenous leukemia. Scand J Haematol. 1986;36:376–78.

273. Rizak MA, Hillman DM. Handbook of Adverse Drug Interactions. New Rochelle, NY: Medical Letter; 1993.

23. METRONIDAZOLE

SYDNEY M. FINEGOLD
GLENN E. MATHISEN

DESCRIPTION

Metronidazole was introduced in 1959 for the treatment of *Tri-chomonas vaginalis* infections. It is now known to be effective against most infections involving anaerobic bacteria and against certain other parasitic infections. Metronidazole diffuses well into all tissues, including the central nervous system. It is well tolerated and has the best bactericidal activity of all drugs active against anaerobic bacteria.

Metronidazole is a nitroimidazole drug with the chemical for-mula 1-(2-hydroxyethyl)-2-methyl-5-nitroimidazole. It has a low molecular weight, 171.

SPECTRUM OF ACTIVITY, RESISTANCE

Table 1 summarizes the activity of metronidazole against 793 strains of anaerobic and microaerophilic bacteria. Note that vir-

TABLE 1. Activity of Metronidazole against Anaerobic and Microaerophilic Bacteria

Bacteria	No. Strains	Cumulative Percentage Susceptible to Indicated Concentration (µg/ml)			
		4	8	16	32
Bacteroides fragilis[a]	161	90	99	100	—
B. melaninogenicus[b]	60	98	100	—	—
Other bacteroides, *Prevotella*, and *Selenomonas* spp.	154	95	98	100	—
Fusobacterium spp.	65	100	—	—	—
Anaerobic gram-negative cocci	24	92	96	100	—
Anaerobic gram-positive cocci	124	98	—	—	—
Clostridium perfringens	18	94	100	—	—
Other *Clostridium* spp.	73	97	99	—	100
Gram-positive nonsporulating bacilli	87	57	60	62	66
Capnocytophaga spp.	27	52	70	93	—

[a] Includes all species of the *B. fragilis* group.
[b] Includes *Prevotello melaninogenica* (formerly *Bacteroides melaninogenicus*) and *Porphyromonas* (formerly *Bacteroides asaccharolyticus* subsp.)
(From Sutter,[1] with permission.)

tually all of the organisms tested were inhibited by 16 µg/ml or less except for one-third of gram-positive non-spore-forming bacilli and 7 percent of *Capnocytophaga* spp. Metabolites are found in serum and urine, and Sutter[1] found that the hydroxy metabolite of metronidazole was slightly less active than was the parent compound against many anaerobes but had equivalent or better activity against some. The acid metabolite has poor activity against anaerobes. In general, studies by other workers have given comparable results in terms of the in vitro activity of metronidazole. Wüst[2] found that seven strains of *Propionibacte-rium acnes* required 100 µg/ml for inhibition. Werner et al.[3] also noted that the hydroxy metabolite of metronidazole was roughly comparable in activity to the parent compound. We found that only about 25 percent of the strains of *Actinomyces* and *Propion-ibacterium propionica* are susceptible to metronidazole at achievable levels. Rosenblatt and Edson[4] noted somewhat less activity against anaerobic gram-positive cocci (a minimum in-hibitory concentration for 70 percent of strains [MIC$_{70}$] of 6.25 and an MIC$_{90}$ of >25 µg/ml). *Propionibacterium acnes* was highly resistant. The study by Chow et al.[5] found significantly more resistance among anaerobes to metronidazole than was indicated by the studies previously cited.

Also sensitive to metronidazole are *Treponema pallidum*, oral spirochetes, *Campylobacter fetus*, *Gardnerella vaginalis*, and *Helicobacter pylori*. In certain animal models, *Escherichia coli* may be inhibited by metronidazole when it is present together in a mixture with *Bacteroides fragilis*. However, in another animal model[6] there was no activity against *E. coli*. We have noted decreased counts of *E. coli* initially present together with anaer-obes in the bypassed loop of patients with ileal bypass for obe-sity who were treated with metronidazole for "bypass enter-opathy."

Resistance to metronidazole develops rarely, and a combina-tion of several mechanisms may be required for emergence of high-level resistance.[7] Although both plasmid-mediated and chromosomally mediated resistance have been described, their transfer to metronidazole-sensitive *Bacteroides* spp. does not appear to be a problem as yet.[8] Resistant strains identified in-clude one strain each of *Bacteroides fragilis*, *Bacteroides dista-sonis*, what was originally described as *Bacteroides melanino-genicus* ss *melaninogenicus* and *Bacteroides bivius*. Phillips et al.[9] note that they have seen occasional marginally resistant isolates of *B. bivius* (now called *Prevotella bivia*), *Bacteroides ureolyticus* and perhaps *B. melaninogenicus* (now called *Prevo-tella melaninogenica*). Tally et al.[10] studied a metronidazole-resistant strain of *B. fragilis*. They found that the uptake of metronidazole by cells was slower than in a sensitive strain. Also, the rate of reduction of metronidazole was four times less than with a sensitive control strain, possibly due to decreased nitroreductase activity. Although rare, case reports suggest that resistant organisms may develop in patients receiving therapy, and this could lead to a clinical relapse of infection.[11,12] *Trichomonas vaginalis* may become resistant to metronidazole, and several case reports have described recalcitrant vaginal trichomoniasis secondary to resistant strains.[13–15]

MODE OF ACTION

Mechanism of Action

It is convenient to think of the action as occurring in four successive steps[16]: *(1)* entry of the drug into the bacterial cell, *(2)* reductive activation, *(3)* toxic effect of the reduced intermediate product(s), and *(4)* release of inactive end products. A key feature is reduction of the nitro group of the drug; the drug acts as a preferential electron acceptor, being reduced by low–redox potential electron transport proteins (ferredoxinlike and flavodoxinlike). Reduction of the drug decreases the intracellular concentration of unchanged drug, thus maintaining a gradient that drives the uptake and generates compounds that are toxic to the cell. The toxicity is due to short-lived intermediate compounds or free radicals that produce damage by interaction with DNA and possibly other macromolecules. The cytotoxic intermediates decompose into nontoxic and inactive end products, including acetamide and 2-hydroxethyl oxamic acid.

Metabolic Products

As noted before, the hydroxy derivative of metronidazole has significant antianaerobic activity; it is more active than metronidazole is on *G. vaginalis*. The acid derivative of metronidazole has relatively little activity, less than one-tenth as much as metronidazole against *B. fragilis* and *Trichomonas*.[16] The drug is also conjugated; the glucuronide has no activity on *Trichomonas* and is not taken up.[16]

Bactericidal Activity

Metronidazole is a potent bactericidal agent. It typically kills organisms at the same concentration or within one twofold dilution of that required for inhibition.[17] Under reduced conditions, metronidazole has a rapid onset of bactericidal activity. Killing rates are not affected by inoculum size, nutritional requirements, or growth rate.[18,19]

Bartlett et al.[20] found metronidazole to be the most effective drug in a *B. fragilis* subcutaneous abscess model in mice even when treatment was delayed for 8–120 hours after challenge.

PHARMACOLOGY

When given orally, metronidazole is absorbed rapidly and almost completely. Serum levels are similar during the elimination phase after equivalent doses by the intravenous and oral routes. Blood levels are proportional to the administered dose. The standard intravenous dosage regimen that has been used in the United States consists of a loading dose of 15 mg/kg of body weight followed by 7.5 mg/kg every 6 hours. This results in peak and trough steady-state plasma levels averaging 25 µg/ml and 18 µg/ml, respectively. There is very little protein binding of metronidazole. The half-life is 8 hours. Absorption of metronidazole is not affected by ingestion of food, but peak levels may be markedly delayed. Metronidazole is absorbed after vaginal administration, but peak serum levels (mean, 1.2 µg/ml) and bioavailability (20 percent) are lower than by oral or intravenous administration.[21] Absorption after rectal administration is quite

good, although peak serum levels occur approximately 3 hours after insertion. Metronidazole is rapidly transferred across the placenta; peak serum levels in the fetus are equivalent to maternal levels after intravenous administration to pregnant women.[22]

There is a large apparent volume of distribution of metronidazole that is equivalent to about 80 percent of body weight; it reaches all tissues and fluids. Therapeutic levels are achieved in amniotic fluid, the unobstructed biliary tract, alveolar bone, cerebrospinal fluid and brain abscess contents, cord blood, pleural empyema fluid, hepatic abscesses, middle ear discharge, middle ear mucosa, breast milk, pelvic tissues (concentrations attained in the myometrium and fallopian tubes are nearly the same as concomitant serum levels), saliva, seminal fluid, and vaginal secretions. Levels achieved in the aqueous humor were between one-third and one-half those attained in the serum.[23]

During metabolization of metronidazole, five major products are formed. The most important one is the hydroxy derivative. In addition, there is an acid metabolite, acetylmetronidazole, metronidazole glucuronide, and the glucuronide conjugate of hydroxy metronidazole. A sulfate conjugate may also be found on occasion. Metronidazole and its metabolites are eliminated primarily in the urine (60–80 percent of the dose). From 6 to 15 percent is excreted in the feces.

The elimination half-life of metronidazole in patients with no renal function is the same as in healthy people. However, the hydroxy metabolite may accumulate in patients with absent renal function, and, although dosage adjustment is usually not considered necessary in the absence of hepatic disease, consideration might be given to dosage adjustment in patients initially receiving large doses. Metronidazole and its metabolites are rapidly removed by hemodialysis; the elimination half-life of metronidazole is reduced to 2.6 hours. Dose reduction is generally not necessary in patients undergoing chronic ambulatory peritoneal dialysis.[24] In patients with impaired hepatic function, even without concomitant renal function impairment, the plasma clearance of metronidazole is delayed. Although data are limited, pharmacokinetic studies in patients with significant liver disease suggest that doses should be reduced by at least 50 percent in this patient population.[25,26]

ADMINISTRATION AND DOSAGE

Table 2 gives dosage recommendations and routes of administration for the major indications for metronidazole therapy. The intravenous route is recommended initially for seriously ill patients. Since oral therapy gives blood levels comparable to those achieved by the intravenous route, we may switch when conditions warrant.

As noted, the standard regimen in the United States for intravenous administration has been a loading dose of 15 mg/kg of body weight followed by a maintenance schedule of 7.5 mg/kg

TABLE 2. Major Indications for Metronidazole: Administration and Dosage

Indication	Route of Administration	Dosage
Susceptible anaerobic infections	iv	Loading dose of 15 mg/kg, then 7.5 mg/kg q6h
	po	1–2 g/day in 2–4 doses q6–12h
Bacterial vaginosis	po	500 mg bid for 7 days
	Intravaginal	5 g of 0.75% intravaginal gel bid × 5 days
Trichomonas vaginitis	po	250 mg tid for 7 days *or* 500 mg bid for 5 days *or* 2 g in single dose
Amebiasis (intestinal or extraintestinal)	iv or po	750 mg tid for 10 days
Giardiasis	po	250 mg bid or tid for 5–7 days *or* 2 g/day for 3 days

every 6 hours. Clearly, the half-life of the drug would warrant administration at longer intervals such as every 8 or even every 12 hours. The manufacturer recommends that intravenous infusions be administered over a period of 1 hour. However, a number of foreign investigators have administered the drug in as little as 20 minutes without any apparent adverse effects. The maximum daily dose recommended is 4 g.

After reconstitution, metronidazole hydrochloride should be diluted with intravenous fluid to a concentration not exceeding 8 mg/ml and should be neutralized to pH 6.0–7.0 with sodium bicarbonate before administration. There is also a metronidazole intravenous solution (Flagyl IV RTU), a ready-to-use isotonic solution that does not require dilution or buffering before infusion.

The duration of therapy will vary according to the entity being treated. Certain recommendations are made in Table 2. For serious infections, however, we may often need to treat the patient for 2–4 weeks or longer.

Comments regarding dosage in patients with impaired renal and/or hepatic function have been noted in the earlier section on pharmacology.

ADVERSE REACTIONS, PRECAUTIONS

In general, metronidazole is well tolerated. The more commonly encountered major and minor adverse reactions are listed in Table 3. There may also be furring of the tongue, glossitis, stomatitis, dry mouth, headache, fever, dizziness, syncope, and occasionally overgrowth of *Candida* in the oral cavity or vagina. Thrombophlebitis has been reported with intravenous infusion but is seldom seen now with proper buffering of the preparation. Gastrointestinal side effects include nausea, epigastric distress, anorexia, and, less commonly, vomiting, diarrhea, or pancreatitis. Although pseudomembranous colitis has been reported rarely with metronidazole therapy, the drug has proved effective therapeutically for this condition and is comparable to vancomycin in effectiveness. The most serious adverse effects are those involving the central nervous system. These are rare unless large doses and/or prolonged therapy is used. If abnormal neurologic symptoms are observed, treatment with the drug must be discontinued immediately. Metronidazole should be used with caution in people with a history of seizures or other central nervous system disorders. The peripheral neuropathy may take a considerable period of time to resolve.

There has been concern about mutagenicity in the Ames *Salmonella* mutant system and carcinogenicity of metronidazole. Reduction of the nitro group of the compound is necessary for both antibacterial activity and mutagenic activity. Mutagenic activity has been detected in the urine of patients receiving 750 mg/day of metronidazole. When a mutant *Salmonella* strain that did not possess nitroreductase was used in the mutagenic testing system, metronidazole could not be demonstrated to be a mutagen. Thus, the drug itself is not mutagenic, but rather it is one

or more reduction products of it. Some protozoa, bacteria (including facultative anaerobes), and fungi possess nitroreductase activity. Eukaryotic tissues have very little nitroreductase activity. It has been suggested that during metronidazole therapy some reduction products of the drug might escape from the bacterial cells and serve as mutagens to the host's mammalian tissue. However, these active derivatives are very short lived and either promptly bind to macromolecules within the bacterial cell or are promptly reduced to compounds that are not mutagenic or carcinogenic. The drug has been studied specifically for mutagenic potential in eukaryotic test systems (human lymphocytes in vitro and lymphocytes of patients receiving metronidazole therapy). No chromosomal aberrations or sister chromatid exchanges could be detected in vitro with metronidazole or its metabolites in concentrations of 1000–10,000 µg/ml. No lymphocyte abnormalities were noted in patients receiving a short course of metronidazole therapy.[27,28] Metronidazole has shown tumorigenic activity in several studies in mice involving lifetime (or almost lifetime) oral administration. Female rats given metronidazole over long periods (sometimes for life) had a significant increase in neoplasms, especially mammary tumors, as compared with controls. Interestingly, in one study drug-fed rats lived longer than did controls. Two lifetime studies in hamsters were negative (see Finegold[29]). It should be noted that acetamide has been found in the urine of patients receiving metronidazole, and prolonged feeding of high doses of this compound to rats has produced hepatocarcinomas.[30] A study in rats[31] with the dimethylhydrazine (DMH) model for colon neoplasia noted that the addition of metronidazole on a long-term basis had an apparent cocarcinogenic effect. As Condon notes in the discussion of this paper, the DMH tumor model is relatively specific and may not be readily extrapolated to humans.[31] Indeed, in another study looking at bile salt–induced colorectal cancer in rats, metronidazole administration appeared to reduce the carcinogenic effect of sodium deoxycholate.[32]

Long-term follow-up of a cohort of 771 women who received metronidazole therapy for the treatment of vaginal trichomoniasis during the 1960s has not shown an increased incidence of malignancy.[33] It should be recognized that these patients received relatively low doses of the drug for brief periods of time (7–10 days). A recent report raises the possibility of carcinogenicity in three patients with Crohn's disease who had received prolonged therapy with metronidazole[34]; these observations remain anecdotal, and further studies are clearly needed. Although metronidazole appears to be safe, the long-term effects of high-dose prolonged therapy are not completely known, and such usage should be avoided if other alternatives are available.

Metronidazole crosses the placental barrier, and concerns have been raised about possible teratogenic effects in light of the evidence for mutagenicity in bacterial systems. To date, there has been little evidence for this in animal models, although one study has raised the possibility of fetal "genotoxicity" in pregnant golden Syrian hamsters fed high doses of metronidazole.[35] Studies in pregnant women who had received metronidazole during pregnancy for the treatment of vaginal trichomoniasis have not shown an increased incidence of stillbirths, small-for-age infants, premature infants, or teratogenicity.[36] Although there is one paper that raises the possibility of a metronidazole-induced teratogenic effect,[37] again, this may well be a coincidence and is not supported by other human or animal studies; nevertheless, the use of metronidazole during pregnancy should be reserved for situations in which it is clearly needed. Metronidazole during the first trimester should be avoided. Because metronidazole is excreted into breast milk, nursing should be discontinued during and for 2 days after therapy with metronidazole.

Drug Interactions, Interference with Laboratory Tests

In patients ingesting alcohol, metronidazole may cause reactions similar to those produced by disulfiram. Patients should

TABLE 3. Adverse Effects Related to Metronidazole Therapy

Major adverse reactions (rare)
  Seizures, encephalopathy
  Cerebellar dysfunction, ataxia
  Peripheral neuropathy
  Disulfiram reaction with alcohol
  Potentiation of effects of warfarin
  Pseudomembranous colitis
  Pancreatitis
Minor adverse reactions
  Minor gastrointestinal disturbances
  Reversible neutropenia
  Metallic taste
  Dark or red-brown urine
  Maculopapular rash, urticaria
  Urethral, vaginal burning
  Gynecomastia

be advised not to drink alcohol when taking this drug. Metronidazole inhibits the metabolism of warfarin and other oral coumarin-type anticoagulants. Therefore, if concomitant use must be carried out, the dosage of the anticoagulant should be reduced to maintain the desired prothrombin time.

Metronidazole interferes with certain chemical analyses for the serum enzyme glutamic oxaloacetic transaminase, which results in falsely low or negative values.

EFFECT ON NORMAL FECAL FLORA

In subjects who have a healthy gastrointestinal tract and are not receiving other drugs, metronidazole has very little effect on the fecal flora.[38] This is thought to be due to the drug being rapidly reduced by the bowel flora under the usual anaerobic conditions in the colon. Why this would not have an impact on the organisms carrying out the reduction, as it does in the course of treating infections, is not at all clear. In patients on high-dosage regimens, in patients with diarrhea, and in patients receiving certain other antimicrobial agents concurrently, there may be a significant impact of metronidazole on the fecal flora. For example, when oral neomycin or kanamycin (active primarily against nonanaerobes) is given with metronidazole, there is a significant impact on both the anaerobic and aerobic flora. Thus, it has been feasible to use metronidazole for therapy in certain conditions such as ileal bypass enteropathy and for preoperative "bowel preparation" along with an oral aminoglycoside.

CLINICAL USES

Parasitic Infections

Metronidazole has been used successfully for therapy for *Trichomonas* vaginitis for many years. It is also an effective agent for therapy of amebic liver abscess and has been used with generally good results in intestinal amebiasis. The drug is also effective against giardiasis, being at least as active as quinacrine for this purpose.

Some workers have felt that metronidazole has been effective in *Balantidium coli* infection and in infection due to *Dracunculus medinensis*, but these indications are certainly not well established. Metronidazole has been used in the treatment of cutaneous leishmaniasis, although it appears to be less effective than are other available agents.[39]

Anaerobic Infections

As is suggested by the spectrum of activity of metronidazole, this drug is useful for the vast majority of anaerobic infections. Certainly actinomycosis is one notable exception, and infections with *P. acnes,* which are uncommon, would be another. There is one other setting in which metronidazole may represent less than optimum therapy—anaerobic infections of the lower respiratory tract. Data from Sanders et al.[40] show a relatively high rate of suboptimal response. Most treatment failures had mixed infections with aerobic bacteria as well as anaerobes. The addition of penicillin G or ampicillin for mixed infections involving streptococci, pneumococci, or *Haemophilus influenzae* or the addition of erythromycin in the case of a penicillin-allergic patient would likely provide an excellent regimen. In the case of aspiration pneumonia involving aerobic and/or facultative gram-negative bacilli and/or *Staphylococcus aureus,* other appropriate therapy to cover these agents would be needed along with metronidazole. Many anaerobic infections are mixed with aerobic or facultative bacteria, of course, and particularly in sicker patients therapy aimed at both categories of organisms is desirable.

The excellent distribution of metronidazole throughout the body, including the central nervous system, and the impressive bactericidal activity of this compound, even against organisms that are not actively multiplying, make it an excellent choice for a number of serious infections, including brain abscess and other central nervous system infections involving anaerobes, endocarditis due to anaerobic bacteria, and, perhaps, any anaerobic infection of serious nature in patients who are immunocompromised.

The *B. fragilis* group of organisms is the one most commonly encountered in anaerobic infections overall. Until recently, there were only three drugs that were consistently active against this group—metronidazole, chloramphenicol, and clindamycin. Recently, a number of medical centers have been encountering varying degrees of resistance of the *B. fragilis* group to clindamycin. Thus, metronidazole may become an even more important part of the armamentarium for the management of anaerobic infections. It should be noted, however, that in intra-abdominal infections, in which *B. fragilis* is almost always involved, comparative studies[18] failed to show any significant difference among metronidazole, clindamycin, chloramphenicol, ticarcillin, or cefoxitin; most of these were used together with an aminoglycoside.

The resistance of a number of clostridia other than *Clostridium perfringens* to cefoxitin and clindamycin again suggests that metronidazole might have an advantage in selected intra-abdominal and obstetric and gynecologic infections. However, there are no specific data to back up this point.

Metronidazole has been useful against other types of anaerobic infections, including bacteremia, infections of bones and joints, soft tissue infections, oral and dental infections, and head and neck infections. Metronidazole has also provided good results in the therapy for bacterial vaginosis, a condition in which various anaerobes, *G. vaginalis,* or both may be important.[41,42] As noted elsewhere, it has been effective in the management of pseudomembranous colitis due to *Clostridium difficile.* Limited studies have shown that fecal levels of metronidazole (up to 1212 μg/g dry weight and 24.2 μg/g wet weight feces) may be attained by using either an oral or a parenteral route in patients with active colitis.[43,44] The parenteral route may be especially useful in patients who have *C. difficile*–induced toxic megacolon and are unable to take oral medications. Recent investigations have linked *Helicobacter pylori* to peptic ulcer disease; metronidazole, in combination with tetracycline and bismuth subsalicylate, appears to be effective therapy and markedly decreases the incidence of relapse.[45] A clinical study suggests that metronidazole may be more effective than penicillin is for antimicrobial therapy for tetanus.[46] Metronidazole is not a suitable alternative to penicillin for syphilis.

Other Therapeutic Uses

Metronidazole has been used experimentally in very high doses as a hypoxic cell sensitizer in radiotherapy for malignancy. It has been useful in a number of types of bowel bacterial overgrowth syndromes such as complications of jejunoileal bypass for obesity[47] and dysfunction of the continent ileostomy,[48] and for the prevention of intrahepatic cholestasis associated with total parenteral nutrition.[49] Although not everyone agrees, it appears that metronidazole has had a beneficial effect in Crohn's disease by producing a lessening of diarrhea (in patients with colonic involvement) and promoting the healing of perianal lesions and erythema nodosum.[50,51] Prolonged use of the drug, however, may result in a significant incidence of metronidazole-induced peripheral neuropathy,[52] and concerns have been raised about possible carcinogenic effects of the drug.[34]

Metronidazole is said to be beneficial in the treatment of acne rosacea whether used orally or topically.[53] An intriguing report[54] notes striking decreases in serum cholesterol and triglyceride levels in patients receiving metronidazole for other indications. Only short courses of therapy were used. There is no information as to the mechanism of this effect.

Prophylactic Use

Several groups have carried out prospective controlled studies of metronidazole, alone or in combination with other agents, for prophylaxis in patients undergoing elective colonic surgery, gynecologic surgery, or emergency appendectomy. In the case of appendectomy, a perforated appendix is an indication for therapy rather than prophylaxis, and in uncomplicated appendicitis the frequency of postoperative infection is quite low. In general, however, in these studies metronidazole has appeared to be as effective as other effective prophylactic agents. It should be kept in mind, however, that the prophylactic use of metronidazole is not an approved indication for the drug in the United States at present.

Finally, it should be appreciated that not all of the prophylactic trials have found metronidazole effective. Metronidazole was not effective prophylactically in one study of hysterectomy[55] and in one study of appendectomy for nonperforated appendictis.[56]

REFERENCES

1. Sutter VL. In vitro susceptibility of anaerobic and microaerophilic bacteria to metronidazole and its hydroxy metabolite. In: Finegold SM, George WL, Rolfe RD, eds. Proceedings of the First United States Metronidazole Conference. Tarpon Springs, FL, February 1982. New York: Biomedical Information Corp; 1982:61.
2. Wüst J. Susceptibility of anaerobic bacteria to metronidazole, ornidazole, and tinidazole and routine susceptibility testing by standardized methods. Antimicrob Agents Chemother. 1977;11:631.
3. Werner H, Schädler G, Krasemann C. In vitro activity of azlocillin, metronidazole and its hydroxy metabolite against anaerobes. Arzneimittelforsch Drug Res. 1983;33:574.
4. Rosenblatt JE, Edson RS. Metronidazole. Mayo Clin Proc. 1983;58:154.
5. Chow AW, Bednorz D, Guze LB. Susceptibility of obligate anaerobes to metronidazole: An extended study of 1,054 clinical isolates. In: Finegold SM, McFadzean JA, Roe FJC, eds. Metronidazole. Proceedings of the International Metronidazole Conference, Montreal, May 1976. Princeton, NJ: Excerpta Medica; 1977:286.
6. Reznikov M, McDonald PJ. Effect of metronidazole on *Escherichia coli* in the presence of *Bacteroides fragilis*: An investigation in mice. Chemotherapy. 1983;29:225.
7. Rasmussen BA, Bush K, Tally FP. Antimicrobial resistance in *Bacteroides*. Clin Infect Dis. 1993;16:S390–S400.
8. Reysset G, Haggoud A, Sebald M. Genetics of resistance of *Bacteroides* species to 5-nitroimidazole. Clin Infect Dis. 1993;16:S401–S403.
9. Phillips I, Warren C, Taylor E, et al. The antimicrobial susceptibility of anaerobic bacteria in a London teaching hospital. J Antimicrob Chemother. 1981; 8:17.
10. Tally FP, Snydman DR, Shimell MJ, et al. Mechanisms of antimicrobial resistance of *Bacteroides fragilis*. In: Phillips I, Collier J, eds. Metronidazole. Proceedings of the Second International Symposium on Anaerobic Infections, Geneva, April 1979. London: The Royal Society of Medicine and Academic Press. New York: Grune & Stratton; 1979:19.
11. Ingham HR, Eaton S, Venables CW, et al. *Bacteroides fragilis* resistant to metronidazole after long-term therapy. Lancet. 1978;1:214.
12. Sprott MS, Ingham HR, Hickman JE, et al. Metronidazole-resistant anaerobes. Lancet. 1983;1:1220.
13. Krajden S, Lossick JG, Wilk E, et al. Persistent *Trichomonas vaginalis* infection due to a metronidazole-resistant strain. Can Med Assoc J. 1986;134: 1373–4.
14. Müller M, Meingassner JG, Miller WA, et al. Three metronidazole-resistant strains of *Trichomonas vaginalis* from the United States. Am J Obstet Gynecol. 1980;138:808–12.
15. Dombrowski MP, Sokol RJ, Bronsteen RA. Intravenous therapy of metronidazole-resistant *Trichomonas vaginalis*. Obstet Gynecol. 1987;69:524–5.
16. Müller M. Mode of action of metronidazole on anaerobic bacteria and protozoa. In: Rhône-Poulenc Pharma Inc, Montreal. Proceedings of the North American Metronidazole Symposium on Anaerobic Infections, Scottsdale, AZ, October 1981. Surgery. 1983;93:165.
17. Nastro LJ, Finegold SM. Bactericidal activity of five antimicrobial agents against *Bacteroides fragilis*. J Infect Dis. 1972;126:104.
18. Tally FP, Sullivan CE. Metronidazole: In vitro activity, pharmacology and efficacy in anaerobic bacterial infections. Pharmacotherapy. 1981;1:28.
19. Corrodi P, Busch DF, Sutter VL, et al. Factors affecting the in vitro antibacterial activity of metronidazole In: Finegold SM, McFadzean JA, Roe FJC, eds. Metronidazole. Proceedings of the International Metronidazole Conference, Montreal, May 1976. Princeton, NJ: Excerpta Medica; 1977:299.
20. Bartlett JG, Dezfulian M, Joiner K. Relative efficacy and critical interval of antimicrobial agents in experimental infections involving *Bacteroides fragilis*. Arch Surg. 1983;118:181.
21. Fredricsson B, Hagström B, Nord C-E, et al. Systemic concentrations of metronidazole and its main metabolites after intravenous, oral and vaginal administration. Gynecol Obstet Invest. 1987;24:200–7.
22. Visser AA, Hundt HKL. The pharmacokinetics of a single intravenous dose of metronidazole in pregnant patients. J Antimicrob Chemother. 1984;13:279–83.
23. Mattila J, Nerdrum K, Rouhiainen H, et al. Penetration of metronidazole and tinidazole into the aqueous humor in man. Chemotherapy. 1983;29:188.
24. Guay DR, Meatherall RC, Baxter H, et al. Pharmacokinetics of metronidazole in patients undergoing continuous ambulatory peritoneal dialysis. Antimicrob Agents Chemother. 1984;25:306–10.
25. Lau AH, Evans R, Chang C-W, et al. Pharmacokinetics of metronidazole in patients with alcoholic liver disease. Antimicrob Agents Chemother. 1987;31: 1662–4.
26. Loft S, Sonne J, Dossing M, et al. Metronidazole pharmacokinetics in patients with hepatic encephalopathy. Scand J Gastroenterol. 1987;22:117–23.
27. Lambert B, Lindblad A, Lindsten J, et al. Genotoxic effects of metronidazole in human lymphocytes in vitro and in vivo. In: Phillips I, Collier J, eds. Metronidazole. Proceedings of the Second International Symposium on Anaerobic Infections, Geneva, April 1979. London: The Royal Society of Medicine and Academic Press. New York: Grune & Stratton; 1979:229.
28. Hartley-Asp B. Chromosomal studies on human lymphocytes exposed to metronidazole in vivo and in vitro. In: Phillips I, Collier J, eds: Metronidazole. Proceedings of the Second International Symposium on Anaerobic Infections, Geneva, April 1979. London: The Royal Society of Medicine and Academic Press; New York: Grune & Stratton; 1979:237.
29. Finegold SM. Metronidazole. Ann Intern Med. 1980;93:585.
30. Koch RL, Chrystal EJT, Beaulieu BB, et al. Acetamide—A metabolite of metronidazole formed by the intestinal flora. Biochem Pharmacol. 1979;28: 3611.
31. Sloan DA, Fleiszer DM, Richards GK, et al. Increased incidence of experimental colon cancer associated with long-term metronidazole therapy. Am J Surg. 1983;145:66.
32. Rainey JB, Maeda M, Williams C, et al. The cocarcinogenic effect of intrarectal deoxycholate in rats is reduced by oral metronidazole. Br J Cancer. 1984; 49:631–6.
33. Beard CM, Noller KL, O'Fallon WM, et al. Cancer after exposure to metronidazole. Mayo Clin Proc. 1988;63:147–53.
34. Krause JR, Ayuyang HQ, Ellis LD. Occurrence of three cases of carcinoma in individuals with Crohn's disease treated with metronidazole. Am J Gastroenterol. 1985;80:978–82.
35. Garry VF, Nelson RL. Host-mediated transformation: Metronidazole. Mutat Res. 1987;190:289–95.
36. Robbie MO, Sweet RL. Metronidazole use in obstetrics and gynecology: A review. Am J Obstet Gynecol. 1983;145:865–81.
37. Cantú JM, Garcia-Cruz D. Midline facial defect as a teratogenic effect of metronidazole. March Dimes Birth Defect Fdn 1982;18:85–8.
38. Lewis RP, Wideman P, Sutter VL, et al. The effect of metronidazole on human fecal flora. In: Finegold SM, McFadzean JA, Roe FJC, eds. Metronidazole. Proceedings of the International Metronidazole Conference, Montreal, May 1976. Princeton, NJ: Excerpta Medica; 1977:307.
39. Chong H. Oriental sore. A look at trends in and approaches to the treatment of leishmaniasis. Int J Dermatol. 1986;25:615–23.
40. Sanders CV, Hanna BJ, Lewis AC, et al. The use of metronidazole in the treatment of anaerobic pleuropulmonary infections. In: Phillips I, Collier J, eds. Metronidazole. Proceedings of the Second International Symposium on Anaerobic Infections, Geneva, April 1979. London: The Royal Society of Medicine and Academic Press. New York: Grune & Stratton, 1979:83.
41. Swedberg J, Steiner JF, Deiss F, et al. Comparison of single-dose vs one-week course of metronidazole for symptomatic bacterial vaginosis. JAMA. 1985;254:1046–9.
42. Biswas NJ. Bacterial vaginosis. Clin Obstet Gynecol. 1993;36:166–76.
43. Kleinfeld DI, Sharpe RJ, Donta ST. Parenteral therapy for antibiotic-associated pseudomembranous colitis. J Infect Dis. 1988;157:389.
44. Bolton RP, Culshaw MA. Faecal metronidazole concentrations during oral and intravenous therapy for antibiotic associated colitis due to *Clostridium difficile*. Gut. 1986;27:1169–72.
45. Graham DY. Treatment of peptic ulcers caused by *Helicobacter pylori*. N Engl J Med. 1993;328:349–50.
46. Ahmadsyah I, Salim A. Treatment of tetanus: An open study to compare the efficacy of procaine penicillin and metronidazole. Br Med J. 1985;291:648–50.
47. Drenick EJ. Extraintestinal complications of jejunoileal bypass for obesity. In: Finegold SM, George WL, Rolfe RD, eds. Proceedings of the First United States Metronidazole Conference, Tarpon Springs, FL, February 1982. New York: Biomedical Information Corp; 1982:371.
48. Kelly DG, Phillips SF, Kelly KA, et al. Dysfunction of the continent ileostomy: Clinical features and bacteriology. Gut. 1983;24:193.
49. Capron J-P, Herve M-A, Gineston J-L, et al. Metronidazole in prevention of cholestasis associated with total parenteral nutrition. Lancet. 1983;1:446.
50. Gilat T. Metronidazole in Crohn's disease (Editorial). Gastroenterology. 1982; 83:702.
51. Bernstein CN, Shanahan F. Metronidazole in Crohn's disease: What's the score? Gastroenterology. 1992;102:1435–6.
52. Duffy LF, Daum F, Fisher SE, et al. Peripheral neuropathy in Crohn's disease patients treated with metronidazole. Gastroenterology. 1985;88:681–4.
53. Nielsen PG. Metronidazole treatment in rosacea. Int J Dermatol. 1988;27: 1–5.
54. Davis JL, Schultz TA, Mosley CA. Metronidazole lowers serum lipids. Ann Intern Med. 1983;99:43.

55. Vincelette J, Finkelstein F, Aoki FY, et al. Double-blind trial of perioperative intravenous metronidazole prophylaxis for abdominal and vaginal hysterectomy. In: Rhône-Poulenc Pharma Inc, Montreal. Proceedings of the North American Metronidazole Symposium on Anaerobic Infections, Scottsdale, AZ, October 1981. Surgery. 1983;93:185.
56. Keiser TA, MacKenzie RL, Feld R, et al. Prophylactic metronidazole in appendectomy: A double-blind controlled trial. In: Rhône-Poulenc Pharma Inc, Montreal. Proceedings of the North American Metronidazole Symposium on Anaerobic Infections, Scottsdale, AZ, October 1981. Surgery. 1983;93:201.

BIBLIOGRAPHY

Finegold SM, McFadzean JA, Roe FJC, eds. Metronidazole. Proceedings of the International Metronidazole Conference, Montreal, May 1976. Princeton, NJ: Excerpta Medica; 1977.
Finegold SM. Metronidazole. Ann Intern Med. 1980;93:585.
Finegold SM, George WL, Rolfe RD, eds. Proceedings of the First United States Metronidazole Conference, Tarpon Springs, FL, February 1982. New York: Biomedical Information Corp; 1982.
Kucers A, Bennett N McK, Kemp RJ, eds. Metronidazole. In: The Use of Antibiotics. Philadelphia: JB Lippincott; 1987.
May & Baker, Ltd. "Flagyl" (Metronidazole) in Anaerobic Infections. Essex, England: May & Baker, Ltd; 1979.
Phillips I, Collier J, eds. Metronidazole. Proceedings of the Second International Symposium on Anaerobic Infections, Geneva, April 1979. London: The Royal Society of Medicine and Academic Press; New York: Grune & Stratton 1979.
Rhône-Poulenc Pharma Inc., Montreal. Proceedings of the North American Metronidazole Symposium on Anaerobic Infections, Scottsdale, AZ, October 1981. Surgery. 1983;93:123.
Rosenblatt JE, Edson RS. Metronidazole. Mayo Clin Proc. 1987;62:1013-17.
Stranz MH, Bradley WE. Metronidazole (Flagyl IV, Searle). Drug Intell Clin Pharm. 1981;15:838.

24. MACROLIDES AND CLINDAMYCIN

NEAL H. STEIGBIGEL

The macrolide antibiotics (erythromycin, azithromycin, clarithromycin, and others) and the lincosamide antibiotics (lincobmycin and clindamycin) are chemically unrelated but possess many similar biologic properties in terms of mechanisms of action and resistance, antimicrobial activity, and clinical pharmacology. Erythromycin, still the most important of the macrolide antibiotics, has a few primary indications in therapy and is often useful as an alternative to penicillin G. It is one of the safest antibiotics in clinical use. Azithromycin and clarithromycin have some advantages over erythromycin in their antimicrobial activity, pharmacokinetics, fewer gastrointestinal side effects and promise in the treatment of certain AIDS-related opportunistic infections. Clindamycin has been restricted in use by its potential gastrointestinal toxicity but remains particularly important in the treatment of certain anaerobic infections. Lincomycin is now mainly of historic interest.

ERYTHROMYCIN

Derivation, Chemistry, and Preparations

Erythromycin was derived in 1952 from a strain of *Streptomyces erythreus* obtained from soil from the Philippines. The structure (Fig. 1) consists of a 14-member macrocyclic lactone ring, therefore the class name *macrolide*, attached to two sugar moieties, desosamine and cladinose. Erythromycin base is poorly soluble in water, has a pK of 8.8, is rapidly inactivated by gastric acid, and is often inconsistently absorbed after oral administration. Pharmaceutical preparations for oral use have been made with an aim to diminish destruction by gastric acid and to promote better absorption. Six preparations for oral use are available:

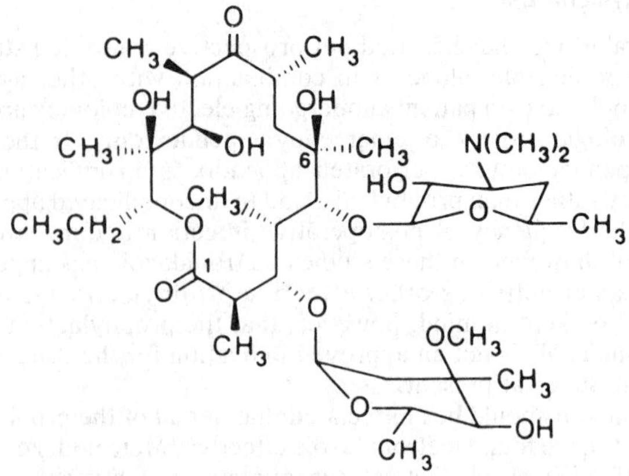

FIG. 1. Erythromycin base.

enteric-coated tablets (Ilotycin, E-mycin, Ery-Tab, Robimycin, and generics), enteric-coated pellets in capsules (Eryc), and "film"-coated tablets of the base (Filmtab, Abbott); stearate salt (formed in association with the amino group on desosamine) and available as film-coated tablets (Erythrocin, Bristamycin, other brand names, and generics); ethylsuccinate ester (formed with the hydroxyl group on desosamine), available in tablet, chewable, and liquid forms (Erythrocin, Eryped, EES, Pediamycin); and lauryl sulfate salt of the propionyl ester (the estolate), available in tablet, capsule, or liquid forms (Ilosone). There are two water-soluble salts of erythromycin prepared for intravenous use, erythromycin gluceptate (Ilotycin gluceptate) and erythromycin lactobionate (Erythrocin lactobionate). The drug is not given intramuscularly because of pain on injection. Erythromycin base is also available in 1.5% and 2% topical solutions, gels, and creams for treatment of acne vulgaris and in an ophthalmic ointment for treatment of bacterial conjunctivitis and prevention of neonatal gonococcal and chlamydial conjunctivitis.

Mechanisms of Action

Erythromycin inhibits RNA-dependent protein synthesis at the step of chain elongation in susceptible prokaryotic organisms. A single molecule of the antibiotic reversibly binds to the 50S ribosomal subunit, resulting in blockage of the transpeptidation and/or translocation reactions.[1-3] In some bacteria erythromycin interferes with the ribosomal binding of other macrolides, lincomycin, and chloramphenicol, suggesting common or overlapping binding sites for these antibiotics.

Antimicrobial Activity and Mechanisms of Resistance

The antimicrobial activity of erythromycin is broad in spectrum, being exhibited against gram-positive and gram-negative bacteria, including actinomycetes and mycobacteria, as well as against treponemes, mycoplasmas, *Chlamydia*, and rickettsia. Depending on the drug concentration, bacterial species, phase of growth, and density of the inoculum, erythromycin may be primarily bacteriostatic or bactericidal. Bacterial killing is favored by higher antibiotic concentrations, lower bacterial density, and rapid growth.[4] The activity of erythromycin, which is a weak base, increases markedly with increasing pH over the range 5.5–8.5 for both gram-positive and gram-negative bacteria,[5,6] possibly reflecting increased entry into the bacterial cell of the un-ionized drug that is more plentiful at the higher pH.

The in vitro susceptibilities of potential pathogens to erythromycin are listed in Table 1.[7-19] Erythromycin shows high activity against the majority of pneumococci and group A streptococci isolated in the United States; however, resistant clinical

TABLE 1. In Vitro Susceptibilities to Erythromycin, Azithromycin, and Clarithromycin

Organism	Erythromycin		Azithromycin		Clarithromycin	
	MIC$_{50}$[a]	MIC$_{90}$[b]	MIC$_{50}$	MIC$_{90}$	MIC$_{50}$	MIC$_{90}$
S. pneumoniae	0.03–0.12	0.015–1	0.06–0.5	0.12–2	0.015–0.06	0.015–0.5
S. pyogenes	0.03–0.12	0.03–4	0.12–1	0.12–4	0.012–0.03	0.012–2
S. agalactiae	0.03–0.12	0.03–0.25	0.12–0.5	0.12–0.5	0.03–0.12	0.03–0.25
Viridans streptococci	0.06	>3.1	8	16	—	0.03
Enterococcus spp.	1.5	>100	8	>32	0.5–1	>32
S. aureus						
Methicillin-sensitive	0.12–0.5	>128	0.12–1	>128	0.06–0.25	>128
Methicillin-resistant	>128	>128	>128	>128	>128	>128
S. epidermidis	8–32	>128	16	>128	4	>128
C. diphtheriae	0.02	3.1	—	—	—	—
L. monocytogenes	0.25–0.5	0.5–4	1–2	2–4	0.12–0.25	0.12–2
M. catarrhalis	0.12–0.5	0.25–2	<0.015–0.12	0.03–0.5	0.06–0.12	0.12–1
H. influenzae	1–8	2–32	0.25–4	0.25–4	1–8	2–16
B. pertussis	—	0.03	0.015	0.06–0.12	—	0.03
N. gonorrhoeae	0.12–0.5	0.25–2	<0.025–0.12	0.03–0.25	0.125–0.25	0.25–2
N. meningitidis	0.4	1.6	0.06	0.12	—	—
C. jejuni	0.5–2	1–4	0.25	0.12–0.5	0.5–2	1–8
H. pylori	0.12	0.25	0.25	0.25	0.03	0.03
M. pneumoniae	0.004–0.01	0.004–0.02	0.01–0.03	0.01–0.12	0.004–0.5	0.03–0.5
C. trachomatis	0.06–1	0.06–2	0.03–0.06	0.12–0.25	0.004–0.06	0.008–0.125
L. pneumophila	0.1–1	0.5–2	0.12–0.5	0.25–2	0.12–0.25	0.25
B. fragilis	2–8	4–32	2–3.2	2–8	1–2	2–8
Peptococcus, Peptostreptococcus	<0.12–2	2–>32	0.25–1	2–4	0.25–2	4–>32
C. perfringens	1	1	0.25–0.78	0.25–0.78	0.25–0.5	0.5–2
P. acnes	<0.03	<0.03–0.03	<0.004–0.015	0.03–0.15	<0.03–0.03	0.03–0.25

[a] Minimum inhibitory concentration for 50 percent of isolates in μg/ml. Values are the ranges reported in the referenced publications.
[b] Minimum inhibitory concentration for 90 percent of isolates in μg/ml. Values are the ranges reported in the referenced publcations.

isolates have been encountered, especially outside of the United States from patient populations recently exposed to erythromycin or clindamycin.[20-26] Of 200 strains of *Streptococcus pneumoniae* isolated from patients with pneumococcal disease in a survey conducted in Spain, 5 were found to be highly resistant to erythromycin and clindamycin.[22] Up to 30 percent of strains of pneumococci isolated in France in 1986 were found to be resistant to these antibiotics.[23] In a study in Japan, 60 percent of strains of group A streptococci isolated from infected children were highly resistant to erythromycin and lincomycin.[24] Almost all of these resistant strains were of type 12, and erythromycin had been widely used to treat respiratory infections in Japan in the several years before the study. A survey of 474 group A streptococcal strains isolated from patients in Oklahoma in 1980 indicated that 5 percent had minimal inhibitory concentrations (MIC) to erythromycin by microtiter broth dilution ≥ 1 μ/ml.[25] In Finland, where there has been a great increase in the use of erythromycin in recent years, resistance to that antibiotic was found in up to 44 percent of clinical isolates of group A streptococci from some communities in 1990.[26] The emergence of resistance to erythromycin encountered in clinical isolates of these organisms from patient populations treated with this antibiotic is consistent with in vitro studies with pneumococci and streptococci subcultured sequentially in the presence of erythromycin, demonstrating the selection of erythromycin resistance and often cross-resistance to other macrolides and lincomycin. Similar in vitro results are obtained with staphylococci.[27] Although resistance to erythromycin by *S. aureus* may be selected by its use in hospitals,[28] most methicillin-sensitive clinical isolates are presently sensitive to this agent.[29] However, there is always a potential for the emergence, during treatment in an individual patient, of erythromycin resistance by *S. aureus*.[7,27,30,31] These strains may demonstrate the emergence of one-step high-level resistance to erythromycin alone or may show cross-resistance to other macrolides and to lincomycin and clindamycin. In addition, staphylococci isolated from patients treated with erythro-

mycin may exhibit a phenomenon called *dissociated resistance* by Garrod.[32] Only a small proportion of the population of such staphylococcal isolates exhibit resistance when grown in large concentrations of erythromycin; however, in the presence of lower concentrations of erythromycin almost the entire population demonstrates resistance to erythromycin, to other macrolides, and often to the lincosamide antibiotics. In the absence of erythromycin these organisms appear sensitive to these antibiotics. Methicillin-resistant strains of *S. aureus* are almost always resistant to erythromycin.[33]

The majority of strains of the "viridans" group of streptococci, *Listeria monocytogenes*, and *Corynebacterium diphtheriae* show appreciable susceptibility to erythromycin. Many strains of *Clostridium perfringens* may be only moderately sensitive.[34] Appreciable in vitro activity has been demonstrated against *Actinomyces israelii*, *Mycobacterium scrofulaceum*, and *Mycobacterium kansasii*[35] and against *Nocardia asteroides* when combined with ampicillin.[36]

With gram-negative bacteria, erythromycin displays consistent and useful activity against *Neisseria meningitidis*, *Neisseria gonorrhoeae*, and *Bordetella pertussis*[8] and somewhat lower activity against *Haemophilus influenzae*.[37] High bacteriostatic and bactericidal activity is demonstrated against over 90 percent of strains of *Campylobacter jejuni*.[10] Erythromycin has activity against some species of gram-negative anaerobes, but *Bacteroides fragilis* strains are usually resistant.[38] The Enterobacteriaceae are usually resistant, except as the pH rises to 8.5.[6]

The extensive spectrum of activity of erythromycin is also demonstrated by its clinically useful activity against such diverse organisms as *Treponema pallidum*, *Legionella pneumophila*,[9] *Mycoplasma pneumoniae*, *Ureaplasma urealyticum*, some strains of *Rickettsia*, and *Chlamydia trachomatis*. Erythromycin is about 50 times more potent against *M pneumoniae* than tetracycline.[39] Erythromycin-resistant variants of *M. pneumoniae* have been isolated in the laboratory and from a patient.[40]

Resistance to erythromycin may be the result of the following:

(1) Decreased permeability of the cell envelope to the drug is exhibited by the Enterobacteriaceae; cell-free systems and protoplasts of these organisms are susceptible to the drug.[29,41,42] This intrinsic resistance is also exhibited by *Pseudomonas* spp. and *Acinetobacter* spp. Plasmid-mediated erythromycin resistance in *S. epidermidis* due to active efflux of the drug has also been described.[29] *(2)* Alteration in a single 50S ribosomal protein of the receptor site confers resistance to erythromycin and often to other macrolides, lincomycin, and clindamycin; in some but not all strains this is associated with a decreased binding affinity for erythromycin.[2] This one-step high-level resistance is the result of chromosomal mutation, has been demonstrated in some strains of *Bacillus subtilis*, *Streptococcus pyogenes*, *Campylobacter* spp. and *Escherichia coli* and probably occurs in *S. aureus*. *(3)* Alteration in the 23S ribosomal RNA of the 50S ribosomal subunit by methylation of adenine.[43] This is associated with resistance to erythromycin and often to other macrolides (M), lincocasamides (L, lincomycin, and clindamycin), and streptogramin type B (S$_B$); this pattern of resistance is referred to as *MLS$_B$ phenotype* and is usually mediated by plasmids or transposons on chromosomes. The resistance is due to decreased binding of the antibiotics to their overlapping targets on the ribosome, which is probably altered in conformation by methylation. It can be exhibited by strains of *S. aureus*, streptococci (including *S. pneumoniae*), *Enterococcus* spp., *C. diphtheriae*, *Campylobacter* spp., *B. fragilis*, *C. perfringens*, *Listeria* spp., *M. pneumoniae* and *Legionella* spp. This phenomenon may be constitutive or inducible by subinhibitory concentrations of erythromycin that bring about induction of the methylating enzyme. The inducible mechanism seems to explain the phenomenon of dissociated resistance already described. Several determinants of MLS$_B$ resistance have been defined, including the erm A, erm B, and erm C genes of *S. aureus*. *(4)* Enzymatic inactivation of erythromycin by esterases or a phosphotransferase in strains of Enterobacteriaceae with high-level resistance has been demonstrated.[29] The esterase genes (ere A and ere B) are probably encoded by a plasmid-mediated determinant.[29]

Clinical Pharmacology

The peak serum levels obtained after single doses of various erythromycin preparations are given in Table 2.[7,8,38,44,45] Erythromycin base is subject to destruction by gastric acid, and preparations of the base have been made with an acid-resistant coating to delay drug dissolution until it reaches the small bowel. The esters and ester salts of erythromycin are more acid stable, form a stable suspension in water, and are tasteless. These characteristics are used in the liquid suspension for children. Erythromycin base (absorbed intact), stearate absorbed as the base), and ethylsuccinate (absorbed both as the intact ester and as the free base after hydrolysis in the intestine) are usually absorbed more completely in the fasting state, although one study demonstrated increased absorption of a stearate preparation when taken with a meal.[45] After absorption, about 45 percent of the ethylsuccinate preparation is present in the serum as the inactive ester and about 55 percent as the active base. Average serum levels achieved under fasting conditions with these preparations are similar; however, results with the base may be erratic. Erythromycin base has become available in a capsule containing enteric-coated granules; this preparation is promoted as giving more uniform absorption.[46,48] but some enteric-coated tablets may provide similar blood levels.[47] The absorption of the estolate is not affected by food, and the resulting peak serum level consists of both free base (20–30 percent) (active form) and estolate (70–80 percent) (much less active); the level of base thus achieved is similar to that achieved by the other oral preparations taken in comparable doses in the fasting state. The clinical significance of the much less active esterified form of the drug that is present in serum in appreciable concentration is controversial. It would seem that in treatment of infections of only moderate severity by organisms highly sensitive to erythromycin (*S. penumoniae*, *S. pyogenes*, *M. pneumoniae*), differences in therapeutic results using the various oral preparations will be insignificant. Limited clinical comparisons confirm that suspicion.[49] However, in the treatment of group A streptococcal pharyngitis in children, substantially higher rates of bacteriologic eradication and lower rates of gastrointestinal side effects have been reported with the estolate preparation in comparison with the ethylsuccinate formulation.[50] Intravenous preparations of erythromycin achieve appreciably higher serum levels and should be used to treat serious infections requiring erythromycin.

Erythromycin is distributed through total body water.[51] Values given for protein binding vary from 40 to 90 percent; however, the significance of such binding is speculative.[52] The drug persists in tissues longer than in the blood. The ratios of tissue or body fluid concentrations to simultaneous serum concentrations (usually at peak) are for aqueous humor, 0.3; ascites, 0.4; bile, 28; middle ear exudate in otitis media, 0.3–0.7; pleural fluid, 0.7; prostatic fluid, 0.4; cerebrospinal fluid without meningitis, 0–0.02, with meningitis, 0.05–0.1; infected maxillary paranasal sinus, 0.4–0.8; tonsil, 0.3. Concentrations achieved in the middle ear in otitis media are adequate to treat pneumococcal and group A streptococcal infections but are not adequate to eradicate consistently *H. influenzae*.[53,54] High concentrations of erythromycin are achieved in alveolar macrophages[55] and polymorphonuclear leukocytes[56] compared to those in extracellular fluid.

There are very limited data on concentrations of erythromycin achieved in the cerebrospinal fluid of patients with meningitis, which suggest that large parenteral doses may be effective against meningeal infection by highly susceptible organisms such as *S. pneumoniae*.[57] Limited data from patients with septic arthritis suggest poor penetration of synovial fluid. Erythromycin is transferred across the placenta; fetal serum concentrations are about 2 percent of those in maternal serum, but higher concentrations accumulate in fetal tissue and amniotic fluid.[58] The drug is excreted in breast milk.

Up to 4.5 percent of an oral dose and 15 percent of a parenteral dose of erythromycin are recoverable in the urine.[7,8] Urine concentrations after oral doses are often high, but quite variable. Erythromycin is concentrated by the liver and excreted into the bile in high concentrations; however, only about 1.5 percent of the dose of the base and 0.2 percent of the ester can be recovered in bile in the first 8 hours, and some of this is reabsorbed from the intestine.[59] The higher serum levels achieved by the estolate have been attributed to both better absorption and lower biliary

TABLE 2. Serum Levels of Erythromycin in Adults

Preparation	Dose (mg)	Route	Peak Serum Level — Hours After Dose	Peak Serum Level — µg/ml
Base	250	Oral	4	0.3–1.0[a]
	500			0.3–1.9
Stearate	250 (fasting)	Oral	3	0.2–1.3
	500 (fasting)		3	0.4–1.8
	500 (after food)		3	0.1–0.4[b]
Ethylsuccinate	500	Oral	0.5–2.5	1.5[c] (0.6[d])
Estolate	250	Oral	2–4	1.4–1.7
	500		3.5–4	4.2[c] (1.1[d])
Lactobionate	200	Intravenous	Immediately	3–4
	500		1	9.9
Gluceptate	250	Intravenous	Immediately	3.5–10.7
	1000		1	9.9

[a] Somewhat higher levels reported with some enteric-coated preparations after repeated doses.[46,47]
[b] One study demonstrated higher levels (to 2.8 µg/ml) with dose taken during a meal.[45]
[c] Total drug (inactive ester and free base.)
[d] Free base.

excretion. After an oral dose, large concentrations of the antibiotic are found in feces, probably representing ingested drug that was never absorbed as well as some that was excreted in bile. A large proportion of absorbed drug cannot be accounted for by urinary or biliary excretion or by tissue binding and may be inactivated in the liver by demethylation.[60]

The normal serum half-life of erythromycin is 1.4 hours, and appreciable serum levels are maintained for 6 hours. In anuric patients, the half-life is only prolonged to about 5 hours, and dosage reduction in patients with renal failure is generally therefore not necessary.[61] Erythromycin is not removed by peritoneal dialysis or hemodialysis.

ADVERSE REACTIONS

Erythromycin is one of the safest antibiotics in clinical use. Untoward reactions except for pseudomembranous colitis and ventricular arrhythmias (with intravenous use) are not life threatening and, with the exception of the irritative reactions, are rare.

1. Irritative reactions are as follows:
   a. Dose-related abdominal cramps, nausea, vomiting, diarrhea, and gas occur more commonly in children and young adults than in older individuals and may be associated with intravenous as well as oral administration. These side effects appear to be due to a gastrointestinal motility-stimulating effect of the 14-member ring macrolides.[62,63] In this regard, erythromycin acts as a motilin receptor agonist in the gut and gallbladder.[64] Enteric coating of erythromycin base in the form of pellets in a capsule (e.g., ERYC) does not reduce the common dose-related gastrointestinal side effects of oral erythromycin.[65]
   b. Thrombophlebitis with intravenous use can be decreased by appropriate dilution of the dose in at least 250 ml of solution and by avoiding rapid bolus infusions (infuse over about 45–60 minutes).
2. Allergic reactions include skin rash, fever, and eosinophilia.
3. Cholestatic hepatitis occurs rarely[66] and almost always with the estolate preparation and chiefly in adults.[67] The syndrome typically begins after 20 days of therapy, but more rapidly in those previously treated, and consists of nausea, vomiting, and abdominal pain followed by jaundice, fever, and abnormal liver function tests consistent with cholestatic hepatitis. These findings are sometimes accompanied by rash, leukocytosis, and eosinophilia. The abnormalities generally clear within days to a few weeks after stopping the drug but may return rapidly on rechallenge. The syndrome appears to represent a hypersensitivity reaction to the specific structure of the estolate compound.[68] However, hepatocyte toxicity induced by the drug or its metabolites, as well as allergy to altered hepatocyte components, may be contributory.[69] Milder forms of the syndrome occur with the estolate and may be more common in pregnant women.[70] It must be distinguished from false-positive serum glutamic-oxaloacetic transaminase (AST) elevations that occur in patients taking the estolate.[71] The latter may be found when AST is determined by colorimetric procedures rather than by an enzymatic method and seems to result from an interfering substance present in the blood in association with estolate administration. Reversible hepatotoxicity has occurred with the stearate salt and the ethylsuccinate ester of erythromycin.[72,73]
4. Transient hearing loss has been reported rarely in association with the use of large intravenous doses of erythromycin lactobionate or large doses of oral erythromycin.[74,75] This may occur more commonly in elderly patients with renal insufficiency.[76–78] The ototoxicity is dependent on the serum concentration of the drug.[79]
5. Polymorphic ventricular tachycardia with QT prolongation (torsade de pointes) has been rarely reported in association with treatment with intravenous erythromycin.[80]
6. Superinfection, especially of the gastrointestinal tract or vagina, with *Candida* species or gram-negative bacilli may occur, as with other antibiotics.
7. Pseudomembranous colitis caused by overgrowth of toxin-producing *Clostridium difficile* occurs rarely with the use of erythromycin.[81,82]

Drug Interactions

Incompatibility during administration between intravenous preparations of erythromycin and other drugs has been reported; the latter include vitamin B complex and vitamin C, cephalothin, tetracycline, chloramphenicol, colistin, heparin, metraminol, and diphenylhydantoin.

Erythromycin may produce interactions with other drugs by interfering with their hepatic metabolism through the cytochrome P-450 enzyme system.[83] This may occur because erythromycin metabolites are capable of forming inactive complexes with cytochrome P-450 enzymes.[84] When oral theophylline and oral erythromycin are used concurrently, increased blood levels of theophylline and potential theophylline toxicity may result.[85] By the same mechanism, erythromycin can increase the anticoagulant effect of warfarin[86] and interfere with the metabolism of methylprednisolone,[87] triazolam, midazolan, afentanil, disopyramidine, bromocriptine,[84] carbamazapine,[88] and cyclosporine,[89] sometimes leading to toxicity with the latter two drugs. Elevations of terfenadine or aztemizole serum concentrations have been associated with the use of erythromycin and have led to serious ventricular arrhythmias.

Erythromycin can increase the bioavailability of digoxin by interfering with its inactivation by gut flora.[83] Erythromycin may inhibit the assay organism used in some determinations of serum folic acid. Sequential use of erythromycin and clindamycin should be avoided when possible because of the potential for the development of cross or "dissociated" resistance.

Uses of Erythromycin

Erythromycin has a few indications for use as the drug of choice and a larger number of important applications as an alternative drug to penicillin G (Table 3).[90] When used in adults by the oral route, preparations other than the estolate are generally preferable because they have less risk of cholestatic hepatitis. Absorption, particularly with the enteric-coated base, stearate, or ethylsuccinate preparations taken in the fasting state or before meals, is usually adequate. The estolate preparation should be particularly avoided during pregnancy, when hepatotoxicity may be more common.[70] When higher serum levels are needed in more severe infections requiring erythromycin therapy, the drug should be given intravenously.

Treatment of *M. pneumoniae* infection with erythromycin, as with tetracycline, shortens the clinical course of the infection; radiologic clearing of pulmonary lesions occurs earlier with erythromycin.[91] Clinical experience and studies in vitro and in guinea pigs suggest that erythromycin is very effective in treating pneumonia caused by *L. pneumophila* or *L. micdadei*.[9,92,93] The use of erythromycin in combination with rifampin is now favored, especially in severe cases.[90,94] Early treatment of pertussis with erythromycin is associated with both clinical improvement and a reduction in secondary transmission in households.[95] Erythromycin treatment of patients with gastroenteritis caused by *C. jejuni* hastens the eradication of the organism from the feces, but it does not appear to alter the clinical course of uncomplicated infection when therapy begins 4 days or more after the onset of symptoms.[96] However, earlier treatment of

TABLE 3. Major Uses of Erythromycin

Indication	Doses of Erythromycin for Adults	Alternative Drug
Infections in which erythromycin is the drug of first choice		
M. pneumoniae infections	0.5 g tid-qid po[a]	Tetracycline
Legionella pneumonia	0.5–1.0 g qid po[a] (plus rifampin)	Trimethoprim-sulfamethoxazole
Diphtheria[b]	Carrier state: 500 mg qid po for 10 days	Penicillin G
	Disease[a]: followed by oral for 10 days	Penicillin G
Pertussis	0.5 g qid po	Ampicillin
Chl. trachomatis pneumonia or conjunctivitis	10 mg/kg qid po	Sulfisoxazole[f]
Chlamydial pelvic infection in pregnancy	0.5–1.0 g qid po[a,c]	Amoxicillin
Prevention of infection after colorectal surgery	1 g po each of neomycin and erythromycin base at 1, 2, and 11 P.M. on the day before surgery combined with vigorous purgation over the 2 days before surgery	Parenteral cephalosporin
Bacillary angiomatosis	0.5 g qid po for at least 6 weeks; with visceral involvement several months of therapy is used	Doxycycline
Infections in which erythromycin is an important alternative drug		*Drug of first choice*
Groups A, C, G streptococcal infection	250–500 mg qid po[a,d]	Penicillin G
S. pneumoniae infection	250–500 mg qid po[a]	Penicillin G
Chlamydia pneumoniae (TWAR) infection	0.5 g tid-qid po[a]	A tetracycline
Rheumatic fever prophylaxis	250 mg bid po	Penicillin G
Prevention of bacterial endocarditis (in dental procedures)	1.0 g po 2 hr before procedure, then 500 mg 6 hr later	Ampicillin
Lymphogranuloma venereum	500 mg qid po for 21 days	Tetracycline
Chancroid	500 mg qid po for 7 days	Ceftriaxone
Nongonococcal urethritis	500 mg qid po for 7 days	Tetracycline
Syphilis 1°, 2°, latent (<1 year) in pregnancy	500 mg qid po for 15 days[e]	Penicillin G
later (>1 year) in pregnancy	500 mg qid po for 30 days[e]	Penicillin G
Bronchopulmonary anaerobic infections	0.5 gm qid po	Penicillin G; clindamycin
C. jejuni gastroenteritis	250 mg qid po	Ciprofloxacin
Acne vulgaris	250 mg qid po or topical preparation	Tetracycline po and a number of topical drugs

[a] Intravenous therapy (2–4 g/day) should be used in serious illness or when oral therapy is not possible or reliable.
[b] Antitoxin is essential primary therapy for disease.
[c] Severe pelvic inflammatory disease is often polymicrobial in origin; treatment of such cases should include other agents more active against likely facultative and anaerobic enteritic bacteria and/or N. gonorrhoeae.
[d] Treatment should be continued for 10 days for group A.
[e] Effectiveness uncertain. Careful follow-up needed when used in pregnancy. Infants should be treated with penicillin at birth.
[f] Only for infants more than 4 wks old.

young children with acute dysentery associated with *C. jejuni* has been shown to shorten the course of diarrhea and fecal excretion of the organism.[97] Nevertheless, in an institutional setting in Thailand, where *C. jejuni* strains were frequently resistant to erythromycin in vitro, early treatment of infants with diarrhea due to this organism was not beneficial.[98] Treatment of infants with erythromycin for pneumonia due to *C. trachomatis* appears to speed recovery and eradication of the shedding of organisms.[99] Erythromycin is preferable to tetracycline in treating chlamydial pelvic infection during pregnancy.[90] Erythromycin base given orally together with neomycin on the day before colorectal surgery and combined with vigorous purgation is about as effective as parenteral cephalosporin administration just before surgery in decreasing the incidence of septic complications.[100] No advantage has been demonstrated for the use of a combination of oral and intravenous antibiotics.[101] In the presence of bowel obstruction or when there is need for emergency surgery, the parenteral antibiotic regimen should be used.[90] Erythromycin has become one of the drugs of choice in treating bacillary angiomatosis in patients with acquired immunodeficiency syndrome (AIDS).[102]

The results of treating syphilis with erythromycin during pregnancy must be considered uncertain at best; fetal syphilis may not be eradicated, and therefore convincing evidence of potentially dangerous penicillin allergy should be obtained before this type of therapy is used.[103] When erythromycin is used to treat syphilis in pregnancy, the infant should be treated with penicillin at birth. Erythromycin may occasionally be useful in treating urinary tract infections due to gram-negative bacilli that might otherwise require the use of more toxic agents.[104] Urine pH must generally be raised to 8.0 or above to achieve effective activity at urinary concentrations against the gram-negative bacilli. Erythromycin may be used as an alternative antibiotic in the treatment of anthrax and in infections by *M. catarrhalis*, *E. corrodens*, and *L. monocytogenes*. Erythromycin is not consistently effective in treatment of infections due to *H. influenzae*,[53,54] and in vitro studies suggest resistance by some strains of *C. perfringens*.[34] In view of the availability of more effective alternative drugs, erythromycin should not be used alone in the treatment of deep-seated staphylococcal infections because of the potential for the emergence of resistant strains during therapy.[27,30,31]

AZITHROMYCIN AND CLARITHROMYCIN

In recent years there has been a search for newer macrolides that have better oral absorption, longer half-life, fewer gastrointestinal side effects, and a greater antimicrobial spectrum of activity than erythromycin. Azithromycin (CP-62,993), clarithromycin (A-56268), and some newer investigational agents have some of these properties.

Derivation, Chemistry, and Preparations

Azithromycin is derived from erythromycin, differing in having a methyl-substituted nitrogen in its 15-member lactone ring (Fig. 2). It is therefore an azalide antibiotic. Clarithromycin, having a 14-member ring structure, is produced by modifying position C6 of the lactone ring of erythromycin to possess a methoxy group (Fig. 3). These changes increase the stability of these compounds in gastric acid, improving absorption by the oral route.[15]

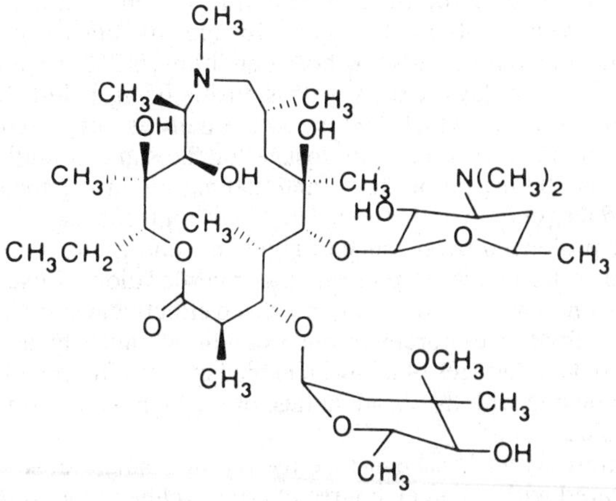

FIG. 2. Azithromycin base.

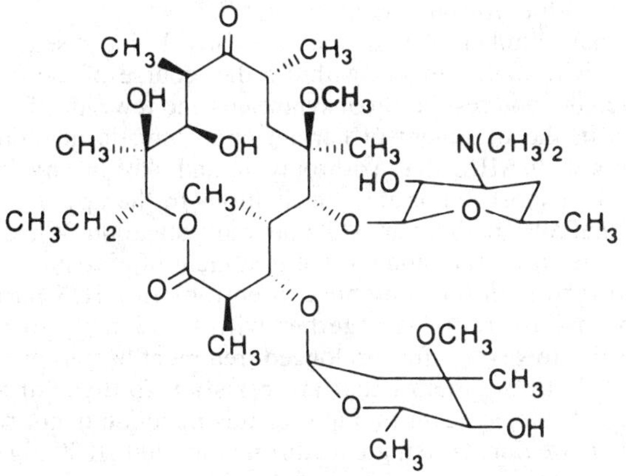

FIG. 3. Clarithromycin base.

Azithromycin is available in capsules for oral use as azithromycin dihydrate equivalent to 250 mg of azithromycin. Clarithromycin is provided in 250 or 500 mg film-coated tablets.

Mechanisms of Action and Resistance

Limited studies suggest that azithromycin, clarithromycin, and erythromycin bind to the same receptor on the bacterial 50S ribosomal subunit and inhibit RNA-dependent protein synthesis by the same mechanism (Abbott Laboratories, personal communication).[14,105] Azithromycin has greater activity than the 14-member macrolides erythromycin and clarithromycin against gram-negative bacteria (especially for *M. catarrhalis* and *H. influenzae*) and therefore appears to better penetrate the outer envelope of those organisms.[17] Similar to other macrolides, azithromycin and clarithromycin are generally considered to be bacteriostatic agents; however, bactericidal activity is easily demonstrated in vitro against such species as *S. pyogenes*, *S. pneumoniae*, and *H. influenzae*.[14,17,105,106] In vitro activity of the new macrolides increases with rising pH as with erythromycin.

There is complete cross-resistance between erythromycin, azithromycin, and clarithromycin for gram-positive organisms showing resistance to erythromycin by the MLS$_B$ phenotype because the methylation mechanism already described operates for all of the 14- and 15-member macrolides.[43,105]

Antimicrobial Activity

Clarithromycin is highly active against gram-positive bacteria, being two- to fourfold more active than erythromycin against most streptococci, including *S. pneumoniae* and *S. pyogenes*

and methicillin-sensitive *S. aureus*.[14,15] However, azithromycin is about two- to fourfold less active than erythromycin against those organisms.[14,15] Streptococci and staphylococci that are resistant to erythromycin are resistant to clarithromycin and azithromycin.[14,17,107] Almost all methicillin-resistant staphylococci are resistant to the new macrolides.[14,16] The activity of clarithromycin against many gram-negative bacteria is similar to that of erythromycin,[14,107] although it is slightly more active against *M. catarrhalis*. An active metabolite of clarithromycin, 14-hydroxyclarithromycin, has slightly greater activity than the parent compound against *H. influenzae* and *M. catarrhalis* and is additive in vitro to the activity of clarithromycin.[107] Azithromycin is more active than erythromycin or clarithromycin against gram-negative bacteria, especially against *H. influenzae* and *M. catarrhalis*.[14,15] The greater activity of azithromycin against the Enterobacteriaceae is of questionable clinical significance.

Azithromycin and clarithromycin have equal or slightly better activities than erythromycin against *L. pneumophila*.[14] All three of those macrolides have good activity against *M. pneumoniae* and *C. pneumoniae*.[14,16,17,19,107] Both of the new macrolides have significantly greater activity than erythromycin against *C. trachomatis*, *U. urealyticum*,[14] and somewhat greater activity for *B. burgdorferi*.[14,17,107]

The macrolides show little activity against *M. tuberculosis*. In contrast, clarithromycin shows substantial activity against *M. leprae* and is superior in this respect to erythromycin and azithromycin.[14,107]

There is currently much interest in the appreciable activities of clarithromycin and azithromycin against *M. avium* complex. Clarithromycin is about fourfold more active than azithromycin against this organism in vitro[108] and is somewhat more active in slowing its replication in infected human macrophages.[109] Both of these new macrolides also have significant and similar activity against *T. gondii* in tissue culture systems.[110,111]

Clinical Pharmacology

Clarithromycin is well absorbed after oral administration, with or without food, and is approximately 50 percent bioavailable.[14] Mean peak serum concentrations in the steady state with oral doses of 250 and 500 mg every 12 hours are 1 and 2–3 µg/ml, respectively. The elimination half-lives for those two regimens are 3–4 hours and 5–7 hours, respectively. Clarithromycin is appreciably metabolized in the liver by oxidation and hydrolysis to a number of compounds, accounting for a recovery of 78 percent. The major metabolite, 14-hydroxyclarithromycin, has antibacterial activity and accounts for 20 percent of the metabolites.[14] With the 250 mg oral dose given every 12 hours, about 20 percent of the drug is excreted into the urine unchanged and 10–15 percent as the hydroxy metabolite. With the 500-mg dose given at the same interval, about 30 percent is excreted into the urine unchanged and 10–15 percent as the major metabolite. At higher doses there is some nonlinearity of half-life, apparently because of saturation of metabolic mechanisms with a higher proportion of unchanged drug eliminated in the urine.[14] About 65–70 percent of the drug is bound to protein in the serum. With renal insufficiency involving creatinine clearances of less than 30 ml/min there is a marked increase in half-life of clarithromycin.[107] Dose adjustment is suggested in patients with severe renal failure, including recommendations for a 500 mg loading dose followed by 250 mg once or twice daily depending on the type of infection being treated.[107] In the face of severe hepatic disease there is an increase in the renal clearance of clarithromycin associated with a decrease in metabolic clearance, to the extent that no dosage adjustment is recommended at present.[107]

Clarithromycin is widely distributed and penetrates well into various tissues, generally exceeding peak maximum serum levels by severalfold.[107] However, there are no data on entry into the cerebrospinal fluid. Clarithromycin, similar to the other macrolides, penetrates well into phagocytic cells.[112]

The oral bioavailability of azithromycin after a single 500 mg dose is 37 percent.[113] Food decreases the absorption by 50 percent; therefore, the dose should be taken at least 1 hour before or 2 hours after a meal.[114] The maximum serum concentration achieved after a single 500 mg oral dose was 0.41 μg/ml; after a 500 mg loading dose on day 1, followed by 250 mg daily for 4 additional days, it was 0.24 μg/ml; after 500 mg twice on day 1, followed by 500 mg daily for 5 additional days, it was 0.62 μg/ml.[14] Protein binding of azithromycin in serum varies between 7 and 50 percent, depending on the drug concentration.[14] Azithromycin is widely distributed in tissues, and for most the drug concentration exceeds that in serum by 10- to 100-fold,[113] particularly in sputum and lung. Very high concentrations were found in alveolar macrophages and neutrophils.[115] The extensive tissue uptake of azithromycin has been attributed to cell uptake of this basic compound into relatively acidic lysosomes because of ionic trapping.[115] Very low concentrations were noted in cerebrospinal fluid in patients without meningitis. The average half-life in many tissues is between 2 and 4 days[113] so that it is estimated that significant antibacterial activity against many pathogens will persist in tissue for at least 5 days after a 5 day course of treatment.[113] The average terminal half-life is 68 hours, consistent with a slow release of drug from tissues followed by elimination from the vascular compartment. About 6 percent of an oral dose appears as unchanged drug in the urine within 1 week of administration, and another small proportion is metabolized to inactive compounds, particularly by demethylation.[113] Most of the drug that is absorbed remains unmetabolized and is probably eliminated in feces by way of biliary excretion and possibly transintestinal elimination.[113] Biliary concentrations of azithromycin are higher than in the serum, and most of the drug in the bile is unchanged.[113] There are no data yet available on dose adjustments required with severe renal or hepatic failure.

Adverse Reactions

Adverse reactions to clarithromycin and azithromycin at the usual doses have been rare.[14,15,114] The most common complaints have been gastrointestinal (diarrhea, nausea, abdominal pain), and discontinuance of therapy was rarely required. This is in contrast to the relatively common abdominal complaints encountered with erythromycin, not infrequently leading to cessation of therapy.[14,15] Abnormalities in liver function and complaints of headache and dizziness have been encountered in occasional patients treated with clarithromycin or azithromycin. With high doses of these drugs used in the treatment of *M. avium-intracellulare,* tinnitus, dizziness and reversible hearing loss have been reported.[116,117] Rarely, severe allergic reactions have occurred with the use of azithromycin. High doses of clarithromycin in animals have been associated with teratogenic effects.

Drug Interactions

Clarithromycin has been reported to be associated with increased concentrations of carbamazepine, theophylline, and terfenadine and decreased concentrations of zidovudine.[14,118] These changes have not been reported as yet with azithromycin, which does not appear to inactivate cytochrome P-450 enzymes.[84]

Uses of Clarithromycin and Azithromycin

Clarithromycin and azithromycin were as effective as other commonly used antimicrobial agents when employed in randomized multicenter trials for the treatment of pharyngitis, sinusitis, community-acquired pneumonia, including that due to *M. pneumoniae,* and skin infections.[14,15,119] In those studies direct comparisons of the effectiveness of azithromycin with clarithromycin were not made. The dosage of clarithromycin recommended for adults for those conditions is 250 mg po twice daily for 7–14 days, except with sinusitis or bronchitis due to *H. influenzae* in which 500 mg twice daily is suggested. The recommended azithromycin dosage for the same conditions in adults is 500 mg po on day 1 and 250 mg on days 2 through 5 for a 5 day course of therapy. The 5 day course is used because of the prolonged persistence of good concentrations of azithromycin in tissues.[14] At present, the consideration to use these new agents, which provide no increased effectiveness over older agents, for those aforementioned conditions must balance the potential advantages of a low incidence of side effects and infrequent dosing with the disadvantage of the higher cost compared with older drugs.

Azithromycin has been as effective in a single dose of 1 g compared with a 1 week course of doxycycline in the treatment of *C. trachomatis* urethritis and cervicitis.[120] There is no reported experience with the use of this drug in pregnancy, and therefore *C. trachomatis* infections in such women should be treated with erythromycin at present.[90]

A small number of patients with early Lyme disease were treated with azithromycin with a 5 day course of the drug. It resulted in good resolution of symptoms and few side effects.[121]

It is in the treatment of certain opportunistic infections of patients with AIDS that azithromycin and clarithromycin may make their most important contributions to therapy; however, their final roles in these are still under investigation. When these macrolides are used alone in the treatment of disseminated *M. avium-intracellulare* complex infections in AIDS patients, symptoms are reduced together with the density of bacteremia.[117] However, after prolonged treatment bacteremia often returns with organisms that are resistant to these drugs.[117] Therefore, single-agent therapy for this infection is not recommended. Regimens using clarithromycin (500–1000 mg twice daily) or azithromycin (500 mg daily) are suggested in combination with at least one other agent such as ethambutol, rifampin, rifabutin, ciprofloxacin or another quinolone, amikacin, or clofazamine.[117] Therapy should continue indefinitely. Gastrointestinal side effects and abnormal liver function tests are reported more commonly in AIDS patients receiving the high doses of clarithromycin or azithromycin than in non-AIDS patients being treated with lower doses for more common infections. Reversible hearing loss has also been noted in some of the patients getting high-dose therapy of the new macrolides.

Limited studies suggest that clarithromycin or azithromycin given alone or with pyrimethamine are effective in treating AIDS patients with *T. gondii* encephalitis,[122,123] but studies comparing these new regimens with older regimens are not yet available. Azithromycin showed substantial activity against cryptosporidia causing intestinal infections in immunosuppressed rats,[124] and preliminary studies with a lactose-free formulation of azithromycin in AIDS patients with this infection are showing promise of effectiveness. There are no reports as yet of the use of clarithromycin in patients for that condition.

Other Macrolides

Trioleandomycin, an ester of the 14-member ring macrolide oleandomycin, is still marketed, although it has no advantages over erythromycin and may occasionally cause cholestatic hepatitis. It is a potent inhibitor of the cytochrome P-450 enzyme system.[84] Roxithromycin and dithromycin are 14-member ring macrolides that represent modifications of erythromycin at the C9 position. The latter two are still investigational drugs with somewhat less or similar in vitro antibacterial activity compared with erythromycin but with longer half-lives.[15]

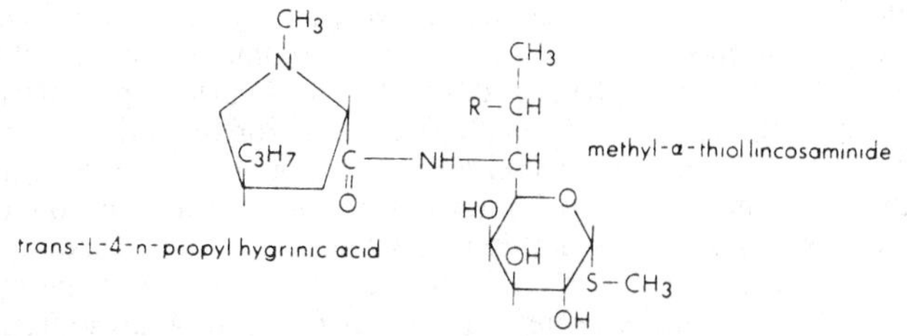

FIG. 4. The lincosamide antibiotics. Lincomycin, R = OH; clindamycin, R = Cl.

LINCOMYCIN AND CLINDAMYCIN

Derivation, Chemistry, and Preparations

Lincomycin was isolated in 1962 from an organism, *Streptomyces lincolnensis*, obtained from soil near Lincoln, Nebraska. Its biologic properties are similar to those of erythromycin, but it is chemically unrelated, consisting of an amino acid linked to an amino sugar (Fig. 2). Chemical modification provided clindamycin (7-chloro-7-deoxy-lincomycin) (Fig. 4) with increased antibacterial potency and absorption after oral administration.[125] Since there are no therapeutic advantages for lincomycin over clindamycin, the discussion will concentrate on the latter, although both are still marketed as pharmaceuticals. Both are weak bases that are readily water soluble when provided as salts.

Lincomycin (Lincocin) is available as the hydrochloride salt in 250- and 500-mg capsules and syrup for oral administration and in solution (300 mg/ml) for parenteral use. Clindamycin (Cleocin) is prepared as the hydrochloride salt of the base in 75-, 150-, and 300-mg capsules and of the palmitate ester for pediatric suspension. It is supplied as the phosphate ester for intramuscular or intravenous use (150 mg/ml). It is also available in a topical solution, gel and lotion for the treatment of acne vulgaris, and in a concentration of 2 percent in a vaginal cream for the treatment of bacterial vaginosis.

Mechanism of Action

The lincosamide antibiotics have, in susceptible organisms, the same or overlapping 50S ribosomal binding sites as those for the macrolides and chloramphenicol, and they may compete with these drugs for binding.[2,3] Protein synthesis is inhibited primarily in early chain elongation by interference with the transpeptidation reaction.[1,3]

Antimicrobial Activity and Mechanisms of Resistance

In vitro susceptibilities to clindamycin are given in Table 4.[7,12,125,126] Clindamycin is more potent than lincomycin but similar in degree of activity to erythromycin against staphylococci, pneumococci, *S. pyogenes*, and streptococci of the "viridans" group. However, while erythromycin demonstrates at least moderate activity against *Enterococcus*, *H. influenzae*, and *N. meningitidis*, clindamycin is generally inactive against these organisms at clinically achievable concentrations. In contrast, clindamycin shows significantly greater activity than erythromycin against most clinically significant anaerobic bacteria, particularly *B. fragilis*,[127,128] and some erythromycin-resistant strains of *S. aureus*.[129] Clindamycin is one of the most active antibiotics available against *B. fragilis*. In a survey of nine hospitals in the United States that provided 750 strains of the *B. fragilis* group in 1981, 6 percent of isolates were resistant to clindamycin (MIC > 4 μg/ml by an agar dilution method); this represented 0–13 percent of strains in individual institutions.[12] In a similar survey by the same group involving eight centers and 678 isolates of the *B. fragilis* group collected in 1984 and 1985, 5 percent were resistant to clindamycin, representing 0–10

TABLE 4. In Vitro Susceptibilities to Clindamycin

Organism	Minimum Inhibitory Concentration (μg/ml)	
	Range	Median
S. pneumoniae	0.002–0.04[a]	0.01
S. pyrogenes	0.02–0.1[a]	0.04
Viridans streptococci	0.005–0.04[a]	0.02
Enterococcus	12.5–>100	100
S. aureus	0.04–>100	0.1
S. epidermidis	0.1–>100	0.1
C. perfringens	<0.1–8	0.8
N. gonorrhoeae	0.01–6.3	3.1
N. meningitidis	6.3–25	12.5
H. influenzae	0.4–50	12.5
B. fragilis group	<0.125–>256	0.25
P. melaninogenicus	≤0.1–1	≤0.1
Fusobacterium spp.	≤0.5[a]	≤0.5
Peptococcus spp.	≤0.1–>100	≤0.5
Peptostreptococcus spp.	≤0.1–0.8	≤0.5
M. pneumoniae	1.6–3.1	3.1

[a] Occasional clinical isolates are more resistant.

percent of the strains in individual institutions.[126] Of the species belonging to the *B. fragilis* group, clindamycin resistance was found in 5 percent of *B. fragilis*, 10 percent of *Bacteroides thetaiotaomicron*, 15 percent of *B. vulgatus*, 6 percent of *B. distasonis*, and 7 percent of *B. ovatus*.[126] Among strains of *Bacteroides* isolated in Los Angeles in 1986, 88 percent of *B. fragilis* species and 16 to 22 percent of nonfragilis species were resistant to clindamycin.[130] Resistance to clindamycin by anaerobes also includes 10–20 percent of clostridial species other than *C. perfringens*, about 10–20 percent of peptostreptococci and peptococci, and most *Fusobacterium varium* strains.[127,128] All the Enterobacteriaceae are resistant to clindamycin.

Clindamycin provides high activity against pneumococci and group A streptococci; however, clinical isolates showing resistance to clindamycin and erythromycin have been increasingly reported from different areas as already discussed in the section on erythromycin. In most hospitals at present, the majority of isolates of *S. aureus* are sensitive to lincomycin or clindamycin[131,132]; however, resistance occurs in 15–45 percent of strains.[29] Lincomycin or clindamycin resistance has been reported in 20 to 84 percent of methicillin-resistant strains[131-133] and in 50 percent of erythromycin-resistant strains[134] of *S. aureus*. Cross-resistance of *S. aureus* between lincomycin and clindamycin is complete. The MIC of clindamycin and erythromycin in vitro are generally similar for *S. aureus* strains that are sensitive to both agents; however, resistance can be selected in vitro by serial subculture in the presence of subinhibitory concentrations of either, and it occurs slowly for clindamycin and more rapidly for erythromycin.[129,135] In contrast, strains that are sensitive to clindamycin and resistant to erythromycin can be rapidly selected for clindamycin resistance by serial subculture on clindamycin. Consistent with these in vitro observations, the emergence of clindamycin-resistant *S. aureus* has been noted in clindamycin-treated patients, in particular when the organisms had demonstrated erythromycin resistance at the onset of treatment.[129] Clindamycin resistance, often crossing to erythromycin, has also emerged from treated patients infected with *S. aureus* that were initially sensitive to erythromycin.[136] Resistance of the "dissociated" type may also emerge during treatment of patients.[135]

The antibacterial activity of lincomycin and clindamycin has been shown, in limited in vitro studies, to be bactericidal for *S. pneumoniae*, *S. pyogenes*, and *S. aureus*. Its killing activity is similar to that of erythromycin and therefore probably varies with the concentration, bacterial species, and inoculum. It is more slowly bactericidal for *S. aureus* than are the penicillins[137] and is inconsistently bactericidal for *B. fragilis*.[138]

Clindamycin has substantial in vitro activity against *Toxoplasma gondii* in infected human fibroblasts.[139]

Mechanisms of resistance to the lincosamide antibiotics include the following: *(1)* Alteration in a single 50S ribosomal protein of the receptor site confers resistance to erythromycin and often to the lincosamides[2]; this mechanism has already been discussed for erythromycin. *(2)* Alteration in the 23S ribosomal RNA of the 50S ribosomal subunit by methylation of adenine[43] has also been discussed. It is usually plasmid mediated and provides the MLS$_B$ type of resistance, which includes that exhibited by some strains of *S. aureus* and *B. fragilis* to clindamycin. *(3)* Inactivation of lincomycin and clindamycin by a few isolates of staphylococci, including *S. aureus,* which possess a plasmid-mediated 3-lincomycin 4-clindamycin 0-nucleotidyltransferase that catalyzes the nucleotidylation of the hydroxyl group in position 4 of clindamycin.[29,140] This adenylation of the lincosamides is associated with high-level resistance to lincomycin, but clindamycin resistance may not be detected by routine methods. The adenylation of clindamycin is associated with impaired bactericidal activity and decreased activity at high inoculum levels. The nucleotide sequences of the plasmid-mediated genes, lin A and lin A', which encode for the inactivating enzymes, have been determined. *(4)* Enterobacteriaceae, *Pseudomonas* spp., and *Acinetobacter* spp. are intrinsically resistant to clindamycin apparently because of poor permeability of the cellular outer envelope to the drug.[29]

Clinical Pharmacology

Peak serum levels achieved after oral administration of clindamycin occur earlier and are at least twice as high as those of lincomycin. Absorption of clindamycin is about 90 percent and is slightly delayed, but not decreased, by ingestion of food, whereas that of lincomycin is markedly decreased.[125] Mean peak serum concentrations of clindamycin in adults after single oral doses of 150 and 300 mg occur at 1 hour and are 2.5 and 3.6 μg/ml, respectively; at 6 hours they are 0.7 and 1.1 μg/ml, respectively. The esters clindamycin palmitate in suspension for oral use and clindamycin phosphate for parenteral use are absorbed as the inactive ester and rapidly hydrolyzed in the blood to the active base. After intramuscular administration, which causes little pain, mean peak serum levels are reached in 3 hours and are about 6 μg/ml after a 300-mg dose and 9 μg/ml after a 600-mg dose; at 12 hours they are 0.7 and 0.9 μg/ml, respectively.[141] In adult healthy volunteers, immediately following 20–45 minute intravenous infusions of 600, 900, or 1200 mg of clindamycin phosphate, serum levels of base are 10, 11, and 14 μg/ml, respectively. Higher levels after intravenous infusion have been reported in infected patients under treatment.[142] Dose regimens of intravenous clindamycin using 900 mg every 8 hours or 600 mg every 6 hours are considered acceptable.[143]

Limited studies have demonstrated good penetration of most tissues by the lincosamides excepting clinically insignificant entry of clindamycin into the cerebrospinal fluid, even with meningitis.[7,144] The concentration in bone in relationship to serum levels is particularly high.[145] Clindamycin administered to pregnant women readily passes the placental barrier and enters fetal blood and tissues.[58] Clindamycin is actively transported into polymorphonuclear leukocytes and macrophages[146] and is present in relatively high concentrations, compared with peak serum levels, in experimental abscesses.[147]

The normal half-life of clindamycin is 2.4 hours. Most of the absorbed drug is metabolized, probably by the liver, to products with variable antibacterial activity, including *N*-demethyl-clindamycin (more active than the parent compound) and clindamycin sulfoxide (less active), which have been detected in bile and urine but not in serum.[141] High bioactivity is found in bile, mostly as the *N*-demethyl metabolite; this represents a minor

route of excretion and accounts for the activity assayed in feces after parenteral administration.[141,148] Clindamycin activity in feces persists for at least 5 days after 48 hours of parenteral administration and is associated with a major reduction in the population of sensitive bacteria in the colon lasting for up to 14 days.[149] Clindamycin concentration in bile is markedly diminished or absent when the common bile duct is obstructed.[150] High clindamycin bioactivity, also mostly in the *N*-demethyl form, is found in the urine and persists for up to 4 days after a single dose, suggesting slow release from tissues.[142] Accurate data on the proportion of absorbed clindamycin that is excreted in the urine are not available because of the variable activity of the metabolites and their unknown proportions in urine.

The half-life of clindamycin is increased from 2.4 to about 6 hours in patients with severe renal failure, and peak blood levels after parenteral administration are about twice those in healthy people.[151] If modified at all, parenteral doses should be halved in such patients. Some prolongation of clindamycin activity in serum is noted in patients with severe liver disease.[152] Appreciable dose modification should be made when there is concomitant severe renal and hepatic disease in the same patient. Neither hemodialysis nor peritoneal dialysis removes significant amounts of clindamycin.

Adverse Reactions

1. Allergic reactions include a variety of rashes, fever, and rare cases of erythema multiforme and anaphylaxis.
2. Diarrhea occurs in up to 20 percent of patients and is more common with oral administration. However, the major toxicity of lincomycin and clindamycin that now appreciably limits their use is the occurrence of pseudomembranous colitis caused by a toxin secreted by *C. difficile* that overgrows in the presence of these antibiotics.[153–155] This has been reported in 0.01–10 percent of clindamycin-treated patients.[128,156] The syndrome may occur in association with administration of other antibiotics but does so less frequently; it is not related to the dose and may occur after oral or parenteral therapy. The variable incidence of colitis in different reports has been ascribed to different diagnostic methods and the variable epidemiology of *C. difficile*.[128,156,157] It may begin during or as long as several weeks after a course of lincomycin or clindamycin therapy and is characterized by diarrhea, sometimes bloody, with fever and cramps and the appearance of yellow-white plaques on the colonic mucosa, seen by proctoscopy. The toxin of *C. difficile* can be detected in the stool of nearly all patients with antibiotic-associated pseudomembranous colitis and in about 20 percent of patients with antibiotic-associated diarrhea by a cytotoxicity assay using tissue culture cells.[82,155,157] The cytotoxic effect can be prevented by neutralization of the toxin in the stool extract with *Clostridium sordelli* antitoxin. The syndrome can be protracted and may end fatally. Prompt cessation of the antibiotic is essential. Use of antiperistaltic drugs should be avoided since they may worsen the condition. Vancomycin given by mouth in doses of 125–500 mg qid and oral metronidazole are effective in treatment.[158,159] Relapse after treatment may occur.
3. Hepatotoxicity: Minor reversible elevation of transaminase levels, unassociated with other evidence of liver abnormality, has been commonly observed in patients receiving clindamycin, especially by the parenteral route. Some of these may have been false-positive reactions associated with colorimetric rather than specific enzymatic measurements.[125] However, rare cases of frank hepatotoxicity, including jaundice associated with hepatocellular damage, have been observed.[160]
4. Isolated cases of reversible neutropenia, thrombocytopenia, and agranulocytosis associated with lincomycin or clinda-

mycin therapy have been reported; their relationship to the antibiotic administration was uncertain.

5. Occasional reports of hypotension, ECG changes, and rarely cardiopulmonary arrest have been reported when large intravenous doses of lincomycin were given rapidly. This has not been reported with clindamycin.

6. Local irritative reactions are rare with these drugs. Intramuscular and intravenous administration is generally well tolerated.

Drug Interactions

Clindamycin may block neuromuscular transmission and may enhance the action of other blocking agents.[161] Clindamycin phosphate in solution is physically incompatible with ampicillin, diphenylhydantoin, barbiturates, aminophylline, calcium gluconate, and magnesium sulfate.

Uses of Clindamycin

The higher activity and absorption properties of clindamycin, along with no greater potential for toxicity, compared with lincomycin, favors the former in all indications for use of these antibiotics. The lincosamides have been used in a variety of infections, often with good effect; however, the appreciation of the potential for serious or even fatal toxicity with pseudomembranous colitis and the availability of safer alternative antibiotics should now generally limit the use of clindamycin to a few indications[90]:

1. Infections that are outside of the central nervous system and are likely to involve *B. fragilis* or other penicillin-resistant anaerobic bacteria. These particularly involve polymicrobial intra-abdominal or gynecologic pelvic infections.[128] Clindamycin is likely to be beneficial where there is spillage of fecal flora associated with tissue damage, as in cases involving bowel damage or perforation. In these situations, studies of experimental animal models and patients with infection suggest that clindamycin decreases the likelihood of abscess formation involving fecal organisms, especially *B. fragilis*.[162,163] In these conditions, clindamycin is administered together with an aminoglycoside, third-generation cephalosporin, or aztreonam because additional activity is required against Enterobacteriaceae. The beneficial effect of clindamycin in preventing or ameliorating morbidity from fecal abscess formation or other infections appears to be superior to that of penicillin, cephalothin, or aminoglycosides.[162,164] However, in comparative trials of therapy for intra-abdominal or pelvic sepsis, clindamycin, cefoxitin, metronidazole, imipenem, ticarcillin-clavulanic acid, and chloramphenicol have shown similar effectiveness.[128,165,166]

   Clindamycin may offer some advantage over penicillin G in the treatment of anaerobic bronchopulmonary infections,[167] and, in addition, it may serve as an alternative in patients allergic to penicillin. In a prospective randomized study of 39 patients with community-acquired putrid lung abscess, clindamycin was more effective than penicillin in terms of the time until eradication of fever and fetid sputum and the "overall response" to treatment.[168] The study involved small numbers of patients and had some flaws in the analysis[169]; however, the superiority of clindamycin for some patients was demonstrated and may relate to observations that 15–25 percent of anaerobic pulmonary infections involve β-lactamase–producing strains of *B. fragilis*, *B. melaninogenica*, *P. ruminicola*, and *B. ureolyticus*, which are resistant to penicillin.[128,169] A more recent and similar study also demonstrated a higher failure rate with penicillin than with clindamycin and attributed it to penicillin-resistant anaerobes.[170] That study was problematic in that penicillin oral therapy was used to complete the course of treatment of some patients in the penicillin group. Nevertheless, clindamycin may be preferable for the treatment of this condition, particularly in seriously ill patients or in those who have responded poorly to penicillin.

2. Clindamycin is useful as an alternative to penicillin in treatment of *C. perfringens* infections.

3. Clindamycin may sometimes be useful as an alternative to a penicillin in the treatment of staphylococcal infections. However, its more limited bactericidal rate for staphylococci than that of the penicillins, and particularly the real potential for the emergence of clindamycin-resistant strains in treated patients, are disadvantages. The latter problem, noted especially but not only with erythromycin-resistant strains, appreciably limits its effectiveness in the therapy of deep-seated staphylococcal infections, particularly endocarditis.[136] Vancomycin or the cephalosporins are usually better alternatives to the penicillins for the latter. Although high concentrations of clindamycin are achieved in bone, an advantage of clindamycin for the treatment of osteomyelitis in patients has not been established.[145]

4. The topical solution of clindamycin may be used to treat acne vulgaris.[171] However, it should be noted that pseudomembranous colitis associated with the use of topical clindamycin has been reported.[172] In the treatment of bacterial vaginosis, clindamycin vaginal cream (2%) appears to be similar in efficacy and in the incidence of side affects to the use of oral metronidazole (both used for 7 days).[173,174]

5. Clindamycin is effective in treating experimental animals and when combined with pyrimethamine in treating patients with toxoplasmosis of the central nervous system.[175,176]

6. Clindamycin in combination with primaquine is an effective and well-tolerated regimen for the treatment of mild and moderately severe *Pneumocystis carinii* pneumonia in patients with AIDS.[177,178]

7. Clindamycin in combination with quinine is effective in the treatment of falciparum malaria.[90,179] That combination has also been reported to be useful in the treatment of babesiosis.[90,180]

8. Several studies have suggested that the coexistence of β-lactamase–producing *S. aureus* or *Bacteroides* species and group A streptococci may be associated with the failure of penicillin to eradicate the latter, resulting in recurrent tonsillitis. These studies suggest that recurrence rates may be lowered when clindamycin is used.[181,182] However, most recurrences of streptococcal pharyngitis are reinfections rather than relapses, and widespread use of clindamycin for this common problem will likely lead to a substantial number of cases of pseudomembranous colitis, as well as selection for clindamycin-resistant strains of group A streptococci.

Doses of clindamycin for adults depend on the site and severity of infection and on the condition of the patient. Oral doses are usually 150–300 mg every 6 hours, and parenteral doses, given every 6–12 hours, usually total 600–2700 mg/day, occasionally higher.

REFERENCES

1. Pestka S. Inhibitors of protein synthesis. In: Weissbach H, Pestka S, eds. Molecular Mechanisms of Protein Biosynthesis. New York: Academic Press; 1977:467.
2. Oleinick NL. The erythromycins. In: Corcoran JW, Hahn FE, eds. Mechanism of Action of Antimicrobial and Antitumor Agents. New York: Springer-Verlag; 1975:396.
3. Franklin TJ, Snow GA. Biochemistry of Antimicrobial Action. 3rd ed. London: Chapman and Hall; 1981:128.
4. Haight TH, Finland M. Observations on mode of action of erythromycin. Proc Soc Exp Biol Med. 1952;81:188–93.
5. Haight TH, Finland M. The antibacterial action of erythromycin. Proc Soc Exp Biol Med. 1952;81:175–83.
6. Sabath LD, Gerstein DA, Loder PB, et al. Excretion of erythromycin and its enhanced activity in urine against gram-negative bacilli with alkalinization. J Lab Clin Med. 1968;72:916–23.

7. Garrod LP, Lambert HP, O'Grady F. Antibiotic and Chemotherapy. 5th ed. Edinburgh: Churchill Livingstone; 1981:183.

8. Washington JA II, Wilson WR. Erythromycin: A microbial and clinical perspective after 30 years of clinical use. I. Mayo Clin Proc. 1984;60:189–203; II. 1985;60:271–8.

9. Edelstein PM, Meyer RD. Susceptibility of Legionella pneumophila to twenty antimicrobial agents. Antimicrob Agents Chemother. 1980;18:403–8.

10. Vanhoff R, Gordts B, Dierickx R, et al. Bacteriostatic and bactericidal activities of 24 antimicrobial agents against Campylobacter fetus subsp. jejuni. Antimicrob Agents Chemother. 1980;18:118–21.

11. Kuo C, Wang S, Grayston T. Antimicrobial activity of several antibiotics and a sulfonamide against Chlamydia trachomitis organisms in cell culture. Antimicrob Agents Chemother. 1977;12:80–3.

12. Tally FP, Cuchural GJ, Jacobus NV, et al. Susceptibility of the Bacteroides fragilis group in the United States in 1981. Antimicrob Agents Chemother. 1983;23:536–40.

13. Ahmad F, McLeod DT, Croughan MJ, et al. Antimicrobial susceptibility of Branhamella catarrhalis isolates from bronchopulmonary infections. Antimicrob Agents Chemother. 1984;26:424–5.

14. Piscitelli SC, Danziger LH, Rodvold KA. Clarithromycin and azithromycin: New macrolide antibiotics. Clin Pharm. 1992;11:137–52.

15. Bahal N, Nahata MC. The new macrolide antibiotics: Azithromycin, clarithromycin, dirithromycin, and roxithromycin. Ann Pharmacother. 1992; 26:46–55.

16. Neu HC. The development of macrolides: Clarithromycin in perspective. J Antimicrob Chemother. 1991;27(Suppl 4):1–9.

17. Neu HC. Clinical microbiology of azithromycin. Am J Med. 1991;91(Suppl 3A):12S–18S.

18. Waites KB, Cassell GH, Canupp KC, et al. In vitro susceptibilities of mycoplasmas and ureaplasmas to new macrolides and aryl-fluoroquinolones. Antimicrob Agents Chemother. 1988;32:1500–2.

19. Renaudin H, Bebear C. Comparative in vitro activity of azithromycin, clarithromycin, erythromycin and lomefloxacin against Mycoplasma pneumoniae, Mycoplasma hominis and Ureaplasma urealyticum. Eur J Clin Microbiol Infect Dis. 1990;9:838–41.

20. Sanders E, Foster MT, Scott D. Group A beta-haemolytic streptococci resistant to erythromycin and lincomycin. N Engl J Med. 1968;278:538–40.

21. Dixon JM. Pneumococcus resistant to erythromycin and lincomycin. Lancet. 1967;1:573.

22. Linares J, Garau J, Dominiquez C, et al. Antibiotic resistance and serotypes of Streptococcus pneumoniae from patients with community acquired pneumococcal disease. Antimicrob Agents Chemother. 1983;23:545–7.

23. Acar JF, Buu-Hoi AY. Resistance patterns of important gram-positive pathogens. J Antimicrob Chemother. 1988;21(Suppl C):41–7.

24. Maruyama S, Yoshioka H, Fujita K, et al. Sensitivity of group A streptococci to antibiotics. Am J Dis Child. 1979;133:1143–5.

25. Istre GR, Welch DF, Marks MI, et al. Susceptibility of group A beta-hemolytic Streptococcus isolates to penicillin and erythromycin. Antimicrob Agents Chemother. 1981;20:244–6.

26. Seppala H, Nissinen A, Jarvinen H, et al. Resistance to erythromycin in group A streptococci. N Engl J Med. 1992;326:292–7.

27. Haight TH, Finland M. Resistance of bacteria to erythromycin. Proc Soc Exp Biol Med. 1952;81:183–8.

28. Lepper MH, Dowling HF, Jackson GG, et al. Effect of antibiotic usage in the hospital on the incidence of antibiotic-resistant strains among personnel carrying staphylococci. J Lab Clin Med. 1953;42:832.

29. Leclercq R, Courvalin P. Intrinsic and unusual resistance to macrolides, lincosamide, and streptogramin antibiotics in bacteria. Antimicrob Agents Chemother. 1991;35:1273–6.

30. Griffith RS, Black HR. Erythromycin. Med Clin North Am. 1970;54: 1199–215.

31. Haight TH, Finland M. Laboratory and clinical studies on erythromycin. N Engl J Med. 1952;247:227–32.

32. Garrod LP. The erythromycin group of antibiotics. Br Med J. 1957;2:57–63.

33. Mapple PAC, Hamilton-Miller JMT, Brumfitt W. World-wide antibiotic resistance in methicillin-resistant Staphylococcus aureus. Lancet. 1989;1: 537–9.

34. Sapico FL, Kwok Y, Sutter V, et al. Standardized antimicrobial disc susceptibility testing of anaerobic bacteria: In vitro susceptibility of Clostridium perfringens to nine antibiotics. Antimicrob Agents Chemother. 1972;2:320–5.

35. Molavi A, Weinstein L. In vitro activity of erythromycin against atypical mycobacteria. J Infect Dis. 1971;123:216–9.

36. Finland M, Bach MC, Garner C, et al. Synergistic action of ampicillin against Nocardia asteroides: Effect of time of incubation. Antimicrob Agents Chemother. 1974;5:344–53.

37. Fernandes PB, Hardy D, Bailer R, et al. Susceptibility testing of macrolide antibiotics against Hemophilus influenzae and correlation of in vitro results with in vivo efficacy in a mouse septicemia model. Antimicrob Agents Chemother. 1987;31:1243–50.

38. Kucers A. Chloramphenicol, erythromycin, vancomycin, tetracyclines. Lancet. 1982;2:425–9.

39. Jao RL, Finland M. Susceptibility of Mycoplasma pneumoniae to 21 antibiotics in vitro. Am J Med Sci. 1967;253:639–50.

40. Niitu Y, Hasegawa S, Kubota H. In vitro development of resistance to erythromycin, other macrolide antibiotics, and lincomycin in Mycoplasma pneumoniae. Antimicrob Agents Chemother. 1974;5:513–9.

41. Mao JC-H, Putterman M. Accumulation in gram-positive and gram-negative bacteria as a mechanism of resistance to erythromycin. J Bacteriol. 1968;95: 1111–7.

42. Taubeneck U. Susceptibility of Proteus mirabilis and its stable L-forms to erythromycin and other macrolides. Nature. 1962;196:195–6.

43. Leclercq R, Courvalin P. Bacterial resistance to macrolide, lincosamide, and streptogramin antibiotics by target modification. Antimicrob Agents Chemother. 1991;35:1267–72.

44. Bechtol LD, Stephens VC, Pugh CT, et al. Erythromycin esters: Comparative in vivo hydrolysis and bioavailability. Curr Ther Res. 1976;20:610–22.

45. Malmborg A. Effect of food on absorption of erythromycin. A study of two derivatives, the stearate and the base. J Antimicrob Chemother. 1979;5: 591–9.

46. McDonald PJ, Mather LE, Story MJ. Studies on absorption of a newly developed enteric-coated erythromycin base. J Clin Pharmacol. 1977;17:601–6.

47. DiSanto AR, Chodos DJ. Influence of study design in assessing food effects on absorption of erythromycin base and erythromycin stearate. Antimicrob Agents Chemother. 1981;20:190–6.

48. Yakatan GJ, Rasmussen CE, Feis PJ, et al. Bioinequivalence of erythromycin ethylsuccinate and enteric-coated erythromycin pellets following multiple oral doses. J Clin Pharmacol. 1985;25:36–42.

49. Janicki RS, Garnham JC, Worland MC, et al. Comparison of erythromycin ethylsuccinate, stearate and estolate treatments of group A streptococcus infections of the upper respiratory tract. Clin Pediatr (Phila). 1975;14: 1098–1107.

50. Ginsburg CM, McCracken GH Jr, Crow SD, et al. Erythromycin therapy for group A streptococcal pharyngitis. Results of a comparative study of the estolate and ethylsuccinate formulation. Am J Dis Child. 1984;138:536–9.

51. Osono T, Umezawa H. Pharmacokinetics of macrolides, lincosamides and streptogramins. J Antimicrob Chemother. 1985;16(Suppl A):151–66.

52. Welling PG. The esters of erythromycin. J Antimicrob Chemother. 1979;5: 633–4.

53. Bass JW, Steele RW, Wiebe RA, et al. Erythromycin concentrations in middle ear exudates. Pediatrics. 1971;48:417–22.

54. Howard JE, Nelson JD, Clahsen J, et al. Otitis media of infancy and early childhood. Am J Dis Child. 1976;130:965–70.

55. Hand WL, Corwin RW, Steinberg TH, et al. Uptake of antibiotics by human alveolar macrophages. Am Rev Respir Dis. 1984;129:933–7.

56. Miller MF, Martin JR, Johnson P, et al. Erythromycin uptake and accumulation by human polymorphonuclear leukocytes and efficacy of erythromycin in killing ingested Legionella pneumophila. J Infect Dis. 1984;149:714–8.

57. Romansky MJ, Nasou JP, Davis DS, et al. The treatment of 171 patients with erythromycin, including 132 with bacterial pneumonia. Antibiotics Annual. New York: Medical Encyclopedia; 1956, 1955–1956:48.

58. Phillipson A, Sabath LD, Charles D. Transplacental passage of erythromycin and clindamycin. N Engl J Med. 1973;288:1219–21.

59. Hammond JB, Griffith RS. Factors affecting the absorption and biliary excretion of erythromycin and two of its derivatives in humans. Clin Pharmacol Ther. 1961;2:308–12.

60. Mao JC-H, Tardrew PL. Demethylation of erythromycin by rabbit tissues in vitro. Biochem Pharmacol 1965;14:1049–58.

61. Kunin CM. A guide to use of antibiotics in patients with renal disease. Ann Intern Med. 1967;67:151–8.

62. Itoh Z, Suzuki T, Nakaya M, et al. Gastrointestinal motor-stimulating activity of macrolide antibiotics and analysis of their side effects on the canine gut. Antimicrob Agents Chemother. 1984;26:863–9.

63. Itoh Z, Suzuki T, Nakaya M, et al. Structure–activity relation among macrolide antibiotics in initiation of interdigestive migrating contractions in the canine gastrointestinal tract. Am J Physiol. 1985;11:G320–5.

64. Catnach SM, Fairclough PD. Erythromycin and the gut. Gut. 1992;33: 397–401.

65. Ellsworth AJ, Christensen DB, Volpone-McMahon MT. Prospective comparison of patient tolerance to enteric-coated vs nonenteric-coated erythromycin. J Fam Pract. 1990;31:265–70.

66. Inman WHW, Rawson NSB. Erythromycin isolate and jaundice. Br Med J. 1983;286:1954–5.

67. Braun P. Hepatotoxicity of erythromycin. J Infect Dis. 1969;119:300–6.

68. Tolman KG, Sannella JJ, Freston JW. Chemical structure of erythromycin and hepatotoxicity. Ann Intern Med. 1974;81:58–60.

69. Pessayre D, Larrey D, Funck-Brentano C, et al. Drug interactions and hepatitis produced by some macrolide antibiotics. J Antimicrob Chemother. 1985; 16(Suppl A):181–94.

70. McCormack WM, George H, Donner A, et al. Hepatotoxicity of erythromycin estolate during pregnancy. Antimicrob Agents Chemother. 1977;12: 630–5.

71. Sabath LD, Gerstein DA, Finland M. Serum glutamic oxalacetic transaminase: False elevation during administration of erythromycin. N Engl J Med. 1968;279:1137–9.

72. Sullivan D, Csuka ME, Blanchard B. Erythromycin ethylsuccinate hepatotoxicity. JAMA. 1980;243:1074.

73. Auckenthaler RW, Zwahlen A, Waldvogel FA. Macrolides. In: Peterson, PK, Verhoef J, eds. The Antimicrobial Agents Annual. v. 2. Amsterdam: Elsevier; 1987:120.

74. Karmody CS, Weinstein L. Reversible sensorineural hearing loss with intravenous erythromycin lactobionate. Ann Oral Rhinol Laryngol. 1977;86:9–11.

75. Eckman MR, Johnson T, Riess R. Partial deafness after erythromycin (Letter). N Engl J Med. 1975;292:649.

76. Mery JP, Kanfer A. Ototoxicity of erythromycin in patients with renal insufficiency (Letter). N Engl J Med. 1979;301:944.

77. Taylor R, Schofield IS, Ramos JM, et al. Ototoxicity of erythromycin in peritoneal dialysis patients (Letter). Lancet. 1981;2:935–6.

78. Haydon RC, Thaelin JW, Davis WE. Erythromycin ototoxicity: Analysis and conclusions based on 22 case reports. Otolaryngol Head Neck Surg. 1984;92:678–84.

79. Swanson DJ, Sung RJ, Fine MJ, et al. Erythromycin ototoxicity: Prospective assessment with serum concentrations and audiograms in a study of patients with pneumonia. Am J Med. 1992;92:61–8.

80. Schoenenberger RA, Haefel WE, Weiss P, et al. Association of intravenous erythromycin and potentially fatal ventricular tachycardia with Q-T prolongation (torsades de pointes). Br Med J. 1990;300:1375–6.

81. Gantz NM, Zawacki JK, Dickerson J, et al. Pseudomembranous colitis associated with erythromycin. Ann Intern Med. 1979;91:866–7.

82. Bartlett JG. Antimicrobial agents implicated in *Clostridium difficile* toxin-associated diarrhea or colitis. Johns Hopkins Med J. 1981;149:6–9.

83. Ludden TM. Pharmacokinetic interactions of the macrolide antibiotics. Clin Pharmacokinet. 1985;10:63–79.

84. Periti P, Mazzei T, Mini E, et al. Pharmacokinetic drug interactions of macrolides. Clin Pharmacokinet 1992;23:106–31.

85. Reisz G, Pingleton SK, Melethil S, et al. The effect of erythromycin on theophylline pharmacokinetics in chronic bronchitis. Ann Rev Respir Dis. 1983;127:581–4.

86. Bachmann K, Schwartz JI, Forney R Jr, et al. The effect of erythromycin on the desposition kinetics of warfarin. Pharmacology. 1984;28:171–6.

87. LaForce CF, Szefler SJ, Miller ME, et al. Inhibition of methylprednisolone elimination in the presence of erythromycin therapy. J Allergy Clin Immunol. 1983;72:34–9.

88. Wong YY, Lundden TD, Bell RD. Effect of erythromycin on carbamazepine kinetics. Clin Pharmacol Ther. 1983;33:460–4.

89. Martell R, Heinrichs D, Stiller CR, et al. The effects of erythromycin in patients treated with cyclosporine. Ann Intern Med. 1986;104:660–1.

90. Handbook of Antimicrobial Therapy. The Medical Letter on Drugs and Therapeutics. New Rochelle, NY: Medical Letter; 1992.

91. Rasch JR, Mogabgab WJ. Therapeutic effect of erythromycin on *Mycoplasma pneumoniae* pneumonia. Antimicrob Agents Chemother. 1965;5:693–9.

92. Kirby BD, Snyder KM, Myer RD, et al. Legionnaires' disease: Report of sixty-five nosocomially acquired cases and review of the literature. Medicine. 1980;59:188–205.

93. Muder RF, Yu VL, Zuravleff MS. Pneumonia due to the Pittsburgh pneumonia agent: New clinical perspective with a review of the literature. Medicine. 1983;62:120–8.

94. Dournon E, Mayaud C, Wolff M, et al. Comparison of the activity of three antibiotic regimens in severe Legionnaires' disease. J Antimicrob Chemother. 1990;26(Suppl B):129–39.

95. Sprauer MA, Cochi SL, Zell ER, et al. Prevention of secondary transmission of pertussis in households with early use of erythromycin. Am J Dis Child. 1992;146:177–81.

96. Anders BJ, Lauer BA, Paisley JW, et al. Double-blind placebo controlled trial of erythromycin for treatment of *Campylobacter* enteritis. Lancet. 1982;1:131–2.

97. Salazar-Lindo E, Sack B, Chea-Woo E, et al. Early treatment with erythromycin of *Campylobacter jejuni*–associated dysentery in children. J Pediatr. 1986;109:355–60.

98. Taylor DN, Blaser MJ, Escheverria P. Erythromycin-resistant *Campylobacter* infections in Thailand. Antimicrob Agents Chemother. 1987;31:438–42.

99. Beem MD, Saxon E, Tipple MA. Treatment of chlamydial pneumonia of infancy. Pediatrics. 1979;63:198–203.

100. Clarke JS, Condon RE, Fenton LJ, et al. Preoperative oral antibiotics reduce septic complications of colon operations: Results of prospective randomized, double-blind clinical study. Ann Surg. 1977;186:251–9.

101. Stellato TA, Danziger LH, Gordon N, et al. Antibiotics in elective colon surgery. A randomized trial of oral, systemic, and oral/systemic antibiotics for prophylaxis. Am Surg. 1990;56:251–4.

102. Berger TG. Dermatologic care in the AIDS patient. In: Sande MA, Volberding PA, eds. The Medical Management of AIDS. Philadelphia: WB Saunders; 1992:151.

103. Fenton LJ, Light IJ. Congenital syphilis after maternal treatment with erythromycin. Obstet Gynecol. 1976;47:492–4.

104. Zinner SK, Sabath LD, Casey JI, et al. Erythromycin and alkalinization of the urine in treatment of urinary tract infections due to gram-negative bacilli. Lancet. 1971;1:1267–8.

105. Retsema J, Giraud A, Schelkly W, et al. Spectrum and mode of action of azithromycin (CP-62,993), a new 15-membered-ring macrolide with improved potency against gram-negative organisms. Antimicrob Agents Chemother. 1987;31:1939–47.

106. Fernardes PB, Bailer R, Swanson R, et al. In vitro and in vivo evaluation of A-56268 (TE-031), a new macrolide. Antimicrob Agents Chemother. 1986;30:865–73.

107. Hardy DJ, Guay DRP, Jones RN. Clarithromycin, a unique macrolide. A pharmacokinetic, microbiological, and clinical overview. Diagn Microbiol Infect Dis. 1992;15:39–53.

108. Naik S, Ruck R. In vitro activities of several new macrolide antibiotics against *Mycobacterium avium* complex. Antimicrob Agents Chemother. 1989;33:1614–6.

109. Perronne C, Gikas A, Truffot-Pernot C, et al. Activities of sparfloxacin, azithromycin, temafloxacin and rifapentine compared with that of clarithromycin against multiplication of *Mycobacterium avium* complex within human macrophages. Antimicrob Agents Chemother. 1991;35:1356–9.

110. Derouin F, Chastang C. Activity in vitro against *Toxoplasma gondii* of azithromycin and clarithromycin alone and with pyrimethamine (Letter). J Antimicrob Chemother. 1990;25:708–11.

111. Chang HR, Pechere JCF. In vitro effects of four macrolides (roxithromycin, spiramycin, azithromycin [CP-62,693], and A-56268) on *Toxoplasma gondii*. Antimicrob Agents Chemother. 1988;32:524–9.

112. Anderson R, Joone G, van Rensburg CEJ. An in vitro evaluation of the cellular uptake and intraphagocytic bioactivity of clarithromycin (A56268, TE-031), a new macrolide antimicrobial agent. J Antimicrob Chemother. 1988;22:923–33.

113. Schentag JJ, Ballow CH. Tissue directed pharmacokinetics. Am J Med. 1991;91(Suppl 3A):5S–11S.

114. Hopkins S. Clinical toleration and safety of azithromycin. Am J Med. 1991;91(Suppl 3A):40S–45S.

115. Ballow CH, Amsden GW. Azithromycin: The first azalide antibiotic. Ann Pharmacother. 1992;26:1253–61.

116. Wallace RJ Jr, Brown BA, Griffith DE. Drug intolerance to high dose clarithromycin among elderly patients. Diagn Microbial Infect Dis. 1993;16:215–21.

117. Inderlied CB, Kemper CA, Bermudez LE. The *Mycobacterium avium* complex. Clin Microbiol Rev. 1993;6:266–310.

118. Honig P, Wortham D, Zamani K, et al. Effect of erythromycin, clarithromycin and azithromycin on the pharmacokinetics of terfenadine (Abstract PI-106). Clin Pharmacol Ther. 1993;53:161.

119. The Medical Letter on Drugs and Therapeutics. Clarithromycin and azithromycin. 1992;34:45–47.

120. Martin DH, Mroczkowski TF, Dalu ZA, et al. A controlled trial of a single dose of azithromycin for the treatment of chlamydial urethritis and cervicitis. N Engl J Med. 1992;327:921–5.

121. Massarotti EM, Luger SW, Rhan DW, et al. Treatment of early Lyme disease. Am J Med. 1992;92:396–403.

122. Fernandez-Martin J, Leport C, Morlat P, et al. Pyrimethamine–clarithromycin combination for therapy of acute *Toxoplasma* encephalitis in patients with AIDS. Antimicrob Agents Chemother. 1991;35:2049–52.

123. Farthing C, Rendel M, Currie B, et al. Azithromycin for cerebral toxoplasmosis. Lancet. 1992;339:437–8.

124. Rehg JE. Activity of azithromycin against *Crytosporidia* in immunosuppressed rats. J Infect Dis. 1991;163:1293–6.

125. McGehee RF Jr, Smith CB, Wilcox C, et al. Comparative studies of antibacterial activity in vitro and absorption and excretion of lincomycin and clindamycin. Am J Med Sci. 1968;256:279–92.

126. Cuchural GJ Jr, Tally FP, Jacobus NV, et al. Susceptibility of the *Bacteroides fragilis* group in the United States: Analysis by site of isolation. Antimicrob Agents Chemother. 1988;32:717–22.

127. Sutter VL: In vitro susceptibility of anaerobes: Comparison of clindamycin and other antimicrobial agents. J Infect Dis. 1977;135(Suppl):S7–12.

128. Bartlett JG. Anti-anaerobic antibacterial agents. Lancet. 1982;2:478–81.

129. McGehee RF, Barrett FF, Finland M. Resistance of *Staphylococcus aureus* to lincomycin, clindamycin and erythromycin. Antimicrob Agents Chemother. 1969;1968:392–7.

130. Appleman MD, Heseltine PNR, Cherubin CE. Epidemiology, antimicrobial susceptibility, pathogenicity, and significance of *Bacteroide fragilis* group organisms isolated at Los Angeles County-University of Southern California Medical Center. Rev Infect Dis. 1991;13:12–8.

131. Reeves DS, Holt HA, Phillips I, et al. Activity of clindamycin against *Staphylococcus aureus* and *Staphylococcus epidermidis* from four UK centres. J Antimicrob Chemother. 1991;27:469–74.

132. McKitrick JC. Antibiotic susceptibility data from the microbiology laboratory for bacterial isolates from 1992 (by the Kirby-Bauer method). Bronx, NY: Montefiore Medical Center, 1992.

133. Barrett FF, McGehee RF Jr, Finland M. Methicillin resistance *Staphylococcus aureus* at Boston City Hospital. N Engl J Med. 1968;279:441–8.

134. Desmyter J, Reybrouck G. Lincomycin sensitivity of erythromycin-resistant staphylococci. Chemotherapia. 1964;9:183–9.

135. Duncan IBR. Development of lincomycin resistance by staphylococci. Antimicrob Agents Chemother—1967; 1968:723–9.

136. Watanakunakorn C. Clindamycin therapy of *Staphylococcus aureus* endocarditis. Clinical relapse and development of resistance to clindamycin, lincomycin and erythromycin. Am J Med. 1976;60:419–25.

137. Sande MA, Johnson ML. Antimicrobial therapy of experimental endocarditis caused by *Staphylococcus aureus*. J Infect Dis. 1975;131:367–75.

138. Nastro LJ, Finegold SM. Bactericidal activity of five antimicrobial agents against *Bacteroides fragilis*. J Infect Dis. 1972;126:104–7.

139. Pfefferkorn ER, Nothnagel RF, Borotz SE. Parasiticidal effect of clindamycin on *Toxoplasma gondii* grown in cultured cells and selection of a drug resistant mutant. Antimicrob Agents Chemother. 1992;36:1091–6.

140. Leclercq R, Brisson-Noel A, Duval J, et al. Phenotypic expression and genetic heterogeneity of lincosamide inactivation in *Staphylococcus* spp. Antimicrob Agents Chemother. 1987;31:1887–91.

141. DeHaan RM, Metzler CM, Schellenberg D, et al. Pharmacokinetic studies of clindamycin phosphate. J Clin Pharmacol. 1973;13:190–209.

142. Fass RJ, Salow S. Clindamycin: Clinical and laboratory evaluations of parenteral therapy. Am J Med Sci. 1972;263:369–82.
143. Townsend RJ, Baker RP. Pharmacokinetic comparison of three clindamycin phosphate dosing schedules. Drug Intell Clin Pharmacol. 1987;21:279–81.
144. Panzer JD, Brown DC, Epstein WL, et al. Clindamycin levels in various body tissues and fluids. J Clin Pharmacol. 1972;12:259–62.
145. Nicholas P, Meyers BR, Levy RN. Concentrations of clindamycin in human bone. Antimicrob Agents Chemother. 1975;8:220–1.
146. Prokesch RC, Hand WL. Antibiotic entry into human polymorphonuclear leukocytes. Antimicrob Agents Chemother. 1982;23:373–80.
147. Joiner KA, Lowe BR, Dzink JL, et al. Antibiotic levels in infected and sterile subcutaneous abscesses in mice. J Infect Dis. 1981;143:487–94.
148. McCall CE, Steigbigel NH, Finland M. Lincomycin: Activity in vitro and absorption and excretion in normal young men. Am J Med Sci. 1967;254:144–55.
149. Kager L, Liljeqvist L, Malmborg AS, et al. Effect of clindamycin prophylaxis on the colonic microflora in patients undergoing colorectal surgery. Antimicrob Agents Chemother. 1981;20:736–40.
150. Brown RB, Martyak SN, Barza M, et al. Penetration of clindamycin phosphate into the abnormal human biliary tract. Ann Intern Med. 1976;84:168–70.
151. Joshi A, Stein R. Altered serum clearance of intravenously administered clindamycin phosphate in patients with uremia. J Clin Pharmacol. 1974;14:140–4.
152. Williams DN, Crossley K, Hoffman C, et al. Parenteral clindamycin phosphate: Pharmacology with normal and abnormal liver function and effect on nasal staphylococci. Antimicrob Agents Chemother. 1975;7:153–8.
153. Rifkin GD, Fekety FR, Silva J Jr, et al. Antibiotic-induced colitis: Implication of a toxin neutralized by Clostridium sordellii antitoxin. Lancet. 1977;11:1103–6.
154. Bartlett JG, Chang TW, Gurwith M, et al. Antibiotic-associated pseudomembranous colitis due to toxin-producing clostridia. N Engl J Med. 1978;298:531–4.
155. Bartlett JG. Antibiotic-associated pseudomembranous colitis. Rev Infect Dis. 1979;1:530–9.
156. Tedesco FJ. Clindamycin and colitis: A review. J Infect Dis. 1977;135(Suppl):S95–8.
157. Knoop FC, Owens M, Crocker IC. Clostridium difficile: Clinical disease and diagnosis. Clin Microbiol Rev. 1993;6:251–65.
158. George WL, Rolfe RD, Finegold SM. Treatment and prevention of antimicrobial agent-induced colitis and diarrhea. Gastroenterology. 1980;79:366–72.
159. Bartlett JG. Treatment of Clostridium difficile colitis. Gastroenterology. 1985;89:1192–5.
160. Elmore M, Rissing JP, Rink L, et al. Clindamycin-associated hepatotoxicity. Am J Med. 1974;57:627–30.
161. Fogdall RP, Miller RD. Prolongation of a pancuronium-induced neuromuscular blockade by clindamycin. Anesthesiology. 1974;41:407–8.
162. Thadepalli H, Gorbach SL, Broido PW, et al. Abdominal trauma, anaerobes, and antibiotics. Surg Gynecol Obstet. 1973;137:270–6.
163. Weinstein WM, Onderdonk AB, Bartlett JG, et al. Antimicrobial therapy of experimental intra-abdominal sepsis. J Infect Dis. 1975;132:282–6.
164. diZerega G, Yonekura L, Roy S, et al. A comparison of clindamycin-gentamicin and penicillin-gentamicin in the treatment of post-cesarean section endometritis. Am J Obstet Gynecol. 1979;134:238–42.
165. Solomkin JS, Dellinger EP, Christou NV, et al. Results of a multicenter trial comparing imipenem/cilastatin to tobramycin/clindamycin for intrabdominal infections. Ann Surg. 1990;212:581–91.
166. Sirinek KR, Levine BR. A randomized trial of ticarcillin and clavulanate versus gentamicin and clindamycin in patients with complicated appendicitis. Surg Gynecol Obstet. 1992;172(Suppl):30–5.
167. Bartlett JG, Gorbach SL. Treatment of aspiration pneumonia and primary lung abscess: penicillin F vs. clindamycin. JAMA. 1975;234:936–7.
168. Levison ME, Mangura CT, Lorber B, et al. Clindamycin compared with penicillin for the treatment of anaerobic lung abscess. Ann Intern Med. 1983;98:466–71.
169. Bartlett JG, Gorbach SL. Penicillin or clindamycin for primary lung abscess? (Editorial). Ann Intern Med. 1983;98:546–8.
170. Gudiol F, Manresa F, Pallares R, et al. Clindamycin vs penicillin for anaerobic lung infections. High rate of penicillin failures associated with penicillin-resistant Bacteroides melaninogenicus. Arch Intern Med. 1990;150:2525–9.
171. Leyden JJ, Shalita AR, Saatjian GD, et al. Erythromycin 2% gel in comparison with clindamycin phosphate 1% solution in acne vulgaris. J Am Acad Dermatol. 1987;16:822–7.
172. Parry MF, Rha CK. Pseudomembranous colitis caused by topical clindamycin phosphate. Arch Dermatol. 1986;122:583–4.
173. Andres FJ, Parker R, Hosein I. Clindamycin vaginal cream versus oral metronidazole in the treatment of bacterial vaginosis: A prospective double-blind clinical trial. South Med J. 1992;85:1077–80.
174. Schmitt C, Sobel JD, Meriwether C. Bacterial vaginosis: Treatment with clindamycin cream versus oral metronidazole. Obstet Gynecol. 1992;79:1020–3.
175. Hofflin JM, Remington JS. Clindamycin in a murine model of toxoplasmic encephalitis. Antimicrob Agents Chemother. 1987;31:492–6.
176. Dannemann B, McCutchan JA, Israelski D, et al. Treatment of toxoplasmic encephalitis in patients with AIDS. A randomized trial comparing pyrimethamine plus clindamycin to pyrimethamine plus sulfadiazine. The California Collaborative Treatment Group. Ann Intern Med. 1992;116:33–43.
177. Black JR, Feinberg J, Murphy RL, et al. Clindamycin and primaquine as primary treatment for mild and moderately severe Pneumocystis carinii pneumonia in patients with AIDS. Eur J Clin Microbiol Infect Dis. 1991;10:204–7.
178. Norskin GA, Murphy RL, Black JR et al. Salvage therapy with clindamycin/primaquine for Pneumocystis carinii pneumonia. Clin Infect Dis. 1992;14:183–8.
179. el Wakeel ES, Homeida MM, Ali HM, et al. Clindamycin in the treatment of falciparum malaria in Sudan. Am J Trop Med Hyg. 1985;34:1065–8.
180. Wittner M, Rowin KS, Tanowitz HB, et al. Successful chemotherapy of transfusion babesiosis. Ann Intern Med. 1982;96:601–4.
181. Brook I, Hirokawa R. Treatment of patients with a history of recurrent tonsillitis due to group A beta-hemolytic streptococci. A prospective randomized study comparing penicillin, erythromycin and clindamycin. Clin Pediatr. 1985;24:331–6.
182. Jensen JH, Larsen SB. Treatment of recurrent acute tonsillitis with clindamycin. An alternative to tonsillectomy? Clin Otolaryngol. 1991;16:498–500.

25. VANCOMYCIN AND TEICOPLANIN

ROBERT FEKETY

VANCOMYCIN

Structure

Vancomycin is a complex soluble glycopolypeptide that has a molecular weight of approximately 1450 daltons. While similar to three new glycopeptide antimicrobials, teicoplanin, daptomycin, and ramoplanin, it is unrelated to other antibiotics. When vancomycin was first introduced, commercial preparations contained as much as 30 percent of another substance of unknown nature that probably contributed to its side effects.[1,2] Current preparations are more pure (although not completely pure) and appear to be less toxic than the early preparations.

Derivation and Nomenclature

Vancomycin (Vancocin, Lilly; and Vancoled, Lederle) is a narrow-spectrum bactericidal antibiotic obtained from *Streptomyces orientales*. Introduced in 1956 because of its effectiveness against penicillin-resistant staphylococci, it was relegated because of its toxicity to the role of alternate therapy when methicillin became available. With spread of methicillin-resistant staphylococci in the United States in recent years, vancomycin underwent a marked increase in frequency of use and popularity, and it is now the drug of choice for treating infections with these organisms. It is also an effective agent for oral treatment of patients with severe antibiotic-associated colitis caused by *Clostridium difficile*.

Mechanism of Action

Vancomycin inhibits synthesis and assembly of the second stage of cell wall peptidoglycan polymers by complexing with the D-alanyl-D-alanine precursor, which fits into a "pocket" in the vancomycin molecule. It may also injure protoplasts by altering the permeability of their cytoplasmic membrane and may impair RNA synthesis. The multiple mechanisms of its action may contribute to the observed low frequency of development of resistance. Rapidly and tightly bound to organisms, vancomycin exerts a bactericidal effect without a lag period, but only on multiplying organisms. Vancomycin continues to exert its antibacterial activity after its concentration falls below the inhibitory level and has a so-called postantibiotic effect of about 2 hours.[3]

Antimicrobial Activity

Both *Staphylococcus aureus* and *Staphylococcus epidermidis* are highly susceptible to vancomycin. Concentrations of 1–5 mg/liter or less are almost invariably inhibitory, even with isolates resistant to methicillin, and most of these organisms are killed at about the same concentrations. A small proportion of strains require 10–20 mg/liter for inhibition, and up to 20 percent of strains are deficient in autolysins and relatively tolerant to the bactericidal action of vancomycin.[4,5] Biofilms of slime produced particularly on plastic foreign bodies by *Staphylococcus epidermidis* can impair penetration of vancomycin to the sites of lodgement of organisms and also may be responsible for tolerance to its bactericidal effect and for treatment failure.[6] A coagulase-negative species, *Staphylococcus haemolyticus,* was shown to be relatively resistant to vancomycin, with the minimum inhibitory concentration (MIC) and minimum bactericidal concentration (MBC) increased fourfold to 8 and 12 mg/liter, respectively, and the MBC with heavy inocula as high as 32 mg/liter, and was associated with failure of treatment until a foreign body was removed. These organisms were also resistant to teicoplanin, but were killed at low concentrations of daptomycin.[7] *Streptococcus pyogenes,* group B streptococci, *Corynebacterium jeikeium, Streptococcus pneumoniae* including penicillin-resistant strains, and *Clostridium difficile* are highly susceptible. *Listeria monocytogenes,* anaerobic or microaerophilic streptococci, clostridia including *Clostridium perfringens, Bacillus anthracis,* Actinomyces, Lactobacilli, Diphtheroids, *Clostridium diphtheriae, Corynebacteria* CDC-D2, and *Neisseria gonorrhoeae* are usually susceptible.[8,9] Viridans streptococci, *Streptococcus agalactiae, Streptococcus bovis,* and *Enterococcus faecalis* (formerly *Streptococcus faecalis*) isolates are usually inhibited at concentrations attainable in serum, but few if any *Enterococcus* isolates are killed at concentrations below 100 mg/liter.[5] Nutritionally deficient variants of streptococci may be killed by vancomycin alone.[10] From 40 to 70 percent of *Enterococcus* isolates show a synergistic bactericidal effect when vancomycin is combined with streptomycin or gentamicin, and the combination of vancomycin plus gentamicin is almost always bactericidal at attainable concentrations[11,12] unless so-called high-level gentamicin-resistant isolates (MIC > 500 mg/liter) are implicated.[13] Vancomycin-resistant isolates of *Enterococcus faecalis, Enterococcus faecium,*[14] *Enterococcus gallinarum,*[15] *Enterococcus casseliflavus,* and *Pediococcus* and *Leukonostoc* spp. (which may be misidentified as streptococci)[16] have been detected. In strains of *Enterococcus faecium* highly resistant to vancomycin and teicoplanin, plasmids that are self-transferable to other gram-positive organisms have been identified.

Three genes and three types of resistance (Van A, Van B, and Van C) have been identified. Van A is the most common type of resistance. The Van A protein is induced by either vancomycin or teicoplanin and may be plasmid encoded.[17,18] Van A strains are resistant to both vancomycin and teicoplanin. The gene for Van A resistance has been cloned and has been found to be part of a cluster of plasmid genes responsible for synthesis of peptidoglycan cell wall precursors containing a pentapeptide instead of the usual D-alanyl-D-alanine terminus. Reduced affinity of glycopeptides to this depsipeptide confers resistance to the antibiotic.[19] Recently it has been found that vancomycin resistance genes can be encoded on a transposon.[20] Van B strains demonstrate inducible synthesis of a 39.5 kD cytoplasmic membrane protein termed *Van B.* This protein is inducible by vancomycin[21] but not by teicoplanin.[22] Van B strains are vancomycin resistant and teicoplanin susceptible. Van C strains demonstrate low-level vancomycin resistance but are susceptible to teicoplanin. Van C is constitutive and chromosomally encoded.[23–25]

Prolonged and/or indiscriminate use of vancomycin or teicoplanin, when given by either the oral or intravenous route, may contribute to the selective pressure encouraging the emergence of glycopeptide-resistant enterococci. There is no cross-resistance between vancomycin and unrelated antibiotics, and significant resistance to vancomycin rarely if ever develops during therapy. Cross-resistance with teicoplanin occurs but is variable. Antibacterial activity of vancomycin varies little between pH 6.5 and 8. Some *Neisseria gonorrheae* isolates are very susceptible and may be missed on culture when vancomycin-containing selective media such as Thayer-Martin are used. *Flavobacterium meningosepticum* (gram-negative) and some *Neisseria meningitis* isolates are also susceptible at attainable concentrations (between 16 and 25 mg/liter), but other gram-negative bacilli, mycobacteria, fungi, and *Bacteroides* are not susceptible. A recent report indicated that *Borrelia burgdorferi* isolates were inhibited at low concentrations of vancomycin (0.5–2 mg/liter) and killed at only slightly higher concentrations and that vancomycin was synergistic with penicillin G at low concentrations against this organism.[26]

Pharmacology

Administration. After being dissolved in sterile water, vancomycin should be given intravenously in 100–250 ml of 5% dextrose or 0.9% NaCl over at least 60 minutes.[1] It can also be given by continuous intravenous drip, but intermittent infusion is preferred by most. Rapid or bolus administration is dangerous, especially if 1 g doses are used, possibly because it causes histamine release by basophils and mast cells.[27] that may cause flushing (the "red-man" or "red-neck" syndrome), anaphylactoid reactions, hypotension, and even cardiac arrest[10]; this is rarely seen except shortly after the rapid administration of vancomycin. Antihistamines may help in preventing this. Hydrocortisone (20 mg) can be added to infusions to reduce side effects, but the mixture may precipitate at high concentrations. Heparin and vancomycin also can precipitate at high concentrations, so they should not be infused simultaneously through the same intravenous line.[28] Because of pain on injection, no satisfactory intramuscular preparation of vancomycin is available. Vancomycin is absorbed poorly from the gastrointestinal tract, even when the colon is inflamed, and it is very nontoxic when used orally for treatment of severe clostridial enterocolitis[1,27–31] and for prevention of infection in leukopenic cancer patients.[32]

Distribution, Excretion, and Protein Binding. Vancomycin is eliminated from the body almost exclusively by glomerular filtration, although a small amount may be metabolized by the liver and appear in active form in the bile. From 80 to 90 percent of an administered dose appears in the urine within 24 hours. The half-life of vancomycin in serum is 6–8 hours in persons with normal renal function. In anuric patients, it may be prolonged to about 9 days and may be detected in serum for as long as 21 days after a single 1 g dose.[33,34] From 10 to 55 percent is protein bound in serum; this is believed to have a negligible effect on clinical results.

Concentrations in Body Fluids and Tissues. Trough serum levels after intravenous administration of 500 mg of vancomycin to adults range from 6 to 10 mg/liter, with an average of 8 mg/liter after repeated dosing. Peak levels of up to 50 mg/liter may be seen, depending on how soon the blood is drawn after the infusion. When 1 g is given slowly intravenously, peak (1 hour after infusion) and trough levels of 20–50 mg/liter and 5–12 mg/liter, respectively, are achieved; these are considered desirable and appropriate concentrations. Some clinicians monitor only trough concentrations and attempt to keep these in the range of about 10 mg/liter,[35] but some patients with severe infections necessitating a bactericidal effect, obesity, and/or less susceptible organisms may not achieve adequate peak levels (25–35 mg/liter, or more) when dosing is based only on trough levels.

Urinary concentrations range from 100 to 300 mg/liter. When vancomycin (0.5 g q6h) is given orally in a dose of 500 mg four

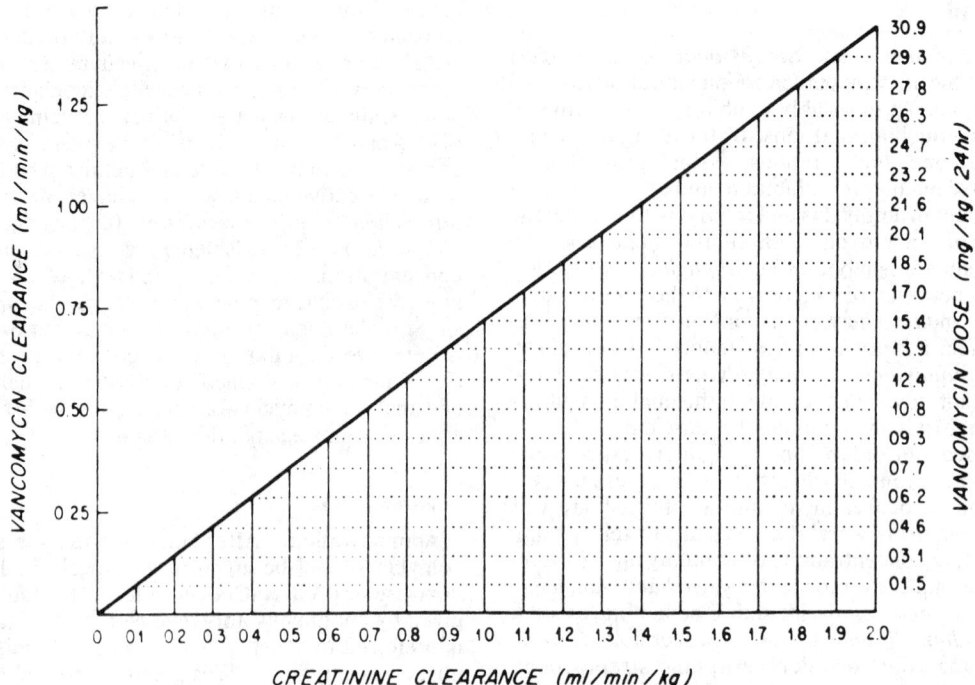

FIG. 1.   Dosage nomogram for vancomycin in patients with impaired renal function. The nomogram is not valid for functionally anephric patients on dialysis. For such patients, the dose is 1.9 mg/kg/24 hr. (From Moellering et al.,[40] with permission.)

times daily, concentrations of 1000–9000 mg/liter may be found in stools, but only trace amounts are ordinarily found in serum[8,9,30]; concentrations as high as therapeutic ones have been found occasionally in the serum of anuric patients given the drug orally for treatment of colitis.[36] When 125 mg is given orally, stool concentrations have ranged from 100 to 800 mg/liter. When vancomycin is given intravenously, concentrations of up to 100 mg/liter may be found in stools of some patients, but the drug is undetectable in stools of most patients[9]; thus, the intravenous route alone is not recommended for treatment of colitis. Vancomycin is not found in cerebrospinal fluid (CSF) of persons without meningitis, but bactericidal levels (<1–7 mg/liter) have been found in the CSF of most (but not all) patients with meningitis.

Small supplemental amounts (3–5 mg) may be given intrathecally in meningitis, particularly if there is no response after 48 hours of intravenous therapy.[37] A larger intrathecal dose may be needed for less susceptible organisms, such as flavobacteria. Vancomycin is irritating when injected into serous or synovial cavities, and peritonitis has been reported following its direct instillation.[38] Adequate concentrations are reached in pleural, pericardial, synovial, and ascitic fluids after intravenous administration, and low levels are found in bile.[8]

It is recommended that an intravenous loading dose of 15 mg/kg be given to adults, regardless of renal function. Since the kidney is the only significant organ of elimination of vancomycin, high and potentially toxic serum levels can be attained in patients with renal insufficiency unless subsequent dosage is reduced appropriately.[32,34,39] To achieve a mean therapeutic concentration of 20 mg/liter in serum of adults with renal impairment, the following simple formula can be used to estimate maintenance dosage: the daily parenteral dose of vancomycin in milligrams should be approximately 150 plus 15 times the creatinine clearance in ml/min.[34] Another strategy is to give 1 g every 36 hours when the serum creatinine concentration is 1.5–5 mg/100 ml and 1 g every 10–14 days when it is greater than 5 mg/100 ml. As little as 1 g may yield effective serum concentrations for 7–14 days in anuric patients.[34] There are nomograms that may be more accurate than the above simple rules for dosing patients with renal failure.[38–41] Most nomograms (such as the one shown in Fig. 1) are designed to provide steady-state trough concentrations of 8–12 mg/liter[40] and are probably the most accurate dosing methods.[41a] In difficult situations, serum concentrations should be monitored, although the data supporting this practice are meager.[41a,41b]

Since hemodialysis does not remove significant amounts of vancomycin (but peritoneal dialysis can),[32,34,38] it is a common practice to dose patients with renal failure with 1 g vancomycin weekly (about 150 mg is removed each day in the average adult by nonrenal mechanisms). Use of newer, more permeable (high-flux) hemodialysis membranes can result in a significant but transient decrease in serum concentrations because of binding to the polyacronitrile membrane,[42] but transfer of the drug from tissues back to blood with a rebound in vancomycin levels occurs, and therapeutic concentrations may still be present for 1 week.[43] Hemofiltration may also be very efficient at removing vancomycin and useful in managing overdosage in patients with renal failure.[44] Serum levels should be monitored at frequent, regular intervals in dialyzed, uremic, or seriously ill patients to ascertain that safe yet adequate concentrations are present. Cardiopulmonary bypass is associated with a fall in serum concentrations because of dilution.[45] When it is used prophylactically, a preoperative vancomycin dose of 15 mg/kg is needed before bypass surgery, and 10 mg/kg should be given after bypass surgery if renal function is normal. Pediatric dosing is discussed below.

Toxicity and Adverse Reactions

With the purified preparations now available, adverse reactions seem to be much less frequent than when vancomycin was first introduced. The most frequent side effects consist of fever, chills, and phlebitis at the site of the infusion. These are less frequent if the drug is infused slowly in a large volume of fluid. Tingling and flushing of the face, neck, and thorax are frequently experienced (the red-neck or red-man syndrome), especially if 1 g doses are given[46] and the drug is infused very rapidly[47]; this is thought to be related to histamine release secondary to local hyperosmolarity and not to allergic hypersensitivity. Maculopapular or diffuse erythematous rashes, presumably due to hypersensitivity, occur in 4–5 percent of patients and may persist for weeks despite discontinuation of vancomycin in patients with marked renal failure. They may respond to steroid or antihistamine therapy. Shock has occurred after rapid intravenous infusion of the drug, especially during surgery. Reversible leukopenia, thrombocytopenia, or eosinophilia sometimes develops,[48] and lacrimation has been reported.[27] One case of antibiotic-induced *C. difficile* colitis has been reported following the intravenous use of vancomycin,[49] and we are aware of other cases that have not been reported.

An important adverse reaction to vancomycin is neurotoxicity, which is manifested primarily by auditory nerve damage and hearing loss. Tinnitus and high-tone hearing loss are often an antecedent to deafness, which is infrequent if serum concentrations are maintained below 30 mg/liter and is more common when concentrations are in the range of 80 mg/liter or more. Hearing occasionally improves when the drug is discontinued, but usually continues to deteriorate and becomes permanent.[50,51] Nephrotoxicity was relatively common with the early impure preparations of vancomycin, especially when given in high doses; it is usually transient or reversible. With appropriate doses selected by monitoring renal function and serum concentrations, nephrotoxicity is now uncommon[51-53] and is usually transient or reversible unless multiple courses are given, high and toxic levels are achieved, or aminoglycosides are also given. Though the preparations of vancomycin now available are more pure and are no longer appreciably nephrotoxic, high doses given by the parenteral route should be avoided, and serum levels should be carefully monitored when other nephrotoxic drugs are being given. The risk of nephrotoxicity appears to be enhanced even with normally safe levels when drugs such as aminoglycosides or ethacrynic acid are given concomitantly.

Drug Interactions

Vancomycin is incompatible with many other drugs in intravenous solutions, especially chloramphenicol, adrenal corticosteroids, and methicillin. Heparin (at very high concentrations) may inactivate vancomycin in intravenous solutions and can be responsible for persistence of bacteremia.[28] Vancomycin is not stable enough for use with Infusaid and certain other implantable pumps.[54]

Major Uses and Doses.　The usual intravenous dose of vancomycin for adults with normal renal function is 1 g every 12 hours (15 mg/kg) or 500 mg (6.5–8 mg/kg) every 6 hours. In severely ill patients with normal renal function, especially patients with obesity or meningitis, 1 g may be given every 8 hours for 2–3 days until the infection is under control. Dosing should be based on actual body weight. Morbidly obese patients with severe infections may require high doses, which should be based on total body weight, creatinine clearance, and the monitoring of serum levels.[55] Various dosage regimens have been proposed for pediatric usage. For newborn infants, 15 mg/kg may be given slowly every 12 hours intravenously during the first week of life or every 8 hours in those 8–30 days of age; 10 mg/kg every 6 hours is recommended for older infants and children and 15 mg/kg every 6 hours for infants and children with staphylococcal central nervous system infections. Monitoring serum levels is desirable, especially in preterm infants.[56] A continuous intravenous drip can be used.[57,58] Oral dosages of 125–500 mg four times per day have been used for treatment of adults with *Clostridium difficile* colitis (but without ileus), with equivalent results.[59] For infants and children with *Clostridium difficile* colitis, an oral dose of 500 mg/1.73 m² every 6 hours has been recommended.[60] Oral therapy is much more reliable than intravenous therapy for treatment of *Clostridium difficile* colitis.

Intravenous dosage must be reduced with renal impairment, and may be monitored to achieve peak serum concentrations no higher than 30–40 mg/liter and troughs ranging from 5 to 10 mg/liter.[41b] If a continuous infusion is used, a steady-state

concentration of 15 mg/liter seems desirable.[37,38,49,61] Recent evidence indicates that impaired liver function may also delay elimination of vancomycin and require dosage modification.[62]

Vancomycin for parenteral use should be reserved for use primarily for serious methicillin-resistant staphylococcal infections. Intravenous vancomycin is the therapy of choice for serious staphylococcal infections in patients with methicillin-oxacillin-nafcillin– or cephalosporin-resistant organisms (MRSA) or in patients who cannot be given these primary drugs.[8,52,63-67] It has also become the most reliable and popular therapy for serious intravenous catheter or device-related coagulase-negative staphylococcal infections.[68]

All strains of methicillin-resistant coagulase-positive staphylococci have been susceptible to low concentrations of vancomycin, but clinical responses in MRSA endocarditis may be slow and may require 1 week or more. Rare isolates show clinically significant tolerance (MBC > 16 times MIC) to its bactericidal action.[5,63,66,69] When treatment of serious MRSA infections with vancomycin alone has failed, addition of gentamicin, rifampin, or both may be successful. Rifampin appears especially beneficial because it penetrates into leukocytes, serous cavities, and other closed spaces. Since antagonism may occur occasionally with some of these combinations of antimicrobials,[63] these combinations should not be used routinely; some experts feel that serum bacteriostatic and bactericidal levels should be monitored as a guide to therapy when they are used. When vancomycin is used for adults in conjunction with an aminoglycoside, some experts believe the former's dosage should rarely exceed 0.5 g every 8 hours.[52] Methicillin-resistant *Staphylococcus epidermidis* endocarditis involving a prosthetic valve is best treated with usual doses of vancomycin for 4 weeks in combination with rifampin, plus an aminoglycoside (the latter for the first 2 weeks).[67] This regimen may also be useful for managing other serious staphylococcal infections involving a foreign body that cannot be removed.

Survival rates of 60–75 percent have been achieved with vancomycin in patients with staphylococcal endocarditis or bacteremia.[1,8] Survival in patients aged 70 or older is about 50 percent. The usual duration of therapy is 4–6 weeks. Success rates of 75 percent or greater have been reported with vancomycin in patients with pneumonia, parotitis, or meningitis.

While vancomycin penetrates into the central nervous system in most ill patients in amounts adequate to treat meningitis and shunt infections, this is not always the case,[37] and removal of foreign bodies or supplemental intraventricular or intrathecal instillation of vancomycin may be required in patients with a poor response.[69-71] Cerebrospinal fluid concentrations need not be greater than about 25 mg/liter, so intrathecal doses of 3–5 mg are usually adequate. Penicillin-resistant *Streptococcus pneumoniae* isolates are usually susceptible to the inhibitory effects of vancomycin, although the concentrations needed for a bactericidal effect may be four- to eightfold higher than inhibitory ones and may not be achievable in the CSF or ventricles of the brain. Penetration into the CSF may be further impaired if adrenal corticosteroids are used and when inflammation subsides. About 40 percent of adults treated with vancomycin for pneumococcal meningitis were reported to experience therapeutic failure,[72] but did respond to therapy with cefotaxime or ceftriaxone. Vancomycin should probably be reserved in meningitis for patients with allergies to other drugs or with organisms resistant to them.

Vancomycin is the treatment of choice for patients with *Enterococcus faecalis* endocarditis who are allergic to penicillin. In this setting it should be given along with an aminoglycoside, since vancomycin is rarely bactericidal by itself against these organisms.[11,12,73,74] Since bactericidal synergism between gentamicin and vancomycin has been uniformly demonstrated until recently with most enterococci,[13,75] gentamicin is preferable to streptomycin, which is not synergistic with as many as 40 percent of these organisms; conversely, streptomycin is only occasionally more active than gentamicin. Laboratory studies of synergism with the patient's organism or by Schlicter tests of the bactericidal activity of their serum may be helpful in determining the best regimen during treatment. A vancomycin dose of 0.5 g every 8 hours intravenously plus either streptomycin, 0.5 g every 12 hours intramuscularly, or gentamicin, 60–80 mg (1 mg/kg) every 8 hours intravenously for 4–6 weeks, is recommended for adults with normal renal function. More vigorous or prolonged therapy may be needed for complicated cases, such as when a prosthetic valve is infected. Patients should be monitored closely for signs of ototoxicity or nephrotoxicity, and drug dosages should be carefully adjusted in renal failure. Viridans streptococcal or *Streptococcus bovis* endocarditis may be treated with vancomycin alone if the MBC for the isolate is no more than 10 mg/liter; otherwise it should be combined with streptomycin, gentamicin, or another aminoglycoside.[8,52] Again, monitoring serum bactericidal activity may be helpful when bactericidal sensitivity tests in combination are not available.

Other serious infections with resistant organisms that have been responsive to vancomycin include *Corynebacterium* endocarditis in patients with prosthetic valves and *Flavobacterium meningosepticum* meningitis.[8,37,70] Vancomycin has been considered the drug of choice for treating acute staphylococcal pseudomembranous enterocolitis, which is now a rare disease. In two series of cases, 67 of 72 patients were cured of the disease (93 percent).[29,76] It was usually given orally, 500 mg diluted in water every 6 hours for adults.

Orally administered vancomycin is considered the drug of choice by most investigators for treating *seriously* ill patients with antibiotic-associated *Clostridium difficile* (pseudomembranous) colitis, although metronidazole is less expensive and usually effective[68] in less severely ill patients. This organism is occasionally resistant to metronidazole, but is always susceptible to vancomycin. Treatment failures are very rare with vancomycin unless treatment is delayed.[29,30,78,79] Dosages of either 125 or 500 mg four times daily have been effective, and the lower and less expensive dose seems as good as the larger one[59] in most patients. Vancomycin is useful in treating relapses of colitis cause by *Clostridium difficile*,[79] but neither it nor metronidazole reliably kills the spores of the organism and eradicates the *Clostridium difficile* carrier state.[80] Vancomycin should be given *orally* for treatment of colitis, since the drug is needed to inhibit toxin production within the lumen of the bowel and not for inhibition of the organism in tissues.[79] Intravenous vancomycin by itself is not reliable for treatment of colitis, since adequate concentrations are seldom achieved within the lumen of the colon when it is given in this way. In patients with ileus, vancomycin should be given orally or by nasogastric tube in 500 mg doses every 6 hours or by a catheter inserted colonoscopically to the proximal cecum.[81,82] A solution containing 200–500/mg vancomycin per liter can be used in the latter situation. Both vancomycin (in full parenteral doses) plus metronidazole may also be given intravenously in this difficult situation. Even though little vancomycin will be absorbed from the intestinal tract,[81] serum levels should be monitored to prevent toxicity when it is used by both routes. When nasogastric tubes are needed for administering vancomycin, they can be clamped for 30–60 minutes after giving it. When patients have ileus, the drug has also been given by enema, via an ileostomy or colostomy, by a long intestinal tube inserted nasogastrically and passed to the distal ileum or cecum, or via catheter inserted per rectum via a colonoscope to the proximal cecum.

Staphylococcal peritonitis occurring during peritoneal dialysis can be treated with intravenous vancomycin alone. One gram given intravenously will yield peritoneal fluid concentrations greater than 5 mg/liter for 1 week or more in this setting.[37,56] Others have noted that peritoneal dialysis may remove vancomycin from the blood and have recommended instilling vancomycin into the peritoneal cavity to a concentration of 25 mg/liter in addition to parenteral vancomycin to ensure good levels in peritoneal fluid.[83] In fact, it may be possible to treat staphylococcal peritonitis in patients undergoing chronic peritoneal dialysis solely by the intraperitoneal administration of vancomycin at a concentration of 50 mg/liter in the dialysate.[83,84] However, vancomycin given intraperitoneally may be irritating,[85] and organisms protected by a biofilm on the catheter may be clinically tolerant to the bactericidal effect of vancomycin and therefore responsible for relapse.[6] The addition of rifampin to vancomycin for treatment of refractory staphylococcal peritonitis in chronic dialysis can be curative.[86]

According to an American Heart Association's Advisory Committee,[87,88] vancomycin is useful for the prevention of bacterial endocarditis in patients who are allergic to penicillin and undergoing dental or respiratory tract procedures.[87] The mechanism of prevention is thought to be either by the bactericidal action of vancomycin or by its ability to interfere with the adherence of the organism to the endocardium. One gram is given slowly intravenously within 60 minutes prior to starting the procedure; no repeat dose is necessary. For genitourinary or gastrointestinal surgery or instrumentation (after which enterococcal endocarditis may develop), vancomycin can be given for prophylaxis as above along with gentamicin, 1.5 mg/kg; these may be repeated once 8–12 hours later.[87] Vancomycin can be used prophylactically for insertion of prosthetic valves, with an initial intravenous dose of 15 mg/ml given over 1 hour just prior to surgery, followed by 10 mg/kg immediately after bypass surgery (if renal function is normal),[45] along with 1.7 mg/kg gentamicin before surgery and 8 hours later. The efficacy of this regimen has not been proven, but it is designed to prevent *Staphylococcus aureus, Staphylococcus epidermidis* enterococcal and coliform infections of the prosthesis and sternum. Vancomycin is often included in empiric therapy for febrile neutropenic patients, but unless there is good evidence to suggest the presence of a staphylococcal infection, its use probably should not be routine,[89] but reserved instead for documented infections.

Vancomycin has been used in prophylactic oral nonabsorbable antibiotic regimens designed to prevent endogenous infections in patients with cancer or leukemia.[32] Such patients also seem to experience a lower rate of *Clostridium difficile* colitis complicating their chemotherapy. Otherwise, these regimens are probably of no value unless protective environments and leukocyte transfusions are available and used, and they may encourage the development of resistance.

Vancomycin has been used prophylactically in patients receiving chronic dialysis in order to prevent staphylococcal infections, but this has resulted in the emergence of vancomycin-resistant enterococci and serious enterococcal infections.[15]

It is obvious that there has been a marked resurgence of use of vancomycin in the last two decades. Many new indications for its use have been established, and much new information has been accumulated. But, because of the emergence of resistance and because of its expense, vancomycin must be used judiciously. An excellent review of vancomycin has been published.[90]

TEICOPLANIN

Teicoplanin (formerly named *teichomycin A*) is a new glycopeptide antibiotic derived from the fermentation products of *Actinoplanes teichomyceticus*.[91] While it is widely used in Europe for treatment of gram-positive infections, it is still investigational in the United States. Teicoplanin is a complex of six analogs having the same linear heptapeptide base and an aglycone containing aromatic amino acids with D-mannose and N-acetyl-D-glycosamine as sugars and a molecular weight ranging from 1562 to 1891. Teicoplanin is chemically similar to vancomycin and daptomycin, but with important differences responsible for the unique physical and chemical properties of the complex.[92] It has greater lipophilicity than vancomycin, which results in rapid and excellent tissue and intracellular phagocytic penetration. Other consequences are a long elimination half-life, slow release from tissues, and water solubility at physiologic pH. It has few if any inactive metabolites.[93]

Mechanism of Action and Pharmacokinetics

Teicoplanin has an antibacterial spectrum and mechanism of action similar to that of vancomycin. It is usually bactericidal (except for enterococci), although tolerance has been observed to its bactericidal action. Staphylococci and enterococci that are resistant to vancomycin are usually resistant to teicoplanin. The development of resistance during treatment has not been reported. Teicoplanin impairs cell wall synthesis by inhibiting polymerization of peptidoglycan in a way similar to that of vancomycin, but at different sites from those inhibited by β-lactams.[94,95] It does this by forming a complex with the terminal D-alanyl-D-alanine precursor, which fits into a "pocket" in the teicoplanin molecule.[96] It has an elimination half-life of 40–70 hours after intravenous administration, a disappearance curve that fits both a two- and a three-compartment model, and a volume of distribution of 0.5–0.8 liter/kg.[97,98] In contrast to the low degree of protein binding of vancomycin, its protein binding is as high as 90 percent,[96] which may account for its slow renal clearance.

Because of its long half-life, it can be given intramuscularly or intravenously once per day.[99] Provided in 200 mg vials, it has usually been given in a daily intravenous dose of 2–3 mg/kg after a loading dose of 6 mg/kg (400 mg).[100] Higher doses may be needed and can be given with better results but with greater toxicity.[101] When single intravenous injections of 3 or 6 mg/kg were given rapidly (over 5 minutes) to healthy volunteers, peak plasma concentrations of 53 and 112 mg/liter were observed, and concentrations of 2.1 and 4.2 μg/ml were observed at 24 hours. Similar concentrations were seen following intramuscular dosing with 3 mg/kg. With these doses, serum levels greater than the MIC-90 for susceptible organisms were sustained for at least 24 hours after a single injection. When 3 mg/kg was given to volunteers at a constant rate over 30 minutes, peak concentrations were about 22 mg/liter. After six intramuscular doses of 200 mg (3 mg/kg) over a 5-day period, absorption was rapid and the initial peak level at 1 hour was 2.8 mg/liter, 5.8 mg/liter at 2 hours, and 7.1 mg/liter at 4 hours. After the last injection, mean peak levels of 12.1 mg/liter were reached. Trough levels at 24 hours on days 2–6 were approximately 5.4–7.3 mg/liter,[98] and the calculated elimination half-life was about 99 hours. Urinary concentrations ranged from 16 to 156 mg/liter from days 1 through 7. About 80 percent of the drug was eliminated in urine.[99] Teicoplanin administered orally was not significantly absorbed from the intestinal tracts of rats, dogs, or human volunteers. In the latter, 40 percent of the administered dose was present in feces in a microbiologically active form.[93]

In patients with renal impairment, serum concentrations are related to creatinine clearance, which can be used for adjusting dosage.[100] Teicoplanin is exchanged bidirectionally across the peritoneum, but is not removed by hemodialysis.[100] In one study, 2.7 percent of a parenterally administered dose was found in feces over the next 8 days.[99] While the evidence suggests teicoplanin penetrates tissues well, the penetration of teicoplanin into bone, peritoneal fluid, and cerebrospinal fluid needs more study. Teicoplanin is well tolerated by children. A dose of 10 mg/kg/day has been recommended for children and 6 mg/kg/day for neonates.[102]

Antibacterial Activity

Teicoplanin has excellent antibactericidal activity against Gram-positive organisms, including *Streptococcus pneumoniae,*

Streptococcus pyogenes, other streptococci, *Enterococcus faecalis, Staphylococcus aureus* (both penicillinase-producing and methicillin-resistant organisms), *Staphylococcus epidermidis, Clostridium species, Corynebacterium jeikeium, Propionibacterium acnes,* and *Listeria monocytogenes.*[103–105] Inhibitory concentrations range from 0.025 to 3.1 mg/liter. Some strains of *Staphylococcus epidermidis* and *Staphylococcus haemolyticus* are relatively resistant to teicoplanin, but susceptible to vancomycin.[106,107] Against many susceptible organisms, teicoplanin is two to four times as active as vancomycin. Teicoplanin was the more active antimicrobial against *Enterococcus faecalis,* but, like vancomycin, it is rarely bactericidal for this species. Teicoplanin-resistant enterococci (usually resistant to vancomycin as well) have been isolated from nosocomial infections. Teicoplanin is more active than vancomycin against *Clostridium difficile,* but it is even more highly bound by cholestyramine.[108] It is not active against gram-negative organisms, including *Neisseria, Mycobacterium* spp., and fungi. Teicoplanin does not give rise to stably resistant mutants in vitro, and it shows no cross-resistance with nonglycopeptide antibiotics, except for aminoglycosides. Like vancomycin, teicoplanin can be synergistic with rifampin or aminoglycosides against staphylococci, enterococci, other streptococci, and *Listeria.*[107,109–112]

Toxicity

Teicoplanin has been well tolerated when given to humans intramuscularly or intravenously. Unlike vancomycin, it produces only mild pain at the site of injection. After slow intravenous infusion, it has not caused thrombophlebitis[113] or adverse effects on platelet function or coagulation.[110] Studies with 100 human volunteers showed no untoward effects at doses of up to 7.5 mg/kg. When used by rapid intravenous infusion in 310 hospitalized infected patients with infections, significant adverse effects were uncommon (2 percent), and no patient developed flushing or the red-man or red-neck syndrome,[115] although the latter has been seen. However, ototoxicity has been reported.[116–118]

Clinical Uses

Teicoplanin is potentially an effective alternate to vancomycin, with the advantage of less frequent dosing (once per day) and, because of its greater potency and therapeutic ratio, less nephrotoxicity and ototoxicity. It may be useful for patients who have had neutropenic or allergic reactions to vancomycin.[11]

Possible uses for teicoplanin include the treatment of serious gram-positive infections, including endocarditis caused by MRSA, pneumonia, septicemia, soft tissue infections, urinary tract infections, and osteomyelitis. It has been more effective than vancomycin in a rabbit model of methicillin-resistant staphylococcal endocarditis.[119] Clinical cures were seen in 96 percent of 88 patients treated with 200–400 mg teicoplanin once daily for coagulase-negative staphylococcal infections[120–122] and in 79–91 percent of 1781 patients with various other gram-positive infections.[117,120] These included MRSA infections, pneumonia, endocarditis,[101] septicemia, and joint infections. Some of these patients developed ototoxicity or nephrotoxicity, but many of them had also received an aminoglycoside.[117]

Given once daily (400 mg) for treatment of mild MRSA infections, teicoplanin was comparable to vancomycin in efficacy. When serious MRSA infections were treated with teicoplanin 200–800 mg/day, in some cases supplemented with another antibiotic, the cure rate was 75 percent. When patients with deep-seated staphylococcal infections were treated with maintenance doses of 200 mg/day, only 44 percent were cured.[123] Treatment failure was related to the presence of foreign bodies and poor tissue concentrations. The high degree of protein binding of teicoplanin may have been an important factor in these low-dose treatment failures. Doses of 400 mg per day or more will probably be needed for successful treatment of severe infections. In combination with an aminoglycoside, teicoplanin could be a suitable alternative to ampicillin, penicillin G, or vancomycin for treatment of serious or refractory enterococcal infections.[124] It could be useful for prophylaxis of endocarditis in penicillin-allergic patients or when vancomycin or other antibiotics are not tolerated.[119] However, when used once daily for prophylaxis in cardiac surgery, teicoplanin was associated with a higher than expected number of sternal wound and urinary tract infections.[125] Other potential indications include shunt infections and treatment of gram-positive peritonitis in chronic dialysis patients.[126,127] Finally, oral administration of teicoplanin may be an alternative for treatment of *Clostridium difficile* colitis or necrotizing staphylococcal enterocolitis. Twenty-two patients with *C. difficile*-associated diarrhea or colitis were treated via the oral route with teicoplanin (400–600 mg/day for 10 days). All patients treated with teicoplanin remained asymptomatic after discontinuation of treatment, while 3 of 23 evaluable patients given vancomycin developed recurrences.[128]

Its potential for safe and effective once daily dosing, by either the intramuscular or intravenous route, may make teicoplanin a useful addition to the antibiotic armamentarium if further clinical studies substantiate its safety and efficacy. Preliminary data suggest caution in its use alone at doses of 400 mg/day or less in patients with endocarditis or other serious deep-seated staphylococcal infections. A recent review of 200 publications indicated teicoplanin needs to be given in significantly larger doses (10–12 mg/kg) than initially thought necessary to maximize clinical efficacy and that its lower incidence of side effects at these dosages as compared with vancomycin is clinically negligible.[129]

REFERENCES

1. Alexander MR. Review of vancomycin after 15 years of use. Drug Intell Clin Pharm. 1974;8:520.
2. Perkins HR, Nieto M. The chemical basis for the action of the vancomycin group of antibiotics. Ann NY Acad Sci. 1974;235:348.
3. Craig WA, Vogelman B. The post-antibiotic effect. Ann Intern Med. 1987; 106:900–902.
4. Gopal V, Bisno AL, Silverblatt FJ. Failure of vancomycin treatment in *Staphylococcus aureus* endocarditis. In vivo and in vitro observations. JAMA. 1976;236:1604.
5. Sabath L, Wheeler N, Laverdiere M, et al. A new type of penicillin resistance in *Staphylococcus aureus*. Lancet. 1977;1:443.
6. Evans RC, Holmes CJ. Effect of vancomycin hydrochloride on *Staphylococcus epidermidis* biofilm associated with silicone elastomer. Antimicrob Agents Chemother. 1987;31:889–94.
7. Schwalke RS, Stapleton JT, Gilligan PH. Emergence of vancomycin resistance in coagulase-negative staphylococci. N Engl J Med. 1987;316:927–31.
8. Geraci JE. Vancomycin. Mayo Clin Proc. 1977;52:631.
9. Geraci JE, Heilman FR, Nichols DR, et al. Some laboratory and clinical experiences with a new antibiotic, vancomycin. Proc Staff Meet Mayo Clin. 1956;31:564.
10. Reimer LG. Measurement of serum bactericidal activity and use of vancomycin for treatment of nutritionally variant streptococcal bacteremia. Diagn Microbiol Infect Dis. 1987;6:319–22.
11. Watanakunakorn C, Bakie C. Synergism of vancomycin-gentamicin and vancomycin-streptomycin against enterococci. Antimicrob Agents Chemother. 1973;4:120.
12. Harwick HJ, Kalmanson GM, Guze LB. In vitro activity of ampicillin or vancomycin combined with gentamicin or streptomycin against enterococci. Antimicrob Agents Chemother. 1973;4:383.
13. Mederski-Samoraj BD, Murray BE. High level resistance to enterococci in clinical isolates of staphylococci. J Infect Dis. 1983;147:751–7.
14. Uttley AC, Collins CH, Naidoo J, et al. Vancomycin-resistant enterococci. Lancet. 1988;1:57–58.
15. Kaplan AH, Gilligan PH, Facklam RR. Recovery of resistant enterococci during vancomycin prophylaxis. J Clin Microb. 1988;26:126–8.
16. Rubin LG, Velozzi E, Shapiro J, et al. Infection with vancomycin-resistant "streptococci," due to *Leuconostoc* species. J Infect Dis. 1988;216.
17. Leclercq R, Deriot E, Weber M, et al. Transferable vancomycin and teicoplanin resistance in *Enterococcus faecium*. Antimicrob Agents Chemother. 1989;33:10–5.
18. Leclercq R, Deriot E, Duval J, et al. Plasmid-mediated resistance to vancomycin and teicoplanin in *Enterococcus faecium*. N Engl J Med. 1988;319: 157–61.
19. Leclercq R, Dutka-Malen S, Brisson-Noel A, et al. Resistance of enterococci to aminoglycosides and glycopeptides. Clin Infect Dis. 1992;15:495–501.
20. Arthur M, Molinas C, Depardieu F, et al. Characterization of Tn *1546*, a Tn-*3* related transposon conferring glycopeptide resistance to synthesis of depsipeptide peptidoglycan precursors in *Enterococcus faecium* BM4147. J Bacteriol. 1993;175:117–27.
21. Williamson R, Al-Obeid S, Shlaes JH, et al. Inducible resistance to vancomycin in *Enterococcus faecium* D366. J Infect Dis. 1989;159:1095–1104.
22. Al-Obeid S, Collatz E, Gutmann L. Mechanism of resistance to vancomycin in *Enterococcus faecium* D366 and *Enterococcus faecalis* A256. Antimicrob Agents Chemother. 1990;34:252–6.
23. Vincent S, Minkler P, Bincziewski R, et al. Vancomycin resistance in *Enterococcus gallinarum*. Antimicrob Agents Chemother. 1992;36:1392–9.
24. Shlaes DM, Etter L, Gutmann L. Synergistic killing of vancomycin-resistant enterococci of classes A, B, and C by combinations of vancomycin, penicillin, and gentamicin. Antimicrob Agents Chemother. 1991;35:776–9.
25. Vincent S, Knight RG, Green M, et al. Vancomycin susceptibility and identification of motile enterococci. J Clin Microbiol. 1991;29:2335–7.
26. Dever L, Jorgensen JH, Barbour A. In vitro activity of vancomycin against the spirochete *Borrelia burgdorferi*. Antimicrol Agents Chemother. 1993;37: 1115–21.
27. Polk RE, Healy DP, Schwartz LB, et al. Vancomycin and the red-man syndrome: Pharmacodynamics of histamine release. J Infect Dis. 1988;157: 502–7.
28. Barg NL, Fekety R, Supena R: Persistant staphylococcal bacteremia in an intravenous drug abuser. Antimicrob Agents Chemother. 1986;29:209–11.
29. Khan MY, Hall WH. Staphylococcal enterocolitis—Treatment with oral vancomycin. Ann Intern Med. 1966;65:1.
30. Tedesco F, Markham R, Gurwith M, et al. Oral vancomycin for antibiotic-associated pseudomembranous colitis. Lancet 1978;2:226–28.
31. Silva J, Batts DH, Fekety R, et al. Treatment of *Clostridium difficile* colitis and diarrhea with vancomycin. Amer J Med 1981;71:815–22.
32. Bodey G. Oral antibiotic prophylaxis in protected environment units: Effect of nonabsorbable and absorbable antibiotics on the fecal flora. Antimicrob Agents Chemother. 1972;1:343.
33. Lindholm DD, Murray JS. Persistence of vancomycin in the blood during renal failure and its treatment by hemodialysis. N Engl J Med. 1966;274: 1047.
34. Eykyn S, Phillip I, Evans J. Vancomycin for staphylococcal shunt infections in patients on regular hemodialysis. Br Med J 1970;3:80.
35. Rice TL. Simplified dosing and monitoring of vancomycin for the burn care clinician. Burns. 1992;18:355–61.
36. Spitzer PC, Eliopoulos GM. Systemic absorption of enteral vancomycin in a patient with pseudomembranous colitis. Ann Intern Med. 1984;100:533–4.
37. Hawley HB, Gump DW. Vancomycin therapy of bacterial meningitis. Am J Dis Child. 1973;126:261.
38. Ayus JC, Enkas JF, Tong TG, et al. Peritoneal clearance and total body elimination of vancomycin during chronic intermittent peritoneal dialysis. Clin Nephrol. 1979;11:129–32.
39. Nielsen HE, Hansen JE, Korsager B, et al. Renal excretion of vancomycin in kidney disease. Acta Med Scand. 1975;197:261.
40. Moellering RC, Krogstad DJ, Greenblatt DJ. Vancomycin therapy in patients with impaired renal function. A nomogram for dosage. Ann Intern Med. 1981;94:343–46.
41. Matzke G, Kovarik JM, Rybak MJ, et al. Evaluation of the vancomycin clearance: Creatinine-clearance relationship for predicting vancomycin dosage. Clin Pharm. 1985;4:311–15.
41a.Cantú TG, Yamanaka-Yuen NA, Lietman PS. Serum vancomycin concentrations: Reappraisal of their clinical value. Clin Infect Dis. 1994;18:533–43.
41b.Moellering RC. Monitoring serum vancomycin levels: Climbing the mountain because it is there? (editorial). Clin Infect Dis. 1994;78:544–6.
42. Quale JM, O'Halloran JJ, De Vincenzo N, et al. Removal of vancomycin by high-flux hemodialysis membranes. Antimicrob Agents Chemother. 1992; 36:1424–6.
43. Bohler J, Reeza-Bonorden P, Keller E, et al. Rebound of plasma vancomycin levels after haemodialysis with highly permeable membranes. Eur J Clin Pharmacol. 1992;42:635–40.
44. Matzke GR, O'Connell MB, Collins AJ, et al. Disposition of vancomycin during hemofiltration. Clin Pharmacol Ther. 1986;40:425–30.
45. Austin TW, Leake J, Coles JC, et al. Vancomycin blood levels during cardiac surgery. Cardiol J Surg. 1981;24:423–25.
46. Healy DP, Polk RE, Garson ML, et al. Comparison of steady-state pharmacokinetics of two dosage regimens of vancomycin in normal volunteers. Antimicrob Agents Chemother. 1987;31:393–97.
47. Newfield P, Roizen MF: Hazards of rapid administration of vancomycin. Ann Intern Med. 1979;91:581.
48. Mordenti J, Ries C, Brooks GF, et al. Vancomycin-induced neutropenia complicating bone marrow recovery in a patient with leukemia. Case report and a review of the literature. Am J Med. 1986;30:333–35.
49. Miller SN, Ringler RP. Vancomycin-induced pseudomembranous colitis. J Clin Gastroenterol. 1987;9:114–15.
50. Traber PG, Levine DP. Vancomycin ototoxicity in a patient with normal renal function. Ann Intern Med. 1981;95:458–60.
51. McHenry MC, Gavan TL. Vancomycin. Pediatr Clin North Am. 1983;30: 31–47.
52. Geraci JE, Hermans PE, Vancomycin. Mayo Clin Proc. 1983;58:88–91.
53. Appel GB, Neu HC. The nephrotoxicity of antimicrobial agents. N Engl J Med. 1977;296:722.
54. Greenberg RN, Saud AMK, Kennedy DJ, et al. Instability of vancomycin in Infusaid drug pump model 100. Antimicrob Agents Chemother. 1987;31: 610–11.

55. Blovin RA, Bauer LA, Miller DD, et al. Vancomycin pharmacokinetics in normal and morbidly obese subjects. Antimicrob Agents Chemother. 1982; 21:575–80.

56. Nagvi SH, Kennan WJ, Reichley RM, et al. Vancomycin pharmacokinetics in small, seriously ill infants. Am J Dis Child. 1986;140:107–110.

57. Riley HD. Vancomycin and novobiocin. Med Clin North Am. 1970;54:1277.

58. Schaad VB, McCracken GH, Nelson JD: Clinical pharmacology and efficacy of vancomycin in pediatric patients. J Pediatr. 1980;96:119–26.

59. Fekety R, Silva J, Kauffman C, et al. Treatment of C. difficile antibiotic-associated colitis with oral vancomycin: Comparison of two dosage regimens. Am J Med. 1989;86:15–19.

60. Batts DH, Martin D, Holmes R, et al. Treatment of antibiotic-associated Clostridium difficile diarrhea with oral vancomycin. J Pediatr. 1980;97:151–53.

61. Rotschafer JC, Crossley K, Zaski DE, et al. Pharmacokinetics of vancomycin. Observations in 28 patients and dosage recommendations. Antimicrob Agents Chemother. 1982;22:391–94.

62. Brown N, Ho DHW, Fong KL, et al. Effects of hepatic function on vancomycin clinical pharmacology. Antimicrob Agents Chemother. 1983;23:603–09.

63. Watanakunakorn C. Treatment of infections due to methicillin-resistant Staphylococcus aureus. Ann Intern Med. 1982;97:376–78.

64. Myers JP, Linnemann CC. Bacteremia due to methicillin-resistant Staphylococcus aureus. J Infect Dis. 1982;4:532–36.

65. Sorrell TC, Packham DR, Shanker S, et al. Vancomycin therapy for methicillin-resistant Staphylococcus aureus. Ann Intern Med. 1982;97:344–50.

66. Levine DP, Cushing R, Jim J, et al. Community-acquired methicillin-resistant Staphylococcus aureus endocarditis in the Detroit Medical Center. Ann Intern Med. 1982;97:330–38.

67. Karchmer AW, Archer GL, Dismukes WE. Staphylococcus epidermidis causing prosthetic-valve endocarditis: Microbiologic and clinical observations as guides to therapy. Ann Intern Med. 1983;98:447–55.

68. Ena J, Dick RW, Jones RN, et al. The epidemiology of intravenous vancomycin usage in a University Hospital: A 10-year study. JAMA. 1993;269:598–602.

69. Sutherlan GE, Palitang EG, Marr JJ, et al. Sterilization of Ommaya reservoir by instillation of vancomycin. Am J Med. 1981;71:1068–70.

70. Gump DW. Vancomycin for treatment of bacterial meningitis. Rev Infect Dis. 3:S289–92.

71. Swayne RS, Rampling A, Newsom SWB. Intraventricular vancomycin for treatment of shunt-associated ventriculitis. J Antimicrob Chemother. 1987;19:249–53.

72. Viladrich PF, Gudiol F, Linares J, et al. Evaluation of vancomycin for therapy of adult pneumococcal meningitis. Antimicrob Agents Chemother. 1991;35:2467–72.

73. Westenfelder GO, Paterson PY, Reisberg BE, et al. Vancomycin-streptomycin synergism in enterococcal endocarditis. JAMA. 1973;223:37.

74. Harwick HJ, Kalmanson GM, Guze LB. Pyelonephritis. XVII. Comparison of combinations of vancomycin, ampicillin, streptomycin, and gentamicin in the treatment of enterococcal infection in the rat. J Infect Dis. 1974;129:358.

75. Zervos MJ, Kauffman CA, Therasse PM, et al. Nosocomial infection by gentamicin-resistant Streptococcus faecalis. Ann Intern Med. 1987;106:687–91.

76. Esposito AL, Gleckman RA: Vancomycin, a second look. JAMA. 1977;238:1756.

77. Teasley DG, Gerding DN, Olson MM, et al. Prospective randomised trial of metronidazole versus vancomycin for Clostridium difficile-associated diarrhea and colitis. Lancet. 1983;2:1043–46.

78. Fekety R, Silva J, Armstrong J, et al. Treatment of antibiotic-associated enterocolitis with vancomycin. Rev Infect Dis. 1981;3:S273–81.

79. Tedesco FJ. Treatment of recurrent antibiotic-associated pseudomembranous colitis. Am J Gastroenterol. 1982;77:220–21.

80. Johnson S, Homann SR, Bettin KM, et al. Treatment of asymptomatic Clostridium difficile carriers (fecal excretors) with vancomycin. A randomized, placebo controlled trial. Ann Intern Med. 1992;117:297–302.

81. Pasic M, Carrel T, Opravil M, et al. Systemic absorption after local intracolonic vancomycin in pseudomembranous colitis. Lancet. 1993;342–443.

82. Pasic M, Jost R, Carrel T, et al. Intracolonic vancomycin for pseudomembranous colitis (Letter). N Engl J Med. 1993;329:583.

83. Nielsen HE, Sorensen I, Hansen HE. Peritoneal transport of vancomycin during peritoneal dialysis. Nephron. 1979;24:274–77.

84. Morse GD, Farolino DF, Apicella MA, et al. Comparative study of intraperitoneal and intravenous vancomycin pharmacokinetics during continuous ambulatory peritoneal dialysis. Antimicrob Agents Chemother. 1987;31:173–77.

85. Piraino B, Bernardini J, Johnston J, et al. Chemical peritonitis due to intraperitoneal vancomycin. Peritoneal Dialys Bull. 1987;7(Suppl):S59.

86. Buggy BP, Schaberg DR, Swartz RD. Intraleukocytic sequestration as a cause of persistent Staphylococcus aureus peritonitis in continuous ambulatory peritoneal dialysis. Am J Med. 1984;76:1035–40.

87. Kaye D. Prophylaxis for infective endocarditis: An update. Ann Intern Med. 1986;104:419–23.

88. Kaplan EL, Anthony BF, Bisno A, et al. Prevention of bacterial endocarditis. Circulation. 1977;56:139A–143A.

89. Rubin M, Hathorn JW, Marshall D, et al. Gram-positive infections and the use of vancomycin in 550 episodes of fever and neutropenia. Ann Intern Med. 1988;108:30–35.

90. Wise RI, Kory M (ed): Reassessments of vancomycin—A potentially useful antibiotic. Rev Infect Dis. 1981;3:S199–S300.

91. Williams AH, Gruneberg RN. Teicoplanin. J Antimicrob Chemother. 1984;14:441–48.

92. Parenti F. Structure and mechanism of action of teicoplanin. J Hosp Infection. 1986;7(Suppl A):79–83.

93. Neville LD, Baillod R, Grady D, et al. Teicoplanin in patients with chronic renal failure on dialysis: Microbiological and pharmacokinetic aspects. Int J Clin Pharm. Res. 1987;VII:485–90.

94. Somma S, Gastaldo L, Corti A: Teicoplanin, a new antibiotic from Actinoplanus teichomyceticus nov sp. Antimicrob Agents Chemother. 1984;26:917–23.

95. Greenwood D. Microbiological properties of teicoplanin. J Antimicrob Agents Chemother. 1988;21(Suppl A):1–13.

96. Parenti F. Glycopeptide antibiotics. J Clin Pharmacol. 1988;28:136–40.

97. McNulty CAM, Garden GMF, Wise R, et al. The pharmacokinetics and tissue penetration of teicoplanin. J Antimicrob Chemother. 1985;16:743–49.

98. Verbist L, Tjandramaga B, Hendrickx B, et al. In vitro activity and human pharmacokinetics of teicoplanin. Antimicrob Agents Chemother. 1984;12:119–28.

99. Buniva G, DelFavero A, Bernareggi A, et al. Pharmacokinetics of ^{14}C-teicoplanin in healthy volunteers. J Antimicrob Chemother. 1988;21(Suppl A):23–28.

100. Bonati M, Traina GL, Rosiva R, et al. Pharmacokinetics of a single intravenous dose of teicoplanin in subjects with various degrees of renal impairment. Antimicrob Chemother. 1988;21(Suppl A):29–37.

101. Presterl E, Graninger W, Georgapoulos A. The efficacy of teicoplanin in the treatment of endocarditis caused by gram-positive bacteria. J Antimicrob Chemother. 1993;31:755–66.

102. Tarral E, Jehl F, Tarral A, et al. Pharmacokinetics of teicoplanin in children. J Antimicrob Chemother. 1988;21(Suppl A):47–51.

103. Domart Y, Pierre C, Clair B, et al. Pharmacokinetics of teicoplanin in critically ill patients with various degrees of renal impairment. Antimicrob Agents Chemother. 1987;31:1600–04.

104. Bauernfeind A. Teichomycin and AM-715 activity on staphylococci and enterococci in comparison to other antibiotic agents (Abstract). Program and Abstracts of the 21st Interscience Conference on Antimicrobioal Agents and Chemotherapy. American Society for Microbiology, Chicago, November 1981.

105. Jadeja L, Fainstein V, LeBlanc B, et al. Comparative in vitro activities of teichomycin and other antibiotics against JK diptheroids. Antimicrob Agents Chemother. 1983;24:145–46.

106. Greenwood D. Microbiological properties of teicoplanin. J Antimicrob Chemother. 1988;21(Suppl A):1–3.

107. Felmingham D, Solomonides K, O'Hare MD, et al. The effect of medium and inoculum on the activity of vancomycin and teicoplanin against coagulase-negative staphylococci. J Antimicrob Chemother. 1987;10:609–19.

108. Pantosti A, Luzzi I, Cardine R, et al. Comparison of the in vitro activities of teicoplanin and vancomycin against Clostridium difficile and their interactions with cholestyramine. Antimicrob Agents Chemother. 1985;28:847–48.

109. Van der Auwera P, Klastersky J. Bactericidal activity and killing rate of serum in volunteers receiving vancomycin or teicoplanin with and without amikacin given intravenously. J Antimicrob Chemother. 1987;19:623–35.

110. Van der Auwera P, Joly P. Comparative in-vitro activities of teicoplanin, vancomycin, coumermycin and ciprofloxacin, alone and in combination with rifampicin or LM427, against Staphylococcus aureus. J Antimicrob Chemother. 1987;19:313–20.

111. Watanakunakorn C. In-vitro activity of teicoplanin alone and in combination with rifampicin, gentamicin or tobramycin against coagulase-negative staphylococci. J Antimicrob Chemother. 1987;19:439–43.

112. Tuazon CU, Washburn D. Teicoplanin and rifampicin singly and in combination in the treatment of experimental Staphylococcus epidermidis endocarditis in the rabbit model. J Antimicrob Chemother. 1987;20:233–37.

113. Shanson DC, Todayon M. Activity of teicoplanin compared with vancomycin alone, and combined with gentamicin, against penicillin tolerant viridans streptococci and enterococci causing endocarditis. J Hosp Infection. 1986;7(Suppl A):65–72.

114. Williams AH, Gruneberg RN, Webster A, et al. Teicoplanin in the treatment of infection caused by Gram-positive organisms. J Hosp Infection. 1986;7(Suppl A):101–03.

115. Agnelli G, Longetti M, Guerciolini R, et al. Effects of the new glycopeptide antibiotic teicoplanin on platelet function and blood coagulation. Antimicrob Agents Chemother. 1987;31:1609–12.

116. Stille W, Sietzen W, Dieterich HA, Fell JJ. Clinical efficacy and safety of teicoplanin. J Antimicrob Chemother. 1988;21(Suppl A):69–79.

117. Maher ER, Hollman A, Gruneberg RN. Teicoplanin induced ototoxicity in Down's syndrome. Lancet. 1986;1:613.

118. Drabu YJ, Walsh B, Blakemore PH, et al. Teicoplanin in infections caused by methicillin-resistant staphylococci. J Antimicrob Chemother. 1988; 21(Suppl A):89–92.

119. Schlemmer B, Falkman H, Boudjadja A, et al. Teicoplanin for patients allergic to vancomycin. N Engl J Med. 1988;318:1127–28.

120. Chambers HF, Rusnak NG, Hackbarth CJ, et al. Treatment of Staphylococcus aureus endocarditis in rabbits with teichomycin (Abstract). Program and Abstracts of the 23rd Interscience Conference on Antimicrobial Agents and Chemotherapy. American Society for Microbiology, Las Vegas, October 1983.

121. Lewis P, Garaud JJ, Parenti F. A multicentre open clinical trial of teicoplanin in infections caused by gram-positive bacteria. J Antimicrob Chemother. 1988;21(Suppl A):61–7.

122. Harding I, Garaud JJ. Teicoplanin in the treatment of infections caused by coagulase-negative staphylococci. J Antimicrob Chemother. 1988;21(Suppl A):93–103.
123. Galanakis N, Giamarellou H, Vlachogiannis N, et al. Poor efficacy of teicoplanin in treatment of deep-seated staphylococcal infections. Eur J Clin Microbiol Infect Dis. 1988;7:130–34.
124. Schmib JL. Efficacy of teicoplanin for enterococcal infections: 63 cases and review. Clin Infect Dis. 1992;15:302–06.
125. Wilson APR, Treasure T, Gruneberg RN, et al. Antibiotic prophylaxis in cardiac surgery: A prospective comparison of two dosage regimens of teicoplanin with combination of flucloxacillin and tobramycin. J Antimicrob Chemother. 1988;21:213–33.
126. Neville LO, Baillod RA, Brumfitt W, et al. Efficacy and safety of teicoplanin in gram-positive peritonitis in patients on peritoneal dialysis. J Antimicrob Chemother. 1988;21(Suppl A):123–31.
127. Bowley JA, Pickering SJ, Scantlebury AJ, et al. Intraperitoneal teicoplanin in the treatment of peritonitis associated with continuous ambulatory peritoneal dialysis. J Antimicrob Chemother. 1988;21(Suppl A):133–39.
128. deLalla F, Privitera G, Rinaldi E, et al. Treatment of *Clostridium difficile*–associated disease with teicoplanin. Antimicrob Agents Chemother. 1989;33:1125–27.
129. Phillips G, Golledge CL. Vancomycin and teicoplanin—Something old, something new. Med J Austral. 1992;156:53–7.

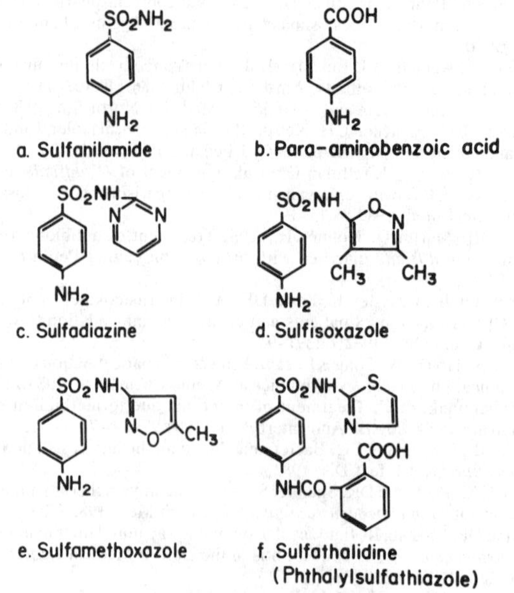

FIG. 1.   (A–F) Structural formulas of selected sulfonamides.

26. SULFONAMIDES AND TRIMETHOPRIM

STEPHEN H. ZINNER
KENNETH H. MAYER

The modern era of antimicrobial chemotherapy began in 1932 with the first reports by Gerhard Domagk of the protective activity of prontosil against murine streptococcal infections. This drug was an outgrowth of the German dye industry and had been commercially available since the early twentieth century. Prontosil (sulfachrysoidine) exerted its antibacterial activity due to the release in vivo of para-aminobenzenesulfonamide (sulfanilamide). This agent was the first antibacterial used in the United States, in an unsuccessful attempt, in July 1935, to treat a 10-year-old girl late in the course of meningitis and sepsis due to *Haemophilus influenzae*.[1] During the late 1930s, the basic sulfanilamide compound was modified to remove unpleasant side effects while expanding its spectrum of activity. More recent modifications have resulted in compounds of specific usefulness, for example, in urinary infections (those compounds that are highly soluble), or those nonabsorbable sulfonamides that act only within the gastrointestinal tract.

Trimethoprim is a 2,4-diamino-pyrimidine and, as such, inhibits the enzyme dihydrofolate reductase, resulting in interference in folic acid and subsequent pyrimidine synthesis in the bacterial cell. Trimethoprim is one of several such compounds synthesized and studied by Hitchings and coworkers in the 1950s and 1960s. The use of trimethoprim as a potentiator of sulfonamide activity was introduced by Bushby and Hitchings[2] in 1968. In the subsequent decade the combination of trimethoprim-sulfamethoxazole was introduced clinically and gained a place in the chemotherapy of many infectious diseases. These agents, available in a fixed drug combination, show true antibacterial synergism against a wide variety of organisms.

SULFONAMIDES

Structure

The clinically useful sulfonamides are derived from sulfanilamide (para-aminobenzenesulfonamide), which is similar in structure to para-aminobenzoic acid (PABA), a factor required by bacteria for folic acid synthesis (Fig. 1).

A free amino group at the 4 position is associated with enhanced activity. Increased activity due to increased PABA inhibition is associated with substitutions at the sulfonyl radical (SO_2)—attached to the 1 carbon, as seen with sulfadiazine, sulfisoxazole, and sulfamethoxazole, all of which are more active than the parent compound, sulfanilamide. The nature of these substitutions determines other pharmacologic properties of the drug such as absorption, solubility, and gastrointestinal tolerance. Substitutions at the 4-amino group result in decreased absorption from the gastrointestinal tract (e.g., phthalylsulfathiazole).

Derivation and Nomenclature

Since the introduction of sulfonamides into clinical medicine, dozens of compounds have been used. However, relatively few survive today, and they can be classified as (1) short- or medium-acting sulfonamides, (2) long-acting sulfonamides, (3) sulfonamides limited to the gastrointestinal tract, and (4) topical sulfonamides.

Short- or Medium-Acting Sulfonamides.   Sulfisoxazole *United States Pharmacopeia* (USP) (sulphafurazole *British Pharmacopeia* [BP], 3,4-dimethyl-5-sulfanilamidoisoxazole; Gantrisin) is a highly soluble drug especially useful in urinary tract infections. Sulfamethoxazole USP (5-methyl-3-sulfanilamidoisoxazole; Gantanol) is somewhat less soluble than sulfisoxazole and yields higher blood levels. It is the sulfonamide presently most frequently combined with trimethoprim. Sulfadiazine USP (2-sulfanilamidopyridine; Microsulfon) is highly active, attains high blood and cerebrospinal fluid levels, and is associated with low protein binding and lower solubility than the above drugs. Sulfamethizole USP (2-sulfanilamide-5-methyl-1:3:4-thiazole; Thiosulfil) is used for urinary tract infections. Sulfadimidine and sulfacarbamide are available in the United Kingdom.

Short-acting sulfonamides are also available in several combinations. Sulfisoxazole and sulfamethoxazole are each combined with phenazopyridine, a urinary analgesic, as Azo Gantrisin and Azo Gantanol or Azo-Urizole and Microsul-A. Phenazopyridine is also present with sulfamethazole and sulfadiazine in Suladyne. Sulfamethizole is also combined with tetracycline and phenazopyridine in Urobiotic, but these two preparations have been classified by the Food and Drug Administration (FDA) as lacking evidence of effectiveness as a fixed drug combination.

Long-Acting Sulfonamides. Sulfamethoxypridazine (3-sulfanilamido-5-methoxy-pyridazine) and sulfameter [4-amino-N-(5-methoxy-2-pyrimidinyl)] benzene-sulfonamide are no longer available for single daily dose therapy, as they were associated with hypersensitivity reactions such as Stevens-Johnson syndrome. Neither sulfadimethoxine (Madribon) nor any other long-acting sulfonamides other than sulfadoxine are currently available in the United States.

Sulfadoxine, originally known as sulformethoxine (N'-[5,6-dimethoxy-4-pyrimidyl]sulfanilamide) is a very long-acting sulfonamide that, combined with pyrimethamine, is available as Fansidar. Sulfadoxine has a half-life of 100–230 hours and reaches a peak serum level of 51–76 µg/ml 2.5–6 hours after an oral dose of 500 mg. Fansidar is active in the treatment and prophylaxis of malaria due to chloroquine-resistant *Plasmodium falciparum*.[3] Due to the unknown teratogenic potential of pyrimethamine, Fansidar should not be recommended for prophylaxis of pregnant women, and its use has been associated with Stevens-Johnson syndrome. Also, some strains of *P. falciparum* from Southeast Asia and South America may be resistant.

Sulfonamides Limited to the Gastrointestinal Tract. Sulfaguanidine (N'-amidinosulfanilamide), sulfasuxidine (2-[para-succinylsulfanilamido]-thiazole, succinylsulfathiazole), and sulfathalidine (2[para-phthalyl-sulfanilamido]-thiazole) are relatively poorly absorbed from the gastrointestinal tract. They have been used in the past to suppress the susceptible bowel flora before surgery.

Salicylazosulfapyridine (sulfasalazine, Azulfidine) is a sulfonamide derivative used in the treatment of ulcerative colitis. This drug is absorbed in its parent form as sulfapyridine, and significant blood levels of this compound are measurable.

Topical Sulfonamides. Mafenide acetate (para-aminomethylbenzene sulfonamide, Sulfamylon cream) is available for use in the topical therapy of burns. However, its use has been limited by metabolic acidosis due to carbonic anhydrase inhibition. Silver sulfadiazine (Silvadene cream) has fewer side effects and is used extensively for burns.[4] Here the sulfonamide acts primarily as a vehicle for release of silver ions that exert an antibacterial effect. Outbreaks of silver-resistant infections in burn units may ultimately limit its usefulness.[5,6] Various combinations of other sulfonamides are available as vaginal creams or suppositories (e.g., Sultrin vaginal cream and tablets, Trysul vaginal cream, AVC cream and suppositories, Vagitrol).

There are a variety of ophthalmic ointments and solutions of sulfacetamide sodium USP (a highly soluble sulfonamide) available for use in treating conjunctivitis due to susceptible bacteria and as adjunctive therapy of trachoma (e.g., Bleph-10, Cetamide, Blephamide, Sulamyd).

Mechanisms of Action

Although a wide variety of chemical modifications of the sulfonamides has been synthesized, all basically share the same mechanism of action. The sulfonamides are bacteriostatic in that they inhibit bacterial growth via interference with microbial folic acid synthesis. More specifically, sulfonamides inhibit competitively the incorporation of PABA into tetrahydropteroic acid,[7–9] and they in turn may be incorporated into dihydropteroate.[10] Sulfonamides may have a higher affinity for the microbial enzyme tetrahydropteroic acid synthetase than the natural substrate PABA. Richmond[11] has suggested that sulfonamides may act on bacterial repressor genes or by feedback inhibition to decrease formation of new enzyme. The ultimate result of decreased folic acid synthesis is a decrease in bacterial nucleotides, with subsequent inhibition of bacterial growth.

TABLE 1. In Vitro Activity of Sulfonamides Against Representative Organisms[a]

	Range of MIC[b] (µg/ml)
Gram-positive	
Staphylococcus aureus	8–64
Streptococcus pneumoniae	4–128
Streptococcus pyogenes	0.5–16
Enterococcus faecalis	25–250
Corynebacterium diphtheriae	25–75
Listeria monocytogenes	3–75
Bacillus anthracis	12–100
Gram-negative	
Escherichia coli	4–64
Klebsiella spp.	8–128
Proteus mirabilis	8–128
Serratia marcescens	25–>1000
Salmonella spp.	16–128
Shigella spp.	2–32
Haemophilus influenzae	1–16
Neisseria gonorrhoeae	4–32
Neisseria meningitidis	0.25–>10
Pseudomonas aeruginosa	>100–200
Other	
Chlamydia trachomatis	0.1
Nocardia asteroides	2–16

[a] The acquisition of plasmids may increase MICs.
[b] Minimum inhibitory concentration. Range is expressed for a variety of sulfonamide compounds.

(Data from Garrod et al.,[30] Bushby,[31] and Bach et al.[32])

Antimicrobial Activity In Vitro

Sulfonamides exhibit in vitro inhibitory activity against a broad spectrum of gram-positive and gram-negative bacteria as well as *Actinomyces, Chlamydia, Plasmodia,* and *Toxoplasma* (Table 1). The in vitro antimicrobial sensitivity of sulfonamides is strongly influenced by the size of the inoculum and the composition of the test media. High concentrations of PABA and thymidine inhibit sulfonamide activity.

Antimicrobial Resistance

Resistance to sulfonamides is widespread and increasingly common in both community and nosocomial strains of bacteria, including streptococci, staphylococci, Enterobacteriaceae, *Neisseria* spp., and *Pseudomonas* spp.[12,13] Cross-resistance between different sulfonamides is common.

Organisms may develop resistance or partial resistance by mutation, resulting in either microbial overproduction of PABA[14] or structural change in dihydropteroate synthetase that results in an enzyme with lowered affinity for sulfonamide.[15] PABA overproduction has been implicated in resistant strains of *Neisseria gonorrhoeae* and *Staphylococcus aureus*[14,16]; altered dihydropteroate synthetase has been found in strains of *Escherichia coli*.[17] Resistance also may be mediated by plasmids that code for the production of drug-resistant enzymes, such as dihydropteroate synthetase,[18] or may result in decreased bacterial cell permeability to sulfonamides.[19] Plasmid transfer can occur in the gastrointestinal tract as well as in vitro and has been seen especially with multiple species of Enterobacteriaceae.[20]

Transformational exchanges of dihydropteroate synthetase among *Neisseria* spp. raise the spectre of wider sulfonamide resistance dissemination by chromosomal and plasmid genes.[21] Sulfonamide resistance genes also have been found in a common *Pseudomonas aeruginosa* integron, which may facilitate the recent spread of resistance among aerobic gram-negative bacilli.[22] More than one resistance mechanism may be operating simultaneously.[23]

Plasmid-mediated sulfonamide resistance has greatly increased in recent years, often in conjunction with trimethoprim resistance. More than one-fourth of the uropathogens and one-half of the clinical *Shigella* isolates studied in Sweden,[24,25] England,[12,26] and the United States[27] were sulfonamide resistant. *Salmonella* resistance to sulfonamides has also increased in the

United States,[28] often in conjunction with resistance to other antibiotic classes. The increase in sulfonamide-resistant *Haemophilus ducreyi* in Asia and Africa has been associated with a plasmid related to those found in Enterobacteriaceae.[29]

Pharmacology

Routes of Administration.   Sulfonamides are usually administered orally, although sulfadiazine and sulfisoxazole are available for use as intravenous or subcutaneous preparations. These latter forms are used rarely, if at all. Sulfacetamide is available as ophthalmic preparations, and silver sulfadiazine and mafenide acetate are applied topically in burn patients and are associated with significant absorption of sulfonamide percutaneously. Vaginal preparations are available for topical application.

Absorption.   Most of the short- and medium-acting sulfonamides are absorbed rapidly and almost completely in the unionized state from the small intestine and stomach. Compounds with N-1 substitutions are absorbed poorly, as are more acidic compounds (e.g., phthalylsulfathiazole, Fig. 1F). Long-acting sulfonamides also are absorbed rapidly but have a much slower excretion rate. Topical sulfonamides are absorbed and may be detectable in blood.

Distribution.   The sulfonamides generally are well distributed throughout the body, entering the cerebrospinal fluid and synovial, pleural, and peritoneal fluids with concentrations approaching 80 percent of serum levels. Blood and tissue levels are related to the degree of protein binding (Table 2) and lipid solubility. Sulfonamides administered in pregnancy readily cross the placenta and are present in the fetal blood and amniotic fluid.[34]

Excretion.   Acetylation and glucuronidation occur in the liver, and free and metabolized drug appears in the urine. Glomerular filtration is probably a route of excretion, although partial reabsorption and active tubular secretion also are involved, especially at low creatinine clearance rates. Urinary excretion is more rapid for those sulfonamides with low pKa values (e.g., sulfamethizole, sulfisoxazole), and alkalinization of the urine increases excretion by this route. Plasma half-lives vary widely and are related inversely to lipid solubility and directly to pKa values but are not clearly related to the degree of protein binding.[33] Small amounts of sulfonamides are found in bile, human milk, prostatic secretions, saliva, and tear.

Protein Binding and Blood or Tissue Levels.   Sulfonamides are bound variably and not irreversibly to plasma albumin, and the bound drug is inactive (Table 2). Levels obtainable in cerebrospinal and other body fluids are inversely related to the degree of protein binding. The amount of free drug in plasma is directly related to pKa.[33]

Use in Renal Insufficiency.   Sulfonamides can be used in renal failure, but therapeutic serum levels will persist longer because of reduced excretion, and the dosage must be reduced

and the interval between doses extended proportional to the degree of renal impairment. Protein binding of sulfonamides is decreased in severe renal insufficiency.[35] The N-4 acetylated metabolite of sulfonamides may accumulate in patients with renal failure, especially during prolonged therapy. This derivative loses its antibacterial effect but still may have toxic properties. Plasma levels of sulfonamide should be measured every 3 days, and peak concentrations of sulfamethoxazole should be less than 120 µg/ml.

Toxicity and Adverse Reactions

Sulfonamides may cause nausea, vomiting, diarrhea, rash, fever, headache, depression, jaundice, hepatic necrosis, and a serum sicknesslike syndrome. Earlier, less soluble compounds (sulfadiazine, sulfathiazole) used in excessively high doses were associated with crystalluria and tubular deposits of sulfonamide crystals. These complications could be minimized by the maintenance of high urine flow and alkalinization of the urine. This complication usually is not seen with modern soluble sulfonamides. Tubular necrosis, interstitial nephritis, or necrotizing angiitis may be associated rarely with sulfonamide sensitivity. Acute pancreatitis has been attributed to sulfonamide.[36]

More serious adverse reactions due to sulfonamides may include acute hemolytic anemia (sometimes related to a deficiency in erythrocyte glucose-6-phosphate dehydrogenase—G6PD), aplastic anemia, agranulocytosis, thrombocytopenia, and leukopenia. A recent study showed that G6PD-deficient patients who received trimethoprim-sulfamethoxazole did not have hemolytic reactions during therapy.[37]

Sulfonamides should not be administered during the last month of pregnancy, because they compete for bilirubin-binding sites on plasma albumin and may increase fetal blood levels of unconjugated bilirubin, increasing the risk of kernicterus. Also, because of the immature fetal acetyltransferase system, blood levels of free sulfonamide may be increased, further adversely affecting the risk of kernicterus.[33]

Finally, significant hypersensitivity reactions may occur due to sulfonamides administered via any route. The most important of these include erythema nodosum, erythema multiforme (including Stevens-Johnson syndrome), drug eruption, vasculitis similar to periarteritis nodosa, and anaphylaxis. Long-acting sulfonamides have been associated with fatal hypersensitivity reactions, especially in children, and this severely limits their use. Locally applied sulfonamides (e.g., to skin) may be associated with any of these adverse reactions. The acute onset of hypotension and fever rarely has been associated with trimethoprim-sulfamethoxazole therapy in human immunodeficiency virus (HIV)-infected patients.[38] Although the reaction resembles IgE-mediated anaphylaxis, the specific etiology and allergen are not clearly known.[39]

Drug Interactions

Sulfonamides may displace from albumin-binding sites drugs such as warfarin, thus increasing the effective activity of the displaced drug. Anticoagulant dosage therefore should be reduced during sulfonamide therapy. Sulfonamides also displace methotrexate from its bound protein, thereby increasing methotrexate toxicity. An increased hypoglycemic effect of chlorpropamide and tolbutamide may occur during sulfonamide therapy, possibly due to the same mechanism or to structural similarities. Sulfonamides may potentiate the action of some thiazide diuretics, phenytoin, and uricosuric agents. Conversely, sulfonamides themselves may be displaced from binding sites by indomethacin, phenylbutazone, salicylates, probenecid, and sulfinpyrazone, resulting in increased sulfonamide activity.

The activity of sulfonamides may be decreased by procaine and other local anesthetics derived from PABA. Methenamine compounds should not be used with sulfonamides because of

TABLE 2. Levels in Blood, Cerebrospinal Fluid (CSF), Plasma Half-Life, and Protein Binding of Some Sulfonamides

Drug	Peak Blood Level[a] (µg/ml)	Serum Level in CSF (%)	Plasma Half-Life (hours)	Protein Binding (%)
Sulfadiazine	30–60	40–80	17	45
Sulfisoxazole	40–50	30–50	5–6	92
Sulfamethoxazole	80–100	25–30	11	70
Sulfadoxine	50–75	20–30	100–230	80–98

[a] Approximate free sulfonamide level after a 2 g oral dose.

(Data from Anand[33] and Garrod et al.[30])

the formation of insoluble urinary precipitates. Intravenous solutions of sulfonamides are physically incompatible with chloramphenicol, aminoglycosides, lincomycin, methicillin, tetracyclines, vancomycin, norepinephrine, insulin, procaine, Ringer lactate solution, and others. Sulfonamides may decrease protein-bound iodine and ^{131}I uptake and may produce false-positive Benedict tests for urine glucose and false-positive sulfosalicylic acid tests for urine proteins.[40–42]

Major Clinical Use

Sulfonamides are primarily used in the treatment of acute urinary tract infections, but increasing resistance has diminished their effectiveness. Most first episodes of infection in the unobstructed urinary tract will be due to *E. coli* that are often sensitive to sulfonamides. Sulfisoxazole is administered orally in a usual dosage of 1 g qid. Since the infecting organism of any urinary tract infection may or may not be sensitive to sulfonamides, the choice of therapy should be based on appropriate sensitivity tests (see Ch. 55).

Sulfonamides are also quite effective in the therapy of infections due to *Nocardia asteroides*. Therapy must include 4–6 g or more daily after a loading dose of 4 g and should be continued for 4–6 months or longer if necessary (see Ch. 234). Sulfonamides may be useful in combination with other antimycobacterial drugs for the management of infections due to rifampin-resistant *Mycobacterium kansasii*.[43]

Sulfonamides are effective in the prophylaxis of patients against recurrent attacks of rheumatic fever associated with group A β-hemolytic streptococcal infections, but they are not effective for therapy for established streptococcal pharyngitis. Sulfonamide prophylaxis of close contacts of patients with meningitis due to *Neisseria meningitidis* is effective if the infecting organism is known to be sulfonamide sensitive (adult dose for sulfadiazine is 1 g q12h for 2 days).

Long-term sulfisoxazole has been efficacious in the management of chronic otitis media.[44] Sulfonamides have been used to treat toxoplasmosis in patients with and without acquired immunodeficiency syndrome (AIDS) and chloroquine-sensitive and -resistant *P. falciparum* malaria (with pyrimethamine). Melioidosis, dermatitis herpetiformis, lymphogranuloma venereum, and chancroid have responded to sulfonamides. Nongonococcal urethritis due to *Chlamydia*, but not to *Ureaplasma urealyticum*, responds well to sulfonamide therapy (see Ch. 55). Sulfasalazine is used in the treatment of inflammatory bowel diseases and has had some success in patients with rheumatoid arthritis and other inflammatory conditions.[45,46] Currently, sulfonamides are used most frequently in combination with trimethoprim (see below).

TRIMETHOPRIM

Structure and Derivation

Trimethoprim is a 2,4-diamino-5-(3',4',5'-trimethoxybenzyl) pyrimidine (Fig. 2). This drug was synthesized by Bushby and Hitchings[2] as a dihydrofolate reductase inhibitor thought to potentiate the activity of sulfonamides by sequential inhibition of

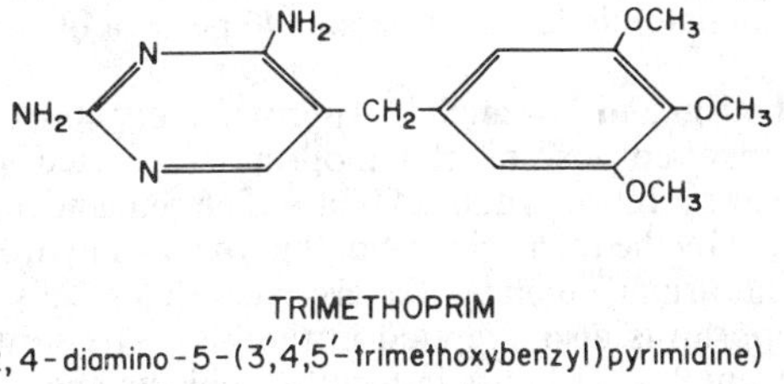

TRIMETHOPRIM

(2,4-diamino-5-(3',4',5'-trimethoxybenzyl)pyrimidine)

FIG. 2 Chemical structure of trimethoprim.

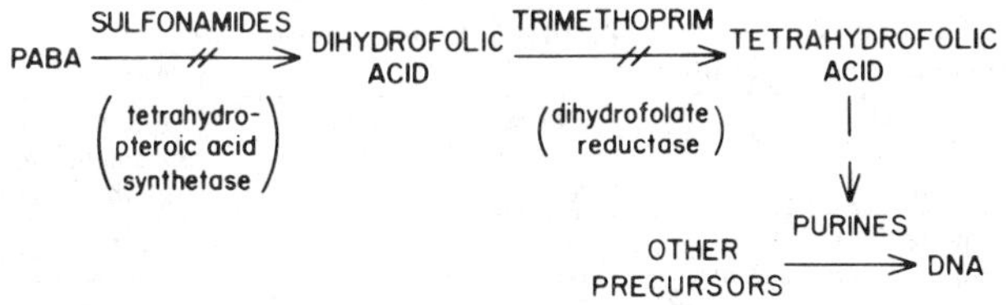

FIG. 3. Action of sulfonamides and trimethoprim on the metabolic pathway of bacterial folic acid synthesis.

folic acid synthesis. In the United States, trimethoprim is now available as a single agent as well as in combination with sulfamethoxazole (see below). Trimethoprim does have antibacterial activity of its own, and its pharmacology will be reviewed.

Mechanism of Action

Trimethoprim owes its activity to powerful inhibition of bacterial dihydrofolate reductase, which is the enzyme step after the step in folic acid synthesis blocked by sulfonamides. Trimethoprim is 50,000–100,000 times more active against bacterial dihydrofolate reductase than against the human enzyme. Trimethoprim interferes with the conversion of dihydrofolate to tetrahydrofolate, the precursor of folinic acid and ultimately purine and DNA synthesis (Fig. 3). The sequential blockage of the same biosynthetic pathway by sulfonamides and trimethoprim results in a high degree of synergistic activity against a wide spectrum of microorganisms. Humans do not synthesize folic acid but require it in their diet, and therefore human purine synthesis is not affected significantly by the enzyme inhibition of trimethoprim.[47,48]

Antimicrobial Activity

Trimethoprim is quite active in vitro against many gram-positive cocci and most gram-negative rods except for *P. aeruginosa* and *Bacteroides* spp. (Table 3). *Treponema pallidum*, *Mycobacterium tuberculosis*, *Mycoplasma* spp., and most anaerobes are resistant. Thymidine will inhibit the in vitro activity of trimethoprim, but the addition of thymidine phosphorylase or 5% lysed horse blood to Mueller-Hinton or other sensitivity media removes this inhibition. The minimum inhibitory concentration (MIC) will vary considerably with the media used.[53]

Potentiation of the action of trimethoprim is seen in combination with sulfamethoxazole (see below and Table 3). Antibacterial synergism has been demonstrated in vitro for trimethoprim and polymyxins[54] and for trimethoprim and aminoglycosides against some gram-negative bacilli.[55] The combination of trimethoprim-sulfamethoxazole is active in vitro against many isolates of tested *S. aureus*,[56] *Streptococcus pyogenes*, *Streptococcus pneumoniae*, *E. coli*, *Proteus mirabilis*, *Shigella* spp., *Salmonella* spp., *Pseudomonas cepacia*, *Pseudomonas pseudomallei*, *Yersinia entercolitica*, *N. gonorrhoeae*,[57] and *Xanthomonas maltophilia*.

Variable bactericidal effects have been noted when enterococci are tested against trimethoprim-sulfamethoxazole.[52,58] The susceptibility of Enterobacteriaceae may vary greatly between locations and within the same location from year to year, due to the spread of trimethoprim-resistant plasmids and transposons.[57] Almost all strains of *P. aeruginosa* are resistant in vitro to trimethoprim-sulfamethoxazole.[56]

Trimethoprim combined with sulfamethoxazole or dapsone has been effective in the treatment of *Pneumocystis carinii* pneumonia in immunocompromised patients (see below). *Listeria monocytogenes*,[59] *Branhamella catarrhalis*,[60] and atypical mycobacteria[61] have been shown to be susceptible to the combination of trimethoprim and sulfamethoxazole.

The optimal ratio for in vitro synergism of trimethoprim-sulfa-

TABLE 3. In Vitro Activity of Trimethoprim Against Representative Organisms

Organism	MIC[a] Alone (µg/ml)	MIC with Sulfamethoxazole (µg/ml, 1:20)[b]
Gram-positive		
Staphylococcus aureus	0.15–2	0.04–1.6
Staphylococcus epidermidis	0.02	—
Streptococcus pneumoniae	0.004–5	0.05–1.5
Streptococcus pyogenes	0.02–1	0.015–0.4
Enterococcus faecalis	0.15–0.5	0.015–0.4[b]
Corynebacterium diphtheriae	0.15–0.5	0.05–0.15
Listeria monocytogenes	0.05–1.5	0.015–0.15
Clostridium perfringens	2–50	—
Propionibacterium acnes	0.07	—
Gram negative		
Escherichia coli	0.01–>5	0.005–>5
Klebsiella spp.	0.15–5	0.05–3.1
Proteus mirabilis	0.15–1.5	0.05–0.15
Serratia marcescens	0.8–50	0.4–50
Salmonella spp.	0.01–0.4	0.05–0.15
Shigella spp.	0.4–0.8	0.02–0.5
Citrobacter freundii	0.2	—
Vibrio cholera	0.2	—
Haemophilus influenzae	0.1–12.5	0.04–50
Neisseria gonorrhoeae	0.2–128	0.15–3.1
Neisseria meningitidis	3.1–50	0.01–1.6
Pseudomonas aeruginosa	50–1000	3.1–100
Pseudomonas cepacia	1–2	—
Xanthomonas maltophilia	1–>32	1–>32
Bacteroides fragilis	≥4.0	—
Other		
Nocardia asteroides	3–100	1.5
Chlamydia trachomatis	20	—

[a] MIC varies with the method, inoculum size, and media used. Acquisition of residence plasmids may increase MICs.
[b] MBC may be much higher.[52]

(Data from refs. 30–32 and 49–51.)

methoxazole in combination is 1:20, but this ratio does not always obtain in vivo. The synergism seen with trimethoprim-sulfamethoxazole depends somewhat on the sensitivity of the organism to each drug. In one study[62] over 95 percent of organisms sensitive to both drugs showed synergism, whereas 60 percent of sulfamethoxazole-resistant strains and 45 percent of trimethoprim-resistant strains showed synergism.

Resistance to Trimethoprim. Bacteria may develop trimethoprim resistance by several mechanisms, which can be chromosomal or plasmid mediated. Clinical resistance has increased. In one hospital in France[57] trimethoprim-resistant Enterobacteriaceae (MIC ≥4 µg/ml) increased from 18 to 25 percent of isolates. A decrease in the ratio of strains resistant to both sulfamethoxazole and trimethoprim compared with strains resistant only to trimethoprim may reflect an increase in independent trimethoprim resistance, and this might be a useful monitoring parameter in hospitals.[63] Concomitant resistance to sulfonamides has increased greatly in East Asia in recent years.[64]

Trimethoprim resistance may be due to changes in cell permeability, loss of bacterial drug-binding capacity, and overproduction of or alterations in dihydrofolate reductase. However, the clinically most important mechanism is due to plasmid-mediated dihydrofolate reductases that are resistant to trimethoprim.[65–67]

Multiple distinctive dihydrofolate reductases have been described in recent years in Enterobacteriaceae, P. aeruginosa, and S. aureus.[67,68] They are frequently plasmid mediated[57,67,69,70] and may be disseminated by highly mobile transposons (such as Tn7) with wide host-species' ranges.[71] Outbreaks due to trimethoprim-resistant conjugative plasmids have been noted in Western and Eastern Europe,[67–69,71–74] East Asia,[75,76] South America,[77] and the United States.[77,78] Many of the outbreaks have occurred in immunocompromised hosts, with the spread of resistance to multiple other antibiotic groups.[79]

Local increases in trimethoprim resistance, particularly among Enterobacteriaceae, have been especially marked in developing countries,[80,81] with up to 20 percent of nosocomial clinical isolates resistant to trimethoprim. Also, fecal isolates from out-patient settings and day care centers are increasingly resistant to trimethoprim.[82,83] With more than one-third of the E. coli and Salmonella resistant to trimethoprim in several South American and Asian nations, the use of this low-cost agent for the treatment of urinary tract infections and serious enteric infections is imperiled. Whether the clinical use of trimethoprim alone in some countries has resulted in increasing resistance to the combination is still unclear. Recent monitoring of data from the Netherlands revealed that almost one-half of Dutch Shigella sonnei isolates were resistant to trimethoprim-sulfamethoxazole.[84] Concomitant trimethoprim and sulfonamide resistance may limit the utility of the combination against methicillin-resistant S. aureus and Staphylococcus epidermidis.[85]

Permeability changes may occur in the bacterial cell and result in resistance to both trimethoprim and sulfonamides. Thymine-requiring auxotrophs may also account for clinically significant resistance to both drugs. These mutants lack thymidylate synthetase and are probably less virulent than are sensitive strains.[86,87]

Pharmacology

Routes of Administration. Trimethoprim is available as 100-mg tablets for oral use. Trimethoprim is absorbed readily and almost completely from the gastrointestinal tract. Peak serum levels after taking 100 mg appear 1–4 hours after ingestion and approach 1 µg/ml. The coadministration of sulfamethoxazole does not affect the rate of absorption of serum levels of trimethoprim.

Trimethoprim is also available in fixed combination with sulfamethoxazole in a ratio of 1:5 for oral use (trimethoprim, 80 mg; sulfamethoxazole, 400 mg; Bactrim, Septra); double-strength and quarter-strength pediatric tablets are available, as is an oral suspension containing 40 mg trimethoprim and 200 mg sulfamethoxazole per 5 ml. Intravenous trimethoprim (16 mg/ml) plus sulfamethoxazole (80 mg/ml) is available. When administered intravenously, 10 ml or 160 mg trimethoprim (with 800 mg sulfamethoxazole) produces a peak serum trimethoprim concentration of 3.4 µg/ml in 1 hour. After repeated doses, the peak trimethoprim concentration may approach 9 µg/ml.[88] Similar peak levels may be reached with oral therapy, but at 2–4 hours after taking the dose.[89,90]

Distribution. Trimethoprim is widely distributed in tissues and may appear in kidney, lung, and sputum in higher concentrations than in plasma, as well as in bile, saliva, human breast milk, and seminal fluid.[91] Trimethoprim is also found in prostatic fluid at two to three times the serum concentration, but lower levels may be present in patients with chronic prostatitis.[92,93] Cerebrospinal fluid levels are about 40 percent of serum levels.

Metabolism and Excretion. Approximately 60–80 percent of an administered dose of trimethoprim is excreted in the urine via tubular secretion within 24 hours. The remainder of the drug is excreted by the kidney in one of four oxide or hydroxyl derivatives. The urinary metabolites are bacteriologically inactive.[88] Trimethoprim is also excreted in the bile. The serum half-life ranges from 9 to 11 hours in healthy subjects and is prolonged in patients with renal insufficiency. Unlike sulfamethoxazole, the excretion rate of trimethoprim is increased with acidification of the urine, and serum protein binding (65–70 percent) does not decrease significantly with increasing degrees of uremia.[35] Urine concentrations in healthy subjects (60–1000 µg/ml) are usually in excess of the MIC of most urinary pathogens.[35] Trimethoprim-sulfamethoxazole can be given in the usual doses to patients with creatinine clearances of 30 ml/min or greater. One-half the usual daily dose can be given to patients with creatinine clearances of 15–30 ml/min, but trimethoprim-sulfamethoxazole is not recommended for use in patients with clearances less than 15 ml/min.[35,94,95] Both trimethoprim and nonacetylated sulfamethoxazole are removed by hemodialysis.[35] Patients needing chronic peritoneal dialysis can receive the equivalent of one double-strength trimethoprim-sulfamethoxazole tablet every 48 hours.

Toxicity and Side Effects

The toxic and undesired effects of trimethoprim-sulfamethoxazole include all those discussed above for sulfonamides. Nausea, vomiting, diarrhea, anorexia, and hypersensitivity reactions are the most frequent.[96,97] Rash and other adverse reactions have been noted frequently in patients with AIDS.[39,98–101] Also, in patients with AIDS, transient diffuse pulmonary infiltrates and hypotension have been described following reexposure to trimethoprim-sulfamethoxazole.[102,103] In addition, impaired folate utilization may be seen in humans with prolonged administration. This is usually manifest as a megaloblastic marrow, with hypersegmented polymorphonuclear leukocytes. Also leukopenia, thrombocytopenia, and granulocytopenia may be seen. One study suggested that this occurs in one case per 18,000 prescriptions and that elderly patients are at greater risk.[104] The administration of folinic acid usually prevents or treats effectively the antifolate effects of trimethoprim, and the latter drug's antibacterial efficacy is not impaired except possibly against enterococci. Pseudomembranous colitis has been described with trimethoprim-sulfamethoxazole but is uncommon.[105] Renal dysfunction may occur in patients with preexisting renal disease, but this is reversible with dose reduction.[106] Trimethoprim-sulfamethoxazole may cause an increase in measured serum creatinine.[107] Drug-induced hepatitis has been reported infrequently,[99] and prolonged cholestasis with pruritis may occur rarely.[108] One case of fulminant hepatic failure and pancreatitis has been reported.[109] Trimethoprim-sulfamethoxazole induced meningitis has been described,[110,111] and renal tubular acidosis has been reported in children during treatment for acute lymphocytic leukemia.[112]

Drug Interactions. Active levels of phenytoin may be increased markedly by trimethoprim-sulfamethoxazole.[113] Also, concomitant administration of trimethoprim-sulfamethoxazole and methotrexate results in decreased renal clearance of free methotrexate.[114] Severe pancytopenia may result.[114] Reversible inhibition of tubular creatinine excretion may be caused by trimethoprim in the presence of cyclosporine.[115] Serum rifampin levels may rise during concomitant therapy with trimethoprim-sulfamethoxazole.[116]

Trimethoprim Plus Other Antimicrobial Agents

Other sulfonamides, such as sulfamoxole, sulfadiazine, sulfadimidine, and sulfametrol, have been combined with trimethoprim, but more clinical studies are needed to recommend their use over the currently administered combination.[117–119] Trimethoprim-sulfadiazine was reported to be less likely to accumulate in the kidneys of elderly patients with impaired renal function than trimethoprim-sulfamethoxazole.[118] Combinations of trimethoprim with other agents such as rifampin[120–122] polymyxin,[54] amikacin,[123] and metronidazole[124] have been suggested or used. Extensive clinical experience with these combinations

is lacking. Recent reports suggest that trimethoprim-dapsone is more efficacious for the treatment of *P. carinii* pneumonia than dapsone alone.[98,125,126]

Clinical Use

Urinary Tract Infections. Trimethoprim-sulfamethoxazole is useful in the treatment of recurrent or chronic urinary tract infections due to sensitive organisms. Many Enterobacteriaceae are sensitive to the combined action of these drugs. The combination is also effective in acute pyelonephritis and cystitis (see Ch. 55), although either antibiotic alone could be appropriate for susceptible isolates.

Because trimethoprim accumulates in prostatic secretions, trimethoprim-sulfamethoxazole is often effective in bacterial prostatitis,[93] as well as in orchitis and epididymitis due to susceptible bacteria.

The usual dosage in an adult for the treatment of acute prostate or urinary infection is two tablets every 12 hours or one double-strength tablet every 12 hours. The pediatric dose for urinary tract infection is 150–185 mg/m² for trimethoprim and 750–925 mg/m² for sulfamethoxazole daily in two divided doses. Single-dose therapy with one or two double-strength tablets may be effective in some women with uncomplicated lower urinary tract infection,[127,128] but a recent trial suggested that 7 days of trimethoprim-sulfamethoxazole was better than single-dose ofloxacin and equivalent to 3-day treatment with the quinolone.[129] However, in patients with chronic tissue invasive urinary infections, longer term therapy of up to 6 weeks might be required.[130]

Trimethoprim-sulfamethoxazole has been shown to be useful in the long-term suppressive therapy of adults and children with chronic or recurrent urinary infections, and extremely low doses (one-half to one tablet at bedtime or every other night) are effective.[131,132] Postcoital prophylactic trimethoprim-sulfamethoxazole effectively reduces recurrent urinary infections following intercourse.[133] Trimethoprim is thought to achieve effective concentrations in the vaginal secretions, and it is believed by some that it exerts its protective effect on reducing the number of recurrent infections in this manner despite the fact that trimethoprim-sulfamethoxazole–resistant organisms may be present in the vaginal and stool flora.[134] Trimethoprim alone is effective therapy for uncomplicated and recurrent urinary infections in women. Usual doses are 100–200 mg bid.[134–136] and nightly doses of 100 mg may be effective suppressive therapy.[136,137] Trimethoprim alone has been felt by some to be preferable to the combination of trimethoprim-sulfamethoxazole for acute urinary tract infections and possibly other infections as well.[138,139] However, trimethoprim-resistant organisms might increase with extended use.

Respiratory Tract Infections. Trimethoprim-sulfamethoxazole is effective in the treatment of acute bronchitis and pneumonitis due to sensitive organisms, although it is not the treatment of choice for any single organism. Trimethoprim-sulfamethoxazole may be as effective as tetracyclines in the reduction of acute exacerbations in patients with chronic bronchitis,[139–141] but full doses should be used. Although not usually considered for use in seriously ill patients with pneumonia, intravenously administered trimethoprim-sulfamethoxazole may be effective in patients with infections due to susceptible gram-negative bacteria.[142]

Consistent with its antibacterial spectrum, trimethoprim-sulfamethoxazole may be as effective as ampicillin for the treatment of sinusitis and otitis media,[143] and ampicillin-resistant strains of *H. influenzae* and *Branhamella catarrhalis* might be susceptible.[60] Trimethoprim-sulfamethoxazole plus prednisone will produce short- but not long-term resolution of otitis media with effusion in children.[144,145]

Gastrointestinal Infections. Although antibiotics per se prolong the carrier state in acute gastroenteritis due to *Salmonella* spp., trimethoprim-sulfamethoxazole may be effective in eliminating chronic *Salmonella* carriage, including carriers of *Salmonella typhi*, especially in patients over 2 years of age. Typhoid fever also may be treated successfully with this combination, although the development of resistant strains has been increasingly reported.[57,80] Trimethoprim-sulfamethoxazole is effective in shigellosis,[146] especially that due to ampicillin-resistant strains; however, susceptibility testing is necessary given reports of plasmid-mediated outbreaks of resistant organisms.[147] Intravenous administration may be necessary for patients with some of these infections. Trimethoprim-sulfamethoxazole also may be effective in the treatment of diarrhea due to enteropathogenic *E. coli* and in the treatment and prophylaxis of traveler's diarrhea with or without loperamide[148–151] if the prevalence of resistant strains in the area to be visited is low. The combination may be a useful adjunct to fluids in the treatment of cholera[152]; however, plasmid-mediated trimethoprim resistance has been reported in East Asia.[153]

Sexually Transmitted Diseases. Trimethoprim-sulfamethoxazole may be effective in the treatment of uncomplicated gonorrhea when used in several dosage regimens (e.g., 2 tablets po bid for 5 days, 4 tablets for 2 days, and a single dose of 8 tabs).[154–156] For pharyngeal gonorrhea, especially that due to penicillinase-producing *N. gonorrhoeae*, 9 tablets/day for 5 days has been recommended.[157] However, almost one-half of the *N. gonorrhoeae* that were chromosomally resistant to penicillin in one study were resistant to trimethoprim-sulfamethoxazole as well.[158] Nongonococcal urethritis due to *Chlamydia trachomatis* may be treatable with the combination, but its activity is due to the sulfonamide.[159] The combination is also effective therapy for chancroid and lymphogranuloma venereum. It is ineffective for syphilis. Trimethoprim plus sulfametrole has been successful as a single-dose regimen for chancroid,[119] but recent reports suggest increasing resistance to trimethoprim-sulfamethoxazole.[160]

Other Infections. Trimethoprim-sulfamethoxazole is useful against brucellosis (long-term therapy for 6 weeks),[161,162] biliary tract infections, acute and chronic osteomyelitis,[163,164] periodontal infection,[165] paracoccidioidomycosis,[166] and nocardiosis[167–169] and is included in some regimens for the treatment of eumycetoma (see Ch. 242). Successful responses to combination therapy have been described for melioidosis,[170] *P. cepacia* bacteremia,[171] Whipple's disease,[172] *Xanthomonas maltophilia* infection, and Wegener's granulomatosis alone or as adjunctive therapy.[173,174] The latter use is controversial.

Intravenous trimethoprim-sulfamethoxazole has been useful in treating gram-negative rod bacteremia and staphylococcal bacteremia and endocarditis, although other agents may be preferred.[124,175–177] Trimethoprim-sulfamethoxazole plus extended spectrum β-lactams and/or aminoglycosides provide effective broad-spectrum antimicrobial coverage in the management of febrile neutropenic patients.[178–180] Meningitis due to susceptible organisms may be successfully treated,[181,182] but other agents are usually preferred. The combination may be effective in meningitis due to *Listeria monocytogenes*.[59]

The *Mycobacterium* species *kansasii*, *marinum*, and *scrofulaceum* are inhibited in vitro by trimethoprim-sulfamethoxazole, and several clinical successes have been reported often in combination with other agents.[43,61,183] Trimethoprim-sulfamethoxazole is being studied in combination with isoniazid and rifampin in the treatment of leprosy.[184]

Trimethoprim plus sulfalene and trimethoprim-sulfamethoxazole have been used in the treatment of susceptible *P. falciparum* infections, although these combinations are not very active against multiple-resistant strains. HIV-infected patients with *Isospora belli* enteritis have had clinical responses after receiving trimethoprim-sulfamethoxazole[185]; however, relapse after treatment is common, necessitating chronic suppressive therapy. Trimethoprim-sulfamethoxazole has no activity against other related coccidial parasites such as *Cryptosporidium parvum*.

Trimethoprim-sulfamethoxazole is active against *Toxoplasma gondii* in vitro[186] and has been used clinically,[187] but is not superior to first-line therapy with pyrimethamine-sulfadiazine. In preliminary studies, low doses (trimethoprim, 160 mg; sulfamethoxazole, 800 mg) appear promising for the prophylaxis of *T. gondii* infection in HIV-infected toxoplasma antibody-positive patients.[188]

PNEUMOCYSTIS CARINII INFECTIONS. Trimethoprim-sulfamethoxazole has been highly efficacious in the treatment of *P. carinii* pneumonia in immunocompromised patients with and without AIDS[98,99,189–193] (see Chs. 105 and 258). Patients with AIDS frequently respond to therapy but have a higher incidence of adverse reactions, particularly neutropenia and rash.[99] Although the toxicities are different, the efficacy and rate of drug reactions associated with systemic pentamidine are comparable.[194,195] Patients were more likely to manifest a hypersensitivity reaction while receiving trimethoprim-sulfamethoxazole if they were less immunocompromised (i.e., had higher CD4 counts) and were treated for more than 2 weeks, suggesting a role for intact cell-mediated immunity in the pathogenesis of these reactions.[196] The toxicities of a 3-week course of parenteral trimethoprim-sulfamethoxazole for *P. carinii* pneumonia may be decreased if serum trimethoprim levels are monitored and maintained between 5 and 8 μg/ml.[197] Trimethoprim also has been used successfully with dapsone for mild to moderate *P. carinii* pneumonia.[126]

Trimethoprim-sulfamethoxazole has been successfully used for the primary and secondary chemoprophylaxis of *P. carinii* pneumonia[99,198–201] and is generally used as the first-line agent, but chronic use may be limited by toxicities such as rash and/or leukopenia.[38,39]

In recent randomized studies trimethoprim, 160 mg, plus sulfamethoxazole, 800 mg, given daily was more effective than monthly aerosolized pentamidine for prophylaxis after an initial episode of *P. carinii* pneumonia,[202] and half of this daily dose was more efficacious in patients with less than 200 CD4 cells/mm[3] and no prior *P. carinii* pneumonia.[203] *P. carinii* pneumonia prophylaxis in conjunction with antiretroviral therapy has been associated with enhanced survival in patients with AIDS.[204]

PROPHYLACTIC THERAPY OF NEUTROPENIC PATIENTS. Several studies have presented evidence of a striking reduction in gram-negative rod bacteremia in neutropenic patients treated prophylactically with trimethoprim-sulfamethoxazole (2 tablets bid or more until stools were free of Enterobacteriaceae) compared with untreated control neutropenic patients.[205–207] Other studies have not universally shown benefit in preventing bacteremia in neutropenic patients with acute myelocytic leukemia.[208] Trimethoprim-sulfamethoxazole plus colistin compared favorably to ciprofloxacin except for gram-negative rod bacteremia in a recent prophylactic trial,[209] but in another study it was less effective than penicillin G in preventing viridans group streptococcal bacteremia.[210] Trimethoprim-sulfamethoxazole may prolong recovery from induction chemotherapy-induced neutropenia, as has been reported in some but not all studies.[211,212] Its effective prophylactic use in chronic granulomatous disease has been reported.[213]

Trimethoprim Use in Pregnancy. The teratogenicity of trimethoprim in humans is not clearly defined, but this drug is not recommended for use in pregnancy. It is, however, well tolerated in pediatric populations.[214]

REFERENCES

1. Carithers HA. The first use of an antibiotic in America. Am J Dis Child. 1974;128–207–11.

2. Bushby SRM, Hitchings GH. Trimethoprim, a sulphonamide potentiator. Br J Pharmacol Chemother. 1968;33:72–90.

3. Pearson RD, Hewlett EL. Use of pyrimethamine-sulfadoxine (Fansidar) in prophylaxis against chloroquine-resistant *Plasmodium falciparum* and *Pneumocystis carinii*. Ann Intern Med. 1987;106:714–18.

4. Ballin JC. Evaluation of a new topical agent for burn therapy. Silver sulfadiazine (Silvadene). JAMA 1974;230:1184–5.

5. Mayer KH, Hopkins JD, Gilleece ES, et al. Molecular evolution, species distribution, and clinical consequences of an endemic aminoglycoside resistance plasmid. Antimicrob Agents Chemother. 1986;29:628–33.

6. McHugh G, Moellering RC Jr, Hopkins CC, et al. *Salmonella typhimurium* resistant to silver nitrate, chloramphenicol and ampicillin: A new threat in burn units? Lancet. 1975;1:235–40.

7. Woods DD. Relation of p-aminobenzoic acid to mechanism of action of sulphamilamide. Br J Exp Pathol. 1940;21:74–90.

8. Fildes P. Rational approach to research in chemotherapy. Lancet. 1940;1:955–7.

9. Miller AK, Bruno P, Berglund RM. The effect of sulfathiazol on the in vitro synthesis of certain vitamins by *Escherichia coli*. J Bacteriol. 1947;54:9.

10. Brown GH. The biosynthesis of pteridines. Adv Enzymol. 1971;35:35–77.

11. Richmond MH. Structural analogy and chemical reactivity in the action of antibacterial compounds. In: Biochemical Studies of Antimicrobial Drugs. Proceedings of the Sixteenth Symposium of the Society of General Microbiology. London: Cambridge University Press; 1966:301.

12. Hamilton-Miller JMT. Mechanisms and distribution of bacterial resistance to diaminopyrimidines and sulphonamides. J Antimicrob Chemother. 1979; 5(Suppl B):61–73.

13. Mennish ML, Salam MA, Hossain MA, et al. Antimicrobial resistance of *Shigella* isolates in Bangladesh, 1983–1990: Increasing frequency of strains multiply resistant to amipicillin, trimethoprim-sulfamethoxazole, and nalidixic acid. Clin Infect Dis. 1992;14:1055–60.

14. Landy M, Larkun NW, Oswald EJ, et al. Increased synthesis of p-aminobenzoic acid associated with the development of resistance in *Staph aureus*. Science. 1943;97:265–7.

15. Wolf B, Hotchkiss RD. Genetically modified folic acid synthesising enzymes in *Pneumococcus*. Biochemistry. 1940;2:145–50.

16. Landy M, Gerstung RB. p-Aminobenzoic acid synthesis by *Neisseria gonorrhoeae* in relation to clinical and cultural sulfonamide resistance. J. Bacteriol. 1944;47:448.

17. Swedberg G, Castenssos S, Sköld O. Characterization of mutationally altered dihydropteroate synthase and its ability to form a sulfonamide-containing dihydrofolate analog. J Bacteriol. 1979;137:129–36.

18. Sköld O. R-factor mediated resistance to sulfonamides by a plasmid-borne, drug resistant dihydropteroate synthase. Antimicrob Agents Chemother. 1976;9:49–54.

19. Kabins SA, Panse MV, Cohen S. Role of R-factor and bacterial host in sulfonamide resistance mediated by R-factor in *Escherichia coli*. J Infect Dis. 1971;123:158–68.

20. Watanabe T. Infective heredity of multiple drug resistance in bacteria. Bacteriol Rev. 1963;27:87–115.

21. Radstrom P, Fermer C, Kristiansen BE, et al. Transformational exchanges in the dihydropteroate synthase gene of *Neisseria meningitidis*: A novel mechanism for acquisition of sulfonamide resistance. J Bacteriol. 1992;174:6386–93.

22. Bissonnette L, Roy PH. Characterization of InO of *Pseudomonas aeruginosa* plasmid pVS1, an ancestor of integrons of multiresistance plasmids and transposons of gram-negative bacteria. J Bacteriol. 1992;174:1248–57.

23. Then RL. Mechanisms of resistance to trimethoprim, the sulfonamides and trimethoprim-sulfamethoxazole. Rev Infect Dis. 1982;4:261–9.

24. Burman LG. Apparent absence of transferable resistance to nalidixic acid in pathogenic gram-negative bacteria. J Antimicrob Chemother. 1977;3:509–14.

25. Hansson HB, Walder M, Juhlin I. Susceptibility of shigellae to mecillinam, nalidixic acid, trimethoprim, and five other antimicrobial agents. Antimicrob Agents Chemother. 1981;19:271–4.

26. Davies JR, Farrant WN, Uttley AHC. Antibiotic resistance of *Shigella sonnei*. Lancet. 1970;2:1157–60.

27. Gordon RC, Thompson TR, Carlson W, et al. Antimicrobial resistance of shigellae isolated in Michigan. JAMA. 1975;231:1159–64.

28. Ryder RW, Blake PA, Murlin AC, et al. Increase in antibiotic resistance among isolates of salmonella in the United States, 1967–1975. J Infect Dis. 1980;142:485–91.

29. Albritton WL, Brunton JL, Slaney L, Maclean I. Plasmid-mediated sulfonamide resistance in *Haemophilus ducreyi*. Antimicrob Agents Chemother. 1982;21:159–66.

30. Garrod LP, Lambert HP, O'Grady F. Antibiotic and Chemotherapy. 4th ed. Edinburgh and London: Churchill Livingstone; 1973.

31. Bushby SRM. Trimethoprim-sulfamethoxazole: In vitro microbiologic aspects. J Infect Dis. 1973;128:S442–62.

32. Bach MC, Finland M, Gold W, et al. Susceptibility of recently isolated pathogenic bacteria to trimethoprim and sulfamethoxazole separately and combined. J Infect Dis. 1973;128:S508–33.

33. Anand N. Sulfonamides and sulfones. In: Corcoran JW, Hahn FE, eds. Antibiotics III: Mechanism of Action of Antimicrobial and Antitumor Agents. Berlin: Springer-Verlag; 1975:668.

34. Sparr RA, Pritchard JA. Maternal and newborn distribution and excretion of sulfamethoxypyridazine (Kynex). Obstet Gynecol. 1958;12:131–4.

35. Craig WA, Kunin CM. Trimethoprim-sulfamethoxazole: Pharmacodynamic effects of urinary pH and impaired renal function. Ann Intern Med. 1973; 78:491–7.

36. Bartels RH, van der Spek JA, Oosten HR. Acute pancreatitis due to sulfamethoxazole-trimethoprim. So Med J. 1992;85:1006–7.

37. Markowitz N, Saravolatz LD. Use of trimethoprim-sulfamethoxazole in a glucose-6-phosphate dehydrogenase-deficient population. Rev Infect Dis. 1987;9:S218–25.

38. Kelly JW, Dooley DP, Lattuada CP, Smith CE. A severe, unusual reaction to trimethoprim-sulfamethoxazole in patients infected with human immunodeficiency virus. Clin Infect Dis. 1992;14:1034–9.

39. Johnson MP, Goodwin SD, Shands JW Jr. Trimethoprim-sulfamethoxazole anaphylactoid reactions in patients with AIDS: Case reports and literature review. Pharmacotherapy. 1990;10:413–6.

40. Dunea G, Freedman P. Proteinuria. JAMA. 1968;203:973–84.

41. Hansten PD. Drug Interactions. 2nd ed. Philadelphia: Lea & Febiger; 1973.

42. Griffin JP, D'Arcy PF. A Manual of Adverse Drug Interactions. Bristol: John Wright and Sons; 1974:63.

43. Ahn CH, Wallace RJ Jr, Steel LC, et al. Sulfonamide-containing regimens for disease caused by rifampin-resistant *Mycobacterium kansasii*. Am Rev Respir Dis. 1987;135:10–6.

44. Bernard PA, Stenstrom RJ, Feldman W, et al. Randomized controlled trial comparing long-term sulfonamide therapy to ventilation tubes for otitis media with effusion. Pediatrics. 1991;88:215–22.

45. Peppercorn MA. Sulfasalazine: Pharmacology, clinical use, toxicity, and related new drug development. Ann Intern Med. 1984;3:377–84.

46. Pullar T, Hunter JA, Capell HA. Sulphasalazine in rheumatoid arthritis: A double-blind comparison of sulphasalazine with placebo and sodium aurothiomalate. Br Med J. 1983;287:1102–6.

47. Burchall JJ. Trimethoprim and pyrimethamine. In: Corcoran JW, Hahn FE, eds. Antibiotics III: Mechanism of Antimicrobial and Antitumor Agents. Berlin: Springer-Verlag; 1975:304.

48. Hitchings GT. The biochemical basis for the antimicrobial activity of septrin. In: Bernstein LS, Salter AJ, eds. Trimethoprim/sulphamethoxazole in Bacterial Infections. Edinburgh and London: Churchill Livingstone, 1973:7–16.

49. Phillips I, Warren C. Activity of sulfamethoxazole and trimethoprim against *Bacteroides fragilis*. Antimicrob Agents Chemother. 1976;9:736–40.

50. Trehane JD, Day J, Yeo CK, et al. Susceptibility of chlamydiae to chemotherapeutic agents. In: Hobsen D, Holmes KK, eds. Nongonococcal Urethritis and Related Infections. Washington, DC: American Society for Microbiology; 1977:214–22.

51. Moody MR, Young VM. In vitro susceptibility of *Pseudomonas cepacia* and *Pseudomonas maltophilia* to trimethoprim and trimethoprim-sulfamethoxazole. Antimicrob Agents Chemother. 1975;7:836–9.

52. Najjar A, Murray BE. Failure to demonstrate a consistent in vitro bactericidal effect of trimethoprim sulfamethoxazole against enterococci. Antimicrob Agents Chemother. 1987;31:808–10.

53. Dornbusch K, Moore WB. The effects of different media on the response of bacteria to sulphonamides and trimethoprim using the disc-diffusion method and regression line analysis. In: Bernstein LS, Salter AJ, eds. Trimethoprim/Sulphamethoxazole in Bacterial Infections. Edinburgh and London: Churchill Livingstone; 1973:39–51.

54. Simmons NA. Colistin, sulphamethoxazole and trimethoprim in synergy against gram-negative bacilli. J Clin Pathol. 1970;23:757–64.

55. Parsley TL, Provonchee RB, Glicksman C, et al. Synergistic activity of trimethoprim and amikacin against gram-negative bacilli. Antimicrob Agents Chemother. 1977;12:349–54.

56. Bushby SRM. Sensitivity patterns and use of a combined disc of trimethoprim-sulphamethoxazole. In: Bernstein LS, Salter AJ, eds. Trimethoprim/Sulphamethoxazole in Bacterial Infections. Edinburgh and London: Churchill Livingstone; 1973:31–8.

57. Goldstein FW, Papadopoulou B, Acar JF. The changing of trimetoprim resistance in Paris, with a review of worldwide experience. Rev Infect Dis. 1986; 8:725–37.

58. Goodhart GL. In vivo versus in vitro susceptibility of enterococcus to trimethoprim-sulfamethoxazole. JAMA. 1984;252:2748–9.

59. Armstrong RW, Slater B. *Listeria monocytogenes* meningitis treated with trimethoprim-sulfamethoxazole. Pediatr Infect Dis J. 1986;5:712–3.

60. Riley TV, Degiovanni C, Hoyne GF. Susceptibility of *Branhamella catarrhalis* to sulphamethoxazole and trimethoprim. J Antimicrob Chemother. 1987;19:39–43.

61. Wallace RJ Jr, Swanson JM, Silcox VA, et al. Treatment of nonpulmonary infections due to *Mycobacterium fortuitum* and *Mycobacterium chelonei* based on in vitro susceptibility. J Infect Dis. 1985;152:500–14.

62. Bohni E. Vergleichende bakteriologishe untersuchungen mit der Kombination Trimethoprim Sulfamethoxazole in vitro and in vivo. Chemotherapy. 1969;14(Suppl):1–21.

63. O'Brien TF, Acar JF, Altmann G, et al. Laboratory surveillance of synergy between and resistance to trimethoprim and sulfonamides. Rev Infect Dis. 1982;4:351–7.

64. Panbangred W, Jayanetra P, Pilantanapak A. Epidemiological study of sulfonamide and trimethoprim resistance genes in Enterobacteriaceae. Southeast Asian J Trop Med Public Health. 1990;21:175–84.

65. Richards HN, Datta N, Sojka NJ, et al. Trimethoprim resistance plasmids and transposons in *Salmonella*. Lancet. 1978;2:1194–5.

66. Burchall JJ, Pelwell L, Fling ME. Molecular mechanisms of resistance to trimethoprim. Rev Infect Dis. 1982;4:246–54.

67. Houvinen P. Trimethoprim resistance. Antimicrob Agents Chemother. 1987; 31:1451–6.

68. Goldstein FW, Labigne-Roussel A, Gerbaud G, et al. Transferable plasmid-mediated antibiotic resistance in *Acinetobacter*. Plasmid. 1983;10:138–47.

69. Sundstrom L. Vinayagamoorthy T, Skold O. Novel type of plasmid-borne resistance to trimethoprim. Antimicrob Agents Chemother. 1987;31:60–6.

70. Jorgensen JH. Update on mechanisms and prevalence of antimicrobial resistance in *Haemophilus influenzae*. Clin Infect Dis. 1992;14:1119–23.

71. Steen R, Sköld O. Plasmid-borne or chromosomally mediated resistance by Tn7 is the most common response to ubiquitous use of trimethoprim. Antimicrob Agents Chemother. 1985;27:933–7.

72. Fleming MP, Datta N, Grüneberg RN. Trimethoprim resistance determined by R factors. Br Med J. 1972;1:726–8.

73. Saroglou G, Parakevopoulou P, Paniara O, Kontomichalou P. Trimethoprim resistance plasmids from Enterobacteriaceae isolated in Greece. In: Mitsuhashi S, Rosival L, Krcméry V, eds. Antibiotic Resistance. Berlin: Springer-Verlag; 1980:267–71.

74. Bratoeva MP, Jorh JF, Barg NL. Molecular epidemiology of trimethoprim-resistant *Shigella boydii* serotype 2 strains from Bulgaria. J Clin Microbiol. 1992;30:1428–31.

75. Agarwal KC, Panhotra BR, Mahanta J, et al. Typhoid fever due to chloramphenicol resistant *Salmonella typhi* associated with R-plasmid. Indian J Med Res. 1981;73:484–8.

76. Goldstein FW, Chumpitaz JC, Guevara JM, et al. Plasmid-mediated resistance to multiple antibiotics in *Salmonella typhi*. J Infect Dis. 1986;153:261–6.

77. O'Brien TF, Hopkins JD, Gilleece ES, et al. Molecular epidemiology of antibiotic resistance in *Salmonella* from animals and human beings in the United States. N Engl J Med. 1982;307:1–6.

78. Mayer KH, Fling ME, Hopkins JD, et al. Trimethoprim resistance in multiple genera of Enterobacteriaceae at a U.S. hospital: Spread of the type II dihydrofolate reductase gene by a single plasmid. J Infect Dis. 1985;5:783–9.

79. Naumovski L, Quinn JP, Miyashiro D, et al. Outbreak of ceftazidime resistance due to a novel extended-spectrum beta-lactamase in isolates from cancer patients. Antimicrob Agents Chemother. 1992;36:1991–6.

80. Murray BE, Alvarado T, Kim K-H, et al. Increasing resistance to trimethoprim-sulfamethoxazole among isolates of *Escherichia coli* in developing countries. J Infect Dis. 1985;152:1107–13.

81. Towner KJ, Slack RCB. Effect of changing selection pressures on trimethoprim resistance in Enterobacteriaceae. Eur J Clin Microbiol. 1986;5:502–6.

82. Heikkila E, Sundstrom L, Skurnik M, et al. Emergence and mechanisms of trimethoprim resistance in *Escherichia coli* isolated from outpatients in Finland. J Antimicrob Chemother. 18:643–4.

83. Reves RR, Fong M, Pickering LK, et al. Risk factors for fecal colonization with trimethoprim-resistant and multiresistant *Escherichia coli* among children in day-care centers in Houston, Texas. Antimicrob Agents Chemother. 1990;34:1429–34.

84. Voogd CE, Schot CS, van Leeuwen WJ, et al. Monitoring of antibiotic resistance in shigellae isolated in The Netherlands 1984–1989. Eur J Clin Microbiol Infect Dis. 1992;11:164–7.

85. Then RL, Kohl I, Burdeska A. Frequency and transferability of trimethoprim sulfonamide resistance in methicillin-resistant *Staphylococcus aureus* and *Staphylococcus epidermidis*. J Chemother. 1992;4:67–71.

86. Smith HW, Tucker JF. The virulence of trimethoprim resistant thymine-requiring strains of *Salmonella*. J Hyg (Lond). 1976;76:97–108.

87. Maskell R, Okubadejo OA, Payne RH, et al. Human infections with thymine-requiring bacteria. J Med Microbiol. 1978;11:33–45.

88. Grose WE, Bodey GP, Loo TL. Clinical pharmacology of intravenously administered trimethoprim-sulfamethoxazole. Antimicrob Agents Chemother. 1979;15:447–51.

89. Bach MC, Gold O, Finland M. Absorption and urinary excretion of trimethoprim, sulfamethoxazole, and trimethoprim-sulfamethoxazole: Results with single doses in normal young adults and preliminary observations during therapy with trimethoprim-sulfamethoxazole. J Infect Dis. 1973;128:S584–98.

90. Kaplan SA, Weinfeld RE, Abruzzo CW, et al. Pharmacokinetic profile of trimethoprim-sulfamethoxazole in man. J Infect Dis. 1973;128:S547–55.

91. Pater RB, Welling PG. Clinical pharmacokinetics of co-trimoxazole (trimethoprim/sulfamethoxazole). Clin Pharmacokinet. 1980;5:405–23.

92. Winningham DG, Nemoy NJ, Stamey TA. Diffusion of antibiotics from plasma into prostatic fluid. Nature. 1968;219:139–43.

93. Meares EM Jr. Prostatitis: Review of pharmacokinetics and therapy. Rev Infect Dis. 1982;4:475–83.

94. Welling PG, Craig WA, Amidon GL, et al. Pharmacokinetics of trimethoprim and sulfamethoxazole in normal subjects and in patients with renal failure. J Infect Dis. 1974;128(Suppl):556–66.

95. Salter AJ. Trimethoprim sulfamethoxazole: An assessment of more than 12 years of use. Rev Infect Dis. 1982;4:196–236.

96. Jick H. Adverse reactions to trimethoprim-sulfamethoxazole in hospitalized patients. Rev Infect Dis. 1982;4:426–8.

97. Lawson DH, Paice BJ. Adverse reactions to trimethoprim-sulfamethoxazole. Rev Infect Dis. 1982;4:429–33.

98. Masur H, Kovacs JA. Treatment and prophylaxis of *Pneumocystis carinii* pneumonia. In: Moellering RC Jr, ed. Infectious Disease Clinics of North America (Medical Management of AIDS). Philadelphia: WB Saunders; 1988: 419–28.

99. Wofsy CB. Use of trimethoprim-sulfamethoxazole in the treatment of *Pneu-mocystis carinii* pneumonitis in patients with acquired immunodeficiency syndrome. Rev Infect Dis. 1987;9:S184–91.

100. Gordin FM, Simon GL, Wofsy CB, et al. Adverse reactions to trimethoprim-sulfamethoxazole in patients with acquired immunodeficiency syndrome. Ann Intern Med. 1984;100:495–9.

101. van der Ven AJ, Koopmans PP, Vree TB, et al. Adverse reaction to co-trimoxazole in HIV infection. Lancet. 1991;338:431–3.

102. Silvestri RC, Jensen WA, Zibrak JD, et al. Pulmonary infiltrates and hypoxemia in patients with the acquired immunodeficiency syndrome re-exposed to trimethoprim-sulfamethoxazole. Am Rev Respir Dis. 1987;136:1003–4.

103. Kelly JW, Dooley DP, Lattuada CP, et al. A severe, unusual reaction to trimethoprim-sulfamethoxazole in patients infected with human immunodeficiency virus. Clin Infect Dis. 1992;14:1034–9.

104. Keisu M, Wiholm BE, Palmblad J. Trimethoprim-sulphamethoxazole-associated blood dyscrasias. Ten years experience of the Swedish spontaneous reporting system. J Intern. Med. 1990;228:353–6.

105. Cameron A, Thomas M. Pseudomembranous colitis and co-trimoxazole. Br Med J. 1977;1:1321.

106. Bailey RR, Little PJ. Deterioration in renal function in association with co-trimoxazole therapy. Med J Aust. 1976;1:914–6.

107. Trollfors B, Wahl M, Alestig K. Co-trimoxazole, creatinine and renal function. J Infect. 1980;2:221.

108. Kowdley KV, Keefe EB, Fawaz KA. Prolonged cholestasis due to trimethoprim-sulfamethoxazole. Gastroenterology. 1992;102:2148–50.

109. Alberti-Flor JJ, Hernandez ME, Ferrer JP, et al. Fulminant liver failure and pancreatitis associated with the use of sulfamethoxazole-trimethoprim. Am J Gastroenterol. 1989;84:1577–9.

110. Escalante A, Stimmler MM. Trimethoprim-sulfamethoxasole induced meningitis in systemic lupus erythematosus. J Rheumatol. 1992;19:800–2.

111. Derhes SJ. Trimethoprim-induced aseptic meningitis, JAMA. 1984;252: 2865–7.

112. Murphy JL. Renal tubular acidosis in children treated with trimethoprim-sulfamethoxazole during therapy for acute lymphoid leukemia. Pediatrics. 1992;89:1072–4.

113. Hansen JM, Kampmann JP, Siersbaek-Nielsen K, et al. The effect of different sulfonamides on phenytoin metabolism in man. Acta Med Scand 1979; 624(Suppl):106–10.

114. Ferrazzini G, Klein J, Sulh H, et al. Interaction between trimethoprim-sulfamethoxazole and methotrexate in children with leukemia. J Pediatr. 1990; 117:823–6.

115. Maki DG, Fox BC, Kuntz J, et al. A prospective, randomized, double-blind study of trimethoprim-sulfamethoxazole for prophylaxis of infection in renal transplantation. Side effects of trimethoprim-sulfamethoxazole, interaction with cyclosporine. J Lab Clin Med. 1991;119:11–24.

116. Bhatia RS, Uppal R, Malhi R, et al. Drug interaction between rifampicin and cotrimoxazole in patients with tuberculosis. Hum Exp Toxicol. 1991; 10:419–21.

117. Bernstein LS. Combination of trimethoprim with sulfonamides other than sulfamethoxazole. Rev Infect Dis. 1982;4:411–8.

118. Bergan T, Allgulander S, Fellner H. Pharmacokinetics of co-trimazine (sulphadiazine plus trimethoprim) in geriatric patients. Chemotherapy. 1986;32: 478–85.

119. Dylewski J, D'Costa LJ, Nsanze H, et al. Single dose therapy with trimethoprim-sulfametrole for chancroid in females. Sex Transm Dis. 1986;13:166–8.

120. Brumfitt W, Hamilton-Miller JMT. Rifamprim (rifampicin plus trimethoprim); Pharmacokinetics and effects on the normal flora of man. Biopharm Drug Dispos. 1981;2:157–66.

121. Kerry DW, Hamilton-Miller JMT, Brumfitt W. Trimethoprim and rifampicin: In vitro activities separately and in combination. J Antimicrob Chemother. 1975;1:417–27.

122. Alvarez S, DeMaria A Jr, Kulkarni R, et al. Interactions of rifampin and trimethoprim in vitro. Rev Infect Dis. 1982;4:390–401.

123. Zinner SH, Lagast H, Kasry A, et al. Synergism of trimethoprim combined with aminoglycosides in vitro and in serum of volunteers. Eur J Clin Microbiol. 1982;1:144–8.

124. Salter AJ. Trimethoprim-sulfamethoxazole in treatment of severe infections. Rev Infect Dis. 1982;4:338–50.

125. Leoung GS, Mills J, Hopewell PC, et al. Dapsone-trimethoprim for *Pneumocystis carinii* pneumonia in acquired immunodeficiency syndrome. Ann Intern Med. 1986;105:48–54.

126. Glatt A, Chirgwin K. *Pneumocystis carinii* pneumonia in human immunodeficiency virus-infected patients. Arch Intern Med. 1990;150:271–9.

127. Tolkoff-Rubin NE, Weber D, Fang LST, et al. Single dose therapy with trimethoprim-sulfamethoxazole for urinary infection in women. Rev Infect Dis. 1982;4:444–8.

128. Counts GW, Stamm WE, McKevitt M, et al. Treatment of cystitis in women with a single dose of trimethoprim-sulfamethoxazole. Rev Infect Dis. 1982; 4:484–90.

129. Hooton TM, Johnson C, Winter C, et al. Single-dose and three-day regimens of ofloxacin versus trimethoprim-sulfamethoxazole for acute cystitis in women. Antimicrob Agents Chemother. 1991;35:1479–83.

130. Gleckman R, Crowley M, Natsios GA. Treatment of recurrent invasive urinary-tract infections of men. N Engl J Med. 1979;301:878–80.

131. Harding GKM, Ronald AR, Nicolle LE, et al. Long-term antimicrobial prophylaxis for recurrent urinary tract infection in women. Rev Infect Dis. 1982; 4:438–43.

132. Stamey TA. Recurrent urinary tract infections in female patients: An overview of management and treatment. Rev Infect Dis. 1987;9:S195–208.

133. Stapleton A, Latham RH, Johnson C, et al. Postcoital antimicrobial prophylaxis for recurrent urinary tract infection. A randomized, double-blind, placebo-controlled trial. JAMA. 1990;264:703–6.

134. Brumfitt W, Pursell R. Double-blind trial to compare ampicillin, cephalexin, co-trimoxazole and trimethoprim in treatment of urinary infection. Br Med J. 1972;2:673–6.

135. Kasanen A, Toivanen P, Sourander L, et al. Trimethoprim in the treatment of long-term control of urinary tract infection. Scand J Infect Dis. 1974;6: 91–6.

136. Iravani A, Richard GA, Baer H. Treatment of uncomplicated urinary tract infection with trimethoprim versus sulfisoxazole with special reference to antibody-coated bacteria and faecal flora. Antimicrob Agents Chemother. 1981;19:842–50.

137. Stamm WE, Counts GW, Wagner KR, et al. Antimicrobial prophylaxis of recurrent urinary tract infections. Ann Intern Med. 1980;92:770–5.

138. Reeves D. Sulphonamides and trimethoprim. Lancet. 1982;2:370–3.

139. Amyes SGB, Doherty CJ, Wonnacott S. Trimethoprim and co-trimoxazole: A comparison of the use in respiratory tract infections. Scand J Infect Dis. 1986;18:561–6.

140. Pandy GJ. Trimethoprim/sulphamethoxazole and doxycycline in acute exacerbations of chronic bronchitis in general practice: A comparative study. Med J Aust. 1979;1:264–6.

141. Pines A. Trimethoprim-sulfamethoxazole in the treatment and prevention of purulent exacerbations of chronic bronchitis. J Infect Dis. 1973;128:S706–9.

142. Schmidt U, Sen P, Kapila R, et al. Clinical evaluation of intravenous trimethoprim sulfamethoxazole for serious infections. Rev Infect Dis. 1982;4:332–7.

143. Shurin PA, Pelton SI, Donner A, et al. Trimethoprim-sulfamethoxazole compared with ampicillin in the treatment of acute otitis media. J Pediatr. 1980; 96:1081–7.

144. Daly K, Giebink GS, Bastalden PB, et al. Resolution of otitis media with effusion with the use of a stepped treatment regimen of trimethoprim-sulfamethoxazole and prednisone. Pediatr Infect Dis J. 1991;10:500–6.

145. Giebink GS, Batalden PB, Le CT, et al. A controlled trial comparing three treatments for chronic otitis media with effusion. Pediatr Infect Dis J. 1990; 9:33–40.

146. Nelson JD, Kusmiesz H, Shelton S. Oral or intravenous trimethoprim-sulfamethoxazole therapy for shigellosis. Rev Infect Dis. 1982;4:546–50.

147. Bannatyne RM, Toma S, Cheung R, et al. Resistance to trimethoprim and other antibiotics in Ontario shigellae (Letter). Lancet. 1980;1:425–6.

148. Thoren A, Wolde-Mariam I, Stintzing G, et al. Antibiotics in the treatment of gastroenteritis caused by enteropathogenic *Escherichia coli*. J Infect Dis. 1980;141:27–31.

149. DuPont HL, Evans DG, Rios N, et al. Prevention of travelers' diarrhea with trimethoprim-sulfamethoxazole. Rev Infect Dis. 1982;4:533–9.

150. DuPont HL, Reves RR, Galindo E, et al. Treatment of travelers' diarrhea with trimethoprim/sulfamethoxazole and with trimethoprim alone. N Engl J Med. 1982;307:841–4.

151. Ericsson CD, Nicholls-Vasquez I, DuPont HL, et al. Optimal dosing of trimethoprim-sulfamethoxazole when used with loperamide to treat traveler's diarrhea. Antimicrob Agents Chemother. 1992;36:2821–4.

152. Francis TI, Lewis EA, Oyediran ABOO, et al. Effect of chemotherapy on the duration of diarrhoea, and on *Vibrio* excretion by cholera patients. J Trop Med Hyg. 1972;74:172–6.

153. Threlfall EJ, Rowe B, Huq I. Plasmid-encoded multiple antibiotic resistance in *Vibrio cholerae* El Tor from Bangladesh (Letter). Lancet. 1980;1:1247–8.

154. Svindland HB. Treatment of gonorrhoea with sulphamethoxazole-trimethoprim. Lack of effect on concomitant syphilis. Br J Vener Dis. 1973;49:50–3.

155. Lawrence A, Phillips E, Nicol C. Various regimens of trimethoprim-sulfamethoxazole in the treatment of gonorrhea. J Infect Dis. 1973;128(Suppl): S673–8.

156. Rahim G. Single dose treatment of gonorrhoea with cotrimoxazole. A report on 1,223 cases. Br J Vener Dis. 1975;51:179–82.

157. Centers for Disease Control and Prevention. 1985 STD treatment guidelines. MMWR. 1985;34(Suppl):4S.

158. Centers for Disease Control and Prevention. Chromosomally mediated resistant *Neisseria gonorrhoeae*—United States. MMWR. 1984;33:408–10.

159. Hammerschlag MR. Activity of trimethoprim-sulfamethoxazole against *Chlamydia trachomatis* in vitro. Rev Infect Dis. 1982;4:500–5.

160. Plourde PJ, D'Costa LJ, Agoki E, et al. A randomized, double-blind study of the efficacy of fleroxacin versus trimethoprim-sulfamethoxazole in men with culture-proven chancroid. J Infect Dis. 1992;165:949–52.

161. Daikos GK, Papapolyzos N, Marketos N, et al. Trimethoprim-sulfamethoxazole in brucellosis. J Infect Dis. 1974;128(Suppl):S731–3.

162. Shehabi A, Shakir K, el-Khateeb M, et al. Diagnosis and treatment of 106 cases of human brucellosis. J Infect 1990;20:5–10.

163. Bajpai J, Chaturvedi SN, Khanuja SPS. Chemotherapy of acute bone and joint infections. Int Surg. 1977;62:172–4.

164. Millard FJC. Trimethoprim/sulphamethoxazole in the treatment of chronic osteomyelitis. In: Bernstein LS, Salter AJ, eds. Trimethoprim-Sulphamethoxazole in Bacterial Infections. Edinburgh: Churchill Livingstone; 1973: 195–9.

165. Lakshamanan CDS. Comparative evaluation of cotrimoxazole and democlocycline in periodontal bacterial infection (Abstract 128). J Dent Res. 1976; 55(Spec Iss):D137.

166. Mahgoub ES. Medical managenment of mycetoma. Bull WHO. 1976;54:303.

167. Welsh O, Sauceda E, Gonzalez J, et al. Amikacin alone and in combination with trimethoprim-sulfamethoxazole in the treatment of actinomycotic mycetoma. J Am Acad Dermatol. 1987;127:443–8.

168. Wallace RJ, Septimus EJ, Williams JH, et al. Use of trimetohoprim-sulfamethoxazole for the treatment of infections due to *Nocardia*. Rev Infect Dis. 1982;4:315–25.

169. Javaly K, Horowitz HW, Wormser GP. Nocardiosis in patients with human immunodeficiency virus infection. Report of 2 cases and review of the literature. Medicine. 1992;71:128–38.

170. Morrison IM. Chronic melioidosis. Proc R Soc Med. 1970;63:239–49.

171. Neu HC, Garvey GJ, Bleach MP. Successful treatment of *Pseudomonas cepacia* endocarditis in a heroin addict with trimethoprim sulfamethoxazole. J Infect Dis. 1973;128(Suppl):768–70.

172. Viteri AL, Greene JF Jr, Chandler JB Jr. Whipple's disease, successful response to sulfamethoxazole-trimethoprim. Am J Gastroenterol. 1981;75: 309–14.

173. Deremee RA, McDonald TJ, Weiland LH. Wegener's granulomatosis: Observations on treatment with antimicrobial agents. Mayo Clin Proc. 1985;60: 27–32.

174. Valeriano-Marcet J, Spiera H. Treatment of Wegener's granulomatosis with sulfamethoxazole-trimethoprim. Arch Intern Med. 1991;151:1649–52.

175. Geddes AM, Ball AP, Farrell ID. Co-trimoxazole for the treatment of serious infections. J Antimicrob Chemother. 1979;5(Suppl B):221–30.

176. Quintiliani R, Levitz RE, Nightingale CH. Potential role of trimethoprim-sulfamethoxazole in the treatment of serious hospital-acquired infections. Rev Infect Dis. 1987;9:S160–5.

177. Sattler FR, Remington JS. Intravenous sulfamethoxazole and trimethoprim for serious gram-negative bacillary infection. Arch Intern Med. 1983;143: 1709–12.

178. Menichetti F, Del Favero A, Guerciolini R, et al. Empiric antimicrobial therapy in febrile granulocytopenic patients. Randomized prospective comparison of amikacin plus piperacillin with and without parenteral trimethoprim sulphamethoxazole. Infection. 1986;14:261–7.

179. Young LS, Hindler J. Use of trimethoprim-sulfamethoxazole singly and in combination with other antibiotics in immunocompromised patients. Rev Infect Dis. 1987;9:S177–81.

180. Engervall PA, Stiernstedt GT, Gunther GC, et al. Trimethoprim-sulfamethoxazole plus amikacin as first-line therapy and imipenem/cilastatin as second empirical therapy in febrile neutropenic patients with hematological disorders. J Chemother. 1992;4:99–106.

181. Levitz RE, Quintilliani R. Trimethoprim-sulfamethoxazole for bacterial meningitis. Ann Intern Med. 1984;100:881–90.

182. Markowitz N, Quinn EL, Saravolatz LD. Trimethoprim-sulfamethoxazole compared with vancomycin for the treatment of *Staphylococcus aureus* infection. Ann Intern Med. 1992;117:390–8.

183. Wallace RJ, Wissk, Bushby MB, et al. In vitro activity of trimethoprim and sulfamethoxazole against nontuberculosis mycobacteria. Rev Infect Dis. 1982;4:326–31.

184. Freerksen E, Alvarenga AE, Legguizamo O, et al. A new short-term combination therapy of leprosy. Chemotherapy. 1991;37:353–63.

185. Gellin BG, Soave R. Coccidian infections in AIDS. Toxoplasmosis, cryptosporidiosis, and isosporiasis. Med Clin North Am. 1992;76:205–34.

186. Israelski DM, Remington JS. Toxoplasmic encephalitis in patients with AIDS. In: Moellering RC Jr, ed. Infectious Disease Clinics of North America (Medical Management of AIDS). Philadelphia: WB Saunders; 1988:429–45.

187. Canessa A, DelBono V, De Leo P, et al. Cotrimoxazole therapy of *Toxoplasma gondii* encephalitis in AIDS patients. Eur J Clin Microbiol Infect Dis. 1992;11:125–30.

188. Carr A, Tindall B, Brew BJ, et al. Low dose trimethoprim sulfamethoxazole prophylaxis for toxoplasmic encephalitis in patients with AIDS. Ann Intern Med. 1992;117:106–11.

189. Sattler FR, Remington JS. Intravenous trimethoprim-sulfamethoxazole therapy for *Pneumocystis carinii* pneumonia. Am J Med. 1981;70:1215–21.

190. Young LS. Trimethoprim-sulfamethoxazole in the treatment of adults with pneumonia due to *Pneumocystis carinii*. Rev Infect Dis. 1982;4:608–13.

191. Kovacs JA, Masur H. Prophylaxis for *Pneumocystis carinii* pneumonia in patients infected with human immunodeficiency virus. Clin Infect Dis. 1992; 14:1005–9.

192. Davey RT, Masur H. Recent advances in the diagnosis, treatment, and prevention of *Pneumocystis carinii* pneumonia. Antimicrob Agents Chemother. 1990;34:499–504.

193. Sattler FR, Feinberg J. New developments in the treatment of *Pneumocystis carinii* pneumonia. Chest. 1992;101:451–7.

194. Wharton JM, Coleman DL, Wofsy CB, et al. Trimethoprim-sulfamethoxazole or pentamidine for *Pneumocystis carinii* pneumonia in the acquired immunodeficiency syndrome. Ann Intern Med. 1985;105:37–44.

195. Klein NC, Duncanson FP, Lenox TH, et al. Trimethoprim-sulfamethoxazole versus pentamidine for *Pneumocystis carinii* pneumonia in AIDS patients: Results of a large prospective randomized treatment trial. AIDS. 1992;6: 301–5.

196. Carr A, Swanson C, Penny R, et al. Clinical and laboratory markers of hypersensitivity to trimethoprim-sulfamethoxazole in patients with *Pneumocystis carinii* pneumonia and AIDS. J Infect Dis. 1993;167:180–5.

197. Sattler FR, Cowan R, Nielsen DM. Trimethoprim-sulfamethoxazole compared with pentamidine for treatment of *Pneumocystis carinii* pneumonia in acquired immunodeficiency syndrome: Prospective, noncrossover study. Ann Intern Med. 1988;109:280–7.

198. Hughes WT, Smith BL. Intermittent chemoprophylaxis for *Pneumocystis carinii* pneumonia. Antimicrob Agents Chemother. 1983;24:300–5.
199. Fischl MA, Dickinson GM. Trimethoprim-sulfamethoxazole prophylaxis of *Pneumocystis carinii* pneumonia in acquired immunodeficiency syndrome (Abstract 436). In: Program and Abstracts of the 25th Interscience Conference on Antimicrobial Agents and Chemotherapy. Washington, DC: American Society for Microbiology; 1985:230.
200. Anonymous. Recommendations for prophylaxis against *Pneumocystis carinii* pneumonia for adults and adolescents infected with human immunodeficiency virus. MMWR. 1992;41:1–11.
201. Martin MA, Cox PH, Beck K, et al. A comparison of the effectiveness of three regimens in the prevention of *Pneumocystis carinii* pneumonia in human immunodeficiency virus-infected patients. Arch Intern Med. 1992; 152:523–8.
202. Hardy WD, Feinberg J, Finkelstein DM, et al. A controlled trial of trimethoprim-sulfamethoxazole or aerosolized pentamidine for secondary prophylaxis of *Pneumocystis carinii* pneumonia in patients with the acquired immunodeficiency syndrome. AIDS Clinical Trials Group Protocol 021. N Engl J Med. 1992;327:1842–8.
203. Schneider MM, Hoepelman IM, Eeftininck Schattenkerk JK, et al. A controlled trial of aerosolized pentamidine or trimethoprim-sulfamethoxazole as primary prophylaxis against *Pneumocystis carinii* pneumonia in patients with human immunodeficiency virus infection. The Dtuch AIDS Treatment Group. N Engl J Med. 1992;327:1836–41.
204. Chaisson RE, Keruly J, Richman DD, et al. *Pneumocystis* prophylaxis and survival in paients with advanced human immunodeficiency virus infection treated with zidovudine. The Zidovudine Epidemiology Group. Arch Intern Med. 1992;152:2009–13.
205. Gurwith M, Brunton J, Lank B, et al. A prospective controlled investigation of prophylactic trimethoprim/sulfamethoxazole in hospitalized granulocytopenic patients. Am J Med. 1979;66:248–56
206. Kauffman CA, Liepman MA, Bergman AG, et al. Trimethoprim/sulfamethoxazole prophylaxis in neutropenic patients: Reduction of infections and effect on bacterial and fungal flora. Am J Med. 1983;74:599–607.
207. Gualtieri RJ, Donowitz GR, Kaiser DC, et al. Double-blind randomized study of prophylactic trimethoprim/sulfamethoxazole in granulocytopenic patients with hematologic malignancies. Am J Med. 1983;74:934–40.
208. EORTC International Antimicrobial Therapy Project Group. Trimethoprim-sulfamethoxazole in the prevention of infection in neutropenic patients. J Infect Dis. 1984;150:372–9.
209. Donnelly JP, Masschmeyer G, Daenen S. Selective oral antimicrobial prophylaxis for the prevention of infection in acute leukaemia-ciprofloxacin versus co-trimoxazole plus colistin. The EORTC-Gnotobiotic Project Group. Eur J Cancer. 1992;28A:873–8.
210. Guiot HF, van der Meer JW, van den Broek PJ, et al. Prevention of viridans-group streptococcal septicemia in oncohematologic patients: A controlled comparative study on the effect of penicillin G and cotrimoxazole. Ann Hematol. 1992;64:260–5.
211. Wade JC, Schimpff SC, Hargadon MT, et al. A comparison of trimethoprim-sulfamethoxazole plus nystatin with gentamicin plus nystatin in the prevention of infections in acute leukemia. N Engl J Med. 1981;304:1057–62.
212. Wade JC, de Jongh CA, Newman KA, et al. Selective antimicrobial modulations as prophylaxis against infection during granulocytopenia: Trimethoprim-sulfamethoxazole vs. nalidixic acid. J Infect Dis. 1983;147:624–34.
213. Margolis DM, Melnick DA, Alling DW, Gallin JI. Trimethoprim-sulfamethoxazole prophylaxis in the management of chronic granulomatous disease. J Infect Dis. 1990;162:723–6.
214. Overturf GD. Use of trimethoprim-sulfamethoxazole in pediatric infections: Relative merits of intravenous administration. Rev Infect Dis. 1987;9: S168–73.

27. QUINOLONES

DAVID C. HOOPER

The first member of the quinolone class of antimicrobial agents, nalidixic acid, is a 1,8-naphthyridine structure that was identified by Lesher and associates in 1962 among the byproducts of chloroquine synthesis. Oxolinic acid and cinoxacin were also developed in the 1970s, but it was the identification in the 1980s of the fluorine- and piperazinyl-substituted derivatives with substantially greater potency and expanded spectrum that began a resurgence in development and a rapid and steady expansion of this class of compounds. A broad spectrum of activity, good

oral absorption, and overall good tolerability have resulted in extensive clinical use of the newer fluoroquinolones.

CHEMICAL STRUCTURES

All current quinolone derivatives in clinical use have a dual ring structure with a nitrogen at position 1, a carbonyl group at position 4, and a carboxyl group attached to the carbon at the 3 position of the first ring (Fig. 1). Several different dual ring structures have been developed (Fig. 2). Quinolones themselves have a carbon at position 8 in the second ring, and naphthyridines contain a nitrogen at position 8. Compounds based on other ring structures such as the cinnoline (nitrogens at positions 1 and 2) and pyridopyrimidine (nitrogens at positions 1, 6, and 8) rings have had fewer derivatives in clinical use in the United States. Derivatives with any of these ring structures, however, are commonly referred to as *quinolones,* and, for simplicity, the numbering of the positions in the ring will follow the convention used for the quinolone ring.

Nalidixic acid is a 1,8-naphthyridine with 1-ethyl and 7-methyl substituents (Fig. 1). Oxolinic acid (quinolone ring) (Fig. 1) and cinoxacin (cinnoline ring) (not shown in Fig. 1) also have 1-ethyl substituents, as well as a dioxolo ring bridging positions 6 and 7. Potency is greatly improved by the addition of a fluorine at position 6, and potency against gram-negative bacteria is further enhanced by the addition of a piperazinyl (norfloxacin, enoxacin, ciprofloxacin), methyl-piperazinyl (pefloxacin, ofloxacin, amifloxacin, lomefloxacin, fleroxacin, temafloxacin), or dimethyl-piperazinyl (sparfloxacin) substituent at position 7. Methyl substituents on the piperazine ring generally result in improved oral bioavailability. These structural features are common to most of the newer quinolone derivatives now in clinical use. Pyrrolidinyl substituents at position 7 (tosufloxacin, clinafloxacin) enhance activity against gram-positive bacteria. Many newer compounds retain the 1-ethyl substituent found in nalidixic acid or contain a similar structure (fleroxacin, 1-fluoroethyl; amifloxacin, 1-methylamino). Notable exceptions are the 1-cyclopropyl group of ciprofloxacin and sparfloxacin, which further enhances potency, the additional ring structure bridging positions 1 and 8 of ofloxacin, and the 1-difluorophenyl group of temafloxacin and tosufloxacin. In sparfloxacin, an amino group replaces the hydrogen found at position 5 in other quinolones.

More recently, quinolones have been chemically linked to cephalosporins. Desacetylcefotaxime has been attached to the 3-carboxyl group of fleroxacin (Ro 23-9424)[1] and ciprofloxacin (Ro 24-6392)[2] by an ester linkage and to the piperazine group of ciprofloxacin by tertiary amino (Ro 24-8138) and carbamate (Ro 24-4383)[2] linkages. The intact ester-linked molecules appear to function as cephalosporins, but spontaneous or β-lactamase–enhanced cleavage of the ester resulted in release of active quinolone. The more stable intact amino- and carbamate-linked derivatives, however, appear to have activities characteristic of both component classes of compounds, and activity was further enhanced in a β-lactamase–producing strain, which may enhance release of the quinolone moiety.[2]

More extensive discussion of the structure–activity relationships of the quinolone class is beyond the scope of this chapter. The reader is referred to recent reviews of this subject.[3,4]

MECHANISM OF ACTION

The quinolones rapidly inhibit bacterial DNA synthesis, an event that is followed by rapid bacterial cell death. The molecular events that underly these actions are understood in part, but key details remain to be defined.[5]

Quinolones inhibit the enzymatic activities of bacterial DNA gyrase and promote the cleavage of DNA within the enzyme–DNA complex. DNA gyrase is an essential bacterial enzyme composed of two A and two B subunits, products of *gyr* A and *gyr* B genes, respectively. DNA gyrase catalyzes the

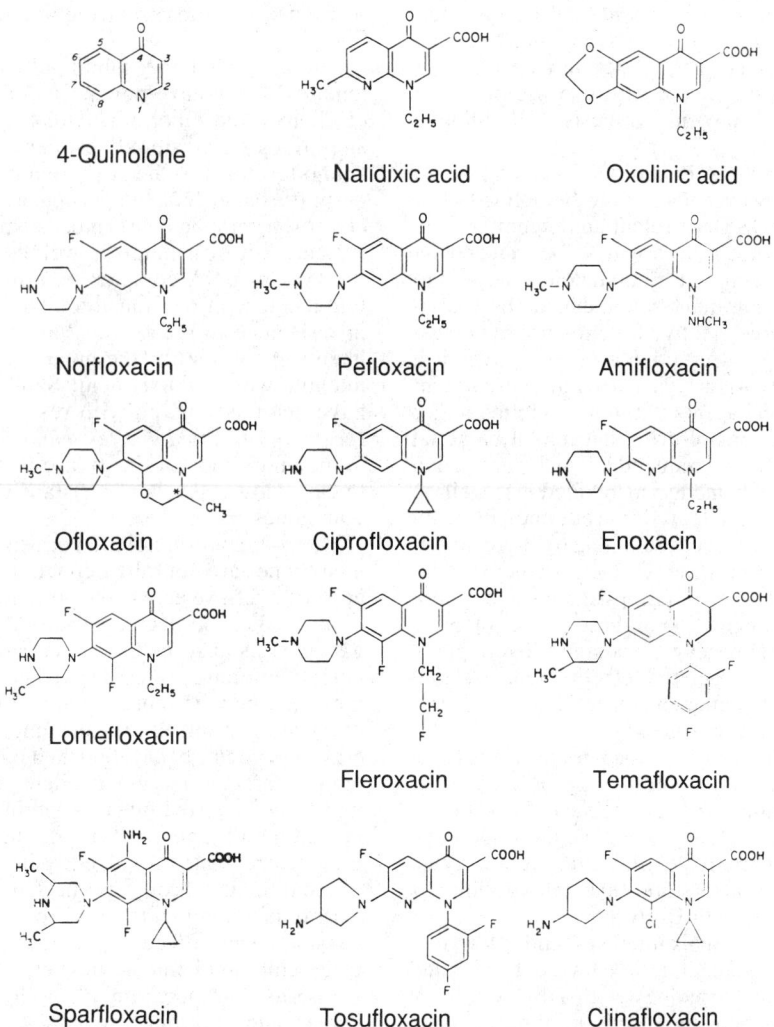

FIG. 1. Quinolone ring structure and numbering and structures of selected quinolones in clinical use or under development.

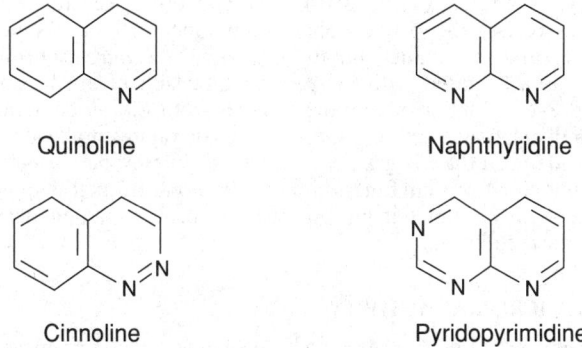

FIG. 2. Dual ring structures that constitute different members of the quinolone class.

introduction of negative superhelical twists into closed covalently circular chromosomal and plasmid DNA within the bacterial cell. The superhelical state of intracellular DNA is regulated by the actions of DNA gyrase and other enzymes of the same class that are called *topoisomerases*. DNA superhelicity affects the initiation of DNA replication and transcription of many genes. DNA gyrase also appears to be involved in the resolution of interlocked (catenated) newly replicated daughter chromosomes. All of these activities result from the enzyme's coordinated breaking of both strands of duplex DNA, passage of an-

other segment of DNA through the break, and resealing of the break.[6]

Quinolones appear to function by trapping or stabilizing the enzyme–DNA complex after strand breakage and before resealing of DNA. This trapped complex appears to function as a cellular poison possibly by generating a DNA break that the cell is unable to repair. Quinolones have been shown to bind specifically to the complex of DNA gyrase and DNA rather than to DNA gyrase alone.[7] The importance of the interaction of quinolones with the gyrase–DNA complex for the antibacterial activities of the quinolones is supported by the strong correlation of quinolone potency in inhibiting DNA gyrase and in inhibiting bacterial growth and by the identification of *gyr A* and *gyr B* bacterial mutants that are resistant to quinolones and produce gyrase–DNA complexes with reduced quinolone binding (see section on mechanisms of resistance).[8] Quinolones also inhibit in vitro the activities of another newly discovered topoisomerase, topoisomerase IV, which has structural similarities to DNA gyrase.[9] It is not yet known, however, whether quinolone interactions with this enzyme within the bacterial cell contribute to antibacterial activity.

Quinolone inhibition of bacterial DNA replication and bacterial killing may be dissociated under some conditions, suggesting that events in addition to the initial interaction of quinolones with the gyrase–DNA complex may be required for cell killing. In particular, inhibitors of RNA and protein synthesis reduce the bactericidal activity of some quinolones but do not affect their ability to inhibit bacterial DNA synthesis.[10] Thus, inhibition of bacterial DNA synthesis per se is not sufficient to account for bacterial killing, and possibly newly synthesized gene products may also be necessary. This effect may account for the observations that at high concentrations of quinolones, which also secondarily inhibit protein synthesis, cell killing is reduced.

The nature of the gene products (in addition to DNA gyrase) that contribute to killing, however, has yet to be defined. The gene products in the RecA-SOS DNA repair and recombination system, the expression of which is known to be induced by the damage to bacterial DNA caused by quinolones, appear to function at least in part to repair quinolone-induced DNA damage, because *rec* mutants with defective function are hypersusceptible to quinolone killing.[11] Certain *hip* mutants exhibit a *hi*gher fraction of *p*ersisters or surviving cells after treatment with bactericidal antimicrobial agents without exhibiting major differences in the concentrations of drug that inhibit bacterial growth. *hip* A mutants selected for reduced killing by ampicillin have alterations in the cell wall and are also killed less well by quinolones, and *hip* Q mutants selected for reduced killing by quinolones also exhibit selective reduced killing by β-lactams.[12] The nature of the *hip* A and *hip* Q gene products are not known, but the overlap in reduced killing by both β-lactams and quinolones suggests that after the interaction of these classes of drugs with their different targets there may be common overlapping pathways that are necessary for bacterial lethality. One possibility, as yet unproved, is that induction of cell autolysins is necessary for killing by both classes of drugs.

Differences among quinolones in the magnitude of bacterial killing in the presence of rifampin (an inhibitor of RNA synthesis), phosphate-buffered saline, and anaerobiasis have led to the suggestions that some quinolones may have more than one mechanism of killing,[13] but the molecular events underlying these phenomena are not yet understood, except that killing is dependent on drug interaction with DNA gyrase.

Eukaryotic cells also contain topoisomerases, and eukaryotic topoisomerase II, which is a homodimeric enzyme, has limited primary amino acid sequence homology with DNA gyrase.[14] Current antibacterial quinolones have only minimal activity against mammalian topoisomerase II,[15] but other recently investigated quinolone structures (containing a 7-hydroxyphenyl substituent or an isothiazolo ring bridging positions 2 and 3) have been shown to have substantially enhanced potency against the mammalian enzyme and are under consideration as potential antitumor agents.[16,17]

MECHANISMS OF ACQUIRED BACTERIAL RESISTANCE

Bacteria acquire resistance to quinolones by spontaneously occurring mutations in chromosomal genes that either alter the target enzyme DNA gyrase or alter drug permeation across the bacterial cell membranes.[18] As yet, no quinolone-degrading or quinolone-inactivating enzymes have been identified, and, although plasmid-mediated resistance has been constructed in the laboratory, no clinical isolates with plasmid-mediated quinolone resistance have been proved.

Resistant chromosomal mutants may be selected in the laboratory by plating bacteria on drug-containing agar. The frequency of occurrence of spontaneous mutants differs with the selecting drug concentration and the drug. For gram-negative bacteria selected with the newer fluoroquinolones, frequencies range, in general, from 10^{-6} or higher at two-fold above the minimum inhibitory concentration (MIC) to undetectable ($<10^{-10}$) at 16–32-fold above the MIC. With a similar selection with nalidixic acid, mutants are detected more frequently. This difference results in part from the ability of certain mutations to confer higher levels of resistance to nalidixic acid than to other quinolones. Serial passage of bacteria on increasing concentrations of quinolones selects mutants with high levels of resistance resulting from the additive effects of several mutations.[19]

Alterations in the A subunit of DNA gyrase that cause quinolone resistance have now been defined in a substantial number of clinical and laboratory isolates of *Escherichia coli*. These alterations are clustered between amino acids 67 and 106 in the amino terminus of the A protein near the active site of the enzyme (tyrosine-122).[6] In particular, changes in serine-83 (to leucine or tryptophan) are most common and cause the largest increment in resistance as well as reduced binding of drug to the gyrase–DNA complex in vitro.[8] Leucine-83 causes a 128-fold increase in resistance to nalidixic acid but lesser increases in resistance to the newer fluoroquinolones (16–32-fold), thus likely accounting for the greater ease of selection of resistant mutants with nalidixic acid. Similar changes in the A subunit have been associated with resistance in *Staphylococcus aureus*[20] and *Campylobacter jejuni*.[21] Single amino acid changes in the midportion of the gyrase B protein have also been found to cause lower levels of resistance to nalidixic acid and fluoroquinolones.[22]

The routes of quinolone permeation across the bacterial cell membranes are not fully defined, but the hydrophilic congeners appear to diffuse across the gram-negative bacterial outer membrane through porin channels. In *E. coli* and *Pseudomonas aeruginosa* resistance mutations in genes that affect expression of outer membrane proteins have been described.[23–25] Resistance, however, may be more complex than reduced diffusion alone, because the reduced drug accumulation in some mutants is energy dependent, being abolished by agents that collapse proton-motive force. Energy-dependent saturable norfloxacin uptake into *E. coli* everted inner membrane vesicles, which have a reversed membrane orientation, suggests that carrier-mediated drug efflux is also involved, possibly acting together with reduced diffusion through porin channels.[26] Resistance associated with reduced amounts of porin outer membrane proteins may be pleiotropic with additional low levels of resistance to tetracycline, chloramphenicol, and some β-lactams.[18]

Information indicating a role for enhanced quinolone efflux in resistance is stronger in *S. aureus,* which lacks an outer membrane. The *S. aureus nor*A gene appears to encode a hydrophobic membrane protein with 12 membrane-spanning segments and with similarities to other drug transport proteins such as TetA, the tetracycline efflux transporter.[27] Cloned *nor*A causes resistance to hydrophilic quinolones in *E. coli* and *S. aureus,* and a resistance mutation *flq*B on the *S. aureus* chromosome is associated with increased expression of *nor*A. Energized everted inner membrane vesicles from *E. coli* containing cloned *nor*A also exhibit saturable norfloxacin uptake that is dependent on the pH gradient across the membrane,[28] suggesting that NorA protein functions as a quinolone efflux transporter energetically coupled in antiport with the proton gradient across the cell membrane.

ANTIMICROBIAL ACTIVITY

Current quinolones are most active against aerobic gram-negative bacilli, particularly members of the family Enterobacteriaceae and *Haemophilus* spp., and against gram-negative cocci such as *Neisseria* spp. and *Moraxella (Branhamella) catarrhalis* (Table 1).[29,30] Relative to nalidixic acid, the fluoroquinolones also have additional activity against gram-negative bacilli such as *P. aeruginosa* (Table 1) and against staphylococci (Table 2). Ciprofloxacin remains the most potent marketed fluoroquinolone against gram-negative bacteria. For norfloxacin, ciprofloxacin, ofloxacin, lomefloxacin, and enoxacin, activity against streptococci and many anaerobes is limited (Tables 2, 3). Some newer agents not yet released in the United States (sparfloxacin, tosufloxacin, clinafloxacin, Bay y 3118, and others), however, have greater potency against these organisms. For the fluoroquinolones that are used for treatment of infections outside the

TABLE 1. Activity of Selected Quinolones Against Selected Gram-Negative, Mycoplasmal, and Chlamydial Pathogens In Vitro

Organism	Nalidixic Acid	Representative MIC₉₀s (range) (μg/ml)[a]							
		Ciprofloxacin	Norfloxacin	Enoxacin	Ofloxacin	Pefloxacin	Lomefloxacin	Fleroxacin	Sparfloxacin
Acinetobacter spp.	32–256	0.25–2 (0.25–>128)	(8–64)	1–2	0.25–1 (0.25–>128)	(1–8)	4	0.5–4 (0.5–32)	0.06–1 (0.06–16)
Aeromonas spp.	0.5	≤0.06 (≤0.06–0.25)	0.03	0.06	0.03–0.5 (0.03–1)	0.03	0.12	0.12–0.25 (0.12–1)	≤0.12 (≤0.12–1)
Campylobacter jejuni	8	(0.12–0.78)	(0.25–2)	(1–32)	(0.12–2)	0.5	(0.125–1)	0.5	0.12–0.25
Chlamydia pneumoniae	—	1–2	—	—	1	—	4	2	0.5
Chlamydia trachomatis	—	1–3.1	≥16	6.3	0.5–1.6	—	2–3.1	(1.5–6.3)	0.06
Citrobacter spp.	8	0.12 (≤0.03–6.25)	0.5 (≤0.25–50)	0.5 (0.25–1.56)	0.5 (0.1–25)	0.4–1	0.5 (0.12–25)	0.12 (≤.06–25)	0.5 (0.6–2)
Enterobacter aerogenes	8	0.06 (≤0.03–0.25)	0.5 (0.2–2)	0.25	0.25 (0.12–1)	0.25	0.5 (≤0.25–1)	0.12–0.25	0.12 (0.12–0.5)
Enterobacter cloacae	8	0.12 (≤0.03–0.5)	0.5 (<0.25–2)	0.5 (0.1–1)	0.25 (0.1–1)	0.5	0.5 (≤0.25–1)	0.25	0.25 (0.12–0.5)
Escherichia coli	4	≤0.06 (≤0.01–0.25)	0.12 (0.01–0.5)	0.25 (0.03–2)	0.12 (0.02–1)	0.12–0.25	0.2 (0.06–1.0)	0.1 (0.03–2)	≤0.06 (≤0.03–0.1)
Haemophilus influenzae	1	(≤0.008–≤0.06)	0.06	0.12	(≤0.06–0.5)	0.06	≤0.06–0.12	(≤0.06–1)	≤0.06
Klebsiella spp.	8–16	0.12 (0.02–1)	0.5 (0.2–2)	1 (0.5–2)	0.25 (0.12–1)	2 (0.5–2)	1 (0.2–6.25)	0.5 (0.12–6.25)	0.12 (≤0.03–1)
Legionella spp.	1	≤0.12	(0.2–2)	0.2	≤0.06	—	≤0.06	≤0.06	≤0.06
Moraxella catarrhalis	2	(≤0.03–0.25)	0.4	0.06	(0.06–0.5)	0.25	(≤0.1–1)	(0.25–2)	(0.01–0.12)
Morganella morganii	8	0.06 (0.01–6.25)	0.12 (≤0.06–25)	0.5 (≤0.12–1.56)	0.25 (0.1–12.5)	(0.25–4)	0.25 (0.25–12.5)	0.12 (<0.06–12.5)	0.5 (0.25–1)
Mycoplasma hominis	>256	0.5–2	8–16	8	1–2	4	2	2	≤0.06
Mycoplasma pneumoniae	—	(1–8)	12	8	(0.78–2)	4	4–8	4	(0.1–0.25)
Neisseria gonorrheae	1	0.01	0.06	0.25	0.06	0.06	0.12	0.2	≤0.06
Neisseria meningitidis	0.5	(0.008–0.12)	0.03	0.03	(≤0.06–0.4)	0.03	(≤0.06–0.42)	(≤0.03–0.25)	≤0.06
Proteus mirabilis	8	0.06 (≤0.03–0.39)	0.1 (0.12–0.5)	0.5 (0.25–1.56)	0.5 (0.12–1)	0.25	0.5–1	0.5 (≤0.12–0.5)	0.5 (0.25–1)
Proteus vulgaris	8	0.06 (0.01–0.25)	0.1 (0.12–0.5)	0.5 (0.25–2)	0.25 (0.06–0.5)	0.25	0.5 (0.25–1)	0.12 (≤0.12–0.25)	0.5–1
Providencia rettgeri	16	1.0(0.03–2)	2 (0.25–3.1)	1 (0.5–6.25)	1 (0.5–8)	0.5	4 (1.6–6.2)	0.5 (0.12–1)	0.5 (0.25–2)
Providencia stuartii	32	0.5 (0.125–2)	2 (≤0.25–2)	1–2	1 (1–8)	(4)	1 (1–4)	1 (0.5–2)	0.5 (0.2–2)
Pseudomonas aeruginosa	16	0.5 (0.25–8)	2 (2–16)	4 (3–32)	2 (2–>50)	2.0	4 (4–>50)	2 (2–>50)	2 (1.6–8)
Pseudomonas cepacia	16	2 (0.5–16)	8 (8–50)	25 (16–25)	3.1 (3–32)	—	16 (16)	4 (4–16)	1.0 (1.0)
Salmonella spp.	2–4	≤0.06	≤0.06 (≤0.06–0.25)	0.12–0.25	0.12–0.25	0.12	0.25	≤0.12–0.25	≤0.06
Serratia marcescens	≥100	0.25 (0.06–12.5)	1 (≤0.25–50)	2 (1–25)	1 (0.5–25)	1 (1–8)	2 (0.25–25)	0.5 (0.25–25)	1 (0.12–12.5)
Shigella spp.	8	≤0.03	≤0.06–0.12	8 (3–16)	(0.06–0.78)	0.25	8 (8–>25)	≤0.125	≤0.06
Xanthomonas maltophilia	16	2 (2–25)	4 (4–>64)	8	3.1 (3–>25)	4.0	(≤0.06–0.25)	3 (3–25)	(0.5–>2)
Yersinia enterocolitica	8	≤0.06	≤0.12	0.12–0.25	(0.06–0.25)	0.25	(≤0.06–0.25)	(≤0.06–2)	≤0.06

[a] MIC₉₀, minimal inhibitory concentration for 90 percent of strains.

(Data from Eliopoulos and Eliopoulos[29] and Wolfson and Hooper.[30])

TABLE 2. Activity of Selected Quinolones Against Selected Gram-Positive Bacteria In Vitro

Organism	Nalidixic Acid	Ciprofloxacin	Norfloxacin	Enoxacin	Ofloxacin	Pefloxacin	Lomefloxacin	Fleroxacin	Sparfloxacin
					Representative MIC$_{90}$s (range) (μg/ml)[a]				
Staphylococcus aureus	100	0.5 (0.25–2)	2 (1–4)	2 (2–4)	0.5 (0.1–2)	0.5 (0.1–2)	2 (0.5–4)	1 (0.125–4)	0.12 (0.006–0.25)
Coagulase-negative staphylococci	100	0.5 (≤0.1–>2)	2 (0.5–>4)	2 (0.5–4)	1 (0.25–2)	1 (0.5–4)	2 (0.5–4)	1 (0.5–8)	0.12 (0.03–>4)
Streptococcus pneumoniae	>128	2 (0.78–6.2)	16 (4–>16)	16 (8–16)	2 (1–8)	12 (8–16)	8 (4–16)	8 (8–25)	0.5 (0.25–1)
Streptococcus pyogenes	>100	1 (0.5–4)	4 (2–16)	>8	2 (1–4)	8 (8–16)	8 (4–12.5)	8 (4–12.5)	1 (0.5–2)
Streptococcus agalactiae	>128	2 (0.5–4)	16 (4–16)	>8	2 (2–4)	32	16 (8–32)	8 (≥8)	0.5 (0.5–2)
Streptococcus bovis	—	4 (1–4)	>8	>8	4 (2–4)	—	—	>8	—
Streptococcus spp.	>64	2 (0.5–4)	16 (4–32)	32 (8–32)	4 (1–6.2)	>12.5	8 (4–16)	4–8	1 (0.25–1)
Enterococcus faecalis	>64	2 (0.5–4)	8 (4–32)	8 (8–16)	4 (2–6.2)	4–8	8 (4–16)	8 (8–>16)	1 (0.25–1)
Enterococcus faecium	>64	4 (2–8)	≥12.5	32	6.2 (2–16)	—	8	8	1 (0.5–4)
Listeria monocytogenes	>64	2 (0.5–2)	8 (4–16)	8–16	2–4	6–8	6.2–8	8 (4–>16)	2 (1–4)
Corynebacterium spp.	—	1 (0.05–128)	4 (4–>128)	8 (4–>128)	1 (0.5–64)	8 (8–>128)	>12.5	2 (1–32)	0.25 (0.25–64)
Bacillus spp.	—	0.25 (0.12–1)	1 (1)	1 (0.5–1)	0.5 (0.5)	—	—	0.5–1	0.25
Nocardia spp.	>128	(1.4–>25)	64	32	(2.6–>25)	64	—	64	—

[a] MIC$_{90}$, minimal inhibitory concentration for 90 percent of strains.
(Data from Eliopoulos and Eliopoulos[29] and Wolfson and Hooper.[30])

TABLE 3. Activity of Selected Quinolones Against Selected Anaerobic Bacteria and Mycobacteria In Vitro

Organism	Nalidixic Acid	Ciprofloxacin	Norfloxacin	Enoxacin	Ofloxacin	Pefloxacin	Lomefloxacin	Fleroxacin	Sparfloxacin
					Representative MIC$_{90}$ (range) (μg/ml)[a]				
Bacteroides fragilis	512	4–128	>128	32	2–12.5	16	8–64	≥16	1–2
Bacteroides spp.	512	1–32	128	16	2–32	—	8–32	2–64	4
Fusobacterium spp.	256	2–8	16	32	2–16	32	16	16	—
Clostridium spp.	256	1–16	2	32	1–8	1	16	2–32	4
Clostridium perfringens	64	0.5–8	8	16	0.5–8	8	2–8	1–4	0.5–2
Clostridium difficile	>128	8–25	128	128	12.5–16	64	≥32	16–32	6.25
Anaerobic gram-positive cocci	256–512	2–6.25	16–64	2–8	2–8	16	4–25	8–12.5	1–4
Mycobacterium tuberculosis	—	1	8	>5	0.8–1.3	8	4	≤0.5	0.2
Mycobacterium avium complex	—	16	≥16	>256	10–100	>64	—	16	12.5
Mycobacterium chelonae	—	8	>16	—	>20	>64	—	>32	6.25–>100
Mycobacterium fortuitum	—	0.3	2	—	1–3.1	2	—	≤0.5	1.56
Mycobacterium kansasii	—	1	8	≥5	1–3.1	4	—	≤0.5	—

[a] MIC$_{90}$, minimal inhibitory concentrations for 90 percent of strains.
(Data from Eliopoulos and Eliopoulos,[29] Wolfson and Hooper,[30] and Leysen et al.[31])

urinary tract, the MIC listed in Table 1 should be interpreted in relation to peak drug concentrations in serum that range from 1.5 to 5.8 μg/ml (with usual dosing) and in relation to concentrations in urine that are manifold higher (see section on pharmacology). For highly susceptible organisms, MIC may be 10–30-fold below achievable serum concentrations.

Fluoroquinolones also have activity against mycobacteria (Table 3).[31] Ciprofloxacin, ofloxacin, and sparfloxacin are active against *Mycobacterium tuberculosis*, *M. fortuitum*, *M. kansasii*, and some strains of *M. chelonae* but have only fair or poor activity against *M. avium-intracellulare*. Ofloxacin and pefloxacin have activity against *M. leprae* in animal models.

Other bacteria are also inhibited by quinolones in vitro (Table 1). Ofloxacin and ciprofloxacin have activity against the agents of atypical pneumonias, including *Legionella pneumophila*, *Mycoplasma pneumoniae*, and *Chlamydia pneumoniae*, and against genital pathogens such as *Chlamydia trachomatis*, *Ureaplasma urealyticum*, and *Mycoplasma hominis*. *Treponema pallidum* is resistant to ofloxacin in animal models.

Activity in vitro is reduced in the presence of urine but generally not in the presence serum. Activity is also reduced at pH values below 7 and in the presence of magnesium concentrations at 8–16 mM. Both of these factors often contribute to the reduced quinolone activity observed in the presence of urine. Low pH and elevated concentrations of magnesium are associated with reduced drug accumulation in *E. coli*.[23]

Minimal bactericidal concentrations of quinolones are usually within two- to fourfold of MIC, and the magnitude of bacterial killing increases with further increases in drug concentration, reaching a maximum at about 30-fold above the MIC. Above this maximal killing concentration, paradoxical reductions in killing are observed and are associated with additional inhibition of protein synthesis by high concentrations of quinolones.[13]

The postantibiotic effect (PAE) is the period of time required for bacteria surviving a brief exposure to an antimicrobial agent to resume growth. Although this parameter may be relevant in estimating the proper interval for drug dosing, its clinical importance, which may be greatest in patients with compromised host defenses, has not been proved. For quinolones, the duration of PAE has been in the range of 1–2 hours and tends to increase with increasing drug concentrations and length of drug exposure.

Combinations of quinolones with other antimicrobial agents have been extensively studied, and interactions with β-lactams and aminoglycosides as measured by fractional inhibitory or bactericidal concentrations or time-kill curve studies have generally been found to be indifferent or additive.[30,32] Synergistic interactions were found in a minority of strains, although for *P. aeruginosa* in some studies synergy with ciprofloxacin in combination with imipenem or azlocillin were seen in a substantial minority, 30–50 percent of strains. Antagonistic interactions of quinolones with other antimicrobial agents have been rare. Rifampin reduced the bactericidal activity of ciprofloxacin and pefloxacin against *S. aureus* in some studies.[33]

PHARMACOLOGY

Absorption

The quinolones are well absorbed from the upper gastrointestinal tract, with bioavailability exceeding 50 percent for all com-

TABLE 4. Pharmacokinetics of Selected Quinolones

Quinolone	Dose (mg)	C_{max} (µg/ml)	Half-life (h)	Bioavailability (%)	V_D (liters)	Cl_r (ml/min)	Renal Excretion[a] (%)
Norfloxacin	400 po	1.5	3.3	(50)	—	234	27
Ciprofloxacin	500 po	2.5	3.2	70	358	358	29
	200 iv	3.2	3.7	—	147	300	—
Ofloxacin	400 po	4.0	5.0	>95	102	195	73
	200 iv	3.2	4.9	—	102	190	—
Pefloxacin	400 po	3.2	10.5	>95	112	13	11[b]
	400 iv	5.8	11.0	—	134	20	—
Enoxacin	400 po	2.3	4.9	88	175	193	44
Lomefloxacin	400 po	3.5	7.8	>95	133	189	66
Fleroxacin	400 po	4.3	11.2	92	97	53	50[c]

Abbreviations: C_{max}: maximum serum concentration; V_D: volume of distribution; Cl_r: renal clearance; po, by mouth; iv, intravenous.
[a] Cumulative percentage of dose in urine after 24 hours.
[b] After 84 hours.
[c] After 72 hours.

(Data from refs. 30, 34–36, 138–140.)

TABLE 5. Body Tissues, Fluids, and Cells in Which Quinolone Concentrations Exceed Quinolone Concentrations in Serum

Site	Fold Increment
Urine	25->100
Kidney	2–10
Prostate tissue	0.9–2.3
Feces	100–1000
Bile	2–20
Lung tissue	1.6–4
Macrophages and neutrophils	2–14

pounds and approaching 100 percent for several (Table 4).[34–37] Peak concentrations in serum are usually attained within 1–3 hours of administering a dose. Food does not substantially reduce quinolone absorption but may delay the time to reach peak drug concentrations in serum.[38,39] Absorption is good when ciprofloxacin is given by nasogastric tube with or without enteral feedings[40] but may be decreased when given by jejunostomy tube.[41]

Peak fluoroquinolone concentrations in serum after a 400-mg dose range from 1.5 µg/ml for norfloxacin to 5.8 µg/ml for pefloxacin. A 1-g dose of nalidixic acid produces concentrations of 20–50 µg/ml of serum. Drug binding to serum proteins is generally low, around 15–30 percent.

Distribution in Tissues

The volumes of distribution of quinolones are high and in most cases exceed the volume of total body water (Table 4), indicating accumulation in some tissues. Concentrations in urine, kidney tissue, prostate tissue, stool, bile, lung, and neutrophils and macrophages usually exceed serum concentrations (Table 5). Concentrations of quinolones in saliva, prostatic fluid, bone, and cerebrospinal fluid are usually lower than drug concentrations in serum.

Penetration into ascitic fluid in patients with liver failure has been found for pefloxacin (72 percent of serum concentration) and ofloxacin (120 percent).[42] Penetration into human breast milk has also been documented for ciprofloxacin, ofloxacin, and pefloxacin.[43]

Elimination

The terminal half-lives of elimination from serum range from 3 hours for norfloxacin and ciprofloxacin to 11 hours for fleroxacin, allowing twice- or once-daily dosing (Table 6). The principle routes of elimination differ among quinolones. Cinoxacin, ofloxacin, and lomefloxacin are eliminated predominantly by the kidneys; and nalidixic acid and pefloxacin are eliminated predominantly by nonrenal pathways. Most other quinolones have substantial excretion by both renal and nonrenal routes.

Renal clearance of norfloxacin, ciprofloxacin, ofloxacin, enoxacin, and lomefloxacin exceeds glomerular filtration rates (GFR), indicating net tubular secretion. In support of tubular secretion, renal clearance of norfloxacin and ciprofloxacin is reduced by probenecid, but drug accumulation did not occur. In contrast, the renal clearance of pefloxacin and fleroxacin is below or equal to GFR, suggesting not tubular reabsorption.[44]

Hepatic metabolism accounts for the majority of the elimination of pefloxacin and nalidixic acid. In these cases, however, active metabolites contribute to antibacterial effects. The desmethylpiperazinyl derivative of pefloxacin is norfloxacin, and hydroxynalidixic acid is more active than its parent compound. These metabolites and inactive glucuronide conjugates to the 3-carboxyl group are excreted in the urine. Conversion of norfloxacin, ciprofloxacin, enoxacin, and fleroxacin to less active metabolites accounts for 10–20 percent of elimination. There is minimal hepatic biotransformation (<10 percent) of ofloxacin and lomefloxacin. In addition to glucuronide conjugates and desmethylpiperazinyl derivatives, other metabolites of quinolones that have been identified have had predominantly alterations of the piperazine ring, including N-oxide, N-sulfo, N-formyl, and desethylene derivatives.[35,44,45]

Transintestinal secretion has been identified after intravenous administration of ciprofloxacin and accounts for about 15 percent of drug excretion.[35]

Dosage Adjustments in Renal and Hepatic Insufficiency

As expected from differences in the routes of excretion, increases in drug half-life in the presence of severe renal insufficiency are greatest for ofloxacin (four- to fivefold) and least for pefloxacin (no change), with other quinolones exhibiting intermediate effects (about twofold) (Table 6). To prevent excessive drug accumulation, dosage reduction (increase in the dose interval from 12 to 24 hours or halving the daily dose for those quinolones normally given once daily) is indicated at creatinine clearances below 50 ml/min for ofloxacin and below 30 ml/min for norfloxacin, enoxacin, and lomefloxacin. No dosage reduction is indicated for nalidixic acid and pefloxacin. Clearance by hemodialysis is low (≤14 percent of plasma clearance) for norfloxacin, ciprofloxacin, ofloxacin, and enoxacin and is slightly greater (28 percent) for pefloxacin. Similarly, peritoneal dialysis contributes little to the clearance of ciprofloxacin and ofloxacin.[46]

Fewer data are available on the effects of hepatic insufficiency on quinolone half-lives. For pefloxacin but not norfloxacin, ciprofloxacin, and ofloxacin, substantial increases (threefold) in half-life were seen in some patients with cirrhosis, but there was substantial variation.[42] Changes in renal function that accompany severe liver disease may, however, affect ciprofloxacin

TABLE 6. Dosage of Quinolones in Patients with Normal and Reduced Renal Function

Quinolone	Normal Renal Function		Renal Failure with GFR (ml/min)		Removal by Dialysis
	Oral	Intravenous	10–50	<10	
Nalidixic acid	500–1000 mg q6h	—	No change	No change	
Cinoxacin	250 mg q6h	—	1× dose q12h	1× dose q24h	
Norfloxacin	400 mg q12h	—	1× dose q24h	1× dose q24h	No (H, P)
Ciprofloxacin	250–750 mg q12h	200–400 mg q12h	1× dose q18h	1× dose q24h	No (H, P)
Ofloxacin	200–400 mg q12h	200–400 mg q12h	1× dose q24h	½× dose q24h	No (H, P)
Pefloxacin	400 mg q12h	400 mg q12h	No change	No change	No (H)
Enoxacin	200–400 mg q12h	—	½× dose q12h	½× dose q24h	No (H)
Lomefloxacin	400 mg q24h	—	½× dose q24h	½× dose q24h	No (H)

Abbreviations: GFR, glomerular filtration rate; H: hemodialysis; P: peritoneal dialysis; 1×: 100%; ½×: 50%.

and ofloxacin elimination to a lesser extent. Specific parameters of liver function that predict effects on pefloxacin clearance have not yet been defined, but in patients with severe liver disease use of quinolones other than pefloxacin or reduction of pefloxacin dose (possibly a twofold increase in dose interval) with monitoring of levels of drug in serum may be indicated.

Interactions with Other Drugs

When coadministered by mouth with aluminum-, magnesium-, or, to a lesser extent, calcium-containing antacids, quinolones have markedly reduced bioavailability, presumably because of the formation of cation–quinolone complexes that are poorly absorbed.[47] Sucralfate, which contains large amounts of aluminum ions, similarly reduces absorption of quinolones. Although staggering of doses of antacids and quinolones may reduce this interaction, there is sufficient variability to suggest that this maneuver may not be fully reliable in an individual patient. Because the histamine receptor antagonists cimetidine and ranitidine may delay absorption, but do not affect the completeness of quinolone absorption, they may be considered as preferred alternatives to antacids and sucralfate in patients receiving oral quinolones who need reductions in gastric acidity. Concurrent administration of quinolones with $FeSO_4$, multivitamin-mineral regimens containing zinc, and the buffered formulation of dideoxyinosine has also been reported to reduce quinolone absorption.[48] Nutritional supplements given by nasogastric tube may reduce the absorption of quinolones given concurrently by the same route, likely because these supplements also contain multivalent cations such as iron and zinc.

For intravenous formulations of ciprofloxacin and pefloxacin, precipitates have been reported when these quinolones were infused through the same intravenous tubing with aminophylline, amoxicillin with and without clavulanate, or floxacillin. Separate infusions are indicated.

Quinolones vary in the extent to which they impair the elimination of the methylxanthines theophylline and caffeine. The effects appear to result from inhibition by some quinolones of hepatic microsomal enzymes involved in theophylline and caffeine metabolism, but it is not yet clear which parts of the quinolone molecules or which metabolites are responsible for inhibition of the microsomal P-450 isozymes involved in methylxanthine metabolism. Enoxacin exhibits the greatest effect and may produce two- to threefold increases in theophylline concentrations in serum associated with a 40–65 percent reduction in total theophylline clearance without alterations in renal clearance of theophylline.[47] An intermediate effect has been reported for ciprofloxacin (30 percent reduction in clearance and 20–90 percent increases in serum concentrations of theophylline) and pefloxacin (30 percent reduction in clearance), but norfloxacin, ofloxacin, fleroxacin, and lomefloxacin had little or no effect (2–11 percent increases in serum concentrations of theophylline).[49] In patients receiving enoxacin or ciprofloxacin in combination with theophylline, serum levels of theophylline should be monitored and reductions in the dose of theophylline

considered. No such adjustments should be needed in patients receiving theophylline concurrently with norfloxacin, ofloxacin, fleroxacin, or lomefloxacin.

Nonsteroidal anti-inflammatory drugs (NSAIDs) may affect the central nervous system stimulant effects of quinolones. Seizures were reported in a group of Japanese patients receiving enoxacin and the NSAID fenbufen. Potentiation of seizures by combinations of quinolones and NSAIDs has also been reported in animals. Assays of the displacement of the inhibitory neurotransmitter γ-aminobutyric acid (GABA) or a related molecule from GABA receptors in rat brain tissue have demonstrated displacement of GABA by quinolones and enhancement of this displacement by fenbufen and by theophylline. It is not clear the extent to which concurrent use of quinolones with other NSAIDs will result in central nervous system toxicities, but patients receiving both classes of drugs should be cautioned about and monitored for these potential adverse effects.

Interactions with other drugs have been studied less extensively. Rifampin appears not to affect the pharmacokinetics of ciprofloxacin. Ciprofloxacin and pefloxacin appear to have little effect on the pharmacokinetics of cyclosporin in some but not all studies. Although probenecid reduces the renal clearance of norfloxacin and fleroxacin, no quinolone accumulation occurred. The effect of probenecid might be predicted to be greater with quinolones such as ofloxacin and lomefloxacin for which renal clearance includes tubular secretion and is the predominant mode of clearance, but data are lacking. Enoxacin has been shown to reduce the clearance of the less active R-enantiomer of warfarin, but had no effect on the more active S-enantiomer.

CLINICAL USES

Earlier quinolones such as nalidixic acid, oxolinic acid, and cinoxacin were used almost exclusively for treatment of urinary tract infections, although nalidixic acid was also used for treatment of shigellosis. With the development of the more potent fluoroquinolones, a broader array of infections can now be treated with members of the fluoroquinolone class.

Urinary Tract Infections

Although the low pH and magnesium concentrations present in urine may reduce quinolone activity, the concentrations of most quinolones in urine are usually sufficient to provide substantial therapeutic ratios of urinary drug concentration to the MIC of most urinary pathogens.

For uncomplicated urinary tract infections, usually in symptomatic young women with cystitis caused by highly susceptible organisms such as *E. coli,* most quinolones are likely to be highly effective when given for brief courses of 3–10 days,[50] and norfloxacin, ciprofloxacin, and ofloxacin have been found to be comparable to trimethoprim-sulfamethoxazole.[51] Usually the lowest dose in the dosage range (Table 6) is sufficient for treatment of these infections. Three-day regimens of norfloxacin and lomefloxacin result in cure rates of 81–96 percent.[52] Limited data on single-dose therapies with ciprofloxacin, ofloxacin, and norfloxacin indicate eradication in 75–96 percent of patients.[53,54] Single-dose norfloxacin (800 mg) was equivalent to a 3-day regimen for *E. coli* infections,[55] but for *Staphylococcus saprophyticus* infections a 7-day regimen is preferred because of failures with shorter courses.[56] Women with uncomplicated pyelonephritis given norfloxacin or ofloxacin for 7–10 days have bacteriologic cure rates comparable to those with trimethoprim-sulfamethoxazole. For prophylaxis of recurrent infections norfloxacin (200 mg qhs) was highly effective and superior to nitrofurantoin.[57]

Complicated urinary tract infections occurring in men and in patients with catheters or structural or functional abnormalities of the urinary tract are often caused by more resistant pathogens and have a higher frequency of relapse and reinfection. Bacteriologic cure rates for ciprofloxacin were superior to those for trimethoprim-sulfamethoxazole and for aminoglycosides shortly after completion of a 7–10 day course, but the low fractions of patients who continued to have sterile urine were similar by 4–6 weeks after therapy.[51,58] In collected noncomparative trials, infections caused by *P. aeruginosa* were eradicated in 70 percent of patients given ciprofloxacin and 83 percent given norfloxacin. Development of bacterial resistance has been associated with therapeutic failure in about 2 percent of patients overall, but resistance rates (10–20 percent) may be higher for *P. aeruginosa* infections.

Prostatitis

Fluoroquinolones concentrate in prostatic tissue with lower levels in prostatic fluid. In one small comparative study of men with predominantly *E. coli* infections, norfloxacin given for 4–6 weeks was superior (92 percent eradication) to trimethoprim-sulfamethoxazole (67 percent eradication) at 1 month follow-up.[59] In open studies, similar courses of norfloxacin, ciprofloxacin, and ofloxacin have produced eradication rates of 67–91 percent at follow-up ranging from 1 to 13 months. With 2-week courses of therapy and infections caused by less susceptible organisms such as *P. aeruginosa* and enterococci, failures appear to be more frequent.[51,60]

Sexually Transmitted Diseases

Quinolones have activity in vitro against the major sexually transmitted pathogens, *N. gonorrhoeae, C. trachomatis,* and *Haemophilus ducreyi,* but appear to lack activity against *T. pallidum.*

Uncomplicated gonococcal urethritis and cervicitis are effectively eradicated by single doses of quinolones (norfloxacin, 800 mg; ciprofloxacin, 250 mg; ofloxacin, 400 mg; fleroxacin, 400 mg.[61] Rectal and pharyngeal infections have also been cured in 99 and 88 percent of patients, respectively. Small numbers of patients with gonococcal salpingitis have been cured with 10–14 day courses of sequential intravenous and oral ciprofloxacin or oral ofloxacin.[62,63]

Single doses of quinolones are ineffective for genital chlamydial infections.[61] Seven-day courses of therapy with norfloxacin and ciprofloxacin have also had unacceptably low response rates, but a similar course of ofloxacin was comparable to doxycycline for treatment of chlamydial infections and nongonococcal urethritis.[64–66] There are only limited data on use of ofloxacin for treatment of patients with chlamydial salpingitis.[63]

In patients with chancroid, *H. ducreyi* was eradicated from genital ulcers by ciprofloxacin, 500 mg bid × 3 days, and enoxacin, 400 mg bid × 3 doses, in 93 percent, a result comparable to that with trimethoprim-sulfamethoxazole.[67,68]

Studies of the use of quinolones for treatment of pelvic inflammatory disease have been few. Gonococcal infections appear to respond, but data on chlamydial and mixed infections that include anaerobic bacteria (likely to be resistant to current quin-

olones in vitro) are too few to allow conclusions. Two cases of gonococcal septic arthritis have responded to ciprofloxacin. Data on treatment of syphilis with quinolones in humans are inadequate, but in animal models ofloxacin has failed.

Gastrointestinal and Abdominal Infections

All bacterial pathogens known to cause gastroenteritis are generally susceptible to quinolones in vitro. Although fecal material may decrease the activity of quinolones, drug concentrations in feces are exceedingly high. The penetration of quinolones into macrophages (Table 5) may also be important for their effectiveness in systemic *Salmonella* infections.

Bacterial gastroenteritis is often a self-limited disease, but in a number of circumstances quinolones have been shown to shorten the duration of diarrhea and to eradicate pathogens from stools. In travelers' diarrhea, which is often caused by enterotoxigenic *E. coli* and *Shigella* spp., norfloxacin, 400 mg bid × 3 days, and ciprofloxacin, 500 mg bid × 5 days, begun shortly after the onset of diarrhea have shortened the duration of loose stools by 1–3 days relative to placebo and have been comparable to trimethoprim-sulfamethoxazole.[69,70] When given as prophylaxis to travelers, quinolones have produced protection rates that ranged from 68 to 92 percent compared with placebo controls, although routine use of quinolones or other antimicrobials is not recommended for prevention of diarrhea in travelers.[71]

In patients with shigellosis, 5-day courses of norfloxacin, ciprofloxacin, and ofloxacin have been highly effective. Addition of loperamide to ciprofloxacin may further shorten the duration of diarrhea.[72] Even a single dose of ciprofloxacin, 750 mg, may be effective in shigellosis, except those cases caused by *Shigella dysenteriae* type 1.[73] In patients with *Salmonella* and *C. jejuni* infections, symptoms may be shortened with ciprofloxacin or norfloxacin, but therapy has been complicated by prolongation or relapse of stool carriage of *Salmonella*[74,75] and by clinical relapse with development of resistant *C. jejuni.*[76,77] Norfloxacin was superior to trimethoprim-sulfamethoxazole and placebo in shortening diarrhea in patients with cholera.[78] In patients with diarrhea caused by *Yersinia enterocolitica, Plesiomonas shigelloides,* and *Aeromonas* spp., quinolones have eradicated the organisms from stool, but have not yet been clearly shown to shorten clinical illness.[51]

In noncomparative studies of patients with enteric fever caused predominantly by *Salmonella typhi,* ciprofloxacin cured 92 percent of patients, and ofloxacin cured 96 percent of patients, with resolution of fever within 5 days.[79,80] Relapses have been reported in some patients with AIDS and bacteremic non-typhoidal *Salmonella* infections. Chronic fecal carriage of *Salmonella typhi* has been eradicated in 83–93 percent of small numbers of patients, including a few with gallstones, given norfloxacin, ciprofloxacin, or ofloxacin for 4 weeks.[81,82]

Although active against *Helicobacter pylori* in vitro, quinolones have failed to eradicate this organism from gastric mucosa, and failures have been associated with acquisition of quinolone resistance.[51] Data are quite limited on use of quinolones for treatment of biliary tract infections. In a single small study, 83 percent of patients with cholecystitis and cholangitis, most associated with *E. coli* bacteremia, responded to intravenous and then oral ciprofloxacin.[86]

Use of quinolones in peritonitis has been evaluated most in patients undergoing chronic ambulatory peritoneal dialysis (CAPD) and in patients with cirrhosis. Oral ofloxacin, 300 mg qd, and ciprofloxacin, 500 mg qd, have cured episodes of peritonitis in CAPD patients, but failures in infections caused by the common coagulase-negative staphylococci have occurred. Higher concentrations of ciprofloxacin have been achieved by adding drug to the dialysate (20–50 μg/ml) with outcomes similar to those with standard regimens of intraperitoneal vancomycin plus gentamicin.[87] In patients with cirrhosis at high risk for recurrent spontaneous bacterial peritonitis, norfloxacin, 400 mg qd, given as prophylaxis reduced recurrences by threefold.[88] The potential risks of selecting resistant enteric bacteria, however, must also be considered before embarking on prolonged use in prophylaxis.

Respiratory Tract Infections

A range of respiratory tract pathogens is susceptible to a number of quinolones in vitro. *Haemophilus influenzae*, *Moraxella catarrhalis*, and enteric gram-negative bacilli are highly susceptible. Ciprofloxacin and ofloxacin also have activity against the agents of atypical pneumonias, *Mycoplasma pneumoniae*, *C. pneumoniae*, and *L. pneumophila*, and against *S. aureus* and *Mycobacterium tuberculosis*. Least susceptible among common pathogens is *S. pneumoniae*.

Patients with acute bacterial bronchitis and acute exacerbations of chronic bronchitis have been evaluated most often in noncomparative studies. Ciprofloxacin, ofloxacin, enoxacin, pefloxacin, lomefloxacin, and fleroxacin have all been effective in eradicating *H. influenzae* from sputum.[30,89,90] In most studies, eradication rates for *S. pneumoniae* and *P. aeruginosa* were lower, and some failures have been associated with the development of bacterial resistance. In comparative trials, clinical responses have usually been similar to or better than those with ampicillin, amoxicillin, and cefaclor.

In patients with community-acquired pneumonias, ciprofloxacin and ofloxacin have consistently eradicated *H. influenzae* and *Moraxella catarrhalis*.[30] Among atypical pneumonias, small numbers of patients with pneumonias caused by *Legionella*,[83,84] *Mycoplasma*,[30] and *C. pneumoniae*[85] have also responded to ciprofloxacin and ofloxacin, but there are no studies comparing treatment with erythromycin or other macrolides. Cures of pneumococcal pneumonias, including a few cases with bacteremia, have been reported with intravenous and then oral ciprofloxacin[91] and ofloxacin[92] and with oral ofloxacin alone,[93] but failures with both drugs have occurred, and pneumococcal bacteremia has developed during ciprofloxacin therapy of pneumonia.[51] There remains concern about the reliability of coverage for serious pneumococcal infections with currently available quinolones. Similarly, quinolones are not considered adequate coverage for aspiration pneumonia in which oral streptococci and anaerobes predominate or for acute sinusitis and otitis media in which pneumococci are frequent pathogens.

Hospital-acquired pneumonias, which are commonly caused by gram-negative bacilli, have responded to intravenous ciprofloxacin[51,94] and ofloxacin,[92] and responses to ciprofloxacin correlated with the level of susceptibility of the infecting organism, with better bacteriologic responses in infections caused by *Haemophilus* spp. and members of the Enterobacteriaceae than in infections caused by the less susceptible *P. aeruginosa*. Similar correlations were seen in patients treated with intravenous pefloxacin.[30] Combination therapy and use of maximum approved doses of ciprofloxacin, 750 mg po or 400 mg iv q12h, may be preferred in patients with *P. aeruginosa* infection. For seriously ill patients, intravenous doses of 400 mg ciprofloxacin every 8 hours are under investigation.[95]

Mild to moderate respiratory exacerbations in patients with cystic fibrosis and *P. aeruginosa* in sputum respond clinically to oral ciprofloxacin, 750 mg bid, and ofloxacin, 400 mg bid, similarly to conventional parenteral therapies that use an antipseudomonal β-lactam and tobramycin.[51] In patients with more severe exacerbations, however, conventional parenteral combination therapy may be superior. Rarely is *P. aeruginosa* eliminated from sputum by any regimen in patients with cystic fibrosis. Rotating the use of different regimens may reduce the selective pressure for persistence of resistant bacteria that may emerge with either type of regimen.

Invasive otitis externa in diabetics is usually caused by *P. aeruginosa* and may respond to oral ciprofloxacin, 750 mg bid,

given for 6 weeks.[51] No studies comparing quinolones with conventional parenteral therapies have been reported.

Bone and Joint Infections

The prolonged antimicrobial therapy usually employed for bone and joint infections is facilitated by effective oral agents, and quinolones may fill this role in some cases.[96] For treatment of chronic osteomyelitis, there have been noncomparative trials using ciprofloxacin, ofloxacin, or pefloxacin in which treatment was usually for 6 or more weeks and follow-up was for at least 6 months after completion of therapy.[30,51] Clinical cures after oral ciprofloxacin, 750 mg bid, were 75 percent overall in infections in which gram-negative bacilli predominanted, and similar rates of cure were reported in the smaller subgroups of patients with *P. aeruginosa* and methicillin-susceptible *S. aureus* (MSSA) infections. Failures were associated with incomplete débridement, the presence of foreign bodies, and the development of resistance in *P. aeruginosa*, *S. aureus*, and *Serratia marcescens*. Three months of treatment with ciprofloxacin produced a cure rate of 60 percent in one study of osteomyelitis in the feet of diabetics.[102]

In four small comparative trials, ciprofloxacin, 750 mg bid, and ofloxacin, 400 mg bid, have generally produced apparent rates of cure similar to those of conventional parenteral therapies using β-lactams with or without an aminoglycoside,[51,97] but the power of these studies to detect differences between the regimens has been small. For ofloxacin, cures of MSSA infections were 80 percent (10 of 12), but cures of *P. aeruginosa* infections were only 25 percent (1 of 4).[97]

There are few data on treatment of septic arthritis with quinolones, most often with ciprofloxacin or ofloxacin[30] and recently fleroxacin.[98] Infections caused by *N. gonorrhoeae* and *E. coli* have responded to oral therapy. Failures have been seen in infections of prosthetic joints and infections caused by *S. aureus* and *P. aeruginosa* infections.

Skin and Soft Tissue Infections

Although the most common causes of cellulitis and pyodermas are streptococci and *S. aureus*, in patients with diabetes and peripheral vascular disease, decubitus ulcers, and some surgical wound infections, soft tissues may become infected with a mixture of bacteria that includes, in addition to streptococci and staphylococci, aerobic gram-negative bacteria and anaerobes. Quinolones have been evaluated as treatment for skin and soft tissue infections in some of these subgroups of patients.[99]

Comparisons of oral ciprofloxacin, 750 mg bid,[100] and ofloxacin, 400 mg bid,[101] with intravenous cefotaxime given for 9 days to patients with mixed infections in which gram-negative bacilli predominated showed similar rates of clinical and bacteriologic efficacy (80–90 percent) in both cases. In these and noncomparative studies[30] failures have been seen with infections caused by *P. aeruginosa* (11 percent), streptococci (6 percent), and *S. aureus* (5 percent) and have been associated with the development of resistant organisms, which for *P. aeruginosa* may be more frequent in diabetic patients.[99] In diabetic foot infections without osteomyelitis, the overall rate for complete healing using ciprofloxacin alone was 50 percent.[102] Use of additional antimicrobial agents with activity against anaerobes should be considered in these patients. Recent studies have shown similar rates of clinical and bacteriologic response to oral fleroxacin, 400 mg qd, and amoxicillin-clavulanate in patients in whom staphylococcal infections with skin abscesses and ulcers and impetigo predominated.[103]

For patients with uncomplicated cellulitis or pyodermas in whom staphylococci and streptococci are the most likely pathogens, conventional therapies with penicillin, semisynthetic penicillins, and cephalosporins, either oral or parenteral, remain the therapy of choice. For infections with methicillin-resistant *S.*

aureus (MRSA) for which the quinolones were initially hoped to be valuable oral therapies, rapid emergence of quinolone resistance has become a particular problem, and resistance is now highly prevalent in some medical centers.[104] Thus, vancomycin remains the therapy of choice for MRSA infections.

Other Uses

There are limited data on the use of quinolones for treatment of mycobacterial infections. In patients with multidrug-resistant pulmonary tuberculosis, ofloxacin, 300 or 800 mg qd, has been used in combination with other second-line agents with sputum conversions and apparent clinical cures,[105] but in cases in which ofloxacin was the only active drug, there was failure of sputum conversion and development of ofloxacin resistance.[105,106] For nontuberculous mycobacteria, ciprofloxacin, 750 mg bid or 500 mg tid, has been used in three-drug (with clarithromycin plus amikacin[107] and four-drug (with rifampin, ethambutol, and clofazimine[108]) regimens in patients with AIDS and *Myobacterium avium-intracellulare* complex bacteremia; improvement in symptoms occurred with both regimens, but clearance of bacteremia appeared better with the clarithromycin-containing three-drug regimen. In cutaneous *Mycobacterium fortuitum* infections, ciprofloxacin used alone was followed by relapse and the development of drug resistance,[51] but ofloxacin has been used successfully in some sternotomy infections caused by *M. fortuitum*.[109] Preliminary studies have also documented bactericidal activity in vivo and clinical improvement in patients with lepromatous leprosy given ofloxacin, 400 mg qd, and pefloxacin, 800 mg qd.[110]

For patients with bacteremias, intravenous ciprofloxacin and ofloxacin have been effective in cases caused by enteric gram-negative bacilli, although responses have been poor for *P. aeruginosa* bacteremias when these drugs were used in relatively low doses of 200 mg bid.[111,112] In neutropenic patients with fever, ciprofloxacin in combination with aminoglycosides produced defervescence and cure of documented infections comparably to standard β-lactam–aminoglycoside combinations,[113] but ciprofloxacin monotherapy was less effective than such combinations[114] and probably should not be used. Although lower doses were used in some studies, in patients with normal renal function doses no less than 400 mg ciprofloxacin bid would be preferred.[95] Use of quinolones in this setting should be cautious and should be considered principally as an alternative regimen when there are reasons for not choosing standard regimens with combinations of β-lactams and aminoglycosides.

Oral ciprofloxacin, 500 mg bid, ofloxacin, 300 mg bid, and norfloxacin, 400 mg bid, given as prophylaxis in neutropenic patients have consistently reduced the occurrence of gram-negative bacteremia and in some cases prolonged the time to first fever, but breakthrough gram-positive bacteremias have occurred.[51] Ciprofloxacin appears superior to norfloxacin for this use.[115]

There is limited experience in using quinolones for treatment of endocarditis. One study has reported good responses in intravenous drug abusers with right-sided *S. aureus* (methicillin-susceptible) endocarditis who complied with the full course of ciprofloxacin, 300 mg iv bid × 1 week, then 750 mg po bid × 3 weeks, plus rifampin, 300 mg po bid × 4 weeks.[116] Drug resistance, however, has occurred in this setting, and there have been failures in patients with left-sided *S. aureus* endocarditis. There have been a number of single case reports of patients with gram-negative bacillary endocarditis whose infections have been suppressed with oral quinolones, but there have been failures. Use of quinolones for endocarditis should currently be limited to circumstances in which established therapies are not possible.

Quinolones vary in their penetration across the blood–brain barrier into cerebrospinal fluid (CSF). In the presence of meningeal inflammation, concentrations in CSF have reached 40, 90,

and 60 percent of serum concentrations for ciprofloxacin, ofloxacin, and pefloxacin, respectively. In two small studies of patients with predominantly gram-negative bacillary meningitis, pefloxacin, 800 mg iv q12h, cured 12 of 16 neurosurgical patients, many of whom had failed to respond to β-lactam therapies,[117] and ciprofloxacin, 200 mg iv q12h, cured 18 of 20 similar patients.[118] Use of these quinolones for treatment of meningitis should only be considered in those circumstances in which standard therapies are not possible or have failed. For eradication of nasopharyngeal carriage of *N. meningitidis*, which is indicated in the setting of close contact with patients with meningococcal meningitis, ciprofloxacin given as a single dose (750 mg) has been highly effective.[119]

Quinolones have been used for treatment of a variety of other infections in small numbers of patients. A few patients with tularemia have responded to ciprofloxacin,[120] and several patients with cat scratch disease improved more rapidly after ciprofloxacin treatment than might be expected without treatment.[121] Patients with Mediterranean spotted fever caused by *Rickettsia conorii* and Q fever caused by *Coxiella burnetii* may respond to ciprofloxacin or ofloxacin, but doxycycline remains the preferred therapy.[122] Attempts to treat patients with brucellosis with quinolones have been complicated by a high frequency of relapses,[123] and patients with falciparum malaria have had inconsistent responses.[124,125]

PROBLEMS WITH RESISTANCE DURING CLINICAL USE

Development of bacterial resistance among pathogens during clinical use of quinolones is predicted to occur more often in settings in which there are large numbers of bacteria at the site of infection and the therapeutic index at this site is below 8,[126] because spontaneous chromosomal resistance mutations causing resistance increments of four- to eightfold for fluoroquinolones may occur at a frequencies of 10^{-8} to 10^{-10}. Therapeutic indices below 8 are more likely in infections caused by less susceptible pathogens such as *P. aeruginosa* and *S. aureus* and at sites of infection at which drug delivery or host eradication mechanisms may be compromised and in patients who receive inadequate drug doses.

General surveys of resistance patterns occurring over time have found resistance to increase following the introduction of fluoroquinolones and to occur most often with *Pseudomonas* spp. and staphylococci and in soft tissue infections and infections associated with foreign bodies.[127,128] In some medical centers ciprofloxacin resistance has increased markedly (to over 80 percent) among MRSA strains. Resistance appears to have been selected in patients colonized with MRSA and given ciprofloxacin for other infections and to have spread within the hospital environment to patients never receiving ciprofloxacin.[129] Possibly reflecting the selective pressures of extensive use, increasing fluoroquinolone resistance has also been noted among strains of *Campylobacter jejuni* in the Netherlands, Finland, and Spain (from 0 to 30 percent)[130] and, surprisingly, even among uropathogenic *E. coli* in Spain (from 0 to 4 percent).[131] Resistance should be monitored, and strategies for minimizing its occurrence, including focused quinolone use, should be considered to avoid compromising the utility of the fluoroquinolones.

ADVERSE EFFECTS

The tolerability of the fluoroquinolones is best assessed in double-blind randomized trials in which the effects of patient populations, methods of ascertainment, and possible bias can be controlled. In a recent analysis of 56 such trials in which fluoroquinolones were compared with placebo or other antimicrobial agents, most studies found similar adverse effect profiles.[132] In six studies, there were significantly fewer adverse events with fluoroquinolones relative to the comparison agent (ciprofloxacin vs. trimethoprim-sulfamethoxazole and ampicillin; norfloxacin vs. trimethoprim-sulfamethoxazole and cefadroxil; ofloxacin vs. erythromycin). Conversely, adverse events were more frequent with the fluoroquinolone in seven studies (ciprofloxacin vs. doxycycline; norfloxacin vs. placebo; temafloxacin vs. cefadroxil; fleroxacin vs. amoxicillin and placebo). In a number of instances increasing doses and durations of therapy were associated with higher rates of adverse effects.

The most frequent category of adverse effect involves the gastrointestinal tract, occurring in 3–13 percent of patients reported in clinical trials. In most patients anorexia, nausea, vomiting, and abdominal discomfort when they occur are mild. Diarrhea is less frequent, and antibiotic-associated colitis has been rare, possibly because most current quinolones have little or no effect on the anaerobic bowel flora.

The next most frequent category of adverse effects involves the central nervous system, occurring in 0.9–7.4 percent of patients. Symptoms of mild headache and dizziness have predominated followed by insomnia and alterations in mood. Hallucinations, delirium, and seizures are rare. Seizures may have resulted in some circumstances from theophylline accumulation or from the ability of theophylline and NSAIDs to augment the ability of quinolones to displace GABA from its receptors.

Allergic and skin reactions have occurred in 0.4–2.2 percent of patients in clinical trials. Unspecified rashes have been most frequent. Phototoxicity reactions also occur in some patients after exposure to UVA (320–400 nm) light and may be more frequent with lomefloxacin, pefloxacin, and fleroxacin.[133–135] Drug fever, urticaria, angioedema, vasculitis, serum sickness-like syndromes, and anaphylactoid reactions have been uncommon. Acute interstitial nephritis likely allergic in origin also occurs infrequently and has been associated with eosinophiluria but generally not crystalluria. Infiltrates of lymphocytes and eosinophils has been found in the renal interstitium on renal biopsies.

Arthropathy with cartilage erosions and noninflammatory effusions occurs in the weight-bearing joints of juvenile animals given quinolones. Experience with use of quinolones in children has been limited, but children receiving nalidixic acid, norfloxacin, and ciprofloxacin have only uncommonly had joint symptoms, which have been reversible.[136] In cystic fibrosis patients given pefloxacin, however, arthralgia and joint swelling developed in 14 percent.[137] Tendonitis has been reported only rarely in adults given norfloxacin, ofloxacin, and pefloxacin. There have as yet been no studies with long-term follow-up of adults given quinolones when they were children. Because of concerns about cartilage toxicity in children, quinolones are not recommended for routine pediatric use, but in some patients, such as those with cystic fibrosis, the benefit of quinolones may outweigh what is probably a relatively small short-term risk of joint toxicity.

Leukopenia and eosinophilia generally occur in less than 1 percent of patients, and mild elevations in serum transaminases occur in less than 1–3 percent of patients receiving quinolones; these abnormalities are rarely of sufficient severity to require cessation of therapy.

Several months after the release of temafloxacin for clinical use in the United States, the U.S. Food and Drug Administration (FDA) through its postmarketing surveillance mechanism received reports of hemolytic anemia in patients given temafloxacin. Subsequent investigations identified patients receiving temafloxacin who developed hemolysis, renal failure, and thrombocytopenia with or without disseminated intravascular coagulation, with an estimated reporting incidence of 1 in 5000 prescriptions (reported at an open meeting of the FDA Anti-Infective Drugs Advisory Committee on 10 July 1992). These occurrences led the manufacturer to remove temafloxacin from the market. In patients given other quinolones, hemolytic anemia, occasionally associated with renal failure, coagulation abnormalities, or both have been reported to the FDA, but the reporting incidence was far lower than that with temafloxacin. The mechanisms of these rare but severe toxic effects are not yet known.

Safety in pregnancy has not been established for any of the quinolones. Because quinolones are excreted in breast milk, they should not be given to nursing mothers.

REFERENCES

1. Jones RN, Barry AL, Thornsberry C. Antimicrobial activity of Ro 23-9424, a novel ester-linked codrug of fleroxacin and desacetylcefotaxime. Antimicrob Agents Chemother. 1989;33:944–50.
2. Georgopapadakou NH, Bertasso A. Mechanisms of action of cephalosporin 3′-quinolone esters, carbamates, and tertiary amines in *Escherichia coli*. Antimicrob Agents Chemother. 1993;37:559–65.
3. Mitscher LM, Davasthale P, Zavod R. Structure–activity relationships. In: Hooper DC, Wolfson JS, eds. Quinolone Antimicrobial Agents. 2nd ed. Washington, DC: American Society for Microbiology; 1993:3–52.
4. Asahina Y, Ishizaki T, Suzue S. Recent advances in structure activity relationships in new quinolones. Prog Drug Res. 1992;38:57–106.
5. Hooper DC, Wolfson JS. Mechanisms of quinolone action and bacterial killing. In: Hooper DC, Wolfson JS, eds. Quinolone Antimicrobial Agents. 2nd ed. Washington, DC: American Society for Microbiology; 1993:53–76.
6. Reece RJ, Maxwell A. DNA gyrase: Structure and function. Crit Rev Biochem Mol Biol. 1991;26:335–75.
7. Shen LL, Kohlbrenner WE, Weigl D, et al. Mechanism of quinolone inhibition of DNA gyrase. Appearance of unique norfloxacin binding sites in enzyme–DNA complexes. J Biol Chem. 1989;264:2973–8.
8. Willmott CJR, Maxwell A. A single point mutation in the DNA gyrase A protein greatly reduces binding of fluoroquinolones to the gyrase–DNA complex. Antimicrob Agents Chemother. 1993;37:126–7.
9. Kato J-I, Suzuki H, Ikeda H. Purification and characterization of DNA topoisomerase IV in *Escherichia coli*. J Biol Chem. 1992;267:25676–84.
10. Dietz WH, Cook TM, Goss WA. Mechanism of action of nalidixic acid on *Escherichia coli*. III. Conditions required for lethality. J Bacteriol. 1966;91:768–73.
11. McDaniel LS, Rogers LH, Hill WE. Survival of recombination-deficient mutants of *Escherichia coli* during incubation with nalidixic acid. J Bacteriol. 1978;134:1195–8.
12. Wolfson JS, Hooper DC, McHugh GL, et al. Mutants of *Escherichia coli* K-12 exhibiting reduced killing by both quinolone and β-lactam antimicrobial agents. Antimicrob Agents Chemother. 1990;34:1938–43.
13. Lewin CS, Morrissey I, Smith JT. The mode of action of quinolones: The paradox in activity of low and high concentrations and activity in the anaerobic environment. Eur J Clin Microbiol Infect Dis. 1991;10:240–8.
14. Lynn R, Giaever G, Swanberg SL, et al. Tandem regions of yeast DNA topoisomerase II share homology with different subunits of bacterial gyrase. Science 1986;233:647–9.
15. Hussy P, Maass G, Tümmler B, et al. Effect of 4-quinolones and novobiocin on calf thymus DNA polymerase α primase complex, topoisomerases I and II, and growth of mammalian lymphoblasts. Antimicrob Agents Chemother. 1986;29:1073–8.
16. Hooper DC. Quinolone mode of action—New aspects. Drugs 1993;45:8–14.
17. Gootz TD, Osheroff N. Quinolones and eukaryotic topoisomerases. In: Hooper DC, Wolfson JS, eds. Quinolone Antimicrobial Agents. 2nd ed. Washington, DC: American Society for Microbiology; 1993:139–60.
18. Hooper DC, Wolfson JS. Mechanisms of bacterial resistance to quinolones. In: Hooper DC, Wolfson JS, eds. Quinolone Antimicrobial Agents. 2nd ed. Washington, DC: American Society for Microbiology; 1993:97–118.
19. Hooper DC, Wolfson JS, Souza KS, et al. Genetic and biochemical characterization of norfloxacin resistance in *Escherichia coli*. Antimicrob Agents Chemother. 1986;29:639–44.
20. Sreedharan S, Oram M, Jensen B, et al. DNA gyrase *gyrA* mutations in ciprofloxacin-resistant strains of *Staphylococcus aureus:* Close similarity with quinolone resistance mutations in *Escherichia coli*. J Bacteriol. 1990;172:7260–2.
21. Wang Y, Huang WM, Taylor DE. Cloning and nucleotide sequence of the *Campylobacter jejuni gyrA* gene and characterization of quinolone resistance mutations. Antimicrob Agents Chemother. 1993;37:457–63.
22. Yoshida H, Bogaki M, Nakamura M, et al. Quinolone resistance-determining region of the DNA gyrase *gyrB* gene of *Escherichia coli*. Antimicrob Agents Chemother. 1991;35:1647–50.
23. Hooper DC, Wolfson JS, Souza KS, et al. Mechanisms of quinolone resistance in *Escherichia coli*: Characterization of *nfx*B and *cfx*B, two mutant resistance loci decreasing norfloxacin accumulation. Antimicrob Agents Chemother. 1989;33:283–90.
24. Cohen SP, McMurry LM, Levy SB. *marA* locus causes decreased expression of OmpF porin in multiple-antibiotic-resistant (Mar) mutant of *Escherichia coli*. J Bacteriol. 1988;170:5416–22.
25. Okazaki T, Hirai K. Cloning and nucleotide sequence of the *Pseudomonas aeruginosa nfxB* gene, conferring resistance to new quinolones. FEMS Microbiol Lett. 1992;97:197–202.
26. Cohen SP, Hooper DC, Wolfson JS, et al. An endogenous active efflux of norfloxacin in susceptible *Escherichia coli*. Antimicrob Agents Chemother. 1988;32:1187–91.

27. Yoshida H, Bogaki M, Nakamura S, et al. Nucleotide sequence and characterization of the *Staphylococcus aureus norA* gene, which confers resistance to quinolones. J Bacteriol. 1990;172:6942–9.

28. Ng EYW, Trucksis M, Hooper DC. Quinolone resistance mediated by *norA*: Physiologic characterization and relationship to *flqB*, a quinolone resistance locus on the *Staphylococcus aureus* chromosome. Antimicrob Agents Chemother. 1994. In press.

29. Eliopoulos GM, Eliopoulos CT. Activity in vitro of the quinolones. In: Hooper DC, Wolfson JS, eds. Quinolone Antimicrobial Agents, 2nd ed. Washington, DC: American Society for Microbiology; 1993:161–94.

30. Wolfson JS, Hooper DC. Fluoroquinolone antimicrobial agents. Clin Microbiol Rev. 1989;2:378–424.

31. Leysen DC, Haemers A, Pattyn SR. Mycobacteria and new quinolones. Antimicrob Agents Chemother. 1989;33:1–5.

32. Eliopoulos GM, Eliopoulos CT. Ciprofloxacin in combination with other antimicrobials. Am J Med. 1989;87(Suppl 5A):22S–22S.

33. Hackbarth CJ, Chambers HF, Sande MA. Serum bactericidal activity of rifampin in combination with other antimicrobial agents against *Staphylococcus aureus*. Antimicrob Agents Chemother. 1986;29:611–3.

34. Mant TGK. Multiple-dose pharmacokinetics of lomefloxacin: Rationale for once-a-day dosing. Am J Med. 1992;92(Suppl 4A):26S–32S.

35. Lode H, Höffken G, Boeckk M, et al. Quinolone pharmacokinetics and metabolism. J Antimicrob Chemother. 1990;26(Suppl B):41–9.

36. Nightingale CH. Overview of the pharmacokinetics of fleroxacin. Am J Med. 1993;94(Suppl 3A):38S–43S.

37. Flor S. Pharmacokinetics of ofloxacin. An overview. Am J Med. 1989; 87(Suppl 6C):24S–30S.

38. Sörgel F, Kinzig M. Pharmacokinetics of gyrase inhibitors, part 1: Basic chemistry and gastrointestinal disposition. Am J Med. 1993;94(Suppl 3A): 44S–55S.

39. Staib AH, Beermann D, Harder S, et al. Absorption differences of ciprofloxacin along the human gastrointestinal tract determined using a remote-control drug delivery device (HF-capsule). Am J Med. 1989;87:66S–9S.

40. Yuk JH, Nightingale CH, Sweeney KR, et al. Relative bioavailability in healthy volunteers of ciprofloxacin administered through a nasogastric tube with and without enteral feeding. Antimicrob Agents Chemother. 1989;33: 1118–20.

41. Sahai J, Memish Z, Conway B. Ciprofloxacin pharmacokinetics after administration via a jejunostomy tube. J Antimicrob Chemother. 1991;28:936–7.

42. Montay G, Gaillot J. Pharmacokinetics of fluoroquinolones in hepatic failure. J Antimicrob Chemother. 1990;26(Suppl B):61–7.

43. Giamarellou H, Kilokythas E, Petrikkos G, et al. Pharmacokinetics of three newer quinolones in pregnant and lactating women. Am J Med. 1989; 87(Suppl 5A):49S–51S.

44. Sörgel F, Kinzig M. Pharmacokinetics of gyrase inhibitors, part 2: Renal and hepatic elimination pathways and drug interactions. Am J Med. 1993; 94(Suppl 3A):56S–69S.

45. Outman WR, Nightingale CH. Metabolism and the fluoroquinolones. Am J Med. 1989;87(Suppl 6C):37S–42S.

46. Fillastre JP, Leroy A, Moulin B, et al. Pharmacokinetics of quinolones in renal insufficiency. J Antimicrob Chemother. 1990;26(Suppl B):51–60.

47. Radandt JM, Marchbanks CR, Dudley MN. Interactions of fluoroquinolones with other drugs: Mechanisms, variability, clinical significance, and management. Clin Infect Dis. 1992;14:272–84.

48. Polk RE, Healy DP, Sahai J, et al. Effect of ferrous sulfate and multivitamins with zinc on absorption of ciprofloxacin in normal volunteers. Antimicrob Agents Chemother. 1989;33:1841–4.

49. Robson RA. The effects of quinolone on xanthine pharmacokinetics. Am J Med. 1992;92(Suppl 4A):22S–5S.

50. Wolfson JS, Hooper DC. Treatment of genitourinary infections with fluoroquinolones. I. Activity in vitro, pharmacokinetics, and clinical efficacy in urinary tract infections and prostatitis. Antimicrob Agents Chemother. 1989; 33:1655–61.

51. Hooper DC, Wolfson JS. Fluoroquinolone antimicrobial agents. N Engl J Med. 1991;324:384–94.

52. Nicolle LE, DuBois J, Martel AY, et al. Treatment of acute uncomplicated urinary tract infections with 3 days of lomefloxacin compared with treatment with 3 days of norfloxacin. Antimicrob Agents Chemother. 1993;37:574–9.

53. Raz R, Rottensterich E, Hefter H, et al. Single-dose ciprofloxacin in the treatment of uncomplicated urinary tract infection in women. Eur J Clin Microbiol Infect Dis. 1989;8:1040–2.

54. Pfau A, Sacks TG. Single dose quinolone treatment in acute uncomplicated urinary tract infection in women. J Urol. 1993;149:532–4.

55. Saginur R, Nicolle LE. Single-dose compared with 3-day norfloxacin treatment of uncomplicated urinary tract infection in women. Arch Intern Med. 1992;152:1233–7.

56. The Urinary Tract Infection Study Group. Coordinated multicenter study of norfloxacin versus trimethoprim-sulfamethoxazole of symptomatic urinary tract infections. J Infect Dis. 1987;155:170–7.

57. Raz R, Boger S. Long-term prophylaxis with norfloxacin versus nitrofurantoin in women with recurrent urinary tract infection. Antimicrob Agents Chemother. 1991;35:1241–2.

58. Fang G, Brennen C, Wagener M, et al. Use of ciprofloxacin versus use of aminoglycosides for therapy of complicated urinary tract infection: Prospective, randomized clinical and pharmacokinetic study. Antimicrob Agents Chemother. 1991;35:1849–55.

59. Sabbaj J, Hoagland VL, Cook T. Norfloxacin versus co-trimoxazole in the treatment of recurring urinary tract infections in men. Scand J Infect Dis. 1986;48(Suppl):48–53.

60. Schaeffer AJ, Darras FS. The efficacy of norfloxacin in the treatment of chronic bacterial prostatitis refractory to trimethoprim-sulfamethoxazole and/or carbenicillin. J Urol. 1990;144:690–3.

61. Hooper DC, Wolfson JS. Treatment of genitourinary tract infections with fluoroquinolones. II. Clinical efficacy in genital infections and adverse effects. Antimicrob Agents Chemother. 1989;33:1662–7.

62. Crombleholme WR, Schachter J, Ohm-Smith M, et al. Efficacy of single-agent therapy for the treatment of acute pelvic inflammatory disease with ciprofloxacin. Am J Med. 1989;87(Suppl 5A):142S–7S.

63. Wendel GD, Cox SM, Bawdon RE, et al. A randomized trial of ofloxacin versus cefoxitin and doxycycline in the outpatient treatment of acute salpingitis. Am J Obstet Gynecol. 1991;164:1390–6.

64. Boslego JW, Hicks CB, Greenup R, et al. A prospective randomized trial of ofloxacin vs. doxycycline in the treatment of uncomplicated male urethritis. Sex Transm Dis. 1988;15:186–91.

65. Hooton TM, Batteiger BE, Judson FN, et al. Ofloxacin versus doxycycline for treatment of cervical infection with *Chlamydia trachomatis*. Antimicrob Agents Chemother. 1992;36:1144–6.

66. Kitchen VS, Donegan C, Ward H, et al. Comparison of ofloxacin with doxycycline in the treatment of non-gonococcal urethritis and cervical chlamydial infection. J Antimicrob Chemother. 1990;26(Suppl D):99–105.

67. Naamara W, Plummer FA, Greenblatt RM, et al. Treatment of chancroid with ciprofloxacin: A prospective, randomized clinical trial. Am J Med. 1987; 82(Suppl 4A):317–20.

68. Naamara W, Kunimoto DY, D'Costa LJ, et al. Treating chancroid with enoxacin. Genitourin Med. 1988;64:189–92.

69. Wiström J, Jertborn M, Hedström SÅ, et al. Short-term self-treatment of travellers' diarrhoea with norfloxacin: A placebo-controlled study. J Antimicrob. Chemother. 1989;23:905–13.

70. Ericsson CD, Johnson PC, DuPont HL, et al. Ciprofloxacin or trimethoprim-sulfamethoxazole as initial therapy for travelers' diarrhea. Ann Intern Med. 1987;106:216–20.

71. Dupont HL, Ericsson CD. Prevention and treatment of traveler's diarrhea. N Engl J Med. 1993;328:1821–7.

72. Murphy GS, Bodhidatta L, Echeverria P, et al. Ciprofloxacin and loperamide in the treatment of bacillary dysentery. Ann Intern Med. 1993;118:582–6.

73. Bennish ML, Salam MA, Khan WA, et al. Treatment of shigellosis: III. Comparison of one- and two-dose ciprofloxacin with standard 5-day treatment. A randomized, blinded trial. Ann Intern Med. 1992;117:727–34.

74. Neill MA, Opal SM, Heelan J, et al. Failure of ciprofloxacin to eradicate convalescent fecal excretion after acute salmonellosis: Experience during an outbreak in health care workers. Ann Intern Med. 1991;114:195–9.

75. Wiström J, Jertborn M, Ekwall E, et al. Empiric treatment of acute diarrheal disease with norfloxacin. A randomized, placebo-controlled study. Ann Intern Med. 1992;117:202–8.

76. Goodman LJ, Trenholme GM, Kaplan RL, et al. Empiric antimicrobial therapy of domestically acquired diarrhea in urban adults. Arch Intern Med. 1990;150:541–6.

77. Petruccelli BP, Murphy GS, Sanchez JL, et al. Treatment of traveler's diarrhea with ciprofloxacin and loperamide. J Infect Dis. 1992;165:557–60.

78. Bhattacharya SK, Bhattacharya MK, Dutta P, et al. Double-blind, randomized, controlled clinical trial of norfloxacin for cholera. Antimicrob Agents Chemother. 1990;34:939–40.

79. Wang F, Gu X-J, Zhang M-F, Tai T-Y. Treatment of typhoid fever with ofloxacin. J Antimicrob Chemother. 1989;23:785–8.

80. Uwaydah AK, Al Soub H, Matar I. Randomized prospective study comparing two dosage regimens of ciprofloxacin for treatment of typhoid fever. J Antimicrob Chemother. 1992;30:707–11.

81. Gotuzzo E, Guerra JG, Benavente L, et al. Use of norfloxacin to treat chronic typhoid carriers. J Infect Dis. 1988;157:1221–5.

82. Ferriccio C, Morris JG Jr, Valdivieso C, et al. Efficacy of ciprofloxacin in the treatment of chronic typhoid carriers. J Infect Dis. 1988;157:1235–9.

83. Unertl KE, Lenhart FP, Forst H, et al. Brief report: Ciprofloxacin in the treatment of legionellosis in critically ill patients including those cases unresponsive to erythromycin. Am J Med. 1989;87(Suppl 5A):128S–31S.

84. Mouton Y, Leroy O, Beuscart C, et al. Efficacy of intravenous ofloxacin: A French multicentre trial in 185 patients. J Antimicrob Chemother. 1990; 26(Suppl D):115–21.

85. Lipsky BA, Tack KJ, Kuo C, et al. Ofloxacin treatment of *Chlamydia pneumoniae* (strain TWAR) lower respiratory tract infections. Am J Med. 1990; 89:722–4.

86. Chrysanthopoulos CJ, Skoutelis AT, Starakis JC, et al. Use of ciprofloxacin in biliary sepsis. Infection. 1988;16:249.

87. Friedland JS, Iveson TJ, Fraise AP, et al. A comparison between intraperitoneal ciprofloxacin and intraperitoneal vancomycin and gentamicin in the treatment of peritonitis associated with continuous ambulatory peritoneal dialysis (CAPD). J Antimicrob Chemother. 1990;26(Suppl F):77–81.

88. Ginés P, Rimola A, Planas R, et al. Norfloxacin prevents spontaneous bacterial peritonitis recurrence in cirrhosis: Results of a double-blind, placebo-controlled trial. Hepatology. 1990;12:716–24.

89. Gotfried MH, Ellison WT. Safety and efficacy of lomefloxacin versus cefaclor in the treatment of acute exacerbations of chronic bronchitis. Am J Med. 1992;92(Suppl 4A):108S–13S.

90. Ulmer W. Fleroxacin versus amoxicillin in the treatment of acute exacerbation of chronic bronchitis. Am J Med. 1993;94(Suppl 3A):136S–41S.

91. Chrysanthopoulos CJ, Starakis JC, Skoutelis AT, et al. Brief report: Sequential intravenous/oral therapy with ciprofloxacin in severe infection. Am J Med. 1989;87(Suppl 5A):225S–7S.

92. Gentry LO, Rodriguez-Gomez G, Kohler RB, et al. Parenteral followed by oral ofloxacin for nosocomial pneumonia and community-acquired pneumonia requiring hospitalization. Am Rev Respir Dis. 1992;145:31–5.

93. Sanders WE Jr, Morris JF, Alessi P, et al. Oral ofloxacin for the treatment of acute bacterial pneumonia: Use of a nontraditional protocol to compare experimental therapy with "usual care" in a multicenter clinical trial. Am J Med. 1991;91:261–6.

94. Peloquin CA, Cumbo TJ, Nix DE, et al. Evaluation of intravenous ciprofloxacin in patients with nosocomial lower respiratory tract infections. Impact of plasma concentrations, organism, minimum inhibitory concentration, and clinical condition on bacterial eradication. Arch Intern Med. 1989;149:2269–73.

95. Echols RM. The selection of appropriate dosages for intravenous ciprofloxacin. J Antimicrob Chemother. 1993;31:783–7.

96. Gentry LO. Oral antimicrobial therapy for osteomyelitis (Editorial). Ann Intern Med. 1991;114:986–7.

97. Gentry LO, Rodriguez-Gomez G. Ofloxacin versus parenteral therapy for chronic osteomyelitis. Antimicrob Agents Chemother. 1991;35:538–41.

98. Putz PA. A pilot study of oral fleroxacin given once daily in patients with bone and joint infections. Am J Med. 1993;94(Suppl 3A):177S–81S.

99. Gentry LO. Review of quinolones in treatment of infections of the skin and skin structure. J Antimicrob Chemother. 1991;28(Suppl C):97–110.

100. Gentry LO, Ramirez-Ronda CH, Rodriguez-Noriega E, et al. Oral ciprofloxacin vs parenteral cefotaxime in the treatment of difficult skin and skin structure infections. Arch Intern Med. 1989;149:2579–83.

101. Gentry LO, Rodriguez-Gomez G, Zeluff BJ, et al. A comparative evaluation of oral ofloxacin versus intravenous cefotaxime therapy for serious skin and skin structure infections. Am J Med. 1989;87(Suppl 6C):57S–60S.

102. Peterson LR, Lissack LM, Canter K, et al. Therapy of lower extremity infections with ciprofloxacin in patients with diabetes mellitus, peripheral vascular disease, or both. Am J Med. 1989;86:801–8.

103. Tassler H. Comparative efficacy and safety of oral fleroxacin and amoxicillin/clavulanate potassium in skin and soft tissue infections. Am J Med. 1993;94(Suppl 3A):159S–65S.

104. Trucksis M, Hooper DC, Wolfson JS. Emerging resistance to fluoroquinolones in staphylococci: An alert. Ann Intern Med. 1991;114:424–6.

105. Yew WW, Kwan SY, Ma WK, et al. In-vitro activity of ofloxacin against Mycobacterium tuberculosis and its clinical efficacy in multiply resistant pulmonary tuberculosis. J Antimicrob Chemother. 1990;26:227–36.

106. Tsukamura M, Nakamura E, Yoshii S, et al. Therapy effect of a new antibacterial substance ofloxacin (DL8280) on pulmonary tuberculosis. Am Rev Respir Dis. 1985;131:352–6.

107. de Lalla F, Maserati R, Scarpellini P, et al. Clarithromycin-ciprofloxacin-amikacin for therapy of Mycobacterium avium–Mycobacterium intracellulare bacteremia in patients with AIDS. Antimicrob Agents Chemohter. 1992;36:1567–9.

108. Kemper CA, Meng T-C, Nussbaum J, et al. Treatment of Mycobacterium avium complex bacteremia in AIDS with a four-drug oral regimen. Ann Intern Med. 1992;116:466–72.

109. Yew WW, Kwan SYL, Ma WK, et al. Ofloxacin therapy of Mycobacterium fortuitum infection: Further experience. J Antimicrob Chemother. 1990;25:880–1.

110. Grosset JH, Ji B, Guelpa-Lauras C-C, et al. Clinical trial of pefloxacin and ofloxacin in the treatment of lepromatous leprosy. Int J Leprosy. 1990;58:281–95.

111. Bouza E, Diaz-López MD, Bernaldo de Quirós JCL, et al. Ciprofloxacin in patients with bacteremic infections. Am J Med. 1989;87(Suppl 5A):228S–31S.

112. Regamey C, Steinbach-Lebbin C. Severe infections with intravenous ofloxacin: A prospective clinical multicenter Swiss study. J Antimicrob Chemother. 1990;26(Suppl D):107–14.

113. Chan CC, Oppendeim BA, Anderson H, et al. Randomized trial comparing ciprofloxacin plus netilmicin versus piperacillin plus netilmicin for empiric treatment of fever in neutropenic patients. Antimicrob Agents Chemother. 1989;33:89–91.

114. Meunier F, Zinner SH, Gaya H, et al. Prospective randomized evaluation of ciprofloxacin versus piperacillin plus amikacin for empiric antibiotic therapy of febrile granulocytopenic cancer patients with lymphomas and solid tumors. Antimicrob Agents Chemother. 1991;35:873–8.

115. The GIMEMA Infection Program. Prevention of bacterial infection in neutropenic patients with hematologic malignancies. A randomized, multicenter trial comparing norfloxacin with ciprofloxacin. Ann Intern Med. 1991;115:7–12.

116. Dworkin RJ, Sande MA, Lee BL, et al. Treatment of right-sided Staphylococcus aureus endocarditis in intravenous drug abusers with ciprofloxacin and rifampicin. Lancet 1989;2:1071–3.

117. Segev S, Rosen N, Joseph G, et al. Pefloxacin efficacy in gram-negative bacillary meningitis. J Antimicrob Chemother. 1990;26(Suppl B):187–92.

118. Schönwald S, Beus I, Lisic M, et al. Brief report: Ciprofloxacin in the treatment of gram-negative bacillary meningitis. Am J Med. 1989;87(Suppl 5A):248S–9S.

119. Dworzack DL, Sanders CC, Horowitz EA, et al. Evaluation of single-dose ciprofloxacin in the eradication of Neisseria meningitidis from nasopharyngeal carriers. Antimicrob Agents Chemother. 1988;32:1740–1.

120. Syrjälä H, Schildt R, Räisänen S. In vitro susceptibility of Franciscella tularensis to fluoroquinolones and treatment of tularemia with norfloxacin and ciprofloxacin. Eur J Clin Microbiol Infect Dis. 1991;10:68–70.

121. Holley HP. Successful treatment of cat-scratch disease with ciprofloxacin. JAMA 1991;265:1563–5.

122. Raoult D, Drancourt M. Antimicrobial therapy of rickettsial diseases. Antimicrob Agents Chemother. 1991;35:2457–62.

123. Lang R, Rubinstein E. Quinolones for the treatment of brucellosis. J Antimicrob Chemother. 1992;29:1063–9.

124. McClean KL, Hitchman D, Shafran SD. Norfloxacin is inferior to chloroquine for falciparum malaria in northwestern Zambia: A comparative clinical trial. J Infect Dis. 1992;165:904–7.

125. Watt G, Shanks GD, Edstein MD, et al. Ciprofloxacin treatment of drug-resistant falciparum malaria. J Infect Dis. 1991;164:602–4.

126. Blaser J, Stone BB, Groner MC, et al. Comparative study with enoxacin and netilmicin in a pharmacodynamic model to determine importance of ratio of antibiotic peak concentration to MIC for bactericidal activity and emergence of resistance. Antimicrob Agents Chemother. 1987;31:1054–60.

127. Parry MF, Panzer KB, Yukna ME. Quinolone resistance: Susceptibility data from a 300-bed community hospital. Am J Med. 1989;87(Suppl 5A):12S–5S.

128. Kresken M, Wiedemann B. Development of resistance to naldixic acid and the fluoroquinolones after the introduction of norfloxacin and ofloxacin. Antimicrob Agents Chemother. 1988;32:1285–8.

129. Blumberg HM, Rimland D, Carroll DJ, et al. Rapid development of ciprofloxacin in methicillin-susceptible and -resistant Staphylococcus aureus. J Infect Dis. 1991;163:1279–85.

130. Reina J, Borrell N, Serra A. Emergence of resistance to erythromycin and fluoroquinolones in thermotolerant Campylobacter strains isolated from feces 1987–1991. Eur J Clin Microbiol Infect Dis. 1992;11:1163–6.

131. Aguiar JM, Chacon J, Canton R, et al. The emergence of highly fluoroquinolone-resistant Escherichia coli in community-acquired urinary tract infections. J Antimicrob Chemother. 1992;29:349–51.

132. Hooper DC, Wolfson JS. Adverse effects. In: Hooper DC, Wolfson JS, eds. Quinolone Antimicrobial Agents. 2nd ed. Washington, DC: American Society for Microbiology; 1993:589–612.

133. Norrby SR. Side-effects of quinolones: Comparisons between quinolones and other antibiotics. Eur J Clin Microbiol Infect Dis. 1991;10:378–83.

134. Stahlmann R. Safety profile of quinolones. J Antimicrob Chemother. 1990;26(Suppl D):31–44.

135. Rizk E. The U.S. clinical experience with lomefloxacin, a new once-daily fluoroquinolone. Am J Med. 1992;92(Suppl 4A):130S–5S.

136. Adam D. Use of quinolones in pediatrics. Rev Infect Dis. 1989;11(Suppl 5):1113–6.

137. Pertuiset E, Lenoir G, Jehanne M, et al. Tolérance articulaire de la péfloxacine et de l'ofloxacine chez les enfants et adolescents atteints de mucoviscidose. Rev Rhum. 1989;56:735–40.

138. Vance-Bryan K, Guay DRP, Rotschafer JC. Clinical pharmacokinetics of ciprofloxacin. Clin Pharmacokinet. 1990;19:434–61.

139. Guay DRP, Opsahl JA, McMahon FG, et al. Safety and pharmacokinetics of multiple doses of intravenous ofloxacin in healthy volunteers. Antimicrob Agents Chemother. 1992;36:308–12.

140. Frydman AM, Le Roux Y, Lefebvre MA, et al. Pharmacokinetics of pefloxacin after repeated intravenous and oral administration (400 mg bid) in young healthy adults. J Antimicrob Chemother. 1986;17(Suppl B):65–79.

28. URINARY TRACT AGENTS: NITROFURANTOIN AND METHENAMINE

DAVID C. HOOPER

Two antimicrobial agents in clinical use are focused exclusively for treatment or prophylaxis of urinary tract infections because of their pharmacologic and chemical properties. At tolerated doses, nitrofurantoin achieves adequate concentrations only in kidney tissues and urine. Methenamine, which lacks antimicrobial activity itself, only becomes active after chemical degradation in the presence of acidic bladder urine to generate its active breakdown product, formaldehyde.

NITROFURANTOIN

Chemical Structure

Nitrofurantoin (N-[5-nitro-2-furfurylidene]-1-aminohydantoin) is a weak acid (pKa 7.2) (Fig. 1) and a member of a group of

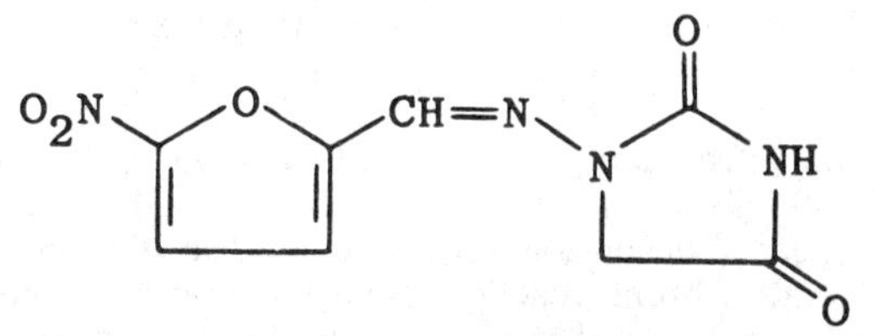

FIG. 1. Chemical structure of nitrofurantoin.

synthetic nitrofuran compounds that also includes furazolidone, which is available in Europe but not the United States. Two oral formulations of nitrofurantoin were developed. A microcrystalline form previously available was introduced in 1953, and a macrocrystalline form (Macrodantin, Norwich-Eaton) has been available since 1967.

Mechanisms of Drug Action and Bacterial Resistance

The mechanism of action of nitrofurantoin is poorly understood, but activity in many cases appears to require enzymatic reduction within the bacterial cell.[1] The reduced derivatives appear to be capable of binding to proteins. Nitrofurans have been shown to inhibit the synthesis of inducible enzymes by blocking translation[2] and also to inhibit bacterial respiration and pyruvate metabolism. These agents, like the quinolones, appear to damage bacterial DNA,[3] and they induce bacterial DNA repair systems.[4] Mutants with defective DNA repair functions are hypersusceptible.[5] Nitrofurantoin may antagonize the bactericidal activity of quinolones against *Proteus* and *Enterobacter*.[6] The principal drug action that determines the bactericidal activity of nitrofurantoin, however, remains to be defined.

Resistant strains of *Escherichia coli* with chromosomal or plasmid-mediated resistance have been associated with reductions in nitrofuran reductase enzyme activities, thereby reducing the production of the active derivative(s).[7-9] In clinical use, however, selection of nitrofurantoin-resistant variants from initially susceptible pathogens has been rare.[10]

Spectrum of Activity

Susceptibility breakpoints are based on urinary concentrations of nitrofurantoin and have been correlated with eradication of bacteriuria in patients with urinary tract infections.[11,12] Bacterial strains with a minimum inhibitory concentration (MIC) of 32 µg/ml or less are considered clinically susceptible. For strains having an MIC of 64 µg/ml, clinical responses may be more variable.[13] MIC of greater than 500 µg/ml uniformly correlates with clinical failure.[11] Based on these criteria, over 90 percent of clinical strains of *E. coli*, *Citrobacter* spp., *Staphylococcus saprophyticus*, and *Enterococcus faecalis* are susceptible. Group B streptococci are also usually susceptible. In contrast, only a minority of strains of *Enterobacter* spp. (20–50 percent), *Klebsiella* spp. (45 percent), and *Enterococcus faecium* (50 percent) are susceptible, and members of the genera *Proteus*, *Providencia*, *Morganella*, *Serratia*, *Acinetobacter*, and *Pseudomonas* are almost always resistant.[12,13] These patterns of susceptibility have generally remained stable in our hospital and others.[14]

Other organisms that are uncommonly associated with urinary tract infections but may be susceptible to nitrofurantoin in vitro include *Salmonella* spp., *Shigella* spp., *Staphylococcus aureus*, coagulase-negative staphylococci, *Streptococcus pneumoniae*, *Streptococcus pyogenes*, *Corynebacterium* spp., and *Bacteroides* spp.[15-17]

Pharmacology

Absorption. The completeness of absorption of orally administered nitrofurantoin as determined from drug recovery in the urine is about 40–50 percent, and absorption is enhanced when the drug is taken with food.[18] Absorption occurs principally and rapidly in the small intestine. Two formulations of nitrofurantoin differ in the rate of drug absorption. The slower rate of dissolution and absorption of the macrocrystalline form relative to the microcrystalline form was associated with a lower occurrence of gastrointestinal adverse effects, a minimal reduction in overall absorption (36 vs. 43 percent), and no change in efficacy (see below). Although parenteral preparations of nitrofurantoin have been evaluated, they are not generally available for clinical use.

Distribution. Serum concentrations of nitrofurantoin are low or undetectable (≤ 1 µg/ml) with standard oral doses of 100 mg qid. After administration of intravenous nitrofurantoin, serum half-life was estimated to be 30 minutes or less. In animals given intravenous nitrofurantoin, a high volume of distribution (0.7 liter/kg) suggested drug distribution into extracellular and intracellular compartments, but enzymatic degradation of nitrofurantoin in situ is thought to contribute to low drug levels in most tissues.[18,19] Therapeutic concentrations are not detected in prostatic secretions,[20] and only low concentrations have been detected in human breast milk.[21] Nitrofurantoin concentrations in bile may be equal to or greater than those in serum.[18] Drug concentrations in urine are substantial (50–250 µg/ml) and exceed the MIC of susceptible organisms.[22]

Excretion. Nitrofurantoin is eliminated predominantly in the urine. Renal elimination involves glomerular filtration, tubular secretion, and tubular reabsorption.[18] Tubular handling is by the weak acid transport system. Reabsorption is reduced in the presence of alkaline urine, because at alkaline pH the equilibrium of nonionized and ionized drug is shifted toward the ionized form, which diffuses back across the renal tubular epithelium less well than the nonionized form. Urine alkalinization does not enhance antibacterial activity in the urine, however, because nitrofurantoin may be less active at alkaline pH.[10] In patients with renal failure, nitrofurantoin excretion is reduced in proportion to reductions in creatinine clearance, and urinary drug concentrations become subtherapeutic.[23] In severe renal failure there may also be modest increases in serum concentrations of nitrofurantoin (≤ 6 µg/ml).[23] Thus, nitrofurantoin should not be used in patients with renal insufficiency (creatinine clearance, <40 ml/min).

With normal renal function, metabolism and biliary excretion are minor pathways of nitrofurantoin elimination that are less well understood.[18] No dosage adjustment is required in patients with liver disease without alterations in renal function.

Dosing. For therapy of established urinary tract infections, nitrofurantoin is given orally at 50–100 mg qid. For use as prophylaxis for recurrent urinary tract infections, it is usually given as 50–100 mg qd.

Clinical Uses

Nitrofurantoin is indicated only for the treatment and prophylaxis of urinary tract infections.

Acute Uncomplicated Cystitis. In earlier noncomparative studies bacteriologic and clinical responses in patients with acute uncomplicated cystitis ranged from 61 to 100 percent,[10] although in a number of these studies follow-up periods were brief. Infections caused by *E. coli* generally responded well, and infections caused by *Proteus* spp. and *P. aeruginosa* responded poorly if at all. When given for 7 days to young women, nitrofurantoin and trimethoprim (200 mg po qd) produced similar rates of eradication of infections caused by *E. coli* (66/78 [84 percent] vs. 72/77 [93 percent]) and *S. saprophyticus* (7/8 [87 percent] vs. 10/12 [83 percent]), but the smaller numbers of infections caused by *Klebsiella* spp. and *Proteus* spp. responded better to trimethoprim.[24] Suppression of potential pathogens in the periurethral and vaginal flora occurred significantly more often with trimethoprim than with nitrofurantoin, a finding that may have contributed to the higher rate of recurrent infections seen in the nitrofurantoin group. Nitrofurantoin has been used for treatment of lower urinary tract infections in pregnant women[25] and children.[16] In young girls with cystitis, responses to nitrofurantoin given for 3 days were similar to responses to a 7-day course.[26] Currently 15–20 percent of urinary isolates causing acute uncomplicated cystitis may be resistant to nitrofurantoin, and responses in infections caused by susceptible pathogens may be less satisfactory than responses to trimethoprim-sulfamethoxazole or fluoroquinolones.[25] Thus, nitrofurantoin should be considered an alternative rather than a first-line therapy for this clinical syndrome.

Acute Uncomplicated Pyelonephritis and Complicated Urinary Tract Infections.   Patients with acute pyelonephritis respond inconsistently to nitrofurantoin, and bacteremias have occurred during nitrofurantoin treatment, presumably because serum concentrations are inadequate.[10] Thus, nitrofurantoin should not be used for treatment of pyelonephritis. In addition, complicated urinary tract infections, which are defined as those associated with structural or functional abnormalities of the urinary tract, are often associated with pyelonephritis and are often caused by pathogens resistant to nitrofurantoin. In general, nitrofurantoin is not indicated for treatment of these infections, and it is specifically contraindicated in cases that are complicated by resistant pathogens, pyelonephritis, renal failure, or prostatic infection. An earlier study of older men with recurring bacteriuria showed that nitrofurantoin given as long-term suppression reduced recurrences of bacteriuria by about 40 percent relative to placebo,[27] but drugs that penetrate the prostate (trimethoprim or fluoroquinolones) are more likely to eradicate bacteriuria in these patients.

Prophylaxis of Recurrent Urinary Tract Infections.   In young women with two or more episodes of symptomatic bacteriuria within 12 months, once daily nitrofurantoin (100 mg) was highly effective and comparable to trimethoprim-sulfamethoxazole (40–200 mg) in preventing recurrent urinary tract infections without selection of resistant organisms.[28] Infections recurred at the same rate when prophylaxis was stopped after 6 months. For women in whom recurrence of infection is associated with sexual intercourse, a single dose of nitrofurantoin (100 mg) taken shortly after intercourse has also been highly effective in preventing symptomatic infection.[29] Postcoital prophylaxis was also effective in pregnant women with a history of recurrent urinary tract infections before pregnancy.[30] Nitrofurantoin has reduced the rates of bacteriuria in patients undergoing intermittent catheterization in some[31] but not all[32] studies. Antimicrobial prophylaxis is not of value in patients with long-term indwelling catheters.[25]

Adverse Effects

Gastrointestinal and Skin Reactions.   The overall tolerability of nitrofurantoin is dominated by gastrointestinal adverse effects, the rates of which are dose related and differ for the two formulations.[22] In a randomized, double-blind comparison, the microcrystalline formulation (100 mg qid) was associated with adverse effects (predominantly nausea or vomiting) in 39 percent of patients as compared with 17 percent of patients receiving the macrocrystalline formulation in the same dose.[33] Slower dissolution of the macrocrystalline formulation is thought to be responsible for its lower frequency of gastrointestinal side effects.

Rashes, presumably of an allergic nature, have been reported in about 1 percent of hospitalized patients receiving nitrofurantoin.[16] Other less common, but more serious toxicities of nitrofurantoin have received considerable attention.[16,22]

Pulmonary Reactions.   Pulmonary reactions have been classified into acute, subacute, and chronic forms[16] and in the United States appear to occur at a frequency of ≤1 in 100,000 courses of treatment.[22] Chronic reactions appear to be less common than acute reactions, at least in part because fewer patients receive the extended courses of therapy that precede chronic reactions.

The acute reaction appears to be a reversible hypersensitivity phenomenon and may occur within hours to weeks of drug exposure, with a shorter time to onset of symptoms after drug reexposure.[34,35] The clinical presentation is characterized by the rapid onset of fever, cough, dyspnea, and myalgia. These symptoms are usually accompanied by peripheral blood eosinophilia (83 percent) and lower lobe infiltrates (94 percent) with (20 percent) or without pleural effusions on chest radiographs. Alveolar exudates, interstitial inflammation, and vasculitis have been found on lung biopsy. In addition, rash, pruritus, chest discomfort, and sputum production may also be present. Improvement is generally rapid after discontinuation of the drug, and acute reactions do not generally progress to chronic reactions.

It is not clear whether the subacute and chronic forms of nitrofurantoin pulmonary reactions are distinct from each other except for onsets after 1 and 6 or more months of drug therapy, respectively.[35] These reactions are thought to result from toxic effects on the lung, possibly related to oxidant injury of the type that has been demonstrated in rat lung explants treated with nitrofurantoin.[36] Both subacute and chronic reactions have the gradual onset of progressive nonproductive cough and dyspnea and findings of interstitial infiltrates on chest radiographs. Fever is variably present. Eosinophilia is uncommon, but abnormalities of liver function tests may be seen in up to 40 percent of patients, and positive tests for antinuclear antibodies have been reported.[34] Regression often occurs with discontinuation of nitrofurantoin, but in the more chronic reactions irreversible pulmonary fibrosis and fatal reactions have occurred. A beneficial effect of corticosteroid therapy has not been convincingly demonstrated in patients with chronic nitrofurantoin pulmonary reactions.

Hepatic Reactions.   Hepatic reactions appear to occur with a frequency similar to that of chronic pulmonary reactions.[37] In some cases both hepatitis and pulmonary infiltrates have occurred together.[38] Acute hepatitis with or without cholestasis associated with short-term use of nitrofurantoin is generally self-limited and reversible.[39] Prolonged use of nitrofurantoin, however, has been associated with chronic active hepatitis, cirrhosis, and death.[38] Hyperglobulinemia and antinuclear antibodies were commonly present, but eosinophilia was variable.

Hematologic Reactions.   Hemolytic anemia has occurred rarely in patients given nitrofurantoin and most often, but not always, in those with deficiency of glucose-6-phosphate dehydrogenase (G6PD).[22,40] Reductions in cellular NADPH in such patients result in diminished cellular levels of reduced glutathione. Nitrofurantoin may inhibit glutathione reductase, further compromising the ability of the cell to generate reduced glutathione,[41] and it may also generate the release of superoxide from oxyhemoglobin in the presence of oxygen,[42] thereby further contributing to oxidant stresses.[16] Patients with deficiencies in enolase and glutathione peroxidases have developed nitrofurantoin-induced hemolysis as well. Folic acid–responsive megaloblastic anemia has also been reported.[43] Eosinophilia is seen as a feature of the acute pulmonary reactions and some hepatic reactions, but leukopenia and aplastic anemia have been only rarely reported.

Peripheral Neuropathy.   A peripheral sensorimotor neuropathy of unclear mechanism has been reported uncommonly and less often than pulmonary reactions. Neuropathy has been seen in patients receiving nitrofurantoin for prolonged periods as well as in patients with renal failure.[22,37] The onset of neuropathy is often insidious with paresthesias and dysesthesias in a stocking-and-glove distribution. Distal weakness with centripetal spread may also occur.[44] Histopathologic findings have included demyelination and axonal degeneration.[45] The reversibility of the deficits after cessation of drug therapy may be slow and variable.

Uses in Pediatrics and in Pregnancy.

Nitrofurantoin appears to have similar toxicities in children and adults,[46] but is not recommended for use in neonates. It may be used for treatment of urinary tract infections in pregnancy when clearly indicated but should not be used at term.[6,25] Nitrofurantoin crosses the placenta, but very low concentrations occur in amniotic fluid.[47] Although it is mutagenic in some bacterial tests in vitro,[48] tests for teratogenicity and carcinogenicity in animals have been negative.[6,22] Reviews of adverse events in a total of 165 pregnant patients who were treated with nitrofurantoin in each of the three trimesters of pregnancy found no increased incidence of fetal loss or fetal abnormality relative to the population in general.[49,50] Healthy infants with G-6-PD deficiency have been born to mothers treated with nitrofurantoin during pregnancy.[22]

METHENAMINE

Chemical Structure

Methenamine (hexamethylenetetramine) (Fig. 2) is currently available as a salt of mandelic acid (α-hydroxybenzene acetic acid) (Mandelamine, Parke-Davis; Uroquid-acid, Beach) or hippuric acid (benzoylamino-acetic acid) (Hiprex, Marion Merrell Dow; Urex, 3M) or without these acids (Uro-Phosphate, Robins).

Mechanism of Action and Antimicrobial Activity

Methenamine itself has little antibacterial activity, but at acid pH each molecule of methenamine that is hydrolyzed generates four molecules of ammonia and six molecules of formaldehyde $(N_4[CH_2])_6 + 6H_2O + 4H^+ \leftrightarrow 4NH_4^- 6HCHO)$.[51,52] Increasing concentrations of H^+ and diffusional loss of NH_3 drive the reaction to the right. Formaldehyde, the active product, is a nonspecific denaturant of proteins and nucleic acids and has broad-spectrum antimicrobial activity. Free formaldehyde concentrations above 25 μg/ml may be bactericidal. Microbial resistance to formaldehyde has not been described.[51] Antimicrobial activity in urine correlates with urinary concentrations of formaldehyde.[53] Although formaldehyde has activity against *Proteus* spp., an alkaline urine may be generated by the urease activity of these organisms, preventing conversion of methenamine to formaldehyde. Inhibitors of urease may prevent this effect in laboratory simulations of *Proteus* growing in urine.[54] Hippuric and mandelic acids themselves have only limited anti-

bacterial activity at concentrations achieved with usual doses of their respective methenamine salts.[55]

Pharmacology

Absorption and Distribution. Methenamine itself is rapidly absorbed after oral administration, and 82–88 percent is recovered in the urine of normal volunteers in the 24 hours after a 1-g dose,[56] indicating excellent bioavailability. Methenamine may be partially degraded in the presence of gastric acid before absorption.[57] This degradation is avoided with enteric-coated formulations, but absorption is slower. The volume of distribution (0.56 liter/kg) is relatively high, suggesting broad distribution in tissues. Methenamine crosses the placenta, and concentrations in breast milk are similar to those in plasma.[58]

Excretion. The half-life of elimination of methenamine from serum is 3–4 hours with normal renal function. Renal clearance is 95 percent of total clearance from serum, indicating a predominant renal route of excretion.[56] Hippuric and mandelic acids are also excreted renally by both glomerular filtration and tubular secretion.[52,59] The extent to which methenamine and hippuric and mandelic acids accumulate in patients with renal failure is not known.

Factors Affecting Formaldehyde Concentrations in Urine. The concentration of formaldehyde in bladder urine determines antimicrobial activity and is a function of *(1)* methenamine concentrations in urine, *(2)* the rate of hydrolysis of methenamine to formaldehyde, and *(3)* the rate of urine loss from the bladder by voiding or drainage. At constant rates of renal clearance methenamine concentrations in urine decrease with increasing urine volumes, but with repetitive dosing concentrations above 150 μg/ml are usually maintained.[56] Conversion of methenamine to formaldehyde occurs as a first-order reaction with higher rates of conversion in the presence of higher concentrations of methenamine.[60] The relative rate constant for conversion increases with decreasing urine pH and is 13-fold higher at pH 5.2 than at pH 6.5[60]; no hydrolysis occurs above pH 6.8. At methenamine concentrations of 1000 μg/ml, the time needed to generate formaldehyde concentrations in excess of 25 μg/ml is more than 6 hours at pH 6.5, 3 hours at pH 5.85, and 1.5–2 hours at pH 5.6.[61] At such concentrations of formaldehyde, bacterial exposure for at least 2 hours was necessary for antibacterial activity. Thus, increases in the frequency of voiding or bladder drainage will reduce antibacterial effects by removing formaldehyde and by reducing the time of exposure of bladder bacteria to formaldehyde.[62] For these reasons methenamine is ineffective in the presence of indwelling bladder catheters and may be ineffective when intermittent catherization is performed frequently. Similarly, the brief time in which methenamine resides in the renal tissues and the upper urinary tract obviates efficacy in pyelonephritis.

Acidification of the Urine During Methenamine Treatment. Maintaining urinary pH below 6 is necessary for generating antibacterial activity from methenamine, and in many patients a sufficiently low urine pH is present without additional measures. The amounts of hippuric and mandelic acids given with usual doses of methenamine hippurate and methenamine mandelate, however, do not contribute importantly to urine acidification.[57] Ascorbic acid has been given to aid urine acidification, but doses as high as 12 g per day may be required.[52] The value of acetohydroxamic acid, an inhibitor of urease, as adjunctive therapy in patients with an alkaline urine associated with *Proteus* infection is suggested by in vitro data[54] but is unclear in vivo.

Dosing. With equimolar mixtures of methenamine and their respective acids, 1 g of methenamine mandelate contains 480

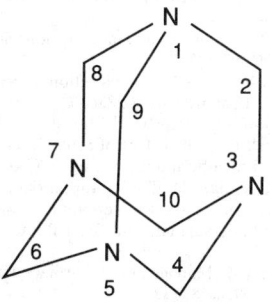

FIG. 2. Chemical structure of methenamine. Numbers are conventional designations of atom positions.

mg methenamine, and 1 g of methenamine hippurate contains 440 mg of methenamine. For adults and children over 12 years, methenamine mandelate and methenamine hippurate are usually given in a dose of 1 g PO twice daily, but up to 4 g per day (1 g qid) may be given. For children between 6 and 12 years, the dose is 500 mg to 1 g twice daily. An oral suspension (methenamine mandelate, 500 mg/5 ml and 250 mg/5 ml) is available for younger children; for children less than 6 years old, the usual dose is 250 mg per 30 lb body weight po qid.

Clinical Uses

The efficacy of methenamine for treatment of established cystitis has not been adequately documented in comparative clinical trials, and methenamine is contraindicated for treatment of pyelonephritis. Methenamine, thus, should not be used for treatment of established urinary tract infections.

Methenamine has been shown, however, to be effective for suppression or prophylaxis of recurrent lower urinary tract infections. In a double-blind, placebo-controlled, cross-over trial in young otherwise healthy women with recurrent cystitis, 1 g of methenamine hippurate twice daily reduced recurrent symptomatic infections by 73 percent.[63] A similar significant reduction (56 percent) was seen in another comparative study of a similar population of young women and girls given methenamine mandelate (500 mg qid) and ascorbic acid (2 g daily).[64] Trimethoprim-sulfamethoxazole (40–200 mg at bedtime), however, was significantly better than methenamine in reducing the frequency of recurrent infections in this study,[64] as was trimethoprim alone in another study.[65] Trimethoprim-sulfamethoxazole was more effective than methenamine in reducing periurethral colonization with gram-negative bacilli, a potential reservoir of recurring pathogens.[64] Although less well tolerated, nitrofurantoin was also more effective than methenamine hippurate in preventing symptomatic infections in another trial.[66]

Methenamine has also prevented episodes of recurring bacteriuria in children[67,68] and has suppressed chronic bacteriuria in men.[27] It has not been shown, however, that methenamine is superior to other agents such as trimethoprim-sulfamethoxazole for these uses.

Attempts to prevent recurring infections in patients with indwelling bladder catheters by use of methenamine have not been successful,[69] as might be expected because of the inability to generate sufficient concentrations of formaldehyde under these conditions. The results of prophylaxis of patients undergoing intermittent catheterization have been variable.[69,70] In a double-blind, randomized, placebo-controlled trial of patients with neurogenic bladders undergoing bladder retraining, urinary acidification was augmented with ammonium chloride in the methenamine group (both given as 1 g every 6 hours), and catheterization (usually every 6 hours), voiding, and drinking schedules were specifically controlled. Over the 21 days of the study there was a significantly lower rate of occurrence of bacteriuria in the methenamine group, 9 of 17 patients (53 percent) in comparison to 19 of 22 patients (86 percent) in the placebo group.[70] For patients undergoing intermittent catheterization for longer periods, however, antimicrobial regimens may only delay episodes of bacteriuria. The effectiveness of methenamine-containing regimens will likely be inversely dependent on the frequency of catheterization and voiding.

Adverse Effects

Methenamine is generally well tolerated,[52,64] and in double-blind studies[70] side effects have been few, mild, reversible, and comparable to placebo. In nonblinded studies, most commonly encountered have been gastrointestinal side effects (nausea, vomiting) and rashes or pruritis.[52] Symptoms of bladder irritation have been reported in patients with sterile urine receiving methenamine suppression.[27] With high doses of methenamine, increased gastrointestinal intolerance and hemorrhagic cystitis[71] may occur, possibly related to increased local concentrations of formaldehyde.

Methenamine salts may predispose to the development of urate crystals in the urine of patients with gout and may cause precipitation of sulfonamides in the urine of patients concurrently treated with these drugs.

Because conversion of methenamine to formaldehyde also releases ammonia, methenamine should be avoided in patients with hepatic insufficiency. The safety of methenamine itself in patients with renal failure is unclear; because of the potential risk of increasing systemic acidosis, acidifying agents should be avoided in such patients.[72] Limited data suggest that methenamine may be given safely in the second and third trimesters of pregnancy.[73]

REFERENCES

1. McCalla DR, Reuvers A, Kaiser C. Mode of action of nitrofurazone. J Bacteriol. 1970;104:1126–34.
2. Herrlich P, Schweiger M. Nitrofurans, a group of synthetic antibiotics, with new mode of action: Discrimination of specific messenger RNA classes. Proc Natl Acad Sci USA. 1976;73:3386–90.
3. Tu Y, McCalla DR. Effect of activated nitrofurans on DNA. Biochim Biophys Acta. 1975;402:142–9.
4. Rahman MdS, Pal AK, Chatterjee SN. Induction of SOS like responses by nitrofurantoin in Vibrio cholerae el tor cells. Arch Microbiol. 1993;159:98–100.
5. Jenkins ST, Bennett PM. Effect of mutations in deoxyribonucleic acid repair pathways on the sensitivity of Escherichia coli K-12 strains to nitrofurantoin. J Bacteriol. 1976;125:1214–6.
6. Shah S, Greenwood D. Interactions between antibacterial agents of the quinolone group and nitrofurantoin. J Antimicrob Chemother. 1988;21:41–8.
7. McCalla DR, Kaiser C, Green MHL. Genetics of nitrofurazone resistance in Escherichia coli. J Bacteriol. 1978;133:10–6.
8. Breeze AS, Obaseiki-Ebor EE. Nitrofuran reductase activity in nitrofurantoin-resistant strains of Escherichia coli K-12: some with chromosomally determined resistance and others carrying R-plasmids. J Antimicrob Chemother. 1983;12:543–7.
9. Breeze AS, Obaseiki-Ebor EE. Transferable nitrofuran resistance conferred by R-plasmids in clinical isolates of Escherichia coli. J Antimicrob Chemother. 1983;12:459–67.
10. Richards WA, Riss E, Kass EH, et al. Nitrofurantoin. Clinical and laboratory studies in urinary tract infections. Arch Intern Med. 1955;96:437–50.
11. Winn WR, Silton J, Finegold SM. In vitro sensitivity to nitrofurantoin compared with clinical bacteriological response. Antimicrob Agents Chemother. 1965;582–90.
12. Turck M, Ronald AR, Petersdorf RG. Susceptibility of Enterobacteriaceae to nitrofurantoin correlated with eradication of bacteriuria. Antimicrob Agents Chemother. 1967;446–52.
13. Barry AL. Nitrofurantoin susceptibility test criteria. J Antimicrob Chemother. 1990;25:711–3.
14. Bulger RJ, Larson E, Sherris JC. Decreased incidences of resistance to antimicrobial agents among Escherichia coli and Klebsiella–Enterobacter: Observations in a university hospital over a 10 year period. Ann Intern Med. 1970;72:65–71.
15. Schroeder SA, Terry PM, Bennett JV. Antibiotic resistance and transfer factor in Salmonella, United States 1967. JAMA. 1968;205:903–6.
16. Gleckman R, Alvarez S, Joubert DW. Drug therapy reviews: Nitrofurantoin. Am J Hosp Pharm. 1979;36:342–51.
17. Brumfitt W, Reynolds AV, Hamilton-Miller JMT. Activity of nitrofurantoin and nifuratel against anaerobic gram-negative bacilli (Letter). Lancet. 1975;1:460.
18. Conklin JD. The pharmacokinetics of nitrofurantoin and its related bioavailability. Antibiot Chemother. 1978;25:233–52.
19. Schmidt FH. Inactivation of nitrofuran derivatives by mammalian tissue. Klin Wochenschr. 1966;44:653–4.
20. Dunn BL, Stamey TA. Antibacterial concentrations in prostatic fluid, 1-nitrofurantoin. J Urol. 1967;97:505–7.
21. Varsano I, Fischl J, Shochet SB. The excretion of orally ingested nitrofurantoin in human milk. J Pediatr. 1973;82:886–7.
22. D'Arcy PF. Nitrofurantoin. Drug Intell Clin Pharm. 1985;19:540–7.
23. Sachs J, Geer T, Noell P, et al. Effect of renal function on urinary recovery of orally administered nitrofurantoin. N Engl J Med. 1968;278:1032–5.
24. Iravani A, Richard GA, Baer H. Trimethoprim once daily vs. nitrofurantoin in treatment of acute urinary tract infections in young women, with special reference to periurethral, vaginal, and fecal flora. Rev Infect Dis. 1982;4:378–7.
25. Stamm WE, Hooton TM. Management of urinary tract infections in adults. N Engl J Med. 1993;329:1328–34.
26. Lohr JA, Hayden GF, Kesler RW, et al. Three-day therapy of lower urinary tract infections with nitrofurantoin macrocrystals: a randomized clinical trial. J Pediatr. 1981;99:980–3.

27. Freeman RB, Smith WM, Richardson JA, et al. Long-term therapy for chronic bacteriuria in men. U.S. Public Health Service Cooperative Study. Ann Intern Med. 1975;83:133–47.

28. Stamm WE, Counts GW, Wagner KF, et al. Antimicrobial prophylaxis of recurrent urinary tract infections. A double-blind, placebo-controlled trial. Ann Intern Med. 1980;92:770–5.

29. Vosti KL. Recurrent urinary tract infections. Prevention by prophylactic antibiotics after sexual intercourse. JAMA. 1975;231:934–40.

30. Pfau A, Sacks TG. Effective prophylaxis for recurrent urinary tract infections during pregnancy. Clin Infect Dis. 1992;14:810–4.

31. Anderson RU. Prophylaxis of bacteriuria during intermittent catheterization of acute neurogenic bladder. J Urol. 1980;123:364–366.

32. Kuhlemeier KV, Stover SL, Lloyd LK. Prophylactic antibacterial therapy for preventing urinary tract infections in spinal cord injury patients. J Urol. 1985;134:514–7.

33. Kalowski S, Radford N, Kincaid-Smith P. Crystalline and macrocrystalline nitrofurantoin in the treatment of urinary-tract infection. N Engl J Med. 1974;290:385–7.

34. Holmberg L, Boman G. Pulmonary reactions to nitrofurantoin. 447 cases reported to the Swedish Adverse Drug Reaction Committee 1966–1976. Eur J Respir Dis. 1981;62:180–9.

35. Sovijärvi ARA, Lemola M, Stenius B, et al. Nitrofurantoin-induced acute, subacute and chronic pulmonary reactions. A report of 66 cases. Scand J Respir Dis. 1977;58:41–50.

36. Martin WJ III. Nitrofurantoin: Evidence for the oxidant injury of lung parenchymal cells. Am Rev Respir Dis. 1983;127:482–6.

37. Holmberg L, Boman G, Böttiger LE, et al. Adverse reactions to nitrofurantoin. Analysis of 921 reports. Am J Med. 1980;69:733–8.

38. Sharp JR, Ishak KG, Zimmerman HJ. Chronic active hepatitis and severe hepatic necrosis associated with nitrofurantoin. Ann Intern Med. 1980;92:14–9.

39. Goldstein LI, Ishak KG, Burns W. Hepatic injury associated with nitrofurantoin therapy. Am J Digest Dis. 1974;19:987–98.

40. Gait JE. Hemolytic reactions to nitrofurantoin in patients with glucose-6-phosphate dehydrogenase deficiency: theory and practice. DICP Ann Pharmacother. 1990;24:1210–3.

41. Buzard JA, Kopko F, Paul MF. Inhibition of glutathione reductase by nitrofurantoin. J Lab Clin Med. 1960;56:885–90.

42. Dershwitz M, Novak RF. Studies of the mechanism of nitrofurantoin-mediated red cell toxicity. J Pharmacol Exp Therapeut. 1982;222:430–4.

43. Shah RR, Wade G. Reappraisal of the risk/benefit of nitrofurantoin: review of toxicity and efficacy. Adverse Drug React Acute Poisoning Rev. 1989;8:183–201.

44. Toole J, Parrish M. Nitrofurantoin polyneuropathy. Neurology. 1973;23:554–9.

45. Yiannikas C, Pollard JD, McLeod JG. Nitrofurantoin neuropathy. Austral NZ J Med. 1981;11:400–5.

46. Corragio MJ, Gross TP, Roscelli JD. Nitrofurantoin toxicity in children. Pediatr Infect Dis J. 1989;8:163–6.

47. Perry JE, LeBlanc AL. Transfer of nitrofurantoin across the human placenta. TX Rep Biol Med. 1967;25:265–9.

48. Wang CY, Benson RC Jr, Bryan GT. Mutagenicity for *Salmonella typhimurium* of urine obtained from humans receiving nitrofurantoin. J Natl Cancer Inst. 1977;58:871–3.

49. Hailey FJ, Fort H, Williams JC, et al. Foetal safety of nitrofurantoin macrocrystals therapy during pregnancy: A retrospective analysis. J Int Med Res. 1983;11:364–9.

50. Kass EH. Pyelonephritis and bacteriuria: A major problem in preventive medicine. Ann Intern Med. 1962;56:46–53.

51. Duca CJ, Scudi JV. Some antibacterial properties of mandelamine (methamine mandelate). Proc Soc Exp Biol Med. 1947;66:123–6.

52. Gleckman R, Alvarez S, Joubert DW, et al. Drug therapy reviews: Methamine mandelate and methenamine hippurate. Am J Hosp Pharm. 1979;36:1509–12.

53. Gandelman AL. Methenamine mandelate: antimicrobial activity in urine and correlation with formaldehyde levels. J Urol. 1967;97:533–6.

54. Musher DM, Griffith DP, Templeton BG. Further observations on the potentiation of the antibacterial effect of methenamine by acetohydroxamic acid. J Infect Dis. 1976;133:564–7.

55. Hamilton-Miller JMT, Brumfitt W. Methenamine and its salts as urinary tract antiseptics. Variables affecting the antibacterial activity of formaldehyde, mandelic acid, and hippuric acid in vitro. 1977;14:287–91.

56. Klinge E, Männistö P, Mäntylä R, et al. Pharmacokinetics of methenamine in healthy volunteers. J Antimicrob Chemother. 1982;9:209–16.

57. Mayrer AR, Andriole VT. Urinary tract antiseptics. Med Clin North Am. 1982;66:199–208.

58. Allgén L-G, Holmberg G, Persson B, et al. Biological fate of methenamine in man. Absorption, renal excretion and passage into umbilical cord blood, amniotic fluid and breast milk. Acta Obstet Gynecol Scand. 1979;58:287–93.

59. Knoefel PK, Huang KC. Biochemorphology of renal tubular transport: Hippuric acid and related substances. J Pharmacol Exp Ther. 1959;126:296–303.

60. Strom JG, Jun HW. Effect of urine pH and ascorbic acid on the rate of conversion of methenamine to formaldehyde. Biopharmaceut Drug Dispos. 1993;14:61–9.

61. Musher DM, Griffith DP. Generation of formaldehyde from methenamine: Effect of pH and concentration, and antibacterial effect. Antimicrob Agents Chemother. 1974;6:708–11.

62. Musher DM, Griffith DP, Richie Y. The generation of formaldehyde from methenamine. Effect of urinary flow and residual volume. Invest Urol. 1976;13:380–2.

63. Cronberg S, Welin C-O, Henriksson L, et al. Prevention of recurrent acute cystitis by methenamine hippurate: Double blind controlled crossover long term study. Br Med J. 1987;294:1507–8.

64. Harding GKM, Ronald AR. A controlled study of antimicrobial prophylaxis of recurrent urinary tract infection in women. N Engl J Med. 1974;291:597–601.

65. Kasanen A, Junnila SYT, Kaarsalo E, et al. Secondary prevention of recurrent urinary tract infections. Comparison of the effect of placebo, methenamine hippurate, nitrofurantoin and trimethoprim alone. Scand J Infect Dis. 1982;14:293–6.

66. Brumfitt W, Cooper J, Hamilton-Miller JMT. Prevention of recurrent urinary tract infections in women: A comparative trial between nitrofurantoin and methenamine hippurate. J Urol. 1981;126:71–4.

67. Holland NH, West CD. Prevention of recurrent urinary tract infections in girls. Am J Dis Child. 1963;105:560–7.

68. Elo J, Sarna S, Ahava K, et al. Methenamine hippurate in urinary tract infections in children: Prophylaxis, treatment and side effects. J Antimicrob Chemother. 1978;4:355–65.

69. Vainrub B, Musher DM. Lack of effect of methenamine in suppression of, or prophylaxis against, chronic urinary tract infection. Antimicrob Agents Chemother. 1977;12:625–9.

70. Kevorkian CG, Merritt JL, Ilstrup DM. Methenamine mandelate with acidification: An effective urinary antiseptic in patients with neurogenic bladder. Mayo Clin Proc. 1984;59:523–9.

71. Ross RR, Conway GF. Hemorrhagic cystitis following accidental overdose of methenamine mandelate. Am J Dis Child. 1970;119:86–7.

72. Kasanen A, Mustakallio EK, Koskinen EH. Methenamine hippurate in the treatment of urinary tract infections. Ann Clin Res. 1974;6:279–84.

73. Furness MB, McDonald PJ, Beasley NV. Urinary antiseptics in asymptomatic bacteriuria of pregnancy. NZ Med J. 1974;81:417–9.

29. TOPICAL ANTIBACTERIALS

ALLAN R. TUNKEL

Topical antibacterial therapy has several advantages over oral or parenteral administration of antibacterial agents (Table 1).[1] Following direct application of small amounts of compounds directly to an infection or wound, very high local drug concentrations are achieved. This broadens the in vitro spectrum of the antibacterial agent, permitting use of compounds that might be too toxic if large amounts or systemic administration were required. Following topical administration, the drug first enters the skin as the target organ, a variable quantity is distributed throughout the body, and then it is eliminated. Concentrations of a topical antibacterial decline from the skin surface to the subcutis, the opposite of which occurs after systemic administration.[2] Therefore, topical antibacterial is favored if the pathologic process is in the epidermis or papillary dermis. For infection in the lower dermis or subcutis, one needs to determine whether topical antibacterial administration yields the necessary drug concentrations to eradicate the infection effectively. Mixtures of antibacterial agents can also be used, which lead to synergistic effects and may delay selection of resistant microorganisms. The following section reviews the general uses of topical antibacterial agents in the therapy and prevention of infections. Although topical agents are also effective in the therapy of eye and ear infections, these indications are reviewed in Chapters 43 and 92.

GENERAL USES OF TOPICAL ANTIBACTERIALS

Disinfecting the Skin

Some topical antibacterial agents are very effective at decreasing the number of bacteria on the skin. The ideal agent should

TABLE 1. Advantages of Topical Antibacterial Therapy

Ease of administration
Lower potential for adverse reactions
Lower risk of noncompliance
Delivery of high drug concentrations to the site of infection
Decreased risk of bacterial resistance or cross-resistance
Cost savings[a]

[a] Depends on agent used.

have the following properties: broad antimicrobial spectrum; rapid bactericidal activity; persistent activity on the skin; absence of irritating, allergic, or toxic reactions; absence of systemic absorption; activity in the presence of body fluids (e.g., blood); and be cosmetically acceptable.[1] Unfortunately, no single compound fulfills all of these criteria. Depending on the specific clinical situation, however, only certain properties may be required. For example, for repeated hand washings (e.g., by medical personnel), lack of irritation and persistence of activity are essential properties. In contrast, for preparation of operative sites, rapid bactericidal activity is needed.

Several topical antibacterial agents have been used as skin disinfectants. Alcohols are rapidly bactericidal, but have a transient action and are irritating, especially with repeated use or when applied to damaged skin. This contrasts with chlorhexidine, a cationic bisbiguanide that derives its activity by causing disruption of microbial cell membranes and precipitation of cell contents; it is the most ideal agent for skin cleaning and surgical scrubs. Its valuable properties include persistent activity on the skin when used regularly, rapid bactericidal activity, a broad antibacterial spectrum, little evidence of irritancy or allergy, activity in the presence of body fluids, and minimal absorption. Hexachlorophene, despite its remarkable persistence on the skin when used regularly, has lost favor as a skin disinfecting agent. It does not have a very effective gram-negative spectrum, and absorption, with resultant toxicity (especially in newborns), has been a concern. Iodophores (e.g., providone iodine) are organic complexes consisting of iodine and a carrier (e.g., poly-vinylpyrrolidone) that slowly liberate iodine on reduction. These agents have a broad antimicrobial spectrum, although antibacterial activity does not persist on the skin and iodophors may be inactivated by body fluids. Their microbicidal effects are the result of cell wall penetration, oxidation, and substitution of microbial contents with free iodine. The iodophors are widely used for preoperative skin preparation, hand scrubbing, and for treatment and prevention of skin infections.[1]

PROPHYLAXIS

Infection in Clean Wounds

When a wound leads to disruption in epidermal integrity (i.e., secondary to abrasions, cuts, or bites), one can consider application of a topical antibacterial agent to prevent infection from developing. However, no antibacterial formulation has ever been proven to be efficacious in the prophylaxis of clean wounds because so few clean wounds become infected. Studies of topical preparations (e.g., neomycin, alone or in combination with bacitracin and/or polymyxin) have shown efficacy in prevention of infection in some circumstances, although these studies have been criticized because of the absence of control groups.[3] Controlled studies are unlikely to be performed, however, because the number of patients required to be studied would be extremely large. To avoid the difficulties in performing a large, randomized controlled trial, a human skin infection model was developed to test the efficacy of topical antibiotic formulations in the prophylaxis of minor skin infections.[3,4] Following induction of abrasion-type wounds in human volunteers, the wounds were inoculated with either 10^5 *Staphylococcus aureus* or 10^7 *Streptococcus pyogenes* and covered with an impermeable dressing for 6 hours. Each site was then treated with a combina-

tion of neomycin-bacitracin-polymyxin or the bland ointment vehicle. Both neomycin and bacitracin were highly effective in preventing infection with both *Staph. aureus* and *Strep. pyogenes*. The treated wounds did not develop pus and reepithelialized within 3–5 days. Other investigators have also found that use of either topical neomycin-bacitracin-polymyxin ointment or bacitracin alone enhanced epidermal healing of wounds.[5,6]

Despite these studies, the efficacy of topical antibacterials in the prevention of infections in clean wounds remains questionable. It is likely that topical antibiotics will continue to be used in this situation. The use of topical antibacterials for a few days in superficial wounds until the integrity of the epidermis is reestablished has been recommended, since the longer the epidermal barrier remains defective, the more likely infection is to occur. An important principle is that the agent does no harm and should not be irritating, toxic, sensitizing, or lead to development of organisms resistant to therapeutically important antimicrobial agents.

Infection in Operative Wounds

There is good evidence from both controlled and uncontrolled trials that topical antibacterials are efficacious in the prevention of postoperative wound infections; a significant decrease in wound infections has been reported in treated patients. In one study involving more than 6000 cases over a 4-year period,[7] a declining rate of infection was documented with the increased use of a neomycin-bacitracin-polymyxin spray during operations. When the neomycin-bacitracin-polymyxin spray was compared with no prophylaxis in 851 surgical wounds,[8] a significant decrease in wound infection was noted in the treatment group. Other investigators have noted similar results in controlled clinical trials,[9,10] indicating the importance of preoperative topical antibacterials in prophylaxis of operative wounds. The iodophors (e.g., providone iodine) are currently the most commonly used topical agents for preoperative skin preparation, producing a rapid, significant reduction in skin microbial counts.[11]

Catheter-Related Infections

Many authorities have recommended the use of topical antibacterial agents for prophylaxis against bacterial colonization of central and peripheral intravascular catheter sites,[12–15] although the efficacy of this practice in prevention of catheter-associated bacteremia remains unclear. In one prospective evaluation if 827 random catheter insertions employing three regimens of catheter care (neomycin-bacitracin-polymyxin at insertion and every 48 hours versus iodophor ointment at insertion and every 48 hours vs. no ointment), no differences in catheter-acquired sepsis (two cases in each group) or local inflammation (38.9 vs. 41.9 vs. 41.7 percent, respectively) were noted.[16] The only differences were in semiquantitative cultures of catheter tips, with six positive cultures in the neomycin-bacitracin-polymyxin group, 10 in the iodophor group, and 18 in the no treatment group. Therefore, the clinical utility of these compounds in prevention of catheter-related infections remains controversial.

THERAPY OF PYODERMAS

The major pyoderma in which topical antibacterials have been utilized is impetigo. Impetigo is a superficial infection of the skin caused by group A streptococci (see Ch. 176) and/or *Staph. aureus*. Bullous impetigo is usually caused by *Staph. aureus*. One of the goals of antimicrobial therapy in impetigo is to prevent spread of infection to uninvolved skin.[1] Early uncontrolled and controlled trials of topical antibacterial therapy in patients with impetigo suggested efficacy of topical antibacterials, although other studies found that systemic antimicrobial therapy was more efficacious.[17] Despite this controversy, it appears that systemic antimicrobial therapy is somewhat superior to topical therapy in the management of streptococcal pyoderma with swifter healing and fewer failures. However, topical therapy may be utilized early in infection when the number of lesions are few and there is a reasonable chance that these agents will be scrupulously and skillfully applied.[17] Exclusions to the use of topical antibacterials in pyodermas include the following: bullous impetigo (because the pathogenesis of this exfoliative infection may lead to continuing infection, rapid spread, and/or recurrence unless *Staph. aureus* is promptly eradicated); extensive pyoderma, regardless of the clinical form or bacterial etiology; and children with poststreptococcal pyodermal nephritis and their infected contacts.[18] However, systemic antimicrobial therapy for streptococcal pyoderma does not guarantee prevention of poststreptococcal glomerulonephritis,[17] although prompt eradication of nephritogenic streptococci may lessen the risk of spread to others, with subsequent prevention of secondary cases. A newer topical antibacterial, mupirocin, has been shown to be as efficacious as systemic antibiotics in the therapy of limited impetigo (see below).

Topical antibacterial agents may have some efficacy in the therapy of secondary pyodermas, although the available studies generally did not include control groups.[17] Despite organism eradication, the underlying process persisted. Therefore, cure, in the sense of complete healing, was not achieved. Since topical antibacterials can lower the bacterial colony counts in acute dermatitis, the use of these agents in combination with topical glucocorticoids is a logical treatment regimen.[1] Topical antibacterials have also been evaluated in the prevention of pyodermas. Prophylactic administration of a neomycin-bacitracin-polymyxin combination has been shown to lead to a significant reduction of streptococcal skin colonization and subsequent infection of small skin traumas in children during the summer season.[18,19] There is no role for topical antibacterials in the treatment of erysipelas, cellulitis, or furuncles; erythrasma may respond.

PREVENTION OF INFECTION OF BURN WOUNDS

Prevention of infection in the burned patient is extremely difficult since burn wound sites are favorable for bacterial overgrowth, the epidermal barrier is often defective for extended periods of time, and the patients are in the hospital where multiple antibiotic-resistant organisms are found.[1] Frequent débridement and establishment of an epidermis, or a surrogate such as skin graft or skin substitute, is essential for prevention of infection. As a result of the pathogenesis and pathophysiology of the burn wound, the delivery of systemic antimicrobial therapy to the deepest, most severely ischemic areas of the wound cannot be relied on because gradient diffusion from the wound periphery is the sole means of access.[20] The use of topical antibacterial agents for burned patients is well established. After administration, high antimicrobial concentrations are found on the wound surface where the risk of bacterial contamination is the greatest. In patients with deep, extensive wounds, dense bacterial colonization, particularly by gram-positive cocci, often occurs within 24 hours; aerobic gram-negative bacilli typically appear within 3–7 days. If this initial bacterial colonization is not treated, deeper spread and ultimate systemic invasion of pathogenic bacteria can occur. Therefore, topical antibacterial therapy should be initiated as soon as possible to delay or prevent these processes.

There is evidence that effective topical antibacterial therapy delays colonization of the burn wound for a variable period (measured in days, not weeks); maintains the wound bacterial density at lower levels than can otherwise be achieved and for appreciable intervals (measured in weeks); and tends to result in a relatively homogeneous and less diverse wound flora than would otherwise be expected.[20] The specific antimicrobial agent chosen for topical therapy should have a broad in vitro spectrum

of activity against gram-positive cocci (staphylococci, streptococci, and enterococci) and the aerobic gram-negative flora (including *Pseudomonas aeruginosa*). Ideally the agent should penetrate the eschar, but may be absorbed so must have low toxicity[21]; the agent must also remain active in the presence of serum and necrotic debris. Successful use of topical agents prevents the bacterial conversion of superficial burns to deeper injury, results in spontaneous healing of wounds that initially appeared clinically to be full thickness, and decreases the frequency of episodes of systemic sepsis.[20] Specific topical agents for use in burned patients are discussed in Chapter 298.

TREATMENT OF ACNE VULGARIS

Topical antibacterials are helpful for inflammatory acne.[22] Benzoyl peroxide exerts its effects by bacteriostatic activity on the proliferation of *Propionibacterium acnes*.[23] Oxygen is liberated when the drug is decomposed by cysteine in the skin, and bacterial proteins are thus oxidized.[24] Following 2 weeks of daily application, a 10% benzoyl peroxide preparation reduces concentrations of free fatty acids by about 50 percent and *Pr. acnes* by about 98 percent, comparable to the results obtained with use of many antibiotics after 4 weeks of use. Gel bases of benzoyl peroxide are more effective vehicles than creams or oil-based lotions.[22] Contact irritation may be a problem.

Topical antibiotics are also used almost universally by dermatologists for the treatment of acne vulgaris[22,25]; these agents also exert their beneficial effects by decreasing the population of *Pr. acnes* in the follicle, although not as effectively or rapidly as benzoyl peroxide.[26] Preparations containing clindamycin and erythromycin are most commonly used[22,27–29]; topical tetracyclines have also been utilized.[30,31]

ELIMINATION OF STAPHYLOCOCCUS AUREUS NASAL CARRIAGE

Approximately 20–40 percent of normal persons carry *Staph. aureus* in their anterior nares.[32] In hospitalized patients, serious infection caused by *Staph. aureus* may occur secondary to autoinoculation onto susceptible sites or transfer of organisms from another patient or staff member who is a carrier.[33–35] Attempts to control these outbreaks have included methods to eradicate nasal carriage of offending staphylococci by means of systemic or topical antimicrobial agents; recolonization is frequent, however, and development of resistance has been reported. Numerous topical antibacterial agents have been utilized in the nasal eradication of *Staph. aureus*, with varying degrees of success (see below).

SPECIFIC TOPICAL ANTIBACTERIALS

Numerous topical antibacterial agents are available for clinical use in various concentrations, vehicles, and mixtures (Table 2). The following sections review in detail the more common topical antibacterials in general use. Antimicrobial agents such as clindamycin, erythromycin, tetracycline, and gentamicin, although utilized as topical agents, are covered in other chapters of this book and will not be discussed here.

Bacitracin

Mechanism of Action.   Bacitracin is a polypeptide antibiotic produced by *Bacillus subtilis*. There are three bacitracins subgrouped as A, B, and C; subgroup A is the major constituent of commercial preparations.[36] Bacitracin contains a thiazolidine ring and peptide side chains. After administration, it forms a complex with C55-prenol pyrophosphate, a component of the bacterial cell wall. This molecule acts as a carrier involved in the transfer of polysaccharides, peptidoglycans, and lipopoly-

TABLE 2. Selected Topical Antibacterial Agents in Clinical Use

Topical Antibacterial (Trade Name)	Concentrations	Frequency	Indications
Benzoyl peroxide	5%, 10%	1–2 times daily	Acne
Chloramphenicol (Chloromycetin)	1%	3–4 times daily	Skin infections
Chlortetracycline (Aureomycin)	3%	2 times daily	Acne vulgaris
Clindamycin (Cleocin)[a]	1%, 2%	2 times daily	Acne vulgaris; bacterial vaginosis
Erythromycin (A/T/S; Emgel; Erycette; Romycin; T-Stat; Theramycin; Erygel; Erymax; Erythra-derm; Akne-mycin)	2%	2 times daily	Acne vulgaris
Erythromycin-benzoyl peroxide	3–5%	2 times daily	Acne vulgaris
Fusidic acid (Fucidin)[b]	2%	3 times daily	Skin infections
Gentamicin (Garamycin; G-myticin)	0.1%	3–4 times daily	Skin infections
Mafenide (Sulfamylon)	10%	2 times daily	Burns
Metronidazole (Metrogel)	0.75%	2 times daily	Inflammatory pustules, papules, and rosacea; bacterial vaginosis
Mupirocin (Bactroban)	2% ointment	3 times daily	Skin infections; elimination of nasopharyngeal carriage of Staph. aureus
Neomycin-dexamethasone (Neodecadron)	3.5 mg/g–0.1%	3–4 times daily	Corticosteroid-responsive dermatoses with secondary infection
Nitrofurazone (Furacin)	0.2%	1 time daily	Burns; skin grafting
Polymyxin B-bacitracin-neomycin (Neosporin)[c]	5000 units/g-400 units/g-3.5 mg/g	1–3 times daily	Prevention of infection in minor cuts, scrapes, burns
Polymyxin B-neomycin-hydrocortisone (Corticosporin)	10,000 units/g-3.5 mg/g-0.5%	2–4 times daily	Corticosteroid-responsive dermatoses with secondary infection
Silver sulfadiazine (SSD; Silvadene)	1%	1–2 times daily	Burns
Tetracycline (Topicycline; Achromycin)	3%	2 times daily	Acne vulgaris

[a] 2% formulation recommended for bacterial vaginosis.
[b] Not licensed in the United States.
[c] Maximum strength formulation contains 10,000 units/g polymyxin B, 500 units/g bacitracin, and 3.5 mg/g neomycin.

saccharides to the growing cell wall.[37] Thus, formation of the bacterial cell wall is stunted.

In Vitro Spectrum of Activity. The spectrum of activity of bacitracin is primarily against gram-positive organisms: staphylococci, streptococci, corynebacteria, and clostridia.[36] Development of resistance to bacitracin is rare, although it has been reported in Staph. aureus.

Clinical Uses. Topical bacitracin has been used for many years, although its efficacy in controlled clinical trials has never been shown. In impetigo, bacitracin ointment was shown to be 80 percent effective in clearing pathogenic organisms,[18] although slow or delayed healing was noted in one-third of those patients cured. Bacitracin was least effective for bullous impetigo in which four of six patients continued to develop new lesions, requiring systemic erythromycin therapy. Bacitracin has also been evaluated in eradication of nasal carriage of Staph. aureus, although its efficacy has never been shown.[38,39] One study demonstrated lack of efficacy of bacitracin in nasal eradication of staphylococci when compared to oral rifampin.[40] For topical use, bacitracin is often formulated with neomycin and/or polymyxin B (Table 2).

Adverse Effects. Toxicity with bacitracin is minimal. Minor skin irritation may occur. Cases of anaphylaxis have been reported after topical administration of bacitracin to open lesions[36,41,42]; these patients had multiple previous exposures to the drug. Itching and swelling were noted prior to the episode of anaphylaxis as a result of direct histamine release.[43] Rarely, an allergic contact dermatitis has been reported.[44] Since bacitracin and polymyxin B are both derived from Bacillus spp., cross-reactivity between the two agents may occur.[45]

Neomycin

Mechanism of Action. Neomycin is an aminoglycoside antibiotic isolated from cultures of Streptomyces fradiae.[36] The mechanism of action involves inhibition of protein synthesis by binding to the 30S subunit of the bacterial ribosome, leading to misreading of the genetic code; neomycin may also inhibit the bacterial DNA polymerase.[46]

In Vitro Spectrum of Activity. Neomycin has in vitro activity against many gram-positive and gram-negative bacteria, including Escherichia coli, Haemophilus influenzae, Proteus spp., Staph. aureus, and Serratia spp. Pseudomonas aeruginosa is generally resistant.[47] There is minimal in vitro activity against streptococci, although at the high concentrations achieved on the skin, Strep. pyogenes are probably killed by topical neomycin preparations.[1] Resistance to neomycin has been reported in both gram-positive and gram-negative bacteria[17,36] and can be plasmid mediated; resistance to other aminoglycosides such as kanamycin and gentamicin may be on the same plasmid. By following sequential acquisition of plasmids of Staph. aureus strains in patients treated with neomycin, the Staph. aureus became resistant by acquisition of plasmids derived from coagulase-negative staphylococci that form part of the normal skin flora.[48]

Clinical Uses. Neomycin is widely used in combination with other antibiotics, antifungals, and corticosteroids because of its availability, relatively low cost, and perceived efficacy.[3,17] There are few well-controlled clinical trials documenting the efficacy and safety of topical neomycin.[18] Neomycin has recently been shown to enhance reepithelialization in wound healing.[6] In view of its well-documented contact sensitivity, possible systemic toxicity, cross-reaction with other antibiotics, and emergence of resistance, it is difficult to recommend the use of topical neomycin in the treatment of superficial skin infections.[36]

Adverse Reactions. Neomycin is not absorbed through intact skin, although application to denuded or damaged epithelium can lead to sensitization and systemic toxicity.[47] Following systemic absorption, neomycin is excreted by the kidney. Patients with decreased renal function may develop ototoxicity that is irreversible and may progress after discontinuation of the drug.

Allergic contact sensitivity is widely reported with a prevalence of 1–6 percent and an incidence of 3–6 percent.[17,47,49] The incidence of hypersensitivity, as assessed by patch testing, in 390 patients with suspected contact dermatitis to topical medications, was approximately 36 percent.[50] Sensitivity is most likely to occur with chronic use on inflamed skin. Sensitivity to neomycin was reported in 49 percent of patients with a history of allergy to any topical agent.[36] Neomycin may also cause mast cell degranulation and histamine release.

Polymyxin B

Mechanism of Action. Polymyxin B is isolated from the aerobic gram-positive rod *Bacillus polymyxa*, a soil organism.[51] The polymyxins are cationic branched cyclic decapeptides that act to destroy bacterial membranes with a surface detergentlike mechanism by interacting with membrane phospholipids and increasing cellular permeability.

In Vitro Spectrum of Activity

The spectrum of activity of polymyxin B is almost exclusively limited to gram-negative organisms.[51] The agent is bactericidal against gram-negative organisms such as *Pseudomonas aeruginosa*, *Proteus mirabilis*, and *Serratia marcescens*[52]; some *Proteus* and *Serratia* may be resistant. There is no in vitro activity against gram-positive organisms. Although *Pseudomonas* is usually sensitive, the in vitro activity of polymyxin B against *Pseudomonas* is promptly neutralized by divalent cations at concentrations in body fluids. Organisms resistant to polymyxin B have cell walls that prevent access of the drug to the bacterial cell membrane. There is no cross-resistance with other antimicrobial agents, and resistance rarely develops during therapy.

Clinical Uses. Polymyxin B is used primarily in the prevention and treatment of minor skin infections.[51] It is most often added to neomycin and bacitracin (see above) to broaden coverage against gram-negative organisms.

Adverse Effects. Because polymyxin B binds to cell membranes with very high affinity, there is little systemic absorption and few reactions even when applied to open wounds. Contact sensitization has been reported.[45]

Mupirocin

Structure and Mechanism of Action. Mupirocin has a unique chemical structure unlike any other antimicrobial agent (Fig. 1).[53–56] It contains a short fatty acid side chain (9-hydroxy nonanoic acid) linked to monic acid by an ester linkage. Mupirocin is formulated in a bland water-miscible ointment base consisting of polyethylene glycol 400 and polyethylene glycol 3350. Mupirocin used to be called *pseudomonic acid* because its major metabolite is derived from submerged fermentation by *Pseudomonas fluorescens*.[57] Pseudomonic acid A represents 90–95 percent of the pseudomonic acid family and is responsible for most of the antibacterial activity; three other minor metabolites of similar chemical structure and antimicrobial spectrum have been denoted as pseudomonic acids B, C, and D.[53] Mupirocin

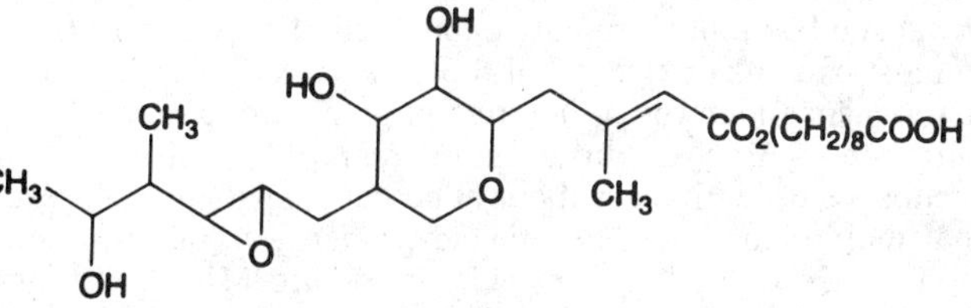

inhibits bacterial RNA and protein synthesis by binding to bacterial isoleucyl-tRNA synthetase, which catalyzes the formation of isoleucyl-tRNA from isoleucine and tRNA.[58,59] This prevents incorporation of isoleucine into protein chains of the bacterial cell wall, leading to arrest of protein synthesis. Only one other naturally occurring substance, furanomycin, which is isolated from a *Streptomyces* spp., also inhibits bacterial isoleucyl-tRNA synthetase, although this agent has no clinical utility.[57] Because of this unique mechanism of action, there is no cross reaction of mupirocin with other antimicrobial agents.

In Vitro Spectrum of Activity. The antibacterial spectrum of mupirocin is shown in Table 3.[53,57,60] Mupirocin is bacteriostatic at low concentrations near the minimal inhibitory concentration (MIC) for *Staph. aureus*, but bactericidal at concentrations achieved by topical administration (20,000 µg/ml with the 2% formulation) after 24–36 hours of exposure.[53,60,61] It is highly active in vitro against methicillin-resistant strains of *Staph. aureus* (MRSA), staphylococcal strains resistant to other antibacterials (e.g., penicillin, streptomycin, neomycin, erythromycin, fusidic acid, lincomycin, chloramphenicol, and tetracycline), and streptococci that are associated with primary and secondary skin infections.[53] The exception to the antistreptococcal activity of mupirocin is the enterococcus.[60] Mupirocin is inactive in vitro against *Pseudomonas aeruginosa*, anaerobes, fungi, and the Enterobacericeae. An important feature of mupirocin's antibacterial spectrum is its weaker in vitro activity against the normal skin flora (e.g., *Micrococcus*, *Corynebacterium*, and *Propionibacterium* spp.), which are part of the skin's natural defense against infection. The in vitro antibacterial activity of mupirocin

TABLE 3. Antibacterial Activity of Mupirocin Against Selected Bacteria

Organism and Strain	MIC (µg/ml)
Gram-positive cocci	
Streptococcus pyogenes 421	0.12
Streptococcus pneumoniae 1959	0.12
Staphylococcus aureus ATCC 25923	0.25
Staphylococcus epidermidis 54815	0.5
Streptococcus agalactiae 9579	0.5
Streptococcus sanguis	1
Peptostreptococcus anaerobius 3395	32
Enterococcus faecium 98-D	32
Enterococcus faecalis I	64
Peptococcus prevotii 372.5	>128
Microboccus luteus ATCC 9341	>128
Gram-positive bacilli	
Bacillus subtilis ATCC 6633	0.12
Erysipelothrix rhusiopathiae	8
Listeria monocytogenes NCTC 5348	8
Clostridium difficile 12328	32
Clostridium sporogenes 532	32
Bacillus anthracis NCTC 8234	64
Corynebacterium hofmannii M8	64
Corynebacterium xerosis 9755	>128
Corynebacterium jekeium	>128
Propionibacterium acnes 10162	>128
Gram-negative cocci	
Neisseria gonorrhoeae WHO V	0.05
Neisseria meningitidis 1990	0.05
Moraxella catarrhalis 1502	0.2
Gram-negative bacilli	
Bordetella pertussis 2420	0.02
Haemophilus influenzae Q1	0.12
Pasteurella multocida 1633	0.25
Proteus vulgaris X	64
Enterobacter cloacae 10005	64
Enterobacter aerogenes T660	128
Citrobacter freundii W18	128
Escherichia coli NCTC 10418	128
Klebsiella pneumoniae A	128
Proteus mirabilis 889	128
Serratia marcescens US9	1600
Morganella morganii F	6400
Pseudomonas aeruginosa R3	6400
Bacteroides fragilis BC4	>6400

(Data from refs. 53, 57, 60.)

FIG. 1. Structure of mupirocin.

is greatest at an acidic pH, which is advantageous because of the low pH of the skin; in one study, mupirocin was four- to eightfold more active in vitro at pH 6 than at pH 7.[60]

Long-term therapy with mupirocin can lead to development of resistant staphylococci,[62–65] an effect that is irreversible. This resistance can be induced in *Staph. aureus* by subculturing the organisms onto media containing increasing concentrations of the drug.[57] Naturally occurring clones of staphylococci with low-level resistance to mupirocin (MIC < 100 µg/ml) have been described,[56] although their clinical significance is unclear since the concentration of mupirocin in ointment exceeds 20,000 µg/ml. High-level mupirocin resistance (MIC > 700 µg/ml) has emerged in both MRSA and *Staph. epidermidis,* associated with clinical treatment failure.[63,66] In one study,[63] resistance emerged in three patients treated with mupirocin for months and, in addition, from patients never treated with mupirocin, suggesting the possibility of cross infection. In another study of 144 patients with epidermolysis bullosa, many of whom received continuous application of mupirocin for as long as 4 consecutive years, five isolates of *Staph. aureus* were resistant to mupirocin[53]; four of the five patients with resistant isolates had a less favorable response to mupirocin and required systemic antistaphylococcal therapy. Most mupirocin-resistant staphylococcal isolates have been found in patients with chronic skin infections, many of whom had been treated with prolonged courses of mupirocin.[56] Therefore, mupirocin should be used intermittently rather than continuously.

Several mechanisms have been advanced to explain mupirocin resistance in staphylococci. Low-level resistance is likely mediated by altered access to binding sites on isoleucyl-tRNA synthetase, whereas high-level resistance appears to be mediated by a transferable plasmid that codes for a modified isoleucyl-tRNA synthetase[56,67]; it has been suggested that high-level resistance may have evolved by the conjugate transfer of plasmids from enterococci,[68–70] which are inherently resistant to mupirocin. A recent study has demonstrated that two different isoleucyl-tRNA synthetase enzymes are present in highly mupirocin-resistant *Staph. aureus* isolates (MIC ≥ 512 µg/ml), whereas only a chromosomally encoded isoleucyl-tRNA synthetase was detected in strains expressing intermediate levels of resistance (MIC between 8 and 256 µg/ml).[71]

Pharmacokinetics. Following systemic administration, mupirocin is immediately metabolized to monic acid, which is bacteriologically inactive and rapidly eliminated (plasma half-life of < 30 minutes).[55] Mupirocin is not appreciably absorbed after topical administration to intact skin. In one study, a mean of 0.24 percent of applied radiolabeled ointment was absorbed through intact skin after 24 hours of occlusion.[72] Greater penetration of mupirocin is expected in damaged or diseased skin. Any drug that is absorbed, however, is converted to monic acid, formed by deesterification of mupirocin at the ester linkage between the side chain and nucleus, and rapidly eliminated in the urine[36]; monic acid is not microbiologically active. Skin can also metabolize mupirocin to its inactive metabolite, but at a rate below 3 percent. Therefore, because only small amounts of mupirocin penetrate skin and equally small amounts are degraded, most of the drug is available to act at skin level. Because mupirocin is highly protein bound (approximately 95 percent), its activity decreases in the presence of serum.[53]

Clinical Uses. Mupirocin is used primarily in skin infections such as impetigo and folliculitis, which are usually caused by *Staph. aureus* and *Strep. pyogenes.* In trials of mupirocin alone in the therapy of impetigo (772 evaluable patients),[73–79] clinical cure rates ranged from 81 to 100 percent and bacterial elimination rates from 67 to 100 percent. Several trials have shown mupirocin to be more effective in the treatment of impetigo than its polyethylene glycol vehicle, which also has antibacterial activity. Clinical cure and bacterial elimination rates have ranged

from 85 to 100 percent and 80 to 95 percent, respectively, for mupirocin vs. 12–84 percent and 12–63 percent, respectively, for the vehicle.[57,73,80–82] Since impetigo is a self-limiting condition, bacteriologic results are a more appropriate assessment of efficacy since elimination of pathogens can be used to ascertain infection resolution. In eight comparative trials of mupirocin vs. several other topical antibacterials (neomycin, fusidic acid, chlortetracycline, polymyxin B-bacitracin-neomycin),[73,83–86] six found mupirocin to be the more effective agent. Multiple studies have also compared topical mupirocin to systemic antibiotics (erythromycin, cloxacillin, dicloxacillin, flucloxacillin, ampicillin) in the therapy of impetigo, in which topical mupirocin was as, or more, effective than the oral agent.[73,87–94] In many of these studies, however, the entry criteria excluded patients who, in the judgment of the investigator, had too many lesions to allow reliable compliance with topical therapy.[95] No studies have shown that topical therapy is as effective as systemic antimicrobial therapy for treatment of widespread, extensive lesions.

Mupirocin is effective for the treatment of secondarily infected eczema, burns, lacerations, and leg ulcers. In one study in which 33 centers contributed a total of 1030 cases,[57] mupirocin ointment produced significantly better bacteriologic and clinical responses than its vehicle in the treatment of secondary skin infections. Of 851 evaluable patients with 1131 pathogens, mupirocin eliminated 87 percent (505/583) of pathogens vs. only 53 percent (288/548) with the vehicle. In a double-blind, vehicle-controlled study, mupirocin successfully eradicated 85 percent of *Staph. aureus* in 33 patients compared with a 6 percent eradication rate in the vehicle-treated group[96]; for all pathogens, the success rate of mupirocin vs. the vehicle was 69 percent vs. 14 percent, respectively. Comparative trials have also demonstrated the efficacy of mupirocin compared with other topical antibacterials and systemic antimicrobial agents in the treatment of secondary skin infections.[85,87,88,94]

Mupirocin can also eliminate nasal carriage of *Staph. aureus.* In three blinded, placebo-controlled trials conducted in health care workers with *Staph. aureus* nasal carriage,[97–99] virtually all persons treated with mupirocin were initially cleared of the carrier state compared with a 0–18 percent rate of clearance following treatment with placebo; in one of the studies, a corresponding effect on eradication of hand carriage at 72 hours of therapy was also found.[98] However, relapse following therapy occurred in 19–59 percent of persons after 4–12 weeks of evaluation. Relapses could have resulted from reinoculation of the nares with staphylococci from an untreated site (e.g., skin, perineum, rectum) or by reinfection with new staphylococcal strains after the completion of therapy. Mupirocin has been evaluated in acute carrier outbreaks of epidemic MRSA.[100–105] Mupirocin was effective in clearing MRSA from nearly all patients and staff, although these studies were uncontrolled and it is difficult to know whether the development of negative cultures in these patients can be attributed to therapy with mupirocin or to a transient carrier state. Recently mupirocin has been evaluated in the control of MRSA in facilities for rehabilitation and long-term care.[106,107] Mupirocin was effective in elimination of chronic nasal MRSA colonization, although in one study transient recolonization occurred in about 44 percent of patients.[107] In another study of 65 patients colonized with MRSA at a Veterans Affairs long-term-care facility, mupirocin (applied to the nares for the first 7 months and to the nares and wounds for the second 5 months) rapidly eliminated MRSA at sites treated in most patients by the end of the first week.[108] Despite weekly maintenance mupirocin therapy, 40 percent of patients had recurrence of MRSA. Furthermore, mupirocin-resistant MRSA strains were identified in about 11 percent of patients, suggesting that mupirocin should be utilized primarily in outbreak situations and not in facilities with endemic MRSA colonization.[56,109,110] Well-controlled clinical trials are needed to clarify these issues.

Adverse Effects. Mupirocin is not associated with substantial toxicity in humans because of its very low affinity for mammalian isoleucyl-tRNA synthetase. The propylene glycol base may irritate mucous membranes and eroded skin. There is minimal potential for inducing allergic contact dermatitis. The drug is not phototoxic. Local effects such as itching, stinging, or rash have been reported when mupirocin is used on broken skin or mucous membranes. No photosensitivity reactions have occurred. In experimental rat and rabbit models, mupirocin has been shown to be without teratogenic effects, embryotoxicity, or effects on fertility and reproduction in doses up to 160 mg/kg/day.[57] Prolonged use may lead to overgrowth of nonsusceptible organisms such as fungi.

Fusidic Acid

Mechanism of Action. Fusidic acid is isolated from culture media of the mold *Fusidium coccineum*.[36] Chemically it is a carboxylic acid belonging to the group of tetracycline triterpenes. Fusidic acid is lipophilic. It penetrates intact epidermis at approximately the same rate as glucocorticoids and penetrates both intact and damaged skin.[111] Fusidic acid inhibits bacterial protein synthesis primarily by interfering with elongation factor G (translocase) (see Ch. 19).[112]

In Vitro Spectrum of Activity. Fusidic acid has a narrow antibacterial spectrum, mainly against gram-positive bacteria; there is an exceptionally high in vitro activity against *Staph. aureus* (MIC range of 0.04–0.16 μg/ml). There is also in vitro activity against corynebacteria and clostridia. Streptococci are 100 times less sensitive (MIC range of 4.2–16 μg/ml) to fusidic acid when compared with staphylococci, but at concentrations given topically it is efficacious against both organisms. Reports from Europe have documented staphylococcal resistance to fusidic acid,[113,114] although general levels of resistance have remained low (about 1–2 percent).[115] In one report of 8176 *Staph. aureus* strains isolated from cases of bacteremia during the years 1963–1987 in Denmark, 1 percent or less of strains were resistant to fusidic acid (MIC ≥ 2 μg/ml).[116] Following topical use of fusidic acid, a rate of staphylococcal resistance of 43 percent has been reported, although other authors have not observed the emergence of resistance.[115] In vitro evidence suggests that resistance to *Staph. aureus* is less likely to occur after exposure to high concentrations of fusidic acid, reflecting the situation with topical use.

Clinical Uses. Fusidic acid has the remarkable ability to penetrate both intact and damaged skin, making it useful for treating deep infections such as paronychia or boils.[36] It also penetrates crust and cellular debris seen in impetigo and pyoderma. In comparative trials of fusidic acid for the therapy of primary and secondary skin infections, fusidic acid has been found to be equivalent or inferior to mupirocin.[73] The drug is unavailable in the United States, but has been used in the United Kingdom and Canada.

Adverse Effects. Because the structure of fusidic acid differs markedly from other antibiotics, it is unlikely to produce cross-sensitivity. There are a few reports of contact sensitivity. Although the ring structure of fusidic acid is remarkably similar to that of the glucocorticoids, there is no evidence of suppressive activity on the pituitary axis.

REFERENCES

1. Feingold DS. Antibacterial agents. In: Fitzpatrick TB, Eisen AZ, Wolff K, et al., eds. Dermatology in General Medicine. 3rd ed. New York: McGraw-Hill; 1987:2550–2.
2. Schalla W, Schaefer H. Pharmacokinetics and topical applications of drugs. In: Fitzpatrick TB, Eisen AZ, Wolff K, et al., eds. Dermatology in General Medicine. 3rd ed. New York: McGraw-Hill; 1987:2525–32.
3. Leyden JJ, Sulzberger MB. Topical antibiotics and minor skin trauma. Am Fam Physician. 1981;23:121–5.
4. Leyden JJ, Stewart R, Kligman AM. Updated in vivo methods for evaluating topical antimicrobial agents on human skin. J Invest Dermatol. 1979;72:165–70.
5. Geronemus RG, Mertz PM, Eaglstein WH. Wound healing—The effects of topical antimicrobial agents. Arch Dermatol. 1979;115:1311–4.
6. Eaglstein WH, Mertz P, Alvarez OM. Effect of topically applied agents on healing wounds. Clin Dermatol. 1984;2:112–5.
7. Forbes GB. Staphylococcal infection of operation wounds with special reference to topical antibiotic prophylaxis. Lancet. 1961;2:505–7.
8. Fielding G, Rao A, Davis NC, et al. Prophylactic topical use of antibiotics in surgical wounds: A controlled clinical trial using "polybactrin." Med J Aust. 1965;2:159–61.
9. Purssey BS. The use of an aerosol antibiotic in minor surgery. Med J Aust. 1970;1:989–92.
10. Gilmore OJA, Martin TDM, Fletcher BN. Prevention of wound infection after appendectomy. Lancet. 1973;1:220–2.
11. Larson E. Guideline for use of topical antimicrobial agents. Am J Hosp Infect. 1988;16:253–66.
12. Maki DG, Goldmann DA, Rhame FS. Infection control in intravenous therapy. Ann Intern Med. 1973;79:867–87.
13. Jarrad MM, Freeman JB. The effects of antibiotic ointments and antiseptics on the skin flora beneath subclavian catheter dressings during intravenous hyperalimentation. J Surg Res. 1977;22:521–6.
14. Maki DG. Infections due to infusion therapy. In: Bennett JV, Brachman PS, eds. Hospital Infections. 2nd ed. Boston: Little, Brown, & Company; 1986:561–80.
15. Maki DG. Epidemic nosocomial bacteremias. In: Wenzel RP, ed. Handbook of Hospital Acquired Infections. Boca Ration, FL: CRC Press; 1981:371–512.
16. Maki DG, Band JD. A comparative study of polyantibiotic and iodophor ointments in prevention of vascular catheter-related infection. Am J Med. 1981;70:739–44.
17. Leyden JJ, Kligman AM. Rationale for topical antibiotics. Cutis. 1978;22:515–28.
18. Dillon HC Jr. Topical and systemic therapy for pyodermas. Int J Dermatol. 1980;19:443–51.
19. Maddox JS, Ware JC, Dillon HC Jr. The natural history of streptococcal skin infection. Prevention with topical antibiotics. J Am Acad Dermatol. 1985;13:207–12.
20. Monafo WW, Freedman B. Topical therapy for burns. Surg Clin North Am. 1987;67:133–45.
21. Andreassi L, Flori L. Pharmacologic treatment of burns. Clin Dermatol. 1992;9:453–8.
22. Melski JW, Arndt KA. Topical therapy for acne. N Engl J Med. 1980;302:503–6.
23. Shalita AR, Leyden JE Jr, Pochi PE, et al. Acne vulgaris. J Am Acad Dermatol. 1987;16:410–2.
24. Fulton JE Jr, Farzad-Bakshandeh A, Bradley S. Studies on the mechanism of action of topical benzoyl peroxide and vitamin A. J Cutan Pathol. 1974;1:191–200.
25. Schachner L, Pestana A, Kittles C. A clinical trial comparing the safety and efficacy of a topical erythromycin-zinc formulation with a topical clindamycin formulation. J Am Acad Dermatol. 1990;22:489–95.
26. Swinyer LJ, Baker MD, Swinyer TA, et al. A comparative study of benzoyl peroxide and clindamycin phosphate for treating acne vulgaris. Br J Dermatol. 1988;119:615–22.
27. Stoughton RB. Topical antibiotics for acne vulgaris. Current usage. Arch Dermatol. 1979;115:486–9.
28. Algra RJ, Rosen T, Waisman M. Topical clindamycin in acne vulgaris: Safety and stability. Arch Dermatol. 1977;113:1390–1.
29. Fisher AA. Erythromycin "free base"—A nonsensitizing topical antibiotic for infected dermatoses and acne vulgaris. Cutis. 1977;20:17–35.
30. Blaney DJ, Cook CH. Topical use of tetracycline in the treatment of acne: A double-blind study comparing topical and oral tetracycline therapy and placebo. Arch Dermatol. 1976;112:971–3.
31. Smith JG, Chalker DK, Wehr RF. The effectiveness of topical and oral tetracycline for acne. South Med J. 1976;69:695–7.
32. Williams RE. Healthy carriage of *Staphylococcus aureus*: Its prevalence and importance. Bacteriol Rev. 1963;27:56–71.
33. Boyce JC. Methicillin-resistant *Staphylococcus aureus*. Infect Dis Clin North Am. 1989;3:901–13.
34. Duckworth GJ, Lothian JL, Williams JD. Methicillin-resistant *Staphylococcus aureus*: Report of an outbreak in a London teaching hospital. J Hosp Infect. 1988;11:1–15.
35. Thompson RL, Cabezudo I, Wenzel RP. Epidemiology of nosocomial infection caused by methicillin-resistant *Staphylococcus aureus*. Ann Intern Med. 1982;97:309–17.
36. Winkelman W, Gratton D. Topical antibacterials. Clin Dermatol. 1989;7:156–62.
37. Sleytr VB, Oliver TC, Thorne KJI. Bacitracin-induced changes in bacterial plasma membrane structure. Biochim Biophys Acta. 1976;419:570–3.
38. Yu VL, Goetz A, Wagener M, et al. *Staphylococcus aureus* nasal carriage and infection in patients on hemodialysis. Efficacy of antibiotic prophylaxis. N Engl J Med. 1986;315:91–6.
39. Bryan CS, Wilson RS, Meade P, et al. Topical antibiotic ointments for staph-

ylococcal nasal carriers: Survey of current practices and comparison of bacitracin and vancomycin ointments. Infect Cont. 1980;1:153–6.

40. McAnally TP, Lewis MR, Brown DR. Effect of rifampin and bacitracin on nasal carriers of *Staphylococcus aureus*. Antimicrob Agents Chemother. 1984;25:422–6.

41. Comaish JS, Cunliffe WJ. Absorption of drugs from varicose ulcers: A cause of anaphylaxis. Br J Clin Pract. 1967;21:97–8.

42. Roupe G, Strannegard O. Anaphylactic shock elicited by topical administration of bacitracin. Arch Dermatol. 1969;100:450–2.

43. Schecter JF, Wilkinson RD, Del Carpio J. Anaphylaxis following the use of bacitracin ointment. Arch Dermatol. 1984;120:909–11.

44. Binnick AN, Clendenning WE. Bacitracin contact dermatitis. Contact Dermatol. 1978;4:180–1.

45. Fisher AA. Adverse reactions to bacitracin, polymyxin, and gentamicin sulfate. Cutis. 1983;32:510–2.

46. Lechevalier HA. The 25 years of neomycin. CRC Crit Rev Microbiol. 1975; 359–97.

47. MacDonald RH, Beck M. Neomycin: A review with particular reference to dermatological usage. Clin Exp Dermatol. 1983;8:249–58.

48. Naidoo J, Noble WC. Acquisition of antibiotic resistance by *Staphylococcus aureus* in skin patients. J Clin Pathol. 1978;31:1187–92.

49. Gette MT, Marks JG Jr, Maloney ME. Frequency of postoperative allergic contact dermatitis to topical antibiotics. Arch Dermatol. 1992;128:365–7.

50. Bajaj AK, Gupta SC. Contact hypersensitivity to topical antibacterial agents. Int J Dermatol. 1986;25:103–5.

51. Hoeprich PD. The polymyxins. Med Clin North Am. 1970;54:1251–65.

52. Eickhoff TC, Finland M. Polymyxin B and colistin: In vitro activity against *Pseudomonas aeruginosa*. Am J Med Sci. 1965;249:172–4.

53. Pappa KA. The clinical development of mupirocin. J Am Acad Dermatol. 1990;22:873–9.

54. Parenti MA, Hatfield SM, Leyden JJ. Mupirocin: A topical antibiotic with a unique structure and mechanism of action. Clin Pharmacol. 1987;6:761–70.

55. Casewell MW, Hill RLR. Mupirocin (''pseudomonic acid'')—A promising new topical antimicrobial agent. J Antimicrob Chemother. 1987;19:1–5.

56. Bradley SF. Effectiveness of mupirocin in the control of methicillin-resistant *Staphylococcus aureus*. Infect Med. 1993;10:23–31.

57. Leyden JJ. Mupirocin: A new topical antibiotic. Semin Dermatol. 1987;6: 48–54.

58. Hughes J, Mellows G. On the mode of action of pseudomonic acid: Inhibition of protein synthesis in *Staphylococcus aureus*. J Antibiot. 1978;31:330–5.

59. Hughes J, Mellows G. Inhibition of isoleucyl-transfer ribonucleic acid synthetase in *Escherichia coli* by pseudomonic acid. Biochem J. 1978;176: 305–18.

60. Sutherland R, Boon RJ, Griffin KE, et al. Antibacterial activity of mupirocin (pseudomonic acid), a new antibiotic for topical use. Antimicrob Agents Chemother. 1985;27:495–8.

61. Casewell MW, Hill RLR. In vitro activity of mupirocin against clinical isolates of *Staphylococcus aureus*. J Antimicrob Chemother. 1985;15:523–31.

62. Baird D, Coia J. Mupirocin-resistant *Staphylococcus aureus*. Lancet. 1987; 2:387–8.

63. Rahman M, Noble WC, Cookson B. Mupirocin-resistant *Staphylococcus aureus*. Lancet. 1987;2:387.

64. Kavi J, Andrews JM, Wise R. Mupirocin-resistant *Staphylococcus aureus*. Lancet. 1987;2:1472.

65. Smith MD, Sanghrijka M, Lock S. Mupirocin-resistant *Staphylococcus aureus*. Lancet. 1987;2:1472–3.

66. Smith GE, Kennedy CTC. *Staphylococcus aureus* resistant to mupirocin. J Antimicrob Chemother. 1988;21:141–2.

67. Capobianco JO, Doran CC, Goldman RC. Mechanism of mupirocin transport into sensitive and resistant bacteria. Antimicrob Agents Chemother. 1989; 33:156–63.

68. Noble WC, Rahman M, Cookson B, et al. Transferable mupirocin-resistance. J Antimicrob Chemother. 1988;22:771–2.

69. Rahman M, Noble WC, Cookson B. Transmissible mupirocin resistance in *Staphylococcus aureus*. Epidemiol Infect. 1989;102:261–70.

70. Cookson BD. Mupirocin resistance in staphylococci. J Antimicrob Chemother. 1990;25:497–503.

71. Gilbart J, Perry CR, Slocombe B. High-level resistance in *Staphylococcus aureus*: Evidence for two distinct isoleucyl-tRNA synthetases. Antimicrob Agents Chemother. 1993;37:32–8.

72. Ward A, Campoli-Richards DM. Mupirocin: A review of its antibacterial activity, pharmacokinetic properties and therapeutic use. Drugs. 1986;32: 425–44.

73. Booth JH, Benrimoj SI. Mupirocin in the treatment of impetigo. Int J Dermatol. 1992;31:1–9.

74. Wuite J, Davies BI, Go M, et al. Pseudomonic acid: A new topical antimicrobial agent. Lancet. 1983;2:394.

75. Wuite J, Davies BI, Go MJ, et al. Pseudomonic acid, a new antibiotic for topical therapy. J Am Acad Dermatol. 1985;12:1026–31.

76. Buchvald J. An evaluation of topical mupirocin in moderately severe primary and secondary skin infections. J Int Med Res. 1988;16:66–70.

77. Phillips LM, Yogev R, Esterly NB. The efficacy of mupirocin (pseudomonic acid) in the treatment of pyoderma in children. Pediatr Emerg Care. 1985; 1:180–3.

78. Bork K, Brauers J, Kresken M. Efficacy and safety of 2% mupirocin ointment in the treatment of primary and secondary skin infections—An open multicentre trial. Br J Clin Pract. 1989;43:284–8.

79. de la Brassinne M, De Bersaques J, Vossaert K, et al. Efficacy of mupirocin 2% ointment in skin infection: Belgian prospective open multicentre study. Dermatologica. 1988;177:397–400.

80. Eells LD, Mertz PM, Piovanetti Y, et al. Topical antibiotic treatment of impetigo with mupirocin. Arch Dermatol. 1986;122:1273–6.

81. Colin M, Avon P. Comparative double-blind evaluation of a new topical antibacterial agent, mupirocin, compared with placebo in the treatment of skin and soft tissue infections. Pharmatherapeutica. 1988;5:198–203.

82. Orecchio RM, Mischler TW. A double-blind multiclinic comparative trial of mupirocin topical and its vehicle in the treatment of bacterial skin infections. Curr Ther Res. 1986;39:82–6.

83. Wilkinson RD, Carey WD. Topical mupirocin versus topical neosporin in the treatment of cutaneous infections. Int J Dermatol. 1988;27:514–5.

84. White DG, Collins PO, Rowsell RB. Topical antibiotics in the treatment of superficial skin infections in general practice: A comparison of mupirocin with sodium fusidate. J Infect. 1989;18:221–9.

85. Gilbert M. Topical 2% mupirocin versus 2% fusidic acid ointment in the treatment of primary and secondary skin infections. J Am Acad Dermatol. 1989;20:1083–7.

86. Morley PA, Munot LD. A comparison of sodium fusidate ointment and mupirocin ointment in superficial skin sepsis. Curr Med Res Opin. 1988;11:142–8.

87. Dux PH, Fields L, Pollock D. 2% topical mupirocin versus systemic erythromycin and cloxacillin in primary and secondary skin infections. Curr Ther Res. 1986;40:933–40.

88. Gratton D. Topical mupirocin versus oral erythromycin in the treatment of primary and secondary skin infections. Int J Dermatol. 1987;26:472–3.

89. Goldfarb J, Crenshaw D, O'Horo J, et al. Randomized clinical trial of topical mupirocin versus oral erythromycin for impetigo. Antimicrob Agents Chemother. 1988;32:1780–3.

90. Barton LL, Friedman AD, Sharkey AM, et al. Impetigo contagiosa. III. Comparative efficacy of oral erythromycin and topical mupirocin. Pediatr Dermatol. 1989;6:134–8.

91. McLinn S. Topical mupirocin vs. systemic erythromycin treatment for pyoderma. Pediatr Infect Dis J. 1988;7:785–90.

92. Mertz PM, Marshall DA, Eaglstein WH, et al. Topical mupirocin treatment of impetigo is equal to oral erythromycin therapy. Arch Dermatol. 1989;125: 1069–73.

93. Arrendondo JL. Efficacy and tolerance of topical mupirocin compared with oral dicloxacillin in the treatment of primary skin infections. Curr Ther Res. 1987;41:121–7.

94. Welsh O, Saenz C. Topical mupirocin compared with oral ampicillin in the treatment of primary and secondary skin infections. Curr Ther Res. 1987; 41:114–20.

95. Leyden JJ. Review of mupirocin ointment in the treatment of impetigo. Clin Pediatr. 1992;31:549–53.

96. Breneman DL. Use of mupirocin ointment in the treatment of secondarily infected dermatoses. J Am Acad Dermatol. 1990;22:886–92.

97. Casewell MW, Hill RLR. Elimination of nasal carriage of *Staphylococcus aureus* with mupirocin (''pseudomonic acid'')—A controlled study. J Antimicrob Chemother. 1986;17:365–72.

98. Reagan DR, Doebbeling BN, Pfaller MA, et al. Elimination of coincident *Staphylococcus aureus* nasal and hand carriage with intranasal application of mupirocin calcium ointment. Ann Intern Med. 1991;114:101–6.

99. Scully BE, Briones F, Gu JW, et al. Mupirocin treatment of nasal staphylococcal colonization. Arch Intern Med. 1992;152:353–6.

100. Dacre JE, Emmerson AM, Jenner EA. Nasal carriage of gentamicin and methicillin-resistant *Staphylococcus aureus* treated with topical pseudomonic acid. Lancet. 1983;2:1036.

101. Davies EA, Emmerson AM, Hogg GM, et al. An outbreak of infection with methicillin-resistant *Staphylococcus aureus* in a special care baby unit: Value of topical mupirocin and of traditional methods of infection control. J Hosp Infect. 1987;1:120–8.

102. Dacre J, Emmerson AM, Jenner EA. Gentamicin-methicillin-resistant *Staphylococcus aureus*: Epidemiology and containment of an outbreak. J Hosp Infect. 1986;7:130–6.

103. Hill RLR, Duckworth GJ, Casewell MW. Elimination of nasal carriage of methicillin-resistant *Staphylococcus aureus* with mupirocin during a hospital outbreak. J Antimicrob Chemother. 1988;22:377–84.

104. Vandenbroucke-Grauls CM, Frenay HME, van Klingeren B, et al. Control of epidemic methicillin-resistant *Staphylococcus aureus* in a Dutch university hospital. Eur J Clin Microbiol Infect Dis. 1991;10:6–11.

105. Barrett SP. The value of nasal mupirocin in containing an outbreak of methicillin-resistant *Staphylococcus aureus* in an orthopedic ward. J Hosp Infect. 1990;15:137–42.

106. Dariouche R, Wright C, Hamill R, et al. Eradication of colonization by methicillin-resistant *Staphylococcus aureus* by using oral minocycline-rifampin and topical mupirocin. Antimicrob Agents Chemother. 1991;35:1612–5.

107. Cederna JE, Terpenning MS, Ensberg M, et al. *Staphylococcus aureus* nasal colonization in a nursing home: eradication with mupirocin. Infect Cont Hosp Epidemiol. 1990;11:13–6.

108. Kauffman CA, Terpenning MS, He X, et al. Attempts to eradicate methicillin-resistant *Staphylococcus aureus* from a long-term-care facility with use of mupirocin ointment. Am J Med. 1993;94:371–8.

109. Neu HC. The use of mupirocin in controlling methicillin-resistant *Staphylococcus aureus*. Infect Cont Hosp Epidemiol. 1990;11:11–2.

110. Muder RR. Mupirocin and MRSA: Current status. Infect Med. 1993;10:21–2.

111. Vickers CFH. Percutaneous absorption of sodium fusidate and fusidic acid. Br J Dermatol. 1969;81:204–7.
112. Verbist L. The antimicrobial activity of fusidic acid. J Antimicrob Chemother. 1990;25:1–5.
113. Anderson JD. Fusidic acid: New opportunities with an old antibiotic. Can Med Assoc J. 1980;122:765–9.
114. Ayliffe AJ, Green W, Livingston R, et al. Antibiotic-resistant *Staphylococcus aureus* in dermatology and burn wards. J Clin Pathol. 1977;30:40–4.
115. Shanson DC. Clinical relevance of resistance to fusidic acid in *Staphylococcus aureus*. J Antimicrob Chemother. 1990;25:15–21.
116. Faber M, Rosdahl VT. Susceptibility to fusidic acid among Danish *Staphylococcus aureus* strains and fusidic acid consumption. J Antimicrob Chemother. 1990;25:7–14.

30. ANTIMYCOBACTERIAL AGENTS

ROBERT H. ALFORD
RICHARD J. WALLACE, JR.

Drugs for mycobacterial infections will be discussed in three groups: those primarily for treatment of infections caused by *Mycobacterium tuberculosis,* drugs for nontuberculous ("atypical") mycobacterial infections, and agents principally for treatment of leprosy.

Approaches to antituberculous chemotherapy have been affected by the recent spread of multidrug-resistant *M. tuberculosis* (MDR-TB), characterized by resistance to at least isoniazid (INH) and rifampin[1–3] and by the special susceptibility to *M. tuberculosis* of those infected with human immunodeficiency virus (HIV).[4,5]

MDR-TB strains having various combinations of resistance to INH, rifampin, streptomycin, or ethambutol have necessitated use of drugs that were considered second-line agents, as well as drugs that must be administered by injection. The list of agents active against MDR-TB is quite limited, emphasizing both the need for supervised therapy when noncompliance is likely[6] and the need for new antituberculous agents.[7]

MDR-TB infections are of increased concern in persons immunologically disabled by HIV with or without acquired immunodeficiency syndrome (AIDS) because the host contribution to controlling the infection is diminished. HIV-infected individuals are especially prone to adverse reactions. For example, thiacetazone has been employed in the treatment of tuberculosis in Africa for a long time because it is inexpensive. However, the drug will have to be abandoned in many populations there because of toxicity in HIV-positive recipients.[6,8] In addition, malabsorption of antituberculous drugs can occur in AIDS patients.[8a]

The advent of AIDS has also greatly increased the prevalence and severity of *Mycobacterium avium-intracellulare* and other nontuberculous mycobacterial infections, especially in their disseminated forms. Fortunately, the new macrolide/azalide and quinolone agents appear to be active against some of these mycobacteria, even in patients with markedly impaired cell-mediated immune defenses. The effects of HIV and AIDS on leprosy and its chemotherapy are as yet unclear but will almost certainly be profound.

Traditionally, antimicrobials for tuberculosis have been classified as "first-line" drugs, having superior efficacy with acceptable toxicity, and "second-line" drugs, having either less efficacy, greater toxicity, or both. Several excellent reviews of antimycobacterial agents and therapy are available,[9–15] including guidelines for therapy of MDR-TB.[15]

Antituberculous drugs differ in mechanism of bactericidal ac-

tion and in delivery to tuberculous lesions.[9] Four first-line agents—INH, rifampin, streptomycin, and ethambutol—are active against the large populations of tubercle bacilli in cavities. Streptomycin, other aminoglycosides, and capreomycin penetrate cells poorly and are inactive at acidic pH. Pyrazinamide (PZA), inactive at the neutral or slightly alkaline pH that may occur extracellularly, is active only in acidic environments. Slowly replicating organisms in necrotic foci are killed by rifampin and somewhat less readily by INH.

First-line antituberculous agents are bactericidal except ethambutol. The bactericidal activities of both INH and rifampin against tubercle bacilli in cavitary, intracellular, or necrotic foci provide the basis for the efficacy of short-course INH-rifampin regimens. A combination of three bactericidal agents active against intracellular organisms—INH, rifampin, and PZA—appears to be fundamental for the shorter 6-month regimen preferred in the United States. A residual population consisting of virtually nonreplicating dormant tubercle bacilli within necrotic foci is especially difficult to eradicate, perhaps explaining the minimum of approximately 4 months of therapy needed even in persons with competent immune defenses.

FIRST-LINE ANTITUBERCULOUS DRUGS

Isoniazid

Derivation and Structure. Isoniazid, isonicotinic acid hydrazide (INH), a synthetic agent, in 1952 was shown to be effective for the treatment of human tuberculosis. Its structure is indicated in Figure 1.

MECHANISM OF ACTION. Isoniazid, bactericidal against actively growing *M. tuberculosis,* is bacteriostatic against nonreplicating organisms. It acts by inhibition of oxygen-dependent synthetic pathways of mycolic acid,[16] an important constituent of mycobacterial cell walls.

Antimicrobial Activity and Resistance. Against *M. tuberculosis,* 0.025–0.05 μg/ml of INH is inhibitory and higher concentrations are bactericidal against replicating organisms. When INH is administered alone, resistance tends to emerge. Initially susceptible isolates become resistant in over 70 percent of cases treated with INH alone for 3 months. Resistance results from selection under antimicrobic pressure of incompletely susceptible variants of *M. tuberculosis* that number 1 in 10^6 among untreated bacillary populations. Surviving tubercle bacilli exhibit decreased INH uptake. Large populations like the $10^9–10^{10}$ bacilli in pulmonary cavities are especially likely to contain significant numbers of inherently resistant tubercle bacilli that regrow because of inadequate therapy to express secondary resistance. Approximately 25 percent of INH-resistant strains have a deletion in the catalase gene. INH resistance (primary resistance) remained at approximately 5–6 percent of isolates from untreated cases in the United States for many years, although higher rates were encountered in isolates from immigrants coming from countries where resistance was more common. Now, MDR-TB is of great concern worldwide, including in the United States. INH resistance rates of greater than 20 percent are being encountered in some population groups in the United States.[1–3] Some groups remain with little INH resistance (e.g., only 2.7 percent of the isolates were resistant in one ethnic Indian subgroup[17]).

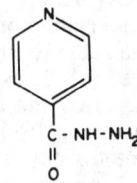

FIG. 1. Structure of isoniazid.

TABLE 1. Dosage Modification for Antituberculous Drugs in Hepatic or Renal Failure

Antimicrobial Drug	Modify in Hepatic Failure	Modify in Renal Failure
Ethionamide	Yes	No
Isoniazid	Yes	Minor
Pyrazinamide	Yes	Yes[a]
Rifampin	Yes	No
Thiacetazone	Yes	Minor
Amikacin	No	Yes
Capreomycin	No	Yes
Cycloserine	No	Yes
Ethambutol	No	Yes
Kanamycin	No	Yes
Para-aminosalicylic acid	No	Yes
Streptomycin	No	Yes
Viomycin	No	Yes

[a] Accumulation of toxic metabolites.

TABLE 2. Age-Related Incidence of Isoniazid Hepatotoxicity

Age (Years)	Serious Hepatotoxicity (% Patients)
<20	"Rare"
20–34	0.3
35–49	1.2
>50	2.3

(From Centers for Disease Control and Prevention,[20] with permission.)

Pharmacology. INH is well absorbed orally or intramuscularly and is distributed throughout the body. Cerebrospinal fluid (CSF) levels are generally about 20 percent of plasma concentrations but may approach plasma levels in the presence of meningeal inflammation. Coadministration with vitamin C appears to inactivate INH suspensions markedly.[18]

Metabolism of INH occurs initally by liver N-acetyltransferase. Diminished acetylation capacity is inherited as an autosomal recessive trait[12] that varies from a 5 percent prevalence rate in Canadian Eskimos to 83 percent in Egyptians. Ten to fifteen percent of Orientals are "slow" acetylators, as are 58 percent of American whites.[12] Six hours after a 4 mg/kg oral dose, slow acetylators exhibit plasma INH levels of more than 0.8 μg/ml and rapid acetylators of less than 0.2 μg/ml.[10] The striking bimodal distribution of plasma half-lives of INH depending on acetylator status generally does not affect outcome with daily therapy, because plasma levels are maintained well above inhibitory concentrations. Rapid acetylators may have poorer outcomes than slow acetylators during weekly intermittent therapy. Metabolically altered INH is principally excreted in urine along with lesser amounts of unaltered drug. Dosage modification in hepatic or renal insufficiency is not usually necessary, but in significant hepatic failure a reduction in dosage by one-half is recommended, and with marked renal failure a dosage reduction to 150–200 mg/day is recommended for slow acetylators. Table 1 summarizes dosage modifications for INH and other antituberculous drugs in hepatic or renal failure.

Adverse Reactions. INH has infrequent major toxicities, most notably hepatitis. Approximately 15 percent of INH recipients have minor asymptomatic elevations in serum aspartate aminotransferase (AST, SGOT) levels that usually resolve with continued therapy. An appreciation of the incidence of major INH hepatotoxicity was gained after the results of a large prophylactic trial were reported in 1972 in which 19 of 2321 recipients developed serious hepatitis and 2 died.[19] Hepatotoxicity can occur at any time but is most likely 4–8 weeks after treatment is begun. INH hepatotoxicity is clearly correlated with age, as indicated in Table 2, presumably due to diminished capacity for repair of INH-induced hepatocellular damage in the elderly. Undernutrition may also play a role in expression of INH hepatoxicity.[21] Hepatoxicity is increased in alcoholics with preexisting liver damage,[19] in pregnant women,[22] with high dosage, and in combination with acetaminophen.[23] Histologically hepatocellular damage that can progress to submassive necrosis usually occurs. Toxic cholestasis is infrequent. Although endemic viral hepatitis has been considered a possible factor contributing to INH hepatoxicity,[24,25] INH has been safely administered to some with acute hepatitis[26] and prophylacticially to persons chronically infected with hepatitis B.[27,28] Educating patients about recognition of symptoms of INH-induced liver disease is key in preventing its progression. Routine monitoring of serum hepatic enzyme concentrations is unnecessary as a rule except in the elderly.[29] Patients should be advised to discontinue INH therapy at the onset of symptoms consistent with incipient hepatitis, such as nausea, loss of appetite, and dull midabdominal pain. Generally hepatotoxicity subsides after INH discontinuation. Cautious readministration of INH after resolution of hepatitis apparently is usually well-tolerated and safe.[30]

Recognition of the frequency and severity[31] of INH hepatotoxicity has not curtailed therapeutic usage but has led to a revision of "prophylactic" indications with special caution indicated in those, especially black women, over 35 years of age.[32]

Neurotoxicity. Peripheral neuropathy has been described in 17 percent of recipients of 6 mg/kg/day of INH but ordinarily is less frequent when adults receive the standard dose of 300 mg/day. Poor nutrition or underlying alcoholism, diabetes mellitus, or uremia predisposes to neuropathy, which is more frequent in slow acetylators who have higher plasma levels of unaltered drug. Increased pyridoxine excretion is promoted by INH. Pyridoxine, 10–50 mg daily, can ameliorate the neuropathy without interfering with the antimycobacterial effect. In one reported case supplemental pyridoxine was thought to contribute to neurotoxicity.[33]

INH-induced central nervous system (CNS) toxicity can produce aberrations ranging from memory loss to psychosis or seizures. Particular caution is indicated when administering INH to those with convulsive disorders. Optic neuropathy has been reported. Toxic CNS reactions are not necessarily related to pyridoxine deficiency but have responded to its administration.[10]

Overdose. Accidental ingestion of INH by children or ingestion during a suicide attempt may result in metabolic acidosis, hyperglycemia, seizures, and coma. Intravenous pyridoxine may be beneficial.

Hypersensitivity Reactions. Fever, which may be sustained or "spiking," skin eruptions, or hematologic abnormalities can occur. A substantial number of INH recipients develop positive antinuclear antibody reactions, and some will manifest an INH-induced lupuslike syndrome that is reversible upon its discontinuation.

Other Reactions. INH-associated arthritic disorders have included Dupuytren's contracture and "shoulder–hand" syndrome. Pellagra can occur in malnourished INH recipients.[10,12,34] Pyridoxine deficiency-related anemia can occur in children or adults.[35]

Significant Drug Interactions. Phenytoin (Dilantin) toxicity is potentiated by INH. Mental changes, nystagmus, and ataxia can result, especially in slow acetylators whose high INH levels inhibit phenytoin metabolism. Similarly mediated theophylline toxicity has been reported with coadministration of INH. In up to 29 percent of recipients combined INH and rifampin therapy predisposes to elevation of plasma hepatic enzymes. Plasma INH concentrations are increased by para-aminosalicylic acid through interference with acetylation.

Usage. INH is indicated for all clinical forms of tuberculosis. Therapeutic regimens must include one or more companion drugs to prevent emergence of INH resistance. INH is used alone for preventive therapy or "chemoprophylaxis" for selected purified protein derivative skin test converters.

Availability and Dosage. Isoniazid is available generically (tablets, syrup, injectable solutions) and under brand names—Isoniazid (tablets) or Nydrazid (injectable solution). Dosage forms include 100 and 300 mg tablets; syrup containing 10 mg/ml; 100 mg/ml solution for parenteral injection; and a capsule combining 150 mg of INH with rifampin (Rifamate). Usual adult dosage is 5 mg/kg/day (preferably 300 mg once daily). A higher dosage (10 mg/kg per day) has been recommended for special situations such as meningitis and for infants and children. Divided doses may result in lower plasma concentrations.

Intermittent, supervised, or observed therapy such as twice-weekly high-dose INH (15 mg/kg po) combined with a streptomycin (25–30 mg/kg im), ethambutol (50 mg/kg po), rifampin (600 mg po), or pyrazinamide is sometimes employed in "consolidation therapy" regimens after an initial period of daily drug administration. Intermittent regimens save money and encourage compliance. A reliable urine test is available to confirm INH ingestion.[36]

Although the preferred parenteral route is intramuscular injection, INH for injection has been administered safely intravenously when other routes are contraindicated.[37]

Rifampin

Derivation and Structure. Rifampin (termed *rifampicin* in the United Kingdom) is a semisynthetic derivative of a complex macrocyclic antibiotic, rifamycin B, produced by *Streptomyces mediterranei*. In 1967, it was introduced for clinical trials in tuberculosis. Rifampin's structure is shown in Figure 2.

Mechanism of Action. Rifampin inhibits mycobacterial DNA-dependent RNA polymerase; human RNA polymerase is insensitive. It is bactericidal against susceptible *M. tuberculosis* strains at 0.005–0.2 µg/ml. Unlike other two-drug combinations, rifampin plus INH sterilizes tissues in experimental murine tuberculosis.

Pharmacology. Rifampin is well absorbed orally, yielding peak plasma concentrations of 7–8 µg/ml after a dose of 600 mg. It is widely distributed throughout the body, including the CSF. CSF concentrations range from undetectable to 0.5 µg/ml in healthy persons and reach 50 percent of plasma concentration with meningeal inflammation. Rifampin's high lipid solubility enhances phagosomal penetration. Rifampin is deacetylated to an active form that undergoes biliary excretion and enterohepatic recirculation. Due to autoinduction of rifampin metabolism (cytochrome P-450-coupled), as evidenced by proliferation of

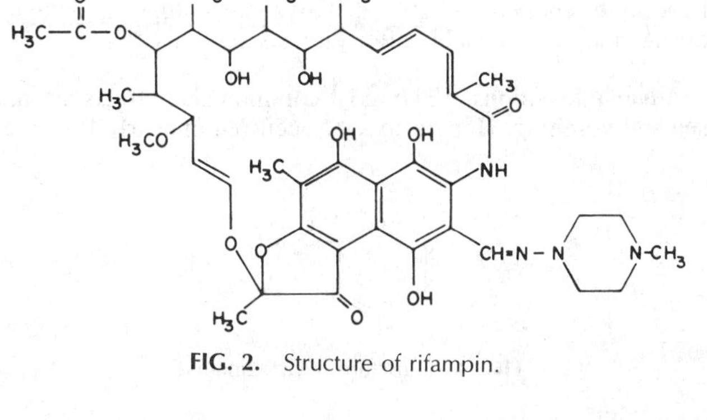

hepatocyte smooth endolasmic reticulum,[38] biliary excretion increases with continued therapy. Induction of rifampin's metabolism with consequent reduction in half-life and plasma concentrations during treatment of tuberculosis becomes maximal after approximately six doses whether administered daily or twice weekly.[39] Excretion is primarily into the gastrointestinal tract, with lesser amounts in the urine. Plasma concentration and urinary excretion increase in hepatic failure. Probenecid blocks hepatic uptake, causing decreased biliary excretion. Liver failure requires moderate dosage reduction, but full dosage can be given in renal insufficiency. Rifampin is removed by hemodialysis or peritoneal dialysis.[40]

Antimicrobial Activity. Rifampin is bactericidal against actively replicating *M. tuberculosis* to a degree comparable to INH. It is also active against intracellular, slowly replicating bacilli and somewhat against nearly dormant organisms in necrotic foci. Rifampin's efficacy is indicated in susceptible pulmonary tuberculosis by sputum conversion 2 weeks earlier with rifampin-containing regimens than those without it. Rapid resistance emerges so frequently as to preclude rifampin's use alone. Frequency of primary resistance among isolates of *M. tuberculosis* remained only 3–5 percent for a long time. Rifampin resistance results from a mutation causing specific amino acid substitutions in RNA polymerase.[41] Rifampin resistance coupled with resistance to INH and other antituberculous agents now characterizes many MDR-TB isolates.[2]

Frequency of Adverse Reactions. Minor adverse reactions are rather frequent with rifampin, but in only 6 of 372 patients taking the drug for 20 weeks was cessation of therapy necessary because of adverse effects.[42]

Hepatotoxicity. Rifampin's major adverse effect is hepatotoxicity, which reportedly caused 16 deaths in 500,000 recipients.[10] Minimal abnormalities in liver function tests are common in those taking rifampin and usually resolve possibly because of autoinduction of its metabolism even with continuation of the drug. Characteristically, elevations of bilirubin and alkaline phosphatase result, whereas elevation of plasma hepatocellular enzyme concentrations can be caused by rifampin, INH, or both. Rifampin-induced toxic liver changes occur earlier and produce patchier cellular reaction with less periportal inflammation than hepatitis caused by INH. Alcoholics with preexisting liver damage appear to be especially prone to serious rifampin-induced liver reactions. Alternative drugs such as PZA, para-aminosalicylic acid, and ethionamide also may be hepatotoxic. Children appear to be at increased risk of serious rifampin hepatotoxicity perhaps because of relatively higher dosage. Jaundice possibly potentiated by phenytoin or other seizure medication was reported in 27 percent of children with tuberculous meningitis receiving rifampin in combination regimens.

Effects on Immune Parameters. Rifampin's widespread effects on humoral and cell-mediated immunity are of uncertain clinical significance. Light-chain proteinuria occurs in 85 percent of rifampin recipients. Blastic transformation of phytohemagglutinin-stimulated lymphocytes is inhibited, and there is interference with cutaneous reactivity to intradermal tuberculin.

Hypersensitivity Reactions. Flushing, fever, pruritus without rash, urticaria, cutaneous vasculitis, eosinophilia, thrombocytopenia, hemolysis, or renal failure due to interstitial nephritis can occur due to rifampin. A systemic flulike syndrome, at times associated with thrombocytopenia, appears to be immunologically mediated and has been described almost exclusively with intermittent, high-dose therapy. Regimens of 600 mg of rifampin twice weekly have infrequently produced the flulike syndrome.

FIG. 2. Structure of rifampin.

TABLE 3. Compounds Having Rifampin-Induced Reduction in Plasma Concentrations

Barbiturates	Itraconazole
Bile acids	Ketoconazole
Chloramphenicol	Methadone
Clofibrate	Metoprolol
Coumadin	Nortryptyline
Cyclosporine	Oral contraceptives
Diazepam	Phenytoin
Digoxin	Prednisone-glucocorticoids
Digitoxin	Propafenone
Diltiazem	Propranolol
Disopyramide	Quinidine
Estrogens	Sulfonylureas
Fluconazole	Theophylline
Haloperidol	Tocainide
	Verapamil

(Data from refs. 37, 44–46.)

Other Adverse Reactions. Widespread systemic distribution of rifampin is reflected in an orange color appearing in urine, feces, saliva, sputum, pleural effusions, tears, soft contact lenses, sweat, semen, CSF, and other body fluids so that recipients of the drug should be appropriately forewarned. With overdosage, a "red-man" syndrome of skin discoloration has been described. Gastrointestinal upset is frequent but is usually ameliorated by temporary reduction in dosage. Lower limb deep venous thrombosis can occur in those receiving rifampin.[43]

Significant Drug Interactions. By potentiating microsomal cytochrome P-450-mediated enzymatic activities, rifampin causes increased hepatic metabolism of many substances. Rifampin interaction with 95 generic drugs has been cataloged.[44] A partial compilation of this expanding list of compounds is given in Table 3. Rifampin–drug interactions can be important clinically.[44–46] Competition for excretion with contrast agents used for biliary tract imaging may cause failure to visualize the gallbladder. Probenecid interferes with excretion, resulting in increased plasma rifampin concentrations. Rifampin crosses placental membranes readily and is not approved for use in pregnancy. PAS preparations interfere with gastrointestinal absorption of rifampin.

Usage. Rifampin is indicated for treatment of all forms of pulmonary and extrapulmonary tuberculosis. Because of rapid emergence of resistance when used alone, rifampin should always be employed in combination. Uses of rifampin for treatment and prophylaxis of bacterial infections are discussed in Chapter 22 and later chapters concerning the individual diseases.

Availability and Dosage. Rifampin is supplied in the United States as Rifadin and Rimactane, available in 150- or 300-mg capsules and in combination 300-mg capsules with 150-mg INH (Rimactane). Rifampin for intravenous infusion (600 mg/vial, Rifadin) should not be used intramuscularly. The usual dosage is 600 mg once daily for adults, which can be given initially in divided doses for better tolerance, and 10–20 mg/kg/day for children (not to exceed 600 mg/day). Twice weekly 900- or 1200-mg dosage regimens have largely been abandoned due to toxic reactions. A 600-mg twice-weekly schedule generally has been well tolerated. Rifampin from opened capsules can be suspended (usually 10 mg/ml) in simple or flavored sugar syrups that should not be co-mixed with ascorbic acid, which can inactivate rifampin.[18] Suspensions can be refrigerated for up to 2 weeks.

Rifabutin

Several spiropiperidyl rifamycins have activity against mycobacteria, including *M. tuberculosis*, *M. avium-intracellulare* complex, and *Mycobacterium fortuitum*.[47] Rifabutin (ansamycin, Mycobutin), a derivative of rifamycin-S, is more active in vitro and more effective in experimental murine tuberculosis than is rifampin.[48–50] It is no more toxic in animals than rifampin. The mechanism of action is inhibition of mycobacterial DNA-dependent RNA polymerase, as is rifampin. It has a long plasma half-life (45 hours) in humans and marked tissue tropism, producing tissue concentrations 5- to 10-fold greater than in plasma. Equivalent doses in humans yield plasma concentrations of rifabutin seven times lower than rifampin.[51] Rifabutin decreases zidovudine plasma concentrations. Fluconazole and probably clarithromycin increase plasma rifabutin concentrations. Arthralgia, arthritis, and uveitis have occurred in patients taking rifabutin, usually at doses exceeding 300 mg daily.[51a,51b] Almost all persons with these side effects have also been receiving clarithromycin or fluconazole. Symptoms of uveitis include unilateral or bilateral ocular pain and blurred vision. Improvement ensues upon discontinuation of rifabutin or use of topical steroids. Less common and milder rifabutin side effects include rash, neutropenia, hepatitis, and gastrointestinal distress. Rifabutin causes an orange-tan discoloration of the skin, urine, saliva, tears, and contact lenses, particularly in doses above 300 mg daily. Rifabutin's potential for treatment of MDR-TB is under investigation.[52,53] Approximately 25 percent of rifampin-resistant tuberculosis strains are inhibited by low concentrations of rifabutin. Its role in *M. avium-intracellulare* infections will be described below and in Chapters 22 and 232.

Pyrazinamide

Derivation and Structure. Pyrazinamide (PZA), a synthetic analog of nicotinamide, has been elevated to first-line usage for "short-course" therapeutic regimens because of its bactericidal activity[9,54,55] and reasonable toxicity at relatively low doses. Its structure is shown in Figure 3.

Mechanism of Action. PZA is bactericidal for tubercle bacilli at 12.5 µg/ml. Its maximal activity in vitro is at acid pH, like that existing intracellularly in phagolysosomes. Its precise action is unknown. Despite good activity at acid pH in vitro and inhibitory concentrations within monocytes,[56] PZA exhibits low activity alone in pretreated macrophages.[57] Resistance rapidly evolves if PZA is used alone. Metabolically inactive tubercle bacilli are resistant to PZA, rendering it inappropriate for long-term therapy.[9] Sporadic primary resistance occurs generally in less that 1 percent of isolates, but nearly one-half of INH-rifampin resistant MDR-TB isolates are reportedly PZA resistant.[2]

Pharmacology. Well absorbed orally, PZA is widely distributed throughout the body, attaining concentrations above that needed to inhibit tubercle bacilli. Peak plasma concentrations are approximately 50 µg/ml, with a half-life of 12–24 hours, making once daily or less frequent dosing practical. PZA crosses inflamed meninges and has been recommended in combination regimens for tuberculous meningitis.[58] It is metabolized by the liver, and metabolic products, including principally pyrazinoic acid, are excreted mainly by the kidneys, requiring dosage modification in renal failure. PZA is dialyzable so that supplemental dosage may be advisable after dialysis sessions.[40]

Adverse Reactions. The most common side effects are nausea and vomiting. Hepatotoxicity occurred in nearly 15 percent

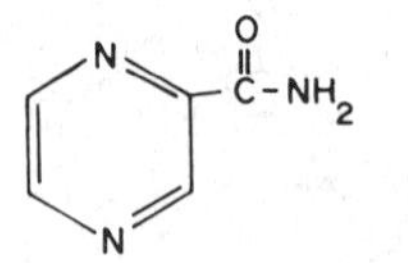

FIG. 3. Structure of pyrazinamide.

of PZA recipients in early trials that employed dosages of 40–50 mg/kg/day for prolonged periods. Current regimens of 20–35 mg/kg/day are much safer.[59] Patients with preexisting liver disease who receive PZA should have symptoms and hepatic function tests monitored closely. PZA-induced interstitial nephritis causing kidney failure has been described,[60] as has rhabdomyolysis with myoglobinuric renal failure.[61] Other side effects include urate retention in 56 percent of PZA recipients[59] and non-incapacitating polymyalgia.[54] Photosensitivity and rash have also been reported.

Usage. PZA is often included as an essential component of multidrug short-course chemotherapy.[9,15,59] Unless PZA is used in the initial phase of 6-month regimens, relapse rates are unacceptable.[55] Efficacy with administration as infrequently as once weekly makes PZA suitable for observed therapy regimens.

Availability and Dosage. PZA is available in 500-mg tablets. Dosage is 20–35 mg/kg/day (often 1.5–2.0 g) orally once or in two divided doses. PZA has been well tolerated in a twice-weekly dosage of 50 mg/kg (not to exceed 3 g/day) for short-course regimens. It has even been administered safely once weekly in a dose of 90 mg/kg.

Ethambutol

Derivation and Structure. Ethambutol was discovered in 1961 among synthetic compounds screened for antituberculous activity. Its structure is indicated in Figure 4.

Mechanism of Action. Ethambutol's precise mechanism of action is unknown. It is bacteriostatic against tubercle bacilli.

Pharmacology. Ethambutol administered orally is 75–80 percent absorbed, yielding peak plasma concentrations of 5 μg/ml after a dose of 25 mg/kg. It is distributed throughout the body, including the CSF. Although little ethambutol crosses normal meninges, levels 10–50 percent of those in plasma occur in CSF with meningeal inflammation. After conversion of approximately 25 percent of absorbed ethambutol to inactive metabolites, 80 percent of the parent together with metabolites is excreted in urine. Consequently, it becomes necessary to modify dosage in significant renal failure.

Antimicrobial Activity. Ethambutol is bacteriostatic in vitro or within macrophages[56] at concentrations of 1 μg/ml against susceptible strains of *M. tuberculosis*. Stepwise resistance occurs whenever ethambutol is administered without companion drugs. Cross-resistance with other antimycobacterial agents was infrequent for years. Thus, ethambutol's principal role has been as a "companion" drug to curtail resistance. However, cross-resistance rates as high as 80 percent for ethambutol in INH-rifampin–resistant isolates from New York City apparently indicate limited utility against MDR-TB.[2]

Adverse Reactions. The major toxicity of ethambutol is neuropathy. Peripheral neuropathy is infrequent; retrobulbar neuritis is more common. Characteristically, visual field constriction or impairment of acuity or color vision develops. Common in association with high-dosage (50 mg/kg/day) or prolonged ad-

ministration, and more common with 25 mg/kg/day than 15 mg/kg/day dosing, retrobulbar neuritis is usually slowly reversible. Blindness has occurred in elderly persons receiving as little as 15 mg/kg/day.[62] Consequently, recipients of ethambutol should be instructed to report optic symptoms promptly and to discontinue the drug until confirmatory visual testing can be done. Visual acuity and color perception testing is recommended every 4–6 weeks, especially in those taking more than 25 mg/kg/day. Gastrointestinal intolerance is infrequent. Hyperuricemia occurs because of decreased renal uric acid excretion. Infrequent hypersensitivity reactions include dermatitis, arthralgias, and fever.

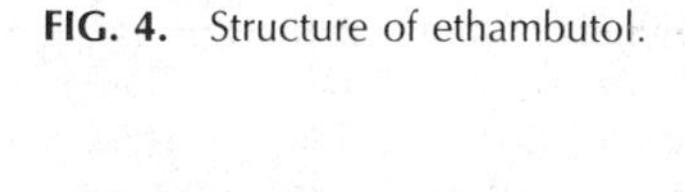

Usage. Ethambutol is indicated as a companion drug for susceptible infections due to *M. tuberculosis*.

Availability and Dosage. Ethambutol is available as ethambutol hydrochloride (Myambutol) supplied in 100- or 400-mg tablets. Usual dosage is 15–25 mg/kg/day initially, followed after 60 days by 15 mg/kg/day as a single daily dose.

Streptomycin

Derivation, Structure, and Pharmacology. Streptomycin, an aminoglycoside antibiotic introduced in the 1940s, was the first drug to reduce tuberculosis mortality. Its structure, mechanism of action, and pharmacology are covered in Chapter 20. Briefly, intramuscular injection of 1 g yields peak plasma concentrations of 25–45 μg/ml. It is virtually excluded from the CNS.

Antimicrobial Activity. Streptomycin is bactericidal against *M. tuberculosis* in vitro, but is inactive against intracellular tubercle bacilli, limiting its activity to suppression in many animal studies. Concentrations of 0.4–10 μg/ml of plasma are inhibitory. Rapid emergence of resistance to streptomycin was quickly recognized as a consequence of single drug therapy. Approximately 1 in 10^6 tubercle bacilli is initially resistant to streptomycin. Primary cross-resistance to streptomycin occurs most often in patient populations having a high incidence of INH resistance. In MDR-TB outbreaks, approximately 80 percent of INH-rifampin–resistant isolates are also streptomycin resistant.[2]

Adverse Reactions. Streptomycin toxicity is like that of other aminoglycoside antibiotics but with less renal and acoustic toxicity and greater vestibular toxicity than more commonly used aminoglycosides. Patients receiving streptomycin should be instructed to be aware of tinnitus, decreased hearing, and problems with balance, and they should be instructed to notify their caregiver immediately if such reactions occur.

Usage. Streptomycin is indicated for multidrug therapy of susceptible tuberculosis. Dosages of greater than 1 g per day should be avoided. Dosage reduction is indicated in patients over 50 years of age, those with low body weight, and when renal function is impaired. Special care must be taken when streptomycin is used in combination with other nephrotoxic or ototoxic drugs. Streptomycin usage for bacterial infections is discussed in Chapter 20.

Availability and Dosage. Streptomycin sulfate for intramuscular injection is provided in 1-g single-injection vials. The recommended dosage in adults with normal renal function is 0.5–1 g daily to 1 g twice weekly. Children receive 20–40 mg/kg/day in divided doses every 12 hours. Currently, streptomycin is commercially available in the United States, but its supply has been interrupted in the past. Information about availability of streptomycin or other antituberculous drugs can be obtained from the centers for Disease Control and Prevention Drug Service ([404] 639–3670).

FIG. 4. Structure of ethambutol.

SECOND-LINE ANTITUBERCULOUS DRUGS

Para-Aminosalicylic Acid

As a calcium or sodium salt, this synthetic compound inhibits growth of tubercle bacilli by impairment of folate synthesis. Para-aminosalicylic acid (PAS) is incompletely absorbed orally. A 4-g oral dose yields plasma concentrations of 70–80 μg/ml. Eighty-five percent of absorbed PAS is excreted in urine as various degradation products.

Adverse Reactions.   Chief among PAS side effects is gastrointestinal intolerance, which is often severe and results in poor compliance. PAS can cause reversible drug-induced lupuslike reactivity and, when given as the sodium salt, sodium overload. It can produce lymphoid hyperplasia, and recipients can develop mononucleosislike syndromes with fever, rash, hepatosplenomegaly, occasionally toxic hepatitis, and adenopathy. Hypersensitivity to PAS is frequent.

Usage.   PAS has retained a limited role in multidrug therapy in developing countries due to its low cost. However, it is becoming less favored because of poor compliance and primary resistance.

Availability and Dosage.   PAS in the United States is available from the Centers for Disease Control and Prevention. Dosage forms include 500-mg tablets or 4-g resin packets. The usual dosage is 10–12 g/day in three or four divided doses for adults (6–8 g/day of the sodium-potassium-free ascorbate) and, in children, 200–300 mg/kg/day in divided doses.

Cycloserine

Derivation.   Initially a fermentation product, cycloserine is now synthesized. By virtue of inhibiting cell wall synthesis, cycloserine possesses antimicrobial activity against a broad range of prokaryotic organisms including mycobacteria. From 5 to 20 μg/ml inhibits susceptible *M. tuberculosis* in vitro.

Pharmacology.   Cycloserine is readily absorbed orally, producing peak plasma concentrations of 20–50 μg/ml. Widely distributed among tissues, no blood-brain barrier exists to cycloserine.[10] Little of the drug is metabolized, and approximately two-thirds is excreted unchanged by the kidneys.

Adverse Reactions.   Cycloserine can cause peripheral neuropathy or CNS dysfunction, including confusion, irritability, somnolence, headache, nervousness, vertigo, dysarthria, and seizures. Behavioral alterations include severe depression with suicidal ideation. Cycloserine is contraindicated in patients with a history of seizures or those with severe underlying depression.

Usage.   Cycloserine is one of several alternatives for re-treatment regimens or for treatment of primary drug-resistant *M. tuberculosis*. It does not appear to have great activity against MDR-TB strains.[2]

Availability and Dosage.   Cycloserine is provided in the United States as Seromycin in 250-mg pulvules. Usual dosage is 500–1000 mg/day in two divided doses, with 500 mg/day commonly used.

Ethionamide

Derivation.   Ethionamide, a derivative of isonicotinic acid, was first synthesized in 1956. It is tuberculostatic at 0.6–2.5 μg/ml against susceptible strains presumably by inhibition of oxygen-dependent mycolic acid synthesis (see discussion of the related drug prothionamide below under "Drugs for Therapy of Leprosy [Hansen's Disease]").[63]

Pharmacology.   Ethionamide is absorbed well orally, yielding peak plasma concentrations of 20 μg/ml. It is widely distributed and penetrates both normal or inflamed meninges to yield CSF concentrations equivalent to those in plasma. It is metabolized by the liver, with metabolites renally excreted. Ethionamide interferes with INH acetylation.

Adverse Reactions.   Gastrointestinal distress with nausea and vomiting frequently leads to poor compliance and drug discontinuance. Various neurologic disorders have been caused by ethionamide, including peripheral neuropathy or psychiatric disturbances. Neurologic side effects have been reported to be alleviated by pyridoxine or nicotinamide. Reversible hepatotoxicity, heralded by increasing levels of plasma hepatic enzymes, occurs in approximately 5 percent of ethionamide recipients. Hypersensitivity-type rash and poor diabetic control are infrequent complications.

Usage.   Ethionamide is among the agents that can be chosen for treatment of resistant tuberculosis. It appears to be active against most MDR-TB isolates.[2]

Availability and Dosage.   Ethionamide is available in the United States as Trecator-SC in 250-mg coated tablets. The initial dosage is 250 mg twice daily (or as a single dose at bedtime), which is increased by 250 mg daily until 1 g/day in divided doses is reached. Usually, 500–750 mg is the maximum tolerated dose.

Capreomycin, Amikacin, Kanamycin, Viomycin

The antimycobacterial drugs capreomycin, amikacin, kanamycin, and viomycin are considered as a group because all are administered by intramuscular injection, have similar pharmacokinetics and toxicities, and are excreted by the renal route. The first three have been used principally as alternative agents for secondarily resistant tuberculosis. All have additive ototoxicity and nephrotoxicity and in that regard should be given cautiously together with streptomycin or other aminoglycosides.

Capreomycin.   Capreomycin, a polypeptide antibiotic obtained from *Streptomyces capreolus*, is active against *M. tuberculosis*, including most MDR-TB strains,[2] at concentrations of 1–50 μg/ml (usually 10 μg/ml), depending on test conditions. Average peak plasma concentrations of 30 μg/ml are achievable. There is no cross-resistance between streptomycin and capreomycin, but some isolates resistant to kanamycin or amikacin will be cross-resistant to capreomycin. Capreomycin can cause hearing loss, tinnitus, and decreased renal function, but is considered less toxic than amikacin, viomycin, and especially kanamycin.[62] Capreomycin is emerging as a first-line injectable agent in multidrug regimens for treatment of drug-resistant tuberculosis, especially when there is streptomycin resistance.

AVAILABILITY AND DOSAGE.   Capreomycin sulfate is supplied as Capastat. The dosage is the same as with streptomycin, with a range in those under age 50 and having normal renal function of 500 mg to 1 g deep intramuscularly 5 times weekly for 2–4 months. The dose is thereafter reduced to 1 g 2–3 times weekly.

Amikacin.   In vitro and in animals, amikacin is among the most active aminoglycosides against *M. tuberculosis*. There is limited experience with amikacin in human tuberculosis. Because of expense and toxicity, it should not replace streptomycin for initial first-line aminoglycoside treatment of susceptible tuberculosis. Except for its cost, it would probably replace kanamycin for resistant infections. Because clinical pathology laboratories are more likely to determine blood levels of amikacin than kanamycin, streptomycin, or capreomycin, amikacin is especially suited when parenteral therapy is required in patients with renal failure or in elderly patients with preexisting hearing loss.

USAGE.   Amikacin is an alternative injectable agent for treatment of resistant *M. tuberculosis* infections. The customary dose is 10 mg/kg (not to exceed 1 g) 5 times weekly.

Kanamycin.   Kanamycin is an aminoglycoside (see Ch. 20) that has activity against most strains of streptomycin-resistant tubercle bacilli. Except for its lower cost, kanamycin offers no advantage over amikacin in combination therapy and has substantial ototoxicity (see "Amikacin," below). In addition, serum levels are not readily available.

AVAILABILITY AND DOSAGE.   Kanamycin sulfate is supplied as Kantrex, 0.5 g/2 ml, 1 g/3 ml, or 75 mg/2 ml (pediatric formulation) for intramuscular injection. The usual dose is 10 mg/kg generally limited to 500 mg/day in adults because of ototoxicity.

Viomycin.   Viomycin is a complex basic polypeptide antibiotic for injection.[11] Many strains of MDR-TB appear to be susceptible.[2] Cross-resistance to viomycin and capreomycin occurs frequently but less between viomycin and kanamycin.[64] Susceptible *M. tuberculosis* strains are inhibited by 1–10 μg/ml.

AVAILABILITY AND DOSAGE.   Viomycin sulfate's usual dosage is 2 g twice weekly, administered as 1 g/12 hr on the days when it is injected. One to two grams daily have been given for no longer than 1–2 weeks. Viomycin is not currently available in the United States but is included herein because of its apparent activity against most MDR-TB strains.[2]

Amithiozone

Amithiozone (thiacetazone), a thiosemicarbazole, is active against many strains of *M. tuberculosis*. Susceptible strains are inhibited by 1 μg/ml.[10,11] Peak plasma concentrations are 1–2 μg/ml. Resistance to amithiozone readily develops with single-drug therapy, necessitating its use in combination regimens. Because of its low cost, amithiozone has been employed as a first-line drug particularly in East Africa.[11] However, because of its serious toxicity in HIV-infected recipients there, its usefulness has come into doubt.[5,8] Amithiozone can be administered orally in a dosage of 150 mg/day or 450 mg twice weekly.

Quinolones

Emerging outbreaks of MDR-TB[1–3] have stimulated investigation of new fluorinated quinolone antibiotics with activity against mycobacteria.[65–71] Some are bactericidal against *M. tuberculosis*, presumably by inhibition of its DNA gyrase at concentrations well within achievable plasma levels.[66] Ciprofloxacin and ofloxacin inhibit 90 percent of strains of susceptible tubercle bacilli at concentrations of 0.5 and 1.0 μg/ml, respectively.[67–69] Pharmacology and dosing of these agents is covered in Chapter 27. Usage as a single agent in animal models has led to resistance. Similarly, human trials using a fluoroquinolone alone or with inactive drugs has led to the rapid emergence of resistance. Fluoroquinolones, particularly sparfloxacin,[72] have produced additive effects with other antituberculous drugs in vitro and in animals. Initial clinical trials of ofloxacin in combination with INH and rifampin indicate activity comparable to ethambutol.[70] Ofloxacin used alone in a dose of 300 mg/day in patients having MDR-TB has produced decreases in sputum colony counts, with sputum conversion in 26 percent.[71] In nonconvertors, ofloxacin resistance emerged. Preliminary trials indicate that there may be a role for ofloxacin in combination with other accompanying active second-line drugs for treatment of resistant tuberculosis.[65]

β-Lactams

All mycobacteria produce one or more β-lactamases. *M. tuberculosis* produces one. Several β-lactamase-resistant β-lactam antibiotics or combinations with β-lactamase inhibitors such as clavulanic acid are active in vitro against *M. tuberculosis*[73] and various nontuberculous mycobacteria.[74] Unfortunately, activity of β-lactam agents against intracellular mycobacteria is generally poor. Ceforanide, active in vitro, was unable in concentrations as high as 50 μg/ml in a macrophage model to inhibit tubercle bacilli.[56] Similarly, cefotaxime, ceftizoxime, and cefoperazone lack intracellular activity against *M. avium-intracellulare* strains that have in vitro susceptibility.[75] However, cefoxitin and to a lesser degree imipenem-cilastatin have proved efficacious in *Mycobacterium fortuitum* and *Mycobacterium abscessus* infections,[76] giving hope that β-lactamase-stable β-lactam antibiotics with activity against resistant *M. tuberculosis* strains could be developed.

DRUGS FOR THE TREATMENT OF NONTUBERCULOUS (ATYPICAL) MYCOBACTERIAL INFECTIONS

Nontuberculous (atypical or environmental) mycobacteria vary greatly in susceptibility to antimicrobics. Some, such as *M. kansasii*, are susceptible to agents used principally for treatment of tuberculosis; others, such as *M. fortuitum* and *Mycobacterium chelonae*, respond to various antibiotics used more commonly for pyogenic bacterial infections; and still others, especially *M. avium-intracellulare*, are broadly resistant. Choosing appropriate therapy for nontuberculous infections is further confounded because methodology for susceptibility testing has not been well standardized, although progress is being made in that direction.[77] Rational chemotherapy for nontuberculous mycobacterial infections based on susceptibility results is now feasible for many species. An important exception is that susceptibility testing has no clinically predictive value in infections due to *M. avium-intracellulare*.[78]

Isoniazid

Drugs used principally for treatment of *M. tuberculosis* such as INH were evaluated relatively early for their activity against nontuberculous mycobacteria. INH inhibits nearly 90 percent of strains of *M. kansasii* at concentrations of 1–5 μg/ml, as contrasted to only 10–30 percent of *M. avium-intracellulare* strains. At present, INH is included routinely in the therapy of *M. kansasii*, *Mycobacterium xenopi*, and *Mycobacterium szulgai*. It has generally been replaced by more active agents for therapy of other species, including *M. avium-intracellulare*.

Rifampin, Rifabutin

Rifampin is employed for treatment of many nontuberculous mycobacterial infections. In vitro, 93–100 percent of strains of *M. kansasii*, *Mycobacterium marinum*, *Mycobacterium haemophilum*, and *M. xenopi* are inhibited by 0.25–1.0 μg/ml.[79] Other species are much less susceptible. Only one-half of *Mycobacterium scrofulaceum* or *M. avium-intracellulare* strains are inhibited in vitro by 4–16 μg/ml of rifampin. *M. fortuitum* complex strains are universally resistant to rifampin. The response of *M. kansasii* and *M. marinum* infections to rifampin-containing regimens has been particularly encouraging. Synergy between rifampin and other agents has been demonstrable for a number of species in vitro. Its role as a single agent is discouraged because resistance rapidly emerges.

Rifabutin is inhibitory against 90 percent of strains of *M. avium-intracellulare* at a concentration of 2 μg/ml.[50,80] It is concentrated severalfold in tissue and, like rifampin, has gastrointestinal toxicity as its major adverse effect. Rifabutin at a dose of 300 mg/day has been shown to reduce by 50 percent the incidence and rate of dissemination of *M. avium-intracellulare* infections in AIDS patients having CD4 counts of less than 200.[81] It is the only drug currently approved in the United States for that indication. Clinical trials are in progress comparing rifabutin with new macrolides and azalides for prevention and therapy of infections with *M. avium-intracellulare*.

Aminoglycosides

Aminoglycoside antibiotics have been used extensively for treatment of nontuberculous mycobacterial infections. Among *M. kansasii* strains, 86 percent demonstrated streptomycin susceptibility, as did 93 percent of *M. scrofulaceum* strains. Forty-four percent of strains of *M. avium-intracellulare* have been streptomycin susceptible. *M. fortuitum* complex is resistant, whereas *M. ulcerans* strains are universally susceptible to streptomycin in vitro. Despite in vitro susceptibility, streptomycin has not been effective in *M. ulcerans* infections.

Amikacin and debekacin, congeners of kanamycin, appear to have greater activity against nontuberculous mycobacteria than the parent compound.[82] However, marked variability exists between mycobacterial species in susceptibility to amikacin. Virtually all strains of *M. marinum*, *M. kansasii*, and *M. fortuitum* are susceptible to 4 μg/ml or less of amikacin.[79,83,84] Isolates of *M. chelonae*, *M. abscessus*, and *M. avium-intracellulare* are more resistant but are usually inhibited by 8–32 μg/ml of amikacin. Tobramycin is the most active aminoglycoside against isolates of *M. chelonae*.[83] Other aminoglycosides are less active and are generally not clinically useful.[85]

Ethambutol, ethionamide, and cycloserine possess variable activity against *M. avium-intracellulare*[86] and have been employed in combination for infections caused by that group.

MISCELLANEOUS ANTIMICROBIALS FOR TREATMENT OF NONTUBERCULOUS MYCOBACTERIA

Macrolides

Nearly all strains of *M. kansasii* and *M. scrofulaceum* and some strains of *M. avium-intracellulare*, *M. chelonae*, and *M. abscessus* (formerly *M. chelonae* subspecies *abscessus*) are susceptible to achievable therapeutic concentrations of erythromycin.[83] Introduction of two new macrolides, clarithromycin and azithromycin, has resulted in a dramatic change in therapy of nontuberculous mycobacteria. Clarithromycin inhibits almost all species with the exception of *M. simiae* at 4 μg/ml or less.[87,88] Initial therapeutic results have indicated that these agents are efficacious especially against *M. avium-intracellulare*. These agents should not be used as monotherapy because of the rapid emergence of resistance.

Tetracyclines

Approximately 50 percent of isolates of the rapidly growing species *M. fortuitum* and 20 percent of *M. chelonae* are tetracycline susceptible.[86] Minocycline and doxycycline are two- to fourfold more active than tetracycline[83] and have been effective in therapy when the isolates were susceptible in vitro. Minocycline and doxycyline are also active against *M. marinum* and have been used successfully in *M. marinum* infections.

Sulfonamides

Sulfamethoxazole is active against *M. fortuitum* but not against *M. chelonae* or *M. abscessus*. Localized infections have been cured with sulfamethoxazole alone or in combination with trimethoprim.[76] *M. marinum* infections have responded to therapy with trimethoprim-sulfamethoxazole, but strains are susceptible in vitro only against a low inoculum.[79,87]

Both *M. marinum* and *M. kansasii* exhibit very similar drug susceptibilities. Sulfamethoxazole is also active against isolates of *M. kansasii*. It has been curative in combination regimens used for treatment of rifampin-resistant *M. kansasii* infections.

Limited experience indicates some in vitro activity and clinical efficacy of sulfonamides against *M. terrae* complex, *M. haemophilum*, *M. simiae*, and *M. avium-intracellulare*.

Clofazimine

Discussed more fully below under "Drugs for Treatment of Leprosy (Hansen's Disease)," clofazimine (Lamprene) possesses in vitro activity against *M. avium-intracellulare*. most strains are inhibited by 1.6–2.0 μg/ml.[49,89] Clinical experience with clofazimine in combination therapy against *M. avium complex* in AIDS has been generally disappointing.

Other Antimicrobics

More active, less toxic oral chemotherapeutic agents are needed for serious *M. abscessus* and *M. avium-intracellulare* infections. Apparently because of their resistance to *M. fortuitum* β-lactamase, cefoxitin, cefmetazole, and imipenem-cilastatin are active in vitro against approximately 80 percent of *M. fortuitum* strains at clinically achievable plasma concentrations.[74,90] Ciprofloxacin is active in vitro against most *M. avium-intracellulare* strains and consequently deserves further study.[66,67]

A summary of in vitro susceptibility data for nontuberculous mycobacteria is recorded in Table 4. It should serve only as a guide because it is a compilation of data from many laboratories, some using nonstandard methodology, or from tests with small numbers of strains. In vitro susceptibility of nontuberculous my-

TABLE 4. Antimicrobials for Nontuberculous Mycobacteria: Likelihood of In Vitro Susceptibilities Being within Range of Achievable Plasma Concentrations

Category	Runyon Group	Mycobacterial Species	Likelihood of Susceptibility to Antimicrobial[a]
Photochromogens	I	*M. kansasii*	Rifampin (4+), streptomycin (4+), ethionamide (4+), clarithromycin (4+), amikacin (3+), cycloserine (3+), ethambutol (3+), INH (2+)
		M. marinum	Rifampin (4+), amikacin (4+), kanamycin (4+), ethambutol (4+), clarithromycin (4+), minocycline or doxycycline (3+)
Scotochromogens	II	*M. scrofulaceum*	Amikacin (4+), erythromycin (4+), streptomycin (4+), rifampin (3+), ethionamide (2+), INH (1+)
Nonchromogens	III	*M. avium-intracellulare*	Clarithromycin (4+), rifabutin (4+), clofazimine (3+), ethionamide (2+), rifampin (2+), streptomycin (2+), amikacin (2+), cycloserine (2+), ethambutol (1+)
Rapid growers	IV	*M. fortuitum*	Amikacin (4+), cefoxitin (4+), cefmetazole (4+), imipenem-cilastatin (4+), ciprofloxacin or ofloxacin (4+), trimethoprim/sulfamethoxazole (4+), clarithromycin (3+), minocycline or doxycycline (2+)
		M. chelonae	Clarithromycin (4+), azithromycin (4+), tobramycin (4+), amikacin (3+), imipenem-cilastatin (2+), doxycycline (1+)
		M. abscessus	Amikacin (4+), clarithromycin (4+), cefoxitin (3+), imipenem-cilastatin (3+)
Other		*M. ulcerans*	Rifampin (4+), streptomycin (4+), clofazimine (2+)

[a] Compilation ranked according to percentage of tested strains susceptible to achievable plasma concentrations of antimicrobials: 81–100%, 4+; 61–80%, 3+; 41–60%, 2+, 21–40%, 2+.

(Data from refs. 74, 76, 78–80, 82, 85–91.)

cobacterial drugs is no guarantee of therapeutic efficacy. Failures cited above of clofazimine in *M. avium-intracellulare* infections and of streptomycin against *M. ulcerans* indicates limitations in extrapolating in vitro data to clinical experience. As a rule, favorable therapeutic results are likely when drugs are used to which nontuberculous mycobacteria are susceptible in vitro, and poor outcomes can be anticipated when there is in vitro resistance. Least predictable are outcomes of *M. avium-intracellulare* infections, for which routine susceptibility testing is *not* recommended.

Clinical trials in *M. avium-intracellular* infections are underway with rifabutin, clarithromycin, and azithromycin alone and in combination both for chemoprophylaxis and for treatment of disseminated infections in AIDS and for treatment of chronic pulmonary infections that usually occur in the elderly without AIDS.[81,92,93] More well-designed clinical trials with additional active antimicrobials are needed. Readily available analyses of plasma concentrations of antimycobacterial drugs are also needed, especially in AIDS patients, where drug interactions and toxicity are common.

DRUGS FOR TREATMENT OF LEPROSY (HANSEN'S DISEASE)

Background

The special parasite-host relationship of *Mycobacterium leprae* (Hansen's bacillus), characterized by persistence of the organism in tissue for years, has mandated prolonged chemotherapy to prevent relapse. Chemotherapy for leprosy for years mainly consisted of dapsone alone, which produced gratifying clinical results and was affordable. However, because of monotherapy, resistance of leprosy bacilli, both secondary and now primary, has become a problem worldwide.[94] Currently, multidrug therapy is the rule for both multibacillary and paucibacillary disease. The principal agents used in therapeutic multidrug regimens are dapsone, rifampin, and clofazimine.

Dapsone

Derivation and Structure. Diaminophenyl sulfone (dapsone, DDS) a synthetic compound, was demonstrated to be effective in rat leprosy in 1941 and soon thereafter was used successfully in human trials. Its structure is shown in Figure 5.

Mechanism of Action. Sulfones inhibit bacterial dihydropteroate synthase, as do sulfonamides, and presumably inhibit *M. leprae* by the same mechanism.

Antimicrobial activity. By mouse footpad inoculation, as little as 0.003 µg/ml of dapsone is estimated to inhibit multiplication of *M. leprae*. Dapsone has been described as "weakly bactericidal" for susceptible leprosy bacilli. In humans, it has been estimated that 99.9 percent of bacillary populations are killed after 3–4 months of dapsone therapy.[95] In lepromatous (multibacillary) patients on monotherapy, secondary dapsone resistance often emerges 5–24 *years* after commencing therapy.[96] Prior to usage of current standard multidrug regimens secondary resistance occurred in approximately 20 percent of cases.

Pharmacology. Dapsone is well absorbed orally. Distributed throughout body fluids, tissue concentrations are approximately 2 µg/ml. The plasma half-life of dapsone is 21–44 hours, with some drug retention for up to 3 weeks. Dapsone becomes acetylated, with 70–80 percent excreted as metabolites in urine. Dosage should be reduced accordingly in renal failure.

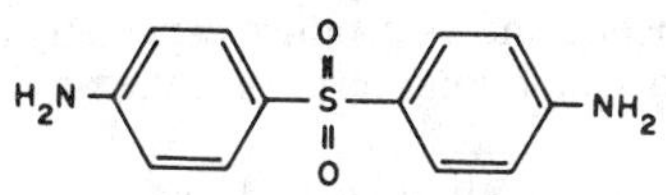

Adverse Reactions. Dapsone, an oxidant drug, produces dose-dependent hemolysis, which is not of clinical consequence in patients without a hematologic disorder taking dapsone 50–100 mg daily. Hemolysis is greatly enhanced in patients with glucose-6-phosphate dehydrogenase (G6PD) deficiency, especially in its severe forms. Gastrointestinal intolerance occurs with resulting anorexia, nausea, or vomiting. Hematuria, fever, pruritus, skin rashes, and granulocytopenia can occur.

Dapsone is now being used in AIDS patients as prophylaxis and treatment of *Pneumocystis pneumoniae* pneumonia. These patients usually have preexisting anemia, making dapsone-induced hemolysis less well tolerated. Conversion of up to 20 percent of erythrocyte hemoglobin to methemoglobin can occur with dapsone doses of 100 mg daily. Although methemoglobinemia is usually asymptomatic, it may become of clinical consequence if the patient develops hypoxemia from lung disease. Rash is common in this patient population. In one study using dapsone, 100 mg daily, for prophylaxis, 33 of 47 patients discontinued the drug.[97]

In leprosy patients, reactions with dapsone may be difficult to extricate from the reactions attendant with the disease itself.[98] A sulfone syndrome occurring 5–6 weeks after initiation of therapy can be characterized by fever, jaundice, dermatitis, and lymphadenopathy—a presentation not unlike infectious mononucleosis.[99] During initial dapsone therapy, erythema nodosum leprosum reactions commonly become manifest in those with multibacillary disease.

Usage. Dapsone and rifampin are the principal therapeutic agents for treatment of both multibacillary and paucibacillary *M. leprae* infections. Usage in pneumocystosis is discussed in Chapter 258. Dapsone is also useful in dermatatitis herpetiformis, a subject beyond the scope of this chapter.

Availability and Dosage. Dapsone is available generically in tablets of 25 or 100 mg. Adult daily dosage is 100 mg, and for children it is 1–1.5 mg/kg/day. It is administered daily for 6 months in paucibacillary disease and for a minimum of 2 years in multibacillary disease.

Rifampin

Mechanism of Action and Resistance. The mechanism of action of rifampin (structure shown in Fig. 2) is presumed to be inhibition of *M. leprae* DNA-dependent RNA polymerase that produces a relatively rapid bactericidal effect. Its inhibitory concentration for human strains of *M. leprae* tested in mice is 0.3 µg/ml. Acquired rifampin resistance is caused by mutational changes in RNA polymerase.[100] A tabulation of relative activity of antileprosy drugs in clearing tissue of viable bacilli is shown in Table 5.

TABLE 5. Efficacy of Antileprosy Agents in Rendering Tissue Free of Viable Bacilli[a]

Antimicrobial Drug	Human Adult Dosage	Days Until Bacilli-Free	
		Range	Median
Rifampin	1500 mg once	<3–<5	<3
Rifampin	600 mg/day	3–<14	<7
Dapsone	50 mg/day[b]	21–>134	61
Clofazimine	200 mg/day[c]	94–138	113
Acedapsone	225 mg/75 days	44–>306	214

[a] By mouse footpad assay.
[b] Dose raised to 50 mg/day over period of 4 weeks.
[c] Dose decreased to 100 mg/day in some patients having excessive skin pigmentation.

(Modified from Shepard et al.,[101] with permission.)

FIG. 5. Structure of dapsone.

Usage. Clinical usage of rifampin has confirmed that it is more bactericidal by several orders of magnitude than all other antileprosy drugs either alone or in combination. It is considered the only rapidly bactericidal drug against *M. leprae*. Using a skin biopsy assay, a single 1500-mg dose of rifampin was determined to reduce the viability of leprosy bacilli to undetectable levels by 3–5 days.[101] Despite such a dramatic impact on numbers of tissue *M. leprae*, rifampin must be employed with one or more companion drugs to prevent development of resistance.[95] The high cost of rifampin has discouraged daily usage in economically disadvantaged regions. However, once-monthly therapy with 600–1200 mg of rifampin in combination drug regimens has produced satisfactory clinical responses with a minimum of adverse reactions.[102] Current recommendations are that rifampin be administered in a single monthly supervised dose of 600 mg. This dosage is continued for 6 months in paucibacillary disease and for a minimum of 2 years in multibacillary disease. In the United States, rifampin is given as a 100-mg daily dose in both of the above settings. Reversal and erythema nodosum leprosum reactions with rifampin have been comparable or less severe than with sulfones alone.

Clofazimine (Lamprene)

Derivation and Structure. The structure of clofazimine, a phenazine dye, is shown in Figure 6.

Mechanism of Action and Antimicrobial Activity. Clofazimine's precise mechanism of action is unknown. Highly lipophilic and bound to mycobacterial DNA, clofazimine is weakly bactericidal against *M. leprae*. Its action may relate to iron chelation with resulting production of nascent oxygen radicals intracellularly.[103] The inhibitory concentration of clofazimine in mouse tissue is between 0.1 and 1 mg/kg. Delay of some 50 days ensues before tissue antimicrobic activity can be demonstrated in humans.

Pharmacology. Clofazimine pharmacokinetics are complex. Absorption is quite variable, with 9–74 percent of an administered dose appearing in feces. Oral administration results in plasma concentrations of 0.4–3 µg/ml with a half-life of approximately 70 days. Clofazimine is widely distributed throughout reticuloendothelial tissues, especially liver, spleen, lung, adrenals, adipose tissue, and skin lesions. Red-orange phagocytized crystals of clofazimine are observed microscopically in macrophages. It is largely unmetabolized and subsequently slowly excreted with less than 1 percent in urine. Biliary excretion appears to be the major route of excretion. Excretion also occurs in breast milk. Dosage of 100 mg/day has been calculated to result eventually in total accumulation of at least 10 g in human tissue.

Adverse Reactions. Gastrointestinal intolerance (anorexia, diarrhea, abdominal pain) is the most common therapy-limiting side effect and is generally dose related. Dry mouth and skin may occur. Skin pigmentation is quite common, resulting from

drug accumulation producing red-brown to nearly black discoloration, especially in dark skinned persons.

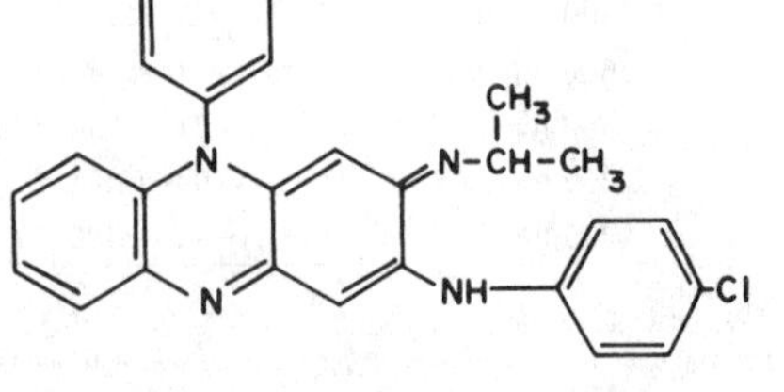

Usage. Clofazimine's current role is principally in combination with rifampin and dapsone for multibacillary disease. It is also used in combination for sulfone-resistant infections and for individuals who are sulfone intolerant, usually because of severe sulfone-associated erythema nodosum leprosum or reversal reactions. Such reactions occur much less with clofazimine than with dapsone,[104] possibly because of anti-inflammatory properties of clofazimine.

Availability and Dosage. Clofazimine (Lamprene) is supplied in 50- and 100-mg capsules. For multibacillary disease, it is administered in a dosage of 50 mg/day for a minimum of 2 years in combination with rifampin and dapsone. A dapsone alternative dosage has usually been 100–300 mg/day.

ADDITIONAL OR SECOND-LINE DRUGS

Thiacetazone (Amithiozone)

Derivation, structure, pharacokinetics, untoward reactions, and dosage of this thiosemicarbazone are described above under "Second-Line Antituberculous Drugs." Thiacetazone's efficacy is greater in tuberculoid (paucibacillary) than in lepromatous (multibacillary) disease. It can be administered when sulfones are not tolerated. Considerable cross-resistance occurs with sulfones. Thiacetazone is unavailable in the United States.

Ethionamide and Prothionamide

Ethionamide (Trecator-SC) has been described above under "Second-Line Antituberculous Drugs." It and its congener prothionamide (not available in the United States) possess similar pharmacokinetics and dosing and provide alternatives to clofazimine in multidrug regimens for multibacillary disease in those who are unable to tolerate clofazimine or refuse it due to skin pigmentation. Ethionamide and prothionamide are apparently weakly bactericidal against *M. leprae*. Ethionamide is provided in 250-mg tablets. Usual dosage is 250 mg daily. Both agents are expensive and cause considerable gastrointestinal intolerance and occasionally drug-induced hepatitis.

Other Substituted Rifamycins

Rifabutin (Mycobutin) and rifapentine are substituted rifamycins active against *M. leprae*. The former is FDA approved in the United States, while the latter remains investigational. In mice, these compounds are even more active than rifampin,[105] which raises interest in human therapeutic trials.

Other Sulfones

Acedapsone. Acedapsone (4,4″-diacetyldiaminodiphenylsulfone) is a long-acting intramuscular repository derivative of dapsone. The parent compound possesses little activity against *M. leprae* but is metabolized into active dapsone. Its half-life is 46 days, and that of the derived dapsone is 43 days.[106] A 300-mg im dose maintains dapsone levels in volunteers above the inhibitory concentration for *M. leprae* for approximately 100 days. Microbiologic and clinical responses are somewhat slower than those for daily dapsone. Long-term studies with acedapsone by injection five times yearly have yielded encouraging results. Acedapsone shows promise especially in regions where or in patients in which long-term oral therapy is not practical.

Sulfoxone. Less well absorbed and more expensive than dapsone, sulfoxone, a disubstituted sulfone, may be better toler-

FIG. 6. Structure of clofazimine.

ated gastrointestinally. It is formulated in 165-mg enteric-coated tablets, with a usual daily dosage of 330 mg.[10]

Newer Agents. Several other agents have shown promising activity against *M. leprae* in mouse foot pad models and early clinical trials. Among these are included minocycline (Minocin), clarithromycin (Biaxin),[107] and fluorinated quinolones—perfloxacin, ofloxacin (Floxin), and especially sparfloxacin.[108] Their roles in shortening therapy or in replacing drugs in existing multidrug regimens remain to be determined, although none of these agents appear to be as bactericidal against *M. leprae* as rifampin.

Chemotherapy-Associated Reactions in Leprosy

Febrile reaction in leprosy can be ameliorated with acetylsalicylic acid (aspirin) in conventional dosage. Immunologic reactions are common during chemotherapy for leprosy. "Reversal" reactions associated with swelling and edema in preexisting skin lesions or peripheral neuropathy in more severe reactions usually occur in the first year of therapy. Corticosteroids such as prednisone 40–80 mg/day initially with subsequent tapering of dosage have been reasonably efficacious for reversal reactions.

For patients with erythema nodosum leprosum reactions, thalidomide in a initial dosage of 400 mg daily may be the treatment of choice. Its beneficial effect for these reactions appears to be mediated by inhibition of tumor necrosis factor-α (TNF-α).[109] It should be tapered over the first week, with a maintenance dose of 50–100 mg/day. Thalidomide is available under an FDA protocol in the United States from the Gillis W. Long Hansen's Diseases Clinic in Carville, LA. Because of its marked teratogenicity, thalidomide should never be administered to women of childbearing age. In patients with erythema nodosum leprosum for whom thalidomide is unavailable or unacceptable, high-dose prednisone offers an alternative. Patients who manifest puzzling or severe reactions are best managed by specialists such as those at the Hansen's Disease Clinic in Carville, LA.[98]

REFERENCES

1. Frieden TR, Sterling T, Pablos-Mendez A, et al. The emergence of drug-resistant tuberculosis in New York City. N Engl J Med. 1993;328:521–6.
2. Goble M, Iseman MD, Madsen LA, et al. Treatment of 171 patients with pulmonary tuberculosis resistant to isoniazid and rifampin. N Engl J Med. 1993;328:527–32.
3. Centers for Disease Control and Prevention. Outbreak of multidrug-resistant tuberculosis at a hospital—New York City, 1991. MMWR. 1993;42:427–34.
4. Laraque F, Riley LW. Tuberculosis in HIV-infected patients. AIDS Reader 1992 (Sept–Oct):171–80.
5. Eriki PP, Okera A, Aisu T, et al. The influence of human immunodeficiency virus infection on tuberculosis in Kampala, Uganda. Am Rev Respir Dis. 1991;143:185–7.
6. Iseman MD, Cohn DL, Sbarbaro JA. Directly observed treatment of tuberculosis. N Engl J Med. 1993;328:576–8.
7. Sensi P. Approaches to the development of new antituberculosis drugs. Rev Infect Dis. 1989;11(Suppl 2):S467–70.
8. Pozniak AL, MacLeod GA, Mahari M, et al. The influence of HIV status on single and multiple drug reactions to antituberculous therapy in Africa. AIDS. 1992;6:809–14.
9. Stead WW, Dutt AK. Chemotherapy for tuberculosis today. Am Rev Respir Dis. 1982;125(Suppl 3):94–101.
10. Mandell GL, Sande MA. Drugs used in the chemotherapy of tuberculosis and leprosy. In: Gilman AS, Rall TW, Nies AS, et al, eds. The Pharmacological Basis of Therapeutics. 8th ed. New York: Pergamon Press; 1990:1146–64.
11. Kucers A, Bennett NM. Drugs mainly for tuberculosis. Part III. In: The Use of Antibiotics. 4th ed. Philadelphia: JB Lippincott; 1987:1351–437.
12. Pratt WB. Chemotherapy of tuberculosis. In: Chemotherapy of Infection. New York: Oxford University Press; 1977:231–62.
13. Davidson PT, Hanh QL. Drug treatment of tuberculosis—1992. Drugs. 1992; 43:651–73.
14. Starke JR, Current chemotherapy for tuberculosis in children. Infect Dis Clin North Am. 1992;6:215–38.
15. Centers for Disease Control and Prevention. Initial therapy for tuberculosis in the era of multidrug resistance. Recommendations of the Advisory Council for the Elimination of Tuberculosis. MMWR. 1993;42:1–8.
16. Herman RP, Weber MM. Site of action of isoniazid on the electron transport chain and its relationship to nicotinamide adenine dinucleotide regulation in *Mycobacterium phlei*. Antimicrob Agents Chemother. 1980;17:450–4.
17. Ormerod LP, Harrison JM, Wright PA. Drug resistance trends in *Mycobacterium tuberculosis:* Blackburn 1985–89. Tubercle. 1990;71:283–5.
18. Seifart HI, Parkin DP, Donald PR. Stability of isoniazid, rifampin and pyrazinaminde in suspensions used for the treatment of tuberculosis in children. Pediatr Infect Dis J. 1991;10:827–31.
19. Kopanoff DE, Snider DE, Caras GJ. Isoniazid-related hepatitis. Am Rev Respir Dis. 1978;117:991–1001.
20. Centers for Disease Control and Prevention. National Consensus Conference on Tuberculosis. Preventive treatment of tuberculosis. Chest. 1985;87(Suppl 2)L128–32.
21. Krishnaswamy K, Prasad CE, Murthy KJ. Hepatic dysfunction in undernourished patients receiving isoniazid and rifampicin. Trop Geogr Med. 1991; 43:156–60.
22. Franks AL, Binkin NJ, Snider DE Jr, et al. Isoniazid hepatitis among pregnant and postpartum Hispanic patients. Public Health Rep. 1989;104:151–5.
23. Murphy R, Swartz R, Watkins PB. Severe acetaminophen toxicity in a patient receiving isoniazid. Ann Intern Med. 1990;113:799–800.
24. Wu JC, Lee SD, Yeh PF, et al. Isoniazid-rifampin-induced hepatitis in hepatitis B carriers. Gastroenterology. 1990;98:502–4.
25. Kumar A, Misra PK, Mehotra R, et al. Hepatotoxicity of rifampin and isoniazid. Is it all drug-induced hepatitis? Am Rev Respir Dis. 1991;143:1350–2.
26. Deshpande DV, Nachne D, Koyande D, et al. Anti-tubercular treatment in patients with hepatitis. J Assoc Physicians India. 1991;39:599–601.
27. McGlynn KA, Lustabader ED, Sharrar RE, et al. Isoniazid prophylaxis in hepatitis B carriers. Am Rev Respir Dis. 1986;134:666–8.
28. Gangadharam PRJ. Isoniazid, rifampin, and hepatotoxicity. Am Rev Respir Dis. 1986;133:963–5.
29. Woo J, Chan HS. Therapeutic problems in the management of elderly patients with tuberculosis. Adverse Drug React Toxicol Rev. 1992;11:13–8.
30. Ansari MM, Beg MH, Haleem S. Hepatitis in patients with surgicial complications of pulmonary tuberculosis. Indian J Chest Dis Allied Sci. 1991;33: 133–8.
31. Centers for Disease Control and Prevention. Severe isoniazid-associated hepatitis—New York, 1991–1993. MMWR. 1993;42:545–7.
32. Jordan TJ, Lewit EM, Reichman LB. Isoniazid preventive therapy for tuberculosis. Decision analysis considering ethnicity and gender. Am Rev Respir Dis. 1991;144:1357–60.
33. Nisar M, Watkin SW, Bucknall RC, et al. Exacerbation of isoniazid induced peripheral neuropathy by pyridoxine. Thorax. 1990;45:419–20.
34. Ishii N, Nishihara Y. Pellagra encephalopathy among tuberculous patients: Its relation to isoniazid therapy. J Neurol Neurosurg Psychiatry. 1985;48: 628–34.
35. Pellock JM, Howell J, Kendig EL Jr, et al. Pyridoxine deficiency in children treated with isoniazid. Chest. 1985;87:658–61.
36. Schraufnagel DE, Stoner R, Whiting E, et al. Testing for isoniazid. An evaluation of the Arkansas method. Chest. 1990;98:314–6.
37. Koestner JA, Jones LK, Polk WH, et al. Prolonged use of intravenous isoniazid and rifampin. DICP. 1989;23:48–50.
38. Venkatesan K. Pharmacokinetic drug interactions with rifampin. Clin Pharmacokinet. 1992;22:47–65.
39. Immanuel C, Jayasankar K, Narayana AS, et al. Induction of rifampicin metabolism during treatment of tuberculous patients with daily and fully intermittent regimens containing the drug. Indian J Chest Dis Allied Sci. 1989;31:251–7.
40. Woo J, Leung A, Chan K, et al. Pyrazinamide and rifampicin regimens for patients on maintenance dialysis. Int J Artif Organs. 1988;11:181–5.
41. Telenti A, Imboden P, Marchesi F, et al. Detection of rifampicin-resistance mutations in *Mycobacterium tuberculosis*. Lancet 1993;341:647–50.
42. Newman R, Doster BE, Murray FJ, et al. Rifampin in initial treatment of pulmonary tuberculosis. A US Public Health Service tuberculosis therapy trial. Am Rev Respir Dis. 1974;109:216–32.
43. White NW. Venous thrombosis and rifampin. Lancet 1989;2:434–5.
44. Mehta M, ed. Physicians Desk Reference Guide to Drug Interactions, Side Effects, Indications. Montvale, NJ: Medical Economics Data; 1992;797–9.
45. Baciewicz AM, Self TH, Bekemeyer WB. Update on rifampin drug interactions. Arch Intern Med. 1987;147:565–8.
46. Borcherding SM, Baciewicz AM, Self TH. Update on rifampin drug interactions II. Arch Intern Med. 1992;152:711–6.
47. Greene JB, Sidhu GS, Lewin S, et al. *Mycobacterium avium intracellulare:* A cause of disseminated life-threatening infection in homosexuals and drug abusers. Ann Intern Med. 1982;97:539–46.
48. Heifets LB, Iseman MD, Lindholm-Levy PJ, et al. Determination of ansamycin MICs for *Mycobacterium avium* complex in liquid medium by radiometric and conventional methods. Antimicrob Agents Chemother. 1985;28: 570–5.
49. Masur H, Tuazon C, Gill V, et al. Effect of combined clofazimine and ansamycin therapy on *Mycobacterium avium-Mycobacterium intracellulare* bacteremia in patients with AIDS. J Infect Dis. 1987;155:127–9.
50. O'Brien RJ, Lyle MA, Snider DE Jr. Rifabutin (ansamycin LM 427): A new rifamycin-S derivative for the treatment of mycobacterial diseases. Rev Infect Dis. 1987;9:519–30.
51. Chan SL, Yew WW, Ma WK, et al. The early bactericidal activity of rifabutin measured by sputum viable counts in Hong Kong patients with pulmonary tuberculosis. Tubercle Lung Dis. 1992;73:33–8.
51a. Shafran SD, Deschenes J, Phillips P, et al. Uveitis and pseudojaundice during

a regimen of clarithromycin, rifabutin and ethambutol. N Engl J Med. 1994; 330:438–9.

52. Hong Kong Chest Service/British Medical Research Council. A controlled study of rifabutin and an uncontrolled study of ofloxacin in the retreatment of patients with pulmonary tuberculosis resisant to isoniazid, streptomycin and rifampicin. Tubercle Lung Dis. 1992;73:59–67.

52a. Frank MO, Graham MB, Wispelway B. Rifabutin and uveitis. N Engl J Med. 1994;330:868.

53. Pretet S, Lebeaut A, Parrot R, et al. and the Group for the Study and Treatment of Resistant Mycobacterial Infections. Combined chemotherapy including rifabutin for rifampicin and isoniazid resistant pulmonary tuberculosis. Eur Respir J. 1992;5:680–4.

54. Steele MA, Des Prez RM. The role of pyrazinamide in tuberculosis chemotherapy. Chest. 1988;94:845–50.

55. Grosset JH. Present status of chemotherapy for tuberulosis. Rev Infect Dis. 1989:S347–52.

56. Crowle AJ. Studies of antituberculosis chemotherapy with an in vitro model of human tuberculosis. Semin Respir Infect. 1986;1:262–4.

57. Nalin R, Potar M, David HL. Pyrazinamide is not effective against intracellulary growing Mycobacterium tuberculosis. Antimicrob Agents Chemother. 1987;31:287.

58. Donald PR, Seifart H. Cerebrospinal fluid pyrazinamide concentrations in children with tuberculous meningitis. Pediatr Infect Dis J. 1988;7:469–71.

59. Zierski M, Bek E. Side effects of drug regimens used in short-course chemotherapy for pulmonary tuberculosis. A controlled clinical study. Tubercle. 1980;61:41–9.

60. Sanwikarja S, Kauffmann RH, teVelde J, et al. Tubulointerstitial nephritis associated with pyrazinamide. Neth J Med 1989;34:40–6.

61. Namba S, Igari T, Nishiyama K, et al. A case of pyrazinamide-associated myoglobinuric renal failure. Jpn J Med. 1991;30:468–72.

62. Chatterjee VK, Buchanan OR, Friedman AI, et al. Ocular toxicity following ethambutol in standard dosage. Br J Dis Chest. 1986;80:288–91.

63. Quemard A, Laneelle G, Lacave C. Mycolic acid synthesis: A target for ethionamide in mycobacteria? Antimicrob Agents Chemother. 1992;36:1316–21.

64. McClatchy JK, Kanes W. Davidson PT, et al. Cross-resistance in M. tuberculosis to kanamycin, capreomycin, and viomycin. Tubercle. 1977;58:29–34.

65. Yew WW, Kwan SY, Ma WK, et al. In-vitro activity of ofloxacin against Mycobacterium tuberculosis and its clinical efficacy in multiply resistant pulmonary tuberculosis. J Antimicrob Chemother. 1990;26:227–36.

66. Leysen DC, Haemers A, Pattyn SR. Mycobacteria and the new quinolones. Antimicrob Agents Chemother. 1989;33:1–5.

67. Gay JD, DeYoung DR, Roberts GD. In vitro activities of norfloxacin and ciprofloxacin against Mycobacterium tuberculosis, M. avium complex, M. chelonei, M. fortuitum, and M. kansasii. Antimicrob Agents Chemother. 1984;26:94–6.

68. Chen CH, Shih JF, Lindholm-Levy PJ, et al. Minimal inhibitory concentrations of rifabutin, ciprofloxacin, and ofloxacin against Mycobacterium tuberculosis isolated before treatment of patients in Taiwan. Am Rev Respir Dis. 1989;140:989–9.

69. Caekenberghe DV. Comparative in vitro activities of ten fluoroquinolones and fusidic acid against Mycobacterium spp. J Antimicrob Chemother. 1990; 26:381–6.

70. Kohno S, Koga H, Kaku M, et al. Prospective comparative study of ofloxacin or ethambutol for the treatment of pulmonary tuberculosis. Chest. 1992;102:1815–8.

71. Tsukamura M, Nakamura E, Yoshii S, et al. Therapeutic effect of new antibacterial substance ofloxacin (DL 8280) on pulmonary tuberculosis. Am Rev Respir Dis. 1985;131:352–6.

72. LaLande V, Truffot-Pernot C, Paccaly-Moulin A, et al. Powerful bactericidal activity of sparfloxacin (AT-4140) against Mycobacterium tuberculosis in mice. Antimicrob Agents Chemother. 1993;37:407–13.

73. Cynamon MH, Palmer GS. In vitro activity of amoxicillin in combination with clavulanic acid against Mycobacterium tuberculosis. Antimicrob Agents Chemother. 1983;24:429–31.

74. Wallace RJ Jr, Brown BA, Onyi GO. Susceptibilities of Mycobacterium fortuitum biovar fortuitum and the two subgroups of Mycobacterium chelonae to imipenem, cefmetazole, cefoxitin, and amoxicillin-clavulanic acid. Antimicrob Agents Chemother. 1991;35:773–5.

75. Nozawa RT, Kato H, Yokota T, et al. Susceptibility of intra- and extracellular Mycobacterium avium-intracellulare to cephem antibiotics. Antimicrob Agents Chemother. 1985;27:132–4.

76. Wallace RJ Jr, Swensom JM, Silcox VA, et al. Treatment of nonpulmonary infections due to Mycobacterium fortuitum and Mycobacterium chelonei on the basis of in vitro susceptibilities. J Infect Dis. 1985;152:500–14.

77. Sommers HM, McClatchy JK. Laboratory diagnoses of the mycobacterioses. Cumitech 16. pp. 1–18. In: Morello JA, ed. Cumulative Techniques and Procedures in Microbiology. Washington, DC: American Society for Microbiology; 1983.

78. Irwin RS, Pratter MR, Corwin RW, et al. Pulmonary infection with Mycobacterium chelonei: Successful treatment with one drug based on disk diffusion susceptibility data. J Infect Dis. 1981;145:772.

79. Sanders WJ, Wolinsky E. In vitro susceptibility of Mycobacterium marinum to eight antimicrobial agents. Antimicrob Agents Chemother. 1980;18:529–31.

80. Woodley CL, Kilburn JO. In vitro susceptibility of Mycobacterium avium

complex and Mycobacterium tuberculosis strains to a spiro-piperidyl rifamycin. Am Rev Respir Dis. 1992;126:586–7.

81. Nightingale SD, Cameron DW, Gordin FM, et al. Two controlled trials of rifabutin prophylaxis against Mycobacterium avium complex infection in AIDS. N Engl J Med. 1993;329:828–33.

82. Nozawa RT, Kato H, Yokota T. Intra- and extracellular susceptibilty of Mycobacterium avium-intracellulare complex to aminoglycoside antibiotics. Antimicrob Agents Chemother. 1984;26:841–4.

83. Swenson JM, Thornsberry C, Silcox VA. Rapidly growing mycobacteria: Testing of susceptibility to 34 antimicrobial agents by broth microdilution. Antimicrob Agents Chemother. 1982;22:186–92.

84. Donta ST, Smith PW, Levitz RE, et al. Therapy of Mycobacterium marinum infections. Use of tetracyclines vs rifampin. Arch Intern Med. 1986;146:902–4.

85. Clegg HW, Foster MT, Sanders WE Jr, et al. Infection due to organisms of the Mycobacterium fortuitum complex after augmentation mammoplasty: Clinical and epidemiologic features. J Infect Dis. 1983;147:427–33.

86. Swenson JM, Wallace RJ Jr, Silcox VA, et al. Antimicrobial susceptibility of five subgroups of Mycobacterium fortuitum and Mycobacterium chelonae. Antimicrob Agents Chemother. 1985;28:807–11.

87. Brown BA, Wallace RJ Jr, Onyi GO. Activities of clarithromycin against eight slowly growing species of nontuberculous mycobacteria, determined by using a broth microdilution MIC system. Antimicrob Agents Chemother. 1992;36:1987–90.

88. Brown BA, Wallace RJ Jr, Onyi GO, et al. Activities of four macrolides, including clarithromycin, against Mycobacterium fortuitum, Mycobacterium chelonae, and Mycobacterium chelonae-like organisms. Antimicrob Agents Chemother. 1992;36:180–4.

89. Gangadharam PRJ, Candler ER. Activity of some antileprosy compounds against Mycobacterium intracellulare in vitro. Am Rev Respir Dis. 1977;115:705–8.

90. Cynamon MH, Palmer GS. In vitro susceptibility of Mycobacterium fortuitum to N-formidoyl thienamycin and several cephamycins. Antimicrob Agents Chemother. 1982;22:1079–81.

91. Stone MS, Wallace RJ Jr, Swenson JM, et al. Agar disk elution method for susceptibility testing of Mycobacterium marinum and Mycobacterium fortuitum complex to sulfonamides and antibiotics. Antimicrob Agents Chemother. 1983;24:486–93.

92. Dautzenberg B, Truffot C, Legris S, et al. Activity of clarithromycin against Mycobacterium avium infection in patients with the acquired immune deficiency syndrome. A controlled clinical trial. Am Rev Respir Dis. 1991;144:564–9.

93. Young LS, Wiviott L, Wu M, et al. Azithromycin for treatment of Mycobacterium avium-intracellulare complex infection in patients with AIDS. Lancet 1991;338:1107–9.

94. Public Health Service Centers for Disease Control and Prevention. Increase in prevalence of leprosy caused by dapsone-resistant Mycobacterium leprae. MMWR. 1982;30:637–8.

95. Hastings RC, Franzblau SG. Chemotherapy of leprosy. Annu Rev Pharmacol Toxicol. 1988;28:231–45.

96. Pearson JMH, Rees RJW, Waters MFR. Sulphone resistance in leprosy. A review of one hundred proven clinical cases. Lancet. 1975;2:69–72.

97. Blum RA, Miller LA, Gaggini LC, Cohn DL. Comparative trial of dapsone versus trimethoprim/sulfamethoxazole for primary prophylaxis of Pneumocystis carinii pneumonia. J Acquir Immune Defic Syndr. 1992;5:341–7.

98. Case records of the Massachusetts General Hospital. Weekly clinicopathological exercises. Case 49-1985. Erythema nodosum leprosum reaction in patient with lepromatous leprosy. N Engl J Med. 1985;313:1464–72.

99. Adverse reactions to dapsone (Editorial). Lancet. 1982;2:184–5.

100. Honore N, Cole ST. Molecular basis of rifampin resistance in Mycobacterium leprae. Antimicrob Agents Chemother. 1993;37:414–418.

101. Shepard CC, Levy L, Fasal P. Further experience with the rapid bactericidal effect of rifampin on Mycobacterium leprae. Am J Trop Med Hyg. 1974;23:1120–4.

102. Yawalkar SJ, Languillon J, Hajra SK, et al. Once-monthly rifampicin plus dapsone in initial treatment of lepromatous leprosy. Lancet. 1982;1:1199–202.

103. Niwa Y, Sakance T, Miyachi Y, et al. Oxygen metabolism in phagocytes of leprotic patients: Enhanced endogenous superoxide dismutase activity and hydroxyl radical generation by clofazimine. J Clin Microbiol. 1984;20:837–42.

104. US Leprosy Panel. Spaced clofazimine therapy of lepromatous leprosy. Am J Trop Med Hyg. 1976;25:437–44.

105. Pattyn SR. Rifabutin and rifapentime compared with rifampin against Mycobacterium leprae in mice. Antimicrob Agents Chemother. 1987;31:134.

106. Peters JH, Murray JF, Gordon GR, et al. Acedapsone treatment of leprosy patients: Response versus drug disposition. Am J Trop Med Hyg. 1977;26:127–36.

107. Ji B, Jamet P, Perani EG, et al. Powerful bactericidal activities of clarithromycin and minocycline against Mycobacterium leprae in lepromatous leprosy. J Infect Dis. 1993;168:188–90.

108. Gelber RH, et al. Activities of various quinolone antibiotics against Mycobacterium leprae in infected mice. Antimicrob Agents Chemother. 1992;36:2522–7.

109. Sampaio EP, Kaplan G, Miranda A. The influence of thalidomide on the clinical and immunologic manifestation of erythema nodosum leprosum. J Infect Dis. 1993;168:404–14.

31. ANTIFUNGAL AGENTS

JOHN E. BENNETT

Both topical and systemic antifungal agents are discussed in this chapter, with the emphasis on pharmacology. Clinical indications are listed, but full details of dose and duration are best sought in the chapters devoted to individual mycoses.

TOPICAL AGENTS

Topical Agents for Cutaneous Use

Use of topical agents is confined to infections of the epidermis, hair, nails, and cornea (Table 1). This form of application is not effective in deeper cutaneous infections, such as sporotrichosis, blastomycosis, or chromomycosis. The choice between treating superficial infections with a topical or systemic agent depends on the fungus and on the site and extent of the lesion. For example, topical therapy is rarely used for ringworm of the scalp, nails, or extensive *Trichophyton rubrum* lesions of the trunk. The efficacy of topical agents in ringworm of the beard or in chronic noninflammatory sole and palm lesions also tends to be poor. Among the topical agents, the choice of formulation is important. Creams or solutions are preferred for fissured or inflamed intertriginous areas such as on the toe webs, groin, or scrotum. Use of powder, whether administered by a shake container or aerosol, is confined to mild lesions in those same areas or to preventive therapy in patients with repeated relapses of tinea pedis. Sprays are not recommended for the face. None of the preparations for cutaneous use should be applied to the vagina or eye. Secondary bacterial infection requires ancillary measures. Despite some antibacterial effect of the imidazoles in vitro, none of the antifungals included here have useful antibacterial activity.

The plethora of agents used for topical application necessitates that older agents with limited indications, such as iodine, sulfur, and gentian violet, not be discussed. Undecylenic acid and its salts, while widely used in nonprescription formulations, have too little efficacy to warrant further comment. While a list of nonprescription drugs would also include tolnaftate, clotrimazole, and miconazole, other agents can be expected to be added.

Changes are also frequent as to which formulations of antifungal agents are marketed in combination with corticosteroids or antibacterial agents.

Details of the treatment of cutaneous mycoses are beyond the scope of this chapter, except to note that the agents listed below are generally applied twice daily and do not differ substantially in the duration of therapy necessary for cure.

Salicylic and Benzoic Acids (Whitfield's Ointment). Salicylic acid is widely used in topical preparations as a keratolytic agent, often combined with other agents. The ointment marketed for nonprescription use in ringworm usually contains 3% salicylic acid and 6% benzoic acid. Although Whitfield's ointment can be used in mild tinea pedis, occlusive effects of the ointment and mild irritation of the salicylic acid make the undiluted preparation inappropriate for inflamed or macerated toe webs or scrotal infections. Except for its low cost, there is little to recommend the use of Whitfield's ointment in ringworm.

Allylamines. Allylamines, including naftifine and terbinafine, are synthetic compounds that inhibit squalene epoxidase, an enzyme essential for the synthesis of ergosterol (Fig. 1). Terbinafine cream 1% has been recently marketed in the United States.[1] These allylamines are effective topical agents for treatment of tinea pedis, tinea cruris, and tinea corporis.

Azoles. Azoles are synthetic compounds and include two classes, imidazoles and triazoles. The latter are named for the presence of three nitrogens in the azole ring, imidazoles having only two (Fig. 1). The primary mechanism of action of azoles is inhibition of α_{14}-demethylase, an enzyme required for the synthesis of ergosterol. At the high concentrations that might be achieved topically, these agents directly damage the cytoplasmic membrane. The antifungal spectrum is extremely broad in vitro but fungistatic. Clinical efficacy has been demonstrated in ringworm of the body, foot, hand, and perineum, as well as in cutaneous candidiasis and tinea versicolor.[2]

Morpholine Derivatives. Not listed in Table 1, amorolfine is available in some European countries as a 5% nail lacquer and a 0.25% cream.[3] Based on limited data, usage may be similar to topical azoles.

TABLE 1. Topical Treatment of Superficial Mycoses[a]

Drug (Trade Name)	Prescription Required	Formulation					Indications	
		Solution or Spray	Lotion	Cream	Ointment	Powder	Ringworm	Candidiasis
Azoles								
Clotrimazole (Lotromin, Mycelex)	No	+	+	+	0	0	+	+
Econazole (Spectazole)	Yes	0	0	+	0	0	+	+
Ketoconazole (Nizoral)	Yes	+	0	+	0	0	+	+
Miconazole (Micatin, Monistat-Derm)	No	+	+	+	0	+	+	+
Sulconazole (Exelderm)	Yes	+	0	0	0	0	+	?
Polyenes								
Amphotericin B (Fungizone)	Yes	0	+	+	+	0	0	+
Nystatin (Mycostatin, Nilstat)	Yes	0	0	+	+	+	0	+
Other								
Ciclopirox (Loprox)	Yes	0	0	+	0	0	+	+
Haloprogin (Halotex)	Yes	+	0	+	0	0	+	+
Naftifine (Naftin)	Yes	0	0	+	+	+	+	0
Terbinafine (Lamisil)	Yes	0	0	+	0	0	+	0
Tolnaftate (Aftate, NP-27, Ting, Tinactin, Zeasorb)	No	+	0	+	0	+	+	0
Undecylenate (Cruex, Desenex)	No	+	0	+	+	+	+	0

[a] Formulations and over-the-counter sales reflect only the U.S. practice and are subject to change. Compounds that have formulations available without prescription often have other preparations that require prescription.

(Adapted from Kwon-Chung,[105] with permission.)

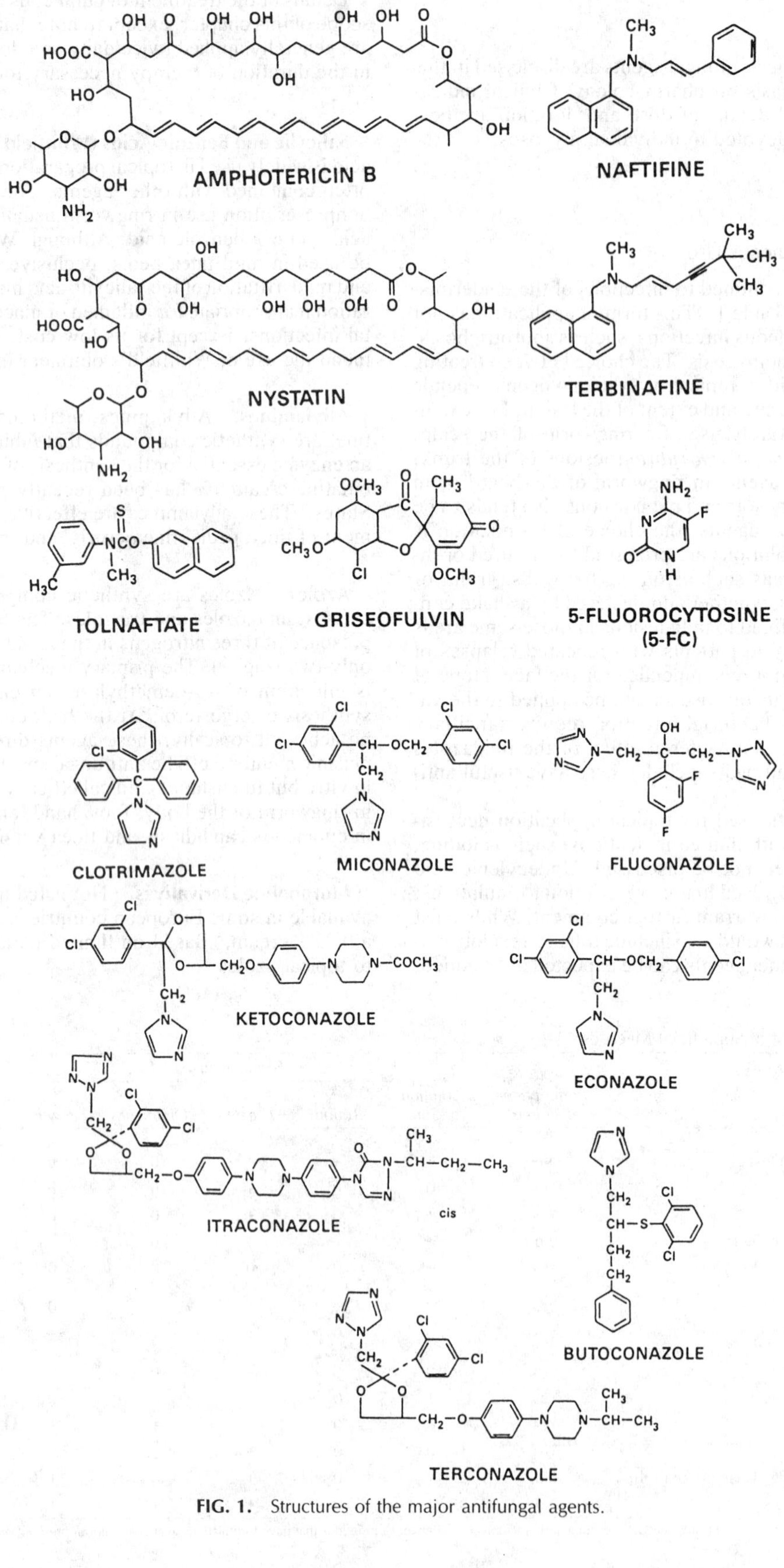

FIG. 1.   Structures of the major antifungal agents.

Polyenes. A large number of macrolide polyene antibiotics are known and have broad-spectrum antifungal activity in vitro.[4] Topically, they are useful only against *Candida,* not ringworm. The hypertrophic skin lesions of chronic mucocutaneous candidiasis do not respond to these antibiotics, although macerated or intertriginous lesions typically respond well. These polyenes are derived by biosynthesis from aerobic actinomycetes, are poorly soluble in water, and share a common mechanism of action. The antifungal activity depends on binding to the cytoplasmic membrane sterols such as ergosterol and thereby increasing membrane permeability.[5] Other pharmacologic properties are discussed later. *Nystatin* and *amphotericin B* are available for topical use in the United States.

Topical Agents for Vaginal Use

Vulvovaginal candidiasis is a common disease that can cause substantial chronic discomfort. Both tablets and creams are marketed for once-a-day use, preferably at bedtime to facilitate retention. If candidiasis has extended onto the vulva or perineum, creams that can be applied topically as well as vaginally may have an advantage over tablets. Cream dispensers are designed to administer 5 g per use. The differences between creams and vaginal troches are less important than correct insertion deep in the vagina. Some preparations have a patient package insert with a clear set of instructions. The duration of therapy is longer for polyene troches than for the imidazoles, leading to increasing use of the latter class. The duration of therapy for the imidazoles, as stated in the literature or in the package insert, seems more dependent on the design of the original clinical studies than on the efficacy of the product. Most of the studies of imidazoles have shown short-term efficacy of roughly 80–90 percent if high-risk patients are excluded, such as patients relapsing from recent treatment.[6–9] Data on late relapse after treatment with these drug are hard to find, although relapse is acknowledged to be common. Ingestion of nystatin tablets to decrease the fecal *Candida* concentration has been recommended to aid treatment and prevent relapse of vulvovaginal candidiasis, but the evidence of efficacy remains unconvincing. Although a fecal reservoir may be one source for relapse, the reduction in fecal colony counts by oral nystatin is small. Even the massive doses of oral nystatin used in laminar flow units usually have not eradicated *Candida* from the feces.

Adverse effects of vaginal therapy are few. Allergy to any one imidazole probably precludes the use of other imidazoles. Local irritation or burning, rarely a serious problem, does vary among preparations. Some systemic absorption, generally less than 10 percent of the dose, has been documented for many of the vaginal imidazoles and may be a general phenomenon. This is of theoretical interest in that it might cause birth defects during the first trimester of pregnancy or alter the metabolism of other medications taken by the patient. However, none of these consequences has been observed. Systemic absorption of vaginal polyenes probably does not occur. A list of agents currently available for vaginal use is given in Table 2. Compounds available in Canada, such as *econazole* (Ecostatin), or only overseas, such as isoconazole, are not listed. *Butoconazole* (Femstat), *miconazole* (Monistat 3 and Monistat 7), and econazole are formulated as the nitrate for vaginal use. The triazole *terconazole* (Terazol 3 and Terazol 7) and the imidazole *clotrimazole* (Gyne-Lotrimin and Mycelex-G) are marketed as the base, not as a salt. Trade names differ in Canada.

ORAL THERAPY FOR SUPERFICIAL MYCOSES

Agents for the Treatment of Oral Candidiasis (Thrush)

Nystatin (Mycostatin, Nilstat, and generic), named for New York State, is produced by *Streptomyces noursei.* The drug is available as an oral suspension of 100,000 units/ml. Adults

TABLE 2. Topical Treatment of *Candida* Vulvovaginitis

Drug	Trade Names	Dose[a]	Duration (Days)
Azoles			
Creams			
Butoconazole 2%	Femstat	5 g	3 or 6[b]
Clotrimazole 1%	Gyne-Lotrimin[c], Mycelex 7[c]	5 g	7–14
Miconazole 2%	Monistat-7[c]	5 g	7
Terconazole 0.4%	Terazole-7	5 g	7
Tioconazole 6.5%	Vagistat	4.6 g	1
Tablets or suppositories			
Clotrimazole	Gyne-Lotrimin[c], Mycelex 7[c]	100 mg	7[d]
Clotrimazole	Gyne-Lotrimin, Mycelex G	500 mg	1
Miconazole	Monistat 7[c]	100 mg	7
Miconazole	Monistat 3	200 mg	3
Terconazole	Terazole 3	80 mg	3
Polyenes			
Suppository			
Nystatin	Mycostatin, Nilstat	100,000 units	14

[a] All medications given at bedtime. Dose of cream refers to total weight, including excipient.
[b] Duration for pregnant patients.
[c] Preparations available in the United States without prescription.
[d] Alternatively, two tablets may be used each night for 3 nights.

(Adapted from Kwon-Chung,[105] with permission.)

should swish 5–10 ml around in the mouth three times a day. Swallowing the suspension rather than expectorating it may help to treat subclinical esophageal candidiasis in immunosuppressed patients. Nystatin suspension is not absorbed from the gastrointestinal tract and, except for its bitter taste, is remarkably free from adverse effects. Vaginal tablets of nystatin can be held in the mouth and used as troches, but these are bitter and not designed for this use. A better alternative is the use of *clotrimazole* troches. These pleasant-tasting 10-mg tablets are effective in oral thrush when used five times a day.[10] Each tablet should not be chewed, but kept in the mouth until it dissolves. Although some absorption occurs after the drug is swallowed, no adverse effects or systemic efficacy occurs. Oral ketoconazole, 200–400 mg/day, is also effective in oral candidiasis.[11–13] The 400-mg dose is recommended for patients in the late stages of acquired immunodeficiency syndrome (AIDS). These patients absorb ketoconazole less well because they have reduced gastric acidity. Fluconazole, 100–200 mg once daily, is more effective than ketoconazole in AIDS patients with oropharyngeal or esophageal candidiasis, possibly because fluconazole is reliably absorbed even in the absence of gastric acid.[14] Chronic administration of fluconazole has led to azole-resistant oropharyngeal candidiasis in a growing number of AIDS patients.[15] Intravenous amphotericin B remains a useful drug in patients who fail fluconazole.

Oral Therapy of Superficial Cutaneous Infections

Systemic therapy of ringworm of the scalp, beard, and nails of the hand is preferred to topical therapy. Chronic noninflammatory ringworm of the soles and palms, as well as extensive ringworm of the trunk or groin, may also require systemic therapy. The preferred drug for these indications is griseofulvin because of its efficacy and low incidence of adverse effects. Although ketoconazole or itraconazole can be used for griseofulvin-resistant ringworm, the chance of serious side effects indicates that readily remedial causes of griseofulvin failures should be sought: erratic drug ingestion, too low a dose, and incorrect diagnosis. Candidiasis of the nail or skin, particularly of the groin, can resemble ringworm closely and does not respond to griseofulvin. None of the currently available topical or systemic agents is very effective against ringworm of the toenail. White superficial onychomycosis, while rare, is more responsive to griseofulvin. For those who are concerned about the cosmetic problem, a 12- to 18-month course of griseofulvin or itraconazole may be worth a trial. Duration of therapy depends on the rate of nail growth, which may be slower than normal.

Griseofulvin. Griseofulvin, derived from a species of *Penicillium,* is active against ringworm but not against *Candida* or tinea versicolor. It is poorly active topically but reaches the skin and hair after ingestion. Absorption is favored by reducing the particle size and perhaps by ingestion with a fatty meal. A microcrystalline form (generic, Fulvicin-U/F, Grifulvin V, and Grisactin) is available as 125-, 250-, and 500-mg tablets, plus a pediatric suspension of 125 mg/5 ml. The ultramicrocrystalline form (Fulvicin-P/G, Gris-PEG, and Grisactin Ultra) comes in 125-, 165-, 250-, and 330-mg tablets. The two forms have comparable efficacy. Griseofulvin is metabolized in the liver with a serum half-life of 24–36 hours. Blood levels can be depressed by phenobarbital therapy and may require increasing the griseofulvin dose. Conversely, metabolism of warfarin anticoagulants is increased by griseofulvin. Adverse reactions to griseofulvin are uncommon. Headache may be observed early in therapy but usually disappears with continued use. Allergic reactions can occur, apparently unrelated to penicillin allergy. Hepatotoxic reactions have been observed in patients with acute intermittent porphyria. A variety of other side effects have also been observed, but a causal relationship is much less clear. Safety during pregnancy has not been established.

The usual daily dose is 500, 750, or 1000 mg daily for the microcrystalline drug, with children receiving 10 mg/kg. The 500-mg/day dose is reserved for mild infections and small adults. A dose of 330 mg daily is recommended for the ultramicrocrystalline form. Either preparation can be given once daily at the end of a meal, but dividing the dose into twice daily administration may help to maintain therapeutic levels in the epidermis and is recommended for refractory infections.

Ketoconazole and Itraconazole. The pharmacologic properties of the oral agents ketoconazole and itraconazole are discussed later. Both drugs are effective for ringworm, chronic mucocutaneous candidiasis, and tinea versicolor. Itraconazole, despite its cost, has become favored over ketoconazole for superficial mycoses because of the latter drug's endocrine side effects and rare but potentially lethal hepatotoxicity. Itraconazole has a number of drug interactions but is a safe drug, a major consideration during the 6–18 months used in treating onychomycosis.[16]

Terbinafine. The oral agent terbinafine, an allylamine structurally related to naftifine, has been evaluated in Europe for treatment of ringworm. In early short-term studies, the agent appeared to be comparable to griseofulvin. Evidence that the drug and its metabolites accumulate substantially during long-term oral administration may limit its use in onychomycosis.

Systemic Therapy of Candida Vulvovaginitis

Ketoconazole, Itraconazole, and Fluconazole. Ketoconazole at 400 mg daily for 5 days is as effective as topical therapy for *Candida* vulvovaginitis and is certainly more convenient, including use during menstruation. However, the potential hepatotoxicity even with a 5-day course and the concern about fetal malformation have prevented widespread acceptance of this regimen. Fluconazole's better safety record, lack of teratogenicity in pregnant rabbits, and equivalent efficacy have made it the preferred oral regimen for this indication. A single 150-mg dose provides a cure rate as good as or better than topical azole therapy. In one study, itraconazole, 400 mg on 1 day, gave equivalent results to fluconazole, 50 mg daily for 3 days.[17]

TREATMENT OF DEEP MYCOSIS

Amphotericin B

Mechanism of Action. Amphotericin B is produced by *Streptomyces nodosus.* The drug is a lipophilic, rodlike molecule (Fig. 1) that exerts its antifungal effect by insertion into the fungal cytoplasmic membrane, probably orienting as head-to-tail oligomers perpendicular to the plane of the membrane.[18] The drug exists as aggregates in the cytoplasmic membrane, bound closely to sterols such as ergosterol. Amphotericin B causes membrane permeability to increase. At lower drug concentrations, K-channel activity is increased.[19] At higher concentrations pores 40–105 nm are formed in the membrane. Loss of intracellular potassium and other molecules impairs fungal viability. Although modest degrees of amphotericin B resistance can be selected under drug pressure in vitro, such strains have altered membrane sterols, reduced growth rates, and decreased virulence.[20] Most clinical isolates of *Candida* spp., particularly *C. lusitaniae,* that have been less susceptible to amphotericin B have been isolated from mucocutaneous surfaces or urine and may not be capable of causing deep infection.[21] The only report said to compare outcome of amphotericin B treatment with amphotericin B minimum inhibitory concentration does in fact not make such a comparison.[22] Absence of a meaningful clinical correlation between outcome of amphotericin B therapy and susceptibility has left in vitro susceptibility determinations as a research tool.

Amphotericin B Deoxycholate (ABD). ABD is insoluble in water at physiologic pH. The drug is marketed for intravenous use as a powder containing amphotericin B, 50 mg, sodium deoxycholate, 41 mg, and sodium phosphate buffer, 25.2 mg. Although a clear yellow solution forms when the powder is hydrated, the colloidal nature of ABD is easy to demonstrate. If a 0.22-μm pore diameter filter is placed in the infusion line, considerable drug is removed by the filter. Addition of electrolyte will aggregate colloids so that a cloudy solution occurs when saline or sodium bicarbonate is added to an ABD solution. Infusion bottles need not be protected from light, as older product brochures advocated.

Investigational Formulations. There are three amphotericin B formulations under investigational use in the United States: amphotericin B colloidal dispersion (ABCD: Amphocil), amphotericin B lipid complex (ABLC), and liposomal amphotericin B (Ambisome).[23–25] The last of these is commercially available in several European countries. All three are less nephrotoxic than ABD. Unfortunately, comparative clinical trials have not been done, leaving open the question as to whether any formulation can provide superior efficacy to ABD. The most logical current indication for requesting one of the investigational formulations is dose-limiting nephrotoxicity rather than failure to respond to conventional doses of ABD.

ABCD contains cholesterol sulfate in equimolar amounts to amphotericin B, forming disclike colloidal particles about 122 ± 48 nm diameter. Like ABD, it forms a clear yellow solution when hydrated. However, pharmacokinetics of ABCD differ substantially, with much lower serum concentrations and, in animals, higher liver amphotericin B concentrations. Rigors have been noted early in the course, much like ABD, but little nephrotoxicity has been seen at doses up to 2.5 mg/kg daily.

ABLC is a complex of almost equimolar concentrations of amphotericin B and lipid, the latter being a 7:3 mixture of dimyristoylphosphatidylcholine and dimyristoylphosphatidylglycerol. The drug is shipped as a cloudy suspension with particles from 1.6 to 11 μm diameter (an erythrocyte is 7 μm diameter). Particle shape is not globular but ribbonlike. Serum concentrations are about one-fifth those of ABD, but the dose being used in clinical trial is currently 5 mg/kg daily (i.e., five times higher than ABD). ABLC is usually well tolerated, with some patients having mild aminotransferase elevations and some AIDS patients having transiently lower leukocyte counts. Infusion of a related preparation has caused transient pulmonary hypertension and hypoxemia, which may be of concern in patients with poor cardiac or pulmonary function.[26]

Ambisome is a unilamellar liposome about 55–75 nm in diameter, containing roughly one molecule of amphotericin B per nine molecules of lipid. The latter is a mixture of hydrogenated soy lecithin:cholesterol:distearoylphosphatidylglycerol in a 10:5:4 ratio. Serum concentrations seem higher than with ABD, though human data are scanty. Doses employed in open trials have ranged from 1 to 5 mg/kg daily. Hypokalemia, but little or no nephrotoxicity, has been observed.[23,27]

Some hospitals in Europe have been mixing ABD with Intralipid (Pharmacia), a parenteral fat emulsion, at an ABD concentration of 1–2 mg/ml of lipid for intravenous infusion. Less nephrotoxicity has been observed with this preparation at a dose of 1 mg/kg daily than infusions of ABD in 5% dextrose.[28] However, serum amphotericin B concentrations were also lower with the fat emulsion, raising the possibility that amphotericin B was simply aggregating in the fat emulsion but the cloudiness could not be perceived in the milky-looking lipid. Microparticulate amphotericin B is known to give lower serum concentrations and less nephrotoxicity than a clear colloidal solution. With ABD, it has long been standard practice to discard cloudy infusion bottles because of concern that aggregated drug would provide less therapeutic effect.

Questions posed by the above formulations underscore our ignorance as to how amphotericin B should be formulated to decrease toxicity without sacrificing efficacy.

Pharmacology. Concentrations of amphotericin B in biologic fluids have usually been measured by bioassay,[29] but high-pressure liquid chromatography,[30] ^{86}Rb release,[31] and radiometric respirometry[32] have been described. Despite the proliferation of methods, routine determination of amphotericin B serum, urine, or cerebrospinal fluid concentration has no definite clinical value. Nonetheless, amphotericin B assays have revealed some remarkable pharmacologic properties of this drug. When colloidal amphotericin B is admixed in serum, desoxycholate separates from amphotericin B,[33] and more than 95 percent of the latter binds to serum proteins,[34] principally to β-lipoprotein.[35] Presumably the drug is bound to the cholesterol carried on this protein. The majority of the drug leaves the circulation promptly, perhaps bound to cholesterol-containing cytoplasmic membranes. Amphotericin B is stored in the liver and other organs; the drug appears to reenter the circulation slowly.[36] Most of the drug is degraded in situ with only a small percentage being excreted in urine[29,37] or bile.[38] Blood levels are uninfluenced by hepatic or renal failure.[34,37] Hemodialysis does not alter blood levels, except in an occasional patient with lipemic plasma who may be losing drug by adherence to the dialysis membrane.[34] Concentrations of amphotericin B in fluids from inflamed areas, such as pleura, peritoneum, joint, vitreous humor,[38] and aqueous humor, are roughly two-thirds of the trough serum level. Cord blood from one infant contained an amphotericin B concentration of 0.37 µg/ml, half the simultaneous maternal trough blood level. Amphotericin B penetrates poorly into either normal or inflamed meninges, vitreous humor, or normal amniotic fluid. Urine concentrations are similar to serum concentrations. Peak serum concentrations with conventional intravenous doses are roughly 0.5–2.0 µg/ml but fall rapidly initially to approach slowly a plateau of roughly 0.2–0.5 µg/ml.[29,39,40]

Toxicity of Amphotericin B Deoxycholate. NEPHROTOXICITY. ABD causes a dose-dependent decrease in glomerular filtrate rate. Amphotericin B has a direct vasoconstrictive effect on afferent renal arterioles, reducing glomerular and renal tubular blood flow.[41] Other primary or secondary effects on the kidney include potassium and bicarbonate wasting and decreased erythropoietin production. Permanent loss of renal function is related to total dose, not to the level of temporary azotemia, and is due to destruction of renal tubular cells, disruption of tubular basement membrane, and loss of functioning nephron units. Saline-deprived rats have more nephrotoxicity than saline-loaded rats.[42] Anecdotally, infusion of 1 liter of saline each day has been thought to decrease nephrotoxicity in some patients.[43] Potassium wasting often requires supplemental oral or intravenous potassium. Renal tubular acidosis from bicarbonate wasting rarely requires base replacement, but patients also given acetazolamide (Diamox) must be watched for significant acidemia.

Azotemia due to amphotericin B is often worse in patients taking other nephrotoxic drugs, such as cyclosporine, ifosfamide, or aminoglycosides.[44] Hypotension, intravascular volume depletion, renal transplantation, and other preexisting renal disease all magnify the management problems attendant on amphotericin B–induced azotemia.

Early in a course of amphotericin B, azotemia may increase rapidly, often fall a little, and then stabilize after several days. Adults with no other renal disease will have an average serum creatinine level of 2–3 mg/dl at a dose of 0.5 mg/kg. Attempting to give amphotericin B to an adult without causing azotemia will usually lead to inadequate therapy.

OTHER CHRONIC TOXICITY. Nausea, anorexia, and vomiting are common. Phlebitis occurs if peripheral vein catheters are used. Normocytic normochromic anemia occurs gradually, with the hematocrit rarely falling below 20–25 percent unless other causes of anemia are present. In one case treated by the author, erythropoietin administration resulted in substantial improvement in amphotericin B–induced anemia. Rarely, thrombocytopenia or modest leukopenia may be observed.

Acute Reactions. About 30–45 minutes after beginning the first several amphotericin B infusions, chills, fever, and tachypnea may occur, peak in 15–30 minutes, and slowly abate over 2–4 hours. A patient with underlying cardiac or pulmonary disease may have hypoxemia or hypotension. These reactions are less common in young children or patients receiving adrenal corticosteroids. Subsequent infusions of the same dose cause progressively milder reactions. Premedication with acetaminophen or addition of hydrocortisone, 25–50 mg, to the infusion solution can diminish the reactions. Meperidine given early in a chill can shorten the rigor. Concern about this kind of reaction in an unstable patient had led some physicians to use a test dose of 1 mg given over 15 minutes to assess the subsequent reaction over 1 hour before deciding whether the next dose should be a full therapeutic dose of at least 0.5 mg or an intermediate dose. Whether or not a test dose is given, patients with rapidly progressive mycoses should receive a full therapeutic dose within 24 hours, without delay entailed by test or intermediate doses. Equally important, this reaction should not be mistaken for anaphylaxis or otherwise considered a contraindication for further amphotericin B. Allergic reactions to amphotericin B are extremely rare.

Administration. ABD is infused in 5% dextrose over a 2–4 hour infusion interval. Infusion over about 1 hour has been tried in small series, but experience is insufficient to recommend this procedure.[45,46] Early in the course of therapy, fever is more pronounced with infusion intervals of only 45 minutes than 4 hours.[47]

Once therapy is well under way, patients receiving the usual dose of 0.5 mg/kg daily may be changed to 1 mg/kg on alternate days. This is largely done as a convenience for outpatient therapy. Doses above 1 mg/kg are not generally given on this schedule because toxicity of such infusions is not well described. Administration of double doses on alternate days does not have a substantial effect on toxicity. A common confusion is that amphotericin B may be switched to alternate-day administration using the same dose as daily therapy. This results in serious underdosing.

Dosage. Daily doses of 0.3 mg/kg often suffice for esophageal candidiasis. A dose of 0.5 mg/kg is appropriate for cryptococcosis, blastomycosis, disseminated histoplasmosis, coccidioidomycosis, and extracutaneous sporotrichosis. Patients with mucormycosis or invasive aspergillosis are given daily doses of 1–1.5 mg/kg until improvement is clearly present. Doses of 0.5–1.0 are often used in neutropenic patients receiving empiric amphotericin B.[48] Local instillation of amphotericin B into the cerebrospinal fluid, joint, or pleura is rarely indicated. One exception is coccidioidal meningitis, which is treated with intrathecal amphotericin B when systemic azole therapy fails. Intraocular administration at the end of a pars plana vitrectomy for fungal endophthalmitis is occasionally used. Corneal baths with 1 mg/ml in sterile water are useful for fungal keratitis but are irritating. Bladder irrigation with 50 mcg/ml in sterile water is useful for patients with *Candida* cystitis and a Foley catheter, particularly as preparation for transurethral resection of the prostate or bladder surgery.

FLUCYTOSINE

Flucytosine (5-fluorocytosine [5-FC]; Ancobon) is the fluorine analog of a normal body constituent, cytosine (Fig. 1). The drug was synthesized as a potential antitumor agent, but that property was lacking. Routine screening discovered the antifungal effect, which became the sole use of this drug. Flucytosine is a white powder, moderately soluble in water, very stable on dry storage, and marketed as 250- and 500-mg capsules. Absorption from the gastrointestinal tract is rapid and complete. Approximately 90 percent is excreted unchanged in the urine. Protein binding is barely measurable.[34] Cerebrospinal fluid concentrations approximate 74 percent of simultaneous serum concentrations. The drug is readily cleared by hemodialysis.[34] Peritoneal dialysis also removes flucytosine from the body.

The half-life of the drug in the serum of patients with normal renal function is 3–5 hours.[49] Abnormal hepatic function has no influence, but decreased renal function can prolong the half-life to beyond 24 hours.

The mechanism of flucytosine's antifungal action appears to be by deamination to 5-fluorouracil (5-FU) and then conversion through several steps to 5-fluorodeoxyuridylic acid monophosphate, a noncompetitive inhibitor of thymidylate synthetase.[50] This interferes with DNA synthesis. Additional mechanisms of action may also be operative.

Flucytosine is usually given as 150 mg/kg/day in four divided doses. Patients with a serum creatinine level of 1.7 mg/dl or greater usually require dose reduction. As an approximation, the total daily dose should be reduced to 75 mg/kg with a creatinine clearance of 26–50 ml/min and to 37 mg/kg when the creatinine clearance is 13–25 ml/min.[51] Ideally, the blood level should be measured in azotemic patients 2 hours after the last dose and immediately before the next dose. These values should range between 50 and 100 μg/ml. Patients receiving hemodialysis may be given a single postdialysis dose of 37.5 mg/kg. Further doses are adjusted by blood level. Reliable biologic,[52] enzymatic,[53] and physical[54] methods are available to assay flucytosine, even in the presence of amphotericin B.

Flucytosine given alone to patients with normal renal, hematologic, and gastrointestinal function is associated with very infrequent adverse effects. These include rash, diarrhea, and, in about 5 percent, hepatic dysfunction. In the presence of azotemia or concomitant amphotericin B, leukopenia, thrombocytopenia, and enterocolitis may appear and can be fatal. These complications seem to be far more frequent among patients whose flucytosine blood levels exceed 100–125 μg/ml.[51] Patients receiving flucytosine should have their leukocyte count and

platelet count determined twice a week. Serum alkaline phosphatase and transaminase levels should be followed weekly. Appearance of loose stools or dull abdominal pain should prompt withholding of the drug to evaluate the progression of symptoms. Patients with bone marrow and gastrointestinal toxicity from flucytosine often tolerate the drug at reduced dosages. Patients with rash or hepatotoxicity have not been rechallenged. Flucytosine is teratogenic for rats and is contraindicated in pregnancy.

Conversion of flucytosine to 5-FU within the human body occurs in sufficient degree to be a possible explanation for toxicity to bone marrow and gastrointestinal tract.[55] It is possible that secretion of the drug into the colon occurs, where flucytosine becomes deaminated by intestinal bacteria and is reabsorbed as 5-FU.[56]

Flucytosine has a beneficial effect in cryptococcosis, candidiasis, and chromomycosis. It is not the drug of choice for any infection except chromomycosis, because the clinical efficacy in the first two mycoses is inferior to that of amphotericin B and because secondary drug resistance is common in all three infections. Although the frequency and clinical significance of primary drug resistance are debatable, drug resistance arising during therapy is usually profound and accompanied by clinical deterioration. Mechanisms for the drug resistance may include loss of deaminase and decreased permeability to the drug. This problem has been significant enough to cause flucytosine to be used largely in combination with amphotericin B.

Flucytosine and amphotericin B are at least additive in their effects in vitro and in mice experimentally infected with doubly sensitive isolates of *Candida* and *Cryptococcus*.[57,58] Results with *Aspergillus* are contradictory.[59,60] In animals, the combination has never been better than an optimum dose of amphotericin B alone. Flucytosine permitted a lower dose of amphotericin B to be used to gain the same therapeutic effect, and amphotericin B prevented the emergence of secondary drug resistance. The same advantages have been confirmed in two large multicenter studies of cryptococal meningitis.[61] Experience with candidiasis remains limited, but the combination has been recommended in *Candida* meningitis[62] and arthritis.

Physicians not familiar with the combination are more likely to encounter serious toxicity than with amphotericin B alone. This is particularly true in patients with rapidly changing azotemia or poor bone marrow reserve. Leukopenia and diarrhea are common and difficult to manage in patients with AIDS. Oral flucytosine may not be reliably ingested by patients who are confused or vomiting. Intravenous flucytosine is no longer available in the U.S. but is used at the same dose as the capsule formulation. There is no less diarrhea or leukopenia with intravenous administration.

Combination regimens with amphotericin B doses in excess of 0.3 mg/kg/day or 0.6 mg/kg every other day cause sufficient azotemia to make the safe administration of flucytosine difficult. The amphotericin-B–sparing function of flucytosine in this setting is lost. At present, there are no clear indications for adding flucytosine to amphotericin B regimens containing these higher doses.

Flucytosine resistance has occurred, albeit uncommonly, during combination therapy. Use of the combination in such patients incurs the risk of toxicity without evidence that flucytosine adds to the therapeutic effect. Whenever flucytosine is used to treat a patient who has received that drug before, the isolate should be tested for susceptibility. In most laboratories, a minimum inhibitory concentration (MIC) of 15 μg/ml or less is considered sensitive.

IMIDAZOLES

The imidazole ring (Fig. 1) confers antifungal activity on a variety of synthetic organic compounds. Unlike the 5-nitroimidazoles such as metronidazole, activity against bacteria and protozoa, although measurable, has not been clinically significant. Most of the imidazoles reaching clinical trials have had similar in vitro activity, encompassing a broad range of superficial and deep pathogens.[63,64] There are methods for measuring in vitro activity, but there are no firm indications for performing such tests.

N-substitution of imidazoles has created a family of drugs called *triazoles* that have the same antifungal spectrum and mechanism of action as imidazoles but less effect on human sterol metabolism. Both imidazoles and triazoles inhibit 14-α-demethylation of lanosterol in fungi by binding to one of the cytochrome P-450 (cyt. P-450) enzymes. This leads to accumulation of 14-α-methylsterols and reduced concentrations of ergosterol, a sterol essential for a normal fungal cytoplasmic membrane. Inhibition of cyt. P-450 also decreases the synthesis of testosterone and cortisol in mammals. By studying cyt. P-450 inhibition in vitro, new drugs can be selected that are more active in inhibiting fungal ergosterol synthesis and less active in mammalian sterol synthesis. For example, in vitro study of itraconazole found that 14-α-demethylation of lanosterol in *Candida albicans* was inhibited at 100-fold lower concentrations than those required to inhibit mammalian sterol synthesis.[65] It is not surprising, then, that the newer triazoles, such as itraconazole and fluconazole, have not caused decreased cortisol and testosterone levels in patients, as was seen with ketoconazole.

Many of the newer triazoles have properties that may allow them to replace ketoconazole—not only less hormonal inhibition but also fewer drug interactions, a parenteral formulation, better distribution into body fluids, less gastrointestinal distress, and less hepatotoxicity. N-substitution of the imidazole ring is thought to confer greater metabolic stability on the triazoles and to offer the potential for slower elimination. Both itraconazole and fluconazole have longer serum half-lives than ketoconazole.

Ketoconazole

The synthetic agent ketoconazole differs from its closely related congener miconazole in its solubility at pH less than 3. Solubility in acidic aqueous solutions is conferred in large part by the basic piperazine ring.

The pharmacology of ketoconazole has been reviewed.[63,65] The drug is metabolized in the liver and excreted as inactive drug in the bile and, to a small extent, in the urine. Very little biologically active drug appears in urine. Serum protein binding exceeds 90 percent. The drug is not removed significantly by hemodialysis or peritoneal dialysis. Decreased renal or hepatic function does not alter plasma drug levels. Based on studies of oral ingestion by volunteers, the initial half-life is approximately 2 hours, with a β-phase half-life of about 9 hours commencing 8–12 hours after ingestion.

Oral absorption of ketoconazole varies among different individuals. Serious gastrointestinal disease, such as the graft-versus-host reaction,[66] may lead to low blood levels. H_2-receptor blocking agents, such as ranitidine, famotidine, or cimetidine, should not be given to patients taking ketoconazole, because blood levels of the latter drug are drastically reduced. Although oral ingestion of hydrochloric acid along with ketoconazole has been said to reverse this effect in volunteers, acid administration would be contraindicated in patients requiring H_2-blocking agents. Citric acid does not seem acidic enough to overcome the effect of H_2-blocking agents.[65] Antacids can be given to patients taking ketoconazole but should be separated in time. Rifampin causes a substantial lowering of ketoconazole blood levels, probably by accelerating metabolism. Isoniazid possibly has the same effect. Occasional patients have had elevated phenytoin or oral anticoagulant levels while taking ketoconazole. Cyclosporine blood levels should be monitored during ketoconazole therapy, because these levels usually increase, causing nephrotoxicity.[67,68] Penetration into the cerebrospinal fluid is very poor, even in the presence of inflammation.[69] Low concentrations are found in vaginal secretions, saliva, and breast milk.

Ketoconazole is presently available only as scored 200-mg tablets. Used as two tablets daily (400 mg), the drug is effective in nonmeningeal histoplasmosis and blastomycosis of the nonimmunosuppressed host.[70] Therapy is continued for 6–12 months. Improvement may require 2–4 weeks to be evident. Although the dose can be advanced to 600 or 800 mg daily in patients not responding to therapy, there is more evidence of increased toxicity than increased efficacy.[69,70] Both disseminated and chronic pulmonary histoplasmosis respond to ketoconazole therapy.[70] Paracoccidioidomycosis responds well to ketoconazole.[71] Disseminated nonmeningeal coccidioidomycosis may be partially and temporarily controlled by ketoconazole.[72] Among patients with disseminated coccidioidomycosis who respond well, relapse is usual if the drug is stopped. With all these mycoses, patients with grave, rapidly progressing infection should receive amphotericin B. The slow therapeutic response and variable absorption of ketoconazole make it a poor choice in such patients. If the mycosis involves the meninges, ketoconazole is too ineffective to warrant trial.

Ketoconazole is of no value in cryptococcosis. The response is also negligible in chromomycosis and extracutaneous sporotrichosis. Although the response in cutaneous sporotrichosis also tends to be poor, a dose of 400 mg/day may be tried in patients with allergic reactions to iodide, the drug of choice. As will be mentioned later, itraconazole may be a better choice. Ketoconazole has been used in Old World leishmaniasis and was useful in *Leishmania major* but not in *L. tropica* or *L. aethiopica* infections (see Ch. 254). Studies on New World leishmaniasis are not encouraging.

Aspergillosis does not respond to ketoconazole. Additionally, there is concern, based on experience with mice, that subsequent use of amphotericin B may be antagonized.[73] The agents of mucormycosis have all been resistant to imidazoles and triazoles in vitro, discouraging clinical use for that indication.

The most frequent toxic effects of ketoconazole are anorexia, nausea, and vomiting. These reactions occurred in 17 percent of 71 patients taking 400 mg/day and in 29 percent of those receiving 800 mg/day.[70] Gastrointestinal distress is most common when the drug is first begun and can be partially controlled by taking the tablets with food. Dividing doses above 400 mg/day has not been recommended because hormonal suppression is prolonged. Ketoconazole causes a dose-dependent depression of serum testosterone and adrenocorticotropic hormone (ACTH)-stimulated cortisol response.[74,75] While this effect is quite modest at the recommended dose of 400 mg/day, doses of 800–1200 mg/day cause a profound enough effect to have prompted trials in the treatment of ACTH-secreting tumors and prostatic cancer. Hypertension has been seen in a few of these high-dose patients in association with increased deoxycorticosterone, corticosterone, and 11-deoxycortisol levels. Gynecomastia, impotence, decreased libido, oligospermia, azospermia in men, and menstrual irregularities in women may also be seen during prolonged therapy.[70,74] Allergic rash has been seen in 10 percent of patients.[70] Pruritus occurs with equal frequency, sometimes associated with a complaint of dry skin. Perhaps the most grave complication of ketoconazole therapy is hepatitis.[76] Fortunately, this complication is quite rare, estimated to appear in 1 in 15,000 exposed individuals. Asymptomatic slight elevation of transaminases is not rare and is generally transient. This event is distinguished from the potentially lethal hepatitis by the presence of symptoms and the progressive course. Ketoconazole hepatitis begins as anorexia, malaise, nausea, and vomiting. Abnormalities of either or both serum transaminase and alkaline phosphatase become increasingly profound, soon accompanied by jaundice. Eighty percent of cases occur within the first 3 months, but the onset can occur at any time. Progression can be surprisingly swift. Patients should be instructed to discontinue ketoconazole if they experience the above symptoms and to call their physician. If hepatotoxicity is suspected, serum transaminase and alkaline phosphatase should be measured within 1–2 days of discontinuing therapy. Symptomatic patients with abnormal liver function should not be rechallenged with ketoconazole. Of course, if serum chemistries are normal, the drug can be reinstituted. Some authorities have recommended that liver function be measured periodically.[76] This procedure does not protect the patient who has a rapid onset of hepatitis in the interval between tests but does require that all patients with abnormalities be contacted in order to inquire about symptoms and to arrange for repeat testing.

Itraconazole (Sporanox)

Pharmacology. Itraconazole is marketed as a 100-mg capsule. An oral suspension in cyclodextrin is under clinical trial. No parenteral formulation is available. Oral absorption of itraconazole is significantly enhanced by food.[77] Bioavailability of itraconazole is 55 percent when ingested after breakfast. Absorption in the fasting state is 30 percent of that following a substantial meal. Steady state is only achieved after 13–15 days, at which time the β-elimination half-life is about 19–22 hours. Absorption in AIDS patients is about half that in normal volunteers.[78] For deep mycoses, an itraconazole loading dose of 200 mg three times a day is recommended for the first 3 days, because this decreases the number of days required for the drug to reach a steady state. Hydroxyitraconazole, a metabolite of itraconazole, appears in blood in amounts roughly twice that of the parent drug and has some biologic activity.[79] Bioassays of itraconazole give much higher concentrations than HPLC, the difference depending on the susceptibility of the bioassay organism to active metabolites. Tissue concentrations of itraconazole are generally higher than plasma concentrations, but cerebrospinal fluid concentrations are usually unmeasurable, even in patients with meningitis. The drug is metabolized in the liver and excreted in feces as metabolites. No significant amount of bioactive itraconazole appears in urine. Plasma concentrations do not increase in renal insufficiency or decrease with hemodialysis. About 99 percent of serum itraconazole is bound to plasma proteins.

Adverse Effects. The most common adverse effect is dose-related nausea and abdominal discomfort, but symptoms rarely necessitate stopping therapy. Dividing the dose into twice daily administration is usual and may improve tolerance. Hypokalemia and edema may occur at 400 mg per day or higher doses. Allergic rash is seen occasionally. Therapy is contraindicated during pregnancy and in nursing mothers. Unlike ketoconazole, itraconazole does not appear to be hepatotoxic and does not suppress adrenal or testicular function at recommended dosages.

Interactions. Blood levels are reduced by about half in patients taking drugs that decrease gastric acidity, such as H_2 blockers and drugs blocking the gastric proton pump.[80] Simultaneous ingestion of itraconazole with antacids and, most likely, with buffered didanosine, decreases absorption. Rifampin, phenytoin, and carbamazepine decrease itraconazole blood levels. Itraconazole increases blood levels of cyclosporine, digoxin, terfenadine (Seldane), astemizole (Hismanal), and possibly loratidine (Claritin), the last three potentially causing polymorphic ventricular tachycardia (torsades de pointes).[81] Rifampin blood levels are reduced by itraconazole.

Indications. This oral triazole, structurally similar to ketoconazole, is useful for treatment of blastomycosis and histoplasmosis[82] and for prevention of relapse in AIDS patients with disseminated histoplasmosis.[16,83,84] Less extensive data indicate usefulness also in coccidioidomycosis, paracoccidioidomycosis, cutaneous and extracutaneous sporotrichosis,[85,86]

pseudallescheriasis, ringworm (including onychomycosis), vaginal candidiasis, and tinea versicolor. Itraconazole has been used for indolent cases of invasive aspergillosis[87] and for cryptococcal meningitis of AIDS patients,[88] but further studies are needed.

Fluconazole (Diflucan)

Pharmacology. Fluconazole is well absorbed from the gastrointestinal tract.[89] After ingestion of fluconazole, more than 80 percent of the drug can be found in the circulation. Of the oral dose, 60–75 percent appears unchanged in the urine and 8–10 percent appears unchanged in the feces. Oral absorption is not decreased in patients with AIDS or patients taking H_2-blocking agents.[90] Only 11 percent of serum fluconazole is protein bound. Concentrations of fluconazole in the cerebrospinal fluid are approximately 70 percent of simultaneous blood levels, whether or not the meninges are inflamed. Penetration into saliva, sputum, urine and other body fluids has also been excellent.[89] The half-life in patients with normal renal function is 27–34 hours, increasing to 59 and 98 hours in groups with creatinine clearances of 35 and 14 ml/min, respectively. According to the manufacturer, the normal dose should be reduced to 50 percent when the creatinine clearance is reduced to 50 ml/min and to 25 percent when the creatinine clearance is below 20 ml/min. A loading dose of twice the daily dose is recommended. Patients receiving hemodialysis should have one daily dose after each session. A dose of 6 mg/kg every 3 days has been advocated for premature infants in the first week of life, with dosing every 2 days during the second week of life.[91]

Drug Interactions. Fluconazole can cause significant increases in the blood level of phenytoin, glypizide, glyburide, tolbutamide, or cyclosporin. This interaction is most obvious in adults given 400 mg daily or in azotemic patients given lower doses. Rifampin lowers fluconazole blood levels by about one-fourth.[92]

Side Effects. Adverse effects are uncommon.[93] According to the manufacturer, nausea has occurred in 2.5 percent, abdominal pain in 1.7 percent, diarrhea in 1.2 percent, vomiting in 1.0 percent, and rash in 0.9 percent of patients. Rarely, Stevens-Johnson syndrome has been observed. There is a question whether or not acute hepatic necrosis may have occurred in a few patients as a result of fluconazole ingestion. The drug has not been embryotoxic or teratogenic in rabbits. Rarely, anaphylaxis has been observed with the first dose of fluconazole. Alopecia has been seen at doses of 400 mg daily or higher.[94]

Administration. Fluconazole is currently available in 50-, 100-, 150-, and 200-mg tablets, as well as in an intravenous formulation of either 200 or 400 mg, both as 2 mg/ml. The much higher price of the intravenous drug makes the tablets preferred. Local instillation into the cerebrospinal fluid, bladder, or other site is unnecessary because of the excellent penetration of the drug into body compartments.

Indications. CANDIDIASIS. Fluconazole, 50–100 mg once daily, is one of the most effective agents for the treatment of oropharyngeal candidiasis. Daily doses of 100–200 mg are recommended for esophageal candidiasis.[14] Fluconazole has been given once a week as prophylaxis in AIDS patients who have recurrent oropharyngeal candidiasis,[95] but this practice can lead eventually to oropharyngeal and esophageal candidiasis resistant to fluconazole, ketoconazole, clotrimazole, and itraconazole.[15] A single dose of 150 mg is approximately as effective as topical therapy of vulvovaginal candidiasis. Patients with candidemia who are not neutropenic or otherwise seriously immunosuppressed respond as well to intravenous fluconazole therapy as to amphotericin B.[96] Changing potentially infected central intravenous catheters in such patients is an important part of therapy. In a small number of patients with *Candida* endocarditis, long-term fluconazole therapy has been used to prevent relapse after amphotericin B therapy.[97] For the immunosuppressed patient, rapidly progressing or severely ill patient with deep candidiasis, amphotericin B remains the drug of choice.

CRYPTOCOCCAL MENINGITIS. Fluconazole has been used for initial therapy of AIDS patients with cryptococcal meningitis who are neurologically intact and judged to have a good prognosis.[98] Most authorities recommend amphotericin B for at least the first 2 weeks, changed to fluconazole if the patient has remained clinically stabile. The propensity of AIDS patients to relapse has led to life-long fluconazole maintenance therapy.[99,100] Thus far, relapse due to fluconazole resistance has been rare. For patients without AIDS, fluconazole is useful for those who have completed a course of amphotericin B and seem to be a high risk of relapse. At present, there are virtually no studies to define the dose and duration of fluconazole for non-AIDS patients with cryptococcosis.

Other Mycoses. Fluconazole has emerged as the drug of choice for coccidioidal meningitis[101] and is approximately as effective as other azoles for disseminated nonmeningeal coccidioidomycosis. Cutaneous sporotrichosis[102] also may respond to fluconazole. Response in histoplasmosis and blastomycosis has not appeared promising.[83] Fluconazole is not indicated for aspergillosis, mucormycosis, or pseudallescheriasis. Data on ringworm and tinea versicolor are sparse.

Prophylaxis. In a multicenter trial, administration of fluconazole, 400 mg daily, decreased the incidence of death due to deep mycoses in bone marrow transplant recipients, most of whom had received allogeneic transplants, from 10 per 177 placebo recipients to 1 per 179 fluconazole recipients.[103] All the protection afforded seemed to be in deep candidiasis, not aspergillosis. Reduction in deep mycoses has not been convincingly demonstrated in other groups, such as patients with acute leukemia.[104] Curiously, fluconazole has not resulted in decreased use of empiric amphotericin B. Nor has an effect of overall survival been demonstrated, perhaps because death from deep candidiasis is uncommon. In most studies, fluconazole prophylaxis has decreased the incidence of mucocutaneous candidiasis, but this complication can also be diagnosed readily and treated when present.

REFERENCES

1. Topical terbinafine for tinea infections. Med Lett. 1993;35:76–8.
2. Fromtling RA. Imidazoles as medically important antifungal agents: An overview. Drugs Today. 1984;20:325–49.
3. Nolting S, Reinel D, Semig G, et al. Amorolfine spray in the treatment of foot mycoses (a dose-finding study). Br J Dermatol. 1993;129:170–4.
4. Hamilton-Miller JMT. Chemistry and biology of the polyene macrolide antibiotics. Bacteriol Rev. 1973;37:166.
5. Kerridge D, Whelan WL. The polyene macrolide antibiotics and 5-fluorocytosine: Molecular actions and interactions. In: Trinci APJ, Riley JF, eds. Mode of Action of Antifungal Agents. London: British Mycological Society; 1984;343–75.
6. Stern GE, Gurwith D, Mummaw N, et al. Single dose tioconazole compared with 3-day clotrimazole treatment in vulvovaginal candidiasis. Antimicrob Agents Chemother. 1986;29:969–71.
7. Gabriel G, Thin RNT. Clotrimazole and econazole in the treatment of vaginal candidosis. Br J Vener Dis. 1983;59:56–8.
8. Svendsen E, Lie S, Gunderson TH, et al. Comparative evaluation of miconazole, clotrimazole and nystatin in the treatment of *Candida* vulvo-vaginitis. Curr Ther Res. 1978;23:666.
9. Franklin R. Seven day clotrimazole therapy for vulvovaginal candidiasis. South Med J. 1978;71:141.
10. Shechtman LB, Funaro L, Robin T, et al. Clotrimazole treatment of oral candidiasis in patients with neoplastic disease. Am J Med. 1984;76:91.
11. Horsbaugh CR, Kirkpatrick CH. Long-term therapy of chronic mucocutaneous candidiasis with ketoconazole: Experience with twenty-one patients. Am J Med. 1983;74:23.
12. Fazio RA, Wickremesinghe PC, Arsure EL. Ketoconazole treatment of *Can-dida* esophagitis; a prospective study of 12 cases. Am J Gastroenterol. 1983; 78:261.
13. Hughes WT, Bartley DL, Patterson GG, et al. Ketoconazole and candidiasis: A controlled study. J Infect Dis. 1983;147:1060.
14. Laine L, Dretler RH, Conteas CN, et al. Fluconazole compared with ketoconazole for the treatment of *Candida* esophagitis in AIDS. Ann Intern Med. 1992;117:655–60.
15. Sanguineti A, Carmichael JK, Campbell K. Fluconazole resistant *Candida albicans* after long-term suppressive therapy. Arch Intern Med. 1993;153: 1122–4.
16. Itraconazole. Med Lett. 1993;35:7–10.
17. Rees T, Phillips R. Multicenter comparison of one-day oral therapy with fluconazole or itraconazole in vaginal candidiasis. Int J Gynecol Obstet. 1992; 37:33–8.
18. Balakrishnan AR, Easwaran KRK. CD and NMR studies on the aggregation fo amphotericin-B in solution. Biochim Biophys Acta. 1993;1148:269–77.
19. Hsu S, Burnette RR. The effect of amphotericin B on the K channel activity of MDCK cells. Biochim Biophys Acta. 1993;1152:189–91.
20. Fryberg M, Oehlschlager AC, Unrau AM. Sterol biosynthesis in antibiotic sensitive and resistant *Candida*. Arch Biochem Biophys. 1975;173:171–7.
21. Merz WG. *Candida lusitaniae:* Frequency of recovery, colonization, infection, and amphotericin B resistance. J Clin Microbiol. 1984;20:1994–5.
22. Powderly WG, Kobayashi GS, Herzig GP, et al. Amphotericin B-resistant yeast infection in severely immunocompromised patients. Am J Med. 1988; 84:826–43.
23. Ambisome—Liposomal amphotericin B. Drug Ther Bull. 1993;31:93–4.
24. Fielding RM. Liposomal drug delivery. Advantages and limitations from a clinical pharmacokinetic and therapeutic perspective. Clin Pharmacokinet. 1991;21:1155–64.
25. Janknegt R, de Marie S, Bakker-Woudenberg AJM, et al. Liposomal and lipid formulations of amphotericin B. Clinical pharmacokinetics. Clin Pharmacokinet. 1992;23:279–91.
26. Levine SJ, Walsh TJ, Martinez A, et al. Cardiopulmonary toxicity after liposomal amphotericin B infusion. Ann Intern Med. 1991;114:664–6.
27. Coker RJ, Viviana M, Gazzard BG, et al. Treatment of *Cryptococcosis* with liposomal amphotericin B (AmBisome) in 23 Patients with AIDS. AIDS. 1993;7:829–35.
28. Chavanet PY, Garry I, Charlier N, et al. Trial of glucose versus fat emulsion in preparation of amphotericin for use in HIV infected patients with candidiasis. Br Med J. 1992;305:921–5.
29. Bindschadler DD, Bennett JE. A pharmacologic guide to the clinical use of amphotericin B. J Infect Dis. 1969;120:427.
30. Mayhew JW, Fiore C, Murray T, et al. An internally standardized assay for amphotericin B in tissues and plasma. J Chromatog. 1983;274:271.
31. Cosgrove RF, Fairbrother JE. Bioassay method for polyene antibiotics based on the measurement of rubidium efflux from rubidium-loaded yeast cells. Antimicrob Agents Chemother. 1977;11:31.
32. Merz WG, Fay D, Thumar B, et al. Susceptibility testing of filamentous fungi to amphotericin B by a rapid radiometric method. J Clin Microbiol. 1984;19: 54.
33. Jagdis FA, Monji N, Lawrence RM, et al. Distribution of radiolabeled amphotercin B methyl ester and amphotericin B in nonhuman primates (Abstract 305). Sixteenth Interscience Conference of Antimicrobial Agents and Chemotherapy. Washington, DC: American Society of Microbiology; 1976.
34. Block ER, Bennett JE, Livoti LG, et al. Flucytosine and amphotericin B: Hemodialysis effects on the plasma concentration and clearance. Ann Intern Med. 1974;80:613.
35. Bennett JE. Amphotericin B binding to serum betalipoprotein. In: Iwata K, ed. Recent Advances in Medical and Veterinary Mycology. Tokyo: University of Tokyo Press; 1977:107.
36. Atkinson AJ, Bennett JE. Amphotericin B pharmacokinetics in humans. Antimicrob Agents Chemother. 1978;13:271.
37. Craven PC, Ludden TM, Drutz DJ, et al. Excretion pathways of amphotericin B. J Infect Dis. 1979;140:329.
38. Fisher JF, Taylor AT, Clark J, et al. Penetration of amphotericin B into the human eye. J Infect Dis. 1983;147:164.
39. Christiansen KJ, Bernard EM, Gold JWM, et al. Distribution and activity of amphotericin B in humans. J Infect Dis. 1985;152:1037–43.
40. Starke JR, Mason EO, Kramer WG, et al. Pharmacokinetics of amphotericin B in infants and children. J Infect Dis. 1987;155:766–74.
41. Sawaya BP, Weihprecht H, Campbell WE, et al. Direct vasoconstriction as a possible cause of amphotericin B–induced nephrotoxicity in rats. J Clin Invest. 1991;87:2097–107.
42. Ohnishi A, Ohnishi T, Stevenhead W, et al. Sodium status influences chronic amphotericin B nephrotoxicity in rats. Antimicrob Agents Chemother. 1989; 33:1222–7.
43. Branch RA. Prevention of amphotericin B-induced renal impairment. Arch Intern Med. 1988;148:2389–94.
44. Kennedy MS, Deeg HJ, Siegel M, et al. Acute renal toxicity with combined use of amphotericin B and cyclosporine after marrow transplantation. Transplantation. 1982;35:211.
45. Cruz JM, Peacock Jr JE, Loomer L, et al. Rapid intravenous infusion of amphotericin B: A pilot study. Am J Med. 1992;93:123–30.

46. Drutz DJ. Rapid infusion of amphotericin B: Is it safe, effective and wise? Am J Med. 1992;93:119–21.

47. Ellis ME, Al-Hokail AA, Clink HM, et al. Double blind randomized study of the effect of infusion rates on toxicity of amphotericin B. Antimicrob Agents Chemother. 1992;36:172–9.

48. Pizzo PA. Management of fever in patients with cancer and treatment-induced neutropenia. N Engl J Med. 1993;328:1323–32.

49. Cutler RE, Balir AD, Kelly MR. Flucytosine kinetics in subjects with normal renal function. Clin Pharmacol Ther. 1978;24:333.

50. Diasio RB, Bennett JE, Myers CE. Mode of action of 5-fluorocytosine. Biochem Pharmacol. 1978;27:703.

51. Stamm AM, Diasio RB, Dismukes WE, et al. Toxicity of amphotericin B plus flucytosine in 194 patients with cryptococcal meningitis. Am J Med. 1987;83:236–42.

52. Kaspar RL, Drutz DJ. Rapid, simple bioassay for 5-fluorocytosine in the presence of amphotericin B. Antimicrob Agents Chemother. 1975;7:462.

53. Huang CM, Kroll MH, Ruddel M, et al. An enzymatic method for 5-fluorocytosine. Clin Chem. 1988;34:59–62.

54. Harding SA, Johnson GF, Solomon HM. Gas chromatographic determination of 5-fluorocytosine in human serum. Clin Chem. 1976;22:772.

55. Diasio RB, Lakings DE, Bennett JE. Evidence for conversion of 5-fluorocytosine to 5-fluorouracil in humans. Possible factor in 5-fluorocytosine clinical toxicity. Antimicrob Agents Chemother. 1978;14:903.

56. Harris BE, Manning BW, Federle TW, et al. Conversion of 5-fluorocytosine to 5-fluorouracil by human intestinal microflora. Antimicrob Agents Chemother. 1986;29:44–8.

57. Medoff G, Comfort M, Kobayashi GS. Synergistic action of amphotericin B and 5-fluorocytosine against yeast-like organisms. Proc Soc Exp Biol Med. 1971;138:571.

58. Polak A. Synergism of polyene antibiotics with 5-fluorocytosine. Chemotherapy. 1978;24:2.

59. Kitahara M, Seth UK, Medoff G, et al. Activity of amphotericin B, 5-fluorocytosine and rifampin against six clinical isolates of *Aspergillus*. Antimicrob Agents Chemother. 1976;9:915.

60. Polak A, Scholer HJ, Wall M. Combination therapy of experimental candidiasis and aspergillosis in mice. Chemotherapy. 1982;28:461.

61. Dismukes WE, Cloud GC, Gallis HA, et al. Treatment of cryptococcal meningitis with combination amphotericin B and flucytosine for four as compared with six weeks. N Engl J Med. 1987;317:334–41.

62. Smego RA, Perfect JR, Durack DT. Combined therapy with amphotericin B and 5-fluorocytosine for *Candida* meningitis. Rev Infect Dis. 1984;6:791–801.

63. Heel RC, Brogden RN, Carmine A, et al. Ketoconazole: A review of its therapeutic efficacy in superficial and systemic fungal infections. Drugs. 1982;23:1.

64. Custem JV. The antifungal activity of ketoconazole. Am J Med. 1983; 74(Suppl):9.

65. Daneshmend TK, Warnock DW. Clinical pharmacokinetics of ketoconazole. Clin Pharmacokinet. 1988;14:13–34.

66. Van HV, Piens MA, Archimbaud E, et al. Serum levels of ketoconazole in bone marrow transplanted patients. Nouv Rev Fr Hematol. 1983;25:241–4.

67. Schroeder TJ, Melvin DB, Clardy CW, et al. Use of cyclosporine and ketoconazole without nephrotoxicity in two heart transplant recipients. J Heart Transplant. 1987;6:84–9.

68. First MR, Schroeder TJ, Michael A, et al. Cyclosporine-ketoconazole interaction. Transplantation. 1993;55:1000–4.

69. Sugar AM, Alsip SG, Galgiani JN, et al. Pharmacology and toxicity of high-dose ketoconazole. Antimicrob Agents Chemother. 1987;31:1874–8.

70. NIAID Mycoses Study Group. Treatment of blastomycosis and histoplasmosis with ketoconazole. Results of a prospective randomized clinical trial. Ann Intern Med. 1985;103:861–72.

71. Restrepo A, Gomez I, Cano LE, et al. Post-therapy status of paracoccidioidomycosis treated with ketoconazole. Am J Med. 1983;74:53.

72. Galgiani JN, Stevens DA, Graybill JR, et al. Ketoconazole therapy of progressive coccidioidomycosis. Comparison of 400 and 800 mg doses and observations at higher doses. Am J Med. 1988;84:603–10.

73. Schaffner A, Frick PG. The effect of ketoconazole on amphotericin B in a model of disseminated aspergillosis. J Infect Dis. 1985;151:902–10.

74. Pont A, Graybill JR, Craven PC, et al. High-dose ketoconazole therapy and adrenal and testicular function in humans. Arch Intern Med. 1984;144:2150–3.

75. De Coster R, Caers R, Haelterman C, et al. Effect of a single administration of ketoconazole on total and physiologically free plasma testosterone and 17-beta-oestradiol levels in healthy male volunteers. Eur J Clin Pharmacol. 1985;29:489–93.

76. Lewis JH, Zimmerman HJ, Benson GD, et al. Hepatic injury associated with ketoconazole therapy. Gastroenterology. 1984;86:503–13.

77. Barone JA, Koh JG, Bierman RH, et al. Food interaction and steady-state pharmacokinetics of itraconazole capsules in healthy male volunteers. Antimicrob Agents Chemother. 1993;37:778–84.

78. Smith D, Van De Velde V, Woestenborghs R, et al. The pharmacokinetics of oral itraconazole in AIDS patients. J Pharm Pharmacol. 1992;44:618–9.

79. Hostetler JS, Heykants J, Clemons KV, et al. Discrepancies in bioassay and chromatography determinations explained by metabolism of itraconazole to hydroxyitraconazole: Studies of interpatient variations in concentrations. Antimicrob Agents Chemother. 1993;37:2224–7.

80. Lim SG, Sawyer AM, Sercombe J, et al. Short report: The absorption of fluconazole and itraconazole under conditions of low intragastric acidity. Alim Pharma Ther. 1993;7:317–21.

81. Crane JK, Shih H. Syncope and cardiac arrhythmia due to an interaction between itraconazole and terfenadine. Am J Med. 1993;95:445–6.

82. Dismukes WE, Bradsher Jr RW, Cloud GC, et al. NIAID, and the Mycoses Study Group. Itraconazole therapy for blastomycosis and histoplasmosis. Am J Med. 1992;93:489–97.

83. Sharkey-Mathis PK, Velez J, Fetchick R, et al. Histoplasmosis in the acquired immunodeficiency syndrome (AIDS): Treatment with itraconazole and fluconazole AIDS 1993;6:809–19.

84. Wheat J, Hafner R, Wulfsohn M, et al. Prevention of relapse of histoplasmosis with itraconazole in patients with the acquired immunodeficiency syndrome. Ann Intern Med. 1993;118:610–6.

85. Sharkey-Mathis PK, Kauffman CA, Graybill JR, et al., and the Mycoses Study Group. Treatment of sporotrichosis with itraconazole. Am J Med. 1993;95:279–85.

86. Winn RE, Anderson J, Piper J, et al. Systemic sporotrichosis treated with itraconazole. Clin Infect Dis. 1993;17:210–7.

87. Jennings TS, Hardin TC: Treatment of aspergillosis with itraconazole. Ann Pharm. 1993;27:1206–11.

88. Cleary JD, Taylor JW, Chapman SW: Itraconazole in antifungal therapy. Ann Pharm. 1992;26:502–9.

89. Zervos M, Meunier F. Fluconazole (Diflucan): A review. Int J Antimicrob Agents. 1993;3:147–70.

90. DeMuria D, Forrest A, Rich J, et al. Pharmacokinetics and bioavailability of fluconazole in patients with AIDS. Antimicrob Agents Chemother. 1993;37:2187–92.

91. Saxèn H, Hoppu K, Pohjavuori M: Pharmacokinetics of fluconazole in very low birth weight infants during the first two weeks of life. Clin Pharm Ther. 1993;54:269–77.

92. Baciewicz AM, Baciewicz FA: Ketoconazole and fluconazole drug interactions. Arch Intern Med. 1993;153:1970–6.

93. Perfect JR, Lindsay MH, Drew RH. Adverse drug reactions to systemic antifungals. Drug Safety. 1992;7:323–63.

94. Weinroth SE, Tuazon CU. Alopecia associated with fluconazole treatment. Ann Intern Med. 1993;119:637.

95. Just-Nublign G, Gentschew G, Meibner K, et al. Fluconazole prophylaxis of recurrent oral candidiasis in HIV-positive patients. Eur J Clin Microbiol Infect Dis. 1991;917–21.

96. Graninger W, Preseteril LE, Schneeweiss B, et al. Treatment of *Candida albicans* fungemia with fluconazole. J Infect. 1993;26:133–46.

97. Czwerwiec FS, Bilsker MS, Kamerman ML, et al. Long-term survival after fluconazole therapy of candidal prosthetic valve endocarditis. Am J Med. 1993;94:545–6.

98. Saag MS, Powderly WG, Cloud GA, et al. Comparison of amphotericin B with fluconazole in the treatment of acute AIDS-associated cryptococcal meningitis. N Engl J Med 1992;326:83–9.

99. Bozzette SA, Larsen R, Chiu J, et al. A placebo-controlled trial of maintenance therapy with fluconazole after treatment of cryptococcal meningitis in the acquired immunodeficiency syndrome. N Engl J Med. 1991;324:580–4.

100. Powderly WG, Saag MS, Cloud GA, et al. A controlled trial of fluconazole or amphotericin B to prevent relapse of cryptococcal meningitis in patients with the acquired immunodeficiency syndrome. N Engl J Med. 1992;326:793–8.

101. Galgiani JN, Catanzaro A, Cloud GA, et al., and the NIAID Mycoses Study Group. Fluconazole therapy for coccidioidal meningitis. Ann Intern Med. 1993;119:28–35.

102. Castro LGM, Belda Jr W, Cuce LC, et al. Successful treatment of sporotrichosis with oral fluconazole: A report of three cases. Br J Dermatol. 1993; 128:352–6.

103. Goodman JL, Winston DJ, Greenfield RA, et al. A controlled trial of fluconazole to prevent fungal infections in patients undergoing bone marrow transplantation. N Engl J Med. 1992;326:845–51.

104. Winston DJ, Chandrasekar PH, Lazarus HM, et al. Fluconazole prophylaxis of fungal infections in patients with acute leukemia. Ann Intern Med. 1993; 118:495–503.

105. Kwon-Chung KJ, Bennett JE. Medical Mycology. Philadelphia: Lea & Febiger; 1992; pp. 98–9.

32. ANTIVIRAL AGENTS

FREDERICK G. HAYDEN

Antiviral drugs with proven therapeutic (Table 1) and prophylactic effectiveness are currently available for a number of common and, in some instances, life-threatening viral infections. In part as a response to the human immunodeficiency virus (HIV) infection and its sequelae, the search for new antiviral agents and therapeutic approaches for managing viral diseases continues to intensify. New agents added to the therapeutic armamentarium since the last edition of this text include didanosine, zalcitabine, and stavudine for HIV, foscarnet for cytomegalovirus (CMV) and other herpesviruses, famciclovir for varicella-zoster virus (VZV), and rimantadine for influenza A virus infections. In addition, the approved indications for other agents (e.g., acyclovir for VZV infections in normal hosts, interferon for chronic hepatitis B and C, ganciclovir for CMV prevention) have been expanded.

GENERAL PRINCIPLES

Mechanisms of Action

Chemotherapeutic agents for viral infections can be categorized into three broad groups: agents that directly inactivate intact viruses (virucides); those that inhibit viral replication at the cellular level (antivirals); and those that augment or modify the host response to infection (immunodulators). Virucidal agents may cause direct inactivation in a single step, such as detergents, organic solvents like ether or chloroform, and ultraviolet light; or in multiple steps, as with photodynamic inactivation. However, such interventions have not proven clinically useful in the treatment of mucocutaneous herpes simplex virus (HSV) infections. Treatments that destroy both host tissues and virus simultaneously, such as cryotherapy, laser, or podophyllin treatment of warts, are useful only in discrete mucocutaneous infections. One potential use of virucidal agents may be in preventing transmission of certain viral infections.

Antiviral Agents. Since viral replication depends primarily on host cell metabolic functions, useful antiviral agents must inhibit virus-specific events, such as attachment to the cell, uncoating of the viral genome, or assembly of progeny virions, or preferentially inhibit virus-directed, as contrasted to host cell–directed, macromolecular synthesis. Consequently, antiviral agents typically have a restricted spectrum of activity. While many compounds exist that exhibit antiviral activity in vitro, most affect some host cell function and are associated with low therapeutic ratios or unacceptable toxicity in humans. Most current antiviral agents target viral nucleic acid synthesis. In addition, since these agents inhibit ongoing replication at the host cell level, replication may resume when the drug is removed. Similarly, current antiviral drugs are not effective in elimination of nonreplicating or latent viruses.

Susceptibility assays for viruses are not standardized, and results depend on various factors, including the assay system, cell line, viral inoculum, and laboratory.[1] Efforts to develop in vitro susceptibility assays using uniform techniques have begun with regard to HIV,[2] and several commercial laboratories offer sensitivity testing of selected herpesviruses.

Host Immune Responses. Intact host immunologic responses remain essential for recovery from virus infections. Immunosuppression due to transplantation, cancer chemotherapy, or HIV infection has been associated with high rates of recrudescent or chronic viral infections. Responses to antiviral treatment may be delayed, and the risk of selecting drug-resistant viruses

may be higher in such patients. In addition, some antiviral agents may blunt host immune responses by direct immunosuppressive effects[3] or by altering humoral and cellular immune responses indirectly through reductions in viral antigen exposure.[4] Factors other than inhibition of viral replication alone are important in resolving certain viral diseases, such as orofacial HSV infections or rhinovirus colds in normal hosts and CMV pneumonia in bone marrow transplant recipients, in which it has been possible to demonstrate antiviral effects without clinical benefit. Increasingly, antivirals are being used for prevention of viral diseases in high-risk persons.[5,6]

Immunomodulating agents used for treating viral infections include those that replace deficient host immune responses, such as exogenous antibody in chronic echovirus infection or interferon in herpes zoster of immunocompromised hosts, or those that enhance endogenous ones. Chemical agents that appear to augment cell-mediated immune (CMI) responses have been used with variable success and remain investigational.[7] The reports of delayed progression in HIV infections by use of immunomodulators such as ampligen, ditiocarb, isoprinosine, and thymopentin require further confirmation.[8]

Drug Resistance. Drug resistant viruses often can be selected under laboratory conditions and have been recognized increasingly during clinical use of various antivirals. Indeed, the selection of a drug-resistant strain of virus implies that the drug has a specific antiviral mechanism. The development of resistance results from mutations within the viral genome, and the presence of selective drug pressure leads to the emergence of a resistant virus population. Resistant subpopulations often exist naturally in clinical isolates, but spontaneous mutations may also arise during drug exposure. Single nucleotide mutations leading to critical amino acid substitutions in a target protein are often sufficient to cause antiviral resistance. The mechanisms of drug resistance described in bacteria, eukaryotic microorganisms, and malignant cells (e.g., gene amplification or overexpression; changes in drug uptake, efflux, or inactivation) have not been documented in viruses.

The possibility of drug resistance is usually suspected because of a lack of clinical and virologic response to treatment. However, clinical failures of antiviral therapy may occur despite the presence of drug-sensitive virus in immunocompromised hosts. Factors favoring the emergence of resistant variants include high viral replicative load, as in infections with chronic and/or high titer replication; high intrinsic viral mutation rate, which is generally greater in RNA than DNA viruses; and degree of selective drug pressure, which is higher with prolonged or repeated courses of drug therapy. Consequently, most drug-resistant viruses (e.g., HSV, VZV, CMV, HIV-1) are recovered from immunocompromised patients, although influenza A virus is an exception.[9–12]

The consequences of the emergence of resistance may include a reduction or alteration in viral pathogenicity (e.g., different clinical syndromes), although resistant viruses appear able to cause severe disease in immunocompromised hosts. Whether resistant variants are at some biologic disadvantage with respect to transmissibility, ability to establish chronic or latent infections, genetic stability, and persistence in the absence of selective drug pressure is not well defined for most viruses.

Drug Administration

Clinical efficacy depends on achieving effective antiviral concentrations at the site of infection and, specifically, on adequate intracellular concentrations of an agent or its active metabolites. Many antivirals, particularly nucleoside analogs, are inactive until metabolized within cells to phosphorylated derivatives that compete with natural nucleosides for viral and sometimes host cell enzymes. Consequently, the state of activation or stage of differentiation of cells can affect intracellular pools of the phos-

TABLE 1. Antiviral Agents of Established Therapeutic Effectiveness

Viral Infection	Drug	Route	Usual Dosage
Cytomegalovirus			
Retinitis	Ganciclovir	IV	5 mg/kg/12 h in 1 h infusion for 14–21 days[a]
	Foscarnet	IV	60 mg/kg/8 h in 1–2 h infusion for 14–21 days[b]
Pneumonia	Ganciclovir	IV	5 mg/kg/12 h in 1 h infusion + IV immunoglobulin[c] for 14–21 days
Hepatitis viruses			
Chronic hepatitis C	Interferon-α2b	SC/IM	3 MU 3 times/week for 24 weeks
Chronic hepatitis B	Interferon-α2b	SC/IM	5 MU/day or 10 MU 3 times/week for 16 weeks
Herpes simplex virus			
Genital herpes			
First episode	Acyclovir	PO[d]	200 mg 5 times/d or 400 mg tid for 10 days
Recurrence	Acyclovir	PO	200 mg 5 times/d or 400 mg tid for 5 days
Suppression[e]	Acyclovir	PO	400 mg bid or 200 mg tid
Encephalitis	Acyclovir[f]	IV	10 mg/kg/8 h in 1 h infusion for 14–21 days
Mucocutaneous disease in immunocompromised	Acyclovir[g]	IV[h]	5 mg/kg/8 h for 7–14 days[i]
		PO	400 mg 5 times/d for 7–14 days
Neonatal	Acyclovir[j]	IV	10 mg/kg/8 h for 10–21 days
Keratoconjunctivitis	Trifluridine[k]		1 drop of 1% solution topically, q2h up to 9 drops/d
	Vidarabine		½ inch ribbon of 3% ointment 5 times/d
Human immunodeficiency virus-1			
AIDS, advanced ARC	Zidovudine	PO	100 mg/4 h or 200 mg/8 h[l]
	Didanosine	PO	200 mg as tablets or 250 mg as powder bid[m]
	Zalcitabine[n]	PO	0.75 mg/8 h
Asymptomatic, CD4 <500	Zidovudine	PO	100 mg 5 times/d
Influenza A virus	Amantadine	PO	100 mg bid for 5 days[o]
	Rimantadine	PO	200 mg/d for 5 days[p]
Papillomavirus			
Condyloma acuminatum	Interferon-α2b[q]	Intralesional	1 mu/0.1 ml injected in up to 5 warts, 3 times/week for 3 weeks
Respiratory syncytial virus	Ribavirin	Aerosol	Aerosol treatment 12 to 18 hours/d for 3 to 7 days[r]
Varicella-zoster virus			
Varicella in normal children	Acyclovir	PO	20 mg/kg up to 800 mg qid for 5 days
Varicella in immunocompromised	Acyclovir	IV	500 mg/m²/8 h for 7–10 days
Herpes zoster in immunocompromised	Acyclovir[g]	IV	10 mg/kg/8 h in 1 h infusion for 7 days[s]
Herpes zoster in normal hosts	Acyclovir	PO	800 mg 5 times/d for 7–10 days
	Famciclovir[t]	PO	250 or 500 mg tid for 7 days

Abbreviations: IV: intravenous; SC: subcutaneous; IM: intramuscular; PO: oral.

[a] In AIDS and in other highly immunocompromised patients, chronic suppression with a daily infusion of 5 mg/kg given 7 days per week or 6 mg/kg given 5 days per week is recommended after acute treatment. These doses are also approved for prevention of CMV disease in transplant recipients after initial 7–14-day course of 5 mg/kg/12 hours. Dose reduction required for creatinine clearance <80 ml/min.

[b] Chronic suppression with daily infusion of 90–120 mg/kg over 2 hours is recommended after initial treatment in AIDS patients. Use of metered infusion pump to maintain dosing at a maximum of 1 mg/kg/min and close monitoring of renal function with dose reduction for creatinine clearance <1.6 ml/min/kg are required.

[c] Not approved by FDA for this indication. In bone marrow transplant patients, combined use of ganciclovir and intravenous immunoglobulin is necessary for therapeutic benefit.

[d] For severe initial genital herpes or in those unable to tolerate oral medicines, IV acyclovir 5 mg/kg/8 h for 5–7 days is recommended. For mild initial genital HSV, 5 percent acyclovir ointment can be applied to lesions every 3 hours up to six times per day for 14 days (about ½-inch ribbon per 4 square inches), using a finger cot or glove.

[e] Chronic suppression does not eliminate subclinical shedding and risk of transmission. Patients have been successfully managed with chronic acyclovir for more than 6 years.

[f] Vidarabine, 15 mg/kg/day as an iv infusion over 12–24 hours, is a less effective alternative.

[g] In acyclovir-resistant HSV or VZV infections, iv foscarnet 40 mg/kg/8 h appears beneficial. Duration of therapy depends on the clinical response.

[h] For limited cutaneous infections in immunocompromised patients, 5% acyclovir ointment can be applied to lesions every 3 hours up to six times per day for 7 days (about ½-inch ribbon per 4 square inches), using a finger cot or glove.

[i] Dose reductions are indicated for creatinine clearance <50 ml/min. Pediatric dosage is 250 mg/m²/8 h iv for 7–14 days.

[j] Not approved by the FDA for this indicaqtion. For premature infants, 20 mg/kg/day in two divided doses is advised. Vidarabine, 15–30 mg/kg/day as an IV infusion over 12–24 hours, is an FDA-approved alternative.

[k] An ophthalmic ointment of 3 percent acyclovir is available in some countries. Idoxuridine 0.1 percent solution, q1h while awake and q2h at night, or 0.5 percent ointment five times/day is a less effective alternative. Treatment of HSV ocular infections should be supervised by an ophthalmologist.

[l] Some experts recommend 200 mg q4h for the first month of therapy in all patients and indefinitely for those with CNS disease. For children 3 months to 12 years old, the recommended starting dose is 180 mg/m²/6 h (to a maximum of 200 mg).

[m] Based on weight ≥60 kg; dose of 125 mg as tablets or 167 mg as powder for weight <60 kg. Pediatric dosing is based on an average dose of 200 mg/m²/day. Need to chew or disperse in water two tablets and swallow on an empty stomach.

[n] Use concomitantly with zidovudine 200 mg/8 h.

[o] The maximum recommended dose for older adults is 100 mg/day. Dose reductions are indicated for creatinine clearance <80 ml/min. The recommended pediatric dose is 4.4 mg/kg/day up to a maximum of 150 mg/day.

[p] Pediatric dose is 5 mg/kg up to maximum of 150 mg/day. Dose of 100 mg/day is recommended in the elderly and in those with severe hepatic or renal dysfunction.

[q] Interferon-αn1 is also approved for this indication.

[r] Reservoir concentration of 20 mg/ml. Requires special aerosol-generating device available from manufacturer and expert respiratory therapy monitoring for administration.

[s] Dose reductions are indicated for creatinine clearance <50 ml/min. Pediatric dosage is 500 mg/m²/8 h for 7–10 days. Vidarabine 10 mg/kg/day as IV infusion over 12–24 hours is a less effective alternative.

[t] Not approved yet by FDA for this indication. Dose reductions are indicated for creatinine clearance <50 ml/min.

phorylated antiviral and its competing natural substrate and affect inhibitory activity and toxicity.[13]

Pharmacokinetic studies that define absorption, stability in body fluids, tissue distribution, and metabolic fate of antiviral drugs are important in selecting proper doses. However, predictive relationships between drug concentrations active in vitro, those achieved in blood or other body fluids, and clinical response have not been established for most antiviral agents. While animal models are useful in testing of antiviral agents, they may differ from the corresponding human infection with regard to pathogenesis, drug sensitivity of the virus, drug pharmacology, or toxicity.

Topical Administration. Topical application of antivirals to the cornea, skin, mucous membranes, or respiratory tract is intended to provide high concentrations at the site of infection and to avoid the possible toxicity of systemic administration. Topically applied drugs must be able to penetrate such barriers as stratified epithelium or local secretions to reach the site of active viral replication. Several agents are effective in therapy of HSV keratitis (Table 1), and work continues on developing improved formulations for other mucocutaneous herpesvirus infections. Delivery of antiviral drugs to the respiratory tract in the form of small-particle aerosols has been used with some benefit in influenza and particularly in respiratory syncytial virus infections, and the use of intranasally administered interferon has been shown to be protective against colds caused by rhinoviruses.

Combination Chemotherapy. The combined use of antiviral agents with different mechanisms of action has been studied as a means of increasing antiviral activity, reducing drug dosage and the associated risk of toxicity, and preventing or modifying the development of drug resistance.[14,15] Viral isolates from treated patients may be genetically heterogeneous with respect to mixtures of sensitive and resistant viruses or viruses with different resistance mutations, so that combinations may be able to provide broader activity than single agents. In addition, individual drugs may act preferentially on different cell types or tissues. Combination therapy has been used successfully in experimental infections due to enteroviruses, influenza, and various herpesviruses. Numerous clinical trials in HIV infection are being conducted with various combinations of reverse transcriptase inhibitors, other antiretrovirals, immunomodulators such as interferon, and growth factors.[8,14–16] Whether combinations can prevent the development of resistant variants in vivo, or whether they will prove to be clinically superior to the use of individual antiviral agents (monotherapy) is currently under investigation. Specific mutations causing resistance to certain HIV reverse transcriptase inhibitors can suppress zidovudine resistance.[14]

ACYCLOVIR (ACYCLOGUANOSINE, ACV, ZOVIRAX) AND VALACICLOVIR (VALTREX)

Spectrum

Acyclovir (9-{2-hydroxyethoxy}methyl]-9H-guanine) is a deoxyguanosine analog that has an acyclic side chain lacking the 3'-hydroxyl group instead of the cyclic base of natural nucleosides (Fig. 1). Valaciclovir (256U87) is the L-valyl ester of acyclovir. Acyclovir's clinically useful antiviral spectrum is limited to herpesviruses, and it is approximately 10-fold more potent against HSV-1 and -2 than VZV and even less active against CMV (Table 2).[17–21] Acyclovir inhibits the replication of Epstein-Barr virus (EBV) DNA in productively infected cells, but does not affect latent or persistent infection.[20] Acyclovir has shown antiviral activity in experimental HSV infection when administered topically, parenterally, or orally and in simian varicella when given systemically.[22–24] Enhanced anti-herpesvirus activity oc-

curs in combination with various antiviral agents in vitro and in animal models.[25,26]

Uninfected mammalian cell growth is generally unaffected by high acyclovir concentrations. Acyclovir at 20 μg/ml does not reproducibly alter CMI responses of human peripheral blood leukocytes or affect human granulocyte progenitor cell growth in vitro.[3,27–30]

Mechanism of Action

Acyclovir is the prototype of a group of antiviral agents that are activated by viral thymidine kinases to become inhibitors of viral DNA polymerases and block viral DNA synthesis.[17,31] Acyclovir uptake and intracellular phosphorylation to the monophosphate derivative are facilitated by HSV thymidine kinase.[31] Cellular enzymes convert the monophosphate to acyclovir triphosphate, which is present in 40-to 100-fold higher concentrations in HSV-infected than in uninfected cells. Acyclovir triphosphate competitively inhibits viral DNA polymerases, and to a much smaller extent cellular DNA polymerases, with respect to dGTP.[32] The triphosphate is also incorporated into viral DNA, where it acts as a chain terminator because of the lack of a 3'-hydroxyl group. Formation of a complex between the terminated DNA template containing acyclovir and the enzyme may lead to irreversible inactivation of the DNA polymerase.[33] The DNA polymerases of various herpesviruses differ in their degree of inhibition by acyclovir triphosphate; the polymerases of EBV and CMV appear to be especially sensitive.[34]

Resistance

Acyclovir-resistant HSV, often defined by an in vitro inhibitory concentration of greater than 3 μg/ml, can be readily selected by passage in the presence of acyclovir and is also present in native virus populations with an estimated frequency of 1 in 10^3–10^4.[9,10] One study found that 40 percent of HSV isolates from untreated patients contain acyclovir-resistant variants that account for at least 1 percent of the total virus population.[35] Three basic resistance mechanisms have been identified: absent or partial production of viral thymidine kinase (TK); altered TK substrate specificity (e.g., phosphorylation of thymidine but not acyclovir); and altered viral DNA polymerase. Changes in these viral enzymes relate to point mutations or base insertion/deletions in the corresponding genes. The most common mechanism found in clinical HSV isolates is deficient TK activity.[36,37] Less commonly, resistant isolates have altered TK activity, whereas DNA polymerase mutants are rare in clinical strains.[38,39] Heterogeneous populations are commonly found when detailed studies are performed.[40]

Acyclovir-resistant HSV isolates are recovered very uncommonly from normal hosts,[41] and most "breakthrough" isolates recovered during oral suppressive therapy have sensitive phenotypes.[42–44] However, many cases of progressive HSV disease associated with recovery of acyclovir-resistant virus and poor response to acyclovir therapy have now been recognized in AIDS and in transplant patients.[45–49] Ulcerating perirectal lesions, often chronic and necrotizing, due to resistant HSV-2 are the most common pattern in AIDS patients, and chronic or severe orofacial disease due to resistant HSV-1 is seen in transplant patients. Resistant ocular infections have also been described.[50] The risk factors include the degree of immunosuppression, size of lesions, and repeated or prolonged use of acyclovir for treatment rather than prophylaxis. However, resistant isolates have also been recovered from patients whose lesions healed spontaneously. One study of bone marrow transplant patients treated with intravenous acyclovir for recurrent mucocutaneous HSV infections recovered resistant HSV in 1 of 52 first-treatment courses and 2 of 22 second courses.[46] Another survey found that resistant HSV can be recovered from

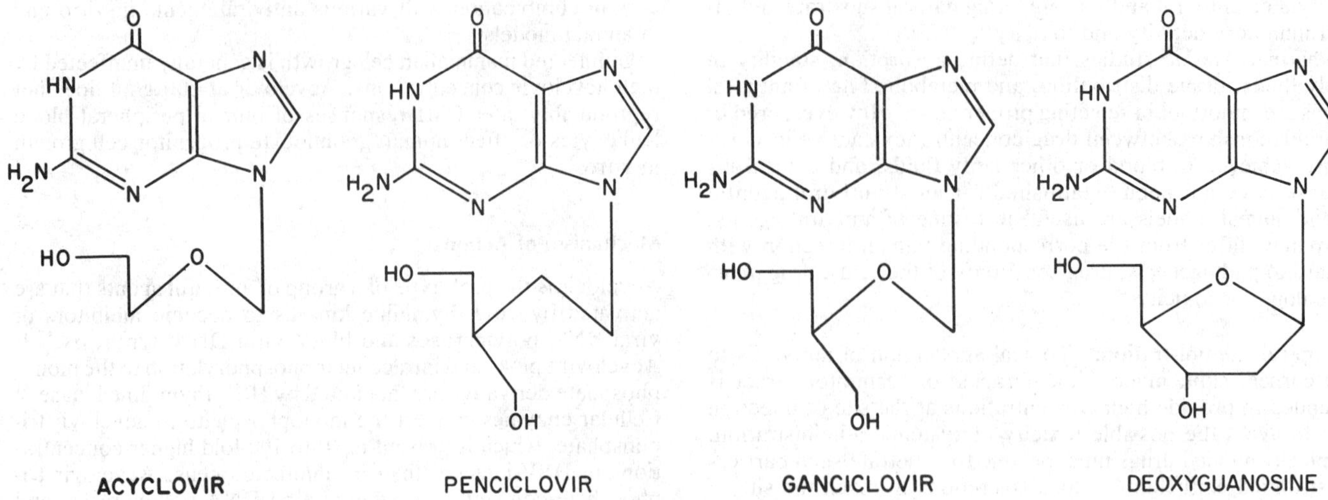

FIG. 1. Chemical structures of acyclovir, penciclovir, ganciclovir, and the nucleoside deoxyguanosine.

TABLE 2. Representative In Vitro Inhibitory Concentrations of Acyclic Nucleosides for Clinical Isolates of Herpesviruses in Human Cells

Virus	Inhibitory Concentration ($\mu g/ml$)		
	Acyclovir	Penciclovir	Ganciclovir
HSV-1	0.02–0.9	0.2–0.6	0.05–0.6
HSV-2	0.03–2.2	0.3–2.4	0.05–0.6
VZV	0.8–4.0	0.9–4.0	0.4–10
CMV	2–57	52	0.2–2.8
EBV	1.6	—	1–5

(Data from refs. 17–20; 291–293; 335–339.)

11–17 percent of AIDS or transplant patients receiving acyclovir treatment for 2 weeks or longer.[51]

Most TK-deficient mutants of HSV are less neurovirulent and less able to be reactivated from latency in animal models, although they may cause extensive mucocutaneous disease in immunocompromised hosts.[9,10] TK-altered or polymerase mutants have variable or minimal decrease in pathogenicity. No recognized person-to-person spread of resistant HSV has been documented yet, and recurrences after cessation of acyclovir are usually due to sensitive virus. However, in AIDS patients, persistent shedding of resistant HSV at the site of initial infection and recurrences with acyclovir-resistant variants have been found in the absence of selective drug pressure.[52,53] Visceral disease may occur uncommonly with resistant variants, and cases of fatal meningoencephalitis in AIDS patients and neonates due to resistant HSV-2, and of HSV-1 pneumonitis in marrow transplant patients, have been reported (R. Whitley, personal communication).[48,49]

The optimal management of infections due to suspected or proven acyclovir-resistant HSV is not certain. Depending on degree of immunosuppression, resistant HSV infections may undergo spontaneous healing following cessation of acyclovir therapy. In patients with progressive disease, intravenous foscarnet therapy is effective, but vidarabine is not.[52,53] High-dose, continuous-infusion acyclovir,[54] topically applied trifluridine,[55] topical interferon-α_2 alone or in combination with topical trifluridine, and topical HPMC[56a] have been used in small numbers of patients. Ganciclovir is not active against TK-deficient mutants.

Acyclovir resistance in VZV isolates, associated with 20- to 40-fold increases in inhibitory concentrations, is related to mutations in VZV TK with inability to phosphorylate acyclovir or less often in viral DNA polymerase. Such isolates are very uncommon[57] but have been recovered from HIV-infected children and adults with chronic, disseminated, hyperkeratotic, or verru-

cous papular lesions that fail to heal with intravenous acyclovir,[58] and rarely from visceral sites.[59] Chronic suppressive therapy with subtherapeutic doses of acyclovir appears to be a risk factor. Clinical isolates with altered TK substrate specificity are more common than for acyclovir-resistant HSV; these VZV isolates may retain in vitro sensitivity to BV-araU or less often penciclovir.[60] Intravenous foscarnet also appears effective for acyclovir-resistant VZV infections.[61]

Pharmacokinetics

The bioavailability of oral acyclovir is low (15–21 percent) and decreases with increasing doses.[62,63] Peak plasma concentrations average 0.4–0.8 $\mu g/ml$ after 200 mg oral doses[64] and increase to about 1.6 $\mu g/ml$ with 800 mg doses.[65] Bioavailability is lower in transplant patients, in whom doses of 400 mg provide peak levels of 0.7–0.9 $\mu g/ml$.[66] A liquid suspension has somewhat lower oral bioavailability; peak plasma concentrations average 1.0 $\mu g/ml$ in children receiving 600 mg/m² doses.[67] Peak and trough plasma concentrations at the end of a 1-hour infusion average 9.8 and 0.7 $\mu g/ml$ after 5 mg/kg/8 h and 20.7 and 2.3 $\mu g/ml$ after 10 mg/kg/8 h, respectively.

Following oral administration, the L-valine ester of acyclovir, valaciclovir, is rapidly and nearly completely converted to acyclovir.[68,69] This is probably due to first-pass enzymatic hydrolysis in the liver and intestine. The relative bioavailability of acyclovir is estimated to be three to five times greater following ingestion of the prodrug valaciclovir. Peak plasma acyclovir levels average 5.0 and 8.5 $\mu g/ml$ after doses of 1000 and 2000 mg of valaciclovir, respectively. The daily AUCs approach levels seen with intravenous acyclovir.

Acyclovir distributes widely in body fluids. Plasma protein binding is less than 20 percent. Cerebrospinal fluid concentrations are approximately one-half of plasma values.[62] After oral administration, salivary concentrations average 13 percent of plasma, but vaginal secretion concentrations range from 15 to 170 percent of plasma.[64] Zoster vesicular fluid levels are similar to those in plasma.[70] Aqueous humor levels average 37 percent of concurrent plasma values.[71] Breast milk concentrations average over threefold higher than those in serum.[72] Percutaneous absorption of acyclovir after topical administration appears to be low. In patients with genital HSV infections treated with topical acyclovir, concentrations in genital lesions at 4–12 hours after application range widely (0.002–38 $\mu g/ml$), and no detectable acyclovir is present in cervicovaginal secretions. Newborn plasma levels are similar to maternal ones, and amniotic fluid and placental concentrations are severalfold higher.[73]

TABLE 3. Acyclovir Dose Adjustments Suggested for Patients with Impaired Renal Function[a]

| Creatinine Clearance (ml/min 1.73 m²) | Intravenous | | Oral[b] | |
	Standard Dose (%)	Dosing Interval (hours)	Dose	Dosing Interval (hours)
>50	100	8	800	4
25–50	100	12	800	4
10–25	100	24	800	8
0–10[c]	50	24	800	12

[a] Recommendations based on Blum et al.[62] and Laskin et al.[75]
[b] Oral acyclovir dose adjustments are needed for severe renal insufficiency. Recommendations are based on high-dose oral regimen (4000 mg/day). For low dose (1000 mg/day) oral regimen, the suggested doses is 200 mg q12h for creatinine clearance <10 ml/min/1.73 m².
An alternative in patients with end-stage renal disease is administration of 14 percent of standard dose every 8 hours after loading with 37 percent of the standard dose.[73] For posthemodialysis administration, 60–100 percent of standard dose should be used.[75] An intravenous dosage of 2.5 mg/kg/day has been suggested in CAPD patients.[79]

The mean plasma elimination half-life ($T_{1/2elim}$) of acyclovir is about 2.5–3 hours (range, 1.5–6.3 hours) in adults with normal renal function, but is slightly longer (3.8 hours) in neonates and increases to 19.5 hours in anuric patients.[62,63,74,75] Renal excretion of unmetabolized acyclovir by glomerular filtration and tubular secretion accounts for 60–91 percent of an administered dose, while less than 15 percent is excreted as 9-carboxymethoxy-methylguanine or minor metabolites.[76] Dosage reductions are indicated in patients with creatinine clearances less than 50 ml/min (see Table 3). Acyclovir is readily hemodialyzable, and plasma concentrations are reduced by about 60 percent during a 6 hour hemodialysis.[75,77] Peritoneal dialysis is much less efficient in removing acyclovir[78,79] so that dosing supplementation is not needed during continuous ambulatory peritoneal dialysis (CAPD). Bioavailability is about 61 percent after intraperitoneal dosing.[80]

Interactions

Severe somnolence and lethargy may occur with combinations of zidovudine and acyclovir.[81] Concomitant cyclosporin and probably other nephrotoxic agents enhance the risk of nephrotoxicity. Probenecid decreases the renal clearance and prolongs the plasma $T_{1/2elim}$. By competing for the organic acid secretory pathway, acyclovir may decrease the renal clearance of other drugs eliminated by active renal secretion, such as methotrexate.[63]

Toxicity

Topical acyclovir may cause transient burning when applied to genital lesions, more commonly in first episodes and in female patients. The polyethylene glycol base of topical acyclovir may cause mucosal irritation and is not approved for intravaginal use.

Intravenous acyclovir is generally well tolerated,[82] although inflammation, phlebitis, and rarely vesicular eruption[83] may occur at the injection site following extravasation of the alkaline solution (pH 9–11). Uncommonly reported side effects include rash, diaphoresis, hematuria, hypotension, headache, and nausea. Approximately 1–4 percent of patients receiving intravenous acyclovir have manifested neurotoxicity characterized by lethargy, confusion, obtundation, tremor, myoclonus, hallucinations, delirium, seizures, extrapyramidal signs, and/or coma.[84–87] Diffuse electroencephalographic (EEG) abnormalities and increased cerebrospinal fluid concentrations of myelin basic protein may occur. Symptoms of neurotoxicity usually develop within 1–3 days of starting treatment. The majority of cases have marked deterioration of renal function or preexisting renal disease and occur in association with high serum acyclovir concentrations (>25 µg/ml). Concurrent interferon administration or intrathecal methotrexate may be risk factors. Neurotox-

icity has been rarely described after oral administration and after prolonged therapy without changes in renal function. Neurologic side effects occur within 1–2 days after maximum acyclovir concentrations and resolve with a comparable delay after decrease in drug concentrations.[87] Hemodialysis may be useful in severe cases.[78,88]

Reversible renal dysfunction has been observed in approximately 5 percent of patients treated with intravenous acyclovir.[85,88] In animals acyclovir can cause a crystalline nephropathy. Acyclovir solubility decreases to 2.5 mg/ml at 37°C, and crystalluria has been described in adult and pediatric patients.[89,90] Obstructive nephropathy may be manifested by nausea, emesis, flank pain, and increasing azotemia. Bolus infusion, dehydration, preexisting renal insufficiency, high doses, and high acyclovir plasma levels are risk factors. Nephrotoxicity usually resolves with drug cessation and volume expansion. Acute interstitial nephritis has also been described.[91]

Oral acyclovir has been associated infrequently with nausea, diarrhea, rash, and headache and rarely with renal insufficiency and neurotoxicity. The safety of long-term acyclovir suppression for frequently recurring genital or mucocutaneous infections has been shown for at least 5 years of continuous use,[92] and no adverse effects on sperm production or peripheral blood lymphocyte cytogenetics have been detected.[93,94] However, chronic oral acyclovir may cause neutropenia in infants (R. Whitley, personal communication). No excess frequency of abnormalities has been recognized in infants born to women exposed to acyclovir during the first trimester of pregnancy.[95]

Acyclovir has shown mutagenic activity in some in vitro assays at high concentrations, but no significant immunosuppressive activity, carcinogenicity, or teratogenicity has been noted in animal studies. High doses decrease spermatogenesis and cause testicular atrophy in animals.

Clinical Studies

Acyclovir is currently the agent of choice for management of many types of HSV and VZV virus infections because of its efficacy, safety, and ease of administration (Table 1).[17] Valaciclovir is currently undergoing evaluation for many of the conditions in which acyclovir is used in both immunocompetent and compromised patients.[68] Comparative trials have found that intravenous acyclovir is superior to vidarabine with regard to efficacy and/or toxicity in HSV encephalitis[96,97] and in varicella[98] or herpes zoster[99] in immunocompromised patients. Vidarabine and acyclovir appear to be comparably active in neonatal HSV infections.[100]

HSV Infections. Acyclovir by various routes is effective in initial genital HSV infections.[101–105] Topical acyclovir is associated with smaller clinical and antiviral effects than oral or intravenous administration (Table 4) and does not influence new lesion formation after treatment. Because some patients treated with topical acyclovir develop new lesions and/or increased symptoms after stopping therapy, longer durations of application (10–14 days) have been advocated.[103] Intravenous acyclovir markedly reduces viral shedding, time to healing, and duration of symptoms in patients hospitalized with severe primary genital HSV infections.[101] Similarly, in outpatients with initial genital HSV infections, oral acyclovir (200 mg five times daily for 10 days) is associated with significant reductions in virus shedding, symptoms, and time to healing.[102,105] Higher doses of oral acyclovir do not appear to increase efficacy.[105a] None of these regimens has been associated with consistent reductions in the rate of recurrent genital lesions. Acyclovir therapy decreases the humoral and cellular immune response to HSV following first-episode genital herpes.[4,106] Higher oral doses (400 mg five times daily for 10 days) provides similar benefit in first-episode HSV proctitis.[107]

Oral acyclovir is associated with reduced shedding but modest

TABLE 4. Relative Effectiveness of Different Acyclovir Formulations in Treating First-Episode or Recurrent Genital Herpes Simplex Virus

	Percent Reduction Compared with Placebo		
	Duration of Viral Shedding	Duration of Pain	Duration of Lesions
First episode			
Intravenous	85	57	57
Oral	80	44	35
Ointment	55	26	29
Recurrent[a]			
Oral	46	12	21
Ointment	45[b]	0	0

[a] Patient-initiated therapy.
[b] Women only; no effect in males.

(Data from refs. 101–105, 108, 109.)

clinical effects (Table 4) in recurrent genital HSV infections.[105,108] When therapy is initiated by patients during the prodrome or at the first sign of lesions, oral acyclovir is associated with a 1.5- 2 to day reduction in the durations of shedding and time to healing, but no difference in the duration of pain. Topical acyclovir offers no significant clinical benefit in recurrent genital herpes.[103,109]

In patients with frequently recurring genital herpes, chronic oral acyclovir (400–1000 mg/day in divided doses) reduces the frequency of recurrences by about 90 percent and protects 65–85 percent of patients from recurrence.[6,92,110–112] Doses of 400 mg twice daily are effective for up to 5 years.[92] Once daily or weekend-only use is unsuccessful.[111,112] Asymptomatic shedding may occur during suppression, and occasional cases of transmission to sexual partners have been documented.[113,114] Following completion of acyclovir administration, patients generally return to their previous pattern of recurrent infection. The possible utility of oral acyclovir for preventing recurrences during pregnancy and reducing caesarean delivery rates requires further study,[115] and failures have occurred.[115a]

Chronic suppression may be useful in other patients with disabling recurrences of herpes whitlow or HSV-related erythema multiforme. In patients with frequently recurring herpes labialis, oral acyclovir (400 mg twice daily for 4 months) reduces the number of clinical recurrences by 53 percent.[116] In patients with a history of sun-induced recurrences, short-term prophylaxis (400 mg twice daily for 1 week) reduces the risk of recurrence by 73 percent.[117] Short-term prophylaxis during day care center outbreaks may be effective in preventing primary infections in children,[118] but the efficacy of postexposure prophylaxis remains to be established.

In recurrent orolabial HSV infections, topical acyclovir reduces virus shedding but is not associated with clinical benefit.[119] Topical application of 5 percent acyclovir in a cream formulation, not currently available in the United States, has been reported to be therapeutically effective in both recurrent labial and genital HSV infections.[120] Oral acyclovir (200–400 mg five times daily for 5 days) provides modest clinical benefit in recurrent orolabial herpes[120] and appears therapeutically efficacious in recurrent whitlow.[122]

Systemic acyclovir in various regimens has been used successfully for both the prevention and treatment of mucocutaneous HSV infections in immunosuppressed patients.[123–130] Intravenous acyclovir (250 mg/m^2/8–12 h), begun prior to transplantation and continuing for several weeks, is highly effective in reducing the incidence of HSV disease in seropositive bone marrow transplant recipients.[123,124] Once daily administration is inadequate. For patients who can tolerate oral medications, oral acyclovir (400 mg five times/daily for 5 weeks) is effective in marrow transplant patients,[66,125] and long-term oral acyclovir (400 mg three times daily for 6 months) also reduces the risk of VZV infection.[124] Low doses of oral acyclovir (200

mg/6–8 h) appear to be effective in renal transplant patients[126] and other immunosuppressed hosts[127] and during periods of intense chemotherapy.[128]

In immunocompromised patients with established mucocutaneous HSV infection, intravenous acyclovir (250 mg/m^2/8 h for 7 days) shortens healing time and duration of pain by 30–60 percent and decreases the period of virus shedding by 60–80 percent.[5,129] Although recurrences are common after cessation of therapy. Oral acyclovir (800 mg five times daily) is also effective.[130] In those with localized labial or facial HSV infections, topical acyclovir diminishes the duration of virus shedding and may shorten the time to loss of pain and healing of lesions. However, topical acyclovir should be used only in limited extraoral mucocutaneous HSV infections in such patients. Anecdotal reports suggest that intravenous acyclovir is beneficial in viscerally disseminating HSV in pregnant and transplant patients.[131,132]

In HSV encephalitis, acyclovir reduces mortality to 19–28 percent compared with 50–54 percent with vidarabine.[96,97] In neonates, immunosuppressed patients, and rarely in apparently healthy persons, early relapses of encephalitis may follow initial acyclovir therapy,[133–135] such that longer courses of treatment may be warranted. Progressive neurologic deterioration in infants has been managed with chronic suppressive oral acyclovir.[134] Acyclovir also appears effective in the acute retinal necrosis syndrome.[136]

VZV Infections. Intravenous acyclovir is currently the treatment of choice for varicella or zoster, both localized and disseminated, in immunocompromised patients. It also appears effective in varicella pneumonia or encephalitis in previously healthy adults.[137–139] In immunocompromised patients with herpes zoster, intravenous acyclovir (10 mg/kg/8 h for 7 days) reduces the risk of cutaneous dissemination (4 vs. 21 percent) and visceral complications (0 vs. 4 percent) compared with placebo.[140] Compared with vidarabine, acyclovir reduces the duration of new lesion formation and time to complete healing by about 3 days and risk of cutaneous dissemination in localized zoster,[99] as well as the length of hospitalization in disseminated zoster.[141] In immunosuppressed children with varicella, intravenous acyclovir is associated with a reduced risk of visceral complications and about a 1-day reduction in the duration of vesicle formation and time to full crusting.[142–144] Early relapses of infection may occur following cessation of therapy, and treatment may be ineffective in visceral disease. Early treatment with oral acyclovir (800 mg 5 times daily for 7 days) may also be effective in immunosuppressed children.[145]

High-dose oral acyclovir is effective treatment for herpes zoster in older adults, for zoster ophthalmicus, and, if begun within 24 hours of onset of rash, for varicella in otherwise normal children,[146] adolescents,[147] and adults.[148] In children, acyclovir's effects include about a 1-day reduction in fever and in 15–30 percent reductions in the severity of other illness measures, so that routine use in uncomplicated varicella is not recommended.[149] In varicella in immunocompetent adults, intravenous acyclovir is associated with reductions in fever and vesicle duration but not in local symptoms.[150] Oral acyclovir (800 mg 5 times daily for 7 days) initiated within 24 hours of the onset of rash reduces the time to total crusting of lesion by approximately 2 days, reduces the maximum number of lesions, and decreases the duration of fever, but does not affect the course of illness if begun later.[148] It is not known whether acyclovir might reduce the risk of complications. Postexposure prophylaxis with oral acyclovir (40–80 mg/kg/d in divided doses) beginning 1 week after exposure may reduce the risk of varicella in household contacts.[150a]

In immunocompetent older adults with herpes zoster, intravenous acyclovir is associated with significant reductions in virus shedding, time to healing of skin lesions, and duration of acute pain.[151,152] Oral acyclovir (600–800 mg five times daily for 7–10 days) also reduces acute pain and healing time in older adults, if treatment can be initiated within 72 hours of rash onset, particularly within 1–2 days.[65,153-6] Lower doses and later initiation of therapy are ineffective. A reduction in ocular complications, particularly keratitis and anterior uveitis, occurs with oral acyclovir treatment of zoster ophthalmicus.[155] However, no consistent effect on the incidence or severity of postherpetic neuralgia has been demonstrated with intravenous or oral acyclovir.[157,158] Topical application of ophthalmic acyclovir is more effective than topical corticosteroids in reducing ocular relapses of zoster ophthalmicus.[159] (Ophthalmic preparations of acyclovir are available in the United States only through a compassionate use protocol from Burroughs Wellcome Co.)

Other Viruses. Although associated with variable effects on CMV shedding, acyclovir is therapeutically ineffective in established CMV infections.[160] High-dose intravenous acyclovir (500 mg/m²/8 h) beginning 5 days before bone marrow transplantation and continuing for 30 days afterwards is associated with an approximate 50 percent lower risk of CMV disease and significantly improves survival compared with placebo in CMV-seropositive patients.[161] High-dose oral acyclovir for 3 months may possibly reduce the risk of CMV disease in renal and liver transplant recipients, including those at risk for primary infection, but appears less effective than ganciclovir.[162-166a] It has not proven effective in liver transplant recipients receiving OKT3 therapy[167] or lung transplant patients.[168]

In infectious mononucleosis of normal hosts, intravenous and oral acyclovir are associated with transient suppression of salivary EBV excretion but no important effects on other illness parameters.[109,170] High-dose acyclovir is not effective in chronic fatigue syndrome patients.[171] Some cases of severe EBV infection or EBV-related lymphoproliferation appear to respond to acyclovir.[172-174] EBV-related oral hairy leukoplakia responds to oral acyclovir.[175] Intravenous acyclovir has been reported to inhibit hepatitis B virus replication, but neither intravenous nor oral therapy enhances the response to interferon in chronic hepatitis B.[176,177]

AMANTADINE (SYMMETREL) AND RIMANTADINE (FLUMADINE)

Spectrum

Amantadine (1-adamantanamine hydrochloride) and rimantadine (α-methyl-1-adamantane methylamine hydrochloride) are symmetric tricyclic amines (Fig. 2) that specifically inhibit the replication of influenza A viruses at low concentrations (<1.0 μg/ml).[178] By plaque assay, inhibitory concentrations of the drugs range from 0.1 to 0.4 μg/ml for human influenza A viruses, including H1N1, H2N2, and H3N2 subtypes.[179,180] Rimantadine is 4- to 10-fold more active than amantadine in several in vitro assays.[181,182] Clinical isolates vary in their susceptibility to the

drugs, but the significance of such differences is not defined. Higher concentrations (10–50 μg/ml) have in vitro inhibitory activity against other enveloped viruses, including parainfluenza, influenza B, rubella, and dengue,[183,184] but these concentrations are too high to be clinically relevant and may also be cytotoxic and immunosuppressive in vitro.

These agents have both prophylactic and therapeutic activity in experimental influenza A virus infection of animals following oral or parenteral dosing.[178,185] Treatment of infected mice limits the extent of virus replication and reduces the risk of transmission to exposed, uninfected animals. Aerosol delivery directly to the respiratory tract has greater efficacy than systemic administration.[186] Amantadine and ribavirin combinations show enhanced antiviral and therapeutic effects in vitro and in experimental influenza.[187] Rimantadine exhibits enhanced antiviral activity in combination with ribavirin, interferon, or protease inhibitors.[187,188]

Mechanism of Action

Amantadine and rimantadine share the same dual mechanisms of antiviral action.[189] One effect involves inhibition of an early step in viral replication, probably viral uncoating. For H7 subtype viruses, a late effect on viral assembly is presumably mediated through alteration of hemagglutinin conformation. Genetic studies indicate that the susceptibility of human isolates to low drug concentrations is a property conferred by the M2 protein, an integral membrane protein with 15–60 copies per virion. A critical transmembrane region of the M2 protein is the site of action of these drugs, which appear to interfere with the ion channel function of M2.[189-192] This action probably accounts for both inhibition of the acid-mediated dissociation of the matrix protein from the ribonucleoprotein (RNP) complex within endosomes early in replication and the potentiation of pH-induced alterations in the hemagglutinin during its transport late in infection.

Amantadine and rimantadine are also concentrated in the lysosomal fraction of mammalian cells. Drug-mediated increases in lysosomal pH may inhibit virus-induced membrane fusion events and account for its broad antiviral spectrum at higher concentrations.[183] However, selective anti-influenza A virus effects are quickly lost upon drug removal from the surrounding medium, which suggests that drug needs to be present in extracellular fluid early in the replicative cycle.[193,194]

Resistance

Contemporary epidemic strains have been drug sensitive,[179,182] but resistant virus is readily selected by virus passage in the presence of drug.[178] Amantadine and rimantadine share cross-susceptibility or resistance. Resistance with over 100-fold increases in inhibitory concentrations has been associated with single nucleotide changes in RNA segment 7 and lead to corresponding amino acid substitutions at one of five critical sites in transmembrane region of M2.[12,189]

When amantadine or rimantadine treatment is given to birds experimentally infected with a pathogenic avian influenza virus, drug-resistant variants emerge and can cause death in the treated animals and in contacts receiving drug prophylaxis.[195] Combined administration of vaccine and amantadine, but not vaccine alone, is protective for contact birds. Resistant viruses are virulent, genetically stable, and able to compete with wild-type virus such that transmission of drug-resistant virus may occur after cessation of drug use.[196]

Resistant variants have also been recovered from treated patients and sometimes their close contacts.[12,197-200] Up to 30 percent of drug-treated children or adults shed resistant virus by the fifth day of therapy. The clinical significance of shedding resistant virus for treated individuals is unclear, since they still resolve their illness promptly,[201] and the duration of shedding

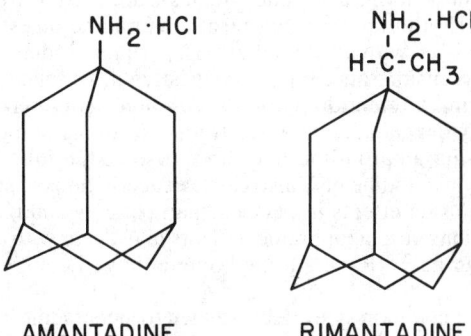

FIG. 2. Chemical structures of amantadine hydrochloride and rimantadine hydrochloride.

is relatively short. However, apparent transmission of resistant virus, associated with failure of drug prophylaxis, has been documented in household contacts of rimantadine-treated index cases[198] and in nursing home residents receiving amantadine.[199,200] Resistant variants appear to be pathogenic and can cause typical disabling influenzal illness in prophylaxis failures. At present, it seems prudent to avoid contact between treated patients and susceptible high-risk contacts and to avoid use of both treatment, specifically of young children, and postexposure prophylaxis in the same household.[12]

Ribavirin is active in vitro against resistant strains, but the efficacy of systemic or aerosolized ribavirin in severe influenza remains to be established.

Pharmacokinetics

Amantadine. Amantadine is well absorbed after oral administration of capsule, tablet, or syrup forms.[202-205] The time to peak plasma levels averages 2–4 hours but varies widely. Steady-state peak plasma concentrations average 0.5–0.8 μg/ml on a 100-mg twice daily regimen in healthy young adults. The elderly require only one-half of the weight-adjusted dose needed for young adults to achieve equivalent trough plasma levels of 0.3 μg/ml.[203] In children with cystic fibrosis, mean plasma concentrations are 0.6 μg/ml during long-term ingestion of 6 mg/kg/day, which suggests that such children require relatively large doses. Although some evidence suggests that amantadine is concentrated in pulmonary tissues,[206] nasal secretion and salivary levels of amantadine approximate those found in the serum. Cerebrospinal fluid levels are about one-half of those in plasma, and amantadine is excreted in breast milk.

Amantadine is excreted unmetabolized in the urine through glomerular filtration and probably tubular secretion.[207] The plasma $T_{1/2elim}$ is about 12–18 hours, but varies widely in apparently healthy young adults. Because of age-related declines in renal function, $T_{1/2elim}$ increases up to twofold in the elderly[202] and even more in patients with impaired renal function.[207] In patients with creatinine clearance less than 10 ml/min, the $T_{1/2elim}$ may be as long as 30 days. Dose reductions are required in renal insufficiency (see Table 5). Amantadine is inefficiently cleared in hemodialysis patients, and additional doses are not required.[207,208] Monitoring of plasma concentrations in such patients is desirable but impractical.

Rimantadine. Rimantadine in tablet form is well but slowly absorbed, with time to peak plasma concentrations averaging 2–6 hours.[209,210] Absorption does not appear to be decreased by the presence of food. A syrup formulation has slightly lower oral bioavailability than the tablet. With multiple doses of 100 mg twice daily, the steady-state peak and trough plasma concentrations in healthy adults are approximately 0.4–0.5 and 0.2–0.4 μg/ml, respectively.[211] In infants receiving doses of 3 mg/kg each day, steady-state peak serum levels range from 0.1 to 0.6 μg/ml.[212] No important age-related changes in plasma levels or pharmacokinetics have been found in healthy elderly adults or in children.[213,214] However, steady-state plasma concentrations in elderly nursing home residents receiving 100 mg twice daily average over twofold higher (mean, 1.2 μg/ml) than those observed in healthy adults, which indicates the need for lower doses in such patients.[215] Rimantadine has a very large volume of distribution, and concentrations in nasal mucus average 50 percent higher than those in plasma.[214]

In contrast to amantadine, rimantadine is extensively metabolized following oral administration. Less than 15 percent of the dose is excreted unchanged in the urine, and 20 percent or more of the dose is excreted in the urine as hydroxylated metabolites.[202,216] The plasma $T_{1/2elim}$ of rimantadine averages 24–36 hours, approximately twofold longer than that of amantadine. No clinically important differences in pharmacokinetics are found in patients with chronic liver disease without significant hepatocellular dysfunction.[217] In hemodialysis patients with severe renal failure, the clearance of rimantadine is decreased by 40 percent and the $T_{1/2elim}$ is about 55 percent longer.[216] Dose reduction by one-half (e.g., 100 mg/day) is suggested for marked hepatic or renal insufficiency (creatinine clearance < 10 ml/min). Hemodialysis removes only a small amount of rimantadine so that supplemental doses are not required.

Interactions

The central nervous system (CNS) effects of amantadine appear to be increased by concomitant ingestion of antihistamines or anticholinergic drugs. Coadministration with anticholinergics in elderly patients may cause toxic delirium and visual hallucinations. Concurrent use of trimethoprim-sulpha or of triamterene-hydrochlorothiazide has been associated with CNS toxicity due to decreased renal clearance in several cases.[218] Drug interactions with rimantadine have not been well studied. Cimetidine is associated with 15–20 percent increases and acetaminophen or aspirin with approximately 10 percent decreases in plasma concentrations of rimantadine, but such changes are unlikely to be of clinical significance.[219] Patients receiving either drug along with drugs affecting CNS function (e.g., antihistamines, antidepressants, and minor tranquilizers) should be monitored closely.

Toxicity

Oral amantadine and rimantadine do not appear to cause clinically important renal, hepatic, or hematopoietic toxicity.[220] In the setting of renal insufficiency or high doses, serious neurotoxic reactions, including tremor, seizures or coma, cardiac arrhythmias, and death may occur in association with high amantadine plasma concentrations (1.0–5.0 μg/ml).[205,221,222] Neurotoxic reactions may be transiently reversed by physostigmine administration, and lidocaine has been used to treat ventricular arrhythmias.[222] Long-term amantadine ingestion has been associated with livedo reticularis, peripheral edema, orthostatic hypotension, and, rarely, congestive heart failure, vision loss, or urinary retention. Patients with preexisting seizure disorders may develop an increased frequency of major motor seizures during amantadine use, and dose reductions are advised.[223] Rimantadine may also cause exacerbations of seizures. Psychiatric side effects in parkinsonian patients and psychotic exacerbations in schizophrenic patients may occur with addition of amantadine.[224] Rash and leukopenia have been described rarely.

The most common side effects related to amantadine ingestion are minor dose-related gastrointestinal and CNS complaints. These include nervousness, lightheadedness, difficulty concentrating, insomnia, and loss of appetite or nausea.[205] CNS side

TABLE 5. Amantadine Dosage Regimens for Prophylaxis and Alterations in Renal Failure

	Suggested Dose
No renal insufficiency	
Children, 1–9 years	4.4 mg/kg/day once daily or in divided doses, up to 150 mg/day
Ages 10–64 years	200 mg once daily or in divided doses
Ages ≥65 years	100 mg/day[a]
Creatinine clearance (ml/min/1.73 m²)[b]	
≥80	200 mg once daily or in divided doses
60–80	200 mg/100 mg alternate days
40–60	100 mg daily
30–40	200 mg twice weekly
20–30	100 mg three times a week
10–20[c]	200 mg/100 mg alternating every 7 days

[a] Further reductions should be considered for weight <50 kg. Doses of 1.4 mg/kg/day have been suggested.[203,231]
[b] Based on adult dose of 200 mg/day. Proportionate reductions should be made for older adults receiving lower doses.
[c] Additional doses are not required during hemodialysis.

(Recommendations based on Horadam.[207])

effects occur in approximately 5–33 percent of amantadine recipients at doses of 200 mg/day, but are significantly less frequent with rimantadine. When used for influenza prophylaxis, doses of 200 mg/day are associated with excess withdrawals in 6–11 percent of recipients because of drug side effects.[225–228] In healthy persons, amantadine doses of 300 mg/day in adults and 6.6 mg/kg/day in children are poorly tolerated.[223,226] Doses of 100 mg/day are better tolerated and may be protective against influenzal illness.[229,230] Amantadine dose reductions are required in older adults (100 mg/day) because of decreased renal function, but 20–40 percent will experience side effects even at this lower dose.[231–233] Trough steady-state plasma concentrations above 0.45 μg/ml or peak concentrations above 1.0 μg/ml are associated with an increased risk of CNS side effects.[234,235] Complaints typically develop within the first week of administration, often resolve despite continued ingestion, and are promptly reversible on discontinuation of the drug. In a large study in young adults, CNS side effects were no more frequent in recipients of 200 mg/day of rimantadine than in the placebo group.[225]

Rimantadine administration is associated with dose-related, reversible side effects qualitatively similar to those observed with amantadine. However, CNS side effects are significantly less frequent with rimantadine at doses of 200 or 300 mg/day.[225,226,236] Rimantadine at 300 mg/day is associated with significantly higher rates of gastrointestinal complaints, but not CNS, sleep, or psychomotor disturbances, than is placebo.[226] During prophylaxis, excess withdrawal rates are usually less than 5 percent.[220,237] However, conventional 200 mg/day doses are associated with higher plasma levels and side effect rates in elderly nursing home residents.[215] The wider therapeutic margin of rimantadine, relative to amantadine, relates to differences in pharmacokinetics between the drugs.[234]

The clinical observations of dry mouth, pupillary dilation, toxic psychosis, and urinary retention in acute amantadine overdose suggest that anticholinergic activity is present in humans.[205] Amantadine demonstrates activity on the adrenergic nervous system by affecting accumulation, release, and reuptake of catecholamines in the central and peripheral nervous systems. Ventricular irritability occurs in animals given high doses of amantadine, and malignant ventricular arrhythmia after amantadine overdose has been described in humans.[221] Amantadine is teratogenic and embryotoxic in animals. Rimantadine is not mutagenic in vitro and does not appear to cause teratogenic effects in rabbits or rats. However, the safety of either drug has not been established in pregnancy.

Clinical Studies

The clinical usefulness of amantadine and rimantadine is limited to the prevention and treatment of influenza A virus infections.[205,225,236,238] Both drugs at a dose of 200 mg/day in adults are about 70–90 percent effective as prophylaxis against clinical illness due to various influenza A subtypes in experimentally induced and naturally occurring infections. One 6-week seasonal prophylaxis trial comparing equivalent 200 mg/day doses of rimantadine and amantadine found that the drugs were 85 and 91 percent effective, respectively, in preventing laboratory-documented influenza A illness.[225] Amantadine prophylaxis is effective in preventing nosocomial influenza and possibly in curtailing established nosocomial outbreaks.[223] Similarly, in immunized nursing home patients, rimantadine is about 75 percent effective in preventing influenza A illness during a community epidemic.[239] Rimantadine (5 mg/kg/day) administration to school-aged children decreases the risk of influenza A illness in recipients (100 percent efficacy) and possibly in their family contacts.[240] However, postexposure prophylaxis with these drugs provides inconsistent protection to family contacts, in part depending on whether ill index children are treated.[198] Doses of 100 mg/day appear to be protective against influenza A illness and well-tolerated in adults.[241]

Seasonal prophylaxis with rimantadine or amantadine is an alternative in high-risk patients, if influenza vaccine cannot be administered because of toxicity or allergy, or if vaccine may be ineffective because the epidemic strain differs substantially from the vaccine strain, or if vaccine is unlikely to induce an adequate immune response, as in patients with immunodeficiency.[242] Because of the additive effect of vaccine-associated protection and that provided by chemoprophylaxis, the combined use of immunization and drug prophylaxis during an outbreak provides optimal protection, particularly for high-risk patients. To prevent the spread of influenza to high-risk patients, chemoprophylaxis can be used in unimmunized health care workers and household members. Prophylaxis should be begun as soon as influenza is identified in a community or region and should be continued throughout the period of risk (usually 4–8 weeks), since any beneficial effects diminish rapidly after discontinuation of the drug. Alternatively, since prophylaxis does not interfere with the response to inactivated vaccine, the drugs can be started in conjunction with immunization and continued for 2 weeks until protective antibody develops.

Amantadine and rimantadine are also effective therapies in uncomplicated influenza A illness.[201,236,243–246] When begun within 1–2 days of onset of symptoms, doses of 200 mg/day reduce the duration of fever and systemic complaints by 1–2 days and in some studies decrease the duration of virus shedding compared with placebo. Treated persons are also able to resume usual activities more rapidly.[201,236] Aspirin-treated patients defervese more rapidly but experience significantly higher rates of drug-related side effects and slower symptomatic improvement than amantadine recipients.[243] In illness due to H3N2 subtype influenza viruses, certain abnormalities of peripheral airway function, but not airway hyperreactivity, resolve more quickly in amantadine-treated patients. However, it remains uncertain whether treatment reduces risk of complications in high-risk patients or is useful in patients with established pulmonary complications.

Oral rimantadine has therapeutic effects in uncomplicated influenza A illness comparable with those of amantadine. One study employing equivalent 100-mg bid dosing found that amantadine-treated patients tended to improve more rapidly than rimantadine-treated patients over the first 24 hours, but that by 48 hours both groups had significantly less fever, greater symptomatic improvement, and lower frequencies of virus shedding than placebo-treated patients.[236] Similar therapeutic benefits occur in elderly influenza patients treated with rimantadine.[244] In children with influenza A/H3N2 subtype infection, rimantadine treatment is associated with lower symptom burden, fever, and viral titers during the first 2 days of treatment compared with acetaminophen administration, but rimantadine-treated children have more prolonged shedding of virus.[245] In children with milder H1N1 subtype infection, reductions in viral shedding and clinical affects comparable to acetaminophen have been found.[246] Treatment generally does not appear to affect immune responses to infection but may blunt secretory antibody levels in children[247] and other immune responses in animal models.[248] The optimal dose and duration of therapy have not been established in children for either agent.

Intermittent aerosol administration of amantadine or rimantadine appears therapeutically useful in experimentally induced, uncomplicated influenza in humans.[249] An injectable formulation of either drug is currently not available.

DIDANOSINE (DDI, VIDEX)

Spectrum

Didanosine (2′,3′-dideoxyinosine) is a purine nucleoside analog (Fig. 3) active against HIV-1 and -2 in vitro, including zidovudi-

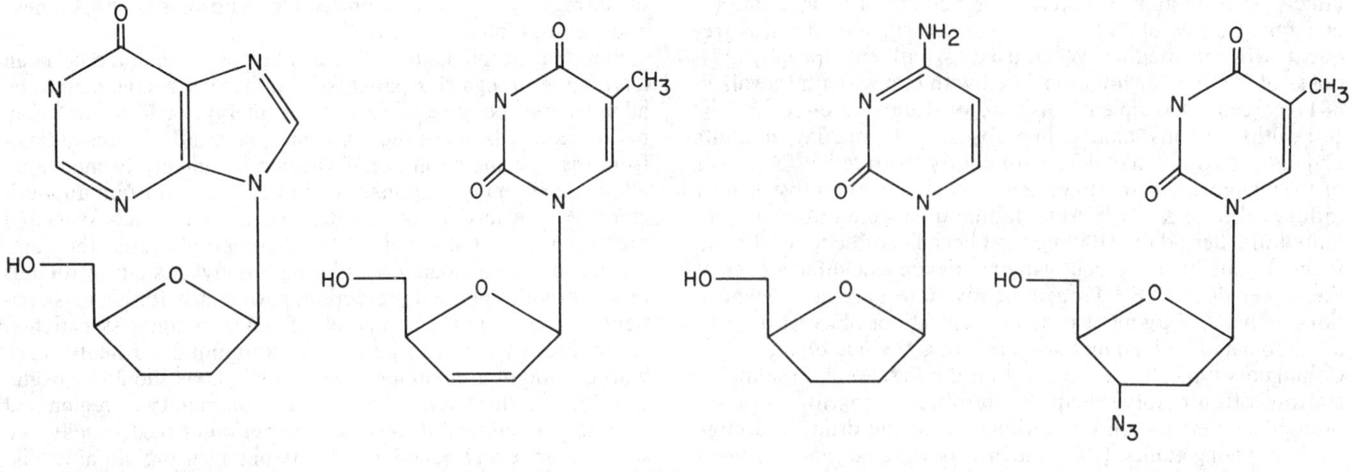

FIG. 3. Chemical structures of antiretroviral dideoxynucleosides: didanosine, stavudine, zalcitabine, and zidovudine.

TABLE 6. Representative In Vitro Inhibitory Concentrations of Dideoxynucleoside Antiviral Agents for HIV-1 in Human Blood Cells

| Agent | Inhibitory Concentration (μg/ml) | |
	PBMC	Macrophage/Monocyte
Zidovudine	<0.001–0.04	0.02–0.2
Didanosine	<1.0–5	0.002–0.02
Stavudine	0.002–0.01	0.02–0.2
Zalcitabine	0.002–0.2	0.0002–0.002

(Data from refs. 13, 251–254, 263, 264.)

ne-resistant isolates. Didanosine is 10- to 100-fold less potent than zidovudine with regard to both antiviral activity and cytotoxicity in activated peripheral blood mononuclear cells (PBMC) but appears more active in quiescent cells and human monocyte/macrophages (Table 6).[250,254] In vitro didanosine is much less toxic for hematopoietic precursor cells[256] or lymphocytes[3] than zidovudine. Combinations of didanosine and zidovudine synergistically inhibit HIV-1 replication in vitro, including zidovudine-resistant strains.[257,258]

Mechanism of Action

Didanosine is taken up intracellularly and converted by 5′-nucleotidase to dd-IMP (dideoxyinosine 5′ monophosphate) and further metabolized by other cellular enzymes to its active derivative 2′-3′-dideoxyadenosine triphosphate (ddATP).[250,259] ddATP functions as a competitive inhibitor of viral reverse transcriptase with respect to dATP and as a chain terminator of viral DNA synthesis. Its selectivity relates to ddATP's higher affinity for viral reverse transcriptase than for cellular DNA polymerases, although it does inhibit mitochondrial DNA polymerase-γ.[260,261] The prolonged intracellular $T_{1/2}$ of ddATP (8–24 hours) may also contribute to didanosine's antiviral activity and provides the basis for its relatively infrequent dosing schedule. The high ratio of ddATP to dATP in resting PBMC may account for the pronounced activity of didanosine in such cells.[253] Inhibitors of IMP dehydrogenase like ribavirin cause increased formation of ddATP and increase the antiviral activity of didanosine. Purine nucleoside phosphorylase catalyzes the cleavage of didanosine to form hypoxanthine, which may be further metabolized to uric acid.

Resistance

HIV-1 isolates from previously untreated patients and those switched from long-term zidovudine to didanosine become progressively less susceptible to didanosine, with 2- to more than 25-fold reductions in sensitivity.[251,262–264] During didanosine therapy, some zidovudine-resistant isolates regain sensitivity over time, while some zidovudine-sensitive ones may become moderately resistant. Susceptibility changes to didanosine have been associated with a mutation at position $74^{\text{leu}\rightarrow\text{val}}$ in the reverse transcriptase[262] and may occur in the absence of mutations conferring zidovudine resistance. One study of AIDS-related complex (ARC) patients, most of whom had received previous zidovudine therapy, found that didanosine therapy for a median of 1 year was associated with 2- to 14-fold decreases in didanosine sensitivity in two-thirds of patients and an average of 10-fold increases in zidovudine susceptibility.[258] Variants with $74^{\text{leu}\rightarrow\text{val}}$ mutation may be rapidly eliminated once didanosine therapy is stopped.[265] Resistance associated with other mutations in the RT at position $184^{\text{met}\rightarrow\text{val}}$ have also been found.[266] Strains resistant to didanosine may show cross-resistance to zalcitabine. The clinical significance of these changes in susceptibility remains to be determined.

Pharmacokinetics

The oral bioavailability of didanosine is about 35–45 percent for doses up to 10 mg/kg but varies widely among patients and is dependent on formulation, gastric acidity, and food.[267–269] Oral absorption may also be lower in children.[270] Didanosine is very acid labile, and food decreases absorption by 50 percent or more.[271] It should be taken at least 1 hour before or 2 hours after a meal. The chewable tablet has about 20 percent greater bioavailability than the powder sachet. Each dose should be administered as two tablets in adults to provide adequate buffering, and weight-adjusted dosing is recommended by the manufacturer. Peak plasma levels after 300 mg tablet doses range from 0.5 to 2.6 μg/ml. Plasma concentrations over time have been positively correlated with antiviral and clinical effects.[270,272] The cerebrospinal fluid to plasma ratio averages 20 percent at 1 hour after administration in adults[268] but may be more variable in children.[270] Didanosine crosses the placenta and is detectable in fetal blood.[273]

After intravenous dosing, about 40–60 percent of the drug is excreted unchanged in the urine through both glomerular filtration and tubular secretion. Plasma $T_{1/2\text{elim}}$ averages 0.6–1.5 hours. Nonrenal pathways of elimination are important but not fully characterized. In uremic patients, the plasma $T_{1/2\text{elim}}$ increases approximately threefold, and the peak plasma concentrations double.[269] Dose adjustments are recommended by the manufacturer for renal insufficiency (serum creatinine >1.5 mg/dl or creatinine clearance [CL_{cr}] <60 ml/min). Didanosine is

TABLE 7. Potential Adverse Drug Interactions with Selected Antiviral Agents

Antiviral Agent	Potential Interactions
Didanosine	Agents associated with peripheral neuropathy[a]
	Agents associated with pancreatitis[b]
	↓ Absorption of ketoconazole, dapsone, quinolones, tetracycline
Foscarnet	Intravenous pentamidine (hypocalcemia)
	Nephrotoxic agents[c]
Ganciclovir	Zidovudine and other agents associated with myelotoxicity[d]
	Nephrotoxic agents[c]
	Imipenem/cilastatin (seizures)
Zalcitabine	Agents associated with peripheral neuropathy[a]
	Agents associated with pancreatitis[b]
	Nephrotoxic agents[c] (increased risk of neuropathy)
Zidovudine	Agents associated with myelotoxicity[d]
Stavudine	Agents associated with peripheral neuropathy[a]

[a] Including other dideoxynucleosides, chloramphenicol, cisplatin, dapsone, disulfram, ethionamide, glutethimide, gold, hydralazine, iodoquinol, isoniazid, metronidazole, nitrofurantoin, phenytoin, ribavirin and vincristine.
[b] Including IV pentamidine, ganciclovir (possibly related to underlying CMV infection), furosemide, cimetidine, ranitidine, sulfonamides, corticosteroids, tetracycline, and ethanol.
[c] Including aminoglycosides, amphotericin B, IV pentamidine, IV acyclovir, cyclosporine, and foscarnet.
[d] Including ganciclovir, zidovudine, sulfonamides, pyrimethamine, interferon, ganciclovir, pentqamidine, flucytosine, amphotericin B, and cancer chemotherapeutic agents.

(Data from Saag[274] and Lee and Safrin.[275])

removed to a limited extent by hemodialysis (approximately 20 percent of dose during 4-hour dialysis), so that replacement doses are not required. However, dosing should be done at the end of a hemodialysis run.[269]

Interactions

The buffered formulations of didanosine can decrease absorption of various drugs, including ketoconazole, dapsone, tetracyclines, and certain quinolones (Table 7).[274,275] Ranitidine increases didanosine bioavilability modestly.[276] The risk of pancreatitis is increased by exposure to intravenous pentamidine and probably other agents (Table 7). Agents associated with peripheral neuropathy should be used cautiously in association with didanosine (Table 7). Coadministration of ganciclovir with the didanosine does not appear to increase the risk of toxicities due to either agent.[277]

Toxicity

Painful peripheral neuropathy and pancreatitis are the major dose-limiting toxicities of didanosine.[278–282] Both usually develop in the first 3–6 months of dosing but may occur later.[283] Neuropathy typically involves the lower extremities, begins acutely with paresthesia, numbness, and/or pain, and usually resolves with cessation of therapy. The risk of neuropathy increases progressively with time and is higher in those with a prior history of the condition. At currently recommended doses, neuropathy does not occur more frequently than observed in a zidovudine treated comparison group.[284]

The risk of pancreatitis, which may rarely be fatal, is increased by a history of prior pancreatitis up to sixfold, exposure to intravenous pentamidine or possibly other agents (Table 7), low CD4 counts, and higher doses (≥750 mg/day). At currently recommended doses, pancreatitis occurs approximately twice as often (7 percent of patients) and hyperamylasemia approximately three times as often (20 percent) with didanosine compared with zidovudine.[284] Glucose intolerance has been associated with didanosine and may precede onset of pancreatitis.[285]

Diarrhea, related to the citrate buffer, appears to be less frequent with tablets than powder. Unusual adverse effects include skin rash, CNS disturbance including headache, insomnia and seizures, retinal depigmentation in children, optic neuritis, increased aminotransferase levels, and rarely hepatic failure[286] or

cardiomyopathy. At currently recommended doses, hematologic abnormalities and hyperuricemia are very uncommon.

Safety during pregnancy has not been determined. Preclinical studies have found gastrointestinal, bone marrow, hepatic, and renal abnormalities in animals given high doses but no adverse effects on fertility or fetal development.[250] Like other nucleoside, didanosine can cause chromosomal damage.

Clinical Studies

Didanosine is currently approved for the treatment of advanced HIV infection in adults and children over 6 months of age who are intolerant of or deteriorating on zidovudine and for use in patients with advanced HIV disease who have been taking zidovudine for 4 months or longer but may otherwise be stable. Initial open trials found that didanosine doses of approximately 3.2 mg/kg/day and above are associated with sustained increases in CD4 counts, decreased p24 antigen levels, symptom reduction, and sometimes improved cognition in AIDS or severe ARC patients, including children and those infected with zidovudine-resistant strains.[278–281,287]

A comparative study of patients with at least 16 weeks of prior zidovudine therapy (ACTG 116b/117) found that didanosine at 500 mg/day is superior to zidovudine at 600 mg/day in reducing new AIDS-defining diagnoses but not in prolonging survival.[284] The therapeutic benefit was observed in patients enrolled with asymptomatic infection and CD4 counts of 200 cells/mm³ or less or ARC. A similar trial in patients with AIDS or ARC and less than 300 CD4 cells/mm³ who exhibited progression after at least 6 months of dizovudine therapy found similar benefits.[288] Didanosine at 750 mg/day is associated with higher rates of pancreatitis and with possibly less overall effectiveness than the lower dose. However, in previously untreated patients (ACTG 116a), didanosine appears to be less effective in preventing clinical progression than zidovudine.[289] In patients with advanced infection who are intolerant of or failing zidovudine, didanosine, and zalcitabine appear comparably effective in slowing disease progression although zalcitabine was associated with slightly prolonged survival.[289a] Simultaneous administration of zidovudine and didanosine appears to be associated with greater effects on CD4 counts and plasma viremia than zidovudine alone in patients with fewer than 400 CD4 cells/mm³ [290] or than sequential administration.[290a] A number of other comparative and combination trials are now in progress (ACTG 143, 175, 193). In patients deteriorating on zidovudine, some experts recommend the addition of didanosine, whereas others advocate substitution of didanosine.

FAMCICLOVIR (FAMVIR) AND PENCICLOVIR

Penciclovir (9-[4-hydroxy-3-hydroxymethylbut-1-yl] guanine) is an acyclic nucleoside analog (Fig. 1) similar to acyclovir in its spectrum of activity against herpesviruses (Table 2).[291–292] Famciclovir is the diacetyl ester prodrug of penciclovir and lacks antiviral activity. The inhibitory activity of penciclovir is cell type dependent.[292] Inhibitory concentrations of penciclovir are about twofold higher than those of acyclovir for HSV-1 and -2 in MRC-5 cells but comparably lower in WISH cells.[291–295] Because of its dependence on viral TK for initial phosphorylation, penciclovir is inactive against TK-deficient strains of HSV or VZV, but may be active against some TK-altered or polymerase mutants resistant to acyclovir.[60,293] Penciclovir is also inhibitory for HBV. Topical and parenteral penciclovir and oral famciclovir are active in experimental HSV infections.[295]

The antiviral activity of penciclovir relates to its selective phosphorylation in herpesvirus-infected cells and inhibition of viral DNA synthesis. In infected cells, penciclovir is preferentially phosphorylated to its active form, penciclovir triphosphate, which serves as a competitive inhibitor of viral DNA polymerase.[296] Unlike acyclovir, it is not an obligate chain terminator. Although penciclovir-triphosphate is approximately 100-fold less potent in inhibiting viral DNA polymerase than acyclovir triphosphate, it is present in much higher concentrations and for more prolonged periods in infected cells. The prolonged intracellular $T_{1/2}$ of penciclovir triphosphate, which ranges from 7 to 20 hours, is associated with a sustained antiviral effect in cell culture and in animal models.[295] This effect allows for infrequent dosing during clinical use. Resistant variants due to TK or DNA polymerase mutations can be selected by passage in vitro, but the occurrence of resistance during clinical use is currently undefined.

Famciclovir is well absorbed orally and rapidly converted to penciclovir by deacetylation and oxidation of the purine during and following absorption through the intestinal wall.[291] Although poorly absorbed itself, the bioavailability of penciclovir exceeds 70 percent following oral administration of famciclovir. After single 250 or 500 mg doses of oral famciclovir, the peak plasma concentration of penciclovir averages 1.9 and 3.5 μg/ml, respectively, in fasting subjects.[297] Food slows absorption and reduces peak plasma concentrations but does not significantly alter overall bioavailability. After intravenous infusion of penciclovir at 10 mg/kg, peak plasma levels average 12 μg/ml.[298] The plasma $T_{1/2elim}$ of penciclovir averages 2 hours, and approximately 70 percent is recovered unchanged in the urine.[298] Its rapid renal clearance suggests elimination by both filtration and active tubular secretion. Nonrenal clearance accounts for about 30 percent of dose, primarily by fecal excretion of penciclovir and its 6-deoxy precursor. In patients with moderately or severely reduced renal function, dose reduction is recommended (creatinine clearance 30–50 ml/min: q 12 hours; 5–29 ml/min: q 24 hours).

Oral famciclovir and topical and intravenous formulations of penciclovir are undergoing clinical trials in various herpes virus infections. Famciclovir is approved for treatment of herpes zoster in the United Kingdom but is investigational in the United States. Famciclovir is generally well tolerated but may be associated with headache and nausea. Randomized double-blind clinical trials involving immunocompetent adults with herpes zoster of 3 days duration or less have found that famciclovir at doses of 250, 500, or 750 mg three times daily is at least as effective as acyclovir 800 mg five times daily and superior to placebo in treating the acute signs and symptoms of zoster.[299,299a–c] In the two studies that followed patients for six months after therapy, famciclovir also significantly shortened chronic pain. Post-herpetic neuralgia, defined as pain persisting after healing of all zoster lesions, resolved 2 months faster in famciclovir patients and more than 3 months sooner in those aged 50 years or older compared with placebo.

FOSCARNET (PFA, FOSCAVIR)

Spectrum

Foscarnet (trisodium phosphonoformate) is an inorganic pyrophosphate analog (Fig. 4) that is inhibitory for all herpesviruses and HIV.[300,301] Depending on the test system, inhibitory concentrations vary widely among clinical isolates but are generally 100–300 μM for CMV and 80–200 μM for other HSV, VZV, and EBV. Foscarnet is inhibitory for most ganciclovir-resistant CMV and acyclovir-resistant HSV and VZV strains. Combinations of foscarnet and ganciclovir or acyclovir synergistically inhibit CMV infection in vitro.[302] Foscarnet also acts synergistically with zidovudine in inhibiting HIV replication.[303]

Concentrations of 500–1000 μM reversibly inhibit the proliferation and/or cellular DNA synthesis of uninfected cells. Foscarnet is active in animal models of herpesvirus and hepadnavirus infection.[300,301]

Mechanism of Action

Unlike nucleosides, foscarnet does not undergo significant intracellular metabolism and directly inhibits herpesvirus DNA poly-

merases or HIV reverse transcriptase. Foscarnet reversibly blocks the pyrophosphate binding site of the viral polymerase in a noncompetitive manner with respect to deoxynucleotide triphosphates (dNTP) and inhibits cleavage of pyrosphosphate from dNTP.[300,301,304] Concentrations that inhibit cell-free viral polymerases are many times lower than those required for inhibition of viral replication in cell culture, and cellular uptake is slow. Foscarnet's selectivity relates to approximately 100-fold greater inhibitory effects against herpesvirus DNA polymerases or HIV reverse transcriptase than cellular DNA polymerase-α.[304]

Resistance

DNA polymerase mutants of HSV and CMV resistant to foscarnet can be selected by passage in the presence of drug.[300,305] Instances in resistance in clinical isolates of HSV, VZV, and rarely CMV with three- to fivefold increases in inhibitory concentrations have been reported during therapeutic use,[55,306] and may be associated with poor responses to foscarnet treatment.[306a] Foscarnet-resistant HSV infections may respond to acyclovir[306a] or topical HPMPC.[56a]

Pharmacokinetics

Oral bioavailability is low and averages less than 20 percent.[307,308] Following an infusion of 60 mg/kg/8 h, peak and trough plasma concentrations range broadly but average approximately 450–575 and 80–150 μM, respectively. Peak concentrations are about 240–650 μM after doses of 90 mg/kg/day.[309] Plasma protein binding is about 15 percent. Cerebrospinal fluid concentrations vary between 13 and 68 percent of plasma but average 66 percent of plasma at steady state in CMV-infected patients.[307,310]

Foscarnet is eliminated by renal mechanisms, and more than 80 percent of the dose is excreted as unmetabolized drug by glomerular filtration and probably tubular secretion. Plasma clearance decreases proportionally with creatinine clearance, and dose adjustments are indicated for small decreases in renal function (Table 8). Plasma elimination is complex, with two initial $T_{1/2elim}$ totaling approximately 4–8 hours, and a prolonged terminal $T_{1/2elim}$ averaging as long as 88 hours. This appears to relate to bone deposition, and sequestration in bone accounts for an estimated 10–20 percent of a dose. Foscarnet is removed by hemodialysis, and plasma levels decrease by about 50 percent with a 3-hour run.[311] Dosing after dialysis is recommended.

Interactions

Administration of foscarnet with amphotericin B[312] and other nephrotoxic agents may cause enhanced renal toxicity (Table 7). The risk of symptomatic hypocalcemia is increased by concomitant intravenous pentamidine. Foscarnet and zidovudine do not affect each other's clearance,[313] but the risk of anemia appears higher with the combination.

Toxicity

Nephrotoxicity with azotemia, mild proteinuria, and possibly acute tubular necrosis is the major dose-limiting side effect.[301,314] Crystalluria and interstitial nephritis have also been described.[315,316] Increases in serum creatinine occur in up to one-half of patients, usually during the second week of therapy, but are reversible within 2–4 weeks of cessation in most patients. High doses, rapid or continuous infusion, dehydration, preexisting renal insufficiency, and concurrent nephrotoxic drugs are risk factors. Saline loading appears to reduce the risk of nephrotoxicity.[314]

Metabolic abnormalities are common and include both hypo- and hypercalcemia, hypo- and hyperphosphatemia, and hypoka-

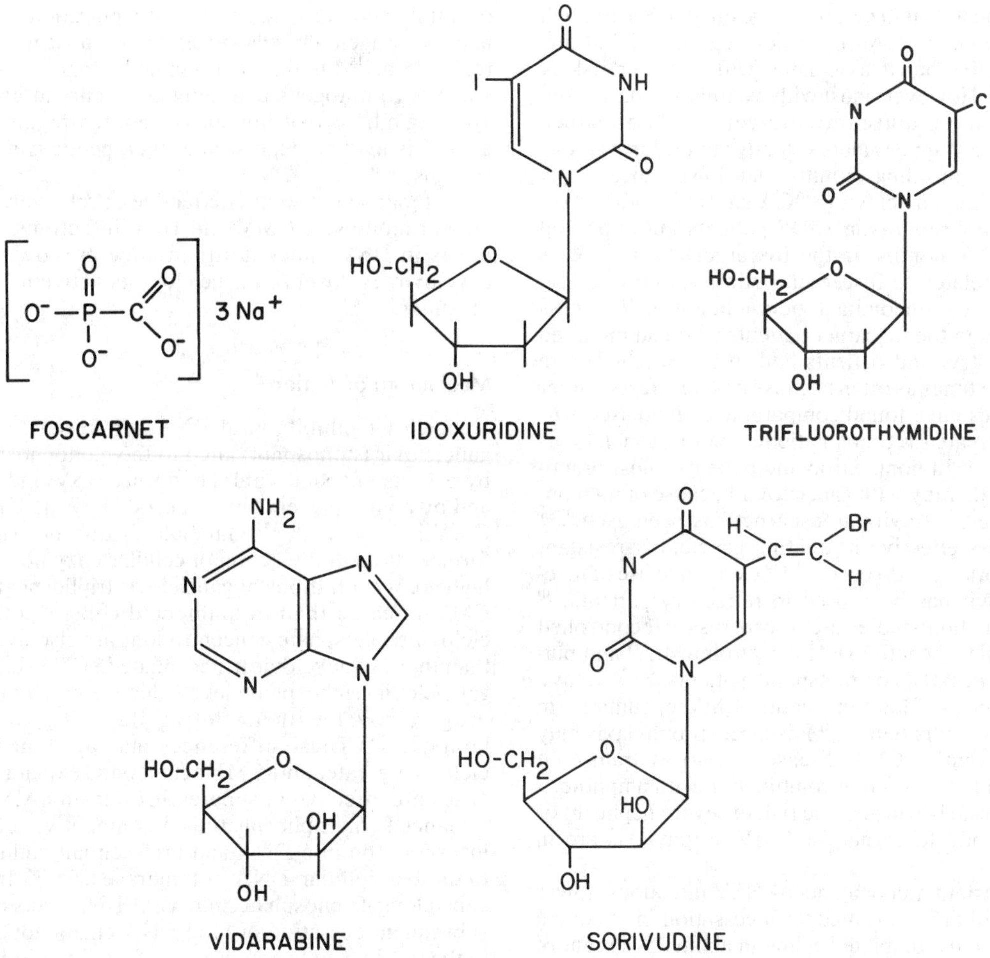

FIG. 4. Chemical structures of antiherpesvirus antiviral agents: foscarnet, idoxuridine, trifluorothymidine, vidarabine, and sorivudine.

TABLE 8. Foscarnet Dose Reduction in Renal Insufficiency

Creatinine Clearance (ml/min/kg)	Induction Dose[a] (mg/kg/8 h)	Maintenance Dose[a,b] (mg/kg/day)	
≥1.6	60	90	120
1.5	57	90	120
1.4	53	78	104
1.3	49	78	104
1.2	46	75	100
1.1	42	75	100
1.0	39	71	94
0.9	35	71	94
0.8	32	63	84
0.7	28	63	84
0.6	25	57	76
0.5	21	57	76
0.4	18	57	76

[a] Dosing based on manufacturer's recommendations. Optimal maintenance dose is under study.
[b] Dosing after hemodialysis (60 mg/kg) is suggested.[311]

lemia. Symptomatic hypocalcemia due to chelation and decreased serum ionized calcium may cause paresthesias, arrhythmias, tetany, seizures, and other CNS disturbances.[317] Intravenous foscarnet should be administered at a fixed rate (maximum of 1 mg/kg/min) by infusion pump to minimize the possibility of acute metabolic abnormalities. Renal function and electrolytes need to be monitored closely, and multiple dose adjustments are often required during induction therapy (Table 8).

Central nervous system side effects include headache in about one-fourth of patients, tremor, irritability, seizures in up to 10 percent, and hallucinosis. Other reported side effects are fever, gastrointestinal intolerance with nausea or emesis in 15–30 percent of patients, abnormal liver function tests, and painful genital ulcerations.[318] These ulcerations may be due to high urinary foscarnet concentrations; they usually resolve within weeks of stopping therapy but may recur upon rechallenge. Although anemia may develop in 20–50 percent of AIDS patients and granulocytopenia in a smaller fraction, foscarnet is less myelosuppressive than ganciclovir and can be used with zidovudine.

Preclinical studies indicate that high concentrations are mutagenic and that foscarnet may cause tooth and skeletal developmental anomalies in animals. Safety in pregnancy or childhood is uncertain. The drug is very expensive, with an estimated pharmacy cost exceeding $25,000 per year, or severalfold that of ganciclovir.

Clinical Studies

Intravenous foscarnet is approved for treatment of CMV retinitis in AIDS patients and is also effective in management of acyclovir-resistant HSV or VZV infections and ganciclovir-resistant CMV retinitis in immunocompromised patients.[319] In patients with non-sight-threatening CMV retinitis, foscarnet treatment plus maintenance significantly prolongs the time to progression of retinitis (approximately 13 weeks) compared with no treatment (approximately 3 weeks).[320] With the usual foscarnet regimen (60 mg/kg/8 h for 14–21 days followed by chronic maintenance at 90–120 mg/kg/day), about 90 percent of patients will experience clinical stabilization, and a smaller portion will cease CMV excretion.[301,309] An induction regimen of 100 mg/kg bid also is effective but is associated with a higher risk of penile ulceration.[323] However, most will eventually progress despite suppression and require retreatment.[323] Maintenance doses of 120 mg/kg/day appear more effective in prolonging survival and possibly controlling retinitis than lower doses.[323] A comparative trial with ganciclovir (SOCA study) found comparable control of CMV retinitis in AIDS patients but improved survival (8.5 vs. 12.6 months) in the foscarnet group.[324] This difference may be related to foscarnet's intrinsic antiretroviral effects[325,326] or greater concomitant zidovudine use.[324] Excess mortality was found in the foscarnet patients who had impaired renal function at entry, and patients had to be switched from foscarnet over three times as often because of side effects. Other retrospective studies have found comparable or increased survival in foscarnet-treated retinitis patients than in ganciclovir-treated patients.[327,328] In nonneutropenic patients, most practitioners still initiate therapy with ganciclovir because of its more predictable toxicities. Intravitreal foscarnet has been used.[328a]

Foscarnet appears effective in treating ganciclovir-resistant CMV retinitis and other syndromes.[319,329] Combined use of foscarnet and ganciclovir has been used in refractory patients,[330] and various combination studies are in progress. Uncontrolled studies suggest clinical benefit in CMV gastrointestinal and pulmonary infections in AIDS or transplant patients.[331,332] However, no clear benefit is found in treating CMV pneumonia in bone marrow transplant patients.[300] Foscarnet prophylaxis may be effective in preventing CMV disease in marrow transplant patients but should not be used in combination with amphotericin B and cyclosporine because of the risk of severe nephrotoxicity.[312] Studies of oral foscarnet for CMV prophylaxis are in progress.

In acylclovir-resistant mucocutaneous HSV infections, lower doses (40 mg/kg/8 h) are associated with cessation of shedding in 100 percent and with complete healing in about 75 percent of patients.[52,53] In contrast, vidarabine is ineffective in such patients. Other dose regimens (90 mg/kg/12 h) appear effective, and the optimal dosages for initial treatment and chronic suppression are under study.[333] Foscarnet also appears effective in acyclovir-resistant VZV infections in AIDS patients.[61] In recurrent orolabial or genital herpes infections of immunocompetent hosts, topically applied foscarnet is not associated with reproducible clinical benefits.[300,334]

In AIDS patients, foscarnet administration significantly reduces p24 antigen titers on a sustained basis, but beneficial effects on CD4 counts and clinical outcomes remain to be established.[326]

GANCICLOVIR (DHPG, CYTOVENE)

Spectrum

Ganciclovir (9-[1,3-dihydroxy-2-propoxymethyl] guanine), is a deoxyguanosine analog that differs from acyclovir in having an additional hydroxymethyl group on the acyclic side chain (Fig. 1). This agent has inhibitory activity against all herpesviruses (Table 2), but its unique characteristic is potent inhibition of CMV replication.[335–340] In vitro inhibitory concentrations are similar to those of acyclovir for HSV and VZV but 10- to over 50-fold lower for human CMV strains. Combinations of ganciclovir and foscarnet synergistically inhibit CMV replication in vitro.[302] Ganciclovir antagonizes the anti-HIV activity of didanosine and zidovudine in vitro,[341] and zidovudine variably inhibits the anti-CMV effects of ganciclovir,[342,343] but the clinical significance of these observations is unknown. Concentrations of less than 10 µg/ml also inhibit adenovirus replication in vitro,[344] and transient suppression of HBV viremia has been observed in patients.

Although high concentrations are needed to inhibit the growth

of uninfected cells, inhibitory concentrations for human bone marrow progenitor cells are similar to those inhibitory for CMV replication.[345] Inhibition of human lymphocyte proliferative responses to mitogens and antigens occurs at concentrations of 1–10 µg/ml, so that immune responses requiring active DNA synthesis may be depressed at therapeutic ganciclovir concentrations.[3,346]

Systemic ganciclovir is effective at relatively low dosages in animal models of CMV and HSV infections.[347,348] Effective doses in HSV encephalitis in mice are lower than those of acyclovir. Aerosolized ganciclovir is active in models of CMV pneumonia.[349]

Mechanism of Action

Ganciclovir inhibits viral DNA synthesis.[335,337] Intracellular ganciclovir is phosphorylated to the monophosphate derivative by a virus-encoded viral TK during HSV and VZV infection, and by a viral protein kinase encoded by the UL97 gene during CMV infection.[350–352] Ganciclovir di- and triphosphates are formed through the action of cellular enzymes. At least 10-fold higher concentrations of ganciclovir triphosphate are present in CMV-infected than in uninfected cells.[339] Intracellular ganciclovir triphosphate concentrations are also over 10-fold higher than those of acyclovir triphosphate in CMV-infected cells, and ganciclovir triphosphate levels decline much more slowly after drug removal with an intracellular $T_{1/2elim}$ exceeding 24 hours.[350,353] These differences may account in part for ganciclovir's greater anti-CMV activity and explain how single daily doses are effective in suppressing human CMV infections.

Ganciclovir triphosphate is a competitive inhibitor of dGPT incorporation into DNA and preferentially inhibits viral rather than host cellular DNA polymerases.[354,355] Incorporation of ganciclovir-triphosphate into viral DNA causes a slowing and subsequent cessation of viral DNA chain elongation.[356] Owing to the two hydroxyl groups on the acyclic side chain, ganciclovir is incorporated into both host cell and viral DNA.[354]

Resistance

Resistance in CMV isolates, often defined by inhibitory concentrations above 3 µg/ml in vitro, has been related to two mechanisms: reduced intracellular ganciclovir phosphorylation due to alteration in a viral enzyme encoded by the UL97 gene[351,352] and point mutations in viral DNA polymerase leading to partial resistance to ganciclovir.[357] Resistant clinical isolates with 4- to 20-fold increases in inhibitory concentrations have been associated with impaired phosphorylation,[358] but some may have DNA polymerase mutations.[359]

Ganciclovir resistance has been recognized clinically by progressive disease and persistent CMV recovery despite therapy.[319,360–362] Viral shedding during ganciclovir therapy has also been found with susceptible virus. One survey found that 8 percent of 72 AIDS patients had progressive disease and shed resistant CMV after at least 3 months of continuous ganciclovir therapy; 38 percent of those shedding virus after 3 months had resistant isolates.[361] The susceptibility of strains recovered before and after therapy in transplant patients is generally unchanged, although instances of emergence of resistance have been described.[329,363,364] The pathogenicity and transmissibility of ganciclovir-resistant CMV strains is undefined, but patients excreting such strains can have progressive disease. Polyradiculopathy associated with CSF isolation of resistant CMV has been described.[365] Foscarnet therapy may benefit patients with ganciclovir-resistant CMV infections.[319,329,362]

Ganciclovir is over 40-fold less active against acyclovir-resistant, TK-deficient HSV strains.[336,337] HSV strains resistant to ganciclovir because of DNA polymerase mutation have been demonstrated in the laboratory, although some HSV strains re-

TABLE 9. Ganciclovir Dose Adjustments in Renal Insufficiency

Creatinine Clearance (ml/min/1.73 m²)	Dose (mg/kg)[a]	Dosing Interval (h)
≥80	5	12
50–79	2.5	12
25–49	2.5	24
<25[b]	1.25	24

[a] The optimal maintenance dose in renal impairment is not known, but proportionate reductions in total dose are recommended. Doses are based on manufacturer's recommendations.
[b] A maximum dose of 1.25 mg/kg/day is suggested for persons on hemodialysis. Dosing should be done after completion of dialysis.

sistant to acyclovir because of DNA polymerase mutations retain sensitivity to ganciclovir.[355]

Pharmacokinetics

The oral bioavailability of ganciclovir is low (<10 percent).[366] Peak and 6-hour trough steady-state plasma levels average about 1.0 and 0.5 µg/ml, respectively, on an oral regimen of 1000 mg/6 hours, which suggests that oral treatment may be feasible. Subcutaneous and intramuscular administration are too irritating for clinical use. Following intravenous administration of 5 mg/kg doses, peak and trough plasma concentrations average 8–11 and 0.6–1.2 µg/ml, respectively.[335,367,368]

Plasma protein binding is only 1–2 percent. Following intravenous dosing, aqueous and subretinal fluid levels are similar to those in serum but intravitreal concentrations average only about 1.0 µg/ml.[369–371] Cerebrospinal fluid levels are 24–70 percent and brain tissue 38 percent of those in plasma.[368,372]

The plasma $T_{1/2elim}$ averages 2–4 hours in patients with normal renal function, but increases almost linearly as creatinine clearance declines.[335] Plasma $T_{1/2elim}$ may increase to 28–40 hours in those with severe renal insufficiency (serum creatinine >4.5).[373] Most ganciclovir is eliminated unmetabolized by renal excretion (>90 percent of dose) by both glomerular filtration and tubular secretion. Dose reductions are necessary in patients with a creatinine clearance of less than 80 ml/min (Table 9). A hemodialysis run reduces the plasma levels of ganciclovir by approximately 50–60 percent, and dosing after dialysis is recommended.[373,374]

Interactions

Zidovudine[375,376] and probably other cytotoxic agents increase the risk of ganciclovir-induced myelosuppression, as do nephrotoxic agents that impair ganciclovir excretion (Table 7). Probenicid and possibly acyclovir reduce renal clearance of ganciclovir. In animals, zidovudine but not amphotericin B, ketoconazole, dapsone, or TMP-sulpha antagonizes the anti-CMV effects of ganciclovir.[342,377] Increases in serum creatinine may occur in patients treated with ganciclovir and either cyclosporine or amphotericin B, and ganciclovir may increase cyclosporine levels.

Toxicity

Myelosuppression is the principal dose-limiting toxicity of ganciclovir. The most common adverse events are neutropenia (<1000 cells/mm³) occurring in about 40 percent of patients and thrombocytopenia (<50,000 platelets/mm³) in up to 20 percent.[335,367] The risk of these toxicities is substantially lower in transplant than AIDS patients. Neutropenia is most commonly observed during the second week of treatment and is reversible in most patients within 1 week of drug cessation, although persistent neutropenia complicated by fatal infections has been reported. Frequent monitoring of blood counts for leukopenia is necessary to adjust doses, and treatment should be temporarily discontinued if the absolute neutrophil count falls below 500 cells/mm³. Recombinant granulocyte/macrophage colony-stim-

ulating factor (GM-CSF) may be useful in treating ganciclovir-induced neutropenia.[378]

CNS side effects including headache, behavioral changes with confusion or psychosis, and rarely convulsions or coma have been described in about 5 percent of patients. About one-third of patients receiving ganciclovir treatment have had to interrupt or prematurely stop therapy because of adverse events. In addition, two to fourfold higher rates of azotemia occur in transplant recipients receiving ganciclovir prophylaxis.[379]

Anemia, rash, fever, liver function test abnormalities, nausea or vomiting, and eosinophilia have also been reported. Phlebitis at the infusion site may be due to the alkalinicity (pH 11) of the solution. In the event of massive overdosage, hemodialysis and hydration may be effective in reducing plasma ganciclovir levels.

Ganciclovir is mutagenic, carcinogenic and immunosuppressive and causes irreversible reproductive toxicity in animals and possibly humans.[335] Teratogenicity, embryotoxicity, testicular atrophy, and bone marrow hypocellularity have been observed in animals at ganciclovir dosages comparable with those used in humans.

Clinical Studies

Ganciclovir is currently approved in the United States for treatment and chronic suppression of CMV retinitis in immunocompromised patients and prevention of CMV disease in transplant patients. Because of its toxicity, ganciclovir use has been limited to patients at risk for or with life- or sight-threatening CMV infections. With initial or induction treatment doses of 5 mg/kg/12 h for 10–21 days, about 85 percent of CMV retinitis patients improve or stabilize their disease.[335,380–385] Ganciclovir is comparable with foscarnet in initial control of retinitis.[324] Fundoscopic improvement is usually evident by 10–14 days. Historical controls indicate that over 90 percent of untreated AIDS patients will have progressive retinal disease leading to blindness, whereas retinitis in transplant patients may resolve spontaneously with reduction in immunosuppression. Approximately 90 percent of treated patients have a conversion of urine, blood, and throat cultures to negative or greater than 100-fold reductions in viral titers in 7–15 days.

Among AIDS patients who respond to initial ganciclovir treatment, almost all will relapse within weeks without suppressive therapy.[367,382,385] High doses of ganciclovir (30 to 35 mg/kg/week), but not low doses (10 to 20 mg/kg/week), are effective for chronic suppression and increase the proportion of subjects free of relapse at 120 days to nearly 60 percent. However, relapse rates are high in AIDS patients despite the use of chronic suppression. Retinal detachments are common during long-term follow-up.[385] Combination of ganciclovir and foscarnet may be effective in patients failing single-agent therapy.[330]

Clinical improvement and virologic responses are also found in CMV pneumonia and gastrointestinal infections in AIDS patients and solid organ transplant recipients.[367,382,385,387–389] Variable responses have been described in CNS syndromes.[367,390] In biopsy-proven CMV colitis in AIDS patients, ganciclovir (5 mg/kg/12 h for 14 days) is associated with significant antiviral effects, improvement in colonoscopy scores, stabilization of weight loss, and lower incidence of extracolonic CMV disease but no differences in symptoms compared with placebo.[391] The value of longer duration therapy remains to be determined. In bone marrow transplant recipients, virologic responses but no reduction in mortality occurs in patients with biopsy-proven CMV pneumonia treated with ganciclovir alone[372] or in combination with corticosteroids.[392] In contrast, ganciclovir combined with intravenous immunoglobulin or CMV immunoglobulin reduces mortality of CMV pneumonia in bone marrow transplant patients from 80–90 percent to 30–50 percent.[393,394] No significant clinical benefit is found in gastrointestinal infection of marrow transplant recipients with ganciclovir monotherapy.[395] Usefulness in congenital CMV disease also remains to be established.

Ganciclovir prophylaxis appears effective and reasonably well-tolerated in preventing CMV disease in bone marrow transplant recipients shedding CMV[396,397] and in seropositive solid organ transplant recipients.[379] Initiation of ganciclovir treatment (5 mg/kg/12 h for 7–14 days followed by 5 mg/kg/day) when CMV is isolated from bronchoalveolar lavage[396] or from other body sites,[397] and continuing ganciclovir to days 100–120 post-transplant, is highly effective in preventing the development of CMV pneumonia and appears to reduce mortality in bone marrow transplant patients. In seropositive bone marrow transplant patients, initiation of ganciclovir at the time of engraftment also markedly reduces CMV shedding and disease rates but does not improve survival, in part because of neutropenia-related infections.[398,399] Such regimens are associated with drug-related neutropenia in 30–35 percent of patients.

Ganciclovir administration for 1 month post-transplantation suppresses CMV excretion and reduces the risk of CMV disease in seropositive allograft recipients following heart, lung, or liver transplantation.[5,168,379,400] However, an effective regimen for prevention of primary CMV disease in seronegative recipients of tissues from seropositive donors remains to be identified. More prolonged administration may provide protection against late-onset CMV disease.[401] When ganciclovir is administered preemptively during antilymphocyte antibody treatment for periods up to 2 weeks, the incidence of CMV disease is reduced over threefold in seropositive renal or liver allograft recipients.[402,403] Ganciclovir prophylaxis is also effective in preventing herpes simplex virus excretion[399] and results in clearance of EBV from oropharyngeal secretions, although a rapid rebound in excretion occurs after cessation.[404] Efficacy of ganciclovir in treatment or prevention of EBV-associated post-transplant lymphoproliferative disease remains to be established.

Intravitreal ganciclovir has been used in limited studies for treating CMV retinitis in patients who are unable to tolerate systemic ganciclovir.[405] The efficacy of oral ganciclovir for CMV prophylaxis or suppression and of ganciclovir-foscarnet combinations for treatment are under study. Prodrugs of ganciclovir with enhanced bioavailability are also under development (e.g., BMS 180194).

IDOXURIDINE (IDU, IUDR, STOXIL, HERPLEX, DENDRID)

Idoxuridine (5-iodo-2′-deoxyuridine) is an iodinated thymidine analog (Fig. 4) that inhibits the in vitro replication of various DNA viruses, particularly herpesviruses and poxviruses.[406] Plaque production by most clinical isolates of HSV-1 is inhibited by concentrations of 2–10 µg/ml. Idoxuridine's antiviral mechanism of action is not completely defined, but the phosphorylated derivatives interfere with various enzyme systems. The triphosphate inhibits viral DNA synthesis and is incorporated into both viral and cellular DNA. Resistance to idoxuridine readily develops under laboratory conditions[407] and occurs in viral isolates recovered from idoxuridine-treated patients with HSV keratitis.

In humans, intravenously administered idoxuridine is rapidly metabolized to iodouracil and uracil. Extremely low plasma concentrations of idoxuridine (0.1–0.4 ppm) are detected in about one-half of patients treated topically with 40 percent idoxuridine in the penetration-enhancing agent dimethylsulfoxide (DMSO). Intravenous idoxuridine is ineffective and toxic in patients with HSV encephalitis. Side effects include liver function abnormalities and serious bone marrow toxicity, and parenteral idoxuridine is no longer considered to be a useful antiviral agent. Idoxuridine is also teratogenic, mutagenic, tumor promoting, and immunosuppressive in preclinical testing. DMSO is teratogenic and can cause adverse ocular effects in laboratory animals.

The therapeutic usefulness of topically applied idoxuridine depends on the site of infection and the vehicle of administration. In the United States, idoxuridine is approved only for topical treatment of HSV keratitis, whereas idoxuridine in DMSO is available in Europe for treatment of herpes labialis, genitalis, and zoster. In ocular HSV infections, topical idoxuridine is more effective in epithelial infections, especially initial episodes, than in stromal infections.[408,409] Adverse reactions include pain, pruritus, inflammation, or edema involving the eye or lids and rarely allergic reactions.

Idoxuridine alone is ineffective in recurrent herpes labialis, varicella, or herpes zoster, whereas frequent topical application of 5–40 percent idoxuridine dissolved in DMSO appears to hasten healing and shorten pain duration in localized herpes zoster. Topical 30 percent idoxuridine in DMSO may shorten the duration of viral shedding in recurrent or primary genital HSV infections, but does not reduce the duration of symptoms or healing time.[410] Topical 15 percent idoxuridine in DMSO reduces the duration of pain and healing time in recurrent herpes labialis, especially in those initiating treatment during the prodrome or early erythema stage.[411] Mild local burning and after-taste are common after topical application of DMSO, and headache, dizziness, sedation, nausea, and localized and generalized dermatitis have also been reported.

INTERFERONS

Classification

Since their discovery in 1957 as mediators of the phenomenon of viral interference, that is, inhibition of growth of one virus by another, interferons (IFN) have become recognized as potent cytokines that are associated with complex antiviral, immunomodulating, and antiproliferative actions.[412] IFN are proteins that are synthesized by eukaryotic cells in response to various inducers and that in turn cause biochemical changes leading to an antiviral state in exposed cells of the same species. Formally designated on the basis of the cell types from which they were derived, three major classes of human interferons are currently recognized (Table 10). Each type is immunologically distinct, has different principal producer cells and biologic effects, as well as unique physicochemical characteristics.[412,413]

IFN-α and -β may be produced by nearly all cells in response to viral infection and a variety of other stimuli, including double-stranded RNA, bacteria, protozoa, mycoplasma, polyanions, several low-molecular-weight organic compounds, and certain cytokines and growth factors (e.g., IL-1, IL-2, and tumor necrosis factor [TNF]). IFN-γ production is restricted to antigenic stimuli, mitogens, and certain cytokines like IL-2. The principal antiviral interferons, IFN-α and -β, are approximately 30 percent homologous at the amino acid level. Human IFN-αs are actually a family of multiple species that share a high degree of amino acid sequence homology (>70 percent) but have differing in vitro antiviral and biologic effects on human cells.[414] Compared with IFN-α/β, IFN-γ has less specific antiviral activity but more potent immunoregulatory effects, particularly with respect to macrophage activation, expression of class II major histocompatibility complex (MHC) antigens, and mediation of local inflammatory responses. IFN in clinical use include those produced by recombinant DNA techniques and native ones purified from stimulated leukocytes or other cells (Table 10).

Mechanisms of Action

A wide range of animal viruses are sensitive to the antiviral actions of IFN, although many DNA viruses are relatively insensitive and considerable differences in potency exist among different viruses and assay systems.[415] Synergistic antiviral effects have been seen with combinations of IFN-α or -β and IFN-γ, various synthetic antivirals, and TNF.[416] Complex interactions occur with other cytokines.[417,418] IFN activity is usually

TABLE 10. Nomenclature and Classification of Human Interferons

	Class		
	α	β	γ
Former designations	Type I, leukocyte	Type I, fibroblast	Type II, immune
No. species	>24	1[a]	1
No. amino acids	165–172	166	143
Apparent MW[b] (kD)	16–27.6	20–23	15.5–25
Disulphide bonds	2	1	0
Glycosylation	Variable[c]	Yes	Yes
Acid stability (pH 2)	Stable[d]	Stable	Labile
Chromosome coding for IFN	9	9	12
Chromosome coding for receptor	21	21	6
Commercial formulations	r-IFN-α-2b	r-IFN-β1b	r-IFN-γ1b
	(Intron A)[e]	(Betaseron)	(Actimmune)[e]
	r-IFN-α2a		r-IFN-γ
	(Roferon A)[e]		(Immunoeron)
	Le-IFN-αn3		
	(Alferon N)[e]		
	Ly-IFN-αn1		
	(Wellferon)		

Abbreviations: r: recombinant; Le: leukocyte derived; Ly: lymphoblastoid cell-derived.
[a] Interleukin-6 (also designatged IFN-β2) has negligible antiviral effects and functions primarily as a β-cell differentiation factor (BSF-2). It has minimal sequence homology with classical IFN-β and is encoded by a different chromosome (12).
[b] Range of molecular weight (MW) relates to post-translation modifications including formation of dimers, glycosylation, protein binding. Molecular weight of nonglycosylated recombinant IFN-α is approximately 19.5 kD.
[c] Generally not, but several minor species are glycosylated.
[d] Acid-labile IFN-α have been described in certain pathologic states, including HIV infection, systemic lupus erythematosus, rheumatoid arthritis, pemphigus.
[e] Currently approved for use in the United States (3/94).
(Data from Zoon[413] and Greenberg.[415])

measured in terms of antiviral effects in cell culture. Typically, one unit of IFN activity is the amount present in a sample dilution that causes a 50 percent reduction in virus replication or expression in certain cell lines and is generally expressed as international units (IU) relative to NIH or WHO reference standards.

IFN are not directly antiviral but cause elaboration of effector proteins in exposed cells, which contribute to a state of viral resistance.[419–421] The initial step involves IFN binding to specific cell surface receptors, which are shared between IFN-α and -β but are different for IFN-γ. The onset of IFN antiviral action occurs in hours and increases in gene transcription occur within minutes. IFN exposure leads to production of over two dozen cellular proteins, some of which appear specifically to inhibit different virus families. Depending on the virus and cell type, IFNs' antiviral effects are mediated through inhibition of viral penetration or uncoating, synthesis or methylation of messenger RNA, translation of viral proteins, and/or of viral assembly and release.

Among IFN-induced proteins are 2'–5' oligoadenylate (2–5[A]) synthetase and a protein kinase, which can inhibit viral protein synthesis in the presence of double-stranded RNA. The 2–5(A) synthetase produces adenylate oligomers that activate a latent cellular endoribonuclease (Rnase L) to cleave both cellular and viral RNAs. Elevated levels of 2–5(A) activity in peripheral white blood cells are also used as a marker for IFN exposure or endogenous release. The protein kinase selectively phosphorylates and inactivates a protein involved in protein synthesis, eukaryotic initiation factor (eIF-2). Interferon may also block mRNA capping by inhibiting transmethylation reactions. IFN induction of a phosphodiesterase, which cleaves a portion of transfer RNA and thus prevents peptide elongation,

also contributes to the inhibition of protein synthesis. Induction of nitric oxide synthase appears to mediate a substantial antiviral effect of interferon-gamma.[422]

However, except possibly for the Mx proteins and influenza viruses and for 2–5(A) synthetase/RNase L and picornaviruses, no consistent correlations exist between induction of a particular enzyme and resistance to specific viruses across a range of cell types.[419–421] A particular virus may be inhibited at several steps, and the principal inhibitory effect for a specific virus differs among virus families. For example, IFN inhibition of HIV-1 replication has been related to decreased proviral DNA formation, 2–5(A) synthetase expression, antagonism of Rev function, and decreased release of infectious particles.[11–13] In addition, certain viruses are able to counter IFN effects by blocking production or activity of selected IFN-inducible proteins.[419–421] IFN exposure may also reduce the expression of certain cellular genes, including selected oncogenes and those involved in collagen synthesis.

Complex interactions exist between IFN and other parts of the immune system.[417,418] For example, IFN-γ enhances the expression of IL-2 receptors on T lymphocytes, and IL-2 modulates IFN-γ production. The induction of cytotoxic T-lymphocyte responses appears to require both IL-2 and IFN-γ. IFN-α is both produced by macrophages and can modify macrophage functions, increasing phagocytosis and cytolytic activity. The effects of IFN include inhibiting delayed-type hypersensitivity responses and lymphocyte blastogenesis and prolonging survival of allogeneic grafts; increasing production of proinflammatory cytokines; enhancing (low-concentration) or suppressing (high-concentration) antibody formation; increasing NK cell activity and antibody-dependent cellular cytotoxicity; enhancing phagocytic and cytolytic activity of macrophages; inhibiting macrophage migration; increasing the expression of MHC antigens on cell surfaces; inhibiting the growth of intracellular parasites; augmenting IgE-mediated histamine release; increasing the expression of Fc receptors on lymphocytes and accessory cells; interfering with attachment of hormones and certain toxins to ganglioside receptors on the cell membrane; inhibiting growth of rapidly dividing cells; and enhancing differentiation (low concentrations) or inhibiting differentiation (high concentrations) of cells.

Thus, IFN may ameliorate viral infections by exerting direct antiviral effects and by modifying the immune response to infection. For example, IFN-induced expression of MHC antigens may contribute to the antiviral actions of IFN by enhancing the lytic effects of cytotoxic T lymphocytes. IFN generally appears at the sites of viral replication just after peak titers of virus and before humoral antibody responses. In contrast to resolution of viral infection, IFN may mediate some of the systemic symptoms associated with viral infections and contribute to immunologically mediated tissue damage in certain viral diseases.[426] High IFN titers are usually followed by a reduction of virus titers, although persistently elevated IFN titers have been recognized in certain chronic and acute (e.g., hemorrhagic fevers) viral infections.

Pharmacokinetics

The prolonged biologic effects of IFN are not easily related to serum concentrations or other conventional pharmacokinetic parameters. After intramuscular or subcutaneous injection of IFN-α, absorption exceeds 80 percent.[427] Plasma levels are dose related, peaking at 4–8 hours and returning to baseline by 18–36 hours. Levels of 2–5(A) synthetase in PBMC, which have been used as an index of biologic responsiveness to IFN, show increases beginning at 6 hours and lasting through 4 days after a single dose.[428] An antiviral state in the same cell is detectable at 1 hour, peaks at 24 hours, and slowly decreases to baseline by 6 days after injection. Neopterin and β2-microglobulin levels also increase in the blood for several days. Absorption of IFN-γ is more variable, and intramuscular or subcutaneous injections of IFN-β result in negligible plasma levels, although increases in 2–5(A) synthetase levels may occur. Oral administration does not result in detectable serum IFN levels or increases in 2–5(A) synthetase activity in PBMC.[429]

After systemic administration, low levels of IFN are detected in respiratory secretions, cerebrospinal fluid, eye, and brain.[415] Following intravenous dosing, cerebrospinal fluid levels average less than 1 percent of serum.[430] IFN-α is relatively stable in most body fluids, whereas IFN-β and -γ appear to lose activity readily. However, it is unknown whether measurable IFN levels at a particular site accurately reflect its antiviral or other biologic activities.

After intravenous dosing, both IFN-α and -β are cleared rapidly in a complex fashion.[431] Leukocyte and recombinant IFN-α species have a plasma $T_{1/2elim}$ of approximately 2–4 hours. The clearance of IFN includes inactivation by various body fluids, cellular uptake, and metabolism by different organs, primarily the kidney and to some extent the liver, heart, skeletal muscle, and lung. Negligible biologically active IFN is excreted in the urine.

Interactions

IFN and its inducers reduce the metabolism of various drugs by the hepatic cytochrome P-450-dependent mixed-function oxidase system and significantly increase plasma $T_{1/2}$ and levels of drugs like theophylline. IFN can increase the bone marrow toxicity of myelotoxic drugs like zidovudine.

Toxicity

Both purified natural and recombinant IFN are associated with dose-related immediate and late-onset toxicities.[432,433] Intramuscular and subcutaneous injection of IFN doses of 1–2 MU and above are usually associated with an acute influenzalike syndrome including fever, chills, headache, myalgia, arthralgia, nausea, vomiting, and diarrhea, especially during the first week of therapy. Symptoms begin several hours after administration, and fever may range over 40°C but usually resolves within 12 hours. Tolerance gradually develops in most patients. Febrile responses are mediated through production of hypothalamic prostaglandins and can be moderated by pretreatment with various antipyretics.

Major toxicities that limit parenteral therapy are bone marrow suppression with granulocytopenia and thrombocytopenia; neurotoxicity manifested by somnolence, confusion, behavioral disturbance, EEG changes, and rarely seizures and coma[434]; reversible neurasthenia with profound fatigue and anorexia, weight loss, and myalgia during long-term use; thyroid dysfunction and autoimmune thyroiditis; and cardiotoxicity with hypotension, arrhythmias, and reversible cardiomyopathy.[435] Psychiatric disturbance and depression are more common in those with preexisting disorders. Elevations in hepatic enzymes and triglyceride levels are common; alopecia, proteinuria, renal insufficiency, interstitial nephritis, autoantibody formation, and hepatotoxicity occur. IFN prophylaxis has been associated with severe leukoencephalopathy in bone marrow transplant recipients[436] and with acute rejection and nephrotic syndrome in kidney transplant recipients.

Up to one-half of patients receiving intralesional therapy for genital warts experience the influenzal illness, although symptoms usually decrease during the first week of therapy. Intralesional IFN may cause discomfort at the injection site and leukopenia. Local reactions consisting of tenderness and erythema also occur after subcutaneous injection. Intranasal administration is associated with mucosal friability and ulceration and complaints of nasal dryness, stuffiness, and bleeding in up to 50 percent of recipients, depending on the dose and duration of administration.[437]

The development of serum neutralizing antibodies to exogenous IFN varies with the IFN type, dose, disease, and route of administration, but may be more common with IFN-α2a.[438] Neutralizing antibodies may be associated infrequently with loss of clinical responsiveness. Those directed against recombinant IFN-α may cross-react with natural IFN-α or other recombinant species, and patients with antibodies against one recombinant IFN-α subtype may respond to natural IFN-α.

IFN may impair fertility and alter hormone levels in females. IFN is an abortifacient in monkeys at high doses, and safety during human pregnancy is not established.

Clinical Studies

Clinical use of IFN has been limited by relative lack of potency, dose-limiting side effects, and availability of competing antiviral agents. Depending on the IFN type, recombinant and natural IFN-α (Table 10) are approved in the United States currently for treatment of condyloma acuminatum, chronic hepatitis C, chronic hepatitis B, Kaposi sarcoma in HIV-infected patients, and/or other malignancies. Recombinant IFN-γ is available for management of chronic granulomatous disease, IFN-β has been approved for multiple sclerosis, and other IFNs are under investigation.

Hepatitis Viruses.   Chronic hepatitis B virus (HBV) infections are associated with deficient IFN production and often decreased responsiveness to IFN. HBV polymerase is able to inhibit cellular responses to IFN-α and -γ in vitro.[439] In patients with chronic hepatitis B, parenteral administration of various IFN is associated with loss of HBV DNA, loss of Hbe antigen and development of anti-Hbe antibody, and biochemical and histologic improvement in about 25–50 percent of patients.[440–446] Lasting responses require moderately high IFN doses and prolonged administration (~5 MU/day or 10 MU three times weekly for 4–6 months). Plasma HBV DNA and polymerase activity decline promptly in most patients, but complete disappearance often requires months of therapy and is sustained in about 30–50 percent. Responses with seroconversion to anti-Hbe are usually associated with a transaminase elevations and often a hepatitislike illness during the second or third month of therapy, presumably related to immune clearance of infected hepatocytes.[440] An increased risk of clinical deterioration exists in patients with poor or decreasing hepatic synthetic function, and lower doses have been suggested for such patients. Factors associated with reduced response rates include high plasma HBV DNA levels (>200 pg/ml), long-standing infection, Asian ethnicity, male gender, low transaminase levels (<2 ULN), chronic persistent hepatitis, immunosuppressive therapy, and HIV infection.

Remissions in chronic hepatitis B induced by IFN are sustained in over 80 percent of patients and are frequently followed by loss of Hbs antigen, histologic improvement or stabilization, and disappearance of plasma HBV DNA and HBV replicative forms in the liver.[447–449] Patients with preexisting anti-HBe may have higher relapse rates.[446,450] IFN-γ is less effective than IFN-α/β, and combinations do not appear to enhance antiviral effects.[451–453] Despite possible short-term enhancement of antiviral effects by combinations of systemic IFN-α with vidarabine, acyclovir, or corticosteroid pretreatment, no dual therapies have yet emerged that provide long-term benefit or reductions in toxicity.[176,177,442,443,454]

IFN may benefit HBV-associated nephrotic syndrome and glomerulonephritis in some patients.[455–457] Antiviral effects and improvements occur in about one-half of chronic hepatitis D virus (HDV) infections,[458] but relapse is common unless Hbs antigen disappears. Long-term treatment (12 months or longer) at doses used for chronic HBV may result in sustained improvement.[442] IFN does not appear beneficial in acute HBV or HDV infections.

In chronic hepatitis C virus infection, subcutaneous IFN-α2b (3 MU three times weekly for 6 months) is associated with an approximate 50 percent rate of biochemical normalization and improvement in liver histopathology.[442] Doses of 1 MU are less effective. Response is associated with loss of detectable serum HCV RNA in 80 percent or more of patients.[463,464] However, at least 50 percent of responding patients have virologic and biochemical relapse 1–2 months after treatment is stopped. A majority respond to retreatment. Reappearance of HCV RNA without biochemical relapse occurs in some patients. Higher doses (6 MU three times weekly) and more prolonged treatment (up to 12 months) may increase sustained response rates.[465] IFN treatment may benefit hepatitis C virus (HCV)–associated cryoglobulinemia and glomerulonephritis.[466,466a]

No reliable clinical predictors of response to IFN have been identified in chronic hepatitis C. Sustained responders have lower pretreatment serum viral titers than nonresponders or those with biochemical relapse.[467] Persistence of HCV RNA occurs in most nonresponders, and virologic relapse occurs in those with sustained biochemical response.[468] Decreases in transaminase levels occur faster than in chronic hepatitis B, and patients who do not respond to IFN within 3 months do not benefit from continued therapy. Safety and efficacy remain to be established in uncompensated liver disease. IFN administration during acute hepatitis C infection may reduce the risk of chronicity[469]; treatment has been suggested for patients with transaminase levels remaining elevated more than 2 months.[442] Patients with autoimmune chronic hepatitis, who may have false-positive EIA tests for anti-HCV antibodies, can worsen if treated with IFN.[470]

Herpesviruses. Although associated with antiviral effects, no consistent reductions in symptoms and lesion duration have been observed with topical or systemic IFN treatment of genital herpes.[415,471–477] Parenteral IFN is frequently associated with systemic side effects and is no better than topical acyclovir in initial genital HSV.[477] It is also less effective than oral acyclovir for treatment or suppression of recurrent genital herpes.[471] Topical application of IFN-α in several formulations modestly reduces viral shedding and symptom duration in recurrent genital herpes.[474–476] Topically applied IFN appears to have some activity in combination with trifluridine in drug-resistant mucocutaneous HSV infections.[56] In superficial HSV keratitis, combined administration of topical IFN-α with trifluridine or acyclovir appears to be more effective than single-agent therapy.[415]

In localized herpes zoster of cancer patients, early treatment with high-dose IFN-α (approximately 36 MU/day for 5–7 days) reduces the risk of cutaneous or visceral dissemination and possibly the severity of postherpetic neuralgia.[478] Lower doses or shorter duration of therapy is less effective, and systemic reactions are frequent. In older adults with acute herpes zoster, treatment with intramuscular IFN-α, 10 MU/day, is similar to intravenous acyclovir in lesion and symptom resolution but associated with more side effects.[479] Prolonged IFN administration reduces the risk of CMV viremia but not HSV shedding in seropositive renal allograft recipients and is not effective in preventing CMV infection or improving survival in bone marrow recipients.[436] IFN is also ineffective in treating CMV pneumonia.

Human Immunodeficiency Virus. HIV-infected patients frequently have detectable IFN levels, and plasma inhibitors of IFN activity are often present during AIDS.[480,481] IFN-α and -γ inhibit HIV replication in vitro, and synergistic inhibition occurs in combination with zidovudine and other antiretroviral agents. High doses of IFN-α induce 10–40 percent response rates in Kaposi sarcoma patients without benefiting concurrent herpes virus infections or immune functions.[482] In HIV infections, IFN treatment has been associated with dose-related antiretroviral effects, particularly in early-stage infection, but also with significant adverse effects.[483] When combined with zidovudine in more advanced infection, only transient antiviral effects without improvements in CD4 counts and excess hematologic toxicity are found.[484–486] Combination studies with various nucleoside reverse transcriptase inhibitors are in progress. Reports that low-dose oral IFN delays progression in HIV infection have not been substantiated.[487] In vitro resistance to IFN has been described in HIV isolates.[488]

Papillomavirus. Both intralesional and systemic administration of IFNs have been shown to produce some regression of anogenital warts.[415,489–495] However, more cost-effective modalities are available and are adequate for most patients.[495] In refractory condylomata acuminata, intralesional injection of various natural and recombinant IFNs is associated with complete clearance of injected warts in 36–62 percent of patients.[491–494] Response rates are two- to threefold higher than those observed in placebo recipients, but uninjected warts do not respond. Further complete responses occur with a second course of therapy. Responding patients generally show lesion involution within 4 weeks and maximal responses at 4–12 weeks after initiating therapy. Complete responders appear to have relatively low relapse rates (21–23 percent) during short-term follow-up. Efficacy has been demonstrated in patients failing conventional therapies, but responsiveness is poor in HIV-infected patients and with chronic lesions. Intralesional IFN may enhance the response to topical podophyllin.[489] Mild to moderate systemic side effects (8–10 percent dropout rate), discomfort at injection site, and leukopenia (up to 30 percent) are common with intralesional IFN.

In extensive or refractory disease, intramuscular or subcutaneous administration has been advocated. Systemic administration is associated with decreased wart size but greater toxicity and no higher complete response rate than placebo in most studies.[490,496–499] Systemic IFN also fails to reduce recurrences reproducibly after ablative therapy.[500,501] The possible usefulness of IFN in managing human papillomavirus–induced cervical dysplasia has not been critically evaluated. Intralesional IFN may clear cervical intraepithelial neoplasia in some patients.[502]

Plantar warts are poorly responsive to intramuscular IFN, but verruca vulgaris may respond to intralesional IFN-α.[503] Responses to intralesional and systemic IFN have also been observed in the rare HPV-related condition of epidermodysplasia verruciformis. Systemic interferon may provide adjunctive benefit in recurrent juvenile laryngeal papillomatosis (JLP). The majority of children have some initial decrease in lesions, but recurrence rates are high after cessation of therapy, and the long-term response to parenteral IFN-α is variable.[504–506] One trial employing intramuscular IFN-α at 2 MU/M^2 three times weekly for 12 months found significant reductions in papilloma growth rates during the first 6 months and in the need for urgent surgical procedures but no long-term benefits.[505] Another trial found prolonged remissions in over one-third of patients treated with higher doses.[506] Laryngeal disease in older patients appears to be more responsive.

Respiratory Viruses. Except for adenovirus, IFN has broad spectrum antiviral activity against respiratory viruses in vitro.[507] In experimentally induced infections in humans, intranasal administration of leukocyte or recombinant IFN-α is protective against rhinovirus, coronavirus, respiratory syncytial, and to a lesser extent influenza virus infections.[508,509] However, under natural conditions, prophylactic intranasal IFN-α is protective only against colds caused by rhinovirus, and chronic use is limited by the occurrence of nasal side effects.[437] When used for postcontact prophylaxis in the family setting, intranasal IFN-α2b (5 MU daily for 7 days) is associated with about 40 percent reductions in secondary respiratory illnesses and nearly 90 percent protection against rhinovirus colds during the period of use.[510,511] However, intranasal IFN-α is therapeutically ineffective in established rhinovirus colds.[512]

RIBAVIRIN (VIRAZOLE)

Spectrum

Ribavirin (1-β-D-ribofuranosyl-1,2,4-thiazole-3-carboxamide) is a guanosine analog (Fig. 5), in which both the base and the D-ribose sugar are necessary for antiviral activity.[513] Ribavirin inhibits the in vitro replication of a wide range of RNA and DNA viruses, including myxo-, paramyxo-, arena-, bunya-, herpes-, adeno-, pox-, and retroviruses and RNA tumor viruses.[513–517] By plaque assay, inhibitory concentrations range from 3 to 10 μg/ml for influenza, parainfluenza, and respiratory syncytial (RSV) viruses.[514,515] High concentrations (30–50 μg/ml) inhibit acute HIV infection of lymphocytes.[516] Ribavirin antagonizes the anti-HIV-1 effects of zidovudine but enhances the activity of purine dideoxynucleosides.[517]

Low concentrations of ribavirin (1–10 μg/ml) reversibly inhibit macromolecular synthesis and the proliferation of certain rapidly dividing, uninfected cells.[3,515] Ribavirin suppresses nucleic acid synthesis in quiescent and mitogen-stimulated human lymphocytes in vitro,[3,519] but does not adversely affect polymorphonuclear leukocyte functions.[520] Inhibition of mast cell secretory responses occurs after in vitro ribavirin exposure.[521]

Aerosol administration is more effective than parenteral dosing in animal models of influenza and RSV infection.[522,523] Parenterally administered ribavirin has antiviral and therapeutic activity in animal models of Lassa virus, other arenaviruses, and bunyavirus infections.[517,524–520] Enhanced therapeutic effects occur in certain animal models when ribavirin is administered in liposomes or with immunomodulators.[526–528] Combinations of ribavirin with immunoglobulin in RSV infection[514] and with amantadine or rimantadine in influenza A infection[184] show enhanced antiviral activity.

Mechanism of Action

The antiviral mechanism of action of ribavirin is not fully defined but relates to alteration of cellular nucleotide pools and of viral messenger RNA formation.[513] The ability of cells to take up ribavirin and to form active metabolites are important determinants of antiviral activity. Intracellular phosphorylation to the mono-, di-, and triphosphate derivatives is mediated by host cell enzymes. In both uninfected and RSV-infected cells, the predominant derivative (>80 percent) is the triphosphate, which is rapidly lost with an intracellular $T_{1/2}$ of less than 2 hours.[529]

Ribavirin monophosphate competitively inhibits inosine-5'-phosphate dehydrogenase (IMPDH) and interferes with the synthesis of GTP and thus nucleic acid synthesis. However, inhibition of this normal cellular enzyme would not fully account for a selective antiviral action, although inhibition of IMPDH and resultant decreased concentrations of competing guanosine could potentiate other antiviral effects. Ribavirin triphosphate may inhibit influenza virus RNA polymerase activity and competitively inhibit the GTP-dependent 5'-capping of viral messenger RNA. Ribavirin triphosphate appears to inhibit the initiation and particularly the elongation of capped mRNA primer fragments by the influenza virus polymerase complex.[530] Ribavirin di- and triphosphates also inhibit HIV reverse transcriptase activity.[531]

Ribavirin has immunosuppressive effects in experimental animals and shows therapeutic activity against transplantable virus-induced tumors and autoimmune diseases.[532] Ribavirin inhibits the serum antibody but not cellular immune responses to inactivated influenza vaccine and diminishes in vivo primary antibody responses and memory cell generation to T-dependent and T-independent antigens.[533]

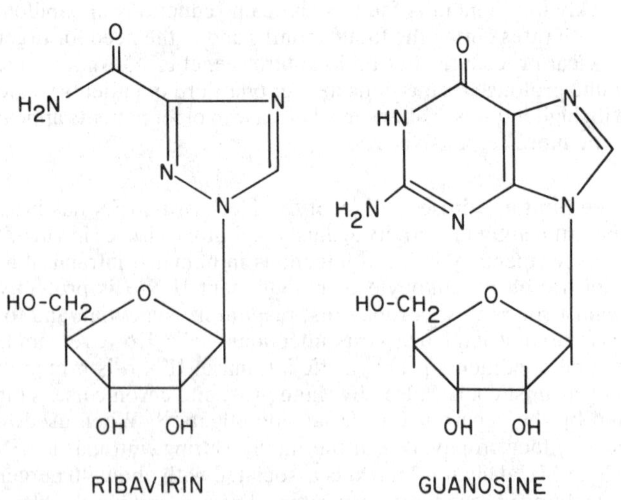

Resistance

In contrast to other nucleoside analogs, resistance to ribavirin has not been recognized, except possibly for Sindbis virus.[534] No ribavirin-resistant RSV have been detected during aerosol therapy of children.[535]

Pharmacokinetics

Following oral administration, bioavailability averages 42–45 percent in adults and children.[536–538] Following single oral doses of 600, 1200, or 2400 mg, peak plasma concentrations occur at 1–2 hours and average 1.3, 2.5, and 3.2 μg/ml, respectively. Tenfold higher peak plasma levels occur 0.5 hour after intravenous administration of equivalent doses.[536] Plasma concentrations average approximately 24 and 17 μg/ml after intravenous doses of 1000 and 500 mg, respectively, in Lassa fever patients.[539] At steady-state cerebrospinal fluid levels are about 70 percent of those in plasma.[537]

The disposition of ribavirin is complex. The β-phase $T_{1/2elim}$ is about 2 hours, but a prolonged terminal phase $T_{1/2elim}$ of 18–36 hours is also present.[536] Ribavirin triphosphate concentrates in erythrocytes with an RBC:ratio of 60:1 or greater, and RBC levels gradually decrease with an apparent $T_{1/2}$ up to several weeks.[537] Renal excretion accounts for approximately 40 percent of ribavirin's clearance, and hepatic metabolism appears to be an important route of elimination. Hemodialysis removes insignificant amounts of drug.[540]

With aerosol administration, plasma levels increase with the duration of exposure. Peak plasma levels range from 0.5 to 2.2 μg/ml after 8 hours exposure and from 0.8 to 3.3 μg/ml after 20 hours in pediatric patients.[539] Respiratory secretion levels often exceed 1000 μg/ml and persist with a $T_{1/2}$ of 1.4–2.5 hours. The amount of ribavirin actually deposited in different regions of the respiratory tract in different pathologic conditions or during mechanical ventilation is not certain. A special aerosol generator utilizing an modified Callison nebulizer is needed to produce particles of proper aerodynamic size to reach the lower respiratory tract (SPAG-2, ICN Pharmaceuticals). Revised estimates indicate that the delivered dose is twice as high in infants (1.8 mg/kg/h) than in adults and that various other factors influence dosage.[541]

Toxicity

Systemic ribavirin causes dose-related anemia due to extravascular hemolysis and, at higher doses, suppression of bone marrow release of erythroid elements.[517,542] Increased reticulocyte counts occur in ribavirin-treated patients after cessation of oral

FIG. 5. Chemical structures of ribavirin and the nucleoside guanosine.

RIBAVIRIN   GUANOSINE

therapy.[543] Reversible increases of serum bilirubin in up to one-fourth of recipients, serum iron, and uric acid concentrations occur during short-term oral administration. Bolus intravenous infusion may cause rigors.[544] In HIV-infected patients, chronic oral therapy is also associated with dose-related lymphopenia and gastrointestinal and CNS complaints, including headache, lethargy, insomnia, and mood alteration.[538,545,546] Aerosolized ribavirin has been well tolerated except for mild conjunctival irritation and rash, transient wheezing, and occasional reversible deterioration in pulmonary function.[535] No adverse hematologic effects have been associated with aerosol ribavirin.

Ribavirin exposure may occur in health care personnel working in the environment of aerosol-treated infants.[547–550] Health care worker exposure is higher during delivery by oxygen hood than by ventilator or vacuum-exhausted hood systems.[550] The use of masks, but not of gloves or gowns, has been recommended.[548]

When used in conjunction with mechanical ventilation, in-line filters, modified circuitry, and frequent monitoring are required to prevent plugging of ventilator valves and tubing with precipitates of ribavirin.[551–554] The possible effects of such modifications on drug delivery to the lower respiratory tract are undefined.

In preclinical studies, ribavirin is teratogenic, embryotoxic, mutagenic, tumor-promoting, and possibly gonadotoxic.[542] Its use is relatively contraindicated during pregnancy, and pregnant women should not directly care for patients receiving ribavirin aerosol.[548]

Clinical Studies

Ribavirin aerosol is approved in the United States for treatment of RSV bronchiolitis and pneumonia in hospitalized children. Aerosolized ribavirin (12–22 hours exposure daily for 3–6 days) variably shortens the duration of virus shedding and improves certain clinical measures, including arterial oxygen saturation, in infants hospitalized with RSV pneumonia.[535,554–557] More rapid improvements in illness severity and oxygenation also occur in high-risk subjects with bronchopulmonary dysplasia or congenital heart disease.[557] In infants receiving mechanical ventilation for RSV-related respiratory failure, one study found that aerosolized ribavirin is associated with an average 4-day reduction in the duration of ventilatory support and a 2-day shortening of the length of hospitalization compared with a water aerosol.[556] Intermittent, high-dose therapy (2-hour exposures tid for 5 days) is under study as a means of simplifying administration and appears to be well tolerated.[558]

Expert opinions vary about the overall clinical value, indications for use, and optimal length of aerosol ribavirin therapy in RSV infections. In particular, infants at high risk for severe or complicated RSV infection (e.g., congenital heart disease, chronic lung disease, immunodeficiency states) and those hospitalized with severe illness ($PaO_2 < 65$ mmHg or increasing $PaCO_2$) should be considered for treatment.[548] Trials to date have not determined whether this costly intervention reduces the likelihood of intubation or death, shortens hospitalization time for nonintubated children, or provides long-term benefit. Decreased RSV-specific serum neutralizing antibody titers, as well as diminished RSV-specific IgE and IgA responses in nasopharyngeal secretion, may occur in ribavirin-treated children,[559] but the clinical significance of these findings is uncertain. Anecdotal reports suggest that aerosolized ribavirin may be effective in severe influenza virus infection.[560] Treatment for an average of 12–18 hours per day for 3 days is associated with reductions in viral titers, fever, and systemic illness in young adults with uncomplicated influenza A or B virus infection in some but not all studies.[560,561] Oral doses of 1.0 g/day have no clinical or antiviral activity in uncomplicated influenza of adults,[529] whereas a high-dose oral regimen (with loading of 3.6 g over 3 hours) may provide clinical benefit.[562] Intravenous ribavirin has been used in treating influenza virus myocarditis.[563] The possible value of aerosolized or intravenous ribavirin in high-risk groups, such as infants or adults hospitalized with influenza, remains to be proven. Intravenous and/or aerosolized ribavirin has also been used in immunosuppressed patients with severe parainfluenza and measles virus infections.[564–566]

Intravenous ribavirin decreases mortality in Lassa fever[567] and in hemorrhagic fever with renal syndrome (HFRS) due to Hantaan virus infection.[568] In Lassa fever patients at high risk of death because of elevated serum aspartate amino-transferase levels or high-titer viremia, intravenous (4 g/day) or oral ribavirin significantly reduces mortality, especially when therapy is initiated during the first 6 days of illness.[567] High-dose intravenous therapy reduces mortality by sevenfold and the risk of oliguria or hemorrhage in HFRS[568] and has also been associated with antiviral effects and clinical benefit in Argentine hemorrhagic fever.[569] Oral ribavirin has been proposed for prophylaxis of Lassa fever and in Congo-Crimean hemorrhagic fever contacts.[570,571] Intravenous ribavirin is being utilized to treat patients with hantavirus pulmonary syndrome in the recently described outbreak in the western United States (see Ch. 142).

In HIV-infected patients, chronic oral ribavirin at tolerable doses has no consistent effects on CD4 count or p24 antigen level.[545,572–574] Higher doses appear to be lymphocytotoxic.[575] Similarly, no consistent reductions in the risk of progression to AIDS have been found. Oral ribavirin has also been reported to provide clinical benefit in measles, acute hepatitis, and mucocutaneous herpes virus infections, but confirmation of such observations is needed. Oral doses up to 1.2 g/day have been associated with temporary reductions in serum aminotransferase activity in chronic hepatitis C infection.[576] One 6-month trial employing escalating doses of 0.6–1.2 g/day found gradual, reversible falls in serum ALT levels and HCV RNA titers but no significant improvement in liver histopathology.[577] Oral and intravenous ribavirin are investigational in the United States.

SORIVUDINE (BV-ARA-U)

Sorivudine (1-β-D-arabinofuranosyl-E-5[2-bromovinyl] uracil), formerly brovavir, is a nucleoside analog (Fig. 4) that has potent inhibitory activity for VZV. In vitro plaque inhibitory concentrations range from 0.0001 to 0.0006 μg/ml, and sorivudine is over 1000-fold more potent than acyclovir against VZV.[578] The inhibitory concentration for clinical VZV isolates averages 0.0013 μg/ml,[579] whereas very high concentrations are required for inhibition of uninfected cell growth. Sorivudine also is active in vitro against HSV-1 and EBV but not against HSV-2 or CMV.[580] Low doses (0.2 mg/kg/day) are active in experimental simian varicella infection.[581]

The uptake of sorivudine by HSV-infected cells is 40-fold or greater than that in uninfected cells.[582] Phosphorylation by viral TK is essential for accumulation and activation of sorivudine, and further metabolism to the diphosphate is dependent on viral TK activity. Sorivudine triphosphate is a competitive inhibitor of viral DNA replication with respect to dTTP, but, unlike acyclovir triphosphate, it is not a substrate for viral DNA polymerase and is not incorporated into viral DNA.[583,584] Resistance to the antiviral action of sorivudine has not yet been detected during clinical use,[579] but TK-deficient mutants of VZV are resistant in vitro.[578]

Sorivudine is well absorbed after oral administration. The oral bioavailability averages approximately 60 percent and is not affected by food.[585] After oral doses of 40 mg once daily, mean peak and trough plasma concentrations are 1.8 and 0.2 μg/ml, respectively. The plasma $T_{1/2\ elim}$ averages 5–7 hours. A 25 mg intravenous dose of sorivudine will produce serum concentrations similar to those achieved with a 40 mg oral dose.[578] In elderly subjects, serum $T_{1/2\ elim}$ and area under the curve values increase by approximately 20–30 percent. Plasma protein binding is over 95 percent. After intravenous dosing, 60–75 percent of the drug is recovered unchanged in the urine and less than 5 percent is excreted as the metabolite BVU. In animals, sorivudine potentiates the toxicity of 5-fluorouracil (5-FU) and possibly cyclophosphamide, and fatalities have occurred in oncology patients treated with both 5-FU and sorivudine.[585] The metabolite BVU may possibly increase 5-FU effects by inhibiting an enzyme required for 5-FU metabolism. No effect on the pharmacokinetics or tolerance of zidovudine or ganciclovir have been recognized in humans.[585]

Oral sorivudine is generally well tolerated, and no serious side effects have been recognized during short-term administration. Gastrointestinal upset with nausea and vomiting, diarrhea, and headache have been the most frequently reported adverse events. A small proportion of patients have had elevations in hepatic enzymes values.

In preclinical testing, long-term administration of high doses (75–750 times the weight-adjusted human dose) of sorivudine has been associated with increased hepatic and testicular neoplasms in rodents.[578,585] Sorivudine is not mutagenic, teratogenic, or embryotoxic in preclinical studies, but safety in pregnancy in humans remains to be established.

Sorivudine has been approved for treatment of VZV infections in Japan but remains investigational in the United States. Oral and intravenous formulations are under development. Clinical trials in localized zoster in immunocompromised patients and in varicella in immunocompetent adults are currently in progress.

STAVUDINE (D4T, ZERIT)

Spectrum

Stavudine (2',3'-didehydro-2'-deoxythymidine) is a thymidine nucleoside analog (Fig. 3) that inhibits HIV-1 replication at concentrations similar to those of zidovudine (Table 6). HIV-2 and most strains of HIV-1 resistant to zidovudine[586] are susceptible to stavudine. Stavudine appears less toxic for certain bone marrow progenitor cells in vitro than zidovudine,[587,588] but is inhibitory for mitochondrial DNA synthesis.[254]

Mechanism of Action

Stavudine rapidly enters cells, but, in contrast to zidovudine, the rate-limiting step in the intracellular metabolism of stavudine is initial phosphorylation by cellular TK.[589] Stavudine is readily converted from the monophosphate to di- and triphosphate forms. The triphosphate, which has an intracellular $T_{1/2}$ of 3–4 hours, acts as both a competitive inhibitor of reverse transcriptase with respect to thymidine triphosphate and a terminator of DNA chain elongation.[590] Unlike zidovudine, stavudine does not significantly inhibit cellular thymidine metabolism, which may explain its lower toxicity for certain cell types.[586] The selectivity of its antiviral action relates to much greater substrate activity of stavudine triphosphate for viral reverse transcriptase than for cellular DNA polymerases,[590] although low concentrations inhibit mitochondrial DNA polymerase-γ.[261]

Resistance

Very limited data are available regarding resistance to stavudine. Most zidovudine-resistant HIV-1 isolates that have been tested are sensitive to stavudine, but some have been reported to have eightfold or greater reductions in stavudine susceptibility as well.[591,592] The propensity for the development of resistance to stavudine in vivo is currently under study.

Pharmacokinetics

Stavudine is acid stable and well absorbed after oral administration with bioavailability of approximately 90 percent.[593] Peak plasma concentrations average 0.7 μg/ml after 1.0 mg/kg doses. Cerebrospinal fluid penetration occurs but is not well characterized. The plasma $T_{1/2\ elim}$ averages about 1 hour. Stavudine appears unchanged in the urine, but approximately 60 percent of its clearance is by nonrenal mechanisms. Dose adjustment guidelines for renal or hepatic insufficiency are not currently available. Formulations include capsules in various strengths, and powder for reconstitution as 1.0 mg/ml solution.

Interactions

Zidovudine may inhibit intracellular phosphorylation of stavudine and antagonize its antiviral effects.[589] Because of the potential for peripheral neuropathy, stavudine should be used with caution in patients receiving other agents associated with neuropathy (Table 7).

Toxicity

The major dose-limiting toxicity of stavudine is painful sensory peripheral neuropathy, which has been observed with doses of 2 mg/kg/day and above. The incidence of neuropathy is dose related.[594] Neuropathic symptoms are usually reversible with withdrawal of the drug, and the majority of patients are able to tolerate further treatment at reduced dosage. At currently studied adult doses of 0.5–1.0 mg/kg/day, neuropathy has occurred in less than 5 percent of patients. Pancreatitis occurs in less than 0.5 percent and has not been directly linked to stavudine therapy. Anemia and elevated transaminase values have been described, but serious bone marrow toxicity or hepatotoxicity appears to be uncommon. Other adverse symptoms of uncertain relationship to stavudine use have included fever, asthenia, headache, depression, and gastrointestinal upset.

Preclinical studies have found that high doses cause bone marrow and hepatic toxicity in animals but not teratogenic or embryotoxic effects. Stavudine can cause chromosomal damage.

Clinical Studies

An initial trial of stavudine in patients with AIDS or ARC and CD4 counts of 400/mm³ or less found that the maximum tolerated dose is 4 mg/kg/day and that stavudine administration is associated with significant improvements in CD4 counts, p24 antigen levels, and clinical symptoms.[594] Doses below 0.5 mg/kg/day appear to be less effective. Stavudine is currently available from the manufacturer under the parallel track guidelines for patients with CD4 counts less than 300/mm³ who are intolerant to or have failed therapy with both zidovudine and didanosine. Studies comparing the safety and efficacy of savudine to zidovudine in patients previously treated with zidovudine are in progress.

TRIFLURIDINE (TFT, TRIFLUOROTHYMIDINE, VIROPTIC)

Trifluridine (5-trifluoromethyl-2'-deoxyuridine) is a fluorinated pyrimidine nucleoside (Fig. 4) that has in vitro inhibitory activity against HSV-1 and -2, CMV, vaccinia, and, to a lesser extent, certain adenoviruses.[595,596] Concentrations of 0.2–10 μg/ml inhibit replication of herpesviruses, including acyclovir-resistant strains.[56]

Its antiviral mechanism of action involves inhibition of viral DNA synthesis. Trifluridine monophosphate irreversibly inhibits thymidylate synthetase, and the triphosphate competitively inhibits DNA polymerases with respect to thymidine triphosphate.[595] Trifluridine is incorporated into viral and, to a lesser extent, cellular DNA and also inhibits cellular DNA synthesis at relatively low concentrations. It also exhibits mutagenic, teratogenic, and antineoplastic activities in experimental systems. Trifluridine-resistant HSV with altered TK substrate specificity can be selected upon laboratory passage.[407] The clinical significance of this observation is uncertain.

Trifluridine's clinical use is limited to topical therapy of HSV infections, and it is approved currently in the United States for treatment of primary keratoconjunctivitis and recurrent epithelial keratitis due to HSV-1 and -2 (Table 1).[408,409,595] Topical trifluridine is more active than idoxuridine in HSV ocular infections, but trials comparing its efficacy with that of topical vidarabine have generally found no important differences.[597] Topical trifluridine is effective in some patients who have not responded clinically to idoxuridine or vidarabine. Adverse reactions include discomfort upon instillation, palpebral edema, and, uncommonly, hypersensitivity reactions, irritation, and superficial punctate or epithelial keratopathy.

Topical trifluridine also appears to benefit some patients with acyclovir-resistant HSV cutaneous infections. Combinations of trifluridine and IFN-α synergistically inhibit HSV replication in vitro and have been used in treating both ocular and drug-resistant mucocutaneous HSV infections.[56,598]

VIDARABINE (ARA-A, ADENINE ARABINOSIDE, VIRA-A)

Spectrum

Vidarabine (9-β-D-ribofuranosyladenine) is an analog of adenosine (Fig. 4) that has in vitro antiviral activity against herpes, pox, rhabdo, and some RNA tumor viruses. Vidarabine inhibits in vitro replication of idoxuridine- or acyclovir-resistant HSV and VZV strains, but has less activity against CMV and EBV.[599–601] Plaque formation by most HSV and VZV strains is completely inhibited by 3.0 μg/ml or less of vidarabine. The carbocyclic analog of vidarabine (cyclaradine) is resistant to the action of adenosine deaminase and has comparable antiviral effects in vitro and in animal models.[602]

Mechanism of Action

The antiviral mechanisms of vidarabine are not completely understood, but it is an inhibitor of viral DNA synthesis.[603] Vidarabine is phosphorylated by cellular enzymes to the triphosphate derivative, which competitively inhibits viral and, to a lesser extent, cellular DNA polymerase activities. Vidarabine triphosphate is incorporated into both cellular and viral DNA, where it may act as a chain terminator.[604] The principal metabolite in vivo and in cell culture is hypoxanthine arabinoside (ara-Hx), which is a compound with 30- to 50-fold less antiviral activity than vidarabine.

Vidarabine triphosphate inhibits other enzyme systems, including ribonucleoside reductase, RNA polyadenylation, and S-adenosylhomocysteine hydrolase (SAHH), which is an enzyme involved in transmethylation reactions. Inhibition of SAHH may result in inhibition of adenosine deaminase and contribute to the antiviral and toxic effects of vidarabine.[605,606]

Resistance

Resistant variants due to mutations in viral DNA polymerase can be selected under laboratory conditions, but drug resistance is not a recognized clinical problem.

Pharmacokinetics

Following intravenous infusion, vidarabine is rapidly deaminated to ara-Hx by adenosine deaminase,[603] an enzyme that is widely distributed through body tissues. During constant infusion (10 mg/kg once a day over 12 hours), plasma ara-Hx, concentrations peak at 3–6 μg/ml and those of vidarabine at only 0.2–0.4 μg/ml.[603,607] Ara-Hx is present in cerebrospinal fluid at

concentrations averaging 35 percent of plasma values, although CSF/plasma ratios over 90 percent occur in infants.[608]

The kidney is the primary route of elimination, and 40–53 percent of the daily dose is recovered in the urine as ara-Hx and 1–3 percent as vidarabine.[603] The serum $T_{1/2elim}$ of ara-Hx is approximately 3.5 hours in adults. Vidarabine may also accumulate in RBC. In patients with impaired renal function, plasma ara-Hx concentrations rise and may be associated with neurologic or other side effects.[609] A dosage reduction of 25 percent has been recommended for patients with severe renal insufficiency, but definitive guidelines have not been established. Ara-Hx is readily cleared during hemodialysis (50 percent over 6 hours), so that dosing should be done after dialysis.[609]

The phosphorylated ester of vidarabine, ara-AMP, or vidarabine phosphate is much more water soluble than the parent drug and can be administered intravenously or intramuscularly on a chronic basis.[610] The antiviral activity and the pharmacokinetics, metabolism, and toxicities of ara-AMP in humans are similar to those of vidarabine.[610,611]

Interactions

Allopurinol may interfere with vidarabine metabolism and possibly increase the risk of toxicity.[612]

Toxicity

Dose-related gastrointestinal toxicity is common with intravenous vidarabine, and 10–15 percent of patients develop anorexia, nausea, vomiting, diarrhea, and/or weight loss.[603] Vidarabine is poorly soluble (<0.45 mg/ml) so that intravenous administration requires infusion of large fluid volumes, often 1.5–2.5 liters/day. Such fluid loads may present problems for patients with impaired renal or cardiac function or cerebral edema. Anemia, leukopenia, or thrombocytopenia, and infusion-related thrombophlebitis, weakness, hypokalemia, rash, elevated transaminases, and SIADH have been described.

Acute and chronic neurotoxicities include tremor, often accentuated by intention and at times associated with facial grimacing, myoclonus, ataxia, or dysgraphia; alterations in behavior or mentation, including disorientation, depression, aphasia, akinetic mutism, agitation, hallucinations, and, rarely, coma or seizures; and pain syndromes, usually in the extremities and sometimes lasting up to 6 months after cessation of therapy.[612–616] High doses, concurrent IFN or possibly allopurinol therapy, and the presence of preexisting hepatic or renal insufficiency may be risk factors. Electroencephalograms have shown diffuse changes consistent with metabolic encephalopathy in some cases.

Vidarabine has been shown to be mutagenic, teratogenic, and oncogenic in preclinical testing. Parenteral use should be restricted to serious infections.

Clinical Studies

Intravenous vidarabine is approved for use in certain life-threatening herpesvirus infections including HSV encephalitis, neonatal herpes, and zoster or varicella in immunocompromised patients. However, acyclovir has replaced it for most indications because of greater efficacy and/or safety.[96–100,141] One comparative trial in varicella of immunocompromised children was stopped because of neurotoxicity, which occurred in 16 percent of vidarabine recipients.[616] Vidarabine is comparably effective to acyclovir in neonatal HSV complicated by visceral dissemination or CNS involvement.[100] However, disseminated HSV infection has occurred in a neonate despite vidarabine prophylaxis.[617] Vidarabine (10 mg/kg/day for 7 days) is of modest usefulness in mucocutaneous HSV infections of immunocompromised hosts,[618] and it is ineffective in acyclovir-resistant HSV infections in AIDS patients.[52,53] Administration to renal transplant patients with CMV-associated illness is associated with no therapeutic effect and with neurologic toxicity in 29 percent of recipients.[615] Combined administration of vidarabine and acyclovir has been used in cases of life-threatening herpesvirus infections.

In chronic hepatitis B virus infection, vidarabine or its monophosphate derivative is associated with reductions in plasma HBV-specific DNA polymerase activity and titers of HBs antigen and HBe antigen in some patients, but no effective and well-tolerated regimens have been identified.[613,619–622]

In HSV keratoconjunctivitis, topical vidarabine is superior to idoxuridine[402,409] (Table 1) and is effective in patients who cannot receive idoxuridine because of allergy, toxicity, or drug resistance.

ZALCITABINE (DDC, HIVID)

Spectrum

Zalcitabine (2′,3′-dideoxycytidine) is a dideoxynucleoside analog (Fig. 3) active against HIV-1 and -2, including strains resistant to zidovudine.[623–628] Zalcitabine has potency similar to zidovudine in PBMC but appears more active in monocytemacrophages and resting cells (Table 6).[253,255] At a well-tolerated dose, zalcitabine is modestly active in a feline model of retrovirus infection.[626] Combinations of zalcitabine and zidovudine synergistically inhibit HIV-1 replication, including zidovudine-resistant strains, in vitro.[627]

Mechanism of Action

Zalcitabine is initially phosphorylated by deoxycytidine kinase and further metabolized by other cellular enzymes to its active metabolite dideoxycytidine 5′-triphosphate (ddCTP).[623–627] ddCTP inhibits reverse transcriptase competitively with respect to dCTP and probably causes chain termination of viral DNA elongation. The intracellular $T_{1/2}$ of ddCTP is approximately 3 hours. Zalcitabine also causes a decrease in intracellular dCTP pool size, which may potentiate antiviral activity,[253] and inhibits mitochondrial DNA synthesis at low concentrations.[260,628] These effects probably contribute to its clinical toxicities.

Resistance

HIV-1 variants with seven- to 14-fold reductions in susceptibility can be selected by in vitro passage in the presence of zalcitabine.[629–631] Clinical isolates with reduced susceptibility have been found to have mutations at position $65^{lys \rightarrow arg}$ of reverse transcriptase.[630,631] One clinical isolate from a patient on long-term zalcitabine had fivefold decreased susceptibility and a reverse transcriptase substitution at position $69^{thr \rightarrow asp}$.[632] Combined ddC and AZT administration does not appear to reduce the emergence of zidovudine-resistant virus. Zalcitabine-resistant strains usually show reduced susceptibility to didanosine.[262,629–633] The clinical significance of resistance is undetermined at present.

Pharmacokinetics

Zalcitabine is well absorbed orally with oral bioavailability exceeding 80 percent in adults.[623,624,634] Food slows absorption and decreases bioavailability by about 15 percent. Bioavailability may also be lower in children.[635] Peak plasma concentrations of 0.02–0.04 μg/ml are observed after oral doses of 0.03 mg/kg. Cerebrospinal fluid concentrations average about 15–20 percent of plasma ones.

Renal excretion is the primary route of elimination, and about 75 percent of drug is found unchanged in the urine after intravenous dosing. The plasma $T_{1/2elim}$ ranges from 1 to 3 hours, but increases up to 8.5 hours in those with renal insufficiency (creatinine clearance <55 ml/min). Dose reductions are recommended

by the manufacturer for clearance of 40 ml/min or less, but guidelines are not well defined.

Interactions

Concomitant use of drugs associated with peripheral neuropathy or pancreatitis should be avoided during zalcitabine administration (Table 7). Similarly, nephrotoxic drugs may interfere with its renal excretion and increase the risk of neuropathy. Zalcitabine and zidovudine do not affect the pharmacokinetics of each other.[636]

Toxicity

The major dose-limiting side effect is painful sensorimotor peripheral neuropathy, which develops in up to 30 percent of patients at currently recommended doses. The risk of neuropathy increases with doses above 0.03 mg/kg/day, duration of continuous therapy, low CD4 counts, and creatinine clearance below 110 ml/min.[624,625,637,638] Symptoms commonly include pain, paraesthesia, and hypoesthesia and are usually reversible upon cessation of therapy or with dose reduction in mild cases.

Pancreatitis occurs in less than percent of cases but may be fatal. Rash, fever, nausea, ulcerative stomatitis, and headache occur particularly during the first month of dosing. Stomatitis usually resolves within 1–2 weeks despite continued administration. Abnormal liver function tests and hepatitis have been described. Hematopoietic toxicities appear uncommon, although granulocytopenia occurs in up to 8–10 percent of recipients. Esophageal ulceration and cardiomyopathy have been described.[639]

High doses of zalcitabine are teratogenic and embryotoxic in rodents. Zalcitabine causes chromosomal alterations in human lymphocytes.

Clinical Studies

Zalcitabine is approved for treatment in combination with zidovudine for adults deteriorating clinically or immunologically with advanced HIV infection and CD4 counts less than 300/mm³ (Table 1).[624] Comparative clinical studies have found that monotherapy with zalcitabine 0.75 mg/8 h is less effective in prolonging survival (82 vs. 90 percent at 1 year) and in reducing opportunistic infections than zidovudine in patients with AIDS or advanced ARC and less than 3 months prior zidovudine therapy (ACTG 114). Moderate or severe neuropathy was observed in 20 percent of zalcitabine recipients, one-half of whom required cessation of therapy. A smaller trial in patients with at least 48 weeks of prior zidovudine found slower CD4 counts and weight declines in zalcitabine recipients but twofold higher side effect rates and no differences in survival or new AIDS diagnoses compared with zidovudine.[638] In patients intolerant of or failing zidovudine, zalcitabine 0.75 mg/8 h appeared to be equivalent to didanosine in delaying disease progression but was associated with a somewhat more prolonged survival.[289a]

A phase I/II dose-finding study of ddC and zidovudine combinations in patients with advanced infection (ACTG 106) found that certain combinations are associated with higher and more sustained CD4 counts than observed in earlier studies of zidovudine alone.[636] A randomized study of patients with CD4 counts of 300/mm³ or less at 4 weeks or less prior zidovudine found higher and more sustained CD4 responses in patients taking zalcitabine 0.75 mg/8 h and zidovudine 200 mg/8 h than in those taking zidovudine alone.[624] Weekly and monthly alternating regimens of high-dose zalcitabine and zidovudine are associated with prolonged antiviral effects and less toxicity than continuous administration.[640] In patients with prolonged prior zidovudine therapy and CD4 counts of 300/mm³, or less, the combination of zalcitabine and zidovudine is associated with better outcomes than monotherapy for those with CD4 counts in the 150–300 range but not for those with counts below 50 (ACTG 155).[641] Other combination trials are in progress.[14,15]

ZIDOVUDINE [AZIDOTHYMIDINE, AZT, ZDV, RETROVIR]

Spectrum

Zidovudine (3'-azido-3'-deoxythymidine) is a thymidine analog (Fig. 3) with antiviral activity against HIV-1, HIV-2, HTLV-1, and other mammalian retroviruses.[642–649] Low concentrations inhibit acute HIV-1 infection in human T-cell lines and peripheral blood lymphocytes (Table 6) but, as with other dideoxynucleosides, are ineffective in chronically infected cells or in inhibiting HIV spread through giant cell formation.[650] Zidovudine is also less active in human monocyte-macrophages or quiescent cells (Table 6)[252,253,651] but inhibits HIV replication in human brain macrophages.[652] Antiviral activity is potentiated in vitro by didanosine, zalcitabine, interferon, several other antiretroviral agents, GM-CSF, and neutralizing antibody, but is antagonized by thymidine or ribavirin.[257,258,629,641,653–655] Zidovudine is also inhibitory for hepatitis B virus and EBV but not for HSV or VZV.[656] Many Enterobacteriaceae and *Vibrio* strains are inhibited at low concentrations (0.03–1.0 μg/ml), but bacterial resistance to zidovudine develops rapidly.[657]

Pharmacologically relevant concentrations inhibit human myeloid and erythroid progenitor cells (0.3–0.6 μg/ml),[3,345] globin chain synthesis in human erythroid progenitor cells,[13] and mitogen-induced blastogenesis of peripheral blood mononuclear cells.[3,643] Uridine partially reverses zidovudine's hematopoietic toxicity for human granulocyte-macrophage progenitor cells without impairing its anti-HIV-1 activity.[658]

In animal models of retroviral infection, early zidovudine administration after virus exposure may suppress the development of infection.[644,659–661] Treatment of pregnant mice delays the onset of virus-induced CNS infection in offspring infected in utero.[659]

Mechanism of Action

Like other dideoxynucleosides, zidovudine's primary antiviral mechanism of action is inhibition of viral RNA-dependent DNA polymerase (reverse transcriptase).[625,662,663] Following diffusion into host cells, the drug is initially phosphorylated by cellular TK, but the rate-limiting step is conversion to the diphosphate by thymidylate kinase. High levels of the monophosphate but much lower levels of di- and triphosphates are present in cells, including PBMC from treated patients.[662,664] Concentrations of the phosphorylated forms of zidovudine are similar in uninfected and infected cells. Zidovudine triphosphate, which has an intracellular $T_{1/2}$ of 3–4 hours, competitively inhibits the viral reverse transcriptase with respect to TTP, and, because the 3'-azido group prevents the formation of 5'-3'phosphodiester linkages, zidovudine acts as a chain terminator of DNA synthesis.[663] The antiviral selectivity of zidovudine is due to its greater affinity for HIV reverse transcriptase than for human DNA polymerases, although low concentrations inhibit DNA polymerase-γ.[259]

Zidovudine monophosphate appears to inhibit the RNase H activity of reverse transcriptase[665] and is also a competitive inhibitor of cellular thymidylate kinase, which may lead to reduced intracellular levels of TTP and enhanced antiviral effects by decreasing competition for zidovudine triphosphate.[662]

Resistance

Isolates of HIV from untreated patients have a narrow range of susceptibility to zidovudine,[11,591,666] although recovery of resistant virus from the PBMC of untreated patients has been described.[667] The definition of resistance depends on the assay method, but clinical isolates with 10- to 100-fold decreases in susceptibility have been recovered from most AIDS patients treated for 6 months or longer. Resistance has been associated with point mutations in the gene encoding viral reverse transcriptase and amino acid substitutions in multiple loci, particularly positions $41^{met \rightarrow leu}$, $67^{asp \rightarrow asn}$, $70^{lys \rightarrow arg}$, $215^{thr \rightarrow tyr/phe}$, and $219^{lys \rightarrow gln}$. The reverse transcriptase mutations associated with zidovudine resistance appear sequentially, and multiple mutations are required to confer high-level resistance.[11,666,668] Substitutions in codon 70 or codon 215, which require two nucleotide changes, are the most common, but in vitro susceptibilities vary 20-fold for clinical isolates with identical mutations.[669] The functional basis of resistance is not fully understood, since reverse transcriptase from resistant viruses is inhibited by zidovudine triphosphate in cell-free systems.

Resistance is a stepwise phenomenon that develops slowly and progressively and culminates in high-level resistance in late-stage infection.[11] The degree of resistance and the frequency with which it develops are both correlated with stage of infection, CD4 count, and duration of therapy, but not with zidovudine dose.[666] It is estimated that after 1 year of therapy, 90 percent of AIDS patients will develop diminished sensitivity to zidovudine compared with 30 percent or less of non- or minimally symptomatic patients. About one-third of isolates from AIDS patients show greater than 100-fold decreases in susceptibility by 1 year.

The clinical significance of the emergence of resistance remains uncertain. Progression from asymptomatic infection to AIDS can occur in treated patients without the emergence of highly resistant variants,[670] and no consistent pattern of p24 antigen change or clinical deterioration has been recognized to date in those with resistant variants. One pediatric study found a correlation between decreased zidovudine susceptibility and poor clinical outcome during the subsequent 6 months of follow-up.[671] In adults with less advanced HIV infection, the development of resistance to zidovudine, as defined by a 50-fold or greater decrease in susceptibility, was found in 64 percent of patients after 180 weeks of therapy and was associated with a twofold higher risk of disease progression.[672] The rate of appearance of the 215 mutation appears to correlate with CD4 counts and viral virulence as reflected by in vitro growth characteristics and possibly by the likelihood of progression to AIDS.[673] High-level zidovudine resistance appears to be an independent marker for disease progression in patients with advanced HIV infection. Primary infection with resistant virus due to transmission from treated contacts or vertically has been documented.[674,675,675a,675b]

A return toward zidovudine sensitivity occurs slowly in isolates from some patients after cessation of drug.[676,677] Following switch to didanosine therapy, 10-fold increases in susceptibility to zidovudine may occur in association with a compensatory mutation at position 74.[261,262] Other agents active in vitro against zidovudine-resistant isolates include didanosine, zalcitabine, stavudine, and foscarnet, although some zidovudine-resistant isolates show decreased susceptibility to didanosine,[264,265] and multidrug-resistant isolates have been recovered from some patients. In vitro studies indicate that resistant HIV is synergistically inhibited by combinations of zidovudine and didanosine or zalcitabine.[257,627]

Pharmacokinetics

Zidovudine is rapidly absorbed from the gastrointestinal tract in most patients. Peak serum concentrations occur at 0.5–1.5 hours, and oral bioavailability averages approximately 60–70 percent.[678,679] Although the range of observed concentrations is broad, mean peak and trough plasma levels are 0.4–0.5 and 0.1 μg/ml, respectively, in those receiving 100 mg every 4 hours.[680] Food intake may delay absorption. Zidovudine plasma protein binding is about 30 percent, and distribution is wide in body fluids. Cerebrospinal fluid concentrations range widely but average approximately 53 percent of those in plasma in adults and

24 percent of plasma in children.[678–682] Semen concentrations are 1.3- to 20-fold higher than serum,[683] and salivary levels are similar to those in plasma.[684] Neonatal blood concentrations are slightly higher and amniotic fluid several times higher than maternal serum levels.[685]

The plasma $T_{1/2elim}$ is approximately 1–1.5 hours. Zidovudine undergoes first-pass metabolism and is rapidly converted to its 5'-O-glucuronide, which has a similar plasma $T_{1/2elim}$ but lacks anit-HIV activity. In addition, another metabolite, 3'-amino-3'-deoxythymidine, is present in plasma at low concentrations and may contribute to marrow toxicity.[686] Following oral administration, the urinary recovery of zidovudine and its glucuronide average 14 and 75 percent, respectively, of the dose. Renal clearance involves both glomerular filtration and tubular secretion.

Renal clearance of zidovudine and its metabolites is markedly decreased in renal failure, and high glucuronide levels can accumulate.[687] Hemodialysis efficiently removes the glucuronide but not zidovudine. In cirrhosis, two- to threefold increases in plasma levels and $T_{1/2elim}$ occur.[688] Reductions in dose frequency to every 8 hours in patients with severely impaired renal or hepatic function have been recommended.

Interactions

Drugs that inhibit glucuronidation and/or renal excretion of zidovudine, such as probenicid[689] and possibly pyrimethamine/sulfadiazine, may increase the risks of marrow toxicity. Many drugs and antimicrobials can inhibit zidovudine glucuronidation in vitro.[690] Rifabutin and rifampin can decrease plasma concentrations of zidovudine.[691] Clarithromycin may interfere with zidovudine absorption. Although associated with an increased risk of marrow toxicity in one study,[692] acetaminophen does not impair zidovudine elimination.[693] Methadone may increase plasma concentrations in some patients.[694] Coadministration with drugs that are nephrotoxic or myelotoxic may increase the risk of hematologic side effects (Table 7). Concomitant ganciclovir increases the risk of severe hematologic toxicity, which occurs in over 80 percent of patients receiving both drugs.[375,376] Neurotoxicity, with severe somnolence in about 4 percent of patients, may occur during concomitant use of zidovudine and acyclovir.[81]

Toxicity

The major toxicities of zidovudine are granulocytopenia and anemia, which occur in up to one-half of recipients at higher doses.[642,692,695] The risk of hematologic toxicities is inversely related to pretreatment CD4, hemoglobin, and granulocyte values and stage of disease and is directly related to the zidovudine dose and duration of therapy. Studies using currently recommended doses have found severe anemia or granulocytopenia in 29 and 37 percent of AIDS patients, respectively, but in only 2 percent of those with asymptomatic infection.[696–699] Granulocytopenia usually occurs after 6–8 weeks, and the incidence remains relatively constant during prolonged treatment. Granulocytopenia has been successfully managed with recombinant G-CSF or GM-CSF but may require dose interruption or reduction.

Anemia associated with erythroid hypoplasia or aplasia and megaloblastic bone marrow changes may occur as early as 2–4 weeks after therapy, but most commonly after the first 6 weeks.[695] Macrocytosis is expected and does not predict transfusion-requiring anemia. Pancytopenia related to partially reversible bone marrow failure has occurred at 14 to 17 weeks after starting therapy in up to 5 percent of patients at higher doses.[700] Significant anemia can be managed by transfusion support, which is required by about 30 percent of patients on higher doses, or with recombinant erythropoietin in patients with low endogenous levels.[701]

Severe headache, nausea, insomnia, and myalgia occur commonly during initiation of zidovudine therapy,[702] but these symptoms often resolve or diminish despite continued use. Other side effects include nail pigmentation,[703] myopathy, CNS toxicities, and, uncommonly, hepatitis, esophageal ulceration, or macular edema. Neurologic syndromes include seizures, acute meningitis after drug cessation, Wernicke's encephalopathy, and a late-onset polymyositis-like illness.[704–709] Myopathy associated with weakness, pain, increased creatine phosphokinase values, an unusual mitochondrial morphology,[708–710] and, less often, cardiomyopathy[711] have been associated with prolonged zidovudine use. Myopathy occurs in up to 6 percent of those treated for more than 6 months but usually resolves slowly after drug cessation.[712] Instances of severe lactic acidosis and hepatomegaly with steatosis, particularly in obese women, have also been described.[713,714] Acute overdose of zidovudine causes CNS depression but apparently no severe marrow toxicity.[715]

Except for instances of anemia and growth retardation, excess fetal morbidity has not been recognized in the offspring of pregnant women treated with zidovudine.[716] However, the teratogenicity of the compound is uncertain, and safety in pregnancy remains to be fully established. Zidovudine is mutagenic in vitro and tumor-promoting and embryotoxic in rodents.

Clinical Studies

Zidovudine is currently the initial agent of choice for treatment of HIV infection in patients with CD4 counts less than 500/mm³.[642,697–699] In AIDS and ARC patients, zidovudine is associated with prolonged survival, weight gain and improved functional status, transient increases in CD4 counts, return of cutaneous delayed-type hypersensitivity reactivity and other cell-mediated immune responses in some patients, improved response to pneumococcal vaccine, and significant decreases in serum HIV p24 core antigen levels as early as 4 weeks.[717–721] Although treatment may reduce viral titers in blood, treated-patients must be regarded as infectious. Follow-up of the cohorts in the initial zidovudine placebo-controlled trial found an 18-month survival rate of approximately 50 percent in AIDS patients and of approximately 80 percent in advanced ARC patients compared with 9 months overall survival of 50 percent in the placebo only group.[718] Doses of 500–600 mg/day are at least as effective and significantly less toxic than doses of 1200 mg/day and above.[699] Doses of 300 mg/day have clinical and antiviral effects similar to those at higher doses, whereas a dose of 150 mg/day appears to have suboptimal anti-HIV affects.[638,722] Doses of 180 mg/m²/day are effective in children with advanced disease,[723] but it is uncertain whether lower doses are effective in CNS disease.

Zidovudine treatment has been shown to slow CD4 decline and delay progression to AIDS in early symptomatic and in asymptomatic HIV-infected patients with less than 500 CD4 lymphocytes/mm³.[697,698,724–726] However, early treatment of such patients does not appear to improve overall survival.[724,725] In asymptomatic patients with CD4 counts below 500/mm³, zidovudine at 500 mg/day decreases the risk of progression to advanced ARC or AIDS-defining illness by about twofold compared with placebo at 1 year.[697] For those with counts from 300–500/mm³, the duration of benefit extends over 2 years but is about 18 months for those with counts less than 300/mm³.[697] One observational study found reduced rates of progression through 24 months and decreased mortality through 18 months of therapy,[727] whereas a prospective trial of early vs. late therapy found no difference in outcome after 3 years of follow-up.[725] Another trial in asymptomatic patients with CD4 counts less than 400/mm³ found that zidovudine (500 mg bid) reduced the probability of disease progression by about one-half at two years.[726]

Studies of the clinical effectiveness of various combinations and dosing regimens are in progress.[8,14,15] In patients with AIDS

TABLE 11. Representative New Antiviral Agents of Investigative Interest

Agents	Principal Spectrum	Comments
3TC (lamivudine)	HIV-1, 2, HBV	Nucleoside reverse transcriptase inhibitor with prolonged intracellular $T_{1/2}$ of triphosphate and good oral bioavailability. Chronic oral use is well tolerated and associated with antiviral effects in chronic hepatitis B.
FTC	HIV1, 2, HBV	Nucleoside reverse transcriptase inhibitor
Nevirapine, atevirdine, BHAPs (U-90152), pyridinones, TIBO derivatives, and others	HIV-1	Non-nucleoside reverse transcriptase inhibitors; rapid emergence of resistance in vitro and in humans; variable cross-resistance among agents; combination studies with other reverse transcriptase inhibitors in progress; dose-limiting skin eruptions
CD4-PE40	HIV-1, 2	*Pseudomonas* exotoxin conjugate with CD4 for iv administration
Ro 31-8959, A80987, L735, 524, and others	HIV-1, 2	Protease inhibitors with better oral bioavailability and longer plasma $T_{1/2\,elim}$; active in chronically infected cells; resistance emergence occurs in vitro and in humans
Ro-24-7429	HIV-1, 2	TAT inhibitor; active in chronically infected cells; modest effects in clinical trials
BW882C87	VZV	Nucleoside analog with good oral bioavailability
HPMPC	CMV, HSV, VZV	Nucleoside analog not dependent on viral TK; prolonged intracellular $T_{1/2}$; active against some acyclovir-resistant HSV and ganciclovir-resistant CMV strains; IV dosing associated with nephrotoxicity; probenecid reduces risk of renal dysfunction; topical formulation also under study.
Fialuridine (FIAU)	HBV, herpesviruses	Nucleoside analog; IV administration associated with inhibition of HBV markers. Associated with severe hepatotoxicity and lactic acidosis
Afovirsen (ISIS 2105)	Papillomavirus	Antisense phosphorotioate oligonucleotide for intralesional injection of genital warts
PMEA	HIV, herpesviruses, HBV	Acyclic nucleotide analog of adenine; IV dosing associated with antiretroviral effects and with neutropenia.

and advanced ARC, the addition of high-dose oral acyclovir to zidovudine at 250 mg/6 h reduces the incidence of herpesvirus infections other than those due to cytomegalovirus and may have increased survival time in one study, but does not decrease the frequency of new AIDS-defining events, increase CD4 counts, or decrease p24 antigen levels compared with monotherapy.[81,728] Combinations of zidovudine with zalcitabine or didanosine appear to be associated with CD4 increases that are in some cases greater and more sustained than those seen with monotherapy.[290a,624,641]

Zidovudine treatment may benefit HIV-associated neurologic disease, thrombocytopenia, psoriasis, and lymphocytic interstitial pneumonia.[681,729–732] Objective improvements in dementia and peripheral neuropathy are apparent within 8 weeks, and up to one-half of patients show sustained neurologic improvement 5–10 months after starting therapy.[681] Rebounds in serum and cerebrospinal fluid p24 antigen levels and development of acute, self-limited meningoencephalitis have occurred shortly after zidovudine dose reductions.[707] Higher doses (1000 mg/day) may be more effective than lower ones in achieving and maintaining platelet responses.[732]

The efficacy of zidovudine for postexposure prophylaxis is unestablished, and anecdotal reports of failures have appeared.[702,733,734] High-dose therapy in primary infection is not associated with clinical benefit compared with historical controls[735] but further studies are in progress. Administration of zidovudine to pregnant women during the second and third trimesters and at delivery and to infants for 6 weeks post delivery reduces neonatal infection risk from 25.5 percent to 8.3 percent (ACTG 076).

AGENTS OF INVESTIGATIVE INTEREST

A large number of viral infections exist for which no effective antiviral treatment is available, either because of a lack of an agent with sufficient potency and selectivity or because active viral replication may not be central to the pathogenesis of disease manifestations. Many current agents have problems with drug-related toxicities, poor oral bioavailability, and/or high cost. Although several current antiviral agents can suppress reactivations of infection, none can eradicate viral latency. Gene inhibition therapy (e.g., antisense oligonucleotides, ribozymes) may be able to accomplish this goal,[736,737] but the feasability of this approach remains to be established.

Current investigation is focused heavily on antiretroviral agents,[8,734] and a substantial number of candidate antiviral agents are in clinical trials (Table 11). In addition to agents with improved pharmacokinetic properties, greater potency, or improved toxicity profiles, the use of drug combinations is receiving greater emphasis.[14,15] The areas in which advances are likely to provide more effective treatments include the identification of new viral targets (e.g., virus-specific enzymes or regulatory proteins); new drug delivery techniques to improve pharmacokinetic properties or target particular tissues; the use of agents to modulate the effects of immunopathologic responses or host inflammatory mediators; and the use of immunomodulators or specific immunotherapies (e.g., monoclonal antibodies, therapeutic vaccines).

REFERENCES

1. Newton AA. Tissue culture methods for assessing antivirals and their harmful effects. In: Field HJ, ed. Antiviral Agents: The Development and Assessment of Antiviral Chemotherapy. v. I. Boca Raton, FL: CRC Press; 1988; 23–67.
2. Japour AJ, Mayers DL, Johnson VA, et al. Standardized peripheral blood mononuclear cell culture assay for determination of drug susceptibilities of clinical human immunodeficiency virus type 1 isolates. Antimicrob Agents Chemother. 1993;37:1095–101.
3. Heagy W, Crumpacker C, Lopez PA, et al. Inhibition of immune functions by antiviral drugs. J Clin Invest. 1991;87:1916–24.
4. Lafferty WE, Brewer LA, Corey L. Alteration of lymphocyte transformation response to herpes simplex virus infection by acyclovir therapy. Antimicrob Agents Chemother. 1984;26:887–91.
5. Rubin RH, Tolkoff-Rubin NE. Minireview. Antimicrobial strategies in the care of organ transplant recipients. Antimicrob Agents Chemother. 1993;37:619–24.
6. Gold D, Corey L. Minireview. Acyclovir prophylaxis for herpes simplex virus infection. Antimicrob Agents Chemother. 1987;31:361–7.
7. Steele RW, Charlton RK. Immune modulators as antiviral agents. In: WL Drew, ed. Clinics in Laboratory Medicine. v. 7. Philadelphia: WB Saunders; 1987:911–24.
8. Connolly KJ, Hammer SM. Minireview. Antiretroviral therapy: Strategies beyond single-agent reverse transcriptase inhibition. Antimicrob Agents Chemother. 1992;36:509–20.
9. Field AK, Biron KK. "The end of innocence" revisited: Resistance of herpes viruses to antiviral drugs. Clin Microbiol Rev. 1994;7:1–13.
10. Chatis PA, Crumpacker CS. Minireview. Resistance of herpesviruses to antiviral drugs. Antimicrob Agents Chemother. 1992;36:1589–95.
11. Richman DD. Minireview. Resistance of clinical isolates of HIV to antiretroviral agents. Antimicrob Agents Chemother. 1993;37:1207–13.
12. Hayden FG, Couch RB. Clinical and epidemiologic importance of influenza A viruses resistant to amantadine and rimantadine. Rev Med Virol. 1992;2:89–96.
13. Sommadossi JP. Nucleoside analogs: Similarities and differences. Clin Infect Dis. 1993;16:S7–15.
14. Caliendo AM, Hirsch MS. Combination therapy for infection due to human immunodeficiency virus type 1. Clin Infect Dis. 1994;18:516–24.
15. McLeod GX, Hammer SM. Nucleoside analogues: Combination therapy. Hosp Pract. 1992;27(Suppl 2):14–25.

16. Chow YK, Hirsch MS, Merrill DP, et al. Use of evolutionary limitations of HIV-1 multidrug resistance to optimize therapy. Nature. 1993;361:650–4.

17. Whitley RJ, Gnann JW, Jr. Acyclovir: A decade later. N Engl J Med. 1992; 327:782–9.

18. Biron KK, Elion GB. In vitro susceptibility of varicella-zoster virus to acyclovir. Antimicrob Agents Chemother. 1980;18:443–7.

19. Colby BM, Shaw JE, Elion GB, et al. Effect of acyclovir [9-(2-hydroxyethoxy-ymethyl) guanine] on Epstein-Barr virus DNA replication. J Virol. 1980;34: 560–8.

20. Lin J-C, Smith MC, Cheng YC, et al. Epstein-Barr virus: Inhibition of replication by three new drugs. Science. 1983;221:578–9.

21. Lang DJ, Cheung K-S. Effectiveness of acycloguanosine and trifluorothymidine as inhibitors of cytomegalovirus infection in vitro. Am J Med. 1982; 73(Suppl):49–53.

22. Kern ER. Acyclovir treatment of experimental genital herpes simplex virus infections. Am J Med. 1982;73(Suppl):100–8.

23. Collins P, Oliver NM. Acyclovir treatment of cutaneous herpes in guinea pigs and herpes encephalitis in mice. Am J Med. 1982;73(Suppl):96–9.

24. Soike KF, Gerone PJ. Acyclovir in the treatment of simian varicella virus infection of the African green monkey. Am J Med. 1982;73(Suppl):112–7.

25. Besser R, Kramer G, Rambow A, et al. Combined therapy with acyclovir and adenosine arabinoside in herpes simplex encephalitis. Eur Neurol. 1987; 27:197–200.

26. Schinazi RF, Peters J, Williams CC, et al. Effect of combinations of acyclovir with vidarabine or its 5′-monophosphate on herpes simplex viruses in cell culture and in mice. Antimicrob Agents Chemother. 1982;22:499–507.

27. Steele RW, Marmer DJ, Keeney RE. Comparative in vitro immunotoxicology of acyclovir and other antiviral agents. Infect Immun. 1980;28:957–62.

28. McGuffin RW, Shiota FM, Meyers JD. Lack of toxicity of acyclovir to granulocyte progenitor cells in vitro. Antimicrob Agents Chemother. 1980;10: 471–3.

29. Levin MJ, Leary PL, Arbeit RD. Effect of acyclovir on the proliferation of human fibroblasts and peripheral blood mononuclear cells. Antimicrob Agents Chemother. 1980;17:947–53.

30. Wingard JR, Hess AD, Stuart RK, et al. Effect of several antiviral agents on human lymphocyte functions and marrow progenitor cell proliferation. Antimicrob Agents Chemother. 1983;23:593–7.

31. Elion GB. History, mechanism of action, spectrum and selectivity of nucleoside analogs. In: Mills J, Corey L, eds. Antiviral Chemotherapy: New Directions for Clinical Application and Research. New York: Elsevier; 1986: 118–37.

32. Derse D, Cheng Y-C, Furman PA, et al. Inhibition of purified human and herpes simplex virus–induced DNA polymerases by 9-(2-hydroxyethoxymethyl)granine triphosphate. J Biol Chem. 1981;256:11447–51.

33. Furman PA, St. Clair MH, Spector T. Acyclovir triphosphate is a suicidal inactivator of the herpes simplex virus DNA polymerase. J Biol Chem. 1984; 259:9575–9.

34. Pagano JS, Datta AK. Perspectives on interactions of acyclovir with Epstein-Barr and other herpes viruses. Am J Med 1982;73(Suppl):18–26.

35. Parris DS, Harrington JE. Herpes simplex virus variants resistant to high concentrations of acyclovir exist in clinical isolates. Antimicrob Agents Chemother. 1982;22:71–7.

36. Hill EL, Hunter GA, Ellis MN. In vitro and in vivo characterization of herpes simplex virus clinical isolates recovered from patients infected with human immunodeficiency virus. Antimicrob Agents Chemother. 1991;35:2322–8.

37. Nugier F, Colin JN, Aymard M, et al. Occurrence and characterization of acyclovir resistant herpes simplex virus isolates: report on a two-year sensitivity screening survey. J Med Virol. 1992;36:1–12.

38. Ellis MN, Keller PM, Fyfe JA, et al. Clinical isolates of herpes simplex virus type 2 that induces a thymidine kinase with altered substrate specificity. Antimicrob Agents Chemother. 1987;31:1117–25.

39. Parker AC, Craig JIO, Collins P, et al. Acyclovir-resistant herpes simplex virus infection due to altered DNA polymerase. Lancet. 1987;2:1461.

40. Sacks SL, Wanklin RJ, Reece DE, et al. Progressive esophagitis from acyclovir-resistant herpes simplex. Ann Intern Med. 1989;111:893–9.

41. Kost RG, Hill EL, Tigges M, Straus SE. Brief report: Recurrent acyclovir-resistant genital herpes in an immunocompetent patient. N Engl J Med. 1993; 329:1777–82.

42. Collins P. Viral sensitivity following the introduction of acyclovir. Am J Med. 1988;85(Suppl 2A):129–34.

43. Straus SE, Takiff HE, Seidlin M, et al. Suppression of frequently recurring genital herpes. N Engl J Med. 1984;310:1545–50.

44. Lehrman SN, Douglas JM, Corey L, et al. Recurrent genital herpes and suppressive oral acyclovir therapy. Ann Intern Med. 1986;104:786–90.

45. Erlich KS, Mills J, Chatis P, et al. Acyclovir-resistant herpes simplex virus infections in patients with acquired immunodeficiency syndrome. N Engl J Med. 1989;320:293–6.

46. Wade JC, McLaren C, Myers JD. Frequency and significance of acyclovir-resistant herpes simplex virus isolated from marrow transplant patients receiving multiple courses of treatment with acyclovir. J Infect Dis. 1983;148: 1077.

47. Norris SA, Kessler HA, Fife KH. Severe, progressive herpetic whitlow caused by an acyclovir-resistant virus in a patient with AIDS. J Infect Dis. 1988;157:209–10.

48. Gateley A, Gander RM, Johnson PC, et al. Herpes simplex virus type 2 meningoencephalitis resistant to acyclovir in a patient with AIDS. J Infect Dis. 1990;161:711–5.

49. Ljungman P, Ellis MN, Hackman RC, et al. Acyclovir-resistant herpes simplex virus causing pneumonia after marrow transplantation. J Infect Dis. 1990;162:244–8.

50. Sonkin PL, Baratz KH, Frothingham R, et al. Acyclovir-resistant herpes simplex virus keratouveitis after penetrating keratoplasty. Ophthalmology. 1992;99:1805–8.

51. Englund JA, Zimmerman ME, Swierkosz EM, et al. Herpes simplex virus resistant to acyclovir. A study in a tertiary care center. Ann Intern Med. 1990;112:416–22.

52. Safrin S, Assaykeen T, Follansbee S, et al. Foscarnet therapy for acyclovir-resistant mucocutaneous herpes simplex virus infection in 26 AIDS patients: Preliminary data. J Infect Dis. 1990;161:1078–84.

53. Safrin S, Crumpacker CS, Chatis P, et al. A randomized comparison of foscarnet versus vidarabine for treatment of acyclovir-resistant mucocutaneous herpes simplex in patients with AIDS. N Engl J Med. 1991;325:551–5.

54. Engel JP, Englund JA, Fletcher CV, et al. Treatment of resistant herpes simplex virus with continuous-infusion acyclovir. JAMA. 1990;263:1662–4.

55. Birch CJ, Tachedjian G, Doherty RR, et al. Altered sensitivity to antiviral drugs of herpes simplex virus isolates from a patient with the acquired immunodeficiency syndrome. J Infect Dis. 1990;162:731–4.

56. Birch CJ, Tyssen DP, Tachedjian G, et al. Clinical effects and in vitro studies of trifluorothymidine combined with interferon-α for treatment of drug-resistant and -sensitive herpes simplex viral infections. J Infect Dis. 1992;166: 108–12.

56a.Snoeck R, Andrei G, Gerard M, et al. Successful treatment of progressive mucocutaneous infection due to acyclovir- and foscarnet-resistant herpes simplex virus with (S)-1-(3-hydroxy-2-phosphonylmethoxypropyl) cytosine (HPMPC). Clin Infect Dis. 1994;18:570–8.

57. Cole NL, Balfour HH Jr. Varicella-zoster virus does not become more resistant to acyclovir during therapy. J Infect Dis. 1986;153:605–8.

58. Jacobson MA, Berger TG, Fikrig S. Acyclovir-resistant varicella-zoster virus infection after chronic oral acyclovir therapy in patients with the acquired immunodeficiency syndrome (AIDS). Ann Intern Med. 1990;112:187–91.

59. Snoeck R, Gerard M, Sadzot-Delvaux C et al. Meningoradiculoneuritis due to acyclovir-resistant varicella-zoster virus in a patient with AIDS. J Infect Dis. 1993;168:1330–1.

60. Talarico CL, Phelps WC, Biron KK. Analysis of the thymidine kinase genes from acyclovir-resistant mutants of varicella-zoster virus isolated from patients with AIDS. J Virol. 1993;67:1024–33.

61. Safrin S, Berger TG, Gilson I, et al. Foscarnet therapy in five patients with AIDS and acyclovir-resistant varicella-zoster virus infection. Ann Intern Med. 1991;115:19–21.

62. Blum RM, Liao SHT, de Miranda P. Overview of acyclovir pharmacokinetic disposition in adults and children. Am J Med 1982;73(Suppl):186–92.

63. Laskin OL. Clinical pharmacokinetics of acyclovir. Clin Pharmacol 1983;8: 187–201.

64. Van Dyke RB, Connor JD, Wyborny C, et al. Pharmacokinetics of orally administered acyclovir in patients with herpes progenitalis. Am J Med 1982; 73(Suppl):172–5.

65. McKendrick MW, McGill JI, White JE, et al. Oral acyclovir in acute herpes zoster. Br Med J. 1986;293:1529–32.

66. Wade JC, Newton B, Flournoy N, et al. Oral acyclovir for prevention of herpes simplex virus reactivation after bone marrow transplantation. Ann Intern Med. 1984;100:823–8.

67. Sullender WM, Arvin AM, Diaz PS, et al. Pharmacokinetics of acyclovir suspension in infants and children. Antimicrob Agents Chemother. 1987;31: 1722–6.

68. Nusinoff-Lehrman S, Smiley L, Szczech, G. Update on acyclovir drugs. In: Mills J, Corey L, eds. Antiviral Chemotherapy, New Directions for Clinical Application and Research. v. 3, 1993. PTR Prentice Hall, Englewood Cliffs, NJ: 97–104.

69. Weller S, Blum MR, Doucette M, et al. Pharmacokinetics of the acyclovir prodrug, valaciclovir, after escalating single- and multiple-dose administration to normal volunteers. Clin Pharmacol Therapeutics. 1993;54:595–605.

70. Peterslund NA, Esmann V, Geil JP, et al. Open study of 2-amino-9-(hydroxyethoxymethyl)-9H-purine (desciclovir) in the treatment of herpes zoster. J Antimicrob Chemother. 1987;20:743–51.

71. Hung SO, Patterson A, Rees PJ. Pharmacokinetics of oral acyclovir (Zovirax) in the eye. Br J Ophthalmol. 1984;68:192–5.

72. Meyer LJ, deMiranda P, Sheth N, et al. Acyclovir in human breast milk. Am J Obstet Gynecol. 1988;158:586–8.

73. Frenkel LM, Brown ZA, Bryson YJ, et al. Pharmacokinetics of acyclovir in the term human pregnancy and neonate. Am J Obstet Gynecol. 1991;164: 569–76.

74. Hintz M, Connor JD, Spector SA, et al. Neonatal acyclovir pharmacokinetics in patients with hepres virus infections. Am J Med. 1982;73(Suppl):210–4.

75. Laskin OL, Longstreth JA, Whelton A, et al. Effect of renal failure on the pharmacokinetics of acyclovir. Am J Med 1982;73(Suppl):197–201.

76. De Miranda P, Good SS, Krasny HC, et al. Metabolic fate of radioactive acyclovir in humans. Am J Med 1982;73(Suppl):215–20.

77. Krasny HC, Liao SHT, de Miranda P, et al. Influence of hemodialysis on acyclovir pharmacokinetics in patients with chronic renal failure. Am J Med. 1982;73(Suppl):202–4.

78. Davenport A, Goel S, Mackenzie JC. Neurotoxicity of acyclovir in patients with end-stage renal failure treated with continuous ambulatory peritoneal dialysis. Am J Kidney Dis. 1992;20:647–9.

79. Boelaert J, Schurgers M, Daneels R. Multiple dose pharmacokinetics of intravenous acyclovir in patients on continuous ambulatory peritoneal dialysis. J Antimicrob Chemother. 1987;20:69–76.

80. Burgess ED, Gill MJ. Intraperitoneal administration of acyclovir in patients receiving continuous ambulatory peritoneal dialysis. Clin Pharmacol. 1990; 30:997–1000.

81. Cooper DA, Pehrson PO, Pedersen C, et al. The efficacy and safety of zidovudine alone or as cotherapy with acyclovir for the treatment of patients with AIDS and AIDS-related complex: A double-blind, randomized trial. AIDS. 1993;7:197–207.

82. Keeney RE, Kirk LE, Bridgen D. Acyclovir tolerance in humans. Am J Med. 1982;73(Suppl):176–81.

83. Sylvester RK, Ogden WB, Draxler CA, et al. Vesicular eruption. JAMA. 986;255:385–6.

84. Wade JC, Meyers JD: Neurologic symptoms associated with parenteral acyclovir treatment after marrow transplantation. Ann Intern Med. 1983;98: 921–5.

85. Bean B, Aeppli D. Adverse effects of high-dose intravenous acyclovir in ambulatory patients with acute herpes zoster. J Infect Dis. 1985;151:362–4.

86. Feldman S, Rodman J, Gregory B. Excessive serum concentrations of acyclovir and neurotoxicity. J Infect Dis. 1988;157:385–8.

87. Haefeli WE, RAZ Schoenenberger, P Weiss, et al. Acyclovir-induced neurotoxicity: Concentration-side effect relationship in acyclovir overdose. Am J Med. 1993;94:212–5.

88. Krieble BF, Rudy DW, Glick MR, et al. Case report: Acyclovir neurotoxicity and nephrotoxicity-the role for hemodialysis. Am J Med Sci. 1993;305:36–9.

89. Potter JL, Krill CE. Acyclovir crystalluria. Pediatr Infect Dis. 1986;5:710–2.

90. Sawyer MH, Webb DE, Balow JE, et al. Acyclovir-induced renal failure: Clinical course and histology. Am J Med 1988;84:1067–71.

91. Rashed A, Azadeh B, Romeh SHA. Acyclovir-induced acute tubulointerstitial nephritis. Nephron. 1990;56:436–8.

92. Goldberg LH, Kaufman R, Kurtz TO, et al. Long-term suppression of recurrent genital herpes with acyclovir. Arch Dermatol. 1993;129:582–7.

93. Clive D, Corey L, Reichman RC, et al. A double-blind, placebo-controlled cytogenetic study of oral acyclovir in patients with recurrent genital herpes. J Infect Dis. 1991;164:753–7.

94. Douglas JM Jr, Davis LG, Remington ML, et al. A double-blind, placebo-controlled trial of chronically administered oral acyclovir on sperm production in men with frequently occurring genital herpes. J Infect Dis. 1988;157: 588–93.

95. Centers for Disease Control and prevention. Pregnancy outcomes following systemic prenatal acyclovir exposure—June 1, 1984–June 30, 1993. MMWR 1993;42:806–9.

96. Whitley RJ, Alford CA, Hirsch MS, et al. Vidarabine versus acyclovir therapy in herpes simplex encephalitis. N Engl J Med. 1986;314:144–9.

97. Skoldenberg B, Alestig K, Burman L, et al. Acyclovir versus vidarabine in herpes simplex encephalitis. Lancet. 1984;2:706–11.

98. Feldman S, Lott L. Varicella in children with cancer: Impact of antiviral therapy and prophylaxis. Pediatrics. 1987;80:465–72.

99. Shepp DH, Dandliker PS, Meyers JD. Treatment of varicella-zoster virus infection in severely immunocompromised patients. N Engl J Med. 1986; 314:208–12.

100. Whitley R, Arvin A, Prober C, et al. A controlled trial comparing vidarabine with acyclovir in neonatal herpes simplex virus infection. N Engl J Med. 1991;324:444–9.

101. Corey L, Fife KH, Benedetti JK, et al. Intravenous acyclovir for the treatment of primary genital herpes. Ann Intern Med. 1983;98:914–21.

102. Bryson YJ, Dillon M, Lovett M, et al. Treatment of first episodes of genital herpes simplex virus infection with oral acyclovir. N Engl J Med. 1983;308: 916–21.

103. Corey L, Nahmias AJ, Guinan ME, et al. A trial of topical acyclovir in genital herpes simplex virus infections. N Engl J Med. 1982;306:1313–9.

104. Mindel A, Adler MW. Intravenous acyclovir treatment for primary genital herpes. Lancet. 1982;1:697–700.

105. Nilsen AE, Aasen T. Efficacy of oral acyclovir in the treatment of initial and recurrent genital herpes. Lancet. 1982;2:571–3.

105a.Wald A, Benedetti J, Davis G, et al. A randomized, double-blind, comparative trial comparing high- and standard-dose oral acyclovir for first-episode genital herpes infections. Antimicrob Agents Chemother. 1994;38:174–6.

106. Bernstein DI, Lovett MA, Bryson YJ. The effects of acyclovir on antibody response to herpes simplex virus in primary genital infections. J Infect Dis. 1984;150:7–13.

107. Rompalo AM, Mertz GJ, Davis LG, et al. Oral acyclovir for treatment of first-episode herpes simplex virus proctitis. JAMA. 1988;259:2879–81.

108. Reichman RC, Badger GJ, Mertz GJ, et al. Treatment of recurrent genital herpes simplex infections with oral acyclovir. A controlled trial. JAMA 1984; 251:2103–07.

109. Luby JP, Gnann JW Jr, Alexander WJ, et al. A collaborative study of patient-initiated treatment of recurrent genital herpes with topical acyclovir or placebo. J Infect Dis 1984;150:1–6.

110. Douglas JM, Critchlow C, Benedetti J, et al. A double-blind study of oral acyclovir for suppression of recurrences of genital herpes simplex virus infection. N Engl J Med. 1984;310:1551–6.

111. Mindel A, Carney O, Freris M, et al. Dosage and safety of long-term suppressive acyclovir therapy for recurrent genital herpes. Lancet. 1988;1:926–8.

112. Straus SE, Seidlin M, Takiff HE, et al. Double-blind comparison of weekend and daily regimens of oral acyclovir for suppression of recurrent genital herpes. Antiviral Res. 1986;6:151–9.

113. Straus SE, Seidlin M, Takiff HE, et al. Effect of oral acyclovir treatment on symptomatic and asymptomatic virus shedding in recurrent genital herpes. Sexually Transmitted Dis 1989;16:107–13.

114. Rooney JF, Felser JM, Ostrove JM, et al. Acquisition of genital herpes from an asymptomatic sexual partner. N Engl J Med. 1986;314:1561–4.

115. Stray-Pedersen B. Acyclovir in late pregnancy to prevent neonatal herpes simplex. Lancet. 1990;2:756.

115a.Haddad J, Langer B, Astruc D, et al. Oral acyclovir and recurrent genital herpes during late pregnancy. Obstet Gynecol. 1993;82:102–4.

116. Rooney JF, Straus SE, Mannix ML, et al. Oral acyclovir to suppress frequently recurrent herpes labialis. Ann Intern Med. 1993;118:268–72.

117. Spruance SL, Hamill ML, Hoge WS, et al. Acyclovir prevents reactivation of herpes simplex labialis in skiers. JAMA. 1988;260:1597–9.

118. Kuzushima K, Kudo T, Kimura H, et al. Prophylactic oral acyclovir in outbreaks of primary herpes simplex virus type 1 infection in a closed community. Pediatrics. 1992;89:379–83.

119. Spruance SL, Schnipper LE, Overall JC Jr, et al. Treatment of herpes simplex labialis with topical acyclovir in polyethylene glycol. J Infect Dis. 1982; 146:85.

120. Kinghorn GR, Turner EB, Barton IG, et al. Efficacy of topical acyclovir cream in first and recurrent episodes of genital herpes. Antiviral Res. 1983; 3:291.

121. Spruance SL, Stewart JCB, Rowe NH, et al. Treatment of recurrent herpes simplex labialis with oral acyclovir. J Infect Dis. 1990;161:185–90.

122. Gill MJ, Bryant HE. Oral acyclovir therapy of recurrent herpes simplex virus type 2 infection of the hand. Antimicrob Agents Chemother. 1991;35:382–3.

123. Saral R, Burns WH, Laskin OL, et al. Acyclovir prophylaxis of herpes-simplex-virus infections. N Engl J Med. 1981;305:63–7.

124. Lundgren G, Wilczek H, Lonnqvist B, et al. Acyclovir prophylaxis in bone marrow transplant recipients. Scand J Infect Dis. 1985;47:137–44.

125. Gluckman E, Devergie A, Melo R, et al. Prophylaxis of herpes infections after bone marrow transplantation by oral acyclovir. Lancet. 1983;2:706–8.

126. Seale L, Jones CJ, Kathpalia S, et al. Prevention of herpesvirus infections in renal allograft recipients by low-dose oral acyclovir. JAMA 1985;254:3435–8.

127. Straus S, Seidlin M, Takiff H, et al. Oral acyclovir to suppress recurrent herpes simplex virus infections in immunodeficient patients. Ann Intern Med. 1984;100:522.

128. Saral R, Ambinder RF, Burns WH, et al. Acyclovir prophylaxis against herpes simplex virus infection in patients with leukemia. Ann Intern Med. 1983;99:773.

129. Wade JC, Newton B, McLaren C, et al. Intravenous acyclovir to treat mucocutaneous herpes simplex infection after marrow transplantation. Ann Intern Med. 1982;96:265.

130. Shepp DH, Newton BA, Dandliker PS, et al. Oral acyclovir therapy for mucocutaneous herpes simplex infections in immunocompromised marrow transplant recipients. Ann Intern Med. 1985;102:783–5.

131. Klein NA, Mabie WC, Shaver DC, et al. Herpes simplex virus hepatitis in pregnancy. Two patients successfully treated with acyclovir. Gastroenterology 1991;100:239–44.

132. Kusne S, Schwartz M, Breinig MK, et al. Herpes simplex virus hepatitis after solid organ transplantation in adults. J Infect Dis. 1991;163:1001–7.

133. Kimura H, Aso K, Kuzushima K, et al. Relapse of herpes simplex encephalitis in children. Pediatrics. 1992;89:891–4.

134. Gutman LT, Wilfert CM, Eppes S. Herpes simplex virus encephalitis in children: Analysis of cerebrospinal fluid and progressive neurodevelopmental deterioration. J Infect Dis. 1986;154:415–21.

135. VanLandingham KE, Marsteller HB, Ross GW, et al. Relapse of herpes simplex encephalitis after conventional acyclovir therapy. JAMA 1988;259: 1051–3.

136. Palay DA, Sternberg P, Davis J, et al. Decrease in the risk of bilateral acute retinal necrosis by acyclovir therapy. Am J Ophthalmol. 1991;112:250–5.

137. Boyd K, Walker E. Use of acyclovir to treat chickenpox in pregnancy. Br Med J. 1988;296:393–4.

138. Johns DR, Gress DR. Rapid response to acyclovir in herpes zoster-associated encephalitis. Am J Med. 1987;82:560–2.

139. Haake DA, Zakowski PC, Haake DL, et al. Early treatment with acyclovir for varicella pneumonia in otherwise healthy adults: Retrospective controlled study and review. Rev Infect Dis. 1990;12:788–98.

140. Balfour HH Jr, Bean B, Laskin OL, et al. Acyclovir halts progression of herpes zoster in immunocompromised patients. N Engl J Med. 1983;308: 1448–53.

141. Whitley RJ, Gnann JW Jr, Hinthorn D, et al. Disseminated herpes zoster in the immunocompromised host: A comparative trial of acyclovir and vidarabine. J Infect Dis. 1992;165:450–5.

142. Prober CG, Kirk LE, Keeney RE. Acyclovir therapy of chickenpox in immunosuppressed children—A collaborative study. J Pediatr. 1982;101:622–5.

143. Nyerges G, Meszner Z, Gyarmati E, et al. Acyclovir prevents dissemination of varicella in immunocompromised children. J Infect Dis. 1988;157:309–13.

144. Balfour HH Jr. Intravenous acyclovir therapy for varicella in immunocompromised children. J Pediatr. 1984;104:134–6.

145. Meszner Z, Nyerges G, Bell AR. Oral acyclovir to prevent dissemination of varicella in immunocompromised children. J Infect. 1993;26:9–15.

146. Dunkle LM, Arvin AM, Whitley RJ, et al. A controlled trial of acyclovir for chickenpox in normal children. N Engl J Med. 1991;325:1539–44.

147. Balfour, HH, Rotbart HA, Feldman S, et al. Acyclovir treatment of varicella in otherwise healthy adolescents. J Pediatr 1992;120:627–33.

148. Wallace MR, Bowler WA, Murray NB, et al. Treatment of adult varicella with oral acyclovir. Ann Intern Med. 1992;117:358–63.

149. Committee on Infectious Diseases. The use of oral acyclovir in otherwise healthy children with varicella. Pediatrics. 1993;91:674–6.

150. Al-Nakib W, Al-Kandari S, El-Khalik DMA, et al. A randomized controlled study of intravenous acyclovir (Zovirax) against placebo in adults with chickenpox. J Infect. 1983;6:49–56.

150a. Asano Y, Yoshikawa T, Suga S, et al. Postexposure prophylaxis of varicella in family contact by oral acyclovir. Pediatrics. 1993;92:219–22.

151. McGill J, MacDonald DR, Fall C, et al. Intravenous acyclovir in acute herpes zoster infection. J Infect. 1983;6:157–61.

152. Bean B, Braun C, Balfour HH Jr. Acyclovir therapy for acute herpes zoster. Lancet. 1982;2:118–21.

153. Huff JC, Bean B, Balfour HH Jr, et al. Therapy of herpes zoster with oral acyclovir. Am J Med. 1988;85(Suppl 2A):84–9.

154. Wood MJ, Ogan PH, McKendrick MW, et al. Efficacy of oral acyclovir treatment of acute herpes zoster. Am J Med. 1988;85(Suppl 2A):79–83.

155. Cobo LM, Foulks GN, Liesegang T, et al. Oral acyclovir in the treatment of acute herpes zoster ophthalmicus. Ophthalmology 1986;93:763–70.

156. Wassilew SW, Reimlinger S, Nasemann T, et al. Oral acyclovir for herpes zoster: A double-blind controlled trial in normal subjects. Br J Dermatol. 1987;117:495–501.

157. McKendrick MW, McGill JI, Wood MJ. Lack of effect of acyclovir on postherpetic neuralgia. Br Med J. 1989;298:431.

158. Wood MJ, Johnson RW, McKendrick MW, et al. A randomized trial of acyclovir for 7 days or 21 days with and without prednisolone for treatment of acute herpes zoster. N Engl J Med. 1994;330:896–900.

159. McGill J, Chapman C. A comparison of topical acyclovir with steroids in the treatment of herpes zoster keratouveitis. Br J Ophthalmol. 1983;67:46–50.

160. Balfour HH Jr, Bean B, Mitchell CD, et al. Acyclovir in immunocompromised patients with cytomegalovirus disease. Am J Med. 1982;73(Suppl):241–8.

161. Meyers JD, Reed EC, Shepp DH, et al. Acyclovir for prevention of cytomegalovirus infection and disease after allogeneic marrow transplantation. N Engl J Med. 1988;318:70–5.

162. Vasquez EM, Sanchez J, Pollak R, et al. High-dose oral acyclovir prophylaxis for primary cytomegalovirus infection in seronegative renal allograft recipients. Transplantation. 1993;55:448–50.

163. Stratta RJ, Shaefer MS, Cushing KA, et al. Successful prophylaxis of cytomegalovirus disease after primary CMV exposure in liver transplant recipients. Transplantation. 1991;51:90–7.

164. Legendre C, Ducloux D, Ferroni A, et al. Acyclovir in preventing cytomegalovirus infection in kidney transplant recipients: A case-controlled study. Transplant Proc 1993;25:1431–33.

165. Balfour HH, Chace BA, Stapleton JT, et al. A randomized, placebo-controlled trial of oral acyclovir for the prevention of cytomegalovirus disease in recipients of renal allografts. N Engl J Med. 1989;320:1381–7.

166. Bailey TC, Ethinger NA, Storch GA et al. Failure of high-dose oral acyclovir with or without immune globulin to prevent primary cytomegalovirus disease in recipients of solid organ transplants. Am J Med. 1993;95:273–8.

166a. Singh N, Yu VL, Mieles L, et al. High-dose acyclovir compared with short-course preemptive ganciclovir therapy to prevent cytomegalovirus disease in liver transplant recipients. A randomized trial. Ann Intern Med. 1994;120:375–81.

167. Stratta RJ, Shaefer MS, Cushing KA, et al. A randomized prospective trial of acyclovir and immune globulin prophylaxis in liver transplant recipients receiving OKT3 therapy. Arch Surg. 1992;127:55–64.

168. Bailey TC, Trulock EP, Ettinger NA, et al. Failure of prophylactic ganciclovir to prevent cytomegalovirus disease in recipients of lung transplants. J Infect Dis. 1991;165:788–92.

169. Andersson J, Britton S, Ernberg I, et al. Effect of acyclovir on infectious mononucleosis: a double-blind, placebo-controlled study. J Infect Dis. 1986;153:283–90.

170. Van der Horst C, Joncas J, Ahronheim G, et al. Lack of effect of peroral acyclovir for the treatment of acute infectious mononucleosis. J Infect Dis. 1991;164:788–92.

171. Straus SE, Dale JK, Tobi M, et al. Acyclovir treatment of the chronic fatigue syndrome: Lack of efficacy in a placebo-controlled trial. N Engl J Med. 1988;319:1692–8.

172. Schooley RT, Carey RW, Miller G, et al. Chronic Epstein-Barr virus infection associated with fever and interstitial pneumonia. Ann Intern Med. 1986;104:636–43.

173. Hanto DW, Frizzera G, Gajl-Peczalska KJ, et al. Epstein-Barr virus-induced B-cell lymphoma after renal transplantation. N Engl J Med. 1982;306:913–8.

174. Sullivan JL, Bryon KS, Brewster FE, et al. Treatment of life-threatening Epstein-Barr virus infections with acyclovir. Am J Med. 1982;73(Suppl):262–6.

175. Resnick L, Herbst JS, Ablashi DV, et al. Regression of oral hairy leukoplakia after orally administered acyclovir therapy. JAMA. 1988;259:384–5.

176. Alexander GJM, Fagan EA, Hegarty JE, et al. Controlled clinical trial of acyclovir in chronic hepatitis B virus infection. J Med Virol. 1987;21:81–7.

177. Berk L, Schalm SW, de Man RA, et al. Failure of acyclovir to enhance the antiviral effect of α lymphoblastoid interferon on HBe-seroconversion in chronic hepatitis B. J Hepatol. 1992;14:305–9.

178. Oxford JS, Galbraith A. Antiviral activity of amantadine: A review of laboratory and clinical data. Pharmacol Ther. 1980;11:181.

179. Hayden FG, Cote KM, Douglas RG Jr. Plaque inhibition assay for drug susceptibility testing of influenza viruses. Antimicrob Agents Chemother. 1980;17:865–70.

180. Browne MJ, Moss MY, Boyd MR. Comparative activity of amantadine and ribavirin against influenza virus in vitro: Possible clinical relevance. Antimicrob Agents Chemother. 1983;23:503–5.

181. Burlington DB, Meiklejohn G, Mostow SR. Anti-influenza A virus activity of amantadine hydrochloride and rimantadine hydrochloride in ferret tracheal ciliated epithelium. Antimicrob Agents Chemother. 1982;21:794–9.

182. Belshe RB, Burk B, Newman F, et al. Resistance of influenza virus to amantadine and rimantadine: Results of one decade of surveillance. J Infect Dis. 1989;159:430–5.

183. Couch RB, Six HR. The antiviral spectrum and mechanism of action of amantadine and rimantadine. In: Mills J, Corey L, eds. Antiviral Chemotherapy: New Directions for Clinical Application and Research. New York: Elsevier, 1986;50–7.

184. Koff WC, Elm JL Jr, Halstead SB. Inhibition of dengue virus replication by amantadine hydrochloride. Antimicrob Agents Chemother. 1980;18:125–9.

185. Hayden FG. Animal models of influenza virus infection for evaluation of antiviral agents. In: Zak O, Sande MA, eds. Experimental Models in Antiviral Chemotherapy. v. 3. London: Academic Press; 1986:353–71.

186. Wilson SZ, Knight V, Wyde PR, et al. Amantadine and ribavirin aerosol treatment of influenza A and B infection in mice. Antimicrob Agents Chemother. 1980;17:642–8.

187. Hayden FG. Combinations of antiviral agents for treatment of influenza virus infections. J Antimicrob Chemother. 1986;18(Suppl B):177–83.

188. Zhirnov OP. High protection of animals lethally infected with influenza virus by aprotinin-rimantadine combination. J Med Virol. 1987;21:161–7.

189. Hay AJ. The action of adamantanamines against influenza A viruses: Inhibition of the M2 ion channel protein. Semin Virol. 1992;3:21–30.

190. Pinto LH, Holsinger LJ, Lamb RA. Influenza virus M2 protein has ion channel activity. Cell. 1992;69:517–28.

191. Grambas S, Hay AJ. Maturation of influenza A virus hemagglutinin—Estimates of the pH encountered during transport and its regulation by the M2 protein. Virology. 1992;190:11–18.

192. Duff KC, Ashley RH. The transmembrane domain of influenza A M2 protein forms amantadine-sensitive proton channels in planar lipid bilayers. Virology. 1992;190:485–9.

193. Richman DD, Yazaki P, Hostetler KY. The intracellular distribution and antiviral activity of amantadine. Virology. 1981;112:81–90.

194. Richman DD, Hostetler KY, Yazaki PJ, et al. Fate of influenza A virion proteins after entry into subcellular fractions of LLC cells and the effect of amantadine. Virology. 1986;151:200–10.

195. Webster RG, Kawaoka Y, Bean WJ, et al. Chemotherapy and vaccination: A possible strategy for the control of highly virulent influenza virus. J Virol. 1985;55:173–6.

196. Bean WJ, Threlkeld SC, Webster RG. Biologic potential of amantadine-resistant influenza A virus in an avian model. J Infect Dis. 1989;159:1050–6.

197. Belshe RB, Smith MH, Hall CB, et al. Genetic basis of resistance to rimantadine emerging during treatment of influenza virus infection. J Virol. 1988;62:1508–12.

198. Hayden FG, Belshe RB, Clover RD, et al. Emergence and apparent transmission of rimantadine-resistant influenza A virus in families. N Engl J Med. 1989;321:1696–702.

199. Mast EE, Harmon MW, Gravenstein S, et al. Emergence and possible transmission of amantadine-resistant viruses during nursing home outbreaks of influenza. Am J Epidemiol. 1991;134:988–97.

200. Degelau J, Somani SK, Cooper SL, et al. Amantadine-resistant influenza A in a nursing facility. Arch Intern Med. 1992;152:390–2.

201. Hayden FG, Sperber SJ, Belshe RB, et al. Recovery of drug-resistant influenza A virus during therapeutic use of rimantadine. Antimicrob Agents Chemother. 1991;35:1741–7.

202. Hayden FG, Minocha A, Spyker DA, et al. Comparative single-dose pharmacokinetics of amantadine hydrochloride and rimantadine hydrochloride in young and elderly adults. Antimicrob Agents Chemother. 1985;28:216–221.

203. Aoki FY, Sitar DS. Amantadine kinetics in healthy elderly men: Implications for influenza prevention. Clin Pharmacol Ther. 1985;37:137–44.

204. Aoki FY, Sitar DS. Clinical pharmacokinetics of amantadine hydrochloride. Clin Pharmacokinet 1988;14:35–51.

205. Tominack RL, Hayden FG. Rimantadine hydrochloride and amantadine hydrochloride use in influenza A virus infections. In: Moellering RC, Knight V, Gilbert BE, eds. Infectious Disease Clinics of North America. Philadelphia: WB Saunders, 1987;1:459–78.

206. Fishaut M, Mostow S. Amantadine for severe influenza A pneumonia in infancy. Am J Dis Child. 1980;134:321.

207. Horadam VW, Sharp JG, Smilack JD, et al. Pharmacokinetics of amantadine hydrochloride in subjects with normal and impaired renal function. Ann Intern Med. 1981;94:454–8.

208. Soung L-S, Ing TS, Daugirdas JT, et al. Amantadine hydrochloride pharmacokinetics in hemodialysis patients. Ann Intern Med. 1980;93:46–9.

209. Wills RJ, Choma N, Buonpane G, et al. Relative bioavailability of rimantadine HCl tablet and syrup formulations in healthy subjects. J Pharmacol Sci. 1987;76:886–8.

210. Wills RJ, Rodriguez LC, Choma N, et al. Influence of a meal on the bioavailability of rimantadine HCl. J Clin Pharmacol. 1987;27:821–3.

211. Wills RJ, Farolino DA, Choma N, et al. Rimantadine pharmacokinetics after single and multiple doses. Antimicrob Agents Chemother. 1987;31:826–8.

212. Nahata MC, Brady MT. Serum concentrations and safety of rimantadine in paediatric patients. Eur J Clin Pharmacol. 1986;30:719–22.

213. Anderson EL, Van Voris LP, Bartram J, et al. Pharmacokinetics of a single dose of rimantadine in young adults and children. Antimicrob Agents Chemother. 1987;31:1140–2.

214. Tominack RL, Wills RJ, Gustavson LE, et al. Multiple-dose pharmacokinetics of rimantadine in elderly adults. Antimicrob Agents Chemother. 1988; 32:1813–9.

215. Patriarca PA, Kater NA, Kendal AP. Safety of prolonged administration of rimantadine hydrochloride in the prophylaxis of influenza A infections in nursing homes. Antimicrob Agents Chemother. 1984;26:101–3.

216. Capparelli EV, Stevens RC, Chow MSS. Rimantadine pharmacokinetics in healthy subjects and patients with end stage renal failure. Clin Pharmacol Ther. 1988;43:536–41.

217. Wills RJ, Belshe R, Tomlinsin D, et al. Pharmacokinetics of rimantadine hydrochloride in patients with chronic liver disease. Clin Pharmacol Ther. 1987;42:449–54.

218. Speeg KV, Leighton JA, Maldonado AL. Case report: toxic delirium in a patient taking amantadine and trimethoprim-sulfamethoxazole. Am J Med Sci. 1989;298:410–2.

219. Willis RJ. Update on rimantadine's clinical pharmacokinetics. J Resp Dis. 1989;10(Suppl 10A):520–5.

220. Soo W. Adverse effects of rimantadine: Summary from clinical trials. J Resp Dis. 1989;10(Suppl 12A):526–31.

221. Sartori M, Pratt CM, Young JB. Malignant cardiac arrhythmia induced by amantadine poisoning. Am J Med. 1984;77:388–91.

222. Pimentel L, Hughes B. Amantadine toxicity presenting with complex ventricular extopy and hallucinations. Pediatr Emerg Care. 1991;7:89–92.

223. Atkinson WL, Arden NH, Patriarca PA, et al. Amantadine prophylaxis during an institutional outbreak of type A (H1N1) influenza. Arch Intern Med. 1986;146:1751–6.

224. Nestelbaum Z, Siris SG, Rifkin A, et al. Exacerbation of schizophrenia associated with amantadine. Am J Psychiatry. 1986;143:1170–1.

225. Dolin R, Reichman RC, Madore HP, et al. A controlled trial of amantadine and rimantadine in the prophylaxis of influenza A infection. N Engl J Med. 1982;307:580–4.

226. Hayden FG, Gwaltney JM Jr, Van de Castle RL, et al. Comparative toxicity of amantadine hydrochloride and rimantadine hydrochloride in healthy adults. Antimicrob Agents Chemother. 1981;19:226–33.

227. Bryson YJ, Monahan C, Pollack M, et al. A prospective double-blind study of side effects associated with the administration of amantadine for influenza A virus prophylaxis. J Infect Dis. 1980;141:543.

228. Pettersson RF, Hellstrom P-E, Penttinen K, et al. Evaluation of amantadine in the prophylaxis of influenza A (H1N1) virus infection: A controlled field trial among young adults and high-risk patients. J Infect Dis. 1980;142: 377–83.

229. Reuman PD, Bernstein DI, Keefer MC, et al. Efficacy and safety of low dosage amantadine hydrochloride as prophylaxis for influenza A. Antiviral Res. 1989;11:27–40.

230. Payler DK, Purdham PA. Influenza A prophylaxis with amantadine in a boarding school. Lancet. 1984;1:502–4.

231. Degelau J, Somani S, Cooper SL, et al. Occurrence of adverse effects and high amantadine concentrations with influenza prophylaxis in the nursing home. J Am Geriatr Soc. 1990;38:428–32.

232. Peters NL, Oboler S, Hair C, et al. Treatment of an influenza A outbreak in a teaching nursing home. Effectiveness of a protocol for prevention and control. J Am Geriatr Assoc. 1989;37:210–18.

233. Stange KC, Little DW, Blatnik B. Adverse reactions to amantadine prophylaxis of influenza in a retirement home. J Am Geriatr Assoc. 1991;39:700–5.

234. Hayden FG, Hoffman HE, Spyker DA. Differences in side effects of amantadine hydrochloride and rimantadine hydrochloride relate to differences in pharmacokinetics. Antimicrob Agents Chemother. 1983;23:458–64.

235. Arden NH, Patriarca PA, Fasano MB, et al. The roles of vaccination and amantadine prophylaxis in controlling an outbreak of influenza A (H3N2) in a nursing home. Arch Intern Med. 1988;148:865–8.

236. Van Voris LP, Betts RF, Hayden FG, et al. Successful treatment of naturally occurring influenza A/USSR/77 H1N1. JAMA. 1981;245:1128–31.

237. Levin M. Experience with amantadine and rimantadine in children. J Respir Dis. 1987;8(Suppl 11A):S60–6.

238. Douglas RG Jr. Drug therapy. Prophylaxis and treatment of influenza. N Engl J Med. 1990;322:443–50.

239. World Health Organization. Current status of amantadine and rimantadine as anti-influenza-A agents. Bull WHO. 1985;63:51–6.

240. Crawford SA, Clover RD, Abell TD, et al. Rimantadine prophylaxis in children: A follow-up study. Pediatr Infect Dis J. 1988;7:379–83.

241. Brady MT, Sears SD, Pacini DL, et al. Safety and prophylactic efficacy of low-dose rimantadine in adults during an influenza A epidemic. Antimicrob Agents Chemother. 1990;34:1633–6.

242. Immunication Practices Advisory Committee (ACIP). Prevention and control of influenza. MMWR. 1992;41:1–14.

243. Younkin SW, Betts RF, Roth FK, et al. Reduction in fever and symptoms in young adults with influenza A/Brazil/78 H1N1 infection after treatment with aspirin or amantadine. Antimicrob Agents Chemother. 1983;23:577–82.

244. Betts RF, Treanor JJ, Graman PS, et al. Antiviral agents to prevent or treat influenza in the elderly. J Respir Dis. 1987;8(Suppl 11A):S56–9.

245. Hall CB, Dolin R, Gala CL, et al. Children with influenza A infection: Treatment with rimantadine. Pediatrics. 1987;80:275–82.

246. Thompson J, Fleet W, Lawrence E, et al. A comparison of acetaminophen and rimantadine in the treatment of influenza A infection in children. J Med Virol. 1987;249–55.

247. Clover RD, Waner JL, Becker L, et al. Effect of rimantadine on the immune response to influenza A infections. J Med Virol. 1991;34:68–73.

248. Hermann JE, West K, Brus M, et al. Effect of rimantadine on cytotoxic T lymphocyte responses and immunity to reinfection in mice. J Infect Dis. 1990;161:180–4.

249. Hayden FG, Zylidnikov DM, Iljenko VI, et al. Comparative therapeutic effect of aerosolized and oral rimantadine HCl in experimental human influenza A virus infection. Antiviral Res. 1982;2:147–53.

250. McLaren C, Datema R, Knupp CA, et al. Review: Didanosine. Antiviral Chem Chemother. 1991;2:321–8.

251. McLeod GX, McGrath JM, Ldd EA, et al. Didanosine and zidovudine resistant patterns in clinical isolates of human immunodeficiency virus type 1 as determined by a replication endpoint concentration assay. Antimicrob Agents Chemother. 1992;36:920–5.

252. Perno C, Yarchoan R, Cooney DA, et al. Replication of human immunodeficiency virus in monocytes. J Exp Med 1989;169:933–51.

253. Gao W, Shirasaka T, Johns DG. Differential phosphorylation of azidothymidine, dideoxycytidine, and dideoxyinosine in resting and activated peripheral blood mononuclear cells. J Clin Invest 1993;91:2326–33.

254. Chu CK, Schinazi RF, Ahn MK, et al. Structure-activity relationships of pyrimidine nucleosides as antiviral agents for human immunodeficiency virus type 1 in peripheral blood mononuclear cells. J Med Chem. 1989;32:612–7.

255. Watson AJ, Wilburn LM. Inhibition of HIV infection of resting peripheral blood lymphocytes by nucleosides. AIDS Res Hum Retroviruses. 1992;8: 1221–7.

256. Molina JM, Groopman JE. Bone marrow toxicity of dideoxyinosine. N Engl J Med. 1989;321:1478.

257. Johnson VA, Merrill DP, Videler JA, et al. Two-drug combinations of zidovudine, didanosine, and recombinant interferon-α A inhibit replication of zidovudine-resistant human immunodeficiency virus type 1 synergistically in vitro. J Infect Dis. 1991;164:646–55.

258. Dornsife RE, St. Clair MH, Huang AT, et al. Anti-human immunodeficiency virus synergism by zidovudine (3′-azidothymidine) and didanosine (dideoxyinosine) contrasts with their additive inhibition of normal human marrow progenitor cells. Antimicrob Agents Chemother. 1991;35:322–8.

259. Johnson MA, Fridland A. Phosphorylation of 2′,3′-dideoxyinosine by cytosolic 5′-nucleotidase of human lymphoid cells. Mol Pharmacol 1989;36: 291–5.

260. Chen C, Vazquez-padua M, Cheng Y. Effect of anti-human immunodeficiency virus nucleoside analogs on mitochondrial DNA and its implication for delayed toxicity. Mol Pharmacol 1991;39:625–8.

261. Ono K, Nakane H, Herdewijn P, et al. Differential inhibitor effects of several pyrimidine 2′,3′-dideoxynucleoside 5′-triphosphates on the activities of reverse transcriptase and various cellular DNA polymerases. Mol Pharmacol 1989;35:578–83.

262. St. Clair MH, Martin JL, Tudor-Williams G, et al. Resistance to ddI and sensitivity to AZT induced by a mutation in HIV-1 reverse transcriptase. Science. 1991;253:1557–9.

263. Reichman RC, Tejani N, Lambert JL, et al. Didanosine (ddI) and zidovudine (ZDV) susceptibilities of human immunodeficiency virus (HIV) isolates from long-term recipients of ddI. Antiviral Res. 1993;20:267–77.

264. Dimitrov DH, Hollinger FB, Baker CJ, et al. Study of human immunodeficiency virus resistance to 2′-3′-dideoxyinosine and zidovudine in sequential isolates from pediatric patients on long-term therapy. J Infect Dis. 1993;167: 818–23.

265. Shirasaka T, Yarchoan R, O'Brien MC, et al. Changes in drug sensitivity of human immunodeficiency virus type 1 during therapy with azidothymidine, dideoxycytidine, and dideoxyinosine: An in vitro comparative study. Proc Natl Acad Sci USA. 1993;90:562–6.

266. Gu Z, Gao Q, Li X et al. Novel mutation in the human immunodeficiency virus type 1 reverse transcriptase gene that encodes cross-resistance to 2′,3′-dideoxyinosine and 2′,3′-dideoxycytidine. J Virol. 1993;66:7128–35.

267. Knupp CA, Shyu WC, Dolin R, et al. Pharmacokinetics of didanosine in patients with acquired immunodeficiency syndrome or acquired immunodeficiency syndrome-related complex. Clin Pharmacol Ther. 1991;49:523–35.

268. Hartman NR, Yarchoan R, Pluda JM, et al. Pharmacokinetics of 2′,3′-dideoxyadenosine and 2′,3′-dideoxyinosine in patients with severe human immunodeficiency virus infection. Clin Pharmacol Ther. 1990;47:647–54.

269. Singlas E, Taburet AM, Lebas FB, et al. Didanosine pharmacokinetics in patients with normal and impaired renal function: Influenza of hemodialysis. Antimicrob Agents Chemother. 1992;36:1519–24.

270. Balis FM, Pizzo PA, Butler KM, et al. Clinical pharmacology of 2′,3′-dideoxyinosine in human immunodeficiency virus-infected children. J Infect Dis. 1992;165:99–104.

271. Shyu WC, Knupp CA, Pittman KA, et al. Food-induced reduction in bioavailability of didanosine. Clin Pharmacol Ther. 1991;50:503–7.

272. Beltangady M, Knupp CA, Gustafson N, et al. Relation between plasma concentrations of didanosine and markers of antiviral efficacy in adults with AIDS or AIDS-related complex. Clin Infect Dis. 1993;16(Suppl 1):S26–31.

273. Pons JC, Boubon MC, Taburet MC, et al. Fetoplacental passage of 2′,3′-dideoxyinosine. Lancet. 1991;1:732.

274. Saag MS. Nucleoside analogues: Adverse effects. Hosp Pract 1992;27(Suppl 2):26–36.

275. Lee BL, Safrin S. Interactions and toxicities of drugs used in patients with AIDS. Clin Infect Dis. 1992;14:773–9.

276. Knupp CA, Graziano FM, Dixon RM, et al. Pharmacokinetic-interaction study of didanosine and ranitidine in patients seropositive for human immunodeficiency virus. Antimicrob Agents Chemother. 1992;36:2075–9.

277. Jacobson MA, Owen W, Campbell J, et al. Tolerability of combined ganciclovir and didanosine for the treatment of cytomegalovirus disease associated with AIDS. Clin Infect Dis. 1993;16(Suppl 1):S69–73.

278. Yarchoan R, Pluda JM, Thomas RV, et al. Long-term toxicity/activity profile of 2′,3′-dideoxyinosine in AIDS or AIDS-related complex. Lancet. 1990;336:526–9.

279. Lambert JS, Seidlin M, Reighman RC, et al. 2′,3′-Dideoxyinosine (ddI) in patients with the acquired immunodeficiency syndrome or AIDS-related complex. A phase I trial. N Engl J Med. 1990;322:1333–40.

280. Cooley TP, Kunches LM, Saunders CA, et al. Once-daily administration of 2′,3′-dideoxyinosine (ddI) in patients with the acquired immunodeficiency syndrome of AIDS-related complex. Results of a phase I trial. N Engl J Med. 1990;322:1340–5.

281. Butler KM, Husson RN, Balis FM, et al. Dideoxyinosine in children with symptomatic human immunodeficiency virus infection. N Engl J Med. 1991;324:138–44.

282. Pike IM, Nicaise C. The didanosine expanded access program: Safety analysis. Clin Infect Dis. 1993;16:S63–8.

283. Liebman HA, Cooley TP. Didanosine in the treatment of AIDS and AIDS-related complex: A critical appraisal of the dose and frequency of administration. Clin Infect Dis. 1993;16:S52–8.

284. Kahn JO, Lagakos W, Richman DD, et al. A controlled trial comparing continued zidovudine with didanosine in human immunodeficiency virus infection. N Engl J Med. 1992;327:581–587.

285. Abrecht H, Arasteh K. Didonosine-induced disorders of glucose tolerance (Letter). Ann Intern Med. 1993;119:1050.

286. Lai KK, Gang KL, Zawacki JK, et al. Fulminant hepatic failure associated with 2′,3′-dideoxyinosine (ddI). Ann Intern Med. 1991;115:283.

287. Connolly KJ, Allan JD, Fitch H, et al. Phase I study of 2′3′-dideoxyinosine administered orally twice daily to patients with AIDS or AIDS-related complex and hematologic intolerance to zidovudine. Am J Med. 1991;91:471–8.

288. Spruance S, Pavia AT, Peterson D, et al. Didanosine compared with continuation of zidovudine in HIV-infected patients with signs of clinical deterioration while receiving zidovudine. A randomized, double-blind clinical trial. Ann Intern Med. 1994;120:360–8.

289. Dolin R, Amato D, Fischl M, et al. Efficiency of didanosine (ddI) versus zidovidine (ZDV) in patients with no or ≤16 weeks of prior ZDV therapy. Abt WS-B24.1 at IXth International Conference on AIDS, June 1993, Berlin, Germany.

289a. Abrams DI, Goldman AI, Launer C, et al. A comparative trial of didanosine or zalcitabine after treatment with zidovudine in patients with human immunodeficiency virus infection. N Engl J Med. 1994;330:657–62.

290. Collier AC, Coombs RW, Fischel MA, et al. Combination therapy with zidovudine and didonosine compared with zidovudine alone in HIV-1 infection. Ann Intern Med. 1993;119:786–93.

290a. Yarchoan R, Lietzau JA, Nguyen B, et al. A randomized pilot study of alternating or simultaneous zidovudine and didanosine therapy in patients with symptomatic human immunodeficiency virus infection. J Infect Dis. 1994;169:9–17.

291. Vere Hodge RA. Review: Antiviral portraits series, Number 3. Famciclovir and penciclovir. The mode of action of famciclovir including its conversion to penciclovir. Antiviral Chem Chemother. 1993;4:67–84.

292. Weinberg A, Bate BJ, Masters HB, et al. In vitro activities of penciclovir and acyclovir against herpes simplex virus types 1 and 2. Antimicrob Agents Chemother. 1992;36:2037–8.

293. Boyd MR, Kern ER, Safrin S. Penciclovir: A review of its spectrum of activity, selectivity and cross-resistance pattern. Antiviral Chem Chemother. 4(Suppl 1):3–11.

294. Safrin S, Phan L. In vitgro activity of penciclovir against clinical isolates of acyclovir-resistant and foscarnet-resistant herpes simplex virus. Antimicrob Agents Chemother. 1993;37:2241–3.

295. Goldthorpe SE, Boyd MR, Field HJ. Effects of penciclovir and famciclovir in a murine model of encephalitis induced by intranasal inoculation of herpes simplex virus type 1. Antiviral Chem Chemother. 1992;3:37–47.

296. Earnshaw DL, Bacon TH, Darlison SJ, et al. Mode of antiviral action of penciclovir in MRC-5 cells infected with herpes simplex virus type 1 (HSV-1), HSV-2 and varicella-zoster virus. Antimicrob Agents Chemother. 1992;36:2747–57.

297. Fowles SE, Pierce DM, Prince WT, et al. Effect of food on the bioavailability and pharmacokinetics of penciclovir, a novel antiherpes agent, following oral administration of the pro-drug, famciclovir. Br J Clin Pharmacol. 1990;3–5:620P–1P.

298. Fowles SE, Pierce DM, Prince WT, et al. The tolerance to and pharmacokinetics of penciclovir (BRL 39123A), a novel antiherpes agent, administered by intravenous infusion to healthy subjects. Eur J Clin Pharmacol. 1992;43:513–6.

299. Gheeraert P. Efficacy and safety of famciclovir (FCV) in the treatment of uncomplicated herpes zoster (HZ) (Abstract 1108). Presented at the 32nd ICAAC Meeting, Anaheim, CA, October 11–14, 1992.

299a. Tyring S, Barbarash R, Nahlik J, et al. Efficacy of famciclovir on herpes zoster rash resolution and postherpetic neuralgia. Antiviral Res. 1994;23(Suppl):73, [Abst 71].

299b. Portnoy J. Famciclovir in the treatment of herpes zoster (HZ) infection. Antiviral Res. 1994;23(Suppl):98, [Abst 119].

299c. Candaele M, Candaele D. Famciclovir: Confirmed efficacy of 250mg t.i.d. for the treatment of herpes zoster (HZ) infection. Antiviral Res. 1994;23(Suppl):98, [Abst 118].

300. Oberg B. Antiviral effects of phosphonoformate (PFA, foscarnet sodium). Pharmacol Ther. 1989;40:213–85.

301. Chrisp P, Clissold SP. Foscarnet. A review of its antiviral activity, pharmacokinetic properties and therapeutic use in immunocompromised patients with cytomegalovirus retinitis. Drugs. 1991;41:104–29.

302. Manischewitz JF, Quinnan GV, Lane HC, et al. Synergistic effect of ganciclovir and foscarnet on cytomegalovirus replication in vitro. Antimicrob Agents Chemother. 1990;34:373–5.

303. Eriksson BFH, Schinazi RF. Combinations of 3′-azido-3′-deoxythymidine (zidovudine) and phosphonoformate (foscarnet) against human immunodeficiency virus type 1 and cytomegalovirus replication in vitro. Antimicrob Agents Chemother. 1989;33:663–9.

304. Crumpacker CS. Mechanism of action of foscarnet against viral polymerases. Am J Med. 1992;92(Suppl 2A):3S–7S.

305. Sullivan V, Coen DM. Isolation of foscarnet-resistant human cytomegalovirus patterns of resistance and sensitivity to other antiviral drugs. J Infect Dis. 1991;164:781–4.

306. Knox KK, Drobyski WR, Carrigan DR. Cytomegalovirus isolate resistant to ganciclovir and foscarnet from a marrow transplant patient. Lancet. 1991;337:1292–3.

306a. Safrin S, Kemmerly S, Plotkin B, et al. Foscarnet-resistant herpes simplex virus infection in patients with AIDS. J Infect Dis. 1994;169:193–6.

307. Sjovall J, Bergdahl S, Movin G, et al. Pharmacokinetics of foscarnet and distribution to cerebrospinal fluid after intravenous infusion in patients with human immunodeficiency virus infection. Antimicrob Agents Chemother. 1989;33:1023–31.

308. Aweeka F, Gambertoglio J, Mills J, et al. Pharmacokinetics of intermittently administered intravenous foscarnet in the treatment of acquired immunodeficiency syndrome patients with serious cytomegalovirus retinitis. Antimicrob Agents Chemother. 1989;33:742–5.

309. Fanning MM, Read SE, Benson M, et al. Foscarnet therapy of cytomegalovirus retinitis in AIDS. J Acquired Immune Deficiency Syndromes. 1990;3:472–9.

310. Hengge UR, Brockmeyer NH, Malessa R, et al. Foscarnet penetrates the blood-brain barrier: Rationale for therapy for cytomegalovirus encephalitis. Antimicrob Agents Chemother. 1993;37:1010–4.

311. MacGregor RR, Graziani AL, Weiss R, et al. Successful foscarnet therapy for cytomegalovirus retinitis in an AIDS patient undergoing hemodialysis: Rationale for empiric dosing and plasma level monitoring. J Infect Dis. 1991;164:785–7.

312. Reusser P, Gambertoglio JG, Lilleby L, et al. Phase I–II trial of foscarnet for prevention of cytomegalovirus infection in autologous and allogeneic marrow transplant recipients. J Infect Dis. 1992;166:473–9.

313. Aweeka FT, Gambertoglio JG, Van der Horst C, et al. Pharmacokinetics of concomitantly administered foscarnet and zidovudine for treatment of human immunodeficiency virus infection (AIDS Clinical Trials Group Protocol 053). Antimicrob Agents Chemother. 1992;36:1773–8.

314. Deray G, Martinez F, Katlama C, et al. Foscarnet nephrotoxicity: Mechanism, incidence and prevention. Am J Nephrol. 1989;9:316–21.

315. Nyberg G, Blohme I, Persson H, et al. Foscarnet-induced tubulointerstitial nephritis in renal transplant patients. Transplant Proc 1990;22:241.

316. Beaufils H, Deray G, Katlama C, et al. Foscarnet and crystals in glomerular capillary lumens. Lancet. 1;336:755.

317. Jacobson MA, Gambertoglio JG, Aweeka FT, et al. Foscarnet-induced hypocalcemia and effects of foscarnet on calcium metabolism. J Clin Endocrinol Metab. 1991;72:1130–5.

318. Van Der Pijl JW, Frissen PHJ, Reiss P, et al. Foscarnet and penile ulceration. Lancet. 1990;1:266.

319. Jacobson MA, Drew LW, Feinberg J, et al. Foscarnet therapy for ganciclovir-resistant cytomegalovirus retinitis in patients with AIDS. J Infect Dis. 1991;163:1348–51.

320. Palestine AG, Polis MA, De Smet MD, et al. A randomized, controlled trial of foscarnet in the treatment of cytomegalovirus retinitis in patients with AIDS. Ann Intern Med. 1991;115:665–73.

321. Jacobsen MA. Maintenance therapy for cytomegalovirus retinitis in patients with acquired immunodeficiency syndrome: foscarnet. Am J Med. 1992;92(Suppl 2A):26S–9.

322. Katlama C, Dohin E, Caumes E, et al. Foscarnet induction therapy for cytomegalovirus retinitis in AIDS: Comparison of twice-daily and three-times-daily regimens. J Acquired Immune Deficiency Syndromes. 1992;5(Suppl 1):S18–24.

323. Jacobson MA, Causey D, Polsky B, et al. A dose-ranging study of daily maintenance intravenous foscarnet therapy for cytomegalovirus retinitis in AIDS. J Infect Dis. 1993;168:444–8.

324. Studies of Ocular Complications of AIDS Research Group. Mortality in patients with the acquired immunodeficiency syndrome treated with either foscarnet or ganciclovir for cytomegalovirus retinitis. N Engl J Med. 1992;326:213–20.

325. Jacobson MA, van der Horst C, Causey DM. In vivo additive antiretroviral

effect of combined zidovidine and foscarnet therapy for human immunodeficiency virus infection (ACTG protocol 053). J Infect Dis. 1991;163:1219–22.

326. Reddy MM, Grieco MH, McKinley GF, et al. Effect of foscarnet therapy on human immunodeficiency virus p24 antigen levels in AIDS patients with cytomegalovirus retinitis. J Infect Dis. 1992;166:607–10.

327. Harb GE, Bacchetti P, Jacobson MA. Survival of patients with AIDS and cytomegalovirus disease treated with ganciclovir or foscarnet. AIDS. 1991; 5:959–65.

328. Polis MA, DeSmet MD, Baird BF, et al. Increased survival of a cohort of patients with acquired immunodeficiency syndrome and cytomegalovirus retinitis who received sodium phosphonoformate (foscarnet). Am J Med. 1993;94:175–80.

328a. Gordon MR, Dick CD, Herzog CA. Efficacy of intravitreal foscarnet in a patient with AIDS. N Engl J Med. 1994;330:868–70.

329. Drobyski WR, Knox KK, Carrigan DR, et al. Foscarnet therapy of ganciclovir-resistant cytomegalovirus in marrow transplantation. Transplantation. 1991;52:155–7.

330. Dieterich DT, Polis MA, Lew EA, et al. Concurrent use of ganciclovir and foscarnet to treat cytomegalovirus infection in AIDS patients. J Infect Dis. 1993;167:1184–8.

331. Youle M, Chanas A, Gazzard B. Treatment of acquired immune deficiency syndrome (AIDS)-related pneumonitis with foscarnet: A double-blind placebo controlled study. J Infect Dis. 1990;20:41–50.

332. Nelson MR, Connolly GM, Hawkins DA, et al. Foscarnet in the treatment of cytomegalovirus infection of the esophagus and colon in patients with the acquired immune deficiency syndrome. Am J Gastroenterol. 1991;86:876–81.

333. Hardy WD. Foscarnet treatment of acyclovir-resistant herpes simplex virus infection in patients with acquired immunodeficiency syndrome: preliminary results of a controlled, randomized, regimen-comparative trial. Am J Med. 1992;92(Suppl 2A):30S–5S.

334. Lawee D, Rosenthal D, Aoki FY, et al. Efficacy and safety of foscarnet for recurrent orolabial herpes: A multicenter randomized double-blind study. Can Med Assoc J. 1988;138:329–33.

335. Faulds D, Heel RC. Ganciclovir. A review of its antiviral activity, pharmacokinetic properties and therapeutic efficacy in cytomegalovirus infections. Drugs. 1990;39:597–638.

336. Field AK, Davies ME, DeWitt C, et al. 9-[2-Hydroxy-1 (hydroxymethyl) ethoxy]methyl guanine: A selective inhibitor of herpes group virus replication. Proc Natl Acad Sci USA. 1983;80:4139–43.

337. Smee DF, Martin JC, Verheyden JPH, et al. Antiherpesvirus activity of the acyclic nucleoside 9-(1,3-dihydroxy-2-propoxymethyl) guanine. Antimicrob Agents Chemother. 1983;23:676–82.

338. Plotkin SA, Drew WL, Felsenstein D, et al. Sensitivity of clinical isolates of human cytomegalovirus to 9-(1,3-dihydroxy-2-propoxymethyl) guanine. J Infect Dis. 1985;152:833–4.

339. Freitas VR, Smee DF, Chernow M, et al. Activity of 9-(1,3-dihydroxy-2-propoxymethyl)guanine compared with that of acyclovir against human, monkey, and rodent cytomegaloviruses. Antimicrob Agents Chemother. 1985;28:240–5.

340. Russler SK, Tapper MA, Carrigan DR. Susceptibility of human herpesvirus 6 to acyclovir and ganciclovir. Lancet. 1989;1:382.

341. Medina DJ, Hsiung GD, Mellors JW. Ganciclovir antagonizes the antihuman immunodeficiency virus type 1 activity of zidovudine and didanosine in vitro. Antimicrob Agents Chemother. 1992;36:1127–30.

342. Feng JS, Crouch JY, Tian PY, et al. Zidovudine antagonizes the antiviral effects of ganciclovir against cytomegalovirus infection in cultured cells and in guinea pigs. Antiviral Chem Chemother. 1993;4:19–25.

343. Freitas VR, Frser-Smith EB, Chiu S, et al. Efficacy of ganciclovir in combination with zidovudine against cytomegalovirus in vitro and in vivo. Antiviral Res. 1993;21:301–15.

344. Taylor DL, Jeffries DJ, Taylor-Robinson D, et al. The susceptibility of adenovirus infection to the anti-cytomegalovirus drug, ganciclovir (DHPG). FEMS Microbiol Lett. 1988;49:337–41.

345. Sommadossi J-P, Carlisle R. Toxicity of 3′-azido-3′-deoxythymidine and 9-(1,3-dihydroxy-2- propoxymethyl)guanine for normal human hematopoietic progenitor cells in vitro. Antimicrob Agents Chemother. 1987;31:452–4.

346. Bowden RA, Digel J, Reed EC, et al. Immunosuppressive effects of ganciclovir on in vitro lymphocyte responses. J Infect Dis. 1987;156:899–903.

347. Shanley JD, Morningstar J, Jordan MC. Inhibition of murine cytomegalovirus lung infection and interstitial pneumonia by acyclovir and 9-(1,3-dihydroxy-2-propoxymethyl)guanine. Antimicrob Agents Chemother. 1985;28:172–5.

348. Fong CKY, Cohen SD, McCormick S, et al. Antiviral effect of 9-(1,3-dihydroxy-2- propoxymethyl)guanine against cytomegalovirus infection in a guinea pig model. Antiviral Res. 1987;7:11–23.

349. Debs RJ, Montgomery AB, Brunette EN, et al. Aerosol administration of antiviral agents to treat lung infection due to murine cytomegalovirus. J Infect Dis. 1988;157:327–31.

350. Smee DF, Boehme R, Chernow M, et al. Intracellular metabolism and enzymatic phosphorylation of 9-(1,3-dihydroxy-2-propoxymethyl)guanine and acyclovir in herpes simplex virus–infected and uninfected cells. Biochem Pharmacol. 1985;34:1049–56.

351. Sullivan V, Talarico CL, Stanat SC, et al. A protein kinase homologue controls phosphorylation of ganciclovir in human cytomegalovirus-infected cells. Nature. 1992;358:162–4.

352. Littler E, Stuart AD, Chee MS. Human cytomegalovirus UL97 open reading frame encodes a protein that phosphorylates the antiviral nucleoside analogue ganciclovir. Nature. 1992;358:160–4.

353. Biron KK, Stanat SC, Sorrell JB, et al. Metabolic activation of the nucleoside analog 9-[2-hydroxy-1-(hydroxymethyl) ethoxy]methyl guanine in human diploid fibroblasts infected with human cytomegalovirus. Proc Natl Acad Sci USA. 1985;82:2473–7.

354. Frank KB, Chiou J-F, Cheng Y. Interaction of herpes simplex virus-induced DNA polymerase with 9-(1,3-dihydroxy-2-propoxymethyl) guanine triphosphate. J Biol Chem. 1984;259:1566–9.

355. St Clair MH, Miller WH, Miller RL, et al. Inhibition of cellular alpha DNA polymerase and herpes simplex virus-induced DNA polymerases by the triphosphate of BW759U. Antimicrob Agents Chemother. 1984;25:191–4.

356. Reid R, Mar E-C, Huang E-S, et al. Insertion and extension of acyclic, dideoxy, and ara nucleotides by herpesviridae and human polymerases. J Biol Chem. 1988;263:3898–904.

357. Lurain NS, Thompson KD, Holmes EW, et al. Point mutations in the DNA polymerase gene of human cytomegalovirus that result in resistance to antiviral agents. J Virol. 1992;66:7146–52.

358. Stanat SC, Reardon JE, Erice A, et al. Ganciclovir-resistant cytomegalovirus clinical isolates: mode of resistance to ganciclovir. Antimicrob Agents Chemother. 1991;35:2191–7.

359. Tatarowicz WA, Lurion NS, Thompson KD. A ganciclovir resistant clinical isolate of human cytomegalovirus exhibiting cross-resistance to other DNA polymerase inhibitors. J Infect Dis. 1992;166:904–7.

360. Erice A, Chou S, Biron KK, et al. Progressive disease due to ganciclovir-resistant cytomegalovirus in immunocompromised patients. N Engl J Med. 1989;320:289–93.

361. Drew WL, Miner RC, Busch DF, et al. Prevalence of resistance in patients receiving ganciclovir for serious cytomegalovirus infection. J Infect Dis. 1991;163:716–9.

362. Jordan MC, Biron KK. Cytomegalovirus resistance to ganciclovir. In: SA Spector, ed. Ganciclovir Therapy for Cytomegalovirus Infection. New York: Marcel Dekker; 1991:185–96.

363. Cole NL, Balfour HH Jr. In vitro susceptibility of cytomegalovirus isolates from immunocompromised patients to acyclovir and ganciclovir. Diagn Microbiol Infect Dis. 1987;6:255–61.

364. Slavin MA, Bindra RR, Gleaves CA, et al. Ganciclovir sensitivity of cytomegalovirus at diagnosis and during treatment of cytomegalovirus pneumonia in marrow transplant recipients. Antimicrob Agents Chemother. 1993;37:1360–3.

365. Tokumoto JIN, Hollander H. Cytomegalovirus polyradiculopathy caused by a ganciclovir-resistant strain. Clin Infect Dis. 1993;17:654–6.

366. Jacobson MA, deMiranda P, Cederberg DM, et al. Human pharmacokinetics and tolerance of oral ganciclovir. Antimicrob Agents Chemother. 1987;31:1251–4.

367. Laskin OL, Cederberg DM, Mills J, et al. Ganciclovir for the treatment and suppression of serious infections caused by cytomegalovirus. Am J Med. 1987;83:201–7.

368. Fletcher C, Sawchuk R, Chinnock B, et al. Human pharmacokinetics of the antiviral drug DHPG. Clin Pharmacol Ther. 1986;40:281–6.

369. Jabs DA, Newman C, deBustros S, et al. Treatment of cytomegalovirus retinitis with ganciclovir. Ophthalmology. 1987;94:824–30.

370. Jabs DA, Wingard JR, deBustros S, et al. BW B759U for cytomegalovirus retinitis: Intraocular drug penetration. Arch Ophthalmol. 1986;104:1436–7.

371. Kuppermann BD, Quiceno JI, Flores-Aguilar M, et al. Intravitreal ganciclovir concentration after intravenous administration in AIDS patients with cytomegalovirus retinitis: Implications for therapy. J Infect Dis. 1993;168:1506–9.

372. Shepp DH, Dandliker DH, deMiranda P, et al. Activity of 9-[(2-hydroxy-1-(hydroxymethyl)ethoxymethyl)]guanine in the treatment of cytomegalovirus pneumonia. Ann Intern Med. 1984;103:368–73.

373. Sommadossi J-P, Bevan R, Ling T, et al. Clinical pharmacokinetics of ganciclovir in patients with normal and impaired renal function. Rev Infect Dis. 1988;10(Suppl 3):S507–14.

374. Swan SK, Munar MY, Wigger MA, et al. Case reports. Pharmacokinetics of ganciclovir in a patient undergoing hemodialysis. Am J Kidney Dis. 1991;17:69–72.

375. Jacobson MA, DeMiranda P, Gordon SM, et al. Prolonged pancytopenia due to combined ganciclovir and zidovudine therapy. J Infect Dis. 1988;158:489–90.

376. Hochster H, Dieterich D, Bozzette S, et al. Toxicity of combined ganciclovir and zidovudine for cytomegalovirus disease associated with AIDS. Ann Intern Med. 1990;113:111–7.

377. Freitas VR, Fraser-Smith EB, Matthews TR. Efficacy of ganciclovir in combination with other antimicrobial agents against cytomegalovirus in vitro and in vivo. Antiviral Res 1993;20:1–12.

378. Hardy WD. Combined ganciclovir and recombinant human granulocyte-macrophage colony-stimulating factor in the treatment of cytomegalovirus retinitis in AIDS patients. J Acquired Immune Deficiency Syndromes. 1991;4:S22–8.

379. Merigan TC, Renlund DG, Keay S, et al. A controlled trial of ganciclovir to prevent cytomegalovirus disease after heart transplantation. N Engl J Med. 1992;326:1182–6.

380. Kotler DP, Culpepper-Morgan JA, Tierney AR, et al. Treatment of disseminated cytomegalovirus infection with 9-(1,3 dihydroxy-2-propoxymethyl)-guanine: Evidence of prolonged survival in patients with the acquired immunodeficiency syndrome. AIDS Res. 1986;2:299–308.

381. Collaborative DHPG Treatment Study Group. Treatment of serious cytomegalovirus infections with 9-(1,3-dihydroxy 2-propoxymethyl)guanine in patients with AIDS and other immunodeficiencies. N Engl J Med. 1986;314: 801–5.

382. Jacobson MA, Mills J. Serious cytomegalovirus disease in the acquired immunodeficiency syndrome (AIDS). Ann Intern Med. 1988;108:585–94.

383. Henderly DE, Freeman WR, Causey DM, et al. Cytomegalovirus retinitis and response to therapy with ganciclovir. Ophthalmology 1987;94:425–34.

384. Holland GN, Sidikaro Y, Kreiger AE, et al. Treatment of cytomegalovirus retinopathy with ganciclovir. Ophthalmology. 1987;94:815–23.

385. Drew WL. Cytomegalovirus infection in patients with AIDS. Clin Infect Dis. 1992;14:608–15.

386. Freeman WR, Henderly DE, Wan WL, et al. Prevalence, pathophysiology, and treatment of rhegmatogenous retinal detachment in treated cytomegalovirus retinitis. Am J Ophthalmol. 1987;103:527–36.

387. Sawyer MD, Mayoral JL, Gillingham MJ, et al. Treatment of recurrent cytomegalovirus disease in patients receiving solid organ transplant. Arch Surg. 1993;128:165–70.

388. Chachoua A, Dieterich D, Krasinski K, et al. 9-(1,3-2-propoxy-methyl)guanine (ganciclovir) in the treatment of cytomegalovirus gastrointestinal disease with the acquired immunodeficiency syndrome. Ann Intern Med. 1987;107: 133–7.

389. Hecht DW, Snydman DR, Crumpacker CS, et al. Ganciclovir for treatment of renal transplant-associated primary cytomegalovirus pneumonia. J Infect Dis. 1988;157:187–90.

390. Fiala M, Cone LA, Cohen N, et al. Responses to neurologic complications of AIDS to 3′-azido-3′-deoxythymidine and 9-(1,3-dihydroxy-2-propoxymethyl) guanine. I. Clinical features. Rev Infect Dis. 1988;10:250–6.

391. Dieterich DT, Kotler DP, Busch DF, et al. Ganciclovir treatment of cytomegalovirus colitis in AIDS: A randomized, double-blind, placebo-controlled multicenter study. J Infect Dis. 1993;167:278–82.

392. Reed EC, Dandliker PS, Meyers JD. Treatment of cytomegalovirus pneumonia with 9-[2-hydroxy-1-(hydroxymethyl)ethoxymethyl]guanine and high-dose corticosteroids. Ann Intern Med 1986;105:214–5.

393. Reed EC, Bowden RA, Dandliker PS, et al. Treatment of cytomegalovirus pneumonia with ganciclovir and intravenous cytomegalovirus immunoglobulin in patients with bone marrow transplants. Ann Intern Med. 1988;109: 783–8.

394. Emanuel D, Cunningham I, Jules-Elysee K, et al. Cytomegalovirus pneumonia after bone marrow transplantation successfully treated with the combination of ganciclovir and high-dose intravenous immune globulin. Ann Intern Med 1988;109:777–82.

395. Reed EC, Wolford JL, Kopecky KJ, et al. Ganciclovir for the treatment of cytomegalovirus gastroenteritis in bone marrow transplant patients. A randomized, placebo-controlled trial. Ann Intern Med. 1990;112:505–10.

396. Schmidt GM, Horak DA, Niland JC, et al. A randomized, controlled trial of prophylactic ganciclovir for cytomegalovirus pulmonary infection in recipients of allogeneic bone marrow transplants. N Engl J Med. 1991;324: 1005–11.

397. Goodrich JM, Mori M, Gleaves CA, et al. Early treatment with ganciclovir to prevent cytomegalovirus disease after allogeneic bone marrow transplantation. N Engl J Med. 1991;325:1601–7.

398. Winston DJ, Ho WG, Bartoni K, et al. Ganciclovir prophylaxis of cytomegalovirus infection and disease in allogeneic bone marrow transplant recipients. Ann Intern Med. 1993;118:179–84.

399. Goodrich JM, Bowden RA, Fisher L, et al. Ganciclovir prophylaxis to prevent cytomegalovirus disease after allogeneic marrow transplant. Ann Intern Med. 1993;118:173–8.

400. Duncan ST, Paradis IL, Dauber JH, et al. Ganciclovir prophylaxis for cytomegalovirus infections in pulmonary allograft recipients. Am Rev Respir Dis. 1992;146:1213–5.

401. Maurer JR, Snell G, deHoyos A, et al. Outcomes of lung transplantation using three different cytomegalovirus prophylactic regimens. Transplant Proc 1993;25:1434–5.

402. Hibbred PL, Tolkoff-Rubin NE, Cosimi AB, et al. Symptomatic cytomegalovirus disease in the cytomegalovirus antibody seropositive renal transplant recipient treated with OKT3. Transplantation. 1992;53:68–72.

403. Lumbreras C, Otero JR, Herrero JA, et al. Ganciclovir prophylaxis decreases frequency and severity of cytomegalovirus disease in seropositive liver transplant recipients treated with OKT3 monoclonal antibodies. Antimicrob Agents Chemother. 1993;37:2450–2.

404. Preiksaitis JK, Diaz-Mitoma F, Mirzayans F, et al. Quantitative oropharyngeal Epstein-Barr virus shedding in renal and cardiac transplant recipients: Relationship to immunosuppressive therapy, serologic responses, and the risk of posttransplant lymphoproliferative disorder. J Infect Dis. 1992;166: 986–94.

405. Henry K, Cantrill H, Fletcher C, Chinnock BJ, Balfour HH Jr. Use of intravitreal ganciclovir (dihydroxy propoxy methyl guanine) for cytomegalovirus retinitis in a patient with AIDS. Am J Ophthalmol. 1987;103:17–23.

406. Prusoff WH. Idoxuridine or how it all began. In: DeClercq E., ed. Clinical Use of Antiviral Drugs. Norwell: Martinus Nijhoff; 1988:15–24.

407. Fardeau C, Langlois M, Mathys B, et al. Emergence of cross-resistant herpes simplex virus following topical drug therapy in rabbit keratitis. Current Eye Res. 1991;10:151–8.

408. Kaufman HE. The treatment of herpetic eye infections with trifluridine and other antivirals. In: DeClercq E, ed. Clinical Use of Antiviral Drugs. Norwell; Martinus Nijhoff, 1988:25–38.

409. Pavan-Langston D. Major ocular viral infections. In: Galasso GJ, Whitley RJ, Merigan TC, ed. Antiviral Agents and Viral Diseases of Man, 3rd ed. New York: Raven Press, 1990:183–233.

410. Silvestri DL, Corey L, Holmes KK. Ineffectiveness of topical idoxuridine in dimethyl sulfoxide for therapy of genital herpes. JAMA. 1982;248:953.

411. Spruance SL, Stewart JCB, Freeman DJ, et al. Early application of topical 15% idoxuridine in dimethyl sulfoxide shortens the course of herpes simplex labialis: A multicenter placebo-controlled trial. J Infect Dis. 1990;161:191–7.

412. Baron S, Coppenhaver DH, Dianzani F, et al. Introduction to the interferon system. In: Baron S, et al, eds. Interferon: Principles and Medical Applications. Galveston, TX: UTMB; 1992:1–15.

413. Zoon KC. Human interferons: Structure and function. In: Interferon 9. London: Academic Press; 1987:1–12.

414. Finter NB. Why are there so many subtypes of alpha-interferons? In: Marcus PI, ed. Journal of Interferon Research, Spec issue. New York: Mary Ann Liebert Publishers; 1991:185–94.

415. Greenberg SB. Human interferon in viral diseases. Infect Dis Clin North Am. 1987;1:383–423.

416. Hall MJ, Duncan IB. Antiviral drug and interferon combinations. In: Field HJ, ed. Antiviral Agents: The Development and Assessment of Antiviral Chemotherapy. v. II. Boca Raton: CRC Press; 1988:29–84.

417. Johnson HM. Interferon-mediated modulation of the immune system. In: Pfeffer LM, ed. Mechanisms of Interferon Actions. v. 2. Boca Raton: CRC Press; 1987:59–77.

418. Heremans H, Billiau A. Interferon Principles and Medical Applications. Baron S, et al, eds. Galveston, TX: UTMB; 1992:361–71.

419. Staeheli P. Interferon-induced proteins and the antiviral state. Adv Virus Res. 1990;38:147–200.

420. Gen GC, Ransohoff RM. Interferon-induced antiviral actions and their regulation. Adv Virus Res. 1993;42:57–102.

421. Sen GC, Lengyel P. The interferon system. J Biol Chem. 1992;267:5017–20.

422. Karupiah G, Xie Q-W, Buller ML, et al. Inhibition of viral replication by interferon-gamma-induced nitric oxide synthase. Science. 1993;261:1445–8.

423. Constantoulakis P, Campbell M, Felber BK, et al. Inhibition of Rev-mediated HIV-1 expression by an RNA binding protein encoded by the interferon-inducible 9-27 gene. Science. 1993;259:1314–8.

424. Meylan PRA, Guatelli JC, Munis JR et al. Mechanisms for the inhibition of HIV replication by interferons-α, -β, and -γ. Virology. 1993;193:138–48.

425. Schroder HC, Ugarkovic D, Merz H, et al. Protection of HeLa-T4+ cells against human immunodeficiency virus (HIV) infection after stable transfection with HIV LTR-2′,5′-oligoadenylate synthetase hybrid gene. FASEB J. 1990;4:3125–30.

426. Hooks JJ, Detrick B. The interferon system and disease. In: Pfeffer LM, ed. Mechanisms of Interferon Actions. v. 2. Boca Raton: CRC Press; 1987: 113–328.

427. Wills RJ. Clinical pharmacokinetics of interferons. Clin Pharmacokinet 1990; 19:390–9.

428. Barouki FM, Witter RF, Griffin DE, et al. Time course of interferon levels, antiviral state, 2′,5′-oligoadenylate synthetase and side effects in healthy men. J Interferon Res. 1987;7:29–39.

429. Witt PL, Goldstein D, Storer BE, et al. Absence of biological effects of orally administered interferon-βser. J Interferon Res. 1992;12:411–3.

430. Smith RA, Norris F, Palmer D, et al. Distribution of alpha interferon in serum and cerebrospinal fluid after systemic administration. Clin Pharmacol Ther. 1985;37:85–8.

431. Bocci V. Physicochemical and biologic properties of interferons and their potential uses in drug delivery systems. Crit Rev Therapeutic Drug Carrier Systems. 1992;9:91–133.

432. Quesada JR. Toxicity and side effects of interferons. In: Baron S, et al, eds. Interferon Principles and Medical Applications. Galveston, TX: UTMB; 1992:426–32.

433. Renault PF, Hoofnagle JH. Side effects of alpha interferon. Semin Liver Dis. 1989;9:273–7.

434. McDonald EM, Mann AH, Thomas HC. Interferons as mediators of psychiatric morbidity. Lancet. 1987;2:1175–8.

435. Deyton LR, Walker RE, Kovacs JA, et al. Reversible cardiac dysfunction associated with interferon alfa therapy in AIDS patients with Kaposi's sarcoma. N Engl J Med. 1989;321:1246–9.

436. Meyers JD, Flournoy N, Sanders JE, et al. Prophylactic use of human leukocyte interferon after allogeneic marrow transplantation. Ann Intern Med. 1987;107:809–16.

437. Hayden FG, Mills SE, Johns ME. Human tolerance and histopathologic effects of long-term administration of intranasal interferon-α2. J Infect Dis. 1983;148:914–21.

438. Antonelli G, Currenti M, Turriziani O, et al. Neutralizing antibodies to interferon-α: Relative frequency in patients treated with different interferon preparations. J Infect Dis. 1991;163:882–5.

439. Foster GR, Ackrill AM, Goldin RD, et al. Expression of the terminal protein region of hepatitis B virus inhibits cellular responses to interferons α and γ and double-stranded RNA. Proc Natl Acad Sci USA. 1991;88:2888–92.

440. Alexander GJM, Fagan EA, Daniels HM, et al. Loss of HBsAg with interferon therapy in chronic hepatitis B virus infection. Lancet. 1988;2:66–9.

441. Wong DKH, Cheung AM, O'Rourke K, et al. Effect of alpha-interferon treatment in patients with hepatitis B antigen-positive chronic hepatitis B. Ann Intern Med. 1993;119:312–23.

442. Hoofnagle JH. Interferon therapy of viral hepatitis. In: Baron S, et al, eds.

Interferon Principles and Medical Applications. Galveston, TX: UTMB; 1992:433–62.

443. Perrillo RP, Schiff ER, Davis GL, et al. A randomized, controlled trial of interferon alfa-2b alone and after prednisone withdrawal for the treatment of chronic hepatitis B. N Engl J Med. 1990;323:295–301.

444. Brook MG, McDonald JA, Karayiannis P, et al. Randomised controlled trial of interferon alfa 2A (Roferon-A) for the treatment of chronic hepatitis B virus (HBV) infection: factors that influence response. Gut. 1989;30:1116–22.

445. Saracco G, Mazzella G, Rosina F, et al. A controlled trial of human lymphoblastoid interferon in chronic hepatitis B in Italy. Hepatology. 1989;10:336–41.

446. Fattovich G, Farci P, Rugge M, et al. A randomized controlled trial of lymphoblastoid interferon-α in patients with chronic hepatitis B lacking HBeAg. Hepatology. 1992;15:584–9.

447. Lok ASF, Ma OCK, Lau JYN. Interferon alfa therapy in patients with chronic hepatitis B virus infection. Gastroenterology. 1991;100:756–61.

448. Korenman B, Baker J, Waggoner JE, et al. Long-term remission of chronic hepatitis B after alpha-interferon therapy. Ann Intern Med. 1991;114:629–34.

449. Perrillo RP, Brunt EM. Hepatic histologic and immunohistochemical changes in chronic hepatitis B after prolonged clearance of hepatitis B e antigen and hepatitis B surface antigen. Ann Intern Med. 1991;115:113–5.

450. Brunetto MR, Oliveri F, Rocca G, et al. Natural course and response to interferon of chronic hepatitis B accompanied by antibody to hepatitis B e antigen. Hepatology. 1989;10:198–202.

451. Di Bisceglie, Rustgi VK, Kassianides C, et al. Therapy of chronic hepatitis B with recombinant human alpha and gamma interferon. Hepatology. 1990;11:266–70.

452. Lau JYN, Lai CL, Chung HT, et al. A randomized controlled trial of recombinant interferon-γ in Chinese patients with chronic hepatitis B virus infection. J Med Virol. 1991;34:184–7.

453. Kakumu S, Ishikawa T, Mizokami M, et al. Treatment with human gamma interferon of chronic hepatitis B: Comparative study with alpha interferon. J Med Virol. 1991;35:32–7.

454. Garcia G, Smith CI, Weissberg JI, et al. Adenine arabinoside monophosphate (vidarabine phosphate) in combination with human leukocyte interferon in the treatment of chronic hepatitis B. Ann Intern Med. 1987;107:278–85.

455. Wong S, Yu ECL, Lok ASF, et al. Interferon treatment for hepatitis B–associated membranous glomerulonephritis in two Chinese children. Pediatr Nephrol. 1992;6:416–20.

456. Lisker-Melman M, Webb D, Di Bisceglie AM, et al. Glomerulonephritis caused by chronic hepatitis B virus infection: Treatment with recombinant human alpha-interferon. Ann Intern Med. 1989;111:479–83.

457. Lai KN, Li PKT, Lui SF, et al. Membranous nephropathy related to hepatitis B virus in adults. N Engl J Med. 1991;324:1457–63.

458. Farci P, Mandas A, Coliana A, et al. Treatment of chronic hepatitis D with interferon alfa-2a. N Engl J Med. 1994;330:88–94.

459. Davis GL, Balart LA, Schiff ER, et al. Treatment of chronic hepatitis C with recombinant interferon alfa. A multicenter randomized, controlled trial. N Engl J Med. 1989;321:1501–6.

460. Bisceglie AM, Martin P, Kassianides C, et al. Recombinant interferon alfa therapy for chronic hepatitis C. A randomized, double-blind, placebo-controlled trial. N Engl J Med. 1989;321:1506–10.

461. Marcellin P, Boyer N, Giostra E, et al. Recombinant human α-interferon in patients with chronic non-A, non-b hepatitis: A multicenter randomized controlled trial from France. Hepatology. 1991;13:393–7.

462. Causse X, Godinot H, Chevallier M, et al. Comparison of 1 or 3 MU of interferon alfa-2b and placebo in patients with chronic non-A, non-B hepatitis. Gastroenterology. 1991;101:497–502.

463. Shindo M, Di Bisceglie AM, Cheung L, et al. Decrease in serum hepatitis C viral RNA during alpha-interferon therapy for chronic hepatitis C. Ann Intern Med. 1991;115:700–4.

464. Hagiwara H, Hayashi N, Mita E, et al. Detection of hepatitis C virus RNA in serum of patients with chronic hepatitis C treated with interferon-α. Hepatology. 1992;15:37–41.

465. Chemello L, Diodati G, Bonetti P, et al. Treatment of chronic hepatitis C with different regimes of interferon alpha-2a (Abstract 196). Antiviral Res. 1993;20:148.

466. Johnson RJ, Gretch DR, Yamabe H, et al. Membranoproliferative glomerulonephritis associated with hepatitis C virus infection. N Engl J Med. 1993;328:465–70.

466a. Misiani R, Bellavita P, Fenili D, et al. Interferon alfa-2a therapy in cryoglobulinemia associated with hepatitis C virus. N Engl J Med. 1994;330:751–6.

467. Lou JYN, Davis GL, Kniffen J, et al. Significance of serum hepatitis C virus RNA levels in chronic hepatitis C. Lancet. 1993;341:1501–4.

468. Lou JYN, Mizokami M, Ohno T, et al. Discrepancy between biochemical and virological responses to interferon-alpha in chronic hepatitis C. Lancet. 1993;342:1208–9.

469. Omata M, Yokosuka O, Takano S, et al. Resolution of acute hepatitis C after therapy with natural beta interferon. Lancet. 1991;338:914–5.

470. Papo T, Marcellin P, Bernuau J, et al. Autoimmune chronic hepatitis exacerbated by alpha-interferon. Ann Intern Med. 1992;116:51–3.

471. Kuhls TL, Sacher J, Pineda E, et al. Suppression of recurrent genital herpes simplex virus infection with recombinant alfa2 interferon. J Infect Dis. 1986;154:437–42.

472. Pazin GJ, Harger JH, Armstrong JA, et al. Leukocyte interferon for treating first episodes of genital herpes in women. J Infect Dis. 1987;156:891–8.

473. Eron LJ, Toy C, Salsitz B, et al. Therapy of genital herpes with topically applied interferon. Antimicrob Agents Chemother. 1987;31:1137–9.

474. Lebwohl M, Sacks S, Conant M, et al. Recombinant alpha-2 interferon gel treatment of recurrent herpes genitalis. Antiviral Res. 1992;17:235–43.

475. Shupack J, Stiller M, Knobler E, et al. Topical alpha-interferon in recurrent genital herpes simplex infection. Dermatologica. 1990;181:134–8.

476. Sacks SL, Varner TL, Davies KS, et al. Randomized, double-blind, placebo-controlled, patient-initiated study of topical high- and low-dose interferon-α with nonoxynol-9 in the treatment of recurrent genital herpes. J Infect Dis. 1990;161:692–8.

477. Levin MJ, Judson FN, Eron L, et al. Comparison of intramuscular recombinant alpha interferon (rIFN-2A) with topical acyclovir for the treatment of first-episode herpes genitalis and prevention of recurrences. Antimicrob Agents Chemother. 1989;33:649–52.

478. Winston DJ, Eron LJ, Ho M, Pazin G, et al. Recombinant interferon alpha-2a for treatment of herpes zoster in immunosuppressed patients with cancer. Am J Med. 1988;85:147–51.

479. Duschet P, Schwarz T, Soyer P, et al. Treatment of herpes zoster. Recombinant alpha interferon versus acyclovir. Int J Dermatol. 1988;27:193–7.

480. Ikossi-O'Connor MG, Chadha KC, Lillie MA, et al. Interferon inactivator(s) in patients with AIDS and AIDS-unrelated Kaposi's sarcoma. Am J Med. 1986;81:783–5.

481. Ambrus JL, Poiesz BJ, Lillie MA, et al. Interferon and interferon inhibitor levels in patients infected with varicella-zoster virus, acquired immunodeficiency syndrome, acquired immunodeficiency syndrome–related complex, or Kaposi's sarcoma, and in normal individuals. Am J Med. 1989;87:405–7.

482. Krown SE. The role of interferon in the therapy of epidemic Kaposi's sarcoma. Semin Oncol. 1987;14:27–33.

483. Lane HC, Davey V, Kovacs JA, et al. Interferon-α in patients with asymptomatic human immunodeficiency virus (HIV) infection. Ann Intern Med. 1990;112:805–11.

484. Berglund O, Engman K, Ehrnst A, et al. Combined treatment of symptomatic human immunodeficiency virus type 1 infection with native interferon-α and zidovudine. J Infect Dis. 1991;163:710–5.

485. Edlin BR, Weinstein RA, Whaling SM, et al. Zidovudine–interferon-α combination therapy in patients with advanced human immunodeficiency virus type 1 infection: Biphasic response of p24 antigen and quantitative polymerase chain reaction. J Infect Dis. 1992;165:793–8.

486. Davey RT Jr, Davey VJ, Metcalf JA, et al. A phase I/II trial of zidovudine, interferon-α, and granulocyte-macrophage colony-stimulating factor in the treatment of human immunodeficiency virus type 1 infection. J Infect Dis. 1991;164:43–52.

487. Katabitra E, et al. IX International Conference on AIDS. Abstract PO-B26-2056. Berlin, 1993.

488. Edlin BR, St. Clair MH, Pitha PM, et al. In-vitro resistance to zidovudine and alpha-interferon in HIV-1 isolates from patients: Correlations with treatment duration and response. Ann Intern Med. 1992;117:457–60.

489. Douglas JM Jr, Eron LJ, Judson FN, et al. A randomized trial of combination therapy with intralesional interferon α2b and podophyllin versus podophyllin alone for the therapy of anogenital warts. J Infect Dis. 1990;162:52–9.

490. Reichman RC, Oakes D, Bonnez W, et al. Treatment of condyloma acuminatum with three different interferon-α preparations administered parenterally: A double-blind, placebo-controlled trial. J Infect Dis. 1990;1270–6.

491. Eron LJ, Judson F, Tucker S, et al. Interferon therapy for condylomata acuminata. N Engl J Med. 1986;315:1059–64.

492. Vance JC, Bart BJ, Hansen RC, et al. Intralesional recombinant alpha-2 interferon for the treatment of patients with condyloma acuminatum or verruca plantaris. Arch Dermatol. 1986;122:272–7.

493. Reichman RC, Oakes D, Bonnex W, et al. Treatment of condyloma acuminatum with three different interferons administered intralesionally. Ann Intern Med. 1988;108:675–9.

494. Friedman-Kien AE, Aeron LJ, Conant M, et al. Natural interferon-alfa for treatment of condylomata acuminata. JAMA. 1988;259:533–8.

495. Kraus SJ, Stone KM. Management of genital infection caused by human papillomavirus. Rev Infect Dis. 1990;12:S620–32.

496. Condylomata International Collaborative Study Group. Recurrent condylomata acuminata treated with recombinant interferon alfa-2a. JAMA. 1991;265:2684–7.

497. Yliskoki M, Syrjanen K, Syrjanen S, et al. Systemic α-interferon (Wellferon) treatment of genital human papillomavirus (HPV) type 6,11,16, and 18 infections: Double-blind, placebo-controlled trial. Gynecol Oncol. 1991;43:55–60.

498. Gall SA, Constantine L, Koukol D. Therapy of persistent human papillomavirus disease with two different interferon species. Am J Obstet Gynecol. 1991;164:130–4.

499. Kirby PK, Kiviat N, Beckman A, et al. Tolerance and efficacy of recombinant human interferon gamma in the treatment of refractory genital warts. Am J Med. 1988;85:183–8.

500. Condylomata International Collaborative Study Group. Randomized placebo-controlled double-blind combined therapy with laser surgery and systemic interferon-α2a in the treatment of anogenital condylomata acuminatum. J Infect Dis. 1993;167:824–9.

501. Greenberg RR, Pizzuti DJ, Omoto KH, et al. Superficial laser vulvectomy. V. Surgical debulking is enhanced by adjuvant systemic interferon. Am J Obstet Gynecol. 1992;166:815–20.

502. Dunham AM, McCartney JC, McCance JC, et al. Effect of perilesional injection of α-interferon on cervical intraepithelial neoplasia and associated human papillomavirus infection. J R Soc Med. 1991;83:490–2.

503. Berman B, Davis-Reed L, Silverstein L, et al. Treatment of verrucae vulgaris with alfa2 interferon. J Infect Dis. 1986;154:238–0.

504. Lusk RP, McCabe BF, Mixon JH. Three-year experience of treating recurrent respiratory papilloma with interferon. Ann Otol Rhinol Laryngol. 1987; 19:158–62.

505. Healy GB, Gerber RD, Trowbridge AL, et al. Treatment of recurrent respiratory papillomatosis with human leukocyte interferon. N Engl J Med. 1988; 319:401–7.

506. Leventhal BG, Kashima HK, Mounts P, et al. Long-term response of recurrent respiratory papillomatosis to treatment with lymphoblastoid interferon alfa-n1. N Engl J Med. 1991;325:613–7.

507. Sperber SJ, Hayden FG. Comparative susceptibility of respiratory viruses to recombinant interferons-α2b and -β. J Interferon Res. 1989;9:285–93.

508. Hayden FG. Intranasal interferons for control of the common cold. In: Revel M, ed. Clinical Aspects of Interferon. Boston, MA: Kluwer Academic; 1988: 3–16.

509. Higgins PG, Barrow GI, Tyrrell DAJ, et al. The efficacy of intranasal interferon-2a in respiratory syncytial virus infection in volunteers. Antiviral Res. 1990;14:3–10.

510. Hayden FG, Albrecht JK, Kaiser KL, et al. Prevention of natural colds by contact prophylaxis with intranasal alpha2-interferon. N Engl J Med. 1986; 314:71–5.

511. Douglas RB, Moore BW, Miles HB, et al. Prophylactic efficacy of intranasal alpha2-interferon against rhinovirus infections in the family setting. N Engl J Med. 1986;314:65–70.

512. Hayden FG, Kaiser KL, Albrecht JK. Intranasal recombinant alfa-2b interferon treatment of naturally occurring common colds. Antimicrob Agents Chemother. 1988;32:224–30.

513. Gilbert BE, Knight V. Minireview: Biochemistry and clinical applications of ribavirin. Antimicrob Agents Chemother. 1986;30:201–5.

514. Hruska JF, Bernstein JM, Douglas RG Jr, et al. Effects of ribavirin on respiratory syncytial virus in vitro. Pharmacol Ther. 1980;6:770.

515. Browne MJ. Comparative inhibition of influenza and parainfluenza virus replication by ribavirin in MDCK cells. Antimicrob Agents Chemother. 1981; 19:712.

516. McCormick JB, Mitchell SW, Getchell JP, et al. Ribavirin suppresses replication of lymphadenopathy-associated virus in cultures of human adult T lymphocytes. Lancet. 1984;2:1367–9.

517. Huggins JW. Prospects for treatment of viral hemorrhagic fevers with ribavirin, a broad-spectrum antiviral drug. Rev Infect Dis. 1989;2:S750–61.

518. Baba M, Pauwels R, Balzarini J, et al. Ribavirin antagonizes inhibitory effects of pyrimidine 2′,3′-dideoxynucleosides but enhances inhibitory effects of purine 2′,3′-dideoxynucleosides on replication of human immunodeficiency virus in vitro. Antimicrob Agents Chemother. 1987;31:1613–7.

519. Peavy DL, Koff WC, Hyman DS, et al. Inhibition of lymphocyte proliferative responses by ribavirin. Infect Immun. 1980;29:583.

520. Steele RW, Crosby DL, Steele RW, et al. Effects of ribavirin on neutrophil function. Am J Med Sci. 1988;295:503–6.

521. Marquardt DL, Gruber HE, Walker LL. Ribavirin inhibits mast cell mediator release. J Pharmacol Exp Ther. 1987;240:145–9.

522. Hruska JF, Morrow PE, Suffin SC, et al. In vivo inhibition of respiratory syncytial virus by ribavirin. Antimicrob Agents Chemother. 1982;21:125.

523. Wyde PR, Wilson SZ, Patrella R, et al. Efficacy of high dose–short duration ribavirin aerosol in the treatment of respiratory syncytial virus infected cotton rats and influenza B virus infected mice. Antiviral Res. 1987;7:211–20.

524. Jahrling PB, Hesse RA, Eddy GA, et al. Lassa virus infection of rhesus monkeys: Pathogenesis and treatment with ribavirin. J Infect Dis. 1980;141: 580.

525. Weissenbacher MC, Calello MA, Merani MS, et al. Therapeutic effect of the antiviral agent ribavirin in junin virus infection of primates. J Med Virol. 1986;20:261–7.

526. Kende M, Lupton HW, Rill WL, Levy HB, Canonico PG. Enhanced therapeutic efficacy of poly(ICLC) and ribavirin combinations against Rift Valley Fever virus infection in mice. Antimicrob Agents Chemother. 1987;31: 986–90.

527. Gangemi JD, Nachtigal M, Barnhart D, et al. Therapeutic efficacy of liposome-encapsulated ribavirin and muramyl tripeptide in experimental infection with influenza or herpes simplex virus. J Infect Dis. 1987;155:510–7.

528. Gruber WC, Wilson SZ, Throop BJ, et al. Immunoglobulin administration and ribavirin therapy: Efficacy in respiratory syncytial virus infection of the cotton rat. Pediatr Res. 1987;21:270–4.

529. Smee DF, Mathews TR. Metabolism of ribavirin in respiratory syncytial virus-infected and uninfected cells. Antimicrob Agents Chemother. 1986;30: 117–21.

530. Wray SK, Gilbert BE, Knight V. Effect of ribavirin triphosphate on primer generation and elongation during influenza virus transcription in vitro. Antiviral Res. 1985;5:39–48.

531. Fernandez-Larsson R, JL Patterson. Ribavirin is an inhibitor of human immunodeficiency virus reverse transcriptase. Mol Pharmacol. 1990;38: 766–70.

532. Potter CW, Phair JP, Vodinelich L, et al. Antiviral, immunosuppressive and antitumour effects of ribavirin. Nature. 1976;259:496–7.

533. Peavy DL, Powers CN, Knight V. Inhibition of murine plaque-forming cell responses in vivo by ribavirin. J Immunol. 1981;126:861.

534. Scheidel LM, Durbin RK, Stollar V. Sindbis virus mutants resistant to mycophenolic acid and ribavirin. Virology. 1987;158:1–7.

535. Hall CB, McBride JT, Walsh EE, et al. Aerosolized ribavirin treatment of infants with respiratory syncytial viral infection. N Engl J Med. 1983;308: 1443.

536. Laskin OL, Longstreth JA, Hart CC, et al. Ribavirin disposition in high-risk patients for acquired immunodeficiency syndrome. Clin Pharmacol Ther. 1987;41:546–55.

537. Connor E, Morrison S, Lane J, et al. Safety, tolerance, and pharmacokinetics of systemic ribavirin in children with human immunodeficiency virus infection. Antimicrob Agents Chemother. 1993;37:531–9.

538. Roberts RB, Laskin OL, Laurence J, et al. Ribavirin pharmacodynamics in high-risk patients for acquired immunodeficiency syndrome. Clin Pharmacol Ther. 1987;42:365–73.

539. Connor JD, Hintz M, Van Dyke R, et al. Ribavirin pharmacokinetics in children and adults during therapeutic trials. In: Smith RA, Knight V, Smith JAD, eds. Clinical Applications of Ribavirin. Orlando: Academic Press; 1984: 107–23.

540. Kramer TH, Gaar GG, Ray CG, et al. Hemodialysis clearance of intravenously administered ribavirin. Antimicrob Agents Chemother. 1990;34: 489–90.

541. Knight V, Yu CP, Gilbert BE, et al. Estimating the dosage of ribavirin aerosol according to age and other variables. J Infect Dis. 1988;158:443–8.

542. Hillyared IW. The preclinical toxicology and safety of ribavirin. In: Smith RA, Kirkpatric W, eds. Ribavirin: A Broad Spectrum Antiviral Agent. New York: Academic Press; 1980:59.

543. Smith CV, Charette RP, Fox JP, et al. Lack of effect of oral ribavirin in naturally occurring influenza A virus (H1N1) infection. J Infect Dis. 1980; 141:548.

544. Fisher-Hock SP, Gborie S, Parker L, et al. Unexpected adverse reactions during a clinical trial in rural West Africa. Antiviral Rev. 1992;19:139–47.

545. Roberts RB, Dickinson GM, Heseltine PNR, et al. A multicenter clinical trial of oral ribavirin in HIV-infected patients with lymphadenopathy. J Acquired Immune Deficiency Syndromes. 1990;3:884–92.

546. Schulof RS, Parenti DM, Simon GL, et al. Clinical, virologic, and immunologic effects of combination therapy with ribavirin and isoprinosine in HIV-infected homosexual men. J Acquired Immune Deficiency Syndromes. 1990; 3:485–92.

547. Rodriguez WJ, Dang Bui RH, Connor JD, et al. Environmental exposure of primary care personnel to ribavirin aerosol when supervising treatment of infants with respiratory syncytial virus infections. Antimicrob Agents Chemother. 1987;31:1143–6.

548. Committee on Infectious Disease, American Academy of Pediatrics. Ribavirin therapy of respiratory syncytial virus. In: Report of the Committee on Infectious Diseases, 22nd ed. Elk Grove, IL: American Academy of Pediatrics; 1991:581–7.

549. Gladu J-M, Ecobichon DJ. Evaluation of exposure of health care personnel to ribavirin. J Toxicol Environ Health. 1989;28:1–12.

550. Bradley JS, Connor JD, Compogiannis LS, et al. Exposure of health care workers to ribavirin during therapy for respiratory syncytial virus infections. Antimicrob Agents Chemother. 1990;34:668–70.

551. Conrad DA, Christenson JC, Waner JL, et al. Aerosolized ribavirin treatment of respiratory syncytial virus infection in infants hospitalized during an epidemic. Pediatr Infect Dis J. 1987;6:152–8.

552. Frankel LR, Wilson CW, Demers RR, et al. A technique for the administration of ribavirin to mechanically ventilated infants with severe respiratory syncytial virus infection. Crit Care Med. 1987;15:1051–4.

553. Outwater KM, Meissner C, Peterson MB. Ribavirin administration to infants receiving mechanical ventilation. Am J Dis Child. 1988;142:512–5.

554. Rodriguez WJ, Parrott RH. Ribavirin aerosol treatment of serious respiratory syncytial virus infection in infants. In: Moellering RC, ed. Infectious Disease Clinics of North America, Antiviral Chemotherapy. Philadelphia: WB Saunders; 1987:425–39.

555. Taber LH, Knight V, Gilbert BE, et al. Ribavirin aerosol treatment of bronchiolitis associated with respiratory syncytial virus infection in infants. Pediatrics. 1983;72:613. .

556. Smith DW, Frankel LR, Mathers LH, et al. A controlled trial of aerosolized ribavirin in infants receiving mechanical ventilation for severe respiratory syncytial virus infection. N Engl J Med. 1991;325:24–9.

557. Hall CB, McBride JT, Gala CL, et al. Ribavirin treatment of respiratory syncytial infection in infants with underlying cardiopulmonary disease. JAMA. 1985;254:3047–51.

558. Englund JA, Piedra PA, Jefferson LS, et al. High-dose, short-duration ribavirin aerosol therapy in children with suspected respiratory syncytial virus infection. J Pediatr. 1990;117:313–20.

559. Rosner IK, Welliver RC, Edelson PJ, et al. Effect of ribavirin therapy on respiratory syncytial virus-specific IgE and IgA responses after infection. J Infect Dis. 1987;155:1043–7.

560. Knight V, Gilbert BE. Ribavirin aerosol treatment of influenza. In: Moellering RC, ed. Infectious Disease Clinics of North America, Antiviral Chemotherapy, Philadelphia: WB Saunders; 1987:441–57.

561. Bernstein DI, Reuman PD, Sherwood JR, et al. Ribavirin small-particle-aerosol treatment of influenza B virus infection. Antimicrob Agents Chemother. 1988;32:761–4.

562. Stein DS, Creticos CM, Jackson GG, et al. Oral ribavirin treatment of influenza A and B. Antimicrob Agents Chemother. 1987;31:1285–7.

563. Ray CG, Icenogle TB, Minnich LL, et al. The use of intravenous ribavirin to treat influenza virus-associated acute myocarditis. J Infect Dis. 1989;159:829–36.

564. Wendt CH, Weisdorf DJ, Jordan MC, et al. Parainfluenza virus respiratory infection after bone marrow transplantation. N Engl J Med. 1992;326:921–6.

565. Kaplan LJ, Daum RS, Smaron M, et al. Severe measles in immunocompromised patients. JAMA. 1992;267:1237–41.

566. Gururangan S, Stevens RF, Morris DJ. Ribavirin response in measles pneumonia. J Infect. 1990;20:219–21.

567. McCormick JB, King IJ, Webb PA, et al. Lassa fever: Effective therapy with ribavirin. N Engl J Med. 1986;314:20–6.

568. Huggins JW, Hsiang CM, Cosgriff TM, et al. Prospective, double-blind, concurrent, placebo-controlled clinical trial of intravenous ribavirin therapy of hemorrhagic fever with renal syndrome. J Infect Dis. 1991;164:1119–27.

569. Enria DA, Maiztegui JI. Antiviral treatment of Argentine hemorrhagic fever. Antiviral Res. 1994;23:23–31.

570. Holmes GP, McCormick JB, Trock SC, et al. Lassa fever in the United States: Investigation of a case and new guidelines for management. N Engl J Med. 1990;323:1120–3.

571. Gasser RA Jr, Magill AJ, Oster CN, et al. The threat of infectious disease in Americans returning from operation Desert Storm. N Engl J Med. 1991;324:859–64.

572. Crumpacker C, Heagy W, Bubley G, et al. Ribavirin treatment of acquired immunodeficiency syndrome (AIDS) and the acquired-immunodeficiency-syndrome-related complex (ARC). Ann Intern Med 1987;107:664–74.

573. Roberts RB, Hollinger FB, Parks WP, et al. A multicenter clinical trial of oral ribavirin in HIV-infected people with lymphadenopathy: Virologic observations. AIDS. 1990;4:67–72.

574. Spanish Ribavirin Trial Group. Comparison of ribavirin and placebo in CDC group III human immunodeficiency virus infection. Lancet. 1991;2:6–9.

575. Roberts RB, Jurica K, Meyer WA III, et al. A phase 1 study of ribavirin in human immunodeficiency virus-infected patients. J Infect Dis. 1990;162:638–42.

576. Reichard O, Anderson J, Schvarcz R, et al. Ribavirin treatment for chronic hepatitis C. Lancet. 1991;37:1058–61.

577. Di Bisceglie AM, Shindo M, Fong TL, et al. A pilot study of ribavirin therapy for chronic hepatitis C. Hepatology. 1992;16:649–54.

578. Gnann JW Jr. BV-araU: Preclinical studies and potential applications. In: Mills J, Corey L, eds. Antiviral Chemotherapy: New Directions for Clinical Application and Research. v. 3. Englewood Cliffs, NJ: Prentice-Hall; 1993:105–15.

579. Machida H, Nishitani M. Drug susceptibilities of isolates of varicella-zoster virus in a clinical study of oral brovavir. Microbiol Immunol. 1990;34:407–11.

580. Lin JC, Machida H. Comparison of two bromovinyl nucleoside analogs, 1-β-D-arabinofuranosyl-E-5-(2-bromovinyl)uracil and E-5-(2-bromovinyl)-2′-deoxyuridine, with acyclovir in inhibition of Epstein-Barr virus replication. Antimicrob Agents Chemother. 1988;32:1068–72.

581. Soike K, Huang JL, Tu JI, Stouffer B, et al. Oral bioavailability and antisimian varicella virus efficacy of 1-β-D-arabinofuranosyl-E-5-(2-bromovinyl)Uracil (BV-araU) in monkeys. J Infect Dis. 1992;165:732–6.

582. Suzutani T, Machida H, Sakuma T, et al. Effects of various nucleosides on antiviral activity and metabolism of 1-β-D-arabinofuranosyl-E-5-(2-bromovinyl)uracil against herpes simplex virus types 1 and 2. Antimicrob Agents Chemother. 1988;32:1547–51.

583. Machida H, Watanabe Y. Inhibition of DNA synthesis in varicella-zoster virus infected cells by BV-araU. Microbiol Immunol. 1991;35:139–45.

584. Yokota T, K Konno, S Mori, et al. Mechanism of selective inhibition of varicella-zoster virus replication by 1-β-D-arabinofuranosyl-E-5-(2-bromovinyl)uracil. Molecular Pharmacol 1989;36:312–6.

585. Bristol-Myers Squibb Company. Investigator Brochure Sorivudine (BVaraU, SQ 32,756), July 1993.

586. Larder BA, Chesebro B, Richman DD. Susceptibilities of zidovudine-susceptible and -resistant human immunodeficiency virus isolates to antiviral agents determined by using a quantitative plaque reduction assay. Antimicrob Agents Chemother. 1990;34:436–41.

587. Mansuri MM, Hitchcock MJM, Buroker RA, et al. Comparison of in vitro biological properties and mouse toxicities of three thymidine analogs active against human immunodeficiency virus. Antimicrob Agents Chemother. 1990;34:637–41.

588. Du D-L, Volpe DA, Grieshaber CK, et al. In vitro toxicity of 3′-azido-3′-deoxythymidine, carbovir and 2′,3′-didehydro-2′,3′-dideoxythymidine to human and murine haematopoietic progenitor cells. Br J Haematol. 1992;80:437–5.

589. Ho H-T, Hitchcock MJM. Cellular pharmacology of 2′,3′-dideoxy-2′,3′-didehydrothymidine, a nucleoside analog active against human immunodeficiency virus. Antimicrob Agents Chemother. 1989;33:844–9.

590. Huang P, Farquhar D, Plunkett W. Selective action of 2′,3′-didehydro-2′,3′-dideoxythymidine triphosphate on human immunodeficiency virus reverse transcriptase and human DNA polymerases. J Biol Chem. 1992;267:2817–22.

591. Larder BA, Darby G, Richman DD. HIV with reduced sensitivity to zidovudine (AZT) isolated during prolonged therapy. Science 1989;243:1731–4.

592. Rooke R, Parniak MA, Tremblay M, et al. Biological comparison of wild-

593. type and zidovudine-resistant isolates of human immunodeficiency virus type 1 from the same subjects: Susceptibility and resistance to other drugs. Antimicrob Agents Chemother. 1991;35:988–91.

593. Bristol-Myers-Squibb Company. Investigator's Brochure—Stavudine. 1992.

594. Browne MJ, Mayer KH, Chafee SBD, et al. 2′,3′-Didehydro-3′-deoxythymidine (d4T) in patients with AIDS or AIDS-related complex: A phase I trial. J Infect Dis. 1993;167:21–9.

595. Carmine AA, Brogden RN, Heel RC, et al. Trifluridine: A review of its antiviral activity and therapeutic use in the topical treatment of viral eye infections. Drugs. 1982;23:329–53.

596. Spector SA, Tyndall M, Kelly E. Inhibition of human cytomegalovirus by trifluorothymidine. Antimicrob Agents Chemother. 1983;23:133.

597. Van Bijsterveld OP, Post H. Trifluorothymidine versus adenine arabinoside in the treatment of herpes simplex keratitis. Br J Ophthalmol. 1980;64:33–6.

598. De Koning EWJ, Van Bijsterveld OP, Cantell K. Combination therapy for dendritic keratitis with human leucocyte interferon and trifluorothymidine. Br J Ophthalmol. 1982;66:509–12.

599. Field H, McMillan A, Darby G. The sensitivity of acyclovir-resistant mutants of herpes simplex virus to other antiviral drugs. J Infect Dis. 1981;143:281–4.

600. Gephart JF, Lerner AM. Comparison of the effects of arabinosyladenine, arabinosylhypoxanthine, and arabinosyladenine 5′-monophosphate against herpes simplex virus, varicella-zoster virus, and cytomegalovirus with their effects on cellular deoxyribonucleic acid synthesis. Antimicrob Agents Chemother. 1981;19:170–8.

601. Biron KK, Fyfe JA, Noblin JE, et al. Selection and primary characterization of acyclovir-resistant mutants of varicella-zoster virus. Am J Med 1982;73(Suppl):383–6.

602. Vince R, Dalarge S, Lee H, et al. Carbocyclic arabinofuranosyladenine (cyclaradine): Efficacy against genital herpes in guinea pigs. Science. 1983;221:1405–6.

603. Whitley R, Alford C, Hess F, et al. Vidarabine: A preliminary review of its pharmacological properties and therapeutic use. Drugs. 1980;20:267–82.

604. Pelling JC, Drach JC, Shipman C Jr. Internucleotide incorporation of arabinosyladenine into herpes simplex virus and mammalian cell DNA. Virology. 1981;109:323–5.

605. Sacks SL, Merigan TC, Kaminska J, et al. Inactivation of S-adenosylhomocysteine hydrolase during adenine arabinoside therapy. J Clin Invest. 1982;69:226–30.

606. Cantoni GL, Aksamit RR, Kim I-K. Methionine biosynthesis and vidarabine therapy. N Engl J Med. 1982;307:1079.

607. Buchanan RA, Kinkel AW, Alford CA Jr, et al. Plasma levels and urinary excretion of vidarabine after repeat dosing. Clin Pharmacol Ther. 1980;27:690–6.

608. Shope TC, Kauffman RE, Bowman D, et al. Pharmacokinetics of vidarabine in infants and children treated for herpes infection. J Infect Dis. 1983;148:721.

609. Aronoff GR, Szwed JJ, Nelson RL, et al. Hypoxanthine-arabinoside pharmacokinetics after adenine arabinoside administration to a patient with renal failure. Antimicrob Agents Chemother. 1980;18:212–4.

610. Weller IVD, Bassendine MF, Murray AK, et al. HBsAg-positive chronic liver disease: Inhibition of viral replication by highly soluble adenine arabinoside 5′-monophosphate (ARA-AMP). Gastroenterology. 1980;79:1129.

611. Whitley RJ, Tucker BC, Kinkel AW, et al. Pharmacology, tolerance, and antiviral activity of vidarabine monophosphate in humans. Antimicrob Agents Chemother. 1980;18:709–15.

612. Friedman HM, Grasela T. Adenine arabinoside and allopurinol—Possible adverse drug interaction. N Engl J Med. 1981;304:423.

613. Garcia G, Smith CI, Weissberg JI, et al. Adenine arabinoside monophosphate (vidarabine phosphate) in combination with human leukocyte interferon in the treatment of chronic hepatitis b. Ann Intern Med. 1987;107:278–85.

614. Etta LV, Brown J, Mastri A, et al: Fatal vidarabine toxicity in a patient with normal renal function. JAMA. 1981;246:1703–5.

615. Marker SC, Howard RJ, Groth KE, et al. A trial of vidarabine for cytomegalovirus infection in renal transplant patients. Arch Intern Med. 1980;140:1441–4.

616. Feldman S, Robertson PK, Lott L, et al. Neurotoxicity due to adenine arabinoside therapy during varicella-zoster virus infections in immunocompromised children. J Infect Dis. 1986;154:889–93.

617. Feder HM Jr. Disseminated herpes simplex infection in a neonate during prophylaxis with vidarabine. JAMA. 1988;259:1054–5.

618. Whitley RJ, Spruance S, Hayden F, et al. Vidarabine therapy of mucocutaneous herpes simplex virus infections in the immunocompromised host. J Infect Dis 1984;149:1–8.

619. Preiksaitis JK, Lank B, Ng PK, et al. Effect of liver disease on pharmacokinetics and toxicity of 9-β-D-arabinofuranosyladenine-5′-phosphate. J Infect Dis. 1981;144:358–64.

620. Hoofnagle JG, Hanson RG, Minuk GY, et al. Randomized controlled trial of adenine arabinoside monophosphate for chronic type B hepatitis. Gastroenterology. 1984;86:150–7.

621. Perrillo RP, Regenstein FG, Bodicky CJ, et al. Comparative efficacy of adenine arabinoside 5′ monophosphate and prednisone withdrawal followed by adenine arabinoside 5′ monophosphate in the treatment of chronic active hepatitis type B. Gastroenterology. 1985;88:780–6.

622. Yokosuka O, Omata M, Imazeki F, et al. Combination of short-term prednis-

olone and adenine arabinoside in the treatment of chronic hepatitis B. Gastroenterology. 1985;89:246–51.

623. Broder S. Pharmacodynamics of 2′,3′-dideoxycytidine: An inhibitor of human immunodeficiency virus. Am J Med. 1990;88(Suppl 5B):2S–7S.

624. Hoffmann-La Roche, Inc., Product Summary: HIVID. June 1992.

625. Yarchoan R, Mitsuya H, Meyers CE, et al. Clinical pharmacology of 3′-azido-2′,3′-dideoxythymidine (zidovudine) and related dideoxy-nucleosides. N Engl J Med. 1989;321:726–38.

626. Polas PJ, Swenson CL, Sams R, et al. In vitro and in vivo evidence that the antiviral activity of 2′,3′-dideoxycytidine is target cell dependent in a feline retrovirus animal model. Antimicrob Agents Chemother. 1990;33:1414–21.

627. Eron JJ Jr, Johnson VA, Merrill DP, et al. Synergistic inhibition of replication of human immunodeficiency virus type 1, including that of a zidovudine resistant isolate, by zidovudine and 2′,3′-dideoxycytidine in vitro. Antimicrob Agents Chemother. 1992;36:1559–62.

628. Lewis LD, Hamzeh FM, Lietman PS. Ultrastructural changes associated with reduced mitochondrial DNA and impaired mitochondrial function in the presence of 2′3′-dideoxycytidine. Antimicrob Agents Chemother. 1992;36:2061–5.

629. Gao Q, Gu Z, Hiscott J, et al. Generation of drug-resistant variants of human immunodeficiency virus type 1 by in vitro passage in increasing concentrations of 2′,3′-dideoxycytidine and 2′,3′-dideoxy-3′-thiacytidine. Antimicrob Agents Chemother. 1993;37:130–3.

630. Gu Zhengxian, Gao Q, Fang H, et al. Identification of a mutation at codon 65 in the IKKK motif of reverse transcriptase that encodes human immunodeficiency virus resistance to 2′,3′-dideoxycytidine and 2′,3′-dideoxy-3′-thiacytidine. Antimicrob Agents Chemother. 1994;38:275–81.

631. Zhang D, Caliendo AM, Eron JJ, et al. Resistance to 2′,3′-dideoxycytidine conferred by a mutation in codon 65 of the human immunodeficiency virus type 1 reverse transcriptase. Antimicrob Agents Chemother. 1994;38:282–7.

632. Fitzgibbon JE, Howell RM, Haberzettl CA, et al. Human immunodeficiency virus Type 1 pol gene mutations which cause decreased susceptibility to 2′,3′-dideoxycytidine. Antimicrob Agents Chemother. 1992;36:153–7.

633. Japour AJ, Chatis PA, Eigenrauch HA, et al. Detection of human immunodeficiency virus type 1 clinical isolates with reduced sensitivity to zidovudine and dideoxyinosine by RNA–RNA hybridization. Proc Natl Acad Sci. 1991;88:3092–6.

634. Klecker RW, Collins JM, Yarchoan RC, et al. Pharmacokinetics of 2′,3′-dideoxycytidine in patients with AIDS and related disorders. J Clin Pharmacol. 1988;28:837–42.

635. Pizzo PA, Butler K, Balis F, et al. Dideoxycytidine alone and in an alternating schedule with zidovudine in children with symptomatic human immunodeficiency virus infection. J Pediatr. 1990;117:799–808.

636. Meng TC, Fischl MA, Boota AM, et al. Combination therapy with zidovudine and dideoxycytidine in patients with advanced human immunodeficiency virus infection. Ann Intern Med. 1992;116:13–20.

637. Merigan TC, Skowron G, Bozzette SA, et al. Circulating p24 antigen levels and responses to dideoxycytidine in human immunodeficiency virus (HIV) infections. Ann Intern Med. 1989;110:189–94.

638. Fischl MA, Olson RM, Follansbee SE, et al. Zalcitabine compared with zidovudine in patients with advanced HIV-1 infection who received previous zidovudine therapy. Ann Intern Med. 1993;118:762–9.

639. Indorf AS, Pegram PS. Esophageal ulceration related to zalcitabine (ddC). Ann Intern Med. 1992;117:133–4.

640. Skowron G, Bozzette SA, Lim L, et al. Alternating and intermittent regimens of zidovudine and dideoxycytidine in patients with AIDS or AIDS-related complex. Ann Intern Med. 1993;118:321–30.

641. Fischl M, Collier A, Stanley JM, et al. The safety and efficacy of zidovudine (ZDV) and zalcitabine (ddC) or ddC versus ZDV (Abstract WS-B25-1). Presented at the IXth International Congress on AIDS, Berlin, Germany, June 1993.

642. Mcleod GX, Hammer SM. Zidovudine: Five years later. Ann Intern Med. 1992;117:487–501.

643. Mitsuya H, Weinhold KJ, Furman PA, et al. 3′-Azido-3′deoxythymidine (BW A509U): An antiviral agent that inhibits the infectivity and cytopathic effect of human T-lymphotropic virus type III/lymphadenopathy-associated virus in vitro. Proc Natl Acad Sci USA. 1985;82:7096–100.

644. Ruprecht RM, O'Brien LG, Rossoni LD, et al. Suppression of mouse viraemia and retroviral disease by 3′-azido-3′-deoxythymidine. Nature. 1986;323:467–9.

645. Dahlberg JE, Mitsuya H, Balm SB, et al. Broad spectrum antiretroviral activity of 2′,3′-dideoxynucleosides. Proc Natl Acad Sci USA. 1987;84:2469–73.

646. Balzarini J, Pauwels R, Baba M, et al. The in vitro and in vivo anti-retrovirus activity, and intracellular metabolism of 3′-azido-2′,3′-dideoxythymidine and 2′,3′-dideoxycytidine are highly dependent on the cell species. Biochem Pharmacol. 1988;37:897–906.

647. Nakashima H, Matsui T, Harada S, et al. Inhibition of replication and cytopathic effect of human T cell lymphotropic virus type III/lymphadenopathy-associated virus by 3′-azido-3′-deoxythymidine in vitro. Antimicrob Agents Chemother. 1986;30:933–7.

648. Matsushita S, Mitsuya H, Reitz MS, et al. Pharmacological inhibition of in vitro infectivity of human T lymphotropic virus type 1. J Clin Invest. 1987;80:394–400.

649. Richman DD. Dideoxynucleosides are less inhibitory in vitro against human immunodeficiency virus type 2 (HIV-2) than against HIV-1. Antimicrob Agents Chemother. 1987;31:1879–81.

650. Nakashima H, Tochikura T, Kobayashi N, et al. Effect of 3′-azido-2′,3′dideoxythymidine (AZT) and neutralizing antibody on human immunodeficiency virus (HIV)-induced cytopathic effects: Implication of giant cell formation for the spread of virus in vivo. Virology. 1987;159:169–73.

651. Richman DD, Kornbluth RS, Carson DA. Failure of dideoxynucleosides to inhibit human immunodeficiency virus replication in cultured human macrophages. J Ex Med. 1987;166:1144–9.

652. Geleziunas R, Arts EJ, Boulerice F, et al. Effect of 3′-azido-3′-deoxythymidine on human immunodeficiency virus type 1 replication in human fetal brain macrophages. Antimicrob Agents Chemother. 1993;37:1305–12.

653. Hartshorn KL, Vogt MW, Chou T-C, et al. Synergistic inhibition of human immunodeficiency virus in vitro by azidothymidine and recombinant alpha A interferon. Antimicrob Agents Chemother. 1987;31:168–72.

654. Hammer SM, Gillis JM. Synergistic activity of granulocyte macrophage colony-stimulating factor and 3′-azido-3′-deoxythymidine against human immunodeficiency virus in vitro. Antimicrob Agents Chemother. 1987;31:1046–50.

655. Vogt MW, Hartshorn KL, Furman PA, et al. Ribavirin antagonizes the effect of azidothymidine on HIV replication. Science. 1987;235:1276–9.

656. Berk L, Schalm SW, Heijtink RA. Zidovudine inhibits hepatitis B virus replication. Antiviral Res. 1992;19:111–8.

657. Elwell LP, Ferone R, Freeman GA, et al. Antibacterial activity and mechanism of action of 3′-azido-3′-deoxythymidine (BW A509U). Antimicrob Agents Chemother 1987;31:274–80.

658. Sommadossi J-P, Carlisle R, Schinazi RJ, et al. Uridine reverses the toxicity of 3′-azido-3′-deoxythymidine in normal human granulocyte-macrophage progenitor cells in vitro without impairment of antiretroviral activity. Antimicrob Agents Chemother. 1988;32:997–1001.

659. Sharpe AH, Jaenisch R, Ruprecht RM. Retroviruses and mouse embryos: A rapid model for neurovirulence and transplacental antiviral therapy. Science. 1987;236:1671–4.

660. Niu MT, Stein DS, Schnitturan SM. Primary human immunodeficiency virus type 1 infection: Review of pathogenesis and early treatment intervention in humans and animal retrovirus infections. J Infect Dis. 1993;168:490–501.

661. Shih CC, Kaneshima H, Rabin L, et al. Postexposure prophylaxis with zidovudine suppresses human immunodeficiency virus type 1 infection in SCID-hu mice in a time-dependent manner. J Infect Dis. 1991;163:625–7.

662. Furman PA, Fyfe JA, St. Clair MH, et al. Phosphorylation of 3′-azido-3′-deoxythymidine and selective interaction of the 5′-triphosphate with human immunodeficiency virus reverse transcriptase. Proc Natl Acad Sci USA 1986;83:8333–7.

663. St. Clair MH, Richards CA, Spector T, et al. 3′-Azido-3′ deoxythymidine triphosphate as an inhibitor and substrate of purified human immunodeficiency virus reverse transcriptase. Antimicrob Agents Chemother. 1987;31:1972–7.

664. Slusher JT, Kuwahara SK, Hamzeh FM, et al. Intracellular zidovudine (ZDV) and ZDV phosphates as measured by a validated combined high-pressure liquid chromatography-radioimmunoassay procedure. Antimicrob Agents Chemother. 1992;36:2473–7.

665. Tan C-K, Civil R, Mian AM, et al. Inhibition of the RNase H activity of HIV reverse transcriptase by azidothymidylate. Biochemistry. 1991;30:4831–5.

666. Richman DD, Grimes JM, Lagakos SW. Effect of stage of disease and drug dose on zidovudine susceptibilities of isolates of human immunodeficiency virus. J Acquired Immune Deficiency Syndromes. 1990;3:743–6.

667. Mohri H, Singh MK, Ching WTW, et al. Quantitation of zidovudine-resistant human immunodeficiency virus type 1 in the blood of treated and untreated patients. Proc Natl Acad Sci USA. 1993;90:25–9.

668. Larder BA, Kemp SD. Multiple mutations in HIV-1 reverse transcriptase confer high-level resistance to zidovudine (AZT). Science. 1989;246:1155–8.

669. Richman DD, Guatelli JC, Grimes J, et al. Detection of mutations associated with zidovudine resistance in human immunodeficiency virus by use of the polymerase chain reaction. J Infect Dis. 1991;164:1075–81.

670. Boucher CA, O'Sullivan E, Mulder JW, et al. Ordered appearance of zidovudine resistance mutations during treatment of 18 human immunodeficiency virus-positive subjects. J Infect Dis. 1992;165:105–10.

671. Tudor-Williams G, St. Clair MH, McKinney RE, et al. HIV-1 sensitivity to zidovudine and clinical outcome in children. Lancet. 1992;1:15–9.

672. Montaner JSG, Singer J, Schechter MT, et al. Clinical correlates of in vitro HIV-1 resistance to zidovudine. Results of the multicenter Canadian AZT trial. AIDS. 1993;7:189–96.

673. Boucher CA, Tersmette M, Lange JMA, et al. Zidovudine sensitivity of human immunodeficiency viruses from high-risk, symptom-free individuals during therapy. Lancet. 1990;1:585–90.

674. Erice A, Mayers DL, Strike DG, et al. Brief report: Primary infection with zidovudine-resistant human immunodeficiency virus Type 1. N Engl J Med 1993;328:1163–5.

675. Fitzgibbon JE, Gaur S, Frenkel LD, et al. Transmission from one child to another of human immunodeficiency virus type 1 with zidovudine-resistance mutation. N Engl J Med. 1993;329:1835–41.

675a. Wahlberg J, Fiore J, Angarano G, et al. Apparent selection against transmission of zidovudine-resistant human immunodeficiency virus type 1 variants. J Infect Dis. 1994;169:611–4.

675b. Conlon CP, Klenerman P, Edwards A, et al. Heterosexual transmission of human immunodeficiency virus type 1 variants associated with zidovudine resistance. J Infect Dis. 1994;169:411–15.

676. Boucher CAB, von Leeuwen R, Kellamin P, et al. Effects of discontinuation of zidovudine sensitivity of human immunodeficiency virus type 1 isolates. Antimicrob Agents Chemother. 1993;37:1525–30.

677. Smith MS, Koerber KL, Pagano JS. Long-term persistence of zidovudine resistance mutations in plasma isolates of human immunodeficiency virus type 1 of dideoxyinosine-treated patients removed from zidovudine therapy. J Infect Dis. 1994;169:184–8.

678. Klecker RW Jr, Collins JM, Yarchoan R, et al. Plasma and cerebrospinal fluid pharmacokinetics of 3'-azido-3'-deoxythymidine: A novel pyrimidine analog with potential application for the treatment of patients with AIDS and related diseases. Clin Pharmacol Ther. 1987;41:407–12.

679. Blum R, Liao SHT, Good SS, et al. Pharmacokinetics and bioavailability of zidovudine in humans. Am J Med 1988;85(Suppl 2A):189–94.

680. Surbone A, Yarchoan R, McAtee N, et al. Treatment of the acquired immunodeficiency syndrome (AIDS) and AIDS-related complex with a regimen of 3'-azido-2',3'-dideoxythymidine (azidothymidine or zidovudine) and acyclovir. Ann Intern Med. 1988;108:534–40.

681. Yarchoan R, Thomas RV, Grafman J, et al. Long-term administration of 3'-azido-2',3'-dideoxythymidine to patients with AIDS-related neurological disease. Ann Neurol. 1988;23:S82–7.

682. Balis FM, Pizzo PA, Eddy J, et al. Pharmacokinetics of zidovudine administered intravenously and orally in children with human immunodeficiency virus infection. J Pediatr. 1989;114:880–4.

683. Henry K, Chinnock BJ, Quinn RP, et al. Concurrent zidovudine levels in semen and serum determined by radioimmunoassay in patients with AIDS or AIDS-related complex. JAMA. 1988;259:3023–6.

684. Rolinski B, Wintergerst U, Matuschke A, et al. Evaluation of saliva as a specimen for monitoring zidovudine therapy in HIV-infected patients. AIDS 1990;5:885–8.

685. Watts DH, Brown ZA, Tartaglione T, et al. Pharmacokinetic disposition of zidovudine during pregnancy. J Infect Dis. 1991;163:226–32.

686. Stagg MP, Cretton EM, Kidd L, et al. Clinical pharmacokinetics of 3'-azido-3'-deoxythymidine (zidovudine) and catabolites with formation of a toxic catabolite, 3'-amino-3'-deoxythymidine. Clin Pharmacol Ther. 1992;51:668–76.

687. Singlas E, Pioger J, Taburet A, et al. Zidovudine disposition in patients with severe renal impairment: Influence of hemodialysis. Clin Pharmacol Ther. 1989;46:190–7.

688. Taburet A, Naveau S, Zorza G, et al. Pharmacokinetics of zidovudine in patients with liver cirrhosis. Clin Pharmacol Ther. 1991;47:731–9.

689. De Miranda P, Good SS, Yarchoan R, et al. Alteration of zidovudine pharmacokinetics by probenecid in patients with AIDS or AIDS-related complex. Clin Pharmacol Ther. 1989;46:494–500.

690. Rajanarison JF, Lacarelle B, Catalin J, et al. 3'-Azido-3'-deoxythymidine drug interactions. Screening for inhibitors in human liver microsomes. Drug Metab Dispos. 1992;20:578–84.

691. Burger DM, Meenharst PL, Koks Ch, Beijnen JH. Pharmacokinetic interaction between rifambin and zidovudine. Antimicrob Agebts Chemother. 1993;37:1426–31.

692. Richman DD, Fischl MA, Grieco NH, et al. The toxicity of azidothymidine (AZT) in the treatment of patients with AIDS and AIDS-related complex. N Engl J Med. 1987;317:192–7.

693. Sattler FR, Ko R, Antoniskis D, et al. Acetaminophen does not impair clearance of zidovudine. Ann Intern Med. 1991;114:937–40.

694. Schwartz EL, Brechbuhl A, Kahl P, et al. Pharmacokinetic interactions of zidovudine and methadone in intravenous drug-using patients with HIV infection. J Acquired Immune Deficiency Syndromes. 1992;5:619–26.

695. Walker RE, Parker RI, Kovacs JA, et al. Anemia and erythropoiesis in patients with the acquired immunodeficiency syndrome (AIDS) and Kaposi sarcoma treated with zidovudine. Ann Intern Med. 1988;108:372–6.

696. Koch MA, Volberding PA, Lagakos SW, et al. Toxic effects of zidovudine in asymptomatic human immunodeficiency virus-infected individuals with CD4+ cell counts of 0.50 × 10⁹/L or less. Arch Intern Med. 1992;152:2286–92.

697. Volberding Pa, Lagakos WS, Koch MA, et al. Zidovudine in asymptomatic human immunodeficiency virus infection. N Engl J Med. 1990;322:941–1002.

698. Fischl MA, Richman DD, Hansen N, et al. The safety and efficacy of zidovudine (AZT) in the treatment of subjects with mildly symptomatic human immunodeficiency virus type 1 (HIV) infection. A double-blind, placebo-controlled trial. Ann Intern Med. 1990;112:727–37.

699. Fischl MA, Parker CB, Pettinelli C, et al. A randomized controlled trial of a reduced daily dose of zidovudine in patients with the acquired immunodeficiency syndrome. N Engl J Med. 1990;323:1009–41.

700. Gill PS, Rarick M, Brynes RK, et al. Azidothymidine associated with bone marrow failure in the acquired immunodeficiency syndrome (AIDS). Ann Intern Med. 1987;107:502–5.

701. Fischl M, Galpin JE, Levine JD, et al. Recombinant human erythropoietin for patients with AIDS treated with zidovudine. N Engl J Med. 1990;322:1488–93.

702. Tokars JI, Marcus R, Culver DH, et al. Surveillance of HIV infection and zidovudine use among health care workers after occupational exposure to HIV-infected blood. Ann Intern Med. 1993;118:913–9.

703. Furth PA, Kazakis AM. Nail pigmentation changes associated with azidothymidine (zidovudine). Ann Intern Med. 1987;107:350.

704. Hagler DN, Frame PT. Azidothymidine neurotoxicity (Letter). Lancet. 1986;2:1392–3.

705. Davtyan DG, Vinters HV. Wernicke's encephalopathy in AIDS patient treated with zidovudine. Lancet. 1987;1:919–20.

706. Bessen LJ, Greene JB, Louie E, et al. Severe polymyositis-like syndrome associated with zidovudine therapy of AIDS and ARC (Letter). N Engl J Med. 1988;318:708.

707. Helbert M, Peddle B, Kocsis A, et al. Acute meningoencephalitis on dose reduction of zidovudine. Lancet. 1988;1:1249–52.

708. Mhiri C, Baudrimont M, Bonne G, et al. Zidovudine myopathy: A distinctive disorder associated with mitochondrial dysfunction. Ann Neurol 1991;29:606–14.

709. Dalakas MC, Illa I, Pezeshpour GH, et al. Mitochondrial myopathy caused by long-term zidovudine therapy. N Engl J Med. 1990;322:1098–105.

710. Arnaudo E, Dalakas M, Shanske S, et al. Depletion of muscle mitochondrial DNA in AIDS patients with zidovudine-induced myopathy. Lancet. 1991;337:508–10.

711. Herskowitz A, Willoughby SB, Baughman KL, et al. Cardiomyopathy associated with antiretroviral therapy in patients with HIV infection: A report of six cases. Ann Intern Med. 1992;116:311–3.

712. Till M, MacDonell KB. Myopathy with human immunodeficiency virus type 1 (HIV-1) infection: HIV-1 or zidovudine? Ann Intern Med. 1990;113:492–4.

713. Freiman JP, Helfert KE, Hamrell MR, et al. Hepatomegaly with severe steatosis in HIV-seropositive patients. AIDS. 1993;7:379–85.

714. Chattha G, Arieff AI, Cummings C, et al. Lactic acidosis complicating the acquired immunodeficiency syndrome. Ann Intern Med. 1993;118:37–9.

715. Pickus OB. Overdose of zidovudine. N Engl J Med. 1988;318:1206.

716. Sperling RS, Stratton P, O'Sullivan MJ, et al. A survey of zidovudine use in pregnant women with human immunodeficiency virus infection. N Engl J Med. 1992;326:857–61.

717. Fischl MA, Richman DD, Grieco MH, et al. The efficacy of azidothymidine (AZT) in the treatment of patients with AIDS and AIDS-related complex. N Engl J Med. 1987;317:185–91.

718. Fischl MA, Richman DD, Causey DM, et al. Prolonged zidovudine therapy in patients with AIDS and advanced AIDS-related complex. JAMA. 1989;262:2405–10.

719. Glaser JB, Volpe S, Aguirre A, et al. Zidovudine improves response to pneumococcal vaccine among persons with AIDS and AIDS-related complex. J Infect Dis. 1991;164:761–4.

720. Rinaldo C, Huang X, Piazza P, et al. Augmentation of cellular immune function during the early phase of zidovudine treatment of AIDS patients. J Infect Dis. 1991;164:638–45.

721. Jackson GG, Paul DA, Falk LA, et al. Human immunodeficiency virus (HIV) antigenemic (p24) in the acquired immunodeficiency syndrome (AIDS) and the effect of treatment with zidovudine (AZT). Ann Intern Med. 1988;108:175–80.

722. Collier AC, Bozzette S, Coombs RW, et al. A pilot study of low-dose zidovudine in human immunodeficiency virus infection. N Engl J Med. 323:1015–21, 1990.

723. McKinney RE, Jr, Maha MA, Connor EM, et al. A multicenter trial of oral zidovudine in children with advanced human immunodeficiency virus disease. N Engl J Med. 1991;324:1018–25.

724. Hamilton JD, Hartigan PM, Simberkoff MS, et al. A controlled trial of early versus late treatment with zidovudine in symptomatic human immunodeficiency virus infection. N Engl J Med. 1992;326:437–43.

725. Aboulker J, Swart AM. Preliminary analysis of the Concorde trial. Lancet. 1993;1:889–90.

726. Cooper DA, Gatell JM, Kroon S, et al. Zidovudine in persons with asymptomatic HIV infection and CD4+ cell counts greater than 400 per cubic millimeter. N Engl J Med. 1993;329:297–303.

727. Graham NMH, Zeger SL, Park LP, et al. The effects on survival of early treatment of human immunodeficiency virus infection. N Engl J Med. 1992;326:1037–42.

728. Pedersen C, Cooper DA, Brun-Vezinet F, et al. The effect of treatment with zidovudine with or without acyclovir on HIV p24 antigenaemia in patients with AIDS or AIDS-related complex. AIDS 1992;6:821–5.

729. Dalakas MC, Yarchoan R, Spitzer R, et al. Treatment of human immunodeficiency virus-related polyneuropathy with 3'-azido-2',3'-dideoxythymidine. Ann Neurol. 1988;23:S92–4.

730. Schmitt FA, Bigley JW, McKinnis R, et al. Neuropsychological outcome of zidovudine (AZT) treatment of patients with AIDS and AIDS-related complex. N Engl J Med. 1988;319:1573–8.

731. Greisman SE, Johnston CA. The effect of azidothymidine on HIV-related thrombocytopenia. N Engl J Med. 1988;318:516–7.

732. Landonio G, Cinque P, Nosari A, et al. Comparison of two dose regimens of zidovudine in an open, randomized, multicentre study for severe HIV-related thrombocytopenia. AIDS. 1993;7:209–12.

733. Lange JMA, Boucher CAB, Hollak CEM, et al. Failure of zidovudine prophylaxis after accidental exposure to HIV-1. N Engl J Med. 1990;322:1375–77.

734. Barzilai A, Sperling RS, Hyatt AC, et al. Mother to child transmission of human immunodeficiency virus 1 infection despite zidovudine therapy from 18 weeks of gestation. Pediatr Infect Dis. 1990;9:931–33.

735. Tindall B, Gaines H, Imrie A, et al. Zidovudine in the management of primary HIV-1 infection. AIDS. 1991;5:477–84.

736. Rossi JJ, Elkins D, Zaia JA, et al. Ribozymes as anti-HIV therapeutic agents: Principles, applications, and problems. AIDS Res Hum Retroviruses. 1992; 8:183–9.
737. Marshall WS, Caruthers MH. Phosphorodithioate DNA as a potential therapeutic drug. Science. 1993;259:1564–70.
738. Schinazi RF, Mead JR, Feorino PM. Insights into HIV chemotherapy. AIDS Res Hum Retroviruses. 1992;8:963–90.

33. IMMUNOMODULATORS

MICHAEL O. FRANK
GERALD L. MANDELL

Traditional strategies for the treatment and prevention of infectious diseases have centered around antimicrobial agents and vaccines, and both have produced considerable success. Yet many infections remain a difficult problem. Treatment is complicated in many cases by a compromised immune system, either secondary to an underlying disease or to the treatment thereof. In these circumstances it may be helpful to enhance the activity of the immune system. In contrast, there are situations such as sepsis in which the body's defense systems have gone awry with an overzealous release of inflammatory cytokines, and here a dampening of activation may be beneficial. This strategy of turning up or down the immune response is the goal in the development of immunomodulators.

Immunomodulators are also known as biologic response modifiers or biologic therapeutics. Fauci[1] has defined an immunomodulator as "a biological or nonbiological substance that directly influences a specific immune function or modifies one or more components of the immunoregulatory network to achieve an indirect effect on a specific immune function." The immunoregulatory network is a very complex and intricate system with a wide variety of cell types and cytokines involved. As our knowledge of this system grows, rational approaches to modulating its activity are becoming possible. At present our attempts in this direction are simple, but basic and clinical investigations into the potential of immunomodulators are progressing at a rapid pace. In the not-too-distant future we may be using cocktails of various cytokines, antibodies, and synthetic compounds to literally "fine tune" the immune response, adjusting it as needed for a given infection. At present many of these products are very expensive, and cost effectiveness will be an important determinant of use.

Immunomodulators can be divided into five main groups: (*1*) naturally occurring cytokines, including the colony-stimulating factors, interferons, and thymic hormones; (*2*) monoclonal antibodies or receptor antagonists that block inflammatory cytokines; (*3*) immunoglobulin, either as replacement in immunoglobulin-deficient individuals or as a true immunomodulator to up- or downregulate the immune response; (*4*) corticosteroids at higher than physiologic replacement doses; and (*5*) synthetic compounds with immunomodulatory effects, such as pentoxifylline.

We focus on agents that have been used to manipulate the immune system for the treatment or prevention of infection. There are a large number of potentially useful immunomodulators that have undergone only in vitro or animal model experiments. Because of the complex interactions of the different components of the immune response, in vitro data often do not correlate with in vivo results. Furthermore, animal models, although useful for preliminary testing, have a number of limitations affecting their applicability to human disease states.[2] We therefore limit our discussion to those agents that have undergone (or are currently undergoing) clinical trials in humans. Table 1 lists those immunomodulators approved by the U.S. Food and Drug Administration for the prevention or therapy of infections.

TABLE 1. U.S. FDA Approved Uses of Immunomodulators for Infection

Immunomodulator	Indication
Granulocyte colony-stimulating factor	Prevention of infection in patients with chemotherapy-induced neutropenia
Granulocyte-macrophage colony-stimulating factor	Prevention of infection after bone marrow transplantation
Erythropoietin	Treatment of zidovudine-associated anemia in AIDS
Interferon α-2a	Treatment of Kaposi sarcoma in AIDS
Interferon α-2b	Treatment of Kaposi sarcoma in AIDS
	Treatment of chronic hepatitis B
	Treatment of chronic hepatitis C
	Treatment of genital warts due to human papillomavirus
Interferon α-n3	Treatment of genital warts due to human papillomavirus
Interferon γ	Prevention of infection in patients with chronic granulomatous disease
Intravenous immunoglobulin	Prevention of infection in primary immunoglobulin deficiency

COLONY-STIMULATING FACTORS

Colony-stimulating factors (CSFs) are a group of naturally occurring glycoproteins that are involved in the production, differentiation, survival, and activation of the myeloid line of blood cells. At present there are five known CSFs with differing degrees of relative activity on the various cell types: granulocyte colony-stimulating factor, granulocyte–macrophage colony-stimulating factor, macrophage colony-stimulating factor, interleukin-3 or multicolony-stimulating factor, and erythropoietin.

Granulocyte Colony-Stimulating Factor

Granulocyte colony-stimulating factor (G-CSF) is a 174-amino acid glycoprotein that predominantly affects the neutrophil cell line and is now available in a recombinant form with the generic name filgrastim and the brand name Neupogen (Amgen). Its most immediate effect is actually a transient decrease in neutrophil count 5–60 minutes after administration; this is followed by a sustained dose-dependent rise in neutrophil levels over a 5–6-day course. Neutrophil counts will stabilize or decrease slightly if continued for a 2-week course and will return to baseline in 4–7 days after discontinuation of G-CSF. The increase in neutrophil count is primarily due to an increase in the rate of production with a shortened maturation time; no change in the half-life of neutrophils in circulation has been noted. At doses above 10 µg/kg/day, slight increases in monocyte and lymphocyte counts are also seen, and doses above 30 µg/kg/day for 2 weeks have been associated with small decreases in number of platelets.[3]

The main use of G-CSF to date (and currently its only U.S. FDA-approved indication) is in neutropenia after cancer chemotherapy, where the risk of infection is related to both the degree and the duration of neutropenia. In a randomized, double-blind, placebo-controlled trial in patients receiving cytotoxic chemotherapy for small cell lung cancer, G-CSF was given for 8–13 days, beginning the day after the last dose of chemotherapy. G-CSF reduced the severity and duration of neutropenia and also decreased the incidence of fever, infections, hospitalization, antibiotic usage, and duration of antibiotic usage and hospitalization. There was no effect on mortality. The benefit was sustained over several cycles of chemotherapy.[4]

G-CSF has also been used after both allogeneic[5] and autologous[6] bone marrow transplantation, where it was found to increase the rate of recovery of neutrophils and to shorten the duration of parenteral antibiotics and time in isolation. However, there are more data with the use of granulocyte-macrophage colony-stimulating factor in this setting, and it is more commonly employed (see below).

Neutropenia is relatively common in human immunodeficiency virus (HIV) infection, especially in patients on zidovudine or ganciclovir. When an alternative therapy cannot be used, G-CSF may raise the neutrophil count sufficiently to allow continuation of these medications in some patients. In 14 patients with acquired immunodeficiency syndrome (AIDS), G-CSF produced a dose-dependent rise in neutrophil levels, with continuation of zidovudine, without affecting CD4 or p24 antigen levels.[7] G-CSF may also be useful in neutropenia associated with AIDS unrelated to medications. In a group of patients with advanced HIV disease, anemia, and leukopenia and not taking either zidovudine or trimethoprim-sulfamethoxazole, G-CSF produced substantial increases in neutrophil counts and also some increase in the erythroid line even without erythropoietin.[8]

Other neutropenic states where G-CSF has been found to raise neutrophil counts and decrease infections include cyclic neutropenia and congenital chronic neutropenia.[9] Whether G-CSF would be of benefit in nonneutropenic patients with serious infections (e.g., in diabetic patients, burn patients, fungal infections, postoperative infections) is not known, and investigation of these potential uses is underway.

Dosage. Recommended dosage of G-CSF for high-risk patients after cytotoxic cancer chemotherapy is 5 µg/kg/day sc starting the day after the last chemotherapy dose and continuing until the absolute neutrophil count reaches 5000–7000.[3] In patients with neutropenia and HIV infection, lower doses are often sufficient, and an initial dose can be 1 µg/kg/day sc with increases up to 10 µg/kg/day as needed. Maintenance doses should be adjusted based on twice-weekly neutrophil counts; often less than 1 µg/kg/day is necessary to maintain an absolute neutrophil count above 1000.

Adverse Effects. G-CSF is usually well tolerated. Bone pain is the most frequent adverse effect, occurring in about 20 percent of patients after chemotherapy.[4] It is usually mild and transient and can be treated with simple analgesics. Other adverse effects have included mild local erythema and swelling at sites of injection; asymptomatic elevations of lactate dehydrogenase, alkaline phosphatase, and leukocyte alkaline phosphatase; splenomegaly (in up to one-third of children on chronic therapy for chronic neutropenia—only 10 percent of these were symptomatic); and isolated reports of Sweets syndrome and leukocytic vasculitis.[10]

Granulocyte-Macrophage Colony-Stimulating Factor

Granulocyte-macrophage colony-stimulating factor (GM-CSF) is a 127-amino-acid glycoprotein also now available as a recombinant product with the generic name sargramostim. The presently approved form of recombinant human GM-CSF is a yeast product manufactured by Immunex and marketed as Leukine (Immunex) and Prokine (Hoechst-Roussel). A recombinant human GM-CSF produced by bacteria and manufactured by Schering-Plough with the trade name Leucomax has not yet been U.S. FDA approved. The yeast product is more glycosylated than the bacterial product and has a lower specific activity in vitro—however, the two products appear to have equal activity in vivo.[3,9] GM-CSF raises counts of monocytes and eosinophils, in addition to neutrophils, in peripheral blood. Like G-CSF, a transient decrease in leukocytes is seen immediately after administration. Unlike G-CSF, it does not appear to shorten the maturation time of neutrophils, but prolongs their half-life in the circulation as well as increases their rate of pro-

duction. A transient decrease in platelets has also been seen, especially at higher doses.[3]

The primary use of GM-CSF to date has been in patients undergoing autologous bone marrow transplantation, for which it has FDA approval. When given for 3 weeks after bone marrow transplantation for lymphoid malignancies, GM-CSF accelerated neutrophil recovery and shortened the duration of antibiotic administration and hospitalization.[11] There was no change in the frequency of infection or fever and no effect on survival. GM-CSF may also be useful after bone marrow transplantation for other (nonlymphoid) malignancies or in peripheral stem cell transplantation when given to increase the collection of peripheral blood progenitor cells for infusion after marrow ablative therapy.[12] A placebo-controlled trial in patients undergoing peripheral stem cell transplantation for lymphoma found that GM-CSF decreased the duration of neutropenia and the incidence of bacterial infections and enhanced engraftment, without affecting relapse or survival rates.[13] Whether GM-CSF is beneficial in allogeneic bone marrow transplantation is less clear, especially when donor and recipient are unrelated. There has been a theoretical concern that GM-CSF therapy may result in an increased incidence of graft-vs.-host disease, but this has not been documented. Several small studies of GM-CSF in allogeneic bone marrow transplantation have not consistently shown a benefit.[9] In HLA-identical sibling transplants, one trial found a difference in outcome depending on the regimen used for prevention of graft-vs.-host disease. In patients who received cyclosporine and prednisone, GM-CSF shortened the time to engraftment and decreased the incidence of early infection (compared with historic controls) without affecting the incidence of graft-vs.-host disease. However, in patients who received cyclosporine and methotrexate, a minimal effect on neutrophil recovery was noted.[14] Randomized controlled trials are underway.

The use of GM-CSF in patients with AIDS has been controversial because of early data showing increased HIV replication in monocytes stimulated with GM-CSF in vitro and increased p24 antigen levels in some patients treated with GM-CSF. However, it appears that this may be offset by the concomitant use of zidovudine. GM-CSF increases intracellular concentrations of zidovudine, and the combination appears to be synergistic in inhibiting HIV replication in vitro.[3] GM-CSF does raise numbers of neutrophils, monocytes, and eosinophils in patients with AIDS, and in some patients, functional neutrophil defects have also been corrected with administration of GM-CSF.[15]

The potential use of GM-CSF in the treatment of infections (as opposed to prevention of infection after bone marrow transplantation) is being investigated. The combination of GM-CSF, granulocyte transfusions, and amphotericin B has been used to treat successfully one patient with invasive *Candida* infection after bone marrow transplant[16] and another with disseminated *Fusarium* infection after chemotherapy for relapse of leukemia.[17] GM-CSF has also been used to treat frequent infections in two children with glycogen storage disease type 1b, although continued administration resulted in severe reactions in one patient.[18]

Dosage. A variety of dosing regimens (generally 0.3–10 µg/kg/day) have been used in the studies after bone marrow transplantation. The current manufacturer's recommendation is a dose of 250 µg/m²/day given as a 2-hour iv infusion starting 2–4 hours after bone marrow infusion and continuing for 21 days—with at least twice weekly blood counts and discontinuation if neutrophil count reaches 20,000/mm³. Other recommendations include a dose of 3–5 µg/kg/day subcutaneously.[9]

Adverse Effects. Toxicity is more common and more severe than with G-CSF, is dose related, and is greater with intravenous than subcutaneous administration. A first dose reaction can occur with flushing, tachycardia, hypotension, dyspnea, hypoxemia, myalgias, and nausea and vomiting. Other adverse effects include fever and chills (especially with doses above 3 μg/kg), lethargy, bone pain, anorexia, and rash; while these occur in one-half or more of patients who received GM-CSF, they are also common after bone marrow transplantation, and the true incidence attributable to GM-CSF is difficult to determine. At doses above 20 μg/kg/day, fluid retention, pleural and pericardial effusions, and venous thrombosis may occur. Reactivation of idiopathic thrombocytopenic purpura, rheumatoid arthritis, autoimmune thyroiditis, and hemolysis have also been reported.[3]

Other Colony-Stimulating Factors

Macrophage colony-stimulating factor (M-CSF) is a glycoprotein that stimulates production of the monocyte–macrophage line and enhances monocyte and macrophage activity in vitro. A phase I trial of recombinant human M-CSF in patients with invasive fungal infections after bone marrow transplantation has been reported.[19] Doses ranged from 100 to 2000 μg/m²/day iv. The only significant toxicity reported was transient dose-related thrombocytopenia. There was no apparent effect on incidence of graft-vs.-host disease or change in numbers of neutrophils, monocytes, or lymphocytes. Of the 12 evaluable patients, 6 had resolution of fungal infections, which was thought to be a better response rate than that of historical controls. A phase III trial is in progress.

Interleukin-3 (IL-3) was formerly known as multicolony-stimulating factor and appears to be a stimulator of multiple cell lineages.[3] Early investigation into possible therapeutic uses and preliminary trials in patients with AIDS have begun. In addition, studies of combinations of growth factors and of a newly created protein called *PIXY321* formed by the fusion of GM-CSF and IL-3[9] are underway.

Erythropoietin (EPO) is available in recombinant form under the generic name epoetin alfa and trade names Procrit (Ortho Biotech) and Epogen (Amgen). It has now received U.S. FDA approval for use in patients infected with HIV who have anemia resulting from zidovudine. A randomized double-blind placebo-controlled trial of EPO in anemic AIDS patients on zidovudine found a statistically significant decrease in the mean number of units of blood transfused in the group receiving EPO, though this benefit was noted only in those patients whose endogenous EPO level was under 500 IU/liter.[20] There was no difference between the EPO and placebo groups in the frequency of adverse effects. The currently recommended initial dosage of EPO in zidovudine-associated anemia is 100 units/kg iv or sc three times a week; dosage should then be adjusted based on weekly hematocrits.

INTERFERONS

Interferons are protein cytokines produced by cells in response to a variety of stimuli, including viral infections and certain intracellular organisms and bacterial toxins. Interferons play a complex role in the immune response, often augmenting the effects of interleukins. There are three main classes of interferons: α and β are produced by many cell types but primarily by leukocytes and fibroblasts, respectively, and γ is produced by T lymphocytes. Though there is overlap and even synergism in activities, interferons α and β are primarily antiviral interferons, while interferon γ is more effective as an activator of macrophages. Interferon β-1b is approved for therapy of relapsing-remitting multiple sclerosis.

Interferon α

The antiviral activity of interferon α is discussed in Chapter 32. Interferon α is not a single molecular entity; in fact, there are at least 17 different human genes for interferon α and the different

activities and roles of the various types are still being elucidated.[21] At present there are three different forms of interferon α available for clinical use: recombinant α-2a (Roferon-A; Roche) and α-2b (Intron A; Schering) and natural α-n3 (Alferon-N; Purdue Frederick). The two recombinant products vary by only one amino acid; the natural product is purified from human leukocytes and consists of 17 different subtypes of interferon α. Interferon α has been shown to be effective in chronic hepatitis B, chronic hepatitic C, condyloma acuminatum, and Kaposi sarcoma in AIDS and is being investigated in HIV infection and viral upper respiratory tract infections.

In chronic hepatitis B, several studies have shown a benefit from parenteral interferon α, if given in sufficient doses for a long enough period of time (see Chs. 97 and 124). The largest study included 169 patients and found that 5 million U/day (but not 1 million U/day) of interferon α for 16 weeks resulted in loss of HBeAg and HBV DNA from serum and histologic and biochemical improvement in about 40 percent of patients.[22] Furthermore, the remissions are often of long duration as shown by a follow-up study at the NIH. Of 23 patients who had responded to above, three relapsed, all within a year. After a mean follow-up of 4.3 years, the other 20 remained asymptomatic with no HBV DNA detectable by blot hybridization, and 13 of the 20 had become negative for HBsAg.[23] The likelihood of response is said to be lower in males and patients with more prolonged infection, coincident HIV infection, or little inflammatory response, as assessed by liver enzymes and histology.[24]

Interferon α-2b has also produced beneficial responses in chronic hepatitis C infection (see Chs. 97 and 132). When given at a dose of 2–3 million U three times a week sc or im for 6 months, improvement in liver enzymes and histology was seen in about half of the patients in two studies—unlike the situation with hepatitis B, however, relapse is common, occurring in 51 percent of the patients in one study[25] and 90 percent in the other[26] by 6 months after completion of therapy. Whether higher doses or more prolonged therapy would lower relapse rates is yet to be determined. α-Interferon is also undergoing trials in hepatitis D virus infection.

Interferon α has been found to be effective for condyloma acuminatum (genital warts) due to human papillomavirus (see Ch. 122). Intralesional interferon α-2b, 1–5 million U (1 million U in each wart, up to five warts at a time) three times a week for 3 weeks, was effective to 60–70 percent of patients with recurrences after other therapeutic modalities.[27] In addition, systemically administered interferon α may be an effective adjunctive therapy for recurrent respiratory papillomatosis.[28] Interferon α is also being investigated as therapy for the common cold (see Chs. 39 and 151). As a nasal spray for prophylaxis, interferon α was able to decrease upper respiratory tract infections due to rhinovirus but not coronaviruses, influenza viruses, or parainfluenza viruses.[29,30] Unfortunately, though, used alone, interferon nasal spray itself causes rhinitis. Combinations of antiviral drugs with interferon α may prove useful in a variety of viral infections. A combination of topical trifluorothymidine and interferon α was reported to be effective in three AIDS patients with severe cutaneous herpes simplex virus infection refractory to acyclovir and foscarnet.[31]

A phase I study of a combination of interferon α and IL-2 in HIV-infected patients with CD4 counts less than 200 has been reported in abstract form.[32] In the study, 15 patients received 5–20 million U/day interferon α. After 2 weeks IL-2, 0.5–2 million U/day by continuous iv infusion, was added. Transient increases in CD4 counts were seen, but four patients dropped out due to toxicity. In general, efficacy of interferon α in HIV infection has been less than that of the nucleoside analog reverse transcriptase inhibitors, with more toxicity. Studies of combinations of interferon α was nucleoside analogs are in progress.

The major adverse effects of systemically administered interferon α are dose related. An influenzalike syndrome of fever, headache, myalgia and arthralgia, nausea, and anorexia is seen in almost all patients; pretreatment with acetaminophen or a nonsteroidal anti-inflammatory agent can lessen its severity, and tolerance to these effects often develops after a few weeks, especially at doses less than 10 million Units daily.[10] At higher doses, bone marrow suppression (seen in 3–69 percent, depending on dose), neuropsychiatric problems (most commonly depression, parasthesias, or change in mental status and seen in about one-fifth of patients), and elevated liver enzymes (frequency of 10–80 percent) can also result. Intralesional interferon has caused local discomfort and inflammation and mild systemic effects, especially with a higher number of injections given concurrently.

Interferon γ

Interferon γ is now available as a recombinant product (Actimmune; Genentech) and has received FDA approval for use in chronic granulomatous disease. The early finding that administration of recombinant human interferon γ to three patients with chronic granulomatous disease resulted in increased bactericidal activity of the patients' monocytes against *Staphylococcus aureus*[33] led to a multicenter double-blind placebo-controlled trial. This study[34] enrolled 128 patients, half of whom received 50 μg/m² interferon γ sc three times a week. The treatment group developed significantly fewer serious infections (14 of 63 interferon patients developed infections vs. 30 of 65 patients given placebo; total number of infections was 20 in the interferon group and 56 in the placebo group), a benefit that was seen regardless of age, use of prophylactic antibiotics, or mode of inheritance. Interestingly, no change in superoxide production by phagocytes from treated patients could be demonstrated, making the mechanism of the benefit unclear. Toxicity was not felt to be serious, requiring withdrawal of only four patients from the treatment group. The major adverse effects noted were fever (in 52 percent of patients), headache (in 33 percent), chills (14 percent), and erythema at the injection site (14 percent).

Interferon γ is being evaluated in an attempt to decrease rates of infection in post-trauma patients with known contamination of wounds. One study of 213 patients given either placebo or interferon γ daily for 10 days after admission found increased HLA-DR expression on monocytes in the treatment group, but no significant difference in infection rates or survival between the two groups.[35] A larger study with a longer duration of treatment is being completed.

Interferon γ has been investigated as adjunctive therapy in several chronic infections caused by intracellular organisms. Badaro et al.[36] reported that interferon γ at a dose of 100–400 μg/m²/day im for 10–40 days given with pentavalent antimony was successful in six of eight patients with visceral leishmaniasis previously unresponsive to pentavalent antimony alone and in eight of nine patients previously untreated. A recent update of their experience[37] added another 22 patients (14 refractory, 8 untreated) with severe pancytopenia and splenomegaly. Though 7 patients required retreatment after relapse (6 of these were in the refractory group), the overall response rate was 17 of 22, with follow-up now at greater than 1 year. The authors feel that these response rates are significantly better than historic controls, but no prospective randomized controlled study has yet been done. Interferon γ plus meglumine antiomonate was effective for cutaneous leishmaniasis.[37a]

Lepromatous leprosy is a chronic indolent infection associated with decreased interferon γ production and macrophage activation. Administration of interferon γ can increase the response of macrophages to *Mycobacterium leprae* and increase clearance of bacteria from skin samples.[38] *Mycobacterium avium* complex (MAC) is another intracellular organism that causes chronic infections and is being seen with increasing frequency, especially in AIDS patients. Since T cells from AIDS patients are deficient in production of interferon γ (yet their mononuclear phagocytes respond normally to it), interferon γ

is being studied for therapy of opportunistic infections. Squires et al.[39] reported six AIDS patients with MAC bacillemia treated with interferon γ. While patients treated with interferon γ alone had only a minimal transient benefit, the three patients being treated concurrently with antimicrobials displayed decreases in the level of bacillemia as measured by colony-forming units per milliliter of blood. Holland et al.[40] recently presented data on six HIV-negative patients with disseminated MAC infection refractory to a multi drug antibiotic regimen who had low levels of γ-interferon and IL-2. When interferon γ 50 μg/m² sc three times weekly, was added to the antibiotics, four patients had dramatic clinical improvement.[40]

INTERLEUKINS

Interleukins are a family of immune system cytokines with a variety of effects on different cell types. They serve primarily as a communication network between inducer and effector cells of the immune response. The number of different interleukins is currently up to 11 and growing; the activities of many of these are only beginning to be elucidated.

Interleukin-1

Clinical interest in IL-1 has centered on mechanisms to dampen its augmentation of the inflammatory response in sepsis (see Ch. 56) and as a nonspecific adjunctive therapy for bacterial infections.[41]

Interleukin-2

IL-2 is currently approved for the treatment of metastatic renal cell carcinoma under the generic name aldesleukin and the brand name Proleukin (Cetus). IL-2 shares many of the same effects as interferon γ and has been used for therapy of some of the same infections. In three patients with disseminated cutaneous leishmaniasis given intralesional injections of 10 μg recombinant IL-2 at 48-hour intervals for 14 days, significant reductions in numbers of amastigotes were seen, and in two of the patients sites became sterile by culture.[42] In leprosy, 10 μg IL-2 intradermally (in the skin of the back) enhanced cell-mediated immunity and decreased the number of organisms in lesions; adverse effects included nontender axillary lymphadenopathy and local site inflammation.[43] In eight patients with HIV infection taking zidovudine, 10 μg recombinant IL-2 or 9 μg of its polyethylene glycol derivative given intradermally daily for 30 days was reported to be nontoxic and resulted in increases in natural killer cell activity, delayed-type hypersensitivity responses, and in vitro proliferative responses to antigens.[44]

IL-2 is being used (often with lymphokine-activated killer cells) as immunotherapy for malignancies.[45] It should be noted that this therapy in cancer patients has been associated with an increased incidence of staphylococcal infections[46] though a recent paper suggests that this increased risk can be adequately dealt with through patient screening, rigorous monitoring, and liberal use of antibiotics for suspected infections.[47] It has been postulated that the increased infections are due to IL-2-induced elevations of tumor necrosis factor with a consequent defect in neutrophil chemotaxis; dexamethasone lowered tumor necrosis factor levels and prevented this defect.[48]

IMMUNOGLOBULINS

Commercially available preparations of immunoglobulin are derived from human blood, and, in addition to the traditional intramuscular route, formulations are now available for intravenous use. There are currently eight preparations of intravenous immunoglobulin marketed in the United States: Gamimmune N, from Miles; Gammagard, from Hyland; Gammar-IV, from Armour; Iveegam, from Immuno-US; Polygam, marketed by the

American Red Cross and manufactured by Hyland with plasma from Red Cross donors; Sandoglobulin, marketed by Sandoz and manufactured by the Swiss Red Cross; and Venoglobulin-I and Venoglobulin-S, from Alpha Therapeutics. They are prepared by somewhat different methods and have different additives for stabilization,[10,49] but for most situations they are felt to be therapeutically equivalent.[50] Gammagard and Polygam have the lowest IgA content, and Gam immune N is supplied as a liquid and does not need to be reconstituted, but also contains 10% maltose as a stabilizer, which may result in a mild diuresis.[10,49,50] All are prepared from plasma from at least 1000 donors per lot and contain greater than 90 percent intact IgG with normal ratios of IgG subclasses.

One of the oldest uses for immunoglobulin is to provide specific antibodies that the recipient is lacking. This is the rationale for its intramuscular use in travelers to prevent hepatitis A and for the use of products such as varicella-zoster immunoglobulin, hepatitis B immunoglobulin, tetanus immunoglobulin, and rabies immunoglobulin in selected patients with a given exposure. The same reasoning has been applied in the well-accepted use of intravenous immunoglobulin in the primary immunoglobulin deficiencies, including X-linked agammaglobulinemia, common variable immunodeficiency, severe combined immunodeficiency, X-linked immunodeficiency with hyperimmunoglobulinemia M, Wiskott-Aldrich syndrome, and ataxia-telangiectasia.[49]

Premature infants are another group that may benefit from administration of immunoglobulin, since there is little transplacental transfer of IgG before 32 weeks gestation. This question was addressed in a double-blind trial involving 588 premature neonates, randomized (with stratification for birth weight) to receive either placebo or periodic infusions of immunoglobulin. The treatment group had fewer infections and fewer days of hospitalization for infection, but there was no difference in morbidity, mortality, or mean duration of hospitalization.[51] Another double-blind study evaluated the use of immunoglobulin for prevention of infection in high-risk postsurgical patients.[52] The study had three arms: placebo, standard immunoglobulin, and hyperimmunoglobulin with high titers of antibody to *Salmonella minnesota* R595 lipopolysaccharide, each given intravenously weekly for up to 4 weeks while in the surgical intensive care unit. A decrease in infections in the standard immunoglobulin group compared with placebo was noted, with the decrease primarily due to fewer episodes of pneumonia (particularly gram-negative pneumonia). Shorter stays in the intensive care unit and hospital were also found in the standard immunoglobulin group vs. placebo. Strangely, the rates of infection in the hyperimmune group were not different from placebo, which is difficult to explain since hyperimmunoglobulin would be expected to be at least as effective as standard immunoglobulin. Furthermore, there was no difference between any of the groups in rates of systemic infection, shock, or death. In an editorial accompanying these two articles, Siber[53] argues against the routine use of immunoglobulin in both premature infants and postsurgical patients, citing problems with the studies and variability between different commercial immunoglobulins and even between different lots by the same manufacturer.

Despite normal or even high serum immunoglobulin levels, infants and young children with AIDS often have decreased antibody responses and a corresponding increased incidence of bacterial and viral infections. A large double-blind placebo-controlled study was performed to assess the value of immunoglobulin in this population.[54] It demonstrated fewer serious infections and hospitalizations in the treatment group among children whose CD4 count was still above 200. Unfortunately, the majority of the study was conducted before zidovudine and *Pneumocystis carinii* pneumonia prophylaxis became widespread, so the applicability to present practice is unknown. Another trial in children with HIV infection receiving zidovudine and *Pneumocystis* prophylaxis is underway.

Intravenous immunoglobulin has been shown to be beneficial in preventing infection in patients with chronic lymphocytic leukemia, though the cost effectiveness has been challenged by Weeks et al.[55] who calculated that each patient would gain only 0.8 quality-adjusted day per year with no change in life expectancy and that it would cost $6 million for each quality-adjusted life-year gained.

In the post bone marrow transplant period, immunoglobulin appears to play an immunomodulatory role besides simply providing antibodies. In a randomized controlled trial of bone marrow transplant patients, administration of 500 mg/kg immunoglobulin iv weekly to day 90 and then monthly to day 360 decreased the incidences of acute graft-vs.-host disease, interstitial pneumonia in cytomegalovirus (CMV) seropositive patients, and gram-negative septicemia and local infection.[56] There were no overall differences in mortality or relapse rates. However, there were significantly fewer deaths due to transplant-related causes in the immunoglobulin-treated group among HLA-identical transplanted patients. The benefit of standard immunoglobulin in prevention of CMV disease after bone marrow transplantation appears to be equivalent to that seen using CMV hyperimmune globulin.[57] In addition, immunoglobulin reduces the incidence of clinical CMV infection after kidney transplantation.[57]

Two studies have found immunoglobulin to be helpful when given with ganciclovir for the treatment of CMV pneumonia after bone marrow transplantation. One study used 400 mg/kg of CMV immunoglobulin iv on days 1, 2, and 7 and 200 mg/kg on days 14 and 21 in addition to ganciclovir in 25 patients and achieved a 52 percent survival rate compared with 15 percent for historical controls.[58] The other study used 500 mg/kg standard immunoglobulin iv every other day for 20 days, then twice a week for 4 weeks, plus ganciclovir, and documented recurrence-free survival in 7 of 10 patients at a median follow up of 10 months compared with no survival in historical controls given ganciclovir alone (2 patients), CMV hyperimmune globulin alone (5 patients), or standard immunoglobulin alone (4 patients).[59]

Intravenous immunoglobulin and aspirin is considered the standard of care for the treatment of Kawasaki syndrome.[60] The mechanism of action is unclear; recent in vitro work showing that intravenous immunoglobulin preparations contain antibodies against staphylococcal toxin superantigens and that these antibodies can block T-cell activation elicited by staphylococcal toxins[61] contributes further evidence to the hypothesis of neutralization of a bacterial toxin.[60] Finally, uncontrolled reports suggest efficacy of immunoglobulin in HIV-related thrombocytopenia.[57]

At present, intravenous immunoglobulin is only U.S. FDA approved for treatment of immune thrombocytopenic purpura and primary antibody immunodeficiency. The recommended dosage of intravenous immunoglobulin for primary immunodeficiency is 100–400 mg/kg, depending on the preparation used, given monthly. If the resulting clinical response or serum level of IgG is inadequate, dosage can be increased to 400–800 mg/kg monthly or the interval between doses can be decreased. Adverse effects are seen in less than 10 percent of patients and are usually related to the rate of administration. Headache is the most frequent adverse effect; others include myalgias, arthralgias, fatigue, and malaise. Immunoglobulin is contraindicated in patients with selective IgA deficiency, since these patients may have anti-IgA antibodies and immunoglobulin preparations contain small amounts of IgA. Rarely, intravenous immunoglobulin causes hypotension with fever, diaphoresis, chest tightness, and other manifestations of anaphylaxis. This reaction is more common when the recommended rate of infusion is exceeded and in patients with hypogammaglobulinemia or agammaglobulinemia who have not received prior immunoglobulin infusion or who have received an infusion within the preceding 8 weeks.

GLUCOCORTICOSTEROIDS

Glucocorticosteroids have marked anti-inflammatory activity on a variety of immune cell types and are potent suppressors of the immune response. When used for infectious diseases, the situation is usually such that an overactive immune response is contributing to the pathology of the infection rather than containing it. A dramatic example of this is in AIDS patients with pneumonia due to *P. carinii,* where patients often suffer worsening oxygenation initially after appropriate antimicrobial therapy. This is thought to be secondary to the increased inflammatory response to the dying organisms. Several studies have shown that, in patients with moderate to severe hypoxia, glucocorticosteroid therapy initiated within 72 hours of initiation of antibiotics increases oxygenation and decreases the incidence of respiratory failure and mortality (see Ch. 258).[62]

In general, steroids are not helpful (and may even be harmful) in septic shock or gram-negative sepsis (see Ch. 56).[63] Severe typhoid fever with shock may, however, be an exception based on a randomized double-blind placebo-controlled trial carried out in Indonesia.[64] Patients with typhoid fever with shock or mental status changes received either placebo or very high doses of dexamethasone (3 mg/kg followed by 1 mg/kg every 6 hours for 8 doses). Mortality in the dexamethasone group was 10 vs. 56 percent in the placebo group, a statistically significant difference. Of note, all patients were treated with chloramphenicol, and there were no intensive care unit facilities available. Bacterial meningitis is another area with some controversy regarding use of steroids. While use of steroids in children with meningitis due to *Haemophilus influenzae* is now well accepted, use in adults or with other bacteria is less straightforward (see Ch. 64).

Complications of tuberculosis are often included as indications for steroid therapy. Tuberculous meningitis is typically a basilar meningitis with considerable inflammation and consequent risk of hydrocephalus. An open label prospective study in Egypt using intramuscular isoniazid, ethambutol, and streptomycin for tuberculous meningitis found that dexamethasone as adjunctive therapy decreased morbidity and mortality.[65] One recommended dosing schedule for patients with increased intracranial pressure, focal neurologic deficits, or change in mental status due to tuberculous meningitis is 60 mg prednisone daily for 1–2 weeks, then tapered over 4–6 weeks.[66] In tuberculous pericarditis, drainage may be necessary to prevent tamponade, and inflammation with scarring can lead to later constriction. A randomized trial in Transkei, South Africa, found that prednisolone as adjunctive therapy for tuberculous pericarditis resulted in faster clinical improvement and decreased mortality.[67] Dosage used in the trial was 60 mg prednisolone daily for 4 weeks, then tapered over the next 7 weeks (see Ch. 230).

INFLAMMATORY CYTOKINE BLOCKERS IN SEPSIS

A variety of different compounds with blocking activity against various inflammatory cytokines are currently being investigated for use in sepsis. These include monoclonal antibodies against endotoxin and tumor necrosis factor, soluble receptors for IL-1 and tumor necrosis factor, IL-1 receptor antagonist, and others. These are discussed in Chapter 56.

PENTOXIFYLLINE

Pentoxifylline is a methylxanthine derivative that in vitro decreases the production of tumor necrosis factor by monocytes stimulated with endotoxin and also counteracts some of the effects of tumor necrosis factor and other inflammatory cytokines on neutrophils.[68] In healthy volunteers pentoxifylline blocked the rise in serum levels of tumor necrosis factor seen in response to an infusion of endotoxin.[69] On the basis of these data and the efficacy in a murine model of malaria, pentoxifylline was administered and thought to be effective for one patient with cerebral malaria.[70] Pentoxifylline is also being evaluated for prevention of renal insufficiency in bone marrow transplant patients receiving amphotericin B and cyclosporine A,[71] for prevention of transplant-related toxicities following bone marrow transplantation,[72,73] and in the treatment of diffuse idiopathic pneumonia complicating bone marrow transplantation.[74]

CIMETIDINE

Cimetidine is a histamine type 2 receptor blocker used primarily for peptic ulcer disease. After in vitro data showed that a histamine-induced factor activated T lymphocyte suppressor cells and that cimetidine reduced this activation, cimetidine was studied in a double-blind trial of patients with herpes zoster.[75] Patients without malignancy and with zoster lesions present for less than 72 hours were randomized to cimetidine 1200 mg or propoxyphene/acetaminophen every 8 hours for 10 days. The cimetidine group had significantly decreased median time to complete healing and time to resolution of pain; no toxicity was noted. There were too few patients to discern any effect on development of postherpetic neuralgia. In vitro, cimetidine reversed the increased activity of suppressor cells from the patients with acute zoster. The authors could not rule out the possibility of confounding due to histamine involvement in pain pathways. Cimetidine has also been shown to decrease symptoms and promote healing of herpes simplex lesions in immunocompromised patients[76] (though this was before the use of acyclovir), and to significantly improve body weight, fever, and diarrhea in patients with HIV infection[77] (though this was before the use of zidovudine).[77]

THYMOSIN

Thymosins are peptides produced by the thymus with effects on the neuroendocrine and immune systems—among these effects are induction of the cytokines IL-1, IL-2, interferon α, and interferon γ. Thymosin fraction 5 (TF5) is a partially purified extract of bovine thymus with at least 40 peptide components. Thymosin α_1 is a 28-amino-acid protein purified from TF5 that is now sequenced and synthesized. Thymosin α-1 has been noted to increase the effectiveness of influenza and hepatitis B vaccines in chronic renal failure patients on hemodialysis.[78] It has also been studied as an adjunct to influenza vaccine in the elderly, another group with poor responses to vaccines. In a phase III double-blind trial[79] 90 men aged 65–99 years were randomized to placebo or 900 μg/m² thymosin α-1 SC twice weekly for 4 weeks, beginning at the same time as the influenza vaccine was administered. No toxicity was noted, and the treatment group demonstrated a greater response to the vaccine at 6 weeks—this difference was due to greater efficacy in the 77 and older age group; the younger groups were not different. The results of a larger trial involving 324 elderly recipients of influenza vaccine are expected soon.

A pilot study suggested efficacy of thymosin in patients with chronic hepatitis B.[80] Patients were randomized in double-blind fashion to TF5 90 mg/m² (four patients), thymosin α-1 900 μg/m² (three patients), or placebo (five patients) administered sc twice weekly for 6 months. The patients receiving one of the thymosin preparations had significantly increased clearance of HBV DNA, decreased transaminase levels, and improved histology compared with those given placebo. The only toxicity was a local reaction at the sites of injection in two patients receiving TF5. A large phase III trial of thymosin α-1 (Alpha One Biomedical) in chronic hepatitis B is in progress. Other ongoing trials of potential uses for thymosin include combination with interferon for hepatitis C, combination with interferon and zidovudine for HIV, and combination with polyethyleneglycol IL-2 and zidovudine for HIV.

Thymopentin is a pentapeptide corresponding to amino acids 32–36 of thymopoietin and sharing its ability to stimulate IL-2 production and activate macrophages. While some uncontrolled or poorly controlled trials seemed to show an increased response to hepatitis B vaccine in hemodialysis patients, better designed studies have found no difference in response to hepatitis B[81] or influenza[82] vaccines in hemodialysis patients.

OTHER IMMUNOMODULATORS UNDER INVESTIGATION

IMREG-1

IMREG-1 (Imreg, Inc.) is a leukocyte-derived product from healthy volunteers prepared by sequential dialysis and high-pressure liquid chromatography. It has been found to contain per dose 4.2 fmol tyr-gly, 0.2 fmol tyr-gly-gly, 30 pmol phenylalanine, and another "immunologically active component . . . whose structure has not been determined."[83] In a randomized double-blind placebo-controlled trial in 143 HIV-infected patients without AIDS, the IMREG-1 group had significantly fewer patients develop an AIDS-defining illness, as well as a smaller mean decrease in CD4 count and improved delayed-type hypersensitivity responses.[83] However, none of the patients took zidovudine or any other antiretroviral agent, or any *Pneumocystis* prophylaxis, calling into question the relevance of the study given the present management of HIV infection.

Ditiocarb

Ditiocarb is the sodium salt of diethyldithiocarbamate, an antioxidant and chelator. After pilot studies found decreases in lymphadenopathy, symptoms, and disease progression in AIDS and AIDS-related complex, a multicenter double-blind placebo-controlled trial of orally administered ditiocarb in 387 patients with AIDS or symptomatic HIV infection was performed.[84] There were 10 patients in the ditiocarb group who developed opportunistic infections compared with 21 in the control group. No significant difference in CD4 counts or mortality occurred, and no significant toxicity was noted. The relevance of this study is less clear now that antiretroviral drugs and prophylaxis for *P. carinii* pneumonia are standard in the management of these patients. Of the 31 opportunistic infections that occurred in the study, 21 were *Pneumocystis* pneumonia.

LF 1695

LF 1695 is a synthetic low-molecular-weight compound. It increases bone marrow recovery after ablative therapy in animals and induces T-cell differentiation, increases lymphocyte proliferative responses, and increases IL-2 production by activated lymphocytes and IL-1 and leukotriene B4 production by macrophages in vitro.[85] It is now undergoing trials in patients with AIDS.

Linomide

Linomide, a quinoline carboxamide also known as LS-2616, has been used in a pilot study of five patients after autologous bone marrow transplantation for acute myelogenous leukemia.[86] Linomide increased natural killer cell numbers and activity, increased number of monocytes, and increased production of tumor necrosis factor, interferon-γ and IL-1. Of concern with regard to allogeneic transplants is that in rats linomide abolishes the protective effect of cyclosporine A on allograft rejection.[87]

REFERENCES

1. Fauci AS. Immunomodulators in clinical medicine. Ann Intern Med. 1987; 106:421–33.
2. Roilides E, Pizzo PA. Modulation of host defenses by cytokines: Evolving adjuncts in prevention and treatment of serious infections in immunocompromised hosts. Clin Infect Dis. 1992;15:508–24.
3. Lieschke GJ, Burgess AW. Granulocyte colony-stimulating factor and granulocyte-macrophage colony-stimulating factor. N Engl J Med. 1992;327:28–35, 99–106.
4. Crawford J, Ozer H, Stoller R, et al. Reduction by granulocyte colony-stimulating factor of fever and neutropenia induced by chemotherapy in patients with small-cell lung cancer. N Engl J Med. 1991;325:164–70.
5. Masaoka T, Takaku F, Kato S, et al. Recombinant human granulocyte colony-stimulating factor in allogeneic bone marrow transplantation. Exp Hematol. 1989;17:1047–50.
6. Sheridan WP, Morstyn G, Wolf M, et al. Granulocyte colony-stimulating factor and neutrophil recovery after high-dose chemotherapy and autologous bone marrow transplantation. Lancet. 1989;2:891–5.
7. Kimura S, Matsuda J, Ikamatsu S, et al. Efficacy of recombinant human granulocyte colony-stimulating factor on neutropenia in patients with acquired immune deficiency syndrome. AIDS. 1990;4:1251–5.
8. Miles SA, Mitsuyasa RT, Lee K, et al. Recombinant human granulocyte-colony-stimulating factor increases circulating burst forming unit-erythron and red blood cell production in patients with severe human immunodeficiency virus infection. Blood. 1990;75:2137–42.
9. Fleischman RA. Southwestern internal medicine conference: Clinical use of hematopoietic growth factors. Am J Med Sci. 1993;305::248–73.
10. American Hospital Formulary Service. AHFS Drug Information. Bethesda, M: American Society of Hospital Pharmacists; 1993.
11. Nemunaitis J, Rabinowe SN, Singer JW, et al. Recombinant granulocyte-macrophage colony-stimulating factor after autologous bone marrow transplant for lymphoid cancer. N Engl J Med. 1991;324:1173–8.
12. Peters WP. Use of cytokines during prolonged neutropenia associated with autologous bone marrow transplantation. Rev Infect Dis. 1991;13:993–6.
13. Advani R, Chao NJ, Horning SJ, et al. Granulocyte-macrophage colony-stimulating factor (GM-CSF) as an adjunct to autologous hemopoietic stem cell transplantation for lymphoma. Ann Intern Med. 1992;116:183–9.
14. Nemunaitis J, Buckner CD, Appelbaum FR, et al. Phase I/II trial of recombinant human granulocyte-macrophage colony-stimulating factor following allogeneic bone marrow transplantation. Blood. 1991;77:2065–71.
15. Baldwin GC, Gasson JC, Quon SG, et al. Granulocyte-macrophage colony stimulating factor enhances neutrophil function in acquired immunodeficiency syndrome patients. Proc Natl Acad Sci USA. 1988;85:2763–6.
16. Montgomery B, Bianco JA, Jacobsen A, et al. Localization of transfused neutrophils to site of infection during treatment with recombinant human granulocyte-macrophage colony-stimulating factor and pentoxifylline. Blood. 1991;78:533–4.
17. Spielberger RT, Falleroni MJ, Coene AJ, et al. Concomitant amphotericin B therapy, granulocyte transfusions, and GM-CSF administration for disseminated infection with *Fusarium* in a granulocytopenic patient. Clin Infect Dis. 1993;16:528–30.
18. Hurst D, Kilpatrick L, Becker J, et al. Recombinant human GM-CSF treatment of neutropenia in glycogen storage disease-1b. Am J Pediatr Hematol Oncol. 1993;15:71–6.
19. Nemunaitis J, Meyers JD, Buckner CD, et al. Phase I trial of recombinant human macrophage colony-stimulating factor in patients with invasive fungal infections. Blood. 1991;78:907–13.
20. Fischl M, Galpain JE, Levine JD, et al. Recombinant human erythropoietin for patients with AIDS treated with zidovudine. N Engl J Med. 1990;322:1488–93.
21. Baron S, Tyring SK, Fleischmann WR Jr, et al. The interferons: Mechanisms of action and clinical applications. JAMA. 1991;266:1375–83.
22. Perillo RP, Schiff ER, Davis GL, et al. A randomized controlled trial of interferon α-2b alone and after prednisone withdrawal for the treatment of chronic hepatitis B. N Engl J Med. 1990;323:295–301.
23. Korenman J, Baker B, Waggoner J, et al. Long-term remission of chronic hepatitis B after alpha-interferon therapy. Ann Intern Med. 1991;114:629–34.
24. Martin P, Friedman LS. Therapies for hepatitis B: Current status and future possibilities. In: Block T, ed. Innovations in Antiviral Development and the Detection of Virus Infection. New York: Plenum Press; 1992;111–20.
25. Davis BL, Balart LA, Schiff ER, et al. Treatment of chronic hepatitis C with recombinant interferon alpha: A multicenter, randomized, controlled trial. N Engl J Med. 1989;321:1501–6.
26. Di Bisceglie AM, Martin P, Kassianides C, et al. Recombinant interferon alpha therapy for chronic hepatitis C: A randomized double-blind placebo-controlled trial. N Engl J Med. 1989;321:1506–10.
27. Reichman RC, Oakes D, Bonnez W, et al. Treatment of condyloma acuminatum with three different alpha interferon preparations administered parenterally: A double-blind, placebo-controlled trial. J Infect Dis. 1990;162:1270–6.
28. Leventhal BG, Kashima HK, Mounts P, et al. Long-term response of recurrent respiratory papillomatosis to treatment with lymphoblastoid interferon α-n1. N Engl J Med. 1991;325:613–7.
29. Hayden FG, Albrecht JK, Kaiser DL, et al. Prevention of natural colds by contact prophylaxis with intranasal alpha 2-interferon. N Engl J Med. 1986;314:71–5.
30. Douglas RM, Moore BW, Miles HB, et al. Prophylactic efficacy of intranasal alpha 2 interferon against rhinovirus infections in the family setting. N Engl J Med. 1986;314:65–70.

31. Birch CJ, Tyssen DP, Tachedjian G, et al. Clinical effects and in vitro studies of trifluorothymidine combined with interferon-alpha for treatment of drug-resistant and -sensitive herpes simplex virus infections. J Infect Dis. 1992; 166:108–12.

32. Schnittman SM, Davey RT, Havelwich S, et al. A phase I study of alpha interferon in combination with interleukin-2 in patients with HIV infection. Clin Res. 1992;40:246A.

33. Sechler JMG, Malech HL, White CJ, et al. Recombinant human interferon gamma reconstitutes defective phagocyte function in patients with chronic granulomatous disease of childhood. Proc Natl Acad Sci USA. 1988;85: 4874–8.

34. The International CGD Cooperative Study Group. A controlled trial of interferon-gamma to prevent infection in chronic granulomatous disease. N Engl J Med. 1991;324:509–16.

35. Polk HC, Cheadle WG, Livingston DH, et al. A randomized prospective clinical trial to determine the efficacy of interferon gamma in severely injured patients. Am J Surg. 1992;163:191–6.

36. Badaro R, Falcoff E, Badaro FS, et al. Treatment of visceral leishmaniasis with pentavalent antimony and interferon gamma. N Engl J Med. 1990;322: 16–21.

37. Badaro R, Johnson WD. The role of interferon-gamma in the treatment of visceral and diffuse cutaneous leishmaniasis. J Infect Dis. 1993;167(Suppl 1): S13–7.

37a.Arana BA, Navim TR, Arana FE, et al. Efficacy of a short course (10 days) of high-dose meglumine antimonate with or without interferon-γ in treating cutaneous leishmaniasis in Guatemala. Clin Inf Dis. 1994;18:381–4.

38. Kaplan G. Recent advances in cytokine therapy in leprosy. J Infect Dis. 1993; 17(Suppl 1):S18–22.

39. Squires KE, Brown ST, Armstrong D, et al. Interferon-gamma treatment for *Mycobacterium avium-intracellulare* complex bacillemia in patients with AIDS. J Infect Dis. 1992;166:686–7.

40. Holland SM, Eisenstein E, Kuhns DB, et al. Disseminated *M. avium* infection without HIV infection is associated with defective interferon-gamma production and responds to treatment with interferon-gamma. Clin Res. 1993;41: 321A.

41. Vogels MTE, Van der Meer JWM. Use of immune modulators in nonspecific therapy of bacterial infections. Antimicrob Agents Chemother. 1992;36:1–5.

42. Akuffo H, Kaplan G, Kiessling R, et al. Administration of recombinant interleukin-2 reduces the local parasite load of patients with disseminated cutaneous leishmaniasis. J Infect Dis. 1990;161:775–80.

43. Kaplan G, Britton WJ, Hancock GE, et al. The systemic influence of recombinant interleukin-2 in the manifestations of lepromatous leprosy. J Exp Med. 1991;173:993–1006.

44. Teppler H, Kaplan G, Smith K, et al. Efficacy of low doses of the polyethylene glycol derivative of interleukin-2 in modulating the immune response of patients with human immunodeficiency virus type 1 infection. J Infect Dis. 1993; 167:291–8.

45. Rosenberg SA, Lotze MT, Muul LM, et al. A progress report on the treatment of 157 patients with advanced cancer using lymphokine-activated killer cells and interleukin-2 or high dose interleukin-2 alone. N Engl J Med. 1987;316: 889–97.

46. Syndman DR, Sullivan B, Gill M, et al. Nosocomial sepsis associated with interleukin-2. Ann Intern Med. 1990;112:102–7.

47. Pockaj BA, Topalian SL, Steinberg SM, et al. Infectious complications associated with interleukin-2 administration: A retrospective review of 935 treatment courses. J Clin Oncol. 1993;11:136–47.

48. Mier JW, Vachino G, Klemper MS, et al. Inhibition of interleukin-2 induced tumor necrosis factor release by dexamethasone: Prevention of an acquired neutrophil chemotaxis defect and differential suppression of interleukin-2 associated side effects. Blood. 1990;76:1933–40.

49. Buckley RH, Schiff RI. The use of intravenous immune globulin in immunodeficiency diseases. N Engl J Med. 1991;325:110–7.

50. Stiehm ER. New uses for intravenous immune globulin. N Engl J Med. 1991; 325:123–5.

51. Baker CJ, Melish ME, Hall RT, et al. Intravenous immune globulin for the prevention of nosocomial infection in low-birth-weight neonates. N Engl J Med. 1992;327:213–9.

52. The Intravenous Immunoglobulin Collaborative Study Group. Prophylactic intravenous administration of standard immune globulin as compared with core-lipopolysaccharide immune globulin in patients at high risk of postsurgical infection. N Engl J Med. 1992;327:234–40.

53. Siber GR. Immune globulin to prevent nosocomial infections. N Engl J Med. 1992;327:269–71.

54. National Institutes of Child Health and Human Development Intravenous Immunoglobulin Study Group. Intravenous immune globulin for the prevention of bacterial infections in children with symptomatic human immunodeficiency virus infection. N Engl J Med. 1991;325:73–80.

55. Weeks JC, Tierney MR, Weinstein MC. Cost effectiveness of prophylactic intravenous immune globulin in chronic lymphocytic leukemia. N Engl J Med. 1991;325:81–6.

56. Sullivan KM, Kopecky KJ, Jocom J, et al. Immunomodulatory and antimicrobial efficacy of intravenous immunoglobulin in bone marrow transplantation. N Engl J Med. 1990;323:705–12.

57. Berkman SA, Lee ML, Gale RP. Clinical uses of intravenous immunoglobulins. Ann Intern Med. 1990;112:278–92.

58. Reed EC, Bowden RA, Dandliker PS, et al. Treatment of cytomegalovirus pneumonia with ganciclovir and intravenous cytomegalovirus immunoglobulin in patients with bone marrow transplants. Ann Intern Med. 1988;109:783–8.

59. Emanuel D, Cunningham I, Jules-Elysee K, et al. Cytomegalovirus pneumonia after bone marrow transplantation successfully treated with the combination of ganciclovir and high-dose intravenous immune globulin. Ann Intern Med. 1988;198:777–82.

60. Dwyer JM. Manipulating the immune system with immune globulin. N Engl J Med. 1992;326:107–16.

61. Takei S, Arora YK, Walker SM. Intravenous immunoglobulin contains specific antibodies inhibitory to activation of T cells by staphylococcal toxin superantigens. J Clin Invest. 1993;91:602–7.

62. The National Institutes of Health—University of California Expert Panel for Corticosteroids as Adjunctive Therapy for Pneumocystis Pneumonia. Consensus statement on the use of corticosteroids as adjunctive therapy for *Pneumocystis* pneumonia in the acquired immunodeficiency syndrome. N Engl J Med. 1990;323:1500–4.

63. McGowan JE, Chesney PJ, Crossley KB, et al. Guidelines for the use of systemic glucocorticosteroids in the management of selected infections. J Infect Dis. 1992;165:1–13.

64. Hoffman SL, Punjabi NH, Kumala S, et al. Reduction of mortality in chloramphenicol-treated severe typhoid fever by high-dose dexamethasone. N Engl J Med. 1984;310:82–8.

65. Girgis NI, Farid Z, Kilpatrick ME, et al. Dexamethasone adjunctive treatment for tuberculous meningitis. Pediatr Infect Dis J. 1991;10:179–83.

66. Molavi A, Lefrock JL. Tuberculous meningitis. Med Clin North Am. 1985; 69:315–31.

67. Strang JIG, Gibson DG, Nunn AJ, et al. Controlled trial of prednisolone as adjuvant in treatment of tuberculous constrictive pericarditis in Transkei. Lancet. 1987;2:1418–22.

68. Sullivan GW, Carper HT, Novick WJ, et al. Inhibition of the inflammatory action of interleukin-1 and tumor necrosis factor (alpha) on neutrophil function by pentoxifylline. Infect Immun. 1988;56:1722–9.

69. Zabel P, Wolter DT, Schonharting MM, et al. Oxpentifylline in endotoxaemia. Lancet. 1989;2:1474–7.

70. Graninger W, Thalhammer F, Locker G. Pentoxifylline in cerebral malaria. J Infect Dis. 1991;164:829.

71. Bianco JA, Almgren J, Kern DL, et al. Evidence that oral pentoxifylline reverses acute renal dysfunction in bone marrow transplant recipients receiving amphotericin B and cyclosporine. Transplantation. 1991;51:925–7.

72. Bianco JA, Appelbaum FR, Nemunaitis J, et al. Phase I–II trial of pentoxifylline for the prevention of transplant-related toxicities following bone marrow transplantation. Blood. 1991;78:1205–11.

73. Kalhs P, Lechner K, Stockschlader M, et al. Pentoxifylline did not prevent transplant-related toxicity in 31 consecutive allogeneic bone marrow transplant recipients. Blood. 1992;80:2683.

74. Bianco JA, Appelbaum FR, Bakke L, et al. A phase II study of intravenous pentoxifylline for the treatment of diffuse idiopathic pneumonia in marrow transplant recipients. In: Mandell GL, Novick WJ Jr, eds. Proceedings of a Workshop: Pentoxifylline, Leukocytes, and Cytokines. Hoechst-Roussel Pharmaceuticals Inc., Somerville, NJ 1992:57–67.

75. Miller A, Harel D, Laor A, et al. Cimetidine as an immunomodulator in the treatment of herpes zoster. J Neuroimmunol. 1989;22:69–76.

76. Kurzrock R, Auber M, Mavlight GM. Cimetidine therapy of herpes simplex infections in immunocompromised patients. Clin Exp Dermatol. 1987;12: 326–31.

77. Brockmeyer NH, Kreuzfelder E, Mertius L, et al. Immunomodulatory properties of cimetidine in ARC patients. Clin Immunol Immunopathol. 1988;48: 50–60.

78. Badamchian M, Goldstein AL, Sztein MB. Immune and neuroendocrine modulation with thymosins: Current status of recent clinical trials in the United States. Int J Neurosci. 1990;51:365–7.

79. Gravenstein S, Duthie EH, Miller BA, et al. Augmentation of influenza antibody response in elderly men by thymosin alpha one. J Am Geriatr Soc. 1989; 37:1–8.

80. Mutchnick ME, Appelman HD, Chung HT, et al. Thymosin treatment of chronic hepatitis B: A placebo-controlled pilot trial. Hepatology. 1991;14: 409–15.

81. Dumann H, Meuer SC, Renschin G, et al. Influence of thymopentin on antibody response, and monocyte and T cell function in hemodialysis patients who fail to respond to hepatitis B vaccination. Nephron. 1990;55:136–40.

82. Beyer WEP, Noordzij TC, Kramer P, et al. Effect of immunomodulator thymopentin on impaired seroresponse to influenza vaccine in patients on hemodialysis. Nephron. 1990;54:296–301.

83. Gottlieb MS, Zackin RA, Fiala M, et al. Response to treatment with the leukocyte-derived immunomodulator IMREG-1 in immunocompromised patients with AIDS-related complex. Ann Intern Med. 1991;115:84–91.

84. Hersh EM, Brewton G, Abrams D, et al. Ditiocarb sodium (diethyldithiocarbamate) therapy in patients with symptomatic HIV infection and AIDS. JAMA. 1991;265:1538–44.

85. Touraine JL. Effect of the immunomodulator LF 1695 on T-lymphocytes and macrophages. Activity in HIV infection. Med Oncol Tumor Pharmacother. 1989;6:59–61.

86. Bengtsson M, Simonsson B, Carlsson K, et al. Stimulation of NK cell, T cell, and monocyte functions by the novel immunomodulator linomide after autologous bone marrow transplantation. Transplantation. 1992;53:882–8.

87. Wanders A, Larsson E, Gerdin B, et al. Abolition of the effect of cyclosporine on rat cardiac allograft rejection by the new immunomodulator LS-2616 (Linomide). Transplantation. 1989;47:216–7.

34. ANTIPARASITIC AGENTS

JOHN A. JERNIGAN
RICHARD D. PEARSON

A comprehensive discussion of antiparasitic chemotherapy must take into account the large number of parasites that can infect humans, the complexity of their life cycles, differences in their metabolism, and the wide array of drugs that have been developed to treat them. Taxonomically, parasites are divided into protozoa and helminths.[1–4] The protozoa often have complex life cycles but are unicellular. Helminths, on the other hand, have highly developed neuromuscular systems, digestive tracts, reproductive organs, and integuments. It is not surprising that many drugs effective against the helminths are not active against protozoa, and vice versa.

The susceptibility of the parasites to chemotherapeutic agents correlates to some degree with taxonomy and metabolism (Table 1). The parasites can be grouped along those two parameters. The protozoa that inhabit the gastrointestinal lumen and vagina form one group. Although they arise from several taxonomic classes,[1] they share a common microenvironment and in many instances have similar metabolic adaptations. Included in this group are the various amebae of the superclass Rhizopodia, the luminal flagellates of the class Zoomastigophorea, and *Balantidium coli* of the class Kinetofragminophorea. The second major group includes members of the phylum Apicomplexa. These protozoa are important causes of morbidity and mortality worldwide. Included are *Plasmodium* spp., which cause malaria, *Babesia* spp., *Toxoplasma gondii*, *Cryptosporidium* spp., and *Isospora belli*. The latter three "coccidians" have emerged as important pathogens in persons with acquired immunodeficiency syndrome (AIDS). The third group of protozoan pathogens include flagellates of the class Zoomastigophorea, family Trypanosomidiae. They are arthropod borne and produce leishmaniasis, Chagas' disease, and African sleeping sickness.

The susceptibility of helminths also correlates to some degree with taxonomy. The helminths can be divided into nematodes (roundworms),[2] which are subdivided into those that live in the lumen of the intestine and those that reside in tissue; trematodes (flukes); and cestodes (tapeworms).[3,4] Chemotherapeutic agents are often active against multiple genera within these groups. Major advances have been made in the treatment of helminthic diseases.

The discussion of antiparasitic drugs that follows is arranged according to these groups. The approach is imperfect in that some drugs are active against pathogens in more than one group. This is particularly true for praziquantel, which is active against a broad spectrum of trematodes and cestodes, and two drugs that are still investigational in the United States, albendazole, with activity against nematodes and cestodes, and ivermectin, with activity against nematodes and blood-sucking arthropods. Nonetheless, the approach taken provides a logical framework in which to organize the data. Drugs that have broad spectrums of activity are discussed in the context of their primary indications.

The dosage and duration of therapy for specific parasitic diseases are provided in Table 2.[5] Not all of these drugs are available through pharmacies in the United States. Some can be obtained only from the manufacturer (indicated by *). Others have not been licensed in the United States but are available only from the CDC Drug Service (**), Centers for Disease Control and Prevention, Atlanta, Georgia 30333. Some cannot be obtained in the United States (***), but they are discussed because they are used elsewhere or hold promise for the future.

DRUGS ACTIVE AGAINST LUMINAL PROTOZOA: AMEBAE, INTESTINAL AND VAGINAL FLAGELLATES, AND THE CILIATE BALANTIDIUM COLI

Metronidazole and Other Nitroimidazoles

Metronidazole (Fig. 1), tinidazole,*** and ornidazole*** have selective toxicity against numerous anaerobic organisms. Only metronidazole, 2-methyl-5-nitroimidazole-1-ethanol, has been licensed in the United States. It is highly effective in the treatment of invasive enterocolitis and liver abscess due to *Entamoeba histolytica*[6,7] and *E. polecki* infections,[8] enteritis due to *Giardia lamblia*,[9,10] and vaginitis due to *Trichomonas vaginalis*.[11,12] It is also considered an alternative drug for the treatment of two other enteric pathogens, *Blastocystis hominis*[13] and *Balantidium coli*.[14] Metronidazole is active against trophozoites of *Entamoeba* species, but it does not invariably eradicate the cysts.[15–17] A luminally active agent is required for this purpose and to treat asymptomatic cyst passers. Metronidazole resistance has been documented in some strains of *Trichomonas vaginalis*.[18] Metronidazole has also been advocated as empiric therapy for presumptive protozoal enterocolitis in areas of the world where laboratory facilities are insufficient to provide a specific diagnosis.[19] Finally, metronidazole is recommended for the treatment of the guinea worm *Dracunculus medinensis*,[20] but its clinical effects are related to a reduction in inflammation rather than to a lethal effect on the worm. The use of metronidazole against anaerobic bacterial pathogens is summarized in Chapter 23.

Metronidazole has Food and Drug Administration (FDA) approval only for the treatment of amebiasis and trichomoniasis. This does not prevent physicians from using metronidazole for diseases like giardiasis, for which data support its efficacy.[21] The cure rate with the doses of metronidazole recommended for giardiasis (Table 2) is slightly lower than with quinacrine,[9,10,19] but metronidazole is generally better tolerated and many physicians prefer it over quinacrine.

Metronidazole is available as 250- and 500-mg tablets for oral use and in vials with 500 mg lyophilized powder for parenteral administration. When it is administered orally, 90–95 percent is absorbed[22,23]; peak serum levels are reached within 1 hour. Metronidazole has limited plasma protein binding. It is widely distributed throughout the body and penetrates well into tissues, abscesses, fluid compartments, vaginal secretions, bone, the central nervous system, and breast milk.[24,25] The elimination half-life is 6.2–11.5 hours. Metronidazole is extensively metabolized in the liver. The principal metabolites result from oxidation of side chains and glucuronide formation and are excreted via the kidney. Although renal failure prolongs the half-life of these metabolites, the hepatic metabolism is such that the drug dosage need not be modified during renal failure, but it should be adjusted in liver failure and in persons with severe malnutrition.[26]

Metronidazole is activated in anaerobic organisms by reduction of the 5-nitro group through a sequence of intermediate steps involving microbial electron transport proteins of low redox potential.[27] This results in a concentration gradient across the membrane of the parasite and permits accumulation of high concentrations of the reduced compound within the cell. Metro-

TABLE 1. Spectrum of Activity of the Major Antiparasitic Drugs Licensed for Use in the United States, Available in the United States Only from the Manufacturer (*), Available from the CDC Drug Service, Centers for Disease Control (**), or Not Currently Available in the United States (***)

Drug	Indications
Amoebae, intestinal and vaginal flagellates, and _Balantidium coli_	
Metronidazole	_Entamoeba histolytica_ (invasive disease)
	Entamoeba polecki
	Trichomonas vaginalis
	Blastocystis hominis
	Giardia lamblia
	Balantidium coli (alternative)
Dehydroemetine** and Emetine***	_Entamoeba histolytica_ (invasive disease)
Iodoquinol	_Entamoeba histolytica_ (luminal infection)
	Dientamoeba fragilis
	Blastocystis hominis
	Balantidium coli (alternative)
Diloxanide furoate**	_Entamoeba histolytica_ (asymptomatic luminal infection)
	Entamoeba polecki (luminal infection)
Paromomycin	_Entamoeba histolytica_ (asymptomatic luminal infection)
	Dientamoeba fragilis
	Cryptosporidium (may be effective)
Quinacrine	_Giardia lamblia_
Furazolidone	_Giardia lamblia_ (alternative)
Tetracycline	_Balantidium coli_
	Dientamoeba fragilis
Amphotericin B	_Naegleria_ spp. (used with miconazole and rifampin)
Apicomplexa	
Chloroquine	Suppressive prophylaxis and treatment of the asexual erythrocytic phase of _Plasmodium vivax, P. ovale, P. malariae,_ and susceptible _P. falciparum._
Primaquine	Radical cure of the exoerythrocytic hypnozoites of _P. vivax_ and _P. ovale._
Quinine	Treatment of chloroquine-resistant _P. falciparum;_ effective against asexual erythrocytic phase of other _Plasmodium_ spp.
Quinidine	Treatment of chloroquine-resistant _P. falciparum_ when parenteral therapy is required; effective against asexual erythrocytic phase.
Mefloquine	Prophylaxis and occasionally treatment of chloroquine-resistant _P. falciparum;_ effective against asexual erythrocytic phase of other _Plasmodium_ spp.
Tetracyclines	
Tetracycline	Used with quinine to treat asexual erythrocytic state of chloroquine-resistant _P. falciparum_ in Southeast Asia.
Doxycycline	Used alone or with chloroquine for suppressive prophylaxis in areas where there is endemic chloroquine-resistant _P. falciparum._
Artemisinin***	Treatment of _Plasmodium_ spp. in the asexual erythrocytic phase including chloroquine-resistant _P. falciparum_ (experimental)
Halofantrine***	Treatment of _Plasmodium_ species in the asexual erythrocytic phase including chloroquine-resistant _P. falciparum_ (alternative)
Pyrimethamine/short-acting sulfonamides	Used with quinine to treat asexual erythrocytic phase of chloroquine-resistant _P. falciparum_ acquired in areas where resistance is not common
	Toxoplasma gondii
Pyrimethamine-sulfadoxime (Fansidar)	Presumptive treatment of chloroquine-resistant _P. falciparum_ in areas where isolates remain sensitive.
Proguanil***	Used with chloroquine for suppressive prophylaxis in areas of East Africa where there is chloroquine-resistant _Plasmodium falciparum_ (failures have been reported)
Trimethoprim-sulfamethoxazole (cotrimoxazole)	_Pneumocystis carinii_
	Isospora belli
Macrolide antibiotics	
Clindamycin	Used with steroids for treatment of ocular _Toxoplasma gondii_ in immunocompetent hosts; used with pyrimethamine for _T. gondii_ encephalitis in persons with AIDS who cannot tolerate sulfonamides.
	Used with quinine for treatment of _Babesia_ spp.
Spiramycin***	_Toxoplasma gondii_ during pregnancy and in the neonate
Pentamidine isethionate	Treatment and prophylaxis of _Pneumocystis carinii_ (alternative when given parenterally)
Atovaquone	Treatment of _Pneumocystis carinii_ (alternative for mild to moderate disease)
	Toxoplasma gondii (experimental)
Members of the family Trypanosomatidae	
Eflornithine*	_Trypanosoma brucei gambiense_ (hemolymphatic and late disease with nervous system involvement)
Suramin**	_Trypanosoma brucei gambiense_ and _Trypanosoma brucei rhodesiense_ (hemolymphatic stage)
Melarsoprol B**	_Trypanosoma brucei gambiense_ and _Trypanosoma brucei rhodesiense_ (late disease with central nervous system involvement)
Nifurtimox**	_Trypanosoma cruzi_
Benznidazole***	_Trypanosoma cruzi_ (alternative)
Stibogluconate sodium**	_Leishmania_ spp.
Meglumine antimoniate***	_Leishmania_ spp.
Amphotericin B	_Leishmania_ spp. (alternative; lipid-complexed amphotericin B*** preparations appear effective but less toxic)
Pentamidine isethionate	_Leishmania_ spp. (alternative)
	Trypanosoma brucei gambiense and _Trypanosoma brucei gambiense_ (alternative for use in the hemolymphatic stage)
Interferon-γ	_Leishmania_ spp. (investigational)
Ketoconazole	_Leishmania_ spp. (investigational)

(Continued)

TABLE 1. *(Continued)*

Drug	Indications
Helminthic diseases: nematodes (roundworms)	
Benzimidazoles	
Mebendazole	*Ascaris lumbricoides*
	Hookworm
	Trichuris trichiura
	Enterobius vermicularis
	Capillaria philippinensis
	Gnathostoma spinigerum (surgical removal is an alternative)
	Mansonella perstans
	Angiostrongylus cantonensis
	Trichostrongylus spp. (alternative)
	Trichinella spiralis (recommended by some; used with steroids)
	Visceral larva migrans (alternative)
	Echinococcus granulosus and *Echinococcus multilocularis* (alternative)
Albendazole*	*Ascaris lumbricoides*
	Hookworm
	Enterobius vermicularis
	Trichuris trichura
	Strongyloides stercoralis
	Cutaneous larva migrans
	Trichostrongylus spp.
	Capillaria philippinensis (alternative)
	Cysticercosis
	Echinococcus granulosus and *Echinococcus multilocularis*
Thiabendazole	*Strongyloides stercoralis*
	Cutaneous larva migrans (effective topically or orally)
	Visceral larva migrans
	Trichostrongylus spp.
	Angiostrongylus costaricensis (surgical intervention is the alternative)
	Dracunculus medinensis (alternative)
	Capillaria philippensis (alternative)
	Trichinella spiralis (alternative, used with steroids)
Pyrantel pamoate	*Enterobius vermicularis*
	Ascaris lumbricoides
	Hookworm
	Trichostrongylus spp.
Piperazine citrate	*Ascaris lumbricoides* (alternative)
Diethylcarbamazine	*Wuchereria bancrofti*
	Brugia malayi
	Mansonella ozzardi
	Loa loa
	Tropical eosinophilia
	Visceral larva migrans
	Onchocerca volvulus
Ivermectin*	*Onchocerca volvulus*
	Strongyloides stercoralis (alternative)
	Wuchereria bancrofti, Brugia malayi (alternative)
	Broad range of nematodes and blood sucking arthropods (use for these indications is investigational)
Metronidazole	*Dracunculus medinensis*
Helminthic diseases: trematodes (flukes) and cestodes (tapeworms)	
Praziquantel	*Schistosoma* spp.
	Clonorchis sinensis
	Opisthorchis viverrini
	Paragonimus westermani
	Fasciolopsis buski
	Heterophytes heterophytes
	Metagonimus yokogawai
	Nanophyetus salmincola
	Diphyllobothrium latum (alternative)
	Taenia solium (adult worm and cysticercosis)
	Taenia saginata (alternative)
	Dipylidium caninum (alternative)
	Hymenolepis nana
Metrifonate	*Schistosoma haematobium* (alternative)
Oxamniquine	*Schistosoma mansoni* (alternative)
Bithionol	*Fasciola hepatica*
	Paragonimus westermani (alternative)
Niclosamide	*Diphyllobothrium latum*
	Taenia saginata
	Taenia solium
	Dipylidium caninum
	Hymenolepis nana (alternative)
	Fasciolopsis buski

TABLE 2. Drugs for Treatment of Parasitic Infections

Infection		Drug	Adult Dosage*	Pediatric Dosage*
AMEBIASES (*Entamoeba histolytica*)				
asymptomatic				
Drug of choice:		Iodoquinol[1]	650 mg tid × 20d	30–40 mg/kg/d in 3 doses × 20d
	OR	Paromomycin	25–30 mg/kg/d in 3 doses × 7d	25–30 mg/kg/d in 3 doses × 7d
Alternative:		Diloxanide furoate[2]	500 mg tid × 10d	20 mg/kg/d in 3 doses × 10d
mild to moderate intestinal disease				
Drugs of choice:[3]		Metronidazole	750 mg tid × 10d	35–50 mg/kg/d in 3 doses × 10d
	OR	Tinidazole[4]	2 grams/d × 3d	50 mg/kg (max. 2 grams) qd × 3d
severe intestinal disease				
Drugs of choice:[3]		Metronidazole	750 mg tid × 10d	35–50 mg/kg/d in 3 doses × 10d
	OR	Tinidazole[4]	600 mg bid × 5d	50 mg/kg (max. 2 grams) qd × 3d
Alternative:		Dehydroemetine[2]	1 to 1.5 mg/kg/d (max. 90 mg/d) IM for up to 5d	1 to 1.5 mg/kg/d (max. 90 mg/d) IM in 2 doses for up to 5d
hepatic abscess				
Drugs of choice:[3]		Metronidazole	750 mg tid × 10d	35–50 mg/kg/d in 3 doses × 10d
	OR	Tinidazole[4]	800 mg tid × 5d	60 mg/kg (max. 2 grams) qd × 3d
Alternatives:		Dehydroemetine[2]	1 to 1.5 mg/kg/d (max. 90 mg/d) IM for up to 5d	1 to 1.5 mg/kg/d (max. 90 mg/d) IM in 2 doses for up to 5d
		followed by chloroquine phosphate	600 mg base (1 gram)/d × 2d, then 300 mg base (500 mg)/d × 2–3 wks	10 mg base/kg (max. 300 mg base)/d × 2–3 wks
AMEBIC MENINGOENCEPHALITIS, PRIMARY				
Naegleria				
Drug of choice:		Amphotericin B[5,6]	1 mg/kg/d IV, uncertain duration	1 mg/kg/d IV, uncertain duration
Acanthamoeba				
Drug of choice:		See footnote 7		
Ancylostoma duodenale, see HOOKWORM				
ANGIOSTRONGYLIASIS				
Angiostrongylus cantonensis				
Drug of choice:		Mebendazole[6,8,9]	100 mg bid × 5d	100 mg bid × 5d
Angiostrongylus costaricensis				
Drug of choice:		Thiabendazole[6,8]	75 mg/kg/d in 3 doses × 3d (max. 3 grams/d)[10]	75 mg/kg/d in 3 doses × 3d (max. 3 grams/d)[10]
ANISAKIASIS (*Anisakis*)				
Treatment of choice:		Surgical or endoscopic removal		
ASCARIASIS (*Ascaris lumbricoides*, roundworm)				
Drug of choice:		Mebendazole	100 mg bid × 3d	100 mg bid × 3d
	OR	Pyrantel pamoate	11 mg/kg once (max. 1 gram)	11 mg/kg once (max. 1 gram)
	OR	Albendazole	400 mg once	400 mg once
BABESIOSIS (*Babesia microti*)				
Drugs of choice:[11]		Clindamycin[6]	1.2 grams bid parenteral or 600 mg tid oral × 7d	20–40 mg/kg/d in 3 doses × 7d
		plus quinine	650 mg tid oral × 7d	25 mg/kg/d in 3 doses × 7d
BALANTIDIASIS (*Balantidium coli*)				
Drug of choice:		Tetracycline[6]	500 mg qid × 10d	40 mg/kg/d in 4 doses × 10d (max. 2 grams/d)[12]
Alternatives:		Iodoquinol[1,6]	650 mg tid × 20d	40 mg/kg/d in 3 doses × 20d
		Metronidazole[6]	750 mg tid × 5d	35–50 mg/kg/d in 3 doses × 5d
BAYLISASCARIASIS (*Baylisascaris procyonis*)				
Drug of choice:		See footnote 13		
BLASTOCYSTIS hominis infection				
Drug of choice:		See footnote 14		
CAPILLARIASIS (*Capillaria philippinensis*)				
Drug of choice:		Mebendazole[6]	200 mg bid × 20d	200 mg bid × 20d
Alternatives:		Albendazole	200 mg bid × 10d	200 mg bid × 10d
		Thiabendazole[6]	25 mg/kg/d in 2 doses × 30d	25 mg/kg/d in 2 doses × 30d

* The letter d stands for day.
1. Dosage and duration of administration should not be exceeded because of possibility of causing optic neuritis; maximum dosage is 2 grams/day.
2. In the USA, this drug is available from the CDC Drug Service, Centers for Disease Control and Prevention, Atlanta, Georgia 30333; telephone: 404-639-3670 (evenings, weekends, and holidays: 404-639-2888).
3. Treatment should be followed by a course of iodoquinol or one of the other intraluminal drugs used to treat asymptomatic amebiasis.
4. A nitro-imidazole similar to metronidazole, but not marketed in the USA; tinidazole appears to be at least as effective as metronidazole and better tolerated. Ornidazole, a similar drug, is also used outside the USA.
5. One patient with a *Naegleria* infection was successfully treated with amphotericin B, miconazole, and rifampin (JS Seidel et al, N Engl J Med, 306:346, 1982).
6. An approved drug, but considered investigational for this condition by the U.S. Food and Drug Administration.
7. Strains of *Acanthamoeba* isolated from fatal granulomatous amebic encephalitis are usually sensitive *in vitro* to pentamidine, ketoconazole (*Nizoral*), flucytosine, and (less so) to amphotericin B (RJ Duma et al, Antimicrob Agents Chemother, 10:370, 1976). For treatment of keratitis caused by *Acanthamoeba*, concurrent topical use of 0.1% propamidine isethionate (*Brolene*-Rhône-Poulence Rorer, Canada) plus neosporin, or oral itraconazole plus topical miconazole, have been successful (MB Moore and JP McCulley, Br J Ophthalmol, 73:271, 1989; Y Ishibashi et al, Am J Ophthalmol, 109:121, 1990). Topical polyhexamethylene biguanide has also been effective in a few patients with keratitis (JH Varga et al, Am J Ophthalmol, 115:466, 1993).
8. Effectiveness documented only in animals
9. Most patients recover spontaneously without antiparasitic drug therapy. Analgesics, corticosteroids, and careful removal of CSF at frequent intervals can relieve symptoms (J Koo et al, Rev Infect Dis, 10:1155, 1988). Albendazole, levamisole (*Ergamisol*), or ivermectin has also been used successfully in animals.
10. This dose is likely to be toxic and may have to be decreased.
11. Exchange transfusion has been used in severely ill patients with high (>10%) parasitemia (V Iacopino and T Earnhart, Arch Intern Med, 150:1527, 1990). One report indicates that azithromycin (*Zithromax*), 500–1000 mg daily, plus quinine may also be effective (LM Weiss et al, J Infect Dis, 168:1289, 1993). Concurrent use of pentamidine and trimethoprim-sulfamethoxazole has been reported to cure an infection with *B. divergens* (D Raoult et al, Ann Intern Med, 107:944, 1987).
12. Not recommended for use in children less than eight years old.
13. Drugs that could be tried include diethylcarbamazine, levamisole, and fenbendazole (KR Kazacos, J Am Vet Med Assoc, 195:894, 1989) and ivermectin. Steroid therapy may be helpful, especially in eye or CNS infection. Ocular baylisascariasis has been treated successfully using laser therapy to destroy intraretinal larvae.
14. Clinical significance of these organisms is controversial, but metronidazole 750 mg tid × 10d or iodoquinol 650 mg tid × 20d anecdotally have been reported to be effective (I Grossman et al, Am J Gastroenterol, 87:729, 1992; PFL Boreham and D Stenzel, Adv Parasitol, 32:2, 1993).

TABLE 2. (Continued)

Infection	Drug	Adult Dosage*	Pediatric Dosage*
Chagas' disease, see TRYPANOSOMIASIS			
Clonorchis sinensis, see FLUKE infection			
CRYPTOSPORIDIOSIS (Cryptosporidium)			
Drug of choice:	See footnote 15		
CUTANEOUS LARVA MIGRANS (creeping eruption, dog and cat hookworm)			
Drug of choice:[16] Thiabendazole		Topically and/or 50 mg/kg/d in 2 doses (max. 3 grams/d) × 2–5d[10]	Topically and/or 50 mg/kg/d in 2 doses (max. 3 grams/d) in 2–5d[10]
OR Albendazole[17]		200 mg bid × 3d	200 mg bid × 3d
CYCLOSPORA infection[18]			
Drug of choice:	Trimethoprime-sulfamethoxazole[19]	TMP 160 mg, SMX 800 mg bid × 3 days	TMP 5 mg/kg, SMX 25 mg/kg bid × 3 days
CYSTICERCOSIS, see TAPEWORM infection			
DIENTAMOEBA fragilis infection			
Drug of choice:	Iodoquinol[1]	650 mg tid × 20d	40 mg/kg/d in 3 doses × 20d
OR	Paromomycin	25–30 mg/kg/d in 3 doses × 7d	25–30 mg/kg/d in 3 doses × 7d
OR	Tetracycline[6]	500 mg qid × 10d	40 mg/kg/d (max. 2 grams/d) in 4 doses × 10d[12]
Diphyllobothrium latum, see TAPEWORM infection			
DRACUNCULUS medinensis (guinea worm) infection			
Drug of choice:	Metronidazole[6,20]	250 mg tid × 10d	25 mg/kg/d (max. 750 mg/d) in 3 doses × 10d
Alternative:	Thiabendazole[6,20]	50–75 mg/kg/d in 2 doses × 3d[10]	50–75 mg/kg/d in 2 doses × 3d[10]
Echinococcus, see TAPEWORM infection			
Entamoeba histolytica, see AMEBIASIS			
ENTAMOEBA polecki infection			
Drug of choice:	Metronidazole[6]	750 mg tid × 10d	35–50 mg/kg/d in 3 doses × 10d
ENTEROBIUS vermicularis (pinworm) infection			
Drug of choice:	Pyrantel pamoate	11 mg/kg once (max. 1 gram); repeat after 2 weeks	11 mg/kg once (max. 1 gram); repeat after 2 weeks
OR	Mebendazole	A single dose of 100 mg; repeat after 2 weeks	A single dose of 100 mg; repeat after 2 weeks
OR	Albendazole	400 mg once; repeat in 2 weeks	400 mg once, repeat in 2 weeks
Fasciola hepatica, see FLUKE infection			
FILARIASIS			
Wuchereria bancrofti, Brugia malayi			
Drug of choice:[21]	Diethylcarbamazine[22]	Day 1: 50 mg, oral, p.c. Day 2: 50 mg tid Day 3: 100 mg tid Days 4 through 21: 6 mg/kg/d in 3 doses[23]	Day 1: 1 mg/kg, oral, p.c. Day 2: 1 mg/kg tid Day 3: 1–2 mg/kg tid Days 4 through 21: 6 mg/kg/d in 3 doses[23]
Loa loa			
Drug of choice:[24]	Diethylcarbamazine[22]	Day 1: 50 mg, oral, p.c. Day 2: 50 mg tid Day 3: 100 mg tid Days 4 through 21: 9 mg/kg/d in 3 doses[23]	Day 1: 1 mg/kg, oral, p.c. Day 2: 1 mg/kg tid Day 3: 1–2 mg/kg tid Days 4 through 21: 9 mg/kg/d in 3 doses[23]
Mansonella ozzardi			
Drug of choice:	See footnote 25		
Mansonella perstans			
Drug of choice:	Mebendazole[6]	100 mg bid × 30d	
Tropical Pulmonary Eosinophilia (TPE)			
Drug of choice:	Diethylcarbamazine	6 mg/kg/d in 3 doses × 21d	6 mg/kg/d in 3 doses × 21d
Onchocerca volvulus			
Drug of choice:	Ivermectin[2]	150 μg/kg oral once, repeated every 6 to 12 months	150 μg/kg oral once, repeated every 6 to 12 months

* The letter d stands for day.

15. Infection is self-limited in immunocompetent patients. In HIV-infected patients with large-volume intractable diarrhea, octreotide (Sandostatin) 300–500 μg tid subcutaneously may control the diarrhea, but not the infection (JD Cello et al, Ann Intern Med, 115:705, 1991). Paromomycin may sometimes be helpful (K Armitage et al, Arch Intern Med, 152:2497, 1992). In unpublished clinical trials, azithromycin, 1250 mg daily for two weeks followed by 500 mg daily, has apparently been effective in some patients.

16. Several reports suggest that ivermectin, 150–200 μg/kg once, is also effective (E Caumes et al, Arch Dermatol, 128:994, 1992).

17. SK Jones et al, Br J Dermatol, 122:99, 1990; HD Davies et al, Arch Dermatol, 129:588, 1993

18. A newly described coccidian parasite, previously designated a cyanobacterium-like body, which causes severe self-limited diarrhea (YR Ortega et al, N Engl J Med, 328:1308, 1993; RP Bendall et al, Lancet, 341:590, 1993)

19. G Madico et al, Lancet, 342:122, 1993

20. Not curative, but decreases inflammation and facilitates removing the worm. Mebendazole 400–800 mg/d for 6d has been reported to kill the worm directly.

21. A single dose of ivermectin, 20–200 μg/kg, has been reported to be effective for treatment of microfilaremia (EA Ottesen et al, N Engl J Med, 322:1113, 1990; M Sabry et al, Trans R Soc Trop Med Hyg, 85:640, 1991; JW Mak et al, Am J Trop Med Hyg, 48:591, 1993).

22. Antihistamines or corticosteroids may be required to decrease allergic reactions due to disintegration of microfilariae in treatment of filarial infections, especially those caused by Loa loa.

23. For patients with no microfilariae in the blood or skin, full doses can be given from day one.

24. Diethylcarbamazine should be administered with special caution in heavy infections with Loa loa because rapid killing of microfilariae can provoke an encephalopathy (B Carme et al, Am J Trop Med Hyg, 44:684, 1991). Ivermectin or albendazole has been used to reduce microfilaremia (Y Martin-Prevel et al, Am J Trop Med Hyg, 48:186, 1993; AD Klion et al, J Infect Dis, 168:202, 1993). Apheresis has been reported to be effective in lowering microfilarial counts in patients heavily infected with Loa loa (EA Ottesen, Infect Dis Clin North Am, 7:619, 1993). Diethylcarbamazine, 300 mg once weekly, has been recommended for prevention of loiasis (TB Nutman et al, N Engl J Med, 319:752, 1988).

25. Diethylcarbamazine has no effect. Ivermectin, 150 μg/kg, may be effective (TB Nutman et al, J Infect Dis, 156:622, 1987).

TABLE 2. *(Continued)*

Infection	Drug	Adult Dosage*	Pediatric Dosage*
FLUKE, hermaphroditic, infection			
Clonorchis sinensis **(Chinese liver fluke)**			
Drug of choice:	Praziquantel	75 mg/kg/d in 3 doses × 1d	75 mg/kg/d in 3 doses × 1d
Fasciola hepatica **(sheep liver fluke)**			
Drug of choice:[26]	Bithionol[2]	30–50 mg/kg on alternate days × 10–15 doses	30–50 mg/kg on alternate days × 10–15 doses
Fasciolopsis buski **(intestinal fluke)**			
Drug of choice:	Praziquantel[6]	75 mg/kg/d in 3 doses × 1d	75 mg/kg/d in 3 doses × 1d
OR	Niclosamide[6]	a single dose of 4 tablets (2 g), chewed thoroughly	11–34 kg: 2 tablets (1 g) >34 kg: 3 tablets (1.5 g)
Heterophyes heterophyes **(intestinal fluke)**			
Drug of choice:	Praziquantel[6]	75 mg/kg/d in 3 doses × 1d	75 mg/kg/d in 3 doses × 1d
Metagonimus yokogawai **(intestinal fluke)**			
Drug of choice:	Praziquantel[6]	75 mg/kg/d in 3 doses × 1d	75 mg/kg/d in 3 doses × 1d
Nanophyetus salmincola			
Drug of choice:	Praziquantel[6]	60 mg/kg/d in 3 doses × 1d	60 mg/kg/d in 3 doses × 1d
Opisthorchis viverrini **(liver fluke)**			
Drug of choice:	Praziquantel	75 mg/kg/d in 3 doses × 1d	75 mg/kg/d in 3 doses × 1d
Paragonimus westermani **(lung fluke)**			
Drug of choice:	Praziquantel[6]	75 mg/kg/d in 3 doses × 2d	75 mg/kg/d in 3 doses × 2d
Alternative:[27]	Bithionol[2]	30–50 mg/kg on alternate days × 10–15 doses	30–50 mg/kg on alternate days × 10–15 doses
GIARDIASIS (*Giardia lamblia*)			
Drug of choice:	Metronidazole[6]	250 mg tid × 5d	15 mg/kg/d in 3 doses × 5d
Alternatives:[28]	Quinacrine HCl	100 mg tid p.c. × 5d	6 mg/kg/d in 3 doses p.c. × 5d (max. 300 mg/d)
	Tinidazole[4]	2 grams once	50 mg/kg once (max. 2 grams)
	Furazolidone	100 mg qid × 7–10d	6 mg/kg/d in 4 doses × 7–10d
	Paromomycin[29]	25–30 mg/kg/d in 3 doses × 7d	
GNATHOSTOMIASIS (*Gnathostoma spinigerum*)			
Treatment of choice:[30]	Surgical removal		
plus	Albendazole[31]	400–800 mg qd × 21d	
HOOKWORM infection (*Ancylostoma duodenale, Necator americanus*)			
Drug of choice:	Mebendazole	100 mg bid × 3d	100 mg bid × 3d
OR	Pyrantel pamoate[6]	11 mg/kg (max. 1 gram) × 3d	11 mg/kg (max. 1 gram) × 3d
OR	Albendazole	400 mg once	400 mg once
Hydatid cyst, see TAPEWORM infection			
Hymenolepis nana, see TAPEWORM infection			
ISOSPORIASIS (*Isospora belli*)			
Drug of choice:	Trimethoprim-sulfamethoxazole[6,32]	160 mg TMP, 800 mg SMX qid × 10d, then bid × 3 wks	
LEISHMANIASIS (*L. mexicana, L. tropica, L. major, L. braziliensis, L. donovani* [Kala-azar])			
Drug of choice:	Sodium stibogluconate[2]	20 mg Sb/kg/d IV or IM × 20–28d[33]	20 mg Sb/kg/d IV or IM × 20–28d[33]
OR	Meglumine antimonate	20 mg Sb/kg/d IV or IM × 20–28d[33]	20 mg Sb/kg/d IV or IM × 20–28d[33]
Alternatives:[34]	Amphotericin B[6]	0.25 to 1 mg/kg IV by slow infusion daily or every 2d for up to 8 wks	0.25 to 1 mg/kg IV by slow infusion daily or every 2d for up to 8 wks
	Pentamidine isethionate[6]	2–4 mg/kg daily or every 2d IM for up to 15 doses[33]	2–4 mg/kg daily or every 2d IM for up to 15 doses[33]
LICE infestation (*Pediculus humanus, capitis, Phthirus pubis*)[35]			
Drug of choice:	1% Permethrin[36]	Topically	Topically
OR	0.5% Malathion	Topically	Topically
Alternatives:	Pyrethrins with piperonyl butoxide	Topically[37]	Topically[37]
	Lindane	Topically[37]	Topically[37]

Loa loa, see FILARIASIS

* The letter d stands for day.

26. Unlike infections with other flukes, *F. hepatica* infections may not respond to praziquantel. Limited data indicate that triclabendazole (*Fasinex*), a veterinary fasciolide, is safe and effective in a single oral dose of 10 mg/kg (L Loutan et al, Lancet, 2:383, 1989; U Bechtel et al, Dtsch Med Wochenschr, 117:978, 1992).
27. Unpublished data indicate triclabendazole may be effective in a dosage of 5 mg/kg once daily for 3 days or 10 mg/kg twice in one day.
28. Albendazole 400 mg daily × 5d has also been reported to be effective against giardiasis (A Hall and Q Nahar, Trans R Soc Trop Med Hyg, 87:84, 1993).
29. Not absorbed and not highly effective, but may be useful for treatment of giardiasis in pregnancy
30. Ivermectin has been reported to be effective in animals (MT Anantaphruti et al, Trop Med Parasitol, 43:65, 1992).
31. P Kraivichian et al, Trans R Soc Trop Med Hyg, 86:418, 1992.
32. In sulfonamide-sensitive patients, such as some HIV-infected patients, pyrimethamine 50–75 mg daily has been effective (LM Weiss et al, Ann Intern Med, 109:474, 1988). In immunocompromised patients, it may be necessary to continue therapy indefinitely.
33. May be repeated or continued. A longer duration may be needed for some forms of visceral leishmaniasis.
34. Limited data indicate that ketoconazole, 400 to 600 mg daily for four to eight weeks, may be effective for treatment of cutaneous and mucosal leishmaniasis (RE Saenz et al, Am J Med, 89:147, 1990; V Ramesh et al, Arch Dermatol, 128:411, 1992). Some studies indicate that *L. donovani* resistant to sodium stibogluconate or meglumine antimonate may respond to recombinant human gamma interferon in addition to antimony (R Badaro and WD Johnson, J Infect Dis, 167 suppl 1:S13, 1993), pentamidine followed by a course of antimony (CP Thakur et al, Am J Trop Med Hyg, 45:435, 1991), or ketoconazole (JP Wall et al, J Infect Dis, 166:215, 1992). Liposomal encapsulated amphotericin B (*AmBisome*, Vestar, San Dimas, CA) has been used successfully to treat multiple-drug-resistant visceral leishmaniasis (RN Davidson et al, Lancet, 337:1061, 1991). Recently, aminosidine (parenteral paromomycin) plus sodium stibogluconate apparently decreased time to clinical and parasitologic cure of visceral leishmaniasis (J Seaman et al, J Infect Dis, 168:715, 1993).
35. For infestation of eyelashes with crab lice, use petrolatum.
36. FDA-approved only for head lice.
37. Some consultants recommend a second application one week later to kill hatching progeny. Seizures have been reported in association with the use of lindane. Do not use higher than recommended doses and avoid warm baths before application (M Tenenbein, J Am Geriatr Soc, 39:394, 1991). Prolonged use of lindane has been associated with aplastic anemia (AE Rauch et al, Arch Intern Med, 150:2393, 1990).

TABLE 2. *(Continued)*

Infection		Drug	Adult Dosage*	Pediatric Dosage*
MALARIA, Treatment of (*Plasmodium falciparum*, *P. ovale*, *P. vivax*, and *P. malariae*)				
Chloroquine-resistant *P. falciparum*[38]				
ORAL				
Drugs of choice:		Quinine sulfate **plus** pyrimethamine-sulfadoxine[40]	650 mg q8h × 3–7d[39] 3 tablets at once on last day of quinine	25 mg/kg/d in 3 doses × 3–7d[39] <1 yr: ¼ tablet 1–3 yrs. ½ tablet 4–8 yrs: 1 tablet 9–14 yrs: 2 tablets
	OR	**plus** tetracycline[6]	250 mg qid × 7d	20 mg/kg/d in 4 doses × 7d[12]
	OR[41]	**plus** clindamycin[6]	900 mg tid × 3d	20–40 mg/kg/d in 3 doses × 3d
Alternatives:[42]		Mefloquine[43,44]	1250 mg once[45]	25 mg/kg once[46] (<45 kg)
		Halofantrine[47]	500 mg q6h × 3 doses; repeat in 1 week	8 mg/kg q6h × 3 doses (<40 kg); repeat in 1 week
PARENTERAL				
Drug of choice:[48,49]		Quinidine gluconate[50]	10 mg/kg loading dose (max. 600 mg) in normal saline slowly over 1 to 2 hrs, followed by continuous infusion of 0.02 mg/kg/min until oral therapy can be started	Same as adult dose
	OR	Quinine dihydrochloride[51]	20 mg salt/kg loading dose in 10 ml/kg 5% dextrose over 4 hrs, followed by 10 mg salt/kg over 2–4 hrs q8h (max. 1800 mg/d) until oral therapy can be started	Same as adult dose
All *Plasmodium* except Chloroquine-resistant *P. falciparum*[38]				
ORAL				
Drug of choice:		Chloroquine phosphate[52,53]	600 mg base (1 gram), then 300 mg base (500 mg) 6 hrs later, then 300 mg base (500 mg) at 24 and 48 hrs	10 mg base/kg (max. 600 mg base), then 5 mg base/kg 6 hrs later, then 5 mg base/kg at 24 and 48 hrs
PARENTERAL				
Drug of choice:[49]		Quinidine gluconate[50]	same as above	same as above
	OR	Quinine dihydrochloride[51]	same as above	same as above
Prevention of relapses: *P. vivax* and *P. ovale* only				
Drug of choice:		Primaquine phosphate[54,55]	15 mg base (26.3 mg)/d × 14d or 45 mg base (79 mg)/wk × 8 wks	0.3 mg base/kg/d × 14d
MALARIA, Prevention of[56,57]				
Chloroquine-sensitive areas				
Drug of choice:		Chloroquine phosphate[58]	300 mg base (500 mg salt) orally, once/week[59]	5 mg/kg base (8.3 mg/kg salt) once/week, up to adult dose of 300 mg base

* The letter d stands for day.

38. Chloroquine-resistant *P. falciparum* infections occur in all malarious areas except Central America west of the Panama Canal Zone, Mexico, Haiti, the Dominican Republic, and the Middle East (including Egypt).
39. In Southeast Asia and possibly in other areas, such as South America, relative resistance to quinine has increased and the treatment should be continued for seven days.
40. *Fansidar* tablets contain 25 mg of pyrimethamine and 500 mg of sulfadoxine. Resistance to pyrimethamine-sulfadoxine has been reported from Southeast Asia, the Amazon basin, East Africa, Bangladesh, and Oceania.
41. In pregnancy
42. For treatment of multidrug resistant *P. falciparum* in Southeast Asia, especially Thailand, where resistance to mefloquine and halofantrine frequently occur, a 7-day course of quinine and tetracycline is recommended (G Watt et al, Am J Trop Med Hyg, 47:108, 1992).
43. At this dosage, adverse effects including nausea, vomiting, diarrhea, dizziness, disturbed sense of balance, toxic psychosis, and seizures can occur. Mefloquine is teratogenic in animals and should not be used in pregnancy. It should not be given together with quinine or quinidine, and caution is required in using quinine or quinidine to treat patients with malaria who have taken mefloquine for prophylaxis. The pediatric dosage has not been approved by the FDA. Resistance to mefloquine has been reported in some areas, such as Thailand.
44. In the USA, a 250-mg tablet of mefloquine contains 228 mg of mefloquine base. Outside the USA, each 275-mg tablet contains 250 mg base.
45. Outside the USA, the manufacturer recommends dividing the 1250-mg dose into 750 mg followed 6–8 hours later by 500 mg (D Kingston, Med J Aust, 153:235, 1990).
46. NJ White, Eur J Clin Pharmacol, 34:1, 1988
47. May be effective in multiple-drug-resistant *P. falciparum* malaria, but treatment failures have been reported (GD Shanks et al, Am J Trop Med Hyg, 45:488, 1991) and the drug causes consistent dose-related lengthening of the PR and QTc intervals (A Castot et al, Lancet, 341:1541, 1993). Several patients have developed first degree block (F Nosten et al, Lancet 341:1054, 1993). It should not be taken one hour before to three hours after meals and probably should not be used for patients with cardiac conduction defects.
48. A recent study found artemether, a Chinese drug, effective for parenteral treatment of severe malaria in children (NJ White et al, Lancet, 339:317, 1992).
49. Exchange transfusion has been helpful for some patients with high-density (>10%) parasitemia, altered mental status, pulmonary edema, or renal complications (JR Zucker and CC Campbell, Infect Dis Clin North Am, 7:547, 1993).
50. EKG and blood pressure monitoring are recommended.
51. Not available in the USA. IV administration of quinine dihydrochloride can be hazardous; constant monitoring of the pulse and blood pressure is necessary to detect arrhythmia or hypotension. Use of parenteral quinine may also lead to severe hypoglycemia; blood glucose should be monitored.
52. If chloroquine phosphate is not available, hydroxychloroquine sulfate is as effective; 400 mg of hydroxychloroquine sulfate is equivalent to 500 mg of chloroquine phosphate.
53. In *P. falciparum* malaria, if the patient has not shown a response to conventional doses of chloroquine in 48–72 hours, parasitic resistance to this drug should be considered. *P. vivax* with decreased susceptibility to chloroquine has been reported from New Guinea (KH Rieckmann et al, Lancet, 2:1183, 1989) and from Indonesia (IK Schwartz et al, N Engl J Med, 324:927, 1991); a single dose of mefloquine, 15 mg/kg, has been recommended to treat these infections.
54. Some relapses have been reported with this regimen; relapses should be treated with chloroquine plus primaquine, 30 mg base/d × 14 days.
55. Primaquine phosphate can cause hemolytic anemia, especially in patients whose red cells are deficient in glucose-6-phosphate dehydrogenase. This deficiency is most common in African, Asian, and Mediterranean peoples. Patients should be screened for G-6-PD deficiency before treatment. Primaquine should not be used during pregnancy.
56. No drug regimen guarantees protection against malaria. If fever develops within a year (particularly within the first two months) after travel to malarious areas, travelers should be advised to seek medical attention. Insect repellents, insecticide-impregnated bed nets, and proper clothing are important adjuncts for malaria prophylaxis.
57. In pregnancy, chloroquine prophylaxis has been used extensively and safely, but the safety of other prophylactic antimalarial agents in pregnancy is unclear. Therefore, travel during pregnancy to chloroquine-resistant areas should be discouraged.
58. For prevention of attack after departure from areas where *P. vivax* and *P. ovale* are endemic, which includes almost all areas where malaria is found (except Haiti), some experts prescribe in addition primaquine phosphate 15 mg base (26.3 mg)/d or, for children, 0.3 mg base/kg/d during the last two weeks of prophylaxis. Others prefer to avoid the toxicity of primaquine and rely on surveillance to detect cases when they occur, particularly when exposure was limited or doubtful. See also footnotes 54 and 55.
59. Beginning one week before travel and continuing weekly for the duration of stay and for four weeks after leaving.

TABLE 2. *(Continued)*

Infection	Drug	Adult Dosage*	Pediatric Dosage*
Chloroquine-resistant areas[38]			
Drug of choice:	Mefloquine[44,58,60]	250 mg oral once/week[59]	15–19 kg: ¼ tablet
			20–30 kg: ½ tablet
			31–45 kg: ¾ tablet
			>45 kg: 1 tablet
OR	Doxycycline[58,61]	100 mg daily[61]	>8 years of age: 2 mg/kg/d orally, up to 100 mg/day[12]
Alternatives:	Chloroquine phosphate[58] **plus** pyrimethamine-sulfadoxine[40] for presumptive treatment	same as above	same as above
		Carry a single dose (3 tablets) for self-treatment of febrile illness when medical care is not immediately available	<1 yr: ¼ tablet
			1–3 yrs: ½ tablet
			4–8 yrs: 1 tablet
			9–14 yrs: 2 tablets
	or **plus** proguanil[62] (in Africa south of the Sahara)	200 mg daily[62]	<2 yrs: 50 mg daily
			2–6 yrs: 100 mg daily
			7–10 yrs: 150 mg daily
			>10 yrs: 200 mg daily
MICROSPORIDIOSIS			
Ocular (*Encephalitozoon hellem, Nosema corneum*)			
Drug of choice:	See footnote 63		
Intestinal (*Enterocytozoon bieneusi, Septata intestinalis*)			
Drug of choice:	See footnote 64		
Disseminated (*Encephalitozoon hellem, Encephalitozoon cuniculi, Pleistophora* sp.)			
Drug of choice:	See footnote 65		
Mites, see SCABIES			
MONILIFORMIS *moniliformis* infection			
Drug of choice:	Pyrantel pamoate[6]	11 mg/kg once, repeat twice, 2 wks apart	11 mg/kg once, repeat twice, 2 wks apart
Naegleria species, see AMEBIC MENINGOENCEPHALITIS, PRIMARY			
Necator americanus, see HOOKWORM infection			
Oesophagostomum bifurcum			
Drug of choice:	See footnote 66		
Onchocerca volvulus, see FILARIASIS			
Opisthorchis viverrini, see FLUKE infection			
Paragonimus westermani, see FLUKE infection			
Pediculus capitis, humanus, Phthirus pubis, see LICE			
Pinworm, see ENTEROBIUS			
PNEUMOCYSTIS *carinii* pneumonia[67]			
Drug of choice:	Trimethoprim-sulfamethoxazole	TMP 15–20 mg/kg/d, SMX 75–100 mg/kg/d, oral or IV in 3 or 4 doses × 14–21d	Same as adult dose
OR	Pentamidine	3–4 mg/kg IV qd × 14–21 days	Same as adult dose
Alternatives:[68]	Trimethoprim[6] **plus** dapsone[6,69]	5 mg/kg PO q6h × 21 days 100 mg PO qd × 21 days	
	Atovaquone[70]	750 mg tid PO × 21 d	
	Primaquine[6,55] **plus** clindamycin[6]	15 mg base PO qd × 21 days 600 mg IV q6h × 21 days, or 300–450 mg PO q6h × 21 days	
	Trimetrexate **plus** folinic acid	45 mg/m² IV qd × 21 days 20 mg/m² PO or IV q6h × 21 days	
Primary and secondary prophylaxis			
Drug of Choice:	Trimethoprim-sulfamethoxazole	1 DS tab PO qd or 3 ×/week	
Alternatives:	Dapsone[6,69]	100 mg PO qd, or 50 mg PO qd plus pyrimethamine 100 mg qid	
	Aerosol pentamidine	300 mg inhaled monthly via *Respirgard II* nebulizer or *System 22 Mizer Jet Nebulizer*	

* The letter d stands for day.

60. The pediatric dosage has not been approved by the FDA, and the drug has not been approved for use during pregnancy. Women should take contraceptive precautions while taking mefloquine and for two months after the last dose. Mefloquine is not recommended for children weighing less than 15 kg, or for patients with cardiac conduction abnormalities. Patients with a history of seizures or psychiatric disorders and those whose occupation requires fine coordination or spatial discrimination should probably avoid mefloquine (Medical Letter, 32:13, 1990). Resistance to mefloquine has been reported in some areas, such as Thailand; in these areas, doxycycline should be used for prophylaxis.

61. Beginning one day before travel and continuing for the duration of stay and for four weeks after leaving. Use of tetracyclines is contraindicated in pregnancy and in children less than eight years old. Doxycycline can cause gastrointestinal disturbances, vaginal moniliasis and photosensitivity reactions.

62. Proguanil (Paludrine—Ayerst, Canada; ICI, England), which is not available in the USA but is widely available overseas, is recommended mainly for use in Africa south of the Sahara. Prophylaxis is recommended during exposure and for four weeks afterwards. Failures in prophylaxis with chloroquine and proguanil have been reported in travelers to Kenya (AJ Barnes, Lancet, 338:1338, 1991).

63. Ocular lesions due to *E. hellem* in HIV-infected patients have responded to fumagillin eyedrops prepared from *Fumidil-B*, a commercial product used to control a microsporidial disease of honey bees, available from Mid-Continent Agrimarketing, Inc., Lenexa, Kansas 66215 (MC Diesenhouse, Am J Ophthalmol, 115:293, 1993). Fumagillin from other sources has also been used successfully (DF Rosberger et al, Cornea, 12:261, 1993). In one report, a keratopathy due to *E. hellem* in an HIV-infected patient was treated successfully with surgical debridement, topical antibiotics, and itraconazole (RW Yee et al, Ophthalmology, 98:196, 1991). For lesions due to *N. corneum*, topical therapy is generally not effective and keratoplasty may be required (RM Davis et al, Ophthalmology, 97:953, 1990).

64. Octreotide (*Sandostatin*) has provided symptomatic relief of *E. bieneusi* infection (JP Cello et al, Ann Intern Med, 115:705, 1991). Albendazole, 400 mg b.i.d., may be helpful for *E. bieneusi* (DT Dieterich et al, J Infect Dis, 1994, in press) and can cure *S. intestinalis* (C Blanshard et al, AIDS, 6:311, 1992).

65. No established treatment

66. Albendazole or pyrantel pamoate may be effective (HP Krepel et al, Trans R Soc Trop Med Hyg, 87:87, 1993).

67. HIV-infected patients should be treated for 21 days. In severe disease with room air PO₂ ≤ 70 mmHg or Aa gradient ≥ 35 mmHg, prednisone should also be used (Medical Letter, 35:79, 1993).

68. For patients who have failed or are intolerant to standard therapy.

69. Assay for G-6-PD deficiency recommended before therapy.

70. Recommended in mild to moderate disease (room air PO₂ > 60 mmHg) (W Hughes, N Engl J Med, 328:1521, 1993).

TABLE 2. *(Continued)*

Infection	Drug	Adult Dosage*	Pediatric Dosage*
Roundworm, see ASCRIASIS			
SCABIES (*Sarcoptes scabiei*)			
Drug of choice:[87]	5% Permethrin	Topically	Topically
Alternatives:	Lindane[37]	Topically	Topically
	10% Crotamiton	Topically	Topically
SCHISTOSOMIASIS (*Bilharziasis*)			
S. haematobium			
Drug of choice:	Praziquantel	40 mg/kg/d in 2 doses × 1d	40 mg/kg/d in 2 doses × 1d
S. japonicum			
Drug of choice:	Praziquantel	60 mg/kg/d in 3 doses × 1d	60 mg/kg/d in 3 doses × 1d
S. mansoni			
Drug of choice:	Praziquantel	40 mg/kg/d in 2 doses × 1d	40 mg/kg/d in 2 doses × 1d
Alternative:	Oxamniquine[71]	15 mg/kg once[72]	20 mg/kg/d in 2 doses × 1d[72]
S. mekongi			
Drug of choice:	Praziquantel	60 mg/kg/d in 3 doses × 1d	60 mg/kg/d in 3 doses × 1d
Sleeping sickness, see TRYPANOSOMIASIS			
STRONGYLOIDIASIS (*Strongyloides stercoralis*)			
Drug of choice:[73]	Thiabendazole	50 mg/kg/d in 2 doses (max. 3 grams/d) × 2d[10,74]	50 mg/kg/d in 2 doses (max. 3 grams/d) × 2d[10,74]
OR	Ivermectin[75]	200 µg/kg/d × 1–2d	
TAPEWORM infection—**Adult** (intestinal stage)			
Diphyllobothrium latum (fish), *Taenia saginata* (beef), *Taenia solium* (pork), *Dipylidium caninum* (dog)			
Drug of choice:	Praziquantel[6]	5–10 mg/kg once	5–10 mg/kg once
OR	Niclosamide	A single dose of 4 tablets (2 grams), chewed thoroughly	11–34 kg: a single dose of 2 tablets (1 gram); >34 kg: a single dose of 3 tablets (1.5 g)
Hymenolepis nana (dwarf tapeworm)			
Drug of choice:	Praziquantel[6]	25 mg/kg once	25 mg/kg once
Alternative:	Niclosamide	A single daily dose of 4 tablets (2 g), chewed thoroughly, then 2 tablets daily × 6d	11–34 kg: a single dose of 2 tablets (1 g) × 1d, then 1 tablet (0.5 grams)/d × 6d; >34 kg: a single dose of 3 tablets (1.5 g) × 1d, then 2 tablets (1 g)/d × 6d
—Larval (tissue stage)			
Echinococcus granulosus (hydatid cyst)			
Drug of choice:	Albendazole[76,77]	400 mg bid × 28 days, repeated as necessary	15 mg/kg/d × 28 days, repeated as necessary
Echinococcus multilocularis			
Treatment of choice:	See footnote 78		
Cysticercus cellulosae (cysticercosis)			
Drug of choice:[79]	Albendazole[80]	15 mg/kg/d in 3 doses × 28d, repeated as necessary	15 mg/kg/d in 3 doses × 28d, repeated as necessary
OR	Praziquantel[6]	50 mg/kg/d in 3 doses × 15d	50 mg/kg/d in 3 doses × 15d
Alternative:	Surgery		
Toxocariasis, see VISCERAL LARVA MIGRANS			
TOXOPLASMOSIS (*Toxoplasma gondii*)[81]			
Drugs of choice:[82]	Pyrimethamine	25–100 mg/d × 3–4 wks	2 mg/kg/d × 3d, then 1 mg/kg/d (max. 25 mg/d) × 4 wks[83]
	plus sulfadiazine[84]	1–2 grams qid × 3–4 wks	100–200 mg/kg/d × 3–4 wks
Alternative:	Spiramycin[85]	3–4 grams/d	50–100 mg/kg/d × 3–4 wks
TRICHINOSIS (*Trichinella spiralis*)			
Drugs of choice:	Steroids for severe symptoms		
	plus mebendazole[6,86]	200–400 mg tid × 3d, then 400–500 mg tid × 10d	

* The letter d stands for day.

71. Neuropsychiatric disturbances and seizures have been reported in some patients (H Stokvis et al, Am J Trop Med Hyg, 35:330, 1986).
72. In East Africa, the dose should be increased to 30 mg/kg, and in Egypt and South Africa, 30 mg/kg/d × 2d. Some experts recommend 40–60 mg/kg over 2–3 days in all of Africa (KC Shekhar, Drugs, 42:379, 1991).
73. In immunocompromised patients it may be necessary to continue therapy or use other agents.
74. In disseminated strongyloidiasis, thiabendazole therapy should be continued for at least five days.
75. C. Naquira et al, Am J Trop Med Hyg, 40:304, 1989; M Lyagoubi et al, Trans R Soc Trop Med Hyg, 86:541, 1992
76. With a fatty meal to enhance absorption. Some patients may benefit from or require surgical resection of cysts (RK Tompkins, Mayo Clin Proc, 66:1281, 1991). Praziquantel may also be useful preoperatively or in case of spill during surgery.
77. Recently, percutaneous drainage with ultrasound guidance plus albendazole therapy has been effective for management of hepatic hydatid cyst disease (MS Khuroo et al, Gastroenterology, 104:1452, 1993).
78. Surgical excision is the only reliable means of treatment, although some reports have suggested use of albendazole or mebendazole (JF Wilson et al, Am J Trop Med Hyg, 37:162, 1987; A Davis et al, Bull WHO, 64:383, 1986).
79. Corticosteroids should be given for two to three days before and during drug therapy for neurocysticercosis. Any cysticercocidal drug may cause irreparable damage when used to treat ocular or spinal cysts, even when corticosteroids are used.
80. Albendazole should be taken with a fatty meal to enhance absorption.
81. In ocular toxoplasmosis, corticosteroids should also be used for an anti-inflammatory effect on the eyes.
82. Pyrimethamine is teratogenic in animals. To prevent hematological toxicity from pyrimethamine, it is advisable to give leucovorin (folinic acid), about 10 mg/day, either by injection or orally. To treat CNS toxoplasmosis in HIV-infected patients, some clinicians use pyrimethamine 50 to 100 mg daily after a loading dose of 200 mg with a sulfonamide and, when sulfonamide sensitivity developed, have given clindamycin 1.8 to 2.4 g/d in divided doses instead of the sulfonamide (JS Remington et al, Lancet, 338:1142, 1991; BJ Luft et al, N Engl J Med, 329:995, 1993). Atovaquone, 750 mg qid, appears to be an effective alternative in sulfa-intolerant patients (JA Kovacs et al, Lancet, 340:637, 1992). Dapsone-pyrimethamine can prevent first episodes of toxoplasmosis (P-M Girard et al, N Engl J Med, 328:1514, 1993). In HIV-infected patients, chronic suppressive treatment should continue indefinitely (Medical Letter, 35:79, 1993).
83. Congenitally infected newborns should be treated with pyrimethamine every two or three days and a sulfonamide daily for about one year (JS Remington and G Desmonts in JS Remington and JO Klein, eds, *Infectious Disease of the Fetus and Newborn Infant*, 3rd ed, Philadelphia: Saunders, 1990, page 89).
84. Available temporarily from the CDC, 404-488-4928.
85. For use during pregnancy, continue the drug until delivery.
86. Albendazole or flubendazole (not available in the USA) may also be effective.

TABLE 2. (Continued)

Infection		Drug	Adult Dosage*	Pediatric Dosage*
TRICHOMONIASIS (Trichomonas vaginalis)				
Drug of choice:[87]		Metronidazole	2 grams once or 250 mg tid orally × 7d	15 mg/kg/d orally in 3 doses × 7d
	OR	Tinidazole[4]	2 grams once	50 mg/kg once (max. 2 grams)
TRICHOSTRONGYLUS infection				
Drug of choice:		Pyrantel pamoate[6]	11 mg/kg once (max. 1 gram)	11 mg/kg once (max. 1 gram)
Alternative:		Mebendazole[6]	100 mg bid × 3d	100 mg bid × 3d
	OR	Albendazole	400 mg once	400 mg once
TRICHURIASIS (Trichuris trichiura, whipworm)				
Drug of choice:		Mebendazole	100 mg bid × 3d	100 mg bid × 3d
	OR	Albendazole	400 mg once[88]	400 mg once[88]
TRYPANOSOMIASIS				
***T. cruzi* (South American trypanosomiasis, Chagas disease)**				
Drug of choice:		Nifurtimox[2,89]	8–10 mg/kg/d orally in 4 doses × 120d	1–10 yrs: 15–20 mg/kg/d in 4 doses × 90d; 11–16 yrs: 12.5–15 mg/kg/d in 4 doses × 90d
Alternative:		Benznidazole[90]	5–7 mg/kg/d × 30–120d	
***T. brucei gambiense; T. b. rhodesiense* (African trypanosomiasis, sleeping sickness) hemolymphatic stage**				
Drug of choice:		Suramin[2]	100–200 mg (test dose) IV, then 1 gram IV on days 1, 3, 7, 14, and 21	20 mg/kg on days 1, 3, 7, 14, and 21
	OR	Eflornithine	See footnote 91	
Alternative:		Pentamidine isethionate[6]	4 mg/kg/d IM × 10d	4 mg/kg/d IM × 10d
late disease with CNS involvement				
Drug of choice:		Melarsoprol[2,92]	2–3.6 mg/kg/d IV × 3 d; after 1 wk 3.6 mg/kg per day IV × 3d; repeat again after 10–21 days	18–25 mg/kg total over 1 month; initial dose of 0.36 mg/kg IV, increasing gradually to max. 3.6 mg/kg at intervals of 1–5d for total of 9–10 doses
	OR	Eflornithine	See footnote 91	
Alternatives:		Tryparsamide	One injection of 30 mg/kg (max. 2g) IV every 5d to total of 12 injections; may be repeated after 1 month	
		plus suramin[2]	One injection of 10 mg/kg IV every 5d to total of 12 injections; may be repeated after 1 month	
VISCERAL LARVA MIGRANS[93]				
Drug of choice:		Diethylcarbamazine[6]	6 mg/kg/d in 3 doses × 7–10d	6 mg/kg/d in 3 doses × 7–10d
Alternatives:		Albendazole[94]	400 mg bid × 3–5d	400 mg bid × 3–5d
		Mebendazole[6,95]	100–200 mg bid × 5d	

Whipworm, see TRICHURIASIS

Wuchereria bancrofti, see FILARIASIS

* The letter d stands for day.
87. Sexual partners should be treated simultaneously. Outside the USA, ornidazole has also been used for this condition. Metronidazole-resistant strains have been reported; higher doses of metronidazole for longer periods are sometimes effective against these strains (J Lossick, Rev Infect Dis, 12:S665, 1990).
88. In heavy infection it may be necessary to extend therapy for 3 days.
89. The addition of gamma interferon to nifurtimox for 20 days in a limited number of patients and in experimental animals appears to have shortened the acute phase of Chagas' disease (RE McCabe et al, J Infect Dis, 163:912, 1991).
90. Limited data
91. In *T. b. gambiense* infections, eflornithine is highly effective in both the hemolymphatic and CNS stages. Its effectiveness in *T. b. rhodesiense* infections has been variable. Some clinicians have given 400 mg/kg/d IV in 4 divided doses for 14 days, followed by oral treatment with 300 mg/kg for 3–4 wks (F Milord et al, Lancet, 340:652, 1992).
92. In frail patients, begin with as little as 18 mg and increase the dose progressively. Pretreatment with suramin has been advocated for debilitated patients. Corticosteroids have been used to prevent arsenical encephalopathy (J Pepin et al, Lancet, 1:1246, 1989).
93. For severe symptoms or eye involvement, corticosteroids can be used in addition.
94. D Stürchler et al, An Trop Med Parasitol, 83:473, 1989
95. One report of a cure using 1 gram tid for 21 days has been published (A Bekhti, Ann Intern Med, 100:463, 1984).
(From ref. 5, with permission.)

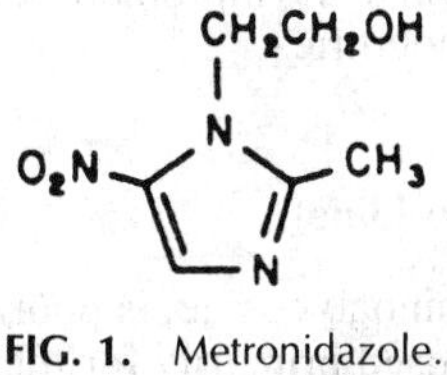

FIG. 1. Metronidazole.

nidazole acts as an electron sink, depriving the anaerobe of reducing equivalents. Furthermore, the reduced form of metronidazole causes loss of the helical structure of DNA, strand breakage, and impaired template function.[28,29]

Side effects are seldom severe enough to cause discontinuation of the drug. They are more likely to occur with higher doses and prolonged administration. Gastrointestinal side effects include nausea, vomiting, diarrhea, and a metallic aftertaste. They are less common with the low doses (250 mg tid) recommended for giardiasis than with the high doses (750 mg tid) used for amebiasis. Other less frequent side effects include headache, dizziness, rash, urethral burning, vaginal or oral candidiasis, and reversible neutropenia.[30] The urine of some persons may become red or brown due to the presence of metabolites. Metronidazole may potentiate the anticoagulant effects of coumarin.[31] Rarely, patients treated with metronidazole experience sensory neuropathies or central nervous system toxicity with vertigo, ataxia, seizures, or encephalopathy.[32] Acute pancreatitis has been reported.[33] Pseudomembranous colitis is also rare. Alcohol should be avoided because of the disulfiram (Antabuse)-like effects of metronidazole and the drug–drug interaction that can result in acute psychosis or a confusional state.[34]

The potential role of metronidazole in human carcinogenesis has been the subject of debate. Metronidazole has not been shown to be carcinogenic in humans, but it is mutagenic for certain strains of *Salmonella typhimurium*.[35] Furthermore, human urine contains metabolites that are carcinogenic in rodents.[36] However, 10-year follow-up of patients who received metronidazole for trichomoniasis has revealed no increase in the prevalence of cancer.[37,38]

Tinidazole and ornidazole, two other 5-nitroimidazole derivatives, have amebicidal, giardiacidal, and trichomonicidal activity similar to that of metronidazole.[7,39–41] On occasion tinidazole has been used successfully to treat metronidazole-resistant *T. vaginalis*.[18] A single 2-gr dose of tinidazole has been used successfully to treat giardiasis. Both tinidazole and ornidazole are well absorbed orally, have good tissue penetration, and are widely distributed in the body. Tinidazole and ornidazole have half-lives of 14 and 12–13 hours, respectively.[42] They are excreted primarily in urine, 50 percent of tinidazole and 96 percent of ornidazole in the form of metabolites.[43] These drugs have a favorable side effect profile in comparison to metronidazole. Reported side effects include anorexia, headache, and dizziness.

Dehydroemetine** and Emetine***

Emetine, for many years the drug of choice for invasive amebiasis, is a tissue-active amebicide prepared from ipecac, which comes from the root of *Cephaëlis ipecacuanha*. The root is still used as a traditional medicine for the treatment of bloody diarrhea in some rural areas of South and Central America. Emetine and dehydroemetine have appreciable toxicity. They are reserved for persons with extraintestinal amebiasis, usually amebic liver abscesses,[44] who do not respond to metronidazole or for the rare person in whom metronidazole cannot be used. They are often given concomitantly with chloroquine, which at high doses is a tissue active amebicide.[45] Iodoquinol or another luminally active agent is necessary to eradicate amebic cysts from the gastrointestinal tract.

Emetine is administered by deep intramuscular injection; oral administration is prevented by severe gastrointestinal irritation. Emetine is well absorbed from muscle and is excreted very slowly.[46] It can be detected in the urine for 1–2 months after completion of treatment. It is distributed to the spleen, kidney, and lung, but the highest concentrations are found in the liver, which enhances its activity in the treatment of amebic liver abscesses.[46] Negligible amounts are detected in the blood. Emetine acts by inhibiting protein synthesis in eukaryotic cells.[46,47]

Emetine is responsible for toxicity in multiple organs. Diarrhea, nausea, and vomiting are frequent. Muscle weakness, aching, tenderness, and stiffness are experienced by the majority of persons who receive a cumulative dose of 1300 mg.[48] The most serious untoward effects are cardiovascular. These include precordial pain, weakness, arrhythmias, hypotension, tachycardia, congestive heart failure, and occasionally death.[49] Electrocardiographic (ECG) changes are characterized by a prolonged Q-T interval, T-wave inversion, and S-T depression. The ECG tends to return to normal 1–2 weeks after cessation of therapy.[50] Emetine has direct toxic effects on skeletal and cardiac muscles.[51] Local toxicity at the site of injection includes muscle pain, tenderness, and stiffness. Less common are urticarial reactions. Persons receiving emetine require hospitalization and careful monitoring for signs of toxicity. Emetine is contraindicated in persons with cardiac and renal disease and is relatively contraindicated in children and pregnant women.

Dehydroemetine has a shorter half-life than emetine, as well as diminished frequency and severity of side effects.[52] It is also less potent then emetine, and higher doses must be used to obtain the desired therapeutic effect.

Iodoquinol

Iodoquinol (diiodohydroxyquin), a halogenated oxyquinoline (5,7-diiodo-8-quinolinol), is a luminally active agent used to eradicate cysts in persons with asymptomatic *E. histolytica* infection or after metronidazole administration in persons with invasive intestinal or extraintestinal disease. Iodoquinol is also recommended for the treatment of *Dientamoeba fragilis* and *Blastocystis hominis,* and it is used as an alternative drug for the treatment of *Balantidium coli.*

Iodoquinol is available in 210- and 250-mg tablets. It is poorly absorbed and best tolerated if given with meals. The mechanism of action is not known. Reported side effects include headache, diarrhea, nausea, vomiting and abdominal pain, fever, itching, seizures, and encephalopathy.[53] Occasionally, the drug is associated with iodine dermatitis (iodine toxicoderma). The high iodine content (63 percent) can interfere with the results of thyroid function tests for months after completion of therapy. Iodoquinol is contraindicated in persons with iodine intolerance.

A related compound, iodochlorhydroxyquin***, which is better absorbed than iodoquinol, gained notoriety as a cause of subacute myelo-optic neuropathy. This syndrome and its relationship to iodochlorhydroxyquin were first described in Japan, where the syndrome occurred in near-epidemic proportions. The discontinuation of iodochlorhydroxyquin led to an almost immediate reduction in the number of cases of subacute myelo-optic neuropathy.[54] Optic nerve damage or inflammation and a peripheral neuropathy may occur with prolonged high doses of iodoquinol as well. The dosage regimen recommended for amebic disease (Table 2) avoids these complications, but the recommended doses and duration of therapy should never be exceeded.[24]

Diloxanide Furoate**

Diloxanide furoate, a substituted acetanilide, 4-(N-methyl-2,2-dichloroacetamido)phenyl-2-furoate, is a luminally active agent used for the treatment of asymptomatic *E. histolytica* infection[55–58] and to eradicate cysts after treatment of invasive disease with metronidazole. It is ineffective in the treatment of extraintestinal amebiasis. Diloxanide furoate is hydrolyzed by intestinal esterases releasing diloxanide, the absorbed form of the amebicide. Delayed or reduced absorption of the ester results in higher concentrations in the large intestine and the desired luminal effect.

Diloxanide furoate is formulated in 500-mg tablets. In experimental animals, 60–90 percent of the drug is excreted in the urine within 48 hours.[49] Excretion in the feces accounts for 4–9 percent. Diloxanide is amebicidal at low concentrations, but the mechanism of action is unknown. There are rarely serious side effects at the recommended dosage. The most common untoward effect is flatulence.[58] Mild gastrointestinal complaints may also occur. The low cost of the drug makes it an excellent alternative for the treatment of asymptomatic intestinal amebic infections in developing countries.

Paromomycin (Aminosidine)

Paromomycin, an aminoglycoside, is poorly absorbed after oral administration. It is used primarily for the treatment of asymptomatic intestinal amebiasis[59,60] and *Dientamoeba fragilis*. Recent reports indicate that paromomycin is effective for the treatment of some persons with cryptosporidiosis, including those with AIDS.[61,62] Paromomycin with methylbenzethonium chloride has been used topically to treat cutaneous leishmaniasis[63] and systemically to treat a small number of cases of visceral leishmaniasis.[64,65] It acts directly on amebae and has antibacterial activity in the colon.

Paromomycin is available in 250-mg capsules. Side effects are primarily gastrointestinal and include nausea, vomiting, abdominal cramps, and diarrhea in some patients. Paromomycin, like other aminoglycosides, is potentially ototoxic and nephrotoxic when administered parenterally. Very little is absorbed from the gastrointestinal tract, but it is contraindicated in persons with renal failure. Paromomycin also has some activity against human tapeworms,[66] but it is rarely used for that purpose.

Quinacrine

Quinacrine (Fig. 2), 3-chloro-7-methoxy-9-(1-methyl-4-diethyl-aminobutylamino)acridine, a yellow dye with a 4-aminoquino-line radical linked to a benzene ring, has been widely used for the treatment of giardiasis.[9,10,67-69] Some experts in the United States consider it the drug of choice for this disease (Table 2). The cure rate in adults is approximately 90 percent,[9] but it may be lower in children.[68] It is the least expensive of the three drugs that are commonly used to treat *G. lamblia*. Quinacrine is also active against adult tapeworms but has been replaced by niclo-samide and praziquantel, which are less toxic. During World War II, quinacrine was used for malaria prophylaxis and treatment.

Quinacrine is available in 100-mg tablets. It is well absorbed from the gastrointestinal tract and is widely distributed through-out the body. Quinacrine can intercalate into DNA and inhibit nucleic acid synthesis.[70] Whether this relates to its antiparasitic activity is unknown. Quinacrine has strong tissue-binding prop-erties and can be detected in urine for up to 2 months after cessation of therapy.

Data on toxicity were accumulated during the widespread use of quinacrine as an antimalarial.[52] Quinacrine has a bitter, un-pleasant taste and can induce nausea and vomiting, especially in children. Other common side effects include headache and dizziness. At high doses, quinacrine can turn the skin and urine yellow. This effect is seen in 4–5 percent of persons treated for giardiasis.[10,71] The sclerae are usually spared. A bright yellow-green fluorescence under Wood's light confirms that the discol-oration is due to quinacrine and not bilirubin. The yellow skin discoloration lasts for periods ranging from a few weeks to sev-eral months.

Uncommon side effects of quinacrine include skin rashes, fever, and reversible acute, toxic psychosis.[72-74] The last occurs in 0.1–1.5 percent of persons receiving the drug and usually lasts for 2–4 weeks.[74] The mechanism is unknown. Quinacrine is contraindicated in patients with a history of psychosis. Very rarely, blood dyscrasias have been reported to follow treatment. Quinacrine is also contraindicated in pregnancy, since it readily crosses the placental barrier. Patients with psoriasis occasion-ally develop extensive exfoliative dermatitis and should not re-ceive the drug.

There are two important potential drug interactions with quin-acrine. First, like metronidazole, quinacrine has a disulfiram-like effect. Adult patients should be warned not to drink alcohol, and children taking quinacrine should not be given ethanol-con-taining medications. Second, quinacrine interferes with the me-tabolism of primaquine and may result in toxic levels of pri-maquine. The inhibitory effect on primaquine metabolism may last for up to 3 months after the last dose of quinacrine is admin-istered.

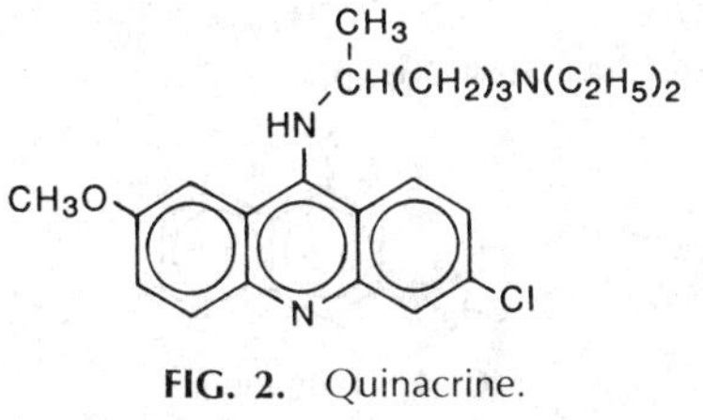

FIG. 2. Quinacrine.

Furazolidone

Furazolidone, 3-[(5-nitro-2-furanyl)methylene-amino]-2-oxazoli-dinone, is a nitrofuran derivative. Like other nitrofurans, it acts by damaging DNA. It is the only anti-*Giardia* drug available as a liquid, and it is commonly used for the treatment of giardiasis in children.[68,75-77] It is as effective as metronidazole. Furazoli-done also has some activity against *I. belli* and a variety of enteropathogenic bacteria.[78]

Furazolidone is available as a suspension containing 25 mg/5 ml and 100-mg tablets. Despite earlier reports to the contrary, furazolidone is well absorbed; greater than 65% is recovered in the urine in the form of metabolites.[79] Common side effects include nausea, vomiting, diarrhea, and fever.[80] Some of the metabolites are brown and may discolor the urine. Other rare side effects are hypotension, urticaria, serum sickness, and hy-persensitivity reactions. A mild to moderate hemolysis may occur in patients with glucose-6-phosphate dehydrogenase (G6PD) deficiency. As with metronidazole and quinacrine, alco-hol should not be ingested because furazolidone has disulfiram-like activity. It is also a monoamine oxidase inhibitor. Furazoli-done should not be administered to mothers who are breast-feeding or to neonates, since hemolytic anemia due to glutathi-one instability may occur.

DRUGS USED AGAINST MEMBERS OF THE PHYLUM APICOMPLEXA

Members of the phylum Apicomplexa pose substantial risks to people throughout the world. *Plasmodium* spp. continue to cause morbidity and mortality throughout the tropics. Attempts to eradicate malaria by mass residual insecticide spraying have failed, and there has been a resurgence of malaria in some areas.[81] Increasing resistance of *Plasmodium* spp. to prophylac-tic and therapeutic regimens has further complicated the situa-tion. The four *Plasmodium* spp. that infect humans are responsi-ble for 100–125 million estimated cases of malaria worldwide each year. It is estimated that between 0.7 and 1 million deaths annually in sub-Saharan Africa alone are due to malaria. As of 1990, 41 percent of the world's population lived in areas where malaria is a serious problem.[82]

As travel has increased, so has the exposure of nonimmune hosts to malaria. Every year approximately 1 million Americans travel to tropical or subtropical areas where they are at risk of acquiring malaria. Prophylaxis is effective, but the evolution of drug resistance among *P. falciparum* continues to pose prob-lems.[83] The erythrocytic stage of malaria is the most sensitive to chemotherapy. The exoerythrocytic stage is difficult to treat, and the sporozoite stage is resistant to all known forms of pro-phylaxis.

Toxoplasma gondii infects people throughout the world.[84] It is an important cause of birth defects, and it has emerged as the most frequent opportunistic pathogen causing encephalitis in persons with AIDS.[85] *Cryptosporidium* spp. and *I. belli* are other coccidians that have emerged as important pathogens among persons with AIDS. They produce chronic diarrhea with weight loss in that setting. *Cryptosporidium* has increasingly been recognized as a cause of self-limited diarrhea in immuno-logically normal hosts as well.[86]

Aminoquinolines Used for the Prophylaxis and Treatment of Malaria

Chloroquine. Chloroquine (Fig. 3), 7-chloro-4-(4-diethy-lamino-1-methylbutylamino)-quinoline, the best known of the 4-aminoquinolines, has been the mainstay of antimalarial chemotherapy and prophylaxis. It is active against the erythro-cytic stages of *P. vivax, P. ovale, P. malaria*, and, in a few

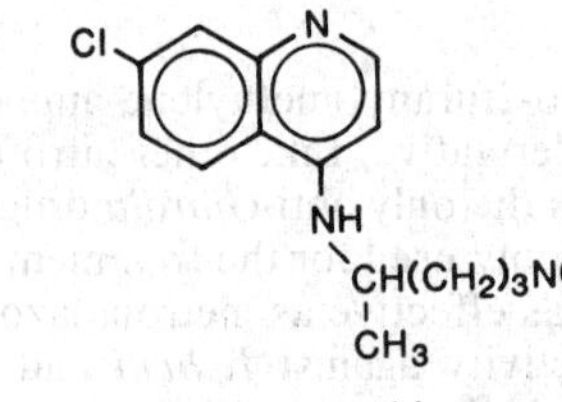

FIG. 3. Chloroquine.

regions, *P. falciparum.* The emergence of resistant strains of *P. falciparum* has been increasing steadily over the past 20 years.[86a,87] The majority of strains in Africa, Southeast Asia, India, and areas of South America are now chloroquine resistant.[87–94] Although not yet a common problem, there have been several reports of chloroquine-resistant *P. vivax* in the southwestern Pacific.[95–98]

Chloroquine has also been used for the treatment of amebic liver abscess concurrently with emetine and for rheumatoid arthritis and systemic lupus erythematosus (SLE). It was once recommended for persons with *Babesia* infection, but it was found to be ineffective.[99]

Chloroquine phosphate is available as a bitter white medication, which is dispensed in tablets containing 250 or 500 mg (150- and 300-mg base, respectively). Chloroquine is rapidly absorbed after oral ingestion and is slowly excreted. The therapeutic blood concentration is reached within 2 or 3 hours. Chloroquine is widely distributed throughout the body but is relatively concentrated in the liver, spleen, kidneys, and erythrocytes. It is metabolized by alkylation in the liver, but approximately 50 percent of the drug is excreted in the urine. The half-life is 4 days, which allows for once-a-week prophylaxis.[100,101] Approximately 50 percent of chloroquine is protein bound. The renal status of the patient does not affect the amount used for acute malaria, but prophylactic doses need to be reduced for those with reduced renal function.[101]

Chloroquine is concentrated in parasitized erythrocytes 100-fold more than in nonparasitized ones.[102] In erythrocytes with schizonts, the concentration of chloroquine is 600-fold greater than in plasma. Chloroquine is toxic for the asexual erythrocytic stages of *Plasmodium* spp. It has a marked and rapid effect on the hemoglobin-containing digestive vesicles of intraerythrocytic parasites. After therapy, there is fusion of adjacent vesicles, followed by sequestration of the fused vesicles and their malaria pigment into a large autophagic vacuole.[103,104] Ferriprotoporphyrin IX, a product of hemoglobin degradation by the parasite, can damage membranes and inhibit a variety of parasitic enzymes in its soluble form. Recent data suggest that the parasite protects itself from this toxin by the activity of a heme polymerase that incorporates ferriprotoporphyrin IX into an insoluble crystalline material.[105] It is now felt that chloroquine and other aminoquinoline drugs act by inhibiting this enzyme.

Attention has also focused on the concentration of chloroquine in the acid-vesicle system of susceptible *P. falciparum.*[106,107] Resistant parasites transport chloroquine out of intraparasitic compartments more rapidly than susceptible strains and maintain lower chloroquine concentrations in their acid vesicles.[107] There is experimental evidence that this can be reversed with phenothiazines, calcium channel blockers, or other agents, raising the theoretical possibility that chloroquine plus an additional agent that blocks the efflux of chloroquine might be effective against chloroquine-resistant strains.[108,109]

Chloroquine is a relatively safe chemoprophylactic and therapeutic drug when used at the recommended doses for malaria. Oral administration is preferred. Occasional temporary side effects include headache, nausea, vomiting, blurred vision, dizziness, fatigue, and confusion.[87,101] Some Africans experience

pruritis, which responds to an antihistamine. Rare side effects include depigmentation of the hair, corneal opacities, weight loss, insomnia, leukopenia, myalgias and exacerbation of psoriasis, and eczema or other exfoliative dermatoses. Extremely rare reactions include blood dyscrasias, toxic psychosis, and photophobia. Permanent retinal damage is rarely associated with malaria prophylaxis and treatment but has occurred with long-term, high-dose therapy given to persons with collagen vascular diseases.[110] Chloroquine is contraindicated in persons with retinal disease, psoriasis, or porphyria.

Chloroquine can also be given by intravenous infusion, but it must be administered slowly and with great caution.[87,111] Respiratory depression, hypotension, cardiovascular collapse, and seizures can follow excessively rapid parenteral administration. These are apparently due to toxic levels of chloroquine in the circulation. Heart block and cardiac arrest are thought to be due to a direct toxic effect on the myocardium at high plasma concentrations. It is recommended that oral administration be substituted for parenteral administration as soon as possible.[87] Deaths from chloroquine toxicity also occur in accidental ingestion by children, in adults who habitually self-medicate, and in those who attempt suicide. The ingestion of 5 g of chloroquine is fatal unless treatment is initiated immediately with mechanical ventilation, diazepam, and epinephrine.[112]

Chloroquine has been implicated in severe cochleovestibular abnormalities in the fetus of a mother taking high doses for the treatment of SLE.[113] There has been no such association between chloroquine administered in antimalarial doses and fetal abnormalities.[101]

Primaquine. Primaquine (Fig. 4) is an 8-aminoquinoline, 8-(4-amino-1-methylbutylamino)-6-methoxyquinoline. It is the only drug available that is effective in eradicating the exoerythrocytic, hypnozoite forms of *P. vivax* and *P. ovale* in the liver.[114] It has some activity against the asexual blood stages of *P. vivax,* but this action is not sufficient to allow it to be used alone for suppressive prophylaxis. The 8-aminoquinolines also have gametocytocidal activity against all four *Plasmodium* spp. that infect humans, but this is not of clinical significance. Primaquine is used after chloroquine to provide a radical cure for persons with acute *P. vivax* or *P. ovale* malaria or after chloroquine prophylaxis in persons exposed to these forms of malaria.[115] Although the relapse rate in persons infected with *P. vivax* is low following primaquine therapy, resistance does occur. Relatively resistant strains were initially limited to the southwestern Pacific. More recently there have been reports of relapse following primaquine therapy in southeast Asia and South America. Persons infected with these relatively resistant strains require higher doses given either daily or at weekly intervals.[116–118]

Primaquine phosphate is supplied in tablets containing 26.3 mg of the salt, which is equivalent to 15 mg of the base. It has a bitter taste, and may be crushed and added to sweet liquid or fruit to make it more palatable. The dosage is usually expressed in terms of the base. Primaquine is readily absorbed when taken orally. Plasma concentrations reach a peak at 6 hours and decline to undetectable levels by 24 hours.

Primaquine interferes with the mitochondrial function of *Plas-*

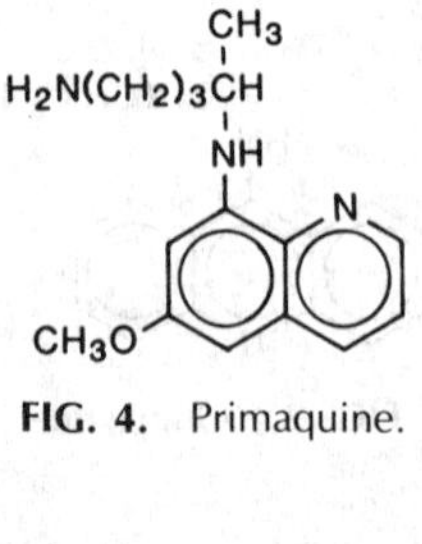

FIG. 4. Primaquine.

modium. It is fully active only after metabolism by the host, but the nature of the active metabolites is not clear. Based on studies with pamoquine***, the first of this series of drugs, the metabolites are thought to affect both the mitochondrial electron transport chain and pyrimidine synthesis.[103] Recent data show that primaquine selectively inhibits the formation of functional cellular transport vesicles *in vitro*, but the significance of this is unknown.[119]

The major toxicity with primaquine is hemolysis in persons with G6PD deficiency.[120,121] G6PD deficiency is rare in whites, but there are more than 100 million people worldwide with this deficiency (1 percent of males in the Middle East, 5 percent of Chinese males, and 10 percent of black males). Persons from these groups should be tested for G6PD deficiency before primaquine is prescribed. Similarly, the administration of primaquine should be discontinued if darkening of the urine or a fall in hematocrit is noted. For persons with the more mild African form of G6PD deficiency, a dose of 45 mg (base) weekly for 8 weeks has been used.[122] For patients with the more severe Mediterranean variety, 30 mg weekly for 30 weeks has been recommended.[121]

Apart from the potential for hemolysis, primaquine is usually well tolerated.[101] Abdominal cramps, epigastric distress, and nausea occur in some patients. Mild anemia, cyanosis (methemoglobinemia), and leukocytosis are observed in some persons given higher doses. Rare complications include granulocytopenia or agranulocytosis, hypertension, and arrhythmia.

Cinchona Alkaloids, Quinine, and Quinidine

Quinine. Quinine (Fig. 5), a cinchona alkaloid, was the first successful agent for the treatment of malaria.[87] It is effective against the asexual blood stages of *Plasmodium* spp. With the introduction of chloroquine, the use of quinine fell dramatically, but with the widespread emergence of chloroquine-resistant *P. falciparum*, quinine has once again become widely used.[87] Progressively decreased sensitivity to quinine has been a problem in Thailand. There have been emerging reports of resistance in West Africa as well.[123,124] Quinine acts rapidly against asexual erythrocytic stages of all four *Plasmodium* spp. that infect humans.

Quinine sulfate is supplied as 260- and 325-mg tablets and in capsules of 130, 200, 260, 300, and 325 mg. The tablets have a very bitter taste. Quinine is rapidly absorbed after oral administration and reaches peak levels in 1–3 hours. Peak serum concentrations after a dose of 10 mg/kg are 7–17 μg/ml; side effects can be seen at concentrations above 10 μg/ml.[101] Quinine is formulated for parenteral use as quinine dihydrochloride*** in 2-ml ampules containing 300 mg/ml. The parenteral preparation is no longer available in the United States. Intravenous quinidine, its dextrostereoisomer, is effective and available in virtually all hospitals. It is now considered the drug of choice for parenteral treatment of complicated *P. falciparum* infection.[125]

Quinine is metabolized in the liver and excreted in the urine,

mainly as metabolites.[126] Only 20 percent of the drug is excreted unchanged.[127] It is not as avidly bound to tissues as chloroquine and has a shorter half-life of 5–15 hours. Monitoring blood levels is recommended for persons with impaired renal or hepatic function, and dose reduction is necessary in severe renal failure.[128]

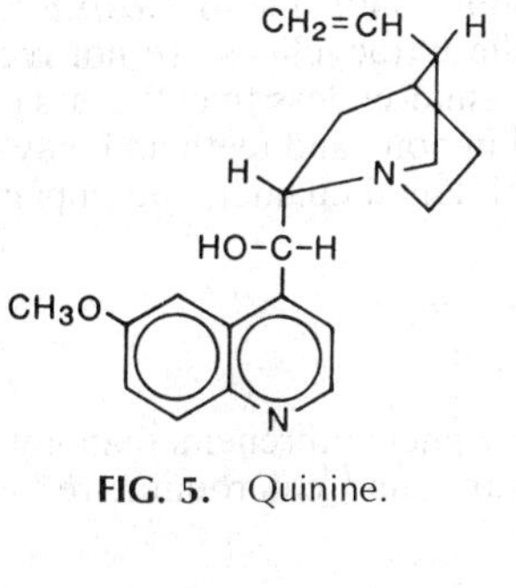

The exact mechanism of action as an antimalarial is unknown, but quinine, like chloroquine, appears to act at the level of the hemoglobin-containing digestive vesicles of the intraerythrocytic parasite. New evidence suggests that quinidine may work by inhibiting heme polymerase, an enzyme responsible for protecting the parasite from toxic hemoglobin degradation products produced by the parasite.[105] Quinine also intercalates into DNA, but this does not appear to be its primary mode of action.

Quinine has the poorest therapeutic-to-toxic ratio of all of the antimalarial drugs.[129] The side effects of quinine are collectively referred to as *cinchonism* and include tinnitis, decreased hearing, headache, dysphoria, nausea, vomiting, and mild visual disturbances.[87,129] These alterations are dose related and reversible. Other less common side effects are skin rashes, including urticaria, angioedema of the face, pruritis, agranulocytosis, hepatitis, and, rarely, massive hemolysis in persons with falciparum malaria (blackwater fever). Quinine can cause respiratory depression in patients with myasthenia gravis. It has a curare-like effect on skeletal muscle and has been useful in the treatment of painful nocturnal leg cramps. Other adverse reactions include hypoglycemia in patients with high *P. falciparum* parasitemia. This is due to the parasites' consumption of glucose and the release of insulin from the pancreas by quinine.[132] It responds to the administration of intravenous glucose. Quinine causes hemolysis in patients with G6PD deficiency. It can stimulate uterine contractions and may produce abortion if given in high doses. However, quinine has been used successfully to treat seriously ill women with malaria in the third trimester of pregnancy.[133] Quinine must be used cautiously by the intravenous route, since rapid intravenous infusion may cause shock due to myocardial depression and peripheral vasodilatation. Overdoses are associated with convulsions, coma, delirium, depressed respiration, circulatory collapse, and death.

Quinidine. Quinidine is the dextrostereoisomer of quinine. Quinidine gluconate is now considered the drug of choice in persons requiring parenteral treatment of chloroquine-resistant falciparum malaria. This new recommendation follows reports of cases in which administration of antimalarial therapy in critically ill persons was delayed by the lack of availability of parenteral quinine.[125] A major advantage of parenteral quinidine over parenteral quinine is that quinidine gluconate is available in virtually every U.S. hospital because of its role in the treatment of cardiac arrhythmias. Recent data have demonstrated the efficacy and safety of parenteral quinidine in the treatment of severe falciparum malaria.[134–137]

Quinidine gluconate is available for intravenous administration. The half-life of quinidine is 12.8 hours. ECG changes including prolonged Q-Tc intervals are common, but life-threatening arrhythmias are rare if proper doses are used. Hypotension may occur if the infusion is too rapid. The rate of infusion, blood pressure, and ECGs of persons receiving intravenous quinidine should be monitored closely,[137] preferably in an intensive care setting.

4-Quinoline-Carbinolamines (Quinoline Methanols): Mefloquine

Mefloquine (Fig. 6), used widely for prophylaxis against chloroquine-resistant *P. falciparum*, is a quinoline-methanol derived chemically from quinine. Mefloquine was the result of a search for a new antimalarial drug by researchers at the Walter Reed Army Institute of Research.[87,88] Like quinine and chloroquine,

FIG. 5. Quinine.

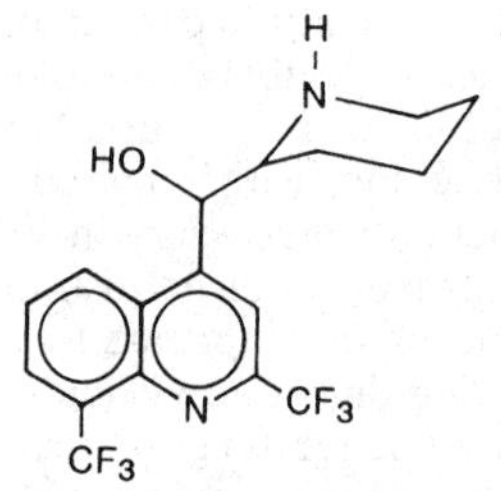

FIG. 6. Mefloquine.

mefloquine is a blood schizontocidal drug and has no effect on exoerythrocytic schizonts or gametocytes.[102] Used as a single dose, it has been effective against all *Plasmodium* spp., including chloroquine-resistant and pyrimethamine-sulfadoxime–resistant isolates of *P. falciparum*.[138–141] Resistance to mefloquine is being increasingly reported, primarily in Thailand and west Africa.[142–147] A unified effort has been made to restrict its use for treatment and prophylaxis to areas with chloroquine-resistant *P. falciparum*.

Mefloquine is available only for oral administration. Administered in tablet form, it is slowly and incompletely absorbed.[148] Mefloquine is widely distributed in the body, and 99 percent of the drug is protein bound. It has a long half-life in humans, ranging from 6 to 23 days, with a mean of 14 days. Mefloquine is given weekly for malaria prophylaxis. It is extensively metabolized and excreted through bile and feces. Mefloquine concentrates on red blood cell membranes and seems to interfere with the food vacuoles of *Plasmodium* in a manner similar to that of quinine.[149] Mefloquine has been administered as a suspension via a nasogastric tube to unconscious patients with cerebral malaria. Absorption was rapid, with an absorption half-life of 1.5 hours. Plasma mefloquine levels were over 200 ng/ml within 3 hours.[150] Mefloquine cannot be administered parenterally because it causes intense local irritation.

Mefloquine is well tolerated by most persons using it for prophylaxis. Side effects are common with treatment doses. Mild transient adverse effects such as nausea and dizziness are not uncommon in patients taking mefloquine, especially with higher doses. Neuropsychiatric reactions such as seizures, acute psychosis, anxiety neurosis, and disturbances of sleep-wake cycles have been estimated to occur in about 0.5 percent of users following treatment doses, but much less frequently following prophylactic doses.[151] Mefloquine is not recommended for individuals with a history of epilepsy or psychiatric disorders. Despite initial concerns, it has not been established that mefloquine is contraindicated for those whose occupation requires fine coordination and spatial discrimination.[86a] Mefloquine can cause alterations in cardiac conduction. Sinus bradycardia and sinus arrythmia are common during therapy, but in the absence of other cardiac medications these changes appear to be transient and benign. However, sudden death has been reported following a single dose of mefloquine in a patient taking propranolol.[152] Therefore, patients with cardiac conduction abnormalities who are taking drugs that alter cardiac conduction (e.g., β-blockers) should not receive mefloquine.[86a] Other isolated reports of adverse effects include exfoliative dermatitis and Stevens-Johnson syndrome, agranulocytosis and parasthesias.[153–156] There is some evidence that mefloquine may be toxic to the live *Salmonella typhi* (Ty21a) oral vaccine at concentrations achieved enterally, and consequently administration of that vaccine should be separated in time from the administration of mefloquine.[157] Mefloquine is teratogenic in animals. Women should avoid pregnancy while taking the drug and for 2 months following the last dose.[152]

Artemisinin (Qinghaosu)***

Artemisinin is a sesquiterpene lactone derived from the wormwood plant *Artemisia annua*. It has been used as a traditional medication by the Chinese for febrile illnesses and is now known to have activity against several *Plasmodium* species, the free-living ameba *Naegleria fowleri*, and the trematodes *Shistosoma japonicum*, *S. mansoni*, and *Clonorchis sinensis*. Its major clinical role, however, is expected to be treatment of chloroquine-resistant *P. falciparum* infection. Preliminary clinical data suggest that artemesinin and its derivatives result in more rapid parasitologic clearance and decreased mortality when compared with aminoquinoline antimalarials. However, there are still insufficient data with which to draw conclusions regarding its role in malaria therapy. Comparative trials are ongoing.[158]

The mode of action is poorly understood, but is thought to involve free radical damage to parasite membrane systems. The drug acts rapidly, arresting parasite development and preventing cytoadherence and rosetting, both thought to be important pathophysiologic mechanisms in severe malaria.[158]

Artemesinin compounds can be administered enterally, intravenously, or intramuscularly. In addition to an oral preparation of the drug, a suppository form is also available, representing a potentially major advantage in treating severe malaria in patients who cannot take oral medications in settings where injections cannot be given.[158]

Early experience with artemesinin suggests that it may be less toxic than the aminoquinoline antimalarials. Adverse effects seen in humans have been transient first-degree heart block, mild decreases in reticulocyte and neutrophil counts, elevated liver transaminases, abdominal pain, diarrhea, and drug fever. No severe adverse effects have occurred in over 4000 patients entered into clinical studies.[158]

Resistance to artemisinin in *P. yoelii* has been produced in mice.[102] Troublesome was the observation that artemisinin-resistant parasites also displayed marked cross-resistance to chloroquine, quinine, and mefloquine, possibly due to a modification of the membrane composition of the parasite. Clinical isolates originating from Africa resistant to artemisinin, mefloquine, and halofantrine have recently been reported.[102a]

Tetracycline and Doxycycline

Tetracycline has been used with quinine to treat acute falciparum malaria acquired in areas such as Thailand where *P. falciparum* is resistant to pyrimethamine, sulfonamides, and chloroquine and has decreased susceptibility to quinine.[159,160] Doxycycline, a long-acting tetracycline, has been used prophylactically in these regions. The Centers for Disease Control and Prevention recommend the use of daily doxycycline while the person is exposed and for 4 weeks after leaving the endemic area.[161]

Tetracyclines are well absorbed orally. Their pharmacology is discussed in Chapter 21. They inhibit protein synthesis in prokaryotic ribosomes, and it is likely that they affect parasite protein synthesis as well.[103] The most common untoward effects are gastrointestinal. Photosensitivity occurs in approximately 3 percent of recipients and is a potential problem for travelers to the tropics. *Candida* vaginitis can complicate tetracycline use. Pseudomembranous colitis due to *Clostridium difficile* can also occur. Finally, the tetracyclines are not recommended during pregnancy or for children less than 9 years of age because they are concentrated in bone and teeth and may cause dental staining, hypoplasia of dental enamel, and impaired bone growth in young children.

Halofantrine***

Halofantrine is a 9-phenanthrenemethanol with activity against chloroquine-sensitive and chloroquine-resistant *P. falciparum* and *P. vivax*. It is a blood schizontocide with selective activity against the intraerythrocytic stages of *Plasmodium* spp. but has no activity against gametocytes or extraerythrocytic schizonts. It has been used primarily for treatment of falciparum malaria in areas where chloroquine and sulfonamide/pyrimethamine resistance are established. Of concern is evidence suggesting that cross-resistance exists between halofantrine and mefloquine. Such cross-resistance will limit its usefulness in areas where mefloquine resistance is being encountered.[162]

Halofantrine is available only in oral form. The recommended dose in adults and children over 40 kg is three 500-mg doses given at 6-hour intervals. A second course after 7 days is recommended in patients who have had minimal or no previous exposure to malaria. In patients less than 40 kg, three doses of 8 mg/kg are given at 6-hour intervals. Halofantrine has poor and variable absorption, but peak serum levels are improved up to 10-fold when the drug is taken with a fatty meal. It is excreted mainly in the feces, with an elimination half-life of 1–2 days and 3–5 days for its active metabolite.[162]

The mechanism of action is poorly understood. Possibilities include inhibition of ferriprotoporphyrin IX sequestration, inhibition of a proton pump present at the host-parasite interface, and mitochondrial injury.[162]

Halofantrine occasionally causes abdominal pain, vomiting, diarrhea, headache, pruritus, or rash. Prolongation of the QT interval and fatal ventricular arrhythmia can occur, usually with higher than recommended doses, recent or concurrent mefloquine therapy, congenitally prolonged QT, or thiamine deficiency.[163] Usage is contraindicated in pregnant or lactating women.[162]

Dihydrofolate Reductase Inhibitors and Sulfonamides

The diaminopyrimidine dihydrofolate reductase inhibitors pyrimethamine and trimethoprim have been used alone or, more commonly, in conjunction with sulfonamides for the prevention and treatment of malaria,[103,163] *I. belli*,[164] *P. carinii* pneumonia,[165–167] and toxoplasmosis.[168–172] They act at sequential steps in the folic acid cycle. *Plasmodium* spp. and presumably other sensitive parasites carry out pyrimidine synthesis de novo, in which reduced folic acid derivatives are essential cofactors. Unlike mammalian cells, these parasites cannot use preformed pyrimidines obtained through salvage pathways. Pyrimethamine is more active than trimethoprim in inhibiting the dihydrofolate reductases of *Plasmodium* spp. and *T. gondii*. Conversely, trimethoprim has greater activity against bacteria. Both of these drugs can inhibit mammalian dihydrofolate reductase at high concentrations. This is more of a problem with pyrimethamine than with trimethoprim. In most instances, a sulfonamide is administered concurrently to inhibit a second step in the folic acid metabolic pathway.

Recent studies indicate that trimetrexate, a low-molecular-weight, lipid-soluble dihydrofolate reductase inhibitor, is active against *T. gondii*.[173] Folinic acid is necessary with trimetrexate to minimize its inhibitory effects on bone marrow.

Pyrimethamine and Short-Acting Sulfonamides. Pyrimethamine (Fig. 7), a 2,4-diaminopyrimidine, was used on a weekly basis for malaria prophylaxis and with sulfadiazine and quinine

FIG. 7. Pyrimethamine.

for the treatment of chloroquine-resistant *P. falciparum*.[5] The usefulness of pyrimethamine with a sulfonamide has been limited by the emergence of resistant *P. falciparum* and *P. vivax*. Pyrimethamine and sulfadiazine are the treatment of choice for toxoplasmosis. The majority of persons who acquire toxoplasmosis have self-limited disease and do not require treatment. In immunocompromised persons, including those with AIDS, toxoplasmic encephalitis is life-threatening. Therapy with high doses of pyrimethamine and sulfonamides is recommended for prolonged periods of time.[168,170] Congenital toxoplasmosis is also treated with pyrimethamine and sulfonamides.[171,172] The optimal treatment for acute toxoplasmosis during pregnancy is uncertain; pyrimethamine is contraindicated, at least for the first trimester, and sulfonamides cannot be used close to the time of delivery because they displace bilirubin from binding sites on albumin. Spiramycin is an alternative, but it is available in the United States only with special approval from the FDA.[174]

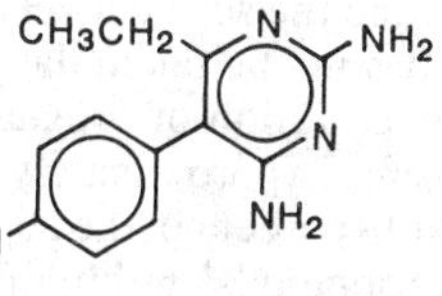

Pyrimethamine is well absorbed orally; the half-life is 4–6 days.[175] It is extensively metabolized; less than 3 percent of the drug is excreted unchanged in the urine in 24 hours. Pyrimethamine acts preferentially to inhibit the parasite's dihydrofolate reductase. It mimics dihydrofolate, competing with this metabolite to inhibit the enzyme. Pyrimethamine is approximately 1000-fold more active against the parasite than the human dihydrofolate reductase.[176]

Pyrimethamine is very well tolerated at a dose of 25 mg/week, which has been used for malaria prophylaxis. Blood dyscrasias, rash, vomiting, seizures, and shock are all rare side effects.[101] Bone marrow suppression with neutropenia, anemia, and thrombocytopenia are seen with the higher doses used for the treatment of toxoplasmosis (25–50 mg/day). Careful follow-up with complete blood counts is necessary, but concurrent administration of folinic acid usually prevents these complications. Pyrimethamine is teratogenic in animals and is contraindicated during the first 16 weeks of pregnancy.[177,178] It has been used to treat pregnant women with primary toxoplasmosis after this period, but concern remains about its safety. Some experts have argued that there has not been unequivocal documentation of pyrimethamine-associated birth defects at the dose levels used for malaria prophylaxis.[179,180]

Sulfonamides decrease the activity of dihydropteroate synthetase and reduce the binding of *p*-aminobenzoic acid (PABA) to this enzyme in several members of the Apicomplexa. The sulfonamides are described in detail in Chapter 26. They are well absorbed orally. The most common untoward effects are allergic reactions and gastrointestinal complaints. Allergic reactions include fever and rash. Less common are toxic epidermal necrolysis, erythema multiforme, Stevens-Johnson syndrome, hepatitis, pneumonitis, bone marrow depression, and serum sickness.[181]

Untoward effects are encountered in 60 percent of persons with AIDS treated for toxoplasmic encephalitis[169] with pyrimethamine and a sulfonamide. These effects include fever, skin rashes, bone marrow suppression, and hepatotoxicity. When these effects occur, pyrimethamine can be used with clindamycin.

Fansidar (Pyrimethamine and Sulfadoxine). Fansidar (each tablet contains pyrimethamine 25 mg and sulfadoxine 500 mg) is used for treatment of chloroquine-resistant falciparum malaria. It was previously recommended as prophylaxis for travelers to areas with chloroquine-resistant *Pl. falciparium*.[162] Fansidar is no longer used for prophylaxis because it can elicit life-threatening allergic reactions. In addition, Fansidar resistance has emerged in many areas. Fansidar has been administered to prevent *P. carinii* pneumonia in patients with AIDS, but the risk of serious untoward allergic reactions has limited its acceptance.[182]

Sulfadoxine, like pyrimethamine, is well absorbed from the gastrointestinal tract. Its half-life is 5–9 days.[175] The severe reactions observed with Fansidar have been attributed to sulfadoxine. Fatalities with prophylactic Fansidar have occurred in 1 in 11,000 to 1 in 26,000 users.[183,184] In 1984, American travelers who took Fansidar as weekly malaria prophylaxis in Kenya were as likely to die from Fansidar toxicity as from malaria. Most of the severe cutaneous reactions, including toxic epidermal necrolysis, erythema multiforme, and the Stevens-Johnson syndrome, have occurred soon after the start of prophylaxis, usually within the first 5 weeks.[183,184] Other serious but unusual side effects with sulfadoxine include serum sickness, bone marrow suppression, hepatitis, hepatic granuloma, and pneumonitis.[163] No fatal reactions have yet been reported when Fansidar (three tablets in a single dose) has been used for the treatment of chloroquine-resistant falciparum malaria. It is still prescribed as empiric treatment for persons who develop symptoms of malaria in areas where they cannot obtain medical evaluation promptly.[5]

Pyrimethamine-Sulfadoxime-Mefloquine (Fansimef)***. The combination of pyrimethamine, sulfadoxine, and mefloquine has been used for the treatment of chloroquine-resistant *Pl. falciparum*.[140,160,185,186] The goal is to reduce the likelihood of developing further resistance. This combination, formulated as Fansimef[186] (pyrimethamine 25 mg, sulfadoxime 500 mg, and mefloquine 250 mg), has also been used prophylactically, but has the potential for the severe allergic cutaneous reactions observed with sulfadoxime.

Trimethoprim-Sulfamethoxazole (Cotrimoxazole). The combination of trimethoprim-sulfamethoxazole, formulated at a ratio of 1:5, is the treatment of choice for *P. carinii*.[165–167,187] The response rate of patients treated for *P. carinii* pneumonia is 80–85 percent and is comparable to that with pentamidine. It has been postulated that trimethoprim–sulfamethoxazole has a static rather than a microbicidal effect on *P. carinii*.[188] Daily prophylactic trimethoprim-sulfamethoxazole has been shown to decrease the incidence of *P. carinii* infection among patients with HIV infection.[189] Intermittent prophylactic trimethoprim–sulfamethoxazole, though not as well studied in HIV-infected patients as daily regimens, is used in this setting by some clinicians based on its efficacy in preventing *P. carinii* infection in immunocompromised children.[190]

Trimethoprim–sulfamethoxazole has been used effectively to treat *I. belli* infections. Although usually a self-limiting illness in immunocompetent hosts, infection with *I. belli* can cause severe, chronic gastroenteritis in patients with AIDS. Relapses are common following therapy in AIDS patients (up to 50 percent), but can be prevented by continued treatment with trimethoprim–sulfamethoxazole.[164]

Both trimethoprim and sulfamethoxazole are well absorbed when administered orally. Peak blood levels are reached in 1–4 hours. The half-lives are similar: 10–12 hours for trimethoprim and 9–11 hours for sulfamethoxazole.[181] Excretion is through the kidney; renal failure prolongs the half-lives of both drugs. Trimethoprim has greater lipid solubility than sulfamethoxazole, and its apparent volume of distribution is five to six times greater. As a result, the drugs are formulated at a trimethoprim/sulfamethoxazole ratio of 1:5. Single-strength tablets contain 80 mg trimethoprim and 400 mg sulfamethoxazole; double-strength tablets have 160 mg trimethoprim and 800 mg sulfamethoxazole. It is also available in suspension for oral use containing 40 mg trimethoprim and 200 mg sulfamethoxazole per 5 ml for children. For intravenous use, trimethoprim-sulfamethoxazole is available as a solution containing 16 mg trimethoprim and 80 mg sulfamethoxazole per milliliter.

In patients without AIDS, common side effects include gastrointestinal upset (4 percent) and skin reactions (3 percent).[191] Rare adverse reactions include agranulocytosis, aplastic anemia, acute interstitial nephritis, Stevens-Johnson syndrome, jaundice, headaches, depression, and hallucinations.[192] Malnourished individuals on prolonged therapy may require concomitant therapy with folinic acid to prevent megaloblastic anemia. The drug combination is not recommended during pregnancy.[181]

For unknown reasons, patients with AIDS have an unusually high incidence of severe adverse reactions when given trimethoprim-sulfamethoxazole. Approximately 65 percent of AIDS patients experience significant drug-related symptoms, half of which are severe enough to result in discontinuation of therapy.[193–195] These adverse reactions include neutropenia, fever, and rashes in up to one-half of these patients and thrombocytopenia, intolerable gastrointestinal effects, and hepatitis in one-tenth.[194,195]

Dapsone and Pyrimethamine. Dapsone, a sulfone that has been widely used in the treatment of leprosy, has been used outside the United States in combination with pyrimethamine as prophylaxis against malaria. Maloprim, a combination of pyrimethamine 25 mg and dapsone 100 mg, has been used weekly for malaria prophylaxis. More recently, dapsone has been used for the prevention of *P. carinii* pneumonia.[196,197]

Like the sulfonamides, dapsone interferes with folic acid metabolism by competitively inhibiting the enzyme dihydropteroate synthetase. Dapsone is available in 25-mg and 100-mg tablets. It is well absorbed after oral administration and is widely distributed in body tissues.[198] About 70–80 percent of the drug is bound to plasma protein. After acetylation and deacetylation, the drug is excreted in the urine as glucuronide or sulfate conjugates. The half-life is variable but averages 25–27 hours.[199] Serious side effects of dapsone include hemolytic anemia, methemoglobinemia, and bone marrow suppression. Very rarely, when maloprim has been used in high doses, the agranulocytosis has been fatal.[200] Uncommon side effects include peripheral neuropathy, anorexia, vomiting, vertigo, blurred vision, tinnitis, fever, headache, pruritis, psychosis, hematuria, and skin rash. Pulmonary eosinophilia has been attributed to maloprim in one report.[201] Dapsone is contraindicated in patients with G6PD deficiency. Complete blood counts should be performed periodically on patients receiving dapsone and pyrimethamine.

Proguanil***. Proguanil, also known as *chloroquanide,* was the first agent found to inhibit plasmodial dihydrofolate reductase. The elucidation of its mechanism of action led to the synthesis of the diaminopyrimidines pyrimethamine and trimethoprim.[202] Proguanil has been used for prophylaxis against *P. falciparum* and *P. vivax*. It acts too slowly to be employed for the treatment of acute malaria. Proguanil has been used with chloroquine as prophylaxis in travelers to East Africa, but failures have been reported.[203] Chloroquine is administered concurrently because of the potential resistance of *P. vivax* to proguanil. The use of proguanil outside of East Africa has been limited by the resistance of *P. falciparum*. However, studies conducted in Thailand have shown it to be effective when combined with a sulfonamide.[204,205] Proguanil is not available in the United States.

Proguanil is formulated in 100-mg tablets. It is slowly absorbed after oral administration. It reaches peak serum concentrations in 2–4 hours, and the serum levels decline to practically zero by 24 hours.[101] It must be taken daily to provide effective prophylaxis. The concentration of proguanil in erythrocytes is six times that in plasma. Approximately 40–60 percent is excreted in the urine and 10 percent in the feces. It is the metabolite 2,4-diamino-1-*p*-chlorophenyl-1,6-dihydro-6,6-dimethyl-1,3,5-triazine that inhibits parasite dihydrofolate reductase.[101]

Proguanil is thought to be very safe at the daily dose levels used for malaria prophylaxis, although rare hematologic effects have been reported.[206] At higher levels, it can produce nausea, vomiting, abdominal pain, and diarrhea. Excessive amounts have been associated with hematuria, proteinuria, and casts in the urine.

Lipid-Soluble Antifolates: Trimetrexate.   Trimetrexate (2,4-diamino 5-methyl-6-[3,4,5-trimethyl-oxyanilino-methyl] quinazoline) is a low-molecular-weight dihydrofolate reductase inhibitor. It was developed as a myelosuppressive agent but was found to have antiparasitic activity. In preliminary studies, trimetrexate was effective in the treatment of *P. carinii*[207] and *T. gondii*.[173] It is 1500 times more potent in inhibiting protozoal dihydrofolate reductase than trimethoprim. Trimetrexate is lipid soluble and readily enters host cells as well as protozoa. Folinic acid (leucovorin) has been administered concurrently to prevent bone marrow suppression. Adverse effects in patients receiving trimetrexate and leucovorin include leukopenia, rash, elevated aminotransferase levels, and reversible peripheral neuropathy.

Hydroxynaphthoquinones: Atovaquone

Hydroxynaphthoquinones (Fig. 8) have been recognized for their antimalarial activity since World War II, but problems with poor absorbtion and rapid metabolism limited their development. Recent work has resulted in the synthesis of newer compounds that overcome these problems. Atovaquone has activity against *P. falciparum*, but in early trials in humans there was a high relapse rate following its use. Its role in the treatment of malaria has not been established.[208]

Atovaquone also has activity against *T. gondii* in a murine model of toxoplasmosis. Its activity is enhanced when used in combination with pyrimethamine or sulfadiazine.[209,210] Early data in humans suggest that it may be effective in the treatment of toxoplasmic encephalitis in patients with AIDS.[211]

Atovaquone has activity against *P. carinii* and has been used to treat *P. carinii* in patients with AIDS.[212] Although it is less effective than trimethoprim–sulfamethoxazole in this setting, it is associated with fewer adverse effects.[213] Atovaquone was recently approved by the FDA for oral treatment of mild to moderate *P. carinii* pneumonia in patients who cannot tolerate trimethoprim–sulfamethoxazole.[214]

Macrolide Antibiotics Active against Apicomplexa

Clindamycin.   Clindamycin has activity against *T. gondii*. When combined with pyrimethamine it is effective in the treatment of toxoplasmic encephalitis in patients with AIDS.[215] This combination is an alternative regimen for those patients who are unable to tolerate the standard regimen of pyrimethamine and sulfadiazine. Clindamycin has also been used along with prednisone for the treatment of ocular toxoplasmosis in immunocompetent patients.[216,217] It has relatively good penetration

FIG. 8.   Atovaquone.

into the eye and inhibits replication of *T. gondii*. Although the outcome of therapy has been good, there are no prospective studies comparing clindamycin with the combination of pyrimethamine and a sulfonamide. Clindamycin also is of potential use with quinine in the treatment of malaria, and this combination is the treatment of choice for symptomatic human babesiosis.[218]

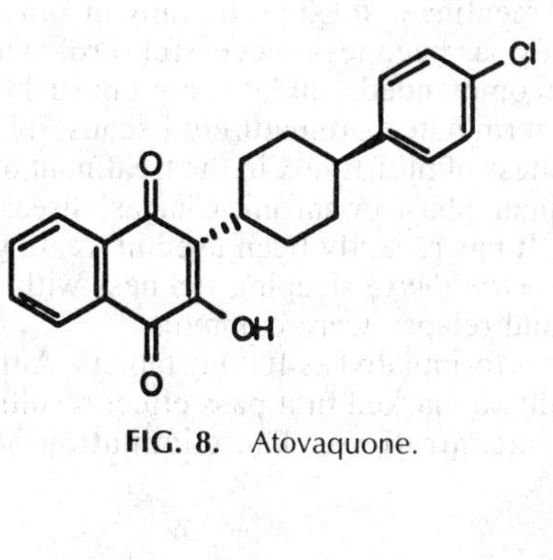

The pharmacokinetics and untoward effects of clindamycin are discussed in Chapter 24. The major concern is the development of pseudomembranous colitis, a side effect that increases in incidence with age.

Spiramycin*, Azithromycin, and Roxithromycin***.   Spiramycin, another macrolide antibiotic, is widely used as an additive in animal feeds. It is active against *T. gondii*, but it has not yet been licensed for use in the United States. Spiramycin has been used to treat primary toxoplasmosis acquired during pregnancy. In a recent study, only 3.7 percent of fetuses became infected in mothers who acquired toxoplasmosis during the first 16 weeks of pregnancy when they received spiramycin.[174] Early data suggested that spiramycin was effective in a few patients with AIDS and cryptosporidiosis; however, in a subsequent controlled trial it was no more effective than placebo.[219]

Azithromycin (see Ch. 24) and roxithromycin have shown activity against *T. gondii* in mice, with azithromycin exhibiting greater activity in comparative in vitro studies.[220–222] Roxithromycin acts synergistically with interferon-γ in the murine model of toxoplasmosis. The role of these agents in treating human toxoplasmosis is not yet defined.[223]

Azithromycin also exhibits activity against *Cryptosporidium* and has been shown to be effective as suppressive therapy in immunosuppressed rodents.[224] Controlled trials are currently underway to evaluate its role in treating cryptosporidiosis in patients with AIDS.

DRUGS FOR TREATMENT OF TRYPANOSOMATIDAE

Members of the genera *Trypanosoma* and *Leishmania* are important pathogens. *Trypanosoma brucei gambiense* and *T. brucei rhodesiense* cause African sleeping sickness. Eflornithine, an inhibitor of ornithine decarboxylase, has been shown to be effective in patients with hemolymphatic and even far-advanced central nervous system involvement with *T. brucei gambiense*.[225–228] It has not been associated with serious toxicity and thus has emerged as the treatment of choice for *T. brucei gambiense*. In the case of *T. brucei rhodesiense*, which is frequently resistant to eflornithine, the early hemolymphatic stage of disease has traditionally been treated with suramin or pentamidine isethionate.[5] Neither of these compounds reaches therapeutic levels in the central nervous system. Once central nervous system involvement is documented, melarsoprol B, a highly toxic trivalent arsenical, has been the treatment of choice. The therapeutic situation is worse with *Trypanosoma cruzi*, the cause of Chagas' disease in Central and South America.[229] The drugs currently available, nifurtimox and benznidazole, are variably effective and frequently associated with sufficiently severe toxicity to necessitate discontinuation of therapy.[229] Efforts continue to identify more effective, less toxic compounds.

The various *Leishmania* spp. produce cutaneous, mucosal, or visceral disease on every continent except Antarctica and Australia. The pentavalent antimonials stibogluconate sodium and meglumine antimoniate have been widely used for the treatment of leishmaniasis, but some *Leishmania* spp. (e.g., *Leishmania ethiopica*) and persons with concurrent AIDS or mucosal or diffuse cutaneous leishmaniasis respond poorly. Resistance is also emerging. Pentamidine isethionate[231–233] and amphotericin B serve as alternative drugs. Several new compounds are currently under study.[230]

Suramin***

Suramin is a nonmetallic compound that is used for the treatment of the hemolymphatic stage of African trypanosomiasis. It has been used on occasion as chemoprophylaxis against *T. brucei gambiense* in persons working in highly endemic regions.[5] Suramin is also active against adult *Onchocerca volvulus*. When used to treat onchocerciasis, it is administered after a course of diethylcarbamazine, which kills microfilariae.

Suramin sodium is a white microcrystalline powder that is readily soluble in water.[234] It is dispensed in 1.0-g vials for parenteral administration. It cannot be given orally. Suramin binds to plasma proteins and persists at low levels in the serum for up to 3 months after infusion. There seems to be negligible metabolism of the drug. Suramin does not penetrate the central nervous system, which limits its usefulness to the hemolymphatic stage of African trypanosomiasis.

Its mechanism of action is uncertain, but at low concentrations suramin is known to inhibit multiple enzymes. It is a polyanion and forms firm complexes with proteins. The antitrypanosomal activity of suramin correlates with its inhibition of glycerol-3-phosphate oxidase and glycerol-3-phosphate dehydrogenase, parasitic enzymes involved in energy metabolism.[235]

Suramin causes a variety of untoward effects.[236] Immediate reactions include nausea, vomiting, shock, loss of consciousness, and occasionally death. Fever and urticaria may also occur. Later reactions, which appear up to 24 hours after administration, include fever, papular rash, exfoliative dermatitis, stomatitis, paresthesias of the palms and soles, photophobia, lacrimation, palpebral edema, and hyperesthesia. These may be followed by renal dysfunction with albuminuria, hematuria, and renal casts. Other reactions include chronic diarrhea and severe prostration. Jaundice, hemolytic anemia, and agranulocytosis are rare. The frequency and severity of side effects are more severe in malnourished hosts.[234] Suramin is relatively contraindicated in persons with preexisting kidney or liver disease.

In persons treated for onchocerciasis, additional side effects occur, apparently due to the release of worm antigens. These include the formation of abscesses around the adult worms, papular eruptions and desquamation, and aggravation of ocular inflammation.

Melarsoprol**

Melarsoprol, or Mel B, is a trivalent arsenical used for the treatment of central nervous system trypanosomiasis. It is effective in some but not all cases. Melarsoprol is also potentially effective in treatment of the hemolymphatic phase, but it is too toxic to be recommended in that setting.

Melarsoprol is only slightly soluble in water, but it is readily soluble in propylene glycol, in which it is dispensed as a 3.6% weight/volume solution.[234] Melarsoprol is administered intravenously. A small but sufficient amount of the drug penetrates the central nervous system, where it can have a lethal effect on trypanosomes. New data indicate that the drug enters the parasite via an adenosine transporter. Resistant strains lack this transport system, suggesting that resistance may be due to lack of drug uptake.[237] Arsenicals react avidly with sulfhydryl groups. They thereby interact with a number of proteins and inactivate enzymes. This is the most likely mechanism of action against trypanosomes, as well as the cause of melarsoprol's pronounced toxicity. There is evidence to suggest that melarsoprol acts differentially on parasite pyruvate kinase, which is a terminal glycolytic enzyme.[238] Melarsoprol is oxidized to a nontoxic or less toxic pentavalent metabolite that is excreted.

Melarsoprol is a highly toxic drug.[239] Febrile reactions are common and may be accompanied by hypertension, abdominal pain, vomiting, and arthralgia. Reactive encephalopathy is the most serious side effect and results in death in approximately 6 percent of recipients.[240] It usually appears in the first 3 or 4 days of therapy. The clinical manifestations include headache, dizziness, mental dullness, confusion, and ataxia with progression to obtundation and seizures. The pathophysiology is felt to be an immune response to trypanosomal antigens released during therapy.[241] Less common untoward effects include hemorrhagic encephalopathy and agranulocytosis. A Guillain-Barré-like syndrome has also been described with melarsoprol use.[242] Allergic reactions including rashes may complicate subsequent courses of therapy. On occasion, the appearance of numerous casts in the urine or evidence of hepatotoxicity necessitates a modification of therapy. Severe hemolysis can occur in patients with G6PD deficiency. The gastrointestinal side effects can be reduced by administering the drug slowly to fasting patients. Melarsoprol therapy may precipitate erythema nodosum in patients who have leprosy.

Eflornithine*

Eflornithine (DL-α-difluoromethylornithine) has proven to be highly effective in the treatment of African sleeping sickness due to *T. brucei gambiense*, even in patients with advanced central nervous system disease.[225–228] Although it is preferred over melarsoprol because it is less toxic, it is not yet available as a first-line agent in West Africa because of economic and logistic reasons.[228] Eflornithine is less useful in east African sleeping sickness because many strains of *T. brucei rhodesiense* are resistant.[243]

Eflornithine hydrochloride can be administered intravenously or orally; 80 percent of the drug is excreted unchanged in the urine.[243] Serum levels during administration of 20 g/day by intravenous infusion approach 1200 nmol/ml; oral administration of 5 g every 4 hours produces levels of approximately 500 nmol/ml.[225] The ratio of cerebrospinal fluid to serum concentration ranges from 0.09 to 0.45.[225] The highest cerebrospinal fluid levels have been found in persons with the most severe central nervous system involvement. Eflornithine is an enzyme-activated, irreversible inhibitor of the enzyme ornithine decarboxylase, which is involved in the first step in the polyamine pathway. Polyamines play an essential role in the growth, differentiation, and replication of the trypanosomatids.[244–247]

Eflornithine is well tolerated. Adverse effects are usually mild and reversible. They include anemia, thrombocytopenia, leukopenia, nausea, vomiting, diarrhea, and transient hearing loss. Eflornithine is a much safer drug than pentamidine, suramin, or melarsoprol, all of which it is likely to replace for the treatment of *T. brucei gambiense*.

Nifurtimox**

Nifurtimox, 4-[(5-nitrofurfurylidene)amino]-3-methylthiomorpholine-1,1-dioxide, a nitrofuran, is the most widely used drug for the treatment of acute Chagas' disease.[229,248] It can reduce the duration of symptoms of acute disease, and it decreases mortality due to myocarditis and meningoencephalitis. The level and duration of parasitemia are also reduced. However, in the clinical trials done to date, there have been significant numbers of treatment failures. There also seems to be geographic variation in responsiveness. Treatment has been found to be most effective in Argentina and Chile; therapy in Brazil and in some other countries has been less successful. Prolonged therapy for 120 days is recommended,[5] and it is not unusual for a treatment course to be terminated prematurely because of drug toxicity. The effectiveness of nifurtimox in the treatment of patients with the indeterminant phase or chronic Chagas' disease has not been documented. It has recently been used in treating arseno-resistant *T. brucei gambiense* sleeping sickness with some success, but toxicity and relapse were common.[249,250]

Nifurtimox is formulated as 100-mg tablets. Although it is well absorbed orally, a marked first pass effect results in low serum and tissue concentrations. The elimination half-life is 2–4 hours.[251] Nifurtimox is active against both the trypomastigote and amastigote forms of *T. cruzi*. The trypanocidal action relates to the ability of nifurtimox to form reactive oxygen radicals that are toxic to the parasite.[248]

Toxicity is experienced by 40–70 percent of persons who receive nifurtimox. This is probably due, at least in part, to free radical formation and oxidative damage to host tissues.[252] Most of the symptoms are related to the gastrointestinal tract and the central and peripheral nervous systems.[234] Nifurtimox seems to be better tolerated by children than adults. Nausea, vomiting, abdominal pain, anorexia, and weight loss are common and may require premature termination of therapy. Neurologic sequelae include restlessness, disorientation, insomnia, twitching, paresthesias, polyneuritis, weakness, and stiffness. Convulsions may occur. Rashes, neutropenia, and decreased sperm counts have also been reported. The side effects are usually reversible with discontinuation of the drug, but they frequently pose a therapeutic dilemma given the prolonged course of therapy that is necessary. More effective, less toxic agents are clearly needed for the treatment of Chagas' disease.

Benznidazole***

Benznidazole, a nitroimidazole derivative, is another relatively toxic drug that has been used for the treatment of Chagas' disease.[229,253] It has not been studied as extensively as nifurtimox, but it seems to be of relatively similar efficacy.[254] Benznidazole is administered orally, usually for several weeks. Therapy is often limited by peripheral neuropathy, rash, or bone marrow suppression. It is not available for use in the United States. In a rabbit model benznidazole was correlated with development of lymphoma.[255]

Pentavalent Antimony; Stibogluconate Sodium** and Meglumine Antimoniate***

The leishmaniases are a group of clinical syndromes caused by multiple *Leishmania* spp. The manifestations of infection and the response to chemotherapy depend on the immune responses of the host, as well as the susceptibility of the causative organism to antimicrobial agents. The pentavalent antimonials stibogluconate sodium and meglumine antimoniate have been widely used for the treatment of leishmaniasis.[230] The compounds are thought to be of comparable efficacy and toxicity. Stibogluconate is the only pentavalent antimonial available in the United States. It has been the most extensively studied and is used in Africa and India.[256–258] Meglumine antimoniate is used in francophone countries, as well as in Central and South America.

The efficacy of the pentavalent antimonials varies with the leishmanial syndrome and the causative *Leishmania* sp. (see Ch. 254). Good responses are observed in the majority of persons with visceral leishmaniasis. Responses in persons with cutaneous leishmaniasis depend on the causative *Leishmania* sp. Treatment failure is becoming increasingly common for all forms of the disease, due at least in part to drug resistance. Some of the resistance is acquired, arising from subcurative therapy that results in selection of resistant parasite strains.[259] Failures are also common in persons with AIDS.[260] Pentamidine isethionate and amphotericin B have been used as alternative drugs when the antimonials fail. Efforts continue to develop new drugs active against the *Leishmania* spp. Attention has focused on the pyrazolopyrimidines allopurinol and allopurinol ribonucleoside[261–266]; on ketaconazole,[267–269] which appears to be effective in the treatment of some forms of New World leishmaniasis; on topical paromomycin with methylbenzethonium chloride for *Leishmania major* infection[270,271]; and on several other drugs. Experience with interferon-γ indicates that it is a useful adjunct to antimonials for severe or refractory cases of visceral leishmaniasis.[272–274]

Sodium stibogluconate is available in sterile aqueous solution for parenteral administration. It is supplied in 10-ml bottles; each milliliter contains 330 mg of drug, which is equivalent to 100 mg of pentavalent antimony. Meglumine antimoniate is available in 5-ml bottles, with 85 mg of antimony per milliliter. These drugs are prescribed on the basis of their antimony content. They can be administered intramuscularly but are usually given intravenously, either undiluted over a 5-minute period or diluted in 50 ml of 5% dextrose in water or saline and administered over 20 minutes. The antimony concentration in blood is best described by a three-compartment model, with a short initial distribution phase followed by biexponential elimination, primarily through the kidney.[275–277] The mean half-lives for the elimination phases have been reported to be 1.7 and 33 hours after intravenous administration and 2 and 766 hours after the drug is given intramuscularly. The slow terminal elimination phase may be due to conversion of pentavalent to trivalent antimony. The latter may be responsible for the toxicity seen with long-term, high-dose therapy. The mechanism of action is uncertain. Pentavalent antimony is concentrated in cells of reticuloendothelial origin, where the drug is thought to affect parasite metabolism.

The pentavalent antimonials are relatively well tolerated.[230,256,257,276,277] Most of the data on toxicity have come from studies of children or adolescents. Common adverse effects include abdominal pain, nausea, vomiting, malaise, headache, elevated transaminase levels, nephrotoxicity, weakness, myalgias, arthralgias, fever, skin rash, cough, and pneumonitis, but these seldom prevent completion of the treatment course. Recent unpublished data show that serum pancreatic enzymes are frequently elevated in patients treated with pentavalent antimonials, and clinically significant pancreatitis is well documented.[278,279] Dose-related changes are observed in the ECG. The most common are ST-T wave changes and prolonged Q-T intervals. Rarer but more serious effects are atrial and ventricular arrhythmias; sudden death has been associated with high-dose therapy. The use of pentavalent antimonials is relatively contraindicated in patients with myocarditis, hepatitis, and pancreatitis.

Pyrazolopyrimidines (Allopurinol and Allopurinol Ribonucleoside***)

Allopurinol, allopurinol riboside, and other purine analogs can inhibit the growth of *Leishmania* spp.[264–266] and *T. cruzi*.[229,280] The metabolism of purines in the kinetoplastids differs significantly from that in humans. The trypanosomatids rely on salvage pathways to obtain purine analogs, whereas humans synthesize purines de novo. Allopurinol, a pyrazolopyrimidine, inhibits *Leishmania* spp. and *T. cruzi* in vitro and in animal models. Allopurinol has been shown to be effective when administered with stibogluconate sodium to persons with visceral leishmaniasis who failed to respond to stibogluconate sodium alone.[266] In a recent randomized, controlled trial oral allopurinol was as effective and less toxic than meglumine antimoniate or a combination of the two drugs in treating cutaneous leishmaniasis due to *L. panamensis*,[261] but others have had less successful experience with allopurinol.[263] The usefulness of allopurinol in humans has been limited by its rapid metabolism by xanthine oxidase. Allopurinol ribonucleoside, an inosine analog, also is active against *Leishmania* spp. and some strains of *T. cruzi*. It is not metabolized as rapidly as allopurinol in humans and is currently being evaluated. Some other purine analogs, such as formycin B, are also lethal for these organisms but are too toxic to be used in humans.[280]

Amphotericin B and Ketaconazole

Amphotericin B has been used as an alternative drug in the treatment of visceral, cutaneous, and mucosal leishmaniasis.[281–283] The precise mechanism of its antiparasitic activity is uncertain, but it probably affects the parasite's surface membrane. Its use in the treatment of leishmaniasis is limited by its appreciable toxicity, the requirement for intravenous administration, and the prolonged course of therapy. Newly developed formulations consisting of amphotericin B complexed with lipids release very little free drug during infusion before being phagocytosed by macrophages, thereby maximizing drug delivery to the infected site and minimizing drug toxicity. Animal data have been promising.[284] Human data are currently limited to case reports, but larger studies are underway.[285] Amphotericin B has also been used with miconazole and rifampin to treat amebic encephalitis due to *Naegleria* spp.[5] The pharmacokinetics and toxicity are detailed in Chapter 31.

Preliminary studies suggest that ketoconazole may be effective against *L. mexicana* and *L. (V.) panamensis*, but not *L. (V.) braziliensis*. The use of ketoconazole in visceral disease has been studied in small numbers of patients with variable results.[286–288] There have been case reports of success in treating cutaneous leishmaniasis with itraconazole, but two out of three small controlled trials failed to show any benefit over placebo.[289–295]

Pentamidine

Pentamidine isethionate (Fig. 9) is a diamidine that has been used as an alternative drug for the treatment of *P. carinii* pneumonia,[165,167] the hemolymphatic stage of *Trypanosoma brucei gambiense* infection,[297] and some forms of leishmaniasis.[231,232,298] Approximately 80–85 percent of patients with *P. carinii* pneumonia respond to intravenously administered pentamidine isethionate, but 50 percent or more suffer untoward effects with the drug.[165,167] Parenteral pentamidine is usually reserved for patients who cannot tolerate trimethoprim–sulfamethoxazole. Aerosolized pentamidine has been used for the prevention of *P. carinii* pneumonia, but a recent comparative study demonstrated that it is less effective than trimethoprim-sulfamethoxazole. It is therefore now considered an alternative regimen.[189,299] The effectiveness of therapy is dependent on the nebulization system and the size of the particles.

Pentamidine isethionate is a white powder that is water soluble; each 1.74 mg contains 1 mg of pentamidine base.[300] It is available in 300-mg ampules for intramuscular or intravenous administration. Intramuscular injections are frequently complicated by pain, swelling, and sterile abscesses at the administration site. Pentamidine is now most commonly given intravenously after being diluted in 100–250 ml of 5% dextrose in water. It must be administered slowly over 1–2 hours.[301] Pentamidine is highly tissue bound and excreted slowly over an extended period of time. It does not penetrate the central nervous system.

The mechanism of action has not yet been defined. Pentamidine is known to bind to DNA in a nonintercalative manner.[302] It interacts selectively with trypanosomal kinetoplast DNA, resulting in swelling and loss of structure of the kinetoplast.[303] Pentamidine also inhibits RNA polymerase,[304] ribosomal function,[305] nucleic acid, protein, and phospholipid synthesis,[306] and polyamine synthesis.[307] It can inhibit folic acid synthesis,[308] but this does not appear to be its mode of action. It can also inhibit trypsin and related proteases.[309] At a high concentration, pentamidine impairs oxygen consumption.[310]

The administration of pentamidine isethionate, by either the intravenous or the intramuscular route, is associated with toxicity in 50 percent of persons.[310] Adverse effects include tachycardia, nausea, vomiting, dizziness, rash, facial flushing, breathlessness, and a metallic taste. Severe hypotension may result after an intramuscular injection or after rapid intravenous infusion.[301] Hypoglycemia has been reported during therapy in 6–9 percent of persons treated in the United States.[311,312] It can be severe and life-threatening, and may even occur after the completion of therapy. It is probably due to a direct toxic effect of pentamidine on pancreatic β-cells.[313,314] The hypoglycemia may be followed by the development of insulin-dependent diabetes mellitus. Severe hypoglycemia may be controlled with diazoxide, but it is not known if this will prevent the subsequent development of diabetes mellitus. Reversible renal failure occurs in approximately 25 percent of persons who receive pentamidine.[312] Although severe renal failure has been reported in a few patients, it has been impossible to attribute the renal toxicity solely to pentamidine because of the concurrent administration of other nephrotoxic agents. Other adverse effects of pentamidine include leukopenia and thrombocytopenia, elevated transaminases, fever, hypocalcemia, confusion, hallucinations, and, rarely, cardiac arrhythmias, particularly polymorphic ventricular tachycardia (torsade de pointes). Rare cases of fatal pancreatitis have been reported in patients with AIDS who received pentamidine.

Aerosolized pentamidine is better tolerated. Only a small amount of drug reaches the systemic circulation. Untoward effects include bronchospasm, particularly in patients with a history of asthma or chronic obstructive pulmonary disease, pharyngeal irritation, and a metallic taste. Pretreatment with inhaled bronchodilators may prevent bronchospasm. Aerosolized pentamidine is less effective for those with underlying bullous or obstructive lung disease. In addition, patients receiving prophylaxis with inhaled pentamidine are at increased risk for developing extrapulmonary pneumocystosis.

Of concern in using aerosolized pentamidine in HIV-infected patients is the potential for spread of pulmonary pathogens (e.g. *M. tuberculosis*) to the environment during treatment. All patients for whom aerosolized pentamidine is prescribed should be screened for tuberculosis before initiating treatment.[315]

DRUGS FOR TREATMENT OF INTESTINAL NEMATODES (ROUNDWORMS)

The intestinal nematodes remain prevalent in areas of the world where sanitation is poor. As many as 80 percent of rural inhabitants in some developing areas may be infected with one or more species. *Enterobius vermicularis* is common in the United States. Other intestinal helminths are most likely to be encountered among immigrants from endemic areas or occasionally in returning travelers who have had intense local exposure. Transmission of intestinal nematodes owing to poor sanitation continues to occur in some areas of North America.

Mebendazole

Mebendazole (Fig. 10), a synthetic benzimidazole, methyl 5-benzoylbenzimidazole-2 carbamate, is widely used for treatment of intestinal nematodes. It is highly effective against *Asca-*

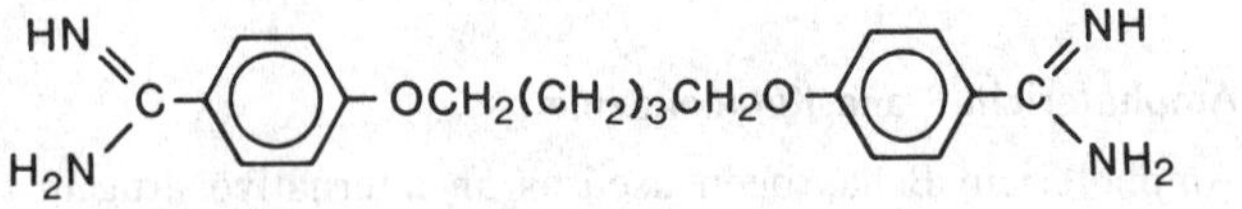

FIG. 9. Pentamidine.

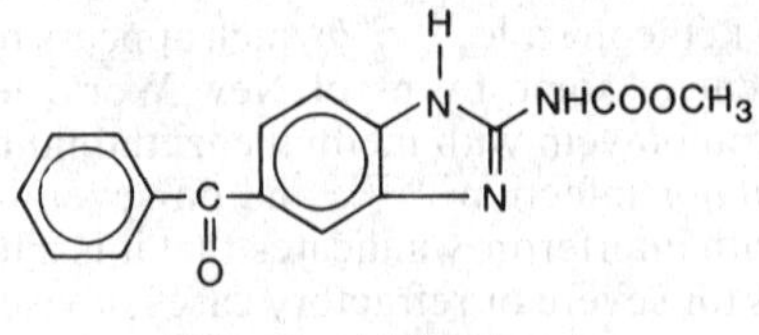

FIG. 10. Mebendazole.

ris lumbricoides, Necator americanus and *Ancylostoma duodenale,* and *Trichuris trichiura*[316] at doses of 100 mg twice a day for 3 days. It is also effective in persons infected with more than one of these nematodes, which is the norm in impoverished areas. Treatment over several days is more effective than a single larger dose of mebendazole for these organisms.[316–318] In contrast, *Enterobius vermicularis* responds to a single dose of 100 mg with a repeat dose given after 2 weeks.[316] The effect of mebendazole on *Strongyloides stercoralis* has been variable[319–321]; thiabendazole remains the drug of choice and in preliminary studies ivermectin has appeared promising.[5] Mebendazole has been used at higher doses, 200 mg twice a day for 20 days, for the treatment of *Capillaria philippinensis,* an uncommon cause of chronic malabsorption in Southeast Asia.[316]

Mebendazole is active against adult *Trichinella spiralis* and has some activity against invading larvae.[322,323] No comparative data are available for humans, but mebendazole has been relatively effective in the treatment of experimental trichinosis in animals and is much less toxic than thiabendazole. It is now recommended for the treatment of human trichinosis. Mebendazole has activity against two filaria species, *Loa loa* and *Mansonella perstans.*[324,325] It is considered the drug of choice, 100 mg twice a day for 30 days, for *M. perstans,*[324] against which diethylcarbamazine is not active. Diethylcarbamazine remains the treatment of choice for *L. loa.* Mebendazole has some activity against *Taenia* sp.[326] but niclosamide and praziquantel are more effective.

Mebendazole has been used at very high doses for prolonged periods of time to treat *Echinococcus granulosus* and *E. multilocularis.*[327–330] Although not usually curative, mebendazole prevents progression of the primary lesion and suppresses or prevents metastasis. Mebendazole has also been used in the perioperative period to decrease the likelihood of peritoneal implants in case cyst contents are accidentally spilled at surgery.[331,332] The major anthelmintic metabolite of albendazole, albendazole sulfoxide, attains higher serum and cyst concentrations than mebendazole, and albendazole has replaced mebendazole for the treatment of echinococcosis.[333–335]

Mebendazole is dispensed in 100-mg tablets. It is only slightly soluble in water and is poorly absorbed from the gastrointestinal tract.[316] This contributes to its low frequency of side effects but limits its usefulness in treating tissue larvae. Up to 10 percent of an orally administered dose of mebendazole is recovered within 48 hours in the urine. Most of the drug excreted by the kidney is the decarboxylated metabolite. Mebendazole selectively binds to helminthic tubulin[336] and blocks microtubule assembly in helminths, and it inhibits glucose uptake.[337] Parasite immobilization and death follow, but it can take several days for susceptible nematodes to be cleared from the gastrointestinal tract. Mebendazole also inhibits the development of the ova of hookworms and *Trichuris.*

Side effects are uncommon when mebendazole is used at low doses (100 mg twice a day for 3 days) for the treatment of the common intestinal helminths.[316,337] Transient abdominal pain and diarrhea occur in a small number of persons, usually those with massive parasite burdens. Migration of adult *A. lumbricoides* to the nose or mouth occurs occasionally. Mebendazole produces embryotoxicity and teratogenicity in animals; it is therefore contraindicated during pregnancy.

At the high doses used for the treatment of echinococcal cysts, systemic side effects such as alopecia, liver enzyme abnormalities, and transient bone marrow suppression with severe but reversible neutopenia have been observed.[316,338,339] The white blood cell count should be followed closely after initiation of high-dose therapy; neutropenia is usually observed within the first 30 days. Accidental poisoning in an infant was associated with respiratory arrest, tachyarrhythmia, and seizures in one instance.[340]

Albendazole*

Albendazole, methyl 5 *n*-propoxythio-2-benzimidazole carbamate, has an exceptionally broad spectrum of antiparasitic activity, but it has not yet been licensed in the United States.[341–372] Albendazole has been widely used throughout the world for the treatment of intestinal nematode infections. It has the advantage of being effective when given as a single dose for the treatment of *Ascaris lumbricoides,* the hookworms, and, to a lesser extent, *Trichuris trichiura.*[341–349] Albendazole is therefore ideally suited for mass treatment programs. Periodic treatment with albendazole has been shown to improve the nutritional status of malnourished children with multiple species of intestinal helminths.[349] Albendazole is also highly effective against *Enterobius vermicularis.* It has been used successfully for the treatment of cutaneous and visceral larva migrans,[350–352] gnathostomiasis,[353] *Capillaria philippinensis,*[354] mixed hookworm and *Oesophagostomum* infections,[355] and *Clonorchis sinensis.*[356] Multiple doses have been used successfully to treat some persons with *Strongyloides stercoralis.*[357] Albendazole has been shown to have activity against *Giardia* species,[358] but its role in the treatment of giardiasis, if any, has yet to be defined. Albendazole has recently been used successfully as palliative treatment for intestinal microsporidiosis in persons with AIDS.[359]

High dose, prolonged therapy with albendazole (cycles of 400 mg twice a day for 28 days, followed by 14 days of rest, for a minimum of three cycles) has emerged as the best approach for the medical treatment of *Echinococcus granulosa, Echinococcus multilocularis,* and *Echinococcus vogeli* infections, replacing mebendazole.[329,333,334,360,361] It is estimated that approximately one-third of persons with echinococcosis are cured with albendazole, and an additional 50 percent show improvement.[361]

Albendazole has also been used successfully for the treatment of neurocysticercosis, and, although it has not been compared with praziquantel in a blinded fashion, albendazole seems to produce higher response rates.[362–370] Corticosteroids are usually administered concurrently to control the inflammatory response elicited by the release of parasite antigens. Albendazole has been used successfully to treat some patients with subarachnoid and ventricular cysticercosis,[369,370] but not all respond. Albendazole has variable activity against adult *Taenia* species in the human gastrointestinal tract.[371,372]

Albendazole is a white, odorless powder that is dispensed as 400-mg tablets.[361] It is practically insoluble in water, and absorption is enhanced when the drug is taken with a fatty meal.[361] Albendazole undergoes extensive first-pass metabolism in the liver, and only albendazole sulfoxide, which is primarily responsible for the systemic anthelmintic effects, is detectable in serum. Sulfoxidation of albendazole also occurs in the gut.[373] Albendazole is not detected in serum; albendazole sulfoxide reaches peak levels after 2.0–2.4 hours, with a half-life of 10–15 hours.[361,374] Plasma levels of albendazole sulfoxide at steady state show great individual variability. Drug concentrations in the central nervous system are approximately 40% that of serum.[375] Concurrent administration of dexamethasone increases the levels of albendazole by approximately 50%.[376] The concentration of albendazole sulfoxide in echinococcal cysts is approximately 25% of the serum concentration.

There is some evidence that bile is the major route of elimination and that enterohepatic recirculation occurs. The mechanism of action is likewise not fully understood. Albendazole, like other benzimidazoles, inhibits the assembly of tubulin into microtubules[377] and impairs the uptake of glucose, leading to the depletion of glycogen stores in helminths. It also inhibits helminthic-specific fumarate reductase.[378]

Albendazole is usually well tolerated when given as a single 400-mg dose for the treatment of intestinal nematodes. Diarrhea, abdominal discomfort, or migration of *Ascaris* through the nose or mouth occur occasionally. High-dose, prolonged therapy for echinococcal disease or neurocyticercosis is occasionally complicated by serum transaminase elevation, bone marrow suppression with neutropenia or thrombocytopenia, or less commonly alopecia.[361,379,380] Liver enzymes and complete blood counts should be monitored at least every 2 weeks. Liver and bone marrow toxicity are reversible with discontinuation of the drug. Occasionally gastrointestinal disturbances, headache, or dizziness occur. Rash and fever are rare. In view of the potential teratogenicity of benzimidazole compounds, albendazole is contraindicated during pregnancy.

Flubendazole***

Flubendazole is the parafluoro analog of mebendazole. It has a spectrum of activity against intestinal helminths that is similar to that of mebendazole. Flubendazole is not as well absorbed. Animal studies suggest that it is teratogenic.[381] Flubendazole has also led to clinical improvement in a small group of persons with neurocysticercosis, but, given its poor absorption and conflicting reports on outcome, it is unlikely that flubendazole will replace albendazole or praziquantel for the treatment of cysticercosis.[382]

Thiabendazole

Thiabendazole, 2-(4'-thiazolyl)-1H-benzimidazole, is among the most potent anthelminthic drugs,[383] but its use has been limited by the high frequency of untoward effects. Thiabendazole is active against a number of adult nematodes that infect the gastrointestinal tract and against larvae in tissues. It is much better absorbed than mebendazole. The most common indication for thiabendazole is the treatment of S. stercoralis[384,385] or S. fuelleborni[386] infection. It has also been used for Trichostrongylus infections,[387] visceral larva migrans,[384] and trichinosis.[5,388,389] It is effective when applied topically[350] or taken orally for cutaneous larva migrans. Some cases of human trichinosis have shown marked clinical improvement with thiabendazole. Antiinflammatory, antipyretic, and analgesic effects of thiabendazole may have contributed to the clinical response. Studies in animals experimentally infected with T. spiralis suggested that some but not all larvae are killed by thiabendazole. Although thiabendazole is active against the hookworms, A. lumbricoides, E. vermicularis, and, to a lesser extent, T. trichiura,[384] mebendazole in general has higher response rates and is far less toxic.

Thiabendazole is available in 500-mg tablets and as an oral suspension of 500 mg/5 ml. It is rapidly absorbed after oral administration; peak concentrations occur in plasma about 1 hour after treatment.[337] It is recommended that the drug be given with meals. Unfortunately, no parenteral preparation is available, which poses a problem for some patients with disseminated S. stercoralis infection. Most of the drug is excreted in urine within 24 hours as 5-hydroxythiabendazole conjugated as the glucuronide or as the sulfate. The precise mechanism of action is not known. Thiabendazole inhibits the fumarate reductase of susceptible helminths.[390] Like mebendazole, it may interfere with microtubule assembly, and it inhibits glucose uptake.[391]

Approximately half of the persons who receive thiabendazole experience one or more side effects. Most frequent are nausea, anorexia, vomiting, and dizziness.[337] Less common are diarrhea, epigastric pain, pruritus, drowsiness, giddiness, and headache. Rare side effects include tinnitus, abnormal sensation in the eyes, numbness, decreased pulse and blood pressure, elevated liver enzymes, and progressive bile duct injury.[337,392] Seizures have been reported in a child with Down syndrome.[393] Transient neutropenia has been observed in some patients. Allergic manifestations such as fever, facial flush, angioneurotic edema, lymphadenopathy, perianal rash, and skin rashes are also observed; some or all of these may be elicited by the release of parasite antigens or the underlying disease process. Thiabendazole can give urine an asparagus-like odor, and crystalluria has been observed. Because of the central nervous system effects, activities requiring alertness should be avoided during therapy. The drug should be used with caution in persons with hepatic disease or decreased hepatic function. Thiabendazole has been found to be genotoxic in in vitro and in vivo assays,[394] and it is contraindicated in pregnancy. Concomitant administration of thiabendazole with theophylline increases the theophylline half-life and has been associated with severe nausea and vomiting.[395]

Pyrantel Pamoate

Pyrantel pamoate is recommended for the treatment of E. vermicularis. It can also be used to treat A. lumbricoides, N. americanus, A. duodenale, and Moniliformis moniliformis.[396–400] It is considered an alternative drug for Trichostrongylus infection. It is not active against the whipworm T. trichura. Oxantel***, an m-oxyphenol derivative that has not been licensed in the United States, is effective against T. trichura.

Pyrantel is available as a suspension (250 mg of pyrantel base/ 5 ml). It is poorly absorbed; less than 15 percent is excreted in the urine as the parent drug or metabolite.[399–401] Pyrantel and its analogs are depolarizing neuromuscular blocking agents. The resulting nicotinic activation results in spastic paralysis of the worm. Pyrantel also inhibits acetylcholinesterases. There is depolarization and increased spike discharge frequency in muscle cells of susceptible nematodes.

Pyrantel pamoate has minimal toxicity at the oral doses used to treat intestinal helminths. Mild, transient gastrointestinal symptoms, headache, drowsiness or insomnia, and dizziness are occasionally encountered. The nitrosated metabolites of pyrantel pamoate are mutagenic in bacteria. Pyrantel pamoate has not been studied in pregnancy, and it is not recommended for pregnant women or children under 1 year of age. Pyrantel and piperazine, which produces hyperpolarization with a reduction in spike wave activity in helminthic muscle cells, appear to be mutually antagonistic and should not be used together.[399,400]

Pyrvinium Pamoate***

Pyrvinium pamoate, a cyanide dye, was used as an alternative drug for the treatment of E. vermicularis,[402,403] but it has been replaced by pyrantel pamoate and mebendazole and is no longer marketed in the United States.

Piperazine

Piperazine citrate is effective in the treatment of A. lumbricoides. It has been replaced in the United States by mebendazole, which is less toxic, but piperazine is less expensive and is still used in some developing areas. Piperazine also has activity against E. vermicularis. Piperazine derivatives have a broad range of pharmacologic activity. Some substituted piperazines are central serotonin agonists; others depress monosynaptic spinal cord excitation, block chloride channels, have antioxidant effects, display antiarrhythmic activity, or act as vasodilators. One derivative, diethylcarbamazine, is effective against filariae, as discussed below.

Piperazine salts are available as tablets containing 250 mg and as syrups and suspensions containing 100 mg/ml.[337] Piperazine is well absorbed orally. Some of the drug is metabolized; the remainder is excreted in the urine. Piperazine causes flaccid paralysis of susceptible intestinal helminths. It acts as a low-potency agonist at extrasynaptic γ-aminobutyric acid (GABA) receptors on the bag region of Ascaris suum.[404] Activation of these receptors gives rise to an increase in chloride conductance. There is also hyperpolarization and suppression of spontaneous action potentials.[405] Worms are excreted alive, usually without migrating.

Piperazine is generally well tolerated. On occasion, there are gastrointestinal symptoms, transient neurologic side effects, or urticarial reactions. Lethal overdoses have been associated with convulsions and respiratory depression. Epileptic activity may be exaggerated, and piperazine is contraindicated in persons with a history of seizures.[406] Neurotoxicity has also been observed in persons with impaired renal function. Visual disturbances, ataxia, and hypotonia occur rarely.[407] The drug has been used during pregnancy without apparent adverse effects, but it has not been thoroughly evaluated in this setting. Although adverse dermatologic reactions are rare, they have been reported in persons sensitized to topical ethylenediamine.[408]

DRUGS FOR TREATMENT OF SYSTEMIC NEMATODES

Diethylcarbamazine*

Diethylcarbamazine (Fig. 11) is a piperazine derivative, N,N-diethyl-4-methyl-1-piperazinecarboxamide dihydrogen citrate. It results in the rapid destruction of microfilariae of *Wuchereria bancrofti*, *Brugia malayi*, and *B. timori*, the three lymphatic-dwelling filariae that infect humans.[409,410] There is strong evidence that it kills adult worms of *W. bancrofti*[411] and, although not as well documented, is felt to be macrofilaricidal against *B. malayi* and *B. timori* as well. It is currently the drug of choice for all three species. It has been successfully used in community-based mass treatment programs.[412-415] Diethylcarbamazine is also the treatment of choice for *Loa loa*[5,416] and has been recommended for *Mansonella ozzardi*,[5] but the results have been variable.[417,418] It has been used successfully to treat persons with pulmonary infiltrates with eosinophilia in the tropics,[419] presumably because this syndrome is in many instances caused by microfilariae in the lungs. Diethylcarbamazine has also been used as an alternative mode of therapy for visceral larva migrans, with variable success.[420]

Diethylcarbamazine rapidly kills microfilariae of *Onchocerca volvulus* in the skin and eye, but the resulting inflammatory reaction can cause severe damage.[421-423] Ocular complications may result in permanent sequelae and include visual field constriction, optic nerve pallor, chorioretinitis, anterior uveitis, and punctate keratitis.[421-428] Diethylcarbamazine does not affect adult *O. volvulus*, and microfilariae reaccumulate after completion of therapy.[424] Ivermectin also is microfilaricidal, but kills slowly and is much less toxic. It has replaced diethylcarbamazine for the treatment of persons with ocular onchocerciasis.

Diethylcarbamazine is available in 50-mg tablets.[337] It is readily absorbed from the gastrointestinal tract. Peak blood levels are reached in 1–2 hours; the serum half-life is approximately 8 hours.[429] The parent compound and its metabolites are cleared through the kidney.[430,431] Diethylcarbamazine is distributed equally throughout all body compartments except adipose tissue, and there is little accumulation even after repeated doses are given.

The drug seems to have two types of effects on microfilariae. First, it is associated with a decrease in muscle activity, leading eventually to immobilization of the worm.[432] The piperazine moiety may result in hyperpolarization, resulting in the observed paralysis.[337] Second, the drug appears to alter the surface membranes of microfilariae, resulting in enhanced killing by the host's immune system.[433,434] Diethylcarbamazine has also been

shown to enhance the adherence properties of eosinophils and polymorphonuclear leukocytes,[435] and there is evidence to suggest that platelets may mediate the action on microfilariae.[436] Recent data suggest that its mechanism of action may in part involve effects on host endothelial and parasite eicosanoid production.[437] Diethylcarbamazine was also found to disrupt microtubules and inhibit their formation *in vitro*.[438] Untoward effects include those produced directly by the drug and inflammatory reactions that follow the release of filarial antigens. Common reactions include headache, malaise, weakness, arthralgia, anorexia, nausea, and vomiting. The gastrointestinal effects are usually dose related. Acute psychotic reactions have been reported but are rare.

During treatment of onchocerciasis with diethylcarbamazine, systemic reactions include severe pruritus, edema of the skin, fever, hypotension, heightened eosinophilia, lymphadenopathy, splenomegaly, and proteinuria.[425,426] The elicitation of such reactions by even low doses of diethylcarbamazine is the basis for the Mazzotti test,[439] which has been used to diagnose onchocerciasis but is potentially dangerous. In *W. bancrofti* and *B. malayi* infections, localized swellings or nodules may develop along lymphatics, and there may be accompanying lymphadenitis.[426] Transient hydrocele formation or lymphedema may be observed. Encephalopathy has occurred rarely in persons treated for *L. loa*.[440]

Ivermectin**

Ivermectin is the 22,23-dihydro derivative of avermectin B1, a macrocyclic lactone, produced by the actinomycete *Streptomyces avermitilis*.[441] It is active at low doses against a broad spectrum of nematodes and blood-sucking arthropod parasites of animals. One of the major recent advances in anthelmintic therapy has been the introduction of ivermectin for treatment of human onchocerciasis.[421-424,441-446] Ivermectin kills microfilariae in the skin as well as in the eye, but the local inflammatory responses are less severe than with diethylcarbamazine. This is particularly important in the eye, where microfilariae disappear slowly after ivermectin therapy. In mass community-based treatment programs ivermectin has proven to be safe, acceptable to indigenous populations, and effective in reducing microfilarial loads and can play a major role in the chemotherapy-based control of onchocerciasis on a broad scale.[447-452] Ivermectin inhibits oviposition in *O. volvulus*, and recent studies show that it may have some effect on the adult worm, though the practical implications of this finding are not clear.[447,453,454] Ivermectin is active against other filarial pathogens such as *W. bancrofti*, *B. malayi* and *Loa loa*.[455-459] Ivermectin has an extremely broad spectrum of antinematodal activity[441] and has an emerging role in the treatment of strongyloidiasis.[460,461] It is now widely used in veterinary practice for control and treatment of helminthic and arthropod infestations.

Ivermectin is odorless and colorless and has been effective when administered as a single oral or parenteral dose. Peak serum concentrations are reached 4–5 hours following an oral dose, and the elimination half-life is 50–60 hours.[462] It is highly protein bound.[463] It is concentrated in the liver and adipose tissues. Only a small percentage of the drug is excreted in the urine; the rest is excreted in the stool. Ivermectin acts by blocking signal transmission from interneurons to excitatory motor neurons. GABA is the neurotransmitter that is blocked, but ivermectin does not appear to compete with GABA for binding and does not bind directly to the GABA-binding site.[441] In animals, GABA-mediated nerves are present only in the central nervous system, whereas they are found in peripheral muscle in susceptible invertebrates. Ivermectin is usually well tolerated. The initiation of therapy in persons with onchocerciasis may be complicated by fever, pruritus, headache, and cutaneous edema, but the side effects are less frequent and less severe than those of diethylcarbamazine or suramin.[421-424,441-446,464] In cattle, 30

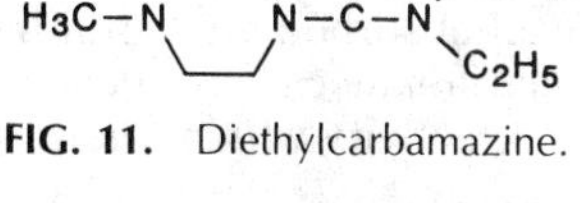

FIG. 11. Diethylcarbamazine.

times the recommended dose was tolerated without signs of toxicity, but death was reported at 40 times the recommended dose. No teratogenicity has been reported in animals, and in a study of 203 children born to women inadvertently treated during pregnancy, no increase in the rate of birth defects was observed.[465]

Amocarzine***

Amocarzine, an experimental drug, has been used to treat a limited number of persons with moderate to severe onchocerciasis.[466] It has the advantage of killing macrofilariae as well as microfilariae. Absorption of amocarzine is enhanced by meals. The drug and its principle metabolite, the N-oxide, are colored and excreted in the urine.[467] Reversible dermal reactions are frequent but mild, and no prohibitive ocular intolerance has been observed. Neurologic side effects including dizziness and a positive Romberg sign are prevalent, but reversible. Further studies are needed to confirm the efficacy of amocarzine and to assess its toxicity more fully.

DRUGS FOR TREATMENT OF PLATYHELMINTHS: TREMATODES (FLUKES) AND CESTODES (TAPEWORMS)

Praziquantel

Praziquantel (Fig. 12), 2-[cyclohexylcarbonyl-(1,2,3,6,7,11b)-hexyahydro-4H-pyrazino(2,1-α)isoquinoline-4-one], is a heterocyclic prazino-isoquinoline derivative with a broad spectrum of activity against trematodes and cestodes. It is well absorbed orally, is given in several doses in 1 or a few days, and has mild untoward effects.[468–470] Praziquantel is highly effective against all of the *Schistosoma* spp. that infect humans including *S. japonicum*, against which there was previously no good form of chemotherapy.[468–477] It has even been effective in the treatment of schistosomiasis of the central nervous system.[476,477] Praziquantel is also the drug of choice for the liver flukes *Clonorchis sinensis* and *Opisthorchis viverrini*, the lung flukes *Paragonimus westermani*, *P. kellicoti*, and other *Paragonimus* spp., and the intestinal flukes *Heterophyes heterophyes*, *Fasciolopsis buski*, *Metagonimus yokogawai*, and *Nanophyetus salmincola*.[464–470,478] Only against the liver fluke *Fasciola hepatica* have praziquantel failures been frequent.[479,480] Despite the effectiveness of praziquantel, cost factors have limited its use in developing countries.[468]

Praziquantel is also highly active against adult and larval forms of the cestodes.[468–470] It has been used successfully for the treatment of neurocysticercosis due to *Taenia solium*.[481–485] It is most effective in the treatment of parenchymal disease. Praziquantel is often ineffective when there is subarachnoid involvement, cysticercal meningitis, or cysts in the ventricular system[485,486] or eye.[487,488] Some prefer praziquantel for the treatment of intestinal *T. solium* infestation.[489] It is highly effective against adult *T. saginata*, *Diphyllobothrium latum*, and *D. pacificum*,[489,490] but niclosamide is equally effective, less expensive, has fewer side effects, and is therefore more widely used against those organisms. In the case of *Hymenolepis nana*, praziquantel can be given as a single dose, whereas niclosamide must be given daily for 6 days. Praziquantel is not effective in the treatment of human hydatid disease. It is active against adult *Echino-*

coccus spp. in the canine gastrointestinal tract and damages protoscolices in hydatids, but the germinal layer of the hydatid is not destroyed.[491,492]

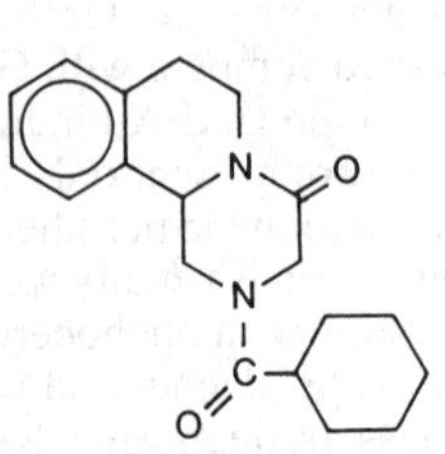

Praziquantel is dispensed as 600-mg tablets that contain a mixture of its two enantiomers.[493,494] The drug is crystalline, colorless, and nearly insoluble in water. Variability has been reported in the bioavailability of different praziquantel preparations.[495] A peak serum concentration of 1 μm/ml is reached 1–2 hours after an oral dose of 50 mg/kg body weight of the standard preparation is administered.[468–470] Praziquantel is approximately 80 percent protein bound. There is pronounced first-pass metabolism.[496,497] Approximately 80 percent of praziquantel is excreted in the urine in 4 days; 90 percent of that amount is excreted within the first 24 hours. The remainder is excreted in the feces. The pharmacokinetics of the drug were not significantly altered in one patient undergoing hemodialysis. The concentration of praziquantel in the cerebrospinal fluid is approximately 14–24 percent of the concentration of free plus protein-bound drug in the plasma.[498] Plasma levels have been decreased in patients with neurocysticercosis receiving dexamethasone simultaneously.

Praziquantel is rapidly taken up by flukes and tapeworms. It is uniformly distributed in these organisms and is not metabolized. Praziquantel increases the permeability of the flukes' tegument to calcium ions.[499–502] In adult schistosomes, an influx of calcium is followed by tetanic contraction and paralysis of the musculature. The initial effects are very rapid, and intense vacuolation of the tegument is observed.[500] Adult worms are then swept to the liver, where they are attacked by phagocytes. Praziquantel also results in increased exposure of parasite antigens including actin on the surface of adult schistosomes.[503,504] In the tapeworm *Hymenolepis diminuta*, praziquantel causes calcium release from endogenous stores, and the worm suffers massive contraction.[505] Expulsion from the gastrointestinal tract follows. The tegument of the neck of the tapeworm develops blebs, but the scolex and proglottids appear to be unaffected.

Praziquantel is generally well tolerated.[468–470] Reactions are common, but are usually mild and transient. The most frequent are nausea, vomiting, abdominal pain, dizziness, headache, and lassitude. Only rarely is vomiting severe. Exudative polyserositis with respiratory failure was reported in one patient.[506] In some instances, adverse effects may be due to allergic responses that follow the release of worm antigens. For example, urticarial reactions have been observed during the treatment of paragonimiasis.[507] Intense abdominal pain and bloody diarrhea have on occasion occurred in patients heavily infected with *Schistosoma mansoni*[508–510] Finally, increased intracranial pressure, cerebral edema, and inflammation have been observed during the treatment of neurocysticercosis, and corticosteroids are often used concomitantly in this setting.[511,512] There has been no evidence of mutagenicity or teratogenicity with praziquantel in vitro, but there is an increase in the abortion rate in rats given three times the single human therapeutic dose. Praziquantel is excreted in breast milk, and it is recommended that women not nurse on the day that praziquantel is given or during the subsequent 72 hours. Cimetidine, ketaconazole and miconazole inhibit the metabolism of praziquantel and increase serum levels.[513]

Metrifonate***

Metrifonate, an organophosphate that is metabolized in humans to dichlorvos,[514] is an alternative to praziquantel for the treatment of *Schistosoma hematobium*. Metrifonate is less expensive than praziquantel and of comparable efficacy, and it has been used in mass treatment programs.[515–517]

Metrifonate is an organophosphate inhibitor of acetylcholinesterase.[518] It is well absorbed after oral ingestion.[519] When given to humans, metrifonate causes a decrease of 95 percent in plasma cholinesterase activity within 6 hours of administration.

FIG. 12. Praziquantel.

This activity usually returns to normal relatively quickly. Erythrocyte cholinesterase is inhibited to approximately 50 percent of pretreatment values but takes 2–2.5 months to return to normal levels.[519] Persons treated with metrifonate should not receive neuromuscular blocking agents or be exposed to insecticides with anticholinesterase effects for at least 48 hours. Although the drug is usually well tolerated, mild vertigo, lassitude, nausea, vomiting, and occasionally bronchospasm have been reported. One limitation for large-scale treatment programs is that metrifonate is given in three doses at 2-week intervals in the standard regimen, which can result in poor compliance and reduced efficacy,[520] whereas praziquantel is administered in 1 day.

Oxamniquine

Oxamniquine, a tetrahydroquinoline, provides an alternative to praziquantel for the treatment of *S. mansoni* infections,[521–527] and it is less expensive than praziquantel. Oxamniquine has been used successfully in mass treatment programs.

Oxamniquine is dispensed in 250-mg capsules. It is well absorbed orally, and the parent drug and its metabolites are excreted in the urine. Peak plasma concentrations are achieved 1–4 hours after dosing, and the elimination half-life is 2.2 hours.[528] It is given as a single dose. Oxamniquine produces marked tegumental alterations in treated adult schistosomes.[529] Side effects include dizziness, which may occur in 40 percent of the treated population, and drowsiness. Convulsions have occasionally been reported, and oxamniquine should not be used in persons with epilepsy. Orange to red discoloration of the urine has been associated with treatment.

Niridazole***

Niridazole, a nitrothiazole derivative, 1-(5-nitro-2-thiazolyl)-2-imidazolidinone was once widely used for the treatment of schistosomiasis.[530,531] It is no longer indicated. It is far more toxic than praziquantel, metrifonate, and oxamniquine and offers no advantage in efficacy.

Bithionol**

Bithionol is the drug of choice for treatment of *F. hepatica* and is an alternative to praziquantel for the treatment of paragonimiasis.[532,533] Bithionol is administered orally, usually on alternate days, for 10–15 doses. It is frequently associated with urticaria, photosensitivity reactions, and gastrointestinal complaints. These allergic reactions may be due, in part or solely, to the release of worm antigens. Leukopenia and toxic hepatitis are rare complications.

Niclosamide

Niclosamide (Fig. 13), *N*-(2′-chloro-4′-nitrophenyl)-5-chlorosalicylamide, given as a single dose, is active against a number of adult tapeworms that reside in the gastrointestinal tract. It is the drug of choice for *T. saginata*, the beef tapeworm; *D. latum*, the fish tapeworm; and *Dipylidium caninum*, the dog tapeworm.[534] Niclosamide is poorly absorbed and less expensive than praziquantel. In the case of *T. solium*, treatment with niclosamide is usually followed by a purge to reduce the theoretical risk of autoinfection since niclosamide results in disintegration

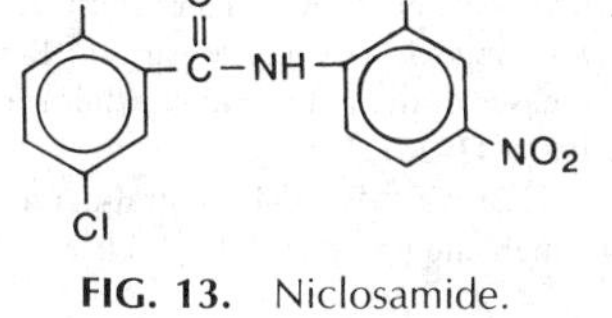

of the adult tapeworm. Some physicians prefer praziquantel for the treatment of *T. solium* because it is active against larvae as well as adults and might prevent cysticercosis if autoinfection occurred. Niclosamide is as active against *H. nana*, the dwarf tapeworm, as is praziquantel, but a single dose of praziquantel is effective, whereas niclosamide must be administered daily for 6 days.[5]

Niclosamide is very poorly absorbed.[534] It is supplied in 500-mg vanilla-flavored tablets, which should be chewed thoroughly and then washed down with water. The anthelmintic mechanisms of niclosamide are not completely understood. The drug appears to uncouple oxidative phosphorylation in the scolex and proximal segments of the adult tapeworm and to stimulate adenosine triphosphatase activity of mitochondria, resulting in death of the worm and rapid disintegration of the scolex.[535] Niclosamide is free of side effects except for occasional mild gastrointestinal complaints, light-headedness, and, rarely, rash. Information on side effects has been collected in an uncontrolled manner, and it is uncertain whether a placebo group would differ significantly in respect to these symptoms.[536] Niclosamide has been found to be genotoxic in vitro,[537] but very little is absorbed. When expulsion of the worm is delayed, neither the scolex nor the proglottids may be identifiable in the stool.

REFERENCES

1. Lee JJ, Hutner SH, Bovee EC. An Illustrated Guide to the Protozoa. Lawrence, KS: Society of Protozoologists; 1985.
2. Levine ND. Nematode Parasites of Domestic Animals and of Man. Minneapolis: Burgess; 1968.
3. Burt DRR. Platyhelminthes and Parasitism. An Introduction to Parasitology. New York: American Elsevier; 1970.
4. Erasmus DA. The Biology of Trematodes. New York: Crane, Russak; 1972.
5. Drugs for parasitic infections. Med Lett Drugs Ther. 1993;35:112–119.
6. Powell SJ, Wilmot AJ, Elsdon-Dew R. Further trials of metronidazole in amoebic dysentery and amoebic liver abscess. Ann Trop Med Parasitol. 1967; 61:511–4.
7. Welsh JS, Rowsell BJ, Freeman C. Treatment of intestinal amoebiasis and giardiasis: Efficacy of metronidazole and tinidazole compared. Med J Aust. 1978;1:469–71.
8. Salaki JS, Shirey JL, Strickland GT. Successful treatment of symptomatic *Entamoeba polecki* infection. Am J Trop Med Hyg. 1979;28:190–3.
9. Wolfe MS. Giardiasis. N Engl J Med. 1978;298:319–21.
10. Lerman SJ, Walker RA. Treatment of giardiasis. Literature review and recommendations. Clin Pediatr. 1982;21:409–14.
11. Lossick JG. Treatment of sexually transmitted vaginosis/vaginitis. Rev Infect Dis. 1990;12(Suppl)6:S665–81.
12. Lossick JG, Kent HL. Trichomoniasis: Trends in diagnosis and management. Am J Obstet Gynecol. 1991;165:1217–22.
13. Wolfe MS. *Blastocystis hominis* infection. In: Strickland GT, ed. Hunter's Tropical Medicine. 6th ed. Philadelphia: Saunders; 1984:513.
14. Walzer PD, Judson FN, Murphy KB, et al. Balantidiasis outbreak in Truk. Am J Trop Med Hyg. 1973;22:33–41.
15. Spillman R, Ayala SC, DeSanchez CE. Double blind test of metronidazole and tinidazole in the treatment of asymptomatic *Entamoeba histolytica* and *Entamoeba hartmanni* carriers. Am J Trop Med Hyg. 1976;25:549–51.
16. Thoren K, Hakansson C, Bergstrom T, et al. Treatment of asymptomatic amebiasis in homosexual men. Clinical trials with metronidazole, tinidazole, and diloxanide furoate. Sex Transm Dis. 1990;17:72–4.
17. Irusen EM, Jackson TF, Simjee AE. Asymptomatic intestinal colonization by pathogenic Entamoeba histolytica in amebic liver abscess: Prevalence, response to therapy and pathogenic potential. Clin Infect Dis. 1992;14: 889–93.
18. Hamed KA, Studemeister AE. Successful response of metronidazole-resistant trichomonal vaginitis to tinidazole. A case report. Sex Transm Dis. 1992; 19:339–40.
19. Dupont HL, Sullivan PS. Giardiasis: The clinical spectrum, diagnosis and therapy. Pediatr Infect Dis. 1986;5:S131–8.
20. Sharma VP, Rathore HS, Sharma MM. Efficacy of metronidazole in dracunculiasis: A clinical trial. Am J Trop Med Hyg. 1979;28:658–60.
21. Weniger BG, Schantz PM. Praziquantel and refugee health. JAMA. 1984; 251:2391–2.
22. Houghton GW, Smith J, Thorpe PS, et al. The pharmacokinetics or oral and intravenous metronidazole in man. J Antimicrob Chemother. 1979;5:621–3.

FIG. 13. Niclosamide.

23. McGilveray IJ, Midha KK, Loo JCK, et al. The bioavailability of commercial metronidazole formulations. Int J Clin Pharmacol. 1978;16:110–5.

24. Norris SM, Ravdin JI. The pharmacology of antiamebic drugs. In: Ravdin JI, ed. Amebiasis: Human Infection by *Entamoeba histolytica*. New York: Wiley;1988:734–40.

25. Lau AH, Lam NP, Piscitelli SC, et al. Clinical pharmacokinetics of metronidazole and other nitroimidazole anti-infectives. Clin Pharmacokinet 1992;23:328–64.

26. Lares-Asseff I, Cravioto J, Santiago P, et al. Pharmacokinetics of metronidazole in severely malnourished and nutritionally rehabilitated children. Clin Pharmacol Ther 1992;51:42–5.

27. Lindmark DG, Müller M. Antitrichomonad action, mutagenicity, and reduction of metronidazole and other nitroimidazoles. Antimicrob Agents Chemother 1976;10:476–82.

28. Knight RC, Skolimowski IM, Edwards DI. The interaction of reduced metronidazole with DNA. Biochem Pharmacol. 1978;27:2089–93.

29. LaRusso NF, Tomasx M, Müller M, et al. Interaction of metronidazole with nucleic acids in vitro. Mol Pharmacol. 1977;13:872–82.

30. Lefebver Y, Hesseltine HC. The peripheral white blood cells and metronidazole. JAMA. 1965;194:15–8.

31. Kazmier FJ. A significant interaction between metronidazole and warfarin. Mayo Clin Proc. 1976;51:782–4.

32. Kusumi RK, Plouffe JF, Wyatt RH, et al. Central nervous system toxicity associated with metronidazole therapy. Ann Intern Med. 1980;93:59–60.

33. Friedman GD, Selby JV. How often does metronidazole induce pancreatitis? Gastroenterology 1990;98:1702–3.

34. Rothstein E, Clancy DD. Toxicity of disulfiram combined with metronidazole. N Engl J Med. 1969;280:1006–7.

35. Rosenkranz HS, Speck WT. Studies on the significance of the mutagenicity of metronidazole for *Salmonella typhimurium*. In: Finegold SM, ed. Metronidazole, Proceedings of the International Metronidazole Conference, Montreal, Quebec, Canada, May 26–28, 1976. Princeton, NJ: Excerpta Medica; 1977:119–25.

36. Koch RL, Beaulieu BB Jr, Chrystal EJT, et al. A metronidazole metabolite in human urine and its risk. Science. 1981;211:398–400.

37. Beard CM, Noller KL, O'Fallon WM, et al. Lack of evidence for cancer due to use of metronidazole. N Engl J Med. 1979;301:519–22.

38. Friedman GD. Cancer after metronidazole (Letter). N Engl J Med. 1980; 302:519.

39. Bassily S, Farid Z, El-Masry NA, et al. Treatment of intestinal *E. histolytica* and *G. lamblia* with metronidazole, tinidazole and ornidazole: A comparative study. J Trop Med Hyg. 1987;90:9–12.

40. Nigam P, Kapoor KK, Kumar A, et al. Clinical profile of giardiasis and comparison of its therapeutic response to metronidazole and tinidazole. J Assoc Phys India. 1991;39:613–5.

41. Gupta JP, Jain AK, Nanivadekar AS. Efficacy of tinidazole (Fasigyn) in giardiasis by parasitologic, biochemical, and gut transit studies. Indian J Gastroenterol. 1989;8:103–4.

42. Goldman P. The development of 5-nitroimidazoles for the treatment and prophylaxis of anaerobic bacterial infections. J Antimicrob Chemother. 1982; 10(Suppl A):23–33.

43. Rossignol JF, Maisonneuve H, Cho YW. Nitroimidazoles in the treatment of trichomoniasis, giardiasis, and amebiasis. Int J Clin Pharmacol Ther Toxicol. 1984;22:63–72.

44. Powell SJ, Wilmot AJ, MacLeod IN, et al. A comparative trial of dehydroemetine and emetine hydrochloride in identical dosage in amoebic liver abscess. Ann Trop Med Parasitol. 1967;61:26–8.

45. Scragg JN, Powell SJ. Emetine hydrochloride and dehydroemetine combined with chloroquine in the treatment of children with amoebic liver abscess. Arch Dis Child. 1968;43:121–3.

46. Yang WCT, Dubick M. Mechanism of emetine cardiotoxicity. Pharmacol Ther. 1980;10:15–26.

47. Grollman AP. Inhibitors of protein synthesis. V. Effects of emetine on protein and nucleic acid biosynthesis in HELA cells. J Biol Chem. 1968;243:4089–94.

48. Klatskin G, Friedman H. Emetine toxicity in man: Studies on the nature of early toxic manifestations, their relation to the dose level, and their significance in determining safe dosage. Ann Intern Med. 1948;28:892–915.

49. Webster LT Jr. Drugs used in the chemotherapy of protozoal infections: Leishmaniasis, trypanosomiasis, and other protozoal infections. In: Gilman AG, Rall TW, Nies AS, et al, eds. The Pharmacological Basis of Therapeutics. 8th ed. New York: Pergamon Press; 1990:1008–17.

50. Pamba HO, Estambale BB, Chunge CN, Donno L. Comparative study of aminosidine, etophamide and nimorazole, alone or in combination, in the treatment of intestinal amoebiasis in Kenya. Eur J Clin Pharmacol 1990;39:353–7.

51. Bradley WG, Fewings JD, Harris JB, et al. Emetine myopathy in the rat. Br J Pharmacol. 1976;57:29–41.

52. Findlay GM. Recent Advances in Chemotherapy. v. II. 3rd ed. London: J & A Churchill; 1951:341–68.

53. Fisher AK, Walter FG, Szabo S. Iodoquinol associated seizures and radiopacity. J Toxicol Clin Toxicol. 1993;31:113–20.

54. Oakley GP Jr. The neurotoxicity of the halogenated hydroxyquinolines. JAMA. 1973;225:395–7.

55. Wolfe MS. The treatment of intestinal protozoal infections. Med Clin North Am. 1982;66:707–20.

56. Krogstad DJ, Spencer HC Jr, Healy GR. Amebiasis. N Engl J Med. 1978; 298:262–5.

57. Pehrson P, Bengtsson E. Treatment of non-invasive amoebiasis. A comparison between tinidazole alone and in combination with diloxanide furoate. Trans R Soc Trop Med Hyg. 1983;77:845–6.

58. Wolfe MS. Nondysenteric intestinal amebiasis: Treatment with diloxanide furoate. JAMA. 1973;224:1601–4.

59. Simon M, Shookhoff HB, Terner H, et al. Paromomycin in the treatment of intestinal amebiasis: A short course of therapy. Am J Gastroenterol. 1967; 48:504–11.

60. Soderman WA Jr. Amebiasis (clinical seminar). Am J Dig Dis. 1971;16:51–60.

61. Fichtenbaum CJ, Ritchie DJ, Powderly WG. Use of paromomycin for the treatment of crytosporidiosis in patients with AIDS. Clin Infect Dis. 1993; 16:298–300.

62. Armitage K, Flanigan T, Carey J, et al. Treatment of cryptosporidoisis with paromomycin. A report of five cases. Arch Intern Med. 1992;152:2497–9.

63. el-On J, Halevy S, Grunwald MH, et al. Topical treatment of old world cutaneous leishmaniasis caused by *Leishmania major*: A double-blind control study. J Am Acad Dermatol 1992;27:227–31.

64. Scott JA, Davidson RN, Moody AH, et al. Aminosidine (paromomycin) in the treatment of leishmaniasis imported into the United Kingdom. Trans R Soc Trop Med Hyg 1992;86:617–9.

65. Thakur CP, Olliaro P, Gothoskar S, et al. Treatment of visceral leishmaniasis (kala-azar) with aminosidine (=paromomycin)–antimonial combinations, a pilot study in Bihar, India. Trans R Soc Trop Med Hyg. 1992;86:615–6.

66. Botero D. Paromomycin as effective treatment of *Taenia* infections. Am J Trop Med. 1970;19:234–7.

67. Smith JW, Wolfe MS. Giardiasis. Annu Rev Med. 1980;31:373–83.

68. Craft JC, Murphy T, Nelson JD. Furizolidone and quinacrine. Comparative study of therapy for giardiasis in children. Am J Dis Child. 1981;135:164–6.

69. Bassily S, Farid Z, Mikhail JW, et al. The treatment of *Giardia lamblia* infection with mepacrine, metronidazole and furazolidone. J Trop Med Hyg. 1970;73:15–8.

70. Rollo IM. Miscellaneous drugs used in the treatment of protozoal infections. In: Gilman AG, Goodman LS, Gilman A, eds. The Pharmacological Basis of Therapeutics. 6th ed. New York: Macmillan; 1980:1070–9.

71. Sokol RJ, Lichtenstein PK, Farrell MK. Quinacrine hydrochloride-induced yellow discoloration of the skin in children. Pediatrics. 1982;69:232–3.

72. Moreno TJ, Green J. Quinacrine-associated mania. Mayo Clin Proc. 1989; 64:129–30.

73. Miller LG, Kraft IA. Quinacrine-induced psychosis in a pediatric patient. J Fam Pract. 1991;32:526–8.

74. Lindenmayer JP, Vargas P. Toxic psychosis following use of quinacrine. J Clin Psychiatry. 1981;42:162–4.

75. Wolfe MS. Giardiasis. JAMA. 1975;233:1362–5.

76. Pratt WB, Fekety R. Chemotherapy in protozoal diseases. In: The Antimicrobial Drugs. New York: Oxford University Press; 1986:385–413.

77. Quiros-Buelna E. Furazolidone and metronidazole for treatment of giardiasis in children. Scand J Gastroenterol. 1989;169(Suppl):65–9.

78. Levi GC, de Avila CA, Neto VA. Efficacy of various drugs for treatment of giardiasis. A comparative study. Am J Trop Med Hyg. 1977;26:564–5.

79. White AH. Absorption, distribution, metabolism, and excretion of furazolidone. A review of the literature. Scand J Gastroenterol. 1989;169(Suppl):4–10.

80. Altamirano A, Bondani A. Adverse reactions to furazolidone and other drugs. A comparative review. Scand J Gastroenterol. 1989;169(Suppl):70–80.

81. Wyler DJ. Malaria—resurgence, resistance, and research. N Engl J Med. 1983;308:875–8, 934–40.

82. Anonymous. World malaria situation in 1990. Bull WHO. 1992;67:161–7.

83. Lobel HO, Campbell CC, Pappaioanou M, et al. Use of prophylaxis for malaria by American travelers to Africa and Haiti. JAMA. 1987;257:2626–7.

84. Remington JS, Desmonts G. Toxoplasmosis. In: Remington JS, Klein JO, eds. Infectious Diseases of the Fetus and Newborn Infant. 2nd ed. Philadelphia: Saunders; 1983:143–263.

85. Wong B, Gold JWM, Brown AE, et al. Central-nervous-system toxoplasmosis in homosexual men and parenteral drug abusers. Ann Intern Med. 1984; 100:36–42.

86. Current WL, Reese NC, Ernst JV, et al. Human cryptosporidiosis in immunocompetent and immunodeficient persons: Studies of an outbreak and experimental transmission. N Engl J Med. 1983;308:1252–7.

86a. Centers for Disease Control and Prevention. Health Information for International Travel 1993. Washington D.C., US Department of Health and Human Services. HHS publication no. (CDC) 93–8280. 1993. p. 110.

87. Krogstad DJ, Herwaldt BL, Schlesinger PH. Antimalarial agents: Specific treatment regimens. Antimicrob Agents Chemother. 1988;32:957–61.

88. Development of mefloquine as an antimalarial drug. Bull WHO. 1983;61:169–78.

89. Chloroquine-resistant *Plasmodium falciparum* malaria in West Africa. JAMA. 1987;257:2556–9.

90. Mulder B, Gazin P, Eggelte TA. Increase in chloroquine resistance in vivo of *Plasmodium falciparum* over two years in Edea, south Cameroon. Trans R Soc Trop Med Hyg. 1992;86:376.

91. Menon A, Otoo N, Herbage EA, et al. A national survey of the prevalence of chloroquine resistant *Plasmadium falciparum* malaria in The Gambia. Trans R Soc Trop Med Hyg. 1990;84:638–640.

92. Sharp BL, Freese JA. Chloroquine resistant *Plasmodium falciparum* malaria in the Kavango region of Namibia. S Afr Med J. 1990;78:322–33.

93. Moran JS, Bernard KW. The spread of chloroquine resistant malaria in Africa. JAMA. 1989;262:245–8.

94. LeBras J, Hatin I, Bouree P, et al. Chloroquine-resistant falciparum malaria in Benin. Lancet. 1986;2:1043–4.

95. Collignon P. Chloroquine resistance in *Plasmodium vivax*. J Infect Dis. 1991;164:222–3.

96. Rieckmann KH, Davis DR, Hutton DC. *Plasmodium vivax* resistant to chloroquine? Lancet. 1989;2:1183–4.

97. Schwartz IK, Lackritz EM, Patchen LC. Chloroquine-resistant *Plasmodium vivax* from Indonesia. N Engl J Med. 1991;324:927.

98. Collignon PJ. Chloroquine-resistant *Plasmodium vivax:* It may be a common problem. Med J Aust. 1993;157:426.

99. Miller LH, Neva FA, Gill F. Failure of chloroquine in human babesiosis (*Babesia microti*): Case report and chemotherapeutic trial in hamsters. Ann Intern Med. 1978;88:200–2.

100. Brohult J, Rombo L, Sirleaf V, et al. The concentration of chloroquine in serum during short and long term malaria prophylaxis with standard and "double" dosage in non-immunes: Clinical implications. Ann Trop Med Parasitol. 1979;73:401–5.

101. Webster LT Jr. Drugs used in the chemotherapy of protozoal infections: Malaria. In: Gilman AG, Rall TW, Nies AS, et al, eds: Goodman and Gilman's. The Pharmacological Basis of Therapeutics. Eighth ed. New York: Pergamon Press; 1990:978–998.

102. Andrews P, Haberkorn A, Thomas H. Antiparasitic drugs: Mechanisms of action, pharmacokinetics, and in vitro and in vivo assays of drug activity. In: Lorian V, ed. Antibiotics in Laboratory Medicine. 2nd ed. Baltimore: Williams & Wilkins; 1986;282–345.

102a. Basco LA, Le Bras J. In vitro activity of artemisinin derivatives against African isolates and clones of *Plasmodiam Falciparum*. Am J Trop Med. 1993;49:301–7.

103. Warhurst DC. Antimalarial drugs: Mode of action and resistance. J Antimicrob Chemother. 1986;18(Suppl B):51–9.

104. Warhurst DC, Homewood CA, Baffaley VC. The chemotherapy of rodent malaria. XX. Autophagic vacuole formation in *Plasmodium berghei* in vitro. Ann Trop Med Parasitol. 1974;68:265–81.

105. Slater AFG, Cerami A. Inhibition by chloroquine of a novel haem polymerase enzyme activity in malaria trophozoites. Nature. 1992;355:167–9.

106. Krogstad DJ, Schlesinger PH. The basis of antimalarial action: Non-weak base effects of chloroquine on acid vesicle pH. Am J Trop Med Hyg. 1987;36:213–20.

107. Krogstad DJ, Schlesinger PH. Acid-vesicle function, intracellular pathogens and the action of chloroquine against *Plasmodium falciparum*. N Engl J Med. 1987;317:542–9.

108. Kyle DE, Milhous WK, Rossan RN. Reversal of *Plasmodium falciparum* resistance to chloroquine in Panamanian *Aotus* monkeys. Am J Trop Med Hyg. 1993;48:126–33.

109. Martin SK, Oduola AMJ, Milhous WK. Reversal of chloroquine resistance in *Plasmodium falciparum* by verapamil. Science. 1987;235:899–901.

110. Marks JS. Chloroquine retinopathy: Is there a safe daily dose? Ann Rheum Dis. 1982;41:52–8.

111. White NJ, Watt G, Bergvist Y, et al. Parenteral chloroquine for treating falciparum malaria. J Infect Dis. 1987;155:192–201.

112. Riou B, Barriot P, Rimailho A, et al. Treatment of severe chloroquine poisoning. N Engl J Med. 1988;318:1–6.

113. Hart CW, Naunton RF. The ototoxicity of chloroquine phosphate. Arch Otolaryngol. 1964;80:407–12.

114. Saxena AK, Saxena M. Advances in chemotherapy of malaria. Prog Drug Res. 1986;30:221–80.

115. Looareesuwan S, White NJ, Chittamas S, et al. High rate of *Plasmodium vivax* relapse following treatment of falciparum malaria in Thailand. Lancet. 1987;2:1052–5.

116. Arias AE, Corredor A. Low response rate of Columbian strains of *Plasmodium vivax* to classical antimalarial therapy. Trop Med Parasitol. 1989;40:21–3.

117. Luzzi GA, Warrell DA, Barnes AJ, Dunbar EM. Treatment of primaquine resistant *Plasmodium vivax* malaria. Lancet. 1992;340:310.

118. Clyde DF, McCarthy VC. Radical cure of Chesson strain vivax malaria in man by 7, not 14, days of treatment with primaquine. Am J Trop Med Hyg. 1977;26:562–3.

119. Hiebsch RR, Raub TJ, Wattenberg BW. Primaquine blocks transport by inhibiting the formation of functional transport vesicles. J Biol Chem 1991;266:20323–8.

120. Kellermeyer RW, Tarlov AR, Brewer GJ, et al. Hemolytic effect of therapeutic drugs: Clinical considerations of the primaquine-type hemolysis. JAMA. 1962;180:388–94.

121. Clyde DF. Clinical problems associated with the use of primaquine as a tissue schizontocidal and gametocytocidal drug. Bull WHO. 1981;59:391–5.

122. Alving AS, Johnson CF, Tarlov AR, et al. Mitigation of the haemolytic effect of primaquine and enhancement of its action against exoerythrocytic forms of the Chesson strain of *Plasmodium vivax* by intermittent regimens of drug administration: A preliminary report. Bull WHO. 1960;22:621–31.

123. Brasseur P, Kouamouo J, Moyou-Somo R, et al. Multi-drug resistant falciparum malaria in Cameroon in 1987–88 I. Stable figures of prevalence of chloroquine- and quinine-resistant isolates in the original foci. Am J Trop Med Hyg. 1992;46:1–7.

124. Lege-Oguntoye L, Abua JU, Werblinska B, et al. Chloroquine-resistant *Plasmodium falciparum* with reduced sensitivity in vitro to mefloquine and quinine in Zaria, Northern Nigeria. J Trop Med Hyg. 1991;94:73–5.

125. Anonymous. Treatment of severe *Plasmodium falciparum* malaria with quinidine gluconate: Discontinuation of quinine from the CDC drug service. MMWR. 1991;40:240–1.

126. Brodie BB, Baer JE, Craig LC. Metabolic products of the cinchona alkaloids in human urine. J Biol Chem. 1951;188:567–81.

127. White NJ, Looareesuwan S, Warrell DA, et al. Quinine pharmacokinetics and toxicity in cerebral and uncomplicated falciparum malaria. Am J Med. 1982;73:564–72.

128. Canfield CJ, Miller LH, Bartelloni PJ, et al. Acute renal failure in *Plasmodium falciparum* malaria. Arch Intern Med. 1968;122:199–203.

129. Pratt WB, Fekety R. Chemotherapy of malaria. In: The Antimicrobial Drugs. New York: Oxford University Press; 1986;355–84.

130. Punukollu RC, Kumar S, Mullen KD. Quinine hepatotoxicity: An underrecognized or rare phenomenon? Arch Intern Med. 1990;150:1112–3.

131. Mathur S, Dooley J, Scheuer PJ. Quinine induced granulomatous hepatitis and vasculitis. Br Med J. 1990;300:613.

132. White JN, Warrell DA, Chanthavanich P, et al. Severe hypoglycemia and hyperinsulinemia in falciparum malaria. N Engl J Med. 1983;309:61–6.

133. Phillips RE, Looareesunwan S, White NJ, et al. Quinine pharmacokinetics and toxicity in pregnant and lactating women with falciparum malaria. Br J Clin Pharmacol. 1986;21:677–83.

134. Phillips RE, Warrell DA, White NJ, et al. Intravenous quinidine for the treatment of severe falciparum malaria. N Engl J Med. 1985;312:1273–8.

135. Rudnitsky G, Miller KD, Padua T, et al. Continuous-infusion quinidine gluconate for treating children with severe *Plasmodium falciparum* malaria. J Infect Dis. 1987;155:1040–3.

136. Miller KD, Greenberg AE, Campbell CC. Treatment of severe malaria in the United States with a continuous infusion of quinidine gluconate and exchange transfusion. N Engl J Med. 1989;321:65–70.

137. Swerdlow CD, Yu JO, Jacobsen E, et al. Safety and efficacy of intravenous quinidine. Am J Med 1983;75:36–42.

138. Botero D, Restrepo M, Montoya A. Prospective double-blind trial of two different doses of mefloquine plus pyrimethamine-sulfadoxine compared with pyrimethamine-sulfadoxine alone in the treatment of falciparum malaria. Bull WHO. 1985;63:731–7.

139. De Sousa JM, Sheth UK, Oliveira RMG, et al. An open, randomized, phase III clinical trial of mefloquine and of quinine plus sulfadoxime–pyrimethamine in the treatment of symptomatic falciparum malaria in Brazil. Bull WHO. 1985;63:603–9.

140. Tin F, Hlaing N, Tun T, et al. Falciparum malaria treated with a fixed combination of mefloquine, sulfadoxine and pyrimethamine: A field study in adults in Burma. Bull WHO. 1985;63:727–30.

141. Chongsuphajaisiddhi T, Sabchareon A, Chantavanich P, et al. A phase-III clinical trial of mefloquine in children with chloroquine-resistant falciparum malaria in Thailand. Bull WHO. 1987;65:223–6.

142. Oduola AM, Sowunmi A, Milhous WK, et al. Innate resistance to new anti-malarial drugs in *Plasmodium falciparum* from Nigeria. Trans R. Soc Trop Med Hyg. 1992;86:123–6.

143. Wongsrichanalai C, Webster HK, Wimonwattrawatee T, et al. Emergence of multidrug-resistant *Plasmodium falciparum* in Thailand: In vitro tracking. Am J Trop Med Hyg. 1992;47:112–6.

144. Karwacki JJ, Webster HK, Limsomwong N, et al. Two cases of mefloquine resistant malaria in Thailand. Trans R Soc Trop Med Hyg. 1989;83:152–3.

145. Nosten F, ter Kuile F, Chongsuphajaisiddhi T, et al. Mefloquine-resistant falciparum malaria on the Thai-Burmese border. Lancet. 1991;337:1140–3.

146. Brasseur P, Kouamouo J, Moyou-Somo R, et al. Multi-drug resistant falciparum malaria in Cameroon in 1987–1988. II. Mefloquine resistance confirmed in vitro and iv vivo and its correlation with quinine resistance. Am J Trop Med Hyg. 1992;46:8–14.

147. Oduola AMJ, Milhous WK, Salako LA, et al. Reduced in-vitro susceptibility to mefloquine in West African isolates of *Plasmodium falciparum*. Lancet. 1987;2:1304–5.

148. Desjardins RW, Pamplin CL III, von Bredow J, et al. Kinetics of a new antimalarial, mefloquine. Clin Pharmacol Ther. 1979;26:372–9.

149. Jacobs GH, Aikawa M, Milhous WK, et al. An ultrastructural study of the effects of mefloquine on malaria parasite. Am J Trop Med Hyg. 1987;36:9–14.

150. Chanthavanich P, Looareesuwan S, White NJ, et al. Intragastric mefloquine is absorbed rapidly in patients with cerebral malaria. Am J Trop Med Hyg. 1985;34:1028–36.

151. Weinke T, Trautmann M, Held T, et al. Neuropsychiatric side effects after the use of mefloquine. Am J Trop Med Hyg. 1991;45:86–91.

152. Anonymous. Mefloquine for malaria. Med Lett Drugs Ther. 1990;31:13–4.

153. Olson PE, Kennedy CA, Morte PD. Parasthesias and mefloquine prophylaxis. Ann Intern Med. 1992;117:1058–9.

154. Van den Enden E, Gompel AV, Colebunders R, et al. Mefloquine induced Stevens-Johnson syndrome. Lancet. 1991;337:683.

155. Hennequin C, Bouree P, Halfon P. Agranulocytosis during treatment with mefloquine. Lancet. 1991;337:984.

156. Martin GJ, Malone JL, Ross EV. Exfoliative dermatitis during malarial prophylaxis with mefloquine. Clin Infect Dis. 1993;16:341.

157. Horowitz H, Carbonaro CA. Inhibition of *Salmonella typhi* oral vaccine strain, Ty21a, by mefloquine and chloroquine. J Infect Dis. 1992;166:1462–1464.

158. Hien TT, White NJ. Qinghaosu. Lancet. 1993;341:603–7.

159. Watanasook C, Singharaj P, Suriyamopngkol V, et al. Malaria prophylaxis with doxycycline in soldiers deployed to the Thai–Kampuchean border. Southeast Asian J Trop Med Public Health. 1989;20:61–4.

160. Meek SR, Doberstyn EB, Gaürzère BA, et al. Treatment of falciparum malaria with quinine and tetracycline or combined mefloquine/sulfadoxine/pyrimethamine on the Thai-Kampuchean border. Am J Trop Med Hyg. 1986;35:246–50.

161. Centers for Disease Control and Prevention. Recommendations for the prevention of malaria in travelers. MMWR. 1988;37:277–84.

162. Bryson HM, Goa KL. Halofantrine: A review of its antimalarial activity, pharmacokinetic properties and therapeutic potential. Drugs. 1992;43:236–58.

163. Drug alert: halofantrine. Change in recommendations for use. Wkly Epidemiol Rec 1993;68:269–70.

164. Pape JW, Verdier RI, Johnson WD. Treatment and prophylaxis of *Isospora belli* infection in patients with the acquired immunodeficiency syndrome. N Engl J Med. 1989;320:1044–7.

165. Hughes WT, Feldman S, Chaudhary SC, et al. Comparison of pentamidine isethionate and trimethoprim-sulfamethoxazole in the treatment of *Pneumocystis carinii* pneumonia. J Pediatr. 1978;92:285–91.

166. Young LS. Trimethoprim-sulfamethoxazole in the treatment of adults with pneumonia due to *Pneumocystis carinii*. Rev Infect Dis. 1982;4:608–13.

167. Siegel SE, Wolff LJ, Baehner RL, et al. Treatment of *Pneumocystis carinii* pneumonitis: A comparative trial of sulfamethoxazole-trimethoprim v. pentamidine in pediatric patients with cancer: Report from Childrens Cancer Study Group. Am J Dis Child. 1984;138:1051–4.

168. Luft BJ, Conley F, Remington JS. Outbreak of central-nervous-system toxoplasmosis in Western Europe and North America. Lancet. 1983;1:781–4.

169. Haverkos HW. Assessment of therapy for toxoplasma encephalitis. The TE study group. Am J Med. 1987;82:907–14.

170. Luft BJ, Remington JS. Toxoplasmic encephalitis. J Infect Dis. 1988;157:1–6.

171. Wilson CB, Remington JS. Toxoplasmosis. In: Feigin RD, Cherry JD, eds. Textbook of Pediatric Infectious Diseases. 2nd ed. Philadelphia: WB Saunders; 1987:2067–78.

172. McCabe R, Remington JS. Toxoplasmosis: The time has come. N Engl J Med. 1988;318:313–5.

173. Kovacs JA, Allegra CJ, Chabner BA, et al. Potent effect of trimetrexate, a lipid-soluble antifolate, on *Toxoplasma gondii*. J Infect Dis. 1987;155:1027–32.

174. Daffos F, Forestier F, Capella-Pavlovsky M, et al. Prenatal management of 746 pregnancies at risk for congenital toxoplasmosis. N Engl J Med. 1988;318:271–5.

175. Weidekamm E, Plozza-Nottebrock H, Forgo I, et al. Plasma concentrations of pyrimethamine and sulfadoxine and evaluation of pharmacokinetic data by computerized curve fitting. Bull WHO. 1982;60:115–22.

176. Jaffe JJ. Dihydrofolate reductase in parasitic protozoa and helminths. In: Van den Bossche H, ed. Biochemistry of Parasites. London: Academic Press; 1972;219–33.

177. Hayama T, Kokue E. Use of the Goettingen miniature pig for studying pyrimethamine teratogenesis. CRC Crit Rev Toxicol. 1985;14:403–21.

178. Petter C, Bourbon J. Foetal red cell macrocytosis induced by pyrimethamine; its teratogenic role. Experientia. 1975;31:369–70.

179. Pyrimethamine combinations in pregnancy. Lancet. 1983;2:1005–7.

180. Harpey JP, Darbois Y, LeFèbvre G. Teratogenicity of pyrimethamine (Letter). Lancet. 1983;2:399.

181. Mandell GL, Sande MA. Antimicrobial agents: Sulfonamides, trimethoprim-sulfamethoxazole, and urinary tract antiseptics. In: Gilman AG, Goodman LS, Rall TW, et al, eds. The Pharmacological Basis of Therapeutics. 7th ed. New York: Macmillian; 1985;1095–114.

182. Navin TR, Miller KD, Satriale RF, et al. Adverse reactions associated with pyrimethamine-sulfadoxine prophylaxis for *Pneumocystis carinii* infections in AIDS (Letter). Lancet. 1985;1:1332.

183. Miller KD, Lobel HO, Satriale RF, et al. Severe cutaneous reactions among American travelers using pyrimethamine-sulfadoxine (Fansidar) for malaria prophylaxis. Am J Trop Med Hyg. 1986;35:451–8.

184. Rombo L, Stenbeck J, Lobel HO, et al. Does chloroquine contribute to the risk of serious adverse reactions to Fansidar? Lancet. 1985;2:1298–9.

185. Karbwang J, Bunnag D, Breckenridge AM, et al. The pharmacokinetics of mefloquine when given alone or in combination with sulphadoxine and pyrimethamine in Thai male and female subjects. Eur J Clin Pharmacol. 1987;32:173–7.

186. De Sousa JM, Sheth UK, Oliveira RMG, et al. A phase I clinical trial of Fansimef (mefloquine plus sulfadoxine-pyrimethamine) in Brazilian male subjects. Bull WHO. 1985;63:611–5.

187. Young LS. Treatment and prevention of *Pneumocystis carinii* infection. In: Young LS, ed. *Pneumocystis carinii* Pneumonia; Pathogenesis, Diagnosis, Treatment. New York: Marcel Dekker; 1984:175–94.

188. Wharton JM, Coleman DL, Wolfsy CB, et al. Trimethoprim-sulfamethoxazole or pentamidine for *Pneumocystis carinii* pneumonia in the acquired immunodeficiency syndrome. Ann Intern Med. 1986;105:37–44.

189. Fischl MA, Dickinson DM, La Voie L, et al. Safety and efficacy of trimethoprim and sulfamethoxazole chemoprophylaxis. JAMA. 1988;259:1185–9.

190. Hughes WT, Rivera GK, Schell MJ, et al. Successful intermittent chemoprophylaxis for *Pneumocystis carinii* pneumonitis. N Engl J Med. 1987;316:1627–32.

191. Jick H. Adverse reactions to trimethoprim–sulfamethoxazole in hospitalized patients. Rev Infect Dis. 1982;4:426–8.

192. Pratt WB, Fekety R. The antimetabolites. In: The Antimicrobical Drugs. New York: Oxford University Press; 1986:229–51.

193. Kaufman DL. *Pneumocystis carinii* pneumonia. Adv Exp Med Biol. 1986;202:153–69.

194. Gordin FM, Simon GL, Wofsy CB, et al. Adverse reactions to trimethoprim–sulfamethoxazole in patients with the acquired immunodeficiency syndrome. Ann Intern Med. 1984;100:495–9.

195. Small CB, Harris CA, Friedland GH, et al. The treatment of *Pneumocystis carinii* pneumonia in the acquired immunodeficiency syndrome. Arch Intern Med. 1985;145:837–40.

196. Kemper CA, Tucker RM, Lang OS, et al. Low dose dapsone prophylaxis of *Pneumocystis carinii* pneumonia in AIDS and AIDS-related complex. AIDS. 1990;4:1145–8.

197. Blum RN, Miller LA, Gaggini C, et al. Comparative trial of dapsone versus trimethoprim/sulfamethoxazole for primary prophylaxis of *Pneumocystis* pneumonia. J AIDS. 1992;5:341–7.

198. Mandell GL, Sande MA. Antimicrobial agents: Drugs used in the chemotherapy of tuberculosis and leprosy. In: Gilman AG, Goodman LS, Rall TW, et al, eds. The Pharmacological Basis of Therapeutics. 7th ed. New York: Macmillan; 1985:1199–218.

199. Pratt WB, Fekety R. Drugs that act on mycobacteria: Isoniazid, rifampin, ethambutol, and streptomycin; the minor antituberculosis drugs; drugs effective against leprosy. In: Pratt WB, Fekety R, eds. The Antimicrobial Drugs. New York: Oxford University Press; 1986:277–314.

200. Cook GC. Prevention and treatment of malaria. Lancet. 1988;1:32–7.
201. Begbie S, Burgess KR. Maloprim-induced pulmonary eosinophilia. Chest. 1993;103:305–6.
202. Rollo IM. The mode of action of sulphonamides, Proguanil and pyrimethamine on *Plasmodium gallinaceum*. Br J Pharmacol Chemother. 1955;10:208–14.
203. Barnes AJ, Ong ELC, Dunbar EM, et al. Failure of chloroquine and proguanil prophylaxis in travellers to Kenya. Lancet. 1991;338:1338–9.
204. Pang LW, Limsomwong N, Singharaj P, et al. Malaria prophylaxis with proguanil and sulfisoxazole in children living in a malaria endemic area. Bull WHO. 1989;67:51–8.
205. Karwacki JJ, Shanks GD, Limsomwong N, et al. Proguanil-sulfonamide for malaria prophylaxis. Trans R Soc Trop Med Hyg. 1990;84:55–7.
206. Ericksson B, Bjorkman A, Keisu M. How safe is proguanil? A post-marketing investigation of side effects. Scand J Infect Dis. 1991;23:489–93.
207. Allegra CJ, Chabner BA, Tuazon CU, et al. Trimetrexate for the treatment of *Pneumocystis carinii* pneumonia in patients with the acquired immunodeficiency syndrome. N Engl J Med. 1987;317:978–85.
208. Hudson AT. Atovaquone—A novel broad-spectrum anti-infective drug. Parasitol Today. 1993;9:66.
209. Araujo FG, Huskinson J, Remington JS. Remarkable in vitro and in vivo activities of the hydroxynaphthoquinone 566C80 against tachyzoites and tissue cysts of *Toxoplasma gondii*. Antimicrob Agents Chemother. 1991;35:293–9.
210. Araujo FG, Lin T, Remington JS. The activity of atovaquone (566C80) in murine toxoplasmosis is markedly augmented when used in combination with pyrimethamine or sulfadiazine. J Infect Dis. 1993;167:494–7.
211. Kovacs JA. Efficacy of atovaquone in treatment of toxoplasmosis in patients with AIDS. The NIAID-Clinical Center intramural AIDS programd. Lancet. 1992;340:637–8.
212. Fallon J, Kovacs J, Hughes W, et al. A preliminary evaluation of 566C80 for the treatment of *Pneumocystis* pneumonia in patients with the acquired immunodeficiency syndrome. N Engl J Med. 1991;325:1534–8.
213. Hughes W, Leoung G, Kramer F, et al. Comparison of atovaquone (566C80) with trimethoprim–sulfamethoxazole to treat *Pneumocystis carinii* pneumonia in patients with AIDS. N Engl J Med. 1993;328:1521–7.
214. Anonymous. Atovaquone for *Pneumocystis* pneumonia. Med Lett Drugs Ther. 1993;35:28–9.
215. Danneman B, McCutchan A, Isrealski D, et al. Treatment of toxoplasmic encephalitis in patients with AIDS: A randomized trial comparing pyrimethamine plus clindamycin to pyrimethamine plus sulfadiazine. Ann Intern Med. 1992;116:33.
216. Lakhanpal V, Schocket SS, Nirankari VS. Clindamycin in the treatment of toxoplasmic retinochoroiditis. Am J Ophthalmol. 1983;95:605–13.
217. Ferguson JG Jr. Clindamycin therapy for toxoplasmosis. Ann Ophthalmol. 1981;13:95–100.
218. Clindamycin and quinine treatment for *Babesia microti* infections. MMWR. 1983;32:65–6.
219. Soave R. Treatment strategies for cryptosporidiosis. Ann NY Acad Sci. 1990;616:442–51.
220. Chan J, Luft BJ. Activity of roxithromycin (RU28965), a macrolide, against *Toxoplasma gondii* infection in mice. Antimicrob Agents Chemother. 1986;30:323–4.
221. Chamberland S, Kirst HA, Current WL. Comparative activity of macrolides against *Toxoplasma gondii* demonstrating utility of an in vitro assay. Antimicrob Agents Chemother. 1991;35:903–9.
222. Deroun F, Chastang C. Activity in vitro against *Toxoplasma gondii* of azithromycin and clarithromycin alone and with pyrimethamine. Antimicrob Agents Chemother. 1990;25:708–11.
223. Hofflin JM, Remington JS. In vivo synergism of roxithromycin (RU965) and interferon against *Toxoplasma gondii*. Antimicrob Agents Chemother. 1987;31:346–8.
224. Rehg JE. Activity of azithromycin against cryptosporidia in immunosuppressed rats. J Infect Dis. 1991;163:1293–6.
225. Taelman H, Schechter PJ, Marcelis L, et al. Difluoromethylornithine, an effective new treatment of Gambian trypanosomiasis. Am J Med. 1987;82:607–14.
226. Di Bari C, Pastore G, Roscigno G, et al. Late-stage African trypanosomiasis and eflornithine (Letter). Ann Intern Med. 1986;105:803–4.
227. Van Nieuwenhove S, Schechter PJ, Declercq J, et al. Treatment of gambiense sleeping sickness in the Sudan with oral DFMO (DL-α-difluoromethylornithine), an inhibitor of ornithine decarbopxylase; first field trial. Trans R Soc Trop Med Hyg. 1985;79:692–8.
228. Milford F, Pepin J, Loko L, et al. Efficacy and toxicity of eflornithine for treatment of *Trypanosoma brucei gambiense* sleeping sickness. Lancet. 1992;340:652–5.
229. Marr JJ, Docampo R. Chemotherapy for Chagas' disease: A perspective of current therapy and considerations for future research. Rev Infect Dis. 1986;8:884–903.
230. Pearson RD, Navin TR, Sousa AQ, et al. Leishmaniasis. In: Kass EH, Platt R, eds. Current Therapy in Infectious Diseases. Toronto: BC Decker; 1990;384–9.
231. Jha TK. Evaluation of diamidine compound (pentamidine isethionate) in the treatment of resistant cases of kala-azar occurring in North Bihar, India. Trans R Soc Trop Med Hyg. 1983;77:167–70.
232. Thakur CP. Epidemiological, clinical and therapeutic features of Bihar kala-azar (including post kala-azar dermal leishmaniasis). Trans R Soc Trop Med Hyg. 1984;78:391–8.
233. Kluge RM, Spaulding DM, Spain AJ. Combination of pentamidine and trimethoprim-sulfamethoxazole in the therapy of *Pneumocystis carinii* pneumonia in rats. Antimicrob Agents Chemother. 1978;13:975–8.
234. Webster LT Jr. Drugs used in the chemotherapy of protozoal infections: Leishmaniasis, trypanosomiasis and other protozoal infections. In: Gilman AG, Goodman LS, Rall TW, et al, eds. The Pharmacological Basis of Therapeutics. 7th ed. New York: Macmillan; 1985:1058–65.
235. Fairlamb AH, Bowman IB. *Trypanosoma brucei:* Suramin and other trypanocidal compounds: Effects on *sn*-glycerol-3 phosphate oxidase. Exp Parasitol. 1977;43:353–61.
236. Fuglsang H, Anderson J. Side effects of suramin. In: Research and Control of Onchocerciasis in the Western Hemisphere. Pan American Health Organization, Scientific Publication No 298:54–7.
237. Carter NS, Fairlamb AH. Arsenical-resistant trypanosomes lack an unusual adenosine transporter. Nature. 1993;361:173–5.
238. Flynn IW, Bowman IBR. Further studies on the mode of arsenicals on trypanosome pyruvate kinase (Abstract). Trans R Soc Trop Med Hyg. 1969;63:121.
239. Robertson DHH. Chemotherapy of African trypanosomes. Practitioner. 1962;188:80–3.
240. Arrox JOL. Melarsoprol and reactive encephalopathy in *Trypanosoma brucei rhodesiense*. Trans R Soc Trop Med Hyg. 1987;81:192.
241. Pepin J, Milord F. African trypanosomiasis and drug induced encephalopathy: Risk factors and pathogenesis. Trans R Soc Trop Med Hyg. 1991;85:222–4.
242. Gherardi RK, Chariot P, Vanderstigel M, et al. Organic arsenic induced Guillain-Barre-like syndrome due to melarsoprol: A clinical, electrophysiological and pathological study. Muscle Nerve. 1990;13:637–45.
243. Bacchi CJ, Nathan HC, Livingston T, et al. Differential susceptibility to DL-α-difluoromethylornithine in clinical isolates of *Trypanosoma brucei rhodesiense*. Antimicrob Agents Chemother. 1990;34:1183–8.
244. Bacchi CJ. Content, synthesis, and function of polyamines in trypanosomatids: Relationship to chemotherapy. J Protozool. 1981;28:20–7.
245. Sjoersdma A, Schechter PJ. Chemotherapeutic implications of polyamine biosynthesis inhibition. Clin Pharmacol Ther. 1984;35:287–300.
246. Brener Z. Present status of chemotherapy and chemoprophylaxis of human trypanosomiasis in the Western Hemisphere. Pharmacol Ther. 1979;7:71–90.
247. Haegele KD, Alken RG, Grove J, et al. Kinetics of alpha-difluoromethylornithine: An irreversible inhibitor of ornithine decarboxylase. Clin Pharmacol Ther. 1981;30:210–7.
248. Docampo R, Morena SNJ. Free radical metabolites in the mode of action of chemotherapeutic agents and phagocytic cells on *Trypanosoma cruzi*. Rev Infect Dis. 1984;6:223–38.
249. Pepin J, Milord F, Mpia B, et al. An open clinical trial of nifurtimox for arseno-resistant *Trypanosoma brucei gambiense* sleeping sickness in Zaire. Trans R Soc Trop Med Hyg. 1989;83:514–7.
250. Pepin J, Milford F, Meurice F, et al. High-dose nifurtimox for arseno-resistant *Trypanosoma brucei gambiense* sleeping sickness: An open trial in central Zaire. Trans R Soc Trop Med Hyg. 1992;86:254–6.
251. Paulos C, Paredes J, Vasquez I, et al. Pharmacokinetics of a nitrofuran compound, nifurtimox, in healthy volunteers. Int J Clin Pharmacol Ther Toxicol. 1989;27:454–7.
252. Moreno SNJ, Palmero DJ, de Palmero KE, et al. Stimulation of lipid peroxidation and ultrastructural alternations by nifurtimox in mammalian tissues. Medicina (B Aires). 1980;40:553–9.
253. Apt W, Arribada A, Arab F, et al. Clinical trial of benznidazole and an immunopotentiator against Chagas' disease in Chile (Letter). Trans R Soc Trop Med Hyg. 1986;80:1010.
254. Andrade SG, Magalhaes JB, Pontes AL. Evaluation of chemotherapy with benznidazole and nifurtimox in mice infected with *Trypanosoma cruzi* strains of different types. Bull WHO. 1985;63:721–6.
255. Teixeira ARL, Cordoba JC, Maior IS, et al. Chagas' disease: Lymphoma growth in rabbits treated with benznidazole. Am J Trop Med Hyg. 1990;43:146–58.
256. Anabwani GM, Ngira JA, Dimiti G, et al. Comparison of two dosage sched-

ules of sodium stibogluconate in the treatment of visceral leishmaniasis in Kenya. Lancet. 1983;1:210–2.

257. Report of a WHO Expert Committee. The leishmaniases. Geneva: WHO Technical Report Series 701; 1984.

258. Ballou WR, McClain JB, Gordon DM, et al. Safety and efficacy of high-dose sodium stibogluconate therapy of American cutaneous leishmaniasis. Lancet. 1987;2:13–6.

259. Grogl M, Thomason TN, Franke ED. Drug resistance in leishmaniasis: Its implications in systemic chemotherapy of cutaneous and mucocutaneous disease. Am J Trop Med Hyg. 1992;47:117–26.

260. Medrano FJ, Hernandez-Quero J, Jimenez E, et al. Visceral leishmaniasis in HIV-1 infected individuals: A common opportunistic infection in Spain? AIDS. 1992;6:1499–503.

261. Martinez S, Marr JJ. Allpurinol in the treatment of American cutaneous leishmaniasis. N Engl J Med. 1992;326:741–4.

262. Saenz RE, Paz HM, Johnson CM, et al. Treatment of American cutaneous leishmaniasis with orally administered allopurinol riboside. J Infect Dis. 1989;160:153–7.

263. Herwaldt BL, Neva FA, Berman JD. Allopurinol in the treatment of American cutaneous leishmaniasis. N Engl J Med. 1992;327:498–9.

264. Marr JJ, Berens RL. Pyrazolopyrmidine metabolism in the pathogenic trypanosomatides. Mol Biochem Parasitol. 1983;7:339–56.

265. Neal RA, Croft SL, Nelson DJ. Anti-leishmanial effect of allopurinol ribonucleoside and the related compounds, allopurinol, thiopurinol, thiopurinol ribonucleoside, and of formycin B, sinefungin and the lepidine WR 6026. Trans R Soc Trop Med Hyg. 1985;79:122–8.

266. Kager PA, Rees PH, Wellde BT, et al. Allopurinol in the treatment of visceral leishmaniasis. Trans R Soc Trop Med Hyg. 1981;75:556–9.

267. Weinrauch L, Livshin R, El-On J. Cutaneous leishmaniasis: Treatment with ketoconazole. Cutis. 1983;32:288–9, 294.

268. Saenz RE, Paz H, Berman JD. Efficacy of ketoconazole against *Leishmania braziliensis panamensis* cutaneous leishmaniasis. Am J Med. 1990;89:147–55.

269. Navin TR, Arana BA, Arana FA, et al. Placebo-controlled clinical trial of sodium stibogluconate (pentostam) versus ketoconazole for treating cutaneous leishmaniasis in Guatemala. J Infect Dis. 1992;165:528–34.

270. El-On J, Weinrauch L, Livshin R, et al. Topical treatment of recurrent cutaneous leishmaniasis in ointment containing paromomycin and methylbenzethionium chloride. Br Med J. 1985;291:704–5.

271. El-On J, Halevy S, Grunwald MH, et al. Topical treatment of old world cutaneous leishmaniasis caused by *Leishmania major:* A double-blind control study. J Am Acad Dermatol. 1992;27:227–31.

272. Badaro R, Johnson WJ. The role of interferon gamma in the treatment of visceral and diffuse cutaneous leishmaniasis. J Infect Dis. 1993;167(Suppl 1):s13–7.

273. Harms G, Zwingenberger K, Sandkamp B, et al. Immunotherapy of visceral leishmaniasis: A pilot trial of sequential treatment with recombinant interferon-gamma and pentavalent antimony. J Interferon Res 1993;13:39–41.

274. Bottasso O, Cabrini J, Falcoff R. Successful treatment of an antimony-resistant American mucocutaneous leishmaniasis: A case report. Arch Dermatol. 1992;128:996–7.

275. Chulay JD, Fleckenstein L, Smith DH. Pharmacokinetics of antimony during treatment of visceral leishmaniasis with sodium stibogluconate or meglumine antimoniate. Trans R Soc Trop Med Hyg. 1988;82:69–72.

276. Information material for physicians—Pentostam (sodium antimony gluconate), HHS, PHS, CDC protocol. Provided by the Centers for Disease Control and Prevention to physicians administering Pentostam in the United States.

277. Berman JD. Chemotherapy for leishmaniasis: Biochemical mechanisms, clinical efficacy, and future strategies. Rev Infect Dis. 1988;10:560–86.

278. Donovan KL, White AD, Cooke DA, et al. Pancreatitis and palindromic arthropathy with effusions associated with sodium stibogluconate treatment in a renal transplant recipient. J Infect. 1990;21:107–10.

279. Halim MA, Alfurayh O, Kalin ME, et al. Successful treatment of visceral leishmaniasis with allopurinol plus ketoconazole in a renal transplant recipient after the occurrence of pancreatitis due to stibogluconate. Clin Infect Dis. 1993;16:397–9.

280. Croft SL, Neal RA. The effect of allopurinol ribonucleoside and formycin B on *Trypanosoma cruzi* infections in mice. Trans R Soc Trop Med Hyg. 1985;79:517–8.

281. Mishra M, Biswas UK, Jha DN, et al. Amphotericin versus pentamidine in antimony-unresponsive kala-azar. Lancet. 1992;340:1256–1257.

282. Sampaio SAP, Godoy JT, Paiva L, et al. The treatment of American (mucocutaneous) leishmaniasis with amphotericin B. Arch Dermatol. 1960;82:627–35.

283. Crofts MAJ. Use of amphotericin B in mucocutaneous leishmaniasis. J Trop Med Hyg. 1976;79:111–3.

284. Berman JD, Ksionski G, Chapman WL, et al. Activity of amphotericin B cholesterol dispersion (Amphocil) in experimental visceral leishmaniasis. Antimicrob Agents Chemother. 1992;36:1978–80.

285. Davidson RN, Croft SL, Scott A, et al. Liposomal amphotericin B in drug-resistant visceral leishmaniasis. Lancet. 1991;337:1061–2.

286. Wali JP, Aggarwal P, Gupta U, et al. Ketoconazole in the treatment of antimony- and pentamidine-resistant kala-azar. J Infect Dis. 1992;166:215–6.

287. Wali JP, Aggarwal P, Gupta U, et al. Ketoconazole in treatment of visceral leishmaniasis. Lancet. 1990;336:810–1.

288. Sundar S, Kumar K, Singh VP. Ketoconazole in visceral leishmaniasis. Lancet. 1990;336:1582.

289. Borrelli D. A clinical trial of itraconazole in the treatment of deep mycoses and leishmaniasis. Rev Infect Dis. 1987;9(Suppl 1):S57–63.

290. Pialoux G, Hennequin C, Dupont B, et al. Cutaneous leishmaniasis in an AIDS patient: Cure with itraconazole. J Infect Dis. 1990;162:1221–2.

291. Dogra J, Aneja N, Behari Lal B, et al. Cutaneous leishmaniasis in India: Clinical experience with itraconazole (R51 211 Janssen). Int J Dermatol. 1990;29:661–2.

292. Albanese G, Giorgetti P, Santagostino L, et al. Cutaneous leishmaniasis: Treatment with itraconazole. Arch Dermatol. 1989;125:1540–2.

293. Akuffo H, Dietz M, Teklemariam S, et al. The use of itraconazole in the treatment of leishmaniasis caused by *Leishmania aethiopica*. Trans R Soc Trop Med Hyg. 1990;84:532–4.

294. Al-Fouzan AS, Al Saleh QA, Najeem NM, et al. Cutaneous leishmaniasis in Kuwait: Clinical experience with itraconazole. Int J Dermatol. 1991;30:519–21.

295. Guderian RH, Chico ME, Rogers MD, et al. Placebo controlled treatment of Ecuadorian cutaneous leishmaniasis. Am J Trop Med Hyg. 1991;45:92–7.

296. Kaufman DL. *Pneumocystis carinii* pneumonia. Adv Exp Med Biol. 1986;202:153–69.

297. King H, Lourie EM, York W. Studies in Chemotherapy: XIX. Further report on new trypanocidal substances. Ann Trop Med Parasitol. 1983;32:117–92.

298. Kager PA, Rees PH, Manguyu FM, et al. Clinical and haematological and parasitological response to treatment of visceral leishmaniasis. Trop Geogr Med. 1984;36:21–35.

299. Hardy WD, Feinberg J, Finkelstein D, et al. A controlled trial of trimethoprim-sulfamethoxazole or aerosolized pentamidine for secondary prophylaxis of *Pneumocystis* pneumonia in AIDS patients. N Engl J Med. 1992;327:1842–8.

300. Pearson RD, Hewlett EL. Pentamidine for the treatment of *Pneumocystis carinii* pneumonia and other protozoal diseases. Ann Intern Med. 1985;103:782–6.

301. Navin TR, Fontaine RE. Intravenous versus intramuscular administration of pentamidine (Letter). N Engl J Med. 1984;311:1701–2.

302. Williamson J. Effects of trypanosides on the fine structure of target organisms. Pharmacol Ther. 1979;7:445–512.

303. Croft SL, Brazil RP. Effect of pentamidine isethionate on the ultrastructure and morphology of *Leishmania mexicana amazonensis* in vitro. Ann Trop Med Parasitol. 1982;76:37–43.

304. Waring MJ. The effects of antimicrobial agents on ribonucleic acid polymerase. Mol Pharmacol. 1965;1:1–13.

305. Wallis OC. The effect of pentamidine on ribosomes of the parasitic flagellate *Crithidia (Strigomonas) oncopelti*. J Protozool. 1966;13:234–9.

306. Gutteridge WE. Some effects of pentamidine di-isethionate on *Crithidia fasciculata*. J Protozool. 1969;16:306–11.

307. Bachrach U, Brem S, Wertman SB, et al. *Leishmania* spp: Effect of inhibitors on growth and on polyamine and macromolecular syntheses. Exp Parasitol. 1979;48:464–70.

308. Waalkes TP, Makulu DR. Pharmacologic aspects of pentamidine. Natl Cancer Inst Monogr. 1976;43:171–7.

309. Geratz JD. Inhibitory effect of aromatic diamidines on trypsin and enterokinase. Experientia. 1969;25:1254–5.

310. Hill GC, Hutner SH. Effect of trypanocidal drugs on terminal respiration of *Crithidia fasciculata*. Exp Parasitol. 1968;22:207–12.

311. Walzer PD, Perl DP, Krogstad DJ, et al. *Pneumocystis carinii* pneumonia in the United States: Epidemiologic, diagnostic, and clinical features. Ann Intern Med. 1974;80:83–93.

312. Western KA, Perera DR, Schultz MG. Pentamidine isethionate in the treatment of *Pneumocystis carinii* pneumonia. Ann Intern Med. 1970;73:695–702.

313. Bouchard P, Sai P, Reach G, et al. Diabetes mellitus following pentamidine-induced hypoglycemia in humans. Diabetes. 1982;31:40–5.

314. Osei K, Falko JM, Nelson KP, et al. Diabetogenic effect of pentamidine: In vitro and in vivo studies in a patient with malignant insulinoma. Am J Med. 1984;77:41–6.

315. Kovacs JA, Masur H. Prophylaxis for *Pneumocystis* pneumonia in patients infected with the human immunodeficiency virus. Clin Infect Dis. 1992;14:1005–9.

316. Keystone JS, Murdoch JK. Mebendazole. Ann Intern Med. 1979;91:582–6.
317. Tankhiwale SR, Kudade AL, Sarmah HC, et al. Single dose therapy of ascariasis—a randomized comparison of mebendazole and pyrantel. J Commun Dis. 1989;21:71–4.
318. Nontasut P, Singhasivanon V, Prarinyanuparp V, et al. Effect of single-dose albendazole and single-dose mebendazole on *Necator americanus*. Southeast Asian J Trop Med Public Health 1989;20:237–42.
319. Abadi K. Single dose mebendazole therapy for soil-transmitted nematodes. Am J Trop Med Hyg. 1985;34:129–33.
320. Pelletier LL Jr, Baker CB. Treatment failures following mebendazole therapy for chronic strongloidiasis. J Infect Dis. 1987;156:532–3.
321. Wilson KH, Kauffman CA. Persistent *Strongyloides stercoralis* in a blind loop of the bowel. Successful treatment with mebendazole. Arch Intern Med. 1983;143:357–8.
322. Levin ML. Treatment of trichinosis with mebendazole. Am J Trop Med Hyg. 1983;32:980–3.
323. Hess JA, Chandrasekar PH, Mortiere M, et al. Comparative efficacy of ketoconazole and mebendazole in experimental trichinosis. Antimicrob Agents Chemother. 1986;30:953–4.
324. Van Hoegaerden M, Ivanoff B, Flocard F, et al. The use of mebendazole in the treatment of filariasis due to *Loa loa* and *Mansonella perstans*. Ann Trop Med Parasitol. 1987;81:275–82.
325. Van Hoegaerden M, Flocard F. Mebendazole treatment of loiasis (Letter). Lancet. 1985;1:1278.
326. Cruz AC. Treatment of human taeniasis in the Philippines: A review. Southeast Asian J Trop Med Public Health 1991;22(Suppl):271–4.
327. Bartoloni C, Tricerri A, Guidi L, et al. The efficacy of chemotherapy with mebendazole in human cystic echinococcosis: Long-term follow-up of 52 patients. Ann Trop Med Parasitol. 1992;86:249–56.
328. Messaritakis J, Psychou P, Nicolaidou P, et al. High mebendazole doses in pulmonary and hepatic hydatid disease. Arch Dis Child. 1991;66:532–3.
329. Wilson JF, Rausch RL, McMahon BJ, et al. Parasiticidal effect of chemotherapy in alveolar hydatid disease: Review of experience with mebendazole and albendazole in Alaskan Eskimos. Clin Infect Dis. 1992;15:234–49.
330. Luder J, Witassek F, Weigand K, et al. Treatment of cystic echinococcosis (*Echinococcus granulosus*) with mebendazole: Assessment of bound and free drug levels in cyst fluid and of parasite vitality in operative specimens. Eur J Clin Pharmacol. 1985;28:279–85.
331. Smego DR, Smego RA Jr. Hydatid cyst: Preoperative sterilization with mebendazole. South Med J. 1986;79:900–1.
332. Sayek I, Cakmakci M. The effect of prophylactic mebendazole in experimental peritoneal hydatidosis. Surg Gynecol Obstet. 1986;163:351–3.
333. Todorov T, Mechkov G, Vutova K, et al. Factors influencing the response to chemotherapy in human cystic echinococcosis. Bull WHO. 1992;70:347–58.
334. Totorov T, Vutova K, Mechkov G, et al. Chemotherapy of human cystic echinococcosis: Comparative efficacy of mebendazole and albendazole. Ann Trop Med Parasitol. 1992;86:59–66.
335. Morris DL. Pre-operative albendazole therapy for hydatid cyst. Br J Surg. 1987;74:805–6.
336. Gill JH, Lacey E. The kinetics of mebendazole binding to *Haemonchus contortus* tubulin. Int. J Parasitol. 1992;22:939–46.
337. Webster LT Jr. Drugs used in the chemotherapy of helminthiasis. In: Gilman AG, Rall TW, Nies AS, et al., eds. Goodman and Gilman's The Pharmacologic Basis of Therapeutics. 8th ed. New York: Pergamon Press; 1990: 959–77.
338. Levin MH, Weinstein RA, Axelrod JL, et al. Severe, reversible neutropenia during high-dose mebendazole therapy for echinococcosis. JAMA. 1983;249: 2929–31.
339. Fernández-Bañares F, González-Huix F, Xiol X, et al. Marrow aplasia during high dose mebendazole treatment. Am J Trop Med Hyg. 1986;35:350–1.
340. el Kalla S, Menon NS. Mebendazole poisoning in infancy. Ann Trop Paediatr. 1990;10:313–4.
341. Rossignol JF, Maisonneuve H. Benzimidazoles in the treatment of trichuriasis: A review. Ann Trop Med Parasitol. 1984;78:135–44.
342. Bassily S, El-Masry NA, Trabolsi B, et al. Treatment of ancyclostomiasis and ascariasis with albendazole. Ann Trop Med Parasitol. 1984;78:81–2.
343. Hui-lan Z, Wei-ji C, Rossignol JF, et al. Albendazole in nematode, cestode, trematode and protozoan (*Giardia*) infections. Chin Med J (Engl). 1986;99: 912–5.
344. Jagota SC. Albendazole, a broad-spectrum anthelmintic, in the treatment of intestinal nematode and cestode infections: A multicenter study in 480 patients. Clin Ther. 1986;8:226–31.
345. Pugh RNH, Teesdale CH, Burnham GM. Albendazole in children with hookworm infection. Ann Trop Med Parasitol. 1986;80:565–7.
346. Raccurt CP, Lambert MT, Bouloumie J, et al. Evaluation of the treatment of intestinal helminthiases with albendazole in Djohong (North Cameroon). Trop Med Parasitol. 1990;41:46–8.

347. Pamba HO, Bwibo NO, Chunge CN, et al. A study of the efficacy and safety of albendazole (Zental) in the treatment of intestinal helminthiasis in Kenyan children less than 2 years of age. East Afr Med J. 1989;66:197–202.
348. Stephenson LS, Latham MC, Adams EJ, et al. Weight gain of Kenyan school children infected with hookworm, *Trichuris trichiura*, and *Ascaris lumbricoides* is improved following once- or twice-yearly treatment with albendazole. J Nutr. 1993;123:656–65.
349. Stephenson LS, Latham MC, Kinoti SN, et al. Improvements in physical fitness of Kenyan schoolboys infected with hookworm, *Trichuris trichiura* and *Ascaris lumbricoides* following a single dose of albendazole. Trans R Soc Trop Med Hyg. 1990;84:277–82.
350. Davies HD, Sakuls P, Keystone JS. Creeping eruption. A review of clinical presentation and management of 60 cases presenting to a tropical disease unit. Arch Dermatol. 1993;129:588–91.
351. Jones SK, Reynolds NJ, Oliwiecki S, et al. Oral albendazole for the treatment of cutaneous larva migrans. Br J Dermatol. 1990;122:99–101.
352. Sturchler D, Schubarth P, Gualzata M, et al. Thiabendazole vs. albendazole in treatment of toxocariasis: A clinical trial. Ann Trop Med Parasitol. 1989; 83:473–8.
353. Kraivichian P, Kulkumthorn M, Yingyourd P, et al. Albendazole for the treatment of human gnathostomiasis. Trans R Soc Trop Med Hyg. 1992;86: 418–21.
354. Chichino G, Bernuzzi AM, Bruno A, et al. Intestinal capillariasis (*Capillaria philippinensis*) acquired in Indonesia: A case report. Am J Trop Med Hyg. 1992;47:10–2.
355. Krepel HP, Haring T, Baeta S, et al. Treatment of mixed *Oesophagostomum* and hook worm infection: Effect of albendazole, pyrantel pamoate, levamisole and thiabendazole. Trans R Soc Trop Med Hyg. 1993;87:87–9.
356. Liu YH, Wang XG, Gao P, et al. Experimental and clinical trial of albendazole in the treatment of *Clonorchiasis senensis*. Chin Med J (Peking). 1991; 104:27–31.
357. Chanthavanich P, Nontasut P, Prarinyanuparp V, et al. Repeated doses of albendazole against strongyloidiasis in Thai children. Southeast Asian J Trop Med Public Health. 1989;20:221–6.
358. Hall A, Nahar Q. Albendazole as a treatment for infections with *Giardia duodenalis* in children in Bangladesh. Trans R Soc Trop Med Hyg. 1993;87: 84–6.
359. Blanshard C, Ellis DS, Tovey DG, et al. Treatment of intestinal microsporidiosis with albendazole in patients with AIDS. AIDS. 1992;6:311–3.
360. Horton RJ. Chemotherapy of *Echinococcus* infection in man with albendazole. Trans R Soc Trop Med Hyg. 1989;83:97–102.
361. Eskazole—Clinical and Technical Review. SmithKline Beecham Pharmaceuticals. 1990:A1–B28.
362. Sotelo J, del Brutto OH, Penagos P, et al. Comparison of therapeutic regimen of anticysticercal drugs for parenchymal brain cysticercosis. J Neurol. 1990; 237:69–72.
363. Escobedo F, Penagos P, Rodriguez J, et al. Albendazole therapy for neurocysticercosis. Arch Intern Med. 1987;147:738–41.
364. Meneghelli UG, Martinelli AL, Bellucci AD, et al. Polycystic hydatid disease (*Echinococcus vogeli*). Treatment with albendazole. Ann Trop Med Parasitol. 1992;86:151–6.
365. Takayanagui OM, Jardim E. Therapy for neurocysticercosis. Comparison between albendazole and praziquantel. Arch Neurol. 1992;49:290–4.
366. Sanchez M, Suastegui R, Gonzalez-Esquivel D, et al. Pharmacokinetic comparison of two albendazole dosage regimens in patients with neurocysticercosis. Clin Neuropharmacol. 1993;16:77–82.
367. Cruz M, Cruz I, Horton J. Clinical evaluation of albendazole and praziquantel in the treatment of cerebral cysticercosis. Southeast Asian J Trop Med Public Health. 1991;22(Suppl):279–83.
368. Cruz M, Cruz I, Horton J. Albendazole versus praziquantel in the treatment of cerebral cysticercosis: Clinical evaluation. Trans R Soc Trop Med Hyg. 1991;85:244–7.
369. del Brutto OH, Sotelo J, Aguirre R, et al. Albendazole therapy for giant subarachnoid cysticerci. Arch Neurol. 1992;49:535–8.
370. del Brutto OH, Sotelo J. Albendazole therapy for subarachnoid and ventricular cysticercosis. Case report. J Neurosurg. 1990;72:816–7.
371. Chung WC, Fan PC, Lin CY, et al. Poor efficacy of albendazole for the treatment of human taeniasis. Int J Parasitol. 1991;21:269–70.
372. de Kaminsky RG. Albendazole treatment for human taeniasis. Trans R Soc Trop Med Hyg. 1991;85:648–50.
373. Lawrenz A, Eglit S, Kroker R. The metabolism of albendazole in the isolated perfused intestine of rats. Deutsche Tierarztliche Wochenschr. 1992;99: 416–8.
374. Jung H, Hurtado M, Sanchez M, et al. Clinical pharmacokinetics of albendazole in patients with brain cysticercosis. J Clin Pharmacol. 1992;32:28–31.
375. Jung H, Hurado M, Sanchez M, et al. Plasma and CSF levels of albendazole

and praziquantel in patients with neurocyticercosis. Clin Neuropharmacol. 1990;13:559–64.

376. Jung H, Hurado M, Medina MT, et al. Dexamethasone increases plasma levels of albendazole. J Neurol. 1990;237:279–80.

377. Ireland CM, et al. The interaction of benzimidazole carbamates with mammalian microtubule protein. Biochem Pharmacol. 1979;28:2680–2.

378. Barrowman MH. The fumarate reductase system as a site of anthelmintic attack in *Ascaris suum*. Biosci Rep. 1984;4:879–83.

379. Morris DL, Smith PG. Albendazole in hydatid disease—Hepatocellular toxicity. Trans R Soc Trop Med Hyg. 1987;81:343–4.

380. Pilar Garcia-Muret M, Sitjas D, Tuneu L, et al. Telogen effluvium associated with albendazole (Letter). Int J Dermatol. 1990;29:669–70.

381. Yoshimura H. Teratogenicity of flubendazole in rats. Toxicology. 1987;43: 133–8.

382. Téllez-Girón E, Ramos MC, Dufour L, et al. Treatment of neurocysticercosis with flubendazole. Am J Trop Med Hyg. 1984;33:627–31.

383. Brown HD, Matzuk AR, Ilves IR, et al. Antiparasitic drugs. IV. 2-(4′-Thiazolyl)-benzimidazole; a new anthelmintic (Letter). J Am Chem Soc. 1961;83: 1764–5.

384. Campbell WC, Cuckler AC. Thiabendazole in the treatment and control of parasitic infections in man. Tex Rep Biol Med. 1969;27(Suppl 2):665–92.

385. Berk SL, Verghese A, Alvarez S, et al. Clinical and epidemiological features of strongyloidiasis—A prospective study in rural Tennessee. Arch Intern Med. 1987;147:1257–61.

386. Barnish G, Barker J. An intervention study using thiabendazole suspension against *Strongloides fulleborni*–like infections in Papua, New Guinea. Trans R Soc Trop Med Hyg. 1987;81:60–3.

387. Gordon HM. Thiabendazole: A highly effective anthelminthic for sheep. Nature. 1961;191:1409–10.

388. Campbell WC, Denham DA. Chemotherapy. In: Campbell WC, ed. *Trichinella* and Trichinosis. New York: Plenum Press; 1983:335–66.

389. Hennekeuser HH, Pabst K, Poeplau W, et al. Thiabendazole for the treatment of trichinosis in humans. Tex Rep Biol Med. 1969;27(Suppl 2):581–96.

390. Criado Fornelio A, Rodriguez Caabeiro F, Jimenez Gonzalez A. The mode of action of some benzimidazole drugs on *Trichinella spiralis*. Parasitology. 1987;95:61–70.

391. Jasra N, Sanyal SN, Khera S. Effect of thiabendazole and fenbendazole on glucose and carbohydrate metabolism in *Trichuris globulosa*. Vet Parasitol. 1990;35:201–9.

392. Manivel JC, Bloomer JR, Snover DC. Progressive bile duct injury after thiabendazole administration. Gastroenterology. 1987;93:245–9.

393. Tchao P, Templeton T. Thiabendazole-associated grand mal seizures in a patient with Down syndrome. J Pediatr. 1983;102:317–8.

394. De Pargament MDM, de Vinuesa ML, Larripa I. Mutagenic bioassay of certain pharmacological drugs. I. Thiabendazole (TBZ). Mutat Res. 1987; 188:1–6.

395. Schneider D, Gannon R, Sweeney K, et al. Theophylline and antiparasitic drug interactions: A case report and study of the influence of thiabendazole and mebendazole on theophylline pharmacokinetics in adults. Chest. 1990; 97:84–7.

396. Austin WC, Courtney W, Danilewicz JC, et al. Pyrantel tartrate, a new anthelmintic effective against infections of domestic animals. Nature. 1966; 212:1273–4.

397. Bumbalo TS, Fugazzoto DJ, Wyczalek JV. Treatment of enterobiasis with pyrantel pamoate. Am J Trop Med Hyg. 1969;18:50–2.

398. Tankhiwale SR, Kukade AL, Sarmah HC, et al. Single dose therapy of ascariasis—A randomized comparison of mebendazole and pyrantel. J Commun Dis. 1989;21:71–4.

399. Aubry ML, Cowell P, Davey MJ, et al. Aspects of the pharmacology of a new anthelmintic: Pyrantel. Br J Pharmacol. 1970;38:332–44.

400. Eyre P. Some pharmacodynamic effects of the nematocides: Methyridine, tetramisole and pyrantel. J Pharm Pharmacol. 1970;22:26–36.

401. Rollo IM. Drugs used in the chemotherapy of helminthiasis. In: Gilman AG, Goodman LS, Gilman A, eds. The Pharmacological Basis of Therapeutics. 6th ed. New York: Macmillan; 1980:1013–37.

402. Royer A. Preliminary report on a new antioxyuritic Poquil. Can Med Assoc J. 1956;74:297.

403. Sawitz WG, Karpinski FE Jr. Treatment of oxyuriasis with pyrrovinyquinium chloride (Poquil). Am J Trop Med Hyg. 1956;5:538–43.

404. Martin RJ. γ-Aminobutyric acid– and piperazine-activated single-channel currents from *scaris suum* body muscle. Br J Pharmacol. 1985;84:445–61.

405. Saz HJ, Bueding E. Relationships between anthelminthic effects and biochemical and physiological mechanisms. Pharmacol Rev. 1966;18:871–94.

406. Nickey LN. Possible precipitation of petit mal seizures with piperazine citrate. JAMA. 1966;195:1069–70.

407. Parsons AC. Piperazine neurotoxicity: "Worm wobble." Br Med J. 1971;4: 792.

408. Wright S, Harman RRM. Ethylenediamine and piperazine sensitivity. Br Med J. 1983;287:463–4.

409. Ottesen EA. Efficacy of diethylcarbamazine in eradicating infection with lymphatic-dwelling filariae in humans. Rev Infect Dis. 1985;7:341–56.

410. Partono F. Treatment of elephantiasis in a community with timorian filariasis. Trans R Soc Trop Med Hyg. 1985;79:44–6.

411. Eberhard ML, Dickerson JW, Hightower AW, et al. Bancroftian filariasis: Long-term effects of treatment with diethylcarbamazine in a Haitian population. Am J Trop Med Hyg. 1991;45:728–33.

412. Kim JS, No BU, Lee WY. Bancroftian filariasis: 10-year follow-up study on the effectiveness of selective chemotherapy with diethylcarbamazine on Che Ju island, Republic of Korea. Bull WHO. 1987;65:67–75.

413. Partono F, Maizels RM, Pumomo. Towards a filariasis-free community: Evaluation of filariasis control over an eleven year period in Flores, Indonesia. Trans R Soc Trop Med Hyg. 1989;83:821–6.

414. Jingyuan L, Zi C, Xiaohang H, et al. Mass treatment of filariasis using DEC-medicated salt. J Trop Med Hyg. 1992;95:132–5.

415. Kimura E, Spears GFS, Singh KI, et al. Long-term efficacy of single dose mass treatment with diethylcarbamazine citrate against diurnally subperiodic *Wuchereria bancrofti:* Eight years' experience in Samoa. Bull WHO. 1992; 70:769–75.

416. Hawking F. Chemotherapy of filariasis. Antibiot Chemother. 1980;30: 135–62.

417. Montestruc E, Blanche R, Laborde R. Action du 1-diethylcarbamyl 4-methylpiperazine sur *Filaria ozzardi*. Bull Soc Pathol Exot. 1950;43:275–8 (cited in Ref. 418).

418. Bartholomew CF, Nathan MD, Tikasingh ES. The failure of diethylcarbamazine in the treatment of *Mansonella ozzardi* infections. Trans R Soc Trop Med Hyg. 1978;72:423–4.

419. Nesarajah MS. Pulmonary function in tropical eosinophilia before and after treatment with diethylcarbamazine. Thorax. 1975;30:574–7.

420. Wiseman RA, Woodruff AW, Pettitt LE. The treatment of toxocaral infection: Some experimental and clinical observations. Trans R Soc Trop Med Hyg. 1971;65:591–8.

421. Taylor HR. Recent developments in the treatment of onchocerciasis. Bull WHO. 1984;62:509–15.

422. Lariviere M, Vingtain P, Aziz M, et al. Double-blind study of ivermectin and diethylcarbamazine in African onchocerciasis patients with ocular involvement. Lancet. 1985;2:174–7.

423. Diallo S, Aziz MA, Lariviere M, et al. A double-blind comparison of the efficacy and safety of ivermectin and diethylcarbamazine in a placebo controlled study of Senegalese patients with onchocerciasis. Trans R Soc Trop Med Hyg. 1986;80:927–34.

424. Dadzie KY, Bird AC, Awadzi K, et al. Ocular findings in a double-blind study of ivermectin versus diethylcarbamazine versus placebo in the treatment of onchocerciasis. Br J Ophthalmol. 1987;71:78–85.

425. Greene BM, Taylor HR, Brown EJ, et al. Ocular and systemic complications of diethylcarbamazine therapy for onchocerciasis: Association with circulating immune complexes. J Infect Dis. 1983;147:890–7.

426. Ottesen EA. Description, mechanisms and control of reactions to treatment in the human filariases. Ciba Found Symp. 1987;127:265–83.

427. Rivas-Alcala AR, Greene BM, Taylor HR, et al. Chemotherapy of onchocerciasis: A controlled comparison of mebendazole, levamisole, and diethylcarbamazine. Lancet. 1981;2:485–90.

428. Dominguez-Varquez A, Taylor HR, Greene BM, et al. Comparison of flubendazole and diethylcarbamazine in treatment of onchocerciasis. Lancet. 1983; 1:139–43.

429. Hawking F. Chemotherapy of filariasis. In: Schnitzer RJ, Hawking F, eds. Experimental Chemotherapy. v. 1. New York: Academic Press; 1963: 893–912.

430. Rée GH, Hall AP, Hutchinson DBA, et al. Plasma levels of diethylcarbamazine in man. Trans R Soc Trop Med Hyg. 1978;71:542–3.

431. Faulkner JK, Smith KJ. Dealkylation and N-oxidation in the metabolism of 1-diethyl-carbamyl-4-methylpiperazine in the rat. Xenobiotica. 1972;2:59–68.

432. Langham ME, Kramer TR. The in vitro effect of diethylcarbamazine on the motility and survival of *Onchocerca volvulus* microfilariae. Tropemed Parasitol. 1980;31:59–66.

433. Hawking F. Diethylcarbamazine and new compounds for the treatment of filariasis. Adv Pharmacol Chemother. 1979;16:129–94.

434. Van den Bossche H. A look at the mode of action of some old and new antifilarial compounds. Ann Soc Belg Med Trop. 1981;16:287–96 (cited in Ref. 387).

435. King CH, Greene BM, Spagnuolo PJ. Diethylcarbamazine citrate, an antifilarial drug, stimulates human granulocyte adherence. Antimicrob Agents Chemother. 1983;24:453–6.

436. Cesbron J-V, Capron A, Vargaftig BB, et al. Platelets mediate the action of diethylcarbamazine on microfilariae. Nature. 1987;325:533–6.

437. Kanesa-thasan N, Douglas JG, Kazura JW. Diethylcarbamazine inhibits endothelial and microfilarial prostanoid metabolism in vitro. Mol Biochem Parasitol. 1991;49:11–20.

438. Fujimaki Y, Ehara M, Kimura E, et al. Diethylcarbamazine, antifilarial drug, inhibits microtubule polymerization and disrupts preformed microtubules. Biochem Pharmacol. 1990;39:851–6.

439. Francis H, Awadzi K, Ottesen EA. The Mazzotti reaction following treatment of onchocerciasis with diethylcarbamazine: Clinical severity as a function of infection intensity. Am J Trop Med Hyg. 1985;34:529–36.

440. Carme B, Boulesteix J, Boutes H, et al. Five cases of encephalitis during treatment of loiasis with diethylcarbamazine. Am J Trop Med Hyg. 1991;44:684–90.

441. Campbell WC, Fisher MH, Stapley EO, et al. Ivermectin: A potent new antiparasitic agent. Science. 1983;221:823–8.

442. Coulaud JP, Lariviere M, Aziz MA, et al. Ivermectin in onchocerciasis (Letter). Lancet. 1984;2:526–7.

443. Taylor H, Pacque M, Munoz B, et al. Impact of mass treatment of onchocerciasis with ivermectin on the transmission of infection. Science. 1990;250:116.

444. Dadzie KY, Remme J, De Sole G. Changes in ocular onchocerciasis after two rounds of community-based ivermectin treatment in a holo-endemic onchocerciasis focus. Trans R Soc Trop Med Hyg. 1991;85:267–71.

445. Taylor HR, Semba RD, Newland HS, et al. Ivermectin treatment of patients with severe onchocerciasis. Am J Trop Med Hyg. 1989;40:494–500.

446. Abiose A, Jones BR, Cousens SN, et al. Reduction in the incidence of optic nerve disease with annual ivermectin to control onchocerciasis. Lancet. 1993;341:130–5.

447. Greene BM. Modern medicine versus an ancient scourge: Progress toward control of onchocerciasis. J Infect Dis. 1992;166:15–21.

448. Pacque M, Munoz B, Greene BM, et al. Safety of and compliance with community-based ivermectin therapy. Lancet. 1990;335:1377–80.

449. Pacque M, Munoz B, Greene BM, et al. Community-based treatment of onchocerciasis with ivermectin: Safety, efficacy, and acceptability of yearly treatment. J Infect Dis. 1991;163:381–5.

450. Somo R, Ngosso A, Dinga JS, et al. A community-based trial of ivermectin for onchocerciasis control in the forest of southwest Cameroon: Clinical and pathologic findings after three treatments. Am J Trop Med Hyg. 1993;48:9–13.

451. Collins RC, Gonzalez-Peralta C, Castro J, et al. Ivermectin: Reduction in prevalence and infection intensity of *Onchcerca volvulus* following biannual treatments in five Guatemalan communities. Am J Trop Med Hyg. 1992;47:156–69.

452. Pacque M, Greene BM, Munoz B, et al. Ivermectin therapy: A 5-year follow-up. J Infect Dis. 1991;164:1035–6.

453. Duke BOL, Pacque MC, Munoz B, et al. Viability of adult *Onchcerca volvulus* after six 2-weekly doses of ivermectin. Bull WHO. 1991;69:163–8.

454. Duke BO, Zea-Flores G, Castro J, et al. Effects of three-month doses of ivermectin on adult *Onchocerca volvulus*. Am J Trop Med Hyg. 1992;46:189–94.

455. Kumaraswami V, Ottesen EA, Vijayasekaran V, et al. Ivermectin for the treatment of *Wuchereria bancrofti* filariasis: Efficacy and adverse reactions. JAMA. 1988;259:3150–3.

456. Ottesen EA, Vijayasekaran V, Kumaraswami V, et al. A controlled trial of ivermectin and diethylcarbamazine in lymphatic filariasis. N Engl J Med. 1990;322:1113–7.

457. Mak JW, Navaratnam V, Grewel JS, et al. Treatment of subperiodic *Brugia malayi* infection with a single dose of ivermectin. Am J Trop Med Hyg. 1993;48:591–6.

458. Hill DR, Pearson RD. Ingestion of *Giardia lamblia* trophozoites by human mononuclear phagocytes. Infect Immun. 1987;55:3155–61.

459. Addiss DG, Eberhard ML, Lammie PJ, et al. Comparative efficacy of clearing-dose and single-dose ivermectin and diethylcarbamazine against *Wuchereria bancrofti* microfilaremia. Am J Trop Med Hyg. 1993;48:178–85.

460. Naquira C, Jimenez G, Guerra JG, et al. Ivermectin for human strongyloidiasis and other intestinal helminths. Am J Trop Med Hyg. 1989;40:304–9.

461. Lyagoubi M, Datry A, Mayorga R, et al. Chronic persistent strongyloidiasis cured by ivermectin. Trans R Soc Trop Med Hyg. 1992;86:541.

462. Okonkowo PO, Ogbuokiri JE, Ofoegbu E, et al. Protein binding and ivermectin estimations in patients with onchocerciasis. Clin Pharm Therapeut. 1993;53:426–9.

463. Klotz U, Ogbuokiri JE, Okonkwo PO. Ivermectin binds avidly to plasma proteins. Eur J Clin Pharmacol. 1990;39:607–8.

464. Chijioke CP, Okonkwo PO. Adverse events following ivermectin therapy for onchocerciasis. Trans R Soc Trop Med Hyg. 1992;86:284–6.

465. Pacque M, Munoz B, Poetschke G, et al. Pregnancy outcome after inadvertent ivermectin treatment during community-based distribution. Lancet. 1990;336:1486–9.

466. Poltera AA, Zea-Flores G, Guderian R, et al. Onchocercacidal effects of amocarzine (CGP 6140) in Latin America. Lancet. 1991;337:583–4.

467. Guderian RH, Anselmi M, Proano R, et al. Onchocercacidal effect of three drug regimens of amocarzine in 148 patients of two races and both sexes from Esmeraldas, Ecuador. Trop Med Parasitol. 1991;42:263–85.

468. King CH, Mahmoud AA. Drugs five years later: Praziquantel. Ann Intern Med. 1989;110:290–6.

469. Pearson RD, Wilson ME. Role of praziquantel in the treatment of helminthic diseases. Int Med Specialist. 1986;7:183–204.

470. Wegner DHG. The profile of the trematodicidal compound praziquantel. Arzneim Forsch. 1984;34:1132–6.

471. Latham MC, Stephenson LS, Kurz KM, et al. Metrifonate or praziquantel treatment improves physical fitness and appetite of Kenyan schoolboys with *Schistosoma haematobium* and hookworm infections. Am J Trop Med Hyg. 1990;43:170–9.

472. Kimura E, Moji K, Uga S, et al. Effects of *Schistosoma haematobium* infection on mental test scores of Kenyan school children. Trop Med Parasitol. 1992;43:155–8.

473. King CH, Muchiri E, Ouma JH, et al. Chemotherapy-based control of schistosomiasis hematobia. IV. Impact of repeated annual chemotherapy on prevalence and intensity of *Schistosoma haematobium* infection in an endemic area of Kenya. Am J Trop Med Hyg. 1991;45:498–508.

474. Simarro PP, Sima FO, Mir M, et al. Effect of repeated targeted mass treatment with praziquantel on the prevalence, intensity of infection and morbidity due to *Schistosoma intercalatum* in an urban community in equatorial Guinea. Trop Med Parasitol. 1991;42:167–71.

475. Homeida MA, el Tom I, Nash T, et al. Association of the therapeutic activity of praziquantel with the reversal of Symmers' fibrosis induced by *Schistosoma mansoni*. Am J Trop Med Hyg. 1991;45:360–5.

476. Watt G, Adapon B, Long GW, et al. Praziquantel in treatment of cerebral schistosomiasis. Lancet. 1986;2:529–32.

477. Richards F Jr, Sullivan J, Ruiz-Tiben E, et al. Effect of praziquantel on the eggs of *Schistosoma mansoni*, with a note on the implications for managing central nervous system schistosomiasis. Ann Trop Med Parasitol. 1989;83:465–72.

478. Fritsche TR, Eastburn RL, Wiggins LH, et al. Praziquantel for treatment of human *Nanophyetus salmincola* (*Troglotrema salmincola*) infection. J Infect Dis. 1989;160:896–9.

479. Farid Z, Trabolsi B, Boctor F, et al. Unsuccessful use of praziquantel to treat acute fascioliasis in children (Letter). J Infect Dis. 1986;154:920–1.

480. Farag HF, Ragab M, Salem A, et al. A short note on praziquantel in human fascioliasis. J Trop Med Hyg. 1986;89:79–80.

481. Botero D, Castano S. Treatment of cysticercosis with praziquantel in Columbia. Am J Trop Med Hyg. 1982;31:811–21.

482. De Ghetaldi LD, Norman RM, Douville AW Jr. Cerebral cysticercosis treated biphasically with dexamethasone and praziquantel. Ann Intern Med. 1983;99:179–81.

483. Sotelo J, Torres B, Rubio-Donnadieu F, et al. Praziquantel in the treatment of neurocysticercosis: Long-term follow-up. Neurology. 1985;35:752–5.

484. Norman RM, Kapadia C. Cerebral cysticercosis: Treatment with praziquantel. Pediatrics. 1986;78:291–4.

485. Vasconcelos D, Cruz-Segura H, Mateos-Gomez H, et al. Selective indications for the use of praziquantel in the treatment of brain cysticercosis. J Neurol Neurosurg Psychiatry. 1987;50:383–8.

486. Joubert J. Cysticercal meningitis—A pernicious form of neurocysticercosis which responds poorly to praziquantel. S Afr Med J. 1990;77:528–30.

487. Santos R, Chavarria M, Aguirre AE. Failure of medical treatment in two cases of intraocular cysticercosis. Am J Ophthalmol. 1984;97:249–50.

488. Kestelyn P, Taelman H. Effect of praziquantel on intraocular cysticercosis: A case report. Br J Ophthalmol. 1985;69:788–90.

489. Groll E. Praziquantel for cestode infections in man. Acta Trop (Basel). 1980;37:293–6.

490. Tesfa-Yohannes TM. Effectiveness of praziquantel against *Taenia saginata* infections in Ethiopia. Ann Trop Med Parasitol. 1990;84:581–5.

491. Heath DD, Lawrence SB. The effect of mebendazole and praziquantel on the cysts of *Echinococcus granulosus, Taenia hydatigena*, and *T. ovis* in sheep. NZ Vet J. 1978;26:11–5.

492. Marshall I, Edwards GT. The effects of sustained release praziquantel on the survival of protoscolices of *Echinococcus granulosus equinus* in laboratory mice. Ann Trop Med Parasitol. 1982;76:649–51.

493. Irie Y, Utsunomiya H, Tanaka M, et al. *Schistosoma japonicum* and *S. mansoni*: Ultrastructural damage in the tegument and reproductive organs after treatment with levo- and dextropraziquantel. Am J Trop Med Hyg. 1989;41:204–11.

494. Staudt U, Schmahl G, Blaschke G, et al. Light and scanning electron microscopy studies on the effects of the enantiomers of praziquantel and its main metabolite on *Schistosoma mansoni* in vitro. Parasitol Res. 1992;78:392–7.

495. Kaojarern S, Nathakarnkikool A, Suvanakoot U. Comparative bioavailability of praziquantel tablets. DICP. 1989;23:29–32.

496. Mandour ME, el Turabli H, Homeida MM, et al. Pharmacokinetics of praziquantel in healthy volunteers and patients with schistosomiasis. Trans R Soc Trop Med Hyg. 1990;84:389–93.

497. Leopold G, Ungethum W, Groll E, et al. Clinical pharmacology in normal volunteers of praziquantel, a new drug against schistosomes and cestodes: An example of a complex study covering both tolerance and pharmacokinetics. Eur J Clin Pharmacol. 1978;14:281–91.

498. Thomas H, Andrews P, Mehlhorn H. New results on the effect of praziquantel in experimental cysticercosis. Am J Trop Med Hyg. 1982;31:803–10.

499. Andrews P. Praziquantel: Mechanisms of anti-schistosomal activity. Pharmacol Ther. 1985;29:129–56.

500. Xiao S-H, Friedman PA, Catto BA, et al. Praziquantel-induced vesicle formation in the tegument of male Schistosoma mansoni is calcium dependent. J Parasitol. 1984;70:177–9.

501. Gardner DR, Brezden BL. The sites of action of praziquantel in smooth muscle of Lymnaea stagnalis. Can J Physiol Pharmacol. 1984;62:282–7.

502. Ruenwongsa P, Hutadilok N, Yuthavong Y. Stimulation of Ca^{2+} uptake in the liver fluke Opisthorchis viverrini by praziquantel. Life Sci. 1983;32:2529–34.

503. Harnett W, Kusel JR. Increased exposure of parasite antigens at the surface of adult Schistosoma mansoni exposed to praziquantel in vitro. Parasitology. 1986;93:401–5.

504. Linder E, Thors C. Schistosoma mansoni: Praziquantel-induced tegumental lesion exposes actin on surface spines and allows binding of actin depolymerizing factor, gelsolin. Parasitology. 1992;105:71–9.

505. Prichard RK, Bachmann R, Hutchinson GW, et al. The effect of praziquantel on calcium in Hymenolepis diminuta. Mol Biochem Parasitol. 1982;5:297–308.

506. Azher M, el-Kassimi FA, Wright SG, et al. Exudative polyserositis and acute respiratory failure following praziquantel therapy. Chest. 1990;98:241–3.

507. Johnson RJ, Jong EC, Dunning SB, et al. Paragonimiasis: Diagnosis and the use of praziquantel in treatment. Rev Infect Dis. 1985;7:200–6.

508. Polderman AM, Gryseels B, Gerold JL, et al. Side effects of praziquantel in the treatment of Schistosoma mansoni in Maniema, Zaire. Trans R Soc Trop Med Hyg. 1984;78:752–4.

509. Farid Z, Wallace CK. Schistosomiasis and praziquantel (Letter). Ann Intern Med. 1983;99:883.

510. Watt G, Baldovino PC, Castro JT, et al. Bloody diarrhoea after praziquantel therapy (Letter). Trans R Soc Trop Med Hyg. 1986;80:345–6.

511. Markwalder K, Hess K, Valavanis A, et al. Cerebral cysticercosis: Treatment with praziquantel. Am J Trop Med Hyg. 1984;33:273–80.

512. Sotelo J, Escobedo F, Rodriguez-Carbajal J, et al. Therapy of parenchymal brain cysticercosis with praziquantel. N Engl J Med. 1984;310:1001–7.

513. Diekmann HW, Schneidereit M, Overbosch D. Inhibitory effects of cimetidine, ketoconazole and miconazole on the metabolism of praziquantel. Acta Leidensia. 1989;57:217–28.

514. Davis A, Bailey DR. Metrifonate in urinary schistosomiasis. Bull WHO. 1969;41:209–24.

515. Omer AHS, Teesdale CH. Metrifonate trial in the treatment of various presentations of Schistosoma haematobium and S. mansoni infections in the Sudan. Ann Trop Med Parasitol. 1978;72:145–50.

516. Feldmeier H, Doehring E, Daffala AA, et al. Efficacy of metrifonate in urinary schistosomiasis: Comparison of reduction of Schistosoma haematobium and S. mansoni eggs. Am J Trop Med Hyg. 1982;31:1188–94.

517. Aden Abdi Y, Gustafsson LL. Field trial of the efficacy of a simplified and standard metrifonate treatments of Schistosoma haematobium. Eur J Clin Pharmacol. 1989;37:371–4.

518. Reiner K, Krauthacker B, Simeon V, et al. Mechanism of inhibition in vitro of mammalian acetylcholinesterase and cholinesterase in solutions of 0,0-dimethyl 2,2,2-trichloro-1-hydroxyethyl phosphonate (Trichlorphon). Biochem Pharmacol. 1975;24:717–22.

519. Nordgren I, Bengtsson E, Holmstedt B, et al. Levels of metrifonate and dichlorvos in plasma and erythrocytes during treatment of schistosomiasis with Bilarcil. Acta Pharmacol Toxicol. 1981;49(Suppl V):79–86.

520. Aden Abdi Y, Gustafsson LL. Poor patient compliance reduces the efficacy of metrifonate treatment of Schistosoma haematobium in Somalia. Eur J Clin Pharmacol. 1989;36:161–4.

521. Katz N, Zicker F, Pereira JP. Field trials with oxamniquine in a schistosomiasis mansoni-endemic area. Am J Trop Med Hyg. 1977;26:234–7.

522. Katz N. Chemotherapy of schistosomiasis mansoni. Adv Pharmacol Chemother. 1977;14:1–70.

523. Omer AHS. Oxamniquine for treating Schistosoma mansoni infection in Sudan. Br Med J. 1978;2:163–5.

524. Kilpatrick ME, Farid Z, Bassily S, et al. Treatment of schistosomiasis mansoni with oxamniquine—Five years' experience. Am J Trop Med Hyg. 1981;30:1219–22.

525. Butterworth AE, Sturrock RF, Ouma JH, et al. Comparison of different chemotherapy strategies against Schistosoma mansoni in Machakos District, Kenya: Effects on human infection and morbidity. Parasitology. 1991;103:339–55.

526. Gryseels B, Nkulikyinka L. Two-year follow-up of Schistosoma mansoni infection and morbidity after treatment with different regimens of oxamniquine and praziquantel. Trans R Soc Trop Med Hyg. 1989;83:219–28.

527. Katz N, Rocha RS, de Sousa CP, et al. Efficacy of alternating therapy with oxamniquine and praziquantel to treat Schistosoma mansoni in children following failure of first treatment. Am J Trop Med Hyg. 1991;44:509–12.

528. Kokwaro GO, Taylor G. Oxamniquine pharmacokinetics in healthy Kenyan African volunteers. E Afr Med J. 1991;68:359–64.

529. Amin A, Mikhail EG. Schistosoma mansoni: Tegumental surface alterations following oxamniquine treatment of infected mice. J Egyptian Soc Parasitol. 1989;19(2 Suppl):815–26.

530. Goble FC, ed. The pharmacological and chemotherapeutic properties of niridazole and other antischistosomal compounds. Ann NY Acad Sci. 1969;160:423–96.

531. Farid Z, Bassily S, Lehman JS Jr, et al. A comparative evaluation of the treatment of Schistosoma mansoni with niridazole and potassium antimony tartrate. Trans R Soc Trop Med Hyg. 1972;66:119–24.

532. Kim JS. Treatment of Paragonimus westermani infections with bithionol. Am J Trop Med Hyg. 1970;19:940–2.

533. Bassiouny HK, Soliman NK, el-Daly SM, et al. Human fascioliasis in Egypt: Effect of infection and efficacy of bithionol treatment. J Trop Med Hyg. 1991;94:333–7.

534. Pearson RD, Hewlett EL. Niclosamide therapy for tapeworm infections. Ann Intern Med. 1985;102:550–1.

535. Hecht VG, Gloxhuber C. Experimentelle Untersuchungen mit N-(2'-Chlor-4'-Nitrophenyl)-5-Chlorsalicylamid, einem neuen Bandwurmmittel: 2. Mitteilung: toxikologische Untersuchungen. Arzneim Forsch. 1960;10:884–5.

536. Perera DR, Western KA, Schultz MG. Nicclosamide treatment of cestodiasis: Clinical trials in the United States. Am J Trop Med Hyg. 1970;19:610–2.

537. de la Torre RA, de la Rua Barcelo R, Hernandez G, et al. Genotoxic effects of niclosamide in Aspergillus nidulans. Mutat Res. 1989;222:337–41.

35. TABLES OF ANTIMICROBIAL AGENT PHARMACOLOGY

GUY W. AMSDEN
JEROME J. SCHENTAG

GENERIC-TRADE NAMES	493
TRADE-GENERIC NAMES	499
ANTIMICROBIAL AGENT PHARMACOLOGY	506
Penicillins	506
Cephalosporins	508
Other β-Lactams	510
Aminoglycosides	510
Tetracyclines	512
Azalides, Macrolides, Lincosamides, Chloramphenicol, and Metronidazole	512
Polymyxins, Vancomycin, Teicoplanin, and Fusidic Acid	514
Sulfonamides and Trimethoprim	514
Quinolones and Urinary Tract Agents	516
Antimycobacterial Agents	516
Antifungal Agents	518
Antiviral Agents	518
ADVERSE DRUG INTERACTIONS INVOLVING ANTIMICROBIAL AGENTS	520
BIBLIOGRAPHY	527

This chapter serves as a centralized source of pharmacologic information on anti-infective agents. If more detailed information is desired on any particular agent, the reader is directed to the appropriate chapter.

Generic and trade name tables for antimicrobial agents are provided. The antimicrobial "family" classification is also included to help the reader locate specific information in subsequent tables.

DOSING GUIDELINES

The selection of an appropriate dose of an antimicrobial agent is based on information such as the site of infection, the identity and known or presumed antibiotic susceptibility of the infecting organism, dose-related drug toxicity, and the patient's ability to eliminate the drug.

Generally, *dosage* selections from the upper end of the dosage range are recommended for severe, life-threatening infections (sepsis, meningitis). Known organisms with intermediate susceptibility (i.e., high minimum inhibitory concentration [MIC]) should also prompt the use of the higher dosages. The lowest dosages are used for urinary tract infections or when the isolated pathogen is extremely susceptible to the antimicrobial. A sizable range in dosing *intervals* exists for some antimicrobial agents, with the longer duration between doses appropriate for less severe infections in which a critical threshold level in serum or other site of infection (e.g., central nervous system) is not mandatory or the drug concentrates significantly at the site of infection (urine, bile). Lower dosages are also appropriate when the patient has impairment in the function of excreting organs.

Dosing recommendations for the following drugs result from preliminary, premarketing clinical trials and at the time of publication have not been officially approved by the U.S. Food and Drug Administration: apalcillin, carumonam, fleroxacin, pefloxacin, teicoplanin, and temocillin. To prevent dosing errors, these recommendations should be checked with recent package inserts or current reference sources.

DOSAGE ADJUSTMENT FOR RENAL IMPAIRMENT

Drug half-life in *adults* with impaired renal function and changes related to dialysis procedures (HD, hemodialysis; PD, peritoneal dialysis) are summarized for the user. An alternative to the elongation of the interval between doses is reduction of the daily dose given at the "usual" dosing interval (Bennett et al.). Antimicrobial serum levels should be determined and patient-specific dosage adjustments made on the basis of these determinations.

Unless otherwise stated, the doses indicated for hemodialysis should supplement "anuric doses." The "usual adult dose" is for parenteral therapy unless designated oral (po).

With the increasing use of chronic ambulatory peritoneal dialysis (CAPD), drug addition to the dialysate solution with direct instillation into the peritoneal cavity is becoming a widely used method of drug delivery. Generally, one adds an amount of drug to dialysate solution to mimic the target concentration. For example, add 5 mg gentamicin per liter of dialysate solution for a desired serum level of 5 μg/ml. A loading dose given IV may be appropriate for severely ill patients, as the addition method is based on steady-state concentrations, and it may not achieve these values for several doses.

BODY FLUID CONCENTRATIONS

In determining the appropriateness of a particular antibiotic for a given site of infection the ultimate concentration of a drug as compared with the MIC for the infecting organism is critical. This is more important than percent penetration as compared with serum. Percent penetration (relationship between peak concentration in a specific body fluid to serum) is, however, a potentially valuable tool for comparisons among similar agents as long as they have similar MIC values.

Generic-Trade Names

Generic	Trade	Class
Acyclovir	Zovirax	Antiviral agent
Acyclovir sodium	Zovirax	Antiviral agent
Albendazole	Zentel	Antiparasitic agent
Amantadine hydrochloride	Symadine	Antiviral agent
	Symmetrel	Antiviral agent
Amdinocillin	Coactin	Penicillin
Amikacin sulfate	Amikin	Aminoglycoside
Aminosalicylate sodium	PAS	Antimycobacterial agent
	Tubasal	Antimycobacterial agent
Amithiozone	Panthrone	Antimycobacterial agent
	Tibione	Antimycobacterial agent
Amoxicillin	Amoxil	Penicillin
	Polymox	Penicillin
	Trimox	Penicillin
	Wymox	Penicillin
Amoxicillin–clavulanate potassium	Augmentin[a]	Penicillin + β-lactamase inhibitor
Amphotericin B	Fungizone	Antifungal agent
Ampicillin	Omnipen	Penicillin
Ampicillin sodium	Omnipen-N	Penicillin
	Polycillin-N	Penicillin
	Totacillin-N	Penicillin
Ampicillin trihydrate	Polycillin	Penicillin
	Principen	Penicillin
	Totacillin	Penicillin
Ampicillin + probenecid	Polycillin-PRB[a]	Penicillin + tubular secretion inhibitor
	Probampacin[a]	Penicillin + tubular secretion inhibitor
Ampicillin + sulbactam	Unasyn	Penicillin + β-lactamase inhibitor
Ansamycin	Mycobutin	Antimycobacterial agent

[a] A combination product.

(Continues)

Generic-Trade Names

Generic	Trade	Class
Apalcillin	—	Penicillin
Atovaquone	Mepron	Antiparasitic agent
Azithromycin	Zithromax	Azalide
Azlocillin	Azlin	Penicillin
Aztreonam	Azactam	Monobactam
Bacampicillin hydrochloride	Spectrobid	Penicillin
Bacitracin	Baci-IM	Polypeptide
Bithionol	Bitin, Lorothidol	Antiparasitic agent
Capreomycin sulfate	Capastat	Polypeptide
Carbenicillin indanyl sodium	Geocillin	Penicillin
Cefaclor	Ceclor	Cephalosporin
Cefadroxil	Duricef	Cephalosporin
	Ultracef	Cephalosporin
Cefamandole nafate	Mandol	Cephalosporin
Cefazolin sodium	Kefzol	Cephalosporin
	Ancef	Cephalosporin
	Zolicef	Cephalosporin
Cefixime	Suprax	Cephalosporin
Cefmetazole sodium	Zefazone	Cephalosporin
Cefonicid sodium	Monocid	Cephalosporin
Cefoperazone sodium	Cefobid	Cephalosporin
Ceforanide	Precef	Cephalosporin
Cefotaxime sodium	Claforan	Cephalosporin
Cefotetan disodium	Cefotan	Cephalosporin
	Apace	Cephalosporin
Cefoxitin sodium	Mefoxin	Cephalosporin
Cefpodoxime proxetil	Vantin	Cephalosporin
Cefprozil	Cefzil	Cephalosporin
Cefsulodin	Cefomonil	Cephalosporin
Ceftazidime	Fortaz	Cephalosporin
	Tazidime	Cephalosporin
	Ceptaz	Cephalosporin
	Pentacef	Cephalosporin
	Tazicef	Cephalosporin
Ceftizoxime sodium	Cefizox	Cephalosporin
Ceftriaxone sodium	Rocephin	Cephalosporin
Cefuroxime axetil	Ceftin	Cephalosporin
Cefuroxime sodium	Kefurox	Cephalosporin
	Zinacef	Cephalosporin
Cefuzonam	Cosmosin	Cephalosporin
Cephalexin	Cefanex	Cephalosporin
	Keflex	Cephalosporin
	Keflet	Cephalosporin
Cephalexin hydrochloride	Keftab	Cephalosporin
Cephaloglycin	Kafocin	Cephalosporin
Cephalothin sodium	Keflin	Cephalosporin
Cephapirin sodium	Cefadyl	Cephalosporin
Cephradine	Velosef	Cephalosporin
Chloramphenicol	Chloromycetin	Chloramphenicol
Chloroquine hydrochloride	Aralen hydrochloride	Antimalarial
Chloroquine phosphate	Aralen phosphate	Antimalarial
Cinoxacin	Cinobac	Quinolone
Ciprofloxacin hydrochloride	Cipro	Fluoroquinolone
Ciprofloxacin lactate	Cipro IV	Fluoroquinolone
Clarithromycin	Biaxin	Macrolide
Clindamycin hydrochloride	Cleocin HCl	Lincosamide
Clindamycin palmitate hydrochloride	Cleocin pediatric	Lincosamide
Clindamycin phosphate	Cleocin phosphate	Lincosamide

ᵃ A combination product.

(Continues)

Generic-Trade Names

Generic	Trade	Class
Clofazimine	Lamprene	Antimycobacterial agent
Clotrimazole	Mycelex	Antifungal agent
	Lotrimin	Antifungal agent
	Lotrisone	Antifungal agent
	Gyne-Lotrimin	Antifungal agent
	FemCare	Antifungal agent
Cloxacillin sodium	Cloxapen	Penicillin
	Tegopen	Penicillin
Co-trimoxazole	Bactrim[a]	Folate antagonists
	Cotrim[a]	Folate antagonists
	Septra[a]	Folate antagonists
	Sulfatrim[a]	Folate antagonists
	Sulfoxaprim[a]	Folate antagonists
	Uroplus[a]	Folate antagonists
Colistimethate sodium	Coly-Mycin M	Polymixin
Colistin sulfate	Coly-Mycin S	Polymixin
Cyclacillin	Cyclapen	Penicillin
Cycloserine	Seromycin	Antimycobacterial
Dapsone	—	Sulfone
Demeclocycline hydrochloride	Declomycin	Tetracycline
Dicloxacillin sodium	Dynapen	Penicillin
	Dycill	Penicillin
	Pathocil	Penicillin
Didanosine	Videx	Antiretroviral agent
Dideoxycytidine (ddC) (see Zalcitabine)	Hivid	Antiretroviral agent
Diethylcarbamazine	Hetrazan	Antiparasitic agent
Diloxanide furoate	Furamide	Antiparasitic agent
Doxycycline calcium	Vibramycin calcium	Tetracycline
Doxycycline hyclate	Doxy-Caps	Tetracycline
	Vibramycin hyclate	Tetracycline
	Doryx	Tetracycline
	Doxy	Tetracycline
Doxycycline monohydrate	Vibramycin monohydrate	Tetracycline
	Monodox	Tetracycline
Econazole nitrate	Spectazole	Antifungal agent
Enoxacin	Penetrex	Fluoroquinolone
Erythromycin	Eryc	Macrolide
	PCE	Macrolide
	E-Mycin	Macrolide
	Ery-Tab	Macrolide
	Robimycin	Macrolide
	E-Base	Macrolide
Erythromycin estolate	Ilosone	Macrolide
Erythromycin ethylsuccinate	EryPed	Macrolide
	E.E.S	Macrolide
Erythromycin ethylsuccinate + sulfisoxazole	Pediazole	Macrolide + sulfonamide
Erythromycin gluceptate	Ilotycin	Macrolide
Erythromycin lactobionate	Erythrocin	Macrolide
Erythromycin stearate	Erythrocin	Macrolide
	Wyamycin	Macrolide
Ethambutol hydrochloride	Myambutol	Antimycobacterial agent
Ethionamide	Trecator	Antimycobacterial agent
Flomoxef	Flumarin	Cephalosporin
Flucloxacillin	Floxapen	Penicillin
Fluconazole	Diflucan	Antifungal agent
Flucytosine	Ancobon	Antifungal agent
Foscarnet sodium	Foscavir	Antiviral agent
Furazolidone	Furoxone	Antiparasitic agent

[a] A combination product.

(Continues)

Generic-Trade Names

Generic	Trade	Class
Ganciclovir sodium	Cytovene	Antiviral agent
Gentamicin sulfate	Garamycin	Aminoglycoside
	Storz-G	Aminoglycoside
	Jenamicin	Aminoglycoside
Griseofulvin	Grisactin	Antifungal agent
	Grifulvin V	Antifungal agent
	Fulvicin-U/F	Antifungal agent
	Fulvicin P/G	Antifungal agent
	Grisactin Ultra	Antifungal agent
	Gris-PEG	Antifungal agent
Halofantrine	Halfan	Antiparasitic agent
Hetacillin	Versapen, Versapen K	Penicillin
Hydroxychloroquine sulfate	Plaquenil sulfate	Antimalarial agent
Imipenem/cilastatin	Primaxin[a]	Carbapenem
Interferon-α-2A recombinant	Roferon-A	Antiviral agent
Interferon-α-2B recombinant	Intron A	Antiviral agent
Interferon-α-N3	Alferon N	Antiviral agent
Iodoquinol	Yodoxin M/	Amebicide
	Diquinol	Amebicide
	Yodoquinol	Amebicide
	Yodoxin	Amebicide
Isoniazid	Laniazid	Antimycobacterial agent
	Tubizid	Antimycobacterial agent
	Nydrazid	Antimycobacterial agent
	Rifamate[a]	Antimycobacterial agent
	Rimactane/INH[a]	Antimycobacterial agent
Itraconazole	Sporanox	Antifungal agent
Ivermectin	Mectizan	Antiparasitic agent
Kanamycin sulfate	Kantrex	Aminoglycoside
Ketoconazole	Nizoral	Antifungal agent
Lincomycin hydrochloride	Lincocin	Lincosamide
Lomefloxacin hydrochloride	Maxaquin	Fluoroquinolone
Loracarbef	Lorabid	Carbacepham
Mafenide	Sulfamylon	Sulfonamide
Mebendazole	Vermox	Antiparasitic agent
Mefloquine	Lariam	Antiparasitic agent
Meglumine antimonate	Glucantime	Antiparasitic agent
Melarsoprol B	Mel B, Arsobal	Antiparasitic agent
Methenamine hippurate	Hiprex	Urinary anti-infective agent
	Urex	Urinary anti-infective agent
Methenamine mandelate	Mandelamine	Urinary anti-infective agent
Methicillin sodium	Staphcillin	Penicillin
Metronidazole	Flagyl	Nitroimidazole
	Metric	Nitroimidazole
	Protostat	Nitroimidazole
	Metro	Nitroimidazole
Mezlocillin sodium	Mezlin	Penicillin
Miconazole	Monistat	Antifungal agent
Minocycline hydrochloride	Minocin	Tetracycline
Moxalactam	Moxam	Cephalosporin
Nafcillin sodium	Unipen	Penicillin
	Nafcil	Penicillin
	Nallpen	Penicillin
Nalidixic acid	NegGram	Quinolone
Neomycin sulfate	Neo-Tabs	Aminoglycoside
	Neo-Fradin	Aminoglycoside
	Neo-Rx Powder	Aminoglycoside
	Mycifradin	Aminoglycoside

[a] A combination product.

(Continues)

Generic-Trade Names

Generic	Trade	Class
Netilmicin sulfate	Netromycin	Aminoglycoside
Niclosamide	Niclocide	Antiparasitic agent
Nifurtimox	Bayer 2502, Lampit	Antiparasitic agent
Niridazole	Ambilhar	Antiparasitic agent
Nitrofurantoin	Macrodantin	Urinary anti-infective agent
	Macrobid	Urinary anti-infective agent
	Furadantin	Urinary anti-infective agent
Norfloxacin	Noroxin	Fluoroquinolone
Novobiocin sodium	Albamycin	Hydroxycoumarin
Nystatin	Nystat-Rx	Antifungal agent
	Nilstat	Antifungal agent
	Mycostatin	Antifungal agent
Ofloxacin	Floxin	Fluoroquinolone
Oxacillin sodium	Bactocill	Penicillin
	Prostaphlin	Penicillin
Oxamniquine	Vansil	Antiparasitic agent
Oxiconazole nitrate	Oxistat	Antifungal agent
Oxolinic acid	Utibid	Quinolone
Oxytetracycline	Terramycin[a]	Tetracycline
Oxytetracycline hydrochloride	Terramycin	Tetracycline
	Uri-Tet	Tetracycline
	Urobiotic	Tetracycline
Para-aminosalicylic acid	PAS, Para, Parasal, Rezipas	Antimycobacterial agent
Paromomycin sulfate	Humatin	Amebicide
Pefloxacin	Peflacine	Fluoroquinolone
Penicillin G Benzathine	Bicillin	Penicillin
	Permapen	Penicillin
Penicillin G + phenoxymethyl penicillin	Kesso-pen	Penicillin
Penicillin G potassium	Pfizerpen	Penicillin
Penicillin G procaine	Crysticillin	Penicillin
	Pfizerpen A.S.	Penicillin
	Wycillin	Penicillin
	Bicillin C-R[a]	Penicillin
Penicillin G sodium	Penicillin G sodium	Penicillin
Penicillin V potassium	Beepen-VK	Penicillin
	Betapen-VK	Penicillin
	Pen-Vee K	Penicillin
	V-Cillin K	Penicillin
	Veetids	Penicillin
	Ledercillin VK	Penicillin
	Robicillin VK	Penicillin
Pentamidine isethionate	NebuPent	Antiparasitic agent
	Pentam	Antiparasitic agent
Phenazopyridine + sulfisoxazole	Azo Gantrisin	Symptomatic bladder therapy + sulfonamide
Phenethicillin	Darcil, Paxipen, Synicillin	Penicillin
Piperacillin sodium	Pipracil	Penicillin
Piperacillin sodium + tazobactam	Zosyn[a]	Penicillin + β-lactamase inhibitor
Piperazine citrate	Antepar	Antiparasitic agent
Polymixin B sulfate	Aerosporin	Polymixin
	Neosporin[a]	Polymixin
Praziquantel	Biltricide	Antiparasitic agent
Primaquine phosphate	—	Antimalarial agent
Proguanil	Paludrine	Antiparasitic agent
Pyrantel pamoate	Antiminth	Antiparasitic agent
	Reese's Pinworm Medicine	Antiparasitic agent
Pyrazinamide	Aldinamid, Tebrazid, Zinamide	Antimycobacterial agent
Pyrimethamine	Daraprim	Antimalarial agent
Pyrimethamine + sulfadoxine	Fansidar[a]	Antimalarial agent

[a] A combination product.

(Continues)

Generic-Trade Names

Generic	Trade	Class
Quinacrine hydrochloride	Atabrine hydrochloride	Antiparasitic agent
Quinine sulfate	Legatrin	Antimalarial agent
	Quin-Amino	Antimalarial agent
	Quinaminoph	Antimalarial agent
	Quinamm	Antimalarial agent
	Quindan	Antimalarial agent
	Quiphile	Antimalarial agent
	M-KYA[a]	Antimalarial agent
	Q-Vel[a]	Antimalarial agent
Ribavirin	Virazole	Antiviral agent
Rifabutin	Mycobutin	Antimycobacterial agent
Rifampin	Rifadin	Antimycobacterial agent
	Rimactane	Antimycobacterial agent
Rifampin-isoniazid	Rifamate[a]	Antimycobacterial agent
	Rimactane/INH[a]	Antimycobacterial agent
Rimantadine	Flumadine	Antiviral agent
Silver sulfadiazine	Silvadene	Sulfonamide
Spectinomycin hydrochloride	Trobicin	Aminocyclitol
Stavudine (d4T)	Zerit	Antiretroviral agent
Stibogluconate	Pentostam	Antiparasitic agents
Streptomycin sulfate	Strycin, Streptolin, Streptoquane	Aminoglycoside
Sufadiazine/sulfamerazine/sulfamethazine	Triple Sulfa[a]	Sulfonamide
Sulfabenzamide/sulfacetamide/sulfathiazole	Dayto-Sulf[a]	Sulfonamide
	Gyne-Sulf[a]	Sulfonamide
	Sulfa-Gyn[a]	Sulfonamide
	Sultrin[a]	Sulfonamide
	Triple Sulfa[a]	Sulfonamide
	Trysul[a]	Sulfonamide
	V.V.S.[a]	Sulfonamide
Sulfadiazine	Microsulfon	Sulfonamide
Sulfadoxine + pyrimethamine	Fansidar[a]	Antiparasitic agent
Sulfamethizole	Thiosulfil Forte	Sulfonamide
	Urobiotic[a]	Sulfonamide
Sulfamethoxazole	Gantanol	Sulfonamide
	Urobak	Sulfonamide
Sulfanilamide	AVC	Sulfonamide
Sulfasalazine	Azulfidine	Sulfonamide
Sulfisoxazole	Gantrisin	Sulfonamide
Sulfisoxazole + phenazopyridine	Azo Gantrisin[a]	Sulfonamide
	Azo-Sulfisoxazole[a]	Sulfonamide
Sulfisoxazole acetyl	Gantrisin	Sulfonamide
Suramin	Germanin	Antiparasitic agent
Teicoplanin	Targocid	Glycopeptide
Terbinafine	Lamisil	Antifungal agent
Terconazole	Terazol	Antifungal agent
Tetracycline	Sumycin	Tetracycline
Tetracycline hydrochloride	Achromycin V	Tetracycline
	Panmycin	Tetracycline
	Robitet	Tetracycline
	Sumycin	Tetracycline
	Tetralan	Tetracycline
Thiabendazole	Mintezol	Antiparasitic agent
Ticarcillin disodium	Ticar	Penicillin
Ticarcillin disodium/clavulanate potassium	Timentin[a]	Penicillin + β-lactamase inhibitor
Tobramycin sulfate	Nebcin	Aminoglycoside
Tolnaftate	Tinactin	Antifungal agent
Trifluridine	Viroptic	Antiviral agent
Trimethoprim	Proloprim	Folate antagonist

[a] A combination product.

(Continues)

Generic-Trade Names

Generic	Trade	Class
	Trimpex	Folate antagonist
Trimethoprim–sulfamethoxazole	Bactrim,[a] Septra[a]	Folate antagonists
Trisulfapyrimidines	Terfonyl	Sulfonamide
Troleandomycin	TAO	Macrolide
Vancomycin hydrochloride	Vancocin	Glycopeptide
	Lyphocin	Glycopeptide
	Vancoled	Glycopeptide
	Vancor	Glycopeptide
Vidarabine	Vira-A	Antiviral agent
Viomycin	Vinactane, Viocin	Antimycobacterial agent
Zalcitabine	HIVID	Antiretroviral agent
Zidovudine	Retrovir	Antiretroviral agent

[a] A combination product.

Trade-Generic Names

Trade	Generic	Class
Achromycin V	Tetracycline hydrochloride	Tetracycline
Aerosporin	Polymyxin B sulfate	Polymyxin
Albamycin	Novobiocin sodium	Hydroxycoumarin
Aldinamid	Pyrazinamide	Antimycobacterial agent
Alferon N	Interferon-α-N3	Antiviral agent
Ambilhar	Niridazole	Antiparasitic agent
Amcill	Ampicillin	Penicillin
Amikin	Amikacin sulfate	Aminoglycoside
Amoxil	Amoxicillin	Penicillin
Ampen	Ampicillin	Penicillin
Ancef	Cefazolin sodium	Cephalosporin
Ancobon	Flucytosine	Antifungal agent
Anspor	Cephradine	Cephalosporin
Antepar	Piperazine	Antiparasitic agent
Antiminth	Pyrantel pamoate	Antiparasitic agent
Apace	Cefotetan	Cephalosporin
Aralen hydrochloride	Chloroquine hydrochloride	Antimalarial agent
Aralen phosphate	Chloroquine phosphate	Antimalarial agent
Arsobal	Melarsoprol B	Antiparasitic agent
Atabrine hydrochloride	Quinacrine hydrochloride	Antiparasitic agent
A/T/S	Erythromycin	Erythromycin
Augmentin[a]	Amoxicillin–clavulanate potassium	Penicillin + β-lactamase inhibitor
AVC[a]	Sulfanilamide	Sulfonamide
Avlosulfon[a]	Dapsone	Sulfone
Azactam	Aztreonam	Monobactam
Azlin	Azlocillin	Penicillin
Azo Gantanol[a]	Sulfamethoxazole	Sulfonamide + symptomatic bladder therapy
Azo Gantrisin[a]	Sulfisoxazole	Sulfonamide
Azo-Sulfisoxazole[a]	Sulfisoxazole	Sulfonamide
Azulfidine	Sulfasalazine	Sulfonamide
Baci-IM	Bacitracin	Polypeptide
Bactocill	Oxacillin sodium	Penicillin
Bactrim[a]	Trimethoprim-sulfamethoxazole	Folate antagonists
Bayer 2502	Nifurtimox	Antiparasitic agent
Beepen-VK	Penicillin V potassium	Penicillin
Benzamycin	Erythromycin	Erythromycin
Betapen-VK	Penicillin V potassium	Penicillin
Biaxin	Clarithromycin	Macrolide
Bicillin	Penicillin G benzathine	Penicillin
Bicillin C-R[a]	Penicillin G procaine	Penicillin

[a] A combination product.

(Continues)

Trade-Generic Names

Trade	Generic	Class
Biltricide	Praziquantel	Antiparasitic agent
Bitin	Bithionol	Antiparasitic agent
Canesten	Clotrimazole	Antifungal agent
Capastat	Capreomycin sulfate	Polypeptide
Ceclor	Cefaclor	Cephalosporin
Cefadyl	Cephapirin sodium	Cephalosporin
Cefanex	Cephalexin	Cephalosporin
Cefatrexail	Cephapirin	Cephalosporin
Cefizox	Ceftizoxime sodium	Cephalosporin
Cefobid	Cefoperazone sodium	Cephalosporin
Cefotan	Cefotetan disodium	Cephalosporin
Ceftin	Cefuroxime axetil	Cephalosporin
Cefzil	Cefprozil	Cephalosporin
Celbenin	Methicillin	Penicillin
Ceptaz	Ceftazidime	Cephalosporin
Chloromycetin	Chloramphenicol	Chloramphenicol
Cipro	Ciprofloxacin hydrochloride	Fluoroquinolone
Cinobac	Cinoxacin	Quinolone
Cipro IV	Ciprofloxacin lactate	Fluoroquinolone
Claforan	Cefotaxime sodium	Cephalosporin
Cleocin HCl	Clindamycin hydrochloride	Lincosamide
Cleocin pediatric	Clindamycin Palmitate hydrochloride	Lincosamide
Cleocin phosphate	Clindamycin phosphate	Lincosamide
Cloxapen	Cloxacillin sodium	Penicillin
Coactin	Amdinocillin	Penicillin
Coly-Mycin M	Colistimethate sodium	Polymixin
Coly-Mycin S	Colistin sulfate	Polymixin
Cosmosin	Cefuzonam	Cephalosporin
Cotrim[a]	Co-trimoxazole	Folate antagonists
Crysticillin	Penicillin G procaine	Penicillin
Cyantin[a]	Nitrofurantoin	Urinary anti-infective agent
Cybis[a]	Nalidixic acid	Quinolone
Cyclapen	Cyclacillin	Penicillin
Cytovene	Ganciclovir Sodium	Antiviral agent
Daraprim	Pyrimethamine	Antimalarial agent
Darcil	Phenethicillin	Penicillin
Dayto-Sulf[a]	Sulfabenzamide/sulfacetamide/sulfathiazole	Sulfonamide
Declomycin	Demeclocycline hydrochloride	Tetracycline
Dendrid	Idoxuridine	Antiviral agent
Diflucan	Fluconazole	Antifungal agent
Dimocillin RT	Methicillin	Penicillin
Diquinol	Iodoquinol	Amebicide
Doryx	Doxycycline hyclate	Tetracycline
Doxy	Doxycycline hyclate	Tetracycline
Doxy-Caps	Doxycycline hyclate	Tetracycline
Doxy II	Doxycycline	Tetracycline
Doxychel	Doxycycline	Tetracycline
Duracillin AS	Penicillin G procaine	Penicillin
Duracillin FA[a]	Penicillin G sodium + penicillin G procaine	Penicillin
Duricef	Cefadroxil	Cephalosporin
Dycill	Dicloxacillin sodium	Penicillin
Dynapen	Dicloxacillin sodium	Penicillin
E.E.S.	Erythromycin ethylsuccinate	Macrolide
E-Base	Erythromycin	Macrolide
E-Mycin	Erythromycin	Macrolide
Ery-Tab	Erythromycin	Macrolide
Eryc	Erythromycin	Macrolide
Erycette[a]	Erythromycin	Macrolide

[a] A combination product.

(Continues)

Trade-Generic Names

Trade	Generic	Class
Eryderm[a]	Erythromycin	Macrolide
Erygel[a]	Erythromycin	Macrolide
Erymax[a]	Erythromycin	Macrolide
EryPed	Erythromycin ethylsuccinate	Macrolide
Erythrocin lactobionate	Erythromycin lactobionate	Macrolide
Erythrocin	Erythromycin stearate	Macrolide
ESP[a]	Erythromycin ethylsuccinate + sulfisoxazole	Macrolide + sulfonamide
Ethril[a]	Erythromycin	Macrolide
ETS-2%[a]	Erythromycin	Macrolide
Fansidar[a]	Pyrimethamine	Antimalarial agent
FemCare	Clotrimazole	Antifungal agent
Flagyl	Metronidazole	Nitroimidazole
Floxapen	Flucloxacillin	Penicillin
Floxin	Ofloxacin	Fluoroquinolone
Flumadine	Rimantadine	Antiviral agent
Flumarin	Flumoxef	Cephalosporin
Fortaz	Ceftazidime	Cephalosporin
Foscavir	Foscarnet sodium	Antiviral agent
Fulvicin P/G	Griseofulvin	Antifungal agent
Fulvicin-U/F	Griseofulvin	Antifungal agent
Fungizone	Amphotericin B	Antifungal agent
Furadantin	Nitrofurantoin	Urinary anti-infective agent
Furamide	Diloxanide furoate	Antiparasitic agent
Furoxone	Furazolidone	Antiprotozoal agent
Gantanol	Sulfamethoxazole	Sulfonamide
Gantrisin	Sulfisoxazole	Sulfonamide
Gantrisin	Sulfisoxazole acetyl	Sulfonamide
Garamycin	Gentamicin sulfate	Aminoglycoside
Geocillin	Carbenicillin indanyl sodium	Penicillin
Geopen	Carbenicillin	Penicillin
Germanin	Suramin	Antiparasitic agent
Glucantime	Meglumine antimonate	Antiparasitic agent
Grifulvin V	Griseofulvin	Antifungal agent
Gris-PEG	Griseofulvin	Antifungal agent
Grisactin	Griseofulvin	Antifungal agent
Grisactin Ultra	Griseofulvin	Antifungal agent
Gyne-Lotrimin	Clotrimazole	Antifungal agent
Gyne-Sulf[a]	Sulfabenzamide/sulfacetamide/sulfathiazole	Sulfonamide
Halfan	Halofantrine	Antiparasitic agent
Herplex	Idoxuridine	Antiviral agent
Hetrazan	Diethylcarbamazine	Antiparasitic agent
Hiprex	Methenamine hippurate	Urinary anti-infective agent
HIVID	Zalcitabine	Antiretroviral agent
Humatin	Paromomycin sulfate	Amebicide
Ilosone	Erythromycin estolate	Macrolide
Ilotycin gluceptate	Erythromycin gluceptate	Macrolide
INH	Isoniazid	Antimycobacterial agent
Intron A	Interferon-α-2b, recombinant	Antiviral agent
Jenamicin	Gentamicin sulfate	Aminoglycoside
Kafocin	Cephaloglycine	Cephalosporin
Kantrex	Kanamycin sulfate	Aminoglycoside
Keflet	Cephalexin	Cephalosporin
Keflex	Cephalexin	Cephalosporin
Keflin	Cephalothin sodium	Cephalosporin
Keftab	Cephalexin hydrochloride	Cephalosporin
Kefurox	Cefuroxime sodium	Cephalosporin
Kefzol	Cefazolin sodium	Cephalosporin
Kesso-mycin[a]	Erythromycin	Macrolide

[a] A combination product.

(Continues)

Trade-Generic Names

Trade	Generic	Class
Kesso-pen[a]	Penicillin G + phenoxymethyl penicillin	Penicillin
Kesso-tetra[a]	Tetracycline	Tetracycline
Lamisil[a]	Terbinafine	Antifungal agent
Lampit[a]	Nifurtimox	Antiparasitic agent
Lamprene	Clofazimine	Antimycobacterial agent
Laniazid	Isoniazid	Antimycobacterial agent
Lariam	Mefloquine	Antiparasitic agent
Larotid	Amoxicillin	Penicillin
Ledercillin VK	Penicillin V potassium	Penicillin
Legatrin	Quinine sulfate	Antimalarial agent
Lincocin	Lincomycin hydrochloride	Lincosamide
Lomidine	Pentamidine	Antiparasitic agent
Lorabid	Loracarbef	Carbacepham
Lorothidol	Bithionol	Antiparasitic agent
Lotrimin	Clotrimazole	Antifungal agent
Lotrisone	Clotrimazole	Antifungal agent
Lyphocin	Vancomycin hydrochloride	Glycopeptide
M-KYA[a]	Quinine sulfate	Antimalarial agent
Macrobid	Nitrofurantoin	Urinary anti-infective agent
Macrodantin	Nitrofurantoin	Urinary anti-infective agent
Mandelamine	Methenamine mandelate	Urinary anti-infective agent
Mandol	Cefamandole hafate	Cephalosporin
Maxaquin	Lomefloxacin hydrochloride	Fluoroquinolone
Maxipen	Phenethicillin	Penicillin
Mectizan	Ivermectin	Antiparasitic agent
Mefoxin	Cefoxitin sodium	Cephalosporin
Mel B	Melarsoprol B	Antiparasitic agent
Mepron	Atovaquone	Antiparasitic agent
Metric	Metronidazole	Nitroimidazole
Metro	Metronidazole	Nitroimidazole
Mezlin	Mezlocillin sodium	Penicillin
Micatin	Miconazole	Antifungal agent
Microsulfon	Sulfadiazine	Sulfonamide
Minocin	Minocycline hydrochloride	Tetracycline
Mintezol	Thiabendazole	Antiparasitic agent
Monistat	Miconazole	Antifungal agent
Monocid	Cefonicid sodium	Cephalosporin
Monodox	Doxycycline monohydrate	Tetracycline
Moxam	Moxalactam	Cephalosporin
Myambutol	Ethambutol hydrochloride	Antimycobacterial agent
Mycelex	Clotrimazole	Antifungal agent
Mycifradin	Neomycin sulfate	Aminoglycoside
Mycobutin	Rifabutin, ansamycin	Antimycobacterial agent
Mycostatin	Nystatin	Antifungal agent
Nafcil	Nafcillin sodium	Penicillin
Nallpen	Nafcillin sodium	Penicillin
Nebcin	Tobramycin sulfate	Aminoglycoside
NebuPent	Pentamidine isethionate	Antiparasitic agent
NegGram	Nalidixic acid	Quinolone
Neo-Fradin	Neomycin sulfate	Aminoglycoside
Neo-Rx Powder	Neomycin sulfate	Aminoglycoside
Neo-Tabs	Neomycin sulfate	Aminoglycoside
Neosporin[a]	Polymixin B sulfate	Polymixin
Netromycin	Netilmicin sulfate	Aminoglycoside
Niadox	Isoniazid	Antimycobacterial agent
Niclocide	Niclosamide	Antiparasitic agent
Niconyl	Isoniazid	Antimycobacterial agent
Nilstat	Nystatin	Antifungal agent

[a] A combination product.

(Continues)

Trade-Generic Names

Trade	Generic	Class
Nizoral	Ketoconazole	Antifungal agent
Noroxin	Norfloxacin	Fluoroquinolone
Nydrazid	Isoniazid	Antimycobacterial agent
Nystat-Rx	Nystatin	Antifungal agent
Omnipen	Ampicillin	Penicillin
Omnipen-N	Ampicillin sodium	Penicillin
Oxamycin	Cycloserine	Antimycobacterial agent
Oxistat	Oxiconazole Nitrate	Antifungal agent
P.A.S.	Aminosalicylate sodium	Antimycobacterial agent
Paludrine	Proguanil	Antiparasitic agent
Panmycin	Tetracycline hydrochloride	Tetracycline
Panthrone[a]	Amithiozone (thiacetazone)	Antimycobacterial agent
Para	Para-aminosalicylic acid	Antimycobacterial agent
Parasal	Para-aminosalicylic acid	Antimycobacterial agent
Pathocil	Dicloxacillin sodium	Penicillin
PCE	Erythromycin	Macrolide
Pediazole[a]	Sulfisoxazole acetyl + erythromycin ethylsuccinate	Sulfonamide + macrolide
Pen-Vee K	Penicillin V potassium	Penicillin
Peflacine	Pefloxacin	Quinolone
PenA	Ampicillin	Penicillin
Penapar VK	Penicillin V potassium	Penicillin
Penbritin	Ampicillin	Penicillin
Penetrex	Enoxacin	Fluoroquinolone
Penicillin G sodium	Penicillin G sodium	Penicillin
Pensyn	Ampicillin	Penicillin
Pentacef	Ceftazidime	Cephalosporin
Pentam	Pentamidine isethionate	Antiparasitic agent
Pentids	Penicillin G	Penicillin
Pentostam	Stibogluconate	Antiparasitic agent
Permapen	Penicillin G benzathine	Penicillin
Pfizerpen	Penicillin G potassium	Penicillin
Pfizerpen A.S.	Penicillin G procaine	Penicillin
Pipracil	Piperacillin sodium	Penicillin
Plaquenil Sulfate	Hydroxychloroquine sulfate	Antimalarial agent
Polycillin	Ampicillin trihydrate	Penicillin
Polycillin-N	Ampicillin sodium	Penicillin
Polycillin-PRB[a]	Ampicillin trihydrate	Penicillin
Polycycline	Tetracycline	Tetracycline
Polymox	Amoxicillin	Penicillin
Precef	Ceforanide	Cephalosporin
Primaquine	Primaquine phosphate	Antiparasitic agent
Primaxin[a]	Imipenem/cilastatin	Carbapenem
Principen	Ampicillin trihydrate	Penicillin
Probampacin[a]	Ampicillin trihydrate	Penicillin
Proloprim	Trimethoprim	Folate antagonist
Prostaphlin	Oxacillin sodium	Penicillin
Protostat	Metronidazole	Nitroimidazole
Pyopen	Carbenicillin	Penicillin
Q-Vel[a]	Quinine sulfate	Antimalarial agent
Quin-Amino	Quinine sulfate	Antimalarial agent
Quinaminoph	Quinine sulfate	Antimalarial agent
Quinamm	Quinine sulfate	Antimalarial agent
Quindan	Quinine sulfate	Antimalarial agent
Quiphile	Quinine sulfate	Antimalarial agent
Reese's Pinworm Medicine	Pyrantel pamoate	Antiparasitic agent
Resistopen	Oxacillin	Penicillin
Retrovir	Zidovudine	Antiretroviral agent
Rezipas	Para-aminosalicylic acid	Antimycobacterial agent
Rifadin	Rifampin	Antimycobacterial agent

[a] A combination product.

(Continues)

Trade-Generic Names

Trade	Generic	Class
Rifamate[a]	Rifampin + isoniazid	Antimycobacterial agents
Rimactane	Rifampin	Antimycobacterial agent
Rimactane/INH[a]	Rifampin + isoniazid	Antimycobacterial agents
Robamox	Amoxicillin	Penicillin
Robicillin VK	Penicillin V potassium	Penicillin
Robimycin	Erythromycin	Macrolide
Robitet	Tetracycline hydrochloride	Tetracycline
Rocephin	Ceftriaxone sodium	Cephalosporin
Roferon-A	Interferon-α-2A, recombinant	Antiviral agent
Septra[a]	Trimethoprim + sulfamethoxazole	Folate antagonists
Seromycin	Cycloserine	Antimycobacterial agent
Silvadene	Silver sulfadiazine	Sulfonamide
Spectazole	Econazole nitrate	Antifungal agent
Spectrobid	Bacampicillin hydrochloride	Penicillin
Sporanox	Itraconazole	Antifungal agent
Staphcillin	Methicillin sodium	Penicillin
Steclin	Tetracycline	Tetracycline
Storz-G	Gentamicin sulfate	Aminoglycoside
Streptoquane	Streptomycin	Aminoglycoside
Streptolin	Streptomycin	Aminoglycoside
Streptomycin sulfate	Streptomycin sulfate	Aminoglycoside
Strycin	Streptomycin	Aminoglycoside
Sulfa-Gyn[a]	Sulfabenzamide/sulfacetamide/sulfathiazole	Sulfonamide
Sulfatrim[a]	Co-trimoxazole	Folate antagonists
Sulamyd	Sulfacetamide	Sulfonamide
Sulfamylon	Mafenide	Sulfonamide
Sulfoxaprim[a]	Co-trimoxazole	Folate antagonists
Sulperazone	Cefoperazone + sulbactam	Cephalosporin + β-lactamase inhibitor
Sultrin[a]	Sulfabenzamide/sulfacetamide/sulfathiazole	Sulfonamide
Sumycin	Tetracycline	Tetracycline
Supen	Ampicillin	Penicillin
Suprax	Cefixime	Cephalosporin
Symadine	Amantadine hydrochloride	Antiviral agent
Symmetrel	Amantadine hydrochloride	Antiviral agent
Synicillin	Phenethicillin	Penicillin
TAO	Troleandomycin	Macrolide
Targocid	Teicoplanin	Glycopeptide
Tazicef	Ceftazidime	Cephalosporin
Tazidime	Ceftazidime	Cephalosporin
Tebrazid	Pyrazinamide	Antimycobacterial agent
Tegopen	Cloxacillin sodium	Penicillin
Terazole	Terconazole	Antifungal agent
Terfonyl	Trisulfapyrimidines	Sulfonamide
Terramycin	Oxytetracycline hydrochloride	Tetracycline
Terramycin[a]	Oxytetracycline	Tetracycline
Tetracyn	Tetracycline	Tetracycline
Tetralan	Tetracycline hydrochloride	Tetracycline
Tetrex	Tetracycline	Tetracycline
Thiosulfil Forte	Sulfamethizole	Sulfonamide
Tibione	Amithiozone (thiacetazone)	Antimycobacterial agent
Ticar	Ticarcillin disodium	Penicillin
Timentin[a]	Ticarcillin disodium/clavulanate potassium	Penicillin + β-lactamase inhibitor
Tinactin	Tolnaftate	Antifungal agent
Totacillin	Ampicillin trihydrate	Penicillin
Totacillin-N	Ampicillin sodium	Penicillin
Trantoin	Nitrofurantoin	Urinary anti-infective agent
Trecator	Ethionamide	Antimycobacterial agent
Trimox	Amoxicillin	Penicillin

[a] A combination product.

(Continues)

Trade-Generic Names

Trade	Generic	Class
Trimpex	Trimethoprim	Folate antagonist
Triple Sulfa[a]	Sulfadiazine/sulfamerazine/sulfamethazine	Sulfonamide
Triple Sulfa[a]	Sulfabenzamide/sulfacetamide/sulfathiazole	Sulfonamide
Trobicin	Spectinomycin hydrochloride	Aminocyclitol
Trojacillin-Plus[a]	Ampicillin probenecid	Penicillin
Trysul[a]	Sulfabenzamide/sulfacetamide/sulfathiazole	Sulfonamide
Tubasal	Aminosalicylate sodium	Antimycobacterial agent
Tubizid	Isoniazid	Antimycobacterial agent
Ultracef	Cefadroxil	Cephalosporin
Unasyn	Ampicillin + sulbactam	Penicillin + β-lactamase inhibitor
Unipen	Nafcillin sodium	Penicillin
Urex	Methenamine hippurate	Urinary anti-infective agent
Uri-Tet	Oxytetracycline hydrochloride	Tetracycline
Urobak	Sulfamethoxazole	Sulfonamide
Urobiotic	Oxytetracycline hydrochloride	Tetracycline
Urobiotic[a]	Sulfamethizole	Sulfonamide
Uroplus[a]	Co-trimoxazole	Folate antagonists
Utibid	Oxolinic acid	Quinolone
Uticillin VK	Penicillin V potassium	Penicillin
V.V.S.[a]	Sulfabenzamide/sulfacetamide/sulfathiazole	Sulfonamide
V-Cillin K	Penicillin V potassium	Penicillin
Vancocin	Vancomycin hydrochloride	Glycopeptide
Vancoled	Vancomycin hydrochloride	Glycopeptide
Vancor	Vancomycin hydrochloride	Glycopeptide
Vansil	Oxamniquine	Antiparasitic agent
Vantin	Cefpodoxime proxetil	Cephalosporin
Vectrin	Minocycline	Tetracycline
Veetids	Penicillin V potassium	Penicillin
Velosef	Cephradine	Cephalosporin
Veracillin	Dicloxacillin	Penicillin
Vermox	Mebendazole	Antiparasitic agent
Versapen	Hetacillin	Penicillin
Versapen K	Hetacillin	Penicillin
Vibramycin calcium	Doxycycline calcium	Tetracycline
Vibramycin hyclate	Doxycycline hyclate	Tetracycline
Vibramycin monohydrate	Doxycycline monohydrate	Tetracycline
Videx	Didanosine	Antiretroviral agent
Vinactane	Viomycin	Antimycobacterial agent
Viocin	Viomycin	Antimycobacterial agent
Vira-A	Vidarabine	Antiviral agent
Virazole	Ribavirin	Antiviral agent
Viroptic	Trifluridine	Antiviral agent
Wyamycin	Erythromycin stearate	Macrolide
Wycillin	Penicillin G procaine	Penicillin
Wymox	Amoxicillin	Penicillin
Yodoquinol	Iodoquinol	Amebicide
Yodoxin	Iodoquinol	Amebicide
Yodoxin M/	Iodoquinol	Amebicide
Yomesan	Niclosamide	Antiparasitic agent
Zefazone	Cefmetazole sodium	Cephalosporin
Zentel	Albendazole	Antiparasitic agent
Zerit	Stavudine (d4T)	Antiretroviral agent
Zinacef	Cefuroxime sodium	Cephalosporin
Zinamide	Pyrazinamide	Antimycobacterial agent
Zithromax	Azithromycin	Azalide
Zolicef	Cefazolin sodium	Cephalosporin
Zosyn[a]	Piperacillin sodium + tazobactam	Penicillin + β-lactamase inhibitor
Zovirax	Acyclovir sodium	Antiviral agent
Zovirax	Acyclovir	Antiviral agent

[a] A combination product.

Antimicrobial Agent Pharmacology: Penicillins

Drug (Oral Absorption, %)	Serum & Urine Concentration; Selected Doses			Dosage Recommendations						
		Peak Serum	Peak or Range, Urine	Adults			Children		Newborn (Parenteral)	
	Dose (g)			Oral	Parenteral	Serious Infection Daily Dose (g)	Oral	Parenteral	Up to 1 wk	1–4 wk
		(µg/ml)		Dose (g)/Interval			Dose/Interval			
Amdinocillin	10 mg/kg	50	1260		10 mg/kg q4–6h			10 mg/kg q4–6h (not approved)		
Amoxicillin[a] (74–92)	0.25 po[b] 0.5 po[b]	3.5–5.0 5.5–11.0		0.25–0.5 q8h		1.5	6.7–13.3 mg/kg q8h[c]			
Amoxicillin/ clavulanate	0.25 po 0.5 po	3.7–4.8 6.0–9.7	381	0.25–0.5 q8h		1.5	6.6–13.3 mg/kg q8h[d]			
Ampicillin[a] (30–55)	0.25 po[b] 0.5 po[b] 2.0 IV	1.8–2.9 3–6 47.6		0.25–0.5 q6h	0.5–2 q4–6h	4 po/12 IV	6.25–25[e] mg/kg q6h	6.25–25[f] mg/kg q6h	25 mg/kg q12h	25 mg/kg q8h
Ampicillin/ sulbactam	1.5 IV 3.0 IV	40–71 109–150			1.5–3.0 q6h	4		25–50 mg/kg q6h		
Apalcillin	2 IV[g]	208	835							
Azlocillin (minimal)	2 IV[g] 3 IV[g]	165 214	2200–8100		2–4 q4–6h	24		75 mg/kg q6h (not approved)[f]	Not recommended	
Bacampicillin[i] (80–98)	0.4 po 0.8 po 1.6 po	5.8–8.3 12.0–15.9 18.6–20.1		0.4–1.6 q12h		1.6	12.5–25 mg/kg q12h			
Carbenicillin	1 IV 3 IV[j]	45–71 278	1000 4165		5–6 q4h	30		25–100 mg/kg q4–6h	66.7–100 mg/kg q8h	400 mg/kg/day q6–8h
Carbenicillin indanyl sodium (30–40)	0.382 po	6.5	0.576–1.13[k]	0.382–0.764 q6h		3				
Cloxacillin[a] (37–60)	0.5 po	6.9–15		0.25–1.0 q6h		2	12.5–25 mg/kg q6h			
Cyclacillin	0.25 po 0.5 po	6–7 11–12		0.25–0.5 q6h		2	12.5–25 mg/kg q6h			
Dicloxacillin[a] (35–76)	0.5 po	10–18		0.125–0.5 q6h		2	3.125–6.25[e] mg/kg q6h			
Hetacillin[l]	0.225 po 0.45 po	1.7–2.1 2.5–2.7		0.225–0.45 q6h		1.8	5.6–11.25 mg/ kg q6h			
Methicillin	1 IV[j] 1 IM 2 IM	59.8 9–18 13.8			1–2 q4–6h	12		25–100 mg/kg q4–6h[m]	25–50 mg/kg q12h	25–50 mg/kg q8h
Mezlocillin	1 IV[j] 2 IV[j] 5 IV[j]	64–143 161–364 199–597	4000		3–4 q4–6h	24		50–75 mg/kg q4h	75 mg/kg q12h	75 mg/kg q6–8h[n]
Nafcillin[a] (36)	1 po 1 IM 0.5 IV[j]	7.7 7.6 40		0.25–1 q4–6h	0.5–2 q4–6h	2 po/9 IV	12.5–25 mg/kg q6h[e]	12.5–25 mg/kg q6h[e]	25 mg/kg q8–12h[o]	25 mg/kg q6–8h[n]
Oxacillin[a] (30–35)	0.25 po 0.5 po 0.5 IV	1.65 2.6–3.9 52–63		0.5–1 q4–6h	0.5–2 q4–6h	4 po/12 IV	12.5–25 mg/kg q6h[e]	12.5–50 mg/kg q6h[e]	25–50 mg/kg q8–12h[o]	25–50 mg/kg q6–8h[n]
Penicillin[a] G (15–30)	400,000 U po 2 mU q2h IV	0.5 U/ml 20		0.5–1 q6h	1–4 mU q4–6h	4 po/24 mU IV	25,000–90,000 U/kg/day in 3–6 doses	25,000–400,000 U/kg/day q4–6h[q]	50,000–150,000 U/kg/day q8–12h[o]	75,000–200,000 U/kg/day q6–8h[n]
Penicillin G benzathine	1.2 mU IM	0.15 U/ml			0.6–1.2 mU IM × 1	2.4 mU		0.6 mU IM × 1[c]		50,000 U/kg IM × 1
Penicillin G procaine	0.6 mU IM 1.2 mU IM	1.6 1.95			0.6–1.2 mU IM q12h	4.8 mU		25,000–50,000 U/kg/day IM[q]		50,000 U/kg/day IM
Penicillin V[a] potassium (60–73)	0.25 po 0.5 po	2.3–2.7 4.9–6.3		0.25–0.5 q6h		2	25,000–100,000 U/kg/day in 3–6 doses			
Piperacillin	2 IV[j] 4 IV[j] 6 IV[j]	159–615 389–484 695–849	8500 14,100		3–4 q4–6h	18		50 mg/kg q4h		
Piperacillin/ tazobactam	3.375 IV[g] 4.5 IV[g]	209 224			3.375 q6–8h	13.5				
Temocillin	0.5 IV[j] 1 IV[j] 2 IV[j]	78 160 236	100–500		0.5–1 q12h					
Ticarcillin	1 IV[j] 2 IV[j] 3 IV[j]	70–100 200–218 257	650–2500[k]		3 q4–6h	18		200–300 mg/kg/ day q4–6h[e]	75 mg/kg q8–12[o]	75 mg/kg q8h if <2 kg; 100 mg/kg q8h if >2 kg
Ticarcillin/ clavulanate	3.1 IV	324	1500		3.1 q4–8h	18.6		50 mg/kg q4–6h		

[a] Decreased rate and/or extent of absorption when given with food.
[b] Fasting.
[c] Children <20–27 kg.
[d] Children <40 kg should not receive the 250 mg film coated tablet.
[e] Children <40–50 kg.
[f] 16.7–33.3 mg/kg q4h for meningitis.
[g] Infusion over 15–30 minutes.
[h] Mean concentration.
[i] 100% of bacampicillin is metabolized to ampicillin.

[j] IV push (over 2–10 minutes).
[k] Over 3 hours.
[l] Hetacillin is rapidly converted to ampicillin.
[m] Depending on severity of infection.
[n] q6h if >2 kg; q8h if <2 kg.
[o] q8h if >2 kg; q12h if <2 kg.
[p] Higher when given with probenecid.
[q] Dosage should not exceed adult dosage.

| Serum Half-life (h) | | | | Usual Adult Dose (g) and Interval Adjustment (h) | | | | | Dosage for Dialysis | | CSF/ Serum (%) Inflamed Meninges | Newborn Serum/ Maternal Serum (%) | Breast Milk/ Maternal Serum (%) | Bile/ Serum (%) | Aqueous Humor/ Serum (%) |
| For Creatinine Clearance (ml/min) | | With Dialysis | | | For Creatinine Clearance (ml/min) | | | | Dose after HD Supplemental to Anuric | Daily Dose During PD | | | | | |
>80	<10	HD	PD	Dose	>80	80–50	50–10	<10 (Anuric)							
0.8–1	3.4–5.6	1.8		10 mg/kg	4	4	6–8	8	10 mg/kg					400	
0.7–1.4	7.4–21			0.25–0.5	8	8	8–12	12–16	0.25–0.5		5–10	25–33	5	100–3000	Negligible
1.1–1.3	7.5			0.25–0.5	8	8	12	12–24	0.25				Low		
0.7–1.4	7.4–21			0.5–2	4–6	4–6	8	12	0.5–2	1–4		100	11	100–3000	2–8
1	9			1.5–3.0	6–8	6–8	8–12	24							
1.5–2															
1	5	1.5–2.6		2–4	4–6	4–6	8	12	3		13.3^h				
0.7–1.4	7.4–21			0.4–1.6	12	12	12					65–75	1.7–3.6	17	
0.78–1	9.4–23.4	6	4.2–7.4	5–6	4	4	2–3 q6h	Avoid	0.75–2	2q6–12h	9.4^i	50–100	0.4	50–75	Up to 3
0.78–1	9.4–23.4														
0.4–0.8	0.8–2.3			0.5–1	6	6	6	6	Usual regimen	Usual regimen					
				0.25–0.5	6	6	12–24	24							
0.6–0.8	1–2.2	1–2.2	1–2.2	0.125–0.5	6	6	6	6	Usual regimen	Usual regimen	Minimal	0–10		5–8	
0.3				0.225–0.45	6										
0.4–0.5	4–6	4–6	4–6	1–2	4–6	6	8	12			10	50–100		≥100	Negligible
0.71–1.3	1.6–14		1.6–14	3–4	4–6	4–6	8	2 g q8h	2–3	3 g q12h	1.2–11.7^i	70–500	Low	1000	
0.5–1.5	1.8–2.8	1.8–2.8	1.8–2.8	0.5–2	4–6	4–6	4–6	4–6	Usual regimen	Usual regimen	9–20	10–15		≥100	Negligible
0.3–0.8	0.5–2	0.5–2	0.5–2	0.5–2	4–6	4–6	4–6	4–6	Usual regimen	Usual regimen		10–15	≤3.5	20–30	0
0.4–0.9	6–20		6–20	1–4 mU	4–6	4–6	4–6	0.5–2 mU q4–6h	500,000 U		0–10	100	6	200–800	
Days											Minimal				
24				0.6–1.2 mU	12	12	12	12							
0.5	7–10			0.25–0.5	6	6	6	6	0.25						
0.6–1.3	2.1–6		2.1–6	3–4	4–6	4–6	8	12	1 g post then 2 g q8h				1	3000–6000	
0.7–1.1	1.9–3.5			2.5–4.5	6–8	6–8								>100	
4.5–5	18–27	4.5		0.5–1	12	12	12–24	36–48	0.5						
0.93–1.3	13.5–16.2			3	4–6	4–6	6–8	2 g q12h	3 g post then 2 g q12h	3 g q12h	39				
1.1–1.5	8.5			3.1	4–6	4–6	2–3.1 g q6–8h	2 g q12h	3.1	3.1 q12			Low		

Antimicrobial Agent Pharmacology: Cephalosporins

Drug (Oral Absorption, %)	Dose (g)	Peak Serum (µg/ml)	Peak or Range, Urine	Adults Oral Dose (g)/Interval	Adults Parenteral Dose (g)/Interval	Serious Infection Daily Dose (g)	Children Oral Dose/Interval	Children Parenteral Dose/Interval	Newborn (Parenteral) Up to 1 wk	Newborn (Parenteral) 1–4 wk
First Generation										
Cefadroxil (100)	0.5 po / 1 po	10–18 / 24–35	1800	0.5–1 q12–24h		2	30 mg/kg/day q12h			
Cefazolin	1 IV / 1 IM	188 / 64–76	4000		0.5–2 q8h	6		25–100 mg/kg/day q6–8h		
Cephalexin (100)	0.25 po / 0.5 po	9 / 15–18	2000	0.25–1 q6h		2	25–100 mg/kg/day in 4 doses			
Cephalothin	1 IM / 1 IV	15–21 / 30	2500		0.5–2 q4–6h	12		80–160 mg/kg/day q6h		
Cephapirin	1 IV	67	2560		0.5–2 q4–6h	12		40–80 mg/kg/day q6h		
Cephradine[a] (>90)	0.25 po / 0.5 po / 1 IV	9 / 15–18 / 86	1600 / 3200	0.25–1.0 q6h	0.5–2 q4–6h	2 po/8 IV	25–100 mg/kg/day q6 or 12h	50–100 mg/kg/day q6h		
Second Generation										
Cefaclor[a] (≥52)	0.25 po / 0.5 po	5–7 / 13–15	600 / 900	0.25–0.5 q8h		1.5	20–40 mg/kg/day q8h[b]			
Cefamandole	1 IV[c] / 2 IV[c] / 3 IV[c]	139 / 214 / 534	750 / 1400		0.5–2 q4–8h	8		50–150 mg/kg/day q4–8h[d]		
Cefmetazole					2 q6–12h	8				
Cefonicid	7.5 mg/kg IV[c] / 0.5 IV / 1 IV	95–156 / 91 / 221	1020		0.5–2 q24h	2				
Cefotetan	1 IV[c] / 2 IV[c]	142–179.6 / 237	1400–2000 / 3500–4000		1–2 q12h	4		40–60 mg/kg/day q12h (not approved)		
Cefoxitin	1 IM / 1 IV[c] / 2 IV[c]	22–24 / 110–125 / 221	3000		1–2 q6–8h	8		80–160 mg/kg/day q4–8h[e]		
Cefprozil (95)	0.25 po / 0.5 po / 1 po	5.6–6.8 / 8.2–10.4 / 15.5–19.9	250 / 1000 / 2900	0.25–0.5 q12–24h		1	15 mg/kg q12h			
Cefuroxime (37–52)[f]	0.5 po / 0.75 IV[g]	7 / 51.1	1150	0.125–0.5 q12h	0.75–1.5 q8h	1 po/4.5 IV	0.125–0.25 q12h[h]	50–100 mg/kg/day q6–8h[i]		10 mg/kg q12h (not approved)
Third Generation										
Cefixime[a] (30–50)	0.4 po tabs / 0.4 po susp	3.7 / 4.6	15.7–305 / 15.7–305	0.4 q24h		0.4	8 mg/kg/day q24h			
Cefoperazone	1 IV[g] / 2 IV[g]	153 / 253	2200		1–2 q6–12h	12		25–100 mg/kg q12h (not approved)		25–100 mg/kg q12h (not approved)
Cefotaxime	0.5 IM / 1 IV[c] / 2 IV[c]	11.7–11.9 / 102.4 / 214.1	90–3261		0.5–2 q8–12h	12		50–200 mg/kg/day q4–8h	50 mg/kg q12h	50 mg/kg q6–8h
Cefpodoxime[k] (50)	0.1 po / 0.2 po / 0.4 po	1.4 / 2.3 / 3.9	60	0.1–0.4 q12h		0.8	5 mg/kg q12h[l]			
Ceftazidime[n]	0.5 IV[g] / 1 IV[g] / 2 IV[g]	42 / 69 / 159–185.5			1–2 q8–12h	6		25–50 mg/kg q8h	30–50 mg/kg q8h[o]	30 mg/kg q8h
Ceftizoxime	1 IV[g] / 2 IV / 3 IV	84.4 / 131.8 / 221.1	>6000		1–3 q6–8h	12		33–50 mg/kg q6–8h[e]		
Ceftriaxone	1 IV[g] / 2 IV[g] / 2 IV[p]	123.2–150.7 / 223–276 / 216–281	504–995		0.5–2 q12–24h	4		50–100 mg/kg/day q12–24h	50 mg/kg q24h	50–75 mg/kg q24h[q]
Moxalactam	1 IV[g] / 2 IV[c]	60–100 / 150–200	2100 / 4200		0.5–4 q8–12h[r]	12[r]		50 mg/kg q6–8h[r,s]	50 mg/kg q12h[r,s]	50 mg/kg q8h[r,s]

[a] Decreased rate and/or extent of absorption when given with food.
[b] Should not exceed 1 g.
[c] IV push (over 2–10 minutes).
[d] Dosage should not exceed adult dosage.
[e] Should not exceed 12 g.
[f] 52% after food.
[g] Infusion over 15–30 minutes.
[h] 0.125 g q12h for children <2 years.
[i] 200–240 mg/kg/day q6–8h for meningitis.
[j] Microbiologic activity in hepatic bile/microbiologic activity serum.
[k] Should be given with food to increase absorption.

[l] No more than 400 mg/d for otitis or 100 mg/d for pharyngitis/tonsillitis.
[m] Creatinine clearance, <30 ml/min.
[n] Arginine component not approved for children <12 years.
[o] 30–50 mg/kg q12h for <2 kg; 30 mg/kg q8h for >2 kg.
[p] 2 g q24h at steady state.
[q] 50 mg/kg/d for <2 kg; 50–75 mg/kg/d for >2 kg.
[r] Bleeding time should be monitored in patients receiving more than 4 g/day for more than 3 days. Prophylactic vitamin K, 10 mg/w should be given to patients treated with moxalactam.
[s] For gram-negative meningitis in children, the manufacturer recommends an initial loading dose of 100 mg/kg.

| Serum Half-life (h) | | | | Usual Adult Dose (g) and Interval Adjustment (h) | | | | | Dosage for Dialysis | | CSF/ Serum (%) Inflamed Meninges | Newborn Serum/ Maternal Serum (%) | Breast Milk/ Maternal Serum (%) | Bile/ Serum (%) | Aqueous Humor/ Serum (%) |
| For Creatinine Clearance (ml/min) | | With Dialysis | | | For Creatinine Clearance (ml/min) | | | | Dose after HD Supplemental to Anuric | Daily Dose During PD | | | | | |
>80	<10	HD	PD	Dose	>80	80–50	50–10	<10 (Anuric)							
1.1–2	20–25			0.5–1	12–24	12–24	0.5 q12–24h	0.5 q36h	0.5–1			50	0.9–1.9	22	
1.2–2.2	18–36			0.5–2	8	8	0.5–1 q8–12h	0.5–1 q18–24h	0.25–0.5		1–4	35–69	3	29–300	<1.7
0.5–1.2	5–30			0.25–1	6	6	8–12	24–48	0.25–1		Minimal	60	2	216	11
0.5–0.9	3–8			0.5–2	4–6	4–6	1–1.5 q6h	0.5 q8h	0.5–2	≤6 mg/ liter to dialysate	1.2–5.6	16–41		22–172	4
0.6–0.9	2.4			0.5–2	4–6	6	8	12	7.5–15 mg/ kg before, then q12 post			60	7		
0.7–2	8–15			0.25–1.0	6	6	0.5 q6h	0.25 q12h	0.25 pre then 12 and 36–48 hr later	0.5 q6h	≤1	9–22	14–20	10–400	5–9
0.5–1	2.8			0.25–0.5	8	8	8	8	0.25–0.5				2	≥60	1–3
0.5–2.1	12.3–18			0.5–2	4–8	6	8	0.5–1 q12h	0.5–1		2		2.4	300–400	1.5
1.2				1–2	6–12	12	16–24	48							
3.5–5.8	50–60			0.5–2	24	8–25 mg/kg q24h	4–15 mg/kg q24–48h	3–15 mg/kg q3–5d	None				<1	<10	0.2
2.8–4.6	12–30			1–2	12	12	24	48	25% nondialysis days, 50% dialysis days				2.3	2–21	
0.7–1.1	13–22			1–2	6–8	8–12	12–24	0.5–1 g q12–48h	1–2		2.8	100	≤3	280	4–7
0.9–1.5	5.9			0.25–0.5	12–24	12–24	50% q12–24h	50% q12–24h							
1–2	20			0.125–0.5 PO / 0.75–1.5 IV	12 / 8	12 / 8	12 / 8–12	0.25 g q24h / 0.75 g q24h	0.75	15 mg/kg post-dialysis	17–88	20–33	≤3	35–80	10–14
2.4–4	11.5	7		0.4	24	24	0.3 q24h	48	None			15–50			
1.6–2.6	2–2.5			1–2	6–12	6–12	6–12	6–12	Schedule dose after dialysis		1.8–3.1	20–50	≤1.5	800–1200	1–6
0.9–1.7				0.5–2	8–12	8–12	12–24	24	0.5–2		27		Up to 3–8	15–75^j	0.5–4
1.9–3.2	9.8			0.1–0.4	12	12	24^m	24	Usual dose 3× wk					102–127	
1.4–2	11.9–35			1–2	8–12	8–12	12–24	0.5 g q24–48h	1 g load then 1 g postdialysis	0.5 g q24h or 250 mg/2 liters dialysate	20–40		7	13–54	3–12
1.4–1.8	25–35			1–3	6–8	0.5–1.5 g q8h	0.25–1 q12h	0.5 q24h	Schedule dose postdialysis	3 g q48h	22.5	28–33	1–6	34–82	3.6–6
5.4–10.9	12.2–18.2	12.2–18.2	12.2–18.2	0.5–2	12–24	12–24	12–24	12–24	None		16–32	18–25	3–4	200–500	
2	20	4	16.7	0.5–4	8–12	3 g q8h	2–3 g q12h	1 g q12–24h	1–2 g post	0.5 g q18–24h	4–55	30–40	2.7	152–224	1–16

Antimicrobial Agent Pharmacology: Other β-Lactams

Drug (Oral Absorption, %)	Serum & Urine Concentration; Selected Doses				Dosage Recommendations						
	Dose (g)	Peak Serum	Peak or Range, Urine		Adults			Children		Newborn (Parenteral)	
					Oral	Parenteral	Serious Infection Daily Dose (g)	Oral	Parenteral	Up to 1 wk	1–4 wk
		(μg/ml)			Dose (g)/Interval			Dose/Interval			
Aztreonam	1 IV[a]	90–164	3000–3500			1–2 q6h	6			30–50 mg/kg q6–12h (NA)		30–50 mg/kg q6–12h (NA)
	2 IV[a]	204–255	5600–6600								
Carumonam	1	190				0.5–2 q8h					
	2	300									
Imipenem	0.25 IV[a]	14–24	50			0.5–1 q6h	2		15–25 mg/kg q6h (NA)		
	0.5 IV[a]	21–58	100								
	1 IV[a]	41–83	≥100								
Loracarbef[c] (90)	0.2 po cap	8			0.2–0.4 q12–24h		0.8	15–30 mg/kg/d q12h			
	0.4 po cap	14									
	0.4 po susp	17									

Abbreviations: NA: not approved.
[a] IV infusion over 15–30 minutes.
[b] 2.7 hours during dialysis.
[c] Decreased rate and/or extent of absorption when given with food.

Antimicrobial Agent Pharmacology: Aminoglycosides

Drug (Oral Absorption, %)	Serum & Urine Concentration; Selected Doses				Dosage Recommendations						
	Dose (g)	Peak Serum	Peak or Range, Urine		Adults			Children		Newborn (Parenteral)	
					Oral	Parenteral	Serious Infection Daily Dose (g)	Oral	Parenteral	Up to 1 wk	1–4 wk
		(μg/ml)			Dose (g)/Interval			Dose/Interval			
Amikacin[a]	0.500 IM	38	832			15 mg/kg/d q8–12h[c]	15 mg/kg		15 mg/kg/d q8–12h[c]	Not approved	Not approved
	7.5 mg/kg IV[b]										
Gentamicin[e]	1 mg/kg IM	4–7.6	113–423			3–5 mg/kg/d q8h[c]	3–5 mg/kg		3–7.5 mg/kg/d q8h[c]	2.5 mg/kg q12h[c]	7.5 mg/kg/d q8h[c]
	1 mg/kg IV[f]	4–7.6									
Kanamycin[a] (1)	7.5 mg/kg IM	22				15 mg/kg/d q8–12h[c]	1.5		15 mg/kg/d q8–12h[c]	15–20 mg/kg/d q12h[c,g]	15 mg/kg/d q8–12h[c]
	7.5 mg/kg IV[b]	22									
Neomycin[h] (3)	4 PO	2.5–6.1			50 mg/kg/d q6h		3 PO				
Netilmicin[i]	2 mg/kg IV[b]	16.6				4–6.5 mg/kg/d q8–12 h[c]	3.9 mg/kg		3–7.5 mg/kg/d q8–12h[c]	4–6.5 mg/kg/d q12h[c,g]	4–6.5 mg/kg/d q12h[c,j]
	2 mg/kg IM	7									
Spectinomycin	2 IM	100				2 g IM/d	2		Not approved	Not approved	Not approved
Streptomycin[k]	0.5 IM	5–12	400			0.5–1 g q12h[c]	1		20–40 mg/kg/d q6–12h[c]		
	1 IM	25–50	≥1000								
Tobramycin[e]	1 mg/kg IM	4–6	75–100			3–5 mg/kg/d q8h[c]	3–5 mg/kg		3–6 mg/kg/d q8h[c]	≤4 mg/kg/d q12h[c]	3–5 mg/kg/d q8h[c]
	1 mg/kg IV[b]	4–6									

[a] Desired concentrations: peak 15–30 μg/ml; trough <5–10 μg/ml.
[b] Infused over 30–60 minutes.
[c] The dosing strategy for aminoglycosides involves the use of ideal (lean) body weight (LBW) for dosage calculation. In obese patients, this approach would result in serum aminoglycoside concentrations less than expected. Alternative dosing recommendations have been proposed that account for the change in drug distribution volume with obesity:
  (1) Lean body weight + 40% of excess weight, defined as total body weight (TBW) minus ideal body weight (IBW) (J Infec Dis 1978; 138:499–505).
  (2) IBW + 58% of excess weight (TBW − IBW) (Clin Pharmacol Ther 1979; 26:508).
  (3) IBW + 38% of excess weight (TBW − IBW) (Am J Hosp Pharm 1980; 37:519–22).
[d] Dosing at CCr ≤10 ml/minute should be assisted with serum concentrations.
[e] Desired concentrations; peak 4–10 μg/ml; trough <2 μg/ml.
[f] Infused over 2 hours.
[g] 15 mg/kg/d q12h for <2 kg; 20 mg/kg/d q12h for >2 kg.
[h] Parenteral administration of neomycin is no longer recommended.
[i] Desired concentrations: peak 6–12 μg/ml; trough <2 μg/ml.
[j] For premature or full term infants <6 weeks.
[k] Desired concentrations; peak 5–25 μg/ml; trough <5 μg/ml.

Serum Half-life (h)				Usual Adult Dose (g) and Interval Adjustment					Dosage for Dialysis		CSF/ Serum (%) Inflamed Meninges	Newborn Serum/ Maternal Serum (%)	Breast Milk/ Maternal Serum (%)	Bile/ Serum (%)	Aqueous Humor/ Serum (%)
For Creatinine Clearance (ml/min)		With Dialysis			For Creatinine Clearance (ml/min)				Dose after HD Supplemental to Anuric	Daily Dose During PD					
>80	<10	HD	PD	Dose	>80	80–50	50–10	<10 (Anuric)							
1.3–2.2	6–9	2.77[b]		1–2	6 h	8–12 h	12–18 h	24 h	⅛ int. dose postdialysis	Usual initial then ¼ usual dose	3–52		0.1–0.6	115–405	5–14
1.3–1.7	11.3			0.5–2 h	8 h	8–12 h	12–24 h	0.25–1 q24h			3				
0.8–1	3.5			0.5–1 h	6 h	0.5 g q6–8h	0.5 g q8–12h	0.25–0.5 g q12h	0.25–0.5 post HD then q12h		1–10			Minimal	3
1	32	4		0.2–0.4 h	12–24 h	12–24 h	24–48 h	3–5 days	0.2–0.4 post HD						

Serum Half-life (h)				Usual Adult Dose (g) and Interval Adjustment					Dosage for Dialysis		CSF Serum (%) Inflamed Meninges	Newborn Serum/ Maternal Serum (%)	Breast Milk/ Maternal Serum (%)	Bile/ Serum (%)	Aqueous Humor/ Serum (%)
For Creatinine Clearance (ml/min)		With Dialysis			For Creatinine Clearance (ml/min)				Dose after HD Supplemental to Anuric	Daily Dose During PD					
>80	<10	HD	PD	Dose	>80	80–50	50–10	<10 (Anuric)							
2–3	30–86			5–7.5 mg/kg	8 h	8–12 h	12–48 h	≥48[d] h	2.5–3.75 mg/kg post	2.5 mg/kg/d	15–24	20		30	Minimal
2–3	24–60			1–1.7 mg/kg	8 h	8–12 h	12–48 h	≥48[d] h	1.0–1.7 mg/kg post-HD	1 mg/2 liters dialysate removed	10–30	30–40		30–60	Minimal
2–4	27–80			7.5 mg/kg	8–12 h	8–12 h	12–48 h	≥48[d] h	4–5 mg/kg post-HD	3.75 mg/kg/d	43	50	35	1	Minimal
2–3	12–24														Minimal
2–2.5	30			2–2.2 mg/kg	8 h	8–12 h	12–48 h	≥48[d] h	2 mg/kg post-HD		21–26				Minimal
1.2–2.8				2	24 h	24 h	24 h	24 h							Minimal
2–3	Up to 110			0.5–1	12 h	7.5 mg/kg q24h	7.5 mg/kg q24	7.5 mg/kg q72–96h	0.5 g post-HD		20	10–40	<25	40–300	Minimal
2–3	5–70			1–1.7 mg/kg	8 h	8–12 h	12–48 h	≥48 h	1 mg/kg post-HD	1 mg/2 liters dialysate removed	14–23	50		10–20	18

Antimicrobial Agent Pharmacology: Tetracyclines[a]

Drug (Oral Absorption, %)	Dose (g)	Peak Serum	Peak or Range, Urine	Adults Oral	Adults Parenteral	Serious Infection Daily Dose (g)	Children Oral	Children Parenteral	Newborn (Parenteral) Up to 1 wk	Newborn (Parenteral) 1–4 wk
		(μg/ml)		Dose (g)/Interval			Dose/Interval			
Chlortetracycline[b] (30)	0.25 po 0.5 po	1.5–2.5 7	320	See tetracycline		2	See tetracycline		Not recommended	
Demeclocycline[b] (60–80)	0.15 po 0.3 po	0.9–1.2 1.5–1.7		0.6/d q6–12h		0.6	6.6–13.2 mg/kg/d q6–12h		Not recommended	
Doxycycline (90–100)	0.1 po 0.1 IV[d]	1.5–2.1 2.5		0.1 q12h	0.1 q12h	0.2	2.2 mg/kg q12–24h	2.2 mg/kg q12–24h	Not recommended	
Methacycline[b] (58)	0.15 po 0.3 po	1.3 2.4		0.15 q6h or 0.3 q12h		1.2	6.6–13.2 mg/kg/d q6–12h		Not recommended	
Minocycline (90–100)	0.2 po	2–3.5		0.1 q12h	0.1 q12h	0.2	2 mg/kg q12h	2 mg/kg q12h	Not recommended	
Oxytetracycline[b] (60)	0.25 po 0.5 po	1.3–1.4 4–4.2		1–2/d q6h	0.25 IM q24h	2	25–50 mg/kg/d q6h	15–25 mg/kg/d q8–12h[e]	Not recommended	
Tetracycline[b] (75–80)	0.25 po 0.5 po 0.5 po[f]	1.5–2.2 3–4.3 2–5		0.25–0.5 q6h		2	25–50 mg/kg/d q6–12h		Not recommended	

[a] The tetracyclines cause a brown discoloration of the teeth and may retard the growth of bone in the human fetus and children. The American Academy of Pediatrics recommends that tetracyclines be used in children who are 9 years of age or older.
[b] All tetracyclines should be given 1 hour before or 2 hours after meals.
[c] Patients in the convalescent stage of poliomyelitis.
[d] Infused over 60 minutes.
[e] No more than 250 mg/day.
[f] At steady-state.

Antimicrobial Agent Pharmacology: Azalides, Macrolides, Lincosamides, Chloramphenicol, and Metronidazole

Drug (Oral Absorption, %)	Dose (g)	Peak Serum	Peak or Range, Urine	Adults Oral	Adults Parenteral	Serious Infection Daily Dose (g)	Children Oral	Children Parenteral	Newborn (Parenteral) Up to 1 wk	Newborn (Parenteral) 1–4 wk
		(μg/ml)		Dose (g)/Interval			Dose/Interval			
Azithromycin[a] (35–40)	0.5 po	.09–0.44	8.64–26.8	0.5 d1 then 0.25 d2–5		1.5/5 days				
Clarithromycin (50–55)	0.25 po[b] 0.5 po[b] 0.5 po[b]	1 2–3 1[c]		0.25–0.5 q12h		1	7.5 mg/kg q12h (not approved)			
Erythromycin base[a,d]	0.25 po	0.1–2		0.25–0.5 q6h		2	30–50 mg/kg/d q6h			
Erythromycin stearate[d]	0.25 po	0.1–2		0.25–0.5 q6h		2	30–50 mg/kg/d q6h			
Erythromycin ethyl succinate[d]	0.4 po	0.1–2		0.4 q6h		2	30–50 mg/kg/d q6h			
Erythromycin lactobionate[e,f]	0.2 IV	3–4			0.5–1 q6h	4		15–20 mg/kg/d q6h		
Erythromycin gluceptate[e]	0.2 IV	3–4			15–20 mg/kg/d q6h	4		15–20 mg/kg/d q6h		
Erythromycin estolate[d]	0.25 po	0.1–2[g]		0.25–0.5 q6h		2	30–50 mg/kg/d q6h			
Clindamycin[a] (90)	0.15 po 0.6 IV[h]	1.9–3.9 10		0.15–0.3 q6h	0.3–0.9 q6–8h	1.2 po/2.7 IV	8–25 mg/kg/d q6–8h	15–40 mg/kg/d q6–8h	15 mg/kg/d q6–8h[j]	15–20 mg/kg/d q6–8h[j]
Lincomycin[a] (20–30)	0.5 po 0.6 IM 0.6 IV[k]	1.8–5.3 9.3–18.5 15.9–20.9		0.5 q6–8h	0.6–1 q8–12h	8	30–60 mg/kg/d q6–8h	10–20 mg/kg/d q8–12h	Not indicated	
Chloramphenicol[l] (75–90)	1 po 1 po[b] 1 IV	11 18 4.9–12		0.25–0.75 q6h	0.25–1 q6h	4	50–100 mg/kg/d q6h	50–100 mg/kg/d q6h	25 mg/kg/d q24h[m]	50 mg/kg/d q12–24h[n]
Metronidazole[a] (80)	0.25 po 7.5 mg/kg[b]	4.6–6.5 26		0.25–0.5 q6–12h	0.5 q6–8h	30 mg/kg				

[a] Denotes decreased rate and/or extent of absorption when given with food.
[b] At steady state.
[c] Of 14-hydroxyclarithromycin (active metabolite).
[d] Erythromycin and its derivatives have varying degrees of bioavailability (18%–45%).
[e] Oral erythromycin therapy should replace IV therapy as soon as possible.
[f] Due to the local irritative effects, the drug must not be administered rapidly by direct IV injection (IV push).
[g] Higher serum concentrations have been reported in patients taking erythromycin estolate vs. other derivatives.
[h] Over 20 minutes.
[i] In premature neonates.
[j] When IV clindamycin is given to neonates and infants, organ system functions should be monitored.
[k] When given over 2 hours.
[l] Chloramphenicol dosage should be administered to maintain plasma concentrations at 5–20 μg/ml.
[m] <2 wks.
[n] >2 wks.

Serum Half-life (h)				Usual Adult Dose (g) and Interval Adjustment					Dosage for Dialysis		CSF/Serum (%) Inflamed Meninges	Newborn Serum/Maternal Serum (%)	Breast Milk/Maternal Serum (%)	Bile/Serum (%)	Aqueous Humor/Serum (%)
For Creatinine Clearance (ml/min)		With Dialysis			For Creatinine Clearance (ml/min)				Dose after HD Supplemental to Anuric	Daily Dose During PD					
>80	<10	HD	PD	Dose	>80	80–50	50–10	<10 (Anuric)							
5.6	6.8–11			0.25–0.5	6 h	Not recommended					2–6[c]		40	333	
10–17	42–68			0.15–0.3	6–12 h	Not recommended					Minimal		70	200–3200	10–30
14–24	18–30	18–30		0.1	12 h	12 h	12 h	12 h	0.1 g q12h	0.1 g q12h	26		30–40	200–3200	10–13
7–15	Up to 44			0.15–0.3	6–12 h	Not recommended									
11–26	12–30			0.1	12 h	12 h	12 h	12 h	0.1 g q12h	0.1 g q12h		77	8–26	200–3200	17
6–10	47–66			0.25–0.5 po / 0.25 IM	6 h / 24 h	6 h / 24 h	Use doxycycline				Minimal		20–140	200–3200	
6–12	57–120			0.25–0.5	6 h	6 h	Use doxycycline				7	60–70	25–150	200–3200	9–11

Serum Half-life (h)				Usual Adult Dose (g) and Interval Adjustment					Dosage for Dialysis		CSF/Serum (%) Inflamed Meninges	Newborn Serum/Maternal Serum (%)	Breast Milk/Maternal Serum (%)	Bile/Serum (%)	Aqueous Humor/Serum (%)
For Creatinine Clearance (ml/min)		With Dialysis			For Creatinine Clearance (ml/min)				Dose after HD Supplemental to Anuric	Daily Dose During PD					
>80	<10	HD	PD	Dose	>80	80–50	50–10	<10 (Anuric)							
79				0.5 Day 1, then 0.25/d × 4 d	Usual	Usual									
5–7				0.25–0.5	12 h	12 h	12–24 h	24 h			Minimal		30	7000	
1.5–2	6			0.25–0.5	6 h	6 h	6 h	6 h	Usual regimen	Usual regimen	2–13	5–20	50		
1.5–2	6			0.25–0.5	6 h	6 h	6 h	6 h	Usual regimen	Usual regimen	2–13	5–20	50		
1.5–2	6			0.4	6 h	6 h	6 h	6 h	Usual regimen	Usual regimen	2–13	5–20	50		
1.5–2	6			0.5–1	6 h	6 h	6 h	6 h	Usual regimen	Usual regimen	2–13	5–20	50		
1.5–2	6			15–20 mg/kg/day	6 h	6 h	6 h	6 h	Usual regimen	Usual regimen	2–13	5–20	50		
1.5–2	6			0.25–0.5	6 h	6 h	6 h	6 h	Usual regimen	Usual regimen	2–13	5–20	50		
2–3	2–3.5			0.15–0.3 po / 0.3–0.9 IV	6 h / 6–8 h	6 h / 6–8 h	6 h / 6–8 h	6 h / 6–8 h	Usual regimen	Usual regimen	Minimal	46	38–50	250–300	
4–6.4	10			0.5 po / 0.6–1 IV	6–8 h / 8–12 h	6–8 h / 8–12 h	6–8 h / 8–12 h	24 h / 24–36 h			18	25	13	250–400	8.75
1.5–4.1	3–7		3–7	0.25–0.75 po / 0.25–1 IV	6 h / 6 h	6 h / 6 h	6 h / 6 h	6 h / 6 h	Schedule dose post-HD	Usual regimen	45–89	30–80	100		
6–14	8–15		8–15	0.25–0.5 po / 0.5 IV	8 h / 6–8 h	8 h / 6–8 h	8 h / 6–8 h	8 h / 6–8 h	Usual regimen	Usual regimen	≥100	97	100	100	33–50

Antimicrobial Agent Pharmacology: Polymixins, Vancomycin, Teicoplanin, and Fusidic Acid

Drug (Oral Absorption, %)	Serum & Urine Concentration; Selected Doses			Dosage Recommendations						
		Peak Serum	Peak or Range, Urine	Adults			Children		Newborn (Parenteral)	
				Oral	Parenteral	Serious Infection Daily Dose (g)	Oral	Parenteral	Up to 1 wk	1–4 wk
	Dose (g)	(µg/ml)		Dose (g)/Interval			Dose/Interval			
Colistimethate^a	0.15 IM	5–7.5	200–270	5–15 mg/kg/d q8h^b	2.5–5 mg/kg/d q6–12h	5 mg/kg	5–15 mg/kg/d q8h^b	2.5–5 mg/kg/d q6–12h	Not recommended	
Polymixin B^c	20,000–40,000 U/kg/IM	1–8			15,000–25,000 U/kg/d q12h			15,000–25,000 U/kg/d q12h	Not recommended	
Vancomycin (minimal)	1 IV	25		0.5–2 g/d q6–8h	1 g q12h	1 po/2 IV	40 mg/kg/d q6–8h^e	40 mg/kg/d q6–12h	15 mg/kg load then 10 mg/kg q12h	10 mg/kg q8h
Teicoplanin	3 mg/kg IV^f 6 mg/kg IV^f	53 112			0.2–0.4 q24h			10 mg/kg q24h	6 mg/kg q24h (preliminary)	6 mg/kg q24h (preliminary)
Fusidic acid	0.5 po	14–38^g	<1	0.5–1 q8h	0.58 q8h^h		6.6–16.6 mg/kg q8h	6.6 mg/kg q8h		

^a Colistimethate is the sulfamethyl derivative of colistin; colistin is absorbed to some extent in infants.
^b Of colistin.
^c Bioavailability can be up to 10% in infants.
^d For CCr 5–20 ml/min dose should be 7500–12,500 U/kg/d q12h.
^e Not to exceed 2 g/d.
^f 5 minute infusion.
^g Accumulation occurs with multiple doses of 0.5 g given q8h; a mean serum concentration of 71 µg/ml has been reported after 96 hours of therapy.
^h Diethanolamine fusidate, 580 mg = 500 mg sodium fusidate.

Antimicrobial Agent Pharmacology: Sulfonamides and Trimethoprim

Drug (Oral Absorption, %)	Serum & Urine Concentration; Selected Doses			Dosage Recommendations						
		Peak Serum	Peak or Range, Urine	Adults			Children		Newborn (Parenteral)	
				Oral	Parenteral	Serious Infection Daily Dose (g)	Oral	Parenteral	Up to 1 wk	1–4 wk
	Dose (g)	(µg/ml)		Dose (g)/Interval			Dose/Interval			
Trimethoprim–Sulfamethoxazole (85–90)^a	0.16/0.8 po 0.16/0.8 IV	1–2/40–60^b 9/105^b		0.16/0.8 q12–24h	3–5 mg/kg q 6–8h^c	1.2 IV^c	6–12 mg/kg/d q6–12h^c	6–12 mg/kg/d q6–12h^c	Not recommended	
Trimethoprim (80)	0.1 po 0.2 po	1 2	30–160	0.1 q12h		0.2	4 mg/kg/d q12h^f			
Sulfisoxazole^a (70–90)	2–4 po 2–4 IM	11.2–25 11.2–25		0.5–1 q6h	25 mg/kg q6h	4	120–150 mg/kg/d q4–6h		Not recommended	
Sulfamethoxazole^a (70–90)	2 po	50–120		1 q8–12h		3	50–60 mg/kg/d q12h		Not recommended	
Sulfamethizole^a (70–90)	2 po	60		0.5–1 q6–8 h		6	30–45 mg/kg/d q6h		Not recommended	
Sulfacytine^a (70–90)	0.25 po	17	420	0.5 load then 0.25 q6h		1	Not recommended		Not recommended	
Sulfadiazine^a (70–90)	3 po	50		2–4 g/day q4–8h		4	120–150 mg/kg/d q4–6h	100 mg/kg/d q6–8h	Not recommended	
Sulfadoxine^a,g (70–90)	0.5 po^h	51–76		1 tablet qwk or 2 tablets qowk		1.5	By age^i		Not recommended	
Sulfasalazine (10–15)	2 po	14/21^j		0.5–1 q4–6h		4^k	30–60 mg/kg/d q4–8h		Not recommended	
Sulfaphenazole^a (70–90)	2 po	100–150		1 q12h.		2	66 mg/kg, then 33 mg/kg q12h		Not recommended	
Dapsone	0.2 po	0.1–7^b		0.05–0.1 q24h		0.1	1–2 mg/kg/d q24h			

^a Denotes decreased rate and/or extent of absorption when given with food.
^b At steady/state.
^c Based on the trimethoprim component.
^d Uninflamed meninges.
^e Amniotic fluid concentration (µg/ml).
^f Not approved for children <12 years.
^g For malaria prophylaxis. The first dose should be given 1–2 days before departure to an endemic area and the course continued throughout the stay and 4–6 weeks thereafter.
^h One tablet = 500 mg sulfadoxine and 25 mg pyrimethamine.
^i Under 4 years: ¼ tablet weekly or ½ tablet every other week; 4–8 years: ½ tablet weekly or 1 tablet every other week; 9–14 years: ¾ tablet weekly or 1½ tablets every other week.
^j Sulfasalazine/sulfapyridine.
^k Although doses up to 12 g have been administered, a daily dosage exceeding 4 g is associated with an increased incidence of adverse effects.
^l Sulfapyridine.

| Serum Half-life (h) | | | | Usual Adult Dose (g) and Interval Adjustment | | | | | Dosage for Dialysis | | CSF/ Serum (%) Inflamed Meninges | Newborn Serum/ Maternal Serum (%) | Breast Milk/ Maternal Serum (%) | Bile/ Serum (%) | Aqueous Humor/ Serum (%) |
| For Creatinine Clearance (ml/min) | | With Dialysis | | | For Creatinine Clearance (ml/min) | | | | Dose after HD Supplemental to Anuric | Daily Dose During PD | | | | | |
>80	<10	HD	PD	Dose	>80	80–50	50–10	<10 (Anuric)							
1.5–8	48–72			2.5–5 mg/kg/d	6–12 h	2.5–3.8 mg/kg/d q12h	2.5 mg/kg/d q12–24h	1.5 mg/kg q36h			Minimal	50	18		25–30
4.3–6	48–72			15,000–25,000 U/kg/d	12 h	12 h	12ᵈ h	2250–3750 U/kg/d q12h			Minimal				
4–6	44.1–406.4			15 mg/kg	12 h	See the nomogram in Chapter 25 or *Antimicrob Agents Chemother* 1984; 25:433			1 g/wk	0.5–1 g/wk	7.21			50	Minimal
40–70	125	163		0.4	24 h	48 h	48 h	72 h							
				0.5–1 po	8 h	8 h	8 h	8 h							

| Serum Half-life (h) | | | | Usual Adult Dose (g) and Interval Adjustment | | | | | Dosage for Dialysis | | CSF/ Serum (%) Inflamed Meninges | Newborn Serum/ Maternal Serum (%) | Breast Milk/ Maternal Serum (%) | Bile/ Serum (%) | Aqueous Humor/ Serum (%) |
| For Creatinine Clearance (ml/min) | | With Dialysis | | | For Creatinine Clearance (ml/min) | | | | Dose after HD Supplemental to Anuric | Daily Dose During PD | | | | | |
>80	<10	HD	PD	Dose	>80	80–50	50–10	<10 (Anuric)							
8–15/7–12	24/22–50			3–5 mg/kg IVᶜ	6–12 h	18 h	24 h	Avoid	4–5 mg/kg post-HDᶜ	0.16/0.8 q48h	50/40ᵈ	80/50ᵉ	125/10	100–200/40–70	10–45/20–30
8–15	24			0.1	12 h	1 h2	18–24 h	Avoid			30–50	70–100	100	100	10
3–7	6–12			1–2	6 h	6 h	1 q8–12h	1 q12–24h			8–57ᵈ	≥50	10	40–70	20–30
7–12	22–50			1	8–12 h						25–30	≥50			
4–8	58			0.5–1	6–8 h							≥50			
4–8				0.25	6 h							≥50			
17	34			0.5–1	4–6 h						50–80	≥50			
100–231				0.5 po / 1 po	q wk / qo wk							≥50			
7.6/10.4ʲ				0.5–1	4–6 h							≥50	30–60ʲ		
				1	12 h							≥50			
20–30				0.05–0.1	24 h	24 h	24 h						69		

Antimicrobial Agent Pharmacology: Quinolones and Urinary Tract Agents

Drug (Oral Absorption, %)	Serum & Urine Concentration; Selected Doses			Dosage Recommendations						
		Peak Serum	Peak or Range, Urine	Adults		Serious Infection Daily Dose (g)	Children		Newborn (Parenteral)	
	Dose (g)	(μg/ml)		Oral	Parenteral		Oral	Parenteral	Up to 1 wk	1–4 wk
				Dose (g)/Interval			Dose/Interval			
Cinoxacin (97)	0.25 po 0.5 po	8 16	400	0.25 q6h or 0.5 q12h[a]		1	Not recommended		Not recommended	
Ciprofloxacin[d] (50–85)	0.5 po 0.75 po 0.4 IV[e]	1.6–2.9 2.5–4.3 4.6	350	0.25–0.75 q12h	0.2–0.4 q8–12h[f]	1.5 PO/1.2 IV	Not recommended		Not recommended	
Enoxacin[d] (80–90)	0.4 po 0.6 po 0.2 IV	2.8–3.6 4 1.8	250–300 337	0.4 q12h	0.4 q12h	0.8	Not recommended		Not recommended	
Fleroxacin (99)	0.4 po 0.1 IV	4.4 2.85	210	0.4 q12–24h[h]			Not recommended		Not recommended	
Lomefloxacin (>95)	0.2 po 0.4 po	2.1 3–4.7	170	0.4 q24h		0.4	Not recommended		Not recommended	
Nalidixic Acid[d] (100)	1 po	20–40		1 q6h		4	Not recommended		Not recommended	
Norfloxacin[d] (30–50)	0.4 po	1.3–1.9	≥200	0.4 q12h		0.8	Not recommended		Not recommended	
Ofloxacin[d] (85–100)	0.4 po 0.2 po 0.4 IV[e]	2.9–5.6 1.5–2.7 4	200	0.2–0.4 q12h	0.2–0.4 q12h	0.8	Not recommended		Not recommended	
Oxolinic acid (poor)	0.75 po	0.9–3.6	45–100	0.75 q12h[a]		2	Not recommended		Not recommended	
Pefloxacin (98)	0.4 po 0.4 IV[e]	3.8–5.6 5.8	100–115	0.4 q12–24h			Not recommended		Not recommended	
Urinary anti-infectives										
Methenamine mandelate[j]	1 po		40 (formaldehyde)	1 q6h[a]		4	12.5–18.75 mg/kg q6h[a]		Not recommended	
Methenamine hippurate[j]	1 po	70–100 μmol/liter	apprx 50 (formaldehyde)	1 q12h[a]		2	12.5–25 mg/kg q12h[a]		Not recommended	
Nitrofurantoin (good but variable)	0.1 po	<2	50–150	0.05–0.1 q6–8h		0.4	5–7 mg/kg/d q6h		Not recommended	

[a] Use primarily for the treatment of urinary tract infections.
[b] Use during pregnancy not recommended.
[c] Animal pharmacology studies indicate the presence of drugs in the milk of lactating rats receiving oral doses of cinoxacin. Human data not currently available.
[d] Denotes decreased rate and/or extent of absorption when given with food.
[e] Infused over 60 minutes.
[f] q8h dosing has not been approved as of yet.
[g] 3.2 hr during dialysis/5.8 hrs in between sessions.
[h] Preliminary data.
[i] For CCr <30 ml/min; for >30 ml/min use normal dose.
[j] Ineffective urinary concentrations expected with compromised renal function.
[k] 8–12 hr during dialysis 13–48 hr in between sessions.

Antimicrobial Agent Pharmacology: Antimycobacterial Agents

Drug (Oral Absorption, %)	Serum & Urine Concentration; Selected Doses			Dosage Recommendations						
		Peak Serum	Peak or Range, Urine	Adults		Serious Infection Daily Dose (g)	Children		Newborn (Parenteral)	
	Dose (g)	(μg/ml)		Oral	Parenteral		Oral	Parenteral	Up to 1 wk	1–4 wk
				Dose (g)/Interval			Dose/Interval			
Ansamycin	0.075–0.3 po	0.2–0.5		0.15–0.3 q24h		0.3				
Capreomycin[a]	1 IM	20–47			1 g IM q24h[b]	1		10–20 mg/kg/d q24h (not approved)		10–20 mg/kg/d q24h (not approved)
Clofazimine[c] (45–70)	0.1 po[d]	0.7[e]		0.1 q24h		0.1				
Cycloserine[g] (70–90)	0.25 po	10		0.25–0.5 q12h		1	10–20 mg/kg/d q12h (not approved)			
Ethambutol (75–80)	25 mg/kg po	2–5		15 mg/kg q24h		15 mg/kg	10–15 mg/kg q24h (not recommended)			
Ethionamide (80)	1 po	20		0.25–0.5 q12h		1	15–20 mg/kg/d q24h[h] (not approved)			
Isoniazid[i,j]	7 mg/kg po	4.5/1[k]		0.3 q24h	0.3 IM q24h	0.3	10–20 mg/kg/d q12–24h	10–20 mg/kg/d q12–24h		
Para-amino salicylic acid	4 po	76–104		150 mg/kg/d q6–12h		12	150–360 mg/kg/d q6–8h[f]			
Pyrazinamide	0.5 po	9–12		15–30 mg/kg q24h		2	30 mg/kg/d q12–24h (not approved)			
Rifabutin (≥20)	0.3 po	0.375		0.3 q24h		0.3	Not approved	Not approved	Not approved	Not approved
Rifampin (100)	0.6 po 0.6 IV[m]	7 17.5		0.6 q24h	0.6 q24h	0.6	10–20 mg/kg/d q12–24h			
Streptomycin	1 IM	25–50	≥1000		1 IM q24h	1		20–40 mg/kg/d q24h		
Viomycin					1 q12h twice weekly	2				

[a] Pharmacokinetics similar to streptomycin.
[b] Administer for 60–120 days followed by 1 q2–3×/wk.
[c] Should be taken with food.
[d] In leprosy patients.
[e] At steady state.
[f] 8-day serum half-life/70-day tissue half-life.
[g] Dosage should be adjusted to maintain plasma concentrations <30 μg/ml.

Serum Half-life (h)				Usual Adult Dose (g) and Interval Adjustment					Dosage for Dialysis		CSF/ Serum (%) Inflamed Meninges	Newborn Serum/ Maternal Serum (%)	Breast Milk/ Maternal Serum (%)	Bile/ Serum (%)	Aqueous Humor/ Serum (%)
For Creatinine Clearance (ml/min)		With Dialysis			For Creatinine Clearance (ml/min)				Dose after HD Supplemental to Anuric	Daily Dose During PD					
>80	<10	HD	PD	Dose	>80	80–50	50–10	<10 (Anuric)							
1.5	8.4	3–4.4		0.25–0.5	6–12 h	0.25 q8h	0.25 q12–24h	Not recommended				—b	<100 (18–78)c		
3–5	5–10	3.2/5.8g		0.25–0.75 po 0.2–0.4 IV	12 h 8–12g h	12 h 8–12f h	0.25–0.5 q12h 0.2–0.4 12–24	0.25–0.5 q18 0.2–0.4 q18–24h	0.25–0.5 q24h post-HD	0.25–0.5 q24h	11–46			2800–4500	3–22
5–7	40	9.8		0.2–0.4	12 h	12 h	0.1–0.2 q12hj	0.1–0.2 q12h			67			900	
9–12	30														
7–8.5	21			0.4	24 h	24 h	0.2 q24h	0.2 q24h	0.4 load then 0.2 q24h					700	
1.1–2.5	21			1	6 h	6 h	6 h	Avoidj			Minimal				
2.3–4	7.6			0.4	12 h	12	24 h	24 h						1000	
4–8	16.9–28.4	8–12/ 13–48k		0.2–0.4 po/IV	12 h	12 h	24 h	0.1–0.2 q24h	0.2 load then 0.1 q24h		28–87		96–112	210–1886	
6–7				0.75	12 h		Not recommended	Not recommended						200–300	
8–12	11–15										52–58			200–600	
3–6				1	6 h	6 h	Avoidj	Avoidj			—m			—m	—m
3–6				1	12 h	12 h	Avoidj	Avoidj			—m	50	70–100	—m	—m
0.3	1			0.05–0.1	6 h	6 h	Avoidj,n	Avoidj,n				100	<25o	200–400	

j Usually coadministered with an acidifying agent to convert the methenimine salts in urine to ammonia and bactericidal formaldehyde (pH ≤5.5). Mandelic and hippuric acid are mildly antiseptic and contribute to urine acidification.
m Methenamine penetrates a number of body fluids, including bile and cerebrospinal fluid. This penetration proves clinically inconsequential since negligible amounts of formaldehyde are generated at physiologic pH.
n Nitrofurantoin accumulates in the serum of patients with a CCr <60 ml/min, which leads to systemic toxicity.
o Although only small amounts of nitrofurantoin have been detected in breast milk, the drug could cause hemolytic anemia in a G-6-PD deficient infant exposed in this manner.

Serum Half-life (h)				Usual Adult Dose (g) and Interval Adjustment					Dosage for Dialysis		CSF/ Serum (%) Inflamed Meninges	Newborn Serum/ Maternal Serum (%)	Breast Milk/ Maternal Serum (%)	Bile/ Serum (%)	Aqueous Humor/ Serum (%)
For Creatinine Clearance (ml/min)		With Dialysis			For Creatinine Clearance (ml/min)				Dose after HD Supplemental to Anuric	Daily Dose During PD					
>80	<10	HD	PD	Dose	>80	80–50	50–10	<10 (Anuric)							
				0.15–0.3	24 h	24 h	0.15 q24h	0.075 q72h							
4–6	29.4–55.5			1	24 h	24 h	7.5 mg/kg q24–48h	7.5 mg/kg 2 × wk						Minimal	
8d/70df				0.1	8 h	8 h	8 h	8 h							
10				0.25–0.5	12 h	12 h	24 h	0.25 q24h			80–100	100	72		
3.3	≥7			15–25 mg/kg	24 h	15 mg/ kg q24h	15 mg/kg q24–36h	15 mg/kg q48h	15 mg/kg/d post-HD	15 mg/kg/ d	25–50	~100			
3	9			0.25–0.5	12 h	12 h	12 h	5 mg/kg q24h			100				
0.5–4	2–10			0.3 po/IM	24 h	24 h	24 h	½ dose in slow acetylators	5 mg/kg post-HD	Daily dose post-dialysis	100	High	100		
1	23			3	6–8 h						10–50				
10–16				15–30 mg/kg	24 h	24 h	24 h	12–20 mg/kg q24h			100				
16–69				0.3	24 h	24 h									
2–5	2–5	Minimal change		0.6	24 h	24 h	24 h	24 h			10–20	33	20–60	10,000	
2–3	Up to 110			1n	24 h	7.5 mg/ kg/d q24h	7.5 mg/kg/d q24–72h	7.5 mg/kg/d q72–96h	0.5 post-HD		20	10–40	<25	40–300	
				1	12h 2×/ wk						Poor				

h Limited evidence suggests that 20 mg/kg daily given as a single dose in children is more likely to produce CSF concentrations exceeding the MIC of 2.5 µg/ml for M. tuberculosis.
i To minimize the risk of polyneuritis from isoniazid-induced pyridoxine deficiency, pyridoxine (15–50 mg) is often given concurrently.
j Decreased rate and/or extent of absorption when given with food.
k 4.5 µg/ml in slow inactivators/1.0 µg/ml in rapid inactivators.
l Should not exceed the adult dose.
m Infused over 30 minutes.
n Desirable serum concentrations: peak 5–25 µg/ml; trough <5 µg/ml.

Antimicrobial Agent Pharmacology: Antifungal Agents

Drug (Oral Absorption, %)	Serum & Urine Concentration; Selected Doses			Dosage Recommendations						
		Peak Serum	Peak or Range, Urine	Adults			Children		Newborn (Parenteral)	
				Oral	Parenteral	Serious Infection Daily Dose (g)	Oral	Parenteral	Up to 1 wk	1–4 wk
	Dose (g)	(µg/ml)		Dose (g)/Interval			Dose/Interval			
Amphotericin B (poor)	0.03 IV[a] 0.05 IV[a]	1 2			0.25–1 mg/kg q24h[b,c]	1 mg/kg[d]		0.25–1 mg/kg q24–48h[b]	0.1–1 mg/kg/d[b]	0.1–1 mg/kg/d[b]
Fluconazole (≥90)	0.4 po 0.1 IV[e]	6.72 3.86–4.96		0.05–0.4 q24h	0.05–0.4 q24h	0.4				
Flucytosine[f,g] (75–90)	2 PO	30–45		50–150 mg/kg/d q6h		150 mg/kg	50–150 mg/kg/d q6h			
Grieseofulvin (50/>50)[h]	0.5/0.25 po[h]	0.4–2/0.4–2		0.5–1 q24/0.33–0.66 q24h		1	15 mg/kg/d q24h			
Itraconazole (99.8)[i,j]	0.2 po[k]	2.3/3.5[l]		0.2–0.4 q24h		0.4				
Ketoconazole[j]	0.2 po	4.2		0.2–0.4 q12–24h		0.8	5–10 mg/kg/d q12–24h			
Miconazole (50)	0.522 IV[n]	6			0.4–1.2 q8h	3.6		20–40 mg/kg/d q8h		
Nystatin (minimal)	All doses	Not detectable		0.4–1 mU q8h		2 mU	0.4–0.6 mU q6h		0.1 mU q6h	0.1 mU q6h

[a] Infused over several hours.
[b] A test dose of 1 mg infused over 15 minutes is often given to assess febrile reactions prior to proceeding to higher doses.
[c] Should be administered by slow infusion; rapid IV infusion should be avoided since potentially serious adverse effects (e.g., hypotension, hypokalemia, arrhythmias, shock) may occur.
[d] Or 1.5 mg/kg every other day.
[e] Infused over 30 minutes; ascertained on day 6–7.
[f] Decreased rate and/or extent of absorption when given with food.
[g] Peak concentrations should be above 25 µg/ml to avoid development of resistance but should not exceed 100–200 µg/ml to avoid side effects.

[h] Microsize/ultramicrosize.
[i] When given with meals.
[j] Gastric acid suppressing agents decrease bioavailability to <5%.
[k] Taken 2× day for 15 days.
[l] Parent drug/active metabolite (hydroxyitraconazole).
[m] Half-life extends as dosing continues.
[n] Infused over 15 minutes.
[o] Triphasic elimination: α = 0.4 h; β = 2.1 h; γ = 24.1 h.

Antimicrobial Agent Pharmacology: Antiviral Agents

Drug (Oral Absorption, %)	Serum & Urine Concentration; Selected Doses			Dosage Recommendations						
		Peak Serum	Peak or Range, Urine	Adults			Children		Newborn (Parenteral)	
				Oral	Parenteral	Serious Infection Daily Dose (g)	Oral	Parenteral	Up to 1 wk	1–4 wk
	Dose (g)	(µg/ml)		Dose (g)/Interval			Dose/Interval			
Acyclovir (15–30)[a]	0.2 po[b] 0.8 po[b] 5 mg/kg IV[e]	0.83 1.61 7.7		0.2–0.8 2–5 ×/d	5–12 mg/kg q8h	4 po/30 mg/kg IV	0.2 5 ×/d	25–50 mg/kg/d q8h		
Amantadine (85–90)	0.1 po[b]	0.302		0.1 q12h		0.2	2.2–4.4 mg/kg q12h			
Didanosine[d] (33–43)[a,e]	0.3 po tab 0.375 po sol.	1.6 1.6		0.167–0.200 q12h		[f]				
Foscarnet	0.16 mg/kg/min IV[g]	134–202			60 mg/kg q8h[h]	120–180 mg/kg				
Ganciclovir	5 mg/kg IV[c]	6.6–8.3			5 mg/kg q12h[i]	5 mg/kg maint.		5 mg/kg q12h[i]		
Ribavirin	0.82 mg/kg/hr[j] 0.82 mg/kg/h[k]	0.275 1.1		—[l]		—[m]				
Vidarabine	10 mg/kg IV	0.2–0.4/3–6[o]			10–15 mg/kg/d over 12 h	15 mg/kg		10–15 mg/kg/d over 12 h	15–30 mg/kg/d over 12 h	15–30 mg/kg/d over 12 h
Zalcitabine[d] (70–88)[e]	0.0005 po 0.005 po	0.0076 0.079		0.75 mg q8h[q]	2.25 mg	2.25 mg	0.75 mg q8h[r]			
Zidovudine (50–76)[s]	0.25 po[b] 5 mg/kg IV[e]	0.62 1.6–2.7		0.100 q4h or 0.200 q8h[t]	1–2 mg/kg q4h[u]	0.6	180 mg/m² q6h			

[a] Bioavailability decreases as dosage is increased.
[b] At steady state.
[c] Infused over 1 hour.
[d] Decreased rate and/or extent of absorption when given with food.
[e] In HIV patients.
[f] Solution doses for children with BSA 1–1.4 m² is 125 mg q12h; BSA 0.8–1 m² is 94 mg q6h; BSA 0.5–0.7 m² is 62 mg q12h; BSA 0.4 m² is 31 mg q12h (manufacturer recommendations although optimum dosage has not been elucidated).
[g] Infused over 3 days.
[h] For 14–21 days as initial induction therapy then 90 mg/kg q24h as maintenance.
[i] For 14–21 days as induction therapy then 5 mg/kg q24h.
[j] Inhaled over 5 hours each day for 3 days.
[k] Inhaled over 8 hours each day for 3 days.

[l] Mist of 190 µg/liter via SPAG-2 aerosol generator; rate of 12.5 liter mist/min × 16–18 h/day 1 of influenza A or B infection; × 12 h/day on days 2 and 3; then ×4 hr on day 4 (not approved in USA).
[m] Mist of 190 µg/liter via SPAG-2 aerosol generator; rate of 12.5 liter mist/min × 12–18 h/day for 3–7 days.
[n] Following administration for 4–7 weeks in AIDS or ARC patients.
[o] Vidarabine/ara-hypoxanthine (less active metabolite).
[p] With purulent meninges.
[q] Should be coadministered with zidovudine 200 mg q8h.
[r] In children 13 years of age or at least 30 kg.
[s] Reaches systemic circulation as unchanged drug.
[t] 0.1 g five times daily is also used.
[u] An IV dose of 1 mg/kg q4h is equivalent to an oral dose of 100 mg q4h.
[v] In asymptomatic patients.

Serum Half-life (h)				Usual Adult Dose (g) and Interval Adjustment					Dosage for Dialysis		CSF/ Serum (%) Inflamed Meninges	Newborn Serum/ Maternal Serum (%)	Breast Milk/ Maternal Serum (%)	Bile/ Serum (%)	Aqueous Humor/ Serum (%)
For Creatinine Clearance (ml/min)		With Dialysis			For Creatinine Clearance (ml/min)				Dose after HD Supplemental to Anuric	Daily Dose During PD					
>80	<10	HD	PD	Dose	>80	80–50	50–10	<10 (Anuric)							
24 or more	24 or more			0.25–1 mg/kg	24 h	24 h	24 h	24 h	Usual regimen	Usual regimen	3	50			25
20–50	48			0.05–0.4	24 h	24 h	50% of dose	25% of dose			50–94				
3–6	30–250			37 mg/kg	6 h	6 h	12–24 h	15–25 mg/kg q24h	20–37.5 mg/kg post-HD		60–100				
24	24			0.5–1/ 0.33–0.66	24/24 h	24/24 h	24/24 h	24/24 h					80		
21–60^m				0.2–0.4	24 h	24 h					<10				
8	8			0.2–0.4	12–24 h	12–24 h	12–24 h	12–24 h	Usual regimen	Usual regimen	Minimal			Minimal	~10
0.4– 24.1^o	0.4–24.1^o			0.4–1.2	8 h	8 h	8 h	8 h			<3–48				
				0.4–1 mU	8 h	8 h	8 h	8 h							

Serum Half-life (h)				Usual Adult Dose (g) and Interval Adjustment					Dosage for Dialysis		CSF/ Serum (%) Inflamed Meninges	Newborn Serum/ Maternal Serum (%)	Breast Milk/ Maternal Serum (%)	Bile/ Serum (%)	Aqueous Humor/ Serum (%)
For Creatinine Clearance (ml/min)		With Dialysis			For Creatinine Clearance (ml/min)				Dose after HD Supplemental to Anuric	Daily Dose During PD					
>80	<10	HD	PD	Dose	>80	80–50	50–10	<10 (Anuric)							
2.1–3.5	19.5		Minimal change	0.2–0.8 po 5–12 mg/ kg IV	2–5 ×/d 8 h	2–5 ×/d 8 h	2–5 ×/d 12–24 h	0.2–0.8 q24h 2.5–6 mg/kg q24h	0.5 Post-HD	2.5 mg/kg/ d	50		≥100		37
15–20	170	7–10.3 days		0.1	12 h	24 h	0.1–0.2 2–3 ×/wk	0.1–0.2 qwk			50				
1.3–1.6	4.5			0.167– 0.375	12 h	Reduction advised		100 mg q24h	No supp but give dose post-HD		12–85				
36–196				90 mg/kg/d maint	90 mg/ kg/d	78–63 mg/kg/d	62–50 mg/ kg/d				43				
2.53–3.6	10			5 mg/kg	12 h	2.5 mg/ kg q12h	2.5 mg/kg q24h	1.25 mg/kg q24h	1.25 mg /kg q24h post-HD		41				40
6.5–11											70^p				
1.5/3.3				15 mg/kg/d	Over 12 h	Over 12 h	Over 12 h	10 mg/kg/d over 12h	Schedule post-HD		33–35^r				
0.5–3	8.5			0.75	8 h	8 h	12 h	24 h			9–37				
0.8–1.9	1.4			0.1^x	4 h	4 h	6 h	6–12 h	100 mg	100 mg q6–12	15–98	100			

Adverse Drug Interactions Involving Antimicrobial Agents

Interacting Drugs	Adverse Effect	Probable Mechanism
Acyclovir with		
Aminoglycosides	Increased nephrotoxicity and/or neurotoxicity	Mechanism not established
Narcotics	Increased meperidine effect	Decreased renal excretion
Probenecid	Possible increased acyclovir toxicity	Decreased renal excretion
Zidovudine	Increased neurotoxicity (profound drowsiness and lethargy)	Additive
Amantadine with		
Anticholinergics	Hallucinations, confusion, nightmares	Mechanism not established
CNS stimulants	Additive CNS stimulant effects	Mechanism not established
Aminoglycoside antibiotics with		
Acyclovir	Increased nephrotoxicity and/or neurotoxicity	Additive
Amphotericin B	Nephrotoxicity	Synergism
Anticoagulants, oral	Potentiation of anticoagulation effects	Decreased GI absorption or synthesis of vitamin K
Bacitracin	Increased nephrotoxicity	Additive
Bumetanide	Increased ototoxicity	Additive
Capreomycin	Increased nephrotoxicity and/or neurotoxicity	Additive
Cephalosporins	Increased nephrotoxicity	Mechanism not established
Cisplatin	Increased nephrotoxicity	Mechanism not established
Colistimethate	Increased nephrotoxicity and/or neurotoxicity	Additive
Cyclosporine	Increased renal toxicity	Possibly additive or synergistic
Digoxin	Probable decreased digoxin effect with oral gentamicin or neomycin	Decreased absorption
Ethacrynic acid	Increased ototoxicity	Additive
Furosemide	Increased ototoxicity and nephrotoxicity	Additive
Magnesium sulfate	Increased neuromuscular blockade	Additive
Methotrexate	Possible increased methotrexate toxicity with kanamycin	Mechanism not established
	Possible decreased methotrexate effect with oral aminoglycosides	Decreased absorption
Methoxyflurane	Increased nephrotoxicity	Additive
Miconazole	Possible decreased tobramycin concentration	Mechanism not established
Neuromuscular blocking agents	Neuromuscular blockade	Additive
Nonsteroidal anti-inflammatory drugs	Possible aminoglycoside toxicity in preterm infants with indomethacin given for patent ductus closure	Decreased renal clearance
Penicillins	Decreased aminoglycoside effect with high concentrations of carbenicillin or ticarcillin	Inactivation
	Falsely low aminoglycoside levels	In vitro inactivation
Polymyxins	Increased nephrotoxicity; neuromuscular blockade	Additive
Vancomycin	Possible increased nephrotoxicity and ototoxicity	Additive
Aminosalicylic acid (PAS) with		
Anticoagulants, oral	Enhanced hypoprothrombinemic effects	Mechanism not established
Ammonium chloride	Increased probability of crystalluria	Acidification of urine
Digoxin	Decreased digoxin effect	Decreased absorption with time
Diphenhydramine	Decreased effect of PAS	Decreases GI absorption
Probenecid	Increased PAS toxicity	Decreased renal excretion
Rifampin	Rifampin effectiveness may be decreased; separate doses by 8–12 h	Decreased GI absorption due to excipient bentonite
Amphotericin B with		
Aminoglycoside antibiotics	Nephrotoxicity	Synergism
Antineoplastics	Possible increased renal toxicity, bronchospasm, and hypotension	Mechanism not established
Capreomycin	Increased nephrotoxicity	Additive
Cisplatin	Increased nephrotoxicity	Additive
Colistin	Increased nephrotoxicity	Additive
Corticosteroids	Increased hypokalemia	Additive
Cyclosporine	Increased renal toxicity	Possible synergism
Digitalis glycosides	Increased digitalis toxicity	Hypokalemia
Imidazole antifungals	Possible antagonism in animal models	Mechanism not established
Methoxyflurane	Increased nephrotoxicity	Additive
Neuromuscular blocking agents	Increased neuromuscular blocking effect	Hypokalemia
Pentamidine	Increased nephrotoxicity	Additive
Polymixins	Increased nephrotoxicity	Additive
Vancomycin	Increased nephrotoxicity	Additive
Azithromycin with		
Aluminum/magnesium antacids	Decreased peak concentrations; does not effect overall absorption	Mechanism not established
Aztreonam with		
Chloramphenicol	Possible in vitro antagonism. Administer a few hours apart	Mechanism not established
Bacitracin with		
Aminoglycosides	Increased nephrotoxicity	Additive
Anaesthetics	Potentiation of neuromuscular blocking effects	Additive
Neuromuscular blocking drugs	Potentiation of neuromuscular blocking effects	Additive
Polymixins	Increased nephrotoxicity	Additive
Capreomycin with		
Aminoglycosides	Increased nephrotoxicity and/or ototoxicity	Additive
Colistin	Increased nephrotoxicity	Additive
Polymixin B	Increased nephrotoxicity	Additive
Vancomycin	Increased nephrotoxicity and/or ototoxicity	Additive

(Continues)

Adverse Drug Interactions Involving Antimicrobial Agents

Interacting Drugs	Adverse Effect	Probable Mechanism
Cephalosporins with		
Alcohol	Disulfiram-like effect with cefamandole, cefmetazole, cefotetan cefoperazone, and moxalactam. Cefonicid also in animals, but not shown in humans.	Inhibition of intermediary metabolism of alcohol
Aminoglycoside antibiotics	Increased nephrotoxicity	Mechanism not established
Ampicillin	In vitro antagonism with ceftazidime vs group B strepto-cocci and listeria	Mechanism not established
Anticoagulants, oral	Possible increased anticoagulant effect with moxalactam cefamandole, cefmetazole or cefoperazone	Mechanism not established
Aspirin	Possible increased bleeding risk with moxalactam	Additive
Chloramphenicol	In vitro antagonism	Mechanism not established
Colistin	Increased nephrotoxicity	Additive
Diuretics	Increased nephrotoxicity with some cephalosporins	Mechanism not established
Ethacrynic acid	Increased nephrotoxicity	Mechanism not established
Furosemide	Increased nephrotoxicity	Mechanism not established
Heparin	Possible increased bleeding risk with moxalactam	Additive
Penicillins	Possible increased cefotaxime toxicity with azlocillin in patients with renal impairment	Decreased excretion
Polymixins	Increased nephrotoxicity	Additive
Probenecid	Higher and prolonged cephalosporin concentrations	Competitive inhibition of tubular secretion
Salicylates	Decreased cefixime concentrations and AUCs	Displacement from protein binding sites
Vancomycin	Increased nephrotoxicity	Additive
Chloramphenicol with		
Acetaminophen	Possible decreased chloramphenicol effect	Increased metabolism
Anticoagulants (oral)	Increased dicumarol effect	Decreased metabolism
Aminoglycosides	In vitro antagonism; not seen in vivo	Mechanism not established
Aztreonam	Antagonism; administer chloramphenicol separately a few hours later	Mechanism not established
Barbiturates	Increased barbiturate effect; decreased chloramphenicol effect	Decreased metabolism Increased metabolism
Cephalosporins	Antagonism	Mechanism not established
Cimetidine	Aplastic anemia	Possibly additive or synergistic
Etomidate	Prolonged anesthesia	Decreased metabolism
Folic acid	Delayed response to folic acid	Mechanism not established
Hypoglycemics, sulfonylurea	Increased hypoglycemic effect	Mechanism not established
Iron	Delayed response to iron	Mechanism not established
Penicillins	In vitro antagonism; not seen in vivo	Mechanism not established
Phenytoin	Increased phenytoin toxicity Possible increased chloramphenicol toxicity	Decreased metabolism Mechanism not established
Rifampin	Decreased chloramphenicol effect	Increased metabolism
Vitamin B_{12}	Delayed response to vitamin B_{12}	Mechanism not established
Chloroquine with		
Rabies vaccine	Decreased vaccine effect	Interference with the antibody response
Clindamycin with		
Neuromuscular blocking agents	Increased neuromuscular blockade	Additive
Clofazimine with		
Dapsone	Possible decrease or nullification of clofazimine's anti-inflammatory activity	Opposing effects on neutrophil motility and lympho-cyte transformation
Isoniazid	Increased clofazimine serum and urine concentrations and decreased skin concentrations	Mechanism not established
Rifampin	Decreased rate of absorption, time to reach peak, and AUC of rifampin	Mechanism not established
Colistimethate, same as polymyxin B		
Cycloserine with		
Alcohol	Increased alcohol effect or convulsions	Mechanism not established
Ethionamide	Increased neurotoxicity	Additive
Isoniazid	CNS effects, dizziness, drowsiness Increased neurotoxicity	Mechanism not established Additive
Phenytoin	Increased phenytoin concentrations	Inhibition of hepatic metabolism
Dapsone with		
Aniline	Increased risk of hemolysis in G6PD deficient patients	Additive
Clofazimine	Decreased or nullification of clofazimine's anti-inflam-matory effects	Opposing effects on neutrophil motility and lympho-cyte transformation in vitro
Didanosine	Increased incidence of PCP recurrence	Mechanism not established
Folic acid antagonists	Increased risk of hematologic toxicity	Additive
Naphthalene	Increased risk of hemolysis in G6PD deficient patients	Additive
Niridazole	Increased risk of hemolysis in G6PD deficient patients	Additive
Nitrite	Increased risk of hemolysis in G6PD deficient patients	Additive
Nitrofurantoin	Increased risk of hemolysis in G6PD deficient patients	Additive
Phenylhydrazine	Increased risk of hemolysis in G6PD deficient patients	Additive
Primaquine	Increased risk of hemolysis in G6PD deficient patients	Additive
Pyrimethamine	Increased risk of hematologic toxicity	Additive
Rifampin	Decreased dapsone serum concentrations	Hepatic enzyme induction
Trimethoprim	Increased dapsone serum concentrations; increased risk of adverse effects	Mechanism not established

(Continues)

Adverse Drug Interactions Involving Antimicrobial Agents

Interacting Drugs	Adverse Effect	Probable Mechanism
Didanosine with		
Benzodiazepines	Increased confusion	Mechanism not established
Co-trimoxazole	Increased risk of pancreatitis	Additive
Dapsone	Increased incidence of PCP recurrence	Antacids necessary for antiviral absorption may have impeded absorption
Ganciclovir	In vitro antiretroviral antagonism	Mechanism not established
Ketoconazole	Decreased absorption; administer ≥2 h before DDI	Antacids necessary for DDI administration raise gastric pH too high for ketoconazole absorption
Pentamidine	Increased risk of pancreatitis	Additive
Quinolones	Decreased absorption; decreased serum concentrations of the quinolones	Concomitant antacids bind quinolones and prevent absorption
Tetracyclines	Decreased absorption; decreased serum concentrations of the tetracyclines	Concomitant antacids bind tetracyclines and prevent absorption
Zalcitabine	Increased neurotoxicity	Additive
Ethionamide with		
Cycloserine	Increased neurotoxicity	Additive
Isoniazid	Increased neurotoxicity	Additive
Fluconazole with		
Amphotericin B	Possible antagonism in animal models	Mechanism not established
Astemizole	Increased QT interval and possible arrhythmias	Inhibition of antihistamine metabolism
Coumarin anticoagulants	Increased prothrombin times	Mechanism not established
Cyclosporine	Increased cyclosporine concentrations	Mechanism not established
Phenytoin	Increased phenytoin concentrations	Inhibition of metabolism
Rifampin	Decreased fluconazole concentrations	Mechanism not established
Sulfonylureas	Increased plasma concentrations and decreased metabolism of tolbutamide, glyburide and glipizide	Mechanism not established
Terfenadine	Increased QT interval and possible arrhythmias	Inhibition of antihistamine metabolism
Thiazides	Increased fluconazole concentrations and AUC	Decreased renal clearance
Fluoroquinolones with		
Antacids	Decreased fluoroquinolone effect with aluminum or magnesium antacids	Decreased absorption
Anticoagulants, oral	Prolonged prothrombin times	Mechanism not established
Chloramphenicol	Inhibition in vitro of norfloxacin bactericidal activity	Mechanism not established
Cyclosporine	Increased risk of nephrotoxicity; increased serum cyclosporine concentrations	Mechanism not established
Iron	Decreased serum fluoroquinolone concentrations	Decreased GI absorption
Nitrofurantoin	Decreased norfloxacin activity	In vitro antagonism
NSAIDs	Possible increased risk of CNS stimulation	Mechanism not established
Pirenzepine	Decreased rate of fluoroquinolone absorption	Mechanism not established
Probenecid	Increased serum concentrations; prolonged AUCs	Decreased tubular secretion
Rifampin	Inhibition in vitro of norfloxacin bactericidal activity	Mechanism not established
Scopolamine	Decreased rate of fluoroquinolone absorption	Mechanism not established
Sucralfate	Decreased serum fluoroquinolone concentrations	Decreased GI absorption
Tetracycline	Inhibition in vitro of norfloxacin bactericidal activity	Mechanism not established
Theophylline	Possible theophylline toxicity	Decreased metabolism
Zinc	Decreased serum fluoroquinolone concentrations	Decreased GI absorption
Foscarnet with		
Acyclovir	Increased nephrotoxicity	Additive
Co-trimoxazole	Increased nephrotoxicity	Additive
Pentamidine	Increased nephrotoxicity; increased hypocalcemia	Additive
Probenecid	Increased foscarnet serum concentrations; increased possibility of adverse effects	Decreased tubular secretion
Suramin	Increased nephrotoxicity	Additive
Furazolidone with		
Alcohol	Disulfiram-like effect	Either inhibition of aldehyde dehydrogenase or inhibition of monoamine oxidase
Ganciclovir with		
Aminoglycosides	Increased nephrotoxicity	Additive
Amphotericin B	Increased nephrotoxicity; replication inhibition of rapidly dividing host cells	Additive; Additive
Co-trimoxazole	Replication inhibition of rapidly dividing host cells	Additive
Cyclosporine	Increased nephrotoxicity	Additive
Cytotoxic antineoplastics	Replication inhibition of rapidly dividing host cells	Additive
Dapsone	Replication inhibition of rapidly dividing host cells	Additive
Didanosine	In vitro antiretroviral antagonism	Mechanism not established
Flucytosine	Replication inhibition of rapidly dividing host cells	Additive
Imipenem	Generalized seizures	Mechanism not established
Immunosuppressives	Increased suppression of bone marrow and immune system	Additive
Nucleoside analogs	Replication inhibition of rapidly dividing host cells	Additive
Pentamidine	Replication inhibition of rapidly dividing host cells	Additive
Probenecid	Increased ganciclovir concentrations; prolonged AUC	Decrease in tubular secretion
Pyrimethamine	Replication inhibition of rapidly dividing host cells	Additive
Zidovudine	In vitro antiretroviral antagonism; increased risk of hematologic toxicity	Mechanism not established; additive
Griseofulvin with		
Alcohol	Increased alcohol effects, tachycardia and flushing	Mechanism not established
Anticoagulants, oral	Decreased anticoagulant effect	Mechanism not established
Contraceptives, oral	Decreased contraceptive effect	Increased metabolism
Phenobarbital	Decreased griseofulvin concentrations	Decreased absorption or hepatic enzyme induction

(Continues)

Adverse Drug Interactions Involving Antimicrobial Agents

Interacting Drugs	Adverse Effect	Probable Mechanism
Hydroxychloroquine with		
Digoxin	Increased digoxin effect	Mechanism not established
Imipenem with		
Aztreonam	Antagonism	β-Lactamase induction
Cephalosporins	Antagonism	β-Lactamase induction
Chloramphenicol	Antagonism; administer a few hours after imipenem	Mechanism not established
Extended spectrum penicillins	Antagonism	β-Lactamase induction
Ganciclovir	Generalized seizures	Mechanism not established
Isoniazid with		
Alcohol	Increased incidence of hepatitis	Mechanism not established
	Decreased isoniazid effect in some alcoholic patients	Increased metabolism
Aluminum antacids	Decreased isoniazid effect	Decreased absorption
Anticoagulants, oral	Possible increased anticoagulant effect	Decreased metabolism
Benzodiazepines	Pharmacologic effects of benzodiazepines may be increased; documented with diazepam and triazolam	Decreased metabolism
BCG vaccine	Vaccine may be ineffective	INH inhibits multiplication of BCG
Carbamazepine	Increased toxicity of both drugs	Altered metabolism
Cycloserine	CNS effects, dizziness, drowsiness	Mechanism not established
Disulfiram	Psychotic episodes, ataxia	Altered dopamine metabolism
Enflurane	Possible nephrotoxicity	Increased metabolism of enflurane caused increased fluoride concentration
Ethionamide	Increased CNS adverse effects	Additive
Ketoconazole	Decreased ketoconazole effect	Decreased concentration
Phenytoin	Increased phenytoin toxicity	Decreased metabolism
Rifampin	Possible increased Isoniazid hepatotoxicity	Possible increased toxic metabolites
Itraconazole with		
Amphotericin B	In vitro antagonism	Mechanism not established
Antacids	Possible decreased itraconazole bioavailability	Mechanism not established
Astemizole	Possible prolongation of QT-interval and arrhythmias	Decreased antihistamine metabolism
Cyclosporine	Possible increase in cyclosporine concentrations	Mechanism not established
H₂ antagonists	Decreased itraconazole bioavailability	Decreased gastric acidity
Omeprazole	Decreased itraconazole bioavailability	Decreased gastric acidity
Rifampin	Decreased systemic bioavailability of itraconazole	Hepatic enzyme induction
Terfenadine	Possible prolongation of QT-interval and arrhythmias	Decreased antihistamine metabolism
Ketoconazole with		
Alcohol	Possible disulfiram-like reaction	Mechanism not established
Antacids	Decreased ketoconazole effect	Decreased absorption
Anticoagulants, oral	Increased anticoagulant effect	Mechanism not established
Astemizole	Increased QT interval and possible arrhythmias	Inhibition of antihistamine metabolism
Corticosteroids	Increased methylprednisolone effect	Decreased metabolism
Cyclosporine	Increased concentration of cyclosporine in blood	Mechanism not established
H₂ antagonists	Possible decreased antifungal effect	Decreased absorption
Hepatotoxic agents	Increased hepatotoxicity	Additive
Isoniazid	Decreased ketoconazole effect	Decreased blood concentrations
Omeprazole	Decreased ketoconazole bioavailability	Decreased gastric acidity
Phenytoin	Altered effects of one or both drugs	Altered metabolism
Rifampin	Decreased rifampin and ketoconazole effects	Decreased blood concentrations
Terfenadine	Increased QT interval and possible arrhythmias	Inhibition of antihistamine metabolism
Theophylline	Decreased theophylline concentrations	Mechanism not established
Macrolides with		
Anticoagulant, oral	Hypoprothrombinemia potentiated	Possible decreased metabolism
Astemizole	Increased QT interval and possible arrhythmias	Decreased antihistamine metabolism
Carbamazepine	Increased carbamazepine toxicity	Possible decreased metabolism
Clindamycin	In vitro antagonism; not documented clinically	Mechanism not established
Corticosteroids	Increased effect and possible toxicity of methylprednisolone	Decreased excretion
Cyclosporine	Increased cyclosporine toxicity	Probably decreased metabolism
Digoxin	Increased digoxin effect	Decreased gut metabolism and increased absorption
Disopyramide	Increased disopyramide concentrations, QT interval prolongation and polymorphic ventricular tachycardia	Mechanism not established
Ergot alkaloids	Increased ergot toxicity	Mechanism not established
Phenytoin	Possible increased or decreased effect	Altered metabolism
Terfenadine	Increased QT interval and possible arrhythmias	Decreased antihistamine metabolism
Theophylline	Increased theophylline effect and possible toxicity	Decreased metabolism
Triazolam	Increased triazolam serum concentrations, increased triazolam effect	Decreased triazolam clearance
Zidovudine	Decreased zidovudine concentrations and AUCs with clarithromycin	Mechanism not established
Mebendazole with		
Carbamazepine	Decreased mebendazole concentrations	Hepatic microsomal enzyme induction
Phenytoin	Decreased mebendazole concentrations	Hepatic microsomal enzyme induction
Methenamine with		
Sulfonamides	Increased risk of crystalluria; precipitate formation between formaldehyde and sulfamethizole	Acidification of the urine
Metronidazole with		
Alcohol	Mild disulfiram-like symptoms	Possible inhibition of intermediary metabolism of alcohol
Anticoagulants, oral	Increased anticoagulant effect	Decreased metabolism

(Continues)

Adverse Drug Interactions Involving Antimicrobial Agents

Interacting Drugs	Adverse Effect	Probable Mechanism
Astemizole	Possible prolongation of the QT interval and arrhythmias	Decreased antihistamine metabolism
Azathioprine	Transient neutropenia	Mechanism not established
Barbiturates	Decreased metronidazole effect with phenobarbital	Probably increased metabolism
Cimetidine	Possible increased metronidazole toxicity	Decreased metabolism
Disulfiram	Organic brain syndrome	Mechanism not established
Fluorouracil	Transient neutropenia	Mechanism not established
Lithium	Lithium toxicity	Mechanism not established
Terfenadine	Possible prolongation of the QT interval and arrhythmias	Decreased antihistamine metabolism
Miconazole with		
Aminoglycosides	Possible decreased tobramycin concentration	Mechanism not established
Amphotericin B	Possible antagonism in in vitro studies	Mechanism not established
Anticoagulants, oral	Increased anticoagulant effect	Mechanism not established
Astemizole	Increased QT interval and possible arrhythmias	Inhibition of antihistamine metabolism
Hypoglycemics, sulfonylurea	Severe hypoglycemia	Mechanism not established
Phenytoin	Increased phenytoin toxicity	Decreased metabolism
Terfenadine	Increased QT interval and possible arrhythmias	Inhibition of antihistamine metabolism
Nalidixic acid with		
Antacids	Decreased nalidixic acid serum concentrations	Impaired absorption
Anticoagulants, oral	Increased anticoagulant effect	Displacement from binding sites
Nitrofurantoin with		
Antacids	Possible decreased nitrofurantoin effect	Decreased absorption
Fluoroquinolones	In vitro antagonism of quinolone activity	Mechanism not established
Probenecid	Increased nitrofurantoin serum concentrations	Inhibition of renal excretion
Sulfinpyrazone	Increased nitrofurantoin serum concentrations	Inhibition of renal excretion
Para-aminosalicylic acid, see aminosalicylic acid		
Penicillins with		
Allopurinol	Increased incidence of rash with ampicillin	Mechanism not established
Aminoglycosides	Decreased aminoglycoside effect with high concentrations of carbenicillin or ticarcillin; falsely low aminoglycoside concentrations in vitro	Inactivation
Anticoagulants, oral	Decreased anticoagulant effect with nafcillin and didoxacillin	Increased metabolism
Bacteriostatic agents	In vitro antagonism	Mechanism not established
β-Adrenergic blockers	Possible decreased atenolol effect with ampicillin	Decreased absorption
β-Lactams	In vitro antagonism	Mechanism not established
Cephalosporins	Possible increased cefotaxime toxicity with azlocillin in patients with renal impairment	Decreased excretion
Colestipol	Decreased concentrations of penicillin G	Decreased absorption
Contraceptives, oral	Decreased contraceptive effect with ampicillin or oxacillin	Decreased enterohepatic circulation of estrogen
Cyclosporine	Decreased cyclosporine concentrations with nafcillin	Increased cyclosporine metabolism
Disulfiram	Possible disulfiram-like reaction when given with bacampicillin	Ethanol is a by-product of bacampicillin metabolism
Lithium	Hypernatremia with ticarcillin	Large sodium load from ticarcillin and decreased renal excretion
Methotrexate	Possible increased methotrexate toxicity	Decreased excretion
Potassium sparing diuretics	Hyperkalemia with penicillin G potassium	Additive
Probenecid	Increased concentrations and AUCs	Inhibition of tubular secretion
Rifampin	Antagonism in vitro with high concentrations of ampicillin, nafcillin and oxacillin	Mechanism not established
Sulfasalazine	Decrease of AUC of the metabolite sulfapyridine when given immediately after oral ampicillin	Mechanism not established
Vecuronium	Extended neuromuscular blockade when given with acylaminopenicillins	Mechanism not established
Pentamidine with		
Aminoglycosides	Increased nephrotoxicity	Additive
Amphotericin B	Increased nephrotoxicity	Additive
Capreomycin	Increased nephrotoxicity	Additive
Colistin	Increased nephrotoxicity	Additive
Cisplatin	Increased nephrotoxicity	Additive
Methoxyflurane	Increased nephrotoxicity	Additive
Polymixins	Increased nephrotoxicity	Additive
Vancomycin	Increased nephrotoxicity	Additive
Piperazine with		
Chlorpromazine	Seizures	Mechanism not established
Pyrantel pamoate	Decreased piperazine and pyrantel pamoate activity	Antagonism
Polymyxin B with		
Aminoglycoside antibiotics	Increased nephrotoxicity; increased neuromuscular blockade	Additive
Neuromuscular blocking agents	Increased neuromuscular blockade	Additive
Parenteral quinidine	Increased neurotoxicity	Additive
Parenteral quinine	Increased neurotoxicity	Additive
Vancomycin	Increased nephrotoxicity	Additive
Primaquine with		
Quinacrine	Increased toxicity to the antimalarial	Additive
Pyrantel pamoate with		
Piperazine	Decreased pyrantel pamoate and piperazine activity	Antagonism

(Continues)

Adverse Drug Interactions Involving Antimicrobial Agents

Interacting Drugs	Adverse Effect	Probable Mechanism
Quinacrine with		
Primaquine	Increased primaquine toxicity	Release from tissue binding sites causing marked increase in primaquine concentrations
Alcohol	Possible disulfiram-like reaction	Accumulation of acetaldehyde
Hepatotoxic agents	Possible increased hepatotoxicity	Additive
Quinine with		
Acetazolamide	Increased quinine serum concentrations; increased toxicity	Decreased clearance from increased urinary pH
Aluminum antacids	Decreased quinine serum concentrations	Decreased absorption
Anticoagulants, oral	Potentiation of hypoprothrombinemic effects	Hepatic suppression of synthesis of vitamin K dependent clotting factors
Cimetidine	Decreased quinine clearance; prolonged AUCs	Hepatic enzyme inhibition
Digoxin/digitoxin	Increased digoxin/digitoxin concentrations	Mechanism not established
Heparin	Decreased anticoagulant effect	Mechanism not established
Mefloquine	Increased cardiac events	Additive
Neuromuscular blocking agents	Potentiation of neuromuscular blocking effects	Additive
Sodium bicarbonate	Increased quinine serum concentrations; increased toxicity	Decreased clearance from increased urinary pH
Ribavirin with		
Zalcitabine	In vitro antiretroviral antagonism	Mechanism not established
Zidovudine	In vitro antiretroviral antagonism	Mechanism not established
Rifabutin with		
Analgesics	Possible decreased concentrations and activity	Rifabutin hepatic enzyme induction
Anticoagulants, oral	Possible decreased concentrations and activity	Rifabutin hepatic enzyme induction
Anticonvulsants	Possible decreased concentrations and activity	Rifabutin hepatic enzyme induction
Barbiturates	Possible decreased concentrations and activity	Rifabutin hepatic enzyme induction
Beta-blockers	Possible decreased concentrations and activity	Rifabutin hepatic enzyme induction
Cardiac glycosides	Possible decreased concentrations and activity	Rifabutin hepatic enzyme induction
Chloramphenicol	Possible decreased concentrations and activity	Rifabutin hepatic enzyme induction
Clofibrate	Possible decreased concentrations and activity	Rifabutin hepatic enzyme induction
Contraceptives, oral	Possible decreased concentrations and activity	Rifabutin hepatic enzyme induction
Corticosteroids	Possible decreased concentrations and activity	Rifabutin hepatic enzyme induction
Cyclosporine	Possible decreased concentrations and activity	Rifabutin hepatic enzyme induction
Dapsone	Possible decreased concentrations and activity	Rifabutin hepatic enzyme induction
Diazepam	Possible decreased concentrations and activity	Rifabutin hepatic enzyme induction
Disopyramide	Possible decreased concentrations and activity	Rifabutin hepatic enzyme induction
Hypoglycemics, oral	Possible decreased concentrations and activity	Rifabutin hepatic enzyme induction
Ketoconazole	Possible decreased concentrations and activity	Rifabutin hepatic enzyme induction
Mexiletine	Possible decreased concentrations and activity	Rifabutin hepatic enzyme induction
Narcotics	Possible decreased concentrations and activity	Rifabutin hepatic enzyme induction
Progestins	Possible decreased concentrations and activity	Rifabutin hepatic enzyme induction
Quinidine	Possible decreased concentrations and activity	Rifabutin hepatic enzyme induction
Theophylline	Possible decreased concentrations and activity	Rifabutin hepatic enzyme induction
Verapamil	Possible decreased concentrations and activity	Rifabutin hepatic enzyme induction
Zidovudine	Decreased zidovudine concentrations and AUCs	Mechanism not established
Rifampin with		
Aminosalicylic acid	Rifampin effectiveness may be decreased; separate doses by 8–12 h	Decreased GI absorption due to excipient bentonite
Anticoagulants, oral	Decreased anticoagulant effect	Increased metabolism
Hypoglycemics, sulfonylurea	Decreased hypoglycemic effect	Increased metabolism
Barbiturates	Decreased barbiturate effect	Increased metabolism
Benzodiazepines	Possible decreased oral and IV diazepam effect	Increased metabolism
β-Adrenergic blockers	Decreased β-blocker effect	Increased metabolism
Chloramphenicol	Decreased chloramphenicol effect	Increased metabolism
Clofazimine	Decreased rate of absorption, slightly decreased AUC	Mechanism not established
Clofibrate	Pharmacologic effects of clofibrate may be decreased	Increased metabolism-enzyme induction
Contraceptives, oral	Decreased contraceptive effect	Increased metabolism
Corticosteroids	Decreased corticosteroid effect	Increased metabolism
Cyclosporine	Decreased cyclosporine effect	Increased metabolism
Dapsone	Decreased dapsone concentrations	Hepatic enzyme induction
Digitalis	Decreased digitoxin and digoxin effect	Increased metabolism
Disopyramide	Decreased disopyramide effect	Probably increased metabolism
Estrogens	Decreased estrogen concentrations	Hepatic enzyme induction
Isoniazid	Possible increased hepatotoxicity	Possible increased toxic metabolites
Ketoconazole	Decreased effect of both drugs	Increased metabolism
Methadone	Methadone withdrawal symptoms	Increased metabolism
Mexiletene	Decreased antiarrhythmic effect	Increased metabolism
Phenytoin	Decreased phenytoin effect	Increased metabolism
Progestins	Decreased norethindrone effect	Increased metabolism
Quinidine	Decreased quinidine effect	Increased metabolism
Theophylline	Decreased theophylline effect	Increased metabolism
Verapamil	Decreased verapamil effect	Increased metabolism
Spectinomycin with		
Lithium	Increased lithium toxicity	Decreased renal excretion
Sulfadoxine/pyrimethamine with		
Lorazepam	Mild hepatotoxicity	Mechanism not established
PABA	Decreased pyrimethamine effect	Interference with pyrimethamine action
Sulfonamides	Increased toxicity	Additive

(Continues)

Adverse Drug Interactions Involving Antimicrobial Agents

Interacting Drugs	Adverse Effect	Probable Mechanism
Sulfonamides with		
Antibiotics	Altered action of sulfasalazine	Alteration of intestinal flora
Anticoagulants, oral	Increased anticoagulant effect	Decreased metabolism and displacement from binding sites
Barbiturates	Increased thiopental effect	Decreased albumin binding
Chloroprocaine	Possible antagonism of sulfonamide action	Competition for PABA site
Cyclosporine	Decreased cyclosporine effect with sulfamethazine	Possible increased metabolism
Digoxin	Possible decreased digoxin effect with sulfasalazine	Decreased digoxin absorption
Folic acid	Decreased absorption, metabolism, and concentrations with sulfasalazine	Inhibition of hepatic folate metabolism, intestinal transport of folic acid, and jejunal brush-border folate conjugase
Hypoglycemics, sulfonylurea	Increased hypoglycemic effect	Mechanism not established
Iron	Decreased sulfasalazine serum concentrations	Chelation
Methenamine	Crystallization of sulfonamides in the urine; precipitate of formaldehyde/sulfamethizole	Acidification of the urine
Methotrexate	Possible increased methotrexate toxicity	Decreased renal clearance and displacement from binding
Monoamine oxidase inhibitors	Possible increased phenelzine toxicity with sulfisoxazole	Decreased metabolism
PABA	Possible antagonism of sulfonamide action	Competition for PABA site
Paraldehyde	Crystallization of sulfonamides in the urine	Acidification of the urine
Phenytoin	Increased phenytoin effect, except possibly with sulfisoxazole	Decreased metabolism
Piperocaine	Possible antagonism of sulfonamide action	Competition for PABA site
Procaine	Possible antagonism of sulfonamide action	Competition for PABA site
Propoxycaine	Possible antagonism of sulfonamide action	Competition for PABA site
Sulfinpyrazone	Increased serum sulfonamide concentrations	Displacement from protein binding sites and inhibition of tubular secretion
Tetracaine	Possible antagonism of sulfonamide action	Competition for PABA site
Thiopental	Increased thiopental effect; decreased dose necessary when given with sulfisoxazole	Plasma protein binding competition
Tetracyclines with		
Alcohol	Decreased doxycycline effect in alcoholics	Increased metabolism
Aminoglycosides	In vitro antagonism; no in vivo support	Mechanism not established
Antacids, oral	Decreased oral tetracycline effects	Decreased tetracycline absorption
Anticoagulants, oral	Increased anticoagulant effect	Mechanism not established
Antidepressants, tricyclic	Localized hemosiderosis with amitriptyline and minocycline	Possible synergism
Barbiturates	Decreased doxycycline effect	Increased metabolism
Bismuth subsalicylate	Decreased tetracycline effect	Decreased absorption
Carbamazepine	Decreased doxycycline effect	Increased metabolism
Contraceptives, oral	Decreased contraceptive effect	Possible decreased enterohepatic circulation of estrogen
Digoxin	Increased digoxin effect	Decreased gut metabolism and increased absorption
Iron, oral	Decreased tetracycline effect, but not with doxycycline	Decreased absorption
	Decreased iron effect	Decreased absorption
Kaolin/pectin	Decreased concentrations of tetracyclines	Decreased absorption
Lithium	Increased lithium toxicity	Decreased renal excretion
Methotrexate	Possible increased toxicity	Mechanism not established
Methoxyflurane	Increased nephrotoxicity	Displacement from binding
Molindone	Decreased tetracycline effect	Calcium as an excipient inhibits absorption
Penicillins	In vitro antagonism; rare in vivo support for this	Mechanism not established
Phenformin	Increased lactic acidosis	Possible decreased phenformin excretion
Phenytoin	Decreased doxycycline effect	Increased metabolism
Rifampin	Possible decreased doxycycline effect	Increased metabolism
Theophylline	Possible theophylline toxicity	Mechanism not established
Zinc sulfate	Decreased tetracycline effect	Decreased absorption
Thiabendazole with		
Theophylline	Increased theophylline toxicity	Decreased metabolism
Trimethoprim with		
Amiloride	Trimethoprim may potentiate hyponatremia caused by the concomitant use of amiloride with thiazide diuretics	Additive
Azathioprine	Leukopenia	Mechanism not established
Cyclosporine	Increased nephrotoxicity	Synergism
Digoxin	Possible increased digoxin effect	Decreased renal excretion and possibly decreased metabolism
Phenytoin	Increased phenytoin serum concentrations—increased risk of phenytoin toxicity; increased risk of folate deficiency	Inhibition of hepatic metabolism; additive
Thiazide diuretics	Trimethoprim may potentiate hyponatremia caused by the concomitant use of amiloride with thiazide diuretics	Additive
Trimethoprim–sulfamethoxazole with		
Anticoagulants, oral	Increased anticoagulant effect	Decreased metabolism
Antidepressants, tricyclic	Recurrence of depression	Mechanism not established
Lidocaine	Methemoglobinemia	Probably additive

(Continues)

Adverse Drug Interactions Involving Antimicrobial Agents

Interacting Drugs	Adverse Effect	Probable Mechanism
Mercaptopurine	Decreased antileukemic effect	Mechanism not established
Methotrexate	Megaloblastic anemia	Additive inhibition of folate metabolism
Phenytoin	Increased phenytoin toxicity; increased incidence of folate deficiency	Probably decreased metabolism; additive
Pimozide	Decreased pimozide effect	Mechanism not established
Vancomycin with		
Aminoglycosides	Possible increased nephrotoxicity and ototoxicity	Possibly additive
Amphotericin B	Increased nephrotoxicity	Additive
Bacitracin	Increased nephrotoxicity	Additive
Cephalosporins	Increased nephrotoxicity	Additive
Cisplatin	Increased nephrotoxicity	Additive
Colistin	Increased nephrotoxicity	Additive
Digoxin	Possible decreased digoxin effect	Possibly decreased absorption
Paromomycin	Increased nephrotoxicity	Additive
Polymyxins	Increased nephrotoxicity	Additive
Vidarabine with		
Allopurinol	Increased neurotoxicity	Decreased metabolism
Theophylline	Increased theophylline effect	Decreased metabolism
Zalcitabine with		
Aminoglycosides	Increased risk of peripheral neuropathy	Decreased clearance of zalcitabine
Amphotericin B	Increased risk of peripheral neuropathy	Decreased clearance of zalcitabine
Chloramphenicol	Increased risk of peripheral neuropathy	Additive
Cisplatin	Increased risk of peripheral neuropathy	Additive
Co-trimoxazole	Increased risk of pancreatitis	Additive
Dapsone	Increased risk of peripheral neuropathy	Additive
Didanosine	Increased risk of peripheral neuropathy	Additive
Disulfiram	Increased risk of peripheral neuropathy	Additive
Ethionamide	Increased risk of peripheral neuropathy	Additive
Foscarnet	Increased risk of peripheral neuropathy	Decreased clearance of zalcitabine
Glutethimide	Increased risk of peripheral neuropathy	Additive
Gold	Increased risk of peripheral neuropathy	Additive
Hydralazine	Increased risk of peripheral neuropathy	Additive
Iodoquinol	Increased risk of peripheral neuropathy	Additive
Metronidazole	Increased risk of peripheral neuropathy	Additive
Nitrofurantoin	Increased risk of peripheral neuropathy	Additive
Pentamidine	Increased risk of pancreatitis	Additive
Phenytoin	Increased risk of peripheral neuropathy	Additive
Ribavirin	Increased risk of peripheral neuropathy; in vitro antiretroviral antagonism	Additive; mechanism not established
Vincristine	Increased risk of peripheral neuropathy	Additive
Zidovudine with		
Acetaminophen	Granulocytopenia	Mechanism not established
Acyclovir	Neurotoxicity	Mechanism not established
Antimycobacterials	Possible increased risk of hematologic toxicity	Possible inhibition of zidovudine glucuronidation
Aspirin	Possible increased risk of hematologic toxicity	Possible inhibition of zidovudine glucuronidation
Cimetidine	Possible increased risk of hematologic toxicity	Possible inhibition of zidovudine glucuronidation
Clarithromycin	Decreased zidovudine concentrations and AUCs	Mechanism not established
Cytotoxic/myelosuppressive agents	Increased risk of hematologic toxicity	Additive
Ganciclovir	In vitro antiretroviral antagonism; increased risk of hematologic toxicity	Mechanism not established; additive
Indomethacin	Possible increased risk of hematologic toxicity	Possible inhibition of zidovudine glucuronidation
Lorazepam	Possible increased risk of hematologic toxicity	Possible inhibition of zidovudine glucuronidation
Nephrotoxic agents	Increased risk of toxicity	Increased serum concentrations; decreased clearance
Nucleoside analogs	Increased risk of hematologic toxicity	Additive
Probenecid	Increased and prolonged zidovudine serum concentration	Inhibition of glucuronidation and/or reduces renal excretion
Ribavirin	In vitro antiretroviral antagonism	Mechanism not established

BIBLIOGRAPHY

Amsden GW, Ballow CH, Schentag JJ. Population pharmacokinetic methods to optimize antibiotic effects. Drug Invest. 1993;5:256–268.

Ballow CH, Amsden GW, Forrest A, et al. Multiple-dose serum and urine pharmacokinetics of oral azithromycin in normal healthy volunteers (Abstract 215). 32nd Interscience Conference on Antimicrobial Agents and Chemotherapy, Anaheim, CA; 1992.

Bartlett JG. Pocketbook of Infectious Disease Therapy. Baltimore: Williams & Wilkins; 1991.

Barza M. Antibacterial agents in the treatment of ocular infections. In: Infectious Disease Clinics of North America—Antibacterial Agents. Philadelphia: WB Saunders; 1989.

Barza M, Thea D. Use of antibacterial agents in infections of the central nervous system. In: Infectious Disease Clinics of North America—Antibacterial Agents. Philadelphia: WB Saunders; 1989.

Bennett WM, Aronoff GR, Morrison G, et al. Drug prescribing in renal failure; dosing guidelines for adults. Am J Kidney Dis. 1983;3:155–193.

Forrest A, Nix DE, Ballow CH, et al. The pharmacodynamics of intravenous ciprofloxacin in seriously ill patients. Antimicrob Agents Chemother. 1993;37:1073–1081.

Forrest A, Ballow CH, Nix DE, et al. Development of a population pharmacokinetic model and optimal sampling strategies for intravenous ciprofloxacin. Antimicrob Agents Chemother. 1993;37:1065–1072.

Gilbert DN, Bennett WM. Use of antimicrobial agents in renal failure. In: Infectious Disease Clinics of North America—Antibacterial Agents. Philadelphia: WB Saunders; 1989.

Mandell GL, Douglas RG Jr, Bennett JE, et al. Principles and Practice of Infectious Diseases Antimicrobial Therapy 1993–1994. New York: Churchill Livingstone; 1993.

Medical Letter Handbook of Antimicrobial Therapy. New York: Medical Letter; 1992.

McCormack JP, Schentag JJ. The potential impact of quantitative susceptibility tests on the design of aminoglycoside regimens. Drug Intell Clin Pharm 1987;21:187–191.

McEvoy GK. American Hospital Formulary Service Drug Information '93. Bethesda, MD: American Society of Hospital Pharmacists; 1993:33–520.

Nelson JD. Pocketbook of Pediatric Antimicrobial Therapy. Baltimore: Williams & Wilkins; 1989.

Nix DE, Goodwin SD, Peloquin CA, et al. Antibiotic tissue penetration and its relevance: Models of tissue penetration and their meaning. Antimicrob Agents Chemother. 1991; 35:1947–1952.

Nix DE, Goodwin SD, Peloquin CA, et al. Antibiotic tissue penetration and its relevance: Impact of tissue penetration on infection response. Antimicrob Agents Chemother. 1991;35:1953–1959.

Norris S, Nightingale CH, Mandell GL. Tables of antimicrobial agent pharmacology. In: Mandell GL, Douglas RG, Bennett JE, eds. Principles and Practice of Infectious Diseases. 3rd ed. New York: Churchill Livingstone; 1990:434–461.

Peloquin CA, Cumbo TJ, Nix DE, et al. Intravenous ciprofloxacin in patients with nosocomial lower respiratory tract infections: Impact of plasma concentrations, organism MIC, and clinical condition on bacterial eradication. Arch Intern Med. 1989;149: 2269–2273.

Schentag JJ. Correlation of pharmacokinetic parameters to efficacy of antibiotics: Relationships between serum concentrations, MIC values, and bacterial eradication in patients with gram negative pneumonia. Scand J Infect Dis 1991;74(Suppl)218–234.

Schentag JJ, Nix DE, Adelman MH. Mathematical examination of dual individualization principles (I). Relationships between AUC above MIC and area under the inhibitory curve for cefmenoxime, ciprofloxacin, and tobramycin. DICP Ann Pharmacother. 1991;25:1050–1057.

MAJOR CLINICAL SYNDROMES

PART **II**

SECTION A. FEVER

36. PATHOGENESIS OF FEVER AND THE ACUTE PHASE RESPONSE

CHARLES A. DINARELLO
SHELDON M. WOLFF

Fever is an elevation of temperature above the normal daily variation. Infections are most commonly associated with fever, but noninfectious causes such as inflammatory, neoplastic, and immunologically mediated diseases may also have fever as their primary clinical presentation. Fever is best understood at the hypothalamic level. The thermoregulatory center located in the anterior hypothalamus regulates internal temperature; orally, this is about 36.8°C (98.2°F). Regulation is primarily by balance of heat loss from the periphery with heat production from tissues, particularly the liver and muscles. During fever, the balance is adjusted to increase internal temperature.

Individuals maintain body temperature at about 37°C despite wide variations in environmental temperatures. For some individuals, normal body temperature can be below or above 37°C without constituting a pathologic process. During a 24-hour period, body temperature varies from a low point in the early morning to the highest levels at 4–6 PM. The amplitude of this daily variation, also called *circadian temperature rhythm*, is about 0.6°C (1°F), and individuals retain their circadian rhythm throughout life despite intervening bouts of prolonged illness. During fever, the morning low and evening high temperature pattern can still be observed. In the occasional situation in which elevated temperature is due to hyperthermia (see below), this rhythm is absent.

Most fevers are induced by polypeptide molecules called *endogenous pyrogens*. Endogenous pyrogens are produced by the host in response to infection, injury, inflammation, or antigenic challenge. These polypeptides cause fever by their ability to trigger biochemical changes in the hypothalamus, particularly to stimulate hypothalamic prostaglandin synthesis. The first endogenous pyrogen described has now been identified as interleukin-1 (IL-1). Recombinant human IL-1 (α or β forms) produce fever in experimental animals or humans[1] at doses of 10 ng/kg kilogram. Interferons (IFN), produced as a consequence of viral infection, are also endogenous pyrogens. Recombinant human IFN-α, IFN-β and IFN-γ produce chills and fever in humans. Another endogenous pyrogen is tumor necrosis factor (TNF), which, like IL-1, produces fever in humans at doses of 10 ng/kg following intravenous injection.[2,3]

Recently, a new class of endogenous pyrogens was described. Although each is a distinct gene product with little or no relationship at the amino acid level, they share the ability to trigger the glycoprotein (gp) 130 cell surface receptor, which is distributed on many cells. This family of gp 130 receptor-activating pyrogens includes IL-6, IL-11, leukemia inhibitory factor (LIF), ciliary neurotropic factor (CNTF), and oncostatin M.[4] IL-6 and IL-11 stimulate bone marrow precursors, and CNTF is a nerve growth factor; each is in clinical trials, and fever has been observed following injection into patients.

PYROGENS

The term *pyrogen* is used to describe any substance that causes fever.[5] Pyrogens may be exogenous or endogenous. Exogenous pyrogens are derived from outside the host, and the vast majority of exogenous pyrogens are microbial products, toxins, or the microbes themselves. The classic example of an exogenous pyrogen is the lipopolysaccharide produced by all gram-negative bacteria and commonly called *endotoxin*. Endotoxins are potent substances not only as pyrogens but also as inducers of various pathologic changes observed in gram-negative infections. Endotoxins are large molecules (>300,000 Daltons). Another group of bacterial substances that are potent pyrogens are produced by gram-positive organisms. There are the enterotoxins of *Staphylococcus aureus* and the groups A and B streptococcal toxins. A staphylococcal toxin of recent clinical importance is the toxic shock syndrome toxin associated with strains of *S. aureus* isolated from patients with the toxic shock syndrome. The gram-positive exotoxins are polypeptides in the 20,000–30,000 dalton range. Like the endotoxins from gram-negative bacteria, the toxins produced by staphylococci and streptococci produce fever in experimental animals when injected intravenously in the submicrogram per kilogram range. Of considerable importance is the fact that endotoxin is a highly pyrogenic molecule in humans, since 2–3 ng/kg produces fever and generalized symptoms of malaise in volunteers.[6]

ENDOGENOUS PYROGENS

In contradistinction to exogenous pyrogens, endogenous pyrogens are polypeptides produced by various host cells, particularly the monocyte/macrophage. They initiate fever by their ability to trigger the hypothalamic thermoregulatory center. Early concepts of the pathogenesis of fever proposed that exogenous pyrogens produced fever by their ability to act directly on the brain. This was later shown to be an unlikely explanation, since there was a requirement for an intermediate role for leukocytes. It was subsequently shown that exogenous pyrogens produce fever by first inducing the release of endogenous pyrogens. Endogenous pyrogens then gain entrance to the circulation, either directly or through the lymph, and reach the hypothalamus. There they initiate a cascade of changes in arachidonic acid metabolites, neurotransmitters, and ions that raise the set-point.

It was originally believed that there was a single endogenous pyrogen, characterized by its ability to produce fever in rabbits and other experimental animals. Following the injection of endogenous pyrogen-containing leukocyte supernatants, there is a rapid rise in body temperature, usually within 5–10 minutes, whereas exogenous pyrogens have a more delayed onset of fever. Initial characterizations of human endogenous pyrogen revealed two polypeptides in the 15,000 dalton range. These have been subsequently renamed IL-1β and IL-1α. Their entire amino acid sequences are known,[7,8] and recombinant IL-1 produce typical endogenous pyrogen fever when injected into animals or humans intravenously. In rabbits, 50 ng/kg induces a peak fever of 0.7–8°C within 50 minutes[5]; in humans, doses as low as 10 ng/kg produce 1.0–1.5°C fever within 90 minutes after the injection.[1,9]

Other molecules have been cloned, and their recombinant forms have produced fever when injected into animals or humans. These are tumor necrosis factor (TNF-α),[10] lymphotoxin (TNF-β), and interferon-α (IFN-α).[11] Other molecules such as IL-6, IL-11, LIF, CNTF, and oncostatin M are grouped together because they each signal the cell through the same gp 130 receptor. In humans, microgram amounts per kilogram of body weight of IL-6, CNTF, or IL-11 produce fever compared with nanogram amounts of IL-1 or TNF. Together with IL-1, TNF, and

TABLE 1. Organisms and Substances Inducing Pyrogenic Cytokines[a]

Viruses
Bacteria
Peptidoglycans (cell walls of all bacteria)
Muramyl peptides (naturally occurring breakdown products of peptidoglycans)
Endotoxins (lipopolysaccharides of gram-negative bacteria)
Enterotoxins (A, B, C, D from *Staphylococcus aureus*)
Toxic shock syndrome toxin-1 (from toxic shock syndrome–associated *S. aureus*)
Erythrogenic toxins (from groups A and B streptococci)
Tuberculin (from *Mycobacterium* in sensitive individuals)
Antigen–antibody complexes (requires activation of complement)
Complement components (C5a, C3a)
Lymphocyte products (IL-2, Interferon-γ[b])
Polynucleic acids (poly I:C)
Pyrogenic steroids (etiocholanolone, bile salts)
Drugs (*via* the production of lymphocyte products in sensitized individuals, for example, penicillin)
Pyrogenic cytokines (IL-1, TNF)
Drugs (bleomycin)

[a] Data are derived from both in vitro and in vivo studies.
[b] IFN-α augments the production of pyrogenic cytokines induced by microbial products.

IFN, the latter substances can be classified as endogenous pyrogens or interchangeably with a more descriptive term rapidly gaining acceptance, *pyrogenic cytokines*. *Cytokine* refers to polypeptides produced by a variety of cells that induce biochemical changes in other cells. Each pyrogenic cytokine is a product of a separate gene; elevated plasma levels of some pyrogenic cytokines are found in humans during fever (discussed below).

IL-1, TNF, IFN, and the gp 130 receptor-triggering family of pyrogenic cytokines possess other biologic properties in addition to producing fever (discussed below under Acute Phase Changes). A wide spectrum of exogenous pyrogens induce the synthesis and release of these pyrogenic cytokines. These are listed in Table 1. Most of the exogenous pyrogenic substances can be recognized for their association with febrile diseases. However, there are clearly substances produced by the host that cause fever because they stimulate the synthesis and release of the endogenous pyrogenic cytokines. For example, antigen-antibody complexes derived from blood incompatability are pyrogens because they induce the production of IL-1, TNF, and IL-1.

THE HYPOTHALAMIC CONTROL OF CORE TEMPERATURE

The control of body temperature in humans takes place at the hypothalamic level. Clusters of neurons located in both the preoptic anterior and posterior hypothalamus receive two kinds of signals. One pathway is from other neurons with connections in the periphery to cold and warm receptors. The other signal is provided by the temperature of the blood bathing the hypothalamic region. These signals are integrated by both "warm" and "cold" neurons whose discharge rates vary with blood temperature and levels of several neurotransmitters. Together, the area is called the *thermoregulatory center*. In health, this center maintains the body temperature of the internal organs between 37°C and 38°C. This is the so-called core temperature, and it is best measured in the esophagus close to the great vessels.

Parts of brain and liver can have a higher temperature, about 38°C, whereas the skin is maintained at a lower temperature. The lower temperature of the skin varies with the state of vasoconstriction and the distance to large arteries. Therefore, axillary temperature tends to be about 1° lower (36°C) than the core temperature. Oral and rectal temperatures reflect core temperature. Oral readings are lower probably because of mouth breathing, which is particularly important in patients with respiratory infections and rapid breathing. Freshly voided urine temperatures also can reflect core temperature. In general, with the exception of young children, correct measurement of oral temperature is a very good approximation of the true core temperature in most clinical settings.

Using vasoconstriction, vasodilation, sweating, and, at times, shivering, the body maintains its temperature in the face of moderate environmental cold or heat. However, these physiologic manipulations cannot overcome severe temperature differences in the environment. Thus the hypothalamic thermoregulatory center also sends signals to the cerebral cortex, where behavioral changes such as seeking less severe environmental temperatures, special posturing, or the use of special clothing to help maintain normal body temperature are initiated. The metabolic rate of humans is constantly producing more heat than is necessary to maintain core body temperature at 37°C; therefore, hypothalamic temperature control is often regulating the amount of heat loss by vasodilation and evaporation. In severe cold, the hypothalamus triggers rapid muscle contractions (shivering) to produce more heat.

HYPERTHERMIA

Despite physiologic and behavioral control of body temperature, excessive heat production or inability to lose heat results in elevated core temperatures. For example, overinsulating clothing can result in elevated core temperature. This is not fever but hyperthermia. Hyperthermia is also observed in persons who work or exercise in hot environments and produce heat faster than the peripheral mechanisms can lose it.

Hyperthermia is an elevation of core temperature at a time when the hypothalamic set-point is at normothermic levels. In hyperthermia, elevation of core temperature occurs because heat loss mechanisms are either prevented or are not adequate. These include heat stroke syndromes in which excessive heat is produced by work or environmental conditions (such as high humidity) which prevent adequate heat loss. Certain metabolic diseases such as hyperthyroidism can result in mild elevations of core temperature. The effects of some pharmacologic agents that interfere with thermoregulation by blocking sweating or vasodilation can also produce elevation of core temperature. Once again, these syndromes represent hyperthermia because they take place in the presence of a normal hypothalamic set-point. Hyperthermia characteristically does not respond to antipyretics. A diagnosis of hyperthermia is often made because of a preceding history of heat exposure or use of certain drugs that interfere with normal thermoregulation. Even overinsulation of children can elevate core temperature, which masks as fever but is, in fact, hyperthermia.

In some patients the hypothalamic set-point is elevated owing to local trauma, hemorrhage, tumor, or intrinsic hypothalamic malfunction. The term *hypothalamic fever* is sometimes used to describe elevated temperature caused by abnormal hypothalamic function. However, the majority of patients with hypothalamic damage have hypothermia or do not respond properly to mild environmental temperature changes. In those few patients in whom hypothalamic fever is suspected, diagnosis depends on demonstrating other abnormal hypothalamic functions, such as production of hypothalamic releasing factors, abnormal response to cold, and absence of circadian temperature and hormonal rhythms. Hyperthermia can also occur when certain anesthetics produce a rapid uncoupling of oxidative phosphorylation in susceptible individuals. This is known as *malignant hyperthermia* and is often fatal. Another form of hyperthermia results in patients taking certain neuroleptic drugs.

There is no rapid way to differentiate elevated core temperature as being fever and not hyperthermia. Clinical history usually plays an important role. However, in addition to the clinical history of the patient, there are several physical aspects of some forms of hyperthermia that may alert the clinician; for example, in heat stroke syndromes and in patients taking drugs that block sweating, the skin is very hot but dry. Antipyretics do not reduce the elevated temperature in hyperthermia, whereas there is usually some decrease in body temperature in patients after adequate doses of either aspirin or acetaminophen.

THE FEBRILE RESPONSE

Fever is due to an upward shift of the set-point in the hypothalamus from "normothermia" to febrile levels. In fever, the hypothalamic set-point is raised and triggers the vasomotor center to commence vasoconstriction. Blood is shunted from the periphery, decreasing the usual heat loss resulting in a steady increase in blood temperature. For most fevers, this is sufficient to raise body temperatures 2–3°C. Shivering is also initiated at this time in order to increase heat production from the muscles, but shivering is frequently not required if heat conservation mechanisms raise blood temperature to the required level.

The processes of heat conservation and heat production continue until the temperature of the blood bathing the hypothalamic neurons matches the new setting. At that point, the hypothalamus maintains the new febrile temperature just as it does at normothermic levels. In fact, studies have shown that the mechanisms of heat balance in fever are the same as in the afebrile state, the only difference being that, in fever, body temperature is maintained at the higher level. When the hypothalamic set-point is reset downward, the processes of heat loss through vasodilation and sweating are initiated. Behavioral changes are also triggered at this time, and removal of insulating clothing or bedding takes place.

Persistent fevers are sometimes classified as "intermittent" or "remittent"; intermittent fevers are characterized as daily fever spikes followed by a return to normal body temperature, whereas remittent fevers do not return to normal body temperature. The biochemical or neurologic basis for these different fever patterns in some infectious diseases remains unknown.

Some hypothalamic substances have been reported to reduce fever; these include various neuropeptides such as somatostatin, arginine vasopressin, and α-melanocyte-stimulating factor. These substances appear to be produced in greater amounts during fever. In animal models, they suppress fever at the hypothalamic level and can be considered from a biologic point of view to function as intrinsic central antipyretics. For example, arginine vasopressin is thought to prevent fever in pregnant animals immediately before and after birth. In the preantibiotic era,

fever due to a variety of infectious diseases rarely exceeded 106°F, and there has been speculation that this natural "thermal ceiling" is mediated by these neuropeptides functioning as central antipyretics. It is possible that absence of production of these natural antipyretics may account for the failure of some fevers to return to baseline body temperature. It is unclear how much of a particular fever pattern observed in some infections is due to the action of these substances and how much is due to sporadic release of the endogenous pyrogenic cytokines.

EFFECT OF ENDOGENOUS PYROGENIC CYTOKINES ON THE HYPOTHALAMUS

Each endogenous pyrogenic cytokine is a product of a separate gene, and each has its own cell surface receptor. IL-1β and IL-1α both recognize IL-1 receptors, and TNF-α and TNF-β also share common receptors. IFN-α and IFN-γ have separate receptors. However, the family of IL-6, IL-11, LIF, CNTF, and oncostatin M share a single cell surface receptor, gp 130, which is associated with the production of fever. Each of these cytokines has its own specific receptor that is "soluble." The soluble part (or extracellular portion) of the receptor is shed and binds to its specific ligand. Unlike other soluble receptors, the binding of the ligand to the soluble receptor enhances rather than suppresses biologic activity because the complex of ligand to soluble receptor then presents the cytokine to the gp 130 receptor.

During fever, hypothalamic tissue and third cerebral ventricle levels of prostaglandin (PG) E_2 are elevated.[12] The highest concentrations of PGE_2 are near the circumventricular vascular organs (organ vasculosum lamina terminalis), which are networks of enlarged capillaries. Destruction of these organs reduces the ability of pyrogens to produce fever. Experiments have not been able to show, however, that pyrogenic cytokines pass from the circulation into the brain substance. Thus, it appears that endogenous pyrogens interact with the endothelium of these capillaries, which is probably the first step in initiating fever (Fig. 1).

The interaction of endogenous pyrogens with the hypotha-

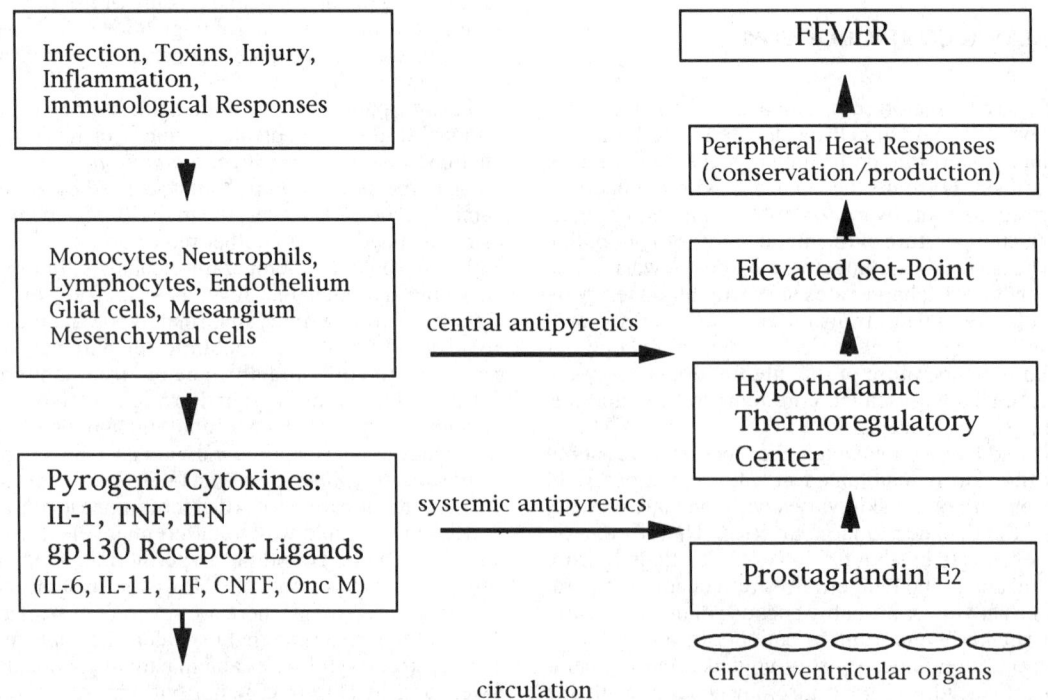

FIG. 1. Scheme for the pathogenesis of fever. IL, interleukin; TNF, tumor necrosis factor; IFN, interferon; LIF, leukemia inhibitory factor; CNTF, ciliary neurotropic factor; Onc M, oncostatin M.

lamic circumventricular vascular organs is poorly understood; however, cultured endothelial cells produce PGE and PGI when stimulated with IL-1 or TNF. In addition, IL-1 and TNF induce a variety of other changes in endothelial cells, including increased adhesion of leukocytes, release of platelet-activating factor, and synthesis of plasminogen activator inhibitor. IFN and the gp 130-triggering family do not induce these latter factors from endothelial cells.

Figure 1 illustrates the key events in the production of fever. Infections via the various toxins and activating molecules produced by microorganisms stimulate the monocyte/macrophage to synthesize and release the various pyrogenic cytokines. As shown, other cells have the potential to produce these endogenous pyrogens. The pyrogenic cytokines cause fever by their ability to initiate metabolic changes in the hypothalamic thermoregulatory center. Of these, the synthesis of prostaglandin E_2 appears to play a critical role. The ability of systemic drugs such as aspirin to inhibit the synthesis of prostaglandins at the hypothalamic level accounts for their antipyretic effect. The elevation in the hypothalamic temperature set-point brought about by elevated prostaglandin triggers the brain centers controlling heat production and peripheral vascular tone. Neuronal transmission delivers this information to the periphery, and core temperatures begins to rise.

FEVER THERAPY

Throughout history, fever therapy has been used to treat a variety of diseases, both physical and psychological. Sometimes these therapies have been quite successful, for example, the treatment of tertiary syphillis with malarial fever. Fever therapies have been replaced with specific drugs for specific infections and diseases. Nevertheless, there is continued interest and investigation into fever therapy. One problem in interpreting the data of such studies is the need to differentiate fever therapy in which a pyrogen or infection induces a fever from that which occurs in hyperthermic therapy in which core temperature is elevated directly by applying heat or preventing its removal. The use of hyperthermia in the treatment of various malignancies has been used with some success. In these situations, microwave energy is delivered to the patient, and core temperature can be raised under controlled conditions. Hyperthermia is particularly successful when combined with chemotherapy or radiation. However, hyperthermia treatment should not be equated with fever therapy. In fever therapy, the inducing agent produces a febrile response but, in addition, a variety of pyrogenic and nonpyrogenic cytokines are produced and can affect host defense. For example, high-dose IL-2 therapy causes fever but also induces TNF, which can directly kill some tumor cells or activate killing mechanisms in cytotoxic T cells.

There is a continuing debate on whether physicians should recommend reducing the elevated temperature that occurs in a variety of infectious diseases. The decision not to treat the fever is usually based on evidence that elevated temperature may offer the patient a benefit because in some animal experiments, host defense mechanisms are enhanced by elevated temperature. Is this evidence sufficient to advise patients not to take antipyretics? Unfortunately, there are few human studies, and those that exist do not show a dramatic difference in recovery from viral upper respiratory infections between groups taking or not taking antipyretics. There is, on the other hand, extensive in vitro data that support the concept that certain immunologic functions are enhanced by elevated temperature. Temperatures of 39°C augment T- and B-cell responses, the generation of cytotoxic T cells, B-cell activity, and immunoglobulin synthesis.[13,14] In addition, in vitro growth of some microbes (e.g., *Plasmodium* spp.) is suppressed at elevated temperatures. But there are no large studies showing that patients not taking antipyretics eliminate their viral infections faster or produce more antibodies. Withholding aspirin from children with viral-like illnesses appears warranted on the basis that this is a risk factor in the development of Reye syndrome. Children with fever, particularly those at risk for a febrile seizure, can be treated with acetaminophen.

An extraordinarily high fever (>41.5°C) is often called *hyperpyrexia*. Hyperpyrexia can be observed in patients with severe infections, but it most commonly occurs in patients with central nervous system hemorrhages. Although antipyretics reduce the fever, cooling blankets and water–alcohol bathing are recommended to accelerate peripheral heat losses. Peripheral cooling can be counterproductive in the absence of antipyretics, since cold receptors in the skin send signals to the spinal cord and brain for reactive vasoconstriction, thus reducing heat loss mechanisms. Similarly, drugs such as atropine and other muscarinics block sweating and make heat loss more difficult.

Studies in patients receiving controlled hyperthermia treatment for various neoplasms have shown that temperatures as high as 42°C can be tolerated for 4 hours without irreversible organ damage. Nevertheless, fever increases the demand for oxygen and can aggravate preexisting cardiac or pulmonary insufficiency. For every increase of 1°C over 37°C there is a 13 percent increase in O_2 consumption. In addition, elevated temperature can induce mental changes in patients with organic brain disease. Therefore, treatment of fever in some patient groups is recommended. Children with a previous febrile or nonfebrile seizure also should be aggressively treated to reduce fever. However, it is unclear what triggers the febrile seizure, since there is no correlation between the absolute temperature elevation and onset of a febrile seizure in susceptible children.

ANTIPYRETICS AND TREATMENT OF FEVER

The ability of the pyrogenic cytokines to induce PGE_2 synthesis is an important event in the production of fever. Numerous experiments have shown that the inhibitors of the cyclooxygenase enzyme system are potent antipyretics. There is a direct correlation of antipyretic potency of various drugs and the inhibition of brain cyclooxygenase.[15] Acetaminophen is a poor cyclooxygenase inhibitor in peripheral tissue and is without noteworthy anti-inflammatory activity; however, in the brain acetaminophen is oxidized, and the oxidized form inhibits cyclooxygenase activity. This oxidation explains the potent antipyretic effect of acetaminophen.

In some studies, there is no difference between oral aspirin and acetaminophen in reducing fever in humans. Nonsteroidal anti-inflammatory agents (e.g., indomethacin, ibuprofen) are also antipyretics and can be used for this purpose. Chronic high-dose antipyretic therapy such as aspirin or nonsteroidal anti-inflammatory agents used in arthritis do not reduce normal core body temperature. Thus, there appears to be no role of PGE_2 in normal thermoregulation.

Corticosteroids are also effective antipyretics. However, they act at two levels: (1) similar to the cyclooxygenase inhibitors, corticosteroids reduce PGE_2 synthesis by inhibiting the activity of phospholipase A_2; and (2) unlike the cyclooxygenase inhibitors, corticosteroids block the transcription of the mRNA for the pyrogenic cytokines. Drugs that interfere with vasoconstriction (phenothiazines, for example) can also act as antipyretics, as can drugs that block muscle contractions. However, these are not true antipyretics as they can also reduce core temperature independently of hypothalamic control.

MEASUREMENT OF CIRCULATING PYROGENIC CYTOKINES

Radioimmunoassay (RIA) and enzyme linked immunoassay (ELISA) kits for most of the pyrogenic cytokines are available commercially. Because pyrogenic cytokines are products of blood leukocytes that are affected by the clotting process, freshly obtained plasma in the presence of protease inhibitors is preferred.[16] Although there are relatively few comprehensive studies in febrile patients, a pattern appears to be emerging: the time of temperature elevation *does not* correlate with the concentration of the cytokine in the circulation. For example, in human volunteers given an injection of endotoxin, the peak of the fever occurs 4 hours after intravenous injection, but the peak elevation in circulating TNF occurs at 90 minutes.[17] In these same studies, IL-1β concentrations in the plasma increase slowly and reach peak elevation after 180 minutes, whereas maximal IL-6 levels occur at 120 minutes. In patients receiving high-dose IL-2 therapy, plasma TNF, IL-1β, and IL-6 are elevated, but, once again, these are not similarly elevated among the patients, and peak plasma levels do not correlate with the peak of the fever. In some studies of septic patients, there is a correlation between the severity of the disease and the level of IL-1β and TNF in the same sample.[18]

Despite no overt evidence of fever or illness, some healthy individuals have elevated plasma TNF, IL-1, or IL-6 levels. Studies do show that some of the pyrogenic cytokines are elevated in burns, sepsis, malaria, exacerbations of rheumatoid arthritis,[19] and during renal allograph rejection. They are also elevated after strenuous exercise and ovulation.[20] Pyrogenic cytokines may be present in the circulation but bound to carrier molecules that reduce or prevent the interaction with the capillary network in the hypothalamic thermoregulatory center. There is evidence to support this concept since IL-1β requires extraction from plasma proteins such as α₂-macroglobulin prior to being assayed.[16] The concentration of cytokine-binding proteins appears to increase in chronic diseases and may be due to increased hepatic acute phase proteins.

Aspirin and nonsteroidal anti-inflammatory agents prevent fever but do not prevent the synthesis and release of pyrogenic cytokines. In fact, the levels of IL-6 in the circulation are elevated in human subjects taking oral cyclooxygenase inhibitors. Hence, it is possible to measure elevated plasma cytokine levels in individuals who are afebrile because of antipyretic therapy.

ACUTE PHASE CHANGES

Infections, trauma, inflammatory processes, and some malignant diseases induce a constellation of host responses that are collectively referred to as the *acute phase response*. This response is associated with characteristic metabolic changes in liver protein synthesis, but, on closer examination, changes also occur in several other systems, including the hematologic, endocrinologic, neurologic, and immunologic systems. These changes are called *acute* because most are observed within hours or days following the onset of infection or injury; however, some acute phase changes also indicate persistent disease. The full spectrum of the response includes dramatic increases in the synthesis of several unique hepatic proteins that are not produced in health. One of these, C-reactive protein, is a marker of the acute phase response and can be used as an indicator of disease. The increased plasma concentrations of acute phase hepatic proteins, glycoproteins, and globulins are responsible for elevated erythrocyte sedimentation rates. Although the liver is producing increasing amounts of a variety of proteins, hepatic albumin synthesis is decreased. Increases in gluconeogenesis, energy expenditure, and muscle proteolysis occur and contribute to weight loss. Increased sleep and lethargy are frequent clinical complaints. Leukocytosis with increased numbers of circulating immature neutrophils is common, and serum iron and zinc levels are depressed while increased ceruloplasmin levels result in elevated serum copper. Thyroid dysfunction can be present, and there is often abnormal glucose tolerance and lipid metabolism. In addition, anemia develops despite adequate stores of iron. This may be due to the suppressive effect of TNF on hematopoiesis. The hypergammaglobulinemia that is often a component of the acute phase response may be mediated by IL-6, one of the pyrogenic cytokines. IL-6 also induces hepatic

acute phase protein synthesis and is a potent B-lymphocyte growth and differentiation factor.

Although the most striking changes in the acute phase response is observed in patients with bacterial infections, burns, or multiple injuries, clinicians also encounter acute phase changes in patients with occult infections or chronic illnesses such as rheumatoid arthritis, Crohn's disease, and several autoimmune diseases. The presence of acute phase changes can also serve as an indicator of silent disease and some cancers, particularly renal cell carcinoma and Hodgkin's disease. The acute phase response has the outstanding characteristic of being a generalized host reaction irrespective of the localized or systemic nature of the inciting disease. The various components of the response are remarkably consistent despite the considerable variety of pathologic processes that induce it.

The patient with a localized bacterial infection represents an excellent example of the development of the acute phase response. At the onset of the infection, blood monocytes and tissue macrophages become activated either by phagocytosis of the invading microbe or by exposure to its products or toxins; the process results in the synthesis and release of the pyrogenic cytokines. These mediators enter the circulation and reach the brain, where they initiate fever. Whereas fever is clearly one of the most obvious signs of the acute phase response, other components of the response can be present without apparent clinical manifestations.

One of the most sensitive measures of the acute phase response is an increase in the number and immaturity of circulating neutrophils. The release of neutrophils is due to the direct action of IL-1 and IL-6 on the bone marrow neutrophil stores. In addition, IL-1, IL-6, and IL-11 stimulates stem cells to become more responsive to various colony-stimulating factors. In human subjects injected with small doses of IL-1, marked neutrophilia and increased circulating stem cells can be measured when fever is suppressed by cyclooxygenase inhibitors.[9] Although not routinely measured, serum zinc and iron levels are depressed. Low serum iron associated with anemia in the face of adequate iron stores is characteristic of the acute phase response. There is a large body of evidence that decreased serum iron probably plays an important role in protecting the host against various bacteria. For example, the reduction in serum iron can suppress the growth rate of several microorganisms and certain tumor cells that have a strict requirement for iron as a growth factor.

Within 8–12 hours after the onset of infection or trauma, the synthetic rate of the liver increases due to acute phase proteins. Several normal plasma proteins increase severalfold during the acute phase response. These include haptoglobin, certain protease inhibitors, complement components, ceruloplasmin, and fibrinogen. However, true acute phase reactants increase several hundredfold. These include serum amyloid A protein, a precursor of the amyloid fibril in secondary amyloidosis, and C-reactive protein. C-reactive protein was named for its ability to interact with the C-polysaccharide of pneumococci and was the first acute phase protein described. Albumin and cytochrome synthesis is depressed during acute phase responses. Of the acute phase proteins, C-reactive protein and serum amyloid A protein are clinically the most important, because their presence serves as an indicator of disease. C-reactive protein is particularly useful as a marker of the acute phase protein response and can be measured easily in most hospital clinical laboratories.

Despite the anabolic processes of the liver, the acute phase response is accompanied by a pronounced catabolism of muscle protein associated with loss of body weight and overall negative nitrogen balance.[21] Fever increases oxygen and caloric demands, and negative nitrogen balance can result from oxidation of amino acids from skeletal muscle, which contributes to wasting. These amino acids are largely used for gluconeogenesis. In addition, there can be demineralization of bone.

Although the metabolic demands of elevated temperature contribute to the increased need for energy substrates, the host also requires a large supply of amino acids for synthesis of new protein at a time when food intake may be severely impaired or appetite reduced. Amino acids are required for immunologic and reparative processes such as the clonal expansion of lymphocytes and the proliferation of fibroblasts. Also, they are needed for synthesis of hepatic acute phase proteins, immunoglobulins, and collagen. The mechanism of providing ample amino acids for these cellular functions seems to be well orchestrated during the acute phase response. The catabolism during infection and inflammation differs from that during starvation. Unlike starvation, in which large amounts of ketones are spilled into the urine, a septic individual excretes protein with small amounts of ketones. IL-1 and TNF inhibit lipoprotein lipase and hence interfere with lipid metabolism. In addition to the biochemical changes during acute phase responses, appetite is depressed. In fact, depressed appetite may play a greater role in the negative nitrogen balance of chronic disease than the mobilization of tissue. IL-1 and TNF are potent suppressors of appetite in animals.[22]

The acute phase response is nonspecific. However, the presence of certain acute phase changes in an otherwise healthy individual can alert the physician to hidden disease. Measuring ACTH, cortisol, growth hormone, and vasopressin is not particularly useful, although levels are elevated during acute phase responses. Measurement of C-reactive protein can assist the physician in determining the presence of disease in patients with vague, constitutional complaints. C-reactive protein levels are usually less than 100 μg per liter but increase within hours 10- to 1000-fold. In severe bacterial infections, the serum level can rise from undetectable to over 100 mg per liter in 48 hours. The presence of elevated levels of C-reactive protein or serum amyloid A protein, even in the absence of fever or neutrophilia, may indicate occult infection or malignant disease. Increases in C-reactive protein and serum amyloid A protein occur in patients of any age and also in immunocompromised patients with opportunistic infections.

Not all inflammatory diseases are associated with elevated C-reactive protein. A refractory state can develop in certain diseases such as scleroderma, ulcerative colitis, and lupus erythematosus. Failure to develop hepatic protein changes and the neutrophilia of the acute phase response seem to be related to the presence of circulating inhibitors of IL-1 and TNF.

Some effects of the acute phase response on the host have an important and vital role in defense against infection and malignant transformation. For example, elevated temperature has a direct effect on immunologic responses in that temperatures of 38 and 39°C augment T- and B-cell responses, the generation of cytolytic T cells, B-cell activity, and immunoglobulin synthesis.[13,14] In addition, these febrile temperatures adversely affect the replication of certain viruses, several bacteria, and some tumors. The requirement for iron as a growth factor for microorganisms increases at elevated temperatures. Therefore, the decision to intervene with antipyretics could, in some diseases, increase host comfort at the expense of host defenses. However, as discussed above, the data for the role of elevated temperature in host defense are based on in vitro and animal experiments; data for humans are lacking.

The role of acute phase proteins in host defense and repair is not entirely clear. Studies suggest that the major role of C-reactive protein is to bind serum lipids or opsonize pneumococci, whereas serum amyloid A is thought to be immunosuppressive. Ceruloplasmin scavenges toxic free-oxygen radicals that are injurious to many tissues. What is clear, however, is that the production and physical structure of these acute phase proteins have been conserved through 400 million years of evolution, and therefore they have presumably been useful to the host. This argues that the acute phase response, like fever, plays a role in survival.

TABLE 2. Biologic Properties of Pyrogenic Cytokines

Biologic Property	IL-1[a]	TNF[b]	gp130R[c]	IFN-α
Endogenous pyrogen	+	+	+	+
Inducer of sleep	+	+	−	+
Inducer of shock syndrome	+	+	−	−
Anorexia	+	+	±	−
Hepatic acute phase proteins	+	+	+	−[d]
Decreased albumin synthesis	+	+	+	−
B-lymphocyte activation	+	+	±	−
T-lymphocyte activation	+	+	±	−
B-lymphocyte immunoglobulin synthesis	+	+	±	−
Hematopoietic stem cell activation	+	−	±	−
Endothelial cell activation	+	+	−	−
Synovial cell stimulation	+	+	−	−
Bone resorption	+	+	±	−
Induction of IL-1, TNF, and IL-6	+	+	−	−

[a] Data are derived from recombinant IL-1β and IL-1α studies.
[b] Similar data are obtained using either TNF-α or TNF-β (lymphotoxin).
[c] gp 130 Receptor-activating family (IL-6, IL-11, LIF, CNTF, oncostatin M). ± Indicates that these biologic properties have not been established experimentally for all members.
[d] IFN-γ stimulates some hepatic protein synthesis.

The pyrogenic cytokines IL-1, TNF, and members of the gp 130 receptor-activating family (IL-6, IL-11, LIF, CNTF, oncostatin M) induce hepatic acute phase protein synthesis.[23,24] IL-6 has been studied in detail.[25] IL-6 and the other cytokines bind to their respective soluble receptors and then bring about the homodimerization of the gp 130 on the cell surface.[26] This results in activation of tyrosine kinases and the initiation of gene transcription for acute phase proteins by the liver.[26] CNTF and LIF also induce hepatic acute phase protein synthesis via a similar mechanism.[23,24]

Although it shares with IL-1 and TNF the ability to produce fever, sleep, and lethargy, IFN-α does not induce hepatic acute phase protein synthesis or other acute phase changes. Thus, elevated erythrocyte sedimentation rates and neutrophilia are not commonly observed during viral infections. IFN-γ, produced during immunologic reactions such as organ transplant rejection and drug fever, induces hepatic acute phase proteins in vitro but, like IFN-α, is a weak inducer of acute phase changes in the liver. The members of the gp 130 receptor-activating family do not appear to induce sleep.

Table 2 compares the multiple biologic effects of the different pyrogenic cytokines. IL-1, TNF, IL-6, IL-11, CNTF, IFN-α, and IFN-γ have been injected into humans intravenously. Only IL-1 and TNF have induced a "shock syndrome" with hypotension and decreased systemic vascular resistance observed at 100 ng/kg.[1,3] High doses of IL-6 have not produced shock despite doses as high as 100 μg/kg. IL-2, given intravenously to treat patients with certain tumors, induces a shock-like state and fever, but neither response is due to a direct action of IL-2; rather, high-dose IL-2 induces IL-1 and TNF. Blocking IL-1 or TNF in experimental animals reduces the toxicity of IL-2.

REFERENCES

1. Smith JW2, Urba WJ, Curti BD, et al. The toxic and hematologic effects of interleukin-1 alpha administered in a phase I trial to patients with advanced malignancies. J Clin Oncol. 1992;10:1141–52.
2. van der Poll T, Bueller HR, ten Cate H, et al. Activation of coagulation after administration of tumor necrosis factor to normal subjects. N Engl J Med. 1990;322:1622–7.
3. Chapman PB, Lester TJ, Casper ES, et al. Clinical pharmacology of recombinant human tumor necrosis factor in patients with advanced cancer. J Clin Oncol. 1987;5:1942–51.
4. Shapiro L, Zhang X-X, Rupp RG, et al. Ciliary neutrophic factor is an endogenous pyrogen. Proc Natl Acad Sci USA. 1993;90:8614–8.
5. Dinarello CA, Cannon JG, Wolff SM. New concepts on the pathogenesis of fever. Rev Infect Dis. 1988;10:168–89.

6. Wolff SM. Biological effects of bacterial endotoxins in man. J Infect Dis. 1973;128(Suppl):733–58.

7. Auron PE, Webb AC, Rosenwasser LJ, et al. Nucleotide sequence of human monocyte interleukin 1 precursor cDNA. Proc Natl Acad Sci USA. 1984;81: 7907–11.

8. Lomedico PT, Gubler R, Hellmann CP, et al. Cloning and expression of murine interleukin-1 cDNA in *Escherichia coli*. Nature (London). 1984;312: 458–62.

9. Tewari A, Buhles WC Jr, Starnes HF Jr. Preliminary report: Effects of interleukin-1 on platelet counts. Lancet. 1990;336:712–4.

10. Dinarello CA, Cannon JG, Wolff SM, et al. Tumor necrosis factor (cachectin) is an endogenous pyrogen and induces production of interleukin 1. J Exp Med. 1986;163:1433–50.

11. Dinarello CA, Bernheim HA, Duff GW, et al. Mechanisms of fever induced by recombinant human interferon. J Clin Invest. 1984;74:906–13.

12. Coceani F, Lees J, Dinarello CA. Occurrence of interleukin-1 in cerebrospinal fluid of the conscious cat. Brain Res. 1988;446:245–50.

13. Duff GW, Durum SK. Fever and immunoregulation: Hyperthermia, interleukins 1 and 2, and T-cell proliferation. Yale J Biol Med. 1982;55:437–42.

14. Hanson DF, Murphy PA, Silicano R, et al. The effect of temperature on the activation of thymocytes by interleukins I and II. J Immunology. 1983;130: 216–21.

15. Flower RJ, Vane JR. Inhibition of prostaglandin synthetase in brain explains the anti-pyretic activity of paracetamol (4-acetamidophenol). Nature. 1972; 240:410–11.

16. Cannon JG, van der Meer JWM, Kwiatkowski D, et al. Interleukin-1β in human plasma: Optimization of blood collection, plasma extraction, and radio-immunoassay methods. Lymphokine Res. 1988;7:457–67.

17. Michie HR, Manogue KR, Spriggs DR, et al. Detection of circulating tumor necrosis factor after endotoxin administration. N Engl J Med. 1988;318: 1481–6.

18. Casey LC, Balk RA, Bone RC. Plasma cytokines and endotoxin levels correlate with survival in patients with the sepsis syndrome. Ann Intern Med. 1993; 119:771–8.

19. Eastgate JA, Symons JA, Wood NC, et al. Correlation of plasma interleukin 1 levels with disease activity in rheumatoid arthritis. Lancet. 1988;2:706–9.

20. Cannon JG, Dinarello CA. Increased plasma interleukin-1 activity in women after ovulation. Science. 1985;227:1247–9.

21. Beisel WR. Magnitude of the host nutritional responses to infection. Am J Clin Nutr. 1977;30:1236–47.

22. Dinarello CA, Wolff SM. The role of interleukin-1 in disease. N Engl J Med. 1993;328:106–113.

23. Schooltink H, Stoyan T, Roch E, et al. Ciliary neurotropic factor induces acute-phase protein expression in hepatocytes. Fed Eur Biochem Soc. 1992; 314:280–4.

24. Baumann H, Wong GG. Hepatocyte-stimulating factor III shares structural and functional identity with leukemia-inhibitory factor. J Immunol. 1989;143: 1163–7.

25. Gauldie J, Richards C, Harnish D, et al. Interferon b₂/B-cell stimulatory factor type 2 shares identity with monocyte-derived hepatocyte-stimulating factor and regulates the major acute phase protein response in liver cells. Proc Natl Acad Sci USA. 1987;84:7251–6.

26. Murakami M, Hibi M, Nakagawa N, et al. IL-6-induced homodimerization of gp130 and associated activation of a tyrosine kinase. Science. 1993;260: 1808–18.

37. FEVER OF UNKNOWN ORIGIN

JEFFREY A. GELFAND
SHELDON M. WOLFF*

Fever is such a common manifestation of illness that it is not surprising to find accurate descriptions of the febrile patient in early recorded history. There is evidence that the symbol of a flaming brazier was used by the ancient Sumerians to denote fever and that cuneiform inscriptions of the sixth century BC had adapted this symbol into a single ideogram for fever and inflammation.[1] By the time of Hippocrates and later during the Roman Empire, physicians were so well acquainted with the signs and symptoms of febrile diseases that their detailed descriptions of typhoid and malarial fevers can still be used as examples of these protracted fevers. However, only some fevers

* Deceased.

of prolonged nature can be diagnosed from descriptive histories, and most patients with long-standing fevers require a careful and thorough investigation. Today, the physician charged with the problem of determining the cause of a prolonged fever must consider the spectrum of febrile diseases, which, through the years, has changed under the influence of nutritional, hygienic, and environmental effects. In addition, age, geographic location, and iatrogenic involvement are also important factors that play a role in determining the cause of prolonged fever.

In most patients with fever lasting 1 or 2 weeks, the underlying cause is soon discovered or the patient recovers spontaneously. In the latter case, a protracted viral illness is usually presumed to be the source of the fever. In other patients, however, fever continues for 2 or 3 weeks during which time physical examination, chest x-ray films, blood tests, and routine cultures do not reveal the cause of fever. In these patients a provisional diagnosis of fever of unknown origin (FUO) is made.

A definition of FUO formulated by Petersdorf and Beeson[2] in 1961 has become a standard: illness of more than 3 weeks duration; documented fevers above 101°F (38.3°C) on several occasions; and lack of a specific diagnosis after 1 week of inpatient investigation. This definition was established for the purpose of comparative retrospective and prospective clinical studies and should not be regarded as absolute. Since the daily rhythm in core temperature varies from individual to individual, we believe that an FUO is best defined when considering the normal temperature rhythm for the patient and the presence of an associated pathologic change. While the "classic" definition of FUO has been used for over 30 years, the enormous changes that have taken place over this period of time have rendered the definition somewhat obsolete; for example, based on the Diagnosis-Related Group for "Pyrexia of Unknown Origin" (ICD9 No. 780.6), Medicare would only allow a patient *5 days* in the hospital. Economic imperatives and constraints, improvements in noninvasive diagnostic methods, and increasing numbers of patients with undiagnosed fevers associated with invasive medical technology, neutropenia, and HIV have led to a newly proposed classification of FUO by Durack and Street.[3] The types of FUO are defined as "classic FUO," nosocomial FUO, neutropenic FUO, and HIV-associated FUO (Table 1).

Classic FUO is an "updated" version of the Petersdorf and Beeson[2] definition of FUO; the requirement of 1 week of investigation in the hospital has been modified to either 3 days of hospital investigation or three outpatient visits, without discovering the source. Petersdorf[4] has recently suggested this might be better modified to encompass "one week of intelligent and intensive investigation, which, in most patients, could be conducted on an outpatient basis." In our opinion, 2 weeks of fever is sufficient to entertain the diagnosis when other criteria have been met.

The designation of *nosocomial FUO* would refer to hospitalized patients receiving acute care in whom infection or fever were absent on admission but in whom a fever of 38.3°C (101°F) or higher occurs on several occasions. Three days of investigation, including at least 2 days incubation of cultures, is required for this diagnosis.

Fever of 38.3°C (101°F) or higher on several occasions in a patient with less than 500 neutrophils/mm³ or a neutrophil level expected to fall below that within 1 to 2 days is considered a *neutropenic FUO*. As in nosocomial FUO, 3 negative days of investigation, including at least 2 days incubation of microbiologic cultures, are required for definition. However, empiric therapy is often indicated, as detailed in Chapter 289.

HIV-associated FUO is defined as a fever of 38.3°C (101°C) or higher on several occasions over a period of more than 3 days in the hospital or of more than 4 weeks duration for an outpatient in an individual with confirmed HIV infection. As with the other categories, appropriate investigation and at least 2 days incubation of cultures are also required.

There are no shortcuts in determining the cause of an FUO.

TABLE 1. Categories of FUO[a]

	"Classic"	Neutropenic	HIV Associated	Nosocomial
Patient type	Patients not in other categories with fevers ≥ 3 weeks	Has ≤500 neutrophils/mm³, or level anticipated in 1–2 days	Confirmed HIV positive	Hospitalized; acute care. No infection when admitted
Duration of illness while under investigation	3 Days[b] or three outpatient visits	3 Days[b]	3 Days[b] or 4 weeks as outpatient	3 Days[b]
Examples of etiologies	Infections, malignancy, inflammatory diseases, drug fever	Perianal infection; *Aspergillosis,* candidemia	*M. avium-intracellulare,* tuberculosis, non-Hodgkin's lymphoma, drug fever	Septic thrombophlebitis, sinusitis, *C. difficile* colitis, drug fever

[a] All require fevers of 38.3°C (101°F) or higher on several occasions.
[b] Includes at least 2 days incubation of microbiology cultures.

(Adapted from Durack and Street,[3] with permission.)

TABLE 2. Fever of Unknown Origin in Children

			Established Causes (%)				
References	Dates of Study	No. of Cases	Infections	Collagen-Vascular Disease	Neoplasms	Miscellaneous	Undiagnosed
McClung[5]	1959–69	99	29	11	8	19	32
Pizzo et al.[6]	1966–72	100	52	20	6	10	12
Lohr and Hendley[7]	1967–74	54	33	18	13	15	19

TABLE 3. Fever of Unknown Origin in Adults

			Established Causes (%)				
References	Dates of Study	No. of Cases	Infections	Collagen-Vascular Disease	Neoplasms	Miscellaneous	Undiagnosed
Petersdorf and Beeson[2]	1952–57	100	36	13	19	25	7
Shoen and Van Ommen[8]	1959–60	60	21	13	6	20	40
Deal[9]	1970	34	35	15	20	9	20
Frayha and Uwaydah[10]	1967–70	49	43	14	27	6	10
Howard et al.[11]	1969–76	100	37	19	31	8	5
Larson et al.[12]	1970–80	105	30	16	31	10	12
Knockaert et al.[13]	1980–89	199	22.5	21.5	7	26.5[a]	22.5[a]

[a] Authors' raw data re-tabulated to conform to prior diagnostic categories.

Only a well-organized systematic approach that is carried out with an awareness of the multiple causes of fever shortens the duration of the investigation. In this regard, reports on patients with the classic form of FUO have been helpful, since they call attention to both the varied causes and incidence of long-standing fevers. From these studies several general conclusions can be made. It is best to divide patients into three age groups: under 6 years, 6–14 years, and over 14 years. Patients under 6 years of age have a high incidence of infection, primarily bacterial and systemic-viral, while collagen—vascular diseases and inflammatory bowel disease are the most prevalent causes in the 6- to 16-year age group (Table 2). Rheumatic fever as a cause of FUO in American children has decreased in the last two decades, although recent reports suggest that the incidence of rheumatic fever in the United States may be rising again. On the other hand, the incidence of tuberculosis as a cause of FUO in children has dropped less sharply.

Based on studies made in the antibiotic era only, Table 3 indicates that infection predominates in most studies as the most frequently diagnosed source of persistent fever. In a recent series, it was suggested that improved noninvasive and microbiologic diagnostic methods have resulted in a greater proportion of classical FUO being due to systemic diseases (Still's disease, sarcoidosis, temporal arteritis) or remaining etiologically undefined. However, it can be generally stated that as the duration of fever increases, the likelihood of an infectious cause decreases. This statement has been substantiated by studies of patients with FUOs lasting for longer than 1 year in which infections were the third most common cause of the FUO.[14] Following infections, malignancies usually compose the next most frequent source of FUO in adults. Recent reviews of patients with FUOs have been reported.[15–17] In general, infectious causes of

FUO are still common, but malignancies are increasingly identified as the cause of FUOs. This is not the case, however, in children. Nevertheless, in both adults and children with neoplastic disease as a source of fever, lymphomas and leukemias are the most prevalent. The third most common diagnosis in adult patients with FUO is collagen-vascular disease. The actual incidence of collagen-vascular disease in patients with FUO is possibly higher than is shown in Table 3 since some studies limit this diagnosis to systemic lupus erythematosus, rheumatoid arthritis, and systemic vasculitis. It may be better to classify these diseases as autoimmune hypersensitivity rather than collagen-vascular. It is useful then to consider the three major causes of FUO, i.e., infection, malignancy, and autoimmune disease, since more than 70 percent of patients fall into one of these three groups. However, there are many diseases that have been grouped in studies as "miscellaneous," and in adults these include drug fever,[18] erythema multiforme, granulomatous hepatitis, regional enteritis, pulmonary embolism, sarcoidosis, familial Mediterranean fever, Fabry's disease, hypertriglyceridemia, alcoholic hepatitis, and factitious fever.[19–22] In children, miscellaneous causes of FUO have been Behçet syndrome and heavy metal intoxication. Although fever can be the presenting sign of the initial infection with human immunodeficiency virus (HIV), most FUOs in these patients are due to other infectious agents.[22] Because of the high incidence of unusual infections in HIV-infected patients, any patient from a high-risk group seeking medical attention for an FUO requires a test for the presence of HIV antibodies.

Other important factors in determining the causes of FUO are the type of institution in which the patient is evaluated. A tertiary care facility may see more unusual illness because of the nature of their referral patterns. Inner city hospitals may have

TABLE 4. Prolonged Fever of Unknown Origin[a]

	Percentage of Cases
No fever[b]	27
FUO	19
Miscellaneous	13
Factitious	9
Granulomatous hepatitis	8
Neoplasm	7
Still's disease	6
Infections	6
Collagen-vascular disease	4
Familial Mediterranean fever	3

[a] Evaluation of 347 patients studied from 1961 to 1977 at the National Institutes of Health. Fever was present for more than 1 year in 75 percent of the cases (mean = 4 years).[14]
[b] Includes patients with exaggerated circadian temperature rhythm.

much higher incidences of infectious disease since patients may lack proper evaluation or therapy before being seen in the hospital. In the same type of hospital, adult patients may be older and thus more likely to have a malignant neoplasm as a cause of their FUO. Thus, other factors such as economics, race, geography, and so forth may determine the distribution of diagnoses in a given report.

In patients in whom fever persists for longer than 6 months without an identifiable source, the spectrum of diagnoses is different. In these patients a high incidence of granulomatous disease has been seen as well as the adult manifestation of Still's disease.[23] The diagnoses in these patients are shown in Table 4. In all studies, there is a group of patients in whom diagnosis cannot be made after years of fever, and the diagnosis remains FUO. A few of these patients may have abnormal hypothalamic thermoregulation, but in most patients this diagnosis remains speculative. Factitious fevers are consistently reported in studies on FUO, and these include adults and children. Also included in the diagnosis of a factitious fever are patients who inject themselves with contaminated materials.[24]

Searching for the underlying cause of prolonged fever requires an open mind and a carefully organized approach by the physician. Since most patients who receive a provisional diagnosis of FUO have no obvious source of fever, we recommend an investigation that includes certain clinical tests that can be considered "routine" for these patients. The work-up may be divided into the following categories: (1) observation of temperature pattern, (2) medical history, (3) physical examinations, (4) laboratory tests, (5) noninvasive procedures, and (6) invasive procedures.

TEMPERATURE PATTERN

It is important to establish that the patient with a presumptive diagnosis of FUO is, in fact, having fever. There are a few patient who seek medical assistance with a chief complaint of persistent fever and, on closer investigation, do not have fever but rather an exaggerated circadian temperature rhythm. This conclusion can be reached by measuring the daily temperature at approximately 6 AM and 6 PM.[25] In the absence of associated symptoms like sweating, chills, and elevated pulse rate and in the absence of abnormal laboratory, radiologic, or physical findings, these patients can be considered to be normal. In a large series of patients referred to us at the National Institutes of Health with a presumptive diagnosis of FUO for longer than 6 months, 27 percent failed to manifest evidence of ongoing disease during the 2–3 weeks of impatient observation.[14] In fact, many patients with so-called benign fever of unknown origin probably belong in this category.[26] It is not uncommon for children of overly concerned parents or from troubled families to seek medical work-up for nonexistent fever that they consider "low grade."

Fever patterns have been classified as continuous, remittent, and intermittent; however, observation and characterization of fever patterns have little or no significance in the diagnosis of prolonged fevers. There are two notable exceptions: malaria and cyclic neutropenia. To a lesser extent the fever associated with Hodgkin's disease (Pel-Ebstein) may be helpful in making this diagnosis. The well-synchronized malarial paroxysm can be used to help make a diagnosis of malaria, although demonstration of the malarial parasite in blood smears is required for diagnostic confirmation. In nonendemic areas, well-synchronized malarial fevers are rarely seen, and this diagnosis is usually suspected on learning of recent travel to malaria-infested areas. Patients with tertian malaria (fever every other day) and quartan malaria (fever on day 1 and day 4 and so forth) can have low-grade fever in between the paroxyms, and most new malarial infections take 1–2 weeks before the paroxyms are synchronized.

The other fever pattern that is most suggestive of a specific diagnosis consists of a 21-day cycle. This fever accompanies cyclic neutropenia in which the peripheral neutrophil count falls to very low levels every 21 days.[27] It is common for these patients to have concurrent ulcers of the mucous membranes.

Other fevers that have been previously considered to be periodic are those of familial Mediterranean fever and Hodgkin's disease. Although such fevers can occur at regular intervals, patients with these diseases do not have a strict periodicity to their fevers like those of malaria or cyclic neutropenia but rather periods of no fevers or irregular fevers.

MEDICAL HISTORY

Clues to the diagnosis of certain febrile diseases may be obtained from historical characteristics and symptoms; examples include transient skin rashes in patients with autoimmune and collagen-vascular disease, the injection of medications in patients with drug fever, and hematuria in patients with renal cell carcinoma. Since patients with FUO often have atypical manifestations of their diseases, many symptoms are present only transiently and are not easily recalled during routine questioning. History of other symptoms such as myalgias, malaise, rigors, sweating, and weight loss may be nonspecific in that they are characteristic of elevation body temperature due to a diversity of causes.

Travel and exposure to certain agents or animals is critical information needed to make a diagnosis of several febrile diseases. For example, in the period from 1970 to 1975 there was a threefold increase in the number of civilian cases of malaria imported into the United States. Clearly, knowledge of travel to regions where malaria is indigenous can be key in suspecting this disease. Knowledge of tick bites is often absent in most cases of tick-transmitted diseases, but awareness of the endemic tick-infested areas is valuable even when the patient denies a tick bite. Certain parts of the United States are endemic areas for *Coccidioides, Histoplasma,* and *Blastomyces,* and the diagnosis of disease due to these organisms can be aided by a history of travel to such areas. Occupational hazards are important aspects of an accurate history. For example, exposure to beryllium can lead to a febrile illness, and knowledge of such exposure should expedite the diagnostic work-up of patients with berylliosis.

PHYSICAL EXAMINATION

There is no substitute for a complete physical examination in evaluating a patient with FUO. Furthermore, these patients require repeated physical examinations on a regular basis during investigation into their disease. Such patients may develop skin lesions, fundoscopic changes, organomegaly, and masses late in the course of their disease. All too often patients receive a thorough physical examination at the time of initial medical evaluation for persistent fever, and subsequently the caring physician focuses on laboratory and other diagnostic procedures, never returning to the bedside to repeat the entire physical examination. There are some areas in particular that require almost daily inspection, and these include examination of the skin, eyes, nail beds, lymph nodes, and abdomen and auscultation of the heart. The rashes of Still's disease are usually faint and fade quickly. The skin lesions of the patients with systemic vasculidites who have an FUO may appear late in the disease and in very few numbers. Atypical areas, for example, under the scrotal and breast folds, must be inspected for a complete examination of the skin. To make a diagnosis of vasculitis, the involved skin lesion must be located and a biopsy must be done.

Regular inspection of the peripheral lymph nodes is necessary. Many febrile diseases involving the lymph nodes that manifest as FUO may involve only a single node. Illnesses such as Hodgkin's disease, toxplasmosis, or infectious mononucleosis can manifest atypically with a single node enlargement. Draining lymph nodes of the head and neck, breast, and pelvic regions can be involved in neoplastic and infectious processes in these areas.

The importance of a complete eye examination in patients with FUO cannot be overstated. Because many FUOs manifest with no apparent localizing symptoms and because the eye is often involved in systemic disease, proper examination of the eye is indicated in every patient with prolonged fevers even in the absence of ophthalmologic symptoms. Examination of the eye can be divided into the orbit, cornea, conjunctiva, uveal tract, and retina. Proptosis due to orbital involvement can be seen in isolated lymphomas of the orbit, retrobital granulomatous disease such as Wegener's granulomatosis, neurofibromas, and metastatic disease to the orbit.

Band keratopathy can be seen in children with Still's disease and sarcoidosis. Punctate epithelial loss associated with tear deficiency and dry eyes is a striking finding of rheumatoid arthritis and can be an initial sign of lupus erythematosus and other collagen-vascular diseases. Marginal ulceration of the cornea can be observed in arteritides as an early manifestation of these diseases.

Conjunctival lesions can be present in several systemic infections, especially viral and chlamydial infections. Frank conjunctivitis can accompany tuberculosis, syphilis, tularemia, fungal infections (particularly histoplasmosis), cat-scratch fever, erythema multiforme, leptospirosis, toxic shock syndrome, and erythema nodosum. Petechial hemorrhages associated with bacterial endocarditis are often observed in conjunctival as well as in retinal vessels.

The uveal tract is often involved in granulomatous as well as nongranulomatous diseases. The latter include lupus erythematosus, vasculidites, serum sickness, and other hypersensitivity diseases. Sarcoidosis, toxoplasmosis, syphilis, tuberculosis, and Still's disease can result in significant uveitis. Thus, a slitlamp examination is desirable in the evaluation of a patient with FUO, even in the absence of ocular complaints. Ophthalmoscopy will reveal diseases that involve the optic nerve, retinal vessels, and choroidal tissues. Many systemic febrile diseases can have retinal as well as uveal manifestations.

LABORATORY TESTS

Cultures, antibody titers, complete blood counts, urine analyses, and direct examination of blood and other body fluids are procedures used in the evaluation of unexplained fevers. Most patients who are given a presumptive diagnosis of FUO have already had some or many laboratory investigations without revealing a specific cause. Some tests need to be repeated at regular intervals during a work-up of a patient with FUO, and these include serum samples for rising antibody titers and, most importantly, repeated cultures of blood and other body fluids for infectious agents. It should be emphasized that in both adults and children the most often encountered cause of unexplained fever is infection. The importance of multiple blood cultures (e.g., up to six over a period of time) cannot be overstressed in

uncovering many infections, especially endocarditis and osteomyelitis. The failure in diagnosing these and other infections sometimes lies with insufficient numbers of blood cultures and to a lesser extent in the inadequacy of cultures taken during concurrent antibiotic therapy. Polymicrobial sepsis often indicates self-induced infection.[24] Multiple urine cultures are also necessary, particularly in the absence of urinary tract symptoms and pyuria. In children, although urine cultures may be difficult to obtain, these are important. Silent urinary tract infections are common in the pediatric age group. In smaller children, direct bladder needle aspiration should be considered if routine procedures fail to yield adequate samples. Urine cultures are also important for the diagnosis of tuberculosis in children and adults. Other body fluids and tissues that may require multiple cultures include sputum, cerebrospinal fluid (CSF), stool, and bone marrow. Morning gastric contents can also be cultured for mycobacteria. It is critical to culture tissues such as liver or lymph nodes that are removed during biopsy. Sputa, CSF, bone marrow, liver, and lymph nodes are cultured for aerobic and anaerobic bacteria, mycobacteria, and fungi. Viral cultures and inoculation of material into embryonated chick eggs, mice, and guinea pigs should also be considered. It is sometimes easier to isolate and to identify some infectious agents using animal and yolk sac inoculation. The recognition of the cause of the legionnaires' disease outbreak of 1976 illustrates an example of the usefulness of such procedures.[29]

Direct examination of the blood is necessary to confirm a diagnosis of malaria, trypanosomiasis, and relapsing fever. Thick and thin smears of blood stained with Giemsa or Wright stain require careful examination, particularly in light infections. Demonstration of *Borrelia* may require multiple smears. Wet mounts using phase contrast microscopy are also useful in the detection of spirochetes. Direct examination of spinal fluid sediment with India ink is a rapid method for detecting cryptococci, although it is less sensitive than antigen detection. Direct examination of stool samples is still the preferred method for demonstrating several parasitic infections. Although schistosomiasis and amebic abscess of the liver can both manifest as FUO, the diagnosis is much more likely to be made by serology than by stool examination.

Rising antibody titers can be diagnostic in many infectious diseases, and it behooves the clinician who is working up a patient for FUO to obtain serum samples from the patient at regular intervals. It is advisable to freeze and to retain a portion of each sample in the event it is necessary to demonstrate a rising antibody titer to an agent isolated or suspected subsequently. Lyme disease is a good example, although some patients with Lyme disease fail to manifest antibodies to the spirochete. This is particularly true of viral and other infectious agents that are difficult to culture on artificial media.

Each antibody determination has its limitations as to specificity in that there are sometimes more false-positive than false-negative results. In addition, some antibody titers may reveal a recent infection with an organism that is not responsible for the prolonged fever. Newer and more specific immunologic and molecular biologic techniques, such as the polymerase chain reaction (PCR), are constantly being developed, and it is the responsibility of the physician to be aware of these while considering which test is most specific in uncovering the underlying cause of an FUO.

Patients with FUO often have elevated serum levels of "acute phase reactants." These may include fibrinogen, haptoglobin, ceruloplasmin, C-reactive protein, and other α_2-globulins. These are part of the nonspecific changes often measurable and elevated with fever. Other nonspecific changes that accompany fever that are frequently found in patients with FUO include elevations in the erythrocyte sedimentation rate, increased ability of neutrophils to reduce nitroblue tetrazolium, low serum iron and zinc concentrations, and an increased peripheral neutrophil count. Recently, plasma cytokine and acute phase reactant levels have been measured in an effort to improve diagnostic specificity.[30] To what degree these determinations are useful in working up a patient with FUO depends on the characteristics of certain disease processes. In general, they are nonspecific and are of little value (see Ch. 36). However, the erythrocyte sedimentation rate, for example, is usually markedly high in patients with temporal arteritis and Still's disease. It must be pointed out, however, that certain acute changes may be absent in some patients with FUO and that these changes are by themselves not indicative of a specific diagnosis. Levels of etiocholanolone do not correlate with fever, and this substance plays no role in causing fever.[31]

NONINVASIVE PROCEDURES

The technical advances in diagnostic radiology, radionuclide scanning, and other methods have reduced the need for invasive procedures in evaluating a patient with FUO. These include plain film contrast studies, tomography, selective cinearteriography, radionuclide scans, computerized tomographic scanning, ultrasonography, and magnetic resonance imaging. There are advantages to using each procedure, depending on the pathologic process. Some radiologic procedures should be considered "routine" in working up patients with FUO and include chest x-ray films, upper gastrointestinal contrast study with small-bowel follow-through, and barium enema. Chest x-ray films should be repeated periodically, and any radiologic study should be repeated if symptoms arise pertaining to a specific area. There are a number of pulmonary diseases that cause prolonged fever and, in rare patients, show no demonstrable involvement on chest x-ray films; for example, in sarcoidosis, mycoses, tuberculosis, many of the pneumoconioses, and infiltrative lung disease, chest x-ray films may be normal in the presence of biopsy-proven disease.[32]

Radionuclide scanning procedures using technetium (Tc) 99m sulfur colloid, gallium (Ga) citrate, or indium-111 are available for the evaluation of many infectious, inflammatory, or neoplastic processes. Success in localizing a process using these radiopharmaceuticals depends on the pathogenic process. [67]Ga was initially used to detect bone tumors, but it now has been shown that the radionuclide concentrates in many neoplastic and inflammatory tissues. The mechanism by which ^{67}Ga localizes in inflammatory tissue is thought to be related to the presence of sequestered leukocytes. Whole body gallium citrate (^{67}Ga) scans are often used as a screening procedure in patients with FUO and can localize abscesses, lymphomas, and infectious and other neoplastic processes. However, there are known false-positive and false-negative results with this procedure, with a wide range of sensitivities (35–75 percent) reported in identifying sources of fever.[33] Technetium 99m sulfur colloid is also used in scanning and seems to be especially useful in the early diagnosis of osteomyelitis. Radiographic abnormalities develop late in this disease, and scanning techniques are able to localize the disease early, probably because of increased blood flow. To reduce false-positive results, it is advisable to use radionuclide scanning techniques in combination with computed tomography (CT) and ultrasonography.[34] [111]Indium-oxine labeled granulocyte scintigraphy in FUO patients has some utility, with sensitivities of 17–55 percent.[33,35]

Recently, ^{111}In-labeled IgG scintigraphy was introduced to delineate focal infections, even in patients with neutropenia. It is not appropriate for detection of lesions in the liver, kidneys, and heart because of high background activity. When lesions in these areas are deleted from calculations, sensitivities may approach 95 percent, with specificity approaching 80 percent.[36,37]

The efficacy of whole body CT scanning in working up a patient with FUO depends on the extent and location of the disease. For example, CT scanning is effective in delineating intra-abdominal abscesses and retroperitoneal, retrosternal, and mes-

enteric lymph nodes that may be the causes of FUO. The procedure can also detect defects in the spleen, liver, kidney, adrenals, pancreas, heart, mediastinum, and pelvis, but radionuclide scanning and ultrasonography are also efficacious in demonstrating disease in these organs and regions. For some patients, more than one noninvasive method may be necessary to demonstrate and to confirm abnormalities. Greater use of CT scanning has reduced the need for invasive procedures.[38]

Magnetic resonance imaging (MRI) is superior to CT scanning for detecting most of the causes of FUO involving the nervous system. The availability of contrast agents for the central nervous system, ability to obtain images in coronal, horizontal, and sagittal planes, the superiority of images in the posterior fossa, middle cranial fossa, of lesions near the vertex seen on coronal views, and of cord and epidural space lesions make MRI the nervous system imaging technique of choice for the majority of lesions that cause FUO. CT is superior to MRI when there are calcifications, as may be present in parasitic or granulomatous lesions, and CT plays a critical role in diagnostic needle-aspiration biopsy of lesions in the brain and spinal cord. Cerebral angiography is no longer a first-line procedure, but may be necessary when cerebral vasculitis or mycotic aneurysm are diagnostic possibilities.[39]

Ultrasonography has been helpful in demonstrating the presence of cardiac abnormalities that may be a cause of fever. Echocardiography can detect valvular vegetations and atrial tumors; it should be included as a potential "screening" procedure in patients with FUO. Two-dimensional imaging, color-flow Doppler imaging, and transesophageal echocardiography have increased the sensitivities for detecting vegetations dramatically (transthoracic may approach 80 percent; transesophageal may exceed 95 percent).[40] However, a negative echocardiogram does not disprove infectious endocarditis, and the diagnosis of infectious endocarditis should not be made exclusively on the basis of echocardiographic findings.[40]

Ultrasonography, CT, and MRI all play a role in imaging the abdomen, pelvis, and retroperitoneum in FUO, in addition to the previously mentioned radioisotope techniques (^{67}Ga, ^{111}In-labeled white blood cells, and IgG). CT is more sensitive than ultrasound for detecting most abdominal abscesses, while MRI may be more sensitive still. Ultrasonography is the current modality of choice for initial imaging of the pelvis.[41] CT is still the best initial imaging technique for the liver, spleen, and retroperitoneum.[41] Ultrasound is especially useful in imaging the kidneys, biliary tract, and pancreas. The pancreas appears to be especially difficult to image by MRI.[42] Endoscopic retrograde cholangiopancreatography may be helpful in further delineating questionable abnormalities of the biliary and pancreatic ducts. Both MRI and CT are superior to routine radiographs in the diagnosis of occult sinusitis as a cause of FUO.

Lymphangiography is a well-established method for demonstrating retroperitoneal, iliac, and periaortic lymph nodes. The involvement of these nodes in patients with lymphomas and Hodgkin's disease that manifest as FUO has been noted in several studies. With the advent of CT scanning, lymphangiography is infrequently used.

SKIN TESTING

With a few exceptions, such as the purified protein derivative (PPD) test for tuberculosis, most skin tests are of limited value in the diagnosis of FUO. Nevertheless, it is important to test for reactivity to tuberculin in patients with FUO. It is necessary at the same time to test for reactivity to other antigens such as mumps, streptodornase streptokinase, or *Candida*. The multitest CMI (Connaught Labs, Swiftwater, PA) consists of an applicator with eight tines, including seven antigens and an antigen-negative tine. The lack of sensitivity to these latter antigens often suggests diseases like miliary tuberculosis or Hodgkin's disease. However, patients with FUO, particularly debilitated patients, may have depressed immunologic reactions secondary to nutritional factors.

INVASIVE PROCEDURES

Biopsy of liver and bone marrow should be considered routine in the work-up of FUO if the studies mentioned above are unrevealing. Other biopsy sites may include skin, pleura, lymph nodes, kidney, muscle, nerve, intestine, or any tissue that may be involved either on physical examination, scans, or radiographs. Bronchoscopy, laparoscopy, and other endoscopies are used for both inspection and obtaining tissues and fluids. Proper disposition of the biopsy material requires an organized plan to divide the tissue for maximal information. This is particularly true with needle biopsy material. Bacterial, viral, fungal, and mycobacterial cultures must be done on appropriate tissue. Reports of unusual organisms cultured from the biopsy material of many patients with FUO underscore the importance of this procedure. There is no substitute for a positive culture in uncovering the cause of fever. Microscopic examination also requires advanced organization. Proper staining may be critical to identification of organisms in tissues as well as in certain tissue and intracellular deposits. For example, formalin-fixed tissue should be stained with Brown-Brenn or Brown-Hopps for bacteria, Fite stain for mycobacteria, methenamine silver and periodic acid-Schiff for fungi, and the Dieterle silver- impregnation method and Warthin-Starry stains for other bacteria and organisms. If possible, a section of the tissue block should always be retained for further sections or stains. Frozen sections can also be used for immunologic procedures. Using anti-IgG, anti-IgM, other anti-immunoglobin and anticomplement sera coupled to fluorescein dyes, these proteins can be identified in certain tissues of patients with autoimmune and collagen-vascular diseases.

Polymerase chain reaction technology and in situ hybridization with nucleic acid probes make it possible to identify and speciate mycobacterial and viral nucleic acids, potentially even in paraffin-embedded, fixed tissues.[43,44]

With the increasing specificity and safety of noninvasive diagnostic methods, the need for diagnostic laparotomy in patients with FUO has markedly decreased. A diagnostic laparotomy may be indicated in patients with FUO and abdominal pain when the approaches outlined above have failed.[45] Percutaneous liver biopsy is a highly valuable procedure and should be performed on all patients with prolonged FUO.[19,46] Liver biopsy provides tissues for microscopic and microbiologic studies and is safe for most patients. A normal finding on liver biopsy is also helpful in that it is reassuring in those cases in which no diagnosis can be made.[46]

CAUSES OF FEVER OF UNKNOWN ORIGIN

Bacterial Infections

Any bacterial infection can be the source of prolonged fever, especially those that produce little or no obvious inflammation. In these situations localizing symptoms that would indicate the site of infection are missing.

Abscesses. Abscesses are frequently encountered as causes of FUO, and intra-abdominal sites are the most common. Liver and subphrenic abscesses are often seen in patients who have had previous abdominal surgery or in whom intestinal disease had resulted in a small perforation with intestinal leakage. Abdominal abscesses are potential complications in patients undergoing colonoscopy or sigmoidoscopy. Similarly, abdominal abscesses can occur in women following certain gynecologic procedures such as culdoscopy or curetage. Abscesses also can occur following ruptured ovarian cysts. Dental and brain abscesses are less common than an abdominal site as causes of unexplained fever because localizing symptoms are usually

present early in the disease; nevertheless, these should be considered as possible causes of a FUO.

Osteomyelitis. Osteomyelitis is a common cause of FUO since symptoms are often masked or are interpreted as nervous or muscular in origin. For example, patients with osteomyelitis of the vertebral bodies or the leg may have symptoms of nerve root compression. Osteomyelitis of the mandible and maxilla can manifest as headache or toothache. Thus, osteomyelitis of any bone can be a cause of FUO because inflammation and pain may occur later in such patients. In this regard, sinusitis can cause prolonged fever without local symptoms except for mild headache.[47]

Infective Endocarditis. Another bacterial source for an FUO in which there may be no localizing symptoms is infective endocarditis (IE). This disease is sometimes a cause of FUO because it may not be diagnosed early due either to insufficient or negative blood cultures or to the absence of characteristic physical findings, both of which may be altered by prior antimicrobial therapy. Modern bacteriologic techniques appear to have reduced the percentage of culture-negative IE cases to approximately 5 percent.[48]

In addition to prior antibiotic therapy (often directed against another putative source of fever), culture-negative IE may be seen with right-sided endocarditis (tricuspid or pulmonic valve), often in intravenous drug users. Culture-negative IE may also be seen with uncommon organism such as the HACEK (*Haemophilus* spp., *Actinobacillus actinomycetemcomitans, Cardiobacterium hominis, Eikenella* spp., *Kingella kingae*) group, nutritionally deficient streptococci (needing media supplemented with pyridoxal or L-cysteine), *Brucella, Rochalimaea, Legionella, Chlamydia, Mycoplasma, Spirillum minus*, and *Coxiella*, as well as fungi such as *Aspergillus* spp.[48] The presence of bacterial endocarditis in the absence of an audible murmur is rare, but some murmurs, particularly in very young and elderly patients, are mistaken as physiologic. In these circumstances, bacterial endocarditis is not considered as a cause of fever, and hence these patients are given a diagnosis of FUO. Increasing use of two-dimensional, Doppler-flow, and transesophageal echocardiography should lead to the diagnosis of IE in these situations.

Biliary System Infections. Bacterial infections of the biliary system include ascending cholangitis, cholecystitis, frank empyema of the gallbladder, and infection of the pancreatic duct. The organisms gain entrance from the duodenum, and in the majority of cases there is a preexisting disease like pancreatitis or cholelithiasis. However, patients with bacterial infections of the biliary system who have been diagnosed as having FUO have little or no right upper quadrant discomfort that would indicate the site of infection. Patients with suppurative biliary tract infection had no localizing physical findings or tenderness before laparotomy.[2,49,50] Furthermore, in these patients liver function tests had been normal and hence the diagnosis had been made primarily at laparotomy. Newer methods such as CT and MRI scanning, radioisotope scintigraphy, and sonography have lessened the need for exploratory operations in these patients.

Urinary Tract Infections. Urinary tract infections due to bacteria are infrequently encountered as causes of FUO because positive urine cultures make this diagnosis early in a febrile illness. Thus, patients with urinary tract infections that manifest as FUO have negative or intermittently positive urine cultures. Perinephric abscesses may spill bacteria into the urine inconsistently, and some urinary tract infections have such a low titer of bacteria (1000–5000 organisms/ml) that the culture results do not suggest the urinary tract as a source of the fever. Obstruction of the infected kidney outflow tract may prevent detection of bacteriuria. In children, particularly in girls with bladder reflux and in boys with posterior urethral valves, urinary tract infections are common causes of FUO. Obtaining urine for culture in some children is difficult, and contaminating organisms are often misleading. Bladder aspiration is indicated in such children with bacteriuria to rule out urinary tract infection as a cause of FUO. In older males, chronic bacterial prostatitis and prostatic abscess are occasionally causes of FUO. When urinary tract infections are a cause of prolonged fever, there usually is absence of symptoms like dysuria, frequency, or lower back pain.

Tuberculosis. *Mycobacterium tuberculosis* is perhaps the single most often cultured organism as a cause of FUO. The worldwide pandemic of AIDS has increased the incidence of tuberculosis in both HIV-infected and uninfected individuals. The rise of AIDS-associated tuberculosis has eliminated the expectation of its virtual eradication in the United States and other highly industrialized nations, and the increase in tuberculosis highest where HIV prevalence is highest. This has been further complicated by the development of multidrug resistant (MDR) strains, which approach 20 percent of isolates in New York City.[51] Tuberculosis is thus likely to increase as a cause of FUO in years to come, even in patients not typically considered immunosuppressed.

There are some patients in whom fever is the only symptom and whose chest x-ray films appear normal. Extrapulmonary tuberculosis is probably the most common manifestation of this infection as an FUO.[52] Miliary tuberculosis including tuberculosis of the spleen, liver, bone, kidney, meninges, peritoneum, and pericardium have all been reported as causes of prolonged fever. Even in cases of overwhelming miliary tuberculosis, the lung fields and other organ sites do not always show signs of involvement until weeks following the onset of fever,[53] and hence diagnosis may be delayed. In addition, the diagnosis of tuberculosis as a cause of fever may not be apparent, since cultures may not become positive before 4–6 weeks. Hopefully, increased availability of PCR-based technology will reduce the delays in diagnosis that are often the norm. Furthermore, a negative skin test may be due to disseminated disease, and, when such is the case, the clinician is often misled by the absence of a positive reaction. Although atypical mycobacteria cause disease, they usually do not manifest as FUO in immunologically normal individuals.

Miscellaneous Infections. Intestinal bacterial infections rarely manifest as prolonged fever in the absence of other symptoms. The notable exception to this is salmonellosis, in which fever may be the only abnormality. The causative agent in Whipple's disease (intestinal lipodystrophy) has been identified by molecular genetic techniques as an actinomycete, *Tropheryma whippelii*,[54] and this disease has been encountered as a cause of prolonged fever.[49,54]

Acute rheumatic fever (ARF) does occur in adults, and in a classic study almost 20 percent of cases were seen in adults over the age of 21 years,[55] some as old as 49 years. The incidence of ARF is clearly on the increase in the United States, as well (56).

Kawasaki syndrome (KS; mucocutaneous lympho node syndrome, [MLNS]) has a fairly typical picture in children, but in adults it may be difficult to distinguish from toxic shock syndrome (TSS).[57] This presumed distinction may prove artificial with the recent demonstration of a TSS toxin-producing *Staphylococcus aureus* from 13 of 16 KS patients, and only 1 of 15 controls. This unusual *S. aureus* was white and easily confused, therefore, with nonpathogenic staphylococci; it was cultured from throat, rectum, groin, and axilla.[58]

Cat scratch disease may produce FUO in non-HIV-infected patients, involving lymph nodes, liver, bone, or brain. The causative organism, detectable in affected tissue by Warthin-Starry stain, is *Rochalimaea (Bartonella) henselae*.[59,60]

The vast majority of bacterial infections causing prolonged, unexplained fever are confined to specific sites, that is, abscess in organs or infection in certain spaces. There are also a few bacterial infections that may cause prolonged fevers and in which the causative organism is disseminated, residing primarily in the reticuloendothelial and lymphatic systems. These include brucellosis, bartonellosis, and Q fever. Of these diseases, brucellosis is clearly most frequently encountered as an FUO. Diagnosis rests, as in all bacterial infections, on positive bacterial cultures as well as on the presence of increasing serum antibody titers.

Spirochetal Infections

Relapsing Fever. Of the three medically important genera of spirochetes, *Treponema*, *Leptospira*, and *Borrelia*, only the last is often associated with prolonged fever and is sometimes called "relapsing fever" because the fever characteristically occurs in paroxysms separated by afebrile intervals. Although louse-borne relapsing fever due to infections of *Borrellia recurrentis* occurs worldwide, it is most prevalent in times of war or famine; the tick-borne form of this disease caused by *B. pakeri*, *B. hermsii*, or *B. turicatae* has been reported in the western and southwestern United States and frequently manifests as an FUO.[61,62] Louse-borne relapsing fever usually occurs in epidemics, and diagnosis is made during the initial febrile episodes. However, tick-borne relapsing fever affects campers and hikers in a sporadic fashion, and patients often are given a provisional diagnosis of FUO until careful direct examination of the blood for the presence of spirochetes or culture in chick embryos suggests the etiology of the infection. The patient may be unaware of a recent tick bite, and during the second or third fever relapse the disease may be overlooked as having an infectious etiology. The initial clinical manifestations of louse-borne relapsing fever can be confused with those caused by tick-borne rickettsiae, but subsequent attacks of relapsing fever may manifest with only fever and no localizing signs.

While Lyme disease is now a common infectious disease in the United States, having been identified in 43 states, as well as in Europe and the former Soviet Union from the Baltic to the Pacific, it is relatively uncommon as a cause of classic FUO.[63] It has been described, however,[64] and is a diagnostic consideration. A positive Lyme serology in a patient with FUO must be interpreted with caution, and the patient's epidemiologic and clinical context must be taken into account. The recent description of a PCR test for the presence of *Borrelia burgdorferi* DNA in synovial fluid once again demonstrates the promise of this new technology in refining diagnostic accuracy.[65]

Leptospirosis. Leptospirosis is a spirochetal infection that can manifest as an FUO, although illness is usually acute and self-limited. During the first phases of leptospirosis, the organisms can be cultured from the blood, but during the second and third phases ("immune phases") organisms may be absent from body fluids and fever may be the only manifestation. In these cases the cause of prolonged fever may be ascertained by serologic tests.

Rat-Bite Fever. *Spirillum minus*, the spirochete that causes rat-bite fever, cannot be cultured on artificial media, but inoculation of the patient's blood into mice confirms a diagnosis in 10 days to 2 weeks. The history of a rat bite should alert the physician to the diagnostic possibility. Rarely, mouse bites have also been shown to cause the disease. Darkfield microscopy of blood may demonstrate the organism; however, in patients with spirochetal infection who appear to have an FUO, the organism may be absent from body fluids, and diagnosis depends on the presence of specific antibody titers.

Rickettsial Infections. Rickettsial infections are rarely encountered as FUOs today. The classic findings of macular rash, often petechial, with profound headache and conjunctivitis, usually suggest Rocky Mountain spotted fever or endemic typhus, depending on epidemiologic setting. Endemic typhus with *Rickettsia typhi* may not be associated with rash, however. Other rickettsiae also lack characteristic rash. Q fever due to *Coxiella burnetii* may cause either infective endocarditis or granulomatous hepatitis; *Ehrlichia chaffeensis* in the United States and *Ehrlichia sennetsu* in Japan can cause ehrlichiosis, with fever and headache[66]; *Rochalimaea quintana* causes trench fever, which may be chronic; *Rochalimaea (Bartonella) henselae* produces bacillary angiomatosis in AIDS patients[67] and cat scratch disease in HIV-infected individuals[68]; a new *Rochalimaea* sp. has been described as a cause of endocarditis.[69] Serology is usually diagnostic; for newer *Rochalimaea* syndromes, Warthin-Starry staining, culture, or PCR may be necessary.

Chlamydial Infections. Psittacosis caused by *Chlamydia psittaci* can occur in the absence of cough and respiratory symptoms and with normal chest x-ray findings. In these situations, fever may be the sole symptom of the disease and splenomegaly the only physical finding. Because fever in psittacosis may be prolonged as long as 3 months, psittacosis has been reported as an infectious cause of FUO in several studies. Isolation of the organism may be difficult in these cases, but diagnosis can be made from a rising titer of complement-fixing antibody. *Chlamydia pneumoniae* (TWAR) may produce a prolonged respiratory illness. In addition to pneumonia, persistent bronchitis and sinusitis may occur, and the disease may be more severe in older adults.[70] Other chlamydial diseases such as trachoma as well as genital tract infections are usually not associated with fever. Lymphogranuloma venereum, although usually diagnosed without difficulty, may manifest as an FUO.

Viral Infections. Viruses can cause prolonged fever in some patients. This is particularly true in children, and the spectrum of infectious causes of FUO in young children includes more viral etiologies than in adults. The proof of a viral agent causing prolonged, unexplained fever rests with two criteria: isolation of the agent and immunologic evidence of infection. Problems arise when the patient does not have a typical immunologic response to the agent and when associated signs and symptoms such as skin rashes and lymphadenopathy are missing or have gone unnoticed. This is particularly true of some viral infections in children. Infectious mononucleosis is perhaps the most commonly encountered viral disease producing prolonged fever without appropriate immunologic response. For example, not all patients develop significant titers of heterophile antibody early in the course of the disease. The disease can thus often be diagnosed by the presence of antibody to Epstein-Barr virus-associated antigens. Rarely, the development of both heterophile and Epstein-Barr virus antibodies is delayed several weeks and diagnosis is difficult. Other viral illnesses associated with FUO include cytomegalovirus infection and hepatitis caused by the hepatitis A, B or C viruses. The full clinical spectrums of human parvovirus[71] and hantavirus infection[72,73] have yet to be defined, and these viruses should be candidates as causes of FUO in appropriate settings.

Fungal Diseases

There is little question that the incidence of fungal diseases, particularly deep mycoses, has increased as a result of the use of antibiotics and immunosuppressive therapy. Many fungal diseases, for example, histoplasmosis, blastomycosis, and coccidiomycosis, manifest primarily as pulmonary infections and are detected early in the disease process. Other fungal diseases, notably cryptococcosis and disseminated histoplasmosis, are less easily detected, and fever may be the major manifestation.

Histoplasmosis involving the reticuloendothelial and lymphatic system may manifest as prolonged, unexplained fever.

The clinical manifestations of this form of histoplasmosis are not unlike that of disseminated tuberculosis. Cryptococcal meningitis is often undiagnosed for several weeks and may manifest as an FUO. Headaches and behavioral changes usually lead to an examination of the spinal fluid. With increasing use of antibiotics, particularly in patients being treated with immunosuppressive agents, some of the indigenous fungi, for example, *Candida albicans,* have caused disseminated disease and fever. Chronic disseminated candidiasis should be suspected in patients who have recovered from profound neutropenia but have persistent fever and focal lesions in the liver or spleen on CT or MRI (see Ch. 237).

Parasitic Disease

Malaria. In endemic areas, malaria is seldom a cause of unexplained fever, but in nonendemic areas this infection has the potential to go undetected. Malaria in particular may cause weeks or months of fever with parasitemia that is low grade and difficult to detect. This may be due to several factors, including the failure of travelers to use prophylactic antimalarials properly, resistant forms, nonsynchronized febrile paroxysms, and the physician's unawareness of travel to endemic areas by the patient. In fact, most reports of malaria as a cause of FUO are due to failure to suspect malaria early in the disease. Blood transfusion as a cause of malarial transmission occurs rarely but increases during periods of war in malarious areas.

Babesiosis. Babesiosis, a related intraerythrocytic protozoan infection, may also cause FUO. In the United States, babesiosis is usually due to *B. microti,* endemic in the northeastern coastal islands around Massachusetts, Connecticut, and New York. Sporadic causes have been identified elsewhere in the United States and Europe (see Ch. 261).

Toxoplasmosis. Toxoplasmosis can manifest as FUO and is often discovered in patients with lymph node enlargement during lymph node biopsy. A few patients have minimal lymph node swelling and may have fever as the predominant symptom. Rising antibody titers can detect the disease when it is suspected.

Trypanosomiasis. Trypanosomiasis due to *Trypanosoma rhodesiense* is carried by the tsetse fly vector in East and Central Africa, and visitors to these areas, even for periods as brief as an overnight flight stop, can contract the disease. The disease is rather acute, accompanied by prominent erythematous rash, central nervous system alterations, and high fever. Trypanosomes can be detected in routine blood smears during the disease. *Trypanosoma gambiense* is found in West and Central Africa and produces a more subtle form of onset. Fever begins irregularly and is accompanied by an evanescent rash, splenomegaly, and lymphadenopathy. The disease is less acute than that caused by *T. rhodesiense* and may be present for months as an FUO before blood smears are examined. Visitors to Africa or natives arriving in the United States from endemic areas can have delayed onset of disease.

Other Parasitic Diseases. Leishmaniasis, trichinosis, and amebic liver abscess are parasitic diseases that can have prominent febrile manifestations and, because of their relative infrequency in the United States, may be missed as a cause of unexplained fever.

NEOPLASTIC DISEASES

Unexplained fever is a common manifestation of many malignancies (Table 5). All solid tumors have the potential to cause obstruction and subsequent infection; hence, malignancy and

TABLE 5. Malignancies Commonly Manifesting as FUO

> Hodgkin's disease
> Non-Hodgkin's lymphoma
> Leukemia (including aleukemia and preleukemia)
> Renal cell carcinoma
> Hepatoma
> Atrial myxomas

fever may coexist. In these situations, the neoplastic process indirectly causes the fever. Color cancer and biliary carcinoma are notable examples. However, even in the absence of infection, certain neoplasms are particularly associated with fever, and when these are treated the fever may disappear. In these cases, the neoplasm is thought to be a direct source of the fever.

The mechanism by which a neoplastic process causes fever may be related to its ability to produce endogenous pyrogens itself or to induce the production of endogenous pyrogens from normal leukocytes. Tissue obtained from patients with Hodgkin's disease, histiocytic lymphomas, and renal cell carcinoma liberate endogenous pyrogens spontaneously in vitro,[74-76] and it is likely that the same process takes place in vivo. In addition to some tumors producing their own endogenous pyrogens, others undergo necrosis as a result of rapid growth, and necrotic debris induces the infiltration of leukocytes in the inflammatory response. Endogenous pyrogens can be the products of inflammatory leukocytes and may be produced in association with tumor necrosis.

Certain neoplasms have a high incidence of manifestation as FUO, and some patients with these malignancies seek medical attention primarily because of recurrent fevers. These neoplasms include lymphoma and other reticuloses, renal cell carcinoma, atrial myxoma, hepatoma, and carcinoma of the intestinal tract. Disseminated carcinomatosis is also a cause of FUO. Nonmalignant neoplasms that are associated with prolonged fever are giant lymph node hyperplasia[77] and infantile cortical hyperostosis.[78] It should be pointed out, however, that these benign neoplasms may have an infectious or inflammatory etiology, although no agent has yet been isolated. Angiomyolipoma is a benign renal tumor that occurs almost exclusively in patients with tuberous sclerosis and can manifest as an FUO.[79]

Lymphomas and Leukemias. Of all the lymphomas, Hodgkin's disease is most commonly associated with recurrent fever, although non-Hodgkin's lymphoma may cause FUO. The likelihood of fever as an initial symptom in Hodgkin's disease increases with the number of lymph nodes involved, and fever is a prominent symptom when disease is present in retroperitoneal nodes. In these latter instances, routine studies to detect a cause of the persistent fever fail, and patients require more specific investigation to uncover the source of fever. Lymphomas that primarily involve the spleen have a high incidence of fever and can manifest along with anorexia, malaise, and weight loss as an FUO.[80] When present, a Pel-Ebstein pattern of fever (3- to 10-day cycles of febrile and afebrile periods) is highly suggestive of Hodgkin's disease.

Acute leukemias may be associated with fever, and sometimes this occurs in the presence of a normal peripheral blood smear, as seen in aleukemic leukemia and preleukemia. In such patients diagnosis is often delayed. Bone marrow aspiration may uncover the aleukemic phase, but in preleukemic forms fever may persist, and bone marrow aspirates remain nondiagnostic for very long periods.[81] The incidence of fever in the preleukemic form of monocytic leukemia is high, and, in general, the number of preleukemias, including myelogenous leukemia, that manifest as FUO varies from 10 to 30 percent in different studies.[81,82] Leukemic persons treated with allogeneic bone marrow transplants may have fever from graft-vs.-host disease as well as from infectious causes.

Renal Cell Carcinoma. Carcinoma of the kidney is often insidious, and many patients do not have hematuria but rather fever as the major symptom.[83] Two large series put the incidence of persistent fever as a manifesting symptom at 11 percent and 12 percent[84] of the cases. There also seems to be a high incidence of a sedimentation rate greater than 100 mm/hr in patients with fever and renal cell carcinoma. In many cases there are no metastases but rather a well-encapsulated neoplasm. Removal of the tumor almost always results in the cessation of fever. Of interest is the fact that investigators have found that the tumor cells synthesize and release endogenous pyrogens spontaneously in vitro, while renal tumor cells taken from patient's who did not have fever did not release endogenous pyrogen.

Tumors of the Liver. There is a greater incidence of metastatic adenocarcinoma to the liver than primary hepatomas, but the latter tumor is often considered as a likely cause of an FUO. Some patients with hepatomas seek medical help because of persistent fever, and several reports of FUO have listed hepatoma as the final diagnosis. Primary or metastatic tumors to the liver that are associated with prolonged fever are not diagnostic problems when accompanied by jaundice or abnormal liver function tests. However, patients with normal liver functions and only fever are admitted to hospitals with the diagnosis of FUO.

Atrial Myxomas. Although myxomas of the atria are very rare neoplasms, they have a high association of fever and manifest as FUO. The mechanism of producing fever is not understood but may be related to embolic phenomena or to the production of interleukin-6. Murmurs may not be present.

Other Tumors. The list of other tumors that can manifest as FUO is varied. Adenocarcinoma of the large intestine, bronchogenic carcinoma, and adenocarcinoma of the breast particularly when they metastasize can cause an FUO. Children tend to have a different spectrum of neoplasms that manifest as FUO. Acute leukemias are most prevalent in children and can manifest as unexplained fever. Solid tumors in children that may manifest as FUO include neuroblastoma and central nervous system tumors.

Hypersensitivity and Autoimmune Diseases. There is a sizable group of diseases that manifest as FUO and that fall into the general categories of hypersensitivity, autoimmune, rheumatic, or collagen-vascular diseases (Table 6). Patients with these diseases may have prolonged, unexplained fever as the prominent symptom of disease, while other clinical manifestations such as cutaneous lesions and joint involvement are either absent or go undetected. Antinuclear antibodies can be found in more than 90 percent of the patients.[86] Fever can be the initial manifestation of the disease in 5 percent of the cases,[87] and such patients are considered to have FUO when they have only fever and no serologic evidence of lupus. Later, additional clinical manifestations such as arthritis may appear, and serologic tests may become positive, which ensures a diagnosis of lupus erythematosus.

Patients with various forms of vasculitis can initially have fever as a prominent sign, and cutaneous manifestations may not occur. Biopsy of affected areas, when they appear, confirms the diagnosis. Drug-induced vasculitis is often associated with

TABLE 6. Hypersensitivity and Autoimmune Diseases Causing FUO

Systemic lupus erythematosus	Polyarteritis nodosa
Still's disease	Erythema multiforme
Polymyalgia rheumatica	Mixed connective tissue disease
Drug fever	Serum sickness
Hypersensitivity vasculitis	Rheumatic fever
Idiopathic vasculitis	

fever and can manifest as FUO.[88] Drugs that are often associated with hypersensitivity vasculitis include penicillin, sulfonamides, isoniazid, and propylthiouracil, but any drug can cause hypersensitivity vasculitis.

Rheumatoid arthritis can be associated with persistent fever, but in adults joint involvement usually indicates the proper diagnosis. In children, however, joint involvement may be minimal or absent, and many patients have an FUO. In fact, of all the autoimmune diseases that manifest as FUO in the pediatric age group, juvenile rheumatoid arthritis is undoubtedly the most common.[89] Still's disease is the diagnosis given to those children who have primarily systemic manifestations in the absence of arthritis. A complex of high fever, evanescent rash, lymphadenopathy, and splenomegaly with varying degrees of arthralgias and myalgias is typical for Still's disease. Because of its acute onset, it may stimulate other diseases and may pose diagnostic difficulties.

Adults with FUO may also have Still's disease. Onset of the adult form of Still's disease occurs most often between ages 20 and 30, but in some patients onset occurs in childhood and is followed by asymptomatic intervals that may be as long as 10 years. The clinical manifestation in adults is almost identical to that in children. However, adults often have other associated symptoms such as sore throat during febrile episodes.[90] Radiologic evidence of joint changes are often absent in the adult form of Still's disease, and there is no rheumatoid factor present. An elevated white blood cell count with an increase in polymorphonuclear leukocytes and an elevated erythrocyte sedimentation rate are characteristic. The diagnosis of Still's disease as the cause of unexplained fever in adults rests with the presence of its symptom complex in the absence of other diseases.[90,91]

There are also patients in whom a diagnosis of an autoimmune or collagen-vascular disease is almost certain, but its classification is difficult. Although these patients may have fever as the prominent symptom, other symptoms and laboratory data suggest unclassified collagen-vascular disease. Mixed connective tissue disease can manifest as FUO, and in such patients elevated titers of extractable nuclear antigen will confirm the diagnosis. Erythema multiforme with fever may be found in this group of illnesses.

Fever may be the only manifestation of hypersensitivity to drugs, including proprietary preparations. Some drugs can cause fever in the absence of an immunologically based hypersensitivity reaction; these include atropine, lysergic acid, some antidepressants, amphotericin B, and bleomycin. The mechanism for atropine and central nervous system–acting drugs causing elevated temperature is through interference with heat regulatory mechanisms, and, as such, the elevated temperature is not fever but rather hyperthermia (see Ch. 36). True drug fever is an immunologically based disease in which, either through previous exposure or recent administration, sensitization takes place to the drug as a foreign antigen. It has been proposed that sensitized T lymphocytes release endogenous pyrogen-inducing substances that cause the fever. Removal of the antigen usually brings about a decrease in the fever within 48 hours.

Fever due to use of amphotericin B or bleomycin is not due to hypersensitivity reactions but rather to the direct ability of these drugs to stimulate production of endogenous pyrogenic cytokines. In some cases, these drugs, which are given parenterally, may contain endotoxins as contaminants.[92,93]

In a study published in 1964, cutaneous manifestations were present in a majority of the cases of drug fever.[94] In a large study of 148 episodes of drug fever in 142 patients, cutaneous manifestations were present in only 18 percent of patients, and less than half of these were urticarial in nature.[95]

The most common manifestation of drug fever is seen in the patient being treated with antibiotics and in whom the protracted fever is due to drug hypersensitivity and not to the infection. Withdrawing the drug usually results in disappearance of the fever. For this reason, the patient's history is critical in establishing a diagnosis of drug fever. Some patients suddenly develop fever to common drugs like isoniazid or other agents that have been taken for years without evidence of any hypersensitivity. The variety of agents that have been reported to be the source of FUO is broad. Some agents, however, tend to be particularly associated with fever in the absence of other clinical manifestations and include salicylates, thiouracil, phenytoin (Dilantin), iodides, isoniazid, methyldopa, and penicillin.

Thyroiditis is usually associated with local pain and fever and does not manifest as FUO. However, a small number of patients with subacute thyroiditis may be unaware of local tenderness and may have persistent fever. Examination of the thyroid gland reveals local tenderness even when there is limited involvement, and appropriate thyroid function tests and serologic measurements ensure the diagnosis.

Granulomatous Diseases

The four major types of granulomatous disease that produce prolonged, unexplained fevers are granulomatous hepatitis, sarcoidosis, inflammatory bowel disease, and temporal arteritis. In general, granulomatous disease can go undetected for many months and yet be the cause of high fevers. In fact, in patients with FUO lasting for longer than 1 year, granulomatous causes were more numerous than neoplasms or autoimmune diseases.[14,23] When the patient has an FUO, localizing symptoms are often absent, while diagnosis requires identification of granulomas in biopsy material or radiologic evidence of lesions typical of the process (e.g., Crohn's disease).

Granulomatous Hepatitis. Granulomatous hepatitis of unknown etiology accounts for a large number of cases of prolonged FUO. Granulomas in the liver represent a pathologic response to injury in that they are induced by many infectious diseases. Some of the diseases that are commonly associated with hepatic granulomas include tuberculosis and other mycobacterial infections, histoplasmosis, syphilis, some parasitic diseases, sarcoidosis, and neoplasms.[23,96–98] It is essential to rule out these and other underlying diseases. However, there is a group of patients with FUO and granulomas in the liver in whom no specific underlying process can be found.[97] The disease is usually associated with high fever intermittently present for periods of months to years and occurs most often during the fifth or sixth decade of life. The only laboratory data that suggest granulomatous hepatitis are mildly elevated alkaline phosphatase levels in many patients and elevated serum transaminase determinations in even fewer. However, these may be normal in a small number of patients, and only liver biopsy confirms the diagnosis.

Sarcoidosis. Sarcoidosis is a systemic granulomatous disease that commonly manifests with pulmonary, skin, or lymphoid involvement. However, a small percentage of patients with sarcoidosis have fever, weight loss, and weakness as initial symptoms without localizing signs or symptoms. In fact, some patients with sarcoidosis have a daily temperature elevation greater than 101°F for months, and in these patients granulomas usually can be found in the liver, while the lung fields remain clear. Fever in sarcoidosis is sometimes associated with erythema nodosum.

Inflammatory Bowel Disease. Crohn's disease or granulomatous colitis are granulomatous processes primarily involving the terminal ileum and colon, and nearly one-third of the patients have fever. A small percentage of these patients can have no gastrointestinal symptoms and only high fevers.[23,99] This is particularly true of young adults in whom fever can be present for months or years without symptoms referable to the gastrointestinal tract. For this reason, it is important to obtain a detailed small bowel contrast study in patients with FUO. Of all gastrointestinal diseases that cause fever, Crohn's disease is the most likely to be a cause of FUO. Ulcerative colitis, although not a granulomatous disease, rarely manifests as an FUO. There have been reports, however, of patients with high fevers and no intestinal symptoms who later have sigmoidoscopic evidence of this disease.

Temporal Arteritis. Giant cell arteritis with polymyalgia rheumatica affects patients usually in the sixth and seventh decades of life and may manifest as FUO. The symptom complex includes headache, visual disturbances, and myalgias and arthralgias. It should be pointed out, however, that none of these symptoms need be present for temporal arteritis to cause prolonged fever. Patients with unexplained recurrent fevers and mild headaches or visual disturbance should be considered for temporal artery biopsy, particularly in the sixth and seventh decades of life.[23] Associated laboratory findings are anemia and very high sedimentation rates. Biopsy specimens of the temporal artery reveal granulomas even in cases in which no temporal artery tenderness was demonstrated. In one series, 44 percent of the patients with biopsy-proven temporal arteritis had no tenderness to palpation,[100] and hence it is important to consider this disease in the absence of clinical signs or symptoms in patients with FUO. Takayasu's disease can also manifest as an FUO.[101]

Inherited Disorders

There are at least four inherited diseases that are associated with intermittent fever, sometimes unexplained for years. These are familial Mediterranean fever, which is inherited in about one-half of the patients as an autosomal recessive trait[102]; Fabry's disease or angiokeratoma corporis difusum, an X-linked disorder[103]; hypertriglyceridemia; and a syndrome of deafness, urticaria, and progressive amyloidosis that is familial or associated with chromosomal aberration.[104]

Familial Mediterranean Fever. Familial Mediterranean fever (FMF) is always associated with unexplained intermittent fever, usually beginning in childhood. Besides fever, FMF has distinct clinical signs and symptoms and laboratory data that, although nonspecific, together suggest this diagnosis in the absence of other disease.[105] These are fever, evidence of serosal inflammation—usually peritoneal or pleural, distinctive skin lesions (painful erythematous swellings), occasional joint pains, and headache. FMF is not periodic but rather a disease characterized by intermittent attacks of fever and serosal pain. In some patients, the attacks may be separated by a number of years, while in others they may occur weekly or more frequently. Spontaneous remissions and recurrence are typical of the disease. Attacks are associated with leukocytosis, elevated sedimentation rate, and elevated levels of several acute phase reactants. Admittedly nonspecific, these usually return to normal following the attacks. Although rarely seen in the United States, amyloidosis is often diagnosed in patients with FMF in the Middle East.

Familial Mediterranean fever is initially diagnosed as FUO because of the misconception that this disease is found only in Sephardic Jews, Armenians, and Arabs. Although there is unquestionably a much higher incidence of this disease in such patients, FMF occurs in patients of other extractions such as western Europeans.[105] The expression of the disease also seems milder in those patients living in the United States in that the skin lesions, joint involvement, and development of amyloidosis are rarely encountered. Most patients primarily have recurrent bouts of abdominal or chest pain with fever. The fever in FMF may be high during some attacks, and during others the temperature may be only minimally elevated. After a careful diagnostic work-up in which no evidence of infectious, hypersensitive, or autoimmune disease can be found in patients with symptoms

and signs of FMF, this diagnosis can be made. A diagnosis of FMF is usually made after years of recurrent attacks. Prophylactic oral colchicine therapy has been shown to prevent attacks of FMF.[106]

Fabry's Disease. Fabry's disease is an X-linked inborn error of glycosphingolipid metabolism resulting from the deficient activity of a specific α-glactosidase.[103] There is a systemic accumulation of the glycosphingolipid substrate trihexosyl ceramide, and this results in vascular and renal insufficiency and death in the third or fourth decade. Clinically, the disease is recognized by punctate skin lesions that are most numerous around the genitals and buttocks. Patients have unexplained attacks of fever and pain and also have severe acroparesthesias. The recurrent fever can manifest as an FUO, particularly when the characteristic lesions are missed. The enzymatic defect can be detected in plasma, urine, and leukocytes.[103]

Hypertriglyceridemia. Hypertriglyceridemia associated with recurrent fever and abdominal pain can present as FUO, and reduction of saturated fat intake results in the disappearance of the fever and pain.[23] Hyperlipidemia type V may be associated with recurrent bouts of abdominal pain, evidence of pancreatitis, and elevated amylase levels and may manifest as FUO.

Deafness, Urticaria, and Amyloidosis. The syndrome of deafness, urticaria, and amyloidosis has been described as a heredofamilial disease that is associated with bouts of high-spiking fever and a nonitching urticarial exanthem.[104] Progressive deafness is usually present since early childhood, and the febrile episodes begin in adolescence. Amyloidosis with renal failure occurs later. During the second decade of life this syndrome can manifest as FUO.

Central Nervous System Causes of FUO

The term *central fever* has been used to describe fever that is due to pathologic processes in or near the thermoregulatory center of the hypothalamus. There are several diseases that can affect the region of the thermoregulatory center, and these include metastatic tumor, primary central nervous system tumors, hemorrhage, degenerative diseases, vascular abnormalities, metabolic disorders, and infectious processes. In addition, such lesions more commonly produce endocrine disturbances. It should be pointed out, however, that lesions in or near the hypothalamus that affect thermoregulation are more likely to produce persistent hypothermia rather than hyperthermia. For example, sarcoid granulomas, degenerative processes,[107] tumor invasion,[108] hemorrhage into the third cerebral ventricle,[109] Wernicke's encephalopathy with hypothalamic hemorrhages,[110] and other hypothalamic lesions are most often associated with hypothermia. Nevertheless, a few patients with hypothalamic disturbances may have persistent or intermittently elevated body temperature.[23,111,112] These patients with fever, like the patients with hypothermia, do not have normal mechanisms of thermoregulation and may exhibit poikilothermia.[111] In addition, these patients may lose their daily temperature rhythm. Patients with local infectious processes, like encephalitis, may have an FUO and minimal changes in the CSF.

Children with central nervous system disease are more likely to develop hyperthermia than are adults. Diencephalic seizure disorders, degenerative brain diseases, chronic heavy metal intoxication, and central nervous system tumors, including central nervous system leukemia, are often associated with fever.[5–7] Nevertheless, hypothalmic lesions or disorders that are thought to be a cause of persistent unexplained fevers are extremely rare.

Factitious Illness

Careful observation of the daily temperature pattern can often lead to a diagnosis of factitious fever, since the circadian temperature rhythm may be absent; in some, the temperature may always be elevated. In addition to abnormal circadian temperature rhythms in patients with factitious fevers, evidence of vasoconstriction, sweating, or increased pulse rate are usually absent despite thermometer readings in excess of 39°C. The use of numbered and electronic thermometers and the simultaneous measurement of urine and body temperature are methods that help in making a diagnosis of factitious fevers.[113,114] Factitious fevers are usually suspected late in the work-up of patients with FUO,[24] but awareness of these methods can alert the attending physician before institution of a costly investigation. Most of these patients have false fevers, and the methods by which they manipulate thermometers is varied and often very ingenious. Others may inject pyrogenic materials or bacteria and induce real fever. Whatever the method used, diagnosis can be difficult, and many patients undergo extensive investigation before the factitious source of their illness is uncovered. There is a high incidence of patients with factitious illness in the health professions, particularly young women.[24] Once the factitious nature of the illness is discovered and the patient is confronted, psychiatric therapy often proves to be very beneficial. In patients with prolonged FUO, usually longer than 6 months, factitious illness accounts for 9 percent of the cases.[14] In addition, there is a higher incidence of association of self-mutilation in those patients with FUO lasting for prolonged periods. Repeated recovery of multiple and unusual organisms from blood and other cultures also suggests factitious illness.

Miscellaneous Causes of FUO

Postoperative fever due to halothane sensitization can persist and can manifest as FUO.[115] Multiple small pulmonary emboli can cause persistent fever with no abnormalities on chest radiographs. VQ scan may be useful in suggesting the diagnosis in such patients. In general, cardiac surgical procedures, particularly those using pump-bypass, are most often followed by prolonged or recurrent fevers that may continue into the second or third postoperative week. Often, in these patients no infectious cause can be found, although approximately 6 percent have a postpericardiotomy syndrome.[116] The pathogenetic mechanisms proposed for these persistent fevers include transfusion-associated cytomegalovirus infection, exacerbation of preexisting rheumatic fever, inflammatory response to blood in the pericardial cavity, and autoimmune response to traumatized cardiac tissue.[116] Neurosurgical procedures are also commonly associated with postoperative fever, and this may be related to the presence of blood in the third cerebral ventricle. A low-grade, aseptic meningitis can manifest as persistent fever after the excision of certain tumors from the central nervous system.[117] Septic thrombophlebitis, particularly of the pelvic veins, and small pulmonary embolization can manifest as FUO.[118] Inflammation resulting from radiation therapy may cause fever.[119] Pheochromocytomas can manifest as FUO years before the tumor is detected.[120] Laennec's cirrhosis is frequently accompanied by fever and is present in over one-third of the patients.[121] Fever due to cirrhosis is moderate but prolonged, and patients with cirrhosis have laboratory and pathologic evidence of active hepatic disease. However, these patients may be diagnosed as FUO only when the evidence of hepatic disease is undetected. The diagnosis of alcoholic hepatitis is frequently made in patients who are admitted to community hospitals with FUOs.

The only true cyclic or periodic cause of fever is cyclic neutropenia, in which the neutrophils are low or absent from the peripheral blood at 21-day intervals.[27] During this time, patients are susceptible to infection. Fever may be prominent during the neutropenic phase, and these patients are considered to have periodic fever before the correct diagnosis is made.

Many patients with the acquired immunodeficiency syndrome (AIDS) initially have an FUO. In the majority, the fever is due to an infection that is often relatively easy to diagnose. Thus, as in all FUO patients, AIDS patients should be evaluated thoroughly, with particular attention to the wide variety of infectious agents that may cause fever.

Exaggerated Circadian Temperature Rhythm

A large number of young children of both sexes, as well as young female adolescents, have been evaluated because of FUO. These persons have often had a previous acute, self-limited febrile illness of infectious origin. The patient or the family then becomes involved in the frequent monitoring of temperature. Following recovery from this illness, it is noted that the temperature (usually in the early evening) never returns to "normal." These persons seem to have exaggerated daily swings, and their normal evening temperature may be 99–100°F. After a minimal work-up, which is completely normal, we observe such persons and encourage them not to take their temperature unless they are ill. Unfortunately, many of these persons have been subjected to unnecessarily expensive, painful, and often dangerous procedures when, in fact, they are normal. Many years of follow-up have substantiated that these patients were not ill but merely had this exaggerated daily swing in temperature brought to their attention by a routine, self-limited infectious illness.

MANAGEMENT

There are a few general principles in approaching the patient with prolonged fever in whom no underlying source can be determined. A significant number of patients with undiagnosed fevers have good prognoses in that they eventually recover. Another group have intermittent bouts of fever for years but are otherwise well. These groups require no therapy, and mortality in the undiagnosed groups has been found in several studies to be low.[23] Nonspecific therapy of those patients with persistent fever and debilitating nutritional and physiologic imbalances may be instituted with caution. Clinical and laboratory evidence suggest that processes of amino acid oxidation contribute to the negative nitrogen balance of chronic fevers and that this may be partially reversed by cyclooxygenase inhibitors. The approach to empiric therapy in a patient with FUO must first consider whether the risk of the therapy outweighs the potential benefit. Thus, there are few, if any, indications for empiric antibiotic or cytotoxic chemotherapy. Our approach is to use antipyretics such as acetylsalicylic acid or acetaminophen first. These are given in maximum dosages, and, if the patient improves, they are continued for varying periods of time. If these drugs fail, then other prostaglandin synthetase inhibitors such as indomethacin or ibuprofen are tried. If these agents prove infective and the patient continues to be ill, then adrenal corticosteroid therapy should be considered if the physician is convinced that the underlying cause of the FUO is not infectious. Initially, we give prednisone around the clock and at a reasonable anti-inflammatory dosage (e.g., 10 mg every 6 hours). If improvement occurs and signs of inflammation recede, then we switch the patient to a single daily dose and eventually to alternate-day therapy. The latter is done to minimize undesirable side effects.

It must be emphasized that if the source of the fever defies diagnosis despite a thorough work-up as outlined, then, depending on the severity of the illness, reevaluation must be done at reasonable intervals. Most empiric therapy is nonspecific, and the patient may have a relapse after treatment. With such patients or with therapeutic failures, it may be necessary to perform complete evaluations as often as every 4–6 months, since in rare patients abnormalities may become apparent only after prolonged periods.

REFERENCES

1. Atkins E, Bodel P. Clinical fever: Its history, manifestations and pathogenesis. Fed Proc. 1979;38:57.
2. Petersdorf R, Beeson P. Fever of unexplained origin: Report of 100 cases. Medicine. 1961;40:1.
3. Durack D, Street A. Fever of unknown origin—reexamined and redefined. In: Remington J, Swartz M, eds. Current Clinical Topics of Infectious Diseases. St. Louis, MO: Mosby-Year Book, Inc.; 1991:35.
4. Petersdorf R. Fever of unknown origin: An old friend revisited. Arch Intern Med. 1992;152:21.
5. McClung HJ. Prolonged fever of unknown origin in children. Am J Dis Child. 1972;124:544.
6. Pizzo PA, Lovejoy FH, Smith DH. Prolonged fever in children: Review of 100 cases. Pediatrics. 1975;55:486.
7. Lohr JA, Hendley JO. Prolonged fever of unknown origin: A record of experiences with 54 childhood patients. Clin Pediatr. 1977;16:768.
8. Shoen RP, Van Ommen RA. Fever of obscure origin. Am J Med. 1963;34:486.
9. Deal WB. Fever of unknown origin. Postgrad Med. 1971;50:182.
10. Frayha R, Uwaydah M. Fever of unknown origin. Leb Med J. 1973;26:49.
11. Howard P Jr, Hahn HH, Palmer PL, et al. Fever of unknown origin: A prospective study of 100 patients. Tex Med. 1977;73:56.
12. Larson EB, Featherstone HJ, Petersdorf RG. Fever of undetermined origin: Diagnosis and followup of 105 cases—1970–80. Medicine. 1982;61:269.
13. Knockaert DC, Vanneste LJ, Vanneste SB, et al. Fever of unknown origin in the 1980s: An update of the diagnostic spectrum. Arch Intern Med. 1992;152:51.
14. Aduan R, Fauci A, Dale D, et al. Prolonged fever of unknown origin. Clin Res. 1978;26:558A.
15. Brusch Jl, Weinstein L. Fever of unknown origin. Med Clin North Am. 1988;72:1247.
16. Kazanjian PH. Fever of unknown origin: Review of 86 patients treated in community hospitals. Clin Infect Dis. 1992;15:968.
17. Knockaert DC, Vanneste LJ, Bobbaers HJ. Recurrent or episodic fever of unknown origin: Review of 45 cases and survey of the literature. Medicine. 1993;72:184.
18. Young EJ, Feinstein V, Mosher DM. Drug-induced fever: Cases seen in the evaluation of unexplained fever in a general hospital population. Rev Infect Dis. 1982;4:69.
19. Jacoby G, Swartz M. Fever of undetermined origin. N Engl J Med. 1973;289:1407.
20. Gleckman R, Crowley M, Esposito A. Fever of unknown origin: A view from the community hospital. Am J Med Sci. 1977;274:21.
21. Oppel TW, Bernstein CA. The differential diagnosis of fevers. Med Clin North Am. 1954;38:891.
22. Sepkowitz KA, Telzak EE, Carrow M, et al. Fever among outpatients with advanced human immunodeficiency virus infection. Arch Intern Med. 1993;153:1909.
23. Wolff SM, Fauci AS, Dale DC. Unusual etiologies of fever and their evaluation. Annu Rev Med. 1975;26:277.
24. Aduan R, Fauci A, Dale D, et al. Factitious fever and self-induced infection. Ann Intern Med. 1979;90:230.
25. Dinarello CA, Cannon JG, Wolff SM. New concepts on the pathogenesis of fever. Rev Infect Dis. 1988;10:168.
26. Weinstein L. Clinically benign fever of unknown origin: A personal retrospective. Rev Infect Dis. 1985;7:692.
27. Wright DG, Dale DC, Fauci AS, et al. Human cyclic neutropenia: Clinical review and long term followup of patients. Medicine. 1981;60:1.
28. Thoft RA. Corneal disease. N Engl J Med. 1978;298:1239.
29. McDade JE, Shepard CC, Fraser DW, et al. Legionnaires' disease. N Engl J Med. 1977;297:1197.
30. Riikonen P, Saarinen UM, Teppo A-M, et al. Cytokine and acute-phase reactant levels in serum of children with cancer admitted for fever and neutropenia. J Infect Dis. 1992;166:432.
31. Wolff SM, Kimball HJ, Perry S, et al. The biological properties of etiocholanolone. Ann Intern Med. 1967;67:1268.
32. Epler GR, McLoud TC, Graensler EA, et al. Normal chest roentgenograms in chronic diffuse infiltrative lung disease. N Engl J Med. 1978;298:934.
33. Becker W, Dolkemeyer U, Gramatzki M, et al. Use of immunoscintigraphy in the diagnosis of fever of unknown origin. Eur J Nucl Med. 1993;20:1078.
34. McNeil BJ, Sanders R, Alderson PO, et al. A prospective study of computed tomography, ultrasound, and gallium imaging in patients with fever. Radiology. 1981;139:647.
35. Schmidt KG, Ramussen JW, Sorensen PG, et al. Indium-111 granulocyte scintigraphy in the evaluation of patients with fever of undetermined origin. Scand J Infect Dis. 1987;19:339.
36. Rubin RH, Fischman AJ, Callahan RJ, et al. Indium-111 labeled nonspecific immunoglobulin scanning in the detection of focal infection. N Engl J Med. 1989;321:935.
37. Oyen WJG, Claessens RAMJ, Raemaekers JMM, et al. Diagnosing infection in febrile granulocytopenic patients with Indium-111-labeled human immunoglobulin G. J Clin Oncol. 1992;10:61.
38. Rowland MD, Del Bene VE. Use of body computed tomography to evaluate fever of unknown origin. J Infect Dis. 1987;156:408.
39. Bowen BC, Donovan-Post MJ. Diagnostic imaging of CNS infection and inflammation. In: Schlossberg D, ed. Infections of the Nervous System. New York: Springer-Verlag; 1990:315.
40. Lukes AS, Bright DK, Durak DT. Diagnosis of infective endocarditis. In: Wilson W, Steckelberg J, eds. Infectious Disease Clinics of North America. v. 7. Philadelphia: WB Saunders Company, 1993:1.
41. Solomon AJB. System imaging in unexplained fever. In: Isaac B, ed. Unexplained Fever. Boca Raton: CRC Press; 1991:495.
42. Stark DD, Moss AA, Goldberg HI, et al. Nuclear magnetic resonance imaging of the pancreas. Normal and pathological findings. Radiology. 1984;159:153.
43. Brisson-Noel A, Gicquel B, Lecossier D, et al. Rapid diagnosis of tuberculosis by amplification of mycobacterial DNA in clinical samples. Lancet. 1989;2:1069.
44. Tenover F. DNA hybridization techniques and their application to the diagnosis of infectious diseases. In: Washington J, ed. Infectious Diseases Clinics of North America. Philadelphia: WB Saunders Company, 1993:171.
45. Rothman DL, Schwartz SI, Adams JT. Diagnostic laparotomy for fever or abdominal pain of unknown origin. Am J Surg. 1977;133:273.
46. Mitchell DP, Hanes TE, Hoyumpa AM, et al. Fever of unknown origin. Arch Intern Med. 1977;137:1001.
47. Katz P, Fauci AS. *Nocardia asteroides* sinusitis. JAMA. 1977;238:2397.
48. Tunkel AR, Kaye D. Endocarditis with negative blood cultures. N Engl J Med. 1992;326:1215.
49. Geraci JE, Weed LA, Nichols DR. Fever of obscure origin. The value of abdominal exploration in diagnosis. JAMA. 1959;169:1302.
50. Fisher HC, White MH Jr. Biliary trace disease in the aged. Arch Surg. 1951;63:536.
51. Frieden TR, Sterling T, Palbos-Mendez A, et al. The emergence of drug-resistant tuberculosis in New York City. N Engl J Med. 1993;328:521.
52. Fung WO, Ong SC, Lee YS. Splenic tuberculosis presenting as pyrexia of unknown origin. Med J Aust. 1973;1:446.
53. Boettinger LE, Nordenstam HH, Wester PO. Disseminated tuberculosis as a cause of fever of obscure origin. Lancet. 1962;1:19.
54. Relman DA, Schmidt TM, MacDermott RP, et al. Identification of the uncultured bacillus of Whipple's disease. N Engl J Med. 1992;327:293.
55. Gordis L, Lilienfeld AM, Rodriguez R. A community-wide study of acute rheumatic fever in adults. JAMA. 1969;210:862.
56. Bisno AL. Group A streptococcal infections and acute rheumatic fever. N Engl J Med. 1991;325:783.
57. Michels TC. Mucocutaneous lymph node syndrome in adults: Differentiation from toxic shock syndrome. Am J Med. 1986;80:724.
58. Leung DYM, Meissner HC, Fulton DR, et al. Toxic shock syndrome toxin-secreting *Staphylococcus aureus* in Kawasaki syndrome. Lancet. 1993;342:1385.
59. Malatack JJ, Jaffe R. Granulomatous hepatitis in three children due to cat-scratch disease without peripheral adenopathy. Am J Dis Child. 1993;147:949.
60. Fretzayas A, Tapratzi P, Kavazarakis E, et al. Multiorgan involvement in systemic cat scratch disease. Scand J Infect Dis. 1993;25:145.
61. Smith L. Relapsing fever: A case history. Calif Med. 1969;110:322.
62. Southern PM Jr, Sanford JP. Relapsing fever. Medicine. 1969;48:129.
63. Steere AC. Lyme disease. N Engl J Med. 1989;321:586.
64. Goellner MH, Agger WA, Burgess JH, et al. Hepatitis due to recurrent Lyme disease. Ann Intern Med. 1988;108:707.
65. Nocton JJ, Dressler F, Rutledge BJ, et al. Detection of *Borrelia burgdorferi* DNA by polymerase chain reaction in synovial fluid from patients with Lyme disease. N Engl J Med. 1994;330:229.
66. Harkess JR. Ehrlichiosis. In: Weinberg A, Weber D, Moellering R, eds. Infectious Disease Clinics of North America. v. 5. Philadelphia: WB Saunders Company; 1991:37.
67. Relman DA, Falkow S, LeBoit PE. The organism causing bacillary angiomatosis, peliosis hepatis, and fever and bacteremia in immunocompromised patients. N Engl J Med. 1991;324:1514.
68. Dolan MJ, Wong MT, Regnery RL, et al. Syndrome of *Rochalimaea henselae* adenitis suggesting cat scratch disease. Ann Intern Med. 1993;118:331.
69. Daly JS, Worthington MG, Brenner DJ. *Rochalimaea elizabethae* sp. nov. isolated from a patient with endocarditis. J Clin Microbiol. 1993;31:872.
70. Grayston J. Chlamydia pneumoniae, strain TWAR. Chest. 1989;95:664.
71. Anderson LJ. Human parvoviruses. J Infect Dis. 1990;161:603.
72. Hjelle B, Jenison S, Torrez-Martinez N, et al. A novel hantavirus associated with an outbreak of fatal respiratory disease in the southwestern United States: Evolutionary relationships to known hantaviruses. J Virol. 1994;68:592.
73. Yanagihara R. Hantavirus infection in the United States: Epizootiology and epidemiology. Rev Infect Dis. 1990;12:449.
74. Cranston WI, Luff RH, Owen D, et al. Studies on the pathogenesis of fever in renal carcinoma. Clin Sci Mol Med. 1973;45:459.
75. Bodel P. Generalized perturbations in the host physiology caused by localized tumors. Tumors and fever. Ann NY Acad Sci. 1974;230:6.
76. Bodel P. Spontaneous pyrogen production by mouse histiocytic and myelomonocytic tumor cell lines *in vitro*. J Exp Med. 1978;147:1503.

77. Miller JS, Miller JJ. Benign giant lymph node hyperplasia presenting as fever of unknown origin. J Pediatr. 1975;87:237.
78. Padfield R, Hicken P. Cortical hyperostosis in infants: A radiological study of sixteen patients. Br J Radiol. 1970;43:231.
79. Campbell EW, Brantley R, Harrold M, et al. Angiomyolipoma presenting as fever of unknown origin. Am J Med. 1974;57:843.
80. Ahmann DL, Kiely JM, Harrison EG, et al. Malignant lymphoma of the spleen. Cancer. 1966;19:461.
81. Zanger B, Dorsey HN. Fever: A manifestation of preleukemia. JAMA. 1976; 236:1266.
82. Kumar S, Bhargava M. Preleukemia acute myelogenous leukemia. Acta Haematol. 1970;43:21.
83. Bowman HS, Martinez E. Fever, anemia and hyperhaptoglobinemia. Ann Intern Med. 1968;68:613.
84. Boettiger LE. Fever of unknown origin: VI. Fever in carcinoma of the kidney. Acta Med Scand. 1957;156:477.
85. Rawlins MD, Luff RH, Cranston WI. Pyrexia in renal carcinoma. Lancet. 1970;1:1371.
86. Wallace D, Hahn B. Dubois' Lupus Erythematosus. Philadelphia: Lea & Febiger; 1993:193.
87. Estes D, Christian CL. The natural history of systemic lupus erythematosus by prospective analysis. Medicine. 1971;50:85.
88. Fauci AS, Haynes B, Katz P. The spectrum of vasculitis. Ann Intern Med. 1978;89:660.
89. Calabro JJ, Marchesano JM. Fever associated with juvenile rheumatoid arthritis. N Engl J Med. 1967;276:11.
90. Bujak JS, Aptekar RG, Decker JL, et al. Juvenile rheumatoid arthritis presenting in the adult as fever of unknown origin. Medicine. 1973;52:431.
91. Yamaguchi M, Ahta A, Tsunematsu T, et al. Preliminary criteria for classification of adults Still's disease. J Rheum. 1992;19:3.
92. Gelfand JA, Kimball K, Burke JF, et al. Amphotericin B treatment of human mononuclear cells in vitro results in secretion of tumor necrosis factor and interleukin-1 (Abstract). Clin Res. 1988;36:456A.
93. Cleary JD, Chapman SW, Nolan RL. Pharmacologic modulation of interleukin-1 expression by amphotericin B-stimulated human mononuclear cells. Antimicrob Agents Chemother. 1992;36:977.
94. Cluff LE, Johnson JE III. Drug fever. Prog Allergy. 1964;8:149.
95. Mackowiak PA. Southwestern Internal Medicine Conference. Drug fever: Mechanisms, maxims, and misconceptions. Am J Med Sci. 1987;294:275.
96. Wolff SM, Simon HB. Granulomatous hepatitis and prolonged fever of unknown origin. Trans Am Climatol Assoc 1973;84:149.
97. Simon HB, Wolff SM. Granulomatous hepatitis and prolonged fever of unknown origin: A study of 13 patients. Medicine 1973;52:1.
98. Fauci AS, Wolff SM. Granulomatous hepatitis. Prog Liver Dis 1976;5:609.
99. Crohn BB, Yarnis H. Regional Ileitis. 2nd ed. New York: Grune & Stratton; 1958.
100. Fauchald P, Rygvold O, Oipstease B. Temporal arteritis and polymyalgia rheumatica. Ann Intern Med. 1972;77:845.
101. Roberts WC, MacGregor RR, DeBlanc HJ, et al. The prepulseless phase of pulseless disease, or pulseless disease with pulses. Am J Med. 1969;46:313.
102. Sohar E, Prass M, Heller J, et al. Genetics of familial Mediterranean fever (FMF). Arch Intern Med. 1961;107:529.
103. Desnick RJ, Allen KV, Desnick SJ, et al. Fabry's disease: Enzymatic diagnosis of hemizygotes and heterozygotes. J Lab Clin Med. 1973;81:157.
104. Andersen V, Buch NH, Jensen MK, et al. Deafness, urticaria and amyloidosis. Am J Med. 1967;42:449.
105. Wolff SM. Familial Mediterranean fever. In: Braunwald E, Wilson J, eds. Harrison's Principles of Internal Medicine. 13 ed. New York: McGraw-Hill; 1994; 81–90.
106. Dinarello CA, Wolff SM, Goldfinger SE, et al. Colchicine therapy for familial Mediterranean fever. N Engl J Med. 1974;291:934.
107. Bauer HG. Endocrine and other clinical manifestations of hypothalamic disease. A survey of 60 cases with autopsies. J Clin Endocrinol. 1954;14:13.
108. Fox RH, Davies TW, Marsh FP, et al. Hypothermia in a young man with an anterior hypothalamic lesion. Lancet. 1970;2:185.
109. Hey EN. Thermal regulation in the newborn. Br J Hosp Med. 1972;8:51.
110. Philip G, Smith JF. Hypothermia and Wernicke's encephalopathy. Lancet. 1973;2:122.
111. Wolff SM, Adler RC, Buskirk ER, et al. A syndrome of periodic hypothalamic discharge. Am J Med. 1964;36:956.
112. Simon HB. Extreme pyrexia. JAMA. 1976;236:2419.
113. Kleinman M. Letter to the editor. N Engl J Med. 1977;296:886.
114. Murray J, Tuazon C, Guerero IC, et al. Urinary temperature. N Engl J Med. 1977;296:23.
115. Dykes MHM. Unexplained postoperative fever. JAMA. 1971;216:641.
116. Ross DF, Rose MR, Rapaport FT. Febrile responses associated with cardiac surgery. J Thorac Cardiovasc Surg. 1974;67:251.
117. Cantu RC, Moses JM, Kjellberg RN, et al. An unusual cause of aseptic postoperative fever in a neurosurgical patient. Clin Pediatr. 1966;5:747.
118. Dunn LJ, Van Voorhis LW. Enigmatic fever and pelvic thrombophlebitis. N Engl J Med. 1967;276:262.
119. Van Herik M. Fever as a complication of radiation therapy for carcinoma of the cervix. Am J Roentgenol Radiol Ther Nucl Med. 1965;93:104.
120. Wallberg AV. Operat phaeochromocytoin med lycklig utgang. Nord Med. 1949;41:470.
121. Tisdale WA, Klatskin G. The fever of Laennec's cirrhosis. Yale J Biol Med. 1960;33:94.

38. THE ACUTELY ILL PATIENT WITH FEVER AND RASH

DAVID J. WEBER
MYRON S. COHEN

A recognizable rash can lead to immediate diagnosis and appropriate therapy. Material isolated from involved skin, when properly handled, can confirm a specific diagnosis. Unfortunately, rashes are often quite bewildering. Dermatologists, who are generally more comfortable with evaluation of the skin, are not always available for immediate consultation. Furthermore, not infrequently, dermatologists and infectious disease specialists differ in their approach to the patient with a rash.

In this chapter we provide a framework emphasizing the following: *(1)* diagnostic approach to patients with fever and rash, *(2)* categories of skin lesions, and *(3)* brief descriptions of the most important febrile illnesses characterized by a rash.

APPROACH TO THE PATIENT

In the initial evaluation of patients with fever and rash three problems are critical. First is whether the patient is well enough to provide further history or immediate cardiorespiratory support is required. Second is whether the nature of the rash (in the context of presentation) demands institution of isolation precautions. Isolation is required primarily for patients whose illnesses allow airborne spread of the pathogen and includes both viral and bacterial disease. Isolation guidelines should be employed with urgency. All patients with undiagnosed infectious diseases should be treated with caution by personnel, who should avoid intimate contact with secretions and employ universal blood and body fluid precautions.[1–7] Third, a skin lesion consistent with meningococcal disease (see below) requires emergent antibacterial therapy. Similar urgency may be warranted when lesions suggest bacterial septic shock, since appropriate use of antibiotics may improve survival.[8]

The history obtained from the patient should elicit the following information:

1. Drug ingestion within the past 30 days
2. Travel outside of the local area
3. Occupational exposures
4. Sun exposure
5. Immunizations
6. Sexually transmitted disease exposure, including risk factors for infection with human immunodeficiency virus (HIV)
7. Immunologic status, including chemotherapy, steroid use, hematologic malignancy, solid organ and bone marrow transplantation, and functional or anatomic asplenia
8. Valvular heart disease
9. Prior illness, including a history of drug and/or antibiotic allergies
10. Exposure to febrile or ill individuals within the recent past
11. Exposure to wild or rural habitats and wild animals
12. Pets and habits

The clinician should pay particular attention to the season of the year, which dramatically affects the epidemiology of febrile rashes. Physical examination should focus on the following:

1. Vital signs
2. General appearance
3. Signs of toxicity
4. Presence and location of adenopathy
5. Presence of genital, mucosal, and/or conjunctival lesions
6. Detection of hepatosplenomegaly
7. Arthritis
8. Signs of nuchal rigidity, meningismus, or neurologic dysfunction

Key ingredients in arriving at a correct diagnosis include *(1)* dermatologic classification of the rash[9–11] (Table 1),[11–16] *(2)* distribution of the rash, *(3)* pattern of progression, and *(4)* timing of the development of rash (relative to the onset of illness and fever) (Table 2). Rashes may be classified by histologic or pathophysiologic criteria,[17] which is generally not of immediate benefit to the clinician. It must be emphasized that noninfectious processes often include skin rash and fever and should be considered strongly during the initial evaluation.[18] Drug reactions, which occur with about 1 in 20 courses of drug therapy, should be considered in any patient presenting with a rash.[19] Rashes associated with occupational exposures,[20] animal exposures,[21] international travel,[22] and athletics[23] have recently been reviewed.

HOST DEFENSE PROPERTIES OF SKIN

The skin is a relatively inhospitable environment for the growth of most pathogenic microorganisms. The hostility of that environment is mainly attributed to two factors. The relative dryness of most cutaneous surfaces provides an insufficient amount of moisture to support significant growth of pathogens, and colonization with strains of bacteria and yeast (normal resident flora), generally regarded as nonpathogenic, appears to exclude more pathogenic species.[24–26] Resident flora may actually produce metabolites that are inhibitory to the growth of more pathogenic species. Examples include bacterial lipases that liberate from sebum free fatty acids that inhibit various strains of *Streptococcus pyogenes* and antibiotic metabolites derived from *Streptococcus epidermidis* that kill strains of *Micrococcus* and *Streptococcus*.[27–29] Eradication of resident flora greatly enhances the survival of *Staphylococcus aureus* and the subsequent development of infection.[30]

Normal skin is an impenetrable barrier to microorganisms. The barrier to penetration is the outermost layer of skin, known as the *stratum corneum*. The stratum corneum is composed of corneified envelopes of dead keratinocytes joined by a relatively impermeable intercellular substance. Together, the cell envelopes and intercellular substance form a physical barrier approximately 10–15 μm thick.[31] The skin is richly supplied with both endogenous and exogenous cellular and humoral mediators of inflammation that subserve host defense functions.[32]

Epidermis and dermis are home to several cell types that may generate soluble factors that initiate and amplify the inflammatory response. Those cells include the keratinocyte, fibroblast, mast cell, Langerhans cell, endothelial cell, and monocyte/macrophage. Recent studies show that keratinocytes are capable of synthesizing a number of proinflammatory and immunostimulatory cytokines (the interleukins IL-1, IL-3, and IL-6; tumor necrosis factor-α; and granulocyte-macrophage colony-stimulating factor), complement proteins, and arachidonate metabolites including prostaglandins and leukotrienes.[33,34] The mast cells that reside around dermal vessels can be stimulated by a variety of factors including those derived from microorganisms to make the release promotors of inflammation such as histamine, arachidonate metabolites, proteinases, and factors that can recruit and activate leukocytes.[35] The skin may play

TABLE 1. Systemic Infections with Prominent Cutaneous Manifestations

Organism (Disease)	Macules, Papules	Vesicles, Bullae	Petechia, Purpura
Viruses			
Human Immunodeficiency (HIV-1) virus	X		
Echoviruses	X	X	X
Coxsackieviruses	X	X	X
Rubeola (measles)	X		
Atypical measles	X		X
Adenovirus	X		X
Lymphocytic choriomeningitis virus	X		
Dengue virus	X		X
Viral hemorrhagic fevers			X
Rubella (German measles)	X		X
Colorado tick fever	X		
Yellow fever			X
Varicella-zoster (disseminated)		X	
Herpes simplex (disseminated)		X	
Varicella (chickenpox)		X	
Vaccinia		X	
Cytomegalovirus	X		
Congenital cytomegalovirus			X
Epstein-Barr virus	X		X
Hepatitis B	X		
Parvovirus B19 (erythema infectiosum)	X		
Human herpes virus 6	X		
Bacteria			
Chlamydia psittaci	X		
Mycoplasma pneumoniae	X	X	
Rickettsia			
R. rickettsii (Rocky Mountain spotted fever)	X		X
R. akari (rickettsialpox)	X	X	
R. prowazekii (epidemic/louse-borne typhus)	X		X
R. typhi (endemic/murine typhus)	X		
R. tsutsugamushi (scrub typhus)	X		
Rochalimaea henselae	X		
Rochalimaea quintana	X		
Salmonella typhi	X		
Francisella tularensis	X		
Streptobacillus moniliformis (rat-bite fever)	X		X
Treponema pallidum (secondary)	X		
Myobacterium haemophilium	X		
Neisseria gonorrhoeae			X
Neisseria meningitidis			X
Leptospira spp.	X		
Listeria monocytogenes		X (rare)	
Bartonella bacilliformis	X		
Borrelia sp. (relapsing fever)	X		X
Borrelia burgdorferi (Lyme)	X (annular)		
Pseudomonas aeruginosa	X		
Spirillum minus (rat-bite fever)	X		
Staphylococcus aureus	X		X
Streptococci—group A (scarlet fever)	X		
Capnocytophaga canimorsus			X
Vibrio vulnificus		X	
Fungi (disseminated)			
Candida spp.	X		
Cryptococcus neoformans	X		
Histoplasma capsulatum	X		
Blastomyces dermatitidis	X		
Coccidioides immitis	X		
Fusarium spp. (agents of mucormycosis)	X		
Protozoa			
Plasmodium falciparum (malaria)			X

(Data from refs. 11–15.)

TABLE 2. Skin Lesions and Systemic Infections

Lesion	Common Pathogens	Histologic Findings	Smears Positive for Pathogens	Time of Appearance (after Onset of Illness)
Symmetric peripheral gangrene, acrocyanosis	Noninfectious or gram-negative bacteria, *Capnocytophaga canimorsus*	Bleeding in skin, vascular thrombosis, perivascular infiltration	No	12–36 hr
Multiple purpuric lesions in seriously ill patients	*Neisseria meningitidis, Capnocytophaga canimorsus, Rickettsia,* other gram-negative bacteria	Vascular thrombosis, perivascular hemorrhage	Yes[a]	12–36 hr[b]
Ecthyma gangrenosum, erythema multiforme, bullous lesions	*Pseudomonas,* other gram-negative bacteria	Veins mainly involved, intima spared, inflammatory reaction	Yes	Several days
Macronodular lesions	*Candida, Cryptococcus neoformans, Histoplasma capsulatum, Fusarium*	Hyphae, mononuclear perivascular reaction	No	Several days
Delayed-onset rash with nonsymmetric scattered maculopapular or vesicular lesions	*Neisseria gonorrhoeae, Neisseria meningitidis*	Perivascular mononuclear infiltrate, immune complex	Occasionally (few bacteria only)	3–10 days
Polymorphous lesions	*Neisseria meningitidis, Neisseria gonorrhoeae, Salmonella*			
Rose spots	*Salmonella,* various bacteria	Perivascular mononuclear inflammation	No	5–10 days
Toxic erythema	*Staphylococcus aureus, Streptococcus*	Dilation and perivascular edema	No	At presentation

[a] Except for Rocky Mountain spotted fever, in which biopsy and immunofluorescent staining are important for early diagnosis.
[b] In Rocky Mountain spotted fever, 1–7 days.

(Adapted from Kingston and Mackey,[17] with permission.)

an active role in the initiation, development, and expression of specific immune responses to microorganisms through a system of skin-associated lymphoid tissues and keratinocytes.[36,37]

PATHOGENESIS OF SKIN RASH

Skin rash with fever can result from a local infectious process due to virtually any class of microbe that has been allowed to penetrate the stratum corneum and multiply locally. However, exanthems are more cogent to this discussion. An exanthem is a cutaneous eruption due to the systemic effects of a microorganism on the skin. An enanthem is an eruption of similar etiology involving the mucous membranes.

Microorganisms produce eruptions by *(1)* multiplication in the skin (e.g., herpesviruses); *(2)* release of toxins that act on skin structures (e.g., scarlet fever, *Pseudomonas aeruginosa*); *(3)* evoking an inflammatory response involving phagocytes and lymphocytes (in this case the microbicidal/tumoricidal metabolism of host defense cells is directed at the skin); and *(4)* via effects on vasculature, including vaso-occlusion and necrosis and/or vasodilation with edema and hyperemia. Obviously, for many eruptions several mechanisms can play a role.

DIFFERENTIAL DIAGNOSIS AND SKIN RASH

There are two ways to approach the investigation of infectious rash: either by the type of lesion visualized or by knowledge of individual pathogens and the rashes they produce. Unfortunately, neither system is inclusive. Accordingly, both approaches are discussed in this section.

Characteristics of the Lesion

Morphologic types of skin lesions include macules, papules, plaques, nodules, vesicles, bullae, and postules. Macules are flat, nonpalpable lesions in the plane of the skin. Papules are small palpable lesions elevated above the plane of the skin. Large papules are referred to as nodules. Vesicles and bullae are small and large blisters, respectively, and pustules are palpable lesions filled with pus. Plaques are large flat lesions that are palpable. In addition to morphology, lesions are characterized by their color and particularly by the presence or absence of

hemorrhage. Lesions may be skin colored, hyperpigmented or hypopigmented, or one of several other colors of which redness is the most common. Blanching erythematous lesions are those in which erythema is due to vasodilation, while nonblanching erythemas may be due to extravasation of blood. Purpuric lesions are those in which there is hemorrhage into the skin and may be small, petechial or large, ecchymotic. We have divided our discussion into rashes that are maculopapular (a rash characterized by flat and elevated lesions), nodular, vesiculobullous, erythematous, and purpuric.

Macular and/or Papular Rash

Macular and/or papular rashes are usually seen in viral illnesses and immune-mediated syndromes. Common viral etiologies include the classic childhood viral diseases such as measles, rubella, erythema infectiosum, and roseola.[38] The etiologic agent of roseola is now known to be human herpesvirus-6.[39] However, infection with this agent may also occur without a rash. Other viral agents that often produce a rash are atypical measles, coxsackieviruses, echoviruses, cytomegalovirus, and hepatitis B. Erythema multiforme is considered a special category of maculopapular rash.

Lesions of erythema multiforme usually begin as round to oval macules and papules that vary in size from less than a centimeter up to 1–2 cm in diameter. Typical lesions have central erythema surrounded by a narrow ring of normal-appearing skin that is in turn surrounded by another thin ring of erythema to form target lesions. The central area may be dark red, blue, or dusky grey in color and may develop into a blister (bullous erythema multiforme). Lesions are typically symmetrically distributed on the trunk and extremities and may show a predilection for knees, elbows, palms, and soles. Mucosal involvement is usually present and painful. The degree of mucosal involvement varies from oral blisters and erosions to a hemorrhagic conjunctivitis and stomatitis. When the latter are present with fever, the term *Stevens-Johnson syndrome* is applied. The distribution, symmetry, tendency to iris formation, and bulla should allow proper identification. Most cases of erythema multiform are idiopathic. In children and adults infections are a leading etiology, but in adults many case are idiopathic or due to drug exposure. Infectious diseases linked to erythema multiforme are

TABLE 3. Differential Diagnosis of Erythema Multiforme

Noninfectious
  Drugs
  X-ray therapy
Infectious
  Herpes simplex infections
  Epstein-Barr virus
  Adenovirus
  Coxsackievirus B5
  Vaccinia (smallpox inoculation)
  Mycoplasma pneumoniae
  Chlamydia (psittacosis, lymphogranuloma venereum)
  Cat scratch (?)
  Salmonella typhi
  Yersinia
  Mycobacterium tuberculosis
  Histoplasma capsulatum
  Coccidioides immitis

TABLE 4. Differential Diagnosis of Erythema Nodosum

Noninfectious
  Systemic lupus erythematosus
  Sarcoidosis
  Ulcerative colitis
  Crohn's colitis
  Behçet's disease
  Drugs
  Pregnancy
Infectious
  Hepatitis C
  Streptococcal infection
  Mycobacterium tuberculosis
  Mycobacterium leprae
  Mycobacterium marinum
  Chlamydia trachomatis (lymphogranuloma venereum)
  Yersinia infection
  Histoplasma capsulatum
  Coccidioides immitis

summarized in Table 3. Atypical rashes suggestive of erythema multiforme may occur in chronic meningococcemia, bacterial endocarditis, secondary syphilis, staphylococcal scalded skin syndrome, Kawasaki disease, toxic shock syndrome, Rocky Mountain spotted fever, collagen vascular disease, and a variety of viral disorders.

Human parvovirus B19 infection is the cause of fifth disease—manifesting as a common exanthem in childhood and as a rheumatic syndrome in adults.[40,41] Other disease manifestations include fever, anorexia, sore throat, abdominal pain, aplastic crisis in patients with hemoglobinopathies (e.g., sickle cell anemia), and hydrops fetalis with a risk of fetal death.[42–44] Erythema infectiosum is characterized by a three-stage rash. The initial stage is that of an erythematous, warm but nontender "slapped cheek" facial rash. Simultaneously up to 4 days later, a variable rash appears on the extremities, which has a morbilliform, confluent, or annular appearance. Later the rash may remit and recur with stress, exercise, sunlight, or bathing. The rash usually disappears within 1–2 weeks. Since by the time the rash has appeared viremia can no longer be detected, patients are likely infective only prior to the appearance of the rash.[45]

Several life-threatening infections may present with blanching erythematous maculopapular lesions before evolving into petechiae. These include meningococcemia, Rocky Mountain spotted fever, and dengue fever. Although rheumatic fever has as one of its diagnostic findings a configurate, migrating erythema known as erythema marginatum, it may also be associated with a maculopapular eruption and subcutaneous nodules. Patients with enteric fever due to *Salmonella* may develop "rose spots," a transient scattering of rose-colored macules over the abdomen.

All physicians should be familiar with the cutaneous manifestations of syphilis, especially as the number of cases of primary and secondary syphilis and congenital syphilis have been rising steadily in the United States since 1986.[46,47] Primary skin lesions (chancres) typically develop about 21 days after exposure. Secondary syphilis is often accompanied by a rash with highly variable morphology. Lesions may be macular, papular, maculopapular, papulosquamous, or pustular. Occasionally all types of lesions may occur in the same person. Condylomata lata characterized by grayish, raised, broad, flat-appearing papular lesions may occur in moist areas, such as the anus, vulva, and scrotum.

Nodular Lesions

A nodule is a palpable, solid round or ellipsoidal lesion, usually resulting from disease in the dermis. Nonerythematous nodules may suggest candidal sepsis (see below), but other fungal disease including blastomycosis, histoplasmosis, coccidiodomycosis, sporotrichosis, and histoplasmosis may produce skin nodules. Bacteria such as *Nocardia* and atypical mycobacteria (especially *Mycobacterium marinum*) may also cause nodular

lesions.[48] Lesions consistent with erythema gangrenosum suggest *Pseudomonas* sepsis. A skin biopsy specimen with appropriate stains and cultures will define the diagnosis.

The lesions of erythema nodosum are characterized by tender, erythematous nodules that vary in diameter from less than a centimeter to several centimeters. They are usually multiple and located on the anterior portions of the legs but may be solitary and occur on the upper part of the body. They typically do not suppurate but rarely may do so. The lesions will often develop in crops and usually heal in days to a few weeks without scarring. Infectious agents are a prominent cause of this lesion (Table 4).

Diffuse Erythema

Diffuse erythema, especially if desquamation or peeling is present, should lead to consideration of scarlet fever, toxic shock syndrome, mucocutaneous lymph node syndrome (Kawasaki disease), staphylococcal scalded skin syndrome, Stevens-Johnson syndrome, and toxic epidermal necrolysis. Desquamation may occur late in all of these syndromes, and its absence early in the disease course should not be considered a reason for excluding any disease process. Most of these disorders can be easily differentiated by the patient's history and appropriate diagnostic tests.

Vesiculobullous Eruptions

A vesicle is a circumscribed, elevated lesion containing free fluid. A vesicular lesion larger than 0.5 cm is termed a bulla. Most vesiculobullous eruptions are immunologic or primarily dermatologic. Infectious diseases to be considered include varicella, disseminated herpes simplex, eczema herpeticum, enteroviruses, and coxsackieviruses (includes A16, the cause of hand, foot, and mouth disease). Herpes simplex infection, the most common infection exhibiting vesicles, is characterized by a cluster of vesicles on an erythematous base that progresses to mucocutaneous ulceration.[49] Viral culture of a scraping from a blister may allow demonstration of a herpes infection.

Vesicles can be confused with pustules. A pustule is an elevation of the skin enclosing a purulent exudate. Vesicular lesions may become pustules, but diffuse pustular diseases usually represent a dermatologic illness (e.g., postular psoriasis) or a cutaneous infection (e.g., pustular *Pseudomonas* lesions after the use of contaminated hot tubs or staphylococcal folliculitis).[50] Pustular skin lesions associated with arthralgias should lead to a consideration of gonococcemia, *Moraxella* bacteremia, chronic meningococcemia, subacute bacterial endocarditis, coxsackie infection, and Behçet syndrome.

Bullous skin lesions with sepsis are suggestive of the following infections: group A streptococcal erysipelas with necrotizing fascitis (gangrenous erysipelas), ecthyma gangrenosum (due to

P. aeruginosa or *Aeromonas*), *Vibrio* infections (especially *V. vulnificus*), staphyloccocal cellulitis or impetigo, streptococcal cellulitis, or toxic epidermal necrolysis (staphylococcal scalded skin syndrome, infections, medication).[51] *Vibrio vulnificus* should be strongly considered in patients with preexisting liver disease or other immunocompromising states who have recently ingested raw seafood.

Vesicopustular eruptions in the neonate may be due to both noninfectious and infectious causes. Infectious etiologies include congenital and neonatal candidiasis, staphylococcal infections, streptococcal infections, *Listeria monocytogenes,* herpes simplex, neonata varicella, and sepsis (various organisms).[52]

Petechial Purpuric Eruptions

Petechiae are lesions less than 3 mm in diameter containing extravasated red blood cells or hemoglobin. Larger lesions are termed *ecchymoses.* Diffuse petechial lesions should always prompt emergent investigation. In critically ill patients these lesions are often associated with symmetric peripheral gangrene, consumptive coagulopathy, and shock. The most common infectious etiologies include gram-negative organisms, especially *N. meningitidis,* and *Rickettsia.* Less commonly *L. monocytogenes* or staphylocci may be associated with a similar clinical picture. Asplenic patients are at an increased risk of overwhelming sepsis, which may be accompanied by symmetric peripheral gangrene.[53–60] About half of the infections are due to *Strep. pneumoniae.*[53,55,60]

Viral illnesses associated with petechial rashes include coxsackievirus A9, echovirus 9, Epstein-Barr virus, cytomegalovirus, atypical measles, and the viral hemorrhagic fevers (see Ch. 142). Children with coxsackievirus and echovirus infections may appear very ill, and differential diagnosis from meningococcemia is difficult.

Rashes are a prominent characteristic of rickettsial disease except for Q fever. Although Rocky Mountain spotted fever is the most common rickettsial disease in the United States, endemic typhus has been noted on the Gulf Coast and epidemic typhus among immigrants and in the mid-Atlantic states. Lesions caused by rickettsiae are usually generalized and symmetric. An eschar (tache noire) characteristically develops at the site of inoculation in the following rickettsial infections: African tick typhus (*R. conorii*), North Asian tick-borne rickettsiosis (*R. sibirica*), Queensland tick typhus (*R. australis*), rickettsialpox (*R. akari*), and scrub- or chigger-borne typhus (*R. tsutsugamushi*).

In patients with an appropriate travel history, infection with *Plasmodium falciparum* must be considered. Heavy parasitization may lead to severe hemolysis, renal failure, central nervous system findings, and petechiae secondary to thrombocytopenia.

The most important causes of noninfectious petechiae are thrombocytopenia, large and small vessel necrotizing vasculitis, and pigmented purpuric eruptions.

Enanthem

While attempting to classify the exanthem, it is critical that a thorough search (including the mouth, conjunctiva, vagina, rectum and glans penis) be made for enanthems. In allergic reactions the mucous membranes are frequently involved. Koplick spots, diagnostic of rubeola, are blue-grey spots on red—a grain of sand on the buccal mucosa opposite the end molar. A strawberry tongue suggests Kawasaki disease, toxic shock syndrome, or scarlet cell. Petechiae of the palate are common in scarlet fever, and with infectious mononucleosis petechiae of the hard and soft palate are common. Oral ulcers occur in a variety of immunologic diseases presenting with exanthems and also with coxsackievirus A16.

PATHOGENS OR INFECTIOUS CONDITIONS STRONGLY ASSOCIATED WITH RASH

Having outlined the general categories by which skin lesions due to infectious agents should be divided, it is worth describing in more detail the spectrum of skin lesions associated with discrete pathogens or pathogenic processes.

Septicemia

Kingston and Mackey[17] have classified the skin lesions associated with septicemia into five pathogenic processes (major infectious etiologies): *(1)* disseminated intravascular coagulation (DIC) and coagulopathy (*Neisseria meningitidis, Streptococcus* spp., enteric gram-negative bacilli); *(2)* direct vascular invasion and occlusion by bacteria and fungi (*N. meningitidis, P. aeruginosa, Candida* spp., *Aspergillus* spp., *Rickettsia* spp.); *(3)* immune vasculitis and immune complex formation (*N. meningitidis, Neisseria gonorrhoeae, Salmonella typhi*); *(4)* emboli from endocarditis (*S. aureus, Streptococcus* spp.); and *(5)* vascular effects of toxins (staphylococcal scalded skin syndrome, toxic shock syndrome, scarlet fever). A variety of bacteria may spread to the skin, generally producing discrete lesions from which bacteria can be isolated or recognized on biopsy.

Cutaneous manifestations of DIC include symmetric peripheral gangrene, purpura fulminans, localized gangrene, acrocyanosis, purpura, ecchymosis, bleeding from wound and venipuncture sites, and subcutaneous hematoma.[17,61] Symmetric peripheral gangrene is defined as ischemic necrosis simultaneously involving the distal portions of two or more extremities without proximal arterial obstruction.[62] Etiologies include cardiogenic shock and other low flow states, disorders that induce severe vasospasm such as ergot poisoning and Raynaud syndrome, disorders that lead to obstruction of small blood vessels such as cold agglutinins or primary polycythemia, snake bites, and infectious agents.[62–64] *Neisseria meningitidis* is the organism most commonly responsible for symmetric peripheral gangrene, but may occur due to *Strep. pneumoniae, Staph. aureus, Streptococcus* spp., *Escherichia coli, Klebsiella* spp., *Proteus* spp., *Aeromonas hydrophila, Aspergillus,* and other gram-negative organisms.[61,63,65] Symmetric peripheral gangrene is preceded by bleeding into the skin, ecchymosis, purpura, and arocyanosis (a grayish cyanosis that does not blanch on pressure and occurs on the lips, legs, nose, ear lobes, and genitalia). Subsequently the ecchymotic lesions become confluent, blister, necrose, and develop into eschars.[17] The histology reveals a Shwartzman-like reaction in the skin with diffuse and extensive hemorrhages, perivascular cuffing, and intravascular thrombosis. Bacteria are usually absent from smears of the lesions. Shock rather than DIC appears to be the major factor in the pathogenesis of symmetric peripheral gangrene.

The term *purpura fulminans* has been used synonymously with *symmetric peripheral gangrene* and in a more restricted sense to describe symmetric bleeding into the skin and subsequent necrosis after a benign infection.[17] This latter syndrome, although most commonly reported in children, may involve adults[66] and usually follows by several days pharyngitis or a viral exanthem.[63,67,68] Common preceding illnesses include scarlet fever, streptococcal pharyngitis, staphylococcal bacteremia, varicella, and measles. Histologically, it resembles an Arthus reaction or localized Shwartzman reaction[69] with deposition of antigen–antibody complexes in tissues. The pathogenesis of purpura fulminans appears to be related to an acquired or transient deficiency of protein C and/or protein S, since identical lesions have been seen in infants with homozygous protein C deficiency and in patients with heterozygous deficiency of protein C or S during the initial phase of coumadin therapy.[66]

Infections Due to Neisseria Species

Neisseria Meningitidis. Purpuric skin lesions have been noted in 80–90 percent of patients with fulminant meningococcemia.[70,71] The lesions characteristically are petechial but may blanch early in the course of infection and resemble a viral exanthem. The petechiae are irregular, small, and often raised with pale centers. Lesions most commonly occur on the extremities and trunk but may also be found on the head, palms, soles, and mucous membranes. Symmetric peripheral gangrene may occur, often in association with DIC. Histology reveals diffuse endothelial damage, fibrin thrombi, necrosis of the vessel walls, and perivascular hemorrhage in the involved skin.[71,72] Aspirates of the involved areas frequently will reveal organisms when Gram stained.[70,73] Meningococcal endotoxin is a potent producer of the dermal Shwartzman reaction in mice and probably plays an important role in the frequency of hemorrhagic cutaneous manifestations in meningococcal infections.[74] Skin lesions and bacteremia are rarely seen in patients with meningococcal pneumonia.[75]

Chronic meningococcemia is a rare disease. The classic clinical constellation of symptoms includes intermittent or sustained fevers; recurring maculopapular, nodular, or petechial eruptions; and migratory arthritis or arthralgias with little systemic toxicity.[76,77] Skin lesions were noted to occur in 93 percent of 148 patients.[77] A variety of skin lesions may occur in chronic meningococcemia. The most frequently reported lesions are pale to pink-colored macular and papular lesions, which occur in over 40 percent of cases. Nodular lesions, mostly on the lower extremities, may occur. These lesions may be distinguished from those of erythema nodosum by their tendency to be less painful and lack the bluish border characteristic of erythema nodosum. Petechiae of variable size may occur with vesicular or pustular centers. Small, irregularly round, subcutaneous hemorrhages with a bluish gray center containing pus cells are a distinctive lesion of this syndrome. Ecchymotic areas or hemorrhagic tender nodules that are located deep in the dermis may also occur. Lesions associated with chronic meningococcemia tend to appear in showers in association with the onset of fever. In contrast to the lesions associated with fulminant meningococcemia, the lesions associated with chronic meningococcemia rarely include organisms demonstrable by Gram-stained smear or biopsy.[78]

Neisseria Gonorrhoeae. Disseminated gonococcal infection (DGI) follows untreated mucosal infection in about 0.5–3 percent of patients.[79-82] Skin lesions are the most common manifestation of DGI and occur in 50–70 percent of patients.[83] The eruption typically appears during the first day of symptoms and may recur with each bout of fever.[84] The skin lesions associated with DGI begin as tiny red papules or petechiae 1–5 mm in diameter, many of which evolve rapidly through vesicular or pustular stages to develop a gray necrotic center, often on a hemorrhagic base.[84,85] Papules, bullae, pustules, and hemorrhagic lesions may all be present simultaneously. The lesions tend to be scanty but widely distributed. The distal portions of the extremities are most commonly involved, with sparing of the scalp, face, trunk, and oral mucous membranes. Histologic examination will reveal local vasculitis, fibrin deposition, necrosis, and neutrophil infiltration.[86] Gram-stained smears of material from skin lesions infrequently reveal organisms, although most smears are positive for gonococci when examined by immunofluorescence techniques. Circulating immune complexes may play a role in the pathogenesis of DGI-associated skin lesions.[87]

Pseudomonas Infection

Skin lesions have been reported to accompany *P. aeruginosa* sepsis in 13–39 percent of patients.[88-90] The dermatologic manifestations of *P. aeruginosa* sepsis include erythema gangrenosum,[89-98] subcutaneous nodules,[89,99-103] vesicular lesions,[89] gangrenous cellulitis, small papules resembling the rose spots of typhoid fever,[104] and grouped petechiae.[97] Ecthyma gangren-

osum, the most characteristic skin lesion caused by *P. aeruginosa,* has generally been reported to occur in 1.3–2.8 percent of septic patients,[88,105,106] but one report noted ecthyma gangrenosum in 28 percent of patients with *Pseudomonas* bacteremia.[90]

Ecthyma gangrenosum lesions begin as a painless round erythematous macule with or without an adherent vesicle that soon becomes indurated and progresses to a hemorrhagic bluish bulla. Later the lesion sloughs to form a gangrenous ulcer with a gray-black eschar and a surrounding erythematous halo. The process evolves rapidly over a period of 12–24 hours. Lesions may be discrete or multiple and are usually found in the groin, axilla, or perianal areas but may occur anywhere on the body. Although most commonly associated with *P. aeruginosa* sepsis, ecthyma gangrenosum has also been reported in sepsis with other pseudomonal species,[107] *A. hydrophila,*[108,109] *Candida* spp.,[110] *Serratia marcescens,*[92] *Staph. aureus,*[92] *Aspergillus* spp.,[92] and *Mucor* spp.[92] It may also result from vasculitis or malignant infiltration.[111] Rarely ecthyma gangrenosum due to *P. aeruginosa* may occur in the absence of sepsis.[98,112,113]

Histologically ecthyma gangrenosum is characterized by three features: bacterial invasion of the media and adventitia of vein walls deep in the dermis, sparing of the intima and lumen, and minimal inflammation.[94,96,108,111] Bacterial invasion results in marked fibrin exudation and frank hemorrhage, followed by ballooning of the upper dermis with resulting bullous formation. Finally, necrosis of the exudated dermis occurs. Bacteria are readily visible in biopsy samples and can be demonstrated in Gram-stained material scraped from the base of the lesion.[93]

Subcutaneous nodules may result from *P. aeruginosa* bacteremia. Characteristically, the nodules are erythematous and warm and may be either fluctuant or nonfluctuant and either tender or nontender. Despite prolonged antibiotic therapy, these lesions may contain viable bacteria weeks after the blood has been cleared of infection. The absence of fluctuance may be due to either the lack of pus in neutropenic patients and/or the deep location of the abscess. Although therapy may require incision and drainage,[101,102] prolonged therapy with drainage may result in a cure.[99,103]

Subacute Bacterial Endocarditis

Skin lesions have been reported to accompany bacterial endocarditis in 15–50 percent of cases in recent series.[114-117] Skin lesions include Osler nodes, Janeway lesions, and petechiae. The prevalence of embolic and hypersensitivity lesions in skin and mucous membranes (50 percent) in heroin-associated infective endocarditis is similar to that described in patients with nonheroin infective endocarditis.[118]

Osler nodes occur in about 5–15 percent of patients with subacute bacterial endocarditis. They are tender, indurated, erythematous nodules with a pale center about 1.0–1.5 mm in diameter.[119,120] Osler nodes most commonly occur on the pads of the fingers or toes but may occur on the thenar and hypothenar eminences and over the arms. Pain may be elicited by palpating the tips of the digits. They tend to occur in crops, are rarely numerous, and tend to be transient. The lesions usually resolve without necrosis or suppuration 1–3 days after antibiotic therapy. Histologically, Osler nodes show microabscesses with microemboli in adjacent arterioles. Osler nodes are most commonly associated with subacute bacterial endocarditis due to infection with streptococci but may occur in endocarditis due to fungi and gram-negative bacilli[120] or in systemic lupus erythematosus, typhoid, and gonococcemia.[17] Osler nodes probably represent microemboli leading to vascular occlusion with localized vasculitis.[121]

Janeway lesions consist of small erythematous macules or less commonly small nodular hemorrhages in the palms and soles. Although they may be seen in subacute bacterial endocarditis, they are more common in acute endocarditis, especially that due to *Staph. aureus*. Unlike Osler nodes, they are painless. Histologically they show microabscesses with neutrophil infiltration of capillaries.

Petechiae are the most common skin and mucous membrane lesions in endocarditis and occur in about 50 percent of patients. The lesions are small, flat, reddish brown lesions that do not blanch on pressure. Mucous membrane involvement is common. Petechiae frequently occur in small crops. Lesions usually are transient.

Infections Due to Staphylococcus Aureus

Staphylococcus aureus is responsible for a variety of infectious syndromes that may produce local or diffuse skin lesions.[122-128] Skin lesions arise from *(1)* production of toxins (staphylococcal scalded skin syndrome, toxic shock syndrome),[129,130] *(2)* shock, and *(3)* vascular invasion often in association with endocarditis.

Staphylococcal Scalded Skin Syndrome. *Staphylococcus aureus* belonging to phage group II (types 3A, 3B, 3C, 55, 71) may produce exfoliative toxins. These toxins are capable of causing a clinical spectrum of disease that includes bullous impetigo, a generalized scarlatiniform eruption without exfoliation, and exfoliative disease (staphylococcal scalded skin syndrome [SSSS]).[124,126,131-134] Bullous impetigo, the most limited variant that results from toxin-producing *Staph. aureus,* is characterized by discrete, flaccid bullae containing clear or cloudy yellow fluid. Lesions are frequently localized to the umbilicus or axillae, and the surrounding skin is normal or mildly erythematous. The bullae rapidly rupture and leave raw, denuded areas that reepithelialize in 5–7 days. Affected infants are afebrile and lack constitutional signs.

SSSS usually occurs in neonates (Ritter's disease) or young children but may occur in older children or rarely in adults. Most cases in adults occur in association with renal impairment or immunosuppression.[135-139] Unlike bullous impetigo, in which the staphylococcal infection is in the skin at the site of the lesion, in SSSS the infection begins abruptly with a diffuse, blanchable erythema in association with marked skin tenderness, fever, and irritability. Light stroking of the ill-defined bullae will cause rupture and separation of the upper portion of the epidermis (Nikolsky sign). Generalized desquamation usually occurs. Unless secondary infection intervenes, the skin heals within 10–14 days. A skin biopsy (or a frozen section for presumptive diagnosis) may be studied to distinguish between SSSS and toxic epidermal necrolysis (TEN). In SSSS the cleavage plane of the early intraepidermal bulla is just beneath the granular cell layer, whereas in TEN the bulla is subepidermal and is seen at the basement membrane zone. Early distinction between these two diseases is important because the therapy for SSSS includes antistaphylococcal antibiotics, whereas in TEN discontinuation of treatment with the offending drug may be lifesaving.

A mild form of SSSS is characterized by a generalized scarletiniform eruption with exfoliation (staphylococcal scarlet fever). The skin has a sandpaper roughness, and Pastia's lines are present, but the strawberry tongue and palatal enanthem of streptococcal scarlet fever are not present.

Toxic Shock Syndrome. Toxic shock syndrome (TSS) is an acute febrile illness characterized by a generalized erythematous eruption that is due to in vivo production of a toxin at the site of localized, often relatively asymptomatic or unnoticed infection caused by *Staph. aureus* capable of toxin production.[124] The multisystem effects observed in TSS patients are induced by TSS toxin-1, which has been shown to be identical[140] to enterotoxin F[141] and exotoxin C.[142] TSS toxin 1 (TSST-1) has been purified, cloned, and sequenced. It has been demonstrated to be a potent, nonspecific inducer of interleukin (IL)-1 and tumor necrosis factor; to be a potent, nonspecific T-cell mitogen; and to induce the suppression of a number of immune responses. Recent work has established that TSST-1 acts as a superantigen that stimulates T cells to proliferate nonspecifically through interaction with class II major histocompatibility complex products on antigen-presenting cells and then with variable regions on the β-chain of the T-cell receptor complex.[143]

Other superantigens include staphylococcal enterotoxins, designated serotypes A, B, C_n, D, E, and G, and the group A streptococcal pyrogenic exotoxins (SPE) serotypes A–C, which are associated with streptococcal toxic shock-like syndrome (see below).[143] All of these toxins share the ability to cause symptoms via release of immune cytokines leading to high fever and enhanced host susceptibility to lethal endotoxin shock.[143]

TSST-1–producing coagulase-negative staphylococci have also been described.[144] In the early 1980s most cases of TSS occurred in menstruating females, often in association with tampon use.[145,146] Currently about 300 cases of TSS are reported each year of which only half are associated with menstruation.[147] Nonmenstrual TSS has been associated with a variety of infections, including postoperative wounds, cutaneous infections, burn wounds, postpartum complications, and *Staph. aureus* respiratory infections, often after viral influenza.[148-154]

TSS may vary from a relatively mild disease, often misdiagnosed as a viral syndrome, to a severe life-threatening illness. The most common symptoms include a temperature greater than 40°C, hypotension, and diffuse erythroderma with desquamation 1–2 weeks after the onset of illness. Additional early features include conjunctival, oropharyngeal, and/or vaginal hyperemia; vomiting and diarrhea; and myalgias.[155-158] Most patients have abnormalities in three or more organ systems: *(1)* muscular—rhabdomyolysis; *(2)* central nervous system—toxic encephalopathy; *(3)* renal—azotemia; *(4)* liver—abnormal transaminases; and *(5)* hematologic—thrombocytopenia. The rash of TSS is almost always present within the first 24 hours of illness. Desquamation occurs after 7–10 days, most prominently on the hands and feet. Histologically, the epidermis exhibits cleavage in the basilar layers, which differentiates TSS from SSSS and from viral and drug eruptions.[159]

Staphylococcus aureus septicemia may be associated with erythematous, petechial, or pustular lesions.[160] In addition, lesions associated with endocarditis such as Osler nodes, Janeway lesions, and splinter hemorrhages may occur. Such skin lesions have been reported in 10–64 percent of patients with staphylococcal septicemia.[161] Purpuric lesions may at times be so extensive as to mimic meningococcemia or Rocky Mountain spotted fever.[162-165] Gram-stained smears of the material in these lesions will usually reveal gram-positive cocci.

Streptococcal Infections

Group A streptococcal infections are associated with several cutaneous presentations, including impetigo (pyoderma), scarlet fever, erysipelas, cellulitis, lymphangitis, gangrene, and perianal cellulitis.[166] These manifestations of streptococcal infection occur via three distinct mechanisms[167]: *(1)* direct infection of the skin, *(2)* immunologically mediated disease, and *(3)* toxin-mediated disease. Rheumatic fever affects up to 3 percent of people with untreated group A β-hemolytic streptococcal infections of the nasopharynx. Cutaneous manifestations include erythema marginatum (10–20 percent), subcutaneous nodules (up to 30 percent), and erythema papulatum (rare). Case reports and informal surveys suggest that the incidence of acute rheumatic fever is rising. A high proportion of strain isolated in recent outbreaks have a highly mucoid appearance of the streptococcal colonies. The resurgence of acute rheumatic fever in the United States has been accompanied by an increase in reports of severe and at times life-threatening group A streptococcus infections. The term *toxic strep syndrome* has been suggested to describe many of these patients with hypotension and multiorgan failure similar to TSS. Many, but not all, patients will have a rash at the time of presentation.[168-170] Skin manifestations include generalized erythroderma with desquamation and localized cellulitis with vesiculation or bullae.[168] Unlike TSS, a focus of pyogenic inflammation is usually present, and a large proportion of the patients have documented bacteremia.[166]

Rickettsial Infections

Rickettsiae are obligate intracellular parasites whose primary target in humans appears to be the endothelial cell.[171] After parasitization of the endothelial cell, necrosis of the media and intima results in thrombosis, microinfarcts, and extravasation of blood. The end result is increased vascular permeability and vasculitis.

Rash is a hallmark of Rocky Mountain spotted fever,[172-176] the most common rickettsial disease in the United States. Initially, the patient develops a maculopapular rash that may not be appreciated by the patient or the physician. Subsequently, the rash becomes more definite and petechial. Characteristically, the rash appears between the second and sixth days of illness (average, 4 days). However, the rash may be absent in 5–17 percent of patients, and in up to 50 percent it may not appear within the first 3 days of illness.[172,173,175,177,178] Most commonly, the rash begins on the extremities, often around the wrists and ankles, and spreads centripetally to the trunk, with relative sparing of the face. However, the rash may begin on the trunk (10 percent) or have a diffuse onset (10 percent). Characteristically, the rash involves the palms and/or soles in the later stages of infection. Over time, the rash, which begins as maculopapular lesions, may progress to become petechial or ecchymotic. Rarely, gangrene and skin necrosis may occur that require amputation.[179] The rash may occasionally be urticarial or pruritic. Since the mortality of infection may be decreased from 15 to 3 percent[173] with appropriate therapy, antibiotics should never be delayed by the absence of rash. Symptoms similar to Rocky Mountain spotted fever may occur with erlichiosis. Rash is usually not present, but, when observed, it is described as petechial or macular, occurring on the trunk or extremities.[180] Rashes are often not present until several days after the onset of illness or initial presentation and may be very limited in distribution or short-lived.

Capnocytophaga canimorsus

Capnocytophaga canimorsus (dysgonic fermentor-2, DF-2) is a fastidious, gram-negative, opportunistic pathogen that can cause serious multiorgan disease in humans. The organism is found worldwide. Studies suggest that it is part of the normal gingival flora of cats and dogs.

Over 50 cases have been described in recent reviews.[181-186] Although infected patients have ranged in age from 5 months to 77 years, most infections have been reported in adults over 40 years. Approximately 80 percent of patients reported in the literature have a predisposing condition, most commonly splenectomy. Other predisposing conditions have included Hodgkin's disease, trauma, idiopathic thrombocytopenic purpura, alcohol abuse, steroid therapy, and chronic lung disease.

Infection is strongly associated with dog bites. More than 50 percent of patients have reported dog bites prior to clinical infection. Infections has also followed cat bites or scratches,[187] scratches from dogs, and contact with wild animals. An additional 20 percent of patients have reported exposure to dogs without a history of an actual bite or scratch.

The clinical syndrome in humans is characterized by fever, DIC, cellular necrosis in certain organs such as kidneys and adrenal glands, thrombocytopenia, hypotension, and renal failure with oliguria and anuria. Dermatologic lesions occur in about 50 percent of patients and may include petechiae, a macular/papular eruption, eschar formation, or painful erythema. Patients frequently develop a hemorrhagic diathesis with purpuric skin lesions and petechiae that may progress to cutaneous gangrene.

The case fatality rate is approximately 25 percent. Death has not been confined to immunocompromised patients. Infection with *C. canimorsus* should be considered in patients who have a compatible clinical syndrome with a history of a dog bite or animal exposure. Definitive diagnosis requires isolation of the organism from blood or other body fluids or tissues. Empiric therapy should be instituted based on the clinical presentation. In patients who show high-grade bacteremia the organism has been demonstrated in peripheral blood smears. Therefore, all patients suspected of having *C. canimorsus* sepsis, especially splenectomized patients, should have a Gram stain of their buffy coat.

Borrelia burgdorferi

Lyme disease is a tick-borne borreliosis with broad distribution and myriad manifestations.[188] Skin lesions are prominent clinical manifestations of all stages of Lyme disease.[189-193] Approximately 50–75 percent of infected patients will develop the classic lesion of erythema migrans (EM) at the site of the tick bite (Stage 1). The initial lesion is usually homogeneous and may remain so until it heals. More commonly the lesion partly or totally clears centrally, leaving an annular erythema that spreads centrifugally. Erythema migrans may develop anywhere, but the most frequent site is the lower leg. Although the lesion may last from a few days to about 1 year, it usually disappears within a few weeks to months. In about half of the patients, itching, dysesthesia/hyperesthesia, or sensations of heat may develop at the site of erythema. Many patients who developed disseminated infection (stage 2) will exhibit EM-like lesions. The disseminated lesions are usually smaller than the primary lesion and often multiple. These lesions may be ring shaped but are often homogeneous and nonmigrating. In Europe borrelial lymphocytomas have been described during stage 2 illness. Acrodermatis chronica atrophicans (ACA) has been more commonly described in Europe but may occur in the United States and is a manifestation of chronic infection (stage 3). ACA begins with an inflammatory phase with a bluish-red erythema, usually on the lower leg or foot. The course is chronic, with persistence of inflammatory lesions for years and gradual conversion to atrophic skin lesions.

Candidiasis

The incidence and relative frequency of *Candida* as a nosocomial pathogen appear to be increasing.[194-200] Disseminated candidiasis is frequently fatal and is a major cause of death in immunocompromised patients.[201,202] Predisposing factors are malignancy with cytotoxic therapy, neutropenia, antimicrobial therapy, hyperalimentation, severe burn injuries, very-low-weight neonates, intravenous catheters, systemic adrenocortical steroids, and gastrointestinal surgery.[201,202]

Disseminated candidiasis may be accompanied by a characteristic macronodular skin rash in up to 13 percent of patients.[202] The lesions are discrete, firm, nontender, subcutaneous raised erythematous areas or nodules.[203-205] Nodules may have a pale center, and some may become hemorrhagic. Often the lesions are diffuse, but they may be localized to a small area. The face is usually spared. Histologically the middle and lower dermis are involved and show vessels distended by fungal pseudohyphae, platelet aggregates, and fibrin. Scant lymphocytic perivenular infiltrate may be present.

The diagnosis of disseminated candidiasis may be established by biopsy and culture of these lesions. However, the diagnosis may be missed unless multiple sections of the subcutaneous tissue are carefully examined.

Chronic mucocutaneous candidiasis results from impaired function of the T-lymphocyte system and may be a manifestation of a variety of cutaneous syndromes.[206]

Many other fungi produce nodular lesions identical to *Can-*

dida and must be considered in the immunocompromised host. In patients with the acquired immunodeficiency syndrome (AIDS), cryptococci may cause umbilicated nodules that look like molluscum contagiosum.

Immunocompromised Patients

The diagnosis of skin lesions in the immunocompromised patient is complex because of the wide range of potential microbial pathogens that may occur in patients with abnormal immune responses.[207–209] In addition in immunocompromised persons common infections may present with unusual manifestations.[210] Cutaneous lesions of suspected infectious etiology should undergo biopsy. Biopsy samples should be processed by using the most rapid and sensitive methods for detecting microbes both histologically and immunologically, and appropriate stains and cultures should be obtained to optimize the chance for identifying the pathogen. Biopsy samples should be divided into two portions: the first should be sent to histology for evaluation by routine and special stains to detect fungi, mycobacteria, and bacteria. The second portion should be sent to microbiology and cultured for aerobic and anaerobic bacteria, mycobacteria, and fungi. Direct fungal touch preparations and Gram, acid-fast, and modified acid-fast stains should be performed. Viral culture should be considered when herpesviruses are considered.

HIV infection commonly results in dermatologic disorders in both adults[211–226] and children.[227–232] Clinically the skin lesions associated with HIV infection may be classified by morphologic appearance, stage of HIV infection, pathophysiology (infectious, neoplastic, vascular, miscellaneous), and, for infectious diseases, by etiologic agent.

Skin disorders are clearly related to the stage of HIV infection. Initial infection with HIV may result in development of the acute retroviral syndrome characterized by transient fever, myalgias, headache, urticaria, aseptic meningitis, and rash.[233–237] The rash is maculopapular and usually confined to the trunk.

The Centers for Disease Control and Prevention (CDC) uses several dermatologic disorders in its definition of symptomatic but not AIDS category of HIV infection.[238] These conditions may provide an early clue to unsuspected HIV infection and include bacillary angiomatosis (see below); oropharyngeal candidiasis in a patient who has not received recent antibiotics, immunosuppressive medication, or chemotherapy; vulvovaginal candidiasis that is persistent, frequent, or poorly responsive to therapy; oral hairy leukoplakia; herpes zoster involving at least two distinct episodes or more than one dermatome; and idiopathic thrombocytopenic purpura. HIV infection should also be considered in persons with herpes simplex infection that is unusually prolonged or poorly responsive to acyclovir.

Several dermatologic conditions have been incorporated into the CDC's diagnostic criteria of AIDS. These include disseminated or extrapulmonary coccidioidomycosis, herpes simplex virus infection characterized by a mucocutaneous ulcer that persists longer than 1 month, extrapulmonary or disseminated histoplasmosis, Kaposi sarcoma, and extrapulmonary or disseminated *Mycobacterium avium*-intracellulare or *Mycobacterium kansasii* infection.[238]

As with other immunocompromised patients, persons with AIDS develop infections with "opportunistic" pathogens that rarely if ever cause infection in immunocompetent individuals. Furthermore, common pathogens may present with clinical manifestations that are unusual, more severe, more prolonged, or poorly responsive to therapy. Skin lesions often yield multiple pathogens.[239–241]

Several common pathogens may present with unusual manifestations. Severe, chronic herpes simplex lesions have been reported.[237] These ulcers are frequently perianal in homosexual men but may also involve the lips and perioral area. Severe herpetic whitlow may be confused with osteomyelitis or other

chronic ulcerative conditions. Herpes zoster occurs with a higher than expected frequency in HIV-infected persons.[213] Chronic varicella-zoster infection has been reported[242–245] that may lead to severe scarring.[215] Molluscum contagiosum may involve both the genital area and face. The number and size of the lesions and their response to therapy tend to correlate with the degree of immunosuppression.[216]

Staphylococcus aureus is the most common cutaneous bacterial pathogen in HIV-infected persons. Infection usually presents as folliculitis of the face, trunk, or groin. Cutaneous staphylococcal infections may progress to botryomycosis, a rare condition characterized by aggregates of bacteria in skin. Syphilis is common in HIV-infected persons, and any stage of syphilis may occur. Primary infection is manifested by a chancre. Secondary syphilis may manifest as a generalized maculopapular eruption with or without scaling; palmoplantar vesicles, papules, or macules; hypopigmented axillary macules; and oral lesions.[223] Unusual patterns of syphilis have been reported in the HIV-infected person, including coexistent lesions of secondary syphilis and tertiary gummas and noduloulcerative lesions with lymphadenopathy in precocious tertiary syphilis. In patients with AIDS, typical serologic tests (i.e., VDRL and fluorescent treponemal antibody absorption test [FTA-ABS]) for syphilis may be unreliable, and a biopsy of the skin with silver staining to show the spirochetes may be required for diagnosis.[246] Scabies may be widespread and manifest as an erythematous papulosquamous eruption in which numerous mites can easily be found in the skin scrapping. Less commonly, classic Norwegian scabies with marked hyperkeratosis may occur.

Unusual pathogens that involve the skin include cytomegalovirus[238,247] nontuberculous mycobacteria (*M. avium* complex, *M. haemophilium, M. fortuitum*), disseminated candidiasis, *Acanthamoeba castellani, Pneumocystis carinii,* and *Toxoplasma gondii*). Dissemination to the skin may occur with histoplasmosis, cryptococcosis, and coccidioidomycosis.[248] Cutaneous histoplasmosis may present as slightly pinkish to red papules with little or no induration or inflammation, a cellulitis-like eruption, and ulcerations and acneiform papules.[215] The most common cutaneous presentation of cutaneous cryptococcus is that of widespread dome-shaped papules with slight central umbilication and waxy translucence.[215] As these may mimic the papules of molluscum contagiosum, biopsy should be considered for diagnosis.[249] Papulopustular lesions may be the presenting sign of disseminated coccidioidomycosis.[250] Gradon and colleagues[222] have classified the unusual skin and soft tissue manifestations of opportunistic infections in AIDS as follows: nodular lesions—*Sporothrix schenckii, M. tuberculosis, Corynebacterium jekeium, Demodex* mites, *Sarcoptes scabiei;* ulcerating lesions—*M. haemophilum,* herpes simplex and cytomegalovirus; scalded skin syndrome—*Staph. aureus;* and pyomyositis—*Staph. aureus,* group C streptococci.

The treatment of infectious disorders of the skin in HIV-infected persons has been reviewed.[217]

Bacillary angiomatosis (BA) is a newly recognized infectious disease of the skin and viscera characterized by angiomatous lesions.[251–257] Skin lesions are the most common clinical finding of BA. Several different skin lesions have been described in BA, including elevated, friable, firm, bright red papules (approximately 67 percent); subcutaneous nodules (approximately 50 percent); and cellulitic plaques (5–10 percent). Lesions may be located anywhere on the body, and patients may have multiple forms of lesions at the same time or sequentially. BA may be clinically and histologically similar to Kaposi sarcoma, and hence biopsy specimens and special stains may be required to confirm the diagnosis. Soft tissue and visceral disease may accompany the cutaneous lesions. Rarely BA may occur in apparently immunologically healthy persons.[258] The agents of BA have been identified by comparison of the 16S ribosomal RNA gene as *Rochalemaea quintana,* the agent of trench fever, and

Rochalemaea henselae, a newly described pathogen.[259–261] *Rochalemaea* spp. are closely related to *Bartonella bacilliformis,* which also causes an angioproliferative host response and is more distantly related to *Afipia felis.*[262] *Rochalemaea quintana* and *R. henslae* have been successfully cultured from the blood or cutaneous lesions of patients with BA.[261,263]

Well-described primary dermatologic disorders not associated with fever but associated with HIV infection include seborrheic dermatitis,[215,223] papular eruptions,[220] ichthyosis,[162] infectious eczemoid dermatitis,[264,265] yellow nail syndrome,[220] vitiligo,[220] telangiectasias of the anterior portion of the chest,[223,263] and alopecia.[215,223] Several patients have developed an eosinophilic pustular rash, responsive to ultraviolet therapy.[223]

Drug reactions are common in patients with AIDS.[220,223] Up to 50 percent of patients treated with trimethoprim-sulfamethoxazole will develop a rash, usually an erythematous, maculopapular rash involving the entire body that is commonly associated with fever. Stevens-Johnson syndrome may develop. Rash may also accompany pentamidine therapy or dapsone-trimethoprim.

REFERENCES

1. Garner JS, Simmons BP. CDC guidelines for isolation precautions in hospitals. Infect Control. 1983;4:245–325.
2. Garner JS, Simmons BP. CDC guidelines for isolation precautions in hospitals. Am J Infect Control. 1983;103–63.
3. Centers for Disease Control and Prevention. Recommendations for prevention of HIV transmission in the health-care setting. MMWR. 1987;36(Suppl 2):3–18.
4. Centers for Disease Control and Prevention. Management of patients with suspected viral hemorrhagic fever. MMWR. 1988;37(S3):1–16.
5. Centers for Disease Control and Prevention. Risks associated with human parvovirus B19 infection. MMWR. 1989;38:8188, 8193–7.
6. Centers for Disease Control and Prevention. Update: Universal precautions for prevention of transmission of human immunodeficiency virus: Hepatitis B virus, and other bloodborne pathogens in health-care settings. MMWR. 1988;37:377–88.
7. Centers for Disease Control and Prevention. Guidelines for prevention of transmission of human immunodeficiency virus and hepatitis B virus to health-care and public-safety workers. MMWR. 1989;38, No. S-6.
8. Kreger BE, Craven DE, McCabe WR. Gram-negative bacteremia. IV. Reevaluation of clinical features and treatment in 612 patients. Am J Med. 1980; 68:344–55.
9. Valman HB. Common rashes. Br Med J. 1981;283:970–1.
10. Fitzpatrick TB, Bernhard JD. The structure of skin lesions and fundamentals of diagnosis. In: Jefferes JD, Scott E, White J, eds. Dermatology in General Medicine. Textbook and Atlas. 3rd ed. New York: McGraw-Hill; 1987; 20–49.
11. Lazarus GS, Goldsmith LA, Tharp MD. Diagnosis of Skin Disease. Philadelphia: FA Davis; 1980.
12. Fitzpatrick TB, Johnson RA. Differential diagnosis of rashes in the acutely ill febrile patient and in life-threatening diseases. In: Jeffers JD, Scott E, White J, eds. Dermatology in General Medicine. Textbook and Atlas. 3rd ed. New York: McGraw-Hill; 1987;21–2.
13. Johnson M-L. Dermatologic problems. In: Samily AH, ed. Textbook of Diagnostic Medicine. Philadelphia: Lea & Febiger; 1987:768–89.
14. Corey L, Kirby P. Rash and fever. In: Braunwald E, Isselbacher KJ, Petersdorf RG, et al, eds. Harrison's Principles of Internal Medicine. 11th ed. New York: McGraw-Hill; 1987:240–4.
15. Oblinger MJ, Sande MA. Fever and Rash. In: Stein JH, ed. Internal Medicine. Boston: Little, Brown; 1983:1173–8.
16. Kline PP. Fever and rash. Emerg Decisions. 1988;April:27–37.
17. Kingston ME, Mackey D. Skin clues in the diagnosis of life-threatening infections. Rev Infect Dis. 1986;8:1–11.
18. Lazar AP. Cutaneous manifestations of systemic diseases. Comprehensive Ther. 1992;18:5–9.
19. Swinyer LJ. Drug eruptions in an emergency department setting. Emerg Med Clin North Am. 1985;3:717–35.
20. Veraldi S, Rizzitelli G, Schianchi-Veraldi R. Occupational cutaneous infections. Clin Dermatol. 1992;10:225–30.
21. Conklin RJ. Common cutaneous disorders in athletes. Sports Med. 1990;9: 100–19.
22. Thomsett L. Zoonotic skin diseases. Practitioner. 1990;234:52–55.
23. Kelsall BL, Pearson RD. Evaluation of skin problems. Infect Dis Clin North Am. 1992;6:441–72.
24. Fitzpatrick TB. Bernhard JD, Soter NA. Correlation of pathophysiology of skin. In: Jeffers JD, Scott E, White J, eds. Dermatology in General Medicine. Textbook and Atlas. 3rd ed. New York: McGraw-Hill; 1987:69–73.
25. Kligman AM, Leyden JJ, McGinley KJ. Bacteriology. J Invest Dermatol. 1976;67:160–8.
26. Leyden JJ, McGinley KJ, Nordstrom KM, et al. Skin microflora. J Invest Dermatol. 1987;88(Supl):65–72.
27. Aly R, Maiback HI, Strauss WG, et al. Survival of microorganisms on human skin. J Invest Dermatol. 1972;58:205–10.
28. Selwyn S, Ellis H. Skin bacteria and skin disinfection reconsidered. Br Med J. 1972;1:136–40.
29. Milyani RM, Selwyn S. Quantitative studies on competitive activities of skin bacteria growing on solid media. J Med Microbiol. 1977;11:379–86.
30. Singh G, Marples RR, Kligman AM. Staphylococcus infections in humans. J Invest Dermatol. 1971;57:149–62.
31. Blank IH. The skin as an organ of protection. In: Fitzpatrick TB, Eisen AZ, Wolff K, et al, eds. Dermatology in General Medicine. 3rd ed. New York: McGraw-Hill; 1987:337–42.
32. Ray TL, Wuepper KD. Experimental cutaneous candidiasis in rodents. Arch Dermatol. 1978;114:539–43.
33. Sauder DN, Wong D, McKenzie R, et al. The pluripotent keratinocyte: Molecular characterization of epidermal cytokines (Abstract). Clin Res. 1988; 36:692.
34. Grabbe J, Rosenback T, Czarnetzki BM. Production of LTB4-like chemotactic arachidonate metabolites from human keratinocytes. J Invest Dermatol. 1985;85:527–30.
35. Siraganian RP. Mast cells and basophils. In: Gallin JI, Goldstein IM, Snyderman R, eds. Inflammation, Basic Principles and Clinical Correlates. New York: Raven Press; 1988:513–42.
36. Streilein JW. Circuits and signals of the skin-associated lymphoid tissues (SALT). J Invest Dermatol. 1985;85(Suppl):10–13.
37. Morhenn VB, Nickoloff BJ, Mansbridge JN. Induction of the synthesis of triton-soluble proteins in human keratinocytes by gamma interferon. J Invest Dermatol. 1985;85(Suppl):27–9.
38. Valman HB. Infectious diseases. Br Med J. 1981;283:1038–9.
39. Leach CT, Sumaya CV, Brown NA. Human herpesvirus-6: Clinical implications of a recently discovered, ubiquitous agent. J Pediatr. 1992;121:173–81.
40. Anderson LJ. Human parvoviruses. J Infect Dis. 1990;161:603–8.
41. Thurn J. Human parvovirus B19: Historical and clinical review. Rev Infect Dis. 1988;10:1005–11.
42. Kurtzman GJ, Ozawa K, Cohen B, et al. Chronic bone marrow failure due to persistent B19 parvovirus infection. N Engl J Med. 1987;317:287–94.
43. Frickhofen N, Abkowitz JL, Safford M, et al. Persistent B19 parvovirus infection in patients infected with human immunodeficiency virus type 1 (HIV-1): A treatable cause of anemia in AIDS. Ann Intern Med. 1990;113: 926–33.
44. Faden H, Gary GW, Anderson LJ. Chronic parvovirus infection in a presumably immunologically healthy women. Clin Infect Dis. 1992;15:595–7.
45. Anderson MJ, Higgins PG, Davis LR, et al. Experimental parvoviral infection in humans. J Infect Dis. 1985;152:257–64.
46. Hook EW, Marra CM. Acquired syphilis in adults. N Engl J Med. 1992;326: 1060–9.
47. Centers for Disease Control and Prevention. Summary of notifiable diseases, United States, 1990. MMWR. 1990;39(53):1–61.
48. Street ML, Umbert-Millet IJ, Roberts GD, et al. Nontuberculous mycobacterial infections of the skin. J Am Acad Dermatol. 1991;24:208–15.
49. Arbesfeld DM, Thomas I. Cutaneous herpes simplex virus infections. Am Fam Physician. 1991;43:1655–64.
50. Williams R. Pustular skin disease. Practitioner. 1991;235:332–9.
51. Koenig KL. *Vibrio vulnificus:* Hazard on the half shell. West J Med. 1991; 155:400–3.
52. Esterly NB. Vesicopustular eruptions in the neonate. Australas J Dermatol. 1991;32:1–12.
53. Baccarani M, Fiacchini M, Galieni P, et al. Meningitis and septicaemia in adults splenectomized for Hodgkin's disease. Scand J Haematol. 1986;36: 492–8.
54. Scully RE, Mark EJ, McNeely BU, eds. Case records of the Massachusetts General Hospital. Case 29-1986. N Engl J Med. 1986;315:241–9.
55. Scully RE, Mark EJ, McNelly BU, eds. Case records of the Massachusetts General Hospital. Case 20-1983. N Engl J Med. 1983;308:1212–8.
56. O'Neal BJ, McDonald JC. The risk of sepsis in the asplenic adult. Ann Surg. 1981;194:775–8.
57. Sekikawa T, Shatney CH. Septic sequelae after splenectomy for trauma in adults. Am J Surg. 1983;145:667–73.
58. Zarrabi MH, Rosner F. Serious infections in adults following splenectomy for trauma. Arch Intern Med. 1984;144:1421–4.
59. Green JB, Shackford SR, Sise MJ, et al. Late septic complications in adults following splenectomy for trauma: A prospective analysis in 144 patients. J Trauma. 1986;26:999–1004.
60. Evans D. Postsplenectomy sepsis 10 years or more after operation. J Clin Pathol. 1985;38:309–11.
61. Robboy SJ, Mihm MC, Colman Rw, et al. The skin in disseminated intravascular coagulation. Prospective analysis of thirty-six cases. Br J Dermatol. 1973;88:221–9.
62. Goodwin JN, Berne TV. Symmetrical peripheral gangrene. Arch Surg. 1974; 108:780–4.
63. Chu DZJ, Blaisdell FW. Purpura fulminans. Am J Surg. 1982;143:356–62.
64. McGouran RCM, Emmerson GA. Symmetrical peripheral gangrene. Br Heart J. 1977;39:569–72.
65. Thisyakorn U, Ningsanond V. Purpura fulminans produced by *Aeromonas hydrophila:* A case report. Southeast Asian J Trop Med. 1985;16:532–3.
66. Chasan PE, Hansbrough JF, Cooper ML. Management of cutaneous mani-

festations of extensive purpura fulminans in a burn unit. J Burn Care Rehabil. 1992;13:410–3.

67. Dudgeon DL, Kellogg DR, Gilchrist GS, et al. Purpura fulminans. Arch Surg. 1971;103:351–8.

68. Hjort PF, Rapaport SI, Jorgensen L. Purpura fulminans. Report of a case successfully treated with heparin and hydrocortisone. Review of 50 cases from the literature. Scand J Haematol. 1964;1:169–92.

69. Hjort PF, Rapaport SI. The Shwartzman reaction: Pathogenetic mechanisms and clinical manifestations. Annu Rev Med. 1965;16:135–69.

70. Hill WR, Kinney TD. The cutaneous lesions in meningococcemia: A clinical and pathologic study JAMA. 1947;134:513–8.

71. DeVoe IW. The meningococcus and mechanisms of pathogenicity. Microbiol Rev. 1982;46:162–90.

72. Sotto MN, Langer B, Hoshimo-Shimizu S, et al. Pathogenesis of cutaneous lesions in acute meningococcemia in humans: Light, immunofluorescent, and electron microscopic studies of skin biopsy specimens. J Infect Dis. 1976; 133:506–14.

73. Bernhard WG, Jordan AC. Purpuric lesions in meningococcic infections. 1944;29:273–81.

74. Davis CE, Arnold K. Role of meningococcal endotoxin in meningococcal purpura. J Exp Med. 1974;140:159–71.

75. Koppes GM, Ellenbogen C, Gebhart RJ. Group Y meningococcal disease in United States Air Force recruits. Am J Med. 1977;62:661–6.

76. Leibel RL, Fangman JJ. Chronic meningococcemia in childhood. Am J Dis Child. 1974;127:94–8.

77. Benoit FL. Chronic meningococcemia. Am J Med. 1963;35:103–12.

78. Ognibene AJ, Dito WR. Chronic meningococcemia. Arch Intern Med. 1964; 114:29–32.

79. Barr J, Danielsson D. Septic gonococcal dermatitis. Br Med J. 1971;1:482–5.

80. Holmes KK, Weisner PJ, Pederson AHB, et al. The gonococcal arthritis–dermatitis syndrome. Ann Intern Med. 1971;75:470–1.

81. Kerle K, Mascola JR, Miller TA. Disseminated gonococcal infection. Am Fam Physician. 1992;45:209–14.

82. Buntin DM, Rosen T, Lesher JL, et al. Sexually transmitted diseases: Bacterial infections. J Am Acad Dermatol. 1991;25:287–99.

83. Handsfield HH. Disseminated gonococcal infection. Clin Obstet Gynecol. 1975;18:131–42.

84. Abu-Nassar H, Hill N, Fred HL, et al. Cutaneous manifestations of gonococcemia. Arch Intern Med. 1963;112:731–7.

85. Holmes KK, Counts GW, Beaty HN. Disseminated gonococcal infection. Ann Intern Med. 1971;74:979–93.

86. Tronca E, Handsfield HH, Wiesner PJ, et al. Demonstration of *Neisseria gonorrhoeae* with fluorescent antibody in patients with disseminated gonococcal infection. J Infect Dis. 1974;129:583–6.

87. Walker LC, Ahlin TD, Tung KSK, et al. Circulating immune complexes in disseminated gonorrheal disease. Ann Intern Med. 1978;89:28–33.

88. Flick MR, Cluff LE. *Pseudomonas* bacteremia. Am J Med. 1976;60:501–8.

89. Forkner CE, Frei E, Edgcomb JH, et al. *Pseudomonas* septicemia. Am J Med. 1958;25:877–89.

90. Whitecar JP, Luna M, Bodey GP. *Pseudomonas* bacteremia in patients with malignant diseases. Am J Med Sci. 1970;260:216–23.

91. Anderson MG. *Pseudomonas* septicaemia and ecthyma gangrenosum. S Afr Med J. 1979;55:504–9.

92. Bodey GP, Bolivar R, Fainstein V, et al. Infections caused by *Pseudomonas aeruginosa*. Rev Infect Dis. 1983;5:279–313.

93. Curtin JA, Petersdorf RG, Bennett IL. *Pseudomonas* bacteremia: Review of ninety-one cases. Ann Intern Med. 1961;54:1077–107.

94. Dorff GJ, Geimer NF, Rosenthal DR, et al. *Pseudomonas* septicemia. Arch Intern Med. 1971;128:591–5.

95. Fast M, Woerner S, Bowman W, et al. Ecthyma gangrenosum. Can Med Assoc J. 1979;120:332–4.

96. Greene SL, Su WPD, Muller SA. Ecthyma gangrenosum: Report of clinical, histopathologic, and bacteriologic aspects of eight cases. J Am Acad Dermatol. 1984;11:781–7.

97. Hall JH, Callaway JL, Tindall JP, et al. *Pseudomonas aeruginosa* in dermatology. Arch Dermatol. 1968;97:312–24.

98. van den Broek PJ, van der Meer JWM, Kunst MW. The pathogenesis of ecthyma gangrenosum. J Infect. 1979;1:263–7.

99. Bagel J, Grossman ME. Subcutaneous nodules in *Pseudomonas* sepsis. Am J Med. 1986;80:528–9.

100. Llistosella E, Revella A, Moreno A, et al. Panniculitis in *Pseudomonas aeruginosa* septicemia. Acta Derm Venereol (Stockh). 1984;64:447–9.

101. Picou KA, Jarratt MT. Persistent subcutaneous abscesses following *Pseudomonas* sepsis. Arch Dermatol. 1979;115:459–60.

102. Reed RK, Larter WE, Sieber OF, et al. Peripheral nodular lesions in *Pseudomonas* sepsis: The importance of incisions and drainage. J Pediatr. 1976; 88:977–9.

103. Schlossberg D. Multiple erythematous nodules as a manifestation of *Pseudomonas aeruginosa* septicemia. Arch Dermatol. 1980;116:446–7.

104. Stanley MM. Bacillus pyocyaneus infections. Am J Med. 1947;9:253–367.

105. Baltch AL, Griffin PE. *Pseudomonas aeruginosa* bacteremia: A clinical study of 75 patients. Am J Med Sci. 1977;274:119–29.

106. Bodey GP, Jadeja L, Elting L. *Pseudomonas* bacteremia. Arch Intern Med. 1985;145:1621–9.

107. Mandell IN, Feiner HD, Price NM, et al. *Pseudomonas cepacia* endocarditis and ecthyma gangrenosum. Arch Dermatol. 1977;113:199–202.

108. Ketover BP, Young LS, Armstrong D. Septicemia due to *Aeromonas hydrophila:* Clinical and immunologic aspects. J Infect Dis. 1973;127:284–90.

109. Shackelford PG, Ratzan SA, Shearer WT. Ecthyma gangrenosum produced by *Aeromonas hydrophilia*. J Pediatr. 1973;83:100–1.

110. Fine JD, Miller JA, Harrist TJ, et al. Cutaneous lesions in disseminated candidiasis mimicking ecthyma gangrenosum. Am J Med. 1981;70:1133–5.

111. Musher DM. Cutaneous and soft-tissue manifestations of sepsis due to gram-negative enteric bacilli. Rev Infect Dis. 1980;2:854–66.

112. El Baze P, Ortonne J-P. Ecthyma gangrenosum. J Am Acad Dermatol. 1985; 13:299–300.

113. Huminer D, Siegman-Igra Y, Morduchowicz G, et al. Ecthyma gangrenosum without bacteremia. Arch Intern Med. 1987;147:299–310.

114. Von Reyn CF, Levy BS, Arbeit RD, et al. Infective endocarditis: An analysis based on strict case definitions. Ann Intern Med. 1981;94:505–18.

115. Venezio FR, Westenfelder GO, Cook FV, et al. Infective endocarditis in a community hospital. Arch Intern Med. 1982;142:789–92.

116. Terpenning MS, Buggy BP, Kauffman CA. Infective endocarditis: Clinical features in young and elderly patients. Am J Med. 1987;83:626–34.

117. King K, Harkness JL. Infective endocarditis in the 1980s. Part 1. Aetiology and diagnosis. Med J Aust. 1986;144:536–40.

118. Dreyer NP, Fields BN. Heroin-associated endocarditis. Ann Intern Med. 1973;78:699–702.

119. Alpert JS, Krous HF, Dalen JE, et al. Pathogenesis of Osler's nodes. Ann Intern Med. 1976;85:471–3.

120. Yee J, McAllister CK. Osler's nodes and the recognition of infective endocarditis: A lesion of diagnostic importance. South Med J. 1987;80:753–7.

121. Cardullo AC, Silvers DN, Grossman ME. Janeway lesions and Osler's nodes: A review of histopathologic findings. J Am Acad Dermatol. 1990;22:1088–90.

122. Harvey D. Staphylococcal infections. J Antimicrob Chemother. 1979; 5(Suppl. A):21–26.

123. Sheagren JN. *Staphylococcus aureus.* The persistent pathogen (first of two parts). N Engl J Med. 1984;310:1368–73.

124. Sheagren JN. *Staphylococcus aureus.* The persistent pathogen (second of two parts). N Engl J Med. 1984;310:1437–42.

125. Sheagren JN. Staphylococcal infections of the skin and skin structures. Cutis. 1985;361:2–6.

126. Wickboldt LG, Fenske NA. Streptococcal and staphylococcal infections of the skin. Hosp Pract. 1986;21:41–7.

127. Williams RE, MacKie RM. The staphylococci. Dermatol Clin. 1993;11: 201–206.

128. Aly R. The pathogenic staphylococci. Semin Dermatol. 1990;9:292–299.

129. Arbuthnott JP, Coleman DC, de Azavedo JS. Staphylococcal toxins in human diseases. J Appl Bacteriol Symp Suppl 1990;19:101S–7S.

130. Ginsburg CM. Staphylococcal toxin syndromes. Pediatr Infect Dis J. 1991; 10:319–21.

131. Dowsett EG. The staphylococcal scalded skin syndrome. J Hosp Infect. 1984;5:347–54.

132. Elias PM, Fritsch P, Epstein EH. Staphylococcal scalded skin syndrome. Arch Dermatol. 1977;113:207–19.

133. Hebert AA, Esterly NB. Bacterial and candidal cutaneous infections in the neonate. Dermatol Clin. 1986;4:3–21.

134. Melish ME, Glasgggow LA. Staphylococcal scalded skin syndrome: The expanded clinical syndrome. J Pediatr. 1971;78:958–67.

135. Borchers SL, Gomez EC, Isseroff RR. Generalized staphylococcal scalded skin syndrome in anephric boy undergoing hemodialysis. Arch Dermatol. 1984;120:912–8.

136. O'Keefe R, Dagg JH, MacKie RM. The staphylococcal scalded skin syndrome in two elderly immunocompromised patients. Br Med J. 1987;295: 179–80.

137. Richard M, Mathieu-Serra A. Staphylococcal scalded skin syndrome in a homosexual adult. J Am Acad Dermatol. 1986;15:385–9.

138. Beers B, Wilson B. Adult staphylococcal scalded skin syndrome. Int J Dermatol. 1990;29:428–9.

139. Donohue D, Robinson B, Goldbert NS. Staphylococcal scalded skin syndrome in a woman with chronic renal failure exposed to human immunodeficiency virus. Cutis 1991;47:317–8

140. Igarashi H, Fujikawa H, Usami H, et al. Purification and characterization of *Staphylococcus aureus* FRI 1169 and 587 toxic shock syndrome exotoxins. Infect Immun. 1984;44:175–81.

141. Bergdoll MS, Crass BA, Reiser RF, et al. A new *Staphylococcus* enterotoxin, enterotoxin F, associated with toxic-shock syndrome *Staphylococcus aureus* isolates. Lancet. 1981;1:1017–21.

142. Schlievert PM, Shands KN, Dan BB, et al. Identification and characteristics of an exotoxin from *Staphylococcus aureus* associated with toxic-shock syndrome. J Infect Dis. 1981;143:509–16.

143. Schlievert PM. Role of superantigens in human disease. J Infect Dis. 1993; 167:997–1002.

144. Crass BA, Bergdoll MS. Involvement of coagulase-negative staphylococci in toxic shock syndrome. J Clin Microbiol. 1986;23:43–5.

145. Davis JP, Chesney PJ, Wand PJ, et al. Toxic shock syndrome. Epidemiologic features, recurrence, risk factors, and prevention. N Engl J Med. 1980;303: 1429–35.

146. Fisher RF, Goodpasture HC, Peterie JD, et al. Toxic shock syndrome in menstruating women. Ann Intern Med. 1981;94:156–63.

147. Centers for Disease Control and Prevention. Summary of notifiable diseases, United States, 1990. MMWR. 1990;39:1–61.

148. Holt PA, Armstrong AM, Norfolk GA, et al. Toxic-shock syndrome due to staphylococcal infection of a burn. Br J Clin Pract. 1987;41:582–3.
149. Reingold AL, Dan BB, Shands KN, et al. Toxic-shock syndrome not associated with menstruation. Lancet. 1982;1:1–4.
150. Reingold AL, Hargrett NT, Dan BB, et al. Nonmenstrual toxic shock syndrome. A review of 130 caes. Ann Intern Med. 1982;96:871–4.
151. Bates I. Characteristic rash associated with staphylococcal pneumonia. Lancet. 1987;2:1026–7.
152. Center for Disease Control and Prevention. Toxic shock syndrome associated with influenza-Minnesota. MMWR. 1986;35:143–4.
153. Center for Disease Control and Prevention. Toxic shock syndrome following influenza-Oregon; Update on influenza activity—United States. MMWR. 1987;36:64–5.
154. Wilkins EGL, Ney F, Roberts C, et al. Probable toxic shock syndrome with primary staphylococcal pneumonia. J Infect. 1985;11:231–2.
155. Finch R, Whitby M: Toxic shock syndrome. J R Coll Physicians Lond. 1985; 19:219–23.
156. Tofte RW, Williams DN. Clinical and laboratory manifestations of toxic shock syndrome. Ann Intern Med. 1982;96:843–7.
157. Tofte RW, Williams DN. Toxic shock syndrome: Clinical and laboratory features in 15 patients. Ann Intern Med. 1981;94:149–56.
158. Tofte RW, Williams DN. Toxic shock syndrome. Recognition and management of a diverse disease. Postgrad Med. 1983;73:275–88.
159. Todd J, Fishaut M, Kapral F, et al. Toxic-shock syndrome associated with phage–group-1 staphylococci. Lancet. 1978;2:1116–7.
160. Plaut MD. Staphylococcal septicemia and pustular purpura. Arch Dermatol. 1969;99:82–5.
161. Musher DM, McKenzie SO. Infections due to *Staphylococcus aureus*. Medicine (Baltimore). 1977;56:383–409.
162. Aach R, Kissane J, eds. A thirty-eight year old woman with overwhelming sepsis. Am J Med. 1972;53:233–41.
163. Murray HW, Tuazon CU, Sheagren JN. Staphylococcal septicemia and disseminated intravascular coagulation. Arch Intern Med. 1977;137:844–7.
164. Milunski MR, Gallis HA, Fulkerson WJ. *Staphylococcus aureus* septicemia mimicking fulminant Rocky Mountain spotted fever. Am J Med. 1987;83:801–3.
165. Rahal JJ, MacMahon E, Weinstein L. Thrombocytopenia and symmetrical peripheral gangrene associated with staphylococcal and streptococcal bacteremia. Ann Intern Med. 1968;69:35–43.
166. Bisno AL. Group A staphylococcal infections and acute rheumatic fever. N Engl J Med. 1991;325:783–93.
167. Bryan BO, Frieden I. Streptococcal skin disease in children. Semin Dermatol. 1992;11:3–10.
168. Stevens DL, Tanner MH, Winship J, et al. Severe group A streptococcal infections associated with toxic shock-like syndrome and scarlet fever toxin A. N Engl J Med. 1989;321:1–7.
169. Drabick JL, Lennox JL. Group A streptococcal infections and toxic shock-like syndrome (Letter). N Engl J Med. 1989;321:1545.
170. Hess EV, Grant KD. Group A streptococcal infections and toxic shock-like syndrome (Letter). N Engl J Med. 1989;321:1545–6.
171. Walker DH. Rickettsial disease: An update. In: Majno G, Cotran RS, Kaufman N, eds. Current Topics in Inflammation and Infection. Baltimore: Williams & Wilkins; 1982:188–204.
172. Kirk JL, Fine DP, Sexton DJ, Muchmore HG. Rocky Mountain spotted fever: A clinical review based on 48 confirmed cases, 1943–1986. Medicine. 1990;69:35–45.
173. Helmick CG, Bernard KW, D'Angelo LJ. Rocky Mountain spotted fever: Clinical, laboratory, and epidemiological features of 262 cases. J Infect Dis. 1984;150:480–8.
174. Hazard GW, Ganz RN, Nevin RW, et al. Rocky Mountain spotted fever in the Eastern United States. N Engl J Med. 1969;280:57–62.
175. Kaplowitz LG, Fischer JJ, Sparling PF. Rocky Mountain spotted fever: A clinical dilemma. In: Remington JS, Swartz MN, eds. Current Clinical Topics in Infectious Diseases. New York: McGraw-Hill; 1981:89–108.
176. Sexton DJ, Burgdorfer W. Clinical and epidemiologic features of Rocky Mountain spotted fever in Mississippi, 1933–1973. South Med J. 1975;68:1529–35.
177. Cohen JI, Corson AP, Corey GR. Late appearance of skin rash in Rocky Mountain spotted fever. South Med J. 1983;76:1457–8.
178. Ramsey PG, Press OW. Successful treatment of Rocky Mountain "spotless" fever. West J Med. 1984;140:94–6.
179. Kirkland KB, Marcom PK, Sexton DJ, et al. Rocky Mountain spotted fever complicated by gangrene: Report of six cases and review. Clin Infect Dis. 1993;16:629–34.
180. Harkess JR. Ehrlichiosis. Infect Dis Clin North Am. 1991;5:37–52.
181. Hicklin H, Verghese A, Alvarez S. Dysgonic fermenter 2 septicemia. Rev Infect Dis. 1987;9:884–90.
182. Zumla A, Lipscomb G, Corbett M, et al. Dysgonic fermenter-type 2: An emerging zoonosis: Report of two cases and review. Q J Med. 1988;257:741–52.
183. Job L, Horman JT, Grigor JK, Israel E. Dysgonic fermenter-2: A clinico-epidemiologic review. J Emerg Med. 1989;7:185–92.
184. Krol-van Staaten MJ, Landheer JE, de Maat CEM. *Capnocytophaga canimorsus* (formerly DF-2) infections: Review of the literature. Neth J Med. 1990;36:304–9.
185. Kullberg B-J, Westendorp RGJ, van't Wout JW, Meinders AE. Purpura fulminans and symmetrical peripheral gangrene caused by *Capnocytophaga*

canimorsus (formerly DF-2) septicemia—A complication of dog bite. Medicine. 1991;70:287–92.
186. Bilgrama S, Bergstron SK, Peterson DE, et al. *Capnocytophaga* bacteremia in a patient with Hodgkin's disease following bone marrow transplantation: Case report and review. Clin Infect Dis. 1992;14:1045–9.
187. Mahrer S, Raik E. *Capnocytophaga canimorsus* septicemia associated with cat scratch. Pathology. 1992;24:194–6.
188. Buchstein SR, Gardner P. Lyme disease. Infect Dis Clin North Am. 1991; 5:103–16.
189. Trevisan G, Cinco M. Lyme disease. Int J Dermatol. 1990;29:1–8.
190. Thyresson N. Historical notes on skin manifestations of Lyme borreliosis. Scand J Infect Dis. 1991;77:9–13.
191. Hercogova J, Tomankova M, Bartak P. Contributions to the treatment of dermatologic manifestations of Lyme borreliosis. Cutis. 1992;49:409–11.
192. Asbrink E. Cutaneous manifestations of Lyme borreliosis. Scand J Infect Dis. 1991;77(Suppl):44–50.
193. Asbrink E, Hovmark A. Lyme borreliosis: Aspects of tick-borne *Borrelia burgdorferi* infection from a dermatologic viewpoint. Semin Dermatol. 1990; 9:277–91.
194. Centers for Disease Control and Prevention. Nosocomial infection surveillance. MMWR. 1984;35(Suppl):17–29.
195. Drutz DJ, Jarvis WR, de Repentigny L, et al. Severe nosocomial yeast infections. Conservations Infect Control. 1985;6:1–12.
196. Morrison AJ, Freer CV, Searcy MA, et al. Nosocomial bloodstream infections: Secular trends in a statewide surveillance program in Virginia (Abstract 452). In: Proceedings of the 25th Interscience Conference on Antimicrobial Agents nad Chemotherapy. Minneapolis: American Society for Microbiology; 1985.
197. Weber DJ, Rutala WA. Epidemiology of nosocomial fungal infections. In: McGinnis MR, ed. Current Topics in Medical Mycology. v. 2. New York: Springer Publishing; 1988:305–37.
198. Schaberg DR, Culver D. Major trends in the microbial etiology of nosocomial infection. Am J Med. 1991;91(Suppl 3B):72–75.
199. Banerjee SN, Emori TG, Culver DH, et al. Secular trends in nosocomial primary bloodstream infections in the United States, 1980–1989. Am J Med. 1991;91(Suppl 3B):86–89.
200. Weber DJ, Rutala WA, Samsa GP, et al. Relative frequency of nosocomial pathogens at a university hospital during the decade 1980 to 1989. Am J Infect Control. 1992;20:192–7.
201. Bodey GP. Fungal infection and fever of unknown origin in neutropenic patients. Am J Med. 1986;80:112–9.
202. Maksymiuk AW, Thongprasert S, Hopfer R, et al. Systemic candidiasis in cancer patients. Am J Med. 1984;77(Suppl):20–7.
203. Bodey GP. Candidiasis in cancer patients. Am J Med. 1984;77(Suppl):13–9.
204. Balandran L, Rothschild H, Pugh N, et al. A cutaneous manifestation of systemic candidiasis. Ann Intern Med. 1973;78:400–3.
205. Jacobs MI, Magid MS, Jarowski CI. Disseminated candidiasis. Arch Dermatol. 1980;116:1277–9.
206. Kirkpatrick CH. Host factors in defense against funcal infections. Am J Med. 1984;77(Suppl):1–12.
207. Dreizen S, McCredie KB, Bodey GP, et al. Unusual mucocutaneous infections. Postgrad Med. 1986;79:287–94.
208. Wolfson JS, Sober AJ. Dermatologic manifestations of infection in the compromised host. In: Rubin RH, Young LS, eds. Clinical Approach to Infection in the Compromised Host. New York: Plenum; 1988:115–30.
209. Parker C. Skin lesions in transplant patients. Dermatol Clin. 1990;8:313–25.
210. Hoppenjans WB, Bibler MR, Orme RL, Solinger AM. Prolonged cutaneous Herpes zoster in acquired immunodeficiency syndrome. Arch Dermatol. 1990;126:1048–50.
211. Valle S. Dermatologic findings related to human immunodeficiency virus infection in high-risk individuals. J Am Acad Dermatol. 1987;17:951–61.
212. Trianan AF, Shapiro RS, Polk BF, et al. Mucocutaneous findings in acquired immunodeficiency syndrome/AIDS-related complex patients. J Am Acad Dermatol. 1987;16:888–9.
213. Kaslow RA, Phair RP, Freidman HB, et al. Infection with the human immunodeficiency virus: Clinical manifestations and their relationship to immune deficiency. Ann Intern Med. 1987;107:474–80.
214. Matis WL, Triana A, Shapiro R, et al. Dermatologic findings associated with immunodeficiency virus infection. J Am Acad Dermatol. 1987;17:746–51.
215. Cockerell CJ. Cutaneous manifestations of HIV infection other than Kaposi's sarcoma: Clinical and histologic aspects. J Am Acad Dermatol. 1990;22:1260–9.
216. Berger TG, Obuch ML, Goldschmidt RH. Dermatologic manifestations of HIV infection. Am J Fam Physician. 1990;41:1729–1742.
217. Cockerell CJ. Human immunodeficiency virus infection and the skin. Arch Intern Med. 1991;151:1295–303.
218. Berger TG, Greene I. Bacterial, viral, fungal, and parasitic infections in HIV disease and AIDS. Dermatol Clin. 1991;9:465–92.
219. Dover JS, Johnson RA. Cutaneous manifestations of human immunodeficiency virus syndrome. Part I. Arch Dermatol. 1991;127:1383–1391.
220. Dover JS, Johnson RA. Cutaneous manifestations of human immunodeficiency virus syndrome. Part II. Arch Dermatol. 1991;127:1549–57.
221. LeBoit PE. Dermatopathologic findings in patients infected with HIV. Dermatol Clin. 1992;10:59–71.
222. Gradon JD, Timpone JG, Schnittman SM. Emergence of unusual opportunistic pathogens in AIDS: A Review. Clin Infect Dis. 1992;15:134–57.

223. Zalla MJ, Su WPD, Fransway AF. Dermatologic manifestations of human immunodeficiency virus infection. Mayo Clin Proc. 1992;67:1089–1108.

224. Stratigos AJ, Johnson RA, Dover JS. Cutaneous manifestations of human immunodeficiency virus infection. Semin Neurol. 1992;12:299–311.

225. Kurgis BS. Skin manifestations of human immunodeficiency virus (HIV): Part 1. Infectious manifestations. J Am Osteopath Assoc 1993;93:106–117.

226. McCrossin I, Wong D. HIV-related skin disease. Med J Aust. 1993;158: 179–85.

227. Prose NS. HIV infection in children. J Am Acad Dermatol. 1990;22:1223–31.

228. Torre D, Zeroli C, Fiori GP, et al. Dermatologic manifestations of AIDS in children. Pediatrician. 1991;18:195–203.

229. Nance KV, Smith ML, Joshi VV. Cutaneous manifestations of acquired immunodeficiency syndrome in children. Int J Dermatol. 1991;30:531–9.

230. Prose NS. Mucocutaneous disease in pediatric human immunodeficiency virus infection. Pediatr Clin North Am. 1991;38:977–90.

231. Prose NS. Cutaneous manifestations of pediatric HIV infection. Pediatr Dermatol. 1992;9:326–8.

232. Lim W, Sadick N, Gupta A, et al. Skin diseases in children with HIV infection and their association with degree of immunosuppression. Int J Dermatol. 1990;29:24–30.

233. Calabrese LH, Proffitt MR, Levin KH, et al. Acute infection with the human immunodeficiency virus (HIV) associated with acute brachial neuritis and exanthematous rash. Ann Intern Med. 1987;107:849–51.

234. Denning DW, Amos A, Wall RA. Oral and cutaneous features of acute human immunodeficiency virus infection. Cutis. 1987;40:171–5.

235. Ho DD, Sarngadharan MG, Resnick L, et al. Primary human T-lymphotropic virus type III infection. Ann Intern Med. 1985;103:880–3.

236. Boyko WJ, Schechter MT, Craib KJP, et al. The Vancouver lymphadenopathy–AIDS study: 7. Clinical and laboratory features of 87 cases of primary HIV infection. Can Med Assoc J. 1987;137:109–113.

237. Goodman DS, Teplitz ED, Wishner A, et al. Prevalence of cutaneous disease in patients with acquired immunodeficiency syndrome (AIDS) or AIDS-related complex. J Am Acad Dermatol. 1987;17:210–20.

238. Centers for Disease Control and Prevention. 1993 revised classification system for HIV infection and expanded surveillance case definition for AIDS among adolescents and adults. MMWR. 1992;41(RR-17):1–19.

239. Pierard G, Pierard-Franchimont C, Estrada JA, et al. Cutaneous mixed infections in AIDS. Am J Dermatopathol. 1990;12:63–6.

240. Kwan TH, Kaufman HW. Acid-fast bacilli with cytomegalovirus and herpes inclusions in the skin of an AIDS patient. Am J Clin Pathol. 1986;85:236–8.

241. Gretzula J, Penneys NS. Complex viral and fungal skin lesions of patients with acquired immunodeficiency syndrome. J Am Acad Dermatol. 1987;16: 1151–4.

242. Gulick RM. Varicella-zoster virus disease in patients with human immunodeficiency virus infection. Arch Dermatol. 1990;126:1086–8.

243. Janier M, Hillion B, Baccard M, et al. Chronic varicella zoster infection in acquired immunodeficiency syndrome. J Am Acad Dermatol. 1988;18:584–5.

244. Disler R, Dover JS. Chronic localized herpes zoster in the acquired immunodeficiency syndrome. Arch Dermatol. 1990;126:1101–6.

245. Leibovitz E, Kaul A, Rigaud M, et al. Chronic varicella zoster in a child infected with human immunodeficiency virus: Case report and review of the literature. Cutis. 1992;49:27–31.

246. Hicks CB, Benson PM, Lupton GP, et al. Seronegative secondary syphilis in a patient infected with the human immunodeficiency virus (HIV) with Kaposi's sarcoma. Ann Intern Med. 1987;107:492–5.

247. Bournerias I, Boisnic S, Patey O, et al. Unusual cutaneous cytomegalovirus involvement in patients with immunodeficiency syndrome. Arch Dermatol. 1989;125:1234–6.

248. Angeles AM. Fungal and mycobacterial skin infections. Clin Dermatol. 1991; 9:65–9.

249. Manrique P, Mayo J, Alvarex JA, et al. Polymorphous cutaneous cryptococcosis: Nodular, herpes-like, and mulluscum-like lesions in a patient with the acquired immunodeficiency syndrome. J Am Acad Dermatol. 1992;26:122–3.

250. Prichard JG, Sorotzkin RA, James RE. Cutaneous manifestations of disseminated coccidioidomycosis in the acquired immunodeficiency syndrome. Cutis. 1987;39:203–5.

251. LeBoit PE, Berger TG, Egbert BM, et al. Epithelioid haemangioma-like vascular proliferation in AIDS: Manifestation of cat scratch disease Bacillus infection? Lancet. 1988;1:960–3.

252. Jimenex-Acosta F, Pardo RJ, Cohen RJ, et al. Bacillary angiomatosis and acquired immunodeficiency syndrome: Case report and literature review. J Am Acad Dermatol. 1990;22:525–9.

253. Cockerell CJ. The clinicopathologic spectrum of bacillary (epitheloid) angiomatosis. Prog AIDS Pathol. 1990;2:111–26.

254. Cockerell CJ, LeBoit PE. Bacillary angiomatosis: A newly characterized, pseudoneoplastic, infectious, cutaneous vascular disorder. J Am Acad Dermatol. 1990;22:501–12.

255. Schwartzman WA, Marchevsky A, Meyer RD. Epithelioid angiomatosis or cat scratch disease with splenic and hepatic abnormalities in AIDS: Case report and review of the literature. Scand J Infect Dis. 1990;22:121–33.

256. LeBoit PE. Bacillary angiomatosis: A systemic opportunistic infection with prominant cutaneous manifestations. Semin Dermatol. 1991;10:194–8.

257. Schwartzman WA. Infections due to Rochalimaea: The expanding spectrum clinical spectrum. Clin Infect Dis. 1992;15:893–902.

258. Tappero JW, Koehler JE, Berger TM, et al. Bacillary angiomatosis and bacillary splenitis in immunocompetent adults. Ann Intern Med. 1993;118:363–5.

259. Relman DA, Loutit JS, Schmidt TM, et al. The agent of bacillary angiomatosis: An approach to the identification of uncultured pathogens. N Engl J Med. 1990;323:1573–80.

260. Koehler JE, Quinn FD, Berger TG, et al. Isolation of Rochalimaea species from cutaneous and osseous lesions of bacillary angiomatosis. N Engl J Med. 1992;327:1625–31.

261. Welch DF, Pickett DA, Slater LN, et al. Rochalimaea henselae sp. nov., a cause of septicemia, bacillary angiomatosis, and parenchymal bacillary peliosis. J Clin Microbiol. 1992;30:275–80.

262. Tompkins DC, Steigbigel RT. Rochalimaea's role in cat scratch disease and bacillary angiomatosis. Ann Intern Med. 1993;118:388–9.

263. Slater LN, Welch DF, Hensel D, et al. A newly recognized fastidious gram-negative pathogen as a cause of fever and bacteremia. N Engl J Med. 1990; 323:1578–93.

264. Brenner S. Acquired ichthyosis in AIDS. Cutis. 1987;39:421–3.

265. Young LY, Steinman HK. Acquired ichthyosis in a patient with acquired immunodeficiency syndrome and Kaposi's sarcoma. Cutis. 1987;39:395–6.

SECTION B. UPPER RESPIRATORY INFECTIONS

39. THE COMMON COLD

JACK M. GWALTNEY, JR.

While the designation "the common cold" is the traditional term used by both physician and lay persons for acute minor coryzal illness, current scientific knowledge has disclosed that there is no basis for the concept of a single entity implied by the term. Instead, "the common cold" is a group of diseases caused, for the most part, by members of five families of viruses. The viruses in these families have distinctive biochemical properties that govern their differing pathogenic and epidemiologic behavior. In addition, the immunotypes found in the different viral families have antigenic variations that are of biologic importance to the immune system of their human host. The problem of controlling acute respiratory disease presents a complex challenge that requires approaches suitable for the properties of the individual virus groups. Thus the hope for the development of a single "cure for the common cold" is an unrealistic expectation that has led to the diversion of resources into attempts at simplistic and unrealistic solutions to the problem.

As a clinical entity, the common cold is a mild, self-limited, catarrhal syndrome that is the leading cause of acute morbidity and of visits to a physician in the United States. It is also a major cause of industrial and school absenteeism.[1] A small proportion of colds is complicated by bacterial infections of the paranasal sinuses and the middle ear, which require antimicrobial therapy.

Based on early observations of their contagious nature, colds have long been thought to be due to infectious agents. However, it was not until the isolation of a number of new respiratory viruses in cell culture in the 1950s that the specific etiology of colds was known. The first of these, a parainfluenza virus, was shown in 1955 to cause acute respiratory disease.[2] In 1956, the first of the rhinoviruses was isolated from adults with common colds.[3,4] The following year, respiratory syncytial virus was associated with acute respiratory illness in infants,[5] and, in 1958, one of the enteroviruses, coxsackievirus A21, was recovered from military recruits with mild respiratory disease.[6] The latest group of common cold viruses to be discovered, the coronaviruses, was first reported in the 1960s.[7,8] Since that time, no new cold viruses have been found, although the specific cause of some colds remains unknown. Other respiratory viruses, such as influenza virus and adenovirus, produce the common cold syndrome but are characteristically associated with a more severe illness, which often involves the lower respiratory tract.

ETIOLOGY

The major respiratory viruses causing colds and similar upper respiratory illnesses are found in the myxovirus, paramyxovirus, adenovirus, picornavirus, and coronavirus groups (Table 1).[9–12] Within three groups of viruses are many different antigenic types. The rhinovirus group, which accounts for approximately 40 percent of colds in adults, has 100 immunotypes. The percentage of colds caused by the coronavirus group and the number of immunotypes of this virus have not been fully determined, but it is believed that these viruses are an important cause of colds. The three parainfluenza viruses and the respiratory syncytial virus each account for a proportion of colds on an annual basis. Influenza virus and adenovirus produce a spectrum of illness that overlaps the common cold syndrome. Some of the enteroviruses produce coryza,[13] as do some viruses that usually produce more characteristic findings, such as exanthems. Because mild streptococcal pharyngitis cannot be differentiated from viral pharyngitis on clinical grounds, it also is included as a cause of "colds." The etiology of approximately one-third to one-fourth of colds in adults remains unknown. Some undiagnosed illnesses may result from the insensitivity of methods currently used for detection of known viruses, and others may be due to undiscovered agents. Colds in children are caused by the same viruses in roughly the same proportion, but the total number of colds that can be diagnosed in children is usually lower. In some studies, as high as 70 percent of acute respiratory illnesses in children could not be assigned as etiology.

Colds are a frequent illness because of the large number of different causative viruses and also because reinfections may occur with the same virus type. Second infections probably occur with members of all the viral groups; with some, such as coronavirus, reinfections appear to be particularly common. Up to 80 percent of persons infected with coronavirus OC43 have had prior neutralizing antibody to the virus.[14]

SEASONAL INCIDENCE

The respiratory viruses have a worldwide distribution. Annual epidemics of upper respiratory tract disease occur in the colder months in temperate areas and during the rainy season in the tropics. In the United States the respiratory disease season begins in late August to mid-September.[15,16] Respiratory illness rates rise sharply over a few weeks and then remain elevated until spring. During March, April, and May, rates decline to the low summer level.

The events controlling the seasonal variation in attack rates of acute respiratory disease are not well understood. Adding to the complexity of the problem has been the discovery that some of the virus groups have their own seasonal pattern within the overall respiratory disease season. Rhinovirus outbreaks occur in the early fall and in mid- to late spring,[16] and coronaviruses are most prominent in the winter.[14] Studies with a specific virus, rhinovirus type 15, showed that chilling of volunteers did not increase their susceptibility to infection and illness.[17] Thus the effect of thermal cold per se on the host does not appear to be the explanation for the seasonal outbreaks of colds.

Undoubtedly, among the responsible variables for seasonal fluctuations in colds are the bringing together of children during school periods and the increased crowding indoors of populations during colder months.[18] Also, seasonal changes in relative humidity may be an important variable controlling prevalence of the different virus families because of the effect of differing relative humidities on virus survival. In general, enveloped viruses survive better under conditions of low relative humidity, as found in colder months of the year, while the converse is true for nonenveloped viruses.

ATTACK RATES

During peak months in the respiratory disease season in the United States, adults average six to eight colds per 1000 persons per day.[16] In the summer, rates fall to two or three colds per 1000 per day. Overall, adults in the United States average two to four colds per year and children six to eight.[15,16] In one 10-year study of illness in families, young children in nursery school averaged up to nine colds for the period of September through May! Illness rates decline in older children and reach adult levels in adolescence. Males have slightly more colds than females up to the age of adolescence, but after that the incidence is slightly higher in women, perhaps reflecting their exposure to young children.[12] Adults with children in the home have more colds than those without this exposure.[15,19] Tonsillectomy does not reduce the incidence of colds.[15] Cigarette smokers have the same incidence of colds as nonsmokers, but the severities of their illnesses are greater.[16,20]

TRANSMISSION

The main reservoir of respiratory viruses is in young children. Spread of colds takes place most commonly in the home,[15,19] school,[21] and day care centers.[22] Children acquire new viral strains from their schoolmates, which they then bring home and pass to other family members. One- to 5-day intervals occur between cases. Secondary attack rates of family members vary, depending on age, position in the family, and prior immunity to the virus. Age and immunity are related risk factors. Young children and mothers have high secondary attack rates as a result of close and prolonged exposure to school children in the family. The secondary attack rate of fathers is relatively low.

The natural mechanisms for the spread of cold viruses have not been well established. Possible means of transmission include (1) direct contact with infectious secretions on skin and

TABLE 1. Viruses Associated with the Common Cold

	Antigenic Types	Percentage of Cases[a]
Rhinoviruses	100 types and 1 subtype	30–40
Coronavirus	3 or more types	≥10
Parainfluenza virus	4 types	
Respiratory syncytial virus	2 types	
Influenza virus	3 types	10–15
Adenovirus	47 types	
Other viruses (enteroviruses, rubeola, rubella, varicella)		5
Presumed undiscovered viruses		25–30
Group A β-hemolytic streptococci[b]		5–10

[a] Estimated percentage of colds annually.
[b] Included because differentiation of streptococcal and viral pharyngitis is not possible by clinical means.

environmental surfaces, (2) large particles of respiratory secretions that are briefly transported in air, (3) infectious droplet nuclei suspended in air, and (4) combinations of these methods.[23] For some viruses, such as rhinovirus, close physical contact appears necessary for efficient spread. Infectious rhinovirus is produced primarily in the nose and is shed in highest concentrations in nasal secretions. Peak viral titers in nasal mucus occur on the second to fourth days of experimental infection and coincide with the period of maximum communicability.[23] A high proportion of persons with natural and experimental rhinovirus colds have recoverable virus on their hands. With experimental rhinovirus infection, brief hand contact permits ready transfer of virus-contaminated nasal secretions from the hands of infected subjects to the hands of susceptible subjects. When the contaminated fingers of the susceptible subjects are then placed in contact with nasal and conjunctival mucosa, infection results in a high percentage of cases.[24] In one study conducted in the home setting, treatment of fingers with a virucidal solution reduced the rate of infection in mothers exposed to other family members with fresh colds.[25] This latter study provides direct evidence of the mechanisms of common cold transmission under natural conditions and suggests that a proportion of colds are spread by a hand contamination/self-inoculation route.

Another rhinovirus transmission model has been developed in which virus is reliably transmitted through the air in large- and/or small-particle aerosol.[26] This model demonstrates the feasibility of the aerosol route of spread but does not prove that it occurs under natural conditions. Studies conducted in the field with intervention techniques specific for aerosol transmission are needed to address that question. There is epidemiologic evidence that influenza and adenovirus may spread, at least in part, by small airborne droplets. Thus, all the respiratory viruses may not behave in the same way, and further studies are necessary to determine which routes of transmission are important in the natural dissemination of these viruses.

PATHOGENESIS

Viral invasion of the upper respiratory tract is the basic mechanism in the pathogenesis of colds, but the specific events leading to clinical illness have only recently been investigated. Infection with common cold viruses is characteristically of short duration and self-limited. For example, maximum rhinovirus shedding lasts 3 weeks or less in young adults with experimental colds,[27,28] and coronavirus excretion has been detected for only 1–4 days.[14] Cold viruses are not usually present in asymptomatic persons,[29] although subclinical infections do occur and viral carriage may be somewhat prolonged in children.[30]

Characteristic changes have been described in sloughed columnar epithelial cells in nasal secretions of persons with natural colds of unknown etiology.[31] Cells with persistent ciliary activity have been found in nasal secretions in the first through the third day of illness. Also, some exfoliated cells show degenerative changes characterized by progressive nuclear pyknosis and the formation of apparent inclusion bodies. Ciliated epithelial cells containing viral antigen have been found in the nasal mucus of volunteers with experimental rhinovirus colds.[32]

Attempts to demonstrate specific histopathologic changes in nasal biopsy specimens of volunteers with rhinovirus colds have not been successful.[33,34] Examination by light and electron microscopy of nasal biopsy specimens from young adults with natural colds also confirmed the absence of destruction of the nasal epithelium.[35] In this study there was a significant increase in the number of neutrophils in the epithelium and in the lamina propria. The number of epithelial mast cells was not increased. The findings with rhinovirus contrast with the destructive changes to the respiratory epithelium that are seen with influenza virus infection.

With rhinovirus colds, the period of maximum viral excretion in nasal secretions coincides with the peak of clinical illness[36] and of appearance of ciliated epithelial cells in nasal mucus.[32] At that time, large quantities of protein, including immunoglobulins, are present in nasal secretions. In addition to any direct destructive effect that the virus may have on the respiratory mucous membrane, there is increasing evidence that chemical mediators and neurologic reflexes play a role in the pathogenesis of the common cold. Bradykinin,[37,38] prostaglandin,[38,39] histamine,[38,40,41] and interleukin-1 (Gwaltney, Proud, personal communication) have been associated with rhinovirus pathogenesis as well as parasympathetic[42] and α-adrenergic nerve pathways.[43] Pathogenic mechanisms for the various respiratory viruses are undoubtedly somewhat different.

The self-limited cold virus infection may lead to changes that affect the resident bacterial flora of the upper respiratory tract and result in secondary bacterial infection. Bacteria become able to invade normally sterile areas such as the sinuses, middle ear, and perhaps the tracheobronchial tree. The variable involved in triggering invasive bacterial infection are unknown but probably include obstruction of outlet areas and damage to the mucociliary cleansing mechanism of the upper respiratory tract. Recently, it was discovered that experimental and natural colds routinely lead to acute, reversible abnormalities of the ostiomeatal area and sinus cavities.[44,45] It is currently unknown whether direct viral invasion of the sinus, middle ear, and tracheobronchial tree is necessary for subsequent bacterial infection to occur or whether the viral involvement can remain localized to the nasal and pharyngeal mucous membrane. However, respiratory viruses have been recovered from sinus[46] and middle ear[9,47] aspirates obtained by direct puncture from patients with acute infections at these sites. Abnormalities in eustachian tube function and middle ear pressures have been consistently observed in volunteers with experimental rhinovirus infection.[48] During colds, increases have also been noted in titers of resident bacterial populations of the upper airways, but the significance of this is unknown.[49,50]

CLINICAL CHARACTERISTICS

The incubation period of the common cold varies somewhat with the different viruses but is usually between 24 and 72 hours. The symptoms of experimental rhinovirus colds have a mean onset within 16 hours of viral inoculation into the nose.[37] The cardinal symptoms are nasal discharge, nasal obstruction, sneezing, sore or "scratchy" throat, and cough.[15,20] Slight fever may be found, but temperature elevation of more than a degree is distinctly uncommon in the adult. Infants and young children may have more frequent temperature elevation. The early symptoms may be minimal, with only mild malaise and nasal complaints. With rhinovirus infection, sneezing, nasal discharge, and nasal obstruction usually begin simultaneously on the first day of illness and rapidly increase to maximum severity by the second or third day. Paralleling the nasal symptoms are sore, dry, or "scratchy" throat. Cough and hoarseness may also begin early in the course of illness and, when present, tend to persist until the end of the first week of symptoms by which time nasal and pharyngeal complaints have usually subsided. Limited information is available suggesting that symptom patterns are similar with coronavirus colds.[14]

The median duration of rhinovirus colds is 1 week, but in approximately one-fourth the illnesses last up to 2 weeks. In cigarette smokers with rhinovirus colds, cough is increased and prolonged. Other complaints include mild burning of the eyes; true conjunctivitis is not seen except in some adenovirus and enterovirus infections. There may also be loss of sense of smell and taste and a feeling of pressure in the ears or sinuses due to obstruction and/or mucosal swelling. The voice may have a nasal quality. Painful maceration of the skin around the nostrils is often bothersome when rhinorrhea has been profuse and persistent.

On physical examination, the findings may be few despite the subjective discomfort of the patient. A red nose and a dripping nasal discharge are the characteristic features of the cold sufferer, but many patients have minimal outward manifestations of the infection. The nasal mucous membrane may have a glassy appearance due to the exudation of serum proteins and increased mucus secretions. It is difficult to judge accurately the presence of increased erythema of the mucous membrane of the nose and throat due to normal variations in the color of these structures. Marked pharyngeal erythema and exudate are not seen with rhinovirus and coronavirus infections, but they do occur with pharyngoconjunctival fever of adenovirus infection. Examination of the chest may reveal the presence of rhonchi.

The clinical picture of the common cold is similar in children and adults. However, in young children, parainfluenza virus and respiratory syncytial virus infection may lead to viral pneumonia, croup, and bronchiolitis, while in adults these viruses usually cause only colds. In both adults and children, the upper airway manifestations of rhinovirus, coronavirus, parainfluenza virus, and respiratory syncytial virus infections are indistinguishable in the individual patient.

DIAGNOSIS

The manifestations of the common cold are so typical that self-diagnosis by the patient is usually correct. Hay fever and vasomotor rhinitis may give similar nasal symptoms, but the recurrent and chronic nature of these diseases is soon recognized by the patient and easily diagnosed by the physician from the patient's history. Diagnosis of the specific virus involved is usually not possible on the basis of clinical observation. Some acute respiratory infections, such as influenza and pharyngoconjunctival fever, when seen in a typical epidemiologic setting, can be recognized without benefit of viral culture or serologic tests. Knowledge of the characteristic seasonal patterns for the different virus groups may also aid in the identification of a particular virus.

The main challenge to the physician is to distinguish the uncomplicated cold from the approximately 0.5 percent of cases with secondary bacterial sinusitis and the 2 percent with otitis media.[15] This is not easy because of the lack of inexpensive and noninvasive diagnostic tests for these infections. A complete examination should be performed on the pharynx, nasal cavity, ears, and sinuses. In the pharynx, marked injection or exudate should raise suspicion of streptococcal or adenovirus infection, Vincent's angina, mononucleosis, or diphtheria. Occasionally, patients have small vesicles on the palate due to coxsackievirus A infections. The presence of nasal polyps is suggestive of an underlying allergic problem. In children, a foreign body may lead to persistent and nasal discharge. Examination of the ears is directed at finding changes in the appearance of the tympanum, indicating infection (see Ch. 43). The use of the pneumatic otoscope is helpful in determining if fluid is present behind the ear drum. The sinuses should be examined by transillumination under optimal conditions (see Ch. 44).

Imaging studies, including sinus radiographs and computed tomography scans, are considerably more sensitive than physical examination and transillumination for detecting acute anatomic changes in the sinuses of patients with cold symptoms.[45] The cost of these procedures precludes their use in most routine cases. Also, imaging techniques cannot distinguish with certainty between cases with and without bacterial infection. The most valuable laboratory test in patients with pharyngeal complaints is rapid antigen detection for group A β-hemolytic streptococci. Many of the respiratory viruses can be isolated in cell culture, although specific virologic diagnosis is not usually available in clinical practice. Rhinoviruses grow in human embryonic lung cells (WI-38), myxo- and paramyxoviruses in primary rhesus monkey kidney cells, and respiratory syncytial virus in Hep2 cells. Isolation of coronavirus in cell culture has proved difficult

with currently available techniques. The sensitivity of the tests for isolating viruses can vary widely with changes in the sensitivity of the cell cultures. Nucleic acid probes are being developed for detecting common cold viruses, but their utility in clinical practice has not been established.[51–53]

The serologic diagnoses of influenza, parainfluenza, respiratory syncytial, and adenovirus infection are available in some state health department laboratories. Serum specimens should be obtained in the acute phase of illness and approximately 3 week later and tested simultaneously. A fourfold or greater rise in antibody titer is indicative of infection. Serologic diagnosis of rhinovirus infection is not practical because of the many different antigenic types. Rapid techniques using fluorescent antibody or other immunodiagnostic procedures on respiratory secretions are being used in clinical laboratories for the diagnosis of influenza virus, parainfluenza virus, respiratory syncytial virus, and adenovirus.

TREATMENT

Only symptomatic treatment is available for the uncomplicated common cold.[54] Individual measures directed at controlling nasal and pharyngeal complaints and cough are more effective than the all-inclusive cold remedies currently available. Direct application to the nasal membrane of vasoconstrictors such as 0.5 or 0.25% phenylephrine or 1% ephedrine drops or sprays are recommended to provide symptomatic relief of nasal obstructions and to promote drainage of nasal secretions. Patients should be instructed to place themselves in a head down position when administering decongestants to achieve penetration of the drug to inaccessible areas of the nasal cavity. An interval of approximately 1 minute should be allowed between three separate applications of drops or spray. Decongestants may be used every 4 hours on a regular basis. Patients should be cautioned on the rebound effect that results if decongestants are used continuously for more than 3 or 4 days. Nasal secretions accompanying colds have been reduced by the intranasal use of the topically active parasympatholytic compounds ipratropium and atropine methonitrate.[42,55,56] Nonsedating antihistamines reduce sneezing and also have a modest, suppressive effect on nasal secretions.[40,41,54,57]

Cough can be controlled with preparations containing dextromethorphan or codeine. Recently, some nonsteroidal anti-inflammatory compounds, sulindac,[58] indomethacin,[59] and naproxen[39] have shown effectiveness in reducing cough, presumably through blocking prostaglandin action.[38] Naproxen reduced cough in volunteers with experimental rhinovirus colds,[39,60] but the usefulness of these compounds in treating cough associated with colds in clinical practice has not been determined.

Sore throat can be relieved with warm saline gargles or lozenges containing a topical anesthetic. The regular application of an ointment containing a petrolatum base is useful in controlling painful maceration of the nares. Aspirin or acetaminophen and bed rest are of value when headache and constitutional symptoms are prominent. The patient should restrict his activities during the height of the illness, at which time he is most contagious to others. Regular hand-washing and care to avoid contamination of the environment with nasal secretions may also help to prevent spread.

Antibiotics have no place in the treatment of uncomplicated colds. Until truly effective and specific treatment becomes available, there will continue to be fads in the use of unproven cold remedies. The ingestion of large doses of vitamin C has been widely used as a preventive or therapeutic measure for colds. In some instances, controlled studies have shown a modest beneficial effect of vitamin C for colds. However, a careful analysis of the studies had indicated that a placebo effect could not be ruled out. In one study, many participants correctly surmised from the taste of the contents of the capsules used whether they were receiving vitamin C or a placebo.[61] In volunteers experimentally infected with rhinovirus, vitamin C in doses of 3 g/day was not effective in preventing infection and illness.[62,63]

PROSPECTS FOR VACCINES, NEW TREATMENTS, AND INTERRUPTION OF TRANSMISSION

Vaccine development has reached an impasse because of the discovery of the many different cold viruses, particularly the 100 rhinoviruses. Unless ways are found to combine large numbers of viral antigens effectively or to take advantage of minor antigenic cross-relationships that exist, prospects for common cold vaccines are not good. A number of chemical compounds have inhibitory activity against respiratory viruses in tissue culture systems, and attempts are being made to develop antiviral agents for clinical use. The activity of such compounds tends to be relatively group specific, but some have shown activity against most of the rhinoviruses.[64]

The most promising approach to prevention of colds has come through the development of interferon. Topically applied intranasal recombinant human interferon-α_{2b} has a highly effective prophylactic activity against experimental rhinovirus infection.[65–67] When given therapeutically in the same manner, interferon has reduced viral excretion, but its effect on development of illness has been of only minimal benefit.[68] In addition, the chronic use of topically applied intranasal interferon is associated with local side effects in the nose, such as stuffiness, dryness, discomfort, and pinpoint areas of ulceration.[69,70] To avoid these problems, a strategy has been tested that employs short-term contact prophylaxis by family members exposed to individuals with colds of recent onset. Using this approach, two field studies have observed an approximately 40 percent reduction of total colds and a virtual elimination of rhinovirus-specific infections in exposed individuals.[71,72] Side effects were avoided by the short duration of the use of the interferon.

The failure of potent antivirals like interferon-α_{2b}[68] and the capsid binders, which block viral attachment and uncoating,[73,74] to provide therapeutic activity in the rhinovirus challenge model suggests that treatment with antiviral compounds alone may be insufficient to provide clinically useful benefits. The lack of a treatment effect with antivirals may be the result of the inflammatory events accompanying the infection that would not be expected to respond to the antiviral. To test this hypothesis, an experimental treatment has been developed that combines a compound with antiviral activity with other compounds that block selected pathways of inflammation. Promising results were obtained in a study in which volunteers with early rhinovirus colds were given interferon-α_{2b} and ipratropium topically into the nose combined with oral naproxen.[60] Symptoms disappeared in some treated subjects, and mean symptom scores were significantly reduced in the treated group, suggesting the benefits of this approach.

Another approach to control of colds that has been studied is to interrupt the person-to-person transmission of the viruses. A virucidal hand treatment used in the home by mothers exposed to children with new colds reduced the mothers' incidence of total colds by 60 percent and eliminated laboratory-proven rhinovirus colds.[25] In another study, children trained to avoid self-inoculatory behavior had reduced cold-associated asthmatic attacks and laboratory-proven respiratory virus infections.[75] Since these studies suggest that spread of some cold viruses may occur by direct hand contact/self-inoculation, handwashing and avoiding finger-to-nose and finger-to-eye contact should be practiced, particularly with exposure to a cold sufferer. Also, covering coughs and sneezes with disposable nasal tissues is recommended as a means of controlling aerosol transmission.

REFERENCES

1. Rice DP, Feldman JJ, White KL. The current burden of illness in the United States. Occasional Papers of the Institute of Medicine. Washington, DC: National Academy of Sciences; 1976:1.
2. Chanock RM. Association of a new type of cytopathogenic myxovirus with infantile croup. J Exp Med. 1956;104:55.
3. Pelon W, Mogabgab WJ, Phillips IA, et al. A cytopathogenic agent isolated from naval recruits with mild respiratory illness. Proc Soc Exp Biol Med. 1957;94:262.
4. Price WH. The isolation of a new virus associated with respiratory clinical disease in humans. Proc Natl Acad Sci USA. 1956;43:892.
5. Chanock RM, Roizman B, Myers R. Recovery from infants with respiratory illness of a virus related to Chimpanzee Coryza Agent (CCA). I. Isolation, properties, and characterization. Am J Hyg. 1957;66:281.
6. Lennette EH, Fox VL, Schmidt NJ, et al. The COE virus: An apparently new virus recovered from patients with mild respiratory disease. Am J Hyg. 1958;68:272.
7. Tyrrell DAJ, Bynoe ML. Cultivation of a novel type of common-cold virus in organ cultures. Br Med J. 1965;1:1467.
8. Hamre D, Procknow JJ: A new virus isolated from the human respiratory tract. Proc Soc Exp Biol Med. 1966;121:190.
9. Gwaltney JM Jr. Virology of middle ear. Ann Otol Rhinol Laryngol. 1971;80: 365.
10. Stuart-Harris CH, Andrewes C, Andrews BE, et al. A collaborative study of the aetiology of acute respiratory infection in Britain 1961–4. A report of the Medical Research Council working party on acute respiratory virus infections. Br Med J. 1965;2:319.
11. Hamre D, Connelly AP Jr, Procknow JJ. Virologic studies of acute respiratory disease in young adults. IV. Virus isolations during four years of surveillance. Am J Epidemiol. 1966;83:238.
12. Monto AS, Bryan ER, Ohmit S. Rhinovirus infections in Tecumseh, Michigan: Frequency of illness and number of serotypes. J Infect Dis. 1987;156:43–9.
13. Kepfer PD, Hable KA, Smith TF. Viral isolation rates during summer from children with acute upper respiratory tract disease and health children. AJCP. 1974;16:1–5.
14. Monto AS. Coronaviruses. In AS Evans (ed). Viral Infections of Humans. Epidemiology and Control. 3rd ed. New York: Plenum; 1989:153–67.
15. Dingle JH, Badger GF, Jordan WS Jr. Illness in the Home: Study of 25,000 Illnesses in a Group of Cleveland Families. Cleveland: The Press of Western Reserve University; 1964:1.
16. Gwaltney JM Jr, Hendley JO, Simon G, et al. Rhinovirus infections in an industrial population. I. The occurrence of illness. N Engl J Med. 1966;275:1261.
17. Douglas RG Jr, Lindgren KM, Couch RB. Exposure to cold environment and rhinovirus common cold: Failure to demonstrate effect. N Engl J Med. 1968;279:743.
18. Gwaltney JM Jr. The Jeremiah Metzger Lecture. Climatology and the common cold. Trans Am Clin Climatol Assoc. 1984;96:159.
19. Hendley JO, Gwaltney JM Jr, Jordan WS Jr. Rhinovirus infections in an industrial population. IV. Infections within families of employees during two fall peaks of respiratory illness. Am J Epidemiol. 1969;89:184.
20. Gwaltney JM Jr, Hendley JO, Simon G, et al. Rhinovirus infections in an industrial population. II. Characteristics of illness and antibody response. JAMA. 1967;202:494.
21. Beem MO. Acute respiratory illness in nursery school children: A longitudinal study of the occurrence of illness and respiratory viruses. Am J Epidemiol. 1969;90:30.
22. Frenck RW, Glezen WP. Respiratory tract infections in children in day care. Semin Pediatr Infect Dis. 1990;1:234–44.
23. Gwaltney JM Jr. Epidemiology of the common cold. Ann NY Acad Sci. 1980; 353:54.
24. Gwaltney JM Jr, Moskalski PB, Hendley JO. Hand-to-hand transmission of rhinovirus colds. Ann Intern Med. 1978;88:463.
25. Hendley JO, Gwaltney JM Jr. Mechanisms of transmission of rhinovirus infections. Epidemiol Rev. 1988;10:242.
26. Dick EC, Jennings LC, Mink KA, et al. Aerosol transmission of rhinovirus colds. J Infect Dis. 1987;156:442.
27. Cate TR, Couch RB, Johnson KM. Studies with rhinoviruses in volunteers: Production of illness, effect of naturally acquired antibody, and demonstration of a protective effect not associated with serum antibody. J Clin Invest. 1964; 43:56.
28. Winther B, Gwaltney JM Jr, Mygind N, et al. Sites of rhinovirus recovery after point inoculation of the upper airway. JAMA. 1986;256:1763.
29. Hamre D, Rhinoviruses. In: Melnick JL, ed. Monographs in Virology 1. Basel: Karger; 1968:1.
30. Frank AL, Taber LH, Wells CR, et al. Patterns of shedding of myxoviruses in children. J Infect Dis. 1981;144:433.
31. Bryan WTK, Bryan MP, Smith CA. Human ciliated epithelial cells in nasal secretions. Transactions of the 85th Annual Meeting of the American Laryngological Association. 1964:145.
32. Turner RB, Hendley JO, Gwaltney JM Jr. Shedding of infected ciliated epithelial cells in rhinovirus colds. J Infect Dis. 1982;145:849.
33. Douglas RG Jr, Alford BR, Couch RB. Atraumatic nasal biopsy for studies of respiratory virus infection in volunteers. Antimicrob Agents Chemother. 1968;8:340.
34. Winther B, Farr B, Turner RB, et al. Histopathologic examination and enumeration of polymorphonuclear leukocytes in the nasal mucosa during experimental rhinovirus colds. Acta Otolaryngol (Stockh). 1984;413(Suppl):19–24.
35. Winther B, Brofeldt S, Christensen B, Mygind N. Light and scanning electron microscopy of nasal biopsies from patients with naturally acquired common colds. Acta Otolaryngol. 1984;97:309.

36. Douglas RG Jr, Cate TR, Gerone PJ, et al. Quantitative rhinovirus shedding patterns in volunteers. Am Rev Respir Dis. 1966;94:159.
37. Naclerio RM, Proud D, Lichtenstein LM, et al. Kinins are generated during experimental rhinovirus colds. J Infect Dis. 1988;157:133.
38. Doyle WJ, Boehm S, Skoner DP. Physiologic responses to intranasal dose-response challenges with histamine, methacholine, bradykinin, and prostaglandin in adult volunteers with and without nasal allergy. J Allergy Clin Immunol. 1990;86:924–35.
39. Sperber SJ, Hendley JO, Hayden FG, et al. Effects of naproxen on experimental rhinovirus colds. A randomized, double-blind, controlled trial. Ann Intern Med. 1992;117:37–41.
40. Doyle WJ, McBride TP, Skoner DP, et al. A double-blind, placebo-controlled clinical trial of the effect of chlorpheniramine on the response of the nasal airway, middle ear and eustachian tube to provocative rhinovirus challenge. Pediatr Infect Dis J. 1988;7:229–38.
41. Gaffey MJ, Gwaltney JM Jr, Sastre A, et al. Intranasal and oral antihistamine treatment of experimental rhinovirus colds. Am Rev Respir Dis. 1987;136:556–60.
42. Gaffey MJ, Hayden FG, Boyd JC, et al. Ipratropium bromide treatment of experimental rhinovirus infection. Antimicrob Agents Chemother. 1988;32:1644–47.
43. Sperber SJ, Sorrentino JV, Riker DK, et al. Evaluation of an alpha agonist alone and in combination with a nonsteroidal anti-inflammatory agent in the treatment of experimental rhinovirus colds. Bull NY Acad Med. 1989;65:145–60.
44. Turner BW, Cail WS, Hendley JO, et al. Physiologic abnormalities in the paranasal sinuses during experimental rhinovirus colds. J Allergy Clin Immunol. 1992;90:474–8.
45. Gwaltney JM Jr, Phillips CD, Miller RD, et al. Computed tomographic study of the common cold. N Engl J Med. 1994;330:25–30.
46. Evans FO Jr, Sydnor JB, Moore WEC, et al. Sinusitis of the maxillary antrum. N Engl J Med. 1975;293:735.
47. Arola M, Ruuskanen O, Ziegler T, et al. Clinical role of respiratory virus infection in acute otitis media. Pediatrics. 1990;86:848–55.
48. Doyle WJ, McBride TP, Skoner DP, et al. A double blind placebo-controlled clinical trial of the effect of chlorpheniramine on the response of the nasal airway, middle ear and eustachian tube to provocative rhinovirus challenge. Pediatr Infect Dis J. 1988;7:222.
49. Straker E, Hill AB, Lovell RA. A study of the nasopharyngeal bacterial flora of different groups of persons observed in London and south-east England during the years 1930 to 1937. Reports on Public Health and Medical Subjects, no. 90. London: His Majesty's Stationery Office; 1939:7.
50. Brimblecombe FSW, Cruickshank R, Master P, et al. Family studies of respiratory infections. Br Med J. 1958;1:119.
51. Myint S, Harmsen D, Raabe T, et al. Characterization of a nucleic acid probe for the diagnosis of human coronavirus 229E infections. J Med Virol. 1990;31:165–72.
52. Johnston SL, Sanderson G, Pattemore PK, et al. Use of polymerase chain reaction for diagnosis of picornavirus infection in subjects with and without respiratory symptoms. J Clin Microbiol. 1993;31:111–7.
53. Arruda E, Hayden FG. Detection of human rhinovirus RNA in nasal washings by PCR. Mol Cell Probes. 1993;7:373–9.
54. Smith MBH, Feldman W. Over-the-counter cold medications. A critical review of clinical trials between 1950 and 1991. JAMA. 1993;269:2258–63.
55. Borum P, Olsen L, Winther B, and Mygind N. Ipratropium nasal spray: A new treatment for rhinorrhea in the common cold. Am Rev Respir Dis. 1981;123:418.
56. Gaffey MJ, Gwaltney JM Jr, Dressler WE, et al. Intranasally administered atropine methonitrate treatment of experimental rhinovirus colds. Am Rev Respir Dis. 1987;135:241–4.
57. Howard JC Jr, Kantner TR, Lilienfield LS, et al. Effectiveness of antihistamines in the symptomatic management of the common cold. JAMA. 1979;242:2414.
58. Nozhat JRM, Choudry B, Fuller RW. The effect of sulindac on the abnormal cough reflex associated with dry cough. J Pharmacol Exper Ther. 1990;255:161–4.
59. Fogari R, Zoppi A, Tettamanti F, et al. Effects of nifedipine and indomethacin on cough induced by angiotensin-converting enzyme inhibitors: A double-blind, randomized, cross-over study. J Cardiovas Pharmacol. 1992;19:670–3.
60. Gwaltney JM Jr. Combined antiviral and antimediator treatment of rhinovirus colds. J Infect Dis. 1992;166:776–82.
61. Chalmers TC. Effects of ascorbic acid on the common cold. An evaluation of the evidence. Am J Med. 1975;58:532.
62. Walker GH, Bynoe ML, Tyrrell DAJ. Trial of ascorbic acid in prevention of colds. Br Med J. 1967;1:603.
63. Schwartz AR, Togo Y, Hornick RB, et al. Evaluation of the efficacy of ascorbic acid in prophylaxis of induced rhinovirus 44 infection in man. J Infect Dis. 1973;128:500.
64. Sperber SJ, Hayden FG. Chemotherapy of rhinovirus colds. Antimicrob Agents Chemother. 1988;32:409–19.
65. Scott GM, Phillpotts RJ, Wallace J, et al. Purified interferon as protection against rhinovirus infections. Br Med J. 1982;284:1822.
66. Hayden FG, Gwaltney JM Jr. Intranasal interferon-alpha₂ for prevention of rhinovirus infection and illness. J Infect Dis. 1983;148:543.
67. Samo T-C, Greenberg SB, Couch RB Jr, et al. Evaluations of efficacy and tolerance to intranasally applied recombinant leukocyte A interferon in normal volunteers. J Infect Dis. 1983;148:535.
68. Hayden FG, Gwaltney JM Jr. Intranasal interferon-α₂ treatment of experimental rhinoviral colds. J Infect Dis. 1984;150:174.
69. Douglas RM, Albrecht JK, Miles HB, et al. Intranasal interferon-α₂ prophylaxis of natural respiratory virus infection. J Infect Dis. 1985;151:731.
70. Hayden FG, Gwaltney JM Jr, Johnson ME. Prophylactic efficacy and tolerance of low-dose intranasal interferon-alpha₂ in natural respiratory viral infections. Antiviral Res. 1985;5:11.
71. Hayden FG, Albrecht JK, Kaiser DL, et al. Prevention of natural colds by contact prophylaxis with intranasal alpha₂-interferon. N Engl J Med. 1986;314:71.
72. Douglas RM, Moore BW, Miles HB, et al. Prophylactic efficacy of intranasal alpha₂-interferon against rhinovirus infections in the family setting. N Engl J Med. 1986;314:65.
73. Al-Nakib W, Higgins PG, Barrow GI, et al. Suppression of colds in human volunteers challenged with rhinovirus by a new synthetic drug (R61837). Antimicrob Agents Chemother. 1989;33:522–5.
74. Hayden FG, Andries K, Janssen PAJ. Safety and efficacy of intranasal pirodavir (R77975) in experimental rhinovirus infection. Antimicrob Agents Chemother. 1992;36:727–32.
75. Corley DL, Gevirtz R, Nideffer R, Cummins L. Prevention of postinfectious asthma in children by reducing self-inoculatory behavior. J Pediatr Psychol. 1987;12:242–58.

40. PHARYNGITIS

JACK M. GWALTNEY, JR.

Acute pharyngitis is an inflammatory syndrome of the pharynx caused by several different groups of microorganisms. Most cases are of viral etiology and occur as part of common colds and influenzal syndromes. The most important of the bacterial infections is due to the group A β-hemolytic streptoccoccus (*Streptococcus pyogenes*). It is important to differentiate streptococcal from viral pharyngitis because of the response of streptococcal infection to penicillin therapy and the ineffectiveness of antibiotic therapy in the viral infections. Also streptococcal pharyngitis may be complicated by acute rheumatic fever and acute glomerulonephritis. There are other uncommon or rare types of pharyngitis, and for some of these treatment is also available. The list of microorganisms known to cause pharyngitis continues to grow as new etiologic associations are established.

ETIOLOGY

The known microbial causes of pharyngitis are listed in Table 1, which shows the syndromes of respiratory illness caused by the various agents[1–4] and their estimated contribution to all cases of pharyngitis.[5,6] The relative importance of the different agents is not fully defined, and it is still not possible to determine the cause of a sizable proportion of cases. The results of epidemiologic investigations are influenced by the season of the year, the age of the population, the severity of illness, and the diagnostic methods used to detect cases. A large amount of mild pharyngitis is associated with rhinovirus and coronavirus colds. Adenovirus and herpes simplex virus pharyngitis, although less common, are important because of their clinical severity. Others of the known respiratory viruses each account for a small proportion of cases. Primary human immunodeficiency syndrome (HIV) infection has joined the list of viral infections associated with acute pharyngitis.[7]

Approximately 15 percent of all cases of pharyngitis are due to *S. pyogenes*. In children with sore throat, *S. pyogenes* may cause up to half of the cases during some periods. The importance of non-group A β-hemolytic streptococci as a cause of pharyngitis is not entirely clear. Non-group A β-hemolytic streptococci in groups C and G have long been associated with foodborne outbreaks of pharyngitis.[8,9] Recently, group C β-hemo-

TABLE 1. Microbial Causes of Acute Pharyngitis

	Syndrome/Disease	Estimated Importance[a]
Viral		
Rhinovirus (100 types and 1 subtype)	Common cold	20
Coronavirus (3 or more types)	Common cold	≥5
Adenovirus (types 3, 4, 7, 14, 21)	Pharyngoconjunctival fever, ARD	5
Herpes simplex virus (types 1 and 2)	Gingivitis, stomatitis, pharyngitis	4
Parainfluenza virus (types 1–4)	Common cold, croup	2
Influenza virus (types A and B)	Influenza	2
Coxsackievirus A (types 2, 4–6, 8, 10)	Herpangina	<1
Epstein-Barr virus	Infectious mononucleosis	<1
Cytomegalovirus	Infectious mononucleosis	<1
Human immunodeficiency virus −1	Primary HIV infection	<1
Bacterial		
Streptococcus pyogenes (group A β-hemolytic streptococcus)	Pharyngitis/tonsillitis, scarlet fever	15–30
Group C β-hemolytic streptococci	Pharyngitis/tonsillitis	5–10
Mixed anaerobic infection	Gingivitis, pharyngitis (Vincent's angina)	<1
	Peritonsillitis/peritonsillar abscess (quinsy)	<1
Neisseria gonorrhoeae	Pharyngitis	<1
Corynebacterium diphtheriae	Diphtheria	≥1
Corynebacterium ulcerans	Pharyngitis, diphtheria	<1
Arcanobacterium hemolyticum (*Corynebacterium hemolyticum*)	Pharyngitis, scarlatiniform rush	<1
Yersinia enterocolitica	Pharyngitis, enterocolitis	<1
Treponema pallidum	Secondary syphilis	<1
Chlamydial		
Chlamydia pneumoniae	Pneumonia/bronchitis/pharyngitis	Unknown
Mycoplasmal		
Mycoplasma pneumoniae	Pneumonia/bronchitis/pharyngitis	<1
Mycoplasma hominis (type 1)	Pharyngitis in volunteers	Unknown
Unknown		30

[a] Estimated percentage of cases of pharyngitis due to indicated organism in civilians of all ages.

lytic streptococci have been associated with endemic pharyngitis in college students[10] and other adults.[11] Other non-group A β-hemolytic streptococci have not been definitely implicated as a cause of endemic pharyngitis.[12–16] Mixed anaerobic bacterial infections (Vincent's angina) cause occasional cases of acute pharyngitis as do *Corynebacterium diphtheriae*, *Arcanobacterium hemolyticum*, *Yersinia enterocolitica*, and *Neisseria gonorrhoeae*. *Mycoplasma pneumoniae* has been associated with pharyngitis since the late 1950s, but in epidemiologic studies of unselected patients, *M. pneumoniae* has not been an important cause of the disease.[5,6,12,13,17] The recognition of the role of *Chlamydia pneumoniae* (TWAR strain) in acute respiratory disease[18] has added another agent to the list of those causing pharyngitis, but its relative importance has yet to be determined.[19,20]

EPIDEMIOLOGY

Most cases of pharyngitis occur during the colder months of the year, during the respiratory disease season. Viral agents such as rhinoviruses tend to have annual periods of peak prevalence, which are most important in the fall and spring; coronaviruses have been found most often in the winter. Influenza appears in epidemics, which in the United States usually occur between December and April. In military recruits adenoviruses cause the syndrome of acute respiratory disease (ARD) during the colder months. In civilians wintertime ARD occurs as well as epidemics of pharyngoconjunctival fever in the summer. Streptococcal pharyngitis occurs during the respiratory disease season, with peak rates of infection in late winter and early spring. Spread among family members in the home is a prominent feature of the epidemiologic behavior of most of these agents, with children being the major reservoir of infection. For details on the epidemiologic behavior of these organisms, the reader is referred to the chapters dealing with each.

PATHOGENESIS

Symptoms of sore or scratchy throat occur in approximately 50 percent of people with rhinovirus colds[21] and in 20–70 percent of people with respiratory illness due to coronavirus.[22,23] Pharyngeal complaints are present in up to 80 percent of people with parainfluenza virus illness[24] and in approximately 50 percent of people with type A influenza[21] and adenovirus illness.[24] Other viral respiratory illnesses with pharyngitis occur with coxsackievirus A21, echoviruses 6 and 20,[24] herpes simplex virus,[25] Epstein-Barr (EB) virus, and cytomegalovirus infections.

The pathogenic mechanisms are different for the various organisms. Nasal epithelial biopsies obtained from volunteers with experimental rhinovirus infections have shown little or no evidence of viral cytopathic effect.[26,27] However, it has recently been discovered that bradykinin and lysylbradykinin are generated in the nasal passages of persons with experimental and natural rhinovirus colds.[28,29] These inflammatory mediators are potent stimulators of pain nerve endings. Also, volunteers given experimental intranasal challenge with bradykinin have developed symptoms of sore throat.[30] With other respiratory virus infections, such as adenovirus and coxsackievirus, there is evidence that direct invasion of pharyngeal mucosa occurs.

The events leading to invasive streptococcal infection of the pharynx and tonsil are also not well understood. Pharyngeal carriage of *S. pyogenes* is commonly observed in asymptomatic people. Factors that influence the balance between colonization and invasive infection may include natural and acquired host immunity and interference among the bacteria present in the oropharynx. *Streptococcus pyogenes* elaborates a number of extracelluar factors, including erythrogenic toxin, hemolysins, streptokinase, deoxyribonuclease, proteinase, and hyaluronidase, which are of known or possible pathogenic importance. Certain M serotypes (1, 2, 4, and 12) of streptococci have been most frequently isolated from patients with uncomplicated pharyngitis, and others (1, 3, and 12) from patients with serious invasive infection.[31] However, epidemiologic analyses of disease association and geographic prevalence have suggested strain-associated virulence rather than virulence broadly related to a given serotype.

The usual pathologic changes occurring in viral pharyngitis are edema and hyperemia of the tonsils and the pharyngeal mucous membrane. An inflammatory exudate may be present with adenovirus and EB virus infections; with the latter, nasopharyngeal lymphoid hyperplasia also occurs. Vesiculation and mucosal ulceration may occur with herpes simplex virus and some coxsackievirus A infections. With streptococcal pharyngitis there is an intense, inflammatory response in the pharyngeal membrane, and there may be exudate and hemorrhage of the tonsils and pharyngeal walls. With diphtheria a fibrous pseudomembrane containing necrotic epithelium, leukocytes, and bacterial colonies develops on the epithelial surface. For a more detailed discussion of the pathogenic events associated with infection by the wide variety of microorganisms that cause pharyngitis, the reader is referred to the chapters describing the individual agents.

CLINICAL PRESENTATION

Pharyngitis with the Common Cold

Mild to moderate pharyngeal discomfort is frequently present during a cold but is usually not the primary complaint. The symptom is characterized as soreness, scratchiness, or irritation. Severe pharyngeal pain and odynophagia are not characteristic of this type of pharyngitis. Nasal symptoms and cough are also usually present. Systemic complaints of feverishness, chilliness, malaise, and myalgia are not prominent, and a temperature elevation is unusual in adults and older children. On examination, the pharynx may appear normal or show a mild amount of edema and erythema. Rhinorrhea and postnasal discharge are usually present. Pharyngeal and tonsillar exudates and painful lymphadenopathy are not seen. Pharyngeal complaints usually subside over 3 or 4 days, and most patients have recovered by the end of a week (see Ch. 39).

Pharyngitis with Influenza

Sore throat is a major complaint in some patients with influenza. It is usually associated with other manifestations of the disease, such as myalgia, headache, and cough.[12,21] Coryzal symptoms and hoarseness may also be present. Temperature elevations are common in both adults and children, reaching levels of 38.3°C or higher. Edema and erythema of the pharyngeal mucosa may be present but are not marked. Pharyngeal exudates and painful cervical adenopathy are not part of influenzal pharyngitis. Defervescence occurs in 3–4 days on the average, but in some uncomplicated cases fever may last up to 1 week (see Ch. 141).

Pharyngoconjunctival Fever

The clinical presentation of adenoviral pharyngitis is usually more severe than pharyngitis associated with the common cold. Malaise, myalgia, headache, chills, and dizziness often accompany adenovirus infections. Temperature elevations persist for 5–6 days in studies of recognized cases. Sore throat is often marked. On examination, pharyngeal erythema and exudate may be present, mimicking streptococcal pharyngitis. A distinguishing feature of adenovirus pharyngitis, when present, is conjunctivitis, which occurs in one-third to one-half of cases. The conjunctivitis is of the follicular type and is bilateral in about one-fourth of the cases when it occurs. Cough, hoarseness, and substernal pain occur in ARD in military recruits but are usually not prominent features of pharyngoconjunctival fever in civilian populations (see Ch. 121).

Acute Herpetic Pharyngitis

Primary infection with herpes simplex virus may present as an acute pharyngitis. Mild cases are indistinguishable from those caused by other respiratory viruses. In severe cases of herpetic pharyngitis, the presence of inflammation and exudate may mimic full-blown streptococcal pharyngitis. Vesicles and shallow ulcers of the palate are characteristic of herpetic infection and when present are helpful in the differential diagnosis. Tender cervical adenopathy and fever are seen in some cases. Vesicles or ulcers are present on the labial and buccal mucosa when there is an associated gingivostomatitis. Acute primary herpetic infection should be distinguished from chronic mucocutaneous infection of the oropharynx due to herpes simplex virus. The chronic form of the disease is seen exclusively in patients with impaired immunity and is characterized by large shallow, painful ulcers that slowly progress unless the patient's immune status improves or antiviral therapy is given (see Ch. 115).

Herpangina

Herpangina is an uncommon type of pharyngitis caused by coxsackieviruses and is distinguished by the presence of small vesicles (1–2 mm) on the soft palate, uvula, and anterior tonsillar pillars. The lesions rupture to become small white ulcers. Herpangina has been recognized primarily in children, in whom it may manifest as a severe febrile illness with marked sore throat and dysphagia. In some cases anorexia and abdominal pain mimic acute appendicitis (see Ch. 149).

Infectious Mononucleosis

Exudative tonsillitis or pharyngitis occurs in approximately one-half of the cases of infectious mononucleosis due to the EB virus. Fever and cervical adenopathy are characteristically present. The pharyngeal complaints of mononucleosis are usually associated with other features of the disease, such as headache and persistent malaise and fatigue. Generalized adenopathy may be present, and there is enlargement of the spleen in approximately half the cases. The mononucleosis syndrome is also associated with cytomegalovirus infection. Some patients with cytomegalovirus mononucleosis have pharyngeal soreness, but examination of the pharynx is usually unremarkable (see Chs. 117 and 118).

HIV Infection

Febrile pharyngitis is a characteristic feature of primary infection with HIV.[32,33] Following an incubation period of 3–5 weeks, patients have developed fever and pharyngitis associated with varying amounts of myalgia, arthralgia, lethargy, and in some cases nonpruritic maculopapular rash. This has been followed in approximately 1 week by the development of lymphadenopathy. Pharyngeal hyperemia, sometimes marked, has been noted as well as mucosal ulcerations, but exudate has not been described (see Ch. 102).

Streptococcal Pharyngitis

The severity of illness associated with *S. pyogenes* infection of the pharynx varies greatly.[12] In severe cases, there is marked pharyngeal pain, odynophagia, and a temperature of 39.4°C or greater. Headache, chills, and abdominal pain may occur. The pharyngeal membrane is a fiery red, and a thick exudate covers the posterior pharynx and tonsillar area. Edema of the uvula is often pronounced. Tender, enlarged cervical nodes and a leukocyte count of over 12,000/mm³ complete the picture of an acute suppurative bacterial infection. Rhinorrhea and cough are more characteristic of viral infection but may occur.[21] At the other extreme are those streptococcal infections that are so mild as to go unrecognized by the patient or that are indistinguishable from pharyngitis caused by the common respiratory viruses. Infection with strains of *S. pyogenes* that produce erythrogenic toxin results in the characteristic erythematous rash of scarlet fever, which involves the face and skin folds and is followed by desquamation. The tongue is red, and the papillae are enlarged (strawberry tongue). It has recently been recognized that noninvasive pharyngitis due to *S. pyogenes* may be the cause of streptococcal toxic shock syndrome (see Ch. 176).[34,35]

The clinical features of pharyngeal infection with strains of groups C and G streptococci are similar to those of *S. pyogenes*, including the occurrence of purulent exudates, fever, and anterior cervical adenopathy.[10,11] In group C–associated pharyngitis, the signs and symptoms on average are less severe than in group A pharyngitis but more so than in patients with negative bacterial cultures. Cases of groups C and G infection occur in the setting of a common source food epidemic; cold hard-boiled eggs have been recognized as an important vehicle.

Anaerobic Pharyngitis (Vincent's Angina)/ Peritonsillitis/Peritonsillar Abscess (Quinsy)

Pharyngeal and tonsillar infection with a mixture of anaerobic bacteria and spirochetes, while uncommon, still occurs. *Streptococcus pyogenes* and *Staphylococcus aureus* may play a role in some cases. With this infection, a purulent exudate coats the membrane, and there may be a foul odor to the breath. Postanginal septicemia (Lemierre's disease) is a specific form of the condition caused by *Fusobacterium necrophorum*.[36] It is associated with jugular vein septic thrombophlebitis and metastatic infection to the lung and other sites. The disease is most common in adolescents and young adults. Exudative tonsillitis or peritonsillar abscess may be present but in some patients will have subsided by the time the patient is seen. With jugular vein thrombophlebitis, there is pain, swelling, neck stiffness, and dysphagia.

With development of an abscess, pharyngeal pain is usually severe, and dysphagia and low grade fever are common. On examination, there is inflammation and swelling of the peritonsillar area with medical displacement of the tonsil. The infection is usually limited to one side, but when the condition is bilateral, partial obstruction of the pharynx occurs. Rarely, there is extension of the infection along the carotid sheath and into the mediastinum (see Ch. 46).[37]

Gonorrheal Pharyngitis

The incidence of gonococcal infections of the pharynx has increased in recent years. Most infections are asymptomatic, but gonorrheal infection may be responsible for an occasional case of mild pharyngitis[38] (see Ch. 190).

Diphtheria

Although uncommon today, diphtheria still occurs in unvaccinated populations in the United States. The disease characteristically has a slow onset, and pharyngeal discomfort is usually not marked. Temperature elevation is present but is low grade. The characteristic tonsillar or pharyngeal membrane varies from light to dark gray and is firmly adherent to the tonsil and pharyngeal mucosa. Human infection with *Corynebacterium ulcerans* is a rare cause of human pharyngeal infection. It is associated with the consumption of raw milk and has presented as mild pharyngitis but in one case presented as serious diphtheria (see Ch. 184).[39]

Arcanobacterial Pharyngitis

Arcanobacterium hemolyticum has been increasingly identified as a cause of exudative pharyngitis, clinically similar to that caused by β-hemolytic streptococci.[40–43] Characteristically, the infection has been recognized in children, adolescents, and young adults and is associated with a diffuse, sometimes pruritic, erythematous maculopapular skin rash on the extremities and trunk. Cases of *A. hemolyticum* with membranous pharyngitis that mimics diphtheria[44] and with peritonsillar abscess[45] have also been reported.

Yersinial Pharyngitis

Yersinia enterocolitica causes exudative pharyngitis, which in adults may occur without the typical enterocolitis seen in children. Fever, prominent cervical lymphadenopathy, and abdominal pain with or without diarrhea have been reported.[46,47] A fulminant course with high mortality has been associated with reported cases of yersinial pharyngitis, making recognition important.

Chlamydial Pharyngitis

The new species *Chlamydia pneumoniae* (strain TWAR) has been established as an etiologic agent of acute infections of the respiratory tract, some of which have pharyngeal manifestations.[20] Pharyngitis with or without fever has occurred as a separate illness and also in association with pneumonia or bronchitis.[19] Distinguishing clinical features of the pharyngitis have not been described, but chronicity of infection despite antimicrobial therapy has been noted.

Mycoplasmal Pharyngitis

Epidemiologic studies of pharyngitis have associated some cases with *Mycoplasma pneumoniae* infection. The illnesses observed have been relatively mild and have had no distinguishing clinical features. *Mycoplasma pneumoniae* characteristically causes bronchitis and primary atypical pneumonia (see Ch. 161).

Noninfectious Pharyngitis

Occasional cases presenting as an inflammatory pharyngitis may have noninfectious causes. These include conditions such as bullous pemphigoid, systemic lupus erythematosis, Behçet's disease, and paraquat ingestion. Kawasaki syndrome may present as a febrile sore throat without exudate. It occurs in children and is associated with characteristic findings of the lips, tongue, and skin.

DIAGNOSIS

The primary objectives in the diagnosis of acute pharyngitis are to distinguish cases of common viral etiology from those due to *S. pyogenes* and to detect and identify the occasional case due to an unusual or rare cause for which treatment is available. In the majority of cases, an etiologic diagnosis is not possible on clinical grounds alone. The presence of pharyngeal or tonsillar exudates, tender adenopathy, skin rash, or conjunctivitis aids in the differential diagnosis, but these findings are not entirely specific and are not present with sufficient frequency to be helpful in most cases.

The list of etiologic agents associated with the presence of pharyngeal exudate include groups A, C, and G streptococci; the anaerobic bacteria; *C. diphtheriae; A. hemolyticum; Y. enterocolitica;* adenovirus; herpes simplex virus; and EB virus. However, pharyngeal exudate is not always present with these infections so that its absence does not exclude them from consideration. On the other hand, exudate is rarely, if ever, seen in the large group of cases of pharyngitis due to the common cold viruses and influenza. The presence of skin rash suggests the possibility of infection with *S. pyogenes, A. hemolyticum,* HIV, and EB virus. Toxic shock syndrome should also be considered. The presence of conjunctivitis suggests infection with adenovirus and some types of enterovirus.

The development of rapid antigen detection tests, using a specimen collected by throat swab, has been a significant advance in the diagnosis of streptococcal pharyngitis. When used in clinical practice, the reported specificity of such tests has been over 90 percent, but the sensitivity has been lower (60 to 95 percent), depending in part on the sensitivity of the culture method used as a control.[48,49]

The sensitivity of culture methods to detect *S. pyogenes* in pharyngeal secretions has recently been reviewed.[50] No single combination of medium and atmosphere was thought likely to detect all possible isolates of the bacteria, but four methods were judged capable of detecting 90–95 percent from symptomatic patients. These were sheep blood agar incubated anaerobically for 48 hours; sheep blood agar incubated aerobically (without CO_2 supplementation) for 48 hours, using a cover glass to reduce oxygen tension on the primary inoculum zone; and sheep blood agar containing sulfamethoxazole and trimethoprim incubated aerobically (5–10 percent CO_2) or anaerobically for 48 hours. The use of anaerobic conditions may improve recovery of group C streptococci.

The performance characteristics of the antigen detection tests have dictated a strategy in which a positive test establishes the diagnosis of streptococcal pharyngitis, while a negative test should be followed by a throat culture on sheep blood agar. Among the advantages of routinely performing an antigen detection test and/or culture in patients with pharyngitis are that the test results may influence the management of family members and other close contacts who subsequently become ill, and a negative test should prompt consideration of the more unusual, and sometimes serious, causes of pharyngeal infection, especially in patients with fever and exudative disease.

The patient's history and a consideration of epidemiologic factors may be helpful in suggesting a specific etiologic diagnosis in cases in which the antigen detection test is negative. Other family members frequently have common colds and influenzal illnesses. The season of the year and the occurrence of known epidemics may provide clues of diagnosis. Rhinovirus infections predominate in the fall and spring and coronavirus infections in the winter. The occurrence of an influenza epidemic in the community is usually known to the physician. Patients with pharyngoconjunctival fever, a summer illness, may give a history of swimming, and they or a family member may have conjunctivitis. The diagnosis of infectious mononucleosis, primary HIV infection, and diphtheria may be suggested by the nonpharyngeal manifestations of these infections.

Examination of the structures of the pharynx should be thorough and should include examination of the nasopharynx and larynx when diphtheria is suspected. In children under the age of 3 years, the presence of an exudate is a less reliable indicator of streptococcal infection than it is in older children and adults. Diphtheria produces a pseudomembrane that may be mistaken for an exudate. The presence of small vesicles or ulcers suggests herpes simplex virus infection or herpangina. The mucosal lesions of herpangina are less numerous and more confined to the area of the palate than are those of herpes simplex virus, which may involve the entire oropharynx. Aphthous stomatitis, a benign condition of unknown cause, produces small painful mucosal ulcers that are sometimes confused with those of herpetic infection. Aphthosis tends to be recurrent, in contrast to acute herpetic pharyngitis, and with the usual case of aphthosis there are fewer lesions, which are usually located in the anterior part of the mouth.

Medial displacement of one or both tonsils is seen with peritonsillitis or peritonsillar abscess, and dysphagia may be present. Patients with postanginal septicemia with jugular vein thrombophlebitis will have malaise, fever, and chills, suggestive of serious illness. Also pain, tenderness, and swelling at the angle of the jaw and stiff neck are characteristic, but these findings may be subtle. Patients with infectious mononucleosis usually have generalized adenopathy and may have enlargement of the spleen. Severe sore throat and odynophagia in an adult in the absence of findings in the pharynx should suggest epiglottitis (see Ch. 45).

Laboratory tests are available to help in the diagnosis of some of the above-mentioned infections. *Neisseria gonorrhea* may be detected on Thayer-Martin or other suitable media. Vincent's angina is diagnosed by a crystal violet–stained smear of the pharyngeal or tonsillar exudate showing the presence of numerous fusobacteria and spirochetes. Blood cultures should be obtained in cases of suspected postanginal septicemia, and radiographic examination of the lungs, bones, and large joint may detect metastatic infection. A throat culture using Loeffler's medium should be obtained in all suspected cases of diphtheria (see Ch. 183). The hemolysis associated with *A. hemolyticum* becomes maximal at 48–72 hours and is more prominent on rabbit and human blood agar than sheep blood agar; thus this organism may be missed on standard throat culture.[41,43] The diagnosis of infectious mononucleosis can be confirmed by specific serologic tests (see Ch. 118). HIV antigen has been detected in the serum of patients with pharyngitis due to primary HIV infection.[28] Also, suspected cases of this infection should be followed for appearance of serum antibody to HIV. Cultures and rapid diagnostic tests for influenza virus, adenovirus, herpes simplex virus, cytomegalovirus, and *M. pneumoniae* are now available in some laboratories. Acute and convalescent (3-week) serum specimens are necessary for serologic tests for these agents. Laboratory tests for the common cold viruses are not readily available. Diagnostic tests for *C. pneumoniae* are being developed[20] but are not commercially available at present.

Pharyngitis due to noninfectious causes may sometimes present a diagnostic problem. Pemphigus, bullous pemphigoid, and systemic lupus erythematosus are among the diseases that can cause pharyngeal inflammation and discomfort. Also drug reactions are sometimes manifest by pharyngeal soreness, as is agranulocytosis. The presence of other manifestations of these diseases, particularly involvement of the skin, is helpful in leading to the diagnosis.

TREATMENT AND PREVENTION

Antimicrobial Therapy

Streptococcal Pharyngitis.   Patients with pharyngitis due to *S. pyogenes* should receive a 10-day course of penicillin[51–54] or an equivalent antibiotic if the patient is allergic to penicillin. The recommended oral dose of penicillin V in adults is 200,000 or 250,000 units every 6–8 hours and in children 50,000 units/kg/24 hours divided into three or four equal doses. An injection of long-acting benzathine penicillin is an excellent, although painful, form of therapy because it does not require patient compliance. The adult dose of benzathine penicillin is 1.2 million units. In patients who are allergic to penicillin, a 10-day course of erythromycin is recommended. In some areas of the world, erythromycin resistance of *S. pyogenes* is sufficiently prevalent to be a problem, but this has not occurred in the United States.[52] For patients who are allergic to penicillin, erythromycin is recommended as an alternative for treatment. First-generation cephalosporins such as cephalexin and cefadroxil are also suitable for treating streptococcal pharyngitis. Although a number of new antimicrobial drugs have activity against *S. pyogenes,* they offer no advantage over penicillin or the first-generation cephalosporins and are more expensive.

The availability of rapid antigen detection tests for *S. pyogenes* has reduced, but not eliminated, the dilemma of when to begin antimicrobial therapy in the suspected case. In patients with a positive antigen test, treatment should be started immediately, with the goals of providing maximal symptomatic relief for the acute illness, eradicating or suppressing the infection to prevent transmission, and preventing suppurative and nonsuppurative complications.[52,55-57] In patients with a negative test in which the clinical diagnosis of streptococcal pharyngitis is still entertained, either of two strategies is recommended. One strategy is to await the results of throat culture before starting treatment; the other is to begin therapy when the patient is originally seen and to discontinue treatment if the culture is negative. Both of these approaches have advantages and disadvantages. Withholding treatment until culture results are known limits the immediate therapeutic benefit of antimicrobial therapy but reduces unnecessary drug use. Beginning treatment before the results of culture are known provides maximal therapeutic benefit but exposes many patients to an antimicrobial drug unnecessarily. Initiation of treatment within 1 week of the onset of streptococcal pharyngitis will prevent subsequent acute rheumatic fever,[58] and either of the two approaches will achieve this goal (see Ch. 177). Also, a 48-hour delay in the initiation of penicillin therapy for patients with *S. pyogenes* pharyngitis did not reduce the rate of recurrence with homologous serotypes compared to that in patients in whom treatment was started at the time of diagnosis.[59]

Reports of therapeutic failure with penicillin therapy as manifested by recurrent symptomatic illness do not warrant the abandonment of penicillin as the drug of choice for streptococcal pharyngitis at the present time.[51-54] Penicillin is the only drug that has been demonstrated to prevent rheumatic fever. Also, it has long been known that a 10-day course of penicillin does not necessarily eradicate carriage of the organism from the pharynx. However, the clinical importance of these bacteriologic failures in asymptomatic persons has not been established. Patients with recurrent pharyngitis associated with the documented presence of *S. pyogenes* in the pharynx require antimicrobial therapy. It is unavoidable that some "cases" of streptococcal pharyngitis, initial or recurrent, that are diagnosed by currently available means in reality represent persons with viral pharyngitis who are merely colonized with *S. pyogenes*. A recent study found that using an antibiotic effective against β-lactamase–producing bacteria to treat patients with *S. pyogenes* pharyngitis did not reduce the bacteriologic treatment failure rate.[60]

Because the incidence of acute rheumatic fever had declined to a low level in the United States, the need for *any* antimicrobial treatment of streptococcal pharyngitis was questioned. However, the resurgence of rheumatic fever in some areas of the United States[61-63] and its continuing prevalence in other areas of the world are sufficient reasons not to abandon the general policy of using antimicrobials in the treatment of streptococcal pharyngitis. Discounting the benefit in rheumatic fever prevention and in reduction of acute morbidity, treatment is still important for prevention of suppurative complications of streptococcal pharyngitis, which include sinusitis, otitis media, mastoiditis, lateral sinus thrombosis, bacteremia, and pneumonia.

Anaerobic Pharyngitis/Peritonsillitis/Peritonsillar Abscess. Oral penicillin in the doses recommended for streptococcal pharyngitis has been successfully used in the treatment of anaerobic pharyngitis and peritonsillitis. The use of early antimicrobial therapy has reduced but not eliminated the cases that require surgical drainage of an abscess. Suspected cases of postanginal septicemia require hospitalization and appropriate diagnostic evaluation.[36] Parenteral treatment with high doses of penicillin or another antimicrobial with activity against *F. necrophorum* should be given for a prolonged course.

Diphtheria. The treatment of diphtheria is described in Chapter 183.

Arcanobacterial Pharyngitis. *Arcanobacterium hemolyticum* pharyngitis has been reported not to respond to a standard 10-day course of penicillin V but did respond to one injection of benzathine penicillin or a course of oral erythromycin.[40,41,43]

Yersinial Pharyngitis. *Yersinia enterocolitica* is usually susceptible to aminoglycosides, trimethoprim-sulfamethoxazole, and third-generation cephalosporins but resistant to penicillin (see Ch. 208).

Gonorrheal Pharyngitis. The treatment of gonococcal infections is described in Chapter 190.

Mycoplasma Pharyngitis. The treatment of *M. pneumoniae* is described in Chapter 161.

Viral Pharyngitis. Amantadine, if given early in the course of illness, has a therapeutic effect for type A influenza. It is recommended for cases of presumed influenzal pharyngitis occurring during a known influenza type A epidemic (see Ch. 141). Acyclovir and foscarnet are available for the treatment of oropharyngeal herpes simplex virus infection (see Ch. 32).

Symptomatic Therapy

Treatment is directed at relieving pharyngeal discomfort and associated systemic or respiratory symptoms. Warm saline gargles and supportive measures such as rest, analgesics, and liquids are sufficient in most cases of viral pharyngitis. Ibuprofen was superior to acetaminophen in relieving throat pain associated with tonsillitis and pharyngitis in 6- to 12-year-old children.[64] Symptomatic therapy is also helpful in relieving symptoms of streptococcal pharyngitis. Patients with severe streptococcal pharyngitis or peritonsillitis may be in extreme discomfort and require liberal use of analgesics during the early course of illness. Hospitalization is necessary with some types of pharyngitis that are associated with systemic illness or that have serious or life-threatening complications.

Prevention

Tonsillectomy has been shown to reduce the incidence of throat infections in children who were severely affected with recurrent pharyngitis.[65] However, it is not recommended as a routine practice.[66] Penicillin prophylaxis for *S. pyogenes* infection is required for patients at risk of recurrent rheumatic fever (see Ch. 177). Active immunization is available for types A and B influenza and for diphtheria (see Chs. 141 and 300). The prophylactic administration of amantadine is also effective against type A influenza. Prophylactic intravenous and oral acyclovir are effective in preventing mucocutaneous herpes simplex virus infection in immunosuppressed patients (see Ch. 32). Live adenovirus vaccines have been used successfully in military populations but are not available for civilian use (see Ch. 121). There has been work on experimental vaccines for a number of the agents that cause pharyngitis, including *S. pyogenes,* but these vaccines are still in the experimental stage of development.

REFERENCES

1. Stuart-Harris CH, Andrewes C, Andrews BE, et al. A collaborative study of the aetiology of acute respiratory infection in Britain 1961–4. A report of the Medical Research Council working party on acute respiratory virus infections. Br Med J. 1965;2:319.
2. Gwaltney JM Jr. Virology of middle ear. Am Otol Rhinol Laryngol. 1971;80:365.
3. Hamre D, Connelly AP Jr, Procknow JJ. Virologic studies of acute respiratory disease in young adults. IV. Virus isolations during four years of surveillance. Am J Epidemiol. 1966;83:238.
4. Monto AS, Ullman BM: Acute respiratory illness in an American community: The Tecumseh study. JAMA. 1974;227:164.

5. Evans AS, Dick EC. Acute pharyngitis and tonsillitis in University of Wisconsin students. JAMA. 1964;190:699.

6. Glezen WP, Clyde WA Jr, Senior RJ, et al. Group A streptococci, mycoplasmas, and viruses associated with acute pharyngitis. JAMA. 1967;202:455.

7. Valle S-L. Febrile pharyngitis as the primary sign of HIV infection in a cluster of cases linked by sexual contact. Scand J Infect Dis. 1987;19:13–7.

8. Stryker WS, Fraser DW, Facklam RR. Foodborne outbreak of group G streptococcal pharyngitis. Am J Epidemiol. 1982;116:533–40.

9. Cohen D, Ferne M, Rouach T, et al. Foodborne outbreak of group G streptococcal sore throat in an Israeli military base. Epidemiol Infect. 1987;99:249–55.

10. Meier FA, Centor RM, Graham L Jr, et al. Clinical and microbiological evidence for endemic pharyngitis among adults due to group C streptococci. Arch Intern Med. 1990;150:825–9.

11. Turner JC, Hayden GF, Kiselica D, et al. Association of group C β-hemolytic streptococci with endemic pharyngitis among college students. JAMA. 1990;264:2644–7.

12. McMillan JA, Sandstrom C, Weiner LB, et al. Viral and bacterial organisms associated with acute pharyngitis in a school-aged population. J Pediatr. 1986;109:747–52.

13. Reed BD, Huck W, Lutz LJ, et al. Prevalence of *Chlamydia trachomatis* and *Mycoplasma pneumoniae* in children with and without pharyngitis. J Fam Pract. 1988;26:387–92.

14. Hofkosh D, Wald ER, Chiponis DM. Prevalence of non-group-A β-hemolytic streptococci in childhood pharyngitis. South Med J. 1988;81:329–31.

15. Hayden GF, Murphy TF, Hendley JO. Non-group A streptococci in the pharynx. Pathogens or innocent bystanders? Am J Dis Child. 1989;143:794–7.

16. Gerber MA, Randolph MF, Martin NJ, et al. Community-wide outbreak of group G streptococcal pharyngitis. Pediatrics. 1991;87:598–603.

17. Gwaltney JM Jr, Hendley JO, Simon G, et al. Rhinovirus infections in an industrial population. I. The occurrence of illness. N Engl J Med. 1966;275:1261.

18. Grayston JT, Kuo C-C, Wang S-P, et al. A new *Chlamydia psittaci* strain, TWAR, isolated in acute respiratory tract infections. N Engl J Med. 1986;315:161–8.

19. Hammerschlag MR, Chirgwin K, Roblin PM, et al. Persistent infection with *Chlamydia pneumoniae* following acute respiratory illness. Clin Infect Dis. 1992;14:178–82.

20. Grayston JT. Infections caused by *Chlamydia pneumoniae* strain TWAR. Clin Infect Dis. 1992;15:757–63.

21. Gwaltney JM Jr. Rhinoviruses. In: Evans AS, ed. Viral Infections of Humans: Epidemiology and Control. 3rd ed. New York: Plenum; 1989:593–611.

22. Hendley JO, Fishburne HB, Gwaltney JM Jr. Coronavirus infections in working adults. Am Rev Respir Dis. 1972;105:805.

23. Wenzel RP, Hendley JO, Davies JA, et al. Coronavirus infections in military recruits. Three-year study with coronavirus strains OC43 and 229E. Am Rev Respir Dis. 1974;109:621.

24. Tyrrell DAJ: Common Colds and Related Diseases: Baltimore: Williams & Wilkins; 1965.

25. Glezen W, Fernald GW, Lohr JA. Acute respiratory disease of university students with special reference to the etiologic role of herpesvirus hominis. Am J Epidemiol. 1975;101:111.

26. Douglas RG Jr, Alford BR, Couch RB: Atraumatic nasal biopsy studies of respiratory virus infections in volunteers. Antimicrob Agents Chemother. 1968;8:340–2.

27. Winther B, Farr B, Turner RB, et al. Histopathologic examination and enumeration of polymorphonuclear leukocytes in the nasal mucosa during experimental rhinovirus colds. Acta Otolaryngol (Stockh) 1984;413(Suppl):19–24.

28. Naclerio RM, Proud D, Lichtenstein, et al. Kinins are generated during experimental rhinovirus colds. J Infect Dis. 1988;157:133–42.

29. Proud D, Naclerio RM, Gwaltney JM, et al. Kinins are generated in nasal secretions during natural rhinovirus colds. J Infect Dis. 1990;161:120–3.

30. Proud D, Reynolds CJ, Lacapra S, et al. Nasal provocation with bradykinin induces symptoms of rhinitis and a sore throat. Am Rev Respir Dis. 1988;137:613–6.

31. Johnson DR, Stevens DL, Kaplan EL. Epidemiologic analysis of group A streptococcal serotypes associated with severe systemic infections, rheumatic fever, or uncomplicated pharyngitis. J Infect Dis. 1992;166:374–82.

32. Valle S-L. Febrile pharyngitis as the primary sign of HIV infection in a cluster of cases linked by sexual contact. Scand J Infect Dis. 1987;19:13–7.

33. Kessler HA, Blaauw B, Spear J, et al. Diagnosis of human immunodeficiency virus infection in seronegative homosexuals presenting with an acute viral syndrome. JAMA. 1987;258:1196–9.

34. Herold AH. Group A beta-hemolytic streptococcal toxic shock from a mild pharyngitis. J Fam Pract. 1990;31:549–51.

35. Chapnick EK, Gradon JD, Lutwick LI, et al. Streptococcal toxic syndrome due to noninvasive pharyngitis. Clin J Infect Dis. 1992;14:1074–7.

36. Moreno S, Altozano JG, Pinilla B, et al. Lemierre's disease: Postanginal bacteremia and pulmonary involvement caused by *Fusobacterium necrophorum*. Rev Infect Dis. 1989;11:319–24.

37. Scully RE, Galdabini JJ, McNeely BU: Case records of the Massachusetts General Hospital. N Engl J Med. 1978;298:894.

38. Hutt DM, Judson FN. Epidemiology and treatment of oropharyngeal gonorrhea. Ann Intern Med. 1986;104:655.

39. Hart RJC. *Corynebacterium ulcerans* in humans and cattle in North Devon. J Hyg Camb. 1984;92:161–4.

40. Banck G, Nyman M. Tonsillitis and rash associated with *Corynebacterium haemolyticum*. J Infect Dis. 1986;154:1037–40.

41. Miller RA, Brancato F, Holmes KK. *Corynebacterium hemolyticum* as a cause of pharyngitis and scarlatiniform rash in young adults. Ann Intern Med. 1986;105:867–72.

42. Greenman JL. *Corynebacterium hemolyticum* and pharyngitis. Ann Intern Med. 1987;106:633.

43. Karpathios T, Drakonaki S, Zervoudaki, et al. *Arcaneobacterium haemolyticum* in children with presumed streptococcal pharyngotonsillitis or scarlet fever. J Pediatr. 1992;12:735–7.

44. Green SL, LaPeter KS. Pseudodiphtheritic membranous pharyngitis caused by *Corynebacterium hemolyticum*. JAMA. 1981;245:2330.

45. Kovatch AL, Schuit KE, Michaels RH. *Corynebacterium hemolyticum* peritonsillar abscess mimicking diphtheria. JAMA. 1983;249:1757.

46. Rose FB, Camp CJ, Antes EJ. Family outbreak of fatal *Yersinia enterocolitica* pharyngitis. Am J Med. 1987;82:636–7.

47. Cover TL, Aber RC. *Yersinia enterocolitica*. N Engl J Med. 1989;321:16–24.

48. Rapid diagnostic tests for group A streptococcal pharyngitis. Med Lett. 1991;33:40–41.

49. Wegner DL, White DL, Schrantz RD. Insensitivity of rapid antigen detection methods and single blood agar plate culture for diagnosing streptococcal pharyngitis. JAMA. 1992;267:695–7.

50. Kellog JA. Suitability of throat culture procedures for detection of group A streptococci and as reference standards for evaluation of streptococcal antigen detection kits. J Clin Microbiol. 1990;28:165–9.

51. Peter G. Streptococcal pharyngitis: Current therapy and criteria for evaluation of new agents. Clin Infect Dis. 1992;14(Suppl):S218–23, S231–2.

52. Denny FW. Current management of streptococcal pharyngitis. J Fam. Pract. 1992;35:619–20.

53. Paradise JL. Etiology and management of pharyngitis and pharyngotonsillitis in children: A current review. Ann Otol Rhinol Laryngol. 1992;155:51–7.

54. Pichichero ME. The rising incidence of penicillin treatment failures in group A streptococcal tonsillopharyngitis: An emerging role for the cephalosporins? Pediatr Infect Dis J. 1991;10:S50–5.

55. Nelson JD. The effect of penicillin therapy on the symptoms and signs of streptococcal pharyngitis. Pediatr Infect Dis. 1984;3:10.

56. Krober MS, Bass JW, Michels GN. Streptococcal pharyngitis. Placebo-controlled double-blind evaluation of clinical response to penicillin therapy. JAMA. 1985;253:1271.

57. Randolph MF, Gerber MA, DeMeo KK, et al. The effect of antibiotic therapy on the clinical course of streptococcal pharyngitis. J Pediatr. 1985;106:870.

58. Caranzaro FJ, Stetson CA, Morris AJ, et al: The role of the streptococcus in the pathogenesis of rheumatic fever. Am J Med. 1954;17:749.

59. Gerber MA, Randolph MF, DeMeo KK, et al. Lack of impact of early antibiotic therapy for streptococcal pharyngitis on recurrence rates. J Pediatr. 1990;117:853–8.

60. Tanz RR, Shulman ST, Sroka PA, et al. Lack of influence of beta-lactamase–producing flora on recovery of group A streptococci after treatment of acute pharyngitis. J Pediatr. 1990;117:859–63.

61. Wald ER, Dashefsky B, Feidt C, et al. Acute rheumatic fever in western Pennsylvania and the tristate area. Pediatrics. 1987;80:371.

62. Congeni B, Rizzo C, Congeni J, et al. Outbreak of acute rheumatic fever in northeast Ohio. J Pediatr. 1987;111:176.

63. Papadimos T, Escamilla J. Acute rheumatic fever at a Navy training center—San Diego, California. Leads from the MMWR. JAMA. 1988;259:1787.

64. Bertin L, Pons G, d'Athis P, et al. Randomized, double-blind, multicenter, controlled trial of ibuprofen versus acetaminophen (paracetamol) and placebo for treatment of symptoms of tonsillitis and pharyngitis in children. J Pediatr. 1991;119:811–4.

65. Paradise JL, Bluestone CD, Bachman RZ, et al. Efficacy of tonsillectomy for recurrent throat infection in severely affected children. Results of parallel randomized and nonrandomized clinical trials. N Engl J Med. 1984;310:674.

66. Hendley JO. Tonsillectomy: Justified but not mandated in special patients. N Engl J Med. 1984;310:717.

41. ACUTE LARYNGITIS

JACK M. GWALTNEY, JR.

Acute laryngitis usually occurs in association with the common cold and influenzal syndromes. Lowering of the normal pitch of the voice, hoarseness, and occasionally aphonia are the characteristic complaints[1,2]; obstruction of the airway is rare in adults. In young children, airway obstruction due to infection of the larynx and tracheobronchial tree is more common, and acute laryngitis must be distinguished from acute bacterial su-

TABLE 1. Occurrence of Hoarseness with Acute Respiratory Infections

Infectious Agent	Incidence of Hoarseness (%)
Viruses	
Influenza virus	22–37 (3, 4)[a]
Rhinovirus	10–25 (4, 5)
Adenovirus	6–25 (5, 6)
Parainfluenza virus	2–18 (5)
Respiratory syncytial virus	10 (5)
Coxsackievirus A21	9 (5)
Coronavirus	Not determined[b]
Bacteria	
Streptococcus pyrogenes	10 (4)
Moraxella catarrhalis	Not determined[7,8,13]

[a] Numbers in parentheses are reference numbers.
[b] In one small study of hospitalized Marine recruits, hoarseness was present in 7 of 11 patients with coronavirus infection diagnosed by seroconversion to coronavirus OC43.[14]

praglottitis (epiglottitis) (see Ch. 45) Acute supraglottitis has been recognized with increasing frequency in adults, but is still unusual.

Hoarseness is present in 20 percent of cases of common respiratory illness.[3] It occurs most frequently with midwinter illnesses and correlates with the occurrence of cough and, to a lesser extent, sore throat. All the major respiratory viruses have been reported to cause hoarseness (Table 1).[3–6] Influenza virus, rhinovirus, and adenovirus have most often been the cause of laryngitis in reported studies. The role of secondary bacterial invasion in acute laryngitis is not clear; however, *Moraxella catarrhalis* has been recovered from the nasopharynx of 50 to 55 percent of adults with acute laryngitis compared with 6 to 14 percent of controls.[7,8] Hoarseness was also reported by approximately 10 percent of adults with streptococcal pharyngitis.[4] Unusual causes of laryngitis include syphilis, tuberculosis,[9] herpes zoster,[10] histoplasmosis, blastomycosis, and candidiasis. Candidal laryngitis has been recognized chiefly in patients with impaired immunity.[11,12]

Diagnosis of acute laryngitis is usually appeared from the history and clinical characteristics of the illness. Eighty-seven percent of patients with laryngitis reporting to an otolaryngology clinic had preceding upper respiratory tract infection symptoms, and 13 percent reported prior voice abuse.[8] Examination of the larynx reveals hyperemia, edema, or vascular injection of the vocal cords, and there may be superficial mucosal ulcerations. The presence of an exudate or membrane on the pharyngeal or laryngeal mucosa should arouse the suspicion of streptococcal infection, mononucleosis, or diphtheria. In acute epiglottitis, the epiglottis is characteristically intensely red and greatly swollen. Patients with traumatic aphonia usually give a history of excessive use of the voice.

A recent controlled trial of erythromycin versus placebo was conducted in adults with acute laryngitis.[13] After the first week of treatment, the isolation rate of *M. catarrhalis* was reduced from 60 to 10 percent in the erythromycin-treated group compared with 37 to 27 percent in the placebo group. Treated patients had significantly lower scores of subjective voice disturbance after 1 week, although laryngologic examination and voice evaluation did not show differences between the groups. An earlier double-blind study failed to show a beneficial effect of penicillin V in the treatment of adults with acute laryngitis.[8] Symptomatic treatment consists of resting the voice until hoarseness and aphonia have subsided. Inhalation of moistened air on a regular basis may also give relief. Diphtheritic laryngitis and acute bacterial supraglottitis require specific antimicrobial therapy. Patients with hoarseness persisting longer than 10 days to 2 weeks should have a laryngoscopic examination to exclude tumors and other chronic diseases of the larynx.

REFERENCES

1. Proctor DF: The upper airways. II. The larynx and trachea. Am Rev Respir Dis. 1977;115:315.
2. Vaughan CW. Current concepts in otolaryngology. Diagnosis and treatment of organic voice disorders. N Engl J Med. 1982;307:863.
3. Dingle JH, Badger GF, Jordan WS Jr: Illness in the Home. A study of 25,000 Illnesses in a Group of Cleveland Families. Cleveland: The Press of Western Reserve University; 1964:66.
4. Gwaltney JM Jr: Rhinoviruses. In: Evans, AS, ed. Viral Infections of Humans: Epidemiology and Control. 3rd ed. New York: Plenum; 1989:593–615.
5. Tyrrell DAJ: *Common Colds and Related Diseases.* Baltimore: Williams & Wilkins; 1965:95.
6. McNamara MJ, Pierce WE, Crawford YE, et al. Patterns of adenovirus infection in the respiratory diseases of naval recruits. A longitudinal study of two companies of naval recruits. Am Rev Respir Dis. 1962;86:485.
7. Schalén L, Christensen P, Kamme C, et al. High isolation rate of *Branhamella catarrhalis* from the nasopharynx in adults with acute laryngitis. Scand J Infect Dis. 1980;12:277.
8. Schalen L, Christensen P, Eliasson I, et al. Inefficacy of penicillin V in acute laryngitis in adults. Evaluation from results of double-blind study. Ann Otol Laryngol. 1985;94:14.
9. Bachman AL, Zizmor J, Noyek AM. Tuberculosis of the larynx. Semin Roentgenol. 1979;14:325.
10. Lederer FJ, Soboroff BJ. Medical problems related to diseases of the larynx. Otolaryngol Clin North Am. 1970;3:599.
11. Lawson R, Bodey G, Luna M. *Candida* infection presenting as laryngitis. Am J Med Sci. 1980;280:173.
12. Dudley JP, Byrne WJ, Kobayashi R, et al. *Candida* laryngitis in chronic mucocutaneous candidiasis. Its association with *Candida* esophagitis. Ann Otol Rhinol Laryngol. 1980;89:574.
13. Schalen L, Eliasson I, Fex S, et al. Acute laryngitis in adults: Results of erythromycin treatment. Acta Oto-Laryngol 1992;492(Suppl):55–7.
14. Wenzel RP, Hendley JO, Davies JA, et al. Coronavirus infections in military recruits. Three-year study with coronavirus strains OC43 and 229E. Am Rev Respir Dis. 1974;109:621.

42. ACUTE LARYNGO-TRACHEOBRONCHITIS (CROUP)

CAROLINE BREESE HALL

... the sharp stridulous voice which I can resemble to nothing more nearly than the crowing of a cock ... is the true diagnostic sign of the disease.—Francis Home, 1765[1]

Croup, or acute laryngotracheobronchitis, is an age-specific viral infection of the upper and lower respiratory tract that produces inflammation in the subglottic area and results in the striking picture of dyspnea accompanied on inspiration by the characteristic stridulous notes of croup. Croup demonstrates perhaps best the piquant interaction of host and microorganism. Age, sex, an undefined predisposition of the child, and the type of virus all appear to influence the susceptibility and severity of the infection.

Francis Home of Edinburgh first introduced the word *croup* in his famous treatise *An Inquiry into the Nature, Cause and Cure of Croup,* in which he describes 12 patients with croup.[1] The term *croup* has been traced to an Anglo-Saxon word *kropan*[2] and to the old Scottish term *roup,* which meant "to cry out in a shrill voice."

Croup at that time and for the next century was the term often applied to a number of disease entities including diphtheria. John Cheyne,[3] however, appeared to describe not only diphtheria, cynache trachealis, but also croup that appeared most similar to the viral laryngotracheobronchitis of today. Bretonneau in 1859 argued that diphtheria was a separate and specific disease.[4] However, the confusion between "membranous" or "true croup" and "spasmodic" or "false croup" continued. Differentiation awaited Klebs' discovery of *Corynebacterium diphtheriae* in 1883. In 1948, Rabe[5] classified the forms of infectious croup according to etiology—bacterial or nonbacterial—and suggested that the latter, larger group may be viral in origin. In only 15 percent of his 347 patients was he able to identify a pathogen, namely, *C. diphtheriae* or *Haemophilus influenzae* type b.

The term *croup* now generally refers to an acute laryngotracheitis or laryngotracheobronchitis caused by a viral infection. Many children develop croup only once during childhood despite multiple infections with the viruses that are the prime etiologic agents. In some children, however, such viral infections may be manifest as repeated episodes of croup in early childhood. In such children the illness is often called *spasmodic croup*. An episode of spasmodic croup, however, cannot be differentiated from a single episode of the usual case of croup in its clinical manifestations, nor in its etiology, which is usually viral.

INCIDENCE

Croup is a relatively common illness in young children, accounting for about 10–15 percent of lower respiratory tract disease in children. In Hoekelman's prospective study[6] of infectious diseases occurring in pediatric practice in the first year of life, 1.2 percent of the infants studied developed croup. However, the peak occurrence of croup is in the second year of life, with most cases occurring between 3 months and 3 years of age.[7–10] In a Seattle prepaid group practice, the annual incidence of croup per 1000 children under 6 years of age was 7.[7] In the first 6 months of life the rate was 5.2, and in the second 6 months of life the rate was 11. The peak incidence was 14.9 in the second year of life, and fell to half that rate in the third year of life. In a group practice in North Carolina, the incidence was about three to five times higher, with a peak of 47 per 1000 each year for children in the second year of life.[10] Even in the first 6 months of life the incidence was 24, and after 6 years of age it was 4.6. In series of hospitalized or outpatient cases of croup, boys predominate, although the attack rates of upper respiratory illnesses by the same viral agents show no sex preference.[7,9–13]

ETIOLOGY

Acute laryngotracheobronchitis may be caused by a variety of viral agents and occasionally by *Mycoplasma pneumoniae* (Table 1).[7,8,10–16] Parainfluenza type 1 virus is the most common cause of croup in the United States and Great Britain (Table 1). Parainfluenza type 3 virus is usually the second most frequently associated agent. In infants this virus more commonly tends to

cause bronchiolitis and pneumonia. However, the more frequent manifestation in children 2–3 years of age is croup, and in older children it is tracheobronchitis.[11,17] Outbreaks with both influenza A and B viruses may result in appreciable numbers of croup cases, especially with influenza A virus. Although influenza, because of its unpredictable nature and fluctuating seasonal occurrence, may be a less frequent instigator of croup than the parainfluenza viruses, some studies have reported it to be more severe,[18–20] while others have not.[10] Influenza A virus may produce croup in a broader age range of children and sometimes with a higher frequency of hospitalization. In Washington, DC, between 1957 and 1976, 14.3 percent of the croup patients had influenza A or B viral infection.[14] Influenza A virus more commonly caused croup than did influenza B virus, and the frequency of croup appeared to be related to the particular strain of influenza. Croup was more frequently observed in H_3N_2 than in H_2N_2 epidemics.[20]

Only a small proportion (approximately 5 percent) of respiratory syncytial viral infections results in croup, but anywhere from 1 to 11 percent of the reported croup cases have been associated with this virus (Table 1). The mean age of croup cases associated with respiratory syncytial virus tends to be younger, in the first year of life, especially in hospitalized cases, and the course may be more severe and prolonged. Adenoviral infection infrequently results in croup, although laryngitis is a relatively common manifestation of adenoviral infection. In contrast, croup is the characteristic manifestation of parainfluenza type 2 viral infection. However, the total proportion of croup cases produced by parainfluenza type 2 virus is less than that associated with types 1 and 3. This is because type 2 virus tends to be a less frequent visitor to a community, and sizable outbreaks of infection with parainfluenza type 2 virus are unusual in comparison to outbreaks with type 1.[9–11,17] Rhinoviruses, enteroviruses, and *M. pneumoniae* all contribute a small, but variable proportion of cases.

The proportion of croup cases caused by the different agents varies somewhat according to age. The parainfluenza viruses remain the major agents at all ages, but, in the first few months of life, respiratory syncytial virus ascends in importance, and the influenza viruses and *M. pneumoniae* predominately cause croup in children older than 5 years of age.[10]

Of all these agents, only parainfluenza type 1 virus and influenza viruses occur in epidemics and have a great enough predilection for causing croup to produce an appreciable rise in the number of community croup cases during their season of activity.[7,10,13,20,21] Outbreaks of respiratory syncytial virus rarely are

TABLE 1. Percentage of Croup Cases Associated with Various Agents

Agent	Cramblett 1977[14] (%)	Parrott et al. 1962[15] (%)	Loda et al. 1968[16] (%)	Glezen et al. 1971[11] (%)	Foy et al. 1973[7] (%)		Buchan et al. 1974[13] (%)	Downham et al. 1974[8] (%)	Denny et al. 1983[10] (%)
Parainfluenza virus									
Type 1	8	21	39	21	13[a]	6.4[b]	25	26	18
Type 2	6	8	1.6	4	1.4	7.3	1.7	6	3
Type 3	14	10	1.6	9	3	13	8	10	6.6
Influenza A	6			2	1	3.7	10	6	1.4
Influenza B				1	1	2			1.2
Respiratory syncytial		8	11.4	6	1	9	1.7	6	3.8
Adenovirus	4	9	3	1	4	4.6	1.7	3	
Rhinovirus				0.6	2		1	6	
Enterovirus	12			1	1		1		
Other viruses							5		2
Mycoplasma pneumoniae			5	1.4	0.5	2		1	1.4
Total percentage of cases with identified agent	50	64	62	47	56		54	64	37.6

[a] Identified by isolation of agent.
[b] Identified by serology.

associated with a similar notable rise of community cases. Parainfluenza type 2 viruses frequently produce croup, but outbreaks with parainfluenza type 2 virus are erratic and often minimal in size.[17]

Recent outbreaks of measles in the United States have been an unfortunate reminder that rubeola in the prevaccine era often resulted in severe and complicated croup. In the recent upsurge of measles cases, laryngotracheobronchitis complicated approximately 20 percent of the hospitalized measles cases in Los Angeles and Houston.[22,23] Children with croup as a complication of measles tended to be younger, and their course more severe, with 17–22 percent requiring intubation. In some the outcome was fatal.

EPIDEMIOLOGY

The epidemiologic patterns of croup mainly reflect the seasonal patterns of the major agents. Since parainfluenza type 1 virus causes the largest proportion of croup cases, the major peak of cases occurs when this virus is prevalent in the community. In recent years, parainfluenza type 1 virus has tended to cause outbreaks of infection every other year in the fall.[9,11,13,17] Outbreaks of croup that occur in the winter to early spring are most apt to be related to influenza A and B viral activities and, to a lesser extent, to respiratory syncytial virus activity.[9–11,21] Sporadic cases of croup commonly are associated with parainfluenza type 3 virus. This virus previously tended to be present throughout much of the year, but more recently has been observed to have swells of activity during the warmer months of late spring and summer.[8,11,13,17] Sporadic cases of croup may also be caused by any of the less commonly associated agents such as the adenoviruses, rhinoviruses, and *M. pneumoniae,* which may be prevalent through many months of the year. Croup from enteroviruses, although uncommon, tends to occur in the summer and early fall. Parainfluenza type 2 virus tends to produce smaller outbreaks of infection at less predictable intervals, commonly in the fall and early winter.[8–10,13]

PATHOPHYSIOLOGY

The viral infection initially affects the upper respiratory tract, usually producing inflammation of the nasal passages and nasopharynx. Subsequently, the infection spreads downward to involve essentially all levels of the respiratory tract. The classic signs of croup—the stridor, hoarseness, and cough—arise mostly from the inflammation occurring in the larynx and trachea. However, involvement of the lower respiratory tract is also present in most cases requiring hospitalization.[24] The inflammation and obstruction are greatest at the subglottic level. This is the least distensible part of the airway since it is encircled by the cricoid cartilage with the narrow anterior ring and the larger posterior quadrangular lamina, forming a "signet ring."

Inflammation at the subglottic level results in the characteristic obstruction observed in viral croup. The impeded flow of air through this narrowed area produces the classic high-pitched vibratory sounds, or stridor. This is most apparent on inspiration since the negative pressure tends to narrow the extrathoracic airway further, much as sucking on a partially occluded paper straw causes it to collapse inwardly. This is enhanced in young children as their airway walls are relatively compliant.[25] In 1836, Ley[26] described the characteristic findings of croup:

> The shrill sonorous inspiration so characteristic of this complaint, marks very unequivocally its seat. . . . From some cause there is an unusual approximation of the sides of the glottis . . . the influence being very analogous to that produced by too strong compression of the reed against the mouthpiece of the clarionet by the lips of one who has made no great proficiency in that instrument, when a harsh, squeaking sound is produced abundantly discordant and grating to the ear.

In histologic sections, inflammatory changes may be seen in the epithelium, the mucosa, and the submucosa of the larynx, trachea, and the linings of the bronchi, bronchioles, and even the alveoli.[27] Small areas of atelectasis may also be present.

Why children in the second year of life are particularly prone to develop croup is not entirely clear. However, a partial explanation is that most of these children are experiencing primary infection with the viral agent, which is more likely to result in spread of the virus to the lower respiratory tract. The anatomy of the young child also may be important in the age predilection. The diameters of the larynx and glottis are relatively small in the young child, and inflammation of the membranes lining these passages causes an appreciably greater degree of obstruction. Airway resistance is highly sensitive to even small changes in the diameter of the airway. In fact, the resistance to airflow is inversely related to the fourth power of the radius of the airway. The mucous membrane is also relatively looser, as well as more vascular, and the cartilage ring is less rigid. Furthermore, nasal obstruction and crying can aggravate the dynamic narrowing of the child's airway.

Immunologic mechanisms may also be involved in the pathogenesis of croup. Urquhart and colleagues[28] have suggested that the pathogenesis of croup may be different in children with abrupt vs. gradual onset. Noting a different serologic response in such children, they hypothesized that croup of sudden onset resulted from a hypersensitivity to parainfluenza type 1 virus in children with previous infection with a closely related paramyxovirus, such as parainfluenza type 3. In the children with a more gradual onset of prodromal upper respiratory tract symptoms for more than 1 day, antibody to parainfluenza viruses in acute-phase serum was less often present and in lower titers than in acute sera of patients with a sudden onset of croup.

Greater concentrations of IgE antibody to parainfluenza viral antigen and histamine have been detected in children with parainfluenza viral infections whose illness was manifested as croup, wheezing, or both, in comparison to those with only upper respiratory tract illness.[29] Furthermore, the lymphoproliferative responses of peripheral blood lymphocytes from children with parainfluenza viral croup were significantly greater than those from children with upper respiratory tract illness; and the histamine-induced suppression of the lymphoproliferative response of children with croup was diminished.[30] From these findings, Welliver et al.[29,30] have suggested that a defect in regulation of the immune response, similar to that found in atopic subjects, contributes to the pathogenesis of croup.

PHYSIOLOGIC CORRELATIONS

When the infection produces obstruction at the subglottic level, the child's tidal volume initially declines. This, however, is compensated by an increase in the respiratory rate to maintain adequate alveolar ventilation (Fig. 1). However, if the degree of obstruction increases, the work of breathing may increase such that the child tires and can no longer maintain the necessary compensatory respiratory effort. The tidal volume may then further decrease, and, as the respiratory rate declines, hypercarbia and secondary hypoxemia ensue.

Hypoxemia, however, occurs in 80 percent of the children hospitalized with croup.[24] The hypoxemia may arise from the inflammation in the lung parenchyma, which results in an abnormally low ratio of ventilation to perfusion and an increased alveolar-to-arterial gradient (Fig. 1). In some children hypoxemia may result from transient airway hyperreactivity or from pulmonary edema from the marked negative intrathoracic pressures exerted during inspiration in an attempt to compensate for obstruction of the upper airway.

CLINICAL MANIFESTATIONS

The disease generally comes on in the evening after the little patient has been exposed to the weather during the day and often after a

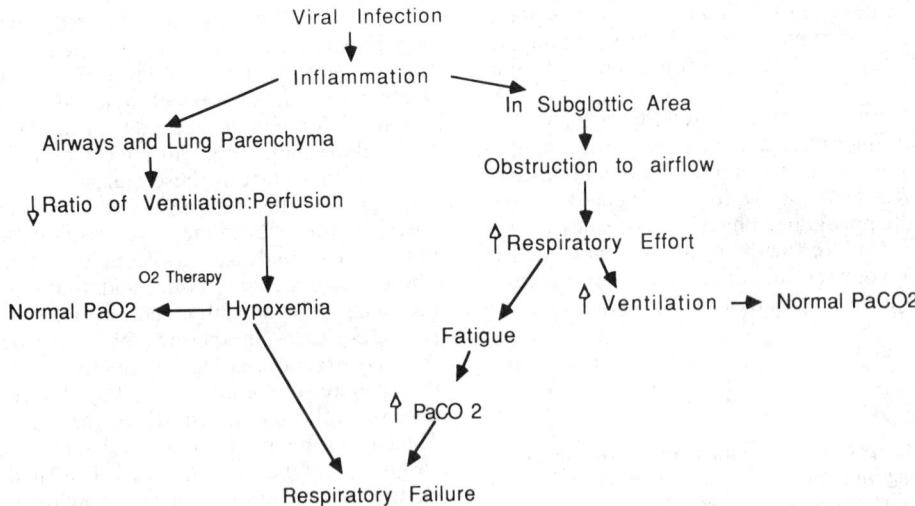

FIG. 1. Physiologic abnormalities in croup.

slight catarrh of some days' standing. At first his voice is observed to be hoarse and pulling . . . he awakens with a most unusual cough, rough, and stridulous. And now his breathing is laborious, each inspiration being accompanied by a harsh, shrill noise.—John Cheyne, 1814[3]

Most children with croup have a history of an upper respiratory tract infection for one to several days previously. Commonly the child has had rhinorrhea, a sore throat, and mild cough. Most children have fever, either initially during the upper respiratory tract infection or at the onset of croup. Children with croup from influenza and parainfluenza viruses commonly have fevers with temperatures ranging from 38–40°C.[31] Fever with respiratory syncytial viral infection tends not to be as high.

The onset of croup commonly is heralded by hoarseness and a deepening cough. The cough is usually not productive but has the striking brassy tone that has earned it the sobriquet "seal's bark." The child may awaken at night with this distinctive cough, tachypnea, and the characteristic inspiratory stridor. In 1836, Ley[26] described the stridor as "the crowing of a cock, the yelping of a fox, the barking of a dog, the braying of an ass, or a ringing sound, as if the voice came from a brazen tube." The child may sit forward in bed and appear apprehensive. Often accompanying the stridor are retractions of the chest wall, usually most marked in the supraclavicular and suprasternal areas.

In children who are more severely affected, auscultation of the chest may reveal not only the inspiratory stridor but also rales, rhonchi, and/or wheezing. Occasionally, a markedly distressed child will have stridor on expiration as well as inspiration. The respiratory rate is commonly elevated to 35–45/min. However, respiratory rates much above 50/min are unusual in children with croup, in contrast to the marked tachypnea often evident in bronchiolitis. With progression of the disease, auscultation of the chest may reveal poor exchange of air with diminished breath sounds.

One of the hallmarks of croup is its fluctuating course. A child may appear clinically to worsen or improve within an hour. In milder cases of croup, children commonly improve in the morning, only to worsen again at night. In most children the course of croup is 3–4 days, although the cough may persist for a longer period.

LABORATORY FINDINGS

In most cases of croup the white blood cell and differential counts are not particularly abnormal or helpful. In the more severely stressed child the white blood cell count may be somewhat elevated, and, if hypoxemia is present, an increase in the proportion of immature polymorphonuclear cells may be observed.

Hypoxemia ($PaO_2 < 85$ mmHg) occurs in most hospitalized children, and hypercapnea is present in over half.[24] In the study of Newth et al.,[24] most children hospitalized with croup had PaO_2 values between 50 and 80 mmHg, and about half had $PaCO_2$ values in the normal range below 40 mmHg. The rest had $PaCO_2$ levels between 40 and 50 mmHg. Only 1 of the 35 children manifested hypercarbia of greater than 50 mmHg. Few other pulmonary function studies have been obtained in children with croup, but in five out of six children in one study the functional residual capacity was found to be increased.[32]

DIAGNOSIS

The diagnosis of croup is usually based on the characteristic clinical picture. However, differentiation from noninfectious causes of stridor such as foreign body aspiration or an allergic reaction and from *H. influenzae*-induced epiglottitis usually may be made on the basis of both the history and the anterior–posterior and lateral roentgenograms of the neck.[33,34]

Characteristically the course of epiglottitis is much more rapidly progressive, and the children appear to be in a more toxic state. The history of an upper respiratory tract infection with rhinorrhea and laryngitis is usually not present in epiglottitis. The absence of the distinctive cough or "seal's bark" and the presence of marked dysphagia with drooling are often two of the more helpful differentiating clinical signs. In viral laryngotracheobronchitis the anterior–posterior view of the neck (Fig. 2) shows the characteristic subglottic swelling, sometimes described as the "hourglass" or "steeple" sign. In epiglottitis, the lateral neck view may show the edematous epiglottis without subglottic narrowing (see Ch. 45). The roentgenographic picture may not, however, always be diagnostic for croup or epiglottitis, and controversy exists about their reliability and usefulness in the acute situation.[35–37]

Identification of the specific viral agent may be accomplished by isolation in tissue culture or by one of the newer techniques of rapid viral diagnosis.[38] Serologic diagnosis generally may be made only retrospectively, and for some of the major agents of croup serologic rises are variable and unreliable. With parainfluenza viral infections, heterotypic antibody rises are frequent among the various types of the parainfluenza viruses and related viruses such as mumps.[15,39] Furthermore, during reinfection no measurable antibody response may occur.[39]

In reported series, the cause has been determined in approximately one-third to two-thirds of the cases of croup (Table 1),

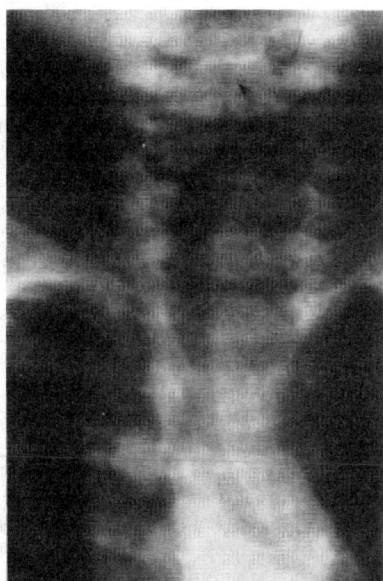

FIG. 2. Roentgenogram of the neck of a child with viral croup that shows the characteristic narrowing of the air shadow of the trachea in the subglottic area.

which is higher than that generally reported for other respiratory tract syndromes. Viral isolation has usually been accomplished from throat, tracheal, and nasal wash specimens.[7,8,10,11,13,16,31] A variety of rapid diagnostic techniques, such as the enzyme-linked immunosorbent assay (EIA) and immunofluorescent techniques, have also been successfully used.[10,38,40–46]

COMPLICATIONS

The severity of croup appears to be influenced by both virus and host factors. Some children appear predisposed to croup, with repetitive episodes from a variety of agents. John Cheyne[3] noted that "... the first attack establishes a predisposition to the disease. I have observed, that after the first attack, a slighter cause will produce Croup a second time than is required originally."

Children with repeated episodes of croup are sometimes diagnosed as having *spasmodic croup*.[47] An allergic diathesis or hyperreactivity of the airway may contribute to the illness in these children, since positive intradermal skin tests and family members with allergy have been frequently seen in children with recurrent versus single episodes of croup.[48–50] A tendency toward lower serum IgA levels has also been noted in children with recurrent croup.[51] Nevertheless, a viral infection initiates the croup even in these children, and the disease cannot be distinguished clinically.

Boys are particularly prone to develop croup for reasons that are not entirely clear.[9–11,13,48–52] However, recently Taussig[53] has shown that young girls had significantly larger flow rates than did boys. This suggests that there are differences anatomically or in intrinsic airway resistance that are related to sex, which might in part explain why young boys tend to develop lower respiratory tract disease more frequently or more severely than do young girls.

Severe croup has sometimes been reported as more frequent with influenza A viral infection than with the other viral agents.[18,19] In the study of Howard et al.,[18] made during an outbreak of influenza A infection, 10 out of 25 infants hospitalized with croup required tracheotomy. This complication has been estimated to occur in about 5–12 percent of the cases of croup.[52,54,55] In Adair and coworkers' review[54] of reported cases of laryngotracheobronchitis, the percentage requiring tracheot-

omy varied between 0 and 13 percent. The associated mortality rate in these series ranged from 0 to 2.7 percent. Of the major acute complications, respiratory failure necessitating such airway intervention is the most frequent. Subglottic stenosis after intubation occasionally occurs in children with complicated and prolonged courses.[52,54–57]

Pneumonia cannot truly be considered a complication of croup but should rather be thought of as a part of the disease. Parenchymal involvement, as evidenced by hypoxemia, is present in most hospitalized children, whether it is visible on the chest roentgenogram or not. Less common complications include pneumothorax, pulmonary edema, and aspiration pneumonia. Aspiration of gastric contents is most likely to occur during emergency intubation. Transient pulmonary edema without evidence of cardiac enlargement has been described in children with croup.[57–59] The mechanism leading to this complication is not completely understood, but it may arise from a neurogenic effect on the pulmonary vasculature, as a direct result of alveolar hypoxia, or possibly from an increased alveolar–capillary gradient causing a leakage of intravascular fluids.

Whether long-term complications can follow croup is currently speculative. The disease is self-limited, and recovery appears clinically to be complete. However, several follow-up studies of children with croup early in life have shown an increased frequency of hyperreactivity of the airways and altered pulmonary function that, in some children, may be clinically occult.[32,55,60,61] In one study of 12-year-old children who had a history of hospitalization for croup, elevated residual volumes and significant reductions in forced vital capacity (FVC), forced expiratory volume in 1 second (FEV_1), and maximal expiratory flow between 25 and 75 percent of vital capacity ($FEF_{25–75\%}$) were found.[61] Hyperreactivity of the airways has been observed in each of these follow-up studies of children with croup.[32,55,60,61]

THERAPY

Despite a Pandora's box of home therapies for croup, none has proved to be consistently effective. The natural fluctuations in the course of croup make evaluation of many therapies difficult. Vaporizers and other means of producing steam or mist in the home have long been advised. In the past century steaming tea kettles were the integral, if not primary, mode of therapy.[62] The beneficial effects of these devices, nevertheless, have not been proved. These methods certainly provide humidification of the upper airway, but the droplet size produced is generally too large to reach the lower respiratory tract. The advantages of such home humidification devices must be balanced against the discomfort or fear they may produce in the child.[63] Crying and lack of rest may aggravate the condition.

In hospitalized patients the essence of successful management is close observation and good supportive care based on a thorough understanding of the physiologic changes associated with croup. Clinical estimation of the severity of croup is difficult. Cyanosis may not be present despite compromising degrees of hypoxemia.[64] Of the clinical signs, an increasing respiratory rate is often the best indication of hypoxemia. The severity of the stridor and retractions reflects more the degree of subglottic obstruction and is not indicative of the arterial oxygen saturation. Oximetry offers a simple, noninvasive means of following the child's arterial oxygen saturation.[65] In the more severely ill child, the PCO_2 also needs to be assessed. In most cases, however, blood drawing and other frightening procedures should be kept to a minimum to avoid compounding the dyspnea and respiratory obstruction. Inspirations that are rapid and shallow, as commonly accompany anxiety and crying, aggravate the narrowing of the airway and further increase the metabolic demand for gas exchange. Most children with hypoxemia who are not hypercarbic will respond to the relatively low concentrations of supplemental oxygen since the hypoxemia primarily results from an abnormal ratio of ventilation to perfusion.[55,66,67]

In the hospital humidification of the airway may be administered by an ultrasonic nebulizer fitted to a mask or an oxygen tent. Although humidification may aid the upper airway secretions, a beneficial effect on the subglottic swelling and on the lower parenchymal abnormalities has not been shown, and few controlled studies have examined this therapy. In one small, controlled trial of 16 children, humidification did not result in discernible improvement.[68] In another study nebulized water administered to five children did not produce a change in the measured total respiratory resistance.[69]

In one of the few animal studies of croup, cold-dry, cold-moist, and dry air were more effective in the dog model in decreasing airway resistance.[70] All of these types of air contain little humidification as compared with warm-moist air, which was least effective. These findings correlate with the clinical observation that many children with croup improve when taken out into cold night air, which would contain little moisture.

A variety of pharmacologic agents has been evaluated in the treatment of croup. Nebulized racemic epinephrine has appeared to provide clinical improvement to many children with marked stridor.[54,71-74] L-Epinephrine, which contains only the active isomer, has been shown to be as effective and may have fewer side effects.[75,76] The α-adrenergic effect of racemic epinephrine, local vasoconstriction, and diminished subglottic inflammation is probably the mechanism by which the stridor is ameliorated. The arterial oxygen saturation is not affected, and the clinical improvement is only transient, lasting usually for a couple of hours.[72,77] Children improving from such treatment should not be discharged, but continued to be observed as rebound mucosal vasodilatation and dyspnea may occur. Despite this and the lack of benefit on arterial oxygen saturation, nebulized racemic epinephrine has resulted in fewer children requiring intubation by alleviating the work of breathing and progression toward respiratory failure.[54,71-74]

Therapy with systemic corticosteroids in croup has been controversial and a subject of interest and investigation over several decades. At least 15 controlled trials have been reported, which have been summarized and reviewed.[73,78-80] Analyses of these studies indicate that corticosteroid therapy in children hospitalized with moderately severe or severe croup may result in significant clinical improvement and fewer intubations if administered in larger doses, 0.3–0.6 mg/kg of dexamethasone (or its equivalent) given once or every 6 hours for two to four doses. Studies using lesser doses of corticosteroids generally failed to show a beneficial effect.

Despite the general acknowledgment that viruses are the perpetrators of croup, antibiotics are frequently used.[73,81] Bacterial infection superimposed or following croup is uncommon, and administering antibiotics to children with croup prophylactically or without evidence of concomitant bacterial infection is not warranted.[73,81]

A few children, despite adequate supportive therapy, may fatigue and develop respiratory failure, demonstrated by a climbing PaCO$_2$ level. If a mechanical airway becomes necessary, nasotracheal intubation is the preferred method, provided personnel skilled in this technique are available.[55-57] Complications with nasotracheal intubation are less than with tracheotomies. In Schuller and Birck's 8-year follow-up study[55] of children receiving nasotracheal intubation for croup and epiglottitis, the rate of immediate and reversible complications was 7 percent, and for the delayed, irreversible complications the rate was 1.6 percent. The average period of intubation for children with croup was 88 hours as compared with 55 hours for those with epiglottitis.

BACTERIAL TRACHEITIS

An atypical form of croup with a clinical picture more similar to epiglottitis than to the usual case of laryngotracheobronchitis has been described and designated as *bacterial tracheitis*.[82-88] Although this entity appears to have been described before 1940, it received little attention until it was rediscovered toward the end of the 1970s. This relatively uncommon disease tends to affect somewhat older children, but may affect any age, and produces a dramatic, acute onset marked by high fever, stridor, and dyspnea with copious amounts of purulent sputum. The clinical picture may progress rapidly, requiring endotracheal intubation. The primary area of inflammation and obstruction is subglottic and is covered with a thick exudate, while the epiglottis and supraglottic structures tend to be minimally inflamed. The lateral soft tissue roentgenogram of the neck characteristically reveals a normal epiglottis with subglottic narrowing within which a shaggy membrane may sometimes be visible.

The organisms most commonly recovered from this exudate are *S. aureus,* group A β-hemolytic streptococci, and, at least prior to widespread immunization, *H. influenzae* type b.[82-88] The pathogenesis of this entity, nevertheless, is not clear. The syndrome appears to develop in children who are predisposed by previous conditions, especially those associated with injury to the trachea. Children who have been intubated recently and sometimes those with a preceding viral infection appear to be at greater risk, suggesting that mucosal damage or impairment of local immune mechanisms may predispose to invasive infections with common pyogenic organisms. In one reported case, *Chlamydia trachomatis* was isolated from the tracheal exudate along with *S. aureus.*[85]

The rapidly progressive course of this disease demands its prompt diagnosis and differentiation from viral croup by its clinical and roentgenographic pictures. Direct laryngoscopy can confirm the diagnosis and provide specimens of the localized exudate for culture. These children do not respond to nebulized racemic epinephrine. Initial antibiotic therapy should be broad enough to cover the associated major pathogens.

REFERENCES

1. Home F. An Inquiry into the Nature, Cause and Cure of Croup. Edinburgh, 1765.
2. Cherry JD. Croup. In: Kiple KF, ed. Cambridge History and Geography of Human Disease Project. Bowling Green, OH: University of Cambridge Press; 1990:654–7.
3. Cheyne J. Essays on the Diseases of Children, with Cases and Dissections. Philadelphia: Anthony Finley Merritt; 1814:20.
4. Semple RH. Memoirs on diphtheria. From the Writings of Bretonneau, Guersant, Trousseau, Bouchut, Empis, Daviot. London: New Sydenham Society Publication; 1859:5.
5. Rabe EF. Infectious croup: I. Etiology. Pediatrics. 1948;2:255–65.
6. Hoekelman RA. Infectious illness during the first year of life. Pediatrics. 1977; 59:119–21.
7. Foy HM, Cooney MK, Maletzky AJ, et al. Incidence and etiology of pneumonia, croup and bronchiolitis in pre-school children belonging to a prepaid medical care group over a four year period. Am J Epidemiol. 1973;97:80–92.
8. Downham MAPS, McQuillan J, Gardner PS. Diagnosis and clinical significance of parainfluenza virus infections in children. Arch Dis Child. 1974;49: 8–15.
9. Glezen WP, Denny FW. Epidemiology of acute lower respiratory disease in children. N Engl J Med. 1973;288:498–505.
10. Denny FW, Murphy TF, Clyde WA Jr, et al. Croup: An 11 year study in a pediatric practice. Pediatrics. 1983;71:871–6.
11. Glezen WP, Loda FA, Clyde WA Jr, et al. Epidemiological patterns of acute lower respiratory disease of children in a pediatric group practice. J Pediatr. 1971;78:397–406.
12. Loda FA, Glezen WP, Clyde WA Jr. Respiratory disease in group day care. Pediatrics. 1972;49:428–37.
13. Buchan KA, Marten KW, Kennedy DH. Aetiology and epidemiology of viral croup in Glasgow, 1966–72. J Hyg (Camb). 1974;73:143–50.
14. Cramblett HG. Croup (epiglottitis, laryngitis, laryngotracheobronchitis). In: Kendig EL Jr, Chernick V, eds. Disorders of the Respiratory Tract in Children. 3rd ed. Philadelphia: WB Saunders; 1977:353.
15. Parrott RH, Vargosko AJ, Kim HW, et al. Acute respiratory diseases of viral etiology. III. Myxoviruses: Parainfluenza. Am J Public Health. 1962;52: 907–17.
16. Loda FA, Clyde WA Jr, Glezen WP, et al. Studies of the role of viruses, bacteria, and *M. pneumoniae* as causes of lower respiratory tract infections in children. J Pediatr. 1968;72:161–76.
17. Knott A, Long CE, Hall CB. Parainfluenza viral infections in pediatric outpatients: Seasonal patterns and clinical characteristics. Pediatr Infect Dis J. 1994; 13:269–73.

18. Howard JB, McCracken GH Jr, Luby JP. Influenza A 2 virus as a cause of croup requiring tracheotomy. J Pediatr. 1972;81:1148–50.

19. Eller JJ, Fulginiti VA, Plunket DC, et al. Attack rates for hospitalized croup in children in a military population: Importance of A₂ influenza infection. Pediatr Res. 1972;6:126.

20. Kim HW, Brandt CD, Chanock RM, et al. Influenza A and B virus infection in infants and young children during the years 1957–1976. Am J Epidemiol. 1979;109:464–79.

21. Hall CB, Douglas RG Jr. Respiratory syncytial virus and influenza: Practical community surveillance. Am J Dis Child. 1976;130:615–20.

22. Ross LA, Mason WH, Lanson J, Deakers TW, Newth CJL. Laryngotracheobronchitis as a complication of measles during an urban epidemic. J Pediatr. 1992;121:511–5.

23. Fortenberry JD, Mariscalco M, Louis PT, et al. Severe laryngotracheobronchitis complicating measles. Am J Dis Child 1992;146:1040–3.

24. Newth CJ, Levison H, Bryan AC. The respiratory status of children with croup. J Pediatr. 1972;81:1068–73.

25. McBride JT. Stridor in childhood. J Fam Pract. 1984;19:782–90.

26. Ley H. An essay on the Laryngismus Stridulus or Croup-like Inspiration of Infants. London: Churchill; 1836:6.

27. Szpunar J, Glowacki J, Laskowski A, et al. Fibrinous laryngotracheobronchitis in children. Arch Otolaryngol. 1971;93:173–8.

28. Urquhart GED, Kennedy DH, Ariyawansa JP. Croup associated with parainfluenza type 1 virus: Two subpopulations. Br Med J 1979;1:1604.

29. Welliver RC, Wong DT, Middleton E Jr, et al. Role of parainfluenza virus-specific IgE in pathogenesis of croup and wheezing subsequent to infection. J Pediatr. 1982;101:889–96.

30. Welliver RC, Sun M, Rinaldo D. Defective regulation of immune responses in croup due to parainfluenza virus. Pediatr Res. 1985;19:716–20.

31. Hall CB, Geiman JM, Breese BB, et al. Parainfluenza viral infections in children: Correlation of shedding with clinical manifestations. J Pediatr. 1977;91:194–8.

32. Loughlin G, Taussig LM. Pulmonary function in children with a history of laryngotracheobronchitis. J Pediatr. 1979;94:365–9.

33. Rapkin RH. The diagnosis of epiglottitis: Simplicity and reliability of radiographs of the neck in the differential diagnosis of the croup syndrome. J Pediatr. 1972;80:96–8.

34. Wildin SR, Chonmaitree T, Swischuk LE. Roentgenographic features of common pediatric viral respiratory tract infections. Am J Dis Child. 1988;142:43–6.

35. Currarino G, Williams B. Lateral inspiration and expiration radiographs of the neck in children with laryngotracheobronchitis (croup). Radiology. 1982;195:365–6.

36. Jones JL. False positives in lateral neck radiographs used to diagnose epiglottitis (Letter). Ann Emerg Med. 1983;12:797.

37. Stankiewicz JA, Bowes AK. Croup and epiglottitis: A radiologic study. Laryngoscope. 1985;95:1159–60.

38. Richman D, Schmidt N, Plotkin S, et al. Summary of a workshop on new and useful methods in rapid viral diagnosis. J Infect Dis. 1984;150:941–51.

39. Bloom HH, Johnson KM, Jacobsen R, et al. Recovery of parainfluenza viruses from adults with upper respiratory illness. Am J Hyg. 1961;74:50–59.

40. McIntosh K, Wilfert C, Chernesky M, et al. Summary of a workshop on new and useful techniques in rapid viral diagnosis. J Infect Dis. 1980;142:793–802.

41. Grauballe PC, Johnsen NJ, Hornsleth A. Rapid diagnosis by immunofluorescence of viral infections associated with the croup syndrome in children. Acta Pathol Microbiol Scand [B]. 1974;82:41–7.

42. Gardner PS, McQuillin J, McGuckin R, et al. Observations on clinical and immunofluorescent diagnosis of parainfluenza virus infections. Br Med J. 1971;2:7–12.

43. Gardner PS, McGuckin R, McQuillin J. Adenovirus demonstrated by immunofluorescence. Br Med J. 1972;3:175.

44. Marks MI, Nagahama H, Eller JJ. Parainfluenza virus immunofluorescence. In vitro and clinical application of the direct method. Pediatrics. 1971;48:73–8.

45. Dennehy PH. Rapid diagnosis of viral infections. Contemp Pediatr. 1987;4:61–76.

46. Drew LW. Direct detection of viruses. Pan American Group for Rapid Viral Diagnosis. 1992;18:1–6.

47. McLain LG. Croup syndrome. Am Fam Physician. 1987;36:207–14.

48. Hide DW, Guyer BM: Recurrent croup. Arch Dis Child. 1985;60:585–6.

49. Laufer P. The relationship of respiratory allergies to croup. J Asthma. 1986;23:9–10.

50. Zach M, Erban A, Olinsky A. Croup, recurrent croup, allergy, and airways hyper-reactivity. Arch Dis Child. 1981;56:336–41.

51. Zach M. Serum IgA in recurrent croup. Am J Dis Child. 1983;137:184–5.

52. Postma DS, Jones RD, Pillsbury HC III. Severe hospitalized croup: Treatment trends and prognosis. Laryngoscope. 1984;94:1170–5.

53. Taussig LM. Maximal expiratory flows at functional residual capacity: A test of lung function for young children. Am Rev Respir Dis. 1977;116:1031–8.

54. Adair JC, Ring WH, Jordan WS, et al. Ten year experience with IPPB in the treatment of acute laryngotracheobronchitis. Anesth Analg (Cleve). 1971;50:649–55.

55. Schuller DE, Birck HG. The safety of intubation in croup and epiglottitis: An eight-year follow-up. Laryngoscope. 1975;85:33–46.

56. Hen J Jr. Current management of upper airway obstruction. Pediatr Ann. 1986;15:274–94.

57. Kilham H, Gillies J, Benjamin B. Severe upper airway obstruction. Pediatr Clin North Am 1987;34:1–14.

58. Broniatowski M. Croup. Ear Nose Throat J. 1985;64:12–21.

59. Travis KW, Todres ID, Shannon DC. Pulmonary edema associated with croup and epiglottitis. Pediatrics. 1977;59:695–8.

60. Zach MS, Schnall RP, Landau LI. Upper and lower airway hyperreactivity in recurrent croup. Am Rev Respir Dis. 1980;121:979–83.

61. Gurwitz D, Corey M, Levison H. Pulmonary function and bronchial reactivity in children after croup. Am Rev Respir Dis. 1980;122:95–9.

62. Baugh R, Gilmore BB Jr. Infectious croup: A critical review. Otolaryngol Head Neck Surg. 1986;95:40–6.

63. Henry R. Moist air in the treatment of laryngotracheitis. Arch Dis Child. 1983;58:577.

64. Hall CB, Hall WJ, Speers DM. Clinical and physiological manifestations of bronchiolitis and pneumonia: Outcome of respiratory syncytial virus. Am J Dis Child. 1979;133:798–802.

65. Gussack GS, Tacchi EJ. Pulse oximetry in the management of pediatric airway disorders. South Med J. 1987;80:1381–4.

66. Barker GA. Current management of croup and epiglottitis. Pediatr Clin North Am. 1979;26:565–79.

67. Newth CJL, Levison H. Diagnosing and managing croup and epiglottitis. J Respir Dis. 1981;2:22–41.

68. Bourchier D, Dawson KP, Fergusson DM. Humidification in viral croup: A controlled trial. Aust Paediatr J. 1984;20:289–91.

69. Lenney W, Milner AD. Treatment of acute viral croup. Arch Dis Child. 1978;53:704–6.

70. Wolfsdorf J, Swift DL. An animal model simulating acute infective upper airway obstruction of childhood and its use in the investigation of croup therapy. Pediatr Res. 1978;12:1062–5.

71. Westley CR, Cotton EK, Brooks JG. Nebulized racemic epinephrine by IPPB for the treatment of croup: A double-blind study. Am J Dis Child. 1978;132:484–7.

72. Taussig LM, Castro O, Beaudry PH, et al. Treatment of laryngotracheobronchitis (croup). Use of intermittent positive-pressure breathing and racemic epinephrine. Am J Dis Child. 1975;129:790–3.

73. Skolnik NS. Treatment of croup. Am J Dis Child. 1989;143:1045–9.

74. Kuusela A-L, Vesikari T. A randomized double-blind, placebo-controlled trial of dexamethasone and racemic epinephrine in the treatment of croup. Acta Paediatr Scand. 1988;77:99–104.

75. Davis HW, Gartner JC, Galvis AG, et al. Acute airway obstruction: croup and epiglottitis. Pediatr Clin North Am. 1981;28:859–80.

76. Waisman Y, Klein BL, Boenning DA, et al. Prospective randomized double-blind study comparing L-epinephrine and racemic epinephrine aerosols in the treatment of laryngotracheitis (croup). Pediatrics. 1992;89:302–306.

77. Fanconi S, Burger R, Maurer H, et al. Transcutaneous carbon dioxide pressure for monitoring patients with severe croup. J Pediatr. 1990;117:701–5.

78. Bass JW, Bruhn FW, Merrit WT. Corticosteroids and racemic epinephrine with IPPB in the treatment of croup. J Pediatr. 1980;96:173–4.

79. Tunnessen WW Jr, Feinstein AR. The steroid-croup controversy: An analytic review of methodologic problems. J Pediatr. 1980;96:751–6.

80. Kairys SW, Olmstead EM, O'Connor GT. Steroid treatment of laryngotracheitis: A meta-analysis of the evidence from randomized trials. Pediatrics. 1989;83:683–93.

81. Pianosi P, Feldman W, Robson MG, et al. Inappropriate use of antibiotics in croup at three types of hospitals. Can Med Assoc J 1986;134:357–9.

82. Jones R, Santos JI, Overall JC. Bacterial tracheitis. J Am Med Assoc. 1979;242:721–6.

83. Liston SL, Gehrz RC, Jarvis CW. Bacterial tracheitis. Arch Otolaryngol. 1981;107:561–4.

84. Davidson S, Barzilay Z, Yahav J, et al. Bacterial tracheitis: A true entity? J Laryngol Otol. 1982;96:173–5.

85. Miller BP, Arthur JD, Parry WH, et al. Atypical croup and chlamydia trachomatis (Letter). Lancet. 1982;1:1022.

86. Donnelly BW, McMillan JA, Weiner LB. Bacterial tracheitis: Report of eight new cases and review. Rev Infect Dis. 1990;12:729–35.

87. Dudin AA, Thalji A, Rambaud-Cousson A. Bacterial tracheitis among children hospitalized for severe obstructive dyspnea. Pediatr Infect Dis J. 1990;9:293–5.

88. Long SS. Bacterial tracheitis. Rep Pediatr Infect Dis. 1992;2:29–31.

43. OTITIS EXTERNA, OTITIS MEDIA, MASTOIDITIS

JEROME O. KLEIN

OTITIS EXTERN

Infection of the external auditory canal (otitis externa) is similar to infection of skin and soft tissue elsewhere. Unique problems occur because the canal is narrow and tortuous; fluid and foreign objects enter, are trapped, and cause irritation and maceration of the superficial tissues. The pain and itching that results may be severe because of the limited space for expansion of the inflamed tissue. Infections of the external canal may be subdivided into four categories: acute localized otitis externa, acute diffuse otitis externa, chronic otitis externa, and malignant otitis externa. Reviews by Senturia et al.,[1] Bergstrom,[2] and Rubin and Yu[3] provide more complete information.

Pathogenesis

The external auditory canal is approximately 2.5 cm long from the concha of the auricle to the tympanic membrane. The lateral half of the canal is cartilaginous; the medial half tunnels through the temporal bone. A constriction, the isthmus, present at the juncture of the osseous and cartilaginous portions, limits entry of wax and foreign bodies to the area near the tympanic membrane. The skin of the canal is thicker in the cartilaginous portion and includes a well-developed dermis and subcutaneous layer. The skin lining the osseous portion is thinner and firmly attached to the periosteum and lacks a subcutaneous layer. Hair follicles are numerous in the outer third and sparse in the inner two-thirds of the canal.

The microbial flora of the external canal is similar to the flora of skin elsewhere. There is a predominance of *Staphylococcus epidermidis*, *S. aureus*, *Corynebacteria*, and, to a lesser extent, anaerobic bacteria such as *Propionibacterium acnes*.[4–6] Pathogens responsible for infection of the middle ear (*Streptococcus pneumoniae*, *Haemophilus influenzae*, or *Moraxella catarrhalis*) are uncommonly found in cultures of the external auditory canal when the tympanic membrane is intact.

The epithelium absorbs moisture from the environment. Desquamation and denuding of the superficial layers of the epithelium may follow. In this warm, moist environment, the organisms in the canal may flourish and invade the macerated skin. Inflammation and suppuration follow. Invasive organisms include those of the normal skin flora and gram-negative bacilli, particularly *Pseudomonas aeruginosa*. Invasive otitis media is a necrotizing infection frequently associated with *P. aeruginosa*. The organism gains access to the deeper tissues of the ear canal and causes a localized vasculitis, thrombosis, and necrosis of tissues. Diabetic microangiopathy of the skin overlying the temporal bone results in poor local perfusion and a milieu for invasion by *P. aeruginosa*.

Clinical Manifestations and Management

Acute localized otitis externa may occur as a pustule or furuncle associated with hair follicles; it is due to *Staphylococcus aureus*. Erysipelas caused by group A *Streptococcus* may involve the concha and the canal. Pain may be severe. Bluish red hemorrhagic bullae may be present on the osseous canal walls and also on the tympanic membrane. Adenopathy in the lymphatic drainage areas is often present. Local heat and systemic antibiotics are usually curative. Incision and drainage may be necessary to relieve severe pain.

Acute diffuse otitis externa (swimmer's ear) occurs mainly in hot, humid weather. The ear itches and becomes increasingly painful. The skin of the canal is edematous and red. Gram-negative bacilli, mainly *P. aeruginosa*, may play a significant role. A severe hemorrhagic external otitis due to *P. aeruginosa* was associated with mobile redwood hot tub systems.[7] Gentle cleansing to remove debris including irrigation with hypertonic saline (3%) and cleansing with mixtures of alcohol (70–95%) and acetic acid should be used initially. Hydrophilic solutions such as 50% Burrow solutions may be used for 1–2 days to reduce inflammation. Ear drops of topical antibiotics (including neomycin and polymyxin) combined with a steroid in an acid vehicle serve to diminish local inflammation and infection. Systemic antibiotics may be necessary if there is significant tissue infection.

Chronic otitis externa is due to irritation of drainage from the middle ear in patients with chronic suppurative otitis media.

Itching may be severe. Management is directed to treatment of the middle ear disorder. Rare causes of chronic otitis externa include tuberculosis, syphilis, yaws, leprosy, and sarcoidosis.

Invasive ("malignant") otitis externa is a severe, necrotizing infection that spreads from the squamous epithelium of the ear canal to adjacent areas of soft tissue, blood vessels, cartilage, and bone.[3,8] Severe pain and tenderness of the tissues around the ear and mastoid is accompanied by drainage of pus from the canal. The elderly, diabetic, immunocompromised, and debilitated patients are at particular risk. Life-threatening disease may result from spread to the temporal bone and then on to the sigmoid sinus, jugular bulb, base of the skull, meninges, and brain. Permanent facial paralysis is frequent, and cranial nerves 9, 10, and 12 may also be affected.[9] *Pseudomonas aeruginosa* is almost always the causative agent. The extent of damage to soft tissue and bone may be identified and monitored by use of CT and MRI.[3] Diagnostic tests for underlying disease should be instituted. The canal should be cleansed, devitalized tissue removed, and ear drops with antipseudomonal antibiotics combined with steroid instilled, and systemic therapy with regimens including activity for *Pseudomonas* spp. should be used for 4–6 weeks. The combination of a ceftazidime or an antipseudomonal penicillin (ticarcillin or piperacillin) with an aminoglycoside (gentamicin or tobramycin) should be considered. Oral quinolones with activity against *Pseudomonas* spp., such as ciprofloxacin, have been effective therapy early in the course of invasive external otitis.[10]

Fungal otitis may be part of a general or local fungal infection. *Aspergillus* spp. are responsible for most cases of fungal otitis.[11] *Candida albicans* is a frequent cause of external otitis in children with chronic mucocutaneous candidiasis.

OTITIS MEDIA

Otitis media, or inflammation of the middle ear, is defined by the presence of fluid in the middle ear accompanied by signs or symptoms of illness. In 1990, there were an estimated 24.5 million visits made to offices of physicians in the United States at which the principal diagnosis was otitis media. For children under age 15 years, otitis media was the most frequent diagnosis in physician office practices. Office visits with a principal diagnosis of otitis media increased from 9.9 million visits in 1975 to 25.5 million visits in 1990.[12] The peak incidence occurs in the first 3 years of life. The disease is less common in the school-aged child, adolescent, and adult. Nevertheless, infection of the middle ear may be the cause of fever, significant pain, and impaired hearing in these age groups. In addition, adults suffer from the sequelae of otitis media of childhood: hearing loss, cholesteatoma, adhesive otitis media, and chronic perforation of the tympanic membrane. A comprehensive review of otitis media is included in the text, *Otitis Media in Infants and Children*.[13]

Epidemiology

By 3 years of age, more than two-thirds of children have had one or more episodes of acute otitis media, and one-third have had three or more episodes.[14] The highest incidence of acute otitis media occurs between 6 and 24 months of age. Subsequently, the incidence declines with age except for a limited reversal of the downward trend between 5 and 6 years of age, the time of school entry. Otitis media is infrequent in adults, but the bacteriology and therapy is similar to that in children.[15,16]

Longitudinal studies have provided information about the characteristics of children who have recurrent and severe episodes of acute otitis media. The vast majority of children have no obvious defect responsible for severe and recurrent otitis media, but a small number have anatomic changes (cleft palate, cleft uvula, submucous cleft), alteration of normal physiologic defenses (patulous eustachian tube), or congenital or acquired immunologic deficiencies. Children with AIDS have a higher age-specific incidence of otitis media, beginning at 6 months of age, than uninfected children or children who initially were positive for HIV antibody but who seroreverted.[17]

As is true for most infectious diseases of childhood, acute otitis media occurs more often in males than females. Correlation of the index child with severe or recurrent acute otitis media in a sibling or parent identifies a likely genetic susceptibility. Age at the time of the first episode of acute otitis media appears to be among the most powerful predictors of recurrent middle ear infections. Breast-feeding for three or more months is associated with decreased risk for acute otitis media in the first year of life.[18] Race and ethnicity provide additional data suggesting a genetic basis for recurrent middle ear infections; Native Americans, Alaskan and Canadian Eskimos, and Australian Aborigines have an extraordinary incidence and severity of otitis media.

The role of increased exposure to infectious agents and the importance of environmental pollutants are identified in studies of incidence of infection in group day care and the effects of passive smoking on children. Introduction of infants into large day care groups increases the incidence of respiratory infections, including otitis media.[19] Passive smoking documented by a biochemical marker, serum nicotine, increased the incidence of new episodes of otitis media with effusion and the duration of effusion.[20]

Pathogenesis

The middle ear is part of a continuous system that includes, medially and anteriorly, the nares, nasopharynx, and eustachian tube and, posteriorly, the mastoid air cells. These structures are lined with a respiratory epithelium that contains ciliated cells, mucus-secreting goblet cells, and cells capable of secreting local immunoglobulins.

Anatomic or physiologic dysfunction of the eustachian tube appears to play a critical role in the development of otitis media. The eustachian tube has at least three physiologic functions with respect to the middle ear: protection of the ear from nasopharyngeal secretions, drainage into the nasopharynx of secretions produced within the middle ear, and ventilation of the middle ear to equilibrate air pressure with that in the external ear canal. When one or more of these functions is compromised, the results may be development of fluid and infection in the middle ear. Congestion of the mucosa of the eustachian tube may result in obstruction. Secretions that are constantly formed by the mucosa of the middle ear accumulate behind the obstruction, and if a bacterial pathogen is present, a suppurative otitis media may result.

Microbiology

Bacteria. The bacteriology of otitis media has been documented by appropriate cultures of middle ear effusions obtained by needle aspiration. Many studies of the bacteriology of acute otitis media have been performed. The results are remarkably consistent in demonstrating the importance of *S. pneumoniae* and *H. influenzae* in all age groups (Table 1).[21,22]

TABLE 1. Bacterial Pathogens Isolated from Middle Ear Fluid in Children with Acute Otitis Media—1980–1987[a]

Microorganism	Mean Percentage of Children with Pathogen
Streptococcus pneumoniae	39
Haemophilus influenzae	27
Streptococcus, group A	3
Staphylococcus aureus	2
Moraxella catarrhalis	10
Miscellaneous bacteria	8
None or nonpathogens	28

[a] Nine reports from centers in the United States and Canada.

(Modified from Bluestone and Klein,[21] with permission.)

Streptococcus pneumoniae is the most important bacterial cause of otitis media. Relatively few types are responsible for most disease. The most common types in order of decreasing frequencies are 19, 23, 6, 14, 3, and 18.[23–25] All are included in the currently available 23-type pneumonococcal polysaccharide vaccine.

Otitis media due to *H. influenzae* is associated with nontypable strains in the vast majority of patients. In approximately 10 percent, the otitis is due to type b; some of these patients appear to be a very toxic state, and about one-quarter have concomitant bacteremia or meningitis.[26] Until recently, *H. influenzae* appeared to be limited in importance to preschool children; however, recent studies indicate that *H. influenzae* is a significant cause of otitis media in older children, adolescents, and adults.[15,16]

Recent studies indicate an increasing importance of *Moraxella catarrhalis*.[27,28] The organism was isolated from the middle ear fluids of 19 percent of 200 middle ear specimens from 146 Pittsburgh children with acute otitis media.[27] Prior to 1970 almost all strains of *M. catarrhalis* were sensitive to penicillin. Today most strains produce β-lactamase and are resistant to penicillin G, ampicillin, and amoxicillin.

Viruses. Virologic and epidemiologic data suggest that viral infection is frequently associated with acute otitis media.[29–31] In a study of children attending a day care program, isolation of viruses from the upper respiratory tract was correlated with a clinical diagnosis of otitis media. Virus outbreaks coincided with epidemics of otitis media. Recent studies identify respiratory viruses[29] or viral antigens[30] in approximately one-quarter of middle ear fluids of children with acute otitis media. Respiratory syncytial virus, influenza virus, enteroviruses, and rhinoviruses were the most common viruses found in middle ear fluids. Many patients with virus in middle ear fluid have a mixed viral-bacterial infection. Respiratory signs may be prolonged in children with dual infection.[32,33]

Mycoplasma, Chlamydia, and Unusual Organisms. *Mycoplasma pneumoniae* was responsible for hemorrhagic bullous myringitis in a study of nonimmune volunteers inoculated with the organism.[34] However, the middle ear fluid of a large number of patients (771) has been studied, and *M. pneumoniae* was isolated in only one case.[35,36] Although mycoplasmas do not appear to play a significant role in acute otitis media, some patients with lower respiratory tract disease due to *M. pneumoniae* may have concomitant otitis media.

Chlamydia trachomatis is associated with acute respiratory infections in infants under age 6 months and is a cause of acute infection of the middle ear in this age group. The organism has been isolated from middle ear fluid of infants with acute infection.[37]

Uncommon forms of otitis include diphtheritic otitis, tuberculous otitis, otogenous tetanus, otitis due to *Mycobacterium chelonae*,[38] and otitis due to *Ascaris lumbricoides* or Wegener's granulomatosis.

Immunology

The middle ear is the site of a secretory immune system similar to those of other areas of the respiratory tract. Local and systemic immune responses occur in patients with acute or chronic otitis media with effusion. In the middle ear, immunologically active antigen interacts with immunocompetent cells in the lamina propria to produce a local immune response. The middle ear effusion that results from acute or chronic infection contains all the major classes of immunoglobulins, complement, cells, immune complexes of antigen and antibody, and various chemical mediators of inflammation. The role of these substances in the course of otitis media is uncertain. The immune response to various antigens may prevent subsequent infection, assist in clearance of fluid during the acute episode, or contribute to the accumulation and persistence of fluid in the middle ear cavity, which becomes the culture medium for the next infection.

Diagnosis and Clinical Course

Acute otitis media is defined by the presence of fluid in the middle ear along with signs or symptoms of acute illness. Signs and symptoms may be specific, such as ear pain, ear drainage, or hearing loss, or may be nonspecific, such as fever, lethargy, or irritability. Vertigo, nystagmus, and tinnitus may occur. Redness of the tympanic membrane is an early sign of otitis media, but erythema alone is not diagnostic of middle ear infection since it may be caused by inflammation of the mucosa throughout the upper respiratory tract.

The presence of fluid in the middle ear is determined by the use of pneumatic otoscopy, a technique that permits an assessment of the mobility of the tympanic membrane. The motion of the tympanic membrane is proportional to the pressure applied by gently squeezing and then releasing the rubber bulb attached to the head of the otoscope. Normal mobility is apparent when positive pressure is applied and the tympanic membrane moves rapidly inward; with release of the bulb and the resulting negative pressure, the membrane moves outward. Fluid or high negative pressure in the middle ear dampens the mobility of the tympanic membrane. Tympanometry uses an electroacoustic impedance bridge to record compliance of the tympanic membrane and middle ear pressure. This technique presents objective evidence of the status of the middle ear and the presence or absence of fluid. Acoustic reflectometry measures sound reflectivity from the middle ear and is able to distinguish an air- or fluid-filled space.

Fluid persists in the middle ear for prolonged periods after the onset of acute otitis media even though symptoms usually resolve within a few days after initiation of antimicrobial therapy. About 70 percent of children with otitis media have fluid in the middle ear 2 weeks after the onset of disease, 40 percent still have fluid 1 month after onset, and 10 percent still have fluid 3 months after the first signs of middle ear infection.[14]

Patients with middle ear effusion suffer from hearing loss of variable severity. On average, a patient with fluid in the middle ear has a 25 dB (pure tone average) loss.[39] Since development is dynamic during infancy when the incidence of acute otitis media is highest, there is concern that any impediment to reception or interpretation of auditory stimuli might have an adverse effect. Recent studies suggest that children with histories of recurrent episodes of acute otitis media score lower in tests of speech, language, and cognitive abilities than do their disease-free peers.[40,41]

The results of microbiologic studies of middle ear effusions in patients with otitis media are so consistent that the choice of antimicrobial agents may be based on knowledge of the bacteriology acquired from the many investigations rather than the results of cultures from other sites such as the throat or nasopharynx (Table 1). If the patient is toxic or has focal infection elsewhere, culture of the blood and culture of the focus are warranted. Needle aspiration of the middle ear effusion (tympanocentesis) to define the microbiology should be considered in selected patients: the patient who is critically ill at the onset, the patient who has not responded to initial antimicrobial therapy in 48–72 hours and is toxic, and the patient with altered host defenses (e.g., immunologic defect, including the newborn infant).

Management

Acute Otitis Media. ANTIMICROBIAL AGENTS. The preferred antimicrobial agent for the patient with otitis media must be active against *S. pneumoniae*, *H. influenzae*, and, in some areas, *M. catarrhalis*. Group A streptococci and *S. aureus* are infrequent causes of acute otitis media and need not be considered in initial therapeutic decisions. Gram-negative enteric ba-

cilli must be considered when otitis media occurs in the newborn infant, in the patient with a depressed immune response, and in the patient with suppurative complications of chronic otitis media. Amoxicillin is the current drug of choice for initial treatment, since it is effective against the two major pathogens and is less expensive than alternative regimens. The current incidence of ampicillin-resistant *H. influenzae* and *M. catarrhalis* is not high enough to require a change in initial therapy.

The rationale for the continued use of amoxicillin is as follows. *H. influenzae* and *M. catarrhalis* are responsible for about 30 and 10 percent of acute otitis media, respectively. If 30 percent of the former and 75 percent of the latter are β-lactamase producing, then 16 percent of acute otitis media is caused by β-lactamase–producing organisms. If 40 percent improve spontaneously or despite β-lactamase activity, then a 10 percent failure rate could be anticipated due to failure of amoxicillin to be active against β-lactamase–producing organisms. Although this incidence is not high enough to prompt abandonment of amoxicillin, parents should be alerted to call the physician if a child does not respond to therapy.

Other drugs are satisfactory and of value if the incidence of β-lactamase–producing organisms increases, including amoxicillin-clavulanate, cefaclor, cefuroxime-axetil, cefixime, cefprozil, cefpodoxime-proxetil, loracarbef, trimethoprim-sulfamethoxazole, and erythromycin plus sulfisoxazole. The sulfonamide combinations or perhaps a cephalosporin are acceptable for a child with penicillin allergy. If the child has had a major reaction to a penicillin (an immediate or accelerated reaction with urticaria, bronchospasm, or hypotension), cross-reactivity of penicillins and cepalosporins must be considered possible, and the use of a cephalosporin should be avoided.

Some children with acute otitis media due to a bacterial pathogen improve without the use of antimicrobial agents. Clinical resolution may occur because the contents of the middle ear are discharged through the eustachian tube or after spontaneous perforation of the tympanic membrane. The cases of spontaneous resolution of acute otitis media are important to the investigator, who must consider this factor in any analysis of the results of new therapeutic regimens, but they do not weigh against the use of appropriate antimicrobial agents for the treatment of acute otitis media to resolve the clinical signs uniformly and prevent suppurative complications.[42,43]

With appropriate antimicrobial therapy, most children with acute otitis media are significantly improved within 48–72 hours. If there is no improvement, the patient should be examined. Toxicity with persistent or recurrent fever or otalgia should prompt reevaluation of the patient. The child may have developed a new focus of infection or have received inadequate therapy. In the absence of a new focus, an antibacterial drug that is effective for less common organisms, including β-lactamase-producing *H. influenzae* and *M. catarrhalis*, should be considered. If amoxicillin was given initially, then amoxicillin-clavulanate, TMP-SMZ, erythromycin-sulfisoxazole, or a cephalosporin should be administered.

DECONGESTANTS AND ANTIHISTAMINES. Nasal and oral decongestants, administered either alone or in combination with an antihistamine, are used extensively for treatment of otitis media with effusion. The use of the drugs is based on the consideration that they reduce congestion of the respiratory mucosa and relieve the obstruction of the eustachian tube that results from inflammation caused by respiratory infection. The results of clinical trials, however, indicate no significant evidence of efficacy of any of these preparations, used alone or in combination, for relief of signs of disease or decrease in time spent with middle ear effusion.[44,45]

Chronic Otitis Media. The term *chronic otitis media* includes recurrent episodes of acute infection and prolonged duration of middle ear effusion usually resulting from a previous episode of acute infection. For the prevention of recurrent episodes of acute otitis media, management includes the consideration of chemoprophylaxis (the use of antimicrobial agents) and immunoprophylaxis (the use of pneumococcal vaccine). For the management of persistent middle ear effusions, three surgical methods are considered: myringotomy, adenoidectomy, and placement of tympanostomy tubes.

Chemoprophylaxis has been shown to be of value for the prevention of acute illness in children who have suffered from recurrences of middle ear infections.[46–48] The results are persuasive in that a reduction of episodes of acute febrile illnesses due to otitis media occurred. On the basis of available information,[48] a protocol has been suggested that uses a once-a-day regimen of amoxicillin or sulfisoxazole during winter and spring, the periods of high incidence of infections of the respiratory tract. Children should be considered for prophylaxis if they have had two episodes of acute otitis media in the first year of life or, in older children, three episodes in 6 months or four episodes in 1 year. Amoxicillin, 20 mg/kg, or sulfisoxazole, 50 mg/kg, may be administered once a day. Chemoprophylaxis may suppress symptoms of otitis media, but middle ear effusion may persist (though without apparent symptoms). The physician who chooses to use chemoprophylaxis to prevent acute recurrent disease must examine the patient at approximately 1-month intervals for middle ear effusion.

Pneumonococcal vaccines have been evaluated for the prevention of recurrences of acute otitis media in children.[49–51] As in previous studies, children less than 2 years of age had unsatisfactory responses to single-dose regimens. The vaccine reduced the number of episodes of acute otitis media due to types of *S. pneumoniae* present in the vaccine, but the reduction was not sufficient to alter the experience of the children with middle ear infections. The basis for failure of the vaccine was due to the poor immunologic response to the polysaccharide antigens in the young infants enrolled in the trials. The data suggested that the vaccine was likely to be more effective in children over the age of 2 years.[51] Vaccines composed of pneumococcal capsular polysaccharides conjugated to proteins promise increased immunogenicity in young infants and are currently undergoing clinical evaluation.

Surgical management of the persistent effusion of the middle ear includes the use of myringotomy, adenoidectomy, and the placement of tympanostomy tubes. Myringotomy, or incision of the tympanic membrane, is a method of draining middle ear fluid. Before the introduction of antimicrobial agents, myringo-

tomy was the major method of managing suppurative otitis media. Today, the use of myringotomy is limited to the relief of intractable ear pain, hastening resolution of mastoid infection, and drainage of persistent middle ear effusion that is unresponsive to medical therapy.

Enlarged adenoids may obstruct the orifice of the eustachian tube in the posterior portion of the nasopharynx and interfere with adequate ventilation and drainage of the middle ear. Studies of the use of adenoidectomy in children with prolonged effusions in the middle ear identify in selected children a beneficial effect in reducing time spent with effusion.[52,53]

Tympanostomy tubes resemble small collar buttons. They are placed through an incision in the tympanic membrane to provide drainage of fluid and ventilation of the middle ear. The placement of these tubes is now one of the most common surgical procedures in children. The criteria for the placement of tubes include persistent middle ear effusions unresponsive to adequate medical treatment over a period of 3 months and persistent negative pressure. Hearing improves dramatically after placement of the ventilating tubes. The tubes have also been of value in patients who have difficulty maintaining ambient pressure in the middle ear such as would occur due to barotrauma in airline personnel. The liabilities of the placement of tubes include those of anesthesia associated with the procedure, persistent perforation, scarring of the tympanic membrane, development of cholesteatoma, and otitis media caused by swimming with ventilating tubes in place, but these occur infrequently.

MASTOIDITIS

The proximity of the mastoid to the middle ear cleft suggests that most cases of suppurative otitis media are associated with inflammation of the mastoid air cells (Fig. 1). The incidence of clinically significant mastoiditis, however, is low since the introduction of antimicrobial agents. Nevertheless, acute and chronic disease still occurs and may be responsible for significant morbidity and life-threatening disease.

Pathogenesis

At birth, the mastoid consists of a single cell, the antrum, connected to the middle ear by a small channel. Pneumatization of the mastoid bone takes place soon after birth and is extensive by 2 years of age. The clinical importance of the mastoid is

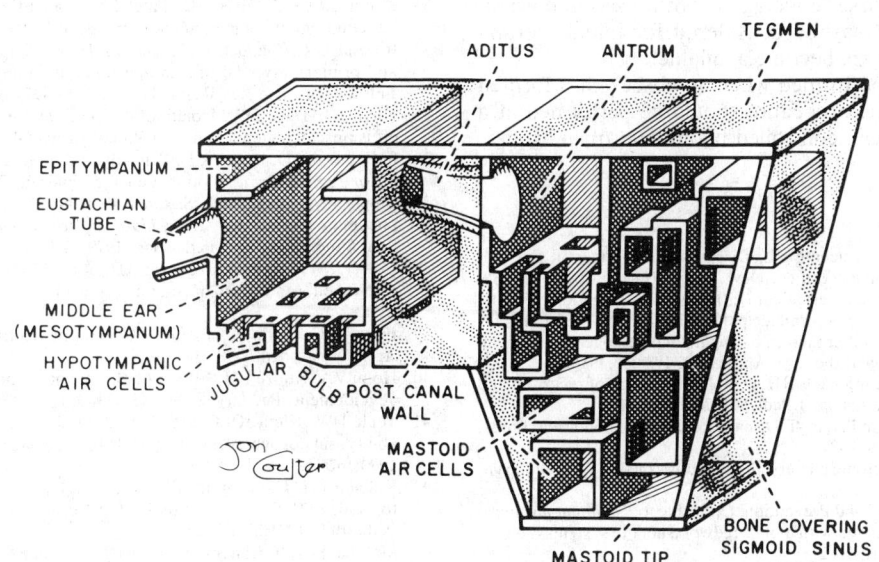

FIG. 1. Diagrammatic representation of the anatomy of the middle and mastoid air cell system showing the narrow connection (aditus and antrum) between the two.

related to contiguous structures including the posterior cranial fossa, the middle cranial fossa, the sigmoid and lateral sinuses, the canal of the facial nerve, the semicircular canals, and the petrous tip of the temporal bone. The mastoid air cells are lined with modified respiratory mucosa, and all are connected with the antrum.

Infection in the mastoid follows middle ear infection. Initially, there is hyperemia and edema of the mucosal lining of the air cells. Serous, then purulent exudate collects in the cells. Necrosis of bone due to pressure of the purulent exudate on the thin bony septa follows. Coalescence of pus in contiguous areas results in abscess cavities.

Clinical Manifestations

Acute mastoiditis is usually accompanied by acute infection in the middle ear. During early stages, the signs are those of acute otitis media with hearing loss, otalgia, and fever. Subsequently, swelling, redness, and tenderness is present over the mastoid bone. The pinna is displaced outward and downward. A purulent discharge may emerge through a perforation in the tympanic membrane.

Chronic otitis media with mastoiditis can erode through the roof of the antrum, causing temporal lobe abscess, or extend posteriorly, causing septic thrombosis of the lateral sinus.

Diagnosis

Radiographs of the mastoid area may show a loss of sharpness of the shadows of cellular walls due to demineralization of bony septa and cloudiness of areas of pneumatization due to inflammatory swelling of the air cells. Computed tomography is very helpful in delineating extent of disease.

Cultures for bacteria from ear drainage fluid must be taken with care to distinguish fresh drainage fluid from material in the external canal. The canal must be cleaned and fresh pus obtained as it exudes from the tympanic membrane. If the tympanic membrane is not perforated, tympanocentesis should be performed to obtain material from the middle ear.

Management

The antimicrobial drugs of choice for acute infection are similar to those for acute otitis media: antibiotics with activity against *S. pneumoniae* and *H. influenzae*. If the disease in the mastoid has had a prolonged course, coverage for *S. aureus* and gram-negative enteric bacilli may be considered for initial therapy until the results of cultures become available.

A mastoidectomy is performed when an abscess has formed in the mastoid bone. The procedure should be performed at a time when sepsis has been controlled by antimicrobial agents.

REFERENCES

1. Senturia BH, Marcus MD, Lucente FE. Diseases of the External Ear. An Otologic Dermatologic Manual. 2nd ed. New York: Grune & Stratton; 1980.
2. Bergstrom L. Disease of the external ear. In Bluestone CD, Stook SE, eds. Pediatric Otolaryngology. 2nd ed. Philadelphia: WB Saunders; 1990:310–19.
3. Rubin J, Yu VL. Malignant external otitis: Insights into pathogenesis, clinical manifestations, diagnosis, and therapy. Am J Med. 1988;85:391–8.
4. Riding KH, Bluestone CD, Michaels RH, et al. Microbiology of recurrent and chronic otitis media with effusion. J Pediatr 1978;93:739–43.
5. Pelton SI, Teele DW, Shurin PA, et al. Disparate cultures of middle ear fluids. Am J Dis Child. 1980;134:951–3.
6. Brook I, Schwartz R. Anaerobic bacteria in acute otitis media. Acta Otolaryngol. 1981;91:111–4.
7. Centers for Disease Control and Prevention. Otitis due to *Pseudomonas aeruginosa* serotype 0:10 associated with mobile redwood hot tub systems—North Carolina. MMWR. 1982;31:541–2.
8. Doroghazi RM, Nadol JB, Hyslop NE, et al. Invasive external otitis. Am J Med. 1981;71:603–13.
9. Johnson MP, Ramphal R. Malignant external otitis: Report on therapy with ceftazidime and review of therapy and prognosis. Rev Infect Dis. 1990;12:173–80.
10. Rapoport Y, Shalit I, Redianu C, Himmelfarb MZ: Oral ofloxacin therapy for invasive external otitis. Ann Otol Rhinol Laryngol. 1991;100:632–7.
11. Phillips P, Bryce G, Shepherd J: Invasive external otitis caused by *Aspergillus*. Rev Infect Dis. 1990;12:277–81.
12. Schappert SM: Office visits for otitis media: United States, 1975–90. In: Vital and Health Statistics of the Centers for Disease Control/National Centers for Health Statistics. Atlanta: Centers for Disease Control and Prevention, 1992; 214:3–18.
13. Bluestone CD, Klein JO, eds. Otitis Media in Infants and Children. Philadelphia: WB Saunders; 1987.
14. Wald ER, Dashefsky B, Byers C, et al. Frequency and severity of infections in day care. J Pediatr. 1968;112:540–6.
15. Celin S, Bluestone C, Stephenson J, et al. Bacteriology of acute otitis media in adults. JAMA. 1991;266:2249–52.
16. Schwartz LE, Brown RB: Purulent otitis media in adults. Arch Intern Med. 1992;152:2301–4.
17. Barnett ED, Klein JO, Pelton SI, Luginbuhl LM: Otitis media in children born to human immunodeficiency virus–infected mothers. Pediatr Infect Dis J. 1992;11:360–4.
18. Teele DW, Klein JO, Rosner B: Epidemiology of otitis media during the first seven years of life in children in greater Boston: A prospective, cohort study. J Infect Dis. 1989;160:83–94.
19. Klein JO: Microbiology. In: Bluestone CD, Klein JO, eds.: Otitis Media in Infants and Children. Philadelphia: WB Saunders; 1988:45–58.
20. Etzel RA, Pattishall EN, Haley NJ, et al. Passive smoking and middle ear effusion among children in day care. Pediatrics. 1992;90:228–32.
21. Bluestone CD, Klein JO: Otitis media, atelectasis, and eustachian tube dysfunction. In: Bluestone CD, Stool SE. Pediatric Otolaryngology. 2nd ed. 1990: 373.
22. Del Baccaro MA, Mendelman PM, Inglis AF, et al. Bacteriology of acute otitis media: A new perspective. J Pediatr. 1992;120:81–4.
23. Kamme C, Ageberg M, Lundgren K. Distribution of *Diplococcus pneumoniae* types in acute otitis media in children and influence of the types on the clinical course in penicillin V therapy. Scand J Infect Dis. 1970;2:183–90.
24. Austrian R, Howie VM, Ploussard JH. The bacteriology of pneumococcal otitis media. Johns Hopkins Med J. 1977;141:104–11.
25. Gray BM, Converse GM, Dillion HC. Serotypes of *Streptococcus pneumoniae* causing disease. J Infect Dis. 1979;140:979–83.
26. Harding AL, Anderson P, Howie VM, et al. *Haemophilus influenzae* isolated from children with otitis media. In: Sell SHW, Karzon DT, eds. *Haemophilus influenzae*. Nashville: Vanderbilt University Press; 1973:21.
27. Van Hare GF, Shurin PA, Marchant CD, et al. Acute otitis media caused by *Branhamella catarrhalis*: Biology and therapy. Rev Infect Dis. 1987;9:16–27.
28. Kovatch AL, Wald ER, Michaels RH: β-Lactamase–producing *Branhamella catarrhalis* causing otitis media in children. J Pediatr. 1983;102:261–4.
29. Chonmaitree T, Howie VM, Truant AL. Presence of respiratory viruses in middle ear fluids and nasal wash specimens from children with acute otitis media. Pediatrics. 1986;77:698–702.
30. Klein BS, Dallette ER, Volken RH. The role of respiratory syncytial virus and other viral pathogens in acute otitis media. J Pediatr. 1982;101:16–20.
31. Henderson FW, Collier AM, Sanyal MA, et al. A longitudinal study of respiratory viruses and bacteria in the etiology of acute otitis media with effusion. N Engl J Med. 1982;306:1377.
32. Arola M, Ziegler T, Ruuskanen O: Respiratory virus infection as a cause of prolonged symptoms in acute otitis media. J Pediatr. 1990;116:697–701.
33. Chonmaitree T, Owen MJ, Patel JA, et al. Effect of viral respiratory tract infection on outcome of acute otitis media. J Pediatr. 1992;120:856–62.
34. Rifkind DR, Chanock RM, Kravetz H, et al. Ear involvement (myringitis) and primary atypical pneumonia following inoculation of volunteers with Eaton agent. Am Rev Respir Dis. 1962;85:497–99.
35. Klein JO, Teele DW. Isolation of viruses and mycoplasma from middle ear effusions: A review. Ann Otol Rhinol Laryngol. 1976;85:140–4.
36. Sobeslavsky O, Syrucek L, Bruckoya M, et al. The etiological role of *Mycoplasma pneumoniae* in otitis media in children. Pediatrics. 1965;35:652–7.
37. Tipple MA, Beem MO, Saxon EM. Clinical characteristics of the afebrile pneumonia associated with *Chlamydia trachomatis* infection in infants less than 6 months of age. Pediatrics. 1979;63:192–7.
38. Lowry PW, Jarvis WR, Oberle AD, et al. *Mycobacterium chelonae* causing otitis media in an ear-nose-and-throat practice. N Engl J Med. 1988;391:978–82.
39. Fria TJ, Cantekin EI, Eichler JA. Hearing acuity of children with effusion. Arch Otolaryngol. 1985;111:10–6.
40. Holm VA, Kunze LH. Effects of chronic otitis media on language and speech development. Pediatrics. 1969;43:833–9.
41. Teele DW, Klein JO, Chase C, et al. Otitis media in infancy and intellectual ability, school achievement, speech and language at age 7 years. J Infect Dis. 1990;162:685–94.
42. Kaleida PH, Casselbrant ML, Rockette HE, et al. Amoxicillin or myringotomy or both for acute otitis media: Results of a randomized clinical trial. Pediatrics. 1991;87:466–74.
43. Marchant CD, Carlin SA, Johnson CE, Shurin PA: Measuring the comparative efficacy of antibacterial agents for acute otitis media: The "Pollyanna phenomenon." J Pediatr. 1992;120:72–7.
44. Cantekin EI, Mandel EM, Bluestone CD. Lack of efficacy of a deconges-

tant–antihistamine combination for otitis media with effusion (''secretory'' otitis media) in children. N Engl J Med. 1983;308:297–301.

45. Bluestone CD, Connell JT, Doyle WJ, et al. Symposium: Questioning the efficacy and safety of antihistamines in the treatment of upper respiratory infection. Pediatr Infect Dis J. 1988;7:15–42.
46. Perrin JM, Charney E, MacWhinney JB, et al. Sulfisoxazole as chemoprophylaxis for recurrent otitis media: A double-blind crossover study in pediatric practice. N Engl J Med. 1974;291:664–7.
47. Maynard JE, Fleshman JK, Tschopp CF. Otitis media in Alaskan Eskimo children: Prospective evaluation of chemoprophylaxis. JAMA. 1972;219:597–9.
48. Klein JO, Bluestone CD. Acute otitis media: Management of pediatric infectious diseases in office practice. Pediatr Infect Dis. 1982;1:66–73.
49. Teele DW, Klein JO, the Greater Boston Collaborative Study Group. Use of pneumococcal vaccine for preventive of recurrent acute otitis media in infants in Boston. Rev Infect Dis. 1981;3(Suppl):113.
50. Sloyer JL, Ploussard JH, Howie VM. Efficacy of pneumococcal polysaccharide vaccine in preventing acute otitis media in infants in Huntsville, Alabama. Rev Infect Dis. 1981;3(Suppl):119.
51. Makela PH, Leinonen M, Pukander J, et al. A study of the pneumococcal vaccine in prevention of clinically acute attacks of recurrent otitis media. Rev Infect Dis. 1981;3(Suppl):124.
52. Paradise JL, Bluestone CD, Rogers KD, et al. Efficacy of adenoidectomy in recurrent otitis media: Historical overview and preliminary results from a randomized, controlled trial. Ann Otol Rhinol Laryngol. 1980;89:319–21.
53. Gates GA, Avery CA, Prihoda TJ, et al. Effectiveness of adenoidectomy and tympanostomy tubes in the treatment of chronic otitis media with effusion. N Engl J Med. 1987;317:1444–51.

44. SINUSITIS

JACK M. GWALTNEY, Jr.

Acute sinusitis is an infection of one or more of the paranasal sinuses that usually complicates a common cold or other viral infection of the upper respiratory tract. A minor proportion of cases are associated with dental infection. Acute sinusitis may also occur in patients with allergic rhinitis or anatomic abnormalities of the nose that interfere with normal mucociliary clearance of the sinus cavity. Sinusitis in turn may be complicated by serious intracranial infections such as bacterial meningitis, epidural and subdural abscess, and brain abscess.

ETIOLOGY

The paranasal sinuses are normally sterile[1–4] and should be considered as a closed space. Although transient microbial contamination of the sinus cavity is thought to occur via the natural ostia, in the setting of acute disease the recovery of microorganisms from the sinus cavity indicates that infection is present. Quantitative cultures of sinus aspirates are particularly useful in establishing bacterial etiology. Sample collection by sinus endoscopy has not been shown to avoid specimen contamination and is not acceptable for etiologic studies.

The infectious agents responsible for most cases of acute community-acquired maxillary sinusitis are listed in Table 1. The information is from studies in which specimens for culture were obtained by direct sinus puncture and aspiration to avoid contamination by nasopharyngeal flora.[3,5–11] *Streptococcus pneumoniae* and unencapsulated strains of *Haemophilus influenzae* accounted for approximately one-half of all cases. Mixtures of anaerobic bacteria were associated with 6 percent of infections in adults. Sinusitis due to anaerobic bacteria was usually found in patients with associated dental disease. *Staphylococcus aureus, Streptococcus pyogenes, Moraxella catarrhalis*, and other gram-negative bacteria were each associated with a proportion of the total cases. α-Hemolytic and other streptococci have also been recovered in pure culture in high titers from aspirates of acute infected sinuses. In children with acute disease, anaerobic

TABLE 1. The Microbial Etiology of Acute Community-Acquired Antral Sinusitis

Microbial Agent	Percent of Cases Mean (Range)	
	Adults	Children
Bacteria		
S. pneumoniae	31 (20–35)	36
H. influenza (unencapsulated)	21 (6–26)	23
S. pneumoniae and H. influenzae	5 (1–9)	—
Anaerobic bacteria (Bacteroides, Peptostreptococcus, Fusobacterium spp., and so forth)	6 (0–10)	—
S. aureus	4 (0–8)	—
S. pyogenes	2 (1–3)	2
M. catarrhalis	2	19
Gram-negative bacteria[a]	9 (0–24)	2
Viruses		
Rhinovirus	15	—
Influenza virus	5	—
Parainfluenza virus	3	2
Adenovirus	—	2

[a] One study had a 24 percent isolation of gram-negative bacteria, but in four other studies the recovery rate was not over 5 percent. Gram-negative bacteria recovered included *P. aeruginosa, K. pneumoniae*, and *E. coli*.

infections are uncommon, presumably due to less frequent dental infections, and *M. catarrhalis* was recovered almost as frequently as *H. influenzae*.[12,13]

Rhinovirus, influenza virus, and parainfluenza virus were recovered alone or in combination with bacteria in approximately one-fifth of the adult cases of acute sinusitis.[3,10] Whether the sequence was for the viral infection to precede the bacterial infection or for a simultaneous invasion by both organisms was not clear.

A newly discovered agent that appears to have a role in community-acquired sinusitis is *Chlamydia pneumoniae* (strain TWAR).[14] The clinical diagnosis of sinusitis was present in 16 percent of 19 children and adults with *C. pneumoniae* infection.[15] *Chlamydia pneumoniae* is of particular interest because it does not respond to currently recommended antimicrobial treatment for acute sinusitis and because of the reported chronicity of the disease in some patients.[16] Recovery of *C. pneumoniae* from sinus aspirates is not well documented, but it should be considered among the etiologic causes of community-acquired sinus infection.

Nosocomial sinusitis has been most often associated with *Staphylococcus aureus, Pseudomonas aeruginosa, Klebsiella pneumoniae, Enterobacter* spp., and *Proteus mirabilis* and was often polymicrobic.[17–21] *Pseudomonas aeruginosa* was also the most frequent isolate in sinus aspirates from patients with cystic fibrosis.[22] *Legionella pneumophila* was identified in sinus tissue from a patient with acquired immunodeficiency syndrome.[23]

Sinus disease acquired in the community and that of immunoimpaired patients may also be caused by fungal infections. An increasing number of fungal groups has been associated with sinus infection (Table 2).[3,24–37] Most groups have been implicated in both community-acquired disease and that of impaired hosts. Also, some *Aspergillus* species and members of the phaeohyphomyces group are associated with an allergic syndrome.

EPIDEMIOLOGY

In studies of minor illness in the home, approximately 0.5 percent of common upper respiratory infections were complicated by acute sinusitis.[38] Sinusitis undoubtedly causes a larger percentage of the cases of acute upper respiratory illness seen by physicians, but accurate figures on the incidence in this setting are not available. The incidence of sinusitis parallels the inci-

TABLE 2. Fungal Etiology of Paranasal Sinusitis

Fungi	Community Acquired	Impaired Host
Aspergillus (A. fumigatus, A. flavus, A. niger, A. oryzae, A. nidulans)	Yes	Yes
Cryptococcus (C. neoformans)		Yes
Pseudallescheria (P. boydii)	Yes	Yes
Sporothrix (S. schenckii)	Yes	
Homobasidiomytes (Schizophyllum commune)	Yes	Yes
Hyalohyphomytes (Penicillium melini)	Yes	Yes
Phaeohyphomytes (Bipolaris hawaiiensis, B. spicifera, Exserohilum rostratum, E. mcginnisii, Alternaria alternata, Curvularia lunata)	Yes	Yes
Zygomytes (Mucor spp., Rhizophus spp., Cunninghamella bertholletiae)	Yes	Yes

dence of acute infections of the upper respiratory tract, being most prevalent during the fall, winter, and spring months. Sinus infection in the summer is often associated with swimming. Sinusitis is more common in adults than in children. Full development of the maxillary, frontal, and sphenoidal sinuses is not reached until adolescence. Some physicians have the clinical impression that the incidence of acute sinusitis is increased in cigarette smokers, but studies of this risk factor are not available.

PATHOGENESIS

Most acute sinusitis cases are thought to be bacterial complications of viral colds. This idea is supported by studies in which viruses were recovered from sinus aspirates of patients with maxillary sinusitis.[3,10] The exact pathogenic mechanisms involved are unknown. The sinuses are normally sterile as a result of continuous mucociliary cleansing of particulate matter that enters the sinus cavity. However, respiratory viruses are efficient in eluding the protection provided by the mucous blanket of normal respiratory epithelium and in initiating infection.

Recent studies have revealed that acute common colds are routinely associated with abnormalities of the ostiomeatal complex of the nose and abnormalities of the sinus cavities.[39,40] In 31 adults with early natural common colds, some of which were due to rhinovirus, acute reversible occlusion of the infundibulum of the maxillary sinus was seen by computed tomography (CT) scan in 77 percent.[40] Also, in these patients, acute reversible abnormalities of the cavities of the maxillary, ethmoid, frontal, and sphenoid sinuses occurred in 87, 64, 32, and 39 percent, respectively. Thus, viral upper respiratory infections frequently produce conditions in the ostiomeatal area and sinuses that would favor a secondary bacterial infection, particularly if bacteria happen to become trapped in a sinus cavity.

From 5 to 10 percent of the cases of acute maxillary sinusitis result from infection originating from a dental source. The floor of the maxillary sinus is close to the roots of the molars and bicuspids, and infection at these sites may spread to the sinus cavity.

During acute sinusitis, the sinus mucosal lining is characteristically inflamed and swollen. Mucosal erosion may occur with some viral infections, such as influenza, but pathologic descriptions of the findings in specific infections are not available. An exudate develops in the sinus cavity containing polymorphonuclear leukocytes that are usually present in concentrations greater than 5000 cells/mm[3].[3,19] The bacterial titers in exudates from acutely infected sinuses are greater than 10^5 cfu/ml and may reach levels of 10^8 cfu/ml.

Noninfectious conditions that predispose to acute sinusitis include anatomic abnormalities such as congenital choanal atresia, septal deviation, foreign bodies, and tumors. Allergic reac-

tions in the nose cause mucosal swelling and polyp formation that also may lead to infection. In recent years, attention has been called to nosocomial sinusitis in hospitalized patients, resulting from indwelling nasal tubes of various types, or nasal packing.[17–21]

Prolonged and repeated episodes of infection in untreated or inadequately treated patients may lead to irreversible changes in the mucosal lining of the sinus, resulting in chronic sinus disease. The normal ciliated epithelium is replaced by stratified squamous epithelium that may eventually fill the sinus lumen. Sterility is no longer maintained in the sinus cavity. Cultures of surgical specimens obtained aseptically from patients with chronic sinus disease have grown a wide variety of gram-positive and gram-negative bacteria.[41] Anaerobic bacteria, S. aureus, and Streptococcus of the viridans group were recovered most often. The ongoing bacterial growth is secondary to the structural damage, which leads to a loss of the sinus membranes' capacity for self-cleansing. Thus, infection is not thought to be the basic problem in chronic sinus disease, although acute infectious exacerbations due to organisms such as S. pneumoniae and H. influenzae do occur.

CLINICAL PRESENTATION

Acute sinusitis usually develops during the course of a common cold or influenzal illness and is often difficult to distinguish from the primary illness. Criteria for the clinical diagnosis of acute bacterial sinusitis have recently been developed by two groups.[42,43] While these criteria are useful in providing a perspective on the clinical presentation of acute sinusitis, they have not been validated by comparison with quantitative bacterial culture of sinus aspirates, the gold standard of diagnosis, and therefore are of uncertain value. One set of criteria, proposed by experts in the field, places emphasis on purulent nasal or pharyngeal discharge and cough lasting greater than 7 days.[42] The other clinical predictors of acute sinusitis, which were validated by four-view sinus radiographs, were maxillary toothache, history of colored nasal discharge, poor response to nasal decongestants, abnormal sinus transillumination, and purulent secretions on examination.[43] The known insensitivity of radiographs compared with CT scans in diagnosing sinus abnormalities, especially of the ethmoid sinuses, must be considered in evaluating the latter set of predictors.

The most consistent clinical feature of acute community-acquired sinusitis is the persistence of respiratory symptoms for longer than 1 week or for longer than the usual course of colds experienced by the individual patient. Symptoms most often present include purulent nasal and postnasal discharge, a feeling of "tightness" or "pressure" over sinus areas of the face, cough, and a nasal quality to the voice. Other complaints include headache, nasal obstruction, and disorders of smell. It the nose has not been recently cleared, a purulent nasal and/or postnasal discharge is usually present on examination. Maxillary sinusitis pus is characteristically observed in the middle meatus on examination of the nose. In a small proportion of cases, erythema and tenderness are present over the involved sinus, but the absence of such external manifestations of inflammation should not exclude the diagnosis of acute sinusitis. Edema of the eyelids and excessive tearing occur with ethmoid sinusitis. Appearance of chemosis, proptosis, or limited extraocular movement should suggest the possibility of orbital extension from the ethmoidal infection. In maxillary sinusitis of dental origin, toothache and signs of an associated dental infection may be present. Temperature elevation has been reported in only approximately one-half of adults and children with acute maxillary sinusitis diagnosed by sinus puncture. In children with an acute upper respiratory illness, persistent symptoms and severe symptoms suggest a diagnosis of acute sinusitis.[13] In this setting, cough and a fetid breath are also characteristics of the infection. In some studies, patients with acute sinusitis have become asymptomatic despite

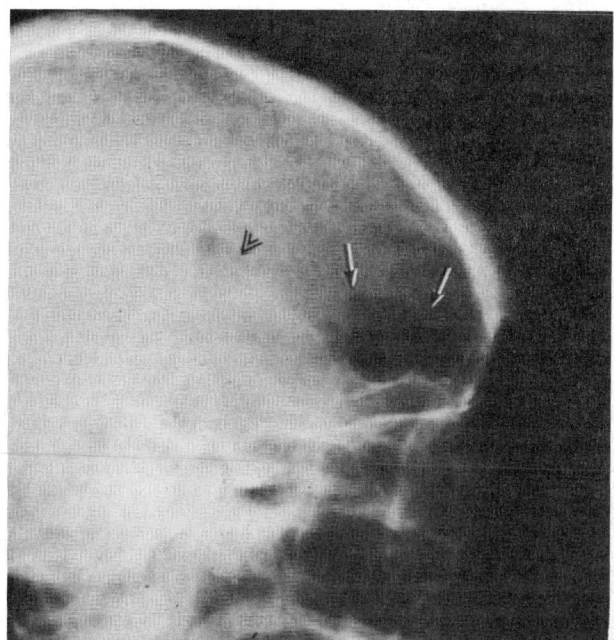

FIG. 1. Lateral sinus roentgenogram of a patient with acute frontal sinusitis complicated by abscess of the frontal lobe of the brain. Destruction of the posterior wall of the frontal sinus resulted in air in the abscess cavity (arrows) and in the lateral ventricle arrowhead). The infection was caused by *S. aureus*.

the persistence of pus and active infection in the sinus cavity as determined by sinus puncture.[3]

Patients who develop intracranial extension of infection, such as meningitis and brain abscess, usually show the characteristic signs of these infections. It may be difficult to determine when acute frontal sinusitis has progressed to a frontal lobe abscess of the brain. Inflammation and tenderness over the frontal sinus is often lacking with this infection. Patients may become apathetic and have a minimum of complaints because of destruction of the frontal lobe cortex (Fig. 1).

Osteomyelitis of the frontal bone may occur by spread from the frontal or ethmoid sinuses. Pus may collect under the periosteum of the frontal bone, causing swelling and edema over the forehead, a condition known as *Pott puffy tumor*.[44]

Nosocomial sinusitis resulting from indwelling nasal tubes has occurred most often during the second week of hospitalization.[19] Unilateral maxillary sinusitis was most common, followed by bilateral maxillary disease and pansinusitis. Fever and leukocytosis were common. Unexplained fever in patients with indwelling nasal tubes is an indication for evaluation for sinus infection.

Community-acquired fungal sinusitis tends to have a more insidious onset than its bacterial counterpart, with pressure symptoms often being the predominant complaint. Bony erosion is present in some cases, and sinus exudates of a dark or "peanut butterlike" appearance are characteristic. Allergic fungal sinusitis is characterized by nasal polyps, asthma, peripheral eosinophilia, and "allergic mucin," a pale eosinophilic or basophilic material containing eosinophils and crystals.

DIAGNOSIS

Diagnostic evaluation should include a history and an examination of the pharynx, nose, ears, sinuses, and teeth. Information should be obtained on the occurrence of coryzal and influenzal illnesses and of respiratory allergies. As discussed above, the duration and severity of the illness as disclosed in the history is often more useful in distinguishing acute sinusitis from an uncomplicated cold or influenzal illness than are the presence

of any particular symptom or symptoms. In any acute upper respiratory illnesses that lasts longer than 7 to 10 days, the diagnosis of acute sinusitis should be considered. The finding of purulent nasal or postnasal secretions in such patients is characteristic but not diagnostic of sinus infection.

The most useful procedure on examination, although it can only be applied to the frontal and maxillary sinuses, is transillumination. The examination should be performed with a sinus transilluminator in a completely darkened room. In patients with previously normal sinuses, the finding of complete opacity on transillumination correlated well with the presence of active infection.[3] Conversely, the finding of normal transillumination was equally good evidence that no infection was present. The finding of diminished light transmission, "dullness" but not complete opacity, was less helpful. Approximately one-fourth of the patients with this finding were found to have active infection as determined by sinus puncture, while the remaining three-fourths were normal. It should be emphasized that sinus transillumination is less helpful in patients with heavy bone structure or with chronic sinusitis in whom absent or reduced light transmission may be a persistent finding.

With the availability of sensitive, new imaging techniques, especially CT scanning, considerable new knowledge has been gained about the diagnosis of acute sinusitis. While standard four-view sinus radiographs are considerably more sensitive and specific for detecting acute anatomic abnormalities of the sinuses than physical examination and transillumination, it is now recognized that they are considerably less sensitive than sinus CT scans. The latter provide exquisitely detailed views of all of the paranasal sinuses and reveal many acute changes that are not detected by standard radiography. In some hospitals and clinics, the cost of limited CT scans of the sinuses has become equivalent to that of standard sinus radiographs.

Despite their relative insensitivity, standard sinus radiographs correlated well with bacterial cultures of sinus aspirates in adults with acute but prolonged upper respiratory illness who were suspected of having acute sinusitis. In such a setting, the presence of radiologic opacity, an air-fluid level, or mucosal thickening was strong evidence for the presence of active infection (Fig. 2).[3,10,45,46] Although somewhat controversial, when allowance is made for the presence of recent respiratory symptoms and for the severity of radiographic abnormalities, sinus radiography appears to be of equal value in the diagnosis of acute sinusitis in children.[13,47,48] Sinus radiology is less useful in diagnosing active infection in patients with chronic sinus disease because of persistent radiologic abnormalities in such patients.

The major deficiency of all currently available imaging techniques for diagnosing acute sinusitis is their inability to distinguish bacterially infected sinuses from those with inflammation due to a viral infection or other nonbacterial cause. The recent discovery by CT scan of the frequent occurrence of acute reversible abnormalities in the sinus cavities of patients with early and presumed uncomplicated common colds[40] has revealed a new complexity to the use of imaging techniques for diagnosing acute sinusitis. Most of the sinus cavity abnormalities observed in the patients with acute colds had resolved or markedly improved on follow-up examination at approximately 2 weeks, a time when the development of acute bacterial sinusitis is likely.

The presence of a bacterial infection of the sinus cavity and its specific microbial etiology can be determined only by culture of an exudate or a rinse obtained directly from the sinus by puncture and aspiration. Cultures of nasal pus or of sinus exudates obtained by rinsing through the natural sinus ostium or by endoscopy give unreliable information because of contamination with resident bacterial flora in the nose. Since the microbial etiology of acute sinusitis has been well described in studies using direct puncture, there is no indication for using sinus puncture in the management of the average case of acute sinusitis. However, sinus puncture should be performed for bacterial diagnoses in patients with unusually severe sinusitis, particularly

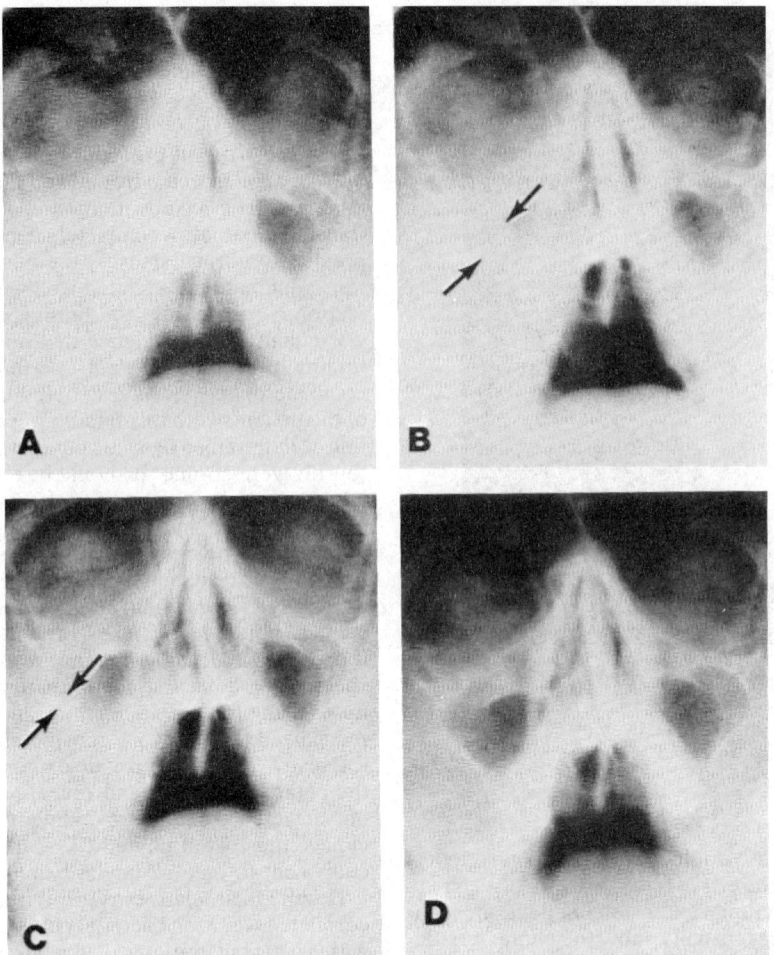

FIG. 2. Serial roentgenograms of a patient with acute infection of the right maxillary antrum (occipitomental views). The patient received ampicillin from February 18 to February 26. (**A**) February 18, complete opacity of the antrum. Culture of sinus aspirate yielded *H. influenzae* in a titer of 10^6 cfu/ml. (**B**) February 25, marked thickening of the mucosal lining. (**C**) March 4, diminished thickening of the mucosal lining. (**D**) March 18, normal.

if intracranial extension of the infection is suspected. Also, sinus puncture is of value in patients who have not responded to empiric antimicrobial therapy, those with severe immunosuppression, and those with nosocomial sinusitis when it is not possible to predict the identity and antimicrobial sensitivity of the causative agent.

The antral sinus is punctured below the inferior turbinate of the nose and the frontal sinus below the infraorbital rim of the eye. Thorough cleansing of the puncture site with an antiseptic solution such as povidone–iodine is important to prevent contamination of the specimen with surface bacteria. Specimens for culture should be aspirated through the puncture needle and should not be obtained by collecting material that has been rinsed through the natural sinus ostium. When free fluid cannot be obtained from the sinus cavity, 1 ml of antibiotic-free normal saline or Ringer's lactate solution can be instilled and aspirated to provide a specimen. The syringe containing the specimen should be transported to the laboratory for examination by Gram stain and aerobic and anaerobic bacterial culture. When available, quantitative culture of the specimen is useful to help detect bacterial contaminants accidentally introduced into the specimen. Most bacteria causing active sinus infection are present in titers of at least 10^5 cfu/ml, while titers of contaminants in a freshly processed specimen are usually considerably less.

In patients with acute sinusitis in whom intracranial complications, such as bacterial meningitis and brain abscess, are suspected, appropriate diagnostic evaluations should be conducted promptly (see Chs. 64 and 68).

Noninfectious causes of persistent sinus disease that enter the differential diagnosis include nasal and sinus tumors, foreign bodies in the nose, Wegener's granulomatosis, and midline granuloma. Rhinoscleroma, a chronic granulomatous disease of the mucosa of the upper airway caused by *Klebsiella rhinoscleromatis,* can also lead to bony invasion and obstruction of the nasal passages. The availability of CT scanning of the nasal passages and sinuses and of endoscopic examination of the nasal cavity has greatly facilitated the differential diagnosis of these conditions.

TREATMENT

Antimicrobial Therapy

Although viruses may play a role in the initiation of acute sinusitis, the disease should be treated as a bacterial infection. The effectiveness of antimicrobial treatment in shortening the course of acute sinusitis has been proven in studies employing pre- and post-treatment cultures of sinus aspirates.[49,50] Antimicrobial therapy must be selected on an empiric basis, since in the usual case sinus puncture to determine a specific microbial diagnosis is not indicated. Therapy should ideally cover all the bacteria listed in Table 1, but primarily it should be effective for both *S. pneumoniae* and *H. influenzae*.

A number of antimicrobial agents have been shown to be effective against the major bacterial causes of acute community-acquired sinusitis in studies employing quantitative cultures of

TABLE 3. Antimicrobials Tested by Pre- and Post-Therapy Sinus Puncture Cultures in Adults with Acute Sinusitis

Antimicrobial Agent	Oral Dose in Adults
Ampicillin[a]	500 mg q6h
Amoxicillin[a]	500 mg q8h
Cyclacillin[a]	500 mg q8h
Bacampicillin[a]	800 mg bid
Trimethoprim-sulfamethoxazole (80 mg/400 mg)	2 tablets bid
Cefaclor	500 mg q6h
Cefuroxime axetil	250 mg q12h
Amoxicillin–clavulanate	500/125 mg q8h
Loracarbef	400 mg q12h
Cefixime	200 mg q12h

[a] No longer recommended because of frequency of β-lactamase–producing bacteria.

pre- and post-therapy sinus aspirates. Data based on puncture results are necessary to evaluate efficacy, because the measurement of antimicrobial concentrations in the paranasal sinuses has not been standardized.[49,51,52] These drugs and the doses for a recommended 14 day course of treatment are listed (Table 3).[11] The ampicillinlike drugs in Table 3 were tested before the widespread prevalence of β-lactamase–producing *H. influenzae* and, with the exception of amoxicillin–clavulanate, are not recommended. Selecting an appropriate drug from the remainder of the list requires balancing cost versus frequency of side effects. Trimethroprim-sulfamethoxazole is quite inexpensive but has the disadvantage of causing relatively frequent skin rashes. Cefuroxime axetil and amoxicillin–clavulanate are considerable more expensive than trimethroprim-sulfamethoxazole but are better tolerated. The cost of some of the other drugs on the list, *in the doses that are required for effective treatment of acute sinusitis,* is a serious disadvantage to their routine use.

The etiologic role of *C. pneumoniae* in community-acquired sinusitis is not well defined. However, in the small percentage (10 percent or less) of patients who do not show a response to the therapy recommended above, treatment with a tetracycline, macrolide, or azalide, to which *C. pneumoniae* is sensitive, may be a reasonable consideration. It should be remembered that tetracycline is not effective for some strains of pneumococci and that the new macrolide and azalide antibiotics, in the doses recommended, are of unproven effectiveness for sinus infection due to *H. influenzae*. Until the effectiveness of the new macrolide and zalide antibiotic for *H. influenzae* is established, initial treatment should consist of one of the antibiotics of proven effectiveness for sinusitis due to *S. pneumoniae* and *H. influenzae*.

Community-acquired fungal sinusitis in persons with normal immunity has been effectively treated with surgical débridement of the affected sinus cavities. Complicated cases and those in patients with immunodeficiencies should be evaluated on an individual basis for appropriate antifungal therapy.

Supportive Therapy

Nasal decongestants should be used in the supportive treatment of acute sinusitis. Phenylephrine nose drops, 0.25 or 0.5%, are recommended for use on a regular basis as described in Chapter 39. Most patients with acute sinusitis can be successfully treated as outpatients. For patients with severe infection and for those in whom intracranial extension of infection is a consideration, hospitalization is advisable for parenteral antimicrobial therapy, close observation, and prompt initiation of diagnostic tests when needed.

Surgical Therapy

Patients with severe sinus infection or those suspected of developing intracranial or orbital complications should be evaluated with CT for emergency or early surgical drainage. Infection of the orbit and of the frontal[53] and sphenoid[54] sinuses should be

recognized as conditions in which surgical intervention may be required.

Subacute and Chronic Sinusitis

Sinus lavage has been used traditionally for the treatment of patients with acute sinusitis in whom complaints have persisted. An irrigation or series of irrigations of the affected sinus appears to be beneficial. When lavage is performed via direct sinus puncture, a sample of the sinus contents should be aspirated and cultured quantitatively for bacterial identification and antibiotic sensitivities. Evaluation for allergy[55,56] or immunodeficiency[57] states is sometimes helpful in the management of patients who have reached this stage of the disease.

Once sinusitis has reached a chronic state, bacterial colonization of the sinus cavity is usual, but the condition no longer responds to antimicrobial treatment. Patients with chronic sinus disease may have acute exacerbations of infection, which should be treated as an acute infection, but the primary problem is impaired drainage of the sinus cavity. It is now recognized that obstruction of the ostiomeatal area in the nose is a major contributing factor to the development of chronic sinus disease. Correction of target areas of obstruction in the ostiomeatal complex by traditional or functional endoscopic sinus surgery is rapidly replacing earlier surgical procedures for promoting sinus drainage.[58] These new techniques are useful for controlling symptoms in many patients with chronic sinus disease and have been associated with reversal of chronic changes and return of mucociliary function in some patients.

MEASURES TO PREVENT ACUTE OR CHRONIC SINUSITIS

There are no proven ways to prevent acute sinusitis. When control of colds and influenzal illness becomes practical, the incidence of sinusitis should decline. For the present, prompt and regular use of vasoconstrictors in nasal drops or sprays for the treatment of colds may help to reduce the incidence of secondary bacterial infection of the sinuses, but this is unproven. Control of nasal allergies and corrective surgery for nasal abnormalities may promote normal sinus drainage and thus lessen the risk of sinus infection. Good dental hygiene and prompt treatment of tooth root infection may help to reduce the incidence of acute infection of the maxillary sinus secondary to dental disease.

Effective antimicrobial therapy for patients with acute sinusitis may help to reduce the incidence of chronic sinus disease, although this is not established. The diversity of bacteria responsible for acute sinusitis limits the choice of antimicrobials that have an adequate spectrum of activity, particularly for both *S. pneumoniae* and *H. influenzae*. Penicillin, tetracyclines, and first-generation cephalosporins, which have been widely used in the past to treat acute sinusitis, do not provide optimum coverage of both of these organisms. Undoubtedly, many patients with acute sinusitis who were given one of these drugs did not receive effective treatment. This may have resulted in the infection causing damage to the sinus and may have been a preventable cause of chronic sinus disease.

REFERENCES

1. Bjuggren G, Kraepelien S, Lind J. Sinusitis in children at home and in day-nurseries. Ann Paediatr. 1949;173:205–21.
2. Björkwall T. Bacteriological examination in maxillary sinusitis: Bacterial flora of the maxillary antrum. Acta Otolaryngol (Stockh). 1964;188(Suppl):390–9.
3. Evans FO, Sydnor JB, Moore WEC, et al. Sinusitis of maxillary antrum. N Engl J Med. 1974;293:735.
4. Shapiero ED, Wald ER, Doyle WJ, et al. Bacteriology of maxillary sinuses of the rhesus monkey. Ann Otol Rhinol Laryngol. 1982;91:150–1.
5. Urdal K, Berdal P. The microbial flora in 81 cases of maxillary sinusitis. Acta Otolaryngol. 1949;37:20.
6. Björkwall T. Bacteriologic examinations in maxillary sinusitis: Bacterial flora of the maxillary antrum. Acta Otolaryngol. 1950;83(Suppl):33.

7. Lystad A, Berdal P, Lung-Iversen L. The bacterial flora of sinusitis with in vitro study of the bacterial resistance to antibiotics. Acta Otolaryngol. 1964; 188(suppl):390.

8. Rantanen T, Arvilommi H. Double-blind trial of doxycycline in acute maxillary sinusitis: A clinical and bacteriological study. Acta Otolaryngol. 1973; 76:58.

9. Axelsson A, Broson JE. The correlation and maxillary sinus in acute maxillary sinusitis. Laryngoscope. 1973;83:2003.

10. Hamory BH, Sande MA, Sydnor A Jr, et al. Etiology and antimicrobial therapy of acute maxillary sinusitis. J Infect Dis. 1979;139:197–202.

11. Gwaltney JM Jr, Scheld WM, Sande MA, et al. The microbial etiology and antimicrobial therapy of adults with acute community-acquired sinusitis: A fifteen-year experience at the University of Virginia and review of other selected studies. J Allergy Clin Immunol. 1992;90:457–62.

12. Wald ER, Milmoe GJ, Bowen A'D, et al. Acute maxillary sinusitis in children. N Engl J Med. 1981;304:749.

13. Wald ER. Sinusitis in children. N Engl J Med. 1992;326:319–23.

14. Grayston JT. Infections caused by *Chlamydia pneumoniae* strain TWAR. Clin Infect Dis. 1992;15:757–63.

15. Hahn DL, Dodge RW, Golubjatnikov R. Association of *Chlamydia pneumoniae* (strain TWAR) infection with wheezing, asthmatic bronchitis, and adult-onset asthma. JAMA. 1991;266:225–30.

16. Hammerschlag MR, Chirgwin K, Roblin PM, et al. Persistent infection with *Chlamydia pneumoniae* following acute respiratory illness. Clin Infect Dis. 1992;14:178–82.

17. Pope TL, Stelling CB, Leitner YB. Maxillary sinusitis after nasotracheal intubation. South Med J. 1981;74:610–2.

18. Via-Reque E, Rattenborg CC. Prolonged oro- or nasotracheal intubation. Crit Care Med. 1981;9:637–9.

19. Caplan ES, Hoyt NJ. Nosocomial sinusitis. JAMA. 1982;247:639–41.

20. Deutschman CS, Wilton PB, Sinow J, et al. Paranasal sinusitis: a common complication of nasoracheal intubation in neurosurgical patients. Neurosurgery. 1985;17:296–9.

21. Linden BE, Aguilar EA, Allen SJ. Sinusitis in the nasotracheally intubated patient. Arch Otolaryngol Head Neck Surg. 1988;114:860–1.

22. Shapiro ED, Milmoe, Wald ER, et al. Bacteriology of the maxillary sinuses in patients with cystic fibrosis. J Infect Dis. 1982;146:589.

23. Schlanger G, Lutwick LI, Kurzman M, et al. Sinusitis caused by *Legionella pneumophila* in a patient with the acquired immune deficiency syndrome. Am J Med. 1984;77:957–60.

24. Morriss FH Jr, Spock A. Intracranial aneurysm secondary to mycotic orbital and sinus infection. Report of a case implicating penicillium as an opportunistic fungus. Am J Dis Child. 1970;119:357–62.

25. McGuirt WF, Harril JA. Paranasal sinus aspergillosis. Laryngoscope. 1979; 89:1563.

26. Stevens MH. Primary fungal sinusitis. Am J Otolaryngol. 1981;2:348–57.

27. Romett J, Newman R. Aspergillosis of the nose and paranasal sinuses. Laryngoscope. 1982;92:764–6.

28. Rinaldi MG, Invasive aspergillosis. Rev Infect Dis. 1983;5:1061.

29. Morgan MA, Wilson WR, Neel B III, et al. Fungal sinusitis in healthy and immunocompromised individuals. Am J Clin Pathol. 1984;82:597–601.

30. Padhye AA, Ajello L, Wieden MA, et al. Phaeohyphomycosis of the nasal sinuses caused by a new species of *Exserohillum*. J Clin Microbiol. 1986;24: 245.

31. Parfrey NA. Improved diagnosis and prognosis of mucormycosis. A clinico-pathologic study of 33 cases. Medicine. 1986;65:113.

32. Kern ME, Uecker FA. Maxillary sinus infection caused by the homobasidiomycetous fungus *Schizophyllum commune*. J Clin Microbiol. 1986;23:1001.

33. MacMillan RH III, Cooper PH, Body BA, et al. Allergic fungal sinusitis due to *Curvularia lunata*. Hum Pathol. 1987;18:960–4.

34. Washburn RG, Kennedy AW, Begley MG, et al. Chronic fungal sinusitis in apparently normal hosts. Medicine. 1988;67:231–47.

35. Killingsworth SM, Wetmore SJ. *Curvularia/Dreschslera* sinusitis. Laryngoscope. 1990;100:932–7.

36. Aviv J, Lawson W, Bottone E, et al. Multiple intracranial mucoceles associated with phaeohyphomycosis of the paranasal sinuses. Arch Otolaryngol Head Neck Surg. 1990;116:1210–3.

37. Zieske LA, Kipke RD, Hamill R. Dematiaceous fungal sinusitis. Otolaryngol Head Neck Surg. 1991;105:567–77.

38. Dingle JH, Badger GF, Jordan WS Jr. Illness in the Home. A Study of 25,000 Illnesses in a Group of Cleveland Families. Cleveland: The Press of Western Reserve University; 1964;292.

39. Turner BW, Cail WS, Hendley JO, et al. Physiologic abnormalities in the paranasal sinuses during experimental rhinovirus colds. J Allergy Clin Immunol. 1992;90:474–8.

40. Gwaltney JM Jr, Phillips CD, Miller RD, et al. Computed tomographic study of the common cold. N Engl J Med. 1994;330:25–30.

41. Frederick J, Braude AI. Anaerobic infection of the paranasal sinuses. N Engl J Med. 1974;290:135.

42. Shapiro GG, Rachelefsky GS. Introduction and definition of sinusitis. J Allergy Clin Immunol. 1992;90:417–8.

43. Williams JW Jr, Simel DL, Roberts L, et al. Clinical evaluation for sinusitis. Making the diagnosis by history and physical examination. Ann Intern Med. 1992;117:705–10.

44. Wells RG, Sty JR, Landers AD. Radiological evaluation of Pott puffy tumor. JAMA. 1986;255:1331–3.

45. Lusted LB, Keats TE. Atlas of Roentgenographic Measurement. 4th ed. Chicago: Year Book Medical Publishers; 1978.

46. Kovatch AL, Wald ER, Ledesma-Medina J, et al. Maxillary sinus radiographs in children with non-respiratory complaints. Pediatrics. 1984;73:306.

47. Arruda LK, Mimica IM, Solé D, et al. Abnormal maxillary sinus radiographs in children: Do they represent bacterial infection? Pediatrics. 1990;85:553–8.

48. Diament MJ. The diagnosis of sinusitis in infants and children: X-ray, computed tomography, and magnetic resonance imaging. J Allergy Clin Immunol. 1992;90:442–4.

49. Carenfelt C, Eneroth C-M, Lundberg C, et al. Evaluation of the antibiotic effect of treatment of maxillary sinusitis. Scand J Infect Dis. 1975;7:259–64.

50. Gwaltney JM Jr, Sydnor A, Sande MA. Etiology and antimicrobial treatment of acute sinusitis. Ann Otol Rhinol Laryngol 1981;90:68.

51. Gullers K. Penicillin in paranasal sinus secretions. Chemotherapy 1969;14: 303–7.

52. Scheld WM, Sydnor A Jr, Farr B, et al. Comparison of cyclacillin with amoxicillin in the therapy of acute maxillary sinusitis. Antimicrob Agents Chemother. 1986;30:350–3.

53. Middleton WG, Briant TDR, Fenton RS. Frontal sinusitis—A 10 year experience. J Otolaryngol. 1985;14:197.

54. Lew D, Southwick FS, Montogomery WW, et al. Sphenoid sinusitis. A review of 30 cases. N Engl J Med. 1983;309:1149.

55. Furukawa CT. The role of allergy in sinusitis in children. J Allergy Clin Immunol. 1992;90:515–7.

56. Spector SL. The role of allergy in sinusitis in adults. J Allergy Clin Immunol. 1992;90:518–20.

57. Polmar SH. The role of the immunologist in sinus disease. J Allergy Clin Immunol. 1992;90:511–5.

58. Lanza DC, Kennedy DW. Current concepts in the surgical management of chronic and recurrent acute sinusitis. J Allergy Clin Immunol. 1992;90:505–11.

45. EPIGLOTTITIS

JAMES E. BURNS
J. OWEN HENDLEY

Acute epiglottitis (supraglottitis) is a rapidly progressive cellulitis of the epiglottis and adjacent structures that has the potential for causing abrupt, complete airway obstruction.

The typical patient is a 2- to 4-year-old boy having at anytime of the year a 6- to 12-hour history of fever, irritability, dysphonia, and dysphagia. Sore throat is the most prominent symptom in older children and adults. At the time medical attention is sought, varying degrees of respiratory distress may be evident. The pediatric patient usually prefers to sit leaning forward while drooling oral secretions. Respirations tend to be tentative and careful without marked tachypnea. Tachycardia is usually commensurate with fever, but may be related to hypoxia and be out of proportion to fever.[1] Inspiratory stridor and hoarseness may occur, but the barking cough and aphonia that may occur in croup syndrome are rare. The diagnosis is established by visualizing an edematous "cherry-red" epiglottis. The course of acute epiglottitis may be fulminating, as emphasized by the report of a patient who progressed from being completely asymptomatic to having complete airway obstruction in 30 minutes.[2] The course may be more languid in adults, but the disease is potentially no less serious.[3–5]

Laboratory data include moderate leukocytosis with a "shift to the left," positive cultures of blood and epiglottis, and evidence of pneumonia on chest x-ray in up to 25 percent of cases.[4,5] A radiograph of the lateral neck may show an enlarged epiglottis, ballooning of the hypopharynx, and normal subglottic structures (Fig. 1).[6] However, use of radiographs in the diagnosis of epiglottitis is questionable because of both the delay in securing an airway while the films are being obtained and the variable sensitivity (as low as 31 percent) and specificity (as low as 44 percent) of this procedure.[3,7,8] Although careful analysis of the films may be able to improve their diagnostic efficiency, their clinical usefulness is limited.[9] The epiglottis should be visu-

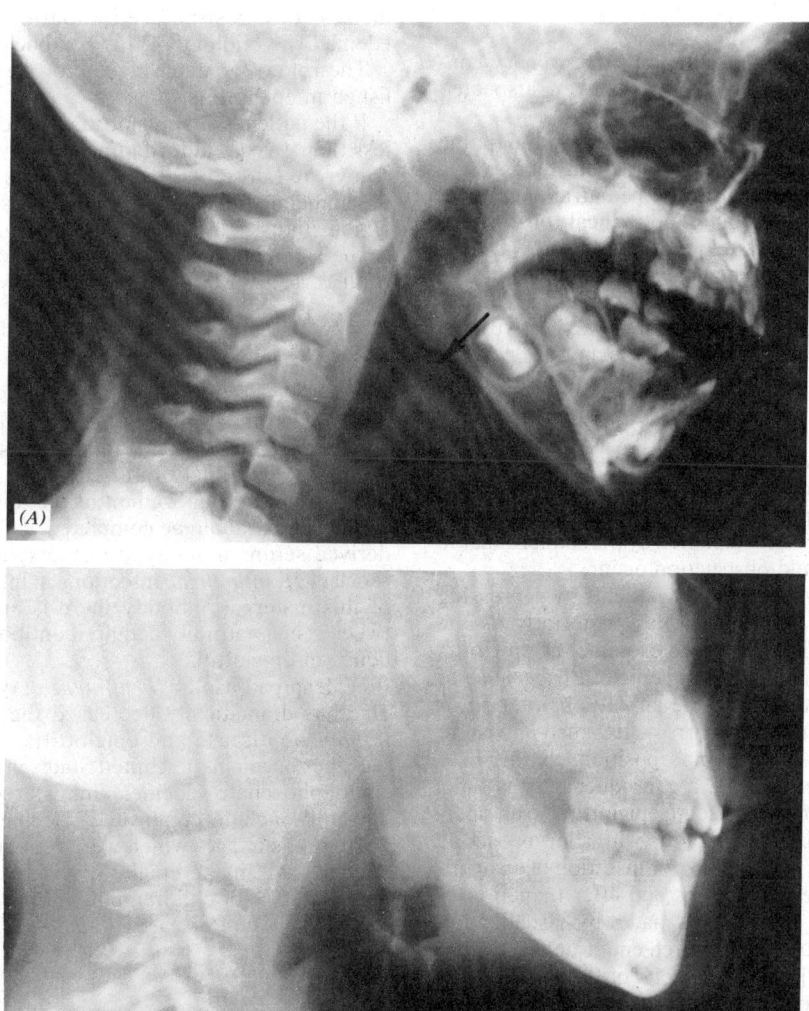

FIG. 1. Lateral neck radiographs. **(A)** Enlarged epiglottis—the thumb sign[6]—in a patient with acute epiglottitis. Arrows indicate epiglottitis. **(B)** Normal epiglottis—the little finger sign—in a patient with croup syndrome. (Courtesy of Dr. Caroline B. Hall, University of Rochester School of Medicine, Rochester, NY.)

alized directly, even if the radiograph is negative, in those patients in whom there is a strong suspicion of epiglottitis. This examination should be performed only when one is prepared to immediately secure the airway. In adults, examination of the epiglottis may be safer than in children.[3,10,11] *Haemophilus influenzae* type b is isolated from cultures of blood and/or epiglottis in most pediatric and in up to 26 percent of adult patients with epiglottitis,[12] an association first demonstrated by Le Mierre et al[13] in 1936. Other agents occasionally implicated are pneumococci, staphylococci, and streptococci.[2,14,15] The role of viruses in epiglottitis is not established.

H. influenzae bacteremia occurs in up to 100 percent of children with epiglottitis.[1,14–16] Significantly, this bacteremia has been associated with only a small number of metastatic infections such as meningitis and arthritis.[1,17,18]

DIFFERENTIAL DIAGNOSIS

The croup syndrome is the most frequent differential consideration in pediatric epiglottitis. Although the barking cough typical of croup is an infrequent feature of epiglottitis, differentiation from croup is sometimes difficult unless the epiglottis is visual-

ized. In contrast to epiglottitis, croup is frequently preceded by an upper respiratory infection, has a more gradual onset, involves somewhat younger children (aged 3 months to 3 years) and may last up to a week. The etiology is usually viral, and the area of obstruction is subglottic while the epiglottis is normal. Children with croup are more likely to prefer to lie supine and do not have the dysphagia and drooling that are characteristic of epiglottitis. In croup, radiographs of the lateral neck may show the airway narrowed in the subglottic region (Fig. 1) and are likely to reveal a normal epiglottis.[6] However, such films may be falsely read as showing epiglottitis in up to 24 percent of patients.[7]

Diphtheria can be differentiated from epiglottitis by the presence of a pseudomembrane in the respiratory tract and by the presence of typical organisms on direct smear and culture of the membrane. Allergic laryngeal edema (angioneurotic edema) and foreign body aspiration lack the toxic manifestations of epiglottitis and often have a history that is helpful in suspecting the correct diagnosis. Retropharyngeal abscess, peritonsillar abscess, and lingual tonsillitis are other rare causes of upper airway obstruction; these can usually be differentiated from epiglottitis on physical examination.

THERAPY

Maintenance of an adequate airway should be the primary concern as soon as the diagnosis of epiglottitis is even suspected in a child or an adult.

After many years of controversy over the necessity and timing of intervention and over the use of endotracheal tubes vs. a tracheostomy, current management of the pediatric patient requires the immediate insertion of an endotracheal (or nasotracheal) tube. In adults a staging system may allow more variability in diagnostic maneuvers and management if the patient is free of any signs of airway obstruction or tachypnea.[19,20] Observation of a child with epiglottitis for signs of airway obstruction cannot be recommended, since the mortality is up to 25 percent in those observed and 80 percent in those in whom obstruction occurs.[2,21]

Because of the potential for rapid deterioration to complete respiratory obstruction, pediatric patients even suspected of having acute epiglottitis should be handled as a medical emergency. Patients being transported between medical facilities and within such facilities must be accompanied by personnel capable of securing the airway should obstruction occur.

The epiglottis can be visualized in most patients by depressing the tongue with a depressor placed as far posteriorly as the tonsillar pillars. However, it is unwise to examine the epiglottis of a pediatric patient suspected of having epiglottitis because of the possibility of precipitating complete airway obstruction or a vagally mediated cardiopulmonary arrest. It is also unwise to restrain pediatric patients in the supine position, as this may also lead to airway obstruction.[22] As a consequence, it is safer to transfer a patient thought to have acute epiglottitis to an operating room and then visualize the epiglottis with a laryngoscope or bronchoscope after all is in readiness for insertion of an artificial airway under controlled conditions and after induction of anesthesia. As soon as the diagnosis is made, by visualization of the "cherry-red" epiglottis, an uncuffed endotracheal (or nasotracheal) tube should be inserted. In spite of theoretical difficulties with insertion of an endotracheal tube through the region of the inflamed epiglottis, this has not proved to be a problem. In rare circumstances in which difficulty is encountered, a bronchoscope may be used to secure the airway; it should be dilated prior to intubation.[5,23] If the epiglottis is normal, the patient may be managed in a manner appropriate for croup or laryngotracheobronchitis. If difficulty is encountered or if obstruction occurs while transporting the patient or while trying to establish the airway, the possibility of ventilating the apneic patient by bag and mask or mouth-to-mouth ventilation should not be overlooked.[24,25]

After establishment of an airway, blood and the epiglottis should be cultured, and the patient should be given intravenous antibiotic therapy directed at *H. influenzae*. In view of the risk of infection with ampicillin-resistant *H. influenzae*,[26,27] cefotaxime (50–180 mg/kg/day in four divided doses), ceftriaxone (80–100 mg/kg/day in two divided doses), or ampicillin (200 mg/kg/day in four divided doses) plus chloramphenicol (75–100 mg/kg/day in four doses) should be given as initial therapy.

Patients with acute epiglottitis usually improve 12–48 hours after initiation of appropriate antibiotic therapy. Depending on the patient's progress, the artificial airway can usually be removed within this period.[5,28] Before extubation the patient should be afebrile, alert, and clinically improved. The decision to extubate may be based on the clinical condition of the patient,[28] evidence of resolution by direct visualization with a fiberoptic laryngoscope,[29] or presence of an air leak around the endotracheal tube. Antibiotics should be continued for 7–10 days. The route by which the antibiotic is administered after extubation should be dictated by the clinical response and status of the patient.

A small number of patients experiencing severe respiratory distress or arrest before intubation will develop pulmonary edema. The etiology of this complication is not known.[28,30]

The role of epinephrine and/or steroids has not been established in epiglottitis.

If the patient with epiglottitis has household contacts who are less than 4 years old, rifampin prophylaxis given once daily for 4 days in a dose of 20 mg/kg/day (maximum of 600 mg/day) is recommended for all household contacts regardless of immunization status.[31] In addition, the patient should receive rifampin in the same dosage before discharge to prevent reintroduction of the organism into the household (see Ch. 202).

IMMUNITY

An episode of *H. influenzae* epiglottis usually results in high levels of serum antibody to capsular polysaccharide.[32] This response appears to provide immunity, since second cases of epiglottitis are extremely rare. However, when epiglottitis occurs in children less than 24 months old, an age-appropriate immunization series should be completed.[31] The presence of maternally derived serum antibody at birth explains the infrequent occurrence of *H. influenzae* infections in infants. After disappearance of this maternal antibody there is an inverse relationship between rising naturally acquired antibody and the declining incidence of epiglottitis.[33]

Widespread use of *H. influenzae* type b polysaccharide vaccine has dramatically decreased the incidence of invasive *H. influenzae* disease and epiglottitis.[34,35] Introduction of these vaccines began in the United States in 1985 with the polyribosylribitol phosphate vaccine administered at 18 months of age and currently include conjugated vaccines administered beginning at 2 months of age, which were first licensed in 1990.[34,35] These vaccines will make epiglottitis increasingly rare among vaccinated cohorts of children but will probably have little effect on the frequency of disease in adults.

REFERENCES

1. Sendi K, Crysdale WS. Acute epiglottitis: Decade of change—A 10-year experience with 242 children. J Otolaryngol. 1987;16:196–202.
2. Bass JW, Steele RW, Wiebe RA. Acute epiglottitis: A surgical emergency. JAMA. 1974;229:671–5.
3. MayoSmith MF, Hirsch PJ, Wodzinski SF, et al. Acute epiglottitis in adults: An eight-year experience in the state of Rhode Island. N Engl J Med. 1986; 314:1133–9.
4. Denholm S, Rivron RP. Acute epiglottitis: A potentially lethal cause of sore throat. J R Coll Surg Edinb. 1992;37:333–5.
5. Andreassen UK, Baer S, Nielsen TG, et al. Acute epiglottitis—25 years experience with nasotracheal intubation, current management policy, and future needs. J Larngol Otol. 1992;106:1072–5.
6. Podgore JK, Bass JW. The "thumb sign" and "little finger sign" in acute epiglottitis. J Pediatr. 1976;88:154–5.
7. Stankiewicz JA, Bowes AK. Croup and epiglottitis: A radiologic study. Laryngoscope. 1985;95:1159–60.
8. Jones JL, Holland P. False positives in lateral neck radiographs used to diagnose epiglottitis. Ann Emerg Med. 1983;12:797.
9. Rothrock SG, Pignatiello GA, Howard RM. Radiologic diagnosis of epiglottitis: Objective criteria for all ages. Ann Emerg Med 1990;19:978–82.
10. Rivron Rp, Murry JA. Adult epiglottitis: Is there a consensus on diagnosis and treatment? Clin Otolaryngol. 1991;16:338–44.
11. Crosby E, Reid D. Acute epiglottitis in the adult: Is intubation necessary? Can J Anaesth. 1991;38:914–8.
12. Mustoe T, Strome M. Adult epiglottitis. Am J Otolaryngol. 1983;4:393–9.
13. Le Mierre A, Meyer A, Laplane R. Les septicemies a bacille de pfeiffer. Ann Med. 1936;39:97–119.
14. Trollfors B, Nylén O, Strangert K. Acute epiglottitis in children and adults in Sweden 1981–3. Arch Dis Child. 1990;65:491–4.
15. Losek JD, Dewitz-Zink BA, Melzer-Lange M, Havens PL. Epiglottitis: Comparison of signs and symptoms in children less than 2 years old and older. Ann Emerg Med. 1990;19:55–8.
16. Alexander HE, Ellis C, Leidy G. Treatment of type-specific *Hemophilus* infections in infancy and childhood. J Pediatr. 1942;20:673–98.
17. Dajani AD, Asmar BI, Thirumoorthia MC. Systemic *Haemophilus influenzae* disease: An overview. J Pediatr. 1979;94:355–64.
18. Branfors-Helander P, Jeppsson P-H. Acute epiglottitis: A clinical, bacteriological and serological study. Scand J Infect Dis. 1975;7:103–11.
19. Friedman M, Toriumi DM, Grybauskas V, Applebaum EL. A plea for uni-

formtiy in the staging and management of adult epiglottitis. Ear Nose Throat J. 1988;67:873–80.
20. Cox GJ, Bates GJ, Drake-Lee AB. The use of flexible nasoendoscopy in adults with acute epiglottitis. Ann R Coll Surg Engl. 1988;70:361–2.
21. Rapkin RH. Tracheostomy in epiglottitis. Pediatrics. 1973;52:426–9.
22. Bass JW, Fajardo JE, Brien JH, et al. Sudden death due to acute epiglottitis. Pediatr Infect Dis. 1985;4:447–9.
23. Walker P, Crysdale WS. Croup, epiglottitis, retropharyngeal abscess, and bacterial tracheitis: Evolving patterns of occurrence and care. Int Anesth Clin. 1992;30:57–70.
24. Adair JC, Ring WH. Management of epiglottitis in children. Anesth Analg. 1975;54:622–5.
25. Blanc VF, Weber ML, Ludec C, et al. Acute epiglottitis in children: Management of 27 consecutive cases with nasotracheal intubation with special emphasis on anaesthetic considerations. Can Anaesth Soc J. 1977;24:1–11.
26. McCracken GH Jr. Commentary. J Pediatr. 1979;94:987.
27. Kessler A, Wetmore RF, Marsh RR. Childhood epiglottitis in recent years. Int J Pediatr Otorhinolaryngol. 1993;25:155–62.
28. Butt W, Shann F, Walker C, et al. Acute epiglottitis: A different approach to management. Crit Care Med. 1988;16:43–7.
29. Gonzalez C, Reilly JS, Kenna MA, et al. Duration of intubation in children with acute epiglottitis. Otolaryngol Head Neck Surg. 1986;95:477–81.
30. Bonadio WA, Losek JD. The characteristics of children with epiglottitis who develop the complication of pulmonary edema. Arch Otolaryngol Head Neck Surg. 1991;117:205–7.
31. Committee on Infectious Diseases, *Haemophilus influenzae* infections. In: Peter G, ed. Report of the Committee on Infectious Diseases. Evanston, IL: American Academy of Pediatrics; 1991;220–229.
32. Whisnant JK, Rogentine GN, Gralnick MA, et al. Host factors and antibody response in *Haemophilus influenzae* type b meningitis and epiglottitis. J Infect Dis 1976;133:448–55.
33. Schneerson R, Rodrigues LP, Parke JC Jr, et al. Immunity to disease caused by *Hemophilus influenzae* type b. J Immunol. 1971;107:1081–9.
34. Adams WG, Deaver KA, Cochi SL, et al. Decline of childhood *Haemophilus influenzae* type b (Hib) disease in the Hib vaccine era. JAMA. 1993;269:221–6.
35. Broadhurst LE, Erickson RL, Kelley PW. Decrease in invasive *Haemophilus influenzae* diseases in US Army children, 1984 through 1991. JAMA. 1993;269:227–31.

46. INFECTIONS OF THE ORAL CAVITY, NECK, AND HEAD

ANTHONY W. CHOW

Infections of the oral cavity most commonly are odontogenic in origin and include dental caries, pulpitis, periapical abscess, gingivitis, and periodontal and deep fascial space infections. Although rare, such life-threatening complications as intracranial, retropharyngeal, or pleuropulmonary extension and hematogenous dissemination to heart valves, prosthetic devices, and other metastatic foci clearly indicate the potentially serious nature of these infections. Nonodontogenic infections of the oral cavity include ulcerative and gangrenous stomatitis and infection of the major salivary glands. Suppurative orofacial infections can also arise from the middle ear, oronasopharynx, and mastoids and paranasal sinuses; these have been discussed in Chapters 43 and 44, respectively.

Infections of the neck and head in the adult most commonly result from human or animal bites, trauma, irradiation, and surgical procedures. In children, cervical adenitis or thyroiditis due to bacterial or viral causes are more common. Rarely do embryologic cysts in the neck region become secondarily infected. These are considered separately from oral infections, since they frequently involve a different microflora and require alternative approaches to diagnosis and therapy.

OROFACIAL ODONTOGENIC INFECTIONS

Microbiologic Considerations

The microbiota associated with odontogenic infections is complex and generally reflects the indigenous oral flora. Despite this complexity, recent evidence strongly supports a causative role of specific microorganisms in different forms of odontogenic infections. This emerging concept of specific microbial cause has created a considerable dilemma in our traditional approach to the diagnosis and management of such infections. Since the microflora associated with these infections is typically polymicrobial, it does not necessarily follow that each component of this complex flora has equal pathogenic potential or that the numerically predominant cultivatable microflora are the most important. Furthermore, it may not be necessary to eradicate the complete microflora for effective therapy. An appreciation of the indigenous oral flora and the host factors that may modify its composition and knowledge of the specific microorganisms implicated in different odontogenic infections should therefore greatly assist in a more rational approach to such infections arising from the oral cavity.

Indigenous Oral Flora. The oral cavity cannot be regarded as a single, uniform environment. Although representative species of microorganisms can be isolated from most areas of the mouth, certain sites such as the tongue, tooth surface, gingival crevice, and saliva tend to favor colonization by specific organisms[1–3] (Table 1). Quantitative studies indicate that obligate anaerobes constitute a large and important part of the residential oral flora. In the gingival crevice of healthy adults, for example, the total microscopic counts averaged 2.7×10^{11} microorganisms per gram wet weight.[4] The total cultivatable anaerobic bacteria averaged 1.8×10^{11} microorganisms per gram, whereas facultative bacteria averaged 2.2×10^{10} microorganisms per gram, an eightfold difference. Overall, *Streptococcus, Peptostreptococcus, Veillonella, Lactobacillus, Corynebacterium,* and *Actinomyces* account for more than 80 percent of the total cultivatable oral flora. Facultative gram-negative rods are uncommon in healthy adults but may be more prominent in seriously ill, hospitalized, and elderly patients.[5,6] Unique ecologic niches are observed. For example, *Streptococcus sanguis, S. mutans,* and *S. mitis* as well as *Actinomyces viscosus* preferentially colonize the tooth surface.[7] In contrast, *S. salivarius* and *Veillonella* sp. have a predilection for the tongue and buccal mucosa.[2] *Fusobacterium,* pigmented *Bacteroides,* (*Porphyromonas* and *Prevotella*) and anaerobic spirochetes appear concentrated in the gingival crevice.[2] Factors that appear to govern these localization patterns include selective adherence characteristics of certain bacteria for various types of cells, local environmental conditions such as oxygen tension, oxidation–reduction potential (Eh) and pH, interbacterial coaggregation, and microbial inhibition.[2,8,9] Apart from anatomic considerations, numerous factors such as age, diet and nutrition, eruption of deciduous dentition, oral hygiene, smoking habits, the presence of dental caries or periodontal disease, antimicrobial therapy, hospitalization, pregnancy, as well as genetic and racial factors may influence the composition of the oral flora.[2,7–9]

Microbial Specificity in Odontogenic Infections. Although it had been recognized for some time that odontogenic infections are initiated by microorganisms through the establishment of dental plaques, the microbial specificity of these infections was not fully appreciated until recently. This breakthrough was brought about by technologic advances in sampling and anaerobic culture of specimens as well as by improved methods for species identification and taxonomy. Important differences in bacterial compositions have been noted for dental caries, gingivitis, and different forms of periodontitis when compared with cultures from healthy tissues.[10–12] An etiologic association of *S. mutans* in dental caries has been firmly established.[13,14] *Streptococcus mutans* is the only organism consistently isolated from all decayed dental fissures and is the only organism consistently found in greater numbers in carious teeth as compared with noncarious teeth. The infectious and transmissible nature of this organism in dental caries has been demonstrated in both

TABLE 1. Predominant Cultivable Bacteria from Various Sites of the Oral Cavity

Type	Predominant Genus or Family	Total Viable Count (Mean %)			
		Gingival Crevice	Dental Plaque	Tongue	Saliva
Facultative					
Gram-positive cocci	Streptococcus	28.8	28.2	44.8	46.2
	S. mutans	(0–30)	(0–50)	(0–1)	(0–1)
	S. sanguis	(10–20)	(40–60)	(10–20)	(10–30)
	S. mitior	(10–30)	(20–40)	(10–30)	(30–50)
	S. salivarius	(0–1)	(0–1)	(40–60)	(40–60)
Gram-positive rods	Lactobacillus	15.3	23.8	13.0	11.8
	Corynebacterium				
Gram-negative cocci	Moraxella	0.4	0.4	3.4	1.2
Gram-negative rods	Enterobacteriaceae	1.2	ND	3.2	2.3
Anaerobic					
Gram-positive cocci	Peptostreptococcus	7.4	12.6	4.2	13.0
Gram-positive rods	Actinomyces Eubacterium Lactobacillus Leptotrichia	20.2	18.4	8.2	4.8
Gram-negative cocci	Veillonella	10.7	6.4	16.0	15.9
Gram-negative rods		16.1	10.4	8.2	4.8
	Fusobacterium	1.9	4.1	0.7	0.3
	Prevotella or Porphyromonas	4.7	ND	0.2	ND
	Bacteroides	5.6	4.8	5.1	2.4
	Campylobacter	3.8	1.3	2.2	2.1
Spirochetes	Treponema	1.0	ND	ND	ND

Abbreviation: ND: not detected.

(Data from Chow et al.,[1] Hardie,[2] and Hamada et al.[3])

experimental animals and longitudinal studies in humans. Similarly, in gingivitis and periodontitis, a unique and specific bacterial composition of the subgingival plaque has been identified. In the healthy periodontium, the microflora is sparse and consists mainly of gram-positive organisms such as *S. sanguis* and *Actinomyces* spp. In the presence of gingivitis, the predominant subgingival flora shifts to a greater proportion of anaerobic gram-negative rods, and *Prevotella intermedia* (formerly *Bacteroides intermedius*) is most commonly isolated.[11,12,15] With established periodontitis, the flora further increases in complexity, with a preponderance of anaerobic gram-negative and motile organisms. *Porphyromonas gingivalis* (formerly *Bacteroides gingivalis*) is most commonly isolated. In juvenile periodontitis, a clinical variant seen primarily in adolescents, the subgingival plaque mainly consists of saccharolytic organisms, with *Actinobacillus actinomycetemcomitans* and *Capnocytophaga* spp. as the most common identifiable species. *P. gingivalis* is rarely found in this condition.[12,16] In suppurative odontogenic infections such as periapical abscesses or deep fascial space infections, a polymicrobial flora is usually present, with *Fusobacterium nucleatum*, pigmented *Bacteroides*, *Peptostreptococcus*, *Actinomyces*, and *Streptococcus* as the most predominant isolates.[1,17] Except in selected patients with serious underlying illnesses, facultative gram-negative bacilli and *Staphylococcus aureus* are uncommonly isolated.[18,19]

This microbial specificity demonstrated for different odontogenic infections probably reflects the acquisition of a unique microflora during the development of a supragingival dental plaque and its progression to a subgingival dental plaque.[20] Plaques that accumulate above the gingival margin are composed mainly of gram-positive facultative and microaerophilic cocci and rods; plaques that accumulate below the gingival margin are composed mainly of gram-negative anaerobic rods and motile forms including spirochetes (Fig. 1). Microorganisms residing within the supragingival plaque are characterized by their ability to adhere to the tooth surface and by their saccharolytic activity. Microorganisms in the subgingival plaque are frequently asaccharolytic and need not be adherent.

Pathogenetic Mechanisms

Suppurative orofacial infections are usually preceded by dental caries or periodontal disease. The pathogenetic mechanisms of cariogenesis remain poorly defined. The most universally accepted theory is that originated by W.D. Miller in 1882, which proposes that bacterial action on carbohydrates produces acidic substances that cause demineralization and dissolution of the hard tissues of the tooth.[21,22] In order for dental caries to develop three factors need to be present: *(1)* a susceptible tooth surface (host factors), *(2)* acidogenic (acid-producing) and aciduric (able to grow at low pH) bacteria within a dental plaque (microbial factors), and *(3)* carbohydrates and simple sugars (dietary factors). In the healthy host, at least three mechanisms serve to protect the tooth from carious decay: *(1)* the cleaning action of the tongue and buccal membranes, which acts to remove any food particles from the proximity of the tooth; *(2)* the buffering effect of saliva, which has a neutral pH, washes away bacterial acids, and provides essential substrates for remineralization and repair of damaged tooth surfaces; and *(3)* the protective effect of an acellular bacteria-free coating of salivary origin on the tooth surface, known as the *acquired pellicle,* which acts as a surface barrier to most dietary and bacterial acids and other proteolytic substances. In the absence of tooth brushing and flossing, the acquired pellicle becomes rapidly colonized and is replaced by the bacterial plaque. It is not surprising, therefore, that carious lesions occur most often in areas inaccessible to the self-cleaning mechanisms of the mouth and on the occlusal surfaces and interproximal sites that are protected from the reaches of the toothbrush.

Unlike dental caries, diet does not appear to have a significant

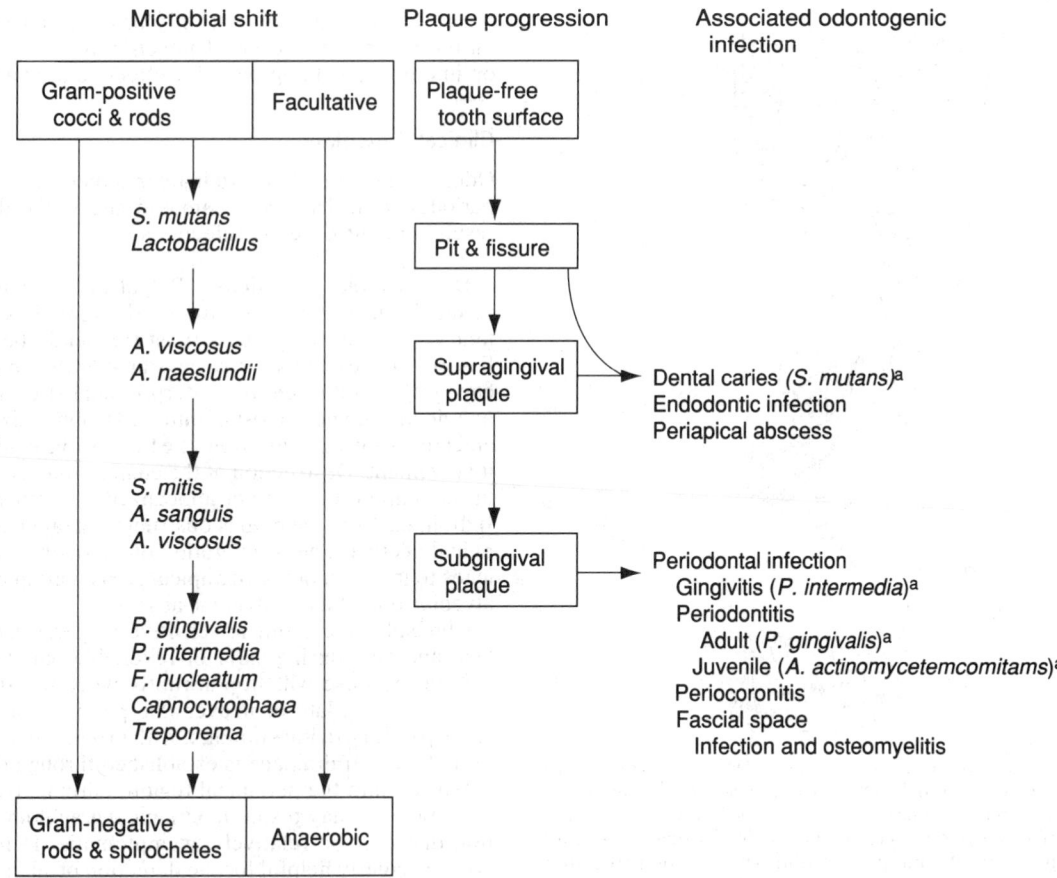

FIG. 1. Microbial specificity in odontogenic infections. A unifying hypothesis demonstrating a microbial shift from a plaque-free tooth surface and progression to supragingival and subgingival plaque organisms. (From Chow,[21] with permission.)

role in the pathogenesis of periodontal disease. The periodontal microflora associated with the subgingival plaque have the ability to penetrate the gingival epithelium and elicit an inflammatory host response that ultimately results in destruction of the periodontium.[11,16,20,22] Two major predisposing factors are poor oral hygiene and increasing age. Other factors include hormonal effects, with exacerbation of disease activity during puberty, menstruation, and pregnancy. Diabetes causes an increased incidence, particularly in juvenile diabetics. Finally, various genetic disorders are associated with an increased incidence of periodontal disease. In particular, those with neutrophil defects (such as Chédiak-Higashi syndrome, agranulocytosis, cyclic neutropenia, and Down syndrome) have a higher incidence of periodontal disease.[22]

It is a tribute to the local defenses in the healthy host that infections within the oral cavity are not more common. Establishment of the normal resident flora appears to be particularly important in providing a strong mucosal defense against colonization and invasion by potential pathogens ("colonization resistance").[23,24] Other nonspecific local defenses include the continuous cell shedding and turnover of the mucosal epithelium and the constant flow of saliva containing lysozyme, lactoferrin, β-lysin, lactoperoxidase, and other antimicrobial systems.[23] Various salivary glycoproteins and histidine-rich polypeptides have been reported to inhibit bacteria and fungi and may prevent infection by the inhibition of microbial attachment to oral epithelium by way of competition for cellular receptor sites or clumping of microorganisms. The epithelial barrier may be affected by radiation therapy, cancer chemotherapy, or trauma. A reduced turnover rate of the epithelial cells will allow retention of adherent organisms. A reduction in saliva volume will also have significant effects on the oral environment and predispose to micro-

bial invasion. In addition to nonspecific host defenses, specific humoral and cellular immune mechanisms are also important. Specific antibodies are present in saliva, with secretory IgA as the predominant immunoglobulin.[25] Salivary antibodies may affect the oral flora by aggregation of organisms and prevention of their attachment to mucosal epithelium. Cell-mediated immunity is important in oral defense against intracellular pathogens, including viruses, fungi, and bacteria. In the severely immunocompromised patient, a reactivation of viral infection involving the oral cavity is common, often with potentially life-threatening complications.[26] In addition to humoral and cellular immunity, various phagocytic cells in the oral mucosa also appear important. Phagocytic cells such as lymphocytes, granulocytes, and macrophages are abundant in the lamina propria and presumably contribute to the removal of foreign matter that has breached the epithelial barrier. Unique defects in host defenses have been identified in periodontal infections.[20] For example, impairment of neutrophil chemotaxis has been demonstrated in patients with juvenile periodontitis.[27,28] A number of oral anaerobes and streptococci implicated in periodontitis including *P. gingivalis, Prevotella intermedia, Prevotella melaningogenica, Capnocytophaga* spp., *S. sanguis*, and *S. mitis* are found to secrete IgA proteases.[29,30] The pathogenic significance of this finding is uncertain at present; it has been suggested that cleavage of IgA by microbial IgA proteases may impair local mucosal immunity of the host. It remains to be seen if similar or other defects of host resistance can be identified in different forms of destructive odontogenic infections.

Anatomic Considerations

Soft tissue infections of odontogenic origin tend to spread along planes of least resistance from the supporting structures of the

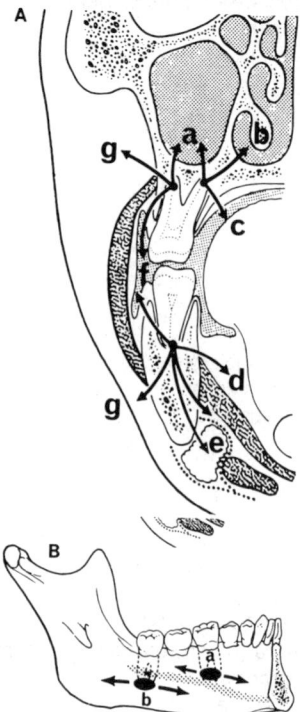

FIG. 2.   Routes of spread of odontogenic orofacial infections along planes of least resistance. **(A)** Coronal section in the region of the first molar teeth: a: maxillary antrum; b: nasal cavity; c: palatal plate; d: sublingual space (above the mylohyoid muscle); e: submandibular space (below the mylohyoid muscle); f: intraoral presentation with infection spreading through the buccal plates inside the attachment of the buccinator muscle; g: extraoral presentation to buccal space with infection spreading through the buccal plates outside the attachment of the buccinator muscle. **(B)** Lingual aspect of the mandible: a: apices of the involved tooth above the mylohyoid muscle, with spread of infection to the sublingual space; b: apices of involved tooth below the mylohyoid muscle, with spread of infection into the submandibular space. (From Chow et al.,[1] with permission.)

affected tooth to various potential spaces in the vicinity. Accumulated pus, therefore, must generally perforate bone at the site where it is thinnest and weakest before it extends into the periapical areas or deeper fascial spaces. In the mandible, this is usually in the region of the molar teeth on the lingual aspect and more anterior on the buccal aspect.[31,32] In the maxilla, the bone is weakest on the buccal aspect throughout and relatively thicker on the palatal aspect. If pus perforates through either the maxillary or mandibular buccal plate, it will present intraorally if inside the attachment of the buccinator muscle to the maxilla or mandible and extraorally if outside this muscle attachment (Fig. 2). When a mandibular infection perforates lingually, it presents in the sublingual space if the apices of the involved teeth lie above the attachment of the mylohyoid muscle (e.g., mandibular incisor, canines, premolars, and first molars) and in the submandibular space if below the attachment of this muscle (e.g., second and third molars) (Fig. 2). Thus, these local anatomic barriers of bone, muscle, and fascia predetermine the routes of spread, extent, and clinical manifestations of many orofacial infections of odontogenic origin. The clinically important "fascial spaces" most often involved are illustrated in Figures 3 and 4. These are potential spaces between layers of fascia normally bound together by loose connective tissue. The breakdown of these attachments by a spreading infective process results in a fascial space infection. These spaces intercommunicate with one another to varying degrees, and the potential pathways of extension from one space to another are illustrated in Figure 5. A thorough understanding of the potential *anatomic*

routes of infection will not only provide valuable information on the nature and extent of infection but will also suggest the optimum surgical approach for effective drainage.

Clinical Presentations

Odontogenic infections originate in either the dental pulp or the periodontium. The most common site is the dental pulp and results in dentoalveolar infections.

Dentoalveolar Infections.   Pulpal infection most frequently results from carious exposure, rarely from physical or chemical injury. The carious process most frequently begins in pits and fissures on the occlusal surfaces of molars and premolars, which encourage food retention. Interproximal sites and the gingival margin are the next most common. Demineralization of the enamel results in discoloration, the first visible evidence of carious involvement. Destruction of the enamel and dentin and invasion of the pulp produce either a localized or a generalized pulpitis. If drainage from the pulp is obstructed, a rapid progression with pulpal necrosis and proliferation of endodontic microorganisms leads to invasion of the periapical areas (periapical abscess) and alveolar bone (acute alveolar abscess).

Clinically, the tooth is sensitive to percussion and to both heat and cold during early or reversible pulpitis, although the painful response will stop abruptly when the stimulus is withdrawn. During late or irreversible pulpitis, the tooth is exquisitely painful to a hot stimulus, with prompt relief by the application of cold. If drainage is established through the tooth before extension into the periapical region, chronic irritation from the necrotic pulp may result in periapical granuloma or cyst formation that may be relatively asymptomatic. Dental radiographs are particularly helpful for the detection of silent lesions, particularly those caused by interproximal caries, which are difficult to detect clinically.

The principles of treatment in dentoalveolar infections include prompt elimination of the infected pulp, deep periodontal scaling, or extraction of the affected tooth. Dentoalveolar abscess should be surgically drained at the same time. Other supportive measures include hydration, a soft diet, analgesics, and oral hygiene. Antibiotic therapy is indicated primarily if drainage cannot be adequately established or when infection has perforated the cortex and spread into surrounding soft tissue.

Gingivitis and Periodontal Infections.   *Periodontal disease* is a general term that refers to all diseases involving the supporting structures of the teeth (periodontium), which include the gingiva, periodontal ligament, alveolar bone, and cementum. In the early phase of periodontal disease, infection is confined to the gingiva (gingivitis). Later, the underlying supporting tissues are affected (periodontitis), ultimately leading to complete destruction of the periodontium and a permanent loss of teeth. Periodontal infections tend to localize in intraoral soft tissues and seldom spread into deeper structures of the face or neck.

GINGIVITIS.   Acute and chronic inflammation of the gingiva is initiated by local irritation and microbial invasion.[11,16,22] Subgingival plaque is always present. In simple gingivitis, there is a bluish red discoloration, with swelling and thickening of the free gingival margin. A tendency for bleeding of the gums after eating or toothbrushing may be one of the earliest findings. There is usually no pain, but a mild fetor oris may be noticed. In acute necrotizing ulcerative gingivitis (Vincent's disease, or trench mouth), the patient typically experiences a sudden onset of pain in the gingiva that interferes with normal mastication. Necrosis of the gingiva occurs mainly in the interdental papilla and results in a marginated, punched-out, and eroded appearance. A superficial grayish pseudomembrane is formed, and a characteristic halitosis with altered taste sensation is present. There is usually associated fever, malaise, and regional lymphadenopathy. Treatment includes local débridement and la-

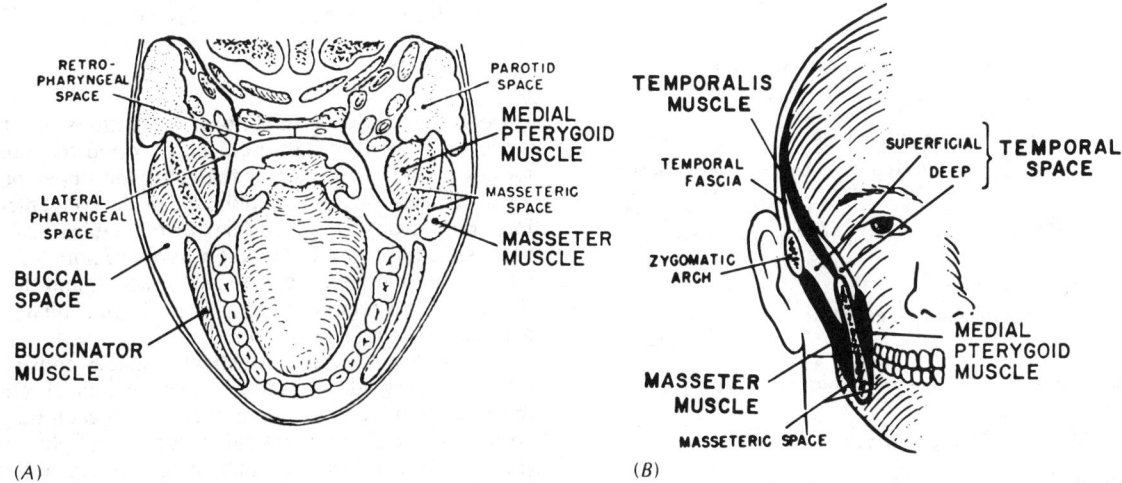

FIG. 3. Fascial spaces around the mouth and face. **(A)** Horizontal section at the level of the occlusal surface of the mandibular teeth. **(B)** Frontal view of the face. (From Chow et al.,[1] with permission.)

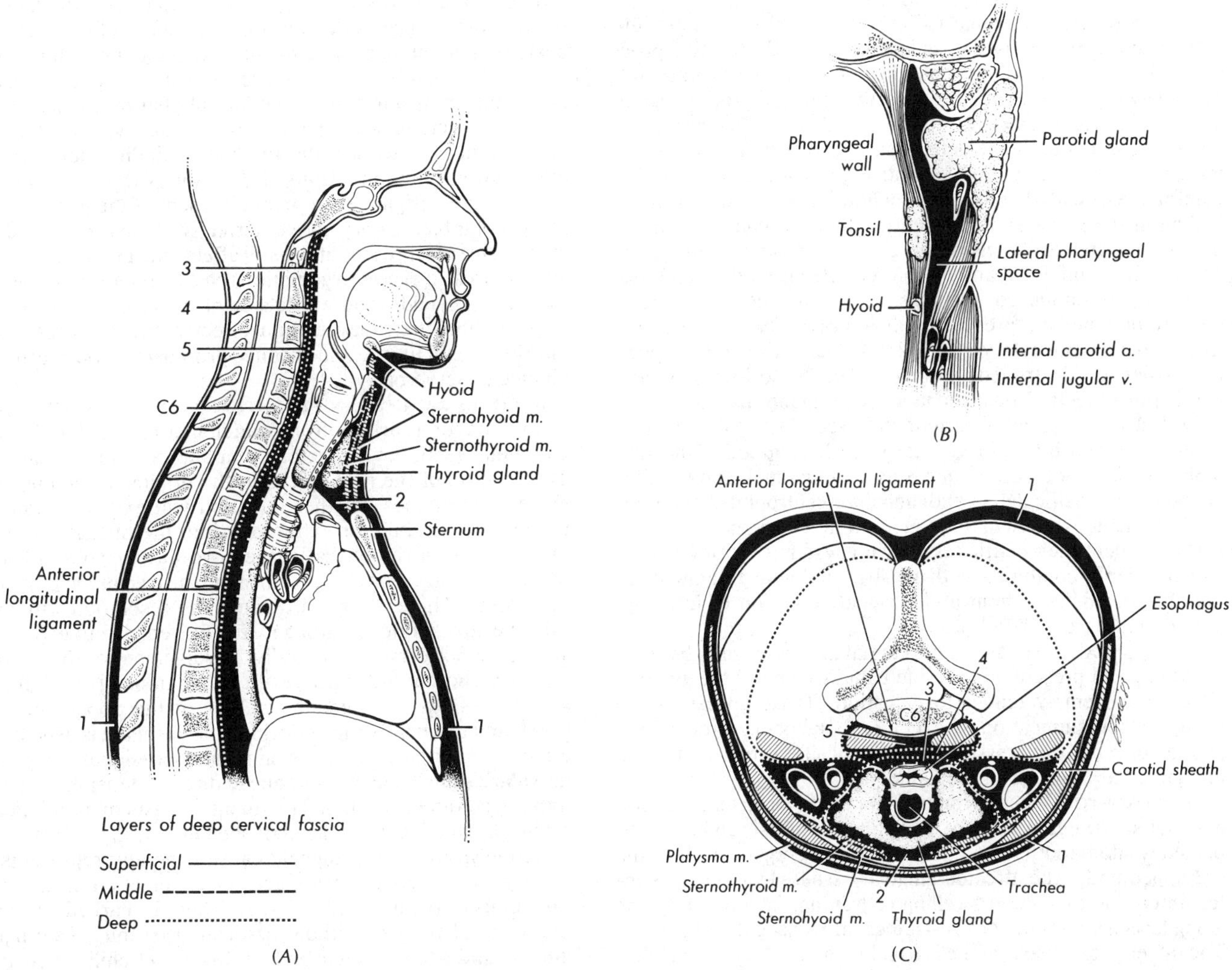

FIG. 4. Relation of lateral pharyngeal, retropharyngeal, and prevertebral spaces to the posterior and anterior layers of the deep cervical fascia. 1: Superficial space; 2: pretracheal space; 3: retropharyngeal space; 4: "danger" space; 5: pre-vertebral space. **(A)** Midsagittal section of the head and neck. **(B)** Coronal section in the suprahyoid region of the neck. **(C)** Cross section of the neck at the level of the thyroid isthmus.

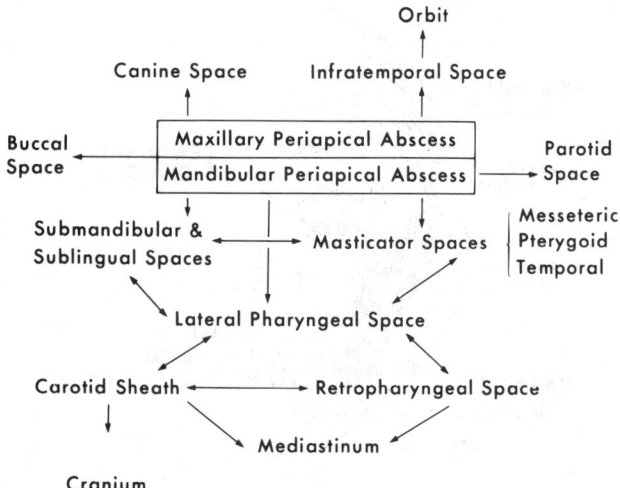

FIG. 5.   Potential pathways of extension in deep fascial space infections.

vage with oxidizing agents, which usually brings relief from pain within 24 hours. Antibiotic therapy with penicillin or metronidazole is indicated and is highly effective.[33,34]

PERIODONTITIS.   Chronic inflammation of the periodontium is the major cause of tooth loss in adults. The destructive process proceeds insidiously, usually beginning in early adulthood. Subgingival plaque is always present, and both supragingival and subgingival calculi are usually abundant. Unlike pulpal infection in which drainage is frequently obstructed, periodontal infections drain freely, and patients experience little or no discomfort. Associated sensations include pressure and an itchy feeling in the gums and between the teeth, a bad taste in the mouth, hot and cold sensitivity, and vague pains in the jaws. The gingiva is inflamed and discolored, bleeds readily, and presents as periodontal pockets around the affected teeth. Frank pus can be readily expressed by digital pressure or may exude freely from the pockets. As periodontitis advances, the supporting tissues are destroyed, ultimately leading to loosening and exfoliation of teeth. Localized juvenile periodontitis is a particularly destructive form of periodontitis seen in adolescents and is characterized by rapid vertical bone loss affecting the first molar and incisor teeth. Plaque is usually minimal, and calculus is absent. A specific defect with impaired neutrophil chemotaxis has been demonstrated in this condition. Recent experience suggests excellent therapeutic results with systemic tetracycline or metronidazole combined with local periodontal treatment involving root débridement and surgical resection of inflamed periodontal tissues.[20,35-37]

PERIODONTAL ABSCESS.   Periodontal abscesses may be focal or diffuse and present as red, fluctuant swelling of the gingiva, which is extremely tender to palpation. These abscesses are always in communication with a periodontal pocket from which pus can be readily expressed after probing. Treatment is surgical and aimed at drainage of loculated pus.

PERICORONITIS.   Pericoronitis is an acute localized infection associated with gum flaps overlying a partially erupted or impacted wisdom tooth. Food debris and microorganisms become entrapped under the affected gingival tissues. If drainage is interrupted due to sudden swelling or trauma, infection extends along fascial planes of least resistance into adjacent soft tissues. The underlying alveolar bone is usually not involved. Clinically, the pericoronal tissues are erythematous and swollen. Digital pressure will produce a small amount of exudate from under the infected flap. Since the masticator spaces are often involved, marked trismus secondary to irritation of the masseter or medial pterygoid muscle is a prominent presenting feature. Treatment of pericoronitis includes gentle débridement and irrigation under the tissue flap. The use of antibiotics and incision and drainage

may be necessary if cellulitis of fascial planes occurs. Excision of the operculum or extraction of the involved tooth may also be considered.

Deep Fascial Space Infections.   Infections of either odontogenic or oropharyngeal origin may extend to potential fascial spaces of the lower part of the head and upper portion of the neck. These "space infections" can be conveniently divided into those around the face (masticator, buccal, canine, and parotid spaces), those in the suprahyoid region (submandibular, sublingual, and lateral pharyngeal spaces), and those involving the infrahyoid region or the total neck (retropharyngeal, "danger," and pretracheal spaces).[19,31,32]

MASTICATOR SPACES.   Masticator spaces consist of the masseteric, pterygoid, and temporal spaces, all of which are well differentiated but intercommunicate with each other as well as with the buccal, submandibular, and lateral pharyngeal spaces (Fig. 3). Infection of the masticator spaces occurs most frequently from molar teeth, particularly the third molars (wisdom teeth). Clinically, the hallmark of masticator space infection is trismus and pain in the area of the body or ramus of the mandible. Swelling may not be a prominent finding, especially in the masseteric compartment, since infection exists deep in large muscle masses, which obscures or prevents clinically apparent swelling. When present, swelling tends to be brawny and indurated, which suggests the possibility of cervicofacial actinomycosis or mandibular osteomyelitis. If infection extends internally, it can involve an area close to the lateral pharyngeal wall and result in dysphagia. A true lateral pharyngeal space infection, however, is accompanied by displacement of the lateral pharyngeal wall toward the midline, a finding not present in masticator space infections. Infection of the deep temporal space usually originates from involvement of the posterior maxillary molar teeth. Very little external swelling is observed early in the course; if present, it usually affects the preauricular region and an area over the zygomatic arch. As infection progresses, the cheek, eyelids, and whole side of the face may be involved (Fig. 6). Infection may extend directly into the orbit via the inferior orbital fissure and produce proptosis, optic neuritis, and abducens nerve palsy.

BUCCAL, CANINE, AND PAROTID SPACES.   As noted previously, infections arising from mandibular or maxillary bicuspid and molar teeth tend to extend in a lateral or buccal direction. The relation of the root apices to the origins of the buccinator muscle determines whether infection will exit intraorally into the buccal vestibule or extraorally into the buccal space (Fig. 2). Infection of the buccal space is readily diagnosed because of marked cheek swelling with minimal trismus and systemic symptoms. There is a great tendency to resolution with antibiotic therapy alone. Drainage, if required, is superficial and should be performed extraorally. Involvement of the maxillary incisors and canines may result in a canine space infection, which presents as dramatic swelling of the upper lip, canine fossa, and frequently the periorbital tissues. Pain is usually moderate, and systemic signs are minimal. Occasionally, a purulent maxillary sinusitis may result due to direct extension of infection into the adjoining antrum. Treatment consists of antibiotics and drainage, which can be accomplished intraorally. Parotid space infection from an odontogenic cause generally represents secondary spread from a masseteric space infection in the area of the ramus of the mandible (Fig. 3). There is marked swelling of the angle of the jaw without associated trismus. Pain may be intense and accompanied by high fever and chills. Because of its close relationship with the posterior aspect of the lateral pharyngeal space, a parotid space infection carries the potential risk of direct extension into the "danger" and visceral spaces and hence to the posterior mediastinum (Fig. 4).

SUBMANDIBULAR AND SUBLINGUAL SPACES.   These two spaces are separated by the mylohyoid muscle (Fig. 2), and the submandibular space is further divided into the submaxillary

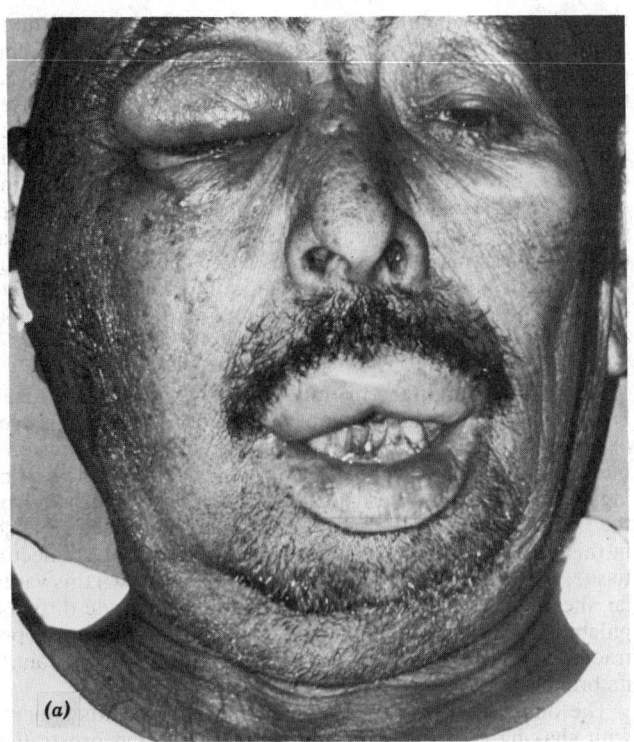
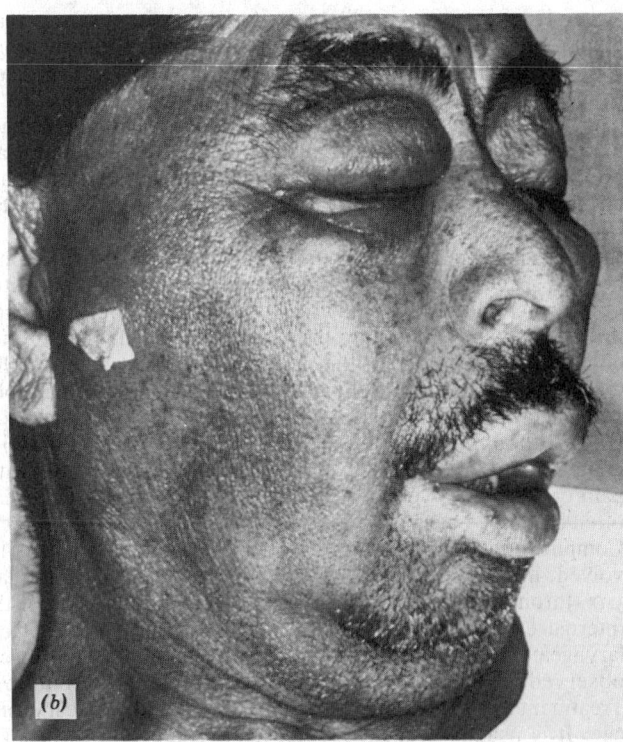

FIG. 6.   Deep temporal space infection with spread to the right parotid space and the orbit. This patient developed right optic neuritis with permanent loss of vision in that eye. **(A)** Frontal view. **(B)** Lateral view. (From Chow et al.,[1] with permission.)

and submental spaces. Infection in these spaces usually arises from the second and third mandibular molar teeth since their root apices lie inferior to the mylohyoid muscle. There is typical swelling, although much less trismus in contradistinction to masseteric space infection, since the major muscles of mastication are usually not involved. Submandibular odontogenic infection should be distinguished from submandibular sialadenitis and lymphadenitis that are due to other causes. Therapy includes antibiotics, dental extraction, and extraoral surgical drainage. Infection of the sublingual space generally arises from mandibular incisors, since their root apices lie above the mylohyoid muscle. Clinically, this space infection presents as a brawny, erythematous, tender swelling of the floor of the mouth that begins close to the mandible and spreads toward the midline or beyond. Some elevation of the tongue may be noted in late states. Surgical drainage of the sublingual space should be performed intraorally by an incision through the mucosa parallel to Wharton's duct. If the submandibular space is also to be drained, both spaces can be reached through a submandibular approach.

The term *Ludwig's angina* has been loosely applied to a heterogenous array of infections involving the sublingual, submaxillary, and submandibular spaces.[38] However, for therapeutic and prognostic purposes, it is desirable to restrict this diagnosis to cases that conform to the following classic description: *(1)* the infection is always bilateral, *(2)* both the submandibular and sublingual spaces are involved, *(3)* the infection is a rapidly spreading indurated cellulitis without abscess formation or lymphatic involvement, and *(4)* the infection begins in the floor of the mouth. A dental source of infection has been found in 50–90 percent of reported cases. The second and third mandibular molars are most commonly involved. Clinically, patients present with a brawny boardlike swelling in the submandibular spaces that does not pit on pressure (Fig. 7). The mouth is usually held open and the floor elevated, which pushes the tongue to the roof of the mouth. Eating and swallowing are difficult, and respiration may be impaired by obstruction from the tongue. A rapid progression of the infection will result in edema of the neck and glottis and may precipitate asphyxiation. Fever and

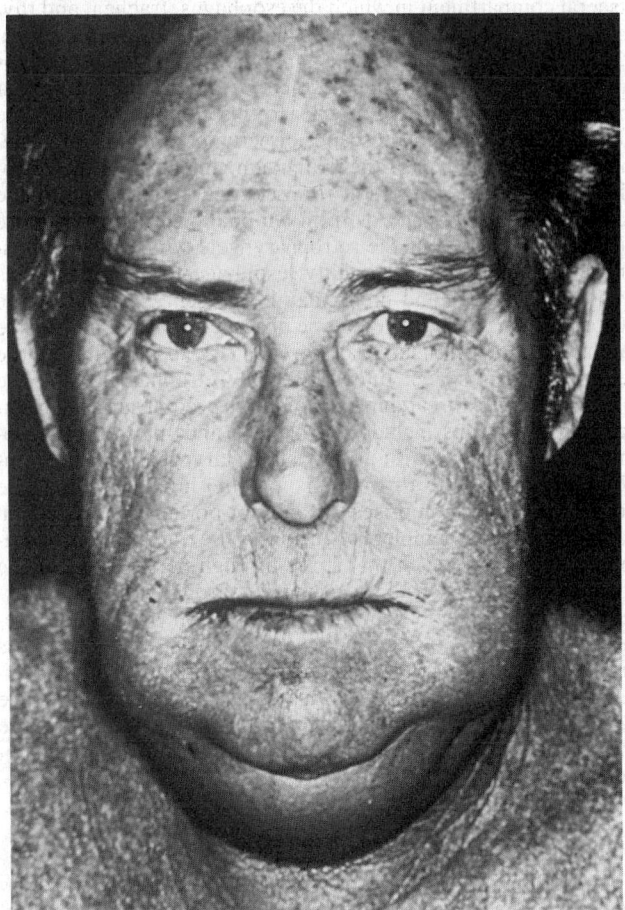

FIG. 7.   Early appearance of a patient with Ludwig's angina with a brawny, boardlike swelling in the submandibular spaces. (From Chow et al.,[1] with permission.)

systemic toxicity are usually present and may be severe. Treatment requires high doses of parenteral antibiotics, airway monitoring, early intubation or tracheostomy when required, soft tissue decompression, and surgical drainage.

LATERAL PHARYNGEAL SPACE.   The lateral pharyngeal space (also known as the pharyngomaxillary space) in the lateral aspect of the neck is shaped like an inverted cone, with its base at the skull and its apex at the hyoid bone (Fig. 4). Its medial wall is contiguous with the carotid sheath, and it lies deep to the pharyngeal constrictor muscle. Infection of the lateral pharyngeal space may result from pharyngitis, tonsillitis, parotitis, otitis, mastoiditis, as well as odontogenic infection, especially if the masticator spaces are primarily involved. If the anterior compartment is infected, the patient will exhibit fever, chills, marked pain, trismus, swelling below the angle of the mandible, dysphagia, and medial displacement of the lateral pharyngeal wall. Although not prominent, dyspnea can occur. Posterior compartment infection is characterized by septicemia with little pain or trismus. Swelling is usually internal and deep and can often be missed because it is behind the palatopharyngeal arch. Complications, particularly if the posterior compartment is involved, include respiratory obstruction from edema of the larynx, thrombosis of the internal jugular vein, and erosion of the internal carotid artery. Because respiratory obstruction from laryngeal edema can occur suddenly, the patient must be closely observed, and prophylactic tracheostomy may be required. Treatment includes high levels of antibiotics and surgical drainage. It is usually prudent to wait for the infection to localize before drainage is attempted unless respiratory obstruction or hemorrhage necessitates early surgical intervention.

RETROPHARYNGEAL, DANGER, AND PRETRACHEAL SPACES. The retropharyngeal space comprises the posterior part of the visceral compartment in which the esophagus, trachea, and thyroid glands are enclosed by the middle layer of deep cervical fascia (Fig. 4). It lies behind the hypopharynx and the esophagus and extends inferiorly into the superior mediastinum to about the level from T1 to T2. Posterior to this compartment lies the "danger" space, which descends directly into the posterior mediastinum to the level of the diaphragm. Infection of the retropharyngeal space may result from contiguous infection of the lateral pharyngeal space or from lymphatic spread from more distant sites to involve the retropharyngeal lymph nodes. Dysphagia, dyspnea, nuchal rigidity, esophageal regurgitation, as well as high fever and chills may be present. Bulging of the posterior pharyngeal wall may be observed. Lateral soft tissue radiographs of the neck may reveal marked widening of the retropharyngeal space. Infection of the retropharyngeal space is potentially life threatening and requires prompt surgical drainage. Complications include hemorrhage and spontaneous rupture into the airway with asphyxiation, laryngeal spasm, bronchial erosion, and thrombosis of the jugular vein. The pretracheal space comprises the anterior portion of the visceral compartment and completely surrounds the trachea. Most commonly, infections reach this space through perforations of the anterior esophageal wall, occasionally through contiguous extension from a retropharyngeal space infection. The clinical presentation is characterized by severe dyspnea, but hoarseness may be the first complaint. Swallowing is difficult, and regurgitation of fluids through the nose may occur. A pretracheal space infection is always serious because of possible extension into the mediastinum, and prompt surgical drainage is critically important.

Complications of Odontogenic Infections

Complications of odontogenic infections can occur either by hematogenous spread or by direct extension. Transient bacteremia is common during or after various dental procedures, especially extraction of infected teeth.[39] The temporal relationship between these procedures and subsequent bacterial endocardi-

tis and cardiovascular prosthetic infections is well documented.[10] Reports of infected total hip replacements after dental procedures add further concern.[22,40] Prophylactic antibiotic treatment during dental procedures, although frequently used, remains a controversial issue, especially in the absence of preexisting valvular heart disease. Complications of odontogenic infections secondary to direct extension include mediastinal spread,[41] intracranial suppuration (especially cavernous sinus thrombosis),[42] suppurative jugular thrombophlebitis, carotid artery erosion,[43] maxillary sinusitis,[1] and osteomyelitis.[44] Acute mediastinitis and intracranial suppuration secondary to odontogenic infections are relatively uncommon in the postantibiotic era.

Suppurative Jugular Thrombophlebitis and Carotid Artery Erosion.   These are uncommon complications of oropharyngeal or odontogenic infections in the postantibiotic era. Extension of infection to the carotid sheath, which encloses both the internal jugular vein and the internal carotid artery, usually arises from the lateral pharyngeal space.[43] Since the carotid sheath space in this area is relatively compact with little areolar connective tissue, there is little tendency of spread up and down this vascular sheath, with the exception of possible retrograde thrombophlebitis and intracranial extension. The major concern is protracted septicemia and erosion of the carotid artery or one of its branches.

The onset of suppurative jugular thrombophlebitis is acute, with shaking chills, spiking fevers, and profound prostration. Localizing signs of pain and swelling at the angle of the jaw, tenderness and induration along the sternocleidomastoid muscle, and swelling of the lateral pharyngeal wall with dysphagia and neck ridigity are usually present. However, these findings may be subtle, and their clinical significance may not be fully recognized until postmortem. Systemic evidence of infection such as septic pulmonary emboli and metastatic abscesses to the brain, lungs, kidneys, and joints is not infrequent. The usual recommended treatment consists of external drainage of the lateral pharyngeal space and ligation of the internal jugular vein. *Fusobacterium necrophorum* has been the organism most frequently isolated from blood cultures,[45,46] and mortality remains high. Important warning signals that may herald major hemorrhage due to erosion of the carotid artery include multiple episodes of minor bleeding from the oral cavity or ear and ecchymosis of oral and cervical tissue. With the onset of major hemorrhage, primary considerations are maintenance and protection of the airway because death may occur more rapidly from asphyxiation than from hemorrhagic shock. Appropriate treatment consists of emergency carotid ligation after the restoration of blood volume and pressure. Hemorrhage is controlled by local compression until ligation can be attempted. The mortality for emergency ligation ranges from 30 to 50 percent. Cerebrovascular accident is a significant complication in survivors.

Septic Cavernous Sinus Thrombosis.   This dreaded complication is fortunately rare in the postantibiotic era. Facial furuncles and purulent paranasal sinusitis were the major predisposing conditions. Infection of the maxillary teeth was the most common dental cause. Eagleton[47] described six criteria for the diagnosis of septic cavernous sinus thrombosis to help distinguish it from other less lethal infections, particularly those of the ethmoid sinus and the orbit: *(1)* a known site of infection; *(2)* evidence of blood stream invasion; *(3)* early signs of venous obstruction in the retina, conjunctiva, and eyelid; *(4)* paresis of the third, fourth, and sixth cranial nerves resulting from inflammatory edema; *(5)* abscess formation in neighboring soft tissue; and *(6)* evidence of meningeal irritation. Before the antibiotic era, septic cavernous sinus thrombosis was virtually always fatal. Mortality since 1970 has been markedly reduced to 15–30 percent.[43,48,49] Treatment requires early recognition, high-dose intravenous antibiotics, and surgical decompression of the underlying predisposing infection. Anticoagulation and steroids are not indicated.

Maxillary Sinusitis.   In many people, the roots of the maxillary molars lie proximate to the maxillary antrum. At times, congenital bony defects occur, with the root adjacent to the sinus membrane. In these cases, sinusitis can result from direct extension of an odontogenic infection or from perforation of the sinus floor during extraction of a maxillary tooth.[49,50] The clinical presentation of secondary sinus involvement is similar to that of primary sinus disease.

Osteomyelitis of the Jaws.   The mandible is much more susceptible to osteomyelitis than is the maxilla, mainly because the cortical plates of the latter are thin and its medullary tissues are relatively poor in vascular supply.[44] In view of the large number of odontogenic infections and the intimate relationship of teeth to the medullary cavity, it is surprising that osteomyelitis of the jaws is not more frequent. When osteomyelitis occurs, there is usually a predisposing condition that affects host resistance such as a compound fracture, previous irradiation, osteopetrosis, Paget's disease, diabetes mellitus, or steroid therapy. With initiation of infection, the intramedullary pressure markedly increases, further compromising blood supply and leading to bone necrosis. Pus travels through the haversian and perforating canals, accumulates beneath the periosteum, and elevates it from the cortex. If pus continues to accumulate, the periosteum is eventually penetrated, and mucosal and cutaneous abscesses and fistulas may develop. As the inflammatory process becomes more chronic, granulation tissue is formed. Spicules of necrotic and nonviable bone may become either totally isolated (sequestrum) or encased in a sheath of new bone (involucrum). Severe mandibular pain is a common symptom and may be accompanied by anesthesia or hypoesthesia on the affected side. In protracted cases, mandibular trismus may develop. A clinical variant is chronic sclerosing osteomyelitis associated with a proliferative periostitis. Clinically, it is characterized by a localized, hard, nontender swelling over the mandible. Actinomycosis and radiation necrosis are two common causes of this form of osteomyelitis of the jaws.

Treatment of osteomyelitis of the jaws is complicated by the presence of teeth and persistent exposure to the oral environment. Antibiotic therapy needs to be prolonged, often requiring weeks to months. Adjunctive therapy with hyperbaric oxygen may prove beneficial in hastening the healing process, particularly for the chronic sclerosing variety.[44] Surgical management including sequestrectomy, saucerization, decortication, and closed-wound suction irrigation may occasionally be necessary. Rarely, in advanced cases the entire segment of the infected jaw may have to be resected.

Diagnostic Approaches

Specimen Collection and Processing.   It is imperative that the normal resident oral flora be excluded during specimen collection in order that culture results be appropriately interpreted. For closed-space infections, needle aspiration of loculated pus by an extraoral approach is desirable, and specimens should be transported immediately to the laboratory under anaerobic conditions. For intraoral lesions, direct microscopic examination of stained smears often provides more useful information than do culture results from surface swabs. Gram and acid-fast stains for bacteria and potassium hydroxide preparations for fungi should be routinely performed. Tissue biopsy specimens examined for typical histopathology and the presence of microbial antigens by immunofluorescence are particularly useful in suspected mycobacterial, fungal, and viral infections. In chronic osteomyelitis, soft tissue swelling and draining fistulas are frequently present. Aspirates from the adjacent soft tissue swellings may be valuable, but cultures from the sinus tracts may

be misleading, since these sinus tracts are often colonized by organisms that do not reflect what is actually occurring within the infected bone.[51] Bone biopsies for histopathology and culture are often required for a definitive diagnosis.

Imaging Techniques for the Localization of Infection.   Ultrasonography, radionuclide scanning, and computed tomography (CT) are particularly useful for the localization of deep fascial space infections of the head and neck.[52,53] A lateral radiograph of the neck may demonstrate compression or deviation of the tracheal air column or the presence of gas within necrotic soft tissues.[54] In retropharyngeal infections, lateral radiographs of the cervical spine or CT scanning can help determine whether the infection is in the retropharyngeal space or the prevertebral space.[55] The former suggests an odontogenic source, whereas the latter suggests involvement of the cervical spine. Technetium bone scanning used in combination with gallium- or indium-labeled white blood cells is particularly useful for the diagnosis of acute or chronic osteomyelitis and for the differentiation of infection or trauma from malignancy. In acute osteomyelitis, both the bone scan and gallium scan are likely to have positive findings. In chronic osteomyelitis, the gallium or indium scans may be negative, but the technetium may be positive. Similarly, both scans may be positive during infection and trauma, while neoplasms in the bone may be associated only with a positive bone scan but negative gallium or indium scan results.

Therapeutic Considerations

Dental Caries and Periodontitis.   For both caries prevention and treatment of periodontitis, the clinical goal must continue to be control of the supragingival and subgingival plaques. With the emerging concept of microbial specificity in these infections, the prospect of specific antimicrobial therapy appears increasingly promising.[10,20,37,56,57] In localized juvenile periodontitis, for example, systemic tetracycline therapy directed against *Actinobacillus actinomycetemcomitans* and combined with local periodontal treatment has yielded excellent results.[35,36] Unfortunately, the administration of tetracycline to children under 9 years of age can cause staining of the permanent dentition and is not generally recommended. Furthermore, tetracycline resistance among periodontal pathogens has been increasingly recognized.[57] In advanced periodontitis, several double-blind studies have indicated that systemic metronidazole plus mechanical débridement of the root surfaces is more effective than placebo treatment plus mechanical débridement.[37] The successful treatment of acute necrotizing ulcerative gingivitis with metronidazole has been well documented, and in fact such treatment by Shinn et al.[33] led to the discovery of metronidazole as a unique anaerobicidal agent.

Several topical agents appear to have cariostatic effects in humans. By far the most effective is fluoride. Fluoride forms a complex with the apatite crystals in dentin by replacing the hydroxyl group, thereby lending strength to the entire structure.[10] Further, fluoride promotes remineralization of the carious lesions and also exerts a bacteriostatic effect. Topical chlorhexidine is another compound with useful anticariogenic properties. It acts as a cationic detergent killing a wide range of bacteria and is retained on the oral surfaces for prolonged periods to prevent plaque advancement.[22] Unfortunately, it has a bitter taste and stains the enamel and tongue. Prolonged application may also promote the emergence of resistant microorganisms. Among the antibiotics, although both penicillin and tetracycline have cariostatic effects in animal models, only topical application of vancomycin has been shown to reduce dental caries with some degree of success in humans.[10] Other important approaches to caries and periodontitis prevention include the adoption of improved oral hygiene through more effective educational programs,[13] a reduction of cariogenic oral flora by diet modification with sucrose substitutes, and active immunization against caries by the use of vaccines prepared from *S. mutans*.[58,59]

Suppurative Odontogenic Infections. The most important therapeutic modality for pyogenic odontogenic infections is surgical drainage and removal of necrotic tissue. Needle aspiration by the extraoral route can be particularly helpful both for microbiologic sampling and for evacuation of pus. The need for definitive restoration or extraction of the infected tooth, the primary source of infection, is readily apparent. Deep periodontal scaling and endodontic treatments with root filling may be required in most instances. Effective surgical management requires a thorough understanding of the most likely anatomic routes of spread. The neighboring potential fascial spaces should be carefully and systematically surveyed. The optimum timing for incision and drainage is equally important. Premature incision into an unlocalized cellulitis in an ill-conceived search for pus can disrupt the normal physiologic barriers and cause further diffusion and extension of infection.

Antibiotic therapy is important in halting the local spread of infection and in preventing hematogenous dissemination. Antimicrobial agents are generally indicated if fever and regional lymphadenitis are present or when infection has perforated the bony cortex and spread into surrounding soft tissue. Severely immunocompromised patients are particularly at risk for unhalted and spreading orofacial infections, and empirical broad-spectrum antimicrobial therapy in these patients is warranted.[60,61] The choice of specific antibiotics for the treatment of odontogenic infections requires not so much the results of bacterial culture and sensitivity as knowledge of the indigenous organisms that colonize the teeth, gums, and mucous membranes. By far most of these organisms, including both anaerobes and aerobes, are sensitive to penicillin.[60-63] Thus, penicillin monotherapy in doses appropriate for the severity of infection remains a good choice. The problem of β-lactamase production and penicillin resistance among *Bacteroides* spp. and *Prevotella melaninogenica* has been increasingly recognized, and treatment failure with penicillin in odontogenic infections due to such β-lactamase–producing strains has been reported.[64-66] Thus, in patients with life-threatening deep fascial space infections and in patients who have had an unfavorable or delayed response to penicillin, alternative therapy with a broader spectrum against anaerobes as well as facultative gram-negative bacilli may be considered. Penicillin-allergic patients may be treated with clindamycin, cefoxitin, or imipenem. Ambulatory patients with less serious odontogenic infections may be treated with amoxicillin with or without a β-lactamase inhibitor, or with either penicillin or ciprofloxacin in combination with metronidazole. Erythromycin and tetracycline are not preferred in orofacial odontogenic infections because of emergence of resistance among oropharyngeal anaerobes and some strains of streptococci.[57,60] Metronidazole, although highly active against anaerobic gram-negative bacilli and spirochetes, is only moderately active against anaerobic cocci and is not active against aerobes, including streptococci.[1,61,67] Except in acute necrotizing gingivitis and in advanced periodontitis,[33,34,37] it should not be used as a single agent in odontogenic infections. In the compromised host such as the patient with leukemia and severe neutropenia after chemotherapy, it is prudent to cover for facultative gram-negative bacilli as well, and agents with broad-spectrum activity against both aerobes and anaerobes are desirable (Table 2).

OROFACIAL NONODONTOGENIC INFECTIONS

Nonodontogenic infections of the oral cavity most frequently occur secondary to chemical, thermal, or traumatic injury. Virtually all infectious microorganisms can present with intraoral manifestations, particularly sexually transmitted agents and childhood viral enanthems. Cancer patients with mucositis from cytotoxic drugs are especially prone to acute and chronic oppor-

TABLE 2. Empirical Antibiotic Regimens for Odontogenic Soft Tissue Infections

Normal host
Penicillin G, 1–4 million U iv q4–6h
Clindamycin, 600 mg iv q6–8h
Cefoxitin, 1–2 g iv q6h
Ceftizoxime, 1–2 g iv q8–12h
Compromised host (each of following ± an aminoglycoside)
Piperacillin, 3 g iv q4h
Cefoxitin, 1–2 g iv q6h
Ceftizoxime, 1–2 g iv q8–12h
Imipenem/cilastatin, 500 mg iv q6h
Ticarcillin/clavulanate, 3.0 g/0.1 g iv q4–6h

tunistic infections of the oral cavity, particularly candidiasis, aspergillosis, mucormycosis, herpetic gingivostomatitis, and mixed gram-negative infections.[68,69] In this section, some of the conditions affecting primarily the oral mucosa and salivary glands in which an infectious cause is either proved or suspected will be briefly discussed.

Infections of the Oral Mucosa

Noma, or Gangrenous Stomatitis. Noma, or gangrenous stomatitis, also known as cancrum oris, is an acute, fulminating, and gangrenous infection of the oral and facial tissues. It usually occurs in the presence of severe debilitation and malnutrition, and children are most often affected. The earliest lesion is a small, painful, red spot or vesicle on the attached gingiva in the premolar or molar region of the mandible. A necrotic ulcer rapidly develops and undermines the deeper tissue. Painful cellulitis of the lips and cheeks is observed as the lesion extends outward in a conelike fashion. Within a short period, sloughing of necrotic soft tissues occurs and exposes underlying bone, teeth, and deeper tissues.

Fusospirochetal organisms such as *Borrelia vincentii* and *Fusobacterium nucleatum* are consistently cultured from noma lesions. *Prevotella melaninogenica* may also be present. Biopsy specimens of tissue from the advancing lesion show a mat of predominantly gram-negative threadlike bacteria that cannot be positively identified.[70] Thus, this lesion bears a similarity to acute necrotizing ulcerative gingivitis in several respects but appears to be more focal and destructive, involving deeper tissues beyond the gingiva. Treatment of noma requires high doses of intravenous penicillin. Every effort should be directed to correct the dehydration and underlying malnutrition and debility. Loose teeth and sequestra may be removed, but saucerization should be avoided. Healing is by secondary intention. Serious mutilation and facial deformity may require subsequent cosmetic surgery.

Aphthous Stomatitis. Aphthous ulcers are the most common cause of recurrent oral lesions. This entity must be distinguished from oral ulceration due to herpes simplex, coxsackievirus, agranulocytosis, and Behçet's and other diseases. Three major clinical variants are recognized: (1) minor aphthous ulcers, (2) major aphthous ulcers, and (3) herpetiform aphthous ulcers.[71] The true cause of aphthous ulcerations is not known, although a number of infectious agents including viruses have been implicated. The most prevailing hypothesis suggests that the mechanism causing the ulceration is autoimmune in nature. Circulating humoral antibodies and sensitized T lymphocytes active against oral mucosa have been demonstrated in patients with aphthous ulcers.[71] Furthermore, the active T lymphocytes undergo a phase of rapid proliferation just before the onset of ulceration. The origin of the autoantibodies is not clear, and no common antigenic factor between oral epithelium and the indigenous microflora has been demonstrated.

In their most characteristic form, minor aphthous ulcers appear as a number of small ulcers on the buccal and labial mucosa, the floor of the mouth, or the tongue. The palatal soft tissues are rarely involved. Moreover, the ulcers are concentrated in the anterior part of the oral cavity, whereas the pharynx and tonsillar fauces are rarely implicated. A prodromal stage is usually present. The ulcers appear gray-yellow, often with a raised and erythematous margin, and are exquisitely painful. Lymph node enlargement is seen only with secondary bacterial infection. The course of ulceration varies from a few days to a little over 2 weeks and is followed by spontaneous healing. Major aphthous ulcers are more protracted and last up to several months. All areas of the oral cavity including the soft palate and tonsillar areas may be involved. Long periods of remission may be followed by intervals of intense ulcer activity. Herpetiform aphthous ulcers are small and multiple and characteristically affect the lateral margins and tip of the tongue. The ulcers are gray, without a delineating erythematous border, and are extremely painful, which makes eating and speaking difficult. Despite its name, there is little clinical resemblance to an acute herpetic gingivostomatitis. Although intranuclear inclusions have been demonstrated in herpetiform aphthous ulcers, there is no evidence to suggest that these inclusions bear any relationship to presence of viruses.

The treatment of aphthous ulcers is primarily symptomatic. Strict oral hygiene should be maintained, and the use of antiseptic mouthwashes may be helpful in temporarily reducing secondary infection. Local anesthetic lozenges or gels may be used as a last resort for brief periods of pain relief. Topical or systemic steroids may be beneficial in selected people with extensive disease, but caution must be exercised in their administration.

Mucositis and Stomatitis in the Severely Immunocompromised. Much of what is known about management of oromucosal infections has been studied in cancer patients being treated with radiotherapy, chemotherapy, and bone marrow transplantation.[68,72] Other patient groups that develop oromucosal complications include those undergoing solid organ transplantation, patients with the acquired immunodeficiency syndrome (AIDS),[73] and those with autoimmune diseases associated with xerostomia and systemic immunosuppression. The underlying mechanism appears to be a breakdown of the mucosal epithelium that leads to mucositis, secondary bacterial or fungal infection, or reactivation of latent viral infection. Oral candidiasis, herpes simplex, varicella-zoster, and cytomegalovirus infections are the most common manifestations. Mucositis that complicates radiation or chemotherapy most commonly involves the nonkeratinized oral epithelium, including the buccal and labial mucosa, soft palate, oropharynx, floor of the mouth, and ventral and lateral surfaces of the tongue. Ulceration and pseudomembrane formation are evident usually between 4 and 7 days after the initiation of chemotherapy when the rate of destruction of the basal epithelium exceeds that of proliferation of new cells. The clinical manifestations may be quite variable. The lesions are often protracted in duration and may not be associated with an inflammatory reaction, thereby masking the usual signs and symptoms. Pain or tenderness may be the only abnormal finding. Since the etiologic agents of infection cannot be readily predicted on clinical grounds alone in such patients, specific microbiologic diagnosis by culture, histopathology, or antigen detection techniques is critical for appropriate treatment. Topical as well as systemic antimicrobial agents may be indicated along with antiseptic (e.g., chlorhexidine) and anesthetic (e.g., benzydamine, viscous lidocaine, etc.) applications.[74] Frequent saline rinses may reduce mucosal irritation, remove thickened secretions or debris, and increase moisture in the mouth.[68] Coating agents such as milk of magnesia or aluminum hydroxide gel (Amphojel) have been useful for the symptomatic relief of painful oral lesions. Topical or oral cytoprotective agents (e.g., sucralfate) or nonsteroidal anti-inflammatory analgesics (e.g., benzydamine, salicylates, etc.) may provide additional benefit, but further controlled clinical trials are required to assess their ap-

propriate indications and efficacy.[74,75] Meticulous oral and dental hygiene, effective management of xerostomia, selective suppression of oropharyngeal microbial colonization, and early control of reactivation by latent viral infections appear to be the critical steps to prevent and reduce the overall morbidity of oromucosal infections in the severely immunocompromised.[68,76]

Infections of the Salivary Gland

Sialadenitis, or infection of salivary tissue, is a relatively common disease. Sialolithiasis in elderly patients leads to ductal obstruction and secondarily to suppuration of the salivary gland and appears to be a major predisposing condition. In this regard, stones of Wharton's duct are much more common than are those of Stensen's duct, and obstructive sialadenitis is much more frequent with the submandibular than the parotid gland.[77] Other predisposing factors for sialadenitis include dehydration, general debility, sialogogic drugs, and trauma.

Suppurative Parotitis. Acute bacterial parotitis is a specific clinical entity primarily affecting the elderly, malnourished, dehydrated, or postoperative patient. Clinically, there is a sudden onset of firm, erythematous swelling of the pre- and postauricular areas that extends to the angle of the mandible. This is associated with exquisite local pain and tenderness. Systemic findings of high fevers, chills, and marked toxicity are generally present. Progression of the infection may lead to massive swelling of the neck, respiratory obstruction, septicemia, and osteomyelitis of the adjacent facial bones. Staphylococci have been the predominant isolates, and antibiotic therapy should include an antistaphylococcal agent. Enterobacteriaceae, other gram-negative bacilli, and anaerobes have also been reported to cause parotitis. Early surgical drainage and decompression of the gland are generally required since spontaneous drainage is uncommon.

Chronic Bacterial Parotitis. In this condition, parotitis is recurrent with intermittent acute exacerbations. There is chronic, low-grade, bacterial infection resulting in functional destruction of the salivary gland. Pus, when obtained directly from the gland, usually reveals the growth of staphylococci or mixed oral aerobes and anaerobes. Sialography during remission may reveal a sialectatic pattern of pooling of contrast medium that suggests multiple cystic cavities in place of the normal acinar pattern. Chronic parotitis may be confused with Sjögren syndrome, a noninfectious illness characterized by the triad of xerostomia, keratoconjunctivitis, and systemic autoimmune disease such as rheumatoid arthritis, lupus erythematosus, scleroderma, periarteritis nodosa, and polymyositis. The presence of associated temporomandibular arthritis or arthralgia should strongly suggest Sjögren syndrome rather than chronic bacterial parotitis.

Therapy for chronic parotitis should initially be conservative and consist of systemic antibiotics and ductal saline or antibiotic irrigations. Parotidectomy may eventually be required for people with long-standing infection.

Viral Parotitis. Mumps parotitis is characterized by the rapid, painful swelling of one or both parotid glands within 2–3 weeks after exposure. A prodromal phase of preauricular pain, fever, chills, and headache may be present. Other viral causes of parotitis include influenza and enteroviruses, and specific neutralizing antibody titers may be required for distinguishing these from true mumps. Mumps parotitis usually resolves spontaneously in 5–10 days. Symptomatic relief of pain and fever is necessary, and prevention of dehydration and secondary bacterial infection is essential.

MISCELLANEOUS INFECTIONS OF THE NECK AND HEAD

In the antibiotic era, dental causes have surpassed oropharyngeal and tonsillar sources of deep neck infections.[49,78–80] Other miscellaneous infections of the neck and head include suppurative cervical adenitis, infected embryologic cysts of the neck, various infections secondary to human and animal bites, maxillofacial trauma, irradiation, and surgical procedures of the head and neck.

Cervical Adenitis

Cervical adenitis, which presents unilaterally in association with warm, tender, enlarged, and fluctuant lymph nodes, is usually due to pyogenic infections. Its anatomic location in relationship to major cervical landmarks will provide the clinical clues to the primary source of infection.[31,81] Bilateral acute cervical adenitis generally suggests a nonspecific or viral cause, toxoplasmosis, or group A streptococcal infection. A more chronic or recurrent cervical adenitis should suggest the possibility of typical or atypical mycobacteriosis, human immunodeficiency virus infection, Epstein-Barr virus or cytomegalovirus mononucleosis, cat-scratch fever, actinomycosis, sarcoidosis, as well as lymphoproliferative and neoplastic disorders.

Infected Embryologic Cysts

Three distinct embryologic abnormalities can present with infection in the neck. They are (1) cystic hygroma or lymphangioma, (2) pharyngeal and bronchial cleft cysts, and (3) thyroglossal duct cysts. Cystic hygroma is associated with a diffuse tumor mass usually evident within the first 2 years of life. It commonly involves the lower aspect of the neck, but it can appear anywhere in the cervical region. It is probably an abnormal development of lymphatic vessels from the jugular lymphatic sacs. Sudden enlargement by infection or hemorrhage into a lymphangioma may cause obstruction of the upper airways. Pharyngeal cleft cysts can develop from the first, second, or third pharyngeal clefts, although the second is most common. They usually present in childhood as fistulas or masses just posterior to the angle of the mandible along the anterior border of the sternocleidomastoid muscle. The mass can fluctuate in size, and enlargement can be associated with upper respiratory infection. Thyroglossal duct cysts originate from the foramen cecum of the tongue and descend through the body of the hyoid bone into the anterior portion of the neck. Any residual secretory lining may give rise to a thyroglossal duct cyst that is midline in location. It can cause respiratory obstruction or fistula formation if secondarily infected. Treatment of these congenital abnormalities during secondary bacterial infection requires broad-spectrum antibiotics such as a cephalosporin. Definitive surgical excision to prevent recurrence should be performed after complete resolution of the acute process.

Suppurative Thyroiditis

Although infections of the thyroid gland are rare, they are potentially life threatening. Such infections may arise by a variety of pathways, including hematogenous dissemination, direct spread from an adjacent deep fascial space infection, an infected thyroglossal fistula, or anterior perforation of the esophagus. Preexisting diseases of the thyroid gland such as a goiter or adenoma are frequently present.[82,83] Acute suppurative thyroiditis is characterized by fever, local pain, tenderness, warmth, erythema, and symptoms of dysphagia, dysphonia, hoarseness, or pharyngitis. The infection may involve single or both lobes, and fluctuance may not be apparent until late in the course. Subacute thyroiditis may have similar local findings, but systemic manifestations are not as severe and tend to be more self-limiting.

Laboratory investigation of thyroid infections should include ultrasonography, radionuclide scanning, and lateral radiographs or CT scanning of the neck for evidence of peritracheal extension; thyroid function tests; and diagnostic needle aspiration for microbiologic diagnosis. *Staphylococcus aureus*, *S. pyogenes*, and *S. pneumoniae* are most frequently isolated. Other pathogens include *Haemophilus influenzae*, viridans streptococci, *Eikenella corrodens*, and *Bacteroides*, *Peptostreptococcus*, and *Actinomyces* spp. Treatment requires specific antimicrobial agents and appropriate surgical drainage.

Infections from Bites, Maxillofacial Trauma, Irradiation, and Surgical Wounds

Human and Animal Bites. Human and animal bite wounds to the head and neck are relatively common. Although they may look innocuous initially, serious complications can occur. For this reason, empirical antibiotic therapy is recommended when the bite wound involves the face, head, or neck. Recent studies that used adequate anaerobic culture techniques indicate indigenous oral flora rather than the skin flora to be the major source of bite wound infections.[84] Streptococci, *E. corrodens*, and *S. aureus* are the most prevalent facultative organisms, and *Bacteroides* and *Peptostreptococcus* are the most common anaerobic isolates. Penicillin-resistant gram-negative rods are infrequent. *Eikenella corrodens* is unique in that it is susceptible to penicillin and ampicillin but resistant to oxacillin, methicillin, nafcillin, and clindamycin.[63] In animal bite wounds, *Pasteurella multocida* has been a common cause of infection.[85] It is susceptible to penicillin. In view of these findings, penicillin remains the antibiotic of choice for initial therapy for both human and animal bite wounds.

Maxillofacial Trauma. Automobile and motorcycle accidents cause the most severe maxillofacial trauma. Particular attention should be paid to fractures that may traverse sinus cavities and teeth-bearing areas of the maxilla or mandible, since secondary infection rates at these sites are particularly high. Treatment is aimed not only at correcting the fracture but also at prevention of infection and subsequent osteomyelitis. Early stabilization of the fracture and the jaws is generally required to protect the airway. Tracheostomy with use of inflated, cuffed endotracheal tubes may prevent aspiration of blood and other foreign materials. The occurrence of otorrhea or rhinorrhea with a persistent cerebrospinal fluid leak should be carefully observed.

Irradiation and Postsurgical Wounds. Malignancies of the head and neck are frequently treated with a combination of irradiation, chemotherapeutic agents, and surgical resection. Infectious complications are particularly common after such procedures. Pharyngocutaneous fistulas, osteonecrosis of the mandible, or radionecrosis of the laryngeal cartilage may occur. *Staphylococcus aureus* and *Pseudomonas aeruginosa* are frequent pathogens.[85] Prolonged courses of intravenous antibiotics selected according to culture and sensitivity data as well as frequent wound débridement and cleansing are indicated. Although some controversy still exists, immunocompromised patients undergoing oropharyngeal surgery for cancer should receive perioperative antibiotics since they are at particular high risk for infection. A broad-spectrum antibiotic such as cefazolin, cefuroxime, cefoxitin, or ceftizoxime appears appropriate in this setting.[18,86,88]

REFERENCES

1. Chow AW, Roser SM, Brady FA. Orofacial odontogenic infections. Ann Intern Med. 1978;88:392.
2. Hardie J. Microbial flora of the oral cavity. In: Schuster GS, ed. Oral Microbiology and Infectious Disease. Baltimore: Williams & Wilkins; 1983:162.

3. Hamada S, Slade HD. Biology, immunology and cariogenicity of *Streptococcus mutans*. Microbiol Rev. 1980;44:331.
4. Gordon DF, Stutman M, Loesche WJ. Improved isolation of anaerobic bacteria from the gingival crevice area of man. Appl Microbiol. 1971;21:1046.
5. Valenti WM, Trudell RB, Bentley DW. Factors predisposing to oropharyngeal colonization with gram-negative bacilli in the aged. N Engl J Med. 1978; 298:1108.
6. Rosenthal S, Tager IB. Relevance of gram-negative rods in the normal pharyngeal flora. Ann Intern Med. 1975;83:355.
7. Schuster GS. The microbiology of oral and maxillofacial infections. In: Topazian RG, Goldberg MH, eds. Oral and Maxillofacial Infections. 2nd ed. Philadelphia: WB Saunders; 1987:33.
8. Hardie JM, Bowden GH. The normal microbial flora of the mouth. In: Skinner FA, Carr JG, eds. The Normal Microbial Flora of the Mouth. London: Academic Press; 1974:47.
9. Geddes DAM, Jenkins GN. Intrinsic and extrinsic factors influencing the flora of the mouth. In: Skinner FA, Carr JG, eds. The Normal Microbial Flora of the Mouth. London: Academic Press; 1974:85.
10. Schachtele CF. Dental caries. In: Schuster GS, ed. Oral Microbiology and Infectious Diseases. Baltimore: Williams & Wilkins; 1983:197.
11. Loesche WJ. Bacterial mediators in periodontal disease. Clin Infect Dis. 1993; 16(Suppl 4):S203.
12. Tanner A, Stillman N. Oral and dental infections with anaerobic bacteria: Clinical features, predominant pathogens, and treatment. Clin Infect Dis. 1993;16(Suppl 4):S304.
13. Shaw JH. Causes and control of dental caries. N Engl J Med. 1987;317:996.
14. Loesche WJ. Role of *Streptococcus mutans* in human dental decay. Microbiol Rev. 1986;50:353.
15. Moore WEC, Holdeman LV, Smibert RM, et al. Bacteriology of experimental gingivitis in young adult humans. Infect Immun. 1982;38:651.
16. Socransky SS, Tan ACR, Haffajee AD, et al. Present status of studies on the microbial etiology of periodontal disease. In: Genco RJ, Mergenhagen SE, eds. Host–Parasite Interactions in Periodontal Diseases. Washington, DC: American Society for Microbiology; 1982:1.
17. Willams BL, McCann GF, Schoenknecht FD. Bacteriology of dental abscesses of endodontic origin. J Clin Microbiol. 1983;18:770.
18. Greenberg RN, James RB, Marier RL, et al. Microbiologic and antibiotic aspects of infections in the oral and maxillofacial region. J Oral Surg. 1979; 37:873.
19. Baker AS, Montgomery WW. Oropharyngeal space infections. Curr Clin Top Infect Dis. 1987;8:227.
20. Newman MG. Anaerobic oral and dental infection. Rev Infect Dis. 1984;6: 107.
21. Chow AW. Odontogenic infections. In: Schlossberg D, ed. Infections of the Head and Neck. New York: Springer Publishing; 1987:148.
22. Kureishi K, Chow AW. The tender tooth—Dentoalveolar, pericoronal, and periodontal infections. Infect Dis Clin North Am. 1988;2:163.
23. Roscoe DL, Chow AW. Normal flora and mucosal immunity of the head and neck. Infect Dis Clin North Am. 1988;2:1.
24. Sutter VL. Anaerobes as normal oral flora. Rev Infect Dis. 1984;6(Suppl):62.
25. McGhee JR, Michalek SM. Immunobiology of dental caries—Microbial aspects and local immunity. Annu Rev Microbiol. 1981;35:595.
26. Saral R, Ambinder RF, Burns WH, et al. Acyclovir prophylaxis against recrudescent herpes simplex virus infections in leukemia patients. A randomized double-blind placebo controlled study. Ann Intern Med. 1983;99:773.
27. Van Dyke TE, Horoszewicz HU, Cianciola LJ, et al. Neutrophil chemotaxis dysfunction in human periodontitis. Infect Immun. 1980;27:124.
28. Cianciola LJ, Genco RJ, Patters MR, et al. Defective polymorphonuclear leukocyte function in human periodontal disease. Nature. 1977;265:445.
29. Genco RJ, Plaut AG, Moellering RC Jr. Evaluation of human oral organisms and pathogenic *Streptococcus* for production of IgA protease. J Infect Dis. 1975;131(Suppl):17.
30. Kilian M. Degradation of immunoglobulins A1, A2, and G by suspected principal periodontal pathogens. Infect Immun. 1981;34:757.
31. Goldberg MH, Topazian RG. Odontogenic infections and deep fascial space infections of dental origin. In: Topazian RG, Goldberg MH, eds. Oral and Maxillofacial Infections. 2nd ed. Philadelphia: WB Saunders; 1987:156.
32. Thadepalli H, Mandal AK. Anatomic basis of head and neck infections. Infect Dis Clin North Am. 1988;2:21.
33. Shinn DLS, Squires S, McFadzean JA. The treatment of Vincent's disease with metronidazole. Dent Pract. 1965;15:275.
34. Stephen KW, McLatchie MF, Mason DK, et al. Treatment of acute ulcerative gingivitis (Vincent's type). Br Dent J. 1966;121:313.
35. Lindhe J. Treatment of localized juvenile periodontitis. In: Genco RJ, Mergenhagen SE, eds. Host–Parasite Interactions in Periodontal Disease. Washington, DC: American Society for Microbiology; 1982:382.
36. Slots J, Reynolds HS, Genco RJ. *Actinobacillus actinomycetemcomitans* in human periodontal disease: A cross-sectional microbiological investigation. Infect Immun. 1980;29:1013.
37. Loesche WJ. Rationale for the use of antimicrobial agents in periodontal disease. Int J Technol Assess Health Care. 1990;6:403.
38. Finch RG, Snider GE, Sprinkle PM. Ludwig's angina. JAMA. 1980;243:1171.
39. Crawford JJ, Sconyers JR, Moriarty JD, et al. Bacteremia after tooth extractions studied with the aid of prereduced anaerobically sterilized culture media. Appl Microbiol. 1974;27:927.
40. Rubin R, Solvate EA, Lewis R. Infected total hip replacement after dental procedures. Oral Surg. 1976;41:18.
41. McCurdy JA, MacInnis EL, Hays LL. Fatal mediastinitis after a dental infection. J Oral Surg. 1977;35:726.
42. Yoshikawa TT, Quinn W. The aching head—Intracranial suppuration due to head and neck infections. Infect Dis Clin North Am. 1988;2:265.
43. Blomquist IK, Bayer AS. Life-threatening deep fascial space infections of the head and neck. Infect Dis Clin North Am. 1988;2:237.
44. Topazian RG. Osteomyelitis of the jaws. In: Topazian RG, Goldberg MH, eds. Oral and Maxillofacial Infections. 2nd ed. Philadelphia: WB Saunders; 1987:204.
45. Chow AW, Guze LB. Bacteroidaceae bacteremia—Clinical experience with 112 patients. Medicine (Baltimore). 1974;53:93.
46. Sinave CP, Hardy GJ, Fardy PW. The Lemierre syndrome: Suppurative thrombophlebitis of the internal jugular vein secondary to oropharyngeal infection. Medicine (Baltimore). 1989;68:85.
47. Eagleton WP. Cavernous Sinus Thrombophlebitis and Allied Septic and Traumatic Lesions of the Basal Venous Sinuses. A Clinical Study of Blood Stream Infection. New York: Macmillan; 1926.
48. Harbour RC, Trobe JD, Ballinger WE. Septic cavernous sinus thrombosis associated with gingivitis and parapharyngeal abscess. Arch Ophthalmol. 1984;102:94.
49. Chow AW. Life-threatening infections of the head and neck. Clin Infect Dis. 1992;14:991.
50. Chow AW, Vortel JJ. Infections of the sinuses and parameningeal structures. In: Gorbach SL, Barlett JC, Blacklow NR, eds. Infectious Diseases. Philadelphia: WB Saunders; 1991:431.
51. Mackowiak PA, Jones SR, Smith JW. Diagnostic value of sinus-tract cultures in chronic osteomyelitis. JAMA. 1978;239:2772.
52. Salit IE. Diagnostic approaches to head and neck infections. Infect Dis Clin North Am. 1988;2:35.
53. Holt GR, McManus K, Newman RK, et al. Computed tomography in the diagnosis of deep-neck infections. Arch Otolaryngol. 1982;108:693.
54. Wholey MH, Bruwer AJ, Baker HL. The lateral roentgenogram of the neck. Radiology. 1958;71:350.
55. Bryan CS, King BG Jr, Bryant RE. Retropharyngeal infection in adults. Arch Intern Med. 1974;134:127.
56. Slots J, Rams TE. Antibiotics in periodontal therapy: Advantages and disadvantages. J Clin Periodontol. 1990;17:479.
57. Olsvik B, Tenover FC. Tetracycline resistance in periodontal pathogens. Clin Infect Dis. 1993;16(Suppl 4):S310.
58. Gregory RL, Filler SJ. Protective secretory immunoglobulin A antibodies in humans following oral immunization with *Streptococcus mutans*. Infect Immun. 1987;55:2409.
59. Russell RRB, Johnson NW. The prospects of vaccination against dental caries. Br Dent J. 1987;162:29.
60. Heimdahl A, Nord CE. Treatment of orofacial infections of odontogenic origin. Scand J Infect Dis Suppl. 1985;46:101.
61. Hill MK, Sanders CV. Principles of antimicrobial therapy for head and neck infections. Infect Dis Clin North Am. 1988;2:57.
62. Busch DF, Kureshi LA, Sutter VL, et al. Susceptibility of respiratory tract anaerobes to orally administered penicillins and cephalosporins. Antimicrob Agents Chemother. 1976;10:713.
63. Tami TA, Parker GS. *Eikenella corrodens*—An emerging pathogen in head and neck infections. Arch Otolaryngol. 1984;110:752.
64. Edson RS, Rosenblatt JE, Lee DT, et al. Recent experience with antimicrobial susceptibility of anaerobic bacteria—Increasing resistance to penicillin. Mayo Clin Proc. 1982;57:737.
65. Heimdahl A, von Konow L, Nord CE. Isolation of β-lactamase producing *Bacteroides* strains associated with clinical failures with penicillin treatment of human orofacial infections. Arch Oral Biol. 1980;25:687.
66. Murray PR, Rosenblatt JE. Penicillin resistance and penicillinase production in clinical isolates of *Bacteroides melaninogenicus*. Antimicrob Agents Chemother. 1977;11:605.
67. Hood FJC. The place of metronidazole in the treatment of acute orofacial infection. Antimicrob Agents Chemother. 1978;15:71.
68. Epstein JB. The painful mouth—Mucositis, gingivitis and stomatitis. Infect Dis Clin North Am. 1988;2:183.
69. Barrett AP. A long-term prospective clinical study of oral complications during conventional chemotherapy for acute leukemia. Oral Surg. 1987;63:313.
70. Topazian RG. Uncommon infections of the oral and maxillofacial regions. In: Topazian RG, Goldberg MH, eds. Oral and Maxillofacial Infections. 2nd ed. Philadelphia: WB Saunders; 1987:317.
71. Tyldesley WR. Recurrent oral ulcerations. In: Tyldesley WR, ed. Oral Medicine. Oxford: Oxford University Press; 1981:49.
72. Epstein JB, Gangbar SJ. Oral mucosal lesions in patients undergoing treatment for leukemia. J Oral Med. 1987;42:132.
73. Lee PL, Kiviat N, Truelove EL, et al. Oral manifestations in patients with AIDS or AIDS-related disorders. J Dent Res. 1987;66:183.
74. Epstein JB, Stevenson-Moore P. Benzydamine hydrochloride in prevention and management of pain in oral mucositis associated with radiation therapy. Oral Surg. 1986;62:145.
75. Adams S, Toth B, Dudley BS. Evaluation of sucralfate as a compounded oral suspension for the treatment of stomatitis. Clin Pharmacol Ther. 1985;2:178.
76. Epstein JB, Schubert MM. Synergistic effects of sialogogues in management of xerostomia following radiation therapy. Oral Surg. 1987;64:179.
77. Goldberg MH. Infections of the salivary glands. In: Topazian RG, Goldberg MH, eds. Oral and Maxillary Infections. 2nd ed. Philadelphia: WB Saunders; 1987:239.
78. Brook I, Finegold SM. Acute suppurative parotitis caused by anaerobic bacteria: Report of two cases. Pediatrics. 1978;62:1019.
79. Whiting JL, Chow AW. Life-threatening infections of the mouth and throat. J Crit Illness. 1987;2:36.
80. Pruett TL, Simmons RL. Nosocomial gram-negative bacillary parotitis. JAMA. 1984;251:252.

81. Brook I. The swollen neck—Cervical lymphadenitis, parotitis, thyroiditis and infected cysts. Infect Dis Clin North Am. 1988;2:221.
82. Berger SA, Zonszein J, Villanema P, et al. Infectious diseases of the thyroid gland. Rev Infect Dis. 1983;5:108
83. Freidig EE, McClure SP, Wilson WR, et al. Clinical-histologic-microbiologic analysis of 419 lymph node biopsy specimens. Rev Infect Dis. 1986;8:322.
84. Goldstein EJC, Citron DW, Wield B, et al. Bacteriology of human and animal bite wounds. J Clin Microbiol. 1978;8:667.
85. Brook I, Hirokawa R. Microbiology of wound infection after head and neck cancer surgery. Ann Otol Rhinol Laryngol. 1989;98:323.
86. Gerard M, Meunier F, Dor P, et al. Antimicrobial prophylaxis for major head and neck surgery in cancer patients. Antimicrob Agents Chemother. 1988;32:1557.
87. Zide MF, Sanders CV, Marier RL, et al. Cefuroxime therapy for maxillofacial infections. Curr Ther Res. 1986;40:278.
88. Aldridge KE, Weeks LS, Stratton CW, Sanders CV. Differences in the in vitro inhibitory and bactericidal activity of ceftizoxime, cefoxitin, cefotetan, and penicillin G against *Bacteroides fragilis* group isolates. Comparison of time-kill kinetic studies with MIC values. Diagn Microbiol Infect Dis. 1990;13:311.

SECTION C. PLEUROPULMONARY AND BRONCHIAL INFECTIONS

47. ACUTE BRONCHITIS

JACK M. GWALTNEY, JR.

Acute bronchitis is an inflammatory condition of the tracheobronchial tree that is usually associated with a generalized respiratory infection. It occurs most commonly during the winter months when acute respiratory tract infections are prevalent. Patients seen in general practices in Great Britain had annual attack rates of acute bronchitis that varied between 40 and 54 percent 100,000.[1] Weekly attack rates peaked (117–171/100,000) in January and February and fell to trough levels (26–42/100,000) in August. The diagnosis was made most often in children under 5 years of age.

The syndrome of acute bronchitis is most often associated with respiratory viruses, both common cold viruses, such as rhinovirus and coronavirus, and those more invasive of the lower respiratory tract such as influenza and adenovirus. Nonviral causes of acute bronchitis also exist and include *Bordetella pertussis, Mycoplasma pneumoniae,* and the recently discovered *Chlamydia pneumoniae.* Secondary invasion with the common respiratory bacteria such as *Streptococcus pneumoniae* and *Haemophilus influenzae* may play a role in acute bronchitis, but this is uncertain.

ETIOLOGY

Cough occurs in approximately 50 percent of the cases of common respiratory illness in persons of all ages.[2] Cough is the localizing symptom in the respiratory tract that is most frequently associated with fever and is also highly associated with the occurrence of hoarseness. Infection with members of all the major respiratory virus groups causes cough (Table 1).[2–9] Cases of acute bronchitis are particularly common during influenza epidemics. While rhinovirus infections do not produce as severe an involvement of the tracheobronchial tree as influenza, rhinovirus infections, because of their frequency, are an important cause of acute bronchitis. In populations of military recruits, adenovirus infections ar a major cause of acute bronchitis. Among the other respiratory viruses that cause acute bronchitis, measles virus has been recognized as causing a particularly severe form of the disease.

A small proportion of cases are of nonviral etiology. *Mycoplasma pneumoniae* and *Bordetella pertussis* are among the nonviral causes of acute bronchitis. Recently, a new *Chlamydia pneumoniae* strain, TWAR,[10] was associated with acute respiratory tract infections that include cases with the clinical features of acute bronchitis.[11,12]

The etiologic role of *S. pneumoniae* and *H. influenzae* in acute bronchitis is not clear. Since these bacteria are carried in the resident flora of the upper respiratory tract of normal persons, it is difficult to evaluate studies in which expectorated sputum specimens have been cultured. To examine the role of secondary bacterial infection in the pathogenesis of acute bronchitis, it is necessary to conduct studies in which samples are collected from the tracheobronchial tree without contamination by nasopharyngeal flora.

PATHOGENESIS

The pathogenesis of acute bronchitis has not been investigated for all the causative agents. During acute bronchial infection, the mucous membrane of the tracheobronchial tree is hyperemic and edematous, and there are increased bronchial secretions. Destruction of respiratory epithelium may be extensive in some infections, such as influenza,[15,16] but appears to be minimal in others, such as rhinovirus colds.[17,18] Bronchial mucociliary function may be diminished in infections in which overt mucosal damage is limited.[19] With *M. pneumoniae* infection, bronchial irritation results from the attachment of the organism to the respiratory mucosa, with eventual sloughing of affected cells.[20]

It is also possible that severity of attacks of acute bronchitis may be increased by exposure to cigarette smoke and air pollutants. These substances, in association with recurrent acute bronchial infection, may result in permanent injury to the bronchial tree. Epidemiologic studies support the idea that acute respiratory infections play a role in the pathogenesis of chronic obstructive lung disease.[21,22] Also, studies of pulmonary func-

TABLE 1. Cough Associated with Acute Viral Infections of the Respiratory Tract

Virus	Percent of Cases with Cough (Refs)
Influenza	75–93 (2, 3)
Adenovirus	45–90 (4, 6)
Rhinovirus	32–60 (3, 5)
Coronavirus	10–50 (7, 8)
Parainfluenza virus	2–45 (5)
Respiratory syncytial virus	61 (9)
Coxsackievirus A21	26 (5)
Miscellaneous (rubeola, rubella, and so forth)	—

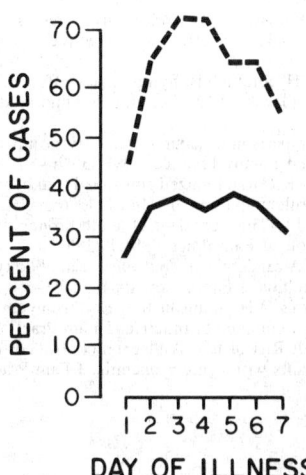

FIG. 1. Occurrence of cough in rhinovirus colds (139 cases) (solid line) and type A$_2$ influenza (33 cases) (broken line) in young adults. (Modified from Gwaltney,[3] with permission.)

tion in adults with acute bronchitis have shown abnormalities in airway resistance and reactivity.[23,24]

There has been recent interest in examining the relationship between acute bronchitis and heightened airway reactivity. Mild bronchial asthma was found to be increased in patients with a history of recurrent acute bronchitis over that seen in the general population.[25] Also, in a case–control study, patients with acute bronchitis were more likely to have a previous history of asthma and a history, or diagnosis, of atopic disease.[26] These findings have raised the question of the possible role of bronchospasm in some cases of prolonged cough associated with acute respiratory infection.

CLINICAL PRESENTATION

Cough begins early in the course of many acute respiratory infections and tends to become more prominent as the illness progresses (Fig. 1). In the usual cold and influenzal illness, nasal and pharyngeal complaints subside after 3 or 4 days, while the cough tends to persist and to achieve greater prominence.[3] Persons presenting for medical care who are diagnosed as having acute bronchitis probably represent a subset of all patients with acute respiratory infection. In one prospective study of acute respiratory disease, 45 percent of patients were still coughing 2 weeks after presentation and 25 percent were still coughing after 3 weeks.[27] With a variety of different respiratory virus infections, sputum production was reported in approximately one-half of the cases in which cough occurred.[4,5] An initially dry cough may later result in mucoid sputum, which characteristically develops a more purulent character in the later stages of illness. A study of natural rhinovirus infections in young adults has shown that the frequency and duration of cough is prolonged in cigarette smokers.[27]

With severe tracheal involvement, there may be burning substernal pain associated with respiration and coughing. Dyspnea and cyanosis are not seen in adults unless the patient has underlying chronic obstructive pulmonary disease or other conditions that impair lung function. Rhonchi and coarse rales may be heard on examination of the chest. Signs of consolidation and alveolar involvement are not present in uncomplicated bronchitis. The frequency with which fever occurs depends on the specific infectious agent involved and the age of the patient. In adults, influenza virus, adenovirus, and *M. pneumoniae* infections are commonly associated with temperature elevations. Fever is unusual in adults with bronchitis associated with cold viruses, like rhinovirus and coronavirus.

DIAGNOSIS

Bronchitis may be suspected in the patient with an acute respiratory infection with cough, but because a large number of more serious diseases of the lower respiratory tract cause cough, bronchitis must be considered a diagnosis of exclusion. A complete history should be obtained, including information on exposure to toxic substances and cigarette use. Complaints involving other organ systems should be sought. Epidemiologic considerations and vaccination history may aid in the diagnosis of specific causes of bronchitis, such as influenza, *M. pneumoniae*, and whooping cough.

Included in a complete physical examination should be a careful evaluation of the chest for evidence of pneumonia and signs of cardiovascular and thromboembolic diseases. Radiologic examination of the chest may be required in the occasional patient in whom the question of parenchymal disease of the lung remains after the physical examination. Cultures of respiratory secretions for influenza virus, *M. pneumoniae*, and *B. pertussis* should be obtained when these diseases are suspected. Cultures and other diagnostic tests for the other respiratory viruses are available in some clinical microbiology laboratories. Culture methods and a microimmunofluorescence test have been developed for the laboratory diagnosis of *C. pneumoniae*.[10] The use of an IgM-specific conjugate helps detect current infections. Routine bacterial cultures of expectorated sputum are not helpful because of the sampling problem of avoiding nasopharyngeal flora and because of the unknown importance of bacterial infection in the etiology of acute bronchitis. Patients in whom cough persists beyond the expected duration of the acute illness should have further diagnostic examinations, including chest x-ray films, sputum cytology, and bronchoscopy to exclude foreign body aspiration, tuberculosis, tumors, and other chronic diseases of the tracheobronchial tree and lungs.

TREATMENT

Treatment of most cases of acute bronchitis is symptomatic and is directed primarily at the control of cough. Otherwise, healthy patients do not require hospitalization except in cases of unusual severity. Patients with underlying chronic cardiopulmonary diseases who contract influenzal or other severe forms of bronchitis may develop serious ventilatory abnormalities that require hospitalization with ventilatory assistance and oxygen therapy. In the average case, cough suppressants such as dextromethorphan 15 mg po every 6 hours are the main form of treatment required. With severe cough, preparations containing codeine are useful.[28] The value of expectorants is not well established,[29] and in patients with a good cough reflex, maintaining hydration is probably the most effective way to prevent drying of bronchial secretions. Aspirin or acetaminophen and bed rest are beneficial in influenzal syndromes in which malaise and fever are prominent. Because of the apparent bronchospastic component in some cases of acute bronchitis there has been a recent interest in treatment with β_2-adrenergic bronchodilators.[30,31]

The value of antibiotics in the treatment of otherwise healthy patients with acute bronchitis is uncertain, and the use of these agents is not recommended as a general practice. Controlled trials comparing antibiotic treatment to placebo[32–36] have given conflicting results, which could result from a number of variables, including type of antibiotic and dosage schedule used, duration of follow-up, season of the year (reflecting prevalence of different pathogens), and adequacy of subject blinding related to drug side effects. With a self-limited disease like acute bronchitis, therapeutic trials that compare one antibiotic with another but do not have a placebo group are difficult to interpret.

Mycoplasma pneumoniae infection should be treated with erythromycin or tetracycline (see Ch. 161), *B. pertussis* infection with erythromycin (see Ch. 209), and *C. pneumoniae* infection with tetracycline, erythromycin, or one of the newer macrolide or azalide antibiotics (see Ch. 24). During epidemics known to be due to influenza A virus, treatment with amantadine (100 mg po bid) is recommended for patients with suspected influenza if the illness is less than 48 hours in duration. Also annual immunization with influenza vaccine or prophylaxis with amantadine is recommended in patients with chronic cardiopulmonary problems (see Ch. 141). Children should receive pertussis vaccine as part of their routine immunizations. It is particularly important to discourage cigarette smoking in patients in whom acute respiratory tract infections are associated with protracted cough and sputum production.

REFERENCES

1. Ayres JG. Seasonal pattern of acute bronchitis in general practice in the United Kingdom 1976–83. Thorax. 1986;41:107–10.
2. Dingle JH, Badger GF, Jordon WS Jr. Illness in the Home: A Study of 25,000 Illnesses in a Group of Cleveland Families. Cleveland: The Press of Western Reserve University; 1964;68.
3. Gwaltney JM Jr. Rhinoviruses. In: Evans AS, ed. Viral Infections of Humans: Epidemiology and Control. 3rd ed. New York: Plenum; 1989:593–615.
4. Dascomb HE, Hilleman MR. Clinical laboratory studies in patients with respiratory disease caused by adenovirus (RI-APC-ARD agents). Am J Med. 1956; 21:161.
5. Tyrrell DAJ. Common Colds and Related Diseases. Baltimore: Williams & Wilkins; 1965.
6. Bloom HH, Forsyth BR, Johnson KM, et al. Patterns of adenovirus infections in Marine Corps personnel. I. A 42-month survey in recruit and nonrecruit populations. Am J Hyg. 1964;80:328.
7. Kaye HS, Marsh HB, Dowdle WR. Seroepidemiologic survey of coronavirus (strain OC43) related infections in a children's population. Am J Epidemiol. 1971;94:43.
8. Hendley JO, Fishburne HB, Gwaltney JM Jr. Coronavirus infections in working adults. Eight-year study with 229E and OC43. Am Rev Respir Dis 1972; 105:805.
9. Knight V, Kapikian AZ, Kravetz MH, et al. Ecology of a newly recognized common respiratory agent RS-virus. Ann Intern Med. 1961;55–507.
10. Grayston JT. Infections caused by Chlamydia pneumoniae strain TWAR. Clin Infect Dis. 1992;16:757–63.
11. Grayston JT, Kuo C-C, Wang S-P, et al. A new Chlamydia psittaci strain, TWAR, isolated in acute respiratory tract infections. N Engl J Med. 1986; 315:161–8.
12. Grayston JT, Kuo C-C, Wang S-P, et al. Clinical findings in TWAR respiratory tract infections. In: Oriel JD, Ridgway G, Schacter J, et al, eds. Chlamydial Infections. Cambridge: Cambridge University Press; 1986;337–40.
13. Hahn DL, Dodge RW, Golubjatnikov R. Association of Chlamydia pneumoniae (strain TWAR) infection with wheezing, asthmatic bronchitis, and adult-onset asthma. JAMA. 1991;266:225–30.
14. Hammerschlag MR, Chirgwin K, Roblin PM, et al. Persistent infection with Chlamydia pneumoniae following acute respiratory illness. Clin Infect Dis. 1992;14:178–82.
15. Loosli CG, Stinson SF, Ryan DP, et al. The destruction of type 2 pneumocytes by airborne influenza PR8-A virus: Its effect on surfactant and lecithin content of the pneumonic lesions of mice. Chest. 1975;67(Suppl):7S.
16. Mulder J, Hers JFPh. Influenza. Groningen: Wolters-Noordhoff; 1972;1–300.
17. Douglas RG Jr, Alford BR, Cough RB: Atraumatic nasal biopsy for studies of respiratory virus infection in volunteers. Antimicrob Agents Chemother. 1968;8:340.
18. Winther B, Farr B, Turner RB, et al. Histopathologic examination and enumeration of polymorphonuclear leukocytes in the nasal mucosa during experimental rhinovirus colds. Acta Otoaryngol [Suppl] (Stockh) 1984;413:19–24.
19. Sasaki Y, Togo Y, Wagner NH Jr, et al. Mucociliary function during experimentally induced rhinovirus infection in man. Ann Otol. 1973;82:203.
20. Powell DA, Hu PC, Wilson M, et al. Attachment of Mycoplasma pneumoniae to respiratory epithelium. Infect Immun 1976;13:959.
21. Lebowitz MD, Burrows B. The relationship of acute respiratory illness history to the prevalence and incidence of obstructive lung disorders. Am J Epidemiol. 1977;105:544.
22. Monto AS, Ross HW. The Tecumseh study of respiratory illness. X. Relation of acute infections to smoking, lung function and chronic symptoms. Am J Epidemiol. 1978;107:57.
23. Hall WJ, Hall CB, Speers DM. Respiratory syncytial virus infection in adults. Clinical, virologic, and serial pulmonary function studies. Ann Intern Med. 1978;88:203.
24. Boldy DAR, Skidmore SJ, Ayres JG. Acute bronchitis in the community: Clinical features, infective factors, changes in pulmonary function and bronchial reactivity to histamine. Respir Med. 1990;84:377–85.
25. Hallett JS, Jacobs RL. Recurrent acute bronchitis: The association with undiagnosed bronchial asthma. Ann Allergy. 1985;55:568–70.
26. Williamson HA, Jr, Schultz P. An association between acute bronchitis and asthma. J Fam Pract. 1987;24:35–8.
27. Gwaltney JM Jr, Hendley JO, Simon G, et al. Rhinovirus infections in an industrial population. II. Characteristics of illness and antibody response. JAMA. 1967;202:494.
28. Eddy NB. Codeine and its alternates for pain and cough relief. Ann Intern Med. 1969;71:1209.
29. Kuhn JJ, Hendley JO, Adams KF. Antitussive effect of guaifenesin in young adults with natural colds. Objective and subjective assessment. Chest. 1982; 82:713.
30. Melbye H, Aasebo U, Straume B. Symptomatic effect of inhaled fenoterol in acute bronchitis: a placebo-controlled double-blind study. Family Practice. 1991;8:216–22.
31. Hueston WJ. A comparison of albuterol and erythromycin for the treatment of acute bronchitis. J Family Practice. 1991;33:476–80.
32. Stott NC, and West RR. Randomized controlled trial of antibiotics in patients with cough and purulent sputum. Br Med J. 1976;2:556.
33. Franks P, Gleiner JA. The treatment of acute bronchitis with trimethoprim and sulfamethoxazole. J Fam Pract. 1984;19:185–90.
34. Williamson HA Jr. A randomized, controlled trial of doxycycline in the treatment of acute bronchitis. J Fam Pract. 1984;19:481–6.
35. Brickfield FX, Carter WH, Johnson RE. Erythromycin in the treatment of acute bronchitis in a community practice. J Fam Pract. 1986;23:119–22.
36. Dunlay J, Reinhardt R, Roi LD. A placebo-controlled, double-blind trial of erythromycin in adults with acute bronchitis. J Fam Pract. 1987;25:137–41.

48. CHRONIC BRONCHITIS AND ACUTE INFECTIOUS EXACERBATIONS

HERBERT Y. REYNOLDS

Chronic bronchitis is a condition in which cough and excessive secretion of mucus occur in the tracheobronchial tree that are not due to other specific diseases such as bronchiectasis, asthma, or tuberculosis. The label *chronic bronchitic* is often applied loosely to patients and is very much a clinical diagnosis. By definition, the diagnosis is given to patients who report coughing up sputum on most days during at least 3 consecutive months for more than 2 successive years.[1] Some clinical surveys have added to the definition the occurrence of attacks of cough with sputum in the previous 2 years that have prevented the patient from working for a total of at least 3 weeks. If wheezing and bronchospasm occur with the disease, the designation *chronic* or *recurrent asthmatic bronchitis* (also *hyperactive airways disease*) may be used. Emphysema often complicates the clinical presentation. Although the precise diagnosis of emphysema is a morbid and anatomic one, its coexistence is usually inferred. The two diagnoses are usually lumped together and used to identify patients as having "chronic obstructive lung disease with bronchitis and emphysema."

ETIOLOGY AND PATHOLOGY

Three factors contributing to chronic bronchitis are of particular importance: cigarette smoking, infection, and inhalation of dust or fumes in the workplace environment. Chronic bronchitis is common and affects about 10–25 percent of the adult population. Bronchitis is more common in men than in women and more common after age 40 than before. Smoking, cigarette smoking in particular, is the most important factor associated with the disease. Related diseases that impair mucociliary transport in the lung may be important in susceptible people. The clinician must be alert for the possibility that recurrent respiratory infections and persistent chronic bronchitis might signal that the patient has a defect in pulmonary host defenses[2,3] or an immunodeficiency syndrome. This association may become evident in teenagers or young adults and not only in young children as generally expected. Investigation for cystic fibrosis, an intrinsic defect in the structure of epithelial cilia, immunoglobulin deficiency involving IgA or selective IgG subclasses,[4,5] and rarely abnormal polymorphonuclear (PMN) granulocyte function should be considered. Long-term, low-dose corticosteroid therapy in patients with asthma or with chronic bronchitis/emphysema can cause IgG subclass level deficiencies in serum, particularly IgG_1.[6]

Cigarette smoking is a significant airway irritant for most patients.[6a,b] Not all patients with chronic bronchitis, however, have a history of smoking; an average of 6–10 percent of nonsmoking men will have persistent cough and phlegm production. In light-to-moderate smokers (20 or fewer cigarettes per day), the frequency of chronic bronchitis is approximately 25 percent; for heavy smokers (greater than a 40–60 pack-year history) it increases to almost 50 percent. The frequency is less in ex-smokers. Investigators who have performed bronchoalveolar lavage to obtain respiratory cells from human lungs have uniformly found a tremendous increase in the recovery of alveolar macrophages from cigarette smokers as compared with nonsmokers.[7,8] "Normal" smokers usually yield a small percentage of inflammatory cells (PMN granulocytes) as well. A modest degree of smoking (2–5 pack-years) induces cellular and lavage fluid immunoglobulin changes similar to those found in heavy smokers. Postmortem examination of lungs obtained from young accident victims showed evidence of inflammation involving respiratory bronchioles in smokers but not in nonsmokers. The lesion consisted of clusters of pigmented macrophages in association with edema, fibrosis, and epithelial hyperplasia of the bronchiolar and alveolar walls.[9] Thus, cigarette users, even those who smoke minimally, initiate irritative stimuli that may insidiously culminate years later as chronic bronchitis and possibly other forms of degenerative lung diseases. The realization that cigarette smoke can inactivate the antiprotease function of α_1-antitrypsin in lung secretions further supports this sequence of destructive lung disease.[10,11]

One striking change noted in the lungs of patients with chronic bronchitis is the increase in the number of goblet (mucus-secreting) cells in the surface epithelium of major and smaller bronchi. Whereas goblet cells normally account for one-fourth of the epithelial cells lining the larger bronchi and are virtually absent from the smaller ones, particularly bronchioles,[12] in chronic bronchitis the epithelium may consist almost entirely of such cells. In addition, mucous glands in the walls of the larger bronchi undergo hypertrophy. Normally, the ratio of the mucous glands compared with the bronchial wall (the latter measured from the surface of the epithelium to the inner surface of the cartilaginous plates) is about 0.3, but with enlargement of the mucous glands, as found in chronic bronchitis, the ratio is greater and on the order of 0.6 (Reid index).[13] Besides mucous gland enlargement, people with chronic bronchitis have irritation of the airway mucosa and more mucus in their peripheral airways. The irritated airways respond by producing extra secretions, exposing sensitive stretch receptors (which aggravates cough) and making more neuropeptides, which promote bronchospasm. Inflammation of the mucosa causes swelling and edema, infiltration of PMN granulocytes in response to chemotaxins such as interleukin-8 produced by epithelial cells,[14] hyperplasia of goblet cells, and enlargement of bronchial mucous glands as observed in the pathology. Surprisingly, tracheal mucus produced by asymptomatic smokers is better hydrated and may have better mucociliary clearability than in nonsmokers.[15]

Explants of human airways (2–10 mm in diameter from the second- to fifth-generation bronchi) can be established and cultured for 2–3 days. Such explants contain normal-appearing mucosal surfaces and goblet cells and intact submucosal glands.[16] In this in vitro system, secretion of mucous glycoproteins can be stimulated with a variety of factors: histamine, various leukotrienes, IgE antibody, and methacholine. Products of mast cell degranulation and pharmacologic agents can enhance the output of mucous glycoproteins as well as neuropeptides. In addition, human blood monocytes and alveolar macrophages produce a mucus secretogog, after a phagocytic stimulus, that causes the release of mucous glycoprotein from cultured human airways.[17,18] This is more relevant now that airway macrophages are recognized and can be selectively characterized.[19]

CLINICAL PRESENTATION

Incessant cough marks most advanced bronchitics. Patients may clear their throats frequently, and, during conversation, an outburst of laughter or animated speech can precipitate a loud, raspy, coughing episode. Many patients expectorate sputum throughout the day, but most cough up the largest amount in the morning on arising. Sputum may be tenacious and sticky and vary in appearance from mucoid or whitish to yellowish green and obviously purulent. Many patients have associated nasal problems and often complain of a postnasal drip or sinus congestion. A bad taste in the mouth and halitosis are frequent complaints. Most patients with chronic bronchitis are not incapacitated by their respiratory disorder unless an acute infection or some other illness occurs.

As mentioned, emphysema is often present, and some patients with advanced chronic bronchitis have complications that are determined for the most part by the degree and type of associated emphysema. The use of descriptive terms to separate patients with chronic obstructive lung disease into groups such as *blue bloaters* (or type B) and *pink puffers* (or type A) is often an oversimplification.[20] However, the separation may be useful in understanding the clinical course of the patient with chronic bronchitis and recurrent respiratory infections.

The blue bloater is characterized by severe obstructive lung disease with serious and persistent blood gas abnormalities and an impaired air flow that is worse than predicated from the forced expiratory volume of the first second (FEV_1). Frequent tracheobronchial infections (bacterial and viral) occur and occasionally lead to bronchopneumonia. Dyspnea, although a prominent symptom, is less intense than in the pink puffer. As a consequence of the blood gas derangements, a number of associated features may follow. Somnolence and lethargy can develop. Pulmonary vasospasm induced by the combination of hypoxemia and respiratory acidosis increases pulmonary vascular resistance, which in turn increases the work load of the right ventricle of the heart. Cor pulmonale with peripheral edema and its other attendant consequences may occur. Patients often cough up copious amounts of sputum and do not show radiologic evidence of emphysema. These patients are thought primarily to be severe bronchitics with little evidence of emphysema. In contrast, pink puffers, despite severe airway obstruction, maintain relatively normal blood gases because of high minute ventilation. These patients, frequently underweight and barrel chested, do not appear cyanotic or plethoric and do not develop cor pulmonale except terminally. Radiologically, emphysema is present. These are considered patients with severe emphysema and little bronchitis. It is now apparent that the clinical distinction between these two syndromes is not clear-cut and that many patients (perhaps the majority) have features of both.

The bronchitic maintains normal body weight and tends to be obese. Normal vesicular breath sounds are diminished, and inspiratory and expiratory rales, rhonchi, and mild wheezing may be heard instead. The chest is noisy rather than quiet, as is observed with emphysema. If pulmonary artery pressure is elevated, cardiac signs may reflect it. With advanced bronchitis and emphysema, the patient may have acrocyanosis, plethoric complexion, and manifestations of overt heart failure. Digital clubbing is not a finding in the uncomplicated bronchitic.

Evidence of an Acute Infectious Exacerbation

Objective signs that bronchitis has worsened in temporal relationship to a documented infection are not always evident. Reliance is placed on the patients' observation that their sputum has changed in color and consistency or has increased in amount. In some patients the development of an increased amount of purulent sputum without eosinophil cells is presumptive evidence of infection. However, other patients consistently produce purulent sputum without other evidence of infection. Patients may note increasing cough and dyspnea, but during an acute illness most will not have symptoms suggesting systemic toxicity such as chills and fever, nor will they develop a blood leukocytosis. Patients often experience chest tightness and increased fatigue. As no uniform definition for an acute exacerbation of chronic bronchitis exists, it is difficult to determine just when one has occurred or ended.

Sputum Analysis

Cellular analysis[21,22] or a fresh sputum specimen (early morning sample) is necessary in the evaluation of every patient with chronic bronchitis. Continual bronchial irritation is indicated by the presence of many PMN granulocytes, even during quiescent periods of the disease. It is important to determine the number of eosinophils. Ciliated epithelial cells can be recognized, and their number correlates reasonably well with the degree of vigorous coughing that was needed to produce the sputum specimen. A few alveolar macrophages may be identified that in the cigarette smoker characteristically contain yellowish brown cytoplasmic inclusions. Gram stain will often show a mixture of gram-positive and gram-negative bacteria that is consistent with contamination by normal mouth flora or with tracheal colonization by species of *Haemophilus influenzae*, *Streptococcus pneumonia*, and *Moraxella (Branhamella) catarrhalis*.

The mucus secreted in chronic bronchitis contains various glycoproteins, mucopolysaccharide acids, and albumin. Small amounts of a number of immunoglobulin species are present, including secretory IgA, IgG, occasionally IgM and IgE, or proteolytic fragments derived from them. Other proteins present include transferrin, complement components, and enzyme inhibitors such as α_1-antiprotease. With high degrees of bronchial irritation and inflammation, any of the intravascular proteins may be identified in purulent mucus; however, the protein is likely to be fragmented or denatured because of the effect of pH or the action of lysosomal enzymes and other degradative substances in sputum.[23,24] Immunologic analysis of IgA in sputum may help in diagnosing the presence of infection in patients with a flare-up of chronic bronchitis. With active infection, the content of 75 IgA is increased, and free-secretory component is all used; without infection, 11S IgA is increased, and excess secretory component exists.[25]

Radiologic Evidence

Standard chest radiographic films contribute little to the definitive diagnosis of chronic bronchitis, but they serve the essential purpose of excluding other diseases that may mimic or contribute to chronic bronchitis. The chest film can appear normal in chronic bronchitis and may not undergo change during infectious exacerbations; therefore, it is not a very sensitive or helpful way of following most patients.

RELATIONSHIP OF INFECTION TO ACUTE EXACERBATIONS

The most enigmatic problem in chronic bronchitis is the role of bacterial infection.[26] Although its exact place is uncertain, bacterial infection does not appear to initiate the disease except possibly in the patient with a history of frequent childhood respiratory infections.[27] However, bacteria are probably significant in perpetuating the disease and may be critical in producing the characteristic exacerbations.

It is generally accepted that the bronchi of nonbronchitic patients who are free of other lung diseases are almost always sterile, although methods of culture are not perfect and may not exclude oral flora.[28–30] Pathogenic bacteria can be cultured from the bronchi in up to 82 percent of chronic bronchitic patients. Pathogenic organisms have also been cultured from the airways of nonbronchitics who have carcinoma of the lung or tuberculosis or after radiation to the lung. Thus, various forms of damage to the lung may predispose to bacterial infection. Routine sputum cultures from patients with chronic bronchitis commonly contain nonencapsulated *H. influenzae*, *S. pneumoniae*, and other oropharyngeal commensal flora. In most clinical series, one or both of these species is recovered from approximately 30–50 percent of the sputum specimens and rightfully can be considered as the baseline microbial flora as many patients with chronic bronchitis. *Moraxella catarrhalis* is also considered a potential pathogen and can be recovered in sputum as well.[26] Anaerobic bacteria could be recovered in only 17 percent of transtracheal aspirate specimens.[31] However, sputum carriage of *H. influenzae* and pneumococci does not seem to be of particular significance. These bacteria tend to persist in sputum during quiescent intervals, and the frequency of recovery is not greatly increased during infectious episodes. The development of purulent sputum is not correlated specifically with the presence of one or the other of these bacteria. However, evidence suggests that purulence is associated with a quantitative increase in the number of pneumococci cultured from sputum.[32] *Mycoplasma pneumoniae* does not seem to be of great importance, for some studies[32,33] attribute only 1–10 percent of acute infections to this organism. Respiratory illness produced by *Chlamydia pneumoniae* (TWAR) may be associated with a subacute form of bronchitis in which symptoms last for days or weeks.[34]

As mentioned, it is often impossible to judge when an acute infection has supervened, microbiologically as well as clinically. This is particularly true of patients who always experience symptoms of cough and produce sputum that is purulent. One study[32] that monitored infectious episodes on the basis of changes in monthly serum antibody titers to a large number of microorganisms indicated that infection could occur frequently without a clinical exacerbation of bronchitis. Of those viral infections documented to have occurred on the basis of significant changes in serum antibody titers, 40 percent were not associated with a clinical exacerbation. It has been suggested that some of the older studies that attempted to document infectious exacerbations by monitoring antibody responses should be reassessed using newer microbial antigens and techniques.[26]

The following statements generally summarize the relationship between causative agents[26,35] and acute flare-ups of infection in chronic bronchitis: (*1*) Chronic colonization of the airways and sputum with unencapsulated strains of *H. influenzae* and with pneumococci occurs in at least one-half of the affected patients. Microbiologically, it is difficult to incriminate one or both of these bacteria as the specific cause of an acute infection. However, many physicians usually attribute acute infectious exacerbations to one or the other, and antibiotic selection is often based on this probability. As noted, *M. catarrhalis* is also frequent. (*2*) Other bacteria such as hemolytic species of streptococci, *Staphylococcus aureus*, and gram-negative enteric bacilli are infrequent causes of acute infection in chronic bronchitis. Only 5–10 percent of the sputum specimens will contain significant numbers of these other bacteria. Since sputum may be contaminated by oropharyngeal flora, it is uncertain whether these bacteria originate in the lower airways. Other sampling methods such as transtracheal aspiration may be necessary to make this distinction.[31] (*3*) *Mycoplasma pneumoniae* infections can be sporadic and may be responsible for some acute exacerbations. (*4*) Viruses are frequent causes of acute infection. Fully 25–50 percent of acute exacerbations are related to these agents, including influenza, parainfluenza, respiratory syncytial virus, rhinovirus, and coronavirus. Viral infections are seasonal and occur more frequently in winter. (*5*) It is difficult to document the microbial cause of many respiratory infections with optimal methods of culture and conscientious diagnostic evaluation. For only 50 percent of acute pneumonia episodes in hospitalized patients was a specific etiology found.[36]

MANAGEMENT

General Considerations[36a,b]

Attempts should be made to have the patient stop smoking or at least reduce the amount of smoking. During the patient's initial evaluation, analysis of the cellular content of a sputum specimen is indicated; if eosinophils are among the inflammatory cells present, an allergic component to the illness should be investigated. Some asthmatics cough instead of wheeze, so it is not infrequent to encounter an asthmatic who has symptoms of chronic cough rather than audible wheezing.[37] Since excessive mucus secretion is common to both asthma and bronchitis, eosinophils in the sputum and in the peripheral blood can be a diagnostic clue. Initial pulmonary function tests to assess expiratory airflow should also include tests performed after the aerosol administration of a bronchodilator, unless a contraindication exists. It is useful to establish whether the patient has a reversible component of bronchospasm to the airway obstruction. Appropriate bronchodilator therapy may improve breathing and may improve exercise tolerance. Patients who develop wheezing during an acute infectious exacerbation may profit from a bronchodilator as well. Consultation with an ear, nose, and throat specialist and radiographic films of the sinuses may help to identify a deviated nasal septum, nasal polyps, or chronic sinusitis. A program of weight reduction and a suitable exercise regimen can be considered. Patients should receive a yearly immunization with the current influenza vaccine. Indications for the use of pneumococcal vaccine need individual consideration.[38,39]

The accumulation and clearance of secretions can be a real problem for some patients, and postural drainage maneuvers are indicated, especially during acute infections. The yield of secretions from postural drainage can sometimes be improved by the addition of two procedures: (1) the initial use of an aerosol bronchodilator to achieve maximum dilation and opening of the airways and then (2) humidification or wetting of respiratory secretions. Patients who are plagued with copious secretions and gain benefit from postural drainage should receive instruction in the technique from a qualified respiratory therapist. Other therapy aimed at liquifying respiratory secretions or controlling cough are not of particular value. Mucolytic agents designed to loosen and dissolve tenacious secretions are often irritative and actually may serve to increase mucus production. Cough-suppressant drugs are rarely indicated. The effect of sedatives contained in many preparations is generally not desirable, especially for patients with chronic obstructive lung disease. Cough is an efficient way of removing secretions. The use of an intermittent positive-pressure breathing device is rarely justified; if aerosol administration of medications is deemed necessary, a hand-held or motorized nebulizer will provide adequate drug distribution in the airways. A spacer compartment attached to the metered dose inhaler is often helpful for patients who have arthritis, incoordination, or visual problems that interfere with activation of the inhaler and taking optimal inspiratory breaths of the aerosol medication.

Spirometry and expiratory airflow values may not improve even though the patient has achieved a quiescent and "infection-free" stage. Actually, bronchiolar inflammation and airway resistance may have decreased, but the routine pulmonary tests are generally insensitive to this improvement.

Since most chronic bronchics continue to be cigarette smokers, they remain in a group that is statistically at increased risk to develop primary lung cancer. Early detection of cancer that is still localized provides the best hope for cure. Therefore, periodic sputum specimens for cytology and chest films can be justified.

Finally, the use of corticosteroid therapy should be mentioned. At some point the bronchitic patient will not rebound from an acute infection despite a vigorous and optimal treatment regimen that includes antibiotics and other ancillary drugs in maximal doses. In such a circumstance, a trial of corticosteroids may be indicated with moderate doses of the drug (e.g., 20–30 mg/day equivalent of prednisone). Current preference still favors the use of a systemically administered drug instead of a topical aerolized preparation. Because mucus plugging and diffuse areas of obstruction are present in the airways, a systemically absorbed steroid will achieve more even distribution throughout the lung tissue. The steroid effect is often not immediate, so a drug course of 3–6 weeks may be necessary. For many patients with chronic obstructive lung disease, a trial of corticosteroids and inhaled β_2-agonist drugs is worthwhile and may improve dyspnea and the FEV_1 value.[40] Moreover, the use of inhaled atropine can be helpful also, not only for bronchospasm but also to inhibit the formation of mucus and secretions.

Antimicrobial Therapy

Although prophylactic treatment with tetracycline decreased the number of exacerbations in patients who had many episodes, it did nothing for those who ordinarily had few exacerbations. Antibiotic treatment did not alter the rate of decline in pulmonary function.[41] However, prophylactic antibiotic therapy may have some usefulness in highly selected patients who experience frequent exacerbations (four or more per year). A number of oral antibiotics will suffice for prophylactic use or as treatment of an acute exacerbation and a selection is based on considerations of microbial sensitivity (or lack of such by secretion of inhibitors such as β-lactamases), patient tolerance, dosing interval, and cost. Because bacteria such as *H. influenzae* can inactivate β-lactam antibiotics by secreting β-lactamases, inhibitors such as clavulanate have been combined with amoxicillin. The use of such a combination is appropriate if β-lactamase–producing bacteria are causing infection. Several different strategies appear to be effective. Patients may receive antibiotics daily the winter months, 4 days per week during the winter or a 7-day course at the first sign of a "chest cold."

The effectiveness of the short-term use of antibiotics for acute exacerbations is difficult to assess.[26,32,33,42–44] Infection can cause acute decompensation and is the most common identifiable cause of death in these patients. The usual strategy is to institute a course of antimicrobial therapy for a 7- to 10-day period and hope that the acute flare-up subsides; an objective endpoint for success is usually lacking. The oral administration of antibiotics is sufficient for most of the acute bacterial flare-ups. Questions still exist about the overall benefit of antimicrobial therapy in exacerbations of chronic bronchitis, although they may improve symptoms and reduce disability. As initial choices, trimethoprim-sulfamethoxazole (160/800 mg bid po), amoxicillin (500 mg qid po) or amoxicillin/clavulanate (250/125 mg tid po), or erythromycin (250 mg qid or 500 mg bid po) can be used. Ampicillin, heretofore a mainstay antibiotic in this situation, is not active for some isolates of *H. influenzae* and for many isolates of *M. catarrhalis*. Trimethoprim-sulfamethoxazole may not inhibit a very few isolates of *S. pneumoniae* and *H. influenzae*, but on balance it is a very satisfactory drug for the bronchitis patient. Various oral cephalosporins (cefuroxime axetil, cefprozil) and newer macrolide antibiotics (azithromycin, clarithromycin) are available also and are often recommended because of their broad spectrum. They are usually not used as the first-line antibiotic in simple flare-ups of chronic bronchitis.

REFERENCES

1. Dantzker DR, Pingleton SK, Pierce JA, and other Task Force Members. Standards for the diagnosis and care of patients with chronic obstructive pulmonary disease and asthma—American Thoracic Society. Am Rev Respir Dis. 1987;136:225–44

2. Reynolds HY. Respiratory infections may reflect deficiencies in host defense mechanisms. Dis Mon. 1985;31:1–98.
3. Reynolds HY. Immunologic system in the respiratory tract. Physiol Rev. 1991; 71:1117–33.
4. Beck GS, Heiner DC. Selective immunoglobulin G4 deficiency and recurrent infections of the respiratory tract. Am Rev Respir Dis. 1981;124:94.
5. Reynolds HY. Immunoglobulin G and its function in the human respiratory tract. Mayo Clin Proc. 1988;63:161–74.
6. Klaustermeyer WB, Gianos ME, Kurohara ML, et al. IgG subclass deficiency associated with corticosteroids in obstructive lung disease. Chest. 1992;102: 1137–42.
6a. Linden M, Rasmussen JB, Piitulainen E, et al. Airway inflammation in smokers with nonobstructive and obstructive chronic bronchitis. Am Rev Respir Dis. 1993;148:1226–32.
6b. Thompson AB, Huerta G, Robbins RA, et al. The bronchitis index. A semiquantitative visual scale for the assessment of airways inflammation. Chest. 1993;103:1482–8.
7. Reynolds HY, Merrill WW. Airway changes in young smokers that may antedate chronic obstructive lung disease. Med Clin North Am. 1981;65:667–89.
8. Sibille Y, Reynolds HY. Macrophages and polymorphonuclear neutrophils in lung defense and injury—State of the art. Am Rev Respir Dis. 1990;141: 471–501.
9. Nieworehner DE, Kleinerman J, Rice DB. Pathologic changes in the peripheral airways of young cigarette smokers. N Engl J Med. 1974;291:755.
10. Gadek JE, Fellis GA, Crystal RG. Cigarette smoking induces functional antiprotease deficiency in the lower respiratory tract of humans. Science. 1979; 206:1315.
11. Crystal RG. Alpha 1-antitrypsin deficiency, emphysema, and liver disease. J Clin Invest. 1990;85:1343–52.
12. Gail DB, Lenfant CJM. Cells of the lung: biology and clinical implications. Am Rev Respir Dis. 1983;127:366–87.
13. Reid L. Measurement of the bronchial mucous gland layer: A diagnostic yardstick in chronic bronchitis. Thorax. 1960;15:132.
14. McElvaney NG, Nakamura H, Birrer P, et al. Modulation of airway inflammation in cystic fibrosis—in vitro suppression of interleukin-8 levels on the respiratory epithelial surface by aerosolization of recombinant secretory leukoprotease inhibitor. J Clin Invest. 1992;90:1296–301.
15. Rubin BK, Ramirez O, Zayas JG, et al. Respiratory mucus from asymptomatic smokers is better hydrated and more easily cleared by mucociliary action. Am Rev Respir Dis. 1992;145:545–7.
16. Marom Z, Shelhamer JH, Bach NK, et al. Slow-reacting substances (LTC$_4$ and LTD$_4$) increase the release of mucus from human airways in vitro. Am Rev Respir Dis. 1982;126:449–51.
17. Marom Z, Shelhamer JH, Kaliner M. Human pulmonary macrophage-derived mucus secretagogue. J Exp Med. 1984;159:884–60.
18. Marom Z, Shelhamer JH, Kaliner M. Human monocyte-derived mucus secretagogue. J Clin Invest. 1985;75:191–8.
19. Rankin JA, Marcy T, Rochester CL, et al. Human airway macrophages—A technique for their retrieval and a descriptive comparison with alveolar macrophages. Am Rev Respir Dis. 1992;145:928–33.
20. Burrows B, Niden AH, Fletcher CM, et al. Clinical types of chronic obstructive lung disease in London and Chicago. Am Rev Respir Dis. 1964;90:14.
21. Chodosh S. Examination of sputum cells. N Engl J Med. 1970;282:854.
22. Baigelman W, Chodosh S. Sputum "wet preps": Window on the airways. J Respir Dis. 1984;59–70.
23. Wiggins J, Hill SL, Stockley RA. The secretory IgA system of lung secretions in chronic obstructive bronchitis: Comparison of sputum with secretions obtained during fiberoptic bronchoscopy. Thorax. 1984;39:517–23.
24. Niederman MS, Merrill WW, Polomski LM, et al. Influence of sputum IgA and elastase on tracheal cell bacterial adherence. Am Rev Respir Dis. 1986; 133:255.
25. Stockley RA, Afford SC, Burnett D. Assessment of 7S and 11S immunoglobulin A in sputum. Am Rev Respir Dis. 1980;122:956.
26. Murphy TF, Sethi S. Bacterial infection in chronic obstructive pulmonary disease—State of the art. Am Rev Respir Dis. 1992;146:1067–83.
27. Leeder SR. Role of infection in the cause and course of chronic bronchitis and emphysema. J Infect Dis. 1975;131:731.
28. Laurenzi GG, Potter RT, Kass EH. Bacterial flora of the lower respiratory tract. N Engl J Med. 1961;265:1273.
29. Potter RT, Totman F, Fernandez R, et al. The bacteriology of the lower respiratory tract. Bronchoscopic study of 100 clinical cases. Am Rev Respir Dis. 1968;97:1051.
30. Halperin SA, Suratt PM, Gwaltney JM Jr, et al. Bacterial cultures of the lower respiratory tract in normal volunteers with and without experimental rhinovirus infection using a plugged double catheter system. Am Rev Respir Dis. 1982;125:678.
31. Hass H, Morris JF, Samson S, et al. Bacterial flora of the respiratory tract in chronic bronchitis. Comparison of transtracheal, fiber-bronchoscopic and oropharyngeal sampling methods. Am Rev Respir Dis. 1977;116:41.
32. Gump DW, Phillips CA, Forsyth BR, et al. Role of infection in chronic bronchitis. Am Rev Respir Dis. 1976;113:465.
33. Tager I, Speizer FE. Role of infection in chronic bronchitis. N Engl J Med. 1975;292:583.
34. Grayston JT. Infections caused by *Chlamydia pneumoniae* strain TWAR—State of the art clinical article. Clin Infect Dis. 1992;15:757–63.
35. Reynolds HY. Bacterial adherence to respiratory tract mucosa—a dynamic interaction leading to colonization. Semin Respir Infect. 1987;2:8–19.
36. Bates JH, Campbell GD, Barron AL, et al. Microbial etiology of acute pneumonia in hospitalized patients. Chest 1992;101:1005–12.

36a. Reynolds HY, Swisher JW. Preoperative management of chronic bronchitis. Infect Med. 1993;10:21–9.
36b. Griffith DE, Kronenberg RS. Chronic bronchitis. Choosing the optimal treatment. Postgraduate Medicine. 1993;9:8.
37. Corrao WM, Bramen SS, Irwin RS. Chronic cough as the sole presenting manifestation of bronchial asthma. N Engl J Med. 1979;300:633.
38. Centers for Disease Control and Prevention. Pneumococcal polysaccharide vaccine. MMWR 1989;38:64–76.
39. LaForce FM, Eickhoff TC. Pneumococcal vaccine: An emerging consensus. Ann Intern Med. 1988;108:757–9.
40. Mendella LA, Manfreda J, Warren CPW, et al. Steroid response in stable chronic obstructive lung disease. Ann Intern Med. 1982;96:17.
41. Fletcher CM, Oldham PD. Value of chemoprophylaxis and chemotherapy in early chronic bronchitis. A report to the medical research council by their working party on trials of chemotherapy in early chronic bronchitis. Br Med J. 1966;1:1317.
42. Nicotra MB, Rivera M, Awe RJ. Antibiotic therapy of acute exacerbations of chronic bronchitis. Ann Intern Med. 1982;97:18.
43. Bates JH. The role of infection during exacerbations of chronic bronchitis. Ann Intern Med. 1982;97:130.
44. Anthonisen NR, Manfreda J, Warren CPW, et al. Antibiotic therapy in exacerbations of chronic obstructive pulmonary disease. Ann Intern Med. 1987;106: 196.

BIBLIOGRAPHY

Cherniack NS, ed. Chronic Obstructive Pulmonary Disease. Philadelphia: WB Saunders; 1991.

49. BRONCHIOLITIS

CAROLINE BREESE HALL
WILLIAM J. HALL

In bronchiolitis we must now contend
  with both the disease of the "now" and the "then";
For many such infants a mold has been cast,
  perhaps by their unborn and unknown past,
  which destines that they shall in time wheeze again.
For them this disease
  is the distant, boding knell
Of vulnerable lungs
  to a microbe's mystic spell.

                                                    C.B.H.

Bronciolitis is an acute viral lower respiratory tract illness occurring within the first 2 years of life. The characteristic clinical findings include an acute onset of wheezing and hyperaeration, most commonly associated with cough, rhinorrhea, tachypnea, and respiratory distress. The term *bronchiolitis* appears to have been born from a long lineage of confusing sobriquets, including *acute catarrhal bronchitis*, *interstitial bronchopneumonia*, *spastic bronchopneumonia*, *capillary* or *obstructive bronchiolitis*, and *asthmatic bronchiolitis*.[1] Bronchiolitis, however, did not become recognized as a separate entity until the 1940s.[2]

ETIOLOGY

Although bronchiolitis was initially thought to be caused by bacteria, viruses and occasionally *Mycoplasma pneumoniae* are now known to be the instigators. Respiratory syncytial virus

TABLE 1. Agents Causing Bronchiolitis

Agent	Cases (%)	Epidemiology
Respiratory syncytial virus	45–75	Yearly epidemics winter to spring
Parainfluenza viruses		
Type 3	8–15	Predominantly spring to fall
Type 1	5–12	Epidemics in the fall every other year
Type 2	1–5	Fall
Rhinoviruses	3–8	Endemic, all seasons
Adenoviruses	3–10	Endemic, all seasons
Influenza viruses	5–8	Epidemic, winter to spring
Mycoplasma pneumoniae	1–7	Endemic, all seasons
Enteroviruses	1–5	Summer to fall

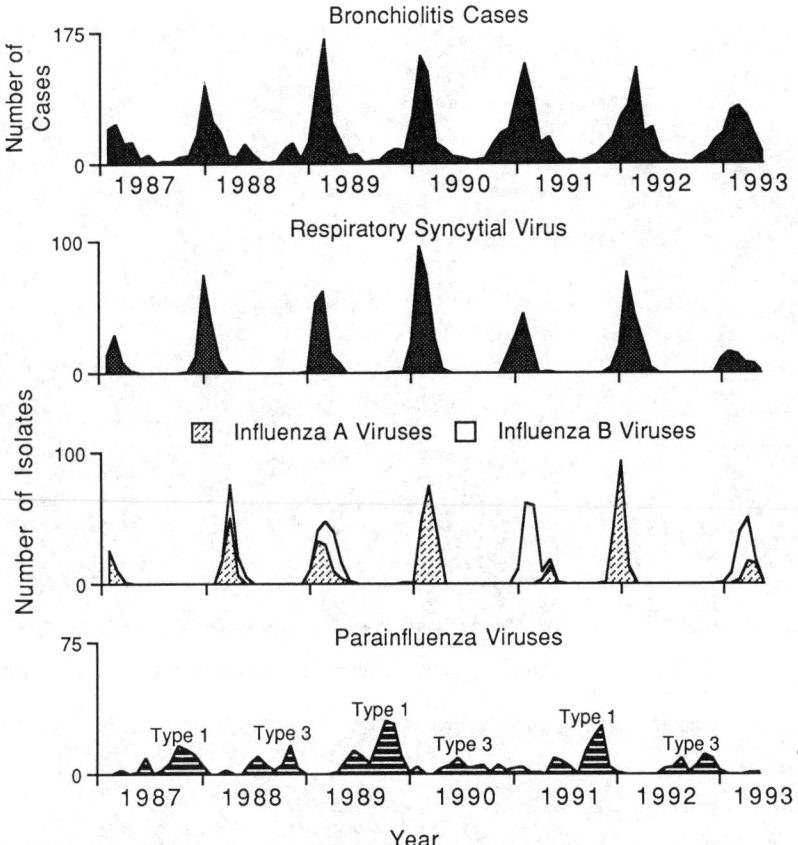

FIG. 1. Patterns of reported cases of bronchiolitis shown in relation to the activity of the major respiratory viruses in Monroe County, New York. Data were obtained from a weekly community surveillance program for infectious diseases.

(RSV) is clearly the major cause, the parainfluenza viruses being the second most commonly isolated agents (Table 1, Fig. 1).[3–12] A long-term study of respiratory illnesses associated with wheezing in children from a private practice in Chapel Hill, North Carolina, showed that RSV, parainfluenza viruses types 1 and 3, adenoviruses, rhinoviruses, and *M. pneumoniae* make up 87 percent of the isolates obtained from children of all ages.[3] Within the first 2 years of life, RSV accounted for 44 percent of the isolates, with the parainfluenza viruses types 1 and 3 and adenoviruses each accounting for about 13 percent. Similarly, RSV has comprised 55 percent of the isolates obtained from children with bronchiolitis from two group practices in Rochester, New York, over a 6-year period.[13] The second most frequently identified agent was parainfluenza type 3, accounting for 11 percent of the cases. The proportion of these agents may change, depending on the population and whether the cases occur as part of an epidemic. In hospitalized cases, the contribution of RSV is even higher, as demonstrated by the Newcastle-upon-Tyne studies in which 74 percent of the infants hospitalized with bronchiolitis had infection with this agent.[10]

EPIDEMIOLOGY

Bronchiolitis shows a definite seasonal pattern in temperate climates, with a yearly upsurge of cases in winter to early spring.[3,7–10,13,14] This pattern mirrors that of its prime agent, RSV. Lesser swells of activity are seen during the fall and spring, when the parainfluenza viruses are active.

Bronchiolitis is a common illness during the first year of life, with the peak attack rate occurring between 2 and 10 months of age.[3,5,10,12,14–17] In the Chapel Hill studies, the incidence of bronchiolitis was about 11 cases per hundred children for both the first and second 6 months of life.[3,14] In the second year of life the incidence fell to approximately one-half. A much higher

incidence, however, has been reported[17] in long-term studies of children in a day care center who were examined regularly. Since even the mildest cases were detected, the rate rose to 115 cases per 100 children aged 6 months or less per year. By the second year of life this rate had declined to 32 cases per 100 children per year.

An appreciable proportion of hospital admissions for infants within the first year of life are caused by bronchiolitis, especially those resulting from RSV. In the review by Breese et al.[18] of their group practice, 4 percent of their patients of all ages requiring hospitalization for medical illnesses were bronchiolitis cases. In the Seattle prepaid medical care group, the rate of infants hospitalized with bronchiolitis during the first 6 months of life was 6 per 1000 children per year.[5] Bronchiolitis is more common in boys, especially in those requiring hospitalization, with a ratio of about 1.5 to 1.[3,16,19]

A number of factors in addition to male sex have been described as risk factors for more severe illness and for hospitalization.[3,12,16,17,20–24] Among these are young age of the infants, especially the first several months of life, as well as young maternal age, living in crowded and polluted surroundings, the number of siblings, lack of breast-feeding, an atopic predisposition, and the illness being caused by RSV.

PATHOPHYSIOLOGY

The term *bronchiolitis* was first used by Engle and Newns[2] in 1940 for the lower respiratory tract disease they observed in young infants which tended to be severe, often fatal, and probably viral. They carefully described the pathologic findings in these infants dying of bronchiolitis, which over the subsequent half century have been confirmed and expanded.[1,25–29]

The pathology of bronchiolitis is characteristically focused on the respiratory epithelium. The virus initially replicates in the

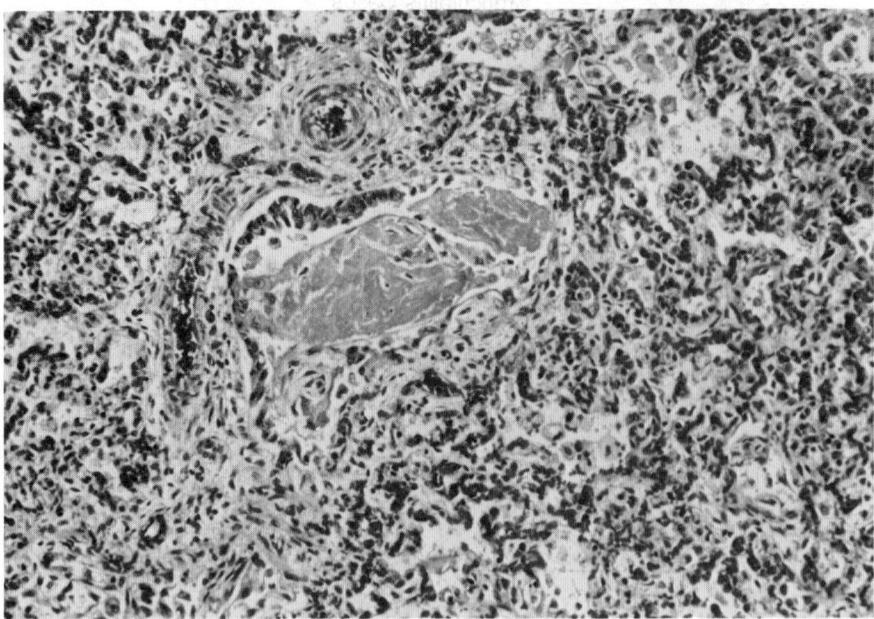

FIG. 2. Inflammation and necrosis in bronchiolitis resulting in obliteration of the bronchiolar lumen.

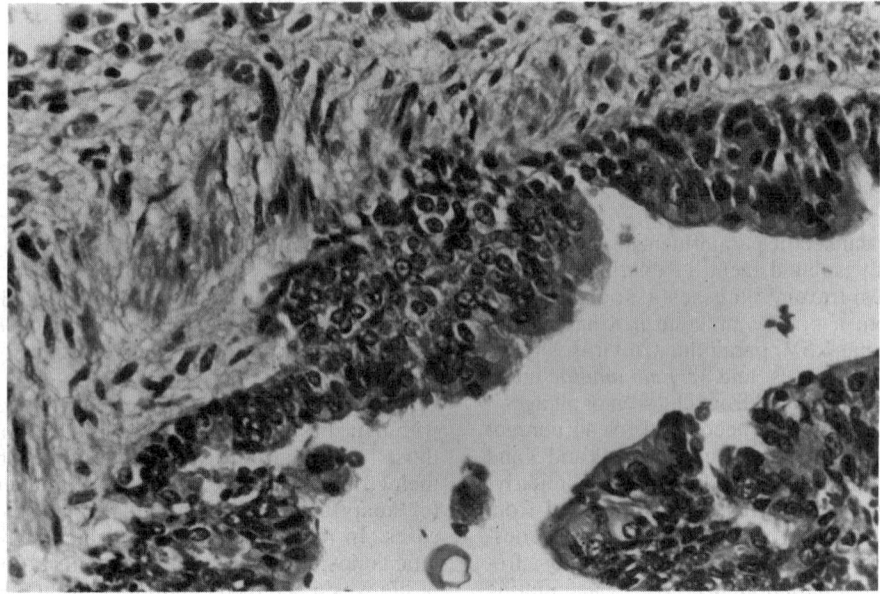

FIG. 3. Inflammation of the bronchiole with regenerating epithelium.

epithelium of the upper respiratory tract, but in the young infant it tends to spread rapidly to the lower tract airways. Early inflammation of the bronchial and bronchiolar epithelium progresses rapidly to necrosis. Subsequently, the epithelium may proliferate and demonstrate cuboidal cells without cilia. Peribronchiolar infiltration, mostly with mononuclear cells, and edema of the submucosa and adventitia are observed. Necrosis of the bronchiolar epithelium and sloughing subsequently result (Figs. 2 and 3).

The pathologic findings of viral bronchiolitis are also characteristically generalized. Inflammatory changes are observed in most small bronchi and bronchioles, but of varying severity. Since resistance to the flow of air is related inversely to the cube of the radius, this inflammation and edema make the small lumens of an infant particularly vulnerable to obstruction. Plugs of necrotic material and fibrin may obstruct completely or partially the small airways.

Smooth muscle constriction does not appear to be important in the obstruction.[28] In areas peripheral to sites of partial obstruction, air becomes trapped by a process similar to a "ball-valve" mechanism. The negative intrapleural pressure exerted during inspiration allows air to flow beyond the point of partial obstruction. However, on expiration, the size of the lumen decreases with the positive pressure, thereby resulting in increased obstruction and hyperinflation. Thus, although airflow is impeded during both inspiration and expiration, the latter is more affected and prolonged. In areas peripheral to complete obstruction, the trapped air eventually becomes absorbed, which results in multiple areas of total atelectasis. The degree of atelectasis or hyperinflation that develops is related to the amount of collateral ventilation present.

The physiologic correlates of this resistance to air flow are dyspnea, tachypnea, and a diminished tidal volume. The distribution of ventilation within the infant's lung also is altered markedly. The low ratio of ventilation perfusion of the lung parenchyma produces arterial hypoxemia. With progression of the disease, hypercarbia may ensue. The pathologic process may progress to involve the alveolar walls and spaces and produce an interstitial pneumonitis. Recovery tends to be slow, requiring several weeks.

An abnormal immune response may contribute to the pathogenesis of bronchiolitis and to the subsequent hyperreactivity of the airways that has been noted so frequently in children who have had bronchiolitis, particularly those who required hospitalization. Roles for IgE and histamine, as well as an abnormal cellular response, have been suggested in the development of bronchiolitis with both RSV and parainfluenza viral infections by Welliver and colleagues.[30-33] In infants with lower respiratory tract disease due to RSV, this group found that IgE antibody to RSV and histamine were present in the nasopharyngeal secretions more frequently and in higher titers in those infants who manifest wheezing as part of their lower respiratory tract disease.[30,31] Furthermore, the amount of specific IgE antibody and histamine in the secretions correlated with the severity of illness as determined by the degree of hypoxemia. However, not all infants with wheezing during the acute illness or with subsequent recurrent wheezing developed specific IgE antibody to RSV.[34] Infants with RSV-induced wheezing also tended to demonstrate higher degrees of whole-blood lymphocyte transformation to RSV,[32] and the number of suppressor cells (OKT8 antigen-positive cells) were observed to be diminished in infants convalescing from bronchiolitis and correlated with higher titers of specific IgE antibody in their secretions.[31] In infants with lower respiratory tract disease from one of the parainfluenza viruses, similar correlations have been made between illness manifested by wheezing and increased titers of virus-specific IgE antibody in the secretions an an increased lymphocyte transformation response to parainfluenza virus.[33]

Other mediators that are known to play a role in inflammation of the airway and bronchospasm have also been detected in the secretions of infants with bronchiolitis. Leukotriene C_4 has also been shown to be present in the respiratory secretions of children with wheezing and in higher titers in those children with proven viral infection.[35] In children with proven RSV infection, leukotriene C_4 has appeared in maximal concentrations during the first 3–8 days of illness and was present most frequently in those with RSV bronchiolitis and in those who developed IgE antibody to RSV.[36] Eosinophil cationic protein (ECP), a cytotoxic protein contained in the granules of eosinophils and implicated in the pathogenesis of asthma, similarly has been implicated in the development of bronchiolitis.[37] In children with RSV infection, high levels of ECP predicted the development of bronchiolitis and correlated with more severe illness.

These studies suggest that the development of wheezing in an infant with viral, especially RSV, lower respiratory tract disease may result from or be augmented by an impaired suppression of the cell-mediated immune response. Exaggerated production of IgE antibody and other cellular responses that evoke the mediators of airway inflammation and bronchospasm may then follow.[31,38] These findings also may help to explain the high rate of persistent hyperreactivity of the airway and recurrent episodes of bronchospasm in children who have had bronchiolitis.

CLINICAL MANIFESTATIONS

Upper respiratory tract signs, especially coryza and cough, usually herald the onset of bronchiolitis. During a prodromal period of 1–7 days fever, usually mild, is common. Lower respiratory tract involvement most frequently appears 2–3 days from the onset of the illness. The progression of the disease initially may be reflected in the development of a prominent cough and subsequently by an increase in the respiratory rate and in nonspecific systemic symptoms such as irritability, lethargy, and anorexia. With progression, the tachypnea and tachycardia may be

marked, although fever may no longer be present. Retractions of the chest walls, flaring of the nasal alae, and grunting are evidence of the increased work of breathing. Cyanosis rarely is evident, even though moderate to severe hypoxemia may be present.[28,39] Auscultatory findings, which may vary from hour to hour, demonstrate wheezing with or without crackles. Increasing dyspnea with decreasing auscultatory findings and movement of air may indicate progressive obstruction and impending respiratory failure.

A recent study of 21 infants with acute bronchiolitis, 18 caused by RSV and 3 caused by parainfluenza virus, demonstrated that bronchiolitis may result in significant cardiovascular effects in infants without underlying cardiac or pulmonary disease.[40] During the acute phase of the illness, the 21 infants were evaluated by cross-sectional and Doppler echocardiography, and 11 had tricuspid valve regurgitation, usually accompanied by increased pulmonary artery systolic pressure. The frequency of these findings correlated with the clinical severity of the bronchiolitis. Subsequent serial evaluation indicated that these abnormalities disappeared as the infants recovered.

Dehydration is a common accompaniment of bronchiolitis, resulting from paroxysms of coughing that may trigger vomiting and from a poor oral intake related to the respiratory distress and lethargy. The tachypnea further increases the fluid requirement. Otitis media, occurring in 10–30 percent of infants, mild conjunctivitis, and occasionally diarrhea may also be present.

For most infants, the acute course lasts 3–7 days. Most show improvement within 3–4 days, with a gradual recovery period of 1–2 weeks, but in some it may be prolonged.[39,41]

LABORATORY FINDINGS

The total white blood cell count is usually within the normal range or slightly elevated.[41,42] In hospitalized infants, however, who are more seriously ill and hypoxemic, the white blood cell count may be elevated, and the differential may show a left shift.[39,42] Almost all hospitalized infants with bronchiolitis are hypoxemic, but the degree of hypoxemia is difficult to assess clinically.[39] The degree of wheezing and retractions cannot be assumed to be indicative of the level of oxygenation. An inverse correlation, however, appears to exist between the respiratory rate and the arterial oxygen saturation.[39,43] Only the most severely ill children develop hypercarbia, as most are able to compensate for the increased work of breathing with an elevated respiratory rate.[39,43,44]

The hallmark of the chest roentgenogram in acute bronchiolitis is the characteristic hyperinflation with the associated depressed diaphragms, hyperlucency of the parenchyma, and decreased costophrenic angles.[45-51] The bronchovascular markings are usually prominent, with linear densities radiating out from the hila. Multiple areas of atelectasis of varying degrees also are commonly present and are difficult to differentiate from the infiltrates of pneumonia. Indeed, both bronchiolitis and pneumonia frequently are present, especially with RSV infection.

The abnormalities observed on the chest roentgenogram in acute bronchiolitis often do not correlate with the degree of clinical illness. The child may be severely ill despite minimal findings on the chest roentgenogram.

DIAGNOSIS

The diagnosis of bronchiolitis is made most frequently on the basis of the characteristic clinical and epidemiologic findings. However, considerable confusion exists over the exact definition of bronchiolitis.[29,52,53] A variety of entities may cause a similar picture of dyspnea and wheezing in the infant. Asthma is not easily differentiated, particularly if it is the infant's first episode. Furthermore, the two diseases may be combined. An appreciable proportion of wheezing episodes occurring in a child with an atopic diathesis may arise from viral infections.[54] Respiratory syncytial virus in particular has a propensity to induce wheezing in young children. Even in adults with acute RSV infection clinically manifested as an upper respiratory tract infection, hyperreactivity of the airways may be detected by pulmonary function testing and may last for 1–2 months.[55] Children who first wheeze during an epidemic of RSV infection, therefore, may be less likely to have an atopic predisposition than do children who develop bronchiolitis during nonepidemic periods.[56]

The differential diagnosis of wheezing in an infant is broad and requires a careful history and examination.[53] Gastric reflux and aspiration may produce a picture that is indistinguishable clinically from acute bronchiolitis. Other considerations include obstruction of the airway from a foreign body, vascular rings, retropharyngeal abscess, and even enlarged adenoids. Wheezing may also be associated with cystic fibrosis, immunodeficiency, and congestive heart failure in young infants.

A specific diagnosis of the agent of acute bronchiolitis can be made in an appreciable proportion of infants by viral isolation from respiratory secretions, preferably from a nasal wash.[3,5–10,57] In most cases the viruses associated with bronchiolitis can be identified in tissue culture within 3–7 days. Newer rapid viral diagnostic techniques are available, especially for RSV, that allow identification of the viral antigen in the respiratory secretions within hours to 1 day.[58–61] Serologic determination of the etiologic agent is rarely helpful. Antibody determinations in convalescent serum specimens provide information too late to be of help in clinical management. Also, maternally acquired antibody to many of the viral agents of bronchiolitis will be present in the sera of infants and will confound interpretation of antibody tests.

THERAPY

Over two decades ago Reynolds and Cook[62] noted that "oxygen is vitally important in bronchiolitis, and there is little convincing evidence that any therapy is consistently or even occasionally useful." Today the mainstay of therapy for the hospitalized child remains oxygen administration with careful supportive care.[1] Although mist therapy is also commonly employed, its use has not been proved beneficial and chest physiotherapy has been shown to be of no help.[63]

A variable, but sometimes high, proportion of hospitalized infants, especially those with RSV infection, may require mechanical ventilation.[64,65] This often requires high tidal volumes with high peak inspiratory pressures and low respiratory rates to achieve a high minute ventilation.[64] Even though infants with bronchiolitis generally have hyperexpanded lungs, most benefit from positive end-expiratory pressure.

Specific therapy is available for bronchiolitis caused by RSV with ribavirin (1-β-D-ribafuranysol-1,2,4-triazole-3-carboxamide), a synthetic nucleoside.[66] This broad-spectrum antiviral agent has been approved only for infants hospitalized with RSV infections and is administered as a small particle aerosol for 12–20 hours each day, usually for 2–5 days.[66–73] Shorter or intermittent periods of administration may be as beneficial, especially since very high levels of drug are achieved in the respiratory secretions by aerosol administration.[74,75] In all of the controlled studies thus far reported, clinical benefit has been demonstrated, with a faster rate of improvement in severity of illness and in arterial blood gases, and without evidence of toxicity.[66–73] The aerosolized drug does not appear to aggravate wheezing or airway hyperreactivity in these infants, as evidenced by improvement in arterial blood gases and by serial pulmonary function testing, including carbachol challenge, of RSV-infected volunteers treated with ribavirin.[70]

Bronchodilator therapy for infants with bronchiolitis is controversial. In most young infants the major cause of the airway obstruction is the inflammation caused by the viral infection,

rather than smooth muscle contraction, but hyperreactive airways may compound the obstruction.[1,28,76] Studies evaluating bronchodilators administered in a variety of routes have given conflicting results. The majority of studies have not shown benefit in clinical signs and in pulmonary function.[77–83] Several studies evaluating nebulized salbutamol have demonstrated a paradoxical, detrimental response.[84–86] Other studies, mostly using nebulized bronchodilators, have indicated improvement.[28,87–90] Therapy with a combination of α- and β-receptor agonists has been suggested as giving a more beneficial response.[1,91] A trial of aerosolized or parenteral bronchodilators, therefore, has been recommended by some for those infants who require hospitalization and who can be carefully monitored.[76,87,92]

Several studies have evaluated the use of steroids in bronchiolitis in terms of clinical response and lung function and have shown no benefit during the acute phase of the bronchiolitis or in the subsequent outcome.[93–97] The Committee of Drugs of American Academy of Pediatrics has thus advised against the use of corticosteroid therapy in bronchiolitis. However, studies have shown a beneficial effect of nebulized beclomethasone dipropionate on the recurrent episodes of wheezing occurring after acute bronchiolitis.[98–100]

Antibiotics should not be administered routinely to infants with bronchiolitis, since bacteria have no role in the etiology. Furthermore, secondary bacterial infection rarely is observed after bronchiolitis.[101]

COMPLICATIONS

A number of studies have attempted to predict the epidemiologic and clinical characteristics of children with acute bronchiolitis who are most likely to have complicated or severe courses. Infants with underlying diseases, especially cardiac, pulmonary, and immunodeficiency diseases, and those who were premature are most at risk for prolonged or complicated illnesses.[21,22,28,64,102,103] Clinical characteristics at the onset of the acute illness such as respiratory rate or auscultatory finding have not been of consistent prognostic value, but the arterial oxygen saturation has been associated with complicated illness.[103,104] With the currently available technical and pharmacologic methods of management, the mortality from bronchiolitis is very low. Respiratory failure and prolonged hypoxemia are most likely to occur in infants with compromising underlying conditions and in very young infants.[39,105] Apnea is a relatively common complication of bronchiolitis, especially in very young infants with RSV infection.[39,106–108]

The long-term effects of bronchiolitis on the immature and developing lung have not been clarified entirely.[28,109] However, infants who have been hospitalized with bronchiolitis appear to be at risk for recurrent wheezing and long-term pulmonary function abnormalities.[80,110–117]

Some studies have shown that as many as 75% of infants hospitalized with acute bronchiolitis will have recurrent episodes of bronchospasm within the first 2 years after discharge.[80] However, over subsequent years, the rate of children with continued clinical episodes of bronchospasm tends to diminish.[115,117,118] Children who had milder bronchiolitis not requiring hospitalization do not have the same degree of risk.[110,119,120] Functional abnormalities of the small airways in some studies persist for years, but may be clinically silent. The pathogenesis of these long-term effects is not clear, and the relative roles of the direct effect of the virus on the lung during its critical stages of development and pre-existing host factors is controversial.[1,110,121,122] A genetic predisposition may play an important role resulting in smaller airways, an atopic diathesis, or hyperreactivity of the airways to viral infections, as well as to other stimuli.[122–126]

BRONCHIOLITIS OBLITERANS

Rarely a chronic type of bronchiolitis, bronchiolitis obliterans, has been reported in both adults and children. In adults, bronchiolitis obliterans has most recently been reported as a complication, often severe, of heart-lung and bone marrow transplantation.[127-129] This unusual disease has also been noted in association with collagen vascular diseases.[130,131] In infants and young children, bronchiolitis obliterans may also complicate transplantation, but it primarily occurs as a rare, frequently devastating sequelae of acute viral bronchiolitis. The major association has been with adenovirus in infants with a certain undefined genetic predisposition.[127,132-134] The disease has appeared to be particularly prevalent in Indian populations in central Canada and in Polynesians in New Zealand.[127,132-134] Such infants commonly have bronchopneumonia along with signs of bronchiolitis that continue for weeks to months with fluctuating severity. Approximately 60 percent of these children develop chronic disease with atelectasis, bronchiectasis, intermittent pneumonia, and hyperinflation. These sequelae are accompanied by severe pathologic abnormalities involving the occlusion and destruction of the bronchi and bronchioles.

REFERENCES

1. Wohl MEB. Bronchiolitis. In: Chernick V, Kendig EL Jr, eds. Kendig's Disorders of the Respiratory Tract in Children. 5th ed. Philadelphia: WB Saunders; 1990:360–70.
2. Engle S, Newns GH. Proliferative mural bronchiolitis. Arch Dis Child. 1940; 15:219–29.
3. Henderson FW, Clyde WA Jr, Collier AM, Denny FW. The etiologic and epidemiologic spectrum of bronchiolitis in pediatric practice. J Pediatr. 1979; 95:183–90.
4. Chanock R, Chambon L, Chang W, et al. WHO respiratory disease survey in children. A serologic study. Bull WHO. 1967;37:363–9.
5. Foy HM, Cooney MK, Maletzky AJ, et al. Incidence and etiology of pneumonia, croup and bronchiolitis in preschool children belonging to a prepaid medical care group over a four year period. Am J Epidemiol. 1973;97:80–92.
6. Glezen WP, Loda FA, Clyde WA Jr, et al. Epidemiologic patterns of acute lower respiratory tract disease of children in a pediatric group practice. J Pediatr. 1971;79:397–406.
7. Kim HW, Arrobio JO, Brandt CD, et al. Epidemiology of respiratory syncytial virus infection in Washington, D.C. I. Importance of the virus in different respiratory disease syndromes and temporal distribution of infection. Am J. Epidemiol. 1973;98:216–225.
8. Loda FA, Glezen WP, Clyde WA Jr. Respiratory disease in group day care. Pediatrics. 1972;49:428–37.
9. Macasaet FF, Kidd PA, Bolano CR, et al. The etiology of acute respiratory infections. II. The role of viruses and bacteria. J. Pediatr. 1968;72:829–39.
10. Gardner PS. How etiologic, pathologic, and clinical diagnosis can be made in a correlated fashion. Pediatr Res. 1977;11:254–61.
11. Chang T-C, Wang C-L, Han H-L: Etiologic and clinical investigation of bronchiolitis. Chin Med J 1978;4:135–41.
12. Everard ML, Milner AD. The respiratory syncytial virus and its role in acute bronchiolitis. Eur J Pediatr. 1992;151:638–51.
13. Hall CB. Infect Dis Newslett. 1982;29:1, 1983;31:1.
14. Denny FW, Clyde WA Jr. Acute lower respiratory tract infections in non-hospitalized children. J Pediatr. 1986;108:635–46.
15. Glezen WP. Pathogenesis of bronchiolitis: Epidemiologic considerations. Pediatr Res. 1977;11:239–43.
16. Parrott RH, Kim HW, Arrobio JO, et al. Epidemiology of respiratory syncytial virus infection in Washington, D.C. II. Infection and disease with respect to age, immunologic status, race and sex. Am J Epidemiol. 1973;98:289–300.
17. Denny FW, Collier AM, Henderson FW, Clyde WA Jr. The epidemiology of bronchiolitis. Pediatr Res. 1977;11:234–6.
18. Breese BB, Disney FA, Talpey W. The nature of a small pediatric group practice. Part I. Pediatrics. 1966;38:264–77.
19. Kravits H. Sex distribution of hospitalized children with acute respiratory diseases, gastroenteritis and meningitis. Clin Pediatr. 1965;4:484–91.
20. Report to the Medical Research Council Subcommittee on Respiratory Syncytial Virus. Respiratory syncytial virus infection: Admission to hospital in industry urban and rural areas. Br Med J. 1978;2:796–8.
21. Carlsen K-H, Larsen S, Bjerve O, Leegaard J. Acute bronchiolitis: Predisposing factors and characterization of infants at risk. Pediatr Pulmonol. 1987; 3:153–60.
22. Holberg CJ, Wright AL, Martinez FD, et al. Risk factors for respiratory syncytial virus–associated lower respiratory illnesses in the first year of life. Am J Epidemiol. 1991;133:1135–51.
23. Simpson H, Matthew DJ, Inglis JM, George EL. Virological findings and blood gas tensions in acute lower respiratory tract infections in children. Br Med J. 1974;2:629–632.
24. Martinez FD, Wright AL, Holberg CJ, et al. Maternal age as a risk factor for wheezing lower respiratory illnesses in the first year of life. Am J Epidemiol. 1992;136:1258–68.
25. Aherne W, Bird T, Court SDM, et al. Pathological changes in virus infections of the lower respiratory tract in children. J Clin Pathol. 1970;23:7–18.
26. McLean KH. The pathology of bronchiolitis. A study of its evolution. I. The exudative phase. Aust Ann Med. 1956;5:254.
27. McLean KH. The pathology of bronchiolitis. A study of its evolution. II. The repair phase. Aust Ann Med. 1957;6:29.
28. Wohl MEB. Bronchiolitis. Pediatr Ann. 1986;15:307–13.
29. Price JF. Acute and long-term effects of viral bronchiolitis in infancy. Lung 1990;168(Suppl):414–21.
30. Welliver RC, Wong DT, Sun M, et al. The development of respiratory syncytial virus specific IgE and the release of histamine in nasopharyngeal secretions after infection. N Engl J Med. 1981;305:841–6.
31. Welliver RC, Kaul TN, Sun M, et al. Defective regulation of immune responses in respiratory syncytial virus infection. J Immunol. 1984;133: 1925–30.
32. Welliver RC, Kaul A, Ogra PL: Cell-mediated immune response to respiratory syncytial virus infection: Relationship to the development of reactive airway disease. J Pediatr. 1979;94:370–5.
33. Welliver RC, Wong DT, Sun M, McCarthy N. Parainfluenza virus bronchiolitis: Epidemiology and pathogenesis. Am J Dis Child. 1986;14:34–40.
34. Welliver RC, Sun M, Rinaldo D, Ogra PL. Predictive value of respiratory syncytial virus specific IgE responses for recurrent wheezing following bronchiolitis. J Pediatr. 1986;109:776–80.
35. Volovitz B, Faden H, Ogra PL. Release of leukotriene C$_4$ in respiratory tract during acute viral infection. J Pediatr. 1988;112:218–22.
36. Volovitz B, Welliver RC, de Castro G, et al. The release of leukotrienes in the respiratory tract during infection with respiratory syncytial virus: Role in obstructive airway disease. Pediatr Res. 1988;24:504–7.
37. Garofalo R, Kimpen JLL, Welliver RC, Ogra PL: Eosinophil degranulation in the respiratory tract during naturally acquired respiratory syncytial virus infection. J Pediatr. 1992;120:28–32.
38. Welliver RC, Ogra PL. Immunology of respiratory viral infections. Annu Rev Med. 1988;39:147–62.
39. Hall CB, Hall WJ, Speers DM. Clinical and physiologic manifestations of bronchiolitis and pneumonia. Am J Dis Child. 1979;133:798–802.
40. Sreeram N, Watson JG, Hunter S. Cardiovascular effects of acute bronchiolitis. Acta Paediatr Scand. 1991;80:133–6.
41. Ackerman BD: Acute bronchiolitis: A study of 207 cases. Clin Pediatr. 1962; 1:75–81.
42. Portnoy B, Haynes B, Salvatore MA, et al. The peripheral white blood count in respirovirus infection. J Pediatr. 1966;68:181–8.
43. Reynolds EOR. Arterial blood gas tensions of babies with bronchiolitis. Br Med J. 1963;1:1192–5.
44. Downes JJ, Wood DW, Striker TW, et al. Acute respiratory failure in infants with bronchiolitis. Anesthesiology. 1968;29:426–34.
45. Simpson W, Hacking PM, Court SDM, Gardner PS. The radiological findings in respiratory syncytial virus infection in children. Pediatr Radiol. 1974;2: 97–100.
46. Simpson W, Hacking PM, Court SDM, Gardner PS. The radiological findings in respiratory syncytial virus infection in children. Part II. The correlation of radiological categories with clinical and virological findings. Pediatr Radiol. 1974;2:155–60.
47. Rice RP, Loda F. A roentgenographic analysis of respiratory syncytial virus pneumonia in infants. Radiology. 1966;87:1021–7.
48. Koch DA. Roentgenologic considerations of capillary bronchiolitis. Am J Roentgenol Rad Ther Nucl Med. 1959;82:433–6.
49. Khamapirad T, Glezen WP. Clinical and radiographic assessment of acute lower respiratory tract disease in infants and children. Semin Respir Infect. 1987;2:130–44.
50. Wildin SR, Chonmaitree T, Swischuk LE. Roentgenographic features of common pediatric viral respiratory tract infections. Am J Dis Child. 1988; 142:43–6.
51. Friis B, Eiken M, Hornsleth A, Jensen A. Chest x-ray appearances in pneumonia and bronchiolitis. Acta Paediatr Scand. 1990;79:219–25.
52. McConnochie K. Bronchiolitis: What's in the name? Am J Dis Child. 1983; 137:11–3.
53. Mahesh VK, Taussig LM. When an infant wheezes: Clues to the differential. J Respir Dis. 1990;11:739–50.
54. McIntosh K, Ellis EF, Hoffman LS, et al. The association of viral and bacterial respiratory infections with exacerbations of wheezing in young asthmatic children. J Pediatr. 1973;82:578–90.
55. Hall WJ, Hall CB, Speers DM. Respiratory syncytial virus infections in adults: Clinical, virologic and serial pulmonary function studies. Ann Intern Med. 1978;88:203–5.
56. Polmar SH, Robinson LD Jr, Minnefor AB. Immunoglobulin E in bronchiolitis. Pediatrics. 1972;50:279–84.
57. Hall CB, Douglas RG Jr. Clinically useful method for the isolation of respiratory syncytial virus. J Infect Dis. 1975;131:1–5.
58. Drew LW. Direct detection of viruses. Pan Am Group Rapid Viral Diagn. 1992;18:1–6.
59. Dennehy PH. Rapid diagnosis of viral infections. Contemp Pediatr. 1987; Sept:61–76.
60. Stout C, Murphy MD, Lawrence S, Julian S. Evaluation of a monoclonal

antibody pool for rapid diagnosis of respiratory viral infections. J Clin Microbiol. 1989;27:448–52.

61. Kellogg JA. Culture vs direct antigen assays for detection of microbial pathogens from lower respiratory tract specimens suspected of containing the respiratory syncytial virus. Arch Pathol Lab Med. 1991;115:451–8.

62. Reynolds EOR, Cook CD. The treatment of bronchiolitis. J Pediatr. 1963; 63:1205–7.

63. Webb MSC, Martin GA, Cartlidge PHT, et al. Chest physiotherapy in acute bronchiolitis. Arch Dis Child. 1985;60:1078–9.

64. Frankel LR, Lewiston NJ, Smith DW, Stevenson DK: Clinical observations on mechanical ventilation for respiratory failure in bronchiolitis. Pediatr Pulmonol. 1986;2:307–11.

65. Outwater KM, Crone RK. Management of respiratory failure in infants with acute viral bronchiolitis. Am J Dis Child. 1984;138:1071–5.

66. Knight V, Gilbert BE. Chemotherapy of respiratory viruses. Adv Intern Med. 1986;31:95–118.

67. Hall CB, McBride JT, Walsh EE, et al. Aerosolized ribavirin treatment of infants with respiratory syncytial virus infection: A randomized double-blind study. N Engl J Med. 1983;308:1443–7.

68. Smith DW, Frankel LR, Mathers LH, et al. A controlled trial of aerosolized ribavirin in infants receiving mechanical ventilation for severe respiratory syncytial virus infection. N Engl J Med 1991;325:24–9.

69. Taber LH, Knight V, Gilbert BE, et al. Ribavirin aerosol treatment of bronchiolitis due to respiratory syncytial virus infection in infants. Pediatrics. 1983;72:613–8.

70. Hall CB, Walsh EE, Hruska JF, et al. Ribavirin aerosol treatment of experimental respiratory syncytial viral infection in young adults: A controlled double-blind study. JAMA. 1983;249:2666–70.

71. Rodriguez WJ, Kim HW, Brandt CD, et al. Aerosolized ribavirin in the treatment of patients with respiratory syncytial virus disease. Pediatr Infect Dis J. 1987;6:159–63.

72. Groothuis JR, Woodin WA, Katz R, et al. Early ribavirin treatment of respiratory syncytial viral infection in high-risk children. J Pediatr. 1990;117: 792–8.

73. Barry W, Cockburn F, Cornall R, et al. Ribavirin aerosol for acute bronchiolitis. Arch Dis Child. 1986;61:593–4.

74. Englund JA, Piedra PA, Jefferson LS, et al. High-dose, short-duration ribavirin aerosol therapy in children with suspected respiratory syncytial virus infection. J Pediatr. 1990;117:313–20.

75. Connor J. Ribavirin pharmacokinetics. Pediatr Infect Dis J. 1990;9:S91–2.

76. Mahesh VK, Taussig LM. The wheezing infant: Acute and long-term management. J Respir Dis. 1990;11:799–810.

77. Silverman M. Bronchodilators for wheezy infants? Arch Dis Child. 1984;59: 84–7.

78. Phelan PD, Williams HE. Sympathomimetic drugs in acute viral bronchiolitis. Their effect on pulmonary resistance. Pediatrics. 1969;44:493–7.

79. Rutter N, Milner AD, Hiller EJ. Effect of bronchodilators on respiratory resistance in infants and young children with bronchiolitis and wheezy bronchitis. Arch Dis Child. 1975;50:719–22.

80. Henry RL, Milner AD, Stokes GM. Ineffectiveness of ipratropium bromide in acute bronchiolitis. Arch Dis Child. 1983;58:925–6.

81. Lenney W, Milner AD. Alpha and beta adrenergic stimulants in bronchiolitis and wheezy bronchitis in children under 18 months of age. Arch Dis Child. 1978;53:707–9.

82. Radford M. Effect of salbutamol in infants with wheezy bronchitis. Arch Dis Child. 1975;50:535–8.

83. Sly PD, Lanteri CJ, Raven JM: Do wheezy infants recovering from bronchiolitis respond to inhaled salbutamol? Pediatr Pulmonol. 1991;10:36–9.

84. Hughes DM, Lesouef PN, Landau LI. Effect of salbutamol on respiratory mechanics in bronchiolitis. Pediatr Res 1987;22:83–6.

85. O'Callaghan C, Milner AD, Swarbrick A. Paradoxical deterioration in lung function after nebulized salbutamol in wheezy infants. Lancet 1986;2:1424–5.

86. Prendiville A, Green S, Silverman M. Paradoxical response to nebulized salbutamol in wheezy infants, assessed by partial expiratory flow-volume curves. Thorax 1987;42:86–91.

87. Soto M, Sly PD, Uren E, et al. Bronchodilator response in acute viral bronchiolitis. Pediatr Pulmonol. 1985;2:85–90.

88. Schuh S, Canny G, Reisman JJ, et al. Nebulized albuterol in acute bronchiolitis. J Pediatr. 1990;117:633–7.

89. Mallory GB, Motoyama EK, Koumbourlis AC, Mutich RL: Bronchial reactivity in infants in acute respiratory failure with viral bronchiolitis. Pediatr Pulmonol. 1989;6:253–9.

90. Klassen TP, Rowe PC, Sutcliffe T, et al. Randomized trial of salbutamol in acute bronchiolitis. J Pediatr. 1991;118:807–11.

91. Sanchez I, DeKoster J, Powell RE, et al. Effect of racemic epinephrine and salbutamol on clinical score and pulmonary mechanics in infants with bronchiolitis. J Pediatr. 1993;122:145–51.

92. Ellis EF. Therapy of acute bronchiolitis. Pediatr Res. 1977;11:263–4.

93. Stecenko MA. Treatment of viral bronchiolitis: Do steroids make sense? Contemp Pediatr. 1987;April:121–30.

94. Connolly JH, Field CMB, Glasgow JFT, et al. A double blind trial of prednisolone in epidemic bronchiolitis due to respiratory syncytial virus. Acta Paediatr Scand. 1969;58:116.

95. Leer JA, Green JL, Heimlich EM, et al. Corticosteroid treatment in bronchiolitis. A controlled collaborative study in 297 infants and children. Am J Dis Child. 1969;117:495–503.

96. Yaffe SJ, Weiss CF, Cann HM, et al. Should steroids be used in treating bronchiolitis? Pediatrics. 1970;46:640–2.

97. Springer C, Bar-Yishay E, Uwayyed K, et al. Corticosteroids do not affect the clinical or physiological status of infants with bronchiolitis. Pediatr Pulmonol. 1990;9:181–5.

98. Maayan C, Itzhaki T, Bar-Yishay E, et al. The functional response of infants with persistent wheezing to nebulized beclamethasone dipropionate. Pediatr Pulmonol. 1986;2:9–14.

99. Carlsen K-H, Leegaard J, Larsen S, Orstavik I: Nebulized beclomethasone dipropionate in recurrent obstructive episodes after acute bronchiolitis. Arch DisChild. 1988;63:1428–33.

100. Inhaled steroids and recurrent wheeze after bronchiolitis. Editorial. Lancet 1989;1:999.

101. Hall CB, Powell KR, Schnabel KC, et al. The risk of secondary bacterial infection in infants hospitalized with respiratory syncytial viral infection. J Pediatr. 1988;113:266–71.

102. Milner AD, Murray M. Acute bronchiolitis in infancy: Treatment and prognosis. Thorax. 1989;44:1–5.

103. Shaw KN, Bell LM, Sherman NH. Outpatient assessment of infants with bronchiolitis. Am J Dis Child. 1991;145:151–5.

104. Mulholland EK, Olinsky A, Shann FA. Clinical findings and severity of acute bronchiolitis. Lancet 1990;335:1259–61.

105. Wohl MEB, Stigol LC, Mead J. Resistance of the total respiratory system in healthy infants and infants with bronchiolitis. Pediatrics 1969;43:495–509.

106. Bruhn FW, Mokrohisky ST, McIntosh K. Apnea associated with respiratory syncytial virus infection in young infants. J Pediatr. 1977;90:382–6.

107. Anas N, Boettrich C, Hall CB, Brooks JG. The association of apnea and respiratory syncytial virus in infants. J Pediatr. 1982;101:65–8.

108. Church NR, Anas NG, Hall CB, Brooks JG. Respiratory syncytial virus related apnea in infants: Demographics and outcome. Am J Dis Child. 1984; 138:247–50.

109. Workshop on Bronchiolitis, sponsored by the National Heart, Blood and Lung Institute, Division of Lung Diseases, National Institutes of Health. Pediatr Res. 1977;11:209–70.

110. Twiggs JT, Larson LA, O'Connell EJ, Illstrup DM. Respiratory syncytial virus infection: Ten-year follow up. Clin Pediatr. 1981;20:187–90.

111. Kattan M, Keens TG, Lapierre JG, et al. Pulmonary function abnormalities in symptom free children after bronchiolitis. Pediatrics. 1977;59:683–8.

112. Sims DG, Gardner PS, Weightman D, et al. Atopy does not predispose to RSV bronchiolitis or postbronchiolitic wheezing. Br Med J. 1981;282:2086–8.

113. McConnochie KM, Roughman KJ. Bronchiolitis as a possible cause of wheezing in childhood: New evidence. Pediatrics. 1984;74:1–10.

114. Duiverman EJ, Neijens HJ, van Strik R, et al. Lung function and bronchial responsiveness in children who had infantile bronchiolitis. Pediatr Pulmonol. 1987;3:38–44.

115. Hall CB, Hall WJ, Gala CL, et al. A long term prospective study of children following respiratory syncytial virus infection. J Pediatr. 1984;105:358–64.

116. Webb MSC, Henry RL, Milner AD, et al. Continuing respiratory problems three and a half years after acute viral bronchiolitis. Arch Dis Child. 1985; 60:1064–7.

117. Mok JY, Simpson H. Outcome of acute lower respiratory tract infection in infants: Preliminary report of seven-year follow-up study. Br Med J. 1982; 285:333–7.

118. Pullan CR, Hey EN. Wheezing, asthma, and pulmonary dysfunction 10 years after infection with respiratory syncytial virus in infancy. Br Med J. 1982; 284:1665–9.

119. McConnochie KM, Mark JD, McBride JT, et al. Normal pulmonary function measurements and airway reactivity in childhood after mild bronchiolitis. J Pediatr. 1985;107:54–8.

120. Morgan WJ. Viral respiratory infection in infancy: Provocation or propagation? Semin Respir Med. 1990;11:306–313.

121. McConnochie KM, Roughman KJ. Breast feeding and maternal smoking as predictors of wheezing in children age 6 to 10 years. Pediatr Pulmonol. 1986; 2:260–7.

122. Taussig LM. The conundrum of wheezing and airway hyperreactivity in infancy. Pediatr Pulmonol. 1992;13:1–3.

123. Martinez FD, Morgan WJ, Wright AL, et al. Diminished lung function as a predisposing factor for wheezing respiratory illness in infants. N Engl J Med. 1988;319:1112–1117.

124. Martinez FD; Morgan WJ, Wright AL, et al. Initial airway function is a risk factor for recurrent wheezing respiratory illnesses during the first three years of life. Am Rev Respir Dis. 1991;143:312–6.

125. Stick SM, Arnott J, Turner DJ, et al. Bronchial responsiveness nad lung function in recurrent wheezy infants. Am Rev Respir Dis. 1991;144:1012–5.

126. Tepper RS, Rosenberg D, Eigen H. Airway responsiveness in infants following bronchiolitis. Pediatr Pulmonol. 1992;13:6–10.

127. Ralph DD, Springmeyer SC, Sullivan KM, et al. Rapidly progressive airflow obstruction in marrow transplant recipients. Am Rev Respir Dis. 1984;129: 641–4.

128. Chan CK, Hyland RH, Hutcheon MA, et al. Small-airways disease in recipients of allogeneic bone marrow transplants. Medicine. 1987;66:327–40.

129. McGregor CG, Jamieson SW, Baldwin JC, et al. Combined heart-lung trans-

plantation for end-stage Eisenmenger's syndrome. J Thorac Cardiovasc Surg. 1986;91:443–50.

130. Geddes DN, Corrin B, Brewerton DA, et al. Progressive airway obliteration in adults and its association with rheumatoid disease. Q J Med 1977;46:427.

131. Nadorra RL, Landing BH. Pulmonary lesions in childhood onset systemic lupus erthematosus: Analysis of 26 cases, and summary of literature. Pediatr Pathol. 1987;7:1–18.

132. Gold R, Wilt JC, Adhikari PK, Macpherson RI: Adenoviral pneumonia and its complications in infancy and childhood. J Can Assoc Radiol. 1969;20: 218–24.

133. Lang WR, Howden CW, Lars J, Burton JF: Bronchopneumonia with serious sequelae in children with evidence of adenovirus type 21 infections. Br Med J 1969;1:73–9.

134. Chernick V, Macpherson RI: Respiratory syncytial and adenovirus infections of the lower respiratory tract in infancy. Clin Notes Respir Dis. 1971;10:3.

50. ACUTE PNEUMONIA

GERALD R. DONOWITZ
GERALD L. MANDELL

In 1901, Sir William Osler noted in the fourth edition of his book *The Principles and Practice of Medicine* that "the most widespread and fatal of all acute diseases, pneumonia, is now Captain of the Men of Death."[1] Over 90 years later, the prominence of pneumonia as a clinical entity remains. It is the sixth most common cause of death in the United States and the most common cause of infection-related mortality.[2] The challenge confronting most clinicians is not in detecting the presence of the disease but rather in identifying its etiology. A wide array of microbial agents may cause acute pneumonia (Table 1), and no single antimicrobial regimen can be expected to cover all the possibilities. A specific diagnosis is an often unachieved goal, and empiric therapy is usually necessary. An understanding of the pathogenesis of disease, evaluation of relevant data from a careful history and physical examination, recognition of common clinical patterns of infection, and information from the microbiology laboratory all aid in narrowing down the possible etiologic agents of pneumonia, thereby allowing reasonable empiric therapy to be selected.

HOST DEFENSES AND PATHOGENESIS

In the absence of disease, normal pulmonary defense mechanisms maintain essentially sterile infralaryngeal airways and parenchyma. The development of acute pulmonary infection indicates a defect in host defenses, challenge by a particularly virulent microorganism, or an overwhelming inoculum. Infectious agents gain entry to the lower respiratory tract through inhalation of aerosolized material or aspiration of upper airway resident flora. Less frequently, pneumonia results from metastatic seeding of the lungs from the blood stream.

Pulmonary host defenses involve anatomic and mechanical barriers, humoral immune activity, cell-mediated immune function, and phagocyte activity (Table 2).[3–11] The upper airways, including the nasopharynx, oropharynx, and larynx, represent the outer perimeters of host defense and are the sites first exposed to inhaled microorganisms. Particles greater than 10 μm are efficiently filtered by the hair in the anterior nares or impact onto mucosal surfaces due to the configuration of the upper airways and the nasal turbinates. The nasal mucosa contains ciliated epithelium and mucus-producing cells, which form the first mucociliary barrier of the pulmonary host defense system. Mechanical clearance of entrapped organisms occurs through the nasopharynx via expulsion or through the oropharynx via swallowing. In the oropharynx, flow of saliva, sloughing of epi-

TABLE 1. Etiologic Agents of Acute Pneumonia

Bacterial
  Common
    Streptococcus pneumoniae
    Staphylococcus aureus
    Haemophilus influenzae
    Mixed anaerobic bacteria
      (aspiration)
        Bacteroides spp.
        Fusobacterium spp.
        Peptostreptococcus spp.
        Peptococcus spp.
    Enterobacteriaceae
        Escherichia coli
        Klebsiella pneumoniae
        Enterobacter spp.
        Serratia spp.
    Pseudomonas aeruginosa
    Legionella spp. (including *L. pneumophila* and *L. micdadei*)
  Uncommon
    Acinetobacter var. *anitratus*
    Actinomyces and *Arachnia* spp.
    Aeromonas hydrophilia
    Bacillus spp.
    Moraxella catarrhalis
    Campylobacter fetus
    Eikenella corrodens
    Francisella tularensis
    Neisseria meningitidis
    Nocardia spp.
    Pasteurella multocida
    Proteus spp.
    Pseudomonas pseudomallei
    Salmonella spp.
    Enterococcus faecalis
    Streptococcus pyogenes
    Yersinia pestis
Viral
  Children
    Common
      Respiratory syncytial virus
      Parainfluenza virus types 1, 2, 3
      Influenza A virus
    Uncommon
      Adenovirus types 1, 2, 3, 5
      Influenza B virus
      Rhinovirus
      Coxsackievirus
      Echovirus
      Measles virus
      Hantavirus
  Adults
    Common
      Influenza A virus
      Influenza B virus
      Adenovirus types 4 and 7
        (in military recruits)
    Uncommon
      Rhinovirus
      Adenovirus types 1, 2, 3, 5
      Enteroviruses
        Echovirus
        Coxsackievirus
        Poliovirus
      Epstein-Barr virus
      Cytomegalovirus
      Respiratory syncytial virus
      Varicella-zoster virus
      Parainfluenza virus
      Measles virus
      Herpes simplex virus
      Hantavirus

Fungal
  Aspergillus spp.
  Candida spp.
  Coccidioides immitis
  Cryptococcus neoformans
  Histoplasma capsulatum
  Agents of mucormycosis
    Rhizopus spp.
    Absidia spp.
    Mucor spp.
    Cunninghamella spp.
Rickettsial
  Coxiella burnetii
  Rickettsia rickettsiae
Bacteria-like agents
  Mycoplasma pneumoniae
  Chlamydia spp.
    C. psittaci
    C. trachomatis
    C. pneumoniae (TWAR)
Mycobacterial
  Mycobacterium tuberculosis
  Nontuberculosis mycobacterium
Parasitic
  Ascaris lumbricoides
  Pneumocystis carinii
  Strongyloides stercoralis
  Toxoplasma gondii
  Paragonimus westermani

thelial cells, pH, local production of complement, and bacterial interference from resident flora serve as important factors in local host defense. Immunoglobulin secretion also plays a role in the upper airways. Secretory IgA is the major immunoglobulin produced here and accounts for 10 percent of the total protein of nasal secretions.[9] It possesses antibacterial and antiviral activity despite being a relatively poor opsonin. Low IgA levels have been associated with increased bacterial adherence.[13] IgG and IgM enter the airways predominantly via transudation from the

TABLE 2. Pulmonary Host Defenses

Location	Host Defense Mechanism
Upper airways	
Nasopharynx	Nasal hair
	Turbinates
	Anatomy of upper airways
	Mucocilliary apparatus
	IgA secretion
Oropharynx	Saliva
	Sloughing of epithelial cells
	Bacterial interference
	pH
	Complement production
Conducting airways	
Trachea, bronchi	Cough, epiglottic reflexes
	Sharp angled branching of airways
	Mucocilliary apparatus
	Immunoglobulin production (IgG, IgM, IgA)
Lower respiratory tract	
Terminal airways, alveoli	Alveolar lining fluid (surfactant, fibronectin, immunoglobulin, complement, free fatty acid, iron-binding proteins)
	Cytokines (TNF, IL-1, IL-8)
	Alveolar macrophages
	Polymorphonuclear leukocytes
	Cell-mediated immunity

blood. Their roles in bacterial opsonization, complement activation, agglutination, and neutralization activity are similar to those noted in serum.

Adherence of microorganisms to epithelial surfaces of the upper airways is a critical initial step in colonization and subsequent infection. Changes in fibronectin secretion and in binding characteristics of epithelium for various lectins occur as a response to underlying diseases. This may help to explain why colonization occurs in some clinical settings and not in others.[14,15] Microbes possess surface adhesions, pili, exotoxins, and proteolytic enzymes that can degrade IgA, which serves to overcome host defenses and allow colonization.[10]

The cough and epiglottic reflexes serve to keep most large particulate matter from reaching the central airways. The trachea and conducting airways are usually effective in entrapping particles from 2 to 10 μm. The sharp angles at which the central airways branch cause particles to impact on mucosal surfaces, where they are entrapped by endobronchial mucus. Once entrapped, particles are removed by ciliated epithelium to the oropharynx. This represents the second major mucociliary apparatus in the respiratory tract.

Particles in the range of 0.5–1.0 μm may reach the terminal airways and alveoli. No mucociliary apparatus exists at this level, yet a variety of humoral and cell-mediated host defenses function here. The alveolar lining fluid contains surfactant, fibronectin, IgG, and complement, all of which are effective opsonins. Free fatty acids, lysozyme, and iron-binding proteins are also present and may be directly microbicidal. The resident phagocytic cells in the lower airway are the alveolar macrophages. They represent a morphologically and functionally diverse group of cells that play several roles in host defense.[5] As phagocytic cells, the alveolar macrophages can eliminate certain organisms. If the numbers of organisms increase beyond the macrophages' capability to handle them or if the organisms involved are particularly virulent (i.e., *Pseudomonas aeruginosa*), the macrophage becomes a mediator of an inflammatory response by producing cytokines that recruit neutrophils into the lung.[8,12,16,17] A variety of cytokines have been identified that appear to play an important role in this regard and include tumor necrosis factor (TNF) and interleukin-1 (IL-1). In addition, cytokines that demonstrate chemoattractant activity such as IL-8, the fifth component of complement (C5), leukotriene B₄, and formyl methionyl peptides of bacterial cell walls are present in the lower airways and probably serve to recruit neutrophils into areas of inflammation. Furthermore, it has recently become clear that nonphagocytic cells such as pulmonary endothelial

cells, epithelial cells, and fibroblasts produce IL-8 and therefore play a role in the generation and maintenance of the pulmonary inflammatory response.[18,19]

The series of events involved in the inflammatory response in the lung have been thought to occur sequentially. As recently reviewed, a pathogen arriving in the lower airways is coated with alveolar lining fluid.[2] The complement cascade is activated by the alternate pathway or, if specific IgG is present, by the classical pathway with the generation of C5a. Phagocytosis by alveolar macrophages occurs and, depending on the nature and number of the organisms, cytokines such as IL-1 and TNF are released that mediate the inflammatory response. IL-8 is produced, and, in coordination with other cytokines and chemoattractants, neutrophils are recruited into the lung and serve as the "professional phagocyte," which ingests and kills the infecting organisms.

Cell-mediated immunity also plays an important role in pulmonary host defense against certain pathogens, including viruses and intracellular parasites that can survive within resident macrophages (i.e., *Mycobacterium* spp., *Legionella* spp.). Activation of T cells via the recognition of foreign antigens by the T-cell receptor/CD3 complex requires the presence of antigen-presenting cells. In the lung, the identity of these accessory cells is not clear. One attractive possibility is the dendritic cell found in the columnar epithelium in bronchi, in the interstitium of the lung, and in the pleura.[20] It has been postulated that cell-mediated immune responses in the lung are compartmentalized.[21] Antigens in the alveoli that are ingested by macrophages will not be presented and therefore will not serve as stimulants for cell-mediated immune function. If the antigen is recognized by dendritic cells or other antigen-presenting cells, cell-mediated immune function can be stimulated. Both CD4 and CD8 lymphocytes are present in the lung and are associated with generating cell-mediated host responses.

A number of factors are known to interfere with normal host defenses and to predispose to infection.[3] Alterations in the level of consciousness from any cause (stroke, seizures, drug intoxication, anesthesia, alcohol abuse, and even normal sleep) can compromise epiglottic closure and lead to aspiration of oropharyngeal flora into the lower respiratory tract.[22,23] Cigarette smoke, perhaps the most common agent involved in compromising natural pulmonary defense mechanisms, disrupts both mucociliary function and macrophage activity.[24]

Viruses not only cause infection of the upper and lower respiratory tract, but may also inhibit important host defenses.[11,25] Viruses may actually destroy respiratory epithelium and may disrupt normal ciliary activity. Neutrophil function, including chemotaxis, phagocytosis, and stimulation of oxidative metabolism, may be inhibited by certain viral infections. Similarly, alveolar macrophage function may be inhibited.[25] Sepsis associated with extrapulmonary infections may also undermine lung defense mechanisms. In animal models, exposure to lipopolysaccharide or endotoxin decreases lung clearance of a bacterial challenge.[21,26] Alcohol not only serves to impair the cough and epiglottic reflexes leading to an increased risk of aspiration, but also has been associated with increased colonization of the oropharynx with aerobic gram-negative bacilli.[27] Alcohol has also been associated with decreased mobilization of neutrophils,[28] abnormal phagocyte oxidative metabolism, and abnormal chemotaxis.[29] Alcohol in animal models effectively blocks TNF response to endotoxin.[30] The associated findings of decreased recruitment of neutrophils to the lung after endotoxin challenge suggests that endotoxin-induced stimulation of TNF is important in neutrophil mobilization of the lung and that alcohol may inhibit this component of the inflammatory response. Iatrogenic manipulations that bypass the usual host defenses of the upper airways (endotracheal tubes, nasogastric tubes, and respiratory therapy machinery) all predispose to infection.[31] A variety of commonly prescribed drugs have been shown to inhibit host defenses in vitro or in models, but the clinical significance of this is uncertain. These agents include aspirin,[32] erythromycin,[33] and aminophylline.[34] Other factors that impair pulmonary host defenses include hypoxemia,[35] acidosis, toxic inhalations,[36,37] pulmonary edema,[38] uremia, malnutrition, immunosuppressive agents,[27,39] and viral and mechanical obstruction.[4]

The effect of HIV infection on host defenses in the upper airways remains incompletely defined, although no consistent impairment has been noted. In the lower airways, the most clear-cut defects in host defense related to HIV infection are related to lymphocyte function and cell-mediated immunity. Mitogeninduced proliferation of T and B cells, cytokine elaboration by T cells (interferon-γ, IL-2), and immunoglobulin secretion by B cells are all decreased in patients infected with HIV.[40]

The elderly appear at increased risk for the development of pneumonia (see Ch. 295). While a variety of factors play an important role in this regard, including increased number and severity of underlying diseases and increased hospitalization, there are age-related impairments in host defense that also may be playing a role.[41–43] Less effective mucociliary clearance and abnormal elastic recoil may lead to less effective coughing and clearing of the upper airways. Changes in humoral immunity and cell-mediated immune function have been documented in the elderly, though their exact roles as factors for infection remain unclear.

Recurrent episodes of bacterial pneumonia suggest the presence of specific predisposing factors.[44–47] In children and young adults, recurrent pneumonias are associated with defects in host defenses, including leukocyte function[48] and immunoglobulin production.[48–51] Congenital defects in cilia activity including the immotile-cilia syndrome,[52] Kartagener syndrome (ciliary dysfunction, situs inversus, sinusitis, bronchiectasis),[53] Young syndrome (azospermia, sinusitis, pneumonia),[54] and cystic fibrosis are other clinical entities associated with recurrent pneumonia in the young. Structural lung abnormalities such as bronchiectasis and pulmonary sequestration[55] are also important predisposing factors for both younger and older patient populations.

While most congenital defects in host defense present in childhood, common variable hypogammaglobulinemia may first present in adulthood with recurrent pneumonia. Acquired host defense defects are more varied and include malignancies (lymphoma, chronic lymphocytic leukemia, myeloma) infection (acquired immune deficiency syndrome [AIDS]) and iatrogenic measures (immune suppression associated with solid organ or marrow transplantation). Underlying respiratory tract disorders such as chronic obstructive pulmonary disease, bronchiectasis, adult-onset cystic fibrosis, bronchopulmonary sequestration, and tracheobronchiomegaly may present with pneumonia. Bronchial obstruction due to intrinsic compression (adenocarcinoma) or extrinsic compression (lymphadenopathy due to sarcoid or malignancy) has also been associated with recurrent episodes of pneumonia. Underlying diseases that predispose to aspiration lead to an increased incidence of pneumonia. These may be associated with gastrointestinal diseases (tracheoesophageal fistula, esophageal diverticula, esophageal reflex, esophageal stricture[56]), neuromuscular disorders (myasthenia gravis, dementia, amyotrophic lateral sclerosis), and cancer of the head and neck. Some systemic illnesses, including Weber-Christian disease, chronic renal failure, diabetes, and sickle cell disease, have been associated with pneumonia.[47]

CLINICAL EVALUATION

History

The history should attempt to define (1) the clinical setting in which the pneumonia is taking place, (2) defects in host resistance that could predispose to the development of pneumonia, and (3) possible exposure to specific pathogens. Although age and race are usually of little diagnostic value, it should be remembered that mycoplasmal pneumonia occurs more often in younger people,[57,58] that gram-negative pneumonia tends to occur in the elderly,[59] and that tuberculosis has re-emerged as an important cause of pulmonary disease regardless of age or race and should be suspected in the homeless, in those infected with HIV, and in those who come from developing countries where tuberculosis is prevalent.[60,61]

Pneumonia has been noted to occur with increased frequency in patients with a variety of underlying disorders such as congestive heart failure, diabetes, alcoholism, and chronic obstructive pulmonary disease.[59,62,63] In one series of 292 patients with pneumonia, only 18 percent were found to have no underlying disease.[59] A history of upper respiratory tract infection has been elicited in 36–50 percent of patients with acute pneumonia, especially in those with pneumococcal disease.[62,64] Recent dental manipulations, sedative overdoses, seizures, alcoholism, or loss of consciousness for any reason should raise the suspicion of anaerobic infection due to aspiration of oral contents.[21]

Specific etiologic agents of pneumonia have been associated with certain underlying diseases. An increased incidence of staphylococcal pneumonia has been noted during epidemics of influenza.[65]

Special note needs to be made of the relationship between pneumonia and patients with chronic obstructive pulmonary diseases (COPD).[66,67] While well-controlled studies are lacking, it does appear that patients with COPD have an increased incidence of pneumonia. However, since the tracheobronchial tree is often colonized with *Streptococcus pneumoniae* and *Haemophilus influenzae*, it has been difficult to distinguish clearly between colonization and infection in many studies. While these organisms play an important role as etiologic agents of pneumonia in this patient population, most of the clinical studies were carried out before it was recognized that other less common pathogens also play a significant role in causing disease. The roles of *Moraxella catarrhalis, Legionella* spp., and aerobic gram-negative rods including *Pseudomonas aeruginosa* have recently been acknowledged.[67–69] Cystic fibrosis is associated with *Pseudomonas* and staphylococcal pulmonary infections.[70] Pulmonary alveolar proteinosis has been associated with *Nocardia* infection.[71]

Patients infected with HIV are at high risk for the development of pneumonia.[72–74] While *Pneumocystis carinii* remains the major pulmonary pathogen, *Mycobacterium tuberculosis, Mycobacterium avium* complex, as well as common bacterial pathogens such as *S. pneumoniae* and *H. influenzae* must be considered. The incidence of pneumococcal pneumonia including bacteremic disease is 7–10 times higher in the HIV-infected population.[75] The incidence of *H. influenzae* is 100-fold higher in HIV-infected individuals.[76] Bacterial agents such as *Legionella* spp., *Nocardia* spp., aerobic gram-negative bacilli, and *Rhodococcus equi* are important causes of pneumonia.[74] The wide range of pulmonary infections for those infected with HIV is discussed in Chapters 102 and 105.

Pneumonia developing in hospitalized patients often involves Enterobacteriaceae, *Pseudomonas aeruginosa,* and *Staphylococcus aureus,* agents that are unusual in community-acquired disease.[77] Similarly, pneumonia in the elderly, especially those living in nursing homes or extended care facilities, is more often associated with gram-negative bacilli than is pneumonia in younger populations.[75–78]

Occupational history, history of exposure to animals, travel history, and sexual history are all important in suggesting specific potential infectious agents (Table 3). The presence of noninfectious pulmonary disease such as tumors or pulmonary emboli, which may masquerade as pneumonia, may also be suggested by a careful history.

Physical Examination

Fever is usually present and may be sustained, remittent, or at times hectic. Fever patterns per se, however, are not useful

TABLE 3. Important Environmental Factors in Pneumonia

Pneumonia Associated with	Environmental History
Anthrax	Exposure to cattle, swine, horses, goat hair, raw wool, animal hides
Brucellosis	Exposure to cattle, goats, pigs; ingestion of unpasteurized dairy products; employment as abattoir worker or veterinarian
Melioidosis	Travel to W. Indies, Australia, Guam, S.E. Asia, South and Central America
Plague	Exposure to ground squirrels, chipmunks, rabbits, prairie dogs, rats
Tularemia	Exposure to tissue or body fluids of infected animals during trapping, hunting, or skinning (rabbits, hares, foxes, squirrels) or to bites of an infected arthropod (flies, ticks)
	Handling or ingesting poorly cooked meat from an infected animal
Psittacosis	Exposure to birds (parrots, budgerigars, cockatoos, pigeons, turkeys)
Leptospirosis	Exposure to wild rodents, dogs, cats, pigs, cattle, horses, or exposure to water contaminated with animal urine
Coccidioidomycosis	Reside in or travel to San Joaquin Valley, S. California, S.W. Texas, S. Arizona, New Mexico
Histoplasmosis	Exposure to bat droppings or dust from soil enriched with bird droppings
Q fever	Exposure to infected goats, cattle, sheep, domestic animals and their secretions (milk, amniotic fluid, placenta, feces)
Legionnaires' disease	Exposure to contaminated aerosols (e.g., air coolers, hospital water supply)
Pasteurella multocida	Exposure to infected dogs and cats
Hantavirus	Exposure to rodent droppings, urine, and saliva

for establishing a specific diagnosis. The temperature should be taken rectally to reduce error due to rapid mouth breathing. Recording of postural changes in blood pressure and pulse rate is useful in assessing hydration and intravascular fluid volume. The pulse usually increases by 10 beats/min for every degree (C) of temperature elevation. A pulse temperature deficit (i.e., a relative bradycardia for the amount of fever) should suggest viral infection, mycoplasmal infection, chlamydial infection, tularemia, or infection with *Legionella* spp. Cyanosis, rapid respiratory rate, the use of accessory muscles of respiration, sternal retraction, and nasal flaring suggest serious respiratory compromise.

Furuncles are rarely secondary to staphylococcal pneumonia acquired by the respiratory route but may signal a source of bacteremia with subsequent hematogenous pneumonia. Herpes labialis is seen in up to 40 percent of the patients with pneumococcal pneumonia.[79] Bullous myringitis is an infrequent although significant finding in mycoplasmal pneumonia.[58] The presence of poor dentition should suggest a mixed infection due to aspiration of anaerobes and aerobes that colonize the oropharynx. While edentulous people may develop anaerobic pneumonia due to aspiration, it is uncommon.[80]

Examination of the thorax may reveal "splinting" or an inspiratory lag on the side of the lesion that is suggestive of bacterial pneumonia. Early in the disease process, definite signs of pulmonary involvement may be lacking or may be manifest only as fine, crackling rales. Chest examination may reveal these early signs of pneumonia even though the chest film is normal. Evidence of consolidation (dullness on percussion, bronchial breath sounds, and E to A changes) is highly suggestive of bacterial infection. Patients with mycoplasmal or viral infection may exhibit few abnormalities on physical examination despite the presence of impressive infiltrates on the chest film.

SPUTUM EXAMINATION

Microscopic examination and culture of expectorated sputum remain the mainstays of the laboratory evaluation of pneumonia despite ongoing controversy concerning their sensitivity and specificity.[80–84] Procurement of expectorated sputum is a noninvasive technique that can be carried out at no risk to the patient, provides samples of lower respiratory tract secretions for immediate evaluation, and in the majority of cases allows the clinician to make a presumptive diagnosis.

Examination of the sputum should include observation of the color, amount, consistency, and odor of the specimen. Mucopurulent sputum is most commonly found with bacterial pneumonia or bronchitis. Sputum of a similar nature has been described in one-third to one-half of patients with mycoplasma[58] or adenovirus infections.[85,86] However, scant or watery sputum is more often noted with these and other atypical pneumonias. "Rusty" sputum suggests alveolar involvement and has been most commonly (although not solely) associated with pneumococcal pneumonia.[87] Dark red, mucoid sputum (currant-jelly sputum) suggests Friedlander's pneumonia caused by encapsulated *Klebsiella pneumoniae*.[88] Foul-smelling sputum is associated with mixed anaerobic infections most commonly seen with aspiration.[80]

Where possible, frankly purulent material should be selected for microscopic examination. In all cases of acute pneumonia, a Gram stain of the sputum should be prepared. To maximize the diagnostic yield of the sputum examination, only samples free of oropharyngeal contamination should be reviewed. As a guide, the number of neutrophils and epithelial cells should be quantitated under low power ($\times 100$), with further examination reserved for samples containing 25 or more neutrophils and 10 or fewer epithelial cells. Such samples contain minimal oropharyngeal contamination.[89] Samples with more epithelial cells and fewer neutrophils are nondiagnostic and should be discarded. The morphologic and staining characteristics of any bacteria seen should be recorded and an estimate made of the predominant organisms (Figs. 1–4). Where no bacterial predominance exists, this should be noted as well.

In the appropriate clinical setting, a predominance of gram-positive, lancet-shaped diplococci should suggest pneumococcal infection (Fig. 1). When strict criteria for Gram stain positivity are used (predominant flora and/or more than 10 gram-positive, lancet-shaped diplococci per oil immersion field [$\times 1000$]), the specificity of the Gram stain for identifying pneumococci has been shown to be 85 percent, with a sensitivity of 62 percent.[90] The diagnostic yield of the sputum examination for pneumococci can be maximized by the use of the quellung reaction. Anticapsular antiserum reacts with capsular polysaccharide, and this may be seen as a distinctly outlined capsule. Rare false-positive results may occur with α-hemolytic streptococci. Occasional false-negative results may occur as well. An 89 percent correlation between pneumococcal isolation by cul-

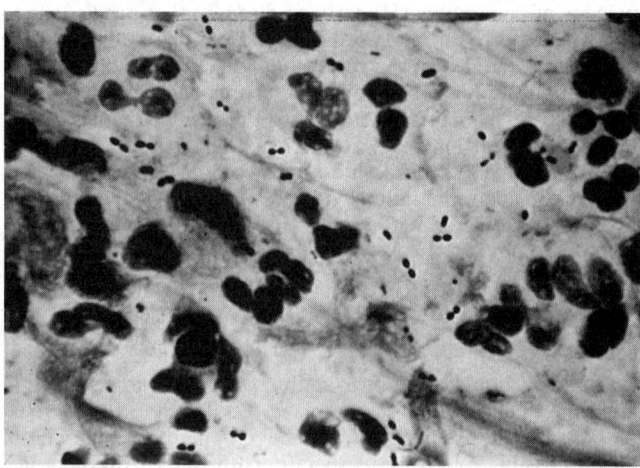

FIG. 1. Expectorated sputum with gram-positive, lancet-shaped diplococci from a patient with pneumococcal pneumonia.

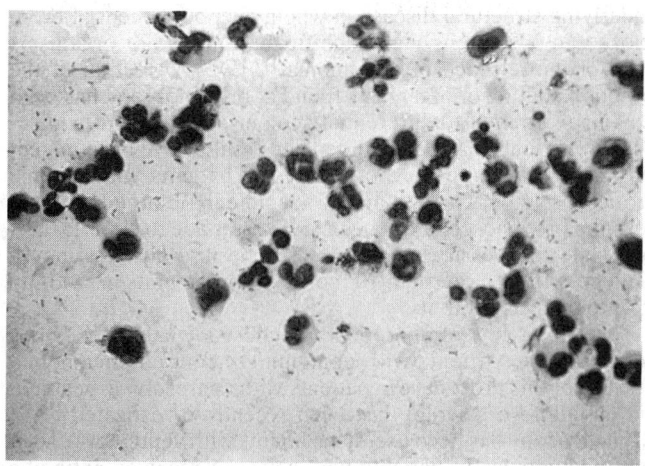

FIG. 2. Expectorated sputum with gram-negative coccobacillary forms from a patient with *Haemophilus influenzae* pneumonia.

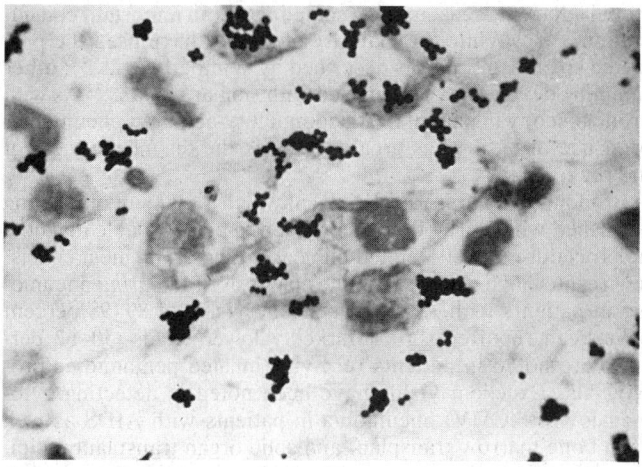

FIG. 3. Expectorated sputum with gram-positive cocci in clumps from a patient with staphylococcal pneumonia.

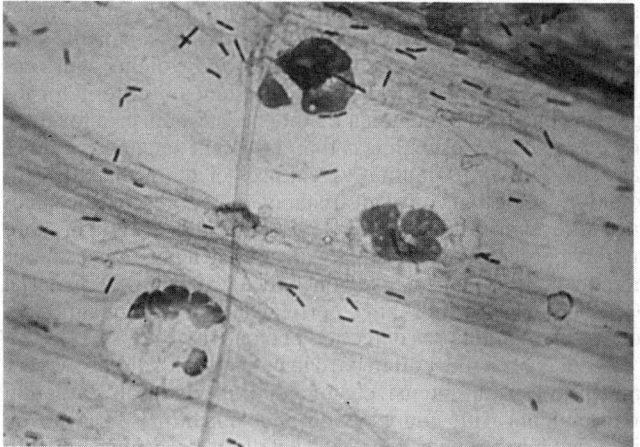

FIG. 4. Expectorated sputum with gram-negative rods in a patient with *Escherichia coli* pneumonia.

ture and a positive sputum quellung test has been demonstrated.[82]

Since pneumococci may be part of the nasopharyngeal flora in up to 50 percent of healthy adults and may colonize the lower airways in patients with chronic bronchitis, identification of the organism does not always mean that it is the cause of disease.[91-93] However, it is our experience that the large number of pneumococci necessary to produce a positive Gram stain or quellung reaction is unusual in carriers.

The sputum Gram stain is helpful to identify organisms other than pneumococci. Small gram-negative coccobacillary organisms are characteristic of *H. influenzae* (Fig. 2). However, the sensitivity of sputum Gram stain for detecting *H. influenzae* is usually less than that for *Streptococcus pneumoniae* and has been reported to be 40–80 percent.[94,95] Staphylococci appear as gram-positive cocci in tetrads and grapelike clusters (Fig. 3). Organisms of mixed morphology are characteristic of anaerobic infection. Few bacteria are seen with legionnaires' disease, mycoplasma pneumonia, and viral pneumonia. When the criteria of greater than 25 neutrophils and less than 10 squamous epithelial cells per low-power ($\times 100$) magnification are met, and when a predominant morphology is observed, the sensitivity of sputum Gram stain in detecting organisms found in the blood was reported as 85 percent in patients with community-acquired pneumonia.[94] Sputum examination has been a useful means of diagnosing *P. carinii* pneumonia in patients with AIDS. Use of commercially available monoclonal antibodies or Giemsa, Gomori methanamine silver, or toluidine blue O stain has led to a diagnosis in over 50 percent of cases, making more aggressive diagnostic procedures unnecessary.[97,98]

A variety of diagnostic techniques have been recently introduced that provide the potential for more accurate and rapid identification of the etiologic agents of pneumonia. Nucleic acid hybridization techniques have been used to detect herpes simplex virus, cytomegalovirus, mycoplasma, *Legionella* spp., *Mycobacterium tuberculosis*, and nontuberculosis mycobacteria. Monoclonal antibodies in the immunofluorescence assay and the enzyme-linked immunosorbent assay (ELISA) have been used to rapidly detect a variety of viruses, *Chlamydia* spp., and *Legionella* spp. in respiratory secretions.[99-103] While many of these techniques are of great interest, their general applicability has yet to be determined.

Antibody coating bacteria in respiratory secretions has been used as a means of differentiating infection from colonization in intubated patients.[104] While the assay has been reported as specific for the presence of lower respiratory infection, sensitivity is only 46 percent, and it cannot clearly differentiate purulent bronchitis from pneumonia.

The utility of the sputum culture as a means of diagnosing pneumonia has been questioned. Patients with bacteremic pneumococcal pneumonia have been reported to have negative sputum cultures in 45–50 percent of cases, even when large numbers of organisms have been noted on Gram stain.[105,106] Similarly, 34–47 percent of sputum cultures are negative with proven *H. influenzae* pneumonia.[107,108] Furthermore, sputum cultures have frequently been shown to yield more bacterial species than more invasive methods of obtaining respiratory tract secretions.[109,110] Contamination with gram-negative bacilli from the oropharynx has been noted in 32 percent of sputum cultures.[111]

Several key parameters have been identified in efforts to maximize the diagnostic yield from sputum culture. Procurement of adequate sputum samples is an essential first step. When fewer than 10 epithelial cells and more than 25 neutrophils per low-power field are noted, oropharyngeal contamination is minimal and sputum samples are comparable to transtracheal aspirates in terms of the number of bacterial species isolated.[86] With increasing numbers of epithelial cells and decreasing numbers of neutrophils, an increased amount of oropharyngeal contamination is present, as indicated by the isolation of more bacterial species.

The presence of alveolar macrophages does not alter the bacteriologic findings when substantial numbers of epithelial cells are present, indicating that otherwise adequate samples of sputum can be contaminated with oropharyngeal contents and thereby rendered nondiagnostic. This type of initial screening has proven helpful in differentiating adequate sputum samples from saliva, thereby increasing the diagnostic yield of sputum culture.

When culture of sputum is delayed, isolation of pneumococci is less likely due to overgrowth of the organism by oropharyngeal flora. Rapid processing of samples is therefore another important factor leading to higher diagnostic yields.

Laboratory techniques for maximizing the useful information from sputum cultures have included quantitative cultures, washing of samples to remove contaminating mouth flora, and the use of mucolytic agents. The varying results noted have not warranted the increased efforts required. Furthermore, washing samples does not guarantee that adequate samples of lower respiratory tract secretions are present.[112] Some reports suggest that, with adequate sputum samples and prompt culture of specimens, the diagnostic yield of the sputum culture may approach 100 percent.[81,113,114]

TRANSTRACHEAL ASPIRATION

Although the sputum examination should always be included in the initial evaluation of patients with pneumonia, it may be inadequate for a presumptive diagnosis. In cases in which *(1)* no sputum is produced, *(2)* no clear predominance of a potential pathogen exists on sputum Gram stain or culture, *(3)* there has been a poor response to antibiotics chosen on the basis of expectorated sputum, *(4)* gram-negative rods or yeast forms are found in the sputum, or *(5)* the possibility of superinfection exists, a more direct method of obtaining lower respiratory tract secretions may be necessary.

In the past, transtracheal aspiration had been used as a means of obtaining lower respiratory tract secretions with minimal oropharyngeal contamination.[67,69,73,74] However, because of the fear of adverse reactions, most clinicians now use other methods of obtaining lower respiratory tract secretions.

FIBEROPTIC BRONCHOSCOPY

Initial studies concerning the usefulness of fiberoptic bronchoscopy for the diagnosis of bacterial pneumonia demonstrated that the procedure was limited by contamination of specimens by oropharyngeal flora. Cultures obtained via the bronchoscope averaged two to three more bacterial isolates than samples from paired transtracheal aspirates.[115] In patients without lower respiratory tract infections, cultures of aspirates obtained at bronchoscopy produced an average of five different bacterial strains.[116] The development of the protected brush catheter (a brush within two catheters sealed at the end with a polyethylene glycol plug) has significantly decreased but not eliminated this problem.[117,118] Quantitative culturing has been used to differentiate contaminants from true infecting agents.[117,119,120]

Approximately 10^6–10^8 organisms/ml are present in areas of pneumonia.[84] Accounting for dilution of samples, bacterial growth of more than 10^3–10^4 has been used as a breakpoint for determining the clinical significance of an isolate.

Studies employing the protected brush catheter have proven experimentally and clinically to be both sensitive (70–97 percent) and specific (95–100 percent) for the diagnosis of bacterial pneumonia.[119–122] However, not all series using this technique have produced impressive results,[123–125] and in some patient groups this technique is not useful. These include patients receiving prior antibiotics, patients with purulent bronchitis in whom bacterial counts above 10^3 are noted, and patients with

underlying structural disease in whom over 50 percent of bronchoscopic specimens yield significant numbers of organisms even in the absence of pneumonia.[117,122,126] Detection of the antibody coating of organisms found at bronchoscopy has been used in an attempt to differentiate colonization from true infection. Experience has been limited and results have been mixed, with a high false-positive rate noted in patients with chronic bronchitis.[127,128] Gram stain of specimens obtained from fiberoptic bronchoscopy has been used as a guide to empiric therapy while cultures are pending.[126,129] A positive Gram stain predicts growth of more than 10^3 colony-forming units/ml with up to 78 percent sensitivity.

The role, if any, of fiberoptic bronchoscopy has not yet been determined in patients with community-acquired pneumonia. The use of this procedure in patients with nonresolving pneumonia or failure of therapy has been recently investigated.[130,131] Bronchoscopy has been useful in patients with ventilator-associated pneumonia. In patients who have not received antibiotic therapy, bronchoscopy with quantitative culture has yielded sensitivities of detection of infecting microbes of 41–100 percent.[132–135] Positive predictive values have ranged from 75 to 83 percent. Reported false-negative findings are seen in almost 15 percent of patients, which may reflect the fact that bacterial counts may differ 50-fold in areas of infected lung vs. noninfected adjacent areas, making sampling site an important consideration.[123,133] While the majority of studies have used the protected specimen brush as described by Wimberly et al.,[117] other sampling devices have been used with similar results.[137] As with bronchoscopy in patients with community-acquired pneumonia, prior use of antibiotics greatly reduces the diagnostic yield of the procedure.[138]

Bronchoalveolar lavage (BAL) in which a segment of the lung is washed with sterile fluid has proven to be a valuable diagnostic procedure in well-defined clinical settings. The most consistent results have been seen in the diagnosis of *P. carinii* pneumonia in patients with AIDS. Diagnostic yields of 89–98 percent have been reported.[139,140] Markedly lower yields (50–62 percent) are noted in patients receiving inhaled pentamidine prophylaxis. Excellent yields have been noted in detecting cytomegalovirus (CMV) pneumonia in patients with AIDS as well as in bone marrow transplant and solid organ transplant recipients.[141–143] By using immunofluorescent monoclonal antibodies to viral antigens or centrifuging lavage material into tissue culture preparations, the diagnosis of CMV pneumonia may be made within hours rather than weeks.[144,145]

The use of BAL for diagnosis of pneumonia in other clinical settings and with other pathogens is less well defined.[146,147] By using cytologic screening, quantitative cultures of BAL fluid, or Gram stain criteria, bacterial pneumonia has been identified in non-AIDS-related immunosuppressed patients, patients with severe community-acquired pneumonia, and patients with ventilator-associated pneumonia.[145] While standard criteria for diagnosing bacterial pneumonia has not been established for BAL procedures, samples with less than 1 percent squamous epithelial cells and with quantitative cultures of more than 10^3–10^5 colony-forming units (cfu)/ml are thought to represent true infection rather than colonization.[149–151] Gram stain criteria of more than 25 percent of neutrophils with intracellular organisms or more than one organism noted on cytocentrifuged BAL material at $\times 1000$ magnification have correlated well with quantitative culture breakpoints for detecting pneumonia.[150,151]

BAL has been most often used in patients with disease severe enough to warrant intensive care and/or mechanical ventilation or in patients with nonresolving pneumonia.[131,136] Diagnostic yields have been lower than that noted for bronchoscopy with the protected brush catheter.[136] False-positive values of up to 31 percent and a lack of clear breakpoints between infected and noninfected specimens have diminished the role of quantitative cultures of BAL fluid for patients with ventilator-associated pneumonia; using criteria of more than 10^3 or 10^4 cfu/ml, sensitivities of 53–59 percent have been reported.[129,135,148,151,152]

Newer techniques continue to be developed to minimize oropharyngeal contamination of BAL specimens in an attempt to increase specificity. Nonbronchoscopic BAL and protected BAL either with or without bronchoscopy have been utilized in small numbers of patients. Their roles remain undefined.[153–156] In addition to quantitative culture and Gram stain of BAL fluid, quantitation of endotoxin has been used to detect the presence of gram-negative pneumonia.[157] This has been shown to be a very sensitive technique in small numbers of patients, but its overall usefulness again remains unclear.

While the risks of bronchoscopy are relatively small, hypoxia occurs in 13–28 percent of patients on ventilators undergoing BAL.[129,158] In patients with gram-negative pneumonia, the procedure may be followed by a sepsislike picture with increased temperature and decreased mean arterial pressure.[159]

BAL has proven especially useful for diagnosing pneumonia caused by *Mycobacterium tuberculosis*.[160–162] Culture of BAL material has a sensitivity of 85 percent, even in the presence of negative cultures of expectorated sputum and gastric aspirate. In patients with miliary tuberculosis where sputum culture yields are low (25 percent), culture of BAL fluid approximates 100 percent. In addition to culture and staining, adenosine deaminase levels and ELISA assays for antibodies to *Mycobacterium tuberculosis* have been studied.[148,163–165] BAL has also been used for diagnosis of atypical pneumonias, including those caused by *Legionella* spp. and *Mycoplasma pneumoniae*.[148]

Lung Biopsy

Direct means of obtaining diagnostic material in patients with pneumonia include percutaneous lung aspiration, transbronchial lung biopsy, thoracoscopy, and open lung biopsy.[166] These procedures are usually reserved for cases of pneumonia in impaired hosts and in pediatric populations, in whom sputum is not routinely available.[167]

Biopsy procedures are rarely indicated in the normal person with acute pneumonia. The indications and usefulness of these invasive procedures remain controversial. Lung aspiration has provided a diagnostic yield of 30–82 percent in adults and children, though false-negative rates of up to 18 percent have been reported.[168–172] Bleeding and pneumothorax have been reported as the major complications in 5–39 percent of procedures.[171–174] The use of transbronchial biopsy in the diagnosis of pneumonia has been reviewed, revealing similar diagnostic yields though somewhat lower complication rates.[175]

Thoracoscopy, in which the pleura and underlying lung are visualized through a thorascope before biopsy, has been used in several series of children and adults with pneumonia. Despite a diagnostic yield of over 90 percent and low complication rates, there has not been extensive experience with this procedure.[176,177]

Open lung biopsy remains the definitive invasive procedure for making an etiologic diagnosis of pneumonia in immunosuppressed patients, with diagnostic yields of 60–100 percent.[174,175,178] The incidence of pneumothorax and bleeding is usually less than 10 percent, even in patients who are thrombocytopenic.[175] Some have questioned whether open lung biopsy provides meaningful information that significantly affects patients' clinical outcome.[179,180]

Examination of Pleural Effusions

The characteristics of pleural effusions and their importance in the differential diagnosis of pulmonary disease are discussed in Chapter 51. It should be noted that the incidence of pleural effusions associated with pneumonia varies with the etiologic agent, from approximately 10 percent with pneumococci to 50–70 percent with gram-negative bacilli to up to 95 percent with group A streptococcal disease.[87,181,182] Pleural fluid cultures, when positive, are specific for the etiology of the underlying pneumonia. Furthermore, analysis of pleural fluid may play a major role in differentiating other causes of pulmonary infiltrates that may mimic pneumonia, including tuberculosis, tumors, pulmonary emboli, and collagen vascular diseases.[183] Pleural biopsy specimens from patients with acute bacterial pneumonia are nonspecific and are therefore of little use in the differential diagnosis. Analysis of pleural fluid may be of prognostic significance. A pleural fluid pH of less than 7.0 or a pleural fluid glucose level below 40 mg/100 ml has been associated with the presence of a complicated parapneumonic effusion and the need for a tube thoracostomy.[184]

Blood Culture, Serologic Studies, and Antigen Detection

Approximately 20–30 percent of patients with bacterial pneumonia are bacteremic. Positive blood cultures offer definitive proof of the etiology of an associated pneumonia, and blood should be cultured from all patients suspected of having bacterial pneumonia.

Streptococcus pneumoniae produce a variety of antigens and surface markers that are type or species specific.[185] Since the demonstration by Dorff et al.[186] that pneumococcal-related antigens could be detected by counterimmunoelectrophoresis (CIE), a variety of techniques have been used to identify pneumococci in urine, serum, sputum, and pleural fluid. Most recent assays have involved recognition of one of two pneumococcal polysaccharides. Pneumococcal C polysaccharide is a teichoic acid constituent of the bacterial cell wall that is species but not type specific. Pneumococcal capsular polysaccharide antigens are constituents of the outer surface of the pneumocci that are type specific. Three immunoassays have been used for antigen identification, including CIE, agglutination, and ELISA. ELISA has proven to be the most sensitive, but is most expensive and time consuming. Latex agglutination, while easy to perform, is less sensitive for detecting urinary antigen. CIE may miss positively charged capsular polysaccharide antigen. Yields have been highest for antigen detection in sputum, with sensitivities of 72–94 percent.[187–191] Antigen detection in urine has been consistently less sensitive, with yields of 40–60 percent. Antigen detection in serum is unacceptably low, with sensitivities of 3–41 percent. Antigen may persist long after the onset of pneumonia, even in patients who are adequately treated and in whom cultures are no longer positive. Specificity of pneumococcal antigen in sputum remains a problem.[190,192] False-positive rates of 18–20 percent are reported.[185,193] Distinguishing colonization and oropharyngeal contamination from infection remain unresolved problems with the technique.

Serologic assays have been used to detect antibodies against four pneumococcal antigens: pneumococcal C polysaccharide, capsular polysaccharide, phosphorylcholine, and the protein toxin pneumolysin. Antibody detection against the capsular polysaccharide and C polysaccharide have reported sensitivities of 89 and 97 percent, respectively.[192]

CIE and latex agglutination techniques have been used for the detection of *H. influenzae* and *Pseudomonas* antigens in patients with pneumonia, though clinical experience has been limited and the results inconsistent.[194]

Serologic tests have been used to diagnose a variety of other pulmonary pathogens, including *Legionella pneumophila*, *Legionella micdadei*, *Mycoplasma pneumoniae*, *Chlamydia* spp., and *Coxiella burnetii*.[132] The sensitivities and specificities of these assays are variable, and many assays have not been completely standardized. Since many of these tests are not routinely

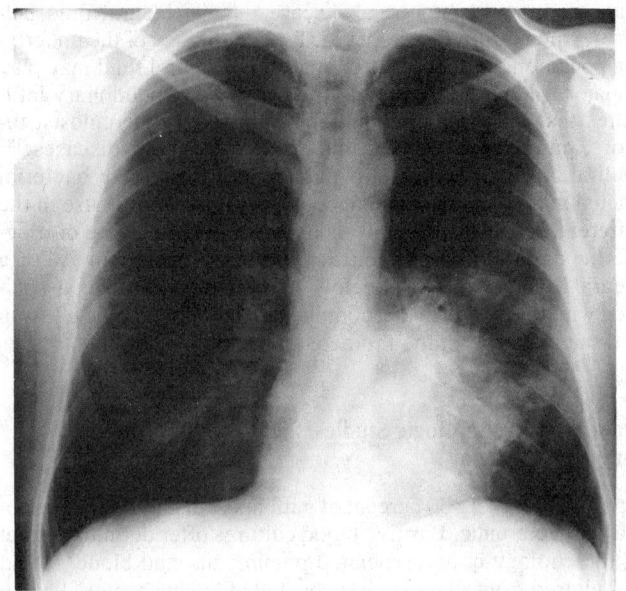

FIG. 5.   Patchy infiltrate representing bronchopneumonia in a patient with *S. pneumoniae* infection.

done, their usefulness in making a rapid diagnosis is limited. They are of more help in confirming a clinical diagnosis.

A variety of assays have been utilized to detect agents that have been difficult to isolate using routine culture techniques. Serologic assays have been used to diagnose infections caused by *Legionella* spp., *Mycoplasma pneumoniae*, *Chlamydia* spp., and *Coxiella burnetii*.[195] The sensitivity and specificity of the

assays vary, and, since they may not be available routinely, their usefulness in making a rapid diagnosis is limited. Soluble *L. pneumophila* antigen can be detected in urine using a radioimmunoassay, though it is useful for detecting only *L. pneumophila* serogroup 1.[196] DNA probes and polymerase chain reaction (PCR) techniques have been used to detect *C. pneumoniae* and *Legionella* spp.[197,198]

RADIOLOGIC EXAMINATION

The chest film most frequently shows a bronchopneumonia pattern that is not very helpful in making a specific etiologic diagnosis (Fig. 5). However, certain features may be of some diagnostic aid. Lobar consolidation, cavitation, and large pleural effusions support a bacterial etiology (Fig. 6). In cases in which bilateral diffuse involvement is noted, *P. carinii* pneumonia, *Legionella* pneumonia, or a primary viral pneumonia should be suspected. Staphyloccal pneumonia may result from infection metastasizing from a primary focus unrelated to the lung. In these cases, multiple nodular infiltrates throughout the lung may be seen. Staphylococci may cause marked necrosis of lung tissue with ill-defined thin-walled cavities (pneumatoceles), bronchopleural fistulas, and empyema, especially in children (Fig. 7).[199–201] Although pneumatoceles are diagnostically significant findings in staphylococcal pneumonia, they may be seen in pneumonias of other etiologies, including *K. pneumoniae, H. influenzae, S. pneumoniae,* and, more rarely, *P. carinii.*[202–204] Pulmonary infections due to *Pseudomonas* may cavitate. *Pseudomonas* and other gram-negative bacillis most commonly cause lower lobe pneumonia.[205]

Aspiration pneumonia should be considered along with gram-negative and staphyloccal pneumonias as a source of necrotizing pneumonia, cavitation, and empyema. Aspiration pneumonia commonly involves either the superior segment or the basilar

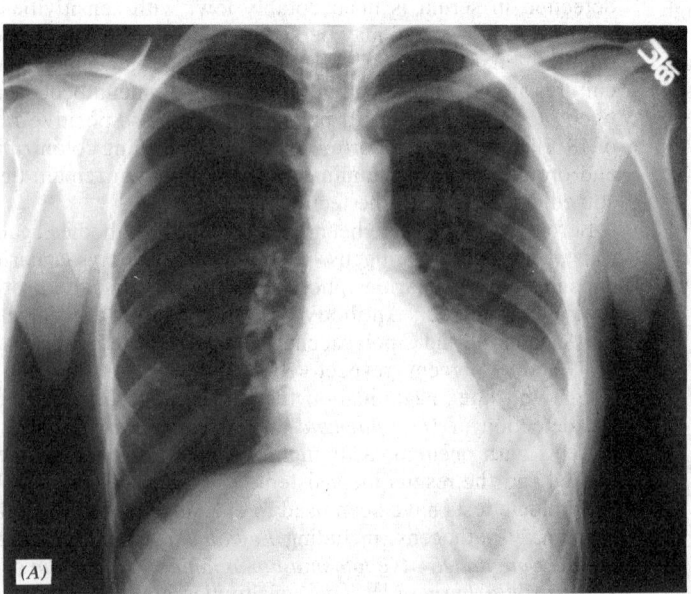

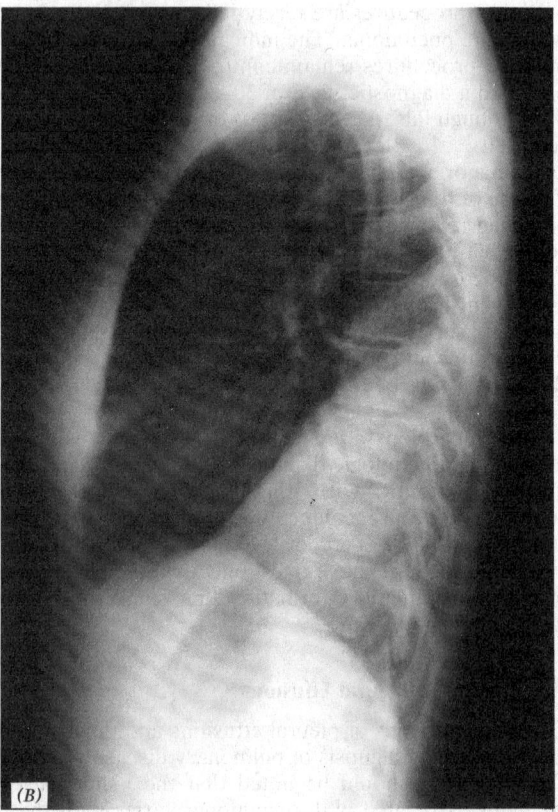

FIG. 6.   **(A)** Posteroanterior film showing dense left lower consolidation consistent with bacterial pneumonia, in this case caused by *S. pneumoniae.* **(B)** Lateral film of patient with left lower lobe pneumococcal pneumonia.

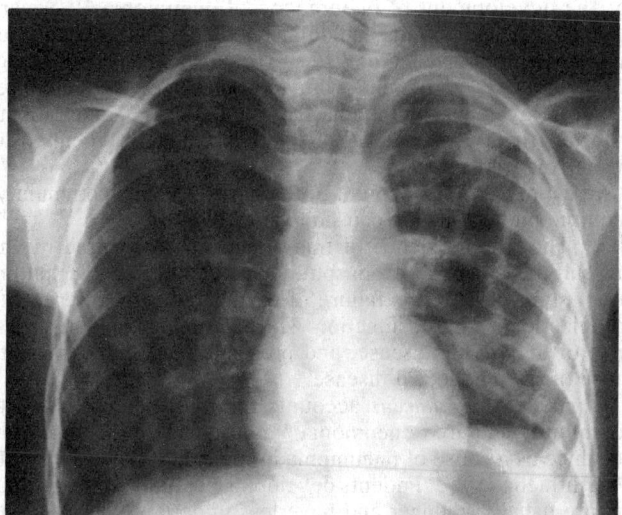

FIG. 7.   Pneumatocele formation in the left upper lobe of a patient with staphylococcal pneumonia.

segment of either lower lobe or the posterior segment of the upper lobes, depending on whether aspiration occurred in the dependent or upright position.[206] Chronic aspiration most commonly results in a bilateral lower lobe pneumonia, although it often may involve one side more than the other.[205]

Many viral pneumonias involve generalized destruction of ciliated epithelium with little radiologic distinction between the various viral etiologies. Initially, ciliated epithelial cells, goblet cells, and bronchial mucous gland cells are destroyed. Subsequent involvement may include terminal bronchioles and alveoli. Diffuse hemorrhagic congestion of alveolar septa with red blood cells and inflammatory edema fluid may be seen, especially with primary influenza pneumonia.[207] The x-ray film concomitants of these pathologic findings are varied and may be confusing if a secondary bacterial infection complicates the initial process. Diffuse and localized involvement with both interstitial and alveolar patterns have been noted (Fig. 8).[208] Peribronchial involvement with nodular infiltrates is a pattern often seen with varicella.

Mycoplasmal pneumonia often manifests with an interstitial pattern in a peribronchial distribution. As more edema fluid is elaborated, there may be rapid progression to lobar or sublobar consolidation. Once this consolidation stage is reached, radiologic differentiation between bacterial and mycoplasmal pneumonia is difficult. *Mycoplasma* is usually associated with lower lobe disease. Cavitation is rare, although pleural effusion may be seen in 20 percent of the cases.[209]

Legionnaires' disease may initially present with an x-ray picture similar to that of mycoplasmal pneumonia. A patchy interstitial or finely nodular pattern is seen in the lower lobe.[210] However, unlike mycoplasmal pneumonia, pneumonia with more than two-lobe involvement is commonly seen. Rapid progression and pleural effusions are also common.[211] Pneumonia caused by *L. micdadei* (Pittsburgh pneumonia agent) may present with pulmonary nodules, either single or multiple, as well as with segmental infiltrates. As in pneumonia caused by *L. pneumophila*, rapid radiologic progression of the disease is characteristic.[212]

It must be recognized that x-ray films are most helpful in conjunction with the clinical history and physical examination. This point was clearly shown by Tew et al.,[213] who evaluated readings of x-ray films of patients with pneumonia made without clinical information. Pneumonia was correctly identified as bacterial only 67 percent of the time and as viral only 65 percent of the time. Mycoplasmal pneumonia was incorrectly identified as bacterial 81 percent of the time.

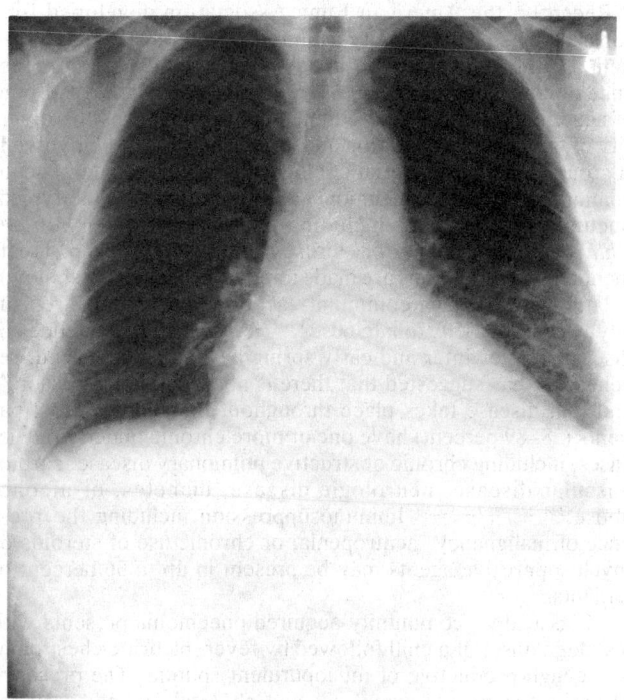

FIG. 8.   Bilateral involvement with a mixed interstitial-alveolar pattern in a patient with viral pneumonia.

Nuclear medicine procedures have been used to detect pneumonia. These procedures include ^{67}Ga-citrate scans, ^{111}In-labeled granulocytes, and ^{99m}Tc-DTPA aerosol clearance.[214] In general, these procedures have been utilized in patients with AIDS to define the presence of lung infection in the absence of abnormal chest radiographs. In patients with AIDS, diffuse uptake of gallium is usually seen with *Pneumocystis carinii* infection, but may also be seen with infection caused by *Mycobacterium avium* complex, CMV, *Cryptococcus neoformans,* and lymphoma. Localized uptake may be associated with bacterial disease. Focal uptake corresponding to lymph node areas has been associated with *Mycobacterium avium* complex, *Mycobacterium tuberculosis,* and lymphoma.

PNEUMONIA SYNDROMES

Acute Community-Acquired Pneumonia

As discussed previously, a long list of bacterial, fungal, viral, and protozoal agents may cause pneumonia. Since the most accessible assay (sputum Gram stain) is not definitive, and since all other assays require time, antibiotic therapy is usually begun empirically. Defining a series of pneumonia syndromes based on clinical, epidemiologic, radiographic, and laboratory parameters with a limited number of organisms commonly associated with each syndrome has helped the clinician to select rational empiric therapy based on the most likely organisms involved. It must be recognized that one cannot determine etiology based on any specific clinical, radiographic, or laboratory parameter. However, recognition of pneumonia syndromes continues to be an important first step in clinical practice.

The characteristics of the syndrome of acute community-acquired pneumonia as defined 20 years ago[59,62,63] and revised more recently[215–217] are changing.[218–228a] The patient population is becoming more elderly, includes more patients with significant coexistent diseases, and more patients who are immunosuppressed. Microbial agents now recognized as potential causes of community-acquired pneumonia were not recognized a decade ago.[223,226] As a result, community-acquired pneumonia has become somewhat more difficult to characterize.

Recently, the American Lung Association developed four subgroupings of community-acquired pneumonia based on patient age, need for hospitalization, severity of illness, and presence of coexisting disease.[228] This "splitting" of the syndrome of acute community-acquired pneumonia recognizes the diversity of the patient population and organisms presently involved. It groups together bacterial etiologies usually involved in acute community-acquired pneumonia and those involved in atypical pneumonia syndromes including *Mycoplasma pneumoniae, Chlamydia* spp., respiratory viruses, and *Legionella* spp. Treatment recommendations are made for each subgroup (see below).

Patients with acute community-acquired pneumonia are usually in their mid-50s to late 60s.[219–222] While peak incidences of disease in midwinter and early spring have been described, recent work has suggested that there is no "pneumonia season," and that disease takes place throughout the year.[223] Most patients (58–89 percent) have one or more chronic underlying diseases, including chronic obstructive pulmonary disease, cardiovascular disease, neurologic disease, diabetes, or alcohol abuse.[221,225–227,229,230] Immunosuppression including the presence of malignancy, neutropenia, or chronic use of steroids or myelosuppresive agents may be present in up to 36 percent of patients.[226]

"Classically" community-acquired pneumonia presents with a sudden onset of a chill followed by fever, pleuritic chest pain, and cough productive of mucopurulent sputum. The presence of various signs and symptoms and physical findings vary according to the age of the patient, therapy with antibiotics prior to presentation, and severity of illness. These classic findings in some combination are present in approximately 81 percent of patients with community-acquired pneumonia. Patients usually present after having been ill for a mean of 6 days.[224] Cough is noted in over 80 percent of patients and is productive in 60–80 percent.[223,226–230] Chest pain is present in approximately 30 percent of cases, chills in 40–50 percent, and true rigors in 15 percent.[221,223,226]

Physical examination reveals fever in 68–78 percent of patients, but may be seen less commonly in older populations. Tachypnea (respiratory rate greater than 24 breaths/min) is noted in 45–69 percent of patients, and tachycardia (pulse rate greater than 100 beats/min) is noted in 45 percent.[4,9] Rales are noted in 78 percent of patients, but signs of consolidation are noted in 29 percent.

Most commonly, the white blood cell count is in the range of 15–35,000/mm^3, and the differential cell count reveals an increased number of juvenile forms.[231] Leukopenia may be noted and is a poor prognostic sign.[232] The hematocrit and the red blood cell indices are usually normal. Sputum is thick and purulent and may be rust colored. The sputum Gram stain reveals numerous neutrophils and bacteria, usually with a single organism predominating. Chest films show areas of parenchymal involvement, usually in a bronchopneumonic pattern. There is moderate hypoxemia due to ventilation perfusion abnormalities. Even with rigorous laboratory evaluation, a microbiologic diagnosis may be made in only 50–70 percent of cases of community-acquired pneumonia.[217,223,226,229–231]

In the past, 50–90 percent of the cases of acute community-acquired pneumonia were caused by *S. pneumoniae*.[62,63,233] More recently, the relative importance of the *Pneumococcus* has been reported to be decreased. Various series report that 16–60 percent of the cases of acute community-acquired pneumonia are pneumococcal in origin.[215,217–227,234–236] The *pneumococcus* remains the leading cause of the syndrome of acute community-acquired pneumonia (as described above) in virtually all series.

Advanced age, cigarette smoking, institutionalization, dementia, seizures, malnutrition and the presence of chronic illnesses such as chronic obstructive pulmonary disease, chronic liver and kidney disease, congestive heart failure, and cerebrovascular disease have been identified as significant risk factors for the development of pneumococcal pneumonia.[237] Severe pneumococcal infections, including pneumonia, have been associated with prior splenectomy due to trauma or staging for Hodgkin's disease,[238,239] patients with abnormal immunoglobulin responses (myeloma, lymphoma, HIV infection),[240] and patients with functional asplenia due to systemic lupus erythematosus or marrow transplant.

An estimated 4–15 percent of the cases of acute community-acquired pneumonia are caused by *H. influenzae*.[59,63,217,234–236,241,242] The true incidence of this organism is obscured by the difficulty in isolating it from sputum and identifying it in sputum Gram stain, and by the failure of early studies to differentiate colonization from true infection. The mean age of patients, presence of underlying disease, and presentation are all similar to those of pneumococcal disease.

Staphylococcus aureus accounts for 2–10 percent of acute community-acquired pneumonia[243] and takes on increased importance as a cause of pneumonia in the elderly and in patients with influenza.[244,245] Patients developing postinfluenza pneumonia are usually younger and have less underlying disease than most other patients with community-acquired pneumonia. Clinical signs and symptoms of influenza are present but appear to resolve over several days. After a variable period of time ranging from 2 to 14 days, symptoms suddenly reappear, with the onset of shaking chills, pleuritic chest pain, and cough productive of purulent sputum. An elevated white blood cell count with a shift to the left, physical signs of pulmonary consolidation, and radiographic evidence of focal parenchymal disease appear. The sputum Gram stain is consistent with bacterial pneumonia. Although the pneumococcus still represents the most common etiologic agent, staphylococcal disease occurs with a higher frequency that that noted in noninfluenza-related, community-acquired pneumonia.[244,245]

Aerobic gram-negative bacteria, exclusive of *H. influenzae,* and mixed aerobic and anaerobic infections cause most of the remaining cases of acute community-acquired pneumonia. Gram-negative rods may cause 7–18 percent of pneumonia[234–236] and are particularly important pathogens in the elderly.

The importance of *Legionella* spp. in causing pneumonia varies greatly in different geographic areas. While incidences as high as 17–30 percent have been reported,[233,246] many centers report significantly lower rates.[222,223,226] No clinical features reliably distinguish *Legionella* spp. pneumonia from that caused by other bacteria. However, the presence of a high fever (>40°C), multilobar involvement, rapid progression of radiographic abnormalities, need for intensive care, gastrointestinal and neurologic abnormalities, elevated liver enzymes, and creatinine have all been associated with *Legionella* pneumonia.[226,246–248]

Recently, *Moraxella catarrhalis* has been identified as a cause of pneumonia.[249–251] The overall incidence of disease due to this bacterium is low, but it is an important pathogen in elderly patients with chronic obstructive pulmonary disease and various forms of immunosuppression.

In contrast to disease patterns in adults, viruses are the most important cause of pneumonia in young children. Respiratory syncytial virus and parainfluenza virus type 3 are the major pathogens. Other parainfluenza viruses and low-numbered adenovirus serotypes are also important.

Community Acquired Pneumonia in the Elderly

Pneumonia in the elderly is a major cause of morbidity and mortality and in some series represents the leading cause of death (see Ch. 295).[252] The clinical presentation may be more subtle than in younger populations, with more gradual onset, less frequent complaints of chills and rigors, and less fever.[226,253–256]

The classic findings of cough, fever, and dyspnea may be absent in over half of elderly patients.[253] Patients may present with a decline in functional status, weakness, subtle changes in mental status, anorexia, or abdominal pain.

While the incidence of fever appears to be similar in elderly vs. younger populations, the degree of fever appears to be lower in the older age groups.[223,226] Tachypnea (respiratory rate greater than 24 breaths/min) is noted in up to 69 percent of patients, and tachycardia (pulse greater than 100 beats/min) is noted in 45 percent.[221,226] While rales are common and are noted in 78 percent of patients, signs of true consolidation are found in only 29 percent.

Bacteremia, metastatic foci of infection, and death are more frequent in older populations.[59,78,232] While the etiologies of pneumonia in the elderly follow the general pattern noted in younger patients, aerobic gram-negative bacilli and *Staphylococcus aureus* play a more important role, especially in patients in nursing homes and extended care facilities.[253–257] Of the gram-negative organisms, *K. pneumoniae* and *H. influenzae,* including nontypeable strains, appear especially important. The elderly also appear to be at high risk of infection from organisms such as group B streptococci, *Moraxella catarrhalis,* and *Legionella* spp.[249–251,258] Polymicrobial infections have also been noted to be increased in the elderly.[78] Increased oropharyngeal colonization with aerobic gram-negative bacilli has been documented in the elderly, with this increase in colonization paralleling the level of care needed by the patient.[259] Other factors that have been associated with increased colonization include prior use of antibiotics, serious underlying disease, decreased activity, diabetes, alcohol abuse, and incontinence.[254,259–261]

Community-Acquired Pneumonia in Patients with AIDS

The etiology of community-acquired pneumonia in patients with AIDS is also different from that noted in other populations. Prior to the development of effective prophylactic regimens, *Pneumocystis carinii* pneumonia occurred in approximately 85 percent of patients at some time during their course.[262,263] While prophylaxis has significantly reduced the incidence of both primary and secondary episodes of *Pneumocystis* pneumonia, it remains a significant pathogen in AIDS patients.[264] Bacterial agents such as *S. pneumoniae* and *H. influenzae* are frequent pathogens, and a greater incidence of bacteremic disease is associated with community-acquired pneumonia. Cytomegalovirus, *Mycobacterium tuberculosis, Cryptococcus neoformans,* and *Rhodococcus equi*[264] also play important roles as etiologic agents (see Chs. 102 and 105).

Severe Community-Acquired Pneumonia

Approximately 10 percent of community-acquired pneumonias are severe enough to require intensive care and/or mechanical ventilation. These cases of "severe community-acquired pneumonia" have been recently reviewed.[221,265,267] *Streptococcus pneumoniae* and *Legionella pneumophila* are the organisms most commonly involved in causing severe community-acquired pneumonia. Gram-negative bacilli, especially *Klebsiella* spp., must be considered in patients who have significant underlying disease such as chronic obstructive pulmonary disease, diabetes, and alcohol abuse.[265,266] In some series, *Mycoplasma pneumoniae,* one of the agents causing atypical pneumonia to be discussed below, may be involved in up to 11 percent of community-acquired pneumonias requiring intensive care.

A series of criteria have been developed that aid in identifying patients who may have severe community-acquired pneumonia and may require intensive care.[221,268–270] These include

1. Respiratory frequency above 30 breaths/min
2. PaO_2/FIO_2 less than 250 or PO_2 less than 50–60 mmHg breathing room air
3. Need for mechanical ventilation

4. Chest radiographs showing bilateral involvement, multilobar involvement, and/or significant progression of disease in the first 48 hours of admission
5. Hypotension (systolic BP <90 mmHg or diastolic BP <60 mmHg)
6. Requirement for vasopressors
7. Urine output less than 20 ml/hr or less than 80 ml over a 4-hour period
8. Abnormal mental status

Mortality rates in patients with severe pneumonia have ranged from 20–53 percent, which is higher than the 6–24 percent noted in all community-acquired pneumonias.[221,265–267] Tachypnea (>30 breaths/min), diastolic blood pressure less than 60 mmHg, and blood urea nitrogen above 7 mmol/liter have been shown to be independently associated with death from pneumonia.[269,270] Other parameters identified with increased mortality include underlying neoplastic disease, age above 65 years, absence of pleuritic chest pain, change in mental status, and pneumonia caused by *S. aureus* or gram-negative bacilli.[270]

Slowly Resolving Community-Acquired Pneumonia

The natural history of adequately treated community-acquired pneumonia is usually that of prompt resolution.[271] In healthy young military personnel recovering from *Pneumococcal* pneumonia, fever resolved after 2.5 days, cough after 7.9 days, and "crackles" on physical examination of the chest by 8 days.[272] Normalization of the white blood cell count occurred by day 4. Patients who are older or who have significant coexisting underlying disease have more gradual resolution of signs and symptoms. Radiographic abnormalities may take 4–10 weeks to normalize, with younger (<50 years of age) patients resolving more quickly.[273–275] Patients who fail to resolve their radiographic abnormalities by day 30, despite clearing of signs and symptoms, usually have significant underlying pulmonary disease such as emphysema, chronic bronchitis, pneumoconiosis, or asthma. Pneumonia caused by certain agents such as *Legionella* spp. will resolve slowly, even in the absence of underlying pulmonary disease or coexistent disease. Clearing of 8–12 weeks or longer is usually seen.[275]

Slowly resolving pneumonia has been defined as less than 50 percent clearing of radiographic abnormalities at 2 weeks and less than complete clearing of abnormalities by 4 weeks.[274,275] Host factors such as age above 50 years, history of alcoholism, and presence of significant underlying diseases (COPD, diabetes, congestive heart failure, asthma, malignancy) have been found to be associated with slow resolution of pneumonia. *Streptococcus pneumoniae* and *Legionella* spp. are the organisms most often associated with slowly resolving pneumonia. In the setting of these host factors or these organisms, slow resolution of pneumonia should not necessitate a vigorous reevaluation looking for another disease process, but rather watchful waiting.[276]

Atypical Pneumonia Syndrome

By the late 1930s most of the main bacterial etiologies of pneumonia had been defined. In 1938, Hobart Reiman[277] described a small number of patients with a clinical picture that was "atypical" in that episodes began as a mild respiratory tract illness that was followed by an atypical pneumonia with dyspnea and cough without sputum.[278] This complex has been associated with a variety of agents, but most commonly associated with *Mycoplasma pneumoniae.*

The older child (>5 years of age), the adolescent, and young adult are at greatest risk for developing infection with *M. pneumoniae.* This agent accounts for 1–10 percent of cases of community-acquired pneumonia. The majority of cases are in patients less than 40 years old. Increased incidence of disease and true epidemics have been documented in relatively enclosed populations of young adults at military bases, colleges, and boarding schools.[279–281] Mycoplasmal infection occurs throughout the year, although a relative increase in incidence is noted in the late summer and fall. In contrast, adenovirus infection, another cause of atypical pneumonia, most commonly occurs between January and April, outbreaks occurring primarily in military recruit camps.[279,281,282]

The course of the atypical pneumonias is characterized by up to 10 days of symptoms before presentation.[224]

In its classic form, mycoplasma presents itself with constitutional symptoms and a progression from the upper to lower respiratory tract. Sore throat is often the initial finding. Bullous myringitis is seen in only about 5 percent of cases, but when present is suggestive of mycoplasmal infection. Fever, malaise, coryza, headache, and cough represent the major clinical findings. Pleuritic chest pain, splinting, and respiratory distress are not usually seen. Moist or crepitant rales may be heard. Sputum production is variable, and although it is purulent in one-third to one-half of the cases, Gram stain and culture of sputum usually reveal mouth flora. White blood cell counts greater than 10,000/mm^3 are uncommon, occurring in approximately 20 percent of the patients.[86] An elevated sedimentation rate is noted in about 25 percent of the cases.[224] Pulmonary involvement seen on x-ray films is commonly more extensive than the physical examination would indicate. Unilateral or bilateral patchy infiltrates in one or more segments, usually in the lower lobes, are noted in a bronchial or peribronchial distribution. Upper lobe involvement and pleural effusions are rare. Progression of the x-ray picture, despite a stable clinical picture, may be seen. The overall clinical course in most cases is benign. Disappearance of constitutional symptoms is usually noted in the first and second weeks, although cough and x-ray changes may persist for several weeks. Occasionally, *Mycoplasma pneumoniae* infection may present as severe community-acquired pneumonia requiring intensive care.[221] A large number of extrapulmonary manifestations may occur with *Mycoplasma pneumoniae*, including involvement of skin, central nervous system, blood, and kidneys. These are reviewed in Chapter 161.

Other etiologic agents involved in the atypical pneumonia syndrome include *Coxiella burnetti* (Q fever), *Chlamydia psittaci* (psittacosis), *Chlamydia trachomatis*, and *Chlamydia pneumoniae* (TWAR).

Chlamydia trachomatis has been described as a pulmonary pathogen in immunocompromised as well as healthy hosts.[283–285] Productive cough, myalgias, and fever associated with diffuse nonsegmental infiltrates appear most commonly. The agent has also been associated with chronic pneumonia in neonates and infants. Onset occurs at 2–3 weeks of age and is associated with tachypnea, a staccato cough with periods of cyanosis and emesis, lack of fever, and diffuse interstitial and patchy alveolar infiltrates on chest films. Elevated IgG and IgM levels and absolute eosinophilia have also been noted.

Chlamydia pneumoniae (TWAR) has emerged as an important cause of atypical pneumonia and may account for up to 6–12 percent of community-acquired pneumonias.[286–289] Though disease is uncommon in those less than 5 years of age, serologic evidence of infection has been noted in over 50 percent of adults.[290] Disease usually occurs sporadically, though several epidemics have been well documented. The majority of infections are either asymptomatic or produce mild symptoms.[291] As with mycoplasmal infection, sore throat and hoarseness herald the onset of pneumonia, though the progression of symptoms appears slower than that noted with mycoplasma or viral pneumonia.[290,291] Cough may begin after several days to weeks, suggesting a biphasic illness. Hoarseness and sinus tenderness appear more commonly than in patients infected with mycoplasma or viruses.[290] The white blood cell count is rarely elevated. Pneumonia with *C. pneumoniae* is usually mild, though complete recovery may be slow. Cough and malaise may persist for

weeks to months. Reinfection occurs and appears to be more mild than primary infection and is usually not associated with pneumonia. Chronic and latent infection have also been described. *Chlamydia pneumoniae* infections have been associated with extrapulmonary manifestations, including bronchitis, otitis, sinusitis, pericarditis, myocarditis, and endocarditis.[292] Most recently, chlamydial infection has been associated seroepidemiologically with coronary artery disease. Furthermore, *C. pneumoniae* organisms have been demonstrated in atheromatous plaques.[293,294] Despite these interesting findings, no clear cause and effect relationship has been established.

Of the viral agents associated with atypical pneumonia in adults, influenza A and B, adenovirus types 3, 4, and 7 (especially in military recruits), parainfluenza virus,[295] and respiratory syncytial virus (especially in the elderly and immune-suppressed) are the most common.[296–298] Reports of other viral agents causing pneumonia are scant but have included rhinovirus,[192] enterovirus,[193] coronavirus,[299] and the herpes viruses.[300]

Legionnaires' disease may present as either an acute, community-acquired pneumonia or an atypical pneumonia. Although early symptoms of malaise, muscle aches, headache, and nonproductive cough resemble the onset of a "viral syndrome," the rapid progression of pulmonary symptoms is noteworthy. Abdominal pain and gastrointestinal symptoms, especially diarrhea and mental status changes, have been noted. Physical examination reveals only rales; x-ray films show patchy interstitial or nodular infiltrates that may progress rapidly to more widespread consolidation. Approximately 50 percent of cases have bilateral involvement. Transient impairment of renal and liver function, abnormally low serum phosphorus levels, and elevated serum creatinine phosphokinase levels have been described.[210,111,301,302] For the most part, it is not possible to distinguish clinically legionnaires' disease from other bacterial pneumonias.[246]

Pneumonia in the Setting of Aspiration

The clinical setting in which aspiration occurs involves any disease state in which consciousness is altered and the normal gag and swallowing reflexes are abnormal.

Three major syndromes are recognized as a consequence of aspiration: chemical pneumonitis, bronchial obstruction secondary to aspiration of particulate matter, and bacterial aspiration pneumonia.[303,304] Although chemical pneumonitis and mechanical obstruction usually cause acute symptoms, aspiration pneumonia is more insidious, with symptoms usually occurring gradually several days after the initial episode of aspiration. Pneumonitis, necrotizing pneumonia, abscess, and empyema are common. Symptoms often include fever, weight loss, and productive cough. Putrid sputum is produced in 50 percent of the cases.[80,206] Anemia and an elevated white blood cell count are frequently associated findings. The bacteriologic findings in aspiration pneumonia reflect the flora of the oropharynx, and the importance of periodontal disease in this regard has been noted. Anaerobic bacteria, alone (45–58 percent of the cases) or in combination with aerobes (41–46 percent), are most commonly seen when adequate culture techniques are used.[21,80]

Bacteroides spp., *Porphyromonas* spp., *Prevotella melaninogenica*, *Fusobacterium* spp., and anaerobic gram-positive cocci are the predominant anaerobes isolated. In community-acquired aspiration pneumonia, *Streptococcus* spp. are the most common aerobic isolates.[21,304,305] *Moraxella catarrhalis* and *Eikenella corrodens* may also be involved.[306] In contrast, gram-negative bacilli and *Staphylococcus aureus* are the most commonly isolated aerobes from nosocomial aspiration pneumonia.[304,305]

Pulmonary Infiltrates with Eosinophilia

Pulmonary infiltrates with eosinophilia (PIE) is a syndrome associated with a variety of clinical entities, only some of which are infectious in etiology.[308-310] Pulmonary eosinophilia with transient, peripheral pulmonary infiltrates and minimal symptoms has been associated with *Ascaris* and *Strongyloides* infections. Prolonged pulmonary eosinophilia associated with weight loss, fever, cough, and dyspnea may be due to tuberculosis, brucellosis, psittacosis, coccidioidomycosis, histoplasmosis, and parasitic infections including ascariasis, strongyloidiasis, paragonomiasis, echinococcosis, visceral larva migrans, cutaneous larva migrans, *Schistosoma, Dirofilaria immitis, Entamoeba histolytica,* and infection with *Ancylostoma* spp. Noninfectious etiologies include drug allergy, sarcoidosis, eosinophilic leukemia, Hodgkin's disease and hypersensitivity pneumonitis (i.e., pigeon breeders' disease).[206,311] A PIE syndrome has been associated with *Pneumocystis carinii* pneumonia in AIDS patients.[312]

It has been suggested that chronic eosinophilic pneumonia may represent a unique clinical entity that is a form of collagen-vascular disease or an infection in a hyperimmune patient.[313-315] Interstitial infiltrates, focal interstitial fibrosis, bronchiolitis obliterans, microabscesses, and sarcoid-like granulomas are characteristic pathologic features. A rapid response to steroids has been reported.[315]

Tropical eosinophilia consists of myalgia, fatigue, weight loss, and anorexia associated with cough, frequently with nocturnal exacerbations, dyspnea, and peripheral eosinophilia in patients who have lived in or visited the tropics. X-ray film changes are distinctive and include increased interstitial markings with 2- to 4-mm nodules throughout the lungs with preferential involvement of the bases. Most cases represent microfilarial infection and can be treated with diethylcarbamazine.

Other causes of PIE syndrome include bronchopulmonary *Aspergillus*, which should be suspected when PIE presents with asthma and pulmonary vasculitis. Patients with the Churg-Strauss syndrome[309] frequently have eosinophilia along with allergic angiitis and granulomatosis and present with asthma and diffuse pulmonary infiltrates.

Nosocomial Pneumonia and Pneumonia in the Immunosuppressed Host

Nosocomial pneumonia accounts for approximately 10–20 percent of all nosocomial infections and is the leading cause of infection-related mortality (20–50 percent) in hospitalized patients.[316-319] Important risk factors for the development of disease include advanced age, severity of underlying disease, intubation, use of respiratory equipment, presence of nasogastric tubes, altered mental status, surgery, and previous use of antibiotics.[320-323] Use of antacids and histamine type 2 blockers that raise the gastric pH have been shown to increase stomach colonization with aerobic gram-negative rods. Whether this leads to an increase in nosocomial pneumonia is uncertain.[324-329] Approximately 60 percent of cases of nosocomial pneumonia are caused by aerobic gram-negative bacilli, with members of the family Enterobacteriaceae *(K. pneumoniae, E. coli, Serratia marcescens, Enterobacter* spp.) and *Pseudomonas* spp. accounting for the majority of these. *Staphylococcus aureus* causes 13–20 percent of nosocomial pneumonia and appears to be more common in burn units and in patients with wound infections.[330] In contrast to its prominent role in community-acquired pneumonia, *S. pneumoniae* causes only 3–8 percent of nosocomial pneumonias.[77,331] Anaerobic bacteria have been isolated in up to 35 percent of cases of nosocomial pneumonia, though usually fewer than 5 percent of infections are thought to be due to these organisms.[332,333] Pneumonia caused by *Legionella* spp. has been reported and may occur sporadically and as part of outbreaks.[334] Nosocomial viral infections have been increasingly recognized in children and adults. Respiratory syncytial virus, influenza, and parainfluenza make up the majority of etiologies.[335]

Pneumonia in the immunosuppressed host represents an important subset of nosocomial pneumonia and deserves special emphasis.[6,336] In patients with nonlymphocytic leukemia, 25 percent of all documented infections are pulmonary.[337] In patients with acute leukemia, 64 percent of fatal bacteremias of known cause originate in the lung, the majority of episodes caused by enteric gram-negative bacilli.[337,338] Approximately 8–16 percent of renal transplant recipients, up to 25 percent of liver transplant recipients, and up to 50 percent of bone marrow transplant patients will develop pneumonia at some time during their course.[339-343] Again, the most common bacterial pathogens are gram-negative bacilli. As with other nosocomial pneumonias, pneumonias in the compromised host are most commonly caused by *K. pneumoniae, E. coli,* or *Pseudomonas aeruginosa.* In some series these organisms cause 50 percent of all infections, with mixed gram-negative infections accounting for another 20 percent.[344,345]

In addition to bacterial pathogens, a variety of nonbacterial agents are of etiologic importance. These include fungi *(Aspergillus* spp., agents of mucormycosis, *Candida* spp.), protozoa *(Pneumocystis carinii, Toxoplasma gondii)*, parasites *(Strongyloides)*, and viruses (varicella-zoster virus, CMV). Chapter 282 and Part IV, Section B discuss more fully nosocomial pneumonia and infections in the compromised host, respectively.

THERAPY OF PNEUMONIA

The challenge involved in selecting empiric antibiotic therapy for a patient with pneumonia is difficult because there is no sure way to distinguish between disease caused by agents that cause "typical" acute bacterial pneumonia and those involved with "atypical" pneumonia.[224,227,346] Certain features characterize pneumonia caused by *Streptococcus pneumoniae* (older patients, more underlying disease, more lower respiratory tract symptoms, elevated white blood cell count) vs. that caused by *Mycoplasma pneumoniae* (younger patients, fewer underlying diseases, more upper respiratory tract findings, lower white count), or *Legionella* spp. (older patients, higher temperatures, more rapidly progressive disease, tendency for development of neurologic problems, liver enzyme abnormalities, and renal abnormalities). However, the great degree of overlap makes use of these criteria limited for the individual patient. Despite these problems, the goal of therapy remains to treat as specifically as possible while covering the most likely organisms.

The first decision confronting the clinician is whether the patient needs to be hospitalized. Patients with respiratory distress, high fever, hypotension (systolic blood pressure <100 mmHg), hypoxemia (PO$_2$ <55 mmHg on room air), altered mental status, suppurative or metastatic infectious complications, the presence of significant coexistent disease, and/or severe laboratory abnormalities (metabolic acidosis, increased blood urea nitrogen/creatinine ratio, hypernatremia with a serum sodium >155 mEq/liter) should be considered for hospitalization.[347,348] Issues such as the patients' ability to return to the clinic and their reliability in taking oral medications need to be considered in this evaluation as well.

The next problem is determining the most likely etiology of the pneumonia. If diagnostic studies, as described above, yield a likely etiologic organism, then specific therapy should be initiated. However, most patients will fall into a group where a specific diagnosis cannot be established with certainty.

For a patient who does not require hospitalization and who is relatively young (<50 years old) and for whom no clear distinction between typical (e.g., bacterial) or atypical (mycoplasmal, chlamydial) pneumonia can be made, both types of organisms should be covered (Table 4). Antibacterial therapy should address the possibility of infection with *Streptococcus pneumoniae* and *H. influenzae.* An oral second-generation cephalosporin such as cefuroxime axetil or an oral β-lactam/β-lactamase inhibitor combination such as amoxicillin-clavulanic acid both in combination with erythromycin would be reasonable choices.

TABLE 4. Strategies for Emperic Therapy of Patients with Pneumonia

Outpatient Therapy (Oral Antibiotics)		Inpatient Therapy (Parenteral Antibiotics)		
Signs and Symptoms Consistent with Bacterial, Mycoplasmal, or Chlamydial Etiology	Signs and Symptoms Strongly Suggesting Bacterial Etiology	Moderately Severe Illness	Debilitated Elderly	ICU Admission
Second-generation cephalosporin[a] + erythromycin OR Amoxicillin/clavulanic acid + erythromycin OR Newer macrolide/azalide[b]	Second-generation cephalosporin[a] OR Amoxicillin/ clavulanic acid	Second- or third-generation cephalosporin[c] ± erythromycin OR Ampicillin/sulbactam ± erythromycin	Third-generation cephalosporin[d] ± aminoglycoside ± erythromycin OR Extended-spectrum penicillin[e] + aminoglycoside ± erythromycin OR β-Lactam/β-lactamase inhibitor combination[f] + aminoglycoside ± erythromycin	Third-generation cephalosporin[d] ± aminoglycoside + erythromycin OR Extended-spectrum penicillin + aminoglycoside + erythromycin OR β-Lactam/β-lactamase inhibitor combination[f] + aminoglycoside + erythromycin

Other agents within the same class may be used.
[a] Cefuroxime axetil.
[b] Clarithromycin/azithromycin.
[c] Cefuroxime (second-generation); cefotaxime, ceftriaxone (third generation).
[d] If Pseudomonas is suspected, use ceftazadime.
[e] Ticarcillin, piperacillin, mezlocillin.
[f] Ticarcillin-clavulanic acid.

Recent reports of significant resistance of *Streptococcus pneumoniae* for trimethoprim-sulfamethoxazole have made this choice for the antibacterial component of combination therapy less attractive.[349] Newer azalide and macrolide compounds (azithromycin and clarithromycin) provide broader antibacterial coverage than does erythromycin and provide activity against *H. influenzae* as well as *Mycoplasma pneumoniae, S. pneumoniae,* and *Chlamydia* spp. They may therefore be used as monotherapy in this situation. Erythromycin or tetracycline monotherapy, choices suggested by the American Thoracic Society,[228] are less attractive. Erythromycin has limited activity against *H. influenzae* and significant resistance of *Streptococcus pneumoniae* for tetracycline has been reported.[240]

In older patients (>50 years old), in whom atypical pneumonia is unlikely and a bacterial etiology is strongly suspected and who are not ill enough to be hospitalized, a second-generation oral cephalosporin or β-lactam/β-lactamase inhibitor combination (without erythromycin) would represent reasonable therapeutic options.

Hospital admission is required for a seriously ill patient with acute community-acquired pneumonia. Those with a nondiagnostic sputum examination should be treated for *Streptococcus pneumoniae, H. influenzae, Staphylococcus aureus,* and perhaps *Legionella pneumophila.* Parenteral therapy is indicated. A second-generation cephalosporin such as cefuroxime or a third-generation cephalosporin such as cefotaxime or ceftriaxone or a β-lactam/β-lactamase inhibitor combination such as ampicillin-sulbactam could be utilized with erythromycin added for *Legionella* coverage.

Elderly or debilitated patients with significant underlying disease and patients from nursing homes may have infection caused by aerobic gram-negative rods. Combination therapy with a third-generation cephalosporin (cefotaxime, ceftriaxone, or ceftazidine if infection with *Pseudomonas aeruginosa* is suspected) or an extended-spectrum penicillin (ticarcillin, mezlocillin) or β-lactam/β-lactamase inhibitor combinations (ticarcillin-clavulanic acid, or piperacillin/tazobactam) all plus an aminoglycoside would be reasonable regimens. A paucity of organisms in the sputum should suggest the possible presence of *Legionella* and the need for erythromycin therapy.

In patients with community-acquired pneumonia for whom intensive care monitoring is necessary, antibiotic therapy should be directed toward *Streptococcus pneumoniae,* aerobic gram-negative bacilli, and *Legionella.* Erythromycin should therefore be added to the regimens noted above.

Aspiration pneumonia and lung abscess are discussed in Chapter 52. Therapy for nosocomial pneumonia is discussed in Chapter 282.

REFERENCES

1. Osler W. The Principles and Practice of Medicine. 4th ed. New York: D. Appleton; 1901:108.
2. Advanced Report of Final Mortality Statistics. v. 42. National Center for Health Statistics; 1992.
3. Johanson WG Jr, Gould KG Jr. Lung defense mechanisms. Basics RD. 1977; 6:1–6.
4. Green G. In defense of the lung. Am Rev Respir Dis. 1970;102:691–703.
5. Sibille Y, Reynolds HY. Macrophage and polymorphonuclear neutrophils in lung defense and injury. Am Rev Respir Dis. 1990;141:471–501.
6. Shelhamer JH (moderator), Toews GB, Masur H, et al. Respiratory disease in the immunosuppressed patient. Ann Intern Med. 1992;117:415–31.
7. Reynolds HY. Pulmonary host defenses. Chest. 1989;95(Suppl):223S–30S.
8. Mason CM, Nelson S. Normal host defenses and impairments associated with the delayed resolution of pneumonia. Semin Respir Infect. 1992;7: 243–55.
9. Reynolds H. Normal and defective respiratory host defense. In: Pennington JE, ed. Respiratory Infections: Diagnosis and Management. 2nd ed. New York: Raven Press; 1988:1–33.
10. Coonrod J. The role of extracellular bactericidal factors in pulmonary host defense. Semin Respir Infect. 1986;1:118–29.
11. Busse WW. Pathogenesis and sequelae of respiratory infections. Rev Infect Dis. 1991;13(Suppl 6):S477–85.
12. Reynolds HY. Lung inflammation: Normal host defense or a complication of some diseases. Annu Rev Med. 1987;38:295–323.
13. Neiderman MS, Merrill WW, Polonski LM, et al. Influence of sputum IgA and elastase on tracheal cell bacterial adherence. Am Rev Respir Dis. 1981; 133:255–60.
14. Neiderman MS, Merrill WW, Ferrante RD, et al. Nutritional status and bacterial binding in the lower respiratory tract in patients with chronic tracheostomy. Ann Intern Med. 1984;100:795–800.
15. Palmer LB, Merrill WW, Neiderman MS, et al. Bacterial adherence to respiratory tract cells—relationship between in vivo and in vitro pH and bacterial attachment. Am Rev Respir Dis. 1986;133:784–8.
16. Lipscomb MF, Onofrio JM, Nash EJ, et al. A morphological study of the role of phagocytes in the clearance of *Staphylococcus aureus* from the lung. J Reticuloendothel Soc. 1983;33:429–42.
17. MacNee W, Selby C. Neutrophil kinetics in the lung. Clin Sci. 1990;79: 97–107.
18. Standiford TJ, Kunkel SL, Basha MA, et al. Interleukin-8 gene expression by a pulmonary epithelial cell line—A model for cytokine networks in the lung. J Clin Invest. 1990;86:1945–53.
19. Strieter RM, Kunkel S, Showell H, et al. Endothelial cell gene expression of a neutrophil chemotactic factor by TNF-α, LPS, and IL-Iβ. Science. 1989; 243:1467–9.
20. Suntil K, Takemura T, Tschachlea E, et al. Dendritic cells with antigen-presenting capability reside in airway epithelium, lung parenchyma and viceral pleura. J Exp Med. 1986;163:436–51.
21. Harris SE, Nelson S, Astry CL, et al. Endotoxin-induced suppression of pulmonary antibacterial defenses against *Staphylococcus aureus.* Am Rev Respir Dis. 1988;138:1439–43.
22. Bartlett J, Gorbach S, Finegold S. The bacteriology of aspiration pneumonia. Am J Med. 1974;56:202–7.
23. Huxley EJ, Viroslav J, Gray WR, et al. Pharyngeal aspiration in normal adults and patients with depressed consciousness. Am J Med. 1978;64:564–8.
24. Green GM, Carolin D. The depressant effect of cigarette smoke on the in vitro antibacterial activity of alveolar macrophages. N Engl J Med. 1967; 276:421–7.
25. Warshauer D, Goldstein E, Akers T, et al. Effect of influenza viral infection

on the ingestion and killing of bacteria by alveolar macrophages. Am Rev Respir Dis. 1977;115:269–77.

26. Nelson S, Chidiac C, Bagby G, et al. Endotoxin-induced suppression of lung host defenses. J Med. 1990;21:85–103.

27. Green GM, Kass EH. The role of the alveolar macrophage in the clearance of bacteria from the lung. J Exp Med. 1964;119:167–76.

28. MacGregor RR. Alcohol and immune defense. JAMA. 1986;256:1474–9.

29. Schopf RE, Trompter M, Bork K, et al. Effects of ethanol and acetaldehyde on phagocytic function. Arch Dermatol Rev. 1985;277:131–7.

30. Nelson S, Bagby GJ, Bainton BG, et al. The effects of acute and chronic alcoholism on tumor necrosis factor and the inflammatory response. J Infect Dis. 1989;160:422–9.

31. Mason CM. The pathogenesis and presentation of nosocomial pneumonia. Crit Care Rev. 1991;2:145–55.

32. Espesito AL. Aspirin impairs antibacterial mechanisms in experimental pneumococcal pneumonia. Am Rev Respir Dis. 1984;130:857–62.

33. Nelson S, Summer WR, Terry PB, et al. Erythromycin-induced suppression of pulmonary antibacterial defenses: A potential mechanism of superinfection in the lung. Am Rev Respir Dis. 1987;136:1207–12.

34. Nelson S, Summer WR, Jakab EJ. Aminophylline-induced suppression of pulmonary antibacterial defenses. Am Rev Respir Dis. 1985;131:923–7.

35. Green GM, Kass EH. The influence of bacterial species on pulmonary resistance to infection in mice subjected to hypoxia, cold stress and ethanolic intoxication. Br J Exp Pathol. 1965;46:360–6.

36. Coffin DL, Gardner DE, Holzman RS, et al. Influence of ozone on pulmonary cells. Arch Environ Health. 1968;16:633–6.

37. Ehrich R, Henry MC. Chronic toxicity of nitrogen dioxide. 1. Effect on resistance to bacterial pneumonia. Arch Environ Health. 1968;17:860–5.

38. LaForce FM, Mullane JF, Boehme RF, et al. The effect of pulmonary edema on antibacterial defenses of the lung. J Lab Clin Med. 1973;82:634–48.

39. Huber GL, LaForce FM, Mason RJ, et al. Impairment of pulmonary bacterial defense mechanisms by immunosuppressive agents. Surg Forum. 1970;21: 285–6.

40. Davis L, Beck JM, Shellito J. Update: HIV infection and pulmonary host defenses. Semin Respir Infect. 1993;8:75–85.

41. Gyetko MR, Toews GB. Immunology of the aging lung. Clin Chest Med. 1993;14:379–91.

42. Simons RJ, Reynolds HY. Altered immune status in the elderly. Semin Respir Infect. 1990;5:251–9.

43. Granton JT, Grossman RF. Community-acquired pneumonia in the elderly patient. Clin Chest Med. 1993;14:537–53.

44. Winterbauer RH, Bedon GA, Bal WC Jr. Recurrent pneumonia: Predisposing illness and clinical patterns in 158 patients. Ann Intern Med. 1969;70: 689–700.

45. Roth RM, Gleckman RA. Recurrent bacterial pneumonia: A contemporary perspective. South Med J. 1985;78:573–9.

46. Ekdahl K, Braconier JH, Rollof J. Recurrent pneumonia: A review of 90 adult patients. Scand J Infect Dis. 1992;24:71–6.

47. Geppert EF. Chronic recurrent pneumonia. Semin Respir Infect. 1992;7: 282–8.

48. Donowitz GR, Mandell GL. Clinical presentation and unusual infections. In: Gallin JI, Fauci AS, eds. Advances in Host Defense Mechanisms. v. 3. New York: Raven Press; 1983;55–75.

49. Donabedian H, Gallin JI. The hyperimmunoglobulin E recurrent infection (Jobs) syndrome. Medicine. 1983;62:195–208.

50. Beck S, Heiner DC. Selective immunoglobulin G₄ deficiency and recurrent infections of the respiratory tract. Am Rev Respir Dis. 1981;124:94–6.

51. Ammann AJ, Hong R. Selective IgA deficiency: Presentation of 30 cases and a review of the literature. Medicine. 1971;50:223–36.

52. Eliasson R, Mossberg B, Camner P, et al. The immotile-cilia syndrome. N Engl J Med. 1977;297:1–6.

53. Kartagener M. Zur Pathologie der Bronchiektasien: Bronkiektasien lei situs inversus. Beitr Klin Tuberk. 1933;83:489–501.

54. Handelsman DJ, Conway AJ, Boylan LM, et al. Young's syndrome: Obstructive azospermia and chronic sinopulmonary infections. N Engl J Med. 1984; 310:3–9.

55. Savic B, Birtel FJ, Tholen W, et al. Lung sequestration: Report of seven cases and review of 540 published cases. Thorax. 1979;34:96–101.

56. Iverson LIG, May IA, Samson PC. Pulmonary complications in benign esophageal disease. Am J Surg. 1973;126:223–8.

57. Grayston JT, Alexander ER, Kenny GE, et al. Mycoplasma pneumoniae infections: Clinical and epidemiological studies. JAMA. 1965;191:369–74.

58. Murray HW, Masur H, Senterfit L, et al. The protean manifestations of mycoplasma pneumoniae infection in adults. Am J Med. 1975;58:229–42.

59. Dorff GJ, Rytel MW, Farmer SG, et al. Etiologies and characteristic features of pneumonias in a municipal hospital. Am J Med Sci. 1973;266:349–58.

60. Bloch AB, Rieder HL, Kelly CD, et al. The epidemiology of tuberculosis in the United States. Semin Respir Infect. 1989;4:157–70.

61. Braun MM, Coté TR, Rabkin CS. Trends in death with tuberculosis during the AIDS era. JAMA. 1993;269:2865–8.

62. Fekety FR, Caldwell J, Grump D, et al. bacteria, viruses, and mycoplasmas in acute pneumonia in adults. Am Rev Respir Dis. 1971;104:499–507.

63. Sullivan RJ, Dowdle WR, Marine WM, et al. Adult pneumonia in a general hospital: Etiology and host risk factors. Arch Intern Med. 1972;129:935–42.

64. Lepow ML, Balassanian N, Emmerich A, et al. Interrelationships of viral, mycoplasmal and bacterial agents in uncomplicated pneumonia. Am Rev Respir Dis. 1968;97:533–45.

65. Martin CM, Kunin CM, Gottlieb LS, et al. Asian influenza A in Boston, 1957–1958. II. Severe staphylococcal pneumonia complicating influenza. Arch Intern Med. 1959;103:532–42.

66. Sprunt K. Infection in chronic lung disease. Bull NY Acad Med. 1972;48: 698–703.

67. Griffith DE, Mazurek GH. Pneumonia in chronic obstructive lung disease. Infect Dis Clin North Am. 1991;5:467–84.

68. Davies BI. *Moraxella catarrhalis:* Clinical significant therapeutic problems. Infect Dis Newslett. 1991;10:73–7.

69. Wright PW, Wallace RJ, Shepard JR. A descriptive study of 42 cases of *Branhamella catarrhalis* pneumonia. Am J Med. 1990;88(Suppl 5A): SA25–75.

70. Hoiby N. Epidemiological investigations of the respiratory tract bacteriology in patients with cystic fibrosis. Acta Pathol Microbiol Scand B. 1974;82: 541–50.

71. Burbank B, Marrione TG, Cutler SS. Pulmonary alveolar proteinosis and nocardiosis. Am J Med. 1960;28:1002–7.

72. Murray JF, Mills J. Pulmonary infections: Complication of human immunodeficiency virus infection. Am Rev Respir Dis. 1990;141:1356–72, 1582–98.

73. Meduri GU, Stein DS. Pulmonary manifestation of acquired immunodeficiency syndrome. Clin Infect Dis. 1992;14:98–113.

74. Daley CL. Bacterial pneumonia in HIV-infected patients. Semin Respir Infect. 1993;8:104–15.

75. García-Leoni ME, Moreno S, Rodeñó P, et al. Pneumococcal pneumonia: Adult hospitalized patients infected with the human immunodeficiency virus. Arch Intern Med. 1992;152:1808–12.

76. Steinhart R, Reingold AL, Taylor F, et al. Invasive *Haemophilus influenzae* infection in men with HIV infection. JAMA. 1992;268:3350–2.

77. Gross PA. Epidemiology of hospital-acquired pneumonia. Semin Respir Infect. 1987;2:2–7.

78. Marrie TJ, Haldane EV, Faulkner RS, et al. Community acquired pneumonia requiring hospitalization: Is it different in the elderly? J Am Geriatr Soc. 1985;33:671–80.

79. Heffron R. Pneumonia. New York: Commonwealth Fund; 1939:505.

80. Bartlett JG, Finegold SM. Anaerobic infections of the lung and pleural space. Am Rev Respir Dis. 1974;110:56–77.

81. Thorsteins son SB, Musher DM, Fagan T. The diagnostic value of sputum culture in acute pneumonia. JAMA. 1975;233:894–5.

82. Merrill C, Gwaltney JM, Hendley JO, et al. Rapid identification of pneumococci. N Engl J Med. 1973;288:510–2.

83. Drew WL. Value of sputum culture in diagnosis of pneumococcal pneumonia. J Clin Microbiol. 1977;6:62–5.

89. Bartlett RC, Melnick A. Usefulness of Gram stain and routine and quantitative culture of sputum in patients with and without acute respiratory infection. Conn Med. 1970;34:347–51.

85. Bryant RE, Rhoades ER. Clinical feature of adenoviral pneumonia in Air Force recruits. Am Rev Respir Dis. 1967;717–23.

86. Goerge RB, Ziskind MM, Rasch JR, et al. Mycoplasma and adenovirus pneumonias—Comparison with other atypical pneumonias in a military population. Ann Intern Med. 1966;65:931–42.

87. Reimann H. The Pneumonias. Philadelphia: WB Saunders; 1938:67.

88. Solomon S. Primary Friedlander pneumonia. JAMA. 1937;108:937–47.

89. Murray PR, Washington JA III. Microscopic and bacteriologic analysis of expectorated sputum. Mayo Clin Proc. 1975;50:339–44.

90. Rein MF, Gwaltney JM, O'Brien WM, et al. Accuracy of the Gram's stain in identifying pneumococci in sputum. JAMA. 1978;239:2671–3.

91. Hendley JO, Sande MA, Stewart PM, et al. Spread of *Streptococcus pneumoniae* in families. I. Carriage rates and distribution of types. J Infect Dis. 1975;132:55–61.

92. Finland M. Recent advances in the epidemiology of pneumococcal infections. Medicine. 1942;21:307–44.

93. Lees AW, McNaught W. Bacteriology of lower-respiratory tract secretions, sputum and upper-respiratory tract secretions in "normals" and "chronic bronchitis." Lancet. 1959;2:1112–5.

94. Gleckman R, DeVita J, Hibert D, et al. Sputum Gram's stain assessment in community-acquired bacteremic pneumonia. J Clin Microbiol. 1988;26: 846–9.

95. Fine MJ, Orloff JJ, Rihs JD, et al. Evaluation of housestaff physician's preparation and interpretation of sputum Gram's stain for community-acquired pneumonia. J Gen Intern Med. 1991;6:189–98.

96. Zaman MK, Wooten OH, Suprahmonya B, et al. Rapid non-invasive diagnosing of *Pneumocystis carinii* from induced liquified sputum. Ann Intern Med. 1988;109:7–10.

97. Bigby TD, Margolskee D, Curtis JL, et al. The usefulness of induced sputum in the diagnosis of *Pneumocystis carinii* pneumonia in patients with the acquired immunodeficiency syndrome. Am Rev Respir Dis. 1986;133:515–8.

98. Pitchenik AE, Ganjei P, Torres A, et al. Sputum examination for the diagnosis of *Pneumocystis carinii* pneumonia in the acquired immunodeficiency syndrome. Am Rev Respir Dis. 1986;133:226–9.

99. Tenover FC. Diagnostic deoxyribonucleic acid probes for infection. Dis Clin Microbiol Rev. 1988;1:82–101.

100. Peterson LR, Shanholtzer CJ. Using the microbiology laboratory in the diagnosis of pneumonia. Semin Respir Infect. 1988;3:106–12.

101. Sullivan RJ, Joran ML. Diagnosis of viral pneumonia. Semin Respir Infect. 1988;3:148–61.

102. Oldach DW, Gaydos CA, Mundy LM, et al. Rapid diagnosis of *Chlamydia psittaci* pneumonia. Clin Infect Dis. 1993;17:338–43.

103. Sills M, White P. Rapid identification of *Chlamydia psittaci* and TWAR *(C. pneumoniae)* in sputum samples using an amplified enzyme immunoassay (Letter). J Clin Pathol. 1990;43:260.

104. Wonderink RG, Russell GB, Mezger E, et al. The diagnostic utility of the antibody-coated bacteria test in intubated patients. Chest. 1991;99:84–8.

105. Barrett-Connor E. The non-value of sputum culture in the diagnosis of pneumococcal pneumonia. Am Rev Respir Dis. 1971;103:845–8.

106. Rathbun HK, Govani I. Mouse inoculation as means of identifying pneumococci in the sputum. Johns Hopkins Med J. 1967;120:46–8.

107. Wallace RJ, Musher DM, Martin RR. *Hemophilus influenzae* pneumonia in adults. Am J Med. 1978;64:87–93.

108. Levin D, Schwarz M, Matthay R, et al. Bacteremic *Hemophilus influenzae* pneumonia in adults. A report of 24 cases and a review of the literature. Am J Med. 1977;62:219–24.

109. Davidson M, Tempest B, Palmer DL. Bacteriologic diagnosis of acute pneumonia, comparison of sputum, transtracheal aspirates, and lung aspirates. JAMA 1976;235:158–63.

110. Geckeler RW, Gremillion DH, McAllister CK, et al. Microscopic and bacteriological comparison of paired sputa and transtracheal aspirates. J Clin Microbiol. 1977;6:396–9.

111. Kalinske RW, Parker RH, Brandt D, et al. Diagnostic usefulness and safety of transtracheal aspiration. N Engl J Med. 1967;276:604–8.

112. Hoeprich PD. Etiologic diagnosis of lower respiratory tract infections. Calif Med. 1970;112:1.

113. Tillotson JR, Lerner AM. Pneumonias caused by gram negative bacilli. Medicine. 1966;45:65–76.

114. Saadah HA, Nasr FL, Shagoury ME. Washed sputum gram stain and culture in pneumonia. J Okla State Med Assoc. 1980;73:354–9.

115. Jordan GW, Wong GA, Hoeprich PD. Bacteriology of the lower respiratory tract as determined by fiber-optic bronchoscopy and transtracheal aspiration. J Infect Dis. 1976;134:428–35.

116. Bartlett JG, Alexander J, Mayhew J, et al. Should fiberoptic bronchoscopy aspirates be cultured? Am Rev Respir Dis. 1976;114:73–8.

117. Wimberly N, Faling LJ, Bartlett JG. A fiberoptic bronchoscopy technique to obtain uncontaminated lower airway secretions for bacterial cultures. Am Rev Respir Dis. 1979;119:337–42.

118. Meden G, Hall GS, Ahmad M. Retrieval of microbiological specimens through the fiberoptic bronchoscope. Cleve Clin Q. 1985;52:495–502.

119. Wimberly NW, Bass JB, Boyd BW, et al. Use of a bronchoscopic protected catheter brush for the diagnosis of pulmonary infections. Chest. 1982;81:556–82.

120. Hays DA, McCarthy LC, Friedman M. Evaluation of two bronchofiberscopic methods of culturing the lower respiratory tract. Am Rev Respir Dis. 1980;122:319–23.

121. Higuchi JH, Coalson JJ, Johanson, WG. Bacteriologic diagnosis of nosocomial pneumonia in primates. Ann Rev Respir Dis. 1982;125:53–7.

122. Pollock HM, Hawkins EL, Bonner JR, et al. Diagnosis of bacterial pulmonary infections with quantitative protected catheter cultures obtained during bronchoscopy. J Clin Microbiol. 1983;17:255–9.

123. Halperin SA, Suratt PM, Gwaltney JM, et al. Bacterial cultures of the lower respiratory tract in normal volunteers with and without experimental rhinovirus infection using a plugged double catheter system. Am Rev Respir Dis. 1982;125:678–80.

124. Bordelon JY Jr, Legrand P, Gewin WL, et al. The telescoping plugged catheter in suspected anaerobic infections: A controlled series. Am Rev Respir Dis. 1983;128:465–8.

125. Wimberly NW, Bass JR Jr, Boyd DW, et al. Bronchial brush specimens from patients with stable chronic bronchitis. Chest. 1986;90:534–6.

126. Bass JB, Hawkins EL, Bonner JR, et al. Use of bronchoscopy protected catheter technique in the clinical evaluation of a new antibiotic. Diagn Microbiol Infect Dis. 1983;1:95–106.

127. Winterbauer RH, Hutchinson JF, Reinhardt GN, et al. The use of quantitative culture and antibody coating of bacteria to diagnose bacterial pneumonia by fiberoptic bronchoscopy. Am Rev Respir Dis. 1983;128:98–103.

128. Vereen L, Smart LM, George RB. Antibody coating and quantitative cultures of bacteria in sputum and bronchial brush specimens from patients with stable chronic bronchitis. Chest. 1986;90:534–6.

129. Guerra LF, Baughman RP. Use of bronchoalveolar lavage to diagnose bacterial pneumonia in mechanically ventilated patients. Crit Care Med. 1990;18:169–73.

130. Ortquist A, Kalin M, Lejdeborn L, et al. Diagnostic fiberoptic bronchoscopy and protected brush culture in patients with community-acquired pneumonia. Chest. 1990;97:576–82.

131. Feinsilver SH, Fein AM, Niederman MS, et al. Utility of fiberoptic bronchoscopy in nonresolving pneumonia. Chest. 1990;98:1322–6.

132. Chastre J, Fagon JY, Soler P, et al. Diagnosis of nosocomial bacterial pneumonia in intubated patients undergoing ventilation: Comparison of the usefulness of bronchoalveolar large at the protected specimen brush. Am J Med. 1988;85:499.

133. Johanson WG, Seidenfeld JJ, Gomez P, et al. Bacteriologic diagnosis of nosocomial pneumonia following prolonged mechanical ventilation. Am Rev Respir Dis. 1988;137:259–69.

134. Mortos JA, Ferrer M, Torres A, et al. Specificity of quantitative cultures of protected specimen brush and bronchoalveolar lavage in mechanically ventilated patients. Am Rev Respir Dis. 1990;161:A276.

135. Broughton WA, Middleton RM, Kirkpatrick MB, et al. Bronchoscopic protected specimen brush and bronchoalveolar lavage in the diagnosis of bacterial pneumonia. Infect Dis Clin North Am. 1991;5:432–52.

136. Sorenson J, Forsberg P, Hakanson E, et al. A new diagnostic approach to the patient with severe pneumonia. Scand J Infect Dis. 1989;21:33–41.

137. Pham LH, Brun-Buisson C, Legrand P, et al. Diagnosis of nosocomial pneumonia in mechanically ventilated patients. Am Rev Respir Dis. 1991;143:1055–61.

138. DeCastro FR, Violan JS, Capuz BL, et al. Reliability of the bronchoscopic protected catheter brush in the diagnosis of pneumonia in the mechanically ventilated patient. Crit Care Med. 1991;19:171.

139. Broaddus C, Dake MD, Stulburg MS, et al. Bronchoalveolar lavage and transbronchial biopsy for the diagnosis of pulmonary infections in the acquired immunodeficiency syndrome. Ann Intern Med. 1986;102:747–52.

140. Jules-Elysee KM, Stover DE, Zaman MB, et al. Aerosolized pentamidine: Effect on diagnosis and presentation of *Pneumocystis carinii* pneumonia. Ann Intern Med. 1990;112:750–87.

141. Crawford SW, Bowden RA, Hackman RC, et al. Rapid detection of cytomegalovirus pulmonary infection by bronchoalveolar lavage and centrifugation culture. Ann Intern Med. 1988;108:180–5.

142. Spector SA. Diagnosis of cytomegalovirus infection. Semin Hematol. 1990;27:11–6.

143. Pisani RJ, Wright AJ. Clinical utility of bronchoalveolar lavage in immunocompromised hosts. Mayo Clin Proc. 1992;67:221–7.

144. Crawford SW, Bowden RA, Hackman RC, et al. Rapid detection of cytomegalovirus pulmonary infection by bronchoalveolar lavage and centrifugation culture. Ann Intern Med. 1988;108:180–5.

145. Emmanuel D, Peppard J, Stover D, et al. Rapid diagnosis of cytomegalovirus pneumonia by bronchoalveolar lavage using human and murine monoclonal antibodies. Ann Intern Med. 1986;104:476–81.

146. Stover DE, Zaman MB, Hajdu SI, et al. Bronchoalveolar lavage in the diagnosis of diffuse pulmonary infiltrates in the immunosuppressed host. Ann Intern Med. 1984;101:1–7.

147. Martin WJ, Smith TF, Sanderson DR, et al. Role of bronchoalveolar lavage in the assessment of opportunistic pulmonary infections: Utility and complications. Mayo Clin Proc. 1987;62:549–57.

148. Meduri GH, Baselski V. The role of bronchoalveolar lavage in diagnosing nonopportunistic bacterial pneumonia. Chest. 1991;100:179–90.

149. Kahn FW, Jones JM. Diagnosing bacterial respiratory infection by bronchoalveolar lavage. J Infect Dis. 1987;155:862–9.

150. Thorpe JE, Baughman RP, Frame PT, et al. Bronchoalveolar lavage for diagnosing acute bacterial pneumonia. J Infect Dis. 1987;155:855–61.

151. Chastre J, Fagon JY, Soler P, et al. Diagnosis of nosocomial bacterial pneumonia in intubated patients undergoing ventilation: Comparing the usefulness of bronchoalveolar lavage and the protected specimen brush. Am J Med. 1988;85:499–506.

152. Torres A, Bellacasa JP, Xaubet A, et al. Diagnostic value of quantitative cultures of bronchoalveolar lavage and telescoping plugged catheters in mechanically ventilated patients with bacterial pneumonia. Am Rev Respir Dis. 1989;140:306–10.

153. Gaussorgues P, Piperno D, Bachman P, et al. Comparison of non-bronchoscopic bronchoalveolar lavage to open lung biopsy for bacteriology diagnosis of pulmonary infection in mechanically ventilated patients. Intensive Care Med. 1989;15:94.

154. Rouby J, Rossignon MD, Nicholas MH, et al. A prospective study of protected bronchoalveolar lavage in the diagnosis of nosocomial pneumonia. Anesthesiology. 1989;71:679–85.

155. Meduri GU, Beals D, Maijub G, et al. Protected bronchoalveolar lavage, a new bronchoscopic technique to retrieve uncontaminated distal airway secretion. Am Rev Respir Dis. 1991;143:855–64.

156. Pugin J, Auckenthaler R, Mili N, et al. Diagnosis of ventilator-associated pneumonia by bacteriologic analysis of bronchoscopic and non-bronchoscopic "blind" bronchoalveolar lavage fluid. Am Rev Respir Dis. 1991;143:1121–9.

157. Pugin J, Auckenthaler R, Delaspre O, et al. Rapid diagnosis of gram-negative pneumonia by assay of endotoxin in bronchoalveolar lavage fluid. Thorax. 1992;47:547–9.

158. Trouillet JL, Guiguet M, Gibert L, et al. Fiberoptic bronchoscopy in ventilated patients: Evaluation of cardiopulmonary risk under midazolam sedation. Chest. 1990;97:927–33.

159. Pugin J, Suter PM. Diagnostic bronchoalveolar lavage in patients with pneumonia produces sepsis-like systemic effects. Intensive Care Med. 1992;18:6–10.

160. Xavier R, Henn L, Costa R. Bronchoalveolar lavage in pulmonary tuberculosis. Chest. 1990;98:975.

161. DeGracia J, Curull V, Vidal R, et al. Diagnostic value of bronchoalveolar lavage in suspected pulmonary tuberculosis. Chest. 1988;93:329–32.

162. Baughman RP, Dohn MN, Loudon RG, et al. Bronchoscopy with bronchoalveolar lavage in tuberculosis and fungal infection. Chest 1991;99:92–7.

163. Bovornkittz S, Pushpakom R. Adenosine deceminase in bronchoalveolar lavage fluid. Chest. 1988;94:1113.

164. Levy H, Wadee AA, Feldman C, et al. Enzyme-linked immunosorbent assay for detection of antibodies against *Mycobacterium tuberculosis* in bronchial washings and serum. Chest. 1988;93:762–6.

165. Raja A, Baughman RP, Daniel TM. The detection by immune assay of antibody to mycobacterial antigens in bronchoalveolar lavage fluid from patients with tuberculosis and control subjects. Chest. 1988;94:133–7.

166. Busk MF, Rosenow EC III, Wilson WR. Invasive procedures in the diagnosis of pneumonia. Semin Respir Infect. 1988;3:113–22.
167. Manresa F, Dorca J. Needle aspiration techniques in the diagnosis of pneumonia. Thorax. 1991;46:601–3.
168. Mimica I, Donoso E, Howard JE, et al. Lung puncture in the etiological diagnosis of pneumonia. Am J Dis Child. 1971;122:278–82.
169. Klein JO. Diagnostic lung puncture in the pneumonias of infants and children. Pediatrics. 1969;44:486–92.
170. Bartlett JG. Invasive diagnostic techniques in respiratory infections. In: Pennington JE, ed. Respiratory Infections: Diagnosis and Management. New York: Raven Press; 1983:55–77.
171. Palmer DL, Davidson M, Lusk R. Needle aspiration of the lung in complex pneumonias. Chest. 1980;78:16–21.
172. Torees A, Jiménez, de la Bellacasa JP, et al. Diagnostic value of nonfluoroscopic percutaneous lung needle aspiration in patients with pneumonia. Chest. 1990;98:840–4.
173. Bandt PD, Blank N, Castellino RA. Needle diagnosis of pneumonitis, value in high risk patients. JAMA. 1972;220:1578–80.
174. Greenman RL, Goodall PT, King D. Lung biopsy in immune compromised hosts. Am J Med. 1975;59:488–96.
175. Cockerill FR III, Wilson WR, Carpenter HA, et al. Open lung biopsy in immunocompromised patients. Arch Intern Med. 1985;145:1398–404.
176. Dijkman JH, van der Meer JWM, Bakker W, et al. Transpleural lung biopsy by the thoracoscopic route in patients with diffuse interstitial pulmonary disease. Chest. 1982;82:76–83.
177. Rodgers BM. Thoracoscopy in children. Poumon-Coeur. 1981;37:301–6.
178. Springmeyer SC, Silvestri RC, Sale GE, et al. The role of transbronchial biopsy for the diagnosis of diffuse pneumonias in immunocompromised marrow transplant recipients. Am Rev Respir Dis. 1982;116:763–5.
179. McCabe RE, Brooks RG, Mark JBD, et al. Open lung biopsy in patients with acute leukemia. Am J Med. 1985;78:609–16.
180. McKenna RJ, Mountain CF, McMurtrey MJ. Open lung biopsy in immunocompromised patients. Chest. 1984;86:671–4.
181. Lowell JR. Pleural Effusions—A Comprehensive Review. Baltimore: University Park Press; 1977:96.
182. Unger JD, Rose HD, Unger GF. Gram-negative pneumonia. Diagn Radiol. 1973;107:283–91.
183. Light RW. Pleural diseases. Disease-A-Month. 1992;38:266–331.
184. Light RN, Girard WM, Jenkinson SG, et al. Parapneumonic effusions. Am J Med. 1970;69:507–12.
185. Venkatesan P, MacFarlane JT. Editorial. Thorax. 1992;47:329–31.
186. Dorff GJ, Coonrod JD, Rytel MW. Detection of immunoelectrophoresis of antigen in sera of patients with pneumococcal bacteremia. Lancet. 1971;1:578–9.
187. Örtquist A, Jonsson I, Kalin M, et al. Comparison of three methods for detection of pneumococcal antigen in sputum of patients with community-acquired pneumonia. Eur J Clin Microbial Infect Dis. 1989;8:956–61.
188. Woodheard MA, MacFarlane JT, Finch RG, et al. A comparison of counter-current immunoelectrophoresis and latex agglutination for the detection of pneumococcal antigen in community based pneumonia study. Serodiagn Immunother Infect Dis. 1990;4:159–65.
189. Lenthe-Ebua S, Brighouse G, Auckenthaler R, et al. Comparison of immunological methods for diagnosis of pneumococcal pneumonia in biological fluids. Eur J Clin Microbiol. 1987;6:28–34.
190. Boermsa WG, Lowenberg A, Holloway Y, et al. Pneumococcal capsular antigen detection and pneumococcal serology in patients with community-acquired pneumonia. Thorax. 1991;46:902–6.
191. Tugwell P, Greenwood BM. Pneumococcal antigen in lobar pneumonia. J Clin Pathol. 1975;28:118–23.
192. Burman LA, Trollfors B, Andersson B, et al. Diagnosis of pneumonia by cultures, bacterial and viral antigen detective tests and serology with special reference to antibodies against pneumococal antigens. J Infect Dis. 1991;163:1087–95.
193. Boermsa WG, Lowenberg A, Holloway Y, et al. Pneumococcal antigen persistence in sputum from patients with community-acquired pneumonia. Chest. 1992;102:422–7.
194. Martin SJ, Hogansan DA, Thomas ET. Detection of Streptococcus pneumoniae and Haemophilus influenzae type B antigens in acute nonbacteremic pneumonia. J Clin Microbiol. 1987;25:248–50.
195. Campbell JF, Spika JS. The serodioagnosis of nonpneumococcal bacterial pneumonia. Semin Respir Infect. 1988;3:123–30.
196. Ruf B, Schurmann D, Horbach, et al. Frequency and diagnosis of Legionella pneumophila: A 3 year prospective study with emphasis on application of urinary antigen detection. J Infect Dis. 1990;162:1341–7.
197. Grayston JT. Infections Caused by Chlamydia pneumoniae strain TWAR. Clin Infect Dis. 1992;15:757–63.
198. Pasculle AW, Veto GE, Krustofiak S, et al. Laboratory and clinical evaluation of a commercial DNA probe for the detection of Legionella sp. J Clin Microbiol. 1989;27:2350–8.
199. Lerner AM, Jankauskas K. The classic bacterial pneumonias. Disease-A-Month. Feb 1975:1–46.
200. Willman VL, Lewis JE, Hanlon CR. Staphylococcal pneumonia—Surgical considerations in cases in infants and children. Arch Surg. 1961;83:93–7.
201. Highman JH. Staphylococcal pneumonia and empyema in childhood. Am J Roentgenol. 1996;103:4–9.
202. Dines DE. Diagnostic significance of pneumatoceles of the lung. JAMA. 1968;204:1169–72.
203. Warner JO, Gordon I. Pneumatocoeles following Haemophilus influenzae pneumonia. Clin Radiol. 1981;32:99–105.
204. Luddy RE, Champion LA, Schwartz AD. Pneumocystis carinii pneumonia with pneumatocele formation. Am J Dis Child. 1977;131:470.
205. Scanlon GT, Unger JD. The radiology of bacterial and viral pneumonias. Radiol Clin North Am. 1973;11:317–38.
206. Bartlett JG, Finegold SM. Anaerobic pleuropulmonary infections. Medicine. 1972;51:413–50.
207. Lindsay MI, Morrow GW. Primary influenzal pneumonia. Postgrad Med. 1971;49:173–8.
208. Conte P, Heitzman ER, Markarian B. Viral pneumonia. Roentgen pathological correlations. Radiology. 1970;95:267–72.
209. Fine NL, Smith LR, Sheedy PF. Frequency of pleural effusions of mycoplasma and viral pneumonias. N Engl J Med. 1970;283:790–3.
210. Fraser DW, Tsai TR, Orenstein W, et al. Legionnaire's disease. Description of an epidemic of pneumonia. N Engl J Med. 1977;297:1189–97.
211. Kirby BD, Snyder KM, Meyer RD, et al. Legionnaire's disease—A cluster of cases (Abstract). Clin Res. 1978;26:A399.
212. Pope TL, Armstrong P, Thompson R, et al. Pittsburgh pneumonia agent chest film manifestations. AJR. 1982;138:237–41.
213. Tew J, Calenoff L, Berlin BS. Bacterial or nonbacterial pneumonia: Accuracy of radiographic diagnosis. Radiology. 1977;124:607–12.
214. Kramer EL, Chaitanya RD. Pulmonary applications of nuclear medicine. Clin Chest Med. 1991;12:55–75.
215. Pennington JE. Community-Acquired Pneumonia and Acute Bronchitis in Respiratory Infections: Diagnosis and Management. New York: Raven Press; 1994.
216. Garibaldi RA. Epidemiology of community acquired respiratory tract infections in adults: Incidence, etiology, and impact. Am J Med. 1985;78(Suppl 6B):32–7.
217. Kerttula Y, Leinonen M, Koskela M, et al. The aetiology of pneumonia. Application of bacterial serology and basic laboratory methods. J Infect. 1987;14:21–30.
218. Gleckman R, DeVita J, Hibert D, et al. Sputum Gram's stain assessment in community-acquired bacteremic pneumonia. J Clin Microbiol. 1988;26:846–9.
219. Woodhead MA, Arrowsmith J, Chamberlain-Webber R, et al. The value of routine microbial investigation in community-acquired pneumonia. Respir Med 1991;85:313–7.
220. Holmberg H, Bodin L, Jönsson I, et al. Rapid aetiological diagnosis of pneumonia based on routine laboratory features. Scand J Infect Dis. 1990;22:537–45.
221. The British Thoracic Society Research Committee and the Public Health Laboratory Service. The aetiology, management and outcome of severe community-acquired pneumonia on the intensive care unit. Respir Med. 1992;86:7–13.
222. Holmberg H. Aetiology of community-acquired pneumonia in hospital-treated patients. Scand J Infect Dis. 1987;19:491–501.
223. Marrie TJ, Durant H, Yates L. Community-acquired pneumonia requiring hospitalization: Five year prospective study. Rev Infect Dis. 1989;11:586–99.
224. Farr BM, Kaiser DL, Harrison BDW, et al. Prediction of microbial aetiology at admission to hospital for pneumonia from the presenting clinical features. Thorax. 1989;44:1031–5.
225. Fine MJ, Orloff JJ, Arisumi D, et al. Prognosis of patients hospitalized with community-acquired pneumonia. Am J Med. 1990;88:5.
226. Fang GD, Fine M, Orloff J, et al. New and emerging etiologies for community-acquired pneumonia with implication for therapy: A prospective multicenter study of 359 cases. Medicine. 1990;69:307–16.
227. Fine M, Smith D, Singer DE. Hospitalization decision in patients with community-acquired pneumonia: A prospective chart. Am J Med. 1990;89:713–4.
228. American Thoracic Society. Guidelines for the initial management of adults with community-acquired pneumonia: Diagnosis, assessment of severity, and initial antimicrobial theapy. Am Rev Respir Dis. 1993;148:1418–26.
228a.Marrie TJ. Community-acquired pneumonia. Clin Infect Dis. 1994;18:501–15.
229. Bates JH, Campbell GD, Barron AI, et al. Etiology of acute pneumonia in hospitalized patients. Chest. 1992;101:1005–12.
230. Karalus NC, Cursons RT, Leng RA, et al. Community-acquired pneumonia: Aetiology and prognostic index evaluation. Thorax. 1991;46:413–8.
231. Chatard JA. The leukocytes in acute lobar pneumonia. Johns Hopkins Hosp Rep. 1910;15:89–98.
232. Austrian R, Gold J. Pneumococcal bacteremia with especial reference to bacteremic pneumococcal pneumonia. Ann Intern Med. 1964;60:759–76.
233. MacFarlane JT, Finch RG, Ward MJ, et al. Hospital study of adult community acquired pneumonia. Lancet. 1982;2:255–8.
234. Klimek JJ, Ajemian E, Fontecchio S, et al. Community acquired bacterial pneumonia requiring admission to hospital. Am J Infect Cont. 1983;11:79–82.
235. Levy M, Dromer F, Brion N, et al. Community-acquired pneumonia: Importance of initial non-invasive bacteriologic and radiographic investigations. Chest. 1988;92:43–8.
236. Stratton CW. Bacterial pneumonia. An overview with emphasis on pathogenesis, diagnosis and treatment. Heart Lung. 1986;15:226–44.
237. Lipsky BA, Boyko EJ, Inui TS, et al. Risk factors for acquiring pneumococcal infections. Arch Intern Med. 1986;146:2179–85.
238. Rosner F, Zarrabi MH. Late infections following splenectomy in Hodgkin's disease. Cancer Invest. 1983;1:57–65.

239. Zarrabi MH, Rosner F. Serious infections in adults following splenectomy for trauma. Arch Intern Med. 1984;144:1421–4.
240. Musher DM. Infections caused by *Streptococcus pneumoniae:* Clinical spectrum, pathogenesis, immunity and treatment. Clin Infect Dis. 1992;14:801–9.
241. Crofton J. The chemotherapy of bacterial respiratory infections. Am Rev Respir Dis. 1970;101:841–59.
242. Hirschmann JV, Everett ED. *Haemophilus influenzae* infections in adults: Report of nine cases and a review of literature. Medicine. 1979;58:80–94.
243. Hausmann W, Karlish AJ. Staphylococcal pneumonia in adults. Br Med J. 1956;2:845–7.
244. Schwarzmann SW, Adler JL, Sullivan RJ, et al. Bacterial pneumonia during the Hong Kong influenza epidemic of 1968–1969. Experience in a city-county hospital. Arch Intern Med. 1971;127:1037–41.
245. Louria DB, Blumenfeld HL, Ellis JT, et al. Studies on influenza. J Clin Invest. 1959;38:213–65.
246. Yu VL, Kroboth FJ, Shonnard J, et al. Legionnaire's disease: New clinical perspective from a prospective pneumonia study. Am J Med. 1982;73:357–61.
247. Falcó V, de Sevilla TF, Alegre J, et al. *Legionella pneumophilia:* A case of severe community-acquired pneumonia. Chest. 1991;100:1007–11.
248. Nguyen MLT, YO VL. *Legionella* infection. Clin Chest Med. 1991;12:257–68.
249. Nicotra B, Rivera M, Luman I, et al. *Branhamella catarrhalis* as a lower respiratory tract pathogen in patients with chronic lung disease. Arch Intern Med. 1986;146:890–3.
250. Slevin NJ, Aitken J, Thornleg PE. Clinical and microbiological features of *Branhamella catarrhalis* bronchopulmonary infections. Lancet. 1987;1:782–3.
251. Wallace RJ Jr, Musher DM. In honor of Dr. Sarah Branham. A star is born: The realization of *Branhamella catarrhalis* as a respiratory pathogen. Chest. 1986;90:447–50.
252. Gross JS, Neufeld RR, Libon LS, et al. Autopsy study of the elderly institutionalized patients: Review of 234 autopsies. Arch Intern Med. 1988;148:173–6.
253. Granton JT, Grossman RF. Community-acquired pneumonia in the elderly patient: Clinical features, epidemiology and treatment. Clin Chest Med. 1993;14:537–53.
254. Musgrave T, Verghese A. Clinical features of pneumonia in the elderly. Semin Respir Infect. 1990;5:269–75.
255. Harper C, Newton P. Clinical aspects of pneumonia in the elderly veteran. Am J Geriatr Soc. 1989;37:867–72.
256. Venkatesan P, Gladman J, MacFarlane JT. A hospital study of community-acquired pneumonia in the elderly. Thorax. 1990;45:254–8.
257. Berk KC, Holtsdan SA, Wiener SL, et al. Nontypeable *Haemophilus influenzae* in the elderly. Arch Intern Med. 1982;142:532–9.
258. Verghese A, Berk SL. Bacterial pneumonia in the elderly. Medicine. 1983;62:271–85.
259. Valenti WM, Trudell RG, Bentley DW. Factors predisposing to oropharyngeal colonization with gram-negative bacilli in the aged. N Engl J Med. 1978;298:1108–11.
260. Mackowiak PA, Martin RM, Jones SR, et al. Pharyngeal colonization by gram-negative bacilli in aspiration-prone persons. Arch Intern Med. 1978;138:1224–47.
261. Nicolle L, McLeod J, McIntyre M, et al. Significance of pharyngeal colonization with aerobic gram-negative bacilli in elderly institutionalized men. Aging. 1986;15:47–52.
262. Murray JF, Felton CP, Garay SM, et al. Pulmonary complications of the acquired immunodeficiency syndrome. Report of a National Heart, Lung and Blood Institute Workshop. N Engl J Med. 1984;310:1682–8.
263. Stover DE, White DA, Romano PA, et al. Spectrum of pulmonary diseases associated with the acquired immune deficiency syndrome. Am J Med. 1985;78:429–37.
264. Kovacs JA, Masur H. Prophylaxis for *Pneumocystis carinii* pneumonia in patients infected with human immunodeficiency virus. Clin Infect Dis. 1992;14:1005–9.
265. Pachon J, Prados D, Capote F, et al. Severe community-acquired pneumonia: Etiology, prognosis, treatment. *Am Rev Respir Dis.* 1990;142:369–73.
266. Torres A, Serra-Batlles J, Ferrer A, et al. Severe community-acquired pneumonia: Epidemiology and prognostic factors. Am Rev Respir Dis. 1991;144:312–8.
267. Potgieter PD, Hammond JMJ. Etiology and diagnosis of pneumonia requiring ICU admission: A discussion. Chest. 1992;101:199–203.
268. Farr BM, Sloman AJ, Fisch MJ. Predicting death in patients hospitalized for community-acquired pneumonia. Am J Med. 1991;115:428–36.
269. The British Thoracic Society Research Committee and the Public Health Laboratory Service. Community-acquired pneumonia in adults in British hospitals in 1982–1983: A survey of aetiology, mortality, prognostic factors and outcome. Q NJ Med. 1987;62:195–220.
270. Fine MJ, Orloff JJ, Arisumi D, et al. Prognosis of patients hospitalized with community-acquired pneumonia. Am J Med. 1990;88:5.
271. Marrie TJ. Normal resolution of community-acquired pneumonia. Semin Respir Infect. 1992;7:256–70.
272. Lehtomaki K. Clinical diagnosis of pneumococcal adenoviral, mycoplasmal and viral pneumonia in young men. Eur Respir J. 1988;1:324–9.
273. Jay SJ, Johnson WG Jr, Pierce WK. The radiographic resolution of *Streptococcus pneumoniae* pneumonia. N Engl J Med. 1991;293:798–801.
274. Winterbauer RH, Bedon GA, Ball WC Jr. Recurrent pneumonia: Predispos-

275. Corley DE, Winterbauer RH. Infectious diseases that result in slowly resolving and chronic pneumonia. Semin Respir Med. 1993;8:3–13.
276. Feinsilver SH, Fein AM, Niederman MS, et al. Utility of fiberoptic bronchoscopy in nonresolving pneumonia. Chest. 1990;98:1322–6.
277. Reiman HA. An acute infection of the respiratory tract with atypical pneumonia. JAMA. 1988;111:2377–84.
278. Luby JP. Pneumonia caused by *Mycoplasma pneumoniae* infection. Clin Chest Med. 1991;12:237–44.
279. Mogabgab WJ. *Mycoplasma pneumoniae* and adenovirus respiratory illness in military and university personnel 1959–1966. Am Rev Respir Dis. 1968;97:345–58.
280. Forsyth BR, Bloom HH, Johnson KM, et al. Etiology of primary atypical pneumonia in a military population. JAMA. 1965;191:364–8.
281. Wenzel RP, McCormick DP, Smith EP, et al. Acute respiratory disease: Clinical and epidemiologic observations of military trainees. Milit Med. 1971;136:873–80.
282. Grayston JT, Kenny GE, Foy HM, et al. Epidemiological studies of *Mycoplasma pneumoniae* infections in civilians. Ann NY Acad Sci. 1967;143:436–46.
283. Sawyer LA, Fishbein DB, McDale JE. Q fever: Current concepts. Rev Infect Dis. 1987;9:935–46.
284. Tack KJ, Peterson PK, Rasp FL, et al. Isolation of *Chlamydia trachomatis* from the lower respiratory tracts of adults. Lancet. 1980;1:116–20.
285. Komaroff AL, Aronson MD, Schachter J. *Chlamydia trachomatis* infections in adults with community acquired pneumonia. JAMA. 1981;245:1319–22.
286. Grayston JT, Diwan VK, Cooney M, et al. Community and hospital acquired pneumonia associated with chlamydia TWAR infection demonstrated serologically. Arch Intern Med. 1989;149:169–73.
287. Grayston JT, Kuo CC, Wang SP, et al. A new *Chlamydia psittaci* strain, TWAR, isolated in acute respiratory tract infection. N Engl J Med. 1986;315:161–8.
288. Marrie TJ, Grayston JT, Wang SP, et al. Pneumonia associated with the TWAR strain of *Chlamydia.* Ann Intern Med. 1987;106:507–11.
289. Thorn DH, Grayston JT. Infections with *Chlamydia pneumoniae* strain TWAR. Clin Chest Med. 1991;12:245–56.
290. Grayston JT, Campbell LA, Kuo CC, et al. A new respiratory tract pathogen: *Chlamydia pneumoniae* strain TWAR. J Infect Dis. 1990;161:618–25.
291. Kleemola M, Saikku P, Viskorpi R, et al. Epidemics of pneumonia caused by TWAR, a new *Chlamydia* organism in military trainees in Finland. J Infect Dis. 1988;157:230–6.
292. Grayston JT. Infection caused by *Chlamydia pneumoniae* strain TWAR. Clin Infect Dis. 1992;15:757–63.
293. Kuo CL, Shor A, Campbell LA, Fukushi H, Patton DL, Grayston JT. Demonstration of *Chlamydia pneumoniae* in atherosclerotic lesions of coronary arteries. J Infect Dis. 1993;167:841–9.
294. Thorn DH, Grayston JT, Siscovick DS, et al. Association of prior infection with *Chlamydia pneumoniae* and angiographically demonstrated coronary artery disease. JAMA. 1992;268:68–72.
295. Wenzel RP, McCormick DP, Beam WE Jr. Parainfluenza pneumonia in adults. JAMA. 1972;221:294–5.
296. Respiratory syncytial virus—Missouri. MMWR. 1977;26:351.
297. Sorvillo FJ, Huie SF, Strassburg MA, et al. An outbreak of respiratory syncytial virus pneumonia in a nursing home for the elderly. J Infect. 1984;9:252–6.
298. Kasupski GJ, Leers WD, Presumed respiratory syncytial virus pneumonia in three immunocompromised adults. Am J Med Sci. 1983;285:28–33.
299. Greenberg SH. Viral pneumonia. Infect Dis Clin North Am. 1991;5:603–21.
300. Ruben FL, Nguyen MLT. Viral pneumonitis. Clin Chest Med. 1991;12:223–35.
301. Legionnaire's disease: Diagnosis and management. Ann Intern Med. 1978;88:363–5.
302. Helms CM, Viner JP, Sturm RH. Comparative features of pneumococcal, mycoplasmal, and Legionnaire's disease pneumonias. Ann Intern Med. 1979;90:543–7.
303. Bartlett JG, Gorbach SL. The triple threat of aspiration pneumonia. Chest. 1979;68:560–6.
304. Wynne JW, Modell JH. Respiratory aspiration of stomach contents. Ann Intern Med. 1977;87:466–74.
305. Lorber B, Swenson RM. Bacteriology of aspiration pneumonia: A prospective study of community and hospital-acquired cases. Ann Intern Med. 1974;81:329–31.
306. Finegold SM. Aspiration pneumonia. Rev Infect Dis. 1991;13(Suppl 9):S737–42.
307. Ludmerer KM, Kissare JM. Pulmonary infiltrates and eosinophilia in a young man. Am J Med. 1986;81:533–40.
308. Chemopathologic conference. Respiratory failure and eosinophilia in a young man. Am J Med. 1993;94:533–42.
309. Lanham JG, Elkon KB, Pusey CD, et al. A clinical approach to the Churg-Strauss syndrome. Medicine. 1984;63:65–81.
310. Allen JN, Davis WB. What is eosinophilic pneumonia. Arch Intern Med. 1992;152:1765–6.
311. Schatz M, Wasserman S, Patterson R. Eosinophils and immunologic lung disease. Med Clin North Am. 1981;65:1055–71.
312. Fleury-Feith J, Van Nhieu JT, Picard L, et al. Bronchoalveolar lavage eosin-

ophilia associated with *Pneumocystis carinii* pneumoritis in AIDS patients. Chest. 1989;95:1198–201.

313. Citro LA, Gordon ME, Miller WT. Eosinophilic lung disease (or how to slice P.I.E.). Am J Roentgenol. 1973;117:787–97.
314. Liebow AA, Carrington CB. The eosinophilic pneumonias. Medicine. 1969; 48:251–85.
315. Jederlinic PJ, Sicilian L., Graenslер EA. Chronic eosinophilic pneumonia. Medicine. 1988;67:154–62.
316. Haley RW, Culver DH, White JW, et al. The nationwide nosocomial infection rate: A new need for vital statistics. Am J Epidemiol. 1985;121:159–67.
317. Simmons BP, Wong ES, CDC guidelines for the prevention and control of nosocomial infections: Guideline for prevention of nosocomial pneumonia. Am J Infect Control. 1983;11:230–3.
318. Scheld WM, Mandell GL. Nosocomial pneumonia: Pathogenesis and recent advances in diagnosis and therapy. Rev Infect Dis. 1991;13(Suppl 9): S743–51.
319. Torres A, Aznar R, Gatell JM, et al. Incidence of risk and prognosis of nosocomial pneumonia in mechanically ventilated patients. Am Rev Respir Dis. 1990;142:523–8.
320. Joshi N, Localio AR, Hamory BH. A predictive risk index for nosocomial pneumonia in the intensive care unit. Am J Med. 1992;93:135–42.
321. Haley RN, Hooton TM, Culver DH, et al. Nosocomial infections in U.S. hospitals 1975–1976. Am J Med. 1981;70:947–59.
322. Toews GB. Nosocomial pneumonia. Clin Chest Med. 1987;8:467–79.
323. Hooten TM, Haley RW, Culver DH, et al. The joint association of multiple role factors with the occurrence of nosocomial infection. Am J Med. 1981; 70:960–70.
324. Donowitz LG, Page MC, Mileur BL, et al. Alteration of normal gastric flora in critical care patients receiving antacid and cimetidine therapy. Infect Control. 1986;7:23–6.
325. Snepar R, Poporad GA, Romano JM, et al. Effect of cimetidine and antacid on gastric microbial flora. Infect Immun. 1982;36:518–24.
326. Driks MR, Craven DE, Celli BR, et al. Nosocomial pneumonia in intubated patients given sucralfate as compared with antacids or histamine type-2 blockers. The role of gastric colonization. N Engl J Med. 1987;317:1376–82.
327. Cook DJ, Laine LA, Guyatt GH, et al. Nosocomial pneumonia and the role of gastric pH: A beta analysis. Chest. 1991;100:7–13.
328. Craven DE, Steger KA, Barber TW. Preventing nosocomial pneumonia: State of the art and perspective for the 1990s. Am J Med. 1991;91(Suppl 3B): 44S–53S.
329. Simms HH, DeMoria E, McDonald L, et al. Role of gastric colonization in the development of pneumonia in critically ill trauma patients: Results of a prospective randomized trail. J Trauma. 1991;31:531–7.
330. Rello J, Ausina V, Cstella J, et al. Incidence, etiology and outcome of nosocomial pneumonia in mechanically ventilated patients. Chest. 1991;100:439–44.
331. Septimus EJ. Nosocomial bacterial pneumonia. Semin Respir Infect. 1989; 4:245–52.
332. A'Court C, Garrard CS. Nosocomial pneumonia in the intensive care unit: Mechanism and significance. Thorax. 1992;47:465–73.
333. Bartlett JG, O'Keefe P, Tally FP, et al. Bacteriology of hospital-acquired pneumonia. Arch Intern Med. 1986;146:868–71.
334. Nguyen MH, Stout JE, Yu VL. Legionellosis. Infect Dis Clin North Am. 1991;5:561–84.
335. Graman PS, Hall CB. Nosocomial viral respiratory infections. Semin Respir Infect. 1989;4:253–60.
336. Wilson WR, Cockerill FR, Rosenow EC III. Pulmonary disease in the immunocompromised host. Mayo Clin Proc. 1985;60:610–31.
337. Schimpff SC, Young VM, Greene WH, et al. Origin of infection in acute nonlymphocytic leukemia: Significance of hospital acquisition of potential pathogens. Ann Intern Med. 1972;77:707–14.
338. Chang HY, Rodriguez V, Narboni G, et al. Causes of death in adults with acute leukemia. Medicine. 1976;55:259–68.
339. Peterson PK, Ferguson R, Fryd DS, et al. Infectious disease in hospitalized renal transplant recipients: A prospective study of a complex and evolving problem. Medicine. 1982;61:360–72.
340. Ramsey PG, Rubin RH, Tolkoff-Rubin NE, et al. The renal transplant patient with fever and pulmonary infiltrates: Etiology, clinical manifestations and management. Medicine. 1980;59:206–22.
341. Winston DJ, Gale RP, Meyer DV, et al. Infectious complications of human bone marrow transplantation. Medicine. 1979;58:1–31.
342. Ettinger NA, Trulock EP. Pulmonary considerations of organ transplantation. Am Rev Respir Dis. 1991;143:1386–405.
343. Ettinger NA, Trulock EP. Pulmonary considerations of organ transplantation. Am Rev Respir Dis. 1991;144:212–23, 433–51.
344. Valdivieso M, Gil-Extremera G, Zoronoza J, et al. Gram-negative bacillary pneumonia in the compromised host. Medicine. 1977;56:241–4.
345. Sickles EA, Young VM, Greene WH, et al. Pneumonia in acute leukemia. Ann Intern Med. 1973;79:528–34.
346. Woodlead MA, MacFarlane JT. Comparative clinical and laboratory features of *Legionella* with pneumococcal and *Mycoplasma* pneumonias. Br J Dis Chest. 1987;81:133–9.
347. Black ER, Mushlin AI, Griner PF, et al. Predicting the need for hospitalization of ambulatory patients with pneumonia. J Gen Intern Med. 1991;6: 394–400.
348. Fine MJ, Smith DN, Singer DE. Hospitalization decision on patients with community-acquired pneumonia: A prospective cohort study. Am J Med. 1990;89:713–21.
349. Henderson FW, Gittigan PH, Wait K, et al. Nasopharyngeal carriage of antibiotic-resistant pneumococci by children in group day care. J Infect Dis. 1988;157:256–63.
350. Donowitz GR, Mandell GL. Beta-lactam antibiotics (parts 1 and 2). N Engl J Med. 1988;318:419–26, 490–500.
351. Levison ME, Mangura CT, Lorber B, et al. Clindamycin compared with penicillin for the treatment of anaerobic lung abscess. Ann Intern Med. 1983; 98:466–71.
352. Bartlett JG, Gorbach SL. Penicillin or clindamycin for primary lung abscess. Ann Intern Med. 1983;98:546–8.

51. PLEURAL EFFUSION AND EMPYEMA

RICHARD E. BRYANT

Pleural empyema is a complex disease with a bad prognosis if the diagnosis is missed or if adequate drainage is not achieved.[1,2] Recent developments in diagnostic imaging have greatly facilitated recognition and management of this disease.[3–5] Microbial contamination of the pleural space is usually secondary to pneumonia but may arise from extrapulmonic infection and complicate neoplasm, collagen vascular disease, trauma, or medical or surgical procedures involving the pleura.[2] The mode of presentation is modified by the origin of the infection, the infecting microorganisms, and the patient's underlying disease(s).

ETIOLOGY

Medical and societal changes have modified the types of organisms causing empyema.[1,2] Fifty to sixty percent of patients develop empyema as a complication of pneumonia.[1,2,6] In otherwise healthy adults with pneumonia, the most common causes of pleural empyema are *Staphylococcus aureus*, *Streptococcus pneumoniae*, and *Streptococcus pyogenes*.[2,7] Empyema caused by *Staph. aureus* and *Haemophilus influenzae* has been common in children.[8] The new conjugate vaccine may reduce the frequency of suppurative complications of *H. influenzae* infection in children.[9]

The increased recognition of anaerobic empyema reflects improved microbiologic techniques and recognition of anaerobic infection associated with aspiration pneumonia, putrid lung abscess, and pleural infection arising from oropharyngeal or gastrointestinal sites.[10,11] Bartlett and Finegold[10] found that pleural empyema was caused by aerobic bacteria in 24 percent, anaerobic bacteria in 35 percent, and both aerobic and anaerobic bacteria in 41 percent of 83 medical service patients without prior antibiotic therapy or surgical procedures. Empyema secondary to subdiaphragmatic disease is often polymicrobial and anaerobic in origin.[12]

Approximately 25 percent of patients develop empyema as a complication of trauma or surgery. There is a high frequency of *Staph. aureus* and aerobic gram-negative bacillary infection in such patients.[7,13] Empyema complicating hemothorax is often staphylococcal, while that associated with pneumothorax or serous effusion is often caused by gram-negative aerobic bacilli.[13] Immunocompromised patients have a higher frequency of empyema caused by fungi and gram-negative bacilli.[14] Organ transplant recipients and patients with the acquired immunodeficiency syndrome may reactivate pleural foci of mycobacterial or fungal infection but will rarely present with empyema without disseminated disease. Unsuccessful resection of cavitary coccidioidomycosis may be complicated by empyema from that organism. The association of fistulous tracts from the pleura suggests the possibility of actinomycosis, nocardiosis, or tuberculosis. Less common causes of empyema include extension of subdiaphragmatic infections caused by *Salmonella*, *Clostridia*, or *Entamoeba histolytica*.

PATHOGENS

Pleural effusions are caused by altered oncotic or capillary pressure from renal, cardiac, hepatic, or metabolic diseases. Pleural effusions may occur in 40–50 percent of patients with pneumonia.[15] However, only a small percentage (≈5 percent) of parapneumonic effusions become exudates with the associated microbiologic, chemical, and physical features of empyema.[2] Microorganisms gain access to the pleura by direct extension from the lung; from blood or lymphatics; by extension from subdiaphragmatic, mediastinal, pericardial, or cervical infection; and by transthoracic entry from trauma, surgery, or manipulative procedures. Patients with trauma to the esophagus, mediastinum, or heart or those who have had surgery in those areas are at increased risk of infection extending to the pleura. Similarly, patients with retropharyngeal or paravertebral suppurative disease may present with pleural empyema. As the efficiency of trauma rescue programs increase, the frequency of empyema associated with chest and head trauma will increase.[13,14]

Empyema fluid is deficient in opsonins and complement needed for optimal phagocytic function and ultimately develops extremes of hypoxia and acidity that further impair local neutrophil activity.[16,17] Endotoxins and other toxic factors elaborated by bacteria suppress the leukocyte host defense function and permit the growth of bacteria to concentrations of 10^8 bacteria per milliliter of empyema fluid.[18]

Inflammatory exudates may become loculated in a relatively small area or may extend to involve virtually the entire hemithorax, leading to ventilatory dysfunction and to the signs and symptoms of overwhelming sepsis and multiple organ failure. The exuberant inflammatory response can on occasion lead to erosion of the chest wall and to spontaneous drainage of the empyema.

Empyema fluid inhibits antimicrobial efficacy by a number of means. Aminoglycoside activity is suppressed by acid pH (minimum inhibitory concentration [MIC] is increased ≥64-fold by a 1-unit drop in pH), hypoxia (membrane transport of aminoglycosides is an oxygen-dependent step), increased concentrations of divalent cations, and binding of aminoglycosides to pus and suppression of bacterial metabolism in abscess fluid.[18,19] β-Lactamase from microorganisms can degrade β-lactamase–susceptible β-lactam antibiotics, and chloramphenicol may be degraded by microbial enzymes in pus.[18] Moreover, late in the course of this chronic suppurative infection, the bacterial growth rate is diminished and bacteria become refractory to antibiotic therapy.

By convention, the phases of empyema formation are divided into the *exudate phase*, during which leukocytes increase until pus is formed; the *fibropurulent phase*, during which fibrin formation begins to limit expansion of the lung; and the *organizing phase*, during which fibroblast formation and scarring produce a thick, leathery encasement that traps the lung.[20]

Microbe-specific factors affect the pathophysiology of pleural space infection. Induction of experimental empyema in guinea pigs requires inoculation of more than 10^6 organisms per milliliter of *Escherichia coli*, or *Staph. aureus* plus *Bacterioides fragilis*, in order to infect more than 50 percent of animals.[21] Use of umbilical tape as a foreign body does not increase lethality, but addition of blood greatly enhances the lethality of challenge with *E. coli* and *B. fragilis* mixtures.[21]

CLINICAL PRESENTATION

The clinical presentation of empyema is largely nonspecific and reflects the findings of pleural fluid accumulation and uncontrolled infection. Patients may have chest pain, dyspnea, weight loss, chills, fever, or night sweats.[15] Development or persistence of fever and leukocytosis, despite appropriate antibiotic therapy of a patient at risk of empyema, is a common clue to its presence. Physical examination often reveals signs of an effusion, but may be unchanged except for altered vital signs. It is unusual to demonstrate loculated pleural fluid on physical examination. A high index of suspicion and recognition of factors that predispose patients to the development of pleural empyema are the keys to its recognition.

Pleural effusion is demonstrated radiologically when 300–500 ml of fluid causes blunting of the costophrenic angles (Fig. 1).[15] Lateral views often show a fluid meniscus and loss of distinct margins of the diaphragm. Lateral decubitus views permit detec-

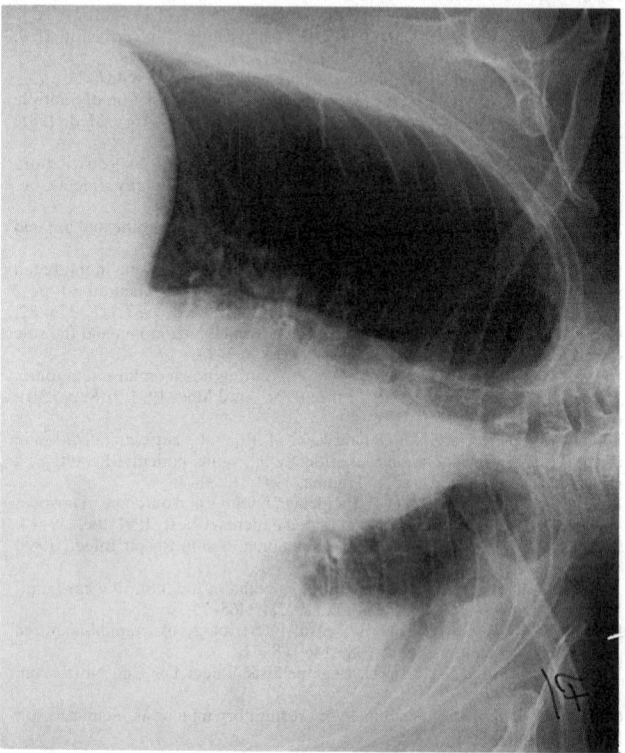

A

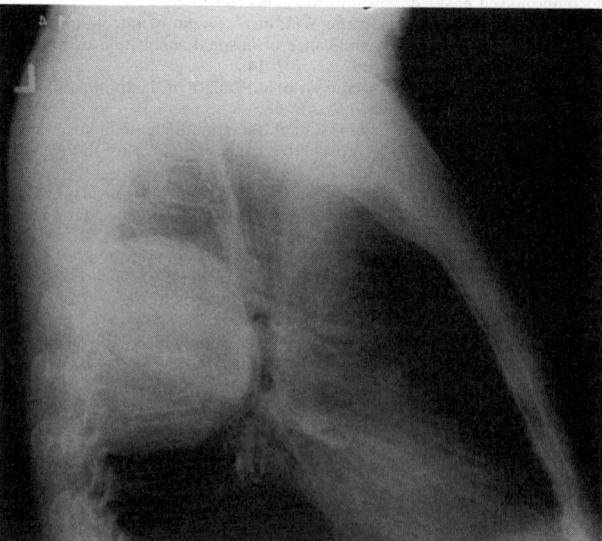

B

FIG. 1. **(A)** Empyema fluid is shown layering out along the dependent chest wall of a patient with left lower lobe pneumonia. **(B)** D-shaped mass representing a loculated empyema at the site of a former right upper lobectomy.

tion of smaller volumes of fluid (100–200 ml) and assessment of loculation if fluid fails to "layer out" along the dependent chest wall.[15] The "disease side up" view often permits recognition of the extent of parenchymal disease. Conventional roentgenograms may not distinguish effusions developing in interlobar or subpulmonic spaces or permit recognition of empyema when pleural volumes are small or when extensive pneumonia is present. Loculated empyema with a bronchopleural fistula may resemble a lung abscess. Fortunately, both ultrasound and computed tomography (CT) provide more sensitive techniques for pleural fluid detection.[3,4] Pleural fluid aspiration under ultrasound guidance provides an accurate and safe means of obtaining infected pleural fluid and is especially helpful when fluid volumes are small or loculated.[5,6] However, it is not necessary to tap all para-pneumonic effusions if the volume of fluid is small (less than 1 cm in depth on lateral decubitus films), the patient is doing well, the fluid moves freely, and the roentgenogram is improving.[15,22,23]

CT is especially helpful for demonstrating pleural fluid accumulation due to extension from mediastinal or subdiaphragmatic disease (Fig. 2).[4,5] This technology can also distinguish between

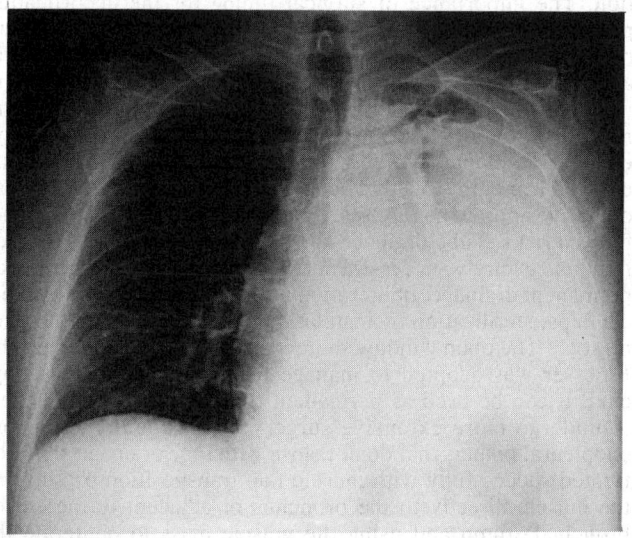

A

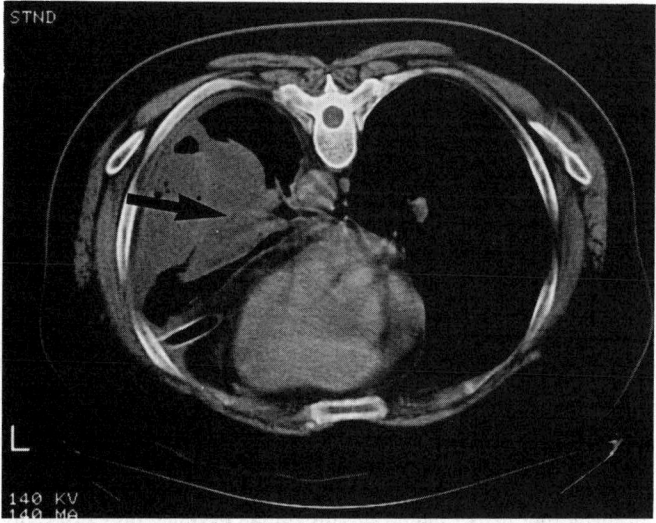

B

FIG. 2. **(A)** The patient's empyema progressed despite percutaneous drainage and appropriate antibiotic therapy. **(B)** Computed tomography showed malposition of chest tubes, but all attempts at tube drainage failed. The arrow indicates the loculated empyema. The patient responded promptly to surgical decortication.

loculated pleural effusions with bronchopleural fistulas and lung abscesses. CT has largely replaced the need for bronchograms to demonstrate bronchopleural fistulas. However, bronchoscopy and contrast-enhanced CT may be needed to define the cause of pleural empyema in patients in whom the etiology of infection is unexplained.[15]

Empyema is documented by finding pus and/or high concentrations of microorganisms in exudative pleural fluid obtained by thoracentesis. The character of the fluid depends on the type and duration of the infection and the associated trauma, surgery, malignancy, or other underlying disease. Initially, the fluid is thin and serous, but it becomes thick and purulent as neutrophil accumulation occurs. The poor correlation between the white blood cell counts in empyema fluid and the clinical features of infection may be due to lysis of neutrophils in pus. Frankly purulent specimens require only smear, culture, and drainage after demonstration that bacteria are present by Gram stain. Less overtly purulent specimens should be assessed for pH, glucose, and lactic dehydrogenase in addition to appropriate smears and cultures.[15,22] Empyema fluid characteristically has a pH of less than 7.2, glucose less than 40 mg/dl, and lactic dehydrogenase activity of at least 1000 mg/dl.[15,22] Demonstration of these features or the presence of large numbers of bacteria on Gram stain indicates that drainage procedures are probably necessary. The pH of empyema fluid has the best correlation with the extent of the inflammatory process. Acid pH is primarily metabolic in origin but affected by local CO_2 retention. It is important to keep pleural fluid specimens tightly capped and on ice to prevent spurious changes in pH or glucose.[15] The mean lactic acid concentration of pus from human abscesses is 30 mg/dl, and pH values may be as low as 5.5. Empyema fluid pH values of 6–6.7 or lower may be associated with esophageal rupture—a condition with a mortality of at least 50 percent when treatment is delayed more than 24 hours.[15] Urgent intervention with measurement of empyema fluid amylase, CT, barium swallow, or endoscopic procedures is required to direct therapy. Systemic acidosis may secondarily lower pleural fluid pH. Pleural fluid pH levels of at least 0.30 below arterial pH levels support the need for chest tube drainage.[15] At the other extreme, frankly purulent empyema fluid can have a disproportionately high pH when infection is caused by urea-splitting *Proteus* strains.[24] Empyema caused by anaerobic bacteria is malodorous in approximately 60 percent of instances.[10] Less specific findings of empyema fluid include a protein concentration of greater than 3.0 mg/dl and a specific gravity of greater than 1.018.[2]

Microorganisms in empyema fluid can usually be seen on Gram stain and grown in culture unless patients have received antibiotic therapy. Occasionally, smears will be positive and cultures will be negative. In those instances, the bacterial origin should be sought by cultures of blood and sputum. When the diagnosis is in question, pleural fluid should be tested for bacterial antigen by countercurrent immunoelectrophoresis or latex agglutination studies. In addition, fluid should be tested for *Legionella* by direct fluorescent antibody stains and culture because that organism will not be seen on conventional Gram stains. Empyema fluid devoid of microorganisms should also be examined for anaerobes, fungi, mycobacteria and amoebae. Patients thought to have pleural or pulmonary amebiasis should have serologic tests for *E. histolytica* and careful search for hepatic abscesses that are almost always present. Patients at risk of developing nocardiosis should have modified acid-fast stains. Acridine orange may permit visualization of organisms in abscess fluid that is smear negative by Gram stain. It should be noted that chylous pleural effusions may resemble purulent material, but lack white cells or microorganisms and remain opaque after centrifugation.[2] Empyema associated with systemic and pleural fluid eosinophilia is a rare condition that is highly suggestive of paragonimiasis. It can be confirmed serologically or by demonstrating eggs in stool, sputum, or, rarely, in pleural fluid.[25]

Potts and coworkers[23] found no bacteria on microscopic examination of 4 of 10 empyema fluids. Two were sterile by culture. Smear-negative sterile empyema fluid has been reported in 6–15 percent of patients, and culture-negative empyema has been described in up to 37 percent of patients.[26] Although improper culture technique, fastidious microorganisms, and prior antibiotic therapy may account for many cases of sterile empyema, it is likely that certain organisms are killed in pus. However, by the time bacterial empyemas become frankly purulent, they must be drained, whether sterile or not.

Pleural tuberculosis may be diagnosed by pleural fluid cultures or stains in 18–23 percent of patients or by cultures, stains, and histologic examination of pleural biopsy specimens in up to 95 percent of patients.[27] Liquid culture media are preferable to solid culture media, and it is rarely necessary to culture more than a single biopsy specimen. Radiometric culture detection methods may increase the speed of diagnosis in patients with pleural tuberculosis. Elevated levels of adenosine deaminase or tuberculostearic acid are indicative of tuberculous pleuritis.[15] A history of exposure, skin test conversion, or symptoms of weight loss, night sweats, and fever are helpful clues to the diagnosis of tuberculosis. However, patients may be both afebrile and anergic.

The pleural fluid of patients with rheumatoid arthritis, pancreatitis, or malignancy will occasionally have features suggestive of empyema.[2] Exudates of rheumatoid or pancreatic origin only rarely have a pH less than 7.2 and can be identified by serologic tests or increased pleural fluid amylase levels, respectively. Pleural fluid from patients with lupus erythematosus or rheumatoid pleuritis characteristically have titers of antinuclear antibody of at least 1:160 or rheumatoid factor of at least 1:320, respectively, with values exceeding those found in serum.[28,29] The rare malignant effusion with a pH of less than 7.0 is readily diagnosed by cytologic examination and is associated with a worse prognosis than that of alkaline pleural fluid.[22]

TREATMENT

The goals of treatment for pleural empyema are eradication of infection, drainage of pus, and expansion of the lung. The primary treatment of empyema is drainage and will be necessary for patients with pleural fluid containing gross pus, a heavy growth of organisms visible by microscopy, a pH less than 7.2, glucose less than 40 mg/dl, and lactic dehydrogenase greater than 1000 mg/dl.[15,22] Those with smear-negative serous pleural fluid and a pH of at least 7.2 and intermediate lactic dehydrogenase and glucose levels may be treated with antibiotics and repeat thoracentesis in 12–18 hours to reassess the need for drainage procedures.[15] Those with improving pleural fluid parameters may be followed and reassessed.[15,22] However, pleural fluid loculation indicates the presence of a complicated para-pneumonic process usually requiring ultrasound or CT-guided tube drainage or thoracoscopy and more aggressive intervention.[15]

Repeated thoracentesis is rarely adequate unless the empyema fluid is quite thin and present in small volume. Percutaneous drainage of thin or serous fluid with small-bore catheters early in the course of empyema has been successful. Closed chest tube drainage with an underwater-sealed system is successful in two-thirds of patients, and the system can be placed by the surgeon, the radiologist, or the pulmonologist.[30,31] One study has suggested that thoracoscopy and irrigation of the pleura hastens healing.[32] Thoracoscopy should increase the accuracy of pleural biopsy but requires further study.[32] Patients failing to respond to tube drainage within 24 hours should have ultrasound examination for loculated fluid and streptokinase infusion. Although streptokinase has not been uniformly satisfactory, current formulations of streptokinase are less toxic and are clearly more likely to be effective when used in the first week of infection.[15] Bronchopleural fistula is an absolute contraindication to intrapleural streptokinase.

The need for continued vacuum or water-sealed drainage is assessed by measuring the volume of fluid drained daily and by the size of the residual pleural cavity. Tubes can usually be withdrawn gradually when drainage is less than 50 ml/day and the cavity is less than 50 ml in size.[1,31]

Drainage of thick pleural pus is largely the province of the chest surgeon, who should be involved early in the course of disease.[31–36] Closed chest tube drainage fails in approximately one-third of patients, who often have more extensive disease or prior chest surgery.[13,14,31] In addition, immunocompromised patients may require more extensive drainage procedures, including early rib resection and open drainage.[14] Management of open drainage tubes with daily irrigation and convalescence for 3–4 months is a tedious and time-consuming but time-honored method. In young adults who are otherwise healthy and are good operative candidates, decortication may be preferable.[30] This procedure provides more rapid recovery and more complete restoration of pulmonary function in adults but may be needed less frequently in children.[1,30] Decortication is traditionally advocated during the second or third week or after the sixth week of the disease in order to minimize the risk of tearing the poorly demarcated pleural peel during the 3–6 weeks of illness. Control of infection is the primary indication for early decortication. The importance of surgical timing for the decortication procedure has been questioned.[34] Although small bronchopleural fistulas may close spontaneously, many are difficult to treat and require surgical closure. There is considerable variation in the frequency with which surgeons at different centers use rib resection, decortication, or empyectomy to manage empyema.[14,35,36] Similarly, several methods are used to treat chronic empyema or empyema that occurs after pneumonectomy. These operative approaches are selected on the basis of expected benefits and risks. Tube drainage has the fewest side effects, is tried first, and is rarely successful in that setting. Alternatives include permanent drainage, obliteration of the empyema space by muscle flaps, sterilization by instillation of antibiotics, and thoracoplasty.[37] The open window thoracostomy procedure devised by Eloesser was adapted to manage postpneumonectomy empyema. It can be used as permanent therapy for patients unable to undergo more extensive surgery.[35–37] Patients with bronchopleural fistulas that do not close with tube drainage are often treated successfully with muscle flap transposition by suturing the muscle directly to the bronchus or adjacent to the closed bronchial stump and using the muscle mass to obliterate the empyema cavity.[37] Patients with empyema and residual lung but without bronchopleural fistulas may respond to decortication or, if that fails, to myoplasty. Thoracoplasty is usually the procedure of last resort.[37]

Tuberculous pleural effusions rarely require more than antibiotic therapy unless a bronchopleural fistula is present. Special care should be taken not to introduce a secondary bacterial infection while performing a diagnostic or therapeutic thoracentesis of a tuberculosis pleural effusion.

The guidelines for optimal antibiotic therapy of bacterial empyema differ little from the recommendations for treatment of suppurative disease at other sites. Antibiotics are selected on the basis of their activity against microorganisms causing infection. Adequate levels of antibiotics are easily achieved in empyema fluid. β-Lactam antibiotics should be used in high doses for prolonged periods (i.e., usually 2–4 weeks for bacterial infection). Patients with nocardiosis, actinomycosis, tuberculosis, or fungal empyema require even more prolonged therapy. In addition, patients with long-standing bacterial empyema may require prolonged therapy. Aminoglycosides should not be used as single-drug therapy of bacterial empyemas because they are toxic drugs with poor activity in the abscess milieu.[17] However, aminoglycosides may be combined with β-lactam antibiotics to achieve a synergistic activity against empyema caused by *Pseudomonas aeruginosa*, *Enterobacter cloacae*, *Acinetobacter calcoaceticus*, and *Serratia marcescens*. Until more information is available, empyema caused by these multiresistant organisms should be treated initially with at least two effective antibiotics. Ciprofloxacin is a potent drug that can be given orally for protracted therapy of gram-negative empyema.

Anaerobic pleural empyema can be treated adequately with clindamycin, imipenem, or combinations of β-lactam and β-lactamase inhibitors. Although metronidazole is an excellent agent for anaerobic infection, it may be ineffective in anaerobic lung abscesses or partially drained empyemas because the drug is not reduced to its active metabolite in a partially oxygenated environment. Furthermore, it has poor activity against streptococci and actinomycetes. Chloramphenicol or tetracycline should not be used to treat empyema caused by anaerobes.

PROGNOSIS

The mortality rate of pleural empyema is affected by the type and severity of infection, the patient's health or associated underlying diseases, and the adequacy of antibiotic therapy and drainage. Although mortality rates of 8–15 percent have been reported in otherwise healthy young patients,[30,36] rates of 40–70 percent have been reported in the elderly and in groups with severe underlying disease.[14,30] Mortality is increased in patients with nosocomial infection or empyema caused by polymicrobial or resistant gram-negative bacteria.[15] Patients with inadequately drained empyemas often die.[10] There are no criteria validating the superiority of a single technique, but in general, the more fragile or compromised patient may need more rapid achievement of adequate drainage by rib resection, lysis of adhesions, and use of a large-bore drainage tube earlier in the illness because such patients are more vulnerable to the serious sequelae of malnutrition, chronic sepsis, and multiple organ failure associated with delayed drainage of pus.[14] There is still controversy over the criteria that indicate it is mandatory to perform pleural fluid drainage, but in general early intervention is preferred.[39–41] Post-traumatic empyema has a worse prognosis and should be considered for early decortication if (*1*) sepsis is not contained despite adequate antibiotic therapy, (*2*) fluid levels persist, (*3*) ventilatory function is compromised by inadequate lung expansion, or (*4*) pleural drainage is inadequate after 2 weeks of therapy.[13,14] An infected hemothorax rarely responds to tube drainage alone because clots obstruct the tube. Polymicrobial or nosocomial infection carries a worse prognosis because such patients have multiple underlying diseases and poor host defense.[7,35] In addition, these patients have an increased frequency of colonization and infection with multiply resistant gram-negative bacilli.[7] Thus, the sickest and most infirm patients often have pus that is hard to drain and organisms that are difficult to treat.

REFERENCES

1. Sherman MM, Subramanian V, Berger RL. Management of thoracic empyema. Am J Surg. 1977;133:474–9.
2. Light RW. Clinical manifestations and useful tests. In: Light RW, ed. Pleural Diseases. Philadelphia: Lea & Febiger; 1983:33–60.
3. O'Moore PV, Mueller PR, Simeone F. Sonographic guidance in diagnostic and therapeutic interventions in the pleural space. AJR. 1987;149:1–5.
4. Mirvis SE, Tobin KD, Kostrubiak I, et al. Thoracic CT in detecting occult disease in critically ill patients. AJR. 1987;148:685–9.
5. Van Sonnenberg E, Nakamoto SK, Mueller PR, et al. CT and ultrasound guided catheter drainage of empyemas after chest-tube failure. Radiology. 1984;151:349–53.
6. Weese WC, Shindler ER, Smith IM, et al. Empyema of the thorax then and now. Arch Intern Med. 1973;131:516–20.
7. Vianna NJ. Nontuberculous bacterial empyema in patients with and without underlying disease. JAMA. 1971;215:69–71.
8. Freij BJ, Kusmiesz H, Nelson JD, McCracken GH. Parapneumonic effusions and empyema in hospitalized children. A retrospective review of 227 cases. Pediatr Infect Dis. 1984;3:578–91.
9. Farley MM, Stephens DS, Brachman PS, et al. Invasive *H. influenzae* disease in adults. A prospective, population-based surveillance. Ann Intern Med. 1992;116:801–12.
10. Bartlett JG, Finegold SM. Anaerobic infections of the lung and pleural space. Am Rev Respir Dis. 1974;110:56–77.

11. Bartlett JG, Thadepalli H, Gorbach SL, et al. Bacteriology of empyema. Lancet. 1974;1:338–40.
12. Ballantyne KC, Sethia B, Reece IJ, et al. Empyema following intra-abdominal sepsis. Br J Surg. 1984;71:723–5.
13. Caplan ES, Hoyt NJ, Rodriguez A, et al. Empyema occurring in the multiply traumatized patient. J Trauma. 1984;24:785–98.
14. Lemmer JH, Botham MJ, Orringer MD. Modern management of adult thoracic empyema. J Thorac Cardiovasc Surg. 1985;90:849–55.
15. Light RW. Management of empyema. Seminars in respiratory medicine. 1992; 13:167–76.
16. Lew P, Zubler R, Vaudauz P. Decreased heat-labile opsonic activity and complement levels associated with evidence of C3 breakdown products in infected pleural effusions. J Clin Invest. 1979;63:326–34.
17. Bryant RE. Pus: Friend or foe? In: Root RK, Trunkey D, Sande MD, eds. Contemporary Issues in Infectious Diseases. v. V: New Surgical and Medical Approaches. New York: Churchill Livingstone, 1987;31–48.
18. Bryant RE. Effect of the suppurative environment on antibiotic activity. In: Root RK, Sand MD, eds. Contemporary Issues in Infectious Diseases. v. 1: New Dimensions in Antimicrobial Therapy. New York: Churchill Livingstone, 1984;313–37.
19. Bryant RE, Fox KE, Oh G, Morthland VH. β-Lactam enhancement of aminoglycoside activity under conditions of reduced pH and oxygen tension that may exist in infected tissues. J Infect Dis. 1992;165:676–82.
20. Andrews NC, Parker EF, Shaw RP, et al. Management of nontuberculous empyema. Am Rev Respir Dis. 1963;3:935–6.
21. Mavroudis C, Ganzel BL, Cox SK, et al. Experimental aerobic-anaerobic thoracic empyema in the guinea pig. Ann Thorac Surg. 1987;43:298–302.
22. Good JA, Taryle DA, Maulitz RM, et al. The diagnostic value of pleural fluid pH. Chest. 1980;78:55–9.
23. Potts DE, Levin DC, Sahn SA. Pleural fluid pH in parapneumonic effusions. Chest. 1976;70:328–31.
24. Pine JR, Hollman JL. Elevated pleural fluid pH in *Proteus mirabilis* empyema. Chest. 1983;84:99–111.
25. Skerrett SJ, Plorde JJ. Parasitic infections of the pleural space. Seminars in respiratory medicine. 1992;13:242–58.
26. Yeh TJ, Hall DP, Ellison RG. Empyema thoracis: A review. Am Rev Respir Dis. 1963;88:785–90.
27. Levine H, Metzger W, Lacera D, et al. Diagnosis of tuberculous pleurisy by culture of pleural biopsy specimen. Arch Intern Med. 1970;126:269–71.
28. Good JT Jr, King TE, Antony VB, et al. Lupus pleuritis: Clinical features and pleural fluid characteristics with special reference to pleural fluid antinuclear antibodies. Chest 1983;84:714–8.
29. Halla JT, Schrohenloher RE, Valanakis JE, et al. Immune complexes and other features of pleural effusions. Ann Intern Med. 1980;92:748–52.
30. Mandal AK, Thadepalli H. Treatment of spontaneous bacterial empyema thoracis. J Thorac Cardiovasc Surg. 1987;94:414–8.
31. Miller KS, Sahn SA. Chest tubes. Chest. 1987;91:258–64.
32. Hutter JA, Harari D, Braimbridge MV. The management of empyema thoracis by thoracoscopy and irrigation. Ann Thorac Surg. 1985;39:517–20.
33. Mittapalli MR. Successful treatment of empyema with thoracenteses and intrapleural antibiotics. South Med J. 1980;73:533–4.
34. Hoover LE, Ross MJ, Webb H, et al. Reappraisal of empyema thoracis. Chest. 1986;90:511–5.
35. Grant DR, Finley RJ. Empyema: Analysis of treatment techniques. Can J Surg. 1985;28:449–52.
36. Mayo P. Early thoracotomy and decortication for nontuberculous empyema in adults with and without underlying diseases. Am Surg. 1985;4:230–6.
37. Le Roux BT, Mohlala ML, Odell JA, et al. Suppurative diseases of the lung and pleural space. Part 1: Empyema thoracis and lung abscess. Curr Probl Surg. 1986;23:4–38.
38. Sahn SA, Light RW. The sun should never set on a parapneumonic effusion. Chest 1989;95:945–6.
39. Poe RH, Marin MG, Israel RH, et al. Utility of pleural fluid analysis in predicting tube thoracostomy/decortication in parapneumonic effusions. Chest 1991; 100:963–67.
40. Himelman RB, Callen PW. The prognostic value of loculations in parapneumonic pleural effusions. Chest 1986;90:852–6.
41. Berger HA, Morganroth ML. Immediate drainage is not required for all patients with complicated parapneumonic effusions. Chest 1990;97:731–5.

52. LUNG ABSCESS

SYDNEY M. FINEGOLD

Lung abscess is a suppurative pulmonary infection involving the destruction of lung parenchyma to produce one or more large cavities with an air–fluid level. A similar process with multiple small cavitations (less than 2 cm in diameter) has been designated *necrotizing pneumonia* by some clinicians. The distinction is arbitrary since lung abscess and necrotizing pneumonia are different expressions of the same fundamental pathologic process. The earliest manifestation of this type of problem is pneumonia without excavation or abscess formation. In the absence of effective therapy, the disease may progress to lung abscess or to necrotizing pneumonia, with or without pleural empyema. Generally, the specific infecting organisms and the predisposing conditions do not influence the type of clinical disease that results. However, the size of the inoculum of organisms and the defense mechanisms of the host are likely to influence the outcome. Most often lung abscess follows aspiration, and anaerobic bacteria are the major organisms involved.

PREDISPOSING CAUSES

By far the most important background factor for abscess of the lung is aspiration,[1] usually related to altered consciousness. Common causes of altered consciousness in such patients are alcoholism, cerebral vascular accident, general anesthesia, drug overdose or addiction, seizure disorder, diabetic coma, shock, and other serious illness. Other factors in aspiration include dysphagia due to either esophageal disease or neurologic disease, intestinal obstruction, and tonsillectomy or tooth extraction. A study by Huxley et al.[2] using a sensitive radioactive tracer technique determined that 70 percent of patients with depressed consciousness and 45 percent of healthy subjects in deep sleep aspirated. Aspiration occurred more frequently and extensively in patients with depressed consciousness. Impairment of normal clearance mechanisms or the overwhelming of such mechanisms by large volumes of aspirated secretions may result in pulmonary infection. Alcoholics and patients who are acutely or chronically ill (whether or not they are hospitalized or in a nursing home) often demonstrate oropharyngeal colonization with gram-negative bacilli, particularly if they undergo endotracheal intubation and especially if they also receive histamine type 2 blockers or antacids.[3,4]

Next to aspiration, the most important factor predisposing to lung abscess or to necrotizing pneumonia is periodontal disease or gingivitis. Lung abscess is rare in an edentulous person and suggests the possibility of an associated bronchogenic carcinoma.[5] Other underlying processes include bronchiectasis, secondary infection of a bland pulmonary embolus with infarction, septic embolization, bacteremia, inhalation of bacteria-containing aerosols, and intra-abdominal infection. Suppurative inflammation behind an obstruction in a bronchus is another important mechanism. Patients receiving immunosuppressive therapy may develop multiple lung abscesses due to *Nocardia* or other organisms.

PATHOGENESIS AND PATHOLOGIC CHARACTERISTICS

Lung abscess is primarily of endogenous origin. Most of the bacteria involved are elements of the normal flora of the upper respiratory tract. Infections involving *Staphylococcus aureus, Klebsiella,* and other organisms may be of nosocomial origin.

The primary site of lung abscess is the posterior segment of the right upper lobe, with the same segment on the left less commonly affected. Next in frequency of involvement are the apical segments of the lower lobes. These segments are dependent in location when the subject is in a horizontal position, and the distribution relates to the fact that aspiration or inhalation is the primary background factor. Normally, aspirated material is handled effectively by ciliary action, cough, and alveolar macrophages. If the protective mechanisms are not effective, as with ethanol ingestion or viral disease, infection may result. Endotracheal tubes impair coughing, impede pulmonary clearance mechanisms, and allow leakage of oropharyngeal secretions into the tracheobronchial tree. Thick or particulate matter and foreign bodies are not easily removed and thus may lead to

bronchial obstruction and atelectasis. With aspiration, gastric acid and enzymes may be the primary offending agents.

Subdiaphragmatic infection may extend to the lung or to the pleural space by way of lymphatics, directly through the diaphragm or defects in it, or by way of the blood stream. Most amebic lung abscesses are located in the right lower lobe adjacent to the diaphragm since they typically arise by direct extension of hepatic abscesses through the diaphragm.

Infection may arise in or behind an obstruction (neoplasm, foreign body, or enlarged mediastinal lymph node). Septic emboli from bacterial endocarditis of the right side of the heart or from pelvic or other deep vein thrombophlebitis may result in a metastatic lung abscess.

Although the virulence of the infecting organism(s) may be a factor determining the nature and extent of the infectious process, this is not usually important in the case of the anaerobes except for *Fusobacterium necrophorum.* Certain other anaerobes, especially *Fusobacterium nucleatum* and the *Bacteroides fragilis* group, are more likely to be present as the sole infecting organism, an indication of virulence. The number of organisms aspirated may well be an important factor. With certain of the nonanaerobes such as *Klebsiella, Staphylococcus,* and group A *Streptococcus,* virulence may play an important role.

The pathologic characteristic is essentially that of necrosis supervened on inflammation with cavitation and abscess formation. The abscess cavity may become partially lined with regenerated epithelium, and localized bronchiectasis and emphysema may develop. There is usually no significant vascular involvement in lung abscess. However, a septic or bland pulmonary embolus may be the initial event. Once underway, the infection itself may give rise to pulmonary arteritis as in infection caused by *Pseudomonas aeruginosa.*

CLINICAL MANIFESTATIONS

Anaerobic Lung Abscess

In patients with lung abscess admitted to a hospital, symptoms have generally been present for at least 2 weeks. At times the patient will have had several weeks or even months of malaise, low-grade fever, and productive cough before seeking medical attention. Weight loss and anemia are common and confirm that the infection is indolent. Often the patient runs a low-grade fever, that is, a temperature about 101–102°F. Sputum production is usually copious. Foul-smelling sputum or empyema fluid occurs in only about one-half of the patients.[1,5,6]

In patients in whom the course of the infection has been followed radiologically, pneumonia appears first and cavitation subsequently. The earliest time of appearance of a cavity is about 7 days after aspiration; the average is about 12 days. Mediastinal adenopathy occasionally accompanies the parenchymal disease in patients with lung abscess or with other types of anaerobic pulmonary infection.[6] There may be a history of a period of unconsciousness, evidence of alcoholism, diseased gums, absence of the gag reflex, or other indications of the predisposing condition.

The physical findings are those of a pneumonia, with or without pleural effusion, early in the course of the illness. Later there may be amphoric or cavernous breath sounds. Clubbing of the fingers is noted on occasion.

Anaerobic Necrotizing Pneumonia

Usually anaerobic necrotizing pneumonia is confined primarily to one pulmonary segment or lobe. However, it may extend to involve an entire lung or even both lungs (Fig. 1). This type of anaerobic pulmonary infection is the most severe of all. There may be an associated empyema. The disease often spreads rapidly and produces destruction that is characterized by ragged,

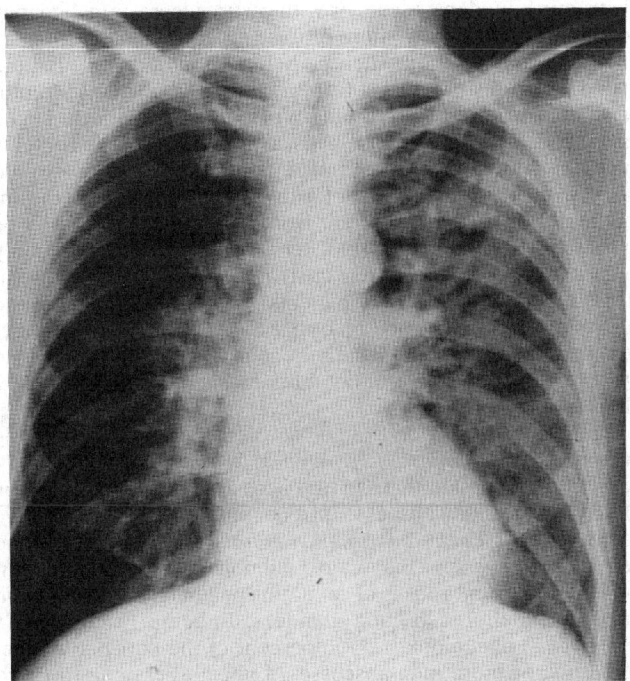

FIG. 1. Posterior–anterior (PA) chest film, anaerobic necrotizing pneumonia, and empyema. There is major involvement of the left lung, less involvement of the right. Note the multiple small excavations and one larger cavity in the left lung and blunting of the left costophrenic angle.

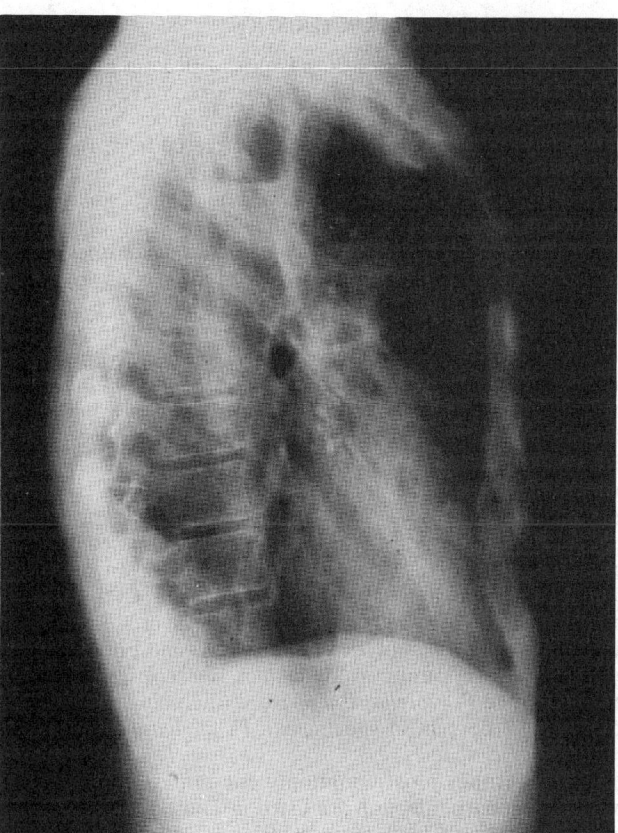

FIG. 2. Lateral chest film, hematogenous staphylococcal lung abscesses and empyema. Note the air–fluid levels.

greenish discoloration of the lung and large putrid sloughs of tissue. This process culminates in "pulmonary gangrene."[5–7]

The patients are generally quite ill, with a temperature of 102–103°F. Leukocytosis is usually pronounced, for example, more than 20,000/mm^3. Most of these patients have putrid sputum or empyema fluid when first seen.

Pulmonary actinomycosis may be manifested as a necrotizing pneumonia; a number of cases will be complicated by extension of the process to the pleural space and to the chest wall.

Nonanaerobic Lung Abscess and Necrotizing Pneumonia

In primary infections due to organisms such as *S. aureus, Streptococcus pyogenes, Nocardia,* or *Klebsiella pneumoniae,* the symptoms are those of a severe pneumonia.

Secondary Lung Abscess and Necrotizing Pneumonia

In cases of secondary lung abscess, the basic process (bacteremia, endocarditis, septic thrombophlebitis, subphrenic infection, and so forth) will usually be evident in addition to the pulmonary process. The most characteristic hematogenous lung abscess is seen in staphylococcal bacteremia, especially in children. These abscesses are commonly multiple and peripheral in location. Empyema is frequently seen in this situation (Fig. 2). Repeated septic emboli should be suspected when multiple lesions appear over an extended period.

Less than 5 percent of bland pulmonary infarcts become secondarily infected. Secondary infection of infarcts should be suspected if fever is persistent, if the temperature rises above 103°F for more than 48 hours, or if the white blood cell count rises to more than 20,000 cells/mm^3. Abscess formation may occur within a necrotic pulmonary tumor or behind an obstructing tumor.

The syndrome of tonsillitis or pharyngitis (Vincent's angina) with septicemia due to *F. necrophorum,* followed by widespread metastatic disease involving the lungs and other organs, is not commonly seen any longer, probably as a result of early antibiotic therapy for upper respiratory tract infections. However, it is important to be aware of this serious illness that occurs in children and young adults.

Amebic Lung Abscess

In patients with amebic lung abscess, the symptoms of the associated liver abscess will often have been present before the rupture through the diaphragm. After perforation of the liver abscess into the lung, there is a gradually developing cough and expectoration of a peculiar chocolaty or anchovy saucelike sputum. There is no odor to the sputum. The development of a pulmonary amebic abscess varies from a very insidious phenomenon to a dramatic onset with a sudden attack of severe cough productive of a large amount of brownish red sputum.[8] There may be a history of diarrhea, and an appropriate travel history may be elicited.

Complications

Approximately one-third of lung abscesses are complicated by empyema. This may be seen with or without bronchopleural fistulas. Brain abscess may also be a complication in patients not receiving appropriate therapy early. A brain abscess is typically solitary. There is virtually never dissemination to other organs. Localized bronchiectasis may occur. Amyloidosis is no longer seen.

Complications of amebic abscess[9] include spontaneous perforation creating a cutaneous sinus, hepatobronchial fistula, empyema, secondary bacterial infection, and amebic abscess of the brain.

MICROBIOLOGIC CHARACTERISTICS

In a prospective study of 26 patients with lung abscesses by Bartlett et al.,[1] anaerobic bacteria were recovered in 24 of the 26 transtracheal aspirate specimens. Only anaerobes (including microaerophilic streptococci) were recovered from 16 of the 24 patients, whereas aerobic or facultative bacteria were recovered along with anaerobes in the other 8. Four patients had a single anaerobe recovered in pure culture, whereas 20 patients had multiple isolates, averaging 3.1 bacteria (2.6 anaerobes) per patient. The most commonly encountered anaerobes were gram-negative rods and gram-positive cocci.

Among 28 cases of anaerobic necrotizing pneumonia,[5] 20 yielded only anaerobes. Overall, there was an average of 2.3 anaerobes and 0.4 aerobes per case. *Fusobacterium nucleatum*, pigmented and other *Bacteroides* (some of which would now be classified as *Prevotella* or *Porphyromonas*), and anaerobic and microaerophilic streptococci and cocci predominated among the anaerobes. Another distinctive cause of necrotizing pneumonia is actinomycosis.

A recent retrospective study of anaerobic or mixed anaerobic pulmonary infections[12] yielded an average of 3.5 anaerobes and 1.7 aerobic or facultative bacteria per specimen. Of the 117 specimens studied, 33 yielded only anaerobes. The predominant nonanaerobes were α-hemolytic *Streptococcus* and Enterobacteriaceae. The predominant anaerobes were pigmented and nonpigmented *Prevotella, Bacteroides* (including the *B. fragilis* group in 4.4 percent of specimens), *F. nucleatum*, and *Peptostreptococcus* species.

The anaerobes most commonly encountered in anaerobic pleuropulmonary infection are listed in Table 1. Although clostridia, including *Clostridium perfringens*, may be recovered from patients with necrotizing pneumonia and empyema or other anaerobic pulmonary infections, there is usually nothing distinctive about the clinical picture in such cases.

There is an important difference in bacterial cause in terms of whether the patient aspirates in the community or in the hospital setting.[6,13] Community-acquired aspiration pneumonia is primarily an anaerobic process, with 35 of 38 cases studied yielding anaerobes and 25 yielding only this type of organism.[13] On the other hand, cultures from patients aspirating in the hospital setting yielded anaerobes in 26 of 32 cases (in pure culture in only 7 cases) and, most importantly, as part of the other infecting flora yielded important nosocomial pathogens such as *S. aureus* and various aerobic and facultative gram-negative bacilli such as *Klebsiella, Pseudomonas,* and *Proteus*.

Nichols and Smith[14] have shown that patients with bleeding or

TABLE 1. Anaerobes Most Commonly Encountered in Pleuropulmonary Infection

Gram-negative bacilli
  Pigmented *Prevotella* or *Porphyromonas*
  Prevotella oralis group
    P. oris
    P. buccae
    P. bivia
  Bacteroides ureolyticus group (especially *B. gracilis*)
  B. fragilis group
  Fusobacterium nucleatum
    F. necrophorum
    F. naviforme
    F. gonidiaformans
Gram-positive cocci
  Peptostreptococcus (especially *P. micros, P. anaerobius, P. magnus,*
    P. asaccharolyticus, P. prevotii, P. intermedius[a])
  Microaerophilic streptococci
Gram-positive spore-forming bacilli
  Clostridium perfringens, C. ramosum
Gram-positive nonspore-forming bacilli
  Actinomyces spp.
  Propionibacterium propionicum
  Bifidobacterium dentium

[a] This organism officially belongs in the genus *Streptococcus*.

(Data from refs. 10–12, 22.)

obstructing duodenal ulcers or with gastric ulcers or malignancy commonly have a much more profuse microflora in the stomach than do people without such pathologic conditions. This flora includes various organisms from the oral flora such as streptococci and anaerobes of various types but also coliform bacilli and, on occasion, *B. fragilis*. Thus, aspiration of gastric contents in people with the aforementioned pathologic conditions would carry with it a greater risk of bacterial infection, and the infecting flora might be different from what would ordinarily be expected. Histamine type 2 blockers or antacids have commonly been used to prevent upper gastrointestinal bleeding due to stress ulcers in critically ill patients. This leads to an elevated gastric pH and gastric and pharyngeal (by the retrograde route) colonization with gram-negative bacilli. This may be avoided by the use of sucralfate in lieu of antacids or histamine type 2 blockers.[3]

There are also several major aerobic causes of necrotizing pneumonia: *S. aureus, S. pyogenes, K. pneumoniae,* and *P. aeruginosa*. It is said that, on rare occasion, pneumococci (type 3) may cause a lung abscess. Infrequently, other gram-negative bacilli such as *Escherichia coli, Legionella pneumophila,* and perhaps *Proteus* spp. may cause pulmonary necrosis. Uncommon but important causes of cavitating pneumonia are *Nocardia* infection, melioidosis, and glanders. In acute Friedländer's (*Klebsiella*) pneumonia, 25–50 percent of the patients will develop one or more lung abscesses. Lung abscess due to *Pseudomonas cepacia* was reported by Poe et al.[15] The source of the organism was determined to be the reservoir of an ultrasonic nebulizer. Such nebulizers have been implicated in gram-negative bacillary pneumonia by several groups of investigators. However, although necrotizing pneumonia is seen in a proportion of these groups, a solitary lung abscess is uncommon. In infants with staphylococcal pneumonia, pneumatoceles occur as frequently as abscesses, whereas in adults the radiolucencies almost always represent abscess formation. Tuberculosis may also cause necrotizing pneumonia, and fungal infection (particularly histoplasmosis, coccidioidomycosis, and aspergillosis) sometimes produces this lesion.

Three major groups of bacteria are involved in hematogenous spread to the lungs: gram-positive cocci, notably staphylococci; gram-negative enteric bacilli; and anaerobic bacteria. Multiple abscesses are likely to be of hematogenous origin, either as a result of bacteremia or of septic embolization. The most characteristic hematogenous lung abscess is seen in staphylococcal bacteremia. Hematogenous pulmonary infection with gram-negative enteric bacilli occurs in association with urinary tract infection or manipulation, after bowel surgery, after septic abortion, or as a nosocomial infection (usually in relation to vascular or urinary tract catheterization). Anaerobic or microaerophilic streptococci and gram-negative anaerobic bacilli may also produce hematogenous necrotizing pulmonary infection secondary to intra-abdominal or pelvic infections. In all of these anaerobic infections, there may be only bacteremia or else a septic thrombophlebitis that results in septic embolization. Uncommon hematogenous necrotizing pulmonary processes are those seen with anthrax, plague, and *Salmonella choleraesuis* infection.

Metastatic lung abscess may occur as a result of septic emboli from bacterial endocarditis of the right side of the heart (*S. aureus* is the major pathogen in this setting) or from pelvic or other deep vein thrombophlebitis. Various anaerobic bacteria and also pyogenic cocci such as *S. aureus* and streptococci not infrequently cause septic thrombophlebitis. As noted earlier, the anaerobes may be involved in this type of process in association with pelvic or intra-abdominal infection or, uncommonly now, with jugular vein thrombophlebitis in association with tonsillopharyngeal infections. Thrombophlebitis of the cavernous sinus most often involves *S. aureus* or streptococci. *Staphylococcus aureus* may also produce septic thrombophlebitis in association with superficial skin or soft tissue infections or in relation to intravenous catheters. The latter setting also may lead to septic thrombophlebitis involving gram-negative bacilli. Various organisms may be involved in secondary infection of bland pulmonary infarcts, including staphylococci, streptococci, pneumococci, gram-negative enteric bacilli, and anaerobes of various types. Infection within a necrotic pulmonary tumor or behind an obstructing tumor may lead to abscess formation. Anaerobic bacteria of various types are commonly involved in such infections, but various other infecting organisms including *Mycobacterium tuberculosis* and fungi, as well as a variety of bacteria, may also be involved.

Unusual organisms may be involved in immunocompromised patients. There is a report[16] of a lung abscess due to *Rhodococcus (Corynebacterium) equi* in a renal transplant recipient.

DIAGNOSIS

The typical lung abscess can be suspected on clinical grounds. Most diagnoses are made from the chest roentgenogram, specifically from the presence of a cavity with an air–fluid level or pneumonitis with multiple small excavations located in a dependent segment. Diagnosis of the specific cause as well as differentiation from similar lesions depends on definitive bacteriologic studies. Because of the presence of large numbers of anaerobes as indigenous flora in the mouth and the common presence in hospitalized people of potential pathogens such as *S. aureus* and *K. pneumoniae* as colonizers in the mouth or the upper respiratory tract, it is necessary to obtain a specimen other than expectorated sputum for bacteriologic diagnosis. Empyema fluid, if available, provides an excellent specimen. On occasion, particularly with a metastatic lung abscess, blood cultures may be positive; however, blood cultures may reveal only part of the infecting flora. In the absence of the aforementioned sources of specimens for diagnosis, percutaneous transtracheal aspiration may be performed to establish the specific cause of the lung abscess or necrotizing pneumonia in patients who are able to cooperate.[17] This procedure should not be used in people with a significant bleeding tendency or in those in whom it is difficult to provide adequate oxygenation. Percutaneous transthoracic aspiration may be useful, particularly in children, but provides a smaller, less satisfactory specimen. Obtaining specimens during fiberoptic bronchoscopy by means of a bronchial brush within a plugged double-lumen catheter[18] is much more widely used now than transtracheal aspiration. It is absolutely essential that the techniques as outlined in detail by Broughton et al.[19] be used exactly as described and that cultures be done quantitatively. Growth at a 10^{-3} dilution is considered significant. The amount of the secretions collected by the brush is 0.001–0.01 ml, so the 10^{-3} dilution represents 10^5–10^6 organisms/ml of lower respiratory tract secretions. The small volume of material obtained and the difficulty one would encounter to arrange for anaerobic transport are a concern; nevertheless, good results appear to have been obtained in a small number of cases of anaerobic pulmonary infection. Quantitative culture of fluid obtained by bronchoalveolar lavage (during bronchoscopy) has provided reliable results in bacterial pneumonia[20] and is rather widely used. There is little information available on recovery of anaerobes from such specimens so far, but limited studies are promising.[21] It is likely that quantitative culture of other respiratory tract specimens (e.g., aspirates from tracheostomies or endotracheal tubes) would provide reliable information.

It is essential that material obtained for culture be placed under anaerobic conditions promptly before transport to the laboratory. It is usually desirable to aspirate the material to be cultured into a syringe, to expel all bubbles of air or gas from the syringe and needle, and then to transfer the specimen to a tube that has been gassed out with oxygen-free gas for transport to the laboratory.[22]

Demonstration of the usual underlying liver abscess is basic to the diagnosis of amebic lung abscess, but one may be able to demonstrate *Entamoeba histolytica* in the patient's sputum.

Charcot-Leyden crystals in the sputum are suggestive of amebic infection. The usual procedures for the diagnosis of intestinal or hepatic amebiasis should be undertaken. The vast majority of patients with extraintestinal amebiasis will have high titers of hemagglutinating or complement-fixing antibodies.

Differential Diagnosis

Factors that would suggest a cavitating carcinoma rather than lung abscess include the absence of predisposing factors for an aspiration abscess (including an edentulous patient), location of an abscess in a nondependent segment, irregular abscess wall, and failure to respond to antibacterial therapy. Tuberculosis may also simulate a lung abscess or necrotizing pneumonia. Patients with infected lung cysts typically lack the systemic symptoms that may be seen in lung abscess, the cavity wall is thin, and there is no surrounding pneumonitis.

THERAPY AND PROGNOSIS

The primary mode of therapy is the administration of antimicrobial agents. Treatment may need to be continued for 2–4 months to achieve cure without relapse. Features to be monitored include fever, sputum production, and radiographic appearance of the abscess.

The anaerobes involved in lung abscess or in necrotizing pneumonia are increasingly resistant to penicillin G. Reports have appeared of less than optimum response or even frank failure to cure anaerobic lung abscesses or necrotizing pneumonia with penicillin therapy,[23–25] primarily because of β-lactamase–producing, gram-negative anaerobic rods. Metronidazole, or clindamycin, supplemented with penicillin G, represents one of the treatments of choice for serious anaerobic pulmonary infections. Since some of the anaerobic cocci may require 8 units/ml or more of penicillin G for inhibition, one should use large doses of this agent (10–20 million units/day intravenously in adults). Thus, penicillin G (or penicillin V, ampicillin, or amoxicillin) is no longer used by the author as the sole initial therapy for patients with a suspected or proven anaerobic lung abscess or necrotizing pneumonia who are moderately or seriously ill. Patients who are not very ill may be treated satisfactorily with penicillin, at times even with an oral penicillin (or cephalosporin). Other penicillins are often considerably less active than is penicillin G.

A significant percentage of strains of most anaerobes are resistant to tetracyclines. Accordingly, these compounds should be used only when susceptibility data are available or when the patient's illness is minor so that a therapeutic trial in the patient can be undertaken safely. Clindamycin is active against most anaerobes with the exception of some strains of *Peptostreptococcus, Bacteroides gracilis, Fusobacterium varium*, and some strains of clostridia other than *C. perfringens*; 20 percent of the *B. fragilis* group are resistant in some centers. The addition of penicillin G would increase the spectrum of coverage except for the *B. fragilis* group and *B. gracilis*. Metronidazole is active against all gram-negative anaerobes including the *B. fragilis* group and other β-lactamase producers except for some *B. gracilis* strains. It is also essentially always active against all clostridia. Some anaerobic cocci and most microaerophilic streptococci, *Actinomyces*, and *Propionibacterium propionicum* strains are resistant. For this reason, metronidazole should ordinarily be used together with penicillin G (or erythromycin) in the treatment of anaerobic pulmonary infections. Certain β-lactam agents are quite active against the *B. fragilis* group and other β-lactamase–producing *Bacteroides* and most other anaerobes, although increasing resistance has been encountered in some centers. Included are cefoxitin, the carboxy penicillins (carbenicillin and ticarcillin), and the piperazine and ureidopenicillins (piperacillin and mezlocillin). Cefoxitin is inactive against one-third of clostridia other than *C. perfringens*. These agents, especially the piperazine and ureidopenicillins and cefoxitin, also have significant activity against various Enterobacteriaceae. Cefoxitin is also active against *S. aureus*, and the penicillins mentioned have activity against *P. aeruginosa*. The third-generation cephalosporins and related new compounds all have less activity against anaerobes, especially the *B. fragilis* group, than do cefoxitin and the broad-spectrum penicillins just discussed. One exception is imipenem, which is active against virtually all anaerobes. Combinations of β-lactam drugs and β-lactamase inhibitors such as ticarcillin plus clavulanic acid and ampicillin plus sulbactam are active against essentially all anaerobes and have good activity vs. *S. aureus* and many gram-negative bacilli. Chloramphenicol is active against essentially all anaerobes of all types and represents another option in a seriously ill patient with necrotizing pneumonia or lung abscess in whom β-lactamase-producing anaerobes may be present.

For staphylococcal infections, a penicillinase-resistant penicillin is preferable, but one of the parenteral cephalosporins or vancomycin may be used in the event of significant allergy. Vancomycin is the drug of choice for methicillin-resistant *S. aureus*. Penicillin G is the drug of choice for group A streptococcal infection. For infections due to *K. pneumoniae* or other facultative or aerobic gram-negative bacilli that may be involved in the type of pulmonary infection under discussion, one of the aminoglycosides would represent a good choice, but the extended-spectrum penicillins, certain newer cephalosporins and aztreonam, and combinations of β-lactam drugs and β-lactamase inhibitors have very good activity against some of these organisms. This is also true of imipenem. Trimethoprim sulfamethoxazole and the newer quinolones have good activity against many nonanaerobic gram-negative rods and may be useful in combination regimens. Gentamicin is ordinarily suitable, but in certain hospitals significant numbers of gram-negative bacilli are resistant to gentamicin; amikacin would then be the aminoglycoside of choice. In seriously ill patients, particularly those who may be immunosuppressed, the use of appropriate β-lactam agents along with the aminoglycoside is desirable.

Postural drainage is an important aspect of the therapy for a lung abscess. Bronchoscopy may be helpful in effecting drainage and for removal of foreign bodies and biopsy diagnosis of tumors. Surgical resection of lung abscesses is rarely required unless there is a coexisting malignant process. Indeed, surgery is contraindicated because of the hazard of the spread of infection or asphyxiation from spillage of abscess contents. Surgical drainage of a lung abscess through the chest wall is rarely indicated. Complicating empyemas do require drainage.

Prognosis

The prognosis varies with the type of underlying or predisposing pathologic process, if any, and, in the case of acute severe necrotizing pneumonias, the speed with which appropriate therapy is instituted. The mortality in anaerobic lung abscess is 15 percent or less. In anaerobic necrotizing pneumonia it is 25 percent. The mortality may be significantly higher in acute pneumonias caused by *S. aureus*, *K. pneumoniae*, and other facultative or aerobic gram-negative bacilli. The prognosis in amebic lung abscess is good when the diagnosis and treatment are prompt. Nocardiosis often has a relatively poor prognosis, especially when it complicates a serious underlying disease.

REFERENCES

1. Bartlett JG, Gorbach SL, Tally FP, et al. Bacteriology and treatment of primary lung abscess. Am Rev Respir Dis. 1974;109:510–18.
2. Huxley EJ, Viroslav J, Gray WR, et al. Pharyngeal aspiration in normal adults and patients with depressed consciousness. Am J Med. 1978;64:564–68.
3. Driks MR, Craven DE, Celli BR, et al. Nosocomial pneumonia in intubated patients given sucralfate as compared with antacids or histamine type 2 blockers. N Engl J Med. 1987;317:1376–82.
4. Tryba M. Risk of acute stress bleeding and nosocomial pneumonia in ventilated intensive care unit patients: Sucralfate versus antacids. Am J Med. 1987; 83(Suppl 3B):117–24.
5. Bartlett JG, Finegold SM. Anaerobic infections of the lung and pleural space. Am Rev Respir Dis. 1974;110:56–77.
6. Finegold SM. Anaerobic Bacteria in Human Disease. New York: Academic Press; 1977.
7. Bartlett JG, Finegold SM. Anaerobic pleuropulmonary infections. Medicine (Baltimore). 1972;51:413–50.
8. Craig DF. The Etiology, Diagnosis and Treatment of Amebiasis. Baltimore: Williams & Wilkins; 1944.
9. Ochsner A, DeBakey ME. Pleuropulmonary complications of amebiasis: An analysis of 153 collected and 15 personal cases. J Thorac Surg. 1936;5:225–58.
10. Kirby BD, George WL, Sutter VL, et al. Gram-negative anaerobic bacilli: Their role in infection and patterns of susceptibility to antimicrobial agents. I. Little-known *Bacteroides* species. Rev Infect Dis. 1980;2:914–51.
11. George WL, Kirby BD, Sutter VL, et al. Gram-negative anaerobic bacilli: Their role in infection and patterns of susceptibility to antimicrobial agents. II. Little-known *Fusobacterium* species and miscellaneous genera. Rev Infect Dis. 1981;3:599–626.
12. Marina M, Strong CA, Civen R, et al. Bacteriology of anaerobic pleuropulmonary infection: A preliminary report. Clin Infect Dis. 1993;16(Suppl. 4): S256–62.
13. Bartlett JG, Gorbach SL, Finegold SM. The bacteriology of aspiration pneumonia. Am J Med. 1974;56:202–07.
14. Nichols RL, Smith JW. Intragastric microbial colonization in common disease states of the stomach and duodenum. Ann Surg. 1975;182:557–61.
15. Poe RH, Marcus HR, Emerson GL. Lung abscess due to *Pseudomonas cepacia*. Am Rev Respir Dis. 1977;115:861–65.
16. Savdie E, Pigott P, Jennis F. Lung abscess due to *Corynebacterium equi* in a renal transplant recipient. Med J Aust. 1977;1:817–19.
17. Bartlett JG, Rosenblatt JE, Finegold SM. Percutaneous transtracheal aspiration in the diagnosis of anaerobic pulmonary infection. Ann Intern Med. 1973; 79:535–40.
18. Wimberly NW, Bass JB Jr, Boyd BW, et al. Use of a bronchoscopic protected catheter brush for the diagnosis of pulmonary infections. Chest. 1982;81: 556–62.
19. Broughton WA, Bass JB, Kirkpatrick MB. The technique of protected brush catheter bronchoscopy. J Crit Ill. 1987;2:63–70.
20. Kahn FW, Jones JM. Diagnosing bacterial respiratory infection by bronchoalveolar lavage. J Infect Dis. 1987;155:862–9.
21. Henriquez AH, Mendoza J, Gonzalez PC. Quantitative culture of bronchoalveolar lavage from patients with anaerobic lung abscesses. J Infect Dis. 1991; 164:414–17.
22. Summanen P, Baron EJ, Citron DM, et al. Wadsworth Anaerobic Bacteriology Manual. 5th ed. Belmont, CA: Star Publishing; 1993.
23. Levison ME, Mangura CT, Lorber B, et al. Clindamycin compared with penicillin for the treatment of anaerobic lung abscess. Ann Intern Med. 1983;98: 466–71.
24. Gudiol F, Manresa F, Pallares R, et al. Clindamycin vs penicillin for anaerobic lung infections. High rate of penicillin failures associated with penicillin-resistant *Bacteroides melaninogenicus*. Arch Intern Med. 1990;150:2525–9.
25. Panwalker AP. Failure of penicillin in anaerobic necrotizing pneumonia. Chest. 1982;82:500–1.

53. CHRONIC PNEUMONIA

WILLIAM E. DISMUKES

For purposes of this chapter, chronic pneumonia syndrome is defined as a pulmonary parenchymal process that may be caused by either an infectious or a noninfectious agent, has been present for weeks to months rather than for days, and is manifested by abnormal chest radiographic findings and by chronic or progressive pulmonary symptoms. The abnormal chest film, which may reveal any one of several radiologic patterns, is probably the most important criterion. In many patients, the diagnosis of chronic pneumonia may be based more on the pulmonary radiographic findings than on the pulmonary symptoms. However, asymptomatic patients who have abnormal findings, for example, a solitary nodule, on routine evaluation should not be considered to have chronic pneumonia.

The major emphasis in this chapter will be on the chronic pneumonias caused by infectious agents; however, it is important to keep in mind that there are noninfectious causes of chronic pneumonia, including vasculitides, neoplasia, drugs, radiation, bronchiolitis obliterans organizing pneumonia,[1,2] and other idiopathic causes.[3,4]

ETIOLOGY

The infectious causes of chronic pneumonia can be divided into two main groups: (*1*) infectious agents that typically cause acute pneumonia and uncommonly cause chronic pneumonia and (*2*) infectious agents that typically cause chronic pneumonia. Among the agents that typically cause acute pneumonia, the anaerobes, *Staphylococcus*, the Enterobacteriaceae, and *Pseudomonas aeruginosa* are the organisms most likely to produce a persistent chronic pneumonia. This is usually a necrotizing process that most commonly occurs in patients with underlying disease such as alcoholism, diabetes mellitus, or chronic obstructive lung disease or in hospitalized patients.[5,6] Acute pneumonias caused by *Streptococcus pneumoniae*, *Mycoplasma pneumoniae*, *Legionella* spp., *Coxiella burnetii*, or *Chlamydia pneumoniae*,[7] or most viruses rarely progress to a chronic pulmonary illness. Table 1 shows the various causes of chronic pneumonia. In the normal host, tuberculosis,[8] other mycobacterial infections,[9] histoplasmosis,[10] coccidioidomycosis (in the appropriate geographic area),[11] mixed aerobic-anaerobic bacterial infection,[5] actinomycosis,[12] blastomycosis,[13] cryptococcosis,[14,15] and sporotrichosis[16] are the infections deserving prime consideration. Adiaspiromycosis, caused by *Emmonsia*, is a rare occurrence.[17] In the compromised host, chronic pneumonia should raise the possibility of tuberculosis, nocardiosis, cryptococcosis, aspergillosis, and, in the appropriate geographic areas, coccidioidomycosis and histoplasmosis.[18,19] In persons with acquired immunodeficiency syndrome (AIDS), a special immunocompromised population, the same infections are frequently seen.[20-26] In addition, in these individuals chronic pneumonia may be caused by *Blastomyces dermatitidis*, atypical mycobacteria, *Rhodococcus equi*, *Pneumocystis carinii*, and cytomegalovirus plus noninfectious disorders such as Kaposi sarcoma, lymphoma, x-ray therapy, and nonspecific interstitial pneumonitis.[27-30] The protozoa and worms listed in Table 1 are uncommon causes of chronic pneumonia disease among people living in the United States, but the diseases caused by these organisms are important considerations in patients who live in or have traveled in areas in which these agents are endemic.

No studies have been done to determine the approximate frequency of the various causes of chronic pneumonia in a large series of patients. This lack of perspective on the incidence of the various etiologies of chronic pneumonia is in contrast to our better understanding of the *acute* pneumonia syndrome. In addition, since the introduction of antibiotics in the 1940s, the overall spectrum of pneumonia has changed; new pathogens have emerged, organisms that were previously considered harmless commensals now cause disease, and powerful immunosuppressive therapies render some patients more susceptible to certain microorganisms. Consequently, in considering the differential diagnosis in an individual patient, emphasis on specific entities must, in general, be based less on statistical likelihood and more on a thorough and methodic analysis of all available clinical, epidemiologic, and laboratory data.

EPIDEMIOLOGY

Age, Sex, Race

Pulmonary tuberculosis over the past two decades has become a disease of the homeless, elderly, and AIDS patient groups.[22,31] In a similar manner, the significance of the age and sex of patients with chronic pneumonia due to other causes usually relates more in an indirect manner to associated epidemiologic factors. For example, an elderly patient is at higher risk of having a cerebrovascular accident, which in turn might predispose to an aspiration episode and subsequent pneumonia and ab-

TABLE 1. Etiology of Chronic Pneumonia Syndrome

Infectious agents that *typically* cause chronic pneumonia
  Bacteria and actinomycetes
    Mixed aerobic–anaerobic bacteria
    Actinomyces spp.
    Propioni bacterium propionicus
    Nocardia spp.
    Rhodococcus equi
    Pseudomonas pseudomallei
  Mycobacteria
    M. tuberculosis
    M. kansasii
    M. avium-intracellulare
  Fungi
    Aspergillus spp.
    Blastomyces dermatitidis
    Coccidioides immitis
    Cryptococcus neoformans
    Emmonsia
    Histoplasma capsulatum
    Sporothrix schenckii
    Paracoccidioides brasiliensis
  Protozoa
    Entamoeba histolytica
  Worms
    Echinococcus granulosus
    Schistosomes—*S. hematobium, S. japonicum, S. mansoni*
    Paragonimus westermani
Noninfectious causes
  Neoplasia
    Carcinoma (primary or metastatic)
    Lymphoma
  Sarcoidosis
  Vasculitis (autoimmune diseases)
    Systemic lupus erythematosus
    Polyarteritis nodosa
    Allergic angitis and granulomatosis (Churg-Strauss syndrome)
    Progressive systemic sclerosis
    Rheumatoid arthritis
    Mixed connective tissue syndrome (Overlap syndrome)
    Wegener's granulomatosis
    Lymphomatoid granulomatosis
  Chemicals, drugs, or inhalation
  Radiation
  Recurrent pulmonary emboli
  Bronchial obstruction with atelectasis (e.g., due to tumor, foreign body)
  Pulmonary infiltration with eosinophilia syndrome
    Löffler syndrome—usually transient
    Tropical eosinophilia
    Pneumonia plus asthma, e.g., allergic bronchopulmonary aspergillosis
    Bronchocentric granulomatosis
    Vasculitis
    Eosinophilic pneumonia—chronic
  Pneumoconiosis
  Chronic form of extrinsic allergic alveolitis (hypersensitivity pneumonitis)
  Other lung disease—unknown cause
    Bronchiolitis obliterans organizing pneumonia
    Chronic interstitial pneumonia (fibrosing alveolitis, idiopathic pulmonary fibrosis)
      Usual interstitial pneumonia (UIP)
      Desquamative interstitial pneumonia (DIP)
      Lymphoid interstitial pneumonia (LIP)
      Giant cell interstitial pneumonia (GIP)
    Eosinophilic granuloma (histiocytosis X)
    Lymphangioleiomyomatosis
    Goodpasture syndrome
    Pulmonary alevolar proteinosis (phospholipoproteinosis)
    Pulmonary alveolar microlithiasis
    Idiopathic pulmonary hemosiderosis
    Angiocentric immunoproliferative lesions

scess. Likewise, older, debilitated patients are at higher risk of developing chronic gram-negative necrotizing pneumonia. In a similar manner, the sex of a given patient is more likely to determine occupation or avocation and, ultimately, the likelihood of exposure to certain infectious agents or other etiologic vehicles. The race of the patient may be a more important factor. For example, pulmonary tuberculosis should be the presumptive diagnosis in a black patient with bilateral upper lobe cavitary disease,[32] coccidioidomycosis is more likely to be severe in dark-skinned persons, including blacks and Filipinos, who have lived or have traveled in the southwestern United States, the endemic area for the disease,[11] and chronic cavitary histoplasmosis is more likely to occur in the white male population.[18]

Occupation and Avocation

Certain occupations or hobbies should arouse the suspicion of certain diseases. Despite the presence of *Cryptococcus neoformans* in pigeon droppings, the vast majority of patients with pulmonary cryptococcosis have no unusual exposure to pigeons. Occupational exposure to plant materials predisposes to cutaneous and, according to some authorities, pulmonary sporotrichosis. Examples of occupationally or avocationally related conditions include coccidioidomycosis among rock collectors, archeologists conducting excavations, construction workers, or others exposed to desert dust in the endemic area; histoplasmosis among persons who are exposed to pigeon or starling roosts, who clean out old chicken houses with dirt floors, who cut and clear hollow trees, or who explore old buildings or caves inhabited by bats; echinococcosis in those who tend sheep; berylliosis along workers in the aircraft, electronics, and nuclear industries[33]; the pneumoconioses, for example, silicosis and asbestosis, among sandblasters and shipyard workers[34]; and chronic as well as acute pulmonary disease resulting from repeated occupational or accidental exposure to agents of extrinsic allergic alveolitis (hypersensitivity pneumonitis)[35] or to irritant gases such as phosgene, ammonia, ozone, and nitrogen dioxide.[36]

Travel

Since the initial exposure to the agents of many chronic and indolent infectious diseases may have occurred months or years before disease, it is necessary to inquire whether a patient has lived in or has traveled to another part of the United States or the world at any time. For example, a patient with bilateral upper lobe infiltrates with or without cavitation who has never traveled or lived in Central America, Mexico, South America, or west of the Mississippi River is unlikely to have coccidioidomycosis. The exceptions include the occasional worker handling dusty material from the endemic areas such as cotton bales. On the other hand, if the patient has lived in the eastern half of the United States, especially the midcentral area, chronic pulmonary histoplasmosis should be considered since histoplasmosis is endemic in this area. Paracoccidioidomycosis is acquired only during residence in Mexico and in South or Central America.

In addition to identifying a state or country visited, there may be a need for detailed questioning about rural or urban exposure, type of lodging, source of drinking water, exposure to native foods, and so forth. For example, any person who has lived or traveled extensively in Southeast Asia, particularly in low-lying or rice-growing areas, and who subsequently develops chronic pneumonia with pulmonary roentgenographic abnormalities resembling tuberculosis or the respiratory mycoses should be suspected of having melioidosis.[37] Similarly, a businessperson who makes frequent trips to Japan and the Philippines, who admits to eating raw or partly cooked crayfish, and who has chronic pulmonary symptoms plus dense, nodular lung opacities and ring shadows should be suspected of having pulmonary paragonimiasis.[38]

Contacts, Habits, and Drugs

In patients in whom tuberculosis is suspected, contacts among companions or relatives with tuberculosis should be sought. Inquiry should be made into the patient's smoking and drinking history as well as other personal habits. The likelihood of cancer of the lung in a patient with coal worker's pneumoconiosis is greater in a smoker than in a nonsmoker. Aspiration pneumonia, chronic gram-negative bacillary pneumonia, and tuberculosis are more likely to occur in an alcoholic than in a nondrinker.

Intravenous drug users who inject heroin or similar agents are at risk of developing not only infection with human immunodeficiency virus (HIV) and subsequently AIDS but also acute pulmonary edema,[39] septic pulmonary emboli followed by necrotizing pneumonia and single or multiple abscesses, or an interstitial granulomatous reaction with pulmonary hypertension.[40] Similarly, frequent use of free-base cocaine has been reported to cause bronchiolitis obliterans organizing pneumonia.[41]

Certain drugs may cause acute and chronic pulmonary symptoms as well as radiographic abnormalities.[42] Early in the course of drug-induced pulmonary disease, the chest roentgenogram findings may be normal; later, an interstitial, nodular, and/or alveolar pattern may be present. Still later, the chest film may reveal only a fibrotic pulmonary process. The drugs that are more likely to cause chronic pulmonary disease include cytotoxic agents such as bleomycin, busulfan, chlorambucil, methotrexate, and nitrosoureas and noncytotoxic agents such as amiodarone, gold salts, nitrofurantoin, and penicillamine. Since drug-induced pulmonary disease may develop after drug therapy has been discontinued, the physician should inquire not only about all drugs the patient is presently taking but also about those taken in the recent past.

Similarly, important questions arise in regard to any previous or current antimicrobial therapy. Did the antimicrobial therapy result in roentgenographic or clinical improvement? If not, was the antimicrobial drug used in sufficient quantity to cure the suspected process or alter its course? Was the appropriate agent used? What effect does the antimicrobial agent have on the results of cultures? Is the report of "normal flora" on the sputum culture the result of antimicrobial therapy eliminating a specific pathogen?

Underlying Disease

Pulmonary complications including both acute and chronic or refractory pneumonia are especially common in persons with AIDS[20–30] (see Ch. 106). Patients with diabetes mellitus or preexisting chronic obstructive pulmonary disease are at high risk for developing chronic or persistent bacterial pneumonia. Similarly, chronic obstructive lung disease commonly precedes fibrocavitary histoplasmosis or *Mycobacterium avium-intracellulare* infection. Recurrent or persistent pneumonia in the same area of the lung raises the suspicion of a local endobronchial lesion that may not be apparent on routine chest films. Since aspiration may predispose to chronic pneumonia, inquiry should be made into any history of recent dental problems or manipulation, sinusitis with chronic postnasal drip, disorders of swallowing resulting from neurologic or esophageal disease, seizure disorders, recent anesthesia, quantity and effect of alcohol, or any illness leading to an unconscious state. Finally, it should be determined whether the chronic pneumonia is community or hospital acquired.

CLINICAL FEATURES

Symptoms

Since there are multiple causes of chronic pneumonia, no single symptom complex is common to all causes. Often, constitutional symptoms including fever, chills, and malaise are present initially. A history of progressive anorexia and weight loss usually indicates chronic illness. Pulmonary symptoms may be present early but frequently appear later in the course of the illness. Any patient with a prolonged illness and nonspecific constitutional complaints plus pulmonary symptoms including a new or persistent cough, sputum production, hemoptysis, chest pain (especially pleuritic pain), or dyspnea deserves medical evaluation, including a chest roentgenogram.

Inquiries should be made to determine whether there is involvement of extrapulmonary organs. For example, skin lesions might suggest coccidioidomycosis, cryptococcosis, blastomycosis, nocardiosis, or Kaposi sarcoma, whereas mucous membrane lesions would suggest histoplasmosis, paracoccidioidomycosis, Wegener's granulomatosis, or Kaposi sarcoma. Mono- or polyarticular arthritis, polyarthralgias, or localized bone tenderness or pain might indicate a vasculitis. A history of persistent headache together with the documentation of abnormal cerebrospinal fluid should raise the suspicion of tuberculosis, cryptococcosis, or coccidioidomycosis involving both the lungs and central nervous system. The presence of focal neurologic symptoms and signs argues strongly for a space-occupying lesion in the central nervous system; such findings in a patient with a cavitary infiltrate seen on a chest film suggest the possibility of a brain abscess associated with chronic suppurative lung disease or pulmonary nocardiosis. Similarly, the triad of skin nodules, pulmonary nodules, and central nervous system abnormalities suggests lymphomatoid granulomatosis.[43]

Signs

Although the findings on physical examination of the chest are usually not helpful in differentiating specific causes of chronic pneumonia, the presence of generalized wheezing or other signs of bronchospasm, in the absence of underlying lung disease, indicates an asthmatic component to the pulmonary illness and raises the possibility of a disorder causing both pneumonia and asthma such as extrinsic allergic alveolitis, allergic bronchopulmonary aspergillosis, or allergic angiitis and granulomatosis (Churg-Strauss syndrome). Similarly, localized wheezes suggest the presence of an endobronchial obstructing lesion. The findings of tachycardia, cardiomegaly, gallop rhythm, and ankle edema provide evidence of cardiac disease and suggest that the pulmonary symptoms and signs are at least in part due to cardiovascular causes. The presence of skin lesions, clubbing, cyanosis, or phlebitis are not specific from any single pulmonary disorder but may help to narrow the differential diagnosis, especially when considered along with other clinical and epidemiologic information. Similarly, the findings of jaundice, adenopathy, hepatomegaly, splenomegaly, or ascites suggest that a systemic disorder involving multiple organs is the cause.

DIAGNOSTIC PROCEDURES

Initial Laboratory Studies

Routine laboratory studies may provide some important clues to diagnosis. Pancytopenia may suggest miliary tuberculosis, disseminated histoplasmosis, or metastatic tumor in the bone marrow. Anemia alone is consistent with too many disorders to suggest a specific cause. A normal white blood cell count does not exclude infection. In particular, mycotic chronic pneumonia is usually associated with a normal or minimally elevated white blood cell count. Leukopenia and/or lymphopenia should raise the suspicion of infection with HIV. In addition, leukopenia should suggest sarcoidosis, systemic lupus erythematosus, tuberculosis, histoplasmosis, or tumor. A leukemoid reaction may be seen in disseminated mycobacteriosis. Leukocytosis is suggestive of but not specific for a bacterial cause.

Laboratory tests that measure the function of other organs may provide more helpful information. Liver function studies including bilirubin, alkaline phosphatase, and serum aspartate aminotransferase determinations and prothrombin time should be obtained in most patients. Urinalysis, with particular attention to the urinary sediment, plus tests of renal function including measurement of blood urea nitrogen and creatinine should also be done. Abnormalities of either liver function, especially elevated enzyme levels, kidney function, or both, should raise the suspicion of disorders that are not limited to the lung but are known to involve multiple organs, including lung, liver, and kidney. Such disorders include disseminated histoplasmosis and

disseminated mycobacteriosis as well as the vasculitides, sarcoidosis, and certain neoplastic diseases, especially the lymphoproliferative types.

An elevated serum globulin level is usually nonspecific and indicates chronic inflammation, although it may indicate an underlying myeloma or another gammopathy predisposing to chronic or recurrent infection. If myeloma is suspected, immunoelectrophoresis of urine and serum is indicated. Similarly, in a patient with an abnormally low serum globulin level, a quantitative serum immunoglobulin determination should be obtained to evaluate the patient for hypogammaglobulinemia. Additional studies that should be performed in patients with suspected vasculitis include serologic tests for antinuclear antibody, rheumatoid factor, and antineutrophil cytoplasmic autoantibody.

Studies to Establish an Etiology

A basic core of studies should usually be performed on all patients with chronic pneumonia, regardless of suspected etiology, but there should be flexibility in choosing additional tests or procedures to confirm a specific diagnosis. The orderly sequence of diagnostic studies that is given below necessarily results in oversimplification and consequently overlooks the unique aspects of a given patient's illness.

Chest Radiographic Studies. The chest radiograph, including a posteroanterior and a lateral film and a computed tomographic (CT) examination of the chest are important diagnostic studies.[22,44] Newer imaging techniques, including high-resolution thin-section chest CT, are being increasingly utilized, especially in the evaluation of the noninfectious cause of chronic pneumonia.[18] Because of the singular importance of these various imaging studies, Table 2 is provided to emphasize the major radiologic patterns that may be seen. In Table 2 the disorders have been grouped according to the type of radiologic abnormality that is characteristic of the disease. Because there are some disorders in which there is a spectrum of radiologic manifestations, these disorders appear more than once in the table. Typical radiographic findings may provide clues to specific diagnoses. For example, documentation of *anterior* mediastinal involvement argues strongly in favor of neoplasia including lymphoma and metastatic carcinoma as the etiology of chronic pneumonia syndrome and argues against an infectious cause.

Tuberculosis and nontuberculous mycobacterial diseases, histoplasmosis, coccidioidomycosis, sporotrichosis, melioidosis, paragonimiasis, and the pneumoconioses, especially silicosis, characteristically produce fibrocavitary disease—a contracted area of lung with linear fibrosis, nodular or rounded densities, and cavitation. In addition, mycobacterial diseases, histoplasmosis, and silicosis characteristically involve the upper lobes. A thin-walled cavity is suggestive of coccidioidomycosis, sporotrichosis, and paragonimiasis, whereas a thick-walled cavity surrounded by an area of pneumonitis is more typical of tuberculosis, nontuberculous mycobacterial diseases, histoplasmosis, aspergillosis, melioidosis, nocardiosis, actinomycosis, pyogenic lung abscess, and lung disease caused by *Rhodococcus equi*. Cavitation is less common in blastomycosis and cryptococcosis. Calcification is typical of tuberculosis, histoplasmosis, and coccidioidomycosis but is rare in actinomycosis, nocardiosis, blastomycosis, and cryptococcosis. Abscess of the chest wall or osteomyelitis of a rib adjacent to the pneumonia and/or pleural effusion may be seen in actinomycosis and nocardiosis. While these radiographic manifestations of selected pulmonary diseases are typical in the majority of patients, experience during the AIDS epidemic has shown that the same pulmonary diseases in AIDS patients may be highly atypical in radiographic appearance and clinical course.[20–30] Representative radiographs are shown in Figures 1–14.

TABLE 2. Radiologic Patterns of Diseases That Commonly Cause Chronic Pneumonia Syndrome

Disease	Radiologic Characteristics
Diseases that cause patchy infiltrates and/or bronchopneumonia or lobar consolidation	
Infectious	
Aspiration pneumonia secondary to mixed aerobic and anaerobic infection	Usually dependent portions: superior or basilar segments of lower lobes or posterior segments of upper lobes
	Pleural involvement with empyema common
Necrotizing pneumonia secondary to Enterobacteriaceae, *P. aeruginosa*, or *S. aureus*	Any lobe or segment
	Chronic *Klebsiella* pneumonia commonly involves upper lobes
	May be multiple sites of pulmonary infection secondary to septic embolization
Actinomycosis	Commonly involves lower lobes
	Cavitation frequently present
	Pleural involvement with empyema common
Nocardiosis	No distinctive pattern
	May involve single or multiple lobes
	Cavitation may be present
	Pleural involvement may occur
	Not restricted to upper lobes
Tuberulous exudative pneumonia	Often bilateral with perihilar distribution
Blastomycosis	Often a dense area of lobar or segmental consolidation
	Cavitation infrequent
Cryptococcosis	Single or multiple patchy infiltrates; less commonly, lobar consolidation
	Occasionally, single or diffuse nodular lesions
Paracoccidioidomycosis	Asymptomatic bilateral fluffy infiltrates
	May be extremely indolent
Noninfectious	
Chronic eosinophilic pneumonia	Rapidly progressive, dense infiltrates
	Usually peripheral (reverse pattern of pulmonary edema)
Bronchiolitis obliterans organizing pneumonia	Patchy nonsegmental areas of consolidation, often subpleural
	Nodular or irregular linear opacities
Diseases that cause pulmonary cavitation	
Infectious	
Pyogenic lung abscess	
Complicating aspiration pneumonia	Usually single cavity
	Location—same as aspiration pneumonia
	Air-fluid level common
Complicating necrotizing pneumonia	May involve any lobe
	Often multiple and bilateral, depending on route of acquisition of pneumonia
Tuberculosis—reactivation or adult type	Usually upper lobes
	Often bilateral
	May be multiple
	Fibrosis and calcification common
Atypical mycobacterial disease	Radiologically indistinguishable from tuberculosis, except that cavitation may be more frequent
Melioidosis	Simulates tuberculosis, but may involve any lobe
Rhodococcal lung disease	Simulates tuberculosis or nocardiosis
	Cavitation common
Histoplasmosis, chronic cavitary	Mimics tuberculosis
	Upper lobes frequently involved but can involve any lobe
Coccidioidomycosis	Unilateral or bilateral
	Usually single thin-walled cavity with minimum involvement of surrounding lung
	Occasionally thick-walled cavity surrounded by extensive parenchymal disease
Sporotrichosis	May mimic tuberculosis but can involve any lobe
	Cavitation is frequent; thin-walled cavity more likely than thick-walled cavity
Aspergillosis	Single or multiple areas of pneumonia with or without central cavitation
	Not to be confused with intracavitary fungus ball
Paragonimiasis	Cystlike lesions as well as cavities, usually associated with linear or patchy infiltrates, fibrosis, and/or calcification
Echinococcosis	Single or multiple discrete, sharply defined round lesions (cysts) with little surrounding inflammatory response
	Cavitation and/or calcification may occur
Noninfectious	
Wegener's granulomatosis and lymphomatoid granulomatosis	Often multiple nodules with cavitation
	May be unilateral or bilateral
Silicosis	Associated with conglomerate nodular densities, frequently in upper lobes
	Usually superimposed on background of diffuse nodulation
	Rarely, eggshell calcification of hilar nodes
Bronchogenic carcinoma	Eccentric cavitation more common in squamous cell type
Lymphoma, especially Hodgkin's disease	Cavitation typically occurs in peripheral parenchymal nodules
Infectious and noninfectious diseases that cause chronic diffuse pulmonary infiltration and fibrosis	
Alveolar cell carcinoma Intrapulmonary bleeding, e.g., Goodpasture syndrome Pulmonary alveolar proteinois	Alveolar pattern
Sarcoidosis Early asbestosis or berylliosis Bronchiolitis obliterans organizing pneumonia	Ground-glass interstitial pattern
Granulomatous infectious diseases, e.g., miliary tuberculosis and disseminated histoplasmosis Sarcoidosis Lymphangitic carcinomatosis Wegener's granulomatosis Lymphomatoid granulomatosis Allergic angiitis and granulomatosis Rheumatoid lung disease Pneumoconiosis, including asbestosis, silicosis, and berylliosis	Nodular interstitial pattern, including miliary spherical nodules
Chronic form of hypersensitivity pneumonitis Idiopathic pulmonary hemosiderosis Radiation injury—chronic Progressive systemic sclerosis Sarcoidosis	Linear interstitial pattern, including fine reticular markings and dense fibrosis
Advanced form of fibrosing alveolitis Bronchiectasis Eosinophilic granuloma Sarcoidosis	Honeycombing (coarse reticular pattern with cystic air spaces)

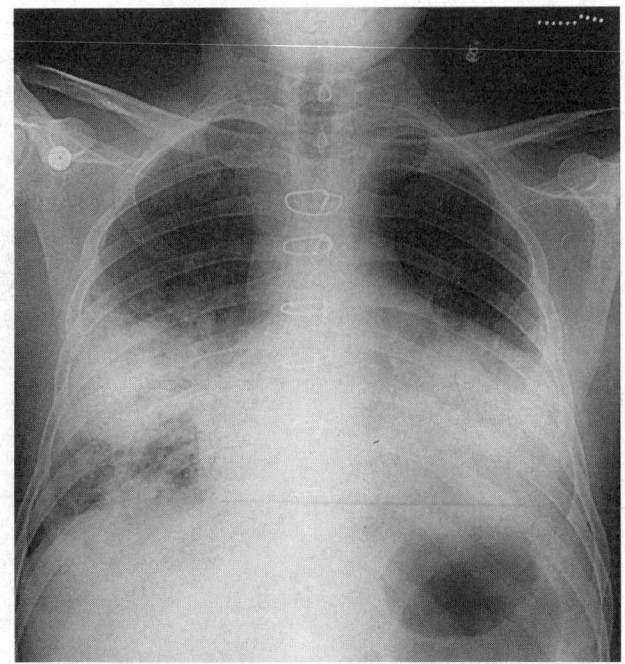
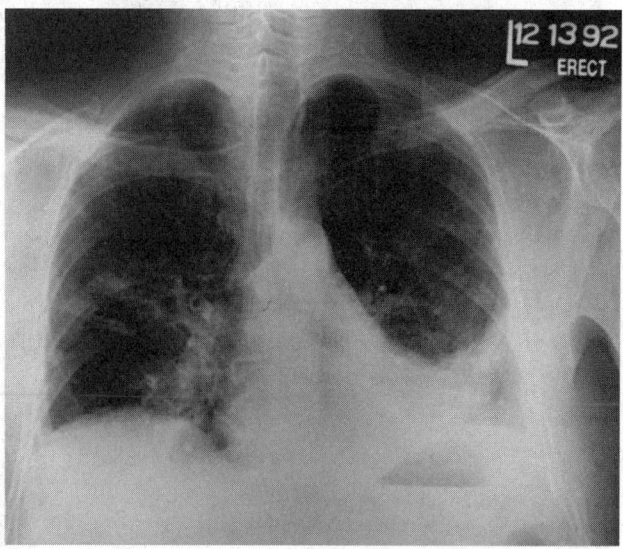

FIG. 1. **(A)** Bronchiolitis obliterans organizing pneumonia (BOOP) in a 32-year-old man who developed progressive chronic pneumonia several weeks after an open pericardiectomy to relieve cardiac tamponade associated with renal failure. Note the bilateral airspace consolidation. Bronchoscopy with transbronchial biopsy was nondiagnostic. The diagnosis of BOOP was established from tissue obtained at open lung biopsy. Corticosteroid therapy was dramatically beneficial. **(B)** BOOP in a 60-year-old man with a 1-month illness manifested by fever, malaise, weight loss, nonproductive cough, dyspnea, and bilateral subpleural nodular opacities. Both symptoms and radiographic abnormalities progressed during antibiotic therapy. A bronchoscopy with transthoracic biopsy was nondiagnostic. The diagnosis of BOOP was made from tissue obtained at open lung biopsy. Corticosteroid therapy was beneficial.

Studies in Patients with Radiographic Evidence of Localized Infiltrates and/or Cavitation. In all patients with radiographic evidence of localized infiltrates and/or cavitation, examination of the sputum is essential. The specimen of sputum must be a representative sample. If the expectorated sputum is a deep, coughed specimen, of adequate volume, and acceptable after cytologic screening, other procedures to obtain sputum may not be necessary. *Microscopic* examination of sputum should include the following:

1. Gram stains for bacteria and actinomyces
2. Acid-fast or fluorochrome stains for *Mycobacteria* and modified acid-fast stain for *Nocardia*
3. Wet mounts for fungi and eggs of *Paragonimus* (calcofluor white-KOH preparation may enhance detection of fungi)
4. Gomori methenamine silver (GMS) stain or periodic acid–Schiff (PAS) stain for fungi
5. Cytologic preparations for neoplastic cells, eosinophils, and fungi

Generous volumes of expectorated sputum (but not 24-hour collections) should also be obtained and sent to the microbiology laboratory for *culture* for bacteria, fungi, and mycobacteria. In addition, it is often diagnostically rewarding if the clinician speaks directly with the personnel in the microbiology laboratory to alert them to specific etiologic considerations. Then the specimens will be inoculated on the most appropriate media, and the microbiologists will be more aware of the suspected pathogens.

In all patients in whom an infectious cause is considered, cultures from sources other than sputum should be obtained. These sources might include the following:

1. Blood
2. Urine
3. Pleural fluid in all patients with pleural effusion (pleural tissue should also be obtained for culture)
4. Cerebrospinal fluid in all patients with central nervous system symptoms or signs
5. Synovial fluid in all patients with joint effusion
6. Skin, mucous membrane, or any tissue obtained at biopsy

To obtain sputum, if adequate sputum cannot be readily produced via spontaneous expectoration by the patient, consider the following:

1. Inducing sputum by the use of hypertonic aerosols (routine or ultrasonic nebulization), hydration, chest physiotherapy, or postural drainage
2. Bronchoscopy for bronchial brushing, transbronchial biopsy, bronchoalveolar lavage, or protected catheter sampling of lower respiratory tract secretions while minimizing upper airway contamination of the sample[18,45–48]

Skin tests should be made in all cases in which an infectious cause is considered. The tuberculin skin test with purified protein derivative (PPD) is the single most important test. If a patient has never had a tuberculin skin test or has had a previously negative response, a 5-tuberculin unit PPD skin test should be used. If the patient has a history of a positive tuberculin skin response, a first-strength PPD may be applied. Skin test antigens for the detection of infection with the atypical mycobacteria are not commercially available.

Skin tests of the tuberculin type are also available for patients with suspected fungal disease; however, these are most valuable when used for epidemiologic studies to determine the prevalence of infection in a given population or in a certain geographic area. Like the tuberculin test, fungal skin tests do not distinguish between current and previous infection. Unlike the tuberculin test, a negative result is common with active disease, even in previously healthy patients. Hence, fungal skin tests are of little diagnostic value in the individual patient. Of the tests available, the coccidioidin antigen is the best, although a negative response does not exclude coccidioidomycosis.

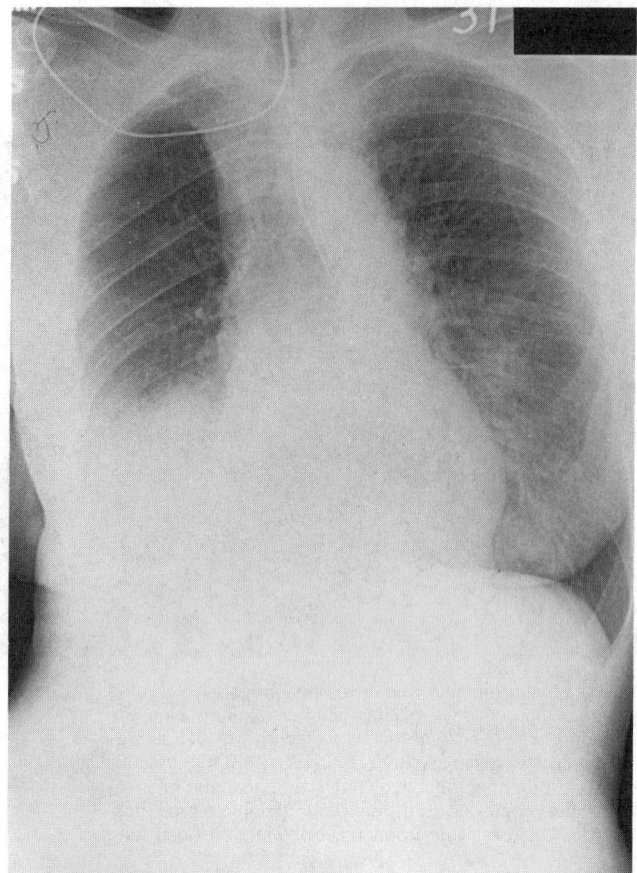

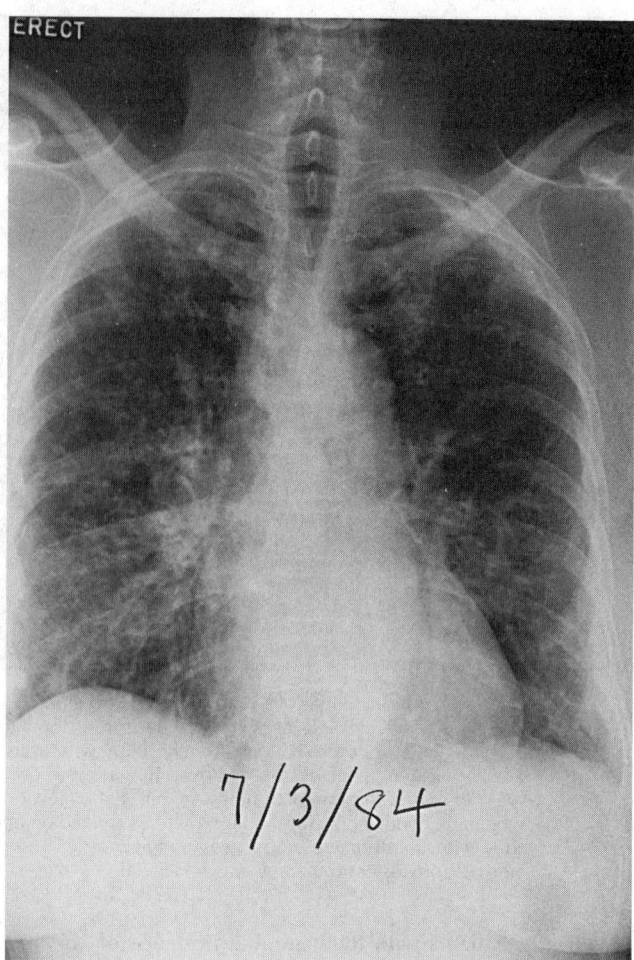

FIG. 2. Bronchioalveolar carcinoma in a 66-year-old nonsmoking woman with a 2-year history of persistent cough productive of up to one cup of clear sputum per day, progressive dyspnea on exertion, and a chronic right lobe infiltrate refractory to multiple courses of antibiotics. Bronchoscopy 1 year earlier revealed only copious secretions and a few atypical cells. Note the dense lobar consolidation of the right lower lobe. There was no pleural effusion. A pathologic diagnosis was made from tissue obtained by transthoracic needle aspiration.

FIG. 3. Pulmonary sarcoidosis in a 51-year-old woman with a 4-month illness characterized by fever, night sweats, nonproductive cough, and progressive dyspnea. Note the bilateral multilobar reticulonodular parenchymal pattern.

Serologic tests for antibodies and antigens are often used when infectious causes, especially fungi, are considered. However, there are problems that include long delays in obtaining results, false-positive results because of cross-reactions to other antigens, and false-negative results. Serologic tests are most helpful in patients when pulmonary mycoses, including coccidioidomycosis, cryptococcosis, histoplasmosis, and paracoccidioidomycosis, are suspected. Similarly, in patients in whom hypersensitivity pneumonitis is suspected, serum should be examined for precipitating antibodies to various inhalant antigens, and, in patients in whom allergic bronchopulmonary aspergillosis is suspected, total serum immunoglobulin E and serum anti-*Aspergillus* antibody should be measured.

Invasive Procedures. Certain clinical situations dictate that a more aggressive diagnostic approach be used. In patients who are unable to raise sputum spontaneously and in whom attempts to induce sputum production are unsuccessful, invasive procedures may become necessary. Bronchoscopy with a flexible fiberoptic bronchoscope usually is the initial procedure and is diagnostically helpful when accompanied by bronchial washings and transbronchial biopsy with appropriate microbiologic and histologic studies.[18,45,46] Analysis of bronchoalveolar lavage fluid may increase the diagnostic yield of bronchoscopy, especially in immunocompromised persons such as AIDS patients with suspected opportunistic infections.[18,47,49] In a patient with extensive pleural involvement, thoracentesis and pleural biopsy may be

more helpful diagnostically then bronchoscopy.[50] In some institutions, open lung biopsy is the procedure of choice and is performed before bronchoscopy in many immunosuppressed patients with pulmonary disease because of the relatively large piece of tissue obtained, expediency of diagnosis, and safety.[51] By contrast, in other institutions with seasoned operators, percutaneous or transthoracic needle aspiration of the lung is preferred over open lung biopsy and associated with a low risk of complications and a high rate of sensitivity, especially in patients with suspected carcinoma or granulomatous disease.[52,53] Although these various invasive procedures frequently are used to obtain lung tissue for diagnosis, especially in compromised hosts, controversy exists as to whether the benefits exceed the risks and whether the findings lead to improved survival.[18,49]

All specimens, regardless of source, should be submitted for microscopic examination and culture, as already described. Any lung or pleural tissue should also be submitted for histopathologic studies including special stains.

In any patient in whom there is extrapulmonary disease, which is likely due to the same cause as the chronic pneumonia, tissue or fluid from the extrapulmonary sites should be obtained for culture and histologic studies. In such patients, consider the following procedures: arthrocentesis, abdominal paracentesis, lumbar puncture, bone marrow biopsy, liver biopsy, lymph node biopsy, and skin and muscle biopsy.

Studies in Patients with Radiographic Evidence of Diffuse Pulmonary Infiltration and Fibrosis.   In patients whose chest films show a predominately diffuse infiltrative pattern, either of the

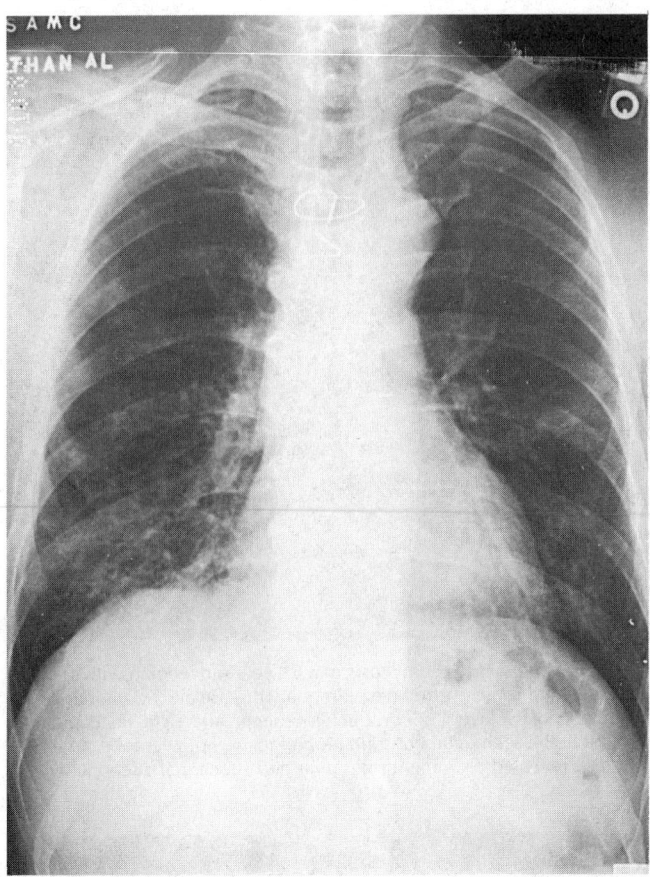

FIG. 4. Drug-induced chronic interstitial lung disease secondary to tocainide in a 68-year-old man with a 6-week illness consisting of fever, nonproductive cough, malaise, and 30-pound weight loss. Three months earlier, the patient underwent coronary artery bypass surgery and was placed on tocainide. Note the bilateral reticulonodular infiltrates, more marked in the lower lung fields.

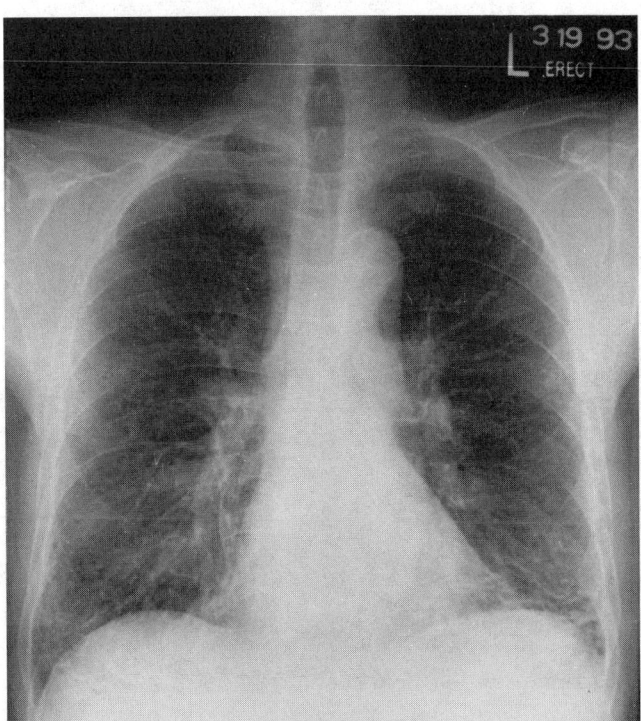

FIG. 5. Desquamative interstitial pneumonia (DIP) in a 76-year-old man with a 2-month history of fatigue, intermittent low-grade fever, and dyspnea on exertion. Note the bilateral interstitial reticular pattern, more prominent at the lung bases. A pathologic diagnosis was made from tissue obtained at open lung biopsy.

alveolar or interstitial type (Table 2), pulmonary function studies may be of greater importance. These studies will not only quantitate the degree of pulmonary insufficiency but may help to delineate the disease processes by virtue of the different patterns of pulmonary function impairment. Accordingly, these tests are particularly useful in characterizing those diseases that impair gas transfer and predispose to ventilation—perfusion inequalities, for example, sarcoidosis or other interstitial lung diseases.

Studies that may be especially useful in this group of patients include the following:

1. Arterial blood gas studies, including resting and postexercise tests
2. Tests of pulmonary function including spirometric measurements, measurements of lung volume, and measurement of pulmonary diffusing capacity
3. Studies on sputum as previously outlined (cytologic examination is especially important)
4. Lung biopsy to make an accurate morphologic diagnosis (transbronchial biopsy via the fiberoptic bronchoscope or open lung biopsy are the procedures of choice)[45,46,51]

THERAPY

Antimicrobial Agents

If a specific infectious agent is readily identified as the cause of the chronic pneumonia, the appropriate antimicrobial agent(s) should be administered. In many patients, no etiologic agent

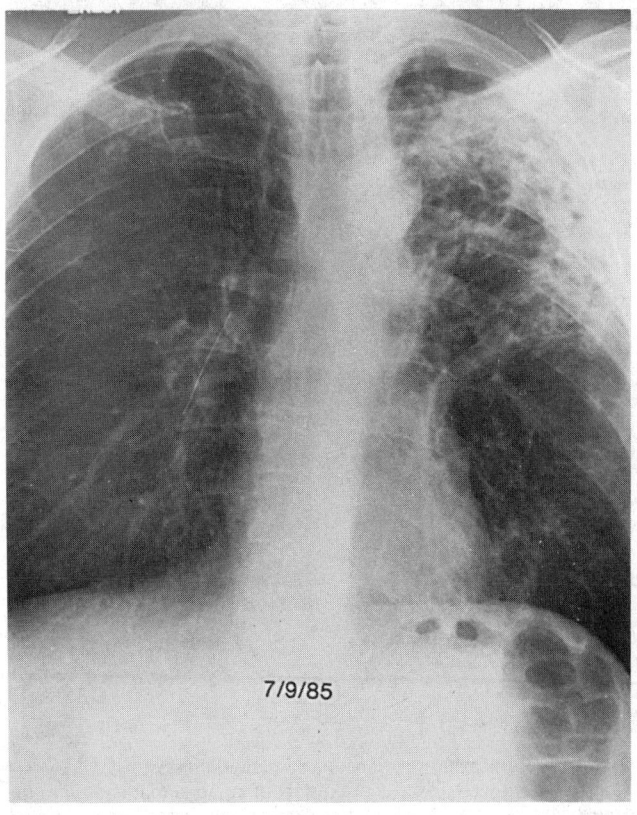

FIG. 6. Chronic cavitary pulmonary histoplasmosis in a 53-year-old man with chronic obstructive pulmonary disease and a 3-month history of low-grade fever, night sweats, cough, progressive dyspnea, and weight loss. Note the bilateral fibrocavitary disease with prominent involvement of the left upper lobe.

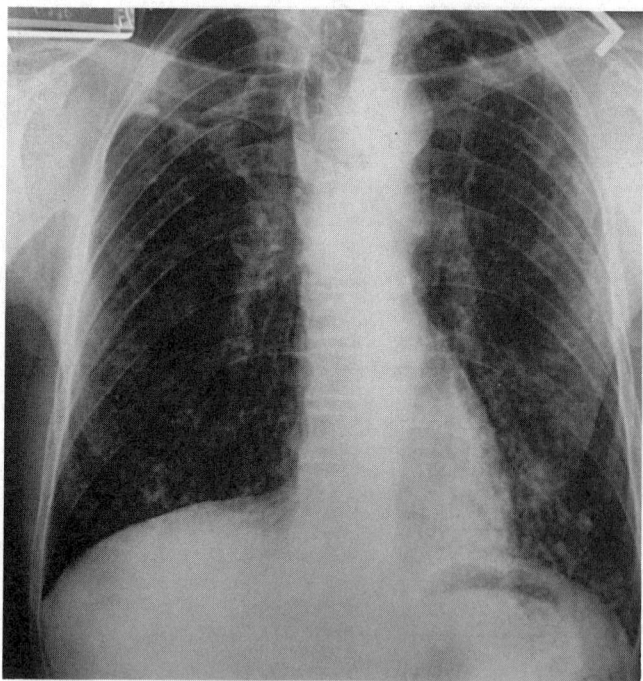

FIG. 7.   Atypical tuberculosis caused by *M. avium-intracellulare* in a 67-year-old with chronic obstructive pulmonary disease and a 2-year history of malaise, anorexia, weight loss, and progressive dyspnea associated with an abnormal chest film. Note the bilateral fibronodular pattern and the large apical cavities, right larger than left.

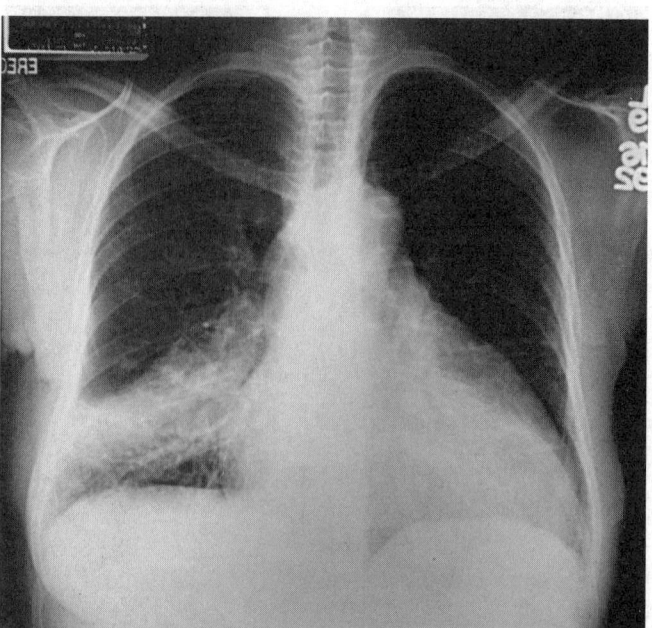

FIG. 9.   Pulmonary blastomycosis in a 51-year-old woman with diabetes mellitus and chronic obstructive pulmonary disease and a 1-month illness characterized by fever, nonproductive cough, and right-sided pleuritic pain. Note the segmental consolidation of the right lower lobe. Chest CT scan also revealed prominent right hilar and subcarinal adenopathy.

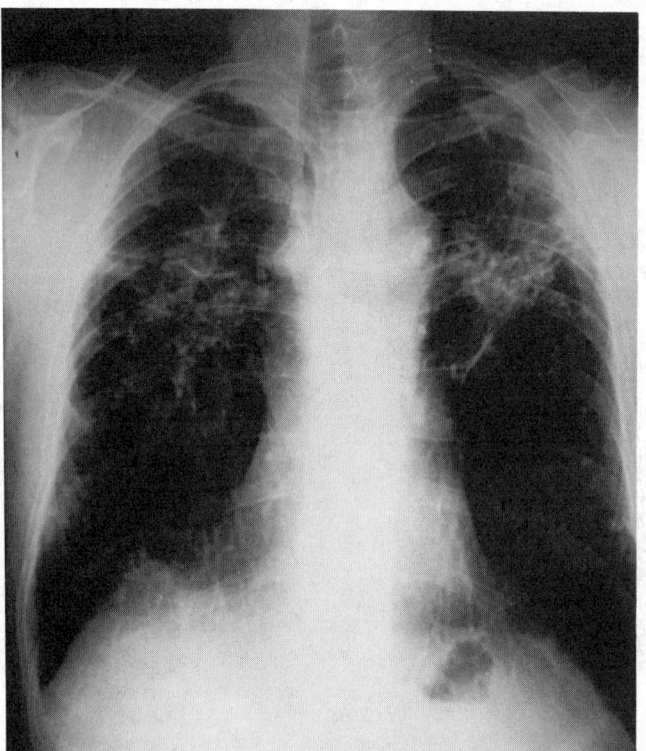

FIG. 8.   Chronic cavitary pulmonary coccidioidomycosis in a 55-year-old rancher from west Texas and a history of an abnormal chest film for the preceding 20 years. He had experienced a single episode of self-limited hemoptysis about 10 years earlier. At the time of this film, the patient noted subcutaneous nodules on his anterior chest. Histopathology of tissue obtained by skin biopsy revealed large, endospore-containing spherules, consistent with *Coccidioides immitis*. Note the bilateral fibrocavitary disease primarily involving the upper lobes.

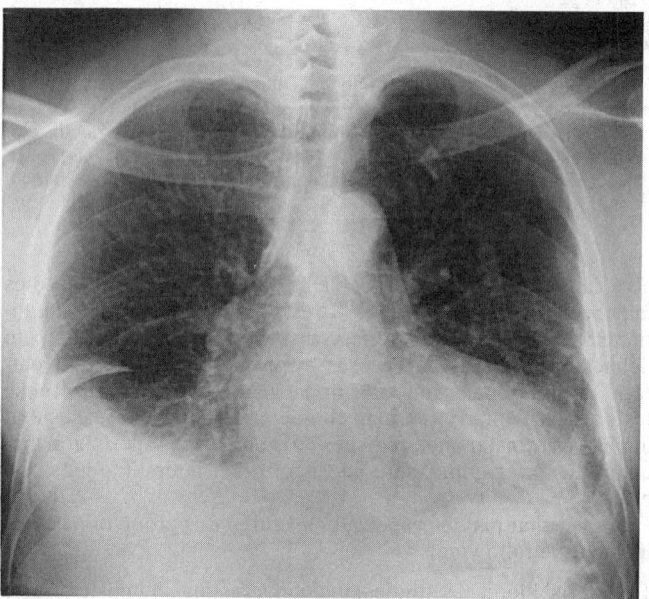

FIG. 10.   Pulmonary cryptococcosis in a 49-year-old renal transplant recipient with a 2-month illness initially manifested by fever, nonproductive cough, and right-sided pleuritic chest pain. Note the bilateral segmental consolidation and the right pleural effusion. During week 6 of illness, the patient became confused. A head CT scan revealed a hypodense mass lesion and culture of cerebrospinal fluid was positive for *Cryptococcus neoformans*. A serum test for cryptococcal antigen was also positive.

will be identified on the basis of the initial stains and cultures, and a definitive diagnosis must await the completion of serologic, histologic, and bacteriologic studies as well as other diagnostic tests. In such situations, if immediate empirical therapy is advisable, the choice of antimicrobial agents must be based on the available epidemiologic, clinical and microbiologic data.

For example, if an otherwise healthy young patient has been ill for a relatively short period (2–3 weeks), the chest film shows

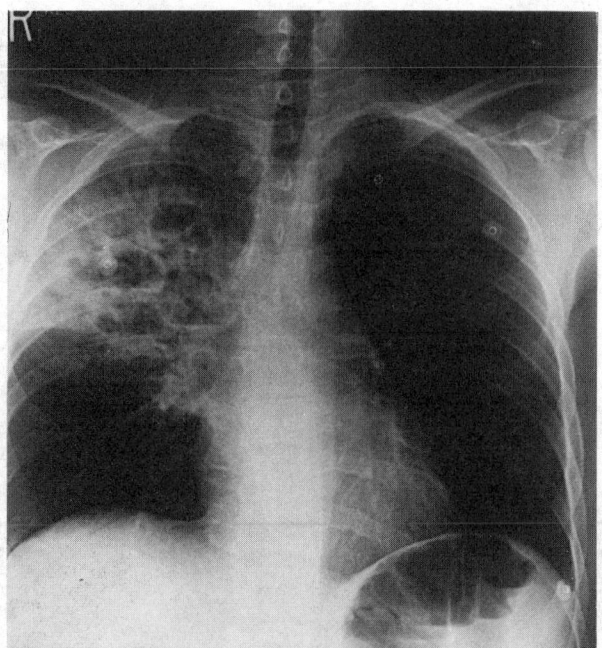

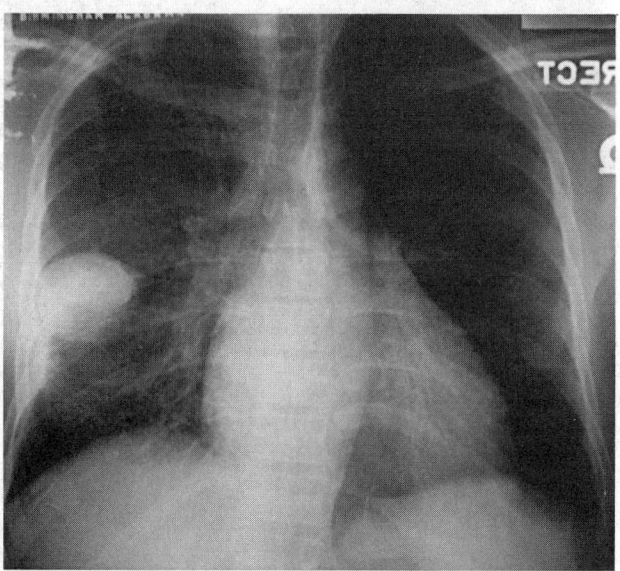

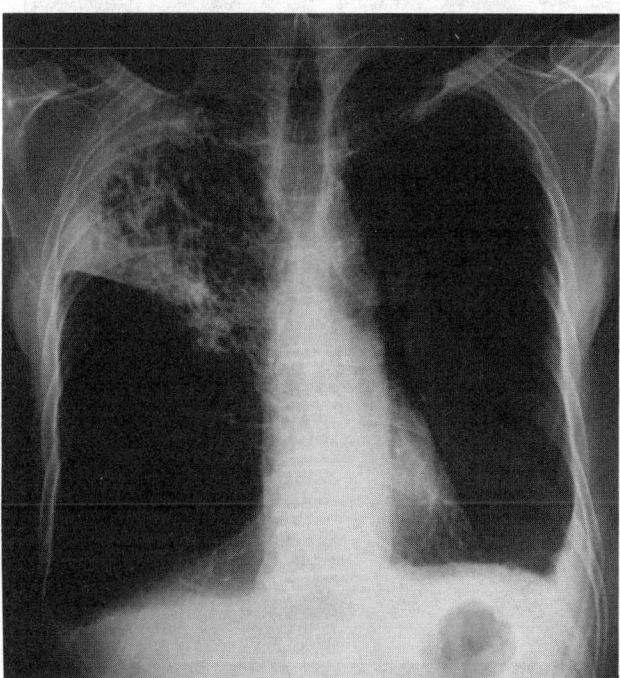

FIG. 12. Invasive pulmonary aspergillosis in a 71-year-old man with a 6-week illness characterized by fever, cough, purulent sputum, and hemoptysis. One year previously, the patient had undergone operative resection and radiation therapy for laryngeal carcinoma. Note the necrotizing pneumonia and small cavities in the right upper lobe.

FIG. 11. (A) *Rhodococcus equi* pneumonia in an AIDS patient with a 2-month progressive illness characterized by fever, night sweats, weight loss, and nonproductive cough. Note the necrotizing, cavitary infiltrate involving the right upper lobe. The microbiologic diagnosis was made from washings and tissue obtained at bronchoscopy. (B) *Rhodococcus equi* pneumonia in an AIDS patient with a 6-week history of fever, weight loss, and right-sided pleuritic pain. Note the pleural-based, well-circumscribed mass lesion. The microbiologic diagnosis was made from tissue obtained at open lung biopsy.

a lobar or patchy pneumonia, especially in the lower lobes, Gram stain of the sputum reveals few-to-moderate polymorphonuclear leukocytes and organisms resembling normal flora, and the patient acquired the infection outside the hospital, the patient may have persistent or chronic pneumonia as a complication of one or more common acute pneumonia syndromes, namely, pneumococcal pneumonia, aspiration pneumonia, *Mycoplasma* pneumonia, or legionnaires' disease. Reasonable empirical therapy in such a patient is erythromycin since this drug, in general, provides effective treatment of these four pneumonias. Azithromycin or clarithromycin may also prove to be useful in the nonseriously ill patient. If, on the other hand, a patient

has chronic pneumonia after thoracotomy, initial antimicrobial therapy should provide broad-spectrum coverage against hospital-acquired mouth flora including anaerobes, *Staphylococcus aureus*, and aerobic gram-negative bacteria. In both of the above cases, once the pathogen(s) have been identified and sensitivity testing completed, appropriate changes in the antibiotic regimen should be made.

If a patient has a more chronic indolent illness, is stable, and does not require immediate empirical therapy, a methodic and thorough diagnostic evaluation is the initial priority. In a patient with bilateral upper lobe cavitary disease in whom the initial microscopic examinations are nonrevealing, the leading considerations include tuberculosis, histoplasmosis, and coccidioidomycosis. In general, in every such patient with a positive tuberculin skin response, tuberculosis should be presumed to be the diagnosis until proved otherwise, and antituberculous therapy should be initiated and continued for at least 8 weeks, pending the final results of the mycobacterial cultures. Similarly, disseminated tuberculosis should be strongly suspected in any patient with unexplained fever and a chest film showing a nodular interstitial pattern; prompt institution of antituberculous therapy may be lifesaving in this otherwise fatal condition. Similarly, empirical antifungal therapy, usually with amphotericin B, may be indicated in an AIDS patient or other immunocompromised hosts with chronic pneumonia, since fungal pulmonary diseases in this setting can be severe and rapidly progressive.[18]

Corticosteroids

The question of when to use corticosteroids in the treatment of a patient with chronic pneumonia frequently arises. If the cause of the illness is an infectious agent, particularly a bacterium or a fungus, steroids are usually not indicated. In contrast, corticosteroids may be beneficial in chronic pneumonia due to noninfectious causes such as the vasculitides, sarcoidosis, chronic eosinophilic pneumonia, radiation injury, bronchiolitis obliter-

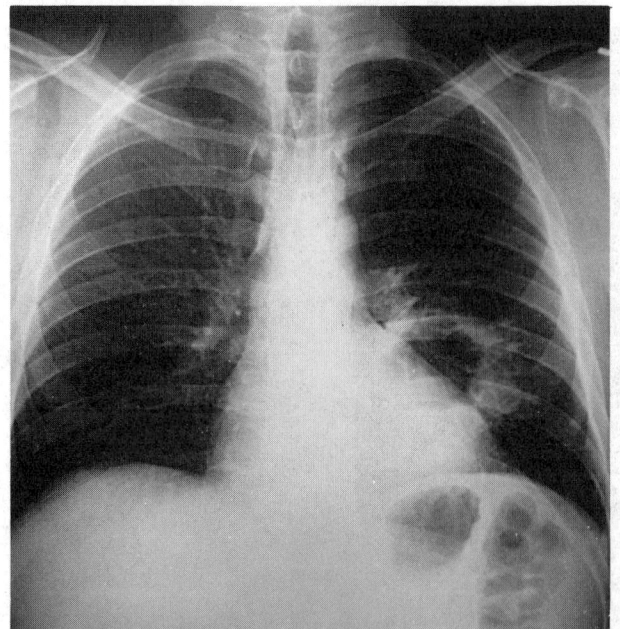

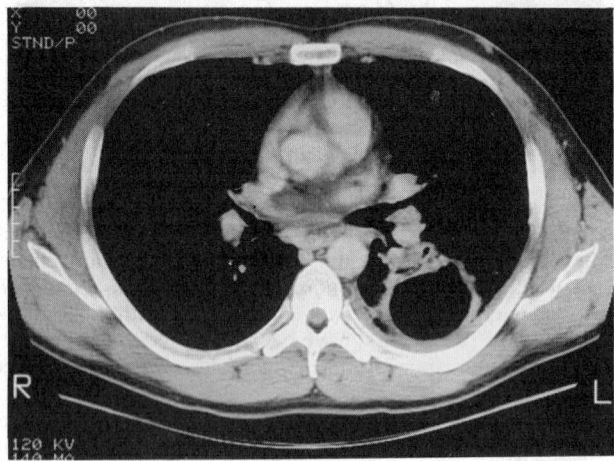

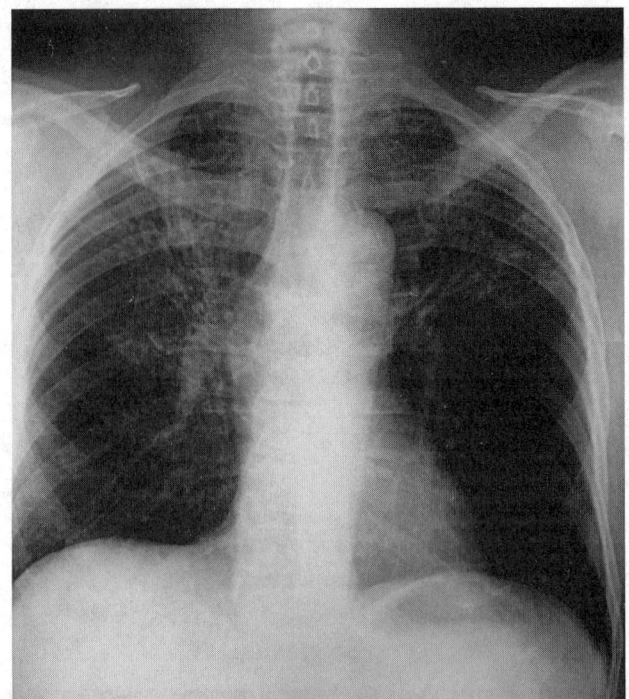

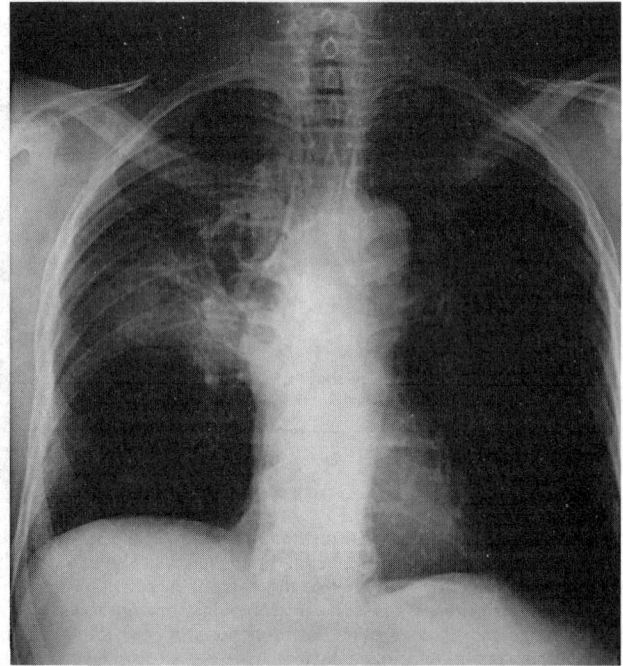

FIG. 13. **(A)** Wegener's granulomatosis in a 35-year-old cattle farmer with a 2-month illness manifested by fever, malaise, weight loss, pleurisy, polyarthralgias, and palpable purpura of the lower extremities. Laboratory studies included a markedly elevated erythrocyte sedimentation rate, a positive test for antineutrophil cytoplasmic autoantibody, and an abnormal urine sediment. Note the large cavitary mass lesion of the left lower lobe. **(B)** A chest CT scan demonstrates the lower lobe cavitary lesion and a small pleural effusion but no other pulmonary parenchymal abnormalities.

FIG. 14. **(A & B)** Squamous cell carcinoma (scar carcinoma) in a 72-year-old man with a history of previously treated pulmonary tuberculosis. In Fig. A, note the fibronodular pattern involving both upper lobes, right greater than left. Fig. B shows a radiographic film taken 2.5 years later; note the new rounded mass lesion in the right upper lobe. A pathologic diagnosis was made from tissue obtained at bronchoscopy.

ans organizing pneumonia, and many of the fibrotic lung diseases including chronic hypersensitivity pneumonitis (along with avoidance of exposure to the offending antigen).

Supportive Measures

Vigorous measures aimed at good bronchopulmonary hygiene should be instituted. Generous fluid intake and humidified air may promote easier expectoration. In patients with chronic cavitary disease or bronchiectasis or in whom there is copious sputum production, postural drainage and chest vibropercussion are important adjuncts. However, these procedures must be carried out with caution in an attempt to prevent infection from spreading to the noninvolved lung. Hypoxia may be a feature of chronic pneumonia; the severity will depend on the cause and the distribution of the pulmonary parenchymal process. Ap-

propriate means of administering oxygen should be used to ensure adequate oxygen supply to the tissues, and alterations in delivery should be made on the basis of sequential arterial blood gas studies.

Bronchoscopy and Surgery

Bronchoscopy may be used as a therapeutic adjunct, especially in patients who have thick tenacious secretions that cannot be raised by noninvasive techniques. In other patients, mucous plugs or foreign bodies may predispose to atelectasis and chronic pneumonia; therapeutic bronchoscopy with a rigid bronchoscope may be necessary to expand the collapsed lung.

Lobectomy or pneumonectomy should be considered in a patient with chronic destructive pneumonia and multiple macro- or microabscesses involving an entire lobe or lung and a ventilation-perfusion scan indicating nonfunction of the involved lung. Thoracotomy may also be indicated for purposes of decortication of the pleura in patients whose chronic pneumonia has involved the pleura with resulting restrictive lung disease.

REFERENCES

1. Epler GR, Colby TV, McCloud TC, et al. Bronchiolitis obliterans organizing pneumonia. N Engl J Med 1985;312:152–8.
2. Müller NL, Guery-Force ML, Staples CA, et al. Differential diagnosis of bronchiolitis obliterans with organizing pneumonia and usual interstitial pneumonia: Clinical, functional and radiologic findings. Radiology. 1987;162:151–6.
3. Carrington CB, Gaensler EA, Coutu RE, et al. Natural history and treated course of usual and desquamative interstitial pneumonia. N Engl J Med. 1978;298:801–9.
4. Crystal RG, Bitterman PB, Rennard SI, et al. Interstitial lung diseases of unknown cause: Disorders characterized by chronic inflammation of the lower respiratory tract (two parts). N Engl J Med. 1984;310:154–66, 235–44.
5. Bartlett JG. Anaerobic bacterial infections of the lung. Chest. 1987;91:901–9.
6. Lerner AM. The gram-negative bacillary pneumonias. Dis Month. 1980;27:1–56.
7. Case records of the Massachusetts General Hospital (Case 48-1990). N Engl J Med. 1990;323:1546–55.
8. Khan MA, Kovnat DM, Bachus B, et al. Clinical and roentgenographic spectrum of pulmonary tuberculosis in the adult. Am J Med. 1977;62:31–8.
9. Rosenweig DU. Pulmonary mycobacterial infections due to *Mycobacterium intracellulare avium* complex—Clinical features and course in 100 consecutive cases. Chest. 1979;75:115–9.
10. Goodwin RA, Owens FT, Snell JD, et al. Chronic cavitary histoplasmosis. Medicine. 1976;55:413–52.
11. Bayer AS. Fungal pneumonias: Pulmonary coccidioidal syndromes. Part 1 and part 2. Chest. 1981;79:575–83, 686–91.
12. Farrell GE, ed. Actinomycosis of the Thorax. St. Louis: Warren H. Green Inc.; 1981:1–90.
13. Halvosen RA, Duncan JD, Merten DF, et al. Pulmonary blastomycosis: Radiologic manifestations. Radiology. 1984;150:1–5.
14. Kerkering TM, Duma RJ, Shadomy S. The evolution of pulmonary cryptococcosis. Clinical implications from a study of 41 patients with and without compromising host factors. Ann Intern Med. 1981;94:611–6.
15. Hammerman KJ, Powell KE, Christianson CS, et al. Pulmonary cryptococcosis: Clinical forms and treatment. Am Rev Respir Dis. 1973;108:1116–23.
16. Plus JL, Opal SM. Pulmonary sporotrichosis: Review of treatment and outcome. Medicine. 1986;65:143–53.
17. Kwon-Chung KJ, Bennett JE, eds. Infections due to miscellaneous molds. In: Medical Mycology. Philadelphia: Lea & Febiger; 1992:733–67.
18. Shelhamer JH, Toews GB, Masur H, et al. Respiratory disease in the immunosuppressed patient. Ann Intern Med. 1992;117:415–31.
19. Cairns MR, Durack DT. Fungal pneumonia in the immunocompromised host. Semin Respir Infect. 1986;1:166–85.
20. Barnes PF, Block AB, Davidson PT, Snider DE Jr. Tuberculosis in patients with human immunodeficiency virus infection. N Engl J Med 1991;324:1644–50.
21. Murray JF, Garay SM, Hopewell PC, et al. Pulmonary complications of the acquired immunodeficiency syndrome: An update. Report of the Second National Heart, Lung and Blood Institute Workshop. Am Rev Respir Dis. 1987;135:504–9.
22. Weinberger SE. Medical progress: Recent advances in pulmonary medicine (two parts). N Engl J Med. 1993;328:1389–98, 1462–70.
23. Cameron ML, Bartlett JA, Gallis HA, Waskin HA. Manifestations of pulmonary cryptococcosis in patients with acquired immunodeficiency syndrome. Rev Infect Dis. 1991;13:64–7.
24. Denning DW, Follansbee SE, Scolaro M, et al. Pulmonary aspergillosis in the acquired immunodeficiency syndrome. N Engl J Med. 1991;324:654–62.
25. Fish DG, Ampel NM, Galgiani JN, et al. Coccidioidomycosis during human immunodeficiency virus infection. A review of 77 patients. Medicine. 1990;69:384–91.
26. Wheat LJ, Connolly-Stringfield PA, Baker RL, et al. Disseminated histoplasmosis in the acquired immunodeficiency syndrome: Clinical findings, diagnosis and treatment, and review of literature. Medicine. 1990;69:361–74.
27. Harvey RL, Sunstrum JC. *Rhodococcus equi* infection in patients with and without human immunodeficiency virus infection. Rev Infect Dis. 1991;13:139–45.
28. Pappas PG, Pottage JC, Powderly WG, et al. Blastomycosis in patients with the acquired immunodeficiency syndrome. Ann Intern Med. 1992;116:847–53.
29. Gill PS, Akil BA, Colletti P, et al. Pulmonary Kaposi's sarcoma: Clinical findings and results of therapy. Am J Med. 1989;87:57–61.
30. Suffredini AF, Ognibene FP, Lack EE, et al. Nonspecific interstitial pneumonitis: A common cause of pulmonary disease in the acquired immunodeficiency syndrome. Ann Intern Med. 1987;107:7–13.
31. Stead WW, Lofgren JP, Warren E, Thomas C. Tuberculosis as an endemic and nosocomial infection among the elderly in nursing homes. N Engl J Med. 1985;312:1483–7.
32. Stead WW, Senner JW, Reddick WT, Lofgren JP. Racial differences in susceptibility to infection by *Mycobacterium tuberculosis*. N Engl J Med. 1990;322:422–7.
33. Kriebel D, Brain JD, Sprince NL, et al. The pulmonary toxicity of beryllium. Am Rev Respir Dis. 1988;137:464–73.
34. Becklake MR. Pneumoconiosis. In: Murray JF, Nadel JA, eds. Textbook of Respiratory Medicine. Philadelphia: WB Saunders; 1988:1556–92.
35. Richerson HB. Hypersensitivity pneumonitis: Pathology and pathogenesis. Clin Rev Allergy. 1983;1:469–86.
36. Evans MJ. Oxidant gases. Environ Health Perspect. 1984;55:85–95.
37. Everett ED, Nelson RA. Pulmonary melioidosis. Am Rev Respir Dis. 1975;112:331–40.
38. Suwanik P, Harinasuta C. Pulmonary paragonimiasis: An evaluation of roentgen findings in 38 positive sputum patients in an endemic area in Thailand. AJR. 1959;81:236–44.
39. Frand UI, Shim CS, Williams MH Jr. Heroin-induced pulmonary edema. Sequential studies of pulmonary function. Ann Intern Med. 1972;77:29–35.
40. Robertson CH, Reynolds RC, Wilson JE. Pulmonary hypertension and foreign body granulomas in intravenous drug abusers. Documentation by cardiac catheterization and lung biopsy. Am J Med. 1976;61:657–64.
41. Patel RC, Dutta D, Schonfeld SA. Free-base cocaine use associated with bronchiolitis obliterans organizing pneumonia. Ann Intern Med. 1987;107:186–7.
42. Cooper JAD Jr, ed. Drug-induced pulmonary disease. Clin Chest Med. 1990;2:1–189.
43. Fauci AS, Haynes BF, Costa J, et al. Lymphomatoid granulomatosis: Prospective clinical and therapeutic experience over 10 years. N Engl J Med. 1982;306:69–74.
44. Müller NL, Miller RA. Computed tomography of chronic diffuse infiltrative lung disease (two parts). Am Rev Respir Dis. 1990;142:1206–15, 1440–8.
45. Fulkerson WJ. Fiberoptic bronchoscopy. N Engl J Med. 1984;311:511–515.
46. Hanson RR, Zavala DC, Rhodes ML et al. Transbronchial biopsy via flexible fiberoptic bronchoscope: Results in 164 patients. Am Rev Respir Dis. 1976;114:67–72.
47. Reynolds HY. Bronchoalveolar lavage. Am Rev Respir Dis. 1987;135:250–63.
48. Wimberly NW, Bass JB, Boyd BW, et al. Use of bronchoscopic protected catheter brush for the diagnosis of pulmonary infections. Chest. 1982;81:556–62.
49. Tenholder MF. Pulmonary infections in the immunocompromised host: Perspectives on procedures (Editorial). Chest. 1988;94:676–7.
50. Sokolowski JW Jr, Burgher LW, Jones FL Jr, et al. Guidelines for thoracentesis and needle biopsy of the pleura (position paper of the American Thoracic Society). Am Rev Respir Dis. 1989;140:257–8.
51. Cockerill FR III, Wilson WR, Carpenter HA, et al. Open lung biopsy in immunocompromised patients. Arch Intern Med. 1985;145:1398–404.
52. Khoun NF, Stitik FP, Erozan YS, et al. Transthoracic needle aspiration biopsy of benign and malignant lung lesions. AJR. 1985;144:281–8.
53. Sokolowski JW Jr, Burgher LW, Jones FL Jr, et al. Guidelines for percutaneous transthoracic needle biopsy (position paper of the American Thoracic Society). Am Rev Respir Dis. 1989;140:255–6.

54. CYSTIC FIBROSIS

M.R. KNOWLES
P.H. GILLIGAN
R.C. BOUCHER

A clearer understanding of cystic fibrosis (CF) as a genetic disorder has evolved since identification of the CF gene in 1989,[1–3] but the molecular pathogenesis is complex, and the clinical syndrome is variable.[4,5] Although CF has been generally regarded as a disease of children, about one-third of currently identified

CF patients are adults. The usual clinical manifestations include chronic obstructive lung disease, characteristic microbiologic flora of sputum (i.e., *Staphylococcus aureus* and mucoid *Pseudomonas aeruginosa*), and pancreatic exocrine insufficiency. The clinical diagnosis is usually supported by the hallmark laboratory abnormality, an elevated sweat chloride concentration. The normal range for sweat chloride values obtained by pilocarpine iontophoresis is greater in adults than in children; whereas values must be less than 40 mEq/liter to be clearly normal in children, healthy adults may have values of up to 70 mEq/liter.[5] The genetic diagnosis can be established by identification of a CF mutation on each allele of the CF gene.[4]

CLINICAL MANIFESTATIONS

The clinical manifestations of CF reflect obstruction of organs by viscous secretions and the presence of chronic bacterial infection in the lung. Although multiple organ systems are involved, chronic airway infection accounts for most disease-related morbidity and mortality. Chronic suppurative airway disease is present in more than 98 percent of adults who have CF, and 95 percent of CF deaths are related to progressive pulmonary insufficiency.[6-9] Most respiratory infections in CF adults are caused by *S. aureus* and *P. aeruginosa*, whereas the incidence of infections with most other infectious agents (e.g., *Mycoplasma pneumoniae* and viruses) is believed to be similar to that in the general population.[10,11] It has been recently noted that up to 20 percent of CF adults in some CF centers may harbor nontuberculous mycobacteria in respiratory secretions[12-14]; the general prevalence and pathogenic role of these organisms are not clearly defined.

The clinical picture of CF is dominated by a chronic cough punctuated by episodes of clinical deterioration characterized by an increased volume and purulence of sputum, dyspnea, and sometimes anorexia and weight loss.[5,8,15] Although adults with CF may exhibit low-grade fever with these exacerbations, a high fever is unusual, and sepsis or bacteremia is uncommon despite the large number of bacteria in the airways (10^8 organisms per milliliter of sputum). Clinical exacerbations are also associated with modest elevations in white blood cell counts and worsening spirometric values. The chest x-ray typically shows diffuse roentgenographic shadowing that reflects airway wall thickening, retained secretions, and cystic bronchiectatic changes. Many adult CF patients exhibit an upper lung zone predominance of these roentgenographic abnormalities, which raises the diagnostic possibility of tuberculosis. Hypoxemia and carbon dioxide retention are uncommon in CF adults during acute exacerbations until the forced expired volume in 1 second (FEV_1) is less than 40 percent of the predicted value. Thus, significant gas exchange abnormalities usually occur only near the terminal stages of the disease and herald a more rapid downhill course.[5]

The pulmonary manifestations of CF in adults are frequently complicated by hemoptysis and pneumothorax.[16] Minor hemoptysis is common in CF patients, and massive hemoptysis occurs in about 1 percent of adult CF patients each year. Fortunately, medical (nonsurgical) intervention is usually sufficient for the treatment of pulmonary hemorrhage. The presence of epithelial dysfunction in the mucosa of the nasal sinuses of CF patients and the frequent occurrence of nasal polyps in adults make symptoms of subacute/chronic sinusitis a major problem in many adult patients. It is important to note that the microbiology of sinusitis is not always reflected by the flora identified in expectorated sputum.[17]

Because most CF patients have progressive destruction and loss of pancreatic function, the prevalence of diabetes mellitus in adult CF populations may be as high as 15 percent.[18] The presence of glucose intolerance may add further difficulty to the treatment of pulmonary infections.

PATHOGENESIS

The clinical syndrome of CF reflects an autosomal recessive genetic disorder. The CF gene was identified in 1989 and is located on the long arm of chromosome 7.[2] It is a relatively large gene, consisting of 27 exons, and codes for a 1480-amino-acid polypeptide known as *cystic fibrosis transmembrane regulator* (CFTR). Three hundred different mutations have been identified in the CF gene.[4] The most common mutation is a three-base-pair deletion that leads to a phenylalanine being absent from the protein at position 508 (ΔF_{508}).

The molecular pathogenesis of cystic fibrosis is complex and varies with the type of CF gene mutation. The CFTR protein appears to reside in the plasma membrane. Molecular modeling predicts that the polypeptide contains, in sequence, a six transmembrane spanning region; a nucleotide (ATP) binding fold that is the site of the ΔF_{508} mutation; a large hydrophilic domain that is the site of a kinase/phosphatase regulation (the "R" domain); another six transmembrane spanner; and another nucleotide binding fold.[2] The full spectrum of functions of CFTR protein is now known. CFTR appears able to function as the cAMP-regulated Cl^- channel in the plasma membrane[9,20] but likely regulates other ion channels in the plasma membrane as well.[21] The common CF mutation (ΔF_{508}) leads to abnormal folding of the CFTR polypeptide in the endoplasmic reticulum and degradation of the protein by intracellular "editing."[22] Thus, the cellular pathogenesis of the ΔF_{508} mutation reflects the absence of protein at the relevant cellular site, e.g., the plasma membrane. Other less common CFTR mutations appear to allow the targeting of CFTR to the plasma membrane but lead to abnormal Cl^- channel regulation and/or abnormal Cl^- ion permeation.

Two general features characterize the pathogenesis of CF at the cellular level: (1) the affected cells in target organs are epithelial, and (2) the abnormality in epithelial cells involves regulation of ion transport. The most prevalent defect is abnormal regulation of the cAMP-dependent plasma membrane Cl^- (CFTR) channels. Defective Cl^- channel activation has been detected in the airways,[23] sweat ducts,[24] and the small intestines[25] of CF patients. A second major defect in ion transport has been detected in CF airway epithelia; the rate of absorption of Na^+ ions from the airway lumen to the interstitium is raised threefold compared with normal.[26,27] The exact relationship between mutations in CFTR and regulation of Na^+ transport are not yet known, but may involve the ion channel regulatory functions of CFTR.

The ion transport abnormalities that characterize CF affect the volume and composition of the secretions that line the airway surfaces. Both accelerated Na^+ absorption and reduced Cl^- secretion would be expected to reduce the water content of secretions and change the electrolyte composition of secretions. Abnormal water and electrolyte composition may alter the hydration of high-molecular-weight glycoconjugates (mucins) on airway surfaces, derange the viscoelastic properties of secretions, and lead to reductions in mucociliary and cough clearance. Whether reduced clearance of thickened secretions from airways is sufficient alone to lead to persistence of staphylococcal and pseudomonal infection is not yet clear. A role for increased bacterial adherence, perhaps through a change in the $SO_4^=$ (i.e., sulfate content of airway surface glycocalyx) has recently been postulated.[28]

The development of persistent bacterial infection generates a complex series of events that lead to airway wall damage and ultimately to destroyed or bronchiectatic airways. Bacterial exoproducts from both *S. aureus* and *P. aeruginosa* have been implicated in airway destruction. In adults, lipopolysaccharides, exotoxin A, and a cell wall–associated rhamnolipid from *P. aeruginosa* have been implicated as important bacterial toxins.[29] The host inflammatory response appears intact in CF, and the vigorous host response contributes to airway damage.[9,30] Chemotactic agents, both bacterial and locally derived (e.g., arachidonic acid metabolites from airway epithelia), attract inflammatory cells into the airway lumen. Polymorphonuclear cell-derived enzymes (e.g., elastase) damage airway wall structures and cleave immune receptors on neutrophils and bacteria,[31] thereby impairing immune function. In addition, chronic antigenic stimulus of persistent airway infections generates immunologically mediated airway wall destruction.[30] Large amounts of neutrophil-derived DNA further thicken and impair clearance of airway secretions.[9] Eventually, the combination of retained secretions and airway damage deranges gas exchange, perturbs cardiac function, and leads to death.

MICROBIOLOGY

Staphylococcus aureus and *P. aeruginosa* are the primary etiologic agents of pulmonary infection in patients with CF.[32] *Staphylococcus aureus* often colonizes the respiratory tract in the first 2 years of life and can be found in approximately 30 percent of patients with CF in the United States. Before the advent of effective antistaphylococcal therapy, lung infection due to this organism was the leading cause of death. Antistaphylococcal penicillins such as oxacillin and nafcillin control infections with this organism, and resistance to these agents is unusual. In patients receiving long-term (>3 months) prophylactic trimethoprim–sulfamethoxazole therapy, approximately 50 percent of *S. aureus* isolates are thymidine dependent.[33] Because thymidine-dependent organisms grow poorly on most commonly used isolation media and because mucoid *P. aeruginosa* may obscure recognition of its growth, mannitol salts agar must be used to ensure reliable recovery of *S. aureus.*

In childhood or early adolescence, patients with CF become chronically infected with *P. aeruginosa.* Up to 80 percent of adolescent and adult patients with CF are infected with this organism.[32] As this chronic infection evolves, isolates of *P. aeruginosa* may produce large amounts of an extracellular mucoid polysaccharide called *alginate.*[34] Molecular studies suggest that environmental factors in the airway of CF patients (high salt concentration and dehydration) switch on a series of genes that regulate production of this virulence factor.[34] Molecular studies also indicate that a large number of different *P. aeruginosa* strains are capable of producing alginate.[35,36] Mucoid colonies that result from alginate production are predominant in infected CF patients but are rarely seen in other patients with chronic airway disease.[37] This mucoid variant is responsible for the formation of microcolonies that are believed to be resistant to both mechanical and immunologic clearance from the airways. The exuberant immune response to these microcolonies is believed to be responsible, in part, for the chronic deterioration in pulmonary function that is the hallmark of this disease.[38]

When first isolated, *P. aeruginosa* is usually susceptible to all antipseudomonal β-lactams, imipenem, quinolones, and aminoglycosides. With increasing antimicrobial pressure due to repeated antimicrobial treatment of pulmonary exacerbations, resistance to these agents may develop, especially if each one is used alone. In airways repeatedly treated for *P. aeruginosa,* the organism may remain susceptible only to polymyxin B and colistin.

As life expectancy has increased in CF patients, a third organism, *Pseudomonas cepacia,* has emerged as an important pathogen in at least some CF centers. Some CF patients infected with *P. cepacia* develop what has been characterized as "the cepacia syndrome."[39] In this syndrome, adolescent and young adult CF patients with relatively mild pulmonary disease become infected, have rapid deterioration in pulmonary function, may develop bacteremia, and die within 6 months. Other CF patients may be infected with *P. cepacia* without a corresponding decline in their clinical status. Molecular epidemiologic studies of *P. cepacia* indicate that it can be spread from person to person during close social contact.[40] Segregation of *P. cepacia*–in-

fected patients is used in some CF centers to prevent spread of the organism to noninfected CF patients.[41]

Pseudomonas cepacia is also a cause of concern in CF patients who receive double lung transplantation. The transplanted lungs of CF patients frequently become reinfected with organisms that infected the native lungs and are still present in the sinuses or trachea of the recipient. At one center, all 10 patients who had *P. cepacia* lung infections pretransplant became infected with *P. cepacia* post-transplant. Five additional CF patients developed nosocomial *P. cepacia* pulmonary infections post-transplant. In the CF lung transplant population, mortality is significantly increased in *P. cepacia*–infected patients.[42]

One of the major problems in managing *P. cepacia*–infected patients is the organism's resistance to antimicrobials. The organism is intrinsically resistant to aminoglycosides. On initial isolation, the organism may be susceptible to trimethoprim–sulfamethoxazole and antipseudomonal β-lactams. However, under antimicrobial pressure, resistance quickly develops and the clinician is frequently given the challenge of managing a patient infected with an organism resistant to all available antimicrobials.[39]

Another problem is detecting *P. cepacia* in the complex microbiologic milieu of CF respiratory secretions. Unless specific isolation media is used, the organism, which grows comparatively slowly,[39] may be obscured, particularly by mucoid *P. aeruginosa.*

The role of mycobacteria in the lung disease of cystic fibrosis patients has recently come under scrutiny. Studies have shown that nontuberculous mycobacteria, usually *Mycobacterium avian-intracellulare,* can be isolated from the respiratory secretions of up to 20 percent of adult CF patients.[12,13,43] Cystic fibrosis patients colonized with these organisms are excluded as transplant candidates at some centers because of the difficulties in treating nontuberculous mycobacterial infections. As with *P. cepacia,* special culture techniques are required to prevent overgrowth of mucoid *P. aeruginosa* reliably and to allow recovery of nontuberculous mycobacteria from CF respiratory secretions.[44]

Other bacteria such as *H. influenzae, Moraxella catarrhalis, Xanthomonas maltophilia, Alcaligenes xylosoxidans,* and Enterobactericeae are recovered from the respiratory tract of CF patients and may play a role in their pulmonary disease. *Aspergillus fumigatus* may be cultured from CF patients.[39] However, the clinical diagnosis of allergic bronchopulmonary aspergillosis (ABPA) should be made using rigorous criteria, because many CF patients have positive immediate hypersensitivity skin tests and serum-precipitating antibodies to *Aspergillus* without the clinical syndrome of ABPA.[45,46]

The role of viruses in the chronic lung disease of CF patients has not been determined. Acute respiratory infections due to respiratory syncytial virus, influenza A, and parainfluenza virus have all been documented.[47–49] The rate and severity of these viral respiratory infections in CF children is similar to that seen in their non-CF siblings.[48]

TREATMENT

The goal of therapy is to retard progressive lung damage by removing viscous/purulent airway secretions, by controlling bacterial infection with antibiotics, and by providing proper nutrition for host defense.[7,8,15] The presence of a large bacterial burden in the bronchiectatic airways of patients dictates that airway clearance techniques be combined with antibacterial therapy to achieve optimal results.[8,11,15] Chest percussion and postural drainage is the time-honored method, but deep breathing, exercise, and voluntary coughing are also effective. Bronchodilators may assist in clearing retained secretions in some patients, but a paradoxical reduction in airflow in some patients[50] and a potential acceleration of abnormal Na$^+$ absorption across airway epithelia[26] suggest that these agents should be used intermittently and with caution in adult CF patients. Anti-inflammatory agents may occasionally be useful in reducing mucosal edema and assisting in airway clearance, but the indications for these agents are poorly defined.[15] There is little role for the use of inhaled mucolytic agents or bronchial lavage.[8,15]

Antibiotics have played a key role in improved survival, and indications for antimicrobial therapy continue to evolve.[7,8,11] Broad-spectrum oral antibiotics (amoxicillin, cephalexin, dicloxacillin, tetracycline, trimethoprim–sulfamethoxazole) can provide useful therapy for acute pulmonary exacerbations despite the presence of *P. aeruginosa* that is resistant to these agents. The clinical benefit may reflect antibiotic activity against pathogens that are difficult to culture in the presence of mucoid *P. aeruginosa (S. aureus, H. influenzae)*, or against airway infection with high concentrations of bacteria ($>10^5$ organisms per milliliter that are not typical pathogens[7]), or inhibition of release of toxic bacterial exoproducts in the absence of bacterial killing.[51–53] High doses and prolonged therapy (3–4 weeks) with oral agents are recommended for treatment of acute illnesses (exacerbations). Oral antibiotics are also of benefit in chronic bacterial sinusitis, which results from pathogens that are frequently sensitive to broad-spectrum antimicrobials.[17] The use of oral antibiotics for prophylactic (maintenance) therapy is controversial but appears to have a useful role in some patients.

Ciprofloxacin is an oral antipseudomonal drug that is useful for intermittent therapy. The emergence of bacterial resistance during monotherapy with this drug limits its usefulness for chronic treatment,[54–56] and the duration of periodic treatment should be limited to 2–4 weeks.[56,57]

Aggressive parenteral therapy is indicated for clinical exacerbations that do not respond to oral antimicrobials.[7–9,11,15] Although sterilization of airway secretions rarely occurs and is not the goal of parenteral therapy, the bacterial burden in airways can be reduced[58] and irreversible lung damage presumably retarded. Whereas parenteral therapy should be guided by sputum bacteriology and drug sensitivity, treatment in adult CF patients usually focuses on *P. aeruginosa*. A combination of antibiotics is indicated because thickened airway secretions present a barrier to drug penetration and because aminoglycoside activity can be reduced by suppurative secretions.[59] A combination of antibiotics also protects against the emergence of resistant strains. Therapy usually includes an aminoglycoside (gentamicin, tobramycin, amikacin), plus another agent effective against *P. aeruginosa*, such as antipseudomonal penicillins, cephalosporins (e.g., ceftazidime[60,61]), or imipenem. If *S. aureus* is clinically suspected or cultured from sputum, addition of a specific antistaphylococcal agent should be considered if the antipseudomonal drug therapy is not adequate for *S. aureus*. Increased plasma clearance of almost all effective antibiotics in CF patients dictates the use of large, frequent doses of antimicrobials.[62] For example, CF adults require 6–15/mg/kg/day of gentamicin to achieve desired peak serum levels of 10 µg/ml in a q8h dosing regimen. Aminoglycoside toxicity is uncommon in CF patients, but trough serum levels should be carefully monitored. Parenteral therapy should be continued for a minimum of 10–14 days or longer, if necessary, to achieve a full clinical and pulmonary functional response. Recent experience indicates that effective parenteral antibiotic therapy can be administered on an outpatient basis.[15,63,64]

Aerosolized antibiotics can be used for subacute pulmonary exacerbations and to assist in the maintenance of a stable clinical status in some patients.[65,66] A recent study demonstrated improved lung function with high dose aerosolized tobramycin in clinically stable patients.[67] Effective aerosol delivery techniques are essential if this approach is to be successful.[68] Colistin is an attractive agent for inhalation therapy.[69] The development of bacterial resistance during prolonged aerosol therapy with colistin does not reduce the response to parenteral alternatives.

Interestingly, despite intensive antibiotic exposure, symptomatic disease with *Clostridium difficile* is uncommon in CF patients despite the presence of the organism in fecal samples.[70,71] The asymptomatic carriage of *C. difficile* may reflect the inability of the CF intestinal epithelium to respond to *C. difficile*–derived secretory toxins.[25]

Chronic malabsorption, coupled with increased caloric requirements due to chronic infection and increased respiratory activity, can induce malnourishment and impaired host-defense mechanisms in CF patients. High caloric intake with supplemental pancreatic digestive enzymes and appropriate fat-soluble vitamins is therefore essential in the treatment of these patients.[5,72]

Although *Aspergillus* spp. are frequently cultured from the sputum of CF adults, treatment is usually not indicated unless the syndrome of allergic bronchopulmonary aspergillosis is established.[45,46] Systemic corticosteroids are usually sufficient, but antifungal therapy may be useful as adjunctive therapy in some patients.[73] The increasing number of adults in the CF patient population is associated with increasing recovery of nontuberculous mycobacteria from sputum cultures.[12,13,43] Although as many as 20 percent of adult CF patients have nontuberculous mycobacteria in respiratory secretions, their pathogenicity is not clearly defined; clinical and radiological studies should be monitored for evidence of possible pathogenic mycobacterial activity.

Annual influenza vaccinations are recommended, but pneumococcal vaccine is not routinely indicated because of the relative absence of *S. pneumoniae* as a pathogen.

Lung transplantation is a viable therapeutic option for patients with end-stage lung disease. In experienced lung transplant centers, the 1-year survival is 80–90 percent, and the 5-year survival may be as high as 50 percent.[74,75]

Recent progress in defining the organ level and molecular pathogenesis of CF has led to the development of new therapeutic approaches. Aerosolized recombinant human DNAse I improves clearance of purulent airway secretions[79–81] and has recently been approved by the FDA; this agent will offer another modality for the treatment of patients with DNA-laden secretions. Anti-inflammatory agents (NSAIDs) and aerosolized antiproteases are being tested as treatment for secondary manifestations of the lung disease.[15,76–78] Therapy of abnormal airway epithelial ion transport, targeting accelerated Na^+ absorption with aerosolized amiloride[82] and reduced Cl^- secretion with UTP,[83] offers the possibility of long-term "preventive" therapy that might impede the development of airway disease; these agents are currently in clinical studies. Finally, gene transfer of normal CFTR cDNA to airway cells offers the promise of treatment at the molecular level[4]; although this technique is some distance from the clinical arena, several pilot studies of gene transfer with adenoviral vectors are underway.

REFERENCES

1. Rommens JM, Iannuzzi MC, Kerem B-T, et al. Identification of the cystic fibrosis gene: Chromosome walking and jumping. Science. 1989;245:1059–65.
2. Riordan JR, Rommens JM, Kerem B-T, et al. Identification of the cystic fibrosis gene: Cloning and characterization of complementary DNA. Science. 1989;245:1066–73.
3. Kerem B-T, Rommens JM, Buchanan JA, et al. Identification of the cystic fibrosis gene: Genetic analysis. Science. 1989;245:1073–80.
4. Collins FS. Cystic fibrosis: Molecular biology and therapeutic implications. Science. 1992;256:774–9.
5. Boat TF, Welsh MJ, Beaudet AL. Cystic fibrosis. In: Scriver CR, Beaudet AL, Sly WS, et al, eds. The Metabolic Basis of Inherited Disease. New York: McGraw-Hill Information Services Company; 1989:2649–80.
6. Davis PB. Cystic fibrosis in adults. In: Lloyd-Still JD, ed. Textbook of Cystic Fibrosis. v. 9, Littleton: John Wright-PSG; 1983:351–66.
7. Myers MG, Koontz FP, Weinberger M. Lower respiratory infections in patients with cystic fibrosis. In: Lloyd-Still JD, ed. Textbok of Cystic Fibrosis. Boston: John Wright, PSG Inc.; 1983:91–107.
8. Taussig LM, Landau LI, Marks MI. Respiratory system. In: Taussig LI, ed. Cystic Fibrosis. New York: Thieme-Stratton; 1984:115–74.
9. David PB. Pathophysiology of the lung disease in cystic fibrosis. In: Davis PB, ed. Cystic Fibrosis (Lung Biology in Health and Disease, v. 64). New York: Marcel Dekker, Inc.; 1993:193–218.

10. Friend PA. Pulmonary infection in cystic fibrosis. J Infect. 1986;13:55–72.
11. Thomassen MJ, Demko CA, Doershuk CF. Cystic fibrosis: A review of pulmonary infections and interventions. Pediatr Pulmonol. 1987;3:334–51.
12. Kilby JM, Gilligan PH, Yankaskas JR, et al. Nontuberculous mycobacteria in adult patients with cystic fibrosis. Chest. 1992;102:70–5.
13. Olivier K, Gilligan P, Yankaskas J, et al. Nontuberculous mycobacteria (NTM) in the respiratory tract of adult cystic fibrosis (CF) patients: Update '92. Pediatr Pulmonol. 1992(Suppl 8):293–294.
14. Aitken ML, Burke W, McDonald G, et al. Nontuberculous mycobacterial disease in adult cystic fibrosis patients. Chest. 1993;103:1096–9.
15. Turpin SV, Knowles MR. Treatment of pulmonary disease in cystic fibrosis. In: Davis PB, ed. Cystic Fibrosis. New York: Marcel Dekker, Inc.; 1993: 277–344.
16. Schidlow DV, Taussig LM, Knowles MR. Cystic Fibrosis Foundation Consensus Conference Report on pulmonary complications of cystic fibrosis. Pediatr Pulmonol. 1993;15:187–98.
17. Shapiro ED, Milmoe GJ, Wald ER, et al. Bacteriology of the maxillary sinuses in patients with cystic fibrosis. J Infect Dis. 1982;146:589–593.
18. Knowles MR, Fernald GW. Diabetes and cystic fibrosis: New questions emerging from increased longevity. J Pediatr. 1988;112:415–6.
19. Anderson MP, Rich DP, Gregory RJ, et al. Generation of cAMP-activated chloride currents by expression of CFTR. Science. 1991;251:679–82.
20. Kartner N, Hanrahan JW, Jensen TJ, et al. Expression of the cystic fibrosis gene in non-epithelial invertebrate cells produces a regulated anion conductance. Cell. 1991;64:681–91.
21. Gabriel SE, Clarke LL, Boucher RC, et al. CFTR and outward rectifying chloride channels are distinct proteins with a regulatory relationship. Nature. 1993;363:263–8.
22. Cheng SH, Gregory RJ, Marshall J, et al. Defective intracellular transport and processing of CFTR is the molecular basis of most cystic fibrosis. Cell. 1990;63:827–34.
23. Knowles MR, Stutts MJ, Spock A, et al. Abnormal ion permeation through cystic fibrosis respiratory epithelium. Science. 1983;221:1067–70.
24. Quinton PM. Chloride impermeability in cystic fibrosis. Nature. 1983;301: 421–2.
25. Berschneider HM, Knowles MR, Azizkhan RG, et al. Altered intestinal chloride transport in cystic fibrosis. FASEB J. 1988;2:2625–9.
26. Boucher RC, Stutts MJ, Knowles MR, et al. Na$^+$ transport in cystic fibrosis respiratory epithelia. Abnormal basal rate and response to adenylate cyclase activation. J Clin Invest. 1986;78:1245–52.
27. Knowles MR, Gatzy J, Boucher R. Increased bioelectric potential difference across respiratory epithelia in cystic fibrosis. N Engl J Med. 1981;305: 1489–95.
28. Cheng P-W, Boat TF, Cranfill K, et al. Increased sulfation of glycoconjugates by cultured nasal epithelial cells from patients with cystic fibrosis. J Clin Invest. 1989;84:68–72.
29. Stutts MJ, Schwab JH, Chen MG, et al. Effects of *Pseudomonas aeruginosa* on bronchial epithelial ion transport. Am Rev Respir Dis. 1986;134:17–21.
30. Konstan MW, Berger M. Infection and inflammation of the lung in cystic fibrosis. In: Davis PB, ed. Cystic Fibrosis (Lung Biology in Health and Disease, v.64). New York: Marcel Dekker, Inc.; 1993:219–76.
31. Tosi MF, Zakem H, Berger M. Neutrophil elastase cleaves C3bi on opsonized *Pseudomonas* as well as CR1 on neutrophils to create a functionally important opsonin receptor mismatch. J Clin Invest. 1990;86:300–8.
32. Fitzsimmons SC. The changing epidemiology of cystic fibrosis. J Pediatr. 1993;122:1–9.
33. Gilligan PH, Cage PA, Welch DF, Muszynski MJ, Wait KR. Prevalence of thymidine-dependent *Staphylococcus aureus* in patients with cystic fibrosis. J Clin Microbiol. 1987;25:1258–61.
34. May TB, Shinabarger D, Maharaj R, et al. Alginate synthesis by *Pseudomonas aeruginosa*: A key pathogenic factor in chronic pulmonary infections of cystic fibrosis patients. Clin Microbiol Rev. 1991;4:191–206.
35. Boukadida J, De Montalembert M, Lenoir G, et al. Molecular epidemiology of chronic colonisation by *Pseudomonas aeruginosa* in cystic fibrosis. J Med Microbiol. 1993;38:29–33.
36. Romling U, Grothues D, Koopmann U, et al. Pulsed-field gel electrophoresis analysis of a *Pseudomonas aeruginosa* pathovar. Electrophoresis. 1992;13: 646–8.
37. McCarthy VP, Rosenberg G, Rosenstein BJ, et al. Mucoid *Pseudomonas aeruginosa* from a patient without cystic fibrosis: Implications and review of the literature. Pediatr Infect Dis. 1986;5:256–8.
38. Fick RB Jr, Sonoda F, Hornick DB. Emergence and persistence of *Pseudomonas aeruginosa* in the cystic fibrosis airway. Semin Respir Infect. 1992;7: 168–78.
39. Gilligan PH. Microbiology of airway disease in patients with cystic fibrosis. Clin Microbiol Rev. 1991;4:35–51.
40. Govan JRW, Brown PH, Maddison J, et al. Evidence for transmission of *Pseudomonas cepacia* by social contact in cystic fibrosis. Lancet. 1993;342: 15–9.
41. Smith DL, Smith EG, Gumery LB, et al. *Pseudomonas cepacia* infection in cystic fibrosis. Lancet. 1992;1:252.
42. Snell GI, de Hoyos A, Krajden M, et al. *Pseudomonas cepacia* in lung transplant recipients with cystic fibrosis. Chest. 1993;103:466–71.
43. Aitken ML. The role of mycobacterial infections in cystic fibrosis pulmonary disease. Pediatr Pulmonol. 1991(Suppl 6):160–1.
44. Whittier S, Hopfer RL, Knowles MR, et al. Improved recovery of Mycobacteria from respiratory secretions of patients with cystic fibrosis. J Clin Microbiol. 1993;31:861–4.
45. Hutcheson PS, Rejent AJ, Slavin RG. Variability in parameters of allergic bronchopulmonary aspergillosis in patients with cystic fibrosis. J Allergy Clin Immunol. 1991;88:390–4.
46. Knutsen AP, Slavin RG. Allergic bronchopulmonary mycosis complicating cystic fibrosis. Semin Respir Infect. 1992;7:179–92.
47. Abman SH, Ogle JW, Butler-Simon N, et al. Role of respiratory syncytial virus in early hospitalizations for respiratory distress of young infants with cystic fibrosis. J Pediatr. 1988;113:826–30.
48. Ramsey BW, Gore EJ, Smith AL, et al. The effect of respiratory viral infections on patients with cystic fibrosis. Am J Dis Child. 1989;143:662–8.
49. Conway SP, Simmonds EJ, Littlewood JM. Acute severe deterioration in cystic fibrosis associated with influenza A virus infection. Thorax. 1992;47: 112–4.
50. Shapiro GG, Bamman J, Kanerek P, et al. The paradoxical effect of adrenergic and methylxanthine drugs in cystic fibrosis. Pediatrics. 1976;58:740–3.
51. Grimwood K, To M, Rabin HR, et al. Subinhibitory antibiotics reduce *Pseudomonas aeruginosa* tissue injury in the rat lung model. J Antimicrob Chemother. 1989;24:937–45.
52. Geers TA, Baker NR. The effect of sublethal levels of antibiotics on the pathogenicity of *Pseudomonas aeruginosa* for tracheal tissue. J Antimicrob Chemother. 1987;19:569–78.
53. Morris G, Brown MRW. Novel modes of action of aminoglycoside antibiotics against *Pseudomonas aeruginosa*. Lancet. 1988;2:1359–60.
54. Scully BE, Nakatomi M, Ores C, et al. Ciprofloxacin therapy in cystic fibrosis. Am J Med. 1987;82(Suppl 4A):196–200.
55. Goldfarb J, Stern RC, Reed MD, et al. Ciprofloxacin monotherapy for acute pulmonary exacerbations of cystic fibrosis. Am J Med. 1987;82(Suppl 4A): 174–8.
56. Stutman HR. Summary of a workshop on ciprofloxacin use in patients with cystic fibrosis. Pediatr Infect Dis J. 1987;6:932–5.
57. Michel BC. Antibacterial therapy in cystic fibrosis: A review of the literature published between 1980 and 1987. Chest. 1988;94:129S–40S.
58. Smith AL, Redding G, Doershuk C, et al. Sputum changes associated with therapy for endobronchial exacerbation in cystic fibrosis. J Pediatr. 1988;112: 547–54.
59. Mendelman PM, Smith AL, Levy J, et al. Aminoglycoside penetration, inactivation, and efficacy in cystic fibrosis sputum. Am Rev Respir Dis. 1985;132: 761–5.
60. Blumer JL, Stern RC, Yamashita TS, et al. Cephalosporin therapeutics in cystic fibrosis. J Pediatr. 1986;108:854–60.
61. Reed MD, Stern RC, O'Brien CA, et al. Randomized double-blind evaluation of ceftazidime dose ranging in hospitalized patients with cystic fibrosis. Antimicrob Agents Chemother. 1987;31:698–702.
62. de Groot R, Smith AL. Antibiotic pharmacokinetics in cystic fibrosis: Differences and clinical significance. Clin Pharmacokinet. 1987;13:228–53.
63. Donati MA, Guenette G, Auerbach H. Prospective controlled study of home and hospital therapy of cystic fibrosis pulmonary disease. J Pediatr. 1987;111: 28–33.
64. Strandvik B, Hjelte L, Malmborg AS, et al. Home intravenous antibiotic treatment of patients with cystic fibrosis. Acta Paediatr. 1992;81:340–4.
65. Stead RJ, Hodson ME, Batten JC. Inhaled ceftazidime compared with gentamicin and carbenicillin in older patients with cystic fibrosis infected with *Pseudomonas aeruginosa*. Br J Dis Chest. 1987;81:272–9.
66. Hodson ME, Penketh ARL, Batten JC. Aerosol carbenicillin and gentamicin treatment of *Pseudomonas aeruginosa* infection in patients with cystic fibrosis. Lancet. 1981;2:1137–9.
67. Ramsey BW, Dorkin HL, Eisenberg JD, et al. Efficacy of aerosolized tobramycin in patients with cystic fibrosis. N Engl J Med. 1993;328:1740–6.
68. Newman SP, Woodman G, Clarke SW. Deposition of carbenicillin aerosols in cystic fibrosis: Effects of nebuliser system and breathing pattern. Thorax. 1988;43:318–22.
69. Jensen T, Pedersen SS, Garne S, et al. Colistin inhalation therapy in cystic fibrosis patients with chronic *Pseudomonas aeruginosa* lung infection. J Antimicrob Chemother. 1987;19:831–8.
70. Welkon CJ, Long SS, Thompson CM Jr, et al. *Clostridium difficile* in patients with cystic fibrosis. Am J Dis Child. 1987;139:805–8.
71. Peach SL, Borriello SP, Gaya H, et al. Asymptomatic carriage of *Clostridium difficile* in patients with cystic fibrosis. J Clin Pathol. 1986;39:1013–8.
72. Hubbard VS. Nutritional considerations in cystic fibrosis. Semin Respir Med. 1985;6:308–13.
73. Denning DW, Van Wye JE, Lewiston NJ, et al. Adjunctive therapy of allergic bronchopulmonary aspergillosis with itraconazole. Chest. 1991;100:813–9.
74. Madden BP, Hodson ME, Tsang V, et al. Intermediate-term results of heart–lung transplantation for cystic fibrosis. Lancet. 1992;339:1583–7.
75. Egan TM. Lung transplantation in cystic fibrosis. Semin Respir Infect. 1992; 7:227–39.
76. Konstan MW, Vargo KM, Davis PB. Ibuprofen attenuates the inflammatory response to *Pseudomonas aeruginosa* in a rat model of chronic pulmonary

infection. Implications for antiinflammatory therapy in cystic fibrosis. Am Rev Respir Dis. 1990;141:186–92.

77. Konstan MW, Hoppel CL, Chai B-L, et al. Ibuprofen in children with cystic fibrosis: Pharmacokinetics and adverse effects. J Pediatr. 1991;118:956–64.

78. McElvaney NG, Hubbard RC, Birrer P, et al. Aerosol alpha 1-antitrypsin treatment for cystic fibrosis. Lancet. 1991;337:392–4.

79. Aitken ML, Burke W, McDonald G, et al. Recombinant human DNAse inhalation in normal subjects and patients with cystic fibrosis. A phase 1 study. JAMA. 1992;267:1947–51.

80. Hubbard RC, McElvaney NG, Birrer P, et al. A preliminary study of aerosol-

ized recombinant human deoxyribonuclease I in the treatment of cystic fibrosis. N Engl J Med. 1992;326:812–5.

81. Ramsey BW, Astley SJ, Aitken ML, et al. Efficacy and safety of short-term administration of aerosolized recombinant human deoxyribonuclease in patients with cystic fibrosis. Am Rev Respir Dis. 1993;148:145–51.

82. Knowles MR, Church NL, Waltner WE, et al. A pilot study of aerosolized amiloride for the treatment of cystic fibrosis lung disease. N Engl J Med. 1990;322:1189–94.

83. Knowles MR, Clarke LL, Boucher RC. Activation by extracellular nucleotides of chloride secretion in the airway epithelia of patients with cystic fibrosis. N Engl J Med. 1991;325:533–8.

SECTION D

55. URINARY TRACT INFECTIONS

JACK D. SOBEL
DONALD KAYE

Bacteriuria is a frequently used term and literally means bacteria in the urine. The probability of the presence of infected urine in the bladder can be ascertained by means of quantitating numbers of bacteria in voided urine and in urine obtained via urethral catheterization. *Significant bacteriuria* is a term that has been used to describe the numbers of bacteria in voided urine that exceed the numbers usually due to contamination from the anterior urethra (i.e., $\geq 10^5$ bacteria/ml). The implication is that in the presence of at least 10^5 bacteria/ml urine, infection must be seriously considered. *Asymptomatic bacteriuria* refers to significant bacteriuria in a patient without symptoms.

Urinary tract infection may only involve the lower urinary tract or may involve both the upper and lower tracts. The term *cystitis* has been used to describe the syndrome involving dysuria, frequency, urgency, and occasionally suprapubic tenderness. However, these symptoms may be related to lower tract inflammation without bacterial infection and can be caused by urethritis (for example, gonorrhea or chlamydial urethritis). Furthermore, the presence of symptoms of lower tract infection without upper tract symptoms by no means excludes upper tract infection, which is also often present.

Acute pyelonephritis describes the clinical syndrome characterized by flank pain and/or tenderness and fever, often associated with dysuria, urgency, and frequency. However, these symptoms can occur in the absence of infection (for example, in renal infarction or renal calculus). A more rigorous definition of acute pyelonephritis is the above syndrome accompanied by significant bacteriuria and acute infection in the kidney.

Urinary tract infection may occur de novo or may be a recurrent infection. Recurrences may be either *relapses* or *reinfections*. Relapse of bacteriuria refers to recurrence of bacteriuria with the same infecting microorganism that was present before therapy was started. This is due to persistence of the organism in the urinary tract. Reinfection is a recurrence of bacteriuria with a microorganism different from the original infecting bacterium. It is a new infection. Occasionally reinfection may occur with the same microorganism, which may have persisted in the vagina or feces. This can be mistaken for a relapse.

The term *chronic urinary tract infection* has little meaning in

many patients. True chronic infection should really mean persistence of the same organism for months or years with relapses after treatment. Reinfections do not mean chronicity any more than repeated episodes of pneumonia indicate chronic pneumonia. However, in spite of the questionable application of the term, some authorities have grouped patients with relapsing infections and frequent reinfections together as having "chronic infection."

The term *chronic pyelonephritis* is difficult to define and means different things to different authors. To some, chronic pyelonephritis refers to pathologic changes in the kidney due to infection only. However, identical pathologic alterations are found in several other entities such as chronic urinary tract obstruction, analgesic nephropathy, hypokalemic nephropathy, vascular disease, and uric acid nephropathy. Pathologic descriptions do not (and cannot) differentiate between the changes produced by infection versus those produced by these other entities.

Papillary necrosis from infection is an acute complication of pyelonephritis usually in the presence of diabetes mellitus, urinary tract obstruction, sickle cell disease, or analgesic abuse. Papillary necrosis can occur in the absence of infection in some of these conditions. The necrotic renal papillae may slough and cause unilateral or bilateral ureteral obstruction. *Intrarenal abscess* may result from bacteremia or may be a complication of severe pyelonephritis. *Perinephric abscess* occurs when microorganisms from either the renal parenchyma or blood are deposited in the soft tissues surrounding the kidneys.

PATHOLOGIC CHARACTERISTICS[1,2]

Acute Pyelonephritis

In severe pyelonephritis the kidney is somewhat enlarged, and discrete, yellowish, raised abscesses are apparent on the surface (Fig. 1). The pathognomonic histologic feature is suppurative necrosis or abscess formation within the renal substance.

Chronic Pyelonephritis (Chronic Interstitial Nephritis)

The pathologic picture of chronic pyelonephritis can be described as follows. One or both kidneys contain gross scars, but, even when involvement is bilateral, the kidneys are not equally damaged. This uneven scarring is useful in differentiating chronic pyelonephritis from diseases that cause symmetric contracted kidneys, for example, chronic glomerulonephritis (Fig. 2). There are inflammatory changes in the pelvic wall with papillary atrophy and blunting. The parenchyma shows intersti-

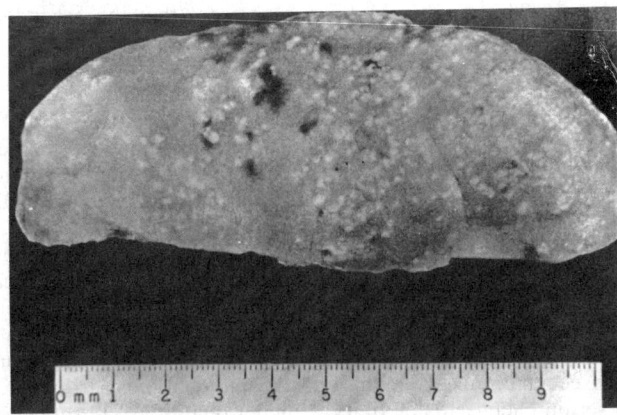

FIG. 1. Acute pyelonephritis in an elderly diabetic man. Note the numerous raised abscesses on the cortical surface. (From Kaye,[3] with permission.)

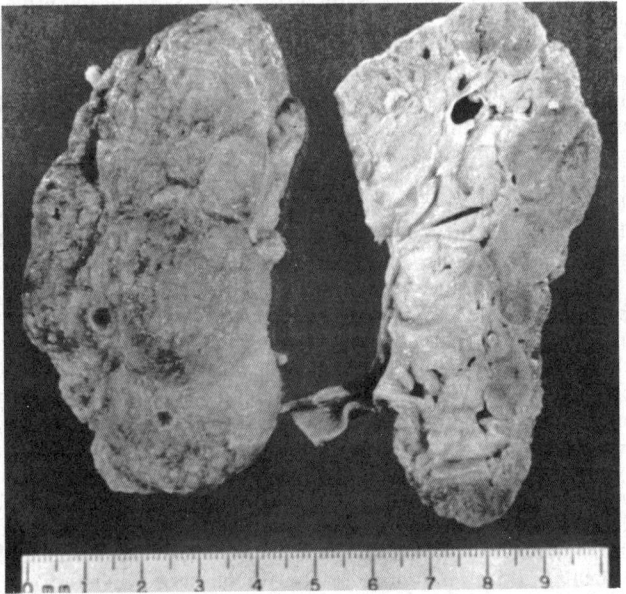

FIG. 2. Chronic pyelonephritis. The kidney is contracted and coarsely scarred, weighing 80 g. Note the thinned cortex and the poorly defined corticomedullary demarcation. (From Kaye,[3] with permission.)

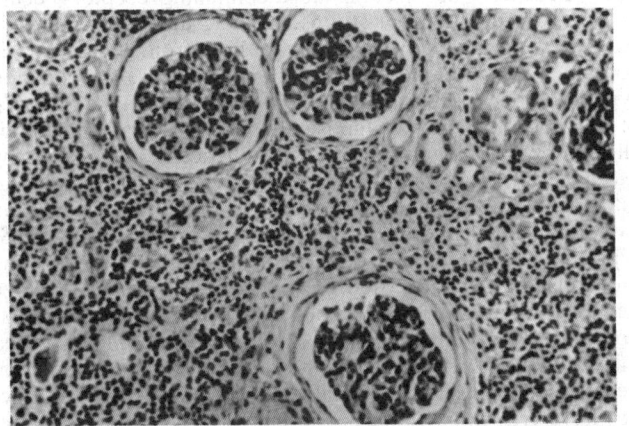

FIG. 3. Chronic pyelonephritis with interstitial and periglomerular fibrosis. Tubules within these scarred areas are atrophic and surrounded by a dense infiltrate of lymphocytes and plasma cells. Glomeruli are well preserved (H&E, ×160). (From Kaye,[3] with permission).

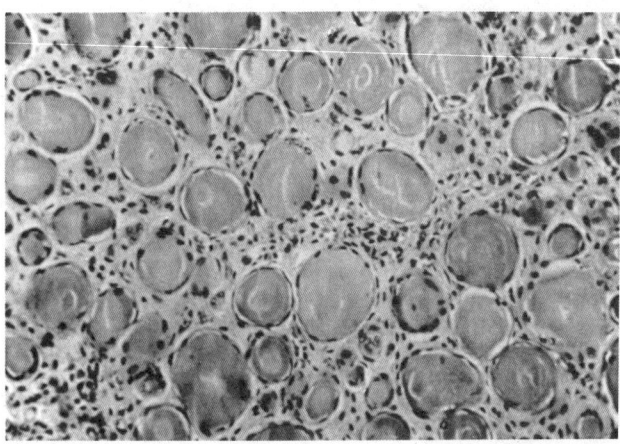

FIG. 4. Chronic pyelonephritis. Tubules are closely packed and filled with eosinophilic casts. Their resemblance to thyroid is striking (H&E, ×160). (From Kaye,[3] with permission).

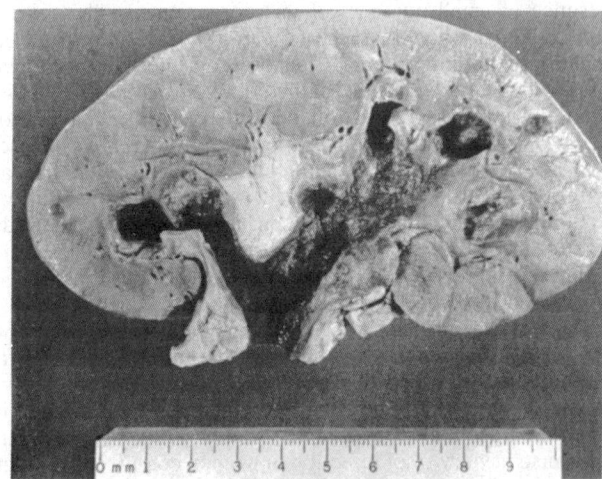

FIG. 5. Papillary necrosis. Necrosis of the renal papillae has resulted in large and irregular defects. The pelvis is hemorrhagic and covered by a granular exudate. (From Kaye,[3] with permission).

tial fibrosis with an inflammatory infiltrate of lymphocytes, plasma cells, and occasionally neutrophils (Fig. 3). The tubules are dilated or contracted with atrophy of the lining epithelium. Many of the dilated tubules contain colloid casts, which suggest the appearance of thyroid tissue ("thyroidization" of the kidney) (Fig. 4). There is also concentric fibrosis about the parietal layer of Bowman capsule (termed *periglomerular fibrosis*) and vascular changes similar to those of benign or malignant arteriolar sclerosis.

Several studies[4–6] have found little correlation between these pathologic findings and evidence for past or present urinary tract infection. Clearly a better term for this pathologic entity would be *chronic interstitial nephritis* to encompass all the clinical states that can cause these changes. To incriminate infection as the sole cause of chronic interstitial nephritis, evidence is required of past or present urinary tract infection and the absence of any other condition that can cause the pathologic picture of chronic interstitial nephritis. These criteria are seldom met, and, even if they are, it is frequently impossible to establish whether infection is complicating interstitial nephritis of some unrecognized etiology.

Papillary Necrosis Caused by Infection

Frequently both kidneys are affected, and one or more pyramids may be involved (Fig. 5). The pyramids are replaced by wedge-shaped areas of yellow necrotic tissue with the base located at the corticomedullary junction. As the lesion progresses, a portion of the necrotic papilla may break off, producing a calyceal deformity that results in a recognizable radiologic filling defect. The sloughed portion may be voided and in some instances can be recovered from the urine. Microscopically, edema is initially seen in the interstitium. Eventually the lesion resembles an infarct with coagulation necrosis involving the entire pyramid. The collecting tubules are filled with bacteria and polymorphonuclear leukocytes.

PATHOGENESIS OF URINARY TRACT INFECTION

There are three possible routes by which bacteria can invade and spread within the urinary tract. These are the ascending, hematogenous, and lymphatic pathways.

Ascending Route

The urethra is usually colonized with bacteria. Studies[7] using suprapubic puncture techniques have revealed the occasional presence of small numbers of microorganisms in the urine of uninfected persons. Massage of the urethra in women[8] and presumably sexual intercourse[9-14] can force bacteria into the bladder. Furthermore, just one catheterization of the bladder will result in urinary tract infection in about 1 percent of ambulatory patients,[15] and infection will develop within 3 or 4 days in essentially all patients with indwelling catheters with open drainage systems.[16] Both the diaphragm with contraceptive jelly in women and condom catheter in men have been shown to predispose to infection.[12,14,17-20] Recent studies have implicated the spermicide rather than the diaphragm. Spermicides increase colonization of the vagina with uropathogens.[21]

The fact that urinary tract infection is much more common in women than men gives support to the importance of the ascending route of infection. The female urethra is short and is in proximity to the warm moist vulvar and perirectal areas, making contamination likely. It has been shown[22] that the organisms that cause urinary tract infection in women colonize the vaginal introitus and the periurethral area before urinary infection results. Once within the bladder, bacteria may multiply and then pass up the ureters, especially if vesicoureteral reflux is present, to the renal pelvis and parenchyma. Animal studies[23] have also confirmed the importance of ascending infection. If bladder bacteriuria is established after unilateral ureteral ligation, only the unligated kidney develops pyelonephritis.

Hematogenous Route

Infection of the renal parenchyma by blood-borne organisms clearly occurs in humans. The kidney is frequently the site of abscesses in patients with staphylococcal bacteremia and/or endocarditis. Experimental pyelonephritis can be produced by intravenous injection of several species of bacteria and even *Candida*.[24] However, production of experimental pyelonephritis by the intravenous route with gram-negative enteric bacilli, the common pathogens in urinary tract infection, is difficult. Additional manipulations such as creation of ureteral obstruction are often necessary.[24] It would appear that, in humans, infection of the kidney with gram-negative bacilli rarely occurs by the hematogenous route.

Lymphatic Route

Evidence for a significant role for renal lymphatics in the pathogenesis of pyelonephritis is unimpressive and consists of the demonstration of lymphatic connections between the ureters and kidneys in animals and the fact that increased pressure in the bladder can cause lymphatic flow to be directed toward the kidney[25]. Thus, it would seem at present that the ascending pathway of infection is the most important.

Host Parasite Interaction

The Organism. Although urinary tract infections are caused by many species of microorganisms, most are due to *Escherichia coli*. However, only a few serogroups of *E. coli*—01, 02, 04, 06, 07, 075, 0150—cause a high proportion of infections.[26] This has led to the concept of uropathogenic *E. coli* clones, whereby certain strains of *E. coli* are selected from the fecal flora by the presence of virulence factors that enhance both colonization and invasion of the urinary tract and the capacity to produce disease.[27] Recognized virulence factors include increased adherence to vaginal and uroepithelial cells,[27] resistance to serum bactericidal activity,[28] higher quantity of K antigen,[28] presence of aerobactin,[29] and hemolysin production.[29] These factors are less frequently observed among serotypes of *E. coli* in the fecal flora that are less likely to produce infection.[27]

In particular, adhesive properties have been suggested to select bacteria capable of reaching and colonizing the normal urinary tract and to influence the level of infection in the urinary tract (i.e., upper vs. only lower tract).[27,30] Accordingly, bacteria with enhanced adherence to vaginal and periurethral cells would be selected to colonize the anatomic regions adjacent to the urethral orifice. Human studies and the mouse model of nonobstructive ascending pyelonephritis have confirmed the significance of the adhesive capacity of the urinary pathogen in causing lower and upper tract infection.[31-33] Svanborg-Eden et al.[33] demonstrated that *E. coli* pyelonephritis isolates adhere better than *E. coli* cystitis isolates, and urinary isolates tend to adhere more strongly to uroepithelial cells than random fecal *E. coli* isolates. The major types of surface adhesins on uropathogenic *E. coli* are fimbrial in nature. Genes encoding the expression of fimbriae on uropathogenic *E. coli* have been found on the chromosomes as opposed to the plasmid-encoded adhesins of enterotoxigenic *E. coli*. Methods such as electron microscopy, as well as erythrocyte agglutination, have been used to characterize fimbriae, and several specific morphologic and functional types have been identified. Numerous uropathogenic strains adhere in the absence of fimbriae. The binding of *E. coli* to epithelial cell receptors containing globoseries glycolipid accounts for the attachment of most strains causing kidney infection and is not inhibited by mannose (MR—for mannose-resistant).[34,35] Fimbriae attaching to globoseries receptors are termed *P fimbriae* since the receptor is a constituent of the P blood group antigen complex present in human erythrocytes and uroepithelial cells.[35] The globoseries glycolipid receptors (gal-gal) are distributed throughout the urinary tract, particularly in the kidney.[35] Binding of *E. coli* to mannose-containing receptors occurs with most uropathogenic strains. In fact, strains from cystitis patients are more likely to bind than those from pyelonephritis patients.[33] Fimbriae attaching to mannosides are the common type 1 fimbriae (pili), and attachment is inhibited in the presence of mannose (MS—for mannose sensitive). Urinary mucus or slime is rich in mannose residues, and hence *E. coli* possessing MS adhesins adhere avidly to urinary slime.[36] The biologic significance of this phenomenon is unclear. Currently, in addition to type 1 and P fimbriae, a variety of adhesins, including S, type 1c, and G fimbriae and M and X adhesins,[37] with differing molecular binding specificities and serologic properties have been identified on uropathogenic strains of *E. coli* and are expressed in vivo in urine (Table 1). Nowicki et al.[38] demonstrated the Dr blood group antigen as the receptor of *E. coli* 075X adhesin. Adherent bacteria not only persist within the urinary tract but have growth advantages and enhanced toxicity due to restricted diffusion of products secreted by eukaryotic cells.[39]

A two-phase concept is postulated regarding adherence kinetics in the pathogenesis of urinary tract infection.[30,31] After entry into the lower urinary tract, MS adhesins, present on the major-

TABLE 1. Uropathogenic *Escherichia coli* Adhesins and Corresponding Epithelial Receptors

Adhesin	Genetic Sequence	Receptor	Comments
Type 1 fimbriae (MS)	*pil, fim*	D-mannose on epithelial cells and PMNs	Bind to Tamm-Horsfall protein (THP) and SIgA
P fimbriae (MR)[a]	*pap*	Gal-α 1–4 gal (P blood group antigen)	Strongly associated with pyelonephritis
S fimbriae (MR)[a]	*sfa*	Sialyl-α 2–3-galactoside	Adherence inhibited by THP
Type 1 C (MR)	*fac*	Undetermined	Possibly associated with pyelonephritis
G fimbriae (MR)	—	Terminal N-acetyl-D-glucosamine	—
M fimbriae (MR)	—	Galactose -N-acetyl-galactosamine Blood group M (glycophoren A)	—
Nonfimbrial adhesins (x)			
F adhesin (MR)[a]	*afa prs (pap*-related)	Gal-N-acetyl-galactose (Forssman ag)	Receptors in renal pelvis
Dr hemagglutinin (075x)	*dra*	Dr blood group antigen	High frequency in cystitis

[a] Associated with pyelonephritis

ity of Enterobacteriaceae, are thought to be important for colonization of the bladder and lower urinary tract.[40] Mannose-resistant P fimbriae and X adhesins, on the other hand, appear to be critical for the organisms to reach the pelvis and renal parenchyma.[35] Experimental studies support these concepts. *E. coli* colonization of the mouse bladder can be prevented by mannose, providing competitive blockade of MS adhesin.[41] Antibodies directed against P fimbriae block adherence to epithelial cells in vitro and prevent upper tract infection in a mouse model of pyelonephritis.[42] In the same model an *E. coli* vaccine utilizing gal-gal pili has been developed that prevents pyelonephritis.[42] There is evidence to suggest that in vivo a urinary pathogen may alter its surface expression or presentation of adhesins so as to ensure survival.[43] Type 1 fimbriae increase the susceptibility of *E. coli* to neutrophil phagocytosis.[30] Therefore, not surprisingly, *E. coli* cease to express these fimbriae on reaching the renal parenchyma.[30] This phenomenon is called *phasic variation*. In contrast to type 1 fimbriae, polymorphonuclear leukocytes lack receptors for P fimbriae, and the latter block phagocytosis.[44] Bacterial adherence to urinary catheters is also type I (MS) fimbrial dependent.[45] MS adhesins also interact with mannose present on SIgA antibodies present in urine.

Studies with other species of bacteria have similarly demonstrated the significance of adherence in the pathogenesis of urinary infections. Silverblatt[43] confirmed the role of fimbriae in *Proteus mirabilis* attachment to the renal pelvic mucosa, and similar observations have been made with *Klebsiella* spp.[46] *Staphylococcus aureus* uncommonly causes cystitis and ascending pyelonephritis; in contrast, *Staphylococcus saprophyticus* is a frequent cause of lower urinary tract infections. *Staphylococcus saprophyticus* adheres significantly better to uroepithelial cells than *S. aureus* or *Staphylococcus epidermidis*.[47] Trimethoprim/sulfamethoxazole, extensively used to prevent urinary infection, at concentrations well below the minimum inhibitory concentration (MIC) reduces synthesis, expression, and adhesive function of type 1 fimbriae.[48]

Evaluation of urinary isolates for virulence characteristics in the presence of underlying structural abnormalities (e.g., severe reflux) frequently fails to demonstrate the typical bacterial virulence factors. Therefore, in complicated urinary tract infections virulence factors are often absent, and a natural selection of uropathogens is not apparent.[30] Similarly, *E. coli* blood isolates obtained from patients with urosepsis following bladder instrumentation lack virulence factors.[49] Virulence determinants are more frequently expressed by urinary isolates of *E. coli* obtained from women with cystitis compared with fecal isolates from healthy women.[50] No difference was found in prevalence of *E. coli* virulence determinants between the subjects with first-time cystitis or those with recurrent cystitis, suggesting that host factors rather than bacteria determine risk for recurrent infection. Of note, Stapleton et al.[50] observed that *E. coli* isolates that caused cystitis in women using diaphragms had fewer virulence determinants than nonusers, suggesting that diaphragm use may allow infection with less virulent *E. coli*.

The importance of adherence as a virulence factor is not complete without consideration of the role of the host. A difference in receptor density linked to variable susceptibility to infection has been proposed. In women and children with recurrent urinary tract infection, an increased avidity of bacterial attachment has been found to vaginal,[51] periurethral,[52] and uroepithelial[53,54] cells. However, several other authors have failed to corroborate these findings.[55] Thus, the role of receptors as biologic risk factors in uncomplicated urinary tract infections remains unsettled.

Certain other characteristics of bacteria may be important in the production of upper tract infection. Motile bacteria can ascend in the ureter against the flow of urine,[56] and the endotoxins of gram-negative bacilli have been shown to decrease ureteral peristalsis,[57] but contribute to the renal parenchymal inflammatory response by phagocytic cell activation.[58] Production of urease by infecting microorganisms such as *Proteus* spp. has been related to ability to cause pyelonephritis.[1] The presence of K antigen protects bacteria from leukocyte phagocytosis. Most uropathogenic strains produce hemolysin, which facilitates tissue invasion and causes renal tubular epithelial and parenchymal cell damage,[60] possibly making iron available to invading *E. coli*. Aerobactin, an iron-scavenging protein or siderophore, is identified with increased frequency in uropathogenic strains of *E. coli*.

Studies have shown that the greater the number of organisms delivered to the kidneys, the greater the chance of producing infection.[61] The kidney itself is not uniformly susceptible to infection, since very few organisms are needed to infect the medulla, whereas 10,000 times as many are needed to infect the cortex.[62] The greater susceptibility of the medulla may be due to the high concentration of ammonia, which may inactivate complement,[63] and to poor chemotaxis of polymorphonuclear leukocytes into an area of high osmolality, low pH, and low blood flow.[64]

The Host. With the exception of urethral mucosa, the normal urinary tract is resistant to colonization by bacteria and for the most part efficiently and rapidly eliminates both pathogenic and nonpathogenic microorganisms that gain access to the bladder. This is achieved by the presence of several lower urinary tract antibacterial defense mechanisms.

Although urine is generally considered to be a good culture medium for most bacteria, it does possess antibacterial activity. Anaerobic bacteria and other fastidious organisms that make up most of the urethral flora generally do not multiply in urine. It has been shown that extremes of osmolality, high urea concentration, and low pH levels are inhibitory for the growth of some of the bacteria that cause urinary tract infection.[65] Furthermore, the pH and osmolality of urine from pregnant women tend to be more suitable for bacterial growth than those of nonpregnant women, which in turn are more suitable for bacterial growth than those of urine from men.[66] The presence of glucose makes urine a better culture medium, whereas the addition of prostatic fluid to urine inhibits bacterial growth.[66,67] Furthermore, urine has been shown to inhibit the migrating, adhering, aggregating, and killing functions of polymorphonuclear leukocytes.[68]

Tamm-Horsfall protein (THP), secreted by cells of the ascending loop of Henle, via its mannose-containing side chains binds strongly to *E. coli* expressing types I (MS) and S fimbriae.[69] THP is the most abundant protein of renal origin in urine, and it has been suggested that THP functions as a urinary antibacterial defense mechanism by binding to MS strains of *E. coli*, preventing them from attaching to epithelial cell receptors.[36] Clinical studies in adults to date have failed to show a relationship between urinary THP concentrations and risk for urinary tract infection, although significantly reduced levels of THP in the elderly occur during episodes of urinary tract infection.[70]

The flushing mechanism of the bladder apparently exerts a protective effect. When bacteria are introduced into the bladders of humans, there is a tendency for spontaneous clearance.[71] Since flushing alone would probably not completely clear the bacteria, there must be additional protective factors. Host factors including bladder catheterization influence susceptibility of uroepithelial cells to attachment by uropathogens, and this in turn increases susceptibility to bacteriuria.[72]

Parsons et al.,[73] in a study of bladder defense mechanisms in dogs, demonstrated an active antiadherence mechanism of bladder mucosa. Pretreatment of the bladder with acid was shown to increase bacterial adherence 20- to 50-fold. The increased adherence was independent of the bacterial species employed. Histochemical studies revealed that bacterial adherence was increased by the removal of a surface mucopolysaccharide, glycosaminoglycan, which seems to be responsible for the natural resistance to adherence.[74] Thus, normally small inocula of bacteria are probably unable to adhere, remain suspended in urine, and are removed by voiding. In the presence of a larger bladder inoculum of bacteria, especially with good adhesive qualities, the primary defense of antiadherence may be overcome, colonization can occur, and subsequent bladder infection may result.[75] With the occurrence of bladder infection, secondary defense mechanisms such as mobilization of leukocytes, phagocytosis, and bacterial destruction are called on to remove bacteria.[75,76]

Colonization of the vaginal introitus and periurethral region by Enterobacteriaceae is thought by some to be important in the pathogenesis of urinary tract infections in women.[22] Several authors have shown that periurethral colonization with the same organism almost invariably precedes episodes of significant bacteriuria.[22,77,78] Microbiologic studies have demonstrated that the urethra, periurethral region, and vaginal vestibule of women with recurrent urinary tract infections tend to be more commonly colonized with coliform bacteria.[51,52,77] Stamey[72] has postulated that such colonization is often the prelude to new infection and that women with recurrent urinary tract infection have a biologic predisposition to infection. The hypothesis is that these women have defective local perineal and vaginal defense mechanisms that result in increased susceptibility to introital and perineal colonization with urinary pathogens such as coliform bacteria.[77] In a series of studies, the effects of several factors in vaginal secretions on colonization were examined.[51,79–84] It appeared that a low vaginal pH level was the most important factor related to lack of colonization. Furthermore, serogroups of *E. coli* that were more likely to cause urinary tract infection were more resistant to low pH levels than serogroups that did not commonly cause infection. It was also found in these studies that *E. coli* was less susceptible to the inhibitory effects of vaginal fluid than *Prot. mirabilis* or *Pseudomonas aeruginosa*. Finally, it was noted that *E. coli* adhered more avidly to vaginal epithelial cells of women with recurrent urinary tract infection, and this was attributed to reduced local production of antibodies in vaginal secretions.[51] Kallenius et al.[52] similarly showed that the periurethral cells of young girls prone to recurrent urinary tract infections were more susceptible to bacterial attachment, and other authors found enhanced attachment of *E. coli* to uroepithelial cells of patients with recurrent urinary

tract infections.[53,54] These observations suggest a genetic predisposition of some women to urinary tract infection. This hypothesis is further supported by the fact that women who are epithelial antigen/receptor nonsecretors may have an increased risk of urinary tract infection, and their uroepithelial cells bind *E. coli* more avidly than do cells from secretors.[85] Sheinfeld et al.[86] in studying women prone to recurrent lower urinary tract infection, found that these patients did not differ from control subjects with regard to distribution of blood groups A, B, O, or P phenotypes, but demonstrated an increased frequency of the Lewis blood group nonsecretor and recessive phenotype. Other endogenous factors, such as estrogenic hormones, may influence bacterial attachment to uroepithelial cells and increase the risk of urinary tract infection.[87] From an acquired or exogenous point of view, both colonization of the vaginal introitus and bacteriuria due to *E. coli* have been strongly associated with diaphragm and spermicide use, which may account for the increased risk of urinary tract infection associated with sexual activity.[14,21] The dominant pathogenic mechanism is probably related to the differential antibacterial effect of nonoxynol-9, whereby more susceptible lactobacilli are replaced by coliform uropathogens.[88] Not all authors agree that introital colonization is the most important factor in the pathogenesis of recurrent urinary tract infection.[78,89–92] They point out that introital colonization with Enterobacteriaceae is as common in women not prone to infection. Furthermore, Parsons and Schmidt[55] found no enhanced bacterial adherence to vaginal epithelial cells in women with recurrent urinary tract infection,[55] and Kurdydyk et al.[93] found no difference in IgG and IgA levels in cervicovaginal washings between women prone to infection and those with no past history of urinary tract infection. These studies failed to confirm the hypothesis that women with recurrent bacteriuria possess a local periurethral and vaginal defect in host resistance. Kunin et al.[78] stated the view that all women who do not have a structural or neurologic problem in the voiding mechanism are approximately at the same risk of having a first urinary tract infection. In their view, once established, each infection sets the stage for the next episode, since infection itself may lead to colonization unless periurethral colonization is eradicated by therapy. Antimicrobial therapy per se may alter periurethral flora in favor of colonization with enteric organisms. Antibiotics, especially β-lactams, also promote introital colonization with *E. coli*.[94] The longer the interval between infections, the less likelihood there is for recurrences. The antagonists to Stamey's hypothesis have concluded that the decisive factor is not the colonization of the periurethral area per se but rather the ability of these organisms to ascend the urethra, including the ability of infecting organisms to adhere to mucosal cells and withstand normal host defense mechanisms.

The role of humoral immunity in the host's defense against infection of the urinary tract, although extensively studied, is poorly understood, as shown in several studies.[95–103] During acute pyelonephritis, there is a systemic antibody response. Antibodies against the O antigen and occasionally the K antigen of the infecting strain have been found, and recently antibodies to type 1 and P fimbriae were described.[97,104] IgM antibodies dominate in the response to the first upper tract infection but not to subsequent episodes. Of note is the observation that high levels of IgG antibodies to lipid A correlate with the severity of renal infection and progression of renal parenchyma destruction.[98] An antibody response consisting of IgG and secretory IgA antibodies can be detected in the urine. In contrast to upper tract infection, lower urinary infection is usually associated with a reduced or nondetectable serologic response reflecting the superficial nature of the infection. The reduced immunologic response to the infecting organism in cystitis may explain the phenomenon of reinfection with the same strain. Hopkins et al.,[105] however, using a monkey model, reported the production of systemic and urinary IgG and IgA that accompanied experimental cystitis.

In particular, antipili antibodies are absent in the urine in lower tract infection.[103] Systemic serologic response has been used to distinguish between upper and lower urinary tract infection, but is not practical because of too many false-negative and false-positive results. However, local coating of bacteria with antibodies within the kidney (and prostate) has formed the basis of modern localization techniques.

In spite of the impressive systemic and local urinary antibody production that follows acute pyelonephritis, the protective role of these antibodies is unclear. When bacteria persist in the kidney for several months, antigenic drift may occur.[99] Nevertheless, antibodies against several bacterial structures, including O and K antigen and more recently fimbrial antigens, have been found to protect against hematogenous or ascending pyelonephritis in experimental animals.[96,97,100] Animal recipients of Pap A pilus-based vaccines were protected against experimental pyelonephritis caused by homologous and heterologous gal-gal–binding uropathogenic *E. coli* strains.[106]

Antibodies may be of value in limiting the damage incurred within the kidney or preventing colonization preceeding recurrence. Svanborg-Eden and Svennerholm[101] reported that the urine of patients with pyelonephritis inhibited the adherence of *E. coli* to uroepithelial cells and that this activity was removed by absorption with O antigen. Antibodies have not been shown to protect against bladder infection.[102,103] Cell-mediated immunity has not been shown to play a major role in host defenses against urinary tract infection. However, IL-6 is secreted by renal tubular epithelial cells[107] and may contribute to mucosal antibacterial activity by increasing IgA secretion by committed B cells.

During pyelonephritis, an acute inflammatory exudate consisting predominantly of polymorphonuclear leukocytes is present. Although the inflammatory reaction is directed at limiting bacterial spread and persistence within the kidney, it has been suggested that the infiltrating phagocytic cells may contribute to tissue damage and renal scarring, as evidenced by reduced parenchymal kidney destruction in experimental neutropenia.[108] It has been suggested that chronic pyelonephritis and persistent renal damage may develop following successful eradication of bacterial pyelonephritis with antimicrobial therapy. According to these concepts, bacterial remnants or antigen persistence induces a chronic humoral immunologic response resulting in cryptogenic renal scarring.[109] Another theory suggests that during acute pyelonephritis Tamm-Horsfall protein, normally present within intact renal tubules only, gains access to the renal interstitial space and induces a chronic autoimmune process leading to renal cortical scarring.[110] Neither of these theories has been substantiated or influences clinical management.

There are several abnormalities of the urinary tract that interfere with its natural resistance to infection. Obstruction to urine flow is the most important of these. Extrarenal obstruction can result from congenital anomalies of the ureter or urethra, such as valves, stenosis, or bands; calculi; extrinsic ureteral compression from a variety of causes; benign prostatic hypertrophy; and others. Intrarenal obstruction may be produced by entities such as nephrocalcinosis, uric acid nephropathy, analgesic nephropathy, polycystic kidney disease, hypokalemic nephropathy, and the renal lesions of sickle cell trait or disease..[111] Obstruction inhibits the normal flow of urine, and the resulting stasis is probably important in increasing susceptibility to infection.

In animals, obstruction of a ureter markedly increases susceptibility to hematogenous infection.[111] Intrarenal obstruction, experimentally produced by scars in a variety of ways, also increases susceptibility of the kidney to infection. Medullary scars, which produce greater amounts of obstruction than cortical scars, increase the susceptibility of animals to infection more than cortical scars.[112] Furthermore, the intravenous injection of *E. coli* in animals with renal scars from prior staphylococcal pyelonephritis produces pyelonephritis in the regions of intrarenal hydronephrosis caused by the old scars.[113] Men of any age

and pregnant women are the most prone to lesions that result in obstruction to the free flow of urine.

Calculi may increase susceptibility to urinary tract infection by producing obstruction. However, not all stones obstruct, and local irritative phenomena may also be important. Furthermore, calculi may develop secondary to infection. It has been observed clinically and experimentally that *Proteus* spp. and other urea-splitting organisms (e.g., *Klebsiella*) are most likely to produce calculi.[114] Furthermore, bacteria survive deep within the calculi and are extremely difficult to eradicate even by artificial means such as by incubating in solutions containing antibiotics or iodine and alcohol.[115] This may account for the well-known difficulties encountered clinically in trying to cure urinary tract infection in the presence of stones.

Vesicoureteral reflux and urinary tract infection are also intricately related. Reflux due to a congenital abnormality, bladder overdistension, or unknown etiology probably contributes to upper tract infection via the ascending route. On the other hand, clinical observations have demonstrated that infection may, in fact, produce reflux especially in children.[116] Reflux tends to perpetuate infection by maintaining a residual pool of infected urine in the bladder after voiding. It is probable that reflux, especially in young children, plays an important role in the production of upper tract infection and subsequent scarring.[117] Patients with incomplete emptying of the bladder for either mechanical reasons (bladder neck obstruction, urethral valves, urethral strictures, prostatic hypertrophy) or neurogenic malfunctions (poliomyelitis, tabes dorsalis, diabetic neuropathy, cord injuries) are prone to frequent urinary tract infections. These patients are subject to bladder overdistension, which may interfere with local defense mechanisms, and, most importantly, frequent instrumentation of the urinary tract.

EPIDEMIOLOGY OF URINARY TRACT INFECTION

Infecting Organisms

More than 95 percent of urinary tract infections are caused by a single bacterial species. There is a great difference between the bacterial flora of the urine in patients with an initial episode of urinary tract infection as compared with the flora from those with frequent recurrences of infection. *Escherichia coli* is by far the most frequent infecting organism in acute infection.[118] In recurrent urinary tract infections, especially in the presence of structural abnormalities of the urinary tract (such as obstructive uropathy, congenital anomalies, neurogenic bladder, and fistulous communication involving the urinary tract), the relative frequency of infection caused by *Proteus, Pseudomonas, Klebsiella,* and *Enterobacter* spp., and by enterococci and staphylococci increases greatly. In the presence of structural abnormalities, it is also relatively common to isolate multiple organisms from the urine. Since instrumentation and repeated courses of antimicrobial therapy are common in these patients, antibiotic-resistance isolates might be expected.

The hospital environment is an important determinant of the nature of the bacterial flora in urinary tract infection. *Proteus, Klebsiella, Enterobacter,* and *Pseudomonas* spp. and staphylococci and enterococci are more often isolated from inpatients, as compared with a greater preponderance of *E. coli* in an outpatient population.[119,120] Cross-infections are important in the pathogenesis of hospital-related urinary tract infections, especially with indwelling catheters.[120,121] *Corynebacterium* group D2 has recently been recognized as an important nosocomial pathogen. This gram-positive, urea-splitting, slow-growing bacillus may cause acute or chronic cystitis and pyelonephritis and is highly resistant to antimicrobials, although usually sensitive to vancomycin.[122] It should be considered in the presence of high urine pH, urologic problems, previous urinary tract infection, and recent antibiotic treatment.

Anaerobic organisms are rarely pathogens in the urinary

tract.[123] A variety of bacteria may be found in the urine of specific clinical settings. Fungi (particularly *Candida* spp.) occur in patients with indwelling catheters who are receiving antimicrobial therapy. Coagulase-negative staphylococci are a common cause of urinary tract infection in some reports.[124] *Staphylococcus saprophyticus* tends to cause infection in young, sexually active females,[125,126] accounting for 5–15 percent of acute cystitis episodes in the United States. Coagulase-positive staphylococci most often invade the kidney from the hematogenous route, resulting in intrarenal or perinephric abscesses. DNA typing of *E. coli* has substantially aided in the epidemiologic study of urinary tract infection.

Adenoviruses (particularly type 11) have been strongly implicated as causative agents in hemorrhagic cystitis in pediatric patients, especially boys.[127] Cell wall–deficient bacteria have been demonstrated in urine from patients with pyelonephritis, particularly in association with therapy using cell wall active antibiotics.[128] However, these forms have not been consistently isolated form either urine or renal tissue despite the use of adequate techniques and are probably not of major importance.

Although Maskell et al.,[129] using special media, have isolated fastidious microaerophilic organisms from women with lower tract symptoms, their causal role is controversial. Similarly *Gardnerella vaginalis* is frequently isolated from the urine of women with and without urinary tract symptoms, but its pathogenic role is unclear. *Ureaplasma urealyticum* and *Mycoplasma hominis* are possible but unproven causes of pyelonephritis and cystourethritis.[130,131]

Bacteriuria in Children

The problem of urinary tract infection spans all age groups, beginning with neonates.[132–136] The frequency of urinary tract infection in infants is about 1–2 percent. It is much more common in boys during the first 3 months and thereafter occurs more often in girls. Bacteremia is common in association with urinary tract infection in male newborns. Autopsy series have revealed a predominance of infant boys with pyelonephritis.[132] Lack of circumcision predisposes to urinary tract infection in infants and young males.[136]

During the preschool years, urinary tract infection is more common in girls than in boys. When infection occurs in preschool boys it is frequently associated with serious congenital abnormalities. With repeated study over a period of 1 year, the period prevalence of significant bacteriuria in this age group is 4.5 percent for girls and about 0.5 percent for boys. Infections during this period often are symptomatic, and it is believed that much of the renal damage that occurs from urinary tract infection takes place at this time.[133,137,138]

Much information on the natural history and epidemiology of urinary tract infection has been gleaned from the studies of Kunin[139,140] and associates[141] with school children from central Virginia. It was found that bacteriuria is common in girls in this population, is often asymptomatic, and frequently recurs. For example, the prevalence of bacteriuria among school girls was about 1.2 percent, and about 5 percent of the girls had significant bacteriuria at some time before leaving high school. About one-third of these patients had some symptom referable to the urinary tract when the bacteriuria was first detected. It was shown that each year about 0.3 to 0.4 percent of the female population (25 percent of those infected) was cured either spontaneously or with antimicrobial agents and was replaced by an equal number who developed bacteriuria. Bacteriuria was rare in school boys (prevalence, 0.03 percent).

These studies also provided an opportunity to treat the patients and follow their clinical course. Patients were initially treated for 10 days to 2 weeks. Girls with frequent infections were given longer courses of therapy (1–3 months). White girls tended to have frequent reinfections, whereas black girls became reinfected less frequently. With each course of therapy,

about 20 percent of white girls went into long-term remission. However, when many of these girls were married or became pregnant, bacteriuria recurred at a rate far above that expected for the general population. Over 50 percent developed bacteriuria within 3 months after marriage. Thus, the presence of bacteriuria in childhood defines a population at higher risk for the development of bacteriuria in adulthood.

Bacteriuria in Adults

Once adulthood is reached, the prevalence of bacteriuria increases in the female population. The prevalence of bacteriuria in young nonpregnant women is about 1–3 percent.[142] Each year about 25 percent of bacteriuric women clear their bacteriuria and are replaced by an equal number who have become infected (often women who have had urinary infection previously). At least 10–20 percent of the female population experience a symptomatic urinary tract infection at some time during their life.[142] Frequency of sexual intercourse, diaphragm use, and lack of urination after intercourse are risk factors for urinary infection in women.[12,14,17–19] The diaphragm can cause urinary obstruction in some women, but its main effect is probably a change in vaginal flora due to the spermicide.[19,21] The risk of a second urinary tract infection in young women is greater than the first, with at least 20 percent developing a recurrent infection within 6 months follow-up.[143]

The prevalence of bacteriuria in adult men is low (0.1 percent or less) until the later years, when it rises. The increase in bacteriuria in older men is probably mainly related to prostatic disease and the resultant instrumentation. Men with bacteriuria frequently have anatomic abnormalities of the urinary tract. Lack of circumcision increases the risk of urinary tract infection in young men caused by uropathogenic strains of *E. coli*, including the development of symptomatic urethritis.[144]

Bacteriuria in the Elderly

At least 10 percent of men and 20 percent of women over 65 have bacteriuria. In contrast to young adults, in whom bacteriuria is 30 times more frequent in women than men, over the age of 65 the ratio alters dramatically, with a progressive decrease in the female/male ratio.[145,146] In both sexes, the prevalence of bacteriuria rises substantially. Possible reasons for the high frequency of urinary tract in the elderly include obstructive uropathy from the prostate and loss of bactericidal activity of prostatic secretions in men, poor emptying of the bladder due to prolapse in women, soiling of the perineum from fecal incontinence in demented women, and neuromuscular diseases and increased instrumentation and bladder catheter usage in both sexes.[146] There is a high rate of spontaneous cure and reinfection in both women and men.[146] The spectrum of microorganisms is unaltered in the elderly.

Bacteriuria in Patients with Other Conditions

There is a higher prevalence of bacteriuria in hospitalized patients than in outpatients.[147] It is stated that the general ill health of hospitalized patients as well as the higher probability of urinary tract instrumentation are the major contributors to these differences.

A single catheterization causes urinary tract infection in only about 1 percent of ambulatory persons.[15] However, after catheterization of hospitalized patients, infection occurs in at least 10 percent. Race apparently does not appreciably affect the prevalence of bacteriuria. However, socioeconomic status is important, with pregnant women from lower socioeconomic groups having a higher prevalence of bacteriuria.[148]

Various underlying diseases have also been associated with an increased frequency of urinary tract infection. Diabetic women but not men have been found to have a higher prevalence of bacteriuria than nondiabetic people.[149]

Black women with sickle cell trait have a higher prevalence of bacteriuria during pregnancy than black women without sickle trait.[150] Other conditions stated to be associated with urinary tract infection (but without documentation) include chronic potassium deficiency, gout, hypertension, and other conditions causing interstitial renal disease.

CLINICAL MANIFESTATIONS

Symptoms

Urinary tract infection in children tends to manifest with different symptoms depending on the age of the child. Symptoms in neonates and children less than 2 years of age are nonspecific.[133–135] Failure to thrive, vomiting, and fever seem to be the major manifestations. When children over 2 years of age (and more consistently above 5) develop infection, they are more likely to display localizing symptoms such as frequency, dysuria, and abdominal or flank pain.

The manifestations of urinary tract infection in adults are usually easy to recognize. The lower tract symptoms result from bacteria producing irritation of urethral and vesical mucosa, causing frequent and painful urination of small amounts of turbid urine. Patients sometimes complain of suprapubic heaviness or pain. Occasionally the urine is grossly bloody or shows a bloody tinge at the end of micturition. Fever tends to be absent in infection limited to the lower tract.

The classic clinical manifestation of upper urinary tract infection includes fever (sometimes with chills), flank pain, and frequently lower tract symptoms (e.g., frequency, urgency, and dysuria). At times the lower tract symptoms antedate the appearance of fever and upper tract symptoms by 1 or 2 days. It should be recognized that the symptoms described, while classic, may vary greatly. In fact, pyelonephritis may show protean clinical manifestations in adults as well as in children. Flank tenderness or discomfort is frequent in upper tract infection in adults and is more intense when there is obstructive disease. Severe pain with radiation into the groin is rare in acute pyelonephritis per se and suggests the presence of a renal calculus. The pain from the kidney is occasionally felt in or near the epigastrium and may radiate to one of the lower quadrants. These manifestations may offer difficulties in differential diagnosis and suggest gallbladder disease or appendicitis.

The vast majority of elderly patients with urinary infection are asymptomatic; in addition, pyuria may be absent.[145,146] Symptoms, when present, are often not diagnostic, since noninfected elderly patients often experience frequency, dysuria, hesitancy, and incontinence. Nevertheless, typical symptoms may occur, and less frequently acute pyelonephritis develops, usually necessitating hospitalization. Gleckman et al.[151] found a much higher frequency of bacteremia (61 percent) associated with pyelonephritis in the elderly than is found in the young, and shock commonly supervened. Most of the patients had significant urologic abnormalities. The effect of asymptomatic bacteriuria on the general sense of well-being, appetite, and urinary continence has been studied, and in one investigation no association could be demonstrated.[152]

The clinical manifestations of recurrent or persistent urinary tract infection are more difficult to define. Patients with lower urinary tract involvement tend to have repeated bouts of transient symptomatic or asymptomatic infection. Patients with upper tract infection may have episodes of fever, pain in the renal regions, and dysuria during acute exacerbations or new bouts of infection. However, upper tract infection may result in only lower tract symptoms or no symptoms at all. Patients with urinary tract infection in the presence of an indwelling urinary catheter usually have no lower tract symptoms, but flank pain or fever are common. Urinary tract infection is the most

common source of bacteremia produced by gram-negative bacilli. Bacteremia may occur with no urinary symptoms, especially in the presence of an indwelling catheter.

Alterations in Renal Function

In experimentally produced pyelonephritis, the only consistent abnormality of renal function is the inability to concentrate the urine maximally.[153,154] The mechanism of the concentrating defect is not clear, but seems to be related in experimental animals to inflammation and perhaps to increased production of prostaglandins.[154,155] The concentrating defect occurs early in the course of experimental infection and is rapidly reversible with antimicrobial therapy and following the administration of prostaglandin inhibitors.[153,154] The same phenomenon occurs in humans.[156]

Progressive destruction of the kidney (particularly in the presence of obstruction) may occur and give rise to clinical manifestations of renal insufficiency. Bilateral papillary necrosis occasionally can lead to rapidly progressive renal failure.[157]

DIAGNOSIS

Presumptive Diagnosis of Urinary Tract Infection

Microscopic examination of the urine is the first step in laboratory diagnosis of urinary tract infection A clean-catch midstream urine specimen is centrifuged for 5 minutes at 2000 rpm, and then the sediment is examined under high power. Each leukocyte seen represents about 5–10 cells/mm^3 of urine; 10–50 white cells/mm^3 have been stated to be the upper limit of normal.[158] With this criterion 5–10 leukocytes per high-power field in the sediment from a clean-catch midstream urine specimen is the upper limit of normal, as they represent 50–100 cells/mm^3. Although more elaborate and precise methods for determining the urinary concentration of leukocytes have been evaluated, it is generally not necessary to use these clinically.[158] It should be emphasized that the finding of pyuria is nonspecific, and patients with and without pyuria may or may not have infection.[159] However, the vast majority of patients with symptomatic infection have significant pyuria.[160] Using a stricter definition of pyuria (at least 10 leukocytes per mm^3 of midstream urine by counting chamber), the vast majority of patients with either symptomatic or asymptomatic bacteriuria will have pyuria. However, pyuria without infection remains common.[161] The dipstick leukocyte esterase test is a rapid screening test for detecting pyuria. It is both sensitive (75–96 percent) and specific (94–98 percent) for detecting more than 10 white blood cells/mm^3 of urine.[162–165]

Microscopic or sometimes gross hematuria is occasionally seen in patients with urinary tract infection (i.e., hemorrhagic cystitis). However, red blood cells may be indicative of other disorders such as calculi, tumor, vasculitis, glomerulonephritis, and renal tuberculosis. White cell casts in the presence of an acute infectious process are strong evidence for pyelonephritis, but the absence of white cell casts does not rule out upper tract infection. White cell casts can also be seen in renal disease in the absence of infection.

Proteinuria is a common although not universal finding in urinary tract infection. Most patients with urinary tract infection excrete less than 2 g of protein in 24 hours; excretion of 3 g or more suggests glomerular disease.

One of the most useful tests for presumptive diagnosis of urinary tract infection is the microscopic examination of a specimen for bacteria. The ability to identify bacteria in the urine depends on whether the specimen has been centrifuged and on whether it has been stained with Gram or methylene blue stain

TABLE 2. Correlation of Methods of Direct Examination of Urine for Bacteria with Quantitative Cultures

	Unstained	Stained
Uncentrifuged	$\geq 10^6$ (400×)	$\geq 10^5$ (1000×)
Centrifuged	$\geq 10^5$ (400×)	$\geq 10^4$ (1000×)

(Table 2).[162,166] Smaller numbers of bacteria can be detected microscopically in a stained than in an unstained specimen, and smaller numbers can be detected in centrifuged than in uncentrifuged urine. Presence of at least one bacterium per oil-immersion field in a midstream, clean-catch, Gram-stained, uncentrifuged urine correlates with 10^5 bacteria or more per milliliter of urine. As this titer is regarded to represent significant bacteriuria, Gram staining of an uncentrifuged specimen is an easy, rapid, and relatively reliable way to detect significant numbers of organisms. The absence of bacteria in several fields in a stained sedimented specimen indicates the probability of less than 10^4 bacteria/ml.

A number of rapid indirect methods have been devised to detect bacteriuria for presumptive diagnosis. Most common are tests that detect the presence of nitrite in the urine that is formed when bacteria reduce the nitrate that is normally present.[162–165] False-negative tests are common, but false-positive results are unusual. The detection of subnormal urinary glucose in urine; filtration of urine with staining of bacteria trapped on the filter; bioluminescence caused by reaction of bacterial ATP with luciferin and luciferase; photometric detection of bacterial growth; and the *Limulus* endotoxin test for gram-negative bacilli have all been utilized as screening tests for bacteriuria.[162,165] Recently, automated rapid screening tests have become available that may be cost effective for processing large numbers of samples.[162]

Diagnosis of Urinary Tract Infection by Culture

Urine in the bladder is normally sterile. Since the urethra and periurethral areas are very difficult to sterilize, even the most carefully collected specimens (including those obtained by catheterization) are frequently contaminated. By quantitating bacteria in midstream, clean-voided urine, it is possible statistically to separate contamination from urinary tract infection. Patients with infection usually have at least 10^5 bacteria/ml in urine in the bladder, and therefore voided urine usually contains at least 10^5 bacteria/ml.[16] Patients without infection have sterile bladder urine, and, with proper collection, voided urine usually contains less than 10^4 bacteria/ml. However, it is important to remember that about one-third of young women with symptomatic lower tract infection have less than 10^5 bacteria/ml urine (see below under "Urinary Tract Infection with Low Numbers of Organisms"). It is likely that a significant proportion of other patients with both symptomatic and asymptomatic infection have less than 10^5 bacteria/ml urine.

Calibrated loops serve as a simple inexpensive way to examine quantitatively the bacteriologic characteristics of urine specimens.[165] Platinum loops that deliver 0.01 ml and 0.001 ml are used to streak urine onto agar plates. After incubating at 37°C for 24 hours the number of colony-forming units are counted, and the total number of organisms originally present in the specimen is estimated by multiplying the colony count by 10^2 or 10^3, respectively. A further refinement of the technique involves the use of differential agars to allow isolation from mixed cultures and more rapid identification.

Other methods of quantitative culture include (1) the flood plate method, which is similar to the calibrated loop method but involves pipetting a volume of urine onto a plate; (2) the filter paper method in which a given volume of urine is absorbed in a piece of filter paper and then put on a plate; and (3) the dip inoculum method in which an agar-coated glass slide is dipped into urine.[150,167] The dip inoculum method and its variants have

excellent correlation with pour plate techniques and are available for office use at inexpensive prices.

Acceptable methods for urine collection include (1) midstream clean catch, (2) catheterization, and (3) suprapubic aspiration. The clean-catch method is preferred for routine collection of urine for culture. It avoids the risk of infection inherent in catheterization. The patient must be instructed in the proper technique of obtaining the urine; this is especially important in women. The woman should wash her hands, straddle the commode (facing the back of the commode), wash the vulva from front to back four times with four different sterile gauze pads soaked in green soap or another appropriate cleansing agent and then rinse with two more sponges soaked in sterile distilled water. She should then spread the labia and void, discarding the first portion of urine and collecting the second. The urine should be processed immediately or, if refrigerated at 4°C, can be cultured within 24 hours. In men the prepuce should be retracted, and thereafter the technique is similar. In infants and small children sterile bags have been used for collection of urine, but contamination is common.[134,167]

In patients unable to cooperate, such as those with an altered sensorium, or those who are unable to void for neurologic or urologic reasons, catheterization may be necessary. When catheterization is performed, scrupulous aseptic technique should be observed.

The suprapubic aspiration method has been established as a safe technique in premature infants, neonates, children, adults, and even pregnant patients.[7,134,150,167] With this method the bladder must be full. The patient refrains from voiding until the bladder can be percussed above the pubic, and suprapubic pressure causes the urge to void. After preparation of the skin, the bladder is then punctured above the symphysis pubis with a 22-gauge needle on a syringe (local anesthesia is not required). Following the procedure self-limited hematuria may be observed. Suprapubic aspiration may be indicated in special clinical situations such as in pediatric practice when urine is difficult to obtain. Another situation is the rare adult in whom infection is suspected, results obtained from more routine procedures have been confusing or equivocal, and diagnosis is critical.

If there are more than 10^5 bacteria/ml in a clean-catch urine specimen from an asymptomatic woman, there is an 80 percent probability that this represents true bacteriuria. If two different specimens demonstrate at least 10^5 of the same bacterium per milliliter, the probability increases to 95 percent. Thus two clean-catch specimens should be obtained in an asymptomatic woman to confirm the diagnosis. When the number of bacteria per milliliter is between 10^4 and 10^5 in an asymptomatic woman, a confirmatory second specimen will contain 10^5 or more bacteria/ml in only 5 percent of instances. Thus in asymptomatic women 95 percent of the time 10^4–10^5 bacteria/ml represents contamination, with occasional infection manifested by less than 10^5 bacteria per milliliter urine. In men, in whom contamination is less likely, 10^3 or more organisms/ml is more suggestive of infection.[168] False-positive cultures are caused by contamination or incubation of urine before processing. False-negative cultures may be due to use of antimicrobial agents, soap from the preparation falling in the urine, total obstruction below the infection, infection with a fastidious organism, renal tuberculosis, and diuresis.

These criteria apply only to the Enterobacteriaceae. Gram-positive organisms, fungi, and bacteria with fastidious growth requirements may not reach titers of 10^5/ml in patients with infection and may be in the 10^4–10^5/ml range. The organism recovered often helps to distinguish contamination from true bacteriuria. Samples with counts of less than 10^4 organisms/ml often contain saprophytic skin organisms such as diphtheroids, *Neisseria,* and staphylococci. Pure growth of Enterobacteriaceae is uncommonly found in low-titer specimens but is present in over 90 percent of the urines containing more than 10^5 bacteria/ml. High colony counts containing more than one species of bacteria from urine of asymptomatic persons often represent contamination but may be more significant in the presence of symptoms. Mixed infection occurs in about 5 percent of the cases.

In patients with symptoms of urinary tract infection, one titer of 10^5 or more bacteria per milliliter urine carries a 95 percent probability of true bacteriuria. With titers below 10^5/ml but in the presence of frequency, urgency, and dysuria, women have a one-third chance of having bacterial infection (see "Urinary Tract Infection with Low Numbers of Organisms," below). Presence of low numbers of Enterobacteriaceae (i.e., 10^2–10^5/ml) in such women correlates highly with infection. Presence of less than 10^2/ml Enterobacteriaceae is evidence against urinary tract infection.

Samples obtained by catheterization from noninfected patients are less likely to become contaminated enough to demonstrate 10^5 bacteria/ml. For example, one catheterized specimen in an asymptomatic patient that contains 10^5 or more organisms/ml has a 95 percent chance of indicating infection, and counts between 10^4 and 10^5/ml (which are uncommon) are significant at least 50 percent of the time. The contamination is presumably from the urethra. Bladder urine obtained by suprapubic aspiration is either sterile or contains significant growth even if bacterial numbers are below 10^5 ml. The practice of forcing fluids before the procedure tends to reduce numbers of organisms.[169] In fact, almost 50 percent of such specimens contain less than 10^5 organisms/ml. However, small numbers of bacteria may be found in aspirated urine from presumably noninfected persons.[5] This suggests that bladder urine may be occasionally contaminated from the urethra.

Urinary Tract Infection with Low Numbers of Organisms. Most women with acute onset of frequency, urgency, and/or dysuria have urinary tract infection with 10^5 or more bacteria/ml urine (Fig. 6). However, up to half are found to have less than 10^5 bacteria/ml urine, and the term *urethral syndrome* has been used to refer to this entity. Stamm et al.[170–173] have demonstrated that many of these women have urinary tract infection but with low titers. Using suprapubic bladder aspirates compared with voided midstream urine in acutely dysuric women, they found that 10^2 or more coliforms/ml in midstream urine had a sensitivity and specificity of 95 percent and 85 percent, respectively for urinary tract infection. These women have urinary infections mainly restricted to the lower tract. Furthermore, about one-fourth of young women with symptomatic infection localized to the lower urinary tract have less than 10^5/ml bacteria in urine. Pyuria (defined as 8 or more leukocytes/

mm^3 uncentrifuged urine) is found in these patients with bacteria in the bladder but less than 10^5 ml in voided urine.

The remaining patients with the urethral syndrome (after excluding those with bacteria in the bladder and those with genital herpes infection or vaginitis) can be divided into two groups: *(1)* those with sterile pyuria from urethritis due to *Chlamydia trachomatis* and less frequently *Neisseria gonorrhoeae* infection and *(2)* those without pyuria in whom all cultures are negative. The pathogenesis of this symptom complex is unknown, but *Ureaplasma urealyticum* as well as noninfectious factors (traumatic, psychological, allergic, and chemical) have been suggested as causes. Patients with *C. trachomatis* and *N. gonorrhoeae* urethritis respond to antimicrobial therapy. Komaroff et al.[174] reported that vaginitis was a common cause of dysuria, and, accordingly, patients should be questioned regarding vaginal symptoms particularly if the complaint of burning is external, such as pain felt in the inflamed vaginal labia during micturition. Dysuria has also been described in 10 percent of women with initial genital herpes infection.[175]

While symptoms and the clinical settings cannot reliably distinguish between causes of frequency, urgency, and dysuria, they can be suggestive. Bacterial urinary tract infections tend to have a sudden onset of symptoms; suprapubic pain and hematuria may be present. Clinical clues to chlamydial infection include a gradual onset of internal dysuria, a sexually active patient with a recent new sexual partner, and no hematuria.

Strong consideration should be given to performing a pelvic examination in sexually active women with dysuria to evaluate for vaginitis and herpes virus infection. The diagnosis of chlamydial infection is best confirmed by culture, but rapid diagnostic techniques such as a direct fluorescent antibody test, an ELISA, and a DNA probe are available. In the absence of a culture or the other methods, the findings of pyuria, less than 10^5/ml bacteria in urine, a negative gonococcal culture, and a negative pelvic examination in a sexually active woman with frequency/dysuria should suggest consideration of therapy for *C. trachomatis* urethritis. Doxycycline would also constitute adequate therapy for the other major possibility—urinary tract infection with less than 10^5/ml bacteria in urine.

Localization of Site of Infection

Localization of the site of infection to the kidney vs. the bladder is not important in any given patient but has been useful in understanding the epidemiology and response to therapy of urinary tract infection. Several methods have been used to deter-

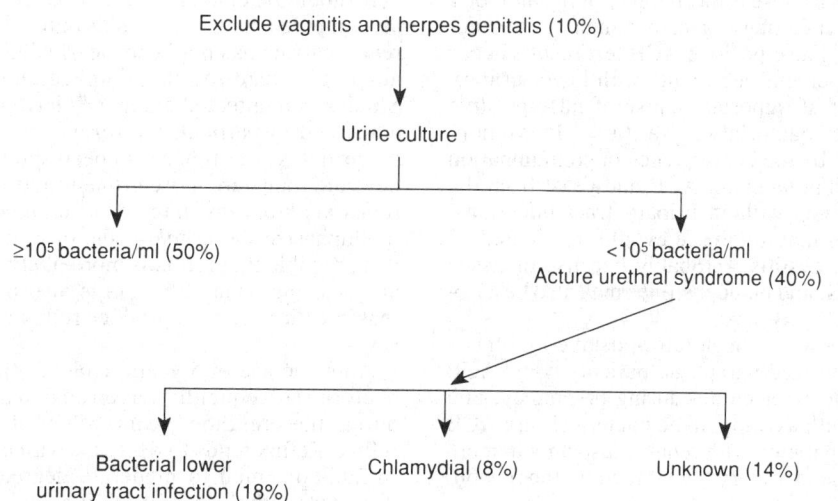

FIG. 6. Relative frequencies of causes of acute onset of frequency/dysuria in young women. (Adapted from Stamm et al.,[170] with permission.)

mine if infection is restricted to the urinary bladder or if the upper tract is also involved. Needle biopsy of the kidney is an unreliable approach, because pyelonephritis is a focal disease and specimens obtained by needle biopsy may miss the area of infection.

The most reliable method of localization of infection involves obtaining urine directly from the ureter for quantitative cultures. In one study[176] using this method 95 women and 26 men with bacteriuria were evaluated. Approximately one-half had infection limited to the bladder. History and physical examination were of little value in predicting the site of infection. Turck et al.,[177] using similar techniques, demonstrated that in women with recurrent urinary tract infection relapse was associated with upper tract involvement and reinfection with lower tract infection.

Fairley and colleagues[178] devised a technique for assessing ureteral bacteriuria that involves Foley catheterization only. However, results are equivocal in about 10–20 percent of patients.[179] As in the ureteral catheterization studies, about 50 percent of the patients have renal infection regardless of signs or symptoms.[179] Methods are also available for localization of bacteria in the prostate gland[180] and are discussed later.

Several studies[181,182] have reported the association of a defect in renal concentrating ability with upper tract infection, and the presence of high titers of serum antibody directed against the infecting organism has been correlated with the presence of upper tract infection.[183] However, there are too many false-positive and false-negative responses to allow the use of these techniques for localization of infection. Urinary levels of various enzymes such as lactic dehydrogenase, alkaline phosphatase, β-glucuronidase, catalase, transaminase, leucine amino peptidase, and lysozyme have been evaluated for their utility in localizing infection to the upper tract.[165,184] However, other inflammatory processes as well as lower tract infection can elevate enzyme levels. Elevated urinary β_2-microglobulin levels have been associated with upper tract infection, but technical problems preclude its widespread use.[165,185]

Detection of antibody coating of bacteria (ACB) in urine has been used to localize infection to the kidney.[186,187] Fluorescein-conjugated antihuman globulin is added to urine containing bacteria, and the bacteria are examined for fluorescence. The sensitivity of the test for ACB has been established collectively by several studies as 88 percent (range, 72–100 percent) with a specificity of 76 percent (range, 50–100 percent).[188] Discrepancies have resulted from lack of standardization of criteria of what constitutes a positive test result. False-negative results occur in 20 percent of patients with early acute pyelonephritis, because it may take several days for adequate antibody titers to develop.[188] An additional cause is the inability of the antibody to combine with certain infecting organisms such as mucoid-coated pseudomonads.[188] False-positive ACB test results occur in approximately 20–30 percent of patients with lower urinary infection. In men, the most important cause of false-positive results is the presence of bacterial prostatitis.[188] In women, false-positive results may be the consequence of contamination of urine samples by small numbers of ACB and yeast from the vaginal vestibule of patients without urinary tract infections. Yeast and pseudomonads may fluoresce even if not coated.[189] Proteinuria, hemorrhagic cystitis—probably because of tissue invasion—bladder tumors, and bladder stones may also be associated with false-positive ACB tests.[188]

Several studies have observed high false-positive and false-negative results in catheterized paraplegic patients.[188,190] ACB testing has been found to be accurate during pregnancy, and one-half of the patients with asymptomatic bacteriuria are ACB positive.[191,192] Although patients with renal transplants demonstrate an immune response to urinary tract infection, the reliability of ACB testing is as yet unconfirmed.[193]

There has been a major discrepancy in children between ACB localization and direct as well as other indirect localization techniques.[194–196] Difficulty obtaining clean-voided specimens, particularly in small girls, could result in contamination with small numbers of ACB of perineal origin.[194] However, Hellerstein et al.,[195] using catheter-obtained specimens, still observed high false-positive and false-negative rates. Currently, ACB testing is not widely available to physicians, nor is there good evidence to conclude that this assay has a major role in the routine management of patients with urinary tract infections.

Outcome of therapy can also be used in a crude but useful manner to separate those with upper and lower tract infection. Virtually all patients with infection restricted to the lower tract can be cured with a short course of antimicrobial therapy.[197] However, the relapse rate with upper tract infection is appreciable, even with 7–10 days of therapy.

At present, only ureteral catheterization studies can reliably predict the site of infection in the urinary tract. However, this procedure is not without risk and cannot be justified for routine use. The Fairley bladder washout procedure is also quite reliable but gives equivocal results in about 10–20 percent of the patients. However, it also involves catheterization. The determination of presence of antibody-coated bacteria in the urine is practical and noninvasive. However, in the clinical management of patients, it is rarely important to localize infection to either the upper tract or the lower tract other than by symptoms.

NATURAL HISTORY OF URINARY TRACT INFECTION

Children

In general, children with urinary tract infections without obstruction or vesicoureteral reflux have a very good prognosis.[133,136,137] In the presence of obstruction (e.g., urethral valves), severe destruction of renal parenchyma can occur.

Reflux is found in 30–50 percent of the children with asymptomatic or symptomatic bacteriuria (Fig. 7).[133,136,137] Reflux can be caused by obstruction with increased pressure in the bladder, delayed development of the ureterovesical junction, a short intravesical ureter, and/or inflammation of the vesicoureteral junction. Reflux in the presence of infection is associated with the development of scarring detected by intravenous pyelography.[137,138,167] Infants and young children (preschool age group) are at the highest risk for the development of progressive renal scarring.[133,137,138] These children frequently have severe degrees of reflux with repeated infections, and some develop end-stage renal disease and hypertension. Obstruction (most commonly in infant boys with congenital anomalies) is likely to be associated with marked reflux.

It should be emphasized that the contribution of reflux alone as compared with reflux plus infection in the progression of renal scarring has not been clearly delineated. Reflux alone can apparently lead to renal damage and insufficiency.[184,198,199] Studies in uninfected animals[200] have demonstrated that reflux alone and in particular *intrarenal reflux* can produce "pyelonephritic" scars. It has also been shown that the immature kidneys of infants are more prone to intrarenal reflux.[201] The term *reflux nephropathy,* infected or uninfected, has been suggested to emphasize the primary role of reflux in scarring. However, it is probable that reflux is more likely to lead to severe damage and scarring when infection is also present.[200] It is also clear that infection tends to produce reflux or at least to make it more severe.

After the age of 5 years, children (predominantly girls) with bacteriuria frequently have renal scars presumably acquired during the preschool years. Many of these children also have reflux. Reflux tends to decrease with elimination of bacteriuria. In addition, mild to moderate degrees of reflux are likely to disappear with the passage of time, probably in relation to maturation of the vesicoureteral junction.[202] Progression of scar already present or development of new ones are uncommon after

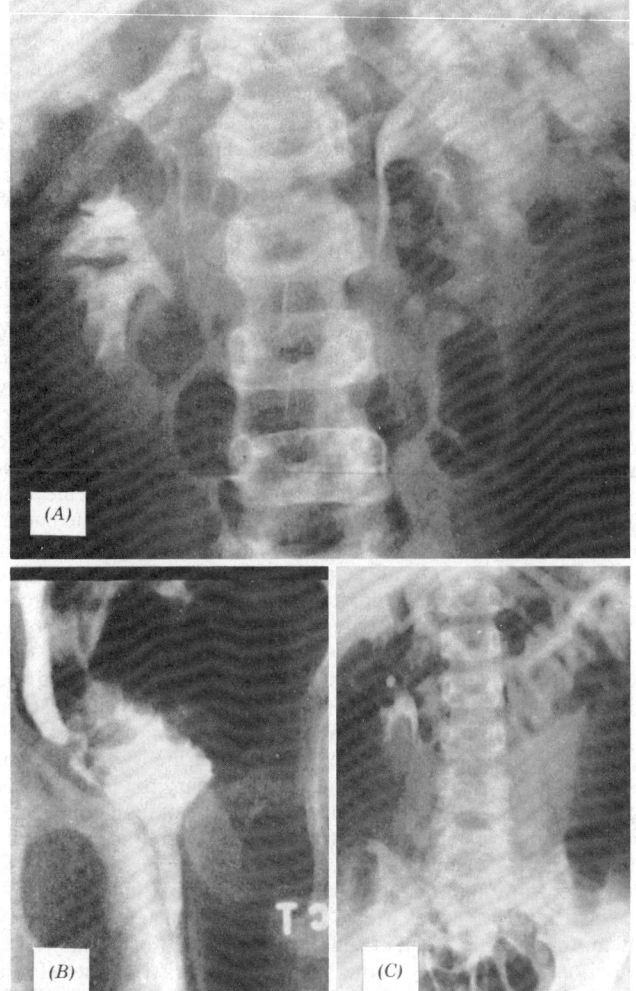

FIG. 7. Vesicoureteral reflux in a 3-year-old girl with recurrent urinary tract infection. **(A)** An intravenous urogram demonstrates duplication of the right renal collecting system with a mild increase in fullness of the right lower renal unit. Although the presence of reflux on the basis of this finding might be suspected, such an inference is not justified since the fullness could be within normal limits. **(B)** A voiding cystourethrogram demonstrates reflux into a dilated right ureter. **(C)** An immediate postvoiding film of the abdomen reveals the reflux to be confined to the lower renal unit on the right. Although in some cases it is possible to suspect the presence of reflux on the basis of the intravenous urogram alone, many cases of reflux are associated with a perfectly normal urogram. (From Kaye,[3] with permission).

the age of 5 years.[202,203] In fact, some investigators have questioned the need for detecting and treating bacteriuria in school-aged children (or, for that matter, in any asymptomatic children).[204] However, it is clear that progression does occur in some of these children, especially in the presence of severe reflux.[202]

Adults

Urinary tract infections are much more common in women than in men. Many of these patients previously had urinary tract infections as children and continue to have infections as adults.[203] Once a woman develops infection, she is more likely to develop subsequent infections than a patient who has had no previous infections.

The courses of women with symptomatic recurrent urinary tract infections were described by Kraft and Stamey.[205] How-

ever, it was not defined whether these recurrences were reinfections or relapses. Twenty-three patients were followed over a total of 800 months, and each episode of urinary tract infection was treated. The overall attack rate was about 0.2 infections per month. Of interest is that even in these women (i.e., with recurrent urinary tract infections), significant bacteriuria (i.e., $\geq 10^5$ bacteria/ml urine) was present in only 70 percent of symptomatic episodes. Infections tended to occur in clusters with an increased attack rate of 0.5 percent per month. These periods of more frequent infection were followed by a remission or infection-free interval that averaged about 13 months. However, most remissions were followed by further clusters of infection. Thus, in many women it is more correct to use the term *remission* rather than *cure* of urinary tract infection. It may be a simple matter to cure an individual episode, but recurrence is common.

It is clear that urinary tract infection in adults can lead to progressive renal damage in the presence of obstruction. However, recurrent infection in adults in the absence of obstruction rarely, if ever, leads to renal failure.[142]

Autopsy studies[203] have shown that it is difficult to implicate infection per se (i.e., in the absence of other renal abnormalities) as an important pathogenetic factor in the production of severe renal disease in adults. One exception might be severe papillary necrosis secondary to infection. In fact, one group of investigators[206] was unable to find any case of uncomplicated pyelonephritis that progressed to end-stage renal disease among 173 patients admitted to dialysis programs. In prospective studies,[141,207–211] hundreds of patients have been followed for years with persistent or recurrent infections without documenting progression of renal disease from infection alone.

The role of infection in the progression of clinically or radiographically diagnosed interstitial renal disease has also been examined.[142,212,213] In general, these studies indicate that infection is rarely, if ever, the major factor leading to further renal decompensation. However, infection may occasionally accelerate the progression of the primary underlying disease process.[212] In summary, except for perhaps rare instances there is no evidence to indicate that uncomplicated urinary tract infection alone produces renal failure in adults.

Some studies have demonstrated decreased survival among elderly people with bacteriuria.[214,215] However, other studies have not confirmed this association.[215,216] At present, it seems unlikely that asymptomatic bacteriuria in the elderly has any deleterious effects. Furthermore, there is no evidence to suggest that treatment of asymptomatic bacteriuria in the elderly has any beneficial effects. Therefore, routine treatment of asymptomatic bacteriuria in the elderly is not advocated by most experts.

Hypertension

It is clear that severe renal disease may cause hypertension. The entity of chronic interstitial renal disease (not necessarily related to infection) has also been related to hypertension.[213] It has been suggested that patients with bacteriuria in the absence of other renal disease are more likely to have hypertension, but the data have not shown a clear-cut relationship. No definite cause and effect relationships have been documented.

MANAGEMENT OF URINARY TRACT INFECTION

General Considerations

Ideally antimicrobial agents should only be administered when there is reasonable evidence of infection in the urinary tract. Symptoms are not a reliable indication of infection. The diagnosis of infection in the asymptomatic patient should be made on no fewer than two cultures of clean-voided, midstream urine in which the same microorganism is present in significant titers.

If the patient is symptomatic, one specimen will suffice, and therapy should be started.

There has been much controversy as to how vigorously chemotherapy should be pursued. A rational approach to the treatment of urinary tract infection depends on an appreciation of the prognosis of the untreated infection and the long-term results to be expected from therapy. The side effects, cost, and inconvenience of different therapeutic regimens must also be considered. As the prognosis of urinary tract infection in nonpregnant adult women seems to be quite good and reinfection is common, therapy probably makes little contribution to the patient's well-being other than eradicating symptoms.

While bacteriuria in the elderly is associated with degenerative and debilitating diseases and in some reports with mortality, there is no convincing evidence for a cause and effect relationship.[146,215,217] There certainly is no evidence that treatment of the urinary tract infection alters the patient's course. Urinary tract infection serves as a marker for debilitating diseases, which in turn may contribute to mortality. In addition, urinary tract infection is very common in the elderly, and many of these patients become reinfected or relapse after antimicrobial therapy. Furthermore, a higher frequency of side effects from chemotherapy would be expected in an older age group because of preexisting renal, auditory, and other diseases. Considering the large numbers of patients involved, intensive antimicrobial therapy may lead to an unwarranted financial burden and the danger of drug toxicity and thus may do more harm than good in elderly patients.

In contrast, bacteriuria in preschool children with vesicoureteral reflux (especially if congenital anomalies are present) can result in stunted growth of the kidney, scar formation, and, rarely, renal failure. Bacteriuria in pregnancy may also have serious implications. Treatment of children and pregnant women is most likely to be beneficial. Furthermore, it is feasible to treat all these patients since the prevalence of bacteriuria is relatively low in these groups.

Hospitalized patients with bacteriuria have higher mortality rates than those without bacteriuria.[218,219] This observation may be related to deaths from bacteremia in patients with indwelling urinary catheters.

It is usually necessary to treat all symptomatic patients regardless of age, even when infection is likely to recur. Some patients have such frequent symptomatic episodes (either relapses or reinfections) that they are almost chronically incapacitated. In these patients it may be necessary to give prolonged therapy or prophylaxis to prevent recurrent symptoms.

Nonspecific Therapy

Hydration. Forcing fluids has been advocated in the therapy of urinary tract infection. There is some theoretical support for this modality of treatment. Hydration produces rapid dilution of the bacteria and removal of infected urine by frequent bladder emptying, which in the presence of minimal residual volume may offset the logarithmic growth of gram-negative bacilli. Forcing fluids usually results in a rapid reduction of bacterial counts. Permanent loss of bacteriuria has been reported in a few patients with rapid hydration, but in most patients bacterial counts return to original levels when hydration is stopped (e..g, overnight when urine flow rate and frequency of micturition are reduced).[220]

Medullary hypertonicity tends to inhibit leukocytic migration into the renal medulla, and the high concentration of ammonia tends to inactivate complement.[63,64] Abolition of medullary hypertonicity by diuresis would be expected to reverse these effects. In addition, a reduction in bacterial counts in the urine by hydration would enhance the effect of factors otherwise overwhelmed by large numbers of bacteria (e.g., bladder mucosal defenses or the effect of relatively low concentrations of antimicrobial drugs).

Hydration may also have some disadvantages. Increased fluid intake could theoretically result in increased vesicoureteral reflux and possibly cause acute urinary retention in the partially obstructed bladder. The larger urine output results in dilution of antibacterial substances normally present in the urine as well as lower urinary concentrations of antimicrobial agents. Water diuresis also decreases urinary acidification, which enhances the antibacterial activity of urine and certain antimicrobial agents.

As there is no evidence that hydration improves the results of appropriate antimicrobial therapy, and because continuous hydration is inconvenient, we are not in favor of this approach.

Urinary pH. Antibacterial activity of urine results mainly from high urea concentration and osmolality and is pH dependent, being greater at a lower pH.[65] the pH-dependent activity may be related to a high concentration of various weakly ionizable organic acids, such as hippuric and β-hydroxybutyric acids.[221] The antibacterial activity of these organic acids is related to the concentration of the undissociated molecule that probably penetrates better than the ionized form into the bacterial cell. As these organic acids have a relatively low pKa (the pH at which 50 percent of the molecules are undissociated), the lower the urinary pH, the greater the concentration of undissociated molecules and the greater the antibacterial activity of the organic acid.

Hippuric acid is a common constituent of urine, being the glycine conjugate of dietary benzoic acid, and is bacteriostatic in proportion to the concentration of undissociated molecules. The production of antibacterial activity in urine by ingestion of large volumes of cranberry juice (if the urinary pH level is kept low) results from the appearance in the urine of high concentrations of hippuric acid derived form precursors in the berry. The successful use of mandelic acid, another organic acid, is also dependent on maintenance of a low urinary pH level.

The urinary pH level affects the antibacterial activity of many chemotherapeutic agents used in the treatment of urinary tract infections. The activity of methenamine results from the release of formaldehyde as the urinary pH level is decreased below 5.5. Clinically, methenamine is used in the form of its mandelic acid salt (methenamine mandelate) or its hippuric acid salt (methenamine hippurate). The antibacterial activity of these salts is related to the formation of the un-ionized organic acid and formaldehyde, which is highly dependent on maintenance of a urinary pH of 5.5 or less. The effectiveness of nitrofurantoin (pKa 7.2) is also greater at low urinary pH level. In contrast, the aminoglycoside antibiotics such as gentamicin, tobramycin, and amikacin are more effective in alkaline urine.

Although different antimicrobial agents have maximum effectiveness at different pH levels, most agents exhibit adequate antibacterial activity at usual urinary pH levels. Maintenance of urine at the low pH level required for effective antibacterial activity of organic acids and methenamine can be accomplished by administration of ascorbic acid or methionine. Acidification of the urine can result in precipitation of urate stones, and, since oxalate is a metabolite of ascorbic acid, large doses of ascorbic acid can cause formation of oxalate stones.

To acidify the urine, it is often necessary to modify the diet by restriction of agents that tend to alkalinize the urine, for example, milk, fruit juices (except cranberry juice), and sodium bicarbonate. Another major problem with acidification is that patients with renal insufficiency are unable to excrete an acid load and may become systemically acidotic when urinary acidification is attempted. It may be impossible to acidify urine infected with urea-splitting organisms such as *Proteus* species because of production of ammonia from urea. Acidification for long-term antimicrobial therapy should only be used with concomitant use of organic acids or methenamine. Urinary acidification is frequently difficult to achieve[222] and is rarely if ever necessary at present.

Analgesics. Urinary analgesics such as phenazopyridine hydrochloride (Pyridium) have little place in the routine management of symptomatic infections. The dysuria of urinary tract infection usually responds rapidly to antibacterial therapy and requires no local analgesia. If flank pain or dysuria is severe, systemic analgesics can be used. Analgesics such as phenazopyridine hydrochloride may be useful in the management of certain patients with dysuria but without infection.

Principles of Antimicrobial Therapy

Selection of an appropriate antimicrobial agent has become complex because of the increasing number of compounds available, each with its characteristic spectrum and toxic properties. However, in most cases, any of many available agents are perfectly satisfactory. Given two or more drugs with equivalent activity against the infecting microorganism, the agent with the least toxicity should be chosen.

There is no evidence to support any superiority of bactericidal drugs over bacteriostatic agents in urinary tract infection. However, there may be theoretical reasons for using bactericidal drugs in the treatment of relapsing urinary tract infection.

Serum, Tissue, and Urine Concentrations of Antimicrobial Agents. A poor correlation exists between response of bacteriuria and blood levels of antimicrobial agents.[176,223,224] Many oral antimicrobial agents, in the dosages commonly used for urinary tract infection, do not achieve serum levels above the MIC for most urinary pathogens.

Disappearance of bacteriuria is closely correlated with the sensitivity of the microorganism to the concentration of the antimicrobial agent achieved in the urine.[176,223,224] Inhibitory urinary concentrations are achieved after oral administration of essentially all commonly used antimicrobial agents. While blood levels do not seem to be important in the treatment of urinary tract infection, they may be critical in patients with bacteremia and may be important in the cure of patients with renal parenchymal infection who relapse.

In patients with renal insufficiency, dosage modifications are necessary for agents that are excreted primarily by the kidneys and cannot be cleared by any other mechanism. In renal failure, the kidney may not be able to concentrate an antimicrobial agent in the urine, and difficulty in eradicating bacteriuria may occur. This may be an important factor in failure of therapy for urinary tract infection with aminoglycosides.

In addition, high concentrations of magnesium and calcium as well as a low pH level can raise the MIC of aminoglycosides for gram-negative bacilli to levels above those achievable in the urine of patients with renal failure.[225] In general the penicillins and cephalosporins attain adequate urine concentrations despite severely impaired renal function and are the agents of choice in renal insufficiency.[226]

Response to Therapy. The objective of antimicrobial therapy is to eliminate bacteria from the urinary tract. Symptoms usually abate spontaneously without chemotherapy, even though bacteriuria may persist. Therefore, the results of therapy can only be determined by follow-up urine cultures.

There are four patterns of response of bacteriuria to antimicrobial therapy: cure, persistence, relapse, and reinfection. Quantitative bacterial counts in urine should decrease within 48 hours after initiation of an antimicrobial agent to which the microorganism is sensitive in vitro. If titers do not decrease within this time, the therapy being given will almost invariably be unsuccessful.

Cure is defined as negative urine cultures on chemotherapy and during the follow-up period (usually 1–2 weeks). However, it must be understood that many of these patients will develop reinfection at a later time.

Persistence has been used in two ways to describe response

to therapy: *(1)* persistence of significant bacteriuria after 48 hours of treatment and *(2)* persistence of the infecting organism in low numbers in urine after 48 hours. Significant bacteriuria usually persists only if urinary levels of the antimicrobial agent are below the concentration of the drug needed to inhibit the microorganism. This can occur when the infecting strain is resistant to the urinary levels usually attained (i.e., a resistant organism) or because levels are inordinately low (i.e., from not taking the agent, insufficient dosage, poor intestinal absorption, or poor renal excretion as in renal insufficiency). Persistence of the infecting microorganism in low titers in voided urine may mean persistence in the urinary tract or contamination from the urethra or vagina. Bladder puncture cultures would be needed to evaluate the significance of low titers of bacteria obtained in therapy, and we do not routinely recommend this procedure. Also worth noting is the fact that bacteria may persist within the urinary tract during therapy without excretion of organisms in the urine. Sites of persistence within the urinary tract are the renal parenchyma, calculi, and the prostate. The simplest way of determining the significance of persistence of the organism in low titers in the urine is to obtain follow-up urine cultures after therapy has been stopped. Prompt relapse of significant bacteriuria usually follows persistence of the organism in the urinary tract.

Relapse usually occurs within 1–2 weeks after cessation of chemotherapy and is often associated with renal infection, with structural abnormalities of the urinary tract, or with chronic bacterial prostatitis. Relapse indicates that the infecting microorganism has persisted in the urinary tract during therapy. However, an apparent relapse can be related to reinfection (new infection) with the same microorganism. In spite of eradication from the urinary tract, the original infecting organism may still be present in the intestine, vagina, or external urethra and then may cause a new infection. Markedly delayed relapses (more than 1 month after stopping therapy) are much more likely due to this phenomenon or to chronic bacterial prostatitis than to true relapse. Relapses occurring within 1–2 weeks are usually true relapses. One postulated but unsubstantiated mechanism of relapse following treatment with cell wall active antibiotics (e.g., penicillins and cephalosporins) is persistence of osmotically fragile, cell wall–deficient forms in the hypertonic renal medulla during therapy, with reversion to normal bacterial forms after therapy is stopped.[128]

After initial sterilization of the urine, *reinfection* may occur during administration of chemotherapy (also called *superinfection*) or at any time thereafter. Reinfection is easy to identify when there is a change in bacterial species. However, there may be reinfection with a different serotype of the same species (usually *E. coli*) or even the same serotype.

Classification and Antimicrobial Therapy for Different Groups

Symptomatic Urinary Tract Infection. The majority of patients classified as having symptomatic urinary tract infection are women, usually of child-bearing age. The onset of symptoms is frequently related to sexual intercourse. The patient may have upper urinary tract symptoms, lower urinary tract symptoms, or both. As mentioned previously, patients with only lower urinary tract symptoms may also have upper urinary tract infection.

ACUTE PYELONEPHRITIS. Patients who are severely ill with pyelonephritis should be hospitalized. Although mild to moderate illness responds well to orally administered antimicrobial agents, nausea and vomiting may preclude oral treatment, necessitating parenteral therapy. If the patient is reliable, compliant, and tolerates oral therapy, the patient may be treated with a variety of oral antimicrobial agents. At the time of antibiotic selection, a Gram stain of the urine should have indicated the morphology of the infecting organism (e.g., gram-negative bacillus, gram-positive coccus), but the precise identity and antimicrobial susceptibility are usually unknown. Therefore, selection of antimicrobial therapy is usually empiric. When streptococci are seen on Gram stain, ampicillin or amoxicillin is probably the agent of choice. When staphylococci are implicated on Gram stain, cephalosporins (such as cephalexin) are appropriate agents.

Although ampicillin and amoxicillin have been mainstays of oral therapy for gram-negative bacillus infection for many years, these agents can no longer be recommended as reliable agents, since 25–35 percent of *E. coli* are now resistant.[227] Accordingly, oral antimicrobial agents currently advocated for gram-negative bacillus urinary infection include trimethoprim, trimethoprim–sulfamethoxazole, cephalexin, amoxicillin–clavulanic acid, and the fluoroquinolones (e.g., norfloxacin and ciprofloxacin). The doses are listed under "Lower Urinary Tract Infection," below. In all patients with symptoms of upper tract infection, therapy should be preceded by culture of a clean-catch midstream urine sample.

In hospitalized patients, particularly those with suspected gram-negative bacillary bacteremia complicating pyelonephritis (high fever, shaking chills, hypotension), parenteral therapy should be use and is directed at the life-threatening bacteremia. In these seriously ill patients the spectrum of antibacterial activity of the initial agents should include all potential pathogens. In seriously ill patients with community-acquired acute pyelonephritis, when the gram stain reveals gram-negative bacilli, empiric therapy includes a wide selection of antimicrobial agents (e.g., parenteral trimethoprim–sulfamethoxazole; aminoglycosides (such as gentamicin, 3–5 mg/kg/day,; aztreonam, 3–6 g/day; ureido-penicillins—mezlocillin, azlocillin, or piperacillin, 18 g/day; the ampicillin—sulbactam combination, as 12 g ampicillin/day), the ticarcillin–clavulanic acid combination (as 18 g ticarcillin/day), third-generation cephalosporins (e.g., cefotaxime or ceftriaxone, or a parenteral fluoroquinolone. In patients with hospital-acquired gram-negative bacillary infection, particularly when seriously ill, the initial selection of antibiotics should not leave any hiatus in the spectrum of activity and should anticipate the possibility of resistant microorganisms. Under these circumstances ceftazidine (3–6 g/day), ticarcillin–clavulanic acid, aztreonam, or imipenem (2 g/day), often used in combination with aminoglycosides or a parenteral fluoroquinolone, are recommended. When the susceptibility pattern of the infecting organism is known, therapy can be altered to less expensive single-agent therapy, and oral treatment can be used once response has occurred.

Effective therapy results in a marked decrease in bacterial titers in the urine within 48 hours after onset of treatment. Antimicrobial agents are sometimes effective in vivo even when disk sensitivity tests indicate drug resistance, because most antimicrobials are excreted in the urine in concentrations much higher than tested for by disk sensitivity testing.

If bacteriologic response does not occur by 48 hours, there is no point in continuing the same regimen. Therapy is then changed to an alternate drug on the basis of susceptibility tests (e.g., from the initial solate). The finding of continuing positive blood cultures or persistent fever and toxicity past the first 3 days suggests the need for investigation to exclude urinary obstruction or intrarenal or perinephric abscess formation. Investigation should include renal ultrasound, computed tomographic or magnetic resonance scan, and, according to the findings, perhaps an intravenous pyelogram (IVP) examination. The availability of sensitive noninvasive studies has resulted in early diagnosis of intrarenal or perinephric abscess formation that may respond to antibiotic therapy alone. In uncomplicated pyelonephritis after clinical response and defervesence occurs, oral therapy is initiated and should be continued to complete a course of 14 days of antimicrobial therapy.[228] When upper tract infection is complicated by abscesses, more prolonged therapy and perhaps drainage is indicated (see "Perinephric Abscess" and "Intrarenal Abscess," below). All patients with acute pyelone-

phritis should have at least an ultrasound examination to evaluate for obstruction and/or stones. Follow-up urine cultures are mandatory within 1–2 weeks of completion of therapy in pregnant women, children, and patients with recurrent symptomatic pyelonephritis in whom suppressive maintenance therapy is planned. In the majority of nonpregnant adults who remain asymptomatic, follow-up cultures are optional.

Renal infection is a special problem in adults with hereditary polycystic disease. Although parenchymal infections respond well to appropriate antibiotics, cyst infections frequently fail to improve and may require lipid-soluble antibiotics (e.g., trimethoprim–sulfamethoxazole[229] or surgical aspiration/drainage). Emphysematous pyelonephritis is most often seen in elderly female diabetics with chronic urinary infections and renal vascular disease. Because of the extraordinarily high mortality rate of 70 percent in spite of appropriate antibiotics and supportive therapy, immediate nephrectomy is indicated for this condition[230] (Fig. 8).

LOWER URINARY TRACT INFECTION.   *Conventional Therapy.*   In the past, 7–10 days of therapy was routinely recommended for patients with lower tract symptoms. However, in recent years it has become apparent that most women with lower tract infection have only a superficial mucosal infection and can be cured with much shorter courses of therapy and in fact with only a single dose of an antimicrobial agent.

Short Course Therapy.   Single-dose therapy achieves high urinary concentrations that are prolonged for at least 12–24 hours and eliminate infection when presumably confined to the bladder. The most widely used regimens have been oral doses of 3 g amoxicillin or one double-strength tablet of trimetho-

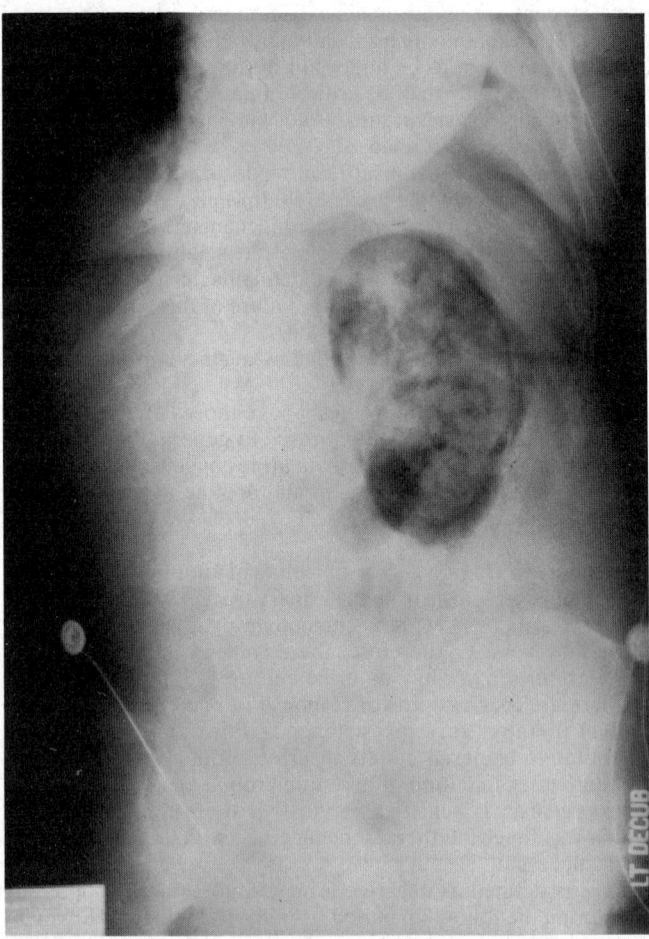

FIG. 8.   Flat plate radiograph of abdomen showing emphysematous pyelonephritis.

prim–sulfamethoxazole.[231] Other regimens have included sulfonamides (e.g., 2 g sulfisoxazole orally), aminoglycosides (e.g., 150 mg netilmicin intramuscularly), 2 g tetracycline orally, 400 mg trimethoprim orally, 200 mg nitrofurantoin orally, cephalosporins (e.g., 0.5 g ceftriaxone intramuscularly), and fluoroquinolones (e.g., 800 mg norfloxacin orally),[231–235] Cure rates have ranged from 65 to 100 percent.

The advantages of single-dose therapy include lesser expense, assured compliance, fewer side effects, and perhaps less intensive selective pressure for emergence of resistant organisms in gut, urinary, or vaginal flora. Possible deleterious effects include a poorer outcome of infections that are actually in the upper tract and are first treated with single-dose therapy, for example, a delay in appropriate therapy may result in more deeply seated infection and impair the response to subsequent more prolonged therapy. Finally, it should not be assumed that every antibiotic administered as a single dose will be effective even with regard to susceptible organisms. Results depend on high sustained urinary concentrations of the antimicrobial agent. For example, a 2-g oral dose of cefaclor resulted in a 57 percent failure rate.[236] Before using single-dose therapy, certain factors should be evaluated, including frequency of attacks, poor response to single-dose therapy in the past, known structural abnormalities, history of childhood infection, symptoms longer than 7 days, pyelonephritis during the past year, diabetes, and so forth. Any of these factors increases the likelihood of upper tract infection and might mitigate against using single-dose therapy.

A by-product of single-dose therapy is that failure to eradicate a urinary tract infection after a single dose of an agent may indicate in which patient further investigation should be considered. Response to single-dose therapy appears comparable with the ACB test in localizing the site of infection.[197,237]

Single-dose therapy gives basically 1 day of therapy with regard to antimicrobial activity in the urine. The same results should be achievable with 1 day of standard-dose antimicrobial therapy; however, the data to support this do not exist. Three reviews concluded that 3 days of therapy are superior to single-dose therapy.[231,238,239] It is our preference to use 3 days of therapy with standard doses. It seems clear that, with either a single dose or 3 days of therapy, trimethoprim–sulfamethoxazole (and perhaps fluoroquinolones) are superior to β-lactam antibiotics in terms of both early (i.e., <2 weeks) and late (i.e., >2 weeks) follow up.[227,231,232] Some of the preferred agents for 3 days of therapy are trimethoprim–sulfamethoxazole (one double-strength tablet twice a day), trimethoprim (100 mg twice a day), norfloxacin (400 mg twice a day), ciprofloxacin (500 mg twice a day), or other fluoroquinolones.

We do not advocate use of sulfonamides, ampicillin, or amoxicillin because of the relatively high frequency of *E. coli* resistant to these agents among community-acquired urinary tract infections.[227]

The approach to management of lower urinary tract infection has evolved to where short course therapy should become the standard for most female patients with suspected lower tract infection. Some studies in pediatric populations have shown similar good results, but others have not.[134] Short course therapy has not been adequately evaluated in men and is not recommended at present. Short course therapy is not appropriate for women who have a history of previous urinary infection caused by antibiotic-resistant organisms or more than 7 days of symptoms.[240] In these patients (who have an increased likelihood of upper tract infection) and in males, 7–10 days of therapy are recommended.

If symptoms do not respond or if they recur, a urine culture should be obtained. In pregnant women, children, and patients at high risk for renal damage who remain asymptomatic, follow-up cultures should be obtained 1–2 weeks after discontinuation of therapy to detect relapses.

OFFICE STRATEGY FOR FREQUENCY, URGENCY, AND DYSURIA SYNDROME. When a sexually active woman is first seen with frequency, urgency, dysuria, urine culture is not mandatory,

and the therapeutic decision is based on the clinical presentation and the presence or absence of pyuria. If pyuria (defined as ≥10 leukocytes/mm³) is present, antimicrobial therapy is warranted for urinary tract infection. Short course therapy is a reasonable first approach in adult females except in settings in which occult pyelonephritis is more likely, as described above. An agent likely to be effective against most pathogens (e.g., trimethoprim, trimethoprim–sulfamethoxazole, amoxicillin–clavulanic acid, norfloxacin, ciprofloxacin) should be used. If clinical response does not occur, a culture should be obtained (for the possibility of a resistant organism), and therapy should be changed and directed at *Chlamydia,* 100 mg doxycycline twice a day for 7 days.

In the nonsexually active female with symptoms of lower tract infection and pyuria, there is a high probability of urinary tract infection. Lack of response to therapy probably indicates a resistant organism and mandates a urine culture.

In the absence of pyuria, symptomatic urinary tract infection is unlikely in any patient. Symptomatic response followed by recurrence after therapy is discontinued indicates the probability of upper tract infection and the need for a culture and at least 2 weeks of therapy. Men and children should have a urine culture, and males should receive 7–10 days of treatment.

Asymptomatic Bacteriuria. Most patients with asymptomatic bacteriuria are women and are in the older age groups. Although cure may result following treatment, relapse and especially reinfection are common. The approach to asymptomatic bacteriuria depends on the age of the patient. In children, therapy should be given as described for symptomatic infection. A trial of short course therapy is reasonable. In contrast, therapy for asymptomatic bacteriuria in the adult is by no means mandatory in the absence of obstruction except during pregnancy. Nonpregnant women can be treated providing that a nontoxic antimicrobial agent is used. If the infecting microorganism is resistant to all but toxic agents, then treatment should not be instituted in the nonobstructed patient.

At present, most physicians believe that asymptomatic bacteriuria in the elderly is a benign disease and need not be treated, especially since with vigorous treatment a great many people will be exposed to drug toxicity.

When dealing with asymptomatic bacteriuria, there is no urgency in treating. Therapy should be delayed until two cultures have been obtained for confirmation of presence of bacteriuria. By that time, the identity and antimicrobial susceptibility pattern of the infecting organism will have been determined.

Relapsing Urinary Tract Infection. If the patient relapses after therapy for symptomatic urinary tract infection or for asymptomatic bacteriuria, the most likely possibilities are that the patient has *(1)* renal involvement, *(2)* a structural abnormality of the urinary tract (e.g., calculi), or *(3)* chronic bacterial prostatitis.

Relapses, especially in the absence of structural abnormalities, may be related to renal infection that may require a longer duration of therapy. Patients who relapse after a short course or 7–10 days of therapy should be considered for a 2-week course. Turck and colleagues[177] demonstrated that a 6-week course of therapy resulted in a higher cure rate than a 2-week course in patients who relapsed after 2 weeks of therapy.

Structural abnormalities of the urinary tract predispose to relapse. Urinary tract infection in the presence of obstruction is likely to be associated with renal involvement, a tendency for renal functional impairment, and bacteremia. Obstructive lesions can be corrected surgically and should be sought in the evaluation of patients with relapsing infection. Calculi may be a cause of relapse of urinary tract infection. Ultimate success of chemotherapy is dependent on the removal of stones.

Some patients continue to relapse despite surgical correction of urologic abnormalities. In others, surgical correction may not be indicated or feasible, or no abnormalities may be found. In these patients who relapse after 2 weeks of chemotherapy, a repeat course of 2 weeks should be considered. Following another relapse a 4–6 week course should be considered. In men, chronic bacterial prostatitis should first be ruled out.

If relapse occurs after a 6-week course, therapy lasting 6 months or even longer may be considered. Only carefully selected patients, such as children, adults who have continuous symptoms, or adults who are at high risk of developing progressive renal damage (e.g., those with obstruction not amenable to surgery), should be considered for 4-week or longer courses of therapy. Asymptomatic adults without obstruction should not receive these longer courses. Some of the agents that can be used for long-term therapy are amoxicillin (250 mg three times a day), cephalexin, trimethoprim–sulfamethoxazole, trimethoprim, norfloxacin, and ciprofloxacin, in usual doses and nitrofurantoin in full dosage for 1 week and then half the usual dose.

An antimicrobial agent being used for long-term therapy is continued only as long as significant bacteriuria is absent. If bacteriuria persists or relapses during chemotherapy (indicating that the infecting organism is now resistant to that agent), the agent is altered. The aim is to achieve continuous suppression of bacteriuria for the entire course of therapy. If relapse occurs after discontinuation of the antimicrobial agent, therapy is reinstituted with the same or another drug. If deemed necessary, this agent is administered for an additional 6–12 months (if bacteriuria remains suppressed). All patients are followed with urine cultures at least monthly while on therapy.

Long-term therapy or even repeated 2-week courses should be reserved for children, symptomatic patients of any age, and patients at high risk of developing progressive renal damage. A creatinine clearance determination and imaging studies of the kidneys initially and yearly (or at least every 2 years) should be obtained on patients receiving long-term therapy to determine glomerular filtration rate and structural changes in the kidneys. Blood counts, urinalyses, and liver chemistries (when indicated) are also obtained periodically as tests for drug toxicity.

Reinfection of the Urinary Tract. Patients with reinfection can generally be divided into two groups: (1) those who have relatively infrequent reinfections, perhaps only once every 2 or 3 years to several times a year and (2) those who develop frequent reinfections. An extreme example of the latter group is patients who become reinfected during or shortly after each course of antimicrobial therapy. With infrequent reinfections, each episode can be approached with therapy as if it were a new episode of either symptomatic or asymptomatic infection. Short course therapy should be used in women with lower tract symptoms. Women with reinfections associated with lower tract symptoms can be managed with self-administration of short course therapy with onset of symptoms.[241]

Many patients with frequent reinfections after therapy are middle-aged or elderly women in whom infection is limited to the lower urinary tract. Most asymptomatic reinfections in this group should not be treated, because the frequent use of antimicrobial agents in this group is apt to result in toxic side effects and because progressive destruction of the kidneys is rare. If, however, the episodes are symptomatic or if the likelihood of renal damage is increased, these patients should be treated.

Occasionally patients of any age develop symptomatic reinfection so frequently that they can be incapacitated. In some women, these symptomatic reinfections are associated with sexual activity. Voiding immediately after intercourse may help prevent reinfection. However, single-dose prophylactic chemotherapy taken after sexual intercourse is a more effective method of decreasing episodes.[242]

In other patients with frequent symptomatic reinfections, no precipitating event is apparent; in these patients, when symptoms are severe, long-term chemoprophylaxis may be instituted. Although these courses seem to decrease the frequency of rein-

fections and symptoms in most patients, it is impossible to prevent completely reinfection in many patients. When reinfection occurs on therapy, the prophylactic agent must be changed.

Long-term chemoprophylaxis should be considered for asymptomatic patients who reinfect frequently and are at risk of developing renal parenchymal damage with each reinfection (e.g., young children with vesicoureteral reflux and children and adults with obstruction uropathy). In these groups, keeping the patient antibacteriuric helps to protect the kidneys. Several studies in patients with frequent reinfections indicate that such prolonged chemotherapy reduces the frequency of reinfections.

Long-term prophylactic antimicrobial agents have reduced the frequency of symptomatic infections of the urinary tract in older men, women, and children.[237,243–245] Before prophylaxis is initiated, the patient should receive a course of therapy with an appropriate antimicrobial agent. Trimethoprim–sulfamethoxazole, nitrofurantoin, or trimethoprim alone are particularly useful for long-term prophylaxis, because these drugs are inexpensive and are unlikely to allow the emergence of antimicrobial-resistant bacteria with prolonged use.[244–247]

Full antimicrobial dosage is not necessary for successful prophylaxis. One 50-mg tablet of nitrofurantoin or one-half table of trimethoprim–sulfamethoxazole (40 mg trimethoprim, 200 mg sulfamethoxazole) nightly will suffice. Fluoroquinolones and other agents have been used with good results.[227]

Patients receiving long-term prophylaxis should be followed with urine cultures monthly or more often if interim symptomatic episodes develop. Therapy is continued with the same agent as long as the patient remains abacteriuric. If bacteriuria persists or recurs during administration of an antimicrobial agent, therapy is altered using response of bacteriuria as a parameter of adequacy of therapy. Long-term prophylaxis can be undertaken only if urine cultures are obtained periodically and therapy altered if bacteriuria recurs.

URINARY TRACT INFECTION IN PREGNANCY

Physiologic Alterations in the Urinary Tract

During pregnancy there is dilatation of the ureters and renal pelves with markedly decreased ureteral peristalsis. These changes begin as early as the seventh week of gestation and progress to term.[248] The bladder also decreases in tone so that late in gestation it can contain twice its normal contents without causing discomfort. These changes vary from patient to patient. They are more marked on the right side and are more likely to occur during the first pregnancy or when pregnancies occur in rapid succession (Fig. 9). The urinary tract tends to revert to normal by the second month following delivery.[248,249]

Changes similar to those of pregnancy have been described in the urinary tracts of women taking oral contraceptives.[250] Because of this observation, it has been suggested that the urinary tract alterations may be at least in part related to hyperestrogenism.[248] Other possible explanations for the alterations are obstruction of the ureters by the gravid uterus and hypertrophy of muscle bundles at the lower end of the ureter.[248] To investigate the effects of estrogens on these changes, Andriole and Cohn[251] treated nonpregnant female and male rats with estrogens and obtained intravenous pyelograms before and during treatment. Hydroureter and marked increased susceptibility to *E. coli* pyelonephritis are observed in both male and female animals.

Epidemiology

The microbiology of bacteriuria during gestation is similar to that seen in nonpregnant women. The prevalence of asymptomatic bacteriuria in pregnancy ranges from 4 to 7 percent.[252,253] It is unclear if *U. urealyticum* and *G. vaginalis*, reported by some to be in bladder urine of an additional 10–15 percent of

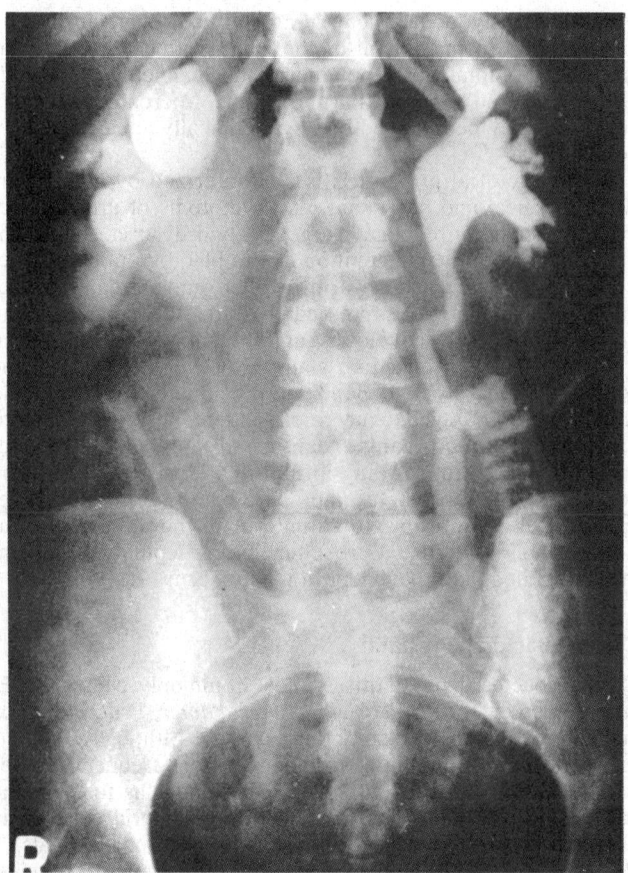

FIG. 9. Urogram in pregnancy. Urography was performed during the seventh month of pregnancy because of severe right-sided pyelonephritis. Although the right hydronephrosis is pronounced, no cause for it other than pregnancy could be found. Following delivery the urogram reverted to normal. Physiologic changes such as these make it difficult to detect superimposed pathologic disorders such as small ureteral calculi when they occur during pregnancy. (From Kaye,[3] with permission).

pregnant women, play a significant pathogenic role.[248,254] Pregnant women of higher socioeconomic status have a lower frequency of bacteriuria of pregnancy than women of lower socioeconomic status.[148] The prevalence of bacteriuria also rises with parity, age, sexual activity, in diabetes mellitus, in women with sickle cell trait, and past history of urinary tract infection.[255,256] For example, in low-income populations, the prevalence of bacteriuria is about 2 percent in primiparas under age 21 as compared with 8–10 percent in grandmultiparas over age 35.[253] Most women who develop bacteriuria during pregnancy have infection at the first prenatal visit. However, 1–1.5 percent of pregnant women or about 25 percent of those with bacteriuria of pregnancy develop infection in the later trimesters.[252,253] The development of symptomatic pyelonephritis late in pregnancy is usually an expression of asymptomatic bacteriuria that was present early in parturition. The marked dilatation of the ureters during the later stages apparently allows bacteria in the bladder to reach the upper tract and to produce symptomatic pyelonephritis.

About 20–40 percent of the patients with bacteriuria early in gestation develop acute symptomatic pyelonephritis later in pregnancy.[254,255,257,258] In contrast, less than 1 percent of patients whose urine is uninfected early in gestation develop acute infection. Therefore, over 75 percent of the cases of acute pyelonephritis can be prevented by eliminating asymptomatic bacteriuria in the early stages of pregnancy.[248,252,253] It has also been noted that those whose bacteriuria fails to respond to treatment

are at highest risk of developing symptomatic infection.[281] Lack of cure is probably an indication of upper vs. lower tract infection.

An association between acute pyelonephritis of pregnancy and premature delivery was well known in the preantibiotic era.[248] The rate of prematurity can be as high as 20–50 percent. Kass[255] in 1959 reported that there was an association between asymptomatic bacteriuria and prematurity and that the eradication of bacteriuria significantly reduced the rate of premature delivery. Since then there have been conflicting studies both supporting and denying these observations.[248,253,259] In general, it seems that prematurity and low birth weight[260] are increased in patients with asymptomatic bacteriuria and, more specifically, in those women with renal involvement. However, it does not necessarily follow that asymptomatic bacteriuria is a cause of prematurity. It is possible that certain patients are predisposed both to bacteriuria and to deliver premature infants. Some investigators have reported that elimination of bacteriuria decreases the frequency of prematurity.[248,253,259] However, other studies have failed to show a decrease in prematurity or fetal wastage with elimination of asymptomatic bacteriuria.[248,253,254] Neonates of patients refractory to multiple courses of therapy have been reported to have a significantly lower birth weight than infants of those who respond; this phenomenon may be related to the presence of upper tract infection in these patients.[191,259,261] There have been several studies that have attempted to relate asymptomatic bacteriuria to the development of hypertension in pregnancy, but results have been unclear.[253]

Even though the data relating bacteriuria of pregnancy to prematurity are not clear cut, the relationship of asymptomatic bacteriuria to later development of acute pyelonephritis is indisputable. As acute pyelonephritis has possible serious consequence for both mother and fetus, screening for and treatment of bacteriuria of pregnancy seem justified. Quantitative urine cultures should be obtained in all pregnant patients at the initial prenatal visit.

Postpartum studies of patients with bacteriuria of pregnancy demonstrate a high frequency of bacteriuria even with treatment during the pregnancy.[262] Postpartum intravenous pyelography of these patients has shown that 10–30 percent have radiologic changes of "chronic pyelonephritis" and other abnormalities.[211,262] These abnormalities are most common in patients in whom renal bacteriuria has been demonstrated or in whom bacteriuria during pregnancy was difficult to eradicate with antimicrobial therapy.[263] However, pyelographic abnormalities should not necessarily be attributed to the infection that occurred during the pregnancy. In fact, these abnormalities probably antedate the pregnancy and in most cases are related to childhood infection. Treatment of bacteriuria of pregnancy has little effect on the long-term course of the patient. When patients who had bacteriuria of pregnancy were studied 10–14 years later, there were no differences between those who were treated and those who were not. About 25 percent of the women in each group had bacteriuria at time of follow-up.[211]

Management of Bacteriuria of Pregnancy

Treatment with an appropriate antimicrobial agent is recommended for all pregnant patients found to have significant bacteriuria.[184,248,253,254,258] The goal of therapy is to maintain sterile urine throughout gestation and thereby to avoid the complications associated with urinary tract infection during pregnancy. The administration of a relatively nontoxic drug for 7 days (e.g., a sulfonamide, amoxicillin, amoxicillin-clavulanate, cephalexin, nitrofurantoin) eradicates bacteriuria in 70–80 percent of patients.[184,248,253] Failure of treatment is most commonly seen in patients with renal infection or radiologic abnormalities of the urinary tract.[184,248,253] Sulfonamides should not be administered in the last few weeks of gestation because of hyperbilirubinemia and kernicterus in the newborn. Tetracyclines and quinolones should be avoided during pregnancy.

There are relatively few studies evaluating the efficacy of single-dose or 3 days of antimicrobial therapy for asymptomatic bacteriuria during pregnancy. In general, results of single-dose therapy appear to be inferior to conventional therapy.[248,264] However, 3 days of therapy may be a reasonable first option both in symptomatic and in asymptomatic infection in an attempt to decrease drug administration in pregnancy.

Urine cultures should be obtained 1–2 weeks after discontinuing therapy and at regular intervals (e.g., monthly) for the remainder of gestation. If bacteriuria recurs, therapy should be given for relapse or reinfection, as already discussed. Catheterization should be avoided at the time of delivery. If relapses or multiple reinfections occurred during pregnancy, radiologic evaluation should be considered postpartum. Effective prophylaxis for recurrent urinary infection in pregnancy can be achieved by postcoital prophylaxis consisting of a single oral dose of either cephalexin (250 mg) or nitrofurantoin macrocrystals (50 mg).[265]

PROSTATITIS

Bacterial prostatitis can manifest as either an acute or a chronic disease. Although the manner by which bacteria reach the prostate is unknown,[266] possibilities include the hematogenous route, ascending infection from the urethra, and lymphatic spread from the rectum. Reflux of infected urine may also play a role in the pathogenesis of bacterial prostatitis.[267] Urethral instrumentation and prostatic surgery are known causes of prostatitis, but many patients have no history of a precipitating event.

Stamey[268] has noted that male sex partners of women with vaginal colonization by gram-negative bacilli may develop transient urethral colonization with the same organisms. They postulated that sexual intercourse might play an important role in infection of the prostate. Prostatic fluid constituents, notably zinc, normally have substantial antibacterial properties.[67,269] However, the prostatic secretions of some patients with chronic bacterial prostatitis have been shown to lack such activity.[269] Bacterial prostatitis infrequently develops after transurethral prostatectomy in men who have infected urine.[266]

The syndromes of acute and chronic bacterial prostatitis are different and distinct. Acute prostatitis does not usually result in chronic prostatitis, and chronic bacterial prostatitis is not usually antedated by acute prostatitis. Acute prostatitis is an acute infectious disease and is similar to an acute localized infection in any other organ, producing local heat, tenderness, and fever. In contrast, chronic bacterial prostatitis often produces few or no symptoms related to the prostate, which just serves as a nidus of low-grade infection. Some patients with chronic bacterial prostatitis have persistent symptoms such as perineal pressure, low back pain, or difficulty urinating. Symptoms of acute cystitis or pyelonephritis occur when bacteria, which are repeatedly invading the bladder, overcome the defense mechanisms of the bladder.

Bacteria originating in the prostate may be coated with antibody and, therefore, are a cause of a false-positive ACB test.[189] Following acute bacterial prostatitis, a serum and local immune response is elicited, with the presence of IgA and IgG bacteria-specific immunoglobulins being detected in prostatic secretions. More prolonged prostatic secretion of antigen-specific IgG and IgA is observed in chronic bacterial prostatitis.[270]

Acute Prostatitis

Most cases of acute bacterial prostatitis in the preantibiotic era were caused by *N. gonorrhoeae*. Gram-negative enteric organisms are now the most frequent pathogens.[266] *Neisseria gonorrhoeae* is currently an unusual cause.

Pathologically, acute bacterial prostatitis is characterized by inflammation of part or all of the gland with marked cellular infiltrate (predominantly polymorphonuclear leukocytes), diffuse edema, and hyperemia of the stroma. Microabscesses may occur and may be followed by large, clinically apparent collections of pus.

Acute bacterial prostatitis is characterized by high fever, chills, perineal and back pain, and symptoms of urinary tract infection such as frequency, urgency, and dysuria.[266] The patient may have urinary retention due to bladder outlet obstruction. The prostate gland is warm, swollen, and extremely tender on rectal examination. Expressed prostatic fluid contains many polymorphonuclear leukocytes, and the infecting organism can frequently be seen on Gram stain. However, massage of the acutely infected prostate gland can precipitate bacteremia and should be discouraged. Since most patients also have bacteriuria, the infecting organism can usually be isolated by midstream urine culture. Many antibiotics diffuse well into the acutely inflamed prostate, and acute bacterial prostatitis responds well to appropriate antimicrobial therapy. Complications such as bacteremia, prostatic abscess, epididymitis, seminal vesiculitis, and pyelonephritis may occur.

Chronic Bacterial Prostatitis

Chronic bacterial prostatitis is most commonly caused by *E. coli* (80 percent), but *Klebsiella, Enterobacter, Prot. mirabilis*, and enterococci are also common causes.[266] Although *S. epidermidis, S. aureus*, and diphtheroids have been frequent isolates in some series,[271] there is considerable doubt as to their real pathogenic role, and most gram-positive bacteria cultured in association with prostatitis represent urethral commensals.[266] Reported rare causes of prostatitis include *Candida* species, *Blastomyces dermatitidis, Histoplasma capsulatum, Mycobacterium* tuberculosis, and nontuberculous *Mycobacteria*. The prostate gland has been identified as an important subclinical focus of *C. neoformans* infection. Occasionally histologic specimens of prostatic tissue reveal granulomatous prostatitis of unknown etiology.

The histologic findings of chronic bacterial prostatitis are focal, nonacute inflammation. Similar findings may be noted in patients without evidence of bacterial infection and are therefore not diagnostic of bacterial prostatitis.

Many men with chronic infection of the prostate are totally asymptomatic. However, some have perineal discomfort, low back pain, or dysuria. Symptoms of acute urinary tract infection may appear periodically. In fact, chronic bacterial prostatitis is probably the most common cause of relapsing urinary tract infection in men. Fever, if present, tends to be low grade unless pyelonephritis occurs. The results of rectal examination and intravenous pyelogram are unremarkable unless the patient also has an enlarged prostate gland from benign prostatic hypertrophy or carcinoma.

Because of the focal nature of chronic bacterial prostatitis, needle biopsy of the prostate gland for culture of tissue is unreliable.[272] Demonstration of leukocytes in prostatic fluid is not specific for bacterial prostatitis. Most clinicians agree that more than 15 leukocytes per high-power field represents an abnormal number of leukocytes in prostatic fluid.[266] Provided that simultaneous urethral and midstream specimens show insignificant pyuria, this finding would indicate prostatic inflammation irrespective of the etiology. Meares and Stamey[180] have described a quantitative localization technique for making the bacteriologic diagnosis. Because bacteria present in the urethra can contaminate prostatic secretions obtained by prostatic massage, accurate diagnosis requires simultaneous quantitative cultures of *(1)* urethral urine (VB$_1$), *(2)* midstream urine (VB$_2$), *(3)* prostatic secretions expressed by massage (EPS), and *(4)* the urine voided after massage (VB$_3$).

The specimens must be cultured immediately after collection, and methods of quantitating small numbers of bacteria must be used. The study should be done at a time the patient does not have significant bacteriuria. If bacteriuria is present, ampicillin, cephalexin, or nitrofurantoin should be given for 2–3 days to sterilize the urine; these agents will not affect bacterial counts in the prostate in chronic bacterial prostatitis. If chronic bacterial prostatitis is present, the number of bacteria in EPS or ejaculate will exceed those in VB_1 or VB_2 urine by at least 10-fold. If no EPS or ejaculate can be obtained, the bacterial counts in the VB_3 specimen should be at least 10-fold higher than the VB_1 or VB_2 samples.

Chronic bacterial prostatitis is very difficult to cure since few antimicrobial agents penetrate well into the noninflamed prostate. Furthermore, the nidus of infection in some patients may be small prostatic calculi or abscesses that presumably are difficult to sterilize. Chronic bacterial prostatitis is therefore likely to persist and cause relapsing urinary tract infection. Unlike classic urinary tract infection, relapses may occur after long periods without bacteriuria (e.g., months). Management may be difficult (see "Therapy," below).

Nonbacterial Prostatitis

This syndrome is the most common type of prostatitis and represents an inflammatory condition of unknown cause.[266] The symptoms are perineal pressure, dysuria, urgency, and/or low back pain, symptoms that can also be caused by chronic bacterial prostatitis. However, bacterial pathogens cannot be demonstrated using sequential quantitative cultures. Urinary tract infection does not occur, although prostatic secretions contain excessive numbers of leukocytes and fat-laden macrophages. The most controversial putative agent of nonbacterial prostatitis is *C. trachomatis*. The problem has been in distinguishing urethral colonization with *Chlamydia* from prostatic infection.[266,273,274] Similarly, the role of *U. urealyticum* is obscure. The term *prostadynia* or *prostatosis* refers to a similar clinical syndrome in the absence of any objective signs of prostatic inflammation. Some feel that the symptoms may be caused by spasm of the pelvic floor musculature.[275] Others feel that there may be a major psychological component. Because the etiology of both entities is unknown, therapy is difficult (see "Therapy," below).

Therapy

A dog model has been used to measure diffusion of antimicrobial agents into the noninflamed prostate.[276] In this system, antimicrobial agents are infused, giving high and constant plasma levels, and prostatic secretions are simultaneously collected. Although the basic macrolides such as erythromycin penetrated well into prostatic secretions, penicillins, cephalosporins, tetracyclines, nitrofurantoin, and vancomycin did not. The explanation given was that only lipid-soluble and basic compounds are capable of entering the acid milieu of the prostate gland. Trimethroprim and fluoroquinolones have been shown to diffuse into prostatic fluid in high concentrations.[277]

Acute bacterial prostatitis frequently responds dramatically to antibacterial therapy. It is thought that the intense diffuse inflammatory reaction of acute bacterial prostatitis allows the passage of antimicrobial agents from plasma into the prostate.[266] Therefore, in management of acute prostatitis, antimicrobial agents should be given to the patient in doses that achieve therapeutic concentrations in the blood. Appropriate treatment of coliform infections includes trimethoprim–sulfamethoxazole, cephalosporins, amoxicillin, or any of the fluoroquinolones. Ciprofloxacin, 500 mg bid, is suitable for the occasional episodes caused by *Ps. aeruginosa*. Rarely parenteral antibiotics are required. Following a favorable clinical response, antimicrobial therapy should be continued for a minimum of 4 weeks to prevent the development of chronic bacterial prostatitis. Measures

such as hydration, analgesics, best rest, and stool softeners may be helpful. Urethral instrumentation should be avoided. If acute urinary retention occurs, suprapubic drainage of urine is required through a suprapubic catheter. Prostatic abscess is rarely cured by antimicrobial agents alone and requires surgical drainage. Computed tomography (CT) studies or transrectal ultrasonography are important advances in diagnosis of abscess formation.[278] Drainage can often be achieved by an ultrasound-guided needle.

Chronic bacterial prostatitis is very difficult to cure. Partial transurethral prostatectomy is curative only if all the infected tissue is removed; about one-third of the patients are cured by this procedure.[266] However, a higher percentage is cured if a complete transurethral prostatectomy is performed.[266] Complete prostatectomy is contraindicated because of the complications of sexual impotence and incontinence.

The primary approach to chronic bacterial prostatitis is an attempt at cure with antimicrobial therapy. Although occasional cures have been achieved with penicillins, cephalosporins, tetracyclines, or aminoglycosides, the focus of infection in the prostate has usually persisted, resulting in relapse after therapy was discontinued. Better results have been reported in limited trials with trimethoprim–sulfamethoxazole (one double-strength tablet twice a day). Cure rates have varied from one-third to most of the patients treated 1–3 or more months. The sulfonamide component of trimethoprim–sulfamethoxazole probably contributes little and rifampin may be more suitable than sulfamethoxazole as a partner for trimethroprim.[280] Although prospective comparative studies are needed, clinical series indicate that the new fluoroquinolones, ciprofloxacin, 500 mg bid, norfloxacin, 400 mg bid, ofloxacin, 300 mg bid, and lomefloxacin, 400 mg once daily for 30 days, achieve comparable if not superior results to trimethoprim–sulfamethoxazole.[266,281–283] At present, our initial regimen of choice is trimethoprim–sulfamethoxazole or a quinolone. If therapy fails on these regimens, the patient should be managed either with treatment of acute exacerbations of urinary tract infection or with chronic suppressive therapy using low daily doses (e.g., half-normal doses) of an antimicrobial agent. Nonbacterial prostatitis can be treated empirically with erythromycin or tetracycline relying on clinical response to justify a further trial of therapy. Reassurance is important.

PERINEPHRIC ABSCESS AND INTRARENAL ABSCESS

Perinephric Abscess

Perinephric abscess is an uncommon complication of urinary tract infection.[284] The most common predisposing factors are urinary tract calculi and diabetes mellitus. It usually occurs secondary to obstruction of an infected kidney or calyx or occasionally secondary to bacteremia. It may occur insidiously, and up to one-third of cases may not be diagnosed until autopsy. The infecting bacteria are usually gram-negative enteric bacilli and occasionally gram-positive cocci when the infection is of hematogenous origin. Multiple bacterial species are present in about 25 percent of cases and occasionally fungi, especially *Candida* spp., can be cultured from the abscess. The abscess is usually confined by Gerota's fascia to the perinephric space but may extend throughout the retroperitoneum to affect adjacent structures.[285]

The patients have a syndrome suggestive of acute pyelonephritis, with fever, abdominal and flank pain (usually unilateral), and often symptoms of lower tract infection. However, presenting symptoms are often nonspecific. The patient has often been ill for 2 or more weeks. The diagnosis should be strongly considered in any patient with a febrile illness and unilateral flank pain who does not respond to therapy for acute pyelonephritis. A palpable mass may or may not be present. About one-half of the patients have an abnormal plain film of the abdomen (e.g., abdominal mass, enlarged kidney with indistinct outlines, loss of psoas margin, a calculus, a poorly defined renal shadow), and 85 percent have abnormal intravenous pyelograms. Pyuria and proteinuria are frequently found, but about 30 percent of patients have a normal urinalysis and about 40 percent have sterile urine cultures.[285]

Intrarenal Abscess

Intrarenal abscess may occur as a consequence of bacteremia (often caused by coagulase-positive staphylococci). However, these lesions are being recognized with increasing frequency as a complication of classic acute pyelonephritis. The clinical setting is usually that of acute pyelonephritis with high fever, severe flank pain, and tenderness, but with no response or very slow response to appropriate antimicrobial therapy. CT may detect intense parenchymatous inflammation and necrosis in a lobe of the kidney, termed lobar nephronia. Although antibiotics may arrest progression at this stage, coalescence of microabscesses can lead to intrarenal abscess. Most patients with intrarenal abscess respond, although slowly, to antimicrobial therapy, but fever and severe flank pain may persist for days. Occasionally drainage becomes necessary.

Diagnosis and Therapy

The introduction of renal ultrasound and in particular computed tomography (CT) scans have added a new dimension of sensitivity and specificity permitting the early diagnosis of intrarenal and perinephric abscesses (Figs. 10 and 11).[286–289] The most common CT findings include thickening of Gerota's fascia, renal enlargement, focal parenchymal decreased attenuation, and fluid and/or gas in and around the kidney.[290]

In patients with a clinical or radiographic suspicion of perinephric abscess, diagnostic needle aspiration can be safely performed by using ultrasound or CT scan guidance. When an abscess is confirmed, small catheters can be introduced

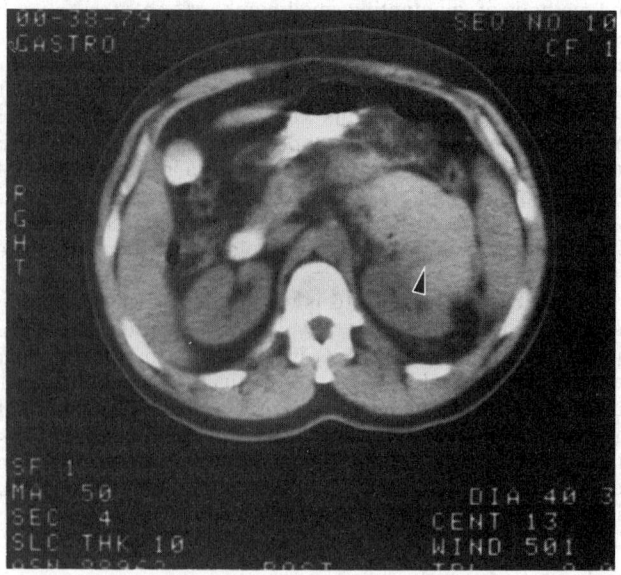

FIG. 11. CT scan showing a perinephric abscess (arrow). (Courtesy of Dr. George Popky, Philadelphia, PA.)

percutaneously via the diagnostic aspiration route to provide immediate decompression as well as continuous and definitive drainage without need for surgery.[286,287,289] Advantages to guided percutaneous drainage compared with open surgical drainage include earlier diagnosis and treatment, avoidance of general anesthesia and surgery, less expensive therapy, easier nursing care, and greater patient acceptance of closed drainage. Accordingly, it is now recommended that after starting antimicrobial therapy directed against the most likely pathogens, a trial of percutaneous drainage should be the initial mode of therapy for perinephric abscess. Surgical intervention should be undertaken only when percutaneous drainage fails or is contraindicated. While parenteral antimicrobial therapy directed against the infecting organism isolated from blood or urine should be initiated before drainage, if additional organisms are isolated at the time of surgery, treatment directed against these organisms must be added. Therapy must also be used for the underlying disease (e.g., obstructive uropathy).

Percutaneous drainage has been equally effective in drainage of renal abscesses and infected renal cysts, often avoiding the previous approach of open surgical drainage or nephrectomy.[286,289,291,292]

Successful percutaneous treatment has been reported in 90 percent of patients with renal or perinephric abscess formation.[289] In the past, delay and missed diagnosis resulted in mortality rates of 20–50 percent, with approximately one-third of cases diagnosed only postmortem. Today, with early recognition utilizing modern imaging techniques, together with prompt drainage and antibiotic therapy the mortality is extremely low.[285]

RADIOLOGIC EVALUATION OF PATIENTS WITH URINARY TRACT INFECTION

Radiologic procedures play an important role in the management of patients with urinary tract infection,[289,293] both in control of complicated episodes of acute pyelonephritis as well as in the investigation of patients of all ages in whom the clinician suspects the presence of underlying structural abnormalities that may be surgically correctable.

Radiologic assessment should commence with a plain film of the abdomen for detection of urinary tract calculi, calcification,

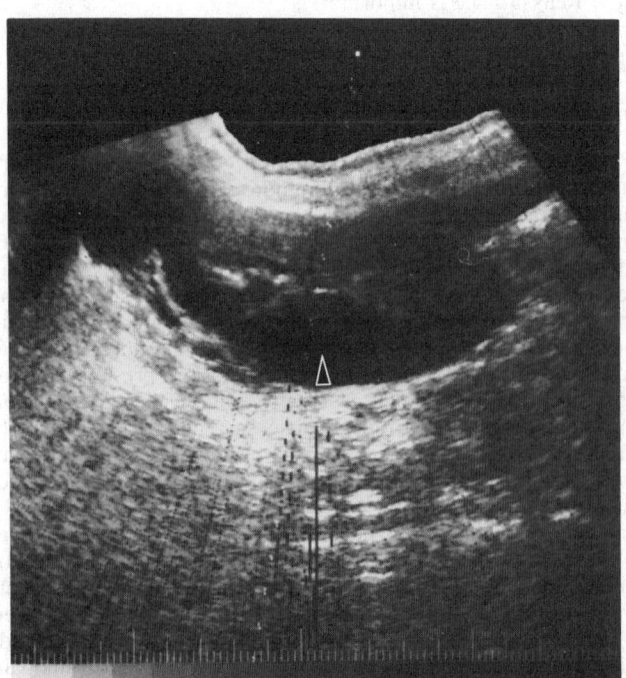

FIG. 10. Ultrasound examination of the kidney showing an intrarenal abscess (arrow). (Courtesy of Dr. George Popky, Philadelphia, PA.)

soft tissue masses, and abnormal gas collections in the past, excretory urography in the form of intravenous pyelography was the initial and definitive investigatory study but has been largely replaced by both ultrasonography and CT scans. In general, sonography serves as a rapid, noninvasive, and relatively inexpensive means of evaluating the renal collecting system, parenchyma, and surrounding retroperitoneum.[208] Ultrasound is more sensitive than IVP for detecting parenchymal changes associated with renal infection.

Recently Johnson et al.[294] confirmed that ultrasonographically demonstrable renal swelling characteristically occurs in almost all women with acute pyelonephritis. Enlargement may be unilateral or bilateral and correlates with protracted pretreatment symptoms, leukocytosis, high fever, focal suppurative complications and prolonged hospitalization. The study also indicated that the frequency of underlying abnormalities and focal complications is low.[294] Several large studies have now confirmed that ultrasonography, especially when combined with a plain film of the abdomen, has become the radiological investigation of choice in young women with urinary tract infection,[295,296] replacing excretory urography.

CT is the most sensitive technique of all. Compared with CT, sonography offers several advantages, including no irradiation, portability, and relative accessibility.[293] Both CT and ultrasound are sensitive in diagnosing intrarenal and perirenal suppuration. When an abscess reaches 2–3 cm in size, it is easily detected by ultrasound.[288] Ultrasound demonstrates a well-marginated, hypoechoic mass with good through transmission, an irregular interior wall margin, and scattered echogenic foci within the mass representing debris. Gas formation is highly echogenic. On CT, most abscesses appear as low-density masses in a nonlobar distribution, with abscess wall enhancing after contrast injection resulting in the "rind sign" owing to the presence of inflamed dilated vessels.[286] When detected, gas within a low-density mass is pathognomonic for abscess formation. Both these procedures may be used for guidance of percutaneous needle aspiration. IVP remains useful for detecting lesions of the collecting system and ureters. Contrast-enhanced CT provides physiologic information similar to that obtained with IVP, with much better parenchymal delineation but less optimal delineation of the collecting system.[290] All studies requiring parenteral administration of contrast material are associated with some risk of allergy or contrast-induced renal insufficiency. Predisposing factors for renal insufficiency include myeloma, diabetes mellitus, preexisting renal failure, severe intravascular volume depletion, and recent administration of large doses of iodinated contrast material. MRI offers no advantage over CT in the diagnosis of intrarenal or perinephric abscess. Radioisotope studies play only a small role, if any, in the investigation of the urinary tract. Gallium-67 citrate scanning and indium-111–labeled white blood cell studies occasionally prove useful in localizing inflammation or infection to the kidneys in patients with fever of unknown origin and may be of value, after ultrasound or CT scans have identified a solid renal mass, in suggesting the inflammatory nature of the lesion.

Radiologic or ultrasound investigation may be indicated in patients with nonresponsive pyelonephritis (particularly if bacteremic) to identify local complications such as renal and perinephric abscess formation. The most important contribution provided by these modalities is the detection of surgically correctable abnormalities of the urinary tract. Investigation should be considered in patients at greatest risk of having surgically correctable abnormalities. Persons with urinary tract infection included in this high-risk category are all children, men of any age, patients who relapse after therapy, and patients whose infection has been complicated by bacteremia. In the past, excretory urography was indicated for all these categories and for adult women only after multiple episodes of urinary tract infection. As mentioned above, given the value of ultrasonography, its availability, and its safety, it is reasonable to study all

patients with upper tract infection by this method. However, as indicated by Johnson et al.,[294] even the routine use of noninvasive renal ultrasonography in women with acute uncomplicated pyelonephritis appears excessive since focal complications are rare and underlying structural abnormalities occur in only about 5 percent of cases. Women with bacteriuria of pregnancy in whom eradication of infection is difficult should be evaluated. Whereas ultrasonography can be safely performed during pregnancy, accurate delineation of the urinary tract should be delayed until at least 2 months after delivery, by which time the physiologic alterations to the urinary tract that occur during pregnancy should be reversed.[248,249] Ultrasound examination is also useful in diagnosing lower urinary tract obstruction and detecting residual urine in the bladder. A radionuclide DTPA scan with furosemide to increase urine flow is useful in determining if there is structural as opposed to functional ureteropelvic junction obstruction.

In addition to delineating lesions amenable to surgical correction, urography frequently provides information previously unknown to the patient or physician. For example, unsuspected renal scarring may be seen, suggesting the presence of undiagnosed urinary tract infection in childhood (Fig. 12). Occasionally an unusual or unsuspected type of renal infection such as tuberculosis, papillary necrosis (Figs. 13 and 14), or xanthogranulomatous pyelonephritis may be discovered.[297] The last is a severe and chronic form of kidney inflammation in which areas of renal parenchyma are replaced by an inflammatory granulomatous reaction characterized by lipid-laden macrophages (foam cells).[297] Renal calculi and obstruction are often associated with this lesion.[249] Two major radiologic patterns are seen: that of a localized mass and that of diffuse nodularity. When a mass lesion is present, differentiation from pyogenic abscess, tuberculous abscess, or avascular carcinoma may not be possible.

Ultrasonography and voiding cystourethrography are recommended in all boys after the first episode of urinary infection and in preschool girls at least after the second infection.[298–300] Investigation is indicated since the incidence of vesicoureteral reflux in this population has been reported to be 20–35 percent. Reflux is associated with renal scar formation, and surgery may be indicated in some of these children and infants. Ultrasonography is as sensitive and has replaced IVP as the initial study in

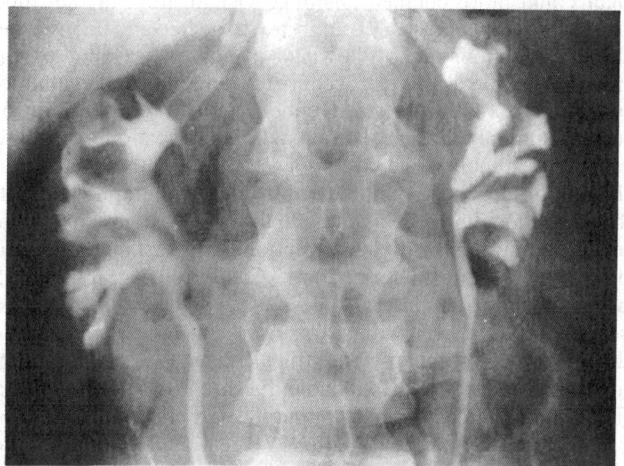

FIG. 12. Bilateral chronic pyelonephritis (retrograde pyelogram). Severe renal insufficiency precluded adequate visualization by excretory urography. Note the severe caliectasis bilaterally with marked left renal atrophy. There is moderate atrophy on the right. While retrograde pyelography is not infrequently required to demonstrate the collecting system in severely diseased kidneys, it is probably best to avoid the performance of bilateral simultaneous retrograde pyelography in the azotemic patient. (From Kaye,[3] with permission).

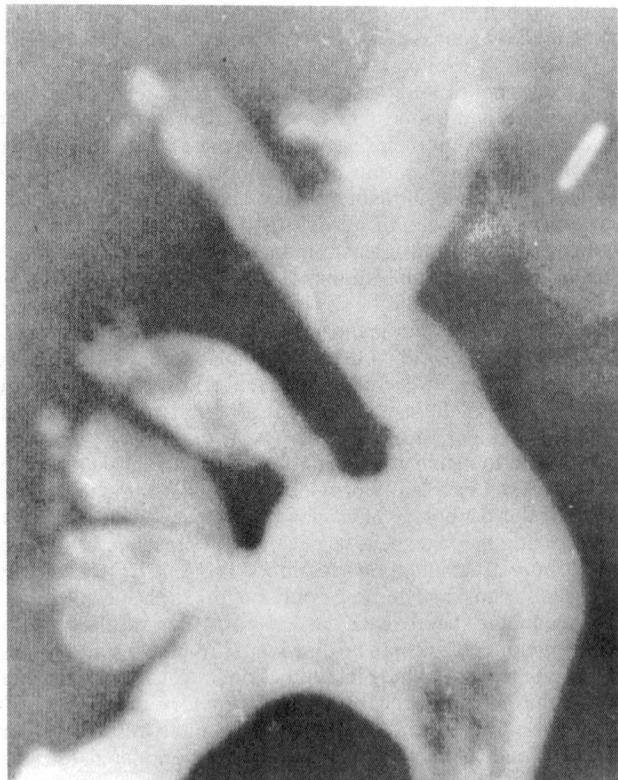

FIG. 13.   Renal papillary necrosis (medullary type). Medullary cavities are seen involving almost all the visualized calyces. The cavities tend to be located within the central portion of the medulla rather than at the calyceal fornices. This is the medullary type of papillary necrosis so frequently associated with sickle cell disease, as was the case in this patient. Filling defects within the renal pelvis are attributable to a combination of sloughed papillas, mucus, and pus. (From Kaye,[3] with permission).

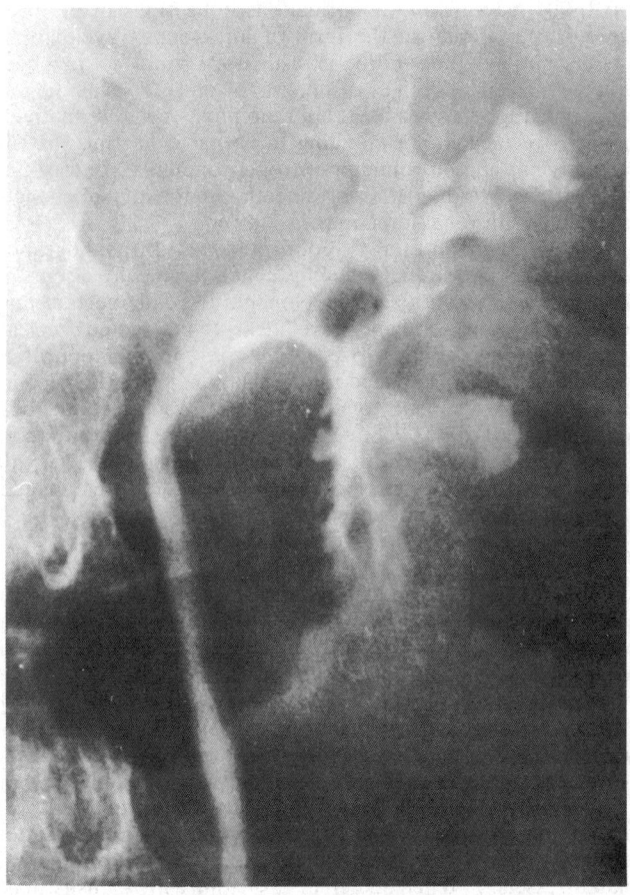

FIG. 14.   Renal papillary necrosis (papillary type). The filling defects in the upper calyces represent sloughed papillas that have completely detached from the medulla. This has been referred to as the *ring sign* and indicates the papillary type of renal papillary necrosis. (From Kaye,[3] with permission).

evaluating children with urinary tract infections and detecting children who require corrective surgery.[298–304] In children, IVP should still be used when other imaging methods show an abnormality and more detailed anatomic visualization of the upper tract is required or urinary calculi are suspected and finally when urinary infections recur following a negative ultrasound examination.[301] As an elective procedure for detection and evaluation of vesicoureteral reflux, conventional cystourethrography or, more commonly, high-resolution radionuclide voiding cystography is still required, especially since reflux with urinary tract dilatation is frequently undetected by ultrasonography and IVP. The use of radionuclide cystography involves less irradiation and is better tolerated than conventional contrast material introduced by bladder catheterization.[301] Cystourethrography should be avoided in older children unless IVP shows evidence of renal scars. However, even with scars, if serial urographic evaluation demonstrates stability of upper tract lesions, the need for studying the lower tract is questionable. Fairley[305] has suggested that it may be possible to avoid cystourethrography by taking a late roentgenogram (4–6 hours) after IVP. By this time the ureters should no longer contain contrast material, but the bladder will be filled. A voiding film taken at this time may then demonstrate presence or absence of reflux. Fairley feels that if no reflux is demonstrated by this method, it is doubtful that cystourethrography will add much in older children and adults. When reflux is found, it should be graded as minimal (grade I) to severe (grade IV), so progression or improvement can be quantitated and decisions on surgery can be made.[138]

SURGICAL MANAGEMENT

Surgical therapy in the management of urinary tract infection consists of the elimination of obstructive lesions or calculi and the reimplantation of ureters in the bladder for reflux. An obstruction may be intrinsic (such as renal cysts), or it may be extrinsic anywhere along the urinary conduit from the ureteropelvic junction to the external urethral meatus. Surgical therapy should be directed toward eliminating the obstruction and preserving renal function. After the obstruction is eliminated, the patient should be followed with urine cultures. Urinary tract infection should be treated before surgery to render the urine sterile at the time of surgery; this decreases the possibility of bacteremia occurring in association with the surgery. For management of perinephric or intrarenal abscess see "Perinephric Abscess" and "Intrarenal Abscess," above.

CATHETER-ASSOCIATED URINARY TRACT INFECTION

See Chapter 282.

SUMMARY FLOW SHEET

Figure 15 summarizes the approach to management of urinary tract infection.

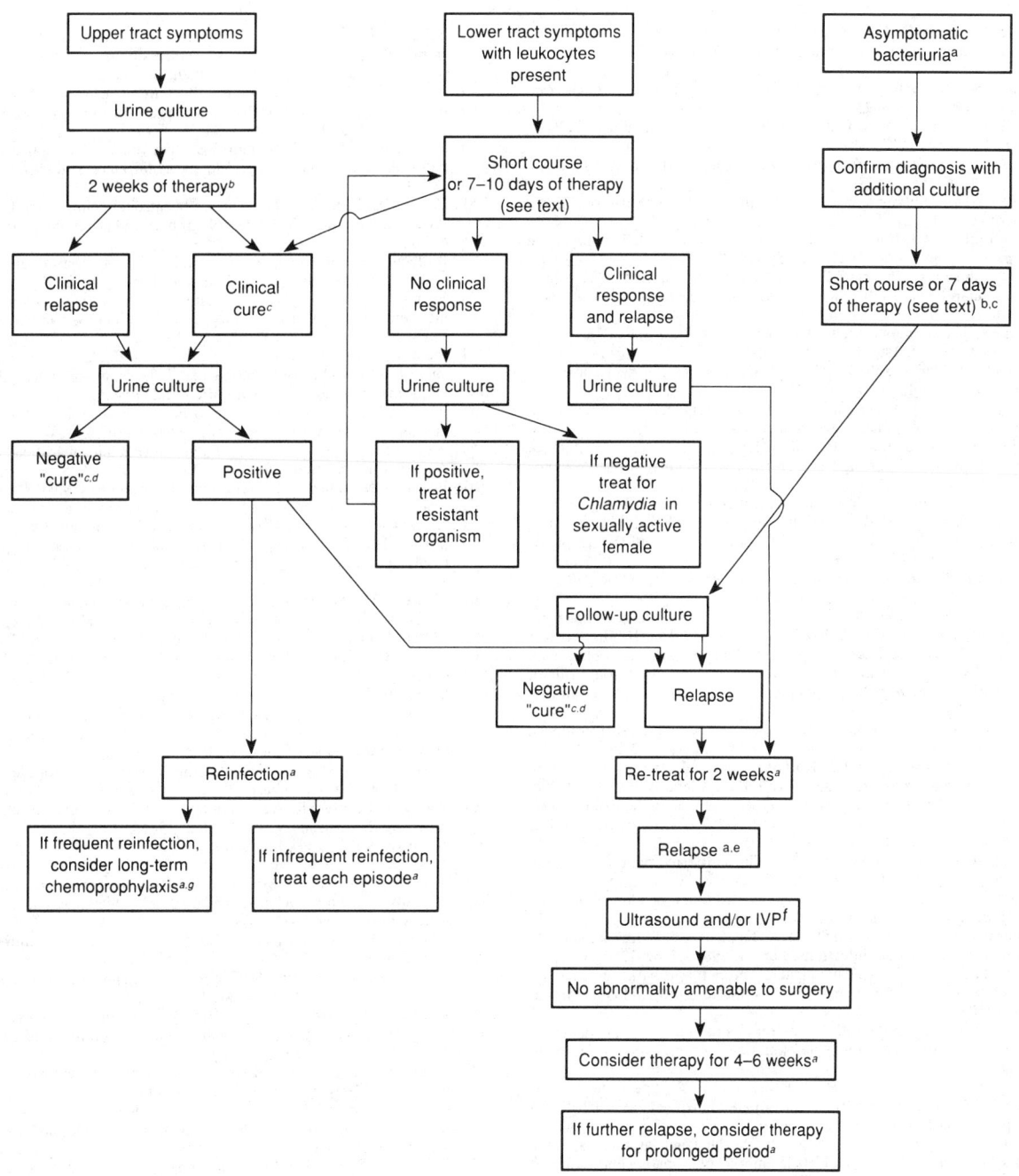

FIG. 15. Management of urinary tract infection.

[a] Consider no therapy in nonpregnant adults without obstructive uropathy or symptoms of urinary tract infection.

[b] Consider ultrasound and/or intravenous pyelogram (IVP) in all children and men with correction of significant lesions.

[c] Follow-up culture required only in pregnancy, in children, and in adults with obstructive uropathy.

[d] Follow-up cultures monthly in pregnant women and at 6 weeks and 6 months in children.

[e] Evaluate men for chronic bacterial prostatitis.

[f] Delay 2 months postpartum in pregnant women.

[g] Consider ultrasound and/or IVP after three to four reinfections in women.

REFERENCES

1. Heptinstall RH. Urinary tract infection and clinical features of pyelonephritis. In: Pathology of the Kidney. 4th ed. v. 3. Boston: Little, Brown and Co.; 1992:1433–88.
2. Heptinstall RH. Pyelonephritis: Pathologic features. In: Pathology of the Kidney. 4th ed. v. 3. Boston: Little, Brown and Co; 1992:1489–561.
3. Kaye D. Urinary Tract Infection and Its Management. St. Louis: CV Mosby; 1972.
4. Freedman L. Chronic pyelonephritis at autopsy. Ann Intern Med. 1967;66:697–710.
5. Huland H, Busch R. Chronic pyelonephritis as a cause of end stage renal disease. J Urol. 1982;127:642–3.
6. Kunin CM. Natural history of lower urinary tract infections. Infection. 1990;18(Suppl 2):S44–9.
7. Monzon OT, Ory EM, Dobson HL, et al. A comparison of bacterial counts of the urine obtained by needle aspiration of the bladder, catheterization and midstream-voided methods. N Engl J Med. 1958;259:764–7.
8. Bran JL, Levison ME, Kaye D. Entrance of bacteria into the female urinary bladder. N Engl J Med. 1972;286:626–9.
9. Buckley RM, McGuckin M, MacGregor RR. Urine bacterial counts following sexual intercourse. N Engl J Med. 1978;298:321–4.
10. Kelsey MC, Mead MG, Gruneberg RN, et al. Relationship between sexual intercourse and urinary tract infection in women attending a clinic for sexually transmitted diseases. J Med Microbiol. 1979;12:511–2.
11. Nicolle LE, Harding GKM, Preiksaitis J, et al. The association of urinary tract infection with sexual intercourse. J Infect Dis. 1982;116:579–83.
12. Foxman B, Frerichs RR. Epidemiology of urinary tract infection: I. Diaphragm use and sexual intercourse. Am J Public Health. 1985;75:1308–13.

13. Leibovici L, Alpert G, Laor A, et al. Urinary tract infections and sexual activity in young women. Arch Intern Med. 1987;147:345–7.

14. Strom BL, Collins M, West SL, et al. Sexual activity, contraceptive use, and other risk factors for symptomatic and asymptomatic bacteremia. Ann Intern Med. 1987;107:816–23.

15. Turck M, Goffe B, Petersdorf RG. The urethral catheter and urinary tract infection. J Urol. 1962;88:834–7.

16. Kass EH. Asymptomatic infections of the urinary tract. Trans Assoc Am Physicians. 1956;69:56–64.

17. Gillespie L. The diaphragm an accomplice in recurrent urinary tract infections. Urology. 1984;24:25–30.

18. Fihn SD, Latham RH, Roberts P, et al. Association between diaphragm use and urinary tract infection. JAMA. 1985;254:240–5.

19. Fihn SD, Johnson C, Pinkstaff C, et al. Diaphragm use and urinary tract infections: analysis of aerodynamic and microbiological factors. J Urol. 1986;136:853–6.

20. Johnson ET. The condom catheter: Urinary tract infection and other complications. South Med J. 1983;76:579–82.

21. Hooton TM, Hillier S, Johnson C, et al. Escherichia coli bacteriuria and contraceptive method. JAMA. 1991;265:64–9.

22. Stamey TA, Timothy M, Millar M, et al. Recurrent urinary infections in adult women. The role of introital enterobacteria. Calif Med. 1971;115:1–19.

23. Vivaldi E, Cotran R, Zangwill DP, et al. Ascending infection as a mechanism in pathogenesis of experimental non-obstructive pyelonephritis. Proc Soc Exp Biol Med. 1959;102:242–4.

24. Measley RE, Levison ME. Host defense mechanisms in the pathogenesis of urinary tract infection. Med Clin North Am. 1991;75:275–86.

25. Murphy JJ, Schoenberg HW, Rattner WH, et al. The role of the lymphatic system in pyelonephritis. Surg Forum. 1960;10:880–3.

26. Roberts AP, Phillips R. Bacteria causing symptomatic urinary infection or bacteriuria. J Clin Pathol. 1979;32:492–6.

27. Svanborg-Eden C, Hagberg L, Hanson LA, et al. Adhesion of Escherichia coli in urinary tract infection. CIBA Found Symp. 1981;80:161–87.

28. Bjorksten B, Kaijser B. Interaction of human serum and neutrophils with Escherichia coli strains: Differences between strains isolated from urine of patients with pyelonephritis or asymptomatic bacteriuria. Infect Immun. 1978;22:308–11.

29. Johnson JR, Moseley SL, Roberts PL, et al. Aerobactin and other virulence factor genes among strains of E. coli. Infect Immun. 1983;40:265–72.

30. Svanborg-Eden C, Gotschlich EC, Korhonen TK, et al. Aspects of structure and function of pili of uropathogenic E. coli. Prog Allergy. 1983;33:189–202.

31. Iwahi T, Abe Y, Nakao M, et al. Role of type 1 fimbriae in the pathogenesis of ascending urinary tract infection induced by Escherichia coli in mice. Infect Immun. 1983;40:265–15.

32. Hagberg L, Hull S, et al. Contribution of adhesin to bacterial persistence in the mouse urinary tract. Infect Immun. 1983;40:265–72.

33. Svanborg-Eden C, Eriksson B, Hanson LA. Adhesion of Escherichia coli to human uroepithelial cells in vitro. Infect Immun. 1977;18:767–74.

34. Kallenius G, Molby R, Svensson SB, et al. Occurrence of P-fimbriated Escherichia coli in urinary tract infections. Lancet. 1981;2:1369–72.

35. Leffler H, Savnborg-Eden C. Glycolipid receptors for uropathogenic Escherichia coli binding to human erythrocytes and uroepithelial cells. Infect Immun. 1981;34:920–9.

36. Orskov I, Ferencz A, Orskov F. Tamm-Horsfall protein or uromucoid is the normal urinary slime that traps type 1 fimbriated Escherichia coli. Lancet. 1980;1:887.

37. Pere A, Nowicki B, Saxen H, et al. Expression of P_1 type-1 and type 1_c fimbriae of Escherichia coli in the urine of patients with acute urinary tract infection. J Infect Dis. 1987;156:567–74.

38. Nowicki B, Labigne A, Mosely S, et al. The Dr hemagglutinin, afimbial adhesins AFA-1 and AFA-III, and F1845 fimbriae of uropathogenic and diarrhea-associated Escherichia coli belong to a family of hemagglutinins with Dr receptor recognition. Infect Immun. 1990;58:279–81.

39. Zafriri D, Gron Y, Eisenstein BI, et al. Growth advantages and enhanced toxicity of Escherichia coli adherent to tissue culture cells due to restricted diffusion of products secreted by the cells. J Clin Invest. 1987;79:1210–6.

40. Schaeffer AJ, Schwan WR, Hulgren SJ, et al. Relationship of type 1 pilus expression in Escherichia coli to ascending urinary tract infections in mice. 1987;55:373–80.

41. Aronson M, Medalia O, Schori L, et al. Prevention of colonization of the urinary tract of mice with Escherichia coli by blocking of bacterial adherence with methyl-α-D-mannopyranoside. J Infect Dis. 1979;139:329–32.

42. Moayeri N, Collins M, O'Hanley P. Efficacy of a Proteus mirabilis outer membrane protein vaccine in preventing experiments Proteus pyelonephritis is a BALB/c mouse model. Infect Immun. 1991;59:3778–86.

43. Silverblatt FS. Host–parasite interaction in the rat renal pelvis: A possible role of pili in the pathogenesis of pyelonephritis. J Exp Med. 1974;140:1696.

44. Svanborg-Eden C, Bjursten LM, Hull R, et al. Influence of adhesins on the interaction of Escherichia coli with human phagocytes. Infect Immun. 1984;44:672–80.

45. Mobley HCT, Chipperdale GR, Teriney JH, et al. MR Haemagglutination of Providencia stuartii correlates with adherence to catheters and with persistence of catheter-associated bacteriuria. J Infect Dis. 1988;157:264.

46. Fader RC, Davis CP. Effect of piliation on Klebsiella pneumoniae infection in rat bladders. Infect Immun. 1980;30:554–61.

47. Mardh PA, Colleen S, Hovelius B. Attachment of bacteria to exfoliated cells from the urogenital tract. Invest Urol. 1979;16:322–6.

48. Schifferli DM, Abraham SN, Beachey EH. Influence of trimethoprim and sulfamethoxazole on the synthesis, expression and function of type 1 fimbriae of Escherichia coli. J Infect Dis. 1986;154:490–6.

49. Johnson JR, Roberts PL, Stamm WE. P fimbriae and other virulence factors in Escherichia coli urosepsis: Association with patient's characteristics. J Infect Dis. 1987;156:225–9.

50. Stapleton A, Mosely S, Stamm WE. Urovirulence determined in Escherichia coli isolates causing first-episode and recurrent cystitis in women. J Infect Dis. 1991;163:773–9.

51. Fowler JE Jr, Stamey TA. Studies of introital colonization in women with recurrent infections. VII. The role of bacterial adherence. J Urol. 1977;117:472–6.

52. Kallenius G, Winberg J. Bacterial adherence to periurethral epithelial cells in girls prone to urinary tract infection. Lancet. 1978;2:540–3.

53. Svanborg-Eden C, Jodal U. Attachment of Escherichia coli to urinary sediment epithelial cells from urinary tract infection prone and healthy children. Infect Immun. 1979;26:837–40.

54. Jacobson S, Carstensen A, Kallenius G, et al. Fluorescence-activated cell analyses of P-fimbriae receptor accessibility on uroepithelial cells of patients wtih renal scarring. Eur J Clin Microbiol. 1986;5:649–54.

55. Parsons CL, Schmidt JD. In vitro bacterial adherence to vaginal cells of normal and cystitis prone women. J Urol. 1980;123:184–7.

56. Weyrauch HM, Bassett JB. Ascending infection in an artificial urinary tract. An experimental study. Stanford Med Bull. 1951;9:25–9.

57. Boyarsky S, Labay P. Ureteral motility. Annu Rev Med. 1969;20:383–94.

58. Svanborg-Eden C, Hagberg L, Hull R, et al. Bacterial virulence versus host resistance in the urinary tracts of mice. Infect Immun. 1987;55:1224–32.

59. Musher DM, Griffith DP, Yawn D, et al. Role of urease in pyelonephritis resulting from urinary tract infection with Proteus. J Infect Dis. 1975;131:177–81.

60. Mobley HLT, Green DM, Triffilis AL, et al. Pyelonephritogenic Escherichia coli and killing of cultured humans renal proximal tubular epithelial cells: Role of hemolysin in some strains. Infect Immun. 1990;58:1281–9.

61. Guze LB, Goldner BH, Kalmanson GM. Pyelonephritis. I. Observation on the course of chronic non-obstructed enterococcal infection in the kidney of the rat. Yale J Biol Med. 1961;33:372–85.

62. Freedman LR, Beeson PB. Experimental pyelonephritis. IV. Observations on infections resulting from direct inoculation of bacteria in different zones of the kidney. Yale J Biol Med. 1958;30:406–14.

63. Beeson PB, Rowley D. The anticomplementary effect of kidney tissue. Its association with ammonia production. J Exp Med. 1959;110:685–97.

64. Rocha H, Fekety FR. Acute inflammation in the renal cortex and medulla following thermal injury. J Exp Med. 1964;119:131–8.

65. Kaye D. Antibacterial activity of human urine. J Clin Invest. 1968;47:2374–90.

66. Asscher AW, Sussman M, Weiser R. Bacterial growth in human urine. In: O'Grady F, Brumfitt W, eds. Urinary Tract Infection. London: Oxford University Press; 1968:3–13.

67. Stamey TA, Fair WR, Timothy MM, et al. Antibacterial nature of prostatic fluid. Nature. 1968;218:444–7.

68. Bryant RE, Sutcliffe MC, McGee FA. Human polymorphonuclear leukocyte function in urine. Yale J Biol Med. 1973;46:113–24.

69. Reinhart H, Obedeanu N, Sobel JD. Quantitation of Tamm-Horsfall protein binding to uropathogenic Escherichia coli and lectins. J Infect Dis. 1990;162:1335.

70. Reinhart H, Obedeanu N, Kaye D, et al. Urinary excretion of Tamm-Horsfall protein in elderly women. J Urol. 1991;146:806–8.

71. Cox CE, Hinman F Jr. Experiments with induced bacteriuria, vesical emptying and bacterial growth on the mechanism of bladder defense to infection. J Urol. 1961;86:739–48.

72. Daifuku R, Stamm WE. Bacterial adherence to bladder uroepithelial cell in catheter associated urinary tract infections. N Engl J Med. 1986;314:72–6.

73. Parsons CL, Greenspan C, Mulholland SG. The primary antibacterial defense mechanism of the bladder. Invest Urol. 1975;13:72–6.

74. Parsons CL, Mulholland SG, Anwar H. Antibacterial activity of bladder surface mucin duplicated by exogenous glycosaminoglycan (heparin). Infect Immun. 1979;24:552–7.

75. Mulholland SG. Lower urinary tract antibacterial defense mechanisms. Invest Urol. 1979;17:93–7.

76. Cobbs CG, Kaye D. Antibacterial mechanisms in the urinary bladder. Yale J Biol Med. 1967;40:93–108.

77. Stamey TA. The role of introital enterobactereria in recurrent urinary infections. J Urol. 1973;109:467–72.

78. Kunin CM, Polyak F, Postel E. Periurethral bacterial flora in women. Prolonged intermittent colonization with Escherichia coli. JAMA. 1980;243:134–9.

79. Stamey TA, Timothy MM. Studies of introital colonization in women with recurrent urinary infections. I. The role of vaginal pH. J Urol. 1975;114:261–3.

80. Stamey TA, Kaufman MF. Studies of introital colonization in women with recurrent urinary infections. II. A comparison of growth in normal vaginal fluid of common versus uncommon serogroups of E. coli. J Urol. 1975;114:264–7.

81. Stamey TA, Timothy MM. Studies of introital colonization in women with recurrent urinary infections. III. Vaginal glycogen concentrations. J Urol. 1975;114:268–70.

82. Stamey TA, Howell JJ. Studies of introital colonization in women with cur-

rent urinary infections. IV. The role of local vaginal antibodies. J Urol. 1976; 115:413–5.

83. Stamey TA, Mihara G. Studies of introital colonization in women with recurrent urinary infections. V. The inhibitory activity of normal vaginal fluid on *Proteus mirabilis* and *Pseudomonas aeruginosa*. J Urol. 1976;115:416–7.

84. Stamey TA, Mihara G. Studies of introital colonization in women with recurrent urinary infections. VI. Analysis of segmented leukocytes on the vaginal vestibule in relation to enterobacterial colonization. J Urol. 1976;116:72–3.

85. Kinane DF, Blackwell CC, Brettle RP, et al. ABO blood group, secretor state, and susceptibility to recurrent urinary tract infection in women. Br Med J. 1982;285:7.

86. Sheinfeld J, Schaeffer AJ, Cordon-Cardo C, et al. Association of the Lewis blood group phenotype with recurrent urinary tract infections in women. N Engl J Med. 1989;320:773–7.

87. Reid G, Brooks HJK, Bacon DF. In vitro attachment of *E. coli* to human epithelial cells: Variations in receptivity during the menstrual cycle and pregnancy. J Infect Dis. 1983;148:412.

88. McGroarty FA, Chong S, Reid G, et al. Influence of the spermicidal compound nonoxynol-9 on the growth and adhesion of urogenital bacteria in vitro. Curr. Microbiol. 1990;21:219–23.

89. Marsh FP, Murray M, Panchamia P. The relationship between bacterial cultures of the vaginal introitus and urinary infection. Br J Urol. 1972;44:368–75.

90. Elkins IB, Cox CE. Vaginal and urethral bacteriology of young women. I. Incidence of gram negative colonization. J Urol. 1974;111:88–92.

91. Cattell WR, McSherry MA, Northeast A, et al. Periurethral enterobacterial carriage in pathogenesis of recurrent urinary infection. Br Med J. 1974;4:136–9.

92. Brumfitt W, Gargan RA, Hamilton-Miller JMT. Periurethral enterobacterial carriage preceding urinary infection. Lancet. 1987;1:824–6.

93. Kurdydyk LM, Kelly K, Harding GMK, et al. Role of cervicovaginal antibody in the pathogenesis of recurrent urinary tract infection in women. Infect Immun. 1980;29:76–82.

94. Hovelius BM, Hedstrom KG, Mollby R, et al. Pathogenesis of urinary tract infections-amoxicillin induces genital *E. coli* colonization. Infection. 1988;5:263.

95. Hanson LA, Ahlstedt S, Fasth A, et al. Antigens of *Escherichia coli*, human immune response, and the pathogenesis of urinary tract infections. J Infect Dis. 19797;136:S144–9.

96. Kaijser B, Larson P, Olling S, et al. Protection against acute pyelonephritis caused by *Escherichia coli* in rats, using isolated capsular antigen conjugated to bovine serum albumin. Infect Immun. 1983;39:142–6.

97. Hanson LA, Fasth A, Jodal U, et al. Biology and pathology of urinary tract infection. J Clin Pathol. 1981;34:695–700.

98. Mattsby-Baltzer I, Claesson I, Hanson LA, et al. Antibodies to lipid A during urinary tract infection. J Infect Dis. 1981;144:319–28.

99. Mattsby-Baltzer I, Hanson LA, Kaijser B, et al. Experimental *Escherichia coli* ascending pyelonephritis in rats: Changes in bacterial properties and the immune response to surface antigens. Infect Immun. 1982;35:639–46.

100. Mattsby-Baltzer I, Hanson LA, Olling S, et al. Experimental *Escherichia coli* ascending infection in rats: Active peroral immunization with live *Escherichia coli*. Infect Immun. 1982;35:647–53.

101. Svanborg-Eden, Svennerholm AM. Secretory immunoglobulin A and G antibodies prevent adhesion of *Escherichia coli* to human urinary tract epithelial cells. Infect Immun. 1978;22:790–7.

102. Rene P, Dinolfo M, Silverblatt FJ. Serum and urogenital antibody response to *Escherichia coli* pili in cystitis. Infect Immun. 1982;38:542–7.

103. Rene P, Silverblatt FJ. Serological response to *Escherichia coli* pili in pyelonephritis. Infect Immun. 1982;37:749–52.

104. DeRee JM, Van DenBosch JF. Serological response to the P fimbriae of uropathogenic *Escherichia coli* in pyelonephritis. Infect Immun. 1987;55:2204–7.

105. Hopkins WJ, Uehling DT, Balish E. Local and systemic antibody responses accompany spontaneous resolution of experimental cystitis in cynomolgus monkeys. Infect Immun. 1987;55:1951–6.

106. Denich K, Blyn LB, Craiu A, et al. DNA sequences of three pap A genes from uropathogenic *Escherichia coli* strains: Evidence of structural and serological conservation. Infect Immun. 1991;59:3849–58.

107. Hedges S, Anderson P, Liden-Janson G, et al. Interlocking response to deliberate colonization of the human urinary tract with gram negative bacteria. Infect Immun. 1991;59:421–7.

108. Bille J, Glauser MP. Protection against chronic pyelonephritis in rats by suppression of acute suppuration. Effect of colchicine and neutropenia. J Infect Dis. 1982;146:220–6.

109. Aoki S, Imamura S, Aoki M, et al. Abacterial and bacterial pyelonephritis. Immunofluorescent localization of bacterial antigen. N Engl J Med. 1969;281:1375–82.

110. Hanson LA, Fasth A, Jodal U. Autoantibodies to Tamm-Horsfall protein, a tool for diagnosing the level of urinary-tract infection. Lancet. 1976;1:226–8.

111. Rocha H. Pathogenesis and clinical manifestations of urinary tract infection. In: Kaye D, ed. Urinary Tract Infection and Its Management. St. Louis: CV Mosby; 1972:6–27.

112. Rocha H, Guze LB, Freedman LR, et al. Experimental pyelonephritis. III. The influence of localized injury in different parts of the kidney on susceptibility to bacillary infection. Yale J Biol Med. 1958;30:341–54.

113. DeNavasquez SJ. Further studies in experimental pyelonephritis produced by various bacteria, with special reference to renal scarring as a factor in pathogenesis. J Pathol Bacteriol. 1956;71:27–32.

114. Cotran TS, Vivaldi E, Zangwill DP, et al. Retrograde pyelonephritis in rats. Am J Pathol. 1963;43:1–31.

115. Rocha H, Santos LCS. Relapse of urinary infection in the presence of urinary tract calculi: The role of bacteria within the calculi. J Med Microbiol. 1969; 2:372–6.

116. Smellie JM, Normand ICS. Experience of follow-up of children with urinary tract infection. In: O'Grady F, Brumfitt W, eds. Urinary Tract Infection. London: Oxford University Press; 1968:123–38.

117. Smellie JM, Normand ICS. Bacteriuria, reflux, and renal scarring. Arch Dis Child. 1975;50:581–5.

118. Gould JC. The comparative bacteriology of acute and chronic urinary tract infection. In: O'Grady F, Brumfitt W, eds. Urinary Tract Infection. London: Oxford University Press; 1968:43–50.

119. Teles E, Rocha H. Epidemiologia de bacteriuria: prevalencia em pacientes hospitalizados e de ambulatorio. In: Rocha H, ed. Temas de Nefrologia. Salvador: Fundacao Goncalo Moniz; 1967:51.

120. Turck M, Stamm WE. Nosocomial infection of the urinary tract. Am J Med. 1981;70:651–4.

121. Kippax PW. A study of *Proteus* infections in a male urological ward. J Clin Pathol. 1957;10:211–4.

122. Soriano F, Aguado JM, Ponto C, et al. Urinary tract infection caused by *Corynebacterium* group D2: Report of 82 cases and review. Rev Infect Dis. 1990;12:1019–28.

123. Finegold SM, Miller LG, Merrill SL, et al. Significance of anaerobic and capnophilic bacteria isolated from the urinary tract. In: Kass EH, ed. Progress in Pyelonephritis. Philadelphia: FA Davis; 1965:159.

124. Paed L, Crump J, Maskell R. Staphylococci as urinary pathogens. J Clin Pathol. 1977;30:427–31.

125. Jordan PA, Iravani A, Richard GA, et al. Urinary tract infection caused by *Staphylococcus saprophyticus*. J Infect Dis. 1980;142:510–5.

126. Hovelius B, Mardh P. *Staphylococcus saprophyticus* as a common cause of urinary tract infections. Rev Infect Dis. 1984;6:328–37.

127. Numazaki YN, Kumasaka T, Yana N, et al. Further study on acute hemorrhagic cystitis due to adenovirus 11. N Engl J Med. 1973;289:344–7.

128. Gutman LT, Turck M, Petersdorf RG, et al. Significance of bacterial variants in urine of patients with chronic bacteriuria. J Clin Invest. 1965;44:1945–2.

129. Maskell R, Pead L, Sanderson RA: Fastidious bacteria and the urethral syndrome. Lancet. 1983;2:1277.

130. Thomsen AC. Mycoplasmas in human pyelonephritis. Demonstration of antibodies in serum and urine. J Clin Microbiol. 1978;8:197.

131. Pickering WJ, Birch DF, Kincaid-Smith P. Biochemical and histologic findings in experimental pyelonephritis due to *Ureaplasma urealyticum*. Infect Immun. 1990;58:3401–6.

132. Neumann CG, Pryles CV. Pyelonephritis in infants and children. Autopsy experience at the Boston City Hospital, 1933–1960. Am J Dis Child. 1962; 104:215–29.

133. McCracken GH. Diagnosis and management of acute urinary tract infections in infants and children. Pediatric Infect Dis. 1987;6:107–12.

134. Sherbotie JR, Cornfeld D. Management of urinary tract infections in children. Med Clin North Am 1991;75:327–38.

135. Jones KV. Urinary tract infections in childhood. Practitioner 1991;235: 135–43.

136. Stull TL, LiPuma JJ. Epidemiology and natural history of urinary tract infections in children. Med Clin North Am. 1991;75:287–97.

137. Huland H, Bush R. Pyelonephritis scarring in 213 patients with upper and lower urinary tract infections: Long-term follow-up. J Urol. 1984;132:936–9.

138. Smellie JM. Reflections on 30 years of treating children with urinary tract infections. J Urol. 1991;146:665–8.

139. Kunin CM. The natural history of recurrent bacteriuria in school girls. N Engl J Med. 1970;282:1443–8.

140. Kunin CM. Urinary tract infections in children. Hosp Pract. 1976;11:91–8.

141. Gillenwater JY, Harrison RB, Kunin CM. Natural history of bacteriuria in school girls. A long-term case–control study. N Engl J Med. 1979;301:396–9.

142. Ronald AR, Patrillo ALS. The natural history of urinary infection in adults. Med Clin North Am. 1991;75:299–312.

143. Foxman B. Recurrent urinary tract infection: Incidence and risk factors. Am J Public Health. 1990;80:331–3.

144. Spach DH, Stapleton AE, Stamm WE. Lack of circumcision increases the risk of urinary tract infection in young men. JAMA. 1992;267:679–81.

145. Nordenstam G, Sundh V, Lincoln K, et al. Bacteriuria in representative population samples of persons aged 72–79 years. Am J Epidemiol. 1989;130: 1176–86.

146. Baldassarre JS, Kaye D. Special problems of urinary tract infection in the elderly. Med Clin North Am. 1991;75:375–90.

147. Kaitz AL, Williams EJ. Bacteriuria and urinary tract infections in hospitalized patients. N Engl J Med. 1960;262:425–30.

148. Turck M, Goffe B, Petersdorf RG. Bacteriuria of pregnancy. N Engl J Med. 1962;266:857–60.

149. Zhanel GG, Harding GKM, Nicolle LE. Asymptomatic bacteriuria in patients with diabetes mellitus. Rev Infect Dis. 1991;13:150–4.

150. Andriole VT, Patterson TF. Epidemiology, natural history, and management of urinary tract infections in pregnancy. Med Clin North Am. 1991;25: 359–73.

151. Gleckman R, Blagg N, Hilbert D, et al. Acute pyelonephritis in the elderly. South Med J. 1982;75:551–4.

152. Boscia JA, Kobasa WB, Abrutyn E, et al. Lack of association between bacteriuria and symptoms in the elderly. Am J Med. 1986;81:979–82.
153. Kaye D, Rocha H. Urinary concentrating ability in early experimental pyelonephritis. J Clin Invest. 1970;49:1427–37.
154. Levison SP, Levison ME. The effect of indomethacin and sodium meclofenamate on the renal concentrating defect in experimental enterococcal pyelonephritis in rats. J Lab Clin Med. 1976;88:958–64.
155. Levison SP, Pitsakis PG, Levison ME. Free water reabsorption during saline diuresis in experimental enterococcal pyelonephritis in rats. J Lab Clin Med. 1982;99:474–80.
156. Norden CW, Tuttle EP. Impairment of urinary concentrating ability in pregnant women with asymptomatic bacteriuria. In: Kass EH, ed. Progress in Pyelonephritis. Philadelphia: FA Davis; 1965:73–80.
157. Hellebusch AA. Renal papillary necrosis. A urological emergency. JAMA. 1969;210:1098–100.
158. Brumfitt W. Urinary cell counts and their value. J Clin Pathol. 1965;18:550–5.
159. Thysell H. Evaluation of chemical and microscopical methods for mass detection of bacteriuria. Acta Med Scand. 1969;185:393–400.
160. Brumfitt W, Percival A. Pathogenesis and laboratory diagnosis of non-tuberculous urinary tract infection: A review. J Clin Pathol. 1964;17:482–91.
161. Boscia JA, Levison ME, Abrutyn E, et al. Correlation of pyuria and bacteriuria in elderly ambulatory women. Ann Intern Med. 1989;110:404–5.
162. Pezzlo M. Detection of urinary tract infections by rapid methods. Clin Microbiol Rev. 1988;1:268–88.
163. Pels RJ, Bor D, Woolhandler S, et al. Dipstick urinalysis screening of asymptomatic adults for urinary tract disorders. JAMA. 1989;262:1221–4.
164. U.S. Preventive Services Task Force. Screening for asymptomatic bacteriuria, hematuria and proteinuria. AFP. 1990;42:389–395.
165. Pappas PG. Laboratory in the diagnosis and management of urinary tract infections. Med Clin North Am. 1991;75:313–25.
166. Cobbs CG. Presumptive tests for urinary tract infections. In: Kaye D, ed. Urinary Tract Infection and Its Management. St. Louis: CV Mosby; 1972:43–51.
167. Leung AKC, Robson WLM. Urinary tract infection in infancy and childhood. Adv Pediatr. 1991;38:257–85.
168. Lipsky BA. Urinary tract infections in men. Ann Intern Med. 1989;110:138–50.
169. Goldberg LM, Vosti KL, Rantz LA. Microflora of the urinary tract examined by voided and aspirated urine culture. In: Kass EH, ed. Progress in Pyelonephritis. Philadelphia: FA Davis; 1965:545.
170. Stamm WE, Wagner KF, Amsel R, et al. Causes of the acute urethral syndrome in women. N Engl J Med. 1980;303:409–15.
171. Stamm WE, Running K, McKuvitt M, et al. Treatment of the acute urethral syndrome. N Engl J Med. 1981;304:956–8.
172. Stamm WE. Quantitative urine cultures revisited. Eur J Clin Microbiol. 1984;3:279–81.
173. Stamm WE, Counts GW, Running R, et al. Diagnosis of coliform infection in acutely dysuric women. N Engl J Med. 1982;307:463–8.
174. Komaroff AL, Pass TM, McCue JD, et al. Management strategies for urinary and vaginal infections. Arch Intern Med. 1978;138:1069–73.
175. Stamm WE. Management of the acute urethral syndrome. Drug Ther. 1982;12:155–9, 162–3, 166.
176. Stamey TA, Govan DE, Palmer JM. The localization and treatment of urinary tract infections: The role of bactericidal urine levels as opposed to serum levels. Medicine. 1965;44:1–36.
177. Turck M, Ronald AR, Peterdorf RG. Relapse and reinfection in chronic bacteriuria. II. The correlation between site of infection and pattern of recurrence in chronic bacteriuria. N Engl J Med. 1968;278:422–7.
178. Fairley KF, Bond AG, Brown RB, et al. Simple test to determine the site of urinary tract infection. Lancet. 1967;2:427–8.
179. Fairley KF, Carson NE, Gutch RC, et al. Site of infection in acute urinary tract infection in general practice. Lancet. 1971;2:615–8.
180. Meares EM, Stamey TA. Bacteriologic localization patterns in bacterial prostatitis and urethritis. Invest Urol. 1968;5:492–518.
181. Clark H, Ronald AR, Cutler RE, et al. The correlation between site of infection and maximal concentrating ability in bacteriuria. J Infect Dis. 1969;120:47–53.
182. Ronald AR, Cutler RE, Turck M. Effect of bacteriuria on renal concentrating mechanisms. Ann Intern Med. 1969;70:723–30.
183. Reeves DS, Brumfitt W. Localization of urinary tract infection. In: O'Grady F, Brumfitt W, eds. Urinary Tract Infection. London: Oxford University Press; 1968:53–67.
184. Andriole VT. Advances in the treatment of urinary infections. J Antimicrob Chemother. 1982;(Jan) 9(Suppl A):163–72.
185. Sheldon CA, Gonzalez RD. Differentiation of upper and lower urinary tract infections: How and when? Med Clin North Am. 1984;68:321–33.
186. Thomas V, Shelokov A, Forland M. Antibody-coated bacteria in the urine and the site of urinary tract infection. N Engl J Med. 1974;290:588–90.
187. Jones SR, Smith JW, Sanford JP. Localization of urinary tract infections by detection of antibody-coated bacteria in urine sediment. N Engl J Med. 1974;290:591–3.
188. Thomas VL, Forland M. Antibody coated bacteria in urinary tract infections. Kidney Int. 1982;21:1–7.
189. Jones SR. The current status of urinary tract infection localization by the detection of antibody-coated bacteria in the urinary sediment. In: Gilbert DN, Sanford JP, eds. Infectious Diseases. Current Topics. v. 1. New York: Grune & Stratton; 1979:97–106.
190. Merritt JL, Keys TF. Limitations of the antibody-coated bateria test in patients with neurogenic bladders. JAMA. 1982;247:1723–5.
191. Harris RE, Thomas VL, Shelokov A. Asymptomatic bacteriuria in pregnancy: Antibody-coated bacteria, renal function and intrauterine growth retardation. Am J Obstet Gynecol. 1975;126:20–5.
192. Thomas VL, Harris RE, Gilstrap LC III, et al. Antibody-coated bacteria in the urine of obstetrical patients with acute pyelonephritis. J Infect Dis. 1975;131(Suppl):557–61.
193. Riedash G, Ritz E, Dreikorn K, et al. Antibody-coating of urinary bacteria in transplanted patients. Nephron. 1978;20:267–72.
194. Montplaisir S, Cote P, Martinelli B, et al. Localization du site de l'infection urinaire chez l'enfant par la recherche des bacteries recouvretes d'anticorps. Can Med Assoc J. 1976;115:1096–9.
195. Hellerstein S, Kennedy E, Nussbaum L, et al. Localization of the site of urinary tract infections by means of antibody-coated bacteria in the urinary sediment. J Pediatr. 1978;92:188–93.
196. Kwasnik I, Klauber G, Tilton RC. Clinical and laboratory evaluation of the antibody-coated bacteria test in children. J Urol. 1979;121:658–61.
197. Ronald AR, Conway B, Zhanel GG. The value of single-dose therapy to diagnose the site of urinary infection. Chemotherapy 1990;36(Suppl 1):2–9.
198. Bakshandeh K, Lynne C, Carrion H. Vesicoureteral reflux and end stage renal disease. J Urol. 1976;557:8.
199. Salfatierra O, Tangaho E. Reflux as a cause of end stage kidney disease. Report of 32 cases. J Urol. 1977;117:441–3.
200. Hodson J, Maling TMJ, McManamon PS, et al. Reflux nephropathy. Kidney Int. 1975;8:S50–8.
201. Rolleston GI, Maling TMJ, Hodson CJ. Intrarenal reflux and the scarred kidney. Arch Dis Child. 1974;49:531–9.
202. Edwards D, Normand ICS, Prescod N, et al. Disappearance of vesicoureteric reflux during long-term prophylaxis of urinary tract infection in children. Br Med J. 1977;2:285–8.
203. Kunin CM. Natural history of ''lower'' urinary tract infections. Infection. 1990;18(Suppl 2):S44–9.
204. Kemper KJ. The case against screening urinalyses for asymptomatic bacteriuria in children. Am J Dis Child. 1992;146:343–6.
205. Kraft JK, Stamey TA. The natural history of symptomatic recurrent bacteriuria in women. Medicine (Baltimore). 1977;56:55–60.
206. Schechter H, Leonard CD, Cribner BH. Chronic pyelonephritis as a cause of renal failure in dialysis candidates. JAMA. 1971;216:514–7.
207. Bullen M, Kincaid-Smith P. Asymptomatic pregnancy bacteriuria: A followup study 4–7 years after delivery. In: Renal Infection and Renal Scarring. Melbourne: Mercedes Publishing; 1970:33.
208. Gower PE, Haswell B, Sidaway ME, et al. Follow-up of 164 patients with bacteriuria of pregnancy. Lancet. 1968;1:990–4.
209. Asscher AW, Chick S, Radford N, et al. Natural history of asymptomatic bacteriuria in non-pregnant women. In: Brumfitt W, Asscher AW, eds. Urinary Tract Infection. London: Oxford University Press; 1973:51–61.
210. Gaches CGC, Miller KW, Roberts BM, et al. The Bristol pyelonephritis registry: 10 years on. Br J Urol. 1976;47:721–5.
211. Zinner S, Kass EH. Long term (10 to 14 years) follow-up of bacteriuria of pregnancy. N Engl J Med. 1971;285:820–4.
212. Gower PE. A long-term study of renal function in patients with radiological pyelonephritis and other allied radiological lesions. In: Brumfit W, Asscher AW, eds. Urinary Tract Infection. London: Oxford University Press; 1973:74–80.
213. Murray T, Goldberg MD. Etiologies of chronic interstitial nephritis. Ann Intern Med. 1975;82:453–9.
214. Dontas AS, Kasviki-Charvati P, Panayiotis CL, et al. Bacteriuria and survival in old age. N Engl J Med. 1981;304:939–43.
215. Boscia JA, Abrutyn E, Kaye D. Asymptomatic bacteriuria in elderly persons. Treat or do not treat? Ann Intern Med. 1987;106:764–6.
216. Nordenstam GR, Brandberg CA, Oden AS, et al. Bacteriuria and mortality in an elderly population. N Engl J Med. 1986;314:1152–6.
217. Boscia JA, Kaye D. Asymptomatic bacteriuria in the elderly. Infect Dis Clin North Am. 1987:1893–905.
218. Platt R, Polk BF, Murdock B, et al. Reduction of mortality associated with nosocomial urinary tract infection. Lancet. 1983;1:893–7.
219. Platt R. Adverse consequences of asymptomatic urinary tract infections in adults. Am J Med. 1987;82(Suppl 6B):47–52.
220. O'Grady F, Gauci CL, Watson BW, et al. In vitro models simulating conditions of bacterial growth in the urinary tract. In: O'Grady F, Brumfitt W, eds. Urinary Tract Infection. London: Oxford University Press; 1968:80–92.
221. Kass EH, Zangwill DP. Principles in the long-term management of chronic infection of the urinary tract. In: Quinn EL, Kass EH, eds. Biology of Pyelonephritis. Boston: Little, Brown; 1960:663–72.
222. Vainrub B, Musher DM. Lack of effect of methenamine in suppression of or prophylaxis against, chronic urinary infection. Antimicrob Agents Chemoterh. 1977;12:625–9.
223. McCabe WR, Jackson GG. Treatment of pyelonephritis: Bacterial, drug and host factors in success or failure among 252 patients. N Engl J Med. 1965;272:1037–44.
224. Stamey TA, Fair WR, Timothy MM, et al. Serum versus urinary antimicrobial concentrations in case of urinary tract infections. N Engl J Med. 1974;291:1159–63.

225. Minuth JN, Masher DM, Thorsteinsonn SB. Inhibition of the antibacterial activity of gentamicin by urine. J Infect Dis. 1976;133:14–21.

226. Kunin CM, Finkelberg Z. Oral cephalexin and ampicillin: Antimicrobial activity, recovery in urine, and persistence in blood of uremic patients. Ann Intern Med. 1970;72:349–56.

227. Hooton TM, Stamm WE. Management of acute uncomplicated urinary tract infection in adults. Med Clin North Am. 1991;75:339–57.

228. Stamm WE, McKevitt M, Counts GW. Acute renal infection in women: Treatment with trimethoprim–sulfamethoxazole or ampicillin for two or six weeks. A randomized trial. Ann Intern Med. 1987;106:341–5.

229. Schwab SJ, Bander S, Klahr S. Renal infection in autosomal dominant polycystic kidney disease. Am J Med. 1987;82:714–8.

230. Michaeli J, Mogle D, Perlberg S, et al. Emphysematous pyelonephritis. J Urol. 1984;131:203–8.

231. Norrby SR. Short-term treatment of uncomplicated lower urinary tract infections in women. Rev Infect Dis. 1990;12:458–67.

232. Saginur R, Nicolle LE. Single-dose compared with 3-day nonfloxacin treatment of uncomplicated urinary tract infection in women. Arch Intern Med. 1992;152:1233–7.

233. Rosenstock J, Smith LP, Gurney M, et al. Comparison of single-dose tetracycline hydrochloride to conventional therapy of urinary tract infection. Antimicrob Agents Chemother. 1985;27:652–4.

234. Harbord RB, Gruneberg RN. Treatment of urinary tract infection with a single dose of amoxycillin, cotrimoxazole or trimethoprim. Br Med J. 1981;283:1301–2.

235. Grossius G. Single dose nitrofurantoin therapy for urinary tract infections in women. Curr Ther Res. 1984;35:925–31.

236. Greenberg RN, Sanders CV, Lewis AC. Single-dose therapy for urinary tract infection with cefaclor. Am J Med. 1981;71:841–5.

237. Stamm WE. Single-dose treatment of cystitis. JAMA. 1980;244:591–2.

238. Philbrick JT, Bracikowski JP. Single-dose antibiotic treatment for uncomplicated urinary infections. Less for less? Arch Intern Med. 1985;145:1672–8.

239. Stamey TA. Recurrent urinary tract infections in female patients: An overview of management and treatment. Rev Infect Dis. 1987;9(Suppl 2):S195–208.

240. Johnson J, Stamm W. Diagnosis and treatment of acute urinary tract infection. Infect Dis Clin North Am. 1987;1:773–91.

241. Wong ES, McKevitt M, Running K, et al. Management of recurrent urinary tract infections with patient-administered single-dose therapy. Ann Intern Med. 1985;102:302–7.

242. Vosti K. Recurrent urinary tract infection: Prevention by prophylactic antibiotics after sexual intercourse. JAMA. 1975;231:934–40.

243. Nicolle LE, Ronald AR. Recurrent urinary tract infection in adult women: Diagnosis and treatment. Infect Dis Clin North Am 1987;1:793–806.

244. Stamey TA, Condy M, Mihara G. Prophylactic efficacy of nitrofurantoin macrocrystals and trimethoprim–sulfamethoxazole in urinary infection. N Engl J Med. 1977;296:780–3.

245. Light RB, Ronald AR, Harding GKM, et al. Trimethoprim alone in the treatment and prophylaxis of urinary tract infection. Arch Intern Med. 1981;141:1807–10.

246. Gruneberg RN, Smellie JM, Leaky A, et al. Long-term low-dose, co-trimoxazole in prophylaxis of childhood urinary tract infection. Bacteriologic aspects. Br Med J. 1976;2:206–8.

247. Brumfitt W, Smith GW, Hamilton-Miller JMT, et al. A clinical comparison between macrodantin and trimethoprim for prophylaxis in women with recurrent urinary infections. J Antimicrob Chemother. 1985;16:111–20.

248. Patterson TF, Andriole VT. Bacteriuria in pregnancy. Infect Dis Clin North Am. 1987;1:807–22.

249. Popky GL, Pollack HW. Radiologic evaluation of patients with urinary tract infection. In: Kaye D, ed. Urinary Tract Infection and Its Management. St. Louis: CV Mosby, 1972:84–123.

250. Guyer PB, Delaney D. Urinary tract dilatation and oral contraceptives. Br Med J. 1970;4:588–90.

251. Andriole VT, Cohn GL. The effect of diethystilbestrol on the susceptibility of rats to hematogenous pyelonephritis. J Clin Invest. 1973;43:1136–45.

252. Norden CW, Kass EH. Bacteriuria of pregnancy: A critical appraisal. Annu Rev Med. 1968;19:431–70.

253. Norden CW. Significance and management of bacteriuria in pregnancy. In: Kaye D, ed. Urinary Tract Infection and Its Management. St. Louis: CV Mosby; 1972:171–87.

254. Pedler SJ, Bint AJ. Management of bacteriuria in pregnancy. Practical Therapeutics. 1987;33:413–21.

255. Kass E. Bacteriuria and pyelonephritis of pregnancy. Trans Assoc Am Physicians. 1959;72:257–64.

256. Golan A, Wexler S, Amit A, et al. Asymptomatic bacteriuria in normal and high risk pregnancy. Eur J Obstet Gynecol Reprod Biol. 1989;33:101–8.

257. Kincaid-Smith P, Bullen M. Bacteriuria in pregnancy. Lancet. 1965;1:395–9.

258. Krieger JN. Complications and treatment of urinary tract infections during pregnancy. Urol Clin North Am. 1986;13:685–93.

259. Condie AP, Williams JD, Reeves DS, et al. Complications of bacteriuria in pregnancy. In: O'Grady F, Brumfitt W, eds. Urinary Tract Infection. London: Oxford University Press; 1968:148–59.

260. Schultz R, Read AW, Straton JA, et al. Genitourinary tract infections in pregnancy and low birth weight: Case–control study in Australian aboriginal women. Br Med J. 1991;303:1369–73.

261. Gruneberg R, Leigh D, Brumfitt W. Relation of bacteriuria to acute pyelonephritis, prematurity and fetal mortality. Lancet. 1969;2:1–3.

262. Leigh D, Gruneberg R, Brumfitt W. Long term followup of bacteriuria in pregnancy. Lancet. 1968;1:603–5.

263. Williams JD, Reeves DS, Condie AD, et al. The treatment of bacteriuria in pregnancy. In: O'Grady F, Brumfitt W, eds. Urinary Tract Infection. London: Oxford University Press; 1968:160–9.

264. Adelson MD, Graves WL, Osborne NG. Treatment of urinary infections in pregnancy using single versus 10-day dosing. J Natl Med Assoc. 1992;84:73–5.

265. Pfau A, Sacks TG. Effective prophylaxis for recurrent urinary tract infections during pregnancy. Clin Infect Dis. 1992;14:810–4.

266. Meaves EM Jr. Prostatitis. Med Clin North Am. 1991;75:405–24.

267. Kirby RS, Lowe ED, Bultitude MI, et al. Intraprostatic urinary reflux: An aetiological factor in abacterial prostatitis. Br J Urol. 1982;54:729–31.

268. Stamey TA. Urinary infections in males. In: Pathogenesis and Treatment of Urinary Tract Infections. Baltimore: Williams & Wilkins; 1980:342–429.

269. Fair WR, Cough J, Wehner N. The purification and assay of the prostatic antibacterial factor (PAF). Biochem Med. 1973;8:329–39.

270. Shortliffe LM, Wehner N. The characterization of bacterial and nonbacterial prostatitis by prostatic immunoglobulins. Medicine. 1986;65:399–414.

271. Drach GW. Prostatitis: Man's hidden infection. Urol Clin North Am. 1975;2:499–520.

272. Kohnen PW, Drach GW. Patterns of inflammation in prostatic hyperplasia: A histologic and bacteriologic study. J Urol. 1979;121:755–60.

273. Weidner W, Brunner H, Krause W. Quantitative culture of *Ureaplasma urealyticum* in patients with chronic prostatitis. J Urol. 1980;124:62–7.

274. Abdelatif OM, Chandler FW, McGuire BS Jr. *Chlamydia trachomatis* in chronic abacterial prostatitis: Demonstration by colorimetric in situ hybridzation. Hum Pathol. 1991;22:41–4.

275. Segura JW, Opitz J, Green LF. Prostatosis, prostatitis, or pelvic floor tension myalgia? J Urol. 1979;122:168–9.

276. Winningham DF, Nemoy NJ, Stamey TA. Diffusion of antibiotics from plasma into prostatic fluid. Nature. 1968;219:139–43.

277. Stamey TA, Bushby SRM, Bragonse J. The concentration of trimethoprim in prostatic fluid: nonionic diffusion or active transport. J Infect Dis. 1973;128(Suppl):S686–90.

278. Mears EM Jr. Editorial: Prostatic abscess. J Urol. 1986;136:1281–2.

279. Meares EM. Long-term therapy of chronic bacterial prostatitis with trimethoprim–sulfamethoxazole. Can Med Assoc J. 1975;112(Spec. No):22–5.

280. Giamarellou H, Kosmidis J, Leonidas M, et al. A study of the effectiveness of rifampin in chronic prostatitis caused mainly by *Staphylococcus aureus*. J Urol. 1982;128:321–4.

281. Naber KG. The role of quinolones in the treatment of chronic bacterial prostatitis. Infection. 1991;19(S3):S170–7.

282. Weidner W, Schiefer HG, Brahler E. Refractory chronic bacterial prostatitis: A re-evaluation of ciprofloxacin treatment after a median followup of 30 months. J Urol. 1991;146:350–2.

283. Pfau A. The treatment of chronic bacterial prostatitis. Infection. 1991;19(Suppl 3):S160–4.

284. Thorley JD, Jones SR, Sanford JP. Perinephric abscess. Medicine (Baltimore). 1974;53:441–51.

285. Steinfeld J, Erturk E, Spataro Rd, et al. Perinephric abscess: Current concepts. J Urol. 1987;137:191–204.

286. Gerzof SG, Gale ME. Computed tomography and ultrasonography for diagnosis and treatment of renal and retroperitoneal abscesses. Urol Clin North Am. 1982;9:185–93.

287. Rauschkolb EN, Sandler CM, Patel S, et al. Computed tomography of renal inflammatory disease. J Comp Assist Tomogr. 1982;6:502–6.

288. Hoddick W, Jeffery RB, Goldberg HI. CT and sonography of severe renal and perirenal infections. AJR. 1983;140:517–20.

289. Huligowska E, Newman B, White S, et al. Interventional ultrasound in detection and treatment of renal inflammatory disease. Radiology 1983;147:521–6.

290. Bova JG, Potter JL, et al. Renal and perirenal infection. The role of computerized tomography. J Urol. 1985;133:375–8.

291. Costello AJ, Blandy JP, Hately W. Percutaneous aspiration of renal cortical abscess. Urology. 1983;21:201–4.

292. Finn DJ, Palestrant AM, DeWolf WC. Successful percutaneous management of renal abscess. J Urol. 1982;127:425–6.

293. Piccirello M, Rigsby C, Rosenfield AT. Contemporary imaging of renal inflammatory disease. Infect Dis Clin North Am. 1987;1:927–64.

294. Johnson JR, Vincent LM, Wang K, et al. Renal ultrasonagraphic correlates of acute pyelonephritis. Clin Infect Dis. 1992;14:15–22.

295. McNicholas MM, Griffin JF, Cantwell DF. Ultrasound of the pelvis and renal tract combined with a plain film of the abdomen in young women with urinary tract infection: Can it replace intravenous urography? A prospective study. Br J Radiol. 1991;64:221–4.

296. Spencer J, Lindsell D, Mastorakou I. Ultrasonography compared with intravenous urography in investigation of urinary tract infection in adults. Br Med J. 1990;301:221–4.

297. Grainger RG, Longstaff AJ. Xanthogranulomatous pyelonephritis: A reappraisal. Lancet. 1982;1:1398–401.

298. Hellerstein S, Wald ER, Winberg J, et al. Consensus: Roentgenographic evaluation of children with urinary tract infections. Pediatr Infect Dis. 1984;3:291–3.

299. Koff SA. A practical approach to evaluating urinary tract infection in children. Pediatr Nephrol. 1991;5:398–400.

300. Hanbury DC, Whitaker RH, Sherwood T, et al. Ultrasound and plain x-ray screening in childhood in urinary tract infection. Br J Urol. 1989;64:638–40.

301. Honkinen O, Ruuskanen O, Rikalairen H, et al. Ultrasonography as a screening procedure in children with urinary tract infection. Pediatr Infect Dis. 1986;5:633–5.
302. Leonidas JC, McCauley RG, Klauber G, et al. Sonography as substitute for excretory urography in children with urinary tract infection. Am J Roentgenol. 1985;144:815–9.
303. Mason WG Jr. Urinary tract infections in children: Renal ultrasound evaluation. Radiology. 1984;153:109–11.
304. Kangarloo H, Gold RH, Fine RN, et al. Urinary tract infection in infants and children evaluated by ultrasound. Radiology. 1985;154:367–73.
305. Fairley KF. The investigation and treatment of urinary tract infection. Med J Aust. 1976;2:305–7.

SECTION E

56. SEPSIS SYNDROME

LOWELL S. YOUNG

Sepsis syndrome has been defined as the earliest stage during an infectious process at which evidence of altered organ perfusion can be detected.[1,2] However, this concept is mired in controversy. Clinicians, intensivists, and infectious disease specialists have employed different terminologies for similar but overlapping clinical conditions. Additional difficulties relate to the challenge of establishing the etiology and extent of an apparent infection. Some noninfectious clinical states (e.g., pancreatitis) may mimic an acute infectious process and be equally catastrophic.[3] While infectious diseases specialists have focused on bacterial infections (both gram positive and gram negative), for much of the last four decades, it is well recognized that fulminant parasitic infections, miliary tuberculosis, and systemic fungal disease can present with the same manifestations as gram-negative septicemia. Indeed, one of the major gains of the last few years of clinical research has been the identification of mediators or cytokines that appear to be responsible for the pathophysiologic changes associated with the systemic manifestations of infection.[4,5] These cytokines are produced upon interaction between host cells such as monocytes and macrophages and microorganisms and/or their products, which may or may not be present in the peripheral circulation. Not surprisingly, as in the case of tumor necrosis factor-α (TNF-α), a specific molecule has been associated with the pathophysiologic changes observed in such diverse states as gram-negative bacillary septicemia, meningococcemia, staphylococcal toxic shock syndrome, pulmonary tuberculosis, and cerebral malaria.[6] In this sense, the sepsis syndrome may be considered a constellation of signs and symptoms that represents the host's response to infection, whereby the effects of cytokines (or substances triggered by cytokines) are responsible for most of the clinical manifestations.

With respect to the issue of definitions, Table 1 is an attempt to modify some of the concepts recently advanced by a committee of the American College of Chest Physicians/Society of Critical Care Medicine.[3] *Infection*, as defined by the presence of organisms in a normally sterile site, can be symptomatic, but it may also be inapparent or subclinical. It is important to recognize that *bacteremia*—the presence of organisms that can be cultured from the blood—is probably a transient phenomenon for virtually every bacterial infection except endocarditis or severe intravascular infection. *Septicemia* is a term that traditionally has been used interchangeably with *bacteremia*, but many clinicians feel that it implies greater severity. To confuse matters further, the term *sepsis* has often been used by many clinicians in a manner synonymous with the term *infection* but without

specifying culture positivity of the blood or body fluids. Increasingly, *septic* refers to individuals who are felt to have systemic infection or who have clinical and laboratory changes consist with a systemic infection but who do not have positive blood cultures. Thus, the term *sepsis* has been used for a clinical situation in which there is evidence of infection plus a systemic response as manifested by an elevated temperature, tachycardia, increased respiration, leukocytosis or an impaired peripheral leukocyte response, and/or the presence of immature band forms in the peripheral circulation. Emphasizing a degree of increased severity, the term *sepsis syndrome* has been defined as sepsis with evidence of altered organ perfusion with at least one of the following: hypoxemia, elevated lactate levels, oliguria, and altered mentation. All of these functions imply some degree of organ dysfunction. *Severe sepsis* clearly represents a

TABLE 1. Some Definitions of Sepsis, Sepsis Syndrome, Bacteremia, and Related Disorders

Disorder	Definition
Infection	Presence of organisms in a normally sterile site that is usually, but not necessarily, accompanied by an inflammatory host response
Bacteremia	Bacteria present in blood, as confirmed by culture; may be transient
Septicemia	Same as bacteremia, but implies greater severity
Sepsis	Clinical evidence of infection, plus evidence of a systemic response to infection. This systemic response is manifested by two or more of the following conditions: Temperature >38°C or <36°C; Heart rate >90 beats/min; Respiratory rate >20 breaths/min or $PaCO_2$ <32 mmHg (<4.3 kPa); WBC >12,000 cells/mm³, <4000 cells/mm³, or >10% immature (band) forms
Sepsis syndrome	Sepsis plus evidence of altered organ perfusion with at least one of the following: hypoxemia, elevated lactate, oliguria, altered mentation
Hypotension	A systolic blood pressure of <90 mmHg or a reduction of >40 mmHg from baseline in the absence of other causes of hypotension
Severe sepsis	Sepsis associated with organ dysfunction, hypoperfusion, or hypotension. Hypoperfusion and perfusion abnormalities may include, but are not limited to, lactic acidosis, oliguria, or an acute alteration in mental status
Septic shock	Sepsis with hypotension despite adequate fluid resuscitation along with the presence of perfusion abnormalities that may include, but are not limited to, lactic acidosis, oliguria, or an acute alteration in mental status. Patients who are on inotropic or vasopressor agents may not be hypotensive at the time that perfusion abnormalities are measured
Refractory septic shock	Septic shock that lasts for more than 1 hour and does not respond to fluid administration or pharmacologic intervention
Systemic inflammatory response syndrome	Response to a wide variety of clinical insults, which can be infectious, as in sepsis, but can be noninfectious in etiology (e.g., burns, pancreatitis)

(Data from refs. 1–3.)

more advanced degree of organ compromise. Tissue hypoperfusion in severe sepsis may include, among other manifestations, lactic acidosis, oliguria, or changes in mental status.

Clinically, one of the most frequently obtained bedside measurements is that of blood pressure. Often we do not know what the normal blood pressure is of an individual who is admitted to hospital through an emergency room or to a critical care unit. A widely used breakpoint for *hypotension* is a systolic blood pressure of less than 90 mmHg or a reduction of greater than 40 mmHg from baseline in the absence of other causes of hypotension. Again, it must be recognized that blood pressure is a fluctuating variable and that some patients may have significant changes over a period of hours. Hypotension may be readily corrected by a fluid challenge, and thus the term *septic shock* should be reserved for patients who have sepsis syndrome and hypotension despite an attempted fluid resuscitation of at least 500 ml of saline. Some patients who are receiving inotropic or vasopressor agents who may not be hypotensive at the time that perfusion abnormalities are measured may yet have evidence for septic shock.

Refractory septic shock refers to septic shock that lasts for more than 1 hour and does not respond to fluid administration or pharmacologic intervention with pressor agents. The 1 hour dividing point is admittedly arbitrary.

Finally, a term that is being increasingly used by intensivists is that of *systemic inflammatory response syndrome* (SIRS). This is perhaps the broadest category of all and includes a wide variety of clinical conditions that are essentially infectious in nature, such as the sepsis syndrome, but also encompasses noninfectious entities such as burns and pancreatitis when fever and organ hypoperfusion may be present.[3] The sepsis syndrome can be considered a subset of patients with SIRS.

In an era of increasingly widespread use of antibiotics in the out-patient or home care setting, culture negativity in febrile patients with many of the hallmarks of bacterial infection is very common by the time such patients reach an acute treatment facility. The rationale for not requiring that bacteremia be present in the definition of the sepsis syndrome derives from a prospective study of sepsis and septic shock.[7] Shock occurred in 47 percent of bacteremic patients and in 30 percent of nonbacteremic patients, but the overall mortality and the ability to reverse shock were the same for the two groups. Thus, the nonmicrobiologic terms like *sepsis, sepsis syndrome,* and *SIRS,* while confusing, represent common clinical situations that prompt diagnostic measures and usually result in the initiation of antimicrobial therapy, depending on the severity of disease.

EPIDEMIOLOGIC CONSIDERATIONS

Terms such as *sepsis* and *sepsis syndrome* are clinical definitions and thus have no direct relationship to microbiologic information. However, voluntary surveillance networks such as the National Nosocomial Infection System (NNIS) provide data from selected American hospitals on the relative occurrence of blood stream infections.[8] Prior to the institution of this voluntary (and therefore selective) surveillance system, information on important blood stream infections was inferred from the experience of teaching hospitals. An often quoted study by McCabe some two decades ago estimated that there were some 300,000 episodes of gram-negative bacillary bacteremia in the United States each year.[9] This estimate may have reflected data from large university hospitals primarily and a special task force collecting data from the Centers for Disease Control and Prevention (CDC) estimated that 71,000–140,000 cases occur annually.[10] A population-based estimate of aerobic gram-negative bacteremia in one U.S. county was 42 cases per 100,000 persons per year.[11] Applying similar techniques to the CDC and McCabe estimates, one derives an estimate of between 34 and 145 cases per 100,000 population per year, respectively. More recent data from the National Hospital Discharge survey collected from a stratified sample of U.S. acute care hospitals and weighted to reflect national distribution, demonstrated a dramatic increase in the rate of septicemia from 73.6 per 100,000 population (164,000 cases) in 1979 to 176 per 100,000 or 425,000 cases in 1987.[12] The total number of septicemia discharges was 2,570,000 for the 9-year period. Over the same period, the percentage of all hospital discharges that included septicemia as a diagnosis increased from 0.5 to 1.3%. The proportion of cases due to gram-negative vs. gram-positive bacteria was not specified in this survey. Septicemia was the thirteenth leading cause of death in the United States according to this survey of discharge diagnosis.

Data from NNIS as well as from intrainstitutional surveys indicate an upsurge in gram-positive infections occurred during the past decade and a half.[13] Hospital-wide surveillance performed by NNIS indicates that the highest rates for hospital-acquired blood stream infection—1.0, 1.4, and 3.9 per 100 discharges—were observed for oncology, burn/trauma, and high risk nursery services, respectively.[14] In the summary of the 1985–1988 period, staphylococci and streptococci were the leading causes of blood stream infection, but *Escherichia coli, Enterobacter* spp., and *Pseudomonas aeruginosa* were the fourth, fifth, and sixth leading causes of bacteremia.[8]

CLINICAL MANIFESTATIONS

Table 1 represents an attempt to categorize a set of overlapping clinical states, and includes clinical conditions that may evolve from one stage to another. The clinician faces the task of determining the likely cause of the clinical state so that appropriate therapy can be instituted. Table 2 is an attempt to summarize some of the common signs and symptoms seen in the bacterial infections with either gram-positive or gram-negative organisms, recognizing that such findings are by no means restricted to bacterial processes. Such findings should prompt careful culture of blood, cultures of likely sources of infection, and prompt consideration of the initiation of antimicrobial therapy. The distinction between primary manifestations and complications is arbitrary; indeed, complications such as hypotension, bleeding, hypoxia, acidosis, and jaundice may be the major clues that first suggest the diagnosis. Although fever and chills are typically encountered, some patients who develop systemic bacterial infections are debilitated and do not exhibit striking changes such as rigors early during the course of infection. Paradoxically, hypothermia rather than hyperthermia can occasionally be the manifestation of a systemic bacterial process, and this is associated with a poor prognosis. While neutropenia definitely predisposes to systemic infection, a precipitous decline in the neutrophil count from a normal or an already depressed level may commonly be seen in immunosuppressed patients. The clinician should be alert to the possibility that hypotension, a fall in urine output, a decrease in circulating platelet levels, and evidence for bleeding even in the absence of fever and chills could be manifestations of a systemic infectious process or be the result of the systemic absorption of bacterial toxins from a focal infectious process.

Even before elevation of temperature or the onset of chills, bacteremic patients may begin to hyperventilate. Continuous

TABLE 2. Signs and Symptoms Suggesting a Systemic Bacterial Infection as the Cause of the Sepsis Syndrome

Primary	Complications
Fever	Hypotension
Chills	Bleeding
Hyperventilation	Leukopenia
Hypothermia	Thrombocytopenia
Skins lesions	Organ failure
Change in mental status	Lung: cyanosis, acidosis
	Kidney: oliguria, anuria, acidosis
	Liver: jaundice
	Heart: congestive failure

monitoring of patients in intensive care units has indicated that the earliest clinical finding is apprehension and hyperventilation; thus, the earliest metabolic change in the sepsis syndrome and in gram-negative bacillary infections in particular is a resultant respiratory alkalosis.[15] In the critically ill patient, a sudden change of status manifested by hyperventilation should lead to obtaining blood cultures and to a careful evaluation for the possibility of infection. Change in mental status can also be an important clinical clue: while the most common pattern is lethargy or obtundation, an occasional patient may become excited, agitated, or combative or display bizarre behavior.[16]

Cutaneous manifestations of the septic process can be seen with bacterial, viral, fungal, and even parasitic processes. In bacterial infections, it has long been recognized that staphylococcal or streptococcal disease can result in metastatic infection of the skin and thus provide an opportunity for early diagnosis and initiation of specific antimicrobial treatment. In addition to causing cellulitis, the gram-positive pathogens can cause a diffuse erythroderma that is the result of the pathophysiologic action of pyrogenic or erythrogenic toxins.[17] As with the gram-negative endotoxins, these substances can cause multiorgan damage. From the viewpoint of clinical manifestations, erythroderma can be striking, and it may not be possible to distinguish between the advancing edge of a cellulitic process and the manifestations of one of these erythrogenic toxins. Aspiration of the leading edge of an advancing erythematous process may be clinically useful and may provide material for an early diagnosis.

Cutaneous manifestations of gram-negative bacillary bacteremia, usually colorful skin lesions, were described as early as the previous century.[18] Skin lesions have been most commonly associated with *P. aeruginosa* bacteremia. The so-called pathognomonic skin lesion of *P. aeruginosa* bacteremia was described and given the name *ecthyma gangrenosum*.[19] Ecthyma gangrenosum lesions are round or oval, vary from 1 to 5 cm, and have a raised halo or rim of erythema and induration that surround a central area that may begin as vesicle but usually evolves into a necrotic ulcer (Fig. 1). The appearance of these "bull's-eye"–type lesions strongly suggests *P. aeruginosa* infection and has been observed in 5–25 percent of all *Pseudomonas* bacteremias. In the thrombocytopenic patient, the periphery of these lesions may become ecchymotic. Biopsy specimens

of the lesions indicate that the underlying process is infectious, with direct vascular invasion by bacilli and thrombosis on the venous side of the capillary bed.[19] It seems likely that extracellular products of bacteria such as proteases (elastases) and/or exotoxins are responsible for tissue damage. Nonetheless, there are some reports attributing this phenomenon to local manifestations of Schwartzman reactions in the skin, that is, a localized area of consumption coagulopathy where venous thrombosis triggered perhaps by endotoxin is the initiator of tissue injury. By and large, however, most of these ecthyma lesions appear to be infectious because organisms can be directly aspirated or cultured from these lesions and histopathologic sections reveal organisms invading blood vessel walls. Thus, the presence of ecthyma lesions can be considered indicative of bacteremia.

It has become clear that, while ecthyma-type lesions are strongly suggestive of *P. aeruginosa* infection, the latter are not the only organisms that can cause this characteristic lesion. *Aeromonas hydrophila* can produce a clinical picture similar to that of *P. aeruginosa* infection, and a large proportion of bacteremic patients have had ecthyma-like skin lesions.[20,21] Additionally, cutaneous lesions have been observed in *E. coli*,[22] *Klebsiella, Enterobacter,* and *Serratia* septicemia. Besides ecthyma lesions, colorful vesicular or bullous lesions, cellulitis, diffuse erythematous reactions (similar to scarlet fever), or showers of petechial lesions (not unlike meningococcemia) can be cutaneous manifestations of gram-negative bacteremia.[23] Thus, cutaneous lesions should not lead the clinician to make a specific etiologic diagnosis (although ecthyma-type lesions in the neutropenic patient are most often due to *P. aeruginosa*) but to alert medical personnel to the possibility of a systemic gram-negative bacillary infection, the need for diagnostic measures, and therapeutic intervention. The availability of a lesion from which a biopsy specimen can be obtained and that is easily aspirated, cultured, and processed with Gram stain may provide the basis for an initial microbiologic diagnosis before the isolation and characterization of organisms from blood cultures.

Some patients may have a fulminating bacteremia manifested by shock or rapidly progressing to the stage of shock in a matter of hours. The latter course may be indistinguishable from meningococcemia and is often due to *P. aeruginosa* or *Aeromonas* infection. More typically, however, the onset of shock is slower

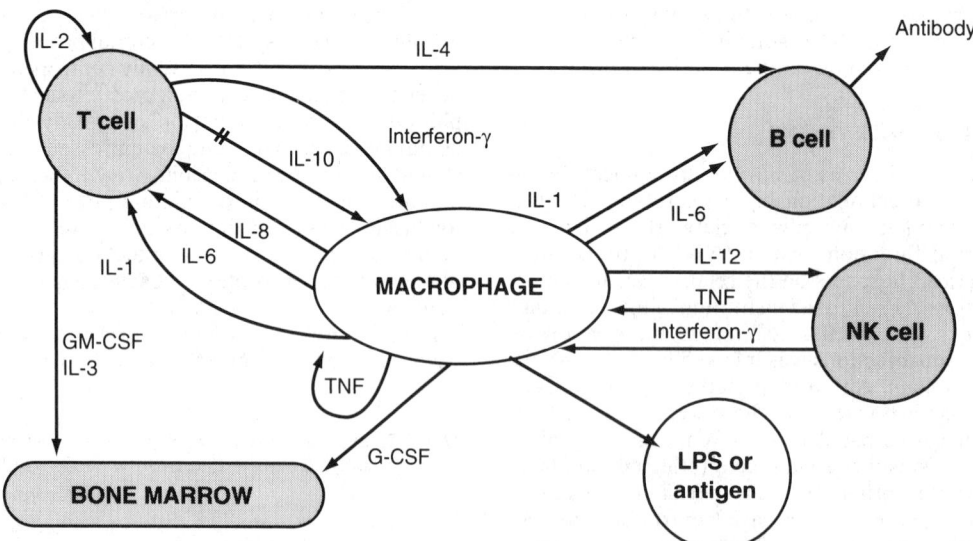

FIG. 1 The interaction between an antigen such as bacterial lipopolysaccharide (LPS or endotoxin) triggers an inflammatory cascade of cytokines that include two potent pyrogenic peptides that can induce hypotension and shock: TNF-α and IL-1 (see text). Other peptides with proinflammatory effects include IL-2 (which stimulates T-cell growth), IL-6, IL-8, and IFN-γ. Hematopoietic colony-stimulating activity is manifested by IL-3, granulocyte colony-stimulating factor (G-CSF) and granulocyte macrophage colony-stimulating factor (GM-CSF). IL-4 and IL-10 (and to some degree IL-6) have downregulating effects on inflammation, while IL-12 activates natural killer (NK) cells.

TABLE 3. Comparison Between Hemodynamic Values during Septic Shock in 19 Patients with Gram-Positive Organisms and 31 Patients with Gram-Negative Organisms Cultured from Blood

	MAP (mmHg)	CVP (mmHg)	HR (per min)	CI (liter/min/m²)	SVR (mmHg/liter/min)	LVEDP (mmHg)
Gram-positive	57 ± 2[a]	3.5 ± 0.06	119 ± 4	3.8 ± 0.3	8.5 ± 1.1	6.7 ± 1.3
Gram-negative	57 ± 3	5.1 ± 0.7	100 ± 4	2.9 ± 0.2	11.5 ± 0.9	9.8 ± 1.6
p (unpaired)	NS	NS	<.01	<.05	NS	NS

Abbreviations: MAP: mean arterial pressure; CVP: central venous pressure; HR: heat rate; CI: cardiac index; SVR: systemic vascular resistance; LVEDP: left ventricular end-diastolic pressure; NS: not significant.
[a] Mean ± SE.
(From Gunnar et al.,[15] with permission.)

and follows a period of several hours of hemodynamic instability.

Oliguria as defined by hourly urine outputs of less than 20 ml, often follows the onset of hypotension. The hallmark of shock is tissue hypoperfusion resulting from a decrease in intravascular fluid volume, diminished vascular resistance, or both. Both vasodilatation and increased vascular permeability of some compartments of the circulation may be an initial manifestation of certain pathophysiologic processes (see section on pathophysiology, below), and the net effect is a reduction in circulating blood volume.

Many patients may have transient hypotension or oliguria that is quickly ameliorated by prompt corrective measures such as fluid administration. Others progress from an initial phase of hypotension, tachycardia, and peripheral vasodilatation ("warm shock") to a moribund phase of deep pallor, intense vasoconstriction, and anuria ("cold shock"). The latter state clearly reflects the inability of compensatory mechanisms to maintain perfusion even to vital organs. The onset of shock is seen in perhaps 20–35 percent of patients with gram-negative bacillary bacteremia and increases the mortality to perhaps twice that figure.

While clinical findings are likely to reflect the severity and stage of shock rather than a specific microbial etiology, there exists some evidence for hemodynamic differences between shock complicating gram-positive bacteremia and gram-negative bacillemia. Gunnar and colleagues[15] have conducted prospective hemodynamic studies in patients in shock associated with both gram-positive cocci and gram-negative rods. Patients were hospitalized in the intensive care unit of a large municipal hospital, and most had procedures involving urinary tract instrumentation. As shown in Table 3, a number of variables were monitored, including heart rate, cardiac index, left ventricular end-diastolic pressure, systemic vascular resistance, and mean arterial pressure. Of these parameters, the cardiac rate and cardiac index (which parallels the former) were significantly lower in patients developing shock secondary to gram-negative bacillary infection. These findings were felt to be consistent with release of a vasodilator substance early during the course of gram-negative bacteremia, but ultimately vasoconstriction was more common in patients with gram-negative infections. Myocardial function was also depressed. While changes in both cardiac rate and index reflect decreased tissue perfusion, it should be noted that the differences were small, with considerable overlap between the two groups. In the individual patient, a single measurement of either heart rate or cardiac index is likely to be of limited value in distinguishing whether the patient has gram-negative or gram-positive infection. For this reason, it still seems prudent in the critically ill patient with septic shock to initiate empiric antimicrobial therapy aimed at both gram-positive and gram-negative causes until the results of cultures are known.

There has been increasing interest in pulmonary complications of the sepsis syndrome.[24,25] Some patients, although probably a minority, have bacteremia originating from the lung. These subjects develop infection secondary to aspiration (bronchial embolism) whereby material from the upper respiratory tract containing organisms is aspirated into the lung parenchyma, and pneumonitis and bacteremia develops subsequently.[26,27] More commonly, however, diffuse pneumonitis can develop secondary to bacteremia and is often of overwhelming severity. The attention of pulmonary physiologists and clinicians has been focused on this complication, which is often referred to as the adult respiratory distress syndrome (ARDS) or "shock lung." It is likely that ARDS reflects a wide variety of pathophysiologic mechanisms and clearly has no single etiology, but can be caused by gram-negative rod bacteremia.[24] The mechanism for the diffuse infiltrates may entail direct involvement of the lung by a bacteremic necrotizing pneumonia or a combination of pulmonary edema (diffuse alveolar/capillary leak) associated with evidence for macro- and microembolization to the lung (consumption coagulopathy). That bacterial products can trigger intrinsic clotting and (pari passu) that the body has mechanisms for resorption of thrombi (activation of the fibrinolytic system) is well known. The complexity of the clinical situation probably relates to multiple events that are triggered by bacterial invasion of the blood stream and by the ensuing host responses that are described in the following section. The characteristic clinical findings include hypoxia, evidence for a right-to-left shunt, and diffuse pulmonary infiltrates. The most important finding is the relatively normal pulmonary wedge pressure (left ventricular end-diastolic pressure) in the face of a high pulmonary arterial pressure and marked hypoxia (PaO_2 < 60 mmHg). This indicates that the diffuse pulmonary capillary leak syndrome and mechanical alterations in lung function are not secondary to left-sided cardiac failure, that is, that they represent "noncardiogenic" pulmonary edema.

PATHOPHYSIOLOGY

Bacterial invasion of the host is the usual setting for the sepsis syndrome. The best studied situation, both in experimental animal systems and in humans, involves systemic disease caused by gram-negative bacteria. The most consistent virulence factor of these gram-negative organisms is bacterial endotoxin or lipopolysaccharide (LPS).

It has become clear during the past two decades of intensive research that LPS triggers humoral enzymatic mechanisms involving the complement, clotting, fibrinolytic, and kinin pathways.[28] Fever and inflammation are mediated by cytokines (peptide hormones acting on cells) that are released in response to the lipid A moiety of LPS (Fig. 1). Some cytokines, such as TNF-α, interleukin-1 (IL-1), interferon-γ (IFN-γ), and various colony-stimulating factors, are produced within minutes to hours of contact between LPS and host defense cells such as monocytes and macrophages.[4,6,29–33] Interleukin-1 is the so-called classic endogenous pyrogen and in some animals can induce shock,[34] but TNF-α has potent fever-inducing properties as well.

Of all of the cytokines identified thus far, TNF-α appears to be the most potent mediator of the pathophysiology of the gram-negative sepsis syndrome. Its biologic properties, which are described as "proinflammatory," are summarized in Table 4. Evidence for the pivotal role of TNF-α in the pathophysiology of the

TABLE 4. Effects of the Proinflammatory Cytokine TNF-α

Inflammation
   Fever
   Leukocyte mobilization
Cardiovascular
   Tachycardia
   Hypotension
   Myocardial depression
   Capillary leak
   Endothelial changes
Central nervous system
   Anorexia
   Fever
   Headache
Metabolic-hormonal
   Acidosis
   Bone resorption
   Catabolic state leading to cachexia
   Increased pituitary and stress hormone production
Hematologic
   Inhibition of erythropoiesis and inhibition of myelopoiesis
   Leukopenia
   Disseminated intravascular coagulation
Renal
   Oliguric renal failure
   Renal cortical necrosis

(Data from refs. 5, 6, 55.)

gram-negative sepsis syndrome is derived from studies showing that (1) mice that are genetically unresponsive to endotoxin lack the capacity to produce murine TNF-α from their macrophages[35]; (2) the administration of endotoxin to human volunteers results in the liberation of free TNF-α in plasma accompanied by many symptoms typical of gram-negative infection[36] (IL-1 and IFN-γ were not detected at challenge doses of 4 ng/kg); (3) high levels of free TNF-α in plasma have been associated with morbidity and increased mortality in human meningococcemia[37] and human gram-negative bacteremia accompanied by shock[4]; (4) the administration of purified recombinant TNF-α to humans[36,38,39] and animals[40,41] mimics most of the clinical, laboratory, and histopathologic findings seen in the gram-negative sepsis syndrome and shock; and (5) antibodies directed against TNF, particularly when given before endotoxin challenge, significantly increased the survival of experimental animals.[42,43] Protection studies have now employed monoclonal antibodies specific for TNF-α epitopes.[43] Infusion of anti-TNF-α murine monoclonal antibodies into primates who were bacteremic abrogated the development of signs of endotoxicity. TNF-α can also act directly on cellular components of blood and vascular epithelium,[44] and TNF-α appears to trigger the release of prostaglandins that can act as "second messengers" of systemic toxicity.[45]

Although TNF-α is a potent pyrogen,[46] when used alone it may be insufficient to induce lethality in experimental animals.[47] However, TNF-α plus bacterial products or whole bacteria induces hemorrhagic necrosis of tissues and murine lethality.[4]

TNF-α plus IL-1, when given in doses that by themselves are not lethal for the host, rapidly induce animal lethality.[34,48] Similarly, IFN-γ can be measured during the course of human and experimental disease but does not appear to induce shock by itself.[49] However, markedly enhanced lethality is observed experimentally when IFN-γ and TNF-α are administered together. Thus, cytokines that are not lethal per se can exact a lethal effect in combination. The inhibition of one or more of these cytokines could abrogate the inflammatory response that leads to the sepsis syndrome.

The effects of cytokines are certainly pleiotropic and sometimes paradoxical. In low doses, cytokines such as IL-1 and TNF-α prime for host defense, but in larger quantities, such as might result from a massive invasion of the host, these cytokines appear to be lethal.[4,50]

The pathophysiology of the sepsis syndrome involves an inflammatory cascade of reactions, with TNF-α as the principal mediator working synergistically with other biologically active products released by host cells. Clearly, other infectious processes such as parasitic or gram-positive infections can lead to TNF-α release, so its detection is not specific for gram-negative infection.[51] Thus, the identification of TNF-α as an important mediator of septic shock suggests that the sepsis syndrome is an example of immune system "over-responsiveness" to invading pathogens[52,53] or to large doses of provocative antigens (e.g., LPS) in a manner analogous to anaphylaxis.

IL-6 and IL-8 can also be measured during the course of gram-negative infection and may have diagnostic, prognostic, or therapeutic importance. IL-6 is a mild endogenous pyrogen but relatively nontoxic per se. It may function to downregulate TNF-α production.[54] IL-8 is primarily a chemotactic and activating factor for neutrophils.[55] IL-10 is a cytokine that acts on macrophages to downregulate TNF-α release.[56] Table 5 compares some of the biologic activities of these cytokines.[55]

Cytokine release by itself is not the final pathway leading to host injury. Effects on tissue metabolism, cardiac function, and vascular tone are three major mechanisms for the damage exerted by TNF-α.[32] It has been shown that the combination of TNF-α with other cytokines such as IFN-γ and IL-1 can induce enzymes known collectively as nitric oxide synthases in many cells and tissues.[57,58] The labile but toxic nitric oxide molecule (also known previously as *endothelial relaxing factor*) is a potent vasodilator.[57,59] The production of nitric oxide by inducible nitric oxide synthases has been postulated for a mechanism of hypotension after administration of lps or tnf-α.[60,61] It has been shown in a variety of animal systems that nitric oxide is responsible for the microbicidal activity of macrophages, but this effect has not been convincingly demonstrated for human phagocytes.[57] Nonetheless, nitric oxide is probably produced in human liver and endothelial cells and released into the circulation.[58]

There are some provocative animal experiments that indicate

TABLE 5. Biologic Activities of Cytokines That May Contribute to Septic Shock

	IL-1	IL-2	GM-CSF	IL-4	IL-5	IL-8	TNF	IFN-γ
In vivo								
Hypotension	+	+					+	+
Fever	+	+	+		+		+	
Edema	+	+				+	+	
Leukocytosis	+		+		+			
Wasting	+						+	
In vitro								
Direct cytotoxicity	+	+	+				+	
Cell-mediated cytotoxicity	+			+			+	+
Proteases, O₂ radicals				+		+	+	
Chemotaxis			+	+		+		
Vascular adhesion	+			+			+	

(Adapted from Cannon,[55] with permission.)

that pretreatment of animal hosts with IL-1 or TNF-α actually induces protection against a bacterial challenge applied hours later.[50,62] The apparent mechanism for this effect is that the host responds by the production of antagonists (IL-1-Ra) or soluble receptors of TNF-α and IL-1, or is capable of downregulating receptors for these proinflammatory cytokines.[33,63,64]

COAGULOPATHY IN THE SEPSIS SYNDROME

Disseminated intravascular coagulopathy may become evident in several ways. Systemic activation of coagulation generates the deposition of fibrin in small blood vessels and microvascular thrombosis in critical target organs, leading to organ failure. Consumption of clotting proteins may lead to bleeding, and thus both clotting and bleeding can occur simultaneously in the same patient. The most convenient laboratory measurements include a decline in the platelet count and serum fibrinogen levels, with an increase in measurable components of fibrin (fibrin split products, D-dimers). Recent studies carried out in humans or in nonhuman primates have cast new light on the mechanisms involved in infection-triggered coagulopathy. Previously published experiments in rodents and in rabbits have their limitations because of intraspecies differences in the production of mediators or mediator-induced by-products, and cogent reservations have been expressed about applying animal data to humans. Lipopolysaccharide infusions into human volunteers have demonstrated the sequential appearance of TNF-α, IL-1, IL-6, and IL-8.[65] The appearance of these cytokines was then followed by markers for the generation of thrombin, as illustrated in Figure 2. Other markers of fibrinogen to fibrin conversion such as fibrinopeptide A have also been documented. The use of recombinant TNF-α in cancer patients and healthy volunteers has shown a parallel activation of coagulation, and inhibition of endotoxin-induced TNF release in chimpanzees results in inhibition of the activation of coagulation.[66,67] Taken together, these studies confirm the central role of TNF-α in endotoxin-triggered coagulopathy. Understanding of the role of other cytokines such as IL-1, IL-6, and IL-8 is incomplete but studies indicate that cytokines other than TNF significantly affect blood coagulation in vitro. IL-6 is a potent stimulus for platelet production.[55]

The well-established compartmentalization of clotting pathways into the intrinsic or contact-activation dependent pathway, and the extrinsic or tissue factor-dependent pathway, is summarized in Figure 2. Studies using large concentrations of LPS showed that Factor XII or Hageman factor can be activated in vitro, which is an initial important event in the contact activation of the intrinsic clotting system. Additionally, clinical studies showed low levels of Factor XII are present in bacteremic patients, thereby supporting the role of the intrinsic pathway for activation. However, in experimental endotoxemia or after cytokine administration with TNF-α, highly sensitive assays have shown that the initial activation of coagulation in septic states appears to be primarily dependent on activation of the extrinsic pathway.[66,67] The lines of evidence supporting this conclusion are as follows: *(1)* After endotoxin administration to healthy human volunteers or chimpanzees, or the administration of TNF-α to volunteers or cancer patients, substantial Factor X–mediated generation of thrombin is observed. At the same time, plasma markers for intrinsic pathway clotting factor activation remain normal. *(2)* In vitro studies show that TNF-α induces the expression of tissue factor on monocytes, and tissue factor binds and activates Factor VII, thereby forming a complex that can convert Factor X and activate it. *(3)* Children with meningococcemia have increased tissue factor expression on circulating monocytes. *(4)* Studies of experimental bacteremia or endotoxemia in nonhuman primates in which the extrinsic clotting system was blocked by the simultaneous infusion of monoclonal antibodies directed either against tissue factor or against Factor VII showed that LPS-induced thrombin and fibrin conversion was completely blocked. Thus, current evidence favors the concept that LPS-induced activation of coagulation is mediated in large part by TNF-α and is initially dependent on activation of the extrinsic pathway of coagulation.

Low levels of Factor XII and prekallikrein and high plasma levels of complexes between kallikrein and C1 inhibitor and between Factor XII and C1 inhibitor are measurable in septic patients. However, experimental studies indicate that activation of the contact system does not necessarily contribute to activation of the coagulation system in sepsis.[68] In experimental studies of *E. coli* bacteremia in baboons, blockade of the contact

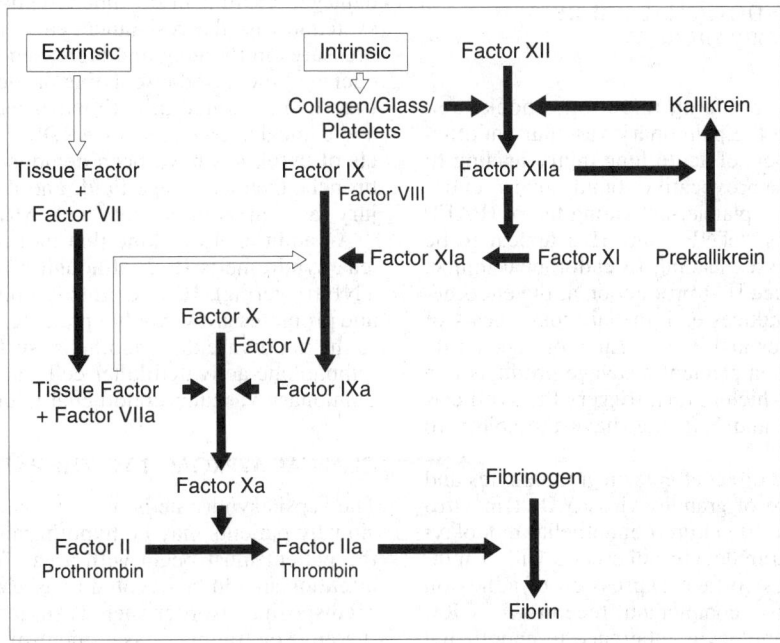

FIG. 2. The coagulation system. Activation of the intrinsic or the extrinsic pathway results in the generation of thrombin and ultimately in fibrinogen-to-fibrin conversion. The tissue factor–factor VIIa complex is also able to directly activate Factor IX, which may be an important connecting link between both pathways. (From Levi et al.,[65] with permission.)

system by the simultaneous administration of anti-Factor XII or anti-Hageman factor antibodies, had no effect on the development of disseminated intravascular coagulation.[65] However, inhibition of contact activation system resulted in a reduction of *E. coli*–induced lethal hypotension. Thus, the contact activation system of hemodynamic effects still appears important and is probably mediated by the generation of kinins, such as bradykinin, during activation of the contact system. Kinins have hypotension-inducing effects and have long been suspected of playing a role in septic shock.[69]

As might be anticipated, activation of the contact system can affect the fibrinolytic system. Activation of the contact system triggers plasminogen activator activity, and thus fibrinolysis is initiated. Activation of the contact system in septic patients does not appear truly to trigger coagulation but does seem to play an important role in the development of hypotension, which ultimately brings about activation of the fibrinolytic system.

With respect to fibrinolysis, low plasma levels of fibrinolytic proteins and inhibitors and increased plasma levels of fibrin degradation products indicate extensive activation of this system.[65] In response to coagulation, the fibrinolytic system initially becomes activated and subsequently inhibited. Healthy human volunteers given LPS or TNF-α show an increase in plasminogen activator activity.[66,67] Both tissue-type plasminogen activator and urokinase-type plasminogen activator have been demonstrated.

The temporal relationship between the appearance of TNF-α and the increase in fibrinolytic activity suggests that TNF-α is a mediator of this effect, but IL-1 may also contribute. In studies of chimpanzees given LPS in which endotoxin-induced TNF-α release was blocked, there was no activation of the fibrinolytic system after endotoxemia. In experiments in which the endotoxin-induced activation of coagulation was blocked by monoclonal antibodies inhibiting the extrinsic pathway, endotoxin-induced effects on fibrinolysis were unaffected. This supports the concept that fibrinolytic responses to endotoxin can be separated from activation of coagulation. Thus, endotoxemia results in rapid activation and subsequent inhibition of fibrinolysis, and the response of the fibrinolytic system to endotoxin is mediated by TNF-α, resulting in inadequate removal of intravascular fibrin deposition.

PULMONARY VASCULAR ENDOTHELIAL INJURY AND THE ADULT RESPIRATORY DISTRESS SYNDROME

Different clinical settings, including infection, shock, and trauma, can trigger injury to the pulmonary vascular endothelium leading to ARDS. Models of acute lung injury leading to the development of ARDS use provocative stimuli such as endotoxin, thrombin, complement, platelet-activating factor (PAF), and arachidonate metabolites.[70] TNF-α and IL-1 appear to be central to the diverse processes leading to endothelial injury. Both LPS and thrombin induce IL-1 production at the endothelial surface.[71] IL-1 in turn induces endothelial biosynthesis of both arachidonate metabolites and PAF.[72] Lipopolysaccharide activates complement, and complement cleavage products can induce TNF-α production, which in turn triggers the synthesis of arachidonate metabolites and PAF that have the ability to initiate lung injury.

Both IL-1 and TNF-α have direct effects on granulocytes and endothelial cells.[73] Exposure of granulocytes to IL-1 in vitro does not facilitate adherence to cultured endothelial monolayers, but TNF-α increases granulocyte adherence within minutes. TNF-α rapidly induces surface expression of adhesion molecules, CDW18, which is a complement receptor for CR3. Thus, cytokine effect on granulocyte adherence to endothelial surfaces may explain the rapid margination phenomenon and granulocytopenia that follow infusion of substances such as LPS or cytokines.

Cytokines induce surface expression of an antigen, the endothelial leukocyte adhesion molecule, or ELAM-1.[70] This molecule also augments endothelial surface procoagulant activity.[71] Thus, both IL-1 and TNF-α interact with endothelial receptors to stimulate synthesis and expression of surface proteins that recognize granulocyte surface adhesion molecules and enhance the endothelial "stickiness" for granulocytes. This stimulation is energy dependent, but once the antigen is expressed on the endothelial cell surface, endothelial metabolism is not required. In addition to direct effects on granulocyte-endothelial interactions, cytokine administration can recruit granulocytes. Thus, pulmonary vascular endothelial injury appears to be facilitated by leukostasis and sequestration of granulocytes within the pulmonary vasculature. Coadministration of both recombinant IL-1 and TNF-α synergistically enhances pulmonary leukostasis in rabbits. Neutrophil release from the bone marrow is further facilitated and results in the release of mature neutrophils into the circulation. However, the presence of granulocytes adherent to pulmonary endothelium or in sequestered vascular channels is not essential for the development of noncardiogenic pulmonary edema. Even in neutropenic patients, complications such as ARDS occur, probably as a result of the direct effect of endotoxin-induced cytokines on endothelial surface integrity.[74]

The effects of cytokines on endothelium involve direct activities because they bind to specific endothelial cell receptors and cause morphologic changes. TNF-α also stimulates angiogenesis and neovascularization. IL-1 can enhance superoxide anion release from cultured endothelial cells. Thus, endothelial cell-generated toxic oxygen radicals and granulocyte-derived oxygen intermediates can add to endothelial injury.

ROLE OF CYTOKINE-INDUCED PLATELET-ACTIVATING FACTOR SYNTHESIS

Cytokines act by triggering other peptide molecules that can act on host tissues, and PAF can be produced following induction of phospholipase A_2 activity by antigens such as LPS.[73] Both IL-1 and TNF-α stimulate biosynthesis of PAF, and TNF-α–induced systemic hypotension and bowel necrosis can be prevented by PAF receptor antagonism. Since TNF-α can induce hypotension, acute lung injury or "shock-lung" can contribute to hypotension and further damage to pulmonary cells. This damage, resulting in sustained hypotension as well as decreased systemic vascular resistance, can lead to increased hydrostatic pressures in the lung and increased noncardiogenic pulmonary edema.[73] Increased circulating or local levels of cytokines have been demonstrated in both experimental models of lung injury and clinical antecedents of ARDS. Furthermore, increased levels of cytokines have been demonstrated in lung parenchyma, bronchoalveolar lavage fluid, and during experimental lung injury, as well as in patients with ARDS.

An additional cytokine that induces the pulmonary vascular leak syndrome is IL-2 (although its effects might be related to TNF triggering). IL-2 recruits lymphoid elements to lung tissue and promotes growth of lymphocytes, and these cells can adhere to the microvascular endothelial surface.[55] Thus, both IL-2 and lymphokine-activated killer cells have the potential to mediate pulmonary vascular endothelial injury as well.

CLINICAL APPROACH TO THE PATIENT

The sepsis syndrome is usually manifested by fever, but occasionally patients may be hypothermic. The initial evaluation of the patient must begin with a carefully taken history. Special attention should be devoted to assessment of any underlying or predisposing disorder such as surgery, transplantation, chemotherapy, or trauma. Assessment of the treatment given to the underlying disorder and its clinical stage should also be carried out. A history of previous infections and antimicrobial treatment along with any microbiologic data that may be available from previous studies in the antecedent few weeks may often be particularly useful for the selection of therapy. Additionally, the presence of symptoms or signs such as pain, erythema, tenderness, or headache can all be important clues to the source and extent of an infectious process. An accurate dietary history, travel history, and exposure history, with special attention to infectious agents in contacts or in the environment, may be extremely valuable to the clinician in identification of an infectious process. Knowledge of the complications of previous treatment such as drug reactions can also be useful in the selection of therapy.

It is likely that a systemic infectious process, such as bacteremia or the sepsis syndrome with fever and other manifestations of systemic disease, has an initial focal source. However, a number of bacteremic infections have no known or easily identified source and are classified by the CDC as "primary bacteremias." In many immunosuppressed patients, these primary bacteremias probably originate in the gastrointestinal tract.[75] The sepsis syndrome can emanate from a localized focus of infection before bacteremia develops, and, if blood cultures are drawn early during the course of the infectious process, the bacteremia may not be documented. The administration of antimicrobial therapy can paradoxically exacerbate fever secondary to a bacteriolytic effect, which leads to endotoxin release or pyrogen release.[76]

The bedside approach to the patient involves not only an integration of the history with physical findings but a search for the clues to infection even though the patient may not have any localizing signs. A vigorous attempt should be made to obtain infected secretions or body fluids or to aspirate an area that is suspicious for infection, such as the advancing edge of cellulitis. Microbiologic studies should include not only blood cultures but study of any potential source of a systemic infection. If the patient has diarrhea, examination of the stool for fecal leukocytes and stool cultures may be appropriate, even studies for the detection of *Clostridium difficile* toxin since fever and a systemic response to infection can be associated with *C. difficile* pseudomembranous colitis.

A complete physical examination should be undertaken as expeditiously as possible. Immunosuppressed and neutropenic patients may have a blunted inflammatory response, and typical signs of infection such as induration, fluctuance, local heat, reactive lymphadenopathy, and exudation of pus may not be present. Immunosuppressed patients may also have suppressed cough mechanisms and not produce purulent sputum or other exudates. Even with urinary tract infection, neutropenic or immunosuppressed patients may not have classic localizing symptoms or pyuria. In immunosuppressed patients with meningitis, the signs of nuchal rigidity may be absent, but two important clues remain: headache and impaired mental status. Erythema is a reliable clue to the presence of infection irrespective of the absolute white count and, along with pain, may be more useful in the detection of a localized infectious process than swelling and warmth in immunosuppressed patients.

The selection of laboratory studies should be based on the physical findings and the overall clinical manifestations. Since the sepsis syndrome implies systemic disease, at least two sets of blood cultures taken at different sites should be obtained to detect bacteremia. In addition to sampling any potential focus of infection, the patient who has an altered mental status or more specific signs of central nervous system infection should have a lumbar puncture performed, providing there is no evidence of increased intracranial pressure or of a focal supratentorial lesion.

If the clinical situation is deteriorating and the patient appears to be seriously ill, it is wise to obtain as many diagnostic studies as possible expeditiously and to initiate empiric antimicrobial therapy. Treatment can subsequently be modified if necessary for those patients who have positive blood cultures. In practice, much of the therapy given in hospitals today is empiric, based on

TABLE 6. Factors Affecting the Outcome of Systemic Bacterial Infection

Underlying conditions
   Neutropenia
   Hypogammaglobulinemia
   Diabetes
   Alcoholism ± cirrhosis
   Renal failure
   Respiratory failure
Complications of the infectious event at the onset of treatment (e.g., shock, anuria)
Antimicrobial chemotherapy
Grade (severity) of bacteremia (polymicrobial bacteremia)
Source of infection
Interval after initiation of treatment
Age

history, intuition, and bedside identification of the most likely infecting pathogens, but without confirmation for several days. The presence of the sepsis syndrome, with the potential for shock and other severe complications, usually mandates prompt treatment.

Clearly, the status of host defense mechanisms and the ability to maintain function of vital organs are the factors that determine the outcome of any blood stream infection. Table 6 summarizes, in order of estimated importance, some of the factors that affect prognosis. In addition to underlying diseases and complications, several other factors have significant effects. Although quantitative blood cultures are now less frequently performed, several studies indicate that mortality is greater with high-grade bacteremia and with polymicrobial bacteremia.[77,78] The absence of a discernible focus of infection may also be associated with a poorer prognosis. Age may also have an impact on outcome, since a poorer survival is seen in the very young and the older age groups. The selection of antimicrobial therapy and the rapidity with which it is administered can also affect outcome.[79] Detectable cytokine levels may be ephemeral, but sustained elevations of serum TNF-α (as well as LPS) have been linked to decreased survival in meningococcemia and gram-negative bacteremia.[80–82]

ANTIMICROBIAL THERAPY FOR THE SEPSIS SYNDROME

Early clinical suspicion, rigorous diagnostic measures, aggressive initiation of appropriate antimicrobial therapy, comprehensive supportive care, and measures aimed at reversing predisposing causes are the cornerstones of successful management. While diagnostic microbiologic techniques are covered elsewhere in more detail (see Ch. 11), it is obvious that the clinical suspicion of the bacterial sepsis syndrome should be promptly confirmed by rapid identification and antimicrobial susceptibility testing of disease-causing organisms.

Antimicrobial therapy remains the mainstay of treatment of the sepsis syndrome, but approaches aimed at correcting the predisposition to this complication have a critical bearing on the outcome of the infection. Amelioration of an underlying disease such as achievement of remission in leukemia is usually the major factor determining recovery irrespective of the choice of antimicrobial agents. The removal of foreign bodies that predispose to or potentiate infection, such as intravascular or urinary catheters, may by themselves cause resolution of symptoms and lead to a cure. Transient bacteremia is a well-documented event, particularly with urinary tract manipulation, and the latter accounts for a number of instances where bacteremic patients have been cured either with inappropriate antibiotics or with no antimicrobial therapy at all.[79,83] A major corollary of the latter observation is that attempts to drain abscesses or to remove obvious sources of infection such as obstructed abdominal viscera are of paramount importance in determining recovery. Antimicrobial sterilization of large abscesses seems futile, although it is possible that small foci of infection could be sterilized by aggressive antimicrobial therapy.

There have been relatively few well-controlled, comparative human clinical trials of the efficacy of new antimicrobial regimens as well as definitive studies of the adjunctive measures that have been advocated to support patients during complications of sepsis. Clearly, it is not possible to conduct clinical trials of antibacterial therapy vs. no therapy, but what is lacking are comparisons of the efficacy and toxicity of some of the popular therapeutic regimens.

An analysis of the status of host factors, the severity of underlying disease, and the outcome of gram-negative bacillary bacteremia has consistently demonstrated increasing mortality in patients with "nonfatal," "ultimately fatal," and "rapidly fatal" diseases.[84–86] The classification of underlying disease as proposed by McCabe and Jackson[84] and others[85] assumes critical importance in attempting to compare treatment results due to the heterogeneity of predisposing or underlying conditions. It is clearly unfair and unscientific to compare therapeutic results in patients with transient bacteremia secondary to a kidney stone (usually these are patients with nonfatal underlying disease) with results in patients developing bacteremia during chemotherapy for acute unremitting leukemia (the usual example of a rapidly fatal disease). Classifying patients with postsurgical or post-traumatic conditions is more difficult, but for the most part intra-abdominal infections complicating surgical procedures or traumatic injury occur in nonimmunosuppressed patients without obvious derangement in host defense mechanisms.

During the 1960s, several major published reports indicated that appropriate antimicrobial therapy for gram-negative bacillary bacteremia (as defined by antimicrobials that inhibited the infecting strain) significantly reduced mortality in patients with nonfatal or ultimately fatal disease.[84,85] It was not possible, however, to show that appropriate antimicrobial therapy significantly improved the chances of recovery in patients with the most adverse host factors, namely, those with rapidly fatal diseases such as acute leukemia in relapse.[85,86] For instance, mortality in three combined series[84,85,87] for patients with rapidly fatal disease who were treated appropriately (the antimicrobial inhibited their infecting strain) was 84 vs. 85 percent for patients treated "inappropriately." In contrast, the results of studies carried out since 1968 in patients with cancer and neutropenia have shown a general overall improvement in clinical response rates.[86,88–90] Most of the studies of patients with neutropenia reported since 1968 show survival rates ranging from 40 to 85 percent, especially with some of the most potent modern treatment regimens.[91–94] These clinical trials have enrolled neutropenic patients because of their increased risk for sepsis and the relative ease in organizing evaluations of drug treatments in this patient population.

Many factors besides the introduction of new antimicrobial agents could account for the improved therapeutic results observed in certain classes of patients or within the experience of a single institution. These factors would include more aggressive approaches to diagnosis and the initiation of treatment, overall improvements in supportive care, and many of the adjunctive measures detailed in subsequent sections of this chapter. Because of institutional and demographic differences, it seems most fair to assess trends within the experience of a single institution or single observers, and these in selected instances have shown a reduction in mortality.[79,95]

One attitude that has become widely prevalent in the therapeutic approaches to suspected infection in the critically ill has been the willingness to begin empirical broad-spectrum therapy before the results of cultures are obtained.[96] This approach has inherent dangers such as the selection for antimicrobial resistance as well as the risk of drug toxicity. There are some patients with apparently intact host defenses in whom empirical therapy may not be indicated because there is adequate time to obtain material for culture and sensitivity testing (e.g., subacute bacterial endocarditis in a patient without congestive heart failure or

emboli). Nonetheless, one definite change in attitude in the last two decades in the approach to the critically ill patient with presumed infection has been to initiate empirical therapy with the intention of making subsequent therapeutic adjustments.

It is only logical that clinicians have used combinations of antimicrobial agents for serious infections, particularly for those patients with the most adverse prognostic factors. The supporting arguments for combination therapy are multiple and not mutually exclusive: (1) Combination therapy makes it possible to cover a broad range of diagnostic possibilities including both gram-positive and gram-negative infection, which may be difficult to distinguish clinically. (2) Polymicrobial bacteremia may be present, so, rather than being an "either/or" type of choice, the use of two agents may give appropriate therapy for dual infections. (3) The use of two agents may prevent the emergence of resistance by eliminating small subpopulations that are resistant to one of the components of the combination. (4) Two antimicrobials may interact either additively or synergistically, thus enhancing the sum of antimicrobial activity or (in the case of synergy) permitting a reduction in dosage of one component of the combination such as the agent that is potentially more toxic. While there is no universally accepted definition of antimicrobial synergy and in practice dosage reduction is not usually carried out, there has been considerable investigative interest in determining whether the use of so-called synergistic combinations is associated with improved clinical results in humans.

The role of synergy between antimicrobial agents used to treat bacillary infections has been difficult to assess because of the problems in initiating randomized, prospective human clinical trials comparing the results of synergistic with nonsynergistic combinations. Experimental studies in animals with normal circulating granulocyte counts or in those rendered neutropenic have shown that use of synergistic combinations leads to a more favorable outcome in *P. aeruginosa* infections.[97,98] Several human studies have shown an association between the use of combinations that interact synergistically against infecting strains and improved clinical results.[99,100] In one study, an association was noted between the use of synergistic combinations and improved clinical results in the face of adverse clinical factors such as neutropenia, rapidly fatal underlying disease, and shock.[99] Because multiple agents are usually given on different dosage schedules, it has been difficult to ensure that the drug concentrations that are achieved in vivo reflect test concentrations used in in vitro studies. The finding of serum inhibitory titers by one group equal to or exceeding 1:8 has been associated with a favorable clinical outcome.[101] Still, it is possible that good clinical results obtained when using combinations of antimicrobial agents may not be related to synergistic interactions. For instance, with such commonly used agents as aminoglycosides and penicillins, which often interact synergistically in vitro, "peak" blood levels that are used to gauge in vitro susceptibility are actually maintained for rather short periods of time followed by periods of rapid "decay." The use of a broad-spectrum penicillin with an aminoglycoside may merely ensure a more sustained interval of serum inhibitory or bactericidal activity or may avoid too low "trough" levels of such activity. Some investigators believe the latter is a cause of treatment failure and have given continuous infusions of antibiotics to maintain a "constant" blood level.[102] However, it is still unclear whether continuous vs. intermittent administration of antimicrobial agents is superior for a variety of infectious conditions. Factors such as tissue penetration, protein binding, rapidity of killing, and post-antibiotic effects are likely to influence the outcome as well as the timing and duration of drug infusion. For critically ill patients with septicemia it is implicit that the administration of all pharmacologic agents should be via the intravenous route.

A principle empiric therapy is to provide broad initial cover-

TABLE 7. Recommended Antimicrobial Regimens for Initial (Presumptive) Therapy for the Sepsis Syndrome[a]

1. Community-acquired infection in the non-neutropenic patient (neutrophil count ≥1000/mm³)
    a. Suspected urinary tract source: a third-generation cephalosporin or piperacillin, mezlocillin, azlocillin, ticarcillin or a quinolone; all ± an aminoglycoside
    b. Nonurinary tract source: third-generation cephalosporin + metronidazole, or ticarcillin-clavulanate or ampicillin-sulbactam or piperacillin-tazobactam; all ± an aminoglycoside
2. Hospital-acquired infection, non-neutropenic patient: a third-generation cephalosporin + metronidazole, or ticarcillin-clavulanate or ampicillin-sulbactam or piperacillin-tazobactam, or imipenem; all + an aminoglycoside
3. Hospital-acquired infection, neutropenic patient: ticarcillin-clavulanate, piperacillin-tazobactam; all + an aminoglycoside; or imipenem ± an aminoglycoside or ceftazidime + metronidazole + an aminoglycoside
4. Thermal injury to at least 20% of the body surface area: ceftriaxone + an aminoglycoside; or vancomyin + antipseudomonal penicillin + an aminoglycoside
5. Established or suspected gentamicin resistance: use amikacin as the aminoglycoside
6. Suspicion of indwelling vascular catheter infection: add vancomycin

[a] Regimens are choices for initial therapy and should be modified on the basis of culture results.

age. Table 7 summarizes recommendations for initial empiric therapy for presumed gram-negative infection as the cause of the sepsis syndrome, but these regimens also provide coverage for *Staphylococcus aureus* and streptococci (except enterococci). First- and second-generation cephalosporins alone may be justified for community-acquired bacteremia secondary to urinary tract infection in the non-neutropenic host where *E. coli* and *Klebsiella* are the main concerns. For the patient with nosocomial infection, initial therapy should consist of an aminoglycoside initially paired with a β-lactam agent. Preference is expressed for a cephalosporin as the β-lactam agent in the non-neutropenic patient because of the greater likelihood of *Klebsiella* and *Staphylococcus*. The regimen of an aminoglycoside paired with a penicillin or cephalosporin having antipseudomonal activity is preferred for the neutropenic patient, the patient receiving assisted ventilation, or the patient with an extensive burn injury.

If organisms are equally susceptible to all aminoglycosides and adequate therapeutic levels are achieved, the clinical results are likely to be similar. Recommended doses of gentamicin, tobramycin, or netilmicin are 1.7 mg/kg q8h and for amikacin either 5 mg/kg q8h or 7.5 mg/kg q12h. More potent semisynthetic penicillins like ticarcillin, mezlocillin, azlocillin, and piperacillin may be given in doses varying from 40 mg/kg q4h to 60 mg/kg q6h.

The third-generation cephalosporins, related β-lactam agents like moxalactam, carbapenems like imipenem, and monobactam agents like aztreonam have markedly augmented activity against enteric bacteria but variable bactericidal effect against *P. aeruginosa*. The potency of cefotaxime, ceftizoxime, and ceftriaxone against *E. coli* and *Klebsiella* (minimum inhibitory concentrations [MICs] often 0.5 μg/ml or less with achievable blood levels 100-fold or more higher) suggests that single-agent therapy directed against those bacteria may be quite successful even in severely compromised hosts. In contrast, resistance among *Pseudomonas*, *Serratia*, and *Enterobacter* spp. may emerge rapidly on monotherapy. Ceftazidime appears most active against *P. aeruginosa*. Monotherapeutic regimens (e.g., ceftazidime, imipenem, or intravenous quinolones) may be effective for fevers of undetermined origin in neutropenic patients and for documented infections due to highly susceptible gram-negative bacteria.[103] However, successful treatment for bacteremic patients with profound persistent neutropenia (e.g., neutrophil counts less than 100/μl) still appears to be linked to the use of two agents that inhibit the infecting strain (irrespective of synergistic interactions). In view of excellent responses associated with the initial use of combination therapy, it still seems prudent to begin treatment of the critically ill patient with two agents that are likely to be active[104,105] and to modify treatment

on the basis of antibiotic susceptibility test results and changes in the status of the host.

There is no evidence that a three-drug regimen, for example, aminoglycoside/penicillin/cephalosporin, is superior to an aminoglycoside/β-lactam combination.[106] Combining bactericidal with bacteristatic agents is generally avoided because some clinical evidence argues against their combined use.

Clinicians should not assume that the administration of apparently adequate doses of antimicrobial agents consistently ensures therapeutic levels. Aminoglycosides have a narrow therapeutic ratio, and there is marked individual variability in the individual peak blood levels of gentamicin.[107] Studies of patients with recurrent or breakthrough bacteremia have indicated an association with subinhibitory blood levels of agents such as gentamicin.[108] In view of the variations in blood pharmacokinetics of aminoglycosides, it would seem prudent in the critically ill patient to monitor blood levels frequently. There is some evidence that such monitoring may also avert potentially toxic complications.[109] The measurement of aminoglycoside blood levels is usually not indicated in patients with bacteremia from the genitourinary tract inasmuch as the levels of many agents excreted in the urine are high. The average duration of treatment in normal hosts experiencing gram-negative sepsis is 10–14 days, but this may be longer if the patient has persistent infection at the source of bacteremia. Treatment of the neutropenic or immunocompromised patient may require an even longer duration. Patients in the latter group should be afebrile for a minimum of 4–7 days and have evidence of resolving infection at the source of bacteremia, and the neutrophil count should be rising and in excess of 500/μl before drug therapy is stopped. The exception to this guideline would be patients with marrow failure syndromes who are unlikely to generate white counts as high as 500/μl; in these subjects clinical defervescence alone should suffice.

Oral therapy is ill advised for the bacteremic patient with fever, hemodynamic instability, and factors that might limit absorption and antimicrobial agents from the gut. On the other hand, a change to an effective oral agent (as determined by in vitro testing) is often justified after defervescence if the patient's overall condition is improving. Potentially useful agents include the quinolones, oral cephalosporins, and trimethoprim-sulfamethoxazole.

ADJUNCTIVE MEASURES IN THERAPY OF THE SEPSIS SYNDROME

Maintenance of Adequate Tissue Perfusion with Volume Replacement

Management of fluid and electrolyte balance is a crucial aspect of the care of the patient with the sepsis syndrome, particularly the person whose course is complicated by shock. Perfusion of vital organs such as the brain and kidney must be maintained. It is clear that the body has an order of priorities that results in distribution of blood preferentially to vital organs; this causes splanchnic vasoconstriction as well as a marked reduction of circulation to the skin. When these compensatory changes are inadequate to maintain adequate perfusion, central arterial pressures will fall. The first goal of management of the patient with the sepsis syndrome, particularly in the incipient stages of shock, is adequate monitoring of vital signs so that any hemodynamic changes can be readily counteracted. Insertion of a central venous pressure monitoring device, an arterial catheter, and Swan-Ganz catheters to determine the left atrial end-diastolic pressure are useful measures in the critically ill patient, although it is clear that they present certain infection hazards per se. These monitoring devices are not used to determine optimal therapy but rather the limits of therapy. In other words, normal or low central venous pressure and left atrial end-diastolic pressures (pulmonary wedge pressures) in the presence of a declining systemic arterial blood pressure are an indication for further volume replacement. On the other hand, it is clear that these parameters may rise to dangerously elevated levels without being able to restore adequate arterial perfusion, and cautious use of inotropic agents should be considered in that setting (see below).

There are a number of solutions that can be used to expand intravascular fluid volume and colloid oncotic pressure, including normal saline, fresh frozen plasma, albumin of the regular type or salt depleted, and various dextran preparations. If the patient is anemic, as well as hypotensive, the transfusion of whole blood in the face of a low central venous pressure is justified. If there is no need for erythrocytes, one of the plasma fractions will suffice. With evidence for bleeding and consumption coagulopathy, the use of fresh frozen plasma may be indicated. There has been a tendency to avoid dextran preparations because of an association with hemorrhagic tendencies. Other authorities have preferred to use crystalloid solutions in preference to colloid.[110]

Use of Sympathomimetic Amines

Sympathomimetic amines have been widely used to treat the hemodynamic complications of shock, but there have been no controlled or comparative studies of the efficacy of different compounds. For many years, norepinephrine and epinephrine were the principal agents available. Norepinephrine has intense peripheral vasoconstricting activity, the extravasation around intravenous infusion sites has led to ischemic necrosis of tissues. There is justifiable concern that its use compromises the perfusion of vital organs. Both norepinephrine and epinephrine increase myocardial irritability. Alternative agents like isoproterenol, dopamine, and dobutamine have largely supplanted norepinephrine. They have an inotropic effect on myocardial function but because of β-adrenergic activity are capable of enhancing peripheral tissue perfusion. Isoproterenol increases the cardiac index but has little effect on mean arterial pressure.[111] Dopamine causes vasodilatation of renal, coronary, and cerebral blood flow while causing an increase in systolic blood pressure and heart rate and an effective reduction in the blood supplied to skeletal muscle. Dobutamine has little chronotropic activity and is otherwise quite similar to dopamine. Presently norepinephrine should be reserved only for those patients in whom it is not possible to support systemic blood pressure and vascular perfusion with dopamine or isoproterenol. Table 8 is a summary of recommended doses and techniques for administering sympathomimetic amines.

Sympathomimetic agents have a wide range of effects, particularly on pulmonary airway passages, regulation of blood sugar, and so forth. None of these considerations is as important as perfusion of vital organs during septic shock. Perhaps the critical factor that is often neglected in the management of patients with sympathomimetic amines is the relationship between fluid therapy and the use of these agents. It is inappropriate to use dopamine and isoproterenol before aggressive volume replace-

ment. If they are used in the presence of a reduced intravascular fluid volume, the vasodilatation secondary to β-adrenergic stimulation can cause a paradoxical decline in blood pressure and decreased tissue perfusion because of the sudden drop in effective intravascular volume. Because of this danger, constant monitoring of central venous pressure and pulmonary wedge pressure is indicated; some authors advocate fluid replacement to the point that either or both of the latter begin to rise to the upper limits of normal. At that juncture it would be appropriate to use an agent such as dopamine, dobutamine, or isoproterenol if the patient remains hypotensive.

In spite of volume replacement and sympathomimetic amine administration, significant metabolic acidosis may ensue. While primary efforts should still be aimed at enhancing tissue perfusion, temporary correction of acidosis may be achieved with infusions of sodium bicarbonate.

Role of Corticosteroids in the Treatment of Gram-Negative Rod Septicemia and Its Complications

Since the clinical availability of corticosteroids, there has been controversy over their effectiveness as adjunctive therapy in the management of infection. Corticosteroids have a variety of metabolic, anti-inflammatory, and immunosuppressive effects, and it is commonly observed that the short-term administration often results in defervescence, thus leading to a clinical impression of improvement. Weitzman and Berger[112] emphasized the lack of convincing evidence from controlled studies that corticosteroids accelerate the rate of recovery or lower mortality from sepsis. Nonetheless, there has been widespread belief that corticosteroids are beneficial as adjunctive therapy in gram-negative infections, particularly those complicated by shock. Much of the belief is derived from animal studies wherein healthy experimental subjects of varying susceptibility to the effects of bacterial endotoxin were given large doses of these substances to induce shock. Such doses are questionably associated with the pathogenesis of the complications of shock in humans. Furthermore, the animals used in such studies have almost always been immunologically intact or physiologically normal before the induction of shock.

One of the major issues relating to the efficacy of corticosteroids in human sepsis complicated by shock has been that of dosage. Since relatively low doses (up to 1 mg/kg of betamethasone or roughly 25–30 mg/kg equivalent of hydrocortisone) were used in one well-controlled, prospective study[113] and showed no beneficial effect, advocates of corticosteroid therapy have escalated their recommendations so that one study reported a beneficial effect of corticosteroids in doses of 30 mg/kg of methylprednisolone or 2 mg/kg of dexamethasone.[114] Doses in this range were found to improve survival in one controlled clinical trial in patients with typhoid fever.[115] Another comparative study found that large doses of corticosteroids (2 g of methylprednisolone for the 70-kg patient) actually reversed septic shock in a significant number of patients. While a transient, "early" effect in increased survival was noted, mortality at the conclusion of the study was similar in both groups, and steroid recipients had a higher incidence of superinfection.[116] Despite these aforementioned studies, however, the largest and most comprehensive controlled clinical trials in the United States have failed to confirm the beneficial effect of corticosteroids in septic shock. This conclusion was reached in the final report of a multicenter collaborative trial involving the Veterans Administration Hospitals[117] and a multihospital collaborative group.[118] Additionally, two other controlled human trials employed similar doses of corticosteroids for ARDS patients and obtained negative results.[119,120] In view of these findings, large doses of prednisone/prednisolone/dexamethasone cannot be recommended as adjunctive therapy for sepsis or shock. Replacement doses of corticosteroids are clearly justified in suspected adrenal insufficiency.

TABLE 8. Sympathomimetic Amines for Support of the Circulation in Septic Shock[a]

1. Dopamine, 2–25 μg/kg/min: increase the rate of infusion (D₅W or saline) q15–20min until systolic blood pressure exceeds 90 mmHg and the urine output exceeds 30 ml/hr
2. Dobutamine, 2–25 μg/kg/min: titrate as with dopamine
3. Isoproterenol, 5 μg/ml/min: observe the effect within 15–25 min and double the rate of infusion if necessary
4. Norepinephrine: give a test dose of 0.1–0.2 μ/kg and observe the response (usually in minutes). The normal maintenance dose is 0.05 μg/kg/min delivered via a plastic catheter into a large peripheral or central vein

Abbreviations: ECG: electrocardiographic; CVP: central venous pressure; BP: blood pressure; D₅W: 5% dextrose in water.
[a] Listed in order of preference, to be used after volume replacement and with careful ECG, CVP, and BP monitoring.

Anticoagulation

The use of anticoagulation, particularly heparinization, to treat septicemic states associated with DIC is logical because there is strong experimental and human clinical evidence that coagulopathy can be terminated by heparinization. At present, however, it is unclear whether anticoagulation has any effect in prolonging survival, however desirable it may be to abolish the sequence of events leading to clotting, consumption of clotting factors, and the onset or aggravation of bleeding. In both human and experimental studies the use of agents such as heparin has failed to decrease significantly the mortality from bacteremic gram-negative infections.[121,122] In human infection, the failure to show a difference may be related to the overall poor prognosis of the underlying disease that is complicated by bacteremia. Until it can be shown that a reduction in mortality is consistent, the use of routine anticoagulation in the management of patients with DIC should be avoided. This is particularly true for normotensive people. If bleeding in such patients is associated with depressed levels of platelets or a specific factor, replacement therapy may be required to control the hemorrhage.

For hypotensive septicemic patients, measures aimed at controlling the infection and correcting hemodynamic alterations (volume replacement and sympathomimetic amines) are of primary importance. If the blood pressure responds to such measures (an effect is usually observed within 4 hours), consumption coagulopathy will usually cease. If the patient has bleeding because of the coagulopathy and not from another cause such as an associated gastrointestinal ulcer, replacement therapy is indicated. This should consist of platelet transfusions for thrombocytopenia, cryoprecipitate preparations for hypofibrinogenemia, and fresh frozen plasma for depleted coagulation factors. While this approach theoretically could aggravate coagulopathy by providing additional substrate for clotting, this complication is not commonly observed when replacement therapy is used in conjunction with measures aimed at controlling shock and infection.[123]

For patients with refractory shock and coagulopathy in spite of the preceding measures, heparin therapy may be beneficial in terminating DIC (without evidence that this prolongs life). Other patients who should be considered for anticoagulation are those who appear to have pulmonary embolic phenomena. This includes patients with pelvic thrombophlebitis. Heparin may be given by either intermittent or continuous infusion. The dose for intermittent infusion is 50–100 units/kg of aqueous heparin given by bolus infusion every 4 hours. For continuous infusion the recommended dose of heparin in adult therapy is 10,000 units made up in 500 ml of 5% dextrose in water (D_5W) delivered over a period of approximately 4–6 hours. Since reversal of coagulation tendencies has an immediate effect, it would appear judicious to terminate therapy as soon as possible after the subsidence of fever.

Therapeutic Role of Granulocyte Transfusion and Colony-Stimulating Factors

Granulocyte transfusions were once popular for treatment of infections in neutropenic subjects, and their use was supported by clinical trials.[124–127] Subsequently, a much larger study randomizing patients with documented gram-negative bacteremia to receive or not to receive neutrophil transfusions showed no difference in recovery rates or survival, even in the subset of patients without evidence of bone marrow recovery.[128] Survival was quite good in the control group as compared with previous studies, and this may have been due to better antimicrobial therapy. The complications of white cell transfusion, particularly viral infections and pulmonary complications, plus the outcome of this more recent study, have discouraged granulocyte transfusions in septicemic, neutropenic patients if appropriate antimicrobial therapy is given. Use of recombinant colony-stimulating factors, G-CSF and GM-CSF, has largely supplanted white cell transfusions. There is still a paucity of data indicating that these CSFs improve outcome in documented infections or increase patient survival.[129]

Diuretics

Diuretics are commonly used in the management of the early oliguric or anuric phases of bacteremic shock. The use of agents such as furosemide is controversial, however, since there is no controlled study demonstrating that acute renal failure may be avoided by the aggressive use of such agents. The action of potent loop diuretics such as furosemide usually results in a significant increase in the output of dilute urine, but it is unclear whether the aggressive use of diuretics in the early oliguric phases of shock makes the ensuing renal failure less severe. What has been observed is that some agents such as furosemide may cause deafness, and there may be enhanced toxicity when these agents are simultaneously used with agents that can damage eighth nerve or renal function such as aminoglycoside antibiotics. In view of these effects it seems prudent to monitor the patient's vital signs and central venous or left atrial pressure and to use diuretics only when volume expansion is not adequate to maintain urine output.

Other Pharmacologic Agents Used to Treat Patients in Septic Shock

Naloxone, an antagonist of opiates and β-endorphins, has been shown to reverse the course of endotoxic and hypovolemic shock in experimental animals.[130,131] In a small study of humans with prolonged hypotension, an intravenous dose of 0.4–1.2 mg of naloxone resulted in a 45 percent increase in systolic blood pressure that lasted at least 45 minutes.[132] Before naloxone infusion, patients had been treated with fluids, dopamine, and appropriate antibiotics. Nonresponders were subjects who had previously been treated with corticosteroids or phenothiazines. Thus, it appears that naloxone has a transient pressor effect in human shock with the added appeal of no immunosuppressive complications (unlike corticosteroids). However, a small controlled study of naloxone therapy in gram-negative infections complicated by shock failed to demonstrate any benefit.[133]

A wide variety of pharmacologic agents including phenothiazines, antihistamines, anti-inflammatory agents such as indomethacin and ibuprufen, glucagon, α-adrenergic blocking agents, and vasodilators have been used experimentally as adjunctive therapy for septic shock complicating gram-negative infections. Among the more interesting observations is the finding that cyclooxygenase inhibitors can inhibit the effects of TNF.[45,49] Other pharmacologic agents such as pentoxyfylline can inhibit the effect of TNF on neutrophils.[134] Controlled studies are now underway to examine the use of agents such as ibuprufen and pentoxyfylline in septic shock in humans.

THERAPEUTIC ANTISERUM IN THE SEPSIS SYNDROME

The use of antiserum to treat bacterial infections antedates the antimicrobial era, but was all but abandoned more than four decades ago. Resurgent interest in the therapeutic applications of antibody stems for the persistently high mortality associated with the gram-negative sepsis syndrome complicated by shock in spite of the use of appropriate antimicrobials.[135] There have been anecdotal reports of the successful use of convalescent serum for *P. aeruginosa* bacteremia[136] or *Pseudomonas* immune globulin in surgical patients.[137] Zeigler and associates[138] reported the results of a large multicenter, double-blind, controlled trial of therapeutic antiserum prepared by immunizing donors with the "J5" mutant of *E. coli* 0111 (a "rough mutant" with an endotoxin core analogous to an Rc mutant). Mortality was 22 percent in 103 bacteremic recipients of antiserum as opposed to 39 percent in 109 subjects randomized to control serum therapy.[137] An even more significant difference was noted in the ability of antiserum to reverse profound shock. Therapeutic antiserum did not, however, significantly affect survival in patients with cancer and/or neutropenia, and no protective antibody titer or level could be inferred. A clinical trial of intravenous IgG was unsuccessful, possibly because of low titer or because IgG antibodies are not protective.[138] Monoclonal antibodies of IgM isotype have been produced that can abrogate the effect of endotoxins and may increase survival above that obtained with antimicrobial therapy.[140,141] Human clinical trials with these antibodies indicate that they are generally well tolerated.[142]

Of two large human clinical trials that have been reported thus far, both suggested a benefit when such antibodies were used to treat some patients with gram-negative infections, but the antibodies had no impact on the outcome of gram-positive disease.[143,144] Nonetheless, analysis of these two large trials has indicated that "on an intention to treat" basis no overall benefit could be derived from the use of these antibodies.[145,146] Indeed, closer analysis of the use of one of these compounds, HA-1A, suggested that the quality of antibiotic treatment in the control group was sufficiently inappropriate to influence the overall outcome of the trial (a potential bias that improved survival in the antibody-treated group).[145] It was only in certain subgroups (in the HA-1A trial in patients with bacteremic shock, and in the E5 trial in patients with documented gram-negative infections and sepsis syndrome who were not in refractory shock) that therapeutic benefit could be claimed.[147] Additional studies are now underway to examine the potential benefit of anti-endotoxin monoclonal antibodies.

In addition, numerous other alternative therapeutic strategies have been conceptualized and are also in various stages of clinical assessment. These include attempts to block some of the events in the inflammatory cascade that are mediated by cytokines during the sepsis syndrome. A naturally occurring receptor antagonist for interleukin-1 (IL-1-Ra) has been identified and prepared by recombinant techniques.[148] A phase II study was encouraging, but a phase III trial was not. Monoclonal antibodies have been produced that bind to TNF-α, and a clinical trial suggested that some therapeutic benefit might be present in patients with shock, but this was not statistically significant.[149] Additional studies are also underway with this approach.

Another attempt to block the effect of TNF-α involves the construction of a hybrid molecule of TNF-α receptor linked to IgG, a compound with a long half-life. Other strategies have included production of monoclonal antibodies directed against other cytokines in the inflammatory cascade, the use of antiinflammatory cytokines such as IL-10, the use of soluble receptors, or the use of endotoxin-binding proteins or antibodies directed against endotoxin-binding proteins.[150] Viewing all of these therapeutic approaches in the appropriate clinical context may be difficult. Application of blocking strategies might be therapeutically useful early in the clinical stages of infection, but after the development of full-blown septic shock such approaches may well be ineffective. Since most of these new approaches involve expensive new technologies, clinicians have insisted that their introduction in the clinical practice should be accompanied by unequivocal evidence of clinical efficacy as well as conclusive benefit with respect to cost.

PROPHYLAXIS OF SEPSIS

Measures to prevent sepsis have included meticulous efforts aimed at limiting the spread of infection within the hospital, the use of prophylactic antimicrobial agents of a topical or systemic form, management of high-risk patients in so-called protective environments, active or passive immunoprophylaxis with type-specific or cross-reactive antibodies, augmentation of the host

granulocyte pool with prophylactic granulocyte transfusions, and stimulation of bone marrow with CSFs. It seems reasonable that the simplest and most cost-effective measures for the prophylaxis of gram-negative bacillary infections would involve minimizing the infection hazard associated with such procedures as Foley catheterization and prolonged intravascular catheterization. Logical applications of antimicrobial prophylaxis include topical application to the skin, the use of an oropharyngeal spray, and orally ingested nonabsorbable antibiotics to suppress the fecal flora. The application of topical agents such as silver nitrate, silver sulfadiazine, or sulfamylon to burned skin appears to have significantly reduced the incidence of burn wound sepsis caused by organisms such as *P. aeruginosa*.[151] The application of a polymyxin spray to the posterior portion of the pharynx appears to have limited gram-negative bacillary colonization of the oropharynx and prevented some cases of nosocomial gram-negative pneumonia.[152] However, such efforts offer the potential hazard of selecting for the emergence of organisms resistant to the prophylactic agent, as has been amply documented with the use of polymyxin sprays.[153]

Since the gastrointestinal tract is a vast reservoir of gram-negative bacilli, an essentially topical approach to prophylaxis is the use of oral nonabsorbable antimicrobial agents. Sterilization of bowel contents is unrealistic, but suppression of the aerobic fecal flora has been achieved to varying degrees with regimens that use polymyxin[154] or gentamicin[155] orally with vancomycin and nystatin. Randomized studies have shown a significant reduction in bacterial sepsis in neutropenic subjects given a polymyxin-containing regimen as compared with placebo.[154] The efficacy of gentamicin-vancomycin-nystatin has been assessed in a three-arm study with management of neutropenic patients in "protected environments" with laminar airflow and under regular ward care.[156] The reduction in infection was similar for both groups receiving oral antimicrobials and was not significantly greater for those additionally managed in laminar airflow rooms.

Regimens containing oral nonabsorbable agents are unpalatable, and patient compliance has been variable. Better-tolerated alternatives include trimethoprim-sulfamethoxazole[157] and the newer quinolones. Trimethoprim-sulfamethoxazole has been used to prevent both *Pneumocystis carinii* pneumonia and bacterial infection. Unfortunately, it has no effect against *P. aeruginosa* and may predispose to superinfection with fungi and resistant bacilli. Some studies have suggest a significant reduction in gram-negative infections occurring in neutropenic patients given prophylactic norfloxacin[158] or ciprofloxacin.[159] Even more aggressive approaches have included both orally and systemically administered antibiotics to achieve "gut decontamination." These approaches are controversial because no consistent benefit has been demonstrated, and there is concern about selection of resistant organisms.[160]

AUGMENTATION OF HOST DEFENSES: GRANULOCYTE TRANSFUSIONS, COLONY STIMULATING FACTORS, AND IMMUNOPROPHYLAXIS

In patients who are neutropenic or likely to become so, use of prophylactic granulocyte transfusions has been replaced by prophylactic CSF. Benefit has been variable, but some studies show a decreased incidence of fevers, diminished use of systemic antibiotics, and shortened hospitalizations.[129]

With respect to the feasibility of immunoprophylaxis in the prevention of gram-negative bacteremia, the impetus for this approach is the convincing evidence that some bacterial infections can be prevented by active or passive immunization with either cell wall components of certain bacteria or toxoid preparations of extracellular toxins. Particularly with toxoid immunization, as in the case of tetanus, immunity appears to be lifelong. With some of the polysaccharide bacterial vaccines there is evidence that active immunization prevents bacterial disease in immunodeficient patients.[161] Immunization of experimental animals or healthy people with a *Pseudomonas* LPS vaccine has led to some augmentation of circulating antibody levels against these seven LPS antigens.[162] Some evidence exists, from the study of patients with burn injuries, that this vaccine is protective, but definitive double-blind controlled studies are lacking.[163] Other *Pseudomonas* LPS antigens have been used in controlled studies in burn patients, and the results have been significantly in favor of immunization.[164] A randomized, prospective study of *Pseudomonas* immunization in cancer patients showed some overall reduction in *Pseudomonas* infections as well as *Pseudomonas*-associated mortality but no significant reduction in bacteremic *P. aeruginosa* infections.[162]

Thus, it appears that immunization alone is not likely to be successful in the prevention of gram-negative bacteremia in markedly immunosuppressed patients, particularly those who are neutropenic. Passive immunization with transfused antibodies is an alternative. Immunoglobulins appear appropriate for hypogammoglobulinemic patients, but convincing evidence of prophylactic efficacy in preventing sepsis and related disorders is lacking.[165]

REFERENCES

1. Bone RC. The pathogenesis of sepsis. Ann Intern Med. 1991;115:457–69.
2. Bone RC, Balk RA, Cerra FB, et al. Definitions for sepsis and organ failure and guidelines for the use of innovative therapies in sepsis. Chest. 1992;101:1644–55.
3. American College of Chest Physicians/Society of Critical Care Medicine Consensus Conference Committee. Definitions for sepsis and organ failure and guidelines for the use of innovative therapies in sepsis. Crit Care Med. 1992;20:864–74.
4. Billiau A, Vandekerckhove F. Cytokines and their interactions with other inflammatory mediators in the pathogenesis of sepsis and septic shock. Eur J Clin Invest. 1991;21:559–73.
5. Kimball ES, ed. Cytokines and Inflammation. Boca Raton: CRC Press; 1991.
6. Beutler B, ed. Tumor Necrosis Factors: The Molecules and Their Emerging Role in Medicine. New York: Raven Press; 1992.
7. Bone RC. Toward an epidemiology and natural history of SIRS (systemic inflammatory response syndrome). JAMA. 1992;268:3452–5.
8. Banerjee SN, Emori TG, Culver DH, et al. Secular trends in nosocomial primary bloodstream infections in the United States, 1980–1989. Am J Med. 1991;91(Suppl 3B):86–9.
9. McCabe WR, Kreger BE, Johns M. Type-specific and cross reactive antibodies in gram-negative bacteremia. N Engl J Med. 1972;287:262.
10. Wolff SM, Bennett JV. Gram-negative rod bacteremia (Editorial). N Engl J Med. 1974;291:733.
11. Martin MA. Epidemiology and clinical impact of gram-negative sepsis. Infect Dis Clin North Am. 1991;5:739–52.
12. Centers for Disease Control and Prevention. Increase in national hospital discharge survey rates for septicemia—United States, 1979–1987. MMWR. 1990;39:31–4.
13. Koll BS, Brown AE. The changing epidemiology of infections at cancer hospitals. Clin Infect Dis. 1993;17(Suppl 2):S322–8.
14. National Nosocomial Infections Surveillance (NNIS) System. Nosocomial infection rates for interhospital comparison: Limitations and possible solutions. Infect Control Hosp Epidemiol. 1991;12:609–21.
15. Gunnar RM, Loeb HS, Winslow EJ, et al. Hemodynamic measurements in bacteremic and septic shock in man. J Infect Dis. 1973;128:287.
16. Sprung CL, Peduzzi PN, Shatney CH, et al. Impact of encephalopathy on mortality in the sepsis syndrome. Crit Care Med. 1990;18:801–6.
17. Stevens DL, Tanner MH, Winship J, et al. Reappearance of scarlet fever toxin among streptococci in the Rocky Mountain West: Severe group A streptococcal infections associated with a toxic shock-like syndrome. N Engl J Med. 1989;321:1–7.
18. Waisbren BA. Gram-negative shock and endotoxin shock. Am J Med. 1964;36:819.
19. Dorff GJ, Geimer NF, Rosenthal Dr, et al. *Pseudomonas* septicemia. Arch Intern Med. 1971;128:591.
20. Ketover BP, Young LS, Armstrong D. Septicemia due to *Aeromonas hydrophilia*: Clinical and immunologic aspects. J Infect Dis. 1973;127:284.
21. Davis II WA, Kane JG, Garagusi VF. Human *Aeromonas* infections: A review of the literature and a case report of endocarditis. Medicine (Baltimore). 1978;57:267.
22. Fisher KW, Berger B, Keusch GT. Subepidermal bullae due to *E. coli*. Arch Dermatol. 1974;110:105.
23. Forkner CE, Frei III E, Edgcomb JH, et al. *Pseudomonas* septicemia. Observations on twenty-three cases. Am J Med. 1958;25:877.
24. Hopewell PC, Murray JS. The adult respiratory distress syndrome. Annu Rev Med. 1976;181:343.
25. Rothstein JL, Schreiber H. Synergy between tumor necrosis factor and bacterial products causes hemorrhagic necrosis and lethal shock in normal mice. Proc Natl Acad Sci USA. 1988;85:607–11.
26. Tillotson JR, Lerner AM. Characteristics of nonbacteremic *Pseudomonas* pneumonia. Ann Intern Med. 1968;68:308.
27. Tillotson JR, Lerner AM. Characteristics of pneumonias caused by *Bacillus proteus*. Ann Intern Med. 1968;68:287.
28. Young LS, Proctor RA, Beutler B, et al. University of California/Davis Interdepartmental Conference on Gram-Negative Septicemia. Rev Infect Dis. 1991;13:666–87.
29. Cannon JG, Tompkins RG, Gelfand JA, et al. Circulating interleukin-1 and tumor necrosis factor in septic shock and experimental endotoxin fever. J Infect Dis. 1990;161:79–97.
30. Heremans H, Van Damme J, Dillen C, et al. Interferon-γ, a mediator of lethal lipopolysaccharide-induced Shwartzman-like shock reactions in mice. J Exp Med. 1990;171:1853–69.
31. Martich GD, Danner RL, Ceska M, et al. Detection of interleukin 8 and tumor necrosis factor in normal humans after intravenous endotoxin: The effect of anti-inflammatory agents. J Exp Med. 1991;173:1021–4.
32. Parrillo JE. Pathogenetic mechanisms of septic shock. N Engl J Med. 1993;328:1471–7.
33. van Deuren M, van der Ven-Jongekrijg J, Demacker PNM, et al. Differential expression of proinflammatory cytokines and their inhibitors during the course of meningococcal infections. J Infect Dis. 1994;169:157–61.
34. Okusawa S, Gelfand JA, Ikejima T, et al. Interleukin 1 induces a shock-like state in rabbits. Synergism with tumor necrosis factor and the effect of cyclooxygenase inhibition. J Clin Invest. 1988;81:1162–72.
35. Beutler B, Krochin N, Milsark IW, et al. Control of cachectin (tumor necrosis factor) synthesis: Mechanisms of endotoxin resistance. Science. 1986;232:977–80.
36. Michie HR, Manogue KR, Spriggs DR, et al. Detection of circulating tumor necrosis factor after endotoxin administration. N Engl J Med. 1988;318:1481–6.
37. Waage A, Halstensen A, Espevik T. Association between tumor necrosis factor in serum and fatal outcome in patients with meningococcal disease. Lancet. 1987;1:355–7.
38. Tracey KJ, Lowry SF, Cerami A. Cachectin/TNF mediates the pathophysiological effects of bacterial endotoxin/lipopolysaccharide (LPS). In: Levin J, Buller HR, tenCate JW, et al., eds. Bacterial Endotoxins: Pathophysiological Effects, Clinical Significance, and Pharmacological Control. New York: Alan R. Liss; 1988:77–88.
39. Blick M, Sherwin SA, Rosenblum M, et al. Phase I study of recombinant tumor necrosis factor in cancer patients. Cancer Res. 1987;47:2986–9.
40. Mathison JC, Wolfson E, Ulevitch RJ. Participation of tumor necrosis factor in the mediation of gram-negative bacterial lipopolysaccharide-induced injury in rabbits. J Clin Invest. 1988;81:1925–37.
41. Stephens KE, Ishizaka A, Larrick JW, et al. Tumor necrosis factor causes increased pulmonary permeability and edema. Am Rev Respir Dis. 1988;137:1364–70.
42. Beutler B, Milsark IW, Cerami A. Passive immunization with cachectin/tumor necrosis factor (TNF) protects mice from the lethal effects of endotoxin. Nature. 1985;229:869–71.
43. Tracey KJ, Fong Y, Hesse DG, et al. Anti-cachectin/TNF monoclonal antibodies prevent septic shock during lethal bacteremia. Nature. 1987;330:662–4.
44. Nawroth PP, Bank I, Handley D, et al. Tumor necrosis factor/cachectin interacts with endothelial cell receptors to induce release of interleukin-1. J Exp Med. 1986;163:1363–75.
45. Kettelhut IC, Fiers W, Goldberg AL. The toxic effects of tumor necrosis factor in vivo and their preventive by cyclooxygenase inhibitors. Proc Natl Acad Sci USA. 1987;84:4273–7.
46. Dinarello CA, Cannon JG, Solff SM, et al. Tumor necrosis factor (cachectin) is an endogenous pyrogen and induces production on interleukin 1. J Exp Med. 1986;163:1433–50.
47. Neilson IR, Neilson KA, Yunis EJ, et al. Failure of tumor necrosis factor to produce hypotensive shock in the absence of endotoxin. Surgery. 1989;106:439–43.
48. Waage A, Espevik T: Interleukin 1 potentiates the lethal effect of tumor necrosis factor α/cachectin in mice. J Exp Med. 1988;167:1987–92.
49. Talmadge JE, Bowersox O, Tribble H, et al. Toxicity of tumor necrosis factor is synergistic with gamma-interferon and can be reduced with cyclooxygenase inhibitors. Am J Pathol. 1987;128:410–25.
50. Ozaki Y, Ohashi T, Minami A, et al. Enhanced resistance of mice to bacterial infection induced by recombinant human interleukin-1α. Infect Immun. 1987;55:1436–40.
51. Scuderi P, Sterling KE, Lam KS, et al. Raised serum levels of tumor necrosis factor in parasitic infections. Lancet. 1986;2:1364–8.
52. Tracey KJ, Beutler B, Lowry SF, et al. Shock and tissue injury induced by recombinant human cachectin. Science. 1986;234:470–4.
53. Ulich TR, Kaizhi G, del Castillo J. Rapid communication. Endotoxin-induced cytokine gene expression in vivo. I. Expression of tumor necrosis factor mRNA in visceral organs under physiologic conditions and during endotoxemia. Am J Pathol. 1989;134:11–14.
54. Aderka D, Le J, Vilcek J. IL-6 inhibits lipopolysaccharide-induced TNF production in cultured human monocytes, U937 cells, and in mice. J Imunol. 1989;143:3517–23.
55. Cannon JG. Cytokines and shock. In: Kimball ES, ed. Cytokines and Inflammation. Boca Raton: CRC Press; 1991:307–29.
56. De Waal MR, Abrams J, Bennet B, et al. Interleukin 10 (IL-10) inhibits cytokine synthesis by human monocytes: An autoregulatory role of IL-10 produced by monocytes. J Exp Med. 1991;174:1209–20.

57. Moncada S, Higgs A. The L-arginine-nitric oxide pathway. N Engl J Med. 1993;329:2002–12.
58. Nussler AK, DiSilvio M, Billiar TR, et al. Stimulation of the nitric oxide synthase pathway in human hepatocytes by cytokines and endotoxin. J Exp Med. 1992;176:261–4.
59. Pepke-Zaba J, Higenbottam TW, Dinh-Xuan AT, et al. Inhaled nitric oxide as a cause of selective pulmonary vasodilatation in pulmonary hypertension. Lancet. 1991;338:1173–4.
60. Petros A, Bennett D, Vallance P. Effect of nitric oxide synthase inhibitors on hypotension in patients with septic shock. Lancet. 1991;338:1557–8.
61. Kilbourn RG, Gross SS, Jubran A, et al. N^G-methyl-L-arginine inhibits tumor necrosis factor-induced hypotension: Implications for the involvement of nitric oxide. Proc Natl Acad Sci USA. 1990;87:3629–32.
62. Wallach D, Holtmann H, Engelmann H, et al. Sensitization and desensitization to lethal effects of tumor necrosis factor and IL-1. J Immunol. 1988;140:2994.
63. Van Zee KJ, Kohno T, Fischer E, et al. Tumor necrosis factor soluble receptors circulate during experimental and clinical inflammation and can protect against excessive tumor necrosis factor α in vitro and in vivo. Proc Natl Acad Sci USA. 1992;89:4845–9.
64. Alexander RH, Doherty GM, Buresh CM, et al. A recombinant human receptor antagonist to interleukin 1 improves survival after lethal endotoxemia in mice. J Exp Med. 1991;173:1029–2.
65. Levi M, ten Cate H, van der Poll T, et al. Pathogenesis of disseminated intravascular coagulation in sepsis. JAMA. 1993;270:975–9.
66. van der Poll T, Buller HR, ten Cate H, et al. Activation of coagulation after administration of tumor necrosis factor to normal subjects. N Engl J Med. 1990;322:1622–7.
67. Bauer KA, ten Cate H, Barzegar S, et al. Tumor necrosis factor infusions have a procoagulant effect on the hemostasis mechanism of humans. Blood. 1989;74:165–72.
68. Warr TA, Mohan-Rao LV, Rapaport SI. Disseminated intravascular coagulation in rabbit induced by administration of endotoxin or tissue factor: Effect of anti-tissue factor antibodies and measurement of plasma extrinsic pathway inhibitor activity. Blood. 1990;75:1481–9.
69. O'Donnell TF, Clowes GHA, Talamo RC, et al. Kinin activation in the blood of patients with sepsis. Surg Gynecol Obstet. 1976;143:539.
70. Bevilacqua MP. Endothelial-leukocyte adhesion molecules. Annu Rev Immunol. 1993;11:767–804.
71. Bevilacqua MP, Pober JS, Majeau GR, et al. Recombinant tumor necrosis factor induces procoagulant activity in cultures of vascular endothelium: Characterization and comparison with the actions of interleukin 1. Proc Natl Acad Sci USA. 1986;83:4533–7.
72. Dinarello CA, Wolff SM. The role of interleukin-1 in disease. N Engl J Med. 1993;328:106.
73. Goldblum SE. The role of cytokines in acute pulmonary vascular endothelial injury. In: Kimball ES, ed. Cytokines and Inflammation. Boca Raton: CRC Press; 1991:191–234.
74. Parsons PE, Worthen GS, Moore EE, et al. The association of circulating endotoxin with the development of the adult respiratory distress syndrome. Am Rev Respir Dis. 1989;140:294–301.
75. Young LS. Nosocomial infections in the immunocompromised adult. Am J Med. 1981;70:398–402.
76. Shenep JL, Flynn PM, Barrett FF, et al. Serial quantitation of endotoxemia and bacteremia during therapy for gram-negative bacterial sepsis. J Infect Dis. 1988;157:565–8.
77. Dietzman DE, Fischer GW, Schoenknecht FD. Neonatal E. coli septicemia: Bacterial counts in blood. J Pediatr. 1974;85:128.
78. DuPont HL, Spink WW. Infections due to gram-negative organisms: An analysis of 860 patients with bacteremia at the University of Minnesota Medical Center, 1958–1966. Medicine (Baltimore). 1969;48:307.
79. Kreger BE, Craven DE, Carling P, et al. Gram-negative bacteremia. III. Reassessment of etiology, epidemiology, and ecology in 612 patients. Am J Med. 1980;68:332.
80. Brandtzaeg P, Kierulf P, Gaustad P, et al. Plasma endotoxin as a predictor of multiple organ failure and death in systemic meningococcal disease. J Infect Dis. 1989;159:195–204.
81. Waage A, Brandtzaeg P, Halstensen A, et al. The complex pattern of cytokines in serum from patients with meingococcal septic shock. J Exp Med. 1989;169:333–8.
82. Calandra T, Baumgartner JD, Grau GE, et al. Prognostic values of tumor necrosis factor/cachectin, interleukin-1, alpha interferon and gamma interferon in the serum of patients with septic shock. J Infect Dis. 1990;149:982–7.
83. Anderson ET, Young LS, Hewitt WL. Antimicrobial synergism in the therapy of gram-negative bacteremia. Chemotherapy. 1978;24:45.
84. McCabe WR, Jackson GG. Gram-negative bacteremia. II. Clinical, laboratory and therapeutic observations. Arch Intern Med. 1962;110:856.
85. Bryant RE, Hood AF, Hood CE, et al. Factors affecting mortality of gram-negative rod bacteremia. Arch Intern Med. 1971;127:120.
86. Young LS, Martin WJ, Meyer RD, et al. Gram-negative rod bacteremia: Microbiologic immunologic, and therapeutic considerations. Ann Intern Med. 1977;86:456.
87. Freid MA, Vosti KL. Importance of underlying disease in patients with gram-negative bacteremia. Arch Intern Med. 1968;121:418.
88. Young LS. Treatment of infections due to gram-negative bacilli: A perspective of past, present and future. Rev Infect Dis. 1985;7(Suppl 4):572.
89. Young LS. Combination or single drug therapy for gram-negative sepsis. In: Remington JS, Swartz MN, eds. Curr Clin Topics Infect Dis. 1982;3:177.
90. Calandra T, Cometta A. Antibiotic therapy for gram-negative bacteremia. Infect Dis Clin North Am. 1991;5:817–34.
91. EORTC Antimicrobial Therapy Project Group. Ceftazidime combined with a short or long course of amikacin for empirical therapy of gram-negative bacteremia in cancer patients with granulocytopenia. N Engl J Med. 1987;317:1692–98.
92. Klastersky J, Glauser MP, Schimpff SC, et al. Prospective randomized comparison of three antibiotic regimens for empirical thearpy of suspected bacteremia infection in febrila granulocytopenic patients. Antimicrobial Agents Chemother. 1986;29:263–70.
93. Young LS. Empirical antimicrobial therapy in the neutropenic host. N Engl J Med. 1986;315:580.
94. Pizzo PA, Hawthorn JW, Hiemenz J, et al. A randomized trial comparing ceftazidime alone with combination antibiotic therapy in cancer patients with fever and neutropenia. N Engl J Med. 1986;315:552–8.
95. Spengler RF, Geenough WB III, Stolley PD. A descriptive study of nosocomial bacteremias at The Johns Hopkins Hospital, 1968–1974. Johns Hopkins Med J. 1978;142:77.
96. Schimpff S, Satterlee W, Young VM, et al. Therapy with carbenicillin and gentamicin in febrile cancer patients. N Engl J Med. 1971;284:1061.
97. Lumish RM, Norden CW. Therapy of neutropenic rats infected with Pseudomonas aeruginosa. J Infect Dis. 1976;133:538.
98. Robson HG. Synergistic activity of carbenicillin and gentamicin in experimental pseudomonas bacteremia in neutropenic rats. Antimicrob Agents Chemother. 1976;10:646.
99. Young LS. Review of clinical significance of synergy in gram-negative bacteremic infections at the UCLA hospital. Infection. 1978;10:247–54.
100. Klastersky J, Meunier-Carpentier F, Prevost JM. Significance of antimicrobial synergism for the outcome of gram-negative sepsis. Am J Med Sci. 1977;273:157.
101. Sculier JP, Klastersky J. Significance of serum bactericidal activity in gram-negative bacillary bacteremia in patients with and without granulocytopenia. Am J Med. 1984;76:429–35.
102. Feld R, Valdivieso M, Bodey GP, et al. A comparative trial of sisomicin therapy by intermittent versus continuous infusion. Am J Med Sci. 1977;274:179.
103. Rolston KVI, Berkey P, Bodey GP, et al. A comparison of imipenem to ceftazidime with or without amikacin as empiric therapy in febrile neutropenic patients. Arch Intern Med. 1992;152:283–91.
104. DeJongh CA, Joshi JH, Newman KA, et al. Antibiotic synergism and response in gram-negative bacteremia in granulocytopenic cancer patients. Am J Med. 1986;80:96–100.
105. Hughes WT, Armstrong D, Bodey GP, et al. Guidelines for the use of antimicrobial agents in neutropenic patients with unexplained fever. J Infect Dis. 1990;161:381–96.
106. International Antimicrobial Therapy Project Group of the European Organization for Research and Treatment of Cancer. Combination of amikacin and carbenicillin with or without cefazolin as empirical treatment of febrile neutropenic patients. J Clin Oncol. 1983;1:597–603.
107. Kaye D, Levison ME, Labovitz ED. The unpredictability of serum concentrations of gentamicin. Pharmacoclinetics of gentamicin in patients with normal and abnormal renal function. J Infect Dis. 1974;130:150.
108. Anderson ET, Young LS, Hewitt WL. Simultaneous antibiotic levels in "breakthrough" gram-negative bacteremia. Am J Med. 1976;61:493.
109. Smith CR, Maxwell RR, Edwards CQ, et al. Nephrotoxicity induced by gentamicin and amikacin. Johns Hopkins Med J. 1978;142:85.
110. Shine K, Silver M, Young LS, et al. Aspects of the management of shock. Ann Intern Med. 1980;93:723–34.
111. Winslow EJ, Loeb HS, Pahimtoola SH, et al. Hemodynamic studies and results of therapy in 50 patients with bacteremic shock. Am J Med. 1973;54:421.
112. Weitzman S, Berger S. Clinical trial design in studies of corticosteroids for bacterial infections. Ann Intern Med. 1974;81:36.
113. Klastersky J, Cappel R, Debusscher L. Effectiveness of betamethasone in management of severe infections. N Engl J Med. 1971;284:1248.
114. Schumer W. Steroids in the treatment of clinical septic shock. Ann Surg. 1976;184:333.
115. Hotfman SL, Punjabi NH, Kumala S, et al. Reduction of mortality in chloramphenicol-treated severe typhoid fever by high-dose dexamethasone. N Engl J Med. 1981;301:456–7.
116. Sprung CL, Caralis PV, Marcial EH, et al. The effects of high-dose corticosteroids in patients with septic shock: A prospective controlled study. N Engl J Med. 1984;311:1137–43.
117. Veterans Administration Systemic Sepsis Cooperative Study Group. Effect of high dose glucocorticoid therapy on mortality in patients with clinical signs of systemic sepsis. N Engl J Med. 1987;317:659–6.
118. Bone RC, Fisher CJ, Clemmer TP, et al. A controlled clinical trial of high-dose methylprednisolone in the treatment of severe sepsis and septic shock. N Engl J Med. 1987;317:653–8.
119. Bernard GR, Luce JM, Sprungs CL, et al. High-dose corticosteroids in patients with the adult respiratory distress syndrome. N Engl J Med. 1987;317:1565–70.
120. Luce JM, Montgomery AB, Marks JD, et al. Ineffectiveness of high-dose methylprednisolone in preventing parenchymal lung injury and improving mortality in patients with septic shock. Am Rev Respir Dis. 1988;138:62–8.
121. Corrigan JJ Jr, Ray WL, May N. Change in blood coagulation system associated with septicemia. N Engl J Med. 1968;279:851.
122. Corrigan JC, Kiernat JF. Effect of heparin in experimental gram-negative septicemia. J Infect Dis. 1975;131:138.
123. Corrigan JJ. Heparin therapy in bacterial septicemia. J Pediatr. 1977;91:695.

124. Higby DJ, Yates JW, Henderson ES. Filtration leukopheresis for granulocyte transfusion therapy. N Engl J Med. 1975;292:761.

125. Herzig RH, Herzig GP, Graw RG Jr, et al. Successful granulocyte transfusion therapy for gram-negative septicemia. N Engl J Med. 1977;296:701.

126. Alavi JB, Root RK, Djerassi I, et al. A randomized clinical trial of granulocyte transfusions for infection in acute leukemia. N Engl J Med. 1977;296:706.

127. Vogler WR, Winston EF. A controlled study of the efficacy of granulocyte transfusions in patients with neutropenia. Am J Med. 1977;63:548.

128. Winston DJ, Ho WG, Gale RP. Therapeutic granulocyte transfusions for documented infections. Ann Intern Med. 1982;97:509.

129. Pizzo PA. Drug therapy: Management of fever in patients with cancer and treatment-induced neutropenia. N Engl J Med. 1993;328:1323–32.

130. Faden AI, Holaday JW. Experimental endotoxin shock. The pathophysiologic function of endorphins and treatment with opiate antagonists. J Infect Dis. 1980;142:229.

131. Faden AI, Holaday JW. Opiate antagonists: A role in the treatment of hypovolemic shock. Science. 1979;205:317.

132. Peters WP, Johnson MW, Friedman PA, et al. Pressor effect of naloxone in septic shock. Lancet. 1981;1:529.

133. DeMaria A, Craven DE, Heffernan JJ, et al. Naloxone versus placebo in treatment of septic shock. Lancet. 1985;1:1363–5.

134. Sullivan GW, Carper HT, Novick WJ, et al. Inhibition of the inflammatory action of interleukin-1 and tumor necrosis factor (alpha) on neutrophil function by pentoxifylline. Infect Immun. 1988;56:1722–9.

135. Young LS. Immunoprophylaxis and serotherapy of bacterial infections. Am J Med. 1984;76:664–71.

136. Feingold DS, Oski F. *Pseudomonas* infection. Treatment with immune human plasma. Arch Intern Med. 1965;116:326.

137. Jones CE, Alexander JW, Fisher MW. Clinical evaluation of *Pseudomonas* hyperimmune globulin. J Surg Res. 1973;14:87.

138. Ziegler EJ, McCutchan JA, Fierer J, et al. Treatment of gram-negative bacteremia and shock with human antiserum to a mutant *Escherichia coli*. N Engl J Med. 1982;307:1225.

139. Calandra T, Glauser MP, Schellekens J, et al. Treatment of gram-negative septic shock with human IgG antibody to *Escherichia coli* J5: A prospective, double-blind, randomized trial. J Infect Dis. 1988;158:312–9.

140. Young LS, Gascon R, Alam S, et al. Monoclonal antibodies for treatment of gram-negative infections. Rev Infect Dis. 1989;11(Suppl 7):S1564–71.

141. Teng NH, Kaplan HS, Hebert JM, et al. Protection against gram-negative bacteremia and endotoxemia with human monoclonal IgM antibodies. Proc Natl Acad Sci USA. 1985;82:1790–4.

142. Harkonen S, Scannon P, Mischak RP, et al. Phase I study of a murine monoclonal anti-lipid antibody in bacteremic and nonbacteremic patients. Antimicrob Agents Chemother. 1988;32:710–6.

143. Ziegler EFJ, Fisher CJ Jr, Sprung CL, et al. Treatment of gram-negative bacteremia and septic shock with HA-1A human monoclonal antibody against endotoxin. N Engl J Med. 1991;324:429–36.

144. Greenman RL, Schein RMH, Martin MA, et al. A controlled clinical trial of E5 murine monoclonal IgM antibody to endotoxin in the treatment of gram-negative sepsis. JAMA. 1991;266:1097–102.

145. Warren HS, Danner RL, Munford RS. Anti-endotoxin monoclonal antibodies. N Engl J Med. 1992;326:1153–7.

146. Wenzel RP. Anti-endotoxin monoclonal antibodies—A second look. N Engl J Med. 1992;326:1151–2.

147. Bone RC. A critical evaluation of new agents for the treatment of sepsis. JAMA. 1991;266:1686–91.

148. Arend SP. Interleukin-1 receptor antagonist: A new member of the interleukin-1 family. J Clin Invest. 1991;88:1445–51.

149. Pennington JE. Therapy with antibody to tumor necrosis factor in sepsis. Clin Infect Dis. 1993;17(Suppl):S515–9.

150. Gallay P, Heumann D, LeRoy D, et al. Lipopolysaccharide-binding protein as a major plasma protein responsible for endotoxemic shock. Proc Natl Acad Sci USA. 1993;90:9935–8.

151. Lindberg RB, Moncrief JA, Mason AD Jr. Control of experimental and clinical burn wound sepsis by topical application of sulfamylon compounds. Ann NY Acad Sci. 1968;50:950.

152. Greenfield S, Teres D, Bushnell LS, et al. Prevention of gram-negative bacillary pneumonia using aerosol polymixin as prophylaxis. J Clin Invest. 1973;52:2935.

153. Feeley TW, du Moulin GC, Hedley-Whyte J, et al. Aerosol polymixin and pneumonia. N Engl J Med. 1975;293:471.

154. Storring RA, McElwain TJ, Jameson B, et al. Oral non-absorbed antibiotics prevent infection in acute non-lymphoblastic leukaemia. Lancet. 1977;2:837.

155. Schimpff SC, Greene WH, Young VM, et al. Infection prevention in acute nonlymphocytic leukemia. Laminar air flow room reverse isolation with oral, nonabsorbable antibiotics prophylaxis. Ann Intern Med. 1975;82:351.

156. Young LS. Trimethorprim-sulfamethoxazole and bacterial infections during leukemic therapy. Ann Intern Med. 1981;95:508.

157. Young LS. Antimicrobial prophylaxis against infection in neutropenic patients. J Infect Dis. 1983;147:611.

158. Karp JE, Merz WG, Hendricksen C, et al. Oral norfloxacin for prevention of gram-negative bacterial infections in patients with acute leukemia and granulocytopenia: A randomized, double-blind, placebo-controlled trial. Ann Intern Med. 1987;106:1–7.

159. Dekker AW, Rozenberg-Arska M, Verhoef J. Infection prophylaxis in acute leukemia: A comparison of ciprofloxacin with trimethoprim-sulfamethoxazole and colistin. Ann Intern Med. 1987;106:7–12.

160. Young LS. Antimicrobial prophylaxis against infection in neutropenic patients. J Infect Dis. 1983;147:611–4.

161. Ammann AJ, Addiego J, Wara D, et al. Polyvalent pneumococcal polysaccharide immunization of patients with sickle cell anemia and patient with splenectomy. N Engl J Med. 1977;297:897.

162. Young LS, Meyer RD, Armstrong D. *Pseudomonas aeruginosa* vaccine in cancer patients. Ann Intern Med. 1973;79:518.

163. Alexander JW, Fisher MW, MacMillan BG. Immunological control of *Pseudomonas* infection in burn patients. A clinical evaluation. Arch Surg. 1971;102:31.

164. Jones RJ, Roe EA, Gupta JL. Low mortality in burned patients in a *Pseudomonas* vaccine trial. Lancet. 1978;2:401.

165. Dwyer JM. Manipulating the immune system with immune globulin. N Engl J Med. 1992;326:106–16.

SECTION F

57. PERITONITIS AND OTHER INTRA-ABDOMINAL INFECTIONS

MATTHEW E. LEVISON
LARRY M. BUSH

Intra-abdominal infection may take several forms. Infection may be in the retroperitoneal space or within the peritoneal cavity. Intraperitoneal infection may be diffuse or localized into one or more abscesses. Intraperitoneal abscesses may form in dependent recesses such as the pelvic space or Morison's pouch, in the various perihepatic spaces, within the lesser sac, and along the major routes of communication between intraperitoneal recesses, such as the right paracolic gutter. In addition, infection may be contained within the intra-abdominal viscera, such as hepatic, pancreatic, splenic, tuboovarian, or renal abscesses. Abscesses also frequently form about diseased viscera—pericholecystic, periappendiceal, pericolic, and tuboovarian—and between adjacent loops of bowel (i.e., interloop abscesses).

ANATOMY

The anatomic relationships within the abdomen are important in determining possible sources as well as routes of spread of infection. The peritoneal cavity extends from the undersurface of the diaphragm to the floor of the pelvis. In men the peritoneal cavity is a closed space. In women it is perforated by the free ends of the fallopian tubes. The stomach, jejunum, ileum, cecum, appendix, transverse and sigmoid colons, liver, gallbladder, and spleen lie within the peritoneal cavity, some being suspended by a mesentery.

The peritoneal reflections and mesenteric attachments compartmentalize the intraperitoneal space and route, spreading exudate to sites that are often distant from the source (Fig. 1). The transverse mesocolon (14, in Fig. 1) divides the peritoneal cavity horizontally into an upper and a lower space. The greater omentum, extending from the transverse mesocolon and lower border of the stomach, covers the lower peritoneal cavity and further separates the upper from the lower peritoneal cavity (Fig. 2). The small bowel mesentery divides the lower peritoneal space.

The peritoneal cavity has several recesses into which exudate may become loculated. The most dependent recess of the peritoneal cavity in the supine position is in the pelvis. Between the rectum and bladder in men is a pouch of peritoneal cavity that extends slightly below the level of the seminal vesicles. In women, the uterus and fallopian tubes project into the pelvic recess. Between the rectum and body of the uterus is the pouch of Douglas, which lies above the posterior fornix of the vagina. On either side of the rectum and bladder are the pararectal and paravesical fossae. The pelvic recess is continuous with both the right and left paracolic gutters.

The phrenicocolic ligament, which fixes the splenic flexure of the colon to the diaphragm, partially bridges the junction between the left paracolic gutter and the left perihepatic space. In contrast, the right paracolic gutter is continuous with the right subhepatic space and the right subphrenic space. A posterior superior extension of the right subhepatic space, Morison's pouch, is the most dependent portion in the supine position of

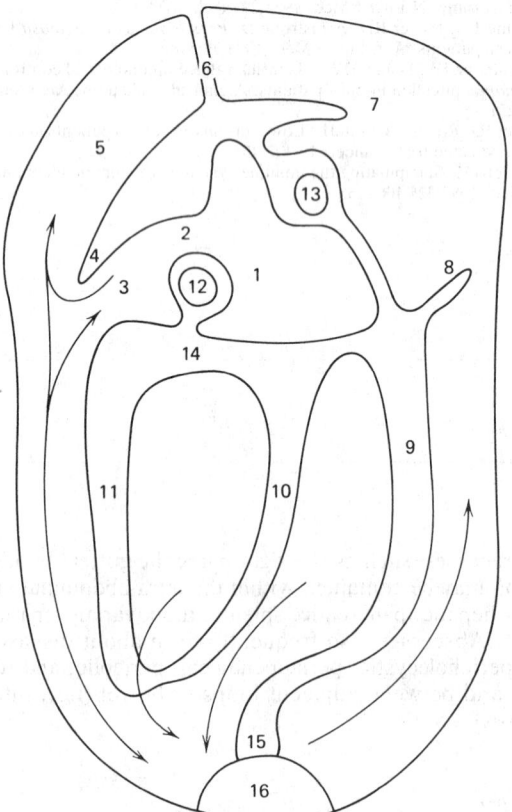

FIG. 1. Schema of the posterior peritoneal reflections and recesses of the peritoneal cavity. 1: Lesser sac; 2: foramen of Winslow; 3: Morison's pouch; 4: right triangular ligament; 5: right subphrenic space; 6: falciform ligament; 7: left subphrenic space; 8: phrenico-colic ligament; 9: bare area of the descending colon; 10: root of the small bowel mesentery; 11: bare area of ascending colon; 12: duodenum; 13: esophagus; 14: root of the transverse mesocolon; 15: bare area of rectum; 16: bladder.

the right paravertebral groove and lies just above the beginning of the transverse mesocolon. The horizontal posterior reflection of the serosal surface of the liver onto the diaphragm (the right triangular and coronary ligaments) and vertical reflection (the falciform ligament) divide the right perihepatic space into right subphrenic and right subhepatic spaces (Figs. 1 and 2A). The left subphrenic and subhepatic spaces communicate freely around the smaller left lobe of the liver and its more superiorly placed left triangular ligament[1,2] (Figs. 1 and 2B). The right and left subphrenic spaces are separated by the falciform ligament, which probably prevents the spread of pus to the opposite side and explains why only about 5–15 percent of subphrenic abscesses are bilateral.[2] The left subhepatic space is divided by the gastrohepatic omentum into an anterior space and the lesser sac (Fig. 2B). Abscesses within the perihepatic spaces become localized by pyogenic membranes. In the right subphrenic space they lie anteriorly or posteriorly and in the subhepatic space superiorly or inferiorly.[1,2] Abscesses of the left perihepatic space are either in the single left subphrenic space or in the lesser sac.[1,2]

The lesser sac, the largest recess of the peritoneal cavity, is connected to the main peritoneal space by the foramen of Winslow, an opening situated between the free border of the gastrohepatic omentum and the posterior parietal peritoneum. The lesser sac is surrounded posteriorly by the pancreas and kidneys, anteriorly by the stomach, and laterally by the liver and spleen. It may also extend to a variable extent between the folds of the greater omentum. Because of the limited communication from the lesser sac to the major cavity via the foramen of Winslow, suppuration in the lesser sac may exist with little or no involvement of the major cavity. Abscesses in the lesser sac lie between the stomach and pancreas but may spread to the right and lie anterior to the right kidney and inferior to the liver.

After intraperitoneal injection of water-soluble contrast material selectively into various intraperitoneal spaces, Myers[3] has demonstrated that the right paracolic gutter is the main communication between the upper and lower peritoneal cavities. Fluid introduced into the right upper peritoneal space gravitates toward Morison's pouch and then into the right subphrenic space and along the right paracolic gutter into the pelvic recess (Fig. 3). Flow of fluid in the left upper peritoneal space is mainly into the left subphrenic space. The phrenicocolic ligament limits flow inferiorly into the left paracolic gutter. Fluid introduced into the lower peritoneal cavity first gravitates to the pelvic recess and then ascends, whether in the supine or erect position, along the right paracolic gutter into the right subhepatic space, especially into Morison's pouch, and into the right subphrenic space. Ascension of fluid from the pelvic space along the left paracolic gutter is minimal and limited by the phrenicocolic ligament. Although gravity would account for the pooling of fluid in the dependent peritoneal recesses, such as the pelvic recess and Morison's pouch, ascension of fluid from the pelvis to the subphrenic space is probably due to hydrostatic pressure differences between the upper and lower peritoneal cavities created by diaphragmatic motion. Normal intestinal and abdominal wall motion would also account for some spread of intraperitoneal fluid.

The retroperitoneal space lies between the posterior peritoneal membrane and the transversalis fascia, extending from the diaphragm to the pelvic brim. In the anterior retroperitoneal space between the peritoneum and anterior renal fascia lie the ascending and descending colons, duodenum, and pancreas. The kidneys and ureters lie within the posterior retroperitoneal (perinephric) space, between the anterior and posterior renal fasciae. The renal fascia encloses the kidneys and adrenals superiorly and laterally, but not inferiorly, favoring spread of infection in this space inferiorly.[4]

The parietal peritoneum, mainly the anterior portion, is well supplied by somatic afferent nerves and is sensitive to all forms of stimuli. The ability of the anterior parietal peritoneum to

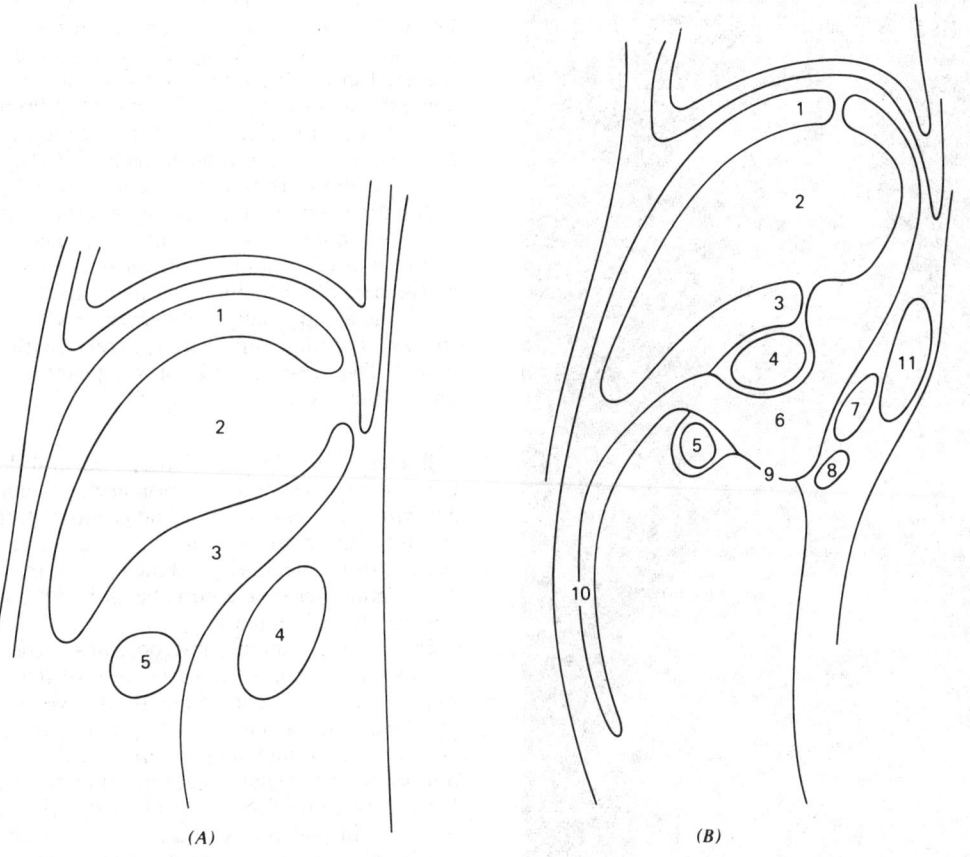

FIG. 2. Schema of a sagittal section of the peritoneal cavity. **(A)** Right upper quadrant. 1: Subphrenic space; 2: liver; 3: subhepatic space; 4: right kidney; 5: transverse colon. **(B)** Left upper quadrant. 1: Subphrenic space; 2: liver, left lobe; 3: subhepatic space; 4: stomach; 5: transverse colon; 6: lesser sac; 7: pancreas; 8: duodenum; 9: transverse mesocolon; 10: omemtum; 11: left kidney.

sense sharp, well-localized pain in response to local inflammation is of primary importance in diagnosing abdominal infection and may be associated with involuntary abdominal muscle contraction, tenderness, and rebound tenderness. Irritation of the peripheral diaphragmatic peritoneum is felt as pain near the adjacent body wall, and irritation of the central portion is felt as pain referred to the shoulder. Stimulation of the visceral peritoneum, usually due to distension of an organ, causes poorly localized, somewhat dull, pain.

The peritoneal cavity is lined by a serous membrane. The surface area of this membrane approximates that of the skin. The membrane consists of a monolayer of flat polygonal cells beneath which are lymphatics, blood vessels, and nerve endings. Normally, the peritoneal space contains only sufficient fluid to maintain moistness of the surface, facilitating movements of the viscera. Noninflamed serous fluid is clear yellow with a low specific gravity (<1.016) and low protein content (usually <3 g/dl). The protein is predominantly albumin. Fibrinogen is not present, and serous fluid will not clot. Solute concentrations are nearly identical to those in plasma. A few leukocytes (<300/mm^3), mostly mononuclear cells, and desquamated serosal cells may be found.

The peritoneal membrane is highly permeable. Bidirectional transfer of substances across this membrane is rapid and, because of the large surface area involved, is potentially great in quantity. In fact, the peritoneal surface has been used extensively as a dialyzing membrane for the treatment of uremia and has also been used for the administration of fluid, electrolytes, antibiotics, and even blood. The effective serum oncotic pressure and the hydrostatic pressure in the portal veins and lymphatics are major determinants of the rate and direction of fluid

movement. The rate of movement of water and solutes between blood and peritoneal fluid is also dependent on concentration gradients between these compartments and has been studied in detail.[5,6] Water and solutes diffuse via blood capillaries and to a lesser extent by lymphatics. Lymphatics are primarily involved in removal of nonirritating colloids and particles into the blood stream. Absorption into lymphatics of particulate matter is thought to take place mostly from the diaphragmatic surface and is aided by the pumping action of diaphragmatic motion.[7] Following infusion of ^{51}Cr-labeled red blood cells into the peritoneal cavity of dogs, Rochlin et al.[8] reported absorption of about 70 percent of the labeled red blood cells by 48–96 hours. This absorption occurred mostly via the lymphatics. In humans, two-thirds of intraperitoneally injected red blood cells in anticoagulated blood have been found in the circulation 8–12 days after infusion.[9] The quantity of resorbed cells was less when no anticoagulant was used with the transfused cells, presumably due to trapping of red blood cells in intraperitoneal clots.[9] Transport of other particulate matter, such as intraperitoneal bacteria, may be similarly impeded because of trapping in fibrinous intraperitoneal exudate.[10]

In addition, there are communications between the peritoneal and pleural cavities that are independent of the blood stream. In patients with Meigs syndrome, for example, radioactive colloidal gold instilled into the peritoneal cavity appears in the pleural space probably as a result of transdiaphragmatic lymphatic transport.[11]

PERITONITIS

Inflammation of the peritoneum may be the result of contamination of the peritoneal cavity with microorganisms, irritating

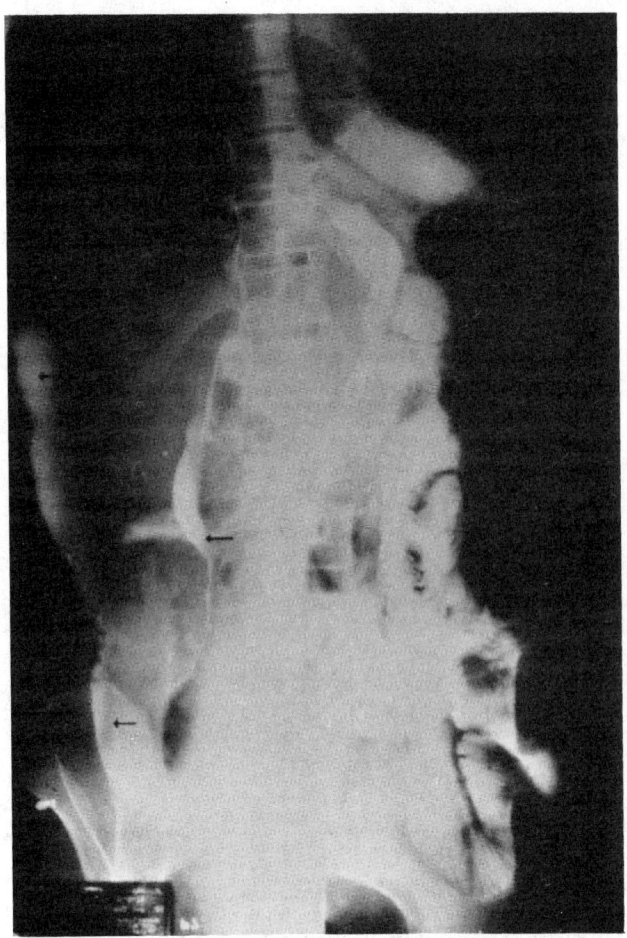

FIG. 3. Abdominal radiograph (right decubitis) after oral administration of gastrografin to a patient with dehiscence of an esophageal-gastric anastomosis. Radiopaque gastrografin (arrows) can be seen in the subhepatic space, right paracolic gutter, and right subphrenic space, as well as within the lumen of the intestinal tract.

chemicals, or both. There are two major types of infective peritonitis: (1) the primary (so-called spontaneous or idiopathic) variety, in which no primary focus of infection is evident; and (2) the secondary variety, in which a primary intra-abdominal process, such as a ruptured appendix or perforated peptic ulcer, is evident.

Primary Peritonitis

Etiology. Primary peritonitis is probably not a specific entity with a common cause but represents a group of diseases with different causes having in common only infection of the peritoneal cavity without an evident source. Primary peritonitis occurs at all ages. The prevalence of primary peritonitis in children apparently has been decreasing.[12] In the preantibiotic era, primary peritonitis occurred in about 10 percent of all pediatric abdominal emergencies; it now accounts for less than 1–2 percent.[13,14] The decline has been attributed to widespread use of antibiotics for minor upper respiratory tract illness. Although primary peritonitis may occur in children without predisposing disease,[12] it is known to occur particularly in children with postnecrotic cirrhosis[13,15] and in 2 percent of children with the nephrotic syndrome.[12,16] In one study, it was also frequently associated with urinary tract infections.[13] In some nephrotic children, repeated episodes of peritonitis occur, and peritonitis may precede other manifestations of nephrosis.[12]

In adults, primary peritonitis usually has been reported in patients with alcoholic cirrhosis and ascites. In 1971, Conn and Fessel[17] summarized their experience with 32 episodes in 28 patients and, in addition, reviewed 46 episodes in 42 patients reported in the literature. Subsequent reports have confirmed and extended their initial findings.[18–24] Primary peritonitis was found to occur in about 10 percent of the patients with alcoholic cirrhosis collected retrospectively.[17,18] Among 63 consecutive patients with cirrhosis and ascites studied prospectively using optimal aerobic and anaerobic bacteriologic techniques, primary peritonitis was found in 5.[21] Primary peritonitis has also been reported in adults with postnecrotic cirrhosis,[15] chronic active hepatitis,[25] acute viral hepatitis,[26] congestive heart failure,[27] metastatic malignant disease,[28] systemic lupus erythematosus,[29] lymphedema,[30] and, rarely, with no underlying disease.[31] The presence of ascites appears to be the common link among these various conditions.

Bacteriologic Characteristics. Several decades ago, the organisms reported to cause primary peritonitis in children were *Streptococcus pneumoniae* and group A streptococci.[12–14] More recently, the number of nephrotic children with streptococcal peritonitis has declined, and the relative frequency of peritonitis due to gram-negative enteric bacilli[13,14,16] and staphylococci[12,14] apparently has increased.

In cirrhotic patients, microorganisms presumably of enteric origin account for up to 69 percent of the pathogens.[32] *Escherichia coli* is the most frequently recovered pathogen, followed by *Klebsiella pneumoniae*, *S. pneumoniae*, and other streptococcal species, including enterococci.[17,20,32–34] *Staphylococcus aureus* is an unusual isolate in primary peritonitis, accounting for 2–4 percent of the cases in most series, and has been noted to occur in patients with an erosion of an umbilical hernia.[33] Anaerobes and microaerophilic organisms are infrequently reported.[20,24] Possible explanations include the intrinsic bacteristatic activity of ascites against *Bacteroides* spp.,[35] the relatively high PO_2 of ascitic fluid,[36] and the lack of optimal anaerobic bacteriologic techniques used to study patients with primary peritonitis in the past. In a review of 126 cases of primary peritonitis in cirrhotic patients recorded in the literature, only 6 percent (eight patients) were due to anaerobic or microaerophilic bacteria, including *Bacteroides* spp., *Bacteroides fragilis*, *Clostridium perfringens*, *Peptostreptococcus* spp., *Peptococcus* spp., and *Campylobacter fetus*.[20] Polymicrobial infection was present in four of these eight cirrhotic patients with peritonitis due to anaerobes, in contrast to the relatively low frequency of polymicrobial infection (only 10 of 118 cases of peritonitis) when aerobes alone were involved.

Ascitic fluid with positive cultures but few leukocytes in patients without clinical findings of peritonitis has been noted and called *bacterascites*.[34] This may represent early colonization before a host response.[24] However, patients with a low leukocyte response have the same mortality as those with a greater response.[23] Conversely, several series have identified cases of primary peritonitis with negative ascitic fluid cultures.[17,24] In one series, sterile cultures occurred in 35 percent of patients with clinical findings consistent with primary peritonitis, ascitic fluid leukocyte counts of above 500/mm³, and no evident source of intra-abdominal infection.[37] Blood cultures were positive in one-third of these patients. This variant of primary peritonitis has been termed *culture-negative neutrocytic ascites*.[37] The frequency of culture-negative ascitic fluid may be decreased by inoculating blood culture bottles with ascitic fluid at the bedside.[38]

Bacteremia is present in up to 75 percent of patients with primary peritonitis due to aerobic bacteria,[32] but is rarely found in those with peritonitis due to anaerobes.[20] Usually the same organisms isolated from the peritoneal fluid are recovered from the blood.[17,20]

Occasionally, primary peritonitis may be caused by *Mycobac-*

terium tuberculosis, Neisseria gonorrhoeae, or *Chlamydia trachomatis.*

Pathogenesis. The route of infection in primary peritonitis is usually not apparent, and often it is presumed to be either hematogenous, lymphogenous, transmural migration through an intact gut wall from the intestinal lumen, or, in women, from the vagina via the fallopian tubes. Conn and Fessel[17] have postulated that the hematogenous route is most likely in cirrhotic patients: either *(1)* organisms removed from circulation by the liver may contaminate hepatic lymph and pass through the permeable lymphatic walls into the ascitic fluid or *(2)* portosystemic shunting greatly diminishes hepatic clearance of bacteremia in the portal circulation, which would tend to perpetuate bacteremia and increase the opportunity to cause metastic infection at susceptible sites such as the ascitic collection. The infrequency of primary peritonitis in all forms of ascites except that secondary to liver disease emphasizes the importance of intrahepatic shunting in the pathogenesis of this disease. The hepatic reticuloendothelial system is known to be a major site for removal of bacteria from blood,[39] and animal studies have suggested that destruction of blood-borne bacteria by the reticuloendothelial system is impaired in experimental cirrhosis[40] and in alcoholic liver disease.[41] The decrease in phagocytic activity seen in alcoholic cirrhosis is proportional to the severity of the liver disease.[42] Additionally, alcohol abuse and cirrhosis have been reported to be associated with impaired intracellular killing by monocytes and neutrophils,[43] as well as impaired opsonization[44] and low levels of serum complement.[45] The characteristics of ascitic fluid in nephrosis and cirrhosis predispose to infection. Opsonic activity, as reflected by low levels of complement and immunoglobulins, is reduced in the ascitic fluid of patients with the nephrotic syndrome and cirrhosis.[46,47] Primary bacteremia, usually due to coliforms, is a common complication in cirrhosis,[48] and metastatic infection in the pleural space has also been reported in cirrhotic patients.[49] An increased frequency of gram-negative endocarditis has also been noted in cirrhotics.[50]

Enteric bacteria may also gain access to the peritoneal cavity by directly traversing the intact intestinal wall. This has been demonstrated in animals. Schweinburg et al.[51] demonstrated that in dogs ^{14}C-labeled *E. coli* passed from the bowel into the peritoneal cavity after the introduction of hypertonic solutions into the peritoneum. A similar mechanism may explain the enteric bacterial peritonitis that frequently complicates peritoneal dialysis.[52] The infrequent occurrence of bacteremia and the multiplicity of species in peritoneal fluid when anaerobic bacteria are involved suggest that transmural migration of bacteria is the probable route of infection of ascitic fluid in the majority of these patients.[20] In addition, the occurrence of polymicrobial anaerobic peritonitis in two patients after infusion of vasopressin into the superior mesenteric or gastroduodenal arteries suggests that arterial vasoconstriction decreased the intestinal mucosal barrier and permitted transmural migration of enteric organisms.[19] Colonic microorganisms have been reported to colonize the upper small bowel in cirrhotic patients.[53]

The simultaneous presence of pneumococci in vaginal secretions and peritoneal fluid in girls[54] makes an ascending infection of genital origin likely in these patients. The alkaline vaginal secretions of prepubertal girls may be less inhibitory to bacterial growth than the acidic secretions of postpubertal females. Transfallopian spread is also suggested by the development of primary peritonitis in women with intrauterine devices (IUDs).[55,56] The route of spread in women with gonococcal or chlamydial perihepatitis (Fitz-Hugh-Curtis syndrome) is presumably from the fallopian tubes and paracolic gutters to the subphrenic space, but may also be hematogenous. In the one man with this syndrome, *N. gonorrhoeae* was recovered from a liver biopsy specimen, and the route of spread was presumably via bacteremia.[57]

Although tuberculous peritonitis may result from direct entry

into the peritoneal cavity of tubercle bacilli (from the lymph nodes, intestine, or genital tract in patients with active disease of these organs), it is more likely to be disseminated hematogenously from remote foci of tuberculosis, most commonly in the lung. Tuberculous peritonitis may become clinically evident after the initial focus has completely healed.

Clinical Manifestations. Primary peritonitis is an acute febrile illness often confused with acute appendicitis in children. Fever, abdominal pain, nausea, vomiting, and diarrhea are usually present with diffuse abdominal tenderness, rebound tenderness, and hypoactive or absent bowel sounds. In cirrhotic patients with primary peritonitis, preexisting ascites is present. In some patients, the clinical manifestations may be atypical. The onset, for example, may be insidious, and findings of peritoneal irritation may be absent in an abdomen distended with ascites. Fever (>100°F) is the most common presenting sign, occurring in 50–80 percent of cases,[17,23] and may be present without abdominal signs or symptoms, or the process may be completely silent. Primary peritonitis in cirrhotic patients is generally associated with other features of end-stage liver disease (hepatorenal syndrome, progressive encephalopathy, and variceal bleeding).

The ascitic fluid protein concentration may be low[17] in abdominal inflammation for the following reasons: *(1)* hypoalbuminemia[58] and *(2)* dilution of ascitic fluid with transudate from the portal system when there is cirrhosis or the portal vein is obstructed.[59] The leukocyte count in peritoneal fluid usually is greater than 300/mm[3] (in 85 percent of cases, >1000/mm[3]), with granulocytes predominating in more than 80 percent of cases.[22] However, the total leukocyte count of some patients with ascites uncomplicated by infection may be similarly elevated.[21] Indeed, an increase in ascites leukocyte counts has been noted during diuresis in patients with chronic liver disease.[60] Some studies of other parameters of ascitic fluid that may help in diagnosing primary bacterial peritonitis have found the lactate concentration and pH to be useful.[61–63] Ascitic fluid pH less than 7.35 and lactate more than 25 mg/dl were more specific but less sensitive than a leukocyte count above 500/mm[3], and using all three parameters together increased the diagnostic accuracy.[62,63] Gram stain of the sediment when positive is diagnostic, but it may be negative in about 60–80 percent of cases with cirrhosis and ascites.[17,22]

Gonococcal perihepatitis (Fitz-Hugh-Curtis syndrome) most often occurs in women. It manifests with sudden onset of pain in the right upper quadrant of the abdomen, at times referred to the right shoulder. There may be low-grade fever, right upper quadrant tenderness, guarding, and a friction rub over the liver.[64] Gonococcal cervicitis and/or salpingitis may or may not be clinically evident. Chlamydial and gonococcal perihepatitis are clinically indistinguishable.

Primary tuberculous peritonitis usually is gradual in onset, with fever, weight loss, malaise, night sweats, and abdominal distension. The abdomen may not be rigid and is often characterized as being "doughy" on palpation. The findings at operation or laparoscopy consist of multiple nodules scattered over the peritoneal surface and omentum. Adhesions and a variable amount of peritoneal fluid are usually present. Ascitic fluid may have an elevated protein concentration (>3 g/dl) and a lymphocytic pleocytosis, but neither may be present, especially in cirrhotic patients.[65] Similarly, *Coccidioides immitis* can cause a granulomatous peritonitis with a variable clinical manifestation.[66]

Diagnosis. The diagnosis of primary peritonitis is one of exclusion of a primary intra-abdominal source of infection and can be made with certainty only after a thorough laparotomy. However, under certain circumstances, laparotomy may be avoided on the basis of findings in peritoneal fluid obtained by paracentesis.[67] For example, if gram-positive organisms are obtained after paracentesis, a diagnosis of primary peritonitis can usually be made and exploratory laparotomy deferred. In children, if gram-negative organisms, a mixed flora, or no organisms are obtained, full exploratory laparotomy is indicated to rule out possible intra-abdominal sources of continuing peritoneal contamination. However, in end-stage cirrhotic patients, exploratory laparotomy may be life-threatening, and the likelihood of finding a primary intra-abdominal focus may be small. Laparotomy performed on cirrhotic patients with sepsis in an attempt to find the source of infection has been reported to have a mortality rate of 80 percent.[68] Surgery in these patients can be deferred while awaiting the response to antimicrobial therapy. Patients with primary peritonitis usually respond within 48–72 hours to appropriate antimicrobial therapy.[69] The observation of an exponential rate of decline in the number of ascitic fluid leukocytes after the initiation of antimicrobial therapy for primary peritonitis has also been found to help differentiate primary from secondary bacterial peritonitis.[70]

Recovery of pneumococci from peritoneal fluid may not indicate primary peritonitis, as illustrated by a case report of appendicitis and secondary peritonitis due to pneumococci.[71] For this reason, some surgeons have considered the differential diagnosis in children between appendicitis and primary peritonitis too difficult to make without operative examination, even when gram-positive bacteria are identified in peritoneal fluid.[14] Paracentesis for smear and culture is indicated in all cirrhotic patients with ascites and in children with gross proteinuria and abdominal pain, whether or not the diagnosis of nephrotic syndrome was previously established. However, paracentesis is not without hazard, especially in patients with hemorrhagic tendencies or bowel distension. In a retrospective analysis of 242 consecutive diagnostic abdominal paracenteses in patients with liver disease and ascites, major complications were reported in 7, including perforation of the bowel with generalized peritonitis or abdominal wall abscess and serious hemorrhage.[72]

The diagnosis of tuberculous peritonitis can usually be made at operation or laparoscopy and confirmed by the histologic characteristics of the peritoneal biopsy specimen[73] and by bacteriologic examination of the peritoneal biopsy specimen and fluid.[74] The diagnosis of *C. immitis* peritonitis can be made by finding *C. immitis* on a wet mount of ascitic fluid, culture, and histologic examination.[66]

Prognosis. The treatment of primary peritonitis has been reported to be successful in more than one-half of the cirrhotic patients, but, because of the frequency of accompanying endstate cirrhosis, the overall mortality in cirrhotic adults has been as high as 95 percent.[17] However, more recent studies have reported lower mortality rates of 70 and 57 percent, with 28 and 40 percent dying from the primary peritonitis, respectively.[22,23] Those patients with the poorest prognosis were found to have renal insufficiency, hypothermia, hyperbilirubinemia, and hypoalbuminemia. The lower mortality rates in these series can perhaps be explained by the less frequent occurrence of hepatic encephalopathy in these later series. The lowest hospitalization mortality of 37.8 percent and infection-related mortality of 2.2 percent reported even more recently has been attributed to early diagnosis and treatment.[69] Treatment of peritonitis caused by gram-positive organisms, as well as early infections, has been more frequently successful than treatment of gram-negative or late infections. In nephrotic patients with gram-positive infections or in patients who do not have a preterminal underlying illness, the survival rate is over 90 percent.[12]

Treatment. Because the Gram stain is frequently negative in primary bacterial peritonitis, the initial choice of antimicrobial drug is often empiric, based on the most likely pathogens. The antimicrobial regimen can be modified once the results of the culture and susceptibility tests are available.

Some of the third-generation cephalosporin antibiotics have been demonstrated to be as efficacious as the combination of ampicillin plus an aminoglycoside in primary bacterial peritonitis.[75] They also avoid the risk of nephrotoxicity, which is sufficiently frequent in this group of patients to warrant the avoidance of aminoglycosides if an equally effective alternative antimicrobial regimen can be used.[23,76] Other antimicrobial agents such as the broad-spectrum penicillins (e.g., mezlocillin, ticarcillin, piperacillin), carbapenems (e.g., imipenem), and β-lactam antibiotic/β-lactamase inhibitor combinations (e.g., ticarcillin-clavulanate, ampicillin-sulbactam) are potential alternatives.

Primary bacterial peritonitis due either to *S. pneumoniae* or to group A streptococci is best treated with penicillin G. Peritonitis suspected of being due to methicillin-sensitive *Staph. aureus* should be treated with a penicillinase-resistant penicillin (e.g., nafcillin) or with a first-generation cephalosporin (e.g., cefazolin) or, if the strain is methicillin resistant or the patient is allergic to penicillin, vancomycin. If *Pseudomonas aeruginosa* is isolated, an aminoglycoside antibiotic combined with an antipseudomonal penicillin or cephalosporin, aztreonam, or imipenem, or ciprofloxacin alone or combined with another antipseudomonal antibiotic[77] should be used. For those situations in which the Gram stain is suggestive of *Bacteroides* or polymicrobial peritonitis is evident, antimicrobials with activity against *B. fragilis* and other anaerobic organisms should be added (e.g., metronidazole, clindamycin).

In those cases in which there is a strong clinical suspicion of primary bacterial peritonitis but all cultures are sterile, antimicrobial therapy should be continued. Clinical improvement together with a significant decline in the ascitic fluid leukocyte count should occur after 24–48 hours of antimicrobial therapy if the diagnosis is correct.[69,70,78] The lack of the expected clinical response or the persistence of an elevated ascitic fluid leukocyte count should make other diagnoses a consideration. Antimicrobial therapy should be continued for 10–14 days if improvement is noted; however, shorter course (5 day) therapy has been shown to be as efficacious.[69] The administration of intraperitoneal antimicrobials is not necessary.

Secondary Peritonitis

Etiology. The primary intra-abdominal processes that may give rise to peritonitis are numerous. These include diseases or injuries of the gastrointestinal tract such as perforation of a peptic ulcer; traumatic perforation of the uterus, urinary bladder, stomach, or small or large bowel; spontaneous perforation associated with typhoid, tuberculous,[79] amebic, *Strongyloides*, and cytomegalovirus ulcers; appendicitis, diverticulitis, or intestinal neoplasms; gangrene of the bowel from strangulation, bowel obstruction, or mesenteric vascular obstruction; suppurative cholecystitis; bile peritonitis; pancreatitis; operative contamination of the peritoneum or disruption of a surgical anastomosis site; lesions of the female genital tract such as septic abortion, puerperal sepsis, postoperative uterine infection, endometritis complicating an IUD,[80] and gonococcal salpingitis or gonococcal vulvovaginitis in children; lesions of the male genital tract such as suppurative prostatitis; and rupture of an intraperitoneal or visceral abscess (e.g., renal or perinephric, tuboovarian, liver, splenic, or pancreatic abscess). Peritonitis is a major hazard of peritoneal dialysis used in the management of renal failure, fluid and electrolytic imbalance, and certain intoxications.[52] Not uncommonly, bacterial peritonitis can occur secondary to the use of peritoneovenous and ventriculoperitoneal shunts.[81,82]

Microbiologic Characteristics. Infrequently, secondary peritonitis is caused by exogenous microorganisms, for example, *Staph. aureus*, *N. gonorrhoeae*, or *M. tuberculosis*, which have caused infection in intra-abdominal or adjacent viscera and have spread to involve the peritoneum. Most cases of secondary peritonitis, however, are endogenous in origin due to the large number and variety of microorganisms that normally colonize mucous membranes lining certain viscera within the abdominal cavity. Although forming a continuous surface, the mucous membranes of the stomach, upper small bowel, lower small bowel, and large bowel each has a characteristic microflora. The vagina also has a distinct microflora. Normally, invasive activities of indigenous bacteria are controlled by the intact mucosa of the gastrointestinal tract and vagina. Disturbances in this mucosal barrier may occur as a result of spontaneous disease, trauma, or surgical operations that permit escape of indigenous bacteria and may result in infection of the peritoneum, the abdominal viscera, or the retroperitoneal space. The frequency with which various indigenous organisms are recovered from intra-abdominal infection varies according to the site of the primary process and whether the primary process is associated with an alteration of the indigenous microflora.[83]

The stomach normally contains up to 10^3 colony-forming units (cfu) of microorganisms/ml in the fasting state. If bacteria are present, they are mostly facultative, gram-positive, salivary microorganisms, such as lactobacilli and streptococci. The numbers of these organisms in stomach contents transiently increase after a meal.[84] Gastric flora is more numerous and may be composed of different organisms when there is achlorhydria (e.g., from cimetidine) or blood in the stomach.[84,85] The flora of the upper small intestine is normally sparse and consists of salivary microorganisms.[86] But in the presence of achlorhydria,[84] intestinal obstruction, or other processes affecting intestinal motility or absorption, the flora of the small intestine is more profuse and varied. Conditions that favor small bowel stasis include scleroderma, regional enteritis, small bowel strictures, nontropical sprue, tropical sprue, duodenal and jejunal diverticula, presence of an afferent loop of the Bilroth II gastrojejunostomy, and intestinal pseudo-obstruction.[87] Large bowel flora has been found in the proximal small bowel of cirrhotic patients.[53] The ileum normally contains *E. coli*, enterococci, and an equal number of microorganisms that are obligately anaerobic, such as *B. fragilis*.[86] It is the colon, however, in which a profuse microflora exists in concentrations of about 10^{11} bacteria/ml of feces, a wet sludge of practically pure bacteria.[88] The colonic flora is predominantly composed of the obligate anaerobes *B. fragilis* and *Bifidobacterium* spp., which outnumber facultative microorganisms, primarily *E. coli*, by 10^3–10^4 to 1. Other colonic bacteria are viridans streptococci, enterococci, *Eubacterium* spp., *Klebsiella* spp., *Proteus* spp., *Enterobacter* spp., and *C. perfringens*. The large bowel flora is relatively stable[88] but may be significantly altered by antibiotic therapy.[89]

As would be anticipated from the nature of the gastrointestinal flora, Altemeier[90] reported anaerobes in 96 percent of 100 cases of peritonitis secondary to acute appendicitis with perforation. *Prevotella melaninogenica* and anaerobic gram-positive cocci were the most frequent isolates. Studies of the bacteriologic characteristics of intra-abdominal infections,[91–93] using modern bacteriologic techniques that provide an anaerobic environment during collection, transport, and incubation, have confirmed the findings of Altemeier that anaerobes play a major role. Finegold[91] reported that in a series of 73 intra-abdominal infections including 16 cases of peritonitis, there were an average of 4.5 isolates per case (range, 1–12 organisms), with 2.5 anaerobes and 2 aerobes or facultatives. The most frequent isolate was *E. coli*, followed by *B. fragilis* (the most common anaerobic isolate), enterococci, other *Bacteroides* spp., *Fusobacterium*, *C. perfringens*, other clostridia, *Peptococcus*, *Peptostreptococcus*, and *Eubacterium*. Similar findings have been reported by Gorbach et al.[92] in a series of 43 patients, which included 10 cases of peritonitis, in 93 percent of whom anaerobes or a mixture of anaerobes and facultatives were recovered, and by Swenson et al.[94] in a series of 64 patients, which included 26 cases of peritonitis, in 81 percent of whom anaerobes were recovered.

In these series, bacteremia was reported in about 20–30 percent of patients. Organisms recovered from blood frequently included *B. fragilis* or *E. coli*. In series of patients with *Bacteroides* bacteremia, 14–62 percent had a gastrointestinal source.[95–98]

Together with highly antibiotic-resistant strains of *Serratia* and *Acinetobacter*, *P. aeruginosa* is more frequently isolated from patients who develop their intra-abdominal infection while in the hospital, after having received broad-spectrum parenteral antimicrobials.[99] However, two studies have noted that *P. aeruginosa* comprises a more significant portion of the aerobic isolates in community-acquired intra-abdominal infection[100,101] than had been noted in previous series.[102]

Penetrating injuries to the liver and spleen are rarely followed by infection due to the usual sterility of these organs.[103]

Quantitative studies[104–106] in sexually active women during the childbearing period have revealed that the predominant vaginal microflora is composed of five to seven different microorganisms and that anaerobes are approximately 10 times more numerous than facultative organisms. There are about 10^8–10^9 cfu of anaerobes and about 10^7–10^8 cfu of facultatives per milliliter of vaginal secretions. The most frequent isolates in titers of 10^5/ ml or more are obligate or facultative anaerobic lactobacilli, nonenterococcal streptococci, anaerobic gram-positive cocci, Bacteroidaceae other than *B. fragilis* (e.g., *P. melaninogenica*, *P. bivia*, and *P. ruminicola*), and a group of unidentified catalase-negative facultative bacilli. Diphtheroids and *S. epidermidis* have also been reported to be frequent vaginal isolates.[106] When specifically looked for, *Gardnerella vaginalis* in high counts has also been found to be only slightly less frequent than lactobacilli in the vaginal secretions of normal women.[104,105] Colonic organisms, such as *B. fragilis*, Enterobacteriaceae, and enterococci, are rarely found as predominant components of the normal vaginal flora and probably proliferate at this site only under exceptional circumstances. For example, these organisms have been reported to appear in vaginal secretions in the immediate postoperative periods after vaginal operations,[107] and *C. perfringens* has been reported more frequently in vaginal secretions after difficult labor or abortions.[108] Hite et al.[109] noted the relative infrequency of *Bacteroides* and anaerobic gram-positive cocci in the vagina of normal prenatal women, whereas during the puerperium in both women with postpartum endometritis and noninfected women, these organisms were found to be more prevalent.[109,110] Factors favoring colonization by these anaerobes after surgery and in the puerperium are unknown but are possibly related to blood or necrotic tissue that provides the reduced, enriched environment required by these anaerobes.

Sequential sampling of vaginal secretions during the menstrual cycle has been reported to show constant levels of anaerobes, although recovery of specific organisms varies from specimen to specimen in each woman.[106] In contrast, levels of facultatives decrease 100-fold in the premenstrual week.[106] This variation in microflora may reflect cyclic fluctuation in the vaginal environment due to changes in hormonal activity during the menstrual cycle. Because the vaginal flora varies under certain conditions and members of this flora have differing pathogenicity, the frequency of endogenous intra-abdominal infections of gynecologic origin, as well as the types of pathogens involved, vary accordingly. For example, the frequency of vaginal colonization with group B streptococci increases during pregnancy, and infections due to these organisms are relatively common in the postpartum period.[111] In addition, in women with trichomoniasis, *Bacteroides* spp. more frequently may be found in vaginal secretions.[105,109] Postpartum infection, presumably due to anaerobes, has been reported to be more frequent in women who have trichomoniasis during pregnancy.[112]

The bacteriologic characteristics of intra-abdominal infection that complicates female genital tract infections are quite similar to those of secondary peritonitis due to a gastrointestinal source, except for the occurrence of *N. gonorrhoeae* in cul-de-sac aspirates.[113] Data compiled by Swenson et al.,[114] Thadepalli et al.,[115] and Chow et al.[116] indicate that anaerobes were found in 72 percent of 200 gynecologic infections. Anaerobes were especially frequent (92 percent) in closed-space infections such as tuboovarian and pelvic abscesses. *Bacteroides*, in particular *B. fragilis, P. melaninogenica,* and anaerobic gram-positive cocci, were the most frequently isolated anaerobes. *Escherichia coli* and streptococci were the most prevalent facultatives. Apparently, even in acute salpingitis, bacteriologic studies have demonstrated in the majority of patients the presence of anaerobes, usually gram-positive cocci in cul-de-sac aspirates, despite the recovery of gonococci from the endocervix.[117-119] The data are interpreted as supporting the concept of superinfection with anaerobes late in the course of this disease after initial infection with *N. gonorrhoeae*.[120] In children, gonococcal peritonitis has been rarely reported with gonococcal vulvovaginitis.[121,122]

Intraperitoneal rupture has been reported in 10 percent of the cases of amebic liver abscess and may cause acute generalized peritonitis or a less commonly localized intraperitoneal abscess with a mortality of about 18 percent.[123] Perforation of the colon with bacterial peritonitis due to fulminant amebic colitis is also unusual but often fatal.[124] Similarly, *Strongyloides stercoralis* infestation of the small bowel may rarely cause fatal peritonitis, with or without concurrent bacterial contamination.[125] *Candida* has been isolated from the abdominal fluid in patients undergoing peritoneal dialysis, as has *Staph. aureus*, Enterobacteriaceae, and *P. aeruginosa*.[126] *Candida* peritonitis has also been observed as a complication of gastrointestinal surgery or in perforation of a viscus,[127,128] and its occurrence is related to numerous factors that increase the rate of *Candida* colonization in the gastrointestinal tract. These include immunosuppression, prolonged hospitalization, and antimicrobial and/or antacid therapy. *Candida* is most commonly isolated from the peritoneum after perforation of a gastric or duodenal peptic ulcer, or after spillage of colonic contents into the peritoneum due to trauma, mesenteric artery occlusion, or dehiscence of a surgical anastomosis.

Pathogenesis. The virulence of the bacteria that cause peritonitis is enhanced when certain microorganisms either are combined intraperitoneally with substances such as mucus, enzymes, or hemoglobin or are combined with certain other microorganisms.

Chemical peritonitis can be produced by escape of bile or of gastric or pancreatic secretions into the peritoneal cavity. When gastric acid escapes into the peritoneal cavity, there is an outpouring of serum protein and electrolytes from the blood into the peritoneal cavity. The acidity is quickly neutralized by these buffers and by diffusion of hydrogen ions into the body fluids.[129,130] Widespread necrosis may result from enzymatic digestion after intraperitoneal spillage of potent pancreatic enzymes. Escape of bile into the peritoneal cavity is generally considered to be a very grave, often fatal situation.[131,132] The severity of peritonitis after escape of these intestinal secretions is due in part to subsequent bacterial peritonitis. Indeed, in the dog with experimentally produced partial biliary diversion into the peritoneal cavity, fatal effects were reduced by oral nonabsorbable or parenteral antibiotics.[133] Bacteria may enter the peritoneal cavity with contaminated intestinal secretions through perforations in the gastrointestinal wall, as well as by migration through the wall of the intact gastrointestinal tract, in response to the irritation of bile and possibly other intestinal tract secretions on the serosal surface.[51]

Nemir et al.[134,135] demonstrated that after experimental strangulation obstruction of a loop of bowel in the dog, the animal usually died within 36 hours, and the peritoneal fluid at first was light pink and eventually became black. When this black fluid was removed and injected into the peritoneal cavity of a normal animal, the recipient also developed a similar fatal peritonitis, but the early peritoneal fluid was nontoxic.[134-136] The toxicity could be largely counteracted by instilling antibiotics into the obstructed loop of intestine or by giving antibiotics simultane-

ously when the fluid was injected into normal animals.[137,138] Many workers in the past have shown that intraperitoneal injection of large numbers of organisms in pure culture is incapable of producing peritonitis unless some additional factor is present, such as gum tragacanth, talc, mucin, turpentine, or other irritants. It seemed unlikely, therefore, that the toxicity of strangulation obstruction fluid was due to its bacterial content alone. Evidence has been reported that viable bacteria in addition to the presence of free hemoglobin in the peritoneal fluid are necessary to account for the lethality both of bowel strangulation and of the fluid that collects in the peritoneal cavity after bowel strangulation.[139-141] The mechanism by which free hemoglobin enhances peritoneal infection is unknown but perhaps is related to free iron. Iron is required for bacterial metabolism and, in amounts that leave an excess of free iron after having saturated transferrin, may greatly enhance infections due to certain microorganisms, such as Enterobacteriaceae and *C. perfringens*.[142] Hau et al.[143] demonstrated that intraperitoneal hemoglobin depresses the influx of granulocytes into the peritoneal cavity in response to intraperitoneal bacteria, and hemoglobin depresses in vitro the chemotactic response of granulocytes and monocytes.

Intraperitoneal fluid and fibrin that enter the peritoneal cavity as a result of the increased vascular permeability due to local trauma or bacterial infection are important components of the inflammatory response and play adjuvant roles. It has been shown that low numbers of *E. coli* in small volumes of saline infused intraperitoneally are innocuous, but these numbers of *E. coli* can become lethal in direct proportion to the increase in the volume of saline infused. This is thought to be related to the resultant dilution of opsonic proteins.[144] Trapping of bacteria beneath layers of fibrin may limit their spread but may also lead to abscess formation and isolation of bacteria from host defense mechanisms.[145-147]

A number of other substances such as hog gastric mucin, bile salts,[148] and barium sulfate[149,150] have been used as adjuvants in producing lethal intraperitoneal infections. The mechanisms of their respective effects have been the subject of numerous studies. It has been postulated that hog gastric mucin coats bacteria, thus protecting them from intraperitoneal phagocytosis.[151]

Cuevas and Fine[152] have attributed the lethality of bowel strangulation and infectious or chemical irritation of the serosal surface of the bowel to endotoxemia. Endotoxin was thought to escape from the gut lumen, to cross the intact bowel wall into the peritoneal cavity, and then to be absorbed into the systemic circulation. Within minutes after experimental superior mesenteric artery occlusion, endotoxin has been detected in the systemic circulation, before its appearance in the portal vein.[152] Similarly, endotoxin levels are reported to be elevated in plasma or peritoneal fluid of patients with severe intra-abdominal infection, but was not of prognostic significance in these patients.[153]

Secondary peritonitis is usually a mixed infection involving predominantly obligate and facultative anaerobes. Obligate anaerobes are sensitive to oxygen in the molecular form and also to bound oxygen, as in organic peroxides. Survival and growth of anaerobes are also dependent on the oxidation-reduction potential, that is, the oxidizing capacity of their environment. Most pathogenic anaerobes require a negative potential of at least -150 mV. Low oxidation-reduction potentials are thought to occur in many abscesses,[154] and oxidation-reduction potentials of -150 mV or less are measured in abscesses from which anaerobes are recovered.[155] Some anerobic organisms have additional requirements, such as vitamin K, arginine, serum, blood pigments, or bile, before growth is obtained. Thus, establishment of an anaerobic infection requires an environment in which the oxygen tension is very low, the oxidation-reduction potential is low, and abundant nutrients are available to support anaerobic metabolism. These requirements are usually met by devitalized tissue as a consequence of ischemia, trauma, or neoplastic growth. Once proper conditions are obtained, anaerobic organisms can achieve doubling rates equivalent to those seen with aerobic enteric bacilli. In vivo, the rapidly expanding bacterial and inflammatory cell mass, frequently accompanied by gas production, can interrupt the blood supply to the immediately surrounding tissue and cause further tissue necrosis.

Gram-negative anaerobic cocci and bacilli (including *B. fragilis* and *P. melaninogenica*) possess endotoxins with much weaker biologic activity in comparison with those extracted from their aerobic counterparts and have low or absent 2-keto-3-deoxyoctanoate content.[156] In addition, certain anaerobes elaborate collagenase,[157] other proteolytic enzymes, and deoxyribonuclease.[158] Certain Bacteroidaceae are capable of degrading heparin,[159] which may be responsible for the suppurative thrombophlebitis frequently seen in infections due to these microorganisms.[160] These factors tend to provide more areas well adapted to the growth requirements of the anaerobe, with the result that the infection progresses.

In addition, anaerobes may be resistant to host defenses. For example, although leukocytes have been shown to have bactericidal activity under both aerobic and anaerobic conditions against several anaerobic species, including *B. fragilis*, presumably by mechanisms other than those dependent on the superoxide anion O_2^- or H_2O_2,[161] Keusch and Douglas[162] found that granulocytic killing of *C. perfringens* was impaired under anaerobic conditions. Also, a capsule has been demonstrated on *B. fragilis*[163] and *Porphyromonas asaccharolytica* (formerly *B. melaninogenicus* ssp. *asaccharolyticus*)[164] that might protect the organisms from phagocytosis and favor abscess formation.[165–167] Some anaerobes, especially *B. fragilis*, may be resistant to the normal bactericidal activity of serum.[161]

Many anaerobic infections appear to be synergistic. Although it is probable that the majority of bacteria isolated in mixed infections are nonpathogenic by themselves, their presence may nevertheless be essential for the pathogenicity of the bacterial mixture. Such examples of bacterial synergism in infection have been demonstrated in periodontal infection by Socransky and Gibbons[168] and in peritonitis by Altemeier.[169]

Facultative organisms in mixed infections may be essential by providing a sufficiently reduced environment for the growth of obligate anaerobic organisms. Another mechanism of bacterial synergy is the generation of a substance by one organism, which is essential for the growth of another, for example, the production of vitamin K (a required growth factor for *P. melaninogenica*) by diphtheroids. Anaerobes such as *Bacteroides* spp. have also demonstrated the ability to protect aerobic bacteria from phagocytic killing[170,171] and from otherwise effective antibiotic therapy (e.g., via β-lactamase production).[172]

In addition, each component of the pathogenic mixture may contribute in different ways to the clinical picture. After implantation of fecal contents intraperitoneally into rats, Onderdonk et al.[173] observed that *E. coli* initially predominated in the peritoneal exudate. Bacteremia, due to *E. coli* during this phase, was uniformly present and frequently fatal. In rats that survived, indolent intra-abdominal abscesses developed in which *B. fragilis* predominated. Elimination of *E. coli* by early administration of gentamicin reduced early mortality but did not prevent late intra-abdominal abscess due to obligate anaerobes, whereas elimination of obligate anaerobes with clindamycin did not prevent early mortality due to *E. coli* bacteremia but reduced late abscess formation in survivors. These findings indicate that, although *E. coli* is responsible for early mortality, anaerobes are responsible for late abscess formation in this model.[174,175]

Pathophysiologic Responses. Whatever the initiating cause of peritonitis, a similar series of reactions takes place, both locally and systemically.

LOCAL RESPONSE. The local inflammatory response of the peritoneum is similar to that in other tissues, but the peritoneal lining presents a large exudative and absorptive surface. At sites of irritation, there is an outpouring of fluid into the peritoneal cavity that, in contrast to normal serous fluid, has a high protein content (>3 g/dl) and many cells, primarily granulocytes, that phagocytize and kill organisms. The exudate contains fibrinogen that polymerizes, and plaques of fibrinous exudate form on the inflamed peritoneal surfaces. This exudate glues adjacent bowel, mesentery, and particularly omentum to each other. Localization is further aided by inhibition of motility in involved intestinal loops. Experimentally, radiopaque medium injected intraperitoneally at one locus can be demonstrated to have spread over much of the greater peritoneal sac within a short time. The extent and rate of intraperitoneal spread of contamination are undoubtedly dependent on the volume and nature of the exudate[10] and on the effectiveness of the localizing processes.

If peritoneal defenses aided by appropriate supportive measures control the inflammatory process, the disease may resolve spontaneously. A second possible outcome is a confined abscess. A third course results when the peritoneal and systemic defense mechanisms are unable to localized the inflammation, which then progresses to spreading diffuse peritonitis. Some of the factors favoring spread of the inflammatory process are *(1)* greater virulence of bacteria, *(2)* greater extent and duration of contamination, or *(3)* impaired host defenses.

SYSTEMIC RESPONSE. Peritonitis leads to changes not only locally in the peritoneal cavity but throughout the body.

Gastrointestinal Tract. Initially in peritonitis there is hypermotility, followed by paralysis of the bowel. Accumulation of fluid and electrolytes in the lumen of the adynamic bowel continues until distension is sufficient to inhibit capillary inflow and secretion ceases.

Cardiovascular. Because of the large surface area of the peritoneum, shifts of fluid into the peritoneal cavity, combined with fluid shifts into the bowel lumen, can produce a profound fall in circulating blood volume and elevation of the hematocrit.[176,177] Fluid and electrolyte loss is further exaggerated by coexistent fever, vomiting, diarrhea, and loss of aspirated gastrointestinal fluid. As the process continues, the decreased venous return to the right side of the heart results in a drop in cardiac output, with resulting hypotension.[177] In addition, the patient may be exposed to the circulatory effects of endotoxin, namely, progressive pooling of blood within tissue capillary beds, producing a further decrease in venous return. Usually, there is evidence of increased adrenergic activity—sweating, tachycardia, and cutaneous vasoconstriction (i.e., cold moist skin, mottled and cyanotic extremities).

With adequate replacement of blood volume, cardiac output may be maintained above normal.[177] Cardiac output of two or even three times normal may be required to satisfy the increased metabolic needs of the body in the presence of infection. Failure to sustain increased cardiac output results in progressive lactic acidosis, oliguria, hypotension, and ultimately death if the infection cannot be controlled.

Respiratory. The intraperitoneal inflammation results in relatively high and fixed diaphragms and considerable pain on respiration. This results in basilar atelectasis with intrapulmonary shunting of blood. Satisfactory compensation is possible only if the increase in energy demands does not exceed the respiratory reserve. Heavy cigarette smoking, chronic bronchitis, emphysema, and obesity compound the problem. With decompensation in respiratory function, hypoxemia is accompanied first by hypocapnia (respiratory alkalosis) and later by hypercapnia (respiratory acidosis). In some patients, pulmonary edema develops, due not to left ventricular failure but perhaps to increased pulmonary capillary leakage as a consequence of hypoalbuminemia or direct effects of bacterial toxins (adult respiratory distress syndrome). In these patients, progressive hypoxemia develops with decreasing pulmonary compliance. This requires volume-cycled ventilatory assistance with increasingly higher concentrations of inspired oxygen and positive end-expiratory pressure.

Renal. Low renal perfusion may be followed by acute tubular necrosis and progressive azotemia.

Metabolic. During the first few days, the excretion of cortisol is increased and subsequently returns to normal.[178] The increased energy demands of infection rapidly deplete body stores of glycogen, followed by catabolism of protein (muscle) and fat, thus accounting for the rapid weight loss of severely infected patients. Prolonged intra-abdominal infection is associated with extreme wasting. Heat production may eventually fail, and body temperature then falls. Exhaustion and death may ensue.

Clinical Manifestations. SYMPTOMS. The early manifestations of peritonitis secondary to disease of abdominal viscera are frequently those of the primary disease process. Moderately severe abdominal pain is almost always the predominant symptom. The pain is aggravated by any motion, even respiration. The progression of abdominal pain is a function of the rate of dissemination of the material producing the pain stimulus. Rupture of a peptic ulcer with massive spillage of gastric contents produces severe epigastric pain that, within minutes, may spread to involve the entire abdomen. In contrast, the spread of pain from a lesion such as a ruptured appendix is much more gradual. Decreased intensity and extent of pain with time usually suggest localization of the inflammatory process.

Anorexia, nausea, and vomiting commonly accompany abdominal pain. Patients may also complain of feverishness, sometimes with chill, thirst, scanty urination, inability to pass feces or flatus, and abdominal distension.

The formation and progression of an intraperitoneal abscess is often gradual: The patient who seemed to be recovering from peritonitis or an abdominal operation stops improving; fever returns, and localizing symptoms may develop.

PHYSICAL FINDINGS. Patients with peritonitis characteristically lie quietly in bed, supine, with the knees flexed and with frequent limited intercostal respirations, since any motion intensifies the abdominal pain. Early in the course the patient is alert, restless, and irritable, but later may become apathetic or delerious.

Body temperatures may reach 42°C. Subnormal temperatures in the range of 35°C are often seen in the early stages of chemical peritonitis and late in the course of patients with continuing intra-abdominal sepsis or septic shock and are a grave sign.

Increasing tachycardia with weak, thready peripheral pulses reflects decreased effective blood volume. The blood pressure is maintained within normal limits early in the disease process. As peritonitis progresses, the blood pressure lowers to shock levels. Respiration is increasingly rapid and shallow.

Marked abdominal tenderness to palpation is present, usually maximally over the organ in which the process originated. Rebound tenderness, both direct and referred, signifies parietal peritoneal irritation. This finding is sometimes more accurate than direct palpation in locating the point of maximal tenderness as well as in delineating the extent of peritoneal irritation.

Muscular rigidity of the abdominal wall is produced both by voluntary guarding and by reflex muscular spasm. Hyperresonance due to gaseous intestinal distension can usually be demonstrated by percussion. Pneumoperitoneum from a ruptured hollow viscus may produce decreased liver dullness to percussion. Bowel sounds, initially hypoactive, later disappear. Rectal and vaginal examination may reveal tenderness and the presence of a pelvic abscess and may indicate a primary focus in the female pelvic organs.

Abdominal pain and muscle spasm may be deceptively absent in some patients. Those with lax abdominal musculature (e.g., patients in the postpartum period, patients with ascites due to cirrhosis, patients with marked cachexia) may not have abdominal rigidity. Similarly, patients in shock, on glucocorticosteroid therapy, or in whom loculated intra-abdominal abscesses are not in contact with the anterior abdominal wall (e.g., subphrenic, lesser sac, pelvic) may not exhibit marked abdominal pain and spasm. Absent bowel sounds may be the only manifestation of peritonitis in such patients, and a high index of suspicion is necessary.

Diagnostic Studies. The differential diagnosis in patients with symptoms and signs of peritonitis includes pneumonia, sickle cell anemia, herpes zoster, diabetic ketoacidosis, tabes dorsalis, porphyria, familial Mediterranean fever, plumbism, lupus erythematosus, and uremia.

A peripheral blood leukocyte count of 17,000–25,000 white blood cells/mm^3 is usual in acute peritonitis, the differential count showing polymorphonuclear predominance and a moderate to marked shift to the left. However, reliance on the significance of the total white blood cell count may be misleading. Massive peritoneal inflammation may mobilize leukocytes into the diseased area, so there may be, for example, fewer than 5000 white blood cells/mm^3 in the circulating blood, but the differential smear in this situation may show an extreme shift to immature polymorphonuclear forms.

Hemoconcentration and dehydration are reflected by elevated hematocrit and blood urea nitrogen values. Hyperglycemia and glycosuria usually are not present in peritonitis but may be seen in diabetic acidosis and acute pancreatitis, which may manifest with signs suggesting peritonitis. Hematuria and pyuria without bacteriuria may reflect intra-abdominal inflammatory disease such as appendicitis adjacent to the urinary tract. Elevated serum amylase levels may be seen in peritonitis due to almost any cause, but very high levels are seen only in acute pancreatitis. Hyponatremia may be seen in patients given water to replace isotonic fluid losses but is also characteristic of porphyria. Acidosis, both metabolic and respiratory, is present in severe and late peritonitis. Supine, upright, and lateral decubitus radiographs of the abdomen may reveal distension of both the small intestine and the colon with adynamic loops of bowel or features of mechanical intestinal obstruction, volvulus, intussusception, or vascular occlusion. Inflammatory exudate and edema of the intestinal wall produces a widening of the space between adjacent loops. Peritoneal fat lines and psoas shadows may be obliterated. Free air may be visible if there is a ruptured viscus. Chest radiographs should always be taken to rule out a pulmonary or thoracic problem as the cause of the abdominal distress. The presence of air beneath the diaphragm may be best defined in these pictures. Trapped gas with a fluid level or mottling due to gas may also be visible in intraperitoneal or visceral abscesses. Calcification in the gallbladder or other organs may also be noted on radiographs.

Needle aspiration of the peritoneal cavity is often helpful. If no fluid can be aspirated, peritoneal lavage with Ringer's lactate solution should be done to obtain fluid for examination. In performing a tap, the region of abdominal scars where bowel may be adherent to the underside of the scar should be avoided. The aspirate is examined grossly for content of blood, pus, bile, or digested fat; chemically for amylase content; and microscopically, with Gram stain, for bacteria. A positive tap is meaningful; a dry or negative tap is of little significance. Guidance for the tap may be obtained by ultrasound or computed tomography (CT) scan.

Prognosis. Survival of a patient with secondary peritonitis depends on many factors, including the age of the patient, the duration of peritoneal contamination, the presence of foreign material (bile or pancreatic secretions, barium), the primary intra-abdominal process, and the microorganisms involved.[179,180] Altemeier[90] has shown that the more organisms present in peritoneal exudate, the worse the prognosis, although there was no correlation between severity of infection and any particular organism. Mortality increases with more distal gastrointestinal sources of contamination.[181] The age of the patient also influences the mortality from peritonitis. In the very young patient, because of the relatively small omentum, the walling-off process is less effective, so diffuse peritonitis occurs more frequently than in the adult. In the elderly, preexisting conditions such as emphysema, diabetes, or cardiovascular disease reduce the capacity of the patient to meet the demands on the cardiovascular, respiratory, and renal systems during this period of intense metabolic activity.[179] Mortality rates range from 3.5 percent in those with early infection following penetrating abdominal trauma to more than 60 percent in patients with established intra-abdominal infection and secondary organ failure.[182] Persistent peritoneal contamination, leakage of pancreatic enzymes, septicemia, fluid and electrolyte abnormalities, pneumonia,[183] and cardiovascular, renal, and respiratory failure[184] are the principal causes of death.

Treatment. ANTIMICROBIAL THERAPY.   Secondary peritonitis is typically polymicrobial, and the pathogens in the majority of patients with secondary peritonitis are derived from the gastrointestinal tract even in patients with a primary gynecologic process. Typically, the facultative microorganisms are *E. coli*, *Klebsiella/Enterobacter* spp., *Proteus* spp., and enterococci, and the obligate anaerobes are *B. fragilis*, *P. melaninogenica*, *Peptococcus*, *Peptostreptococcus*, *Fusobacterium*, *Eubacterium lentum*, and *Clostridium*. Other less commonly isolated pathogens include *Staph. aureus*, *P. aeruginosa*, and *Candida*.

The role of antimicrobial therapy in the outcome of infection due to anaerobes or due to a mixture of anaerobes and facultative microorganisms is extremely difficult to assess. This is primarily because of the often dramatic response to surgical drainage and débridement alone when there is localized infection. Nevertheless, appropriate antimicrobial therapy has been shown to reduce significantly mortality among patients with bacteremic infections due to Bacteroidaceae or Enterobacteriaceae.[98,185,186] Antimicrobial drugs are expected to control bacteremia and early metastatic foci of infection, to reduce suppurative complications if given early, and to prevent local spread of existing infection. Once suppuration has occurred, it may be difficult to cure the infection if antimicrobial drugs are used without drainage; also, antimicrobial drugs used alone may mask some of the clinical manifestations of abscess formation. However, some intra-abdominal abscesses can be treated successfully with antibiotics alone.[187,188]

Antimicrobial therapy should be started immediately after appropriate specimens (e.g., blood and peritoneal fluid) are obtained for culture. This means that antimicrobial therapy is often started before the completion of in vitro antimicrobial sensitivity testing of the specific facultative pathogens. In addition, rapid isolation, identification, and in vitro sensitivity testing of anaerobes, in contrast to testing of facultatives, are often not possible in many community hospitals. Several factors account for the delay in obtaining anaerobic bacteriologic results. For example, infections due to anaerobes are frequently caused by mixtures of five or more microorganisms, and cultures require long periods for growth and isolation. In addition, in vitro sensitivity testing by the conventional disk diffusion technique has not been standardized for anaerobes.[155] Such tests are influenced to a large extent by the growth rate of the bacteria, inoculum size, pH and type of medium, duration of incubation, and CO_2 concentration in the atmosphere.[189,190] In vitro studies of the stability of the β-lactam antibiotics when exposed to reducing agents such as mercaptoamines (cysteine), which are frequently incorporated in media used for the growth of anaerobes, have shown that these compounds are able to open the β-lactam ring and to inactivate penicillins.[191] However, susceptibility of anaerobic organisms can be reliably determined by the broth or agar dilution techniques with appropriate media.[192] Because these tests are generally performed by research laboratories, knowledge of the antimicrobial susceptibility of anaerobes is gained from periodically published reports on anaerobic isolates by centers that specialize in performing these tests. Therefore, initial chemotherapy is usually empiric, based on the use of the most

reliable and least toxic antimicrobial agents for the most probable anaerobic and facultative pathogens. In vitro sensitivity reports (usually reliable only for the facultative or aerobic organisms) allow subsequent adjustment of the initial regimen to more specific therapy.

Because these infections are commonly polymicrobial, a broad spectrum of antimicrobial activity is required. Indeed, recent data suggest that survival in patients with intra-abdominal infection is diminished if initial therapy is inadequate, regardless of the adequacy of subsequent treatment.[193] The ideal regimen remains controversial, but must be active against both anaerobic and facultative pathogens. Drugs active against anaerobic bacteria may be quite inactive against the accompanying aerobic or facultative pathogens in the mixed infections, and vice versa. For this reason, combinations of usually two or three drugs are used. These combinations of antimicrobial agents are selected for their activity against most of the more virulent pathogens in the infective mixture (e.g., the Enterobacteriaceae and *B. fragilis*). The Enterobacteriaceae in the mixture are significant and frequently cause bacteremia in these patients, as in the rat model of intra-abdominal infection of Onderdonk et al.[173] However, antibiotics need not be active against every pathogen isolated. It is apparent that if only some of the organisms can be eliminated, the synergistic effect may be removed, and the patient's defenses may be able to eradicate the remaining organisms. For example, clindamycin alone (which has no activity against Enterobacteriaceae and enterococci) has been reported to be sufficient treatment for some patients with infections resulting from a mixture of Enterobacteriaceae, enterococci, and anaerobes.[194] Experimental evidence in the rat model of intraperitoneal infection suggests that the enterococcus is not a primary pathogen, although in the presence of anaerobes it may aid in abscess formation.[195] In several clinical studies of anaerobic infections, patients were treated successfully with both gentamicin and clindamycin despite absence of activity of this therapeutic regimen against enterococci.[196,197] However, more recent reviews emphasize the role of the enterococcus in intra-abdominal infections.[198] In some reports, this organism has been noted to emerge as the sole intra-abdominal pathogen, at times associated with enterococcal bacteremia,[199,200] especially if patients with polymicrobial intra-abdominal infection were treated with an antimicrobial agent that lacked activity against the enterococcus.[201,202] Indeed enterococci, both *E. faecalis* and *E. faecium*, have emerged as major nosocomial pathogens with high-level resistance to multiple antibiotics, including aminoglycosides, ampicillin, and vancomycin.[203–206]

When combinations of antibiotics are used, synergism or antagonism may occur. Chloramphenicol has been shown to impair early bactericidal activity of gentamicin in vitro, and antagonism was demonstrated in mice with experimental *Proteus mirabilis* infection when phagocytic function was impaired (i.e., in neutropenic mice).[207] Two studies suggest that clindamycin inhibits early in vitro killing of *E. coli* and *K. pneumoniae* by gentamicin.[208] However, in an in vivo study of aminoglycoside therapy of *E. coli* peritonitis and bacteremia in normal and neutropenic mice, prior or simultaneous administration of clindamycin with the aminoglycoside did not inhibit the therapeutic effect of the aminoglycoside.[209] Clindamycin combined in vitro with gentamicin has been reported to have indifferent or synergistic activity against Enterobacteriaceae after 18 hours of incubation.[210] The activities of various antimicrobial agents against the usual peritoneal pathogens and the results of various clinical trials are discussed in the sections that follow.

Chloramphenicol.   At a concentration of 16 μg/ml, chloramphenicol has activity against over 99 percent·of the anaerobic pathogens involved in intra-abdominal infection, especially *B. fragilis*.[211] However, the availability of equally effective and potentially less toxic antimicrobial agents to treat anaerobic infections (e.g., clindamycin, metronidazole, imipenem) has all but eliminated the need for chloramphenicol,[212] except perhaps for significant infection owing to strains of enterococci resistant to all other antimicrobial agents.

Clindamycin.   Clindamycin has been reported to inhibit over 95 percent of the anaerobes, including *B. fragilis*, at a concentration of 8 μg/ml.[211] About 15 percent of the strains of *Clostridium* spp. other than *C. perfringens*, *Peptococci* spp., and rare strains of *Fusobacterium* spp. have been reported to be resistant to clindamycin. Most strains of *B. fragilis* have remained highly susceptible to clindamycin during the past decade.[213,214] Plasmid-mediated, transferable clindamycin resistance in *B. fragilis* has been demonstrated,[213] and clindamycin resistance among *B. fragilis* has become a problem at certain medical centers. Clindamycin is active against only certain facultative gram-positive cocci, such as *Staph. aureus* and *S. pyogenes*, but not *faecalis*, and has virtually no activity against Enterobacteriaceae.

Diarrhea is reported to be the most frequent side effect of clindamycin therapy and occurs at an incidence of 2–20 percent.[215] The severity of the diarrhea varies but may be associated with pseudomembranous colitis in up to one-half of the patients with diarrhea, as reported in one study.[216] Toxic megacolon, colonic perforation, and death on rare occasions have been reported. The cause has been attributable to an exotoxin produced by clindamycin-resistant strains of *Clostridium difficile*.[215]

Metronidazole.   Metronidazole is active against strict anaerobes, inhibits most *B. fragilis*, *Fusobacterium* spp., and *Clostridium* spp., and has a unique bactericidal action against *B. fragilis* and *C. perfringens*.[217] Its in vitro activity, however, is poor against aerobes, microaerophiles, and anaerobes that may become somewhat aerotolerant on subculture (i.e., certain anaerobic gram-positive cocci and sporeless gram-positive rods).[211,218] Despite the poor in vitro activity demonstrated against aerobic and microaerophilic organisms, there is now some in vivo evidence in animal models and humans that metronidazole has activity against *E. coli* and other aerobes in mixed aerobic–anaerobic infections.[219,220] The mechanism for this is poorly understood but may be related to the conversion by *B. fragilis* of metronidazole into active metabolites with activity against *E. coli* and other aerobes.[219] Nonetheless, metronidazole should be used clinically in combination with other antimicrobial agents in the treatment of mixed infections.

Tetracyclines.   The large number of resistant anaerobes, especially *B. fragilis*, precludes the use of these drugs,[221,222] except perhaps for significant infection owing to strains of enterococci resistant to all other antimicrobial agents.

Cephalosporins.   *Bacteroides fragilis* and other *Bacteroides* spp. are usually resistant to the so-called first-generation cephalosporins (e.g., cefazolin) and to some second-generation cephalosporins (e.g., cefamandole, cefuroxime). However, cefoxitin is distinctly more active than any of the other second-generation cephalosporins against *Bacteroides* spp.,[211,223,224] but cefoxitin resistance has become a problem at certain medical centers.[214] Cefotetan has activity similar to that of cefoxitin, except that it is less active against the *B. fragilis* group (not including *B. fragilis*).[223,224] These first- and second-generation cephalosporins are also active against the majority of the strains of *E. coli*, *P. mirabilis*, and *K. pneumoniae*. The third-generation cephalosporins (e.g., cefotaxime, ceftizoxime, cefoperazone, ceftriaxone, and ceftazidime) have demonstrated significantly better activity against the Enterobacteriaceae. Only ceftazidime, and less so cefoperazone, have activity against *P. aeruginosa*. With a few exceptions, the third-generation cephalosporins have relatively poor activity against *B. fragilis* and other *Bacteroides* spp.[225] Ceftizoxime is reported to have good in vitro activity against *B. fragilis* and other *Bacteroides* species in some studies,[224,226] but has been found to be inadequate against *Bacteroides* species, including *B. fragilis*, in other in vitro studies.[223,227] Because the activity of ceftizoxime is greatly affected by the inoculum of *Bacteroides* in in vitro studies,[211] this antibiotic would most likely be inadequate in treating severe intra-abdominal infections where the inoculum of organisms is great.

Penicillins.   Penicillin G and ampicillin have excellent activity against all anaerobes, with the exception of *Bacteroides* spp. (especially *B. fragilis*) and *Fusobacterium* spp. other than *F. nucleatum*. Ampicillin also is active against 70–80 percent of the strains of *E. coli* and almost all *P. mirabilis*. Although *B. fragilis* has been considered to be resistant to penicillins, in vitro sensitivity testing reveals that over 90 percent of *B. fragilis* isolates may be sensitive to ticarcillin, mezlocillin, and piperacillin in concentrations of 125 μg/ml or less. In fact, these antibiotics have been reported to be rapidly bactericidal against *B. fragilis*.[228,229] The clinical experience with these broad-spectrum penicillins in the treatment of anaerobic bacterial infection has been reported to be favorable.[230,231] A prospective controlled study has shown that the therapeutic response to ticarcillin was similar to that of clindamycin or chloramphenicol, each in combination with an aminoglycoside in the therapy of intra-abdominal infection.[232]

Because sensitive strains of *B. fragilis* may require up to 125 μg of the broad-spectrum penicillins per milliliter for inhibition, these antibiotics should be used in high dosages (300–500 mg/kg/day) to treat these infections. However, because up to 20 percent of the strains of *B. fragilis* are resistant to concentrations of the broad-spectrum penicillins[233] that can be achieved in serum, use of the broad-spectrum penicillins as the initial therapy for suspected *B. fragilis* infection should be undertaken with caution. In addition, there is some evidence to suggest that penicillin G may fail to achieve concentrations at the site of *B. fragilis* infection, because of both a reduction in penetration of penicillin into infected sites and inactivation of the drug by *B. fragilis*.[234] It is unknown if this is also true for broad-spectrum penicillins. Therapeutic failures despite high doses of penicillin for *B. fragilis* bacteremia have been well documented.[95] Resistance of *B. fragilis* to penicillins is frequently due to production of β-lactamase.[235]

The spectrum of antibacterial activity of the older broad-spectrum penicillin, ticarcillin, includes the majority of aerobic gram-negative bacilli (including *P. aeruginosa*) commonly isolated from patients with intra-abdominal infections with the exception of most *Klebsiella* and many *Serratia* spp. However, ticarcillin is considerably less active than ampicillin and penicillin G against enterococci. The newer broad-spectrum penicillins (e.g., mezlocillin, azlocillin, piperacillin) are more active than ticarcillin against the Enterobacteriaceae group, including many strains of *Klebsiella*, and against *P. aeruginosa* and enterococci.[236]

The combination of a β-lactamase inhibitor, such as clavulanic acid or sulbactam, with a penicillin increases the activity of the penicillin against certain β-lactamase producers.[237,238] Ticarcillin-clavulanic acid inhibits 60–80 percent of ticarcillin-resistant strains of Enterobacteriaceae, including most *E. coli* and *Klebsiella* spp., as well as all β-lactamase-producing *Bacteroides* species.[239] However, the combination will not inhibit the inducible β-lactamase produced by *P. aeruginosa*, *Serratia* spp., *Citrobacter freundii*, or *Enterobacter cloacae*.[240] Ampicillin-sulbactam is active against many β-lactamase-producing bacteria resistant to ampicillin, including *E. coli*, *Klebsiella*, and *Bacteroides* spp.[241,242]

Other β-Lactams.   Imipenem, a carbapenem antibiotic, has the broadest antimicrobial spectrum of any current antibiotic,[243] with activity against almost all aerobic and anaerobic bacteria. It is resistant to most β-lactamases, including chromosomal inducible β-lactamases of bacteria such as *P. aeruginosa*, *Serratia*, and *E. cloacae*,[244] except those produced by rare strains of *B. fragilis*[245] and *Xanthomonas maltophilia*. Aztreonam, a monobactam antibiotic, has a spectrum of activity limited to aerobic gram-negative bacilli.[246] It would be necessary to use an antibiotic with activity both against anaerobes and against microaerophilic and aerobic gram-positive cocci (i.e., clindamycin) rather than metronidazole, which has poor activity against these common pathogens, along with aztreonam in the treatment of secondary intra-abdominal infections.

Aminoglycosides. Aminoglycosides, except for their excellent spectrum of activity against Enterobacteriaceae and *P. aeruginosa*, do not have much advantage over penicillins or cephalosporins against sensitive strains of these organisms for many reasons. For example, the serum concentrations of gentamicin are unpredictable after a dose based on the body weight, so peak and trough serum levels must be confirmed by any of the various assay methods available.[247] In addition, the therapeutic range of peak serum concentrations of 4–8 μg/ml is narrow: Levels below 4 μg/ml may likely be below the inhibiting concentration for the pathogen, and levels greater than 10–12 μg/ml may be toxic. Thus, the peak serum levels are either equal to or only slightly greater than the minimum inhibitory concentration (MIC) for the aminoglycoside in vitro.

Aminoglycosides are inactive against obligate anaerobes, and their activity against sensitive pathogens is antagonized by an anaerobic environment[248] and by reducing substances such as sulfhydryl compounds. Aminoglycosides are also not active in acidic conditions. Both anaerobic and acidic conditions are frequently present in intra-abdominal abscesses. The β-lactams, in contrast, are relatively nontoxic, can be used in concentrations that are many times higher than the MIC for the pathogen, and are active under anaerobic or acidic conditions. For these reasons, the efficacy of aminoglycosides in intra-abdominal infection has been questioned.[249] The β-lactams are probably more reliable antibiotics than the aminoglycosides against sensitive pathogens. Therefore, if indicated on the basis of in vitro sensitivity testing, β-lactams should be used in preference to aminoglycosides. An aminoglycoside is usually included with a β-lactam antibiotic in the initial antimicrobial regimen for patients who are critically ill or in whom a resistant pathogen (e.g., *P. aeruginosa*) is suspected.

Quinolones. The fluoroquinolones (e.g., norfloxacin, ciprofloxacin, enoxacin, ofloxacin, and lomefloxacin) are a new class of antimicrobial agents related to nalidixic acid.[250] They are active against almost all aerobic gram-negative bacilli. They are generally less active against most gram-positive cocci, including some enterococci.[251] Their ability to kill bacteria in both the exponential and the stationary phases of growth, along with the lack of development of plasmid-mediated resistance, make the fluoroquinolones potentially valuable antimicrobial agents for the treatment of intra-abdominal infections, including abscesses. Currently two fluoroquinolones, ciprofloxacin and ofloxacin, are available for intravenous administration. The fluoroquinolones are well absorbed after oral administration, except for nonfloxacin, and are concentrated in many tissues so that tissue levels are well in excess of the MICs of many sensitive pathogens. However, with current fluoroquinolone dosing regimens, these tissue levels may be inadequate to treat susceptible pathogens with relatively high MICs (e.g., ≥0.5 μg/ml of ciprofloxacin), which may include some strains of *P. aeruginosa, S. pneumoniae*, staphylococci, and enterococci.[252] If such organisms can be anticipated (e.g., in nosocomial infections) additional antimicrobial agents may be necessary to broaden the spectrum of an empiric regimen. The addition of an antimicrobial agent active against anaerobic bacteria and aerobic or microaerophilic gram-positive cocci (e.g., clindamycin, ampicillin–sulbactam, or amoxicillin–clavulanic acid) would be required if the use of a quinolone was considered for secondary intra-abdominal infection.

Controlled Clinical Trials. There is no one antimicrobial regimen applicable to every clinical situation. However, it is clear that for an antimicrobial regimen to be efficacious in the treatment of secondary peritonitis and other secondary intra-abdominal infections, the agents chosen must have significant antibacterial activity against *B. fragilis* and enteric gram-negative bacilli.[253–255] Therapy with an agent with activity against *P. aer-*

uginosa would be desired if the infectious process developed while in the hospital or after a course of broad-spectrum antibiotics. The need to add specific agents active against the enterococcus remains controversial.[198] Although the results of many antimicrobial trials for treatment of intra-abdominal infections have been published, caution must be exercised when interpreting these studies because of the possibility of inadequate study design and analysis of data.[256] Some of the variables that must be considered are (*1*) differences in patient populations, (*2*) types and severity of underlying illnesses, (*3*) community- vs. hospital-acquired infection, and (*4*) the pathogens isolated.

The standard antimicrobial regimen against which most new regimens are compared is an aminoglycoside in combination with clindamycin.[257–259] The risk of renal toxicity and ototoxicity, along with the need to monitor serum aminoglycoside levels, may limit the use of aminoglycosides as newer agents prove to be useful alternatives.[249] Development of β-lactam antibiotics, such as imipenem, as well as cefoxitin, cefotetan, ampicillin-sulbactam, and ticarcillin-clavulanic acid, which have activity against both *B. fragilis* and facultative enteric gram-negative bacilli, have made single drug therapy possible.[260] Table 1 lists many of the antimicrobials regimens that have been found to be efficacious for the treatment of intra-abdominal infections in clinical trials. The majority of second- or third-generation cephalosporins have limited activity against the *B. fragilis* group, and their use as single antimicrobial agents for the treatment of intra-abdominal infections has had variable results.[100,271–274] However, combining one of these cephalosporins with clindamycin or metronidazole would likely be an adequate antimicrobial regimen in this setting.[275]

Although the need for treatment is controversial,[276,277] clearly *Candida* species, either as part of a polymicrobial peritoneal infection or as a single isolate, have the potential to cause peritonitis, intraperitoneal abscesses, and subsequent candidemia.[127,278] The dominant clinical view today favors aggressive early therapy of all intra-abdominal isolates of *Candida* species in symptomatic patients with peritonitis, usually with the parenteral administration of at least 375–500 mg amphotericin B over 10–14 days.[279]

The duration of therapy is usually prolonged to prevent relapse, because host defenses cannot be relied on to eradicate completely the pathogens from sequestered areas of extensive tissue necrosis and abscess formation. Not all of these areas are accessible to adequate surgical drainage. Antibiotic therapy should be given before, during, and after surgery to ensure tissue and blood drug levels that can combat local and metastatic spread of the infection. Therapy should be continued until the patient's temperature and white blood cell and differential counts have normalized and all drains have been removed, although penetrating abdominal trauma with bowel perforation in otherwise healthy patients can be treated for 48–72 hours. The dose, the frequency, and usually the route of administration of the antimicrobial agents are maintained to achieve adequate blood and tissue drug concentrations during the entire treatment period and are not necessarily changed as the patient improves. The antibiotic regimen should be adjusted to include the most efficacious, least toxic, and least expensive agents, once cultures have been finalized, with the proviso that therapy must have activity against anaerobes, even when not isolated, be-

TABLE 1. Comparative Antimicrobial Trials for Treatment of Intra-Abdominal Infections

Regimen	Reference
Cefoxitin ± aminoglycoside vs. clindamycin + aminoglycoside	261–263
Ticarcillin + aminoglycoside vs. clindamycin + aminoglycoside	264
Piperacillin vs. cefoxitin	265
Ampicillin-sulbactam vs. clindamycin + aminoglycoside	266
Imipenem vs. clindamycin + aminoglycoside	260, 267–269
Aztreonam + clindamycin vs. clindamycin + aminoglycoside	270

cause anaerobic bacteriologic techniques are frequently inadequate.

The intravenous route of antibiotic administration is preferred, especially in shock, when poor perfusion of the gut and muscle preclude use of the oral or intramuscular routes. When gastrointestinal function returns to normal those drugs that are well absorbed after oral administration (e.g., ciprofloxacin, ofloxacin, metronidazole, trimethoprim-sulfanethroazole, clindamycin, or amoxicillin-clavulanic acid) can be given orally. Blood levels may be less satisfactory after intramuscular administration of certain antibiotics, for example, chloramphenicol. Although some surgeons use antibiotics intraperitoneally at the time of operation in irrigating fluid,[280] others do not.[281] Decreases in the rate of wound infection but not in the rate of intraperitoneal sepsis have been shown with the use of intraperitoneal irrigation.[282] Respiratory arrest may occur after peritoneal absorption of aminoglycosides, and lavage of the peritoneal cavity at the time of surgery with large amounts of saline alone may be sufficient.[283] Also, intravenous or intramuscular antibiotics in adequate doses reach the peritoneum without additional intraperitoneal administration.

The effect of irrigation of the peritoneal cavity with agents such as povidone-iodine has also been studied. In one study, there was a decreased frequency of intra-abdominal abscess formation in the povidone-iodine group compared with that of the saline group.[284] However, povidone-iodine has been shown to be a potent inactivator of such neutrophil functions as chemotaxis and phagocytosis and thus may have a detrimental effect.[285]

Another technique is to place a plastic catheter through the abdominal wall at the time of the operation so that antibiotics can be injected directly postoperatively into the peritoneal cavity. The method is said to be beneficial clinically,[286] but its superiority over intravenous antibiotics alone has not been proven in clinical peritonitis. Recent comparative studies showed no significant difference in clinical outcome between patients who had irrigation of the peritoneal cavity and those who did not.[287,288] However, when peritoneal dialysis is being done in the presence of peritonitis, antibiotics in therapeutic doses should be included in the dialysis fluid to maintain antibiotic levels in the rapidly exchanged peritoneal fluid.[289] If intraperitoneal antibiotics are used, systemic antibiotics may be necessary as well to maintain adequate blood levels.

HYPERBARIC OXYGEN.   Increased oxygen tension attainable with hyperbaric oxygen therapy inhibits and kills *C. perfringens*[290] and reduces the production of *C. perfringens* α-toxin. Hyperbaric oxygenation has been used clinically and experimentally for clostridial myonecrosis, with some reported success.[291] Because *C. perfringens* is a relatively oxygen-tolerant anaerobe in comparison to other obligate anaerobic pathogens, it would be reasonable to assume that hyperbaric oxygen therapy would be at least equally efficacious with anaerobic infections due to these more oxygen-sensitive anaerobes. Except for a few reports,[292] almost no clinical or experimental data, however, are available. Hill[293] reported suppression of experimental liver abscesses due to anaerobes in mice treated with hyperbaric oxygen therapy alone. In one study, it appeared that the use of hyperbaric oxygen therapy favorably affected the outcome of experimental sepsis in a rat model, perhaps by enhancing host defense mechanisms.[294] Consideration should also be given to the hazards of hyperbaric oxygen therapy.

GASTROINTESTINAL DRAINAGE.   In the presence of peritonitis, the patient should receive nothing by mouth. If no distension is present when treatment is instituted, continuous gastric suction is usually sufficient. For those patients who are distended when treatment is started and for those who become distended in spite of gastric drainage, small intestinal intubation should be instituted.

WATER AND ELECTROLYTE ADMINISTRATION.   The type of fluid replacement is determined in large part by the chemical abnormalities found. In general, hypovolemia, dehydration, and metabolic acidosis predominate, so plasma or albumin, Ringer's lactate solution, and 5% dextrose in water usually suffice. The amount to be given in the 2–4-hour period before anticipated surgery is determined by watching vital signs, hematocrit values, hourly urinary output, and central venous pressure.

BLOOD AND PLASMA TRANSFUSION.   Although many patients recover from an illness satisfactorily with a hemoglobin of 8 or 10 g/dl, some surgeons recommend that the patient be transfused to maintain levels as high as 12–13 g/dl in order to provide a margin of safety should some complication such as septic shock or upper gastrointestinal hemorrhage supervene.

RESPIRATORY SUPPORT.   Fluid sequestered in the abdomen and loops of bowel distended by gas may elevate the diaphragm. Inflammation of the parietal peritoneum, including the diaphragmatic surface, leads to guarding and splinting of the muscular wall, which interferes with deep breathing or coughing. A subphrenic abscess may be responsible for splinting of the diaphragm. Retained bronchial secretions may lead to atelectasis and subsequent pneumonitis. These factors that impair the ability to augment respiratory exchange in the face of the increased expenditure of energy required by the inflammatory process produce hypoxemia and respiratory alkalosis. When the patient tires, the combination of metabolic and respiratory acidosis may develop and prove fatal.

Arterial blood gas studies are necessary to detect and quantitate respiratory decompensation. Measures aimed primarily at gastrointestinal decompression, elevation of the head of the bed, and control of the inflammation may sufficiently improve respiration. Administration of oxygen may improve arterial oxygen saturation. If these measures are inadequate, endotracheal intubation or tracheostomy should be done without delay. A volume-cycled respirator should be used and adjusted to give a P_{O_2} of 80–100 mmHg and a normal pH. If the P_{CO_2} is not then normal, metabolic acidosis or alkalosis may need to be treated. As the intra-abdominal process subsides, the patient may be able to breathe spontaneously again and may be weaned from the ventilator. In certain severe cases, positive end-expiratory pressure may also be necessary.

OPERATIVE APPROACH.   The aims of an operation for spreading peritonitis are to stop continuing contamination, to remove foreign material from the peritoneal cavity, and to provide drainage of purulent collections. Operation is generally not indicated (1) in primary peritonitis, (2) in moribund patients who continue to deteriorate despite vigorous supportive therapy, (3) in patients in whom the disease process subsides and localizes while they are being prepared for surgery, (4) in patients with peritonitis secondary to hemorrhagic pancreatitis, and (5) in patients with peritonitis secondary to pelvic inflammatory disease, since this usually responds to nonsurgical therapy.

There is general agreement as to the necessity of (1) removing all material, such as necrotic tissue, feces, and blood, from the operative field, since the virulence of peritoneal infections is enhanced by the presence of these substances; (2) eliminating any possible anaerobic conditions; and (3) reducing the bacterial count to a minimum. Also, in acute diffuse peritonitis, copious peritoneal irrigation with isotonic saline or Ringer's lactate solution significantly reduces mortality and morbidity.[283] Leaving the peritoneal cavity packed open, facilitated by the use of polypropylene mesh to avoid evisceration, and planned repeated return to the operating room to break up loculations and débride necrotic and purulent material in patients with severe generalized peritonitis[295] has been reported to be effective, but these results are yet to be confirmed by controlled prospective randomized trials. In localized infection, local drainage alone is adequate because the risk of disseminating infection outweighs any possible benefit of removing foreign material that may have escaped mechanical removal.

Use of multiple drains for drainage of the general peritoneal cavity is physically impossible, since exudate and adhesions rapidly isolate and occlude the drains and may increase secondary infections.[296] However, drains are often placed in a dependent point to which fluid can be expected to gravitate or in an area of devitalized tissue that cannot be removed.

Prevention. Prevention of postoperative peritonitis requires avoiding contamination of the peritoneum with gastrointestinal or vaginal secretions. In addition to using good surgical technique, this can be accomplished by early treatment of an intra-abdominal infection. For example, Leigh et al.[297] noted that the rate of wound infection in patients with perforated appendix was over 50 percent if no antimicrobial therapy was used and 15 percent in the group given appropriate therapy. Similarly, two studies demonstrate the efficacy of early use of antibiotics in penetrating wounds of the abdomen, especially involving the colon.[298,299] Surgeons have also used various means to reduce the complex gastrointestinal or vaginal flora before clean, contaminated surgery. Mechanical cleansing of the bowel with a low-residue diet and then a liquid diet, cathartics, and enemas can reduce the total fecal mass and coliform count in the colon, although not necessarily the predominant anaerobic flora.[300] The use of oral antibiotics preoperatively to reduce bowel flora is well accepted. *Escherichia coli* in the colonic flora is sensitive to either oral neomycin or kanamycin, whereas *B. fragilis* frequently is sensitive to erythromycin or metronidazole. Thus, combinations such as neomycin-erythromycin base have been shown to be effective in reducing total bowel flora preoperatively and decreasing the incidence of postoperative infection.[301]

Parenteral antibiotics have also been used in gastrointestinal and vaginal surgery prophylactically when there is a chance of contamination with normal microflora at the operative site (clean, contaminated surgery). Up to 30 percent of these types of operations may be complicated by infections. These involve cutting through the large bowel without significant spillage; compromising the blood supply of the large bowel; cutting through stomach or small bowel when there is anticipated intraluminal bacterial overgrowth; appendectomy for appendicitis without rupture; penetrating wounds of the abdomen; gallbladder surgery in the elderly; cesarian section after rupture of the membranes and labor; vaginal hysterectomy in the premenopausal woman; and radical pelvic surgery for gynecologic malignancy.[302] Several studies have shown significant reduction in the frequency of postoperative infection from about 20–30 percent to about 4–8 percent after prophylactic antibiotic use in clean, contaminated surgery.[303,304] The basic principle of antibiotic prophylaxis is to provide adequate tissue levels at the site of contamination and blood levels during the procedure and for possibly up to 24 hours after the procedure.

Peritonitis During Peritoneal Dialysis

Chronic Peritoneal Dialysis. Peritoneal dialysis has been used successfully to treat uremia in patients with end-stage renal disease since the mid-1940s. Peritonitis was a frequently associated side effect that hindered the acceptance of chronic peritoneal dialysis until an improved access catheter was developed by Tenckhoff in 1968. This catheter significantly decreased the incidence of peritonitis, but initial reports of patients undergoing chronic ambulatory peritoneal dialysis (CAPD) with this catheter had peritonitis rates of more than six episodes per patient-year.[305,306] This rate has appeared to decline with the introduction of collapsible plastic bags, improved adapters, and better techniques. However, peritonitis remains the major complication of CAPD today.[307] It occurs at a rate of about one episode per patient a year, with a range from three or more episodes a year to less than one every 2 years. Forty-five percent of CAPD patients develop peritonitis at least once during their initial 6 months on CAPD. This increases to 60–70 percent during the first year.[308–310] Recurrent peritonitis occurs in 20–30 percent

of patients and is one of the most common reasons for discontinuation of CAPD.[311] A small proportion of patients seem to have an unusually high frequency of peritonitis.[312] This disparity in the frequency of infection has been attributed, at least in part, to faulty sterile technique on the part of the patient when self-administering CAPD.

The origin of infection in most cases appears to be contamination of the catheter by common skin organisms.[306] Alterations of skin flora in CAPD patients[313] may lead to peritoneal contamination with enteric pathogens. A higher incidence of peritonitis has been reported in dialysis patients who are nasal carriers of *Staph. aureus*.[314] Pathogens may also contaminate the peritoneum from exit-site and subcutaneous-tunnel infections, transient bacteremia, and contamination of the dialysate delivery system during bag exchanges. As mentioned previously, it has been demonstrated that enteric bacteria may also gain access to the peritoneal cavity by transmural migration through an intact intestinal wall after the introduction of hypertonic solutions into the peritoneum.[51] This mechanism may account for enteric bacterial peritonitis in dialysis patients.[52] Polymicrobial infection with fecal organisms suggests perforation of the bowel as a complication of catheter placement.

Alterations in peritoneal defenses may increase the risk of peritonitis in CAPD patients. The antimicrobial function of peritoneal macrophages and polymorphonuclear cells generally requires the presence of opsonins. A reduction in the levels of IgG and C3 has been noted in peritoneal dialysis effluents when compared with serum, and the levels of these crucial opsonizing agents are inversely related to the frequency of peritonitis.[315] The addition of IgG to peritoneal dialysis fluid has been found to have a prophylactic effect.[316] Other important factors that impair host defense mechanisms are the low pH and high osmolality of peritoneal dialysis fluid, both of which can impair polymorphonuclear function and antibiotic efficacy.[317]

Gram-positive organisms compose 60–80 percent of isolates, most commonly *Staph. epidermidis* followed by *Staph. aureus*, *Streptococcus* spp., and diphtheroids. Staphylococcal isolates have been noted to grow on polymer surfaces and frequently produce an extracellular slime substance or biofilm that may protect these bacteria from host defenses.[318] Gram-negative organisms are obtained from 15–30 percent of isolates. *Escherichia coli* is the most common, followed by *Klebsiella/Enterobacter*, *Proteus*, and *Pseudomonas* spp. Less common pathogens include *Acinetobacter* spp., *C. albicans*, and anaerobic bacteria. Rare isolates include *Mycobacterium tuberculosis*, *Candida parapsilosis*, *Aspergillus fumigatus*, *Nocardia asteroides*, and *Fusarium* spp.[312,319–321]

Diagnosis of peritonitis is made when microorganisms and an increased number of leukocytes are present in the dialysate combined with a constellation of clinical findings that include abdominal pain and tenderness (found in 60–80 percent of patients), nausea and vomiting (in 30 percent), fever (in 10–20 percent), and diarrhea (in 10 percent).[306,312,320,321] However, not all these criteria need to be met to fulfill the diagnosis.

The dialysate is almost always cloudy, and microscopic examination reveals a leukocyte count greater than 100/mm³, approximately 85 percent being more than 500/mm³, with neutrophils predominating.[312] Gram stain of the fluid reveals organisms in 9–50 percent of cases.[306,312] Peripheral leukocytosis has been reported to be a poor indicator for peritonitis in this group of patients.[320] Blood cultures are rarely positive, in contrast to the 30–50 percent positive rate in other types of intra-abdominal infection.

Peritonitis with negative cultures occurs in 5–10 percent of cases. Constant flow of dialysis fluid into and out of the peritoneal cavity dilutes the microbial density and may falsely lower the rate of positive dialysate culture results. Negative cultures may also be due to infection with fastidious organisms, previous antimicrobial treatment, or inadequate culture technique. One method that has been used to improve the yield of dialysate cultures is the filtration method. A 100 ml aliquot of peritoneal fluid is filtered through a 0.45 μm filter. The filter is then washed with sterile saline and incubated in thioglycolate broth.[320] Rubin et al.[306] compared the filtration method with direct inoculation of blood culture bottles and found no significant difference in positive culture rates. Still others found the inoculation of 2–3 ml of dialysate into thioglycolate broth to be the most sensitive culture technique.[320] A study comparing direct inoculation of dialysate into a biphasic blood culture system, direct inoculation of dialysate into routine blood culture bottles, and centrifugation of 50 ml of dialysate and culture of the sediment failed to demonstrate a significant difference among these methods in the recovery of a pathogen.[322] All cultures should be performed aerobically. Fungal, mycobacterial, and anaerobic cultures should be performed if clinically indicated (e.g., negative aerobic cultures).

The prognosis of peritonitis in dialysis patients is generally favorable. For example, one large series reported less than 1 percent mortality attributed directly to infection.[312] The duration of illness and positive peritoneal fluid cultures after institution of antimicrobial therapy is usually 1–4 days. However, some infections, especially those due to *Staph. aureus*, *Pseudomonas*, or fungus, resolve more slowly and may cause relapse more frequently.[320]

Adequate levels of antimicrobial agents necessary to treat peritonitis successfully can be obtained in the peritoneal fluid by both systemic and intraperitoneal routes.[312,319,320,323] However, because CAPD peritonitis is a localized infection, the intraperitoneal route is preferred, as no therapeutic advantage of intravenously administered antibiotic has been demonstrated.[324] Although a variety of doses can be found in the literature, the initial doses recommended in Table 2 for intraperitoneal administration result in effective peritoneal fluid drug concentrations. Subsequent dosing is used to maintain these levels. The aim of the dosing regimen is to maintain a concentration of the drug in the peritoneal cavity fluid above the MIC of the offending pathogen for most if not all of the dosing interval. Caution must be exercised when reviewing the MIC and minimum bactericidal concentration (MBC) data, since these concentrations have been demonstrated to be markedly increased when peritoneal dialysis effluent is used as the in vitro growth medium.[325]

Because of the lack of comparative, prospective clinical trials, no one antimicrobial regimen can be called superior to another. After cultures are obtained, initial antimicrobial therapy should be based on the Gram stain results or the most likely pathogens if the Gram stain is not helpful. A reasonable initial empiric regimen would be vancomycin in combination with an aminoglycoside. Vancomycin is preferable to a cephalosporin because of the frequency of β-lactam resistance (i.e., methicillin resistance) in staphylococci, which predicts resistance to cephalosporins as well. Initial antibiotic choices should be modified, if necessary, after culture results are obtained. The minimum length of therapy needed for dialysis-related peritonitis has not been determined, but the usual duration ranges from 10 days to 3 weeks. Most patients with CAPD peritonitis show clinical improvement within 48–96 hours of the initiation of antimicrobial therapy. If the signs and symptoms of peritonitis persist after 96 hours of therapy, reevaluation is warranted, with consideration given to the possibilities of resistant pathogens, unusual organisms (e.g., mycobacterial, fungal), and other intra-abdominal processes, as recommended by Keane et al.[324]

Fungal peritonitis, usually caused by *C. albicans*, should be treated with amphotericin B.[326–328] However, *Candida lusitaniae* and some isolates of *C. albicans*, *C. tropicales*, and *Fusarium* spp. may be amphotericin-resistant. If CAPD is continued, amphotericin B should be given intraperitoneally, but it can cause appreciable abdominal pain when given by this route. However, most patients with fungal CAPD infection will fail to respond unless the catheter is removed. Once the catheter is removed, amphotericin B should be given intravenously (30 mg/day). Flucytosine has also been recommended. However, this drug may be difficult to use in end-stage renal disease because of dose-dependent bone marrow toxicity. If this drug is used, serum levels should be monitored closely to prevent the development of toxic levels (>100 μg/ml). There is limited experience with the use of miconazole and ketoconazole in treating fungal peritonitis.[328–331]

Removal of the catheter may be necessary in 10–20 percent of patients. The indications for removal of the catheter include persistent skin exit site or tunnel infection; fungal, fecal, and mycobacterial peritonitis; *P. aeruginosa* peritonitis; persistent peritonitis; recurrent peritonitis with the same organism; and catheter malfunction (e.g., poor flow). The catheter should also be removed in patients with intraperitoneal abscess. Use of oral or intraperitoneal antibiotics has not been shown to be effective in preventing peritonitis during peritoneal dialysis.[51,332]

Acute Peritoneal Dialysis. The incidence of peritonitis during acute peritoneal dialysis has remained stable during the past 20 years. Innovations in technique, which began during the 1960s, reduced the rate of peritonitis from as high as 50 percent to acceptably low levels. These innovations included closed-drainage systems, small-bore catheters, limitation of dialysis to no longer than 48–72 hours, incorporation of a millipore filter into the tubing, and development of closed automatic systems. Also, the use of dry-heat incubators to warm the dialysate decreases the risk of contamination that may occur when water baths are used for this purpose.[333]

Some authorities have recommended that cultures of dialysate be obtained every 8–24 hours during acute peritoneal dialysis and at its termination. Culture of dialysate from the last exchange is more useful than culture of the catheter tip at the end of dialysis because of the frequent contamination of the catheter tip at the time of its removal. However, results of such routine cultures, in the absence of symptoms or cloudy fluid, provide a guide of doubtful value for initiation of therapy. More importantly, dialysate samples should be cultured and examined microscopically (cell count, Gram stain) if the dialysate becomes cloudy or the patient develops signs or symptoms of peritonitis (e.g., fever, abdominal pain). Cultures are best obtained by syringe from the port closest to the catheter.

Peritonitis during acute peritoneal dialysis is frequently caused by antibiotic-resistant, hospital-acquired, gram-negative bacilli and staphylococci. Therefore, it is recommended that therapy be initiated with intraperitoneal vancomycin and gentamicin (or tobramycin), with or without concurrent or subsequent addition of the same antibiotics parenterally, depending on the severity of the illness and the response to initial therapy (see Table 2 for dosages). Modification of the antibiotic regimen should be made when the culture results become available.

TABLE 2. Antibiotic Dosage for Peritonitis during Peritoneal Dialysis

Drug	Intraperitoneal Dosage (mg/liter dialysate)		Intraperitoneal Maintenance Dosage (mg/liter dialysate)	
Amphotericin B[a]	0.007	mg/kg[b]	0.07	mg/kg
Ampicillin	7	mg/kg	0.7	mg/kg
Cefazolin	5	mg/kg	1.3	mg/kg
Ceftazidime	7	mg/kg	3.5	mg/kg
Clindamycin	4.3	mg/kg	0.7	mg/kg
Gentamicin	0.9	mg/kg	0.5	mg/kg q24h
Piperacillin	14	mg/kg	1.5	mg/kg
Trimethoprim-sulfamethoxazole	80 400	mg mg	16 80	mg mg
Vancomycin	9	mg/kg	0.2	mg/kg

[a] A low dose is used initially with progression to a maintenance dose, guided by tolerance to abdominal pain.
[b] Body weight.

(Adapted from Peterson and Keane,[321] with permission.)

The clinical manifestations, prognosis, and response to therapy are similar to those described above for peritonitis associated with chronic peritoneal dialysis.

INTRAPERITONEAL ABSCESSES

Etiology

Intraperitoneal abscess may complicate either primary or secondary peritonitis.[334,335] Diseases causing secondary intraperitoneal abscesses include appendicitis, diverticulitis, biliary tract lesions, pancreatitis, perforated peptic ulcers, inflammatory bowel disease, trauma, and abdominal surgery. The relative frequency of abscess formation associated with appendicitis may be declining, and those of trauma and diverticulitis may be increasing.[335,336] The location of an abscess is generally related to the site of primary disease and the direction of dependent peritoneal drainage. For example, appendicitis has been reported to be most commonly associated with right lower quadrant and pelvic abscesses; colonic diverticulitis with left lower quadrant and pelvic abscesses; and pancreatitis with lesser sac abscesses.[334] In one large series[334] of 194 intraperitoneal abscesses, about 44 percent were in the right lower quadrant, 14 percent in the left lower quadrant, and 14 percent in the pelvis, whereas 20 percent were perihepatic. In a more recent series reported by Saini et al.,[335] the frequency of various abscess locations had changed somewhat, perhaps reflecting the change in the relative frequency of the various etiologic diseases.

Of the various perihepatic (right subphrenic, right subhepatic, left perihepatic, and lesser sac) abscesses, the most common continues to be in the right subphrenic space, but the difference in numbers between the right and left sides has been falling. In fact, in one large series of 267 cases of intra-abdominal abscesses, about one-half were in the subphrenic space, 60 percent of which were noted in the left perihepatic space.[337] This increased frequency of left perihepatic space abscess has also been noted by Ozeran,[338] Sherman et al.,[339] and Sanders.[340] This is in contrast to the series of Ochsner-DeBakey in 1938[341] when right subphrenic abscesses were the most frequent, due to the numerous ruptured appendices.

In children, appendicitis is still responsible for more than 50 percent of the cases of subphrenic abscesses.[342] In contrast, in adults, perihepatic abscesses currently are seen mainly as postoperative complications[338–340,343] rather than in neglected primary intra-abdominal infections, such as appendicitis or perforated peptic ulcer. This may explain the increasing frequency of subphrenic abscesses, especially on the left, in comparison to other intraperitoneal sites.[337] Usually, the surgery has been in the gastroduodenal and biliary tracts. One group of investigators[344] has noted that abscesses that followed gastric operations were left subphrenic if incidental splenectomy had been performed but right subhepatic if splenectomy had not been done. The subhepatic space is less frequently involved than the subphrenic spaces. Lesser sac abscesses generally follow pancreatitis or perforation of the stomach or duodenum. Multiple perihepatic space abscesses have been reported in 5–26 percent of the patients.[338–340,343,344]

Bacteriologic Findings

These infections are typically polymicrobial. In studies in which bacteriologic techniques permitted isolation of anaerobes, anaerobes were found in 60–70 percent of cases.[334,335,343,345] In one study,[343] anaerobes were recovered in 20 of 24 subphrenic abscesses, and *B. fragilis* was the most common pathogen, with anaerobic cocci and clostridia in 50 percent of the patients. Other bacteria frequently recovered are *E. coli*, *Klebsiella/Enterobacter* group, *Proteus* spp., *P. aeruginosa*, *Staph. aureus*, and enterococci.[334,338,339,343]

Pathogenesis

Intraperitoneal abscesses develop as a result of localization of diffuse peritonitis usually in the pelvis, perihepatic spaces, and paracolic gutters. In addition, abscess may develop about diseased organs such as periappendiceal or pericholecystic abscesses or after a penetrating wound (from a stab, gunshot, auto accident, or other trauma) or a surgical procedure. These abscesses are termed *secondary* and account for the majority of these cases. In contrast, the pathogenesis of primary abscesses is unknown and is presumably similar to that of primary peritonitis.

Clinical Manifestations

An acute course, with a high intermittent fever, shaking chills, abdominal pain, and tenderness over the involved area, is characteristic. The clinical pattern may be that of an acute secondary illness occurring after surgery for primary abdominal disease or a prolonged recuperative course in a patient who has been receiving antibiotics after abdominal surgery. Various authors[339–344] have emphasized the occasional chronicity of subphrenic abscesses and have speculated that the course is often modified by antibiotics. Subphrenic abscesses have been described with 6 months or more of an indolent illness.[346]

Local symptoms and signs vary widely with the location and source of the abscess. Subphrenic abscesses are usually accompanied by chest findings with costal tenderness and pleural or pulmonary involvement, whereas subhepatic abscesses have more dominant signs of upper abdominal or subcostal involvement and fewer pulmonary changes.

Diagnosis

Noninvasive diagnostic procedures, including ultrasonography and CT, have provided greater sensitivity and specificity than routine radiography and radionuclide scanning.[347,348] However, these latter techniques remain useful, and often a combination of diagnostic tests is the optimal approach to confirm the diagnosis of intra-abdominal abscess.[349]

Plain radiographs of the abdomen can suggest the location of abscesses in as many as 50 percent of patients.[350] Radiologic findings associated with a subphrenic abscess may include pleural effusion, elevation of the hemidiaphragm, and/or loss of diaphragmatic movement on fluoroscopy. Routine radiography may also reveal displacement of viscera by an abscess. These findings can be enhanced by contrast radiology. The stomach, for example, may be outlined with barium or air to indicate displacement due to a left perihepatic or lesser sac abscess. The presence of gas, either as a single air–fluid level or mottling within the abscess, may aid localization on routine abdominal radiography.

[67]Ga- and ^{111}In-tagged leukocytes are two other radionuclide scans that at times are helpful in detecting intra-abdominal abscesses. Unlike the ^{99m}Tc sulfur colloid liver-spleen scan, which visualizes the entire organ and delineates abnormal areas as "cold" spots due to decreased uptake of the isotope,[67]Ga- and ^{111}In-tagged leukocytes actually accumulate in areas of inflammation, such as abscesses, and appear as areas of increased radioactivity or "hot" spots[351–354] (Fig. 4). Gallium is excreted into the intestinal tract and can accumulate in any inflammatory process, as well as in certain neoplasms. For these reasons, false-positive scan readings may occur when radioactivity within the lumen of the bowel, within the wall of an inflamed bowel, or within a noninfected operative site in the process of healing is misinterpreted as an intra-abdominal abscess.

[111]In-tagged leukocyte scans are as sensitive as but more specific than ^{67}Ga scans because the labeled leukocytes tend to concentrate only in areas of inflammation, since, unlike ^{67}Ga, ^{111}In is not secreted into the bowel.[355,356] Abscesses in the liver

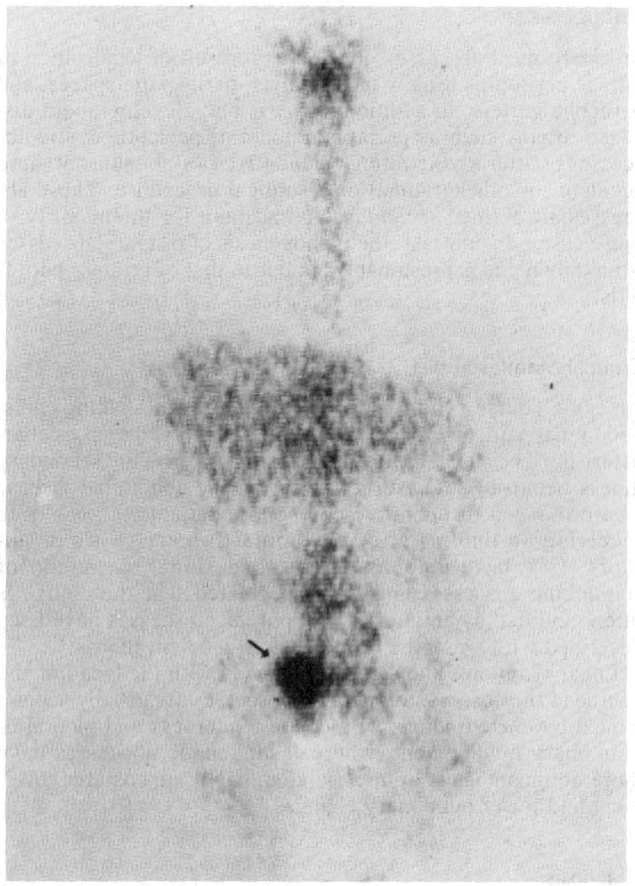

FIG. 4.   [67]Ga scan in a patient with a regional enteritis and signs of an intra-abdominal abscess. Note the area of increased radioactivity in the right lower quadrant (arrow).

Magnetic resonance imaging (MRI) has the potential to display normal anatomy and to show abnormal conditions in many of the body's organ systems and anatomic regions.[365,366] However, only a few trials have compared MRI with older radiologic procedures. In one study, MRI demonstrated a clearer delineation of the extent of inflammatory changes than did computed tomography and better distinguished the abscess from the surrounding structures.[367] In addition, the use of MRI does not require the administration of contrast medium and eliminates exposure to radiation, but it may be more costly than radiologic techniques.

Arteriographic localization has also been helpful. However, overreliance on any one of these techniques is dangerous and should be confirmed by other methods and by the clinical findings (Fig. 5).

Prognosis

The period of morbidity is unusually prolonged in patients with intraperitoneal abscesses. Altemeier et al.[334] reported average hospital stays of 21–47 days. The presence of residual or recurrent infection due to inadequate surgical drainage, more common in patients with multiple or bilateral abscesses, is associated with significantly greater mortality.

Treatment

Although conflicts exist in the literature regarding the proper form of drainage of subphrenic abscesses, all agree that the main therapy for any intraperitoneal abscess is drainage. Effective management is dependent on accurate localization of the abscess, discrimination between single and multiple abscesses, and early and adequate drainage. Conventional therapy for intraperitoneal abscesses has usually included surgical drainage. However, in recent years, successful therapy has been accomplished using percutaneous catheter drainage as an alternative to surgery.[368–370] This method has become possible with the use of refined imaging techniques, especially ultrasonography and computed tomography.[371–373] The general requirements for percutaneous catheter drainage include *(1)* an abscess that can be adequately approached via a safe percutaneous route; *(2)* an abscess that is unilocular; *(3)* an abscess that is not vascular and the patient has no coagulopathy; *(4)* joint radiologic and surgical evaluation, with surgical backup for any complication or failure; and *(5)* the possibility of dependent drainage via the percutaneously placed catheter. Of the patients who fit these criteria, percutaneous drainage has been successful in 80–90 percent.[370,374] In most series, the frequency of complications ranges from 5 to 15 percent[368,375] and include septicemia, hemorrhage, peritoneal spillage, and fistula formation. In addition, failure may occur due to undrained abscesses or pus too viscid to drain via the catheter. Reports indicate that the morbidity and mortality associated with percutaneous drainage may be less than with surgical treatment.[369,376]

Antimicrobial therapy should be started immediately after appropriate specimens (e.g., blood) are obtained for culture; usually this occurs before drainage. Because the pathogens usually are similar to those involved in secondary peritonitis, initial antibiotic therapy is similarly directed at the anaerobes, especially *B. fragilis* and the Enterobacteriaceae. The antimicrobial regimens discussed above in the section on treatment of secondary peritonitis would be appropriate initial therapy. This antibiotic regimen should be adjusted to conform to results of in vitro testing of the infecting organisms isolated from blood or from purulent material obtained at surgery or catheter drainage. During the course of a prolonged illness, repeated cultures of blood and purulent collections, when clinically indicated, should provide a basis for change in antimicrobial therapy.

and spleen may be difficult to detect solely on [67]Ga- or ^{111}In-tagged leukocyte images because normal accumulation of activity in these organs may mask an adjacent inflammatory focus. This problem can be overcome by comparing ^{67}Ga or ^{111}In images with ^{99m}Tc scans.

Ultrasound is a noninvasive technique that is helpful in the determination of the size, shape, consistency, and anatomic relationships of an intra-abdominal mass.[357,358] A pulsed, focused, beam of high-frequency sound is directed into the suspect area of the patient's body by means of a transducer. Echoes are received by the same transducer from skin and tissue planes. The echo pattern is displayed on an oscilloscope as the transducer is moved along the surface of the body. The appearance of abscesses may vary widely from echo-free lesions to highly echogenic masses, but typically appear as a fluid collection with an irregular wall and the presence of a few internal echoes. Ultrasound images may be obscured by overlying gas-filled viscera and by postoperative wounds and drains.

Computed tomography has proven especially well suited for the diagnosis of intra-abdominal abscess.[359–364] Definition is unimpeded by intraluminal gas and postoperative changes, except in the presence of surgical metallic clips or residual barium that may disrupt the image. Observed findings consistent with abscess include a low-density tissue mass and a definable capsule. Computed tomography can detect extraluminal gas, a finding highly suggestive of abscess.[348] Contrast material is commonly administered orally, rectally, and intravenously when attempting to diagnose intra-abdominal abscess. The intraluminal contrast material helps to distinguish loops of bowel from abscess cavities, and the parenteral contrast material may enhance a surrounding capsule, thus allowing for easier identification.

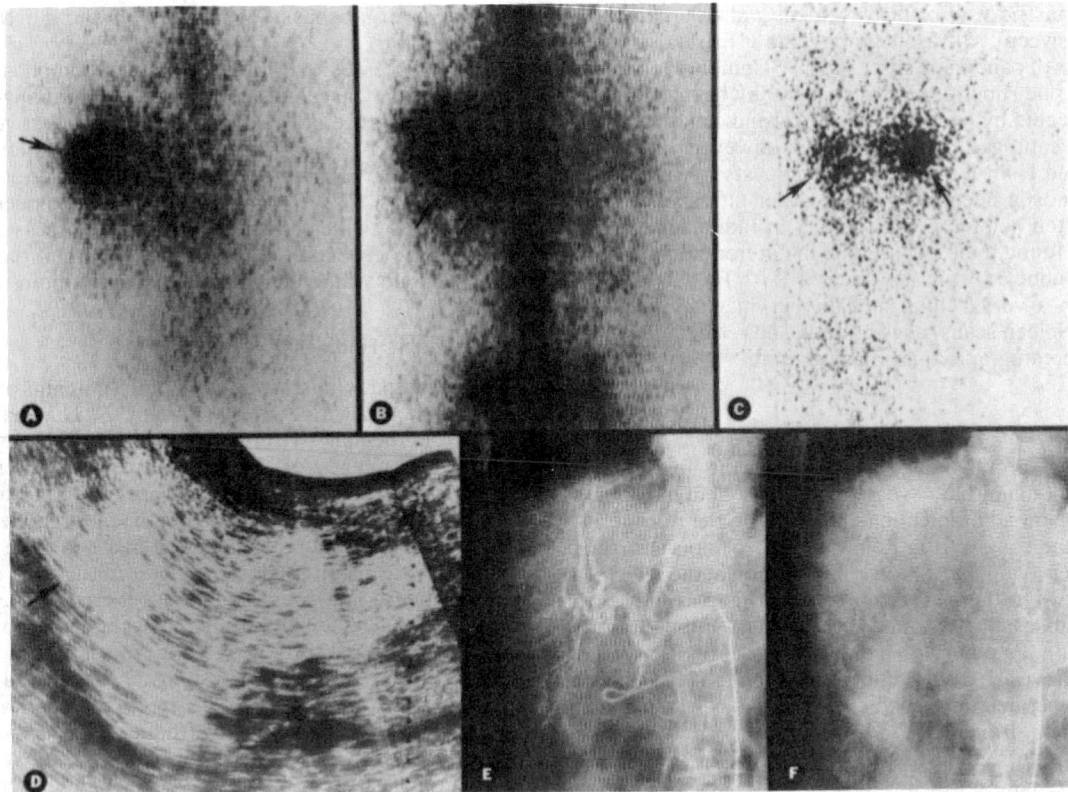

FIG. 5. [67]Ga scan in anterior view (**A**), posterior view (**B**), and right lateral view (**C**) shows increased radioactivity in a dumbell-shaped abscess (arrows) in the right lobe of the liver. Ultrasound examination in this patient (**D**) reveals an echo-free area in the right lobe of the liver (arrow), but both the arterial phase (**E**) and hepatogram (**F**) after selective celic axis arteriography were normal. At laparotomy a large abscess in the right lobe of the liver was drained.

VISCERAL ABSCESS: PANCREATIC ABSCESS

Etiology

Most pancreatic abscesses develop as a complication of pancreatitis, which may be biliary, alcoholic, postsurgical, or post-traumatic in origin. More recently, pancreatitis has been found to be a complication of endoscopic retrograde cholangiopancreatography (ERCP).[377] Pancreatic abscess occurs in about 1–9 percent of the patients after acute pancreatitis.[378–382] The preceding attack of acute pancreatitis has been noted to be frequently severe.[383,384] Occasionally, penetration of a peptic ulcer or secondary infection of a pancreatic pseudocyst may be the cause of a pancreatic abscess.

Bacteriologic Findings

About one-third to one-half of pancreatic abscesses have been reported to be polymicrobial with mainly enteric facultative microorganisms, such as *E. coli* and other Enterobacteriaceae, enterococci, viridans streptococci, and occasionally *Staph. aureus*.[380–383] However, since most studies have not used modern anaerobic bacteriologic techniques, it is unknown how frequently anaerobes are involved. More recent series have documented the presence of anaerobic bacteria in pancreatic abscesses.[379,380,385,386] *Mycobacterium tuberculosis* has also been cultured from pancreatic abscesses,[387] including from a patient with acquired immunodeficiency syndrome (Joseph F. John, Jr., M.D., personal communication).

Pathogenesis

The release of enzymes from an acutely damaged pancreas results in pancreatic necrosis. Infection of pancreatic necrosis is

most likely a secondary event.[388,389] The mixed enteric bacterial etiology of many pancreatic abscesses suggests that bacteria may reach the pancreas by reflux of contaminated bile. The frequency of bactobilia increases with biliary obstruction and with the patient's age, occurring in approximately 50 percent of those over 70 years of age.[390] The hematogenous route may account for some of the monomicrobial infections, especially those due to *Staph. aureus*.

Clinical Manifestations

The clinical manifestations are varied. The patient may fail to respond to therapy for pancreatitis, or 1–3 weeks after the onset of pancreatitis the patient may suddenly deteriorate after an initial response.[380–383] Abdominal pain that frequently radiates to the back, nausea, and vomiting are present in more than 80–90 percent of patients. Temperature of more than 101°F and abdominal tenderness are usually present, although fever may be absent. Less frequently, jaundice, abdominal distension, or an abdominal mass may be present, or the patient may have generalized peritonitis. The serum amylase level is elevated in 21–66 percent of cases and may remain elevated.

Diagnosis

Radiologic, ultrasonic, radionuclide, and CT studies reveal the lesion in 80–90 percent of the cases. Plain films may show diaphragmatic elevation, pleural effusion, presence of a retrogastric mass, forward displacement of the gastric air shadow on cross-table lateral views of the abdomen, widening of the gastrocolic omentum as seen by an increase in the distance between the gastric and colon gas, or mottling and the presence of gas bubbles in the gastrocolic or retrogastric region. Barium studies may show the visceral displacement (e.g., pressure effects in the posterior gastric wall or displacement and enlargement of the duodenal sweep). Ultrasonography and CT are also useful in the diagnosis of pancreatic abscess.[391,392] Computed tomography appears to be superior to ultrasonography because the images are unaffected by overlying bowel gas and can better demonstrate pancreatic gas collections. It is, however, difficult to discern infected from noninfected pseudocysts by both methods, and diagnostic needle aspiration under ultrasound or CT guidance is often helpful.[391] [67]Ga and ^{111}In radionuclide scans have not been found to be very helpful in differentiating pancreatitis or a pseudocyst from an abscess.[393,394] To date, neither has MRI been a very helpful modality in imaging pancreatic abscesses.[395] Spleen scans, angiography, and retrograde duodenoscopic pancreatography may also be useful.[396]

Prognosis

The presence of proteolytic enzymes within the abscess may cause erosion of major blood vessels with intra-abdominal hemorrhage.[382,383] Spread of infection may occur in the retroperitoneum, along the roots of the transverse mesocolon and small bowel mesentery, and may involve suppuration in the lesser sac with extension into the perihepatic spaces. Fistulas may form between the abscess cavity and the stomach, duodenum, or transverse colon. Patients with undrained abscesses seen in surgical practice have a 100 percent mortality.[381] About 53–86 percent of those operated on survive. Survival has been dependent on early surgical drainage.[380,383,385] Higher mortality has occurred in those with infected pancreatic necrosis[397] or biliary tract disease or in those who developed pancreatic abscess postoperatively. These were usually older patients who had ultimately fatal underlying disease. Death may result from septicemia, peritonitis, pleuropulmonary complications, or hepatic or renal failure.

Treatment

Early surgical drainage is most important.[398] Percutaneous drainage alone appears to be inadequate for the majority of pancreatic abscesses.[399,400] However, it may do until the patient can be stabilized for surgical drainage[401,403] and may be definitive therapy in selected patients.[404,405] Optimal treatment appears to require effective surgical débridement and drainage,[406,407] although retroperitoneal laparoscopy has been reported to afford direct access to the pancreas and peripancreatic spaces for exploration and removal of necrotic infected material without the risk of peritoneal contamination.[408] Also, prompt reoperation is often necessary for persistent infection. The prophylactic use of antibiotics early in the course of pancreatitis has been shown to be ineffective in preventing the subsequent development of pancreatic abscess.[409] Initial antibiotic therapy should have adequate activity against *E. coli*, other Enterobacteriaceae, and anaerobic gram-negative bacilli. The regimens discussed in the section on the treatment of secondary peritonitis would be appropriate choices. Antibiotic therapy should be adjusted according to the results of in vitro sensitivity testing. Routine therapy for pancreatitis should also be used.

VISCERAL ABSCESS: HEPATIC ABSCESS

Etiology

Bacterial abscesses of the liver are relatively uncommon lesions, despite the frequency of cholecystitis, appendicitis, diverticulitis, and peritonitis, which frequently are the sources of bacterial infections in the liver. More recently, pyogenic liver abscess has been noted to be one of the infectious complications following liver transplantation,[410] and there is a high frequency of liver abscesses in patients with chronic granulomatous disease.[410]

Bacterial abscesses have been reported to be more frequent than amebic liver abscess, especially in the northern United States.[411–414]

Liver abscesses due to *E. histolytica* complicate about 3–9 percent of the cases of amebic colitis.[411] Although there is no sex predominance in bacterial liver abscesses, over 90 percent of amebic liver abscesses occur in men, and patients with amebic liver abscesses are generally younger than those with bacterial abscesses.[411,414] Pyogenic abscesses have been reported in patients with sickle cell anemia.[415] Liver abscesses occur at all ages but are especially rare in children, when they have been noted to follow umbilical vein catheterization in neonates.[416]

Bacteriologic Findings

Pyogenic hepatic abscess is frequently polymicrobial.[414,417–419] Enteric gram-negative bacilli, usually *E. coli*, have been cultured from the majority of pyogenic hepatic abscesses.[414,419,420] The high frequency of "sterile" abscesses, reported in some series to be about 50 percent, is probably due to inadequate anaerobic cultivation.[419,421,422] As a result of modern anaerobic bacteriologic techniques, anaerobic bacteria have become recognized as a major cause of hepatic abscesses. In reports in which modern anaerobic techniques were used, about 50 percent of all pyogenic liver abscesses were caused by anaerobes, and blood cultures were positive for anaerobes in up to 54 percent of these cases.[421,423] These anaerobes included anaerobic gram-positive cocci, *Bacteroides* spp., *Fusobacterium* spp., and *Actinomyces* spp. Although the frequency of recovery of *Staph. aureus* or group A streptococci from liver abscesses varies among reports, these organisms occur in 20 percent or less of the cases.[411,419,422] *Staph. aureus* is noted to be more frequently isolated in children, primarily in those under 5 years of age,[419,424] and is presumably of hematogenous origin.

Staphylococcus aureus microabscesses in the liver may be associated with microabscesses in other organs as part of generalized hematogenous dissemination in children with impaired host defenses (e.g., in acute leukemia).[425]

On rare occasions, *Yersinia enterocolitica* has been isolated from liver abscesses.[426] It most commonly produces an acute gastroenteritis, especially in children, and a right iliac fossa syndrome due to inflammation of the terminal ileum, mesenteric lymphadenitis, or both.

Candida may invade the liver as part of a systemic infection. However, a marked increase in cases has been observed in which the infection is confined to the liver and/or the spleen.[427,428] Most of these patients have acute leukemia, usually granulocytic, and the microabscesses in the liver are probably secondary to intestinal *Candida* colonization and portal fungemia.[279] The diagnosis is most often delayed because of a nonspecific clinical presentation while the patient is neutropenic. Fever occurs with right upper quadrant abdominal pain and abdominal distension. During this phase of the illness, ultrasound and CT are not helpful, and blood and liver biopsy cultures are usually negative. The diagnosis can be made by histopathologic findings in the liver biopsy. Even when the patient's neutropenia resolves, fever and abdominal pain persist. At this point, ultrasonography or CT may reveal characteristic "bull's-eye" lesions.[428] The response to amphotericin therapy has been noted to be poor, sometimes requiring 2 or 3 months for defervescence, but response to fluconazole has reportedly been better, even in those patients who previously failed amphotericin β therapy.[429–431] However, until these reports are confirmed, amphotericin should be considered the initial therapy of choice.

The specific types of microorganisms that cause hepatic abscess probably vary with the underlying disease. For example, anaerobic abscesses are more frequently cryptogenic or portal in origin, whereas gallbladder disease has been noted in one series in only 2 of 25 patients with anaerobic liver abscesses.[421] Group A streptococcal and *Staph. aureus* abscesses probably result from bacteremia due to these organisms. In the past, it was believed that about 10–20 percent of amebic liver abscesses were secondarily infected with bacteria, usually of enteric origin.[413] However, in more recent series, superinfection was found to have occurred in 0–4 percent of cases.[414] Echinococcal hepatic cysts may also become secondarily infected.

Pathogenesis

The source of infection in the liver may be *(1)* biliary, in which disease of the extrahepatic biliary tract is due to a calculus, stricture, or malignancy and results in ascending cholangitis; *(2)* portal, in which a pathologic process such as appendicitis, diverticulitis,[432] or inflammatory bowel disease[433] is in the bed of the portal venous circulation and may be associated with pylephlebitis (acute suppurative thrombophlebitis in the portal venous system; *(3)* infection in a contiguous structure, such as the gallbladder, which spreads directly to the liver; *(4)* infected foci anywhere in the body via the hepatic artery; *(5)* infection secondary to penetrating wounds and even nonpenetrating trauma to the liver; or *(6)* cryptogenic, in which no source is evident. About one-fourth of the liver abscesses are cryptogenic and are thought to be caused by infection of infarcted portions of the liver.[434] Although a portal venous source, mainly appendicitis, was a common cause of liver diseases in the past, biliary disease is now the most common source.[419,435]

Pyogenic abscesses may be single or multiple. Multiple abscesses are more apt to be due to biliary tract disease,[422] whereas abscesses arising via the portal vein are usually solitary[422]; the right lobe is more commonly involved than the left. Amebic abscesses are predominantly solitary in the right lobe.

Clinical Manifestations

The predominant symptoms of pyogenic hepatic abscess include fever and chills of several days to weeks duration. Characteristically, multiple abscesses associated with ascending cholangitis give rise to spiking temperatures. Right upper quadrant pain may be dull, and abscesses high in the right lobe may cause respiratory symptoms such as cough and pleuritic pain with radiation to the right shoulder and an associated pleural rub. Tender hepatomegaly is present in 50–70 percent of the patients. Jaundice is not often present unless ascending cholangitis is a cause of the abscesses or there is extensive hepatic involvement usually associated with multiple abscesses.[411,419,421] Either the

indolence of the illness in some patients or the minimal physical findings (no hepatomegaly or abdominal tenderness) may account for some of these patients having a "fever of unknown origin."[419]

Clinical differentiation of an amebic from a pyogenic abscess is difficult; a history of diarrhea, the presence of chest findings, or the lack of spiking temperatures has been reported in some series to be more common in patients with amebic abscesses, but these characteristics have not been especially frequent in other series of patients with amebic abscesses. Pain in the left upper quadrant of the abdomen in patients with amebic abscess is infrequent but may indicate a left lobe abscess that can extend into the pericardium.[123] Swelling may occur over the right chest wall, or there may be point tenderness that localizes abscesses due to ameba.[123]

The serum alkaline phosphatase is the most frequently elevated serum liver enzyme test. Blood cultures have been reported to be positive in about one-half of the patients with pyogenic abscesses.[421,422] The presence of viridans streptococcus in several blood cultures in patients with an indolent clinical course and elevated hepatic enzymes without evidence of endocarditis may be an important clue to the diagnosis of liver abscess (Fig. 6).[436] Persistent recovery of viridans streptococci from liver also has been reported in the absence of bacteremia in a patient with an indolent clinical course and persistent serum alkaline phosphatase elevation.[437]

Diagnosis

Elevation and limitation of motion of the right diaphragm, basilar atelectasis, right pleural effusion, or gas within the abscess cavity may be noted on plain films of the abdomen or chest.[438] Scintigraphy with ^{99m}Tc, ultrasonography, CT, and MRI are highly sensitive techniques for the detection of liver abscesses.[439] ^{99m}Tc sulfur colloid liver scan is capable of detecting about 85 percent of lesions greater than 2 cm in diameter.[439] Anteroposterior and lateral views should reveal decreased isotope concentration in both pyogenic and amebic abscesses (Fig. 6).[439] ^{67}Ga- or ^{111}In-tagged leukocyte scans can reveal areas of increased isotope concentration of pyogenic abscesses (Fig. 5). Because the amebic abscess is not really a purulent lesion, it may show decreased central gallium concentration and may be surrounded by a zone of increased activity in the hypervascular abscess rim.[439]

The hepatic angiographic findings in liver abscess are the

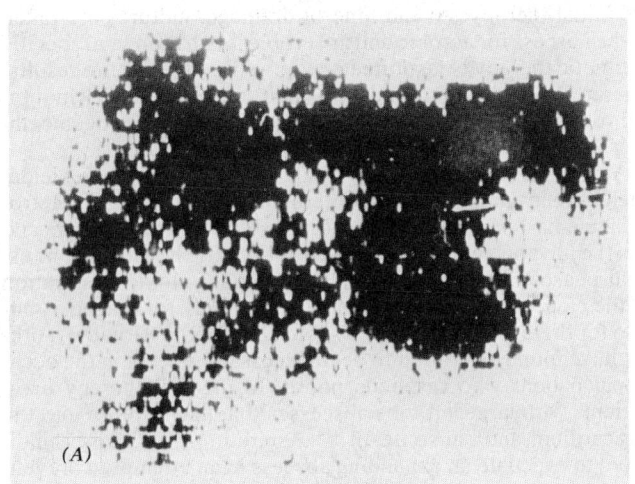

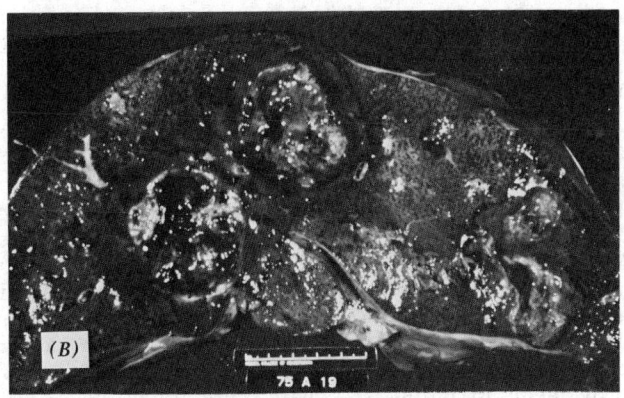

FIG. 6.   **(A)** ^{99m}Tc scan of the liver in a patient who had an α-hemolytic streptococcal bacteremia. **(B)** At autopsy, cut section of the liver revealed several large abscesses that correspond to areas of decreased radionuclide uptake in Fig. A. At laparotomy, needle aspiration failed to yield pus, perhaps because of its viscosity, as evidenced at necropsy.

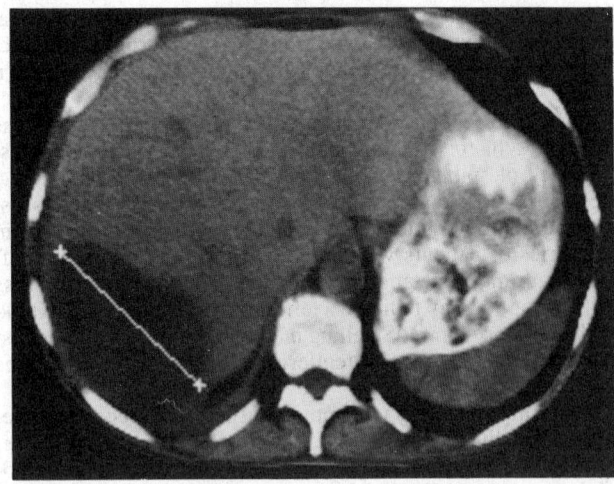

FIG. 7. Abdominal CT scan reveals a liver abscess (arrow) due to a mixture of anaerobic and aerobic pathogens. The abscess developed following drainage of an appendiceal abscess.

mass effect with stretching or displacement of blood vessels and an avascular area surrounded by a blush of contrast seen during the capillary-venous phase of the angiogram.[440]

The effectiveness of ultrasonography for the detection of liver abscess is now well documented.[420,435,441] It has proven especially useful for the evaluation of right upper quadrant structures, primarily because of the absence of air-filled viscera that often impede visualization in other areas of the abdomen. As mentioned previously, the appearance of abscesses may vary from echo-free lesions to highly echogenic masses within the liver. Sonography, as opposed to ^{99m}Tc scintigraphy, can often distinguish abscess from tumor and other solid focal lesions. Computed tomography is also a highly sensitive technique for the diagnosis of liver abscess.[420,442,443] Abscesses produce areas of decreased attenuation on CT (Fig. 7). Both ultrasound and CT may be used to guide needle aspiration for diagnostic and therapeutic purposes.[369,443,444] The aspirated material should be cultured aerobically and anaerobically.

Ultrasound- or CT-guided percutaneous aspiration in patients suspected of having amebic abscess has been recommended to rapidly rule out a pyogenic etiology. Aspiration of sterile fluid that is brownish and without a foul odor is characteristic of an amebic abscess. However, fluid in amebic abscesses may frequently be yellow or green, and possibly is secondarily infected with enteric bacteria. Diagnosis is confirmed by finding *E. histolytica* on direct microscopy or culture of the aspirate or wall of the abscess. In endemic areas, aspiration is usually not performed if amebic abscess is suspected clinically because of the favorable response to drug therapy. Serologic tests indicative of past or present amebiasis are positive in over 90 percent of amebic liver abscesses but may be misleading in endemic areas.[414]

Prognosis

The prognosis of pyogenic liver abscesses depends on the rapidity with which the diagnosis is made and treatment is started. High mortality is also associated with advanced age and serious underlying disease. In the past, the mortality from pyogenic abscesses ranged from about 24 to 79 percent,[419,421,422] and undrained abscesses had a reported mortality of up to 100 percent.[445,446] More recent series, however, have shown an improvement in prognosis, with cure rates of 88–100 percent.[187,188,444] Traditional therapy for pyogenic liver abscesses has been surgical drainage and antibiotics; however, the recently reported high success rates have occurred in patients

treated with either antibiotics plus percutaneous drainage or antibiotics alone. The older series reporting high mortality for undrained abscesses may have included patients who were not candidates for surgical drainage because of poor clinical condition or extensive infection (i.e., multiple small abscesses). The apparent improvement in prognosis during more recent years may be related to earlier diagnosis afforded by the use of ultrasonography and CT. Mortality of uncomplicated amebic abscesses is reported to be less than 1 percent in recent series.[123,414] However, amebic abscesses that rupture into the peritoneal or pericardial cavity carry an 18 or 30 percent mortality, respectively, and amebic abscesses that rupture into the bronchi or pleura carry a 6 percent mortality.[123]

Treatment

The treatment of pyogenic liver abscesses has changed during recent years as the use of ultrasonography and CT has become common for diagnosis and therapy.[447] These imaging procedures offer the ability to follow closely the resolution of the abscess during therapy and allow precise placement of percutaneous catheters for single or continuous drainage. Some series have reported high cure rates after antibiotic treatment without concomitant percutaneous drainage.[187,188] However, most other reports have emphasized the necessity of some drainage procedure to ensure a good outcome.[444,445,448,449] Most patients will defervesce within 2 weeks of the start of medical therapy and drainage.[414] However, some patients who are cured by medical and drainage therapy may still take up to 4 weeks to defervesce.[414] It has been recommended that surgery be considered for patients whose fever persists for more than 2 weeks despite percutaneous catheter drainage and appropriate antimicrobial therapy.[414]

The abscess should decrease in size following percutaneous catheter drainage. Should the patient's condition not improve and fever not resolve within 48 hours after catheter drainage, repeat ultrasound or CT scan should be performed to assess for undrained loculations of pus. Surgery is required for hepatic abscesses secondary to biliary obstruction. Loculated or highly viscous abscesses also usually require surgical incision and drainage.

Antibiotic therapy should be started as soon as the diagnosis is suspected and should be directed at the expected pathogens. Because the pathogens usually are similar to those involved in secondary peritonitis, initial antibiotic therapy is similarly directed at the anaerobes (especially *B. fragilis*) and the Enterobacteriaceae. The antimicrobial regimens outlined earlier in the section on treatment of secondary peritonitis would be appropriate initial therapy. At the time of drainage, cultures are taken of the abscess for aerobic and anaerobic incubation, and specific antibiotic therapy is instituted on the basis of the culture results. Therapy should be prolonged, usually for more than 1 month. Up to 4 months of antibiotic therapy for multiple pyogenic abscesses has been recommended to prevent relapses.[421]

Amebic abscess is usually treated with a tissue amebicide, such as metronidazole or parenteral dehydroemetine.[450] Metronidazole has cure rates similar to those of dehydroemetine and has the advantage of being active for both the hepatic and intestinal phases of the disease and of being less toxic. Aspiration of the cavity has been recommended not only for diagnosis but also for therapeutic drainage by some authors.[123] However, others have found aspiration to be unnecessary, except in the occasional patient who responds poorly to medical therapy or in patients with large left lobe abscesses that may rupture into the pericardium and cause death.[414] Aspiration may also be indicated to evacuate an expanding abscess in an attempt to prevent imminent rupture. Repeated aspiration has been recommended if more than 250 ml is obtained initially.[123] If a solitary right lobe abscess occurs in a male, despite the finding of bacteria in the aspirate, additional antiamebic therapy has been recommended initially because of the likelihood of a secondarily infected amebic abscess.

VISCERAL ABSCESS: SPLENIC ABSCESS

Etiology

Splenic abscesses are uncommon lesions and may occur in patients with sickle hemoglobinopathies, trauma, or bacteremia or in intravenous drug abusers.[451] Usually multiple small abscesses develop as a complication of hematogenous dissemination. One-fourth of these abscesses have been reported to be solitary.[452]

Bacteriologic Characteristics

Splenic abscesses that develop during the course of bacterial endocarditis are usually due to *Staph. aureus* or streptococcus. Enterobacteriaceae (e.g., *Salmonella*) and anaerobic microorganisms have also been recovered.[451–453] In one series, the bacteriology of the abscess was polymicrobial in 25 percent and included anaerobes.[451] The proportion of splenic abscesses reported to have sterile cultures has declined as anaerobic culture techniques have improved. Fungi (mostly *Candida* species) have been isolated from splenic abscesses with greater frequency during the past decade as the population with conditions predisposing to infections with *Candida* has increased (e.g., patients on high-dose corticosteroids or cancer chemotherapy). Fungal splenic abscesses are often part of the syndrome of hepatosplenic candidiasis.[427,432] Blood cultures have been reported to be positive in 70 percent of patients with multiple splenic abscesses but in only 14 percent with solitary abscesses.[451]

Pathogenesis

Splenic abscesses most likely develop as a metastatic process, for example, as a complication of bacterial endocarditis,[454] disseminated tuberculosis,[455] or *Salmonella* bacteremia in HIV-infected patients.[456,457] Some are related to infection in contiguous organs and others from infected traumatic hematomas or infarcts, for example, in patients with sickle hemoglobinopathies.

Manifestations

Left upper quadrant abdominal pain is usual. Irritation of the adjacent diaphragm may result in pain referred to the left shoulder. Splenic enlargement and tenderness are often present, with high, spiking temperatures and perhaps a splenic rub. No clinical findings to suggest splenic involvement may occur in some patients with multiple small splenic abscesses.[451,452]

Diagnosis

Radiographic examination may reveal an elevated left hemidiaphragm, basilar pulmonary infiltrates, atelectasis, or left pleural effusion. Shift of the colon and stomach down and to the right and extraintestinal gas, either diffusely mottled or producing an air–fluid level in the left upper quadrant, may also be seen.[451,452] Radionuclide imaging with ^{99m}Tc sulfur colloid may also be helpful. However, ^{67}Ga- and ^{111}In-tagged leukocyte scans may have relatively low sensitivity, in part due to the inherent normal splenic uptake of these isotopes.[453,458] Ultrasonography, CT, and MRI are the preferred diagnostic techniques for the evaluation of suspected splenic abscess (Fig. 8).[459,460] Computed tomography appears to be somewhat superior to ultrasound for visualization of the spleen because of adjacent gas-filled viscera and inconstant position in the left upper quadrant.[458]

Treatment

In untreated cases, the mortality rate with splenic abscess is 100 percent.[458] Initial antibiotic therapy should have a broad spectrum of activity. A combination of antibiotics that has activity against streptococci and both aerobic and anaerobic gram-negative bacilli would be appropriate initial antimicrobial therapy. Subsequent modifications of antibiotic therapy may be based on results of blood cultures or cultures of material obtained at the time of surgery. With multiple, small abscesses, and with some large solitary abscesses when feasible, splenectomy is the treatment of choice; otherwise, when the spleen is surrounded by extensive adhesions, incision and drainage may be preferred.[451–453,461] Percutaneous drainage was successful in some patients,[451,462] but its indications, efficacy, and safety remain to be determined.[463,464]

SPECIFIC SOURCES OF INTRA-ABDOMINAL INFECTION

Acute Appendicitis

Appendicitis manifests as right lower quadrant abdominal pain accompanied by anorexia, nausea, and vomiting. When the inflamed appendix lies in the anterior position, tenderness is often maximal at or near McBurney's point with low-grade fever, rebound tenderness, voluntary guarding at first, and then abdominal rigidity. Variations in the anatomic location of the appendix may result in variations in the location of the pain and physical findings. For example, a retrocecal appendix may cause principally flank or back pain and tenderness; a pelvic appendix may cause suprapubic pain; and on rectal examination pain may be felt locally and suprapubically.

Persistent obstruction of the appendiceal lumen, usually due to a fecalith, leads to gangrene and rupture of the pus-filled organ. During the several hours between onset of acute appendicitis and rupture, adjacent viscera and omentum may wall off and confine the subsequent spill to the periappendiceal area, with development of an inflammatory mass felt in the right lower quadrant. If the walling-off process is incomplete, spreading diffuse peritonitis occurs. The two sites for loculation of intraperitoneal spread are the pelvic recess and the right subhepatic space. Pylephlebitis and liver abscess may complicate the picture. Colonic microflora, namely, a mixture of *B. fragilis*, *P. melaninogenica*, anaerobic gram-positive cocci, and Enterobacteriaceae, are the primary pathogens in appendicitis and its complications.

The therapy for appendicitis without rupture and for ruptured appendicitis with local or diffuse peritonitis is surgery. If perforation is suspected to have occurred, antibiotic therapy is initiated while the patient is being prepared for surgery. For recommendation of specific antimicrobial agents, see the section on therapy for secondary peritonitis. The severity of appendicitis is related to the development of the rupture of the appendix, which is more common in children and the elderly. Meckel's diverticulitis may manifest in a manner identical to that of acute appendicitis, and the therapeutic approach is similar.

Although not a source of intra-abdominal infection, nonspecific mesenteric lymphadenitis is often confused with appendicitis in children and may account for the symptoms suggestive of appendicitis in up to 20 percent of these patients. It is a self-limited, sometimes recurrent illness in childhood of unknown etiology that primarily involves mesenteric nodes in the right iliac fossa. The nodes are enlarged and discrete. The adjacent

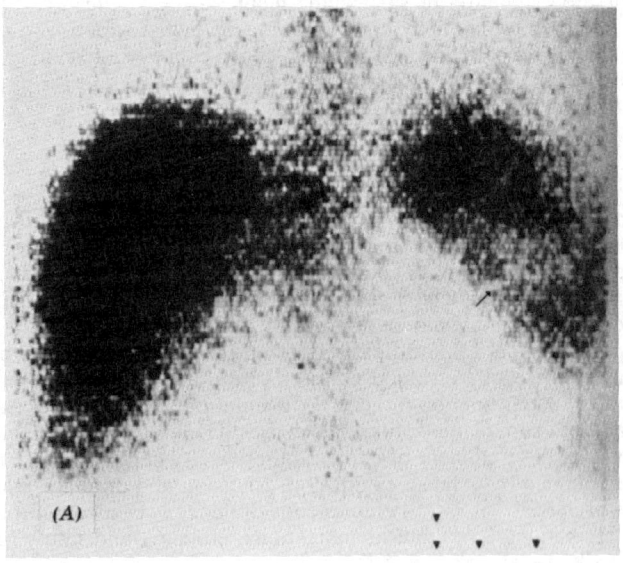

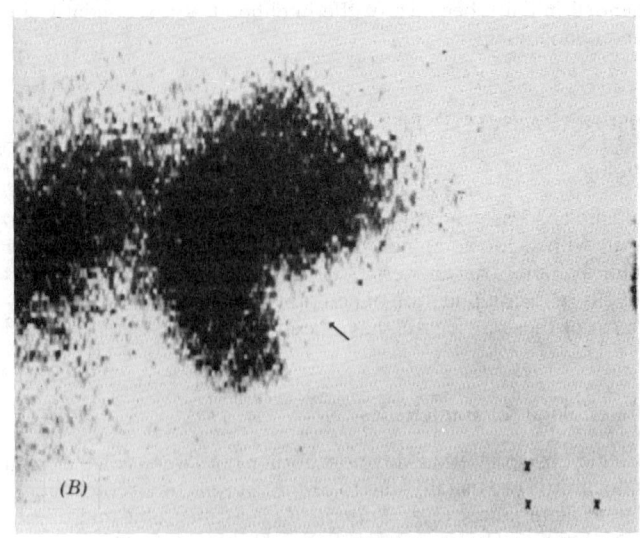

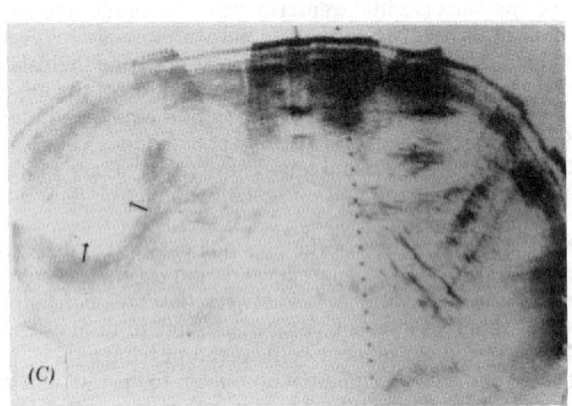

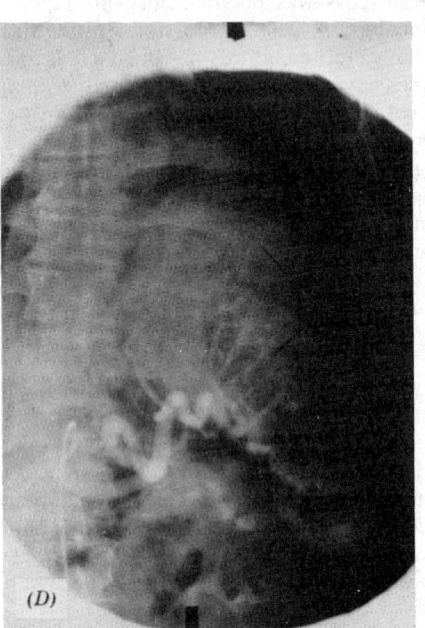

FIG. 8. **(A)** ^{99m}Tc sulfur colloid liver-spleen posterior scan in a patient with fever of unknown origin, high left hemidiaphragm, and left pleural effusion. Note the area of decreased splenic radioactivity (arrow) in an otherwise enlarged spleen. **(B)** Left lateral scan of the same patient. **(C)** Ultrasound examination of the same patient revealing echo-free area (arrows) in the spleen surrounded by an echo-dense border due to increased transmission of the sound. **(D)** Splenic arteriography in the same patient. Note the avascular area (arrows) and surrounding area of increased vascularity.

bowel and peritoneum are at most mildly inflamed, and a small amount of clear serous peritoneal fluid is frequently present. The patient has fever, poorly localized right lower quadrant tenderness, rebound tenderness, and voluntary guarding, but rarely abdominal rigidity. On occasion, leukocytosis is present.

Since the clinical manifestation of nonspecific mesenteric lymphadenitis is so similar to that of acute appendicitis, the therapeutic approach is surgical to rule out appendicitis. Even though the appendix may appear normal, an appendectomy should be done, since a recurrent episode of mesenteric adenitis may again lead to misinterpretation. An identical clinical picture can be caused by rubeola, infectious mononucleosis, and *Yersinia* spp.

Diverticulitis

Diverticula of the colon are herniations of the mucosa and submucosa through the circular muscular layer. Diverticula are usu-

ally located in the sigmoid and descending colons, and usually occur after 35 years of age. Inflammation is the most frequent complication of diverticulosis. The pathogenesis is similar to that of appendicitis. Diverticulitis is more frequent in patients with widespread diverticulosis, and the frequency of the complication increases with age and perhaps with use of nonsteroidal anti-inflammatory drugs.[465] The inflammation may remain localized to the bowel wall as a simple diverticulitis. Complications such as confined perforation with pericolic abscess to which adjacent viscera and omentum are adherent,[466] fistula formation, or, less commonly, free perforation with spreading peritonitis may occur.[467] The clinical picture of uncomplicated sigmoid diverticulitis resembles that of appendicitis, but with findings on the left side of the abdomen. Urinary symptoms are sometimes present as a result of inflammation close to the bladder or ureter and may be followed by fistulization. Pneumaturia and fecaluria often accompanied by chills and fever indicate fistulization between the colon and urinary tract. Passage of flatus and feces through the vagina indicates fistulas into the uterus or vagina. With uncomplicated diverticulitis, low-grade fever and mild leukocytosis are usually found with tenderness, some rigidity in the left lower quadrant and/or suprapubic area, and normal bowel sounds. Perforation produces clinical findings of an intraperitoneal abscess or of diffuse peritonitis.

It is advisable to defer the barium enema until the process has abated with conservative therapy. Nonoperative therapy should be tried for the first few attacks of acute uncomplicated diverticulitis or for well-localized pericolic abscesses. For confined perforation, conservative treatment that may include percutaneous catheter drainage can resolve an inflammatory mass sufficiently to permit a one-stage resection of the diseased portion of the colon.[468-471] Initial nonoperative treatment consists of parenteral fluids, broad-spectrum antibiotics, and nasogastric suction. Antibiotic recommendations are similar to those discussed in the section on therapy for secondary peritonitis.

There are several procedures advocated for surgical management of perforated diverticulitis. The optimal procedure has not been clearly defined[472] because of the absence of properly controlled studies and the variety of complications of diverticulitis and patient characteristics that may influence outcome. Patients who are poor medical risks have traditionally had a three-stage procedure of proximal diverting colostomy and drainage of the area of perforation alone in the first stage, followed by resection and anastomosis in the second stage and closure of the proximal colostomy in the third stage, a prolonged and costly course of events. Primary resection, proximal colostomy and a mucous fistula or Hartmann's pouch, has been advocated more recently as a safe and effective two-stage procedure, even in the presence of diffuse peritonitis or abscess.[472] Elective resection of the involved segment and primary anastomosis with no colostomy (one-stage procedure) has been advocated as a safe and effective procedure for some patients with diverticulitis who are good medical risks and can be operated on after adequate bowel preparation, even in the presence of localized peritonitis or abscess.[473] Operative intervention is also indicated if the patient with acute diverticulitis fails to respond promptly to conservative management in 48–72 hours, if there is a colonic fistula or persistent colonic obstruction, or if carcinoma is suspected.

Regional Enteritis

The onset of regional enteritis may be acute, especially in the young, and may mimic acute appendicitis. The correct diagnosis of early regional enteritis may be made only at operation, which reveals a thickened bowel wall and mesenteric lymph node involvement. Usually, however, the diagnosis is established by contrast radiography.

Perforation as the result of an ulcer burrowing through the entire thickness of the bowel wall may occur.[474] Usually the perforation is confined and may result in abscesses or internal fistulas. Rarely does the ulcer perforate freely into the peritoneal cavity. Perianal or perirectal abscesses and fistulas are also common manifestations of regional enteritis.

Systemic antibiotics are often of value in the management of suppurative complications (see the section on antimicrobial therapy for secondary peritonitis). Surgery is indicated to drain abdominal abscesses, to correct fistulas, and for free perforation. The principal complications of surgery are enterocutaneous fistula, intraperitoneal or wound sepsis, and prolonged postoperative ileus.

Necrotizing Enterocolitis in Neutropenic Patients (Typhlitis)

Necrotizing enterocolitis occurs in patients who are severely granulocytopenic from any cause, including acute leukemia,

aplastic anemia, cyclic neutropenia, Felty syndrome, and chemotherapy for various neoplasms.[475-477]

Pathologically, the bowel is edematous, with marked thickening of the wall. The luminal surface has discrete areas of punctate ulceration, which at times may coalesce. There is also transmural inflammation with hemorrhagic necrosis and degeneration of the muscularis mucosae. The inflammatory cells found in histologic specimens are almost always mononuclear. It is thought that bacteria found in the normal gut flora opportunistically invade the ulcerations in the bowel during periods of profound neutropenia. Due to the lack of granulocytes, these organisms proliferate and cause local destruction by elaboration of exotoxins.[475]

Initially, the signs and symptoms are similar to those of acute appendicitis. These patients present with a new fever, abdominal pain, rebound tenderness in the right lower quadrant (because of the predominance of cecal involvement), and diarrhea. Rapid progression to the development of an acute abdomen is not uncommon.

Plain radiographs of the abdomen may demonstrate a thickened cecum and possibly the presence of gas within the wall of the colon.[478]

The mortality rate with neutropenic enterocolitis is greater than 50 percent.[479] Although the management of this disease is somewhat controversial,[480,481] antimicrobial therapy with activity against the aerobic and anaerobic gut bacteria, together with surgical resection of the necrotic bowel, is generally recommended.

Actinomycosis

Actinomycosis is an uncommon suppurative infection produced by the anaerobe *Actinomyces israelii* or one of several closely related species. The cecal area is most frequently the site of abdominal actinomycosis. Typically, the history begins with an attack of acute appendicitis or with recurrent bouts of right lower quadrant pain and fever, which prompts surgery for a presumptive diagnosis of appendicitis. At surgery an indurated pericecal mass is found with sinus tracts. After appendectomy, persistent draining sinuses form. The diagnosis of actinomycosis is made by demonstration of "sulfur granules" in the purulent sinus discharge and by histologic examination of the tissues. Treatment is discussed in Chapter 235.

ACUTE CHOLECYSTITIS

Pathogenesis

In over 90 percent of patients with acute cholecystitis, gallstones are impacted in the cystic duct.[482] Thus, it is generally assumed that a sudden change in the degree of obstruction leads to a sudden increase in intraductal pressures, which produces distension of the gallbladder, compromising the blood supply and lymphatic drainage. This is followed by tissue necrosis and proliferation of bacteria present in calculous gallbladders. Although infection may not be a primary cause of acute cholecystitis, it develops in over half of the cases. Infective complications include empyema or gangrene of the gallbladder, emphysematous cholecystitis, pericholecystic abscess, intraperitoneal abscess, peritonitis, cholangitis, liver abscess, and bacteremia. A detailed schema for the proposed pathogenesis of acute cholecystitis is shown in Figure 9.

Pathologic Findings

Acute cholecystitis is usually superimposed on a histologic picture of chronic cholecystitis. Ninety-five percent of the gallbladders removed for acute cholecystitis exhibit fibrosis, flattening of the mucosa, and clusters of chronic inflammatory cells as sequelae of previous disease. Rokitansky-Aschoff sinuses are

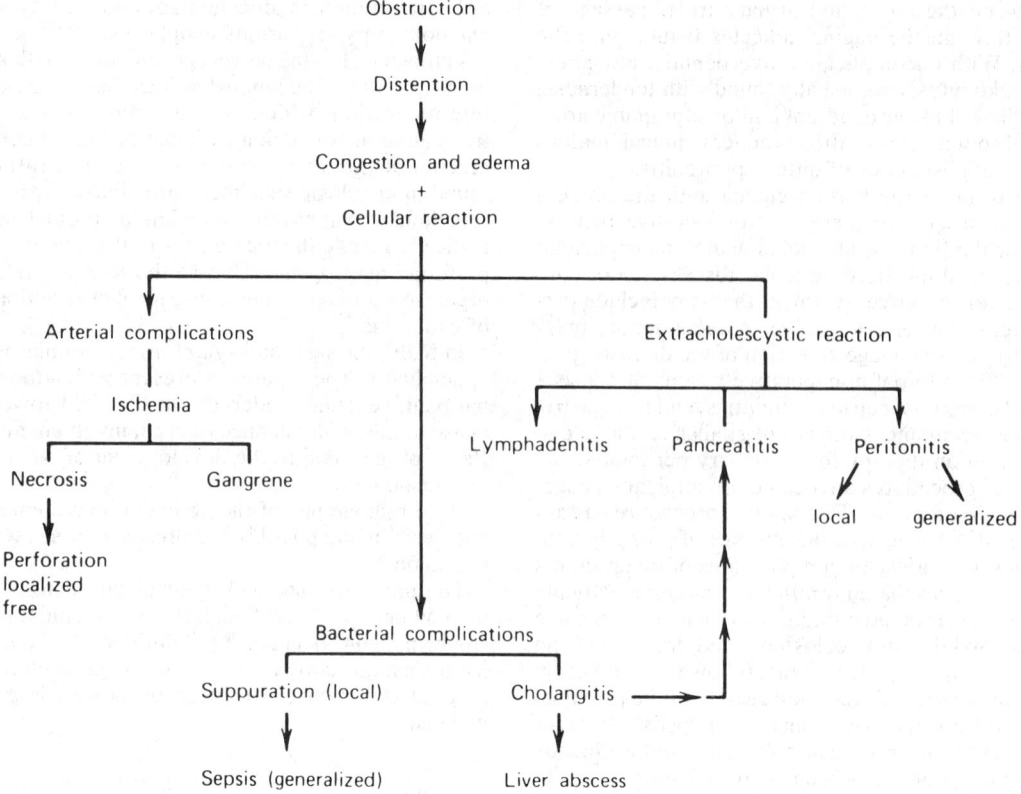

FIG. 9. Pathogenesis of acute cholecystitis.

TABLE 3. Pathologic Classification of Acute Cholecystitis

Edema
Edema and congestion
Focal necrosis
Suppuration {Intramural, Intraluminal, Pericholecystic}
Gangrene
Perforation {Localized, Free}

present in 56 percent of the cases. These sinuses represent mucosal herniations presumably related to increased hydrostatic pressure during previous episodes of cystic duct obstruction. The early acute changes may be only edema and venous congestion. This is followed by focal necrosis and an influx of neutrophils as secondary bacterial proliferation occurs. This may then be followed by actual gangrene or perforation (Table 3).

Symptoms and Signs

Initial obstruction of the cystic duct may be accompanied by only mild epigastric pain followed by reflex nausea and vomiting. If the obstruction is transient, these symptoms subside within 1–2 hours. With persistent obstruction the findings of acute cholecystitis evolve. Pain shifts to the right upper quadrant and becomes increasingly severe. Signs of peritoneal irritation may be present, and in a small number of patients the pain may radiate to the right shoulder or scapula. The gallbladder is palpable in 30–40 percent of the cases.[483] Moderate temperature elevations are common and minimal icterus may occur. However, repeated chills and fever, jaundice, or hypotension would suggest suppurative cholangitis as a consequence of common duct obstruction (see below under "Bacteriologic Findings"). Most patients with acute cholecystitis have a complete remis-

sion within 1–4 days. However, approximately 25–30 percent of patients require surgery or develop some complication.

Laboratory Findings

The laboratory data obtained rarely are required to make the diagnosis of acute obstructive cholecystitis, but they may be indicative of further complications (see the next section). The leukocyte count is usually moderately elevated, with a slight increase in early segmented forms. About 50 percent of the patients have mild hyperbilirubinemia; 40 percent have a mild elevation of serum aspartate aminotransferase (AST) levels; 25 percent have elevated alkaline phosphatase levels; and only 10 percent have mild elevations of serum amylase levels.[484]

Bacteriologic Findings

In the presence of cholecystitis and cholelithiasis, appreciable numbers of various bacteria may be found in the bile and walls of the gallbladder, even in the absence of symptoms. The frequency of bactibilia is higher *(1)* the longer the duration and severity of symptoms, *(2)* in the elderly (>60–70 years of age), *(3)* in the jaundiced patient, *(4)* in acute cholecystitis (up to 94 percent of patients) in comparison to chronic cholecystitis, and *(5)* especially when the common duct is obstructed.[390,485]

The organisms found in the biliary tract are commonly the same as the normal intestinal flora, namely, the enteric gram-negative bacilli, including *E. coli, Klebsiella/Enterobacter,* and *Proteus* spp., as well as the enterococci.[390,486] In addition, studies have demonstrated the frequent recovery of anaerobic organisms including *Bacteroides, Clostridia,* and *Fusobacterium* spp.[486] When present, these anaerobes are frequently involved in polymicrobic infections, mixed with other anaerobes and aerobic gram-negative bacilli.[487]

Patients from whom anaerobes have been recovered were reported more likely to have had prior multiple, complex, biliary tract surgical procedures, especially biliary-intestinal anastomoses and common duct manipulations. These patients often have severe symptoms and a high incidence of postoperative infectious complications, especially wound infections.[488]

The source of bactibilia is unknown, but has been assumed to be the duodenum, and spread is assumed to occur via an ascending route.[487] Although the duodenum normally has a sparse flora in the fasting state, higher counts occur transiently after meals and in conditions that allow bacterial overgrowth in the stomach (achlorhydria or gastric obstruction) or in the small bowel (obstruction, diverticula, or blind loops).

Radiographic and Related Studies

An upright chest film is of limited value. In two-thirds of the cases the right hemidiaphragm is elevated. Since subdiaphragmatic free air cannot originate in the biliary tract, if present, it indicates another disease process. In only about 10–15 percent of cases are calcified gallstones seen on plain films of the abdomen, but this finding in any case indicates only cholelithiasis. Occasionally, a diffusely calcified gallbladder ("porcelainized gallbladder") may be seen. Since this rarely, if ever, develops into acute cholecystitis, its presence should strongly suggest another diagnosis. The demonstration of gas limited to the gallbladder wall or lumen is diagnostic of emphysematous cholecystitis.

Oral cholecystography is of little value in diagnosing acute cholecystitis, because it requires too long a preparation time and is not applicable in jaundiced or vomiting patients. Intravenous cholangiography has been replaced by more sensitive and specific techniques. Recent advances in ultrasonography and nuclear medicine have made these modalities the diagnostic studies of choice for acute cholecystitis. Both imaging modalities are noninvasive, with little reported morbidity, and have been reported to have sensitivity and specificity values of greater than 90 percent. Sonographic findings consistent with acute cholecystitis include the presence of stones, thickened gallbladder wall, dilated lumen of the gallbladder, or a pericholecystic collection.[489,490] Hepatobiliary scanning with one of the ^{99m}Tc-labeled acetanilide iminodiacetic acid derivatives (IDA) is also a sensitive and rapid study for the diagnosis of acute cholecystitis.[489–491] Even in the presence of moderately severe liver dysfunction,[491] the IDA nuclide is concentrated in the liver and excreted into the bile, resulting in visualization of the functioning hepatobiliary system, including the gallbladder and duodenum, within the first hour. In acute cholecystitis, however, since the cystic duct is occluded by a stone or mucosal inflammation, the gallbladder is not visualized, despite common duct and small bowel visualization. During the first hour, nonvisualization of the gallbladder also occurs in more than 50 percent of patients with chronic cholecystitis, but usually the gallbladder is visualized in delayed images obtained up to 4 hours after IDA administration. In chronic cholecystitis and cholelithiasis, a normal cholescintigram may also occur if the cystic duct is patent.

Findings consistent with acute cholecystitis may also be demonstrated with CT, but this technique should not be used for initial screening.[492] MRI has been found to provide both functional and anatomic information and is sensitive in detecting gallbladder disease in patients with suspected cholecystitis.[493]

Complications

Perforation occurs in 10–15 percent of the cases. A small percentage of these are acute free perforations into the peritoneal cavity. These cases are readily recognizable, since they have the catastrophic symptoms and signs of diffuse peritonitis. More frequently, the omentum and serosa of contiguous viscera localize the perforation early. In such cases, there is persistent fever, often a palpable mass that may be in a somewhat atypical location, and occasionally a friction rub. Acute emphysematous cho-

lecystitis is seen most commonly in elderly diabetic men. Systemic symptoms are more severe, and the classic radiographic picture of the abdomen reveals gas within the gallbladder lumen, frequently with a gas-fluid level, and gas in a ring along the contours of the gallbladder wall.[494] Cholangitis is described in detail below. Pancreatitis may also complicate cholecystitis. Here the pain is more midline and may radiate to the back. Urine and serum amylase are often elevated.

Differential Diagnosis

In addition to the complications noted above, the differential diagnosis should include myocardial infarction, perforating ulcer, right lower lobe pneumonia, intestinal obstruction, hepatitis, perihepatitis, and acute disease involving the right kidney. Radiographs of the chest and abdomen, electrocardiograms, and urinalysis can exclude these in the majority of cases.

Antimicrobial Therapy in Acute Obstructive Cholecystitis

Certainly in severely ill or elderly patients or in patients with infectious complications such as emphysematous cholecystitis, perforation with peritonitis or a pericholecystic collection and cholangitis should be treated early for infection possibly due to enteric gram-negative bacilli and anaerobic bacteria, including *B. fragilis*.[381,485,486] An appropriate initial antibiotic regimen includes an aminoglycoside (gentamicin or tobramycin) and ampicillin or piperacillin, in addition to an agent such as clindamycin or metronidazole, to treat for *B. fragilis*. The antimicrobial regimens discussed in the section on treatment of secondary peritonitis would be appropriate alternatives. A more specific antibiotic regimen should be substituted when results of antimicrobial sensitivity testing of the isolated pathogens become available.

The role of antibiotics for the treatment of uncomplicated acute cholecystitis remains unclear. A large retrospective study has demonstrated that routine antibiotic therapy for acute cholecystitis did not appear to affect the outcome of the attack or to decrease the incidence of local infectious complications such as empyema or pericholecystic abscess formation.[495] These results could be due to the fact that, although high concentrations of antibiotics may be present in blood, tissues, and common duct bile, these levels do not appear in the gallbladder bile, blocked by the almost universal presence of cystic duct obstruction in acute cholecystitis, and thus are unable to eradicate bactobilia.

Available evidence suggests that perioperative antibiotics are a helpful adjunct to surgery to prevent postoperative infectious complications.[496] Because wound infection is thought to be due to contamination of the incision with infected bile at the time of operation, prophylactic antibiotics should be given in a manner that will achieve high blood and tissue concentrations at the time of surgery.

Perioperative antibiotics have been recommended in situations in which the frequency of bactibilia is high (such as in the elderly and in those with either a history of jaundice or jaundice at operation, common duct obstruction from stones, chills and fever, or previous biliary tract surgery). Also, it has been recommended that administration of prophylactic antibiotics be dependent on the results of an intraoperative Gram stain of bile.[390] Although ineffective against enterococci and some anaerobes, a cephem antibiotic appears to be a reasonable choice,[496] but antibiotics such as ampicillin-sulbactam would have a broader spectrum of activity.

Surgery

Immediate surgery is indicated for gangrenous (emphysematous) cholecystitis, perforation with peritonitis, and suspected pericholecystic abscess. In these patients, cholecystectomy with intraoperative cholangiography is the procedure of choice.

However, in patients with severe clinical deterioration, a cholecystostomy and removal of cystic duct stones may prove to be a temporizing life-saving measure until a second definitive procedure can be performed,[497,498] provided there is no evidence of suppurative cholangitis (i.e., repeated chills, fever, jaundice, and hypotension), which would require immediate decompression of the common bile duct. Cholecystostomy is not an adequate operation for acute suppurative cholangitis unless the common duct is clearly decompressed through a large patent cystic duct.

The timing of surgery in patients with uncomplicated acute cholecystitis has been controversial. Supporters of delayed surgery after the acute attack has subsided following conservative management feel that morbidity is decreased and that the delay may lower the frequency of unnecessary surgery when the diagnosis is unclear.[499] However, many series have supported early surgery, reporting that a deceptively benign presentation, especially in the elderly, may actually mask the presence of complications and prompt an inappropriate delay in surgery. Also, no difference in morbidity has been reported between early and delayed surgery, and advances in diagnostic studies have markedly decreased the incidence of misdiagnosis.[500,501] The disadvantages of delayed surgery include prolonged hospitalization and a significant incidence of recurrent symptoms that may precipitate urgent surgery under less favorable conditions.

CHOLANGITIS

Cholangitis may be defined as varying degrees of inflammation and/or infection involving hepatic and common bile ducts. Since the mucosa of the gallbladder is continuous with that of the common bile duct via the cystic duct, it is not surprising that varying degrees of choledochitis occur as a limited cholangitis with cholecystitis. In fact, specimens of the common duct taken at the time of cholecystectomy for acute cholecystitis usually show localized edema and inflammation. However, this disease is indistinguishable from uncomplicated acute cholecystitis. In this section, we focus on the more severe entities of ascending cholangitis and acute obstructive suppurative cholangitis.

Pathogenesis

In a manner similar to that described for cholecystitis, obstruction of the common duct results in increased pressure, edema, congestion, and necrosis of the walls of the biliary tree followed by rapid proliferation of bacteria within the biliary tree. In most instances, obstruction is due to gallstones.[502] However, obstruction may be due to prior biliary tract surgery, tumor, chronic calcific pancreatitis, and parasitic infections. Fulminant cholangitis has also been reported as a complication of ERCP.[503]

Pathogenic Findings

Microscopic examination of the common duct reveals marked fibrous thickening and focal areas of chronic inflammation. Superimposed on this is necrosis of the mucosa and dense infiltration of acute inflammatory cells. In the liver, portal inflammation is uniformly seen. Usually, this is a dense neutrophilic infiltrate. In 40 percent of the cases, numerous microabscesses are present. Bile duct dilatation and cholestasis are also present.

Symptoms and Signs

Patients usually have an antecedent history compatible with gallbladder disease. The onset is usually acute, with high fever, chills, and diffuse pain and tenderness over the liver. Jaundice is usually prominent. In some cases, shock and other findings of gram-negative bacteremia may be present; altogether, 85 percent of the patients fulfill Charcot's triad of fever, chills, and jaundice.[504]

Laboratory Findings

There is usually marked leukocytosis with an increase in immature forms. The serum bilirubin level is often higher than 4 mg/dl, and the serum alkaline phosphatase level is significantly higher than that encountered in acute cholecystitis. Serum AST level is modestly elevated. Biochemical and even clinical evidence of disseminated intravascular coagulation may be present.

Bacteriologic Findings

Little adequate data are available on the bacteriologic findings in cholangitis. Studies using detailed aerobic and anaerobic culture techniques suggest that the bacteriologic findings in cholangitis are similar to those in acute obstructive cholecystitis. Gram-negative enteric bacilli and anaerobic bacteria are the most common isolates. Those patients with a stent in their bile duct may harbor resistant flora such as *P. aeruginosa*. Unlike uncomplicated cholecystitis, bacteremia occurs in approximately 50 percent of the cases. *Escherichia coli* (52 percent of the isolates), *B. fragilis* (22 percent), and *C. perfringens* (16 percent) are the most frequent isolates from blood cultures.

Radiographic and Related Studies

An upright chest film is of limited value. The right hemidiaphragm is frequently elevated. Other findings are similar to those described above for acute cholecystitis and are nonspecific. Oral cholecystography is of no value. Intravenous cholangiography is usually not helpful, since the serum bilirubin level is frequently higher than 4.0 mg/dl and the technique has been replaced by less morbid and more sensitive techniques. Ultrasonography can easily be used to evaluate gallbladder size, the presence of stones, and the degree of bile duct dilatation. Marked bile duct dilatation in a patient with the clinical picture described above corroborates this diagnosis. It is important to note that not all patients with obstructive cholangitis have a grossly dilated biliary tree because of chronic inflammation of the biliary tract, and ultrasonography is unlikely to be helpful in these cases. Obstruction of the common bile duct can be diagnosed by hepatobiliary scanning with one of the ^{99m}Tc-labeled derivatives of IDA. In this case, no component of the biliary system or small bowel is visualized, despite adequate hepatic uptake. In obstructive cholangitis, however, ultrasonography is the preferred study due to its ability to visualize dilated ducts and the decreased dependability of IDA scintigraphy in the presence of severe jaundice.[505] Percutaneous transhepatic cholangiography and endoscopic retrograde cholangiography are extremely valuable in evaluating bile duct obstruction. However, it is seldom feasible to use these techniques in the acutely ill patient with cholangitis.

Complications

Bacteremia and shock occur commonly and perhaps are best included as part of the clinical picture of obstructive cholangitis. Perforation of the gallbladder may occur and is described under complications of acute cholecystitis. In some less acute cases, macroscopic hepatic abscesses may develop. This clinical picture may be similar to cholangitis alone. However, ultrasonography, CT, or technetium or gallium scans may visualize multiple defects in the hepatic parenchyma. Finally, pancreatitis may occur as a complication.

Differential Diagnosis

Acute cholecystitis and its complications, hepatic abscess, perforating ulcer, pancreatitis, intestinal obstruction, right lower lobe pneumonia, acute disease involving the right kidney, and bacteremic shock related to another focus of infection, should all be considered in the differential diagnosis. In acute cholecystitis the patient is usually less ill; in addition, the serum bilirubin level is usually less than 4.0 mg/dl, the serum alkaline phosphatase level is not markedly elevated, and ultrasonography or cholescintigraphy usually demonstrates a patent, nondilated hepatic and common duct. Patients with hepatic abscesses not due to obstructive cholangitis are usually not as acutely ill; hepatic tenderness, when present, is also not as severe, and liver function tests may be only minimally abnormal. Diagnostic studies usually detect a macroscopic parenchymal defect. In pancreatitis, the pain and tenderness are more midline and may radiate to the back. Serum and urine amylase levels are significantly elevated, but liver function tests are not markedly abnormal. Finally, radiographs of the chest and abdomen and urinalysis exclude the majority of other possibilities.

Antimicrobial Therapy in Cholangitis

Prompt institution of appropriate antibiotic therapy is mandatory, since these severe infections are frequently complicated by bacteremia and shock. Based on the bacteriologic findings described above and on the known in vitro susceptibilities of these organisms, the antimicrobial regimens discussed in the section on treatment of secondary peritonitis would be appropriate choices. This antibiotic regimen is directed primarily at the complicating bacteremia, since antibiotics alone will not sterilize the biliary tract in the face of obstruction.[486]

Surgery

Prompt operative intervention with decompression of the common duct is mandatory in all but those few patients who respond promptly to antibiotics.[506] In all patients who undergo surgery, regardless of the procedure, operative cholangiography should be performed. The simplest but least satisfactory procedure is simple cholecystostomy if patency of the cystic duct is assured. However, if at all possible, a cholecystectomy should be performed, followed by common duct exploration and T-tube drainage. In more complicated cases, choledochoduodenostomy or cholecystoduodenostomy may have to be performed.

REFERENCES

1. Whalen JP, Bierny JP. Classification of perihepatic abscesses. Radiology. 1969;92:1427–37.
2. Sanders RC, James AE Jr, Fischer K. Correlation of liver scans and images with abdominal radiographs in perihepatic sepsis. Am J Surg. 1972;124:346–52.
3. Myers MA. The spread and localization of acute intraperitoneal effusions. Radiology. 1970;95:547–54.
4. Altemeier WA, Culbertson WR, Fullen WD, et al. Intra-abdominal abscesses. Am J Surg. 1973;125:70–9.
5. Shear L, Swartz C, Shinaberger JA, et al. Kinetics of peritoneal fluid absorption in adult men. N Engl J Med. 1965;272:123–7.
6. Boen ST. Kinetics of peritoneal dialysis: A comparison with artificial kidney. Medicine. 1961;40:243–87.
7. Tsilibury EC, Wissig SL. Absorption from the peritoneal cavity: SEM study of the mesothelium covering the peritoneal surface of the muscular portion of the diaphragm. Am J Anat. 1977;149:127–33.
8. Rochlin DB, Zill H, Blakemore WS. Studies of the resorption of chromium-51 tagged erythrocytes from the peritoneal cavity; the absorption of fluids and particulate matter from the peritoneal cavity. Int Abstr Surg. 1958;107:1–14.
9. Pritchard JA, Adams RH. The fate of blood in the peritoneal cavity. Surg Gynecol Obstet. 1957;105:621–9.
10. Zinsser HH, Pryde AW. Experimental study of physical factors, including fibrin formation, influencing the spread of fluids and small particles within and from the peritoneal cavity of the dog. Ann Surg. 1952;136:818–27.
11. Macbeth RA, Mackenzie WC. The abdominal wall, umbilicus, peritoneum, mesenteries, and retroperitoneum. In: Sabiston DC Jr, ed. Davis-Christopher Textbook of Surgery. 10th ed. Philadelphia: WB Saunders; 1972:773–95.
12. Nohr CW, Marshall DG. Primary peritonitis in children. Can J Surg. 1984;27:179–81.
13. McDougal WS, Izant RJ, Zollinger RM Jr. Primary peritonitis in infancy and childhood. Ann Surg. 1975;181:310–3.
14. Golden GT, Shaw A. Primary peritonitis. Surg Gynecol Obstet. 1972;135:513–6.
15. Epstein M, Calia FM, Gabuzda GJ. Pneumococcal peritonitis in patients with postnecrotic cirrhosis. N Engl J Med. 1968;278:69–71.
16. Speck WT, Dresdale SS, McMillan RW. Primary peritonitis and the nephrotic syndrome. Am J Surg. 1974;127:267–9.
17. Conn HO, Fessel JM. Spontaneous bacterial peritonitis in cirrhosis: Variations on a theme. Medicine. 1971;50:161–97.
18. Conn HO. Spontaneous bacterial peritonitis, multiple revisitations. Gastroenterology. 1976;70:455–7.
19. Bar-Meir S, Conn HO. Spontaneous bacterial peritonitis induced by intra-arterial vasopressin therapy. Gastroenterology. 1976;70:418–21.
20. Targan SR, Chow AW, Guze LB. Role of anaerobic bacteria in spontaneous peritonitis of cirrhosis: Report of two cases and review of the literature. Am J Med. 1977;62:397–403.
21. Kline MM, McCallum RW, Guth PH. The clinical value of ascitic fluid culture and leukocyte count studies in alcoholic cirrhosis. Gastroenterology. 1976;70:408–12.
22. Weinstein MP, Iannini PB, Stratton CW, et al. Spontaneous bacterial peritonitis: A review of 28 cases with emphasis on improved survival and factors influencing prognosis. Am J Med. 1978;64:592–8.
23. Hoefs JC, Canawati HN, Sapico FL, et al. Spontaneous bacterial peritonitis. Hepatology. 1982;2:399–407.
24. Pinzello G, Simonetti R, Craxi A, et al. Spontaneous bacterial peritonitis: A prospective investigation in predominantly nonalcoholic cirrhotic patients. Hepatology. 1983;3:545–9.
25. Conn HO. Cirrhosis. In: Schiff L, Schiff ER, eds. Diseases of the Liver. 5th ed. Philadelphia: JB Lippincott; 1982:847–977.
26. Thomas FB, Fromkes JJ. Spontaneous bacterial peritonitis associated with acute viral hepatitis. J Clin Gastroenterol. 1982;4:259–62.
27. Runyon BA. Spontaneous bacterial peritonitis with cardiac ascites. Am J Gastroenterol. 1984;79:796.
28. Isner J, MacDonald JS, Schein PS. Spontaneous *Streptococcus pneumoniae* peritonitis in a patient with metastatic gastric cancer. Cancer. 1979;39:2306–9.
29. Shesol BF, Rosato EF, Rosato FE. Concomitant acute lupus erythematosus and primary pneumococcal peritonitis. Am J Gastroenterol. 1975;63:324–6.
30. Friedland JA, Harris MN. Primary pneumococcal peritonitis in a young adult. Am J Surg. 1970;119:737–9.
31. Golden GT, Stevenson TR, Ritchie WP Jr. Primary peritonitis in adults. South Med J. 1975;68:413–4.
32. Wilcox CM, Dismukes WE. Spontaneous bacterial peritonitis: A review of pathogenesis, diagnosis and treatment. Medicine. 1987;66:447–56.
33. Correia JP, Conn HO. Spontaneous bacterial peritonitis in cirrhosis: Endemic or epidemic? Med Clin North Am. 1975;59:963–81.
34. Hoefs JC, Runyon BA. Spontaneous bacterial peritonitis. Dis Mon. 1985;31:1–48.
35. Fromkes JJ, Thomas FB, Mekhjian HS, et al. Antimicrobial activity of human ascitic fluid. Gastroenterology. 1977;73:668–72.
36. Scheckman P, Onderdonk AB, Bartlett JG. Anaerobes in spontaneous peritonitis. Lancet. 1977;2:1223.
37. Runyon BA, Hoefs JC. Culture-negative neutrocytic ascites: A variant of spontaneous peritonitis. Hepatology. 1984;4:1209–11.
38. Runyon BA, Umland ET, Merlin T. Inoculation of blood culture bottles with ascitic fluid: Improved detection of spontaneous bacterial peritonitis. Arch Intern Med. 1987;147:73–5.
39. Beeson PB, Brannon ES, Warren JU. Observations on the sites of removal of bacteria from the blood in patients with bacterial endocarditis. J Exp Med. 1945;81:9–23.
40. Rutenburg AM, Sonnenblick F, Koven I, et al. Comparative response of normal and cirrhotic rats to intravenously injected bacteria. Proc Soc Exp Biol Med. 1959;101:279–81.
41. Lahnborg G, Friman L, Berghem L. Reticuloendothelial function in patients with alcoholic liver disease. Scand J Gastroenterol. 1981;16:481–9.
42. Rimola A, Soto R, Bory F, et al. Reticuloendothelial system phagocytic activity in cirrhosis and its relation to bacterial infections and prognosis. Hepatology. 1984;4:53–8.
43. Rajkovic IA, Williams R. Abnormalities of neutrophilic phagocytosis, intracellular killing and metabolic activity in alcoholic cirrhosis and hepatitis. Hepatology. 1986;6:252–62.
44. Wyke RJ, Rajkovic IA, Eddleston WF, et al. Defective serum opsonization in patients with chronic liver disease (Abstract). Gut. 1979;20:A931.
45. Yousif-Kadura AGM, Rajkovic IA, Wyke RJ, et al. Defects in serum attractant activity in different types of chronic liver disease. Gut. 1984;25:79–84.
46. Simberkoff MS, Moldover NH, Weiss G. Bactericidal and opsonic activity of cirrhotic ascites and nonascitic peritoneal fluid. J Lab Clin Med. 1978;91:831–9.
47. Runyon BA, Hoefs JC. Ascitic fluid analysis in the differentiation of spontaneous bacterial peritonitis from gastrointestinal perforation into ascitic fluid. Hepatology. 1984;4:447–50.
48. Whipple RL Jr, Harris JF. E. coli septicemia in Laennec's cirrhosis of the liver. Ann Intern Med. 1950;33:462–9.
49. Murray HW, Marks SJ. Spontaneous bacterial empyema, pericarditis and peritonitis in cirrhosis. Gastroenterology. 1977;72:772–3.
50. Snyder N, Atterbury CE, Correia JP, et al. Increased concurrence of cirrhosis and bacterial endocarditis. Gastroenterology. 1977;73:1107–13.
51. Schweinburg FB, Seligman AM, Fine J. Transmural migration of intestinal

bacteria: A study based on the use of radioactive *Escherichia coli*. N Engl J Med. 1950;242:747–51.

52. Schwartz FD, Kallmeyer J, Durea G, et al. Prevention of infection during peritoneal dialysis. JAMA. 1967;199:79–81.

53. Gorbach SL, Lai D, Levitan R. Intestinal microflora in Laennec's cirrhosis. J Clin Invest. 1970;49:36a.

54. McCartney JE, Fraser J. Pneumococcal peritonitis. Br J Surg. 1922;9:479–89.

55. Herbert TJ, Mortimer PP. Recurrent pneumococcal peritonitis associated with an intrauterine contraceptive device. Br J Surg. 1974;61:901–2.

56. Brinson RR, Kolts BE, Monif GRG. Spontaneous bacterial peritonitis associated with an intrauterine device. J Clin Gastroenterol. 1986;8:82–4.

57. Kimball MW, Knee S. Gonococcal perihepatitis in a male. The Fitz-Hugh-Curtis syndrome. N Engl J Med. 1970;282:1082–4.

58. Luetscher JA Jr. Electrophoretic analysis of the proteins of plasma and serous effusions. J Clin Invest. 1941;20:99–106.

59. Witte MH, Witte CL, Davis WM, et al. Peritoneal transudate: A diagnostic clue to portal system obstruction in patients with intra-abdominal neoplasms or peritonitis. JAMA. 1972;221:1380–3.

60. Hoefs JC. Increase in ascites white blood cell and protein concentrations during diuresis in patients with chronic liver disease. Hepatology. 1981;1:249–54.

61. Stassen WN, McCullough AJ, Bacon BR, et al. Immediate diagnostic criteria for bacterial infection of ascitic fluid: Evaluation of ascitic fluid polymorphonuclear leukocyte count, pH, and lactate concentration, alone and in combination. Gastroenterology. 1986;90:1247–54.

62. Garcia-Tsao G, Conn HO, Lerner E. The diagnosis of bacterial peritonitis: Comparison of pH, lactate concentration and leukocyte count. Hepatology. 1985;5:91–6.

63. Yang C-Y, Liaw F, Chu E-M, et al. White count, pH and lactate in ascites in the diagnosis of spontaneous bacterial peritonitis. Hepatology. 1985;5:85–90.

64. Vickers FN, Maloney PJ. Gonococcal perihepatitis: Reports of three cases with comments on diagnosis and treatment. Arch Intern Med. 1964;114:120–3.

65. Burack WR, Hollister RM. Tuberculous peritonitis: A study of forty-seven proved cases encountered by a general medical unit in twenty-five years. Am J Med. 1960;28:510–23.

66. Saw EC, Shields SJ, Comer TP, et al. Granulomatous peritonitis due to *Coccidioides immitis*. Arch Surg. 1974;108:369–71.

67. Hoefs JC. Diagnostic paracentesis: A potent clinical tool. Gastroenterology. 1990;98:230–6.

68. Harrison RN, Cryer HM, Howard DA, et al. Clarification of risk factors for abdominal operations in patients with hepatic cirrhosis. Ann Surg. 1984;199:648–65.

69. Runyon BA, McHutchison JG, Antillon MR, et al. Short-course versus long-course antibiotic treatment of spontaneous bacterial peritonitis. A randomized controlled study of 108 patients. Gastroenterology. 1991;100:1737–42.

70. Runyon BA, Hoefs JC. Spontaneous vs. secondary bacterial peritonitis: Differentiation by response of ascitic fluid neutrophil count to antimicrobial therapy. Arch Intern Med. 1986;146:1563–5.

71. Dimond M, Proctor HJ. Concomitant pneumococcal appendicitis, peritonitis and meningitis. Arch Surg. 1976;111:888–9.

72. Mallory A, Schaefer JW. Complications of diagnostic paracentesis in patients with liver disease. JAMA. 1978;239:628–30.

73. Levine H. Needle biopsy of peritoneum in exudative ascites. Arch Intern Med. 1967;120:542–5.

74. Dineen P, Homan WP, Grafe WR. Tuberculous peritonitis: 43 years experience in diagnosis and treatment. Ann Surg. 1976;184:717–22.

75. Felisart J, Rimona A, Arroyo V, et al. Cefotaxime is more effective than is ampicillin-tobramycin in cirrhotics with severe infections. Hepatology. 1985;5:457–62.

76. Cabrera J, Arroyo V, Ballesta AM, et al. Aminoglycoside nephrotoxicity in cirrhosis: Value of urinary β_2-microglobulin to discriminate functional renal failure from acute tubular damage. Gastroenterology. 1982;82:97–105.

77. Forrest A, Nix DE, Ballow CH et al. Phamacodynamics of intravenous ciprofloxacin in seriously ill patients. Antimicrob Agents Chemother. 1993;37:1073–81.

78. Runyon BA, Hoefs JC. Ascitic fluid chemical analysis before, during and after spontaneous bacterial peritonitis. Hepatology. 1985;5:257–9.

79. Porter JM, Snowe RJ, Silver D. Tuberculous enteritis with perforation and abscess formation in childhood. Surgery. 1972;71:254–7.

80. Rowland TC Jr. Severe peritonitis complicating an intrauterine contraceptive device. Am J Obstet Gynecol. 1971;110:786–7.

81. Prokesch RC, Rimland D. Infectious complications of the peritoneovenous shunt. Am J Gastroenterol. 1983;78:235–40.

82. Reynold M, Sherman JO, Mclone DG. Ventriculoperitoneal shunt infections masquerading as an acute abdomen. J Pediatr Surg. 1983;18:951–4.

83. Nichols RL. Intra-abdominal infections: An overview. Rev Infect Dis. 1985;7(Suppl 4):S709–15.

84. Drasar BS, Shiner M, McLeod GM. Studies on the intestinal flora. I. The bacterial flora of the gastrointestinal tract in healthy and achlorhydric persons. Gastroenterology. 1969;56:71–9.

85. Nichols RL, Smith JW. Intragastric microbial colonization in common disease states of the stomach and duodenum. Ann Surg. 1975;182:557–61.

86. Gorbach SL, Plaut AG, Nahas L, et al. Studies of intestinal microflora. II.

Microorganisms of the small intestine and their relations to oral and fecal flora. Gastroenterology. 1967;53:856–67.

87. Drasar BS, Shiner M. Studies on the intestinal flora. Part II. Bacterial flora of the small intestine in patients with gastrointestinal disorders. Gut. 1969;10:812–9.

88. Gorbach SL, Nahas L, Lerner PI, et al. Studies of intestinal microflora. I. Effects of diet, age, and periodic sampling of numbers of fecal microorganisms in man. Gastroenterology. 1967;53:845–55.

89. Finegold SM. Interaction of antimicrobial therapy and intestinal flora. Am J Clin Nutr. 1970;23:1466–71.

90. Altemeier WA. The bacterial flora of acute perforated appendicitis with peritonitis. Ann Surg. 1938;107:517–28.

91. Finegold SM. Abdominal and perineal infections. In: Finegold SM, ed. Anaerobic Bacteria in Human Disease. New York. Academic Press; 1977;257–313.

92. Gorbach SL, Thadepalli H, Norsen J. Anaerobic microorganisms in intra-abdominal infections. In: Balows A, de Haan RM, Dowell VR Jr, et al, eds. Anaerobic Bacteria: Role in Disease. Springfield, IL: Charles C. Thomas; 1974:399–407.

93. Lorber B, Swenson RM. The bacteriology of intra-abdominal infections. Surg Clin North Am. 1975;55:1349–54.

94. Swenson RM, Lorber B, Michaelson TC, et al. The bacteriology of intra-abdominal infections. Arch Surg. 1974;109:398–9.

95. Bodner SJ, Koenig MG, Goodman JS. Bacteremic *Bacteroides* infections. Ann Intern Med. 1970;73:537–44.

96. Gelb EF, Seligman SJ. Bacteroidaceae bacteremia. Effect of age and focus of infection upon clinical course. JAMA. 1970;212:1038–41.

97. Fry DE, Garrison RN, Polk HC Jr. Clinical implications in *Bacteroides* bacteremia. Surg Gynecol Obstet. 1979;149:189–92.

98. Chow AW, Guze LB. Bacteroidaceae bacteremia: Clinical experience with 112 patients. Medicine. 1974;53:93–126.

99. Tally FP, McGowan K, Kellum JM, et al. A randomized comparison of cefoxitin with or without amikacin and clindamycin plus amikacin in surgical sepsis. Ann Surg. 1981;193:318–23.

100. Aronoff SC, Olson MM, Gaudierer MWL, et al. *Pseudomonas aeruginosa* as a primary pathogen in children with bacterial peritonitis. J Pediatr Surg. 1987;22:861–4.

101. Heseltine PNR, Yellin AE, Applebaum MD, et al. Perforated and gangrenous appendicitis: An analysis of antibiotic failures. J Infect Dis. 1983;148:322–9.

102. Dunn DL, Simmons RL. The role of anaerobic bacteria in intra-abdominal infections. Rev Infect Dis. 1984;6(Suppl 1):S139–46.

103. Nichols RL, Smith JW, Klein DB, et al. Risk of infection after penetrating abdominal trauma. N Engl J Med. 1984;311:1065–70.

104. Levison ME, Korman LC, Carrington ER, et al. Quantitative microflora of the vagina. Am J Obstet Gynecol. 1977;127:80–5.

105. Levison ME, Trestman I, Quach R, et al. Quantitative bacteriology of the vaginal flora in vaginitis. Am J Obstet Gynecol. 1979;133:139–44.

106. Bartlett JG, Onderdonk AB, Drude E, et al. Quantitative bacteriology of the vaginal flora. J Infect Dis. 1977;136:271–7.

107. Ohm M, Galask RP. The effect of antibiotic prophylaxis on patients undergoing vaginal operations: II. Alteration of microbial flora. Am J Obstet Gynecol. 1975;123:597–604.

108. Ramsay AM. The significance of *C. welchii* in the cervical swab and blood serum in postpartum and postabortum sepsis. J Obstet Gynecol. 1949;56:247–58.

109. Hite KE, Hesseltine HC, Goldstein L. A study of the bacterial flora of the normal and pathologic vagina and uterus. Am J Obstet Gynecol. 1947;53:233–40.

110. Gibbs RS, O'Dell TN, MacGregor RR, et al. Puerperal endometritis: A prospective microbiologic study. Am J Obstet Gynecol. 1975;121:919–25.

111. Baker CJ, Barrett FF, Yow MD. The influence of advancing gestation on group B streptococcal colonization in pregnant women. Am J Obstet Gynecol. 1975;122:820–3.

112. Penza JF. Moniliasis and trichomoniasis. In: Charles D, Finland M, eds. Obstetric and Perinatal Infections. Philadelphia: Lee & Febiger; 1973:209.

113. Finegold SM. Female genital tract infections. In: Finegold SM, ed. Anaerobic Bacteria in Human Disease. New York: Academic Press; 1977:350–85.

114. Swenson RM, Michaelson TC, Daly MJ, et al. Anaerobic bacterial infections of the female genital tract. Obstet Gynecol. 1973;42:538–41.

115. Thadepalli H, Gorbach SL, Keith L. Anaerobic infections of the female genital tract: Bacteriologic and therapeutic aspects. Am J Obstet Gynecol. 1973;117:1034–40.

116. Chow AW, Marshall JR, Guze LB. Anaerobic infections of the female genital tract: Prospects and perspectives. Obstet Gynecol Surg. 1975;30:477–94.

117. Chow AW, Malkasian KI, Marshall JR, et al. The bacteriology of acute pelvic inflammatory disease. Value of cul-de-sac cultures and relative importance of gonococcal and other aerobic or anaerobic bacteria. Am J Obstet Gynecol. 1975;122:876–9.

118. Eschenbach DA, Buchanon TM, Pollock HM, et al. Polymicrobial etiology of acute pelvic inflammatory disease. N Engl J Med. 1975;293:166–71.

119. Wasserheit JN, Bell TA, Kiviat NB, et al. Microbial causes of proven pelvic inflammatory disease and efficacy of clindamycin and tobramycin. Ann Intern Med. 1986;104:187–93.

120. Monif GRG, Welkos SI, Baer H, et al. Cul-de-sac isolates from patients with endometritis-salpingitis-peritonitis and gonococcal endocervicitis. Am J Obstet Gynecol. 1976;126:158–61.

121. Burry VF. Gonococcal vulvovaginitis and possible peritonitis in prepubertal girls. Am J Dis Child. 1971;121:536–7.
122. Fuld GL. Gonococcal peritonitis in a prepubertal child. Am J Dis Child. 1968;115:621–2.
123. Adams EB, MacLeod IN. Invasive amebiasis. II. Amebic liver abscess and its complications. Medicine. 1977;56:325–34.
124. Turner GR, Millikan M, Carter R, et al. Surgical significance of fulminating amebic colitis. Report of perforation of the colon with peritonitis. Am Surg. 1965;31:759–63.
125. Lintermans JP. Fatal peritonitis, an unusual complication of *Strongyloides stercoralis* infestation. Clin Pediatr. 1975;14:974–5.
126. Eisenberg ES, Leviton I, Soeiro R. Fungal peritonitis in patients receiving peritoneal dialysis: Experience with 11 patients and review of the literature. Rev Infect Dis. 1986;3:309–21.
127. Bayer AS, Blumenkrantz MJ, Montgomerie JZ, et al. Candida peritonitis: Report of 22 cases and review of the English literature. Am J Med. 1976;61:832–40.
128. Solomkin JS, Flohr AB, Quie PG, et al. The role of *Candida* in intraperitoneal infections. Surgery. 1980;88:524–30.
129. Howard JM, Singh LM. Peritoneal fluid pH after perforation of peptic ulcers. Arch Surg. 1963;87:483–4.
130. Mortez WH, Erickson WG. Neutralization of hydrochloric acid in the peritoneal cavity. Arch Surg. 1957;75:834–7.
131. Santschi DR, Huizenga KA, Scudamore HH, et al. Bile ascites. Arch Surg. 1963;87:851–6.
132. Diamonon JS, Barnes JP. Choleperitoneum. Am Surg. 1964;30:331–4.
133. Cohn I, Cotlar AM, Atik M, et al. Bile peritonitis. Ann Surg. 1960;152:827–35.
134. Nemir P Jr, Hawthorne HR, Cohn I, et al. I. The cause of death in strangulation obstruction. An experimental study. Ann Surg. 1949;130:857–73.
135. Nemir P Jr, Hawthorne HR, Cohn I, et al. II. The lethal action of the peritoneal fluid. Ann Surg. 1949;130:874–80.
136. Barnett WO, Hardy JD. Observations concerning the peritoneal fluid in experimental strangulated intestinal obstruction: The effects of removal from the peritoneal cavity. Surgery. 1958;43:440–4.
137. Barnett WO, Doyle RS. The effects of neomycin upon the toxicity of peritoneal fluid resulting from strangulation obstruction. Surgery. 1958;44:442–6.
138. Barnett WO, Messina AJ. The influence of massive antibiotics in experimental strangulation obstruction. Gastroenterology. 1959;36:534–6.
139. Davis JH, Yull AB. A possible toxic factor in abdominal surgery. J Trauma. 1962;2:291–300.
140. Filler RM, Sleeman HK, Hendry WS, et al. Lethal factors in experimental peritonitis. Surgery. 1966;60:671–8.
141. Lee JT Jr, Ahrenholz DN, Nelson RD, et al. Mechanisms of the adjuvant effect of hemoglobin in experimental peritonitis. V. The significance of the coordinated iron component. Surgery. 1979;86:41–8.
142. Weingerg ED. Roles of iron in host–parasite interactions. J Infect Dis. 1971;124:401–10.
143. Hau T, Nelson RD, Fiegel VD, et al. Mechanisms of the adjuvant action of hemoglobin in experimental peritonitis—2. Influence of hemoglobin on human leukocyte chemotaxis in vitro. J Surg Res. 1977;22:174–80.
144. Dunn DL, Barke RA, Ahrenholz DH, et al. The adjuvant effect of peritoneal fluid in experimental peritonitis. Ann Surg. 1984;199:37–43.
145. Rotstein OD, Pruett TL, Simmons RD. Fibrin in peritonitis. V. Fibrin inhibits phagocytic killing of *Escherichia coli* by human polymorphonuclear leukocytes. Ann Surg. 1986;203:413–9.
146. McRitchie DI, Girotti MJ, Glynn MF, et al. Effect of systemic fibrinogen depletion on intraabdominal abscess formation. J Lab Clin Med. 1991;118:48–55.
147. Dubrow T, Schwartz RJ, Kissock J, Wilson SE. Effect of aerosolized fibrin solution in intraperitoneal contamination. Arch Surg. 1991;126:80–3.
148. Schneierson SS, Amsterdam D, Perlman E. Enhancement of intraperitoneal staphylococcal virulence for mice with different bile salts. Nature. 1961;190:829–30.
149. Sisel RJ, Donovan AJ, Yellin AE. Experimental fecal peritonitis. Influence of barium sulfate or water-soluble radiographic contrast material on survival. Arch Surg. 1972;104:765–8.
150. Westfall RH, Nelson RH, Musselman MM. Barium peritonitis. Am J Surg. 1966;112:760–3.
151. Olitzki L. Mucin as a resistance-lowering substance. Bacteriol Rev. 1948;12:149–72.
152. Cuevas P, Fine J. Role of intraintestinal endotoxin in death from peritonitis. Surg Gynecol Obstet. 1972;134:953–7.
153. Fugger R, Hamilton G, Rogy M, et al. Prognostic significance of endotoxin determination in patients with severe intraabdominal infection. J Infect Dis. 1990;161:1314–5.
154. Bieluch VM, Tally FP. Pathophysiology of abscess formation. Clin Obstet Gynecol. 1983;10:93–103.
155. Gorbach SL, Bartlett JG. Anaerobic infections (third of three parts). N Engl J Med. 1974;290:1289–94.
156. Hofstad T. Endotoxins of anaerobic gram-negative microorganisms. In: Balows A, de Haan RM, Dowell VR Jr, et al., eds. Anaerobic Bacteria: Role in Disease. Springfield, IL: Charles C. Thomas; 1974:295.
157. Gibbons RJ, MacDonald JB. Degradation of collagenous substrates by *Bacteroides melaninogenicus*. J Bacteriol. 1961;81:614–21.
158. Bjornson HS. Enzymes associated with the survival and virulence of gram-negative anaerobes. Rev Infect Dis. 1984;6(Suppl 1):S21–4.
159. Gesner BM, Jenkin CR. Production of heparinase by bacteroides. J Bacteriol. 1961;81:595–604.
160. Bjornson H, Hill EO. Bacteroidaceae in thromboembolic disease. Effects of cell wall components on blood coagulation in vivo and in vitro. Infect Immun. 1974;9:337–41.
161. Casciato DA, Rosenblatt JE, Goldberg LS, et al. In vitro interaction of *Bacteroides fragilis* with polymorphonuclear leukocytes and serum factors. Infect Immun. 1975;11:337–42.
162. Keusch GT, Douglas SD. Intraleukocytic survival of anaerobic bacteria. Clin Res. 1974;22:445A.
163. Kasper DL. The polysaccharide capsule of *Bacteroides fragilis* subspecies fragilis: Immunochemical and morphologic definition. J Infect Dis. 1976;133:79–87.
164. Mansheim BJ, Orderdonk AB, Kasper DL. Immunochemical characterization of surface antigens of *Bacteroides melaninogenicus*. Rev Infect Dis. 1979;1:263–77.
165. Onderdonk AB, Kasper DL, Cisneros RL, et al. The capsular polysaccharide of *Bacteroides fragilis* as a virulence factor: Comparison of the pathogenic potential of encapsulated and unencapsulated strains. J Infect Dis. 1977;136:82–9.
166. Ingham HR, Tharagonnet D, Sisson PR, et al. Inhibition of phagocytosis in vitro by obligate anaerobes. Lanct. 1977;2:1252–4.
167. Simon GL, Klempner MS, Kasper DL, et al. Alterations in opsonophagocytic killing by neutrophils of *Bacteroides fragilis* associated with animal and laboratory passage: Effect of capsular polysaccharide. J Infect Dis. 1982;145:72–7.
168. Socransky SS, Gibbons RJ. Required role of *Bacteroides melaninogenicus* in mixed anaerobic infections. J Infect Dis. 1965;115:247–53.
169. Altemeier WA. The pathogenicity of the bacteria of appendicitis peritonitis. Surgery. 1942;11:374–84.
170. Namavar FA, Verweij MJ, Bal M, et al. Effects of anaerobic bacteria on killing of *Proteus mirabilis* by human polymorphonuclear leukocytes. Infect Immun. 1983;40:930–5.
171. Rotstein OD, Nasmith PE, Grinstein S. The bacteroides by-product succinic acid inhibits neutrophil respiratory burst by reducing intracellular pH. Infect Immun. 1987;55:864–70.
172. Brook I. Anaerobic infections in childhood. Rev Infect Dis. 1984;6(Suppl 1):S187–92.
173. Onderdonk AB, Weinstein WN, Sullivan NM, et al. Experimental intraabdominal abscess in rats: Quantitative bacteriology of infected animals. Infect Immun. 1974;10:1256–9.
174. Weinstein WM, Onderdonk AB, Bartlett JG, et al. Antimicrobial therapy of experimental intraabdominal sepsis. J Infect Dis. 1975;132:282–6.
175. Onderdonk AB, Bartlett JG, Louie T, et al. Microbial synergy in experimental intra-abdominal abscess. Infect Immun. 1976;13:22–6.
176. Rosoff L, Weil M, Bradely EC, et al. Hemodynamic and metabolic changes associated with bacterial peritonitis. Am J Surg. 1967;114:180–9.
177. MacLean LD, Mulugan WG, McLean APH, et al. Patterns of septic shock in man: A detailed study of 56 patients. Ann Surg. 1967;166:543–62.
178. Davis JH. Current concepts of peritonitis. Am Surg. 1967;33:673–81.
179. Pine RW, Wertz MJ, Lennard ES, et al. Determinants of organ malfunction or death in patients with intra-abdominal sepsis. Arch Surg. 1983;118:242–9.
180. Nystrom PO, Bax R, Dellinger EP, et al. Proposed definitions for diagnosis, severity scoring, stratification, and outcome for trials on intraabdominal infection. Joint Working Party of SIS North America and Europe. World J Surg. 1990;14:148–58.
181. Dellinger EP, Wertz MJ, Meakins JL, et al. Surgical infection stratification system for intra-abdominal infection. Arch Surg. 1985;120:21–9.
182. Meakins JL, Solomkin JS, Allo MD, et al. A proposed classification of intra-abdominal infections. Stratification of etiology and risk for future therapeutic trials. Arch Surg. 1984;119:1372–8.
183. Mustard RA, Bohnen JM, Rosati C, et al. Pneumonia complicating abdominal sepsis: An independent risk factor for mortality. Arch Surg. 1991;126:170–5.
184. Runcie C, Ramsey G. Intraabdominal infection: Pulmonary failure. World J Surg. 1990;14:196–203.
185. Nobles ER Jr. Bacteroides infections. Ann Surg. 1973;177:601–6.
186. Young LS, Martin WJ, Meyer RD, et al. Gram-negative rod bacteremia. Microbiologic, immunologic and therapeutic considerations. Ann Intern Med. 1977;86:456–71.
187. Maler JA Jr, Reynolds TB, Yellin AE. Successful medical treatment of pyogenic liver abscess. Gastroenterology. 1979;77:618–22.
188. Herbert DA, Fogel DA, Rothman J, et al. Pyogenic liver abscesses: Successful nonsurgical therapy. Lancet. 1982;1:134–6.
189. Stalons DR, Thonsberry C, Dawell VR. Effect of culture medium and carbon dioxide concentration on growth of anaerobic bacteria commonly encountered in clinical specimens. Appl Microbiol. 1974;27:1098–104.
190. Rosenblatt JE, Schoenknecht F. Effect of several components of anaerobic incubation on antibiotic susceptibility test results. Antimicrob Agents Chemother. 1972;1:433–40.
191. Wagoner ES, Gorman M. The reaction of cysteine and related compounds with penicillins and cephalosporins. J Antibiot. 1971;24:647–58.
192. Wilkins TD, Chalgren S. Medium for use in antibiotic susceptibility testing of anaerobic bacteria. Antimicrob Agents Chemother. 1976;10:926–8.
193. Mosdell DM, Morris DM, Voltura A, et al. Antibiotic treatment for surgical peritonitis. Ann Surg. 1991;214:543–549.
194. Gorbach SL, Thadepalli H. Clindamycin in pure and mixed anaerobic infections. Arch Intern Med. 1974;134:87–92.

195. Bartlett JG, Louie TJ, Onderdonk AB, et al. Whither the enterococcus? 15th ICACC. Abstract No. 297. Washington, DC; September 24–26, 1975.
196. Fass RJ, Scholand JF, Hodges GR, et al. Clindamycin in the treatment of serious anaerobic infections. Ann Intern Med. 1973;78:853–9.
197. Levison ME, Santoro J, Bran JL, et al. In vitro activity and clinical efficacy of clindamycin in the treatment of infections due to anaerobic bacteria. J Infect Dis. 1977;135:S49–53.
198. Dougherty SH. Role of enterococcus in intra-abdominal sepsis. Am J Surg. 1984;148:303–12.
199. Weinstein MP, Reller LB, Murphy J, et al. The clinical significance of positive blood cultures: A comprehensive analysis of 500 episodes of bacteremia and fungemia in adults. I. Laboratory and epidemiologic observations. Rev Infect Dis. 1983;5:35–53.
200. Shales DM, Levy J, Wolinsky E. Enterococcal bacteremia without endocarditis. Arch Intern Med. 1981;141:578–81.
201. Dougherty SH, Flohr AB, Simmons RL. Breakthrough enterococcal septicemia in surgical patients. Arch Surg. 1983;118:232–7.
202. Salzer W, Pegram PS, McCan CE. Clinical evaluation of moxalactam: Evidence of decreased efficacy in gram-positive aerobic infection. Antimicrob Agents Chemother. 1983;23:565–70.
203. Livornese LL Jr, Dias S, Samel C, et al. Hospital-acquired infection with vancomycin-resistant Enterococcus faecium transmitted by electronic thermometers. Ann Intern Med. 1992;117:112–6.
204. Murray BE. The life and times of the Enterococci. Clin Microbiol Rev. 1990; 3:46–65.
205. Courvalin P. Resistance of enterococci to glycopeptides. Antimicrob Agents Chemother. 1990;34:2291–6.
206. Moellering RC. Emergence of enterococci as a significant pathogen. Clin Infect Dis. 1992;14:1173–8.
207. Sande MA, Overton JW. In vivo antagonism between gentamicin and chloramphenicol in neutropenic mice. J Infect Dis. 1973;128:247–50.
208. Zinner SH, Provonchee RB, Elias KS. Effect of clindamycin on the in vitro activity of amikacin and gentamicin against gram negative bacilli. Antimicrob Agents Chemother. 1976;9:661–4.
209. Ekwo E, Peter G. Effect of clindamycin on aminoglycoside activity in murine model of Escherichia coli infection. Antimicrob Agents Chemother. 1976; 10:893–8.
210. Fass RJ, Rotilie CA, Prior RB. Interaction of clindamycin and gentamicin in vitro. Antimicrob Agents Chemother. 1974;6:582–7.
211. Cuchural GJ Jr, Tally FB, Jacobus NV, et al. Susceptibility of the Bacteroides fragilis group in the United States: Analysis by site of isolation. Antimicrob Agents Chemother. 1988;32:717–22.
212. Van Scoy RE, Wilkowske CJ, O'Fallon WM, et al. Clindamycin versus chloramphenicol in treatment of anaerobic infections: A prospective, randomized double-blind study. Mayo Clin Proc. 1984;59:842–6.
213. Tally FB, Sosa A, Jacobus NV, et al. Clindamycin resistance in Bacteroides fragilis. J Antimicrob Chemother. 1981;8(Suppl):43–8.
214. Tally FP, Cuchural GH Jr, Jacobus NV, et al. Nationwide study of the susceptibility of the Bacteroides fragilis group in the United States. Antimicrob Agents Chemother. 1985;28:675–7.
215. Wilson WR, Cockerhill FR III. Tetracyclines, chloramphenicol, erythromycin and clindamycin. Mayo Clin Proc. 1987;62:906–15.
216. Tedesco FJ, Barton RW, Alpers DH. Clindamycin associated colitis: A prospective study. Ann Intern Med. 1974;81:429–33.
217. Ralph ED, Kirby WMM. Unique bactericidal action against Bacteroides fragilis and Clostridium perfringens. Antimicrob Agents Chemother. 1975; 8:409–14.
218. Chow AW, Patten V, Guze LB. Susceptibility of anaerobic bacteria to metronidazole: Relative resistance of non-spore-forming gram-positive bacilli. J Infect Dis. 1975;131:182–5.
219. Onderdonk AB, Louie TJ, Tally FP, et al. Activity of metronidazole against Escherichia coli in experimental intra-abdominal sepsis. J Antimicrob Chemother. 1979;5:201–10.
220. Bartlett JG, Louie TJ, Gorbach SL, et al. Therapeutic efficacy of 29 antimicrobial regimens in experimental intra-abdominal sepsis. Rev Infect Dis. 1981;3:535–42.
221. Sutter VL, Kwoh Y-Y, Finegold SM. Standardized antimicrobial disc susceptibility testing of anaerobic bacteria. I. Susceptibility of Bacteroides fragilis to tetracyclines. Appl Microbiol. 1972;23:268–75.
222. Sutter VL, Finegold SM. Susceptibility of anaerobic bacteria to 23 antimicrobial agents. Antimicrob Agents Chemother. 1976;10:736–52.
223. Wexler HM, Finegold SM. In vitro activity of cefotetan compared with that of other antimicrobial agents against anaerobic bacteria. Antimicrob Agents Chemother. 1988;32:601–4.
224. O'Keefe JP, Vlenezio FR, Divincenzo CA, et al. Activity of newer beta-lactam agents against clinical isolates of Bacteroides fragilis and other Bacteroides species. Antimicrob Agents Chemother. 1987;31:2002–4.
225. Rolfe RD, Finegold SM. Comparative in vitro activity of new beta-lactam antibiotics against anaerobic bacteria. Antimicrob Agents Chemother. 1981; 200:600–9.
226. Aldridge KE. Comparison of the activities of penicillin G and new beta-lactam antibiotics against clinical isolates of Bacteroides species. Antimicrob Agents Chemother. 1984;26:410–3.
227. Chow AW, Finegold SM. In vitro activity of ceftizoxime against anaerobic bacteria and comparison with other cephalosporins. J Antimicrob Chemother. 1982;10(Suppl c):45–50.
228. Schoutens E, Yourassowsky E. Speed of bactericidal action of penicillin G, ampicillin and carbenicillin on Bacteroides fragilis. Antimicrob Agents Chemother. 1974;6:227–31.
229. Trestman I, Kaye D, Levison ME. Activity of semisynthetic penicillins and synergism with mecillinam against Bacteroides species. Antimicrob Agents Chemother. 1979;16:283–6.
230. Swenson RM, Lorber B. Clindamycin and carbenicillin in treatment of patients with intra-abdominal and female genital tract infections. J Infect Dis. 1977;135:S40–5.
231. Winston DJ, Murphy W, Young LS, et al. Piperacillin therapy for serious bacterial infections. Am J Med. 1980;69:255–61.
232. Harding GKM, Buckwalk FJ, Ronald AR, et al. Prospective, randomized comparative study of clindamycin, chloramphenicol, and ticarcillin, each in combination with gentamicin, for therapy of intra-abdominal and female genital tract sepsis. J Infect Dis. 1980;142:384–93.
233. Levison ME, Trestman I, Egert J, et al. Evaluation of ticarcillin in anaerobic infections. 17th ICAAC. Abstract No. 176. New York; October 12–14, 1977.
234. O'Keefe JP, Tally FP, Barza M, et al. Inactivation of penicillin G during experimental infection with Bacteroides fragilis. J Infect Dis. 1978;137: 437–42.
235. Sykes RB, Squibb Institute for Medical Research. The classification and terminology of enzymes that hydrolyze beta-lactam antibiotics. J Infect Dis. 1982;145:762–5.
236. Eliopoulos GM, Moellering RC Jr. Azlocillin, mezlocillin and piperacillin: New broad-spectrum penicillins. Ann Intern Med. 1982;97:755–60.
237. Gould IM, Wise R. Beta-lactamase inhibitors. In: Peterson PK, Verhoef J, eds. The Antimicrobial Agents Annual. 2nd ed. New York: Elsevier; 1987: 58–69.
238. Wise R, Andrews JM, Bedford KA. Clavulanic acid and CP-45, 899: A comparison of their in vitro activity in combination with penicillins. J Antimicrob Chemother. 1980;6:197–206.
239. Donowitz GR, Mandell GL. Beta-lactam antibiotics (first of two parts). N Engl J Med. 1988;313:419–26.
240. Bansal MB, Chuah SK, Thadepalli H. In vitro activity and in vivo evaluation of ticarcillin plus clavulanic acid against aerobic and anaerobic bacteria. Am J Med. 1985;79(Suppl 5B):33–8.
241. Retsema JA, English AR, Girard A, et al. Sulbactam/ampicillin: In vitro spectrum, potency and activity in models of acute infection. Rev Infect Dis. 1986;8(Suppl 5):S528–42.
242. Reinhardt JF, Johnston L, Ruane P, et al. A randomized double blind comparison of sulbactam/ampicillin and clindamycin for the treatment of aerobic and aerobic-anaerobic infections. Rev Infect Dis. 1986;8(Suppl 5):S569–75.
243. Jones RN. Review of the in vitro spectrum of activity of imipenem. Am J Med. 1985;78(Suppl 6A):22–32.
244. Sanders CC, Sanders WE Jr. Clinical significance of inducible beta-lactamase in gram-negative bacteria. Eur J Clin Microbiol. 1987;6:435.
245. Yotsuji A, Minami S, Inoue M, et al. Properties of a novel beta-lactamase produced by Bacteroides fragilis. Antimicrob Agents Chemother. 1983;24: 925–9.
246. Jacobus NV, Ferreira MC, Barza M. In vitro activity of aztreonam, a monobactam antibiotic. Antimicrob Agents Chemother. 1982;22:832–8.
247. Kaye D, Levison ME, Labovitz ED. The unpredictability of serum concentrations of gentamicin: Pharmacokinetics of gentamicin in patients with normal and abnormal renal function. J Infect Dis. 1974;130:150–4.
248. Verklin RM Jr, Mandell GL. Alteration of effectiveness of antibiotics by anaerobiosis. J Lab Clin Med. 1977;89:65–71.
249. Ho JL, Barza M. Minireview. Role of aminoglycoside antibiotics in the treatment of intra-abdominal infection. Antimicrob Agents Chemother. 1987;31: 485–91.
250. Wolfson JS, Hooper DC. The fluoroquinolones: Structures, mechanisms of action and resistance, and spectra of activity in vitro. Antimicrob Agents Chemother. 1985;28:581–86.
251. Neu HE. New antibiotics: Areas of appropriate use. J Infect Dis. 1987;155: 403–17.
252. Forrest A, Nix DE, Ballow CH, et al. Phamacodynamics of intravenous ciprofloxacin in seriously ill patients. Antimicrob Agents Chemother. 1993; 37:1073–81.
253. Finegold SM, Wexler HM. Therapeutic implications of bacteriologic findings in mixed aerobic-anaerobic infections. Antimicrob Agents Chemother. 1988; 32:611–6.
254. David IB, Buck JR, Filler RM. Rational use of antibiotics for perforated appendicitis in childhood. J Pediatr Surg. 1982;17:494–500.
255. Norwegian Study Group for Colorectal Surgery. Should antimicrobial prophylaxis in colorectal surgery include agents effective against both anaerobic and aerobic microorganisms? A double blind multicenter study. Surgery. 1984;97:402–7.
256. Solomkin JS, Meakins JC, Allo MD, et al. Antibiotic trials in intra-abdominal infections. A critical evaluation of study design and outcome reporting. Ann Surg. 1984;200:29–39.
257. Stone HH. Metronidazole in the treatment of surgical infections. Surgery. 1983;93:230–4.
258. Aoki FY, Biron S, Doris PJ, et al. Prospective, randomized comparison of metronidazole and clindamycin, each with gentamicin, for the treatment of serious intra-abdominal infection. Surgery. 1983;93:217–20.
259. Canadian Metronidazole-Clindamycin Study Group: Prospective, randomized comparison of metronidazole and clindamycin, each with gentamicin, for the treatment of serious intra-abdominal infections. Surgery. 1983;93: 221–9.

260. Solomkin JS, Dellinger EP, Christou NV, et al. Results of a multicenter trial comparing imipenem cilastatin to tobramycin-clindamycin for intra-abdominal infections. Ann Surg. 1990;212:581–91.

261. Drusano GL, Warren WJ, Saah AJ, et al. A prospective randomized controlled trial of cefoxitin versus clindamycin-aminoglycoside in mixed aerobic-anaerobic infections. Surg Gynecol Obstet. 1982;154:715–20.

262. Tally FP, McGowan K, Kellum JM, et al. A randomized comparison of cefoxitin with or without amikacin and clindamycin plus amikacin in surgical sepsis. Ann Surg. 1981;193:318–23.

263. Nichols RL, Smith JW, Klein DB, et al. Risk of infection after penetrating abdominal trauma. N Engl J Med. 1984;311:1065–70.

264. Tally FP, Kellum JM, Ho TF, et al. Randomized prospective study comparing moxalactam and cefoxitin with or without tobramycin for treatment of serious surgical infections. Antimicrob Agents Chemother. 1986;29:244–9.

265. Najem AZ, Kaminski CR, Spiller CR, et al. Comparative study of parenteral piperacillin and cefoxitin in the treatment of surgical infections of the abdomen. Surgery. 1983;157:423–5.

266. Study Group of Intra-Abdominal Infections: A randomized controlled trial of ampicillin plus sulbactam vs gentamicin plus clindamycin in the treatment of intra-abdominal infections. Rev Infect Dis. 1986;8(Suppl 5):S533–88.

267. Scandinavian Study Group. Imipenem-cilastatin versus gentamicin-clindamycin for treatment of serious bacterial infections. Lancet. 1983;1:868–71.

268. Solomkin JS, Fant WK, Rivera JO, et al. Randomized trial of imipenem-cilastatin versus gentamicin and clindamycin in mixed flora infections. Am J Med. 1985;78(Suppl 6A):85–91.

269. Guerra JG, Casaline GE, Plomina JC, et al. Imipenem-cilastatin versus gentamicin-clindamycin for treatment of moderate to severe infections in hospitalized patients. Rev Infect Dis. 1985;7(Suppl 3):463–70.

270. Birolini D, Moraes MF, Soare de Souza O. Aztreonam plus clindamycin vs tobramycin plus clindamycin for the treatment of intra-abdominal infections. Rev Infect Dis. 1985;7(Suppl 4):S724–8.

271. Harding GJ, Vincelette A, Rachlis I, et al. A preliminary report on the use of ceftizoxime vs clindamycin/tobramycin for the therapy of intra-abdominal and pelvic infections. J Antimicrob Chemother. 1982;10(Suppl C):191–2.

272. Lou MA, Chen DF, Bansal M, et al. Evaluation of ceftizoxime in acute peritonitis. J Antimicrob Chemother. 1982. (Suppl C):183–9.

273. Berne TV, Yellin AW, Applebaum MC, et al. Antibiotic management of surgically treated or perforated appendicitis: Comparison of gentamicin and clindamycin versus cefamandole versus cefoperazone. Am J Surg. 1982;144:8–12.

274. Lau WY, Fan ST, Chu KW, et al. Randomized, prospective and double-blind trial of new beta-lactams in the treatment of appendicitis. Antimicrob Agents Chemother. 1985;28:639–42.

275. Saurio IH, Aruilommi C, Silvola H. Comparison of cefuroxime and gentamicin in combination with metronidazole in the treatment of peritonitis due to perforation of the appendix. Acta Chir Scand. 1983;149:423–6.

276. Peoples JB. Candida and perforated peptic ulcers. Surgery. 1986;100:758–64.

277. Rutledge R, Mandel SR, Wilde RE. Candida species. Insignificant contaminant or pathogenic species? Am Surg. 1986;52:299–302.

278. Marsh PK, Tally FP, Kellum J, et al. Candida infections in surgical patients. Ann Surg. 1983;198:42–7.

279. Sobel JD. Candida infections in the intensive care unit. Crit Care Clin North Am. 1988;4:325–44.

280. Hau T, Nishilawa R, Phuangsab A. Irrigation of the peritoneal cavity and antibiotics in the treatment of peritonitis. Surg Gynecol Obstet. 1983;156:25–30.

281. Rambo WM. Irrigation of the peritoneal cavity with cephalothin. Am J Surg. 1972;123:192–5.

282. Nichols RL. Management of intra-abdominal sepsis. Am J Med. 1985;80(Suppl 6B):204–9.

283. Hudspeth AS. Radical surgical debridement in the treatment of advanced generalized bacterial peritonitis. Arch Surg. 1975;110:1233–6.

284. Sindelar WF, Mason GR. Intraperitoneal irrigation with povidone-iodine solution for the prevention of intra-abdominal abscess in the bacterially contaminated abdomen. Surg Gynecol Obstet. 1979;148:409–11.

285. Ahrenholz DH, Simmons RL. Povidone-iodine in peritonitis. I. Adverse effects of local instillation in experimental E. coli peritonitis. J Surg Res. 1979;26:458–63.

286. Bhushan C, Mital VK, Elhence IP. Continuous postoperative peritoneal lavage in diffuse peritonitis using balanced saline antibiotic solution. Int Surg. 1975;60:526–8.

287. Hallerback B, Anderson C, Englund N, et al. A prospective randomized study of continuous peritoneal lavage postoperatively in the treatment of purulent peritonitis. Surg Gynecol Obstet. 1986;163:433–6.

288. Leiboff AR, Soroff HS. The treatment of generalized peritonitis by closed postoperative peritoneal lavage: A critical review of the literature. Arch Surg. 1987;122:1005–10.

289. Smithivas T, Hyams PJ, Matalon R, et al. The use of gentamicin in peritoneal dialysis. I. Pharmacologic results. J Infect Dis. 1971;124:S77–83.

290. Hill GB, Osterhout S. Experimental effects of hyperbaric oxygen on selected clostridial species. In vitro studies. J Infect Dis. 1972;125:17–25.

291. Holland JA, Hill GB, Wolfe WG, et al. Experimental and clinical experience with hyperbaric oxygen in the treatment of clostridial myonecrosis. Surgery. 1975;77:75–85.

292. Schreiner A, Tonjum S, Digranes A. Hyperbaric oxygen therapy in bacteroides infections. Acta Chir Scand. 1974;140:73–6.

293. Hill GB. Hyperbaric oxygen exposures for intrahepatic abscesses produced in mice by nonsporeforming anaerobic bacteria. Antimicrob Agents Chemother. 1976;9:312–7.

294. Thom SR, Lavermann MW, Hart GB. Intermittent hyperbaric oxygen therapy for reduction of mortality in experimental polymicrobial sepsis. J Infect Dis. 1986;154:504–10.

295. Aprahamian C, Wittman DH. Operative management of intraabdominal infection. Infection. 1991;19:453–5.

296. Haller JA Jr, Shaker IJ, Donahoo JS, et al. Peritoneal drainage versus nondrainage for generalized peritonitis from ruptured appendicitis in children: A prospective study. Ann Surg. 1973;177:595–600.

297. Leigh DA, Simmons K, Norman E. Bacterial flora of the appendix fossa in appendicitis and postoperative wound infection. J Clin Pathol. 1974;27:997–1000.

298. Follen WD, Hunt J, Altemeier WA. Prophylactic antibiotics in penetrating wounds of the abdomen. J Trauma. 1972;12:282–8.

299. Fabian TC, Boldreghini SJ. Antibiotics in penetrating abdominal trauma. Comparison of ticarcillin plus clavulanic acid with gentamicin plus clindamycin. Am J Med. 1985;79(Suppl 5B):157–60.

300. Nichols RL, Gorbach SL, Condon RE. Alteration of intestinal microflora following preoperative mechanical preparation of the colon. Dis Colon Rectum. 1971;14:123–7.

301. Condon RE, Bartlett JG, Greenlee H, et al. Efficacy of oral and systemic antibiotic prophylaxis in colorectal operations. Arch Surg. 1983;118:496–502.

302. Kaiser AB. Antibiotic prophylaxis in surgery. N Engl J Med. 1986;315:1129–38.

303. Baum ML, Anish Ds, Chalmers TC, et al. A survey of clinical trials of antibiotic prophylaxis in colon surgery: Evidence against further use of nontreatment controls. N Engl J Med. 1981;305:795–9.

304. Guglielmo BJ, Hohn DC, Koo PJ, et al. Antibiotic prophylaxis in surgical procedures: A critical analysis of the literature. Arch Surg. 1983;118:943–55.

305. Holph KD, Sorkin M, Rubin J, et al. Continuous ambulatory peritoneal dialysis: Three-year experience at one center. Ann Intern Med. 1980;92:609–13.

306. Rubin J, Rogers WA, Taylor HM, et al. Peritonitis during continuous ambulatory peritoneal dialysis. Ann Intern Med. 1980;92:7–13.

307. Fenton SSA, Pei Y, Delmore T, et al. The CAPD peritonitis rate is not improving with time. Trans Am Soc Artif Intern Organs. 1986;32:546–9.

308. Vas SL. 2. Peritonitis of peritoneal dialysis patients: Pathogenesis and treatment. Med Microbiol. 1986;5:21–43.

309. Peterson PK, Matzke GR, Keane WF. Current concepts in the management of peritonitis in continuous ambulatory peritoneal dialysis patients. Rev Infect Dis. 1987;9:604–12.

310. Everett ED. Diagnosis, prevention and treatment of peritonitis. Perit Dialy Bull. 1984;4(Suppl):139–42.

311. Steinberg SM, Cutler SJ, Novak JK, et al. Report of the national CAPD registry of the National Institutes of Health: Characteristics of participants and selected outcome measures for the period January 1, 1981 through August 31, 1984. In: National CAPD Registry of the National Institute of Arthritis, Diabetes, and Digestive and Kidney Diseases. Washington, DC: US Public Health Services; 1985.

312. Kraus ES, Spector DA. Characteristics and sequelae of peritonitis in diabetics and non-diabetics receiving chronic intermittent peritoneal dialysis. Medicine. 1983;62:52–7.

313. Fenton S, Wu G, Cattran D, et al. Clinical aspects of peritonitis in patients on CAPD. Perit Dialy Bull. 1981;1(Suppl):4–8.

314. Sewell CM, Clarridge J, Lacke C, et al. Staphylococcal nasal carriage and subsequent infection in peritoneal dialysis patients. JAMA. 1982;248:1493–5.

315. Keane WJ, Comty CM, Verbrugh HA, et al. Opsonic deficiency of peritoneal dialysis effluent in CAPD. Kidney Int. 1984;25:539–43.

316. Lamperi S, Carozzi S, Nasini MG. Intraperitoneal immunoglobulin treatment in prophylaxis of bacterial peritonitis in CAPD. In: Khanna R, Nolph KD, Provant B, et al., eds. Advances in CAPD. Toronto: University of Toronto Press; 1986:110.

317. Duwe AK, Vas SI, Weatherhead IW. Effects of composition of peritoneal dialysis fluid on chemiluminescence, phagocytosis and bacterial activity in vitro. Infect Immun. 1981;33:130–5.

318. Marrie TJ, Noble MA, Costerton JW. Examination of the morphology of bacteria adhering to peritoneal dialysis catheters by scanning and transmission electron microscopy. J Clin Microbiol. 1983;18:1388–98.

319. Arfania D, Everett ED, Nolph KD, et al. Uncommon causes of peritonitis in patients undergoing peritoneal dialysis. Arch Intern Med. 1981;141:61–4.

320. Vas SI. Microbiologic aspects of chronic ambulatory dialysis. Kidney Int. 1983;23:83–92.

321. Peterson PK, Keane WF. Infections in chronic peritoneal dialysis patients. In: Remington JS, Swartz MN, eds. Current Clinical Topics in Infectious Diseases. New York: McGraw-Hill; 1985:239–60.

322. Woods GL, Washington JA II. Comparison of methods for processing dialysate in suspected continuous ambulatory peritoneal dialysis-associated peritonitis. Diagn Microbiol Infect Dis. 1987;7:155–7.

323. Gokal R, Ramos JM, Francis DM, et al. Peritonitis in continuous ambulatory peritoneal dialysis: Laboratory and clinical studies. Lancet. 1982;2:1388–91.

324. Keane WF, Everett ED, Fine RN, et al. CAPD related peritonitis management and antibiotic therapy recommendations: Travenol Peritonitis Management Advisory Committee. Perit Dialy Bull. 1987;7:55–68.

325. Verbrogh HA, Keane WF, Conroy WE, et al. Bacterial growth and killing in chronic ambulatory peritoneal dialysis fluids. J Clin Microbiol. 1984;20:199–203.

326. Eisenberg ES, Leviton I, Soeiro R. Fungal peritonitis in patients receiving peritoneal dialysis: Experience with 11 patients and review of the literature. Rev Infect Dis. 1986;8:309–21.

327. Rubin J, Kirchner K, Walsh D, et al. Fungal peritonitis during continuous ambulatory peritoneal dialysis: A report of 12 cases. Am J Kidney Dis. 1987; 10:361–8.

328. Vargemezis V, Papadopoulov ZL, Llamos H, et al. Management of fungal peritonitis during continuous ambulatory peritoneal dialysis (CAPD). Perit Dialy Bull. 1986;6:17–20.

329. McNeely DJ, Vas SI, Dambros N, et al. *Fusarium* peritonitis: An uncommon complication of continuous ambulatory peritoneal dialysis. Perit Dialy Bull. 1981;1:94–6.

330. Chapman JR, Warnock DW. Ketoconazole and fungal CAPD peritonitis. Lancet. 1983;2:510–1.

331. McGuire NM, Port FK, Kauffman CA. Ketoconazole pharmacokinetics in continuous peritoneal dialysis. Perit Dialy Bull. 1984;4:199–201.

332. Axelrod J, Meyers BR, Hirschman SZ, et al. Prophylaxis with cephalothin in peritoneal dialysis. Arch Intern Med. 1973;132:368–71.

333. Abrutyn E, Goodhart GL, Roos K, et al. *Acinetobacter calcoaceticus* outbreak associated with peritoneal dialysis. Am J Epidemiol. 1978;107:328–35.

334. Altemeir WA, Culbertson WR, Fullen WD, et al. Intra-abdominal abscesses. Am J Surg. 1973;125:70–9.

335. Saini S, Kellum JM, O'Leary MP, et al. Improved localization and survival in patients with intra-abdominal abscesses. Am J Surg. 1983;145:136–42.

336. Gibson DM, Feliciano DV, Mattox KL, et al. Intra-abdominal abscess after penetrating abdominal trauma. Am J Surg. 1981;142:699–703.

337. Patterson HC. Left subphrenic abscesses. Am Surg. 1977;43:430–3.

338. Ozeran RS. Subdiaphragmatic abscess: Diagnosis and treatment. Am Surg. 1967;33:64–7.

339. Sherman NJ, Davis JR, Jesseph JE. Subphrenic abscess: A continuing hazard. Am J Surg. 1969;117:117–23.

340. Sanders RC. The changing epidemiology of subphrenic abscess and its clinical and radiological consequences. Br J Surg. 1970;57:449–55.

341. Ochsner A, DeBakey M. Subphrenic abscess. Collective review of 3608 collected and personal cases. Surg Gynecol Obstet. 1939;66:426.

342. Mackenzie M, Fordyle J, Young DG. Subphrenic abscess in children. Br J Surg. 1975;62:305–8.

343. Wang SMS, Wilson SE. Subphrenic abscess. The new epidemiology. Arch Surg. 1977;112:934–6.

344. DeCosse JJ, Poulin TL, Fox PS, et al. Subphrenic abscess. Surg Gynecol Obstet. 1974;138:841–6.

345. Gorbach SL. Treatment of intra-abdominal infection. Am J Med. 1984; 76(Suppl 5A):107–10.

346. Milne GAC, Geere IIW. Chronic subphrenic abscess: The missed diagnosis. Can J Surg. 1977;20:162–5.

347. Mueller PR, Simeone JF. Intra-abdominal abscesses: Diagnosis by sonography and computed tomography. Radiol Clin North Am. 1983;21:425–43.

348. Ferrucci JT Jr, Van Sonnenberg E. Role of ultrasound and computed tomography in the diagnosis and treatment of intraabdominal abscess. In: Remington JS, Swartz MN, eds. Current Clinical Topics in Infectious Diseases. New York: McGraw-Hill; 1982:136–59.

349. Kerlan RK Jr, Pogany AC, Jeffrey RB, et al. Radiologic management of abdominal abscesses. AJR. 1985;144:145–9.

350. Connell TR, Stephens DH, Carlson HC, et al. Upper abdominal abscess: A continuing and deadly problem. AJR. 1980;134:759–65.

351. Caffee HH, Watts G, Mena I. Gallium 67 citrate scanning in the diagnosis of intra-abdominal abscess. Am J Surg. 1977;133:665–9.

352. Tsan M. Mechanism of gallium 67 accumulation in inflammatory lesions. J Nucl Med. 1985;26:88–92.

353. Disbro M, Datz F, Cook P, et al. Indium-111 labeled leukocytes: Clinical utility and accuracy. Clin Nucl Med. 1982;7:44–6.

354. Froelich JW, Krasicky GA. Radionuclide imaging of abdominal infections. Curr Concepts Diagn Nucl Med. 1985;2:12–6.

355. Coleman RE, Brack RE, Welch DM, et al. Indium-111 labeled leukocytes in the evaluation of suspected abdominal abscess. Am J Surg. 1980;139: 99–104.

356. Sfakianakis GN, A-Sheitch W, Heal A, et al. Comparisons of scintigraphy with In-111 leukocytes and Ga⁶⁷ in the diagnosis of occult sepsis. J Nucl Med. 1982;23:618–26.

357. Hill BA, Yamaguchi K, Flynn JJ, et al. Diagnostic sonography in general surgery. Arch Surg. 1975;110:1089–94.

358. Goudie E, Andrew WK. The role of diagnostic ultrasound in the assessment of masses in the left upper quadrant of the abdomen. S Afr Med J. 1976;50: 1391–4.

359. Knochel JQ, Koehler PR, Lee TG, et al. Diagnosis of abdominal abscesses with computed tomography, ultrasound and ¹¹¹In leukocyte scans. Radiology. 1980;137:425–32.

360. Koehler PR, Moss AA. Diagnosis of intraabdominal and pelvic abscesses by computerized tomography. JAMA. 1980;224:49–52.

361. Gisi P, Graham DB. Splenic abscess: Two case reports. SD J Med. 1992;45: 37–40.

362. Ooi LL, Nambiar R, Rauff A, et al. Splenic abscess. Aust NZ J Surg. 1992; 62:780–4.

363. Balthazar EJ, Robinson DL, Megibow AJ, et al. Acute pancreatitis: Value of CT in establishing diagnosis. Radiology. 1990;174:331–6.

364. Brock JS, Pachter HL, Schreiber J, et al. Surgical diseases of the falciform ligament. Am J Gastroenterol. 1992;87:757–8.

365. Baker HL Jr, Berquist TN, Kispert DB, et al. Magnetic resonance imaging in a routine clinical setting. Mayo Clin Proc. 1985;60:75–90.

366. Cammoun D, Hendee WR, Davis KA. Clinical applications of magnetic resonance imaging—Current status. West J Med. 1985;143:793–803.

367. Wall SD, Fisher MR, Amparo EG, et al. Magnetic resonance imaging in the evaluation of abscesses. AJR. 1985;144:1217–21.

368. Gerzof SG, Robbins AH, Johnson WC. Percutaneous catheter drainage of abdominal abscesses. N Engl J Med. 1981;305:653–7.

369. Mandel SR, Boyd D, Jaques PF, et al. Drainage of hepatic, intra-abdominal and mediastinal abscesses guided by computerized axial tomography: Successful alternative to open drainage. Am J Surg. 1983;145:120–5.

370. Pruett TL, Simmons RL. Status of percutaneous catheter drainage of abscesses. Surg Clin North Am. 1988;68:89–105.

371. Jaques P, Mauro M, Safrit H, et al. CT features of intraabdominal abscesses: Prediction of successful percutaneous drainage. Am J Radiol. 1986;146: 1041–5.

372. Malangioni MA. Pathogenesis and treatment of intraabdominal infection. Surg Gynecol Obstet. 1990;171:31–4.

373. Fornari F, Buscarini L. Ultrasonically guided fine-needle biopsy of gastrointestinal organs: Indications, results and complications. Dig Dis. 1992;10: 121–33.

374. Brolin RE, Nosher JL, Leiman S, et al. Percutaneous catheter versus open surgical drainage in the treatment of abdominal abscesses. Am Surg. 1984; 50:102–8.

375. Van Sonnenberg E, Ferruci JT Jr, Mueller PR, et al. Percutaneous drainage of abscesses and fluid collections: Technique, results and applications. Radiology. 1982;142:1–10.

376. Olak J, Christov NV, Stein LA, et al. Operative vs percutaneous drainage of intra-abdominal abscesses. Arch Surg. 1986;121:141–6.

377. Hurley JE, Vargish T. Early diagnosis and outcome of pancreatic abscesses in pancreatitis. Am J Surg. 1987;53:29–33.

378. Kodesch R, DuPont HL. Infectious complications of acute pancreatitis. Surg Gynecol Obstet. 1973;136:763–8.

379. Becker JM, Pemberton JH, Diamgno EP, et al. Prognostic factors in pancreatic abscess. Surgery. 1984;96:455–60.

380. Shi ECP, Yeo BW, Ham JM. Pancreatic abscesses. Br J Surg. 1984;71: 689–91.

381. Altemeier WA, Alexander JW. Pancreatic abscess. A study of 32 cases. Arch Surg. 1963;87:80–9.

382. Holden JL, Berne TV, Rosoff LSR. Pancreatic abscess following acute pancreatitis. Arch Surg. 1976;111:858–61.

383. Miller TA, Lindenauer SM, Frey CF, et al. Pancreatic abscess. Arch Surg. 1974;108:545–51.

384. Ransom JHC, Balthazar E, Caccavale R, et al. Computed tomography and the prediction of pancreatic abscess in acute pancreatitis. Ann Surg. 1985; 201:656–63.

385. Aranha GU, Prinz RA, Greenlee HB. Pancreatic abscess: An unresolved surgical problem. Am J Surg. 1982;144:534–8.

386. Bradley EL, Fulenwider JT. Open treatment of pancreatic abscess. Surg Gynecol Obstet. 1984;159:509–13.

387. Stambler JB, Klibaner MI. Tuberculous abscess of the pancreas. Gastroenterology. 1982;83:922–5.

388. Sostre CF, Flournoy JG, Bova P, et al. Pancreatic phlegmon: Clinical features and course. Dig Dis Sci. 1985;30:918–27.

389. Berger HG, Krautzberger W, Bittner R, et al. Results of surgical treatment of necrotizing pancreatitis. World J Surg. 1985;9:972–9.

390. Keighley MRB, Drysdale RB, Quoraiski AH, et al. Antibiotic treatment of biliary sepsis. Surg Clin North Am. 1975;55:1379–90.

391. Crass RA, Meyer AA, Jeffrey RB, et al. Pancreatic abscess: Impact of computerized tomography on early diagnosis and surgery. Am J Surg. 1985;150: 127–31.

392. Williford ME, Foster WL Jr, Halversen RA, et al. Pancreatic pseudocyst: Comparative evaluation of sonography and computed tomography. Am J Roentgenol. 1983;140:53–7.

393. Bicknell TA, Kohatsu S, Goodwin DA. Use of indium-111 labeled autologus leukocytes in differentiating pancreatic abscess from pseudocyst. Am J Surg. 1981;142:312–6.

394. Tanaka T, Miskin FS, Buozas DJ, et al. Pancreatic uptake of gallium-67 citrate in acute pancreatitis. Appl Radiol. 1978;1:163–5.

395. Paushter DM, Modic MT, Borkowski GP, et al. magnetic resonance: Principles and applications. Med Clin North Am. 1984;68:1393–1421.

396. Weiss HD, Anacker H, Kramann B, et al. The diagnosis of necrotizing pancreatic lesions by means of duodenoscopic pancreatography. Its value for the surgical procedure. Am J Gastroenterol. 1975;64:26–33.

397. Fedorak IJ, Ko TC, Djuricin G, et al. Secondary pancreatic infections: Are they distinct clinical entities? Surgery. 1992;112:824–30.

398. D'Egidio A, Schein M. Surgical strategies in the treatment of pancreatic necrosis and infection. Br J Surg. 1991;78:133–7.

399. Rotman N, Mathieu D, Anglade MC, et al. Failure of percutaneous drainage of pancreatic abscesses complicating severe acute pancreatitis. Surg Gynecol Obstet. 1992;174:141–4.

400. Brolin RE, Flancbaum L, Ercoli FR, et al. Limitations of percutaneous catheter drainage of abdominal abscesses. Surg Gynecol Obstet. 1991;173:203–10.

401. Karlson KB, Martia EC, Fankochen EL, et al. Percutaneous drainage of pancreatic pseudocysts and abscesses. Radiology. 1982;142:619–24.

402. Pruett TC, Rotstein OD, Crass J, et al. Percutaneous aspiration and drainage for selected abdominal infections. Surgery. 1984;96:731–7.

403. Lang EK, Paolini RM, Pottmeyer A. The efficacy of palliative and definitive percutaneous versus surgical drainage of pancreatic abscesses and pseudocysts: A prospective study of 85 patients. *South Med J* 1991;84:55–64.

404. Adams DB, Harvey TS, Anderson MC. Percutaneous catheter drainage of infected pancreatic and peripancreatic fluid collections. Arch Surg. 1990; 125:1554–7.

405. Lumsden A, Bradley EL 3rd. Secondary pancreatic infections. Surg Gynecol Obstet. 1990;170:459–67.

406. Ranson JH, Spencer FC. Prevention, diagnosis and treatment of pancreatic abscess. Surgery. 1977;82:99–106.

407. Warshaw AL, Jin G. Improved survival in 45 patients with pancreatic abscess. Ann Surg. 1985;202:408–15.

408. Van Vyve EL, Reynaert MS, Lengele BG, et al. Retroperitoneal laparostomy: Surgical treatment of pancreatic abscesses after acute necrotizing pancreatitis. Surgery. 1992;111:369–75.

409. Finch WT, Sawyers JL, Schenker S. A prospective study to determine the efficacy of antibiotics in acute pancreatitis. Ann Surg. 1976;183:667–71.

410. Kusne S, Dummer JS, Singh N, et al. Infections after liver transplantation. An analysis of 101 consecutive cases. Medicine. 1988;67:132–43.

411. Barbour GL, Juniper K Jr. A clinical comparison of amebic and pyogenic abscesses of the liver in sixty-six patients. Am J Med. 1972;53:323–34.

412. Dietrich RB. Experience with liver abscess. Am J Surg. 1984;147:288–91.

413. Ribaudo JM, Ochsner A. Intrahepatic abscesses: Amebic and pyogenic. Am J Surg. 1973;125:570–4.

414. Barnes PF, DeLock KM, Reynolds TN, et al. A comparison of amebic and pyogenic abscess of the liver. Medicine. 1987;66:472–83.

415. Shulman ST, Beem MO. A unique presentation of sickle cell disease. Pyogenic hepatic abscess. Pediatrics. 1971;47:1019–22.

416. Williams JW, Rittenberry A, Dillard R, et al. Liver abscess in newborn: Complications of umbilical vein catheterization. Am J Dis Child. 1973;125: 111–3.

417. Gyorffy EJ, Frey CF, Silva J Jr, et al. Pyogenic liver abscess. Diagnostic and therapeutic strategies. Ann Surg. 1987;206:699–705.

418. Sabbaj J. Anaerobes in liver abscess. Rev Infect Dis. 1984;6(Suppl 1):152–5.

419. Rubin RH, Swartz MN, Malt R. Hepatic abscess: Changes in clinical, bacteriologic and therapeutic aspects. Am J Med. 1974;57:601–10.

420. McDonald MI, Corey GR, Gallis HA, et al. Single and multiple pyogenic liver abscesses. Medicine. 1984;63:291–302.

421. Sabbaj J, Sutter VL, Finegold SM. Anaerobic pyogenic liver abscess. Ann Intern Med. 1972;77:629–38.

422. Lazarchick J, de Souza E, Silva NA, et al. Pyogenic liver abscess. Mayo Clin Proc. 1973;48:349–55.

423. Perera MR, Kirk A, Noone P. Presentation, diagnosis and management of liver abscess. Lancet. 1980;2:629–32.

424. Loh R, Wallace G, Thong Y. Successful non-surgical management of pyogenic liver abscess. Scand J Infect Dis. 1987;19:137–40.

425. Kaplan SL. Pyogenic liver abscess. In: Feigin RD, Cherry JD, eds. Textbook of Pediatric Infectious Disease. Philadelphia: WB Saunders; 1981:537–40.

426. Rabson AR, Koornhof HJ, Notman J, et al. Hepatosplenic abscesses due to *Yersinia enterocolitica*. Br Med J. 1972;4:341.

427. Haron E, Feld R, Tuffnell P, et al. Hepatic candidiasis: An increasing problem in immunocompromised patients. Am J Med. 1987;83:17–26.

428. Thaler M, Pastakia B, Shawker T, et al. Hepatic candidiasis in cancer patients: The evolving picture of the syndrome. Ann Intern Med. 1988;108: 88–100.

429. Flannery MT, Simmons DB, Saba H, et al. Fluconazole in the treatment of hepatosplenic candidiasis. Arch Intern Med. 1992;152:406–8.

430. Anaissie E, Bodey GP, Kantarjian H, et al. Fluconazole therapy for chronic disseminated candidiasis in patients with leukemia and prior amphotericin B therapy. Am J Med. 1991;91:142–50.

431. Kauffman CA, Bradley SF, Ross SC, et al. Hepatosplenic candidiasis: Successful treatment with fluconazole. Am J Med. 1991;91:137–41.

432. Wallack MK, Brown AS, Austrian R, et al. Pyogenic liver abscess secondary to asymptomatic sigmoid diverticulitis. Ann Surg. 1976;184:241–3.

433. Sparberg M, Gottschalk A, Kirsner JB. Liver abscess complicating regional enteritis: Report of two cases. Gastroenterology. 1965;49:548–51.

434. Lee JF, Block GE. The changing clinical pattern of hepatic abscesses. Arch Surg. 1972;104:465–70.

435. Miedema BW, Dineen P. The diagnosis and treatment of pyogenic liver abscesses. Ann Surg. 1984;200:328–35.

436. Williams RA, Finegold SM. Pyogenic and amebic liver abscess and splenic abscess. In: Wilson SE, Finegold SM, Williams RA, eds. Intra-Abdominal Infection. New York: McGraw-Hill; 1982:139–56.

437. Weinstein L. Bacterial hepatitis: A case report on an unrecognized cause of fever of unknown origin. N Engl J Med. 1978;299:1052–4.

438. Foster SC, Schneider B, Seaman WB. Gas-containing pyogenic intra-hepatic abscesses. Radiology. 1970;94:613–8.

439. Stenson WF, Eckert T. Pyogenic liver abscess. Arch Intern Med. 1983;143: 126–8.

440. Madayag MA, LeFleur RS, Braunstein P, et al. Radiology of hepatic abscesses. NY State J Med. 1975;75:1417–23.

441. Reynolds TB. Medical treatment of pyogenic liver abscesses. Ann Intern Med. 1982;96:373–4.

442. Callen PW. Computed tomographic evaluation of abdominal and pelvic abscesses. Radiology. 1979;131:171–5.

443. Koehler PR, Moss AA, Diagnosis of intraabdominal and pelvic abscesses by computerized tomography. JAMA. 1980;244:49–52.

444. Gerzof SG, Johnson WC, Robbins AH, et al. Intrahepatic pyogenic abscesses: Treatment by percutaneous drainage. Am J Surg. 1985;149:487–94.

445. Altemeier WA, Schowenserdt CG, Whiteby DH. Abscesses of the liver: Surgical consideration. Arch Surg. 1970;101:258–66.

446. DeBakey ME, Jordan GL Jr. Hepatic abscesses, both intra- and extra-hepatic. Surg Clin North Am. 1977;57:325–37.

447. Do H, Lambiase RE, Deyoe L, et al. Percutaneous drainage of hepatic abscesses: Comparison of results in abscesses with and without intrahepatic biliary communication. Am J Roentgenol. 1991;157:1209–12.

448. Attar B, Levendoglu H, Cuasay N. CT-guided percutaneous aspiration and catheter drainage of pyogenic liver abscesses. Am J Gastroenterol. 1986;81: 550–5.

449. McCorkell SJ, Niles NC. Pyogenic liver abscess: Another look at medical management. Lancet. 1985;1:803–6.

450. Abramowicz M, ed. Drugs for parasitic infections. Med Lett. 1988;30:15–24.

451. Nelken N, Isnatius J, Skinner M, et al. Changing clinical spectrum of splenic abscess. A multicenter study and review of the literature. Am J Surg. 1987; 154:27–34.

452. Gadacz T, Way LW, Dunphy JE. Changing clinical spectrum of splenic abscess. Am J Surg. 1974;128:182–7.

453. Chun CH, Raff MJ, Contreras L, et al. Splenic abscess. Medicine. 1980;59: 50–63.

454. Robinson SL, Saxe JM, Lucas CE, et al. Splenic diseases associated with endocarditis. Surgery. 1992;112:781–6.

455. Khalil T, Uzoaru I, Nadimpalli V, et al. Splenic tuberculous abscess in patients positive for human immunodeficiency virus: Report of two cases and review. Clin Infect Dis. 1992;14:1265–6.

456. Torres JR, Rodriquez Casas J, Balda E, et al. Multifocal *Salmonella* splenic abscess in an HIV-infected patient. Trop Geograph Med. 1992;44:66–8.

457. Drugas D, Duarte B, Barrett J. *Salmonella typhi* splenic abscess in an intravenous drug abuser following splenorrhaphy: Case report. J Trauma. 1992;33: 143–4.

458. Linos DA, Nagorney DM, McIlrath DC. Splenic abscess: The importance of early diagnosis. Mayo Clin Proc. 1983;58:261–4.

459. Grant E, Mertens MA, Mascatello VJ. Splenic abscess: Comparison of four imaging methods. AJR. 1979;132:465–6.

460. Pawar S, Kay CJ, Gonzalez R, et al. Sonography of splenic abscess. AJR. 1982;138:259–62.

461. Sarr MG, Zuidema GD. Splenic abscess: Presentation, diagnosis and treatment. Surgery. 1982;92:480–5.

462. Chou YH, Hsu CC, Tiu CM, et al. Splenic abscess: Sonographic diagnosis and percutaneous drainage or aspiration. Gastrointestinal Radiol. 1992;17: 262–6.

463. Quinn SF, von Sonnenberg E, Casola G, et al. Interventional radiology in the spleen. Radiology. 1986;161:289–91.

464. Levison MA. Percutaneous versus open operative drainage of intra-abdominal abscesses. Infect Dis Clin North Am. 1992;6:525–44.

465. Campbell K, Steele RJ. Non-steroidal anti-inflammatory drugs and complicated diverticular disease: A case–control study. Br J Surg 1991;78:190–1.

466. Byrne RV. Localized perforated diverticulitis. Arch Surg. 1964;88:552–5.

467. Lozon AA, Duff JH. Acute perforation of the colon. Can J Surg. 1976;19: 48–51.

468. Rodkey GV, Welch CE. Colonic diverticular disease with surgical treatment. A study of 338 cases. Surg Clin North Am. 1974;54:655–74.

469. Elfrink RJ, Miedema BW. Colonic diverticula. When complications require surgery and when they don't. Postgrad Med. 1992;92:97–8, 101–2.

470. Hemming A, Davis NL, Robbins RE. Surgical versus percutaneous drainage of intra-abdominal abscesses. Am J Surg. 1991;161:593–5.

471. Stabile BE, Puccio E, von Sonnenberg E, et al. Preoperative percutaneous catheter drainage of diverticular abscesses. Am J Surg. 1990;159:99–104.

472. Peoples JB, Vilk DR, Maguire JP, et al. Reassessment of primary resection of the perforated segment for severe colonic diverticulitis. Am J Surg. 1990; 159:291–3.

473. Moreaux J, Vons C. Elective resection for diverticular disease of the sigmoid colon. Br J Surg. 1990;77:1036–8.

474. Tugwell P, Southcott D, Walmesley P. Free perforation of the colon in Crohn's disease. Br J Clin Pract. 1972;26:44–5.

475. Prolla JC, Kirsner JB. The gastrointestinal lesions and complications of the leukemias. Ann Intern Med. 1964;61:1084–1103.

476. Pokorney BH, Jones JM, Skaikh BS, et al. Typhlitis: A treatable cause of recurrent septicemia. JAMA. 1980;243:682–3.

477. Mulholland MW, Delaney JP. Neutropenic colitis and aplastic anemia: A new association. Ann Surg. 1983;197:84–90.

478. Archibald RG. Nelson JA. Necrotizing enterocolitis in acute leukemia: Radiographic findings. Gastrointestinal Radiol. 1987;3:63–5.

479. Alt B, Glass NR, Sallinger H. Neutropenic enterocolitis in adults: Review of the literature and assessment of surgical intervention. Am J Surg. 1985; 149:405–8.

480. Shaked A, Shinar E, Freund H. Neutropenic typhlitis: A plea for conservatism. Dis Colon Rectum. 1983;26:351–2.

481. Varki AP, Armitage JO, Feagler JR. Typhlitis in acute leukemias: Successful treatment by early surgical intervention. Cancer. 1979;43:695–7.

482. Berk JE, Zinbers SS. Acute cholecystitis: Medical aspects. In: Berk JE, Haubrich WS, Kalser MH, et al., eds. 4th ed. Gastroenterology. Philadelphia: WB Saunders; 1985;6:3597–616.

483. Bailey HA, Thrush LB. Consideration of acute cholecystitis: An analysis of seventy-six cases. Am J Surg. 1951;82:328–33.

484. Schein CJ. Acute Cholecystitis. New York: Harper & Row; 1972:63–5.
485. Truedson H, Elmros T, Holm S. The incidence of bacteria in gallbladder bile at acute and elective cholecystectomy. Acta Chir Scand. 1983;149:307–13.
486. Pitt HA, Postier RG, Cameron JC. Biliary bacteria: Significance and alteration after antibiotic therapy. Arch Surg. 1982;117:445–9.
487. Finegold S. Anaerobes in biliary tract infection. Arch Intern Med. 1979;139:1338–9.
488. Bourgalt AM, England DM, Rosenblatt JE, et al. Clinical characteristics of anaerobic bactibilia. Arch Intern Med. 1979;139:1346–9.
489. Samuels BI, Freitas JE, Bree RL, et al. A comparison of radionuclide hepatobiliary imaging and real-time ultrasound for the detection of acute cholecystitis. Radiology. 1983;147:207–10.
490. Gill PT, Dillon E, Leahy AL, et al. Ultrasonography, HIDA scintigraphy or both in the diagnosis of acute cholecystitis? Br J Surg. 1985;72:267–8.
491. Johnson DG, Coleman RE. New techniques in radionuclide imaging of the alimentary system. Radiol Clin North Am. 1982;20:635–51.
492. Kane RA, Costello P, Duszlak E. Computed tomography in acute cholecystitis: New observations. AJR. 1983;141:697–701.
493. McCarthy S, Hricak H, Cohen M, et al. Cholecystitis: Detection with MR imaging. Radiology. 1986;158:333–6.
494. Mentzer RM, Golden CT, Chandler JG, et al. A comparative appraisal of emphysematous cholecystitis. Am J Surg. 1975;125:10–5.
495. Kune GA, Burdon JGW. Are antibiotics necessary in acute cholecystitis? Med J Aust. 1975;2:627–30.
496. Hirschmann JV, Inui TS. Antimicrobial prophylaxis: A critique of recent trials. Rev Infect Dis. 1980;2:1–23.
497. Bulow S, Dronberg O, Lung-Kristenson K. Reappraisal of surgery for suppurative cholecystitis. Arch Surg. 1977;112:282–4.
498. Moore EE, Kelly GL, Driver T, et al. Reassessment of simple cholecystostomy. Arch Surg. 1979;114:515–8.
499. Naitove A. When cholecystectomy? Hosp Pract. 1978;13:121–8.
500. Jarvinen HJ, Hastbacka J. Early cholecystectomy for acute cholecystitis: A prospective randomized study. Ann Surg. 1980;191:501–5.
501. Morrow DJ, Thompson J, Wilson SE. Acute cholecystitis in the elderly: A surgical emergency. Arch Surg. 1979;113:1149–52.
502. Thompson JE Jr, Tompkins RK, Longmire WP Jr. Factors in the management of acute cholangitis. Ann Surg. 1982;117:437–44.
503. Bilboa MK, Dotter CT, Lee TG, et al. Complications of endoscopic retrograde cholangiopancreatography. A study of 10,000 cases. Gastroenterology. 1976;70:314–20.
504. Hinshaw DB. Acute obstructive cholangitis. Surg Clin North Am. 1973;53:1089–94.
505. Ralls PW, Colletti PM, Halls JM, et al. Prospective evaluation of ^{99m}TC-IDA cholescintigraphy and gray-scale ultrasound in the diagnosis of acute cholecystitis. Radiology. 1982;144:369–71.
506. Welch JP, Donaldson G. The urgency of diagnosis and surgical treatment of suppurative cholangitis. Am J Surg. 1976;131:527–32.

SECTION G.　CARDIOVASCULAR INFECTIONS

58. ENDOCARDITIS AND INTRAVASCULAR INFECTIONS

W. MICHAEL SCHELD
MERLE A. SANDE

INFECTIVE ENDOCARDITIS

The term *infective endocarditis* (IE) denotes infection of the endocardial surface of the heart and implies the physical presence of microorganisms in the lesion. Although the heart valves are most commonly affected, the disease may also occur on septal defects or on the mural endocardium. Infection of arteriovenous shunts, arterioarterial shunts (patent ductus arteriosus), and coarctation of the aorta are also included under this heading since the clinical manifestations are similar. The term *infective endocarditis,* first used by Thayer in the Gibson lectures of 1930 and later popularized by Lerner and Weinstein,[1,2] is preferable to the old term *bacterial endocarditis,* since chlamydiae, rickettsiae, mycoplasma, fungi, and perhaps even viruses may be responsible for the syndrome.

In the past, the disease has been classified as "acute" or "subacute." This was based on the usual progression of the untreated disease and is mainly of historic interest. The acute form follows a fulminant course, usually with high fever, systemic toxicity, and leukocytosis, with death occurring in several days to less than 6 weeks. It is classically associated with infection caused by *Staphylococcus aureus, Streptococcus pyogenes, Streptococcus pneumoniae,* and *Neisseria gonorhoeae.* The subacute (death in 6 weeks to 3 months) and "chronic" (death in greater than 3 months) forms are usually considered together. They commonly occur in the setting of prior valvular disease and are characterized by a slow, indolent course with ˄ low-grade fever, night sweats, weight loss, and vague systemic complaints. This form of the disease is classically caused by the viridans streptococci. Although useful conceptually, this classification ignores the nonbacterial forms of IE and the frequent overlap in manifestations by individual organisms such as the enterococci. A classification based on the etiologic agent responsible is preferable, since it has implications for the course usually followed, the likelihood of preexisting heart disease, and the appropriate antimicrobial agent(s) to employ.

Although relatively uncommon, IE has received considerable attention by both clinicians and scientists for the past century. The clinical manifestations of the disease are so varied that they may be encountered in any of the medical subspecialities. Successful management is dependent on the close cooperation of medical and surgical disciplines. Indeed, endocarditis services have been created at several tertiary care centers in the United States. This collaboration has markedly improved the outlook of a disease that was universally fatal 50 years ago. The disease has attracted considerable investigative interest. Although the factors that influence its development are now more clearly identified, many questions remain about the unique aspects of this infection. For example, *(1)* why do organisms lodge specifically on the cardiac valves rather than elsewhere in the vascular tree; *(2)* what enables the microorganisms to survive on the valve surface after colonization; *(3)* why do only a relatively small number of strains of bacteria produce the vast majority of cases of endocarditis, while many others produce only bacteremia; *(4)* what factors are responsible for the marked variations in the manifestation of the disease; and *(5)* why is the infection so difficult to eradicate with antibiotics even though the infecting organisms are often exquisitely sensitive to the drugs in vitro? These questions will be discussed in detail in the following sections.

Epidemiology

The incidence of IE is difficult to determine since the criteria for diagnosis and the methods of reporting vary with different series.[3,4] An analysis based on strict case definitions often reveals that only a small proportion (≈20 percent) of clinically diagnosed cases are categorized as definite. Nevertheless, IE accounted for approximately 1 case/1000 hospital admissions with a range of 0.16–5.4 cases/1000 admissions in a review of 10 large surveys.[3,5] This incidence has not changed in the past 30 years.[6] The mean annual incidence was 3.8/100,000 person-years in Olmstead County, Minnesota, from 1950 to 1981 with no significant change during this interval.[7] A similar figure of 1.7/100,000 person-years was reported from a prospective survey in Louisiana[8] and is analogous to results from the United Kingdom.[9] A series of 210 episodes of IE seen at a large community hospital in Youngstown, Ohio, from 1980 through 1990 documented an annual rate of 0.32–1.30 (mean 0.75) episodes per 1000 admissions per year.[10] In an autopsy study[11] there was no change in the yearly number of cases of IE in the United Kingdom from 1939 to 1967. The proportion of acute cases has increased from approximately 20 percent in the preantibiotic era to 33 percent.[5,6] Despite these changes in the disease spectrum, IE remains a prevalent disease with a significant mortality in the antibiotic era.[10,12,13]

The mean age of patients with IE has gradually increased in the antibiotic era. In 1926, the median age was less than 30 years;[14] this had increased to 39 years by 1943, and currently over 50 percent of the patients are older than 50 years.[6,10,15,16] At the present time, approximately 54 percent (range, 41–69 percent) of the cases occur in patients aged 31–60, 26 percent (range, 12–40 percent) in patients less than 30 years of age, and 21 percent (range, 8–38 percent) in people older than 60 years.[2] The mean age of patients with IE caused by group D streptococci is even higher: 61–67 years.[17] The disease remains uncommon in children and is associated primarily with (1) underlying structural congenital heart disease, particularly septal defects or complex lesions involving septal defects; (2) surgical repair of these defects; or (3) nosocomial catheter-related bacteremia, especially in infants.[18,19] The mean age for men is 6–7 years older than that for women, and men are more commonly affected (54–69 percent of the cases; the mean male:female ratio is 1.7:1 with a range of 1.0–3.0:1 in 18 large series).[5] In patients under the age of 35 years, more cases occur in women. A number of factors may relate to this shift in age distribution. First, there has been a change in the substrate of the underlying heart disease due to a decline in the incidence of acute rheumatic fever and rheumatic heart disease countered by the increasing importance of degenerative heart disease in elderly patients. Second, the age of the population has been steadily increasing, and people with rheumatic or congenital heart disease are surviving longer. A new form of the disease (nosocomial endocarditis) secondary to new therapeutic modalities (intravenous catheters, hyperalimentation lines, pacemakers, dialysis shunts, and so forth) has emerged.[3] Of 125 cases of endocarditis reviewed in Seattle, 35 were nosocomial in origin (28 percent).[20] Although nosocomial endocarditis accounted for only 14.3 percent of cases in another recent study, 64 percent of patients were over 60 years of age, and mortality was high.[21] It is interesting, however, that the age-adjusted incidence for the most common organisms (viridans streptococci) has not appreciably changed.[22]

The heart valve involved by the infection varies considerably with the proportion of acute cases reported in each series. The distribution ranges from 28 to 45 percent for the mitral valve alone, 5 to 36 percent for the aortic valve alone, and 0 to 35 percent for the aortic and mitral valves combined. The tricuspid valve is rarely involved (0–6 percent), and the pulmonary valve even less (<1 percent).[15,17,20,23] Both right- and left-sided disease is present in 0–4 percent.[2] Involvement of the aortic valve alone is increasing in frequency and correlates with the increase in acute cases; the incidence was 5 percent in 1938 and rose to 39 percent by 1978.[15] The aortic valve is involved in 61 percent of the male cases but in only 31 percent of the female cases.[20]

Almost any type of structural heart disease may predispose to IE, especially when the defect results in turbulence of blood flow. Rheumatic heart disease has been the underlying lesion in 37–76 percent of the infections in the past, and the mitral valve is involved in more than 85 percent of these cases.[5] If the mitral valve is solely involved, women outnumber men by 2:1. The aortic valve is affected in approximately 50 percent of these cases, and, if involved alone, men outnumber women by 4:1. Right-sided endocarditis is rare and accounts for fewer than 10 percent of all cases occurring in patients with rheumatic heart disease. The proportion of cases related to rheumatic heart disease has continued to decline to ≤25 percent in the past two decades.[24]

Congenital heart disease (especially patent ductus arteriosus, ventricular septal defect, coarctation of the aorta, bicuspid aortic valve, tetralogy of Fallot, and, rarely, pulmonic stenosis) is responsible in 6–24 percent of the cases.[5] Endocarditis is uncommon in the secundum atrial septal defects, probably because this lesion results in a low-pressure shunt with little turbulence. The congenitally bicuspid aortic valve, erroneously attributed to rheumatic carditis in the past,[25] is now recognized as an important condition in elderly patients (especially men), is the underlying lesion in over 20 percent of the cases occurring over the age of 60, and is associated with a poor prognosis despite rapid valve replacement.[26] Marfan's syndrome, when associated with aortic insufficiency, has also been associated with IE. Surgical closure of a ventricular septal defect lowers the risk of IE.[27]

The "degenerative" cardiac lesions (calcified mitral annulus, calcific nodular lesions secondary to arteriosclerotic cardiovascular disease, postmyocardial infarction thrombus, and so forth) assume the greatest importance in the 30–40 percent of the patients without any demonstrable underlying valvular disease. The actual contribution made by these lesions is unknown, but they occur with an increased incidence in the elderly. In one series, degenerative lesions were present in 50 percent of patients over 60 years old with native valve endocarditis.[28] The contribution of these degenerative cardiac lesions to the development of IE is apparent in an analysis of 148 patients treated in London since 1970.[29,30] The underlying structural cardiac defects were as follows: rheumatic heart disease, 39; congenital defects, 13; and normal or degenerate valves, 65. Similarly, only 31 percent of patients with IE in another series[31] had known cardiac disease. Although a calcified mitral annulus is fairly frequent in elderly women, this lesion is rarely complicated by IE (only 3 of 80 in one report).[32] When acute cases of IE are considered separately, over 50 percent have no recognized underlying cardiac disease.[10]

Many other conditions such as luetic heart disease, arterioarterial fistulas, hemodialysis shunts or fistulas, intracardiac pacemaker wires, and intracardiac prostheses may predispose to endocarditis. Prosthetic valve endocarditis is rising in incidence in proportion to other forms of endocarditis and is discussed in Chapter 59. Infective endocarditis also occurs more frequently in seriously ill hospitalized patients who are compromised hosts and who are subjected to invasive intravascular access procedures (intravenous catheters, including central venous pressure monitoring lines, hyperalimentation lines, intracardiac pacemaker wires, and so on).[15] Another group with an increased risk of IE are intravenous ("mainlining") drug abusers. (This group will be considered in detail in a later section.) In this population, there is the added problem of a rapidly rising prevalence of IE in patients with human immunodeficiency virus (HIV) infection. In addition, intravenous drug users are also the group at greatest risk for recurrent IE.[5,23] Although the contribution of invasive procedures (e.g., sigmoidoscopy or colonoscopy) has been debated, native valve IE appears to be more frequent in patients with active inflammatory bowel disease (6 of 213 patients in one recent report[34]).

Although idiopathic hypertrophic subaortic stenosis (IHSS) or asymetric hypertrophy of the interventricular septum has not classically been recognized as a condition leading to bacterial endocarditis, by 1982, 32 such cases had been reported in the literature.[35–37] In seven cases examined histologically, the infection was found on the aortic valve in three cases, mitral valve in two, both valves in one, and the subaortic endocardium in one. This distribution is likely related to the associated mitral regurgitation due to the displacement of the anterior leaflet by the abnormal ventricular architecture and by the turbulence of the jet stream affecting the aortic valve distal to the intraventricular obstruction. The age of patients developing endocarditis ranged from 20 to 66 years, and in most cases (70 percent) the disease was produced by viridans streptococci. Approximately 5 percent of patients with IHSS develop IE.[37] Infective endocarditis is more common in the subset of patients with IHSS who have hemodynamically severe forms of the disease manifested by a higher peak systolic pressure gradient and a high prevalence of symptoms. New murmurs develop in 36 percent of patients with IHSS complicated by IE, and this new physical finding correlates with a higher mortality rate.[37]

The association of the mitral prolapse syndrome and endocarditis has also been recognized. Of 87 consecutive cases of IE reported from Stanford University, 10 (11 percent) occurred in patients with well-documented mitral valve prolapse.[33] These 10 cases represented over one-third of the 28 cases in which isolated mitral regurgitation was the predisposing condition. Four additional cases occurred in patients who were not studied by echocardiography or angiography but who had clinical evidence of the mitral prolapse syndrome. Thus, 40–50 percent of the cases of IE associated with isolated insufficient mitral valves probably occurred in patients with the mitral prolapse syndrome. In one series[23] of 63 cases of native valve endocarditis diagnosed in Memphis from 1980 to 1984, mitral valve prolapse was the most common underlying lesion (29 percent). In another study,[39] 5 of 58 patients with mitral valve prolapse followed prospectively for 9–22 years developed endocarditis. This syndrome should be suspected in patients with midsystolic clicks with or without a late systolic murmur. The condition is common and has been recognized in 0.5–20 percent of otherwise healthy people, especially young women. It has become apparent that mitral valve prolapse is only one component of a developmental syndrome. This lesion is often associated with a distinct habitus in women,[40] von Willebrand's disease, or ophthalmoplegia. Some of these characteristics may be useful in identifying patients at high risk for IE. It is important to emphasize that all 25 patients who developed IE on a prolapsing mitral valve had a holosystolic murmur, and none had the isolated click without a murmur.[38] The risk of IE appears to be increased in the subset of patients with mitral valve prolapse who exhibit valvular redundancy.[28] Nevertheless, the risk of IE is clearly higher in patients with mitral valve prolapse. In a careful retrospective epidemiologic matched case control analysis, the odds ratio (8.2; 95 percent confidence interval, 2.4–28.4) indicates a substantially higher risk for the development of IE in these patients than in controls.[41] It appears that once IE develops in people with mitral valve prolapse, the symptoms and signs are more subtle and the mortality rate less when compared with left-sided IE of other types.[42]

Pathogenesis and Pathophysiology

In vitro observations and studies in experimental animals have demonstrated that the development of IE most likely requires the simultaneous occurrence of several independent events, each of which may be influenced by a host of separate factors. The valve surface must first be altered to produce a suitable site for bacterial attachment and colonization. Surface changes may be produced by various local and systemic stresses, including blood turbulence. These alterations result in the deposition of platelets and fibrin and in the formation of so-called nonbacterial thrombotic endocarditis (NBTE). Bacteria must then reach this site and adhere to the NBTE to produce colonization. Cer-

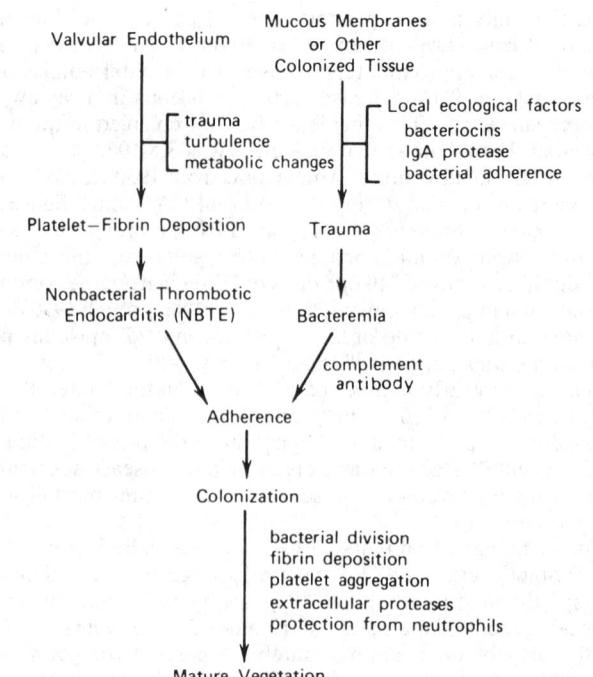

FIG. 1. Proposed scheme for the pathogenesis of infective endocarditis.

tain strains appear to have a selective advantage in adhering to platelets and/or fibrin and thus produce the disease with a lower inoculum. After colonization, the surface is rapidly covered with a protective sheath of fibrin and platelets to produce an environment conducive to further bacterial multiplication and vegetation growth. The interaction of these events is depicted in Figure 1. In the following sections, these factors will be considered independently (see refs. 43–46 for in-depth discussions).

Nonbacterial Thrombotic Endocarditis. Luschka, in 1852, first suggested that endocarditis resulted when septic coronary emboli lodged in the vessels of the cardiac valve.[47] This hypothesis was discarded since cardiac valves are poorly vascularized and only in the proximal portion, which does not coincide with the area of infection.[45,48,49] It is now clear that the initial colonization occurs on the endothelial surface of the valve. In experimental animals it is nearly impossible to produce IE with intravenous injections of bacteria unless the valvular surface is first damaged or otherwise altered. When a polyethylene catheter is passed across the aortic valve of a rabbit, endocarditis is readily produced with intravenously injected bacteria or fungi.[50,51] Microscopic examination of this early lesion demonstrates the organisms intimately adherent to fibrin-platelet deposits overlying interstitial edema and mild cellular distortion that have formed in areas of valvular trauma.[52] Scanning electron micrographs of the damaged valvular surface confirm the adhesion of microorganisms to these areas of fibrin-platelet deposition early in the disease course.[53] The organisms are rapidly covered by fibrin.[54] Opossums and pigs are the only animals known to develop endocarditis readily without experimentally induced valvular alteration.[46,55] The stress of captivity is apparently sufficient in these animals to produce subtle valvular changes that lead to both spontaneous endocarditis and a markedly increased susceptibility to the disease after the intravenous injection of bacteria. In other animals and probably in humans, alteration of the valve surface is a prerequisite for bacterial colonization. Angrist first recognized the importance of these deposits as the critical factor in allowing bacterial colonization of valve surfaces and suggested the term *nonbacterial thrombotic endocarditis*. Many forms of exogenous stress produce these lesions experimentally, including infection, hypersensitivity states, cold exposure, simulated high altitude, high cardiac output states, cardiac lymphatic obstruction, and hormonal manipulations.[46] These procedures all increase the susceptibility of the animals to IE.

Nonbacterial thrombotic endocarditis has been found in patients with malignancy (particularly pancreatic, gastric, or lung carcinoma) or other chronic wasting diseases, rheumatic or congenital heart disease,[48] uremia, connective tissue diseases such as systemic lupus erythematosus, after the placement of intracardiac catheters (e.g., Swan-Ganz), and even after a self-limited acute illness, and it generally reflects two pathogenic mechanisms, hypercoagulability and/or endothelial damage. In a careful analysis performed in Japan, NBTE was found in 2.4 percent of 3404 autopsies, especially in elderly people with chronic wasting disease.[56] Importantly, NBTE was most frequent on the low-pressure side of the cardiac valves along the line of closure, precisely the site most often involved in IE. Whether this lesion is always essential for the development of endocarditis in humans is unknown.

Hemodynamic Factors. Infective endocarditis characteristically occurs on the atrial surface of the mitral valve and the ventricular surface of the aortic valve when associated with valvular insufficiency. Rodbard[57] showed that this localization is related to a decrease in lateral pressure (presumably with decreased perfusion of the intima) immediately "downstream" from the regurgitant flow. Lesions with high degrees of turbulence (small ventricular septal defect with a jet lesion, valvular stenosis < insufficient valves) readily create conditions that lead to bacterial colonization, whereas defects with a large surface area (large ventricular septal defect), low flow (ostium secundum atrial septal defect), or attenuation of turbulence (chronic congestive heart failure with atrial fibrillation) are rarely implicated in IE. Cures of IE achieved with ligation alone of an arteriovenous fistula or patent ductus arteriosus also stress the importance of hemodynamic factors. A hyperdynamic circulation itself, such as that created after experimentally induced arteriovenous fistulas in dogs or fistulas and shunts in hemodialysis patients, indirectly may lead to IE by producing NBTE.[45,46]

The degree of mechanical stress exerted on the valve also affects the location of the endocarditis.[58] In 1024 autopsy cases of IE reviewed through 1952, the incidence of valvular lesions was as follows: mitral, 86 percent; aortic, 55 percent; tricuspid, 19.6 percent; and pulmonic, 1.1 percent. This correlates with the pressure resting on the closed valve: 116, 72, 24, and 5 mmHg, respectively.

Transient Bacteremia. In the setting of preexistent NBTE, transient bacteremia may result in the colonization of these lesions and to the development of IE.[59] Transient bacteremia occurs whenever a mucosal surface heavily colonized with bacteria is traumatized, such as with dental extractions and other dental procedures and gastrointestinal, urologic, and gynecologic procedures (Table 1).[59,60] The degree of bacteremia is proportional to the trauma produced by the procedure and to the number of organisms inhabiting the surface, and the organisms isolated reflect the resident microbial flora. The bacteremia is usually low grade ($\leq$10 colony-forming units [cfu]/ml) and transient; the blood stream is usually sterile in less than 15–30 minutes. It is noteworthy that in two studies where blood cultures were drawn from patients with severe gingival disease before the dental procedure, spontaneous bacteremia was identified in 9–11 percent. Other studies have demonstrated an even higher frequency of spontaneous bacteremia. Of the blood cultured from healthy people, 60–80 percent were positive when filters and anaerobic techniques were used.[61] The degree of bacteremia, however, was low, with only 2–10 cfu/5 ml of blood isolated. "Nonpathogenic" organisms such as *Propionibacterium acnes, Actinomyces viscosus, Staphylococcus epidermidis*, and other *Actinomyces* or streptococcal species were responsible.

TABLE 1. Incidence of Bacteremia after Various Procedures

Procedure/Manipulation	Percentage of Positive Blood Cultures
Dental	
Dental extraction	18–85
Periodontal surgery	32–88
Chewing candy or paraffin	17–51
Tooth brushing	0–26
Oral irrigation device	27–50
Upper airway	
Bronchoscopy (rigid scope)	15
Tonsillectomy	28–38
Nasotracheal suctioning/intubation	16
Gastrointestinal	
Upper GI endoscopy	8–12
Sigmoidoscopy/colonoscopy	0–9.5
Barium enema	11
Percutaneous needle biopsy of liver	3–13
Urologic	
Urethral dilatation	18–33
Urethral catheterization	8
Cystoscopy	0–17
Transurethral prostatic resection	12–46
Obstetric/gynecologic	
Normal vaginal delivery	0–11
Punch biopsy of the cervix	0
Removal/insertion of an IUD	0

(From Everett and Hirschmann,[60] with permission.)

Frequent episodes of silent bacteremia are also suggested by the identification of circulating humoral antibodies to the resident oral flora and by the noted increase in sensitized peripheral T cells to the flora of dental plaque.

Another factor of critical importance during the transient bacteremia stage is susceptibility of the potential pathogen to complement-mediated bactericidal activity. Only "serum-resistant" gram-negative aerobic bacilli (e.g., *Escherichia coli, Pseudomonas aeruginosa, Serratia marcescens*) reliably produce experimental IE in rabbits,[62,63] and this property is found in all isolates from human cases of IE. Although experimental IE can be induced in rats with "serum-sensitive" *E. coli*, the organisms are eliminated rapidly upon catheter removal.[63]

Microorganism–Nonbacterial Thrombotic Endocarditis Interaction. The ability of certain organisms to adhere to NBTE is a critical early step in the development of endocarditis. Gould et al.[64] showed that organisms frequently associated with IE (enterococci, viridans streptococci, *Staphylococcus aureus, Staphylococcus epidermidis, P. aeruginosa*) adhered more avidly to normal canine aortic leaflets in vitro than did organisms uncommon in IE (*Klebsiella pneumoniae, E. coli*). In addition, *Staphylococcus aureus* and the viridans streptococci produce IE more readily than does *E. coli* in the rabbit model of IE.[65] This observation correlates with the relative frequency with which these organisms produce the disease in humans. The rarity of IE due to gram-negative aerobic bacilli may also be related to their "serum sensitivity," as above.

Differences in the propensity to cause endocarditis are apparent even within a single species. Eleven capsular serotypes of *Staphylococcus aureus* have been described to date; highly mucoid strains (e.g., serotypes 1 and 2) are rarely recovered from clinical isolates, whereas types 5 and 8 account for approximately 75 percent of isolates. Nevertheless, mutant strains devoid of microencapsulation had significantly lower ID$_{50}$ values in a rat (catheter-induced NBTE) endocarditis model[66] than wild-type parent strains. Thus, microcapsule expression may attenuate *Staphylococcus aureus* endocarditis production by blocking bacterial cell surface adhesins, but this hypothesis requires confirmation.

Recent studies with an elegant experimental model of IE after dental extraction in rats with periodontitis, which closely resembles the presumed pathogenetic sequence in humans, also suggest an important role for bacterial adhesion to NBTE in the early events. Although viridans streptococci were much more commonly isolated than were group G streptococci in blood cultures obtained 1 minute postextraction, the latter strains caused 83 percent of the IE episodes in this rat model.[67,68] This propensity to cause IE was associated with an increased adhesion of group G streptococci to fibrin-platelet matrices in vitro.[68]

The adherence of oral streptococci to NBTE may depend on the production of a complex extracellular polysaccharide, dextran. This polymer plays an essential role in the pathogenesis of dental caries by *Streptococcus mutans*.[69] It allows the organism to adhere tightly to the surface of dental enamel. The enhanced ability to adhere to inert surfaces may also be important in IE. In an analysis of 719 cases of streptococcal infections in the United Kingdom, 317 cases of IE were found.[70] The most common etiologic agents were *Streptococcus sanguis* (16.4 percent of the cases), previously called "streptococcus SBE," and *Streptococcus mutans* (14.2 percent). When a ratio denoting endocarditis to nonendocarditis bacteremia was derived (Table 2), the relative propensity for a particular organism to cause endocarditis could be predicted. The ratios range from 14.2:1 for *Streptococcus mutans* to a reversed ratio of 1:32 for *Streptococcus pyogenes*. Only the first four organisms listed in Table 2 (all with ratios greater than 3:1) produce extracellular dextran. This suggests that dextran production may also be a virulence factor in the pathogenesis of IE.

The role of dextran in the adherence of oral streptococci to NBTE has also been studied in vitro by using artificial fibrin-platelet matrices (simulating NBTE). The amount of dextran produced by the organism in broth correlated with adherence and was increased by incubating the organism in sucrose (which stimulates dextran production) and was decreased by the addition of dextranase (which removes the dextran from the cell surface). The addition of exogenous dextran to *Streptococcus sanguis* grown in sucrose-free media increased adherence. Dextran production also correlated directly with the ability of these organisms to produce endocarditis in vivo in the rabbit model.[71] The strain of *Streptococcus sanguis* produced endocarditis less readily when incubated in dextranase than did control strains, and a strain that produced large quantities of dextran produced endocarditis more easily than did a strain that produced relatively small quantities of dextran. Dextran production also increases the adherence of *Streptococcus mutans* to traumatized canine aortic valves in vitro,[72] an effect dependent on polymers of higher molecular weight.[73] Thus, dextran formation (or, more properly exopolysaccharide or glycocalxy production) by oral streptococci may be a virulence factor for the production of IE by these organisms.[74] Furthermore, continued in vivo synthesis of exopolysaccharide during experimental IE correlates with vegetation size and resistance to antimicrobial therapy.[75,76] Measurement of cell-adherent glycocalyx by a quantitative spectrophotometric tryptophan assay among viridans streptococci isolated from blood cultures has potential value as an independent predictor of the likelihood of endocarditis.[77] It is clear, however, that non-dextran-producing streptococci may produce endocarditis in humans and adhere to artificial fibrin-platelet surfaces in vitro,[78] which suggests that other microbial surface characteristics are instrumental for this early event. Whatever the role of the extracellular glycocalyx in microbial adhesion, its presence may retard antimicrobial therapy for streptococcal endocarditis (see below).[75,76,79]

A similar important role of adhesion to NBTE in the pathogenesis of IE has also been shown for yeasts. *Candida albicans* adheres readily to NBTE in vitro and produces IE in rabbits more readily than does *Candida krusei*, a nonadherent yeast rarely implicated in IE in humans.[80] Although microbial adhesion is a crucial early event in the pathogenesis of IE, the precise intracardiac loci are unknown and may differ among organisms. Most organisms probably adhere initially to a constituent of NBTE; some evidence implicates fibronectin as the host receptor within NBTE.[81] Recent studies[82,83] support this concept. Low fibronectin-binding mutants of *Staphylococcus aureus* and *Streptococcus sanguis* had decreased ability to produce endocarditis in rats compared with high fibronectin-binding parent strains. Other normal constituents of damaged endothelium or NBTE (e.g., fibrinogen, laminin, type 4 collagen, and so forth)[84] may also serve to bind circulating bacteria. For example, *Streptococcus defectivus* (the major species isolated in cases of endocarditis due to "nutritionally variant streptococci" [NVS]; see below) bound the extracellular matrix of both fibroblasts and endothelial cells in a saturable specific manner, whereas *Streptococcus adjacens* and serotype III NVS strains did not bind.[85] A study also documented binding of *Streptococcus mutans*, *Streptococcus mitis*, *Streptococcus sanguis*, and *Enterococcus faecalis* to this extracellular matrix. Laminin-binding proteins (e.g., a 145-kD protein found in *Streptococcus gordonii* [formerly *S. sanguis* I]) have been found on the cell walls of organisms recovered from patients with endocarditis,[86] and the level of protein expression appeared to be regulated by the presence of extracellular matrix proteins. Other organisms may bind directly to, or become ingested by, endothelial cells as the initial event[87–89]; this sequence appears important in the initiation of IE by *Staphylococcus aureus* on "normal" cardiac valves. Although the specific microbial surface-host receptor ligand relationship remain obscure, this is an active area of investigation because inhibition of these events may provide novel prophylactic strategies.

The importance of adherence characteristics in the development of endocarditis has also been examined by using preincubation of organisms with antibiotics. Many classes of drugs, after incubation even at subinhibitory concentrations, decrease the adhesion of streptococcal species to fibrin-platelet matrices and damaged canine valves in vitro.[90] Several elegant studies in animal models have verified the significance of this in vitro observation, since preincubation of the organism in subinhibitory antibiotic concentrations prevents the development of endocarditis in vivo.[91,92] This has direct relevance to the chemoprophylactic prevention of IE (see Ch. 60). In one study, subinhibitory concentrations of penicillin were found to result in a loss of streptococcal lipoteichoic acid with reduced adhesion to NBTE and an impaired ability to produce IE in vivo.[93] Thus, antibiotics may prevent IE by at least two mechanisms: *(1)* bacterial killing and *(2)* inhibition of adhesion to NBTE.[94]

Since platelets are (with fibrin) the major constituents of NBTE, the role of the platelet in the pathogenesis of endocarditis has also been studied. Some strains of bacteria have been found to be potent stimulators of platelet aggregation and the release reaction.[95] In general, endocarditis-producing strains of staphylococci and streptococci more actively aggregate platelets than do other bacteria that less frequently produce IE. Platelet-bacterial aggregates have been found in the peripheral blood in patients with bacteremia. The importance of these bacterial-platelet aggregates in the formation of the vegetation or, con-

TABLE 2. Ratio of Infective Endocarditis Cases to Nonendocarditis Bacteremia for Various Streptococci

Bacteria	Endocarditis:Nonendocarditis
S. mutans	14.2:1
S. bovis I	5.9:1
DX + S. mitior[a]	3.3:1
S. sanguis	3.0:1
S. mitior	1.8:1
Unclassified "viridans"	1.4:1
Enterococcus faecalis	1:1.2
Miscellaneous streptococci	1:1.3
S. bovis II	1:1.7
S. anginosus	1:2.6
Group G streptococci	1:2.9
Group B streptococci	1:7.4
Group A streptococci	1:32.0

[a] DS +: dextran-positive.

(Modified from Parker and Ball,[70] with permission.)

versely, in the effect of the aggregation on the rate of removal of organisms from the circulation is unknown. Even small numbers of platelets greatly increased the adherence of oral streptococci to fibrin in vitro.[71] Recent studies[96] have shown that *Streptococcus sanguis,* an important cause of IE, aggregates platelets and adheres to these blood components by protease-sensitive components, not dextrans. A platelet receptor for ligands on certain strains of *Streptococcus sanguis* was suggested. This platelet aggregation by viridans streptococci, however, requires both direct platelet binding and plasma components.[97] Other experiments implicate IgG in this specific streptococcal-platelet interaction and suggest that platelet activation is mediated through the platelet surface, 40,000 molecular weight Fc receptor.[98]

Once the colonization of the valve occurs and a critical mass of adherent bacteria develops, the vegetation enlarges by further platelet-fibrin deposition and continued bacterial proliferation. The complex interplay among factors responsible for bacterial-platelet adhesion and aggregation have only been recently recognized. The ability of *Streptococcus sanguis* to induce platelet aggregation in vitro is conferred by two bacterial cell surface antigens: *(1)* class I antigen, which promotes adhesion of *Streptococcus sanguis* to platelets (adh[+]); and *(2)* coexpression of class II antigen, which promotes platelet adhesion or platelet aggregation (agg[+]). At least nine adh agg phenotypes have been identified among naturally occurring variants, reflecting a range of platelet interactivity. Furthermore, intravenous inoculation of agg[+] *Streptococcus sanguis* strains into rabbits with catheter-induced aortic valve trauma leads to larger vegetations, a more severe clinical course, more gross lesions in major organs, and greater mortality than inoculation with a agg[−] strain or the agg[+] strains pretreated with FAb fragments specific for the platelet interactivity phenotype.[99] Platelet aggregation induced by *Streptcoccus sanguis* in vivo appears to be an important virulence determinant of vegetation development and disease progression. Furthermore, streptococcal exopolysaccharide production inversely correlates with platelet adhesion while inhibiting aggregation,[100] indicating that these surface molecules may enhance endocarditis at some pathogenic steps, but not others.

Platelets may also play a role in host defense within the cardiac vegetation during IE. Following specific exposure to thrombin, release of α-granule-derived platelet microbicidal proteins (PMP or thrombodefensins) with bactericidal activity against some gram-positive cocci has been shown.[101] Although the ability of *Staphylococcus aureus* to adhere to and aggregate platelets are related properties, the resistance to PMP is an independent phenotypic characteristic and a potential virulence factor.[102] PMP are low-molecular-weight (approximately 8–10 kD) cationic proteins and may act primarily on the bacterial cell membrane or cell wall synergistically with antibiotics to kill bacteria. PMP may also demonstrate fungicidal activity against some yeasts in vitro.[103] Microbial resistance to the cidal activity of PMP may contribute to the pathogenesis of IE. This hypothesis is supported by a reduction in vegetation weight and bacterial concentration in rabbits with experimental aortic valve *Staphylococcus aureus* endocarditis when treated with aspirin.[104]

The bacterial colonies are found beneath the surface of the vegetation (variable, depending on the intracardiac location[105]), and infiltration by phagocyte cells in minimal; hence the vegetation creates an environment of impaired host resistance. These conditions allow for relatively unimpaired bacterial growth resulting in extremely high colony counts of 10^9–10^{11} bacteria/g of tissue. Bacteria deep within the fibrin matrix have been shown by autoradiography to reach a state of reduced metabolic activity.[106] Recent studies by Freedman and others suggest that impairment of host defenses (e.g., neutropenia, corticosteroids) potentiates progression of the disease when the tricuspid but not the aortic valve is involved[107,108] but is largely dependent on the intracardiac location of the vegetation.[109] The role of granulocytes within the vegetation is unsettled. When vegetation formation is retarded with anticoagulants in experimental animals with IE, the organisms appear to divide on the surface, total bacterial titers are lower, and the clinical disease is more explosive.[110,111] In addition, it has been suggested that phagocytosis of microorganisms by monocytes on or within the vegetation generates tissue thromboplastin formation that then acts as a stimulant to fibrin deposition and growth of the vegetation.[112] The best evidence, however, suggests that coagulation activation initiated by tissue factor,[113] with subsequent local thrombus formation, is responsible for the initiation of vegetation growth and persistence on the cardiac valve. It appears that some organisms (i.e., *Staphylococcus aureus*) induce tissue factor production by endothelium without the necessity for host cytokines.[114]

Immunopathologic Factors. Infective endocarditis causes the stimulation of both humoral and cellular immunity as manifested by hypergammaglobulinemia, splenomegaly, and the presence of macrophages in the peripheral blood. The possibility that preformed antibody increased the likelihood of the development of IE was suggested by the spontaneous occurrence of IE in horses receiving repeated immunizations with live pneumococci.[115] It was suggested that these antibodies produced bacterial agglutination in vivo that increased the chances of valvular colonization. Studies in animals have suggested a protective role for circulating antibody. Rabbits preimmunized with heat-killed streptococci plus Freund's adjuvant had a significantly higher median infective dose (ID_{50}) than did nonimmunized controls after aortic valve trauma.[116] Others have found similar results with *Streptococcus sanguis, S. mutans,* and *S. pneumoniae.*[117,118] In other experiments, antibody directed against cell surface components (including mannan) reduced the adhesion of *Candida albicans* to fibrin and platelets in vitro and endocarditis production in vivo.[119] This effect may be dependent on the infecting organism, however, since antibody to *Staphylococcus epidermidis* and *Staphylococcus aureus* does not prevent the development of endocarditis in immunized animals or result in reduced bacterial concentrations in infected vegetations or kidneys,[120] perhaps due to the inability of immune sera to enhance opsonophagocytosis of staphylococci. Therefore, the role of preformed antibody in the pathogenesis of IE remains unclear. Intravascular agglutination of bacteria may, in fact, decrease the frequency of endocarditis by reducing the actual number of circulating organisms, but cross protection is not achieved by passive transfer of high-titer immune globulin from *Streptococcus defectivus*–immunized rabbits to control animals.[118] Furthermore, nitrogen mustard–treated immunized rabbits lose their ability to efficiently clear *Streptococcus defectivus* from the circulation, a process partially restored by neutrophil transfusion.[121]

Rheumatoid factor (anti-IgG IgM antibody) develops in about 50 percent of patients with IE of greater than 6 weeks duration.[122] Rheumatoid factors have been found at the time of admission in 24 percent of the patients with acute staphylococcal endocarditis (less than 6 weeks duration), and the frequency increased to 40 percent if fever persisted for 2 weeks after the initiation of antibiotic therapy.[123] Over two-thirds of the patients became seronegative after 6 weeks of therapy, and two patients with a second episode of acute IE promptly redeveloped positive rheumatoid factors. The titers correlate with the level of hypergammaglobulinemia and decrease with therapy. Rheumatoid factor may play a role in the disease process by blocking IgG opsonic activity (by reacting with the Fc fragment), stimulating phagocytosis, and/or accelerating microvascular damage. Rheumatoid factor (IgM) has not been eluted from the immune complex glomerulonephritis associated with IE.[124] Antinuclear antibodies also occur in IE and may contribute to the musculoskeletal manifestations, low-grade fever, or pleuritic pain.[125]

Infective endocarditis, like malaria, schistosomiasis, syphilis, kala-azar, and leprosy, is associated with a constant intravascular antigenic challenge; therefore, the development of several classes of circulating antibody is not unexpected. Opsonic (IgG), agglutinating (IgG, IgM), and complement-fixing (IgG, IgM) antibodies, cryoglobulins (IgG, IgM, IgA, C3, fibrinogen), various antibodies to bacterial heat-shock proteins and macroglobulins have all been described in IE.[126–128] By using the sensitive Raji cell or Clq deviation techniques, circulating immune complexes have been found in high titer in virtually all patients with IE.[129] Circulating immune complexes are found with increased frequency in connection with a long duration of illness, extravalvular manifestations, hypocomplementemia, and right-sided IE. Levels fall and become undetectable with successful therapy. Patients with IE and circulating immune complexes may develop a diffuse glomerulonephritis that is analogous to the nephritis seen with infected ventriculoatrial shunts.[130] Immune complexes plus complement are deposited subepithelially along the glomerular basement membrane to form a "lumpy-bumpy" pattern. Immunoglobulin eluted from these lesions has been shown to cross react with bacterial antigens.[131] In addition, bacterial antigens have actually been demonstrated within circulating immune complexes.[132] Some of the peripheral manifestations of IE, such as Osler nodes, may also result from a deposition of circulating immune complexes. Pathologically these lesions resemble an acute Arthus reaction. However, the finding of positive culture aspirates in Osler nodes[133] suggests that they may in fact be due to septic emboli rather than immune complex deposition. In some diffuse purpuric lesions in IE, immune complex deposits (IgG, IgM, and complement) have been demonstrated in the dermal blood vessels by immunofluorescence.[134] Quantitative determinations of serum immune complex concentrations are useful in gauging the response to therapy. Effective treatment leads to a prompt decrease, with eventual disappearance of circulating immune complexes.[135] Conversely, therapeutic failures or relapses are characterized by rising titers or a reappearance of circulating immune complexes.[136]

Pathologic Changes

Heart. The classic vegetation of IE is usually located along the line of closure of a valve leaflet on the atrial surface for atrioventricular valves or the ventricular surface for semilunar valves. Vegetations may be single or multiple, are a few millimeters to several centimeters in size, and vary in color, consistency, and gross appearance. Microscopically, the lesion consists primarily of fibrin, platelet aggregates, and bacterial masses; neutrophils and red blood cells are rare. Destruction of the underlying valve may coexist. With treatment, healing occurs by fibrosis and occasionally calcification. The vegetation in acute cases is larger, softer, and more friable and may be associated with suppuration, more necrosis, and less healing than in subacute cases.[47,137] This infection may lead to perforation of the valve leaflet, rupture of the chordae tendinae, interventricular septum, or papillary muscle. Staphylococcal endocarditis frequently results in valve ring abscesses[138] with fistula formation into areas of the myocardium or pericardial sac. Aneurysms of the valve leaflet or sinus of Valsalva are also common. Valvular stenosis may result from large vegetations. Myocarditis, myocardial infarction, and pericarditis[137,138] are frequently found at autopsy. Myocardial abscesses are found in 20 percent of the autopsy cases and are associated primarily with acute staphylococcal endocarditis with hectic fever, a rapid onset of congestive heart failure, and conduction disturbances. Myocardial infarcts are found in as many as 40–60 percent of the autopsied cases, often without diagnostic changes in the electrocardiogram. Pericarditis is much more common in acute IE.

Although echocardiographic abnormalities are common in patients with the acquired immunodeficiency syndrome (AIDS), pericardial disease (pericarditis, effusions), myocardial disease

leading to heart failure or arrhythmias, NBTE, and Kaposi sarcoma are all more frequent than IE.[137,139] AIDS patients with IE are usually intravenous drug users with right-sided involvement, with an increase in the prevalence of cases due to *Staphylococcus aureus* or fungi.[139,140] The clinical course in AIDS patients is often more fulminant than IE in intravenous drug users without AIDS; pneumonia and sepsis are common. IE has also been described in the transplanted heart.

Embolic phenomena are common in IE. In the preantibiotic era, 70–95 percent of the patients had clinically demonstrable embolic events, but this has decreased to 15–35 percent today. Pathologic evidence of embolization is still detected in 45–65 percent of autopsies, most frequently involving the renal, splenic, coronary, or cerebral circulation. Emboli and immune complex deposition contribute to the extracardiac manifestations of IE and may involve virtually any organ system. When large emboli occlude major vessels, fungal endocarditis, marantic endocarditis, or an intracardiac myxoma should be suspected.

Kidney. Three pathologic processes may be found in the kidney in IE: abscess, infarction, or glomerulonephritis. Abscesses are infrequent, but infarctions have been seen in 56 percent of the autopsy cases.[1] The kidney is usually normal in size but may be slightly swollen, and petechiae may be found in the capsule. When renal biopsies are done during active IE, the renal architecture is abnormal in *all* cases,[141] even in the absence of clinical or biochemical evidence of renal disease. "Focal" glomerulonephritis is found in 48–88 percent of the cases but is rare in acute IE. It is a focal, local, and segmental process characterized by endothelial and mesangial proliferation, hemorrhage, neutrophilic infiltration, fibrinoid necrosis, crescent formation, and healing by fibrosis. Diffuse glomerulonephritis is found in 17–80 percent of the cases and consists of generalized cellular hyperplasia in all glomerular tufts. A less common condition called *membranoproliferative glomerulonephritis* is associated with endocarditis due to *Streptococcus epidermidis* and characterized by marked mesangial proliferation and by splitting of the glomerular basement membrane. Renal interstitial cellular infiltration is common.[141]

Of the patients with IE, 10–15 percent will exhibit an immune complex glomerulonephritis similar to that seen in lupus erythematosus.[130,131,135,136] The evidence for immune complex deposition rather than recurrent embolic phenomenon as the primary pathogenic mechanism includes the following:

1. Bacteria are rarely if ever seen in the lesions.
2. Glomerulonephritis occurs with right-sided IE.
3. Glomerulonephritis is rare in acute IE even though large, friable vegetations result in widespread metastatic abscess formation.
4. Immunofluorescent staining with anti-immunoglobulin antibody reveals the typical lumpy-bumpy distribution seen in other forms of immune complex nephritis.
5. In diffuse glomerulonephritis, subepithelial electron-dense deposits are seen by electron microscopy, with IgG, IgM, IgA, and/or complement demonstrated in these deposits by immunofluorescence.
6. Specific antibacterial antibody can be eluted from the lesions.[131]
7. Antiglomerular basement membrane antibody has been found in a single case of IE with nephritis.
8. The glomerulonephritis is often accompanied by hypocomplementemia and a positive rheumatoid factor in serum.
9. All these abnormalities usually resolve with successful antimicrobial therapy as the concentration of circulating immune complexes declines.

Mycotic Aneurysms. Mycotic aneurysms usually develop during active IE but are occasionally detected months or years after successful treatment. They are more common with viridans streptococcal infections and are found in 10–15 percent of the autopsied cases. They may arise by any of the following mechanisms: *(1)* direct bacterial invasion of the arterial wall with subsequent abscess formation and/or rupture, *(2)* septic or bland embolic occlusion of the vasa vasorum, or *(3)* immune complex deposition with resultant injury to the arterial wall. The aneurysms tend to occur at bifurcation points. They are found in the cerebral vessels (primarily the peripheral branches of the middle cerebral artery), but they also occur in the abdominal aorta, sinus of Valsalva, a ligated patent ductus arteriosus, and the splenic, coronary, pulmonary, and superior mesenteric arteries. Myoctic aneurysms are usually clinically silent until rupture occurs; consequently, their true incidence in active IE is unknown.[142]

Central Nervous System.   Cerebral emboli occur in at least one-third of all cases[47] and most commonly affect the middle cerebral artery and its branches. Three percent of the cerebral emboli from all causes are secondary to IE. Cerebral infarction, arteritis, abscesses, mycotic aneurysms, intracerebral or subarachnoid hemorrhage, encephalomalacia, cerebritis, and meningitis have all been reported.[143] Hemorrhagic transformation of an ischemic infarct due to septic emboli is the most frequent mechanism leading to fatal intracerebral hemorrhage during IE.[144] True acute purulent meningitis is rare except in pneumococcal endocarditis, but multiple microabscesses (cerebritis) are relatively common in acute staphylococcal endocarditis.

Spleen.   Splenic infarctions have been reported in 44 percent of the autopsy cases but are rarely detected clinically.[47] Abscess formation and rupture have been described but are uncommon. Splenic enlargement is common, and virtually all cases are associated with hyperplasia of the lymphoid follicles, an increase in secondary follicles, proliferation of reticuloendothelial cells, and scattered focal necrosis.[137]

Lung.   When right-sided IE is present, pulmonary emboli with or without infarction, acute pneumonia, pleural effusion, or empyema are common and are due to septic or bland emboli.

Skin.   Petechiae are found in 20–40 percent of the cases (Fig. 2) (see below). Osler nodes microscopically consist of arteriolar intimal proliferation with extension to venules and capillaries and may be accompanied by thrombosis and necrosis. A diffuse perivascular infiltrate consisting of neutrophils and monocytes surrounds the dermal vessels. Immune complexes have been demonstrated in the dermal vessels. Janeway lesions consist of bacteria, neutrophilic infiltration, necrosis, and subcutaneous hemorrhage (Fig. 3). Janeway lesions are due to septic emboli and reveal subcutaneous abscesses on histologic examination.[145]

Eye.   "Roth spots" consist microscopically of lymphocytes surrounded by edema and hemorrhage in the nerve fiber layer of the retina (Fig. 4).[146]

Clinical Manifestations

The interval between an event likely to produce bacteremia (e.g., dental extraction) and the onset of symptoms of IE, contrary to older estimates, is actually quite short. The so-called "incubation period" in 84 percent of 76 cases of streptococcal endocarditis was less than 2 weeks.[147] However, the time from the onset of symptoms to diagnosis in the subacute form of IE is quite long, with a median interval of approximately 5 weeks. Symptom duration of cases managed in community hospitals is often shorter than in patients referred to a tertiary care center.[4]

The symptoms and signs (Table 3) are protean, and essentially any organ system may be involved. Four processes contribute

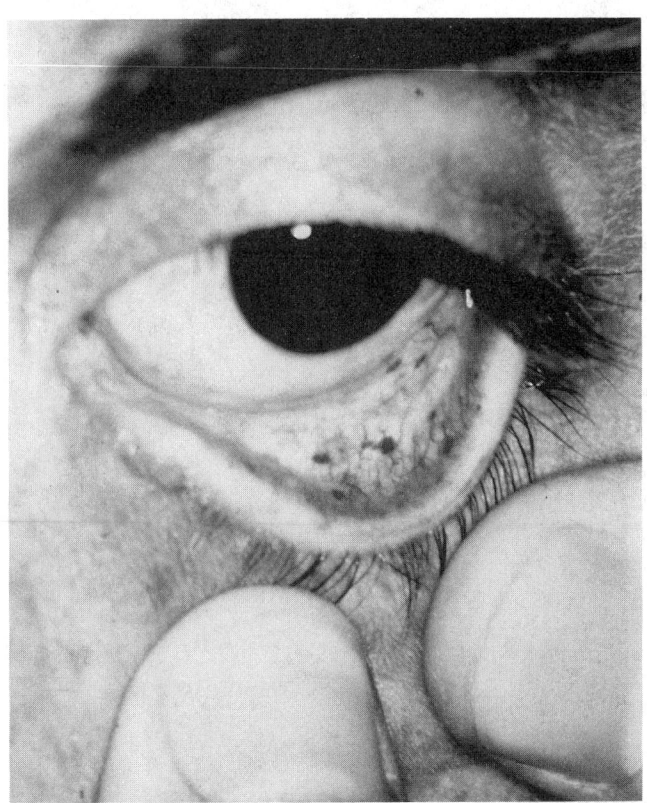

FIG. 2.   Conjunctival petechiae in a patient with bacterial endocarditis.

to the clinical picture[47]: *(1)* the infectious process on the valve, including the local intracardiac complications; *(2)* bland or septic embolization to virtually any organ; *(3)* constant bacteremia, often with metastatic foci of infection; and *(4)* circulating immune complexes and other immunopathologic factors.[43–47,148,149] As a result, the clinical presentation of patients with IE is highly variable and the differential diagnosis often broad.[150]

Fever is common but may be absent (5 percent of the cases), especially in the setting of congestive heart failure (CHF), renal failure, a terminal disease, old age,[151] or previous antibiotic therapy. The fever pattern is usually remittent, and the patient's temperature rarely exceeds 103°F except in acute IE.[148] Persistent fever during antimicrobial therapy of IE is relatively infrequent but may be an ominous sign. In a review[152] of 123 patients with IE managed in Cleveland from 1972 to 1984, approximately one-half became afebrile within 3 days of the initiation of antibiotics; approximately 75 percent and approximately 90 percent had defervesced after 1 and 2 weeks of treatment, respectively. Prolonged fever (≥2 weeks) is associated with specific etiologic agents (*Staphylococcus aureus,* gram-negative bacilli, fungi), culture-negative endocarditis, but, perhaps more importantly, microvascular phenomena, embolization of major vessels, intracardiac (e.g., myocardial abscess) or peripheral complications, tissue infarction, a need for cardiac surgery, and a higher mortality rate.[152,153] Pulmonary emboli (bland), drugs, and nosocomial infection are also causes of prolonged fever in this patient population.

Nonspecific symptoms such as anorexia, weight loss, malaise, fatigue, chills, weakness, nausea, vomiting, and night sweats are common, especially in subacute cases.[20] These nonspecific symptoms often result in an incorrect diagnosis of malignancy, collagen vascular disease, tuberculosis, or other chronic diseases.

Heart murmurs occur in over 85 percent of the cases but may be absent with right-sided or mural infection. The classic

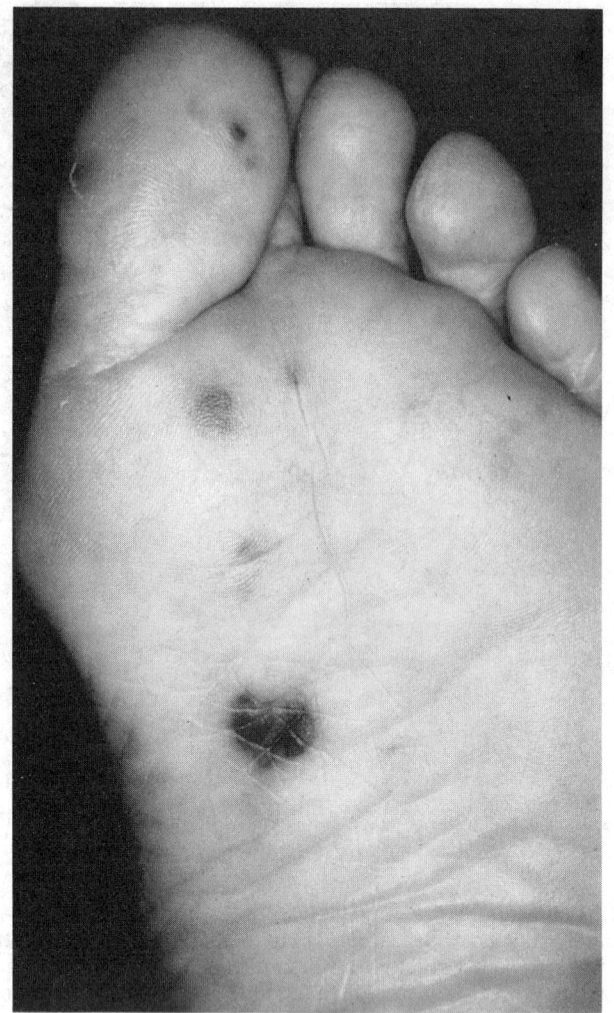

FIG. 3. Janeway lesions in a patient with *Staphylococcus aureus* endocarditis. (From Sande et al.,[676] with permission.)

TABLE 3. Clinical Manifestations of Infective Endocarditis

Symptoms	Percentage	Physical Findings	Percentage
Fever	80	Fever	90
Chills	40	Heart murmur	85
Weakness	40	Changing murmur	5–10
Dyspnea	40	New murmur	3–5
Sweats	25	Embolic phenomenon	>50
Anorexia	25	Skin manifestations	18–50
Weight loss	25	Osler nodes	10–23
Malaise	25	Splinter hemorrhages	15
Cough	25	Petechiae	20–40
Skin lesions	20	Janeway lesion	<10
Stroke	20	Splenomegaly	20–57
Nausea/vomiting	20	Septic complications	20
Headache	20	(pneumonia,	
Myalgia/arthralgia	15	meningitis, etc.)	
Edema	15	Mycotic aneurysms	20
Chest pain	15	Clubbing	12–52
Abdominal pain	15	Retinal lesion	2–10
Delirium/coma	10–15	Signs of renal failure	10–5
Hemoptysis	10		
Back pain	10		

(Data from refs. 1, 20, 31, 148.)

"changing murmur" and the development of a new murmur (usually aortic insufficiency) are uncommon and occur in 5–10 percent and in 3–5 percent of the cases, respectively. When present, these are diagnostically useful signs and usually complicate acute staphylococcal disease. New or changing murmurs are less common in the elderly and often lead to diagnostic confusion.[151,154] Over 90 percent of patients who demonstrate a new regurgitant murmur will develop CHF. The incidence of CHF appears to be increasing (approximately 25 percent in 1966 and 67 percent in 1972)[20] and is now the leading cause of death in IE. Pericarditis is rare but, when present, is usually accompanied by myocardial abscess formation as a complication of staphylococcal infection. Although valvular regurgitation is the most important hemodynamic complication of IE, hemodynamically significant valvular obstruction requiring surgery may occur rarely, even without a prior history of valvular stenosis.[155]

The classic peripheral manifestations are found in up to one-half of the cases, but the prevalence has decreased in recent years. Clubbing is present in 10–20 percent, especially if the disease is of long duration, and may recede with therapy. The complete syndrome of hypertrophic osteoarthropathy is rare. Splinter hemorrhages are linear red to brown streaks in the fingernails or toenails and are commonly found in IE. They are a nonspecific finding and are often seen in the elderly or in people experiencing occupation-related trauma. These lesions are most suggestive of IE when located proximally in the nailbed. Petechiae are found in 20–40 percent of the cases, particularly after a prolonged course, and usually appear in crops on the conjunctivae (Fig. 2), buccal mucosa, palate, and extremities. These lesions are initially red and nonblanching but become brown and barely visible in 2–3 days. Petechiae may result from either local vasculitis or emboli. Osler nodes are small, painful, nodular lesions usually found in the pads of fingers or toes and occasionally in the thenar eminence. They are 2–15 mm in size and are frequently multiple and evanescent, disappearing in hours to days. Osler nodes are rare in acute cases of IE but occur in 10–25 percent of all the cases. They are not specific for IE since they may be seen in systemic lupus erythematosus, marantic endocarditis, hemolytic anemia, and gonococcal infections and in extremities with cannulated radial arteries. Janeway lesions (Fig. 3) are hemorrhagic, macular, painless plaques with a predilection for the palms or soles. They persist for several days and are thought to be embolic in origin and occur with greater

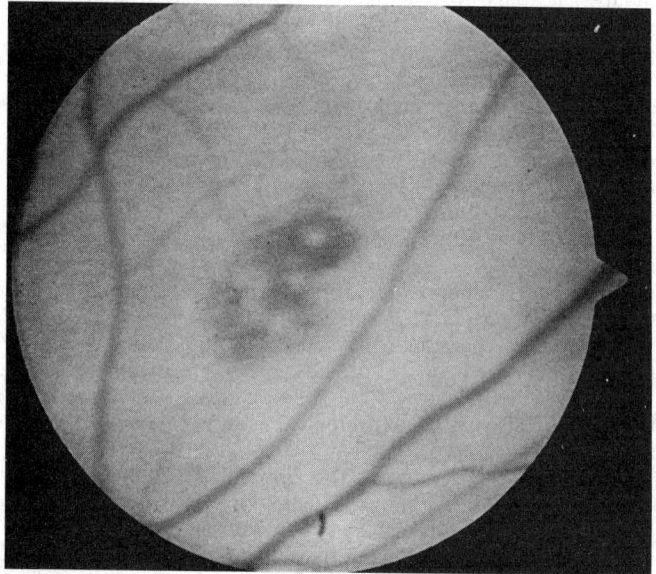

FIG. 4. Retina from a patient with viridans streptococcal endocarditis showing Roth spots. (From Sande et al.,[676] with permission.)

frequency in staphylococcal endocarditis. Roth spots (Fig. 4) are oval, pale, retinal lesions surrounded by hemorrhage and are usually located near the optic disk. They occur in less than 5 percent of the cases of IE and may also be found in anemia, leukemia, and connective tissue disorders such as systemic lupus erythematosus.

Splenomegaly has been reported in 25–60 percent of all the cases and is more common in patients with endocarditis of prolonged duration. The incidence of splenomegaly appears to be progressively decreasing since the advent of antibiotics. Splenic septic emboli are common during IE, but localized findings may be absent in approximately 90 percent of patients with this complication.[156] Abdominal computed tomography is highly sensitive and should be employed in cases with prolonged fever or sepsis.

Musculoskeletal manifestations are common in IE. In a review of 192 cases,[157] 44 percent of the patients had musculoskeletal symptoms. These symptoms usually occurred early in the disease and were the only initial complaint in 15 percent of the cases. They included proximal oligo- or monoarticular arthralgias (38 percent), lower extremity mono- or oligoarticular arthritis (31 percent), low back pain (23 percent), and diffuse myalgias (19 percent). The back pain may be severe, limiting movement, and the initial complaint in 5–10 percent of cases.[10] These findings may mimic rheumatic disease and result in a diagnostic delay.

Major embolic episodes, as a group, are second only to congestive heart failure as a complication of IE and occur in at least one-third of cases. Splenic artery emboli (as above) with infarction may result in left upper quadrant abdominal pain with radiation to the left shoulder, a splenic or pleural rub, or a left pleural effusion. Renal infarctions may be associated with microscopic or gross hematura, but renal failure, hypertension, and edema are uncommon. Retinal artery emboli are rare (fewer than 2 percent of the cases) and may be manifested by a sudden complete loss of vision. A panophthalmitis has been reported with pneumococcal endocarditis. Pulmonary emboli arising from right-sided endocarditis is a common feature in narcotic addicts (see below). Coronary artery emboli usually arise from the aortic valve and may cause myocarditis with arrythmias or myocardial infarction. This finding may be overlooked, especially given the time constraints of interventions such as thrombolytic therapy or angioplasty during acute myocardial infarction resulting in serious complications in patients with IE presenting as an acute myocardial infarction.[158] Major vessel emboli (femoral, brachial, popliteal, or radial arteries) are more frequent in fungal endocarditis.

Neurologic manifestations occur in 20–40 percent of the cases and may dominate the clinical picture, especially in staphylococcal endocarditis. A sudden neurologic event in a young person should suggest IE. Major cerebral emboli afflict 10–30 percent of the patients and may result in hemiplegia, sensory loss, ataxia, aphasia, or an alteration in mental status.[143,159] Of those patients with neurologic complications, up to 50 percent present with these signs and symptoms as the heralding features of their illness.[160,161] The development of clinical neurologic deterioration during IE is associated with a two- to fourfold increase in mortality rate for the implicated etiologic microbe.[161] Mycotic aneurysms of the cerebral circulation occur in 2–10 percent of the cases. They are usually single, small, and peripheral and may lead to devastating subarachnoid hemorrhage. Other features include seizures, severe headache, visual changes, choreoathetoid movements, mononeuropathy, and cranial nerve palsies. A toxic encephalopathy with symptoms ranging from a mild change in personality to frank psychosis may occur, especially in elderly patients.

Patients with IE may have symptoms of uremia. In the preantibiotic era, renal failure developed in 25–35 percent of the cases, but presently fewer than 10 percent are affected. When uremia does develop, diffuse glomerulonephritis with hypocomplementia is usually found, but focal glomerulonephritis has also been implicated. Renal failure is more common with long-standing disease but usually subsides with appropriate antimicrobial treatment alone. IE may be confused with thrombotic thrombocytopenic purpura when neurologic signs, fever, renal failure, anemia, and thrombocytopenia are present.[162]

Infective Endocarditis in Drug Addicts. Acute infection accounts for approximately 60 percent of hospital admissions among intravenous drug abusers; IE is implicated in 5–8 percent of these episodes.[163] It has proved difficult to predict accurately the presence of IE in the febrile drug addict,[164] especially from physical examination findings alone,[165] although cocaine use by the intravenous drug user should heighten the suspicion of IE.[166] Cocaine was strongly associated with the presence of IE in 102 intravenous drug users in San Francisco when analyzed by logistic regression analysis in comparison with febrile addicts from other causes. The most reliable predictors of IE in febrile parenteral drug users are visualization of vegetations by echocardiography and the presence of embolic phenomena.[165] Although many of the aforementioned clinical manifestations are seen in addicts with endocarditis, several distinctions are worthy of emphasis. In this group of patients, two-thirds have no clinical evidence of underlying heart disease, and there is a predilection for the infection to affect the tricuspid valve. Only 35 percent of addicts ultimately proven to have IE demonstrate heart murmurs on admission.[163] The frequency of valvular involvement is as follows: tricuspid alone or in combination with others, 52.2 percent; aortic alone, 18.5 percent; mitral alone, 10.8 percent; and aortic plus mitral, 12.5 percent,[2] although left-sided involvement has been more frequent in some series.[167] Of these patients with tricuspid valve infection, 30 percent have pleuritic chest pain, pulmonary findings may dominate the clinical picture, and the chest roentgenogram will document abnormalities (infiltrates, effusion, and so forth) in 75–85 percent of patients.[168] Roentgenographic evidence of septic pulmonary emboli is eventually present in 87 percent of cases.[169] Signs of tricuspid insufficiency (gallop rhythm, systolic regurgitant murmur louder with inspiration, large V waves, or a pulsatile liver) are present in only one-third of the cases. Most of these patients are 20–40 years old (80 percent), and men predominate 4–6:1. The course of acute staphylococcal endocarditis in the addict tends to be less severe than in nonaddicts,[168] although this may not be true in AIDS patients. Almost two-thirds of these patients have extravalvular sites of infection that are helpful in the diagnosis.[168–170]

Laboratory Findings

Hematologic parameters are often abnormal in IE, but none are diagnostic. Anemia is nearly always present (70–90 percent of the cases) and has the characteristics of the anemia of chronic disease with normochromic, normocytic indices, a low serum iron concentration, and a low iron-binding capacity. The anemia tends to worsen with the duration of the illness. Thrombocytopenia occurs in 5–15 percent of the cases but is common in neonatal IE. Leukocytosis is present in 20–30 percent of cases but is rare in the subacute variety, whereas counts of 15,000–25,000/mm^3 are not uncommon in acute IE. The differential count is usually normal, but there may be a slight shift to the left. Leukopenia is uncommon (5–15 percent) and, when present, is usually associated with splenomegaly. Large mononuclear cells (histiocytes) can be detected in the peripheral blood in approximately 25 percent of the patients, but the yield is higher in blood taken from an earlobe puncture. This finding is nonspecific, since similar cells have been found in malaria, typhus, typhoid fever, and tuberculosis.

The erythrocyte sedimentation rate (ESR) is nearly always (90–100 percent) elevated, with a mean value of 57 mm/hr found in one large series.[20] In the absence of renal failure, congestive heart failure, or disseminated intravascular coagulation, a normal ESR is evidence against a diagnosis of IE. Hypergammaglobulinemia is detected in 20–30 percent of the cases and may be accompanied by a plasmacytosis in the bone marrow aspirate. A positive rheumatoid factor is found in 40–50 percent of the cases, especially when the duration of the illness is greater than 6 weeks.[122] Hypocomplementemia (5–15 percent) parallels the incidence of abnormal renal function test results (elevated creatinine level in 5–15 percent). A false-positive Venereal Disease Research Laboratory (VDRL) test is uncommon (0.2 percent). Lyme serologic tests may be positive in patients with IE living in endemic areas for Lyme disease and may lead to diagnostic delay.[171]

The urinalysis is frequently abnormal; proteinuria occurs in 50–65 percent of the cases and microscopic hematuria in 30–60 percent. Red cell casts may be seen in as many as 12 percent of the cases[20]; gross hematuria, pyuria, white cell casts, and bacteriuria may also be found.

Circulating immune complexes can be detected in most cases of IE but are also found in 32 percent of the patients with septicemia but without endocarditis, in 10 percent of the healthy controls, and in 40 percent of noninfected narcotic addicts.[122] However, levels greater than 100 μg of aggregated human γ-globulin equivalent per milliliter were found only in IE (35 percent of the cases). Detection of high levels of immune complexes may be useful in the diagnosis of right-sided IE in narcotic addicts or in culture-negative cases. In addition, since the levels fall with appropriate treatment, serial measurement of immune complexes may assist in management of the disease.[135,136] Mixed-type cryoglobulins are detectable in 84–95 percent of the patients with IE but are also a nonspecific finding. Although nonspecific and virtually always elevated in IE, serial determination of the serum C-reactive protein concentration may be useful to monitor therapy and detect intercurrent complications or infections.[172]

The detection of vegetations by ^{67}Ga myocardial imaging initially appeared to be a useful diagnostic tool. Of 11 patients in one study,[173] 7 had infected vegetations localized by scans including one culture-negative case that was confirmed at autopsy. Further studies are needed to determine the potential value of noninvasive imaging of cardiac vegetations by using a radiolabeled compound, for example, ^{99m}Tc-labeled antibacterial antibody[174] or ^{111}In-labeled platelets,[175] because both have shown promise in experimental endocarditis. At present, these techniques must be considered investigational. Radiographic techniques are occasionally useful in the diagnosis or in decisions regarding surgical intervention. For example, computed tomography (CT) of the abdomen detected splenic infarcts in 6 of 25 (24 percent) consecutive patients with IE in one series[176]: 2 of 6 were asymptomatic.

The blood culture is the single most important laboratory test performed in a diagnostic work-up for IE. The bacteremia is usually continuous and low grade (80 percent of the cases have less than 100 cfu/ml of blood).[177] In approximately two-thirds of the cases, all the blood cultures drawn will be positive.[20] When bacteremia is present, the first two blood cultures will yield the etiologic agent more than 90 percent of the time. In a review of 206 cases of IE seen over a 15-year period at The New York Hospital,[178] 95 percent of the blood cultures were positive. In streptococcal endocarditis, the first blood culture was positive in 96 percent of cases, and one of the first two cultures was positive in 98 percent. When antibiotics had been administered in the previous 2 weeks, the rate of positive cultures declined from 97 to 91 percent ($p < 0.02$). The influence of outpatient antibiotic administration on blood culture positivity was more significant in another retrospective analysis[179]; 64 percent of 88 cultures were positive in 17 patients receiving antibiotics before hospitalization vs. 100 percent in 15 patients without antibiotic exposure. In nonstreptococcal endocarditis, the first blood culture was positive in 86 percent of the cases

and when two cultures were taken, in 100 percent. Most blood cultures contained only a few organisms; over 50 percent of the cultures contained 1–30 bacteria/ml. Only 17 percent of the cultures yielded more than 100 bacteria/ml. The bacteremia was also constant with little variation in quantitative culture determinations in any individual patient. The sensitivity of blood cultures for the detection of streptococci is particularly susceptible to prior antibiotic therapy and/or the media employed.[180]

On the basis of these studies, the following procedures for culturing blood are recommended. At least three blood culture sets (no more than two bottles per venipuncture) should be obtained in the first 24 hours. More cultures may be necessary if the patient has received antibiotics in the preceding 2 weeks. At least 10 ml of blood (when feasible) should be injected into both trypticase soy (or brain-heart infusion) and thioglycollate broth.[181,182] Trypticase soy bottles should be transiently "vented." Pour plates may be made at the bedside for an estimate of the degree of bacteremia. Supplementation with 15% sucrose (in an attempt to isolate cell wall-deficient forms) or the use of prereduced anaerobic media is unrewarding.[183] The newer commercial media are also effective, but comparative data are few. In general, culture of arterial blood offers no advantage over venous blood. Inspection for macroscopic growth should be performed daily and routine subcultures done on days 1 and 3. The cultures should be held for at least 3 weeks. When gram-positive cocci grow on the initial isolation but fail to grow on subculture, nutritionally variant (thiol-dependent) streptococci should be suspected.[184] In this event, subculture should be onto media supplemented with either 0.05%–0.1% L-cysteine or 0.001% pyridoxal phosphate.

Intraleukocytic bacteria have been visualized in peripheral blood in approximately 50 percent of the cases[185] by a simple "monolayer" technique. This may be helpful in culture-negative cases or when patients have been receiving antibiotics.[186]

Ribitol teichoic acids are major constituents of the cell wall of staphylococci. Gel diffusion and counterimmunoelectrophoresis techniques have been used to detect teichoic acid antibodies in the serum of patients suspected of having *Staphylococcus aureus* endocarditis. Teichoic acid antibodies can be detected by counterimmunoelectrophoresis in over 95 percent of the patients,[187] but the rate of false-positive tests may exceed 10 percent. Serial titrations of serum with the double-agar diffusion technique can be used to detect the low titers found in some healthy people. Antibody titers of 1:4 or more are indicative of disseminated staphylococcal disease (endocarditis, multiple metastatic abscesses, or hematogenous osteomyelitis). Since these conditions all require prolonged antimicrobial therapy, this test may be of practical value if the results are positive. The value of a negative result is controversial; some authorities suggest that a short course of antimicrobial therapy is justified in this instance,[188] while others find a negative test response helpful only if all clinical signs are indicative of "benign" (i.e., superficial) staphylococcal bacteremia.[189] This issue is unresolved; we view this test as confirmatory of clinical suspicions only. The detection of other circulating staphylococcal antigens (e.g., capsular polysaccharide by enzyme-linked immunosorbent assay [ELISA]) has been documented in experimental animal models of IE,[190] but experience in humans in scant. Detection of antibodies against *Staphylococcus aureus* capsular polysaccharide types 5 and 8 (responsible for approximately 75 percent of clinical isolates; see above), especially in conjunction with serotyping of the patient's isolate, appears promising for the diagnosis of IE due to this organism. In one series,[191] positive ELISA results were recorded as follows: 7 of 8 with *Staphylococcus aureus* endocarditis, 0 of 28 nonendocarditis bacteremia patients, 1 of 12 non-*Staphylococcus aureus* endocarditis cases, and in 3 of 37 febrile controls. Further testing appears warranted.

Special Diagnostic Tests.   Special diagnostic tests are not routinely used (with the exception of echocardiography) in all cases of IE but may be useful in two situations: *(1)* in the diagnostic approach to culture-negative IE and *(2)* in decisions about surgical intervention during active infection.

The incidence of so-called blood culture-negative endocarditis has varied from 2.5 to 31 percent in published series.[192,193] If the patients have not received previous antibiotic therapy and the blood cultures are obtained as outlined, these cases should represent fewer than 5 percent of the total.[3] Some of the aforementioned tests (rheumatoid factor, teichoic acid antibodies, earlobe histiocytes, monolayer technique for intraleukocytic bacteria) may be helpful in identifying such cases, but other procedures are often necessary. If the patient has received antibiotics, blood cultures in hypertonic media may allow detection of cell wall-defective organisms. Supplementation of media with vitamin B_6 or with cysteine may assist the recovery of nutritionally variant streptococci. The lysis-centrifugation blood culture technique assists in the detection of staphylococci[194] and fungi, but nutritionally variant streptococci do not survive this procedure, and yields of pneumococci and anaerobes are decreased.[195] Routine use of this technique is not indicated, but it may be helpful in suspected culture-negative cases of IE. Since some anaerobes, *Brucella* spp., and members of the HACEK group (see below) are slow-growing organisms, holding cultures for 4 weeks may increase the recovery rate. Removal of antibiotics from blood with a resin device may facilitate microbial recovery in patients previously on antimicrobial agents. Cultures of bone marrow or urine may rarely be positive when blood cultures are negative. Serologic studies are necessary for the diagnosis of Q fever or murine typhus.[196] Psittacosis endocarditis is usually diagnosed with serologic methods but one recent case[197] yielded positive blood and pharyngeal cultures. Special culture techniques (e.g., for *Legionella* spp.[198]) are indicated in patients with suspected prosthetic valve endocarditis when initial cultures are "negative" (Chapter 60). Other tests to exclude collagen vascular diseases are usually necessary in patients undergoing evaluation for culture-negative, native-valve IE.[199]

Blood cultures are negative in over 50 percent of the cases of fungal endocarditis.[200] The lysis-centrifugation method of blood culture is also useful in detecting fungi. This disease is increasing in frequency and usually affects narcotic addicts, patients with prosthetic valves, or hospitalized patients receiving antibiotics and/or hyperalimentation. The Castaneda principle (a culture of blood in a bottle containing both agar and liquid broth) has been shown to increase the yield of fungal cultures.[183] Blastospores and pseudohyphae have been found in Wright-stained peripheral blood in at least one case of *Candida*-induced endocarditis.[201] Various serologic procedures have been used in an attempt to substantiate a diagnosis of fungal endocarditis. Tests for the determination of antifungal antibody are poorly standardized, variably sensitive, often nonspecific, and difficult to interpret.[202] In a rabbit model of *Candida*-induced endocarditis, both precipitating and agglutinating antibodies were detected after 12 days of active infection, and titers rose progressively until death of the animals.[203] In contrast, animals without endocarditis developed only a transient rise in antibody titers after a single intravenous injection of viable *Candida albicans*. Tests for mannan antigenemia (a constituent of the cell wall of *Candida*) or enolase by hemagglutination inhibition or by the ELISA method[204,205] have been reported as helpful in the diagnosis of disseminated candidiasis. In addition, a reliable radioimmunoassay for the detection of *Aspergillus* antigenemia is currently under investigation. When embolism to major vessels occurs, an embolectomy should be performed, and the material should be examined by both special fungal stains and culture. Identification of the fungus by either technique is diagnostic of fungal endocarditis even when blood cultures are sterile.

The use of echocardiography in the diagnosis of IE was first reported in 1973.[206] Echocardiograms have correctly identified vegetations on all valves. Most reports have focused on left-

sided disease. The sensitivity and specificity of this technique is uncertain; however, two studies correctly identified 33 of 52 vegetations documented surgically or at autopsy.[207,208] The characteristic finding is a shaggy dense band of irregular echoes in a nonuniform distribution on one or more leaflets with full unrestricted motion of the valve. The smallest vegetation detected was approximately 2 mm, but the acoustic impedance of the mass relative to the surrounding structures is a more important factor than size in identifying the vegetation. The use of two-dimensional cross-sectional real-time techniques improves the diagnostic accuracy over M-mode methods.[209] If the vegetation is calcified (which may occur early and independent of the healing process), the sensitivity of echocardiography may be increased. Echocardiography has correctly localized vegetations in culture-negative cases. Echocardiography may be of special value in the detection of the large friable vegetations characteristic of fungal endocarditis. However, use of M-mode or two-dimensional transthoracic techniques with prosthetic heart valves has been disappointing because of the difficulty in resolution around the prosthetic device. Many reports have appeared[210] that have evaluated the role of transthoracic echocardiography in the diagnosis and management of suspected IE and were summarized in cogent analyses.[211,212] These studies suggest the following: *(1)* variable sensitivity for the detection of vegetations (<50 to >90 percent positive), and therefore a negative study does not exclude IE; *(2)* false-positive results are extremely rare; *(3)* only technically adequate studies are really valuable, a characteristic heavily dependent on the experience of the person performing the examination; *(4)* echocardiography is extremely valuable in assessing local complications of IE, especially surrounding the aortic valve; and *(5)* patients with a "vegetation" identified by echocardiography are at an increased risk for subsequent systemic emboli, congestive heart failure, the need for emergency surgery, and death, especially with aortic valve involvement. This apparent influence on prognosis has hastened earlier surgery in some cases,[213] but this point remains controversial.[212,214] A positive echocardiogram in a patient with IE should serve as an adjunctive piece of evidence, together with clinical parameters, in indicating surgical intervention. In one analysis from the Mayo Clinic,[215] emboli were not statistically more common in patients with left-sided native valve IE and echocardiographically documented vegetatious within 72 hours of beginning antimicrobial therapy when compared to those without vegetatious by transthoracic techniques. The occurrence of emboli correlated with the infecting microorganism, being more common in IE due to viridans streptococci than *Staphylococcus aureus* disease. Visualization of vegetations by echocardiography is not sufficient alone to prompt early surgery.[212,216] Serial echocardiograms often reveal the persistence of vegetations after successful therapy, but sequential studies may be useful in the timing of surgical intervention. Short-term changes in vegetation size during therapy do not correlate well with clinical outcome.[217] However, a new technique, digital image processing of two-dimensional echocardiograms, may differentiate active from healed lesions.[218] If substantiated, this method may be useful in "culture-negative" cases (particularly with suspected recurrent IE) or when the response to therapy is suboptimal or inconclusive.

Transesophageal echocardiography (TEE) is a relatively new technique[212] that has altered the diagnostic approach to some patients with suspected IE.[219–221] It utilizes a 5-mHz phased array transducer with Doppler and color flow encoding capabilities mounted on the tip of a flexible endoscope. Biplane (horizontal and longitudinal) imaging is improved over transthoracic echocardiography because of *(1)* better spatial resolution with a higher frequency transducer; *(2)* lack of acoustic interference from the lungs, chest wall, and so forth; and *(3)* proximity to posterior structures (e.g., mitral valve, left atrium, interatrial septum, descending aorta).[221] Transesophageal echocardiography has proven useful in a wide variety of clinical situations, including detection of possible sources of emboli, diagnosis of thoracic aortic dissection, detection of prosthetic valve dysfunction, and evaluation of IE.[212,219–221]

Transesophageal echocardiography is more sensitive than conventional transthoracic echocardiography in the detection of intracardiac vegetations (approximately 95 percent and 60–65 percent, respectively), particularly in the setting of prosthetic valves (see Ch. 59). For example,[222] in one report of 96 patients with IE, the sensitivity of TEE was 100 vs. 63 percent, for the transthoracic approach, with identical specificity (98 percent). The advantage of TEE was particularly evident for vegetations less than 10 mm in diameter. In another study,[223] vegetations were detected by TEE in 82 vs. 69 percent for transthoracic echocardiography. Although a negative TEE does not exclude IE,[219–221,224] the procedure should be considered in patients with suspected IE and a negative transthoracic study. Transesophageal echocardiography has also become the procedure of current choice for the detection of perivalvular extension of infection in patients with IE.[225,226] For example, Daniel et al.[226] reported diagnostic sensitivity of 87 and specificity of 95 percent for TEE for detection of IE-related abscess vs. 28 and 99 percent for transthoracic echocardiography. TEE should be performed (unless contraindicated, e.g., by significant esophageal disease) in all IE patients with a complicated course when perivalvular extension is suspected. Magnetic resonance imaging also appears promising for the detection of these complications,[225] but clinical experience is limited. TEE is not a screening or noninvasive procedure, but is generally safe[227] in experienced hands, and it may alter management in selected patients with proven or suspected IE.

In conjunction with the physical examination, phonocardiography, and electrocardiography, the echocardiogram may play an important role in assessing the severity of acute aortic insufficiency in cases of active IE.[228] In this setting, classic physical findings such as a wide pulse pressure and bounding pulses are often absent; however, there is usually a reduction in intensity of the first heart sound, and Austin Flint murmurs may be audible. The chest roentgenogram and electrocardiogram may be normal. The degree of mitral valve preclosure (as determined by echocardiography) correlates with the elevation in left ventricular end-diastolic pressure. If this event occurs before the Q wave on the electrocardiogram, rapid surgical intervention is recommended.

Cardiac catheterization with quantitative blood cultures proximal and distal to suspected sites of infection has been useful in the localization of vegetations in both right-sided and left-sided IE.[229] Multiple specimens from identical sites are necessary, since minor fluctuations in bacteremia do occur. However, this technique is potentially dangerous and has been associated with rapid clinical deterioration when used in the setting of acute aortic insufficiency complicated by progressive congestive heart failure.[229] Cardiac catheterization does provide valuable hemodynamic and anatomic information in patients with IE when considering surgical intervention.[170] Properly performed, the procedure is safe, as demonstrated by the lack of postcatheterization emboli or hemodynamic deterioration in 35 consecutive patients in one series.[230]

Cineangiography is the definitive procedure in determining the anatomic alterations resulting from the infection. It is of value in determining the degree of aortic regurgitation, in assessing the contribution of left ventricular dysfunction in congestive heart failure, in visualizing ventricular and aortic aneurysms, and in gauging the patency of the coronary arteries. Magnetic resonance imaging also appears promising for detection of perivalvular infection.[225] This information may be critically important in determining a surgical approach, especially if multivalvular involvement is documented. The additional information gained from obtaining right- and left-heart pressures with complete cardiac catheterization are not useful in decisions on therapy in acute IE.[229] Furthermore, intraoperative TEE imaging

TABLE 4. Proposed New Criteria for Diagnosis of IE

Definite infective endocarditis
  Pathologic criteria
    Microorganisms: demonstrated by culture *or* histology in a vegetation, or in a vegetation that has embolized, or in an intracardiac abscess, *or*
    Pathologic lesions: vegetation or intracardiac abscess present, confirmed by histology showing active endocarditis
  Clinical criteria (using specific definitions for these terms as listed in Table 5)
    2 major criteria, *or*
    1 major and 3 minor criteria, *or*
    5 minor criteria
Possible infective endocarditis: findings consistent with infective endocarditis that fall short of *Definitive*, but not *Rejected*
Rejected
  Firm alternate diagnosis explaining evidence of infective endocarditis, *or*
  Resolution of endocarditis syndrome, with antibiotic therapy for 4 days or less, *or*
  No pathologic evidence of IE at surgery or autopsy, after antibiotic therapy for 4 days or less

(Adapted from Durack et al.,[231] with permission.)

TABLE 5. Terminology Used in the Proposed New Criteria for IE

Major criteria
  Positive blood culture for infective endocarditis
    Typical microorganism for infective endocarditis from 2 separate blood cultures
      Viridans streptococci, *S. bovis*, HACEK group, *or*
      Community-acquired *S. aureus* or enterococci, in the absence of a primary focus, *or*
    Persistently positive blood culture, defined as microorganism consistent with infective endocarditis from
      Blood cultures drawn more than 12 hours apart, *or*
      All of 3, or majority of 4 or more separate blood cultures, with first and last drawn at least 1 hour apart
  Evidence of endocardial involvement
    Positive echocardiogram for infective endocarditis
      Oscillating intracardiac mass on valve or supporting structures or in the path of regurgitant jets, or on iatrogenic devices, in the absence of an alternative anatomic explanation, *or*
      Abscess, *or*
      New partial dehiscence of prosthetic valve, *or*
    New valvular regurgitation (increase or change in preexisting murmur *not* sufficient)
Minor criteria
  Predisposition: predisposing heart condition *or* intravenous drug use
  Fever: ≥38.0°C (100.4°F)
  Vascular phenomena: arterial embolism, septic pulmonary infarcts, mycotic aneurysm, intracranial hemorrhage, Janeway lesions
  Immunologic phenomena: glomerulonephritis, Osler nodes, Roth spots, rheumatoid factor
  Echocardiogram: consistent with infective endocarditis but not meeting major criterion above
  Microbiologic evidence: positive blood culture but not meeting major criterion above, *or* serologic evidence of active infection with organism consistent with infective endocarditis

(Adapted from Durack et al.,[231] with permission.)

has become a valuable new tool, often providing real-time feedback to the surgical team during the procedure.

The currently accepted diagnostic criteria for IE were published in 1982[3] and do not use echocardiographic findings in the case definitions, despite major improvements in echocardiographic technology (see above). In addition, the isolation of a "typical" IE pathogen from blood cultures is not considered in the von Reym definitions. Thus, many cases are classified as not "definite." With improved methodology *and* recognizing the central role of echocardiography in the evaluation of suspected IE, new case definitions and diagnostic criteria have been proposed recently (Tables 4 and 5).[231] The new definitions retain, in slightly modified form, the pathologic criteria of von Reym et al.[3] (Table 4). Echocardiographic and blood culture results are among the major and minor clinical criteria (Table 5) and have been validated in at least one large series of patients. Although refinements may be necessary with wider usage, the newer criteria are more flexible, reflect current clinical practice more realistically, yield a higher proportion of definite cases, and should be useful for more accurate classification of IE, for epidemiologic studies, and as entry criteria for clinical trials.

TABLE 6. Etiologic Agents in Infective Endocarditis

Agent	Percentage of Cases
Streptococci	60–80
Viridans streptococci	30–40
Enterococci	5–18
Other streptococci	15–25
Staphylococci	20–35
Coagulase-positive	10–27
Coagulase-negative	1–3
Gram-negative aerobic bacilli	1.5–13
Fungi	2–4
Miscellaneous bacteria	<5
Mixed infections	1–2
"Culture negative"	<5–24

Etiologic Agents

Streptococci. A plethora of microorganisms have been implicated in IE, but streptococci and staphylococci account for 80–90 percent of the cases in which identification is made. The most common etiologic agents are outlined in Table 6. The streptococci still cause most of the cases of IE.[31] Although many community hospitals still report viridans streptococci as the most common isolates among patients with IE,[233] and series from large tertiary care centers still represent these organisms among the major pathogens, staphylococci have assumed increasing importance among isolates in community hospitals in recent years (see below).[10,223] Viridans streptococci remain the major cause of IE in children. The disease usually runs a classic subacute course with multiple nonspecific symptoms as outlined in Table 3. Over 80 percent of these patients have underlying heart disease. Infective endocarditis in a young woman with isolated mitral valve involvement is almost universally caused by streptococci. Approximately 20 percent of the cases are seen because of embolic phenomena. With modern medical and surgical management, the cure rate should exceed 90 percent in cases of nonenterococcal streptococcal endocarditis, although complications may ensue in more than 30 percent of cases.[232]

The nomenclature of the streptococci is confusing, and various authors differ in terminology used. As detailed in Chapters 181 and 182, current names for the α-hemolytic streptococci other than *Streptococcus pneumoniae* (i.e., "viridans streptococci") causing endocarditis are *S. mitis, S. sanguis, S. mutans, S. salivarius*, the "nutrionally variant streptococci (*S. adjacens* and *S. defectivus*), and some isolates of the "*S. intermedius* group" (*S. intermedius* and *S. anginosus*). *Streptococcus morbillorum* is now classified as *Gemella morbillorum; S. mitior* is now considered to be a "genospecies" of *S. mitis*. However, *S. mitior* is so deeply imbedded in the endocarditis literature that this name will be retained in the discussion that follows. Group D streptococci are sometimes α-hemolytic, depending on the conditions and the isolate, but are not included among the viridans streptococci. Streptococci of the viridans group (not a true species) are α-hemolytic and usually nontypeable by the Lancefield system. The most common streptococci isolated from cases of endocarditis are *Streptococcus sanguis, S. bovis, S. mutans*, and *S. mitior*.[70] In a series of 317 cases of streptococcal endocarditis, the breakdown was as follows: α-hemolytic, 45 percent; nonhemolytic, nongroup D, 21 percent; group D, 25 percent; pyogenic (groups A, B, C, G), 5 percent; miscellaneous, 3 percent; and aerococci, 1.3 percent. The α-hemolytic strains included *S. sanguis* (16.4 percent of all cases of IE), nondextran-producing *S. mitior* (13.2 percent), dextran-positive *S. mitior* (7.3 percent), and an unclassified group (7.9 percent). Some isolates of *S. sanguis*, formerly called "*Streptococcus* SBE," are in Lancefield group H; however, most are nontypeable. *Streptococcus mutans* (14.2 percent), *S. anginosus* (5.4 percent), and *S. salivarius* (1.3 percent) comprised the nonhemolytic, non-group D strains. Group D organisms included the enterococci (8 percent) and *S. bovis* (17 percent). In another analysis,[234] viridans streptococci caused 58 percent of cases of

IE at the New York Hospital from 1970 to 1978. The various responsible species were as follows: *Streptococcus mitior*, 31 percent; *S. bovis*, 27 percent; *S. sanguis*, 24 percent; *S. mutans*, 7 percent; vitamin B_6–dependent *S. mitior*, 5 percent; *S. anginosus*, 4 percent; and others, 2 percent—all of which are slightly different from the experience in the United Kingdom. A similar species distribution was observed in 48 patients (with 51 episodes of IE) reported from Washington, DC.[235] There appears to be no correlation, however, between the clinical outcome and the species involved,[232,235] with the exception of nutritionally deficient strains (see below). Viridans streptococci remain the most commonly isolated pathogens in IE cases associated with mitral valve prolapse.[236] The relative role of each species overall is problematic, however, since species designations of identical strains among laboratories are often disparate,[232] and most blood and cerebrospinal fluid isolates of viridans and/or nonhemolytic streptococci are not from patients with IE.[237]

Streptococcus mutans, the etiologic agent in 14.2 percent of the cases in the review of Parker and Ball,[70] is microaerophilic, pleomorphic, and fastidious. Two-thirds of strains will hydrolyze bile-esculin,[238] a test used to identify group D organisms, and thus may be confused with enterococci. Other characteristics of *S. mutans* include the absence of group D antigen (some strains are positive for group E), production of acid from mannitol, a failure to hydrolyze hippurate, and the formation of gelatinous deposits (dextran) in media containing 5% sucrose. This organism may be difficult to isolate and to identify. It often requires over 3 days for primary isolation, grows best on horse blood agar in 5%–10% CO_2 on subculture, and is very pleomorphic, resulting in confusion with diphtheroids. *Streptococcus mutans* was first isolated in 1924 by Clark from dental caries lesions of humans and was first reported in 1928 to cause IE. The central importance of this organism in dental caries has been amply documented.

Streptococcus bovis is a normal inhabitant of the gastrointestinal tract of humans and many animal species. It is important to separate this organism from the other members of group D (the enterococci) because their respective therapeutic approaches are different (see below). Group D organisms are presumptively identified by bile-esculin hydrolysis.[239,240] However, only the enterococci (*E. faecalis* and its varieties *zymogenes* and *liquifaciens, E. faecium*, and *E. durans*) grow in 6.5% NaCl, whereas *S. bovis* and *S. equinus* (a very rare cause of IE) are salt sensitive. Seventy-five percent of strains of *S. bovis* are heat tolerant, and they may also grow and produce acid in "*E. faecalis* broth"; therefore, these methods are unreliable for separation.[241] Arginine hydrolysis by enterococci and starch hydrolysis by *S. bovis* are other means for reliable separation. The association of bacteremia due to *S. bovis* with carcinoma of the colon and other lesions of the gastrointestinal tract suggests that colonoscopy and/or a barium enema be performed when this organism is isolated from blood cultures.[292,293]

Enterococci are normal inhabitants of the gastrointestinal tract and occasionally the anterior urethra or mouth. All enterococci are in Lancefield's group D; are catalase-negative and nonmotile; and may exhibit α-, β-, or γ-hemolysis on blood agar. They grow well in sodium azide ("SF broth"), 40% bile, 6.5% NaCl, and 0.1% methylene blue and can survive at 56°C for 30 minutes or at a pH of 9.6.[244] They should be separated from *S. bovis*. The enterococcus group is responsible for 5–18 percent of the cases of IE, and the incidence appears to be increasing,[233,245,246] The disease usually runs a subacute course and affects older (mean age, 59) men after genitourinary manipulation or younger (mean age, 37) women after obstetric procedures. The mean duration of nonspecific symptoms such as malaise, fatigue, anorexia, and weight loss was 140 days in one review. Over 40 percent of the patients have no underlying heart disease, although more than 95 percent develop a heart murmur during the course of the illness. Classic peripheral manifestations are uncommon (fewer than 25 percent of the cases). Bacteriuria with enterococci is a helpful diagnostic clue and was found in 4 of 15 patients[244] in one study. Cure is difficult because of resistance to antibiotics, and a high mortality persists in this disease. With the increasing usage of third-generation cephalosporins, which are relatively inactive vs. enterococci in vitro, and other factors, recent reports[246–248] emphasize an alarming increase in enterococcal bacteremias during the past two decades. Most enterococcal bacteremias are nosocomial in origin, often polymicrobial (42 percent in one large series[249]), and are associated with serious underlying disorders. Factors that suggest IE in patients with enterococcal bacteremia include *(1)* community acquisition, *(2)* preexistent valvular heart disease, *(3)* a cryptogenic source, and *(4)* the absence of polymicrobial bacteremia.[249] Antibiotic usage patterns, the aging of the population, and more invasive procedures in hospitalized adults all portend a continued increase in serious enterococcal infections, including IE, in the future.

Before 1945, *Streptococcus pneumoniae* was responsible for approximately 10 percent of cases of IE, but this has decreased to approximately 1–3 percent currently.[198] The course is usually fulminant and is often (in approximately one-third of cases) associated with perivalvular abscess formation and/or pericarditis. Left-sided involvement is the rule, and there is a predilection for the aortic valve (≈70 percent). Many patients with pneumococcal endocarditis are alcoholics (≈40 percent), and concurrent meningitis is present in about 70 percent of cases.[250–252] The overall mortality remains at approximately 50 percent (≈60–65 percent in children[253]) usually due to rapid valvular destruction and hemodynamic compromise although indolent presentations of pneumococcal endocarditis with a favorable outcome have been described.[254]

Nutritionally variant streptococci (usually *S. defectivus* and *S. adjacens*) may cause difficulties in isolation and were implicated in 5.4 percent of the cases of streptococcal endocarditis at The New York Hospital.[255] The organisms do not grow on subculture unless L-cysteine or pyridoxal (vitamin B$_6$) is supplemented. Infective endocarditis due to nutritionally deficient streptococci is virtually always indolent in onset and associated with prior heart disease.[256] Therapy remains difficult because systemic embolization, relapse, and death are not infrequent (17–27 percent of cases). A closely related species, *Streptococcus mitis,* although not nutritionally deficient, also causes serious infections, including IE, in adults[257] and has emerged as an important causative agent of IE among drug addicts in some areas (i.e., New York City[258]). Group B streptococci (*S. agalactiae*) are normal inhabitants of the mouth, vagina, and anterior urethra in 5–12 percent of the general population. In 149 patients with group B streptococcal infections, the serotypes isolated were Ia in 46 percent, II in 22 percent, and III in 11 percent.[259] Although long recognized as a cause of bacteremia and meningitis in neonates, serious *Streptococcus agalactiae* infections in adults have been emphasized recently.[260] Risk factors for group B streptococcal sepsis and IE in adults include diabetes mellitus, carcinoma, alcoholism, hepatic failure, elective abortion, and intravenous drug use.[260–262] Like *Streptococcus bovis,* occasional cases occur in association with villous adenomas of the colon.[263] Over 70 cases of group B streptococcal IE have been reported.[261–264] Underlying heart disease is common, the male-to-female ratio is 1.4:1, the mean age is approximately 54 years, and left-sided involvement predominates. The overall mortality is nearly 50 percent. The organism does not produce fibrinolysin, which may be responsible for the large crumbling vegetations and frequent major systemic emboli. A similar clinical picture with a destructive process, left-sided predominance, frequent complications, and high mortality (≈40 percent) has been observed in the 47 cases of group G streptococcal endocarditis reported in the literature.[265,266] Most human infections with *Streptococcus suis* have presented as meningitis (with a striking predilection for deafness among sequelae) and sepsis with accompanying arthritis and/or endophthalmitis, but two cases of

endocarditis due to serotype 2 have been described.[267] Pig or raw pork contact was present in both patients. Group A streptococci remain a very rare cause of IE in both adults and children.[268]

Streptococcus anginosus is a rare cause of IE (≈6–7 percent of cases) but is unusual among these streptococci in that it has a predilection for suppurative complications including brain, liver, perinephric and other abscesses, cholangitis, peritonitis, and empyema.[269–271] Some of these complications occur during IE with this organism and may require surgical attention. Approximately 50 percent of *S. anginosus* strains carry the group F antigen.[270] Infective endocarditis caused by *S. anginosus* may result in "virulent" intracardiac complications (e.g., myocardial abscess, purulent pericarditis) more typical of *S. aureus* infections.[272]

Infective endocarditis due to *Gemella haemolysans* was recognized recently.[273] This organism is now placed in genus V of the family Streptococcaceae. *Gemella* should be suspected if blood cultures reveal a variable morphology (resembling diphtheroids) and an indeterminate Gram stain. The antimicrobial susceptibility of *Gemella* spp. is similar to that of the viridans streptococci. Although misidentification in the microbiology laboratory is presumably common, six cases of IE due to *Gemella haemolysans* have been reported since 1982.[274]

Staphylococci. Staphylococci cause at least 20–30 percent of the cases of IE, and 80–90 percent of these are due to coagulase-positive *S. aureus. Staphylococcus aureus* is the causative agent in most cases of acute IE, but only a minority of patients with *S. aureus* bacteremia seen currently have IE.[275,276] The organism attacks normal (no clinically detectable cardiac disease) heart valves in approximately one-third of the patients. The course is frequently fulminant when it involves the mitral or aortic valve, with widespread metastatic infection, and results in death in approximately 40 percent of the cases.[277–280] As stated above, the proportion of cases of IE due to *S. aureus* appears to be increasing at both community and university hospitals.[10,232,233,281]

Myocardial abscesses (with conduction disturbances), purulent pericarditis, and valve ring abscesses are more common in staphylococcal endocarditis than in other forms. Peripheral foci of suppuration (lung, brain, spleen, kidney, and so forth) are common and afflict over 40 percent of these patients.[277,280,281] These extravascular sites of involvement may offer clues for an early diagnosis, especially in addicts.[168,169] This disease is often unsuspected and therefore not clinically recognized in elderly patients, and mortality rates often exceed 50 percent in patients over 50 years of age, especially when nosocomially acquired.[154,281,282] The rare entity of neonatal endocarditis is also often caused by *S. aureus*[283]; survival is unusual.

Infective endocarditis in narcotic addicts is usually due to *S. aureus,* but the disease tends to be less severe, with mortality rates of 2–6 percent.[168,169] The recent emergence of methicillin-resistant strains (MRSA) in addicts with staphylococcal IE in the Detroit area is disturbing.[163,284] Among 180 bacteremic addicts admitted to the Detroit Medical Center in 1 year, 24 percent grew MRSA, and 41 percent of the patients overall had IE. Previous hospitalizations, long-term addiction (particularly in males), and nonprescribed antibiotic use were predictive of MRSA acquisition (odds ratio, 8.6:1[284]).

Staphylococcus epidermidis is an important agent in prosthetic valve endocarditis (see Ch. 59) and in infants with umbilical venous catheters in neonatal intensive care units.[285] Although still rare, recent reports[286–288] have emphasized the importance of coagulase-negative staphylococci in native-valve IE, particularly in patients with mitral valve prolapse.[286] Approximately two-thirds of patients have preexistent valvular disease. Although indolent in onset, complications of IE were frequent; despite this, medical and/or surgical therapy was usually successful. Males predominate among the 85 patients reported, and the incidence of emboli, skin manifestations, and CHF is low.[289] Separation of IE from uncomplicated bacteremias due to *S. epidermidis* (implicated in ≈50 percent of native-valve coagulase-negative staphylococcal endocarditis) may be difficult, but a solid-phase radioimmunoassay for the detection of IgG antibodies is promising.[290] Extensive laboratory evaluation[291] reveals that most *S. epidermidis* endocarditis isolates are distinct and do not represent common-source outbreaks despite the frequent shift to a small-colony variant by many strains in vivo.[292] Rare cases of IE due to other coagulase-negative staphylococci (e.g., *S. saprophyticus* and *S. capitis*) have been reported.[293,294]

Gram-Negative Bacilli. Gram-negative aerobic bacilli have been reported to cause 1.3–4.8 percent of the cases of IE, but in two reports[295,296] they accounted for over 10 percent of the cases. In the latter reports, approximately two-thirds of the cases coexisted with or followed serious gram-positive infections. In spite of an increasing incidence of gram-negative bacillary septicemia, IE due to these organisms remains uncommon, but the incidence is increasing. Only 1.7 percent of 452 valvular infections reported in the 1960s were caused by gram-negative organisms vs 7 to 15 percent in more recent series.[232,297] A total of 56 cases of IE due to gram-negative bacteria were seen at the Mayo Clinic from 1958 to 1975, 35 in the last decade alone.[298] Most cases were due to "fastidious" nonenteric organisms (see below); this group caused 10 percent of the IE cases seen at this institution. Narcotic addicts, prosthetic valve recipients, and patients with cirrhosis[299] appear to be at an increased risk for the development of gram-negative bacillary endocarditis. The duration of illness is usually less than 6 weeks, most patients are aged 40–50 years, and the sex distribution is equal.[300] In gram-negative septicemia, the blood stream is usually cleared readily with appropriate antimicrobial agents. In contrast, in gram-negative bacillary endocarditis persistent bacteremia is common even with high levels of antimicrobial activity. Congestive heart failure is common, and the prognosis is poor. Most series report a mortality approaching 75–83 percent,[20,300] but recent experience indicates a better prognisis[298] with a cure rate of 62 percent in 21 patients infected with aerobic enteric bacilli. A heart murmur noted during an episode of gram-negative sepsis with unexplained anemia or the persistence of positive blood cultures despite adequate antibiotics may indicate endocarditis. In the early postoperative period after prosthetic valve replacement, sustained gram-negative bacillary bacteremia does not necessarily imply IE,[301] and other foci of infection (sternal wound, pneumonia, urinary tract, IV catheters, and so forth) should be carefully sought (see Ch. 59).

Among the Enterobacteriaceae, *Salmonella* spp. were most common in early reports. These organisms have an affinity for abnormal cardiac valves, usually on the left side of the heart.[300,302] Although many serotypes have been implicated, most cases are due to *S. chloraesuis*, *S. typhimurium*, and *S. enteritidis*. Valvular perforation and/or destruction, atrial thrombi, myocarditis, and pericarditis are common, and the outlook is grave. Salmonellae may also produce endarteritis in aneurysms of major vessels (see below).

In a review of 44 cases of Enterobacteriaceae endocarditis due to species other than *Salmonella*,[300] the following organisms were identified: *E. coli*, 17; *Citrobacter* sp., 1; *Klebsiella–Enterobacter* spp., 9; *Serratia marcescens*, 13; *Proteus* spp. 2; and *Providencia* spp., 2. There were 19 additional cases of endocarditis due to *Serratia marcescens* reported from San Francisco[303]; 17 occurred in narcotic addicts. Two-thirds of these patients had previously normal heart valves, and most of the infections occurred on the aortic and mitral valves. The cases are characterized by large vegetations with near-total occlusion of the valve orifice in the absence of significant underlying valvular destruction. The overall mortality ranges from 68 to 73 percent, since a cure of left-sided IE due to the Enterobacteria-

ceae is uncommon with medical therapy alone. Since 1974, 17 more cases of IE due to *Serratia marcescens* have been observed in the San Francisco area; 15 occurred in intravenous drug abusers. As above, only 3 of 10 patients with left-sided involvement survived despite antimicrobial combination therapy and high serum bactericidal activity. Valve replacement after approximately 7–10 days of antibiotics was recommended for these difficult infections.[304] Approximately 12 cases of IE due to *Campylobacter fetus* have been reorted since the first case in 1955.[305]

The first case of *Pseudomonas*-induced endocarditis was recognized in 1899; over 200 cases have subsequently been reported.[163,284,299,306–309] Most (95 percent) of the patients have abused intravenous drugs.[284,306–309] Males predominate by a ratio of 2.5:1, and the mean age is 30 years. The organism affects normal valves in most cases. Major embolic phenomena, inability to sterilize valves, neurologic complications (53 percent), ring and annular abscesses, splenic abscesses, bacteremic relapses, and rapidly progressive congestive heart failure are common. Ecthyma gangrenosum, the necrotizing cutaneous lesion characteristic of *Pseudomonas* bateremia, has occasionally been noted, especially in cases of IE due to *Pseudomonas cepacia*.[310] The disease carries the highest mortality in patients over 30 years of age (73 percent mortality vs. 33 percent in younger patients), when the duration of illness is less than 5 days (raises the mortality from 41 percent to 76 percent), and when there is left-sided cardiac involvement.[307,309,311] Due to the gloomy outlook and frequent complications,[163] early surgery is recommended by many authorities for *Pseudomonas* endocarditis.[308,309] Nearly all addicts with *P. aeruginosa* endocarditis in recent reports[63,284,308,309] have abused pentazocine and tripelennamine ("T's and blues").

Unusual Gram-Negative Bacteria. Endocarditis produced by several other gram-negative species has received recent attention. *Neisseria gonorrhoeae* was responsible for at least 5–10 percent of the cases of IE before the introduction of penicillin but is now rarely implicated. In the older series, one-half of the patients with gonococcal endocarditis had involvement of the right side of the heart and exhibited the characteristic double quotidian fever pattern. Of the 46 cases of gonococcal endocarditis reported since 1949,[312–314] most occurred in young men. Skin manifestations consistent with the gonococcal arthritis–dermatitis syndrome or endocarditis are documented in only 20 percent of cases. Most of the cases of gonococcal endocarditis now follow an indolent course, in contrast to the often fulminant progression in the preantibiotic era. Aortic valve involvement, large vegetations on transthoracic echocardiography, associated valve ring abscesses, congestive heart failure, and nephritis are quite common. Recently[314] a high frequency of late-complement component deficiencies have been noted in patients with gonococcal endocarditis. Sudden hemodynamic deterioration despite appropriate therapy may occur,[312–314] and the mortality rate remains approximately 20 percent. Nonpathogenic *Neisseria* spp. (*N. perflava*, *N. flava*, *N. pharyngis*, *N. mucosa*, *N. sicca*, *N. flavesceus*, and especially *Moraxella* [*Neisseria*] *catarrhalis* and *Neisseria elongata* subsp. *nitroreducens* [CDC group M-6]) are now isolated more frequently in IE than are gonococci, but they usually produce infection on abnormal or prosthetic heart valves.[315–317] *Haemophilus* spp., predominantly *H. paraphrophilus*, *H. parainfluenzae*, and *H. aphrophilus*, account for 0.8–1.3 percent of all cases of IE.[318–321] This disease usually runs a subacute course and occurs in the setting of preexisting valvular disease. Emboli to major peripheral arteries were found in six of seven cases of *H. parainfluenzae* endocarditis,[318] and major central nervous system complications are relatively frequent.[321] *Haemophilus aphrophilus* produced a similar clinical pattern and has been transmitted from dogs to humans. Single cases of IE due to *H. segnis* and *H. aegyptius* have been reported from Denmark and Israel, respectively.[322,323] A closely related organism, *Actinobaccillus actinomycetemcomitans,* is a rare cause of subacute endocarditis (approximately 35 cases reported) with a mortality of 34 percent.[324,325] Infective endocarditis due to *Cardiobacterium hominis*[326] resembles the disease caused by *Haemophilus* spp.; 26 cases of IE due to this organism were reported by 1983. Only one extravascular infection due to *C. hominis* has been documented (meningitis during IE). At least 28 cases of *Kingella* endocarditis (*K. kingae,* 25; *K. denitrificans,* 2; *K. indologenes,* 1) have been reported.[327] Approximately 50 percent develop complications, including acute stroke in approximately 25 percent of cases. A dozen cases of IE due to *Eikenella corrodens* have been reported; intravenous drug use (especially amphetamines) was implicated in five patients.[328,329] Dental infections or a history of dental procedures may be present, and drug users have often "cleaned" the injection site with saliva; *E. corrodens* is a usual habitant of the oropharynx. The disease is generally indolent but may present acutely.[329] All these organisms (the HACEK group) are fastidious and may require 2–3 weeks for primary isolation. Routine subculturing onto supplemented chocolate agar or incubation in atmospheres of 5%–10% CO_2 is necessary for the isolation of these organisms and should be performed in all culture-negative cases of IE. Granular growth in broth is characteristic and should suggest their presence. In addition, the clinical syndrome produced by this group is virtually identical with a subacute course of IE: large friable vegetations, frequent emboli, and the development of congestive heart failure and often eventual valve replacement.[330]

Gram-Positive Bacilli. Infective endocarditis due to various species of corynebacteria (diphtheroids) is uncommon and usually occurs on damaged or prosthetic valves,[331] although native-valve infections (e.g., *Arcanobacterium* [*corynebacterium*] *haemolyticum* in an addict) are rarely reported. About 19 cases of IE due to *Corynebacterium pseudodiphtheriticum* (previously *C. hofmannii*) have been reported; native valves were involved in approximately 50 percent of these cases.[332] *Corynebacterium xerosis* is a very rare cause of native valve IE. Nontoxigenic *C. diphtheriae* IE has been reported in more than 40 patients. A recent cluster of seven cases in 1 year from New South Wales, Australia,[333] emphasized the aggressive nature of the infection, including major vascular complications, the frequent occurrence of septic arthritis (four of seven patients), and involvement of native valves. Intravenous drug use is also a predisposing factor. *Listeria monocytogenes* has been isolated from 44 cases of IE.[334,335] Most cases of IE due to *Listeria* have occurred in patients without any underlying defect in host defenses, although preexistent heart disease is present in approximately 50 percent. The mean age was 51 years, and the overall mortality was 48 percent.[335] Lactobacilli have also been reported to cause a subacute form of IE and are rare, with only 41 cases reported.[336,337] Despite an initial response to therapy, relapse of this infection is not unusual (≈60 percent of cases). Most cases occur on structurally abnormal native valves following dental manipulation.[337] Therapy with single agents is often unsatisfactory, as lactobacilli, like enterococci, are tolerant to penicillins. Medical cure has been difficult to achieve in the past. These organisms also may take several weeks for isolation on blood culture. Over 90 percent of 49 serious infections caused by *Erysipelothrix rhusiopathiae* were characterized as endocarditis.[338] Occupational or vocational animal or fish exposure is a major risk factor, and approximately one-third of patients are alcoholics. Most patients are male, a characteristic erysipeloid skin lesion is present in ≈40 percent of cases, and the organism exhibits significant aortic valve tropsim (involved in 70 percent of patients).[338] The overall mortality was 38 percent. Most cases of *Bacillus* endocarditis involve the tricuspid valve in addicts but nonaddicts and prosthetic valve recipients have also been affected.[339] *Rothia dentocariosa* is a rare cause of IE (six re-

ported cases) but has led to significant central nervous system complications.[340,341]

Anaerobic Bacteria. Nonstreptococcal anaerobic bacteria were responsible for 1.3 percent of all the cases of IE in 1970.[342] *Bacteroides fragilis* was the predominant pathogen in a review of 67 cases from the literature.[343] The following organisms were isolated: *B. fragilis,* 35.8 percent; *B. oralis,* 3.0 percent; *P. melaninosenica* (*B. melaninogenicus*), 3.0 percent; *Fusobacterium necrophorum,* 13.4 percent; *Fusobacterium nucleatum,* 9.0 percent; *Clostridium* spp., 13.4 percent; *Propionibacterium acnes,* 7.5 percent; *Dialister granuliformans,* 1.5 percent; and unidentified, 16.4 percent. Over one-third of the unidentified cases were also thought by the authors to represent *B. fragilis.* Approximately 25 percent of these cases were polymicrobial, usually mixed with anaerobic or microaerophilic streptococci. The portal of entry for *B. fragilis* was most likely the gastrointestinal tract, while *B. oralis, P. melaninogenica* (*B. melaninogenicus*) or fusobacteria originated from the mouth or upper respiratory tract. Two-thirds of the patients were over 40 years of age and had preexisting heart disease. The course is usually subacute except for *F. necrophorum,* which characteristically produces a more fulminant disease. These organisms usually cause extensive valve destruction, CHF, and major systemic emboli (in 60–70 percent of the cases). Thromboembolic episodes are especially common in cases caused by *B. fragilis,* a phenomenon that may be related to the heparinase produced by this organism. The mortality in cases of anaerobic endocarditis has ranged from 21 to 46 percent,[343] but one series from California noted no deaths in seven patients with anaerobic or microaerophilic endocarditis,[344] which constituted 10.6 percent of the IE cases seen. This is similar to a 7.7 percent incidence reported by others[3] and suggests that anaerobic endocarditis may be more prevalent now than it was in 1970.[345] Isolation of these organisms may be improved by the newer culture techniques currently in use.

Other Bacteria. Many other genera of bacteria have been described in cases of IE; however, consideration of these organisms separately is beyond the scope of this review. These include *Acinetobacter* (approximately 20 cases reported, a mamlopapular rash on the palms and soles may be present),[346] *Actinomyces,*[347] *Alcaligenes, Bordetella, Flavobacterium, Micrococcus, Moraxella, Paracolon, Stomatococcus mucilaginosus* (four cases of IE),[348] *Streptobacillus moniliformis* (approximately 16 cases, usually on damaged native valves),[349] *Vibrio,* and *Yersinia. Brucella* spp. continue as important etiologic agents in Spain and in Saudi Arabia where these organisms are responsible for approximately 10 percent of IE cases.[350] Aggressive medical therapy with valve replacement is usually necessary for a cure of *Brucella* endocarditis.

Etiology of Infective Endocarditis in Addicts. The organisms responsible for IE in narcotic addicts require separate consideration since the distribution differs from other patients with IE. The frequencies of the etiologic agents isolated before 1977 in seven major series were as follows[2]: *Staphylococcus aureus,* 38 percent; *Pseudomonas aeruginosa,* 14.2 percent; *Candida* spp., 13.8 percent; enterococci, 8.2 percent; viridans streptococci, 6.0 percent; *Staphylococcus epidermidis,* 1.7 percent; gram-negative aerobic bacilli, 1.7–15 percent; other bacteria, 2.2 percent; mixed infections, 1.3 percent; and culture-negative, 12.9 percent. In addition, there appears to be an unexplained geographic variation in the causal agents of narcotic-associated IE. *Staphylococcus aureus* predominated in New York City, Washington, D.C., Chicago, and Cincinnati; *Pseudomonas aeruginosa* was commonly isolated in Detroit, but methicillin-resistant *S. aureus* now predominates. The most recent compilation from Detroit indicates the distribution of causative agents in addicts with IE (n = 74) as follows: *S. aureus,* 60.8 percent; streptococci, 16.2 percent; *P. aeruginosa,* 13.5 percent; polymicrobial,

8.1 percent; and *Corynebacterium* JK, 1.4 percent. Polymicrobial endocarditis (as eight different pathogens have been recovered from blood cultures of an individual patient) is fairly common among addicts. Some authors have speculated that HIV infection predisposes intravenous drug users to IE due to unusual bacteria, including *Corynebacterium* or *Neisseria* spp.[351] Although *Staphylococcus aureus* IE in this population was usually tricuspid, streptococci infected left-sided valves significantly more often than the other pathogens. Biventricular and multiple-valve infections occurred most commonly in *Pseudomonas* endocarditis; all of these addicts abused "T's and blues." Left-sided IE due to *Pseudomonas aeruginosa* is a devastating disease and usually presents as an acute illness refractory to seemingly optimal antimicrobial regimens. Complications including ring and annular abscesses, neurologic sequelae (≥53 percent), congestive heart failure, and splenic abscesses are frequent; surgery is often necessary for cure,[352] but overall mortality rate still approaches 60 percent. There is an increased incidence of enterococcal endocarditis in Cleveland. *Serratia marcescens* was once an important pathogen in San Francisco[304] but currently *Staphylococcus aureus* is the most common (≅85 percent) etiologic agent (M. Sande, personal communication). These differences do not correlate with contamination of "street" heroin.[353] The high incidence of staphylococcal endocarditis may be partially explained by an increase in nasal and/or oral carriage of this organism.[354] Heroin usage in the previous week was associated with a *Staphylococcus aureus* isolation rate of 35 percent from skin, nose, or throat cultures; this declined to 11 percent (not significantly different from controls) if heroin had not been injected in the preceding 2 weeks. This suggests an endogenous source for the infecting organism, since *Staphylococcus aureus* is infrequently (<5 percent) isolated from street heroin or injection paraphernalia. The exact incidence of IE in narcotic addicts is unknown. A conservative estimate is 1.5–2 cases of IE per 1000 addicts at risk per year.[355] Moreover, intravenous drug use is the most common risk factor for the development of recurrent native-valve IE; 43 percent of 281 patients surveyed from 1975 to 1986 with this syndrome were addicts[366] (see above).

Fungi. Most of the cases of fungal endocarditis can be grouped into three categories: *(1)* narcotic addicts, *(2)* patients after reconstructive cardiovascular surgery, and *(3)* patients after prolonged intravenous and/or antibiotic therapy. In a review of 24 patients with fungal endocarditis seen at the New York University Medical Center from 1968 to 1973,[200] 11 were heroin addicts, 9 had undergone cardiac surgery, and 5 had other serious illnesses requiring antibiotics or hyperalimentation. Underlying heart disease and a tendency for major systemic embolization were noted in two-thirds of these patients. *Candida parapsilosis* and *C. tropicalis* predominated in the addicts, whereas *C. albicans* and *Aspergillus* spp. caused most cases in nonaddicts. In 23 addicts reviewed, *C. parapsilosis* was responsible in 12 patients (52 percent), and other *Candida* spp. (*C. guillermondii, C. stellatoidea, C. krusei, C. tropicalis*) caused most of the remaining cases. *Candida albicans* was isolated in only 1 of the 23 addicts. In contrast, in 82 patients who developed fungal endocarditis after cardiac surgery, the reported distribution of causative organisms was different. *Candida albicans* and *Aspergillus* spp. each accounted for approximately one-third of the isolates. *Candida parapsilosis* was found in fewer than 10 percent. Fungal endocarditis was documented in 29 patients after prolonged intravenous therapy, and in 17 it developed during the treatment of bacterial endocarditis. One-half of this group of patients was infected with *C. albicans*. The overall cure rate in cases of fungal endocarditis is poor (14.5 percent in cases treated since 1968). The poor prognosis may be due to *(1)* the large bulky vegetations, *(2)* the tendency for fungal invasion of the myocardium, *(3)* widespread systemic septic emboli, *(4)* the poor penetration of antifungal agents into the vegeta-

tion,[357] *(5)* the low toxic/therapeutic ratio of the available antifungal agents, and *(6)* the usual lack of fungicidal activity with these compounds. A cure is virtually impossible without surgical intervention (see below). Fatal endocarditis due to *Candida* spp. has also followed Swan-Ganz catheterization.

In a review of 25 cases of *Aspergillus*-induced endocarditis in which cultures were made,[358] the organisms isolated were as follows: *A. fumigatus*, 14; *A. flavus*, 4; *A. niger*, 3; and *A. ustus, A. sydowi, A. terreus,* and *A. glaucus*, 1 each. Only 5 of 34 patients in this series had positive blood cultures, and only 1 patient survived. A few cases, usually fatal, of *Aspergillus* endocarditis after coronary artery bypass surgery have been described. *Aspergillus clavatus* was isolated in one case. Other fungi that have caused IE include *Histoplasma, Blastomyces, Coccidioides, Cryptococcus, Hansenula, Fonsecaea (Hormodendrum), Scedosporium prolificans, Mucor, Paecilomyces,* and *Phialophora*. Of the eight reported cases of IE due to *Trichosporon beigelii*, six occurred on prosthetic valves; only two have survived a combined medical-surgical approach.[359] *Pseudallescheria boydii* has caused IE in approximately five reported patients; all were immunosuppressed (e.g., liver transplant, AIDS) or previous recipients of prosthetic heart valves.[360] Fungal endocarditis was unknown before 1945, and the incidence is increasing; currently 1.2–2.6 percent of all cases of IE are due to fungi. Endocarditis has also been caused by higher bacteria such as *Actinomyces, Oerskoviai, Nocardia,* and *Mycobacterium* spp.

Other Microorganisms. Five cases of IE due to *Spirillum minor,* a spirochete, have been reported.[361] This organism is widely distributed in nature, especially in fresh or salt water with organic debris. *Spirillum minor* is the etiologic agent of "rat-bite fever" (sodoku), but rodent transmission was not documented in the cases of endocarditis. Preexistent heart disease or severe underlying disease (e.g., aplastic anemia) is usually present, although one case occurred in an otherwise healthy person.

Infective endocarditis due to *Coxiella burnetii* (the cause of Q fever) is well documented in the United Kingdom, Canada, and Australia, with over 200 recognized cases, and was recently reported in the United States.[362] Ten cases of Q fever endocarditis were recognized in four Dublin teaching hospitals in only 3 years.[362] Q fever is usually a self-limited respiratory illness due to the inhalation of infected aerosols, especially from animal products. The first endocarditis cases were reported in 1959. Males outnumber females by a ratio of 6:1, and 90 percent have preexisting heart disease. Most cases of IE are chronic, with a history of an influenza-like illness occurring 6–12 months previously. Risk factors may include exposure to parturient cats or rabbits. The aortic valve is involved in over 80 percent of the cases. Hematuria is uncommon, even though it is frequently observed in acute Q fever. Hepatosplenomegaly and hepatitis, common features in other types of Q fever, are usual in IE caused by this organism. Other important clues are thrombocytopenia (90 percent) and hypergammaglobulinemia. Immune complex-mediated glomerulonephritis develops in approximately 25 percent of cases.[363] The rickettsiae were demonstrated histologically in the valve tissue in 62 percent of the cases, and the organism was isolated in 83 percent, although this poses a significant laboratory hazard. The diagnosis is best made serologically; a positive antibody titer by complement fixation or ELISA to the phase I antigen is indicative of chronic infection, whereas a fourfold rise in titer to the phase II antigen is associated with active current infection. A phase I antibody titer (generally IgG and/or IgA) greater than 1:200 is considered virtually diagnostic of Q fever endocarditis and may be useful to follow the response to therapy.[364] Isolation of *Coxiella burnetii* by inoculation of valve suspensions into a human fetal diploid fibroblast cell line appears to be a promising technique.[365] DNA probes are under development. The prognosis with medical therapy alone is poor, and valve replacement is often necessary for a cure (see below). This agent may also cause endarteritis. A single case of IE due to the causative agent of murine typhus has been reported.[196]

Chlamydia psittaci, the agent of psittacosis, has been implicated in at least 10 well-documented cases of IE.[366] This organism may also cause myocarditis or pericarditis. Most of the cases have been associated with psittacine bird exposure; in one case, chlamydiae were found in the liver of the suspected budgerigar. However, transmission from pet cats has also been proposed. The course is subacute, and the diagnosis is often made retrospectively. Most patients had preexisting heart disease with a striking propensity for aortic valve involvement, and rapid valvular destruction leading to surgical interventions and/or death. A diagnosis can be established with the demonstration of complement-fixing antibodies. Cure usually requires valve replacement and prolonged antibiotic therapy. The mortality in this small group was 40 percent. Two well-documented cases of IE due to *Chlamydia trachomatis* have been reported.[367] Microimmunofluorescence tests are necessary for a diagnosis. A single case of probable *Chlamydia pneumoniae* endocarditis has been reported.[368] IE due to *Mycoplasma pneumoniae* was proposed in one case report, but cultural confirmation was lacking.[369]

The role of viruses in IE is unknown. Experimentally, coxsackie B virus has been shown to produce valvular and mural endocarditis in mice and cynomolgus monkeys.[370] In these studies the viral antigen was demonstrated in the valvular tissue by immunofluorescent techniques. Although the enteroviruses are commonly implicated in cases of myocarditis or pericarditis in humans, there is no proof that viral infections produce IE in the human. Adenoviruses are also capable of producing IE in mice.[371] Persand has described a case of "cytomegalovirus endocarditis," but bacteria were also cultured from a mural lesion.

"Culture-Negative" Endocarditis. As discussed earlier, sterile blood cultures have been noted in 2.5–31 percent of the cases of IE.[372,373] This may be due to several factors: (1) subacute right-sided endocarditis; (2) cultures taken toward the end of a chronic course (longer than 3 months); (3) uremia supervening in a chronic course; (4) mural endocarditis as in ventricular septal defects, postmyocardial infarction thrombi, or pacemaker wires; (5) slow growth of fastidious organisms such as anaerobes, *Haemophilus* spp., *Actinobacillus* spp., *Cardiobacterium* spp., nutritionally variant streptococci, or *Brucella* spp; (6) the prior administration of antibiotics[372,373]; (7) fungal endocarditis; (8) endocarditis caused by obligate intracellular parasites such as rickettsiae, chlamydiae, and perhaps viruses; or (9) noninfective endocarditis or an incorrect diagnosis. Attention to the proper collection of blood cultures, serologic tests, and newer diagnostic techniques may reduce the proportion of "culture-negative" cases.

Polymicrobial Endocarditis. The proportion of IE cases due to more than one pathogen may be increasing. In a literature review spanning the decade of the 1980s,[374] 101 cases of polymicrobial IE were found. The mean age was only 36.5 years, the male to female ratio was nearly 2 to 1, and 71 patients used intravenous drugs (as expected, tricuspid valve involvement with septic pulmonary emboli were frequent). Left-sided involvement, two organisms (vs. three or more), and older ages were associated with a greater mortality rate.

THERAPY FOR INFECTIVE ENDOCARDITIS

The response to antimicrobial therapy for IE is unique among bacterial infections. Although the organisms may be exquisitely sensitive to the antibiotics used, complete eradication takes weeks to achieve, and relapse of disease is not unusual. There are a few possible explanations for these phenomena: (1) the

infection exists in an area of impaired host resistance and is tightly encased in a fibrin meshwork where the bacterial colonies are free to divide relatively free from interference from phagocytic cells, and (2) the number of bacteria in these vegetations reaches tremendous population densities (often 10^9–10^{10} cfu/g). At these high populations, the organisms may exist in a state of reduced metabolic activity and cell division, as was suggested by Durack and Beeson[106] in studies of L-alanine incorporation into bacterial cell walls. A similar finding is observed in broth in vitro after 18 hours of incubation. In both situations the bacteria are less susceptible to the bactericidal action of penicillin or other drugs that require cell wall synthesis and division for maximum activity. The relative importance of antimicrobial penetration into vegetations and the response to therapy is unresolved. Although multiple studies have examined antibiotic concentrations in human cardiac valve tissue obtained during surgery,[375] usually in close agreement with concurrent serum concentrations, the relevance of these data to therapy for IE is unknown and has not altered current recommendations. Information on antimicrobial concentration in vegetations, either in experimental models or in humans with IE, is sparse. Recent experiments after a single dose of radiolabeled antimicrobial agents with autoradiographic analysis of drug dispersion within vegetations of animals with experimental IE revealed three patterns[376]: (1) concentration at the periphery of the vegetation without diffusion into the core (e.g., teicoplanin); (2) progressive diffusion but with a high gradient from periphery to core (e.g., ceftriaxone); or (3) homogenous diffusion throughout the vegetation (e.g., several fluoroquinolones). The predictive value of these observations on therapeutic efficacy is unknown, however. Analysis of pharmacodynamic variables (e.g., concentration-dependent bactericidal activity, postantibiotic effect) may also assist in the rational selection of regimens for the therapy of IE.[376] Agents that are selectively localized in vegetations (vs. normal endocardium), such as porphyrins,[377] may be useful in the diagnosis and/or drug delivery to the site of infection as carriers for other compounds. Studies in animals have confirmed that when vegetation formation is inhibited with anticoagulants the organisms are eradicated more rapidly with penicillin treatment than in control animals with larger vegetations.[110] Furthermore, enzymatic modification of the glycocalyx in the vegetations of experimental streptococcal endocarditis by in vivo dextranase administration facilitates the bactericidal activity of penicillin by more rapid sterilization of the lesion.[378] In contrast, tissue-type plasminogen activator produced a concentration-dependent lysis of fibrin clots or vegetations infected with *Staphylococcus epidermidis* or *Streptococcus sanguis* but did not enhance antimicrobial activity in in vitro models.[379,380]

Certain general principles have been accepted that provide the framework for the current recommendations for treatment of endocarditis. Parenteral antibiotics are recommended over oral drugs because of the importance of sustained antibacterial activity. Erratic absorption makes oral drugs less desirable. Short-term therapy has been associated with relapse of disease, and all current recommendations emphasize extended drug administration. Early studies by the British Medical Research Council[381] first emphasized the necessity for prolonged treatment. Bacteriostatic antibiotics are generally ineffective in the treatment of bacterial endocarditis. Their use has been associated with frequent relapses and/or a failure to control the infection. A symptomatic response to such agents as tetracycline, erythromycin, or, in some cases, clindamycin should not be accepted as indicative of successful treatment, since once treatment with these agents is discontinued relapse is common. Likewise, antibiotic combinations should produce a rapid bactericidal effect. This is seen with synergistic combinations such as penicillin plus an aminoglycoside against most viridans streptococci or enterococci. In experimental animals it has been shown that the rate of bactericidal action expressed by a drug or combination of drugs in broth is predictive of the relative rate that the organisms will be eradicated from the cardiac vegetations in vivo. Antagonistic combinations such as penicillin plus chloramphenicol, which are less rapidly bactericidal, are less effective in experimental endocarditis than is the single bactericidal drug (penicillin) alone.[382] General guidelines for the evaluation of new antimicrobial agents for the therapy of IE were published recently.[383]

Patients with IE may have an associated myocarditis complicated by cardiac arrhythmias and congestive heart failure and require close observation in an intensive care environment with electrocardiographic monitoring. As discussed below, the selection of antibiotics should be based on antimicrobial susceptibility tests and the treatment monitored with periodic determinations of serum bactericidal activity and/or antimicrobial blood levels when indicated. Blood cultures should be obtained during the early phase of therapy to ensure eradication of the bacteremia. The use of anticoagulants during therapy for native valve endocarditis has been associated with fatal subarachnoid hemorrhage and other bleeding complications. Most authorities agree that anticoagulant administration is this setting is contraindicated, but this area remains controversial.

All patients with IE should be managed in facilities with rapid access to cardiothoracic surgery. Although persistent or recurrent fever despite appropriate antimicrobial therapy may be due to pulmonary or systemic emboli or drug hypersensitivity, the most common cause is extensive valve ring or adjacent structure infection.[384] These patients and many others with IE require surgery, often emergently. Close monitoring and early surgical consultation is therefore essential.

Tests Useful for Antimicrobial Treatment Monitoring

Management of IE demands careful considerations of the choice, dose, and duration of antimicrobial therapy. The following laboratory tests can help the physician to monitor treatment and can aid in rational therapeutic decisions. In every case of bacterial endocarditis, the etiologic agent must be isolated in pure culture, and the minimum inhibitory concentration (MIC) and the minimum bactericidal concentration (MBC) must be determined for the usual antibiotics used (see below). Standard disk sensitivity testing is unreliable, and results may be misleading without the quantitative information provided by determining the MIC and MBC. During therapy the serum can be monitored for bactericidal activity against the offending organism as originally described by Schlicter and MacIlean.[385] The performance of this test varies greatly, and consequently there are disagreements in interpretation. The inoculum size, composition of the broth, timing of samples ("peak" vs. "trough"), methods of dilution and subculture, and criteria for determination of the bactericidal end point are among the important variables. Perhaps because of these problems and the frequent adverse events unrelated to bactericidal effects, the serum bactericidal titer (SBT) often correlates poorly with the clinical outcome in patients with IE. There is still intense disagreement regarding the value of this test in monitoring therapy for IE. A retrospective review[386] of 17 reports published between 1948 and 1980 failed to confirm any correlation between and SBT of 1:8 or greater and therapeutic success.[387] Controversy regarding the usefulness of "peak" vs. "trough" SBT abounds.[388] When all of these variables are standardized,[389,390] the SBT test may be useful in selected patients with IE. A recent prospective multicenter study[391] evaluated a standardized SBT method in 129 patients with bacterial endocarditis. Peak and trough SBT ratios of 1:64 or greater and 1:32 predicted bacteriologic cure in all patients, but specific levels could *not* be used to predict bacteriologic failure or clinical outcome accurately. Although there are problems with this study,[387] other data[391] support a role for the SBT when standardized and performed in the presence of 50% human serum: all patients with a peak SBT of 1:32 or greater were cured, whereas 7 of 21 (33 percent) with an SBT

of 1:16 or less failed treatment.[392] Unless precluded by drug toxicity, it seems reasonable to attempt to achieve this level (1:8–1:16) of activity in patients, although this goal may be unattainable in some forms (e.g., gram-negative bacillary, enterococcal) of IE. Performance of the SBT test is usually unnecessary in patients with viridans streptococcal endocarditis but may be useful when *(1)* the organism is inherently resistant or tolerant to one of the drugs administered or *(2)* the response to therapy is suboptimal.

In some forms of IE, combinations of antibiotics are used routinely.[393] These regimens are based on synergy studies performed in vitro and results obtained in experimental animal models of IE. In difficult cases with a slow therapeutic response or in those due to unusual organisms, a determination of synergistic combinations of antibiotics may be helpful. In these cases, tests for bactericidal synergism may be undertaken by standard techniques such as broth dilution, microtiter "checkerboards," or "time-kill" curves in broth. Proper attention to standardized techniques, especially inoculum size, are critically important for a meaningful interpretation of the results.

When aminoglycosides are used in therapy, the concentration of antibiotic in the serum should be periodically determined. These agents have a low toxic-therapeutic ratio, especially in elderly patients or in those with renal disease. Peak and trough concentrations should be measured, and the dose should be altered accordingly. This method is superior to reliance solely on nomograms for dosage changes. When synergy with another agent is demonstrable, serum concentrations of the aminoglycosides lower than those generally considered "therapeutic" may be adequate, thus lessening the potential for toxicity.

Antimicrobial Therapy

"Penicillin-Sensitive" Streptococcal Endocarditis. Most strains of viridans streptococci, "other" streptococci (including *S. pyogenes*), and nonenterococcal group D streptococci (primarily *S. bovis*) are exquisitely sensitive to penicillins with an MIC of less than 0.2 μg/ml. However, 15–20 percent of viridans streptococci are "resistant" to this arbitrary concentration of penicillin.[234,255] In addition,[238] approximately 15 percent of the strains of *S. mutans* demonstrate a low MIC to penicillin (<0.1 μg/ml), but the MBC is considerably higher (1.25–50 μg/ml). These organisms should probably be considered "penicillin tolerant" and should be treated accordingly. Although dependent on the in vitro methodology employed, studies suggest that tolerance to penicillin among viridans streptococci is more prevalent than previous reports suggested.[394] For example, 19 percent of viridans streptococci cultured from gingiva and blood after dental procedures were tolerant,[395] especially among *S. mutans* (27 percent) and *S. mitior* (20 percent) isolates. Almost identical figures were reported among blood culture isolates of viridans streptococci,[396] with tolerance defined as a penicillin MBC-to-MIC ratio exceeding 10:1. Nearly all strains of nutritionally dependent streptococci are tolerant to penicillin.[397,398] The influence of the tolerance phenomenon on the response to penicillin therapy in experimental endocarditis is not known; two studies yielded conflicting results.[399,400] Data on human infections with tolerant strains and the therapeutic results are unavailable. Except for nutritionally variant streptococci, we do not believe that the demonstration of tolerance by an isolate of viridans streptococci influences therapeutic decisions.

By broth dilution susceptibility tests, the usual MBC for these so-called penicillin-sensitive streptococci are as follows: penicillin, 0.1–1.0 μg/ml; cephalothin, 0.15–1.25 μg/ml; vancomycin, 0.15–0.4 μg/ml; streptomycin, 6.25–50 μg/ml; and gentamicin, 1.56–3.12 μg/ml.[401,402] *Streptococcus bovis* is 10–5000 times more susceptible to penicillin than are the other group D species (enterococci). They are also relatively susceptible to oxacillin, methicillin, and lincomycin, while the enterococci are resistant.[240] Most streptococci in this group demonstrate synergism in vitro between penicillin or vancomycin and streptomycin, gentamicin, or kanamycin (see below).[403,404] The first strains of viridans streptococci with high-level streptomycin resistance (MIC ≥ 1000 μg/ml) were reported in 1982 from Paris. Although these strains are rare (2–8 percent of isolates in some locales[405]) the documentation of aminoglycoside-modifying enzymes and the lack of penicillin–streptomycin synergy in vitro and in experimental animal models[405,406] is alarming. These penicillin-susceptible strains are killed synergistically by penicillin-gentamicin combinations. Significant antibiotic antagonism has been shown with the combination of clindamycin and gentamicin for *S. mutans*. The in vitro synergism between penicillin and aminoglycosides has been found to correlate with a more rapid rate of eradication of bacteria from cardiac vegetations in vivo in the rabbit endocarditis model[407,408] for the common viridans streptococci. All of these studies have been summarized in recent reviews.[409–411] Low-level penicillin resistance (MIC 0.2–2.0 μg/ml) was found in 31 percent of viridans streptococci in Madrid in 1988–1989, and an additional 17 percent of strains demonstrated high-level resistance.[412] Perhaps most importantly, streptomycin and cefotaxime resistance was also "common."[411] The authors suggest a vancomycin-gentamicin regimen for IE due to viridans streptococci in Spain.

The combination of penicillin and streptomycin has been used in over 200 cases at the New York Hospital–Cornell Medical Center since 1959 without a documented relapse.[403] This clinical experience has been confirmed elsewhere,[2] but the overall reported relapse rate is 1.4 percent.[410] This regimen is as follows: aqueous penicillin G, 10–20 million units IV qd, or procaine penicillin G, 1.2 million units im q6h for 4 weeks, combined with streptomycin, 0.5 g IM q12h for the first 2 weeks. Studies by Wilson and colleagues at the Mayo Clinic[413,414] demonstrated that a 2-week course of intramuscular procaine penicillin (1.2 million units q6h) and streptomycin (0.5 g q12h) cured at least 99 percent of patients with penicillin-sensitive streptococcal endocarditis. These results are similar to those obtained with therapy consisting of β-lactams alone for a total of 4 weeks[415,416] but significantly better than penicillin alone for 2 weeks; the latter regimen was associated with a 50 percent relapse rate when low doses of penicillin were used and improved to 17 percent with higher penicillin dosages. The 2-week penicillin-streptomycin regimen is the most cost-effective and is the preferred therapy among the three regimens in uncomplicated penicillin-sensitive (MIC ≤0.1 μg/ml) streptococcal endocarditis in young patients. Four weeks of penicillin (or ceftriaxone; see below) alone is recommended in patients with impaired renal function or those particularly susceptible to the low risk of streptomycin-induced ototoxicity (the elderly). The "Cornell regimen" of 4 weeks of penicillin plus an initial 2 weeks of streptomycin is recommended in patients with a complicated course, a history of disease exceeding 3 months' duration, or prosthetic valve endocarditis due to these sensitive strains or when susceptibility testing reveals the rare penicillin-resistant streptococci.[417] The preferred regimen for IE due to penicillin-"tolerant" streptococci is unsettled. These concepts have been recently summarized[411] and serve as a basis for the recommendations of the American Heart Association on therapy for penicillin-sensitive streptococcal endocarditis.[418] We believe that gentamicin, at a dosage of 1.0 mg/kg (not to exceed 80 mg) IM or IV q8h, can be substituted for streptomycin in the aforementioned regimens when combination therapy is deemed advisable. A penicillin-gentamicin regimen is indicated for viridans streptococcal endocarditis if high-level streptomycin resistance is present[405,406] or for strains with a penicillin MIC more than 0.2 and less than 0.5 μg/ml.[418] Strains with a penicillin MIC above 0.5 μg/ml should be treated as for enterococcal endocarditis (see below). Due to the enhanced rate of bacterial killing in animal models[419,420] and the high relapse rates of about 17 percent,[421] we also believe the "Cornell regimen" should be employed for all patients with IE due to nutritionally variant

streptococci. The aminoglycoside component of the penicillin-combination regimen may be administered once (rather than thrice) daily or at "low" synergistic dosages,[422] but this remains controversial. Although temafloxacin plus tobramycin was as effective as penicillin plus tobramycin in the therapy of experimental *Streptococcus adjacens* (a nutritionally variant streptococcal species) in rabbits,[423] quinolones are best avoided for IE due to streptococci pending further data. Other regimens for the treatment of this disease (e.g., vancomycin plus rifampin) deserve further study.[421] In the penicillin-allergic patient when a cephalosporin is deemed safe, several regimens are acceptable: cephalothin, 2 g IV q4h, or cefazolin, 1–2 g IM or IV q8h for 4 weeks, combined with streptomycin, 0.5 g IM q12h, or gentamicin, 1 mg/kg (≤80 mg) IM or IV q8h for the initial 2 weeks or ceftriaxone 2q IV or IM daily alone for 4 weeks. The latter regimen has proven efficacy for the therapy of penicillin-sensitive streptococcal endocarditis.[424,425] For example, 55 of 59 patients in one uncontrolled trial in Europe completed treatment with 4 months to 5 years of follow-up. Treatment was completely uneventful in 71% of patients while valve replacement was eventually required in 10 patients. Ceftriaxone administered once daily may permit outpatient therapy in a majority of stable patients with this disease. In addition, ceftriaxone plus an aminoglycoside demonstrates in vivo synergy in experimental viridans streptococcal endocarditis[426] and a combination regimen may allow shortened courses (approximately 2 weeks) of once-daily administration for this disease; a randomized clinical trial to evaluate this possibility is currently ongoing. When treatment with β-lactams are contraindicated, the regimen of choice is vancomycin, 1 g IV q12h (or 500 mg IV q6h) for 4 weeks. A 4-week regimen of high-dose teicoplanin has been successful in a small number of patients with streptococcal endocarditis,[427] but the occurrence of drug fever and infection with teicoplanin-tolerant *Streptococcus bovis* are cause for concern. It is doubtful that daptomycin will be developed for the therapy of IE.

"Penicillin-Resistant" Streptococcal and Enterococcal Endocarditis (e.g., MIC for Penicillin ≥0.5 μg/ml).[418] Infective endocarditis due to the enterococcus is the third most common form of the disease and is the most resistant to therapy. The mortality still approximates 20 percent,[244] and relapses are not uncommon. By broth dilution susceptibility tests, the MIC determinations for many enterococci are as follows: penicillin, 0.4–12.5 μg/ml; ampicillin, less than 0.4–3.1 μg/ml; cephalothin, 12.5–25 μg/ml; vanomycin, 0.78–3.1 μg/ml; streptomycin, 3.1 to more than 50 μg/ml; and gentamicin, 6.25–25 μg/ml. Ampicillin is approximately twice as active as penicillin by weight. In contrast, the usual MBC are as follows: penicillin, greater 6.25 μg/ml (80 percent are >100 μg/ml); cephalothin, more than 100 μg/ml; streptomycin, more than 25 μg/ml; vancomycin, more than 100 μg/ml; and gentamicin, 25 μg/ml or less.[428] *Enterococcus faecium* strains are more resistant to β-lactams than *Enterococcus faecalis* strains.[429] Thus, in general these agents are bacteriostatic against the enterococci and should not be administered alone in this disease. This bacteriostatic action of agents known to inhibit cell wall synthesis is due to a defective bacterial autolytic enzyme system.[430,431] As stated before, all β-lactams, including imipenem, are bacteriostatic against enterococci in vitro, and combination regimens are always employed.[432] A new mechanism of penicillin-resistance among *E. faecalis* was described in 1983: plasmid-mediated β-lactamase production. These strains remain relatively rare[433,434]; *E. faecalis* predominates, but β-lactamase production was recently documented in *E. faecium*.[435] Ampicillin-sulbactam overcomes the β-lactamase production and appears equivalent to vancomycin[436,437] (or teicoplanin[438]) in experimental IE due to these organisms and superior to therapy with ticarcillin-clavulanate.[437] Unfortunately, most β-lactamase–producing organisms also display high-level aminoglycoside resistance, thus further compromising the choice of available regimens (see below). Still other enterococci, particularly *E. faecium* or *E. raffinosus,* may display high-level penicillin resistance in the absence of β-lactamase production; experimental IE due to these organisms responds to therapy with daptomycin or vancomycin.[439] It should be noted that the traditional view of β-lactam tolerance among enterococci has been challenged[440] in that some strains demonstrate "paradoxical" tolerance (i.e., a higher percentage of survivors at higher antibiotic concentrations.) This phenomenon is more easily demonstrated in vitro at high bacterial densities in stationary growth phase, a situation presumably reflecting the in vivo conditions in the vegetation, and may be important in bacterial persistence and/or relapse during or following therapy of enterococcal endocarditis.

Cell wall–active antibiotics plus an aminoglycoside are synergistic and produce a bactericidal effect in vitro against most enterococcal strains. Successful treatment of enterococcal endocarditis requires such combinations. Studies in experimental models[441] suggest that "low-dose" streptomycin (peak serum concentrations of 9.1 μg/ml) in combination with penicillin is sufficient to treat streptomycin-susceptible enterococcal endocarditis. "High-level" streptomycin resistance (MIC >2000 μg/ml) is demonstrable in at least 40 percent of the enterococcal strains. This resistance correlates with an inability to demonstrate in vitro synergism between penicillin and streptomycin.[442] These highly resistant strains demonstrate synergism between a penicillin and gentamicin in vitro[443,444] at clinically achievable serum concentrations. Enhanced activity with the penicillin and gentamicin combination was seen in vivo for both streptomycin-resistant and streptomycin-sensitive enterococci in the rabbit model of IE. No differences in results were seen when penicillin was combined with low- vs. high-dose gentamicin (peak serum levels of 3.06 and 8.05 μg/ml, respectively) in the treatment of experimental streptomycin-resistant enterococcal endocarditis.[445] Early reports[446,447] revealed high-level gentamicin resistance among enterococci in up to 14 percent of isolates beginning in 1979. This phenomenon has become increasingly prevalent in many areas[448–450] beginning among *E. faecalis,* but now includes *E. faecium* as well.[450–452] High-level gentamicin resistance (MIC ≥ 2000 μg/ml) now accounts for at least 35 percent of enterococcal blood isolates in many hospitals. The resistance is plasmid mediated via the production of aminoglycoside-modifying enzymes and can be readily transferred among strains. A clonal dissemination is not the cause of the increased frequency of these resistant strains, since gentamicin resistance appears in a wide variety of different conjugative and nonconjugative plasmids among enterococci.[450] Although these strains seldom cause IE, they present major problems in nosocomial infections[450] and, since resistance to multiple aminoglycosides is common, represent a formidable therapeutic challenge.[453] In addition, penicillin- or vancomycin-aminoglycoside synergy is not apparent against these organisms in vitro. The optimal therapy for IE due to these highly resistant strains has not been established. None of the currently recommended regimens is bactericidal against these isolates, and valve replacement[454] may be necessary for a cure. When these isolates are encountered, all available aminoglycosides must be tested separately because the organism may be susceptible to one while resistant to others. Some isolates are sensitive to quinolones or daptomycin, but these agents have received scant attention in human infections. At this time, we favor long-term therapy (8–12 weeks) with high dosages of penicillin (20–40 million units IV daily in divided doses) or ampicillin (2–3 g IV q4h) or by continuous intravenous infusion for IE due to these multiply aminoglycoside-resistant enterococci, pending further data. Although results vary among experimental animal models of IE due to these strains,[453,455] continuous infusions of high-dose ampicillin throughout the 24-hour period may be more effective than divided doses and deserve a trial in recalcitrant cases. Even higher dose aminoglycosides and trimethoprim-sulfamethoxazole were ineffective in animal models[456,457] and cannot be recommended.

Vancomycin is also bacteriostatic against enterococci and exhibits synergy with the aminoglycosides in vitro. The vancomycin-streptomycin combination synergistically kills 40–80 percent of enterococcal strains, whereas the vancomycin-gentamicin combination demonstrates synergy against 93–98 percent.[458] Vancomycin therapy alone was ineffective in eradicating enterococci from cardiac vegetations in the rabbit model of endocarditis, but the combination of vancomycin plus gentamicin rapidly achieved a bactericidal effect.[445] Vancomycin combined with rifampin has an indifferent effect against enterococci (43/48 strains) in vitro; antagonism is observed rarely.[459] Of some concern, outbreaks of infection due to vancomycin-resistant enterococci have been described recently.[460] Glycopeptide-resistant strains of enterococci were first isolated in France in 1986. Such strains have emerged rapidly in recent years in certain areas (e.g., New York City[461]) as important causes of nosocomial infections. The genetics of vancomycin resistance[462] is described elsewhere (see Ch. 179), but multiple phenotypes exist that may confer cross-resistance to related agents (e.g., teicoplanin, daptomycin). Molecular analyses suggest that a highly mobile genetic element (e.g., a transposon) is responsible for the rapid spread of vancomycin-resistant enterococci.[461] The molecular basis for some forms of this resistance (substitutions of D-alanine-D-lactate for D-alanine-D-alanine in the terminal pentapeptide chain) has been defined. IE due to vancomycin-resistant enterococci has, so far fortunately, been unusual[463] but has occurred in transplanted hearts.[464]

The therapy of vancomycin-resistant enterococcal IE is unsettled. All suspected strains should be tested quantitatively (e.g., MIC, MBC) in vitro for susceptibility to glycopeptides, penicillins, and aminoglycosides. Teicoplanin (or potentially daptomycin)[465–467] may be useful, in combination with gentamicin, against some isolates with low-level vancomycin resistance that do not exhibit cross-resistance. Ramoplanin, a cyclic lipoglycopeptide, is active against more than 90 percent of highly vancomycin-resistant enterococci in vitro,[468] but clinical experience is virtually nonexistent for IE. A triple combination of high-dose penicillin plus vancomycin plus gentamicin appears very promising in animal models of IE induced by resistant enterococci[469,470] and should be employed if in vitro susceptibility results suggest multiply resistant isolates. The cephalosporins are relatively inactive against enterococci, even in combination with an aminoglycoside, and should not be used in this disease. The quinolones (i.e., ciprofloxacin) do not appear promising for the treatment of enterococcal endocarditis.[471]

Although controlled trials are lacking, clinical experience would dictate that enterococcal endocarditis be treated with combination antimicrobial therapy for at least 4–6 weeks.[417] The recommended regimen is as follows: aqueous penicillin G, 20 million units IV qd, combined with streptomycin, 0.5 g IM q12h, or gentamicin, 1 mg/kg IM or IV q8h, for 4–6 weeks. If toxicity (vestibular, aural, or renal) occurs, the streptomycin dose is divided into a q6h regimen. If the streptomycin MIC determined for the infecting strain is 2000 μg/ml or higher, gentamicin should be substituted for streptomycin, although relapses or therapeutic failures are unusual with penicillin plus streptomycin. We recommend penicillin plus gentamicin as the initial therapy. If the peak serum bactericidal level is less than 1:8, the penicillin dose may be increased, or the aminoglycoside drug may be changed in accordance with in vitro tests. Wilson et al.[472] analyzed the experience at the Mayo Clinic of 56 patients treated for 4 weeks with aqueous penicillin G (20 million units IV qd) combined with either streptomycin, 0.5 g IM q12h, for enterococcal IE due to streptomycin-sensitive strains or with gentamicin (1 mg/kg IM q8h) for IE due to streptomycin-resistant strains. Relapse rates were high (12.5 percent) for both regimens; however, all patients who relapsed had had symptoms suggestive of IE for longer than 3 months. Relapses also only occurred in patients with mitral valve involvement. All patients who received over 3 mg/kg qd of gentamicin developed reversible nephrotoxicity (defined as a twofold increase in serum creatinine concentration), and 19 percent of patients receiving streptomycin for 4 weeks developed irreversible vestibular toxicity. Although this was not a prospective randomized trial, we believe that selected patients with enterococcal endocarditis may be treated with 4 weeks of combination therapy. The exceptions include mitral valve involvement, symptomatic illness exceeding 3 months, enterococcal prosthetic valve endocarditis (PVE), and patients with relapse(s) of enterococcal endocarditis.

The penicillin-allergic patient presents the clinician with a difficult therapeutic dilemma. Vancomycin as a single drug at 1 g IV q12h has been used in the treatment of enterococcal endocarditis. However, experience is limited, and, because of its lack of bactericidal activity in vitro and poor performance in experimental endocarditis, vancomycin should be combined with streptomycin or gentamicin. Unfortunately, this combination is potentially more nephrotoxic, and clinical proof of the superiority of this regimen over vancomycin alone is not available. The other therapeutic option in the allergic patient is "penicillin desensitization" followed by the administration of penicillin and an aminoglycoside. The therapy of enterococcal IE due to highly aminoglycoside- or glycopeptide-resistant strains is discussed above.

Staphylococcal Endocarditis.   The mortality in acute staphylococcal endocarditis still approximates 40 percent, and the preferred antibiotic regimen is controversial. Mortality is highest for men, patients over 50 years of age, and patients with left-sided involvement and/or central nervous system manifestations. In addition, narcotic addicts appear to have a lower mortality than do nonaddicts. Most *S. aureus* isolates, whether community or hospital acquired, are now resistant to penicillin G (MIC >0.2 µg/ml). The current recommended regimen includes a penicillinase-resistant penicillin (nafcillin or oxacillin, 1.5–2 g IV q4h) or a cephalosporin (cephalothin, 2 g IV q4h, or cefazolin, 1–2 g IV or IM q8h) given for 4–6 weeks.[417,473] The addition of gentamicin produces a synergistic effect against *S. aureus* in vitro and in experimental staphylococcal endocarditis in rabbits.[474] However, the combination did not improve the survival rate (60 percent) over that observed with a penicillin derivative alone in a small group of patients.[280] Combination therapy did not improve the results of therapy for staphylococcal IE in addicts,[475] but the mortality rate is low in this subgroup of patients (≃2–8 percent) with this disease. Combination therapy may permit a shorter duration of therapy in addicts with *S. aureus* endocarditis. Two weeks of nafcillin plus tobramycin (1 mg/kg IV q8h) cured 47 of 50 (94 percent) intravenous drug abusers with right-sided endocarditis[476] without evidence of renal failure, extrapulmonary metastatic infectious complications, aortic or mitral involvement, meningitis, or infection by MRSA. In addition, anecdotal case reports in nonaddicts with staphylococcal endocarditis suggest a beneficial response by the addition of gentamicin in patients failing to respond to nafcillin therapy.[477] This issue was addressed in a multicenter prospective trial comparing nafcillin alone with nafcillin plus gentamicin (for the initial 2 weeks) in the treatment of endocarditis due to *S. aureus*.[478] Although the combination resulted in a more rapid rate of eradication of the bacteremia, the incidence of nephrotoxicity was increased, and no improvement in mortality was achieved. Despite these results, many authorities still use combination therapy for short periods (e.g., 3–5 days), especially in fulminant cases. If the organism is susceptible to penicillin (MIC, <0.1 µg/ml), then this agent in a dose of 20 million units IV qd should be used. The response to treatment may be slow, often with fever and positive blood cultures lasting up to 1 week.[277]

The therapy of staphylococcal endocarditis in penicillin allergic patients, or when the isolate is methicillin resistant (MRSA), is problematic. First-generation cephalosporins (as above) are generally recommended in patients with nonlife-threatening

penicillin allergy, but nafcillin is more active in experimental methicillin-susceptible *S. aureus* endocarditis[479] and is preferred if skin tests are negative. With the exception of ceftazidime, the in vivo efficacy of cephalosporins in experimental *S. aureus* endocarditis correlates with in vitro activity (MIC) and the time (percentage) during the dosing interval exceeding the MIC.[479] Vancomycin is still recommended for the therapy of *S. aureus* endocarditis in patients with life-threatening penicillin allergy or when MRSA are involved, but recent experience suggests caution as suboptimal outcomes have been associated with the use of this agent. Vancomycin is less rapidly bactericidal than nafcillin in vitro against *S. aureus*, especially at high inocula (approximately 10^7 cfu), mimicking intravegetation densities. Furthermore, failure rates of approximately 40 percent have been documented in patients with *S. aureus* endocarditis treated with vancomycin[480] despite right-sided involvement. In another study[481] utilizing vancomycin-based regimens, blood cultures were still positive after 7 days of therapy in approximately 50 percent of patients, again despite right-sided involvement and a large number of negative-echocardiographic studies. Daptomycin or teicoplanin are unlikely to be acceptable substitutes due to unfavorable pharmacokinetics[482] or the development of resistance[483,484] during therapy. For MSSA endocarditis in patients with β-lactam allergy and suboptimal response to vancomycin, careful consideration of performing β-lactam desensitization should be entertained.[485,486]

Clindamycin has been used to treat over 60 cases of staphylococcal endocarditis but is associated with an unacceptable relapse rate, and its use is not recommended.[487] The optimal therapy for IE due to "tolerant" strains of *S. aureus* is controversial.[488,489] One retrospective study[490] suggested that patients with IE due to these tolerant strains had a more complicated course; however, combination therapy did not appear to be of benefit. Tolerance does appear to influence the response to therapy in some experimental animal models of *S. aureus* endocarditis,[491] and combination regimens appear prudent when these strains are recovered from patients, but this is not universally accepted. Another controversial area is the adjunctive role of rifampin, the most active antibiotic currently available against *S. aureus* in vitro in therapy for IE. Due to the emergence of resistant strains, this drug is ineffective alone. Unfortunately, in vitro studies on rifampin combinations with either β-lactam agents or vancomycin are frequently contradictory, and the results in experimental IE induced by *S. aureus* are dependent on which drug in the combination exerts the greatest bactericidal activity in vivo.[492] At present, rifampin should be reserved for patients demonstrating poor serum bactericidal activity during therapy with a β-lactam or vancomycin or in those with suppurative complications (e.g., valve-ring abscesses) although rifampin-ciprofloxacin was effective therapy for right-sided *S. aureus* endocarditis in 10 intravenous drug users.[493] Resistance to both drugs has emerged during therapy of this condition, however.[494] The therapy of IE due to *S. aureus* displaying borderline susceptibility to antistaphylococcal penicillins, first described by McDougal and Thornsberry in 1986, is also a matter of debate. Experimental models of IE induced with these isolates suggest, however, that nafcillin (or oxacillin) or ampicillin–sulbactam should be effective.[495,496] Several new agents, including teicoplanin, fosfomycin, and fluoroquinolones, are active against MRSA in vitro and are as rapidly bactericidal as vancomycin in experimental animal models of IE due to MRSA,[497,498] although resistance to the quinolones has emerged during therapy and frank failures have been recorded.[486,499,500] For patients with MRSA endocarditis not responding to vancomycin, several choices are available, including the addition of rifampin and/or gentamicin, or other regimens including minocycline, trimethoprim-sulfamethoxazole, or ciprofloxacin-rifampin. Experience with these drugs in humans with *S. aureus* endocarditis is scant.

Some authors[501] have felt that when *S. aureus* bacteremia occurs in a patient with a removable focus of infection the risk of concurrent endocarditis is low, and treatment schedules may be shortened to 2–3 weeks, thus avoiding the high costs, risks of suprainfection, and/or antibiotic reactions associated with prolonged therapy. In another study, 8 of 21 patients with an infected intravenous catheter as the suspected source of *S. aureus* bacteremia developed endocarditis.[502] We concur with the findings of Bayer et al.,[486,503] who identified four parameters predictive of the presence of IE in 72 patients with *S. aureus* bacteremia in a prospective study: *(1)* the absence of a primary site of infection; *(2)* community acquisition of infection; *(3)* metastatic sequelae; and *(4)* valvular vegetations detected by echocardiography. Therefore, short-term therapy should be used only if endocarditis can be reasonably excluded by methods previously discussed. Nevertheless, the presence of occult IE in patients with nosocomial *S. aureus* bacteremia is low.[485] Screening all patients with nosocomial *S. aureus* bacteremia by transthoracic echocardiography is not cost-effective and should be reserved for those with peripheral manifestations, known underlying valvular heart disease, persistent fever, and/or bacteremia after removal of the presumed primary focus, or with new or significant heart murmurs.[485,486]

Staphylococcus epidermidis is the most common etiologic agent in cases of prosthetic valve endocarditis. Most of these strains (87 percent) are methicillin resistant when isolated within 1 year of valve implantation. Recent studies[504] suggest that the optimal antimicrobial therapy of these infections is vancomycin plus rifampin, usually with the addition of an aminoglycoside as well. The recent emergence of vancomycin resistance among coagulase-negative staphylococci[505] is cause for concern. These concepts are discussed further in Chapter 59.

Endocarditis Due to Enterobacteriaceae or Pseudomonas Species. Of 125 cases of IE reported from Seattle, 4.8 percent were due to gram-negative aerobic bacilli.[20] These patients had a mortality of 83 percent, and none treated without surgery survived. The prognosis is especially poor with left-sided cardiac involvement. Determinations of tube dilution MBC are necessary to guide therapy. Certain combinations of penicillins or cephalosporins and aminoglycosides have been shown to be synergistic against many of these strains and are usually recommended. For IE due to most strains of *E. coli* or *Proteus mirabilis* a combination of a penicillin, either ampicillin (2 g IV q4h) or penicillin (20 million units IV qd) with an aminoglycoside, usually gentamicin (1.7 mg/kg q8h) or a broad-spectrum cephalosporin is suggested. Third-generation cephalosporins are extremely active against *E. coli* in vitro, and some (e.g., ceftriaxone) have proved effective in experimental animal models of *E. coli* endocarditis,[506] even when long dosing intervals were used. This group of agents deserves further evaluation in humans for IE due to susceptible gram-negative bacilli. A combination of a third-generation cephalosporin and an aminoglycoside (either gentamicin or amikacin) is recommended for *Klebsiella* endocarditis. Certain β-lactam/β-lactamase inhibitor combinations (e.g., piperacillin-tazobactam[507] but not ceftriaxone-sulbactam[508]) are active in vivo in experimental models of *Klebsiella* endocarditis in animals induced by TEM-3–producing isolates and deserve further evaluation in combination with an aminoglycoside in humans with this disease. The specific aminoglycoside employed is a critical variable and cannot be totally predicted from MIC data alone, as pharmacodynamic characteristics differ markedly in animal models of IE due to gram-negative aerobic bacilli.[509,510] Endovascular *Salmonella* infections, including IE, may also respond to third-generation cephalosporins (see below).[511] Left-sided IE due to *S. marcescens* is refractory to medical therapy alone; valve replacement is invariably required to effect a cure.[304]

Pseudomonas aeruginosa remains an important pathogen in addicts with IE. Medical therapy may be successful in *P. aeruginosa* endocarditis involving the right side of the heart. If the disease is refractory to antibiotics, tricuspid valvulectomy or

"vegetectomy"[512] without valve replacement is indicated.[513] Although valve replacement is often necessary for a cure of left-sided IE due to *P. aeruginosa*,[514] recent experience[163] with 10 patients (7 with left-sided involvement alone or in combination with tricuspid disease) suggests that medical therapy alone is occasionally curative. Studies in animals with experimental *Pseudomonas* endocarditis[515] offer an explanation for these disparate results: the penetration into vegetations and the time antibiotic concentrations exceeded the MBC were both significantly greater in tricuspid than in aortic vegetations for both ceftazidime and tobramycin.

The optimal antimicrobial regimen for *P. aeruginosa* endocarditis is evolving; the most extensive experience has been at the Detroit Medical Center. Problems have emerged with all potential regimens in animal models of this disease, as extensively studied by Bayer, Levison, and colleagues: *(1)* therapy with β-lactams (e.g., ceftazidime) has failed due to the constitutive hyperproduction of type Id β-lactamase[516]; *(2)* aminoglycoside-resistant isolates due to permeability defects emerge during therapy[517]; *(3)* no postantibiotic effect of β-lactams against *P. aeruginosa* is evident in vivo,[518] thus necessitating frequent (or continuous) drug administration; and *(4)* inhibition by the alginate exopolysaccharide of clearance of mucoid strains from the vegetation via cellular or antimicrobial mechanisms. This can be partially reversed by the coadministration of alginase in animal models of *Pseudomonas* endocarditis.[519] Treatment failures of *Pseudomonas* endocarditis in humans have been due to the selection of isolates with an enhanced production of type Id β-lactamase.[520] Based on clinical experience,[163,284,306,307] however, the preferred regimen for IE due to *P. aeruginosa* is high-dose tobramycin (8 mg/kg/day IV or IM in divided doses q8h) with maintenance of peak and trough concentrations of 15–20 and 2 μg/ml or less, respectively, in combination with an extended-spectrum penicillin (e.g., ticarcillin, piperacillin, azlocillin) or ceftazidime in full doses. The toxicity associated with this regimen is surprisingly low; treatment should be combined for a minimum of 6 weeks. The quinolones are promising for the treatment of *Pseudomonas* endocarditis on the basis of favorable results in animal models[516] and in humans,[521] but the development of stepwise resistance during therapy may limit the efficacy of this class of drugs in the future. Based on limited experimental data,[522] ceftazidime–tobramycin is preferred over aztreonam–tobramycin for this disease. Approximately seven cases of *P. aeruginosa* endocarditis have been successfully treated with imipenem plus an aminoglycoside,[523] but the potential for the development of resistance exists with any of these regimens.

Infective endocarditis due to *Haemophilus* spp. is usually responsive to ampicillin alone[293] administered for 3 weeks. However, therapy for IE due to these (and other) fastidious gram-negative organisms must be individualized on the basis of in vitro susceptibility data; in practice, β-lactam–aminoglycoside combinations are usually employed for approximately 1 month. The role of the newer third-generation cephalosporins in the treatment of IE due to gram-negative bacilli is unknown despite excellent in vitro activity and the potential for the avoidance of aminoglycoside-induced toxicity. Similarly, the place for quinolones (if any) in the therapy of these infections is not known.[524] It is important to emphasize that the above recommendations offer only a rough guide for initial treatment. However, it is imperative that each isolate be subjected to quantitative sensitivity testing in vitro to ensure the optimal selection of antibiotics.

Endocarditis Due to Anaerobic Bacilli. Although IE caused by anaerobic bacilli is uncommon, the mortality is high. *Bacteroides fragilis* is isolated in many of these cases and is responsible for most fatalities. Most strains of anaerobic bacilli, with the exception of *B. fragilis*, are sensitive to penicillin in vitro, and this agent, in a dose of 20 million units IV qd, is the recommended therapy.[342,343] In addition, 33 percent of the strains of *B. fragilis* demonstrate an MIC of penicillin that is less than 25 μg/ml, and increasing resistance to penicillin among multiple anaerobic genera is evident. However, penicillin is only bacteriostatic against these strains (MBC invariably greater than 100 μg/ml), and relapse of the disease is common. Although clindamycin, carbenicillin, and chloramphenicol readily inhibit most strains of *B. fragilis*, they lack bactericidal activity, and they are poor therapeutic choices even though several patients have been cured with either high-dose penicillin, chloramphenicol (1 g IV q6h), clindamycin (600 mg IV q6h), or carbenicillin (5 g IV q3h). Due to excellent bactericidal activity in vitro and the serum concentrations attained, metronidazole, ticarcillin plus clavulanic acid, or imipenem are reasonable choices for therapy for anaerobic endocarditis.[344]

Pneumococcal, Gonococcal, and Meningococcal Endocarditis. Infective endocarditis caused by these organisms is now very rare. Pneumococcal endocarditis must be considered in any patient with pneumococcal bacteremia, especially if meningitis is present. Most common in alcoholics, the organism generally attacks the aortic valve and results in valvular insufficiency, often with perivalvular abscess formation and/or pericarditis. Type 12 pneumococci cause over 20 percent of the cases of pneumococcal endocarditis but are a rare (5 percent of the cases) cause of pneumococcal pneumonia. Penicillin, 20 million units IV qd or a third-generation cephalosporin for 4 weeks, is recommended for the treatment of pneumococcal endocarditis.

The gonococci that cause systemic infection are usually susceptible to penicillin.[525] These organisms as well as the meningococci can be effectively treated with the same penicillin regimen recommended for pneumococcal endocarditis. Although endocarditis due to penicillin-resistant gonococci (PPNG or chromosomally mediated) has not been reported, ceftriaxone has been used successfully to treat gonococcal endocarditis.[526]

Fungal Endocarditis. The incidence of IE caused by fungi has undergone a striking increase in the past decade. Fungal endocarditis occurs principally in a setting of narcotic addiction, after cardiac surgery, after the prolonged intravenous administration of drugs (especially broad-spectrum antibiotics), and in the compromised host. The overall survival rate in patients treated since 1968 is only 14.5 percent.[200] The preferred mode of therapy is unknown. The use of antifungal agents alone has been almost universally unsuccessful in achieving a cure of this disease. The addition of surgical measures to antifungal therapy may result in an improvement in prognosis, but to date there is insufficient clinical experience. When fungal endocarditis is diagnosed, a combined medical/surgical approach should be undertaken.

The mainstay of antifungal drug therapy is amphotericin B. This agent is toxic and produces multiple side effects, including fever, chills, phlebitis, headache, anorexia, anemia, hypokalemia, renal tubular acidosis, nephrotoxicity, nausea, and vomiting. Drug toxicity is frequent and commonly necessitates alterations in the regimen. Dosages and the technique of administration are given in Chapter 31.

After 1–2 weeks of amphotericin B therapy at "full" dosages, surgery should probably be performed. If isolated tricuspid endocarditis is present, as in a narcotic addict, total tricuspid valvulectomy can usually be performed. Rarely, removal of the vegetation alone is curative. Most of these patients tolerate the valvulectomy without the development of significant right-sided heart failure. Valve replacement is necessary for left-sided fungal endocarditis. The duration of antifungal therapy after surgery is empirical, but 6–8 weeks is usually recommended.

It is possible that combination antifungal therapy may improve the poor survival from fungal endocarditis. Some strains of *Candida* spp. and *Cryptococcus neoformans* are inhibited in vitro by concentrations of 5-fluorocytosine achieved with the oral administration of 150 mg/kg/day in six divided doses. Synergism between 5-fluorocytosine and amphotericin B has been documented for these yeasts in vitro and in the treatment of cryptococcal meningitis. This combination was fungicidal and perhaps instrumental in the cure of one case of *Aspergillus* endocarditis. However, in the rabbit model of endocarditis due to *Candida albicans*[203] the addition of 5-fluorocytosine did not improve the rate of eradication of fungal organisms from the vegetation when compared with amphotericin B alone. Potentiation of amphotericin B activity by rifampin has been noted for virtually all strains tested of *Candida* spp. and for a few isolates of *Histoplasma capsulatum*. The therapeutic advantage of the addition of 5-fluorocytosine or rifampin to amphotericin for fungal endocarditis requires further investigation, but initial results in animal models of disseminated candidiasis are not encouraging.[527] On the basis of animal model data,[528] high-dose intraconazole may be of value in the treatment of *Aspergillus* endocarditis, but valve replacement will likely remain imperative for a cure. Amphotericin B is more effective than fluconazole for the prophylaxis and/or treatment of experimental *Candida* endocarditis[529] and remains the agent of choice. Fluconazole has apparently, however, led to long-term cures of *Candida* endocarditis in a few patients[530,531] when valve replacement was considered to be contraindicated. This agent should be tried after an initial course of amphotericin B in this setting. The role of amphotericin-lipid/liposomal complexes in the treatment of fungal endocarditis is unknown.

Q Fever Endocarditis. More than 200 well-documented cases of Q fever have been reported, and the mortality exceeds 65 percent.[361,362,364] Prolonged therapy with doxycycline and either trimethoprim–sulfamethoxazole or rifampin is considered to be the regimen of choice (see Ch. 166). The fluoroquinolones may be a useful addition to doxycycline.[534] Valve replacement is often required, and long-term prognosis is guarded. A careful follow-up for recrudescence of infection is essential.

Infective Endocarditis Due to Chlamydiae. Albeit based on limited experience, a combination of valve replacement and prolonged (greater than 3 months) tetracycline therapy seems justified in these cases. Rifampin has cured at least one case of chlamydial IE after therapy with tetracyclines had failed, but exposure to this agent rapidly induces the emergence of rifampin resistance of *C. trachomatis* in tissue culture.[540] The role of combination regimens (e.g., rifampin plus erythromycin or tetracycline) deserves further study.

Culture-Negative Endocarditis. The therapy for culture-negative endocarditis is controversial, but the regimen usually used will "cover" the enterococcus and fastidious gram-negative bacilli and consists of a combination of penicillin, 20 million units IV qd in divided doses, or ampicillin, 2 g IV q4h, plus streptomycin, 0.5 g IM q12h, or gentamicin, 1.7 mg/kg IM or IV q8h. When staphylococcal endocarditis is a strong consideration (for narcotic addicts or after cardiac surgery), a penicillinase-resistant penicillin or a cephalosporin in full dosage should be added to this regimen. If clinical improvement occurs, some authorities recommend discontinuation of treatment with the aminoglycoside after 2 weeks. The other agent(s) should be continued for a full 6 weeks of treatment. Continued surveillance for an etiologic agent and careful follow-up are mandatory. An analysis of any correlation between the response to empirical antimicrobial therapy and survival was performed in 52 patients with culture-negative endocarditis:[372] 92 percent of the patients who became afebrile within the first week of therapy survived vs. only 50 percent if fever persisted longer than 7 days. Most deaths were caused by major systemic emboli or uncontrollable congestive heart failure due to valvular insufficiency.

Surgical Therapy

In recent years, valve replacement has become an important adjunct to medical therapy in the management of IE and is now used in at least 25 percent of the cases. The generally accepted indications for surgical intervention during active IE are as follows: *(1)* refractory congestive heart failure; *(2)* more than one serious systemic embolic episode; *(3)* uncontrolled infection; *(4)* valve dysfunction as demonstrated by fluoroscopy; *(5)* ineffective antimicrobial therapy (e.g., fungal endocarditis); *(6)* resection of mycotic aneurysms; *(7)* most cases of prosthetic valve endocarditis; and *(8)* local suppurative complications including perivalvular or myocardial abscesses with conduction system abnormalities, heart block, and so forth. The major indications in the past have been persistent infection and congestive heart failure[536–538] in both adults and children.[539] For example, congestive heart failure during active IE was the indication for surgery in 86 percent of 108 patients undergoing valve replacement at Stanford from 1963 to 1984.[538]

The most frequent causes of death in IE, in approximate order, are neurologic and septic complications,[540] congestive heart failure, embolic phenomena, rupture of a mycotic aneurysm, complications of cardiac surgery, lack of response to antimicrobial therapy, and prosthetic valve endocarditis.[2,3,6–9,11,12,14–17,20] Failure to make a diagnosis or renal failure are rare causes of death. In a recent review from Seattle,[20] congestive heart failure was present in 91 percent of the patients who died. Overall, two-thirds of the patients in this series of 125 cases developed congestive heart failure, and this complication appears to be increasing in frequency. The overall mortality in this group of patients was 37 percent.

When acute aortic regurgitation complicated by congestive heart failure supervenes in IE, the mortality still exceeds 50 percent. The classic physical findings of chronic aortic regurgitation are often absent in these patients.[228] The current trend is to advise early surgery in this group of patients, since nothing is gained by delay. In a series of 28 patients from Birmingham, Alabama, with acute aortic regurgitation, 4 had no congestive heart failure and were treated medically, and all survived. In contrast, 7 of 11 patients with mild congestive heart failure and 7 of 8 with moderate to severe congestive heart failure died during medical therapy, often suddenly and with pathologic evidence of coronary emboli and myocardial infarction. Four of five patients with moderately severe congestive heart failure who underwent surgery survived. This suggests that early surgical intervention may improve the survival statistics in this setting. Valvular regurgitation on Doppler echocardiography is not predictive of death in the absence of congestive heart failure.[541] Similar results were obtained at the Mayo Clinic (3/11 deaths). The hemodynamic status of the patient, not the activity of the infection, is the critical determining factor in the timing of cardiac valve replacement.[542] The hemodynamic severity of the acute aortic regurgitation may be assessed by determining the degree of mitral valve preclosure by echocardiography. If premature closure of the mitral valve occurs before the Q wave of the electrocardiogram, then the left ventricular end-diastolic pressure is very high, and surgical intervention is urgently required. Nothing is gained by temporizing, even if only a few hours of antibiotics can be administered. When congestive heart failure persists despite digoxin, diuretics, and other therapeutic modalities, surgery is also indicated. In 80 patients subjected to aortic valve replacement for IE, the surgical cure rate was 72 percent. There were no instances of subsequent infection of the prosthesis, but 16 percent developed paravalvular regurgitation. This latter complication was usually easily controlled medically. Organisms visible on Gram stain, positive cultures, or annular abscesses at the time of surgery are associated with late complications.[540] When left-sided IE is present and the clinical assessment implicates more than one valve or extravalvular extension

of the disease, then cardiac angiography is useful in delineating the proper surgical approach (see above).

In contrast to left-sided IE where congestive heart failure is the usual indication for surgical intervention, in right-sided IE persistent infection is the indication for surgery in over 70 percent of the patients. Most of the patients are narcotic addicts, with IE caused by organisms that are difficult to eradicate with antimicrobial therapy alone (e.g., fungi, gram-negative aerobic bacilli). Tricuspid valvulectomy or "vegetectomy" with valvuloplasty is now the procedure of choice for refractory right-sided IE.[543,544] Valve replacement at a second operation is advised only when medical management fails to control the hemodynamic manifestations and the patient has ceased using illicit drugs. Combination antimicrobial therapy with optimal serum bactericidal activity should be continued for 4–6 weeks postoperatively. These patients may develop mild to moderate right-sided heart failure, but this is easily tolerated, and the success rate of this approach is over 70 percent. Persistent fever, recurrent pulmonary emboli, or vegetations demonstrable by echocardiography usually do not require tricuspid valvulectomy in this setting.[545] In addition, many surgeons contend that a return to the use of illicit drugs and reinfection of the valve after initial cure is a contraindication to reoperation.[546]

Outstanding reviews on the indications for surgery during therapy for IE are available.[537,547] The rationale for surgical intervention, including major and minor criteria for valve replacement, are discussed in detail. A point system weighting multiple factors has been devised by Alsip and colleagues to assist in decision making concerning surgery in patients with active IE.[547] The value of this system remains to be defined. It has become apparent that most patients with prosthetic valve endocarditis (except those with late disease caused by penicillin-sensitive viridans streptococci) require valve replacement for consistent cures (see Ch. 59). Valve replacement is also necessary in a large proportion of patients with IE on native valves after a medical cure; aortic involvement is a predictor of the need for surgery.[548]

SUPPURATIVE THROMBOPHLEBITIS

Suppurative thrombophlebitis is an inflammation of the vein wall due to the presence of microorganisms and is frequently associated with thrombosis and bacteremia. Suppuration of the vein wall is usually absent in intravenous catheter-related sepsis and bacteremia secondary to contaminated intravenous fluid but does occur. Suppurative thrombophlebitis may be classified into four forms: superficial, central (including pelvic), cavernous sinus, and infection of the portal vein (pylophlebitis). The last two conditions have become rare since the introduction of antibiotics. Cavernous sinus thrombosis and thrombosis of the intracranial dural sinuses are discussed in Chapters 71 and 95. In contrast, superficial suppurative thrombophlebitis has been steadily increasing in incidence since the introduction of the plastic intravenous cannula. Superficial suppurative thrombophlebitis secondary to intravenous fluid therapy was first described in 1947[549] when 93 cases were reported, 43 of which were amenable to surgical therapy.

Epidemiology

In 1973, approximately one of every four hospitalized patients received intravenous therapy, for a total of over 10 million patients annually in the United States.[550] Suppurative thrombophlebitis accounts for up to 10 percent of all nosocomial infections and is a particular problem in burned patients, for whom it represents a common cause of death due to infection. In several large series of burned patients,[551–554] suppurative thrombophlebitis developed in 4–8 percent and increased in frequency if cutdowns were performed. Suppurative thrombophlebitis is also found in other hospitalized patients (especially those with cancer and/or those receiving steroid therapy).[555,556] Seven such cases were recognized in an 18-month period in Charleston, South Carolina, and 35 cases were identified in 7 years in Louisville, Kentucky. Suppurative thrombophlebitis may also be increasing in frequency. Eight cases were encountered during an 8-month period in Johannesburg; suppurative thrombophlebitis was estimated to represent a minimum incidence of 0.12 percent of all admissions.[558] When using strict criteria, 29 episodes of suppurative thrombophlebitis in 27 patients were identified in a large Air Force hospital within 4 years.[559] Based on data from the National Nosocomial Infection Study, Rhame and associates[560] estimate the overall incidence of suppurative thrombophlebitis as 88 per 100,000 discharges, but this disease is underreported. Suppurative thrombophlebitis is also common in abusers of intravenous drugs.[561] This condition is unusual during childhood[562] but may occur as a complication related to intravenous therapy. Catheter-related sepsis without suppurative thrombophlebitis is more common and affects at least 25,000 patients per year in the United States.[563] The risk of this complication is approximately 40 times higher with plastic cannulas (8 percent) than with steel or "scalp vein" cannulas (0.2 percent). Irritation to the vein wall and the subsequent development of suppurative thrombophlebitis is greater with polyethylene catheters than those constructed of Teflon or Silastic materials. Central venous catheterization has been employed for over 30 years for hemodynamic monitoring, total parenteral nutrition (TPN), and infusion of drugs. The exact incidence of suppurative thrombophlebitis of the central veins commonly cannulated (i.e., jugulars, subclavian, venae cavae) is unknown. Catheter-induced thrombosis is relatively common. Autopsy series have revealed central venous thrombosis in 37 percent of catheterized subjects, but this diagnosis is rarely recognized because most patients are asymptomatic. When examined by phlebography at the time of catheter withdrawal, 42 percent of catheters have sleeve thrombi, and another 8 percent revealed veno-occlusive thrombi.[564] In addition, sepsis has been reported in approximately 7 percent of patients receiving TPN and other medications by the central route. When thrombosis and bacterial or fungal contamination/sepsis coexist, suppurative thrombophlebitis may intervene. At least 50 cases of suppurative thrombophlebitis of the great thoracic veins have been reported in the literature,[565–567] but this is almost certainly a gross underestimate of the problem. Eight cases in 8 years due to *Candida* spp. alone were observed at the University of Wisconsin.[568] As another example, 53 cancer patients with catheter-related *Staphylococcus aureus* bacteremia were identified over a 3-year period (1986–1989) at the M.D. Anderson Cancer Center; septic thrombosis was diagnosed in 12 (23 percent) and suspected in another 3 (6 percent) patients. Five of these 12 patients developed deep-seated complications, including septic pulmonary emboli and endocarditis, vs. 2 of 38 without septic thrombosis (p < 0.01). Persistent fever despite appropriate antistaphylococcal agents was an early clue to the diagnosis.[569] Septic atrial thrombosis, occasionally with a coexistent Budd-Chiari syndrome, has complicated Broviac catheter insertion in infants.[570]

Superficial suppurative thrombophlebitis is a complication of either a dermal infection or an indwelling intravenous catheter. Pelvic suppurative thrombophlebitis is associated with parturition, abortion, gynecologic surgery, or a pelvic abscess. Therefore, this is a disease of women of the childbearing age, with most cases occuring between the ages of 15 and 40 years (mean, 20 years). In 123 cases in two reports,[571,572] the predisposing conditions were as follows: vaginal delivery, 39 cases; cesarean section, 19 cases; abortion, 33 cases; and major gynecologic surgery, 32 cases. During a 9-year period in Atlanta, 27 cases of postpartum septic pelvic thrombophlebitis were identified in over 54,000 deliveries.[572] The relative risks for this condition were as follows: parturition, 1/2000 (highest in the inner-city population); septic abortion, 1/200; and major gynecologic sur-

gery, 1/800. The incidence of suppurative thrombophlebitis rises proportionally with the degree of trauma to the pelvic tissues.

Pathogenesis

The pathogenesis of suppurative thrombophlebitis is poorly understood. A thrombus may act as a nidus for local entrapment and colonization of bacteria that gain access to the site from another focus. This is analogous to the proposed role of nonbacterial thrombotic endocarditis in the pathogenesis of IE. When superficial suppurative thrombophlebitis is associated with intravascular cannulae, the route of infection may be *(1)* migration from the skin between the catheter wall and perivascular tissue, *(2)* in contaminated IV fluid, and *(3)* hematogenous dissemination from an infected focus elsewhere. The relative contribution(s) of these three routes is unknown. The observation that the predominant organism in burn wounds, *Pseudomonas aeruginosa,* is a rare cause of suppurative thrombophlebitis and that suppurative thrombophlebitis usually develops days to weeks after the cutdown incision is healed[552,554] argues against a local cutaneous source in burn patients.

The venous system draining the pelvis includes the intervertebral venous plexus, the lumbar venous plexus, the superficial and deep veins of the abdominal wall, and the hemorrhoidal plexus. Any component of this system may be affected in pelvic suppurative thrombophlebitis, but the veins draining the uterus, including the ovarian veins and the inferior vena cava, are most often involved.[573] Thrombus formation may result from stasis of blood flow due to the gravid uterus and by the hypercoagulable state of parturition. Normal residents of the vaginal or perineal bacterial flora gain access to the thrombus via the blood stream and/or regional lymphatics. There is often an associated endometritis or parametritis. Septic pulmonary emboli and metastatic abscess formation are common. Septic thrombosis of the portal vein is often associated with hepatic abscess (five of seven patients in one series[574]); an obvious extrahepatic source of intrabdominal infection is usually absent.

Pathologic Changes

Regardless of the vein involved, the pathologic changes are similar. The vein is enlarged, tortuous, and thickened. There may be associated perivascular suppuration and/or hemorrhage, and the vein lumen usually contains both pus and thrombus. Microscopically, endothelial damage, fibrinoid necrosis, and thickening of the vein wall are evident. Microabscesses may be present in the vein wall or in the surrounding tissue.[557,575] Gross periphlebitic abscesses are not unusual and may be evident on physical examination. Thrombi frequently extend beyond the area of suppuration. In an autopsy series of peripheral suppurative thrombophlebitis in burned patients, extension of the clot into the great central veins was found in 18 percent of the cases.[552,554] Metastatic abscess formation and septic pulmonary emboli with infarction are found in over 50 percent of the fatal cases. This may result from bacterial liquefaction and fragmentation of affected thrombi within the vein, since clot liquefaction is noted commonly in autopsy series.

Clinical Manifestations

Superficial suppurative thrombophlebitis is often difficult to identify since local findings of inflammation may be absent. The disease occurs more frequently when plastic catheters are inserted in the lower extremities, a common practice in burn patients. In 132 cases reported from the burn center at Fort Sam Houston, Texas, the distribution of superficial suppurative thrombophlebitis was as follows: lower extremity (predominantly saphenous system), 100; upper extremity (predominantly antecubital fossa), 32; jugular, 7; and iliac, 4. The mean duration of preceding venous cannulation was 4.81 days, and the latent interval from removal of the catheter to the development of symptoms ranged from 2 to 10 days.[551,553] Fever was present in over 70 percent of the cases, but rigors were rare. Local findings such as warmth, erythema, tenderness, swelling, or lymphangitis were present in only 32 percent of these patients; however, bacteremia with signs of systemic sepsis were found in 84 percent. Septic pulmonary emboli with secondary pneumonia occurred in 44 percent and were often the first diagnostic clue. Thus, pneumonia, sepsis, or metastatic abscess formation was the only manifestation of this disease in two-thirds of the cases. These authors emphasize that the late onset of pneumonia or sepsis in a burned patient demands the careful inspection of all previously cannulated veins since untreated suppurative thrombophlebitis is associated with a high mortality. In these series, fewer than 50 percent of the cases were diagnosed antemortem.[552]

In contrast to the experience with suppurative thrombophlebitis in burn patients, most medical and postoperative patients develop superficial suppurative thrombophlebitis in the upper extremities, and signs of local inflammation are more commonly present (94 percent in one series).[561] Many of these patients are elderly (20/35 over 50 years old) with debilitating diseases and are often receiving antibiotics when superficial suppurative thrombophlebitis intervenes. As above, the duration of intravenous catheterization is an important risk factor; 68 percent of implicated cannulae had been left in place for at least 5 days in patients reported.[560,561]

Subperiosteal abscesses of adjacent long bones may complicate superficial suppurative thrombophlebitis in children.[576] The local findings of this condition, including bone tenderness, erythema, warmth, and limitation of motion with occasional extension into the joint space, may overshadow the suppurative thrombophlebitis itself. Septic deep vein thrombosis of the femoral vessels with swollen, tender, and inflamed inguinal areas has been described in intravenous users of heroin and cocaine. Contiguous pelvic bone osteomyelitis is unusual.

Suppurative thrombophlebitis of the thoracic central veins occurs in critically ill patients with central catheters in place, in those receiving TPN, or in patients after long-term cannulation with Broviac, Hickman, and other devices. The systemic findings of sepsis overshadow any local findings of venous occlusion (e.g., superior vena cava syndrome), which are rare in this setting. This syndrome should be suspected in any septic patient when bacteremia and/or fungemia fail to resolve upon removal of the central catheter and institution of appropriate antimicrobial therapy.

Pelvic suppurative thrombophlebitis usually develops 1–2 weeks postpartum or postoperatively and is associated with high fever, chills, anorexia, nausea, vomiting, abdominal pain, and a protracted course.[572] Flank pain may result from ureteral obstruction by enlarged veins. Abdominal tenderness, usually in the right lower quadrant, may be mild to severe. Approximately 80 percent of cases are unilateral on the right side, 14 percent are bilateral, and only 6 percent are unilateral and left sided. This distribution is thought to result from compression of the right ovarian vein at the pelvic brim by the enlarged uterus with retrograde flow on the left and protection from ascending infection. However, the physical examination may be normal. A tender vein can be palpated in 30 percent of the cases on pelvic or abdominal examination.[557] The uterus is usually freely movable. Spread of the process to the femoral vein with edema and tenderness of the lower extremity is unusual. Many of these patients are extremely ill with an acute or chronic course characterized by little or no response to antibiotics and the development of multiple, small, septic pulmonary emboli. Since many of the manifestations are nonspecific, the differential diagnosis is broad and includes acute appendicitis, ureteral obstruction, torsion of an ovarian cyst, pyelonephritis, broad ligament hematoma, parametritis, endometritis, perinephric abscess, pelvic

abscess, small bowel volvulus, pelvic inflammatory disease, sickle cell crisis, and ectopic pregnancy.

Laboratory Findings

Bacteremia occurs in 80–90 percent of the cases of superficial suppurative thrombophlebitis. Gross pus within the vein lumen is found in about one-half of the cases, and this finding establishes a diagnosis of suppurative phlebitis. When infection of a venous catheter is suspected, it should be removed and cultured. The results, however, may be misleading, since even though bacteria will be isolated in up to 60 percent of the cases a positive culture does not correlate with inflammation.[577] The following semiquantitative culture technique has been developed in an attempt to differentiate catheter-related sepsis from suppurative thrombophlebitis. After preparing the skin with alcohol, the catheter is removed with sterile forceps (avoiding skin contact) and is placed in a sterile tube for transport. The catheter is then aseptically cut into 5.7 cm pieces, and each section is rolled across the surface of a 5% sheep blood agar plate. The growth of more than 15 colonies on the plate correlates well[577] with the presence of venous infection. In the few cases of suppurative thrombophlebitis studied by this technique, all catheters have yielded confluent growth. Since the standard 5.7 cm catheter retains approximately 0.7–1.5 mg of moisture on its surface and the plate growth has exceeded 1000 colonies in every case of suppurative thrombophlebitis, bacterial counts must exceed 10^6 organisms/g in the catheter wound. These titers are similar to those found in other types of infected wounds. This technique is simple, rapid, and inexpensive and may prove useful in establishing the need for exploratory venotomy. Simple needle aspiration of the suspected vein may also be diagnostic.[111] In-labeled leukocyte imaging studies have detected superficial suppurative thrombophlebitis, but experience is limited.

Other laboratory findings in patients with superficial suppurative thrombophlebitis, for example, leukocytosis, are nonspecific. The chest x-ray film may reveal multiple peripheral densities or a pleural effusion consistent with pulmonary emboli, infarction, abscess, or empyema. The diagnosis of an associated subperiosteal abscess is difficult: bone and gallium scans usually reveal hyperperfusion without definite osteomyelitis, routine x-ray films are virtually always negative, and CT often demonstrates only soft tissue swelling with obliteration of tissue planes. High-resolution CT scans may improve these results.[576] The diagnosis of deep central vein suppurative thrombophlebitis in the thorax is established by venography with the demonstration of thrombi in a patient with positive blood cultures, but CT with contrast enhancement is probably as sensitive and is noninvasive. Computed tomography scans are clearly useful in the diagnosis of suppurative phlebitis of the great central veins[578,579] and the portal vein[573]; gas may be detected in the venular lumen, diagnostic of this condition. Experience with magnetic resonance imaging and ^{111}In-labeled leukocytes is meager.

In most cases of pelvic suppurative thrombophlebitis there is a peripheral blood leukocytosis, and the urinalysis is usually normal. The chest x-ray film may reveal multiple septic pulmonary emboli, and abdominal x-ray films may show a pelvic mass. Intravenous pyelography can be useful in disclosing ureteral obstruction. Real-time ultrasonography is very helpful in delineating the location and extent of the thrombus, but the ileus that is often associated with this infection may render interpretation difficult. Computed tomography reveals low attenuation with contrast enhancement in suppurative venous thrombosis and is very sensitive in the diagnosis of pelvic suppurative thrombophlebitis.[580,581] Magnetic resonance imaging may be even more sensitive and can differentiate fresh ($\leq$1-week-old) from organizing or subacute thrombosis.[582] These sensitive and noninvasive techniques may lead to an increased recognition of pelvic suppurative thrombophlebitis, earlier diagnosis, and improved outcome. The role of newer diagnostic techniques such as pelvic venography, transuterine phlebography, ^{111}In-labeled leukocyte scanning, and laparoscopy is still undefined. Since bacteremia is demonstrated in only 20–30 percent[571,572,583] of cases of pelvic suppurative thrombophlebitis, negative blood cultures do not exclude the diagnosis.

Etiologic Agents

Staphylococcus aureus was the causative agent of 65–78 percent of the cases of superficial suppurative thrombophlebitis reported before 1968. In recent years, most have been due to the Enterobacteriaceae, especially *Klebsiella-Enterobacter* spp.[555,561] These agents are acquired nosocomially and are often resistant to multiple antibiotics. Nearly all patients with superficial suppurative thrombophlebitis due to gram-negative aerobic bacilli or fungi are receiving broad-spectrum antibiotics at the time the disease becomes manifested. In a review of 86 cases compiled from the literature reported since 1970, the organisms isolated were as follows: *Klebsiella-Enterobacter* spp., 34; *Providencia* spp., 5; *Proteus* spp., 5; *Serratia* spp., 3; *E. coli*, 6; *Pseudomonas aeruginosa*, 3; *Staphylococcus aureus*, 15; *Candida albicans*, 9; *Staphylococcus epidermidis*, 4; and enterococci, 2.[560,561] Suppurative thrombophlebitis due to gram-negative pathogens and *E. faecalis* is more common (than *Staphylococcus aureus*) in patients with significant intra-abdominal pathology.[559] *Staphylococcus aureus*, other gram-positive cocci, and *Candida* spp. were more frequent when this risk factor was absent. Multiple organisms are isolated in up to 14 percent of cases. Anaerobic isolates are extremely rare. An increase in incidence of superficial suppurative thrombophlebitis due to *Candida* spp. was reported recently;[584,585] all patients were receiving antibiotics without hyperalimentation. None were neutropenic or receiving corticosteroids. In one series of seven patients observed in a 15-month interval,[585] all had concomitant or preceding bacterial infections and had received a median of five antibiotics for at least 2 weeks. Preceding candidal colonization at other sites (e.g., sputum, urine) was often present.[573] *Malassezia furfur* is also seen as an opportunistic pathogen of deep vein catheters, especially in premature infants[586] and others in the pediatric age group receiving lipid emulsions, but this risk factor is not present in all patients. Septic thrombosis, endocarditis, and other metastatic complications are not uncommon in this setting of disseminated *Malassezia* infection.[586] Although not documented by culture, histopathologic evidence suggests that cytomegalovirus may cause suppurative thrombophlebitis in patients with AIDS despite therapy with ganciclovir.[587]

The responsible agents in pelvic suppurative thrombophlebitis are poorly defined, since blood cultures are often negative and most investigators did not use adequate anaerobic techniques. The organisms isolated in approximate order of frequency are *Bacteroides* spp., microaerophilic or anaerobic streptococci, *E. coli* and other coliforms, and β-hemolytic streptococci. The predominance of *Bacteroides* spp. may be related to the heparinase produced by this organism. A prolonged latent period (up to 3 weeks) may occur before blood cultures become positive. The more extensive use of anaerobic isolation techniques and the routine culturing of surgical specimens may serve to clarify the role of anaerobic bacteria in this entity.

Presumptive Therapy

Superficial suppurative thrombophlebitis is a lethal iatrogenic disease, and surgery is often necessary for cure. The first reported successful cure of suppurative thrombophlebitis followed surgical ligation of the vein by John Hunter in 1784.[588] All investigators strongly endorse surgical excision as an integral part of the management. In a review of 24 patients,[552] 14 were treated medically alone, and all died either directly from suppurative thrombophlebitis with persistent bacteremia or secondary to metastatic complications. However, of 10 patients who underwent surgical exploration, 7 survived, and only 1 of the 3 deaths was attributable to suppurative thrombophlebitis. Antibiotics should also be used in the treatment of this disease; initial treatment with a semisynthetic penicillin (e.g., nafcillin, 2 g IV q4–6h) plus an aminoglycoside (e.g., gentamicin, 1.0–1.7 mg/kg IV or IM q8h) is recommended, since the Enterobacteriaceae and/or staphylococci are the usual etiologic agents. The optimum duration of therapy is unknown and largely empirical. The role of antifungal therapy for superficial suppurative thrombophlebitis due to *Candida albicans* is controversial.[584,585] Although most of these infections can be cured by vein excision, a short course of amphotericin B (approximately 200 mg) is advised postoperatively, pending further data. Antifungal therapy is mandatory in the immunosuppressed patient or if signs of metastatic complications (e.g., endophthalmitis) develop.

When superficial suppurative thrombophlebitis is considered, an exploratory venotomy is necessary. This procedure should be performed proximal to the suspected site; the vein should be ligated and then "milked" in an attempt to express purulent material for inspection by Gram stain and culture. If no pus is apparent, an exploratory venotomy is necessary to establish the diagnosis. Simple ligation was thought to be sufficient 30 years ago, but the rate of relapse with ongoing sepsis was high. Therefore, the segment of vein and all its involved tributaries should be totally excised. Radical surgery from the ankle to the groin may be required in some burn patients. Nevertheless, local or regional anesthesia alone is often sufficient (approximately 90 percent of cases) for vein excision. Backbleeding, indicative of a patent lumen, should be evident at the point of vein transection. Vein excision is usually followed by prompt (≤24 hours) defervescence. If systemic symptoms, bacteremia, and/or marked local findings persist after vein excision, reexploration is necessary with careful attention to total removal of all involved veins and drainage of contiguous (e.g., periphlebitic, subperiosteal) abscesses. It should be stressed, however, that the role of less radical surgery in therapy for superficial suppurative thrombophlebitis has not been addressed adequately. Although the literature supports vein excision, this experience stems largely from burn centers. Despite infection with gram-negative bacilli or *Candida* spp., six of eight children with superficial suppurative thrombophlebitis were cured by local incision and drainage of the involved site plus parenteral antimicrobials.[559] Radical surgery with extensive excision can perhaps be reserved for patients failing these measures. Delayed closure is preferred over primary wound closure. If osteomyelitis is documented in the adjacent long bones, antimicrobial therapy should be continued for at least 6 weeks. Resection of the involved vasculature in most patients with suppurative thrombophlebitis of the great central veins is technically impossible. Fortunately, medical therapy is usually sufficient.[565,568,589] The recommended approach is catheter removal, full-dose anticoagulation with heparin,[589] and parenteral antibiotics. Although tissue plasminogen activator therapy has been used successfully in this setting,[590] experience is limited and its use must be considered experimental. Septic thrombosis of the portal vein usually responds to systemic antimicrobial therapy directed at bowel flora with or without percutaneous drainage of associated hepatic abscess(es).[573] The duration of therapy is unsettled; 2–3 weeks after catheter removal is suggested, with at least 4 weeks for *Staphylococcus aureus* disease.[569] The antibiotics employed are the same as for superficial suppurative thrombophlebitis. Experience with more potent agents (e.g., third-generation cephalosporins) for suppurative thrombophlebitis due to gram-negative bacilli is scant, but trials are indicated. Because heparin may precipitate vancomycin with a partial loss of antibacterial activity at concentrations present in intravenous lines,[591] these drugs should not be administered simultaneously by the same intravenous access when MRSA, *S. epidermidis*, *E. faecalis*, and so forth, are suspected or grown. Unlike *Candida* IE, suppurative thrombophlebitis of the great central veins due to *Candida* spp. is curable medically, but antifungal regimens must be continued longer than those usually adequate for superficial suppurative thrombophlebitis. Based on limited data,[568] amphotericin B at a daily dose of 0.7 mg/kg to a total dosage of at least 22 mg/kg plus 5-fluorocytosine (100–150 mg/kg/day in four divided doses, if tolerable) is recommended after catheter removal. Surgery may, however, be essential in patients with suppurative thrombophlebitis of the thoracic or neck veins when perivascular collections are present.

The optimal therapy for pelvic suppurative thrombophlebitis is still controversial. Because anaerobic streptococci and *Bacteroides* spp. predominate, the initial antibiotics of choice are aqueous penicillin G, 20 million units IV qd, plus either clindamycin, 450–600 mg IV q6h, or metronidazole, 500–750 mg IV q8h. The use of heparin is debated. The addition of heparin after several days of unsuccessful treatment with antibiotics may itself produce an antipyretic effect.[583] In one series of 46 patients with pelvic suppurative thrombophlebitis,[572] including 7 with massive ovarian vein involvement and 15 with septic pulmonary emboli, 42 patients become afebrile within 7 days (mean, 2.5 days) while receiving penicillin, chloramphenicol, and heparin. Four patients required exploratory laparotomy, and pelvic abscesses were found in three. These results argue strongly that medical therapy alone is often effective, but no controlled studies on the use of heparin have been done. When medical therapy is unsatisfactory, surgery with drainage of abscesses and usually ligation of the implicated venous system must be performed. Some authorities[573] feel that inferior vena cava and/or ovarian vein ligation should be performed in all these cases, but the evidence for this approach is inconclusive.

Prevention

The incidence of superficial suppurative thrombophlebitis can be reduced by the same preventive procedures that are used for intravenous cannulae in general. These include the use of "scalp vein" cannulae whenever possible, the avoidance of lower extremity cannulations, insertion under aseptic conditions, secure anchoring of the cannula, and frequent replacement (at least every 48–72 hours) of intravenous fluid bottles, cannulae, and connecting tubing. Although neomycin-polymixin B-bacitracin ointment is effective in reducing the incidence of cutdown infections,[592] this modality has not demonstrated consistent benefit with intravenous cannulae.[593] When clinical signs of bacteremia occur in a patient receiving intravenous fluids, the following steps should be taken: *(1)* blood cultures should be obtained, *(2)* intravenous administration should be discontinued and all cannulae removed, *(3)* the intravenous fluid itself should be cultured, *(4)* the cannula should be cultured semiquantitatively on blood agar as described by Maki et al.,[577] and *(5)* appropriate antibiotic therapy should be initiated. If clinical signs of sepsis and bactermia persist despite appropriate antibiotic therapy, then an intravascular focus (including suppurative thrombophlebitis at a previously cannulated vein) should be sought as discussed above.

INFECTIVE ENDARTERITIS AND "MYCOTIC ANEURYSMS"

The term *mycotic aneurysm* was coined by Osler in the Gulstonian lectures of 1885 to describe a mushroom-shaped aneurysm that developed in a patient with subacute bacterial endocarditis. At that time *mycotic* was used to refer to all microorganisms. Presently, the use of *mycotic* has been restricted specifically to fungal infections, but the term *mycotic aneurysm* is still used for all extra- (or intra-) cardiac aneurysms of infectious etiology except for syphilitic aortitis. Unfortunately, this term has also been used to describe preexisting aneurysms secondarily in-

TABLE 7. Classification of "Mycotic Aneurysms"

Preexistent Arterial Status	Source of Infection
Normal	Intravascular
Atherosclerotic	Embolism
Aneurysm	Bacteremia with "seeding"
Arterial prosthesis	Extension from adjacent endocardial focus or erosion
	Extravascular
	Contiguous site of infection
	Iatrogenic

fected from contiguous or distant foci or pseudoaneurysms arising from trauma or iatrogenic causes. *Endarteritis* refers to inflammation of the arterial wall, which may occur with or without coexistent aneurysmal dilatation. Unless an aneurysm or coarctation of the aorta is present, infective endarteritis is usually a postmortem diagnosis. Since infected aneurysms differ in their pathogenesis, the various classifications, given in Table 7, will be examined separately.[594] Infections of arterial prosthetic devices are dealt with in detail in Chapter 59 and are not considered here.

Epidemiology

Although incidence figures are unavailable, a localized suppurative process of the arterial wall is rare. Estimates derived from autopsy series of aortic aneurysms are available but ignore infections at other locations in the arterial tree. In a review of over 22,000 autopsies performed at the Boston City Hospital from 1902 to 1951,[595] aortic aneurysms were found in 1.5 percent. However, mycotic aneurysms constituted only 2.6 percent of these lesions. In another review of 178 aneurysms found among more than 20,000 autopsies at the Mayo Clinic from 1925 to 1954,[596] only 6 were felt to be of infectious origin. Similarly, in a review[597] of 77 pure iliac aneurysms in 48 patients detected over a 21-year period, only 2 (4.2 percent) were mycotic in origin. In the preantibiotic era, infected aneurysms were predominantly confined to patients with IE; in a series of 217 cases reported in 1923,[598] 86 percent were associated with IE. With the advent of antibiotics, mycotic aneurysms in IE have become less prevalent, and hematogenous seeding of a previously damaged arteriosclerotic vessel constitutes the most common mechanism. There is also evidence to suggest that this entity is increasing in frequency. In reviewing four large series,[142,559–561] 78 lesions of this type were discovered from 1946 to 1975. Only eight of these were reported before 1957. Because most of these lesions arise in areas of severe atherosclerosis, males predominate by a ratio of 3 : 1, and the average age has been 65 years. The mean age for mycotic aneurysms that occur with IE is younger (approximately 40 years), and the sex distribution is nearly equal. Estimates of the incidence of mycotic aneurysms in patients with IE range up to 15 percent.[142,602] Approximately 2–4 percent of IE patients develop intracranial mycotic aneurysms,[603] although a neurologic presentation is not uncommon in patients with IE (approximately 16–23 percent of cases), and at least 30 percent of cases develop neurologic findings.[604,605] As discussed above, neurologic manifestations during IE have an adverse effect on the ultimate mortality rate. These lesions remain a significant cause of morbidity and mortality due to intracerebral and subarachnoid hemorrhage, especially in young people in developing countries where acute rheumatic fever, rheumatic heart disease, and resultant IE are still prevalent.[606] Nine intracranial mycotic aneurysms associated with IE were treated in one neurosurgical unit in South Africa in a recent 18-month period, with five deaths.[606] In addition, aortic root complications, including abscess and/or mycotic aneurysm, are associated with a poor outcome from IE. For example, in one review,[607] aortic root complications were documented in 23 of 50 cases of aortic valve IE (46 percent) over a 6-year period; prosthetic valve involvement was common, and surgical mortality and postoperative aortic regurgitation were more frequent in the group with root complications.

Mycotic aneurysms are extremely rare in childhood[608] and, when present, are usually associated with IE, cardiovascular malformations, or connective tissue disorders. However, a new disease entity, first described in 1970, has become apparent—aneurysms associated with umbilical artery catheterizations of newborn infants.[609] Usually of staphylococcal etiology, 34 cases have now been reported with the following distribution: [609] descending thoracic aorta, 14; abdominal aorta, 10; iliac arteries, 6; and multiple sites, 4.

Pathogenesis

Four different mechanisms have been postulated to produce infection of the arterial wall: *(1)* embolomycotic aneurysm secondary to septic microemboli to the vasa vasorum, *(2)* extension from a contiguous infected focus, *(3)* hematogenous seeding of the intima during bacteremia originating from a distant infection, and *(4)* trauma to the arterial wall with direct contamination.[610] Embolomycotic aneurysms usually occur in patients with active IE, and the incidence of this type has declined in the antibiotic era. The source of infection is the cardiac vegetation with production of arterial emboli that lodge in the vasa vasorum, often at points of bifurcation of the affected artery. Contiguous foci of infection such as a caseous tuberculous lymph node or pyogenic vertebral osteomyelitis may extend directly to major vessels with subsequent aneurysm formation. The normal arterial intima is very resistant to infection. However, when this lining is altered by congenital malformations (e.g., coarctation of the aorta) or acquired disease (especially atherosclerotic plaques and/or ulcers), resistance to infection is lowered, and the surface may become colonized by blood-borne organisms. This hypothesis is analogous to the central role of nonbacterial thrombotic endocarditis in the pathogenesis of IE. An intraluminal thrombus associated with an atherosclerotic vessel may also serve as a nidus for colonization. Atherosclerosis accounts for over 74 percent of secondarily infected aneurysms. Luetic arteritis and cystic medial necrosis have also been associated with secondary infection.[599] Trauma to the arterial wall with subsequent infection has been associated with narcotic addicts due to needle trauma,[611] as well as with gunshot wounds, vascular surgery, cardiac catheterization, percutaneous transluminal coronary angioplasty,[612,613] and even puncture of a femoral artery for analysis of arterial blood gases.[594] These events, if associated with contamination, usually lead to pseudoaneurysm formation in a peripheral artery and a contiguous abscess in extravasated blood.

Pathologic Changes

Infection of the arterial tree has been recognized by pathologists for more than a century. Virchow first demonstrated local dilatation of the arterial wall at the site of a septic embolus in 1847. Infection superimposed on an atherosclerotic aorta was first reported by Koch in 1851. Stengel and Wolfroth[598] collected 217 cases of mycotic aneurysms in 1923. Since these lesions are probably underreported, pathologic material has been scant in recent years.

Most mycotic aneurysms that develop during the course of IE are situated in the sinus of Valsalva or in the supravalvular proximal thoracic aorta (>70 percent develop proximal to the aortic arch). Aneurysms are more frequent in the right and/or posterior sinus and may be complicated by acquired shunts (rupture into the right ventricle is the most common), tamponade, coronary artery occlusion, or an atrioventricular conduction block.[614] Less commonly, major visceral, intracranial, and peripheral arteries are involved. Intracranial mycotic aneurysms characteristically develop in the distribution of the middle cerebral artery at peripheral bifurcation points[604,605] vs. a more prox-

imal location for most congenital aneurysms. Multiple intracranial lesions may be present. Mycotic aneurysm of the extracranial carotid arteries is rare (26 case reports[615]), but most develop in association with IE, usually due to *Staphylococcus aureus*. Fewer than 10 percent are found in the upper extremities, but these arteries are usually not examined adequately by pathologic or radiologic techniques. Infrafemoral aneurysms during IE or following its treatment[616] are also unusual. Multiple lesions are identified in many IE patients with mycotic aneurysms.[617] Saccular forms appear to be more common than fusiform ones are.[596] The aneurysms vary in size from 1 mm to more than 10 cm. As mentioned before, many of these aneurysms arise from emboli to the vasa vasorum, and occasionally the embolus can be demonstrated grossly and microscopically. Acute and chronic inflammation is found diffusely through the arterial wall; necrosis, hemorrhage, abscess formation, and bacterial colonies may all be present in the sections. The elastica and muscularis layers are usually obliterated, but the intima is often intact. Rupture with surrounding hemorrhage and infection may be present.

Secondary infection of a preexisting aneurysm is most commonly found in the abdominal aorta (70 percent of the cases), since this is the area most frequently and severely damaged by atherosclerosis. Ascending and descending aortic aneurysms each account for about 15 percent of the cases. The primary bacteremia most commonly originates from distal infections in soft tissue, lung, bone, or joint. The arterial infection usually begins in the distal abdominal aorta or iliac arteries as a focus of inflammation on an ulcerated atheromatous plaque. The wall of the aneurysm is thinned, and there is focal acute and chronic inflammation that may lead to arterial rupture. Even "bland" aortic aneurysms commonly have some mild inflammation (predominantly lymphocytes and mononuclear cells) in the wall; however, infected atherosclerotic aneurysms are characterized by acute polymorphonuclear inflammation, necrosis, abscess formation, hemorrhage, and visible bacterial colonies. This lesion is probably underreported, since the focal suppuration may be limited in extent and overlooked unless routine culture and histologic sections are examined on every aortic aneurysm specimen. Erosion and rupture may be present without aneurysmal dilatation. Lumbar or thoracic osteomyelitis is present in up to one-third of the cases[599] and may either precede the aneurysm or develop secondary to contiguous spread from the vascular infection.

When contamination accompanies arterial injury, an infected pseudoaneurysm may result. These lesions are located in the extremities in over 80 percent of the cases and are characterized by more extensive local tissue inflammation than are the two types mentioned previously. Infection as a cause of pseudoaneurysm formation is increasing; 17 of 57 (30 percent) such lesions seen in the past decade[618] were infected. When endarteritis develops following angioplasty, it usually follows a repeat procedure or repuncture, and this scenario should suggest this diagnosis; all cases have been due to *Staphylococcus aureus*.[612,613] Distal emboli, pseudoaneurysm formation, and coexistent osteomyelitis are present in more than 50 percent of these cases. Infective aortic root aneurysm has also followed coronary artery bypass grafting with disastrous results.[617] Subclavian artery aneurysms may be present with systemic findings plus unilateral upper extremity rash or splinter hemorrhages.[620] Nineteen cases of intracavernous carotid artery aneurysms have been reported,[621] usually occurring with meningitis with or without IE.

Of special interest are mycotic aneurysms in renal transplant patients. In 640 renal transplants performed at the University of Minnesota over a period of 8 years, perinephric infections developed in 28 patients, and 8 of these developed mycotic aneurysms.[622] These lesions were evident clinically 1.5–4 months post-transplant. Six were located in the external iliac artery, with one each in the internal iliac artery and aorta. All these lesions were secondary to contiguous foci of infection in the deep tissues of the transplant wound.[622,623]

Clinical Manifestations

When mycotic aneurysms occur during the course of IE, manifestations of the underlying disease may be evident. Peripheral middle cerebral artery aneurysms constitute 2.5–6.2 percent of all intracranial aneurysms[602–606,624] and are usually secondary to infection. Intracranial mycotic aneurysms are usually clinically silent. When hemorrhage occurs, a sudden onset of severe headache with rapid deterioration in the level of consciousness is noted. The time interval from the diagnosis of IE to the onset of hemorrhage is variable (0–35 days), with a mean of 18 days.[603] Some of these lesions produce premonitory or "herald" neurologic findings, including focal deficits and seizures. Unfortunately, these symptoms are relatively common in patients with IE without intracranial aneurysms, and the differential diagnosis as well as decisions regarding arteriography are difficult.[625] A sudden focal deficit consistent with embolism is seen in approximately 23 percent of patients and should prompt arteriography.[625] A high proportion of patients with intracranial mycotic aneurysm with severe, unremitting localized headache, often in association with homonymous hemianopsia, has been reported in some series.[626] As above, stroke syndromes may be seen and manifest as focal neurologic deficit(s), headache, confusion, meningismus, seizures, or coma.[604,605] Contrary to popular belief, the majority of intracranial hemorrhages associated with IE are not due to ruptured mycotic aneurysms but to septic, necrotic arteritis.[604] Symptomatic intracranial hemorrhage was associated with a mortality rate of 60–90 percent in this study. Patients may present with bilateral cortical blindness as well. Unusual location and/or etiology of an intracranial mycotic aneurysm suggests a diagnosis other than IE.[627] Mycotic aneurysms tend to occur more commonly in females of a younger age than does IE in general. They must be differentiated from aneurysms secondary to tumor emboli (especially choriocarcinoma or atrial myxoma), trauma, arteritis, or moyamoya disease and from congenital aneurysms. Visceral artery aneurysms are uncommon but, when present, are almost uniformly due to infection[610] or polyarteritis nodosa. The most common location is in the superior mesenteric artery. Although superior mesenteric artery aneurysms account for only 8 percent of visceral artery aneurysms overall, most are of infectious etiology.[628] Symptoms include an acute onset of colicky abdominal pain, but the presentation is variable. Hepatic artery aneurysms may produce colicky right upper quadrant pain, fever, jaundice, and gastrointestinal hemorrhage[629] or hemobilia.[630] There are over 190 cases of this entity reported in the literature; 75 percent were extrahepatic and 25 percent intrahepatic. Ruptured mycotic aneurysm of the celiac artery may present with hemoptysis and/or hemothorax.[631] When the external iliac artery is involved, a triad of clinical signs may be present: pain in the lower extremity (especially the anterior aspect of the thigh) with quadriceps muscle wasting and a depressed knee jerk; arterial insufficiency of the extremity with coolness, pallor, and depressed pulses; and bacteremia.[632] Distal aneurysms (e.g., femoral) occasionally present with unusual manifestations, including arthritis and purpura in the affected limb.

When more peripheral arteries are involved (usually with a pseudoaneurysm), a tender, diffusely indurated mass is present in 92 percent of cases. The mass is pulsatile with an associated bruit in 50–60 percent of patients, and approximately 20–30 percent are associated with decreased peripheral pulses, skin changes, or even frank gangrene.[611] Local suppuration, petechiae, and purpura are often present, and the lesion may be confused with localized cellulitis or an abscess without consideration of vascular involvement. In abusers of illicit drugs, 80 percent of mycotic aneurysms occur in the lower extremity, with the remainder in the radial, brachial, or occasionally ca-

rotid arteries. Only 50 percent of these patients are febrile on admission. A superimposed septic arthritis may also be present.[633]

Although most infected aortic atherosclerotic aneurysms occur in elderly men, there are no pathognomonic findings to separate these patients from those with bland uninfected aneurysms. Fever is a helpful differentiating sign (present in over 70 percent of the patients) since it is uncommon in patients with bland aneurysms. Back pain or abdominal pain each occur in about one-third of the cases. A draining cutaneous sinus may be present. Separation of an infected aneurysm from the entity of inflammatory abdominal aortic aneurysms may be difficult. Inflammatory abdominal aortic aneurysms were first described in 1935 and account for 5–10 percent of abdominal aortic aneurysms; the lesions are usually infrarenal and often lead to ureteral obstruction due to the densely adherent fibrotic mass surrounding the vessel.[634] In a large series of 2816 patients undergoing repair of abdominal aortic aneurysms, 127 (4.5 percent) had inflammatory abdominal aortic aneurysms.[635] Most patients (123/127) were men and heavy smokers. Inflammatory abdominal aortic aneurysms are associated with an elevated erythrocyte sedimentation rate (73 percent), weight loss, symptoms (back and/or abdominal pain in 30–50 percent), and a higher operative mortality. Continuing bacteremia despite "appropriate" antimicrobial therapy in an elderly (especially diabetic) patient with no signs of IE is suggestive of an infected intravascular site. The aneurysm is palpable in 50–60 percent of the cases.[601,610] In most cases, the onset is insidious, and a low-grade fever may be present for several months before diagnosis. The nonspecificity of the clinical manifestations is reflected by the 75 percent preoperative rupture rate for this entity. Rupture may occur into the retroperitoneal space or peritoneal cavity (56 percent), pleural cavity (9 percent), duodenum (12 percent), esophagus (6 percent), mediastinum (3 percent), or pericardium (3 percent). The most common site of aortoenteric fistulas is between the aorta and the third portion of the duodenum. Short periods of "herald" bleeding are common warning signs before exsanguinating hemorrhage occurs.[636] Severe pain and the rapid onset of shock usually accompany rupture of the aneurysm.

Laboratory Findings

There are no characteristic laboratory abnormalities in this group of diseases. When mycotic aneurysms occur with IE, alterations suggesting the underlying disease may be present. Computed tomography is useful in patients with neurologic manifestations of IE, especially for the demonstration of intracranial hemorrhage. It is not sufficiently sensitive for the detection of intracranial mycotic aneurysms;[604,605] however, these lesions are not likely when the CT scan is completely normal. Diagnosis of intracranial mycotic aneurysm is still best established by four-vessel cerebral arteriography, although magnetic resonance imaging (MRI) angiography[605] or the less dangerous and invasive procedure of intravenous digital subtraction angiography[637] are promising. MRI may detect aneurysms only 2–3 mm in diameter, but false-negative studies occur (8–10 percent) and cannot substitute for selective angiography. Patients with infected aortic aneurysms usually demonstrate a leukocytosis (65–83 percent), but this is nonspecific and may be present when the aneurysm is bland. Bacteremia is found in 53 to more than 90 percent of the cases, is continuous, and usually does not clear with antibiotic therapy alone. Evidence for a primary source of bacteremia (e.g., pneumonia, osteomyelitis) may be evident but is absent in up to 46 percent of the cases.[599] The abdominal aorta is noted to be calcified on abdominal x-ray films in 47 percent,[601] and anterior vertebral body erosion has been demonstrated in 18 percent. A lack of calcification is suggestive of infection, since 70–80 percent of bland aneurysms demonstrate this finding on abdominal x-ray films. Certain procedures (e.g., intravenous pyelography, sonography, CT) may reveal the presence of an aneurysm but are often not satisfactory for preoperative detail. The absence of intimal calcification, an associated perianeurysmal fluid collection or osteomyelitis, or the sudden appearance of an aneurysm in a septic patient are all suggestive features of an infected abdominal aortic aneurysm by CT.[638,639] Gas in the aortic wall is diagnostic, but rare. Although the sensitivity is unknown, ^{67}Ga and ^{111}In leukocyte imaging have been used to localize intra-arterial infections.[640] Occult infected aneurysms have been identified in patients with fever of unknown origin and negative CT and/or MRI studies with gallium[641] or leukocyte scintigraphy[642] and may separate seroma/hematoma from adjacent infection. Leukocyte imaging with ^{99m}Tc-HMPAO–labeled cells also appears promising, but false-positive results have been noted.[643] Nevertheless, preoperative angiography is often preferred to delineate precisely the extent of aneurysmal involvement.[642] This information may alter the operative approach and may minimize the complications. Two-dimensional or M-mode echocardiography is a very useful noninvasive technique for documenting mycotic aneurysms in the vicinity of the aortic valve, (e.g., sinus of Valsalva, supravalvular, subvalvular), and this technique is adjunctive to aortic root angiography preoperatively.[645] Infective endarteritis and/or mycotic aneurysm in the vicinity of a patent ductus arteriosus has also been successfully visualized with two-dimensional and Doppler echocardiography.[646,647] Intraoperative epicardial echocardiography has also been used to facilitate the surgical approach. When a hepatic aneurysm is suspected, liver scans and ultrasonography may be helpful before angiography.[629]

Etiologic Agents

Before the antibiotic era, mycotic aneurysms associated with IE were usually due to the more "virulent" organisms such as the β-hemolytic group A streptococci, pneumococci, or *H. influenzae*. With the decline of these organisms as causal agents in IE, most of these lesions are now due to streptococci or staphylococci (≥60% of cases) and follow the incidence patterns outlined in Table 4 for the underlying disease.

When bacteria "seed" a preexisting atherosclerotic vessel, the etiologic agents are markedly different from those found in mycotic aneurysms associated with IE. Gram-positive organisms cause approximately 60 percent of these lesions, but gram-negative (chiefly *Salmonella*) bacilli are isolated in 35 percent. Staphylococci are implicated in 40 percent of the cases overall,[601] and over two-thirds of these are *Staphylococcus aureus*. Salmonellae cause 20 percent of the cases and involve, in order of frequency, the aorta and femoral and iliac arteries. Only 1 of 24 cases reported before 1974 was above the renal arteries.[648] Lumbar osteomyelitis due to *Salmonella* was present in one-third of cases. The presumed portal of entry is the gastrointestinal tract. *Salmonella enteritidis* strains are isolated in 40 percent of cases, which is proportional to their overall rate of isolation in the United States. *Salmonella chloreaesuis*, an uncommon clinical isolate, appears to be particularly pathogenic for this condition since this species was isolated in 32 percent of the cases.[649] *Salmonella typhi* is very rarely implicated in this disorder (one case report). *Salmonella* infections of aortic aneurysms were first reported in 1948. The predilection for involvement by this organism is not understood, but *Salmonella* organisms tend to "seed" abnormal tissues during bacteremia (e.g., hematomas, malignant tumors, cysts, gallstones, bone infarcts, and altered endothelium; aortic aneurysms). It has been estimated that 25 percent of patients over 50 years of age with *Salmonella* bacteremia have an intravascular focus of infection.[650,651] *Arizona* species (especially *A. hinshawii*) are closely related to *Salmonella* spp., cause similar clinical syndromes, and also infect aortic aneurysms in elderly diabetic males.[652] The following organisms also produce infection in atherosclerotic aneurysms: *E. coli, Pseudomonas aeruginosa, Proteus* spp., *Citrobacter*

freundii, Klebsiella-Enterobacter spp., *Brucella* spp.,[653] *S. marcescens, Campylobacter fetus,*[654] *Listeria monocytogenes,* (10 reported cases[655]), *Bacteroides fragilis,* gonococci, group A or C streptococci, corynebacteria, *Clostridium septicum*[656] enterococci, and pneumococci. Fungal mycotic aneurysms are rare in the intracranial compartment, with only 13 definite cases reported by 1981.[657] The most common etiologic agents are *Aspergillus* spp., agents of mucormycoses, and *Candida* spp. The first two agents may involve intracranial arteries by direct extension from foci of sinusitis. One case of multiple intracranial aneurysms due to *Coccidioides immitis* that occurred during therapy for basilar meningitis has been described. Fungal mycotic aneurysms tend to involve larger, more proximal vessels at the base of the brain (11/18 [61 percent] carotid or basilar) than do bacterial cases with IE.[658] and may complicate intracranial surgery. *Aspergillus* mycotic aneurysms have followed transphenoidal resections. Fungi may also cause endarteritis in the aorta or on aortic grafts, including cases due to *Aspergillus* or *Bipolaris* spp.[659,660] Mycotic aneurysms with subarachnoid bleeding may complicate the course of neurobrucellosis.[661] Tuberculous aneurysms are now uncommon and when present are due to contiguous foci of infection.

Pseudoaneurysms resulting from intra-arterial or perivascular injection of illicit street drugs, often in addicts with sclerosed veins due to repeated intravenous inoculation, are associated with contiguous abscesses. The causative agents are *Staphylococcus aureus* (76 percent), *Pseudomonas aeruginosa* (18 percent), and many others.[611]

Therapy

No uniformly acceptable approach has been devised for the treatment of mycotic aneurysms in IE. The treatment of intracranial mycotic aneurysms is particularly controversial. Some of these lesions appear to resolve with antimicrobial therapy alone. In a review of 56 aneurysms occurring in 45 patients,[662] 3 of 20 patients died when treated with antibiotics alone. Mild to moderate neurologic deficits were observed in 8 of the 17 survivors. Likewise, 6 of 25 patients treated with both antibiotics and surgery died, and 9 of 19 survivors were left with mild to moderate neurologic deficits. Others report a different experience with a higher mortality in the nonsurgical group,[603] but patients were selected only after subarachnoid hemorrhage had occurred. For example, in a review of 13 intracranial mycotic aneurysms,[603] 6/8 patients treated with antibiotics alone died, and no deaths were observed in the surgically treated group. In a review of 85 cases treated between 1954 and 1978, 20 of 38 patients treated solely with antibiotics died vs. 8 of 30 operated upon.[602] The distal location of most intracranial mycotic aneurysms associated with IE may permit ligation and excision with fewer complications when compared with surgery for berry aneurysms in the circle of Willis. Interestingly, the mortality rate was low in patients with multiple aneurysms (4/15) treated with antibiotics alone. In one series, the mortality was 29 percent after rupture of an intracranial mycotic aneurysm. The use of serial angiography may be useful in following these patients, since the aneurysm(s) may change in size or new lesions may develop. In 21 patients subjected to serial angiography, the mycotic aneurysm increased in size in 5, did not change in 1, became smaller in 6, and completely resolved in 11, and new aneurysms developed in 2. Therefore, over 50 percent of these peripheral intracranial aneurysms resolved with antibiotic therapy alone during the treatment of IE.[662] Surgery is indicated for aneurysms increasing in size on repeat angiography[663,664] but may be deferred for 4–6 weeks for those remaining the same size (if the patient is an acceptable medical risk). The definitive treatment for aneurysms decreasing in size on repeat serial angiography every 2 weeks is unclear. Computed tomography is not helpful in localizing the aneurysm but provides important information if hematomas, infarcts, or abscesses develop. The antibiotics used are governed by the etiologic agent of the IE, but therapy of intracranial mycotic aneurysm, especially multiple lesions, must be individualized.[604,605] (see above).

Peripheral vessels are usually involved when arterial trauma (narcotic addict, gunshot wound, iatrogenic) results in pseudoaneurysm formation with infection. Therapy with antibiotics, proximal ligation of the vessel, resection of the pseudoaneurysm, and appropriate drainage result in cures in 75 percent of the cases. Vascular reconstruction through uninfected tissue planes with autogenous grafts is necessary when limb viability is dependent on the affected vessel. This is encountered more frequently in the lower extremity. For example, severe ischemia developed in 9 of 28 patients after excision of mycotic aneurysms of the common femoral artery[611] in one series of 52 cases. Amputation was required in only 11 percent of a large series of 54 aneurysms among drug addicts recently seen at the Henry Ford Hospital; there were no deaths.[665]

The mortality for patients with infected atherosclerotic aneurysms often exceeds 90 percent; approximately 40 long-term survivors have been reported since 1962.[666–669] A high index of suspicion is necessary to intervene surgically before rupture occurs since this complication is uniformly fatal and occurs in about 80 percent of the cases. When gram-negative bacilli are the cause of the infection, "early" (e.g., within 2 weeks after the first positive blood culture) rupture occurs much more frequently (84 percent) than if gram-positive bacteria are isolated (10 percent). Survival after surgery is also more common (75 percent) for patients with aneurysms infected with gram-positive cocci than for those with gram-negative bacilli (25 percent). Antibiotics should be used in this disease; but even if the lesion is sterilized (only three reported cases) the aneurysm may still continue to enlarge and rupture, and therefore surgery is required. At surgery, the aneurysm and any intraluminal thrombus must be sectioned, Gram stained, and cultured. If infection is present, all aneurysmal tissue and surrounding inflammation must be resected before grafting. Basic principles of grafting in this situation include the use of autogenous rather than synthetic grafts and insertion only in clean noninfected tissue planes. If the graft is placed in the infected area, then continued infection, leakage, thrombus formation, abscess formation, and rupture usually result. Although some authorities have achieved a successful result by restoration of vascular continuity in situ after radical débridement,[666,668] this approach is not recommended in most cases. Nevertheless, the type of reconstruction must be individualized, as in situ repair appears to be more favorable when the aortic aneurysm is suprarenal[670–673] than more distal in location if combined with prolonged courses of intravenous antimicrobial agents. Radical resection of intra-abdominal aortic aneurysms without prosthetic material has also been used in small numbers of cases.[674] In a review of 24 patients with abdominal aortic aneurysms infected with *Salmonella* spp., 10 died after rupture without surgery, and another 7 patients survived grafting only to succumb to continued leakage from the anastomosis (only 5 were long-term survivors). If a graft is inserted in situ and persistent fever and bacteremia or emboli to the lower extremities ensue, reoperation with extra-anatomic grafting is mandatory. Since the resected area is contaminated, special bypass techniques (especially thoracoiliac, transpubic, or axillofemoral) are usually required. When an axillofemoral approach is used, a single graft should be inserted for both lower extremities since long-term patency is prolonged under these circumstances.[667,669] Bactericidal antibiotics should be continued for 6–8 weeks postoperatively, and peak serum bactericidal levels of at least 1:8 should be achieved. The actual agents used are dependent on the isolated organism (or the morphologic characteristics of the organisms in the surgical specimen) and on the results of in vitro susceptibility testing. Implantation of antibiotic-releasing carriers with in situ reconstruction has been used[675] but only in small numbers of patients without controlled trials;

use of such carriers remains of unproven benefit in the therapy of mycotic aneurysm.

REFERENCES

1. Lerner PI, Weinstein L. Infective endocarditis in the antibiotic era. N Engl J Med. 1966;274:199.
2. Watanakunakorn C. Changing epidemiology and newer aspects of infective endocarditis. Adv Intern Med. 1977;22:21.
3. Von Reym CF, Levy BS, Arbeit RD, et al. Infective endocarditis: An analysis based on strict case definitions. Ann Intern Med. 1982;94:505.
4. Steckelberg JM, Melton LJ III, Ilstrup DM, et al. Influence of referral bias on the apparent clinical spectrum of infective endocarditis. Am J Med. 1990;88:582.
5. Harris SL. Definitions and demographic characteristics. In: Kaye D, ed. Infective Endocarditis. New York: Raven Press; 1992:1.
6. Durack DT, Petersdorf RG. Changes in the epidemiology of endocarditis. In: Kaplan EL, Taranta AV, eds. Infective Endocarditis. An American Heart Association Symposium. Dallas: American Heart Association; 1977:3.
7. Griffin MR, Wilson WR, Edwards WD, et al. Infective endocarditis. Olmsted County, Minnesota, 1950 through 1981. JAMA. 1985;254:1199–202.
8. King JW, Nguyen VQ, Conrad SA. Results of a prospective statewide reporting system for infective endocarditis. Am J Med Sci. 1988;295:517–27.
9. Shulman ST. Infective endocarditis: 1986. Pediatr Infect Dis. 1986;5:691–4.
10. Watanakunakorn C, Burkert T. Infective endocarditis at a large community teaching hospital, 1980–1990. Medicine 1993;72:90.
11. Hayward GW. Infective endocarditis: A changing disease. Br Med J. 1973;2:706.
12. Anonymous (Editorial). Infective endocarditis. Br Med J. 1981;1:677.
13. Gold MJ. Cure rates and long term prognosis. In: Kaye D, ed. Infective Endocarditis. New York: Raven Press; 1992:455.
14. Thayer WS. Studies on bacterial (infective) endocarditis. Johns Hopkins Hosp Rep. 1926;22:1.
15. Garvey GJ, Neu HC. Infective endocarditis: An evolving disease. Medicine (Baltimore). 1978;57:105.
16. Lien EA, Solberg CO, Kalager T. Infective endocarditis 1973–1984 at the Bergen University Hospital: Clinical feature, treatment and prognosis. Scand J Infect Dis. 1988;20:239–46.
17. Come PC. Infective endocarditis: Current perspectives. Compr Ther. 1982;8:57.
18. Kaplan EL. Infective endocarditis in the pediatric age group: An overview. In Kaplan EL, Taranta AV, eds. Infective Endocarditis. An American Heart Association Symposium. Dallas: American Heart Association; 1977:51.
19. Baltimore RS. Infective endocarditis in children. Pediatr Infect Dis J. 1992;11:907.
20. Pelletier LL, Petersdorf RG. Infective endocarditis: A review of 125 cases from the University of Washington Hospitals, 1963–72. Medicine (Baltimore). 1977;56:287.
21. Terpenning MS, Buggy BP, Kaufmann CA. Hospital-acquired infective endocarditis. Arch Intern Med. 1988;148:1601–3.
22. Cherubin CE, Neu HC. Infective endocarditis at the Presbyterian Hospital in New York City from 1938–1967. Am J Med. 1971;51:83.
23. Roberts WC, Buchbinder NA. Right-sided valvular infective endocarditis. A clinicopathologic study of 12 necropsy patients. Am J Med. 1972;53:7.
24. Kaye D. Changing pattern of infective endocarditis. Am J Med. 1985;78(Suppl 6B):157–62.
25. Roberts WC, Perloff JK, Constantin T. Severe valvular aortic stenosis in patients over 65 years of age. Am J Cardiol. 1971;27:497.
26. Delahaye JP, Loire R, Milon H, et al. Infective endocarditis on stenotic aortic valves. Eur Heart J. 1988;9(Suppl E):43–9.
27. Gersony WM, Hayes CJ, Driscoll DJ, et al. Bacterial endocarditis in patients with aortic stenosis, pulmonary stenosis, or ventricular septal defect. Circulation. 1993;87(Suppl I):I–121.
28. McKinsey DS, Ratts TE, Bisno AL. Underlying cardiac lesions in adults with infective endocarditis. The changing spectrum. Am J Med. 1987;82:681–8.
29. Lowes JA, Hamer J, Williams G, et al. Ten years of infective endocarditis at St. Bartholomew's hospital: Analysis of clinical features and treatment in relation to prognosis and mortality. Lancet. 1980;1:133.
30. Moulsdale MT, Eykyn SJ, Phillips I. Infective endocarditis, 1970–1979. A study of culture-positive cases in St. Thomas' Hospital. Q J Med. 1980;49:315.
31. Venezio FR, Westenfelder GO, Cook FV, et al. Infective endocarditis in a community hospital. Arch Intern Med. 1982;142:789.
32. Fulkerson PK, Beaver BM, Aveson JC, et al. Calcification of the mitral annulus: Etiology, clinical associations, complications and therapy. Am J Med. 1979;66:967.
33. Welton DE, Young JB, Gentry LO, et al. Recurrent infective endocarditis: Analysis of predisposing factors and clinical features. Am J Med. 1979;66:932.
34. Kreuzpaintner G, Horstkotte D, Heyll A, et al. Increased risk of bacterial endocarditis in inflammatory bowel disease. Am J Med. 1992;92:391.
35. Cardelia JV, Befeler B, Hildner FJ, et al. Hypertrophic subaortic stenosis complicated by aortic insufficiency and subacute bacterial endocarditis. Am Heart J. 1971;81:543.

36. Wang K, Gobel FL, Gleason DF. Bacterial endocarditis in idiopathic hypertrophic subaortic stenosis. Am Heart J. 1975;89:359.

37. Chagnac A, Rudniki C, Loebel H, et al. Infectious endocarditis in idiopathic hypertrophic subaortic stenosis. Report of three cases and review of the literature. Chest. 1982;81:346.

38. Corrigan D, Bolen J, Hancock EW, et al. Mitral valve prolapse and infective endocarditis. Am J Med. 1977;63:215.

39. Jeresaty RM. Mitral valve prolapse—click syndrome. Prog Cardiovasc Dis. 1973;15:623.

40. Schutte JE, Gaffney FA, Blend L, et al. Distinctive anthropometric characteristics of women with mitral valve prolapse. Am J Med. 1981;71:533.

41. Clemens JD, Horwitz RI, Jaffe CC, et al. A controlled evaluation of the risk of bacterial endocarditis in persons with mitral-valve prolapse. N Engl J Med. 1982;307:776.

42. Nolan CM, Kane JJ, Grunow WA. Infective endocarditis and mitral prolapse. A comparison with other types of endocarditis. Arch Intern Med. 1981;141:447.

43. Scheld WM. Pathogenesis and pathophysiology of infective endocarditis. In: Sande MA, Kaye D, Root RK, eds. Endocarditis. v. 1. Contemporary Issues in Infectious Diseases. London: Churchill Livingston; 1984:1–32.

44. Freedman LR. The pathogenesis of infective endocarditis. J Antimicrob Chemother. 1987;20(Suppl A):1–6.

45. Livornese LL Jr, Korzeniowski OM. Pathogenesis of infective endocarditis. In: Kaye D, ed. Infective Endocarditis. New York: Raven Press; 1992:19.

46. Tunkel AR, Scheld WM. Experimental models of endocarditis. In: Kaye D, ed. Infective Endocarditis. New York: Raven Press; 1992:37.

47. Weinstein L, Schlesinger JJ. Pathoanatomic, pathophysiologic, and clinical correlations in endocarditis (first of two parts). N Engl J Med. 1974;291:832.

48. Angrist AA, Oka M. Pathogenesis of bacterial endocarditis. JAMA. 1963;183:249.

49. Durack DT, Beeson PB. Pathogenesis of infective endocarditis. In: Rahimtoola SH, ed. Infective Endocarditis. New York: Grune & Stratton, 1978:1.

50. Durack DT, Beeson PB. Experimental bacterial endocarditis. I. Colonization of a sterile vegetation. Br J Exp Pathol. 1972;53:44.

51. Durack DT, Beeson PB, Petersdorf RG. Experimental bacterial endocarditis. III. Production and progress of the disease in rabbits. Br J Exp Pathol. 1973;54:142.

52. Durack DT. Experimental bacterial endocarditis. IV. Structure and function of very early lesions. J Pathol. 1975;115:81.

53. McGowan DA, Gillett R. Scanning electron microscopic observations of the surface of the initial lesion in experimental streptococcal endocarditis in the rabbit. Br J Exp Pathol. 1980;61:164.

54. Ferguson DJP, McColm AA, Ryan DM, et al. Experimental staphylococcal endocarditis and aortitis. Morphology of the initial colonization. Virchows Arch [A] 1986;410:43–8.

55. Sherwood BF, Rowlands DT, Vakilzadeh J, et al. Experimental bacterial endocarditis in the opossum (Didelphis virginiana). Am J Pathol. 1971;64:513.

56. Chino F, Kodama A, Otake M, et al. Nonbacterial thrombotic endocarditis in a Japanese autopsy sample. A review of 80 cases. Am Heart J. 1975;90:190.

57. Rodbard S. Blood velocity and endocarditis. Circulation. 1963;27:18.

58. Lepeschkin E. On the relation between the site of valvular involvement in endocarditis and the blood pressure resting on the valve. Am J Med Sci. 1952;224:318.

59. Okell CC, Elliott SD. Bacteraemia and oral sepsis. With special reference to the aetiology of subacute endocarditis. Lancet. 1935;2:869.

60. Everett ED, Hirschmann JV. Transient bacteremia and endocarditis prophylaxis: A review. Medicine (Baltimore). 1977;56:61.

61. Loesche WJ. Indigenous human flora and bacteremia. In: Kaplan EL, Taranta AV, eds. Infective Endocarditis. An American Heart Association Symposium. Dallas: American Heart Association; 1977:40.

62. Durack DT, Beeson PB. Protective role of complement in experimental Escherichia coli endocarditis. Infect Immun. 1977;16:213.

63. Yersin B, Glauser M-P, Guze L, et al. Experimental Escherichia coli endocarditis in rats: Roles of serum bactericidal activity and duration of catheter placement. Infect Immun. 1988;56:1273–80.

64. Gould IM, Ramirez-Ronda CH, Holmes RK, et al. Adherence of bacteria to heart valves in vitro. J Clin Invest. 1975;56:1364.

65. Freedman LR, Valone J Jr. Experimental infective endocarditis. Prog Cardiovasc Dis. 1979;22:169.

66. Baddour LM, Lowrance C, Albus A, et al. Staphylococcus aureus microcapsule expression attenuates bacterial virulence in a rat model of experimental endocarditis. J Infect Dis. 1992;165:749.

67. Overholser CD, Moreillon P, Glauser MP. Experimental bacterial endocarditis after dental extractions in rats with periodontitis. J Infect Dis. 1987;155:107–12.

68. Moreillon P, Overholser CD, Malinverni R, et al. Predictors of endocarditis in isolates from cultures of blood following dental extractions in rats with periodontal disease. J Infect Dis. 1988;157:990–5.

69. Gibbons RJ, Nygaard M. Synthesis of insoluble dextran and its significance in the formation of gelatinous deposits by plaque-forming streptococci. Arch Oral Biol. 1968;13:1249.

70. Parker MT, Ball LC. Streptococci and aerococci associated with systemic infection in man. J Med Microbiol. 1976;9:275.

71. Scheld WM, Valone JA, Sande MA. Bacterial adherence in the pathogenesis of endocarditis. Interaction of bacterial dextran, platelets, and fibrin. J Clin Invest. 1978;61:1394.

72. Ramirez-Ronda CH. Adherence of glucan-positive and glucan-negative streptococcal strains to normal and damaged heart valves. J Clin Invest. 1978;62:805.

73. Ramirez-Ronda CH. Effects of molecular weight of dextran on the adherence of Streptococcus sanguis to damaged heart valves. Infect Immun. 1980;29:1.

74. Pelletier LL Jr, Coyle M, Petersdorf R. Dextran production as a possible virulence factor in streptococcal endocarditis. Proc Soc Exp Biol Med. 1978;158:415.

75. Pulliam L, Dall L, Inokuchi S, et al. Enzymatic modification of the glycocalyx in experimental endocarditis due to viridans streptococci. J Infect Dis. 1987;156:736.

76. Dall L, Barnes WG, Lane JW, et al. Enzymatic modification of glycocalyx in the treatment of experimental endocarditis due to viridans streptococci. J Infect Dis. 1987;156:736–40.

77. Dall LH, Herndon BL. Association of cell adherent glycocalyx and endocarditis production by viridans group streptococci. J Clin Microbiol. 1990;28:1698.

78. Crawford I, Russell C. Comparative adhesion of seven species of streptococci isolated from the blood of patients with subacute bacterial endocarditis to fibrin-platelet clots in vitro. J Appl Bacteriol. 1986;60:127–33.

79. Dall L, Keilhofner M, Herndon B, et al. Clindamycin effect on glycocalyx production in experimental viridans streptococcal endocarditis. J Infect Dis. 1990;161:1221.

80. Scheld WM, Calderone RA, Alliegro GM, et al. Yeast adherence in the pathogenesis of Candida endocarditis. Proc Soc Exp Biol Med. 1981;168:208.

81. Scheld WM, Strunk RW, Balian G, et al. Microbial adhesion to fibronectin in vitro correlates with production of endocarditis in rabbits. Proc Soc Exp Biol Med. 1985;180:474–82.

82. Kuypers JM, Proctor RA. Reduced adherence to traumatized rat heart valves by a low-fibronectin-binding mutant of Staphylococcus aureus. Infect Immun. 1989;57:2306.

83. Lowrance JH, Baddour LM, Simpson WA. The role of fibronectin binding in the rat model of experimental endocarditis caused by Streptococcus sanguis. J Clin Invest. 1990;86:7.

84. Becker RC, DiBello PM, Lucas FV. Bacterial tissue tropism: An in vitro model for infective endocarditis. Cardiovasc Res. 1987;21:813–20.

85. Tart RC, van de Rijn I. Analysis of adherence of Streptococcus defectivus and endocarditis-associated streptococci to extracellular matrix. Infect Immun. 1991;59:857.

86. Sommer P, Gleyzal C, Guerret S, et al. Induction of a putative laminin-binding protein of Streptococcus gordonii in human infective endocarditis. Infect Immun 1992;60:360.

87. Vercellotti G, Lussenhop D, Peterson PK, et al. Bacterial adherence to fibronectin and endothelial cells: A possible mechanism for bacterial tissue tropism. J Lab Clin Med. 1984;103:34–43.

88. Ogawa SK, Yurberg ER, Hatcher VB, et al. Bacterial adherence to human endothelial cells in vitro. Infect Immun. 1985;50:218–24.

89. Hamill RJ, Vann JM, Proctor RA. Phagocytosis of Staphylococcus aureus by cultured bovine aortic-endothelial cells: Model for post adherence events in endovascular infections. Infect Immun 1986;54:833–6.

90. Scheld WM, Zak O, Vosbeck K, et al. Bacterial adhesion in the pathogenesis of endocarditis. Effect of subinhibitory antibiotic concentrations on streptococcal adhesion in vitro and the development of endocarditis in rabbits. J Clin Invest. 1981;68:1381.

91. Bernard J-P, Francioli P, Glauser MP, et al. Vancomycin prophylaxis of experimental Streptococcus sanguis endocarditis: Inhibition of bacterial adherence rather than bacterial killing. J Clin Invest. 1981;68:1113.

92. Glauser MP, Francioli P. Successful prophylaxis against experimental streptococcal endocarditis with bacteriostatic antibiotics. J Infect Dis. 1982;146:806.

93. Lowry FD, Chang DS, Neuhaus EG, et al. Effect of penicillin on the adherence of Streptococcus sanguis in vitro and in the rabbit model of endocarditis. J Clin Invest. 1983;71:668.

94. Glauser MP, Bernard JP, Moreillon P, et al. Successful single-dose amoxicillin prophylaxis against experimental streptococcal endocarditis. Evidence for two mechanisms of protection. J Infect Dis. 1983;147:568.

95. Clawson CC, Rao Gunda HR, White JG. Platelet interaction with bacteria. IV. Stimulation of the release reaction. Am J Pathol. 1975;81:411.

96. Herzberg MC, Brintzenhofe KL, Clawson CC. Aggregation of human platelets and adhesion of Streptococcus sanguis. Infect Immun. 1983;39:1457.

97. Sullam PM, Valone FH, Mills J. Mechanisms of platelet aggregation by viridans group streptococci. Infect Immun. 1987;55:1743–50.

98. Sullam PM, Jarvis GA, Valone FH. Role of immunoglobulin G in platelet aggregation by viridans group streptococci. Infect Immun. 1988;56:2907–11.

99. Herzberg MC, MacFarlane GD, Gong K, et al. The platelet interactivity phenotype of Streptococcus sanguis influences the course of experimental endocarditis. Infect Immun. 1992;60:4809.

100. Sullam PM, Costerton JW, Yamasaki R, et al. Inhibition of platelet binding and aggregation by streptococcal exopolysaccharide. J Infect Dis. 1993;167:1123.

101. Yeaman MR, Puentes SM, Norman DC, et al. Partial characterization and staphylocidal activity of thrombin-induced platelet microbicidal protein. Infect Immun 1992;60:1202.

102. Yeaman MR, Norman DC, Bayer AS. Staphylococcus aureus susceptibility

to thrombin-induced platelet microbicidal protein is independent of platelet adherence and aggregation in vitro. Infect Immun. 1992;60:2368.

103. Yeaman MR, Ibrahim AS, Edwards JE Jr, et al. Thrombin-induced rabbit platelet microbicidal protein is fungicidal in vitro. Antimicrob Agents Chemother. 1993;37:546.

104. Nicolau DP, Freeman CD, Nightingale CH, et al. Reduction of bacterial titers by low-dose aspirin in experimental aortic valve endocarditis. Infect Immun. 1993;61:1593.

105. Ferguson DJP, McColm AA, Ryan DM, et al. A morphological study of experimental staphylococcal endocarditis and aortitis II. Inter-relationship of bacteria, vegetation and cardiovasculature in established infections. Br J Exp Pathol. 1986;67:679–86.

106. Durack DT, Beeson PB. Experimental bacterial endocarditis. II. Survival of bacteria in endocardial vegetations. Br J Exp Pathol. 1972;53:50.

107. Yersin BR, Glauser MP, Freedman LR. Effect of nitrogen mustard on natural history of right-sided streptococcal endocarditis: Role of cellular host defenses. Infect Immun. 1982;35:320.

108. Meddens MJM, Thompson J, Eulderink F, et al. Role of granulocytes in experimental *Streptococcus sanguis* endocarditis. Infect Immun. 1982;36:325.

109. Meddens MJM, Thompson J, Mattie H, et al. Role of granulocytes in the prevention and therapy of experimental *Streptococcus sanguis* endocarditis in rabbits. Antimicrob Agents Chemother. 1984;25:263–7.

110. Hook EW III, Sande MA. Role of the vegetation in experimental *Streptococcus viridans* endocarditis. Infect Immun. 1974;10:1433.

111. Thorig L, Thompson J, Eulderink F, et al. Effects of monocytopenia and anticoagulation in experimental *Streptococcus sanguis* endocarditis. Br J Exp Pathol. 1980;61:108.

112. van Ginkel CJW, Thorig L, Thompson J, et al. Enhancement of generation of monocyte tissue thromboplastin by bacterial phagocytosis: Possible pathway for fibrin formation on infected vegetations in bacterial endocarditis. Infect Immun. 1979;25:388.

113. Drake TA, Rodgers GM, Sande MA. Tissue factor is a major stimulus for vegetation formation in enterococcal endocarditis in rabbits. J Clin Invest. 1984;73:1750–3.

114. Drake TA, Pang M. *Staphylococcus aureus* induces tissue factor expression in cultured human cardiac valve endothelium. J Infect Dis. 1988;157:749–56.

115. Mair W. Pneumococcal endocarditis in rabbits. J Pathol Bacteriol. 1923;26:426.

116. Scheld WM, Thomas JH, Sande MA. Influence of preformed antibody on experimental *Streptococcus sanguis* endocarditis. Infect Immun. 1979;25:781.

117. Durack DT, Gilliland BC, Petersdorf RG. Effect of immunization on susceptibility to experimental *Streptococcus mutans* and *Streptococcus sanguis* endocarditis. Infect Immun. 1978;22:52.

118. van de Rijn I. Analysis of cross-protection between serotypes and passively transferred immune globulin in experimental nutritionally variant streptococcal endocarditis. Infect Immun. 1988;56:117.

119. Scheld WM, Calderone RA, Brodeur JP, et al. Influence of preformed antibody on the pathogenesis of experimental *Candida albicans* endocarditis. Infect Immun. 1983;40:950.

120. Greenberg DP, Ward JI, Bayer AS. Influence of *Staphylococcus aureus* antibody on experimental endocarditis in rabbits. Infect Immun. 1987;55:3030–4.

121. Sieling PJ, van de Rijn I. Evaluation of the immune response in protection against experimental *Streptococcus defectivus* endocarditis. J Lab Clin Med. 1991;117:402.

122. Williams RC, Kunkel HG. Rheumatoid factors and their disappearance following therapy in patients with SBE. Arthritis Rheum. 1962;5:126.

123. Sheagren JN, Tuazon CV, Griffin C, et al. Rheumatoid factor in acute bacterial endocarditis. Arthritis Rheum. 1976;19:887.

124. Phair JP, Clarke J. Immunology of infective endocarditis. Prog Cardiovasc Dis. 1979;22:137.

125. Bacon PA, Davidson C, Smith B. Antibodies to *Candida* and autoantibodies in subacute bacterial endocarditis. Q J Med. 1974;43:537.

126. Laxdal T, Messner RP, Williams RC. Opsonic, agglutinating, and complement-fixing antibodies in patients with subacute bacterial endocarditis. J Lab Clin Med. 1968;71:638.

127. Horwitz D, Quismorio FP, Friou GJ. Cryoglobulinemia in patients with infectious endocarditis. Clin Exp Immunol. 1975;19:131.

128. Qoronfleh MW, Weraarchakul W, Wilkinson BJ. Antibodies to a range of *Staphylococcus aureus* and *Escherichia coli* heat shock proteins in sera from patients with *S. aureus* endocarditis. Infect Immun. 1993;61:1567.

129. Bayer AS, Theofilopoulos AN, Eisenberg R, et al. Circulating immune complexes in infective endocarditis. N Engl J Med. 1976;295:1500.

130. Gutman RA, Striker GE, Gilliland BC, et al. The immune complex glomerulonephritis of bacterial endocarditis. Medicine (Baltimore). 1972;51:1.

131. Levy RL, Hong R. The immune nature of subacute bacterial endocarditis (SBE) nephritis. Am J Med. 1973;54:645.

132. Inman RD, Redecha PB, Knechtle SJ, et al. Identification of bacterial antigens in circulating immune complexes of infective endocarditis. J Clin Invest. 1982;70:271.

133. Alpert JS, Krous HF, Dalen JE, et al. Pathogenesis of Osler's nodes. Ann Intern Med. 1976;85:471.

134. Lowenstein MB, Urman JD, Abeles M, et al. Skin immunofluorescence in infective endocarditis. JAMA. 1977;238:1163.

135. Cabane J, Godeau P, Herreman G, et al. Fate of circulating immune complexes in infective endocarditis. Am J Med. 1979;66:277.

136. Kauffman RH, Thompson J, Valentijn RM, et al. The clinical implications and the pathogenetic significance of circulating immune complexes in infective endocarditis. Am J Med. 1981;71:17.

137. McFarland MM. Pathology of infective endocarditis. In: Kaye D, ed. Infective Endocarditis. New York: Raven Press; 1992:57.

138. Roberts WC. Characteristics and consequences of infective endocarditis (active or healed or both) learned from morphologic studies. In: Rahimtoola SH, ed. Infective Endocarditis. New York: Grune & Stratton; 1978;55.

139. Coplan NL, Bruno MS. Acquired immunodeficiency syndrome and heart disease: The present and future. Am Heart J. 1989;117:1175.

140. Francis CK. Cardiac involvement in AIDS. Curr Prob Cardiol. 1990;15:571.

141. Morel-Maroger L, Sraer JD, Herreman G, et al. Kidney in subacute endocarditis. Pathological and immunofluorescence findings. Arch Pathol. 1913;94:205.

142. Anderson CB, Butcher HR, Ballinger WF. Mycotic aneurysms. Arch Surg. 1974;109:712.

143. Greenlee JE, Mandell GL. Neurological manifestations of infective endocarditis: A review. Stroke. 1973;4:958.

144. Masuda J, Yutani C, Waki R, et al. Histopathologic analysis of the mechanisms of intracranial hemorrhage complicating infective endocarditis. Stroke. 1992;23:843.

145. Kerr A Jr, Tan JS. Biopsies of the Janeway lesion of infective endocarditis. J Cutan Pathol. 1979;6:124.

146. Silverberg HH. Roth spots. Mt Sinai J Med. 1970;37:77.

147. Starkebaum M, Durack D, Beeson P. The "incubation period" of subacute bacterial endocarditis. Yale J Biol Med. 1977;50:49.

148. Weinstein L, Rubin RH. infective endocarditis—1973. Prog Cardiovasc Dis. 1973;16:239.

149. Freedman LR. Infective endocarditis and other intravascular infections. In: Braude AI, David CE, Fierer J, eds. Medical Microbiology and Infectious Diseases. Philadelphia: WB Saunders; 1981:1511.

150. Hermans PE. The clinical manifestations of infective endocarditis. Mayo Clin Proc. 1982;57:15.

151. Terpenning MS, Buggy BP, Kauffman CA. Infective endocarditis: Clinical features in young and elderly patients. Am J Med. 1987;83:626–34.

152. Lederman MM, Sprague L, Wallis RS, et al. Duration of fever during treatment of infective endocarditis. Medicine. 1992;71:52.

153. Blumberg EA, Robbins N, Adimora A, et al. Persistent fever in association with infective endocarditis. Clin Infect Dis. 1992;15:983.

154. Espersen F, Frimodt-Moller N. *Staphylococcus aureus* endocarditis. A review of 119 cases. Arch Intern Med. 1986;146:1118–21.

155. Charney R, Keltz TN, Attai L, et al. Acute vavular obstruction from streptococcal endocarditis. Am Heart J. 1993;125:544.

156. Ting W, Silverman NA, Arzaman DA, et al. Splenic septic emboli in endocarditis. Circulation. 1990;82(Suppl IV):IV-105.

157. Churchill MA, Geraci JE, Hunder GG. Musculoskeletal manifestations of bacterial endocarditis. Ann Intern Med. 1977;87:754.

158. Herzog CA, Henry TD, Zimmer SD. Bacterial endocarditis presenting as acute myocardial infarction: A cautionary note for the era of reperfusion. Am J Med. 1991;90:392.

159. Lerner PI. Neurologic complications of infective endocarditis. Med Clin North Am. 1985;69:385–98.

160. Tunkel AR, Kaye D. Neurologic complications of infective endocarditis. Neurol Clin. 1993;11:419.

161. Selky AK, Roos KL. Neurologic complications of infective endocarditis. Semin Neurol. 199s;12:225.

162. Bayer AS, Theofilopoulos AN, Eisenberg R, et al. Thrombotic thrombocytopenic purpura-like syndrome associated with infective endocarditis. A possible immune complex disorder. JAMA. 1977;238:408.

163. Levine DP, Crane LR, Zervos MJ. Bacteremia in narcotic addicts at the Detroit Medical Center II. Infectious endocarditis: A prospective comparative study. Rev Infect Dis. 1986;8:374–96.

164. Marantz PR, Linzer M, Feiner CJ, et al. Inability to predict diagnosis in febrile intravenous drug abusers. Ann Intern Med. 1987;106:823–8.

165. Weisse AB, Heller DR, Schimenti RJ, et al. The febrile parenteral drug user: A prospective study in 121 patients. Am J Med. 1993;94:274.

166. Chambers HF, Morris DL, Tauber MG, et al. Cocaine use and the risk for endocarditis in intravenous drug users. Ann Intern Med. 1987;106:833–6.

167. Graves MK, Soto L. Left-sided endocarditis in parenteral drug abusers: Recent experience at a large community hospital. South Med J. 1992;85:387.

168. Chambers HF, Korzeniowski OM, Sande MA, et al. *Staphylococcus aureus* endocarditis: Clinical manifestations in addicts and nonaddicts. Medicine (Baltimore). 1983;62:170.

169. Sklaver AR, Hoffman TA, Greenman RL. Staphylococcal endocarditis in addicts. South Med J. 1978;71:638.

170. Thadepalli H, Francis CK. Diagnostic clues in metastatic lesions of endocarditis in addicts. West J Med. 1978;128:1.

171. Kaell AT, Volkman DJ, Gorevic PD, et al. Positive Lyme serology in subacute bacterial endocarditis. JAMA. 1990;264:2916.

172. McCartney AC, Orange GV, Pringle SD, et al. Serum C reactive protein in infective endocarditis. J Clin Pathol. 1988;41:44–8.

173. Wiseman J, Rouleau J, Rigo P, et al. Gallium-67 myocardial imaging for the detection of bacterial endocarditis. Radiology. 1976;120:135.

174. Wong DW, Dhawan VK, Tanaka T, et al. Imaging endocarditis with technitium 99m-labeled antibody—An experimental study: Concise communication. J Nucl Med. 1982;23:229.

175. Riba AL, Thakur ML, Gottschalk A, et al. Imaging experimental infective

endocarditis with indium-111–labeled blood cellular components. Circulation. 1979;59:336.

176. Haft JI, Altieri J, Smight LG, et al. Computed tomography of the abdomen in the diagnosis of splenic emboli. Arch Intern Med. 1988;148:193–7.

177. Beeson PB, Brannon ES, Warren JV. Observations on the sites of removal of bacteria from the blood of patients with bacterial endocarditis. J Exp Med. 1945;81:9–23.

178. Werner AS, Cobbs CG, Kaye D, et al. Studies on the bacteremia of bacterial endocarditis. JAMA. 1967;202:199.

179. Pazin GJ, Saul S, Thompson ME. Blood culture positivity. Suppression by outpatient antibiotic therapy in patients with bacterial endocarditis. Arch Intern Med. 1982;142:263.

180. McKenzie R, Reimer LG. Effect of antimicrobials on blood cultures in endocarditis. Diagn Microbiol Infect Dis. 1987;8:165–72.

181. Aronson MD, Bos DH. Blood cultures. Ann Intern Med. 1987;106:246–53.

182. Washington JA II, Ilstrup DM. Blood cultures: Issues and controversies. Rev Infect Dis. 1986;8:792–802.

183. Washington JA II. The role of the microbiology laboratory in the diagnosis and antimicrobial treatment of infective endocarditis. Mayo Clin Proc. 1982; 57:22.

184. Carey RB, Gross KC, Roberts RB. Vitamin-B₆–dependent *Streptococcus mitior* (*mitis*) isolated from patients with systemic infections. J Infect Dis. 1975;131:722.

185. Powers DL, Mandell GL. Intraleucocytic bacteria in endocarditis patients. JAMA. 1974;227:313.

186. Whitcomb DC. Bugs in the blood: Acute staphylococcal septicemia and endocarditis diagnosed by staining the buffy coat. NC Med J. 1986;47:293–5.

187. Tuazon CU, Sheagren JW. Teichoic acid antibodies in the diagnosis of serious infections with *Staphylococcus aureus*. Ann Intern Med. 1976;84:543.

188. Bayer AS, Tillman DB, Concepcion M, et al. Clinical value of teichoic acid antibody titers in the diagnosis and management of staphylococcemias. West J Med. 1980;132:294.

189. Kaplan JE, Palmer DL, Tung KSK. Teichoic acid antibody and circulating immune complexes in the management of *Staphylococcus aureus* bacteremia. Am J Med. 1981;70:769.

190. Arbeit RD, Nelles MJ. Capsular polysaccharide antigenemia in rats with experimental endocarditis due to *Staphylococcus aureus*. J Infect Dis. 1987; 155:242–6.

191. Christensson B, Boutonnier A, Ryding V, et al. Diagnosis *Staphylococcus aureus* endocarditis by detecting antibodies against *S. aureus* capsular polysaccharide types 5 and 8. J Infect Dis. 1991;163:530.

192. Cannady PB, Sanford JP. Negative blood cultures in infective endocarditis. A review. South Med J. 1976;69:1420.

193. Tunkel AR, Kaye D. Endocarditis with negative blood cultures. N Engl J Med. 1992;326:1215.

194. Walker RC, Henry NK, Washington JA II, et al. Lysis-centrifugation blood culture technique. Clinical impact in *Staphylococcus aureus* bacteremia. Arch Intern Med. 1986;146:2341–3.

195. Washington JA II. The microbiological diagnosis of infective endocarditis. J Antimicrob Chemother. 1987;20(Suppl A):29–36.

196. Austin SM, Smith SM, Co B, et al. Case report: Serologic evidence of acute murine typhus infection in a patient with culture-negative endocarditis. Am J Med Sci. 1987;293:320–3.

197. Shapiro DS, Kenney SC, Johnson M, et al. *Chlamydia psittaci* endocarditis diagnosed by blood culture. N Engl J Med. 1992;326:1192.

198. Tompkins LS, Roessler BJ, Redd SC, et al. *Legionella* prosthetic-valve endocarditis. N Engl J Med. 1988;318:530–5.

199. Walterspiel JN, Kaplan SL. Incidence and clinical characteristics of "culture-negative" infective endocarditis in a pediatric population. Pediatr Infect Dis. 1986;5:328–32.

200. Rubenstein E, Noreiga ER, Simberkoff MS, et al. Fungal endocarditis: Analysis of 24 cases and review of the literature. Medicine (Baltimore). 1975;54: 331.

201. Kobza K, Steenblock U. Demonstration of candida in blood smears. Br Med J. 1977;1:1640.

202. Merz WG, Evans GL, Shadomy S, et al. Laboratory evaluation of serological tests for systemic candidiasis: A cooperative study. J Clin Microbiol. 1977; 5:596.

203. Sande MA, Bowman CR, Calderone RA. Experimental *Candida albicans* endocarditis: Characterization of the disease and response to therapy. Infect Immun. 1977;17:140.

204. Warren RC, Bartlett A, Bidwell DE, et al. Diagnosis of invasive candidosis by enzyme immunoassay of serum antigen. Br Med J. 1977;1:1183.

205. Scheld WM, Brown RS Jr, Harding SA, et al. Detection of circulating antigen in experimental *Candida albicans* endocarditis by an enzyme-linked immunosorbent assay. J Clin Microbiol. 1980;12:679.

206. Dillan JC, Feigenbaum H, Konecke LL, et al. Echocardiographic manifestations of valvular vegetations. Am Heart J. 1973;86:698.

207. Boucher CA, Fallion JT, Myers GS, et al. The value and limitations of echocardiography in recording mitral valve vegetations. Am Heart J. 1977;94:37.

208. Thomson KR, Nanda NC, Gramiak R. The reliability of echocardiography in the diagnosis of infective endocarditis. Radiology. 1977;125:473.

209. Melvin ET, Berger M, Lutzker LG, et al. Noninvasive methods for detection of valve vegetations. Am J Cardiol. 1981;47:271.

210. Mintz GS, Kotler MN. Clinical value and limitations of echocardiography. Its use in the study of patients with infectious endocarditis. Arch Intern Med. 1980;140:1022.

211. Popp RL. Echocardiography and infectious endocarditis. In: Remington JS, Swartz MN, eds. Current Clinical Topics in Infectious Diseases. v. 4. New York: McGraw-Hill; 1983:98.

212. Popp RL. Echocardiography. N Engl J Med. 1990;323:165.

213. Davis RS, Strom JA, Frishman W, et al. The demonstration of vegetations by echocardiography in bacterial endocarditis. An indication for early surgical intervention. Am J Med. 1980;57:69.

214. Martin RP, Mettzer RS, Chia EL, et al. Clinical utility of two-dimensional echocardiography in infective endocarditis. Am J Cardiol. 1980;46:379.

215. Steckelberg JM, Murphy JG, Ballard D, et al. Emboli in infective endocarditis; the prognostic value of echocardiography. Ann Intern Med. 1991;114: 635.

216. Bayer AS, Blomquist IK, Bello E, et al. Tricuspid valve endocarditis due to *Staphylococcus aureus*. Correlation of two-dimensional echocardiography with clinical outcome. Chest. 1988;93:247–53.

217. Manolis AS, Melita H. Echocardiographic and clinical correlates in drug addicts with infective endocarditis. Implications of vegetation size. Arch Intern Med. 1988;148:2461–5.

218. Tak T, Rahimtoola SH, Kumar A, et al. Value of digital image processing of two-dimensional echocardiograms in differentiating active from chronic vegetations of infective endocarditis. Circulation. 1988;78:116–23.

219. Fisher EA, Goldman ME. Transesophageal echocardiography—Sound diagnostic technique or two-edged sword. N Engl J Med. 1991;324:841.

220. Pearlman AS. Transesophageal echocardiography—Sound diagnostic technique or two-edged sword. N Engl J Med. 1991;324:841.

221. Anonymous. Transesophageal echocardiography. Lancet. 1992;339:709.

222. Erbel R, Rohmann S, Drexler M, et al. Improved diagnostic value of echocardiography in patients with infective-endocarditis by transesophageal approach: A prospective study. Eur Heart J. 1988;9:43.

223. Mügge A, Daniel WG, Frank G, et al. Echocardiography in infective endocarditis: Reassessment of prognostic implications of vegetation size determined by the transthoracic and transesophageal approach. J Am Coll Cardiol. 1989; 14:631.

224. Sochowski RA, Chan K-L. Implication of negative results on a monoplane transesophageal echocardiographic study in patients with suspected infective endocarditis. J Am Coll Cardiol. 1993;21:216.

225. Carpenter JL. Perivalvular extension of infection in patients with infectious endocarditis. Rev Infect Dis. 1991;13:127.

226. Daniel WG, Mügge A, Martin RP, et al. Improvement in the diagnosis of abscesses associated with endocarditis by transesophageal echocardiography. N Engl J Med. 1991;324:795.

227. Daniel WG, Erbel R, Kasper W, et al. Safety of transesophageal echocardiography: A multicenter survey of 10419 examinations. Circulation. 1991;83: 817.

228. Mann T, McLaurin L, Grossman W, et al. Assessing the hemodynamic severity of acute aortic regurgitation due to infective endocarditis. N Engl J Med. 1975;293:108.

229. Mills J, Abbott J, Utley JR, et al. Role of cardiac catheterization in infective endocarditis. Chest. 1977;72:576.

230. Welton DE, Young JB, Raizner AE, et al. Value and safety of cardiac catheterization during active infective endocarditis. Am J Cardiol. 1979;44:1306.

231. Durack DT, Lukes AS, Bright DK, et al. New criteria for diagnosis of infective endocarditis. Am J Med. 1994;96:200–9.

232. Kim EL, Ching DL, Pien FD. Bacterial endocarditis at a small community hospital. Am J Med Sci. 1990;229:87.

233. Kazanjian PH. Infective endocarditis: Review of 60 cases treated in community hospitals. Infect Dis Clin Pract. 1993;2:41.

234. Roberts RB, Krieger AG, Schiller NL, et al. Viridans streptococcal endocarditis: The role of various species, including pyridoxal-dependent streptococci. Rev Infect Dis. 1979;1:955.

235. Tuazon CV, Gill V, Gill F. Streptococcal endocarditis: Single vs. combination antibiotic therapy and the role of various species. Rev Infect Dis. 1986; 8:54–60.

236. Baddour LM, Bisno AL. Infective endocarditis complicating mitral valve prolapse: Epidemiologic, clinical, and microbiologic aspects. Rev Infect Dis. 1986;8:117–37.

237. Hamoudi AC, Hribar MM, Marcon MJ, et al. Clinical relevance of viridans and nonhemolytic streptococci isolated from blood and cerebrospinal fluid in a pediatric population. Am J Clin Pathol. 1990;93:270.

238. Harder EJ, Wilkowske CJ, Washington JA, et al. *Streptococcus mutans* endocarditis. Ann Intern Med. 1974;80:364.

239. Watanakunakorn C. *Streptococcus bovis* endocarditis. Am J Med. 1974;56: 256.

240. Moellering RC, Watson BK, Kunz LJ. Endocarditis due to group D streptococci. Comparison of disease caused by *Streptococcus bovis* with that produced by the enterococci. Am J Med. 1974;57:239.

241. Hoppes WL, Lerner PI. Nonenterococcal group D streptococcal endocarditis caused by *Streptococcus bovis*. Ann Intern Med. 1974;81:588.

242. Klein RS, Reuco RA, Catalano MT, et al. Association of *Streptococcus bovis* with carcinoma of the colon. N Engl J Med. 1977;297:800.

243. Steinberg D, Naggar CZ. *Streptococcus bovis* endocarditis with carcinoma of the colon. N Engl J Med. 1977;297:1354.

244. Mandell GL, Kaye D, Levison ME, et al. Enterococcal endocarditis: An analysis of 38 patients observed at the New York Hospital–Cornell Medical Center. Arch Intern Med. 1970;125:258.

245. Serra P, Brandimarte C, Martino P, et al. Synergistic treatment of enterococcal endocarditis. Arch Intern Med. 1977;137:1562.

246. Mergran DW. Enterococcal endocarditis. Clin Infect Dis. 1992;15:63.

247. Malone DA, Wagner RA, Myers JP, et al. Enterococcal bacteremia in two large community teaching hospitals. Am J Med. 1986;81:601–6.

248. Hoffmann SA, Moellering RC Jr. The enterococcus: "Putting the bug in our ears." Ann Intern Med. 1987;106:757–61.

249. Maki DG, Agger WA. Enterococcal bacteremia: Clinical features, the risk of endocarditis, and management. Medicine (Baltimore). 1988;67:248–69.

250. Ugolini V, Pacifico A, Smitherman TC, et al. Pneumococcal endocarditis update: Analysis of 10 cases diagnosed between 1974 and 1984. Am Heart J. 1986;112:813–19.

251. Powderly WG, Stanley SL Jr, Medoff G. Pneumococcal endocarditis: Report of a series and review of the literature. Rev Infect Dis. 1986;8:786–91.

252. Bruyn GAW, Thompson J, van der Meer JWM. Pneumococcal endocarditis in adult patients. A report of five cases and review of the literature. Q J Med. 1990;74:33.

253. Elward K, Hruby N, Christy C. Pneumococcal endocarditis in infants and children: Report of a case and review of the literature. Pediatr Infect Dis J. 1990;9:652.

254. Gelfand MS, Threlkeld MG. Subacute bacterial endocarditis secondary to Streptococcus pneumoniae. Am J Med. 1992;93:91.

255. Carey RB, Brause BD, Roberts RB: Antimicrobial therapy of vitamin B₆–dependent streptococcal endocarditis. Ann Intern Med. 1977;87:150.

256. Stein DS, Nelson KE. Endocarditis due to nutritionally deficient streptococci: Therapeutic dilemma. Rev Infect Dis. 1987;9:908–16.

257. Catto BA, Jacobs MR, Shlaes DM. Streptococcus mitis. A cause of serious infection in adults. Arch Intern Med. 1987;147:885–8.

258. Rapeport KB, Giron JA, Rosner F. Streptococcus mitis endocarditis. Report of 17 cases. Arch Intern Med. 1986;146:2361–3.

259. Hager WD, Speck EL, Mathew PK, et al. Endocarditis with myocardial abscesses and pericarditis in an adult. Group B streptococcus as a cause. Arch Intern Med. 1977;137:1725.

260. Opal SM, Cross A, Palmer M, et al. Group B streptococcal sepsis in adults and infants. Contrasts and comparisons. Arch Intern Med. 1988;148:641–5.

261. Gallagher PG, Watanakunakorn C. Group B streptococcal endocarditis: Report of seven cases and review of the literature, 1962–1985. Rev Infect Dis. 1986;8:175–88.

262. Scully BE, Spriggs D, Neu HC. Streptococcus agalactiae (group B) endocarditis—A description of twelve cases and review of the literature. Infection. 1987;15:169–76.

263. Wiseman A, Rene P, Crelinsten GL. Streptococcus agalactiae endocarditis: An association with villous adenomas of the large intestine. Ann Intern Med. 1985;103:893–4.

264. Vartrian CV, Septimus EJ. Tricuspid valve group B streptococcal endocarditis following elective abortion. Rev Infect Dis. 1991;13:997.

265. Venezio FR, Gullberg RM, Westenfelder GO, et al. Group G streptococcal endocarditis and bacteremia. Am J Med. 1986;81:29–34.

266. Smyth EG, Pallett AP, Davidson RN. Group G streptococcal endocarditis: Two case reports, a review of the literature and recommendations for treatment. J Infect. 1988;16:169–76.

267. Ho AKC, Woo KS, Tse KK, et al. Infective endocarditis caused by Streptococcus suis serotype 2. J Infect. 1990;21:209.

268. Liu VC, Stevenson JG, Smith AL. Group A Streptococcus mural endocarditis. Pediatr Infect Dis J. 1992;11:1060.

269. Murray HW, Gross KC, Masur H, et al. Serious infections caused by Streptococcus milleri. Am J Med. 1978;64:759.

270. Shlaes DM, Lerner PI, Wolinsky E, et al. Infections due to Lancefield group F and related streptococci (S. milleri, S. anginosus). Medicine (Baltimore). 1981;60:197.

271. Gossling J. Occurence and pathogenicity of the Streptococcus milleri group. Rev Infect Dis. 1988;10:257–85.

272. Hosea SW: Virulent Streptococcus viridans bacterial endocarditis. Am Heart J. 1981;101:174.

273. Buu-Joi A, Sapoetra A, Branger C, et al. Antimicrobial susceptibility of Gemella haemolysans isolated from patients with subacute endocarditis. Eur J Clin Microbiol. 1982;1:102.

274. Frésard A, Michel VP, Rueda X, et al. Gemella haemolysans endocarditis. Clin Infect Dis. 1993;16:586.

275. Mylotte JM, McDermott C, Spooner JA. Prospective study of 114 consecutive episodes of Staphylococcus aureus bacteremia. Rev Infect Dis. 1987;9:891–908.

276. Eykyn SJ. Staphylococcal sepsis. The changing pattern of disease and therapy. Lancet. 1988;1:100–4.

277. Watanakunakorn C, Tan JS, Phair JP. Some salient features of Staphylococcus aureus endocarditis. Am J Med. 1973;54:473.

278. Musher DM, McKenzie SO. Infection due to Staphylococcus aureus. Medicine (Baltimore). 1977;56:383.

279. Bayer AS. Staphylococcal bacteremia and endocarditis. State of the art. Arch Intern Med. 1982;142:1169.

280. Thompson RL. Staphylococcal infective endocarditis. Mayo Clin Proc. 1982; 57:106.

281. Sanabria TJ, Alpert JS, Goldberg R, et al. Increasing frequency of staphylococcal infective endocarditis. Experience at a university hospital, 1981 through 1988. Arch Intern Med. 1990;150:1305.

282. Julander I. Unfavourable prognostic factors in Staphylococcus aureus septicemia and endocarditis. Scand J Infect Dis. 1985;17:179–87.

283. O'Callaghan C, McDougall P. Infective endocarditis in neonates. Arch Dis Child. 1988;63:53–7.

284. Crane LR, Levine DP, Zervos MJ, et al. Bacteremia in narcotic addicts at the Detroit Medical Center. I. Microbiology, epidemiology, risk factors, and empiric therapy. Rev Infect Dis. 1986;8:364–73.

285. Noel GJ, O'Loughlin JE, Edelson PJ. Neonatal Staphylococcus epidermidis right-sided endocarditis: Description of five catheterized infants. Pediatrics. 1988;82:234–9.

286. Baddour LM, Phillips TN, Bisno AL. Coagulase-negative staphylococcal endocarditis. Occurrence in patients with mitral valve prolapse. Arch Intern Med. 1986;146:119–21.

287. Harris LF, O'Shields H. Coagulase-negative staphylococcal endocarditis: A view from the community hospital. South Med J. 1986;79:1379–86.

288. Caputo GM, Archer GL, Calderwood SB, et al. Native valve endocarditis due to coagulase-negative staphylococci. Clinical and microbiologic features. Am J Med. 1987;83:619–25.

289. Arber N, Militano A, Ben-Yehuda A, et al. Native valve Staphylococcus epidermidis endocarditis: Report of seven cases and review of the literature. Am J Med. 1991;90:758.

290. Espersen F, Wheat LJ, Bemis AT, et al. Solid-phase radio-immunoassay for IgG antibodies to Staphylococcus epidermidis: Use in serious coagulase-negative staphylococcal infections. Arch Intern Med. 1987;147:689–93.

291. Etienne J, Brun Y, El Solh N, et al. Characterization of clinically significant isolates of Staphylococcus epidermidis from patients with endocarditis. J Clin Microbiol. 1988;26:613–7.

292. Baddour LM, Simpson WA, Weems JJ Jr, et al. Phenotypic selection of small-colony variant forms of Staphylococcus epidermidis in a rat model of endocarditis. J Infect Dis. 1988;157:757–63.

293. Singh VR, Radd I. Fatal Staphylococcus saprophyticus native valve endocarditis in an intravenous drug addict. J Infect Dis. 1990;162:783.

294. Lina B, Celard M, Vandenesch F, et al. Infective endocarditis due to Staphylococcus capitis. Clin Infect Dis. 1992;15:173.

295. Finland M, Barnes MW. Changing etiology of bacterial endocarditis in the antibacterial era. Experiences at Boston City Hospital 1933–1965. Ann Intern Med. 1970;72:341.

296. Pedersen FK, Petersen EA. Bacterial endocarditis of Blegdamshospitalet in Copenhagen 1944–1973. Scand J Infect Dis. 1976;8:99.

297. Cohen PS, Maquire JH, Weinstein L. Infective endocarditis caused by gram-negative bacteria: A review of the literature, 1945–1977. Prog Cardiovasc Dis. 1980;22:205.

298. Geraci JE, Wilson WR. Endocarditis due to gram-negative bacteria. Report of 56 cases. Mayo Clin Proc. 1982;57:145.

299. Snyder N, Atterbury CE, Correia JP, et al. Increased occurrence of cirrhosis and bacterial endocarditis. Gastroenterology. 1977;73:1107.

300. Carruthers M. Endocarditis due to enteric bacilli other than salmonellae: Case reports and literature review. Am J Med Sci. 1977;273:203.

301. Sande MA, Johnson WD, Hook EW, et al. Sustained bacteremia in patients with prosthetic cardiac valves. N Engl J Med. 1972;286:1067.

302. Schneider PJ, Nernoff J, Gold JA. Acute salmonella endocarditis. Report of a case and review. Arch Intern Med. 1967;120:478.

303. Mills J, Drew D. Serratia marcescens endocarditis. Ann Intern Med. 1976; 85:397.

304. Cooper R, Mills J. Serratia endocarditis. A follow-up report. Arch Intern Med. 1980;140:199.

305. Caramelli B, Mansur AJ, Grinberg M, et al. Campylobacter fetus endocarditis on a prosthetic heart valve. South Med J. 1988;81:802–3.

306. Reyes MP, Brown WJ, Lerner AM. Treatment of patients with Pseudomonas endocarditis with high dose aminoglycoside and carbenicillin therapy. Medicine (Baltimore). 1978;57:57.

307. Reyes MP, Lerner AM. Current problems in the treatment of infective endocarditis due to Pseudomonas aeruginosa. Rev Infect Dis. 1983;5:314.

308. Wieland M, Lederman MM, Kline-King C, et al. Left-sided endocarditis due to Pseudomonas aeruginosa. A report of 10 cases and review of the literature. Medicine (Baltimore). 1986;65:180–9.

309. Komshian SV, Tablan OC, Palutke W, et al. Characteristics of left-sided endocarditis due to Pseudomonas aeruginosa in the Detroit Medical Center. Rev Infect Dis. 1990;12:693.

310. Noriega ER, Rubinstein E, Simberkoff M, et al. Subacute and acute endocarditis due to Pseudomonas cepacia in heroin addicts. Am J Med. 1975;59:29.

311. Reyes MP, Palutke WA, Wylin RF, et al. Pseudomonas endocarditis in the Detroit Medical Center 1969–1972. Medicine (Baltimore). 1973;52:173.

312. Jurica JV, Bomzer CA, England AC III. Gonococcal endocarditis: A case report and review of the literature. Sex Transm Dis. 1987;14:231–3.

313. Wall TC, Peyton RB, Corey GR. Gonococcal endocarditis: A new look at an old disease. Medicine. 1989;68:375.

314. Jackman JD Jr, Glamann DB. Gonococcal endocarditis: Twenty-five year experience. Am J Med Sci. 1991;301:221.

315. Wong JD, Janda JM. Association of an important Neisseria species, Neisseria elongata subsp. nitroreducens, with bacteremia, endocarditis, and osteomyelitis. J Clin Microbiol. 1992;30:719.

316. Ingram RJH, Cornere B, Ellis-Pegler RB. Endocarditis due to Neisseria mucosa: Two case reports and review. Clin Infect Dis. 1992;15:321.

317. Heiddal S, Sverrisson JT, Yngvason FE, et al. Native-valve endocarditis due to Neisseria sicca: Case report and review. Clin Infect Dis. 1993;16:667.

318. Chunn CJ, Jones SR, McCutchan JA, et al. Haemophilus parainfluenzae infective endocarditis. Medicine (Baltimore). 1977;56:99.

319. Lynn DJ, Kane JG, Parker RH. Haemophilus parainfluenzae and influenzae endocarditis: A review of forty cases. Medicine (Baltimore). 1977;56:115.

320. Geraci JE, Wilkowske CJ, Wilson WR, et al. *Haemophilus* endocarditis. Report of 14 cases. Mayo Clin Proc. 1977;52:209.

321. Parker SW, Apicella MA, Fuller CM. *Hemophilus* endocarditis. Two patients with complications. Arch Intern Med. 1983;143:48.

322. Bangsborg JM, Tuede M, Skinhoj P. *Haemophilus seguis* endocarditis. J Infect. 1988;16:81–5.

323. Porath A, Wanderman K, Simu A, et al. Case report: Endocarditis caused by *Haemophilus aegyptius*. Am J Med Sci. 1986;292:110–11.

324. Vandepitte J, DeGeest H, Jousten P. Subacute bacterial endocarditis due to *Actinobacillus actinomycetemcomitans*. Report of a case with a review of the literature. J Clin Pathol. 1977;30:842.

325. AhFat LNC, Patel BR, Pickens S. *Actinobacillus actinomycetemcomitans* endocarditis in hypertrophic obstructive cardiomyopathy. J Infect Dis. 1983; 6:81.

326. Lane T, MacGregor RR, Wright D, et al. *Cardiobacterium hominis:* An elusive cause of endocarditis. J Infect. 1983;6:75.

327. Jenny DB, Letendre PW, Iverson G. Endocarditis due to *Kingella* species. Rev Infect Dis. 1988;10:1065–6.

328. Decker MD, Graham BS, Hunter EB, et al. Endocarditis and infections of intravascular devices due to *Eikinella corrodens*. Am J Med Sci. 1986;292: 209–12.

329. Patrick WD, Brown WD, Bowmer MI, et al. Infective endocarditis due to *Eikinella corrodens:* Case report and review of the literature. Can J Infect Dis. 1990;1:139.

330. Ellner JJ, Rosenthal MS, Lerner PI, et al. Infective endocarditis caused by slow-growing, fastidious, gram-negative bacteria. Medicine (Baltimore). 1979;58:145.

331. Gerry JL, Greenough WB. Diphtheroid endocarditis: Report of nine cases and review of the literature. Johns Hopkins Med J. 1976;139:61.

332. Morris A, Guild I. Endocarditis due to *Corynebacterium pseudodiphthericum:* Five case reports, review, and antibiotic susceptibilities of nine strains. Rev Infect Dis. 1991;13:887.

333. Tiley SM, Kociuba KR, Heron LG, et al. Infective endocarditis due to nontoxigenic *Corynebacterium diphtheriae:* Report of seven cases and review. Clin Infect Dis. 1993;16:271.

334. Bayer AS, Chow AW, Guze LB. *Listeria monocytogenes* endocarditis: Report of a case and review of the literature. Am J Med Sci. 1977;273:319.

335. Carvajal A, Frederiksen W. Fatal endocarditis due to *Listeria monocytogenes*. Rev Infect Dis. 1988;10:616–23.

336. Sussman JI, Baron EJ, Goldberg SM, et al. Clinical manifestations and therapy of *Lactobacillus* endocarditis: Report of a case and review of the literature. Rev Infect Dis. 1986;8:771–6.

337. Griffiths JK, Daly JS, Dodge RA. Two cases of endocarditis due to *Lactobacillus* species: Antimicrobial susceptibility, review, and discussion of therapy. Clin Infect Dis. 1992;15:250.

338. Gorby GL, Peacock JE Jr. *Erysipelothrix rhusiopathiae* endocarditis: Microbiologic, epidemiologic, and clinical features of an occupational disease. Rev Infect Dis. 1988;10:317–25.

339. Steen MK, Bruno-Murtha LA, Chaux G, et al. *Bacillus cereus* endocarditis: Report of a case and review. Clin Infect Dis. 1992;14:945.

340. Shands JW Jr. *Rothia dentocariosa* endocarditis. Am J Med. 1988;85:280–1.

341. Sudduth EJ, Rozich JD, Farrar WE. *Rothia dentocariosa* endocarditis complicated by perivalvular abscess. Clin Infect Dis. 1993;17:772.

342. Felner JM, Dowell UR. Anaerobic bacterial endocarditis. N Engl J Med. 1970;283:1188.

343. Nastro LJ, Finegold SM. Endocarditis due to anaerobic gram-negative bacilli. Am J Med. 1973;54:482.

344. Nastro FL, Sarma RJ. Infective endocarditis due to anaerobic and microaerophilic bacteria. West J Med. 1982;137:18.

345. Jackson RT, Dopp AC. *Bacteroides fragilis* endocarditis. South Med J. 1988; 81:781–2.

346. Gradon JD, Chapnick EK, Lutwick LI. Infective endocarditis of a native valve due to *Acinetobacter:* Case report and review. Clin Infect Dis. 1992; 14:1145.

347. Lam S, Samraj J, Rahman S, et al. Primary actinomycotic endocarditis: Case report and review. Clin Infect Dis. 1993;16:481.

348. Ascher DP, Zbick C, White C, et al. Infections due to *Stomatococcus mucilaginosus:* 10 cases and review. Rev Infect Dis. 1991;13:1048.

349. Rupp ME. *Streptobacillus moniliformis* endocarditis: Case report and review. Clin Infect Dis. 1992;14:769.

350. Al-Kasab S, Fagih MR, Al-Yousef S, et al. *Brucella* infective endocarditis. Successful combined medical and surgical therapy. J Thorac Cardiovasc Surg. 1988;95:862–7.

351. Szabo S, Lieberman JP, Lue YA. Unusual pathogens in narcotic-associated endocarditis. Rev Infect Dis. 1990;12:412.

352. Komshian SV, Tablan OC, Palutke W, et al. Characteristics of left sided endocarditis due to *Pseudomonas aeruginosa* in the Detroit Medical Center. Rev Infect Dis. 1990;12:693.

353. Tuazon CW, Hill R, Sheagren JW. Microbiologic study of street heroin and injection paraphenalia. J Infect Dis. 1974;129:327.

354. Tuazon CW, Sheagren JW. Increased rate of carriage of *Staphylococcus aureus* among narcotic addicts. J Infect Dis. 1974;129:725.

355. Reisberg BE. Infective endocarditis in the narcotic addict. Prog Cardiovasc Dis. 1979;22:193.

356. Baddour LM. Twelve-year review of recurrent native-valve infective endocarditis: A disease of the modern antibiotic era. Rev Infect Dis. 1988;10: 1163–70.

357. Rubenstein E, Noreiga ER, Simberkoff MS, et al. Tissue penetration of amphotericin B in *Candida* endocarditis. Chest. 1974;66:376.

358. Carrizosa J, Levison ME, Lawrence T, et al. Cure of *Asperigillus ustus* endocarditis of prosthetic valve. Arch Intern Med. 1974;133:486.

359. Keay S, Denning DW, Stevens DA. Endocarditis due to *Trichosporon beigelii:* In vitro susceptibility of isolates and review. Rev Infect Dis. 1991; 13:383.

360. Welty FK, McLeod GX, Ezratty C, et al. *Pseudallescheria boydii* endocarditis of the pulmonic valve in a liver transplant recipient. Clin Infect Dis. 1992; 15:858.

361. McIntosh CS, Nickers PJ, Isaqacs AJ. *Spirillum* endocarditis. Postgrad Med J. 1975;51:645.

362. Applefield MM, Billingsley LJ, Tucker HJ, et al. Q fever endocarditis—A case occurring in the United States. Am Heart J. 1977;93:669.

363. Tobin MJ, Cahill N, Gearty G, et al. Q fever endocarditis. Am J Med. 1982; 72:396.

364. Peter O, Flepp M, Bestetti G, et al. Q fever endocarditis: Diagnostic approaches and monitoring of therapeutic effects. Clin Invest. 1992;70:932.

365. Fernandez-Guerrero ML, Muelas JM, Aquado JM. Q fever endocarditis on porcine bioprosthetic valves. Ann Intern Med. 1988;108:209–13.

366. Jones RB, Priest JB, Kuo C-C. Subacute chlamydial endocarditis. JAMA. 1982;247:655.

367. Brearley BF, Hutchinson DN. Endocarditis associated with *Chlamydia trachomatis* infection. Br Heart J. 1981;46:220.

368. Marrie TJ, Harczy M, Mann OE, et al. Culture-negative endocarditis probably due to *Chlamydia pneumoniae*. J Infect Dis. 1990;161:127.

369. Popat K, Barnardo D, Webb-Peploe M. *Mycoplasma pneumoniae* endocarditis. Br Heart J. 1980;44:111.

370. Burch GE, Tsui CY. Evolution of coxsackie viral valvular and mural endocarditis in mice. Br J Exp Pathol. 1971;52:360.

371. Persand V. Two unusual cases of mural endocarditis with a review of the literature. Am J Clin Pathol. 1970;53:832.

372. Van Scoy RE. Culture-negative endocarditis. Mayo Clin Proc. 1982;57:149.

373. Pesanti EL, Smith IM. Infective endocarditis with negative blood cultures. An analysis of 52 cases. Am J Med. 1979;66:43.

374. Baddour LM, Meyer J, Henry B. Polymicrobial infective endocarditis in the 1980's. Rev Infect Dis. 1991;13:963.

375. Daschner FD, Frank V. Antimicrobial drugs in human cardiac valves and endocarditis lesions. J Antimicrob Chemother. 1988;12:776–82.

376. Cremieux A-C, Carbon C. Pharmacokinetic and pharmacodynamic requirements for antibiotic therapy of experimental endocarditis. Antimicrob Agents Chemother. 1992;36:2069.

377. Spokojny AM, Sinclair IN, Schnitt S, et al. Uptake of hematoporphyrin derivative by valvular vegetations in experimental infective endocarditis. Circulation 1985;72:1087–91.

378. Dall L, Barnes WG, Lane JW, et al. Enzymatic modification of glycocalyx in the treatment of experimental endocarditis due to viridans streptococci. J Infect Dis. 1987;156:736–40.

379. Buiting AGM, Thompson J, Emeis JJ, et al. Effects of tissue-type plasminogen activator on *Staphylococcus epidermidis*–infected plasma clots as a model of infected endocardial vegetations. J Antimicrob Chemother. 1987; 19:771–80.

380. Buiting AG, Thompson J, Emeis JJ, et al. Effects of tissue-type plasminogen activator (t-PA) on *Streptococcus sanguis*–infected endocardial vegetations in vitro. J Antimicrob Chemother. 1988;21:609–20.

381. Cates JE, Christie RV. Subacute bacterial endocarditis. Q J Med. 1951;20: 93.

382. Carrizosa J, Kobasa WD, Kaye D. Antagonism between chloramphenicol and penicillin in streptococcal endocarditis in rabbits. J Lab Clin Med. 1975; 85:307.

383. Wilson WR, Gilbert DN, Bisno AL, et al. Evaluation of new anti-infective drugs for the treatment of infective endocarditis. Clin Infect Dis. 1992; 15(Suppl 1):S89.

384. Douglas A, Moore-Gillon J, Eykyn S. Fever during treatment of infective endocarditis. Lancet. 1986;1:1341–3.

385. Schlicter JG, MacIlean H. A method of determining the effective therapeutic level in the treatment of subacute bacterial endocarditis with penicillin. Am Heart J. 1947;34:209.

386. Coleman DL, Horwitz RI, Andriole VT. Association between serum inhibitory and bactericidal concentrations and therapeutic outcome in bacterial endocarditis. Am J Med. 1982;73:260.

387. Mellors JW, Coleman DL, Andriole VT. Value of serum bactericidal test in management of patients with bacterial endocarditis. Eur J Clin Microbiol. 1986;5:67–70.

388. Rahal JJ, Chan Y-K, Johnson G. Relationship of staphylococcal tolerance, teichoic acid antibody, and serum bactericidal activity to therapeutic outcome in *Staphylococcus aureus* bacteremia. Am J Med. 1986;81:43–52.

389. Wolfson JS, Swartz MN. Serum bactericidal activity as a monitor of antibiotic therapy. N Engl J Med. 1985;312:968–75.

390. Reller LB. The serum bactericidal test. Rev Infect Dis. 1986;8:803–8.

391. Weinstein MP, Stratton CW, Ackley A, et al. Multicenter collaborative evaluation of a standardized serum bactericidal test as a prognostic indicator in infective endocarditis. Am J Med. 1985;78:262–9.

392. Stratton CW. The role of the microbiology laboratory in the treatment of infective endocarditis. J Antimicrob Chemother. 1987;20(Suppl A):41–9.

393. Sande MA, Scheld WM. Combination antibiotic therapy of bacterial endocarditis. Ann Intern Med. 1980;92:390.

394. Meylan PR, Francioloi P, Glauser MP. Discrepancies between MBC and actual killing by viridans group streptococci by cell-wall-active antibiotics. Antimicrob Agents Chemother. 1986;29:418–23.

395. Holloway Y, Pankert J, Hess J. Penicillin tolerance and bacterial endocarditis. Lancet. 1980;1:589.

396. Pulliam L, Inokuchi S, Hadley WK, et al. Penicillin tolerance in experimental streptococcal endocarditis. Lancet. 1979;2:957.

397. Gephart JF, Washington JA II. Antimicrobial susceptibilities of nutritionally variant streptococci. J Infect Dis. 1982;146:536.

398. Holloway Y, Dankert J. Penicillin tolerance in nutritionally variant streptococci. Antimicrob Agents Chemother. 1982;22:1073.

399. Lowry FD, Neuhas EG, Chang DS, et al. Penicillin therapy of experimental endocarditis caused by tolerant *Streptococcus sanguis* and nontolerant *Streptococcus mitis*. Antimicrob Agents Chemother. 1983;23:67.

400. Brennan RO, Durack DT. Therapeutic significance of penicillin tolerance in experimental streptococcal endocarditis. Antimicrob Agents Chemother. 1983;23:273.

401. Baker CW, Thornsberry C. Antimicrobial susceptibility of *Streptococcus mutans* isolated from patients with endocarditis. Antimicrob Agents Chemother. 1974;5:268.

402. Thornsberry C, Baker CN, Facklam RR. Antibiotic susceptibility of *Streptococcus bovis* and other group D streptococci causing endocarditis. Antimicrob Agents Chemother. 1974;5:228.

403. Wolfe JC, Johnson WD. Penicillin-sensitive streptococcal endocarditis. In vitro and clinical observations on penicillin-streptomycin therapy. Ann Intern Med. 1974;81:178.

404. Watanakunakorn C, Glotzbecker C. Synergism with aminoglycosides of penicillin, ampicillin, and vancomycin against nonenterococcal group D streptococci and viridans streptococci. J Med Microbiol. 1977;10:133.

405. Enzler MJ, Rouse MS, Henry NK, et al. In vitro and in vivo studies of streptomycin-resistant, penicillin-susceptible streptococci from patients with infective endocarditis. J Infect Dis. 1987;155:954–8.

406. Farber BF, Yee Y. High-level aminoglycoside resistance mediated by aminoglycoside-modifying enzymes among viridans streptococci: Implications for the therapy of endocarditis. J Infect Dis. 1987;155:948–53.

407. Sande MA, Irvin RG. Penicillin-aminoglycoside synergy in experimental *Streptococcus viridans* endocarditis. J Infect Dis. 1974;129:572.

408. Durack DT, Pelletier LL, Petersdorf RG. Chemotherapy of experimental streptococcal endocarditis. II. Synergism between penicillin and streptomycin against penicillin-sensitive streptococci. J Clin Invest. 1974;53:929.

409. Drake TA, Sande MA. Studies of the chemotherapy of endocarditis: Correlation of in vitro, animal model, and clinical studies. Rev Infect Dis. 1983; 5(Suppl):345.

410. Wilson WR, Geraci JE. Treatment of streptococcal infective endocarditis. Am J Med. 1985;78(Suppl 6B):128–137.

411. Scheld WM. Therapy of streptococcal endocarditis: Correlation of animal model and clinical studies. J Antimicrob Chemother. 1987;20(Suppl A): 71–85.

412. Baquero F, Loza E. Penicillin resistance in Spain. Infect Dis Clin Pract. 1992;1:147.

413. Wilson WR, Geraci JE, Wilkowske CJ, et al. Short-term intramuscular therapy with procaine penicillin plus streptomycin for infective endocarditis due to viridans streptococci. Circulation. 1978;57:1158.

414. Wilson WR, Thompson RL, Wilkowske CJ, et al. Short-term therapy for streptococcal infective endocarditis. Combined intramuscular administration of penicillin and streptomycin. JAMA. 1981;245:360.

415. Karchmer AW, Mollering RC Jr, Maki DG, et al. Single antibiotic therapy for streptococcal endocarditis. JAMA. 1979;241:1801.

416. Malacoff RF, Frank E, Andriole VT. Streptococcal endocarditis (nonenterococcal, non-group A). Single vs. combination therapy. JAMA. 1979;241: 1807.

417. Parillo JE, Borst GC, Mazur MH, et al. Endocarditis due to resistant viridans streptococci during oral penicillin chemoprophylaxis. N Engl J Med. 1979; 300:296.

418. Bisno AL, Dismukes WE, Durack DT, et al. Antimicrobial treatment of infective endocarditis due to viridans streptococci, enterococci, and staphylococci. JAMA. 1989;261:1471–7.

419. Bouvet A, Cremieux AC, Contrepois A, et al. Comparison of penicillin and vancomycin, individually and in combination with gentamicin and amikacin, in the treatment of experimental endocarditis induced by nutritionally variant streptococci. Antimicrob Agents Chemother. 1985;28:607–11.

420. Henry NK, Wilson WR, Roberts RB, et al. Antimicrobial therapy of experimental endocarditis caused by nutritionally variant viridans group streptococci. Antimicrob Agents Chemother. 1986;30:465–7.

421. Stein DS, Nelson KE. Endocarditis due to nutritionally deficient streptococci: Therapeutic dilemma. Rev Infect Dis. 1987;9:908–16.

422. Saleh-Mghir A, Cremieux A-C, Vallois J-M, et al. Optimal aminoglycoside dosing regimen for penicillin-tobramycin synergism in experimental *Streptococcus adjacens* endocarditis. Antimicrob Agents Chemother. 1992;36:2403.

423. Cremieux A-C, Saleh-Mghir A, Vallois J-M, et al. Efficacy of temafloxacin in experimental *Streptococcus adjacens* endocarditis and autoradiographic diffusion pattern of [14C]temafloxacin in cardiac vegetations. Antimicrob Agents Chemother. 1992;36:2216.

424. Stramboulian D, Bonvehi P, Arevalo C, et al. Antibiotic management of outpatients with endocarditis due to penicillin-susceptible streptococci. Rev Infect Dis. 1991;13(Suppl 2): 160.

425. Francioli P, Etienne J, Hoigué R, et al. Treatment of streptococcal endocardi-

tis with a single daily dose of ceftriaxone sodium for 4 weeks. Efficacy and outpatient treatment feasibility. JAMA. 1992;267:264.

426. Francioli PB, Glauser MP. Synergistic activity of ceftriaxone combined with netilmicin administered once daily for treatment of experimental streptococcal endocarditis. Antimicrob Agents Chemother. 1993;37:207.

427. Yenditti M, Gelfusa V, Serra P, et al. 4-week treatment of streptococcal native valve endocarditis with high-dose teicoplanin. Antimicrob Agents Chemother. 1992;36:723.

428. Watanakunakorn C. Penicillin combined with gentamicin or streptomycin: Synergism against enterococci. J Infect Dis. 1971;124:581.

429. Moellering RC Jr, Korzeniowski OM, Sande MA, et al. Species-specific resistance to antimicrobial synergism in *Streptococcus faecium* and *Streptococcus faecalis*. J Infect Dis. 1979;140:203.

430. Krogstad DJ, Parquette AR. Defective killing of enterococci: A common property of antimicrobial agents acting on the cell wall. Antimicrob Agents Chemother. 1980;17:965.

431. Storch GA, Krogstad DA, Parquette AR. Antibiotic-induced lysis of enterococci. J Clin Invest. 1981;68:639.

432. Megran DW. Enterococcal endocarditis. Clin Infect Dis. 1992;15:63.

433. Murray BE, Church DA, Wanger A, et al. Comparison of two β-lactamase–producing strains of *Streptococcus faecalis*. Antimicrob Agents Chemother. 1986;30:861–4.

434. Ingerman M, Pitsakis PG, Rosenberg A, et al. β-Lactamase production in experimental endocarditis due to aminoglycoside-resistant *Streptococcus faecalis*. J Infect Dis. 1987;155:1226–32.

435. Coudron PE, Markowitz SM, Wong ES. Isolation of a β-lactamase-producing, highly-gentamicin-resistant isolate of *Enterococcus faecalis*. Antimicrob Agents Chemother. 1992;36:1225.

436. Lavoie SR, Wong ES, Coudron PE, et al. Comparison of ampicillin-sulbactam with vancomycin for treatment of experimental endocarditis due to a β-lactamase-producing, highly-gentamicin-resistant isolate of *Enterococcus faecalis*. Antimicrob Agents Chemother. 1993;37:1447.

437. Thal LA, Vazquez J, Perri MB, et al. Activity of ampicillin plus sulbactam against β-lactamase producing enterococci in experimental endocarditis. J Antimicrob Chemother. 1993;31:182.

438. Yao JDC, Thauvin-Eliopoulos C, Eliopoulos GM, et al. Efficacy of teicoplanin in two dosage regimens for experimental endocarditis caused by a β-lactamase-producing strain of *Enterococcus faecalis* with high level resistance to gentamicin. Antimicrob Agents Chemother. 1990;34:827.

439. Ramos MC, Grayson ML, Eliopoulos GM, et al. Comparison of daptomycin, vancomycin, and ampicillin-gentamicin for treatment of experimental endocarditis caused by penicillin-resistant enterococci. Antimicrob Agents Chemother. 1992;36:1864.

440. Fontana R, Grossato A, Ligozzi M, et al. In vitro response to bactericidal activity of cell wall-active antibiotics does not support the general opinion that enterococci are naturally tolerant to these antibiotics. Antimicrob Agents Chemother. 1990;34:1518.

441. Henry NK, Wilson WR, Geraci JE. Treatment of streptomycin-susceptible enterococcal experimental endocarditis with combinations of penicillin and low- or high-dose streptomycin. Antimicrob Agents Chemother. 1986;30: 725–8.

442. Harwick HJ, Kalmanson GM, Guze LB. In vitro activity of ampicillin or vancomycin combined with gentamicin or streptomycin against enterococci. Antimicrob Agents Chemother. 1973;4:383.

443. Weinstein AJ, Moellering RC. Penicillin and gentamicin therapy for enterococcal infections. JAMA. 1973;223:1030.

444. Moellering RC, Wennersten C, Weinberg AW. Synergy of penicillin and gentamicin against enterococci. J Infect Dis. 1971;124(Suppl):207.

445. Hook EW III, Roberts RB, Sande MA. Antimicrobial therapy of experimental enterococcal endocarditis. Antimicrob Agents Chemother. 1975;8:564.

446. Wright AJ, Wilson WR, Matsumoto JY, et al. Influence of gentamicin dose size on the efficacies of combinations of gentamicin and penicillin in experimental streptomycin-resistant enterococcal endocarditis. Antimicrob Agents Chemother. 1982;22:972.

447. Murray BE, Tsao J, Panida J. Enterococci from Bangkok, Thailand, with high-level resistance to currently available aminoglycosides. Antimicrob Agents Chemother. 1983;23:799.

448. Mederski-Samoraj BD, Murray BE. High-level resistance to gentamicin in clinical isolates of enterococci. J Infect Dis. 1983;147:751.

449. Zervos MJ, Dembinski S, Mikesell T, et al. High-level resistance to gentamicin in *Streptococcus faecalis*: Risk factors and evidence for exogenous acquisition of infection. J Infect Dis. 1986;153:1075–83.

450. Patterson JE, Zervos MJ. High-level gentamicin resistance in *Enterococcus*: Microbiology, genetic basis, and epidemiology. Rev Infect Dis. 1990;12:644.

451. Zervos MJ, Terpenning MS, Schaberg DR, et al. High-level aminoglycoside-resistant enterococci. Arch Intern Med. 1987;1491591–4.

452. Eliopoulos GM, Wennersten C, Zighelboim-Daum S, et al. High-level resistance to gentamicin in clinical isolates of *Streptococcus* (*Enterococcus*) *faecium*. Antimicrob Agents Chemother. 1988;32:1528–32.

453. Eliopoulos GM, Thauvin-Eliopoulos C, Moellering RC Jr. Contribution of animal models in the search for effective therapy for endocarditis due to enterococci with high-level resistance to gentamicin. Clin Infect Dis. 1992; 15:58.

454. Fernandez-Guerrero ML, Barros C, Rodriquez Tudela JL, et al. Aortic endocarditis caused by genamicin-resistant *Enterococcus faecalis*. Eur J Clin Microbiol. 1988;7:525–7.

455. Hellinger WC, Rouse MS, Robadan PM, et al. Continuous intravenous ver-

sus intermittent ampicillin therapy of experimental endocarditis caused by aminoglycoside-resistant enterococci. Antimicrob Agents Chemother. 1992; 36:1272.

456. Fantin B, Carbon C. Importance of the aminoglycoside dosing regimen in the penicillin-netilmicin combination for treatment of *Enterococcus faecalis*-induced experimental endocarditis. Antimicrob Agents Chemother. 1990;34:2387.

457. Grayson ML, Thauvin-Eliopoulos C, Eliopoulos GM, et al. Failure of trimethoprim-sulfamethoxazole therapy in experimental enterococcal endocarditis. Antimicrob Agents Chemother. 1990;34:1792.

458. Watanakunakorn C, Bakie C. Synergism of vancomycin-gentamicin and vancomycin-streptomycin against enterococci. Antimicrob Agents Chemother. 1973;4:120.

459. Watanakunakorn C, Tisone JC. Effects of a vancomycin-rifampin combination on enterococci. Antimicrob Agents Chemother. 1982;22:915.

460. Uttley AH, Collins CH, Naidoo J, et al. Vancomycin-resistant enterococci. Lancet. 1988;1:57–8.

461. Frieden TR, Munsiff SS, Low DE, et al. Emergence of vancomycin-resistant enterococci in New York City. Lancet. 1993;342:76.

462. Courvalin P. Resistance of enterococci to glycopeptides. Antimicrob Agents Chemother. 1990;34:2291.

463. Murray BE. The life and times of the *Enterococcus*. Clin Microbiol Rev. 1990;3:46.

464. Venditti M, Biavasco F, Varaldo PE, et al. Catheter-related endocarditis due to glycopeptide-resistant *Enterococcus faecalis* in a transplanted heart. Clin Infect Dis. 1993;17:524.

465. Leclercq R, Derlot E, Dural J, et al. Plasmid-mediated resistance to vancomycin and teichoplanin in *Enterococcus faecium*. N Engl J Med. 1988;319:157–61.

466. Fantin B, Leclercq R, Arthur M, et al. Influence of low-level resistance to vancomycin on efficacy of teicoplanin and vancomycin for treatment of experimental endocarditis due to *Enterococcus faecium*. Antimicrob Agents Chemother. 1991;35:1570.

467. Caron F, Kitzis M-D, Gutmann L, et al. Daptomycin or teicoplanin in combination with gentamicin for treatment of experimental endocarditis due to a highly glycopeptide-resistant isolate of *Enterococcus faecium*. Antimicrob Agents Chemother. 1992;36:261.

468. Collins LA, Eliopoulos GM, Wennersten CB, et al. In vitro activity of ramoplanin against vancomycin-resistant gram-positive organisms. Antimicrob Agents Chemother. 1993;37:1364.

469. Caron F, Carbon C, Gutmann L. Triple-combination penicillin-vancomycin-gentamicin for experimental endocarditis caused by a moderately penicillin- and highly glycopeptide-resistant isolate of *Enterococcus faecium*. J Infect Dis. 1991;164:888.

470. Caron F, Lemeland J-F, Humbert G, et al. Triple combination penicillin-vancomycin-gentamicin for experimental endocarditis caused by a highly penicillin- and glycopeptide-resistant isolate of *Enterococcus faecium*. J Infect Dis. 1993;168:681.

471. Fernandez-Guerrero M, Rouse MS, Henry NK, et al. In vitro and in vivo activity of ciprofloxacin against enterococci isolated from patients with infective endocarditis. Antimicrob Agents Chemother. 1987;31:430–3.

472. Wilson WR, Wilkowski CJ, Wright AJ, et al. Treatment of streptomycin-susceptible and streptomycin-resistant enterococcal endocarditis. Ann Intern Med. 1984;100:816–23.

473. Karchmer AW. Staphylococcal endocarditis. Laboratory and clinical basis for antibiotic therapy. Am J Med. 1985;78(Suppl B):116–27.

474. Sande MA, Courtney KB. Nafcillin-gentamicin synergism in experimental staphylococcal endocarditis. J Lab Clin Med. 1976;88:118.

475. Abrams B, Sklaver A, Hoffman T, et al. Single or combination therapy of staphylococcal endocarditis in intravenous drug abusers. Ann Intern Med. 1979;90:789.

476. Chambers HF, Miller RT, Newman MD. Right-sided *Staphylococcus aureus* endocarditis in intravenous drug abusers: Two week combination therapy. Ann Intern Med. 1988;109:619–24.

477. Murray HW, Wigley FM, Mann JJ, et al. Combination antibiotic therapy in staphylococcal endocarditis: The use of methicillin sodium-gentamicin sulfate therapy. Arch Intern Med. 1976;136:480.

478. Korzeniowski OM, Sande MA, The National Collaborative Endocarditis Study Group. Combination antimicrobial therapy for *Staphylococcus aureus* endocarditis in patients addicted to parenteral drugs and in nonaddicts. A prospective study. Ann Intern Med. 1982;97:496.

479. Steckelberg JM, Rouse MS, Tallan BM, et al. Relative efficacies of broad-spectrum cephalosporins for treatment of methicillin-susceptible *Staphylococcus aureus* experimental infective endocarditis. Antimicrob Agents Chemother. 1993;37:554.

480. Small PM, Chambers HF. Vancomycin for *Staphylococcus aureus* endocarditis in intravenous drug users. Antimicrob Agents Chemother. 1990;34:1227.

481. Levine DP, Fromm BS, Reddy BR. Slow response to vancomycin or vancomycin plus rifampin in methicillin-resistant *Staphylococcus aureus* endocarditis. Ann Intern Med. 1991;115:674.

482. Rybak MJ, Bailey EM, Lamp KC, et al. Pharmacokinetics and bactericidal rates of daptomycin and vancomycin in intravenous drug abusers being treated for gram-positive endocarditis and bacteremia. Antimicrob Agents Chemother. 1992;36:1109.

483. Kaatz GW, Seo SM, Reddy VN, et al. Daptomycin compared with teicoplanin and vancomycin for therapy of experimental *Staphylococcus aureus* endocarditis. Antimicrob Agents Chemother. 1990;34:2081.

484. Kaatz GW, Seo SM, Dorman NJ, et al. Emergence of teicoplanin resistance during therapy of *Staphylococcus aureus* endocarditis. J Infect Dis. 1990; 162:103.

485. Mortara LA, Bayer AS. *Staphylococcus* bacteremia and endocarditis—New diagnostic and therapeutic concepts. Infect Dis Clin North Am. 1993;7:53.

486. Bayer AS. Infective endocarditis. Clin Infect Dis. 1993;17:313.

487. Watanakunakorn C. Clindamycin therapy of *Staphylococcus aureus* endocarditis. Clinical relapse and development of resistance to clindamycin, lincomycin, and erythromycin. Am J Med. 1976;60:419.

488. Kaye D. The clinical significance of tolerance of *Staphylococcus aureus*. Ann Intern Med. 1980;93:924.

489. Jackson MA, Hicks RA. Vancomycin failure in staphylococcal endocarditis. Pediatr Infect Dis J. 1987;6:750–2.

490. Rajashekaraiah KR, Rice T, Rao VS, et al. Clinical significance of tolerant strains of *Staphylococcus aureus* in patients with endocarditis. Ann Intern Med. 1980;93:796.

491. Voorn GP, Thompson J, Goessens WHF, et al. Role of tolerance in cloxacillin treatment of experimental *Staphylococcus aureus* endocarditis. J Infect Dis. 1991;163:640.

492. Zak O, Scheld WM, Sande MA. Rifampin in experimental endocarditis due to *Staphylococcus aureus* in rabbits. Rev Infect Dis. 1983;5(Suppl):481.

493. Dworkin RJ, Lee BL, Sande MA, et al. Treatment of right-sided *Staphylococcus aureus* endocarditis in intravenous drug users with ciprofloxacin and rifampin. Lancet. 1989;2:1071.

494. Tebas P, Martinez Ruiz R, Roman F, et al. Early resistance to rifampin and ciprofloxacin in the treatment of right-sided *Staphylococcus aureus* endocarditis. J Infect Dis. 1991;163:204.

495. Hirano L, Bayer AS. β-lactam–β-lactamase inhibitor combinations are active in experimental endocarditis caused by β-lactamase-producing oxacillin-resistant staphylococci. Antimicrob Agents Chemother. 1991;35:685.

496. Pefanis A, Thauvin-Eliopoulos C, Eliopoulos GM, et al. Activity of ampicillin-sulbactam and oxacillin in experimental endocarditis caused by β-lactamase–hyperproducing *Staphylococcus aureus*. Antimicrob Agents Chemother. 1993;37:507.

497. Fernandez-Guerrero M, Rouse M, Henry N, et al. Ciprofloxacin therapy of experimental endocarditis caused by methicillin-susceptible or methicillin-resistant *Staphylococcus aureus*. Antimicrob Agents Chemother. 1988;32:747–51.

498. Kaatz GW, Seo SM, Lamp KC, et al. CI-960, a new fluoroquinolone, for therapy of experimental ciprofloxacin-susceptible and resistant *Staphylococcus aureus* endocarditis. Antimicrob Agents Chemother. 1992;36:1192.

499. Kaatz GW, Seo SM, Barriere SL, et al. Development of resistance to fleroxacin during therapy of experimental methicillin-susceptible *Staphylococcus aureus* endocarditis. Antimicrob Agents Chemother. 1991;35:1547.

500. Munoz P, Berenguer J, Rodriguez-Creixems M, et al. Ciprofloxacin and infective endocarditis. Infect Dis Clin Pract. 1993;2:119.

501. Iannini PB, Crossley K. Therapy of *Staphylococcus aureus* bacteremia associated with a removable focus of infection. Ann Intern Med. 1976;84:558.

502. Watanakunakorn C, Baird IM. *Staphylococcus aureus* bacteremia and endocarditis associated with a removable infected intravenous device. Am J Med. 1977;63:253.

503. Bayer AS, Lam K, Ginzton L. *Staphylococcus aureus* bacteremia. Clinical, serologic, and echocardiographic findings in patients with and without endocarditis. Arch Intern Med. 1987;147:757–62.

504. Karchmer AW, Archer GL, Dismukes WE. *Staphylococcus epidermidis* causing prosthetic valve endocarditis: Microbiologic and clinical observations as guides to therapy. Ann Intern Med. 1983;98:447.

505. Schwalbe RS, Stapleton JT, Gilligan PH. Emergence of vancomycin resistance in coagulase-negative staphylococci. N Engl J Med. 1987;316:927–31.

506. Joly V, Parigon B, Vallois J-M, et al. Value of antibiotic levels in serum and cardiac vegetations for predicting antibacterial effect of ceftriaxone in experimental *Escherichia coli* endocarditis. Antimicrob Agents Chemother. 1987;31:1632–9.

507. Caron F, Gutmann L, Bure A, et al. Ceftriaxone-sulbactam combination in rabbit-endocarditis caused by a strain of *Klebsiella pneumoniae* producing extended-broad-spectrum TEM-3 β-lactamase. Antimicrob Agents Chemother. 1990;34:2070.

508. Mentec H, Vallois J-M, Bure A, et al. Piperacillin, tazobactam, and gentamicin alone or combined in an endocarditis model of infection by a TEM-3–producing strain of *Klebsiella pneumoniae* or its susceptible variant. Antimicrob Agents Chemother. 1992;36:1883.

509. Potel G, Caillon J, Fantin B, et al. Impact of dosage schedule on the efficacy of gentamicin, tobramycin, or amikacin in an experimental model of *Serratia marcescens* endocarditis: In vitro–in vivo correlation. Antimicrob Agents Chemother. 1991;35:111.

510. Potel G, Caillon J, LeGallou F, et al. Identification of factors affecting in vivo aminoglycoside activity in an experimental model of gram-negative endocarditis. Antimicrob Agents Chemother. 1992;36:774.

511. Rodriguez C, Olcoz MT, Izquierdo G, et al. Endocarditis due to ampicillin-resistant nontyphoid *Salmonella:* Cure with a third-generation cephalosporin. Rev Infect Dis. 1990;12:817.

512. Hughes CF, Noble N. Vegetectomy: An alternative surgical treatment for infective endocarditis of the atrioventricular valves in drug addicts. J Thorac Cardiovasc Surg. 1988;95:857–61.

513. Arbulu A, Thomas NW, Chiscano A, et al. Total tricuspid valvulectomy without replacement in the treatment of *Pseudomonas* endocarditis. Surg Forum. 1971;22:162.

514. Mammana RB, Levitsky S, Sernaque D, et al. Valve replacement for left-sided endocarditis in drug addicts. Ann Thorac Surg. 1983;35:436.

515. Bayer AS, Crowell DJ, Yih J, et al. Comparative pharmacokinetics and pharmacodynamics of amikacin and ceftazidine in tricuspid and aortic vegetations in experimental Pseudomonas endocarditis. J Infect Dis. 1988;158:355–9.

516. Bayer AS, Hirano L, Yih J. Development of β-lactam resistance and increased quinolone MIC's during therapy of experimental Pseudomonas aeruginosa endocarditis. Antimicrob Agents Chemother. 1988;32:231–5.

517. Parr TR Jr, Bayer AS. Mechanisms of aminoglycoside resistance in variants of Pseudomonas aeruginosa isolated during treatment of experimental endocarditis in rabbits. J Infect Dis. 1988;158:1003–10.

518. Hessen MT, Pitsakis PG, Levison ME. Absence of a post-antibiotic effect in experimental Pseudomonas endocarditis treated with imipenem, with or without gentamicin. J Infect Dis. 1988;158:542–8.

519. Bayer AS, Park S, Ramos MC, et al. Effects of alginase on the natural history and antibiotic therapy of experimental endocarditis caused by mucoid Pseudomonas aeruginosa. Infect Immun. 1992;60:3979.

520. Jimenez-Lucho VE, Saravolatz LD, Medeiros AA, et al. Failure of therapy in Pseudomonas endocarditis: Selection of resistant mutants. J Infect Dis. 1986;154:64–8.

521. Daikos GL, Kathopalia SB, Lolans VT, et al. Long-term oral ciprofloxacin: Experience in the treatment of incurable infective endocarditis. Am J Med. 1988;84:786–90.

522. Pefanis A, Giamarellou H, Karayiannakos P, et al. Efficacy of ceftazidime and aztreonam alone or in combination with amikacin in experimental left-sided Pseudomonas aeruginosa endocarditis. Antimicrob Agents Chemother. 1993;37:308.

523. Fichtenbaum CH, Smith MJ. Treatment of endocarditis due to Pseudomonas aeruginosa with imipenem. Clin Infect Dis. 1992;14:353.

524. Pavicic MJAMP, van Winkelhoff AJ, de Graaff J. In vitro susceptibilities of Actinobacillus actinomycetemcomitans to a number of antimicrobial combinations. Antimicrob Agents Chemother. 1992;36:2634.

525. Weisner PJ, Handsfield HH, Holmes KK. Low antibiotic resistance of gonococci causing disseminated infection. N Engl J Med. 1973;288:1221.

526. Black JR, Brint JM, Reichart CA. Successful treatment of gonococcal endocarditis with ceftriaxone. J Infect Dis. 1988;157:1281–2.

527. Ernst JD, Rusmak M, Sande MA. Combination antifungal chemotherapy for experimental disseminated candidiasis: Lack of correlation between in vitro and in vivo observations with amphotericin B and rifampin. Rev Infect Dis. 1983;5(Suppl):626.

528. Longman LP, Martin MV. A comparison of the efficacy of intraconazole, amphotericin B and 5-fluorocytosine in the treatment of Aspergillus fumigatus endocarditis in the rabbit. J Antimicrob Chemother. 1987;20:719–24.

529. Witt MD, Bayer AS. Comparison of fluconazole and amphotericin B for prevention and treatment of experimental Candida endocarditis. Antimicrob Agents Chemother. 1991;35:2481.

530. Venditti M, De Bernardis F, Micozzi A, et al. Fluconazole treatment of catheter-related right-sided endocarditis caused by Candida albicans and associated with endophthalmitis and folliculitis. Clin Infect Dis. 1992;14:422.

531. Czwerwiec FS, Bilsker MS, Kamerman ML, et al. Long-term survival after fluconazole therapy of candidal prosthetic valve endocarditis. Am J Med. 1993;94:545.

532. Haldane EV, Marrie TJ, Faulkner RS, et al. Endocarditis due to Q fever in Nova Scotia: Experience with five patients in 1981–1982. J Infect Dis. 1983;148:978–85.

533. Street AC, Durack DT. Experience with trimethoprim-sulfamethoxazole in treatment of infective endocarditis. Rev Infect Dis. 1988;10:915–22.

534. Levy PY, Drancourt M, Etienne J, et al. Comparison of different antibiotic regimens for therapy of 32 cases of Q fever endocarditis. Antimicrob Agents Chemother. 1991;35:533.

535. Jones JB, Ridgeway GL, Boulding S, et al. In vitro activity of rifamycins alone and in combination with other antibiotics against Chlamydia trachomatis. Rev Infect Dis. 1983;5(Suppl):556.

536. McAnulty JH, Rahimtoola SH. Surgery for infective endocarditis. JAMA. 1979;242:77.

537. Dinubile MJ. Surgery in active endocarditis. Ann Intern Med. 1980;96:650.

538. D'Agostino RS, Miller DC, Stinson EB, et al. Valve replacement in patients with native valve endocarditis: What really determines operative outcome? Ann Thorac Surg. 1985;40:429–38.

539. Tolan RW Jr, Kleiman MB, Frank M, et al. Operative intervention in active endocarditis in children: Report of a series of cases and review. Clin Infect Dis. 1992;14:852.

540. Mansur AJ, Grinberg M, Lemosdaluz P, et al. The complications of infective endocarditis. Arch Intern Med. 1992;152:2428.

541. Karalis DG, Blumberg AE, Vilaro JF, et al. Prognostic significance of valvular regurgitation in patients with infective endocarditis. Am J Med. 1991;90:193.

542. Wilson WR, Danielson GK, Giuliani ER, et al. Valve replacement in patients with active infective endocarditis. Circulation. 1978;58:585.

543. Arbulu A, Asfaw I. Tricuspid valvulectomy without prosthetic replacement. Ten years of clinical experience. J Thorac Cardiovasc Surg. 1981;82:684.

544. Straumann E, Stulz P, Jenzer HR. Tricuspid valve endocarditis in the drug addict: A reconstructive approach ("vegetectomy"). Thorac Cardiovasc Surg. 1990;38:291.

545. DiNubile M. Surgery for addiction-related tricuspid valve endocarditis: Caveat emptor. Am J Med. 1987;82:811–3.

546. Arbulu A, Asfaw I. Management of infective endocarditis: Seventeen years' experience. Ann Thorac Surg. 1987;43:144–9.

547. Alsip SG, Blackstone EH, Kirklin JW, et al. Indications for cardiac surgery in patients with active infective endocarditis. Am J Med. 1985;78(Suppl 6B): 138–48.

548. Tornos M-P, Permanyer-Miralda G, Olona M, et al. Long-term complications of native valve infective endocarditis in non-addicts. A 15-year follow-up study. Ann Intern Med. 1992;117:567.

549. Neuhof H, Seley GP. Acute suppurative phlebitis complicated by septicemia. Surgery. 1947;21:831.

550. Goldman DA, Maki DG, Rhame FS, et al. Guidelines for infection control in intravenous therapy. Ann Intern Med. 1973;79:848.

551. O'Neill JA, Pruitt BA, Foley FD, et al. Suppurative thrombophlebitis—a lethal complication of intravenous therapy. J Trauma. 1968;8:256.

552. Stein JM, Pruitt BA. Suppurative thrombophlebitis: A lethal iatrogenic disease. N Engl J Med. 1970;282:1452.

553. Pruitt BA, Stein JM, Foley FD, et al. Intravenous therapy in burn patients. Suppurative thrombophlebitis and other life-threatening complications. Arch Surg. 1970;100:399.

554. Pruitt BA, McManus WF, Kim SH, et al. Diagnosis and treatment of cannula-related intravenous sepsis in burn patients. Ann Surg. 1980;191:546.

555. Garrison RN, Richardson JD, Fry DE. Catheter-associated septic thrombophlebitis. South Med J. 1982;75:917.

556. Sacks-Berg A, Strampfer MJ, Cunha BA. Suppurative thrombophlebitis caused by intravenous line sepsis. Heart Lung. 1987;16:318–20.

557. Munster AM. Septic thrombophlebitis. A surgical disorder. JAMA. 1974; 230:1010.

558. Berkowitz FE, Argent AC, Baise T. Suppurative thrombophlebitis: A serious nosocomial infection. Pediatr Infect Dis J. 1987;6:64–7.

559. Johnson RA, Zajac RA, Evans ME. Suppurative thrombophlebitis: Correlation between pathogen and underlying disease. Infect Control. 1986;7:582–5.

560. Rhame FS, Maki DG, Bennett JV. Intravenous cannula-associated infections. In: Bennett JV, Brachman PS, eds. Hospital Infections. Boston: Little, Brown; 1979;433–42.

561. Baker CC, Peterson SR, Sheldon GF. Septic phlebitis: A neglected disease. Am J Surg. 1979;138:97.

562. Sears N, Grosfeld JL, Weber TR, et al. Suppurative thrombophlebitis in childhood. Pediatrics. 1981;68:630.

563. Zinner MJ, Zuidema GD, Lowery BD. Septic nonsuppurative thrombophlebitis. Arch Surg. 1976;111:122.

564. Brismar B, Hardstedt C, Jacobson S. Diagnosis of thrombosis by catheter phlebography after prolonged central venous catheterization. Ann Surg. 1981;194:779–83.

565. Slagle DC, Gates RH Jr. Unusual case of central vein thrombosis and sepsis. Am J Med. 1986;81:351–4.

566. Kaufman J, Demas C, Stark K, et al. Catheter-related septic central venous thrombosis—current therapeutic options. West J Med. 1986;145:200–3.

567. Veghese A, Widrich WC, Arbeit RD. Central venous septic thrombophlebitis—the role of medical therapy. Medicine (Baltimore). 1985;64:394–400.

568. Strinden WD, Helgerson RB, Maki DG. Candida septic thrombosis of the great central veins associated with central catheters. Clinical features and management. Ann Surg. 1985;202:653–8.

569. Raad I, Narro J, Khan A, et al. Serious complications of vascular catheter-related Staphylococcus aureus bacteremia in cancer patients. Eur J Clin Microbiol Infect Dis. 1992;11:675.

570. Haddad W, Idowu J, Georgeson K, et al. Septic atrial thrombosis: A potentially lethal complication of Broviac catheters in infants. Am J Dis Child. 1986;140:778–80.

571. Collins CG, MacCallum EA, Nelson EW, et al. Suppurative pelvic thrombophlebitis. I. Incidence, pathology, and etiology. Surgery. 1951;30:298.

572. Josey WE, Staggers SR. Heparin therapy in septic pelvic thrombophlebitis: A study of 46 cases. Am J Obstet Gynecol. 1974;120:228.

573. Collins CG. Suppurative pelvic thrombophlebitis. A study of 202 cases in which the disease was treated by ligation of the vena cava and ovarian vein. Am J Obstet Gynecol. 1970;108:681.

574. Lim GM, Jeffrey RB Jr, Ralls PW, et al. Septic thrombosis of the portal vein: CT and clinical observations. J Comput Assist Tomogr. 1989;13:656.

575. Barenholtz L, Kaminsky NI, Palmer DL. Venous intramural microabscesses: A cause of protracted sepsis with intravenous cannulas. Am J Med Sci. 1973;265:335.

576. Jupiter JB, Ehrlich MG, Novelline RA, et al. The association of septic thrombophlebitis with subperiosteal abscesses in children. J Pediatr. 1982;101:690.

577. Maki DG, Weise CE, Sarafin HW. A semiquantitative culture method for identifying intravenous-catheter-related infection. N Engl J Med. 1977;296: 1305.

578. Ashkenazi S, Pickering LK, Robinson LH. Diagnosis and management of septic thrombosis of the inferior vena cava caused by Candida tropicalis. Pediatr Infect Dis J. 1990;9:446.

579. Mori H, Fukuda T, Isomoto I, et al. CT diagnosis of catheter-induced septic thrombosis of vena cava. J Comput Assist Tomogr. 1990;14:236.

580. Angel JL, Knuppel RA. Computed tomography in diagnosis of puerperal ovarian vein thrombosis. Obstet Gynecol. 1984;63:61–4.

581. Isada NB, Landy HJ, Larson JW Jr. Postabortal septic pelvic thrombophlebitis diagnosed with computed tomography. J Reprod Med. 1987;32:866–8.

582. Martin B, Molopoulos GP, Bryan PJ. MRI of puerperal ovarian vein thrombosis. AJR. 1986;147:291–2.

583. Josey WE, Cook CC. Septic pelvic thrombophlebitis. Report of 17 patients treated with heparin. Obstet Gynecol. 1970;35:891.
584. Torres-Rojas JR, Stratton CW, Sanders CV, et al. Candidal suppurative peripheral thrombophlebitis. Ann Intern Med. 1982;96:431.
585. Walsh TJ, Bustamente CI, Vlahov D, et al. Candidal suppurative peripheral thrombophlebitis: Recognition, prevention, and management. Infect Control. 1986;7:16–22.
586. Shek YH, Tucker MC, Viciana AL, et al. *Malassezia furfur*—disseminated infection in premature infants. Am J Clin Pathol. 1989;92:595.
587. Peterson P, Stahl-Bayliss CM. Cytomegalovirus thrombophlebitis after successful DHPG therapy. Ann Intern Med. 1987;106:632–3.
588. Miller CJ. Ligation and excision of pelvic veins in treatment of puerperal pyaemia. Surg Gynecol Obstet. 1917;25:431.
589. Topiel MS, Bryan RT, Kessler CM, et al. Treatment of Silastic catheter-induced central vein septic thrombophlebitis. Am J Med Sci. 1986;291:425–8.
590. Schranz D, Haugwitz D, Zimmer B, et al. Successful lysis of a septic thrombosis of the superior vena cava using recombinant tissue-plasminogen activator. Klin Padiatr. 1991;203:363.
591. Barg NL, Supena RB, Fekety R. Persistent staphylococcal bacteremia in an intravenous drug abuser. Antimicrob Agents Chemother. 1986;29:209–11.
592. Moran JM, Atwood RP, Rowe MI. A clinical and bacteriologic study of infections associated with venous cutdowns. N Engl J Med. 1965;272:554.
593. Norden CW. Application of antibiotic ointment to the site of venous catheterization—a controlled trial. J Infect Dis. 1969;120:611.
594. Patel S, Johnston KW. Classification and management of mycotic aneurysms. Surg Gynecol Obstet. 1977;144:691.
595. Parkhurst GF, Decker JP. Bacterial aortitis and mycotic aneurysms of the aorta. A report of 12 cases. Am J Pathol. 1955;31:821.
596. Sommerville RL, Allen EV, Edwards JE. Bland and infected arteriosclerotic abdominal aortic aneurysms: A clinicopathologic study. Medicine (Baltimore). 1959;38:207.
597. Sekkal S, Cornu E, Cristides C, et al. Isolated iliac aneurysms. Seventy-seven cases in forty-eight patients. J Mal Vasc. 1993;18:13.
598. Stengel A, Wolfroth CC. Mycotic (bacterial) aneurysms of intravascular origin. Arch Intern Med. 1923;31:527.
599. Bennett DE, Cherry JK. Bacterial infection of aortic aneurysms. A clinicopathologic study. Am J Surg. 1967;113:321.
600. Cliff MM, Soulen RL, Firestone AJ. Mycotic aneurysms: A challenge and a clue. Arch Intern Med. 1970;126:977.
601. Jarrett F, Darling C, Mundth ED, et al. Experience with infected aneurysms of the abdominal aorta. Arch Surg. 1975;110:1281.
602. Bohmfalk GL, Story JL, Wissenger JP, et al. Bacterial intracranial aneurysm. J Neurosurg. 1978;48:369.
603. Frazee JG, Cahan LD, Winter J. Bacterial intracranial aneurysm. J Neurosurg. 1980;53:633.
604. Selky AK, Roos KL. Neurologic complications of infective endocarditis. Semin Neurol. 1992;12:225.
605. Tunkel AR, Kaye D. Neurologic complications of infective endocarditis. Neurol Clin. 1993;11:419.
606. Bullock R, Van Dellen JR, Van den Heever CM. Intracranial mycotic aneurysms. A review of 9 cases. S Afr Med J. 1981;60:970.
607. John RM, Pugsley W, Treasure T, et al. Aortic root complications of infective endocarditis—influence on surgical outcome. Eur Heart J. 1991;12:241.
608. Hollingworth J, Palmer KS, Simms MH. Ruptured mycotic aneurysm of the abdominal aorta in childhood. Eur J Vasc Surg. 1992;6:665.
609. Cribari C, Meadors FA, Crawford ES, et al. Thoraco-abdominal aortic aneurysm associated with umbilical artery catheterization: Case report and review of the literature. J Vasc Surg. 1992;16:75.
610. Jarrett F, Darling RC, Mundth ED, et al. The management of infected arterial aneurysms. J Cardiovasc Surg. 1977;18:361.
611. Johnson JR, Ledgerwood AM, Lucas CE. Mycotic aneurysm. New concepts in therapy. Arch Surg. 1983;118:577.
612. Brummitt CF, Kravitz GR, Granrud GA, et al. Femoral endarteritis due to *Staphylococcus aureus* complicating percutaneous transluminal coronary angioplasty. Am J Med. 1989;86:822.
613. Frazee BW, Flaherty JP. Septic endarteritis of the femoral artery following angioplasty. Rev Infect Dis. 1991;13:620.
614. Feigl D, Feigl A, Edwards JE. Mycotic aneurysms of the aortic root. A pathologic study of 20 cases. Chest. 1986;90:553–7.
615. Jebara VA, Dervanian P, Acar C, et al. Mycotic aneurysm of the carotid artery secondary to acute bacterial endocarditis. Arch Mal Coeur Vaiss. 1992;85:1615.
616. Akers DL Jr, Fowl RJ, Kempczinski RF, et al. Mycotic aneurysm of the tibioperoneal trunk: Case report and review of the literature. J Vasc Surg. 1992;16:71.
617. Dean RH, Mecham PW, Weaver FA, et al. Mycotic embolism and embolomycotic aneurysms. Neglected lessons of the past. Ann Surg. 1986;204:300–7.
618. Sedwitz MM, Hye RJ, Stabile BE. The changing epidemiology of pseudoaneurysm. Therapeutic implications. Arch Surg. 1988;123:473–6.
619. Morgan MB, Cintron G, Balis JV. Infective "mycotic" aortic root aneurysm following coronary artery bypass grafting. Am J Med. 1993;94:550.
620. Vyas SK, Law NW, Loehry CA. Mycotic aneurysm of the left subclavian artery. Br Heart J. 1993;69:455.
621. Hurst RW, Choi IS, Persky M, et al. Mycotic aneurysms of the intracavernous carotid artery: A case report and review of the literature. Surg Neurol. 1992;37:142.
622. Kyriakides GK, Simmons RL, Najarian JS. Mycotic aneurysms in transplant patients. Arch Surg. 1976;111:472.
623. Smith EJ, Milligan SL, Filo RS. *Salmonella* mycotic aneurysms after renal transplantation. South Med J. 1981;74:1399.
624. Olmsted WW, McGee TP. The pathogenesis of peripheral aneurysms of the central nervous system: A subject review from the AFIP. Radiology. 1977;123:661.
625. Salgado AV, Furlan AJ, Keys TF. Mycotic aneurysm, Subarachnoid hemorrhage, and indications for cerebral angiography in infective endocarditis. Stroke. 1987;18:1057–60.
626. Wilson WR, Lie JT, Houser OW, et al. The management of patients with mycotic aneurysm. Curr Clin Top Infect Dis. 1981;2:151.
627. Barrow DL, Prats AR. Infectious intracranial aneurysms: Comparison of groups with and without endocarditis. Neurosurgery. 1990;27:562.
628. Friedman SG, Pogo GJ, Moccio CG. Mycotic aneurysm of the superior mesenteric artery. J Vasc Surg. 1987;6:87–90.
629. Sukerkar AN, Dulay CC, Anandappa E, et al. Mycotic aneurysm of the hepatic artery. Radiology. 1977;124:444.
630. Khoda J, Lantsberg L, Sebbag G. Hepatic artery mycotic aneurysm as a cause of hemobilia. J Hepatol. 1993;17:131.
631. Carrel D, Cohle SD, Chapman AJ. Fatal hemothorax from mycotic celiac artery aneurysm. Am J Med Pathol. 1992;13:233.
632. Feinsod FM, Norfleet RG, Hoehn JL. Mycotic aneurysm of the external iliac artery. A triad of clinical signs facilitating early diagnosis. JAMA. 1977;238:245.
633. Merry M, Dunn J, Weissmann R, et al. Popliteal mycotic aneurysm presenting as septic arthritis and purpura. JAMA. 1972;221:58.
634. Plate G, Forsley N, Stigsson L, et al. Management of inflammatory abdominal aortic aneurysm. Acta Chir Scand. 1988;154:19–24.
635. Pennell RC, Hollier LH, Lie JT, et al. Inflammatory abdominal aortic aneurysms: A thirty year review. J Vasc Surg. 1985;2:859–69.
636. Morrow C, Safi H, Beall AC Jr. Primary aortoduodenal fistula caused by *Salmonella* aortitis. J Vasc Surg. 1987;6:415–8.
637. Kimura I, Okumura R, Yamashita K, et al. Mycotic aneurysm. Radia Med. 1989;7:121.
638. Vogelzang RL, Sohaey R. Infected aortic aneurysms: CT appearance. J Comput Assist Tomogr. 1988;12:109–12.
639. Blair RH, Resnik MD, Polga JP. CT appearance of mycotic abdominal aortic aneurysms. J Comput Assist Tomogr. 1989;13:101.
640. Rivera JV, Blanco G, Perez M, et al. Gallium-67 localization in a mycotic aneurysm of the thoracic aorta. Clin Nucl Med. 1985;10:814–6.
641. Zwas ST, Lorberboyin M, Schechter M. Occult aortic arch mycotic aneurysm diagnosed by radio gallium scintigraphy. Clin Nucl Med. 1992;17:797.
642. Ben-Haim S, Seabold JE, Hawes DR, et al. Leukocyte scintigraphy in the diagnosis of mycotic aneurysm. J Nucl Med. 1992;33:1486.
643. Ramo OJ, Vorne M, Lantto E, et al. Postoperative graft incorporation after aortic reconstruction-comparison between computerized tomography and Tc-99m-HMPAO labelled leukocyte imaging. Eur J Vasc Surg. 1993;7:122.
644. Brewster DC, Retana A, Waltman AC, et al. Angiography in the management of aneurysms of the abdominal aorta. N Engl J Med. 1972;292:822.
645. Griffiths BE, Petch MC, English TAH. Echocardiographic detection of subvalvular aortic root aneurysm extending to mitral valve annulus as complication of aortic valve endocarditis. Br Heart J. 1982;47:392.
646. Ozkutlu S, Ozbarlas N, Bilgi CA, et al. Mycotic aneurysm of the descending aorta diagnosed by echocardiography. Int J Cardiol. 1992;37:112.
647. Vargas-Barron J, Avila-Rosales L, Romero-Cardenas A, et al. Echocardiographic diagnosis of a mycotic aneurysm of the main pulmonary artery and patent ductus arteriosus. Am Heart J. 1992;123:1707.
648. Kanwar YS, Malhotra U, Anderson BR, et al. Salmonellosis associated with abdominal aortic aneurysm. Arch Intern Med. 1974;134:1095.
649. Cohen JI, Bartlett JA, Corey GR. Extra-intestinal manifestations of *Salmonella* infections. Medicine (Baltimore). 1987;66:349–88.
650. Cohen OS, O'Brien TF, Schoenbaum SC, et al. The risk of endothelial infection in adults with *Salmonella* bacteremia. Ann Intern Med. 1978;89:931.
651. Flamand F, Harris KA, DeRose G, et al. Arteritis due to *Salmonella* with aneurysm formation: Two cases. Can J Surg 1992;35:248.
652. McIntyre KE Jr, Malone JM, Richards E. Mycotic aortic pseudoaneurysm with aortoenteric fistula caused by *Arizona hinshawii*. Surgery. 1982;91:173.
653. Kumar N, Prabhakar G, Kandeel M, et al. *Brucella* mycotic aneurysm of ascending aorta complicating discrete subaortic stenosis. Am Heart J. 1993;125:1780.
654. Anolik JR, Mildvan D, Winter JW, et al. Mycotic aortic aneurysm. A complication of *Campylobacter fetus* septicemia. Arch Intern Med. 1983;143:609.
655. Garto AR, Cone LA, Woodard DR, et al. Arterial infections due to *Listeria monocytogenes*: Report of four cases and review of world literature. Clin Infect Dis. 1992;14:23.
656. Hurley L, Howe K. Mycotic aortic aneurysm infected by *Clostridium septicum*—A case history. Angiology. 1991;42:585.
657. Mielke B, Weir B, Oldring D, et al. Fungal aneurysm: Case report and review of the literature. Neurosurgery. 1981;9:578.
658. Hadley MN, Martin NA, Spetzler RF, et al. Multiple intracranial aneurysms due to *Coccidioides immitis* infection. J Neurosurg. 1987;66:453–6.
659. Ogden PE, Hurley DL, Cain PT. Fatal fungal endarteritis caused by *Bipolaris spicifera* following replacement of the aortic valve. Clin Infect Dis. 1992;14:596.
660. Aguado JM, Valle R, Arjona R, et al. Aortic bypass graft infection due to *Aspergillus*: Report of a case and review. Clin Infect Dis. 1992;14:916.
661. McLean DR, Russell N, Khan MY. Neurobrucellosis: Clinical and therapeutic features. Clin Infect Dis. 1992;15:582.

662. Bingham WF: Treatment of mycotic intracranial aneurysms. J Neurosurg. 1977;46:428.
663. Leipzig MJ, Brown FD. Treatment of mycotic aneurysms. Surg Neurol. 1985;23:403–7.
664. Rodesch G, Noterman J, Thys JP, et al. Treatment of intracranial mycotic aneurysm: Surgery or not. Acta Neurochir. 1987;85:63–8.
665. Reddy DJ, Smith RF, Elliott JP Jr, et al. Infected femoral artery false aneurysms in drug addicts: Evolution of selective vascular reconstruction. J Vasc Surg. 1986;3:718–24.
666. Johansen K, Devin J. Mycotic aortic aneurysms. A reappraisal. Arch Surg. 1983;118:583.
667. Parsons R, Gregory J, Palmer DL. *Salmonella* infections of the abdominal aorta. Rev Infect Dis. 1983;5:227.
668. Bitseff EJ, Edwards WH, Mulherin JL Jr, et al. Infected abdominal aortic aneurysms. South Med J. 1987;80:309–12.
669. Taylor LM Jr, Deitz DM, McConnell DB, et al. Treatment of infected abdominal aneurysms by extra anatomic bypass, aneurysm excision, and drainage. Am J Surg. 1988;155:655–8.
670. Pasic M, Carrel T, von Segesser L, et al. In situ repair of mycotic aneurysm of the ascending aorta. J Thor Cardiovasc Surg. 1993;105:321.
671. Cull DL, Winter RP, Wheeler JR, et al. Mycotic aneurysm of the suprarenal abdominal aorta. J Cardiovasc Surg. 1992;33:181.
672. Robinson JA, Johansen K. Aortic sepsis: Is there a role for in situ graft reconstruction? J Vasc Surg. 1991;13:677.
673. Pasic M, Carrel T, Vogt M, et al. Treatment of mycotic aneurysm of the aorta and its branches: The location determines the operative technique. Eur J Vasc Surg. 1992;6:419.
674. Viglione G, Younes GA, Coste P, et al. Mycotic aneurysm of the celiac trunk: Radical resection and reconstruction without prosthetic material. J Cardiovasc Surg. 1993;34:73.
675. Pasic M, von Segesser L, Turina M. Implantation of antibiotic-releasing carriers and in situ reconstruction for treatment of mycotic aneurysm. Arch Surg. 1992;127:745.
676. Sande MA, Strausbaugh LJ. Infective endocarditis. In: Hook EW, Mandell GL, Gwaltney JM Jr, et al., eds. Current Concepts of Infectious Diseases. New York: Wiley Press, 1977.

59. INFECTIOUS DISORDERS OF PROSTHETIC VALVES AND INTRAVASCULAR DEVICES

MICHAEL G. THRELKELD
C. GLENN COBBS

PROSTHETIC VALVE ENDOCARDITIS

Infection of the intracardiac prosthesis is a serious complication of valve replacement surgery. The intravascular foreign body is inherently more susceptible to bacterial colonization than is native valve tissue, and established infection on a prosthetic device is often difficult to eradicate. Although clinical outcome has improved during the past decade, prosthetic valve endocarditis (PVE) remains a significant cause of morbidity and mortality.

Epidemiology

Early and Late Prosthetic Valve Endocarditis. By convention, PVE occurring within 60 days of valve insertion has been termed "early PVE" and endocarditis occurring more than 60 days after valve replacement, "late PVE." This distinction is justified by the differences in microbiology and pathogenesis of infections during the two time periods. However, illness characteristic of early disease may not always become apparent until 6 months or more after the operation. Some investigators have therefore recommended that the time limit for early disease be extended to 6 months or even 1 year.[1,2]

Incidence. A number of authors have described their experiences with PVE during the past two decades.[1–22] Among 25,923 patients undergoing valve replacement, 740 episodes of PVE were observed (an incidence of 2.9 percent). Incidence peaked in the first few weeks following surgery and then fell to a stable low rate during subsequent months to years. If one uses the traditional 60-day time limit, approximately 37 percent of reported episodes represented early PVE, while 63 percent were late PVE. Of the 459 patients identified by sex, 64 percent were male.

Valves in the aortic position were once believed to be more susceptible to infection than are valves in the mitral position. However, more recent studies have failed to confirm this finding.[21] Of 603 reported cases of PVE, 55 percent involved an aortic prosthesis; 32 percent, a mitral prosthesis; and 12 percent, other valves or combinations of valves.[3,4,6–14,18,19,21,22] These differences presumably reflect the frequency of surgery at the different sites.

Types of Prostheses Involved. There are currently more than two dozen varieties of artificial valves in use.[23] They can be classified as mechanical valves (including ball valves, disk valves, hinged leaflet valves, and tilting disk valves) and bioprosthetic tissue valves (including homografts and porcine heterografts). Based on data from several recent series, the incidence of PVE in patients receiving porcine heterografts is 3.1 percent, and the incidence for mechanical valve recipients is 3.8 percent.[2,19,20]

Microorganisms Responsible. Table 1 lists the microbial etiology of PVE in 272 patients with early infection and 429 patients with late.[4–7,13,19,21,22,24] The most common etiologic microorganism was *Staphylococcus epidermidis*, which accounted for 29 percent of episodes. Viridans streptococci accounted for 17 percent and *Staphylococcus aureus* for 14 percent. These frequencies vary substantially from those seen in native valve endocarditis (NVE), in which the viridans streptococci and *S. aureus* account for approximately 50 and 20 percent of episodes, respectively. Aerobic gram-negative bacilli and fungi (especially *Candida* spp. and *Aspergillus* spp.), uncommon in NVE, are important causes of early PVE.

Diphtheroids, a term used to describe corynebacteria other than *Corynebacterium diphtheriae*, are important causes of early PVE.[25] Recognition of their role in PVE has served to emphasize the pathologic potential of these usually avirulent

TABLE 1. Microorganisms Responsible for Prosthetic Valve Endocarditis

Organism	Early PVE[a] (%)	Late PVE (%)	Overall (%)
Staphylococci			
S. epidermidis	35	26	29
S. aureus	17	12	14
Streptococci			
Group D streptococci (including enterococci)	3	9	7
S. pneumoniae	1	<1	1
Other including viridans streptococci)	4	25	17
Gram-negative bacilli	16	12	13
Diphtheroids	10	4	7
Other bacteria	1	2	2
Candida	8	4	5
Aspergillus	2	1	1
Other fungi	1	<1	1
Culture-negative	1	4	3
Total number			
Microorganisms	292	445	737
Patients	272	429	701

[a] Occurring less than 2 months after surgery.

(Data from refs. 4–7, 13, 19, 21, 22, 24.)

bacteria. Group JK corynebacteria, in particular, are important pathogens of prosthetic devices. A wide variety of other bacterial and fungal species has been reported in individual patients with PVE.

Pathogenesis of Early Prosthetic Valve Endocarditis

Staphylococcus epidermidis is the most common cause of early PVE. Of 16 patients with *S. epidermidis* PVE seen at one medical center, 11 became ill within 6 months of surgery, with a median time of onset of 2 months.[2] These data suggest that *S. epidermidis* PVE may result from valve contamination occurring in the perioperative period. Several studies have emphasized the potential role of intraoperative contamination in the pathogenesis of early PVE. Kluge et al.,[26] during an investigation of microbial contamination occurring during open heart surgery, found tissue surfaces and the valvular prostheses to be the most common sites from which microorganisms could be recovered. An important observation was the frequent recovery of *S. epidermidis* and diphtheroids, presumably shed from the skin of the patient or operating room personnel. Another possible mode of contamination was suggested by Blakemore et al.,[27] who found bacteria contaminating blood in the bypass pump. Identical microorganisms were isolated from the air in the operating room, which suggests that suctioning devices used in the operative field inoculated microorganisms into the blood.

In the immediate postoperative period, the prosthetic valve and sewing ring are not yet endothelialized and are apparently quite susceptible to microbial colonization. Bacteria or fungi originating from infected intravascular catheters, cardiac pacemakers, or pressure monitoring devices may seed the prosthesis. One study of patients undergoing open heart surgery demonstrated that 29 percent of intravenous catheters were contaminated.[28] This rate was reduced to 12 percent when catheters were removed sooner. Another study suggested that *S. epidermidis* is readily introduced into the blood stream during thermodilution cardiac output determinations unless careful aseptic technique is practiced.[29] Bacteremia may also result from postoperative infections at extracardiac sites. Dismukes et al.[3] noted pneumonia, wound infection, or contaminated intravascular catheters in 12 patients who subsequently developed early PVE. Another potential (but uncommon) source of infection is contamination of the prosthesis before implantation such as the contamination of glutaraldehyde-fixed porcine prosthetic valves by *Mycobacterium chelonae*.[30,31]

Pathogenesis of Late Prosthetic Valve Endocarditis

The pathogenesis of late PVE appears similar to that of NVE, with microorganisms from a source of transient bacteremia localizing on a prosthesis or area of damaged endocardium. This is reflected in the much higher incidence of infection due to viridans streptococci in late disease. Late PVE caused by *S. epidermidis* or other organisms that typically cause early PVE may result from a delayed onset of the infection acquired in the perioperative period. Nosocomial bacteremia is a significant risk factor for prosthetic valve endocarditis.[31a]

Pathology of Prosthetic Valve Endocarditis

Valve ring abscess is a serious complication of PVE in both mechanical and bioprosthetic valves.[3,6,12,32,33] Valve ring abscesses occur when infection involves the sutures used to secure the sewing ring to the periannular tissue; this may result in dehiscence of the valve (Fig. 1). The clinical finding of a paravalvular leak in a patient with PVE is presumptive evidence of a valve ring abscess. Arnett and Roberts[33] described the precise pathologic findings in 22 patients with valve ring abscess. The infectious process involved the entire valve circumference in 14 patients; there was partial involvement in the other 8.[33] Exten-

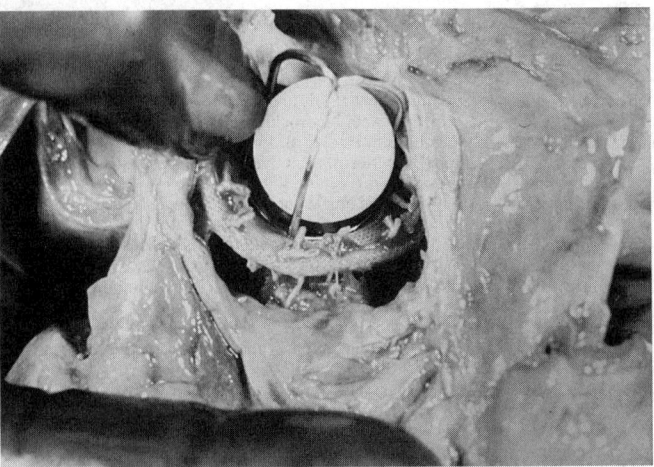

FIG. 1.   Autopsy specimen demonstrates valve dehiscence complicating prosthetic valve endocarditis.

TABLE 2. Clinical Findings in Prosthetic Valve Endocarditis
(228 Patients)

Finding	%
Feve	97
New or changing murmur	56
Systemic embolus	40
Petechiae	39
Splenomegaly	32
Peripheral signs (Osler nodes, Janeway lesions, Roth spots)	15
Anemia (Hct <35)	74
Hematuria	57
Leukocytosis (WBC >12,000)	54

(Data from refs. 6, 11, 40, 42.)

sion of the abscess beyond the valve ring may result in myocardial abscess formation, septal perforation, or purulent pericarditis. In addition to sewing ring abscesses, PVE of bioprostheses may cause leaflet destruction with resulting valvular incompetence.[14,34] Large vegetations occasionally obstruct blood flow and lead to functional valvular stenosis or a combination of stenosis and insufficiency. This complication appears to be more common in mitral PVE than in aortic disease.[14,33,35]

Extracardiac pathologic features classically associated with NVE may also be seen in PVE. Embolic events are common in patients with PVE. Septic emboli to the carotid circulation may lead to a brain infarct, brain abscess, mycotic aneurysm, or hemorrhagic infarct (especially in patients who are excessively anticoagulated). Leport et al.[36] noted that 7 of 17 deaths from their series of patients with late PVE were due to neurologic complications. Peripheral emboli may lead to deep tissue abscesses and mycotic aneurysms.

Immune complex–mediated glomerulonephritis manifested by abnormal urinalysis with or without elevations of serum creatinine levels has been described in patients with PVE.[37–39] Renal pathologic findings are variable but often mimic the diffuse proliferative changes found in poststreptococcal glomerulonephritis. Immunoglobulin and complement deposits can frequently be demonstrated along the glomerular basement membrane (by immunofluorescent staining).

Diagnosis of Prosthetic Valve Endocarditis

Clinical Manifestations.   The symptoms and signs of PVE are protean.[6,11,40–42] As shown in Table 2, fever is the most common sign and occurs in almost all patients. Clinical evidence of systemic embolization has been reported in 40 percent of patients. The frequency of various organ system involvement by emboli is similar to that of NVE. Embolization to the central nervous system (CNS) commonly presents as an acute focal neurologic deficit. Splenomegaly is reported in one-third of patients and may be more common in late PVE, presumably reflecting more prolonged antigenemia. Petechiae have been noted in 39 percent, but other peripheral signs due to small emboli or small vessel vasculitis (Osler nodes, Janeway lesions, Roth spots) are less frequently encountered.

New or changing cardiac murmurs have been reported in 56 percent of patients with PVE. Regurgitant murmurs reflect the hemodynamic consequences of valvular insufficiency due to a paravalvular leak, while muffling of heart sounds or stenosis murmurs result from occlusion or malfunction of the prosthetic valve. Although cardiac murmurs may frequently suggest the diagnosis of PVE, in general it is difficult to predict accurately the extent of valvular pathology by auscultation alone.

Laboratory Findings.   Anemia is present in many patients with PVE. In late PVE, the degree of anemia is probably a function of the duration of infection. The packed cell volume is a less useful finding in the diagnosis of early PVE. Leukocytosis occurs in only 50 percent of the patients; it may be more frequently seen in those with early PVE. Hematuria (secondary to glomerulonephritis) can be a helpful diagnostic sign in the patient with suspected late PVE but is difficult to interpret in a postoperative patient who may have recently required urethral catheterization. A number of investigators have reported elevated levels of circulating immune complexes in patients with PVE, but their utility for diagnosis or prognosis requires further evaluation.[37,38]

Blood Cultures.   The cornerstone of diagnosing PVE is the isolation of an etiologic microorganism from the blood. As in the case of NVE, the bacteremia associated with PVE is continuous. Ninety percent of blood cultures obtained in such patients should reveal the infecting pathogen.[43] Negative blood cultures in a patient who has not received antibiotics is quite unusual in PVE unless the infection is caused by organisms such as *Legionella*, *Mycobacterium*, *Rickettsia*, *Histoplasma capsulatum*, or *Aspergillus* spp., which do not grow readily in routine blood cultures. Fastidious microorganisms such as *Haemophilis* spp. may require prolonged incubation before appearing in blood cultures; therefore, all blood cultures from patients with suspected PVE should be held for a minimum of 3 weeks. Specialized culture techniques such as biphasic media or lysis centrifugation may increase the yield of fungi and other difficult to isolate organisms.[44]

On the other hand, not all instances of bacteremia occurring after valve replacement indicate PVE.[45] Infected wounds and contaminated intravascular catheters may lead to transient bacteremia. Prosthetic valves seem relatively resistant to colonization by gram-negative bacilli, and PVE is rare after transient gram-negative bacteremia. If gram-negative bacteremia clears after the extracardiac source is removed, patients who have no other manifestations of PVE can usually be treated with 2 weeks of intravenous antibiotics.[46] If bacteremia fails to clear or the source of infection is not apparent, the patient should be assumed to have PVE and be treated accordingly. Because gram-positive bacteria are more adherent, their presence in blood cultures usually reflects colonization of the prosthetic device. However, if there is doubt about the significance of a positive blood culture (e.g., a single blood culture growing *S. epidermidis* in the absence of clinical manifestations), antimicrobial therapy may reasonably be withheld while additional cultures are obtained.

Special Studies.   Myocardial damage from ischemia, an abscess, or pericarditis may cause a variety of arrhythmias or conduction defects in patients with PVE. In one series, atrioventricular conduction defects occurred in 44 percent of patients with prosthetic aortic valve infection due to extension of the abscess

into the conduction system.[41] Serial electrocardiograms or continuous cardiac monitoring may be important for some patients.

Standard echocardiography, which is useful in the management of patients with NVE, has been less helpful in patients with PVE. Echoes generated by the prosthesis are intense, and subtle abnormalities such as small vegetations may be obscured. In contrast, transesophageal echocardiography (TEE) appears to be a valuable tool in the assessment of patients with PVE.[47–50] TEE is significantly more sensitive than transthoracic echocardiography in the detection of vegetations and valve complications. Daniel et al.[50] describe 16 patients with prosthetic valve ring abscesses. Fourteen of these were correctly identified before surgery by TEE versus only six by transthoracic echocardiography. Despite its promise, TEE is an invasive technique subject to complications not seen with transthoracic echocardiography.[51] However, TEE should be considered in cases in which the diagnosis is uncertain. Doppler echocardiography also appears to be a useful technique for assessment of valvular dysfunction. In one series, Doppler techniques correctly identified significant regurgitation or obstruction in 15 of 17 patients with malfunctioning prosthetic valves.[52]

Several reports describe the use of indium or gallium scintigraphy with SPECT imaging in the detection of prosthetic valve infections.[53–55] The exact role this technology will play is not clear, as large-scale studies have not been performed.

Cardiac catheterization is often unnecessary in the evaluation of patients with PVE. In some circumstances, however, catheterization can provide valuable information, including an estimation of the degree of valvular dysfunction, the location of the fistula, an evaluation of left ventricular function, delineation of coronary artery anatomy, or an assessment of possible multiple valve involvement.[56]

Computed tomography of the head is indicated in all patients with PVE and neurologic symptoms. Infarction, hemorrhage, or an abscess can usually be differentiated by this technique. In addition, all patients with neurologic symptoms not readily explained by computed tomography should undergo cerebral angiography to exclude the possibility of an intracranial mycotic aneurysm.[57]

Mortality of Prosthetic Valve Endocarditis

The mortality of patients with PVE remains high. Dismukes[58] analyzed 105 cases of PVE treated between 1976 and 1979 at the Massachusetts General Hospital and the University of Alabama Medical Center and reported an overall mortality of 29 percent. The mortality was 41 percent in early PVE and 21 percent in late disease. More recently, Calderwood et al.[1] reported the outcomes of 116 patients with PVE; in-hospital mortality was 23 percent. The authors applied logistic regression analysis and found that "complicated" infection (defined as persistent fever while receiving antibiotics, changing murmurs heard on physical examination, worsening heart failure, or new conduction abnormalities) was the best predictor of death. Keyser et al.[59] noted a 50 percent mortality among patients with neurologic complications; none of three patients with intracranial hemorrhage survived.

The mortality of PVE varies somewhat with the etiologic microorganism. In a group of 184 patients reviewed by Wilson et al.,[60] significantly higher mortality was seen in PVE caused by fungi, gram-negative bacilli, or staphylococci.

Management of Prosthetic Valve Endocarditis

General Principles.   Successful management of patients with PVE depends on the same principles used in treating patients with NVE. All patients should be hospitalized, confined to bed during the acute phase of the illness, and monitored carefully for hemodynamic deterioration and arrhythmias. Patients should undergo careful daily physical examination to detect heart fail-

TABLE 3. Antimicrobial Therapy for Patients with Bacterial Infections of Prosthetic Valves

Organism	Regimen	Duration of Therapy (wk)	Regiment in Penicillin-Allergic Patients[a,b]
Susceptible streptococci (MIC <0.1 μg/ml Pen G)	Aqueous Pen G[c] plus gentamicin[d,e]	4–6 2	Vancomycin[f] plus gentamicin[d,e] or Cephalothin[g] plus gentamicin[d,e]
Resistant streptococci (MIC >0.1 μg/ml Pen G), enterococci	Aqueous Pen G[c] or ampicillin[h] plus gentamicin[d]	6–8 6–8	Vancomycin[f] plus gentamicin[d]
Staphylococcus aureus			
Methicillin susceptible	Nafcillin[i] plus gentamicin[d]	6–8 2	Cephalothin[g] plus gentamicin[d]
Methicillin resistant	Vancomycin[f]	6–8	Not applicable
Staphylococcus epidermidis	Vancomycin[f] plus rifampin[j] and gentamicin[d]	6–8 6–8 2	Not applicable
Diphtheroids	Aqueous Pen G[c] plus gentamicin[d] or Vancomycin[f,k]	6 6	Vancomycin[f,k] Not applicable
Aerobic gram-negative bacilli	β-Lactam[l] plus aminoglycoside—based on in vitro data	6–8 6–8	Consider aztreonam[l] plus aminoglycoside
Empirical regimen, bacteria not identified	Vancomycin[f] plus gentamicin[d]		Not applicable

[a] The duration of therapy is similar to that recommended for non-penicillin-allergic patients.
[b] Cephalosporins are contraindicated when there is history of penicillin anaphylaxis.
[c] Aqueous penicillin G, 24 million units daily in divided doses q4h.
[d] Gentamicin, 1 mg/kg iv q8h.
[e] Streptomycin may be used for sensitive organisms (MIC <1000 μg/ml).
[f] Vancomycin, 0.5 g iv q6h.
[g] Cephalothin, 2 g iv q4h (or equivalent cephalosporin).
[h] Ampicillin, 2 g iv q4h.
[i] Nafcillin, 2 g iv q4h.
[j] Rifampin, 300 mg po q8h.
[k] Preferred agent for gentamicin-resistant strains.
[l] For strains resistant to all β-lactams, consider ciprofloxacin as a single agent.

ure, changes in murmurs, or evidence of embolization or a mycotic aneurysm.

Antibiotic Therapy. Antimicrobial therapy is based on laboratory identification of the etiologic microorganism and in vitro susceptibility testing; bactericidal antibiotics are necessary. In an effort to enhance in vivo activity, combinations of antibiotics that demonstrate synergistic killing of the pathogen in vitro are often used. Whenever possible, intravenous medications should be administered via scalp vein needles rather than indwelling intravenous catheters to reduce the risk of bacteremia from a contaminated intravascular device. Recommended antibiotic regimens are shown in Table 3.

The combination of aqueous penicillin G plus gentamicin[61,62] is recommended to treat patients with PVE caused by penicillin-susceptible streptococci (minimum inhibitory concentration [MIC] ≤0.1 μg/ml). Streptomycin may be used in place of gentamicin if the MIC for streptomycin is less than 1000 μg/ml.

The combination of penicillin (or ampicillin) with an aminoglycoside has been the preferred regimen for most enterococci and resistant streptococci.[62–64] In recent years, however, drug resistance among enterococci has become sufficiently common to warrant careful sensitivity testing of all blood isolates. Some strains are now resistant to high levels of aminoglycosides (>2000 μg/ml) and occasionally to penicillin or vancomycin as well.[64,65] Gentamicin-resistant isolates should be tested with streptomycin since occasional strains will be sensitive. There is no proven treatment regimen for endocarditis caused by high-level aminoglycoside resistant enterococci. If active in vitro, large doses of ampicillin or vancomycin alone may be tried. Ampicillin/sulbactam may be of use for those strains that produce β-lactamase. Early surgery should be considered for patients not responding.

For PVE caused by *S. aureus*, penicillin G is the treatment of choice if the isolate is penicillinase negative and the MIC for penicillin G is 0.1 μg/ml or less. If penicillinase is produced, a semisynthetic antistaphylococcal penicillin (e.g., nafcillin) should be used instead. Because in vitro studies have demonstrated enhanced killing of *S. aureus* by certain antibiotic combi-

nations, many authorities advocate the addition of gentamicin for the first 2 weeks of therapy. Prosthetic valve endocarditis caused by methicillin-resistant isolates of *S. aureus* must be treated with vancomycin. Addition of rifampin can also be considered, but the combination is not synergistic for all strains.

In one study, approximately 80 percent of *S. epidermidis* isolates from patients with PVE were resistant to methicillin.[66] Resistance is not due to β-lactamase production but to alterations in penicillin-binding proteins. Resistance of *S. epidermidis* to methicillin or cephalosporins may not always be apparent by routine in vitro susceptibility testing. Consequently, the use of β-lactam antibiotics alone to treat *S. epidermidis* PVE has resulted in high failure rates.[67] On the basis of currently available data, the combination of vancomycin and rifampin with gentamicin added for the first 2 weeks of therapy appears to be the most effective regimen for *S. epidermidis* PVE.[62,68]

Selection of an antimicrobial regimen for the treatment of diphtheroid PVE is somewhat controversial. If the diphtheroid strain is susceptible to penicillin and gentamicin, therapy with this combination is recommended. The clinical efficacy of penicillin plus gentamicin has also been demonstrated even when the diphtheroid isolate is penicillin resistant,[25] although some would recommend vancomycin in this circumstance. Vancomycin is the therapy of choice for PVE caused by diphtheroid strains (such as group JK corynebacteria) that are resistant to both penicillin and gentamicin.

The design of an antibiotic regimen for PVE caused by aerobic gram-negative bacilli must be based on identification of the organism and careful in vitro susceptibility and synergy studies. Therapy will usually include a β-lactam antibiotic (penicillin, cephalosporin, carbapenem, or monobactam) plus an aminoglycoside. Newer quinolones may be useful in therapy for resistant organisms, but their efficacy in endocarditis has not yet been established in large-scale clinical trials.[69,70]

Fungal PVE is a very serious disorder that requires combined medical and surgical therapy. For *Candida* endocarditis, high doses of intravenous amphotericin B (up to 1 mg/kg/day) is given in combination with oral flucytosine (dose adjusted for renal function). A preoperative induction course of amphotericin B does not seem to improve outcome; prompt valve replacement is mandatory.[71] One patient with *Histoplasma* PVE apparently responded to amphotericin B alone but a combined medical/surgical approach is probably optimal.[72]

When PVE seems clinically apparent but blood cultures are not yet positive, therapy with vancomycin plus gentamicin should be initiated. For patients in whom infection has been demonstrated at an extracardiac site (e.g., wound infection, pneumonia, urinary tract infection), initial antimicrobial therapy should include drugs active against the microorganism present at that site as well. When PVE is considered but the level of clinical suspicion is low, three or four blood cultures should be obtained by separate venipunctures and the patient observed. If valve replacement is imminent, it is reasonable to initiate empirical antimicrobial therapy with vancomycin and gentamicin. The diagnosis of PVE can usually be confirmed or excluded at the time of surgery.

Serum bactericidal activity should be measured during the first few days of therapy to demonstrate the in vivo activity of the antimicrobial regimen being used. Controversy exists regarding the usefulness of the test, the best method of testing, the optimal antimicrobial activity desired, and the timing of testing (peak vs. trough). In general, a serum bactericidal titer of greater than 1:32 against the infecting bacteria (measured at the time of peak antibiotic concentration) appears to correlate with a more favorable clinical response.[73,74] If a titer of at least 1:8 is not achieved, an increase in dosage or change in antibiotics should be considered, particularly if the patient is not responding clinically.

After the initiation of antimicrobial therapy, blood cultures should be obtained daily for the first 3–4 days and weekly thereafter until the completion of therapy. Usually blood cultures will be sterile within 3–5 days of initiating appropriate antimicrobial therapy. After the completion of therapy, blood cultures should be obtained weekly for 1 month. A relapse necessitates reinstitution of antimicrobial therapy, retesting of the microorganism for antimicrobial susceptibility, and strong consideration of valve replacement. Occasionally, a relapse may be due to persistent infection at an extracardiac site; careful consideration should be given to the possibility of an occult abscess or mycotic aneurysm.

Surgical Therapy.   Several general observations can be made regarding the increasingly important role of surgery in the management of PVE. First, the mortality of patients with PVE who undergo valve replacement during active infection is no greater (and may be less) than is the mortality of patients who receive medical therapy alone. Mortality statistics may underestimate the value of surgical intervention in the management of PVE since many of the patients in the medical-surgical treatment group were critically ill and underwent surgery only after failing medical therapy. Second, the risk of recurrent PVE after the surgical removal of an infected prosthesis is real but usually acceptable. The incidence in published series has ranged from 0 to 15 percent, and the microorganisms causing PVE after valve replacement for NVE are usually different from those infecting the native valve.[2,12,75] This perhaps reflects the more complex techniques necessary for repair in these patients. Third, when valve replacement is clinically indicated, there is little to be gained by delaying surgery despite an incomplete course of antibiotic therapy. A delay only increases the chances for serious complications such as refractory heart failure, renal failure, or emboli.[2,12,76]

The objectives of cardiac surgery in PVE are to remove infected tissues and materials and to restore hemodynamic integrity.[77] Other goals include the repair of acquired defects (such as abscesses) and elimination of sources of emboli.[73,78] The decision to proceed with cardiac surgery in the seriously ill patient with PVE is seldom an easy one. To provide some guidelines for physicians and surgeons caring for these patients, we have

TABLE 4. Indications for Valve Replacement during Active Prosthetic Valve Endocarditis

Disorder	Point Rating[a]
Heart failure due to valve dysfunction	
Severe	5
Moderate	5
Mild	2
Acute valve obstruction	5
Fungal etiology	5
Persistent bacteremia	5
Organism other than penicillin-susceptible *Streptococcus*	2
Relapse after appropriate therapy	3
One major embolus	2
Two or more emboli	4
Vegetations by echocardiogram	1
Heart block	3
Ruptured ventricular septal defect or sinus of Valsalva	4
Early PVE (<60 days)	2
Unstable prosthesis by fluoroscopy	5
Paravalvular leak	2
Prior prosthetic valve replacement	−2

[a] The accumulation of 5 or more points suggests the need for valve replacement.

(From Alsip et al.,[79] with permission.)

used a point system to assess the need for valve replacement. If assessment of a patient results in the accumulation of five or more points by the system described in Table 4, we would recommend surgery—emergent surgery in the case of severe heart failure and urgent surgery in the case of other complications. Cardiac transplantation has been utilized in patients with recurrent disease not responding to combined medical and surgical therapy.[80]

The severity of heart failure is a leading prognostic factor in patients with PVE. In patients with moderate to severe heart failure secondary to valvular dysfunction, emergency valve replacement may be lifesaving. Two large series reported by Richardson et al.[12] and Karchmer et al.[13] contain a total of 52 PVE patients with moderate to severe heart failure. The mortality in the medical therapy group was 100 percent, while the combined medical-surgical therapy group had a 49 percent mortality. Valve replacement is therefore recommended in all PVE patients with moderate to severe heart failure. Emergency valve replacement is also required in patients who develop acute prosthetic obstruction due to large vegetations. Hemodynamically stable patients who may later require valve replacement for mild heart failure or a paravalvular leak should receive a full course of antimicrobial therapy before elective surgery.

Valve replacement within 48–72 hours is recommended in cases of fungal PVE because of the poor response to medical therapy and high frequency of major emboli.[62] In patients with bacterial PVE, valve replacement should be considered whenever bacteremia persists for more than a few days after the initiation of the best antimicrobial therapy.

Anticoagulation.   Most patients with mechanical heart valves require long-term anticoagulation to prevent thromboembolic complications. However, the theoretic risks of bleeding at the site of a mycotic aneurysm or embolic infarction raises important questions about the use of anticoagulants in patients with active PVE. Carpenter et al.[81] described 14 patients who received anticoagulants during therapy for PVE. Thirty-six percent had symptomatic episodes of CNS hemorrhage. In contrast, Wilson et al.[82] noted a higher frequency of neurologic complications in PVE patients who did not receive adequate anticoagulation. Although the proper use of anticoagulants remains controversial, most authorities do continue anticoagulation in patients with PVE. However, it may be prudent to monitor patients closely and maintain clotting parameters at the lower end of the therapeutic range.

Prophylaxis

Although there have been no adequate placebo-controlled trials to assess the value of prophylactic antibiotics in valve replacement, they are routinely employed. Several studies have compared first- and second-generation of cephalosporin regimens.[83–85] There was little difference in the incidence of PVE, though some differences in sternal infections were described. Cefazolin or cefuroxime seem to be the most cost-effective agents. The duration of prophylaxis usually should not exceed 2 days. Vancomycin is an appropriate alternative drug for β-lactam–allergic patients or in facilities where there is a high incidence of resistant staphylococci. After hospital discharge, the patient should be aware of the importance of prophylactic antimicrobial agents before any procedure likely to cause transient bacteremia.

INDWELLING RIGHT ATRIAL CATHETERS

Broviac and Hickman catheters are silicone elastomer intravenous devices designed to permit long-term vascular access for hyperalimentation, drug or blood product administration, and blood sampling (see Chs. 58 and 281).[86,87] The distal, intravascular portion of the catheter is inserted into the superior vena cava or right atrium via the external jugular or cephalic vein. The extravascular portion, with a Dacron felt cuff in place, is drawn through a subcutaneous chest wall tunnel that exits between the nipple and sternum. The Dacron cuff is designed to permit fibroblast ingrowth to anchor the catheter and prevent microorganisms from tracking along the outside. Newer implantable catheters (i.e., Port-A-Cath, Pharmacia Deltic, Inc., St. Paul, MN) have a similar intravascular component but end on the chest with an implanted port that is accessed percutaneously.

Four varieties of infectious complication of Broviac or Hickman catheters include (1) exit site infections, (2) tunnel infections, (3) septic thrombophlebitis, and (4) isolated bacteremia or fungemia. Press et al.[88] reviewed the courses of 992 oncology patients with a total of 1088 Hickman catheter placements. One hundred forty-three catheter infections were documented (incidence, 0.14 infections/100 catheter days). Exit site infections, isolated bacteremia, tunnel infections, and septic thrombophlebitis accounted for 46, 31, 20, and 4 percent of all infections, respectively. Later reviews suggest similar infection rates for implantable versus tunnelled catheters among adults. However, implantable catheters may be preferable in pediatric populations.[89–91]

Microbiology

Presently, gram-positive cocci are responsible for most silicone elastomer catheter infections in the United States.[88–96] Coagulase-negative and -positive staphylococci accounted for 31 and 14 percent, respectively, of catheter infections in Clark and Raffin's review.[89] *Staphylococcus epidermidis* accounted for 54.1 percent and *Staphylococcus aureus* for 20 percent of the clinical isolates in the review of 143 catheter infections by Press et al.[88] Gram-negative bacilli, gram-positive bacilli, and fungi such as *Candida albicans*, respectively, accounted for 9, 5, and 7 percent of all clinical isolates.

Pathogenesis

The precise pathogenesis of catheter-related infections is unclear. However, the frequency with which *S. epidermidis* is isolated suggests that microorganisms may track along the catheter from the skin or perhaps are introduced at the time of catheter placement. The risk of hematogenous seeding of the catheter during bacteremia from a distant focus appears to be low.[88]

Clinical Manifestations

The clinical manifestations of catheter infections vary with the sites of involvement. (1) Exit site infections are characterized by local warmth, erythema, and tenderness at the site where the catheter exits from the skin. Purulent drainage around the catheter may or may not be evident. (2) Tunnel infections may resemble exit site infections, but tenderness and erythema extend up the chest along the subcutaneous tract of the proximal portion of the catheter. Both exit site and tunnel infections may be complicated by the presence of concomitant bacteremia (three of four and three of eight patients, respectively, in one series).[88] (3) The manifestations of septic thrombophlebitis reflect bacterial invasion and subsequent thrombosis of the vein that the catheter enters. Patients are almost always bacteremic, and there are local signs of venous insufficiency such as edema of the upper extremity. (4) Finally, patients may be bacteremic in the absence of localizing signs or symptoms. This type of infection may be particularly important in neutropenic individuals who are unable to mount a local inflammatory response to infection.

Diagnosis

The early diagnosis of catheter-related infections requires regular examination of the catheter exit site and the skin overlying the tunnel for signs of tenderness and erythema. If infection is suspected, Gram stain and culture should be performed on any purulent material expressed from around the catheter. In addition, blood cultures should be routinely obtained. Cultures drawn through the catheter will occasionally be positive even though peripheral blood cultures are negative.

Therapy

Therapy for indwelling right atrial catheter infections changed significantly in the 1980s. Previously, clinicians believed that all infected catheters required removal, especially if bacteremia was documented. Many catheters can now be salvaged. Exit site infections with or without associated bacteremia are the type most responsive to antibiotic therapy, with cure rates as high as 85 percent in one series.[88] Bacteremia without evidence of localized catheter infection may also be successfully managed with parenteral antibiotics (see Chs. 58 and 281). Tunnel infections and septic thrombophlebitis are more difficult to eradicate and usually require catheter removal. Similarly, catheters infected with resistant organisms such as gram-negative bacilli or fungi are difficult to salvage. In any case, catheter removal should be considered whenever patients fail to respond to antibiotics as indicated by persistent fever or continued positive blood cultures while receiving therapy. The empirical treatment of catheter-related infections should generally include vancomycin and gentamicin to treat *S. epidermidis*. The therapeutic regimen can be altered on the basis of the antimicrobial susceptibility patterns of organisms isolated. All cases other than mild exit site infections should be treated with approximately 14 days of parenteral antibiotics. Some investigators have advocated the instillation of fibrinolytic agents (streptokinase or urokinase) into the catheter if there is evidence of partial occlusion by a clot. Schuman et al.[97] reported a 90 percent catheter salvage rate when using local fibrinolytic therapy and systemic antimicrobial agents in 28 episodes of bacteremia occurring in 24 patients with indwelling right atrial catheters.

INFECTION OF VASCULAR GRAFTS

Incidence

The reported incidence of vascular prosthesis infection ranges from less than 1 percent to more than 5 percent and varies with the site of graft placement.[98–100] Grafts implanted in the inguinal area (e.g., aortofemoral or femoropopliteal grafts) have a higher rate of infection than do grafts that lie entirely within the abdomen. In one series of 3652 patients receiving primarily aortic, aortoiliac, or aortofemoral grafts, a groin incision was associated with a threefold increase in the incidence of graft infection (1.34 vs. 0.43 percent).[101] Infection rates for grafts in the upper extremities and other sites are less well documented.

Pathogenesis

The mechanisms by which microorganisms colonize vascular grafts include (1) contamination at the time of surgery, (2) direct extension from an adjacent tissue site, and (3) hematogenous seeding during an episode of bacteremia.

Lower extremity grafts are at greatest risk for infection, which may reflect higher rates of perioperative contamination with microorganisms from the skin at the relatively superficial lower extremity graft site. Preoperative extremity infections, postoperative wound infections, and underlying disorders such as diabetes mellitus may also contribute to the high incidence of infections in femoral and popliteal grafts.

Abdominal aortic grafts have a relatively high incidence of infection with gram-negative enteric bacilli, probably reflecting contamination of the graft by bowel microorganisms. Several investigators have suggested that unsuspected infections in aortic aneurysms may be responsible for some cases of postrepair graft infections. In two recent reports, cultures were obtained from 266 clinically uninfected aneurysmectomy specimens. Bacteria were isolated in 33 instances, with *S. epidermidis* the most common organism.[102,103] However, the incidence of subsequent infections in these individuals was quite low, and the significance of these data remains unclear.

Graft infections may result from bacteremia, but the risk of infection diminishes as the graft becomes incorporated in the host tissue.[104] After an initial inflammatory reaction, fibrous tissue accumulates on the outer surface of the graft, and a pseudointima composed of connective tissue and fibrin begins to form on the inner surface of the graft.[105] A true endothelial lining extends from the native artery but rarely grows more than 10 mm beyond the anastomosis.[106] In animal models, resistance of an implanted graft to blood-borne infection correlates with the degree of pseudointima formation.[107,108]

Microbiology

Table 5 lists by site the etiologic microorganisms recovered from 85 patients with graft infections.[99,109,110] *Staphylococcus aureus* and *S. epidermidis* are the most commonly reported causes of graft infections, particularly sites involving the lower extremity.[98,111] Intra-abdominal graft infections are most commonly caused by *E. coli* or other gram-negative enteric bacilli. Data from several large series show that two or more microorganisms were isolated from 37 percent of graft infections; multiple isolates were found in 60 percent of abdominal graft infections and 23 percent of groin infections.[9,109,110,112] Polymicrobial infections most often included a *Staphylococcus* and a gram-negative bacillus or combinations of gram-negative bacilli.

Clinical Features

The local and systemic manifestations of graft infections vary with the location of the prosthesis. Over 70 percent of infections involving groin and popliteal vascular prostheses develop within 2 months of surgery, whereas 70 percent of intra-abdominal graft infections do not become clinically apparent until more than 1 year after surgery.[109,113] The most common presentations of graft infection in the groin or leg are the formation of a localized abscess or draining sinus, the formation of a false aneurysm (which may be associated with pain and a new bruit), thrombosis of the graft, or septic emboli to the distal extremity.[113] Erythema, warmth, or tenderness at a graft site is highly suggestive of infection. Rapid swelling over an area of vascular repair of a hemorrhage from a graft site suggests disruption of the suture line with bleeding or false aneurysm formation. Ischemic changes and a loss of pulse in the distal part of the extremity indicate thrombosis of the arterial implant. Exteriorization of the graft due to a breakdown of overlying tissues is pathognomonic of infection.

The presentation of intra-abdominal graft infections may be subtle. Fever is usually present but may be low grade. Specific findings in aortic graft infections can include abdominal tenderness, retroperitoneal hemorrhage, an abdominal mass due to a false aneurysm, graft thrombosis, ureteral obstruction with hydronephrosis, and septic emboli.[114] Petechiae and splinter hemorrhages similar to those in endocarditis may also occur. Aortoenteric fistula formation due to erosion of the graft into the bowel occurred in 0.36 percent of patients in one series.[101] In 80 percent of cases of aortoenteric fistula, the proximal anastomosis erodes into the third portion of the duodenum.[115] A breakdown of the suture line results in upper or lower gastrointestinal bleeding that may be massive. Melena or hematemesis in a patient with an aortic graft should immediately arouse suspicion of a developing aortoenteric fistula.[109,116]

Diagnosis

A variety of diagnostic techniques are useful in evaluating patients with suspected vascular graft infection. If a draining sinus is present, a careful sinogram may reveal the extent of an underlying infectious process. Abscesses and aneurysms may also be demonstrated by noninvasive techniques such as sonography and CT. Magnetic resonance imaging may prove to be a sensitive technique for diagnosing graft infections. In one report of three patients, MRI clearly delineated the extent of perigraft infection. Abscesses have a high signal intensity that contrasts strongly with the signal of flowing blood.[117] Gallium scanning has not generally been found to be useful; indium-labeled leukocyte scanning may be a sensitive diagnostic technique, but its specificity appears to be low, at least in the perioperative period.[118] Arteriography is the most precise method for documenting suture line leakage or graft thrombosis, but CT imaging may provide similar information as well as demonstrate other complications not visible by angiography.[119]

Cultures and Gram stains should be obtained on all draining wounds, although cultures obtained at the time of surgical inspection provide more reliable microbiologic data. Routine venous blood cultures should also be obtained. No good estimation of the frequency of positive blood cultures is available, but negative blood cultures do occur in an appreciable number of cases when infection has not yet extended to the graft lumen. Material removed at embolectomy, however, should always be cultured.

TABLE 5. Microbial Etiology of Vascular Graft Infections

Organism	Anatomic Location of Infection			
	Abdominal (%)	Groin (%)	Popliteal (%)	Overall (%)
S. aureus	14	40	33	33
S. epidermidis	7	13	17	12
Streptococci	14	8	25	11
E. coli	42	9	0	16
Proteus sp.	3	11	0	8
Other aerobic gram-negative bacilli	0	8	17	7
Other bacteria	10	5	0	6
Candida sp.	3	1	0	1
Unknown	7	5	8	6
Total number				
Microorganisms	29	85	12	126
Patients	17	60	8	85

(Data from refs. 99, 109, 110.)

Morbidity and Mortality

Morbidity and mortality vary with the position of the graft. In a review of 84 patients with vascular graft infection, O'Hara et al.[101] found an overall 30-day mortality rate of 28 percent. The same authors reported a 1-year mortality rate of 46 percent among the 43 patients who received grafts since 1980.[101] In another series of infected aortobifemoral prostheses, mortality was 23 percent.[120] Mortality rates are lower for distal graft infections (14 percent[113] in one series of femoropopliteal grafts), largely due to the ease of earlier diagnosis and the decreased severity of bleeding relative to proximal grafts.

The major morbidity associated with graft infection is loss of the extremity supplied by the prosthesis. In one recent review, the amputation rate among 13 patients with aortofemoral infections was 38 percent.[120]

Management

Successful treatment usually requires a combination of systemic antibiotic administration and surgery. Removal of the entire graft and débridement of infected tissue is almost always necessary for cure. Most attempts to treat graft infection with antibiotics and local wound care alone are unsuccessful. Infections occurring at midpoints of long grafts (e.g., axillofemoral) may be temporarily managed by drainage and antibiotics, but graft removal will ultimately be required for a successful outcome. The viability of distal structures depends on the adequacy of collateral vessels and the feasibility of additional bypass procedures. If the extremity or organ is totally dependent upon flow through the graft, some form of revascularization that bypasses the site of infection should be attempted. For example, axillofemoral grafts may be used to bypass an infected aortic bifurcation graft. If a new graft must be placed in the infected field, some authors have recommended use of autogenous artery or vein grafts, which may be less susceptible to infection than are grafts made of synthetic materials. The only common situation in which removal of a portion of the graft is acceptable occurs when infection involves the distal anastamosis of one branch of an aorto-femoral graft; the infected limb may sometimes be removed and the opposite limb preserved. Identification of the infecting microorganism and in vitro susceptibility testing are also essential for successful therapy. Some graft infections may be temporarily managed by drainage and antibiotics, but graft removal will ultimately be required for a successful outcome. Recommended initial antimicrobial regimens for graft infections are generally the same as those recommended for PVE (Table 3). Antibiotics should be administered parenterally for 4 weeks after the prosthetic device is removed.

Prevention

Strict adherence to principles of asepsis, vigorous preoperative skin decontamination, and meticulous surgical technique are the most important factors in preventing wound and graft infections. Simultaneous procedures that could result in bacteremia or wound contamination should be avoided.

Prophylactic antibiotics are routinely employed in vascular operations. A double-blind study of cefazolin vs. placebo demonstrated a significantly lower rate of postoperative wound and graft infections in patients who receive cefazolin.[121] Some surgeons routinely instill antibiotic solutions into the wound before closure, but the value of this practice is unproved.[122] Grafts containing antibiotics incorporated into the material have been developed but remain investigational.[123]

Little information is available to assess the value of prophylactic antibiotics in patients with vascular grafts who undergo manipulations likely to result in bacteremia. Graft infection resulting from such bacteremia appears to be rare, but some authors have recommended that prophylactic antibiotics be given before dental, genitourinary, or other procedures.[124,125] This may have the greatest value in the first few months after graft placement.[126]

INFECTIONS OF DIALYSIS-ACCESS ARTERIOVENOUS FISTULAS

Because of lower rates of infection and thrombosis, surgically created subcutaneous arteriovenous fistulas (AVFs) have generally replaced external arteriovenous cannulas for vascular access in chronic dialysis patients.[127,128] An AVF may be created by direct artery-to-vein anastomosis (native AVF) or by implantation of a prosthetic conduit. Expanded polytetrafluoroethylene is the most commonly used material.

Infectious complications of native vessel AVFs appear to be uncommon. The incidence of infection has averaged less than 2 percent in several recent studies with follow-ups as long as 5 years.[129,130] Infection occurs more frequently in prosthetic AVFs. In three recent studies, infections developed in 11, 23, and 25 percent of patients receiving expanded polytetrafluoroethylene grafts.[129–131]

Microbiology

Staphylococcus aureus is the most common etiologic microorganism and accounts for 60–90 percent of access site infections.[127,128,132–134] Gram-negative bacilli, especially *Pseudomonas aeruginosa*, are also commonly encountered.[128,132,134] A prosthetic AVF may become infected through a variety of mechanisms. Contamination may occur at the time of implantation, or a relatively superficial wound infection may extend to involve the graft. In addition, access sites are subjected to multiple needle punctures during dialysis, which may result in direct inoculation of the prosthesis. Hematomas or false aneurysms occurring at puncture sites may also become infected. Bacteremia is a possible but apparently uncommon source of AVF infection.

Clinical Manifestations

Arteriovenous fistula infections may present with local pain, tenderness, erythema, abscess formation, or bacteremia. However, as many as one-third of AVF infections have no clinically apparent local findings.[132,135] As with other types of vascular graft infections, involvement of the suture line may result in disruption of the anastomosis and subsequent hemorrhage. Approximately 30 percent of AVF infections are associated with bacteremia. Metastatic infections such as endocarditis or septic pulmonary thromboembolism may occur, especially with staphylococcal AVF infections.[127,135]

Therapy

Management of infected AVFs almost always necessitates the combination of antibiotic administration and surgery. However, there are reports of graft salvage when antimicrobial therapy and surgical débridement are combined. This may be more effective when the infectious process involves only a localized site distant from suture lines.[136] Infection involving native vessel AVFs may respond to antimicrobial therapy alone.[111,132]

Initial empirical antimicrobial therapy for an infected AVF should include agents active against staphylococci and aerobic gram-negative bacilli (e.g., vancomycin, an antipseudomonal β-lactam, and an aminoglycoside). Subsequent therapy must be based on the susceptibility pattern(s) of the isolated pathogen(s). The doses of all agents must be carefully adjusted for the patient's renal function.

PERMANENT PACEMAKER INFECTIONS

Infection is second only to problems with pacing or sensing as a complication of permanent pacemaker insertion. In one series of 457 patients, the reported incidences of pacemaker infections were 3.6 and 2 percent for epicardial and transvenous devices, respectively.[137] Pacemaker infections may involve any portion of the implanted hardware from the generator box to the pacing electrode. Concomitant bacteremia or endocarditis may also be present.

The most common location for pacemaker infections is the subcutaneous pocket containing the generator box. Most such infections present soon after surgery but may not become evident for 2 years or more. Staphylococci are the most common causes of generator box infections. In one large review, *S. epidermidis* was responsible for 44 percent of pacemaker infections, while *S. aureus* was isolated from 29 percent.[138] The most likely pathogenesis of generator box infections is contamination of the device by skin flora at the time of implantation. Wound infection or erosion of the box through the overlying skin may also lead to microbial contamination.

The other major category of pacemaker infection is involvement of the epicardial or transvenous electrodes. This usually results from the direct spread of microorganism along the wires from an infected generator box, but hematogenous seeding occasionally occurs.[139]

The clinical manifestations of pacemaker infection depends on the site of involvement. Generator box infections typically present with fever and local warmth, erythema, and tenderness over the generator pocket. Isolated lead infections are less common but may present similarly to bacterial endocarditis with fever and positive blood cultures. A definite diagnosis of pacemaker infection depends on the isolation of an etiologic microorganism from the pacemaker pocket or the blood stream.

Treatment of pacemaker infections remains controversial. All hardware should be removed in both generator box and electrode infections, particularly when these disorders are accompanied by bacteremia. Parry et al.[140] noted a complication rate of 51 percent when functionless pacer electrodes were left in place after partial system removal for infection. Occasional cures have been reported in generator box infections with parenteral antibiotics and local irrigation alone. Parenteral antimicrobial agents must be chosen carefully on the basis of the identification and susceptibility of the isolated pathogen. The proper duration of therapy is not well established. If any foreign material is left in place, antibiotic administration should be continued for at least 6 weeks, perhaps followed by long-term suppressive therapy. Antimicrobial therapy should continue for approximately 4 weeks after the hardware is removed if bacteremia is documented. Two weeks of antimicrobial therapy may be adequate for nonbacteremic infection if the device is removed.

REFERENCES

1. Calderwood SB, Swinski LA, Karchmer AW, et al. Prosthetic valve endocarditis: Analysis of factors affecting outcome of therapy. J Thorac Cardiovasc Surg. 1986;92:776–83.
2. Ivert TSA, Dismukes WE, Cobbs CG, et al. Prosthetic valve endocarditis. Circulation. 1984;69:223.
3. Dismukes WE, Karchmer AW, Buckley MJ, et al. Prosthetic valve endocarditis: Analysis of 38 cases. Circulation. 1973;48:365.
4. Rossiter SJ, Stinson EB, Oyer PE, et al. Prosthetic valve endocarditis: Comparison of heterograft tissue valves and mechanical valves. J Thorac Cardiovasc Surg. 1978;76:795.
5. Grignon A, Spencer H, Robson HG, et al. Prosthetic valve infections. Can J Surg. 1981;24:615.
6. Masur H, Johnson WD Jr. Prosthetic valve endocarditis. J Thorac Cardiovasc Surg. 1980;80:31.
7. Auger P, Marquis G, Dyrda I, et al. Infective endocarditis update: Experience from a heart hospital. Acta Cardiol. 1981;36:105.
8. Aintablian A, Hilsenrath J, Hamby RJ, et al. Endocarditis in prosthetic valves. NY State J Med. 1976;76:673.
9. Wilson WR, Jaumin PM, Danielson GK, et al. Prosthetic valve endocarditis. Ann Intern Med. 1975;82:751.
10. Slaughter L, Morris JE, Starr A. Prosthetic valvular endocarditis: A 12-year review. Circulation. 1973;47:1319.
11. Petheram IS, Boyce JMH. Prosthetic valve endocarditis: A review of 24 cases. Thorax. 1977;32:478.
12. Richardson JV, Karp RB, Kirklin JW, et al. Treatment of infective endocarditis: A 10 year comparative analysis. Circulation. 1978;58:589.
13. Karchmer AW, Dismukes WE, Buckley MJ, et al. Late prosthetic valve endocarditis: Clinical features influencing therapy. Am J Med. 1978;64:199.
14. Bortotti U, Thiene G, Milano A, et al. Pathological study of infective endocarditis on Hancock porcine bioprostheses. J Thorac Cardiovasc Surg. 1981; 81:934.
15. Magilligan DJ, Quinn EL, Davila JC. Bacteremia, endocarditis, and the Hancock valve. Ann Thorac Surg. 1977;24:508.
16. Isom OW, Spencer FC, Glassman E, et al. Long-term results in 1375 patients undergoing valve replacement with the Starr-Edwards cloth-covered steel ball prosthesis. Ann Surg. 1977;186:310.
17. Downham WH, Rhoades ER. Endocarditis associated with porcine valve xenografts. Arch Intern Med. 1979;139:1350.
18. Gallo JI, Ruiz B, Carrion MF, et al. Heart valve replacement with the Hancock bioprosthesis: A 6-year review. Ann Thorac Surg. 1981;31:444.
19. Rutledge R, Kim BJ, Applebaum RE. Actuarial analysis of the risk of prosthetic valve endocarditis in 1,598 patients with mechanical and bioprosthetic valves. Arch Surg. 1985;120:469.
20. Hammond GL, Geha AS, Kopf GS, et al. Biological versus mechanical valves: Analysis of 1,116 valves inserted in 1,012 adult patients with a 4,818 patient-year and a 5,327 valve-year follow-up. J Thorac Cardiovasc Surg. 1987;93:182.
21. Calderwood SB, Swinski LA, Waternaux CM, et al. Risk factors for the development of prosthetic valve endocarditis. Circulation. 1985;72:31.
22. Horstkotte D, Korfer R, Loogen F, et al. Prosthetic valve endocarditis: Clinical findings and management. Eur Heart J. 1984;5:17.
23. Chun PKC, Nelson WP. Common cardiac prosthetic valves: Radiologic identification and associated complications. JAMA. 1977;238:401.
24. Delgado DG, Cobbs CG. Infections of prosthetic valves and intravascular devices. In: Mandell GL, Douglas RG Jr, Bennett JE, eds. Principles and Practice of Infectious Diseases. New York: Churchill Livingstone; 1979;690.
25. Murray BE, Karchmer AW, Moellering RC Jr. Diphtheroid prosthetic valve endocarditis: A study of clinical features and infecting organisms. Am J Med. 1980;69:838.
26. Kluge RM, Calia FM, McLaughlin JS, et al. Sources of contamination in open heart surgery. JAMA. 1974;230:1415.
27. Blakemore WS, McGarrity GJ, Thurer RJ, et al. Infection by airborne bacteria with cardiopulmonary bypass. Surgery. 1971;70:830.
28. Freeman R, King B. Analysis of results of catheter tip cultures in open-heart surgery patients. Thorax. 1975;30:26.
29. Stiles GM, Singh L, Imazaki G, et al. Thermodilution cardiac output studies as a cause of prosthetic valve bacterial endocarditis. J Cardiovasc Surg. 1984; 88:1035.
30. Centers for Disease Conttrol and Prevention. Follow-up on mycobacterial contamination of porcine heart valve prostheses—United States. MMWR. 1978;27:92.
31. Rumisek JD, Albus RA, Clarke JS. Late *Mycobacterium chelonei* bioprosthetic valve endocarditis: Activation of implanted contaminant? Ann Thorac Surg. 1985;39:277.
31a. Fang G, Keys TF, Gentry LO, et al. Prosthetic valve endocarditis resulting from nosocomial bacteremia. Ann Intern Med. 1993;119:560–7.
32. Anderson DJ, Bulkley BH, Hutchins GM. A clinicopathologic study of prosthetic valve endocarditis in 22 patients: Morphologic basis for diagnosis and therapy. Am Heart J. 1977;94:325.
33. Arnett EN, Roberts WC. Prosthetic valve endocarditis: Clinicopathologic analysis of 22 necropsy patients with comparison of observations in 74 necropsy patients with active infective endocarditis involving natural left-sided cardiac valves. Am J Cardiol. 1976;38:281.
34. Ferrans VJ, Boyce SW, Billingham ME, et al. Infection of glutaraldehyde-preserved porcine valve heterografts. Am J Cardiol. 1979;43:1123.
35. Karchmer AW, Stinson EB. The role of surgery in infective endocarditis. In: Swartz M, Remington J, eds. Current Clinical Topics in Infectious Diseases. New York: McGraw-Hill; 1980:124.
36. Leport C, Vilde JL, Bricaire F, et al. Fifty cases of late prosthetic valve endocarditis: Improvement in prognosis over a 15 year period. Br Heart J. 1987;58:66.
37. Hooper DC, Bayer AS, Karchmer AW, et al. Circulating immune complexes in prosthetic valve endocarditis. Arch Intern Med. 1983;143:2081.
38. Kauffmann RH, Thompson J, Valentijn RM, et al. The clinical implications and the pathogenetic significance of circulating immune complexes in infective endocarditis. Am J Med. 1981;71:17.
39. Neugarten J, Baldwin DS. Glomerulonephritis in bacterial endocarditis. Am J Med. 1984;77:297.
40. Watanakunakorn C. Prosthetic valve infective endocarditis: A review. Prog Cardiovasc Dis. 1979;22:181.
41. Madison J, Wang K, Gobel FI, et al. Prosthetic aortic valvular endocarditis. Circulation. 1975;51:940.
42. Quenzer RW, Edwards LD, Levin S. A comprehensive study of 48 host valve and 24 prosthetic valve endocarditis cases. Am Heart J. 1976;92:15.
43. Washington JA II. The role of the microbiology laboratory in the diagnosis and antimicrobial treatment of infective endocarditis. Mayo Clin Proc. 1982; 57:22.
44. Johnson PG, Lee J, Domanski M, et al. Late recurrent *Candida* endocarditis. Chest 1991;99:1531.
45. Sande MA, Johnson WD Jr, Hook EW, et al. Sustained bacteremia in patients with prosthetic cardiac valves. N Engl J Med. 1972;286:1067.

46. Dismukes WE, Karchmer AW. The diagnosis of infected prosthetic heart valves: Bacteremia versus endocarditis. In: Duma RJ, ed. Infections of Prosthetic Heart Valves and Vascular Grafts. Baltimore: University Park Press; 1977:61.

47. Van Camp G, Vandenbossche JL. Illustration by transesophageal echocardiography of rapid and important pannus formation during infective endocarditis of a prosthetic valve. Acta Cardiol. 1991;46:589.

48. Rogers J, Walker M, Olson JD, et al. Value of transesophageal echocardiography as an adjunct to transthoracic echocardiography in evaluation of native and prosthetic valve endocarditis. Chest. 1991;100:351.

49. Taams MA, Gussenhoven EJ, Bos E, et al. Enhanced morphological diagnosis in infective endocarditis by transesophageal echocardiography. Br Heart J. 1990;63:109.

50. Daniel WG, Mugge A, Martin RP, et al. Improvement in the diagnosis of abscesses associated with endocarditis by transesophageal echochardiography. N Engl J Med. 1991;324:795.

51. Pearlman AS. Transesophageal echocardiography—sound diagnostic technique or two-edged sword? N Engl J Med. 1991;324:841.

52. Panidis IP, Ross J, Mintz GS. Normal and abnormal prosthetic valve function as assessed by Doppler echocardiography. J Am Coll Cardiol. 1986;8:317.

53. Cerqueira MD, Jacobson AF. Indium 111 leukocyte scintigraphy detection of myocardial abscess formation in patients with endocarditis. J Nucl Med. 1989;30:703.

54. Purnell GL, Walker CW, Allison JW, et al. Indium 111 leukocyte localization in infected prosthetic graft. Clin Nucl Med. 1990;15:586.

55. Obrien K, Barnes D, Martin RH, et al. Gallium SPECT in the detection of prosthetic valve endocarditis and aortic ring abscess. J Nucl Med. 1991;32: 1791.

56. Welton DE, Young JB, Raizner AE, et al. Value and safety of cardiac catheterization during active infective endocarditis. Am J Cardiol. 1979;44:1306.

57. Dean RH, Waterhouse G, Meacham PW, et al. Mycotic embolism and emolomycotic aneurysms: Neglected lessons of the past. Ann Surg. 1986;204:300.

58. Dismukes WE. Prosthetic valve endocarditis: Factors influencing outcome and recommendations for therapy. In: Bisno AL, ed. Treatment of Infective Endocarditis. New York: Grune & Stratton; 1981:67.

59. Keyser DL, Biller J, Coffman TT, et al. Neurologic complications of late prosthetic valve endocarditis. Stroke. 1990;21:472.

60. Wilson WR, Danielson GK, Giuliani ER, et al. Prosthetic valve endocarditis. Mayo Clin Proc. 1982;57:155.

61. Bisno AL, Dismukes WE, Durack DT, et al. Treatment of infective endocarditis due to viridans streptococci. JAMA. 1989;261:1471.

62. Bisno AL, Dismukes WE, Durack DT, et al. Antimicrobial treatment of infectious endocarditis due to viridans streptococci, enterococci, and staphylococci. JAMA. 1989;261:1471.

63. Carrizosa J, Kaye D. Antibiotic synergism in enterococcal endocarditis. J Lab Clin Med. 1976;88:132.

64. Rice LB, Calderwood SB, Eliopoulos GM, et al. Enterococcal endocarditis: A comparison of prosthetic and native disease. Rev Infect Dis. 1991;13:1.

65. Mederski-Samoraj BD, Murray BE. High-level resistance to gentamicin in clinical isolates of enterococci. J Infect Dis. 1983;147:751.

66. Archer GL. Antimicrobial susceptibility and selection of resistance among *Staphylococcus epidermidis* isolates recovered from patients with infections of indwelling foreign devices. Antimicrob Agents Chemother. 1978;14:353.

67. Karchmer AW, Archer GL, Dismukes WE. *Staphylococcus epidermidis* causing prosthetic valve endocarditis: Microbiologic and clinical observations as guides to therapy. Ann Intern Med. 1983;98:447.

68. Karchmer AW, Archer GL, Dismukes WE. *Staphylococcus epidermidis* causing prosthetic valve endocarditis: Microbiologic and clinical observations as guides to therapy. Ann Intern Med. 1983;98:447.

69. Sande MA, Brooks-Fournier RA, Gerberding JL. Efficacy of ciprofloxacin in animal models of infection: Endocarditis, meningitis, and pneumonia. Am J Med. 1987;82:63.

70. Fernandez-Guerrero M, Rouse M, Henry N, et al. Ciprofloxacin therapy of experimental endocarditis caused by methicillin-susceptible or methicillin-resistant *Staphylococcus aureus*. Antimicrob Agents Chemother. 1988;32: 747.

71. McLeod R, Remington JS. Fungal endocarditis. In: Rahimtoola SH, ed. Infective Endocarditis. New York: Grune & Stratton; 1978:211.

72. Kanawaty DS, Stalker MJ, Munt PW. Nonsurgical treatment of *Histoplasma* endocartidis involving a bioprosthetic valve. Chest. 1991;99:253.

73. Reller LB. The serum bactericidal test. Rev Infect Dis. 1986;8:803.

74. Weinstein MP. Multicenter collaborative evaluation of a standardized serum bactericidal test as a prognostic indicator in infective endocarditis. Am J Med. 1985;78:262.

75. Baumgartner WA, Miller DC, Reitz BA, et al. Surgical treatment of prosthetic valve endocarditis. Ann Thorac Surg. 1983;35:87.

76. Mayer KH, Schoenbaum SC. Evaluation and management of prosthetic valve endocarditis. Prog Cardiovasc Dis. 1982;25:48.

77. Dinubile MJ. Surgery in active endocarditis. Ann Intern Med. 1982;96:650.

78. Karp RB. Role of surgery in infective endocarditis. Cardiovasc Clin. 1981; 12:157.

79. Alsip SG, Blackstone EH, Kirklin JW, et al. Indications for cardiac surgery in patients with infective endocarditis. Am J Med. 1985;78:138.

80. DiSesa VJ, Sloss LJ, Cohn LH. Heart transplantation for intractable prosthetic valve endocarditis. J Heart Transplant. 1990;9:142.

81. Carpenter JL, McAllister CK, US Army Collaborative Group. Anticoagulation in prosthetic valve endocarditis. South Med J. 1983;76:1372.

82. Wilson WR, Geraci JE, Danielson GK, et al. Anticoagulant therapy and central nervous system complications in patients with prosthetic valve endocarditis. Circulation. 1978;57:1004.

83. Peterson CD, Lake KD, Arom KV, et al. Antibiotic prophylaxis in open heart surgery patients: Comparison of cefamandos and cefuroxime. Drug Intell Clin Pharmacol. 1987;21:28.

84. Slama TG, Sklar SJ, Misinski J, et al. Randomized comparison of cefamandol, cefazolin, and cefuroxime prophylaxis in open heart surgery. Antimicrob Agents Chemother. 1986;29:744.

85. Bayer AS, Nelson RJ, Slama TG. Current concepts in prevention of prosthetic valve endocarditis. Chest. 1990;97:1203.

86. Broviac JW, Cole JJ, Scribner BH. A silicone rubber atrial catheter for prolonged parenteral alimentation. Surg Gynecol Obstet. 1973;136:602.

87. Hickman RO, Buckner CD, Cliff RA, et al. A modified right atrial catheter for access to the venous system in marrow transplant recipients. Surg Gynecol Obstet. 1979;148:871.

88. Press OW, Ramsey PG, Larson EB, et al. Hickman catheter infections in patients with malignancies. Medicine (Baltimore). 1984;63:189.

89. Clark DE, Raffin TA. Infectious complications of indwelling long-term central venous catheters. Chest. 1990;97:966.

90. Mueller BU, Skelton J, Calleneder DP, et al. A prospective randomized trial comparing the infectious and noninfectious complications of an externalized catheter versus a subcutaneously implanted device in cancer patients. J Clin Oncol. 1992;12:1943.

91. La Quaglia MP, Lucas A, Thaler HT, et al. A prospective analysis of vascular access device-related infections in children. J Pediatr Surg. 1992;7:840.

92. Begala JE, Maher K, Cherry JD. Risk of infection associated with the use of Broviac and Hickman catheters. Am J Infect Control. 1982;10:17.

93. Wade JC, Newman KA, Schimpff SC, et al. Two methods for improved venous access in acute leukemia patients. JAMA. 1981;246:140.

94. Abrahm JL. A prospective study of prolonged central venous access in leukemia. JAMA. 1982;248:2868.

95. Thomas JH, MacArthur RI, Pierce GE, et al. Hickman-Broviac catheters: Indications and results. Am J Surg. 1980;140:791.

96. Lowder JN, Lazarus HM, Herzig RH. Bacteremias and fungemias in oncologic patients with central venous catheters. Arch Intern Med. 1982;142: 1456.

97. Schuman ES, Winters V, Gross GF, et al. Management of Hickman catheter sepsis. Am J Surg. 1985;149:627.

98. Liekweg WG, Greenfield LJ. Vascular prosthetic infections: Collected experience and results of treatment. Surgery. 1977;81:335.

99. Szilagyi DE, Smith RF, Elliott JP, et al. Infection in arterial reconstruction with synthetic grafts. Ann Surg. 1972;176:321.

100. Goldstone J, Moore WS. Infection in vascular prostheses: Clinical manifestations and surgical management. Am J Surg. 1974;128:225.

101. O'Hara PJ, Hertzer NR, Beven EG, et al. Surgical management of infected abdominal aortic grafts: Review of a 25-year experience. J Vasc Surg. 1986; 3:725.

102. Ilsenfritz FM, Jordan FT. Microbiological monitoring of aortic aneurysm wall and contents during aneurysmectomy. Arch Surg. 1988;123:506.

103. Schwartz JA, Powell TW, Burnham SJ, et al. Culture of abdominal aortic aneurysm contents. An additional series. Arch Surg. 1987;122:777.

104. Moore WS, Malone JM, Keown K. Prosthetic arterial graft material: Influence on neointimal healing and bacteremic infectibility. Arch Surg. 1980; 115:1379.

105. DeBakey ME, Jordan GL Jr, Abbott JP, et al. The fate of Dacron vascular grafts. Arch Surg. 1964;89:757.

106. Berger K, Sauvage LR, Rao AM, et al. Healing of arterial prostheses in man: Its incompleteness. Ann Surg. 1972;175:118.

107. Malone JM, Moore WS, Campagna G, et al. Bacteremic infectibility of vascular grafts: The influence of pseudointimal integrity and duration of graft function. Surgery. 1975;78:211.

108. Roon AJ, Malone JM, Moore WS, et al. Bacteremic infectibility: A function of vascular graft material and design. J Surg Res. 1977;22:489.

109. Becker RM, Blundell PE. Infected aortic bifurcation grafts: Experience with 14 patients. Surgery. 1976;80:544.

110. Hoffert PW, Gensler S, Haimovici H. Infection complicating arterial grafts: Personal experience with 12 cases and review of the literature. Arch Surg. 1965;90:427.

111. Wilson SE, Van Wagenen P, Passaro E Jr. Arterial infection. Curr Probl Surg. 1978;15:1.

112. Casali RE, Tucker WE, Thompson BW, et al. Infected prosthetic grafts. Arch Surg. 1980;115:577.

113. Liekweg WG Jr, Levinson SA, Greenfield LJ. Infections of vascular grafts: Incidence, anatomic location, etiologic agents, morbidity, and mortality. In: Duma RJ, ed. Infections of Prosthetic Heart Valves and Vascular Grafts. Baltimore: University Park Press; 1977:239.

114. Rich NM, Collins GJ Jr, Andersen CA. Infected grafts: Clinical presentation and diagnosis. In: Duma RJ, ed. Infections of Prosthetic Heart Valves and Vascular Grafts. Baltimore: University Park Press; 1977:253.

115. Elliott JP Jr, Smith RF, Szilagyi DE. Aortoenteric and paraprostheticenteric fistulas. Arch Surg. 1974;108:479.

116. Willwerth BM, Waldhausen JA. Infection of arterial prostheses. Surg Gynecol Obstet. 1974;139:446.

117. Justich E, Amparo EG, Hricak H, et al. Infected aortoiliofemoral grafts: Magnetic resonance imaging. Radiology. 1985;154:133.

118. Sedwitz MM, Davies RJ, Pretorius HT, et al. Indium 111-labeled white blood cell scans after vascular prosthetic reconstruction. J Vasc Surg. 1987;6:476.

119. Vozelzang RL, Limpert JD, Yao JS. Detection of prosthetic vascular complications: Comparison of CT and angiography. Am J Roentgenol. 1987;4:819.

120. Schellack J, Stewart MT, Smith RB III, et al. Infected aortobifemoral prosthesis—A dreaded complication. Am Surg. 1988;54:137.

121. Kaiser AB, Clayson KR, Mulherin JL, et al. Antibiotic prophylaxis in vascular surgery. Ann Surg. 1978;188:283.

122. Pitt HA, Postier RG, MacGowan WA, et al. Prophylactic antibiotics in vascular surgery: Topical, systemic, or both? Ann Surg. 1980;192:356.

123. Moore WS, Chvapil M, Seiffert G, et al. Development of an infection-resistant vascular prosthesis. Arch Surg. 1981;116:1403.

124. Moore WS, Malone JM. Vascular infection. In: Simmons RL, Howard RJ, eds. Surgical Infectious Diseases. New York: Appleton-Century-Crofts; 1982:777.

125. Sweeney TF, Kerstein MD. Management of peripheral vascular infections. In: Kerstein MD, ed. Management of Surgical Infections. New York: Futura; 1980:117.

126. Threlkeld MG, Cobbs CG: Questions and answers: Arterial graft infections—Is antibiotic prophylaxis necessary? JAMA. 1988;259:2608.

127. Ralston AJ, Harlow GR, Jones DM, et al. Infections of Scribner and Brescia arteriovenous shunts. Br Med J. 1971;3:408.

128. Kuruvila KC, Beven EG. Arteriovenous shunts and fistulas for hemodialysis. Surg Clin North Am. 1971;51:1219.

129. Winsett OE, Wolma FJ. Complications of vascular access for hemodialysis. South Med J. 1985;78:513.

130. Kheriakian GM, Roedersheimer LR, Arbaugh JJ. Comparison of autogenous fistula versus expanded polytetrafluoroethylene graft fistula for angioaccess in hemodialysis. Am J Surg. 1986;152:238.

131. Munda R, First MR, Alexander JW, et al. Polytetrafluoroethylene graft survival in hemodialysis. JAMA. 1983;249:219.

132. Dobkin JF, Miller MH, Steigbigel NH. Septicemia in patients on chronic hemodialysis. Ann Intern Med. 1978;88:28.

133. Nsouli KA, Lazarus M, Schoenbaum SC, et al. Bacteremic infection in hemodialysis. Arch Intern Med. 1979;139:1255.

134. Kaslow RA, Zellner SR. Infection in patients on maintenance hemodialysis. Lancet. 1972;2:117.

135. Cross AS, Steigbigel RT. Infective endocarditis and access site infections in patients with hemodialysis. Medicine (Baltimore). 1978;55:453.

136. Bhat DJ, Tellis VA, Kohlberg WI, et al. Management of sepsis involving expanded polytetrafluoroethylene grafts for hemodialysis access. Surgery. 1980;87:445.

137. Oldershaw PJ, Sutton MG, Ward D, et al. Ten-year experience of 359 epicardial pacemaker systems: Complications and results. Clin Cardiol. 5:515, 1982.

138. Bluhm G. Pacemaker infections: A clinical study with special reference to prophylactic use of some isoxazolyl penicillins. Acta Med Scand Suppl. 1985; 699:1.

139. Wade JS, Cobbs CG. Infections in cardiac pacemakers. In: Remington JS, Swartz MN, eds. Current Clinical Topics in Infectious Diseases. v. 9. New York: McGraw-Hill; 1988:44.

140. Parry G, Goudevenos J, Jameson S, et al. Complications associated with retained pacemaker leads. Pacing Clin Electrophysiol. 1991;8:1251.

60. PROPHYLAXIS OF INFECTIVE ENDOCARDITIS

DAVID T. DURACK

Infective endocarditis continues to cause serious morbidity and mortality despite advances in diagnosis and treatment. Even though the etiologic organisms usually can be eradicated by antibiotics, they often leave permanent valvular damage or other major sequelae. Only a minority of patients die during the active phase of endocardial infection, but many suffer later complications and have a shortened life span despite being "cured."[1,2] In the near future, increasing prevalence of antibiotic resistance among gram-positive organisms that commonly cause endocarditis may worsen the prognosis even further. For these reasons, prevention of infective endocarditis remains an important objective.[3–9]

Selection of rational interventions to prevent infective endocarditis has been hampered by a lack of information upon which to base recommendations. For example, reliable data are not available to answer even these basic questions: What is the risk of developing infective endocarditis after procedures that cause bacteremia? What procedures and operations should be covered by antibiotics? Is antibiotic prophylaxis effective? If so, which prophylactic antibiotic regimens give the best results?

It is doubtful that sufficient epidemiologic data can be accumulated to answer these questions definitively. Random bacteremias occur commonly, probably daily[10,11]; thus patients with underlying heart disease are continually at some risk of developing endocarditis, and it is not possible to determine with certainty which one of many bacteremias, including some that may be caused by health care practitioners, is responsible for an episode of endocarditis. Clinical studies on the prophylactic efficacy of antibiotics are also unlikely to provide the answers, because an excessively large number of patients would be required to reach a significant conclusion, as the following example illustrates. Let us make the following assumptions: that the risk of acquiring bacterial endocarditis after dental extraction is approximately 1 in 500,[12,13] that approval for a randomized trial of antibiotic versus a placebo could be obtained from an ethics review committee, and that an antibiotic regimen is available that is 100 percent effective in preventing endocarditis. An imaginary clinical trial under these admittedly arbitrary conditions might yield the following figures:

Treatment Group	Number of Patients	Cases of Endocarditis
Placebo	3000	6
Antibiotic	3000	0
Total	6000	Chi-Square = 4.2
		$p < 0.05$

In this model, at least 6000 patients, *all with preexisting valvular heart disease,* would have to be studied during dental procedures for the results to reach statistical significance. Although these figures are based on arbitrary and unproven assumptions, it is likely that such a large study would be difficult or impossible to perform. However, it may be possible to demonstrate the efficacy of prophylaxis by selecting subgroups of patients at highest risk for endocarditis. Among patients with prosthetic heart valves undergoing various surgical procedures, no cases of endocarditis followed 287 procedures for which antibiotic prophylaxis was given, while 6 occurred after 390 procedures for which it was omitted.[13] This result, which needs to be independently confirmed, just reaches statistical significance.

Attempted prevention of bacterial infections with antibiotics is most likely to be effective and cost-effective when a single antimicrobial drug is directed against a single pathogen and when the disease occurs with fairly high frequency in the absence of prophylaxis.[14] Prevention of endocarditis does not meet these ideals because a variety of antibiotics are used against a variety of organisms and because the disease occurs rarely even if prophylactic antibiotics are not given. Furthermore, only a small proportion (not more than 5–10 percent) of all cases of infective endocarditis can be attributed to bacteremias caused by previous medical, surgical, or dental procedures.[10,15,16] It follows that the proportion of potentially preventable cases is also small.

Because definitive data are lacking, prevention of infective endocarditis remains an empirical practice, characterized by uncertainty and controversy.[6,16,17] Nevertheless, most authorities agree that prophylaxis should be offered to susceptible patients during certain procedures known to be associated with bacteremia.[3–5,8–10]

ESTIMATES OF RISK FOR INFECTIVE ENDOCARDITIS

To determine when antibiotic prophylaxis for infective endocarditis should be given, it is necessary to estimate the relative risk of developing endocarditis after certain procedures. The incidence of transient bacteremia after various manipulations has been extensively studied.[10,11,18–33] It should be noted that incidence of bacteremia varies quite widely between studies. Also, the transient presence in the blood of certain bacterial species associated with endocarditis, especially streptococci, may be more important than the overall frequency of bacteremia. Some representative figures from selected studies are presented in Table 1.

Several hundred cases of endocarditis that were attributed to prior dental procedures have been recorded in the literature. In many of these, the first symptoms of endocarditis appeared within less than 2 weeks.[34] Although the incubation period of endocarditis is not known precisely, the onset of symptoms soon after dental operations in these cases makes a causal relationship seem likely. These case reports provide the basis for the belief that dental procedures often cause endocarditis—a belief that is widely but not universally accepted.[16] The risk of developing infective endocarditis due to a dental extraction certainly must be low because bacteremia usually results from this common operation, yet endocarditis is a relatively rare disease. It has been variously estimated that the risk is as high as 1 in 533,[12] as low as 1 in 115,500,[35] or even zero.[36] Most authorities would agree that dental operations do indeed pose a significant risk to susceptible patients, but it appears that the risk of acquiring infective endocarditis is probably *less than 1 percent* for each procedure, even if no antibiotic prophylaxis is given.

Similarly, more than 100 case reports provide reasonably good evidence that bacteremias originating from the genitourinary tract may cause endocarditis, especially when urologic or gynecologic operations are carried out in the presence of bacterial infections of the urinary or genital systems.[20] Evidence that other medical and surgical procedures cause infective endocarditis is limited to a few case reports. For example, only a handful of cases have been recorded following miscellaneous operations such as drainage of soft tissue infections, abdominal surgery, diagnostic cardiac catheterization, and the use of oral irrigation devices.[10,15,38] The frequency of bacteremia during normal delivery is very low,[39,40] and few cases of endocarditis have been recorded in this setting.[40] Four cases following skin biopsies have recently been reported, two of which were due to *Staphylococcus aureus*.[41] Although bacteremias may occur during the performance of common diagnostic procedures such as endoscopies, barium enemas, and liver biopsies, very few cases of endocarditis attributable to these common procedures have been reported.[24,30,42–46] Estimates of the risk related to procedures that may cause bacteremia are offered in Table 2.

An assessment of risk in relation to the patient's underlying cardiac condition must also be made (Table 3). These estimates are based on the frequency with which various preexisting cardiac defects are found in patients with infective endocarditis.

TABLE 1. Incidence of Transient Bacteremia after Various Procedures

Procedures	%	Range
Dental		
Extraction of one or more teeth	65	18–85
Peridontal surgery	88	60–90
Brushing teeth	30	7–50
Tonsillectomy	35	33–38
Catheter removal after urologic surgery	50	
Prostatectomy (sterile urine)	11	
Prostatectomy (infected urine)	57	
Normal delivery	3	1–113
Diagnostic		
Transesophageal echocardiography	0–1	0–17
Bronchoscopy with flexible scope	0	
Barium enema	10	5–11
Liver biopsy	10	
Upper GI endoscopy	4	
Sigmoidoscopy with flexible scope	0	0–5
Colonoscopy	5	0–5

(Data from multiple studies reviewed in refs. 10, 24, 18–33.)

TABLE 2. Estimate of Risk of Developing Infective Endocarditis after Various Procedures That May Cause Bacteremias

Significant Risk	Very Low or Negligible Risk[a]
Dental procedures likely to cause bleeding (e.g., detailed examinations, scaling, extractions)	Minor dental procedures not causing bleeding (e.g., superficial examinations, simple fillings above the gum line, adjustment of orthodontic appliances)
Oral surgery involving teeth and gums	
Delivery, abortion, insertion or removal of IUD, dilatation and curettage (in the presence of pelvic infection)	Spontaneous loss of deciduous teeth
	Normal delivery, therapeutic abortion, insertion or removal of IUD, dilatation and curettage (in the absence of pelvic infection)
Tonsillectomy, adenoidectomy	Cardiac catheterization
Urinary catheterization, passage of urethral dilators, cystoscopy, prostatectomy (especially with infected urine or bacterial prostatitis)	Insertion of cardiac pacemaker
	Endotracheal intubation
	Diagnostic procedures[a]
Drainage of abscesses, operations involving infected soft tissue; possibly skin biopsy[41]	Endoscopy of upper and lower GI tract
	Barium meal, barium enema
	Liver biopsy
Injection of varices, esophageal dilatation	Bronchoscopy (with flexible bronchoscope)
	Transesophageal echocardiography

[a] The risk for some of these procedures may be significant in patients with prosthetic valves. (Based upon refs. 9, 10, 15, 24, 47.)

TABLE 3. Estimate of Risk of Developing Infective Endocarditis as Related to Underlying Cardiovascular Conditions

Relatively High Risk	Intermediate Risk	Very Low or Negligible Risk
Prosthetic valves	Mitral valve prolapse with regurgitation	Mitral valve prolapse without regurgitation
Previous infective endocarditis	Tricuspid valve disease	Anteriosclerotic plaques
Fallot's tetralogy and other cyanotic congenital heart disease	Asymmetric septal hypertrophy	Coronary artery disease
	Mitral stenosis	Atrial septal defects
Ventricular septal defect	Degenerative valvular disease in the elderly	Cardiac pacemakers
Coarctation of the aorta		Trivial regurgitation by echo without structural abnormality
Aortic valve disease		
Mitral regurgitation		
Marfan syndrome		
Intra-atrial alimentation catheters		
Arteriovenous fistulas		

(Based upon refs. 37, 47, 48, 99–103.)

Certain conditions strongly predispose to endocardial infection; thus a patient with uncorrected patent ductus arteriosus runs approximately a 30 percent risk of developing the disease during his lifetime. Similarly, congenital or acquired aortic valve disease, interventricular septal defects, mitral stenosis or incompetence, and especially prosthetic valves are known to present a relatively high risk of infection.[37,47,48] At the other end of the spectrum, uncomplicated secundum-type atrial septal defects carry such a low risk for infective endocarditis[37,47] that prophylaxis is probably not indicated for these patients.[9]

Mitral valve prolapse presents a special problem because it is so common in the general population, being found in 4 percent or more according to the definition used.[49,50] Mitral valve prolapse increases a person's risk for endocarditis by five- to eightfold,[47,49–51] and underlies 15–25 percent of cases of subacute bacterial endocarditis.[52–54] The risk appears to be greater for those patients with a systolic murmur[51,53] and for those with thickening and redundancy of the mitral leaflets on echocardiography.[50] Nevertheless, infective endocarditis is an uncommon disease, so mitral valve prolapse cannot be regarded as a high-risk lesion,[49] even when a murmur is present. Most authorities currently recommend prophylaxis for patients with prolapse and regurgitation.[9] A study of benefits versus costs by decision analysis indicated that prophylaxis for mitral valve prolapse could prevent some cases, but probably would not be cost-effective.[55] Furthermore, because the incidence of endocarditis when a patient with prolapse undergoes a dental procedure without prophylaxis is very low, the years of life lost from anaphylaxis due to parenteral penicillin could exceed the years of life saved by prevention of endocarditis.[55]

What are the implications of the above for prophylaxis? In the author's opinion, patients with mitral valve prolapse and regurgitation should receive oral antibiotics before dental procedures, because the costs and risks of taking two oral doses of amoxicillin are very low and a serious disease may occasionally be prevented. However, the use of antibiotics could be considered optional rather than mandatory in this setting, and parenteral prophylaxis usually should be avoided.

INDIRECT EVIDENCE OF EFFICACY OF PROPHYLAXIS

In the absence of definitive data, recommendations for the prophylaxis of infective endocarditis must be based on secondary sources of information. These include anecdotal experience with patients, in vitro study of the organisms that cause bacteremia and endocarditis, and evaluation of the prevention of infective endocarditis in experimental animals.

Uncontrolled Clinical Observations

Case reports describing patients who developed endocarditis after a procedure known to cause bacteremia despite the administration of antibiotics provide anecdotal evidence that attempts to prevent endocarditis are not uniformly successful.[54,56] From 1979 to 1982 an American Heart Association committee collected and recorded examples of apparent prevention failures.[54] Among 52 such cases, mitral valve prolapse was the single most common underlying cardiac lesion (33 percent), followed by various congenital abnormalities (29 percent) and rheumatic heart disease (21 percent). Nineteen percent had prosthetic valve endocarditis. Forty-eight cases (92 percent) followed a dental procedure, and 75 percent of cases were caused by viridans streptococci. Symptoms began fairly soon after the procedure suspected to have caused endocarditis: within 2 weeks in 50 percent and within 5 weeks in 79 percent. Most patients received oral penicillin for prophylaxis. Sixty percent of organisms for which antimicrobial susceptibility was known were sensitive to the antibiotic(s) used for prophylaxis. This experience, although anecdotal, indicates that endocarditis prophylaxis failures are not rare and that failures may occur even when the infecting organism is susceptible to the antibiotics used. It confirms that mitral valve prolapse is a common underlying lesion in patients with streptococcal endocarditis.

Case-Control Studies and Decision Analysis

Two case-control studies have been performed. One indicated that prophylaxis appeared to be effective,[57] while the other concluded that prevention was of marginal value.[58] Decision analysis also led the authors of one study to doubt that prophylaxis would be cost-effective, except in the highest risk situations.[55]

In Vitro Studies

A variety of organisms may be found in the blood stream after dental, surgical, and diagnostic procedures, including anaerobes and contaminants from the skin flora.[10,12,19,33,59] However, only gram-positive cocci such as viridans streptococci, enterococci, and staphylococci commonly cause infective endocarditis in this setting. It is therefore appropriate to focus on the antibiotic susceptibilities of these organisms in attempting to formulate rational prophylactic programs. Most of the bacteria in the oral flora that are likely to cause endocarditis are sensitive to penicillin G.[60] In fact, it is widely believed that all strains of viridans streptococci are exquisitely sensitive to penicillin. This is not entirely correct; in some series up to one-third of the strains are partially resistant, with minimal bactericidal concentrations (MBC) for penicillin G of 0.1–1.0 μg/ml or more.[61,62] Ampicillin and amoxicillin both possess good in vitro activity against most streptococci associated with endocarditis[60] and provide high serum concentrations.[63] Almost all strains of viridans streptococci, irrespective of their MBCs, are killed more rapidly and completely by a combination of a penicillin and an aminoglycoside than by a penicillin alone.[62,64] Many strains of enterococci, although more likely to be resistant to both penicillins and aminoglycosides, are killed synergistically by these drugs in combination, in vitro and in vivo.[65,66] Unfortunately, many strains of enterococci have recently developed high-level resistance to penicillins, aminoglycosides, or vancomycin, posing new problems for prophylaxis and treatment.[67]

Experimental Infective Endocarditis

Study of the prevention of experimental infective endocarditis in animal models has provided an important secondary source of information. In 1970, Garrison and Freedman[68] reported that placement of a polyethylene catheter in the rabbit heart led to the development of small sterile vegetations at points of contact between the catheter and endocardium. If staphylococci were placed in the lumen of the catheter, staphylococcal endocarditis resulted. Modification of this model by injecting organisms intravenously[69] provided a suitable in vivo system for examining the efficacy of various antibiotic regimens for the prophylaxis of endocarditis.[66,70–73] A similar model in rats has also been used to investigate antibiotic prophylaxis.[74–79] Under experimental conditions, the time of onset of infective endocarditis is known exactly. Another important advantage is that the incidence of infection in untreated animals can be adjusted easily by altering the inoculum size; thus the problem of very low infection rates in patients can be overcome in animals by choosing an inoculum large enough to infect most of the subjects. Significant differences among antibiotic regimens can then be demonstrated with manageable numbers of animals in each group.[66,70,72–82]

Early experiments comparing the success rates of various antibiotic regimens against viridans streptococci in this model system showed that bacteriostatic antibiotics were usually ineffective, that penicillin in low doses or in high doses of brief duration were often ineffective, that high penicillin concentrations in serum for 12 hours or more were desirable for effective prophylaxis, that the combination of a penicillin plus an aminoglycoside was synergistic against viridans streptococci as well as enterococci, and that vancomycin provided an excellent alternative to regimens using penicillins.[66,70,71,73,80] Other antibiotics that proved effective under controlled experimental conditions were ampicillin, amoxicillin,[72,77,78] erythromycin,[78] clindamycin,[81] and rifampin.[76]

Further experiments have modified the view that bactericidal antibiotic activity is essential for prophylaxis. Streptomycin proved surprisingly effective in the prevention of experimental infection by some strains of enterococci, even though the serum concentrations of streptomycin were far too low to kill them.[66] Subinhibitory concentrations of certain antibiotics, especially vancomycin, can inhibit the adherence of streptococci to fibrin surfaces in vitro.[82] More recent experiments have demonstrated successful prophylaxis for various streptococci with sub-bactericidal doses of vancomycin, clindamycin, erythromycin, and even a tetracycline.[78,80,81] Penicillin was much less effective in the prevention of experimental streptococcal endocarditis if the strain was tolerant to penicillin.[83] However, penicillin exhibited some prophylactic activity even if the strain was so tolerant that bactericidal concentrations of penicillin could not be achieved in serum.[83] All these findings suggest that prevention can sometimes be achieved by antibiotic effects that fall short of total bacterial killing, perhaps by an alteration of surface structures that mediate adherence to fibrin or by other unknown mechanisms. Bactericidal action may be sufficient but not always necessary for prevention of endocarditis. The observation that successful prophylaxis with amoxicillin can be reversed by administration of penicillinase shortly *after* colonization of the vegetation shows that killing of organisms in the blood stream or prevention of their adherence to the endocardium is not essential for antibiotic prophylaxis in every situation. The implications of these experimental findings for humans are uncertain. At present, it still seems prudent to choose bactericidal drugs for the prophylaxis of infective endocarditis whenever possible.

To place these extensive experimental data into perspective, it should be emphasized that direct extrapolation to humans may not be meaningful. Although in vitro models provide a closer simulation of human endocarditis than any in vitro system could, there are at least two important differences. First, a foreign body was present throughout many of these experiments because the intracardiac catheter often was left in place. The presence of a foreign body in tissue lowers the inoculum required to initiate infection and then makes infection harder to eradicate. Therefore, the animal models probably simulate patients with prosthetic valves more closely than they do patients with congenital or rheumatic valvular disease. Second, in many of the experiments a high inoculum was chosen deliberately to make statistical comparisons possible with a relatively small number of animals. Because both the presence of a foreign body and the use of high inocula would tend to make prevention harder to achieve, any regimen that proved effective under these rigorous experimental conditions is likely to provide a margin of safety in clinical use.

With these reservations in mind, what has been the real contribution of experimental studies of prevention? Animal models provide a convenient in vivo method for ranking prophylactic antibiotic regimens in order of efficacy, but they cannot be used to determine whether any particular antibiotic regimen will or will not prevent endocarditis in patients.[73] For example, experimental findings do not exclude the possibility that tetracycline or other bacteriostatic drugs may prevent endocarditis in some patients. They do support the conclusion that one of the optimal bactericidal regimens such as vancomycin, or penicillin plus streptomycin, should provide a much wider margin of safety than does a lower-ranking regimen such as tetracycline.[73]

CARDIAC SURGERY

Most cardiovascular surgeons believe that the use of prophylactic antibiotics has reduced the incidence of postcardiotomy endocarditis.[48] While this may be true, it should be noted that numerous technical improvements, introduced during the period when the incidence of postoperative endocarditis was falling, also may have contributed significantly. In fact, the efficacy of antibiotics for the prevention of postcardiotomy endocarditis has not yet been subjected to an adequate, critically controlled trial. The clinical impression that antibiotic prophylaxis during cardiac surgery is effective is now so widely accepted that ethical consent to perform a placebo-controlled trial probably could no longer be obtained.

Early-onset postcardiotomy endocarditis may be caused by a variety of organisms, including staphylococci, gram-negative bacteria, and fungi. No single antibiotic regimen is effective against all these, and the use of broad-spectrum antibiotics may itself predispose to superinfection with resistant organisms. Therefore, attempts to prevent endocarditis with antibiotics during open heart surgery should probably be limited to a short course of an antistaphylococcal agent such as a cephalosporin or vancomycin.[9] An aminoglycoside may be added in the hope of taking advantage of possible synergism.

Diagnostic cardiac catheterizations (including Swan-Ganz

catheters), insertion of pacemakers, coronary artery surgery, pericardial surgery, and the use of the aortic balloon pump all appear to present little risk, and the administration of antibiotics specifically for the prevention of infective endocarditis is not usually recommended during these operations. Pulmonary artery catheters have been reported to predispose to both nonbacterial and bacterial endocarditis in patients with severe burns, who often develop bacteremias.[84] Antibiotic treatment for infection often is needed in this setting, but prophylaxis for endocarditis is not recommended.

PROSTHETIC HEART VALVES

Extensive clinical experience has established that patients with prosthetic heart valves are at a relatively high risk for infective endocarditis.[13,47,48,85,86] The high mortality and morbidity associated with prosthetic valve endocarditis and re-replacement of valves make its prevention a priority. Although the incidence of endocarditis after cardiac surgery has fallen steadily since these operations first became commonplace, the risk of early-onset endocarditis within 60 days of valve replacement remains in the range of 0.3–0.5 percent, and thereafter approximates 0.5 percent per year.[48,86] For comparison, the incidence of endocarditis is approximately 0.4 percent per year in patients with rheumatic heart disease.[87] It is important to recognize this risk and to take all possible steps to minimize it. Before elective valve replacement, the dental health of every patient should be evaluated and any necessary dental work completed under close observation and with appropriate antibiotic coverage. Thereafter, the patient should maintain good oral hygiene. Healthy teeth should not be extracted, but, if advanced dental or periodontal disease is present, extraction of all teeth should be considered. Consultation between the patient's dentist and physician is important to ensure optimal antibiotic coverage during routine dental procedures. For patients with prosthetic valves, some practitioners choose to administer antibiotic prophylaxis to cover diagnostic procedures such as colonoscopy that present negligible risk in patients without prosthetic valves (Tables 1 and 2).

Late-onset prosthetic valve endocarditis (60 days after the operation) is more likely to be caused by organisms originating in the oral cavity and reaching the valve via the blood stream, just as for native valve endocarditis. Attempted prophylaxis for endocarditis in the setting of a dental procedure should be directed primarily against streptococci, not staphylococci or gram-negative bacilli, just as for patients without prosthetic valves.

Many cardiac patients receive anticoagulant therapy, which may alter the choice of prophylactic antibiotics. Intramuscular injections are contraindicated in patients receiving heparin and should be avoided if possible in patients on coumadin. For some patients an oral regimen may suffice, but for patients with prosthetic valves an intravenous regimen should be chosen.

COMMON ERRORS IN ATTEMPTED PREVENTION OF ENDOCARDITIS

Starting Antibiotic Prophylaxis Too Early

Antibiotics should be administered so as to provide the highest serum levels at the time when the procedure that might cause bacteremia is performed. There is no rationale to support the common practice of beginning antibiotic therapy earlier than is necessary to meet this criterion. Indeed, if antibiotics are given more than a few hours before the procedure, penicillin-sensitive oral flora may be replaced by penicillin-resistant organisms, and endocarditis, should it occur, may be caused by resistant organisms.[56] For most regimens, the administration of antibiotics 30–60 minutes before the procedure is appropriate. If the operation is delayed unexpectedly, doses may have to be repeated.

Continuing Antibiotic Therapy Too Long

Many practitioners continue prophylaxis for longer than necessary.[54,88,89] This wastes antibiotic, may lead to the emergence of resistant organisms, and places the patient at an additional risk of adverse reactions. Moreover, a patient who is feeling perfectly well is unlikely to adhere to an unnecessarily prolonged regimen. As with most other forms of antibiotic prophylaxis, a short course is indicated. Experimental studies provide some evidence that even a single dose may be adequate, providing an optimal antibiotic regimen is chosen,[69–71,73,77] and some recommendations utilize only one dose for humans.[90] There is some evidence of improved practice in the timing of administration in recent years.[91]

Use of Low-Dose Antibiotics

Low-dose prophylactic regimens have often been given for attempted prevention of endocarditis, even though both theoretic considerations and experimental studies indicate that a fairly high serum level of antibiotics is advisable.[54,72,73] For this reason parenteral prophylaxis may be preferred when convenient, for example, when the patient is hospitalized. However, oral amoxicillin gives good serum concentrations in most patients and is appropriate in the majority of cases because it is more convenient for both patient and practitioner. The full dose of amoxicillin should always be given (Table 4).

Prophylaxis for Tooth Extraction but Not for Lesser Dental Procedures

Much of the literature on infective endocarditis after dental procedures has emphasized tooth *extraction*. This is appropriate, but bacteremias may occur after almost any form of dental manipulation.[10,11] One reasonable criterion is to use antibiotic prophylaxis for all procedures likely to cause gingival bleeding.[9] This will exclude examination of the mouth and teeth without scaling, simple fillings above the gum line, and adjustment of orthodontic appliances, but will usually include scaling and cleaning of the teeth by a dentist or hygienist and many other dental operations.

Confusion Between Prevention of Rheumatic Fever and Prevention of Infective Endocarditis

Antibiotics have often been withheld from patients with rheumatic heart disease before dental extractions "because they were already receiving penicillin prophylaxis." Whereas the administration of low-dose penicillin orally or by monthly injection effectively prevents rheumatic fever, it is *inadequate* to prevent infective endocarditis. The incidence of infective endocarditis in children receiving penicillin for the prevention of rheumatic fever is no less than in those with rheumatic heart disease who are not receiving prophylaxis.[87] Because patients taking low-dose oral penicillin for the prevention of rheumatic fever often carry moderately penicillin-resistant streptococci in the mouth, attempted prevention of infective endocarditis with an oral penicillin regimen in these patients is not advisable. They should receive one of the parenteral regimens or clindamycin as an alternative oral regimen that does not include penicillin or amoxicillin (Table 4).

Failure To Use Prophylaxis for Children

Because bacteremia during dental procedures appears to be somewhat less common in children than in adults, it has been suggested that antibiotic prophylaxis for infective endocarditis is unnecessary in children.[92] However, careful studies indicate that bacteremia does indeed occur in a significant proportion of children after dental procedures,[93] and cases of endocarditis

TABLE 4. Current Recommendations for Prophylaxis of Endocarditis

	Indication	Regimen[a]
Standard regimen	For dental procedures; oral or upper respiratory tract surgery; minor GI or GU tract procedures	Amoxicillin, 3.0 g orally 1 hr before, then 1.5 g 6 hr later[b]
Special regimens	Oral regimen for penicillin-allergic patients (oral and respiratory tract only)	Clindamycin, 300 mg orally 1 hr before, then 150 mg 6 hr later[b]
	Parenteral regimen for high-risk patients; also for GI or GU tract procedures	Ampicillin, 2.0 g IM or IV, *plus* gentamicin, 1.5 mg/kg im or iv, 0.5 hr before, followed by amoxicillin, 1.5 g po 6 hr after initial dose; alternatively, the parenteral regimen may be repeated 8 hr after initial dose
	Parenteral regimen for penicillin-allergic patients	Vancomycin, 1.0 g IV slowly over 1 hr, starting 1 hr before; *add* gentamicin, 1.5 mg/kg IM or IV, if GI or GU tract involved[b]
	Cardiac surgery including implantation of prosthetic valves	Cefazolin, 2.0 g IV, at induction of anesthesia, repeated 8 and 16 hr later[b,c] or vancomycin, 1.0 g IV slowly over 1 hr starting at induction, then 0.5 g IV 12 hr later[b–d]

[a] These regimens are empirical suggestions; no regimen has been proved effective for the prevention of endocarditis, and prevention failures may occur with any regimen. These regimens are not intended to cover all clinical situations; practitioners should use their own judgment on safety and cost-benefit issues in each individual case. One or two additional doses may be given if the period of risk for bacteremia is prolonged.
[b] Pediatric dosages: ampicillin, 50 mg/kg; cefazolin, 30 mg/kg; clindamycin, for children who weigh more than 60 lb, use the same as for adults; for children less than 60 lb, use half the adult dose; gentamicin, 2.0 mg/kg; amoxicillin, for children who weigh more than 60 lb, use the same as for adults; for children less than 60 lb, use half the adult dose; vancomycin, 20 mg/kg.
[c] Gentamicin, 1.5 mg/kg iv, may be given with each dose if postoperative gram-negative infections have occurred with significant frequency at that hospital.
[d] This regimen is recommended for units where *Staphylococcus epidermidis* prosthetic valve infection is a problem.
(Data from Dajani et al.[9] and Simmons.[90])

following soon after dental extraction have been reported.[93] The present consensus, therefore, is that children should receive antibiotic prophylaxis for infective endocarditis, with appropriate adjustment of dosages.

Failure To Follow Standard Recommendations

Multiple studies and surveys have shown that most practitioners are aware of current recommendations, regarding them as authoritative. Despite this, practitioners often do not follow them in practice.[94–96] The reasons for this are not clear, since the current recommendations are fairly simple. Although the recommendations are admittedly empiric and of unproven efficacy, it seems desirable to follow standard procedures in this uncertain area.

THE MALPRACTICE DILEMMA

The issue of professional liability in the prophylaxis of endocarditis often has led to allegations of negligence and malpractice suits. Clearly, the lack of basic factual information referred to above makes evaluation of such cases difficult. For example, it is hard to establish that any single procedure known to cause bacteremia was the "proximate cause" in a case of endocarditis. It is even harder to prove that the failure of a physician or dentist to administer antibiotics was the direct cause of a patient acquiring endocarditis. If a strict demonstration of proximate cause were always required, it is doubtful that any claim based on the failure to administer prophylaxis could succeed, but juries are sometimes capricious in deciding liability in malpractice cases. Another common problem for the defense in claims based on failure to administer prophylaxis is our ignorance of the precise duration of the incubation period of infective endocarditis. Damages have been claimed when the first symptoms of endocarditis did not appear for months after tooth extractions without antibiotic cover. The likelihood of proximate cause here is remote, because review of case reports indicates that the incubation period is 2 weeks or less in most cases.[34]

A reasonable standard of care requires that health care professionals are aware of the risk that infective endocarditis may occur under certain circumstances. He or she should question the patient about underlying conditions that may predispose to endocarditis and should inform susceptible patients of the small risk that they may develop the disease. For patients judged to be at significant risk, an antibiotic regimen should be administered before selected dental, surgical, and genitourinary tract manipulations that might cause bacteremia. Indications for prophylaxis outside these areas are less firmly established at present. A failure to use any recognized antibiotic regimen in preference to another should not be construed as negligence, because many different regimens have been published over the past 30 years. Although some authorities recognize evidence that certain antibiotic regimens probably provide a wider margin of efficacy than do others,[9,90] this evidence is not yet firm enough to make the choice of any particular regimen mandatory.

The risks of toxicity from any prophylactic regimen must be considered carefully. Allergic reactions may occur even after low doses of penicillin; this risk is common to all regimens using penicillins as drugs of choice. However, the risk of anaphylaxis to penicillin is higher for parenteral than for oral administration. Other side effects such as ototoxicity and nephrotoxicity from aminoglycosides or vancomycin are extremely unlikely to occur after the very short courses (1 day or less) now used for the prophylaxis of infective endocarditis.

CURRENT RECOMMENDATIONS

Antibiotic Regimens

An American Heart Association Committee,[9] the editors of *Medical Letter*,[97] and others have published recommendations for the prophylaxis of infective endocarditis in the United States. Many other countries have produced similar publications for local use.[90] Current recommendations are listed in Table 4.

Local Oral Prophylaxis

The number of organisms in the mouth and gingival crevices can be temporarily reduced by local irrigation with an antiseptic solution such as iodinated glycerol.[98] Some dental experts recommend routine use of this potentially helpful measure before dental extractions.

REFERENCES

1. Tornos M-P, Permanyer-Miralda G, Olona M, et al. Long-term complications of native valve infective endocarditis in non-addicts. A 15-year follow-up study. Ann Intern Med. 1992;117:567–72.
2. Ormiston JA, Neutze JM, Agnew TM, Lowe JB, Kerr AR. Infective endocarditis: A lethal disease. Aust NZ J Med. 1981;11:620–9.
3. Greenman RL, Bisno AL. Prevention of bacterial endocarditis. In: Kaye D, ed. Infective Endocarditis. 2nd ed. New York: Raven Press. 1992;465–481.
4. McGowan DA. A dental view of controversies in the prophylaxis of infective endocarditis. J Antimicrob Chemother. 1987;20(Suppl A):105–9.
5. Kaye D. Prevention of bacterial endocarditis: 1991. Ann Intern Med. 1991; 114:803–4.
6. Kaplan EL. Bacterial endocarditis prophylaxis—Tradition or necessity? Am J Cardiol. 1986;57:478–9.
7. Finch R. Chemoprophylaxis of infective syndocarditis. Scand J Infect Dis. 1990;70:102–10.
8. Durack DT. Current issues in prevention of infective endocarditis. Am J Med. 1985;78:149–56.
9. Dajani AS, Bisno AL, Chung KJ, et al. Prevention of bacterial endocarditis. Recommendations by the American Heart Association. JAMA. 1990;264: 2919–22.
10. Everett ED, Hirschmann JV. Transient bacteremia and endocarditis prophylaxis. A review. Medicine. 1977;56:61–77.
11. Cobe HM. Oral medicine. Transitory bacteremia. Oral Surg Oral Med Oral Pathol. 1954;7:609–15.
12. Kelson SR, White PD. Notes on 250 cases of subacute bacterial (streptococcal) endocarditis studied and treated between 1927 and 1939. Ann Intern Med. 1945;22:40–60.
13. Horstkotte D, Friedrichs W, Pippert H, Bircks W, Loogen F. Nutzen der endokarditisprophylaxe bei patienten mit prothetischen herzklappen. Z Kardiol. 1986;75:8–11.
14. Sanford JP. Prophylactic use of antibiotics: Basic considerations. South Med J. 1977;70(Suppl 1):2–3.
15. van der Meer JTM, Thompson J, Valkenburg HA, Michel MF. Epidemiology of bacterial endocarditis in the Netherlands. II. Antecedent procedures and use of prophylaxis. Arch Intern Med. 1992;152:1869–73.
16. Guntheroth WG. How important are dental procedures as a cause of infective endocarditis? Am J Cardiol. 1984;54:797–801.
17. Editorial. Chemoprophylaxis for infective endocarditis: faith, hope, and charity challenged. Lancet. 1992;1:525–526.
18. Elliott SD. Bacteraemia and oral sepsis. Proc R Soc Med. 1939;32:747–54.
19. Rogosa M, Hampp EG, Nevin TA, Wagner HN, Driscoll EJ, Baer PN. Blood sampling and cultural studies in the detection of postoperative bacteremias. JADA. 1960;60:171–80.
20. Slade N. Bacteriaemia and septicaemia after urological operations. Proc R Soc Med. 1958;51:331–4.
21. LeFrock JL, Ellis CA, Turchik JB, Weinstein L. Transient bacteremia associated with sigmoidoscopy. N Engl J Med. 1973;289:467–9.
22. LeFrock J, Ellis CA, Klainer AS, Weinstein L. Transient bacteremia associated with barium enema. Arch Intern Med. 1975;135:835–7.
23. Hoffman BI, Kobasa W, Kaye D. Bacteremia after rectal examination. Ann Intern Med. 1978;88:658–9.
24. Shorvon PJ, Eykyn SJ, Cotton PB. Gastrointestinal instrumentation, bacteraemia, and endocarditis. Gut. 1983;24:1078–93.
25. Baltch AL, Pressman HL, Schaffer C, et al. Bacteremia in patients undergoing oral procedures. Study following parenteral antimicrobial prophylaxis as recommended by the American Heart Association, 1977. Arch Intern Med. 1988;148:1084–8.
26. Lamich R, Alonso C, Guma JR, et al. Prospective study of bacteremia during transesophageal echocardiography. Am Heart J. 1993;125:1454–5.
27. Botoman VA, Surawicz CM. Bacteremia with gastrointestinal endoscopic procedures. Gastrointest Endosc. 1986;32:342–6.
28. Low DE, Shoenut JP, Kennedy JK, Harding GKM, Boer BD, Micflikier AB. Risk of bacteremia with endoscopic sphincterotomy. Can J Surg. 1987; 30:421–3.
29. Ho H, Zuckerman MJ, Wassem C. A prospective controlled study of the risk of bacteremia in emergency sclerotherapy of esophageal varices. Gastroenterology. 1991;101:1642–8.
30. Rodriguez W, Levine JS. Enterococcal endocarditis following flexible sigmoidoscopy. West J Med. 1984;140:951–3.
31. Low DE, Shoenut JP, Kennedy JK, et al. Prospective assessment of risk of bacteremia with colonoscopy and polypectomy. Dig Dis Sci. 1987;32: 1239–43.
32. Okell CC, Elliott SD. Bacteriaemia and oral sepsis with special reference to the etiology of subacute endocarditis. Lancet 1935;2:869–72.
33. Roberts GJ, Gardner P, Simmons NA. Optimum sampling time for detection of dental bacteremia in children. Int J Cardiol. 1992;35:311–15.
34. Starkebaum MK, Durack DT, Beeson PB. The "incubation period" of subacute bacterial endocarditis. Yale J Biol Med. 1977;50:49–58.
35. Pogrel MA, Welsby PD. The dentist and prevention of infective endocarditis. Br Dent J. 1975;139:12–16.
36. Schwartz SP, Salman I. The effects of oral surgery on the course of patients with diseases of the heart. Am J Orthod. 1942;28:331–45.
37. van der Meer JTM, Thompson J, Valkenburg HA, Michel MF. Epidemiology of bacterial endocarditis in the Netherlands. 1. Patient characteristics. Arch Intern Med. 1992;152:1863–8.
38. Drapkin MS. Endocarditis after the use of an oral irrigation device. Ann Intern Med. 1977;87:455.
39. Sugrue D, Blake S, Troy P, MacDonald D. Antibiotic prophylaxis against infective endocarditis after normal delivery—Is it necessary? Br Heart J. 1980;44:499–502.
40. Seaworth BJ, Durack DT. Infective endocarditis in obstetric and gynecologic practice. Am J Obstet Gynecol. 1986;154:180–8.
41. Spelman DW, Weinmann A, Spicer WJ. Endocarditis following skin procedures. J Infect. 1993;26:185–9.
42. Logan RF, Hastings JGM. Bacterial endocarditis: A complication of gastroscopy. BMJ. 1988;296:1107.
43. Pritchard TM, Foust RT, Cantey JR, Leman RB. Prosthetic valve endocarditis due to *Cardiobacterium hominis* occurring after upper gastrointestinal endoscopy. Am J Med. 1991;90:516–8.
44. Rigilino J, Mahapatra R, Barnhill J, Gutierrez J. Enterococcal endocarditis following sigmoidoscopy and mitral valve prolapse. Arch Intern Med. 1984; 144:850–1.
45. Norfleet RG. Infectious endocarditis after fiberoptic sigmoidoscopy with a literature review. J Clin Gastroenterol. 1991;13:448–51.
46. Niv Y. Bacterial endocarditis after Hurst bougienage in a patient with a benign esophageal stricture and mitral valve prolapse. Gastrointest Endosc. 1985;31:265–7.

47. Steckelberg JM, Wilson WR. Risk factors for infective endocarditis. Infect Dis Clin North Am. 1993;7:9–19.
48. Braimbridge MV, Eykyn SJ. Prosthetic valve endocarditis. J Antimicrob Chemother. 1987;20:173–80.
49. Clemens JD, Horwitz RI, Jaffe CC, Feinstein AR, Stanton BF. A controlled evaluation of the risk of bacterial endocarditis in persons with mitral-valve prolapse. N Engl J Med. 1982;307:776–81.
50. Marks AR, Choong CY, Sanfilippo AJ, Weyman AE. Identification of high-risk and low-risk subgroups of patients with mitral-valve prolapse. N Engl J Med. 1989;320:1031–6.
51. Danchin N, Briancon S, Mathiew P, et al. Mitral valve prolapse as a risk factor for infective endocarditis. Lancet. 1989;743–5.
52. Nolan CM, Kane JJ, Grunow WA. Infective endocarditis and mitral prolapse: A comparison with other types of endocarditis. Arch Intern Med. 1981;141: 447–50.
53. MacMahon SW, Hickey AJ, Wilcken DEL, Wittes JT, Feneley MP, Hickie JB. Risk of infective endocarditis in mitral valve prolapse with and without precordial systolic murmurs. Am J Cardiol. 1986;58:105–8.
54. Durack DT, Kaplan EL, Bisno AL. Apparent failures of endocarditis prophylaxis: Analysis of 52 cases submitted to a national registry. JAMA. 1983; 250:2318–22.
55. Clemens JD, Ransohoff DF. A quantitative assessment of pre-dental antibiotic prophylaxis for patients with mitral-valve prolapse. J Chronic Dis. 1984; 37:531–44.
56. Garrod LP, Waterworth PM. The risks of dental extraction during penicillin treatment. Br Heart J. 1962;24:39–46.
57. Imperiale TF, Horwitz RI. Does prophylaxis prevent postdental infective endocarditis? A controlled evaluation of protective efficacy. Am J Med. 1990; 88:131–6.
58. van der Meer JTM, van Wijk W, Thompson J, et al. Efficacy of antibiotic prophylaxis for prevention of native-valve endocarditis. Lancet 1992;339: 135.
59. Nikutta P, Mantey-Stiers F, Becht I, et al. Risk of bacteremia induced by transesophageal echocardiography: Analysis of 100 consecutive procedures. J Am Soc Echocardiogr. 1922;5:168–72.
60. Basker MJ, Sutherland R. Activity of amoxycillin, alone, and in combination with aminoglycoside antibiotics against streptococci associated with bacterial endocarditis. J Antimicrob Chemother. 1977;3:273–282.
61. Blount JG. Bacterial endocarditis. Am J Med. 1965;38:909–22.
62. Wilson WR, Geraci JE, Wilkowske CJ, Washington JA. Short-term intramuscular therapy with procaine penicillin plus streptomycin for infective endocarditis due to viridans streptococci. Circulation. 1978;57:1158–61.
63. Shanson DC. The prophylaxis of infective endocarditis. J Antimicrob Chemother. 1978;4:2–4.
64. Wolfe JC, Johnson WD. Penicillin-sensitive streptococcal endocarditis. In-vitro and clinical observations on penicillin-streptomycin therapy. Ann Intern Med. 1974;81:178–81.
65. Russell EJ, Sutherland R. Activity of amoxycillin against enterococci and synergism with aminoglycoside antibiotics. J Med Microbiol. 1973;8:1–10.
66. Durack DT, Starkebaum MK, Petersdorf RG. Chemotherapy of experimental streptococcal endocarditis. VI. Prevention of enterococcal endocarditis. J Lab Clin Med. 1977;90:171–79.
67. Murray BE. The life and times of the enterococcus. Clin Microbiol Rev. 1990;3:46–65.
68. Garrison PK, Freedman LR. Experimental endocarditis I. Staphylococcal endocarditis in rabbits resulting from placement of a polyethylene catheter in the right side of the heart. Yale J Biol Med. 1970;42:394–410.
69. Durack DT, Beeson PB, Petersdorf RG. Experimental bacterial endocarditis. III. Production and progress of the disease in rabbits. Br J Exp Pathol. 1973; 54:142–51.
70. Durack DT, Petersdorf RG. Chemotherapy of experimental streptococcal endocarditis. I. Comparison of commonly recommended regimens. J Clin Invest. 1973;52:592–98.
71. Pelletier LJ, Jr, Durack DT, Petersdorf PG. Chemotherapy of experimental streptococcal endocarditis. J Clin Invest. 1975;56:319–30.
72. McGowan DA, Nair S, MacFarlane TW, MacKenzie D. Prophylaxis of experimental endocarditis in rabbits using one or two doses of amoxycillin. Br Dent J. 1983;155:88–90.
73. Durack DT: Experience with prevention of experimental endocarditis. In: Kaplan EL, Taranta, AV, eds. Infective Endocarditis. An American Heart Association Symposium. American Heart Association Monograph Number 52. Dallas, TX: American Heart Association, Inc.; 1977:28–32.
74. Moreillon P, Francioli P, Overholser P, Meylan P, Glauser MP. Mechanisms of successful amoxicillin prophylaxis of experimental endocarditis due to Streptococcus intermedius. J Infect Dis. 1986;154:801–7.
75. Overholser CD, Moreillon P, Glauser MP. Experimental bacterial endocarditis after dental extractions in rats with periodontitis. J Infect Dis. 1987;155: 107–12.
76. Malinverni R, Bille J, Glauser MP. Single-dose rifampin prophylaxis for experimental endocarditis induced by high bacterial inocula of viridans streptococci. J Infect Dis. 1987;156:151–7.
77. Malinverni R, Francioli PB, Glauser MP. Comparison of single and multiple doses of prophylactic antibiotics in experimental streptococcal endocarditis. Circulation. 1987;76:376–82.
78. Malinverni R, Overholser CD, Bille J, Glauser MP. Antibiotic prophylaxis of experimental endocarditis after dental extractions. Lab Invest. 1988;77: 182–7.
79. Berney P, Francioli P. Successful prophylaxis of experimental streptococcal endocarditis with single-dose amoxicillin administered after bacterial challenge. J Infect Dis. 1990;161:281–5.
80. Bernard J, Francioli P, Glauser MP. Vancomycin prophylaxis of experimental Streptococcus sanguis: inhibition of bacterial adherence rather than bacterial killing. J Clin Invest. 1981;68:1113–16.
81. Glauser MP, Francioli P. Successful prophylaxis against experimental streptococcal endocarditis with bacteriostatic antibiotics. J Infect Dis. 1982;146: 806–10.
82. Scheld WM, Zak O, Vosbeck K, Sande MS. Bacterial adhesion in the pathogenesis of infective endocarditis. Effect of subinhibitory antibiotic concentrations on streptococcal adhesion in vitro and the development of endocarditis in rabbits. J Clin Invest. 1981;68:1381–4.
83. Hess J, Dankert J, Durack DT. Significance of penicillin tolerance in endocarditis. Antimicrob Agents Chemother. 1983;11:555–564.
84. Ehrie M, Morgan AP, Moore FD, O'Connor NE. Endocarditis with the indwelling balloon-tipped pulmonary artery catheter in burn patients. J Trauma. 1978;18:665–6.
85. Horstkotte D, Friedrichs W, Pippert H, Bircks W, Loogen F. Benefits of endocarditis prevention in patients with prosthetic heart valves [in German]. Z Kardiol. 1986;75:8–11.
86. Kaye D: Infective endocarditis. 2nd ed. New York: Raven Press; 1992:1–497.
87. Doyle EF, Spagnuolo M, Taranta A, Kuttner AG, Markowitz M. The risk of bacterial endocarditis during antirheumatic prophylaxis. JAMA. 1967;201: 129–34.
88. Durack DT. Current practice in prevention of bacterial endocarditis. Br Heart J. 1975;37:478–81.
89. Brooks SL. Survey of compliance with American Heart Association guidelines for prevention of bacterial endocarditis. JADA. 1980;101:41–3.
90. Simmons NA. Recommendations for endocarditis prophylaxis. J Antimicrob Chemother. 1993;31:437–53.
91. Brooks RG, Notario G, McCabe RE. Hospital survey of antimicrobial prophylaxis to prevent endocarditis in patients with prosthetic heart valves. Am J Med. 1988;84:617–21.
92. Hurwitz GA, Speck WT, Keller GB. Absence of bacteremia in children after prophylaxis. Oral Surg Oral Med Oral Pathol. 1971;32:891–4.
93. Johnson DH, Rosenthal A, Nadas AS. A forty-year review of bacterial endocarditis in infancy and childhood. Circulation. 1975;51:581–8.
94. Kunzel C, Sadowsky D. Knowledge acquisition processes: Dissemination of expert recommendations to general practice dentists. J Health Soc Behav. 1989;30:330–43.
95. Sadowsky D, Kunzel C. Recommendations for prevention of bacterial endocarditis: Compliance by dental general practitioners. Circulation. 1988;77: 1316–18.
96. van der Meer JTM, Van Wijk W, Thompson J, Valkenburg HA, Michel MF. Awareness of need and actual use of prophylaxis: Lack of patient compliance in the prevention of bacterial endocarditis. J Antimicrob Chemother. 1992; 29:187–94.
97. Anonymous. Prevention of bacterial endocarditis. The Med Let. 1989;112.
98. Bender IB, Naidorf IJ, Garvey GJ. Bacterial endocarditis: A consideration for physician and dentist. JADA. 1984;109:415–50.
99. Durack DT, Lukes AS, Bright DK, et al. New criteria for diagnosis of infective endocarditis: Utilization of specific echocardiographic findings. Am J Med. 1994;96:200–1.
100. Durack DT: Infective and noninfective endocarditis. In: Schlant RC, Alexander RW, eds. Hurst's the Heart. 8th ed. New York: McGraw Hill; 1994: 1681–7.
101. Lerner PI, Weinstein L. Infective endocarditis in the antibiotic era. N Engl J Med. 1966;274:199–206.
102. von Reyn CF, Levy BS, Arbeit RD, Friedland G, Crumpacker CS. Infective endocarditis: An analysis based on strict case definitions. Ann Intern Med. 1981;94:505–517.
103. Pelletier LL, Petersdorf RG. Infective endocarditis: A review of 125 cases from the University of Washington Hospitals, 1963–72. Medicine. 1977;56: 287–313.

61. MYOCARDITIS AND PERICARDITIS

MARIA C. SAVOIA
MICHAEL N. OXMAN

Inflammatory processes affecting the heart frequently involve both the myocardium (myocarditis) and the pericardium (pericarditis). However, involvement of one or the other usually predominates, and the syndromes of myocarditis and pericarditis are sufficiently distinct in clinical presentation, etiology, and pathophysiology to warrant separate consideration.

MYOCARDITIS

Myocarditis, literally inflammation of the myocardium, is a protean disease with a wide variety of infectious and noninfectious etiologies. Postmortem examinations reveal evidence of previously unsuspected myocarditis in 1–4 percent of unselected cases,[1,2] with a higher incidence in young persons who have died suddenly.[3,4] The diagnosis of infectious myocarditis is generally considered when unexplained heart failure or arrhythmias occur in the setting of a systemic febrile illness or after symptoms of an upper respiratory tract infection. In some cases, however, the antecedent systemic illness is mild or long forgotten. In addition, myocarditis has been found histologically in 10–20 percent of cases of idiopathic dilated cardiomyopathy.[5] In myocarditis, the inflammatory process may affect myocytes, vascular elements, the conducting system, autonomic nerves, and/or the interstitium. One or more of at least four mechanisms appear to be involved: (1) direct damage to cells by an infectious agent; (2) cytotoxicity caused by a circulating toxin; (3) cytotoxicity caused by infection-induced immune reactions; and (4) nonspecific damage to myocytes as a result of an adjacent inflammatory process. Damage to the vascular endothelium may also result in indirect myocardial injury.

Etiologic Agents

In most cases of myocarditis, no definite etiology is ever established. Viruses are the most important infectious cause of myocarditis in the United States and Western Europe, and many cases of idiopathic myocarditis are assumed to be viral in origin. Long before the era of modern virology, pericardial and myocardial involvement was recognized during outbreaks of mumps,[6] and influenza,[7] measles,[8–10] poliomyelitis,[11] and enterovirus-associated pleurodynia.[12] In modern times, enteroviruses[13,14] and especially group B coxsackieviruses[15,16] have been the major agents implicated. These small, nonenveloped, single-stranded RNA viruses belonging to the picornavirus family attach to specific receptors on myocardial cells.[13] When sensitive techniques such as in situ hybridization or the polymerase chain reaction are employed, enterovirus genome has been found in approximately 25 percent of cases of myocarditis in 15 percent of samples of patients with dilated cardiomyopathy.[17] Symptomatic myocarditis or myopericarditis has also been reported in persons infected with many other viruses, particularly arboviruses and arenaviruses (Table 1).

Myocardial involvement is the most common cause of death in diphtheria[53]; the toxin produced by *Corynebacterium diphtheriae* severely damages the myocardium and conduction system. The cardiac damage seen in patients with *Clostridium perfringens* may be the result of toxin, metastatic abscess formation, or both.[55,56] The immunologically mediated carditis associated with acute rheumatic fever[57] is discussed in Chapter 177.

Invasion of the blood stream by any bacterial pathogen may result in metastatic foci in the myocardium, and myocarditis has been recognized in the course of meningococcemia,[59] salmonellosis,[60] brucellosis,[62] and streptococcal and staphylococcal bacteremia.[64] More commonly, bacteria invade the myocardium as a complication of endocarditis by contiguous spread from valvular tissue or via septic embolization of the coronary arteries.[99]

Myocarditis is a rare complication during *Legionella* infection.[68] Myocarditis has also been observed in the course of *Mycoplasma pneumoniae*,[69,70] *Chlamydia psittaci*,[72] and *Chlamydia pneumoniae*[73,74] infections and is commonly seen in rickettsial infections,[75] especially scrub typhus.[52,76,77] Approximately 10 percent of patients with Lyme disease develop cardiac abnormalities, most commonly conduction system disturbances.[79,80] In South America, the principal agent responsible for myocarditis is *Trypanosoma cruzi*, the protozoan that causes Chagas disease. The initial infection is often asymptomatic but it sometimes results in an acute illness complicated by myocarditis.[89] Myocarditis is the principal manifestation of chronic Chagas disease, which occurs in approximately 30 percent of infected individuals. These patients typically have cardiomegaly, congestive heart failure (often predominantly right-sided), and conduction disturbances.[90,91] *Trypanosoma gambiense* and *rhodesiense*, the agents of African trypanosomiasis, may also affect the heart with similar results, but central nervous system findings usually predominate.[92] Myocarditis is also observed in trichinosis[93–95] and is responsible for the occasional deaths that occur in severe infections.

In immunocompromised patients, myocarditis occurs as a consequence of a number of disseminated infections. Overt myocarditis is common in disseminated toxoplasmosis,[96–98] and systemic aspergillosis and candidiasis may also involve the heart.[82,83] Cryptococcal, toxoplasma, and aspergillus myocarditis have been reported in patients with the acquired immunodeficiency syndrome (AIDS).[85–88] Cardiac abnormalities in AIDS are common but are usually clinically silent.[100–103] A review of published autopsy series of AIDS cases by Kaul et al. suggests the incidence of myocarditis in AIDS patients may be as high as 46 percent, although a strict definition of myocarditis requiring both myocardial inflammation and necrosis was not uniformly applied.[104] In a prospective study, DeCastro et al. reported the presence of echocardiographic abnormalities in 47 of 72 AIDS patients (65.2 percent) with cardiac involvement usually occurring late in disease.[105] Cardiac dysfunction is appreciated clinically in approximately 20 percent of AIDS patients and frequently takes the form of dilated cardiomyopathy. In more than 80 percent of these patients, no specific etiology is ever found.[104] Although human immunodeficiency virus (HIV) has been cultured from endomyocardial biopsies,[106,107] and identified by Southern blot analysis[108] or in situ hybridization,[109] in most AIDS patients with cardiac pathology, HIV is not detected in cardiac tissue[110] and, when it is, there is often no correlation with histopathologic or clinical evidence of heart muscle disease.[109] A causal relationship between HIV and myocarditis has yet to be clearly established. Patients with AIDS may also be infected with known cardiotropic viruses,[107] such as coxsackieviruses and cytomegalovirus.[107,111] Antimyosin and anticardiac mitochondrial adenine nucleotide translocator antibodies have been identified in some AIDS patients with cardiac dysfunction.[112]

TABLE 1. Infectious Causes of Myocarditis

Viruses	
Coxsackie A[13–15]	Yellow fever[31]
Coxsackie B[13–16]	Argentinian hemorrhagic fever[32]
Echoviruses[18,19]	Bolivian hemorrhagic fever[32]
Polio[11,20,21]	Lymphocytic choriomeningitis[33]
Mumps[6,22,23]	Adenovirus[34,35]
Rubeola[8–10]	Varicella-zoster[36–38]
Influenza A and B[7,24,25]	Cytomegalovirus[39–44]
Rabies[26]	Epstein-Barr[45,46]
Rubella[27,28]	Vaccinia[47]
Dengue[29,30]	Variola[48]
Chikungunya[30]	Hepatitis B[49–51]
Bacteria and Rickettsia	
Corynebacterium diphtheriae[52–54]	*Listeria monocytogenes*[65–67]
Clostridium perfringens[55,56]	*Legionella pneumophila*[68]
Streptococcus pyogenes[52,57,58]	*Mycoplasma pneumoniae*[69–71]
Neisseria meningitidis[59]	*Chlamydia psittaci*[72]
Salmonella[60,61]	*Chlamydia pneumoniae*[73,74]
Brucella[62,63]	*Rickettsia rickettsii*[75]
Staphylococcus aureus[64]	*Rickettsia tsutsugamushi*[56,76–78]
	Borrelia burgdorferi[79–81]
Fungi	
Aspergillus[82–85]	*Cryptococcus*[83,86,87]
Candida[83]	
Parasites	
Trypanosoma cruzi[89–91]	*Trichinella spiralis*[93–95]
Trypanosoma gambiense[92]	*Toxoplasma gondii*[88,96–98]
Trypanosoma rhodesiense[92]	

Pathology and Pathogenesis

Myocardial pathology depends on the infecting agent, the mechanism of pathogenesis, and the duration of the process. The hallmarks of myocarditis are an inflammatory infiltrate and injury to adjacent myocardial cells. Pathologic changes may be acute or chronic and vary markedly in severity, depending on the nature of the disease and the point in its course at which tissue is obtained. Some agents, like the coxsackie B viruses, infect the myocytes themselves, whereas agents like varicella-zoster virus, cytomegalovirus, and hepatitis B virus appear to injure vascular endothelial cells. Although routine histology may help in the differential diagnosis, it rarely provides definitive information regarding the etiologic agent. Early in many viral infections, scattered hypereosinophilic myofibers, widespread edema, and only a few inflammatory cells may be present. Later, there is loss of striation, nuclear degeneration, and fragmentation of myofibers. The degenerating or partially necrotic myofibers are usually surrounded by lymphocytes, plasma cells, and macrophages.[15] The types of lymphocytes and macrophages present vary depending on the etiologic agent and stage of infection.[110,113–115] Polymorphonuclear cells are occasionally seen[3] (Fig. 1). Return to normal cardiac function usually precedes resolution of the histologic abnormalities.[116] The acute process may resolve completely; healing and chronicity are reflected by the development of interstitial fibrosis and loss of myofibers.[117]

The pathogenesis of human viral myocarditis is incompletely understood. Mouse models of myocarditis induced by infection with either coxsackievirus B3 or encephalomyocarditis virus have revealed several possible pathogenetic mechanisms. Susceptibility to coxsackievirus B-induced myocarditis is age-dependent and genetically determined.[118] Mechanisms of injury vary in different mouse strains.[119–122] In susceptible animals acute myocarditis results from direct infection and cytolysis of myocytes.[3,123,124] In surviving animals, neutralizing antibody, perhaps in conjunction with macrophages[125,126] and natural killer (NK) cells,[127] appears to terminate virus replication by 7–9 days after infection.[13,128,129] Exercise[3,13] and corticosteroids[130] markedly enhance mortality during the early stages of infection. Nonsteroidal anti-inflammatory agents may also have deleterious effects,[131] perhaps through inhibition of interferon production.[132] Mice surviving the acute replicative phase of the virus infection may go on to develop severe myocarditis in the absence of recoverable virus. This second phase of virus-induced myocardial destruction is dependent on the presence of cytolytic T cells,[15,133] which appear as productive virus replication

ceases. Some of these cytolytic T cells recognize and lyse both infected and uninfected myocytes,[134] and their presence correlates with myocardial damage.[135,136] The severity of myocardial damage caused by this immune mechanism is greatest in male and in pregnant female mice.[137] In some strains of mice less prone to myocarditis, the cytolytic T-cell response appears to be inhibited by suppressor cells.[138] Variants of coxsackievirus B3 that do not evoke cytolytic T cells directed against both infected and uninfected myocytes fail to cause myocarditis even though they are indistinguishable from myocarditic strains in their ability to replicate and stimulate neutralizing antibodies.[139] Using two strains of coxsackievirus B3 that differ in their ability to produce autoimmunity, Weller et al. demonstrated that the viruses used different receptors for cell entry, indicating that the receptor utilized by a virus may be important in triggering autosensitization.[140] Interleukin-1, tumor necrosis factor, and bacterial lipopolysaccharide all enhance autoimmune injury and cause resistant mice to become susceptible.[141] Data demonstrating enhanced expression of intracellular adhesion molecule-1 in mice and both type I and type II major histocompatibility complex (MHC) antigens in human myocarditis also support the theory that autoimmunity plays a major role in the development of viral myocarditis.[142,142a]

Recent in situ hybridization studies, however, suggest that the enterovirus genome can be found in all stages of acute and chronic infection, and that virus persistence in the heart is characterized by restricted viral RNA and capsid protein synthesis. In mouse strains that developed myocarditis, acute and chronic myocardial lesions were found consistently to be associated with infected myocardial cells, and mouse strains that cleared the virus after acute infection did not develop chronic disease.[143] Whether the persistence of viral genome plays any role in pathogenesis in humans has yet to be determined.

Mice infected with coxsackievirus B3 also develop heart reactive antibodies,[144–146] and these may contribute to myocyte destruction in some strains.[120,147] Of note, Huber et al. have recently demonstrated three monoclonal antibodies to group A streptococcus that also bind to various heart antigens and neutralize a myocarditic strain of coxsackievirus B3.[148]

In human enteroviral infection, direct injury to myocytes appears to play a major role in neonatal infection and some cases of fulminant acute myocarditis in adults.[149] In situ hybridization studies also document the presence of enterovirus genome in 20–30 percent of cases of acute myocarditis and in some cases of dilated cardiomyopathy.[17] Patients with myocarditis also have been found to possess both cytotoxic lymphocytes that react with normal myocytes and high titers of antimyocyte antibodies.[149,152,153]

Another mechanism that may explain the myocardial dysfunction and myocyte necrosis observed in viral myocarditis involves damage to coronary vasculature with luminal narrowing, spasm, and obstruction leading to myocyte ischemia. This has been demonstrated in murine coxsackievirus B3 myocarditis[150] and a similar mechanism appears to underlie the development of dilated cardiomyopathy in some humans after viral or idiopathic myocarditis.

In mouse models of cytomegalovirus myocarditis, genes linked to the H-2 complex influence susceptibility.[151] Cardiac lesions develop in and around the small penetrating blood vessels of the heart. When infected mice are depleted of CD4 and T lymphocytes, myocardial lesions fail to develop even though viral titers may be increased.[154] Cytomegalovirus also induces antibodies that cross react with cardiac myosin.[155] In contrast, in reovirus-induced murine myocarditis, humoral immunity and cellular immunity protect against cardiac damage; myocarditis results from direct virus injury to myocytes.[156]

In acute Chagas disease, pathologic examination often reveals parasites within cardiac myocytes. When rupture of the cysts occurs, there is a marked inflammatory infiltrate consisting of lymphocytes, plasma cells, macrophages, and some eosino-

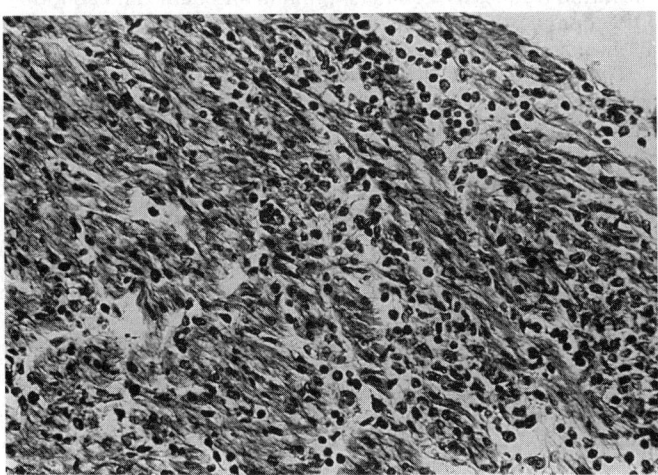

FIG. 1. Coxsackievirus myocarditis with extensive infiltration of mononuclear cells, plasma cells, lymphocytes, and some eosinophils in the interstitial tissue. ($\times$ 250) (From Bloor,[3] with permission.)

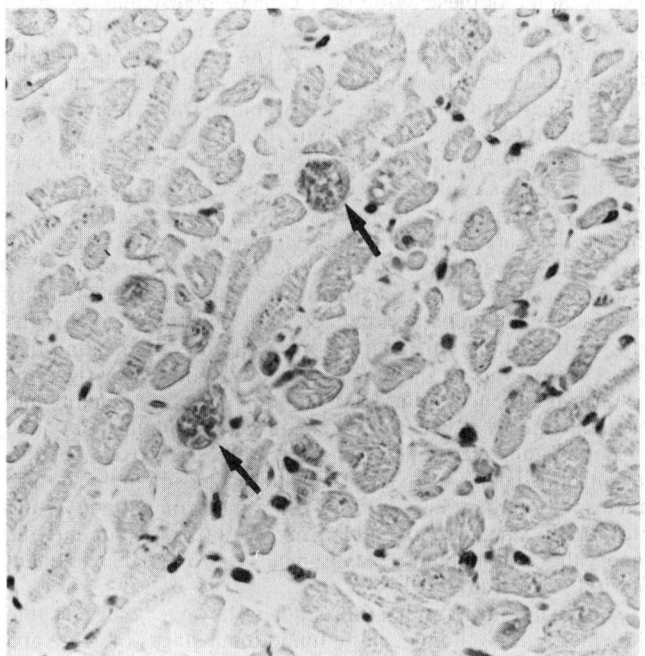

FIG. 2. Cysts of *Toxoplasma gondii* (arrows) are easily visible in the heart of this immunosuppressed patient who died with disseminated toxoplasmosis.

phils.[89,157] In chronic Chagas disease, the heart is often enlarged and flabby. Aneurysm formation may be present at the apex. The conduction system is often also involved, and this is reflected by a high frequency of rhythm disturbances. Microscopic examination reveals focal mononuclear cell infiltrates and fibrosis.[90,157] In this stage, parasites can only be identified in 25 percent of patients.[90] Epitopes shared by *T. cruzi* and cardiac myocytes, and recognized by cytotoxic T cells, may play an important role in the progression of myocarditis late in disease.[158]

The heart, as well as the central nervous system is often prominently involved in disseminated toxoplasmosis. *Toxoplasma* pseudocysts containing numerous organisms may be readily identified in cardiac tissue, and there is a striking absence of cellular response around them (Fig. 2). Rupture of parasitized fibers is followed by infiltration of neutrophils and eosinophils.[157]

Myocardial microabscesses, affecting both myocytes and the conducting system, may occur in the course of systemic bacterial infections with organisms such as *Staphylococcus aureus*, but heart failure is rarely a direct consequence of such lesions.[99] In experimental animals, *Borrelia burgdorferi* has a predilection for connective tissue in the heart base and disease severity correlates with the number of spirochetes found.[159]

Rickettsia and most fungi produce vasculitic lesions with surrounding inflammation. Damage to myocytes may be caused by the adjacent inflammatory process or may reflect anoxia due to occlusion of small blood vessels.

Diphtheria toxin inhibits cellular protein synthesis. This results in hyaline degeneration and necrosis of myocardial fibers, with a secondary inflammatory response.[3,53]

Clinical Manifestations

Patients with myocarditis may be asymptomatic or may have a rapidly progressive fatal disease. The diagnosis of infectious myocarditis is generally considered when a young person develops unexplained heart failure or arrhythmias, or when cardiac abnormalities occur in the course of a recognized systemic infec-

tion. Fever, malaise, arthralgias, upper respiratory tract symptoms, and chest pain may precede or accompany coxsackievirus myocarditis,[149,160] but these symptoms are not specific. Supraventricular tachycardia and ventricular extrasystoles are common.[161] Arrhythmias provide early evidence of involvement of the conduction system and are responsible for the occurrence of sudden death in patients with myocarditis. Myocarditis may mimic acute myocardial infarction,[162–166] but care should be taken not to mistake myocardial infarction occurring in a patient with infection for myocarditis.[167] In acute myocarditis, cardiac enzymes may be elevated and remain so for several days.[168] Symptomatic pericarditis may or may not be present.

Diagnosis

Diagnosis of myocarditis requires a high index of suspicion. In infants, myocarditis is often just one manifestation of a widespread fulminant systemic infection. Involvement of the lungs, liver, and central nervous system, disseminated intravascular coagulation, and circulatory collapse may obscure the clinical signs of cardiac disease.[34,169] Recognition of myocarditis can also present difficulties in older children and adults when it occurs as part of an overwhelming systemic infection. When sought, however, signs of cardiac dysfunction are generally apparent. Even when cardiac signs and symptoms predominate, establishing a firm diagnosis may be difficult.

Nonspecific ST-segment and T-wave abnormalities on electrocardiogram are frequently cited as presumptive evidence of myocarditis. Classically in myocarditis, there are sequential ST-segment elevations and T-wave inversions, which usually resolve in a month or two without the development of Q waves or R-wave depression.[170] The degree of ST-segment elevation and the extent and duration of later T-wave inversion have been reported to correlate with myocardial enzyme release and thus with the amount of cell necrosis.[171] However, similar ST-segment and T-wave changes may also be seen with fever, hypoxia, tachycardia, and electrolyte disturbances, and they frequently occur during uncomplicated childhood viral infection.[172] Failure to reverse such ST-segment and T-wave changes with β-blockade is felt by some to be indicative of myocarditis,[173] but physicians should approach the diagnosis of myocarditis based solely on the presence of nonspecific ST-segment and T-wave abnormalities with skepticism.

Tachycardia out of proportion to the height of the fever, ventricular and supraventricular arrhythmias, and atrioventricular or intraventricular conduction disturbances may also be indicative of myocarditis. In a recent study of 45 patients with active myocarditis, the presence of Q waves in addition to ST-segment elevation frequently heralded a fulminant course and abnormal QRS complexes and left bundle branch block were indicative of an increased risk of sudden cardiac death.[174]

The MB fraction of creatinine kinase is frequently elevated in patients with acute myocarditis and significant ST-segment elevation.[170] Elevated serum levels of troponin T, a component of the myocyte contractile apparatus, provide a more specific indication of myocyte necrosis and appear useful for the diagnosis of myocarditis.[170] In addition, a variety of heart-reactive antibodies have been detected in patients with myocarditis, and their persistence at high titer appears to be a poor prognostic sign. However, the clinical utility of these assays remains to be demonstrated.

Echocardiography is useful in detecting and quantifying impaired systolic function. Inflammation and edema may cause local thickening of the myocardium and regional wall motion abnormalities are often observed.[175–178] Repeated echocardiographic examinations may be used to follow the resolution or progression of myocarditis. Persistent wall motion abnormalities and ventricular dilatation suggest the development of chronic myocarditis or dilated cardiomyopathy, and indicate the need for endomyocardial biopsy (see below).

Indium-111 antimyosin antibody imaging is a promising new technique for the diagnosis of myocarditis. It detects myocardial necrosis rather than inflammation but appears to be more sensitive for diagnosing myocarditis than endomyocardial biopsy.[179–183] Increased myocardial uptake is observed in almost all patients with myocarditis who have positive endomyocardial biopsies, but it is also observed in many comparable patients with negative biopsies.[179–183] A negative indium-111 antimyosin antibody scan is highly predictive of a negative endomyocardial biopsy.[182] However, scans may continue to be positive long after the active phase of myocarditis, and this may account for at least some of the positive scans observed in biopsy-negative patients. However, this highly sensitive test lacks specificity. In one study, 15 of 21 patients with dilated cardiomyopathy had positive scans before cardiac transplantation, but careful examination of their explanted hearts revealed histologic evidence of myocarditis in only 7.[184]

Magnetic resonance imaging (MRI), which can detect small increases in the water content of tissues, has proven reliable in the diagnosis of cardiac allograft rejection.[185,186] Limited experience indicates that MRI provides a sensitive means of detecting acute viral or idiopathic myocarditis, as well.[187] In one study, MRI detected focal myocardial edema in two patients that corresponded anatomically to segmental wall motion abnormalities detected by echocardiography and that normalized after the acute phase.[188] In another study, abnormal myocardial signal intensities indicative of edema were detected in 6 of 6 children with acute myocarditis proven by endomyocardial biopsy, but in none of the 5 biopsy-negative controls.[187] Both MRI and indium-11 antimyosin antibody scans were recently reported to be positive in a patient with endomyocardial biopsy-proven Lyme myocarditis.[189]

The "gold standard" for the premortem diagnosis of myocarditis is endomyocardial biopsy.[190–193] However, biopsy confirmation of the clinical diagnosis of myocarditis has been highly variable, ranging from 16 to 100 percent in different series.[193–198] Results of endomyocardial biopsy have also been highly variable in patients with unexplained congestive heart failure, with evidence of active myocarditis being found in from 2 to 80 percent.[170,190,199–203] Several factors contribute to this variability and make interpretation of the literature difficult. These include lack of uniform clinical and histopathologic criteria for the diagnosis of myocarditis, a high degree of interobserver variability, sampling error, and marked variation in the timing of biopsies with respect to the onset of disease.[117,170,191,204–206] Recent agreement among pathologists on histopathologic criteria for the diagnosis of myocarditis (the *Dallas criteria*) is a helpful development.[207] Scattered small collections of inflammatory cells with focal necrosis of myocytes may occur in response to stress or the administration of vasopressors,[207] and their presence in patients with heart failure may not be indicative of myocarditis. However, a single small focus of myocarditis in the conducting system may be responsible for a fatal arrhythmia in someone without significant myocarditis elsewhere. Timing of endomyocardial biopsy is also critical. Early in enteroviral myocarditis there is necrosis of myocytes but not the lymphocytic infiltration demanded by the Dallas criteria.[208,209] Persistence of myocarditis is also highly variable; in some patients with acute enteroviral or idiopathic myocarditis, histopathologic abnormalities may resolve within a month or two after onset.[163,192]

Dilated cardiomyopathy may, at least in some cases, represent the end stage of viral myocarditis.[5,170,201,210,211] This concept is supported by data from the mouse model, by serial biopsies demonstrating progression to dilated cardiomyopathy in some patients with acute myocarditis, by evidence of active myocarditis in many patients with idiopathic dilated cardiomyopathy who are biopsied soon after the onset of their symptoms, and by the detection of enterovirus RNA in biopsies and explanted hearts.[17,190,191,194,199,210,212–214]

Proof of causation requires the isolation of virus from, or the demonstration of viral proteins or nucleic acids in, the myocardium. Except in neonatal myocarditis and myocarditis occurring in immunocompromised patients, virus has rarely been isolated from cardiac tissue.[17,215] Detection of viral proteins has been difficult, primarily because lack of specificity has led to false-positive results, but the use of antiserum to purified coxsackievirus capsid proteins produced by recombinant DNA technology may overcome this difficulty. To date, diagnosis of viral myocarditis has generally been based on the isolation of virus from another site (e.g., stool), the demonstration of a fourfold or greater rise in antibody titer from acute to convalescent sera, or by the demonstration of a high titer of virus-specific IgM antibody in serum.[13,15,17,149] At best, such data provide only circumstantial evidence of causation of myocarditis and must be interpreted with caution because of the prevalence of asymptomatic infections by the same agents known to cause myocarditis. In a typical prospective study, 26 percent of patients without myocarditis had serologic evidence of infection with agents known to cause myocarditis.[161] These traditional methods have failed to provide a specific diagnosis in most patients with myocarditis of presumed viral etiology.

The development of new techniques for the detection and amplification of viral nucleic acids and their application to cardiac tissue obtained by endomyocardial biopsy is now providing exciting data on the viral etiology of myocarditis and dilated cardiomyopathy.[17,215–218] Cloned DNA fragments complementary to different regions of the enterovirus genome serve as type-specific or broadly cross-reactive hybridization probes or polymerase chain reaction (PCR) primers capable of detecting or amplifying nucleic acid sequences of a specific virus (e.g., coxsackievirus B3) or most of the enteroviruses. In situ hybridization, although somewhat less sensitive than PCR, has the advantage of identifying the specific cells that are infected, whereas PCR can increase the sensitivity of the assay to between 1 and 10 viral genomes per milligram of tissue. Studies carried out to date have yielded interesting, although somewhat confusing results. Overall, enteroviral RNA was detected in approximately 25 percent of specimens from patients with myocarditis and in 15–19 percent of patients with dilated cardiomyopathy.[17,218]

Results from individual studies have varied markedly, however. A large proportion of cases in which coxsackieviruses were implicated serologically did not give positive results by in situ hybridization.[219,220] Furthermore, the cells that contained enteroviral RNA were generally not in areas of myocarditis.[220] Moreover, enteroviral RNA was detected by PCR in cardiac tissue from control patients with a variety of other conditions, including normal heart, although not from noncardiac control tissues.[214] These results raise a number of difficult questions, including the specificity of the assays, the sensitivity and validity of the histopathologic assessments, and the pathogenetic significance of enteroviral RNA in the absence of inflammation or necrosis. Interpretation of such results are even more problematic when the viruses in question are members of the herpesvirus family, which regularly persist in normal persons and which may even be present in the blood.[42]

The criteria for endomyocardial biopsy are evolving. At this time, myocardial biopsy is only clearly indicated in the monitoring of cardiac allograft rejection and anthracycline cardiotoxicity.[170] However, the sensitivity and specificity of PCR, especially when carefully chosen sets of nested primers are used, and the development of antiviral drugs capable of inhibiting enteroviral replication, may eventually justify endomyocardial biopsy during the acute phase of idiopathic myocarditis in patients with positive indium-111 antimyosin antibody scans.

A wide variety of noninfectious diseases and agents may mimic infectious myocarditis and produce identical clinical syndromes (Table 2).

TABLE 2. Noninfectious Causes of Myocarditis

Collagen vascular disease[221–227]
   Systemic lupus erythematosus
   Systemic sclerosis
   Rheumatoid arthritis
   Dermatomyositis/polymyositis
   Still's disease
Thyrotoxicosis[221]
Thrombotic thrombocytopenic purpura[228]
Pheochromocytoma[229]
Peripartum[230]
Radiation-induced[231]
Drug-induced (direct toxic)[232]
   Cocaine
   Alcohol
   Emetine
   Catecholamines
   Arsenic
   Cyclophosphamide
   Daunorubicin
   Adriamycin
Drug-induced (hypersensitivity)[233]
   Methyldopa
   Sulfonamides
   Tetracycline
Scorpion, wasp, and spider stings[229,234]
Agent(s) not yet identified
   Kawasaki disease[235]
   Giant cell myocarditis[236]
   Sarcoid[237]

Treatment

Treatment of myocarditis should be directed at the specific etiologic agent involved whenever possible. Based on inferences from the murine model of coxsackievirus B3 myocarditis, bed rest remains an important part of therapy. Ensuring adequate oxygenation, avoiding and treating fluid overload if it develops, and monitoring for the development of ventricular arrhythmias constitute usual adjunctive care. In severe cases of myocarditis, cardiac assist devices may be lifesaving.[238]

Most patients with viral myocarditis recover completely,[239,240] and the factors that predispose certain patients to a poor outcome are not clear. Glucocorticoids administered during the acute phase of viral myocarditis have been associated with rapid clinical deterioration, and their deleterious effects have been clearly demonstrated in the acute phase of coxsackievirus infection in mice.[130,241] In some uncontrolled trials, patients with myocarditis on endomyocardial biopsy[242,243] or with positive gallium scans[244] who have been given immunosuppressive agents have shown improvement, but others have not,[202,245,246] and interpretation of case reports and uncontrolled trials is very difficult because many patients with acute myocarditis recover spontaneously. In the only double-blind, randomized trial of immunosuppression in myocarditis to date, the American Myocarditis Trial, neither benefit nor harm was demonstrated when a regimen of prednisone and cyclosporine was compared to placebo. In animal models, early therapy with cyclosporine[247] or other immunosuppressive or anti-inflammatory agents[131] increased myocardial damage in some studies. In others, immunosuppressive therapy increased mortality but decreased cardiac pathology when given during the first 3 weeks after experimental infection. No beneficial effects occurred when immunosuppression was given after day 21.[248] Of note, a new antiviral, WIN 54954, has shown some promise in animal models of coxsackievirus B3 myocarditis,[249–251] but data in humans are not yet available. As our knowledge of the pathogenesis of viral myocarditis increases and our ability to detect and identify the agents involved improves, subgroups that might benefit from antiviral therapy or immunosuppression may emerge. Currently, immunosuppressive therapy is not recommended unless patients are enrolled in controlled trials, and antiviral agents effective against the most common offenders are still experimental and unproven.

PERICARDITIS

Pericarditis (inflammation of the pericardium) may be caused by any of a wide variety of infections and noninfectious processes. It may be clinically silent or result in severe hemodynamic compromise and death. In 1892, Sir William Osler called attention to the frequency with which pericarditis was overlooked by the practitioner,[252] and recent series indicate that this is still true today.[253–255] Advances in medicine, including antibiotic therapy, cardiac surgery, hemodialysis, cancer chemotherapy, and organ transplantation, have altered the etiologic spectrum of pericarditis over the course of this century. Idiopathic and viral pericarditis now predominate and usually result in a benign self-limited disease. Purulent bacterial pericarditis and tuberculous pericarditis are now less frequent, but they still cause significant morbidity and mortality, and present a diagnostic challenge.

Etiologic Agents

Because of the difficulty in establishing a specific diagnosis, the etiology of most cases of acute self-limited pericarditis is never determined, and they are classified as idiopathic. In recent series, idiopathic pericarditis accounted for 40–86 percent of patients hospitalized with acute pericarditis.[255–257] There are no clinical or epidemiologic features that distinguish idiopathic pericarditis from acute pericarditis of proven viral etiology. Thus, it is likely that viral infections are responsible for many, if not most, cases of acute pericarditis presently classified as idiopathic.

Most viruses infecting the heart affect both the myocardium and the pericardium (see above). Of the many viruses associated with heart disease, the enteroviruses, especially the coxsackieviruses, are most frequently implicated in pericarditis.[16,258,259] The association of myopericarditis with coxsackieviruses was first demonstrated in neonates with overwhelming fatal systemic infections.[260] Pericarditis has also been recognized in the setting of epidemic coxsackievirus infection.[261,262] A century ago, cases of acute benign pericarditis were recognized during epidemics of Bornholm disease (epidemic pleurodynia), and it was postulated that the etiologic agent of the two diseases was the same.[261] Subsequently, the group B coxsackieviruses were shown to be the principal cause of epidemic pleurodynia, and their etiologic role in the associated cases of pericarditis was well established.[261,262] Coxsackieviruses have only rarely been isolated from pericardial fluid[263,264] and, as with myocarditis, most diagnoses have been based on the isolation of virus from other body sites (e.g., stool) and/or the demonstration of a fourfold or greater rise in antibody titer after the acute illness. A number of other viruses have also been shown to cause pericarditis, but symptomatic involvement of the pericardium is uncommon. When it occurs, it is often a manifestation of severe disseminated infection. Viruses known to cause pericarditis are listed in Table 3.

A wide variety of bacteria can cause pericarditis. In the preantibiotic era, purulent pericarditis occurred primarily as a complication of pneumonia in previously healthy children and adults.[254,291,292,298] Of the 425 cases of purulent pericarditis reported in 1961 by Boyle,[291] 43 percent were associated with pleuropulmonary infections. *Streptococcus pneumoniae* and *Staph. aureus* accounted for more than half of the cases. With the advent of antibiotics, the incidence of purulent pericarditis has decreased markedly. Although staphylococci and streptococci are still etiologic in a substantial number of cases, the incidence of pneumococcal pericarditis has declined substantially, and gram-negative bacilli have assumed a much more important role.[253,254,292,298] Patients with purulent pericarditis are now often older and have an underlying predisposing condition.[253,254,292,298] Purulent pericarditis may occur as a complication of meningococcal meningitis or fulminant meningococ-

TABLE 3. Infectious Causes of Pericarditis

Viruses	
Coxsackie A[265–267]	Epstein-Barr[279–281]
Coxsackie B[16,258,259,261–264]	Varicella-zoster[282]
Echovirus[257,268–271]	Cytomegalovirus[283–287]
Adenovirus[257,266,272–274]	Herpes simplex[288,289]
Mumps[257,275]	Hepatitis B[290]
Influenza[276–278]	

Bacteria	
Streptococcus pneumoniae[291–293]	*Actinomyces* spp.[312,313]
Other *Streptococcus* spp.[294–297]	*Nocardia* spp.[314]
Staphylococcus aureus[291,292,298–300]	*Listeria monocytogenes*[315]
Neisseria meningitidis[301]	*Mycoplasma pneumoniae*[316–319]
Neisseria gonorrhoeae[302,303]	*Legionella pneumophila*[320–324]
Haemophilus influenzae[291,304–306]	*Chlamydia*[325]
Enteric gram-negative rods[292,307,308]	*Borrelia burgdorferi*[79,80,181]
Salmonella spp.[291,309]	*Mycobacterium tuberculosis*[326–331]
Campylobacter spp.[310]	*Mycobacterium avium-*
Brucella spp.[311]	*intracellulare*[332]

Fungi	
Histoplasma capsulatum[333,334]	*Cryptococcus neoformans*[339]
Coccidioides immitis[335–337]	*Candida* spp.[340–342]
Blastomyces dermatitidis[291,338]	*Aspergillus* spp.[298,343–345]

Parasites
Toxoplasma gondii[346–349]
Entamoeba histolytica[350–353]
Schistosomes[354]

cemia, but *Neisseria meningitidis,* especially serogroup C, also causes primary pericarditis.[301] *Mycoplasma pneumoniae* can cause pericarditis, and, although uncommon, this manifestation has been observed in nearly 1 percent of patients hospitalized with this infection.[316–319] *Legionella pneumophila* has been isolated from the pericardial fluid,[320–322] and pericarditis has occurred in association with pneumonia[320–323] and endocarditis.[324] Bacterial infections account for proportionately more pericarditis in children, and after *S. aureus, Haemophilus influenzae* is the second most common etiologic agent.[304] Childhood immunization with *H. influenzae* type b conjugate vaccine has markedly reduced the frequency of *H. influenzae* type b infections in children, and this should result in a comparable reduction in the incidence of *H. influenzae* type b pericarditis.

Acute or chronic pericarditis is reported to occur in approximately 1 percent of patients with pulmonary tuberculosis.[326] Before the AIDS epidemic, because of the declining incidence of primary tuberculosis and the use of effective chemotherapy, *Mycobacterium tuberculosis* accounted for fewer than 5 percent of cases of acute pericarditis in Europe and North America.[256,327,349] In contrast, tuberculous pericarditis is a major cause of heart disease in Africa[355,356] and in patients with AIDS.[105,357,358] Diagnosis is difficult and mortality remains high.[328,359] *Mycobacterium tuberculosis* remains an important treatable cause of chronic pericardial effusion and constrictive pericarditis.[329,355,356,360,361]

Fungi are infrequently recognized as a cause of pericarditis. However, in large recent outbreaks, pericarditis occurred in 6 percent of patients with acute symptomatic histoplasmosis.[333] In most, it appeared to represent a sterile inflammatory response to infection in adjacent mediastinal lymph nodes, and it resolved spontaneously without specific therapy. In disseminated histoplasmosis the pericardium itself may be infected with *Histoplasma capsulatum.*[334] Pericarditis is rarely recognized in acute coccidioidomycosis. Spontaneously resolving cases resembling those seen in acute histoplasmosis have been described,[335] but most reported cases have occurred in the setting of disseminated coccidioidomycosis and represent *Coccidioides immitis* infection of the heart.[336] Fungal pericarditis, (resulting from direct inoculation or extension of mediastinal infection), is seen with increasing frequency as a complication of cardiothoracic surgery.[298] Pericarditis caused by *Candida* spp., *Aspergillus* spp., *Cryptococcus neoformans,* and other fungi occurs as a consequence of disseminated infection in severely debilitated and immunocompromised patients, especially those with prolonged neutropenia receiving multiple courses of antibiotics.[339–343] Per-

icardial effusions occur in 16–40 percent of patients with AIDS.[104,105] Although they are generally idiopathic, a wide variety of viral, bacterial, and fungal agents have been isolated from the pericardial fluid, and malignant effusions have also been observed.[104,358] The rare parasitic causes of pericarditis are referenced in Table 3.

Pathology, Pathogenesis, and Pathophysiology

The pericardium has two opposing mesothelial surfaces. The parietal pericardium forms a flask-shaped sac that encloses the heart and the origins of the great vessels. It consists of a 1-mm thick layer of dense collagen lined by a single layer of mesothelial cells, which are covered by microvilli. The mesothelial cell layer is reflected onto the epicardial surface of the heart to form the visceral pericardium. The parietal pericardium has firm attachments to the sternum, the diaphragm, and the adventitia of the great vessels. The function of the normal pericardium has been a matter of considerable investigation and speculation.[362] It normally contains 15–50 ml of clear fluid, which may act as a lubricant. The pericardium reacts to acute injury by exuding fluid, fibrin, and cells in various combinations.[361] Acute pericarditis may resolve completely or progress to fibrous thickening, with or without constriction.

Cardiotropic viruses generally spread to the myocardium and pericardium hematogenously. Inflammation occurs in both visceral and parietal portions; effusion may develop and be serous, serofibrinous, or serosanguineous. Concomitant myocarditis may or may not be evident. Although most patients with viral pericarditis recover completely, occasional patients have repeated disabling recurrences.[255,363] The pathophysiology of these recurrences has not been established, but it probably involves immunologic mechanisms and not recurrent or persistent virus replication. Rarely, viral pericarditis leads to constriction as a late complication.[364]

Bacterial pericarditis generally results from (1) spread from a contiguous focus of infection within the chest, either de novo or after surgery or trauma; (2) spread from a focus of infection within the heart, most commonly from endocarditis; (3) hematogenous infection; or (4) direct inoculation due to a penetrating injury or cardiothoracic surgery. The incidence of purulent pericarditis arising from a contiguous pneumonia has steadily decreased and now generally occurs only when there has been significant delay in antibiotic therapy.[254,292,293] Pericarditis after cardiothoracic or esophageal surgery often occurs in patients with sternal wound infections and/or mediastinitis[298] and may be overlooked. Mortality is high. Pericarditis not infrequently accompanies fatal endocarditis,[99] especially that caused by *S. aureus.*[64] It often results from extension of a perivalvular abscess into the pericardium.[99] However, pericardial effusions in endocarditis may also be hemorrhagic[365] or sympathetic and sterile.[366] The presence of preexisting nonbacterial pericardial effusion may predispose to the development of purulent pericarditis in bacteremic patients. Although the pericardial fluid may initially be clear,[291,298] it is usually grossly purulent and may be loculated by the time the disease is clinically apparent. Subsequent organization with adhesions, obliteration of the pericardial space, and calcification may occur and result in constrictive pericarditis.

Tuberculous pericarditis may develop from a hematogenous focus present from the time of primary infection, as a result of lymphatic spread from peritracheal, peribronchial, or mediastinal lymph nodes, or by contiguous spread from a focus of infection in lung or pleura. Four pathologic stages in tuberculous pericarditis have been described.[361,367] In the first stage, there is diffuse fibrin deposition, and granulomas with viable mycobacteria are present (Fig. 3). A serous or serosanguineous pericardial effusion then develops, usually quite slowly and often without symptoms. Lymphocytes, monocytes, and plasma cells replace the polymorphonuclear cells present early in infection.

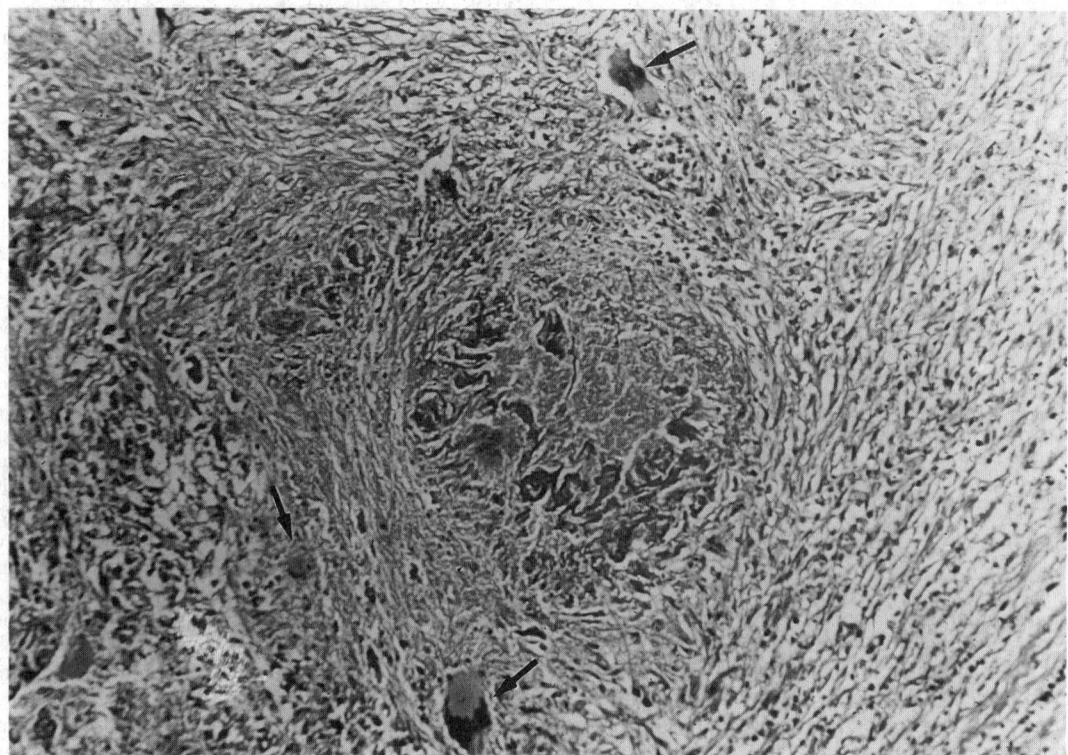

FIG. 3. Tuberculous pericarditis, with a typical granuloma in the pericardium. There is central necrosis with aggregates of epithelioid cells at the periphery. Several multinucleated giant cells (arrows) are present. (× 40) (From Bloor,[3] with permission.)

In the third stage, the effusion is absorbed, the pericardium thickens, granulomas proliferate, and a thick coat of fibrin is deposited on the parietal pericardium. Acid-fast bacilli become difficult to find as dense fibrous tissue and collagen are deposited. In stage four, which is associated with constriction, the pericardial space is obliterated by dense adhesions, the parietal pericardium is markedly thickened, and many granulomas are replaced by fibrous tissue. This is often followed by the accumulation of cholesterol crystals and calcification. Constrictive pericarditis may develop in up to 50 percent of patients with tuberculous pericarditis despite the use of antituberculous chemotherapy.[331,368] Although the incidence of tuberculosis has declined, it remains an important cause of constrictive pericarditis, especially in underdeveloped countries.[355,360,361]

Irrespective of etiology, if fluid accumulates rapidly in the pericardium and intrapericardial pressure rises, cardiac tamponade may result. Tamponade implies a progressive limitation of ventricular diastolic filling, with resultant reduction in stroke volume and cardiac output. In a recent series of medical patients with early cardiac tamponade, the etiology was infectious in 12.5 percent, noninfectious in 74 percent, and undetermined in the remainder.[369]

Clinical Manifestations

The presentation of acute pericarditis varies depending on the etiology. In viral or idiopathic pericarditis, chest pain is an important feature. This pain is often retrosternal, radiating to the shoulder and neck, and typically is aggravated by breathing, swallowing, and lying supine. In Smith's review of coxsackievirus B heart disease in adults,[259] 67 percent of patients had chest pain. Fever was present in 59 percent. A concurrent or prodromal flulike illness with malaise, arthralgias, myalgias, and occasionally cough with sputum was present in 36 percent.

Bacterial pericarditis generally develops in the course of a severe systemic infection.[253,254,298] The patient is usually acutely ill; fever is almost always present and dyspnea is common. However, chest pain is only reported by one-third of patients with purulent pericarditis and a pericardial friction rub, pathognomonic of pericarditis, is also only present in about one-third.[253,254] The symptoms and signs of pericarditis that are present (i.e., fever, dyspnea, and tachycardia), are often attributed to the underlying disease. Consequently, purulent pericarditis is recognized in most patients only at necropsy or after severe hemodynamic compromise has developed.[253,254]

Tuberculous pericarditis most often has an insidious onset. Chest pain is present in 39–76 percent[331] but may be vague in nature. Weight loss, night sweats, cough, and dyspnea are common.

The classic physical finding in acute pericarditis is the three-component pericardial friction rub, which reflects cardiac motion during atrial systole, ventricular systole, and rapid ventricular filling in early diastole. This three-component rub was present in 50 percent of patients with acute pericarditis reported by Spodick.[370] The ventricular systolic component is often the loudest and most frequently appreciated. Rubs are often evanescent and may vary in quality; they are characteristically high-pitched, scratching, or grating. In the presence of significant pericardial effusion, there may be jugular venous distension, the most common physical finding in acute cardiac tamponade. Enlargement of the cardiac silhouette usually does not occur until at least 250 ml of fluid have accumulated in the pericardial space;[371] if fluid accumulates rapidly, tamponade may occur without detectable cardiomegaly. A pulsus paradoxus of more than 10 mmHg and a prominent x descent with loss of the y descent in the jugular venous pressure may present. Dyspnea is common, but signs of left heart failure are usually absent in cardiac tamponade, and clear lung fields may help to differentiate tamponade from cardiogenic shock.

Although the pericardium produces no electrical activity, the electrocardiogram (ECG) is abnormal in 90 percent of patients with acute pericarditis,[371] reflecting diffuse subepicardial inflammation. Characteristic ECG changes are seen in approximately 50 percent of patients.[372,373] Early in pericarditis, ST segment elevation without change in QRS morphology typically occurs in multiple leads. Several days later, the ST segment returns to baseline, and there is T-wave flattening. During these early stages, there may also be depression of the PR segment. In contrast to myocardial infarction, the T-wave inversions in pericarditis do not generally occur until after the ST segment has returned to baseline. These T-wave inversions may last for weeks or months. Large pericardial effusions may be associated with reduced QRS voltage and electrical alternans. Sinus tachycardia is common, but the presence of other arrhythmias suggests preexisting underlying heart disease or significant myocardial involvement.[374]

Echocardiography has been proved to be an extremely useful tool for diagnosis of pericardial effusion and should be performed if the situation is not immediately life-threatening. The size of the effusion can be roughly quantitated, and early hemodynamic compromise can often be detected.[371] Computed tomography has been useful in demonstrating pericardial thickening and, in some cases, in differentiating an uncomplicated transudate from a high-density exudate.[375,376] Magnetic resonance imaging techniques also can easily detect pericardial fluid and thickening[377] but have no particular advantage over echocardiography.

Diagnosis

A wide variety of agents and diseases may cause pericarditis and pericardial effusion (Tables 3 and 4). Low-grade fever is common to many. A careful history, knowledge of the clinical setting in which the pericarditis occurs, and a search for clues outside the cardiovascular system are helpful in establishing a diagnosis. In a young person without underlying illness who presents with acute pericardial pain, the most likely diagnosis is viral or idiopathic pericarditis. However, establishing a specific viral diagnosis is difficult, costly, and often possible only in retrospect. Virus isolation can be attempted from throat and stool, and acute and convalescent sera can be tested for antibodies to potential pathogens (e.g., the coxsackie B viruses and any other enteroviruses prevalent locally at the time), but these approaches frequently fail to yield a specific diagnosis. Viruses are rarely isolated from pericardial fluid, even in patients in whom the diagnosis of viral myocarditis is highly probable.

If the clinical suspicion of viral or idiopathic pericarditis is strong in an otherwise healthy patient with uncomplicated peri-

carditis, pericardiocentesis or other invasive procedures add little diagnostically[349] and carry a small but definite risk.[398] After excluding patients with postpericardiotomy syndrome, myocardial infarction, renal failure, known neoplastic disease, trauma, and irradiation, Soler-Soler et al.[256] prospectively evaluated 256 immunocompetent patients with primary acute pericardial disease. After thorough diagnostic evaluation, 221 (86 percent) were felt to have acute idiopathic pericarditis. Unsuspected neoplastic pericarditis was found in 12 (5 percent), tuberculosis in 11 (4 percent), and collagen vascular disease in 4. Purulent pericarditis and viral pericarditis were each found in 3 patients, and *Toxoplasma gondii* infection was found in 4 patients. The diagnostic yield was substantial when pericardiocentesis or pericardiectomy with biopsy were done to relieve cardiac tamponade (28 percent and 54 percent, respectively), but it was only 5 and 4 percent, respectively, when these procedures were done solely for the purpose of diagnosis. The authors concluded that the presence of a pericardial effusion per se is not an indication for an invasive procedure; in patients with pericardial effusion that has persisted for more than 3 weeks, an invasive procedure may be indicated.

Untreated purulent pericarditis is usually rapidly fatal.[298] In acutely ill patients in whom purulent pericarditis is suspected, the diagnosis should be pursued quickly and aggressively. When possible, pericardiotomy with biopsy and drainage is preferable to pericardiocentesis because of greater diagnostic yield and fewer complications.[371] Noninfectious diseases predominate as causes of significant pericardial effusion and cardiac tamponade,[369] but bacterial and tuberculous effusions are more likely to have serious hemodynamic consequences.[398]

Treatment

Bed rest, symptomatic therapy for pain, and careful monitoring for the development of hemodynamic compromise are the mainstays of treatment for presumed viral or idiopathic pericarditis. Nonsteroidal anti-inflammatory agents are often successful in relieving symptoms. Because myocarditis often accompanies viral pericarditis and steroids enhance myocardial injury during active virus replication, we believe that steroids should be avoided during the acute illness. Viral or idiopathic pericarditis is generally benign and self-limited, but recurrences[363] and late constriction[364] do occur.

Surgical drainage of the pericardium, in addition to appropriate antibiotic therapy, is essential in almost all patients with purulent pericarditis.[291,298,304] Initial pericardiocentesis may be lifesaving, but fluid often reaccumulates, and constriction can develop rapidly.[298,304] There is little rationale for irrigating the pericardium with antibiotics, because penetration from serum is excellent.[399] With early diagnosis and aggressive therapy, *H. influenzae* pericarditis in young patients has a good prognosis.[304] However, overall mortality in bacterial pericarditis remains high, especially when it develops after surgery or occurs in the course of endocarditis.[298]

The treatment of tuberculous pericarditis remains controversial. Antituberculous therapy has reduced mortality substantially.[400] The addition of steroids to reduce inflammation and avoid late constriction is favored by many, including the authors.[356,360] The use of corticosteroids, in addition to antituberculous therapy, is supported by the results of two large controlled trials in Transkei reported by Strang et al.[356,360] In patients with tuberculosis pericardial effusions, the addition of prednisone to a four-drug antituberculosis regimen reduced the risk of death, the need for repeat pericardiocentesis, and the need for open surgical drainage because of rapid reaccumulation of pericardial fluid. Constrictive pericarditis developed in 8 percent of steroid recipients and 12 percent of controls.[356] In a similar trial in patients with active tuberculous constrictive pericarditis, the addition of prednisone increased the rate of clinical improvement.[360] Early surgical intervention is advocated in pa-

TABLE 4. Major Noninfectious Causes of Acute Pericarditis

Acute myocardial infarction[378-380]
Uremia[381,382]
Neoplasia[371]
Primary
Metastatic
Postirradiation[383,384]
Postcardiac injury[385]
Trauma (penetrating or blunt)[371]
Postmyocardial infarction (Dresslers)[386]
Postpericardiotomy[387]
Dissecting aortic aneurysm[371,388]
Sarcoidosis[389]
Collagen vascular diseases
Systemic lupus erythematosus[390]
Rheumatoid arthritis[391-393]
Scleroderma[394,395]
Rheumatic fever[391]
Inflammatory bowel disease[396]
Drug-induced[371]
Procainamide
Hydralazine
Other
Myxedema[397]

tients with hemodynamic compromise from recurrent effusion or progressive pericardial thickening.[368,400]

REFERENCES

1. Saphir O. Myocarditis: A general review with an analysis of two hundred and forty cases. Arch Pathol. 1941;32:1000–51 and 1942;33:88–137.
2. Gravanis MG, Sterby NH. Incidence of myocarditis. Arch Pathol Lab Med. 1991;115:390–2.
3. Bloor CM. Pericarditis and myocarditis. In: Cardiac Pathology. Philadelphia: JB Lippincott; 1978:265–95.
4. Bandt CM, Staley NA, Noren GR. Acute viral myocarditis: Clinical and histological changes. Minn Med. 1979;62:234–7.
5. Sole MJ, Lui P. Viral myocarditis: A paradigm for understanding the pathogenesis and treatment of dilated cardiomyopathy. J Am Coll Cardiol. 1992;22(Suppl A):99A–105A.
6. Bengtsson E, Orndahl G. Complications of mumps with special reference to the incidence of myocarditis. Acta Med Scand. 1954;149:381–8.
7. Lucke B, Wight T, Kime E. Pathologic anatomy and bacteriology of influenza: Epidemic of autumn 1918. Arch Intern Med. 1919;24:154–237.
8. Degen JA Jr. Visceral pathology in measles; clinicopathologic study of 100 fatal cases. Am J Med Sci. 1937;194:104–11.
9. Lucke B. Postmortem findings in measles bronchopneumonia and other acute infections. JAMA. 1918;70:2006–11.
10. Frustaci A, Abdulla AK, Caldarulo M, et al. Fatal measles myocarditis. Cardiologia. 1990;35:347–9.
11. Saphir O, Wile SA. Myocarditis in poliomyelitis. Am J Med Sci. 1942;203:781–8.
12. Sylvest E. Epidemic Myalgia: Bornholm Disease. London: Oxford University Press; 1934.
13. Reyes MP, Lerner AM. Coxsackievirus myocarditis—with special reference to acute and chronic effects. Prog Cardiovasc Dis. 1985;27:373–94.
14. Hirschman SZ, Hammer GS. Coxsackie virus myopericarditis. A microbiological and clinical review. Am J Cardiol. 1974;34:224–32.
15. Woodruff JF. Viral myocarditis. Am J Pathol. 1980;101:427–78.
16. Grist NR, Bell EJ. A six-year study of coxsackievirus B infections in heart disease. J Hyg Camb. 1974;73:165–72.
17. Hyypia T. Etiologic diagnosis of viral heart disease. Scand J Infect Dis. 1993;88(Suppl):25–31.
18. Russell SJM, Bell EJ. Echoviruses and carditis. Lancet. 1970;1:784–5.
19. Bell EJ, Grist NR. ECHO viruses, carditis and acute pleurodynia. Am Heart J. 1971;82:133–8.
20. Jungeblut CW, Edwards JE. Isolation of poliomyelitis virus from the heart in fatal cases. Am J Clin Pathol. 1951;21:601–23.
21. Weinstein L, Shelokov A. Cardiovascular manifestations in acute poliomyelitis. N Engl J Med. 1951;244:281–5.
22. Roberts WC, Fox III SM. Mumps of the heart: Clinical and pathological features. Circulation. 1965;32:342–5.
23. Chaudary S, Jaski BE. Fulminant mumps myocarditis. Ann Intern Med. 1989;110:569–70.
24. Hamburger WW. The heart in influenza. Med Clin North Am. 1938;22:111–21.
25. Verel D, Warrack AJN, Potter CW, et al. Observations on the A2 England influenza epidemic. A clinicopathological study. Am Heart J. 1976;92:290–6.
26. Ross E, Armentrout SA. Myocarditis associated with rabies. Report of a case. N Engl J Med. 1962;266:1087–9.
27. Ainger LE, Lawyer NG, Fitch CW. Neonatal rubella myocarditis. Br Heart J. 1966;28:691–7.
28. Kriseman T. Rubella myocarditis in a 9 year old patient. Clin Pediatr. 1984;23:240–1.
29. Chuah SK. Transient ventricular arrhythmia as a cardiac manifestation in dengue haemorrhagic fever—a case report. Singapore Med J. 1987;28:569–72.
30. Obeyesekere I, Hermon Y. Myocarditis and cardiomyopathy after arbovirus infections (dengue and chikungunya fever). Br Heart J. 1972;34:821–7.
31. Cannell DE. Myocardial degenerations in yellow fever. Am J Pathol. 1928;4:431–43.
32. Milei J, Bolomo NJ. Myocardial damage in viral hemorrhagic fevers. Am Heart J. 1982;104:1385–91.
33. Thiede WH. Cardiac involvement in lymphocytic choriomeningitis. Arch Intern Med. 1962;109:50–4.
34. Henson D, Mufson MA. Myocarditis and pneumonitis with type 21 adenovirus infection: Association with fatal myocarditis and pneumonitis. Am J Dis Child. 1971;121:334–6.
35. Karjalainen J, Heikkila J, Nieminen MS, et al. Etiology of mild acute infectious myocarditis. Relation to clinical features. Acta Med Scand. 1983;213:65–73.
36. Waagner DC, Murphy TV. Varicella myocarditis. Pediatr Infect Dis J. 1990;9:360–3.
37. Woolf PK, Chung T-S, Stewart J, et al. Life-threatening dysrhythmias in varicella myocarditis. Clin Pediatr. 1987;26:480–2.
38. Coppack SW, Doshi R, Ghose AR. Fatal varicella in a healthy young adult. Postgrad Med J. 1985;61:529–31.
39. Tiula E, Leinikki P. Fatal cytomegalovirus infection in a previously healthy boy with myocarditis and consumption coagulopathy as presenting signs. Scand J Infect Dis. 1972;4:57–60.
40. Maisch B, Schonian U, Crombach M, et al. Cytomegalovirus associated inflammatory heart muscle disease. Scand J Infect Dis. 1993;88:135–48.
41. Millett R, Tomita T, Marshall HE, et al. Cytomegalovirus endomyocarditis in a transplanted heart. A case report with in situ hybridization. Arch Pathol Lab Med. 1991;115:511–5.
42. Schonian U, Crombach M, Maisch B. Assessment of cytomegalovirus DNA and protein expression in patients with myocarditis. Clin Immunol Immunopathol. 1993;68:229–33.
43. Ando H, Shiramizu T, Hisanou R. Dilated cardiomyopathy caused by cytomegalovirus infection in a renal transplant recipient. Jpn Heart J. 1992;33:409–12.
44. Arbustini E, Grasso M, Diegoli M, et al. Histopathologic and molecular profile of human cytomegalovirus infections in patients with heart transplants. Am J Clin Pathol. 1992;98:205–13.
45. Webster BH. Cardiac complications of infectious mononucleosis: A review of the literature and report of five cases. Am J Med Sci. 1957;234:62–70.
46. Tyson AA Jr, Hackshaw BT, Kutcher MA. Acute Epstein-Barr virus myocarditis simulating myocardial infarction with cardiogenic shock. S Med J. 1989;82:1184–7.
47. Matthews AW, Griffiths ID. Post vaccinal pericarditis and myocarditis. Br Heart J. 1974;36:1043–5.
48. Anderson T, Foulis MA, Grist NR, et al. Clinical and laboratory observations in a smallpox outbreak. Lancet. 1951;1:1248–52.
49. Mahapatra RK, Ellis GH. Myocarditis and hepatitis B virus. Angiology. 1985;36:116–9.
50. Bell H. Cardiac manifestations of viral hepatitis. JAMA. 1971;218:387–91.
51. Ursell PC, Habib A, Sharma P, et al. Hepatitis B virus and myocarditis. Hum Pathol. 1984;15:481–4.
52. Gore I, Saphir O. Myocarditis. A classification of 1402 cases. Am Heart J. 1947;34:827–30.
53. Gore I. Myocardial changes in fatal diphtheria; summary of observations in 221 cases. Am J Med Sci. 1948;215:257–66.
54. Havaldar PV, Patil VD, Siddibhavi BM, et al. Fulminant diptheretic myocarditis. Indian Heart J 1989;41:265–9.
55. Roberts WC, Berard CW. Gas gangrene of the heart in clostridial septicemia. Am Heart J. 1967;74:482–8.
56. Guneratne F. Gas gangrene (abscess) of heart. NY State J Med. 1975;75:1766.
57. Joshi MK, Kandoth PW, Barve RJ, et al. Rheumatic fever: Clinical profile of 339 cases with long term follow up. Indian Pediatr. 1983;20:849–53.
58. Karjalainen J. Streptococcal tonsillitis and acute nonrheumatic myopericarditis. Chest. 1989;95:359–63.
59. Brasier AR, Macklis JD, Vaughan D, et al. Myopericarditis as an initial presentation of meningococcemia. Unusual manifestation of infection with serotype W135. Am J Med. 1987;82:641–4.
60. Cohen JI, Bartlett JA, Corey GR. Extra-intestinal manifestations of Salmonella infections. Medicine. 1987;66:349–88.
61. Wamder GS, Khurana SB, Puri S. Salmonella myopericarditis presenting with acute pulmonary oedema. Indian Heart J. 1992;44:55–6.
62. Lubani M, Sharda D, Helin I. Cardiac manifestations in brucellosis. Arch Dis Child. 1986;61:569–72.
63. Jubber AS, Gunawardana DR, Lulu AR. Acute pulmonary edema in Brucella myocarditis and interstitial pneumonitis. Chest. 1990;97:1008–9.
64. Watanakunakorn C, Tan JS, Phair JP. Some salient features of Staphylococcus aureus endocarditis. Am J Med. 1973;54:473–81.
65. Tice AD, Nelson JS, Visconti EB. Listeria monocytogenes pericarditis and myocardial abscess. RI Med J. 1979;62:135–8.
66. McCue MJ, Moore EE. Myocarditis with microabscess formation caused by Listeria monocytogenes associated with myocardial infarct. Hum Pathol. 1979;10:469–72.
67. Stamm AM, Smith SH, Kirklin JK, et al. Listerial myocarditis in cardiac transplantation. Rev Infect Dis. 1990;12:820–3.
68. Armengol S, Domingo C, Mesalles E. Myocarditis: A rare complication during Legionella infection. Int J Cardiol. 1992;27:418–20.
69. Chen S-C, Tsai CC, Nouri S. Carditis associated with Mycoplasma pneumoniae infection. AJDC. 1986;140:471–2.
70. Lind K. Manifestation and complications of Mycoplasma pneumoniae disease: A review. Yale J Biol Med. 1983;56:461–8.
71. Karjalainen J. A loud third heart sound and asymptomatic myocarditis during Mycoplasma pneumoniae infection. Eur Heart J. 1990;11:960–3.
72. Dymock IW, Lawson JM, MacLennan WJ, et al. Myocarditis associated with psittacosis. Br J Clin Pract. 1971;25:240–2.
73. Gran JT, Hjetland R, Andreassen AH. Pneumonia, myocarditis and reactive arthritis due to Chlamydia pneumoniae. Scand J Rheumatol. 1993;22:43–4.
74. Wesslen LP, Pahlson C, Friman G, et al. Myocarditis caused by Chlamydia pneumoniae (TWAR) and sudden unexpected death in a Swedish elite orienteer (Letter). Lancet. 1992;340:427–8.
75. Marin-Garcia J, Mirvis DM. Myocardial disease in Rocky Mountain spotted fever: Clinical, functional, and pathologic findings. Pediatr Cardiol. 1984;5:149–54.
76. Brown GW, Shirai A, Jegathesan M, et al. Febrile illness in Malaysia—an analysis of 1629 hospitalized patients. Am J Trop Med Hyg. 1984;33:311–5.
77. Ognibene AJ, O'Leary DS, Czarnecki SW, et al. Myocarditis and disseminated intravascular coagulation in scrub typhus. Am J Med Sci. 1971;262:233–9.
78. Diab SM, Araj GF, Fenech FF. Cardiovascular and pulmonary complications of epidemic typhus. Trop Geog Med. 1989;41:76–9.

79. Steere AC, Batsford WP, Weinberg M, et al. Lyme carditis: Cardiac abnormalities of Lyme disease. Ann Intern Med. 1980;93:8–16.
80. McAlister HF, Klementowicz PT, Andrews C, et al. Lyme carditis: An important cause of reversible heart block. Ann Intern Med. 1989;110:339–45.
81. van der Linde MR. Lyme carditis: Clinical characteristics of 105 cases. Scand J Infect Dis. 1991;77:81–4.
82. Williams AH. Aspergillus myocarditis. Am J Clin Pathol. 1974;61:247–56.
83. Atkinson JB, Connor DH, Robinowitz M, et al. Cardiac fungal infections: Review of autopsy findings in 60 patients. Hum Pathol. 1984;15:935–42.
84. Rogers JG, Windle JR, McManus BM, et al. Aspergillus myocarditis presenting as myocardial infarction with complete heart block. Am Heart J. 1990; 120:430–2.
85. Cox JN, Di Dio F, Pizzolato G-P, et al. Aspergillus endocarditis and myocarditis in a patient with the acquired immunodeficiency syndrome (AIDS): A review of the literature. Virchows Arch A Pathol Anat. 1990;417:255–9.
86. Lewis W, Lipsick J, Cammarosano C. Cryptococcal myocarditis in acquired immune deficiency syndrome. Am J Cardiol. 1985;9:1240.
87. Lafont A, Wolff M, Marche C, et al. Overwhelming myocarditis due to Cryptococcus neoformans in an AIDS patient. Lancet. 1987;2:1145–6.
88. Hofman P, Drici MD, Gibelin P, et al. Prevalence of toxoplasma myocarditis in patients with the acquired immunodeficiency syndrome. Br Heart J. 1993; 70:376–81.
89. Rosenbaum MB. Chagasic myocardiopathy. Prog Cardiovasc Dis. 1964;7: 199–255.
90. Mott KE, Hagstrom JWC. The pathologic lesions of the cardiac autonomic nervous system in chronic Chagas' myocarditis. Circulation. 1965;31:273–86.
91. Mendoza I, Camardo J, Moleiro F, et al. Sustained ventricular tachycardia in chronic Chagasic myocarditis. Am J Cardiol. 1986;57:423–7.
92. Poltera AA, Owor R, Cox JN. Pathological aspects of human African trypanosomiasis in Uganda. Virchows Arch [A] 1977;373:249–65.
93. Barr R. Human trichinosis: Report of 4 cases with emphasis on central nervous system involvement and a survey of 500 consecutive autopsies at the Ottawa Civic Hospital. Can Med Assoc J. 1966;95:912–7.
94. Grey DF, Morse BS, Phillips WF. Trichinosis with neurologic and cardiac involvement. Review of the literature and report of three cases. Ann Intern Med. 1962;57:230–44.
95. Compton SJ, Celum CL, Lee C, et al. Trichinosis with ventilatory failure and persistent myocarditis. Clin Infect Dis. 1993;16:500–4.
96. Yermakov V, Rashid RK, Vuletin JC, et al. Disseminated toxoplasmosis. Case report and review of the literature. Arch Pathol Lab Med. 1982;106: 524–8.
97. Matturri L, Quattrone P, Varesi C, et al. Cardiac toxoplasmosis in pathology of acquired immunodeficiency syndrome. Panminerva Med. 1990;32:194–6.
98. Israelski DM, Remington JS. Toxoplasmosis in the non-AIDS immunocompromised host. Cur Clin Topics Infect Dis. 1993;13:322–56.
99. Buchbinder NA, Roberts WC. Left-sided valvular active infective endocarditis. A study of 45 necropsy patients. Am J Med. 1972;53:20–35.
100. Welch K, Finkbeiner W, Alpers CE, et al. Autopsy findings in the acquired immune deficiency syndrome. JAMA. 1984;252:1152–9.
101. Baroldi G, Carallo S, Moroni M, et al. Focal lymphocytic myocarditis in acquired immunodeficiency syndrome (AIDS): A correlative morphologic and clinical study in 26 consecutive fatal cases. J Am Coll Cardiol. 1988;12: 463–9.
102. Cammarosano C, Lewis W. Cardiac lesions in acquired immune deficiency syndrome (AIDS). J Am Coll Cardiol. 1985;5:703–6.
103. Fink L, Reichek N, St. John Sutton MG. Cardiac abnormalities in acquired immune deficiency syndrome. Am J Cardiol. 1984;54:1161–3.
104. Kaul S, Fishbein MC, Siegel RJ. Cardiac manifestations of acquired immune deficiency syndrome: A 1991 update. Am Heart J. 1991;122:537–44.
105. De Castro S, Migliau G, Silvestri A, et al. Heart involvement in AIDS: A prospective study during various stages of the disease. Eur Heart J. 1992; 13:1452–9.
106. Calabrese LH, Proffitt MR, Yen-Lieberman B, et al. Congestive cardiomyopathy and illness related to the acquired immunodeficiency syndrome (AIDS) associated with isolation of retrovirus from myocardium. Ann Intern Med. 1987;107:691–2.
107. Dittrich H, Chow L, Denaro F, et al. Human immunodeficiency virus, coxsackievirus, and cardiomyopathy (Letter). Ann Intern Med. 1988;108:308–9.
108. Factor S, Flomenbaum M, Vdem S, et al. Proliferative membranopathy and human immunodeficiency virus in AIDS hearts (Abstract). Circulation. 1989; 80(Suppl II):II–535.
109. Grody W, Cheng L, Pang M, et al. Direct infection of the heart by human immunodeficiency virus (HIV) (Abstract). Circulation. 1989;80(Suppl II): II–665.
110. Beschorner WE, Baughman K, Turnicky RP, et al. HIV-associated myocarditis: Pathology and immunopathology. Am J Pathol. 1990;137:1365–71.
111. Wu TC, Pizzorno MC, Hayward GS, et al. In situ detection of human cytomegalovirus immediate-early gene transcripts within cardiac myocytes of patients with HIV-associated cardiomyopathy. AIDS. 1992;6:777–85.
112. Herskowitz A, Ansori A, Neumann D, et al. Cardiomyopathy in acquired immunodeficiency syndrome: Evidence for autoimmunity. Circulation. 1989; 80(suppl)II–322.
113. Parravicini C, Baroldi G, Gaiera G, et al. Phenotype of intramyocardial leukocytic infiltrates in acquired immunodeficiency syndrome (AIDS): A postmortem immunohistochemical study in 34 consecutive cases. Mod Pathol. 1991;4:559–65.
114. Mues B, Brisse E, Zwadlo G, et al. Phenotyping of macrophages with monoclonal antibodies in endomyocardial biopsies as a new approach to diagnosis of myocarditis. Eur Heart J 1990;11:619–27.
115. Chow LH, Ye Y, Linder J, et al. Phenotypic analysis of infiltrating cells in human myocarditis. An immunohistological study in paraffin-embedded tissue. Arch Pathol Lab Med. 1989;113:1357–62.
116. Keogh AM, Billingham ME, Schroeder JS. Rapid histological changes in endomyocardial biopsy specimens after myocarditis. Br Heart J. 1990;64: 406–8.
117. Edwards WD. Myocarditis and endomyocardial biopsy. Cardiol Clin. 1984; 2:647–56.
118. Lyden D, Olszewski J, Huber S. Variation in susceptibility of BALB/c mice to coxsackievirus group B type 3-induced myocarditis with age. Cell Immunol. 1987;105:332–9.
119. Herskowitz A, Wolfgram LJ, Rose NR, et al. Coxsackievirus B$_3$, murine myocarditis: A pathologic spectrum of myocarditis in genetically defined inbred strains. J Am Coll Cardiol. 1987;9:1311–9.
120. Huber SA, Lodge PA. Coxsackievirus B-3 myocarditis. Identification of different pathogenic mechanisms in DBA/2 and BALB/c mice. Am J Pathol. 1986;122:284–91.
121. Wolfgram LJ, Beisel KW, Herskowitz A, et al. Variations in the susceptibility to coxsackievirus B$_3$-induced myocarditis among different strains of mice. J Immunol. 1986;136:1846–52.
122. Khatib R, Probert A, Reyes MP, et al. Mouse strain-related variation as a factor in the pathogenesis of coxsackievirus B3 murine myocarditis. J Gen Virol. 1987;68:2981–8.
123. Chow LH, Beisel KW, McManus BM. Enteroviral infection of mice with severe combined immunodeficiency. Evidence for direct viral pathogenesis of myocardial injury. Lab Invest. 1992;66:24–31.
124. McManus BM, Chow LH, Wilson JE, et al. Direct myocardial injury by enterovirus: A central role in the evolution of murine myocarditis. Clin Immunol Immunopathol. 1993;68:159–69.
125. Rager-Zisman B, Allison AC. The role of antibody and host cells in the resistance of mice against infection by coxsackie B-3 virus. J Gen Virol. 1973;19:329–38.
126. Woodruff JF. Lack of correlation between neutralizing antibody production and suppression of coxsackievirus B-3 replication in target organs: Evidence for involvement of mononuclear inflammatory cells in host defense. J Immunol. 1979;123:31–6.
127. Godeny EK, Gauntt CJ. In situ immune autoradiographic identification of cells in heart tissue of mice with coxsackievirus B3-induced myocarditis. Am J Pathol. 1987;129:267–76.
128. Godeny EK, Gauntt CJ. Murine natural killler cells limit coxsackievirus B3 replication. J Immunol. 1987;139:913–8.
129. Godeny EK, Gauntt CJ. Involvement of natural killer cells in coxsackievirus B3-induced murine myocarditis. J Immunol. 1986;137:1695–702.
130. Kilbourne ED, Wilson CB, Perrier D. The induction of gross myocardial lesions by a coxsackie (pleurodynia) virus and cortisone. J Clin Invest. 1956; 35:362–70.
131. Rezkalla S, Khatib G, Khatib R. Coxsackievirus B3 murine myocarditis: Deleterious effects of nonsteroidal anti-inflammatory agents. J Lab Clin Med. 1986;107:393–5.
132. Khatib R, Reyes MP, Smith F, et al. Enhancement of coxsackievirus B4 virulence by indomethacin. J Lab Clin Med. 1990;116:116–20.
133. Kishimoto C, Abelmann WH. In vivo significance of T cells in the development of coxsackievirus B3 myocarditis in mice. Immature but antigen-specific T cells aggravate cardiac injury. Circ Res. 1990;67:589–98.
134. Huber SA, Lodge PA. Coxsackievirus B-3 myocarditis in BALB/c mice. Evidence for autoimmunity to myocyte antigens. Am J Pathol. 1984;116: 21–9.
135. Guthrie M, Lodge PA, Huber SA. Cardiac injury in myocarditis induced by coxsackievirus group B, type 3 in BALB/c mice is mediated by Lyt 2$^+$ cytolytic lymphocytes. Cell Immunol. 1984;88:558–67.
136. Kishimoto C, Kuribayashi K, Masuda T, et al. Immunologic behavior of lymphocytes in experimental viral myocarditis: Significance of T lymphocytes in the severity of myocarditis and silent myocarditis in BALB/c-nu/nu mice. Circulation. 1985;71:1247–54.
137. Lyden DC, Huber SA. Aggravation of coxsackievirus, group B, type 3-induced myocarditis and increase in cellular immunity to myocyte antigens in pregnant BALB/c mice and animals treated with progesterone. Cell Immunol. 1984;87:462–72.
138. Job LP, Lyden DC, Huber SA. Demonstration of suppressor cells in coxsackievirus group B, type 3 infected female BALB/c mice which prevent myocarditis. Cell Immunol. 1986;98:104–13.
139. Huber SA, Job LP. Differences in cytolytic T cell response of BALB/c mice infected with myocarditic and non-myocarditic strains of coxsackievirus group B, type 3. Infect Immun. 1983;39:1419–27.
140. Weller AH, Simpson K, Herzum M, et al. Coxsackie-virus-B3-induced myocarditis: Virus receptor antibodies modulate myocarditis. J Immunol. 1989; 143:1843–50.
141. Lane JR, Neumann DA, Lafond-Walker A, et al. Role of IL-1 and tumor necrosis factor in coxsackievirus-induced autoimmune myocarditis. J Immunol. 1993;151:1682–90.
142. Seko Y, Matsuda H, Kato K, et al. Expression of intercellular adhesion molecule-1 in murine hearts with acute myocarditis caused by coxsackievirus B3. J Clin Invest. 1993;91:1327–36.
142a. Herskowitz A, Admed-Ansari A, Neumann DA, et al. Induction of major histocompatibility complex antigens within the myocardium of patients with

active myocarditis: A nonhistologic marker of myocarditis. J Amer Col Cardiol. 1990;15:624–32.

143. Kandolf R, Klingel K, Zell R, et al. Molecular pathogenesis of enterovirus-induced myocarditis: Virus persistence and chronic inflammation. Intervirology. 1993;35:140–51.

144. Wolfgram LJ, Beisel KW, Rose NR. Heart-specific autoantibodies following murine coxsackievirus B₃ myocarditis. J Exp Med. 1985;161:1112–21.

145. Neu N, Beisel KW, Traystman MD, et al. Autoantibodies specific for the cardiac myosin isoform are found in mice susceptible to coxsackievirus B3-induced myocarditis. J Immunol. 1987;138:2488–92.

146. Gauntt C, Higdon A, Bowers D, et al. What lessions can be learned from animal model strudies in viral heart disease? Scand J Infect Dis. 1993;Suppl 88:49–65.

147. Neu N, Rose NR, Beisel KW, et al. Cardiac myosin induces myocarditis in genetically predisposed mice. J Immunol. 1987;139:3630–6.

148. Huber S, Polgar J, Moraska A, et al. T-lymphocyte responses in CVR3-induced murine myocarditis. Scand J Infect Dis. 1993;Suppl 88:67–78.

149. See DM, Tilles JG. Viral myocarditis. Rev Infect Dis. 1991;13:951–6.

150. Silver MA, Kowalczyk BS. Coronary microvascular narrowing in acute murine coxsackie B3 myocarditis. Am Heart J. 1989;118:173–4.

151. Lawson CM, O'Donoghue H, Bartholomaeus WN, et al. Genetic control of mouse cytomegalovirus-induced myocarditis. Immunology. 1990;69:20–6.

152. Maisch B, Bauer E, Cirsi M, et al. Cytolytic cross-reactive antibodies directed against the cardiac membrane and viral proteins in coxsackievirus B3 and B4 myocarditis. Characterization and pathogenetic relevance. Circulation 1993;87(Suppl 5):IV49–65.

153. Herzum M, Maisch B. Humoral and cellular immune reactions to the myocardium in myocarditis. Herz. 1992;17:91–6.

154. Craighead JE, Martin WB, Huber SA. Role of CD4 + (helper) T cells in the pathogenesis of murine cytomegalovirus myocarditis. Lab Invest. 1992;66:755–61.

155. Lawson CM, O'Donoghue HL, Reed WD. Mouse cytomegalovirus infection induces antibodies which cross-react with virus and cardiac myosin: A model for the study of molecular mimicry in the pathogenesis of viral myocarditis. Immunology 1992;75:513–9.

156. Sherry B, Li XY, Tyler KL, et al. Lymphocytes protect against and are not required for reovirus-induced myocarditis. J Virol. 1993;67:6119–24.

157. Bloor CM. Protozoal, helminthic and fungal heart disease. In: Cardiac Pathology. Philadelphia: JB Lippincott; 1978:335–66.

158. Felix JC, von Kreuter BF, Santos-Buch CA. Mimicry of heart cell surface epitopes in primary anti-*Trypanosoma cruzi* lyt 2+ T lymphocytes. Clin Immunol Immunopathol. 1993;68:141–6.

159. Armstrong A, Barthold SW, Persing DH, et al. Carditis in Lyme disease: Susceptible and resistant strains of laboratory mice infected with *Borrelia burgdorferi*. Am J Trop Med Hyg. 1992;47:249–58.

160. Abelmann WH. Virus and the heart. Circulation. 1971;44:950–6.

161. Vikerfors T, Stjerna A, Olcen P, et al. Acute myocarditis. Serologic diagnosis, clinical findings and follow-up. Acta Med Scand. 1988;223:45–52.

162. Stratmann HG. Acute myocarditis versus myocardial infarction: Evaluation and management of the young patient with prolonged chest pain—case reports. Angiology. 1988;39:253–8.

163. Miklozek CL, Crumpacker CS, Royal HD, et al. Myocarditis presenting as acute myocardial infarction. Am Heart J. 1988;115:768–76.

164. Spodick DH. Infection and infarction. Acute viral (and other) infection in the onset, pathogenesis, and mimicry of acute myocardial infarction. Am J Med. 1986;81:661–8.

165. Beaufils P, Slama R. Myocarditis confirmed by biopsy presenting as acute myocardial infarction. Br Heart J. 1986;4:420.

166. Dec GW Jr, Waldman H, Southern J, et al. Viral myocarditis mimicking acute myocardial infarction (See comments). J Am Coll Cardiol. 1992;20:85–9.

167. Griffiths PD, Hannington G, Booth JC. Coxsackie B virus infections and myocardial infarction. Results from a prospective, epidemiologically controlled study. Lancet. 1980;1:1387–9.

168. Heikkila J, Karjalainen J. Evaluation of mild acute infectious myocarditis. Br Heart J. 1982;47:381–91.

169. Kaplan MH, Kelin SW, McPhee J, et al. Group B coxsackievirus infection in infants younger than three months of age: A serious childhood illness. Rev Infect Dis. 1983;5:1019–32.

170. Karjalainen J. Clinical diagnosis of myocarditis and dilated cardiomyopathy. Scand J Infect Dis. 1993;Suppl 88:33–43.

171. Karjalainen J, Heikkila J. Acute pericarditis: Myocardial enzyme release as evidence for myocarditis. Am Heart J. 1986;111:546.

172. Scott LP III, Gutelius MF, Parrott RH. Children with acute respiratory tract infections. An electrocardiographic survey. Am J Dis Child. 1970;119:111–3.

173. Karjalainen J. Functional and myocarditis-induced T-wave abnormalities: Effect of orthostasis, beta blockade, and epinephrine. Chest. 1983;83:868–72.

174. Morgera T, Di Lenarda A, Dreas L, et al. Electrocardiography of myocarditis revisited: Clinical and prognostic significance of electrocardiographic changes. Am Heart J. 1992;124:455–67.

175. Weinhouse E, Wanderman KL, Sofer S, et al. Viral myocarditis simulating dilated cardiomyopathy in early childhood: Evaluation by serial echocardiography. Br Heart J. 1986;56:94–7.

176. Nieminen MS, Heikkila J, Karjalainen J. Echocardiography in acute infectious myocarditis: Relation to clinical and electrocardiographic findings. Am J Cardiol. 1984;53:1331–7.

177. Kondo M, Takahashi M, Shimono Y, et al. Reversible asymmetric septal

hypertrophy in acute myocarditis. Serial findings of two-dimensional echocardiogram and thallium-201 scintigram. Jpn Circ J. 1985;49:589–93.

178. Pinamonti B, Alberti E, Cigalotto A, et al. Echocardiographic findings in myocarditis. Am J Cardiol. 1988;62:285–91.

179. Yasuda T, Palacios IF, Dec W, et al. Indium-111 monoclonal antimyosin antibody imaging in the diagnosis of acute myocarditis. Circulation. 1987;76:306–11.

180. Carrio I, Berna L, Ballester M, et al. Indium-111 antimyosin scintigraphy to assess myocardial damage in patients with suspected myocarditis and cardiac rejection. J Nucl Med. 1988;29:1893–900.

181. Casans I, Villar A, Almenar V, et al. Lyme myocarditis diagnosed by indium-111 antimyosin scintigraphy. Eur J Nucl Med. 1989;15:330–1.

182. Dec W, Palacios I, Yasuda T, et al. Antimyosin antibody cardiac imaging: Its role in the diagnosis of myocarditis. J Am Coll Cardiol. 1990;16:97–104.

183. Nakata T, Gotoh M, Noto T, et al. Quantification of antimyosin uptake and infarct size at various stages of myocardial infarction. Int J Cardiol. 1992;34:85–95.

184. Obrador D, Ballester M, Carrio I, et al. Active myocardial damage without attending inflammatory response in dilated cardiomyopathy. J Am Coll Cardiol. 1993;21:1667–71.

185. Aherne T, Tscholakoff D, Finkbeiner W, et al. Magnetic resonance imaging of cardiac transplants: The evaluation of rejection of cardiac allografts with and without immunosuppression. Circulation. 1986;74:145–56.

186. Sasaki H, Sada M, Nishimura T, et al. The expanded scope of effectiveness of nuclear magnetic resonance imaging to determine cardiac allograft rejection. Transplant Proc. 1987;19:1062–4.

187. Gagliardi MG, Bevilacqua M, Di Renzi P, et al. Usefulness of magnetic resonance imaging for diagnosis of acute myocarditis in infants and children, and comparison with endomyocardial biopsy. Am J Cardiol. 1991;68:1089–91.

188. Chandraratna AN, Nimalasuriya A, Reid CL, et al. Left ventricular asynergy in acute myocarditis. Simulation of acute myocardial infarction. JAMA. 1983;250:1428–30.

189. Bergler-Klein J, Sochor H, Stanek G, et al. Indium 111-monoclonal antimyosin antibody and magnetic resonance imaging in the diagnosis of acute Lyme myopericarditis. Arch Intern Med. 1993;153:2696–700.

190. O'Connel JB, Mason JW. Diagnosing and treating active myocarditis. West J Med. 1989;150:431–5.

191. Peters NS, Poole-Wilson PA. Myocarditis—continuing clinical and pathologic confusion. Am Heart J. 1991;121:942–7.

192. Billingham ME. The safety and utility of endomyocardial biopsy in infants, children and adolescents. J Am Coll Cardiol. 1990;15:443–5.

193. Fowles RE, Mason JW. Endomyocardial biopsy. Ann Intern Med. 1982;97:885–94.

194. Nippoldt TB, Edwards WD, Holmes DR, et al. Right ventricular endomyocardial biopsy. Clinicopathologic correlates in 100 consecutive patients. Mayo Clin Proc. 1982;57:407–18.

195. Parrillo JE, Aretz HT, Palacios I, et al. The results of transvenous endomyocardial biopsy can frequently be used to diagnose myocardial diseases in patients with idiopathic heart failure. Endomyocardial biopsies in 100 consecutive patients revealed a substantial incidence of myocarditis. Circulation. 1984;69:93–101.

196. Takahashi O, Kamiya T, Echigo S, et al. Myocarditis in children—clinical findings and myocardial biopsy findings. Jpn Circ J. 1983;47:1298–303.

197. Vasiljevic JD, Kanjuh V, Seferovic P, et al. The incidence of myocarditis in endomyocardial biopsy samples from patients with congestive heart failure. Am Heart J. 1990;120:1370–1377.

198. Herskowitz A, Campbell S, Deckers J. Demographic features and prevalence of idiopathic myocarditis in patients undergoing endomyocardial biopsy. Am J Cardiol. 1993;71:982–6.

199. Dec GW, Palacios IF, Fallon JT, et al. Active myocarditis in the spectrum of acute dilated cardiomyopathies. Clinical features, histologic correlates, and clinical outcome. N Engl J Med. 1985;312:885–90.

200. Zee-Cheng C-S, Tsai CC, Palmer DC, et al. High incidence of myocarditis by endomyocardial biopsy in patients with idiopathic congestive cardiomyopathy. J Am Coll Cardiol. 1984;3:63–70.

201. Fenoglio JJ, Ursell PC, Kellogg CF, et al. Diagnosis and classification of myocarditis by endomyocardial biopsy. N Engl J Med. 1983;308:12–8.

202. Mason JW, Billingham ME, Ricci DR. Treatment of acute inflammatory myocarditis assisted by endomyocardial biopsy. Am J Cardiol. 1980;45:1037–44.

203. Chow LC, Dittrich HC, Shabetai R. Endomyocardial biopsy in patients with unexplained congestive heart failure. Ann Intern Med. 1988;109:535.

204. Shanes JG, Ghali J, Billingham ME, et al. Interobserver variability in the pathologic interpretation of endomyocardial biopsy results. Circulation. 1987;75:401–5.

205. Billingham M. Acute myocarditis: A diagnostic dilemma. Br Heart J. 1987;58:6–8.

206. Kereiakes DJ, Parmley WW. Myocarditis and cardiomyopathy. Am Heart J. 1984;108:1318–26.

207. Aretz HT, Billingham ME, Edwards WD, et al. Myocarditis, a histopathologic definition and classification. Am J Cardiovasc Pathol. 1987;1:3–14.

208. Morita H, Kitaura Y, Deguchi H, et al. Coxsackie B5 myopericarditis in a young adult. Clinical course and endomyocardial biopsy findings. Jpn Circ J. 1983;47:1077–83.

209. Fukuhara T, Konoshita M, Bito K, et al. Myopericarditis associated with echovirus type 3 infection. A case report. Jpn Circ J. 1983;47:1274–80.

210. Friman G, Fohlman J. The epidemiology of viral heart disease. Scand J Infect Dis. 1993;88(Suppl):7–10.
211. Kawai C, Matsumori A, Fujiwara H. Myocarditis and dilated cardiomyopathy. Annu Rev Med. 1987;38:221–39.
212. Kopecky SL, Gersh BJ. Dilated cardiomyopathy and myocarditis: Natural history, etiology, clinical manifestations, and management. In: O'Rourke RA, Crawford MH, eds. Current Problems in Cardiology. Chicago: Year Book Medical Publishers, Inc.; 1987;569–647.
213. Lowry BS. Viruses and heart disease: A problem in pathogenesis. Ann Clin Lab Sci. 1986;16:358–64.
214. Weiss LM, Liu XF, Chang KL, et al. Detection of enteroviral RNA in idiopathic dilated cardiomyopathy and other human cardiac tissues. J Clin Invest. 1992;90:156–9.
215. Weinstein C, Fenoglio JJ. Myocarditis. Hum Pathol. 1987;18:613–8.
216. Rotbart HA, Eastman PS, Ruth JL, et al. Nonisotopic oligomeric probes for the human enteroviruses. J Clin Microbiol. 1988;26:2669–71.
217. Erlich HA, Gelfand DH, Saiki RK. Specific DNA amplification. Nature. 1988;331:461–2.
218. Schwaiger A, Umlauft F, Weyrer K, et al. Detection of enteroviral ribonucleic acid in myocardial biopsies from patients with idiopathic dilated cardiomyopathy by polymerase chain reaction. Am Heart J. 1993;126:406–10.
219. Tracy S, Wiegand V, McManus B, et al. Molecular approaches to enteroviral diagnosis in idiopathic cardiomyopathy and myocarditis. J Am Coll Cardiol. 1990;15:1688–94.
220. Easton AJ, Eglin RP. The detection of coxsackievirus RNA in cardiac tissue by *in situ* hybridization. J Gen Virol. 1988;69:285–91.
221. Fowler NO. The secondary cardiomyopathies. In: Fowler NO. Myocardial Disease. New York: Grune & Stratton; 1973;337–59.
222. Bank I, Marboe CC, Redberg RF, et al. Myocarditis in adult Still's disease. Arthritis Rheum. 1985;28:452–4.
223. Vintila M, Tanaseanu S, Luca R, et al. Is cardiac involvement in collagen diseases important? A clinical study in 917 patients. Med Int. 1990;28:219–27.
224. Goldenberg J, Ferraz MB, Pessoa AP, et al. Symptomatic cardiac involvement in juvenile rheumatoid arthritis. Int J Cardiol. 1992;34:57–62.
225. Askari AD, Huettner TL. Cardiac abnormalities in polymyositis/dermatomyositis. Sem Arthritis Rheum. 1982;12:208–19.
226. Tami LF, Bhasin S. Polymorphism of the cardiac manifestations in dermatomyositis. Clin Cardiol. 1993;16:260–4.
227. Clemson BS, Miller WR, Luck JC, et al. Acute myocarditis in fulminant systemic sclerosis. Chest. 1992;101:872–4.
228. Webb JG, Butany J, Langer G, et al. Myocarditis and myocardial hemorrhage associated with thrombotic thrombocytopenic purpura. Arch Int Med. 1990; 150:1535–7.
229. Myocarditis. In: Braunwald E, ed. Heart Disease, a Textbook of Cardiovascular Medicine. 3rd ed. Philadelphia: WB Saunders; 1988:1440–69.
230. Midei MG, DeMent SH, Feldman AM, et al. Peripartum myocarditis and cardiomyopathy. Circulation 1990;81:922–8.
231. Ikaheimo MJ, Niemela KO, Linnaluoto MM, et al. Early cardiac changes related to radiation therapy. Am J Cardiol. 1988;56:943–6.
232. Isner JM, Chokshi SK. Cardiac complications of cocaine abuse. Ann Rev Med. 1991;42:133–8.
233. Taliercio CP, Olney BA, Lie JT. Myocarditis related to drug hypersensitivity. Mayo Clin Proc. 1985;60:463–8.
234. Brand A, Keren A, Kerem E, et al. Myocardial damage after a scorpion sting: Long-term echocardiographic follow-up. Pediatr Cardiol. 1988;9: 59–61.
235. Matsuura H, Ishikita T, Yamamoto S, et al. Gallium-67 myocardial imaging for the detection of myocarditis in the acute phase of Kawasaki disease (mucocutaneous lymph node syndrome): The usefulness of single photon emission computed tomography. Br Heart J. 1987;58:385–92.
236. Humbert P, Faivre R, Fellman D, et al. Giant cell myocarditis: An autoimmune disease? Am Heart J. 1988;115:485–7.
237. Temple-Camp CR. Sarcoid myocarditis: A report of three cases. N Z Med J. 1989;102:501–2.
238. Moreno-Cabral CE, Moreno-Cabral RJ, McNamara JJ, et al. Prolonged extracorporeal circulation for acute myocarditis. Int J Art Organs. 1992;15: 475–80.
239. Hayakawa M, Inoh T, Yokota Y, et al. A long-term follow-up study of acute viral and idiopathic myocarditis. Jpn Circ J. 1983;47:1304–9.
240. Remes J, Helin M, Vaino P, et al. Clinical outcome and left ventricular function 23 years after acute coxsackie virus myopericarditis. Eur Heart J. 1990;11:182–8.
241. Tomioka N, Kishimoto C, Matsumori A, et al. Effects of prednisolone on acute viral myocarditis in mice. J Am Coll Cardiol. 1986;7:868–72.
242. Ettinger J, Feucht H, Gartner R, et al. Cyclosporine A (CyA) for successful treatment of myocarditis (Letter). Eur Heart J. 1986;7:452.
243. Chan KY, Iwahara M, Benson LM, et al. Immunosuppressive therapy in the management of acute myocarditis in children: A clinical trial. J Am Coll Cardiol. 1991;17:458–60.
244. O'Connell JB, Robinson JA, Henkin RE, et al. Immunosuppressive therapy in patients with congestive cardiomyopathy and myocardial uptake of gallium-67. Circulation. 1981;64:780–6.
245. Hosenpud JD, McAnulty JH, Niles NR. Lack of objective improvement in ventricular systolic function in patients with myocarditis treated with azathioprine and prednisone. J Am Coll Cardiol. 1985;6:797–801.
246. Salvi A, Di Lenarda A, Dreas L, et al. Immunosuppressive treatment in myocarditis. Int J Cardiol. 1989;22:329–38.
247. Monrad ES, Matsumori A, Murphy JC, et al. Therapy with cyclosporine in experimental murine myocarditis with encephalomyocarditis virus. Circulation. 1986;73:1058–64.
248. Kishimoto C, Thorp KA, Abelmann WH. Immunosuppression with high doses of cyclophosphamide reduces the severity of myocarditis but increases the mortality in murine coxsackievirus B3 myocarditis. Circulation. 1990; 82:982–9.
249. Woods MG, Diana GD, Rogge MC, et al. In vitro and in vivo activities of WIN 54954, a new broad-spectrum antipicornavirus drug. Antimicrob Agents Chemother. 1989;33:2069–74.
250. Pauksen K, Ilback NG, Friman G, et al. Therapy of coxsackievirus B3-induced myocarditis with WIN 54954 in different formulations. Scand J Infect Dis. 1993;88(Suppl):125–30.
251. See DM, Tilles JG. Treatment of coxsackievirus A9 myocarditis in mice with WIN 54954. Antimicrob Agents Chemother. 1993;36:425–8.
252. Osler W. The Principles and Practice of Medicine. New York: D Appleton; 1892.
253. Sagrista-Sauleda J, Barrabes JA, Permanyer-Miralda G, et al. Purulent pericarditis: Review of a 20 year experience in a general hospital. J Am Coll Cardiol. 1993;22:1661–5.
254. Park S, Bayer AS. Purulent pericarditis. Curr Clin Topics Infect Dis. 1992; 12:56–82.
255. Ilan Y, Oren R, Ben-Chetrit E. Acute pericarditis: Etiology, treatment and prognosis. Jpn Heart J. 1991;32:315–21.
256. Soler-Soler J, Permanyer-Miralda G, Sagrista-Sauleda J. A systematic diagnostic approach to primary acute pericardial disease. The Barcelona experience. Cardiol Clin. 1990;8:609–20.
257. Johnson RT, Portnoy B, Rogers NG, et al. Acute benign pericarditis: Virologic study of 34 patients. Arch Intern Med. 1961;108:823.
258. Koontz CH, Ray CG. The role of coxsackie group B virus infections in sporadic myopericarditis. Am Heart J. 1971;82:750–8.
259. Smith WG. Coxsackie B myopericarditis in adults. Am Heart J. 1970;80: 34–46.
260. Montgomery J, Gear JHS, Prinslou FR, et al. Myocarditis of the newborn. An outbreak in a maternity home in Southern Rhodesia associated with coxsackie group-B virus infection. S Afr Med J. 1955;29:608–12.
261. Bain HW, McLean DM, Walker SJ. Epidemic pleurodynia (Bornholm disease) due to coxsackie B5 virus. Pediatrics. 1961;27:889–902.
262. Helin M, Savola J, Lapinleimu K. Cardiac manifestations during a coxsackie B5 epidemic. Br Med J. 1968;2:97–9.
263. Brodie HR, Marchessault V. Acute benign pericarditis caused by coxsackie virus group B. N Engl J Med. 1960;262:1278–80.
264. Kagan H, Bernkopf H. Pericarditis caused by coxsackie virus B. Ann Pediatr. 1957;189:44–50.
265. Grist NR, Bell EJ. Coxsackie viruses and the heart. Am Heart J. 1969;77: 295–300.
266. Van Reken D, Strauss A, Henandez A, et al. Infectious pericarditis in children. J Pediatr. 1974;85:165–9.
267. Movitt ER, Lenette EH, Mangum JF, et al. Acute benign pericarditis: Report of 2 cases associated with group A and group B coxsackie viruses. N Engl J Med. 1958;158:1082–6.
268. Russell SJM, Bell EJ. Echoviruses and carditis. Lancet. 1970;1:784–5.
269. Celers J, Celers P, Bertocchi A. Non-polio enterovirus in France from 1974 to 1985. Pathol Biol. 1988;36:1221.
270. Grist NR, Beil EJ, Assaad F. Enteroviruses in human disease. Prog Med Virol. 1978;24:114–57.
271. Roberts R. Viral pericarditis. Med Serv J Can. 1961;17:588.
272. Canas JA, Balsam D, Leggiadro RJ. Adenovirus pericarditis. NY State J Med. 1986;86:269–70.
273. Nahmias AJ, Griffith D, Snitzer J. Fatal pneumonia associated with adenovirus type 7. Am J Dis Child. 1967;114:36–41.
274. Odio C, McCracken GH Jr, Nelson JD. Disseminated adenovirus infection: A case report and review of the literature. Pediatr Infect Dis. 1984;3:46–9.
275. Kleinfeld M, Milles S, Lidsky M. Mumps pericarditis: Review of the literature and report of a case. Am Heart J. 1958;55:153–6.
276. Proby CM, Hacket D, Gupta S, et al. Acute myopericarditis in influenza A infection. Q J Med. 1986;60:887–92.
277. Adams CW. Postviral myopericarditis associated with the influenza virus: Report of 8 cases. Am J Cardiol. 1959;4:56–67.
278. Hildenbrandt HM, Maassab HF, Willis PW III. Influenza virus pericarditis: Report of a case with isolation of Asian influenza virus from the pericardial fluid. Am J Dis Child. 1962;104:579.
279. Cheng TC. Severe chest pain due to infectious mononucleosis. Postgrad Med. 1983;73:149–52.
280. Shugoll GI. Pericarditis associated with infectious mononucleosis. Arch Intern Med. 1957;100:630–4.
281. Satoh T, Kojima M, Ohshima K. Demonstration of the Epstein-Barr genome by the polymerase chain reaction and in situ hybridization in a patient with viral pericarditis. Br Heart J. 1993;69:563–4.
282. Williams AJ, Freemont AJ, Barnett DB. Pericarditis and arthritis complicating chickenpox. Br J Clin Pract. 1983;37:226–7.
283. Kassab A, Demoulin JC, Vanlancker MA, et al. Cytomegalovirus hemopericarditis. Report of 1 case with histologic confirmation. Acta Cardiol. 1987; 42:69–72.
284. Martin V, Miranda ML, Stiefel P, et al. Acute pericarditis caused by cytomegalovirus in a normal host (Letter). Enferm Infec Microbiol Clin. 1989;7: 515.

285. Nathan PE, Arsura EL, Zappi M. Pericarditis with tamponade due to cytomegalovirus in the acquired immunodeficiency syndrome. Chest. 1991;99: 765–6.

286. Powell KF, Bellamy AR, Catton MG. Cytomegalovirus myocarditis in a heart transplant recipient: Sensitive monitoring of viral DNA by the polymerase chain reaction. J Heart Transplant. 1989;8:465–70.

287. Scott PJ, Conway SP, Da Costa P. Cardiac tamponade complicating cytomegalovirus pericarditis in a patient with AIDS. J Infect. 1990;20:92.

288. Freedberg RS, Gindea AJ, Dieterich DT, et al. Herpes simplex pericarditis in AIDS. NY State J Med. 1987;87:304–6.

289. Toma E, Poisson M, Claessens MR, et al. Herpes simplex type 2 pericarditis and bilateral facial palsy in a patient with AIDS (Letter). J Infect Dis. 1989; 160:553–4.

290. Adler R, Takahashi M, Wright, Jr. HT. Acute pericarditis associated with hepatitis B infection. Pediatrics. 1978;61:716–9.

291. Boyle JD, Pearce ML, Guze LB. Purulent pericarditis: Review of literature and report of eleven cases. Medicine. 1961;40:119–44.

292. Klacsmann PG, Bulkley BH, Hutchins GM. The changed spectrum of purulent pericarditis. An 86 year autopsy experience in 200 patients. Am J Med. 1977;63:666–73.

293. Kauffman CA, Watanakunakorn C, Phair JP. Purulent pneumococcal pericarditis. A continuing problem in the antibiotic era. Am J Med. 1973;54: 743–50.

294. Pruitt JL. Group A streptococcal pericarditis in a previously well child (Letter). Pediatr Infect Dis J. 1989;8:338.

295. Karikm MA, Bach RG, Dressler F, et al. Purulent pericarditis caused by group B streptococcus with pericardial tamponade. Am Heart J. 1993;126: 727–30.

296. Halverson KC, Van Etta LL, Langager JH. Group G streptococcal purulent pericarditis. A case report. Minn Med. 1991;74:27–9.

297. Hirata K, Asato H, Maeshiro M. A case of effusive constrictive pericarditis caused by Streptococcus milleri. Jpn Circ J. 1991;55:154–8.

298. Rubin RH, Moellering RC. Clinical, microbiologic and therapeutic aspects of purulent pericarditis. Am J Med. 1975;59:68–78.

299. Kopec JS, Grifka RG, Karpawich PP. Isolated staphylococcal pericarditis following varicella in an adolescent: An unusual age-associated complication. Pediatr Emerg Care. 1990;6:38–9.

300. Demey HE, Eycken M, Vandermast M. Purulent pericarditis due to methicillin-resistant Staphylococcus aureus. A case report. Acta Cardiol. 1991; 46:485–91.

301. Blaser MJ, Reingold AL, Alsever RN, et al. Primary meningococcal pericarditis: A disease of adults associated with serogroup C Neisseria meningitidis. Rev Infect Dis. 1984;6:625–32.

302. Coe MD, Hamer DH, Levy CS, et al. Gonococcal pericarditis with tamponade in a patient with systemic lupus erythematosus. Arthritis Rheum. 1990; 33:1438–41.

303. Wilson J, Zaman AG, Simmons AV. Gonococcal arthritis complicated by acute pericarditis and pericardial effusion. Br Heart J. 1990;63:134–5.

304. Fyfe DA, Hagler DJ, Puga FJ, et al. Clinical and therapeutic aspects of Haemophilus influenzae pericarditis in pediatric patients. Mayo Clin Proc. 1984;59:415–22.

305. Schwartz KV, Guercio CA, Katz A. Haemophilus influenza pericarditis. Conn Med. 1987;51:423–4.

306. Welikovitch L, Knight JL, Burggraf GW, et al. Cardiac tamponade secondary to haemophilus pericarditis: A case report. Can J Cardiol. 1992;8:303–5.

307. Corachan M, Poore P, Hadley GP, et al. Purulent pericarditis in Papua New Guinea: Report of 12 cases and review of the literature in a tropical environment. Trans R Soc Trop Med Hyg. 1983;77:341–3.

308. Lecomte F, Eustache M, Lemeland JF, et al. Purulent pericarditis due to Yersinia enterocolitica (Letter). J Infect Dis. 1989;159:363.

309. Sanchez-Guerrero J, Alarcon-Segovia D. Salmonella pericarditis with tamponade in systemic lupus erythematosus. Br J Rheumatol. 1990;29:69–71.

310. Morrison VA, Lloyd BK, Chia JK, et al. Cardiovascular and bacteremic manifestations of Campylobacter fetus infection: Case report and review. Rev Infect Dis. 1990;12:387–92.

311. Ugartemendia MC, Curos-Abadal A, Pujol-Rakosnik M, et al. Brucella melitensis pericarditis. Am Heart J. 1985;109:1108.

312. Ramsdale DR, Gautam PC, Perera B, et al. Cardiac tamponade due to actinomycosis. Thorax. 1984;39:473–4.

313. O'Sullivan RA, Armstrong JG, Rivers JT, et al. Pulmonary actinomycosis complicated by effusive constrictive pericarditis. Aust N Z J Med. 1991;21: 879–80.

314. Poland GA, Jorgensen CR, Sarosi GA. Nocardia asteroides pericarditis: Report of a case and review of the literature (See comments). Mayo Clin Proc. 1990;65:819–24.

315. Ferguson R, Yee S, Finkle H, et al. Listeria-associated pericarditis in an AIDS Patients. J Natl Med Assoc. 1991;85:225–8.

316. Linz DH, Tolle SW, Elliott DL. Mycoplasma pneumoniae pneumonia. Experience at a referral center. West J Med. 1984;140:895–900.

317. Ponka A. The occurrence and clinical picture of serologically verified Mycoplasma pneumoniae infections with emphases on central nervous system, cardiac and joint manifestations. Ann Clin Res. 1979;24:1–60.

318. Sands MJ, Satz JE, Turner WE Jr, et al. Pericarditis and perimyocarditis associated with active Mycoplasma pneumoniae infection. Ann Intern Med. 1977;86:544–8.

319. Balaguer A, Boronat M, Carrascosa A. Successful treatment of pericarditis associated with Mycoplasma pneumoniae infection. Pediatr Infect Dis J. 1990;9:141–3.

320. Maycock R, Skale B, Kohler RB. Legionella pneumophila pericarditis proved by culture of pericardial fluid. Am J Med. 1983;75:534–6.

321. Reyes RR, Noble RC. Legionnaires' pericarditis. J Ky Med Assoc. 1983;81: 757–8.

322. Luck PC, Helbig JH, Wunderlich E, et al. Isolation of Legionella pneumophila serogroup 3 from pericardial fluid in a case of pericarditis. Infection. 1989;17:388–90.

323. Svendsen JH, Jonsson V, Niebuhr U. Combined pericarditis and pneumonia caused by Legionella infection. Br Heart J 1987;58:663–4.

324. Friedland L, Snydman DR, Weingarden AS, et al. Ocular and pericardial involvement in Legionnaires' disease. Am J Med 1984;77:1105–7.

325. Odeh M, Oliven A. Chlamydial infections of the heart. Eur J Clin Microbiol Infect Dis. 1992;11:885–93.

326. Larrieu AJ, Tyers GFO, Williams EH, et al. Recent experience with tuberculous pericarditis. Ann Thorac Surg. 1980;29:464–8.

327. Sagrista-Sauleda J, Permanyer-Miralda G, Soler-Soler J. Tuberculous pericarditis: Ten year experience with a prospective protocol for diagnosis and treatment. J Am Coll Cardiol. 1988;11:724–8.

328. Rooney JJ, Crocco JA, Lyons HA. Tuberculous pericarditis. Ann Intern Med. 1970;72:73–8.

329. Desai HN. Tuberculous pericarditis. A review of 100 cases. S Afr Med J. 1979;55:877–80.

330. Dalli E, Quesada A, Juan G, et al. Tuberculous pericarditis as the first manifestation of acquired immunodeficiency syndrome. Am Heart J. 1987;114: 905–6.

331. Ortbals DW, Avioli LV. Tuberculous pericarditis. Arch Intern Med. 1979; 139:231–4.

332. Woods GL, Goldsmith JC. Fatal pericarditis due to Mycobacterium avium-intracellulare in acquired immunodeficiency syndrome. Chest. 1989;95: 1355–7.

333. Wheat LJ, Stein L, Corya BC, et al. Pericarditis as a manifestation of histoplasmosis during two large urban outbreaks. Medicine. 1983;62:110–9.

334. Young EJ, Vainrub B, Musher DM. Pericarditis due to histoplasmosis. JAMA. 1978;240:1750.

335. Larson R, Scherb RI. Coccidioidal pericarditis. Circulation. 1953;7:211–7.

336. Chapman MG, Kaplan L. Cardiac involvement in coccidioidomycosis. Am J Med. 1957;23:87–98.

337. Amundson DE. Perplexing pericarditis caused by coccidioidomycosis. So Med J. 1993;86:694–6.

338. Witorsch P, Utz JP. North American blastomycosis: A study of 40 patients. Medicine (Balt). 1968;47:169–200.

339. Duvall CP, Carbone PP. Cryptococcus neoformans pericarditis associated with Hodgkin's diseases. Ann Intern Med. 1966;64:850–6.

340. Kraus WE, Valenstein PN, Corey GR. Purulent pericarditis caused by Candida: Report of three cases and identification of high-risk populations as an aid to early diagnosis. Rev Infect Dis. 1988;10:34–41.

341. Eng RHK, Sen P, Browne K, et al. Candida pericarditis. Am J Med. 1981; 70:867–9.

342. Kaufman LD, Seifert FC, Eilbott DJ, et al. Candida pericarditis and tamponade in a patient with systemic lupus erythematosus. Arch Intern med. 1988; 148:715–7.

343. Walsh TJ, Bulkley BH. Aspergillus pericarditis: Clinical and pathologic features in the immunocompromised patient. Cancer. 1982;49:48–54.

344. Cooper JAD, Weinbaum DL, Aldrich TK, et al. Invasive aspergillosis of the lung and pericardium in a nonimmunocompromised 33 year old man. Am J Med. 1981;71:903–7.

345. Ross EM, Macher AM, Roberts WC. Aspergillus fumigatus thrombi causing total occlusion of both coronary arterial ostia, all four major coronary arteries and coronary sinus and associated with purulent pericarditis. Am J Cardiol. 1985;56:499.

346. Theologides A, Kennedy BJ. Editorial: Toxoplasmic myocarditis and pericarditis. Am J Med. 1969;47:169–74.

347. Sagrista-Sauleda J, Permanyer-Miralda G, Juste-Sanchez C, et al. Huge chronic pericardial effusion caused by Toxoplasma gondii. Circulation. 1982; 66:895–7.

348. Lyngberg KK, Vennervald BJ, Bygbjerg IC, et al. Toxoplasma pericarditis mimicking systemic lupus erythematosus. Diagnostic and treatment difficulties in one patient. Ann Med. 1992;24:337–40.

349. Permanyer-Miralda G, Sagrista-Sauleda J, Soler-Soler J. Primary acute pericardial disease: A prospective series of 231 consecutive patients. Am J Cardiol. 1985;56:623–30.

350. Ibarra-Perez C, Green LS, Calvello-Juarez M, et al. Diagnosis and treatment of rupture of amebic abscess of the liver into the pericardium. J Thorac Cardiovasc Surg. 1972;64:11–7.

351. Rab SW, Alam N, Hoda AN, et al. Amoebic liver abscess. Some unique presentations. Am J Med. 1967;43:811–6.

352. Baid CS, Varma AR, Lakhotia M. A case of subacute effusive constrictive pericarditis with a probable amoebic aetiology. Br Heart J. 1987;58:296–8.

353. Strang JIG. Two-dimensional echocardiography in the diagnosis of amoebic pericarditis. A case report. S Afr Med J. 1987;71:328–9.

354. Van der Horst R. Schistosomiasis of the pericardium. J R Soc Trop Med Hyg. 1979;73:243–4.

355. Strang JIG. Tuberculous pericarditis in Transkei. Clin Cardiol. 1984;5:667.

356. Strang JI, Kakaza HH, Gibson DG, et al. Controlled clinical trial of complete

open surgical drainage and of prednisone in treatment of tuberculous pericardial effusion in Transkei. Lancet. 1988;2:759–64.

357. D'Cruz IA, Sengupta EE, Abrahams C, et al. Cardiac involvement, including tuberculous pericardial effusion, complicating acquired immune deficiency syndrome. Am Heart J. 1986;5:1100.

358. Kwan T, Karve MM, Emerole O. Cardiac tamponade in patients infected with HIV. Chest. 1993;104:1059–62.

359. Fowler NO. Tuberculous pericarditis. (See comments). JAMA. 1991;266:99–103.

360. Strang JI, Kakaza HH, Gibson DG, et al. Controlled trial of prednisolone as adjuvant in the treatment of tuberculous constrictive pericarditis in Transkei. Lancet. 1987;2:1418.

361. Roberts WC, Spray TL. Clinical and morphologic spectrum of pericardial heart disease. Curr Probl Cardiol. 1977;2:1–71.

362. Shabetai R. Function of the pericardium. In: Fowler NO, ed. The Pericardium in Health and Disease. Mount Kisco, NY: Futura; 1985:19–50.

363. Fowler NO, Harbin AD. Recurrent acute pericarditis: Follow-up study of 31 patients. J Am Coll Cardiol. 1986;7:300–5.

364. Matthews JD, Cameron SJ, George M. Constrictive pericarditis following coxsackie virus infection. Thorax. 1970;25:624–6.

365. Utley JR, Mills J. Annular erosion and pericarditis. Complications of endocarditis of the aortic root. J Thorac Cardiovasc Surg. 1972;64:76–81.

366. Ribeiro P, Shapiro L, Nihoyannopoulos P, et al. Pericarditis in infective endocarditis. Eur Heart J. 1985;6:975–8.

367. Peel AAF. Tuberculous pericarditis. Br Heart J. 1948;10:195–207.

368. Carson TJ, Murray GF, Wilcox BR, et al. The role of surgery in tuberculous pericarditis. Ann Thorac Surg. 1974;17:163–7.

369. Guberman BA, Fowler NO, Engel PJ, et al. Cardiac tamponade in medical patients. Circulation. 1981;64:633–40.

370. Spodick DH. Pericardial rub: Prospective multiple observer investigation of pericardial friction rub in 100 patients. Am J Cardiol. 1975;35:357–62.

371. Lorell BH, Braunwald E. Pericardial disease. In: Braunwald E, ed: A Textbook of Cardiovascular Medicine. 4th ed. Philadelphia: WB Saunders; 1992:1465–516.

372. Spodick DH. Electrocardiogram in acute pericarditis. Distributions of morphologic and axial changes by stages. Am J Cardiol. 1974;33:470–4.

373. Shabetai R. Acute pericarditis. Cardiol Clin. 1990;8:639–44.

374. Spodick DH. Frequency of arrhythmias in acute pericarditis determined by holter monitoring. Am J Cardiol. 1984;53:842–5.

375. Isner JM, Carter BL, Bankoff MS, et al. Computed tomography in the diagnosis of pericardial heart disease. Ann Intern Med. 1982;97:473–9.

376. Tomoda H, Hoshiai M, Furuya H, et al. Evaluation of pericardial effusion with computed tomography. Am Heart J. 1980;99:701–6.

377. Sechtem U, Tscholakoff D, Higgins CB. MRI of the abnormal pericardium. AJR. 1986;147:245–52.

378. Krainin FM, Flessas AP, Spodick DH. Infarction associated pericarditis. Rarity of diagnostic electrocardiogram. N Engl J Med. 1984;311:1211–4.

379. Galve E, Garcia-del-Castillo H, Evangelista A, et al. Pericardial effusion in the course of myocardial infarction: Incidence, natural history, and clinical relevance. Circulation. 1986;73:294.

380. Gregoratos G. Pericardial involvement in acute myocardial infarction. Cardiol Clin. 1990;8:601–8.

381. Renfrew R, Buselmeier TJ, Kjeilstrand CM. Pericarditis and renal failure. Annu Rev Med. 1980;31:345–60.

382. Rutsky EA, Rostand SG. Treatment of uremic pericarditis and pericardial effusion. Am J Kidney Dis. 1987;10:2.

383. Brosius FC, Waller BF, Roberts WC. Radiation heart disease. Am J Med. 1981;70:519–30.

384. Stewart JR, Fajardo LF. Radiation-induced heart disease: An update. Prog Cardiovasc Dis. 1984;27:173.

385. Khan AH. The postcardiac injury syndromes. Clin Cardiol. 1992;15:67–72.

386. Dressler W. Post-myocardial infarction syndrome. JAMA. 1956;160:1379–83.

387. Engle MA, Gay WA Jr, Zabriskie JB, et al. The post pericardiotomy syndrome: 25 years experience. J Cardiovasc Med. 1984;4:321–32.

388. Saner HE, Gobel FL, Nicoloff DM, et al. Aortic dissection presenting as pericarditis. Chest. 1987;91:71.

389. Silverman KJ, Hutchins GM, Bulkley BH. Cardiac sarcoid: A clinicopathologic study of 84 unselected cases with systemic sarcoidosis. Circulation. 1978;58:1204–11.

390. Ansari A, Larson PH, Bates HD. Cardiovascular manifestations of systemic lupus erythematosis: Current perspective. Prog Cardiovasc Dis. 1985;27:421–34.

391. Lebowitz WB. The heart in rheumatoid arthritis (rheumatoid disease). A clinical and pathological study of sixty-two cases. Ann Intern Med. 1963;58:102–23.

392. Kelly CA, Bourke JP, Malcolm A, et al. Chronic pericardial disease in patients with rheumatoid arthritis: A longitudinal study. Q J Med. 1990;75:461–70.

393. Goldenberg J, Ferraz MB, Pessoa AP, et al. Symptomatic cardiac involvement in juvenile rheumatoid arthritis. Int J Cardiol. 1992;34:57–62.

394. McWhorter JE, LeRoy RC. Pericardial disease in scleroderma (systemic sclerosis). Am J Med. 1974;57:566–75.

395. Janosik DL, Osborn TG, Moore TL, et al. Heart disease in systemic sclerosis. Semin Arthritis Rheum. 1989;19:191.

396. Abid MA, Gitlin N. Pericarditis—an extraintestinal complication of inflammatory bowel disease. West J Med. 1990;153:314–5.

397. Zimmerman J, Yahalom J, Bar-On H. Clinical spectrum of pericardial effusion as the presenting feature of hypothyroidism. Am Heart J. 1983;106:770–1.

398. Krikorian JG, Hancock EW. Pericardiocentesis. Am J Med. 1978;65:808–14.

399. Tan JS, Holmes JC, Fowler NO, et al. Antibiotic levels in pericardial fluid. J Clin Invest. 1974;53:7–12.

400. Quale JM, Lipschik GY, Heurich AE. Management of tuberculous pericarditis. Ann Thorac Surg. 1987;43:653–5.

62. MEDIASTINITIS

MARK E. RUPP
GORDON L. ARCHER

Acute mediastinitis is an uncommon, but potentially devastating, infection involving the structures of the mediastinum. Prior to the development of sophisticated techniques in cardiovascular and thoracic surgery, most cases resulted from esophageal perforation or contiguous spread from oropharyngeal foci. Currently, mediastinitis occurs most frequently as a postoperative infection following median sternotomy. Regardless of the pathogenesis of acute mediastinitis, a high index of clinical suspicion must be maintained for this serious infection in order to diagnose mediastinitis promptly and institute potentially life-saving medical and surgical therapy. Sclerosing mediastinitis, also known as *fibrosing* or *granulomatous mediastinitis,* often due to *Histoplasma capsulatum,* is also discussed.

ANATOMIC CONSIDERATIONS

The mediastinum is the region within the thorax between the pleural sacs (Fig. 1). It extends from the diaphragm inferiorly to the superior aperture of the thorax. The sternum and costal cartilages make up the anterior boundary, and the 12 thoracic vertebral bodies border the mediastinum posteriorly. The mediastinum is arbitrarily divided into four subdivisions: superior, posterior, anterior, and middle. Structures within the mediastinum include the heart and great vessels, the distal portion of the trachea and mainstem bronchi, esophagus, vagus nerves, phrenic nerves, remains of the thymus, and thoracic duct. These structures are surrounded by adipose tissue, loose connective tissue, and lymph nodes. The mediastinum communicates with the structures of the head and neck via several fascial planes and potential spaces (see Ch. 46, Fig. 4). Detailed descriptions

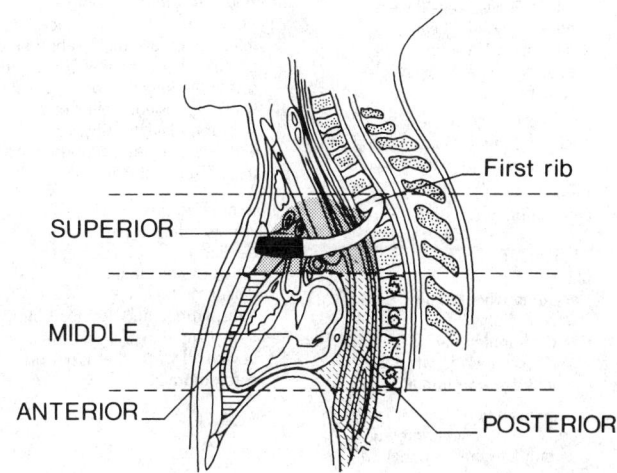

FIG. 1. Anatomic boundaries and divisions of the mediastinum.

of mediastinal anatomy are available,[1-4] and the major points will be reviewed below. The three major routes by which infection spreads from the head and neck to the mediastinum are (1) the pretracheal space, (2) the long fascial planes of the posterior neck, and (3) the viscerovascular or lateral pharyngeal space. The long fascial planes of the posterior neck extend from the base of the skull to the diaphragm and are made up of the retropharyngeal or retrovisceral space, the prevertebral space, and the danger space. Pearse[1] attempted to delineate the relative importance of each route in the pathogenesis of mediastinitis and found the retropharyngeal space to be involved in 71 percent of cases, followed by the lateral pharyngeal space in 21 percent and the pretracheal space in 8 percent.

ACUTE MEDIASTINITIS

Epidemiology and Pathogenesis

Primary infection of the mediastinum is a rare event. Essentially all cases of mediastinitis are secondary to the spread of infection from other sites or direct inoculation due to trauma. The causes of mediastinitis are summarized in Table 1 and can be grouped into the following four categories: esophageal perforation, head and neck infection, infection originating at another site, and cardiothoracic surgery. The pathogenesis, clinical manifestations, and treatment vary according to the underlying cause of mediastinitis.

Mediastinitis Secondary to Infections of the Head and Neck and other Contiguous Structures

Prior to the development of cardiac surgery, perforation of the esophagus was the leading cause of mediastinitis, followed by suppurative infections of the oropharynx.[1] In 1724, Herman Boerhaave described the first case of mediastinitis due to spontaneous rupture of the esophagus in a Dutch admiral who self-induced emesis.[107,108] Subsequently, this entity has been known as Boerhaave syndrome. Currently, esophageal perforation is most frequently due to iatrogenic events.[6] Flexible fibro-optic endoscopy of the upper gastrointestinal tract is complicated by esophageal perforation in 0.074–0.4 percent of procedures.[4,16,109] This occurs more frequently when sclerotherapy or

dilation procedures are performed.[6] Swallowed foreign bodies, esophageal carcinoma, and nonsurgical trauma may also result in perforation of the esophagus and mediastinitis.

Depending on where the esophageal perforation occurs, mediastinitis may result from direct spillage of esophageal contents into the posterior mediastinum or migration into the mediastinum via the fascial planes of the neck. A necrotizing chemical mediastinitis ensues that is followed by an aerobic and anaerobic bacterial mediastinitis. Often a synergistic necrotizing form of mediastinitis is observed.[33] Spread of infection from the neck into the mediastinum is influenced by respiratory dynamics in which the negative intrathoracic pressure generated during respiration tends to force the infection into the mediastinum.[24]

Before antibiotics were widely available odontogenic and pharyngeal infections caused from 10 to 31 percent of cases of mediastinitis.[1,2,110] Fortunately, they are a rare cause of mediastinitis today. The prototypic odontogenic infection leading to mediastinitis is Ludwig's angina. This generally arises from an infection of the second or third mandibular molar to involve the sublingual and submandibular spaces. From there, the infection can spread via the lateral pharyngeal space to involve the retropharyngeal space or carotid sheath and thus track into the mediastinum. During the antibiotic era approximately 3.5 percent of cases of Ludwig's angina have been complicated by mediastinitis.[41] Mediastinitis resulting from infections involving the lateral pharyngeal space may originate from a number of sources, including the teeth, parotid glands, tonsils, or, rarely, from otitis or mastoiditis. Retropharyngeal space infections generally arise from perforation of the esophagus or extension from pharyngitis, epiglottitis, or tonsillitis. From the long fascial planes of the neck these infections easily spread into the superior mediastinum, or, if the danger space is involved, the posterior mediastinum.[33,34] The pretracheal space descends into the anterior mediastinum and most often is involved in mediastinitis complicating surgery of the thyroid or trachea.[1]

Mediastinitis Secondary to Cardiothoracic Surgery

Since the refinement of cardiothoracic surgery in the 1960s and 1970s, mediastinitis has become largely a postsurgical infection. Numerous studies have documented the incidence of mediastinitis following cardiothoracic surgery and the risk factors for development of this serious complication. In 1984, Sar et al.[71] reviewed the available literature and found the incidence of mediastinitis to be from 0.4 to 5 percent of patients undergoing median sternotomy.[71] Since that time studies documenting the experience in over 70,000 patients have been published, with incidence rates ranging from 0.66 to 2.4 percent.[58,63,65–68,72,73, 75,78,83,84] The incidence of mediastinitis during outbreaks has been as high as 5–23.7 percent.[111–115] Patients undergoing heart transplantation are at higher risk of developing mediastinitis, with incidences of 2.5–7.5 percent.[96–98] This increased risk of mediastinitis is particularly true if a mechanical device, such as a left ventricular assist device or a total artificial heart, is used to support a patient while awaiting a suitable donor heart. Incidences of mediastinitis in this situation range from 7.5–35.7 percent.[101–105]

A number of factors have been suggested to increase the risk of mediastinitis. The studies examining these risk factors are primarily retrospective case-control studies and, thus, are limited by the problems inherent in retrospective surveys. Risk factors can be divided into the following groups: preoperative, intraoperative, and postoperative. Risk factors that can be identified preoperatively include diabetes mellitus, obesity, previous sternotomy, chronic obstructive pulmonary disease, cigarette smoking, low cardiac output states, remote infection, method of hair removal, and prolonged preoperative hospitalization.[58,61–63,66–71,74,78,81,85] Intraoperative and surgical factors include complexity of surgery, type of bone saw used, type of sternal closure, use of internal mammary arteries in coronary

TABLE 1. Causes of Acute Mediastinitis

Esophageal perforation	Head and neck infections
Iatrogenic	Odontogenic,[1,4,33–40] Ludwig's
Esophagogastroduodenoscopy,[5–9]	angina,[1,4,41,42] pharyngitis,[43–45]
esophageal dilation,[5–9]	tonsillitis,[46] parotitis,[47]
esophageal variceal	epiglottitis[48]
sclerotherapy,[10,11] nasogastric	
tube,[6] Sengstaken-Blakemore	*Infection originating at another site*
tube,[12] endotracheal	Pneumonia,[49,50] pleural space
intubation,[13] esophageal	infection/empyema,[51] subphrenic
surgery[14] para-esophageal	abscess,[51] pancreatitis,[52] cellulitis/
surgery[6,15]	soft-tissue infection of the chest
	wall,[53–55] osteomyelitis of
Swallowed foreign bodies	sternum, clavicle, ribs, or
bones,[16] coins,[6] can pull-tabs,[6]	vertebrae,[2] hematogenous spread
drug-filled condoms,[17] swords[6]	from distant foci[56,57]
Trauma	*Cardiothoracic surgery*
Penetrating	Coronary artery bypass grafting,[58–93]
Gun shot wound,[18] knife	cardiac valve replacement,[63–93]
wound[18]	repair of congenital heart
Blunt	defect,[94,95] heart
Steering wheel injury,[19] seat-	transplantation,[96–104] heart-lump
belt injury,[20]	transplantation, cardiac assist
cardiopulmonary	devices,[102–106] other types of
resuscitation,[21] whip-lash	cardiothoracic surgery
injury,[22] barotrauma[23]	
Spontaneous/other	
Emesis,[6,24–26] cricoid pressure	
during anesthesia induction,[27]	
heavy lifting,[28] defecation,[29,30]	
parturition,[31] carcinoma[322]	

artery bypass grafting, use of bone wax, prolonged operative time, prolonged time on cardiopulmonary bypass, blood transfusions, indiscriminate use of electrocautery, and antibiotic prophylaxis.[58–67,71,74–83,85,88–91,116] Postoperatively patients at greater risk for mediastinitis have been found to require reexploration to control bleeding, prolonged length of stay in the intensive care unit, mechanical ventilation for greater than 24–48 hours, need for tracheostomy, use of cardiopulmonary resuscitation, and low cardiac-output states.[58,63,64,66,67,69,71,74–78,88,90,93] It should be noted that there is not universal agreement regarding any of these factors. For instance, despite over three decades of surgical experience, it is unclear whether the use of internal mammary artery (IMA) grafts in coronary artery bypass surgery predisposes patients to mediastinitis. In 1972, Arnold[117] suggested that, based on anatomical studies of sternal blood supply, the use of the IMA in coronary artery bypass procedures might lead to significant sternal ischemia and thus predispose patients to sternal osteomyelitis and mediastinitis. This has been supported by several laboratory and clinical studies.[59,64,78,85,88,118] However, other investigators have observed no significant increase in sternal wound infections in patients undergoing coronary artery bypass grafting when the IMA is used.[58,60,61,63,70,119–121]

It is generally believed that the pathogenesis of postcardiac surgery mediastinitis is related to the inoculation of organisms from the patient's endogenous bacterial flora or from the surgical field into the operative wound. Bacteria are able to propagate in the relatively protected avascular area of the surgical wound and cause infection. Thus, factors such as length of time of surgery, complexity of surgery, and need for reexploration might be expected to increase the risk of mediastinitis. Outbreaks of mediastinitis that have been epidemiologically linked to sources such as bacteria from a surgeon's hands or nares lend support to this concept.[115–122] Ferrazzi et al.[82] observed a significant decrease in the incidence of gram-negative mediastinitis but no significant change in gram-positive infections with changes in the operating room environment, supporting the belief that many of these infections arise from a reservoir of gram-positive organisms resident on the patient's skin. Archer and Tenenbaum[123] and Archer and Amstrong[124] have demonstrated that patients are colonized by small numbers of antibiotic-resistant coagulase-negative staphylococci that become the predominant species when subjected to the selective pressure of prophylactic antibiotics. In addition, various postulated immunosuppressive effects of cardiopulmonary bypass may contribute to the pathogenesis of postcardiac surgery mediastinitis.[125,126] Outbreaks of mediastinitis that have been linked to environmental sources and poor hand-washing techniques have indicated the importance of postoperative factors.[111–114,127–129] Controlled prospective studies are needed to define better the factors that influence postcardiac surgery mediastinitis.[130]

Bacteriology

The bacteriology of mediastinitis related to cardiovascular surgery and that secondary to odonotogenic or other head and neck infections is strikingly different, as summarized in Table 2. Mediastinitis secondary to cardiothoracic surgery is primarily due to gram-positive cocci with lesser contributions by gram-negative bacilli. The bacteriology of mediastinitis secondary to extension from head and neck sources is largely polymicrobic. Often a synergistic infection made up of a number of oral anaerobes and gram-negative bacilli is present. The most frequently isolated organisms include viridans streptococci, peptococci, peptostreptococci, *Bacteroides* spp., and *Fusobacterium*. The relative frequency with which these organisms are isolated is uncertain.[131]

Clinical Manifestations and Diagnosis

The clinical manifestations of mediastinitis also differ according to the underlying cause of disease. Patients with mediastinitis

TABLE 2. Microbiology of Mediastinitis

Organisms frequently recovered in mediastinitis secondary to infection of the head and neck or esophageal perforation[a]

Anaerobic	Aerobic or facultative
Gram-positive cocci	Gram-positive cocci
Peptococcus spp.	Streptococcus spp.
Peptostreptococcus spp.	Staphylococcus spp.
Gram-positive bacilli	Gram-positive bacilli
Actinomyces	Corynebacterium
Eubacterium	Gram-negative cocci
Lactobacillus	Branhamella
Gram-negative cocci	Gram-negative bacilli
Veillonella	Enterobacteriaceae
Gram-negative bacilli	Pseudomonas spp.
Bacteroides spp.	Eikenella corrodens
Fusobacterium spp.	Fungi
Prevotella spp.	Candida albicans
Porphyromonas spp.	

Organisms frequently recovered in mediastinitis secondary to cardiothoracic surgery[b]

Organism	Range (%)	Representative Rate (%)
Gram-positive cocci		
S. aureus	7.1–66.7	25
S. epidermidis	6–45.5	30
Enterococcus spp.	8–18.8	10
Streptococci spp.	0–18.2	2
Gram-negative bacilli		
E. coli	0–12.5	5
Enterobacter spp.	4–21.4	10
Klebsiella spp.	0–21.1	3
Proteus spp.	0–7.1	2
Other Enterobacteriaceae	0–20	2
Pseudomonas spp.	0–54	2
Fungi		
Candida albicans	0–14.3	<2
Polymicrobial	0–40	10

Others occasionally reported

Acinetobacter,[74] Legionella spp.,[136] B. fragilis,[137,138] C. tropicalis,[139] Nocardia spp.,[140] Kluyvera,[141] M. fortuitum,[142] M. chelonei,[142] Rhodococcus bronchialis[143]

Other unusual causes of mediastinitis

Anthrax,[144] brucellosis,[145] actinomycoses,[146] paragonimiasis[147]

[a] See refs. 3, 4, 13, 33, 34, 36, 38, 41, 50, 51, 131–133.
[b] See refs. 58, 62–64, 66, 68, 69, 71, 72, 74, 75, 77, 84, 114, 128, 134, 135.

from extension of odontogenic or pharyngeal infections generally have obvious primary infections with significant pain, fever, and swelling at the affected site. Esophageal perforation may be clinically obvious or inapparent. Early in the course of mediastinitis, signs and symptoms may be subtle, but, as the condition progresses, patients note increasing chest pain, respiratory distress, and dysphagia. Chest pain is often the most prominent symptom and may localize depending on which portion of the mediastinum is involved. In anterior mediastinitis, pain is often located in the cervical or substernal region. Pain due to posterior mediastinitis may localize to the epigastric area with radiation to the interscapular region.[16,24,50,110] Pleuritic chest pain may also be experienced due to the relatively frequent complication of pleural effusion. Retroperitoneal extension may be accompanied by acute abdominal signs and may prompt unnecessary exploratory laparotomy.[33] Examination may reveal fever, tachycardia, crepitus, and edema of the chest or neck. Hamman's sign, a crunching rasping sound heard over the precordium synchronous with the cardiac rhythm, due to emphysema of the mediastinum, may be present in up to 50 percent of patients with pneumomediastinum.[148,149] The heart sounds may appear distant and dull. In the later stages of disease, signs of bacteremia and sepsis may predominate. The early diagnosis of mediastinitis in the infant or neonate is particularly challenging. A peculiar, interrupted, staccato type of inspiration has been described in a number of cases.[150] The signs and symptoms of mediastinitis in older children are similar to those observed in adults.[151] Laboratory tests usually reveal a leukocytosis with a leftward shift evident on the differential. Radiographically, plain films of the chest may reveal mediastinal widening, air-fluid levels, and subcutaneous or mediastinal emphysema.[8,9,16,34,]

[38,152] The lateral chest radiograph may be useful in demonstrating superior mediastinal gas not evident on upright films. Approximately 50 percent of cases of pneumomediastinum are not evident without lateral views.[153] Complications of mediastinitis, such as pleural effusion or pneumoperitoneum, may also be evident on the chest radiograph. Esophageal perforation is best demonstrated by contrast esophagography, which reveals extravasation of dye in 59–100 percent of cases.[9,16,154–158] It is recommended that a water-soluble contrast agent be used initially to avoid the inflammation and granuloma formation evoked by extravasated barium.[154] If extravasation is not observed, barium should be used to detect subtle defects, as it provides a better definition of the anatomy.[159] Computed tomography (CT) is often helpful in cases in which the diagnosis is not evident clinically or on plain films.[160,161] Technetium-labeled white blood cell scans have been reported helpful in the diagnosis of mediastinitis in specialized circumstances when CT scan was not readily available.[162] The role of magnetic resonance imaging (MRI) has not been well established.

Postcardiothoracic surgery mediastinitis usually presents within the first 2 weeks following surgery.[69,71–74] However, rare cases have been described occurring up to 416 days postoperatively.[69] Infections due to gram-negative organisms generally present earlier. One study found that all cases of mediastinitis presenting later than 2 weeks postoperatively were due to gram-positive organisms.[69] Mediastinitis may present fulminantly or subtly. Some cases may present as sepsis without localizing signs.[71] Patients may experience greater than normal postoperative pain, which may be pleuritic in nature. Dysphagia is a rare complaint. Fever and an abnormal appearance of the surgical wound, characterized by erythema, cellulitis, or purulent discharge, are the most frequent signs of mediastinitis.[59,69–71,73,74,86,88] Sternal instability, dehiscence, or the observation of bubbles emanating from the sternal wound are less frequent findings. Occasionally chest wall emphysema is observed. Poststernotomy mediastinitis presenting as a deep neck abscess without abnormal findings on chest examination has been reported.[163] Laboratory tests usually show a moderate leukocytosis with a leftward shift on the white blood cell differential. Radiographically, mediastinal widening is a rare finding on plain chest films, and generally routine radiographs are of very little use in the diagnosis of mediastinitis following cardiothoracic surgery.[69,71,161] CT scanning has proven helpful in many cases of postoperative mediastinitis, particularly in differentiating superficial wound infections from deeper retrosternal processes.[160,161,164] However, normal postoperative collections of fluid and gas are at times difficult to differentiate from early signs of mediastinitis.[160] The diagnostic value of nuclear scans has been espoused by several investigators.[165,166] Browdie et al.[167] studied the relative value of CT, [111]I-labeled leukocyte scanning, and epicardial pacer wire cultures in 24 patients being evaluated for possible mediastinitis. They found that CT had a sensitivity of 67 percent and a specificity of 71 percent, [111]Indium-labeled leukocyte scan was 83 percent sensitive and 100 percent specific, and epicardial pacer wire cultures were reported to be 100 percent sensitive and 92 percent specific. Another investigator, however, found epicardial pacer wire cultures to be associated with an unacceptably high false-positive rate.[168] The role of MRI is not well delineated, and it is contraindicated in instances where ferromagnetic metals are used in sternal wires, artificial heart valves, cardiac pacemakers, or vascular clips. Several investigators have found mediastinal needle aspiration useful in the diagnosis of mediastinitis.[63,64,71,86,169] This method, which has been reported positive in 65.8 percent of patients, appears to be particularly useful in diagnosing mediastinitis before it becomes more clinically obvious.[63,64,169]

Treatment

Therapy that includes both medical and surgical techniques should be promptly initiated once the diagnosis of mediastinitis is made. In all cases aggressive supportive and nutritional therapy is required. Barrett[170] is credited with documenting the first successful treatment of mediastinitis due to esophageal perforation. Since then, most authorities recommend aggressive surgical drainage, débridement, and repair in cases of mediastinitis secondary to esophageal perforation.[7–9,16,154,171–173] However, based on experience with eight patients, Cameron et al.[174] identified a subset of patients that could be treated without surgical intervention. These patients should have a well-contained disruption of the esophagus, the abscess should drain back into the esophagus, minimal symptoms should be present, and there should be minimal evidence of clinical toxicity. Shaffer et al.[155] expanded upon these recommendations based on the recognition of patients with esophageal perforation due to instrumentation before major mediastinal contamination had occurred. Santos and Frator[175] have recommended transesophageal irrigation for patients in whom primary repair of the esophagus is not possible due to advanced local infection with extensive tissue necrosis.

As in cases of mediastinitis due to esophageal perforation, cases secondary to descending odontogenic or pharyngeal infection require prompt surgical intervention. Several authors have warned that a transthoracic approach is necessary and that transcervical drainage is often inadequate.[33,40]

Although the importance of supportive therapy and surgical intervention cannot be overemphasized, administration of appropriate antibiotics is an essential component of therapy. Empirical regimens are based on the underlying etiology and should cover the major pathogens listed in Table 2. Penicillin G has traditionally been the antibiotic of choice in the treatment of anaerobic infections arising above the diaphragm and continues to exhibit excellent activity against most oral anaerobic bacteria. However, oral anaerobes such as *Prevotella* and *Porphyromonas* spp. (formerly *Bacteroides* spp.) are often resistant to penicillin G, and, therefore, when infection with those organisms is suspected, treatment with metronidazole, clindamycin, or broad-spectrum β-lactam, antibiotics with activity against penicillin-resistant anaerobes as well as other oropharyngeal anaerobes, may be indicated.[131] In addition, gram-negative enteric bacilli are often implicated in mediastinitis and should be covered in initial empirical therapy. Antibiotic therapy should then be more specifically tailored to the infecting organisms when definitive culture results are available, but therapy directed against anaerobic oropharyngeal organisms should probably be continued due to the difficulty in obtaining reliable anaerobic cultures.[131] Duration of therapy, which may range from weeks to months, is determined by the virulence of the bacteria, host factors, and the patient's response to therapy.

The treatment of postcardiac surgery mediastinitis generally requires aggressive surgical drainage and débridement. A small number of patients have been successfully treated via percutaneous catheter drainage.[176] Two approaches have been utilized in the surgical management of postcardiac surgery mediastinitis—an open technique and a closed technique. The open technique involves débridement of infected tissue and open packing of the wound with delayed closure.[58,63,64,71,83,88] Disadvantages of this technique include respiratory insufficiency due to lack of mechanical support for the thorax, delayed healing and closure of the surgical wound, and hemorrhage from exposed vessels.[62,71,86,88] The closed method involves débridement of affected tissues, closure of the sternum, and postoperative irrigation through drainage tubes within the mediastinum.[58,63,64,71,83,88] Irrigants have included a variety of antimicrobial and antiseptic solutions, such as neomycin, gentamicin, bacitracin, polymyxin B, saline, and Dakin's solution. They have been associated with a variety of complications, including emergence of resistant organisms, pericardial and tissue toxicity, and systemic absorption and toxicity.[87,177–179] The most commonly employed irrigant is povidone-iodine. Use of povidone-iodine has been associated with iodine toxicity, renal failure, metabolic acidosis, and seizures.[180-182] Therefore, this agent must be used with caution, and it has been recommended that serum iodide concentration be measured to ensure that toxic levels are not reached.[180-182] Durandy et al.[183] reported a closed technique successfully utilizing Redon drainage devices in 11 patients that did not require postoperative irrigation. A number of investigators have reported the successful use of muscle flaps and omental grafts, often at the time of initial débridement, to close mediastinal wounds with or without postoperative irrigation.[63,88,94,184-188]

The use of parenteral antibiotics has remained a cornerstone of therapy. Generally, empiric therapy should be directed at staphylococci and gram-negative aerobic bacilli until definitive culture results are available. As with mediastinitis secondary to infection of the head and neck, the duration of therapy is determined by a number of factors and may be quite prolonged. Although controlled studies are lacking, in several cases of mediastinitis recalcitrant to more traditional therapy, packing the wound with granulated sugar or honey has been used successfully to eradicate infection.[189-192] It appears that the sugar lowers the water activity of the tissue substrate to a level at which bacterial growth is inhibited.[190]

Antibiotic Prophylaxis

Although cardiothoracic surgical procedures are classified as clean procedures, and the risk of infection is low, the consequences of infection can be devastating. Therefore, despite the lack of placebo-controlled studies documenting efficacy, antibiotic prophylaxis has become commonplace. Cefazolin has generally been regarded as the drug of choice for prophylaxis.[193] The use of vancomycin or of second-generation cephalosporins such as cefamandole and cefuroxime has also been considered. Studies regarding the relative efficacy of first- and second-generation cephalosporins are conflicting, and no agent has conclusively been shown superior to another. In a comparison between vancomycin, cefazolin, and cefamandole, Maki et al.[194] demonstrated a significant reduction in postoperative wound infection in patients receiving vancomycin prophylaxis. Vancomycin should be considered for prophylaxis in medical centers in which there is a high prevalence of infections due to methicillin-resistant staphylococci.

Complications and Prognosis

Complications of mediastinitis include extension of the infection into a number of contiguous structures and spaces, including the pericardial space, resulting in pericardial effusion and tamponade, the pleural space, and the peritoneum, resulting in peritonitis.[24,33] A major complication of postcardiac surgery mediastinitis is sternal osteomyelitis. Prior to the development of modern surgery and antibiotics, mediastinitis, due primarily to esophageal perforation, was regarded as uniformly fatal. Unfortunately, since the time of Barrett's first successful surgical repair of the esophagus in 1946,[108] morbidity and mortality have remained high, with many studies recording mortality rates of 30–50 percent.[9,33,40,58,69] Survivors of mediastinitis usually have no permanent sequelae. In examining the economic ramifications of mediastinitis, Loop et al.[58] found that the hospital charges for coronary artery bypass surgery patients who experience mediastinitis were 280 percent greater than patients with uncomplicated bypass surgery, and the median length of stay ranged from 38 to 51 days. The most important factor in determining outcome has been the length of time to diagnosis and initiation of definitive therapy.[9,40,50,63,64,154] Other prognostic indicators have included blood urea nitrogen level, white blood cell count, culture positivity, type of surgical repair, and cytomegalovirus shedding.[63,195,196]

SCLEROSING MEDIASTINITIS

Sclerosing, fibrosing, or granulomatous mediastinitis are terms for a chronic form of mediastinitis characterized by an invasive and compressive inflammatory infiltrate. The first report of this entity, which can cause up to 10 percent of all primary mediastinal masses,[197] reportedly dates to a description by Ulmont in 1855.[198] Although the etiology of up to 83 percent of cases of sclerosing mediastinitis remain obscure,[197] many authorities believe that most cases are secondary to infection with *H. capsulatum*.[199-203] Gryboski et al.[201] and Peabody et al.[202] found that up to 73 percent of cases previously characterized as nonspecific granulomatous mediastinitis could be reclassified as secondary to *H. capsulatum* by restaining the tissue with fungal stains and thorough review of the pathologic sections. Other infectious etiologies that have been reported to cause this condition include tuberculosis,[204,205] actinomycoses,[206,207] nocardiosis,[208] blastomycosis,[209] coccidioidomycosis,[209] aspergillosis,[210] and infection with *Rhizopus* spp.[211] Older literature often lists syphilis as a prominent cause of this condition. However this was erroneously based simply on seropositivity without other supporting evidence. Other conditions that closely mimic this entity include sarcoidosis,[197,212] silicosis,[197] lymphoma,[212] mesothelioma,[213] and mediastinal fibrosis associated with idiopathic retroperitoneal fibrosis, Reidel's struma, or sclerosing cholangitis.

Approximately 40 percent of patients with sclerosing mediastinitis are asymptomatic and come to medical attention when a chest roentgenogram incidentally reveals a mediastinal mass.[200] Symptomatic patients usually note symptoms related to invasion or obstruction of structures within or adjacent to the mediastinum (Table 3). Sclerosing mediastinitis is the most common nonmalignant cause of superior vena cava syndrome, responsible for up to 23 percent of cases.[214] These patients generally present with plethora and edema of the face, neck, and upper torso, neck vein distention, headache, and visual disturbances. Patients presenting with obstruction of the pulmonary arteries often note cough, dyspnea, and symptoms consistent with right-sided heart failure. Pulmonary infarction, although rare, has been reported to occur in patients with fibrosing mediastinitis.[215] Pulmonary venous obstruction causes patients to experience cough, dyspnea, and hemoptysis. Patients with airway obstruction due to sclerosing mediastinitis usually present with wheezing, cough, hemoptysis, and recurrent episodes of bacterial bronchitis or pneumonia. Patients complaining of dysphagia may have esophageal obstruction due to posterior extension of the mediastinitis.

Radiographically patients with fibrosing mediastinitis will often be observed to have a mediastinal mass, most frequently located in the superior mediastinum at the level of the bifurcation of the trachea. Kerley B lines may be present.[216] CT often reveals calcification and delineates the extent of infection, while MRI is superior in assessment of the vascular integrity.[217] Ventilation-perfusion lung scans often reveal large perfusion deficits due to obstruction of the pulmonary vessels.

The diagnosis of fibrosing mediastinitis requires pathologic examination. There is a continuum of disease ranging from a predominantly granulomatous entity to an almost completely fibrosing process. Lesions described include caseating granuloma, dense hyalinized collagenous tissue, and infiltrations of lymphocytes, plasma cells, and giant cells. Specific stains for

TABLE 3. Complications and Manifestations of Sclerosing Mediastinitis

Superior vena cava obstruction	Pulmonary infarction
Inferior vena cava obstruction	Cor pulmonale
Esophageal obstruction	Thoracic duct obstruction
Esophagobronchial obstruction	Constrictive pericarditis
Tracheobronchial obstruction	Coronary artery stenosis
Pulmonary venous or arterial obstruction	Mediastinal nerve entrapment
Pulmonary hypertension	Recurrent laryngeal nerve palsy

fungi often reveal organisms consistent with *Histoplasma*, but cultures are usually negative.[197,209]

The pathologic features of this disease suggest a marked inflammatory reaction. Several different mechanisms have been proposed to explain the pathology of fibrosing mediastinitis. Some investigators believe that a caseous lymph node from primary infection with *Histoplasma* ruptures into the mediastinum, invoking an intense inflammatory reaction.[197,209] A second hypothesis is the development of a delayed hypersensitivity reaction due to the spread of soluble *Histoplasma* antigens into the mediastinum.[218] An alternate explanation proposes that fibrosing mediastinitis represents an abnormality of collagen production and organization similar to idiopathic retroperitoneal fibrosis[218] or Riedel's struma.[218] Noguchi et al.[219] have incriminated the eosinophil in the pathogenesis of fibrosing mediastinitis by demonstrating eosinophils or major basic protein in tissue specimens from five of seven patients with fibrosing mediastinitis.[219]

No controlled trials of medical or surgical therapy in the treatment of fibrosing mediastinitis have been conducted. Although there is some anecdotal evidence of a beneficial effect of antifungal agents,[220] most authorities believe that at the time of presentation there is little evidence of an active infection, and antifungal agents are not indicated.[199,209,216] Because the natural history of this disease is variable, with some patients progressing to compression of vital structures while others seem to have self-limited disease,[209] it is difficult to make recommendations regarding the timing of surgical intervention. It has been suggested that early surgical intervention and removal of granulomatous tissue may prevent the development of subsequent end-stage fibrosis and involvement of vital structures.[221] Clearly, patients experiencing obstruction or invasion of mediastinal structures require intervention, even though such surgery is often difficult and results are at times less than optimal.[209] Therapy with corticosteroids does not appear to have a role in the treatment of fibrosing mediastinitis.[222]

REFERENCES

1. Pearse HE Jr. Mediastinitis following cervical suppuration. Ann Surg. 1938; 108:588–611.
2. Neuhof H, Jemerin EE. Acute Infections of the Mediastinum. Baltimore: Wiliams & Wilkins; 1943.
3. de Marie S, Tjon A, Tham RTO, et al. Clinical infections and nonsurgical treatment of parapharyngeal infections complicating throat infection. Rev Infect Dis. 1989;11:975–82.
4. Chow AW. Life-threatening infections of the head and neck. Clin Infect Dis. 1992;14:991–1004.
5. Silvis SE, Nebel O, Rogers G, et al. Endoscopic complications: Results of the 1974 American gastrointestinal endoscopy survey. JAMA. 1976;235: 928–30.
6. Michael L, Grillo HC, Malt RA. Esophageal perforation. Ann Thorac Surg. 1982;33:203–10.
7. Goldstein LA, Thompson WR. Esophageal perforations: A 15 year experience. Am J Surg. 1982;143:495–503.
8. Sarr MG, Pemberton JH, Payne WS. Management of instrumental perforations of the esophagus. J Thorac Cardiovasc Surg. 1982;84:211–8.
9. Moghissi K, Pender D. Instrumental perforations of the oesophagus and their management. Thorax. 1988;43:642–6.
10. Edling JE, Bacon BR. Pleuropulmonary complications of endoscopic variceal sclerotherapy. Chest. 1991;99:1252–7.
11. Baydur A, Korula J. Cardiorespiratory effects of endoscopic esophageal variceal sclerotherapy. Am J Med. 1990;89:477–82.
12. Conn HO. Hazards attending the use of esophageal tamponade. N Engl J Med. 1958;259:701–7.
13. Uram J, Hauser MS. Deep neck and mediastinal necrotizing infection secondary to a traumatic intubation. J Oral Maxillofac Surg. 1988;46:788–91.
14. Aggerholm K, Illum P. Surgical treatment of Zenker's diverticulum. J Laryngology Otol. 1990;104:312–4.
15. Wang RC, Perlman PW, Parnes SM. Near-fatal complications of tracheotomy infections and their prevention. Head Neck. 1989;11:528–33.
16. Wychulis AR, Fontana RS, Payne WS. Noninstrumental perforations of the esophagus. Dis Chest. 1969;55:190–6.
17. Johnson JA, Landreneau RJ. Esophageal obstruction and mediastinitis: A hard pill to swallow for drug smugglers. Am Surgeon. 1991;57:723–6.
18. Miller RH, Duplechain JK. Penetrating wounds of the neck. Otolaryngol Clin North Am. 1991;24:15–29.
19. Gulbrandson RN, Gaspard DJ. Steering wheel rupture of the pharyngoesophagus: A solitary injury. J Trauma. 1977;17:74–7.
20. Micon L, Geis L, Siderys H, et al. Rupture of the distal thoracic esophagus following blunt trauma. J Trauma. 1990;30:214–7.
21. Rotstein OD, Rhame FS, Molina E, Simmons RL. Mediastinitis after whiplash injury. Can J Surg. 1986;29:54–6.
22. Mensah GA, Gold JP, Schreiber T, Isom OW. Acute purulent mediastinitis and sternal osteomyelitis after closed chest cardiopulmonary resuscitation: A case report and review of the literature. Ann Thorac Surg. 1988;46:353–5.
23. Ribet M, Pruvot FR. Barotraumatic rupture of the esophagus. J Chir Paris. 1986;123:164–8.
24. Payne WS, Larson RH. Acute mediastinitis. Surg Clin North Am. 1969;49: 999–1009.
25. Bennett DJ, Deveridge RJ, Wright JS. Spontaneous rupture of the esophagus: A review with reports of six cases. Surgery. 1970;68:766–70.
26. Derbes VJ, Mitchell RE Jr. Rupture of the esophagus. Surgery. 1956;39: 688–709, 865–88.
27. Ralph SJ, Wareham CA. Rupture of the esophagus during cricoid pressure. Anaesthesia. 1991;46:40–1.
28. Mackler SA. Spontaneous rupture of the esophagus. Surg Gynecol Obstet. 1952;95:345–55.
29. Tidman MK, John HT. Spontaneous rupture of the esophagus. Br J Surg. 1967;54:286–92.
30. Beal JM. Spontaneous rupture of the esophagus. Ann Surg. 1949;512–6.
31. O'Connell ND. Spontaneous rupture of the esophagus. Am J Roentgenol. 1967;99:186–203.
32. Kimose HH, Lund O, Hasenkam JM, et al. Independent predictors of operative mortality and postoperative complications in surgically treated carcinomas of the oesophagus and cardia—Is the aggressive surgical approach worthwhile? Acta Chir Scand. 1990;156:373–82.
33. Estrera AS, Landay MJ, Grishom JM, et al. Descending necrotizing mediastinitis. Surg Gynecol Obstet. 1983;157:545–52.
34. Levine TM, Wurster CF, Krespi YP. Mediastinitis occurring as a complication of odontogenic infections. Laryngoscope. 1986;96:747–50.
35. Moncada R, Warpeha R, Pickleman J, et al. Mediastinitis from odontogenic and deep cervical infection. Chest. 1978;73:497–500.
36. Steiner M, Grau MJ, Wilson DL, Snow NJ. Odontogenic infection leading to cervical emphysema and fatal mediastinitis. J Oral Maxillofac Surg. 1982; 40:600–4.
37. Zachariades N, Mezitis M, Stavrinidis P, Agourdaki EK. Mediastinitis, thoracic empyema, and pericarditis as complications of a dental abscess. J Oral Maxillofac Surg. 1988;46:493–5.
38. Rubin MM, Cozzi GM. Fatal necrotizing mediastinitis as a complication of an odontogenic infection. J Oral Maxillofac Surg. 1987;45:529–33.
39. Masgrove BT, Malden NJ. Mediastinitis and pericarditis caused by dental infection. Br J Oral Maxillofac Surg. 1989;27:423–8.
40. Wheatley MJ, Stirling MC, Kirsh MM, et al. Descending necrotizing mediastinitis: Transcervical drainage is not enough. Ann Thorac Surg. 1990;49: 780–4.
41. Moreland LW, Corey J, McKenzie R. Ludwig's angina: Report of a case and review of the literature. Arch Intern Med. 1988;148:461–6.
42. van der Brempt X, Derue G, Severin F, et al. Ludwig's angina and mediastinitis due to *Streptococcus milleri*: Usefulness of computed tomography. Eur Respir J. 1990;3:728–31.
43. Baker AR, Moir AA, Donnelly PK. Life-threatening peripharyngeal sepsis with mediastinitis. Br J Clin Pract. 1990;44:640–1.
44. Zaltman M, Kallenbach J, Hockman M, et al. Fatal intrathoracic sepsis associated with neck space infection. Thorax. 1983;38:143–5.
45. Enquist RW, Blanck RR, Butler RH. Nontraumatic mediastinitis. JAMA. 1976;236:1048–9.
46. Komatsu ES, Costa F, Marchese LT, Filho SV. Abscess of the mediastinum: A case report. J Pediatr Surg. 1989;24:1125.
47. Guardia SN, Cameron R, Phillips A. Fatal necrotizing mediastinitis secondary to acute suppurative parotitis. J Otolarngol. 1991;20:54–6.
48. Chong WH, Woodhead MA, Millard FJC. Mediastinitis and bilateral thoracic empyemas complicating adult epiglottitis. Thorax. 1990;45:491–2.
49. Pane GA, Hamilton GC, Call E. Nontraumatic suppurative mediastinitis presenting as acute mediastinal widening. Ann Emerg Med. 1983;12:777–9.
50. Freidman BC, Pickul DC. Acute mediastinitis: What to do when the cause is nonsurgical. Postgrad Med. 1990;87:273–85.
51. Hardy CC, Raza SN, Isalska B, Barber PV. Atraumatic suppurative mediastinitis and purulent pericarditis due to *Eikenella corrodens*. Thorax. 1988; 43:494–5.
52. Iacono C, Procacci C, Frigo F, et al. Thoracic complications of pancreatitis. Pancreas. 1989;4:228–36.
53. Dreyfuss D, Djedaini K, Lapomme CB, Coste F. Nontraumatic acute anterior mediastinitis in two HIV-positive heroin addicts. Chest. 1992;101:583–5.
54. Duncan GW, Randall WE, Mulholland JH. *Hemophilus influenza* type B, mediastinitis cellulitis, bacteremia, and meningitis in an adult. Am Rev Respir Dis. 1981;123:333–5.
55. Barradas MCR, Muscher DM, Hamill RJ, Dowell M, Bagwell JT, Sanders CV. Unusual manifestations of pneumococcal infection in human immunodeficiency virus–infected individuals: The past revisited. Clin Infect Dis. 1992; 14:192–9.

56. Antreasian B. Mediastinal abscess: Two case reports. Indiana Med. 1988; 81:528–32.

57. Smith A, Sinzobahamvya N. Anterior mediastinal abscess complicating septic arthritis. J Pediatr Surg. 1992;27:101–2.

58. Loop FD, Lytle BW, Cosgrove DM, et al. Sternal wound complications after isolated coronary artery bypass grafting: Early and late mortality, morbidity, and cost of care. Ann Thorac Surg. 1990;49:179–87.

59. Grossi EA, Esposito R, Harris LJ, et al. Sternal wound infections and use of internal mammary artery grafts. J Thorac Cardiovasc Surg. 1991;102:342–7.

60. Sethi GK, Copeland JG, Moritz T, et al. Comparison of postoperative complications between saphenous vein and IMA grafts to left anterior descending coronary artery. Ann Thorac Surg. 1991;51:733–8.

61. Sutherland RD, Martinez HE, Guynes WA, Miller L. Postoperative chest wound infections in patients requiring coronary bypass. J Thorac Cardiovasc Surg. 1977;73:944–7.

62. Nafziger DA, Perl TM, Herwaldt LA, et al. Mediastinitis at a tertiary referral hospital. In: Abstracts of the 32nd Interscience Conference on Antimicrobial Agents and Chemotherapy. Abstract 1259; American Society for Microbiology, Washington, DC, 1992;320.

63. Grossi EU, Culliford AT, Krieger KH, et al. A survey of 77 major infectious complications of median sternotomy: A review of 7949 consecutive operative procedures. Ann Thorac Surg. 1985;40:214–23.

64. Culliford AT, Cunningham JN, Zeff RH, et al. Sternal and costochondral infections following open-heart surgery. J Thorac Cardiovasc Surg. 1976;72: 714–26.

65. Hammermeister KE, Burchfiel C, Johnson R, Grover FL. Identification of patients at greatest risk for developing major complications at cardiac surgery. Circulation. 1990;82(Suppl IV):380–9.

66. Ottino G, De Paulis R, Pansini S, et al. Major sternal wound infection after open-heart surgery: A multivariate analysis of risk factors in 2579 consecutive operative procedures. Ann Thorac Surg 1987;44:173–9.

67. Newman LS, Szczukowski LC, Bain RP, Perlino CA. Suppurative mediastinitis after open heart surgery. Chest. 1988;94:546–53.

68. Nagachinta T, Stephens M, Reitz B, Polk BF. Risk factors for surgical-wound infection following cardiac surgery. J Infect Dis. 1987;156:967–73.

69. Bor DH, Rose RM, Modlin JF, et al. Mediastinitis after cardiovascular surgery. Rev Infect Dis. 1983;5:885–97.

70. Engleman RM, Williams CD, Gouge TH, et al. Mediastinitis following open-heart surgery. Arch Surg. 1973;107:772–8.

71. Sarr MG, Gott VL, Townsend TR. Mediastinal infection after cardiac surgery. Ann Thorac Surg. 1984;38:415–23.

72. Verkkala K, Jarvinen A. Mediastinal infection following open-heart surgery. Scand J Thor Cardiovasc Surg 1986;20:203–7.

73. Kutsal A, Ibrisim E, Catav Z, et al. Mediastinitis after open heart surgery. J Cardiovasc Surg. 1991;32:38–41.

74. Farrington M, Webster M, Fenn A, Phillips I. Study of cardiothoracic wound infection at St. Thomas's hospital. Br J Surg. 1985;72:759–62.

75. Miholic J, Hudec M, Domanig E, et al. Risk factors for severe bacterial infections after valve replacement and aortocoronary bypass operations: Analysis of 246 cases by logistic regression. Ann Thorac Surg. 1985;40: 224–8.

76. Serry C, Bleck PC, Javid H, et al. Sternal wound complications. J Thorac Cardiavasc Surg. 1980;80:861–7.

77. Sanfelippo PM, Danielson GK. Complications associated with median sternotomy. J Thorac Cardiovasc Surg. 1972;63:419–23.

78. Kouchoukos NT, Wareing TH, Murphy SF, et al. Risks of bilateral internal mammary artery bypass grafting. Ann Thorac Surg. 1990;49:210–9.

79. Nishida H, Grooters RK, Soltanzadeh H, et al. Discriminate use of electrocautery on the median sternotomy incision. J Thorac Cardiovasc Surg. 1991; 101:488–94.

80. Doebbeling BN, Pfaller MA, Kuhns KR, et al. Cardiovascular surgery prophylaxis. J Thorac Cardiovasc Surg. 1990;99:981–9.

81. Ko W, Lazenby D, Zelano JA, et al. Effects of shaving methods and intraoperative irrigation on suppurative mediastinitis after bypass operations. Ann Thorac Surg. 1992;53:301–5.

82. Ferrazzi P, Allen R, Crupi G, et al. Reduction of infection after cardiac surgery. Ann Thorac Surg. 1986;42:321–5.

83. Cheung EH, Craver JM, Jones EL, et al. Mediastinitis after cardiac valve operations. J Thorac Cardiovasc Surg. 1985;90:517–22.

84. Lambl B, Lichtenberg D, Melvin Z, Karchmer AW. Deep sternal wound infection complicating cardiac surgery. In: Abstracts of the 1992 Interscience Conference on Antimicrobial Agents and Chemotherapy. Abstract 1260.

85. Harris RL, West MS, Kimball KT, et al. Host risk factors for median sternotomy surgical infections: A case control study. In: Abstracts of the 32nd Interscience Conference on Antimicrobial Agents and Chemotherapy. Abstract 1261. American Society for Microbiology, Washington, DC, 1992;321.

86. Jimenez-Martinez M, Arguero-Sanchez R, Perez-Alvarez JJ, Mina-Casteneda P. Anterior mediastinitis as a complication of median sternotomy incisions. Surgery. 1970;67:929–34.

87. Thurur RJ, Bognolo D, Vargas A, et al. The management of mediastinal infection following cardiac surgery. J Thorac Cardiovasc Surg. 1974;68: 962–8.

88. Grmoljez PF, Barner HK, Willman VL, Kaiser GC. Major complications of median sternotomy. Am J Surg. 1975;130:679–81.

89. Firor WB. Infection following open-heart surgery, with special reference to the role of prophylactic antibiotics. J Thorac Cardiovasc Surg. 1967;53: 371–8.

90. Brown AH, Baimbridge MV, Panagopoulos P, Sabar EF. The complications of median sternotomy. J Thorac Cardiovasc Surg. 1969;58:189–97.

91. Ochsner JL, Mills NL, Woolverton WC. Disruption and infection of the median sternotomy incision. J Cardiovasc Surg. 1972;13:394–9.

92. Macmanus Q, Okies JE. Mediastinal wound infection and aortocoronary graft patency. Am J Surg. 1976;132:558–61.

93. Rutledge R, Applbaum RE, Kim BJ. Mediastinal infection after open heart surgery. Surgery. 1985;97:88–92.

94. Stiegel RM, Beasley ME, Sink JD, et al. Management of postoperative mediastinitis in infants and children by muscle flap rotation. Ann Thorac Surg. 1988;46:45–6.

95. Orringer MB, Murray GF, Haller JA, Gott VL. Median sternotomy and outflow patch infections in total repair of tetralogy of Fallot. J Thorac Cardiovasc Surg. 1972;63:442–8.

96. Miller R, Rudler J, Karwande SV, Burton NA. Treatment of mediastinitis after heart transplantation. J Heart Transplant 1986;5:477–9.

97. Trento A, Dummer GS, Hardesty RL, et al. Mediastinitis following heart transplantation: Incidence, treatment, results. Heart Transplantation. 1984; 3:336–40.

98. Baldwin RT, Radovancevic B, Sweeney MS, et al. Bacterial mediastinitis after heart transplantation. J Heart Lung Transplant. 1992;11:545–9.

99. Pearl SN, Weiner MA, Dibbell DG. Sternal infection after cardiac transplantation. J Thorac Cardiovasc Surg. 1982;83:632–4.

100. Lonchyna VA, Pifarre R, Sullivan H, et al. Successful use of the total artificial heart as a bridge to transplantation with no mediastinitis. J Heart Lung Transplant. 1992;11:803–11.

101. Griffith BP, Kormos RK, Hardesty RL, et al. The artificial heart: Infection-related morbidity and its effect on transplantation. Ann Thorac Surg. 1988; 45:409–14.

102. Pennington DG, McBride LR, Kanter KR, et al. Bridging to heart transplantation with circulatory support devices. J Heart Transplant. 1989;8:116–23.

103. Rooks JR, Burton NA, Lefrak EA, Macmanus Q. Mediastinitis complicating successful mechanical bridge to heart transplantation. J Heart Lung Transplant. 192;11:261–4.

104. Phillips WS, Burton NA, Macmanus Q, Lefrak EA. Surgical complications in bridging to transplantation: The thermo cardiosystems LVAD. Ann Thorac Surg. 1992;53:482–6.

105. Didsheim P, Olsen DB, Farrar DJ, et al. Infections and thromboembolism with implantable cardiovascular devices. Trans Am Soc Artif Intern Organs. 1989;35:54–70.

106. Hazelrigg SR, Auer JE, Seifert PE. Experience in 100 transthoracic balloon pumps. Ann Thorac Surg. 1992;54:528–32.

107. Boerhaave H. Artocis, nec descripti prius Morbi Historia. Secundem Artis Leges Conscripta. Lugdunis Batavorum Bouresteniana; 1724.

108. Barrett NR. Spontaneous perforation of the oesophagus. Thorax. 1946;1: 48–70.

109. Katz D. Morbidity and mortality in standard and flexible gastrointestinal endoscopy. Gastrointest Endosc. 1969;15:134–41.

110. Keefer CS. Acute and chronic mediastinitis. Arch Intern Med. 1938;62: 109–36.

111. deSilva MI, Rissing JP. Postoperative wound infections following cardiac surgery: Significance of contaminated cases performed in the preceding 48 hours. Infect Control. 1984;5:371–7.

112. Dandalides PC, Rutala WA, Sarubbi FA Jr. Postoperative infections following cardiac surgery: Association with an environmental reservoir in a cardio-thoracic intensive care unit. Infect Control. 1984;5:378–84.

113. Palmer DL, Kuritsky JN, Lapham SC, et al. *Enterobacter* mediastinitis following cardiac surgery. Infect Control. 1985;6:115–9.

114. Ehrenkranz NJ, Pfaff SJ. Mediastinitis complicating cardiac operations: Evidence of postoperative causation. Rev Infect Dis. 1991;13:803–14.

115. Boyce JM, Bynoe GP, Opal SM, et al. A common-source outbreak of *Staphylococcus epidermidis* infections among patients undergoing cardiac surgery. J Infect Dis. 1990;161:493–9.

116. Nelson DR, Buxton TB, Luu QN, Rissing JP. The promotional effect of bone wax on experimental *Staphylococcus aureus* osteomyelitis. J Thorac Cardiovasc Surg. 1990;99:977–80.

117. Arnold M. The surgical anatomy of sternal blood supply. J Thorac Cardiovasc Surg. 1972;64:596–610.

118. Lust RM, Sun YS, Chitwood WR Jr. Internal mammary artery use: Sternal revascularization and experimental infection patterns. Circulation. 1991; 84(Suppl 3):285–9.

119. Kay EB, Naraghipour H, Beg RA. Internal mammary artery bypass graft: Long-term patency rate and follow-up. Ann Thorac Surg. 1974;18: 269–79.

120. Green GE. Internal mammary artery-to-coronary artery anastomosis: Three-year experience with 165 patients. Ann Thorac Surg. 1972;14:260–5.

121. Tector AJ, Davis L, Gabiel R, et al. Experience with internal artery grafts in 298 patients. Ann Thorac Surg. 1976;22:515–9.

122. Gaynes R, Marosok R, Hanley JM, et al. Mediastinitis following coronary artery bypass surgery: A 3-year review. J Infect Dis. 1991;163:117–21.

123. Archer GL, Tenenbaum MJ. Antibiotic-resistant *Staphylococcus epider-*

midis in patients undergoing cardiac surgery. Antimicrob Agents Chemother. 1980;17:269–72.

124. Archer GL, Armstrong BC. Alteration of staphylococcal flora in cardiac surgery patients receiving antibiotic prophylaxis. J Infect Dis. 1983;147: 642–9.

125. Chenoweth DE, Cooper SW, Hugli TE, et al. Complement activation during cardiopulmonary bypass. N Engl J Med. 1981;304:497–503.

126. Kirklin JK, Westaby S, Blackstone EH, et al. Complement and the damaging effects of cardiopulmonary bypass. J Thorac Cardiovasc Surg. 1983;86: 845–57.

127. Weinstein RA, Jones EL, Schwarzmann SW, Hatcher CR Jr. Sternal osteomyelitis and mediastinitis after open-heart operation: Pathogenesis and prevention. Ann Thorac Surg. 1976;21:442–4.

128. Rosendorf LL, Daicoff G, Baer H. Sources of gram-negative infection after open-heart surgery. J Thorac Cardiovasc Surg. 1974;67:195–201.

129. Andersen BM, Sorlie D, Hotvedt R, et al. Multiply beta-lactam resistant *Enterobacter cloacae* infections linked to the environmental flora in a unit for cardiothoracic and vascular surgery. Scand J Infect Dis. 1989;21:181–91.

130. Kaiser AB. Risk factors for infection in cardiac surgery: Will the real culprit please stand up? Infect Control. 1984;5:369–70.

131. Murray M, Finegold SM. Anaerobic mediastinitis. Rev Infect Dis. 1984;6: S123–7.

132. Howell HS, Prinz RA, Pickleman JR. Anaerobic mediastinitis. Surg Gynecol Obstet. 1976;143:353–9.

133. Weil RJ. Candidal mediastinitis after surgical repair of esophageal perforation. S Med J. 1991;84:1052–3.

134. Yardena SI, Shafir R, Weiss J, et al. Serious infectious complications of midsternotomy: A review of bacteriology and antimicrobial therapy. Scand J Infect Dis. 1990;22:633–43.

135. Glower DD, Douglas JM, Gaynor JW, et al. *Candida* mediastinitis after a cardiac operation. Ann Thorac Surg. 1990;49:157–63.

136. Lowry PW, Blankenship RJ, Gridley W, et al. A cluster of legionella sternal wound infections due to postoperative topical exposure to contaminated tap water. N Engl J Med. 1991;324:109–13.

137. Czachor JS, Hawley HB. Anaerobic wound infection: *Bacteroides* mediastinitis after cardiovascular surgery. Heart Lung. 1988;17:335–8.

138. Cerat GA, McHenry MC, Loop FD. Median sternotomy wound infection and anterior mediastinitis caused by *Bacteroides fragilis*. Chest. 1976;69: 231–2.

139. Isenberg HD, Tucci V, Cintron F, et al. Single-source outbreak of *Candida tropicalis* complicating coronary bypass surgery. J Clin Microbiol. 1989;27: 2426–8.

140. Thaler F, Gotainer B, Teodori G, et al. Mediastinitis due to *Nocardia asteroides* after cardiac transplantation. Intens Care Med. 1992;18:127–8.

141. Madero JS, Pratt K, Hall GS, et al. *Kluyvera* mediastinitis following open-heart surgery: A case report. J Clin Microbiol. 1990;28:2848–9.

142. Hoffman PC, Fraser DW, Robicsek F, et al. Two outbreaks of sternal wound infections due to organisms of the *Mycobacterium fortuitum* complex. J Infect Dis. 1981;143:533–42.

143. Richet HM, Craven PC, Brown JM, et al. A cluster of *Rhodococcus (Gordona) bronchialis* sternal wound infections after coronary artery bypass surgery. N Engl J Med. 1991;324:104–9.

144. Plotkin SA, Brachman PS, Utell M, et al. An epidemic of inhalation anthrax, the first in the twentieth century. Am J Med. 1960;29:992–1001.

145. Gelfand MS, Kaiser AB, Dale WA. Localized brucellosis: Popliteal artery aneurysm, mediastinitis, dementia, and pneumonia. Rev Infect Dis. 1989; 11:783–8.

146. Morgan DE, Nath H, Sanders C, Hasson JH. Mediastinal actinomycosis. AJR. 1990;155:735–7.

147. Yokogawa S, Cort WW, Yokogawa M. *Paragonimus* and paragonimiasis. Exp Parasitol. 1960;10:139–205.

148. Hamman L. Spontaneous mediastinal emphysema. Bull Johns Hopkins Hosp. 1939;64:1–21.

149. Aragon SB, Dolwick F. Buckley S. Pneumomediastinum and subcutaneous cervical emphysema during third molar extraction under general anesthesia. J Oral Maxillofac Surg. 1986;44:141–4.

150. Feldman R, Gromisch DS. Acute suppurative mediastinitis. Am J Dis Child. 1971;121:79–81.

151. Meade RH. Laryngeal obstruction in children. Pediatr Clin North Am. 1962; 9:233–62.

152. Rossiter JL, Hendrix RA. Iatrogenic subcutaneous cervicofacial and mediastinal emphysema. J Otolaryngol. 1991;20:315–9.

153. Kirshner JA. Cervical mediastinal emphysema. Arch Otolaryngol. 1980;106: 368–75.

154. Burnett CM, Rosemurgy AS, Pfeiffer EA. Life-threatening acute posterior mediastinitis due to esophageal perforation. Ann Thorac Surg. 1990;49: 979–83.

155. Shaffer HA, Valenzuela G, Mittal RK. Esophageal perforation. Arch Intern Med. 152:757–61.

156. Elleson DA, Rowley SD. Esophageal perforation: Its early diagnosis and treatment. Laryngoscope. 1982;92:678–80.

157. Appleton DS, Sandrasagra FA, Flower CDR. Perforated esophagus: Review of twenty-eight consecutive cases. Clin Radiol. 1979;30:493–7.

158. Berry BE, Ochsner JL. Perforation of the esophagus: A 30 year review. J Thorac Cardiovasc Surg. 1973;65:1–7.

159. Vessal K, Mantali RJ, Larson SM, et al. Evaluation of barium and gastrografin as contrast media for the diagnosis of esophageal ruptures or perforations. AJR. 1975;123:307–19.

160. Carrol CL, Jeffrey B Jr, Federle MP, Vernacchia FS. CT evaluation of mediastinal infections. J Comput Assist Tomogr. 1987;11:449–54.

161. Breatnach E, Nath PH, Delany DJ. The role of computed tomography in acute and subacute mediastinitis. Clin Radiol. 1986;37:139–45.

162. Kao CH, Wang SJ. Spread of infectious complications of odontogenic abscess detected by technetium-99m–HMPAO-labeled WBC scan of occult sepsis in the intensive care unit. J Nucl Med. 1992;33:254–5.

163. Simpson LC, Peters GE. Poststernotomy infections presenting as deep neck abscess. Arch Otolaryngol Head Neck Surg. 1988;114:909–12.

164. Kay HR, Goodman LR, Teplick SK, Mundth ED. Use of computed tomography to assess mediastinal complications after median sternotomy. Ann Thorac Surg. 1983;36:706–14.

165. Quirce R, Serano J, Arnal C, et al. Detection of mediastinitis after heart transplantation by gallium-67 scintigraphy. J Nucl Med. 1991;32:860–1.

166. Bahar RH, Shuhaiber HJ, Dayem HMA. The value of gallium-67 scintigraphy in localizing infection following cardiac surgery. Int J Cardiol. 1986;11:125–7.

167. Browdie DA, Bernstein RW, Agnew R, et al. Diagnosis of poststernotomy infection: Comparison of three means of assessment. Ann Thorac Surg 1991; 51:290–2.

168. Robicsek F. Posternotomy infections. Ann Thorac Surg. 1991;52:896–900.

169. Sarr MG, Watkins L Jr, Stewart JR. Mediastinal tap as useful method for the early diagnosis of mediastinal infection. Surg Gynecol Obstet. 1984;159: 79–82.

170. Barrett NR. Report of a case of spontaneous perforation of the oesophagus successfully treated by operation. Br J Surg. 1947;35:216–8.

171. Finley RJ, Pearson FG, Weisel RD, et al. The management of nonmalignant intrathoracic esophageal perforations. Ann Thorac Surg. 1980;30:575–83.

172. Trastek VF. Esophageal perforation: A reassessment of the criteria for choosing medical or surgical therapy. Arch Intern Med. 1992;152:693.

173. Kiernan PD, Conte JV Jr, Petri R, et al. Thoracic esophageal perforations at a Virginia hospital 1979–1990. VA Med Q. 1992;119:102–4.

174. Cameron JL, Kieffer RF, Hendrix TR, et al. Selective nonoperative management of contained intrathoracic esophageal disruptions. Ann Thorac Surg. 1979;27:404–8.

175. Santos GH, Frater WM. Transesophageal irrigation for the treatment of mediastinitis produced by esophageal rupture. J Thorac Cardiovasc Surg. 1986; 91:57–62.

176. Gobien RP, Stanley JH, Gobien BS, et al. Percutaneous catheter aspiration and drainage of suspected mediastinal abscesses. Radiology. 1984;151:69–71.

177. Gruhl VR. Renal failure, deafness, and brain lesions following irrigation of the mediastinum with neomycin. Ann Thorac Surg. 1971;11:376–9.

178. Kopel ME, Riemersma L, Finlayson DC, et al. Gentamicin solution for mediastinal irrigation: Systemic absorption, bactericidal activity, and toxicity. Ann Thorac Surg. 1989;48:228–31.

179. Kratz JM, Metcalf JS, Sade RM. Pericardial injury by antibacterial irrigants. J Thorac Cardiovasc Surg. 1983;86:785–7.

180. Zec N, Donovan JW, Kincaid RL, Demers LM. Seizures in a patient treated with continuous povidone-iodine mediastinal irrigation. N Engl J Med. 1992; 326:1784.

181. Glick PL, Guglielmo BJ, Tranbaugh RF, Turley K. Iodine toxicity in a patient treated by continuous povidone-iodine mediastinal irrigation. Ann Thorac Surg. 1985;39:478–80.

182. Campistol JM, Abad C, Nogue S, Bertran A. Acute renal failure in a patient treated by continuous povidone-iodine mediastinal irrigation. J Cardiovasc Surg. 1988;29:410–2.

183. Durandy Y, Batisse A, Bourel P, et al. Mediastinal infection after cardiac operation: A simple closed technique. J Thorac Cardiovasc Surg. 1989;97: 282–5.

184. Nahai F, Rand RP, Hester TR, et al. Primary treatment of the infected sternotomy wound with muscle flaps: A review of 211 consecutive cases. Plast Reconstr Surg. 1989;84:434–441.

185. Scully HE, Leclerc Y, Martin RD, et al. Comparison between antibiotic irrigation and mobilization of pectoral muscle flaps in treatment of deep sternal infections. J Thorac Cardiovasc Surg. 1985;90:523–31.

186. Majure JA, Albin RE, O'Donnell RS, Arganese TJ. Reconstruction of the infected median sternotomy wound. Ann Thorac Surg. 1986;42:9–12.

187. Miller JI, Nahai F. Repair of the dehisced median sternotomy incision. Surg Clin North Am. 1989;69:1091–102.

188. Heath BJ, Bagnato VJ. Poststernotomy mediastinitis treated by omental transfer without postoperative irrigation or drainage. J Thorac Cardiovasc Surg. 1987;94:355–60.

189. Szerafin T, Vaszily M, Peterffy A. Granulated sugar treatment of severe mediastinitis after open-heart surgery. Scand J Thorac Cardiovasc Surg. 1991;25:77–80.

190. Chirfe J, Scarmato G, Herszage L. Scientific basis for use of granulated sugar in treatment of infected wounds. Lancet. 1982;1:560–1.

191. Efem SEE. Clinical observations on the wound healing properties of honey. Br J Surg. 1988;75:679–81.

192. Trouillet JL, Chastre J, Fagon JY, et al. Use of granulated sugar in treatment of open mediastinitis after cardiac surgery. Lancet. 1985;2:180–4.

193. Antimicrobial prophylaxis in surgery. Abramowicz M, ed. Med Lett. 1992; 34:5–8.

194. Maki DG, Bohn MJ, Stolz SM, et al. Comparative study of cefazolin, cefamandole, and vancomycin for surgical prophylaxis in cardiac and vascular operations. J Thorac Cardiovasc Surg. 1992;104:1423–34.

195. Hoen B, Gerard A, Berne C. Prognostic factors for mediastinitis following cardiac surgery. In: Abstracts of the 32nd Interscience Conference on Antimicrobial Agents and Chemotherapy. Abstract 1258. American Society for Microbiology, Washington, DC, 1992;320.

196. Domart Y, Trouillet JL, Fagon JY, et al. Incidence and morbidity of cytomegaloviral infection in patients with mediastinitis following cardiac surgery. Chest. 1990;97:18–22.

197. Schowengerdt CG, Suyemoto R, Main FB. Granulomatous and fibrous mediastinitis. J Thorac Cardiovasc Surg. 1969;57:365–79.

198. Hache L, Woolner LB, Bernatz PE. Idiopathic fibrous mediastinitis. Dis Chest. 1962;41:9–25.

199. Strimlan CV, Dines DE, Payne WS. Mediastinal granuloma. Mayo Clin Proc. 1975;50:702–5.

200. Dines DE, Payne WS, Bernatz PE, Pairolero PC. Mediastinal granuloma and fibrosing mediastinitis. Chest. 1979;75:320–4.

201. Gryboski WA, Crutcher RR, Holloway JB, et al. Surgical aspects of histoplasmosis. Arch Surg. 1963;87:590–9.

202. Peabody JW, Brown RB, Sullivan MB, Cannon A. Mediastinal granulomas. J Thorac Surg. 1958;35:384–96.

203. Goodwin RA, Loyd JE, Des Prez RM. Histoplasmosis in normal hosts. Medicine. 1981;60:231–66.

204. Ramakantan R, Shah P. Dysphagia due to mediastinal fibrosis in advanced pulmonary tuberculosis. AJR. 1990;154:61–3.

205. Shah P, Ramakantan R. Hoarseness of the voice due to left recurrent laryngeal nerve palsy in tuberculous mediastinitis. Arch Otolaryngol Head Neck Surg. 1990;116:108.

206. Weese WC, Smith IM. A study of 57 cases of actinomycosis over a 36-year period. Arch Intern Med. 1975;135:1562–8.

207. Bennhoff DF. Actinomycosis: Diagnostic and therapeutic considerations and a review of 32 cases. Laryngoscope. 1984;94:1198–217.

208. Poland GA, Jorgensen CR, Sarosi GA. *Nocardia asteroides* pericarditis: Report of a case and review of the literature. Mayo Clin Proc. 1990;65:819–24.

209. Dunn EJ, Ulicny KS Jr, Wright CB, Gottesman L. Surgical implications of sclerosing mediastinitis. Chest. 1990;97:338–46.

210. Ahmad M, Weinstein AJ, Hughes JA, Cosgrove DE. Granulomatous mediastinitis due to *Aspergillus flavus* in a nonimmunocompromised patient. Am J Med. 1981;70:887–90.

211. Leong ASY. Granulomatous mediastinitis due to *Rhizopus* species. Am J Clin Pathol. 1978;70:103–7.

212. Case records of the Massachusetts General Hospital (case 6-1989). N Engl J Med. 1989;320:380–9.

213. Grotty TB, Colby TV, Gay PC, Pisani RJ. Desmoplastic malignant mesothelioma masquerading as sclerosing mediastinitis. Hum Pathol. 1992;23:79–82.

214. Loeb JM, Lombard CM. Idiopathic mediastinitis with superior vena cava obstruction, cardiac tamponade, and cutaneous vasculitis. West J Med. 1991; 155:296–9.

215. Williamson WA, Tronic BS, Levitan N, et al. Pulmonary venous infarction. Chest. 1992;102:937–40.

216. Berry DF, Buccigrossi BS, Peabody J, et al. Pulmonary vascular occlusion and fibrosing mediastinitis. Chest. 1986;89:296–301.

217. Rholl KS, Levitt RG, Glaser HS. Magnetic resonance imaging of fibrosing mediastinitis. AJR. 1985;145:255–9.

218. Feigin DS, Eggleston JC, Siegelman SS. The multiple roentgen manifestations of sclerosing mediastinitis. Johns Hopkins Med J. 1979;144:1–8.

219. Noguchi H, Kephart GM, Colby TV, Gleich GJ. Tissue eosinophilia and eosinophil degranulation in syndromes associated with fibrosis. Am J Pathol. 1992;140:521–8.

220. Urschel HC Jr, Razzuk MA, Netto GJ, et al. Sclerosing mediastinitis: Improved management with histoplasmosis titer and ketoconazole. Ann Thorac Surg. 1990;50:215–21.

221. Zajtchuk R, Strevey TE, Heydorn WH, Treasure RL: Mediastinal histoplasmosis: Surgical considerations. J Thorac Cardiovasc Surg. 1973;66:300–4.

222. Cardasco EM Jr, Ahmad M, Mehta A, Rubio F. The effects of steroid therapy on pulmonary hypertension secondary to fibrosing mediastinitis. Cleve Clin J Med. 1990;57:647–52.

SECTION H. CENTRAL NERVOUS SYSTEM INFECTIONS

63. ANATOMIC CONSIDERATIONS IN CENTRAL NERVOUS SYSTEM INFECTIONS

JOHN E. GREENLEE

The pathogenesis and course of central nervous system infections are greatly influenced by the anatomy of the brain and spinal cord and by the relationships of brain and cord to vessels, cranial nerves, spinal nerve roots, meninges, and overlying skeletal structure.

ANATOMIC RELATIONSHIPS OF THE BRAIN AND SPINAL CORD

Relationships of Brain, Meninges, and Skull

The brain is suspended in cerebrospinal fluid (CSF) and is surrounded by three layers of meninges: the pia mater and arach-

noid, which constitute the leptomeninges, and the dura mater or pachymeninges (Fig. 1).[1] The pia mater is continuous with the external surface of the brain and cord, forming a cuff of meningeal tissue around penetrating vessels and merging with the ependymal lining of the fourth ventricle at the foramina of Luschka and Magendie. The arachnoid encloses the brain more loosely, and between the pia and arachnoid, completely surrounding the brain and cord and communicating with the fourth ventricle, is the CSF-filled subarachnoid space. The outward pressure of brain and CSF holds the arachnoid in contact with the most superficial layer of meninges, the dura mater. The dura mater is adherent to the periosteum and skull except where it invaginates into the cranial cavity to form four rigid septa: the falx cerebri, falx cerebelli, tentorium cerebelli, and diaphragma selli.

Under normal conditions, the only meningeal compartment within the skull is the subarachnoid space. Acute bacterial infections within this space—bacterial meningitis—tend to involve the entire surface of the leptomeninges surrounding brain and spinal cord and frequently also spread inward through the foramina of Luschka and Magendie to produce ventriculitis (Fig. 1).[2] Infections may also involve the outer layers of meninges, by dissecting along tissue planes between the skull and dura. Epidural abscesses—those between the dura mater and the

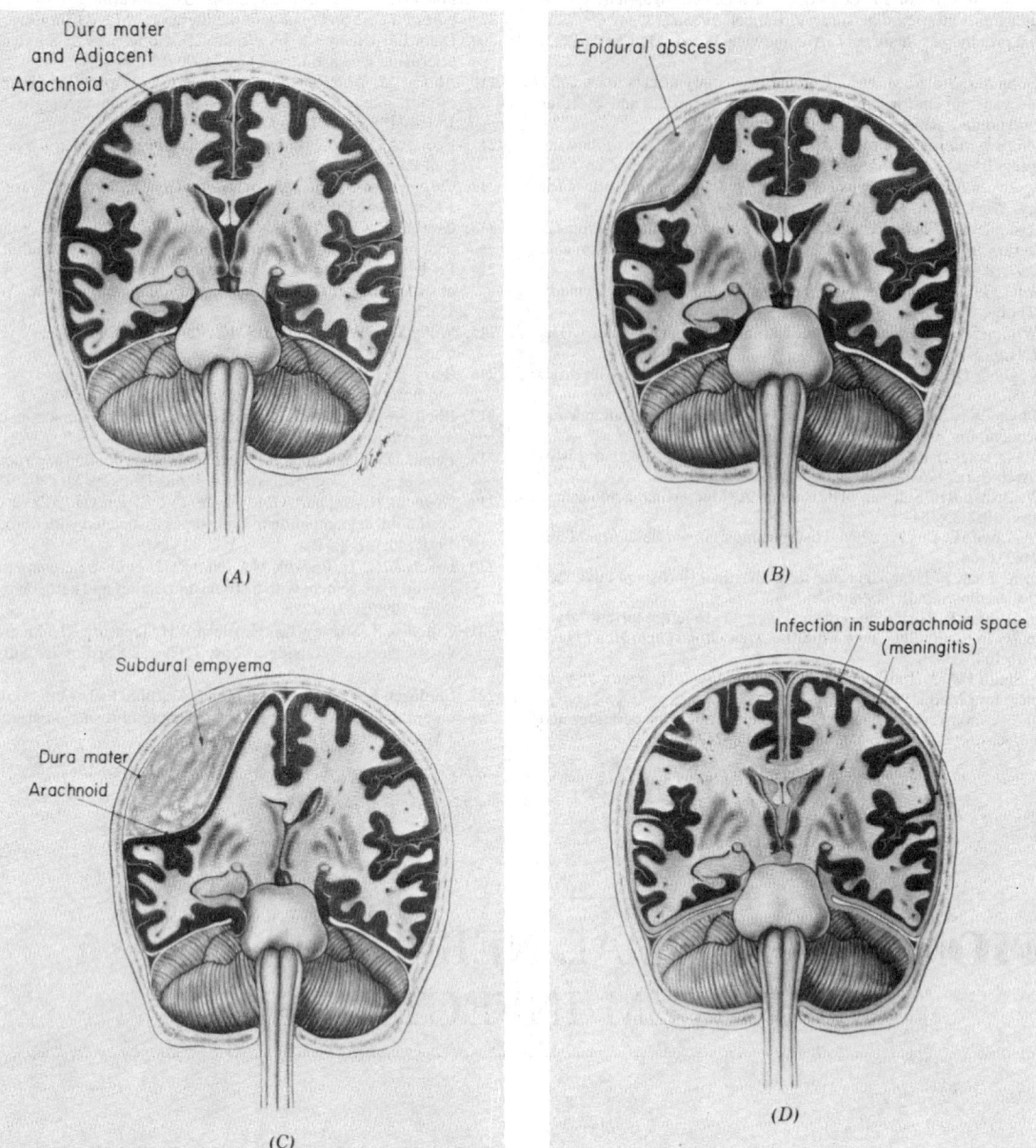

FIG. 1.   The cranial meninges. **(A)** Normal anatomic relationships; **(B)** alterations in epidural abscess; **(C)** subdural empyema; **(D)** and meningitis.

skull—tend to be sharply circumscribed by the tight attachment of the dura to the overlying skull (Fig. 1). Infection within the potential space between dura and arachnoid, on the other hand, results in a subdural empyema that may spread rapidly to cover an entire cerebral hemisphere, or one-half of the posterior fossa.

The location and severity of intracranial infection greatly influence the safety with which lumbar puncture can be performed.[3] Epidural abscess, subdural empyema, and brain abscess all behave as rapidly expanding mass lesions. Early in the course of bacterial meningitis, intracranial pressure may rise significantly, but this increase in pressure is transmitted throughout the subarachnoid space. In this setting, increased intracranial pressure results in little directional displacement of brain and little risk of herniation following lumbar puncture. More fully developed bacterial meningitis, however, is frequently accompanied by extensive cerebral edema as well as hydrocephalus, causing the entire brain to act as a mass lesion.[2,3] In the patient with advanced meningitis, as in the patient with epidural abscess, subdural empyema, or brain abscess,

lumbar puncture may be followed by transtentorial herniation and death.[3]

Relationship of Brain and Meninges to Cranial Structures

The undersurface of the brain rests within the anterior, middle, and posterior cranial fossae. Each fossa abuts on structures from which infection may spread (Fig. 2). The anterior fossa forms the roof of the frontal and ethmoidal sinuses. Infection within either sinus may produce a frontal epidural abscess, subdural empyema over the frontal lobes or falx, or a frontal lobe brain abscess.[4,5] The sella turcica, located between the left and right middle fossae, forms the roof of the sphenoid sinuses. Infection within these sinuses can spread centrally to cause not only epidural abscess and subdural empyema but also palsies of extraocular muscles, optic neuritis, and cavernous sinus thrombophlebitis.[6]

Infections of the middle ear or mastoid within the petrous

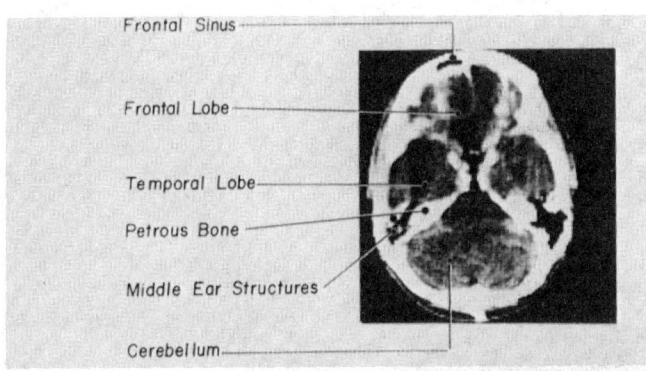

FIG. 2. Anatomic relationships of anterior, middle, and posterior fossa structures as seen on computed tomography. The frontal sinuses lie at the anterior pole of the cerebrum. The petrous bone, containing middle ear structures, lies between temporal lobe and cerebellum. An abscess, arising from the left frontal sinus, is faintly seen within the frontal lobe. (Courtesy of Dr. Frederick Vines, Jacksonville, FL.)

bone may extend into the middle fossa to involve the temporal lobe or may extend into the posterior fossa to involve the cerebellum or brain stem.[5,7] Rarely, infection within the maxillary sinus may cause temporal lobe abscess.

Injury to Cranial Nerves During Infections

All 12 cranial nerves exit through the meninges at the base of the brain and may be injured during meningitis. Cranial nerve deficits are particularly common in chronic infections of the basilar meninges such as those caused by *Mycobacterium tuber-*

culosis, Cryptococcus neoformans, or sarcoidosis.[8-11] Cranial nerves VII and VIII are most often affected, followed by cranial nerves III, IV, VI, IX, and X. Cranial nerve II may also be involved. If meningeal infection is protracted, multiple cranial nerve deficits may develop and may fluctuate during the course of the illness.[12]

Several of the cranial nerves have anatomic characteristics that predispose them to damage during infections or during states of increased intracranial pressure (see Table 1). Of particular importance is the close relationship of cranial nerve III to the tentorium. The parasympathetic fibers that control pupillary constriction are located on the superomedial surface of the third cranial nerve and are the first part of the nerve to be compressed during transtentorial herniation.[13] The clinical manifestations of cranial nerve III involvement during transtentorial herniation thus begin with unilateral pupillary dilatation, followed by lateral deviation of the affected eye as the third nerve fibers supplying the medial rectus, superior rectus, inferior rectus, and inferior oblique muscles are compromised. Cranial nerve VI has the longest intracranial course of any cranial nerve. An isolated paresis of the sixth nerve may indicate either direct involvement of the nerve anywhere along its length or compression due to elevated intracranial pressure.

Anatomic Relationships of the Spinal Cord

The spinal cord extends from the foramen magnum to the level of the L1-L2 intervertebral disk.[14] Below L2 the spinal canal contains the nerve roots that form the cauda equina. Unlike the cerebral hemispheres, where gray matter is most external, the spinal cord has a central core of gray matter and an external layer of white matter containing ascending and descending nerve tracts. Lesions developing within the cord (intramedullary le-

TABLE 1. Cranial Nerve Involvement in CNS Infections

Cranial Nerve or Nerves	Anatomic Features	Significance	Consequence
I	Traverses dura mater and ethmoid bone, surrounded by a cuff of arachnoid; terminates in free nerve endings within the nasal mucosa and nasopharynx.	The only cranial nerve in direct contact with the external environment.	May provide a route of direct CNS inoculation for neurotropic viruses.
II	Develops as a part of the brain and is contained within the subarachnoid space up to its point of entry into the eye.	1. Increased intracranial pressure causes papilledema. Chronic increased pressure results in optic atrophy.	1. Early signs are retinal vascular engorgement, followed by blurring of the optic disk, with hemorrhages appearing later. Initial visual change is enlargement of the physiologic blind spot. If intracranial hypertension persists, transient visual blurring and concentric constriction of visual fields occur. Chronic papilledema progresses to optic atrophy and blindness. Central scotomas may occur but are rare.
	Myelin sheath is composed of central myelin.	2. May be the target of immune response against central myelin in postinfectious encephalitis or encephalomyelitis.	2. Visual field deficit (usually central or centrocecal scotoma).
III	Passes directly beneath the edge of the tentorium cerebelli below the uncus of the temporal lobe.	Is almost always the first structure compressed by the uncus during transtentorial herniation.	Paresis of CN III parasympathetic fibers causes pupillary dilatation. Interruption of nerve supply to all extraocular muscles except lateral rectus and superior oblique causes lateral deviation of the eye and ptosis.
III, IV, V, VI	Travel together in the wall of the cavernous sinus.	All may be affected by cavernous sinus thrombosis.	Total ophthalmoplegia, mid-position fixed pupil, loss of corneal reflex and ipsilateral facial sensation.
V, VI	Travel in close proximity to the tip of the petrous bone.	May be injured in the course of chronic otitis media, especially where osteomyelitis of the petrous tip has developed.	Abducens palsy (lateral rectus weakness) and ipsilateral facial pain or sensory loss (Gradenigo syndrome).
IX–XI	Exit from skull through jugular foramen.	May be injured by thrombosis of the internal jugular vein at the jugular foramen.	Ipsilateral palatal weakness and diminished gag reflex; weakness of trapezius and sternomastoid muscles on the involved side (jugular foramen syndrome)
III–XII	Myelin sheaths composed of peripheral myelin.	May be involved with peripheral nerves and spinal nerve roots in postinfectious polyneuritis (Landry-Guillain-Barré syndrome).	Deficits of any cranial nerve except I or II may occur. Cranial nerve VII is most often involved.

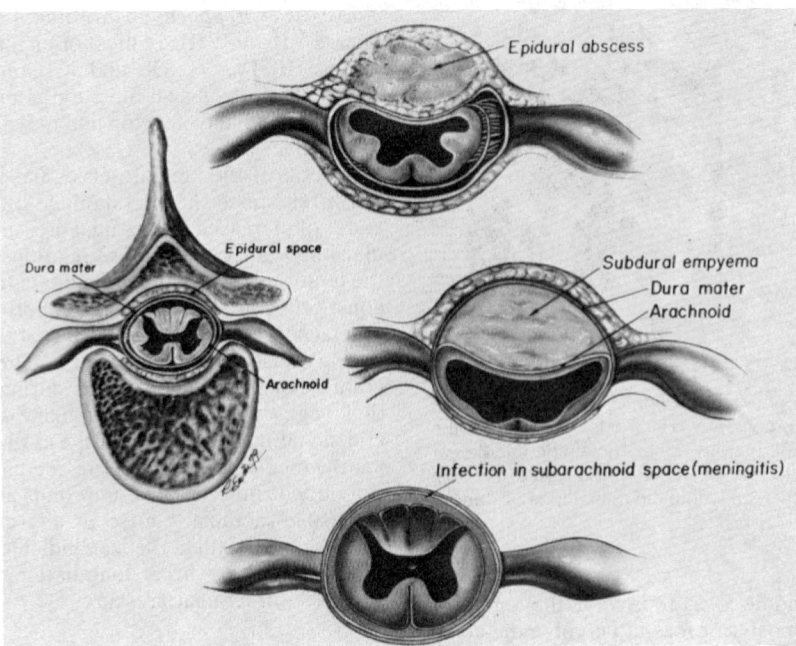

FIG. 3. The spinal meninges and epidural space: normal anatomic relationships and alterations in epidural abscess, subdural empyema, and meningitis.

sions) often produce neuronal injury at one or more spinal cord segments early in their course and only later expand laterally to involve motor and sensory nerve tracts. On the other hand, lesions external to the cord (extramedullary lesions) produce symptoms of nerve root irritation early in their course, followed by long tract signs; injury to central gray matter occurs only later.

The relationships of pia mater, arachnoid, and dura are essentially the same for the spinal cord as for the brain (Fig. 3), and the interface between spinal arachnoid and dura, like its intracranial counterpart, provides a plane along which infection can easily dissect. In contrast to the close adherence of the dura mater to the cranial periosteum and skull, however, the spinal dura and periosteum diverge at the foramen magnum, and by the level of the seventh cervical vertebra are separated by a fat-filled epidural space that offers little resistance to the longitudinal spread of infection. Both spinal subdural empyema and spinal epidural abscess may thus extend over many vertebral segments. Both are often posterior to the cord and may be inadvertently entered during lumbar puncture (see Fig. 3).[15]

ROLE OF THE INTRACRANIAL CIRCULATION IN CENTRAL NERVOUS SYSTEM INFECTIONS

Vascular Anatomy

Arteries. The brain is supplied by two internal carotid arteries and two vertebral arteries that join to form the basilar artery (Fig. 4).[16,17] Each internal carotid supplies the retina via the ophthalmic artery and bifurcates into an anterior cerebral artery that supplies the medial surface of the cerebrum and a middle cerebral artery that supplies the frontal, parietal, and temporal lobes over the cerebral convexity. The vertebrobasilar system supplies the rostral spinal cord, the brain stem, and the cerebellum before terminating in two posterior cerebral arteries. These angle sharply backward over the tentorium cerebelli to supply the occipital lobes, the posterior parietal lobes, and the posterior and mesial portions of temporal lobes. Because the ophthalmic artery is a branch of the internal carotid, emboli within the anterior circulation may produce monocular visual loss or retinal lesions visible by ophthalmoscopy and may give indirect evidence of an embolic source of central nervous system infection.

The major intracranial arteries differ in both caliber and volume of flow. The middle cerebral arteries receive the greatest volume of blood, followed by the anterior cerebrals and vertebrobasilar system. The likelihood of septic embolization, with resultant brain abscess or mycotic aneurysm, is thus greatest in the branches of the middle cerebral and least in the smaller branches of the posterior circulation.[18] The choroid plexuses also receive a large volume of blood.[19]

The major arteries of the brain are connected at the circle of Willis by anterior and posterior communicating branches and are also connected by smaller anastomotic vessels at the meningeal surface. The intracranial circulation communicates with the external carotid system through anastomoses between the ophthalmic and maxillary arteries and between branches of the vertebrals and the occipital arteries. There is also extensive communication with the meningeal branches of the external carotid via the rete mirabile, a network of small vessels that cross the meninges and anastomose with arteries on the surface of the brain.[16,17] Despite this collateral circulation, however, certain parts of the brain are arterial border zones or ''watershed areas,'' receiving their arterial supply from terminal branches of two or more vessels. The most important of these watershed areas lies between middle and posterior cerebral arteries at the junction of parietal, occipital, and temporal lobes. Similar watershed areas exist on the medial surface of the hemispheres, within the internal capsule, and over the cerebellum. These areas, particularly in the elderly patient with extensive vascular disease, are particularly vulnerable to ischemic injury if any of their supplying vessels becomes compromised. The signs and symptoms produced by watershed infarcts often extend beyond the usual distribution of the vessel involved. Cerebral white matter also forms a watershed area, receiving terminal arterial flow from both penetrating cortical and ventricular vessels. For this reason, white matter is more easily rendered ischemic than is gray matter, and abscesses arising within devitalized brain are most common in white matter or at the gray-white junction.[20]

Veins. The intracranial venous system is composed of three groups of vessels: superficial veins that drain the external portions of cerebrum and brain stem; deep veins that drain central white matter, basal ganglia, and thalamus; and venous sinuses

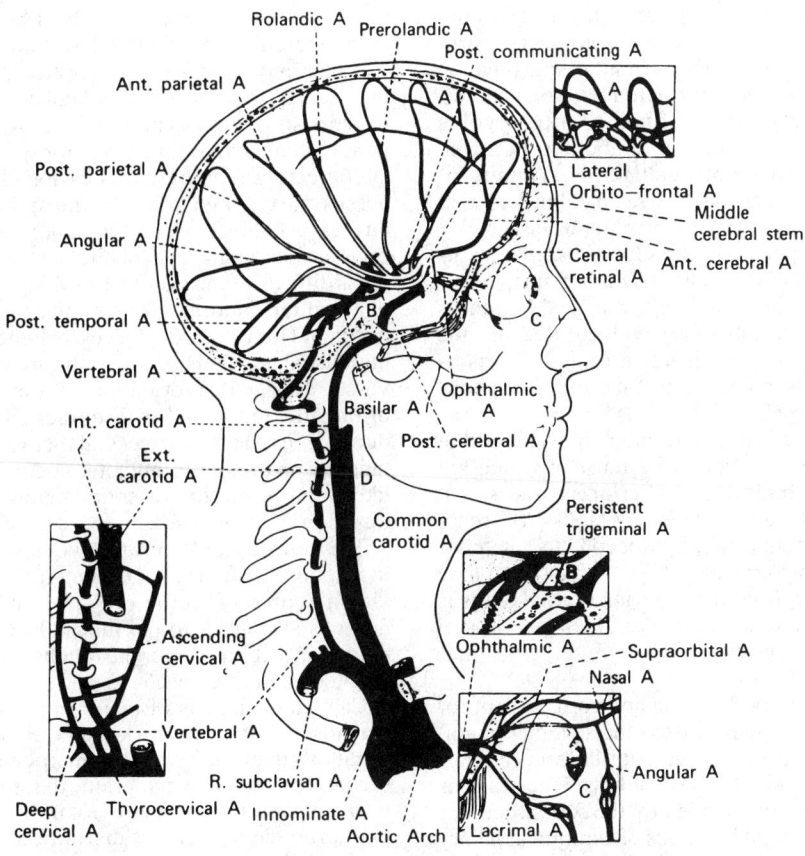

FIG. 4.   Arterial supply of central nervous system. (From Adams and Victor,[61] with permission.)

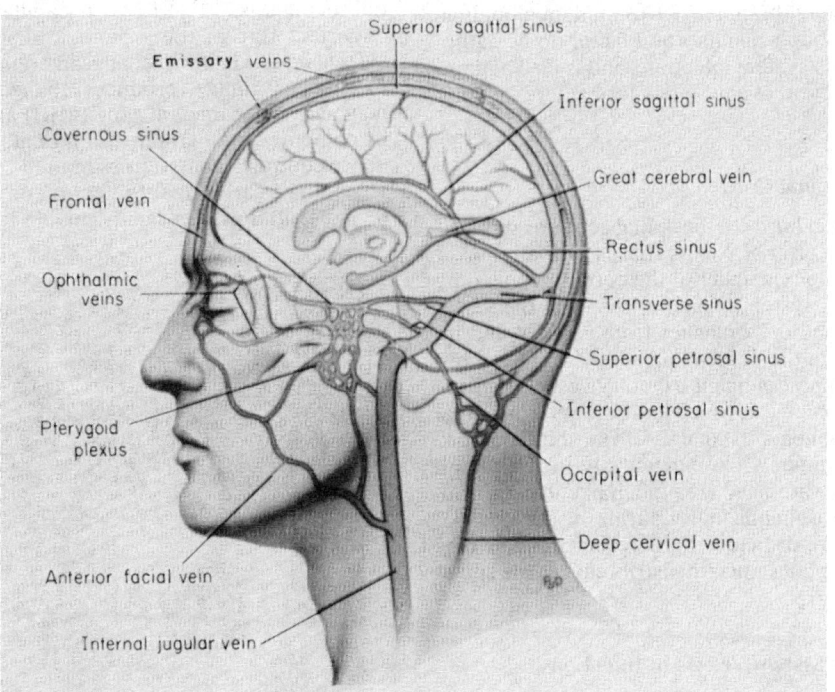

FIG. 5.   Venous supply of the central nervous system. (From Truax and Carpenter,[62] with permission.)

within the dura mater (Fig. 5).[17,21,22] The superficial veins of the cerebrum are divided about a watershed area above the Sylvian fissure into veins that empty upward into the superior sagittal sinus and veins emptying downward into the basilar venous sinuses.[21] The superficial and deep cerebral veins are extensively

interconnected, and anastomoses exist as well among the venous sinuses. There is also communication of superficial veins and venous sinuses with the extracranial venous system via numerous emissary veins that cross the skull and meninges. Neither intracranial veins nor venous sinuses have valves, so the direction of venous flow may reverse in response to hemodynamic changes. Because of these extensive anastomoses, cortical vein thrombosis or even occlusion of a venous sinus may at times be silent or may produce only transient neurologic abnormalities. If infarction results, clinical findings often evolve slowly and in fluctuating fashion as the thrombotic process involves increasing numbers of venous collaterals. Venous infarcts are frequently hemorrhagic, with irregular borders that are determined by remaining collateral venous drainage.[21,22] Thrombosis of the posterior portion of the superior sagittal sinus may produce cortical venous thrombosis of both hemispheres, causing bilateral lower extremity weakness. Cortical blindness may be present if both occipital lobes are involved. Because the hand area on the cerebral convexity has two routes of venous drainage, neurologic deficits referable to this area in venous thrombosis frequently resolve.

The cerebral venous sinuses not only drain venous blood but also reabsorb CSF through arachnoid villi, most of which are located along the anterior third of the superior sagittal sinus. Thrombosis of the superior sagittal sinus may block CSF reabsorption and produce communicating hydrocephalus, at times without other symptoms. Impairment of CSF reabsorption may also occur if venous outflow from the superior sagittal sinus is blocked by occlusion of both lateral sinuses or of one lateral sinus where the other is hypoplastic.[17,22]

Capillaries. The capillaries of the brain and cord, except for those of the pituitary, the choroid plexuses, and several circumventricular structures within the brain stem, differ from capillaries elsewhere in the body in that they do not have fenestrations or intracellular clefts and are surrounded by the foot processes of nearby astrocytes.[3,19] The tight junctions of cerebral capillary endothelial cells and the layer of astrocytic foot processes form a barrier through which molecules spread less by diffusion than by active transport or on the basis of lipid solubility. The relative impermeability of this blood-brain barrier to immunoglobulins, complement, and antibiotics is an important factor in the pathogenesis of central nervous system infections and is also a major consideration in the selection of antibiotics for bacterial meningitis or brain abscess.

Vascular Supply of the Spinal Cord

The posterior columns and horns of the spinal cord are supplied by an irregular posterior arterial plexus that is virtually never involved in infections. The remainder of the cord is supplied by the anterior spinal artery system, which arises from the vertebrals and receives contributory branches from cervical and intercostal arteries and from the descending aorta.[23] In many but not all patients there is a predominant tributary vessel from the aorta, the artery of Adamkiewicz, which joins the anterior spinal artery between cord segments T8 and L4. The thoracic cord above the artery of Adamkiewicz, particularly in the region around T4, may act as a watershed area much like those within the brain and may suffer ischemic injury during systemic hypotension or if vessels above or below it are occluded. The veins of the spinal cord are roughly similar in distribution to the spinal arteries.

Role of Central Nervous System Vessels in Infections

The vessels of the central nervous system provide the most frequent route by which infection reaches the meninges, brain, or cord (see below). In addition, involvement of the vessels themselves may produce ischemic or hemorrhagic injury to the brain or cord, with or without accompanying suppuration.[24] Arteries may be occluded by septic emboli. If the embolus breaks up before irreversible ischemia has occurred, it may produce symptoms of a transient ischemic attack; more protracted ischemia results in infarction. Arterial thrombosis may occur if

the vessel wall becomes involved by meningeal inflammation, as in tuberculous meningitis.[8] Multiplication of organisms within vascular endothelial cells, as in Rocky Mountain spotted fever, may cause thrombosis of small vessels.[25,26] Vasculitis and thrombosis of vessels may also occur as a complication of hepatitis B antigenemia[27] and is responsible for the syndrome of ipsilateral cerebral infarction occasionally seen during ophthalmic herpes zoster infections.[28] Similar but more chronic virus-induced vasculitis may be the major pathogenetic mechanism in progressive rubella encephalitis.[29] Occasionally, in bacterial endocarditis or other states of prolonged bacteremia, hyperplasia of vascular endothelial cells or obliterative endarteritis may occur and may occlude the vessel lumen.[30,31] In addition to causing vascular occlusion, arteritis may produce necrosis of the vessel wall and/or formation of a mycotic aneurysm. Rupture of the affected vessel with intracranial hemorrhage may occur during or even after successful therapy for the infection.[18] Spontaneous resolution of mycotic aneurysms may occur,[32] but the likelihood of rupture or spontaneous resolution cannot be predicted in a given case.

The veins of the central nervous system may also thrombose in response to internal or extramural inflammation and may provide a source of sterile or septic emboli to other parts of the nervous system or to the lungs. The infarcted tissue produced by either arterial or venous occlusion may become the site of single or multiple abscesses.

Capillary injury is of major importance in the pathogenesis, diagnosis, and treatment of central nervous system infections. Capillary damage by septic microemboli may allow escape of organisms into ischemic brain, to initiate brain abscess. Tumor necrosis factor and other cytokines released by bacterial products produce significant disruption in capillary integrity (see below). Cerebral edema, produced by transudation of fluid across injured capillaries, is an important cause of mortality in brain abscess, epidural abscess, subdural empyema, and bacterial meningitis.[24,33,34] Loss of capillary integrity also plays an important role in the radiologic diagnosis of central nervous system infection: focal change in brain water content, secondary to capillary injury, produces changes visible on T2-weighted magnetic resonance imaging (MRI) and in brain density visible by computed tomography (CT). Leakage of gadolinium or radiodense contrast agents across injured capillaries may permit visualization of early foci of infection on MRI or contrast CT (Fig. 6).[35,36] Antibiotics normally unable to cross cerebral or menin-

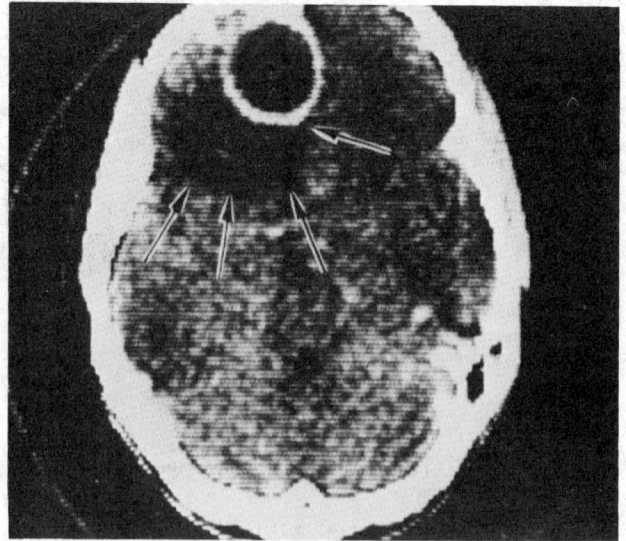

FIG. 6. Brain abscess as seen on computed tomography. The arrows outline an area of cerebral edema equal in size to the abscess itself. This is a more rostral view of the abscess faintly seen in Figure 2. (Courtesy of Dr. Frederick Vines, Jacksonville, FL.)

geal capillaries penetrate brain and CSF across damaged capillaries. As inflammation subsides, capillary integrity is restored, cerebra edema resolves, and CSF antibiotic concentrations fall, even if no alteration is made in antibiotic dose or route of administration.

Spinal vessels are rarely involved by infection. Spinal artery occlusion may occur during bacterial endocarditis, Rocky Mountain spotted fever, or tertiary syphilis. Spinal veins may be involved by epidural abscess or subdural empyema and may produce cord injury more extensive than would be expected on the basis of compression alone.

CEREBROSPINAL FLUID CIRCULATION IN NERVOUS SYSTEM INFECTIONS

Eighty-five percent of the CSF is produced within the lateral, third, and fourth ventricles by the choroid plexuses (see Fig. 7), the remainder forming by diffusion across the meninges.[3] The choroid plexuses resemble renal tubules histologically and produce CSF by secretion rather than passive diffusion. Like renal tubules, the choroid plexuses also contain probenecid-sensitive and other transport mechanisms and are capable of removing weak organic acids, including penicillin and gentamicin, from the CSF against a concentration gradient.[3,19] The direction

of the CSF circulation is outward through the foramina of Luschka and Magendie into the subarachnoid space, where it circulates around the brain and cord by bulk flow. Reabsorption of CSF occurs by vesicular transport through cells of the arachnoid villi along the superior sagittal sinus. A small amount of CSF may be absorbed directly across the meninges. Complete exchange of CSF occurs every 3 to 4 hours.

The CSF circulation is important in the diagnosis, treatment, and complications of central nervous system infections. Chemical and cellular changes in CSF may provide valuable information about infections within the subarachnoid space and, in extensive leptomeningeal infections, may contain the infectious agent in large numbers.[3] However, lumbar CSF may not always give precise information in chronic basilar or other localized meningeal infections and, unless very large volumes of lumbar CSF are studied,[3] may not allow recovery of the infectious agent or contain diagnostic antigens at a time when the causative agent may be isolated by high cervical or cisternal puncture.[3] In subdural or epidural infection or in brain abscess, where infection occurs outside the subarachnoid space, the CSF may be normal or may reveal only a mild, nonspecific lymphocytosis, with a slight elevation of the protein concentration and a normal sugar level; organisms are only rarely present.[37,38]

The physiology of the CSF circulation is important in those

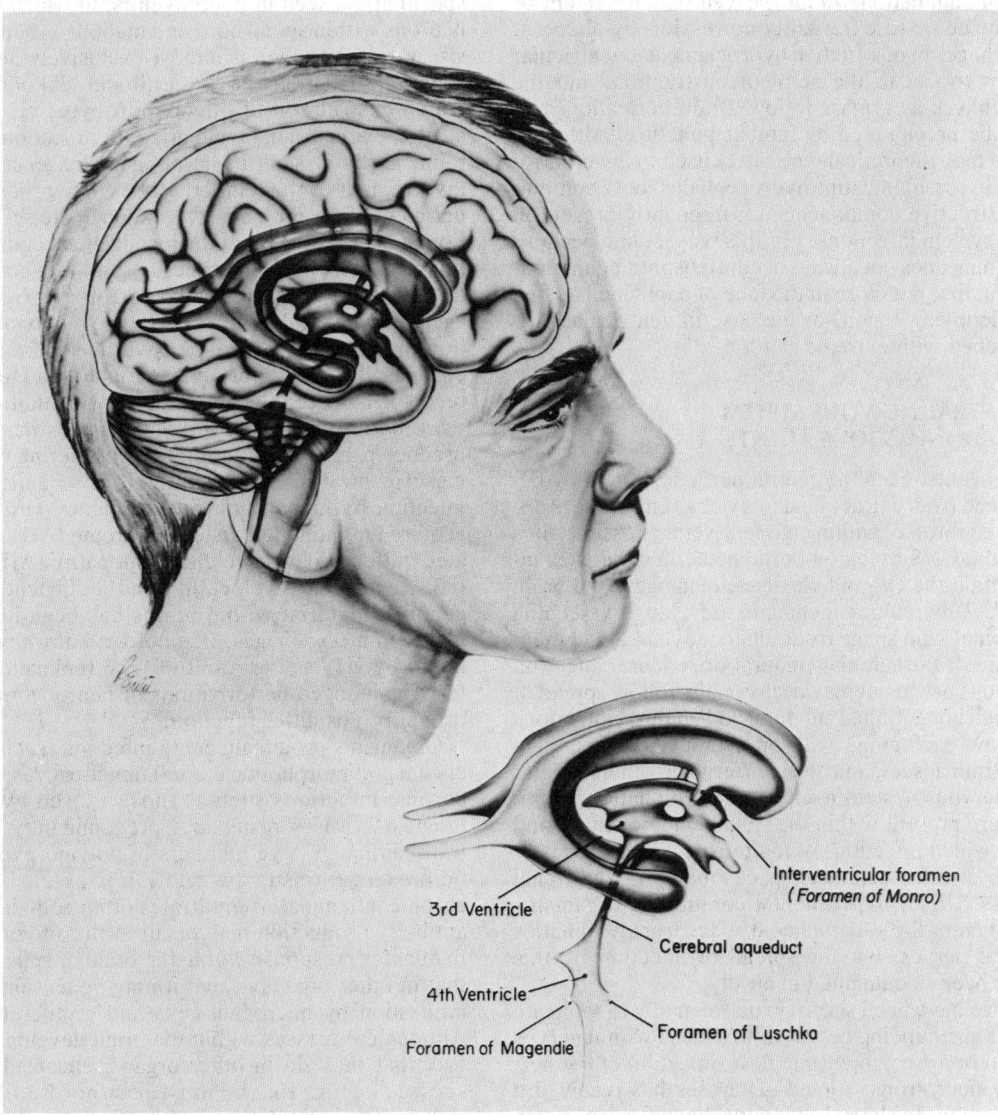

3rd Ventricle

Interventricular foramen (Foramen of Monro)

Cerebral aqueduct

4th Ventricle

Foramen of Luschka

Foramen of Magendie

FIG. 7. The cerebral ventricles. The ventricular system is narrowest and hence most easily obstructed at the foramen of Monro, the cerebral aqueduct (aqueduct of Sylvius), and the foramina of Luschka and Magendie.

instances in which it becomes crucial to treat bacterial or fungal ventriculitis with an aminoglycoside, amphotericin B, or other agents that penetrate into CSF poorly. Although it is possible, under experimental conditions, to produce high ventricular levels of agents by the instillation of large volumes,[39] intrathecal administration of antibiotics in conventional volumes produces unreliable ventricular concentrations, and lumbar administration does not allow measurement of the ventricular concentrations achieved.[40] Because of these factors, therapy with agents that must be instilled directly into the CSF requires direct administration into the ventricles through a subcutaneous reservoir.

Infections involving the nervous system may produce communicating or obstructive hydrocephalus. Communicating hydrocephalus follows impairment of CSF reabsorption across the arachnoid villi and may be due to blood within the subarachnoid space, chronic meningitis, or occlusion of the superior sagittal or lateral sinuses. In communicating hydrocephalus, although ventricular dilatation occurs, the increase in pressure is distributed equally throughout the subarachnoid space and ventricular system. Obstructive hydrocephalus develops when there is compromise of CSF circulation within the ventricles and most often represents occlusion of the ventricular system at its narrowest points: the foramina of Luschka and Magendie, the aqueduct of Sylvius, or, rarely, the foramina of Monro. Occlusion may be due to inflammation within the ventricular system or subarachnoid space or to external compression by abscess, mass, or hemorrhage. In obstructive hydrocephalus, ventricular dilatation occurs rostral to the point of obstruction, and the trapped CSF behaves as a mass lesion. Brain herniation may occur and may be precipitated by lumbar puncture. Although lumbar puncture may theoretically be safely used to lower intracranial pressure in communicating hydrocephalus, both communicating and obstructive components are frequently present in central nervous system infections. For this reason, and because CT or MRI scanning does not always accurately predict impending herniation, lumbar puncture in the face of papilledema, suspected space-occupying lesion, or increase in ventricular size must be approached with extreme caution.[3,41]

ROUTES OF CENTRAL NERVOUS SYSTEM INVOLVEMENT BY INFECTIOUS AGENTS

Most infectious agents reach the central nervous system by hematogenous spread from extracranial foci or by retrograde propagation of infected thrombi within emissary veins. Possible sites for invasion of the CNS by blood-borne bacteria or viruses include vessels within the choroid plexuses, meninges, and brain parenchyma.[29,42] Tuberculous meningitis develops by seeding of the cerebrospinal fluid space from subependymal or submeningeal granulomas.[43] Intracranial epidural or subdural infection is usually of venous origin but may occasionally follow spread of organisms through bone. Spinal subdural and epidural infections more often follow bacteremia with or without accompanying osteomyelitis. Brain abscess may be of arterial or venous origin.

The central nervous system itself has no lymphatic system, but lymphatics are present within the spinal epidural space and form a route by which infections of the retropharyngeal, posterior mediastinal, or retroperitoneal spaces may produce spinal epidural abscess. Under experimental conditions, organisms can be shown to enter the subarachnoid space from lymphatics within peripheral nerves, but the spread of infection by this route has never been documented clinically.[29]

Because viruses have been shown experimentally to replicate in Schwann cells surrounding nerves or to ascend within nerves at a rate equal to reverse axoplasmic flow, infection of the nervous system by neurotropic spread of viruses has received a great deal of attention. In clinical situations, however, neurotropism has been shown to be important only for herpes simplex and zoster, which produce latent infection of sensory ganglia, and rabies, which may bind to or near acetylcholine receptors at the neuromuscular junction and reaches the central nervous system by spread within axons.[44,45] Rare cases of rabies have been reported after exposure to infected aerosols.[29,46] In these instances, the virus is believed to have penetrated free olfactory nerve endings within the nasal cavity, with rapid entry into the central nervous system (Table 1).[29] Infection of the nervous system via cranial nerve I has also been postulated in herpes simplex encephalitis, because of the frequent involvement of olfactory brain, but has never been proven.

RESPONSE OF THE CENTRAL NERVOUS SYSTEM TO INFECTION

The central nervous system is unlike other organs in its unique cellular composition, its sequestration from the rest of the body by physiologic barriers, and its close confinement within rigid skeletal structures. These properties greatly influence the course of infection. Widespread infection of the brain, involving all tissue elements, is characteristic of many viral encephalitides and of the diffuse cortical inflammation that accompanies bacterial meningitis. The functional specialization of different cell populations and of specific neuroanatomic regions, however, enables infections that involve specific cell types or anatomic areas to produce characteristic neurologic syndromes. Cellular specificity is seen in poliomyelitis, in which infection of motor neurons within spinal cord and medulla produces flaccid paralysis; in rabies, which is almost exclusively an infection of neurons; and in progressive multifocal leukoencephalopathy, in which destruction of oligodendrocytes results in multifocal, scattered areas of demyelination. Predilection for particular anatomic areas is seen in herpes simplex encephalitis, in which involvement of the temporal lobes may produce psychosis, impairment of recent memory, and uncinate seizures. Focal infection may also be seen in the localized encephalitis that precedes brain abscess, in brain abscess itself, or in granulomatous infections of tuberculous, fungal, or other origins. Certain viral agents, such as rabies virus, produce severe neurologic dysfunction in the absence of extensive necrosis or other pathologic changes. The ability of rabies virus to bind to the acetylcholine receptor has been discussed above. In addition, evidence from work both in vitro and in vivo suggests that rabies virus may produce part of its symptoms by interfering with receptor binding of central neurotransmitters.[47–49] Central nervous system infection by human immune deficiency virus (HIV) in human acquired immunodeficiency syndrome (AIDS) has been associated with a progressive encephalopathy (AIDS-related dementia), a vacuolar myelopathy, and a subacute meningitis. HIV genomic material within brains has been identified predominantly in macrophages. It is not yet known whether neurologic injury by HIV is the result of viral replication per se or is due to virus-induced perturbations of neuronal metabolic activities or neurotransmitter function.[50,51]

Organisms producing acute infection, such as most bacteria, elicit a polymorphonuclear inflammatory response. Subacute or chronic infections such as those caused by M. tuberculosis, fungi, or viruses result in a predominantly lymphocytic infiltrate, although large numbers of polymorphonuclear cells may be present if tissue destruction is extensive. Subacute and chronic inflammatory infiltrates often contain plasma cells, and antibody production may occur at the site of infection. The inflammatory response within the brain or spinal cord differs from that in other organs in that it may be less intense and includes infiltration by microglial cells and proliferation of astrocytes. Although abscesses within the brain develop in much the same way that they do in other organs, encapsulation of brain abscesses occurs for the most part not by fibrosis but by the slower, less complete process of gliosis. When the brain has suffered previous ischemic injury, the inflammatory response may be minimal, and reactive gliosis may fail to occur.

Recovery from central nervous system infection involves antibody, cell-mediated immunity, and complement. Antibody is normally excluded from the central nervous system. The presence of antibody in brain or spinal fluid thus indicates diffusion of immunoglobulin molecules across an injured blood-brain barrier or local synthesis of antibody by immunocompetent cells that have gained entry into brain parenchyma.[3] Antibody produced within the central nervous system is oligoclonal, suggesting that the plasma cells responsible for local antibody synthesis are derived from a limited number of B cells.[29] Systemic humoral immunity plays a major protective role against bacterial infections of the central nervous system and may play a role in determining survival in bacterial meningitis.[2,29] Demonstration of a rise in antibody titers between acute and convalescent sera is an important retrospective means of identifying infections caused by viruses or other agents that are poorly recovered by culture techniques. Determination of CSF antibody titers to specific agents is of more limited value. Because the blood-CSF barrier is poorly permeable to immunoglobulins, the serum : CSF antibody ratio is normally above 200.[3] Injury to the blood-brain barrier can lower this ratio nonspecifically, and intrathecal synthesis of antibody directed against a particular infectious agent may selectively alter the ratio for that agent. Detection of CSF antibody or proof of intrathecal antibody synthesis has proved useful in the diagnosis of chronic or slow infections such as Lyme disease, subacute sclerosing panencephalitis, or progressive rubella encephalitis.[3] Investigation of CSF antibody titers has also been employed in epidemiologic studies of central nervous system involvement by HIV.[52,53] Penetration of antibody across the blood-brain barrier and intrathecal antibody synthesis develop over time, however, and are not reliable initial diagnostic tests in acute infections such as herpes simplex virus encephalitis.[3] Cell-mediated immunity comprises the major defense of the central nervous system against infections due to fungi or to intracellular parasites such as viruses, *M. tuberculosis, Listeria monocytogenes,* and *Toxoplasma gondii.* Where cell-mediated immunity is impaired, these organisms are particularly likely to involve the central nervous system and may cause fatal disease despite extremely high titers of specific antibody. Humoral and cell-mediated immune responses are closely related, and severe compromise of T-cell-mediated immune response, as in AIDS, may be accompanied by blunting of humoral immune response.[54] Complement has a number of functions, including the ability to lyse infectious agents or cells expressing viral or other foreign antigens on their surfaces. Complement may thus serve as an important mechanism of host defense against infection, but, in experimental circumstances at least, the action of complement on infected cells may be a major cause of neurologic injury.[55]

In certain infections due to virus or *Mycoplasma* or after immunization, the host may develop an immune response not only against the causative agent but also against the basic protein of peripheral or central myelin.[29,56,57] Reaction against peripheral myelin produces segmental demyelination and at times axonal loss within nerve roots and peripheral nerves, causing an ascending motor paralysis (Landry-Guillain-Barré syndrome). Reaction to central myelin results in a monophasic illness characterized by perivascular inflammation and multifocal demyelination of brain, spinal cord, and optic nerve.[29,57] In severe cases, necrosis and/or hemorrhage of white matter may occur.

Role of Edema and Brain Herniation in Central Nervous System Infections

Infection and inflammation produce not only local injury to nervous system parenchyma but also loss of capillary integrity with transudation of intravascular fluid into brain or cord. The cerebral edema that results from this process is an invariable and potentially lethal consequence of central nervous system infections.

Several factors contribute to the development of cerebral edema. Bacterial products such as the endotoxins of Gram-negative organisms and teichoic acid produced by *Staphylococcus aureus* cause release of tumor necrosis factor and cytokines from cerebral capillary endothelial cells and astrocytes.[58] These mediators of inflammation, in turn, produce extensive loss of capillary integrity. The vasogenic cerebral edema produced by this mechanism is a major—and potentially treatable—contributor to patient morbidity and mortality in the early stages of bacterial meningitis (see Ch. 64). Development of cerebral edema can be slowed by administration of corticosteroids and may actually be accelerated following initiation of antibiotic therapy, as bacterial products released from antibiotic-lysed organisms cause further cytokine release.[58] Similar cytokine-mediated processes may also be involved in the cerebral edema that accompanies severe viral encephalitis. In meningitis, encephalitis, or ischemia, additional brain swelling may result from entry of extracellular water into injured cells (cytotoxic edema). Interstitial edema of periventricular structures may develop in hydrocephalus. Although small amounts of edema may be asymptomatic, more extensive cerebral edema may act as a space-occupying lesion.

Inflammation, hemorrhage, hydrocephalus, and edema may all produce displacement of brain or cord. In infections of the nervous system any or all of these conditions may be present simultaneously. Although the nervous system is able to deform greatly beneath gradual compression, both brain and spinal cord are poorly compliant beneath rapidly expanding lesions and, within the rigid confines of the skull or spinal column, have little room in which to be displaced before significant compression occurs. Displacement of one cerebral hemisphere will force brain tissue beneath the falx cerebri and over the tentorium cerebelli (Fig. 8).[13,59] Herniation beneath the falx is usually

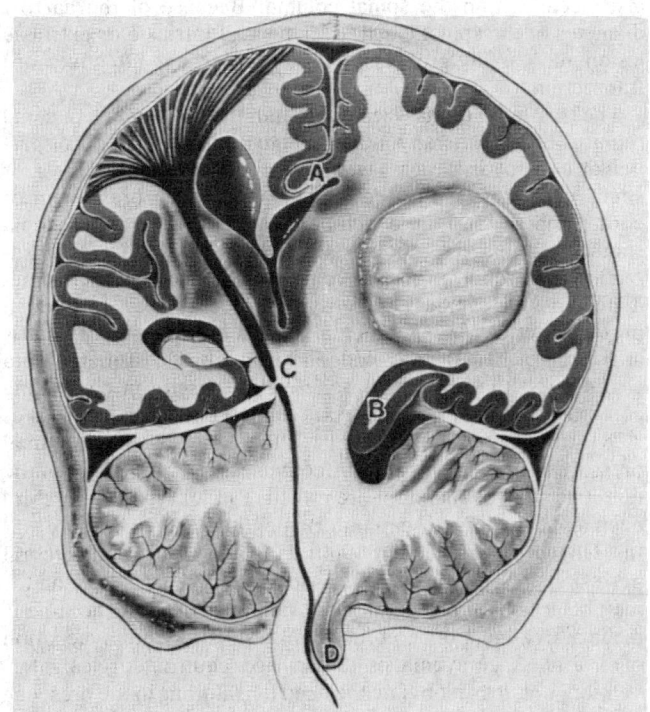

FIG. 8. Consequences of brain displacement by a mass lesion. (*A*) Herniation of cingulate gyrus beneath the falx cerebri; (*B*) herniation of the uncus of the temporal lobe over the tentorium cerebelli, (*C*) with compression of the contralateral corticospinal tract against the tentorium and (*D*) development of false localizing signs; herniation of the cerebellar tonsils through the foramen magnum.

TABLE 2. Short-Term Therapy of Cerebral Edema[a]

Therapy	Mechanism of Action	Dosage or Therapeutic Endpoint	Remarks
Hyperventilation	Causes vasoconstriction with resultant decrease in total intracranial blood volume	PCO_2 should be lowered to 25–30 mmHg. Increase respiratory rate by 20% for 10–20 minutes and return gradually to baseline	Produces almost immediate fall in intracranial pressure but effect rapidly diminishes. Requires intubation and mechanical ventilation
Dexamethasone	Stabilizes capillary integrity and lessens cerebral edema	10 mg IV followed by 4 mg IV at 4–6 hour intervals	Effective in vasogenic edema complicating bacterial meningitis or brain abscess. Role in viral CNS infections uncertain. Has little effect in edema accompanying brain infarction
Mannitol	Hyperosmolar effect, with shift of brain water into the vascular compartment	Give as 20% solution IV 0.5–1 g/kg over 10 minutes followed by 0.25–0.5 g/kg q3–5h as needed	Produces rapid fall in ICP but constitutes a significant metabolic stress. Mannitol-induced intravascular hypervolemia may precipitate congestive heart failure. Patient should undergo urinary catheterization at initiation of therapy. Protracted use of mannitol necessitates measurement of intake and urinary output, serum electrolytes, and serum osmolality. Risk of rebound in ICP from diffusion of mannitol into brain is minimal in first 24 hours of therapy

[a] Medical therapy of increased intracranial pressure (ICP) is never a substitute for evacuation of loculated infection or relief of hydrocephalus. Intracranial pressure monitoring may be essential in assessing efficacy of treatment.

asymptomatic. Herniation of the temporal lobe over the tentorium, however, initially produces paresis of cranial nerve III and may cause corticospinal tract signs ipsilateral to the lesion as the contralateral cerebral peduncle is compressed against the tentorium (Fig. 8). Coma follows, and there is progressive loss of brain stem reflexes culminating in respiratory arrest as the medullary respiratory centers are affected. The characteristic neurologic syndromes that result at successively lower levels of brain stem function are described in detail in the monograph by Plum and Posner[13]; an understanding of these syndromes is crucial to the management of the patient with central nervous system infection. It should be kept in mind, however, that posterior fossa mass lesions such as a cerebellar abscess or hemorrhage may produce rapid compression of the medulla and pons without antecedent midbrain signs. Compressive lesions may also occur within the spinal column. Because of the narrow diameter of the spinal canal, even a small intrinsic or extrinsic lesion may rapidly progress to cord necrosis and effective cord transection.

The treatment of mass lesions within the skull or spinal canal requires prompt therapy in addition to antibiotics and is of particular urgency in patients with lesions of the posterior fossa or spinal canal because of the rapidity with which brain stem or cord compression may develop. Treatment of cerebral edema should be initiated as soon as suspected (see Table 2).[59] Dexamethasone, which in part reverses tumor necrosis factor-mediated loss of capillary integrity, has been shown to exert a protective effect in experimental models of bacterial meningitis and to be of benefit in childhood meningitis.[58,60] Limited data also suggest that dexamethasone may be useful in controlling cerebral edema in brain abscess.[59] Hyperventilation to a CO_2 of <28 torr may provide emergent control of increased intracranial pressure but rapidly loses its effectiveness over time.[59] Osmotic diuretics such as mannitol are effective in all types of cerebral edema but require close monitoring of fluid and electrolyte status. Ongoing measurement of intracranial pressure and cerebral perfusion pressure through a transcranial or ventricular monitor may be crucial in protecting the brain over time. At no time is medical treatment of cerebral edema a substitute for evacuation of an abscess, empyema, or hemorrhage requiring surgical intervention, nor does it obviate the need for shunting in the presence of hydrocephalus. The most urgent priority in bacterial infections of the central nervous system is prompt institution of appropriate antibiotic therapy. Immediately following this, appropriate neuroradiologic studies should be obtained emergently if a mass lesion is suspected, and plans should be made for immediate surgery if indicated.

REFERENCES

1. Bargmann W, Oksche A, Fix JD, et al. Meninges, choroid plexus, ependyma, and their reactions. In: Haymaker W, Adams RD, eds. Histology and Histopathology of the Nervous System. Springfield, IL: Charles C. Thomas; 1982: 560–714.
2. Quagliarello V, Scheld WM. Bacterial meningitis: Pathogenesis, pathophysiology, and progress. N Engl J Med. 1992;327:864–72.
3. Greenlee JE. Cerebrospinal fluid in central nervous system infections. In: Scheld WM, Whitley RJ, Durack DT, eds. Infections of the Central Nervous System. New York: Raven Press; 1991:861–85.
4. Weber AL, Mikulis DK. Inflammatory disorders of the paraorbital sinuses and their complications. Radiol Clin North Am. 1987;25:615–30.
5. Wackym PA, Canalis RF, Feuerman T. Subdural empyema of otorhinological origin. J Laryngol Otol. 1990;104:118–22.
6. Dale BAB, Mackenzie J. The complications of sphenoid sinusitis. J Laryngol Otol. 1983;97:661–70.
7. Morgan DW, Williams B. Posterior fossa subdural empyema. Brain. 1985; 108:983–92.
8. Tandon PN. Tuberculous meningitis. In: Vinken PJ, Bruyn GW, Klawans HL, eds. Handbook of Clinical Neurology. Amsterdm: Elsevier North Holland; 1978:195–262.
9. Lewis JL, Rabinovich S. The wide spectrum of cryptococcal infections. Am J Med. 1972;53:315–22.
10. Dismukes WE. Cryptococcal meningitis in patients with AIDS. J Infect Dis. 1988;157:624–28.
11. Chapelon C, Zisa JM, Piette JC, et al. Neurosarcoidosis: Signs, course, and treatment in 35 confirmed cases. Medicine. 1990;69:261–76.
12. Symonds C. Multiple recurrent cranial nerve palsies. J Neurol Neurosurg Psychiatr. 1958;21:95–100.
13. Plum F, Posner JB. The Diagnosis of Stupor and Coma. 3rd ed. Philadelphia: FA Davis; 1980.
14. DeMyer W. Anatomy and clinical neurology of the spinal cord. In: Baker AB, Joynt RJ, eds. Clinical Neurology. Philadelphia: Harper & Row; 1987:1–24.
15. Darouiche RO, Hamill RJ, Greenberg SB, et al. Bacterial spinal epidural abscess. Review of 43 cases and literature survey. Medicine. 1992;71:369–85.
16. Toole JF. Applied anatomy and embryology of the brain arteries. In: Toole JF, ed. Cerebrovascular Disorders. 4th ed. New York: Raven Press; 1990: 1–27.
17. Stehbens WE. Anatomy of the blood vessels of blood vessels of the brain and spinal cord. In: Stehbens WE, ed. Pathology of the Cerebral Blood Vessels. St. Louis: CV Mosby; 1972:1–59.
18. Roach MR, Drake CG. Ruptured cerebral aneurysms caused by microorganisms. N Engl J Med. 1965;273:240–4.
19. Fishman RA. Cerebrospinal Fluid in Diseases of the Nervous System. 2nd ed. Philadelphia: WB Saunders; 1992.
20. Wispelwey B, Dacey RG, Jr, Scheld WM. Brain abscess. In: Scheld WM, Whitley RJ, Durack D, eds. Infections of the Central Nervous System. New York: Raven Press; 1991:457–86.
21. Toole JF. Anatomy and diseases of the venous system. In: Toole JF, ed. Cerebrovascular Disorders. 4th ed. New York: Raven Press; 1990:503–34.
22. Merwarth HR. The syndrome of the Rolandic vein. Am J Surg. 1942;56: 526–44.
23. Moossy J. Vascular diseases of the spinal cord. In: Joynt RJ, ed. Clinical Neurology. Philadelphia: JB Lippincott; 1993:1–17.
24. Pfister HW, Feiden W, Einhaupl KM. Spectrum of complications during bacterial meningitis in adults. Arch Neurol. 1993;50:575–81.
25. Miller JQ, Price TR. The nervous system in Rocky Mountain spotted fever. Neurology. 1972;22:561–6.
26. Rao AK, Schapira M, Clements ML, et al. A prospective study of platelets

and plasma proteolytic systems during the early stages of Rocky Mountain spotted fever. N Engl J Med. 1988;318:1021–8.

27. Guillevin L, Lhote F, Leon A, et al. Treatment of polyarteritis nodosa related to hepatitis B virus with short term steroid therapy associated with antiviral agents and plasma exchanges. A prospective trial in 33 patients. J Rheumatol. 1993;20:289–98.

28. Reshef E, Greenberg SB, Jankovic J. Herpes zoster ophthalmicus followed by contralateral hemiparesis: Report of two cases and review of the literature. J Neurol Neurosurg Psychiatr. 1985;48:122–7.

29. Johnson RT. Viral Infections of the Nervous System. New York: Raven Press; 1982.

30. Winkelman NW, Eckel JL. The brain in bacterial endocarditis. Arch Neurol Psychiatr. 1930;23:1161–82.

31. Winkelman NW, Eckel JL. Productive endarteritis of the small cortical vessels in severe toxemias. Brain. 1927;50:608–23.

32. Moskowitz MA, Rosenbaum AE, Tyler HR. Angiographically monitored resolution of cerebral mycotic aneurysms. Neurology. 1974;24:1103–8.

33. Goitein KJ, Tamir I. Cerebral perfusion pressure in central nervous system infections of infancy and childhood. J Pediatr. 1983;103:40–3.

34. Rebaud P, Berthier JC, Hartemann E, et al. Intracranial pressure in childhood central nervous system infections. Int Care Med. 1988;14:522–5.

35. Britt RH, Enzmann DR. Clinical stages of human brain abscesses on serial CT scans after contrast enhancement. J Neurosurg. 1983;59:972–89.

36. Sze G, Zimmerman RD. The magnetic resonance imaging of infections and inflammatory diseases. Imaging in neuroradiology part I. Radiol Clin North Am. 1988;26:839–59.

37. Silverberg AL, DiNubile MJ. Subdural empyema and cranial epidural abscess. Med Clin North Am. 1985;69:361–74.

38. Wispelwey B, Scheld WM. Brain abscess. Semin Neurol. 1992;12:273–8.

39. Rieselback RE, Di Chiro G, Freireich EJ, et al. Subarachnoid distribution of drugs after lumbar injection. N Engl J Med. 1962;267:1273–8.

40. Kaiser AB, McGee ZA. Aminoglycoside therapy of gram-negative bacillary meningitis. N Engl J Med. 1975;293:1215–20.

41. Saez-Llorens XJ, Uman MA, Odio CM, et al. Brain abscess in infants and children. Pediatr Infect Dis J. 1989;8:449–58.

42. Iwasaki Y, Liu D-S, Yamamoto T, Konno H. On the replication and spread of rabies virus in the human central nervous system. J Neurol Neurosurg Psychiatr. 1985;44:185–95.

43. Rich AR, McCordock HA. The pathogenesis of tuberculous meningitis. Bull Johns Hopkins Hosp. 1933;52:5–37.

44. Lentz TL, Burrage TG, Smith AL, et al. Is the acetylcholine receptor a rabies virus receptor? Science. 1982;215:182–4.

45. Murphy FA, Bauer SP, Harrison AK, et al. Comparative pathogenesis of rabies and rabies-like viruses: Viral infection and transit from inoculation site to the central nervous system. Lab Invest. 1973;28:361–76.

46. Winkler WG, Fashinell TR, Leffingwell L, et al. Airborn rabies transmission in a laboratory worker. JAMA. 1973;226:1219–21.

47. Tsiang H. Neuronal functional impairment in rabies-infected rat brain. J Gen Virol. 1982;61:277–81.

48. Ceccaldi PE, Fillion MP, Ermine A, et al. Rabies virus selectively alters 5-HT1 receptor subtypes in rat brain. Eur J Pharmacol. 1993;245:129–38.

49. Hanham CA, Zhao F, Tignor GH. Evidence from the anti-idiotypic network that the acetylcholine receptor is a rabies virus receptor. J Virol. 1993;67:530–42.

50. Giulian D, Noonan CA. Secretion of neurotoxins by mononuclear phagocytes infected with HIV-1. Science. 1990;250:1593–6.

51. Pulliam L, Herndier BG, Tang NM, et al. Human immunodeficiency virus-infected macrophages produce soluble factors that cause histological and neurochemical alterations in cultured human brains. J Clin Invest. 1991;87:503–12.

52. Hollander H. Cerebrospinal fluid normalities and abnormalities in individuals infected with human immunodeficiency virus. J Infect Dis. 1988;158:855–8.

53. McArthur JC, Cohen BA, Selnes OA, et al. Low prevalence of neurological and neuropsychological abnormalities in otherwise healthy HIV-1-infected individuals: Results from the multicenter AIDS cohort study. Ann Neurol. 1989;26:601–11.

54. Bowen DL, Lane HC, Fauci AS. Immunopathogenesis of the acquired immunodeficiency syndrome. Ann Intern Med. 1985;103:703–10.

55. Hirsch MS, Griffin DE, Winkelstein JA. The efect of complement depletion on the course of Sindbis virus infection in mice. J Immunol. 1978;121:1276–8.

56. Fisher RS, Clark AW, Wolinsky JS, et al. Postinfectious leukoencephalitis complicating Mycoplasma pneumoniae infection. Arch Neurol. 1083;40:109–13.

57. Johnson RT. The pathogenesis of acute viral encephalitis and postinfectious encephalomyelitis. J Infect Dis. 1987;155:359–64.

58. Saez-Llorens X, Ramilo O, Mustafa MM, et al. Molecular pathophysiology of bacterial meningitis: current concepts and therapeutic implications. J Pediatr. 1990;116:671–84.

59. Ropper AH, Rockoff MA. Treatment of intracranial hypertension. In: Ropper AH, Kennedy SK, eds. Neurological and Neurosurgical Intensive Care. 2nd ed. Rockville: Aspen Publishers, Inc.; 1988:23–41.

60. Lebel MH, Freij BJ, Syrogiannopoulos GA, et al. Dexamethasone therapy for bacterial meningitis. Results of two double-blind, placebo-controlled trials. N Engl J Med. 1988;319:964–71.

61. Adams RD, Victor M. Principles of Neurology. 2nd ed. New York: McGraw-Hill; 1981:532.

62. Truax RC, Carpenter MB. Human Neuroanatomy. 6th ed. Baltimore: Williams & Wilkins; 1969:80

64. ACUTE MENINGITIS

ALLAN R. TUNKEL
W. MICHAEL SCHELD

Meningitis is inflammation of the meninges that is identified by an abnormal number of white blood cells in cerebrospinal fluid (CSF). Acute meningitis is clinically defined as a syndrome characterized by the onset of meningeal symptoms over the course of hours up to several days. Headache is a prominent early symptom, often followed later by confusion or coma. Examination reveals few focal findings early during infection, although signs of meningeal irritation (e.g., Kernig and/or Brudzinski signs) are common. The acute meningitis syndrome blurs imperceptibly into the syndromes of chronic meningitis (see Ch. 65) and encephalitis (see Ch. 66). Chronic meningitis has an onset measured in weeks to months (but is generally defined when symptoms, signs, and the CSF remains abnormal for at least 4 weeks), whereas encephalitis is distinguished by the presence of decreased mentation (i.e., confusion or stupor) early in the course of disease and minimal meningeal signs. The distinction between these syndromes is clinically useful in guiding management, but is obviously artificial in terms of etiology and pathology. For example, tuberculous meningitis may present with a subacute or chronic onset.

The acute meningitis syndrome may be caused by a wide variety of infectious agents and may also be a manifestation of noninfectious diseases (Table 1). Diseases in which meningeal symptoms occur but are not predominant (e.g., measles) are excluded. Many of the causes of chronic meningitis, which can present acutely, have been omitted but are listed in Chapter 65. Here, we review the common infectious causes of acute meningitis with particular emphasis on epidemiology and etiology, pathogenesis and pathophysiology, clinical presentation, diagnosis, treatment, and prevention.

EPIDEMIOLOGY AND ETIOLOGY

Viral Meningitis

Viruses are the major causes of the *acute aseptic meningitis syndrome*, a term used to define any meningitis (infectious or noninfectious), particularly one with a lymphocytic pleocytosis, for which a cause is not apparent after initial evaluation and routine stains and cultures of CSF.[1,2] Over the years 1982–1988, from 8300 to 12,700 cases of aseptic meningitis were reported to the Centers for Disease Control and Prevention,[1] although these figures likely underestimate the importance of this syndrome since not all cases are reported and cases with a nonviral etiology are not reported as aseptic meningitis. In another large retrospective review of all cases of central nervous system (CNS) infection in Olmstead County, Minnesota, from 1950 to 1981,[3] 238 cases met the criteria for definite aseptic meningitis for an adjusted incidence rate of 10.9/100,000 person-years. A specific viral etiology was only established in 33 (11%) of the cases, likely because of limitations of microbiologic techniques in the past and the low frequency of microbiologic searches for the virus in the patient population. The common viral etiologic agents that cause the acute aseptic meningitis syndrome are discussed below.

TABLE 1. Differential Diagnosis of Acute Meningitis

Major infectious etiologies
  Viruses
    Nonpolio enteroviruses[a]
    Mumps virus
    Arboviruses[b]
    Herpesviruses[c]
    Lymphocytic choriomeningitis virus
    Human immunodeficiency virus
    Adenovirus
    Poliovirus
  Rickettsiae
    Rickettsia rickettsii (Rocky Mountain spotted fever)
    Rickettsia conorii
    Rickettsia prowazekii (epidemic or louse-borne typhus)
    Rickettsia typhi (endemic or murine typhus)
    Rickettsia tsutsugamushi (scrub typhus)
    Ehrlichia spp.
  Bacteria
    Haemophilus influenzae
    Neisseria meningitidis
    Streptococcus pneumoniae
    Listeria monocytogenes
    Streptococcus agalactiae
    Propionibacterium acnes
    Staphylococcus aureus
    Staphylococcus epidermidis
    Enterococcus faecalis
    Escherichia coli
    Klebsiella pneumoniae
    Pseudomonas aeruginosa
    Salmonella spp.
    Nocardia spp.
    Mycobacterium tuberculosis
  Spirochetes
    Treponema pallidum (syphilis)
    Borrelia burgdorferi (Lyme disease)
    Leptospira spp.
  Protozoa and helminths
    Naegleria fowleri
    Angiostrongylus cantonensis
    Strongyloides stercoralis (hyperinfection syndrome)
  Other infectious syndromes
    Parameningeal foci of infection[d]
    Infective endocarditis
    Viral postinfectious syndromes
    Postvaccination[e]
Noninfectious and diseases of unknown etiology
  Intracranial tumors and cysts
    Craniopharyngioma
    Dermoid/epidermoid cyst
    Teratoma
  Medications
    Antimicrobial agents[f]
    Nonsteroidal anti-inflammatory agents[g]
    Muromonab-CD3 (OKT3)
    Azathioprine
    Cytosine arabinoside (high dose)
    Carbamazepine[h]
    Immune globulin
    Phenazopyridine
  Systemic illnesses
    Systemic lupus erythematosus
    Vogt-Koyanagi-Harada syndrome
  Procedure-related
    Postneurosurgery
    Spinal anesthesia
    Intrathecal injections[i]
    Chymopapain injection
  Miscellaneous
    Seizures
    Migraine or migraine-like syndromes
    Mollaret's meningitis

[a] Primarily echoviruses and coxsackieviruses.
[b] In the United States, the major etiologic agents are the mosquito-borne California, St. Louis, Eastern equine, Western equine, and Venezuelan equine encephalitis viruses; and the tick-borne Colorado tick fever.
[c] Primarily herpes simplex virus type 2, but also herpes simplex virus type 1, varicella-zoster virus, cytomegalovirus, Epstein-Barr virus, and human herpesvirus-6.
[d] Brain abscess, sinusitis, otitis, mastoiditis, subdural abscess, epidural abscess, venous sinus thrombophlebitis, pituitary abscess, cranial osteomyelitis.
[e] Mumps, measles, polio, pertussis, rabies, vaccinia.
[f] Trimethoprim, sulfamethoxazole, trimethoprim-sulfamethoxazole, ciprofloxacin, penicillin, isoniazid.
[g] Ibuprofen, sulindac, naproxen, tolmetin.
[h] In patients with connective tissue diseases.
[i] Air, isotopes, antimicrobial agents, antineoplastic agents, steroids, radiographic contrast media.

Enteroviruses. Enteroviruses are currently the leading recognizable cause of the aseptic meningitis syndrome, accounting for 80–85 percent of all cases in which a pathogen is identified.[1] Enteroviruses are worldwide in distribution. In temperate climates they appear with a marked summer/fall seasonality, although in tropical and subtropical areas there is a high year-round incidence. Periods of warm weather and wearing sparse clothing may facilitate the fecal-oral spread of these organisms; enteroviruses may also be recovered from houseflies, wastewater, and sewage.[2,4] In the United States, the 15 most commonly occurring enteroviral serotypes account for more than 80 percent of isolates.[5] The predominant enteroviruses isolated from patients with meningitis during the years 1970–1983 were (in decreasing order) echovirus 11; echovirus 9; coxsackievirus B5; echoviruses 30, 4, and 6; coxsackieviruses B2, B4, B3, and A9; echoviruses 3, 7, 5, and 21; and coxsackievirus B1.[5] In one epidemiologic investigation in New York state,[6] 20 percent of isolates were echovirus 30.

Infants and young children are the primary victims of enteroviral meningitis because they are the most susceptible host population (i.e., there is absence of previous exposure and immunity) within the community. In one large cohort study from Finland,[7] children less than 1 year of age had an annual incidence of viral meningitis of 219 cases per 100,000 population versus an incidence of 19 cases per 100,000 population in children between the ages of 1 and 4 years; the incidence dropped even further with advancing age. The vast majority of these viral pathogens were enteroviruses. Immunodeficiency, and possibly physical exercise, also predisposes to enteroviral meningitis.[2]

Arboviruses. The most common arthropod-transmitted cause of aseptic meningitis is St. Louis encephalitis (SLE) virus, a flavivirus.[8] Aseptic meningitis accounts for about 15 percent of all symptomatic cases of SLE and may be as high as 35–60 percent in children.[9] Patients over the age of 60 years rarely present with aseptic meningitis if infected with SLE virus; encephalitis is the more common presentation. These infections are more common in warmer months when contact with the insect vector is more likely. Vector exposure is more likely to occur indoors than outside, because poorly sealed residences appear to be a risk factor.[10] Other arboviruses reported to cause aseptic meningitis include the California encephalitis group of viruses (e.g., La Crosse, Jamestown Canyon, and Snowshoe hare viruses, which are bunyaviruses) and the agent of Colorado tick fever, an orbivirus, which is seen in mountain and western regions of the United States and Canada.[2,11,12]

Mumps Virus. In an unimmunized population, mumps is one of the most common causes of aseptic meningitis and encephalitis; symptomatic meningitis is estimated to occur in 10–30 percent of patients overall.[13] Central nervous system disease caused by mumps virus can occur in patients without evidence of parotitis[2,13,14]; 40–50 percent of patients with mumps meningitis have no evidence of salivary gland enlargement. Meningitis is the most common neurologic manifestation of infection with mumps virus[2,13] and is usually a benign and self-limited process. Males are affected two to five times more often than females, and the peak incidence is in children aged 5–9 years.[13]

Lymphocytic Choriomeningitis Virus. Lymphocytic choriomeningitis virus was one of the earliest and seemingly most significant viruses to be associated with human aseptic meningitis[1,2]; this virus is now rarely reported as an etiologic agent. Lymphocytic choriomeningitis virus is transmitted to humans by contact with rodents (e.g., hamsters, rats, mice) or their excreta[15–17]; the greatest risk of infection is in laboratory workers, pet owners, and persons living in impoverished and nonhygienic situations. A recent outbreak was described in laboratory workers who were caring for nude mice that had been injected with lymphocytic choriomeningitis virus-infected tumor cell lines.[18]

Presumed routes of transmission are ingestion of food contaminated with animal urine and exposure of open wounds to dirt. There is no evidence for human-to-human transmission.

Herpesviruses.   The herpesviruses are DNA viruses that include herpes simplex virus types 1 and 2, varicella-zoster virus, cytomegalovirus, Epstein-Barr virus, human herpesvirus-6, and human herpesvirus-7. Although neurologic complications are known to occur with some of these viruses,[19-25] the complications associated with the herpes simplex viruses are of the most significance. Overall, herpes simplex viruses account for approximately 0.5–3 percent of all cases of aseptic meningitis.[26] In patients beyond the neonatal period, it is critical to differentiate between herpes simplex encephalitis, a potentially fatal form of encephalitis, and herpes simplex meningitis, a self-limited syndrome. The syndrome of herpes simplex virus aseptic meningitis is most commonly associated with primary genital infection with herpes simplex virus type 2[19-21]; in one study, 36 percent of women and 13 percent of men developed an aseptic meningitis syndrome concomitant with primary infection.[21] Meningitis is less likely with recurrences of genital herpes.[27] Primary genital infection with herpes simplex virus type 1 and nonprimary genital infection with herpes simplex virus of either type rarely results in meningitis.[21] Acute aseptic meningitis has also been associated with herpes zoster in patients with or without typical skin lesions,[22,28,29] the latter known as *zoster sine herpete*. Single cases of Mollaret's recurrent meningitis have been associated with herpes simplex virus type 1[30,31] and Epstein-Barr virus.[32] Human herpervirus-6 has also been associated with meningitis,[33] in association with roseola infantum. Cytomegalovirus and Epstein-Barr virus may cause aseptic meningitis in association with a mononucleosis syndrome,[24,34] particularly in the immunocompromised host.

Human Immunodeficiency Virus.   The human immunodeficiency virus (HIV) can infect the meninges early and persist in the CNS after initial infection.[35] Meningitis associated with HIV may occur as part of the primary infection or in an already infected patient[36]; HIV has been isolated from the CSF in some of these cases. However, acute meningitis does not occur in every individual who becomes infected and can be silent. Retrospective studies have noted that an acute meningoencephalitis is observed in 5–10 percent of HIV-infected patients during or after the mononucleosis-like syndrome that heralds initial infection.[37-41]

Bacterial Meningitis

Bacterial meningitis remains a very important disease worldwide. Data defining the incidence of bacterial meningitis in the United States and abroad are shown in Table 2.[42-46] The overall annual attack rate for bacterial meningitis, as defined by a surveillance study of 27 states in the United States from 1978 through 1981, was approximately 3.0 cases per 100,000 population, although there was variability based on age, race, and

sex.[42] The three most common meningeal pathogens, *Haemophilus influenzae*, *Neisseria meningitidis*, and *Streptococcus pneumoniae*, accounted for over 80 percent of cases; respective mortality rates were 6.0, 10.3, and 26.3 percent. Case fatality rates in a subsequent study of cases of bacterial meningitis in five states and in Los Angeles County (population approximately 34 million) were generally lower (e.g., 19 percent for meningitis caused by *S. pneumoniae*),[43] suggesting that improvements in early recognition of the meningitis syndrome and antimicrobial therapy may have occurred in the 1980s.

Bacterial meningitis is also a significant problem in hospitalized patients. In a recent review of 493 episodes of bacterial meningitis in adults 16 years of age or older at the Massachusetts General Hospital from 1962 through 1988,[47] 40 percent of episodes were nosocomial in origin, and these episodes carried a high mortality rate (35 percent for single episodes of nosocomial meningitis). The overall case fatality rate for all patients (community-acquired and nosocomial) was 25 percent and did not vary significantly over the 27 years of the study. Risk factors for death among patients with community-acquired meningitis included age 60 years or older, obtunded mental status on admission, and seizures within the first 24 hours.

In addition, bacterial meningitis is a major problem in other areas of the world. A review of approximately 4100 cases of bacterial meningitis at Hospital Couta Maia in Salvador, Brazil, from 1973 through 1982 revealed an attack rate of 45.8 cases per 100,000 population.[46] The overall case fatality rate was 33 percent, with 50 percent of deaths occurring within 48 hours of hospitalization. *Haemophilus influenzae*, *N. meningitidis*, and *S. pneumoniae* accounted for 62 percent of the cases and 70 percent of the deaths. The case fatality rates for meningitis caused by the Enterobacteriaceae was 86 percent; more than half of these cases in children less than 24 months of age were caused by *Salmonella* spp., an unusual meningeal pathogen in industrialized nations.

The likely etiologic agents of bacterial meningitis vary depending on the age and underlying disease status of the patient (Table 3). The following sections review the epidemiologies and etiologies of specific meningeal pathogens.

Haemophilus influenzae.   *Haemophilus influenzae* is isolated in 45–48 percent of all cases of bacterial meningitis in the United States; the overall mortality rate is 3–6 percent.[42,43] Most episodes of meningitis occur in infants and children under the age of 6 years, with 90 percent of cases caused by capsular type b strains. The peak incidence is between 6 and 12 months of age in the United States.[48] Isolation of this organism in older children and adults should suggest the presence of certain underlying conditions, including sinusitis, otitis media, epiglottitis, pneumonia, diabetes mellitus, alcoholism, splenectomy or asplenic states, head trauma with CSF leak, and immune deficiency (e.g., hypogammaglobulinemia).[49-52] Recently there has been a profound reduction (from 76 to 90 percent) in the incidence of invasive infections caused by *H. influenzae* type b in the United States, specifically in young children.[53-55] This is

TABLE 2. Etiology of Bacterial Meningitis Based on Geographic Locale

Organism	Percentage of Total Cases				
	United States (1978–1981)	United States (1986)	United Kingdom (1980–1984)	Dakar, Senegal (1970–1979)	Salvador, Brazil (1973–1982)
Haemophilus influenzae	48	45	29	20	23
Neisseria meningitidis	20	14	25	11	22
Streptococcus pneumoniae	13	18	20	29	17
Streptococcus agalactiae	3	6	7	4	—
Listeria monocytogenes	2	3	2	<0.5	—
Other	8	14	16	9	20
Unknown	6	—	—	26	18

(Data from refs. 42–46.)

TABLE 3. Common Bacterial Pathogens Based on Predisposing Factor in Patients with Meningitis

Predisposing Factor	Common Bacterial Pathogens
Age	
0–4 weeks	Streptococcus agalactiae, Escherichia coli, Listeria monocytogenes, Klebsiella pneumoniae, Enterococcus spp., Salmonella spp.
4–12 weeks	Streptococcus agalactiae, Escherichia coli, Listeria monocytogenes, Haemophilus influenzae, Streptococcus pneumoniae, Neisseria meningitidis
3 months to 18 years	Haemophilus influenzae, Neisseria meningitidis, Streptococcus pneumoniae
18–50 years	Streptococcus pneumoniae, Neisseria meningitidis
>50 years	Streptococcus pneumoniae, Neisseria meningitidis, Listeria monocytogenes, aerobic gram-negative bacilli
Immunocompromised state	Streptococcus pneumoniae, Neisseria meningitidis, Listeria monocytogenes, aerobic gram-negative bacilli (including Pseudomonas aeruginosa)
Basilar skull fracture	Streptococcus pneumoniae, Haemophilus influenzae, group A β-hemolytic streptococci
Head trauma; postneurosurgery	Staphylococcus aureus, Staphylococcus epidermidis, aerobic gram-negative bacilli (including Pseudomonas aeruginosa)
Cerebrospinal fluid shunt	Staphylococcus epidermidis, Staphylococccus aureus, aerobic gram-negative bacilli (including Pseudomonas aeruginosa), Propionibacterium acnes

attributed, in part, to the recent widespread use of conjugate vaccines against *H. influenzae* type b that have been licensed for routine use in all children beginning at 2 months of age. Similar results have been observed in Finland, where there has been a marked decrease in the number of cases of *H. influenzae* type b meningitis (i.e., from a peak of 43 cases per 100,000 population in the late 1970s to zero cases in 1991 in the greater Helsinki area).[56]

Neisseria meningitidis. *Neisseria meningitidis* most commonly causes meningitis in children and young adults and is isolated in 14–20 percent of cases with an overall mortality rate of 10–13 percent.[42,43] Serogroup B strains account for about 51 percent of meningeal isolates in the United States, usually occurring in sporadic outbreaks. Disease caused by serogroups A and C may occur in epidemics; group Y strains may be associated with pneumonia. There has recently been an overall increase in incidence of serogroup C disease in the United States equaling that caused by serogroup B,[57] suggesting a fluctuation in predominant serogroups over time. Patients with deficiencies in the terminal complement components (C5, C6, C7, C8, and perhaps C9), the so-called membrane attack complex, have a markedly increased incidence of neisserial infections,[58–62] including that caused by *N. meningitidis*, although mortality rates in meningococcal disease are lower than in patients with an intact complement system (3 vs. 19 percent in the general population). An increased risk of invasive meningococcal disease has also been described in a Dutch family with dysfunctional properdin,[63] suggesting a potential role for the alternative pathway in complement-mediated resistance against meningococci.

Streptococcus pneumoniae. *Streptococcus pneumoniae* meningitis is most frequently observed in adults, accounting for 13–17 percent of total cases in the United States and carrying a mortality rate of 19–26 percent.[42,43] Of the 83 known pneumococcal serotypes, 18 are responsible for 82 percent of the cases of bacteremic pneumococcal pneumonia,[64,65] with a close correlation between bacteremic subtypes and those implicated in meningitis.[66–68] Patients often have contiguous or distant foci of pneumococcal infection such as pneumonia, otitis media, mastoiditis, sinusitis, and endocarditis. Serious infection may be observed in patients with various underlying conditions (e.g., splenectomy or asplenic states, multiple myeloma, hypogammaglobulinemia, alcoholism, malnutrition, chronic liver or renal

disease, malignancy, and diabetes mellitus).[69–73] The *Pneumococcus* is the most common etiologic agent of meningitis in patients who have suffered basilar skull fracture with CSF leak.[74]

Listeria monocytogenes. *Listeria monocytogenes* causes only 2–3 percent of cases of bacterial meningitis in the United States, but carries a mortality rate of 22–29 percent.[42,43] Serotypes Ia, Ib, and IVb have been implicated in up to 90 percent of meningitis cases caused by this organism. *Listeria* has been isolated from dust, soil, water, sewage, and decaying vegetable matter (including animal feed and silage). Listerial infection is most common in neonates (up to 10 percent of cases), the elderly, alcoholics, cancer patients, and immunosuppressed adults (e.g., renal transplant recipients).[75–79] Other predisposing conditions include diabetes mellitus, liver disease, chronic renal disease, collagen-vascular diseases, and conditions associated with iron overload. Although colonization rates are low, pregnant women may harbor the organism asymptomatically in their genital tract and rectum and transmit the infection to their infants. Perinatal listeriosis may take two forms: the "early" form, which results from intrauterine infection producing the devastating illness granulomatosis infantisepticum; and the "late" form, presumably acquired during or just after birth, presenting as meningitis in the second or third week of life. *Listeria* meningitis is found infrequently in patients with HIV infection,[80–82] despite its increased incidence in patients with deficiencies in cell-mediated immunity. Meningitis can also occur in previously healthy adults.[83] Outbreaks of *Listeria* infection have been associated with consumption of contaminated cole slaw, raw vegetables, milk, and cheese,[75,84,85] pointing to the intestinal tract as the usual portal of entry. In addition, it has been suggested that gastric acidity may be an important host defense against *Listeria* infection; antacid and cimetidine therapy have been associated with acquisition of listeriosis.

Streptococcus agalactiae. The group B *Streptococcus* is a common cause of meningitis in neonates.[86] In the United States, this organism accounts for 3–6 percent of cases of bacterial meningitis, with a mortality rate ranging from 12 to 27 percent.[42,43] The group B *Streptococcus* has been isolated from vaginal or rectal cultures of 15–40 percent of asymptomatic pregnant women[87–90]; colonization rates do not vary during pregnancy and may be chronic (40 percent), transient, or intermittent.[88] The risk of transmission from the mother to her infant is increased when the inoculum of organisms and number of sites of maternal colonization are increased; the route of delivery does not influence transmission. Horizontal transmission has also been documented from the hands of nursery personnel to the infant. Most cases of neonatal meningitis are caused by subtype III organisms and occur after the first week of life. The group B *Streptococcus* can also cause meningitis in adults.[91,92] Risk factors in adults include age over 60 years, diabetes mellitus, parturient women, cardiac disease, collagen-vascular diseases, malignancy, alcoholism, hepatic failure, renal failure, and corticosteroid therapy; in one review of group B streptococcal meningitis in adults, no underlying illnesses were found in 43 percent of patients.[92]

Aerobic Gram-Negative Bacilli. The aerobic gram-negative bacilli (e.g., *Klebsiella* spp., *Escherichia coli*, *Serratia marcescens*, *Pseudomonas aeruginosa*, *Salmonella* spp.) have become increasingly important as etiologic agents in patients with bacterial meningitis.[93–97] These agents may be isolated from the CSF of patients following head trauma or neurosurgical procedures and may also be found in neonates, the elderly, immunosuppressed patients, and patients with gram-negative septicemia. Some cases have been associated with disseminated strongyloidiasis in the hyperinfection syndrome, in which meningitis caused by enteric bacteria occurs secondary to seeding of the meninges during persistent or recurrent bacteremias associated with the migration of infective larvae.[98,99] Alternatively, the larvae may carry enteric organisms on their surfaces or within their own gastrointestinal tracts as they exit the intestine and subsequently invade the meninges. In patients with *E. coli* meningitis, 75 percent of cases are caused by strains possessing the K1 antigen.[86] Almost half of pregnant women have this organism isolated on rectal culture, and as many as 75 percent of their infants will be colonized during the first days of life; horizontal transmission from nursery staff members or other infants has also been reported.

Staphylococci.   Meningitis caused by *Staphylococcus aureus* is usually found in early postneurosurgical or post-trauma patients and in those with CSF shunts; other underlying conditions include diabetes mellitus, alcoholism, chronic renal failure requiring hemodialysis, injection drug abuse, and malignancies.[100,101] Thirty-five percent of cases are observed in the setting of head trauma or postneurosurgery, and an additional 20 percent of patients have underlying infective endocarditis or paraspinal infection. Other sources of community-acquired *Staphylococcus aureus* meningitis include patients with sinusitis, osteomyelitis, and pneumonia. Mortality rates have ranged from 14 to 77 percent in various series. *Staphylococcus epidermidis* is the most common cause of meningitis in patients with CSF shunts.[102]

Other Bacteria.   A recent review of 28 cases of nocardial meningitis revealed predisposing conditions in approximately 75 percent of patients,[103] including immunosuppressive drug therapy, malignancy, head trauma, CNS procedures, chronic granulomatous disease, and sarcoidosis. Anaerobic meningitis is unusual and is usually associated with contiguous foci of infection (e.g., otitis, sinusitis, pharyngitis, brain abscess, head and neck malignancy, recent head and neck surgery or wound infection, post-trauma, postneurosurgery)[104-107]; in many cases more than one organism may be recovered. Diphtheroids, particularly *Propionibacterium acnes,* have become important etiologic agents of meningitis in patients with CNS shunt infections.[102]

Spirochetal Meningitis

Treponema pallidum.   *Treponema pallidum* disseminates to the CNS during early infection.[108] The organism can be isolated from the CSF of patients with primary syphilis, and CSF laboratory abnormalities are detected in 5 to 9 percent of patients with seronegative primary syphilis. The actual rate of invasion of the CNS during these early stages is likely to be considerably higher, however. Clinical neurosyphilis can be divided into four distinct syndromes[108]; syphilitic meningitis, meningovascular syphilis, parenchymatous neurosyphilis, and gummatous neurosyphilis. There may be some overlap in the clinical and laboratory findings of these syndromes. The incidence of syphilitic meningitis is greatest in the first 2 years following infection and is estimated to occur in only 0.3–2.4 percent of syphilis cases.[109] In contrast, meningovascular syphilis is found in 10 to 12 percent of individuals with CNS involvement,[108,110-112] occurring months to years following syphilis acquisition (peak incidence approximately 7 years). Parenchymatous neurosyphilis has two variants, general paresis and tabes dorsalis. Both are relatively rare today and do not become apparent until 10–20 years following acquisition of infection.[108] Gummata are late manifestations of tertiary syphilis and may occur anywhere[108]; gummatous neurosyphilis is rare.

The overall incidence of neurosyphilis has recently increased, with many of the reported cases seen in patients with HIV infection.[113-115] In one report,[116] 44 percent of all patients with neurosyphilis had acquired immunodeficiency syndrome (AIDS); the remaining patients who may have had HIV infection without AIDS was not addressed in this report. The study also showed that 1.5 percent of AIDS patients were found to have neurosyphilis at some point during the course of their disease.

Borrelia burgdorferi.   The nervous system is eventually involved clinically in at least 10–15 percent of patients with Lyme disease, either while erythema chronicum migrans is still present or 1–6 months later.[117-119] A recent study utilizing polymerase chain reaction (PCR) detected spirochetal DNA in CSF samples from 8 of 12 patients with acute (<2 weeks) disseminated Lyme borreliosis,[120] indicating that *Borrelia burgdorferi* usually invades the CNS early in infection.

Protozoal and Helminthic Meningitis

Amebae.   Despite the hundreds of species of free-living amebae that are known, only a few have been reported to infect humans.[121,122] The most important are in the genera *Naegleria* and *Acanthamoeba. Naegleria fowleri,* the main protozoan causing primary amebic meningoencephalitis in humans, has been recovered from lakes, puddles, pools, ponds, rivers, sewage sludge, tap water, air-conditioner drains, and soil.[121-123] Sporadic cases of primary amebic meningoencephalitis occur when persons, usually children and young adults, swim or play in water containing the amebae or when swimming pools or water supplies have become contaminated, often through failure of chlorination.[122,124] Asymptomatic carriage by humans can also occur. The incidence of infection is unknown, although a study of Florida lakes reported only seven documented cases of primary amebic meningoencephalitis in over one billion swimming episodes.[125] Several cases have recently been reported in HIV-infected patients, all with advanced HIV disease at the time of amebic infection.[126-128]

Angiostrongylus cantonensis.   Infection of humans by the larvae of the nematode *Angiostrongylus cantonensis* can lead to development of an eosinophilic meningitis.[99,129,130] The larvae invade the brain either directly from the blood stream or after migrating through other organs before reaching the spinal cord and brain. Once in the CNS, the larvae mature into adult worms that migrate through the brain. *Angiostrongylus cantonensis* is widespread and human infections are fairly common, reported from many parts of the world (Thailand, India, Malaysia, Vietnam, Indonesia, Papua New Guinea, and the Pacific Islands, including Hawaii).[99,129-132] The parasites may spread to many countries as rats move freely from port to port on ships.[129,133] The rat infection rate in urban Bangkok has reached about 40 percent.[134]

PATHOGENESIS AND PATHOPHYSIOLOGY

Viral Meningitis

Initiation of Infection.   Following colonization by various viruses of mucosal surfaces throughout the body, the host possesses numerous barriers to prevent viral entry.[135] For example, the respiratory tract contains a thin film of mucus and a mucociliary elevator that moves viral particles away from the lower respiratory tract; even if this barrier is crossed, alveolar macrophages are actively phagocytic for viral particles. The gastric acidity inactivates most swallowed viruses, and gastrointestinal enzymes and bile also disrupt viral envelopes, capsid proteins, and the lipoprotein membranes; however, some nonenveloped, acid-resistant viruses (e.g., enteroviruses, adenoviruses, reoviruses, parvoviruses) are adapted for replication in the gastrointestinal tract. When the host has had previous contact with the viral agent, the mucosa of the gastrointestinal and respiratory tracts may be coated with secretory IgA, which neutralizes the virus and prevents attachment and subsequent cell penetration. If certain viruses are able to escape initial host defense mechanisms, they may replicate and disseminate with the potential for CNS invasion.

Viremia and Central Nervous System Invasion. Following hematogenous dissemination of the virus, CNS infection may occur. Most neurotropic viruses initially multiply at extraneural sites (initially at the portal of entry), establish viremia, and then cross the blood-brain barrier (BBB) to invade the CNS. For example, enteroviruses initially multiply in the peritonsillar lymphatics, Peyer's patches, lamina propria of the intestine, and vascular and endothelial cells, depending on the particular agent.[136] M cells may mediate virus penetration from the gut lumen to the lymphoid cells. From this initial site, the virus then disseminates to vascular tissues (e.g., liver, spleen, and muscle) where further multiplication augments the viremia.[137] Following viremia, viral particles are normally cleared by the reticuloendothelial system, with the speed of removal directly related to virus size (i.e., large viruses are cleared more promptly from the blood stream). For example, small enteroviruses may grow in vascular endothelial cells and lymphatic channels maintaining the viremia.[137] Viruses may also elude host clearance by associating with certain cells. Some viruses (e.g., measles, herpes, mumps) grow in human leukocytes, which protects them from phagocytosis by the reticuloendothelial system, neutralization by circulating antibody, and/or inactivation by nonspecific serum inhibitors.[135]

Central nervous system invasion by viruses may occur via several mechanisms. Most viruses invade directly across cerebral capillary endothelial cells, the major site of the BBB. Some viruses directly infect cerebral microvascular endothelial cells prior to infection of adjacent glia and neurons,[137] whereas others initially infect glia without evidence of endothelial cell infection. Still other viruses may be carried between cerebral endothelial cells in infected leukocytes after BBB disruption. Another site of virus entry is the choroid plexus epithelium. Studies of mumps virus in hamsters have shown a sequence of infection from the choroid plexus to ependyma to parenchymal cells; viral nucleocapsids have been found in the choroid plexi and ependymal cells of humans with mumps meningitis.

Viruses may reach the CNS by spread along olfactory nerves.[135–138] In an experimental hamster model,[135] intranasal inoculation of herpes simplex virus and togaviruses led to early infection of the olfactory bulb, which could be inhibited by cutting the olfactory tracts or chemical treatment of the olfactory mucosa. Olfactory spread may explain the frontal and temporal localizations characteristic of herpes simplex virus encephalitis,[137] although spread along neural fibers from the trigeminal ganglia to the base of the middle and frontal fossae is another possibility.[139] Peripheral nerve spread by viruses may also lead to CNS invasion. In an experimental mouse model,[140] rabies virus initially concentrates and binds at the motor end plates before any replication occurs and prior to invasion of ipsilateral anterior horn cells. In addition, a recent study utilizing a transgenic mouse model demonstrated that, following intramuscular inoculation of poliovirus in the limb, infectious poliovirus was first detected in the inferior segment of the spinal cord and then in the superior spinal cord and the brain,[141] suggesting that poliovirus initially spreads to the CNS through peripheral nerve pathways.

Virus Spread within the Central Nervous System. Regardless of the mechanism of CNS invasion, the production of disease requires viral attachment to and penetration of susceptible cells, spread within the nervous system, and induction of cellular changes. Viral entry into the subarachnoid space via the choroid plexus leads to dispersion of virus within CSF contacting meningeal and ependymal cells[135]; sequential spread of virus may then occur in a contiguous fashion to glia and neurons. Other viruses spread through extracellular gaps between cells and CNS processes (e.g., dendrites, axons, or glia), transit along the exten-

sive axonal and dendritic ramifications of neurons by way of the glia, or are carried by mobile leukocytes in the inflammatory response. Experimental evidence supports each mode of transit, and all may be involved to various degrees in different viral infections.

Once viral infection of the CNS occurs, there is usually an accumulation of inflammatory cells, although the mechanisms leading to inflammatory cell recruitment and their role in viral CNS infections are only partially understood.[135,136] It appears that the initial inflammatory response is immunologically specific, consisting of a population of lymphocytes sensitized by the virus. However, an inflammatory response may fail to develop in other viral CNS infections; this may be dependent on host age rather than the virus itself. Sensitized lymphocytes likely respond to a virus-specific protein that diffuses or is transported to the luminal surface of the endothelium with subsequent passage through endothelial cells and release of inflammatory cytokines. In an experimental mouse model of meningitis caused by lymphocytic choriomeningitis virus,[142] elevated CSF concentrations of interleukin-6 (IL-6) and interferon gamma (IFN-γ) were demonstrated. The CSF IL-6 concentrations began to rise 24 hours after intracerebral infection, followed by a rapid increase after day 4. IFN-γ was not detected in CSF until 5–6 days after infection, but then markedly increased. Cerebrospinal fluid concentrations of these cytokines were only slightly and transiently elevated in athymic nude mice. In one review, IFN was also detectable in the CSF in 75 percent of 16 patients with enteroviral meningitis,[143] with more consistent production and higher titers noted with coxsackievirus than echovirus. Elevated CSF IL-6 concentrations were also detected in 12 of 15 samples from patients with acute aseptic meningitis.[142]

Other inflammatory cytokines have been measured in the CSF of patients with aseptic meningitis. In one study,[144] CSF concentrations of tumor necrosis factor alpha (TNF-α) and interleukin-1β (IL-1β) were measured in 36 patients with aseptic meningitis, 13 of whom had culture-proven enteroviral meningitis, and in 14 controls. None of the samples from the patients with aseptic meningitis or controls had detectable TNF-α activity, whereas 86 percent of patients with aseptic meningitis had detectable CSF IL-1β concentrations; only 2 of 14 control patients had elevated concentrations. The increased CSF IL-1β concentrations correlated with CSF white blood cell counts.

After development of a CSF inflammatory response, alterations in the BBB permit the traversal into CSF of serum proteins, including immunoglobulins. In addition, local CNS immunoglobulin synthesis occurs as B cells enter the CSF and differentiate into plasma cells. There is also intracerebral synthesis of immunoglobulins, reflected by an increase in the CSF:serum ratios of specific immunoglobulins that persist for several weeks after infection.[135] The production of oligoclonal IgG proteins within the CNS has been demonstrated in patients with meningitis caused by mumps virus, varicella-zoster virus, and HIV.[22,145–147] Furthermore, elevated CSF concentrations of oligoclonal IgG may persist for up to 1 year in mumps meningitis,[148] suggesting the possibility of viral persistence and ongoing antigenic stimulation.

An intact host immune response appears to be important for clearance of virus from the CNS[135,136]; T-cell responses appear to be more important than B-cell responses. Failure of an immune response to develop may be a result of immunologic tolerance, host immune defects, and/or the ability of the virus to escape immune surveillance. Patients with depressed cell-mediated immunity have developed chronic infections with varicella-zoster virus, cytomegalovirus, adenovirus, and measles virus.

Bacterial Meningitis

Numerous investigators over the last 20 years have elucidated many of the pathogenic and pathophysiologic mechanisms oper-

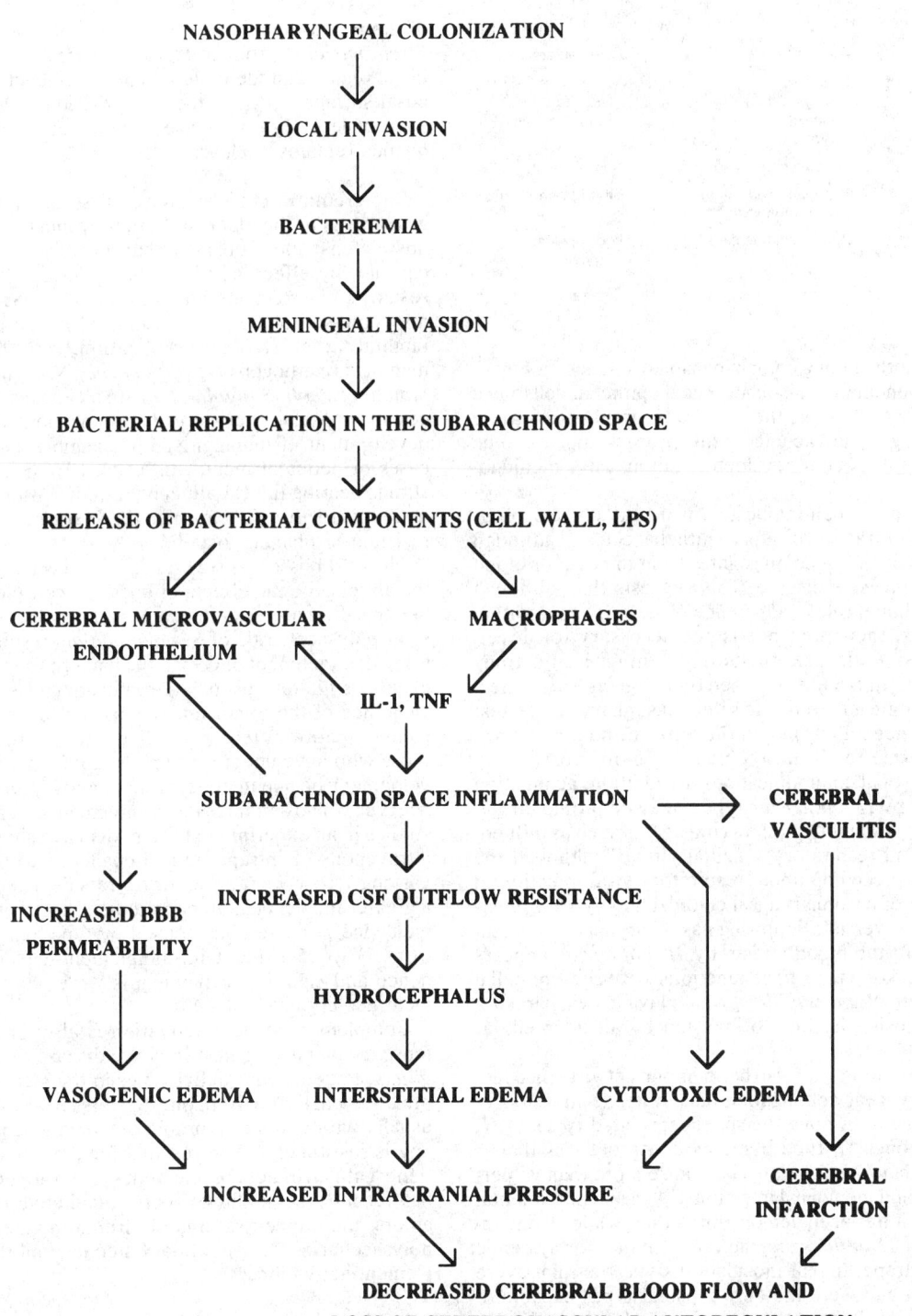

FIG. 1. Pathogenesis and pathophysiology of bacterial meningitis. LPS, lipopolysaccharide; IL-1, interleukin-1; TNF, tumor necrosis factor; BBB, blood-brain barrier. (From Tunkel and Scheld,[153] with permission.)

able in bacterial meningitis.[136,149–153] Figure 1 shows a hypothetical scheme of these mechanisms, which are discussed in greater detail below.

Mucosal Colonization and Systemic Invasion. The early pathogenic events that result in bacterial meningitis depend on an interplay between specific virulence factors and host defense mechanisms (Table 4). The initiation of infection with meningeal pathogens usually begins with host acquisition of a new organism by nasopharyngeal colonization.[154] Many of the major meningeal pathogens possess surface characteristics that enhance

mucosal colonization. For example, the fimbriae (or pili) of *N. meningitidis* mediate adherence of this organism to nasopharyngeal epithelial cells; these fimbriated strains accounted for 80 percent of primary meningococcal isolates from nasopharyngeal carriers and from the CSF of patients with meningococcal meningitis,[153] although all fimbriae were lost on serial subculture in the laboratory. The fimbriae appear morphologically as aggregated bundles or single filaments.[155] The aggregated bundles are found primarily among disease isolates exhibiting a low degree of adherence to human buccal epithelial cells, whereas the single filaments have medium to high adherence characteristics, being

TABLE 4. Factors Involved in the Pathogenesis of Bacterial Meningitis

Pathogenic Event	Bacterial Factors	Host Factors
Mucosal colonization	Fimbriae, polysaccharide capsule, IgA protease production	Mucosal epithelium, secretory IgA, ciliary activity
Intravascular survival	Polysaccharide capsule	Complement
Meningeal invasion	Fimbriae, association with monocytes	Blood-brain barrier
Survival within the subarachnoid space	Polysaccharide capsule	Poor opsonic activity

found predominantly among colonizing isolates. Once meningococci attach to nonciliated nasopharyngeal epithelial cells via a specific cell surface receptor, they are transported across these cells within a phagocytic vacuole[154]; this process appears to be essential for the subsequent development of invasive meningococcal disease.

Fimbriae have also been implicated in the attachment of *H. influenzae* to upper tract respiratory epithelial cells,[153] although fimbriae have not been found on isolates from the CSF or blood of patients with invasive disease. This suggests that, although fimbriae play an initial role in adherence of *H. influenzae* within the nasopharynx, their presence is not necessary for development of invasive disease, including meningitis. Furthermore, the type of fimbriae expressed by *H. influenzae* type b strains may facilitate adherence to select nasopharyngeal sites: α-fimbriae enhance adherence in the anterior nasopharynx, whereas β-fimbriae facilitate the process more posteriorly (A.L. Smith, personal communication). In addition, acquisition and colonization by *H. influenzae* type b may be promoted following respiratory tract infection by viral agents such as influenzae A Victoria and respiratory syncitial virus,[156] although the precise role of a preceding upper respiratory viral infection in the enhancement of nasopharyngeal colonization by *H. influenzae* type b is controversial. Following nasopharyngeal colonization, invasion into the blood stream by *H. influenzae* appears to occur via breakdown in tight junctions between epithelial cells (in contrast to *N. meningitidis,* which invades via parasite-directed endocytosis), leading to invasion by an intercellular mechanism.[154]

Surface encapsulation may also be an important virulence factor for nasopharyngeal colonization and systemic invasion of meningeal pathogens. Among the six encapsulated types of *H. influenzae* (a through f), type b strains constitute less than 5 percent of nasopharyngeal isolates but cause more than 95 percent of systemic and meningeal infections.[156] In an experimental infant rat model, it has been demonstrated that, while all encapsulated strains of *H. influenzae* had the potential for systemic invasion after intraperitoneal inoculation, type b strains were the most virulent and were the only capsular types capable of systemic invasion following intranasal inoculation.[157,158] Indeed, antibodies to type b capsule, which are almost uniformly detected in humans by the age of 4 years even in the absence of known exposure to *H. influenzae* type b, are protective against invasive disease.[153] Polysaccharide capsule may also be an important virulence factor for development of invasive disease by *Streptococcus pneumoniae.* Eighteen of the 83 pneumococcal serotypes are responsible for 82 percent of cases of bacteremic pneumococcal disease,[64,65] with a close correlation between bacteremic subtypes and those implicated in meningitis.[67–69]

The adherence of microorganisms to mucosal surfaces may be inhibited by natural antibodies, such as IgA, found in mucosal secretions. However, it appears that the presence of high concentrations of circulating IgA antibodies to *N. meningitidis* may permit the development or progression of invasive disease by preferentially binding to the organism and blocking the beneficial effects of IgG and IgM antibodies.[153] In addition, species

of many pathogenic bacteria (e.g., *Neisseria, Haemophilus, Streptococcus*) produce IgA1 proteases that cleave IgA in the hinge region and facilitate adherence of bacterial strains to mucosal surfaces through local destruction of IgA. However, the exact role of IgA protease production in this pathogenic sequence remains unclear.

Bacteremia.   Once bacteria cross the mucosal barrier and gain access to the blood stream, they must overcome additional host defense mechanisms to survive. The presence of bacterial capsule, by effectively inhibiting neutrophil phagocytosis and resisting classic complement-mediated bactericidal activity, may enhance blood stream survival of the organism, thereby facilitating intravascular replication.[136,153] The most common meningeal pathogens (*H. influenzae, N. meningitidis, S. pneumoniae, E. coli, S. agalactiae*) are all encapsulated. In addition, certain capsular types are disproportionately associated with development of meningitis. For example, about 84 percent of cases of neonatal meningitis caused by *E. coli* are caused by strains bearing the K1 antigen[159]; in the absence of specific host antibody to the K1 capsule, these organisms are profoundly resistant to phagocytosis.[153]

The host possesses several defense mechanisms to counteract the antiphagocytic effects of bacterial capsule.[136,153] For example, the alternative complement pathway is activated by the capsular polysaccharide of *S. pneumoniae,* resulting in cleavage of C3 with attachment of C3b to the bacterial surface. This series of events facilitates opsonization, phagocytosis, and intravascular clearance of the organism. Impairment of the alternative complement pathway (e.g., in patients with sickle cell anemia and those who have undergone splenectomy) predisposes to the development of pneumococcal meningitis. *Haemophilus influenzae* type b also activates the complement cascade. Experimental studies in an experimental rat model have shown that, following intravenous or intraperitoneal challenge with *H. influenzae* of varying serotypes (a, b, c, or d), rats depleted of C3 developed a greater incidence and magnitude of bacteremia. Although the incidence of bacteremia caused by type b organisms increased from 63 to 95 percent in complement-depleted rats, the incidence and severity of meningitis were unaffected by complement depletion.

Complement system activation is also an essential host defense mechanism against invasive disease caused by *N. meningitidis.* Patients with deficiencies in the membrane attack complex are particularly prone to neisserial infections, though usually with a more favorable outcome when appropriate therapy is instituted.[58] The reasons for the worse outcome in patients with an intact complement system are unclear, although it has recently been shown that a qualitative relationship exists among the concentrations of circulating meningococcal lipopolysaccharide (LPS), a fatal outcome, and the degree of complement activation.[160]

Meningeal Invasion.   The mechanism(s) by which meningeal pathogens gain access to the CNS remain unknown. The development of a sustained, high-grade bacteremia has been suggested as one important factor.[161,162] In one study culture-positive meningitis was produced in an experimental infant rat model only after an intense bacteremia had been present for at least 6 hours.[163] However, sustained bacteremia cannot be the sole factor responsible for meningeal invasion because many other organisms (e.g., viridans streptococci) that produce high-grade bacteremia during infective endocarditis rarely produce meningitis.

The site of CNS invasion by meningeal pathogens is also unclear. Early studies suggested that invasion from the blood stream was via the dural venous sinus system, whereas other experiments suggested that the site of invasion was above the cribriform plate or via the choroid plexi (due to their exceptionally high rate of blood flow of approximately 200 ml/g/min).[162]

Recent experimental studies, however, have demonstrated that receptors for some meningeal pathogens are present on cells of the choroid plexi and cerebral capillaries. In cryostat sections of infant rat brain cortical slices, *E. coli* strains possessing S fimbriae have been shown to bind specifically to the luminal surfaces of the vascular endothelium and the epithelium lining the choroid plexi and brain ventricles.[164] Phase variation to the nonfimbriated form may then be necessary for these bacteria to invade the CNS.[165] Despite these studies, the importance of adherence of meningeal pathogens to sites within the CNS requires further study.

Another pathogenic mechanism postulated to promote CNS invasion by meningeal pathogens is association of the organism with circulating monocytes. Utilizing histologic and scanning microscopic techniques to examine the neuraxes of pigs inoculated with a strain of *Streptococcus suis* type 2,[166] the only pathologic lesions detected were associated with the choroid plexus, manifested as brush border disruption, decrease in the number of Kolmer cells, and exudation of fibrin and inflammatory cells into the ventricles. Intracellular bacteria were demonstrated in the parenchyma of the choroid plexus, in the ventricular monocytes, and within circulating peripheral blood monocytes, suggesting that bacteria may gain access to the CSF in association with monocytes migrating along normal pathways.

Alterations of the Blood-Brain Barrier. Bacterial meningitis has been shown to increase permeability across the BBB, which is composed of the arachnoid membrane, choroid plexus epithelium, and cerebral microvascular endothelium; the cerebral microvascular endothelium has been the site of intensive study in bacterial meningitis. Utilizing an adult experimental rat model, the propensity for meningeal pathogens to induce functional and morphologic alterations of the BBB was examined.[167] Following the intracisternal inoculation of either *E. coli*, *S. pneumoniae*, or *H. influenzae* type b, alterations of the BBB were found with all three pathogens, manifested morphologically by an early and sustained increase in pinocytotic vesicle formation and a progressive separation of intercellular tight junctions; these morphologic changes correlated with the functional penetration of albumin, a molecule normally excluded by an intact BBB, into CSF. Following intracisternal inoculation of an unencapsulated strain of *H. influenzae*, there was an increase in pinocytotic vesicle formation without separation of intercellular tight junctions, suggesting that encapsulation of *H. influenzae* was not essential for BBB injury but facilitated its progression by avoidance of host defense mechanisms. The increased BBB permeability was observed in both normal and leukopenic animals,[168] although permeability was augmented by the presence of leukocytes. The site of BBB injury was subsequently examined by in situ tracer perfusion and immunolabeling procedures to identify the topography and microvascular exit pathways of bovine serum albumin (BSA).[169] Exit of both perfused colloidal gold-BSA and immunodetectable BSA was through open intercellular junctions of venules in the pia-arachnoid specifically and topographically localizing the BBB injury in bacterial meningitis to the meningeal venules.

Since surface encapsulation was not an essential virulence factor for production of BBB injury, BBB permeability was examined following the intracisternal inoculation of purified *H. influenzae* type b LPS.[170] Purified LPS was shown to increase BBB permeability in an experimental rat model in both a dose- and time-dependent manner (maximum change at a dose of 20 ng at 4 hours after intracisternal inoculation), with a close correlation between permeability and CSF pleocytosis 4 hours after intracisternal inoculation. Further experiments demonstrated that LPS did not directly mediate the increased BBB permeability, but did so by inducing the production of various inflammatory cytokines (i.e., IL-1 and TNF) within the CNS; intracisternal inoculation of purified LPS led to increased CSF

concentrations of both IL-1 and TNF within 30–120 minutes.[153] Furthermore, the intracisternal inoculation of human recombinant IL-1β into rats led to a peak increase in BBB permeability about 3 hours after inoculation, earlier than the peak response obtained following inoculation with LPS (4 hours).[171] No permeability changes were induced following the intracisternal inoculation of human recombinant TNF-α, although all available evidence suggests that these cytokines act synergistically, since inoculation with submaximal doses of IL-1β plus TNF-α, at concentrations that produced no changes individually, enhanced BBB permeability. In contrast, in a study of patients with bacterial meningitis,[172] CSF concentrations of TNF-α, but not IL-1β, correlated with BBB disruption (assessed by CSF protein concentrations); synergy between IL-1β and TNF-α was also noted in this study.

The effects of LPS on BBB permeability in the experimental rat model have also been examined in an in vitro model by growing purified preparations of cerebral microvascular endothelium on a semipermeable support.[173–175] Several investigators have demonstrated increased permeability across this monolayer after exposure to *H. influenzae* type b or purified LPS. The mechanism for this increased permeability is unclear, however. It may be related to a direct cytotoxic effect of LPS,[175] through serum components such as LPS-binding protein,[176] on the cerebral microvascular endothelium, or by the LPS-induced formation of various second messengers (e.g., cyclic AMP or cyclic GMP) by the endothelial cells.[153]

Bacterial Survival within the Subarachnoid Space. Once meningeal pathogens enter the subarachnoid space, host defense mechanisms are inadequate to control the infection.[136,153] CSF concentrations of complement components are absent or present in minimal concentrations; meningeal inflammation leads to increased, although low, CSF complement concentrations. This relative complement deficiency may be of critical importance, since specific antibody and/or complement is essential for opsonization of encapsulated meningeal pathogens and efficient phagocytosis. Observations in experimental animal models and in patients with meningitis have revealed absent or barely detectable opsonic and bactericidal activities. The explanation for these low complement components during bacterial meningitis is unclear. It has been suggested that complement components crossing the BBB may be degraded by leukocyte proteases, resulting in inefficient opsonic activity at the site of infection. Indeed, in an experimental rabbit model of pneumococcal meningitis, the intracisternal inoculation of a nonspecific protease inhibitor (phenylmethylsulfonyl fluoride) led to a decline in pneumococcal concentrations in CSF compared with saline-inoculated controls.

Immunoglobulin concentrations are also low in normal CSF (blood:CSF ratio of IgG of about 800:1), and, although concentrations increase during bacterial meningitis, they remain low compared with simultaneous serum concentrations.[136,153] In an experimental rabbit model, the intravenous administration of a bactericidal monoclonal antibody against the polyribosyl-ribitol phosphate of *H. influenzae* type b produced high serum antibody concentrations,[177] but BBB permeability was poor (5.5 percent or less) even in the presence of meningeal inflammation, suggesting that systemic administration of type-specific antibodies alone is likely to be suboptimal in the therapy of bacterial meningitis.

Bacterial meningitis is characterized by the development of a neutrophilic pleocytosis within the CSF, although the precise mechanism of leukocyte traversal across the BBB is undefined.[153] The complement component C5a has been suggested as one chemotactic component, with chemotactic activity appearing 2–4 hours before neutrophil influx into CSF. In an experimental rabbit model, the intracisternal inoculation of C5a led to an influx of leukocytes into CSF 1 hour after inoculation,[178] a response that was attenuated by coadministration of prostaglandin E₂ (PGE₂) in a dose- and time-dependent manner, suggesting a direct anti-inflammatory action of PGE₂ on C5a-induced CSF pleocytosis during bacterial meningitis. Despite this early influx of leukocytes in bacterial meningitis, host defense in CSF remains suboptimal because of the lack of functional opsonic and bactericidal activity. With inefficient phagocytosis, bacteria can multiply to huge concentrations in the CSF during meningitis.

The precise pathway of leukocyte traversal into the CSF is unknown, although adherence to vascular endothelial cells is a likely prerequisite. Pretreatment of noncerebral endothelial cells in culture with cytokines has been shown to induce the formation of specific adhesion molecules such as endothelial leukocyte adhesion molecule 1.[179] In addition, adherence of neutrophils to vascular endothelium is enhanced by pretreatment of the endothelial cells with LPS or cytokines (i.e., IL-1 or TNF),[152,180-182] a mechanism that may also exist in cerebral vascular endothelium. Recent experimental studies have examined these issues in greater detail. In an experimental rabbit model, the intravenous inoculation of a monoclonal antibody (IB4) directed against the CD18 family of receptors on leukocytes blocked the accumulation of leukocytes in CSF despite the intracisternal inoculation of *H. influenzae* type b, *N. meningitidis*, pneumococcal cell wall, or LPS[183]; increased protein concentrations in CSF were also attenuated by IB4. In addition, the monoclonal antibody prevented the development of cerebral edema and death in animals challenged with lethal doses of *S. pneumoniae*. Cerebrospinal fluid penetration of antibiotics, CSF bactericidal concentrations, and bactericidal response to ampicillin therapy were not affected by administration of the monoclonal antibody, although the onset of bacteremia was delayed and there was an attenuated CSF inflammatory response after ampicillin-induced bacterial killing. Therefore, it appears that systemic inoculation of a monoclonal antibody that prevents leukocyte-endothelial cell interactions can block some manifestations of leukocyte-mediated damage during bacterial meningitis.

Induction of Subarachnoid Space Inflammation. The induction of a marked subarachnoid space inflammatory response by meningeal pathogens contributes to many of the pathophysiologic consequences of bacterial meningitis and, therefore, significant morbidity and mortality from this disorder. Recent experimental studies have focused on the virulence factors of meningeal pathogens, and the specific inflammatory mediators they induce (Table 5), to learn more about the mechanisms responsible for subarachnoid space inflammation.

Despite the importance of the polysaccharide capsule of bacteria in the intravascular and subarachnoid space survival of meningeal pathogens, capsular polysaccharides are remarkably noninflammatory even when inoculated in purified form into the CSF of animals. In contrast, the cell walls of *S. pneumoniae* are potent inducers of CSF inflammation,[184] and even the independent intracisternal inoculation of the major components of the pneumococcal cell wall, teichoic acid and peptidoglycan,

TABLE 5. Potential Factors Contributing to Subarachnoid Space Inflammation

Bacterial factors
 Cell wall components
 Lipopolysaccharide
 Outer membrane vesicles
Host factors
 Prostaglandins (PGE₂, prostacyclin)
 Interleukin-1 (α and β)
 Interleukin-6
 Interleukin-8
 Tumor necrosis factor-α
 Platelet-activating factor
 Macrophage inhibitory proteins 1 and 2
 Leukocyte integrins (CD18)
 Endothelial leukocyte adhesion molecule 1

induces CSF inflammation.[185] These findings lend support to the concept that release of pneumococcal cell wall lytic products during antibiotic-induced autolysis during treatment of bacterial meningitis contributes to an accentuated host inflammatory response in the subarachnoid space. Subarachnoid space inflammation is also induced by the intracisternal inoculation of purified *H. influenzae* type b LPS,[170,186] a response blocked by pretreatment of the LPS with polymyxin B or neutrophil acyloxyacyl hydrolase, supporting the importance of the lipid A region of the LPS molecule in the induction of inflammation.

Recently, however, experimental evidence has supported the concept that pneumococcal cell wall or LPS do not directly induce subarachnoid space inflammation, but do so through the local CNS release of inflammatory mediators such as IL-1, TNF, and/or prostaglandins. For example, intact pneumococci, pneumococcal cell wall, or lipoteichoic acid induced IL-1, but not TNF, production by human peripheral monocytes in vitro.[187] In addition, in an experimental rat model, the intracisternal inoculation of purified *H. influenzae* type b LPS led to elevated CSF concentrations of IL-1 and TNF within 30–120 minutes[153]; elevated CSF concentrations of TNF have also been found in an experimental rabbit model,[188] with peak activity at 2 hours and persistence for about 5 hours. Similar results were observed after intracisternal challenge with live *H. influenzae* type b, although TNF activity persisted longer (about 14 hours). The TNF was produced principally within the CNS (i.e., no TNF activity was detected in serum samples) in this experimental animal model system, a finding that has also been observed in patients with bacterial meningitis.[189] In addition, the finding of increased CSF concentrations of TNF-α may be specific for bacterial meningitis. The presence of TNF-α in CSF appears to be indicative of a bacterial etiology,[189-192] although the absence of TNF-α does not exclude the diagnosis of bacterial meningitis. Furthermore, elevated CSF concentrations of PGE₂, prostacyclin, IL-1β, and TNF have been found in the majority of infants and children with bacterial meningitis.[193]

The direct intracisternal inoculation of these inflammatory mediators can also induce CSF inflammation. In an experimental rabbit model, injection of purified rabbit TNF-α or human recombinant IL-1β produced significant CSF inflammation.[194] This effect was synergistic when lower doses of each cytokine were administered simultaneously, with more rapid and significantly increased leukocyte influx than when each cytokine was administered alone. In contrast, in an experimental rabbit model of pneumococcal meningitis, the parameters of CSF leukocytosis, BBB permeability, and brain edema were induced by intracisternal inoculation of human recombinant TNF-α, macrophage inhibitory proteins 1 and 2, and IL-1α, but not by IL-1β.[195] Leukocytosis and brain edema were inhibited by antibodies homologous to each mediator as well as in rabbits treated with a monoclonal antibody to CD18 to render neutrophil-endothelial cell interactions dysfunctional. Platelet-activating factor is also inflammatory in the CNS, causing significant BBB permeability and cerebral edema[196]; at higher doses these effects are accompanied by CSF leukocytosis, which can be inhibited by administration of antibody to the CD18 family of leukocyte adhesion molecules. In an experimental rabbit model, treatment with a platelet-activating factor receptor antagonist decreased CSF cytochemical values induced by intracisternal challenge with pneumococci but not *H. influenzae*,[196] suggesting a specific role for platelet-activating factor in pneumococcal disease. It would appear that these inflammatory mediators have multiple complex and interrelated activities in the CNS that contribute to inflammation and tissue damage during bacterial meningitis.

These findings have importance with regard to outcome in patients with bacterial meningitis. Outcome from gram-negative bacillary meningitis has been correlated with persistence of organisms and higher concentrations of endotoxin (as measured by the *Limulus* lysate assay) in CSF.[197] In children with *H. influenzae* type b meningitis, CSF concentrations of free LPS correlated with the Herson-Todd severity score and number of febrile hospital days.[198] The degree of elevated CSF concentrations of IL-1β also correlated with outcome from neonatal gram-negative bacillary meningitis.[199] Furthermore, in infants and children with predominantly *H. influenzae* type b meningitis, patients with CSF concentrations of IL-1β of 500 pg/ml or more were more likely to develop neurologic sequelae[200]; elevated CSF concentrations of TNF were not associated with outcome. Elevated CSF concentrations of platelet-activating factor have been demonstrated in children with *H. influenzae* meningitis,[201] correlating with bacterial density and with CSF concentrations of LPS and TNF-α; these increased concentrations of TNF-α and platelet-activating factor were associated with severity of disease. Elevated CSF concentrations of IL-6 have also been observed in the CSF of patients with bacterial meningitis[202–204]; these increased concentrations occurred after release of TNF-α and before neutrophilic infiltration into CSF.[205] IL-8, a cytokine with potent chemoattractant and activating effects on neutrophils, was recently detected in CSF of patients with meningococcal meningitis[206]; IL-8 concentrations in serum were significantly higher in patients with meningococcal septic shock without meningitis than in patients with other manifestations. Therefore, it appears that release of inflammatory mediators in the CNS is responsible for induction of a marked subarachnoid space inflammatory response and may correlate with morbidity and mortality in patients with bacterial meningitis.

Increased Intracranial Pressure. Cerebral edema is the major element contributing to the increased intracranial pressure during bacterial meningitis and may result in life-threatening cerebral herniation and other complications.[153] The cerebral edema may be vasogenic, cytotoxic, and/or interstitial in origin; all three elements probably contribute to cerebral edema during bacterial meningitis. Vasogenic cerebral edema is primarily a consequence of increased BBB permeability, cytotoxic cerebral edema results from swelling of the cellular elements of the brain most likely due to release of toxic factors from neutrophils or bacteria or both, and interstitial cerebral edema reflects obstruction of the flow of normal CSF as in hydrocephalus. The last factor has been examined in an experimental rabbit model of pneumococcal or *E. coli* meningitis in which the CSF outflow resistance (defined as factors that inhibit the flow of CSF from the subarachnoid space to the major dural sinuses) was markedly elevated and remained elevated for as long as 2 weeks despite rapid CSF sterilization with penicillin therapy.[207]

These concepts have been examined in greater detail in an experimental animal model of pneumococcal meningitis by measuring the brain water content (indicative of cerebral edema if elevated), CSF lactate concentrations, and CSF pressure.[208] All three parameters were elevated in infected animals. Although treatment with ampicillin rapidly sterilized the CSF and normalized brain water content and CSF pressure, the CSF lactate concentration remained elevated. The bacterial virulence factor responsible for production of brain edema was subsequently examined in an experimental animal model of *E. coli* meningitis in which therapy with cefotaxime, but not chloramphenicol, induced a marked rise in CSF endotoxin concentrations that were associated with increased brain water content.[209] The peptidoglycan of the *H. influenzae* cell wall also induced cerebral edema without perturbing the other parameters of inflammation (i.e., increased BBB permeability),[210] suggesting that peptidoglycan induces cytotoxic rather than vasogenic cerebral edema. Neutrophils appeared to contribute to development of cerebral edema if adequately stimulated,[211] although the parameters of increased intracranial pressure and increased CSF concentrations of lactate and protein were unrelated to the presence of neutrophils. However, this area remains controversial because neutrophils are required for the increased BBB permeability seen in response to the intracisternal inoculation of bacterial virulence factors and inflammatory mediators.[170,171]

Furthermore, it has recently been suggested that oxygen radicals may contribute to the increased brain water content, intracranial pressure, and changes in regional blood flow (see below) in bacterial meningitis. In an experimental rat model of pneumococcal meningitis following intracisternal inoculation of live pneumococci or pneumococcal cell wall components,[212] the increases in brain water content and intracranial pressure were prevented, and the increase in regional blood flow was significantly attenuated by conjugated superoxide dismutase and deferoxamine. Catalase, which eliminates hydrogen peroxide, also significantly attenuated the increase in regional blood flow and brain water content, although there was only a trend in reduction of intracranial pressure.[213] Recently, evidence has suggested that reactive nitrogen intermediates may also play a role in these pathophysiologic events.[214]

Alterations in Cerebral Blood Flow. Bacterial meningitis exerts profound effects on blood vessels coursing through the subarachnoid space,[153] and the resulting vasculitis leads to narrowing and/or thrombosis of cerebral blood vessels and the propensity for ischemia and/or infarction of underlying brain. In combination with increased intracranial pressure, these changes may result in altered cerebral blood flow in patients with bacterial meningitis. It has been demonstrated in an infant rhesus monkey model of *H. influenzae* meningitis that there is cerebral cortical hypoperfusion during meningitis with resultant relative cerebral anoxia.[162] Cerebrovascular autoregulation is also lost during experimental bacterial meningitis, in which cerebral blood flow was increased when systemic pressure was increased and decreased when blood pressure was lowered.[215] Furthermore, studies in an experimental rabbit model of pneumococcal meningitis have demonstrated that animals given a lower intravenous fluid regimen (50 ml/kg per 24 hours) of normal saline had a lower mean arterial pressure, lower cerebral blood flow, and a higher concentration of CSF lactate compared with animals that received a higher fluid regimen (150 ml/kg per 24 hours).[216] In the first 4–6 hours of antibiotic administration, rabbits receiving lower fluid regimens had a significant decrease in mean arterial pressure and cerebral blood flow and a significant increase in CSF lactate concentrations than rabbits receiving higher fluid regimens. These results, in combination with other experimental studies that have noted an increase in cerebral blood flow within the first few hours of intracisternal inoculation of either live pneumococci or pneumococcal cell wall fragments,[217] have suggested that maintenance of adequate intravascular volume and minimization of stimuli that increase systemic blood pressure may be important in the treatment of bacterial meningitis. These findings may also be of potential clinical relevance, since inadvertent increases in mean arterial pressure directly increase cerebral blood flow and intracranial pressure, and depletion of intravascular volume with decreases in mean arterial pressure can cause parallel decreases in cerebral blood flow and reduction of substrate delivery to the brain. Therefore, the brain is at risk from either hypoperfusion or hyperperfusion.

Cerebral blood flow has been measured in patients with bacterial meningitis. In an early study,[218] measurement of cerebral blood flow (by the xenon-133 intra-arterial injection method) revealed a 30–40 percent reduction in average total blood flow in five patients with pneumococcal meningitis (mean age of 54 years), but not in five patients with meningococcal meningitis (mean age of 20 years). An inverse relationship between cerebral blood flow and intracranial pressure has been observed in infants with bacterial meningitis[219]; among eight patients, alterations were noted only in the four older infants (age range of 3–10 months) and not in the four neonates (age range of 5–30 days) in whom no changes in cerebral blood flow velocity were detected.

In a subsequent study in 20 children seriously ill with bacterial meningitis,[220] total and regional cerebral blood flow measured by stable xenon computed tomography revealed a global decrease in flow and even more regional variability. Although autoregulation of cerebral blood flow was preserved in the patients studied, hyperventilation reduced flow below the ischemic threshold, raising important concerns about the routine use of hyperventilation in the management of increased intracranial pressure in patients with bacterial meningitis.[221] In another study of 86 adult patients with bacterial meningitis,[222] cerebral angiography was performed in 27 patients who had focal deficits (either clinically, on cranial computed tomography, or both) and who had persistent coma without explained cause despite 3 days of antimicrobial therapy. Thirteen of the patients who underwent angiography had alterations of the blood vessel system; prognosis in these patients was poor. However, the definitive changes in cerebral blood flow during bacterial meningitis are controversial and may vary with stage of disease. These blood flow alterations may lead to regional hypoxia, increased lactate concentrations in the brain secondary to utilization of glucose by anaerobic glycolysis, and CSF acidosis, which may be a precursor to encephalopathy.[223]

CLINICAL PRESENTATION

Viral Meningitis

Enteroviruses. The clinical manifestations of enteroviral meningitis are dependent on host age and immune status.[2] In neonates (2 weeks of age or younger) with proven enteroviral meningitis, fever is a ubiquitous finding, usually accompanied by vomiting, anorexia, rash, and/or upper respiratory symptoms and signs. Neurologic involvement may be associated with nuchal rigidity and a bulging anterior fontanelle, although infants under 1 year of age are less likely to demonstrate meningeal signs. Mental status may be altered, but focal neurologic signs are uncommon. A more severe meningoencephalitis may be seen in neonates, in which the affected infant appears to be at greatest risk for morbidity and mortality (rates as high as 74 and 10 percent, respectively),[224] particularly when symptoms and signs develop during the first day of life (following presumed transplacental transmission of the virus). With disease progression, hepatic necrosis, myocarditis, and necrotizing enterocolitis may develop. Findings in the CNS are of an encephalitis associated with seizures and focal neurologic findings. Lack of humoral antibody may contribute to the severity of neonatal infection.

This contrasts with the clinical findings of enteroviral meningitis beyond the neonatal period (older than 2 weeks), in which severe disease and poor outcome are rare. In this patient population the onset of illness is usually sudden, with fever present in 76–100 percent of patients[225]; the fever may be biphasic, initially appearing with nonspecific constitutional symptoms, disappearing, and then reappearing with the onset of meningeal signs. More than half of the patients have nuchal rigidity. Headache (often severe and frontal in location) is nearly always present in adults; photophobia is also common. Nonspecific symptoms and signs include vomiting, anorexia, rash, diarrhea, cough, upper respiratory findings (especially pharyngitis), and myalgias. Other clues to the presence of enteroviral disease, in addition to time of year and known epidemic disease in the community, include the presence of exanthems, myopericarditis, conjunctivitis, and specifically recognizable enteroviral syndromes such as pleurodynia, herpangina, and hand-foot-and-mouth disease.[1] In addition, specific clinical stigmata may be associated with certain enteroviral serotypes.[2] For example, echovirus 9 is associated with scattered maculopapular rashes. Herpangina, in particular the finding of painful vesicles on the posterior oropharynx, is associated with coxsackievirus A; the presence of pericarditis or pleurisy may identify coxsackievirus B. The duration of illness in enteroviral meningitis is usually less than 1 week, with many patients reporting improvement after the lumbar puncture,[226] presumably as a result of reduction of intracranial pressure.

A unique clinical situation exists in children and adults with absent or deficient humoral immunity that impairs clearance of enteroviruses. Persons who are agammaglobulinemic may develop chronic enteroviral meningitis or meningoencephalitis lasting several years, often with a fatal outcome.[227] About half of these patients also develop a rheumatologic syndrome, usually dermatomyositis, likely as a direct result of enteroviral invasion of affected tissues.

Mumps Virus. In patients with mumps, CNS symptoms usually follow the onset of parotitis, when present, by about 5 days. The most frequent clinical presentation of mumps CNS infection is the triad of fever, vomiting, and headache (Table 6).[13] The fever is usually high and lasts for 72–96 hours. Salivary gland enlargement is present in only about 50 percent of patients. Other findings include neck stiffness, lethargy or somnolence, and abdominal pain. Most patients have signs of meningitis, but no evidence of cortical dysfunction. Defervescence is usually accompanied by clinical recovery and, in uncomplicated cases, the total duration of illness is 7–10 days. Rarely, mumps may cause encephalitis, seizures, polyradiculitis, polyneuritis, cranial nerve palsies, myelitis, Guillain-Barré syndrome, and fatality.[13]

Lymphocytic Choriomeningitis Virus. Lymphocytic choriomeningitis virus infection begins with nonspecific viral symptoms. Following a brief period of improvement, approximately 15 percent of patients develop severe headache, photophobia, lightheadedness, lumbar myalgias, and pharyngitis.[1] Occasionally orchitis, arthritis, myopericarditis, and alopecia are also seen, usually as late manifestations.

Herpesviruses. Meningitis associated with herpes simplex virus type 2 infection is usually characterized by stiff neck, headache, and fever.[21] In one review of 27 patients with herpes simplex virus type 2 meningitis,[27] neurologic complications were found in 37 percent of cases and consisted of urinary retention, dysesthesias, paresthesias, neuralgia, motor weakness, paraparesis, concentration difficulties of about 3 months duration, and impaired hearing. All, however, subsided within 6 months in all patients. Recurrent meningitis was documented in five patients. Pharyngitis, lymphadenopathy, and splenomegaly should suggest Epstein-Barr virus infection. A diffuse vesicular pustular rash may be seen in meningitis caused by varicella-zoster virus.

Human Immunodeficiency Virus. HIV-infected patients may present with a typical aseptic meningitis syndrome associated with acute infection (i.e., the mononucleosis-like syndrome).[35,36,39] In addition, some patients may present with an atypical aseptic meningitis that is often chronic, tends to recur, and often includes cranial neuropathies (usually cranial nerves V, VII, and VIII) or long tract findings.[40,41,228] The most common features are headache, fever, and meningeal signs. The illness is self-limited or recurrent rather than progressive.

TABLE 6. Presenting Symptoms and Signs in Patients with Central Nervous System Mumps

Symptom or Sign	Relative Frequency (%)
Fever	88–100
Vomiting	68–94
Headache	47–88
Salivary gland swelling	47–62
Meningismus	43–93
Lethargy	28–69
Abdominal pain	14–23
Seizures	14–18

(Adapted from Gnann,[13] with permission.)

Bacterial Meningitis

Patients with bacterial meningitis classically present with fever, headache, meningismus, and signs of cerebral dysfunction (i.e., confusion, delirium, or a declining level of consciousness ranging from lethargy to coma)[69,229,230]; these are found in more than 85 percent of patients (Table 7). The meningismus may be subtle, marked, or accompanied by Kernig's and/or Brudzinski's signs.[231] Kernig's sign is elicited with the patient in the supine position, in which the thigh is flexed on the abdomen with the knee flexed. The leg is then passively extended, and, in the presence of meningeal inflammation, the patient resists leg extension; this differs somewhat from the maneuver as initially described by Kernig, in which the patient was initially placed in the seated position. Several signs were described by Brudzinski, although the best known is the nape-of-the-neck sign, in which passive flexion of the neck results in flexion of the hips and knees. However, these signs are elicited in only about 50 percent of adult patients with bacterial meningitis, and their absence does not rule out the diagnosis. Cranial nerve palsies (especially involving cranial nerves III, IV, VI, and VII) and focal cerebral signs are seen in 10–20 percent of cases. Cranial nerve palsies likely develop as the nerve becomes enveloped by exudate in the arachnoid sheath surrounding the nerve, or may be a sign of increased intracranial pressure. Seizures occur in about 30 percent of patients. Focal neurologic deficits and seizures arise from cortical and subcortical ischemia, resulting from inflammation and thrombosis of blood vessels, often within the subarachnoid space. Hemiparesis may also result from the presence of a large subdural effusion, arising when infection in the adjacent subarachnoid space leads to an increased permeability of the thin-walled capillaries and veins of the inner layer of the dura; this is usually self-limited, although an enlarging effusion can lead to mass effect with resultant hemiparesis. Papilledema is seen in less than 1 percent of cases early in infection, and its presence should suggest an alternative diagnosis. With disease progression, patients may develop signs of increased intracranial pressure including coma, hypertension, bradycardia, and palsy of cranial nerve III.

A specific etiologic diagnosis in patients with bacterial meningitis may be suggested by certain symptoms and/or signs. About 50 percent of patients with meningococcemia, with or without meningitis, present with a prominent rash, located principally on the extremities.[232,233] Early in the course of illness, the rash is typically erythematous and macular, but quickly evolves into a petechial phase with further coalescence into a purpuric form. The rash often matures rapidly, with new petechial lesions appearing during the physical examination. A similar rash may also be seen in splenectomized patients with rapidly overwhelming sepsis caused by *S. pneumoniae* or *H. influenzae* type b. In patients who have suffered a basilar skull fracture in which a dural fistula is produced between the subarachnoid space and nasal cavity, paranasal sinuses, or middle ear, a common presentation is rhinorrhea or otorrhea due to a CSF leak[74]; in these patients meningitis may be recurrent and is most commonly caused by *S. pneumoniae*. Patients with *Listeria monocytogenes* meningitis have an increased tendency to have seizures

TABLE 7. Presenting Symptoms and Signs in Patients with Bacterial Meningitis

Symptom or Sign	Relative Frequency (%)
Headache	≥90
Fever	≥90
Meningismus	≥85
Altered sensorium	>80
Kernig's sign	≥50
Brudzinski's sign	≥50
Vomiting	~35
Seizures	~30
Focal findings	10–20
Papilledema	<1

and focal deficits early in the course of infection, and some patients may present with ataxia, cranial nerve palsies, or nystagmus due to rhomboencephalitis[75,76,79]; however, patients with *Listeria* meningitis may present with no focal signs.

Some categories of patients may not manifest many of the classic symptoms and signs of bacterial meningitis.[234] For example, neonates with bacterial meningitis usually do not have meningismus.[86] The clinical clues to the presence of meningitis in neonates are temperature instability (hypothermia or hyperthermia), listlessness, high-pitched crying, fretfulness, lethargy, refusal to feed, weak suck, irritability, jaundice, vomiting, diarrhea, or respiratory distress. A change in the child's affect or state of alertness is one of the most important signs of meningitis. A bulging fontanelle (seen in one-third of cases) usually occurs late during the course of illness; seizures are observed in 40 percent of neonates with bacterial meningitis. Elderly patients, especially those with underlying conditions (e.g., diabetes mellitus or cardiopulmonary disease), may present insidiously with lethargy or obtundation, no fever, and variable signs of meningeal inflammation. In one review,[235] confusion was very common in elderly patients on presentation, occurring in 92 and 78 percent of those with pneumococcal and gram-negative bacillary meningitis, respectively. The elderly patient may also present with an antecedent or concurrent bronchitis, pneumonia, or paranasal sinusitis. The diagnosis of bacterial meningitis in neutropenic patients requires a high index of suspicion because symptoms and signs may initially be subtle due to the impaired ability of the patient to mount a subarachnoid space inflammatory response.[236,237] In patients with head trauma, the symptoms and signs of meningitis may be present as a result of the underlying injury and not meningitis.[74] In all of these subgroups of patients, an altered or changed mental status should not be ascribed to other causes until bacterial meningitis has been excluded by CSF examination.

Cerebrospinal Fluid Shunt Infections

The clinical presentation of CSF shunt infection can be quite variable and depends on the pathogenesis of infection, organism virulence, and type of shunt.[238–240] The most frequent symptoms are headache, nausea, lethargy, and/or change in mental status; these occur as a result of shunt malfunction. Fever is reported in as low as 14 percent to as high as 92 percent of cases, so its absence cannot be interpreted as a factor against infection.[240] Pain, often related to infection at the peritoneal or pleural endings of the shunt, may be absent in up to 60 percent of infections.[241] Symptoms and signs of CSF shunt infection may be referable to either the proximal or distal portions of the shunt. Infection beginning in the proximal portion of the shunt (i.e., the catheter within the CSF space) results in a meningitis or ventriculitis in about 30 percent of cases.[239,241,242] However, meningeal symptoms should not be expected with infected ventricular shunts, since there is usually a lack of communication between the infected ventricles and the CSF in contact with the meninges. Infections presenting with symptoms referable to the distal portion of the shunt are more specific to terminus location: infected vascular shunts lead to bacteremia, whereas shunts that terminate in the pleural or peritoneal space lead to an inflammatory response in the absorbing tissue (i.e., pleuritis or peritonitis).[240] Furthermore, some shunt infections are insidious, causing few or no symptoms in which patients may have only an intermittent low-grade fever or general malaise.

Spirochetal Meningitis

Treponema pallidum. The described clinical presentations of neurosyphilis are based on studies compiled before the availability of penicillin, and there is some debate as to whether the clinical presentations of symptomatic neurosyphilis have been modified in the antibiotic era and by associated HIV infection.[108]

Although there are numerous clinical presentations of neurosyphilis, patients with acute meningitis and meningovascular syphilis are discussed here.

Patients with syphilitic meningitis usually present similarly to patients with other forms of aseptic meningitis with complaints of headache, nausea, and vomiting; in one series these were present in 91 percent of patients.[109] Meningismus occurred in 59 percent and fever in less than half of patients with syphilitic meningitis. Seizures occurred in 17 percent of patients, whereas cranial nerve palsies were found in 45 percent of cases (most commonly cranial nerves VII and VIII, followed by II, III, VI, and V). Focal abnormalities such as hemiplegia, aphasia, or mental status changes were seen less commonly. Syphilitic meningitis rarely affects the spinal cord.

Meningovascular syphilis is distinguished clinically from syphilitic meningitis temporally and on the basis of focal neurologic findings as a result of focal syphilitic arteritis, which almost always occurs in association with meningeal inflammation.[108,112,243] Most patients experience weeks to months of episodic prodromal symptoms and signs, including headache or vertiginous episodes, personality changes (e.g., apathy or inattention), behavioral changes (e.g., irritability or memory impairment), insomnia, or seizures. Focal deficits, reflecting episodes of ischemia to regions of the brain by involved blood vessels (usually in the distribution of the middle cerebral artery), may also occur; if untreated, this may progress to a stroke syndrome with attendant irreversible neurologic deficits.

Coinfection with HIV may modify the clinical spectrum of syphilis. Case reports and small series have suggested that patients with HIV infection are more likely to progress to neurosyphilis and to show accelerated disease courses.[113–116,244] However, few clinical data currently support these hypotheses. In one study of HIV-infected and noninfected patients with syphilis at sexually transmitted disease clinics in Baltimore,[245] no significant differences were observed in clinical stage or in disease progression.

Borrelia burgdorferi. Meningitis is the most important neurologic abnormality of acute disseminated Lyme disease, usually following erythema chronicum migrans by 2–10 weeks[117]; however, only about 40 percent (range of 10–90 percent) of cases of Lyme meningitis are preceded by this characteristic rash.[119,246] Headache is the single most common symptom (30–90 percent of patients) in Lyme meningitis, whereas neck stiffness is seen in only 10–20 percent of cases.[117] Photophobia, nausea, and vomiting are intermediate in frequency between headache and neck stiffness. About two-thirds of patients have accompanying systemic symptoms, including malaise, fatigue, myalgias, fever, arthralgias, and involuntary weight loss. In untreated cases the duration of symptoms ranges from 1 to 9 months. Patients typically experience recurrent attacks of meningeal symptoms lasting several weeks, alternating with similar periods of milder symptoms.[117–119,246]

About half of patients with Lyme meningitis have mild cerebral symptoms consisting most commonly of somnolence, emotional lability, depression, impaired memory and concentration, and behavioral symptoms.[117–119,246] These symptoms may fluctuate in severity in untreated patients before resolution. Transverse myelitis, spastic paraparesis or quadriparesis, disturbances of micturition, and Babinski signs are also reported during this stage. Approximately 50 percent of patients also have cranial neuropathies. Facial nerve palsy is the most common (80–90 percent) of the cranial nerve palsies overall and occurs with rapid onset (often over 1–2 days), frequently accompanied by slight ipsilateral facial numbness or tingling or ipsilateral ear or jaw pain.[117–119,246,247] The facial palsy is bilateral in 30–70 percent of cases, although the two sides are affected asynchronously in most cases. Other cranial nerves affected less commonly are cranial nerves II, III, the sensory portion of V,

VI, and the acoustic portion of VIII. Recovery usually takes place within 2 months.

Protozoal and Helminthic Meningitis

Amebae. Primary amebic meningoencephalitis presents in two forms.[121,122] In the acute form (incubation period of 3–8 days) there is the sudden onset of high fever, photophobia, headache, and progression to stupor or coma; this is usually indistinguishable from acute bacterial meningitis, although focal signs and seizures are more common in amebic meningoencephalitis. Because of early involvement of the olfactory area, early symptoms of abnormal smell or taste may be reported.[123] Confusion, irritability, and restlessness progress to delirium, stupor, and, finally, coma. Death in untreated patients generally occurs within 2–3 days from the onset of symptoms.

In contrast, the subacute or chronic form of primary amebic meningoencephalitis presents more insidiously with low-grade fever, headache, and focal signs (e.g., hemiparesis, aphasia, cranial nerve palsies, visual field disturbances, diplopia, ataxia, seizures)[121,122]; the olfactory bulbs are usually spared. Deterioration occurs over a period of 2–4 weeks until death. However, longer durations of illness have also been reported (range of 5–18 months).

Angiostrongylus cantonensis. Symptoms of meningitis begin 6–30 days after ingestion of raw mollusks or other sources of the parasite.[99,248] Findings include severe headache (90 percent), stiff neck (56 percent), paresthesias (54 percent), and vomiting (56 percent). Moderate fever is present in about half of the cases.

DIAGNOSIS

Viral Meningitis

Cerebrospinal Fluid Examination. Cerebrospinal fluid pleocytosis is almost always present in enteroviral meningitis, although some enteroviruses have been isolated from young infants with clinical evidence of meningitis but no CSF white blood cells.[1,2] The cell count is usually $100–1000/mm^3$, although counts in the several thousands have also been reported; higher CSF white blood cell counts have been associated with a greater likelihood of isolating the causative enterovirus.[249] Early in infection, neutrophils may dominate the CSF profile, although this quickly gives way to a lymphocytic predominance over the first 6–48 hours. An elevated CSF protein and decreased CSF glucose, if present, are usually mild, although extreme degrees of both have been reported. Specific virologic diagnosis of enteroviral meningitis depends on isolation of the virus from the CSF in tissue culture,[250,251] although the sensitivity for enteroviral serotypes is only 65–75 percent, largely a result of the inability to grow many coxsackievirus A serotypes[252] that require suckling mouse inoculations. The difficulty in isolation of enteroviruses from CSF may also relate to the low titers of enteroviruses in CSF (as low as $10^1–10^3$ TCID$_{50}$/ml of CSF).[2] The mean time for CSF enteroviruses to grow is 3.7–8.2 days.[2,7] Although isolation of a nonpolio enterovirus from the throat or rectum of a patient with aseptic meningitis is suggestive of an etiologic diagnosis, the mean shedding periods from those sites following infection are 1 week and several weeks, respectively. In addition, viral shedding can occur in 7.5 percent of healthy controls during enterovirus epidemics.[1] Therefore, shedding from a past infection cannot be ruled out. Furthermore, a recent study found that non-CSF viral cultures were not helpful in predicting enteroviral CNS infection, in which enteroviruses were isolated at the same frequency from non-CSF sites from infants in whom enteroviruses were cultured from CSF as in hospitalized infants with an acute illness whose CSF was negative.[253] Follow-up acute and convalescent serologic testing for the specific isolated strain may confirm the etiologic diagnosis.[1]

Rapid diagnosis of enterovirus infections by immunoassay techniques has been hampered by the lack of a common antigen among the various serotypes and the low concentrations of virus in body fluids.[1,2] However, several recent studies have reported success with use of polyclonal or monoclonal antibodies. Tests to detect specific IgM enteroviral antibodies has also been attempted,[254] although the specificity of some of the tests has been unsatisfactory. Complementary DNA nucleic acid probes have been prepared and can detect multiple enteroviral serotypes, but the clinical sensitivity was only 33 percent or less,[2] undoubtedly a result of low titers of enteroviruses in CSF specimens from patients with aseptic meningitis. The technique of PCR for detection of enteroviral RNA has also been studied,[255,256] with results positive in 12 of 12 patients in one study of patients with a clinical diagnosis of aseptic meningitis. Polymerase chain reaction has also been utilized to detect enteroviral RNA in fecal samples from patients with aseptic meningitis[257]; results were positive in all patients from whom an enterovirus was isolated from stool.

In patients with mumps meningitis, there is almost always a CSF pleocytosis (usually less than 500/mm³), primarily mononuclear cells (greater than 80 percent lymphocytes in 80–90 percent of patients)[14]; the pleocytosis may persist for weeks. The CSF protein is reported in some series to be normal in more than half of patients with mumps meningitis.[13] The CSF glucose is normal in most patients, but it may be depressed in up to 25 percent of cases.[13,14] Complement fixation and hemagglutination inhibition on serum specimens are the most reliable serologic tests for the diagnosis of mumps. Testing of paired acute and convalescent sera should demonstrate a diagnostic fourfold rise in mumps antibody titer. Mumps virus can be grown from CSF in tissue culture for at least 1 week following the onset of disease, but sensitivity of this technique is highly variable (30–50 percent if collected from CSF early during the course of mumps CNS infection).[13] There are no rapid detection methods.

The CSF of patients with meningitis caused by lymphocytic choriomeningitis virus typically shows a lymphocytic pleocytosis (usually less than 750/mm³, although counts up to several thousand may be seen).[1,258] Hypoglycorrhachia is seen in up to 25 percent of cases. No rapid detection method is available. The virus may be cultured from blood and CSF early in infection and later from urine. The diagnosis is usually made by a fourfold rise between acute and convalescent sera.

In patients with herpes simplex virus type 2 meningitis, there is also a lymphocytic meningitis (less than 500/mm³) and a normal glucose.[1] The virus has been cultured from the CSF and buffy coat of some patients. Polymerase chain reaction appears promising for the diagnosis of CNS infections caused by herpes simplex virus.[259] The CSF in HIV-infected patients typically shows a mild lymphocytic pleocytosis (20–300/mm³), mildly elevated protein, and normal or slightly decreased glucose[39,41,147,228]; HIV has been isolated from the CSF in some patients with neurologic disease,[39,260] although it can be isolated from HIV-infected patients without neurologic symptoms or signs.[260,261] A few mononuclear cells and elevated protein in CSF are commonly documented in HIV-positive patients throughout the course of infection. The CSF findings in patients with arboviral meningitis are similar to those caused by enteroviruses.[1,2] Virus has been cultured from blood and CSF, but the diagnosis is usually made by acute and convalescent serology.

Bacterial Meningitis

Cerebrospinal Fluid Examination. The diagnosis of bacterial meningitis rests on CSF examination by lumbar puncture[262]; the typical CSF findings in acute bacterial meningitis are shown in

TABLE 8. Typical Cerebrospinal Fluid Findings in Patients with Bacterial Meningitis

Cerebrospinal Fluid Parameter	Typical Findings
Opening pressure	>180 mm H₂O
White blood cell count	1000–5000/mm³ (range <100 to >10,000)
Percentage of neutrophils	≥80%
Protein	100–500 mg/dl
Glucose	≤40 mg/dl
Lactate	≥35 mg/dl
Gram stain	Positive in 60–90%
Culture	Positive in 70–85%
Limulus lysate	Positive in gram-negative meningitis
Bacterial antigen detection	Positive in 50–100%
Polymerase chain reaction	Promisingᵃ

ᵃ See text for details.

Table 8.[230] In virtually all cases the opening pressure is elevated, with values over 600 mmH₂O suggesting the presence of cerebral edema, intracranial suppurative foci, or communicating hydrocephalus. The white blood cell count is elevated in untreated bacterial meningitis, usually 1000–5000/mm³ (range of less than 100 to more than 10,000/mm³). There is usually a neutrophilic predominance, although approximately 10 percent of patients with acute bacterial meningitis present with a lymphocytic predominance in spinal fluid; this is more common in neonatal gram-negative bacillary meningitis and meningitis caused by *Listeria monocytogenes* (about 30 percent of cases). Patients with very low CSF white cell counts (0–20/mm³) despite high CSF bacterial concentrations tend to have a poor prognosis. The absence of a CSF pleocytosis can characterize up to 4 percent of cases of bacterial meningitis overall,[263] most commonly in premature neonates (up to 15 percent of cases) and infants younger than 4 weeks of age (17 percent of cases). Therefore, a Gram stain and culture should be performed on all spinal fluid specimens even if the white blood cell count is normal. A decreased CSF glucose concentration less than 40 mg/dl is found in about 60 percent of patients and a CSF:serum glucose ratio less than 0.31 in about 70 percent of patients.[264] The CSF protein is elevated in virtually all patients, presumably due to disruption of the BBB.[167] However, a normal CSF white blood cell count and protein may be seen in specimens obtained at the onset of meningitis, in some cases of neonatal meningitis, and in severely immunocompromised patients. A recent analysis found that a CSF glucose concentration less than 34 mg/dl, a CSF:blood glucose ratio less than 0.23, a CSF protein concentration more than 220 mg/dl, more than 2000/mm³ CSF leukocytes, or more than 1180/mm³ CSF neutrophils were individual predictors of bacterial, rather than viral, meningitis, with 99 percent certainty or better.[265] Elevated CSF lactate concentrations (especially above 35 mg/dl) may also be useful in differentiating bacterial from nonbacterial meningitis in patients who have not received prior antimicrobial therapy.[266]

Gram stain examination of CSF permits a rapid, accurate identification of the causative microorganism in 60–90 percent of patients with bacterial meningitis and has a specificity of nearly 100 percent.[264] The likelihood of detecting the organism by Gram stain correlates with the concentration of bacteria in CSF; concentrations of 10³ or fewer colony-forming units (cfu)/ml are associated with positive Gram stains about 25 percent of the time, whereas CSF concentrations of bacteria of 10⁵ cfu/ml or above leads to positive microscopy in up to 97 percent of cases.[267] The clinical utility of the Gram stain also depends on the bacterial pathogen[268,269]: bacteria have been observed in 90 percent of cases of meningitis caused by *S. pneumoniae*, 86 percent of cases caused by *H. influenzae*, 75 percent of cases caused by *N. meningitidis*, and 50 percent of cases caused by gram-negative bacilli; the CSF Gram stain is positive in less than 50 percent of patients with *L. monocytogenes* meningitis. In addition, the probability of identifying the organism may decrease in patients who have received prior antimicrobial therapy

(40–60 percent and less than 50 percent positivity on Gram stain and culture, respectively).[79,270,271] In studies of infants and children with bacterial meningitis, initially positive CSF cultures became sterile in 90–100 percent of patients within 24–36 hours of administration of "appropriate" antimicrobial therapy.[263] However, in most infants and children with bacterial meningitis who have received prior antimicrobial therapy, no significant differences in the CSF formula occurs, although two studies revealed significantly lower CSF protein concentrations and rates of Gram stain positivity.[270,272]

Several rapid diagnostic tests have been developed to aid in the diagnosis of bacterial meningitis.[269] Counterimmunoelectrophoresis (CIE) may detect specific antigens in CSF when meningitis is caused by meningococci (serogroups A, C, Y, or W135), H. influenzae type b, pneumococci (83 serotypes), type III group B streptococci, and E. coli K1; the sensitivity ranges from 50 to 95 percent, although the test is highly specific. However, more recent tests are now available that are more rapid (15 minutes or less) and 10-fold more sensitive than CIE; these include staphylococcal coagglutination and latex agglutination (Table 9).[269] Currently available latex agglutination techniques detect the antigens of H. influenzae type b, S. pneumoniae, N. meningitidis, E. coli K1, and the group B streptococci. However, many of the test kits do not include tests for group B meningococci, and other kits are probably poor because of the limited immunogenicity of group B meningococcal polysaccharide. One of these rapid diagnostic tests should be performed on all CSF specimens from patients with presumed bacterial meningitis, especially in cases with a negative CSF Gram stain, although it must be emphasized that a negative test does not rule out infection caused by a specific meningeal pathogen. Lysate prepared from the amebocytes of the horseshoe crab Limulus polyphemus may be useful in suspected cases of gram-negative meningitis in which a positive test indicates the presence of endotoxin.[269] A correctly performed Limulus lysate assay can detect about 10^3 gram-negative bacteria/mL of CSF; the sensitivity and specificity of this assay are 93 and 99.4 percent, respectively. However, this test does not distinguish between specific gram-negative organisms, and a negative test does not rule out the diagnosis of gram-negative meningitis. Polymerase chain reaction has been utilized to amplify DNA from patients with meningitis caused by N. meningitidis and L. monocytogenes.[273–275] In one study of CSF samples from patients with meningococcal meningitis,[274] the sensitivity and specificity of PCR were both 91 percent. There are problems with false-positive results when utilizing PCR, although further refinements in this technique may lead to its usefulness in the diagnosis of bacterial meningitis, particularly when CSF Gram stain, bacterial antigen tests, and cultures are negative.

Radiography. Cranial computed tomography (CT scan) or magnetic resonance imaging (MRI) do not aid in the diagnosis of acute bacterial meningitis. However, one of these modalities should be considered during the course of illness in patients who have persistent or prolonged fever, clinical evidence of increased intracranial pressure, focal neurologic findings or seizures, enlarging head circumference (in neonates), persistent neurologic dysfunction, or persistently abnormal CSF param-

TABLE 9. Sensitivity of Assays for Detection of Bacterial Antigens in Cerebrospinal Fluid from Patients with Bacterial Meningitis

Organism	Sensitivity (%)	
	Coagglutination	Latex Agglutination
Haemophilus influenzae type b	66–100	78–100
Neisseria meningitidis	50–78	50–93
Streptococcus pneumoniae	59–93	67–100
Streptococcus agalactiae	62–87	69–100

(Adapted from Gray and Fedorko,[269] with permission.)

eters or cultures (Fig. 2).[86,262] Cranial CT or MRI has been recommended at the end of antimicrobial therapy in newborn infants to be certain that no intracranial complications have occurred.[86] In one review of 107 children with bacterial meningitis who underwent CT scanning,[276] one or more abnormalities were found in 52 percent of cases, although the majority of findings did not require specific intervention. However, children with fever and subdural collections detected by CT may require a drainage procedure.

Radiographic studies may be useful in the subset of patients with meningitis as a result of a basilar skull fracture with CSF leak.[74,102] CT scanning may detect air-fluid levels or opacification of the paranasal sinuses, or intracranial air; CT scanning with sagittal reconstruction can also be used to document or localize fracture sites. Radioisotope cisternography, with cottonoid pledgets placed at the outlet of the sinuses within the nasal passage, can be used to document a CSF leak, although high-resolution CT scanning with water-soluble contrast enhancement of the CSF (metrizamide cisternography) is the best test for defining the site of leakage.

Spirochetal Meningitis

Treponema pallidum. For diagnosis of CNS involvement in patients with syphilis, no single routine laboratory test is definitive. Cerebrospinal fluid cellular and protein abnormalities have been reported to occur in 10–20 percent of patients with primary syphilis, 30–70 percent of patients with secondary syphilis, and 10–30 percent of patients with latent syphilis.[115] Cerebrospinal fluid abnormalities are common in patients with syphilitic meningitis, but are nonspecific. Findings include a mononuclear pleocytosis (more than 10 cells/mm³ in the majority of patients), elevated CSF protein concentrations (78 percent of patients), and mild decreases in CSF glucose concentrations (less than 50 mg/dl in 55 percent of patients).[109] Oligoclonal bands and intrathecally produced antitreponemal antibodies are frequently present. Isolation of T. pallidum from CSF specimens is difficult, expensive, time-consuming, and not routinely performed.[115]

Given the difficulties in the diagnosis of neurosyphilis, other CSF laboratory tests, particularly serologic testing (i.e., venereal disease research laboratory [VDRL] and fluorescent treponemal antibody [FTA] tests) have been utilized.[109,115,277] However, serologic testing of CSF in patients with syphilis is problematic. For example, CSF collected by lumbar puncture is subject to blood contamination in about 10 percent of patients, which may lead to contamination of CSF and, therefore, a false-positive serologic test result[108]; the likelihood of a false-positive test depends on the relative amount of contamination, the antibody titer in blood, and the sensitivity of the test. For patients with a serum VDRL of 1:256 or less, sufficient blood contamination to be visible to the naked eye is required to cause false-positive CSF VDRL results. However, although the specificity of the CSF VDRL for the diagnosis of neurosyphilis is high, the sensitivity is low (reactive tests in only 30–70 percent of patients).[277] Therefore, a reactive CSF VDRL test in the absence of blood contamination is sufficient to diagnose neurosyphilis; a nonreactive result does not exclude the diagnosis. The CSF fluorescent treponemal antibody absorption (FTA-ABS) test has also been examined as a possible diagnostic test for neurosyphilis.[108,277,278] A nonreactive test effectively rules out the likelihood of neurosyphilis, but the specificity of the test is much less than the CSF VDRL because of the possibility of leakage of small amounts of antibody from the serum into CSF. Furthermore, there are no compelling data that define the significance of a reactive CSF FTA-ABS as useful for the diagnosis of neurosyphilis.[108] Polymerase chain reaction has been used to detect T. pallidum DNA in CSF samples in patients with acute symptomatic neurosyphilis.[279] Further large-scale studies are needed to determine the sensitivity and specificity of this tech-

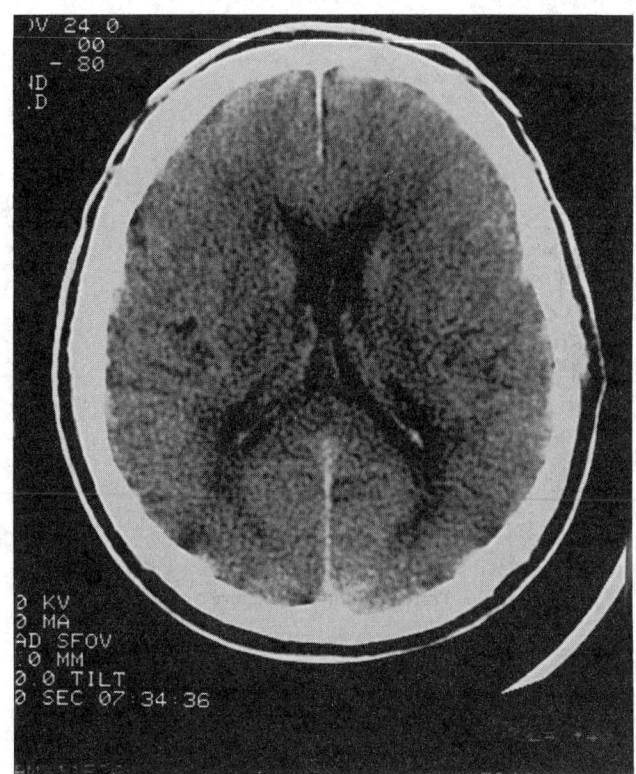
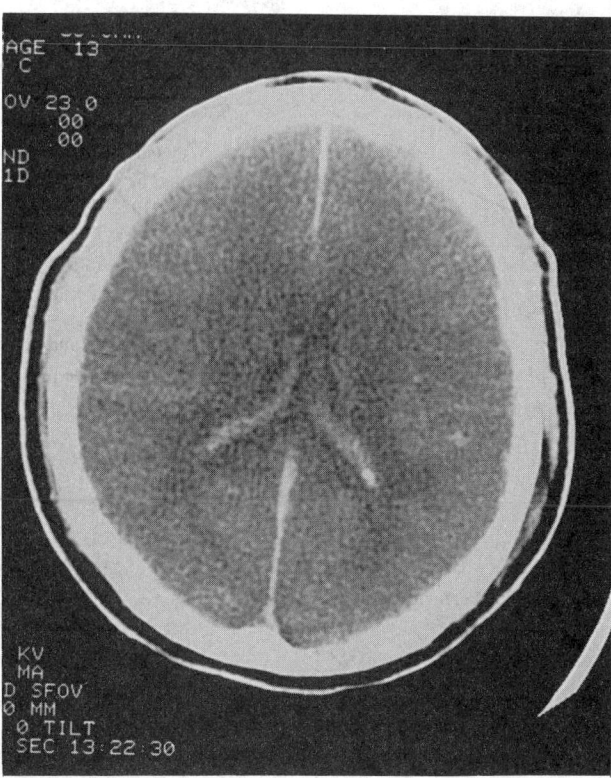

FIG. 2. CT scans of the head in a patient with pneumococcal meningitis. **(A)** CT scan on presentation revealing moderate cortical atrophy; **(B)** CT scan 3 days later revealing diffuse swelling of the cerebral hemispheres bilaterally with effacement of the ventricular system.

nique. Based on the low sensitivity of the CSF VDRL and until further studies demonstrate the usefulness of rapid diagnostic techniques, the diagnosis of neurosyphilis is based on elevated CSF concentrations of white blood cells and/or protein in the appropriate clinical and serologic setting.

Borrelia burgdorferi. Typical CSF changes in patients with Lyme meningitis are a pleocytosis (usually fewer than 500 cells/mm³, but up to 3500 cells/mm³), with more than 90 percent lymphocytes in 75 percent of cases[117]; plasma cells may also be present. There is usually an elevated CSF protein (up to 620 mg/dl) and a normal CSF glucose, although the glucose can be low in patients with illness of long duration. Oligoclonal banding may be present, with the bands reactive to *B. burgdorferi* antigens.

The best currently available laboratory test for the diagnosis of Lyme disease is demonstration of specific serum antibody to *B. burgdorferi*, in which a positive test in a patient with a compatible neurologic abnormality is strong evidence for the diagnosis.[117,280] However, these tests are not standardized, and there is marked variability between laboratories.[281] Most laboratories now use the ELISA with sonicated *B. burgdorferi* as the antigen, although others still utilize the immunofluorescence technique. By the time most patients develop subacute disseminated (i.e., stage II) disease, they have elevated serum concentrations of IgG antibody to *B. burgdorferi*. False-positive reactions have been reported in patients with rheumatoid arthritis, Rocky Mountain spotted fever, infectious mononucleosis, tuberculous meningitis, leptospirosis, yaws, syphilis, and relapsing fever,[117] although high titers of cross-reacting IgG antibodies have only been detected in patients with syphilis or relapsing fever. False-negative results may be obtained from an unreliable assay, early infection, or early antibiotic use that may blunt the normal humoral immune response. Specific antibody against *B. burgdorferi* also appears in CSF and calculation of a specific

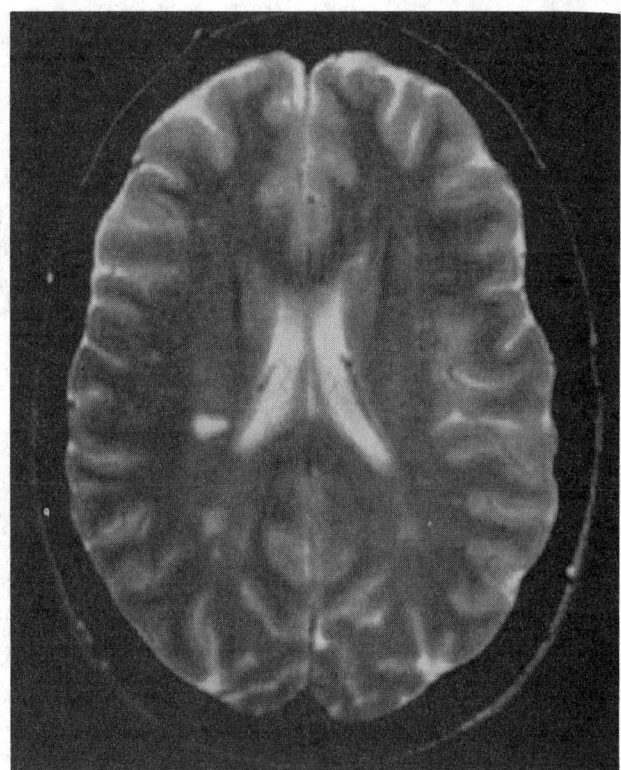

FIG. 3. T2-weighted MRI scan in a patient with Lyme disease revealing areas of increased signal intensity in the cerebral white matter.

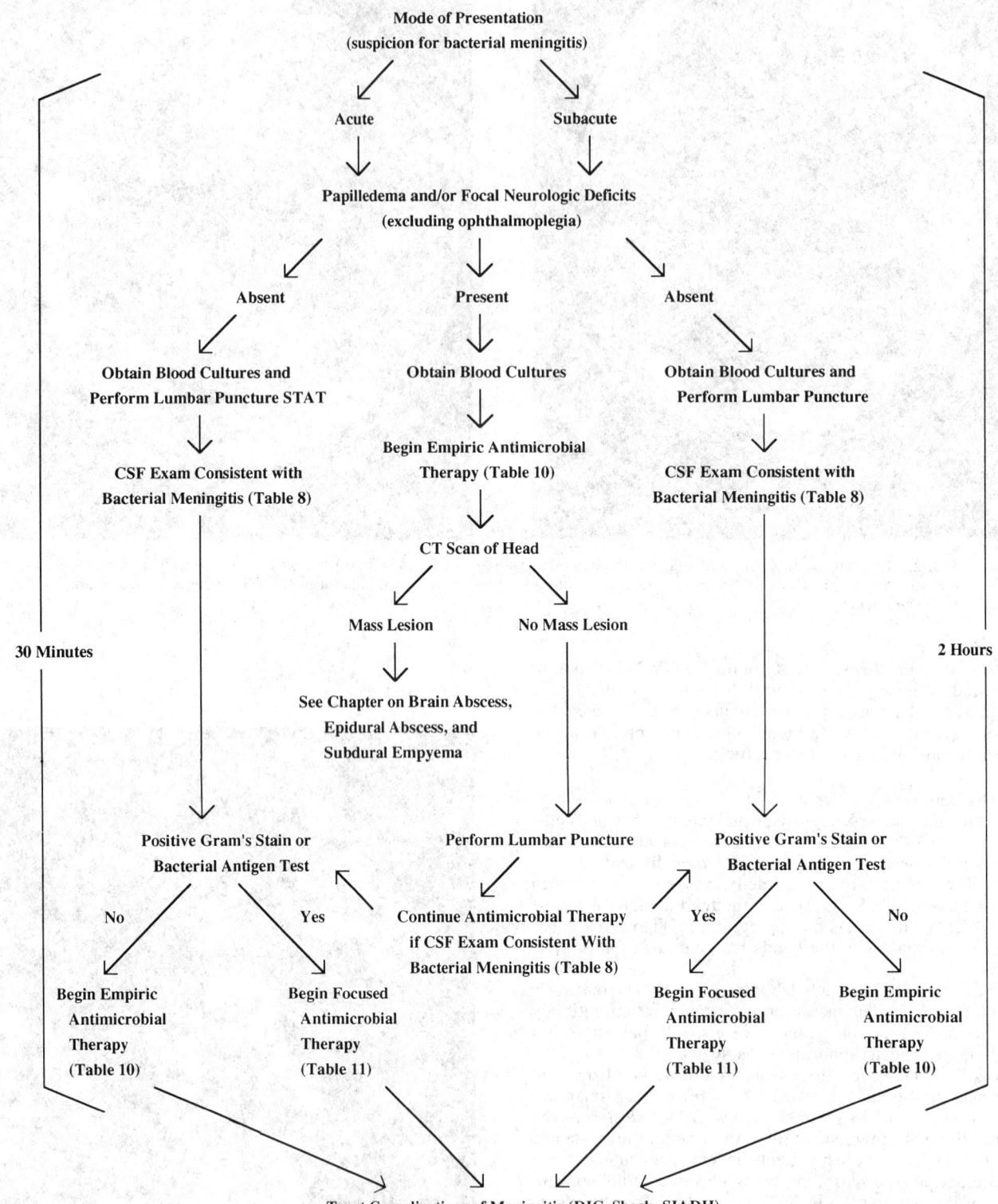

FIG. 4. Algorithm for the initial management of the patient with meningitis.

antibody/IgG index for serum and CSF may indicate intrathecal antibody synthesis.[117] The technique of PCR on CSF samples has also been successfully used to identify *B. burgdorferi* DNA in patients with Lyme neuroborreliosis (see Ch. 219).[282,283]

Radiologic studies may also be useful in patients with CNS manifestations of Lyme disease. Computed tomography has shown both enhancing and nonenhancing low-density lesions, mass effect, and cerebral demyelination. Magnetic resonance imaging may reveal punctate hyperresonant areas, without mass effect, within the cerebral white matter (Fig. 3).

Protozoal and Helminthic Meningitis

Amebae. The CSF formula in patients with the acute form of primary amebic meningoencephalitis reveals a neutrophilic pleocytosis, low glucose, elevated protein, and red blood cells.[121,122] The Gram stain is always negative. However, examination of fresh, warm specimens of CSF can reveal the ameboid movements of the motile trophozoites.[284] After death, trophozoites can be demonstrated by light or electron microscopy of brain tissue.

In patients with the subacute or chronic form of the illness, there is a less florid CSF inflammatory response with a predominant mononuclear leukocytosis. The CSF protein concentration is elevated, and the glucose is often normal or slightly reduced. Because amebae are not found in CSF, the diagnosis usually requires examination of a biopsy or necropsy specimen revealing the characteristic cysts. The value of serologic tests is variable.[121] Serum immunofluorescence, amebic immobilization titers, and complement-fixing antibodies support the diagnosis, although demonstration of rising titers are necessary to establish the diagnosis since some normal persons have circulating antibodies.

Angiostrongylus cantonensis. The combination of history of ingestion of suspected food, moderate to high peripheral eosinophilia, and CSF eosinophilia leads to the suspicion of angiostrongyloidiasis.[121] The CSF leukocytosis is moderate, with 16–72 percent eosinophils and increased protein concentration; larvae are occasionally found in CSF.

INITIAL MANAGEMENT OF THE PATIENT WITH ACUTE MENINGITIS

The initial management of a patient with presumed bacterial meningitis includes performance of a lumbar puncture to determine whether the CSF formula is consistent with that diagnosis (Fig. 4).[150,262,263,285,286] If purulent meningitis is present, empiric antimicrobial therapy should be instituted based on results of Gram staining or rapid bacterial antigen tests. However, if no etiologic agent can be identified by these means or if there is a delay (i.e., longer than 30 minutes) in performance of the lumbar puncture, empiric antimicrobial therapy should be instituted based on the patient's age and underlying disease status. In most patients, antimicrobial therapy should be ordered upon initial clinical impression; in critically ill patients, the first dose may even precede lumbar puncture. In patients who present with a focal neurologic examination or who have papilledema, but in whom bacterial meningitis is suspected, a CT scan of the head should be performed prior to lumbar puncture to rule out the presence of an intracranial mass lesion because of the potential risk of herniation[264]; the true incidence of this problem is unclear but has been suggested to be less than 1.2 percent in patients with papilledema and about 12 percent in patients without papilledema but with elevated intracranial pressure. However, the time involved in waiting for a CT scan significantly delays initiation of antimicrobial therapy, with the potential for increased morbidity and mortality in patients with bacterial meningitis. Therefore, emergent empiric antimicrobial therapy should be initiated before sending the patient to the CT scanner. Although

TABLE 10. Empiric Therapy of Purulent Meningitis[a]

Predisposing Factor	Antimicrobial Therapy
Age	
0–4 weeks	Ampicillin plus cefotaxime; or ampicillin plus an aminoglycoside
4–12 weeks	Ampicillin plus a third-generation cephalosporin[b]
3 months to 18 years	Third-generation cephalosporin[b]; or ampicillin plus chloramphenicol
18–50 years	Third-generation cephalosporin[b] ± ampicillin[c]
>50 years	Ampicillin plus a third-generation cephalosporin[b]
Immunocompromised state	Vancomycin plus ampicillin plus ceftazidime
Basilar skull fracture	Third-generation cephalosporin[b]
Head trauma; postneurosurgery	Vancomycin plus ceftazidime
Cerebrospinal fluid shunt	Vancomycin plus ceftazidime

[a] vancomycin should be added to empiric therapeutic regimens when highly penicillin- or cephalosporin-resistant strains of *Streptococcus pneumoniae* are suspected; see text for details.
[b] cefotaxime or ceftriaxone.
[c] See text for details.

CSF cultures may be sterile after initiation of antimicrobial therapy, pretreatment blood cultures and the CSF formula, Gram stain, and/or bacterial antigen tests will likely provide evidence for or against a diagnosis of bacterial meningitis. In one retrospective review of 177 patients (39 of whom had received prior antimicrobial therapy) with CSF culture-proven bacterial meningitis,[287] the combination of blood culture, CSF Gram strain, and/or latex agglutination identified the causative bacterium in 92 percent of patients. Our choices of empiric antimicrobial therapy based on age and underlying disease status of the patient are shown in Table 10. Once the infecting meningeal pathogen is isolated and susceptibility testing known, antimicrobial therapy can be modified for optimal treatment (Table 11). Recommended dosages of antimicrobial agents in adults for infections of the CNS are shown in Table 12 and for neonates, infants, and children in Table 13.

In addition, certain patients should receive adjunctive dexamethasone therapy when presenting with suspected or proven bacterial meningitis (see Adjunctive Therapy, below, for complete details on adjunctive therapies in bacterial meningitis). Currently, the data support the routine use of adjunctive dexamethasone therapy (0.15 mg/kg every 6 hours for 4 days) in infants and children with meningitis caused by *H. influenzae* type b.[288] In adults or in patients with meningitis caused by other bacteria, dexamethasone is not routinely recommended, although some authors recommend their use in all patients with presumed bacterial meningitis.[152] Patients with severely impaired mental status, cerebral edema, or markedly elevated intracranial pressure may benefit most from adjunctive dexamethasone; we recommend its use in this clinical situation. When adjunctive dexamethasone is to be given, administration just before or concomitant with the first dose of an antimicrobial agent is optimal to obtain maximal attenuation of the subarachnoid space inflammatory response.

ANTIMICROBIAL THERAPY

Viral Meningitis

Specific antiviral chemotherapy for the enteroviruses is not currently available; treatment is supportive. A number of drugs have been developed with efficacy in vitro and in animal models of enteroviral infection, but have not yet reached clinical trials.[2] One of these drugs, disoxaril, protects mice from developing meningoencephalitis due to echoviruses and has also been shown to cure mice of chronic enteroviral meningitis; oral administration has also been shown to reduce the incidence of paralysis due to echovirus 9. No specific antiviral therapy exists for the arboviruses, mumps virus, or lymphocytic choriomeningitis virus.

Recovery of patients with herpes simplex virus type 2 menin-

TABLE 11. Specific Antimicrobial Therapy of Acute Meningitis

Microorganism	Standard Therapy	Alternative Therapies
Bacteria		
Haemophilus influenzae		
β-Lactamase negative	Ampicillin	Third-generation cephalosporin[a]; chloramphenicol; aztreonam
β-Lactamase positive	Third-generation cephalosporin[a]	Chloramphenicol; aztreonam; fluoroquinolone
Neisseria meningitidis	Penicillin G or ampicillin	Third-generation cephalosporin[a]; chloramphenicol
Streptococcus pneumoniae		
Penicillin MIC < 0.1 μg/ml	Penicillin G or ampicillin	Third-generation cephalosporin[a]; chloramphenicol; vancomycin
Penicillin MIC 0.1–1.0 μg/ml	Third-generation cephalosporin[a]	Vancomycin; imipenem[b]
Penicillin MIC ≥ 2.0 μg/ml	Vancomycin[c]	Imipenem[b]; meropenem[d]
Enterobacteriaceae	Third-generation cephalosporin[a]	Aztreonam; fluoroquinolone; trimethoprim-sulfamethoxazole
Pseudomonas aeruginosa	Ceftazidime[e]	Aztreonam[e], fluoroquinolone[e]
Listeria monocytogenes	Ampicillin or penicillin G[e]	Trimethoprim-sulfamethoxazole
Streptococcus agalactiae	Ampicillin or penicillin G[e]	Third-generation cephalosporin[a]; vancomycin
Staphylococcus aureus		
Methicillin-sensitive	Nafcillin or oxacillin	Vancomycin
Methicillin-resistant	Vancomycin	
Staphylococcus epidermidis	Vancomycin[c]	
Spirochetes		
Treponema pallidum	Penicillin G	Doxycycline[f]; ceftriaxone[f]
Borrelia burgdorferi	Third generation cephalosporin[a]	Penicillin G; doxycycline
Protozoa/helminths		
Naegleria fowleri	Amphotericin B[g] plus rifampin plus doxycycline	

[a] Cefotaxime or ceftriaxone.
[b] Use is associated with an increased incidence of seizures.
[c] Addition of rifampin should be considered.
[d] Currently under study in patients with pneumococcal meningitis.
[e] Addition of an aminoglycoside should be considered.
[f] Value of these antimicrobial agents has not been established.
[g] Intravenous and intraventricular administration.

TABLE 12. Recommended Dosages of Antimicrobial Agents for Meningitis in Adults with Normal Renal and Hepatic Function[a]

Antimicrobial Agent	Total Daily Dose	Dosing Interval (Hours)
Amikacin[b]	15 mg/kg	8
Ampicillin	12 g	4
Aztreonam	6–8 g	6–8
Cefotaxime	8–12 g	4–6
Ceftazidime	6 g	8
Ceftriaxone	4 g	12–24
Chloramphenicol[c]	4–6 g	6
Ciprofloxacin	800 mg	12
Doxycycline	200–400 mg	12
Gentamicin[b]	3–5 mg/kg	8
Imipenem	2 g	6
Nafcillin	9–12 g	4
Oxacillin	9–12 g	4
Penicillin G	24 Million units	4
Rifampin[d]	600 mg	24
Tobramycin[b]	3–5 mg/kg	8
Trimethoprim-sulfamethoxazole[e]	20 mg/kg	12
Vancomycin[b,f]	2–3 g	8–12

[a] Unless indicated, therapy is administered intravenously.
[b] Need to monitor peak and trough serum concentrations.
[c] Higher dose recommended for pneumococcal meningitis.
[d] Oral administration.
[e] Dosage based on trimethoprim component.
[f] May need to monitor CSF concentrations in severely ill patients.

gitis is usually complete without neurologic sequelae. It is not clear whether antiviral treatment alters the course of mild meningitis. However, treatment with acyclovir is generally indicated for primary genital herpes infection (see Ch. 115).[26]

Specific antiretroviral therapy (e.g., zidovudine, didanosine, dicalcitrine) is not indicated for the aseptic meningitis of acute HIV infection, although later neurologic involvement may respond to therapy and should be administered to patients with absolute CD4 lymphocyte counts below 500/mm^3 (see Ch. 104).[289]

Bacterial Meningitis

Principles of Therapy. Many factors influence the choice of an antimicrobial agent in the therapy of bacterial meningitis. Utilization of animal models of infection have permitted quantitation of the relative penetration of drug into CSF, the effects of meningitis on this entry parameter, and determination of the relative bactericidal efficacy (defined as the rate of bacterial eradication) within purulent CSF.[290]

The first factor relates to penetration of the antimicrobial agent into CSF, which depends, to a great extent, on the status of the BBB. For example, β-lactam antibiotics such as penicillin penetrate into CSF poorly (about 0.5–2.0 percent of peak serum concentrations) when the BBB is normal.[150,285,290] In the presence of meningeal inflammation, CSF penetration of the antibiotic is enhanced due to increased permeability across the BBB, perhaps as a result of separation of intercellular tight junctions and increased numbers of pinocytotic vesicles in cerebral microvascular endothelial cells.[167] Antimicrobial entry decreases as inflammation subsides, indicating that maximal parenteral doses of antimicrobial agents should be continued throughout the course of therapy to maintain adequate CSF concentrations. Antibiotic entry into CSF is also enhanced by drugs with a high lipid solubility, low molecular weight, low degree of protein binding in serum, and low degree of ionization at physiologic pH.

The second factor is the bactericidal activity of the antimicrobial agent within purulent CSF.[150,285,290] Due to the accumulation of lactate in CSF during bacterial meningitis, the pH of CSF is decreased, thereby inhibiting the bactericidal activity of the aminoglycosides; this has likely contributed to the poor response observed with the aminoglycosides in the therapy of meningitis in experimental animal models and in patients. Elevated CSF protein concentrations may decrease the efficacy of antimicrobial agents that are highly protein bound because free drug is needed for the antibacterial effect. Drug that penetrates

TABLE 13. Recommended Dosages of Antimicrobial Agents for Meningitis in Neonates, Infants, and Children with Normal Renal and Hepatic Function[a]

Antimicrobial Agent	Total Daily Dose (Dosing Interval in Hours)		
	Neonates (0–7 days)[b]	Neonates (8–28 days)[b]	Infants and Children
Amikacin[c]	15–20 mg/kg (12)	20–30 mg/kg (8)	20–30 mg/kg (8)
Ampicillin	100–150 mg/kg (8–12)	150–200 mg/kg (6–8)	200–300 mg/kg (6)
Cefotaxime	100 mg/kg (12)	150–200 mg/kg (6–8)	200 mg/kg (6–8)
Ceftazidime	60 mg/kg (12)	90 mg/kg (8)	125–150 mg/kg (8)
Ceftriaxone	—	—	80–100 mg/kg (12–24)
Chloramphenicol	25 mg/kg (24)	50 mg/kg (12–24)	75–100 mg/kg (6)
Gentamicin[c]	5 mg/kg (12)	7.5 mg/kg (8)	7.5 mg/kg (8)
Nafcillin	100–150 mg/kg (8–12)	150–200 mg/kg (6–8)	200 mg/kg (6)
Penicillin G	0.1–0.15 mU/kg (8–12)	0.15–0.2 mU/kg (6–8)	0.25 mU/kg (4–6)
Rifampin[d,e]	—	—	10–20 mg/kg (12–24)
Tobramycin[c]	5 mg/kg (12)	7.5 mg/kg (8)	7.5 mg/kg (8)
Trimethoprim-sulfamethoxazole[f]	—	—	10 mg/kg (12)
Vancomycin[c]	20 mg/kg (12)	30–40 mg/kg (8)	50–60 mg/kg (6)

[a] Unless indicated, therapy is administered intravenously.
[b] Smaller dosages and longer intervals of administration may be advisable for very low birth weight neonates (<2000 g).
[c] Need to monitor peak and trough serum concentrations.
[d] Oral administration.
[e] Maximum daily dosage of 600 mg.
[f] Dosage based on trimethoprim component.

the CSF may be removed by an active transport system that exists in the choroid plexus (as for the penicillins and cephalosporins), or it may be converted to an inactive metabolite. In addition, other drugs may influence antibiotic activity within purulent CSF. In experimental animal models of meningitis, antagonism has been shown when a bactericidal agent is coadministered with a bacteriostatic antibiotic (e.g., chloramphenicol plus gentamicin). However, in other instances the combination of antibiotics may be synergistic as in the combination of penicillin or ampicillin with gentamicin in *L. monocytogenes* meningitis, and ampicillin plus gentamicin against *S. agalactiae*.

A final factor concerns the need for bactericidal activity in CSF for optimal therapy, because bacterial meningitis represents an infection in an area of impaired host defense. Multiple studies in experimental animal models have shown that rapid bacterial killing is observed in vivo only when CSF concentrations of β-lactams or aminoglycosides exceed the minimal bactericidal concentration (MBC) by about 10- to 20-fold.[291,292] The importance of this rapid bacterial killing has also been examined in patients with bacterial meningitis. One study that compared the outcome in infants and children with bacterial meningitis who had negative or positive CSF cultures 18–36 hours after initiation of antimicrobial therapy revealed an increased rate of neurologic complications (i.e., ataxia, hemiparesis, developmental delay, moderate to severe hearing impairment) in the group in whom the causative organism could still be recovered after this time interval.[293]

Haemophilus influenzae. Therapy of meningitis caused by *H. influenzae* type b has been markedly altered by the emergence of β-lactamase–producing strains. These strains accounted for approximately 24 percent of all CSF isolates in the United States based on a surveillance study of 27 states from 1978 through 1981.[42] A subsequent surveillance study of five states and Los Angeles county in 1986 found the incidence of these β-lactamase–producing strains to be 32 percent.[43] Resistance of *H. influenzae* to chloramphenicol has also been described, although more commonly from areas such as Spain (more than 50 percent of isolates)[294,295] than the United States (less than 1 percent of isolates).[296] Even in patients with chloramphenicol-sensitive isolates, a recent prospective study found chloramphenicol to be bacteriologically and clinically inferior to ampicillin, ceftriaxone, or cefotaxime in the therapy of childhood bacterial meningitis caused predominantly by *H. influenzae* type b.[297] Furthermore, the use of chloramphenicol can be

problematic because of its unpredictable metabolism in young infants and its pharmacologic interactions with other concomitantly administered drugs such as phenobarbital, rifampin, phenytoin, and acetaminophen, which increase the likelihood of toxicity.[298] Several studies have documented similar efficacy of the third-generation cephalosporins (particularly cefotaxime or ceftriaxone) to the combination of ampicillin plus chloramphenicol for bacterial meningitis.[299,300] Based on these findings, the American Academy of Pediatrics has recommended use of the third-generation cephalosporin as empiric antimicrobial therapy for children with bacterial meningitis.[301]

Despite initial studies suggesting that cefuroxime, a second-generation cephalosporins, was as efficacious as the combination of ampicillin plus chloramphenicol for childhood bacterial meningitis,[302] this has recently been questioned. In one study comparing cefuroxime to ceftriaxone, both regimens were efficacious for the treatment of bacterial meningitis, although some patients did not respond as satisfactorily to cefuroxime with slower rates of CSF sterilization (0 vs. 9 percent of CSF cultures positive at 24 hours in patients treated with cefuroxime; $p < 0.001$) and a higher incidence of hearing impairment (18 vs. 11 percent).[303] Another recent prospective randomized study comparing ceftriaxone to cefuroxime for the treatment of childhood bacterial meningitis documented a more rapid CSF sterilization (2 vs. 12 percent of CSF cultures positive at 18–36 hours; $p = 0.11$) and a lower incidence of hearing impairment (4 vs. 17 percent; $p = 0.05$) in the patients receiving ceftriaxone.[304] Furthermore, there have been reports of delayed CSF sterilization in patients receiving cefuroxime for *H. influenzae* meningitis,[302] as well as the development of *H. influenzae* meningitis in patients receiving cefuroxime for nonmeningeal *H. influenzae* disease.[305] The mechanism of this diminished response, as suggested in a recent report analyzing a nontypable β-lactamase–negative strain of *H. influenzae* that was relatively resistant to cefuroxime,[306] may be a result of reduced binding of cefuroxime to penicillin-binding proteins 4 and 5. Therefore, cefuroxime cannot be recommended as a first-line drug for the therapy of bacterial meningitis. In addition, there have been single case reports of delayed CSF sterilization in patients with *H. influenzae* meningitis treated with ceftizoxime or ceftazidime.[307] However, resistance of *H. influenzae* to the third-generation cephalosporins and fluoroquinolones in vitro has not been described to date.[308]

Neisseria meningitidis. Penicillin G and ampicillin are the antimicrobial agents of choice for meningitis caused by *N. men-*

ingitidis. However, these recommendations may change in future years. Meningococcal strains have recently been reported from several areas (particularly Spain) that are relatively resistant to penicillin G with a minimal inhibitory concentration (MIC) range of 0.1–1.0 μg/ml.[309–311] For example, of 3264 strains of *N. meningitidis* isolated from blood and CSF from Spain during 1978–1985,[312] only one resistant isolate was observed, whereas 9 of 168 (5 percent) invasive isolates relatively resistant to penicillin G were found in the first 6 months of 1986; this reached 20 percent in 1989. This resistance has been reported to be mediated by a reduced affinity of the antibiotic for penicillin-binding proteins 2 and 3.[312,313] The clinical significance of these isolates is unclear, however, because patients with meningitis caused by these organisms have recovered with standard penicillin therapy. If an alternative agent is chosen for therapy of meningococcal meningitis caused by these relatively resistant strains, ceftriaxone is recommended based on in vitro susceptibility data.[314] High-level meningococcal resistance to penicillin G (MIC 250 μg/ml or higher) has also been documented for several isolates; the mechanism is secondary to production of β-lactamases.[315]

Streptococcus pneumoniae. The therapy of meningitis caused by the *Pneumococcus* has been recently modified based on current pneumococcal susceptibility patterns. In the past, pneumococci were uniformly susceptible to penicillin with MICs of 0.06 μg/ml or less. Numerous reports from throughout the world have now documented strains of pneumococci that are relatively resistant to penicillin (MIC range of 0.1–1.0 μg/ml) as well as strains that are highly resistant to penicillin (MIC of 2.0 μg/ml or higher).[150,316–321] The mechanism of this resistance is due to alterations in the structure and molecular size of penicillin-binding proteins. Resistance has been reported in several different pneumococcal serotypes, although the overwhelming majority of resistant strains are serotypes 6, 14, 19, and 23.[322] Most of the multiresistant strains isolated in the United States have disseminated from a multiresistant serotype 23F clone of *S. pneumoniae* that was isolated in Spain as early as 1978.[323]

Based on these trends and because sufficient CSF concentrations of penicillin are difficult to achieve with standard high parenteral dosages (initial CSF penicillin concentrations of approximately 1 μg/ml, with a significantly decreased CSF concentration on subsequent days), penicillin can no longer be recommended as empiric antimicrobial therapy when *S. pneumoniae* is considered a likely infecting pathogen in patients with purulent meningitis. In areas of the world in which relatively resistant strains are found, a third-generation cephalosporin (ceftriaxone or cefotaxime) should be used[150,285,286,324,325]; vancomycin should be utilized when highly resistant strains are suspected or isolated. In one review of cases of penicillin-resistant pneumococcal meningitis from Spain,[326] it was suggested that high-dose cefotaxime (250–350 mg/kg/day) was useful (seven cures, one relapse, and one death) against strains with penicillin MBCs of 4 μg/ml or less and cefotaxime MBCs of 2 μg/ml or less. Of great concern is the emergence of pneumococcal resistance to the third-generation cephalosporins in the United States (MIC range of 4–32 μg/ml),[327–331] and that cefotaxime MICs have been increasing in South Africa.[332] Of three patients in the United States with pneumococcal strains that were highly resistant to the third-generation cephalosporins, two responded to initial antimicrobial therapy with vancomycin plus chloramphenicol, followed by chloramphenicol alone.[329] However, clinical failures with chloramphenicol have been reported in patients with penicillin-resistant isolates, likely due to the poor bactericidal activity of chloramphenicol against these strains; 20 of 25 children had an unsatisfactory outcome (i.e., death, serious neurologic deficit, poor clinical response) in one study.[333] These data indicate the need to perform susceptibility testing of all pneumococcal isolates, at which time antimicrobial therapy can be modified for optimal treatment (Table 11).

Of additional concern is the recent report of 11 consecutive patients, with CSF culture-proven pneumococcal meningitis caused by relatively resistant strains, who were treated with intravenous vancomycin.[334] All patients improved, and 10 were eventually cured of their infection, but 4 patients experienced a therapeutic failure with vancomycin, necessitating a change in therapy. Reasons for failure may have included variability in serum vancomycin concentrations and/or impaired CSF vancomycin penetration as a result of adjunctive dexamethasone administration. Nevertheless, these data indicate the need for careful monitoring, perhaps even measurement of CSF vancomycin concentrations, of adult patients receiving vancomycin therapy for pneumococcal meningitis. The utility of intrathecal or intraventricular doses of vancomycin remains a reasonable possibility for treatment of unresponsive cases. Some investigators have recommended the addition of rifampin to vancomycin for therapy of meningitis caused by highly resistant pneumococcal strains, although there are no firm data to support this recommendation. Meropenem, a new carbapenem with less proconvulsive activity than imipenem, is currently under study in patients with pneumococcal meningitis; initial results appear promising.[335]

Listeria monocytogenes. Despite their broad range of in vitro activity, the third-generation cephalosporins are inactive in meningitis caused by *L. monocytogenes.* For patients with *Listeria* meningitis, therapy should consist of ampicillin or penicillin G[75,76,78,79]; the addition of an aminoglycoside should be considered in proven infection due to documented in vitro synergy and enhanced killing in vivo as documented in a variety of animal models of *Listeria* infection. Nevertheless, it is important to emphasize that a controlled clinical trial comparing ampicillin to ampicillin plus gentamicin has never been performed in humans with listeriosis. An alternative agent in the penicillin-allergic patient is trimethoprim-sulfamethoxazole,[336] which is bactericidal against *Listeria* in vitro. Although chloramphenicol has varying activity against *Listeria* in vitro, its use has been associated with an unacceptably high failure rate in patients with *Listeria* meningitis. Vancomycin is also unsatisfactory for *Listeria* meningitis despite favorable in vitro susceptibility results. However, intraventricular administration of vancomycin was successful in one case of recurrent *L. monocytogenes* meningitis.[337] Rifampin is bacteriostatic against *L. monocytogenes* in vitro and was no better than penicillin alone when evaluated in the experimental rabbit model of meningitis.[338] Meropenem is active in vitro and in experimental animal models of *L. monocytogenes* meningitis[339] and may be a useful alternative in the future.

Streptococcus agalactiae. Standard therapy for neonatal meningitis caused by the group B *Streptococcus* is the combination of ampicillin plus an aminoglycoside,[86] which is also recommended for adult patients with meningitis caused by this organism[92]; this combination is recommended due to documented in vitro synergy and recent reports detailing the presence of penicillin-tolerant strains. Alternative agents are the third-generation cephalosporins; vancomycin is reserved for penicillin-allergic patients.

Aerobic Gram-Negative Bacilli. The treatment of bacterial meningitis caused by enteric gram-negative bacilli has been revolutionized by the availability of the third-generation cephalosporins.[340,341] Previous mortality rates with standard regimens (usually an aminoglycoside with or without chloramphenicol) ranged from 40–90 percent vs. cure rates of 78–94 percent with the third-generation cephalosporins.[342,343] Cefotaxime is the preferred over ceftriaxone as the third-generation cephalosporin for use in neonates because it has been used more extensively and is not excreted in the bile, which may have an inhibitory effect on the bacterial flora of the intestinal tract[262]; ceftriaxone also has increased protein binding. One particular third-generation cephalosporin, ceftazidime, has enhanced in vitro activity against *P. aeruginosa* and resulted in the cure of 19 of 24 patients in one study of *P. aeruginosa* meningitis when administered alone or in combination with an aminoglycoside.[344] In another study of 10 pediatric patients with *Pseudomonas* meningitis, 7 patients were cured clinically and 9 were cured bacteriologically when treated with ceftazidime-containing regimens.[345] Concomitant intrathecal or intraventricular aminoglycoside therapy should be considered in patients with gram-negative meningitis who are not responding to conventional parenteral therapy. However, this mode of administration is rarely needed at present and was associated with a higher mortality rate than systemic therapy alone in infants with gram-negative meningitis and ventriculitis.[346]

Several other antimicrobial agents have been used in patients with meningitis caused by aerobic gram-negative bacilli. Aztreonam attains excellent CSF concentrations and has been shown to be efficacious in the therapy of gram-negative meningitis.[347] Imipenem was found to be efficacious in one case of *Acinetobacter* meningitis[348] and in bacterial eradication from CSF in a recent study of 21 children with bacterial meningitis (most cases caused by *H. influenzae* type b and *N. meningitidis*),[349] although a high rate of seizure activity (33 percent) limits its usefulness in the therapy of bacterial meningitis. High-dose meropenem (2 g every 8 hours) given for 18 weeks was successful in a lymphoma patient with *P. aeruginosa* meningitis who had failed therapy with ceftazidime plus gentamicin.[350] Newer cephalosporins (e.g., cefepime, cefpirome) are currently under investigation in clinical trials of meningitis patients. The fluoroquinolones (e.g., ciprofloxacin, pefloxacin) have been used successfully in some patients with gram-negative meningitis.[351] The limited published literature on the use of the fluoroquinolones suggests that the primary area of usefulness of these agents is for therapy of multidrug-resistant gram-negative organisms (e.g., *P. aeruginosa*) or when the response to conventional β-lactam therapy is slow (e.g., meningitis caused by *Salmonella* spp.). The fluoroquinolones are relatively contraindicated in infants and children, the age groups accounting for the majority of cases of bacterial meningitis, because of concerns of cartilage damage. These agents should never be used as first-line empiric therapy in patients with meningitis of unknown etiology because of their poor in vitro activity against pneumococci and *L. monocytogenes*.

Staphylococci. *Staphylococcus aureus* should be treated with nafcillin or oxacillin,[101] with vancomycin reserved for patients allergic to penicillin or when methicillin-resistant organisms are suspected or isolated. The addition of rifampin should be considered in patients not responding to therapy. Meningitis caused by coagulase-negative staphylococci, the most commonly encountered organisms in CSF shunt infections, should be treated with vancomycin; rifampin should be added if the patient fails to improve.[102] Removal of the shunt is often necessary to optimize therapy (see below).

CSF Shunt Infections. Numerous methods of treating CSF shunt infections have been reported, although no randomized, prospective studies have been performed.[102,240] In suspected infection, CSF should be removed from the shunt via the reservoir and sent for cell count, glucose, protein, Gram stain, and culture. Antimicrobial therapy should be initiated prior to culture results if meningeal inflammation is present (Table 10); therapy can then be modified based on culture results (Table 11). Occasionally, direct instillation of antimicrobial agents into the ventricles (i.e., through an external ventriculostomy or shunt reservoir) is necessary in patients with infections that are difficult to eradicate or when the patient is unable to undergo the surgical components of therapy (see below).[240] Vancomycin has been directly instilled into the ventricles to overcome the relatively

meager CSF penetration after intravenous administration; daily dosages have ranged from 4–10 mg. Gentamicin (1–2 mg daily for infants and children and 4–8 mg daily for adults) can be utilized, always in combination with a parenteral agent (e.g., a β-lactam), for infections caused by susceptible gram-negative organisms. Teicoplanin, a new glycopeptide antimicrobial agent, was also found to be successful following intraventricular administration in seven patients with staphylococcal neurosurgical shunt infection.[352] Empiric dosing should initially be used, with subsequent dosage adjustments based on CSF antimicrobial concentrations.

In addition, patients with CSF shunt infections should undergo removal of all components of the infected shunt at the beginning of antimicrobial therapy, with an external ventriculostomy placed to clear the ventriculitis and monitor CSF findings.[102,240] The ability of many organisms to adhere to the prostheses and survive antimicrobial therapy precludes optimal treatment in situ. Furthermore, the propensity for the entire shunt to become contaminated when one portion becomes infected argues against partial revisions. With externalization, treatment success is usually greater than 90 percent.

Duration of Therapy. Traditionally the duration of antimicrobial therapy in patients with bacterial meningitis has been 10–14 days for cases of nonmeningococcal meningitis.[353,354] Several studies, however, comparing 7 with 10 days of treatment in infants and children with *H. influenzae* type b meningitis have documented that 7 days of therapy is safe and effective,[355,356] although therapy must be individualized and some patients may require longer courses. Meningococcal meningitis can be treated for 7 days with intravenous penicillin, and some authors have also suggested that 4 days of therapy are adequate[357]; this study requires confirmation, as only 50 patients were studied and no control group was included. A single dose, or even two to three doses, of long-acting penicillin or chloramphenicol has been used successfully in developing countries to treat meningococcal meningitis,[354] although this is not considered standard therapy. In adults with meningitis caused by enteric gram-negative bacilli, treatment regimens should be continued for 3 weeks due to the high rate of relapse in patients treated with shorter courses of therapy. Ten to 14 days is recommended for therapy of meningitis caused by *S. pneumoniae* and 14–21 days for *L. monocytogenes* and the group B *Streptococcus*.

Spirochetal Meningitis

Treponema pallidum. In syphilis patients with CSF abnormalities but without clinically apparent disease, the goals of therapy are to prevent progression to symptomatic disease and to ameliorate the laboratory abnormalities thought to indicate disease activity.[108] For patients with clinical neurosyphilis syndromes, the goal may be to reverse clinical symptoms and signs or to arrest disease progression. In patients with syphilitic meningitis whose clinical presentation is that of meningeal inflammation as a result of the acute inflammatory response, clinical findings, other than cranial nerve abnormalities, usually resolve without therapy. In patients with meningovascular syphilis, the prognosis following therapy is quite good, except perhaps in patients with larger clinically apparent neurologic deficits prior to therapy; therapy in this situation may halt progression and prevent further ischemic events caused by neurosyphilis.

The drug of choice for the treatment of neurosyphilis is penicillin G (Table 11), although considerable controversy remains as to the most appropriate total dose, formulation, and duration of therapy.[108,115] Therapy with benzathine penicillin (2.4 million units intramuscularly) does not reliably produce CSF penicillin concentrations above 0.018 μg/ml and should not be used for treatment of neurosyphilis. Furthermore, a small but poorly defined proportion of patients with syphilis treated with benzathine penicillin fail therapy, defined as persistent CSF abnormalities of clinically apparent neurosyphilis. However, many patients treated with benzathine penicillin resolve their CSF abnormalities and do not progress, suggesting that factors other than CSF concentrations of penicillin play a role in response to therapy.

The preferred antimicrobial regimen for therapy of CNS syphilis is intravenous aqueous crystalline penicillin G at a dose of 12–24 million units daily in divided doses every 4 hours for 10–14 days.[108] Alternatively, procaine penicillin, at a dose of 2.4 million units intramuscularly daily, plus probenecid (500 mg orally four times daily), both for 10–14 days can be utilized. Some experts also recommend follow-up therapy with 1 injection of benzathine penicillin G (2.4 million units intramuscularly), although there are no data to support this recommendation. No large studies have been performed to evaluate alternative antimicrobial agents for neurosyphilis. The tetracyclines, chloramphenicol, and ceftriaxone have all been described to be of potential clinical utility in the penicillin-allergic patient based on case reports, clinical experience, and extrapolations from experimental animal studies. One experimental study, however, suggested that ceftriaxone may not be adequate therapy for neurosyphilis.[358] Furthermore, a recent study of 43 HIV-infected patients with latent or neurosyphilis treated with ceftriaxone (1 or 2 g daily for 10–14 days) had a 23 percent failure rate,[359] similar to that seen in 13 HIV-infected patients with latent or neurosyphilis treated with benzathine penicillin (30 percent). Erythromycin is not recommended based on failures in erythromycin-treated patients. In HIV-infected patients with neurosyphilis, careful monitoring for response to therapy is needed.[114,360] Follow-up lumbar puncture should be performed every 6 months in all patients until the CSF changes have normalized. There have been several reports of failures in HIV-infected patients receiving standard therapy for neurosyphilis, probably because the patient's immunologic response has an important role in controlling the infection even in the presence of "adequate" antimicrobial therapy.

Borrelia burgdorferi.   Parenteral antimicrobial therapy is usually needed to treat the neurologic manifestations of Lyme disease, including meningitis (Table 11). Initial studies utilized high-dose (15–20 million units daily) intravenous penicillin G for 10–14 days,[117,280] although one author found the benefits limited to patients treated within 5 weeks of the onset of neurologic symptoms. The meningeal and systemic reactions tend to improve within days, whereas radicular pains and motor deficits improve over many weeks. Central nervous system abnormalities are arrested by treatment and may slowly improve, but some residual deficit is common. Some patients have also responded to treatment with intravenous doxycycline. A randomized trial comparing intravenous doxycycline (200 mg for 2 days, followed by 100 mg daily for 8 days) to intravenous penicillin G (20 million units daily for 10 days) found both treatments to be equally efficacious.[361] Patients who have failed to respond to intravenous penicillin have responded to therapy with intravenous cefotaxime, ceftriaxone, or chloramphenicol.[117] In one prospective randomized trial,[362] ceftriaxone was superior to penicillin in the therapy of late Lyme borreliosis. The current recommendation is to treat most patients with Lyme meningitis with intravenous ceftriaxone at a dosage of 2 g daily for 2–4 weeks[117,280]; the literature contains no agreement on the duration of therapy or on the minimal adequate dose of the antimicrobial. There is no evidence to support treatment durations for longer than 4 weeks. However, no regimen has proven to be universally effective. Although one report has indicated that high-dose oral doxycyline may produce inhibitory concentrations against *B. burgdorferi* in CSF,[363] parenteral regimens are generally necessary for CNS infection.

Protozoal and Helminthic Meningitis

Amebae.   Many antimicrobial agents, including amphotericin B, the tetracyclines, the imidazoles, qinghaosu, and rifam-

pin, have in vitro activity against free-living amebae[122]; phenothiazines are amebicidal only at high concentrations (100 μm). Amphotericin B is rapidly amebicidal against *N. fowleri* in vitro, but is much less active against *Acanthamoeba*. Only four patients reported in the literature have survived after therapy for primary amebic meningoencephalitis.[121,364,365] All received amphotericin B along with various other antimicrobial agents. The best documented survivor received amphotericin B and miconazole intravenously and intrathecally, rifampin, sulfizoxazole, and dexamethasone. However, no effective regimen has been established. Therapy with parenteral and intracisternal amphotericin B combined with rifampin and tetracycline has been suggested[122]; addition of experimental therapies such as phenothiazine or qinghaosu may also be justified, considering the extremely poor outcome in patients with primary amebic meningoencephalitis. Therapy is continued over 2–3 weeks if the clinical response is good and no complications occur.

Angiostrongylus cantonensis.   Symptomatic treatment for symptoms such as headache, nausea, and vomiting is indicated for eosinophilic meningitis caused by *A. cantonensis*. Most patients recover within 1–2 weeks.[121] The benzimidazoles have been tried in humans without definite benefit; thiabendazole cleared *A. cantonensis* from rats in one study.[129] Thiabendazole has been used in the early stages of migration of the larvae of *A. cantonensis*, but the drug fails as soon as the worm reaches the CNS.

ADJUNCTIVE THERAPY

Viral Meningitis

Because of the lack of effective antiviral therapy against the enteroviruses, other adjunctive measures have been employed in seriously ill patients with enteroviral meningitis. Since enteroviral clearance from the host is antibody mediated, exogenously administered antibody has been examined.[2] Administration of γ-globulin by multiple routes (including directly into the CNS) has led to stabilization or improvement of agammaglobulinemic patients with chronic enteroviral meningitis or meningoencephalitis. Neonates with overwhelming enteroviral sepsis and meningitis have received intravenous γ-globulin, maternal plasma, and exchange transfusions with occasional success. A trial is currently underway to compare outcome of enteroviral infection in neonates comparing standard therapy alone vs. standard therapy plus intravenous γ-globulin.

Specific hyperimmune globulin has been shown to reduce the incidence of orchitis in a single prospective controlled trial in patients with mumps,[2] but no benefit has been proven for neurologic syndromes. There have been anecdotal reports on the use of corticosteroids in patients with mumps encephalitis,[13] but no benefits have been documented.

Bacterial Meningitis

Anti-Inflammatory Agents.   Despite the availability of effective bactericidal antimicrobial agents in the therapy of bacterial meningitis, morbidity and mortality from this disorder remains unacceptably high. Because the subarachnoid space inflammatory response is a major factor contributing to morbidity and mortality, investigators have examined whether attenuation of this response would improve outcome in bacterial meningitis. As stated above (see Pathogenesis and Pathophysiology), generation of pneumococcal cell wall components in an experimental animal model of pneumococcal meningitis after treatment with bacteriolytic antibiotics may contribute to the inflammatory response in the subarachnoid space.[184,185] The inflammatory response induced by either live pneumococci or pneumococcal cell wall was reduced by agents (e.g., methylprednisolone, oxindanac) that inhibit the cyclooxygenase pathway of arachidonic acid metabolism, and there was a correlation between CSF concentrations of the arachidonic acid metabolite PGE$_2$ and CSF leukocytes.[366] In another study administration of the anti-inflammatory agent indomethacin decreased both the brain water content and CSF concentrations of PGE$_2$ during experimental pneumococcal meningitis, although intracranial pressure was not reduced.[367] In addition, the administration of either dexamethasone or oxindanac lessened the massive influx of serum albumin and other proteins of high and low molecular weight into the CSF during the early stages of experimental pneumococcal meningitis.[368]

Several corticosteroid agents have also been examined in experimental animal models of meningitis. Early studies revealed that methylprednisolone administration led to a significant reduction in the mass of leukocytes within the meninges of rabbits with pneumococcal meningitis.[369] Another study demonstrated that CSF outflow resistance was reduced by methylprednisolone therapy and to a greater extent than in untreated or penicillin-treated rabbits with pneumococcal meningitis.[207] In further studies that examined the effects of corticosteroids (methylprednisolone or dexamethasone) on brain water content, CSF pressure, and CSF lactate in rabbits with pneumococcal meningitis, it was found that both agents completely reversed the development of brain edema, but only dexamethasone led to a reduction in CSF pressure and lactate[208]; however, neither agent was superior to therapy with ampicillin alone in reducing cerebral edema or intracranial pressure, and no comparison was made between ampicillin alone and the combination of ampicillin plus corticosteroids, a comparison that would have been relevant to the potential clinical usefulness of adjunctive corticosteroid therapy in bacterial meningitis. A subsequent study did examine treatment with ceftriaxone vs. ceftriaxone plus dexamethasone in an experimental rabbit model of *H. influenzae* meningitis.[370] Although combination therapy consistently reduced the brain water content, CSF pressure, and CSF lactate to a greater degree than ceftriaxone alone, the differences were not statistically significant. The authors suggested, however, that adjunctive dexamethasone might be more beneficial if administered early, or even before antibiotic-induced bacterial lysis and release of microbial products. In a subsequent analysis using the experimental rabbit model of *H. influenzae* type b meningitis,[371] ceftriaxone administration led to a significant increase in CSF endotoxin concentration 2 hours after administration, which was followed by a rise in CSF TNF concentrations. Simultaneous administration of dexamethasone and ceftriaxone did not affect release of endotoxin into CSF, but markedly attenuated CSF concentrations of TNF measured 8 hours later. Adjunctive dexamethasone therapy also resulted in a significant decrease in CSF leukocytosis and a trend toward earlier improvement in CSF concentrations of glucose, lactate, and protein. These parameters improved without any apparent decrease in the rate of bacterial killing within the CSF in vivo.

On the basis of these observations, several clinical trials were undertaken in the late 1980s to determine the effects of adjunctive corticosteroids on outcome in patients with bacterial meningitis. The first study was a double-blind, placebo-controlled trial of adjunctive dexamethasone therapy in infants and children with bacterial meningitis.[372] The patients were treated with antibiotic (cefuroxime or ceftriaxone) with either dexamethasone or placebo. The patients who received antibiotic plus dexamethasone became afebrile sooner, had a more rapid normalization of CSF parameters (glucose, protein, and lactate), and were significantly less likely to acquire moderate to severe bilateral sensorineural hearing loss (15.5 vs. 3.3 percent). Concentrations of IL-1β, but not TNF-α, were significantly lower 18–36 hours later in patients receiving adjunctive dexamethasone therapy. However, these findings were significant only for patients with meningitis caused by *H. influenzae* type b, and the benefits in terms of morbidity (i.e., sensorineural hearing loss) were statistically significant only in patients receiving cefuroxime and not

ceftriaxone. This feature is important because cefuroxime has been recently shown, in a randomized prospective study of the therapy of childhood bacterial meningitis, to be inferior to ceftriaxone.[304] Four patients who received adjunctive dexamethasone developed gastrointestinal hemorrhage, two of whom required blood transfusions.

In a second trial from the same authors,[373] 31 infants and children with bacterial meningitis were treated with cefuroxime and dexamethasone, and 29 patients received dexamethasone alone. No statistically significant differences in neurologic abnormalities or hearing impairment were noted between the two groups at 6 weeks. However, when the data from these two studies were combined,[372,373] overall support for the benefit of adjunctive dexamethasone was suggested.

A third published trial, from Egypt, in children and adults with bacterial meningitis randomized patients to receive antibiotics (intramuscular ampicillin plus chloramphenicol) with or without adjunctive dexamethasone therapy.[374] The subgroup of patients with pneumococcal meningitis who received adjunctive dexamethasone had a significant reduction in mortality rate and overall neurologic sequelae. However, there were no significant differences between groups in time to afebrility or improvement in CSF parameters, there was no documentation of possible adverse effects, and an extraordinarily high percentage of patients presented in a comatose state. In fact, most patients (370 of 429) received inadequate therapy for 3–5 days prior to hospitalization. No differences in mortality were noted in patients with meningococcal or *H. influenzae* meningitis.

A fourth published trial from Costa Rica randomized infants and children with bacterial meningitis in a placebo-controlled, double-blind fashion to receive cefotaxime with either dexamethasone or placebo.[375] In this study the dexamethasone or placebo was administered 15–20 minutes before the first dose of cefotaxime in an attempt to attenuate maximally the potential bacteriolytic antibiotic-induced CSF inflammatory response. Twelve hours after initiation of therapy, meningeal inflammation and CSF concentrations of TNF-α and platelet-activating factor had decreased more rapidly in patients receiving adjunctive dexamethasone, and, when these patients were monitored for a mean of 15 months, those who had received adjunctive dexamethasone had a significantly decreased incidence of one or more neurologic sequelae, although there was only a trend in reduction of audiologic impairment. No differences in mortality were observed.

In addition, in a review of the records of 97 infants and children with pneumococcal meningitis in Dallas, Texas, from 1984 to 1990,[376] the patients treated with adjunctive dexamethasone had a significant reduction in adverse long-term neurologic outcome, including hearing impairment. However, despite similarities in the demographics and clinical characteristics between the groups that received antibiotics alone and antibiotics plus dexamethasone, the study was retrospective and no data on use of specific antimicrobial agents were presented.

Based on the above studies and on a recently published meta-analysis (including earlier trials not cited here),[377] the data support the routine use of adjunctive dexamethasone (0.15 mg/kg every 6 hours for 4 days) in infants and children with bacterial meningitis caused by *H. influenzae* type b. Adjunctive dexamethasone is likely to be of particular benefit in the subset of patients in high-risk categories (i.e., Herson-Todd score of 4.5 points or higher) or in those with suspected or proven cerebral edema, raised intracranial pressure, or profound alterations of consciousness.[378] When using dexamethasone, the timing of administration is likely to be crucial. Administration before or concomitant with antimicrobial therapy is optimal for attenuating the subarachnoid space inflammatory response. In addition, patients should be carefully monitored for the possibility of gastrointestinal hemorrhage. In adults or in patients with meningitis caused by other bacterial organisms, the routine use of adjunctive dexamethasone cannot be recommended pending results of ongoing studies, although some authors recommend their use in all cases of meningitis with a likely bacterial etiology (i.e., demonstrable bacteria on CSF Gram stain, which may predict the patients at greatest risk of bacteriolysis-induced exacerbation of inflammation)[152]; however, there are no clinical data to support this recommendation. Adults with severely impaired mental status (stupor or coma), documented cerebral edema (e.g., by CT scan), and/or markedly elevated intracranial pressure (i.e., high opening pressure on lumbar puncture, palsy of cranial nerve VI) may benefit from adjunctive dexamethasone. The use of adjunctive dexamethasone is of particular concern in patients with pneumococcal meningitis caused by highly penicillin resistant strains, in which a diminished CSF inflammatory response might significantly reduce vancomycin penetration into CSF and delay CSF sterilization.

Other agents that reduce subarachnoid space inflammation have also been examined as possible adjuncts in the therapy of bacterial meningitis. Pentoxifylline, a phosphodiesterase inhibitor that decreases endotoxin-induced TNF-α production and attenuates the inflammatory action of IL-1 and TNF on leukocyte function[379] and blocks the LPS-induced release of TNF and IL-1 from microglial cell cultures,[380] has been examined in an experimental rabbit model of *H. influenzae* type b meningitis.[381] Administration of pentoxifylline 20 minutes before intracisternal challenge with *H. influenzae* type b LPS significantly reduced CSF concentrations of leukocytes, protein, and lactate. However, dexamethasone was superior to pentoxifylline in modulation of these CSF inflammatory changes, and no appreciable synergism was observed when both agents were administered.

Other studies have examined the effects of a monoclonal antibody (IB4) directed against the CD18 family of receptors on leukocytes to reduce CSF inflammation. The intravenous inoculation of IB4 blocked the accumulation of leukocytes in CSF despite intracisternal challenge with *H. influenzae* type b, *N. meningitidis*, pneumococcal cell wall, or LPS.[183] Furthermore, the monoclonal antibody was effective in preventing the development of cerebral edema and death in animals challenged with lethal doses of *S. pneumoniae*. In a second study utilizing an experimental rabbit model of *H. influenzae* type b meningitis,[382] the concomitant administration of dexamethasone and IB4 led to a marked attenuation of all indices of meningeal inflammation and a reduction in brain water content compared with the results obtained in untreated animals or when each agent was used alone. Clinical trials with this agent, perhaps in conjunction with dexamethasone, will be needed to determine whether outcome (i.e., morbidity or mortality) can be improved by administration of IB4 in patients with bacterial meningitis.

Reduction of Intracranial Pressure. Patients with bacterial meningitis who have signs of increased intracranial pressure (e.g., altered level of consciousness, dilated poorly reactive or nonreactive pupils, and/or ocular movement disorders) and who are stuporous or comatose may benefit from insertion of an intracranial pressure monitoring device.[383,384] Intracranial pressures exceeding 20 mmHg are abnormal and should be treated. Furthermore, there is rationale for treating smaller pressure elevations (i.e., above 15 mmHg) to avoid larger elevations, so-called plateau waves, that can lead to cerebral herniation and irreversible brain stem injury.

Several methods are available to reduce intracranial pressure.[384] These include elevation of the head of the bed to 30° to maximize venous drainage with minimal compromise of cerebral perfusion, hyperventilation to maintain the $PaCO_2$ between 27 and 30 mmHg, which causes cerebral vasoconstriction and reduction in cerebral blood volume, use of hyperosmolar agents (e.g., mannitol) to make the intravascular space hyperosmolar to the brain permitting movement of water from brain tissue into the intravascular compartment, intravenous lidocaine to block the reflex increase in intracranial pressure after tracheal suctioning, and corticosteroids. However, some experts have questioned the routine use of hyperventilation to reduce intracranial pressure in patients with bacterial meningitis.[221] In infants and children with bacterial meningitis who have initially normal CT scans of the head, hyperventilation can safely reduce elevated intracranial pressure because it is unlikely that cerebral blood flow would be reduced to ischemic thresholds. However, in children with cerebral edema on head CT, cerebral blood flow is more likely to be normal or reduced. Although hyperventilation might decrease intracranial pressure, it would do so at the expense of a significant reduction in cerebral blood flow, possibly approaching ischemic thresholds. These patients may benefit more from early use of diuretics, osmotically dehydrating agents (provided that intravascular volume is protected), and corticosteroids; however, controlled trials exploring these issues have yet to be performed.

Patients who continue to have elevated intracranial pressures despite the above measures may be treated with high-dose barbiturate therapy,[384,385] which decreases cerebral metabolic demands and cerebral blood flow. Barbiturates can also cause vasoconstriction in normal tissue, thereby shunting blood to ischemic tissue and protecting the brain from ischemic insult. During administration of pentobarbital, the patient is monitored to measure decreases in intracranial pressure, or the dose can be titrated to development of a burst-suppression pattern on the electroencephalogram. Cardiac parameters also need to be monitored (by placement of a Swan-Ganz catheter) because of the risk of cardiac toxicity (e.g., decreased cardiac output, decreased contractile force, arrhythmias) with high-dose barbiturate therapy. This mode of treatment for meningitis and elevated intracranial pressure is of unproven benefit, however, and must be considered experimental.

Surgery. Surgical intervention may be required in some patients with bacterial meningitis. Patients who have suffered a basilar skull fracture with CSF leak may have persistent dural defects that can lead to recurrent episodes of bacterial meningitis.[74] Many leaks will cease spontaneously, but surgery is indicated for leaks that persist for several weeks or in patients who present with delayed or recurrent infection. Surgery is not indicated in the acute phase (before 7 days) of leakage; there is no difference in outcome when patients with acutely repaired leaks are compared with those whose leaks stop spontaneously within 7 days. Surgical intervention may also be required in patients who develop recurrent meningitis from congenital or acquired cranial defects and dermal sinuses.[102]

PREVENTION

Viral Meningitis: Immunoprophylaxis

The cornerstone of prevention of mumps is active immunization with the live, attenuated mumps vaccine. Administration is in the second year of life, and protective serum antibody concentrations are seen in more than 97 percent of patients.[13] Widespread use of the mumps vaccine has greatly reduced the incidence of mumps and mumps meningoencephalitis. By the mid-1980s mumps was the seventh most common cause of viral encephalitis in the United States (approximately 0.5 percent of cases), whereas it was the leading cause of viral encephalitis through the mid-1960s.[13] Mumps meningitis has been reported in children 11 days to 2 months after vaccine administration,[386,387] although it is not clear whether these cases represented vaccine failure or meningitis due to the vaccine strain of mumps virus.

Bacterial Meningitis

Haemophilus influenzae Chemoprophylaxis. It has become clear in recent years that the spread of several types of bacterial meningitis can be prevented by prophylaxis of contacts of cases with antimicrobial agents. Several studies have documented the transmission of *H. influenzae* type b from patients with meningitis to household contacts.[388,390] The risk is markedly age dependent, highest for children under 2 years of age. Most secondary cases (75 percent) occur within 6 days of onset of the index case, although untreated household contacts remain at increased risk for *H. influenzae* type b disease for at least 1 month after onset in the index case. Day care outside of the home is considered another risk factor for transmission[42]; children younger than 2 years of age are more likely to develop secondary disease. There is controversy, however, as to the magnitude of the risk to children in day care settings, leading to disagreement concerning the recommendation for chemoprophylaxis of children in these facilities.

The rationale for the use of chemoprophylaxis for prevention of secondary disease is eradication of nasopharyngeal colonization of *H. influenzae* type b, thereby preventing transmission to young, susceptible contacts and the development of invasive disease in those already colonized. The recommended chemoprophylactic agent of choice is rifampin (20 mg/kg daily for 4 days) for all individuals, including adults, in households with at least one child younger than 48 months of age.[390,391] One study suggested that 2 days of rifampin therapy was equally efficacious to 4 days' treatment,[392] although this requires further study before a recommendation to shorten duration of prophylaxis can be made. The index patient should also receive rifampin prophylaxis because some antibiotics given for invasive *H. influenzae* type b disease do not necessarily eliminate nasopharyngeal colonization. Prior or pending *H. influenzae* type b immunization should not influence decisions regarding prophylaxis. Rifampin is not recommended for pregnant women who are contacts of infected infants, since the risk of rifampin to the fetus has not been established. Chemoprophylaxis is not currently recommended for day care contacts 2 years of age or older unless two or more cases occur in the day care center within a 60-day period. For children younger than 2 years of age, the Centers for Disease Control and Prevention (CDC) recommends prophylaxis for day care contacts, whereas the American Academy of Pediatrics does not in most cases.[390] The question of whether to administer prophylaxis in this setting needs to be individualized and should be considered more strongly in day care centers that resemble households where children have prolonged contact.

Neisseria meningitidis Chemoprophylaxis. Chemoprophylaxis is also necessary for contacts of patients with invasive meningococcal disease; up to 10 percent of meningococcal meningitis cases have had contact with another known case.[233] The estimated prevalence of meningococcal carriage in the United States is 5–10 percent under nonepidemic conditions. In closed populations, such as military recruits, carriage rates can reach levels of 40–90 percent.[230] In households the secondary attack rate may be as high as 0.4 percent and is substantially higher for children under 5 years of age. Secondary systemic meningococcal disease often develops within 5 days of recognition of the index case. Chemoprophylaxis is recommended for close contacts of the index case, defined as household contacts or day care center members that sleep or eat in the same dwelling, close contacts in a closed community such as a military barracks or boarding school, and medical personnel performing mouth-to-mouth resuscitation.[230,233] Chemoprophylaxis may also need to be administered to the index case prior to hospital discharge because certain antimicrobial agents (e.g., high-dose penicillin or chloramphenicol) do not reliably eradicate meningococci from the nasopharynx of colonized patients.

The optimal chemoprophylactic agent of choice to prevent invasive meningococcal disease is controversial. The CDC currently recommends administration of rifampin at 12-hour intervals for 2 days in the following dosages: adults, 600 mg; children beyond the neonatal period, 10 mg/kg; and infants less than 1 month of age, 5 mg/kg.[230] However, rifampin has several short-

comings, including nasopharyngeal eradication rates of only about 80 percent, adverse events, necessity for multiple doses over 2 days, and emergence of resistant organisms (up to 10–27 percent of isolates) which may then cause invasive disease. In the search for alternative agents, ceftriaxone (intramuscular administration of 250 mg in adults and 125 mg in children) eliminated the serogroup A carrier state in 97 percent of patients in one study for up to 2 weeks,[393] although parenteral administration is required. Additional studies have demonstrated a single dose of oral ciprofloxacin (500 or 750 mg in adults) to be very effective in elimination of the nasopharyngeal carriage of *N. meningitidis*.[351] Ciprofloxacin concentrations in nasal secretions have been shown to exceed the MIC$_{90}$ for meningococci.[394] Ciprofloxacin may well supplant rifampin for chemoprophylaxis in adults. Ciprofloxacin is not recommended for use in children because of concerns regarding cartilage damage. In pregnant patients, ceftriaxone is probably the safest alternative agent for chemoprophylaxis. Widespread chemoprophylaxis to low-risk contacts should be discouraged because of the concerns of emergence of resistant organisms and the possible future limitations on this approach.

Streptococcus pneumoniae Chemoprophylaxis. The risk of secondary pneumococcal disease in contacts of infected patients has not been defined, although outbreaks have been described in closed populations such as gold miners, military recruits, and jail inmates.[391] In one outbreak in a day care center,[395] treatment of 97 percent of the day care center children and staff with rifampin (10 mg/kg twice daily for 2 days) resulted in a 70 percent reduction (i.e., only partial eradication) of positive nasopharyngeal cultures for *S. pneumoniae*, but did not prevent new acquisition of this organism by three children and one family member. Further studies are needed before chemoprophylaxis is recommended for contacts of patients with pneumococcal meningitis. Some authors do recommend prophylaxis with oral penicillin in patients with sickle cell disease in whom therapy has been shown to reduce the incidence of pneumococcal septicemia and meningitis[396]; this practice is not universally accepted, however.

Streptococcus agalactiae Chemoprophylaxis. Administration of ampicillin during labor to mothers with prenatal vaginal or rectal group B streptococcal colonization and obstetric risk factors (e.g., premature labor, prolonged rupture of membranes, or intrapartum fever) has been associated with reduced rates of colonization and early-onset streptococcal sepsis in the neonate.[397] The American Academy of Pediatrics has recently established guidelines for prevention of group B streptococcal infection by chemoprophylaxis.[398] Maternal group B streptococcal carriers, identified either antepartum or intrapartum, should receive chemoprophylaxis if one or more of the following risk factors is present: preterm labor at less than 37 weeks gestation; premature rupture of membranes at less than 37 weeks gestation; fever during labor; multiple births; or rupture of membranes beyond 18 hours during any gestation. Furthermore, previous delivery of a sibling with invasive group B streptococcal disease warrants intrapartum maternal chemoprophylaxis in each subsequent pregnancy. Chemoprophylaxis should consist of intrapartum intravenous ampicillin (2 g initially, then 1–2 g every 4–6 hours) or penicillin G (5 million units every 6 hours) until delivery; intravenous clindamycin or erythromycin should be used in penicillin-allergic patients.

Basilar Skull Fracture. A number of studies have reported on the use of prophylactic antibiotics in patients with basilar skull fractures and CSF leak, based on the premise that in patients with a dural effect, the CSF is exposed to pathogenic organisms from the nasopharynx, nasal or mastoid sinuses, or external auditory canal.[74,102] Interpretation and comparison of the various studies examining this question are confounded by multiple variables, including patient selection, choice of antimicrobial agents, and definition of infection. No prospective controlled trials have examined the efficacy of prophylactic antimicrobial agents in these patients. Despite conflicting studies, the use of prophylactic antibiotics is not recommended for patients with basilar skull fracture and CSF leak. Their use does not appear to change the incidence of post-traumatic bacterial meningitis and may result in selection and growth of resistant organisms.

Haemophilus influenzae Immunoprophylaxis. Vaccination to prevent infection with specific meningeal pathogens is a very useful measure for decreasing the incidence of bacterial meningitis. For *H. influenzae* type b, the initial capsular polysaccharide vaccine, composed of polyribosyl-ribitol phosphate (PRP), was 90 percent effective in preventing *H. influenzae* infections in children vaccinated between 18 and 71 months of age,[230,391] but was not effective in infants, the age group most prone to invasive *H. influenzae* type b disease. To improve immunogenicity, the polysaccharide was coupled with certain protein carriers that are covalently linked directly to a short-chain PRP molecule.[391,399,400] The Immunization Practices Advisory Committee recommendation is to vaccinate all children with one of the conjugate vaccines licensed for infant use (Table 14): *H. influenzae* type b conjugate vaccine (diphtheria CRM_{197} protein conjugate) (HbOC) or *H. influenzae* type b conjugate vaccine (meningococcal protein conjugate) (PRP-OMP).[401] Children over 60 months of age should be vaccinated based on their disease risk (e.g., patients with asplenia, sickle cell disease, or an immunosuppressive malignancy). Use of the vaccine does not preclude recommendations for rifampin chemoprophylaxis in the appropriate setting.

Neisseria meningitidis Immunoprophylaxis. Monovalent vaccines utilizing purified serogroup capsular polysaccharide antigens of *N. meningitidis* have been shown to be immunogenic in humans over the age of 2 years; younger infants and toddlers do not mount an effective immune response.[230] Bactericidal antibody responses are also elicited in adults with the newly licensed quadrivalent vaccine (activity against serogroups A, C, Y, and W135). However, a major obstacle to the control of meningococcal vaccine is the lack of a suitable vaccine against serogroup B, which is responsible for approximately 51 percent of cases of meningococcal meningitis in the United States.[42] Although vaccinated adults can mount an antibody response to serogroup B polysaccharide, the antibodies are not bactericidal in the presence of human complement[230]; furthermore, the antibody response is almost entirely IgM. A trial from Norway of the efficacy of an outer membrane vesicle vaccine to confer protection against group B meningococcal disease revealed that the protection rate or vaccine efficacy was 57 percent.[402] Several approaches are underway in an attempt to enhance the immunogenicity of serogroup B polysaccharide, which would be necessary for development of an effective vaccine.[230,391] Vaccination with the quadrivalent meningococcal vaccine is currently rec-

ommended for patients in certain high-risk groups including those with terminal complement component or properdin deficiency or dysfunction; asplenia; those who travel to areas with hyperendemic or epidemic meningococcal disease (e.g., Nigeria); military recruits; and those who are close contacts of the primary case as an adjunct to chemoprophylaxis, although this is controversial and of unproven efficacy. The vaccine is not recommended for routine use in the United States because of the overall low risk of infection, the inability to protect against serogroup B disease, and the inability to provide lasting immunity to young children. The major use of the meningococcal vaccine is during outbreaks of disease caused by the serogroups represented in the vaccine preparation.

Streptococcus pneumoniae Immunoprophylaxis. The use of the current 23-valent pneumococcal vaccine is currently recommended for prevention of bacteremic pneumococcal disease in certain high-risk groups. Of all the pneumococci isolated from blood cultures in the United States and recently reported to the CDC, 88 percent were from serotypes represented in the 23-valent vaccine.[403] Similar studies from blood and CSF isolates from the United States, Sweden, and South Africa revealed that from 77 to 96 percent of the organisms were represented in the 23-valent vaccine. The efficacy of the vaccine in prevention of pneumococcal meningitis has never been documented, although it would seem prudent to administer the vaccine to certain high-risk groups over 2 years of age who are at increased risk for bacteremic pneumococcal disease: the elderly over the age of 65 years; patients with diabetes mellitus, congestive heart failure, hepatic disease, renal disease, and other cardiopulmonary conditions; chronic alcoholics; patients with asplenia, multiple myeloma, or the Wiskott-Aldrich syndrome; patients with a CSF fistula or leak; and HIV-infected patients.[391,403] Although there are no data to support it, vaccination for persons traveling to an area with a significant incidence of resistance pneumococci may also be warranted.

REFERENCES

1. Connolly KJ, Hammer SM. The acute aseptic meningitis syndrome. Infect Dis Clin North Am. 1990;4:599–622.
2. Rotbart HA. Viral meningitis and the aseptic meningitis syndrome. In: Scheld WM, Whitley RJ, Durack DT, eds. Infections of the Central Nervous System. New York: Raven Press; 1991:19–40.
3. Nicolosi A, Hauser WA, Beghi E, et al. Epidemiology of central nervous system infections in Olmstead County, Minnesota, 1950–1981. J Infect Dis. 1986;154:399–408.
4. Melnick JL. Enteroviruses: Polioviruses, coxsackieviruses, echoviruses, and newer enteroviruses. In: Fields BN, Knipe DM, eds. Virology. New York: Raven Press; 1990:549–605.
5. Strikas RA, Anderson LJ, Parker RA. Temporal and geographic patterns of isolates of nonpolio enterovirus in the United States, 1970–1983. J Infect Dis. 1986;153:346–51.
6. Centers for Disease Control and Prevention. Aseptic meningitis—New York state and United States, weeks 1–36, 1991. MMWR. 1991;40:773–5.
7. Rantakallio P, Leskinen M, von Wendt L. Incidence and prognosis of central nervous system infections in a birth cohort of 12,000 children. Scand J Infect Dis. 1986;18:287–94.
8. Monath TP. Flaviviruses. In: Fields BN, Knipe DM, eds. Virology. New York: Raven Press; 1990:763–814.
9. Tsai TF, Monath TP. Viral diseases in North America transmitted by arthropods or from vertebrate reservoirs. In: Feigin RD, Cherry JD, eds. Textbook of Pediatric Infectious Diseases. 2nd ed. Philadelphia: WB Saunders; 1987: 1417–56.
10. Tsai TF, Canfield MA, Reed CM, et al. Epidemiologic aspects of a St. Louis encephalitis outbreak in Harris County, Texas, 1986. J Infect Dis. 1988;157: 351–6.
11. Emmons RW. Ecology of Colorado tick fever. Annu Rev Microbiol. 1988; 42:49–64.
12. Goodpasture HC, Poland JD, Francy DB, et al. Colorado tick fever: Clinical, epidemiologic, and laboratory aspects of 228 cases in Colorado in 1973–1974. Ann Intern Med. 1978;88:303–10.
13. Gnann JW Jr. Meningitis and encephalitis caused by mumps virus. In: Scheld WM, Whitley RJ, Durack DT, eds. Infections of the Central Nervous System. New York: Raven Press; 1991:113–25.
14. Levitt LP, Rich TA, Kinde SW, et al. Central nervous system mumps. Neurology. 1970;20:829–34.

TABLE 14. Vaccination Schedule for *Haemophilus influenzae* type b Conjugate Vaccines

Vaccine	Age at First Dose (months)	Vaccine Schedule
HbOC[a]	2–6	3 Doses, 2 months apart[b]
	7–11	2 Doses, 2 months apart[b]
	12–14	1 Dose[b]
	15–59	1 Dose
PRP-OMP[b]	2–6	2 Doses, 2 months apart[d]
	7–11	2 Doses, 2 months apart[b]
	12–14	1 Dose[b]
	15–59	1 Dose

[a] Diphtheria CRM_{197} protein conjugate.
[b] Give booster dose at age 15 months, at least 2 months after the previous dose.
[c] Meningococcal protein conjugate.
[d] Give booster dose at age 12 months, at least 2 months after the previous dose.
(Adapted from Immunization Practices Advisory Committee.[401])

15. Deibel R, Woodall JP, Decher WJ, et al. Lymphocytic choriomeningitis virus in man. Serologic evidence of association with pet hamsters. JAMA. 1975;232:501–4.

16. Vanzee BE, Douglas RG Jr, Betts RF, et al. Lymphocytic choriomeningitis in university hospital personnel. Clinical features. Am J Med. 1975;58:803–9.

17. Hirsch MS, Moellering RC Jr, Pope HG, et al. Lymphocytic-choriomeningitis-virus infection traced to a pet hamster. N Engl J Med. 1974;291:610–2.

18. Dykewicz CA, Dato VM, Fisher-Hoch SP, et al. Lymphocytic choriomeningitis outbreak associated with nude mice in a research institute. JAMA. 1992;267:1349–53.

19. Olsen LC, Beuscher EL, Artenstein MS, et al. Herpesvirus infections of the human central nervous system. N Engl J Med. 1967;277:1271–7.

20. Craig CP, Nahmias AJ. Different patterns of neurologic involvement with herpes simplex virus types 1 and 2: Isolation of herpes simplex virus type 2 from the buffy coat of two adults with meningitis. J Infect Dis. 1973;127:365–72.

21. Corey L, Adams HG, Brown ZA, et al. Genital herpes simplex virus infection: Clinical manifestations, course, and complications. Ann Intern Med. 1983;98:958–72.

22. Echevarria JM, Martinez-Martin P, Tellaz A, et al. Aseptic meningitis due to varicella-zoster virus: Serum antibody levels and local synthesis of specific IgG, IgM, and IgA. J Infect Dis. 1987;155:959–67.

23. Barnes DW, Whitley RJ. CNS diseases associated with varicella zoster virus and herpes simplex virus infection. Pathogenesis and current therapy. Neurol Clin. 1986;4:265–83.

24. Causey JQ. Spontaneous cytomegalovirus mononucleosis-like syndrome and aseptic meningitis. South Med J. 1976;69:1384–7.

25. Duchowny M, Caplan L, Siber G. Cytomegalovirus infection of the adult nervous system. Ann Neurol. 1979;5:458–61.

26. Corey L, Spear PG. Infections with herpes simplex viruses (second of two parts). N Engl J Med. 1986;314:749–57.

27. Bergström T, Vahlne A, Alestig K, et al. Primary and recurrent herpes simplex virus type 2-induced meningitis. J Infect Dis. 1990;162:322–30.

28. Mayo DR, Booss J. Varicella zoster-associated neurologic disease without skin disease. Arch Neurol. 1989;46:313–5.

29. Karp SJ. Meningitis and cutaneous disseminated zoster complicating herpes zoster infection. J Neurol Neurosurg Psychiatry. 1983;46:582–90.

30. Steel JG, Dix RD, Baringer JR. Isolation of herpes simplex virus type 1 in recurrent (Mollaret) meningitis. Ann Neurol. 1982;11:17–21.

31. Yamamoto LJ, Tedder DG, Ashley R, et al. Herpes simplex virus type 1 DNA in cerebrospinal fluid of a patient with Mollaret's meningitis. N Engl J Med. 1991;325:1082–5.

32. Graman PS. Mollaret's meningitis associated with acute Epstein-Barr virus mononucleosis. Arch Neurol. 1987;44:1204–5.

33. Huang LM, Lee CY, Lee PI, et al. Meningitis caused by human herpesvirus-6. Arch Dis Child. 1991;66:1443–4.

34. Silverstein A, Steinberg G, Nathanson M. Nervous system involvement in infectious mononucleosis. Arch Neurol. 1972;26:353–8.

35. Evans BK, Donley DK, Whitaker JN. Neurological manifestations of infection with the human immunodeficiency viruses. In: Scheld WM, Whitley RJ, Durack DT, eds. Infections of the Central Nervous System. New York: Raven Press; 1991:201–32.

36. McArthur JC. Neurologic manifestations of AIDS. Medicine. 1987;66:407–37.

37. Friedland GH, Klein RS. Transmission of the human immunodeficiency virus. N Engl J Med. 1987;317:1125–34.

38. Carne CA, Tedder RS, Smith A, et al. Acute encephalopathy coincident with seroconversion for anti-HTLV-III. Lancet. 1985;2:1206–8.

39. Hollander H, Stringari S. Human immunodeficiency virus-associated meningitis. Clinical course and correlations. Am J Med. 1987;83:813–6.

40. Levy RM, Bredesen DE, Rosenblum ML. Neurological manifestations of the acquired immunodeficiency syndrome (AIDS): Experience at UCSF and review of the literature. J Neurosurg. 1985;62:475–95.

41. Snider WD, Simpson DM, Nielsen S, et al. Neurological complications of acquired immune deficiency syndrome: Analysis of 50 patients. Ann Neurol. 1983;14:403–18.

42. Schlech WF III, Ward JI, Band JD, et al. Bacterial meningitis in the United States, 1978 through 1981. The national bacterial meningitis surveillance study. JAMA. 1985;253:1749–54.

43. Wenger JD, Hightower AW, Facklam RR, et al. Bacterial meningitis in the United States, 1986: Report of a multistate surveillance study. J Infect Dis. 1990;162:1316–23.

44. Noah ND. Epidemiology of bacterial meningitis: UK and USA. In: Williams JD, Burnie J, eds. Bacterial Meningitis. London: Academic Press; 1987:93–115.

45. Greenwood BM. The epidemiology of acute bacterial meningitis in tropical Africa. In: Williams JD, Burnie J, eds. Bacterial Meningitis. London: Academic Press; 1987:61–91.

46. Bryan JP, de Silva HR, Tavares A, et al. Etiology and mortality of bacterial meningitis in northeastern Brazil. Rev Infect Dis. 1990;12:128–35.

47. Durand ML, Calderwood SB, Weber DJ, et al. Acute bacterial meningitis in adults. A review of 493 episodes. N Engl J Med. 1993;328:21–8.

48. Broome CV. Epidemiology of Haemophilus influenzae type b infections in the United States. Pediatr Infect Dis J. 1987;6:779–82.

49. Spagnuolo PJ, Ellner JJ, Lerner PI, et al. Haemophilus influenzae meningitis: The spectrum of disease in adults. Medicine. 1982;61:74–85.

50. Crowe HM, Levitz RE. Invasive Haemophilus influenzae disease in adults. Arch Intern Med. 1987;147:241–4.

51. Takala AK, Eskola J, van Alphen L. Spectrum of invasive Haemophilus influenzae type b disease in adults. Arch Intern Med. 1990;150:2573–6.

52. Farley MM, Stephens DS, Brachman PS, et al. Invasive Haemophilus influenzae disease in adults. A prospective, population-based surveillance. Ann Intern Med. 1992;116:806–12.

53. Murphy TV, White KE, Pastor P, et al. Declining incidence of Haemophilus influenzae type b disease since introduction of vaccination. JAMA. 1993;269:246–8.

54. Adams WG, Deaver KA, Cochi SL, et al. Decline of childhood Haemophilus influenzae type b (Hib) disease in the Hib vaccine era. JAMA. 1993;269:221–6.

55. Broadhurst LE, Erickson RL, Kelley PW. Decrease in invasive Haemophilus influenzae diseases in US army children, 1984 through 1991. JAMA. 1993;269:227–31.

56. Peltola H, Kilpi T, Anttila M. Rapid disappearance of Haemophilus influenzae type b meningitis after routine childhood immunisation with conjugate vaccines. Lancet. 1992;340:592–4.

57. Pinner RW, Gellin BG, Bibb WF et al. Meningococcal disease in the United States—1986. J Infect Dis. 1991;164:368–74.

58. Ross SC, Densen P. Complement deficiency states and infection: Epidemiology, pathogenesis and consequences of neisserial and other infections in an immune deficiency. Medicine. 1984;64:243–73.

59. Ellison RT III, Kohler PF, Curd JG, et al. Prevalence of congenital or acquired complement deficiency in patients with sporadic meningococcal disease. N Engl J Med. 1983;308:913–6.

60. Rosen MS, Lorber B, Myers AR. Chronic meningococcal meningitis. An association with C5 deficiency. Arch Intern Med. 1988;148:1441–2.

61. Fijen CAP, Kuijper EJ, Hannema AJ, et al. Complement deficiencies in patients over ten years old with meningococcal disease due to uncommon serogroups. Lancet. 1989;2:585–8.

62. Zoppi M, Weiss M, Nydegger UE, et al. Recurrent meningitis in a patient with congenital deficiency of the C9 component of complement. First case of C9 deficiency in Europe. Arch Intern Med. 1990;150:2395–9.

63. Sjöholm AG, Kuijper EJ, Tijssen CC, et al. Dysfunctional properdin in a Dutch family with meningococcal disease. N Engl J Med. 1988;319:33–7.

64. Austrian R, Gold J. Pneumococcal bacteremia with special reference to bacteremic pneumococcal pneumonia. Ann Intern Med. 1964;60:759–76.

65. Finland M. Excursions into epidemiology: Selected studies during the past four decades at Boston City Hospital. J Infect Dis. 1973;128:76–124.

66. Fraser DW, Geil CC, Feldman RA. Bacterial meningitis in Bernalillo County, New Mexico: A comparison with three other American populations. Am J Epidemiol. 1974;100:29–34.

67. Gray BM, Converse GM III, Dillon HC Jr. Serotypes of Streptococcus pneumoniae causing invasive disease. J Infect Dis. 1979;140:979–83.

68. Broome CV, Facklam RR, Allen JR, et al. Epidemiology of pneumococcal serotypes in the United States. J Infect Dis. 1980;141:119–23.

69. Geiseler PJ, Nelson KE, Levin S, et al. Community-acquired purulent meningitis: A review of 1,316 cases during the antibiotic era, 1954–1976. Rev Infect Dis. 1980;2:725–45.

70. Burman LA, Norrby R, Trollfors B. Invasive pneumococcal infections: Incidence, predisposing factors, and prognosis. Rev Infect Dis. 1985;7:133–42.

71. Olopoenia L, Frederick W, Greaves W, et al. Pneumococcal sepsis and meningitis in adults with sickle cell disease. South Med J. 1990;83:1002–4.

72. Godeau B, Bachir D, Schaeffer A, et al. Severe pneumococcal sepsis and meningitis in human immunodeficiency virus-infected adults with sickle cell disease. Clin Infect Dis. 1992;15:327–9.

73. Musher DM. Infections caused by Streptococcus pneumoniae: Clinical spectrum, pathogenesis, immunity, and treatment. Clin Infect Dis. 1992;14:801–9.

74. Tunkel AR, Scheld WM. Acute infectious complications of head trauma. In: Braakman R, ed. Handbook of Clinical Neurology, Head Injury. Amsterdam: Elsevier Science Publishing Company; 1990:317–26.

75. Gellin BG, Broome CV. Listeriosis. JAMA. 1989;261:1313–20.

76. Cherubin CE, Appleman MD, Heseltine PNR, et al. Epidemiological spectrum and current treatment of listeriosis. Rev Infect Dis. 1991;13:1108–14.

77. Anaissie E, Kontoyiannis DP, Kantarjian H, et al. Listeriosis in patients with chronic lymphocytic leukemia who were treated with fludarabine and prednisone. Ann Intern Med. 1992;117:466–9.

78. Skogberg K, Syrjänen J, Jahkola M, et al. Clinical presentation and outcome of listeriosis in patients with and without immunosuppressive therapy. Clin Infect Dis. 1992;14:815–21.

79. Kessler SL, Dajani AS. Listeria meningitis in infants and children. Pediatr Infect Dis J. 1990;9:61–3.

80. Mascola L, Lieb L, Chiu J, et al. Listeriosis: An uncommon opportunistic infection in patients with acquired immunodeficiency syndrome. A report of five cases and a review of the literature. Am J Med. 1988;84:162–4.

81. Decker CF, Simon GL, DiGioia RA, et al. Listeria monocytogenes infections in patients with AIDS: Report of five cases and review. Rev Infect Dis. 1991;13:413–7.

82. Berenguer J, Solera J, Diaz MD, et al. Listeriosis in patients infected with human immunodeficiency virus. Rev Infect Dis. 1991;13:115–9.

83. Zuniga M, Aguado JM, Vada J. Listeria monocytogenes meningitis in previously healthy adults: Long-term follow-up. Q J Med. 1992;85:911–5.

84. Schuchat A, Deaver KA, Wenger JD, et al. Role of foods in sporadic listeriosis. I. Case-control study of dietary risk factors. JAMA. 1992;267:2041–5.

85. Pinner RW, Schuchat A, Swaminathan B, et al. Role of foods in sporadic

listeriosis. II. Microbiologic and epidemiologic investigation. JAMA. 1992; 267:2046–50.

86. Saez-Llorens X, McCracken GH Jr. Bacterial meningitis in neonates and children. Infect Dis Clin North Am. 1990;4:623–44.

87. Dillon HC Jr, Gray E, Pass MA, et al. Anorectal and vaginal carriage of group B streptococci during pregnancy. J Infect Dis. 1982;145:794–9.

88. Anthony BF, Eisenstadt R, Carter J, et al. Genital and intestinal carriage of group B streptococci during pregnancy. J Infect Dis. 1981;143:761–6.

89. Allardice JG, Baskett TF, Seshia MMK, et al. Perinatal group B streptococcal colonization and infection. Am J Obstet Gynecol. 1982;142:617–20.

90. Regan JA, Klebanoff MA, Nugent RP. The Vaginal Infections and Prematurity Study Group. The epidemiology of group B streptococcal colonization in pregnancy. Obstet Gynecol. 1991;77:604–10.

91. Farley MM, Harvey RC, Stull T, et al. A population-based assessment of invasive disease due to group B streptococci in nonpregnant adults. N Engl J Med. 1993;328:1807–11.

92. Dunne DW, Quagliarello V. Group B streptococcal meningitis in adults. Medicine. 1993;72:1–10.

93. Mangi RJ, Quintiliani R, Andriole VT. Gram-negative bacillary meningitis. Am J Med. 1975;59:829–36.

94. Cherubin CE, Marr JS, Sierra MF, et al. Listeria and gram-negative bacillary meningitis in New York City, 1972–1979. Am J Med. 1981;71:199–209.

95. Gower DJ, Barrows AA, Kelly DL, et al. Gram-negative bacillary meningitis in the adult: Review of 39 cases. South Med J. 1986;79:1499–502.

96. Campbell JR, Diacovo T, Baker CJ. Serratia marcescens meningitis in neonates. Pediatr Infect Dis J. 1992;11:881–6.

97. Unhanand M, Mustafa MM, McCracken GH Jr, et al. Gram-negative enteric bacillary meningitis: A twenty-one-year experience. J Pediatr. 1993;122: 15–21.

98. Owor R, Wamukota WM. A fatal case of strongyloidiasis with Strongyloides larvae in the meninges. Trans R Soc Trop Med Hyg. 1976;70:497–9.

99. Cameron ML, Durack DT. Helminthic infections of the central nervous system. In: Scheld WM, Whitley RJ, Durack DT, eds. Infections of the Central Nervous System. New York: Raven Press; 1991:825–58.

100. Gordon JJ, Harter DH, Phair JP. Meningitis due to Staphylococcus aureus. Am J Med. 1985;78:965–70.

101. Schlesinger LS, Ross SC, Schaberg DR. Staphylococcus aureus meningitis: A broad-based epidemiological study. Medicine. 1987;66:148–56.

102. Kaufman BA, Tunkel AR, Pryor JC, et al. Meningitis in the neurosurgical patient. Infect Dis Clin North Am. 1990;4:677–701.

103. Bross JE, Gordon G. Nocardial meningitis: Case reports and review. Rev Infect Dis. 1991;13:160–5.

104. Heerema MS, Ein ME, Musher DM, et al. Anaerobic bacterial meningitis. Am J Med. 1979;67:219–27.

105. Feder HM Jr. Bacteroides fragilis meningitis. Rev Infect Dis. 1987;9:783–6.

106. Long JG, Preblud SR, Keyserling HL. Clostridium perfringens meningitis in an infant: Case report and literature review. Pediatr Infect Dis J. 1987;6: 752–4.

107. Law DA, Aronoff SC. Anaerobic meningitis in children: Case report and review of the literature. Pediatr Infect Dis J. 1992;11:968–71.

108. Hook EW III. Central nervous system syphilis. In: Scheld WM, Whitley RJ, Durack DT, eds. Infections of the Central Nervous System. New York: Raven Press; 1991:639–56.

109. Merritt HH, Moore M. Acute syphilitic meningitis. Medicine. 1935;14: 119–83.

110. Hoshmand H, Escobar MR, Kopf SW. Neurosyphilis: A study of 241 patients. JAMA. 1972;219:726–9.

111. Hotson JR. Modern neurosyphilis: A partially treated chronic meningitis. West J Med. 1981;135:191–200.

112. Simon RP. Neurosyphilis. Arch Neurol. 1985;42:606–13.

113. Hook EW III. Syphilis and HIV infection. J Infect Dis. 1989;160:530–4.

114. Musher DM, Hamill RJ, Baughn RE. Effect of human immunodeficiency virus (HIV) infection on the course of syphilis and on the response to treatment. Ann Intern Med. 1990;113:872–81.

115. Hook EW III, Marra CM. Acquired syphilis in adults. N Engl J Med. 1992; 326:1060–9.

116. Katz DA, Berger JR. Neurosyphilis in acquired immunodeficiency syndrome. Arch Neurol. 1989;46:895–8.

117. Reik L Jr. Lyme disease. In: Scheld WM, Whitley RJ, Durack DT, eds. Infections of the Central Nervous System. New York: Raven Press; 1991: 657–89.

118. Reik L, Steere AC, Bartenhagen NH, et al. Neurologic abnormalities of Lyme disease. Medicine. 1979;58:281–94.

119. Pachner AR, Steere AC. The triad of neurologic manifestations of Lyme disease: Meningitis, cranial neuritis and radiculoneuritis. Neurology. 1985; 35:47–53.

120. Luft BJ, Steinman CR, Neimark HC, et al. Invasion of the central nervous system by Borrelia burgdorferi in acute disseminated infection. JAMA. 1992; 267:1364–7.

121. Niu MT, Duma RJ. Meningitis due to protozoa and helminths. Infect Dis Clin North Am. 1990;4:809–41.

122. Cegielski JP, Durack DT. Protozoal infections of the central nervous system. In: Scheld WM, Whitley RJ, Durack DT, eds. Infections of the Central Nervous System. New York: Raven Press; 1991:767–800.

123. Chang SL. Etiological, pathological, epidemiological and diagnostical considerations of primary amoebic meningoencephalitis. Crit Rev Microbiol. 1974;3:135–59.

124. John DT. Primary amebic meningoencephalitis and the biology of Naegleria fowleri. Annu Rev Microbiol. 1982;36:101–23.

125. Wellings FM, Amuso PT, Chang SL, et al. Isolation and identification of pathogenic Naegleria from Florida lakes. Appl Environ Microbiol. 1977;34: 661–7.

126. Gardner HAR, Martinez AJ, Visvesvara GS, et al. Granulomatous amebic encephalitis in an AIDS patient. Neurology. 1991;41:1993–5.

127. Di Gregorio C, Rivasi R, Mongiardo N, et al. Acanthamoeba meningoencephalitis in a patient with acquired immunodeficiency syndrome. Arch Pathol Lab Med. 1992;116:1363–5.

128. Gordon SM, Steinberg JP, DuPuis MH, et al. Culture isolation of Acanthamoeba species and leptomyxid amebas from patients with amebic meningoencephalitis, including two patients with AIDS. Clin Infect Dis. 1992;15: 1024–30.

129. Koo J, Pien F, Kliks MM. Angiostrongylus (Parastrongylus) eosinophilic meningitis. Rev Infect Dis. 1988;10:1155–62.

130. Punyagupta S, Juttijudata P, Bunnag T. Eosinophilic meningitis in Thailand. Clinical studies of 484 typical cases probably caused by Angiostrongylus cantonensis. Am J Trop Med Hyg. 1975;24:921–32.

131. Punyagupta S, Bunnag T, Juttijudata P, et al. Eosinophilic meningitis in Thailand. Epidemiologic studies of 484 typical cases and the etiologic role of Angiostrongylus cantonensis. Am J Trop Med Hyg. 1970;19:950–8.

132. Kliks MM, Palumbo NE. Eosinophilic meningitis beyond the Pacific basin: The global dispersal of a peridomestic zoonosis caused by Angiostrongylus cantonensis, the nematode lungworm of rats. Soc Sci Med. 1992;34:199–212.

133. Campbell BG, Little MD. The finding of Angiostrongylus cantonensis in rats in New Orleans. Am J Trop Med Hyg. 1988;38:568–73.

134. Schmutzhard E, Boongird P, Vejjajiva A. Eosinophilic meningitis and radiculomyelitis in Thailand, caused by CNS invasion of Gnathostoma spinigerum and Angiostrongylus cantonensis. J Neurol Neurosurg Psychiatry. 1988;51: 80–7.

135. Johnson RT. Pathogenesis of CNS infections. In: Viral Infections of the Central Nervous System. New York: Raven Press; 1982:37–60.

136. Tunkel AR, Wispelwey B, Scheld WM. Pathogenesis and pathophysiology of meningitis. Infect Dis Clin North Am. 1990;4:555–81.

137. Johnson RT, Mims CA. Pathogenesis of viral infections of the nervous system. N Engl J Med. 1968;278:23–30, 84–92.

138. Kristensson K, Ghetti B, Wisniewski HM. Study on the propagation of herpes simplex virus (type 2) into brain after intraocular injection. Brain Res. 1974;69:189–201.

139. Davis LE, Johnson RT. An explanation for the localization of herpes simplex encephalitis? Ann Neurol. 1979;5:2–5.

140. Watson HD, Tignor GH, Smith AL. Entry of rabies virus into the peripheral nerves of mice. J Gen Virol. 1981;56:371–82.

141. Ren R, Racaniello VR. Poliovirus spreads from muscle to the central nervous system by neural pathways. J Infect Dis. 1992;166:747–52.

142. Frei K, Leist TP, Meager A, et al. Production of B cell stimulatory factor-2 and interferon γ in the central nervous system during viral meningitis and encephalitis: Evaluation in a murine model infection and in patients. J Exp Med. 1988;168:449–53.

143. Chonmaitree T, Baron S. Bacteria and viruses induce production of interferon in the cerebrospinal fluid of children with acute meningitis: A study of 57 cases and review. Rev Infect Dis. 1991;13:1061–5.

144. Ramilo O, Mustafa MM, Porter J, et al. Detection of interleukin 1β but not tumor necrosis factor-α in the cerebrospinal fluid of children with aseptic meningitis. Am J Dis Child. 1990;144:349–52.

145. Forsberg P, Fryden A, Link H, et al. Viral IgM and IgG antibody synthesis within the central nervous system in mumps meningitis. Acta Neurol Scand. 1986;73:372–80.

146. Resnick L, diMarzo-Veronese F, Schüpbach J, et al. Intra-blood-brain-barrier synthesis of HTLV-III-specific IgG in patients with neurologic symptoms associated with AIDS or AIDS-related complex. N Engl J Med. 1985; 313:1498–504.

147. Applebaum ME, Marshall DW, Brey RL, et al. Cerebrospinal fluid abnormalities in patients without AIDS who are seropositive for the human immunodeficiency virus. J Infect Dis. 1988;158:193–9.

148. Vandvik B, Norrby E, Steen-Johnson M, et al. Mumps meningitis: Prolonged pleocytosis and occurrence of mumps virus-specific oligoclonal IgG in the cerebrospinal fluid. Eur Neurol. 1978;17:13–22.

149. Sande MA, Täuber MG, Scheld WM, et al. Pathophysiology of bacterial meningitis: Summary of the workshop. Pediatr Infect Dis J. 1989;8:929–33.

150. Tunkel AR, Wispelwey B, Scheld WM. Bacterial meningitis: Recent advances in pathophysiology and treatment. Ann Intern Med. 1990;112:610–23.

151. Saez-Llorens X, Ramilo O, Mustafa MM, et al. Molecular pathophysiology of bacterial meningitis: Current concepts and therapeutic implications. J Pediatr. 1990;116:671–84.

152. Quagliarello V, Scheld WM. Bacterial meningitis: Pathogenesis, pathophysiology, and progress. N Engl J Med. 1992;327:864–72.

153. Tunkel AR, Scheld WM. Pathogenesis and pathophysiology of bacterial meningitis. Clin Microbiol Rev. 1993;6:118–36.

154. Stephens DS, Farley MM. Pathogenic events during infection of the human nasopharynx with Neisseria meningitidis and Haemophilus influenzae. Rev Infect Dis. 1991;13:22–33.

155. Greenblatt JJ, Floyd K, Philipps MW, et al. Morphologic differences in Neisseria meningitidis pili. Infect Immun. 1988;56:2356–62.

156. Smith AL. Pathogenesis of Haemophilus influenzae meningitis. Pediatr Infect Dis J. 1987;6:783–6.

157. Moxon ER, Vaughn KA. The type b capsular polysaccharide as a virulence determinant of *Haemophilus influenzae:* Studies using clinical isolates and laboratory transformants. J Infect Dis. 1981;143:517–24.

158. Roberts M, Stull TL, Smith AL. Comparative virulence of *Haemophilus influenzae* with a type b or type d capsule. Infect Immun. 1981;32:518–24.

159. Robbins JB, McCracken GH Jr, Gotschlich EL, et al. *Escherichia coli* K1 capsular polysaccharide associated with neonatal meningitis. N Engl J Med. 1974;290:1216–20.

160. Brandtzaeg P, Mollnes TE, Kierulf P. Complement activation and endotoxin levels in systemic meningococcal disease. J Infect Dis. 1989;160:58–65.

161. Moxon ER, Smith AL, Averill DR, et al. *Haemophilus influenzae* meningitis in infant rats after intranasal inoculation. J Infect Dis. 1974;129:154–62.

162. Smith AL, Daum RS, Scheifele D, et al. Pathogenesis of *Haemophilus influenzae* meningitis. In: Sell SH, Wright PF, eds. *Haemophilus influenzae: Epidemiology, Immunology, and Prevention of Disease.* New York: Elsevier Science Publishing Company; 1982:89–109.

163. Ostrow PT, Moxon ER, Vernon N, et al. Pathogenesis of bacterial meningitis. Studies on the route of meningeal invasion following *Haemophilus influenzae* inoculation in infant rats. Lab Invest. 1979;40:678–85.

164. Parkkinen J, Korhonen TK, Pere A, et al. Binding sites in the rat brain for *Escherichia coli* S fimbriae associated with neonatal meningitis. J Clin Invest. 1988;81:860–5.

165. Saukkonen KM, Nowicki B, Leinonen M. Role of type 1 and S fimbriae in the pathogenesis of *Escherichia coli* O18:K1 bacteremia and meningitis in the infant rat. Infect Immun. 1988;56:892–7.

166. Williams AE, Blakemore WF. Pathogenesis of meningitis caused by *Streptococcus suis* type 2. J Infect Dis. 1990;162:474–81.

167. Quagliarello VJ, Long WJ Jr, Scheld WM. Morphologic alterations in the blood-brain barrier with experimental meningitis in the rat. Temporal sequence and role of encapsulation. J Clin Invest. 1986;77:1084–95.

168. Lesse AJ, Moxon ER, Zwahlen A, et al. Role of cerebrospinal fluid pleocytosis and *Haemophilus influenzae* type b capsule on blood brain barrier permeability during experimental meningitis in the rat. J Clin Invest. 1988; 82:102–9.

169. Quagliarello VJ, Ma A, Stukenbrok H, et al. Ultrastructural localization of albumin transport across the cerebral microvasculature during experimental meningitis in the rat. J Exp Med. 1991;174:657–72.

170. Wispelwey B, Lesse AJ, Hansen EJ, et al. *Haemophilus influenzae* lipopolysaccharide-induced blood brain barrier permeability during experimental meningitis in the rat. J Clin Invest. 1988;82:1339–46.

171. Quagliarello VJ, Wispelwey B, Long WJ Jr, et al. Recombinant human interleukin-1 induces meningitis and blood-brain barrier injury in the rat. Characterization and comparison with tumor necrosis factor. J Clin Invest. 1991; 87:1360–6.

172. Sharief MK, Ciardi M, Thompson EJ. Blood-brain barrier damage in patients with bacterial meningitis: Association with tumor necrosis factor-α but not interleukin-1β. J Infect Dis. 1992;166:350–8.

173. Tunkel AR, Scheld WM. Alterations in the blood-brain barrier in bacterial meningitis: In vivo and in vitro models. Pediatr Infect Dis J. 1989;8:911–3.

174. Tunkel AR, Rosser SW, Hansen EJ, et al. Blood-brain barrier alterations in bacterial meningitis: Development of an in vitro model and observations on the effects of lipopolysaccharide. In Vitro Cell Dev Biol. 1991;27A:113–20.

175. Patrick D, Betts J, Frey EA, et al. *Haemophilus influenzae* lipopolysaccharide disrupts confluent monolayers of bovine brain endothelial cells via a serum-dependent cytotoxic pathway. J Infect Dis. 1992;165:865–72.

176. Tobias PS, Mathison JC, Ulevitch RJ. A family of lipopolysaccharide binding proteins involved in responses to gram-negative sepsis. J Biol Chem. 1988; 263:13479–81.

177. Gigliotti F, Lee D, Insel RA, et al. IgG penetration into the cerebrospinal fluid in a rabbit model of meningitis. J Infect Dis. 1987;156:394–8.

178. Kadurugamuwa JL, Hengstler B, Zak O. Inhibition of complement-factor-5a-induced inflammatory reactions by prostaglandin E₂ in experimental meningitis. J Infect Dis. 1989;160:715–9.

179. Bevilacqua MP, Stengelin S, Gimbrone MA Jr, et al. Endothelial leukocyte adhesion molecule 1: An inducible receptor for neutrophils related to complement regulatory proteins and lectins. Science. 1989;243:1160–5.

180. Bevilacqua MP, Pober JS, Wheeler ME, et al. Interleukin 1 acts on cultured human vascular endothelium to increase the adhesion of polymorphonuclear leukocytes, monocytes, and related leukocyte cell lines. J Clin Invest. 1985; 76:2002–11.

181. Schleimer RP, Rutledge BK. Cultured human vascular endothelial cells acquire adhesiveness for neutrophils after stimulation with interleukin 1, endotoxin, and tumor-promoting phorbol diesters. J Immunol. 1986;136:649–54.

182. Moser R, Schleiffenbaum B, Groscurth P, et al. Interleukin 1 and tumor necrosis factor stimulate human vascular endothelial cells to promote transendothelial neutrophil passage. J Clin Invest. 1989;83:444–55.

183. Tuomanen EI, Saukkonen K, Sande S, et al. Reduction of inflammation, tissue damage, and mortality in bacterial meningitis in rabbits treated with monoclonal antibodies against adhesion-promoting receptors of leukocytes. J Exp Med. 1989;170:959–68.

184. Tuomanen E, Tomasz A, Hengstler B, et al. The relative role of bacterial cell wall and capsule in the induction of inflammation in pneumococcal meningitis. J Infect Dis. 1985;151:535–40.

185. Tuomanen E, Liu H, Hengstler B, et al. The induction of meningeal inflam-

186. Syrogiannopoulos GA, Hansen EJ, Erwin AL, et al. *Haemophilus influenzae* type b lipooligosaccharide induces meningeal inflammation. J Infect Dis. 1988;157:237–44.

187. Riesenfeld-Orn I, Wolpe S, Garcia-Bustos JF, et al. Production of interleukin-1 but not tumor necrosis factor by human monocytes stimulated with pneumococcal cell surface components. Infect Immun. 1989;57:1890–3.

188. Mustafa MM, Ramilo O, Olsen KD, et al. Tumor necrosis factor in mediating experimental *Haemophilus influenzae* type b meningitis. J Clin Invest. 1989; 84:1253–9.

189. Moller B, Mogensen SC, Wendelboe P, et al. Bioactive and inactive forms of tumor necrosis factor-α in spinal fluid from patients with meningitis. J Infect Dis. 1991;163:886–9.

190. Leist TP, Frei K, Kam-Hansen S, et al. Tumor necrosis factor α in cerebrospinal fluid during bacterial, but not viral, meningitis. Evaluation in murine model infections and in patients. J Exp Med. 1988;167:1743–8.

191. Nadal D, Leppert D, Frei K, et al. Tumor necrosis factor-α in infectious meningitis. Arch Dis Child. 1989;64:1274–9.

192. Glimaker M, Kragsbjerg P, Forsgren M, et al. Tumor necrosis factor-α (TNFα) in cerebrospinal fluid from patients with meningitis of different etiologies: High levels of TNFα indicate bacterial meningitis. J Infect Dis. 1993; 167:882–9.

193. Mustafa MM, Ramilo O, Saez-Llorens X, et al. Cerebrospinal fluid prostaglandins, interleukin 1β, and tumor necrosis factor in bacterial meningitis. Clinical and laboratory correlations in placebo-treated and dexamethasone-treated patients. Am J Dis Child. 1990;144:883–7.

194. Ramilo O, Saez-Llorens X, Mertsola J, et al. Tumor necrosis factor α/cachectin and interleukin 1β initiate meningeal inflammation. J Exp Med. 1990;172:497–507.

195. Saukkonen K, Sande S, Cioffe C, et al. The role of cytokines in the generation of inflammation and tissue damage in experimental gram-positive meningitis. J Exp Med. 1990;171:439–48.

196. Cabellos C, MacIntyre DE, Forrest M, et al. Differing roles for platelet-activating factor during inflammation of the lung and subarachnoid space. The special case of *Streptococcus pneumoniae.* J Clin Invest. 1992;90:612–8.

197. McCracken GH Jr, Mustafa MM, Ramilo O, et al. Cerebrospinal fluid interleukin 1-beta and tumor necrosis factor concentrations and outcome from neonatal gram-negative enteric bacillary meningitis. Pediatr Infect Dis J. 1989;8:155–9.

198. Arditi M, Ables L, Yogev R. Cerebrospinal fluid endotoxin levels in children with *H. influenzae* meningitis before and after administration of intravenous ceftriaxone. J Infect Dis. 1989;160:1005–11.

199. Mustafa MM, Mertsola J, Ramilo O, et al. Increased endotoxin and interleukin-1β concentrations in cerebrospinal fluid of infants with coliform meningitis and ventriculitis associated with intraventricular gentamicin therapy. J Infect Dis. 1989;160:891–5.

200. Mustafa MM, Lebel MH, Ramilo O, et al. Correlation of interleukin-1β and cachectin concentrations in cerebrospinal fluid and outcome from bacterial meningitis. J Pediatr. 1989;115:208–13.

201. Arditi M, Manogue KR, Caplan M, et al. Cerebrospinal fluid cachectin/tumor necrosis factor-α and platelet-activating factor concentrations and severity of bacterial meningitis in children. J Infect Dis. 1990;162:139–47.

202. Rusconi F, Parizzi F, Garlaschi L, et al. Interleukin 6 activity in infants and children with bacterial meningitis. Pediatr Infect Dis J. 1991;10:117–21.

203. Waage A, Halstensen A, Shalaby R, et al. Local production of tumor necrosis factor α, interleukin 1, and interleukin 6 in meningococcal meningitis. Relation to the inflammatory response. J Exp Med. 1989;170:1859–67.

204. Chavanet P, Bonnotte B, Guiguet M, et al. High concentrations of intrathecal interleukin-6 in human bacterial and nonbacterial meningitis. J Infect Dis. 1992;166:428–31.

205. Waage A, Brandtzaeg P, Halstensen A, et al. The complex pattern of cytokines in serum from patients with meningococcal septic shock. Association between interleukin 6, interleukin 1, and fatal outcome. J Exp Med. 1989; 169:333–8.

206. Halstensen A, Ceska M, Brandtzeg P, et al. Interleukin-8 in serum and cerebrospinal fluid from patients with meningococcal disease. J Infect Dis. 1993;167:471–5.

207. Scheld WM, Dacey RG, Winn HR, et al. Cerebrospinal fluid outflow resistance in rabbits with experimental meningitis. Alterations with penicillin and methylprednisolone. J Clin Invest. 1980;66:243–53.

208. Täuber MG, Khayam-Bashi H, Sande MA. Effects of ampicillin and corticosteroids on brain water content, cerebrospinal fluid pressure, and cerebrospinal fluid lactate levels in experimental pneumococcal meningitis. J Infect Dis. 1985;151:528–34.

209. Täuber MG, Shibl AM, Hackbarth CJ, et al. Antibiotic therapy, endotoxin concentrations in cerebrospinal fluid, and brain edema in experimental *Escherichia coli* meningitis in rabbits. J Infect Dis. 1987;156:456–62.

210. Burroughs M, Prasad S, Cabellos C, et al. The biologic activities of peptidoglycan in experimental *Haemophilus influenzae* meningitis. J Infect Dis. 1993;167:464–8.

211. Täuber MG, Borschberg U, Sande MA. Influence of granulocytes on brain edema, intracranial pressure, and cerebrospinal fluid concentrations of lactate and protein in experimental meningitis. J Infect Dis. 1988;157:456–64.

mation by components of the pneumococcal cell wall. J Infect Dis. 1985; 151:859–68.

212. Pfister HW, Koedel U, Lorenzl S, et al. Antioxidants attenuate microvascular changes in the early phase of experimental pneumococcal meningitis in rats. Stroke. 1992;23:1798–804.

213. Pfister HW, Ködel U, Dirnagl U, et al. Effect of catalase on regional cerebral blood flow and brain edema during the early phase of experimental pneumococcal meningitis. J Infect Dis. 1992;166:1442–5.

214. Pfister HW, Koedel U, Bernatowicz A, et al. Role of nitrogen intermediates in experimental pneumococcal meningitis. In: Program and Abstracts of the 33rd Interscience Conference on Antimicrobial Agents and Chemotherapy. Washington, DC: American Society for Microbiology; 1993:265.

215. Tureen JH, Dworkin SL, Kennedy SL, et al. Loss of cerebrovascular autoregulation in experimental meningitis in rabbits. J Clin Invest. 1990;85:577–81.

216. Tureen JH, Täuber MG, Sande MA. Effect of hydration status on cerebral blood flow and cerebrospinal fluid lactic acidosis in rabbits with experimental meningitis. J Clin Invest. 1992;89:947–53.

217. Pfister HW, Koedel U, Haberl RL, et al. Microvascular changes during the early phase of experimental bacterial meningitis. J Cerebral Blood Flow Metab. 1990;10:914–22.

218. Paulson OB, Brodersen P, Hansen EL, et al. Regional cerebral blood flow, cerebral metabolic rate of oxygen, and cerebrospinal fluid acid-base variables in patients with acute meningitis and with acute encephalitis. Acta Med Scand. 1974;196:191–205.

219. McMenamin JB, Volpe JJ. Bacterial meningitis in infancy: Effects on intracranial pressure and cerebral blood flow velocity. Neurology. 1984;34:500–4.

220. Ashwal S, Stringer W, Tomasi L, et al. Cerebral blood flow and carbon dioxide reactivity in children with bacterial meningitis. J Pediatr. 1990;117:523–30.

221. Ashwal S, Tomasi L, Schneider S, et al. Bacterial meningitis in children: Pathophysiology and treatment. Neurology. 1992;42:739–48.

222. Pfister HW, Borasio GD, Dirnagl U, et al. Cerebrovascular complications of bacterial meningitis in adults. Neurology. 1992;42:1497–504.

223. Guerra-Romero L, Täuber MG, Fournier MA, et al. Lactate and glucose concentrations in brain interstitial fluid, cerebrospinal fluid, and serum during experimental pneumococcal meningitis. J Infect Dis. 1992;166:546–50.

224. Kaplan MH, Klein SW, McPhee J, et al. Group B coxsackievirus infections in infants younger than three months of age: A serious childhood illness. Rev Infect Dis. 1983;5:1019–32.

225. Wilfert CM, Lehrman SN. Enteroviruses and meningitis. Pediatr Infect Dis. 1983;2:333–41.

226. Jaffe M, Srugo I, Tirosh E, et al. The ameliorating effect of lumbar puncture in viral meningitis. Am J Dis Child. 1989;143:682–5.

227. McKinney RE Jr, Katz SL, Wilfert CM. Chronic enteroviral meningoencephalitis in agammaglobulinemic patients. Rev Infect Dis. 1987;9:334–56.

228. Gaduzda DH, Hirsch MS. Neurologic manifestations of infection with human immunodeficiency virus. Clinical feaures and pathogenesis. Ann Intern Med. 1987;107:383–91.

229. Carpenter RR, Petersdorf RG. The clinical spectrum of bacterial meningitis. Am J Med. 1962;33:262–75.

230. Roos KL, Tunkel AR, Scheld WM. Acute bacterial meningitis in children and adults. In: Scheld WM, Whitley RJ, Durack DT, eds. Infections of the Central Nervous System. New York: Raven Press; 1991:335–409.

231. Verghese A, Gallemore G. Kernig's and Brudzinski's signs revisited. Rev Infect Dis. 1987;9:1187–92.

232. Swartz MN, Dodge PR. Bacterial meningitis—a review of selected aspects. I. General clinical features, special problems and unusual meningeal reactions mimicking bacterial meningitis. N Engl J Med. 1965;272:725–31.

233. Scheld WM. Meningococcal diseases. In: Warren KS, Mahmoud AAF, eds. Tropical and Geographical Medicine. 2nd ed. New York: McGraw-Hill; 1990; 798–814.

234. Geiseler PJ, Nelson KE. Bacterial meningitis without clinical signs of meningeal irritation. South Med J. 1982;75:448–50.

235. Gorse GJ, Thrupp LD, Nudleman KL, et al. Bacterial meningitis in the elderly. Arch Intern Med. 1984;149:1603–6.

236. Rubin RH, Hooper DC. Central nervous system infections in the compromised host. Med Clin North Am. 1985;69:281–93.

237. Armstrong D, Wong B. Central nervous system infections in immunocompromised hosts. Annu Rev Med. 1982;33:291–308.

238. George R, Leibrock L, Epstein M. Long-term analysis of cerebrospinal fluid shunt infections—A 25 year experience. J Neurosurg. 1979;51:804–11.

239. Schoenbaum SC, Gardner P, Shillito J. Infections of cerebrospinal fluid shunts: Epidemiology, clinical manifestations, and therapy. J Infect Dis. 1975;131:543–52.

240. Kaufman BA, McLone DG. Infections of cerebrospinal fluid shunts. In: Scheld WM, Whitley RJ, Durack DT, eds. Infections of the Central Nervous System. New York: Raven Press; 1991:561–85.

241. Forward KR, Fewer HD, Stiver HG. Cerebrospinal fluid shunt infections—A review of 35 infections in 32 patients. J Neurosurg. 1983;59:389–94.

242. Odio C, McCracken GH Jr, Nelson JD. CSF shunt infections in pediatrics. Am J Dis Child. 1984;138:1103–8.

243. Holmes MD, Zawadzki B, Simon RP. Clinical features of meningovascular syphilis. Neurology. 1984;34:553–5.

244. Johns DR, Tierney M, Felsenstein D. Alteration in the natural history of neurosyphilis by concurrent infection with the human immunodeficiency virus. N Engl J Med. 1987;316:1569–72.

245. Hutchinson CM, Rompalo AM, Reichart CA, et al. Characteristics of patients with syphilis attending Baltimore STD clinics: Multiple, high-risk subgroups and interactions with human immunodeficiency virus infection. Arch Intern Med. 1991;151:511–6.

246. Reik L, Burgdorfer W, Donaldson JO. Neurologic abnormalities in Lyme disease without erythema chronicum migrans. Am J Med. 1986;81:73–8.

247. Stiernstedt G, Gustafsson R, Karlsson M, et al. Clinical manifestations and diagnosis of neuroborreliosis. Ann NY Acad Sci. 1988;539:46–55.

248. Kuberski T, Wallace GD. Clinical manifestations of eosinophilic meningitis due to Angiostrongylus cantonensis. Neurology. 1979;29:1566–70.

249. Dagan R, Henista JA, Menegus MA. Association of clinical presentation, laboratory findings, and virus serotypes with the presence of meningitis in hospitalized infants with enterovirus infection. J Pediatr. 1988;113:975–8.

250. Wildin S, Chonmaitree T. The importance of the virology laboratory in the diagnosis and management of viral meningitis. Am J Dis Child. 1987;141:454–7.

251. Chonmaitree T, Baldwin CD, Lucia HL. Role of the virology laboratory in diagnosis and management of patients with central nervous system disease. Clin Microbiol Rev. 1989;2:1–14.

252. Lipson SM, Walderman R, Costello P, et al. Sensitivity of rhabdomyosarcoma and guinea pig embryo cell cultures to field isolates of difficult-to-cultivate group A coxsackieviruses. J Clin Microbiol. 1988;26:1298–303.

253. Johnson GM, McAbee GA, Seaton ED, et al. Suspect value of non-CSF viral cultures in the diagnosis of enteroviral CNS infections in young infants. Dev Med Child Neurol. 1992;34:876–84.

254. Glimaker M, Samuelson A, Magnius L, et al. Early diagnosis of enteroviral meningitis by detection of specific IgM antibodies with a solid-phase reverse immunosorbent test (SPRIST) and μ-capture EIA. J Med Virol. 1992;36:193–201.

255. Rotbart HA. Enzymatic RNA amplification of the enteroviruses. J Clin Microbiol. 1990;28:438–42.

256. Rotbart HA. Diagnosis of enteroviral meningitis with the polymerase chain reaction. J Pediatr. 1990;117:85–9.

257. Glimaker M, Abebe A, Johansson B, et al. Detection of enteroviral RNA by polymerase chain reaction in faecal samples from patients with aseptic meningitis. J Med Virol. 1992;38:54–61.

258. Ratzan KR. Viral meningitis. Med Clin North Am. 1985;69:399–413.

259. Rowley A, Lakeman F, Whitley R, et al. Diagnosis of herpes simplex encephalitis by DNA amplification of cerebrospinal fluid cells. Lancet. 1990;335:440–1.

260. Hollander H, Levy JA. Neurologic abnormalities and recovery of human immunodeficiency virus from cerebrospinal fluid. Ann Intern Med. 1987;106:692–5.

261. Chalmers AC, Aprill BS, Shephard H. Cerebrospinal fluid and human immunodeficiency virus. Findings in healthy, asymptomatic, seropositive men. Arch Intern Med. 1990;150:1538–40.

262. Feigin RD, McCracken GH Jr, Klein JO. Diagnosis and management of meningitis. Pediatr Infect Dis J. 1992;11:785–814.

263. Bonadio WA. The cerebrospinal fluid: Physiologic aspects and alterations associated with bacterial meningitis. Pediatr Infect Dis J. 1992;11:423–32.

264. Marton KI, Gean AD. The spinal tap: A new look at an old test. Ann Intern Med. 1986;104:840–8.

265. Spanos A, Harrell FE Jr, Durack DT. Differential diagnosis of acute meningitis. An analysis of the predictive value of initial observation. JAMA. 1989;262:2700–7.

266. Genton B, Berger JP. Cerebrospinal fluid lactate in 78 cases of adult meningitis. Intensive Care Med. 1990;16:196–200.

267. La Scolea LJ Jr, Dryja D. Quantitation of bacteria in cerebrospinal fluid and blood of children with meningitis and its diagnostic significance. J Clin Microbiol. 1984;19:187–90.

268. Greenlee JE. Approach to diagnosis of meningitis. Cerebrospinal fluid evaluation. Infect Dis Clin North Am. 1990;4:583–97.

269. Gray LD, Fedorko DP. Laboratory diagnosis of bacterial meningitis. Clin Microbiol Rev. 1992;5:130–45.

270. Kaplan SL, O'Brian Smith E, Wills C, et al. Association between preadmission oral antibiotic therapy and cerebrospinal fluid findings and sequelae caused by Haemophilus influenzae type b meningitis. Pediatr Infect Dis J. 1986;5:626–32.

271. Blazer S, Berant M, Alon U. Bacterial meningitis: Effect of antibiotic treatment on cerebrospinal fluid. Am J Clin Pathol. 1983;80:386–7.

272. Davis SD, Hill HR, Feigl P, et al. Partial antibiotic therapy in Haemophilus influenzae meningitis. Its effect on cerebrospinal fluid abnormalities. Am J Dis Child. 1975;129:802–7.

273. Kristiansen BE, Ask E, Jenkins A, et al. Rapid diagnosis of meningococcal meningitis by polymerase chain reaction. Lancet. 1991;337:1568–9.

274. Ni H, Knight AI, Cartwright K, et al. Polymerase chain reaction for diagnosis of meningococcal meningitis. Lancet. 1992;340:1432–4.

275. Jaton K, Sahli R, Bille J. Development of polymerase chain reaction assays for detection of Listeria monocytogenes in clinical cerebrospinal fluid samples. J Clin Microbiol. 1992;30:1931–6.

276. Friedland IR, Paris MM, Rinderknecht S, et al. Cranial computed tomographic scans have little impact on management of bacterial meningitis. Am J Dis Child. 1992;146:1484–7.

277. Hart G. Syphilis tests in diagnostic and therapeutic decision making. Ann Intern Med. 1986;104:368–76.

278. Davis LE, Schmitt JW. Clinical significance of cerebrospinal fluid tests for neurosyphilis. Ann Neurol. 1989;25:50–5.

279. Noordhoek GT, Wolters EC, de Jonge MEJ, van Embden JDA. Detection by polymerase chain reaction of *Treponema pallidum* DNA in cerebrospinal fluid from neurosyphilis patients before and after antibiotic treatment. J Clin Microbiol. 1991;29:1976–84.

280. Steere AC. Lyme disease. N Engl J Med. 1989;321:586–96.

281. Corpuz M, Hilton E, Lardis MP, et al. Problems in the use of serologic tests for the diagnosis of Lyme disease. Arch Intern Med. 1991;151:1837–40.

282. Keller TL, Halperin JJ, Whitman M. PCR detection of *Borrelia burgdorferi* DNA in cerebrospinal fluid of Lyme neuroborreliosis patients. Neurology. 1992;42:32–42.

283. Lebech AM, Hansen K. Detection of *Borrelia burgdorferi* DNA in urine samples and cerebrospinal fluid samples from patients with early and late Lyme neuroborreliosis by polymerase chain reaction. J Clin Microbiol. 1992; 30:1646–53.

284. Martinez AJ, Visvesvara GS. Laboratory diagnosis of pathogenic free-living amoebas: *Naegleria, Acanthamoeba,* and *Leptomyxid*. Clin Lab Med. 1991; 11:861–72.

285. Tunkel AR, Scheld WM. Therapy of bacterial meningitis: Principles and practice. Infect Cont Hosp Epidemiol. 1989;10:565–9.

286. Tunkel AR, Scheld WM. Acute therapy of bacterial meningitis. J Intensive Care Med. 1991;6:229–37.

287. Coant PN, Kornberg AE, Duffy LC, et al. Blood culture results as determinants in the organism identification of bacterial meningitis. Pediatr Emerg Care. 1992;8:200–5.

288. McGowan JE Jr, Chesney PJ, Crossley KB, et al. Guidelines for the use of systemic gluocorticoids in the management of selected infections. J Infect Dis. 1992;165:1–13.

289. Volberding PA, Lagakos SW, Koch MA, et al. Zidovudine in asymptomatic human immunodeficiency virus infection. A controlled trial in persons with fewer than 500 CD4-positive cells per cubic millimeter. N Engl J Med. 1990; 322:941–9.

290. Tunkel AR, Scheld WM. Applications of therapy in animal models to bacterial infection in human disease. Infect Dis Clin North Am. 1989;3:441–59.

291. Scheld WM, Sande MA. Bactericidal versus bacteriostatic antibiotic therapy of experimental pneumococcal meningitis in rabbits. J Clin Invest. 1983;71: 411–9.

292. Täuber MG, Sande MA. General principles of therapy of pyogenic meningitis. Infect Dis Clin North Am. 1990;4:661–76.

293. Lebel MH, McCracken GH Jr. Delayed cerebrospinal fluid sterilization and adverse outcome of bacterial meningitis in infants and children. Pediatrics. 1989;83:161–7.

294. Campos J, Garcia-Tornel S, Sanfeliu I. Susceptibility studies of multiply resistant *Haemophilus influenzae* isolated from pediatric patients and contacts. Antimicrob Agents Chemother. 1984;25:706–9.

295. Campos J, Garcia-Tornel S, Gairi JM, et al. Multiply resistant *Haemophilus influenzae* type b causing meningitis: Comparative clinical and laboratory study. J Pediatr. 1986;108:897–902.

296. Givner LB, Abramson JS, Wasilauskas B. Meningitis due to *Haemophilus influenzae* type b resistant to ampicillin and chloramphenicol. Rev Infect Dis. 1989;11:329–34.

297. Peltola J, Anttila M, Renkonen OV, The Finnish Study Group. Randomised comparison of chloramphenicol, ampicillin, cefotaxime, and ceftriaxone for childhood bacterial meningitis. Lancet. 1989;1:1281–7.

298. McCracken GH Jr. Current management of bacterial meningitis in infants and children. Pediatr Infect Dis J. 1992;11:169–74.

299. del Rio M, Chrane D, Shelton S, et al. Ceftriaxone versus ampicillin and chloramphenicol for treatment of bacterial meningitis in children. Lancet. 1983;1:1241–4.

300. Jacobs RF, Wells TG, Steele RW, et al. A prospective randomized comparison of cefotaxime vs ampicillin and chloramphenicol for bacterial meningitis in children. J Pediatr. 1985;107:129–33.

301. American Academy of Pediatrics Committee on Infectious Diseases. Treatment of bacterial meningitis. Pediatrics. 1988;81:904–7.

302. Marks WA, Stutman HR, Marks MI, et al. Cefuroxime versus ampicillin plus chloramphenicol in childhood bacterial meningitis: A multicenter randomized controlled trial. J Pediatr. 1986;109:123–30.

303. Lebel MH, Hoyt MJ, McCracken GH Jr. Comparative efficacy of ceftriaxone and cefuroxime for treatment of bacterial meningitis. J Pediatr. 1989;114: 1049–54.

304. Schaad UB, Suter S, Gianella-Borradori A, et al. A comparison of ceftriaxone and cefuroxime for the treatment of bacterial meningitis in children. N Engl J Med. 1990;322:141–7.

305. Arditi M, Herold BC, Yogev R. Cefuroxime treatment failure and *Haemophilus influenzae* meningitis: Case report and review of the literature. Pediatrics. 1989;84:132–5.

306. Mendelman PM, Chaffin DO, Krilov LR, et al. Cefuroxime treatment failure of nontypable *Haemophilus influenzae* meningitis associated with alteration of penicillin-binding proteins. J Infect Dis. 1990;212:1118–23.

307. Hatch DL, Overturf GD. Delayed cerebrospinal fluid sterilization in infants with *Haemophilus influenzae* type b meningitis. J Infect Dis. 1989;160:711–5.

308. Jorgensen JH. Update on mechanisms and prevalence of antimicrobial resistance in *Haemophilus influenzae*. Clin Infect Dis. 1992;14:1119–23.

309. Campos J, Mendelman PN, Sako MU, et al. Detection of relatively penicillin G-resistant *Neisseria meningitidis* by disk susceptibility testing. Antimicrob Agents Chemother. 1987;31:1478–82.

310. Van Esso D, Fontanals D, Uriz S, et al. *Neisseria meningitidis* with decreased susceptibility to penicillin. Pediatr Infect Dis. 1987;6:438–9.

311. Jones DM, Sutcliffe EM. Meningococci with reduced susceptibility to penicillin. Lancet. 1990;335:863–4.

312. Saez-Nieto JA, Lujan R, Berron S, et al. Epidemiology and molecular basis of penicillin-resistant *Neisseria meningitidis* in Spain: A 5-year history (1985–1989). Clin Infect Dis. 1992;14:394–402.

313. Mendelman PM, Campos J, Chaffin DO, et al. Relatively penicillin G resistance in *Neisseria meningitidis* and reduced affinity of penicillin-binding protein 3. Antimicrob Agents Chemother. 1988;32:706–9.

314. Trallero EP, Garcia Arenzana JM, et al. Comparative activity in vitro of 16 antimicrobial agents against penicillin-susceptible meningococci and meningococci with diminished susceptibility to penicillin. Antimicrob Agents Chemother. 1989;33:1622–3.

315. Dillon JR, Pauze M, Yeung KH. Spread of penicillinase-producing and transfer plasmids form the gonococcus to *Neisseria meningitidis*. Lancet. 1983; 1:779–81.

316. Fenoll A, Bourgon CM, Munoz R, et al. Serotype distribution and antimicrobial resistance of *Streptococcus pneumoniae* isolates causing systemic infections in Spain, 1979–1989. Rev Infect Dis. 1991;13:56–60.

317. Garcia-Leoni ME, Cerenado E, Rodeno P, et al. Susceptibility of *Streptococcus pneumoniae* to penicillin: A prospective microbiological and clinical study. Clin Infect Dis. 1992;14:427–35.

318. Mason EO Jr, Kaplan SL, Lamberth LB, et al. Increased rate of isolation of penicillin-resistant *Streptococcus pneumoniae* in a children's hospital and in vitro susceptibilities to antibiotics of potential therapeutic use. Antimicrob Agents Chemother. 1992;36:1703–7.

319. Marton A, Gulyas M, Munoz R, et al. Extremely high incidence of antibiotic resistance in clinical isolates of *Streptococcus pneumoniae* in Hungary. J Infect Dis. 1991;163:542–8.

320. Appelbaum PC. Antimicrobial resistance in *Streptococcus pneumoniae:* An overview. Clin Infect Dis. 1992;15:77–83.

321. Caputo GM, Appelbaum PC, Liu HH. Infections due to penicillin-resistant pneumococci. Clinical, epidemiologic, and microbiologic features. Arch Intern Med. 1993;153:1301–10.

322. Klugman KP. Pneumococcal resistance to antibiotics. Clin Microbiol Rev. 1990;3:171–96.

323. McDougal LK, Facklam R, Reeves M, et al. Analysis of multiply antimicrobial-resistant isolates of *Streptococcus pneumoniae* from the United States. Antimicrob Agents Chemother. 1992;36:2176–84.

324. Friedland IR, Istre GR. Management of penicillin-resistant pneumococcal infections. Pediatr Infect Dis J. 1992;11:433–5.

325. Tan TQ, Mason EO Jr, Kaplan SL. Systemic infections due to *Streptococcus pneumoniae* relatively resistant to penicillin in a children's hospital: clinical management and outcome. Pediatrics. 1992;90:928–33.

326. Viladrich PF, Gudiol F, Linares J, et al. Characteristics and antibiotic therapy of adult meningitis due to penicillin-resistant pneumococci. Am J Med. 1988;84:839–46.

327. Bradley JS, Connor JD. Ceftriaxone failure in meningitis caused by *Streptococcus pneumoniae* with reduced susceptibility to beta-lactam antibiotics. Pediatr Infect Dis J. 1991;10:871–3.

328. Tenover FC, Swenson JM, McDougal LK. Screening for extended-spectrum cephalosporin resistance in pneumococci. Lancet. 1992;340:1420.

329. Sloas MM, Barrett FF, Chesney PJ, et al. Cephalosporin treatment failure in penicillin- and cephalosporin-resistant *Streptococcus pneumoniae* meningitis. Pediatr Infect Dis J. 1992;11:622–6.

330. Figueiredo AMS, Connon JD, Severin A, et al. A pneumococcal clinical isolate with high-level resistance to cefotaxime and ceftriaxone. Antimicrob Agents Chemother. 1992;36:886–9.

331. Friedland IR, Shelton S, Paris M, et al. Dilemmas in diagnosis and management of cephalosporin-resistant *Streptococcus pneumoniae* meningitis. Pediatr Infect Dis J. 1993;12:196–200.

332. Friedland IR, Klugman KP. Antibiotic-resistant pneumococcal disease in South African children. Am J Dis Child. 1992;146:920–3.

333. Friedland IR, Klugman KP. Failure of chloramphenicol therapy in penicillin-resistant pneumococcal meningitis. Lancet. 1992;339:405–8.

334. Viladrich PF, Gudiol F, Linares J, et al. Evaluation of vancomycin for therapy of adult pneumococcal meningitis. Antimicrob Agents Chemother. 1991; 35:2467–72.

335. Pelser HH. Meropenem or cephalosporins for bacterial meningitis. In: Program and Abstracts of the 18th International Congress of Chemotherapy. June–July 1993.

336. Levitz RE, Quintiliani R. Trimethoprim-sulfamethoxazole for bacterial meningitis. Ann Intern Med. 1984;100:881–90.

337. Richards SJ, Lambert CM, Scott AC. Recurrent *Listeria monocytogenes* meningitis treated with intraventricular vancomycin. J Antimicrob Chemother. 1992;29:351–3.

338. Scheld WM. Evaluation of rifampin and other antibiotics against *Listeria monocytogenes* in vitro and in vivo. Rev Infect Dis. 1983;5:S593–9.

339. Nairn K, Shepard G, Turner PJ, et al. Evidence of the activity of meropenem in a model of experimental meningitis caused by *Listeria monocytogenes* (Abstract 814). In: Program and Abstracts of the 6th European Congress of Clinical Microbiology and Infectious Diseases. March 1993.

340. Cherubin CE, Eng RHK, Norrby R, et al. Penetration of newer cephalosporins into cerebrospinal fluid. Rev Infect Dis. 1989;11:526–48.

341. Kaplan SL, Patrick CC. Cefotaxime and aminoglycoside treatment of meningitis caused by gram-negative enteric organisms. Pediatr Infect Dis J. 1990; 9:810–4.

342. Cherubin CE, Corrado ML, Nair SR, et al. Treatment of gram-negative bacillary meningitis: Role of the new cephalosporin antibiotics. Rev Infect Dis. 1982;4:S453–64.

343. Landesman SH, Corrado ML, Shah PM, et al. Past and current roles of cephalosporin antibiotics in treatment of meningitis. Emphasis on use in gram-negative bacillary meningitis. Am J Med. 1981;71:693–703.

344. Fong IW, Tomkins KB. Review of *Pseudomonas aeruginosa* meningitis with special emphasis on treatment with ceftazidime. Rev Infect Dis. 1985;7: 604–12.

345. Rodriguez WJ, Khan WN, Cocchetto DM, et al. Treatment of *Pseudomonas* meningitis with ceftazidime with or without concurrent therapy. Pediatr Infect Dis J. 1990;9:83–7.

346. McCracken GH Jr, Mize SG, Threlkeld N. Intraventricular gentamicin therapy in gram-negative bacillary meningitis of infancy: Report of the second neonatal meningitis cooperative study group. Lancet. 1980;1:787–91.

347. Kilpatrick M, Girgis N, Farid Z, et al. Aztreonam for treating meningitis caused by gram-negative rods. Scand J Infect Dis. 1991;23:125–6.

348. Rodriguez K, Dickinson GM, Greenman RL. Successful treatment of gram-negative bacillary meningitis with imipenem/cilastatin. South Med J. 1985; 78:732–3.

349. Wong VK. Wright HT Jr, Ross LA, et al. Imipenem/cilastatin treatment of bacterial meningitis in children. Pediatr Infect Dis J. 1991;10:122–5.

350. Donnelly JP, Horrevorts AM, Sauerwein RW, et al. High-dose meropenem in meningitis due to *Pseudomonas aeruginosa*. Lancet. 1992;339:1117.

351. Tunkel AR, Scheld WM. Treatment of bacterial meningitis. In: Wolfson JS, Hooper DC, eds. Quinolone Antimicrobial Agents. Washington, DC: American Society for Microbiology; 1993:481–95.

352. Cruciani M, Navarra A, Di Perri G, et al. Evaluation of intraventricular teicoplanin for the treatment of neurosurgical shunt infections. Clin Infect Dis. 1992;15:285–9.

353. Radetsky M. Duration of treatment in bacterial meningitis: A historical inquiry. Pediatr Infect Dis J. 1990;9:2–9.

354. O'Neill P. How long to treat bacterial meningitis. Lancet. 1993;341:530.

355. Jadavji T, Biggar WD, Gold R, et al. Sequelae of acute bacterial meningitis in children treated for seven days. Pediatrics. 1985;78:21–5.

356. Lin TY, Chrane DF, Nelson JD, et al. Seven days of ceftriaxone therapy is as effective as ten days' treatment for bacterial meningitis. JAMA. 1985;253: 3559–63.

357. Viladrich PF, Pallares R, Ariza J, et al. Four days of penicillin therapy for meningococcal meningitis. Arch Intern Med. 1986;146:2380–2.

358. Marra CM, Slatter V, Tartaglione TA, et al. Evaluation of aqueous penicillin G and ceftriaxone for experimental neurosyphilis. J Infect Dis. 1991;165: 396–7.

359. Dowell ME, Ross PG, Musher DM, et al. Response of latent syphilis or neurosyphilis to ceftriaxone therapy in persons infected with human immunodeficiency virus. Am J Med. 1992;93:481–8.

360. Hook EW III. Management of syphilis in human immunodeficiency virus-infected patients. Am J Med. 1992;93:477–9.

361. Kohlhepp W, Oschmann P, Mertens HG. Treatment of Lyme borreliosis: Randomized comparison of doxycycline and penicillin G. J Neurol. 1989; 236:464–9.

362. Dattwyler RJ, Halperin JJ, Volkman DJ, et al. Treatment of late Lyme borreliosis—randomised comparison of ceftriaxone and penicillin. Lancet. 1988; 1:1191–4.

363. Dotevall L, Hagberg L. Penetration of doxycycline into cerebrospinal fluid in patients treated for suspected Lyme neuroborreliosis. Antimicrob Agents Chemother. 1989;33:1078–80.

364. Sischel JS, Harmatz P, Visvesvara GS, et al. Successful treatment of primary amebic meningoencephalitis. N Engl J Med. 1982;306:346–8.

365. Brown RL. Successful treatment of primary amebic meningoencephalitis. Arch Intern Med. 1991;151:1201–2.

366. Tuomanen E, Hengstler B, Rich R, et al. Nonsteroidal anti-inflammatory agents in the therapy for experimental pneumococcal meningitis. J Infect Dis. 1987;155:985–90.

367. Tureen JH, Täuber MG, Sande MA. Effect of indomethacin on the pathophysiology of experimental meningitis in rabbits. J Infect Dis. 1991;163: 647–9.

368. Kadurugamuwa JL, Hengstler B, Zak O. Cerebrospinal fluid protein profile in experimental pneumococcal meningitis and its alteration by ampicillin and anti-inflammatory agents. J Infect Dis. 1989;159:26–34.

369. Nolan CM, McAllister CK, Walters E, et al. Experimental pneumococcal meningitis. IV. The effect of methylprednisolone on meningeal inflammation. J Lab Clin Invest. 1978;91:979–88.

370. Syrogiannopoulos GA, Olsen KD, Reisch JS, et al. Dexamethasone in the treatment of experimental *Haemophilus influenzae* type b meningitis. J Infect Dis. 1987;155:213–9.

371. Mustafa MM, Ramilo O, Mertsola J, et al. Modulation of inflammation and cachectin activity in relation to treatment of experimental *Haemophilus influenzae* type b meningitis. J Infect Dis. 1989;160:818–25.

372. Lebel MH, Freij BJ, Syrogiannopoulos GA, et al. Dexamethasone therapy for bacterial meningitis. Results of two double-blind, placebo-controlled trials. N Engl J Med. 1988;319:964–71.

373. Lebel MH, Hoyt MJ, Waagner DC, et al. Magnetic resonance imaging and dexamethasone therapy for bacterial meningitis. Am J Dis Child. 1989;143: 301–6.

374. Girgis NI, Farid Z, Mikhail IA, et al. Dexamethasone treatment for bacterial meningitis in children and adults. Pediatr Infect Dis J. 1989;8:848–51.

375. Odio CM, Faingezicht I, Paris M, et al. The beneficial effects of early dexamethasone administration in infants and children with bacterial meningitis. N Engl J Med. 1991;324:1525–31.

376. Kennedy WA, Hoyt MJ, McCracken GH Jr. The role of corticosteroid therapy in children with pneumococcal meningitis. Am J Dis Child. 1991;145: 1374–8.

377. Geiman BJ, Smith AL. Dexamethasone and bacterial meningitis. A meta-analysis of randomized controlled trials. West J Med. 1992;157:27–31.

378. Gary N, Powers N, Todd JK. Clinical identification and comparative prognosis of high-risk patients with *Haemophilus influenzae* meningitis. Am J Dis Child. 1989;143:307–11.

379. Sullivan GW, Carper HT, Novick WJ Jr, et al. Inhibition of the inflammatory action of interleukin-1 and tumor necrosis factor (alpha) on neutrophil function by pentoxifylline. Infect Immun. 1988;56:1722–9.

380. Chao CC, Hu S, Close K, et al. Cytokine release from microglia: Differential inhibition by pentoxifylline and dexamethiasone. J Infect Dis. 1992;166: 847–53.

381. Saez-Llorens X, Ramilo O, Mustafa MM, et al. Pentoxifylline modulates meningeal inflammation in experimental bacterial meningitis. Antimicrob Agents Chemother. 1990;34:837–43.

382. Saez-Llorens X, Jafari HS, Severien C, et al. Enhanced attenuation of meningeal inflammation and brain edema by concomitant administration of anti-CD18 monoclonal antibodies and dexamethasone in experimental *Haemophilus* meningitis. J Clin Invest. 1991;88:2003–11.

383. Dacey RG. Monitoring and treating increased intracranial pressure. Pediatr Infect Dis J. 1987;6:1161–3.

384. Lyons MK, Meyer FB. Cerebrospinal fluid physiology and the management of increased intracranial pressure. Mayo Clin Proc. 1990;65:684–707.

385. Roos KL, Scheld WM. The management of fulminant meningitis in the intensive care unit. Crit Care Med. 1988;4:375–92.

386. Colville A, Pugh S. Mumps meningitis and measles, mumps, and rubella vaccine. Lancet. 1992;340:786.

387. Forsey T, Bentley ML, Minor PD, et al. Mumps vaccines and meningitis. Lancet. 1992;340:980.

388. Ward JI, Fraser DW, Baraff LJ, et al. *Haemophilus influenzae* meningitis: A national study of secondary spread in household contacts. N Engl J Med. 1979;301:122–6.

389. Band JD. Chemoprophylaxis of *Haemophilus influenzae* type b disease: A strategy for preventing secondary cases. In: Sell SH, Wright PF, eds. *Haemophilus influenzae:* Epidemiology, Immunology, and Prevention of Disease. New York: Elsevier Science Publishing Company; 1982:309–15.

390. Peter G. Treatment and prevention of *Haemophilus influenzae* type b meningitis. Pediatr Infect Dis J. 1987;6:787–90.

391. Lieberman JM, Greenberg DP, Ward JI. Prevention of bacterial meningitis. Vaccines and chemoprophylaxis. Infect Dis Clin North Am. 1990;4:703–29.

392. Green M, Li KI, Wald ER, et al. Duration of rifampin chemoprophylaxis for contacts of patients infected with *Haemophilus influenzae* type b. Antimicrob Agents Chemother. 1992;36:545–7.

393. Schwartz B, Al-Tobaiqi A, Al-Ruwais A, et al. Comparative efficacy of ceftriaxone and rifampicin in eradicating pharyngeal carriage of group A *Neisseria meningitidis*. Lancet. 1988;1:1239–42.

394. Darouiche R, Perkins B, Musher D, et al. Levels of rifampin and ciprofloxacin in nasal secretions: Correlation with MIC$_{90}$ and eradication of nasopharyngeal carriage of bacteria. J Infect Dis. 1990;162:1124–7.

395. Rauch AM, O'Ryan M, Van R, et al. Invasive disease due to multiply resistant *Streptococcus pneumoniae* in a Houston, Tex, day-care center. Am J Dis Child. 1990;144:923–7.

396. Gaston MH, Verter JI, Woods G, et al. Prophylaxis with oral penicillin in children with sickle cell anemia. A randomized trial. N Engl J Med. 1986; 314:1593–9.

397. Zangwill KM, Schuchat A, Wenger JD, Group B Streptococcal Disease Study Group. Group B streptococcal disease in the United States, 1990: Report from a multistate active surveillance system. MMWR. 1992;41:25–32.

398. Committee on Infectious Diseases, Committee on Fetus and Newborn. Guidelines for prevention of group B streptococcal (GBS) infection by chemoprophylaxis. Pediatrics. 1992;90:775–8.

399. Eskola J, Käyhty H, Takala AK, et al. A randomized, prospective field trial of a conjugate vaccine in the protection of infants and young children against invasive *Haemophilus influenzae* type b disease. N Engl J Med. 1990;323: 1381–7.

400. Santosham M, Wolff M, Reid R, et al. The efficacy in Navajo infants of a conjugate vaccine consisting of *Haemophilus influenzae* type b polysaccharide and *Neisseria meningitidis* outer-membrane protein complex. N Engl J Med. 1991;324:1767–72.

401. Immunization Practices Advisory Committee. *Haemophilus* b conjugate vaccines for prevention of *Haemophilus influenzae* type b disease among infants and children two months of age and older. MMWR. 1991;40:1–7.

402. Bjune G, Hoiby EA, Gronnesby JK, et al. Effect of outer membrane vesicle vaccine against group B meningococcal disease in Norway. Lancet. 1991; 338:1093–6.

403. Immunization Practices Advisory Committee. Update on adult immunization. MMWR. 1991;40:1–94.

65. CHRONIC MENINGITIS

BARBARA M. GRIPSHOVER
JERROLD J. ELLNER

A large number of infectious and noninfectious diseases can cause the clinical syndrome of chronic meningitis (Tables 1 and 2). The onset of symptoms in such cases typically is subacute to chronic with signs of meningoencephalitis such as fever, headache, lethargy, confusion, nausea, vomiting, and stiff neck. Cerebrospinal fluid (CSF) is abnormal with elevated protein concentrations, a pleocytosis that usually is predominantly lymphocytic, and sometimes a low glucose level. The major difficulty during initial evaluation is in distinguishing the rare patient with chronic meningitis from individuals with the more common syndromes of acute meningitis and encephalitis. If the neurologic symptoms and signs either persist or progress clinically and the CSF remains abnormal for a period of at least 4 weeks, the diagnosis of chronic meningitis is appropriate.[1–5] The diagnosis of chronic meningitis has a number of implications; particularly important are those that relate to etiology, management, and prognosis. This duration of symptoms was derived empirically to optimize the distinction between patients with chronic progressive disease and those with self-limited processes. In practice, patients frequently are seen by a physician within 1–4 weeks of the onset of symptoms. Prompt diagnosis and institution of appropriate treatment, therefore, may abort the neurologic process before the criteria for chronic meningitis are fulfilled.

Central nervous system (CNS) involvement by most diseases causing chronic meningitis has a high morbidity and mortality. Successful intervention requires the early administration of specific, often potentially toxic forms of therapy. Furthermore, drugs appropriate for treating one cause of chronic meningitis may be contraindicated in others. Therefore, a precise etiologic diagnosis is critical in modifying the course of this syndrome, and broad empirical therapeutic regimens are a poor and sometimes hazardous substitute. Whereas exact diagnosis may prove difficult (one-third of cases in a retrospective series of 87 patients with chronic meningitis were undiagnosed),[4] certain aspects of the presentation can be helpful in determining causality or at least in limiting the differential diagnosis.

HISTORY

The exposure history may be important in suggesting certain infectious diseases such as tuberculosis, coccidioidomycosis, histoplasmosis, brucellosis, cysticercosis, syphilis, Lyme disease, and especially acquired immunodeficiency syndrome (AIDS) with its distinctive spectrum of pathogens. The exposure history should direct the evaluation to include specific serologic studies and other diagnostic tests. The presence of HIV infection significantly alters the differential diagnosis, so HIV testing should be done on all patients with chronic meningitis.

The history also is of importance in distinguishing chronic meningitis from two superficially similar syndromes, acute meningitis or encephalitis with a protracted recovery and recurrent meningitis. In chronic meningitis, onset is insidious and symptoms chronic, although they may wax and wane. Episodes of acute neurologic deterioration sometimes punctuate the clinical course and may be caused by cerebral edema, hydrocephalus, cerebrovascular occlusions, and seizures. Even when symptoms temporarily regress, CSF abnormalities persist and reflect continued disease activity. In the protracted recovery period that sometimes follows pyogenic or aseptic meningitis and viral encephalitis, actual progression of disease is confined to the acute stages of the illness; clearing of the signs, symptoms, and CSF abnormalities, although gradual, may occur during observation. The second syndrome that must be differentiated from chronic meningitis is recurrent meningitis.[6,7] Patients with recurrent meningitis usually have repeated episodes of acute disease followed by symptom-free periods during which signs and symptoms are absent and the CSF is normal (Table 3).

The history also is important in defining the cause of meningitis in those instances in which CNS extension typically occurs as a late manifestation of a previously diagnosed systemic disease. These conditions include acute leukemia, lymphoma, blastomycosis, and Behçet's disease.

PHYSICAL EXAMINATION

Diagnostic physical findings are rare. However, physical examination may delineate signs of an associated systemic disease that provide a potential source of rapid diagnosis. Skin lesions, although infrequent, are particularly important for their diagnostic value. Even benign-appearing superficial lesions, subcutaneous nodules and abscesses, or draining sinuses should be cultured and biopsy specimens obtained. Among the causes of chronic meningitis that are notable for presenting with skin le-

TABLE 1. Infectious Diseases That May Be Manifest as Chronic Meningitis: Usual Presentation in the CNS

Meningitis	Focal CNS Lesions	Encephalitis
Acanthamoeba	Actinomycosis	African trypanosomiasis
Angiostrongylus cantonensis	Blastomycosis	Cytomegalovirus
	Coenurosis	Enterovirus (in patients with hypogammaglobulinemia)
Brucellosis	Cysticercosis	
Candidiasis	Molds: aspergillosis,	Measles (SSPE)
Coccidioidomycosis	phaeohyphomycosis,	Rabies
Cryptococcosis	pseudallescheriasis	Viral encephalitis
Histoplasmosis	Nocardiosis	(see Ch. 66)
Lyme disease	Schistosomiasis	
Sporotrichosis	Toxoplasmosis	
Syphilis		
Tuberculosis		

TABLE 2. Noninfectious Causes of Chronic Meningitis

Behcet's disease	Neoplasm
Chronic benign lymphocytic meningitis	Sarcoidosis
Chronic meningitis of unknown etiology	Uveomeningoencephalitis
Granulomatous angiitis	

TABLE 3. Differential Diagnosis of Recurrent Meningitis

Drug-induced (with rechallenge)[8,9]
Parameningeal focus
  Infection (sinusitis, mastoiditis, osteomyelitis, brain abscess)
  Tumor (epidermoid cyst, craniopharyngioma)
Post-traumatic (bacterial)
Mollaret's meningitis[6,7]
Systemic lupus erythematosus

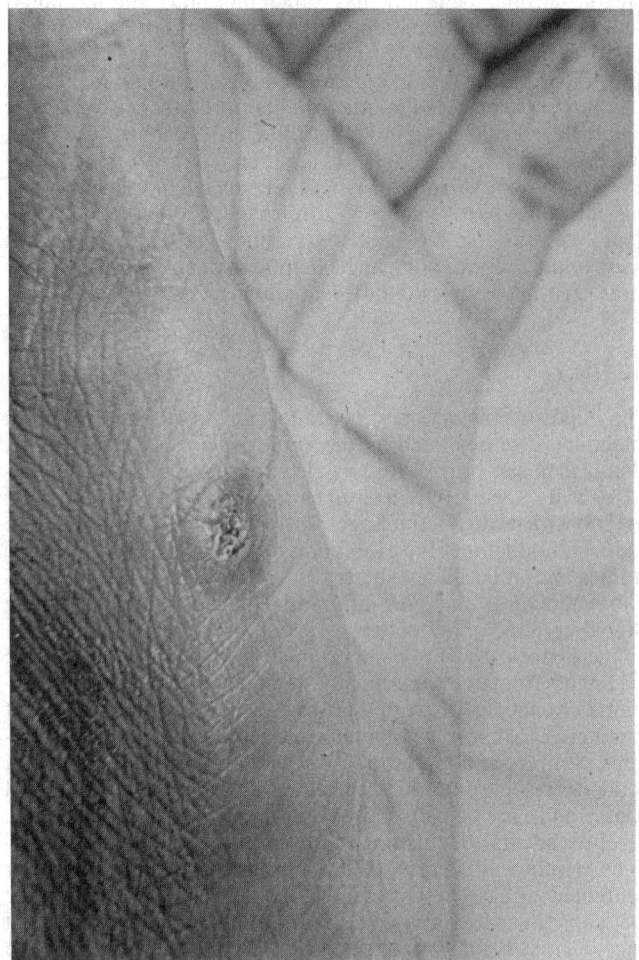

FIG. 1. Skin lesion of a woman with chronic lymphocytic leukemia treated with corticosteroids and cytotoxic drugs, admitted with chronic meningitis. Material expressed from lesion was positive on India ink preparation and culture for *Cryptococcus neoformans*.

sions, one can list cryptococcosis (Fig. 1), sarcoidosis, *Acanthamoeba*, coccidioidomycosis, blastomycosis, and secondary syphilis, as well as the subcutaneous nodules of cysticercosis and metastatic carcinoma (breast, melanoma, etc.) India ink preparations also should be made from expressed material. The eye examination may be helpful if such lesions as choroidal tubercles, sarcoid granulomas, or uveitis are demonstrable. The finding of papilledema also is of significance, since it alters the course of the neurologic work-up and contraindicates lumbar puncture. Hepatomegaly may reflect systemic disease involving the liver and increases the potential diagnostic yield of a liver biopsy.

Neurologic examination is of obvious importance in delineating the extent of CNS involvement. However, it is of limited use in differentiating among specific etiologies, since mental status changes, meningismus, oculomotor palsies, and, less frequently, focal findings, evidence of increased intracranial pressure, and spinal cord signs may be caused by most processes associated with chronic meningitis. Focal signs, however, often reflect a parenchymal mass such as an abscess or granuloma that would dictate specific diagnostic and therapeutic maneuvers. Involvement of multiple levels of the neuraxis is suggestive of meningeal carcinomatosis. Hydrocephalus may complicate chronic meningitis, and appropriate neuroradiographic evaluation should be initiated when the constellation of headache, nausea, vomiting, mental changes, ataxia, incontinence, and papilledema is present. The finding of hydrocephalus, particularly

with associated cranial neuropathies, is suggestive of an infectious etiology with basilar leptomeningitis, although hydrocephalus also may complicate sarcoidosis and CNS tumor. Peripheral neuropathy is noted uncommonly in chronic meningitis and is suggestive of sarcoidosis or Lyme disease.

LABORATORY EVALUATION

The etiology of chronic meningitis ultimately must be established in the laboratory (Table 4). Abnormalities on chest x-ray films may reflect systemic involvement by the underlying infectious process, carcinoma, or sarcoidosis. These findings should be pursued in an attempt to define the etiology of the meningitis. In more enigmatic cases, biopsy of lung lesions may be indicated and is associated with less morbidity and greater yield than is a brain biopsy.

The CSF formula is never itself diagnostic. However, certain abnormalities and patterns are more characteristic of a restricted group of causes of chronic meningitis (Table 5).

Lumbar puncture needs to be repeated periodically both for culture and to follow the course of meningeal inflammation. India ink preparations should be made from the sediment of 3–5 ml of CSF. The entire slide must be examined, since cryptococci may be present in small numbers. As opposed to artifacts that are seen commonly, encapsulated yeast has a regular, round, distinct capsule and a refractile central structure; budding yeast forms also may be found. The India ink preparation is more likely to be positive in patients with relatively acute presentations and/or immunosuppressed patients with lymphoma or AIDS. In the latter setting, yeast organisms often far outnumber leukocytes in the CSF. Cerebrospinal fluid cytologic studies are indicated in all patients with chronic meningitis. Multiple specimens may be necessary for the diagnosis of CNS involvement by tumor, and negative cytologic studies do not preclude this possibility.[12] The demonstration of a clonal origin of CSF lymphocytes using B- and T-cell immunologic markers also is useful in the diagnosis of lymphomatous meningitis[13,14]; consultation with the hospital hematopathologist is useful.

Serologic studies of serum and CSF are extremely important in evaluating the patient for coccidioidomycosis, cryptococco-

TABLE 4. Evaluation of Patients with Chronic Meningitis

Initial evaluation of all patients

  History: travel to Southwestern USA, developing countries, or tropical Africa; new sexual partner, high-risk activity for HIV, household member with tuberculosis, brucellosis exposure such as meat packing, intravenous drug abuse, skin lesion resembling erythema migrans, childhood measles, monkey handler

  Physical examination: complete examination, including search for skin lesions or subcutaneous nodules; ocular examination for retinal lesions, papilledema, uveitis or iritis; lymphadenopathy; hepatosplenomegaly; neurologic examination

  Laboratory tests: complete blood count with differential and sedimentation rate; liver and renal function; PPD; chest x-ray; MRI with gadolinium enhancement or CT (with special attention for parameningeal foci in paranasal sinus or mastoids, intracerebral lesions, ependymoma, and hydrocephalus); blood culture for fungi and mycobacteria by lysis centrifugation; urine culture for fungi and mycobacteria; serology for HIV, syphilis, cryptococcal antigen, and ANA; lumbar puncture for opening pressure, WBC, protein, glucose (simultaneous blood glucose), cytospin cytology, VDRL, cryptococcal antigen, India ink, acid-fast stain, and large volume (3–5 cc) cultures each for fungus and mycobacteria

Tests indicated by appropriate exposure history

  Serum serology for antibody to *Histoplasma*, *Coccidioides*, *Brucella*, and *Borrelia burgdorferi* (Lyme); *Histoplasma* antigen

  CSF antibody to *Histoplasma*, *Coccidioides*, *Taenia solium* (cysticercosis), and measles virus; *Histoplasma* antigen; stain CSF WBC for eosinophils; *Brucella* culture; blood smear for trypanosomes

Enigmatic cases

  Repeat PPD in 2–4 weeks; serum immunoglobulins and angiotensin-converting enzyme; CSF for antibody to *Sporothrix*; enteroviral culture (if low serum IgG), repeat cytology and lymphocyte markers.[a] Consider brain biopsy for diffuse carcinomatosis or gliomatosis, *Acanthamoeba*, or mold infections. PCR assays for increasing number of agents (CMV, Lyme, echovirus, etc) are available in research laboratories

[a] To assess for clonality: B- and T-cell immunologic markers such as light chain (κ and λ); immunoglobulin subclasses, CD20 (B cell markers) and CD3, CD43, and CD45RO (T-cell markers).

TABLE 5. CSF Characteristics of Various Causes of Chronic Meningitis

Pleocytosis <50 cells/μl	Neutrophilic Pleocytosis[10]	Eosinophilic Pleocytosis	Low Glucose
Behcet's disease	Bacteria	Chemical	Bacteria
Benign lymphocytic meningitis	*Actinomyces*	Coccidioides	*Actinomyces*
Carcinoma	*Nocardia*	Lymphoma	*Nocardia*
Cryptococcus in HIV-infected patients	Chemical	Parasites	Carcinoma
Sarcoidosis	CMV in HIV-infected	Angiostrongylus	Cysticercus
Vasculitis	Early *Mycobacterium* tuberculosis	Cysticercus	Fungi (all)
	Fungi	Schistosoma	*Mycobacterium* tuberculosis
	Aspergillus		Postsubarachnoid hemorrhage
	Candida		Sarcoidosis
	Systemic lupus erythematosus		Syphilis
			Toxoplasma
			Viral
			Chronic enterovirus
			CMV in HIV-infected

sis, and syphilis and should be performed routinely. In the case of cryptococcal meningitis, testing for cryptococcal polysaccharide antigen is helpful; testing for antibody is not useful. Serum antibodies to *Brucella* and *Toxoplasma* also may suggest these infections when they are present in high or increasing titers. Serum antibodies to *Histoplasma* are found in 60 percent of patients with *Histoplasma* meningitis.[15] Complement-fixing antibodies to *Histoplasma* are found in the CSF of most patients with CNS histoplasmosis, but the test lacks specificity.[16,17] The EIA for antibody to *Sporothrix schenckii* in CSF has also been useful, though the disease rarely causes meningitis. More promising is the detection of *H. capsulatum* antigen in serum, urine, or CSF by radioimmunoassay.[15,18] Similarly, demonstration of tuberculostearic acid (a component of *Mycobacterium*) in CSF is said to be indicative of tuberculous meningitis.[19,20]

Skin testing should be limited to tuberculin purified protein derivative (PPD) and antigens to test for anergy. Repeated skin testing may be helpful when tuberculosis is a possibility. Fungal skin test antigens are of no use diagnostically and may cause confusion by altering the fungal serologies, particularly in the case of histoplasmosis.

Cultures are mandatory even when a specific diagnosis is suggested by serologies or other studies. Cerebrospinal fluid should be cultured at least three times for bacteria, acid-fast bacilli, and fungi and more numerous samples obtained and cultured in their entirety when the cause of the meningitis remains uncertain after the initial diagnostic evaluation is complete. The low density of fungi in the CSF and difficulty in culturing certain organisms may delay the diagnosis of some mycotic infections. In such cases, the yield can be improved by inoculating Sabouraud agar layered on the bottom of Erlenmeyer flasks with large volumes of CSF. The finding of even a single colony of an organism capable of causing chronic meningitis such as *Sporothrix schenckii* should never be disregarded as a contaminant (Fig. 2).[21] In fact, it may be useful to continue to examine fungal cultures for at least 4–6 weeks because the growth of such organisms can be exceedingly slow. Ventricular CSF may have a higher cultural yield than lumbar CSF in certain infections.[22] Urine, sputum, and blood cultures should be obtained and processed routinely for mycobacteria and fungi even in the absence of clinical evidence of extraneural infection. These ancillary cultures frequently are positive in cases of cryptococcosis, tuberculosis, histoplasmosis, and blastomycosis. Special culture techniques such as anaerobiasis or increased carbon dioxide tension also are appropriate in the search for certain pathogens such as *Actinomyces* species and *Brucella abortus,* respectively. Consultation with a clinical microbiologist may be helpful in difficult cases.

Biopsy of specific tissues should be directed by abnormal findings on physical examination. Skin, lymph node, and liver biopsy specimens may demonstrate granulomas, sometimes with caseation and occasionally with an organism demonstrable on special staining. Caseation is suggestive of tuberculosis, histoplasmosis, and coccidioidomycosis. Focal necrosis may be

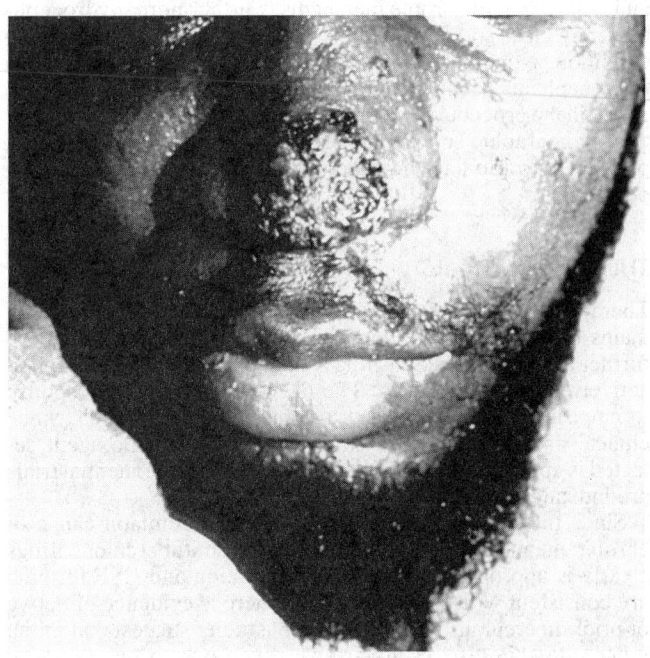

FIG. 2. Skin lesions developed in this patient with enigmatic chronic meningitis after ventriculojugular shunting for hydrocephalus. A discarded CSF culture from earlier admission was found, overgrown with mold subsequently identified as *Sporothrix schenchii*.

found in brucellosis. All biopsy specimens should be cultured for bacteria, fungi, and mycobacteria. Bone marrow biopsy and culture are particularly useful in tuberculosis and histoplasmosis. Liver biopsy is indicated when miliary tuberculosis is suspected, and has a greater yield when liver function tests suggest an infiltrative process (increased alkaline phosphatase and γ glutamyltranspeptidase). Meningeal and brain biopsies should be performed and ventricular fluid sampled at the time of craniotomy for exploration of a mass or other focal lesion or indicated ventricular shunting procedures. Brain and meningeal biopsy also should be considered in undiagnosed patients with a deteriorating course, recognizing that the yield of treatable etiologies is low. In the only published series of unselected patients with chronic meningitis, 14 brain biopsies were done; 10 were nondiagnostic (including 3 patients who ultimately had tuberculosis meningitis and one with carcinomatosis), two showed nonspecific granulomatous inflammation (which were later proven tuberculous), and two biopsies were diagnostic of malignant meningitis.[4] Despite the low yield, patients with hypoglycorrhachia and CSF pleocytosis greater than 50 cells/μl progressing on empiric antituberculosis therapy should be considered for biopsy. Earlier biopsy may be indicated, especially if the PPD skin test is negative (and the patient is not anergic), and the clinical course is deteriorating without a diagnosis.

Additional Radiographic Techniques

Magnetic resonance imaging (MRI) or computed axial tomography (CT) should be performed in all patients with chronic meningitis to search for parameningeal lesions (especially paranasal sinus and mastoids), ependymona, glioma and other parenchymal lesions. Magnetic resonance imaging provides a better evaluation of the meninges than CT; the high density bone of the skull on CT can obscure enhancement in the meninges, whereas bone on MRI is void of signal (and therefore black adjacent to the bright inflamed meninges).[23] However, all etiologies of chronic meningitis will cause meningeal enhancement, so this finding does not help to narrow the differential diagnosis. Hydrocephalus is also detected by imaging; the demonstration of hydrocephalus is not itself a sufficient indication for ventricular shunting, since neurosurgical procedures have a high morbidity and failure rate in chronic meningitis. Furthermore, hydrocephalus may clear spontaneously with treatment of the underlying condition. Nonetheless, if clinical deterioration attributable to hydrocephalus occurs, a surgical approach must be considered.

Ancillary procedures such as mammography and gastrointestinal radiographic series may be appropriate in the search for a primary carcinoma when meningeal carcinomatosis is suspected.

THERAPEUTIC TRIALS

Therapeutic trials are indicated when the specific etiology remains uncertain despite comprehensive evaluation. However, further attempts at establishing a diagnosis should be continued actively during such trials. The interpretation of the response to empirically administered drugs may be quite difficult, since clinical improvement is often slow, even when the agent selected is appropriate. When the patient is stable, sequential trials are indicated.

Since tuberculous meningitis is the most common cause of chronic meningitis,[4] an empirical trial of antituberculous drugs clearly is appropriate when the presentation and CSF formula are consistent with tuberculosis and there is evidence of active or prior tuberculous infection. Recent studies suggest that initial tuberculin skin test results are negative in up to two-thirds of patients with tuberculous meningitis.[24,25] Therefore, empirical antituberculous therapy in fact is indicated in most cases of undiagnosed chronic meningitis. Adequate cultures of CSF, urine, sputum, or gastric aspirates must be obtained before starting therapy and should include biopsy specimens of liver and bone marrow if miliary disease is suspected. Repeat intermediate-strength PPD skin testing after 2–4 weeks also may be of value if the initial studies are negative. The second-strength tuberculin skin test is less frequently negative than are intermediate tests and may be helpful. Positive cultures or a clinical response to antituberculous treatment despite negative cultures would be an indication to complete a full course of therapy.

Fluconazole is potentially useful for empiric therapy of chronic meningitis due to *Cryptococcus neoformans*, *Coccidioides immitis*, *Candida albicans*, and *Histoplasma capsulatum*. No clinical trials have been published to guide empiric use. The diagnostic value of empirical fluconazole would be limited by the slow response known to occur in documented cases. Improvement may not be obvious for several months, during which time meningitis due to other causes may irreversibly deteriorate. If such a trial is attempted, a dose of 400 mg per day would be indicated and repeated CSF examinations done to follow the results of therapy. Should the patient respond but remain undiagnosed, a minimum course would probably be at least 6 months.

Empirical use of amphotericin B should be withheld as long as possible in view of its toxicity and the difficulty in determining the duration of administration even when the causative fungus is known. However, when chronic meningitis is caused by certain fungi (*Histoplasma*, *Blastomyces*, *Sporothrix*), cultures of lumbar CSF often are negative. Generally empirical treatment with amphotericin B should be reserved for patients with progressive chronic meningitis who remain undiagnosed despite meningeal biopsy. Once initiated empirically, amphotericin B should be administered for 10–12 weeks intravenously. The development of nephrotoxicity should indicate a reduction in daily dose rather than discontinuation of the trial. Shorter term trials of this drug are of little value. If patients respond to amphotericin B but relapse, a pattern suggestive of coccidioidal or cryptococcal meningitis, intrathecal therapy must be considered.

Traditionally, empirical trials of corticosteroids have been avoided due to the potential catastrophic adverse effects on unrecognized tuberculosis or fungal meningitis. However, observers in New Zealand noted a subset of patients with chronic meningitis (9 of 87 patients) who were responsive to corticosteroids and required long-term immunosuppression to control symptoms.[4] This group consisted of patients not responding to tuberculosis medications, with negative fungal cultures at 3–4 weeks. Five of these nine patients had nondiagnostic brain biopsy prior to steroid therapy. Two patients relapsed and died when their steroids were tapered off, and four more required long-term therapy to prevent recurrence of symptoms. These authors note that fungal meningitis (other than cryptococcal) is very rare in their country and acknowledge that use of empiric steroids in areas endemic for fungal disease such as histoplasmosis or coccidioidomycosis may be risky. Therefore, despite its low diagnostic yield, brain biopsy should precede empiric glucocorticoids to exclude fungal disease more completely.

DIFFERENTIAL DIAGNOSIS

A number of conditions may cause syndromes resembling chronic meningitis superficially but are usually distinguishable from it on clinical grounds at presentation or during evaluation and observation of the patient (Table 6). In addition, a careful history is important to differentiate between recurrent and chronic meningitis, since the former syndrome connotes a different spectrum of diseases (Table 3).

Those infections causing the syndrome of chronic meningitis (Table 1) are discussed in detail in other chapters. Features that are important in establishing the cause of the chronic meningitis are reviewed here.

Tuberculous Meningitis

Tuberculous meningitis[24–35] results from rupture of a superficial infective focus into the subarachnoid space. In younger patients, this event typically is associated with active, progressive systemic disease. Stigmata of miliary tuberculosis may be present on physical examination and on chest x-ray films. Tuberculin skin test results frequently are negative initially, but conversion is noted on repeated skin testing. The diagnosis of tuberculosis

TABLE 6. Diseases That Sometimes Resemble Chronic Meningitis

Infectious etiologies
  Aseptic meningitis
  Infective endocarditis
  Parameningeal infections
  Partially treated bacterial meningitis
  Viral and nonviral encephalitis
Noninfectious diseases
  Brain tumor
  Giant cell arteritis
  Metabolic and other encephalopathies
  Multiple sclerosis
  Postinfectious encephalitis
  Subarachnoid hemorrhage
  Subdural hematoma
  Systemic lupus erythematosus
  Thrombotic thrombocytopenic purpura

usually is confirmed by smear, biopsy, and cultures obtained from extraneural specimens as well as CSF culture. In contrast, tuberculous meningitis in the adult more frequently results from the discharge of an old tuberculous focus into the subarachnoid space. As a result, physical examination, chest x-ray films, and extraneural cultures often are not helpful; despite presumably long-standing tuberculous infection, recent series indicate that the initial tuberculin skin test result is negative in 50–65 percent of patients.[24,25,34] The diagnosis rests on the outcome of CSF cultures. As a result of the frequent early use of antituberculous therapy empirically, more cases now are "unproved" microbiologically, but the diagnosis of tuberculosis is suggested by an apparent response to treatment.[30] Overall there is nothing about the clinical syndrome of tuberculous meningitis that distinguishes it from other etiologies of chronic meningitis. About one-half of the patients have had symptoms for over 2 weeks. Ocular palsies, particularly due to involvement of nerve VI, are found in 30–70 percent of the cases. The typical CSF findings consist of a lymphocytic pleocytosis, usually of 100–500 cells, increased protein concentration and depressed glucose levels in two-thirds of the patients on the initial lumbar puncture. This formula also is not specific for tuberculous meningitis. However, in unclear cases, progressive decrease in CSF glucose in the absence of specific treatment may be useful in distinguishing tuberculosis from aseptic meningitis and viral encephalitis. Cytologic examination of CSF often shows activated monocytoid cells and rarely Langhans cells.[32] It should be noted that neutrophils may predominate, particularly during the first 10 days of symptoms.[24,36] Cerebrospinal fluid smears contain acid-fast bacilli in 10–22 percent of the cases[24,25,34]; proteinaceous spinal fluid contains fibrinogen and will form a clot or pellicle upon standing; staining of the pellicle may increase the yield of the direct smear.[35] Cerebrospinal fluid cultures are positive in 38–88 percent of the cases, and sputum in about 14–50 percent. Cerebrospinal fluid tests under evaluation for the presumptive diagnosis of tuberculous meningitis include various antibody and antigen detection assays.[33] Adenosine deaminase is released by T lymphocytes, and elevated CSF levels are found in tuberculous meningitis, but not viral or bacterial meningitides.[36,37] Specificity, however, is not perfect, with elevations seen also in lymphomatous meningitis and neurosarcoid. Tuberculostearic acid is a structural component of mycobacteria, and its detection in the CSF using gas liquid chromatography has been highly sensitive and specific.[20] Currently this test is available from the Centers for Disease Control and Prevention (CDC) on request. Polymerase chain reaction to detect mycobacterial DNA in CSF shows some promise, but the two reports so far are limited by small numbers, largely culture-negative (therefore clinically defined) tuberculous meningitis cases, and unacceptably high false-positive results in controls (felt secondary to contamination).[38,39]

Cryptococcal Meningitis

Cryptococcal meningitis[24,40–47] presents in several different fashions, but the most characteristic, that of a subacute to chronic meningoencephalitis, is not at all distinctive among the etiologies of chronic meningitis. Exposure history is of little value clinically since this yeastlike fungus is a widespread saprophyte. Although one-half of patients in the pre-AIDS era lacked clinically apparent immunologic deficits, an underlying cellular immune dysfunction was known to predispose to this infection. The development of chronic meningitis in patients with Hodgkin's disease or lymphosarcoma, in persons receiving high-dose daily corticosteroid therapy, or in individuals at risk for AIDS suggests cryptococcal meningitis. In the previously healthy person, cryptococcal meningitis may cause an extremely indolent illness with gradual progression of dementia. The India ink preparation frequently is negative in such cases. More commonly, the onset of disease is subacute, at times mimicking a

brain tumor, particularly when signs of increased intracranial pressure are present. In patients with hematologic malignancies or AIDS, the initial manifestations of cryptococcosis may be unexplained fever. However, CNS involvement often evolves rapidly. Cerebrospinal fluid abnormalities include a lymphocytic pleocytosis, generally with 40–400 cells, and a depressed glucose level in 55 percent of the cases. In patients with AIDS, the CSF often shows little evidence of an inflammatory response.[44–47] Overall, the India ink preparation suggests the diagnosis of cryptococcal meningitis in over one-half of cases. The yield is highest in patients with an acute syndrome. More than 85 percent of patients have cryptococcal polysaccharide antigen in the CSF. However, serum also should be processed for this antigen; the overlap between significant antigen titers in the serum and CSF allows a presumptive diagnosis of cryptococcosis in 94 percent of the cases. Negative serologies do not exclude a diagnosis of cryptococcal meningitis, and false-positive tests are not rare. Cultural confirmation of the diagnosis is mandatory. The initial CSF culture is positive in three-quarters of patients; additional CSF cultures increase this yield and are indicated. Cultures of urine, sputum, stool, and blood also should be obtained. They have both diagnostic and prognostic value and frequently are positive in the absence of overt signs of extraneural infection. CSF cultures and serologies also are indicated in all patients with extraneural cryptococcal infection since they may have subclinical CNS disease; this is particularly likely in the immunocompromised host.

Coccidioidal Meningitis

Exposure history is important in the diagnosis of coccidioidal meningitis, since this infection is endemic in certain arid and semiarid areas of the Western Hemisphere.[48–54] Central nervous system infection may be a part of generalized coccidioidomycosis or may represent the sole extrapulmonary site of active clinical disease. Headache is the most prominent finding in patients with coccidioidal meningitis; the clinical syndrome is, however, in no way distinctive from the other causes of chronic meningitis. Skin tests with coccidioidin or spherulin are positive in one-third to one-half of patients with meningitis.[53,54] Complement-fixing antibody to the causative organism is found in the CSF of 75–95 percent of such patients. A presumptive diagnosis is possible when chronic meningitis occurs in the presence of demonstrated systemic coccidioidomycosis or a serum complement fixation titer to *Coccidioides immitis* of at least 1:16. Cerebrospinal fluid findings resemble those of cryptococcal meningitis; CSF cultures are positive in one-third to one-half of the cases, and rarely, spherules of *C. immitis* may be present on a smear.

Histoplasma Meningitis

Histoplasma meningitis[15,55–59] is a rare complication of infection with *Histoplasma capsulatum*. However, in one fourth of cases of histoplasma meningitis, disease is limited to the CNS. Clinical presentation is not differentiable from other causes of chronic meningitis; fever is almost universally present.[15] Symptoms may have been present for weeks or many months. Oral mucosal lesions, while found in only 16 percent of patients with *Histoplasma* meningitis, can be diagnostic if present and are more common than skin lesions. CSF cultures are positive in only 27–65 percent of cases making diagnosis problematic. Blood cultures should always be done; use of isolator tubes significantly increased the yield of blood cultures in a study of AIDS patients.[59] As discussed above, detection of serum and CSF antibodies to the fungus is suggestive of histoplasmosis (though not specific, as the antibodies may cross-react with other fungi), and the serum antibody tests are negative in 10–40 percent of proven cases of *Histoplasma* meningitis. *Histoplasma* polysaccharide antigen may be detected in urine, blood, or CSF in 61 percent of patients with histoplasma meningitis[15]; yields are even higher in HIV-infected persons.[59]

Lyme Disease

Infection with the spirochete *Borrelia burgdorferi* frequently involves the central nervous system.[60-63] The spirochete is introduced to its human host by an often unrecognized bite of the small deer tick *Ixodes scapularis* (*dammini*). Early infection is characterized by a flulike syndrome and the pathognomonic rash of erythema chronicum migrans. Neurologic symptoms follow the rash by a median of 4 weeks; headache and lymphocytic pleocytosis are seen in almost all patients with neuroborreliosis. Cranial nerve palsies (especially facial nerve) and peripheral neuropathies may be prominent and help to differentiate Lyme disease from the other chronic meningitides except sarcoidosis, which can present similarly. Exposure history is key in guiding appropriate serologic testing; in the absence of exposure, positive serology is more likely to be a false-positive test than diagnostic for Lyme disease. False-positive tests have been associated with infectious mononucleosis, rheumatoid arthritis, systemic lupus erythematosus, and other spirochetal disease such as syphilis and periodontal disease.[64] However, in endemic areas, up to 25 percent of healthy people are seropositive, so antibody detection in serum alone is not diagnostic. The most specific test is the detection of synthesis of intrathecal antibody to *Borrelia burgdorferi* in the CNS.[65,66]

Cysticercosis

Cysticercosis[67-73] is the most common parasitic disease of the CNS. Highly endemic areas include Mexico, Central and upper South America, China, India, subsaharan Africa, and the Caribbean. In the United States, immigrants from Mexico are the largest infected population and can present with symptoms up to 25 years after leaving Mexico. The infection is acquired by eating food contaminated with stool containing the eggs of the tapeworm *Taenia solium;* these hatch in the small intestine, with the larvae invading the blood stream and infecting muscle, eye, and brain. In these sites the larvae mature into cysts and remain asymptomatic for an average of 4–5 years. The person develops symptoms as the larvae begin to die, inciting an increased inflammatory response. Symptoms vary depending on the part of the brain infected; intraparenchymal neurocysticercosis (the most common) presents with seizures and focal neurologic deficits. Cysts in the subarachnoid space can collect in the basilar cisterns and induce a chronic basilar meningitis with hydrocephalus. Cerebrospinal fluid shows a lymphocytic pleocytosis, and hypoglycorrhachia occurs in up to one-fourth of patients. Cysts can also occur in the ventricles, causing ventriculitis or internal hydrocephalus. Diagnosis is suggested by characteristic multiple cystic or calcified lesions detected by head CT scan in a person who has been in an endemic area; early in infection the calcium may not be present. Subcutaneous cysts were present in one-fourth of patients in a large series with neurocysticercosis; biopsy reveals the larval tapeworm.[70] Skeletal muscle calcification on plain film is also suggestive of cysticercosis; however, the yield was low (<10 percent) in a recent series from the United States.[71] Serologic studies of both serum and particularly CSF are helpful, but negative serology does not rule out neurocysticercosis, as up to 50 percent of cases have negative serum antibodies. The yield in CSF is high (up to 84 percent positive serology) in patients with meningitis or hydrocephalus. Detection of antibodies in a patient from an endemic area with a typical history and characteristic head CT scan confirms the diagnosis.

Other Infectious Etiologies

Candida meningitis[5,74-76] is rare and often associated with widely disseminated disease. Risk factors for meningitis are sim-

ilar to those for candidemia, including prolonged antimicrobial therapy, indwelling venous catheters, hyperalimentation, corticosteroid use, recent intra-abdominal surgery, and intravenous drug abuse. Cerebrospinal fluid shunts or ventricular catheters have also been associated specifically with meningitis. Neonates, and especially premature infants, seem to be at increased risk for candidal meningitis (11 of 17 patients in one series were less than 1 year of age).[76] Presentation ranges from subacute to indolent, with the interval from symptoms to diagnosis ranging from days to months. Spinal fluid shows pleocytosis with predominance of neutrophils in one-half of cases and hypoglycorrhachia in 60 percent. Gram stain reveals yeast in 43 percent of smears, and CSF culture is usually diagnostic.

Syphilitic meningitis[77-79] is a rare but easily diagnosed and treated form of secondary syphilis. The disease is usually subacute, with the symptoms persisting for over 1 month in about one-quarter of the cases. Meningitis is the first overt sign of syphilis in 25 percent of meningitic patients. When extraneural manifestations occur, they generally precede CNS involvement by less than 2 years. The clinical presentation and CSF abnormalities resemble those of the other causes of chronic meningitis; however, cranial nerve palsies are seen in almost one-half of cases, with a special predilection for nerves VII and VIII. Hypoglycorrhachia is present in 55 percent of the cases. The diagnosis of syphilitic meningitis is suggested by positive CSF and serum serologies for syphilis. Transient dramatic deterioration of patients with meningitis after the initiation of penicillin therapy should suggest a Jarisch-Herxheimer reaction and the possibility of syphilis.

A meningoencephalomyelitis may follow the initial manifestations of brucellosis by 2 months to 2 years in fewer than 5 percent of cases.[80-84] Exposure to unpasteurized milk products or contact with cows, goats, sheep, swine, or their carcasses suggests the diagnosis. The patient also may have or have had symptoms and signs of systemic brucellosis such as night sweats, unexplained fever, orchitis, and hepatosplenomegaly. The clinical manifestations of the meningitis and CSF abnormalities usually are nonspecific. However, transient episodes of hemianesthesia or paresthesia can be prominent in neurobrucellosis. Serologic studies often suggest the diagnosis of brucellosis. In chronic cases, calcified foci may be noted in the liver and spleen on abdominal x-ray films. Cultures should be maintained in an increased carbon dioxide atmosphere for 3 weeks. Cerebrospinal fluid cultures are positive for *Brucella* in fewer than one-half of the cases. Blood cultures are occasionally positive.

Sporothrix schenckii has been described as a cause of chronic meningitis, and the CSF may demonstrate *Sporothrix* antibody before the fungus is recovered by culture.[85] *Angiostrongylus cantonensis* is a nematode endemic to southeast Asia and Pacific Islands and is the most common cause worldwide of eosinophilic meningitis.[86] Symptoms develop approximately 1 week after ingestion of raw fish or snails and persist for 2 to 4 weeks, usually resolving spontaneously. Rarely the living larvae may be found in the CSF or eye; however, diagnosis is usually made clinically (eosinophilic meningitis with the correct exposure history).

Central nervous system involvement by a large number of infections commonly is expressed as brain abscesses or other focal lesions occurring by hematogenous seeding or direct extension from clinically apparent extraneural sites. Rarely, the syndrome of chronic meningitis may be caused by these agents, sometimes without other stigmata of the infection. Infectious diseases belonging in this category include North American blastomycosis,[22,87-89] paracoccidioidomycosis,[90] cerebral phaeohyphomycosis,[91] actinomycosis,[92-94] nocardiosis,[95-97] and toxoplasmosis.[98-100]

Several infectious agents have been documented to cause chronic meningitis in unique epidemiologic circumstances (*Coenurus cerebralis*)[1] or in isolated case reports (*Leptospira ictero-*

haemorrhagiae, mucormycosis)[1,101] and will not be discussed here. Other infections in which CNS involvement is a late manifestation with few related symptoms, or leptomeningitis is noted pathologically but not clinically, also will not be reviewed.

Neoplastic Meningitis

The noninfectious diseases causing chronic meningitis may be difficult to diagnose and distinguish from occult infections (Table 2). Primary and metastatic, hematologic, and solid tumors all may involve the meninges diffusely to cause a similar clinical syndrome. In the case of acute leukemia and lymphoma,[102–104] CNS involvement usually occurs in the setting of known underlying malignancy. The major diagnostic problem involves distinguishing CNS involvement by the tumor from superimposed CNS infection and the uncommon paraneoplastic syndromes. Primary brain tumors including gliomas, pinealomas, ependymomas, and choroid plexus tumors may involve the meninges diffusely,[105] sometimes without gross parenchymal involvement. A diagnosis can be difficult in such cases. In metastatic "meningeal carcinomatosis,"[12,106–109] the nature of the meningeal process also may be difficult to ascertain. In one large series, the primary tumor had not been diagnosed at the onset of neurologic symptoms in 75 percent of the patients,[108] although the figure was 8 percent in patients selected by admission to an oncology center.[12] Typically, the onset of symptoms is subacute, with an intractable headache a prominent complaint along with mental changes. Cranial neuropathy occurs in 50 percent of the cases, and meningismus in about 20 percent. Fever usually is absent or when it occurs is associated with an intercurrent infection. Characteristically, neurologic signs far exceed symptoms and indicate widespread neurologic dysfunction; cerebral, cranial nerve, and spinal involvement are noted in one-half of the patients on initial physical examination. Cerebrospinal fluid is abnormal; 72 percent of the patients have a pleocytosis, often minimal, although occasional patients have a marked cellular response. The glucose content is depressed in 38 percent of the patients initially and in 72 percent during serial examinations. The finding of marked hypoglycorrhachia in the presence of minimal pleocytosis should suggest this diagnosis. In one series, CSF cytologies were diagnostic in 42 percent of patients in the first study and in 74 percent when multiple specimens were processed.[12] Of the ancillary neurodiagnostic tests, the myelogram was particularly helpful diagnostically and revealed multiple nodular deposits on nerve roots in 39 percent of the cases. The finding of markedly elevated CSF levels of β-glucuronidase is suggestive of meningeal carcinomatosis.[110] The most frequent primary sites of malignancy causing this syndrome are the breast, lung, stomach, pancreas, and skin (melanoma). Although neurologic signs may fluctuate and even partly regress, the course of meningeal carcinomatosis usually is rapidly progressive with involvement of all parts of the neuraxis. Since the primary tumor may be occult and extraneural metastatic sites lacking, cytologic examination of multiple CSF specimens is appropriate in all patients with undiagnosed chronic meningitis.

Sarcoid Meningitis

Neurologic involvement is seen in 5 percent of patients with sarcoidosis[111–117]; however, in these patients, almost one-third present with neurologic signs as their initial indication of sarcoidosis and 17 percent as their sole manifestation of the disease.[117] The clinical syndrome of sarcoid meningitis often includes cranial nerve palsies, long-tract and cerebellar abnormalities, and changes in mentation. The predilection for the basilar meninges with extension to the hypothalamus results in diabetes insipidus in 14–30 percent of the cases; this is of diagnostic significance because it rarely occurs in other forms of chronic meningitis. In addition, peripheral neuropathies accompany CNS sarcoidosis in 14 percent of patients but generally are unusual in chronic meningitis except for Lyme disease. Characteristic CSF abnormalities consist of a minimal lymphocytic pleocytosis in 60 percent of the patients and hypoglycorrhachia in 10–18 percent. The diagnosis of CNS sarcoidosis in patients with classic systemic manifestations of the disease is complicated by the necessity of excluding superimposed tuberculosis or cryptococcosis both of which occur with increased frequency in sarcoidosis and in patients receiving corticosteroid therapy. The diagnosis is more difficult when disease is limited to the CNS. Even the demonstration of granulomas in meningeal biopsy specimens is not specific. Serum and CSF angiotensin-converting enzyme levels may be elevated in neurosarcoidosis,[118] although elevated levels also are seen in malignant and bacterial meningitis.[119] Prolonged corticosteroid therapy is recommended for the treatment of CNS sarcoidosis; cytotoxic drug therapy may be required in some cases. Low-dose irradiation of the CNS has been used with apparent advantage in several patients.[117,120] Overall prognosis is good.[117]

Other Noninfectious Etiologies

Granulomatous angiitis is a necrotizing vasculitis of small leptomeningeal and perforating arteries and veins.[121–125] The process is usually manifested as a subacute meningoencephalitis in patients over 45 years of age. Cerebrospinal fluid findings include minimal lymphocytic pleocytosis and elevated protein levels. The major involvement by this syndrome has been limited to the CNS, although one patient developed a generalized granulomatous angiitis. The diagnosis can only be made from brain biopsy specimens or at autopsy. Corticosteroids may have had a saluatory effect in some cases, but the disease often is fatal. On clinical and pathologic grounds, this syndrome is distinct from sarcoidosis, giant cell arteritis, and Wegener's granulomatosis. Central nervous system vasculitis also may accompany or follow ophthalmic zoster; in some instances, varicella-zoster virus has been cultured from involved cerebral blood vessels.

A subacute meningoencephalitis usually occurs early in the course of the Vogt-Koyanagi-Harada syndrome (uveomeningoencephalitis).[126–128] The diagnosis is established by the development of severe, protracted, granulomatous uveitis and depigmentary skin changes such as poliosis (whitening of the eyebrows and eyelashes) and vitiligo. The CNS disease gradually resolves spontaneously.

Of the patients with Behçet's disease (recurrent oral and genital ulcerations and iridocyclitis) 10–25 percent develop CNS involvement.[129] The neurologic manifestations are variable, severe, and progressive in most cases. Occasionally, they precede other features of the syndrome. All parts of the neuraxis may be involved. Cerebrospinal fluid abnormalities include a slight elevation of protein levels and minimal pleocytosis.

The syndrome of "chronic benign lymphocytic meningitis"[130] defines a small group of patients with unexplained headache and lymphocytic pleocytosis but no focal signs. In one series, clinical remission occurred in all patients within 7–25 weeks. In the New Zealand series of 87 patients with chronic meningitis, four also recovered without treatment.[4] An additional nine patients were felt to have clinically responded to corticosteroid therapy, but this was an uncontrolled study and these patients may well overlap with the syndrome of chronic benign lymphocytic meningitis.

In contrast to the patients with unexplained minimal, self-limited disease, an additional group of patients have an enigmatic chronic meningitis with significant neurologic involvement, a high CSF protein concentration, and sometimes a depressed glucose level.[1] The prognosis in this group is poor. Therapeutic trials may alter the course of the disease, the cultures, and the pathologic findings. A specific diagnosis may be apparent at autopsy, but this is not always the case. A temporal response to antifungal therapy in some cases has implicated an infectious etiology, and mycotic meningitis too often is associated with negative CSF cultures (as discussed above) and only diagnosed postmortem. Therefore a thorough diagnostic evaluation followed ultimately by meningeal and brain biopsy and, if appropriate, an empirical trial of amphotericin B or fluconazole therapy.

THE IMMUNOCOMPROMISED PATIENT

Chronic meningitis in the immunosuppressed patient with impaired cellular immunity requires special consideration because of the distinctive differential diagnosis. Among renal transplant recipients and patients with lymphoma and leukemia, *Cryptococcus neoformans* is the most common etiology of chronic meningitis.[131] *M. tuberculosis, Toxoplasma gondii, Nocardia, Histoplasma,* and *Coccidioides* also cause chronic meningitis more often in such patients. Progressive multifocal leukoencephalopathy (caused by papovaviruses) may produce profound focal neurologic deficits with minimal or no abnormalities in the CSF. Computed tomographic scans in such cases demonstrate low-density, nonenhancing, progressive lesions in the white matter without mass effect. Hypogammaglobulinemic patients are susceptible to chronic meningoencephalitis secondary to enteroviral infections.[132] Symptoms include headache, seizures, lethargy, weakness, and ataxia; CSF shows lymphocytic pleocytosis with hypoglycorrhachia.

THE HIV-INFECTED PATIENT

Aseptic meningitis with fever, headache, and meningismus is common in primary HIV infection; symptoms resolve rapidly, but CSF pleocytosis can be found in 10 percent of asymptomatic HIV-infected patients.[133] A mild elevation in protein is also seen, but glucose remains normal. Cryptococcus, the most common opportunistic pathogen to cause meningitis in AIDS patients, occurs in 2–9 percent of patients with AIDS. There is often little inflammatory reaction in the CSF, but unlike HIV-negative patients this has not been a risk factor for poor outcome.[46,47] Tuberculous meningitis is a more common complication of tuberculosis in HIV-infected persons, occurring in 10 percent of tuberculosis patients with HIV disease and only 2 percent of tuberculosis patients without HIV infection in Spain.[134] Clinical presentation, CSF findings, and mortality in HIV-infected patients were similar to HIV-negative patients with tuberculous meningitis. Risk factors for poor outcome were duration of symptoms greater than 2 weeks prior to admission and CD_4 <200. Meningitis secondary to *Coccidioides*,[135] *Histoplasma*,[59] and *Blastomyces*[89] has also been reported with HIV. Reactivation of *Toxoplasma gondii* is common in AIDS patients, but usually causes ring-enhancing mass lesions rather than meningitis. Central nervous system lymphoma similarly presents more frequently as mass lesions; lymphocytic meningitis is much less common. End-stage AIDS patients are at risk for cytomegalovirus (CMV) ventriculoencephalitis[136]; presenting symptoms include cranial nerve palsies, nystagmus, and confusion usually in patients with previously diagnosed CMV end-organ disease (such as retinitis). Magnetic resonance imaging scans show ependymal enhancement along the ventricles; CSF has a neutrophilic pleocytosis with hypoglycorrhachia. An associated ascending radiculomyelitis with flaccid weakness and hyporeflexia is often seen. Prognosis is grim, with death occurring a median of 4 weeks from diagnosis despite antiviral chemotherapy. Progression of syphilis is accelerated in HIV-infected patients, with more syphilitic meningitis and uveitis seen[79]; usually routine serologic tests confirm the diagnosis.[137] Negative serologies with frank syphilitic meningitis have been reported, but follow-up serologies were positive.[138,139] Thirty percent of advanced HIV-infected patients with documented previous histories of syphilis have a negative FTA-ABS, questioning the interpretation of negative serologies in AIDS patients.[140] When clinical suspicion for syphilis is high, serologies should be repeated in follow up, looking for delayed seroconversion.

REFERENCES

1. Ellner JJ, Bennett JE. Chronic meningitis. Medicine (Baltimore). 1976;55:341–69.
2. Wilhelm C, Ellner JJ. Chronic meningitis. Neurol Clin. 1986;4:115–41.
3. Swartz M. Chronic meningitis—Many causes to consider. N Engl J Med. 1987;317:957–59.
4. Anderson NE, Willoughby EW. Chronic meningitis without predisposing illness—A review of 83 cases. Q J Med. 1987;63:283–95.
5. Salaki JS, Louria DB, Chmel H. Fungal and yeast infections of the central nervous system: A clinical review. Medicine (Baltimore). 1984;63:108–32.
6. Hermans PE, Goldstein NP, Wellman WE. Mollaret's meningitis and differential diagnosis of recurrent meningitis. Am J Med. 1972;52:128–40.
7. Haynes BF, Wright R, McCracken JP. Mollaret's meningitis: A report of three cases. JAMA. 1976;236:1967–9.
8. Joffle AM, Farley JD, Linden D, et al. Trimethoprim-sulfamethoxazole–associated aseptic meningitis: Case reports and review of the literature. Am J Med. 1989;87:332–8.
9. Marinac JS. Drug-and-chemical-induced aseptic meningitis: A review of the literature. Ann Pharmacother. 1992;26:813–21.
10. Peacock JE Jr, McGinnis MR, Cohen MS. Persistent neutrophilic meningitis: Report of four cases and review of the literature. Medicine (Baltimore). 1984;63:379–95.
11. Sawyer J, Ellner J, Ransohoff DF. To biopsy or not to biopsy in suspected herpes simplex encephalitis: A quantitative analysis. Med Decis Making. 1988;8:95–101.
12. Olson ME, Chernik NL, Posner JH. Infiltration of the leptomeninges by systemic cancer. A clinical and pathologic study. Arch Neurol. 1974;30:122–37.
13. Goodson JD, Strauss GM. Diagnosis of lymphomatous leptomeningitis by cerebrospinal fluid lymphocyte cell surface markers. Am J Med. 1979;66:1057–9.
14. Kranz BR, Thiel E, Thierfelde R. Immunocytochemical identification of meningeal leukemia and lymphoma: Poly-L-lysine–coated slides permit multimarker analysis even with minute cerebrospinal fluid cell specimens. Blood. 1989;73:1942–50.
15. Wheat LJ, Batteiger BE, Sathapatayarongs B. *Histoplasma capsulatum* infections of the central nervous system: A clinical review. Medicine. 1990;69:244–60.
16. Plouffe JF, Fass RJ. *Histoplasma* meningitis. Diagnostic value of cerebrospinal fluid serology. Ann Intern Med. 1980;92:189–91.
17. Wheat J, French M, Batteiger B, et al. Cerebrospinal fluid *Histoplasma* antibodies in central nervous system histoplasmosis. Arch Intern Med. 1985;145:1237–40.
18. Wheat LJ, Kohler RB, Tewari RP. Diagnosis of disseminated histoplasmosis by detection of *Histoplasma capsulatum* antigen in serum and urine specimens. N Engl J Med. 1986;314:83–8.
19. Mardh P-A, Larsson L, Hoiby N, et al. Tuberculostearic acid as a diagnostic marker in tuberculous meningitis. Lancet. 1983;1:367.
20. Brooks JB, Daneshvar MI, Haberberger RL, et al. Rapid diagnosis of tuberculous meningitis by frequency-pulsed-electron-capture gas liquid chromatography detection of carboxylic acids in cerebrospinal fluid. J Clin Microbiol. 1990;28:989–97.
21. Ewing GE, Bose GJ, Petersen PK. *Sporothrix schenckii* meningitis in a farmer with Hodgkin's disease. Am J Med. 1980;68:455–7.
22. Kravitz GR, Davies SF, Eckman MR, et al. Chronic blastomycotic meningitis. Am J Med. 1981;71:501.
23. Sze G. Diseases of the intracranial meninges: MR imaging features. Am J Roentgenol. 1993;160:727–33.
24. Stocksill MT, Kauffman CA. Comparison of cryptococcal and tuberculous meningitis. Arch Neurol. 1983;40:81–5.
25. Klein NC, Damsker B, Hirschman SZ. Mycobacterial meningitis: Retrospective analysis from 1970–1983. Am J Med. 1985;79:29–34.
26. Rich AR, McCordock HA. The pathogenesis of tuberculous meningitis. Bull Johns Hopkins Hosp. 1933;52:5–38.
27. Merritt HH, Fremont-Smith F. Cerebrospinal fluid in tuberculous meningitis. Arch Neurol Psychol. 1935;33:516–36.
28. Lepper MH, Spies HW. The present status of the treatment of tuberculosis of the central nervous system. Ann NY Acad Sci. 1963;106:106–23.
29. Weiss W, Flippin HF. The changing incidence and prognosis of tuberculous meningitis. Am J Med Sci. 1965;250:46–59.
30. Barrett-Connor EB. Tuberculous meningitis in adults. South Med J. 1967;60:1061–7.
31. Kennedy DH, Fallon FJ. Tuberculous meningitis. JAMA. 1979;241:264–8.
32. Jeren T, Beus I. Characteristics of cerebrospinal fluid in tuberculous meningitis. Acta Cytol (Baltimore). 1982;26:678.
33. Daniel TM. New approaches to the rapid diagnosis of tuberculous meningitis. J Infect Dis. 1987;155:599–602.
34. Ogawa SH, Smith MA, Brennessel DJ, et al. Tuberculous meningitis in an urban medical center. Medicine. 1987;66:317–26.
35. Johnson JL, Ellner JJ. Tuberculous meningitis. In: Evans RW, Baskin DS, Vatsu FM, eds. Prognosis in Neurological Disease. New York: Oxford University Press; 1991;209–25.

36. Ribera E, Martinez-Vazquez JM, Ocana I, et al. Activity of adenosine deaminase in cerebrospinal fluid for the diagnosis and follow up of tuberculous meningitis in adults. J Infect Dis. 1987;155:603–7.

37. Petterson T, Klockars M, Weber TH, et al. Diagnostic value of cerebrospinal fluid adenosine deaminase determination. Scand J Infect Dis. 1991;23:97–100.

38. Kaneko K, Onodera O, Miyatake T, et al. Rapid diagnosis of tuberculous meningitis by polymerase chain reaction (PCR). Neurology. 1990;40:1617–18.

39. Shankar P, Manjunath N, Mohan K, et al. Rapid diagnosis of tuberculous meningitis by polymerase chain reaction. Lancet. 1991;339:5–7.

40. Spickard A, Butler WT, Andriole V, et al. The improved prognosis of cryptococcal meningitis with amphotericin B therapy. Ann Intern Med. 1963;58:66–83.

41. Butler WT, Alling DW, Spickard A, et al. Diagnostic and prognostic value of clinical and laboratory findings in cryptococcal meningitis. A follow-up study of forty patients. N Engl J Med. 1964;270:59–66.

42. Littman ML, Walter JE. Cryptococcosis: Current status. Am J Med. 1968;45:922–32.

43. Diamond RD, Bennett JE. Prognostic factors in cryptococcal meningitis. A study of 111 cases. Ann Intern Med. 1974;80:176–81.

44. Kovacs JA, Kovacs AA, Polis M, et al. Cryptococcosis in the acquired immunodeficiency syndrome. Ann Intern Med. 1985;103:533–8.

45. Zuger A, Louie E, Holzman RS, et al. Cryptococcal disease in patients with the acquired immunodeficiency syndrome: Diagnostic features and outcome of treatment. Ann Intern Med. 1986;104:234–40.

46. Chuck SZ, Sande MA. Infections with *Cryptococcus neoformans* in the acquired immunodeficiency syndrome. N Engl J Med. 1989;321:794–9.

47. Clark RA, Greer D, Atkinson W, et al. Spectrum of *Cryptococcus neoformans* infection in 68 patients infected with human immunodeficiency virus. Rev Infect Dis. 1990;12:768–77.

48. Smith CE, Saito MT, Simons SA. Pattern of 39,500 serologic tests in coccidioidomycosis. JAMA. 1956;160:546.

49. Winn WA. The treatment of coccidioidal meningitis. The use of amphotericin B in a group of 25 patients. Calif Med. 1964;101:75–89.

50. Winn WA. Coccidioidal meningitis: A follow-up report. In: Ajello L, ed. Coccidiomycosis. Tucson: University of Arizona Press; 1967:55.

51. Candill RG, Smith CE, Reinarz JA. Coccidioidal meningitis. A diagnostic challenge. Am J Med. 1970;49:360.

52. Deresinski SC, Stevens DA. Coccidioidomycosis in compromised hosts. Medicine (Baltimore). 1974;54:377.

53. Bouza E, Dreyer JS, Hewitt WL, et al. Coccidioidal meningitis. An analysis of 31 cases and review of the literature. Medicine (Baltimore). 1981;60:139–71.

54. Vincent T, Galgiani JN, Huppert M, et al. The natural history of coccidioidal meningitis: VA–Armed Forces cooperative studies 1955–1958. Clin Infect Dis. 1993;16:247–54.

55. Tynes BS, Crutcher JC, Utz JP. Histoplasma meningitis. Ann Intern Med. 1963;59:615–21.

56. Smith JW, Utz JP. Progressive disseminated histoplasmosis. Ann Intern Med. 1972;76:557.

57. Gilden DH, Miller EM, Johnson WG. Central nervous system histoplasmosis after rhinoplasty. Neurology (Minn). 1974;24:874–7.

58. Gelfand JA, Bennett JE. Active *Histoplasma* meningitis of 22 years duration. JAMA. 1975;233:1294–5.

59. Wheat LJ, Connolly-Stringfield PA, Baker RJ, et al. Disseminated histoplasmosis in the acquired immunodeficiency syndrome: Review of the literature. Medicine. 1990;69:361–74.

60. Pachner AR, Steere AC. The triad of neurologic manifestations of Lyme disease: Meningitis, cranial neuritis, and radiculoneuritis. Neurology (NY). 1985;35:47–53.

61. Pachner AR. Neurologic manifestations of Lyme disease, the new "Great Imitator." Rev Infect Dis. 1989;11:S1482–6.

62. Halperin JJ, Volkeman DJ, Wu P. Central nervous system abnormalities in Lyme neuroborreliosis. Neurology. 1991;41:1571–82.

63. Finkel MJ, Halperin JJ. Nervous system Lyme borreliosis—Revisited. Arch Neurol. 1992;49:102–7.

64. Rahn DW, Malawista SE. Lyme disease: Recommendations for diagnosis and treatment. Ann Intern Med. 1991;114:472–81.

65. Wilske B, Schierz G, Preac-Mursic V, et al. Intrathecal production of specific antibodies against *Borrelia burgdorferi* in patients with lymphocytic meningoradiculitis (Bannworth's syndrome). J Infect Dis. 1986;153:304–14.

66. Steere AC, Berrardi VP, Weeks KE, et al. Evaluation of the intrathecal antibody response to *Borrelia burgdorferi* as a diagnostic test for Lyme neuroborreliosis. J Infect Dis. 1990;761:1203–9.

67. Denti JH. Cysticercosis cerebri-cestode infestation of the human brain. JAMA. 1957;164:401.

68. Lombardo LL, Mateos JH. Cerebral cysticercosis in Mexico. Neurology (Minn). 1961;11:824–6.

69. Loo L, Braude A. Cerebral cysticercosis in San Diego. A report of 23 cases and a review of the literature. Medicine (Baltimore). 1982;61:341–59.

70. Nash TE, Neva FA. Recent advances in the diagnosis and treatment of cerebral cysticercosis. N Engl J Med. 1984;311:1492–6.

71. Earnest MP, Reller LD, Filley CM, et al. Neurocysticercosis in the United States: 35 cases and a review. Rev Infect Dis. 1987;9:961–79.

72. Del Brutto OH, Sotelo J. Neurocysticercosis: An update. Rev Infect Dis. 1988;10:1075–87.

73. Bandres JC, White AC, Samo T, et al. Extraparenchymal neurocysticercosis—Report of five cases and review of management. Clin Infect Dis. 1992;15:799–811.

74. DeVita VT, Utz JP, Williams T, et al. *Candida* meningitis. Arch Intern Med. 1966;117:527–35.

75. Bayer AS, Edwards JE Jr, Seidel JS, et al. *Candida* meningitis. Medicine (Baltimore). 1976;55:477–86.

76. Somego RA, Perfect JR, Durach DT. Combined therapy with amphotericin B and 5-fluorocytosine for candida meningitis. Rev Infect Dis. 1984;6:791–801.

77. Merritt HH, Adams RD, Solomon HC. Neurosyphilis. New York: Oxford University Press; 1946:24.

78. Hooshmand H, Escobar MR, Kopf SW. Neurosyphilis, a study of 241 patients. JAMA. 1972;219:726–9.

79. Katz DA, Berger JR, Duncan RC. Neurosyphilis: A comparative study of the effects of infection with human immunodeficiency virus. Arch Neurol. 1993;50:243–9.

80. Nelson-Jones A. Neurologic complications of undulant fever. Lancet. 1951;1:495.

81. Nichols E. Meningoencephalitis due to brucellosis. Ann Intern Med. 1951;35:673.

82. Fincham RW, Sahs AL, Joynt RJ. Protean manifestations of nervous system brucellosis. JAMA. 1963;184:97–103.

83. Reddin JL, Anderson RK, Jenness R, et al. Significance of 7S and macroglobulin brucella agglutinins in human brucellosis. N Engl J Med. 1965;272:1263.

84. Bouza E, Garcia de la Torre M, Parras F, et al. Brucellar meningitis. Rev Infect Dis. 1987;9:810–22.

85. Scott EN, Kauman L, Brown AC, et al. Serologic studies in the diagnosis and management of meningitis due to *Sporothrix schenckii*. N Engl J Med. 1987;317:935–40.

86. Koo J, Pien F, Kliks MM. *Angiostrongylus (Parastrongylus)* eosinophilic meningitis. Rev Infect Dis. 1988;10:1155–62.

87. Wilhelmj CM. The primary meningeal form of systemic blastomycosis. Am J Med Sci. 1925;169:172.

88. Buechner HA, Clawson CM. Blastomycosis of the central nervous system. II. A report of nine cases from the Veterans Administration Cooperative Study. Am Rev Respir Dis. 1967;95:820.

89. Pappas PG, Pottage JC, Powderly WF, et al. Blastomycosis in patients with the acquired immunodeficiency syndrome. Ann Intern Med. 1992;116:847–53.

90. Pereira WC, Raphael A, Tehuto RA, et al. Localizacao encefalica da blastomicose sul-Americana: Consideracoes a proposito de 9 casos. Arq Neuropsiquiat. 1965;23:113.

91. Bennett JE, Bonner H, Jennings AE, et al. Chronic meningitis caused by *Cladosporium trichoides*. Am J Clin Pathol. 1973;59:398–407.

92. Bolton CF, Ashenhurst EM. Actinomycosis of the brain. Case report and review of the literature. Can Med Assoc J. 1964;90:922–28.

93. Brown JR: Human actinomycosis. Hum Pathol. 1973;4:319–30.

94. Smego RA Jr. Actinomycosis of the central nervous system. Rev Infect Dis. 1987;9:855–65.

95. King RB, Stoops WL, Fitzgibbons J, et al. *Nocardia asteroides* meningitis. A case successfully treated with large doses of sulfadiazine and urea. J Neurosurg. 1966;24:749.

96. Richter RW, Silva M, Neu HC, et al. The neurological aspects of *Nocardia asteroides* infection. Infect Nervous System. 1968;44:424.

97. Bross JE, Gordon G. Nocardial meningitis: Case reports and review. Rev Infect Dis. 1991;13:160–5.

98. Kramer W. Frontiers of neurological diagnosis in acquired toxoplasmosis. Psychiatr Neurol Neurochirg. 1966;69:43.

99. Townsend JJ, Wolinsky JS, Baringer JR, et al. Acquired toxoplasmosis. A neglected cause of treatable nervous system disease. Arch Neurol. 1975;32:335–43.

100. Grines C, Plouffe JF, Baird IM, et al. *Toxoplasma* meningoencephalitis with hypoglycorrhachia. Arch Intern Med. 1981;141:935.

101. Jones PG, Gilman RM, Medeiros AA, et al. Focal intracranial mucormycosis presenting as chronic meningitis. JAMA. 1981;24:2063.

102. Moore EW, Thomas LB, Shaw RK, et al. The central nervous system in acute leukemia. Arch Intern Med. 1960;105:451.

103. Hyman CB, Boyle JM, Brubaker CA, et al. Central nervous system involvement by leukemia in children. Blood. 1965;25:1.

104. Griffin JW, Thompson RW, Mitchinson MJ, et al. Lymphomatous leptomeningitis. Am J Med. 1971;51:200–8.

105. Berg L. Hypoglycorrhachia of noninfectious origin: Diffuse meningeal neoplasia. Neurology (Minn). 1953;3:811–24.

106. Fischer-Williams M, Bosanquet FD, Daniel P. Carcinomatosis of the meninges. Brain. 1955;78:42–58.

107. Dinsdale HB, Taghavy A. Carcinomatosis of the meninges. Can Med Assoc J. 1964;90:505–12.

108. Vital C, Bruno-Martin F, Henry P, et al. La carcinomatose méningée. Bordeaux Med. 1970;12:2927–44.

109. Gonzalez-Vitale JC, Garcia-Bunvel R. Meningeal carcinomatosis. Cancer. 1976;37:2906.

110. Shuttleworth E, Allen N. CSF β-glucuronidase assay in the diagnosis of neoplastic meningitis. Arch Neurol. 1980;37:684–7.

111. Wiederholt WC, Siekert RB. Neurological manifestations of sarcoidosis. Neurology (Minn). 1965;15:1147–54.

112. Mathews WB. Sarcoidosis of the nervous system. J Neurol Neurosurg Psychiatry. 1965;28:23.

113. Gaines JD, Eckman PB, Remington JS. Low CSF glucose level in sarcoidosis involving the central nervous system. Arch Intern Med. 1970;125:333–6.

114. Douglas AC, Maloney AFJ. Sarcoidosis of the central nervous system. J Neurol Neurosurg Psychiatry. 1973;36:1024.

115. Delaney P. Neurological manifestations in sarcoidosis. Ann Intern Med. 1977;87:336–45.

116. Stern BJ, Knumholz A, Scott P, et al. Sarcoidosis and its neurological manifestations. Arch Neurol. 1985;42:909–19.

117. Chapelon C, Ziza JM, Piette JC, et al. Neurosarcoidosis: Signs, course and treatment in 35 confirmed cases. Medicine. 1990;69:261–76.

118. Chan Seu CP, Norfolk G, Spokes EG. CSF angiotensin-converting enzyme in neurosarcoidosis. Lancet. 1985;1:456–7.

119. Oksaner V, Fyhrquist F, Somer H, et al. Angiotensin converting enzyme in cerebrospinal fluid: a new assay. Neurology. 1985;35:1220–3.

120. Grizzanti JN, Knapp AB, Schecter AJ, et al. Treatment of sarcoid meningitis with radiotherapy. Am J Med. 1982;73:605–8.

121. Kolodny EM, Rebeiz JJ, Caviness VS, et al. Granulomatous angiitis of the central nervous system. Arch Neurol. 1968;19:510–24.

122. Nurick S, Blackwood W, Mair WGP. Giant cell granulomatous angiitis of the central nervous system. Brain. 1972;95:133–42.

123. Mohr JP, Powell HC. Clinicopathologic conference. Headache and progressive mental deterioration in a 45-year-old man. N Engl J Med. 1976;295:944.

124. Cupps TR, Moore PM, Fauci AS. Isolated angiitis of the central nervous system. Prospective diagnostic and therapeutic experience. Am J Med. 1983;74:97–105.

125. Reik L, Grunnet ML, Spencer RP, et al. Granulomatous angiitis presenting as chronic meningitis and ventriculitis. Neurology (NY). 1983;33:1609–12.

126. Cowper AR. Harada's disease and Vogt-Koyanagi syndrome. AMA Arch Ophthalmol. 1951;45:367.

127. Pattison EM. Uveomeningoencephalitis syndrome. Arch Neurol (Chicago). 1965;12:197–205.

128. Riehl J-L, Andrews JM. The uveomeningoencephalitis syndrome. Neurology (Minn). 1966;16:603–9.

129. Schotland DL, Wolf SM, White HH, et al. Neurologic aspects of Behçets disease. Am J Med. 1963;34:544–52.

130. Hopkins AP, Harvey PKP. Chronic benign lymphocytic meningitis. J Neurol Sci. 1973;18:443–53.

131. Hooper DC, Pruitt AA, Rubin RH. Central nervous system infection in the chronically immunosuppressed. Medicine (Baltimore). 1982;61:166–88.

132. McKinney RE, Katz SL, Wilfert CM. Chronic enteroviral meningoencephalitis in agammaglobulinemic patients. Rev Infect Dis. 1987;9:334–56.

133. Appleman ME, Marshall DW, Porey RL, et al. Cerebrospinal fluid abnormalities in patients without AIDS who are seropositive for the human immunodeficiency virus. J Infect Dis. 1988;158:193–9.

134. Berenguera J, Moreno S, Laguna F, et al. Tuberculous meningitis in patients infected with the human immunodeficiency virus. N Engl J Med. 1992;326:668–72.

135. Fish DG, Ampel NM, Galgiani JN, et al. Coccidioidomycosis during human immunodeficiency virus infection: A review of 77 patients. Medicine. 1990;69:384–91.

136. Kalayjian RC, Cohen MC, Bonomo RA, et al. Cytomegalovirus ventriculoencephalitis in AIDS: A syndrome with distinct clinical and pathological features. Medicine. 1993;72:67–77.

137. Matlow AG, Rachlis AR. Syphilis serology in human immunodeficiency virus-infected patients with symptomatic neurosyphilis—Case report and review. Rev Infect Dis. 1990;12:703–7.

138. Feraru ER, Aronow HA, Lipton RB. Neurosyphilis in AIDS patients: Initial CSF VDRL may be negative. Neurology. 1990;40:541–3.

139. Hicks CB, Benson PM, Lupton GP, et al. Seronegative secondary syphilis in a patient infected with the human immunodeficiency virus (HIV) with Kaposi's sarcoma. Ann Intern Med. 1987;107:492–5.

140. Haas JS, Bolan G, Larse SA, et al. Sensitivity of treponenal tests for detecting prior treated syphilis during human immunodeficiency virus infection. J Infect Dis. 1990;162:862–6.

66. ENCEPHALITIS, MYELITIS, AND NEURITIS

DIANE E. GRIFFIN

Encephalitis, myelitis, and *neuritis* mean inflammations of brain, spinal cord, and peripheral nerves, respectively. If sensory or motor spinal roots are specifically involved, the term *radiculitis* may be used. Since meningeal inflammation often accompanies these inflammatory processes, compounded terms

such as *meningoencephalitis* and *meningoencephalomyelitis* are sometimes used. None of these terms, however, differentiates between the inflammatory diseases caused by direct invasion of agents and the post- or parainfectious demyelinating processes that may involve the brain, spinal cord, or peripheral nerves. Because of the diversity of clinical symptoms and signs that can occur with these inflammatory diseases, infectious or parainfectious causes must be entertained in the differential diagnosis of a great variety of neurologic diseases. As in the diagnosis of all neurologic disease, the differential diagnosis will be determined by the temporal evolution of signs and symptoms and by the localization of the disease process to one or more anatomic sites by physical findings. Systemic involvement of skin, lung, salivary glands, gastrointestinal tract, and so forth, or fever may suggest an infectious cause, but these may also be absent.

ENCEPHALITIS AND MYELITIS

This section deals with infectious and postinfectious encephalitis and myelitis together since they are often considered in the same differential diagnosis and have considerable overlap in manifestation and causation. Peripheral neuropathies due to infectious agents are considered, along with tetanus, in a separate section.

Pathogenesis and Pathologic Characteristics

Infectious agents can produce clinical symptoms and signs within the central nervous system (CNS) by either direct or indirect involvement of neural tissue. Infectious agents can invade the CNS by several pathways. The most common is via the blood. This is best documented for viral infections but probably is also important in rickettsial, bacterial, and fungal infections.[1-3] The initial site of entry of a pathogen and the primary site of replication may be the respiratory tract (measles, mumps, influenza, and varicella-zoster viruses, *Mycobacterium tuberculosis, Cryptococcus neoformans*), gastrointestinal tract (poliovirus, coxsackievirus, echovirus), or subcutaneous tissue (arthropod-borne viruses, *Rickettsia rickettsia, Rickettsia typhi,* trypanosomes). Involvement of the CNS is, for the most part, an infrequent consequence of common infections.[1]

In certain viral infections, entry into the CNS occurs by way of the peripheral nerves. Transport systems within motor and sensory axons carry substances from the cell body to the periphery (anterograde transport) and from the periphery to the cell body (retrograde transport). The neural route of entry is important in viral infections such as rabies[4] and occasionally poliomyelitis.[5] Retrograde transport from the skin or mucous membranes moves herpes simplex and varicella-zoster viruses into sensory ganglia at the time of primary infection, and anterograde transport carries reactivated virus from the ganglia to the periphery during exacerbations.[6] On occasion reactivated virus may also be carried retrograde to the CNS.

Entry of infectious agents into the CNS by way of the exposed olfactory nerves in the nasal mucosa has been demonstrated in experimental animals[7,8] but is of proven clinical importance only in the entry of free-living amebas into the olfactory and frontal lobes through the nasal mucosa and across the cribriform plate.[9]

Once within the CNS, only selected cells may be infected, giving rise to variations in clinical manifestations. Neuronal infection may cause seizure activity, which, depending on the areas involved, may be focal or generalized. Infection of oligodendroglia may cause demyelination alone. Cortical infection or reactive parenchymal swelling may give rise to changes in the state of consciousness,[10] and infection of specific brain stem neurons can cause coma or respiratory failure.[11] Infection of microglia and macrophages may lead to neurologic dysfunction through indirect effects on neuronal function.[12,13]

In fatal viral encephalitis, an inflammatory reaction is usually prominent in the meninges and in a perivascular distribution within the brain. Although the perivascular inflammatory reaction is composed predominantly of mononuclear cells, polymorphonuclear cells may be evident. Neural cells may show degenerative changes, and apparent phagocytosis of neurons by macrophages or microglial cells (neuronophagia) is often found. Multinucleated giant cells containing viral antigen are found in the brains of patients with encephalitis induced by human immunodeficiency virus (HIV).[14] CNS lesions in HIV infections may also include myelin pallor, vacuolar myelopathy, and gracile tract degeneration.[14,15] Whether these pathologic changes are direct or indirect consequences of virus infection is not yet clear. Intranuclear inclusion bodies are seen in herpesvirus,[6] adenovirus,[16] and subacute and chronic forms of measles virus infections.[17] Cytomegalovirus infections produce characteristic pathologic changes with the induction of cytomegalic cells containing inclusion bodies.[18] Negri bodies are found in rabies virus encephalitis.[19]

Rickettsiae tend to invade and to multiply in vascular endothelial cells, resulting in widespread vasculitis of capillaries, arterioles, and small arteries,[20] including the retina.

Infectious agents can give rise to signs or symptoms suggesting encephalitis or myelitis without actually invading CNS parenchyma. One mechanism is by the development of adhesive meningitis and vasculitis during the course of subacute or chronic leptomeningeal infections. In chronic tuberculosis, fungal or syphilitic meningitis, or in untreated or partially treated bacterial meningitis, the chronic meningeal reaction may cause obstruction of cerebrospinal fluid (CSF) flow, causing hydrocephalus, cranial nerve palsies, or gliosis in the underlying cerebral cortex. In addition, the vasculitis involving large vessels may lead to infarctions of brain and focal neurologic deficits. This sequence of events is frequently observed in tuberculosis,[21] aspergillosis,[22] meningovascular neurosyphilis,[23] and occasionally in coccidioidomycosis[24] and herpes zoster.[25] Syphilis of the meningovascular type appears relatively early in the course of this disease, and, in contrast to the parenchymatous manifestations (tabes dorsalis and paresis) that appear later, is inflammatory and often reversible. *Cryptococcus* produces a chronic meningitis with little inflammatory reaction even in the immunologically normal host.[26] In chronic bacterial or fungal meningitis, organization of a subarachnoid exudate at the base of the brain may lead to communicating hydrocephalus and cranial nerve palsies.[27]

In the acute demyelinating disease complicating viral exanthems or respiratory or gastrointestinal infections, it is not known whether invasion into the CNS is a prerequisite to disease. The pathogenesis of this syndrome is thought to be related to a sensitization of the infected person to central myelin.[28] This mechanism is analogous to neurologic complications of neural tissue-derived rabies vaccines.[29]

The pathologic changes of postinfectious and postvaccinal encephalomyelitis are characterized by perivascular infiltration of mononuclear inflammatory cells and perivenous demyelination. Acute hemorrhagic leukoencephalitis, characterized by fibrinoid necrosis of arterioles and hemorrhage, as well as the perivenular demyelination, is thought to represent a more severe form of postinfectious encephalomyelitis.[30]

On the other hand, Reye syndrome is a distinct acute encephalopathy of unknown cause that usually follows a viral infection. This syndrome affects children and is characterized by acute fatty liver and noninflammatory cerebral edema. Reye syndrome has been most commonly associated with varicella and influenza A and B virus infections and is epidemiologically related to administration of salicylates during infection.[31]

Neurotoxins produced by bacteria infecting gastrointestinal and respiratory sites have been postulated to cause the acute CNS diseases seen occasionally with shigellosis[32] and melioidosis.[33] The role of the organism in the encephalopathy associated with cat-scratch disease is unknown.[34]

Clinical Findings

Infections limited to the leptomeninges manifest with signs and symptoms of meningeal irritation: headache, stiff neck, and pleocytosis. If the meningeal process is chronic, as in tuberculosis, manifesting symptoms and signs may be of a communicating hydrocephalus (headache, nausea and vomiting, mental deterioration, or spastic paraparesis) and/or of localized infarction secondary to vasculitis.[35] The chronic form of cryptococcal meningitis may manifest as progressive mental deterioration and headache rather than with fever and meningismus, as is seen in the more acute form.[27,36]

Patients with viral encephalitis usually have signs and symptoms of meningeal inflammation, but, in addition to headache, fever, and nuchal rigidity, encephalitis is characterized by alterations of consciousness: Mild lethargy may progress to confusion, stupor, and coma. Focal neurologic signs usually develop, and seizures are common. Motor weakness, accentuated deep tendon reflexes, and extensor plantar responses may be observed. Abnormal movements are seen in some cases of encephalitis, and, rarely, a tremor characteristic of Parkinson's disease may develop. The hypothalamic pituitary area may be involved, causing severe hyperthermia or poikilothermia, diabetes insipidus, and inappropriate antidiuretic hormone secretion. Involvement of the spinal cord can lead to flaccid paralysis, depression of tendon reflexes, and paralysis of bowel and bladder. Increased intracranial pressure can cause papilledema and third and sixth cranial nerve palsies.

In herpes simplex encephalitis signs often include bizarre behavior, hallucinations, and aphasia, suggesting the temporal lobe localization typical of that infection.[37] Rabies may begin with local paresthesia at the site of the bite.[38] A parkinsonian syndrome is common in Japanese encephalitis.[38] Acute contralateral hemiparesis may occur after herpes zoster ophthalmicus related to a localized cerebral angiitis, causing frontal lobe infarction.[25] With Lyme neuroborreliosis, both peripheral system and CNS complications occur, ranging from severe meningoencephalitis to isolated cranial nerve palsies.[40,41]

Myelitis can occur, with or without encephalitis. Transverse myelitis simulates acute transection of the cord with rostral limb weakness, sensory level, and loss of bowel and bladder control. Ascending myelitis leads to an ascending flaccid paralysis and rising sensory deficit and is characterized by early bowel and bladder involvement. Poliomyelitis, in which anterior horn cells are involved primarily, typically causes flaccid paralysis and muscular pain without sensory loss or bladder dysfunction.

In postinfectious encephalomyelitis the time lapse between manifestations of the primary viral infection and the onset of symptoms referable to the nervous system ranges between 2 and 12 days. The onset is often abrupt, with depression of consciousness or seizure.[28,30]

Systemic findings of particular importance are the rashes of Lyme disease, Rocky Mountain spotted fever (palms and soles), typhus, varicella, herpes B virus and herpes zoster. An exanthem is also occasionally seen with *Mycoplasma*, coxsackievirus, and echovirus infections. A history of tick bite is often obtained in Rocky Mountain spotted fever, Lyme disease, ehrlichiosis, and Colorado tick fever. A history of animal or bat bite may be obtained in rabies, although most patients in the United States never give such a history.[42]

Mycobacterial and fungal infections often present as chronic and, on occasion, fluctuating disease, but in certain cases (including mucormycosis) they may progress very rapidly.

Bacterial infections usually manifest with an acute onset, but certain infections such as neurosyphilis, Lyme disease, relapsing fever, brain abscess, trypanosomiasis, and Whipple's disease may have an insidious onset and an indolent, chronic, or even fluctuating course. The neurologic features of Whipple's disease may include dementia, supranuclear ophthalmoplegia, myoclonus, spastic paresis, ataxia, and papilledema. The patient may have neurologic signs and symptoms without significant manifestations of malabsorption.[43] The rickettsial diseases are usually acute in onset with fever, headache, and myalgias. Rocky Mountain spotted fever is associated with a rash before or after neurologic disease,[44] while there is rarely a rash in ehrlichiosis.[45]

Viral infections also may be acute, subacute, or chronic. Encephalitis due to adenovirus and enteroviruses has occurred both as acute disease in immunologically healthy individuals[1,46] and as subacute disease in immunologically compromised individuals.[16,47] Certain of the "slow virus infections" such as Creutzfeldt-Jakob disease, subacute sclerosing panencephalitis, rubella panencephalitis, HIV encephalopathy and myelopathy, tropical spastic paraparesis, and progressive multifocal leukoencephalopathy are slowly progressive diseases with an insidious onset and absence of fever.[1,48–50]

Laboratory Findings

Peripheral blood counts are rarely helpful in this group of diseases since they may be normal or show a moderate leukocytosis or leukopenia. Peripheral blood smears may show atypical lymphocytes in Epstein-Barr virus infections, the diagnostic gametocytes of *Plasmodium falciparum* malaria, the morulae of *Ehrlichia*, the borreliae in relapsing fever, or the trypanosomes in trypanosomiasis. The serum amylase level may be elevated in mumps virus infection. Pulmonary infiltrates may accompany lymphocytic choriomeningitis virus, typhus, and *Mycoplasma* infections.

CSF examination is essential. The pleocytosis of viral encephalomyelitis is variable (10–2000 cells/mm³), and mononuclear cells usually predominate, although early in any of these diseases there may be no cells, or polymorphonuclear cells may be present in considerable numbers. Repeat examination of the CSF in 24 hours is often useful.[51] Significant numbers of red blood cells may be found in herpes simplex encephalitis,[52] acute necrotizing hemorrhagic leukoencephalitis,[53] and *Naegleria* encephalitis.[54] In the chronic fungal and bacterial meningitides a moderate mononuclear pleocytosis is usually found. Meningoencephalitis due to *Naegleria*, *Nocardia*, *Actinomyces*, *Candida*, and *Aspergillus* elicit a polymorphonuclear response.[54,55]

The CSF protein level is usually elevated, and in chronic infections an increased proportion of this protein is IgG (normal is <12 percent).[56] Under normal conditions, CSF IgG is derived primarily from the serum, but antibodies are present at about $\frac{1}{200}$ of the concentration.[57] During acute inflammatory reactions a transudate of protein occurs, including serum immunoglobulins. During convalescence plasma cells may produce a specific IgG within the CNS, as seen after mumps,[58] herpes simplex,[52] and zoster[59] encephalitides. In chronic infection examination of the CSF for specific antibody can be diagnostic in syphilis,[60] Lyme disease,[61] tropical spastic paraparesis,[50] subacute sclerosing,[62] and rubella panencephalitis[63] and may be useful, when compared with serum levels, in the viral, rickettsial, fungal, and bacterial encephalitides for which antibody tests are available. If antibody to a particular pathogen is present at a comparable or higher amount in CSF than in serum and the CSF protein is only moderately elevated, it is indicative of CNS infection with the agent.

For diagnosis by serum antibodies, it is important to obtain serum early in the course (acute phase) for comparison with serum taken after 1–3 weeks of illness to demonstrate a significant antibody increase.[64] Tests for specific IgM in serum and CSF often allow for earlier diagnoses.[65,66] This diagnosis is often of more than academic interest since presumptive therapy begun early may then be discontinued if a diagnosis is established. Tests for cold agglutinins and heterophile antibody may yield false negatives in the diagnosis of *Mycoplasma* and Epstein-Barr virus infections, respectively; therefore, organism-specific antibody tests need to be done.

The CSF glucose level is usually within the normal range during viral or rickettsial infections of the CNS, although a mild depression may be seen. The glucose level is usually low in tuberculous,[67] fungal,[27] bacterial, or amebic infections.[54]

Direct examination of the CSF by Gram stain for bacteria, by acid-fast stain for mycobacteria, and by India ink for *Cryptococcus* should be performed and may be diagnostic. Wet preparation of CSF may reveal free-living amebae, and Giemsa stain will identify trypanosomes. Bacteria, mycobacteria, fungi, amebae, and viruses may also be recovered from the CSF by appropriate culture techniques. Microbial antigen detection methods have proved particularly useful in cryptococcal disease.[36]

The EEG is often abnormal in acute and chronic forms of herpes simplex encephalitis and may provide early localizing information in herpesvirus encephalitis. The computed tomographic (CT) scan is useful for ruling out space-occupying lesions, but is often unrevealing in encephalitis and myelitis. The magnetic resonance imaging (MRI) scan allows better visualization of the spinal cord, is a sensitive indicator of demyelination, and can detect the edematous changes that are often an early feature of encephalitis.

Etiology of Encephalomyelitis

Table 1 lists the viruses known to cause acute encephalitis or myelitis, as well as the viruses associated with postinfectious encephalomyelitis. Many of these infections have distinct seasonal variations that are helpful in narrowing the differential diagnosis (Fig. 1). The togavirus, flavivirus, and bunyavirus encephalitides (except rubella) are arthropod borne and therefore occur when their insect vectors are biting. The mosquito-borne encephalitides peak in late summer in temperate regions.[68] The tick-borne diseases occur most often in spring and early summer.[69–71] Enteroviruses are the most common cause of viral encephalitis and occur primarily in late summer and fall. In contrast, the herpesvirus encephalitides occur throughout the year. Lymphocytic choriomeningitis virus is most frequent in the winter when rodents come indoors, and leptospirosis is more common in the warm months when rodents and people are in contact with ponds and streams.[64]

In addition to the season, geographic and travel histories may be helpful in the diagnosis of vector-borne encephalitides. For instance, eastern equine encephalitis is most common along the Atlantic and Gulf Coasts, while western equine encephalitis is most common in the Western states. LaCrosse and St. Louis encephalitides are widespread in the United States.[1,72] Lyme disease is endemic in the Northeast and the upper Midwestern United States and Europe.[74] Japanese encephalitis is found in most of Asia,[74] and tick-borne encephalitis occurs over a wide area of eastern Europe and the Soviet Union.[75]

Infections with eastern equine encephalitis virus produce clinically evident encephalitis with high frequency in all age groups,[76] in contrast to the other causes of viral encephalitis, in which a large majority of the infections are subclinical. Clinical disease with St. Louis and western equine encephalitis viruses occurs in about 1 percent of infections, and infants and adults over age 50 are most likely to develop encephalitis.[72,77] California virus infects persons of all ages but produces encephalitis predominantly in children.[78] Venezuelan equine encephalitis virus primarily causes a flulike illness in humans but can produce encephalitis in any age group.[79]

Nonviral causes of encephalomyelitis are listed in Table 2. Some of these diseases are of known and others of unknown cause. They include drug reactions such as the neuroleptic malignant syndrome[80] and chemotherapy-induced leukoencephalopathy,[81] which may be confused with infection. Many are treatable. One of the most important concerns in evaluating a patient with encephalomyelitis is to rule out treatable entities.

The cause of encephalitis is frequently different in immunode-

TABLE 1. Viral Causes of Acute Encephalomyelitis

Direct Infection	Postinfection
Togaviridae	Togaviridae
Alphaviruses	Rubivirus
Eastern equine	Rubella
Western equine	Orthomyxoviridae
Venezuelan equine	Influenzavirus
Flaviviridae	Mumps
St. Louis	Morbillivirus
Murray Valley	Measles
West Nile	Poxviridae
Japanese	Orthopoxvirus
Dengue	Vaccinia
Tick-borne complex	Herpesviridae
Bunyaviridae	Herpesvirus
La Crosse	Varicella-zoster virus
Rift Valley	Epstein-Barr virus
Toscana	
Paramyxoviridae	
Paramyxovirus	
Mumps	
Morbillivirus	
Measles	
Arenaviridae	
Arenavirus	
Lymphocytic choriomeningitis	
Machupo	
Lassa	
Junin	
Picornaviridae	
Enterovirus	
Poliovirus	
Coxsackievirus	
Echovirus	
Hepatitis A	
Reoviridae	
Colorado tick fever	
Rhabdoviridae	
Lyssavirus	
Rabies	
Filoviridae	
Ebola	
Marburg	
Retroviridae	
Lentivirus	
Human immunodeficiency	
Herpesviridae	
Herpesvirus	
Herpes simplex virus types 1 and 2	
Varicella-zoster virus	
Herpes B virus	
Epstein-Barr virus	
Cytomegalovirus	
Human herpesvirus 6	
Adenoviridae	
Adenovirus	

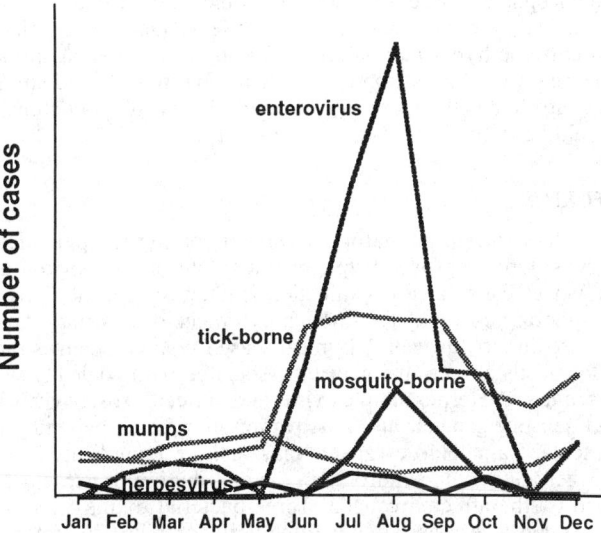

FIG. 1. Seasonal variation in temperate zones of the northern hemisphere in the encephalitides caused by mosquito-borne viruses, enteroviruses, mumps virus, herpesvirus, and tick-borne diseases.

TABLE 2. Nonviral Causes of Encephalomyelitis

Rocky Mountain spotted fever	Tuberculosis
Typhus	*Cryptococcus*
Ehrlichia canis	*Histoplasma*
Q fever	*Naegleria*
Mycoplasma	*Acanthamoeba*
Brucellosis	*Toxoplasma*
Subacute bacterial endocarditis	*Plasmodium falciparum*
Listeria	Trypanosomiasis
Syphilis (meningovascular)	Whipple's disease
Relapsing fever	Behçet's disease
Lyme disease	Cat-scratch disease
Leptospirosis	Vasculitis
Nocardia	Carcinoma
Actinomycosis	Drug reactions

ficient patients. Patients with hypogammaglobulinemia may have chronic encephalitis with enterovirus.[47] Patients with defects in cell-mediated immunity have unusual forms of encephalitis or myelitis with herpesviruses,[18,82,83] a subacute inclusion body encephalitis with measles,[17] meningoencephalitis with adenovirus,[16] and *Acanthamoeba*.[85] In acquired immunodeficiency syndrome (AIDS) a number of unusual agents, principally *Toxoplasma, Cryptococcus, Histoplasma,* cytomegalovirus, *Nocardia,* and papovavirus (progressive multifocal leukoencephalopathy), may cause CNS disease, either singly or in combination.[18,36,48,84–86]

Transverse myelitis caused by a vasculitis of the anterior spinal artery has been seen in tuberculosis, syphilis, and schistosomiasis.[87] Postinfectious transverse myelitis has been associated with measles, rubella, mumps, and upper respiratory diseases, as well as with immunizations.[88,89] Direct infection of the spinal cord with varicella-zoster virus or Lyme borrelia may also produce a transverse myelitis.[90] Infection with human T-lymphotropic virus type I causes disease primarily in the tho-

racic cord, leading to progressive spastic paraparesis.[49,50] Infection with HIV causes myelopathy manifested by spastic paraparesis and sensory ataxia.[48] Dumb rabies after lower extremity bites by rabid vampire bats has also been described as producing an ascending myelitis.[91] The lower motor neuron variety of myelitis causing flaccid paralysis may be produced by a number of enteroviruses, particularly poliovirus and enterovirus 71.[92]

Presumptive Treatment

Specific therapy is available for most of the diseases listed in Table 2 and should be instituted as soon as possible if a presumptive diagnosis can be made. For herpes simplex encephalitis, effective therapy is available with acyclovir. Varicella-zoster virus encephalitis may also be treated with acyclovir and cytomegalovirus encephalitis with ganciclovir or foscarnet, but the effectiveness of therapy for these encephalitides has not yet been established.[93–96] HIV-associated neurologic disease may improve with zidovudine treatment.[97] None of these treatments eliminates the latent state of these viruses. Other antiviral drugs are under development.[98]

Patients in coma caused by encephalitis or postinfectious encephalomyelitis may make remarkable recoveries even after prolonged periods of unconsciousness. For this reason vigorous supportive treatment is indicated, and the complications of ventilator therapy, catheters, intravenous lines, and so forth should be avoided if possible and should be treated vigorously if they occur. Blood glucose levels and electrolytes should be monitored closely, since the hypothalamic area may be involved in the encephalitic process. Seizures should be controlled, if they occur, with diphenylhydantoin. Some fever may be beneficial, but extreme hyperthermia, as well as hypoxia, may aggravate seizures. Cerebral edema can be damaging in itself and should be controlled with glycerol or mannitol, if possible, but steroids should be used if necessary for this purpose.

NEURITIS

Neuritis is an inflammatory disease involving the peripheral nerves. Only leprosy, trypanosomes, and microsporidia are known to cause a direct infection leading to clinical signs of peripheral neuropathy, although cytomegalovirus may cause disease directly as well.[99] Lyme disease frequently causes radiculoneuritis and cranial neuritis associated pathologically with vasculitis.[100] Herpes simplex virus and varicella-zoster virus infect sensory ganglia, and reactivation may be associated with radicular pain. Herpes zoster may also be complicated by a postherpeutic pain syndrome in the distribution of nerves supplied by the affected ganglia. Three bacterial toxins affect peripheral nerves either directly (diphtheria) or indirectly (tetanus, botulism), each causing distinct syndromes. The Guillain-Barré syndrome is a postinfectious inflammatory process of peripheral nerves that can involve destruction of axons or myelins.

Pathologic Characteristics and Pathogenesis

In lepromatous leprosy the immunologic response does not effectively control the infection. There is a widespread distribution of *Mycobacterium leprae*. Nerves in the skin may exhibit only minor changes, but larger peripheral nerves contain many leprosy bacilli in Schwann cells. The organisms grow best in the cooler parts of the body, and nerves close to skin surface and distal nerves are affected preferentially. In late stages of the disease extensive axonal degeneration may occur.[101]

Tuberculoid leprosy is characterized by a marked granulomatous reaction to the infection and few demonstrable bacilli. Cutaneous nerves beneath the depigmented skin macules are destroyed, producing anesthesia. The peripheral nerves are nodular and thickened, with destruction of the normal architecture. Segmental demyelination and axonal degeneration result in nerve destruction and severe fibrosis.

Trypanosoma cruzi, T. gambiense, and *T. rhodesiense* all can invade and replicate in tissue of the peripheral as well as the central nervous system. *Trypanosoma cruzi* preferentially damages cells of the autonomic nervous system by replication in the supporting Schwann cells, satellite cells, and capsular fibroblasts rather than in the neurons. In Africa, trypanosomiasis patients dying with encephalomyelitis often have evidence of neuritis.[102] The microsporidia *Nosema connori* can invade the nerve fibers of Auerbach plexus, causing nerve dysfunction.[102]

Tetanus toxin, produced by *Clostridium tetani* under anaerobic conditions, is transported up the axon and binds to the presynaptic endings on motor neurons in the anterior horns of the spinal cord, blocking inhibitory input.[103,104] This results in uncontrolled motor input to skeletal muscle and the spasms typical of this disease. Because of this transport mechanism for entry into the CNS, patients may have only localized disease in the area of the *Clostridium*-containing wound.

Botulinum toxin is produced during anaerobic metabolism of *Clostridium botulinum* and may either be ingested as performed toxin (food botulism) or produced by organisms in the intestine (infant botulism) or introduced into a wound (wound botulism). Botulinum toxin binds to the presynaptic axon terminal of the neuromuscular junction, preventing release of acetylcholine and thus producing a flaccid paralysis.[104,105] Little, if any, histologic abnormality is seen in either tetanus or botulism.

Diphtheria toxin is produced by *Corynebacterium diphtheriae* lysogenized by a phage coding for this toxin. The toxin is a protein with two subunits; one (A) inhibits protein synthesis by blocking the adenosine diphosphate (ADP) ribosylation of elongation factor 2, whereas the second (B) binds to cell membranes and therefore enables the active subunit A to enter the cell.[106] The effect of this toxin on peripheral nerves is to cause a noninflammatory demyelination. Both cranial and peripheral nerves may be demyelinated, although cranial nerves are more frequently affected.

The Guillain-Barré syndrome often follows within 4 weeks of a respiratory or gastrointestinal infection, immunization, trauma, or metabolic insult. Infections with a wide spectrum of viruses as well as *Mycoplasma pneumoniae* and *Campylobacter jejuni* have been associated with this syndrome. *C. jejuni* is emerging as the most common preceding infection, particularly in patients with axonal degeneration and in children.[107,108] Particular strains may be involved.[109] Nerves show segmental inflammation and demyelination. Low-grade perivascular inflammation may persist for months to years after the episode.[110] It is not yet clear whether disease is induced by molecular mimicry, a toxin, or immune dysregulation. Both macrophages and lymphocytes are involved with the lesion.[111]

Clinical Findings

Leprosy has two distinctive manifestations, depending on whether the disease is of the tuberculoid or the lepromatous type. Tuberculoid leprosy produces a mononeuropathy beneath the sharply demarcated, hypopigmented skin patches. Peripheral nerves may be palpably and visibly enlarged, and the neurologic involvement is a prominent part of the disease. In lepromatous leprosy a distal hypesthesia with a selective loss of pain and temperature is most common, although a mononeuropathy may be present. Cooler areas of the body are more strikingly affected, and the loss of pain sensation results in mutilation and eventual loss of digits.[101]

Tetanus usually manifests with rigidity of muscles, which may be painful. The initial manifestation may be of "local tetanus" in which the rigidity affects only one limb or area of the body in which the *Clostridium*-containing wound is located. Stiffness of the jaw muscles causes trismus, and stiffness of the facial muscles may cause a change of expression. This mild picture may progress to generalized rigidity with reflex spasms and dysphagia. The history of a soil-contaminated puncture wound should be sought. The wound may have seemed insignificant at the time of the injury and may appear well healed at the time of the neurologic disease.[112]

Botulism characteristically manifests 12–36 hours after the ingestion of the toxin with weakness, dizziness, and dryness of the mouth. Neurologic symptoms follow within 12–72 hours with blurred vision, diplopia, dysphonia, dysphagia, and muscle weakness. On examination sensation is preserved, the tendon reflexes are depressed or absent, and the paralysis is flaccid.[113] The same picture can develop more gradually in a patient with wound botulism. The original wound is usually of a rather severe traumatic nature and may appear to be healing well at the time of neurologic disease.[114]

The earliest sign of pharyngeal diphtheria (5–12 days) is paralysis of the palate, which produces a nasal quality of the voice and an increasing tendency to regurgitate fluids through the nose. Other cranial nerves (particularly the third, sixth, seventh, ninth, and tenth) may become involved, with blurring of vision and inability to accommodate as early symptoms. Later in the course of the disease, when previous symptoms may have subsided (4–8 weeks), a predominantly motor polyneuropathy involving initial symmetrical weakness of distal extremities may appear similar to Guillain-Barré syndrome. There is a flaccid paralysis with loss of deep tendon reflexes that may be accompanied by the signs and symptoms of a diphtheritic myocarditis.[115]

Neuropathies associated with human immunodeficiency virus infection include acute and chronic inflammatory demyelinating polyneuropathies, sensory ganglioneuritis, and polyradiculopathy early in infection, and a distal symmetrical primarily sensory neuropathy later when AIDS has developed.[116]

In approximately 60 percent of the cases, Guillain-Barré syndrome follows an infection or immunization. Clinically it manifests with subjective paresthesias and/or weakness, which may continue to progress for up to 4 weeks.[117] Examination typically reveals a flaccid paralysis with loss of deep tendon reflexes. Involvement of the autonomic nervous system resulting in lability of blood pressure, inappropriate antidiuretic hormone secretion, and inability to compensate for volume changes occurs in approximately 20 percent of the cases.[118] These problems frequently necessitate the management of patients in an intensive care unit even though they may not require ventilatory assistance. The condition of an individual patient may change rapidly either during progression or during recovery. Improvement is often slow, however, and may continue for up to 12 months.[117]

Laboratory Findings

Routine blood chemistries are not helpful in this group of diseases. If botulism is suspected, serum for mouse inoculation should be procured. Cerebrospinal fluid should also be obtained. In Guillain-Barré syndrome or diphtheritic polyneuritis, an increased protein level with few cells (albuminocytologic dissociation) in the CSF is the characteristic finding; some patients, however, may have a normal protein level particularly early in the disease, and others, especially those with human immunodeficiency virus infection, will have a moderate pleocytosis.[119,120] The CSF findings are normal in tetanus, botulism, and leprosy. Neurometric tests that aid in localization of the pathologic changes and thus the diagnosis are *(1)* the measurement of nerve conduction times to look for the slowed conduction found in the peripheral nerve lesions of Guillain-Barré syndrome and diphtheria (F wave measurements may allow the identification of abnormalities if lesions are very proximal) and *(2)* the recording from muscle during repetitive nerve stimulation to look for the incremental response characteristic of botulism[113] and not found in Guillain-Barré syndrome. Nerve biopsies may be useful in identifying the granulomas and/or acid-fast bacilli of leprosy and the inflammatory demyelination of Guillain-Barré syndrome.

Presumptive Treatment

In this group of clinically distinctive diseases it is important to recognize the disease and to treat it appropriately. Most patients with Guillain-Barré syndrome benefit from plasmapheresis or intravenous immunoglobulin especially when performed or given early in the disease.[119,121] Patients must be closely monitored for vital capacity, electrolytes, blood pressure, temperature, and heart rate, and those with respiratory failure should be ventilated mechanically. Patients with autonomic nervous system dysfunction should be treated with short-acting drugs, since autonomic function in these patients may be very labile. A patient who is hypertensive in the morning may be distressingly hypotensive in the evening and vice versa. Patients may not adjust to abrupt changes in intravascular volume, so intravenous fluids should be carefully controlled.

REFERENCES

1. Johnson RT. Viral Infections of the Nervous System. New York: Raven Press; 1982.
2. Mims CA. The Pathogenesis of Infectious Diseases. 3d ed. New York: Academic Press; 1987.
3. Moxon ER, Murphy PA. *Hemophilus influenzae* bacteremia and meningitis resulting from survival of a single organism. Proc Natl Acad Sci USA. 1978; 75:1534–6.
4. Tsiang H. Pathophysiology of rabies virus infection of the nervous system. Adv Virus Res. 1993;42:375–412.
5. Wyatt HV. Incubation of poliomyelitis as calculated from the central nervous system via the peripheral nerve pathways. Rev Infect Dis. 1990;12:547–56.
6. Baringer JR. Herpes simplex virus infection of nervous tissue in animals and man. Prog Med Virol. 1975;20:1–26.
7. Monath TP, Cropp CP, Harrison AK. Mode of entry of a neurotropic arbovirus into the central nervous system. Reinvestigation of an old controversy. Lab Invest. 1983;48:399–410.
8. Barnett EM, Perlman S. The olfactory nerve and not the trigeminal nerve is the major site of CNS entry for mouse hepatitis virus, strain JHM. Virology. 1993;194:185–191.
9. Ma P, Visvesvara GS, Martinez AJ, et al. *Naegleria* and acanthamoeba infections: Review. Rev Infect Dis. 1990;12:490–513.
10. Johnson RT. Selective vulnerability of neural cells to viral infection. Brain. 1980;103:447.
11. Johnson RT, Burke DS, Elwell M, et al. Japanese encephalitis: Immunocytochemical studies of viral antigen and inflammatory cells in fatal cases. Ann Neurol. 1985;18:567–73.
12. Epstein LG, Gendelman HE. Human immunodeficiency virus type 1 infection of the nervous system: Pathogenetic mechanisms. Ann Neurol. 1993;33: 429–36.
13. Eilbott DJ, Peress N, Burger H, et al. Human immunodeficiency virus type 1 in spinal cords of acquired immunodeficiency syndrome patients with myelopathy: Expression and replication in macrophages. Proc Natl Acad Sci USA 1989;86:3337–41.
14. Budka H. Neuropathology of human immunodeficiency virus infection. Brain Pathol. 1991;1:163–75.
15. Rance NE, McArthur JC, Cornblath DR, et al. Gracile tract degeneration in patients with sensory neuropathy and AIDS. Neurology. 1988;38:265–71.
16. Davis D, Henslee PJ, Markesbery WR. Fatal adenovirus meningoencephalitis in a bone marrow transplant patient. Ann Neurol. 1988;23:385–9.
17. Roos RP, Graves MC, Wollmann RL, et al. Immunologic and virologic studies of measles inclusion body encephalitis in an immunosuppressed host: The relationship to subacute sclerosing panencephalitis. Neurology. 1981; 31:1263–70.
18. Kalayjian RC, Cohen ML, Bonomo RA, et al. Cytomegalovirus ventriculoencephalitis in AIDS: A syndrome with distinct clinical and pathologic features. Medicine. 1993;72:67–77.
19. Dupont JR, Earle KM. Human rabies encephalitis: A study of forty-nine fatal cases with a review of the literature. Neurology. 1965;15:1023.
20. Miller JQ, Price TR. The nervous system in Rocky Mountain spotted fever. Neurology. 1972;22:561.
21. Dastur DK, Lalitha VS, Udani PM, et al. The brain and meninges in tuberculous meningitis: Gross pathology in 100 cases and pathogenesis. Neurol India. 1970;18:86.
22. Young RC, Bennett JE, Vogel CL, et al. Aspergillosis: The spectrum of disease in 98 patients. Medicine. 1970;49:147–73.
23. Greenfield JG. Infectious diseases of the central nervous system: Neurosyphilis. In: Blackwood W, McMenemey WH, Meyer A, et al, eds. Greenfield's Neuropathology. Baltimore: Williams & Wilkins; 1963:164.
24. Williams PL, Johnson R, Pappagianis D, et al. Vasculitic and encephalitic complications associated with *Coccidioides immitis* infection of the central nervous system in humans: Report of 10 cases and review. Clin Infect Dis. 1992;14:673–82.
25. Hilt DC, Buchholz D, Krumholz A, et al. Herpes zoster ophthalmicus and delayed contralateral hemiparesis due to cerebral angiitis: Diagnosis and management approaches. Ann Neurol. 1983;14:543.
26. Baker RD, Haugen RK. Tissue changes and tissue diagnosis in cryptococcosis: A study of 26 cases. J Clin Pathol. 1955;25:14.
27. Ellner JJ, Bennett JE. Chronic meningitis. Medicine. 1976;55:341.
28. Johnson RT, Griffin DE, Hirsch RL, et al. Measles encephalomyelitis—Clinical and immunologic studies. N Engl J Med. 1984;310:137–41.
29. Hemachudha T, Griffin DE, Giffels JJ, et al. Myelin basic protein as an encephalitogen in encephalomyelitis and polyneuritis following rabies vaccination. N Engl J Med. 1987;316:369–74.
30. Hart MN, Earle KM. Haemorrhagic and perivenous encephalitis: A clinical pathologic review of 38 cases. J Neurol Neurosurg Psychiatry. 1975;38: 585–91.
31. Hurwitz ES, Barrett MJ, Bregman D, et al. Public health service study on Reye's syndrome and medications: Report of the main study. JAMA. 1987; 257:1905–11.
32. Goren A, Freier S, Passwell JH. Lethal toxic encephalopathy due to childhood shigellosis in a developed country. Pediatrics. 1992;89:1189–93.
33. Woods ML II, Currie BJ, Howard DM, et al. Neurological melioidosis: Seven cases from the Northern Territory of Australia. Clin Infect Dis. 1992; 15:163–9.
34. Lewis DW, Tucker SH. Central nervous system involvement in cat scratch disease. Pediatrics. 1986;77:714–21.
35. Osuntokun BO, Adeuja AOG, Familusi JB. Tuberculous meningitis in Nigerians: A study of 194 patients. Trop Geogr Med. 1971;23:225.
36. Kovacs JA, Kovacs AA, Polis M, et al. Cryptococcosis in the acquired immunodeficiency syndrome. Ann Intern Med. 1985;103:533–8.
37. Whitley RJ, Soong S-J, Linneman C, et al. Herpes simplex encephalitis: Clinical assessment. JAMA. 1982;247:317.
38. Hattwick MAW. Human rabies. Public Health Rep. 1981;96:580–4.
39. Dickerson RB, Newton JR, Hansen JE. Diagnosis and immediate prognosis of Japanese B encephalitis. Am J Med. 1952;12:277–88.

40. Halperin JJ, Volkman DJ, Wu P. Central nervous system abnormalities in Lyme neuroborreliosis. Neurology. 1991;41:1571–82.
41. Halperin J, Golightly M, Andriola M, et al. Lyme borreliosis in Bell's palsy. Neurology. 1992;42:1268.
42. Centers for Disease Control and Prevention. Human rabies—Texas, Arkansas, and Georgia, 1991. MMWR. 1991;40:765–9.
43. Knox DL, Bayless TM, Pittman FE. Neurologic disease in patients with treated Whipple's disease. Medicine. 1976;55:467–76.
44. Helmick CG, Bernard KW, D'Angelo LJ. Rocky Mountain spotted fever: Clinical, laboratory, and epidemiological features of 262 cases. J Infect Dis. 1984;150:480–8.
45. McDade JE. Ehrlichiosis—A disease of animals and humans. J Infect Dis. 1990;161:609–17.
46. Kelsey DS. Adenovirus meningoencephalitis. Pediatrics. 1978;61:291.
47. McKinney RE Jr, Katz SL, Wilfert CM. Chronic enteroviral meningoencephalitis in agammaglobulinemic patients. Rev Infect Dis. 1987;9:334–56.
48. McArthur JC. Neurologic manifestations of human immunodeficiency virus infection. Medicine. 1987;66:407–37.
49. Bucher B, Poupard JA, Vernant J-C, et al. Tropical neuromyelopathies and retroviruses: A review. Rev Infect Dis. 1990;12:890–9.
50. Höllsberg P, Hafler DA. Pathogenesis of diseases induced by human lymphotropic virus type I infection. N Engl J Med. 1993;328:1173–82.
51. Feigin RD, Shackelford PG. Value of repeat lumbar puncture in the differential diagnosis of meningitis. N Engl J Med. 1973;289:571.
52. Koskiniemi M, Vaheri A, Taskinen E. Cerebrospinal fluid alterations in herpes simplex virus encephalitis. Rev Infect Dis. 1984;6:608–18.
53. Adams RD, Victor M. Multiple sclerosis and allied demyelinating diseases. In: Principles of Neurology, 3rd ed. New York: McGraw-Hill; 1985:699.
54. Carter RF. Primary amoebic meningoencephalitis: An appraisal of present knowledge. Trans R Soc Trop Med Hyg. 1972;66:193–208.
55. Peacock JE Jr, McGinnis MR, Cohen MS. Persistent neutrophilic meningitis: Report of four cases and review of the literature. Medicine. 1984;63:379–95.
56. Link H, Muller R. Immunoglobulins in multiple sclerosis and infections of the nervous system. Arch Neurol. 1971;25:326–44.
57. Tourtellotte W. On cerebrospinal fluid immunoglobulin-G (IgG) quotients in multiple sclerosis and other diseases. J Neurol Sci. 1970;10:279.
58. Vandvik B, Nilsen RE, Vartdal F, et al. Mumps meningitis: Specific and nonspecific antibody responses in the central nervous system. Acta Neurol Scand. 1982;65:468–87.
59. Vartdal F, Vandvik B, Norrby E. Intrathecal synthesis of virus-specific oligoclonal IgG, IgA, and IgM antibodies in a case of varicella-zoster meningoencephalitis. J Neurol Sci. 1982;57:121–32.
60. Vartdal F, Vandvik B, Michaelson TE, et al. Neurosyphilis: Intrathecal synthesis of oligoclonal antibodies to *Treponema pallidum*. Ann Neurol. 1982; 11:35.
61. Steere AC, Berardi VP, Weeks KE, et al. Evaluation of the intrathecal antibody response to *Borrelia burgdorferi* as a diagnostic test for Lyme neuroborreliosis. J Infect Dis. 1990;161:1203–9.
62. Salmi AA, Norrby E, Panelius M. Identification of different measles virus-specific antibodies in the serum and cerebrospinal fluid from patients with subacute sclerosing panencephalitis and multiple sclerosis. Infect Immun. 1972;6:248.
63. Townsend JJ, Baringer JR, Wolinsky JS, et al. Progressive rubella panencephalitis: Late onset after congenital rubella. N Engl J Med. 1975;292: 99.
64. Meyer HM, Johnson RT, Crawford IP, et al. Central nervous system syndromes of "viral" etiology: A study of 713 cases. Am J Med. 960;29:334–47.
65. Calisher CH, Berardi VP, Muth DJ, et al. Specificity of immunoglobulin M and G antibody responses in humans infected with eastern and western equine encephalitis viruses: Application to rapid serodiagnosis. J Clin Microbiol. 1986;23:369–72.
66. Burke DS, Nisalak A, Ussery MA, et al. Kinetics of IgM and IgG responses to Japanese encephalitis virus in human serum and cerebrospinal fluid. J Infect Dis. 1985;151:1093–9.
67. Ogawa SK, Smith MA, Brennessel DJ, et al. Tuberculous meningitis in an urban medical center. Medicine. 1987;66:317–26.
68. Lennette EH, Longshore WA. Western equine and St. Louis encephalitis in man. California 1945–1950. Calif Med. 1951;75:189.
69. Spruance SL, Bailey A. Colorado tick fever: A review of 115 laboratory confirmed cases. Arch Intern Med. 1973;131:288.
70. Wilfert CM, MacCormack JN, Kleeman K, et al. Epidemiology of Rocky Mountain spotted fever as determined by active surveillance. J Infect Dis. 1984;150:469–79.
71. Ciesielski CA, Hightower AW, Horsley R, et al. The geographic distribution of Lyme disease in the United States. Ann NY Acad Sci. 1989;539:283–8.
72. Centers for Disease Control and Prevention. Arboviral disease—United States, 1991. MMWR. 1992;41:545–8.
73. Schmid GP. The global distribution of Lyme disease. Rev Infect Dis. 1985; 7:41–50.
74. Rosen L. The natural history of Japanese encephalitis virus. Annu Rev Microbiol. 1986;40:395–414.
75. Monath TP. Flaviviruses. In: Fields BN, Knipe DM, Channock RM, et al, eds. Virology 2nd ed, New York: Raven Press; 1990;763–814.
76. Przelomski MM, O'Rourke E, Grady GF, et al. Eastern equine encephalitis in Massachusetts: A report of 16 cases, 1970–1984. Neurology. 1988;38: 736–9.
77. Southern PM, Smith JW, Luby JP, et al. Clinical and laboratory features of epidemic St. Louis encephalitis. Ann Intern Med. 1969;71:681.
78. Woodruff BA, Baron RC, Tsai TF. Symptomatic LaCrosse virus infections of the central nervous system: A study of risk factors in an endemic area. Am J Epidemiol. 1992;136:320–7.
79. Ventura AK, Buff EE, Ehrenkranz NJ. Human Venezuelan equine encephalitis virus infection in Florida. Am J Trop Med Hyg. 1974;23:507.
80. Guze BH, Baxter LR Jr. Neuroleptic malignant syndrome. N Engl J Med. 1985;313:163–6.
81. Glass JP, Lee YY, Bruner J, et al. Treatment-related leukoencephalopathy: A study of three cases and literature review. Medicine. 1986;65:154–62.
82. Jemsek J, Greenberg SB, Taber L, et al. Herpes zoster–associated encephalitis: Clinicopathologic report of 12 cases and review of the literature. Medicine. 1983;62:81–96.
83. Linnemann CC, First MR, Alvira MM, et al. Herpes virus hominis type 2 meningoencephalitis following renal transplantation. Am J Med. 1976;61:703.
84. Gordon SM, Steinberg JP, DuPuis MH, et al. Culture isolation of *Acanthamoeba* species and leptomyxid amebas from patients with amebic meningoencephalitis, including two patients with AIDS. Clin Infect Dis. 1992;15: 1024–30.
85. Luft BJ, Remington JS. Toxoplasmic encephalitis in AIDS. Clin Infect Dis. 1992;15:211–22.
86. Gillespie SM, Chang Y, Lemp G, et al. Progressive multifocal leukoencephalopathy in persons infected with human immunodeficiency virus, San Francisco, 1981–1989. Ann Neurol. 1991;30:597–604.
87. Cohen J, Capildeo R, Rose FC, et al. Schistosomal myelopathy. Br Med J. 1977;1:1258.
88. Altrocchi PH. Acute transverse myelopathy. Arch Neurol. 1963;9:111.
89. Lipton HL, Teasdall RD. Acute transverse myelopathy in adults. Arch Neurol. 1973;28:252.
90. Devinsky O, Cho E-S, Petito CK, et al. Herpes zoster myelitis. Brain. 1991; 114:1181–96.
91. Hurst EW, Pawan JL. A further account of the Trinidad outbreak of acute rabic myelitis: Histology of the experimental disease. J Pathol Bacteriol. 1932;35:301.
92. Melnick JL. Enterovirus type 71 infections. A varied clinical pattern sometimes mimicking paralytic poliomyelitis. Rev Infect Dis. 1984;6(Suppl 2): S387–90.
93. Whitley RJ, Alford CA, Hirsch MS, et al. Viradabine versus acyclovir therapy in herpes simplex encephalitis. N Engl J Med. 1986;314:144–9.
94. Weigler BJ. Biology of B virus in macaque and human hosts: A review. Clin Infect Dis. 1992;14:555–67.
95. Whitley RJ, Gnann JW Jr, Hinthorn D, et al. Disseminated herpes zoster in the immunocompromised host: A comparative trial of acyclovir and vidarabine. J Infect Dis. 1992;165:450–5.
96. AIDS Clinical Trials Group: Mortality in patients with the acquired immunodeficiency syndrome treated with either foscarnet or ganciclovir for cytomegalovirus retinitis. N Engl J Med. 1992;326:213–20.
97. Schmitt FA, Bigley JW, McKinnis R, et al. Neuropsychological outcome of zidovudine (AZT) treatment of patients with AIDS and AIDS-related complex. N Engl J Med. 1988;319:1573–8.
98. Griffin DE. Therapy of viral infections of the central nervous system. Antiviral Res. 1991;15:1–10.
99. Said G, Lacroix C, Chemouilli P, et al. Cytomegalovirus neuropathy in acquired immunodeficiency syndrome: A clinical and pathological study. Ann Neurol. 1991;29:139–46.
100. Meurers B, Kohlhepp W, Gold R, et al. Histopathological findings in the central and peripheral nervous systems in neuroborreliosis. J Neurol. 1990; 237:113–6.
101. Sabin TD, Swift TR, Jacobson RR. Leprosy. In: Dyck PJ, Thomas PK, Griffin JW, et al, eds. Peripheral Neuropathy. Philadelphia: WB Saunders: 1993;1354–79.
102. Connor DH, Manz HJ. Parasitic infections of the peripheral nervous system. In: Peripheral Neuropathy. Dyck PJ, Thomas PK, Griffin JW, et al, eds. Philadelphia: WB Saunders: 1993;1380–1400.
103. Price DL, Griffin J, Young A, et al. Tetanus toxin: Direct evidence for retrograde intraaxonal transport. Science. 1975;188:945.
104. Simpson LL. Molecular pharmacology of botulinum toxin and tetanus toxin. Annu Rev Pharmacol Toxicol. 1986;26:427–53.
105. Black JD, Dolly JO. Interaction of ^{125}I-labelled botulinum neurotoxins with nerve terminals. II. Autoradiographic evidence for uptake into motor nerves by acceptor-mediated endocytosis. J Cell Biol. 1986;103:535–44.
106. Pappenheimer AM. Diphtheria toxin. Annu Rev Biochem. 1977;46:69–94.
107. Winer JB, Hughes RAC, Osmond C. A prospective study of acute idiopathic neuropathy. 2. Antecedent events. J Neurol Neurosurg Psychiatry. 1988;51: 613–8.
108. McKhann GM, Cornblath DR, Griffin JW, et al. Acute motor axonal neuropathy: A frequent cause of acute flaccid paralysis in China. Ann Neurol. 1993; 33:333–42.
109. Kuroki S, Saida T, Nukina M, et al. *Campylobacter jejuni* strains from patients with Guillain-Barré syndrome belong mostly to Penner serogroup 19 and contain B-N-acetylglucosamine residues. Ann Neurol. 1993;33:243–7.
110. Asbury AK, Arnason BG, Adams RD. The inflammatory lesion in idiopathic polyneuritis: Its role in pathogenesis. Medicine. 1969;48:173–215.
111. Thomas PK. The Guillain-Barré syndrome: No longer a simple concept. J Neurol. 1992;239:361–2.
112. Weinstein L. Tetanus. N Engl J Med. 1973;289:1293.

113. Cherington M. Botulism: Ten-year experience. Arch Neurol. 1974;30:432.
114. Merson MH, Dowell VR Jr. Epidemiologic, clinical and laboratory aspects of wound botulism. N Engl J Med. 1973;289:1005.
115. McDonald WI, Kocen RS. Diphtheritic neuropathy. In: Dyck PJ, Thomas PK, Griffin JW, et al, eds. Peripheral Neuropathy. Philadelphia: WB Saunders; 1993;1412–7.
116. Parry GJ. Peripheral neuropathies associated with human immunodeficiency virus infection. Ann Neurol. 1988;23(Suppl):S49–S53.
117. Masucci EF, Kurtzke JF. Diagnostic criteria for the Guillain-Barré syndrome: An analysis of 50 cases. J Neurol Sci. 1971;13:483.
118. Lichtenfeld P. Autonomic dysfunction in the Guillain-Barré syndrome. Am J Med. 1971;50:772–80.
119. Cornblath DR, McArthur JC, Kennedy PGE, et al. Inflammatory demyelinating peripheral neuropathies associated with human T cell lymphotropic virus type III infection. Ann Neurol. 1987;21:32–40.
120. Wiederholt WC, Mulder DW, Lambert EH. The Landry-Guillain-Barré-Strohl syndrome or polyradiculoneuropathy: Historical review, report on 97 patients, and present concepts. Mayo Clin Proc. 1964;39:427.
121. The Guillain-Barré Syndrome Study Group: Plasmapheresis and acute Guillain-Barré syndrome. Neurology. 1985;35:1096–1104.

67. PRION DISEASES OF THE CENTRAL NERVOUS SYSTEM (TRANSMISSIBLE NEURODEGENERATIVE DISEASES)

KENNETH L. TYLER

The concept of "atypically slow infections" was introduced in 1954 by Sigurdsson,[1] based on his observations of the naturally occurring diseases of visna, maedi, and scrapie in sheep. By adapting his criteria, a slow infection may be defined as a progressive pathologic process caused by a transmissible agent that remains clinically silent during a prolonged incubation period of months to years, after which progressive clinical disease appears, usually ending months later in profound disability or death.

Interest in slow infections of the human central nervous system (CNS) has been particularly keen since the experimental transmission of several of these diseases from humans to experimental animals and the elucidation of prions as putative agents with unconventional biologic properties. This group of diseases includes the human disorders of Creutzfeldt-Jakob disease (CJD), Gerstmann-Straussler syndrome, and fatal familial insomnia, as well as the animal diseases of scrapie, transmissible mink encephalopathy, chronic wasting disease of elk and deer, bovine and feline spongiform encephalopathy, and exotic ungulate encephalopathy.[2–7] These disorders share certain pathologic features and are referred to as *transmissible neurodegenerative diseases* (TNDs). The human TNDs noted above will be discussed in this chapter. Two slow infections of the CNS of known viral etiology (subacute sclerosing panencephalitis and progressive multifocal leukoencephalopathy) are described in Chapters 137 and 123. The subject of prions is discussed in Chapter 155.

KURU

Kuru was the first of the human TNDs to be studied in detail.[4a,8–16] It was originally endemic within the Fore linguistic tribal group of the Eastern Highlands of Papua-New Guinea.

Epidemiologic studies suggested that the disease may have been transmitted through the practice of ritual cannibalism,[17] and no one born since the cessation of these practices has developed kuru. The disease typically begins insidiously with a prodromal phase of headaches and arthralgia. This is followed by the development of an inexorably progressive neurologic disease resulting in death within 2 years of onset. The cardinal clinical features include cerebellar ataxia, action tremor, and involuntary movements (choreoathetosis, myoclonic jerks, coarse fasciculations), followed in the later stages of the illness by progressive dementia. Cranial nerve findings, motor weakness, and sensory loss remain absent or occur only in the late stages of the disease. Laboratory tests are rarely helpful in making the diagnosis. The cerebrospinal fluid (CSF) profile is unremarkable, and the EEG does not show the characteristic periodic sharp wave complexes typical of CJD (see below).[18] Although studies have been limited by the lack of recent cases, there are no reports of mutations in the PrP gene associated with cases of kuru. However, patients with kuru may show a higher than expected incidence of homozygosity at a polymorphic codon, 129, of the PrP gene (see below).[6]

CREUTZFELDT-JAKOB DISEASE

Although CJD remains a rare disease with a prevalence and incidence of ~1 case/million population worldwide, it is the most commonly encountered of the TNDs and has been responsible for much of our current knowledge concerning the clinical, pathologic, and laboratory features of TNDs.[2,3,4,4a,6,7] The overwhelming majority (85–95 percent) of cases are sporadic. Familial cases, although accounting for only a minority of patients, have proven to be invaluable in establishing the role played by the PrP gene in the pathogenesis of this disease (see below). Familial CJD is typically an autosomal dominant disorder, although the penetrance may be variable.

Cases of CJD show no sex predilection. Mean age at onset is between 57 and 62 years, although patients as young as 17 years have been reported.[19] Early onset of CJD should prompt a thorough search for iatrogenic sources of illness, such as administration of cadaveric human growth or gonadotropic hormones or the transplantation of potentially infected human material.

Despite fears to the contrary, CJD is not contagious. Examples of iatrogenic person-to-person spread are exceedingly rare[20] but have followed transplantation of infected corneas,[21] dural grafts,[22–29] and use of contaminated neurosurgical instruments or stereotactic depth electrodes.[30–32] An increasing number of cases have recently been described in young patients who received human cadaveric growth hormone (GH) for treatment of endocrine disorders including panhypopituitarism[33–38] or cadaveric pituitary gonadotropin for infertility.[39–41] Patients with GH-associated CJD typically received injections of GH, prepared from pools of up to 15,000 pituitary glands, several times weekly for several years. Creutzfeldt-Jakob disease developed after a variable incubation period (range, 3–22 years) and often presented with a clinical picture reminiscent of kuru. Ataxia and associated incoordination and extrapyramidal features are often prominent, and dementia may be minimal or absent in the early stages. There have only been two reported cases of gonadotropin-associated CJD, but the clinical features appear similar to those described in GH-associated CJD.

Isolated cases of CJD have occurred in approximately 24 physicians and other health care workers,[42] including two neurosurgeons,[43,44] one pathologist,[45] nine nurses,[19,44] and two histology technicians.[46,47] Despite the natural concern these reports produce among some health professionals, it is important to recognize that the incidence of CJD in this group does not exceed what would be expected by chance alone. There have been no documented reports of clear-cut transmission of disease from patients to hospital or mortuary staff. Similarly, although isolated cases of conjugal CJD have been reported, there does not appear to be any increased risk to spouses or other family members from exposure to CJD. As noted earlier, the presence of familial cases of CJD appear invariably to result from genetic factors rather than person-to-person spread of illness.

Creutzfeldt-Jakob disease typically presents as a rapidly progressive dementing illness with associated myoclonus, although these characteristics are hardly apparent in the original descriptions of the disease.[48–51] There is a great deal of variability in the clinical manifestations of CJD, and this has led to attempts to describe a variety of clinical subtypes, including those with predominance of visual (Heidenhain[52]), cerebellar (Brownell-Oppenheimer[53]), and thalamic (Stern[54]) and striatal (Garcin[55]) features (see Kirschbaum[56] for review). The primary importance of these syndromes is that they indicate that CJD may at times predominantly affect particular brain regions disproportionately. In the majority of patients CJD begins with mental deterioration, which may be manifested as dementia, behavioral disturbances, or other deficits in higher cortical function.[57,58] In about one-third of patients predominant initial visual or cerebellar symptoms may overshadow dementia. Mental deterioration is typically rapidly progressive, and the average duration of illness from onset of symptoms to death is 7–9 months. Unusual cases of longer duration have been described.[59] In addition to profound and rapidly progressive mental deterioration, another almost invariant feature of the disease is the presence of myoclonus. This is frequently aggravated or induced by startle. Extrapyramidal symptoms and signs including hypokinesia and rigidity, and cerebellar signs and symptoms including nystagmus, tremor, and ataxia ultimately develop in about two-thirds of patients. About 40–80 percent of patients will have signs of corticospinal tract dysfunction, including hyperreflexia, spasticity, and extensor plantar responses. Fifty percent of CJD patients will have prominent visual disturbances, which can include visual field cuts, cortical blindness, and visual agnosia. There are some neurologic disturbances that only rarely occur as prominent features in CJD, and their presence should prompt consideration of other diagnostic possibilities. Although seizures occur in 10–20 percent of cases, they are rarely a dominant feature and are typically amenable to therapy. Some patients have vague sensory complaints, but prominent sensory signs almost never occur. Cranial nerve involvement is never prominent, although rare cases with involvement of the pupils, extraocular movements, and auditory and vestibular systems have been reported. CJD does not affect the peripheral nervous system to any significant degree and is not associated with neuropathies.

A subgroup of patients (10 percent) develop prominent lower motor neuron signs and symptoms, including prominent muscular atrophy and fasciculations.[60] These patients frequently have a slowly progressive, longer duration illness that is atypical for classic CJD. Unlike classic CJD,[61,62] this "amyotrophic" variant of CJD is only rarely transmissible to primates, suggesting that most cases are not truly cases of TND or prion disease, but are probably more closely related to syndromes of amyotrophic lateral sclerosis plus dementia (ALS–dementia complex).

Routine laboratory and diagnostic tests are rarely of help in establishing the diagnosis of CJD, but may be useful in excluding other diagnostic possibilities. The blood count, differential, and sedimentation rate are all normal. A few patients have had abnormalities in liver function.[62,63] The CSF is acellular, with a normal glucose and a normal or mildly elevated protein. The presence of a significant pleocytosis or hypoglycorrhachia should prompt a search for other diagnostic possibilities. Abnormalities in the protein profile after two-dimensional isoelectric focusing have been described,[64,65] but this test has not been utilized with enough frequency for its diagnostic value to be determined. Levels of a variety of proteins including neuron-specific enolase, creatinine kinase BB, and ubiquitin[66,67] may be elevated in the CSF, although it remains to be seen if these abnormalities are

characteristic enough to be clinically useful. PrP^C has been detected in human CSF, but as yet there is no available CSF-based diagnostic test for the presence of PrP^{Sc}, which is diagnostic for CJD.

Computed tomography scans may be abnormal in CJD, but the changes are nonspecific and nondiagnostic.[68,69] However, the presence of a profound and rapidly progressive dementia in association with a CT scan without evidence of significant atrophy should suggest the possibility of CJD, as patients with advanced Alzheimer's disease typically have prominent atrophy. In some patients with CJD, serial CT scans[70,71] may show rapidly progressing cerebral atrophy and associated ex vacuo ventricular enlargement. This type of rapid evolution of CT scan changes is only rarely encountered in other forms of dementia. Magnetic resonance imaging (MRI) appears to be more sensitive than CT in detecting abnormalities in patients with CJD. A number of reports describe MRI findings in isolated cases or small series of patients.[72–78] Abnormally increased T_2 signals in the striatum and thalamus are commonly reported. Less commonly seen are signal abnormalities limited to peripheral cortex.[79] It is important to recognize that the MRI may be entirely normal. There are too few reported studies with other imaging techniques, such as positron emission tomography,[80] to determine whether there are typical or diagnostically useful patterns in CJD.

Patients with CJD often have characteristic electroencephalographic (EEG) abnormalities,[32,70,81–85] and this test may be extremely helpful as a diagnostic tool. The classic EEG pattern, which ultimately appears in 75–90 percent of patients, consists of a slow background interrupted by generalized bilaterally synchronous bi- or triphasic periodic sharp wave complexes (PSWCs).[81,82,86] These occur at intervals of 0.5–2.5 seconds and have a duration of 200–600 msec. They may be absent early in disease, may disappear in the terminal stages, and are often more dramatic during periods of alertness, but may disappear during sleep or under the influence of certain drugs including barbiturates, benzodiazepines, and methylphenidate.[87] During sleep many patients will have almost complete absence of the REM stage, as well as other disturbances in sleep architecture.[88] Obtaining serial EEGs in patients suspected of CJD may be extremely useful if PSWCs are absent on an initial EEG.[83,84,89] Lack of this typical EEG pattern in a patient whose illness has lasted for more than 4 months should cast doubt on the diagnosis of CJD. However, it is important to recognize that typical EEG findings may be absent in cases of familial CJD[90] and are not typically seen in Gerstmann-Straussler-Scheinker syndrome (GSS) or fatal familial insomnia (FFI) (see below).

For definitive diagnosis of sporadic cases, examination of brain material remains the gold standard. The presence of the typical neuropathologic features of neuronal loss, reactive gliosis, and neuronal vacuolation (spongiform change), with an absence of inflammatory responses, are typical features and consistent with the diagnosis. It is important to recognize that CJD may occasionally coexist with Alzheimer's disease or other forms of dementia.[91,92] Demonstration of transmissibility of the characteristic disease and associated neuropathology to animals (now typically mice or hamsters rather than primates) confirms the diagnosis of TND.

More recently, the availability of monoclonal and polyclonal antibodies against prion proteins[93,94] has allowed for the identification of PrP^{Sc} by Western immunoblotting of brain material obtained at autopsy or by biopsy. Immunologic tests appear to be both sensitive and specific[95,96] and have largely replaced transmission experiments. A variety of techniques have also been developed to immunostain for PrP^{Sc} in paraffin-embedded brain material[97] or cryostat preparations blotted onto nitrocellulose membranes (histoblots). Hydrolytic autoclaving or proteolysis disrupts the normal PrP^C isoform but leaves abnormal and still immunoreactive PrP^{Sc}. With these techniques, a variety of PrP staining patterns have been identified in CJD brains. Brains may show positive PrP staining limited to plaques or a more diffuse pattern of staining that colocalizes with synaptic markers (e.g., synaptophysin) throughout the grey matter, or a combination of both patterns.[97] In cases of familial CJD, distinct neuropathologic and immunostaining features often correlate with particular PrP gene mutations (see below).

There has been an explosion of reports identifying mutations in the PrP gene in the inherited prion diseases, including familial CJD, GSS, and FFI (see refs. 6, 98, 99 for review). No consistent mutation in the PrP gene has been identified in patients with sporadic (nonfamilial) CJD.[100] However, a number of reports suggest that polymorphisms at codon 129 of the PrP gene may play a role in disease expression in sporadic and iatrogenic CJD, including cases resulting from administration of cadaveric GH. Fifty-one percent of normal individuals will be heterozygous at codon 129 of the PrP gene (Met/Val), with the remainder being homozygous (37 percent Met/Met, 12 percent Val/Val). It has been reported that up to 95 percent of patients who develop sporadic (nonfamilial) CJD will be homozygous (73 percent Met/Met, 22 percent Val/Val) at this locus.[101] Similarly, five of seven studied cases of GH-related CJD showed homozygosity at codon 129 (four Val/Val, one Met/Met).[102] Particular patterns of codon 129 polymorphism in patients with sporadic CJD may also be associated with particular patterns of PrP^Sc immunostaining in brain tissues.[97]

A number of mutations within the PrP gene have now been reported in cases of familial CJD. One of the most interesting features of these cases is that specific mutations in the PrP gene are often associated with particular clinical and pathologic disease phenotypes. It appears that particular mutations may influence the age of onset and duration of disease, the prominence of certain clinical features including dementia, myoclonus, and ataxia, the presence of typical EEG abnormalities, the degree of spongiform neuropathologic change, and the regional distribution and pattern of accumulation of PrP^Sc within the brain. Perhaps the most commonly encountered is a lysine (Lys) for glutamate (Glu) mutation in codon 200. This mutation has been found in geographic clusters of familial CJD in Slovakia, Chile, and among Sephardic Jews in Greece, Libya, Tunisia, and Israel.[6,103–106] At least one family with this particular mutation presented with a disease resembling progressive supranuclear palsy that was not associated with myoclonus or EEG findings typical of CJD.[107] It has been reported that immunostaining for PrP^Sc in familial CJD cases with this mutation tends to show PrP accumulation in a dense synaptic pattern in the grey matter rather than within plaques.[97]

Additional mutations reported in familial CJD include an asparagine (Asn) for aspartic acid (Asp) mutation in codon 178.[108,109] This mutation has been described in kindreds from Finland and Europe.[108,110] Some of these patients have had disease characterized by earlier age at onset, longer duration of illness, and absence of typical periodic EEG changes.[109] Mutations in this codon have also been described in patients with GSS and FFI (see below). It has recently been suggested that the phenotype expression of the codon 178 mutation may be influenced by the nature of the associated codon 129 polymorphism. Patients with a Val 129 present as familial CJD, whereas those with a Met 129 present as FFI (see below). In addition to mutations resulting in amino acid substitutions in the PrP, a number of basepair insertions have been described within the PrP gene in cases of familial CJD.[6,111–113]

GERSTMANN-STRAUSSLER-SCHEINKER SYNDROME

The GSS syndrome is an exceedingly rare TND, with an incidence of 1–10 cases/100 million population per year. The majority of reported cases are familial, with an autosomal dominant pattern of inheritance and virtually complete penetrance. Approximately two dozen independent kindreds have been identified worldwide to date.

The basic clinical features are those of a midlife progressive spinocerebellar degeneration with associated dementia.[114–116] The average duration of disease is 5 years, with mean age of onset of 43–48 years (range, 24–66 years). In typical cases, cerebellar features dominate the clinical picture, with dementia a late or minor accompaniment. Cerebellar dysfunction manifests as incoordination, clumsiness, and difficulty walking. Associated clinical findings include ataxia, dysmetria, tremor, nystagmus, and dysarthria. Some families have more prominent dementia, or associated extrapyramidal or other findings. In contrast to CJD, myoclonus is only rarely a prominent feature and is often entirely absent. Much of the clinical heterogeneity of the disease may be the result of the variable phenotypic effects of different PrP gene mutations associated with the disease (see below).

Laboratory tests are rarely helpful in the diagnosis, but may be of value in excluding other diagnostic possibilities. Like kuru, but unlike CJD, the EEG in GSS does not show periodic sharp wave complexes.[115] The CT may show evidence of cerebellar and/or brain stem atrophy and MRI studies have been limited,[115,117] but some patients have had decreased T_2-signal in the striatum, substantia nigra, and red nucleus.

Definitive diagnosis requires the examination of brain material. Like the other prion diseases, GSS may be transmitted to animals by brain material from infected cases.[118] Neuropathologic findings are typical of other TNDs with the exception that many patients have amyloid plaques reminiscent of those of kuru (kuru plaques) found throughout the brain, but in largest concentration within the cerebellum. In some families, spongiform changes are minimal or absent. Atypical kindreds have been reported in which prion amyloid plaques are prominent throughout the telencephalon and not limited to the cerebellum and in which neurofibrillary tangles are prominent.[119] Cases of this type may have been previously mischaracterized as familial Alzheimer's disease. The availability of immunostaining now allows the amyloid plaques associated with prion diseases to be clearly distinguished from the senile plaques characteristic of Alzheimer's disease. Prion plaques immunostain with antibodies against PrP^Sc and do not stain with antibodies to β-amyloid protein, whereas senile plaques have the opposite characteristics.[3,120]

A number of PrP gene mutations have been identified in patients with familial GSS.[6,98,99,111,121,122] The most common appears to be a leucine (Leu) for proline (Pro) substitution in codon 102.[121,123,124] This mutation was found in descendants of the original family described by Gerstmann, Straussler, and Scheinker.[125,126] Transgenic mice with this codon 102 mutation spontaneously develop a neurodegenerative disease indistinguishable from scrapie,[127] providing additional evidence that PrP gene mutations are responsible for familial GSS. Affected families have been described with valine (Val) for alanine (Ala) mutations in codon 117, double mutations involving codons 117 and 129,[128] serine (Ser) for phenylalanine (Phe) mutations in codon 198, and basepair inserts.[129] It has been suggested that GSS (102 mutation) may present predominantly as ataxia,[124] whereas patients with GSS (117 mutation) and GSS (198 mutation) have more prominent dementia. An additional feature in GSS (198 mutation) is the presence of prominent neurofibrillary tangles.

FATAL FAMILIAL INSOMNIA

Fatal familial insomnia is the most recently recognized of the familial human prion diseases,[130–132] although there is some clinical and pathologic overlap with cases previously described as thalamic dementia.[133] Onset of disease is in middle or late life (35–61 years), with an average disease duration of 13 (range, 7–25) months.[131] Inheritance follows an autosomal dominant pattern.[131] In this unusual disorder patients present with progressive insomnia, dysautonomia (hyperhidrosis, hyperthermia, tachycardia, hypertension), and motor disturbances that can include ataxia, myoclonus, spasticity, hyperreflexia, and dysarthria.[130,131,134] Mental status abnormalities can include hallucinations, confusion, memory deficits, and decreased attention, but frank dementia is rarely encountered.[134] Many patients have endocrine disturbances, including decreased adrenocorticotropic hormone secretion, increased cortisol secretion, and loss of the normal circadian pattern of growth hormone, prolactin, and melatonin secretion. Neuropathologic changes including neuronal loss and gliosis are consistently found in the anterior and mediodorsal nuclei of the thalamus and at times in the olivary nucleus and cerebellar and cerebral cortex.[130,131] Spongiform changes have only been reported in a single case. Immunostaining of brain material is positive for PrP^{Sc}.[130] Periodic sharp wave complexes in the EEG, characteristic of CJD, have only been described in one patient. Although the disease has not yet been successfully transmitted to animals, all the reported cases have had an Asn for an Asp mutation in codon 178.[130,135] As discussed earlier, polymorphism at codon 129 may determine whether patients with codon 178 mutations present with familial CJD or with FFI.[136]

TREATMENT OF TNDs

Kuru, CJD, GSS, and FFI appear to be invariably fatal diseases from which there is virtually no hope of recovery. One documented patient with CJD has apparently recovered, but all other confirmed cases have ended fatally. There is no known currently available effective form of therapy. Treatment with agents such as idoxuridine,[137,138] acyclovir,[139,140] interferons,[141] polyanions,[142] and amphotericin B[143] have all been unsuccessful. Anecdotal reports of stabilization or improvement following treatment with amantadine,[144-147] vidarabine,[148] and methisoprinol[149] have not been confirmed by other studies[150] or in unpublished trials in individual patients. Further unraveling of the genetics, mechanism, and site of conversion of PrP^C to PrP^{Sc} may provide insights into new forms of therapy in the future.

HANDLING OF POTENTIALLY INFECTIOUS MATERIAL

As noted earlier, there is no evidence that prion diseases are contagious in the usual sense of the term, although instances of person-to-person spread have been documented. Almost without exception these iatrogenic cases have required the direct inoculation, implantation, or transplantation of infectious material. Kuru appears to have been transmitted by ingestion, and both kuru and CJD have been transmitted to primates by this route, although it is quite inefficient.[151] Despite this fact, there is no evidence that ingestion is an important route of spread for CJD, GSS, or FFI. Based on studies in animals,[4,4a] it can be expected that the highest concentration of the infectious agent in human tissues occurs in the brain, spinal cord, and eye. Other organs or body fluids occasionally found to contain infectious material include CSF, lymphoreticular organs, kidney, and lung. The infectious agent is almost never found in blood or urine, and blood transfusions do not appear to be a major risk factor for the acquisition of CJD.[152] There are no reported isolations of infectious material from human feces, saliva, sputum, vaginal secretions, or milk.[4,4a]

From a practical viewpoint it appears that the universal system of precautions now widely employed in most health care settings are more than adequate for dealing with patients suspected of having TNDs. Gloves should be worn when handling blood, CSF, urine, feces, and material soiled by these fluids and when performing invasive procedures including venipuncture and lumbar puncture. Masks, gowns, and protective eyewear should be employed if extensive exposure to blood, CSF, body fluids, or neural tissue is anticipated. Gloves should be discarded after single patient use, and hands should be thoroughly washed. Potentially infectious material should be placed in appropriate containers, bagged to reduce the risk of accidental spills, and clearly marked. Individuals transporting this material should wear gloves. Care should be taken to avoid autoinoculation with needles, surgical instruments, or other sharp objects.

Controversy continues concerning the best procedures for fully sterilizing instruments, tissues, or other materials known to contain prions. The Committee on Health Care Issues of the American Neurological Association has suggested either steam autoclaving (1 hour × 132°C) or immersion into 1 N NaOH (1 hour at room temperature).[153] Prusiner and Hsiao[154] and Prusiner et al.[2] have suggested more rigorous decontamination protocols for steam autoclaving (4.5 hours, 121°C, 15 psi) or 1 N NaOH immersion (30 minutes for three treatments). Prion infectivity is not reliably reduced by exposure to ultraviolet light, alcohol solutions, phenol, bleach, or formalin.

REFERENCES

1. Sigurdsson B. Rida, a chronic encephalitis of sheep: With general remarks on infections which develop slowly and some of their special characteristics. Br Vet J. 1954;110:341–354.
2. Prusiner SB, Hsiao KK, Bredesen DE, DeArmond SJ. Prion disease. In: McKendall RR, ed. Viral Disease. (Handbook of Clinical Neurology, vol 12/56.) Amsterdam: Elsevier; 1989:543–580.
3. Prusiner SB. Prions and neurodegenerative diseases. N Engl J Med. 1987;317:1571–1581.
4. Asher DM. Slow viral infections of the nervous system. In: Scheld WM, Whitley RS, Durack DT, eds. Infections of the Central Nervous System: New York: Raven Press; 1991:145–166.
4a. Brown P, Gibbs CJ Jr, Rodgers-Johnson P, et al. Human spongiform encephalopathy: The National Institutes of Health series of 300 cases of experimentally transmitted disease. Ann Neurol. 1994;20:513–29.
5. Gajdusek DC. Subacute spongiform encephalopathies: Transmissible cerebral amyloidoses caused by unconventional viruses. In: Fields BN, Knipe DM, eds. Virology. 2nd ed. New York: Raven Press; 1990:2289–2324.
6. Hsiao K, Prusiner SB. Inherited human prion diseases. Neurology. 1990;40:1820–1827.
7. Ravilochan K, Tyler KL. Human transmissible neurodegenerative diseases (prion diseases). Semin Neurol. 1992;12:178–192.
8. Gajdusek DC. Unconventional viruses and the origin and disappearance of kuru. Science. 1977;197:943–60.
9. Zigas V. Laughing Death. The Untold Story of Kuru. Clifton, NJ: Humana Press; 1990.
10. Zigas V, Gajdusek DC. Kuru: Clinical study of a new syndrome resembling paralysis agitans in natives of the Eastern Highlands of Australian New Guinea. Med J Aust. 1957;2:745–54.
11. Gajdusek DC, Gibbs CJ Jr, Alpers MP. Experimental transmission of a kuru syndrome to chimpanzees. Nature. 1966;209:794–6.
12. Gajdusek DC, Zigas V. Degenerative disease of the central nervous system in New Guinea. The endemic occurrence of "kuru" in the native population. N Engl J Med. 1957;257:974–78.
13. Gajdusek DC, Zigas V. Clinical, pathological and epidemiological study of an acute progressive degenerative disease of the central nervous system among natives of the Eastern Highlands of New Guinea. Am J Med. 1959;26:442–69.
14. Scrimgeour EM, Masters CL, Alpers MP, et al. A clinico-pathologic study of a case of kuru. J Neurol Sci. 1983;59:265–275.
15. Hornabrook RW. Kuru: A subacute cerebellar degeneration—the natural history and clinical features. Brain. 1968;91:53–74.
16. Klatzo I, Gajdusek DC, Zigas V. Pathology of kuru. Lab Invest. 1959;8:799–847.
17. Alpers MP. Epidemiology and ecology of kuru. In: Prusiner SB, Hadlow WJ, eds. Slow Transmissible Diseases of the Nervous System. New York: Academic Press; 1979:67–90.
18. Cobb WA, Hornabrook RW, Sanders S. The EEG of kuru. Electroencephalogr Clin Neurophysiol. 1973;34:419–27.
19. Brown P, Cathala F, Rabertas RB, et al. The epidemiology of Creutzfeldt-Jakob disease. Conclusions of a 15 year investigation in France and review of the world literature. Neurology. 1987;37:895–909.
20. Brown P. Iatrogenic Creutzfeldt-Jakob disease. Aust NZJ Med. 1990;20:633–635.
21. Duffy P, Wolf J, Collins G, et al. Possible person to person transmission of Creutzfeldt-Jakob disease (Letter). N Engl J Med. 1974;290:692–693.
22. Thadani V, Penar PL, Partington J, et al. Creutzfeldt-Jakob disease probably acquired from a cadaveric dural graft. J Neurosurg. 1988;69:766–769.
23. Nisbet TJ, MacDonaldson I, Bishara SN. Creutzfeldt-Jakob disease in a second patient who received a cadaveric dura mater graft. J Am Med Assoc. 1989;261:1118.
24. Masullo C, Pocchiari M, Macchi G, et al. Transmission of Creutzfeldt-Jakob disease by dural cadaveric graft (Letter). J Neurosurg. 1989;71:954–955.
25. Willison HJ, Gale AN, McLaughlin JE. Creutzfeldt-Jakob disease following cadaveric dura mater graft [Letter]. J Neurol Neurosurg Psychiatry. 1991;54:940.

26. Harvey I, Coyle E. Creutzfeldt-Jakob disease after non-commercial dura mater graft (Letter). Lancet. 1992;340:615.

27. Pocchiari M, Masullo C, Salvatore M, et al. Creutzfeldt-Jakob disease after non-commercial dura mater graft (Letter). Lancet. 1992;340:614–615.

28. Weber T, Tumani H, Holdorff B, et al. Transmission of Creutzfeldt-Jakob disease by handling of dura mater graft (Letter). Lancet. 1993;341:123–124.

29. Miyashita K, Inuzuka T, Kondo H, et al. Creutzfeldt-Jakob disease in a patient with a cadaveric dural graft. Neurology. 1991;41:940–941.

30. Will RG, Matthews WB. Evidence for case-to-case transmission of Creutzfeldt-Jakob disease. J Neurol Neurosurg Psychiatry. 1982;45:235–238.

31. Nevin S, McMenemey WH, Behrman S, Jones DP. Subacute spongiform encephalopathy–a subacute form of encephalopathy attributable to vascular dysfunction (spongiform cerebral atrophy). Brain. 1960;83:519–564.

32. Jones DP, Nevin S. Rapidly progressive cerebral degeneration (subacute vascular encephalopathy) with mental disorder, focal disturbances, and myoclonic epilepsy. J Neurol Neurosurg Psychiatry. 1954;17:148–159.

33. Gibbs CJ Jr, Joy A, Heffner R, et al. Clinical and pathological features and laboratory confirmation of Creutzfeldt-Jakob disease in a recipient of pituitary derived human growth hormone. N Engl J Med. 1985;313:734–738.

34. Brown P, Gajdusek DC, Gibbs CJ jr, Asher DM. Potential epidemic of Creutzfeldt-Jakob disease from human growth hormone therapy. N Engl J Med. 1985;313:728–731.

35. Brown P. The decline and fall of Creutzfeldt-Jakob disease associated with human growth hormone therapy. Neurology. 1988;38:1135–1137.

36. Ellis CJ, Katifi H, Weller RO. A further British case of growth hormone induced Creutzfeldt-Jakob disease. J Neurol Neurosurg Psychiatry. 1992;55:1200–1202.

37. Gibbs CJ jr, Asher DM, Brown PW, et al. Creutzfeldt-Jakob disease infectivity of growth hormone derived from human pituitary glands (Letter). N Engl J Med. 1993;328:358–359.

38. Markus HS, Duchen LW, Parkin EM, et al. Creutzfeldt-Jakob disease in recipients of human growth hormone in the United Kingdom: A clinical and radiographic study. Q J Med. 1992;82:43–51.

39. Cochius JI, Hyman N, Esiri MM. Creutzfeldt-Jakob disease in a recipient of human pituitary-derived gonadotrophin: A second case. J Neurol Neurosurg Psychiatry. 1992;55:1094–1095.

40. Dumble LJ, Klein RD. Creutzfeldt-Jakob legacy for Australian women treated with human pituitary gonadotropins (Letter). Lancet. 1992;340:847–848.

41. Cochius JI, Burns RJ, Blumbergs PC, et al. Creutzfeldt-Jakob disease in a recipient of human pituitary-derived gonadotropin. Aust NZJ Med. 1990;20:592–593.

42. Berger JR, David NJ. Creutzfeldt-Jakob disease in a physician: A review of the disorder in health care workers. Neurology. 1993;43:205–206.

43. Schoene WC, Masters CL, Gibbs CJ jr, et al. Transmissible spongiform encephalopathy (Creutzfeldt-Jakob disease): Atypical clinical and pathological findings. Arch Neurol. 1981;38:473–477.

44. Masters CL, Harris JO, Gajdusek DC, et al. Creutzfeldt-Jakob disease: Patterns of worldwide occurrence and significance of familial and sporadic clustering. Ann Neurol. 1979;5:177–188.

45. Gorman DG, Benson DF, Vogel DG, Vinters HV. Creutzfeldt-Jakob disease in a pathologist (Letter). Neurology. 1992;42:463.

46. Miller DC. Creutzfeldt-Jakob disease in histopathology technicians (Letter). N Engl J Med. 1988;318:853–854.

47. Sitwell L, Lach B, Atack E, et al. Creutzfeldt-Jakob disease in a histopathology technician (Letter). N Engl J Med. 1988;31:854.

48. Creutzfeldt HG. Eber eine eigenartige herdformige erkrankung des zentralnervensystems (vorlaufuge mitteilung). Z Ges Neurol Psychiatry. 1920;57:1–18.

49. Creutzfeldt HG. On a particular focal disease of the central nervous system (preliminary communication). In: Rottenberg DA, Hochberg FH, eds. Neurological Classics in Modern Translation. New York: Hafner; 1977:97–112.

50. Jakob A. Uber eigenartige erkrankungen des zentralnervensystems mit bemerkenswertem anatomischem befunde (spastische pseudosklerose-encephalomyelopathie mit disseminierten degenerationsherden). Deutsch Z Nervenheilkd. 1921;70:132–146.

51. Jakob A. Concerning a disorder of the central nervous system clinically resembling multiple sclerosis with remarkable anatomic findings (spastic pseudosclerosis). Report of a fourth case. In: Rottenberg DA, Hochberg FH, eds. Neurological Classics in Modern Translation. New York: Hafner; 1977:113–125.

52. Heidenhain A. Klinische und anatomische untersuchungen uber eine eigenartige erkrankung des zentralnervensystems im praesenium. Z Ges Neurol Psychiatry. 1928;118:49.

53. Brownell B, Oppenheimer DR. An ataxic form of subacute presenile polioencephalopathy (Creutzfeldt-Jakob disease). J Neurol Neurosurg Psychiatry. 1965;28:350–361.

54. Stern K. Severe dementia associated with bilateral symmetrical degeneration of the thalamus. Brain. 1939;62:157–171.

55. Garcin R, Brion S, Khochneviss AA. Le syndrome de Creutzfeldt-Jakob et les syndromes corticostries du presenium (a l'occasion de 5 observations anatomo-cliniques). Rev Neurol (Paris). 1963;109:419–441.

56. Kirschbaum WR. Jakob-Creutzfeldt Disease. New York: Elsevier; 1968:

57. Brown P, Cathala F, Castaigne P, Gajdusek DC. Creutzfeldt-Jakob disease: Clinical analysis of a consecutive series of 230 neuropathologically verified cases. Ann Neurol. 1986;20:597–602.

58. Cathala F, Baron H. Clinical aspects of Creutzfeldt-Jakob disease. In: Prusiner SB, McKinley MP, eds. Prions-Novelinfectious Pathogens Causing Scrapie and Creutzfeldt-Jakob Disease. Orlando: Academic Press; 1987:467–509.

59. Brown P, Rodgers-Johnson P, Cathala F, et al. Creutzfeldt-Jakob disease of long duration: Clinicopathological characteristics, transmissibility, and differential diagnosis. Ann Neurol. 1984;16:295–304.

60. Salazar AM, Masters CL, Gajdusek DC, Gibbs CJ Jr. Syndromes of amyotrophic lateral sclerosis and dementia: Relation to transmissible Creutzfeldt-Jakob disease. Ann Neurol. 1983;14:17–26.

61. Gibbs CJ Jr, Gajdusek DC, Asher DM, et al. Creutzfeldt-Jakob disease (spongiform encephalopathy): Transmission to chimpanzee. Science. 1968;161:388–389.

62. Roos R, Gajdusek DC, Gibbs CJ jr. The clinical characteristics of transmissible Creutzfeldt-Jakob disease. 1973;96:1–20.

63. Tanaka M, Iizuko O, Yuasa T. Hepatic dysfunction in Creutzfeldt-Jakob disease. Neurology. 1992;42:1249.

64. Blisard KS, Davis LE, Harrington MG, et al. Pre-mortem diagnosis of Creutzfeldt-Jakob disease by detection of abnormal cerebrospinal fluid proteins. J Neurol Sci. 1990;99:75–81.

65. Harrington MG, Merril CR, Asher DM, Gajdusek DC. Abnormal proteins in the cerebrospinal fluid of patients with Creutzfeldt-Jakob disease. N Engl J Med. 1986;315:279–283.

66. Jimi T, Wakayama Y, Shibuya S, et al. High levels of nervous system-specific proteins in cerebrospinal fluid in patients with early stage Creutzfeldt-Jakob disease. Clin Chim Acta. 1992;21:37–46.

67. Manaka H, Kato T, Kurita K, et al. Marked increase in cerebrospinal fluid ubiquitin in Creutzfeldt-Jakob disease. Neurosci Lett. 1992;139:47–49.

68. Galvez S, Cartier L. Computed tomographic findings in 15 cases of Creutzfeldt-Jakob disease with histological verification. J Neurol Neurosurg Psychiatry. 1984;47:1244–1246.

69. Berciano J, Diez C, Polo JM, et al. CT appearance of panencephalopathic and ataxic type of Creutzfeldt-Jakob disease. J Comput Assist Tomogr. 1991;15:332–334.

70. Hayashi R, Hanyu N, Kuwabara T, Moriyama S. Serial computed tomographic and electroencephalographic studies in Creutzfeldt-Jakob disease. Acta Neurol Scand. 1992;85:161–165.

71. Schlenska GK, Walter GF. Serial computed tomography findings in Creutzfeldt-Jakob disease. Neuroradiology. 1989;31:303–306.

72. Kovanen J, Erkinjuntti T, Livanainen M, et al. Cerebral MR and CT imaging in Creutzfeldt-Jakob disease. J Comp Assist Tomogr. 1985;9:125–128.

73. Gertz H-J, Henkes H, Cerros-Navarro J. Creutzfeldt-Jakob disease: Correlation of MRI and neuropathological findings. Neurology. 1988;38:1481–1482.

74. Milton WJ, Atlas SW, Lavi E, Mollman JE. Magnetic resonance imaging of Creutzfeldt-Jakob disease. Ann Neurol. 1991;29:438–440.

75. Rother J, Schwartz A, Harle M, et al. Magnetic resonance imaging follow-up in Creutzfeldt-Jakob disease. J Neurol. 1992;239:404–406.

76. Esmonde TFG, Will RG. Magnetic resonance imaging in Creutzfeldt-Jakob disease (Letter). Ann Neurol. 1992;31:230–231.

77. Johns DW, Drazkowski JF, Drayer BP, Lieberman AN. Appearance of striatal signal hyperintensity on MRI preceding classic symptoms in ataxic Creutzfeldt-Jakob disease: Case report. BNI Q 1993;9:14–17.

78. Yamamoto K, Morimatsu M. Increased signal in basal ganglia and white matter on magnetic resonance imaging in Creutzfeldt-Jakob disease. Ann Neurol. 1992;32:114.

79. Falcone S, Quencer RM, Bowen B, et al. Creutzfeldt-Jakob disease: Focal symmetrical cortical involvement demonstrated by MR imaging. Am J Neuroradiol. 1992;13:403–406.

80. Holthoff VA, Sandmann J, Pawlik G, et al. Positron emission tomography in Creutzfeldt-Jakob disease. Arch Neurol. 1990;47:1035–1038.

81. Levy RS, Chiappa KH. Clinical neurophysiology. In: Bastian FO, ed. Creutzfeldt-Jakob Disease and Other Transmissible Spongiform Encephalopathies. St. Louis: Mosby; 1991:185–202.

82. Levy RS, Chiappa KH, Burke CJ, Young RR. Early evolution and incidence of electroencephalographic abnormalities in Creutzfeldt-Jakob disease. J Clin Neurophysiol. 1986;3:1–21.

83. Chiofalo N, Fuentes A, Galvez S. Serial EEG findings in 27 cases of Creutzfeldt-Jakob disease. Arch Neurol. 1980;37:143–145.

84. Aguglia U, Farnarier G, Tinuper P, et al. Subacute spongiform encephalopathy with periodic paroxysmal activities: clinical evolution and serial EEG findings in 20 cases. Clin Electroencephalogr. 1987;18:147–158.

85. Burger LJ, Rowan AJ, Goldensohn ES. Creutzfeldt-Jakob disease. An electroencephalographic study. Arch Neurol. 1972;26:428–433.

86. Traub RD, Pedley TA. Virus induced electrotonic coupling: Hypothesis on the mechanism of periodic EEG discharges in Creutzfeldt-Jakob disease. Ann Neurol. 1981;10:405–410.

87. Elliott F, Gardner-Thorpe C, Barwick DD, Foster JB. Jakob-Creutzfeldt disease: Modification of clinical and electroencephalographic activity with methylphenidate and diazepam. J Neurol Neurosurg Psychiatry. 1974;37:879–887.

88. Donnet A, Farnarier G, Gambarelli D, et al. Sleep electroencephalogram at the early stage of Creutzfeldt-Jakob disease. Clin Electroencephalogr. 1992;23:118–125.

89. Schlenska GK, Walter GF. Temporal evolution of electroencephalographic abnormalities in Creutzfeldt-Jakob disease. J Neurol. 1989;236:456–460.

90. Tietjen GE, Drury I. Familial Creutzfeldt-Jakob disease without periodic EEG activity. Ann Neurol. 1990;28:585–588.

91. Brown P, Jannotta F, Gibbs CJ Jr, et al. Coexistence of Creutzfeldt-Jakob disease and Alzheimer's disease in the same patient. Neurology. 1990;40:226–228.

92. Muramoto T, Kitamoto T, Koga H, Tateishi J. The coexistence of Alzheimer's disease and Creutzfeldt-Jakob disease in a patient with dementia of long duration. Acta Neuropathol. 1992;84:686–689.

93. Barry RA, Prusiner SB. Monoclonal antibodies to the cellular and scrapie prion proteins. J Infect Dis. 1986;154:518–521.

94. Bendheim PE, Barry RA, DeArmond SJ, et al. Antibodies to a scrapie prion protein. Nature. 1984;310:418–421.

95. Bockman JM, Kingsbury DT, McKinley MP, et al. Creutzfeldt-Jakob disease prion proteins in human brains. N Engl J Med. 1985;312:73–78.

96. Brown P, Coker-Vann M, Pomeroy K, et al. Diagnosis of Creutzfeldt-Jakob disease by Western blot identification of a marker protein in human brain tissue. N Engl J Med. 1986;314:547–551.

97. Kitamoto T, Doh-ura K, Muramoto T, et al. The primary structure of the prion protein influences the distribution of abnormal prion protein in the central nervous system. Am J Pathol. 1992;141:271–277.

98. Brown P. The phenotypic expression of different mutations in transmissible human spongiform encephalopathy. Rev Neurol (Paris). 1992;148:317–327.

99. Collinge J. Inherited prion diseases. Adv Neurol. 1993;61:155–165.

100. Goldfarb LG, Brown P, Goldgaber D, et al. Creutzfeldt-Jakob disease and kuru patients lack a mutation consistently found in the Gerstmann-Straussler-Scheinker syndrome. Exp Neurol. 1990;108:247–250.

101. Palmer MS, Dryden AJ, Hughes JT, Collinge J. Homozygous prion protein genotype predisposes to sporadic Creutzfeldt-Jakob disease [published erratum appears in Nature 1991 Aug 8;352(6335):547]. Nature. 1991;352:340–342.

102. Collinge J, Palmer MS, Dryden AJ. Genetic predisposition to iatrogenic Creutzfeldt-Jakob disease. Lancet. 1991;337:1441–1442.

103. Hsiao K, Meiner Z, Kahana E, et al. Mutation of the prion protein in Libyan Jews with Creutzfeldt-Jakob disease. N Engl J Med. 1991;324:1091–1097.

104. Brown P, Galvez S, Goldfarb LG, et al. Familial Creutzfeldt-Jakob disease in Chile associated with the codon 200 mutation of the PRNP amyloid precursor gene on chromosome 20. J Neurol Sci. 1992;112:65–67.

105. Goldfarb LG, Mitrova E, Brown P, et al. Mutation in codon 200 of scrapie amyloid protein gene in two clusters of Creutzfeldt-Jakob disease in Slovakia (Letter). Lancet. 1990;336:514–515.

106. Goldfarb LG, Korczyn AD, Brown P, et al. Mutation in codon 200 of scrapie amyloid precursor gene linked to Creutzfeldt-Jakob disease in Sephardic Jews of Libyan and non-Libyan origin (Letter). Lancet. 1990;336:637–638.

107. Bertoni JM, Brown P, Goldfarb LG, et al. Familial Creutzfeldt-Jakob disease (codon 200 mutation) with supranuclear palsy. J Am Med Assoc. 1992;268:2413–2415.

108. Goldfarb LG, Brown P, Haltia M, et al. Creutzfeldt-Jakob disease cosegregates with the codon 178 Asn PRNP mutation in families of European origin. Ann Neurol. 1992;31:274–281.

109. Brown P, Goldfarb LG, Kovanen J, et al. Phenotypic characteristics of familial Creutzfeldt-Jakob disease associated with the codon 178 Asn PRNP mutation. Ann Neurol. 1992;31:282–285.

110. Goldfarb LG, Haltia M, Brown P, et al. New mutation in scrapie amyloid precursor gene (at codon 178) in Finnish Creutzfeldt-Jakob disease kindred (Letter). Lancet. 1991;337:425.

111. Prusiner SB, McKinley MP, Bolton DC, et al. Methods for assay, purification and characterization. in: Maramorosch K, Koprowski H, eds Methods in Virology, v. 8. New York: Academic Press; 1984:293–345.

112. Brown P, Goldfarb LG, McCombie WR, et al. Atypical Creutzfeldt-Jakob disease in an American family with an insert mutation in the PRNP amyloid precursor gene. Neurology. 1992;42:422–427.

113. Collinge J, Brown J, Hardy J, et al. Inherited prion disease with a 144 base pair gene insertion. 2. Clinical and pathological features. Brain. 1992;115:687–710.

114. Brown P, Goldfarb LG, Brown WT, et al. Clinical and molecular genetic study of a large German kindred with Gerstmann-Straussler-Scheinker syndrome. Neurology. 1991;41:375–379.

115. Farlow MR, Yee RD, Dlouhy SR, et al. Gerstmann-Straussler-Scheinker disease. I. Extending the clinical spectrum. Neurology. 1989;39:1446–1452.

116. Kuzuhara S, Kanazawa I, Sasaki H, et al. Gerstmann-Straussler-Scheinker's disease. Ann Neurol. 1983;14:216–225.

117. Wimberger D, Uranitsch K, Schindler E, Kramer J. Gerstmann-Straussler-Scheinker syndrome: MR findings. J Comput Assist Tomogr. 1993;17:326–327.

118. Masters CL, Gajdusek DC, Gibbs CJ Jr. Creutzfeldt-Jakob disease virus isolations from the Gerstmann-Straussler-Scheinker syndrome. With an analysis of the various forms of amyloid plaque deposition in the virus-induced spongiform encephalopathies. Brain. 1981;104:559–588.

119. Amano N, Yagishita S, Yokoi S, et al. Gerstmann-Straussler syndrome—a variant type: Amyloid plaques and Alzheimer's neurofibrillary tangles in cerebral cortex. Acta Neuropathol. 1992;84:15–23.

120. Nolchin D, Sumi SM, Bird TD, et al. Familial dementia with PrP positive amyloid plaques: A variant of Gerstmann-Straussler syndrome. Neurology. 1989;39:910–918.

121. Hsiao KK, Baker HF, Crow TJ, et al. Linkage of prion protein missense variant to Gerstmann-Straussler syndrome. Nature. 1989;338:342–345.

122. Hsiao KK, Cass C, Schellenberg GD, et al. A prion protein variant in a family with the telencephalic form of Gerstmann-Straussler-Scheinker syndrome. Neurology. 1991;41:681–684.

123. Doh-ura K, Tateishi J, Sasaki H. Pro–Leu change at position 102 of prion protein is the most common but not the sole mutation related to Gerstmann-Straussler syndrome. Biochem Biophys Res Commun. 1989;163:974–979.

124. Kretzschmar HA, Kufer P, Riethmuller G, et al. Prion protein mutation at codon 102 in an Italian family with Gerstmann-Straussler-Scheinker syndrome. Neurology. 1992;42:809–810.

125. Gerstmann J, Straussler E, Scheinker I. Uber eine eigenartige hereditar-familiare erkrankung des zentralnervensystems. Zugleich ein beitrag zur frage des vorzeitigen lokalen alterns. Z Ges Neurol Psychiatry. 1936;154:736–762.

126. Kretzschmar HA, Honold G, Seitelberger F, et al. Prion protein mutation in family first described by Gerstmann, Straussler, Scheinker (Letter). Lancet. 1991;337:1160.

127. Hsiao KK, Scott M, Foster D, et al. Spontaneous neurodegeneration in transgenic mice with mutant prion protein. Science. 1990;250:1587–1590.

128. Tranchant C, Doh-ura K, Warter JM, et al. Gerstmann-Straussler-Scheinker disease in an Alsatian family: Clinical and genetic studies. J Neurol Neurosurg Psychiatry. 1992;55:185–187.

129. Goldfarb LG, Brown P, Vrbovska A, et al. An insert mutation in the chromosome 20 amyloid precursor gene in a Gerstmann-Straussler-Scheinker family. J Neurol Sci. 1992;111:189–194.

130. Medori R, Tritschler H-J, LeBlanc A, et al. Fatal familial insomnia, a prion disease with a mutation at codon 178 of the prion protein gene. N Engl J Med. 1992;326:444–449.

131. Manetto V, Medori R, Cortelli P, et al. Fatal familial insomnia: Clinical and pathologic study of five new cases. Neurology. 1992;42:312–319.

132. Lugaresi E, Medori R, Montagna P, et al. Fatal familial insomnia and dysautonomia with selective degeneration of thalamic nuclei. N Engl J Med. 1986;315:997–1003.

133. Petersen BB, Tabaton M, Berg L, et al. Analysis of the prion protein gene in thalamic dementia. Neurology. 1992;42:1859–1863.

134. Galassi R, Morreale A, Montagna P, et al. Fatal familial insomnia: A neuropsychological study of a disease with thalamic degeneration. Cortex. 1992;28:175–187.

135. Medori R, Montagna P, Tritschler HJ, et al. Fatal familial insomnia: A second kindred with mutation of prion protein gene at codon 178. Neurology. 1992;42:669–670.

136. Goldfarb LG, Petersen RB, Tabaton M, et al. Fatal famial insomnia and familial Creutzfeldt-Jakob disease: Disease phenotype determined by a DNA polymorphism. Science. 1992;258:806–808.

137. Goldhammer Y, Bubis JJ, Sarova-Pinhas I, Braham J. Subacute spongiform encephalopathy and its relation to Creutzfeldt-Jakob disease: Report on six cases. J Neurol Neurosurg Psychiatry. 1972;35:1–10.

138. Herishanu Y. Antiviral drugs in Jakob-Creutzfeldt disease. J Am Geriatr Soc. 1973;21:229–231.

139. David AS, Grant R, Ballantyne JP. Unsuccessful treatment of Creutzfeldt-Jakob disease with acyclovir. Lancet. 1984;1:512–513.

140. Newman PK. Acyclovir in Creutzfeldt-Jakob disease (Letter). Lancet. 1984;1:793.

141. Kovanen J, Haltia M, Cantell K. Failure of interferon to modify Creutzfeldt-Jakob disease. Br Med J. 1980;280:902.

142. Brown P. Biologic and chemotherapeutic forays into the field of unconventional viruses. In: DeClercq E, Walker RT, eds. Targets for the Design of Antiviral Agents. New York: Plenum Press; 1984:131–157.

143. Masullo C, Macchi G, Xi YG, Pocchiari M. Failure to ameliorate Creutzfeldt-Jakob disease with amphotericin B therapy (Letter). J Infect Dis. 1992;165:784–785.

144. Braham J. Jakob-Creutzfeldt disease: Treatment by amantadine. Br Med J. 1971;4:212–213.

145. Sanders WL, Dunn TL. Creutzfeldt-Jakob disease treated with amantadine. J Neurol Neurosurg Psychiatr. 1973;36:581–584.

146. Sanders WL. Creutzfeldt-Jakob disease treated with amantadine. J Neurol Neurosurg Psychiatr. 1979;42:960–961.

147. Terzano MG, Montanari E, Calzetti S, et al. The effect of amantadine on arousal and EEG patterns in Creutzfeldt-Jakob disease. Arch Neurol. 1983;40:555–559.

148. Furlow TW Jr, Whitley RJ, Wilmes FJ. Repeated suppression of Creutzfeldt-Jakob disease with vidarabine. Lancet. 1982;2:564–565.

149. Villa G, Caltagirone C, Macchi G. Unusual clinical course in a case of Creutzfeldt-Jakob disease. Ital J Neurol Sci. 1982;2:155–158.

150. Ratcliffe J, Rittman A, Wolf S, Verity MA. Creutzfeldt-Jakob disease with focal onset unsuccessfully treated with amantadine. Bull LA Neurol Soc. 1975;40:18–20.

151. Gibbs CJ Jr, Amyx HL, Bacote A, et al. Oral transmission of kuru, Creutzfeldt-Jakob disease and scrapie to non-human primates. J Infect Dis. 1980;142:205–208.

152. Esmonde TF, Will RG, Slattery JM, et al. Creutzfeldt-Jakob disease and blood transfusion. Lancet. 1993;341:205–207.

153. Committee on Health Care Issues American Neurological Association. Precautions in handling tissues, fluids and other contaminated materials from patients with documented or suspected Creutzfeldt-Jakob disease. Ann Neurol. 1986;19:75–77.

154. Prusiner SB, Hsiao KK. Prions causing transmissible neurodegenerative diseases. In: Schlossberg D, ed. Infections of the Nervous System. New York: Springer-Verlag; 1990:153–168.

68. BRAIN ABSCESS

BRIAN WISPELWEY
W. MICHAEL SCHELD

Brain abscess is a focal suppurative process within the brain parenchyma. A description of the disease together with a therapeutic proposal was found in an article dating back to the sixteenth century[1]; however, it was not until the late nineteenth century that the first encouraging results of surgical intervention were reported. MacEwen[2] reported the remarkable figure of an 80 percent (8 of 10) survival rate after neurosurgical drainage of temporal lobe abscesses.

Since that time, surgical techniques have continued to improve, and antibiotics have been introduced, but diagnostic delay has continued to be the major obstacle in the success of therapeutic intervention. Significant improvement in the mortality and morbidity of brain abscess has only occurred within the last 15–20 years. These improvements reflect advances in noninvasive imaging techniques that allow earlier diagnosis and more precise localization. Later in the disease, cerebral edema and mass effect lead to intracranial shifts, irreversible brain damage, and death. Optimal management of a brain abscess requires cooperation between the medical physician and neurosurgeon.

EPIDEMIOLOGY

The incidence of brain abscess has remained relatively stable in the antibiotic era.[3–5] Brain abscess is generally regarded as a rare disease, with large autopsy series reporting occurrence rates of 0.18–1.3 percent.[6] Although some series report a mild increase in cases diagnosed during life,[7,8] this may represent a bias due to more sensitive diagnostic techniques.[9] In contrast, two series, which span greater than four decades, have noted a decline in brain abscess recently.[6,10] It is estimated that brain abscess accounts for approximately 1 in 10,000 general hospital admissions and that 4–10 cases are seen yearly on active neurosurgical services in hospitals of developed countries.[11–14] The advent of the acquired immunodeficiency syndrome (AIDS) has led to increased numbers in most parts of the world of individuals with focal intracranial infections. Estimates of the prevalence of cerebral toxoplasmosis alone, in patients with AIDS, have ranged from 2.6 to 30.8 percent.[15]

The etiology and incidence of brain abscesses vary among different geographic areas. In China, 65 percent of brain abscesses are thought to be secondary to otitis media but only 0.5 percent secondary to paranasal sinusitis.[16] This is contrasted to a 20–40 percent incidence secondary to otitis media and a 15–25 percent incidence secondary to paranasal sinusitis reported in series from Northern European countries.[17,18]

Several authors[5,7,19] reported a male predominance (3:1) among patients with brain abscesses; more recently a series of 45 patients diagnosed between 1970 and 1983 revealed a male-to-female ratio of 2.7:1.7 In another series of 257 patients (1973–1977), the ratio was only 1.2:1.[20,21] Two series of brain abscess diagnosed exclusively in the computed tomography (CT) era and excluding AIDS patients lend further support to the observations of brain abscesses being twice as common in males.[13,14]

The median age of patients is 30–45 years[13,14,16,22,23]; however, the predominant age may vary somewhat by etiology. In some series, brain abscess due to otitis media displays a bimodal age distribution, with peaks in the pediatric age group and after 40 years of age,[24] whereas abscesses secondary to paranasal sinusitis more commonly occur between 10 and 30 years of age.[24,25] Approximately 25 percent of all brain abscesses occur in children less than 15 years of age,[7] with a peak incidence between ages 4 and 7 years.[26] A male predominance (2:1) has again been observed in most pediatric series.[27,28] A brain abscess before the age of 2 years is extremely rare.[27]

PATHOGENESIS

Brain abscesses develop in four clinical settings: *(1)* in association with a contiguous suppurative focus; *(2)* after hematogenous spread from a distant focus; *(3)* after trauma (e.g., open cranial fracture with a dural breach, postneurosurgery, pencil-tip injuries to the eye in children,[29] and, more recently, after lawn dart injuries to the head[30]; and *(4)* cryptogenic (no focus is recognized in approximately 15–20 percent of cases).[3,5,7,19,23,31] Data compiled from 19 series of brain abscesses from 1927 to 1980[9,10,16] have revealed that abscesses related to contiguous infections accounted for 47 percent of more than 3500 cases. Metastatic or hematogenous abscesses accounted for 25 percent, and no predisposing factor could be determined in 15 percent.

In approximate decreasing order of frequency, a solitary abscess may involve various regions: frontal ≈ temporal > frontoparietal > parietal > cerebellar > occipital.[7] This distribution reflects the associated, often contiguous, focus of infection. Understanding the predisposing condition(s) in a given brain abscess case has important implications for its therapy (Table 1). Intrasellar, brain stem, basal ganglia, and thalamic abscesses are rare. Intrasellar abscesses are most common in the setting of preexisting pituitary adenomas; however, cases have occurred in their absence.[32] Sinusitis, particularly sphenoid sinusitis, is a most important predisposing condition, with one series revealing pituitary abscesses in 16 of 126 patients with sphenoid sinusitis.[33] Brain stem abscesses arise most often from hematogenous spread from a distant focus; rare cases occur in association with a contiguous infection. In one-third of the 48 reported cases, no source was defined. These abscesses are often fusiform and extend over several levels of the brain stem; therefore, the clinical findings can be confusing. Before 1974, brain stem abscesses were uniformly fatal, but recent improvements in diagnosis and aggressive neurosurgical drainage have led to occasional survival.[34] Inflammatory lesions (especially when solitary) of the thalamus or basal ganglia are also somewhat unusual. One series reported five such solitary thalamic abscesses among a total of 135 cases. Most often they were hematogenous in origin.[35] The incidence of multiple brain abscesses was only 1–15 percent in older series; however, with the advent of CT scanning, the frequency of multiple lesions has increased to 10–50 percent.[36] Prior to more recent therapeutic modalities, the mortality from multiple brain abscesses approached 100 percent.

Approximately 40 percent of brain abscesses were associated with otitis media and/or mastoiditis. This source of brain abscess is decreasing in most parts of the world. However, in areas where otitis media continues to be neglected or therapy is delayed, intracranial complications still present a serious threat.[37,38] As stated, a bimodal age distribution of brain abscess as a complication of otitis media is often seen, with cases in the youngest age groups often secondary to acute otitis media as opposed to the overwhelming preponderance of associated chronic otitis media in the older age group.[24] Overall, chronic otitis media and/or mastoiditis leads to intracranial extension four to eight times more frequently than does acute disease. Before the availability of antibiotic therapy it was estimated

TABLE 1. Brain Abscess: Predisposing Condition, Site of Abscess, and Microbiology

Predisposing Conditions[a]	Site of Abscess	Usual Isolate(s) from Abscess
Contiguous site or primary infection		
Otitis media and mastoiditis	Temporal lobe or cerebellar hemisphere	Streptococci (anaerobic or aerobic), *Bacteroides fragilis*, Enterobacteriaceae
Frontoethmoidal sinusitis	Frontal lobe	Predominantly streptococci; *Bacteroides*, Enterobacteriaceae, *S. aureus*, and *Haemophilus* spp.
Sphenoidal sinusitis	Frontal or temporal lobe	Same as in frontoethmoidal sinusitis
Dental sepsis	Frontal lobe	Mixed *Fusobacterium*, *Bacteroides*, and *Streptococcus* spp.
Penetrating cranial trauma or postsurgical infection	Related to wound	*S. aureus*; streptococci, Enterobacteriaceae, *Clostridium*
Distant site of primary infection		
Congenital heart disease	Multiple abscess cavities; middle cerebral artery distribution common but may occur at any site	Viridans, anaerobic, and microaerophilic streptococci; *Haemophilus* spp.
Lung abscess, empyema, bronchiectasis	Same as in congenital heart disease	*Fusobacterium*, *Actinomyces*, *Bacteroides*, streptococci, *Nocardia asteroides*
Bacterial endocarditis	Same as in congenital heart disease	*S. aureus*, streptococci
Compromised host (AIDS, immunosuppressive therapy or malignancy)	Same as in congenital heart disease	*Toxoplasma*, fungi, Enterobacteriaceae, *Nocardia*

[a] Predisposing conditions are identified in approximately 80 percent of cases.

(Data from Dacey and Winn.[31])

that about 3–6 percent of patients with otogenic suppuration developed an intracranial complication, with approximately 15 percent of those complications presenting as brain abscesses.[27,39] Current risk estimates are more difficult to assess; however, epidemiologic data from Scotland suggest that only 1 in 3500 cases of otitis media is complicated by intracranial spread.[40] In a 10-year study of otogenic brain abscess, the annual risk in an adult with chronic otitis media of developing a brain abscess was 1 in 10,000.[41] Most otogenic brain abscesses are located in the temporal lobe; next is the cerebellum, but cases of frontal lobe and rare brain stem localizations have been reported. It has been noted that 85–99 percent of cerebellar abscesses are secondary to otogenic infections. Most otogenic brain abscesses are solitary lesions.[3–5,7,12,19,23]

Brain abscess secondary to paranasal sinusitis also appears to be decreasing in incidence; however, sinusitis continues to be the major predisposing condition leading to subdural empyema. In a recent British review, sinusitis accounted for 15 percent of brain abscesses over a 30-year period.[25] The frontal lobe is almost exclusively involved as a complication of sinusitis; however, particularly with sphenoid sinusitis, the temporal lobe or sella turcica has been affected. Sphenoid sinusitis, despite its relative rarity when compared with frontoethmoidal or maxillary disease, has seemingly more frequent and severe complications. This stems from the difficulty in making this diagnosis and/or the lack of appropriately aggressive therapy for this condition.[42] Some reports implicate cocaine inhalation as a risk factor for sphenoid sinusitis and subsequent brain abscess development.[43]

Dental infection is a less frequent site of infection that can be complicated by brain abscess. Some series, however, noted that dental infections have been implicated in greater than 10 percent of cases.[9,44] Brain abscess appears more likely after infection of the molar teeth. A large majority of intracranial infections in this setting follow a recent tooth extraction. The site of the abscess is most commonly frontal, but temporal lobe localization can also occur.[45] Four recently described cases of occipital lobe abscesses 2–4 weeks after dental manipulations suggest the potential for hematogenous spread from a dental source as well.[46] Many cases of cryptogenic brain abscess may be secondary to dental foci of infection. Facial or scalp infections are also important since they may lead to cavernous sinus thrombosis and attendant intracranial complications.

Brain abscess rarely complicates meningitis; however, it should be strongly considered as an associated possibility in the neonate with meningitis, particularly meningitis due to gram-negative organisms. Abscess formation has been associated

with more than 70 percent of cases of *Citrobacter diversus* meningitis in the infant,[47] and therefore it can be argued that any infant in whom this organism is isolated from either blood or spinal fluid should undergo a scanning procedure of the head. Brain abscesses are fortunately infrequent complications of neurosurgical procedures or cranial trauma. It has been observed that central nervous system infections occur in only 0.6–1.7 percent of clean neurosurgical procedures, and brain abscess accounts for only 10 percent of these.[48] However, because of the decline in other predisposing factors as causes of brain abscesses recently, the relative contribution of intracranial surgery as a cause of brain abscess has increased in some recent series.[49] Brain abscess has been noted to complicate approximately 3 percent of penetrating cranial injuries, with increased risk noted in the setting of gunshot wound complications. Retained bone fragments have been consistently noted as an important risk factor.[48,49]

Brain abscesses from contiguous infection may occur by two major mechanisms: (1) direct extension through areas of associated osteitis or osteomyelitis and (2) retrograde thrombophlebitic spread via diploic or emissary veins into the intracranial compartment. Additional possibilities in the case of otogenic infection include spread through preexisting channels (such as the internal auditory canal, cochlear and vestibular aqueducts, or between temporal suture lines). Hematogenous dissemination is occasionally implicated, particularly in cases of sinus or odontogenic origin.[11,12,45,50,51] None of these hypotheses explains the relative rarity of intracranial infection with sinusitis or otitis, how bacteria traverse an intact dura, the striking age and sex predominance of subdural empyema, or what determines the form of intracranial complication that eventually evolves (e.g., epidural abscess vs. brain abscess vs. subdural empyema) in the individual case with the same predisposing condition.

Hematogenous brain abscesses often share the following characteristics: (1) distant foci of infection, most often within the chest; (2) location in the distribution of the middle cerebral artery; (3) initial location at the gray–white matter junction, where brain capillary flow is slowest; (4) poor encapsulation; and (5) high mortality. These abscesses are more commonly multiple and multiloculated than those that have an origin in foci of contiguous infection.[3–5,7,11,12,19,23,51,52] Chronic pyogenic lung diseases (especially lung abscess, bronchiectasis, empyema, and cystic fibrosis) remain important diagnostic considerations.[7,11,12,53] Other distant foci of infection may be associated with brain abscesses and include wound and skin infections, osteomyelitis, pelvic infection, cholecystitis, and other forms of intraabdominal sepsis. More recently, brain abscess has been described as a complication of esophageal dilation of caustic strictures and endoscopic sclerosis of varices, both of which can produce bacteremia.[54–56] Brain abscess rarely develops after bacteremia in the presence of a normal blood-brain barrier. Thus, brain abscess is rare in bacterial endocarditis, despite the presence of persistent bacteremia. In a series of 218 patients with infective endocarditis, only 9 cases of brain abscess were noted. In 8 of these cases, the brain abscesses were less than 1 cm³, and in all cases multiple lesions were found.[57] In addition, only 4 of 148 brain abscesses in two large series were due to endocarditis.[5,23] Hereditary hemorrhagic telangiectasia is complicated by brain abscess with striking regularity, almost always presenting in those patients with pulmonary arteriovenous malformations. These abnormalities presumably allow septic microemboli to pass through the pulmonary circulation and avoid the normal pulmonary capillary filter, thereby affording direct access to the cerebral circulation. Cyanosis, clubbing, polycythemia, and hypoxemia were also found in those patients most likely to develop a brain abscess[58] and was believed to be a necessary substrate. Recent cases have documented the occurrence of brain abscesses in the setting of asymptomatic pulmonary arteriovenous malformations (AVM), and therefore occult pulmonary AVM need to be considered in cryptogenic brain abscesses.[59] Cyanotic congenital heart disease (CCHD) is found in 5–10 percent of brain abscess cases, with some pediatric series revealing it to be the most common underlying condition. As many as 25 percent of all brain abscesses in children are attributable to CCHD. Between 2 and 6 percent of children with CCHD develop a brain abscess, with tetralogy of Fallot and transposition of the great vessels being the most commonly cited.[1,7,27,60,61] The polycythemia associated with CCHD increases the viscosity, thus reducing brain capillary flow and perhaps leading to microinfarction and reduced tissue oxygenation. This may be the final common pathway of brain abscess from many etiologies. These insults can be caused by polycythemic thrombosis and hypoxia (as described), septic emboli, or a suppurative vasculitis from a contiguous infection. Experimental data suggest that infection is extremely difficult to establish in normal brain tissue.[62]

PATHOLOGY

Established infection recruits inflammatory cells and alters local vascular permeability. The evolution of an abscess includes four somewhat arbitrary histopathologic stages.[63] This staging process, described in animal models of brain abscess, correlates well with human brain abscess evolution.[64] An important feature of this description is its correlation with CT findings, which has direct implications for subsequent therapy. The four stages include early cerebritis (days 1–3), late cerebritis (days 4–9), early capsule formation (days 10–13), and late capsule formation (day 14 on).

Recent work has criticized the above model's utility in describing a uniform mode of brain abscess evolution.[65] The authors, utilizing the same dog model and inoculum, were unable to detect viable organisms in the brain lesions after 3 days, and in all the animals the lesions spontaneously resolved. Further work is necessary to reconcile this descrepancy. Nonetheless, a brain abscess model in rats recently described supports the above-mentioned histologic progression.[66] This sequence of events may be altered in the immunosuppressed host. Dogs immunosuppressed by azathioprine and prednisone therapy showed a decreased early inflammatory response and edema formation followed by a delayed increase in abscess size as compared with healthy controls.[67]

Two repeated observations regarding encapsulation deserve special attention. First, capsule formation is frequently more complete on the cortical than on the ventricular side of the abscess.[51,63] Second, encapsulation is less extensive in abscesses

from hematogenous spread than in those arising from a contiguous focus of infection.[68] These observations may be related to the requirement of oxygen for pro-α-chains of collagen to form triple-helix strands.[69] Normal cortical gray matter is more vascular than is adjacent white matter, perhaps allowing greater fibroblast proliferation and collagen helix formation. This discrepancy probably explains the propensity for abscesses to rupture medially into the ventricles rather than into the subarachnoid space. Similarly, the infarct resulting from a septic embolus might impede optimal collagen formation by fibroblasts.[63]

Two experimental models using organisms other than α-hemolytic streptococci, however, indicate that this view of abscess evolution may be overly stereotyped. In a model of *Bacteroides fragilis* brain abscess,[70] the same stages of evolution were observed, but the early and late capsule stages could not be differentiated due to a delay in encapsulation. *Staphylococcus aureus* inoculation in the same experimental model[71] resulted in larger lesions, earlier ependymitis, and delayed progress toward healing. Again, separation of the previously described stages was not as distinct. Additionally, the abscess reached maximum size in the late cerebritis stage, which suggests that the host was able to contain the infection before capsule formation and thereby contradicts the assumption that the capsule serves to contain infection.

Brain abscess formation is a continuum from cerebritis to a collagen-encapsulated necrotic focus; however, maturation is dependent on many factors, including local oxygen concentration, the offending organism, and the host immune response.

ETIOLOGIC AGENTS

In the preantibiotic era, analysis of intracranial pus revealed *S. aureus* in 25–30 percent of cases, streptococci in 30 percent, coliforms in 12 percent, and no growth in about 50 percent.[20,21] With proper attention to techniques, the role of anaerobic agents in brain abscesses has become apparent. In one earlier study,[72] 14 of 18 abscesses grew anaerobes on culture, predominately streptococci in 66 percent with *Bacteroides* spp. in 60 percent. Series from the United Kingdom have stressed the role of anaerobic bacteria in brain abscesses, especially of otic origin.[20,21,73] In addition, some reports suggest that the proportion of abscesses due to staphylococci are decreasing in frequency, whereas those due to Enterobacteriaceae are now more prevalent.[3,7]

The current pattern of microbial isolates from brain abscesses is shown in Table 2. Pyogenic brain abscesses are often (30–60 percent) mixed infections.[6,8,13,14,20,21,73–77] *Staphylococcus aureus* causes 10–15 percent of brain abscesses, usually in pure culture, and is the most common pathogen in abscesses after trauma. The Enterobacteriaceae are found, usually in mixed culture, in 23–33 percent of cases.[20,21,78] *Proteus* spp., *Escherichia coli*, and *Pseudomonas* spp. appear in approximate order of decreasing frequency. Bacteria associated with pyogenic meningitis (*Streptococcus pneumoniae*, *Haemophilus influenzae*) cause fewer than 1 percent of brain abscesses. Various streptococci are implicated in 60–70 percent of cases. These streptococci are often microaerophilic but yield aerobic patterns

TABLE 2. Microbiologic Etiology of Brain Abscess

Organism	Isolation Frequency (%)
S. aureus	10–15
Enterobacteriaceae	23–33
S. pneumoniae	<1
H. influenzae	<1
Streptococci (S. intermedius group, including S. anginosus)	60–70
Bacteroides and Prevotella spp.	20–40
Fungi	10–15
Protozoa, helminths[a]	<1

[a] Heavily dependent on geographic locale (see the text).

by gas liquid chromotographic analysis.[20,21] The *Streptococcus intermedius* group ("milleri"; *S. anginosus, S. constellatus,* and *S. intermedius*) has a predilection for causing focal suppurative disease, including brain abscesses.[79,80] These organisms were found in 13 of 16 (approximately 80 percent) cases in one recent analysis.[81] Some of the *Streptococcus intermedius* group are placed within Lancefield group F and possess the group O III antigen,[20,21,80] a potential virulence factor for the suppuration characteristic of these organisms. *Bacteroides* and *Prevotella* spp., including *B. fragilis,* are isolated in 20–40 percent of cases of brain abscess, often in mixed culture.[20,21,73,77] Many other bacteria are occasionally found in brain abscess pus,[21,82] including *Clostridium* spp. (often trauma related), *Haemophilus* spp., *Fusobacterium* spp., other anaerobes,[12,20,21,83,84] *Actinomyces* spp., *Listeria monocytogenes,*[85,86] *Nocardia asteroides,*[87] and others. When *Citrobacter* spp.[88] and *Eikenella corrodens*[52] invade the central nervous system (CNS), abscess formation is very commonly present. *Citrobacter diversus* is the most common pathogen isolated from cerebral abscesses of neonates.[89] *Salmonella* brain abscess is rare, with the most common serotypes being *typhi, typhimurium,* and *enteritidis.*[90] It occurs more commonly in adults, with precipitating factors being meningitis, trauma, and intracranial hematoma. *Streptobacillus moniliformis,* the cause of the streptobacillary form of rat-bite fever, has also been reported as a rare cause of brain abscess.[91] *Brucella* spp. have been implicated in CNS infections, especially meningitis and meningoencephalitis. A case of multiple brain abscesses due to *B. melitensis* has been reported.[92] *Propionibacterium acnes* has been observed as a cause of brain abscess, especially in the post-trauma neurosurgery patient.[93] *Bacillus cereus* has been implicated in at least three cases of brain abscess in the immunocompromised host.[94] Space-occupying lesions due to *Mycobacterium tuberculosis* were thought to be rare, but, since the advent of CT scanning and AIDS, focal lesions (tuberculomas) have been observed in a substantial minority of cases of tuberculous meningitis.[95] Tuberculosis accounted for 11 percent of focal intracranial infections in Mexico.[12]

Yeasts and dimorphic fungi have assumed an increasing role, causing 9–17 percent of cases in a series from San Francisco.[96] Most cases occur in immunocompromised patients, and mortality remains extremely high.[97] A partial list of fungi causing intracerebral mass lesions includes *Aspergillus* spp.,[98] agents of mucormycosis, *Candida* spp.,[99] *Cryptococcus neoformans, Coccidioides immitis, Cladosporium trichoides (Xylohypha bantianum,*[100] *C. bantianum*[101]*), Pseudallescheria boydii, Bipolaris* spp., *Curvularia* spp., *Exophiala dermatitidis,*[102] agents of chromoblastomycosis, *Blastomyces dermatitidis,* and, rarely, *Histoplasma capsulatum.* Other unusual fungal organisms have been recently described as the cause of brain abscess and include *Ramichloridium obovoideum* and *Dactylaria gallopava (Ochroconis gallopavum).*[103,104] In addition to the rhinocerebral form found in diabetes with ketoacidosis or leukopenic hosts, cerebral mucormycosis with brain abscess formation also occurs in parenteral drug abusers.

Various protozoa and helminths may cause brain abscesses. In a well-documented case of multiple abscesses caused by *Strongyloides stercoralis,*[105] bacteria carried within the gut of the nematode were implicated in the abscesses found in the distribution of the middle cerebral artery. Brain abscesses caused by *Entamoeba histolytica, Schistosoma japonicum,* other schistosomes, and *Paragonimus* spp. remain uncommon in the United States, but are seen in other countries.[106,107] *Acanthamoeba* spp. have been increasingly implicated as a cause of focal intracranial infections, most notably in patients with AIDS.[108] Cysticercosis is a major cause of brain lesions in the developing world. For example, cysticercosis accounted for 85 percent of all brain infections in Mexico City.[12] Other helminthic infections that can occasionally lead to focal intracranial lesions include echinococcosis, trichinosis,[109] and sparganosis.[110]

The patient's immune status is an important determinant of the microbiology of a brain abscess. The infecting organism can be predicted with some degree of certainty, or the differential diagnosis can be narrowed significantly by knowing which arm of the immune system is more severely altered.[111] Patient's with T-lymphocyte or mononuclear phagocytic defects are commonly encountered in most hospital settings. Common causes of brain abscess in this patient group are *Toxoplasma gondii* and *Nocardia asteroides.* Less common but still possible etiologies are other *Nocardia* species, *Cryptococcus neoformans, Mycobacterium* spp., and *Listeria monocytogenes. Nocardia asteroides* infection almost always has a pulmonary portal of entry, so patients with nocardial brain abscesses usually have a concomitant pulmonary lesion.[111,112] Central nervous system involvement with this organism has been reported in 18–44 percent of patients with nocardial infection elsewhere in the body. Nocardial abscesses are most often single, but multiple abscesses have been reported. *Toxoplasma gondii* is the most common cause of brain abscess in patients with AIDS (see below).[112] *Cryptococcus neoformans* more commonly causes meningitis in the compromised host, but mass lesions have been described. *Listeria monocytogenes* is also more commonly associated with meningitis or meningoencephalitis, but single large abscesses as well as disseminated small abscesses with this organism have also been reported.[86,114] Neutrophil defects are most often due to chemotherapy-induced neutropenia. An increased incidence of brain abscess secondary to Enterobacteriaceae and *Pseudomonas aeruginosa* is seen to parallel their increased presence as a cause of meningitis in this group of patients.[111] Neutrophil abnormalities also lead to an increased occurrence of CNS fungal disease. Multiple agents have been described, as seen above, and prominent among these are infections with *Aspergillus* spp., Mucoraceae, or *Candida* spp. A fungal etiology of a brain abscess should be suspected in a patient with a protracted hospital course who has been neutropenic for more than 1 week and has been treated with broad-spectrum antibiotics.[112]

Focal CNS lesions of several etiologies can occur in patients with AIDS, and multiple pathologic processes commonly coexist.[115] In one series, CNS toxoplasmosis occurred in 103 of 366 (28 percent) AIDS patients with CNS complications.[116] Single or multiple abscesses are characteristic and are difficult to distinguish from pyogenic lesions by CT. Unlike the situation in non-AIDS patients, serologic studies are rarely helpful; cases of CNS toxoplasmosis have been documented even in serology-negative patients.[115] In the same series, primary CNS lymphoma was the next most prevalent complication and occurred in 11 percent. Progressive multifocal leukoencephalopathy occurs in a significant minority, and abnormal focal CT findings are observed; however, the lack of mass effect, surrounding edema, or contrast enhancement and the confinement of the lesions to white matter helps to differentiate this process from toxoplasmosis or lymphoma. Additional less common infectious etiologies of mass lesions in this patient population include *Mycobacterium tuberculosis,*[117] *Mycobacterium avium* complex, *Cryptococcus neoformans, Candida* spp., *Aspergillus* spp., *Nocardia asteroides, Listeria monocytogenes, Salmonella* group B,[115,118] *Rhodococcus equi,*[119] and *Acanthamoeba* spp.[108] Recently, four cases of pneumococcal brain abscesses in the setting of AIDS were reported, underscoring the increased pathogenicity of this organism in this setting.[120]

Location within the brain can predict the etiologic agent(s) (Table 1). For example, a frontal lobe abscess in association with sinusitis often yields one of the *Streptococcus intermedius* group in pure culture.[20,21,77] Post-traumatic abscesses are usually caused by staphylococci, and abscesses from otitis media are virtually always polymicrobial in origin, with streptococci, *Bacteroides* spp., and gram-negative aerobic bacilli (particularly *Proteus* spp.) most often isolated in combination.[20,21,73,77] Thus, the location of the abscess may have important implications for antimicrobial therapy.

CLINICAL MANIFESTATIONS AND DIFFERENTIAL DIAGNOSIS

The clinical course for a brain abscess patient may range from indolent to fulminant; in approximately 75 percent of patients, the duration of symptoms is 2 weeks or less.[9,13,19,22] Only a minority (≤50 percent) of patients display the classic triad of fever, headache, and focal neurologic deficit. The prominent clinical manifestations of brain abscesses are due to the space-occupying mass rather than to infection. A moderate to severe headache, often hemicranial but also generalized, is the most common symptom (approximately 70 percent of cases).[5,7,19,73] Fever occurs in only 45–50 percent of patients,[4,7,13,19] but may be more commonly observed in children (up to 80%).[121] A change in mental status ranging from lethargy to frank coma occurs in most patients.[5,9,19] Focal neurologic findings are present in approximately 50 percent of cases and are dependent on the location and size of the lesion and concurrent surrounding edema; hemiparesis is the most common manifestation.[3–5,7,11,12,19] Nausea and vomiting afflict one-half of patients, presumably due to raised intracranial pressure. Seizures occur in 25–35 percent of patients at the time of presentation; they most often appear generalized and are common with frontal lobe lesions.[7,11,12,13,19] Nuchal rigidity and papilledema each are present in about 25 percent of cases.[7,11,12,19,23] The clinical manifestations of a brain abscess, on rare occasions, may closely mimic pyogenic meningitis with a rapidly fulminant course. Other symptoms and signs are dependent on the intracranial location. Abscesses of the cerebellar hemispheres (10–18 percent of intracranial abscesses) often produce nystagmus, ataxia, vomiting, and dysmetria.[74,78]

The clinical presentation of frontal lobe abscesses is often dominated by headache, drowsiness, inattention, and a generalized deterioration in mental function. Hemiparesis with unilateral motor signs and a motor speech disorder are the most common focal neurologic signs. A temporal lobe abscess may present with an early ipsilateral headache. If the abscess is in the dominant hemisphere, aphasia may be present. An upper homonymous quadrantanopia may also be demonstrated and may be the only sign of a temporal lobe abscess.[122] Intrasellar abscesses often simulate a pituitary tumor and present with headache, visual field defects, and various endocrine disturbances.[32,123] Brain stem abscesses most frequently present with facial weakness, fever, headache, hemiparesis, dysphagia, and vomiting.[34] The symptoms and signs of the extracerebral focus of infection may be present and dominate the clinical picture. Neurologic findings, however subtle, in a patient with a predisposing condition outlined in Table 1, mandate investigation of the CNS to exclude a brain abscess and other intracranial complications of these disorders.[7,11,17,19]

The differential diagnosis of brain abscesses is broad and includes subdural empyema, epidural abscess, pyogenic meningitis, primary or metastatic cerebral neoplasms, viral (especially herpes simplex) encephalitis, hemorrhagic leukoencephalitis, echinococcosis, cysticercosis, cryptococcosis, cerebral infarction, CNS vasculitis, mycotic aneurysms, and chronic subdural hematoma. Computed tomography is often necessary but frequently not sufficient to accomplish this differentiation. A recent study also suggested that occasionally multiple sclerosis may mimic a brain abscess on clinical presentation and by magnetic resonance imaging (MRI).[124]

LABORATORY FINDINGS AND DIAGNOSIS

A moderate peripheral blood leukocytosis may be present in patients with abscesses but exceeds $20,000/mm^3$ in only 10 percent of patients, while 40 percent display a completely normal leukocyte concentration.[5,7,84] The erythrocyte sedimentation rate is usually elevated, with a mean of 45–50 mm/hr. Serum C-reactive protein, an acute phase protein produced in the liver, has recently been evaluated in the differential diagnosis between brain abscess and neoplasm. The serum C-reactive protein was elevated in seven of nine brain abscess patients compared with none of 11 patients with the final diagnosis of brain tumor.[125] Similarly, only 3 of 23 patients with a brain abscess had a normal C-reactive protein in a second study.[44] Finally, C-reactive protein was elevated in 9 of 10 recently published cases of brain abscess; however, an elevated level was also noted in 3 of 13 patients with the eventual diagnosis of a neoplasm.[126] Hyponatremia may be seen as a reflection of the syndrome of inappropriate antidiuretic hormone secretion.

Lumbar puncture is contraindicated in patients with a suspected or proven cerebral abscess, since the diagnostic yield is poor and the procedure is dangerous. The cerebrospinal fluid (CSF) profile is nonspecific in patients with brain abscesses: hypoglycorrhachia in 25 percent; elevated protein in 67–81 percent; and a pleocytosis, usually $<500/mm^3$ and predominantly mononuclear, in 60–70 percent of cases.[5,7,12,19] Fewer than 10 percent of CSF cultures are positive, only increasing to 20 percent after ventricular rupture.[9] In addition, the removal of CSF may result in herniation. In one series,[3] 41 of 140 patients subjected to lumbar puncture deteriorated clinically in less than 48 hours; 25 of these 41 patients died (11 of these were fully alert or only mildly drowsy at the time of the procedure). Similarly, 7 of 44 patients deteriorated in less than 24 hours after lumbar puncture, and 6 died.[85] In the analysis of Samson and Clark,[19] 22 of 44 patients with brain abscesses underwent lumbar puncture; 5 of the 22 developed signs of midbrain compression within 2 hours of the procedure. These sobering figures have been confirmed in a series of patients observed from 1970 to 1983. Sixty percent (27/45) of these patients were subjected to a lumbar puncture, and 4 of these 27 patients died within 24 hours of the procedure.[9] The poor diagnostic yield and significant morbidity of lumbar puncture in brain abscess has been confirmed by two series.[44,121] For these reasons, a lumbar puncture should be delayed in patients with a febrile CNS disorder with focal neurologic signs.[31,127] However, if pyogenic meningitis is also a strong consideration, blood cultures should be obtained and appropriate antibiotics started parenterally before obtaining the CT scan. In this case, if the CT scan findings are negative, a lumbar puncture is then performed.

The skull roentgenogram is usually normal in patients with brain abscesses but may show a pineal shift, signs of raised intracranial pressure, an effaced dorsum sellae (with intrasellar abscess), or pathognomonic collections of air within a cavity.[3–5,7,11,12,19,23] The electroencephalogram (EEG) is usually abnormal in patients with brain abscess and lateralizes to the side of the lesion.[5,7,19,23,84] In developing countries, the EEG is a useful (and often the only) screening procedure for the detection of brain abscesses.[12]

Arteriography and ventriculography are rarely necessary in the evaluation of patients with suspected brain abscesses since the advent of CT and MRI. Arteriograms are abnormal in about 80 percent of brain abscess patients and may show a "ring shadow" in 20–40 percent; the usual pattern is an avascular mass with surrounding hyperemia.[3–5,7,11,12,19,128] The absence of neovascularity may be helpful in excluding a necrotic tumor. Arteriography is essential if mycotic aneurysms due to endocarditis are suspected.

A technetium-99 (^{99m}Tc) brain scan is a very sensitive test for the detection of brain abscess and remains the procedure of choice in areas where CT or MRI scanning is unavailable. The results are abnormal in less than 95 percent of patients, and a "doughnut" lesion is detected in 25–35 percent.[129] Unfortunately, this radiographic appearance is also compatible with a necrotic tumor or infarction. The results of some series suggest that the brain scan is more sensitive than CT in the early cerebritis stage of a brain abscess, but more information is necessary.[130] Compared with CT and MRI, localization is not as accurate; posterior fossa lesions are more difficult to visualize, and postoperative uptake can obscure the recognition of persistent or recurrent abscesses.[131]

The introduction of CT revolutionized the diagnostic (and perhaps therapeutic) approach to brain abscess. CT has been shown to be superior to standard radiologic procedures for the evaluation of the paranasal sinuses, mastoids, and the middle ear; scans of these areas should be obtained, along with chest x-ray films, in all patients with suspected brain abscesses.[132] This technique is more sensitive (95–99 percent) than are traditional brain scans beyond the cerebritis stage and yields more information—the extent of surrounding edema, the presence of a midline shift, hydrocephalus, or imminent ventricular rupture.[133,134] The characteristic appearance (Figs. 1 and 2) is a hypodense center (leukocytes and necrotic debris) with an outlying uniform ring enhancement surrounded by a variable hypodense region of brain edema. Contrast enhancement is essential. The impressive sensitivity of CT is not paralleled by an equivalent specificity; a similar appearance is seen with neoplasms, granulomas, cerebral infarction, or resolving hematoma.[135,136] In addition, this characteristic appearance may be lost after ventricular rupture (Fig. 3). Additionally, the presence of pyocephalus strongly suggests an associated brain abscess and probable ventricular rupture.[137] Features thought to discriminate abscesses from malignant tumors (thinner, more regular contrast-enhancing rim, and homogeneous enhancement of the capsule after infusion of contrast medium) do not always permit a precise diagnosis. Ependymal enhancement, when present, is indicative of ventriculitis and favors a diagnosis of brain abscess.[9] Holtas et al.[138] reported a series of 26 patients with brain abscesses wherein the CT and clinical findings in 8 were interpreted as representing a malignant tumor instead of abscess. In an effort to improve the diagnostic accuracy of CT, Coulam and associates[139] selected six parameters that could be used to differentiate between abscess and tumor, including patient age, ring thickness variability, outside ring diameter, lesion-to-ring ratio, maximum ring thickness, and CT mean value in the ring center. The overall classification accuracy in their study was still only 86 percent (84 percent for abscesses, 96 percent for tumors).

A diagnostic modality that may prove to be complimentary

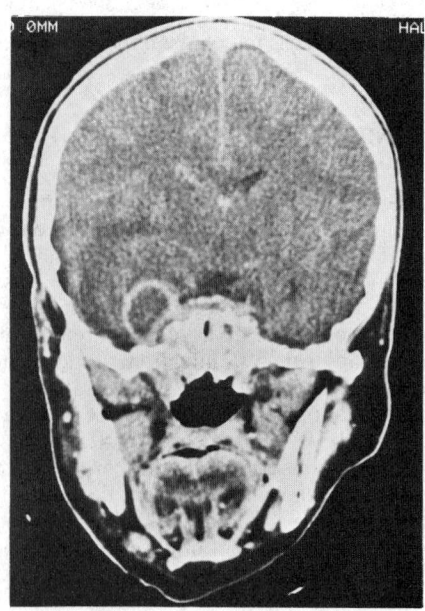

FIG. 2. CT scan after contrast administration in the coronal projection from the same patient shown in Figure 1. Note the ring enhancement of the inferomedial left temporal lobe abscess, edema in the temporal lobe white matter, and effacement of the left lateral ventricle. Also note the proximity of the abscess to the petrous ridge and cavernous sinus. After abscess aspiration, drainage of sphenoid sinusitis, and 4 weeks of parenteral penicillin, the patient made a complete recovery without sequelae.

to CT is ^{111}In-labeled leukocyte scintigraphy, which has been studied for the diagnosis of occult abscesses elsewhere in the body and has been recently evaluated in the diagnosis of brain abscess. Radiolabeled leukocytes migrate to and accumulate in a focus of active inflammation, thus differentiating a brain abscess from other causes of mass lesions in the brain. In a study of 16 patients for whom CT was felt to be inconclusive in making a differentiation between tumor or abscess, leukocyte scintigraphy correctly predicted tumor in 10 of 11 patients and abscess in 4 of 5 patients, for an overall diagnostic accuracy of 88 percent.[140] A second study of 20 patients yielded a sensitivity of 100 percent, specificity of 94 percent, and overall accuracy of 96 percent in making this differentiation.[141] Three other reports, totalling 17 additional patients, confirm this high degree of diagnostic accuracy.[142] Potential problems illustrated in these studies are that necrotic tumors can occasionally yield a false-positive result and that the concomitant use of steroids may be responsible for a false-negative scan finding. A second isotope, ^{99}Tc-hexamethylpropyleneamine oxime, has recently been evaluated in leukocyte scintigraphy. This technique was evaluated in 23 patients with intracranial mass lesions. It correctly detected all 10 confirmed brain abscesses, and, importantly, there were no false-positive results noted.[126]

Data regarding the utility of MRI (Fig. 4) in the diagnosis of a brain abscess continue to accumulate and are very encouraging. MRI appears to be more sensitive than CT in the early detection of cerebritis as well as in detecting cerebral edema in healthy brain tissue adjacent to a cerebritic focus.[143–145] This increased sensitivity may be of limited clinical usefulness, since there is already an obvious CT lesion when most brain abscess patients seek help. However, MRI may detect satellite lesions earlier. Additionally, MRI is more accurate than CT in differentiating the central liquefactive necrosis of a brain abscess from other fluid accumulations. On CT, the central region is isodense with CSF, whereas on MRI it is usually hyperintense relative to the CSF. Also, concentric rings of intensity, or a target appearance, have been observed frequently in the necrotic center with MRI, which appears to be specific for abscess rather than for necrotic or cystic malignancies.[146] Contrast-enhanced MRI scans using

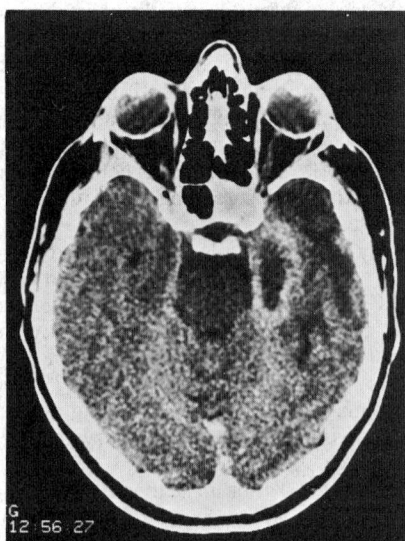

FIG. 1. CT scan after contrast administration in the axial projection from a 44-year-old woman with a history of chronic otitis media and documented sphenoid sinusitis. Note the ring synhancement around a hypodense lesion in the left medial temporal lobe with hypodense edema in the white matter. Aspiration revealed *S. anginosus* in pure culture.

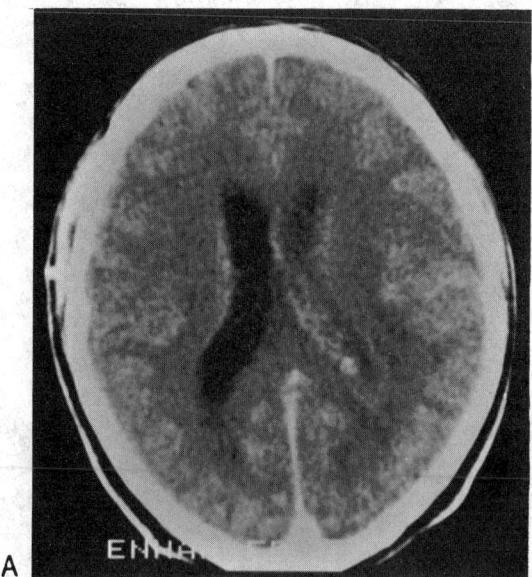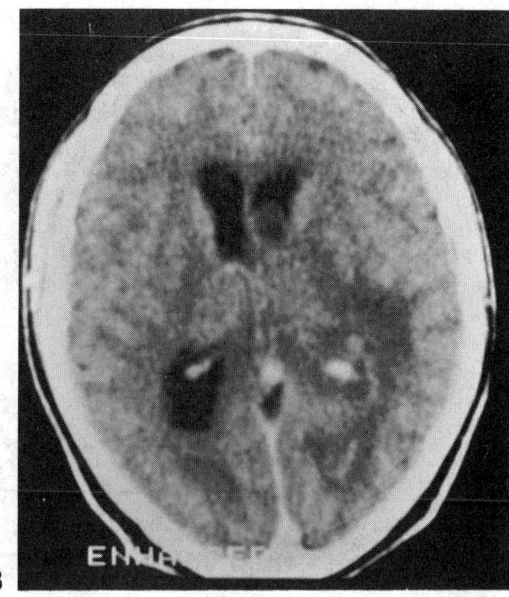

FIG. 3. CT scan after contrast administration in the axial projection. Note the loss of contrast enhancement in the original right hemispheric abscess after rupture into the right lateral ventricle. **(A)** Abscess enhancement is replaced by ependymal enhancement. **(B)** Abscess fluid/CSF interface in the right lateral ventricle.

the paramagnetic agent gadolinium diethylenetriamine penta-acetic acid (Gd-DTPA) increase the information obtained by MRI. This agent crosses a damaged blood-brain barrier and enhances proton relaxation, which in turn increases T1 signal intensity at the site of its accumulation. Gd-DTPA yields consistently increased enhancement of lesions relative to that seen with enhanced CT scans. Additionally, it differentiates three regions with greater accuracy: (1) the central abscess, (2) the surrounding enhancing rim, and (3) cerebral edema around the abscess.[144–147] The potential devastating complication of extra-parenchymal extension of a brain abscess (such as ventricular rupture) is more easily detected by MRI, because the abscess fluid will again appear hyperintense relative to the CSF. Reports indicate that MRI is superior to CT for the detection and characterization of a cerebral abscess, particularly in early stages of evolution.[148,149] Its lack of ionizing radiation, greater tissue characterization, lack of bone artifact (which improves its sensitivity in posterior fossa lesions), and the decreased toxicity of Gd-DTPA as compared with CT contrast agents make MRI the procedure of choice in the evaluation of brain abscesses.

ANTIBIOTIC THERAPY

Antibiotic Entry into Brain Abscess Pus

The various factors that determine the passage of an antibiotic into the CSF[150] may not predict entry into brain tissue or abscess pus. The blood-brain barrier is altered in proximity to areas of cerebritis or an encapsulated abscess[151] and permits increased permeation of normally excluded antibiotics such as penicillin into the brain parenchyma. Few studies have addressed this issue in the treatment of brain abscesses.

An early study[152] examined brain tissue, CSF, and serum antibiotic concentrations in 27 patients subjected to a prefrontal lobotomy, presumably with an intact blood-brain barrier. After collection at various intervals after dosing, tetracycline entered both the CSF and the brain, streptomycin and erythromycin were found in the CSF but not in the brain, and penicillin was not present at either site, perhaps reflecting the low dose (600,000 units) and serum concentrations attained (0.06–2.0 μg/ml) 4 hours later when brain samples were analyzed. In patients undergoing excision of an intracranial neoplasm, a parenteral

bolus of 2 g led to the following calculated brain-blood ratios: chloramphenicol, 9:1; cephalothin, 1:10; penicillin G, 1:23; and ampicillin, 1:56.[153] On the basis of this evidence and activity against anaerobic bacteria, chloramphenicol has often been included in older regimens for the treatment of brain abscesses.

Black et al.[154] analyzed antibiotic concentrations in brain abscess pus from 6 patients. Chloramphenicol, methicillin, and penicillin were detectable in the pus after standard dosages, whereas nafcillin was not. All six patients deteriorated clinically during medical treatment, and all cultures were still positive at surgery, thus indicating the need for surgical intervention. In the best analysis to date, de Louvois et al.[155] examined antibiotic concentrations in brain abscess pus obtained from 32 patients. Penicillin G was detectable consistently if the dose exceeded 24 million units daily (adults); however, the drug was at least 90 percent inactivated after incubation in pus for 1 hour in vitro[156] in 4 of 22 specimens. Fusidic acid entered the brain abscess pus readily, but concentrations of various cephalosporins and cloxacillin were low.[155] CSF and brain concentrations of clindamycin are low after conventional dosages[156]; however, potentially therapeutic concentrations in abscess fluid may be attainable.[157] Metronidazole attains high concentrations (approximately 35–45 μg/g) in brain abscess pus,[73] often exceeding serum concentrations after a dose of 400–600 mg every 8 hours. Due to these results and the bactericidal activity of metronidazole against strict anaerobes, this agent is often a component of antimicrobial regimens for brain abscesses.[158]

Trimethoprim-sulfamethoxazole, effective in cerebral nocardiosis[159,160] and gram-negative meningitis,[161] may have a role when susceptible organisms are present. In two studies, this drug combination was found to attain adequate brain abscess pus concentrations for the organisms being treated (*Proteus mirabilis* and *Nocardia asteroides*) and yielded successful results when combined with surgery.[160,162] In a recent report,[163] vancomycin also attained acceptable concentrations in a single brain abscess.

Little information is currently available on the penetration of newer antimicrobial agents into brain abscesses or their clinical efficacy in this infection. Cefotaxime, ceftizoxime, ceftriaxone, ceftazidine, and moxalactam have been shown to penetrate the CSF in therapeutic concentrations, but this does not necessarily predict activity in a brain abscess. A recent report demonstrated

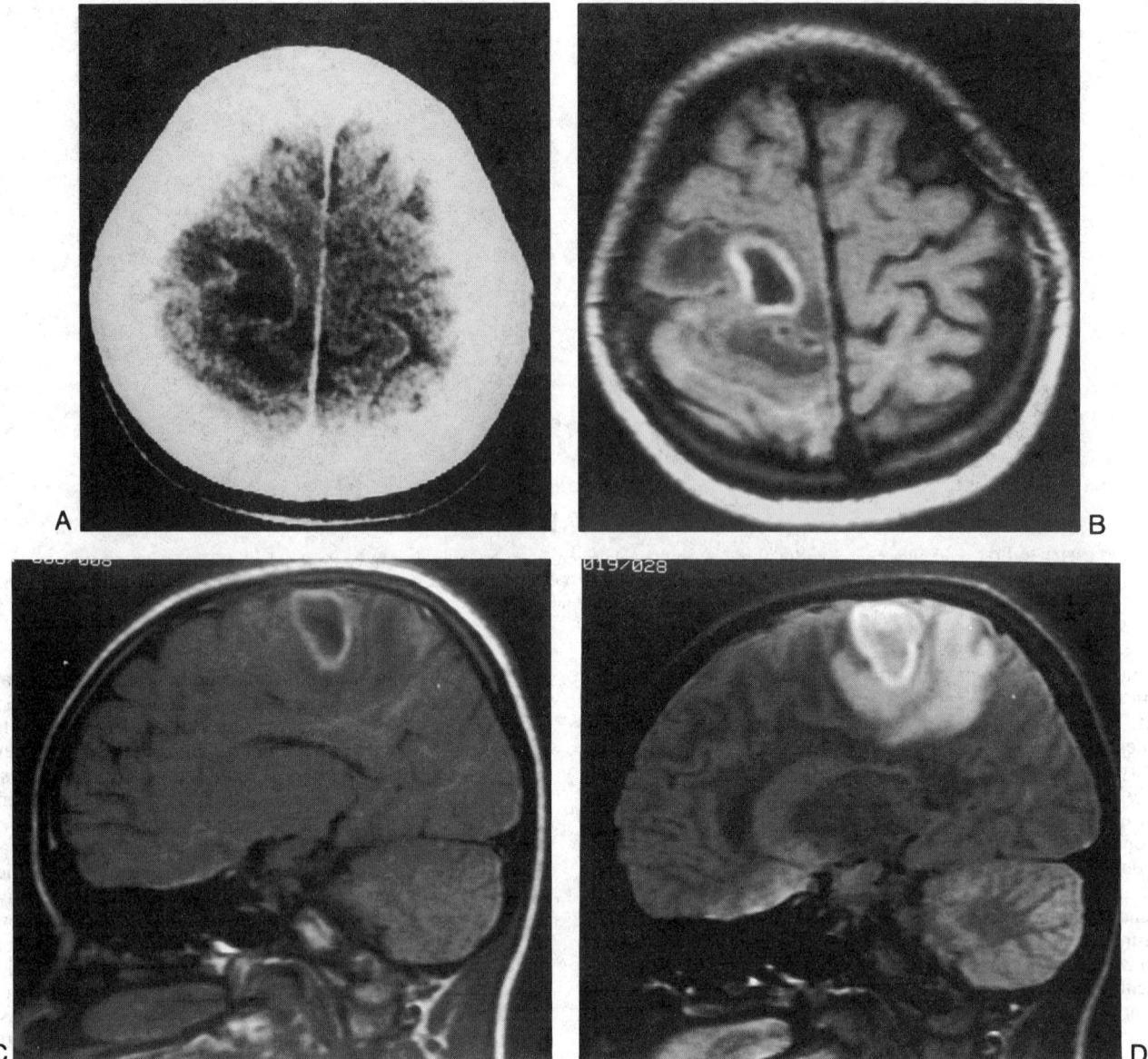

FIG. 4. MRI of a brain abscess in a teenage girl who developed seizures several days after esophageal dilation. **(A)** Contrast CT shows a thin-walled enhancing cystic lesion in the right parietal subcortical region. **(B)** T1-weighted MRI of a 5-mm-thick axial section shows a thin-walled hyperintense rim abscess with surrounding hypointensity. Note, in comparison to the opposite side, the effacement of the sulci on the right. **(C)** Sagittal T1-weighted image of a 5-mm-thick section shows the hyperintense thin-walled abscess. **(D)** Sagittal T2-weighted image of a 5-mm-thick section shows a hyperintense abscess wall with high-signal contents (pus) and high-signal surrounding edema. (Courtesy of Dr. Robert Zimmerman, Department of Radiology, Hospital of the University of Pennsylvania, Philadelphia, PA.)

good penetration of moxalactam into brain abscess fluid,[164] and this agent has been used successfully in the treatment of neonatal brain abscess.[165] Cefotaxime penetration into human brain abscess pus was recently evaluated in 8 patients.[166] When given in high dose (3 g q8h), both cefotaxime and its active metabolite were present in abscess fluid in concentrations above the minimal inhibitory concentrations of the majority of gram-positive and gram-negative aerobic organisms for which it is normally used systemically. Aztreonam, a new monobactam derivative, has recently been shown to be effective in the treatment of experimental cerebritis,[167] but its penetration into brain tissue has not been evaluated, and it has not yet been evaluated in human brain abscesses. A single case report details a successful outcome in the treatment of a polymicrobial brain abscess with imipenem-cilastatin.[168] A concentration in the abscess greater than the minimal inhibitory concentration for the isolated organ-

isms was attained with a dose of 2.0 g/day. A major concern, however, is that the use of imipenem may be associated with an increased incidence of seizures, which may limit its use in brain abscess patients, who are already seizure prone.[169] An open prospective study evaluated the efficacy of ampicillin-sulbactam in the treatment of 21 patients with brain abscesses.[170] Seventeen patients were cured, including all five treated without surgery, suggesting the potential utility of this agent in the treatment of brain abscess.

Any study evaluating antibiotic penetration into the CNS must be interpreted cautiously. Considerable variation in tissue concentrations among different patients is often present, as well as conflicting results between studies. A single tissue concentration may not represent the dynamics of antibiotic movement into the brain in the presence of inflammation.[171,172] The relevance of brain and abscess pus antibiotic concentrations or the necessity of bactericidal activity at the site of infection remains unknown. In addition, the role of osmotic manipulation of the blood-brain barrier in order to increase the penetration of various antibiotics into a brain abscess, while promising in experimental animal models, is uncertain.[173]

Choice of Antibiotic

The antimicrobial regimens commonly recommended for therapy of brain abscesses are empirical and reflect the considerations already noted, as well as their in vitro activity against the usual pathogens. No controlled trials on the relative efficacy of various regimens have been performed. Since the early 1960s, a combination of penicillin G (20–24 million units/day) plus chloramphenicol (1.0–1.5 g IV q6h) has been advocated. Penicillin remains a mainstay of therapy[20,21,77] due to its excellent activity against streptococci in vitro and the favorable results obtained in experimental models of brain abscess.[174] The introduction of penicillin in the 1940s may have been instrumental in reducing brain abscess mortality from 50–80 percent to 20–30 percent by 1950.[175-178] Due to the important role of streptococci (especially the *S. intermedius* group) in brain abscesses complicating contiguous foci of infection and pyogenic lung disease, penicillin should be employed in all such cases. As noted above, cefotaxime appears to be adequate for the majority of streptococcal isolates, with the advantage of a broad gram-negative spectrum of activity, and therefore could be considered as an alternative to penicillin in combination regimens.[166,179] Most anaerobes are also susceptible to penicillin with the notable exception of *Bacteroides fragilis*.

Chloramphenicol has been administered concurrently with penicillin because its high lipid solubility results in concentrations in brain tissue often exceeding those in serum, and its activity against anaerobic bacteria is significant. The use of metronidazole in brain abscesses has increased greatly in recent years because *(1)* metronidazole is bactericidal against *B. fragilis,* where chloramphenicol is frequently bacteriostatic; *(2)* metronidazole attains reproducibly excellent concentrations in brain abscess pus[73]; *(3)* metronidazole's entry into brain abscess pus is not affected by concomitant steroid treatment, unlike several other antibiotics[178]; *(4)* chloramphenicol may be degraded in pus (shown in experimental intra-abdominal abscesses); and *(5)* metronidazole may have a salutary effect on mortality, as suggested by retrospective experience.[151] Metronidazole, when substituted for chloramphenicol, may lead to more rapid healing and lower mortality[57,158,180]; however, these two agents have never been compared in a prospective, randomized trial. Additionally, metronidazole may cause CNS side effects that are difficult to differentiate from clinical deterioration in brain abscess patients. An antianaerobic agent (e.g., chloramphenicol or metronidazole) is indicated in brain abscesses complicating otitis media, mastoiditis, or pyogenic lung disease, since anaerobes (particularly *B. fragilis*) are often present. These agents may not be required in abscesses secondary to frontoethmoidal sinusitis because *B. fragilis* is an uncommon isolate.

When staphylococci are suspected (Table 1) or grown, nafcillin (1.5 g q4h) is indicated.[181] Vancomycin should be substituted if the patient is either allergic to penicillin or a methicillin-resistant strain is isolated. European investigators favor fusidic acid for this indication,[20,21] but experience with this agent by physicians in the United States is limited.

The frequent isolation of Enterobacteriaceae in brain abscesses of otitic origin prompts many authorities to add a third-generation cephalosporin or trimethoprim-sulfamethoxazole to the regimen pending culture results. Given the increased frequency of *P. aeruginosa* in the setting of chronic middle ear disease, ceftazidime is a logical empirical choice as part of a combination regimen. Finally, the duration of therapy with any of the regimens as outlined remains unknown.

SURGICAL THERAPY

Although some patients with brain abscess respond to prolonged medical therapy alone, most require surgery for optimal management. The timing and type of surgical procedure remain controversial. Aspiration of the abscess after burr hole placement and complete excision after craniotomy have both been advocated, but no prospective randomized trial has ever been performed. By retrospective analysis, the two procedures appear to be equivalent as judged by outcome.[3-5,21] It would be inappropriate, based on currently available data, to proclaim the superiority of either method.[3-5,19,182-186] However, patients considered for excision are more often in a satisfactory neurologic condition, whereas aspiration is more often performed in the deteriorating neurologically compromised patient or for the drainage of inaccessible lesions (brain stem, thalamus, basal ganglia, and so forth) where mortality is significant.[12] The procedure employed must be individualized in each patient and is dependent on the clinical course, size, and location of the abscess; CT scan appearance; and other factors. Emergent surgery is mandatory when there is a progression of neurologic signs. Young and Frazee[187] advocate that abscesses exhibiting gas by CT or plain film should be considered for complete excision. In a review of five such patients, three of whom had unsuccessful aspiration procedures, a total excision was required, and a persistent extracranial communication was discovered. A brain abscess in a comatose patient carries a grave prognosis regardless of the form of treatment,[7,188] and surgery is indicated before this stage. Incomplete drainage of a multiloculated abscess is a major disadvantage of aspiration and is an important reason why reoperation is required more frequently after this procedure.[12] Excision is preferred for posterior fossa lesions and in fungal brain abscesses, for which the efficacy of antifungal therapy is likely to be limited; however, one recent case report detailed a successful outcome of an *Aspergillus* brain abscess treated by aspiration.[189]

The incidence of postoperative seizures or other deficits is not clearly different after excision as compared with aspiration[12,190]; however, since the advent of CT, the data appear to favor more conservative surgical procedures (i.e., aspiration).[185] This suggestion has been recently supported in a study of 28 cases of brain abscess in children where a trend toward a decreased incidence of post-treatment seizures and other neurologic sequelae was noted in the patients treated by aspiration.[28] Instillation of antibiotics into the abscess cavity during aspiration (often bacitracin or penicillin) is sometimes employed, although its efficacy and toxicity have never been clearly evaluated. Antibiotics given in this manner may potentially diffuse into surrounding brain tissue in high concentrations and cause seizures.[21,154,176,191] In cases in which *Pseudomonas* spp. are implicated, direct instillation of specific antibiotics is probably warranted because adequate local antibiotic concentrations for this organism after systemic administration are difficult to obtain, with the possible exception of ceftazidime or aztreonam.[9] A recent case report of successful therapy of an *Aspergillus* brain abscess utilized continual intracavitary administration of amphotericin B in conjunction with systemic therapy.[192] This approach is fraught with hazard due to the toxicity of amphotericin B for brain tissue and is not currently recommended.

Aspiration may now be accomplished by stereotaxic CT guidance.[193] This procedure affords the surgeon rapid, accurate (within 1 mm), and safe access to virtually any intracranial point. In a recent review of its use in 80 patients, recovery of tissue specific to establish a histologic diagnosis or the etiologic factors related to each disease process was realized in 94 percent of cases. There was no associated mortality and only 4 percent transient morbidity. The diagnosis of 20 cases of infection was made, 6 of which were pyogenic brain abscess, and in most instances the choice of antimicrobial therapy was significantly affected. In addition, this procedure allowed for successful drainage, even in two cases of multicompartment abscesses.[194] A second series of 102 patients[195] showed a diagnostic yield of 96 percent by this technique. There was no mortality and a 5.9 percent transient morbidity. The five abscesses that were encountered were definitively drained. Several recent evaluations confirm the efficacy and low morbidity of this procedure.[196–198] Two issues deserve comment. As noted previously, the incidence of multiple abscesses can be as high as 50 percent, and, prior to the availability of CT, the mortality could approach 100 percent. With the advent of CT-guided stereotactic surgery, multiple, deep seated lesions can now be successfully managed with a resultant reduction in mortality to 0–8 percent.[199] Secondly, brain stem abscesses also resulted in an almost uniformly fatal outcome previously, and open operative procedures may be associated with an unacceptably high morbidity. Several cases of successful drainage of brain stem abscesses by CT-guided aspiration have now been reported, suggesting that this is the therapy of choice for these lesions.[200,201] The risk of stereotaxic aspiration may be less than the risk of incorrect diagnosis and suboptimal choice of antibiotics, which makes it, in many cases, more difficult to support empirical therapy. Serial CT is useful in individual cases and may permit improved decisions regarding the need, timing, and type of surgery.

GENERAL MANAGEMENT

The CT scan, as noted earlier, has dramatically altered the diagnosis and treatment of brain abscesses. The results in animal models and humans suggest that focal bacterial infections of the brain parenchyma may be "staged" by sequential CT scans.[63,202] Cerebritis is characterized by an area of low density surrounded by ring enhancement (often thick and diffuse) that does not decay on delayed contrast scans obtained 60 minutes later (Table 3). In contrast, encapsulation is characterized by a faint ring on the unenhanced scan and ring enhancement that decays in the delayed CT scan. These parameters may prove useful in planning the combined medical-surgical approach.

Since 1971 it has been recognized that early antibiotic therapy alone could cure cerebritis without the later development of an encapsulated abscess.[203] Between 1975 and 1985, 67 cases of presumably established brain abscesses were reported to be cured by medical therapy alone.[204] These studies share the following features: (1) the initial diagnosis and resolution of brain abscess(s) were documented by sequential CT scans, (2) prolonged courses of high-dose antibiotic therapy (8 weeks or longer parenterally) were administered, and (3) there was a lack of surgical or histopathologic evidence of encapsulation.[12,185,205–210] Careful studies in animal models of brain abscess[13,211] and clinical observations[64,136,202,212] have clearly shown, however, that ring enhancement on the CT scan and focal edema on MRI may be observed during the cerebritis stage. Thus, it is possible that these results with antimicrobial therapy represent successful resolution of bacterial cerebritis rather than a well-encapsulated abscess in some cases. Also, in several of these cases, a "diagnostic" aspiration was performed, which may have biased the results. Nonetheless, it appears certain that some brain abscesses may be cured without surgical intervention. This problem requires further study.

TABLE 3. "Staging" of Brain Abscesses with Computed Tomography

		Contrast Enhancement at	
Stage[a]	Precontrast	10 min	60 min
Cerebritis	Low density	Ring enhancement	No decay
Abscess	Capsule-faint ring around low density	Ring enhancement	Decay in contrast enhancement

[a] Both lesions may be surrounded by low-density areas of edema.

(Data from Britt and Enzmann.[64])

Approach to the Patient with Suspected Brain Abscess

Patients who present with altered consciousness, focal central nervous system signs, or seizures usually are candidates for contrast-enhanced CT or MRI. In hospitals where these imaging techniques are not available, ^{99m}Tc brain scan can be employed. Lumbar puncture is usually postponed until a space-occupying CNS lesion is excluded. If rapid clinical progression is occurring, blood cultures for bacteria and fungi may be done and empiric antimicrobial therapy begun prior to neuroimaging. In every case, management should be done in conjunction with a neurosurgeon. A probable focus in the paranasal sinus or middle ear should prompt consultation also with an otolaryngologist. Empiric treatment depends on the presence or absence of immunosuppression, particularly AIDS, as follows.

Nonimmunosuppressed Patients. Patients with a lesion on CT or MRI consistent with bacterial brain abscess are begun on empiric antibiotic therapy even if urgent neurosurgical intervention is indicated. The most frequently recommended regimen for adults is to begin with penicillin G, 4 million units IV q4h, plus metronidazole, 7.5 mg/kg (often rounded out to 500 mg) q6h. Chloramphenicol is less frequently utilized currently. As noted previously, cefotaxime, 2 g IV q4–6h, is an acceptable and perhaps favored replacement for penicillin in this regimen.[213] Antibiotic therapy should not preclude efforts to isolate the organism by aerobic and anaerobic culture of surgical material obtained later.

Nonoperative management is most often considered when the patient is neurologically stable and CT or MRI is consistent with cerebritis. The decision for nonoperative management is also influenced by the following: (1) medical conditions that greatly increase the risk of surgery; (2) the presence of multiple abscesses, especially remotely distant from one another; (3) abscesses in a deep or dominant location; (4) concomitant meningitis or ependymitis; (5) early abscess reduction and clinical improvement attributable to antibiotic therapy; and (6) abscess size under 3 cm.[26,135,207,208] As noted, these criteria may be altered by the availability of stereotaxic CT-guided aspiration. Neurologic deterioration mandates surgery, usually aspiration.[12] If the patient remains stable and the abscess is accessible, aspiration (CT guided, if possible) is desirable to make a specific bacteriologic diagnosis and narrow the antimicrobial regimen. Although this delay may render cultures negative, aspiration during the cerebritis stage may be dangerous with resultant hemorrhage.[212] Certain poor prognostic parameters, clinical or radiographic, may necessitate earlier aspiration.[188] If the lesion appears encapsulated by CT scan criteria, antibiotic treatment can be started and aspiration (for diagnosis and drainage) performed without delay.[64,202] Subsequent management is dependent on clinical and radiographic (CT) parameters. Later neurologic deterioration or failure of the abscess to decrease in size as detected by CT scan are indications for further surgery, often excision, if feasible. The duration of antimicrobial therapy remains unsettled. Many authorities treat parenterally for approximately 4–6 weeks. Duration cannot be determined by resolution of all CT or MRI abnormalities. A cured brain abscess may continue to appear as nodular contrast enhancement on CT scans for 4–10 weeks to up to 6 months[64,135,136] after completion of successful therapy. No empiric regimen consisting solely of oral agents is recommended, even in the later stages of therapy.

AIDS Patients. Patients with advanced HIV infection or AIDS and who have CNS lesions on MRI or contrast-enhanced CT consistent with toxoplasmosis are usually begun on empiric therapy with pyrimethamine and sulfadiazine. Pyrimethamine is given to adults as a single loading dose of 75–100 mg followed by 25–50 mg daily. Folinic acid is given as 10 mg daily to decrease bone marrow suppression from pyrimethamine. Sulfadiazine is given as 1 g PO every 6 hours. If sulfadiazine is not available, clindamycin is an acceptable substitute (600 mg IV q6h). Low-grade fever and a gradual onset also prompt this approach. The limitation of empiric therapy is that radiologic distinction between toxoplasmosis and other lesions is not accurate. Progressive deterioration, an atypical CT or MRI, or failure to show clinical and imaging improvement during 2 weeks of therapy generally prompts biopsy or aspiration.[214] Some physicians would also use a negative *Toxoplasma* serology to prompt early neurosurgical intervention. Patients taking trimethoprim-sulfamethoxazole prophylaxis for pneumocystosis may be at a lower risk of toxoplasmosis and are therefore more likely to have an alternative diagnosis (for further details, see Ch. 257).

Other Immunosuppressed Patients.   The range of etiologic agents for brain abscess is so broad in these patients that empiric therapy has limited value. Early neurosurgical intervention is usually indicated.

Corticosteroids

Steroids are often employed as adjunctives in the management of brain abscess, but their role remains controversial. These agents may be deleterious by reducing antibiotic entry into the CNS,[215,216] decreasing collagen formation and glial response,[217] or altering the CT scan appearance of ring enhancement as inflammation subsides,[218,219] which may obscure information from sequential studies or an assessment of cure. Two recent studies in experimental animal models of brain abscess, however, noted no increase or decrease in mortality in those animals receiving dexamethasone.[220,221] However, steroids may prove life-saving in the patient with rapid neurologic deterioration and raised intracranial pressure. In this circumstance, intracranial pressure monitoring is advisable, and elevations in pressure should be controlled with steroids, forced hyperventilation, and mannitol if necessary. Anticonvulsants are appropriate in the patient having seizures and are frequently started empirically.

PROGNOSIS

The mortality of brain abscesses was 40–60 percent in the preantibiotic era; some series report a decline after the introduction of penicillin.[3–5,7,11,12,19,23,84] An adverse prognosis is associated with (1) delayed or missed diagnosis; (2) poor localization, especially in the posterior fossa before the availability of CT scans; (3) multiple, deep, or multiloculated lesions; (4) ventricular rupture (80–100 percent mortality); (5) coma (Table 4) (80–100 percent mortality); (6) fungal etiology; and (7) inappropriate antibiotics.[7,12,188] Additional negative factors often cited include extremes of age, large abscesses, and metastatic abscesses.[9] More recently, a decreased mortality ranging between 0 and 24 percent has been reported in numerous series and is attributed to the introduction of CT scanning.[24,131,158,222] Two series found that the most important risks of death in cases in the CT and MRI era were a shorter duration and more rapid progression of symptoms prior to presentation. Therefore, earlier recognition of predisposing conditions may be the only way to improve the outcome in this subgroup of patients.[6,13] The incidence of neuro-

logic sequelae ranges between 30 and 55 percent.[6,7,13] Most sequelae are mild, but up to 17 percent of patients may be incapacitated, with the severity of sequelae more often correlating with the patient's neurologic condition on admission than the form of treatment employed.[9,19,61,131] The likelihood of seizures is variable and ranges from 35 to more than 90 percent; these differences may relate to the length of follow-up. Anticonvulsant therapy appears to reduce this complication.[223,224] There is a recent suggestion that lesions treated conservatively (i.e., with antibiotics and/or aspiration vs. complete excision) have a lower incidence of post-treatment sequelae, correlating with less visible abnormalities on follow-up CT scans.[28,185] Earlier diagnosis, refinements in technology, and an aggressive medical-surgical approach may lead to a more consistent reduction in the morbidity and mortality of this still serious disease.

REFERENCES

1. Theophilo F, Markakis E, Theophilo L, et al. Brain abscess in childhood. Child Nerv Syst. 1985;1:324–8.
2. MacEwen W. Pyogenic Infective Diseases of the Brain and Spinal Cord. Glasgow: James MacLehose & Sons; 1893.
3. Garfield J. Management of supratentorial intracranial abscess: A review of 200 cases. Br Med J. 1969;2:7–11.
4. Beller AJ, Sahar A, Praiss I. Brain abscess. Review of 89 cases over 30 years. J Neurol Neurosurg Psychiatry. 1973;36:757–68.
5. Morgan H, Wood M, Murphy F. Experience with 88 consecutive cases of brain abscess. J Neurosurg. 1973;38:698–704.
6. Nicolosi A, Hauser WA, Musicco M, et al. Incidence and prognosis of brain abscess in a defined population: Olmstead County, Minnesota, 1935–1981. Neuroepidemiology. 1991;10:122–31.
7. Nielsen H, Glydensted C, Harmsen A. Cerebral abscess: Aetiology and pathogenesis, symptoms, diagnosis and treatment. Acta Neurol Scand. 1982;65:609–22.
8. Duel P, Siboni K, Jensen TG. Intracranial abscesses in Odense. Dan Med Bull. 1991;38:407–10.
9. Chun CH, Johnson JD, Hofstetter M, et al. Brain abscess. A study of 45 consecutive cases. Medicine (Baltimore). 1986;65:415–31.
10. Arseni C, Ciurea AV. Cerebral abscesses secondary to otorhinolaryngological infections. A study of 386 cases. Zentralbl Neurochir. 1988;49:22–36.
11. Garvey G. Current concepts of bacterial infections of the central nervous system. Bacterial meningitis and bacterial brain abscess. J Neurosurg. 1983;59:735–44.
12. Carey ME. Brain abscesses. Contemp Neurosurg. 1982;3:1.
13. Seydoux C, Francioli P. Bacterial brain abscesses: Factors influencing mortality and sequelae. Clin Infect Dis. 1992;15:394–401.
14. O'Donoghue MAT, Green HT, Shaw DM. Cerebral abscess on Merseyside, 1980–1988. J Infect. 1992;25:163–72.
15. Levy RM, Janssen RS, Bush TJ, et al. Neuroepidemiology of the acquired immunodeficiency syndrome. J AIDS. 1988;1:31–40.
16. Yang SH. Brain abscess: A review of 400 cases. J Neurosurg. 1981;55:794–9.
17. Bradley PJ, Shaw MDM. Three decades of brain abscess in Merseyside. J R Coll Surg Edinb. 1983;28:223–8.
18. Van Alphen HAM, Driessen JJR. Brain abscess and subdural empyema. J Neurol Neurosurg Psychiatry. 1976;39:481–90.
19. Samson DS, Clark K. A current review of brain abscess. Am J Med. 1973;54:201–10.
20. de Louvois J, Gortvai P, Hurley R. Bacteriology of abscesses of the central nervous system. A multicentre prospective study. Br Med J. 1977;2:981–4.
21. de Louvois J. The bacteriology and chemotherapy of brain abscess. J Antimicrob Chemother. 1978;4:395–413.
22. Harrison MJG. The clinical presentation of intracranial abscesses. Q J Med. 1982;51:461–8.
23. Brewer NS, MacCarty CS, Wellman WE. Brain abscess: A review of recent experience. Ann Intern Med. 1975;82:571–6.
24. Small M, Dale BAB. Intracranial suppuration 1968–1982—A 15 year review. Clin Otolaryngol. 1984;9:315–21.
25. Bradley PJ, Manning KP, Shaw MDM. Brain abscess secondary to paranasal sinusitis. J Laryngol Otol. 1984;98:719–25.
26. Kaplan K. Brain abscess. Med Clin North Am. 1985;69:345–60.
27. Spires JR, Smith RJH, Catlin FI. Brain abscesses in the young. Otolaryngol Head Neck Surg. 1985;93:468–74.
28. Aebi C, Kaufmann F, Schaad UB. Brain abscess in childhood-long term experience. Eur J Pediatr. 1991;150:282–6.
29. Foy P, Skarr M. Cerebral abscesses in children after pencil-tip injuries. Lancet. 1980;2:662–3.
30. Tay JS, Garland JS. Serious head injuries from lawn darts. Pediatrics. 1987;79:261–3.
31. Dacey RG Jr, Winn HR. Brain abscess and perimeningeal infections. In: Stein JH, Cline MJ, Daly WJ, eds. *Internal Medicine* Boston: Little, Brown; 1983:1213.
32. Berger SA, Edberg SC, David G. Infectious disease of the sella turcica. Rev Infect Dis. 1986;8:747–55.

TABLE 4. Brain Abscess: Influence of Preoperative Mental Status on Mortality

Mental Status	Patients (No.)	Mortality (%)
Grade I (fully alert)	33	0
Grade II (drowsy)	55	4
Grade III (response to pain only)	61	59
Grade IV (coma, no pain response)	51	82

(Data from Nielsen et al.[7])

33. Teed RW. Meningitis from the sphenoid sinus. Arch Otolaryngol. 1938;28: 589–619.

34. Dake MD, McMurdo SK, Rosenblum ML, et al. Pyogenic abscess of the medulla oblongata. Neurosurgery. 1986;18:370–2.

35. Naidu MRC. Solitary thalamic abscess. Clin Neurol Neurosurg. 1988;90: 245–7.

36. Rousseaux M, Lesoin F, Destee A, et al. Developments in the treatment and prognosis of multiple cerebral abscesses. Neurosurgery. 1985;16:304–8.

37. Samuel J, Fernandes CMC, Steinberg JL. Intracranial otogenic complications: A persisting problem. Laryngoscope. 1986;96:272–8.

38. Matthews TJ, Marcus G. Otogenic intracranial complications: A review of 37 patients. J Laryngol Otol. 1988;102:121–4.

39. Gower D, McGuirt WF. Intracranial complications of acute and chronic infectious ear disease: A problem still with us. Laryngoscope. 1983;93: 1028–33.

40. Browning GG. The unsafeness of safe ears. J Laryngol Otol. 1984;98:23–6.

41. Nunez DA, Browning GG. Risks of developing an otogenic intracranial abscess. J Laryngol Otol. 1990;104:468–72.

42. Lew D, Southwick FS, Montgomery WW, et al. Sphenoid sinusitis. A review of 30 cases. N Engl J Med. 1983;309:1149–54.

43. Rao AN. Brain abscess: A complication of cocaine inhalation. NY State J Med. 1988;88:548–50.

44. Schlaimser SE, Backman K, Norrby SR. Intracranial abscess in adults: An analysis of 54 consecutive cases. Scand J Infect Dis. 1988;20:1–9.

45. Hollin SA, Hayashi H, Gross SW. Intracranial abscesses of odontogenic origin. Oral Surg. 1967;23:277–93.

46. Wohl TA, Kattah JC, Kolsky MP, et al. Hemianopsia from occipital lobe abscess after dental care. Am J Ophthalmol. 1991;112:689–94.

47. Foreman SD, Smith EE, Ryan NJ, et al. Neonatal *Citrobacter* meningitis: Pathogenesis of cerebral abscess formation. Ann Neurol. 1984;16:655–9.

48. Tenney JH. Bacterial infections of the central nervous system in neurosurgery. Neurol Clin. 1986;4:91–114.

49. Rish BL, Caveness WF, Dillon JD, et al. Analysis of brain abscess after penetrating craniocerebral injuries in Vietnam. Neurosurgery. 1981;9: 535–41.

50. Brand B, Caparosa RJ, Lubic LG. Otorhinological brain abscess therapy—Past and present. Laryngoscope. 1984;94:483–7.

51. Waggener JD. The pathophysiology of bacterial meningitis and cerebral abscesses: An anatomical interpretation. Adv Neurol. 1974;6:1–17.

52. Bronitsky R, Heim CR, McGee ZA. Multifocal brain abscesses: Combined medical and neurosurgical therapy. South Med J. 1982;75:1261–3.

53. Kline MW. Brain abscess in a patient with cystic fibrosis. Pediatr Infect Dis. 1985;4:72–3.

54. Schlitt M, Mitchem L, Zorn G, et al. Brain abscess after esophageal dilation for caustic stricture: Report of three cases. Neurosurgery. 1985;17:947–51.

55. Cohen FL, Koerner RS, Taub SJ. Solitary brain abscess following endoscopic injection sclerosis of esophageal varices. Gastrointest Endosc. 1985; 31:331–3.

56. Algoed L, Boon P, DeVos M, et al. Brain abscess after esophageal dilatation for stenosis. Clin Neurol Neurosurg. 1992;94:169–72.

57. Pruit AA, Rubin RHJ, Karchmer AW, et al. Neurologic complications of bacterial endocarditis. Medicine (Baltimore). 1978;57:329–43.

58. Press OW, Ramsey PG. Central nervous system infections associated with hereditary hemorrhagic telangiectasia. Am J Med. 1984;77:86–92.

59. Caroli M, Arienta C, Rampini PM, Balbi S. Recurrence of brain abscess associated with asymptomatic arteriovenous malformations of the lung. Neurochirurgia. 1992;35:167–70.

60. Fischbein CA, Rosenthal A, Fischer EG, et al. Risk factors for brain abscess in patients with congenital heart disease. Am J Cardiol. 1974;34:97–102.

61. Fischer EG, McLennan JE, Suzuki Y. Cerebral abscess in children. Am J Dis Child. 1981;135:746–69.

62. Molinari GF, Smith L, Goldstein MN, et al. Brain abscess from septic cerebral embolism: An experimental model. Neurology. 1973;23:1205–10.

63. Britt RH, Enzmann DR, Yeager AS. Neuropathological and computerized tomographic findings in experimental brain abscess. J Neurosurg. 1981;55: 590–603.

64. Britt RH, Enzmann DR. Clinical stages of human brain abscesses on serial CT scans after contrast infusion. Computerized tomographic, neuropathological, and clinical correlations. J Neurosurg. 1983;59:972–89.

65. Kurzydlowski H, Wollenschlager C, Venezie FR, et al. Reevaluation of an experimental streptococcal canine brain abscess model. J Neurosurg. 1987; 67:717–20.

66. Flaris NA, Hickey WF. Development and characterization of an experimental model of brain abscess in the rat. Am J Pathol. 1992;141:1299–307.

67. Obana WG, Britt RH, Placone RC, et al. Experimental brain abscess development in the chronically immunosuppressed host. Computerized tomographic and neuropathological correlations. J Neurosurg. 1986;65:382–91.

68. Wood JH, Doppman JL, Lightfoote WE. Role of vascular proliferation on angiographic appearance and encapsulation of experimental traumatic and metastatic brain abscesses. J Neurosurg. 1978;48:264–73.

69. Prockop DJ, Kivirikko KI, Tuderman L, et al. The biosynthesis of collagen and its disorders. Part I. N Engl J Med. 1979;301:13–23.

70. Britt RH, Enzmann DH, Placone RC, et al. Experimental anaerobic brain abscess. J Neurosurg. 1984;60:1148–59.

71. Enzmann DR, Britt RH, Obana WG, et al. Experimental *Staphylococcus aureus* brain abscess. AJNR. 1986;7:395–402.

72. Heinnemann HS, Braude AI. Anaerobic infection of the brain. Observations on eighteen consecutive cases of brain abscess. Am J Med. 1963;35:682–97.

73. Ingham HR, Selkon JB, Roxby CM. Bacteriological study of otogenic cerebral abscesses: Chemotherapeutic role of metronidazole. Br Med J. 1977;2: 991–3.

74. Arseni C, Ciurea AV. Cerebellar abscesses. A report on 119 cases. Zentralbl Neurochir. 1982;43:359–70.

75. Arseni C, Ciurea AV. Etiological data on cerebral abscesses. Zentralbl Neurochir. 1982;43:1.

76. Arseni C, Ciurea AV. Rhinogenic cerebral abscesses. Zentralbl Neurochir. 1982;43:12.

77. de Louvois J. Antimicrobial chemotherapy in the treatment of brain abscess. J Antimicrob Chemother. 1983;11:205–7.

78. Shaw MDM, Russell JA. Cerebellar abscess—A review of 47 cases. J Neurol Neurosurg Psychiatry. 1975;38:429–35.

79. Murray HW, Gross KC, Masur H, et al. Serious infections caused by *Streptococcus milleri*. Am J Med. 1978;64:759–64.

80. Shlaes DM, Lerner PM, Wolinsky E, et al. Infections due to Lancefield group F and related streptococci (*S. milleri, S. anginosus*). Medicine (Baltimore). 1981;60:197–207.

81. Parker MT, Ball LC. Streptococci and aerococci associated with systemic infection in man. J Med Microbiol. 1976;9:275–302.

82. de Louvois J. Bacteriological examinations of pus from abscesses of the central nervous system. J Clin Pathol. 1980;33:66–71.

83. Brook I. Bacteriology of intracranial abscess in children. J Neurosurg. 1981; 54:484–8.

84. Carey ME, Chou SN, French LA. Experience with brain abscesses. J Neurosurg. 1972;36:1–9.

85. Lechtenberg R, Sierra MF, Pringle GF, et al. *Listeria monocytogenes:* Brain abscess or meningoencephalitis. Neurology. 1979;29:86–90.

86. Nieman RE, Lorber B. Listeriosis in adults: A changing pattern. Report of eight cases and review of the literature. Rev Infect Dis. 1980;2:207–27.

87. Norden CW, Ruben FL, Selker R. Nonsurgical treatment of cerebral nocardiosis. Arch Neurol. 1983;40:594–5.

88. Levy RL, Saunders RL. *Citrobacter* meningitis and cerebral abscess in early infancy: Cure by moxalactam. Neurology. 1981;31:1575–7.

89. Curless RG. Neonatal intracranial abscess: Two cases caused by *Citrobacter* and a literature review. Ann Neurol. 1980;8:269–72.

90. Rodriquez RE, Valero V, Watanakunakorn C. *Salmonella* focal intracranial infections: Review of the world literature (1884–1984) and report of an unusual case. Rev Infect Dis. 1986;8:31–41.

91. Dijkmans BAC, Thomeer RTWM, Vielvoye GJ, et al. Brain abscess due to *Streptobacillus moniliformis* and *Actinobacterium meyerii*. Infection. 1984; 12:262–4.

92. Guvene H, Korabay K, Okten A, Bektas S. Brucellosis in a child complicated with multiple brain abscesses. Scand J Infect Dis. 1989;21:333–6.

93. Berenson CS, Bia FJ. *Propionibacterium acnes* causes postoperative brain abscesses unassociated with foreign bodies: Case reports. Neurosurgery. 1989;25:130–4.

94. Jensen HB, Levy SR, Duncan C, McIntosh S. Treatment of multiple brain abscesses caused by *Bacillus cereus*. Pediatr Infect Dis J. 1989;8:795–8.

95. Sheller JR, Des Prez RM. CNS tuberculosis. Neurol Clin. 1986;4:143–57.

96. Bell WE. Treatment of fungal infections of the central nervous system. Ann Neurol. 1981;9:417.

97. Chernik NL, Armstrong D, Posner JB. Central nervous system infections in patients with cancer. Medicine (Baltimore). 1973;52:563–81.

98. Beal MF, O'Carroll CP, Kleinman GM, et al. Aspergillosis of the nervous system. Neurology. 1982;32:473.

99. Parker JC Jr, McCloskey JJ, Lee RS. The emergence of candidosis. The dominant postmortem cerebral mycosis. Am J Clin Pathol. 1978;70:31.

100. Heney C, Song E, Kellen A, et al. Cerebral phaeohyphomycoses caused by *Xylohypha bantiana*. Eur J Clin Microbiol Infect Dis. 1989;8:984–8.

101. Sandhyamani S, Bhalia R, Mohapatra LN, et al. Cerebral cladosporiosis. Surg Neurol. 1981;15:431.

102. Kenney RT, Kwan-Chung KJ, Waytes AJ, et al. Successful treatment of systemic *Exophiala dermatitidis* infection in a patient with chronic granulomatous disease. Clin Infect Dis. 1992;14:235–42.

103. Rahman N, Mahgoub E, Chagla AH. Fatal brain abscesses by *Ramichloridium obovoideum:* Report of three cases. Acta Neurochir. 1988;93:92–5.

104. Sides EH, Bensen JD, Paybye AA. Phaeohyphomycotic brain abscess due to *Ochroenis gallopavum* in a patient with malignant lymphoma of a large cell type. J Med Vet Mycol. 1991;29:317–22.

105. Masdeu JC, Tantulavanich S, Gorelick PP, et al. Brain abscess caused by *Strongyloides stercoralis*. Arch Neurol. 1982;39:62–3.

106. Becker GL Jr, Knep S, Lance KP, et al. Amebic abscess of the brain. Neurosurgery. 1980;6:192.

107. Schmutzhard E, Mayr U, Rumpl E, et al. Secondary cerebral amebiasis due to infection with *Entamoeba histolytica*. Eur Neurol. 1986;25:161.

108. Gordon SM, Steinberg JP, et al. Culture isolation of *Acanthamoeba* species and leptomyxid amebas from patients with amebic meningoencephalitis, including two patients with AIDS. Clin Infect Dis. 1992;15:1019–30.

109. Bia FJ, Barry M. Parasitic infections of the central nervous system. Neurol Clin. 1986;4:171–206.

110. Mitchell A, Scheithauer BW, Kelly PJ, et al. Cerebral sparganosis. J Neurosurg. 1990;73:147–50.

111. Armstrong D. Central nervous system infections in the immunocompromised host. Infection. 1984;12(Suppl 1):58–64.

112. Hooper DC, Pruitt AA, Rubin RH. Central nervous system infection in the chronically immunosuppressed. Medicine (Baltimore). 1982;61:166–88.

113. Horowitz SL, Bentson JR, Benson F, et al. CNS toxoplasmosis in acquired immunodeficiency syndrome. Arch Neurol. 1983;40:649–52.

114. Stamm SM, Dismukes WE, Simmons BP, et al. Listeriosis in renal transplant recipients: Report of an outbreak and review of 102 cases. Rev Infect Dis. 1982;4:589–619.

115. McArthur JC. Neurologic manifestations of AIDS. Medicine (Baltimore). 1987;66:407.

116. Levy RM, Bredesen DE, Rosenblum ML. Neurological manifestations of the acquired immunodeficiency syndrome (AIDS): Experience at UCSF and review of the literature. J Neurosurg. 1985;62:475.

117. Bishburg E, Sunderan EG, Reichman LB, et al. Central nervous system tuberculosis with the acquired immunodeficiency syndrome and its related complex. Ann Intern Med. 1986;105:210.

118. Helweg-Larsen S, Jakobsen J, Boesen F, et al. Neurological complications and concomitants of AIDS. Acta Neurol Scand. 1986;74:467.

119. Obana WG, Scanell KA, Jacobs R, Greco G, Rosenblum ML. A case of *Rhodococcus equi* brain abscess. Surg Neurol. 1991;35:321–4.

120. Barradas MC, Musher DM, Hamill RJ, et al. Unusual manifestations of pneumococcal infection in human immunodeficiency virus-infected individuals: The past revisited. Clin Infect Dis. 1992;14:192–9.

121. Saez-Llorens XJ, Umann MA, Odio CM, et al. Brain abscess in infants and children. Pediatr Infect Dis J. 1989;8:449–58.

122. Adams RD, Victor M. Nonviral infections of the nervous system. In: Adams RD, Victor M, eds. Principles of Neurology. New York: McGraw-Hill; 1985: 552–6.

123. Domingue JN, Wilson CB: Pituitary abscesses. Report of seven cases and review of the literature. J Neurosurg. 1977;46:601–8.

124. Giang DW, Poduri KR, Eskin TA, et al. Multiple sclerosis masquerading as a mass lesion. Neuroradiology 1992;34:150–4.

125. Hirschberg H, Bosnes V. C-reactive protein levels in the differential diagnosis of brain abscesses. J Neurosurg. 1987;67:358–60.

126. Grimstad IA, Hirschberg H, Rootwelt K. ^{99}Tc Hexamethylpropyleneamine oxime leukocyte scintigraphy and C-reactive protein levels in the differential diagnosis of brain abscesses. J Neurosurg. 1992;77:732–6.

127. Yoshikawa TT, Goodman SJ. Brain abscess. West J Med. 1974;121:207.

128. Nielsen H, Halaburt H. Cerebral abscess with special reference to the angiographic changes. Neuroradiology. 1976;12:73.

129. Crocker EF, McLaughlin AF, Morris JG, et al. Technetium brain scanning in the diagnosis and management of cerebral abscess. Am J Med. 1974;56: 192.

130. Mascucci EF, Sauerbrunn BJL. The evolution of a brain abscess. The complementary roles of radionuclide and computed tomography scans. Clin Nucl Med. 1982;7:166.

131. Rosenblum ML, Hoff JT, Norman D, et al. Decreased mortality from brain abscesses since advent of computerized tomography. J Neurosurg. 1978;49: 658.

132. Potter GD, ed. CT of the ear, nose and throat. Radiol Clin North Am. 1984; 22:1.

133. New PFJ, Davis KR, Ballantine HT Jr. Computed tomography in cerebral abscess. Radiology. 1976;121:641–6.

134. Whelan MA, Hilal SK. Computed tomography as a guide in the diagnosis and follow-up of brain abscesses. Radiology. 1980;135:663–71.

135. Weisberg L. Clinical-CT correlations in intracranial suppurative (bacterial) disease. Neurology. 1984;34:509–10.

136. Dobkin JF, Healton EB, Dickinson T, et al. Nonspecificity of ring enhancement in medically cured brain abscess. Neurology. 1984;34:139–44.

137. Chapman ME, Sellar RJ, Whittle IR. Pyocephalus: A valuable CT finding in cerebral abscess. Clin Radiol. 1992;45:195–7.

138. Holtas S, Tornquist C, Cronqvist S. Diagnostic difficulties in computed tomography of brain abscesses. J Comput Assist Tomogr. 1982;6:683–8.

139. Coulam CM, Seshul M, Donaldson J. Intracranial ring lesions: Can we differentiate by computed tomography? Invest Radiol. 1980;15:103–12.

140. Rehncrona S, Brismar J, Holtas S. Diagnosis of brain abscesses with indium-111 labeled leukocytes. Neurosurgery. 1985;16:23–36.

141. Bellotti C, Aragno MG, Medina M, et al. Differential diagnosis of CT-hypodense cranial lesions with indium-111-oxine–labeled leukocytes. J Neurosurg. 1986;64:750–3.

142. Kock-Jensen C, Anderson B, Sogaard I. Leukocyte scanning: A valuable tool in diagnosing cerebral abscess-a survey. Acta Neurochir. 1986;83:121–4.

143. Brant-Zawadzki M, Enzmann DR, Placone RC, et al. NMR imaging of experimental brain abscess: Comparison with CT. AJNR. 1983;4:250–3.

144. Runge VM, Clanton JA, Price AC, et al. Evaluation of contrast-enhanced MR imaging in a brain-abscess model. AJNR. 1985;6:139–47.

145. Grossman RI, Joseph PM, Wolf G, et al. Experimental intracranial septic infarction: Magnetic resonance enhancement. Radiology. 1985;155:649–53.

146. Zimmerman RD, Haimes AB. The role of MR imaging in the diagnosis of infections of the central nervous system. In: Remington JS, Swartz MN, eds. Current Clinical Topics in Infectious Diseases. Boston: Blackwell; 1989: 82–108.

147. Davidson MD, Steiner RE. Magnetic resonance imaging in infections of the central nervous system. AJNR. 1985;6:499–504.

148. Wispelwey B, Scheld WM. Brain abscess. Semin Neurol. 1992;12:273–8.

149. Latchaw RE, Hirsch WL, Yock DH. Imaging of intracranial infection. Neurosurg Clin North Am. 1992;3:303–22.

150. Scheld WM. Experimental animal models of bacterial meningitis. In: Zak O,

151. Oftedahl PR, Winn G, Rodeheaver G, et al. Changes in regional cerebral blood flow and blood brain barrier permeability in experimental brain abscess. J Cereb Blood Flow Metab. 1981;1(Suppl):38.

152. Wellman WE, Dodge HW, Heilmann FR, et al. Concentration of antibiotics in the brain. J Lab Clin Med. 1954;43:275–9.

153. Kramer PW, Griffith RS, Campbell RL. Antibiotic penetration of the brain. A comparative study. J Neurosurg. 1969;31:295–302.

154. Black P, Graybill JR, Charache P. Penetration of brain abscess by systemically administered antibiotics. J Neurosurg. 1973;38:705–9.

155. de Louvois J, Gortvai P, Hurley R. Antibiotic treatment of abscesses of the central nervous system. Br Med J. 1977;2:985–7.

156. Picardi JL, Lewis HP, Tan JS, et al. Clindamycin concentrations in the central nervous system of primates before and after head trauma. J Neurosurg. 1975;43:717.

157. de Louvois J, Hurley R. Inactivation of penicillin by purulent exudates. Br Med J. 1977;1:998–1000.

158. Alderson D, Strong AJ, Ingham HR, et al. Fifteen year review of the mortality of brain abscess. Neurosurgery. 1981;8:1–6.

159. Smego R, Moeller MS, Gallis HA. Trimethoprim-sulfamethoxazole therapy for *Nocardia* infections. Arch Intern Med. 1983;143:711–8.

160. Maderazo EG, Quintiliani R. Treatment of nocardial infection with trimethoprim and sulfamethoxazole. Am J Med. 1974;57:671–5.

161. Levitz R, Quintiliani R. Trimethoprim-sulfamethoxazole for bacterial meningitis. Ann Intern Med. 1984;100:881–90.

162. Greene BM, Thomas FE Jr, Alford RH. Trimethoprim-sulfamethoxazole and brain abscess. Ann Intern Med. 1975;82:812–3.

163. Levy RM, Gutin PH, Baskin DS, et al. Vancomycin penetration of a brain abscess: Case report and review of the literature. Neurosurgery. 1986;18: 633–6.

164. Preheim LC, McCracken GH, Jubeliver DP. Moxalactam penetration into brain abscess (Abstract 738). In: Proceedings of the 21st Interscience Conference on Antimicrobial Agents and Chemotherapy. Chicago: American Society for Microbiology (ASM); 1981.

165. Marcus MG, Atluru VL, Epstein N, et al. Conservative management of *Citrobacter diversus* meningitis with brain abscess. NY State J Med. 1984;84: 252–4.

166. Sjolin J, Eriksson N, Arneborn P, et al. Penetration of cefotaxime and desacetylcefotaxime into brain abscesses in humans. Antimicrob Agents Chemother. 1991;35:2606–10.

167. Scheld WM, Brodeur JP, Foresman PA, et al. Comparative evaluation of aztreonam in therapy for experimental bacterial meningitis and cerebritis. Rev Infect Dis. 1985;7(Suppl 4):635–47.

168. Carton JA, Perry F, Maradona JA, et al. Successful treatment of recurrent cerebral empyema and brain abscesses with imipenem. Eur J Clin Microbiol. 1989;6:578–80.

169. Rice LB, Eliopoulos GM. Imipenem and aztreonam: Current role in antimicrobial therapy. In: Remington JS, Swartz MN, eds. Current Clinical Topics in Infectious Diseases Boston: Blackwell; 1989:109–39.

170. Akova M, Akal'in HE, Korten V, et al. Treatment of intracranial abscesses: Experience with sulbactam/ampicillin. J Chemother. 1993;5:181–5.

171. Neu HC. Uses of antimicrobial agents in brain abscesses. In: Nelson JD, Grassi C, eds. Current Chemotherapy and Infectious Disease, v. 1. Washington, DC: American Society for Microbiology; 1980:41–2.

172. Norrby R. A review of the penetration of antibiotics into CSF and its clinical significance. Scand J Infect Dis. 1978;14(Suppl):296–309.

173. Neuwelt EA, Enzmann DR, Pagel MA, et al. Bacterial and fungal brain abscess and the blood-brain barrier. In: Neuwelt EA, ed. Implications of the Blood-Brain Barrier and Its Manipulation New York: Plenum Press; 1989: 263–305.

174. Haley EC Jr, Costello GT, Rodeheaver GT, et al. Treatment of experimental brain abscess with penicillin and chloramphenicol. J Infect Dis. 1983;148: 737–44.

175. Ballantine HJ, White JC. Brain abscess. Influence of the antibiotic on therapy and morbidity. N Engl J Med. 1953;248:14–9.

176. Jooma OV, Pennybacker JB, Tutton GT. Brain abscess: Aspiration, drainage or excision? J Neurol Neurosurg Psychiatry. 1951;14:308–13.

177. Tutton GK. Cerebral abscess. The present position. Ann R Coll Surg Engl. 1953;13:281–311.

178. Holm S, Kourtopoulos H. Penetration of antibiotics into brain tissue and brain abscesses. An experimental study in steroid treated rats. Scand J Infect Dis. 1985;44(Suppl):68–70.

179. Sjoln J, Lilja A, Eriksson N, et al. Treatment of brain abscess with cefotaxime and metronidazole: prospective study on 15 consecutive patients. Clin Infect Dis. 1993;17:857–63.

180. Warner J, Perkins RL, Cordero L. Metronidazole therapy of anaerobic bacteremia, meningitis, and brain abscess. Arch Intern Med. 1979;139:167–9.

181. Frame PT, Watanakunakorn C, McLaurin RL, et al. Penetration of nafcillin, methicillin, and cefazolin into human brain tissue. Neurosurgery. 1983;12: 14.

182. Stepanov S. Surgical treatment of brain abscess. Neurosurgery. 1988;22: 724–30.

183. Westcombe DS, Dorsch NWC, Teo C. Management of cerebral abscess in adolescents and adults. Acta Neurochir. 1988;95:85–9.

184. Taylor JC. The case for excision in the treatment of brain abscess. Br J Neurosurg. 1987;1:173–8.

Sande MA, eds. Experimental Models in Antimicrobial Chemotherapy. v. 1. Orlando, FL: Academic Press; 1986:139.

185. Rousseaux M, Lesoin F, Destee A, et al. Long term sequelae of hemispheric abscesses as a function of treatment. Acta Neurochir. 1985;74:61–7.
186. Stroobandt G, Zech F, Thauvoy C, et al. Treatment by aspiration of brain abscesses. Acta Neurochir. 1987;85:138–47.
187. Young RF, Frazee J. Gas within intracranial abscess cavities: An indication for surgical excision. Ann Neuro. 1984;16:35–9.
188. Karandanis D, Shulman JA. Factors associated with mortality in brain abscess. Arch Intern Med. 1975;135:1145–50.
189. Goodman ML, Coffey RJ. Stereotactic drainage of *Aspergillus* brain abscess with long term survival: Case report and review. Neurosurgery. 1989;24:96–9.
190. Ohaegbulam SC, Saddeqi NU. Experience with brain abscesses treated by simple aspiration. Surg Neurol. 1980;13:289–91.
191. LeBeau J, Creissard P, Harispe L, et al. Surgical treatment of brain abscess and subdural empyema. J Neurosurg. 1973;38:198–203.
192. Camarata PJ, Dunn DL, Farney AC, et al. Continued intracavitary administration of amphotericin B as an adjunct in the treatment of *Aspergillus* brain abscess: Case report and review of the literature. Neurosurgery. 1992;31:575–9.
193. Lunsford LD, Nelson PB. Stereotactic aspiration of a brain abscess using the therapeutic CT scanner. Acta Neurochir. 1982;62:25–9.
194. Apuzzo MLJ, Sabshin JK. Computed tomographic guidance stereotaxis in the management of intracranial mass lesions. Neurosurgery. 1983;12:277–85.
195. Lunsford D, Martinez AJ. Stereotactic exploration of the brain in the era of computed tomography. Surg Neurol. 1984;22:222–30.
196. Nauta HJW, Conteras FL, Weiner RL, et al. Brain stem abscess managed with computed tomography—guided stereotactic aspiration. Neurosurgery. 1987;20:476.
197. Itakura T, Yokote H, Ozaki F, et al. Stereotactic operation for brain abscess. Surg Neurol. 1987;28:196.
198. Hall WA, Martinez AJ, Dummer JS, et al. Nocardial brain abscess: Diagnostic and therapeutic use of stereotactic aspiration. Surg Neurol. 1987;28:114.
199. Dyste GN, Hitchon PW, Menezes AH, et al. Stereotaxic surgery in the treatment of multiple brain abscesses. J Neurosurg. 1988;69:188–94.
200. Nauta HJW, Conteras FI, Weiner RI, et al. Brain stem abscess managed with computed tomography-guided stereotactic aspiration. Neurosurgery. 1987;20:476.
201. Rossitch E, Alexander E, Schiff SJ, et al. The use of computed tomography-guided stereotactic techniques in the treatment of brain stem abscesses. Clin Neurol Neurosurg. 1988;90:365–8.
202. Enzmann DR, Britt RH, Placone R. Staging of human brain abscess by computed tomography. Radiology. 1983;146:703–8.
203. Heinnemann HS, Braude AI, Osterholm JL. Intracranial suppurative disease. Early presumptive diagnosis and successful treatment without surgery. JAMA 1971;218:1542–7.
204. Rosenblum ML, Mampalam TJ, Pons VG. Controversies in the management of brain abscesses. Clin Neurosurg. 1986;33:603.
205. Berg B, Franklin G, Cuneo R, et al. Nonsurgical cure of brain abscess: Early diagnosis and follow-up with computerized tomography. Ann Neurol. 1978;3:474–8.
206. Rotheram EB Jr, Kessler LA. Use of computerized tomography in nonsurgical management of brain abscess. Arch Neurol. 1979;36:25–6.
207. Rosenblum ML, Hoff JT, Norman D, et al. Nonoperative treatment of brain abscesses in selected high-risk patients. J Neurosurg. 1980;52:217–25.
208. Boom WH, Tuazon CU. Successful treatment of multiple brain abscesses with antibiotics alone. Rev Infect Dis. 1985;7:189–99.
209. Daniels SR, Price JK, Towbin RB, et al. Nonsurgical cure of brain abscess in a neonate. Child Nerv Syst. 1985;1:346–8.
210. Keren G, Tyrrell DLJ. Nonsurgical treatment of brain abscesses: Report of two cases. Pediatr Infect Dis. 1984;3:331–4.
211. Enzmann DR, Britt RH, Yeager AS. Experimental brain abscess evolution: Computed tomographic and neuropathologic correlation. Radiology. 1979;133:113–22.
212. Epstein F, Whelan M. Cerebritis masquerading as brain abscess: Case report. Neurosurgery. 1982;10:757–9.
213. Sjölin J, Lilja A, Eriksson N, et al. Treatment of brain abscess with cefotaxime and metronidazole: Prospective study of 15 consecutive cases. Clin Infect Dis. 1993;17:857–63.
214. Luft BJ, Remington JS. Toxoplasmic encephalitis. J Infect Dis. 1988;157:106.
215. Scheld WM, Brodeur JP. Effect of methylprednisolone on entry of ampicillin and gentamicin into the cerebrospinal fluid in experimental pneumococcal and *E. coli* meningitis. Antimicrob Agents Chemother. 1983;23:108–12.
216. Kourtopoulos H, Holm SE, Norrby SR. The influence of steroids on the penetration of antibiotics into brain tissue and brain abscesses. An experimental study in rats. J Antimicrob Chemother. 1983;11:245–9.
217. Neuwelt EA, Lawrence MS, Blank NK. Effect of gentamicin and dexamethasone on the natural history of the rat *Escherichia coli* brain abscess model with histopathologic correlation. Neurosurgery. 1984;15:475.
218. Enzmann DR, Britt RH, Placone RC Jr, et al. The effect of short-term corticosteroid treatment on the CT appearance of experimental brain abscesses. Radiology. 1982;145:79.
219. Black KL, Farhat SM. Cerebral abscess: Loss of computed tomographic enhancement with steroids. Neurosurgery. 1984;14:215–7.
220. Schroeder KA, McKeever PE, Schaberg DR, et al. Effect of dexamethasone on experimental brain abscess. J Neurosurg. 1987;66:264–9.
220. Yildizhan A, Pasoglu A, Kandemir B. Effect of dexamethasone on various stages of experimental brain abscess. Acta Neurochir. 1989;96:141–8.
221. Gruszkiewicz J, Doron Y, Peyser E, et al. Brain abscess and its surgical management. Surg Neurol. 1982;18:7–17.
222. Calliauw WL, dePraetere P, Verbeke L. Postoperative epilepsy in subdural suppurations. Acta Neurochir. 1984;71:217–23.
223. Koszewski W. Epilepsy following brain abscess. The evaluation of possible risk factors with emphasis on a new concept of epileptic focus formation. Acta Neurochir. 1991;113:110–17.

69. SUBDURAL EMPYEMA

JOHN E. GREENLEE

The outer two layers of meninges, the dura and arachnoid, enclose a potential subdural space crossed by numerous small veins. Anatomic barriers to extension of infection within this space exist only at the falx cerebri, the tentorium cerebelli, the base of the brain, the foramen magnum, and the anterior spinal canal where arachnoid and dura are joined by penetrating nerves and vessels.[1] These structures divide the subdural space into several large compartments, within each of which subdural infection can spread but in which the infection will be confined to behave as a rapidly expanding mass lesion. Infection of the spinal subdural space is rare, but subdural empyema constitutes 13–23 percent of localized intracranial bacterial infections.[2,3] LeBeau et al.[4] have described subdural empyema as "the most imperative of all neurosurgical emergencies."

ETIOLOGY AND PATHOGENESIS

In most cases, infection reaches the subdural space through emissary veins or by extension of an osteomyelitis of the skull, with accompanying epidural abscess.[2,3,5–8] In over half the cases, the source of infection is the paranasal sinuses, with the frontal and ethmoidal sinuses involved in 50–80 percent of the cases.[5,8–11] The middle ear and mastoid are the source in 10–20 percent. In 5 percent of the cases, the infection is metastatic, principally from the lung.[3] Subdural empyema may also follow skull trauma, surgical procedures, or infection of a preexisting subdural hematoma.[2,12,13]

BACTERIOLOGIC CHARACTERISTICS

Aerobic streptococci have been isolated in 35 percent of reported cases and staphylococci in 17 percent. A variety of other organisms including *Streptococcus pneumoniae, Haemophilus influenzae,* and gram-negative organisms have been recovered in 14 percent of cases.[2,6,15] Anaerobic organisms, including anaerobic and microaerophilic streptococci (in particular the *Streptococcus anginosus–Streptococcus milleri* group), and *Bacteroides fragilis* are recovered in up to 100 percent of cases.[2,3,5,14–17] Polymicrobial infections are common.

PATHOLOGIC CHARACTERISTICS

The infection may involve one or both hemispheres and may occur at the base of the brain, over the convexity, or along the falx cerebri.[1,5–7,18,19] The posterior fossa is rarely involved. The subdural space contains an inflammatory exudate that is largest over the frontal lobes if the empyema follows sinusitis or over the temporal and occipital lobes if it follows otitis.[8,20,21] The empyema may be multiloculated and may be contralateral to the associated sinusitis. A focal, inflammatory reaction is frequently present within the subarachnoid space, but purulent meningitis occurs in only 14 percent of the cases. Focal osteomyelitis and/or epidural abscess is present in as many as 50 percent of the cases.[1,5,7,18,19] Septic thrombosis of veins within the empyema may extend into venous sinuses or cortical veins, causing hemorrhagic infarction and superficial abscess formation. Cerebral edema rapidly develops and may contribute greatly to mass effect early in the course of infection. Transtentorial herniation occurs unless there is prompt surgical intervention and may be precipitated by lumbar puncture.[3,22]

CLINICAL FEATURES

Subdural empyema may develop at any age but is most common in the second and third decades. Males are affected four times more frequently than are females.[2,3,5,23] In 60–90 percent of the cases there is an accompanying, frequently asymptomatic sinusitis or otitis. Extension of infection into the subdural space produces fever, focal headaches that later become generalized, vomiting, and signs of meningeal irritation.[2,3,17,24] Alteration in mental status may be insidious in onset and is present in 50 percent of the patients early in the infection.[2,24] Within 24–48 hours focal neurologic signs appear and progress rapidly to those of dysfunction of an entire cerebral hemisphere,[2,24] with hemiparesis, hemisensory deficit, and hemianopsia. Seizures, usually focal,[2,3,23] occur in 50 percent of the cases, and aphasia is common when the dominant hemisphere is involved.[3] Unless treatment is instituted, neurologic signs worsen, and signs of increased intracranial pressure appear, with transtentorial and tonsillar herniation. The course of the illness is sufficiently rapid that papilledema develops in less than 50 percent of the patients.[2,3]

Several exceptions exist to this clinical picture. Symptoms may be fulminant in onset or may develop over a period of several weeks. Development of symptoms in cases arising after craniotomy may be extremely insidious.[25] Prior antibiotic therapy may minimize systemic symptoms and may mask sinusitis

or otitis, to make the clinical presentation that of brain abscess.[13,22] Infections metastatic to the subdural space or to a preexisting subdural hematoma may fail to produce sinus tenderness or systemic symptoms.[22,26] In such cases, particularly in the alcoholic with an infected subdural hematoma, the patient often is seen late in the illness, and mortality is higher.

DIAGNOSIS

Subdural empyema should be suspected in any patient with meningeal signs and a focal neurologic deficit, particularly where the deficit indicates extensive dysfunction of one cerebral hemisphere. Sinusitis followed by meningeal signs should also suggest the diagnosis, for bacterial meningitis per se is rarely due to sinusitis.[27]

Magnetic resonance imaging (MRI) with gadolinium enhancement is the diagnostic procedure of choice and may detect empyemas not seen on contrast-enhanced computed tomography (CT)[28–34] (Fig. 1). Sinusitis or otitis is present on skull x-rays or CT in over two-thirds of patients.[2,8,28] Spinal fluid changes are nonspecific, and the danger of transtentorial herniation represents an absolute contraindication to lumbar puncture.[3,23]

THERAPY

Aerobic and anaerobic cultures of blood and other material should be obtained, and antibiotics should be begun as described in Table 1. Increased intracranial pressure may necessitate the preoperative use of mannitol, 0.5–1.0 g/kg infused over 10–15 minutes; hyperventilation to a PCO_2 of 30 mmHg; or dexamethasone, 10 mg IV, to be followed postoperatively by 4 mg every 6 hours (see Ch. 63). MRI may detect subdural empyemas too small to be surgically drained, and early subdural empyemas may sometimes be treated with antibiotics alone.[35–37] In most instances, however, the rapidly progressive nature of the infec-

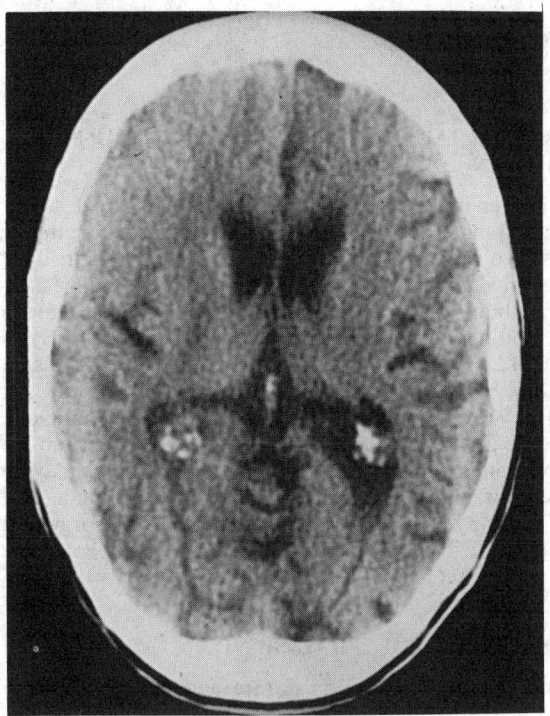
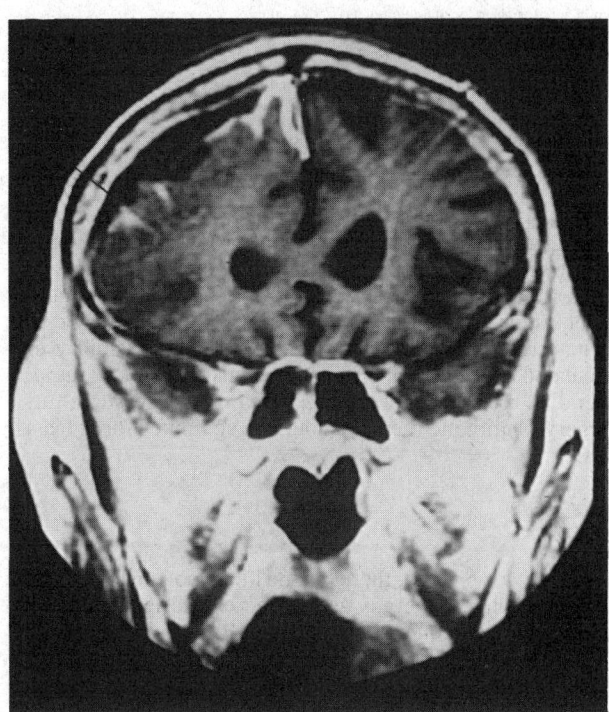

FIG. 1. Computed tomography scan and gadolinium-enhanced MRI of patient with subdural empyema. **(A)** CT scan. There is effacement of sulci over the right hemisphere, without obvious fluid collection or evidence of empyema. **(B)** Gadolinium-enhanced coronal MRI obtained shortly after CT, showing a large subdural empyema. (Courtesy of Dr. Rick Harnsberger, University of Utah.)

TABLE 1. Bacterial Etiology and Initial Antibiotic Therapy of Subdural Empyema, Epidural Abscess, and Septic Intracranial Thrombophlebitis

Condition	Site of Primary Infection	Probable Organisms	Initial Therapy for Patients with Normal Renal Function	
			Suggested Initial Therapy	Suggested Initial Therapy if Immediate Type Penicillin Allergy Present
Subdural empyema, epidural absecess, or septic intracranial thrombophlebitis: older children or adults	Paranasal sinuses (especially frontal, ethmoidal, or sphenoidal sinuses)	Aerobic, microaerophilic and anaerobic streptococci (especially *S. milleri*, i.e., *S. intermedius*) *Bacteroides fragilis* and other anaerobes *Staphylococcus aureus* Enterobacteriaceae *Haemophilus* spp.	Metronidazole[b] *plus* ceftriaxone or cefotaxime *plus* nafcillin or oxacillin	Vancomycin[a] *plus* metronidazole *plus* aztreonam or gentamicin[c]
	Otitis media or mastoiditis	Aerobic, microaerophilic, and anaerobic streptococci *Bacteroides fragilis* and other anaerobes *Staphylococcus aureus* Enterobacteriaceae	Metronidazole *plus* ceftriaxone or cefotaxime *plus* nafcillin or oxacillin	Vancomycin *plus* metronidazole *plus* aztreonam or gentamicin
	Following cranial surgery or trauma	*Staphylococcus aureus* *Staphylococcus epidermidis* *Clostridium* spp. Enterobacteriaceae	Vancomycin *plus* ceftazidime	Vancomycin *plus* aztreonam or gentamicin
	Following dental sepsis	Mixed *Fusobacterium*, *Bacteroides*, and aerobic and anaerobic streptococci	Penicillin,[d] ceftriaxone, or cefotaxime *plus* metronidazole	Vancomycin *plus* metronidazole
Subdural empyema in neonates	Associated with meningitis	Enterobacteriaceae Group B streptococci	Ceftriaxone or cefotaxime[e]	
Subdural empyema in older infants and small children	Associated with meningitis	*Haemophilus influenzae*, *Streptococcus pneumoniae*, *Neisseria meningitidis*	Ceftriaxone or cefotaxime[e]	
Spinal epidural abscess or subdural empyema	Hematogenous spread; extension from osteomyelitis or paravertebral infection	*Staphylococcus aureus*, *Streptococcus* spp. (Enterobacteriaceae)	Oxacillin or nafcillin[c] (add ceftriaxone or cefotaxime *plus* gentamicin if gram-negative infection suspected)	Vancomycin (add ceftriaxone or cefotaxime *plus* gentamicin if gram-negative infection suspected)

[a] Vancomycin in adults is given 1.0–1.25 g q12h.
[b] Metronidazole therapy in adults is initiated with a loading dose of 15 mg/kg over 1 hour followed by 7.5 mg/kg q6h (30 mg/kg/24 h). The drug must be diluted and neutralized before intravenous use and is administered by slow intravenous infusion.
[c] Aztreonam is given as 2 g IV q8h; gentamicin is given as 1.5 mg/kg IV q8h.
[d] Penicillin in adults is given as 20 million units over 24 hours.
[e] Subdural empyema in neonates and infants is most frequently associated with meningitis. See Chapter 64 for discussion of therapy.
[f] Nafcillin or oxacillin in adults is given as 1.5 g IV q4h. Oxacillin is somewhat less likely to cause thrombophlebitis.

tion and the fact that neuroradiologic studies may understate the actual size of the empyema necessitate emergency surgical as well as medical intervention. Craniotomy is believed by many workers to have a lower rate of complications than use of burr holes and may be essential in posterior fossa subdural empyema.[38–40] Use of burr holes and irrigation of the subdural space may be possible in early cases.[41] Empyema fluid should be submitted for culture, including culture for anaerobes. Otitis or sinusitis may require simultaneous surgery. The possibility of multiloculated or parafalcine infection must be kept in mind. Postoperative recurrence of the empyema may necessitate further surgery. Antibiotic therapy should be continued for at least 3 weeks.

PROGNOSIS

When treatment is prompt, there is good likelihood of neurologic recovery, but delay in therapy greatly increases the risk of permanent neurologic sequelae.[24,38,41] Overall mortality is 14–18 percent. If the patient is alert, mortality is 4–8 percent but if comatose, 75 percent. Prognosis is poor in the aged or when the infection is precipitous in onset. Late focal or generalized seizures develop in 42 percent of patients surviving subdural empyema and usually appear within 16 months. The likelihood of developing late seizures is not influenced by the presence or absence of seizures during the acute illness.[42]

SUBDURAL EMPYEMA IN INFANTS AND YOUNG CHILDREN

In children under 5 years of age,[38,43,44] intracranial subdural empyema almost invariably follows bacterial meningitis, and the causative organism is that of the meningitis itself, most often *H. influenzae*, or, in neonates, gram-negative bacilli. Early signs of irritability, poor feeding, or increase in head size are nonspecific and may cause delay in seeking medical help. By the time the child is seen by a physician, hemiparesis, convulsions, stupor, and coma are common, but fever may be absent. Examination may reveal increased head size and bulging fontanelle. Papilledema is unusual. The empyema fluid is often too turbid to allow transillumination. In infants, the diagnosis may be made by subdural taps, although this procedure will not detect a parafalcine empyema. Radiographic diagnosis and surgical therapy are as described for adults. Initial antibiotic therapy is that of the meningitis itself (see Ch. 64).

SPINAL SUBDURAL EMPYEMA

Spinal subdural empyema is rare and virtually always metastatic.[24,45] Etiologic organisms are usually *Staphylococcus aureus* and, less often, streptococci, gram-negative organisms, or *Staphylococcus epidermidis*.[24,45] The empyema is usually posterior to the cord and involves the thoracic and lumbar cord more often than the cervical. Radicular pain and symptoms of cord compression may occur at multiple levels. Spinous process tenderness is often absent and vertebral osteomyelitis rare. High-resolution CT may detect the lesion at one level but cannot, with the equipment presently available, give accurate information as to the extent of the empyema. Magnetic resonance imaging (MRI) is the diagnostic procedure of choice.[46,47] Experience with MRI in spinal subdural empyema is still limited, however, and myelography should be considered if spinal subdural empyema is strongly suspected and MRI is suboptimal or negative.[48] Myelography should be employed when MRI is not available. Both MRI and myelography will reveal cord compression, block, or multiple extra-axial defects. Myelography, however, may not delineate the entire length of the empyema if complete obstruction of the subarachnoid space is present at multiple levels. If lower thoracic or lumbar empyema is suspected, myelography should be performed using a lateral cervical or cisternal route to avoid producing infection of the subarachnoid space. Therapy involves surgical drainage and antibiotics against penicillinase-producing staphylococci and streptococci, with coverage for gram-negative or other organisms if indicated (Table 1). Unless therapy is begun early, cord necrosis is likely, and prognosis for recovery is poor.

REFERENCES

1. Courville CB. Subdural empyema secondary to purulent frontal sinusitis. Arch Otolaryngol. 1944;39:211–39.
2. Silverberg AL, DiNubile MJ. Subdural empyema and cranial epidural abscess. Med Clin North Am. 1985;69:361–74.
3. Kaufman DM, Miller MH, Steigbigel NH. Subdural empyema: Analysis of 17 recent cases and review of the literature. Medicine. 1975;54:485–98.
4. Le Beau J, Creissard P, Harispe L, et al. Surgical treatment of brain abscess and subdural empyema. J Neurosurg. 1973;38:198–203.
5. Kaufman DM, Litman N, Miller MH. Sinusitis: Induced subdural empyema. Neurology. 1983;33:123–32.
6. Mauser HW, Van Houwelingen HC, Tulleken CAF. Factors affecting the outcome in subdural empyema. J Neurol Neurosurg Psychiatry. 1987;50:1136–41.
7. Stephanov S, Joubert MJ, Welchman JM. Combined convexity and parafalx subdural empyema. Surg Neurol. 1979;11:147–51.
8. Wackym PA, Canalis RF, Feuerman T. Subdural empyema of otorhinological origin. J Laryngol Otol. 1990;104:118–22.
9. Dale BAB, Mackenzie J. The complications of sphenoid sinusitis. J Laryngol Otol. 1983;97:661–70.
10. Maniglia AJ, Goodwin WJ, Arnold JE, et al. Intracranial abscesses secondary to nasal, sinus, and orbital infections in adults and children. Arch Otolaryngol Head Neck Surg. 1989;115:1424–9.
11. Skelton R, Maixner W, Isaacs D. Sinusitis-induced subdural empyema. Arch Dis Child. 1992;67:1478–80.
12. Takoro K, Yamataki A, Nakajima F. Subdural empyema occurring 20 years after trauma: Case report. Neurosurgery. 1987;21:724–6.
13. Luken MG III, Whelan MA. Recent diagnostic experience with subdural empyema. J Neurosurg. 1980;52:764–71.
14. Brook I. Aerobic and anaerobic bacteriology of intracranial abscesses. Pediatr Neurol. 1992;8:210–4.
15. Yoshikawa TT, Chow AW, Guze LB. Role of anaerobic bacteria in subdural empyema: Report of four cases and review of 327 cases from the English literature. Am J Med. 1975;58:99–104.
16. Harris LF, Haws FP, Triplett JN Jr. Subdural empyema and epidural abscess: Recent experience in a community hospital. South Med J. 1987;80:1254–8.
17. Blayney AW, Frootko NJ, Mitchell RG. Complications of sinusitis caused by Streptococcus milleri. J Laryngol Otol. 1984;98:895–9.
18. Schiller F, Cairns H, Russell DS. The treatment of purulent pachymeningitis and subdural suppuration with special reference to penicillin. J Neurol Neurosurg Psychiatry. 1948;11:143–82.
19. Kubik CS, Adams RD. Subdural empyema. Brain. 1943;66:18–42.
20. Courville CB. Fatal complications of otitis media: With particular reference to the intracranial lesions in a series of ten thousand autopsies. Arch Otolaryngol. 1934;19:451–501.
21. Kaplan RJ. Neurological complications of infections of the head and neck. Otol Clin North Am. 1976;9:729–49.
22. Coonrod JD, Dans PE. Subdural empyema. Am J Med. 1972;53:85–91.
23. Hitchcock E, Andreadis A. Subdural empyema: A review of 29 cases. J Neurol Neurosurg Psychiatry. 1964;27:422–34.
24. Brock DG, Bleck TP. Extra-axial suppurations of the central nervous system. Semin Neurol. 1992;12:263–72.
25. Post E, Modesti LM. "Subacute" postoperative subdural empyema. J Neurosurg. 1981;55:761–5.
26. Braun CW, Axelrod J. Hematogenous infection of subdural hematoma. Arch Neurol. 1980;37:467–8.
27. Biehl JP. Subdural empyema secondary to acute frontal sinusitis. A neglected but curable emergency complication. JAMA. 1955;158:721–4.
28. Hodges J, Anslow P, Gillett G. Subdural empyema—Continuing diagnostic problems in the CT scan era. Q J Med. 1986;59:387–93.
29. Weingarten K, Zimmerman RD, Becker RD, et al. Subdural and epidural empyemas: MR imaging. AJNR. 1987;10:81–7.
30. Sze G, Zimmerman RD. The magnetic resonance imaging of infections and inflammatory diseases. Imaging in neuroradiology, part I. Radiol Clin North Am. 1988;26:839–59.
31. Komori H, Takagishi T, Otaki E, et al. The efficacy of MR imaging in subdural empyema. Brain Dev. 1992;14:123–5.
32. Weingarten K, Zimmerman RD, Becker RD, et al. Subdural and epidural empyemas: MR imaging. AJR Am J Roentgenol. 1989;152:615–21.
33. Dunker RO, Khakoo RA. Failure of computed tomographic scanning to demonstrate subdural empyema. JAMA. 1981;246:1116–8.
34. Moseley IF, Kendall BE. Radiology of intracranial empyemas, with special reference to computed tomography. Neuroradiol. 1984;26:333–45.
35. Mauser HW, Ravijst AP, Elderson A, et al. Nonsurgical treatment of subdural empyema. J Neurosurg. 1985;63:128–30.
36. Leys D, Christiaens JL, Derambure P, et al. Management of focal intracranial infections: Is medical treatment better than surgery? J Neurol Neurosurg Psychiatry. 1990;53:472–5.
37. Obana WG, Rosenblum ML. Nonoperative treatment of neurosurgical infections. Neurosurg Clin North Am. 1992;3:359–73.
38. Pathak A, Sharma BS, Mathuriya SN, et al. Controversies in the management of subdural empyema. A study of 41 cases with review of literature. Acta Neurochir Wien. 1990;102:25–32.
39. Nussbaum ES, Rigamonti D, Standiford H, et al. Spinal epidural abscess: A report of 40 cases and review. Surg Neurol. 1992;38:225–31.
40. Feuerman T, Wackym PA, Gade GF, et al. Craniotomy improves outcome in subdural empyema. Surg Neurol. 1989;32:105–10.
41. Miller ES, Dias PS, Uttley D. Management of subdural empyema: A series of 24 cases. J Neurol Neurosurg Psychiatry. 1987;50:1415–8.
42. Cowie R, Williams B. Late seizures and morbidity after subdural empyema. J Neurosurg. 1983;58:569–73.
43. Smith HP, Hendrick EB. Subdural empyema and epidural abscess in children. J Neurosurg. 1983;58:392–7.
44. Ogilvy CS, Chapman PH, McGrail K. Subdural empyema complicating bacterial meningitis in a child: Enhancement of membranes with gadolinium on magnetic resonance imaging in a patient without enhancement on computed tomography. Surg Neurol. 1992;37:138–41.
45. Bartels RH, de Jong TR, Grotenhuis JA. Spinal subdural abscess. Case report. J Neurosurg. 1992;76:307–11.
46. Post MJ, Bowen BC, Sze G. Magnetic resonance imaging of spinal infection. Rheum Dis Clin North Am. 1991;17:773–94.
47. Smith AS, Blaser SI. MR of infectious and inflammatory diseases of the spine. Crit Rev Diagn Imaging. 1991;32:165–89.
48. Gelfand MS, Bakhtian BJ, Simmons BP. Spinal sepsis due to Streptococcus milleri: Two cases and review. Rev Infect Dis. 1991;13:559–63.

70. EPIDURAL ABSCESS

JOHN E. GREENLEE

An epidural abscess represents localized infection between the outermost layer of the meninges, the dura mater, and the overlying skull or vertebral column. Within the skull, the dura forms the inner layer of the cranial periosteum, and an intracranial epidural abscess must form by stripping periosteum from bone: such an abscess is almost always sharply confined and accompanied by focal osteomyelitis. Because of the ease with which infection can cross the cranial dura along emissary veins, subdural empyema is often present. Within the spinal canal, however, the dura mater is separated from the vertebrae by an epidural space filled with fat and vascular areolar tissue. Although the spinal dura itself is only rarely breached by bacteria, the spinal epidural space offers little resistance to the longitudinal spread of infection. For this reason, a spinal epidural abscess often occupies several vertebral segments and, within the narrow confines of the vertebral canal, may cause extensive cord compression and necrosis.

INTRACRANIAL EPIDURAL ABSCESS

The etiology, pathogenesis, and bacteriology of intracranial epidural abscess are identical to those described for intracranial subdural empyema (see Ch. 69).[1-11] Virtually all cases follow frontal sinusitis, craniotomy, or mastoiditis. Rare cases may complicate nasopharyngeal malignancies.[12] *Staphylococcus aureus* is a frequent isolate in cases associated with surgical procedures or cranial trauma.[4,11] Individual cases have been associated with *Eikenella*,[13] *Salmonella*,[14] *Aspergillus*,[15] and *Mucor (Rhizopus)*.[16]

Pathologic Characteristics

Epidural abscess most often arises adjacent to the frontal sinuses. In almost all cases, osteomyelitis is present within overlying bones, and there is septic thrombosis of veins bridging skull and meninges. Subdural empyema is present in 81 percent of autopsied cases, with 38 percent of the cases also having meningitis and 17 percent brain abscess.[17] Rarely, infection of the bridging veins may provide venous necrosis and epidural hemorrhage rather than abscess.[18]

Clinical Features

The onset of symptoms may be insidious[1,8-10,19] and at first may be overshadowed by sinusitis or otitis. The abscess produces local pain followed by generalized headache, at times with alteration of mental state.[1,8,9] Focal neurologic signs and focal or generalized seizures then appear. An epidural abscess near the petrous bone may involve cranial nerves V and VI, with unilateral facial pain and lateral rectus weakness (Gradenigo syndrome).[20] A single instance has been reported in which occipital epidural abscess produced obstruction of the superior sagittal sinus.[21] As the abscess enlarges, papilledema and other signs of intracranial hypertension develop. Extension of the infection into the subdural space is accompanied by rapid neurologic deterioration.

Therapy

In most cases, therapy of cranial epidural abscess consists of antibiotic therapy and emergent surgical drainage to prevent development of subdural empyema. Concomitant surgical therapy of sinusitis, otitis, or osteomyelitis may be required as well. Antibiotic therapy should be directed against aerobic and anaerobic streptococci, *Staphylococcus aureus,* and gram-negative aerobic and anaerobic organisms, as outlined in Table 1 of Chapter 69. The ability of magnetic resonance imaging (MRI) to allow repeated, noninvasive imaging of epidural abscess has made it possible, in a limited number of patients, to treat cranial epidural abscess by antibiotics alone. It should also be noted that MRI may sometimes detect epidural abscesses small enough that surgical drainage is not yet possible. In such cases treatment should be initiated with antibiotics alone. If surgery is deferred, MRI should be repeated in 24 hours after initiation of antibiotics and at frequent intervals thereafter to document reduction in abscess size and to avoid missing extension of infection into the subdural space.

Diagnosis

Persistent fever, leukocytosis, elevated erythrocyte sedimentation rate, and focal or generalized neurologic signs in the setting of sinusitis or otitis suggest intracranial infection. Edema or cellulitis of the face or scalp may be present.[1,10] Gadolinium-enhanced MRI is the diagnostic procedure of choice.[22,23] This imaging technique will identify pachymeningeal enhancement or epidural collections of pus not yet detectable by computed tomography (CT) and may also demonstrate the presence of

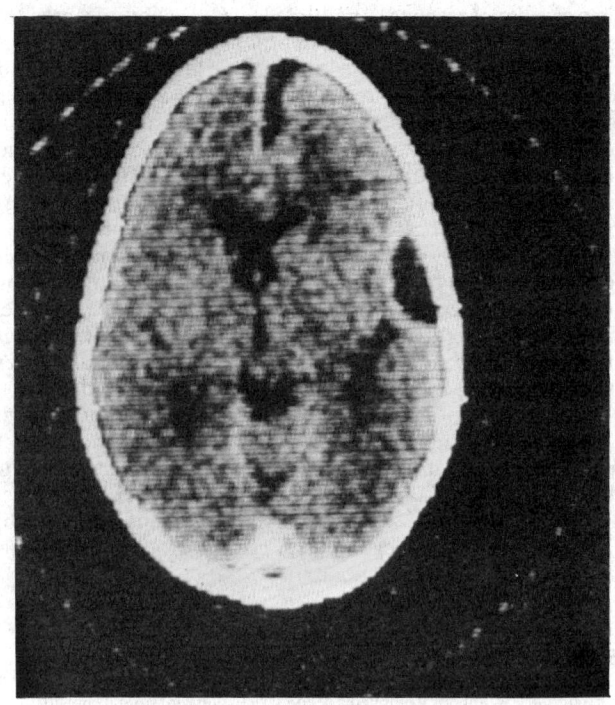

FIG. 1. Computed tomography of right-sided epidural abscess. A subdural empyema is also present between the falx cerebri and the medial aspect of the right frontal lobe. (Courtesy of Drs. D.M. Kaufman, N.E. Leeds, and I. Kricheff; from Kaufman and Leeds,[24] with permission.)

sinusitis or otitis. Computed tomography may be used to image bone and as the major diagnostic study for the abscess itself if MRI is not available (Fig. 1).[24] Routine skull x-rays almost never detect findings not evident on CT and MRI. Angiography is rarely if ever indicated, unless there is a question of concomitant venous sinus thrombosis and MRI is not available. Spinal fluid is usually sterile, and the danger of tonsillar herniation contraindicates lumbar puncture.[1,25]

SPINAL EPIDURAL ABSCESS

Etiology and Pathogenesis

Both acute and chronic spinal epidural abscess follow infection elsewhere in the body.[26-35] In most cases, infection reaches the epidural space by hematogenous spread, either by direct metastasis or by production of a vertebral osteomyelitis with extension into the spinal epidural space. Infection of the epidural space may also be caused by penetrating injuries or by extension of decubitus ulcers or paraspinal abscesses.[1,28,33,34] Epidural abscess has been reported following back surgery, lumbar puncture, and epidural anethesia.[36-40] Occasionally, epidural abscess arises as a complication of abdominal surgery.[41,42] Rarely, infection may spread along a persistent dermal sinus. In 10–30 percent of the cases there is a history of back trauma and, less often, a history of diabetes mellitus, intravenous drug abuse, or pregnancy.[1,28,29,32-34]

Bacteriology

Staphylococcus aureus is the agent in 60–90 percent of both the acute and chronic cases and in some series is the only organism recovered.[1,28,32,34] Aerobic and anaerobic streptococci cause approximately 18 percent of the cases and gram-negative organisms, especially *Escherichia coli* and *Pseudomonas aeruginosa,* 13 percent.[1,28,34] Isolated cases of epidural abscess have been associated with *Staphylococcus epidermidis*,[28] *Streptococcus pneumoniae* during bacterial endocarditis,[35] *Nocardia astero-ides*,[43] *Echinococcus*,[29] *Actinomyces israeli*,[1] and *Aspergillus*.[15] Multiple organisms are found in approximately 10 percent of patients.[27,28,33,34] A mixed flora of *Staphylococcus aureus* and *Cryptococcus neoformans* has been reported in a patient with AIDS.[44] Chronic epidural infection may occur during tuberculo-sis, frequently without other detectable evidence of in-fection.[29,32,45]

Pathology

The abscess involves thoracic spine in 50–80 percent of the cases, lumbar in 17–38 percent, and cervical in 10–25 per-cent.[1,28,33,34] In children, cervical and lumbar spine are more often involved.[47] Abscesses may be posterior to the cord, ante-rior, or circumferential.[1,33,34,48] Anterior abscesses usually occur at cervical levels, except in tuberculosis, in which the anterior thoracic or lumbar epidural spaces may also be in-volved. Diskitis and/or vertebral osteomyelitis, detectable by MRI, may be present in 80–100 percent of cases.[33,48,49] Acute abscesses consist of granulation tissue containing loculated pus; in chronic abscesses there may be a prominent fibroblastic com-ponent. The abscess usually occupies four or five vertebral seg-ments but may extend the length of the cord. Enlargement of the abscess produces myelomalacia or cord necrosis both by compression and by invasion of the spinal venous plexus.[1,28,33,34] Extension of infection into the subarachnoid space occurs in 12–25 percent of cases.[28,33,50]

Clinical Features

Epidural abscess is significantly more common in males and may occur at any age. The abscess may develop acutely within hours to days or may pursue a chronic course over months. Most abscesses, however, pass through four clinical stages, dif-fering only in time course: focal vertebral pain; root pain; defi-cits of motor, sensory, or sphincter function; and paralysis.[51] Acute metastatic infection of the epidural space produces rapid progression with prominent systemic symptoms and severe, focal pain. Patients usually seek medical help within the first few days of illness when radicular signs are already present. When epidural abscess arises following vertebral osteomyelitis, vertebral pain may develop over 2–3 weeks, but progression is rapid once radicular symptoms appear. Chronic epidural ab-scess may manifest with a course indistinguishable from that of an extrinsic neoplasm and without systemic signs. Where cervi-cal cord is involved, respiratory function may be impaired.[52] Rapidly developing cervical epidural abscesses may produce flaccid hyporeflexia to mimic Guillain-Barré syndrome.[33]

Diagnosis

Epidural abscess is a diagnostic consideration in any patient with localized back pain and radicular symptoms, especially when a source of infection is evident. Headache is a common additional complaint. Nuchal rigidity and focal tenderness to percussion are almost universal.[28,33,51] In acute cases the white blood cell count and the erythrocyte sedimentation rate are ele-vated. X-ray films of the spine may show osteomyelitis but may also be normal. Magnetic resonance imaging is the diagnostic procedure of choice (Fig. 2), since it can visualize the cord and epidural space in both sagittal and transverse sections and can identify not only epidural abscess but also osteomyelitis, intra-medullary spinal cord lesions, and joint space infection.[48,49,53,54] Myelography should be employed if MRI is not available or cannot be performed. Computed tomography with contrast en-hancement may be helpful in differentiating subdural from epi-dural infections or in identifying osteomyelitis. Computed to-mography is less sensitive than MRI, however, and may fail to define the longitudinal extent of the abscess. MRI should pre-

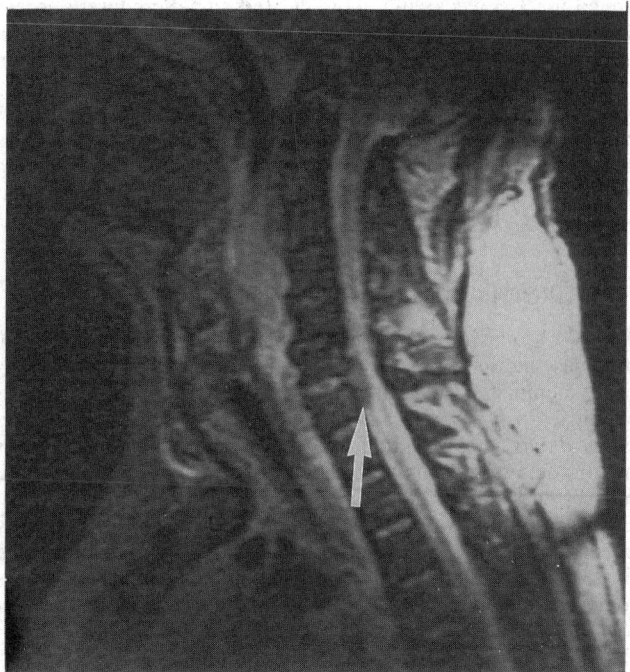

FIG. 2. Magnetic resonance scan of patient with anterior cervical epi-dural abscess. The abscess is seen as an area of diminished attenuation bulging into the spinal canal and compressing the spinal cord (arrow). The infection also involves the adjacent disc space. (Courtesy of Dr. J. Richard Baringer, Salt Lake City, UT.)

cede lumbar puncture when epidural abscess is suspected. In the absence of MRI, lumbar puncture should never be attempted without provision to introduce dye and carry out myelography before the needle is withdrawn. Spinal puncture, if indicated, should be performed well above or below the suspected area of involvement, and the needle should be advanced slowly with frequent aspiration to avoid contaminating the subdural or sub-arachnoid space. Artifacts produced by patient movement may obscure positive findings on MRI, CT, or myelography, and adequate sedation should be employed if required to achieve an optimal study. Positive cultures of cerebrospinal fluid are detected in 12–25 percent of cases. In most of these cases, blood cultures are also positive.[33] Gram stain of cerebrospinal fluid is usually negative.[28,29,33] Blood and abscess material should be submitted for aerobic and anaerobic culture.

Therapy

The danger of spinal cord necrosis requires surgical drain-age—usually by laminectomy—as soon as the diagnosis is made.[55] Antibiotic coverage should be initiated prior to surgery. Minimal coverage should be directed against penicillin-resistant *Staphylococcus aureus*. Gram-negative coverage, consisting of ceftriaxone plus coverage for *Bacteroides* with metronidazole, should be added if there is any suspicion that these organisms might be present. Because the epidural space lies outside the blood-brain barrier, consideration should be given to adding gentamicin in addition to ceftriaxone if gram-negative organisms are suspected. Antibiotic therapy should be modified based on results of culture. In selected patients, CT-guided needle aspira-tion may be used in place of laminectomy. Antibiotic therapy alone, with meticulous serial neurologic examinations and fol-low-up MRI studies, may be considered if the patient has local-ized pain or radicular symptoms, without neurologic deficit. Ap-pearance of neurologic deficit, worsening pain, or increasing temperature and leukocytosis while on antibiotic therapy are indications for surgery.[56,57] Antibiotic coverage should be continued for 3–4 weeks in uncomplicated spinal epidural abscess and for 8 weeks if osteomyelitis is present. Severe destruction of bone may require surgery for stabilization once the infection is cured. Prognosis for neurologic recovery is excellent if therapy is begun before or during the stage of radicular symptoms but worsens rapidly as evidence of cord injury appears. Likelihood of neurologic improvement is poor if surgery is delayed over 24 hours after the onset of paralysis.[33] Mortality in most recent series has been in the range of 5 percent.[33,34]

HYPERTROPHIC SPINAL PACHYMENINGITIS

Rarely, chronic inflammation or infection within the spinal canal involves the dura mater alone, to produce a diffuse, fibrosing pachymeningitis. Cases have been associated with tuberculosis, syphilis, *Streptococcus intermedius (milleri)* infection, *Aspergillus flavus,* and *Pseudallescheria boydii,* but in many cases no etiologic organism can be identified.[58–63] The fibrosis compresses nerve roots and if extensive may injure the spinal cord. Early symptoms are pain, muscle weakness, and muscle atrophy occurring in a radicular pattern. Spinal fluid contains elevated protein but no cells. Electromyography may localize the process to nerve roots. In most cases, diagnosis has been made by myelography with lateral views. At present, the diagnostic procedure of choice is MRI with gadolinium enhancement.[64] Treatment consists of surgical removal of hypertrophied dura producing symptoms and antibiotic therapy of any diagnosed causative infection.

REFERENCES

1. Silverberg AL, DiNubile MJ. Subdural empyema and cranial epidural abscess. Med Clin North Am. 1985;69:361–74.
2. Weber AL, Mikulis DK. Inflammatory disorders of the paraorbital sinuses and their complications. Radiol Clin North Am. 1987;25:615–30.
3. Harris LF, Haws FP, Triplett JN Jr. Subdural empyema and epidural abscess: Recent experience in a community hospital. South Med J. 1987;80:1254–8.
4. Smith HP, Hendrick EB. Subdural empyema and epidural abscess in children. J Neurosurg. 1983;58:392–7.
5. Blayney AW, Frootko NJ, Mitchell RG. Complications of sinusitis caused by *Streptococcus milleri.* J Laryngol Otol. 1984;98:895–9.
6. Dale BAB, Mackenzie J. The complications of sphenoid sinusitis. J Laryngol Otol. 1983;97:661–70.
7. Larrabee WF Jr, Travis LW, Tabb HG. Frontal sinus fractures—Their suppurative complications and surgical management. Laryngoscope. 1980;90:1810–3.
8. Handel SF, Klein WC, Kim YW. Intracranial epidural abscess. Radiology. 1974;111:117–20.
9. Koenig RP, Craigmile TK. Epidural intracranial abscess. USAF Med J. 1956; 8:120–4.
10. French LA, Chou SN. Osteomyelitis of the skull and epidural abscess. In: Gurdjian ES, ed. Cranial and Intracranial Suppuration. Springfield, IL: Charles C. Thomas; 1969:59–72.
11. Maniglia AJ, Goodwin WJ, Arnold JE, et al. Intracranial abscesses secondary to nasal, sinus, and orbital infections in adults and children. Arch Otolaryngol Head Neck Surg. 1989;115:1424–9.
12. Kaplan RJ. Neurological complications of infections of the head and neck. Otol Clin North Am 1976;9:729–49.
13. Akhtar MJ, Chandler JR. Periorbital, subgaleal, and epidural empyema secondary to *Eikenella* sinusitis. Ear Nose Throat J. 1979;58:358–61.
14. Rodriguez RE, Valero V, Watanakunakorn C. *Salmonella* focal intracranial infection: Review of the world literature and report of an unusual case. Rev Infect Dis 1986;8:31–41.
15. Hendrix WC, Arruda LK, Platts Mills TA, et al. *Aspergillus* epidural abscess and cord compression in a patient with aspergilloma and empyema. Survival and response to high dose systemic amphotericin therapy. Am Rev Respir Dis. 1992;145:1483–6.
16. Muresan A. A case of cerebral mucormycosis diagnosed in life, with eventual recovery. J Clin Pathol. 1960;13:34–6.
17. Slager UT. Infection and parainfectious inflammation. In: Slager UT, ed. Basic Neuropathology. Baltimore: Williams & Wilkins; 1970:89–125.
18. Rajput AJ, Rozdilsky B. Extradural hematoma following frontal sinusitis. Arch Otolaryngol. 1971;94:83–5.
19. Reader ME, Eliachar I, McIntire LD, et al. Frontal sinusitis with chronic epidural abscess: A case presentation. Ear Nose Throat J. 1992;71:599–603.
20. Courville CB. Fatal complications of otitis media with particular reference to the intracranial lesions in a series of ten thousand autopsies. Arch Otolaryngol. 1934;19:451–501.

21. Mineura K, Kamisato N, Miura S, et al. Occipital epidural abscess causing superior sagittal sinus obstruction. Clin Neurol Neurosurg. 1990;92:277–81.
22. Sze G, Zimmerman RD. The magnetic resonance imaging of infections and inflammatory diseases. Imaging in neuroradiology part I. Radiol Clin North Am. 1988;26:839–59.
23. Borovich B, Johnston E, Spagnuolo E. Infratentorial subdural empyema: Clinical and computerized tomography findings. Report of three cases. J Neurosurg. 1990;72:299–301.
24. Kaufman DM, Leeds NE. Computed tomography (CT) in the diagnosis of intracranial abscesses. Neurology. 1977;27:1069–73.
25. Greenlee JE. Cerebrospinal fluid in central nervous system infections. In: Scheld WM, Whitley RJ, Durack DT, eds. Infections of the Central Nervous System. New York: Raven Press; 1991:861–85.
26. Browder J, Meyers R. Pyogenic infections of the spinal epidural space. Surgery. 1941;10:296–308.
27. Dus V, Spinal periphachymeningitis (epidural abscess). J Neurosurg. 1960; 17:972–83.
28. Baker AS, Ojemann RG, Swartz MN, et al. Spinal epidural abscess. N Engl J Med 1975;293:463–8.
29. Kaufman DM, Kaplan JG, Litman N. Infectious agents in spinal epidural abscesses. Neurology. 1980;30:844–50.
30. Verner FE, Musher DM. Spinal epidural abscess. Med Clin North Am. 1985; 69:375–84.
31. Elian D, Hassin D, Tomer A, et al. Spinal epidural abscess: An unusual complication of bacterial endocarditis. Infection. 1984;12:258–9.
32. Koppel BS, Tuchman AJ, Mangiardi JR, et al. Epidural spinal infection in intravenous drug abusers. Arch Neurol. 1988;45:1331–7.
33. Darouiche RO, Hamill RJ, Greenberg SB, et al. Bacterial spinal epidural abscess. Review of 43 cases and literature survey. Medicine. 1992;71:369–85.
34. Nussbaum ES, Rigamonti D, Standiford H, et al. Spinal epidural abscess: A report of 40 cases and review. Surg Neurol. 1992;38:225–31.
35. Clark R, Carlisle JT, Valainis GT. *Streptococcus pneumoniae* endocarditis presenting as an epidural abscess. Rev Infect Dis. 1989;11:338–40.
36. Shintani S, Tanaka H, Irifune A, et al. Iatrogenic acute spinal epidural abscess with septic meningitis: MR findings. Clin Neurol Neurosurg. 1992;94:253–5.
37. Ericsson M, Algers G, Schliamser SE. Spinal epidural abscesses in adults: Review and report of iatrogenic cases. Scand J Infect Dis. 1990;22:249–57.
38. Chan ST, Leung S. Spinal epidural abscess following steroid injection for sciatica. Case report. Spine. 1989;14:106–8.
39. Ferguson JF, Kirsch WM. Epidural empyema following thoracic extradural block. J Neurosurg. 1974;41:762–4.
40. Abdel Magid RA, Kotb HI. Epidural abscess after spinal anesthesia: A favorable outcome. Neurosurgery 1990;27:310–1.
41. Wayne DA, Muizelaar PJ. Acute lumbosacral epidural abscess after percutaneous transluminal angioplasty. Am J Med. 1989;87:478.
42. Murr MM, Metcalf AM. Spinal epidural abscess complicationg an ileal J-pouch-anal anastomosis. Report of a case. Dis Colon Rectum. 1993;36:293–4.
43. Siao P, McCabe P, Yagnik P, Nocardial spinal epidural abscess. Neurology. 1989;39:996.
44. Pirofski L, Casadevall A. Mixed staphylococcal and cryptoccal epidural abscess in a patient with AIDS [letter]. Rev Infect Dis. 1990;12:964–5.
45. Latronico N, Tansini A, Gualandi GF, et al. Successful nonoperative treatment of tuberculous spinal epidural abscess with cord compression: The role of magnetic resonance imaging. Eur Neurol. 1993;33:177–80.
46. Baker CJ. Primary spinal epidural abscess. Am J Dis Child. 1971;121:337–9.
47. Schweich PJ, Hurt TL. Spinal epidural abscess in children: Two illustrative cases. Pediatr Emerg Care. 1992;8:84–7.
48. Numaguchi Y, Rigamonti D, Rothman MI, et al. Spinal epidural abscess: Evaluation with gadolinium-enhanced MR imaging. Radiographics. 1993;13: 545–59.
49. Meyers SP. Diagnosis of hematogenous pyogenic vertebral osteomyelitis by magnetic resonance imaging. Arch Intern Med. 1991;151:683–97.
50. Sergent JS, Lockshin MD, Christian CL, et al. Vasculitis with hepatitis B antigenemia. Medicine. 1976;55:1–18.
51. Heusner AP. Nontuberculous spinal epidural infections. N Engl J Med. 1948; 239:845–54.
52. Durity F, Thompson GB. Localized cervical epidural abscess. J Neurosurg. 1968;28:387–90.
53. Teman AJ. Spinal epidural abscess. Early detection with gadolinium magnetic resonance imaging. Arch Neurol. 1992;49:743–6.
54. Kricun R, Shoemaker EI, Chovanes GI, et al. Epidural abscess of the cervical spine: MR findings in five cases. Am J Roentgenol. 1992;158:1145–9.
55. Rea GL, McGregor JM, Miller CA, et al. Surgical treatment of the spontaneous spinal epidural abscess. Surg Neurol. 1992;37:274–9.
56. Hanigan WC, Asner NG, Elwood PW. Magnetic resonance imaging and the nonoperative treatment of spinal epidural abscess. Surg Neurol. 1990;34: 408–13.
57. Wheeler D, Keiser P, Rigamonti D, et al. Medical management of spinal epidural abscesses: Case report and review [see comments]. Clin Infect Dis. 1992;15:22–7.
58. Bucy PC, Freeman W. Hypertrophic spinal pachymeningitis. J Neurosurg. 1952;9:564–78.
59. Carli P, Yao N, Marlier S, et al. [Febrile cervicalgia caused by Streptococcus milleri external pachymeningitis (Letter). Presse Med. 1993;22:33.
60. Murai H, Kira J, Kobayashi T, et al. Hypertrophic cranial pachymeningitis due to *Aspergillus flavus.* Clin Neurol Neurosurgy. 1992;94:247–50.
61. Berenguer J, Diaz Mediavilla J, Urra D, et al. Central nervous system infection caused by *Pseudallescheria boydii:* Case report and review [see comments]. Rev Infect Dis. 1989;11:890–6.

62. Guidetti B, LaTorre E. Hypertrophic spinal pachymeningitis. J Neurosurg. 1967;26:496–503.
63. Oonishi T, Ishiko T, Arai M, et al. Pachymeningitis cervicalis hypertrophica. Acta Pathol Jpn. 1982;32:163–71.
64. Digman KE, Partington CR, Graves VB. MR imaging of spinal pachymeningitis. J Comput Assist Tomogr. 1990;14:988–990.

71. SUPPURATIVE INTRACRANIAL PHLEBITIS

JOHN E. GREENLEE

Septic intracranial thrombophlebitis most frequently follows infection of paranasal sinuses, middle ear, mastoid, face, or oropharynx. The infection spreads centrally along emissary veins.[1–5] Septic thrombophlebitis may also occur in association with epidural abscess, subdural empyema, or meningitis. Occasionally, the infection is metastatic from lungs or other distant sites.[3] The likelihood of thrombosis is increased by states altering blood viscosity or coagulability, including dehydration, polycythemia, pregnancy, oral contraceptive use, sickle cell disease, malignancy, or trauma.[4,6,7] *Staphylococcus aureus* is the most frequent isolate.[1] A minority of cases are due to *Staphylococcus epidermidis*, streptococci including *Streptococcus pneumoniae*, gram-negative bacilli,[1,2] and anaerobic organisms. Multiple infecting organisms may be present.[8]

PATHOLOGIC CHANGES

Septic intracranial thrombophlebitis may begin within veins or venous sinuses and may involve additional vessels by propagation or discontinuous spread.[1,9] The pathologic changes are those of both venous thrombosis and suppuration. Venous occlusion may produce no local injury, but, if collateral veins are compromised, edema and hemorrhagic infarction result. The most common sites of infarction are the area of venous watershed immediately above the Sylvian fissue (see Ch. 63)[3] and the medial surfaces of the cerebral hemispheres.[3,4] Thrombosis of the anterior portion of the superior sagittal sinus or of the lateral sinuses may block reabsorption of cerebrospinal fluid with resultant communicating hydrocephalus. Local suppuration may produce venous necrosis and hemorrhage or may cause epidural abscess, subdural empyema, meningitis, or brain abscess.[1–4] Septic embolization may produce pulmonary infarction, abscesses in lungs or other organs, or mycotic aneurysm.[2–4,9]

CLINICAL FEATURES

Cortical Vein Thrombosis

If collateral venous drainage is adequate, septic venous thrombosis may produce only transient neurologic findings or may be silent except for its metastatic consequences. If the thrombus outstrips collateral flow, however, a progressive neurologic deficit will result and may mimic brain abscess, with impairment of consciousness, focal or generalized seizures, and increased intracranial pressure.[2,3] Focal neurologic findings include hemiparesis, which involves the face and hand if veins over the cerebral convexity are involved.[3] Thrombosis of veins along the falx cerebri may produce unilateral leg weakness, which becomes bilateral if propagation of the thrombus involves the veins of the contralateral hemisphere.[2,3] Aphasia is common when the dominant hemisphere is involved. Transient hemodynamic variation in venous collateral flow may cause considerable fluctuation in neurologic signs.

Venous Sinus Thrombosis

The clinical findings vary with the sinus involved and are summarized in Table 1 (see Ch. 63, Fig. 5). Cavernous sinus, lateral sinus, and superior sagittal sinus are most often involved. Cavernous sinus thrombosis most commonly follows infections of the face or of the sphenoid and ethmoid sinuses.[1,10,11] Onset is abrupt, with diplopia, photophobia, orbital edema, and progressive exophthalmos.[10–12] Involvement of cranial nerves III, IV, V, and VI produces ophthalmoplegia, a midposition fixed pupil, loss of corneal reflex, and diminished sensation over the upper face. Obstruction of venous return from the retina results in papilledema, retinal hemorrhages, and visual loss. Similar findings appear in the opposite eye as the infection spreads to the contralateral cavernous sinus. Engorgement or thrombosis of facial veins may occur.

Thrombosis of the anterior third of the superior sagittal sinus may impair reabsorption of cerebrospinal fluid to produce intracranial hypertension without other signs.[2,3,5,13] More extensive thrombosis of the superior sagittal sinus, however, results in bilateral leg weakness followed by arm weakness and clouding of consciousness as cortical veins are affected.[2,3,5] Occlusion of the lateral sinus produces pain over the ear and mastoid and may cause edema over the mastoid (Griesinger's sign).[4,13,14] Impairment of veins supplying cranial nerves V and VI produces ipsilateral facial pain and lateral rectus weakness (Gradenigo syndrome). Septic cortical vein or venous sinus occlusion may produce subdural empyema, meningitis, or brain abscess. The danger of septic pulmonary embolization is always present.[9]

DIAGNOSIS

Septic intracranial thrombophlebitis may manifest as sepsis without neurologic signs or with stupor and focal neurologic signs in the presence of cranial infection. In the latter instance, septic thrombophlebitis may be indistinguishable from brain abscess or subdural empyema. Fever, leukocytosis, and elevated erythrocyte sedimentation rate are usually present. Skull x-rays should be evaluated for the presence of sinusitis or mastoiditis, with particular attention to frontal, ethmoidal, and sphenoidal sinuses. Lumbar puncture may reveal increased pressure, slight lymphocytic pleocytosis, and mild elevation of protein. Evidence of subarachnoid blood detectable by lumbar puncture is present in less than 15 percent of cases,[1,2] and cerebrospinal fluid is usually sterile. Magnetic resonance imaging (MRI), because of its ability to differentiate between flowing blood and thrombus, is the diagnostic procedure of choice. Sensitivity of MRI can be increased by used of magnetic resonance angiography (Fig. 1).[16–22] Computed tomography (CT) scanning, although considerably less sensitive and reliable than MRI, permits diagnosis of venous sinus thrombosis in many cases and should be employed as the initial diagnostic test when MRI is not available.[23–25] Magnetic resonance imaging and CT also provide information about concomitant subdural or epidural infections and allow visualization of brain infarction, hemorrhage, and edema. Angiography with close attention to the venous phase should be employed when venous sinus thrombosis is suspected despite negative MRI or CT. Blood, spinal fluid, and all infected material should be cultured for both aerobic and anaerobic organisms.

TREATMENT

Appropriate antibiotic therapy, reversal of elevated intracranial pressure, and control of seizures are the goals of therapy. Initial antibiotics should be directed against *Staphylococcus aureus*, aerobic streptococci, and anaerobes (see Ch. 69, Table 1). Con-

TABLE 1. Symptoms of Intracranial Venous Sinus Occlusion

Venous Sinus Involved	Associated Infection	Anatomic Structures Affected	Clinical Findings
Cavernous sinus	Paranasal sinusitis, especially of frontal, ethmoidal or sphenoidal sinuses, infection of face or mouth	Venous drainage from orbit and eye. Cranial nerves III, IV, V, and VI within the cavernous sinus [venous supply of frontal lobe and pituitary]	Unilateral periobital edema, exophthalmos, and chemosis; examination shows papilledema, ocular palsies, diminished pupillary reactivity, frequently diminished corneal reflex, and impaired sensation in the first and second divisions of V; extension to the contralateral sinus may duplicate these findings in the opposite eye [seizures, frontal lobe, deficits, hypopituitarism]
Lateral sinus	Otitis media or mastoiditis; rarely pharyngitis	Cranial nerves V and VI Venous route of CSF reabsorption [venous supply of temporal lobe, jugular bulb, cranial nerves IX, X, XI at jugular foramen]	Lateral rectus weakness; facial pain and altered facial sensation; increased intracranial pressure with papilledema if the other lateral sinus is also compromised [temporal lobe seizures; jugular foramen syndrome with ipsilateral palatal weakness, diminished gag reflex, and weakness of trapezius and sternomastoid]
Superior sagittal sinus	Infections of face, scalp, subdural or epidural spaces; meningitis	Venous drainage from medial portion of cerebral hemispheres; CSF reabsorption	Bilateral leg weakness; intracranial hypertension
Superior petrosal sinus	Otitis media or mastoiditis	Trigeminal ganglion [venous drainage from temporal lobe]	Ipsilateral pain or sensory deficit [temporal lobe seizures]
Inferior petrosal sinus	Otitis media or mastoiditis	Cranial nerves V and VI at tip of petrous bone	"Gradenigo syndrome"; ipsilateral facial pain and sensory deficit; ipsilateral lateral rectus palsy

Note: Brackets indicate structures affected or symptoms produced by extension of the sinus thrombus into cortical veins.

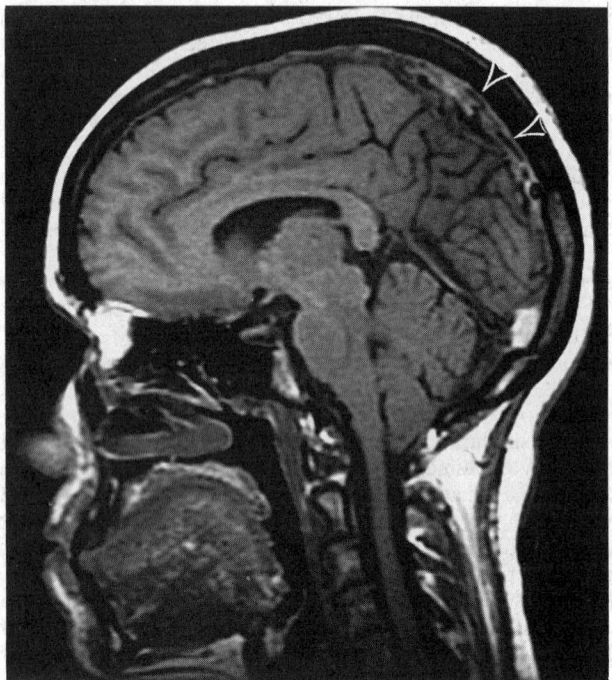
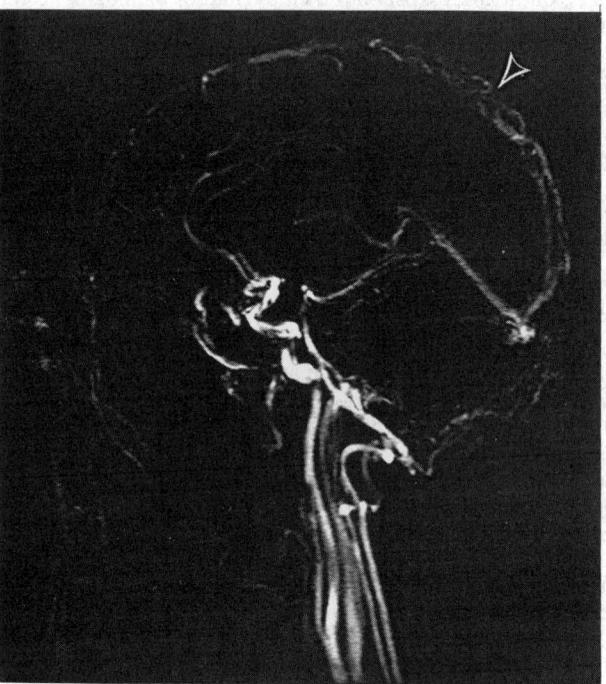

A   *B*

FIG. 1. (**A**) Magnetic resonance image of superior sagittal sinus thrombosis. There is increased signal within the vessel on T2-weighted images (arrows), indicating the presence of thrombus. (**B**) Magnetic resonance angiogram of the same patient, showing nonfilling of the superior sagittal sinus. The sinus is surrounded by tortuous collateral vessels (arrow). (Courtesy of Dr. Wayne Davis, University of Utah.)

trol of infection may require urgent surgery of infected cranial structures or drainage of intra- or extracranial abscess. Intracranial hypertension may require glucocorticoids, osmotic diuretics, or hyperventilation; an intracranial pressure monitor may be essential in assessing efficiency of therapy. Communicating hydrocephalus may require serial lumbar punctures or ventricular drainage. The use of anticoagulants is controversial[26–28] but may be necessary when there is progressive thrombosis or overt embolization in the face of antibiotic therapy. If anticoagulation is used, the danger of intracranial hemorrhage should always be kept in mind. Internal jugular vein ligation has been used with lateral sinus thrombosis.[14,15] Thrombolytic therapy with urokinase or other agents has been employed successfully in uninfected venous sinus thrombosis,[29–31] but the efficacy and safety of this approach in suppurative intracranial

thrombophlebitis have not been determined. In a few instances, thrombectomy has been successful.[32]

PROGNOSIS

Even when an apparently fixed neurologic deficit is present, intracranial venous infarction carries a better likelihood of functional recovery than does arterial infarction, but permanent deficits may occur. Overall mortality in suppurative intracranial thrombophlebitis is 34 percent. Mortality in complete occlusion of the superior sinus, however, is 78 percent.[1,10,32] Ominous prognostic signs are coma, progression of focal seizures to generalized ones, generalized seizures as an initial symptom, and bilateral signs, particularly bilateral flaccid hemiplegia.[1,2,10,27,32]

REFERENCES

1. Southwick FS, Richardson EP, Swartz MN. Septic thrombosis of the dural venous sinuses. Medicine. 1986;65:82–106.
2. Krayenbuhl HA. Cerebral venous and sinus thrombosis. Clin Neurosurg. 1967;14:1–24.
3. Stuart EA, O'Brien FH, McNally WJ. Cerebral venous thrombosis. Ann Otolaryngol. 1951;406–38.
4. Courville CB, Nielsen JM. Fatal complications of otitis media. Arch Otolaryngol. 1934;19:451–9.
5. Strauss SI, Stern NS, Mendelow H, et al. Septic superior sagittal sinus thrombosis after oral surgery. J Oral Surg. 1973;31:560–5.
6. Stehbens WE, ed. Pathology of the Cerebral Blood Vessels. St. Louis: CV Mosby; 1972:188–92.
7. Parsons M. Intracranial venous thrombosis. Postgrad Med J. 1967;43:409–14.
8. Pallares R, Santamaria J, Ariza X, et al. Polymicrobial anaerobic septicemia due to lateral sinus thrombophlebitis. J Laryngol Otolaryngol. 1984;98:895–9.
9. Diaz JM, Schiffman JS, Urban ES, et al. Superior sagittal sinus thrombosis and pulmonary embolism: A syndrome rediscovered. Acta Neurol Scand. 1992;86:390–6.
10. DiNubile MJ. Septic thrombosis of the cavernous sinuses. Arch Neurol. 1988;45:567–72.
11. Thatai D, Chandy L, Dhar KL. Septic cavernous sinus thrombophlebitis: A review of 35 cases. J Indian Med Assoc. 1992;90:290–2.
12. Pascarelli E, Lemlich A. Diplopia and photophobia as premonitory symptoms in cavernous sinus thrombosis. Ann Rhinol Laryngol. 1964;73:210–7.
13. Johnston I, Hawke S, Halmagyi M, et al. The pseudotumor syndrome. Disorders of cerebrospinal fluid circulation causing intracranial hypertension without ventriculomegaly. Arch Neurol. 1991;48:740–7.
14. Jahrsdoerfer RA, Fitz-Hugh GS. Lateral sinus thrombosis. South Med J. 1968;61:1271–5.
15. Teichgraeber JF, Per-Lee JH, Turner JS. Lateral sinus thrombosis: A modern perspective. Laryngoscope. 1982;92:744–51.
16. Sze G, Simmon B, Krol G, et al. Dural sinus thrombosis: Verification with spin-echo techniques. AJNR. 1988;9:679–86.
17. Snyder TC, Sachdev HS. MR imaging of dural sinus thrombosis. J Comput Assist Tomogr. 1986;10:889–92.
18. Chakeres DW, Schmalbrock P, Brogan M, et al. Normal venous anatomy of the brain: Demonstration with gadopentetate dimeglumine in enhanced 3-D MR angiography. AJNR. 1990;11:1107–18.
19. Rippe DJ, Boyko OB, Spritzer CE, et al. Demonstration of dural sinus occlusion by the use of MR angiography. AJNR. 1990;11:199–201.
20. Mattle HP, Wentz KU, Edelman RR, et al. Cerebral venography with MR. Radiology. 1991;178:453–8.
21. Munz M, Farmer JP, Auger L, et al. Otitis media and CNS complications. J Otolaryngol. 1992;21:224–6.
22. Medlock MD, Olivero WC, Hanigan WC, et al. Children with cerebral venous thrombosis diagnosed with magnetic resonance imaging and magnetic resonance angiography. Neurosurgery. 1992;31:870–6.
23. Goldberg AL, Rosenbaum AE, Wang H, et al. Computed tomography of dural sinus thrombosis. J Comput Assist Tomogr. 1986;10:16–20.
24. Virapongse C, Cazenave C, Quisling R, et al. The empty delta sign: frequency and significance in 76 cases of dural sinus thrombosis. Radiology. 1987;162:779–85.
25. Shinohara Y, Yoshitoshi M, Yoshii F. Appearance and disappearance of the empty delta sign in superior sagittal sinus thrombosis. Stroke. 1986;17:1282–4.
26. Einhaupl KM, Villringer A, Meister W, et al. Heparin treatment in venous sinus thrombosis. Lancet. 1991;338:597–600.
27. Bousser M-G, Chiras J, Bories J, et al. Cerebral venous thrombosis: A review of 38 cases. Stroke. 1985;16:199–213.
28. Gettelfinger DM, Kokmen E. Superior sagittal sinus thrombosis. Arch Neurol. 1977;34:2–6.
29. DiRocco C, Iannddelli A, Leone G, et al. Heparin-urokinase treatment in aseptic dural venous sinus thrombosis. Arch Neurol. 1981;38:431–5.
30. Alexander LF, Yamamota Y, Ayoubi S, et al. Efficacy of tissue plasminogen activator in the lysis of thrombosis of the cerebral venous sinus. Neurosurgery. 1990;26:559–64.
31. Persson L, Anders L. Extensive dural sinus thrombosis treated by surgical removal and local streptokinase infusion. Neurosurgery. 1990;26:117–21.
32. Kalbag RM, Woolf AL. Cerebral Venous Thrombosis. London: Oxford University Press; 1967:242–3.

SECTION I. SKIN AND SOFT TISSUE INFECTIONS

72. CELLULITIS AND SUBCUTANEOUS TISSUE INFECTIONS

MORTON N. SWARTZ

CELLULITIS AND SUPERFICIAL INFECTIONS

Major attention should be directed to determination of the specific microbial cause of any infection involving the skin. In this chapter, bacterial and mycotic (exclusive of those due to the common dermatophytes) infections are considered. Classification of cutaneous infections on morphologic and clinical grounds can be most helpful in providing initial clues as to the most likely responsible infectious agents (Table 1).

PRIMARY PYODERMAS

Impetigo

Impetigo is an initially vesicular, later crusted, superficial infection of the skin, usually due to group A streptococci. The majority of cases occur in children. Previously, group A streptococcus was considered the principal cause of impetigo and was isolated from about 80 percent of cases, either alone or mixed with *Staphylococcus aureus.*[1] In the past decade, group A streptococcus has been found less commonly (20–30 percent) in impetigo and appears to have been supplanted by *S. aureus* in frequency.[2–4] Occasional studies, however, continue to implicate group A streptococci as a major cause of impetigo.[5] These differences may well reflect geographic shifts in streptococcal hyperendemicity over time. As a cautionary note, the role of staphylococci may be overestimated, since they are common secondary invaders and since some strains appear to produce bacteriocins that may make it more difficult to isolate group A streptococci in their presence.[6]

Pathologic Characteristics and Pathogenesis. Histopathologically, impetigo consists of a superficial, intraepidermal, unilocular vesicopustule. In epidemiologic studies, group A streptococcal acquisition on normal skin antedates the appearance of impetigo by about 10 days.[1] During that time, minor trauma (insect bites, abrasions) predisposes to the development of infected lesions. Impetigo is most common during hot, humid summer weather. Two to three weeks after skin acquisition of streptococci, pharyngeal colonization by the same organism occurs in about 30 percent of the children with skin lesions. (The sporadic cases of facial impetigo occurring in cooler climates probably result from contiguous spread from an initial nasopharyngeal infection, and the serotypes involved are those commonly causing pharyngeal disease.) In contrast, in the cases of staphylococcal impetigo (where *S. aureus* is the only pathogen),

TABLE 1. Classification of Bacterial and Mycotic Infections of the Skin

Type of Lesion	Etiologic Agents
Primary pyodermas	
Impetigo	Group A streptococcus; *S. aureus*
Folliculitis	*S. aureus; Candida; P. aeruginosa; Pityrosporum ovale*
Furuncles and carbuncles	*S. aureus*
Paronychia	*S. aureus;* Group A streptococcus; *Candida; P. aeruginosa*
Ecthyma	Group A streptococcus
Erysipelas	Group A streptococcus
Chancriform lesions	*T. pallidum; H. ducreyi; Sporothrix; B. anthracis; F. tularensis; M. ulcerans; M. marinum*
Membranous ulcers	*Corynebacterium diphtheriae*
Cellulitis	Group A streptococcus; *S. aureus;* rarely, various other organisms
Infectious gangrene and gangrenous cellulitis	
Streptococcal gangrene and necrotizing fasciitis	Group A streptococcus; mixed infections with Enterobacteriaceae and anaerobes
Progressive bacterial synergistic gangrene	Anaerobic streptococci plus a second organism (*S. aureus, Proteus*)
Gangrenous balanitis and perineal phlegmon	Group A streptococcus; mixed infections with enteric bacteria (*E. coli, Klebsiella,* etc.) and anaerobes
Gas gangrene; crepitant cellulitis	*Clostridium perfringens* and other clostridial species; *Bacteroides,* peptostreptococci, *Klebsiella, E. coli*
Gangrenous cellulitis in immunosuppressed patients	*Pseudomonas, Aspergillus,* agents of murcormycosis
Erythrasma	*Corynebacterium minutissimum*
Nodular lesions	*Candida; Sporothrix; S. aureus* (botryomycosis); *M. marinum; Nocardia brasiliensis; Leishmania brasiliensis*
Hyperplastic (pseudoepitheliomatous) and proliferative lesions (mycetomas, etc.)	*Nocardia, Pseudallescheria boydii, Blastomyces dermatitidis; Paracoccidioides brasiliensis; Phialophora; Cladosporum*
Vascular papules/nodules (bacillary angiomatosis, epithelioid angiomatosis)	*Bartonella (Rochalimaea) henselae; Bartonella (Rochalimaea) quintana*
Annular erythema (erythema chronicum migrans)	*B. burgdorferi*
Secondary bacterial infections complicating pre-existing skin lesions such as the following:	
Burns	*P. aeruginosa; Enterobacter;* various other gram-negative bacilli; various streptococci; *S. aureus; Candida; Aspergillus*
Eczematous dermatitis and exfoliative erythrodermas	*S. aureus;* group A streptococcus
Chronic ulcers (varicose, decubitus)	Coliform bacteria; *P. aeruginosa;* peptostreptococci; enterococci, *Bacteroides, C. perfringens*
Dermatophytosis	*S. aureus;* group A streptococcus
Traumatic lesions (abrasions, animal bites, insect bites, etc.)	*P. multocida; C. diphtheriae; S. aureus;* group A streptococcus
Vesicular or bullous eruptions (varicella, pemphigus)	*S. aureus;* group A streptococcus
Acne conglabata	*Propionibacterium acnes*
Hidradenitis suppurativa	*S. aureus, Proteus* and other coliforms, streptococci, peptostreptococci, *Bacteroides*
Intertrigo	*S. aureus,* coliforms, *Candida*
Pilonidal and sebaceous cysts	Peptostreptococci; *Bacteroides;* coliforms
Pyoderma gangrenosa	*S. aureus;* peptostreptococci; *Proteus* and other coliforms; *P. aeruginosa*
Cutaneous involvement in systemic bacterial and mycotic infections	
Bacteremias	*S. aureus;* group A streptococcus (also other groups such as D); *N. meningitidis; N. gonorrhoeae; P. aeruginosa; S. typhi; H. influenzae*
Endocarditis	Viridans streptococci; *S. aureus;* group D streptococci, etc.
Fungemias	*Candida; Cryptococcus; B. dermatitidis; Fusarium*
Listeriosis	*Listeria monocytogenes*
Leptospirosis (Weil's disease and pretibial fever)	*L. interrogans* serotypes
Rat-bite fever	*Streptobacillus moniliformis; Spirillum minus*
Melioidosis	*P. pseudomallei*
Glanders	*P. mallei*
Carrion's disease (verruga peruana)	*Bartonella bacilliformis*
Scarlet fever syndromes	
Scarlet fever	Group A streptococcus; rarely *S. aureus*
Scalded skin syndrome	*S. aureus* (phage group II)
Toxic shock syndrome	*S. aureus* (pyrogenic toxin-producing strains)
Para- and postinfectious nonsuppurative complications	
Purpura fuminans	Group A streptococcus; *S. aureus;* pneumococcus
Erythema nodosum	Group A streptococcus; *M. tuberculosis; M. leprae; C. immitis; L. autumnalis; Y. enterocolitica; L. pneumophila*
Erythema multiforme-like lesions (rarely)	Group A streptococcus

nasal colonization precedes that of the normal skin; skin lesions then follow such colonization.[7,8]

Impetigo is a highly communicable infection. Spread in families (particularly among preschool children) is facilitated by crowding and poor hygiene.

Clinical Findings. Streptococcal impetigo begins as small vesicles, sometimes with narrow inflammatory halos, that rapidly pustulate and readily rupture. The purulent discharge dries, forming the characteristic thick, golden-yellow "stuck-on" crusts. Exposed areas are the most common sites of lesions. Pruritus is common, and scratching of lesions can spread infec-tion. Occasionally, large crusts are produced by coalescence of smaller pustules. The lesions remain superficial and do not ulcerate or infiltrate the dermis. Mild regional lymphadenopathy is common. Healing occurs without scarring. The lesions are painless, and constitutional manifestations are minimal.

Laboratory Findings. Gram-stained smear of vesicles shows gram-positive cocci. Culture of exudate beneath an unroofed crust reveals group A streptococci, *S. aureus,* or a mixture of streptococci and *S. aureus.* The antistreptolysin O (ASLO) titer after streptococcal impetigo is scant, probably related to the inhibition of streptolysin O by skin lipids at the infection site.

In contrast, the anti-DNase B response readily occurs (elevated titers in 90 percent of patients with nephritis complicating streptococcal skin infections).[9]

Etiologic Agents. Group A streptococci responsible for impetigo usually belong to different M serotypes (e.g., 2, 49, 52, 55, 57, 59–61) than the strains producing pharyngitis (e.g., 1, 2, 4, 6, 25). Groups C and G streptococci rarely may cause impetigo; group B streptococci have been associated with impetigo in the newborn.

Differential Diagnosis. Although the initial vesicular lesions may resemble early varicella, the crusts of the latter are darker brown and harder. The central clearing of a confluent cluster of lesions of impetigo may suggest tinea circinata but can be distinguished by the thick crusts that are not formed in the fungus infection. When the vesicles of herpes simplex become turbid, they may look like impetigo.

Presumptive Therapy. Penicillin has been the drug of choice in the treatment of ordinary impetigo because of the role of group A streptococci and the possible occurrence of acute glomerulonephritis as a sequela. Whether penicillin therapy is effective (because of the delay in seeking medical attention for such a mild infection) in reducing the incidence of pyoderma-associated nephritis remains unclear. Penicillin is administered either as a single intramuscular injection of benzathine penicillin (300,000–600,000 units for children; 1,200,000 units for adults), or as oral penicillin V (25,000–90,000 units/kg/day in divided doses every 6 hours for 10 days), or as amoxicillin. Erythromycin (30–50 mg/kg/day in divided doses every 6 hours for 10 days for children; 250–500 mg orally every 6 hours for adults) is an alternative for the penicillin-allergic patient. Local care (removal of crusts by soaking with soap and water) is helpful.

Mixed streptococcal-staphylococcal impetigo has the same crusted lesions and clinical course as streptococcal impetigo and usually respond well to treatment with penicillin G.[10]

A topical antibiotic, mupirocin ointment in a polyethylene glycol base, has been shown to be as effective as oral erythromycin in the treatment of impetigo,[3] and more effective when erythromycin-resistant *S. aureus* strains were involved.[4] With the recent increased frequency of isolation of *S. aureus* from the lesions of patients with impetigo, some physicians favor alternative (but more expensive) approaches such as the use of cephalexin (25–50 mg/kg orally daily for children in two divided doses), cefadroxil (30 mg/kg orally daily for children in two divided doses), or dicloxacillin (12.5 mg/kg orally daily for children in four divided doses).[11] For most patients with nonbullous impetigo, erythromycin (or penicillin), or topical mupirocin, is appropriate therapy, unless problems in the community with erythromycin-resistant organisms are suspected.

Mupirocin has also been used topically to eradicate methicillin-resistant *S. aureus* from secondarily infected skin lesions and from colonized patients. However, since resistance in *S. aureus* strains has emerged sooner than anticipated after its introduction, particularly where long-term therapy has been employed, prolonged use should probably be avoided.

Bullous Impetigo

Clinical Findings. The bullous form of impetigo is due to *S. aureus* of phage group II (usually type 71), occurs principally in the newborn and younger children, and comprises about 10 percent of all cases of impetigo. The lesions begin as vesicles that turn into flaccid bullae, initially containing clear yellow fluid. There is no erythematous areola, and the Nikolsky sign is absent. The bullae quickly rupture, leaving a moist red surface, and then form thin, "varnish-like" light brown crusts. Bullous impetigo, like the "staphylococcal scalded skin syndrome" (SSSS) and the staphylococcal scarlatiniform syndrome, repre-

sents a form of cutaneous response to the two extracellular exfoliative toxins (ET) produced by *S. aureus* of phage group II. The gene for one of the toxins (ETA) is chromosomal in origin and that of the other (ETB) is located on a plasmid[12]; ETA appears to be a serine protease.[13] Staphylococci are regularly isolated from the skin lesions of bullous impetigo. Streptococcal superinfection rarely complicates bullous impetigo, probably because type 71 strains of *S. aureus* produce a bacteriocin that inhibits streptococci. Fever and constitutional symptoms are uncommon. Healing occurs without scarring.

Presumptive Therapy. Extensive bullous impetigo responds to treatment with a penicillinase-resistant penicillin (e.g., in the child, cloxacillin, 12.5–25 mg/kg, or dicloxacillin, 3.125–6.25 mg/kg, in divided doses orally every 6 hours) or erythromycin in the penicillin-allergic patient.

Staphylococcal Scalded Skin Syndrome

SSSS is the most severe manifestation of infection with *S. aureus* strains producing an exfoliative exotoxin and is characterized by widespread bullae and exfoliation.[14–16] Pemphigus neonatorum (Ritter's disease) is the SSSS in the newborn. The more general term *toxic epidermal necrolysis* (TEN) is often used to encompass both SSSS and a morphologically identical syndrome due to various etiologies (drug reactions, viral illnesses) (see Ch. 172).

Clinical Findings. SSSS usually occurs in younger children, but rarely it can develop in adults. Epidemics have occurred in neonatal nurseries.[17] It begins abruptly (sometimes a few days after a recognized staphylococcal infection) with fever, skin tenderness, and a scarlatiniform rash. The Nikolsky sign can be demonstrated. Large, flaccid, clear bullae form and promptly rupture, resulting in the separation of sheets of skin. New bullae appear over 2–3 days. Exfoliation exposes large areas of bright red skin surface (Fig. 1). With appropriate fluid replacement and antimicrobial therapy, the skin lesions heal within 2 weeks, in contrast to drug-induced TEN, where recovery is more prolonged, since the entire epidermis must be replaced, and where scarring is more frequent.

Presumptive Therapy. Intravenous use of a penicillinase-resistant penicillin (e.g., nafcillin, 50–100 mg/kg/day in the newborn, 100–200 mg/kg/day for older children) is indicated in the initial treatment of SSSS because of the presence of active staphylococcal infection and the rapid progression of the skin lesions. Topical treatment consists of cool saline compresses. Systemic corticosteroids alone should not be used in the treatment of SSSS, although they may be indicated in the therapy of drug-induced TEN.

Staphylococcal Scarlet Fever

Staphylococcal scarlet fever is fundamentally a forme fruste of SSSS (due to ET) that does not progress beyond the initial stage of a generalized erythematous eruption. At that stage the rash is indistinguishable from that of scarlet fever, and Pastia's lines can develop. However, pharyngitis is usually not present, and an enanthem does not develop. Desquamation, beginning on the face and involving most of the body, occurs 2–5 days after the onset of the scarlatiniform rash. Antibiotic treatment with penicillinase-resistant penicillins is indicated.

Toxic Shock Syndrome

The toxic shock syndrome (TSS) is another acute febrile illness with a generalized scarlatiniform eruption associated with *S. aureus* infection. Other elements of the syndrome include *(1)* hypotension (or shock), *(2)* functional abnormalities of three or

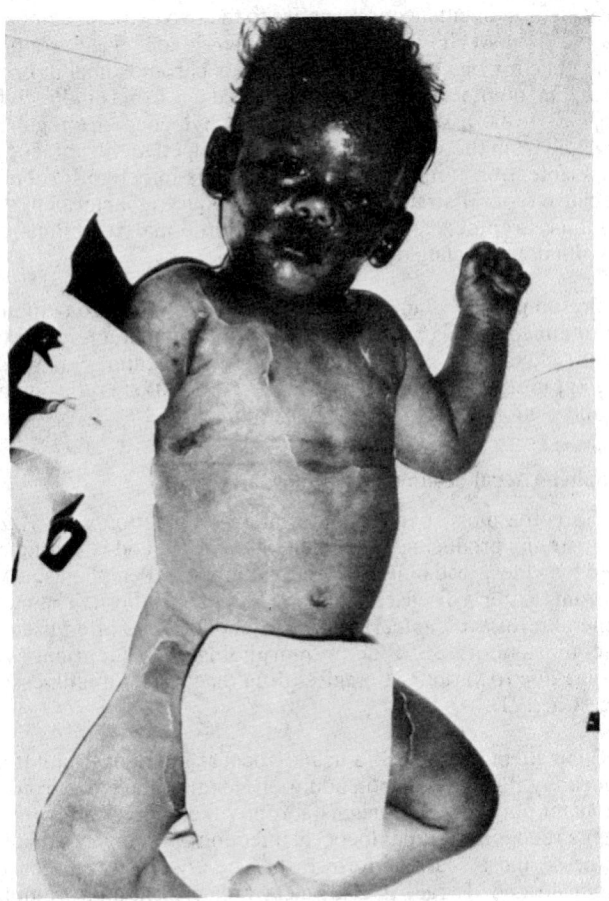

FIG. 1. Staphylococcal scalded skin syndrome in a young infant. Exfoliation has occurred on the face, chest, and groin, exposing areas of bright red skin surface.

more organ systems, and *(3)* desquamation in the evolution of the skin lesions (see Ch. 173).[18-20]

Folliculitis

Folliculitis is a pyoderma located within hair follicles and the apocrine regions. The lesions consist of small (2–5 mm) erythematous, sometimes pruritic, papules often topped by a central pustule. Sycosis barbae is a distinctive form of deep folliculitis, often chronic, occurring on the bearded areas. *Staphylococcus aureus* is the usual etiology of folliculitis. *Pseudomonas aeruginosa* (most often serotype 0-11) has been responsible for folliculitis acquired from swimming pools and whirlpools contaminated with large numbers of these organisms.[21] This type of skin infection produces pruritic papulourticarial lesions (appearing within 48 hours of exposure) that go on to pustule formation. Lesions in different stages of development are present simultaneously. Sites of predilection include the buttocks, hips, and axillae; the palms and soles are spared. Otitis externa is also a common manifestation. Healing occurs spontaneously, either by drainage or regression, within 5 days. Scarring develops rarely when an occasional pustule has progressed to furuncle formation. When acquired in a whirlpool, the lesions are sharply limited to the trunk below the upper chest or neck. Inadequate chlorine levels in whirlpools, hot tubs, and swimming pools have been responsible for many of the reported outbreaks. *Pseudomonas aeruginosa* can also cause superinfection in acne. In granulocytopenic or immunosuppressed hospitalized patients, *P. aeruginosa* 0-11 from tap water used for washing has been implicated in folliculitis that has rapidly progressed to ecthyma gangrenosum.[22]

Folliculitis due to Enterobacteriaceae can occur as a complication in patients with acne, usually during prolonged courses of oral antibiotic therapy.[23]

Candida is sometimes the etiology of folliculitis, producing pruritic satellite lesions surrounding areas of intertriginous candidiasis, particularly in patients on prolonged antibiotic or corticosteroid therapy. *Malassezia furfur,* common skin saprophytes, may also produce a folliculitis with pruritic erythematous papules and papulopustules on the trunk, upper extremities, and face, particularly in the setting of diabetes mellitus, corticosteroid administration, or granulocytopenia.[24,25] These lesions, particularly the early papular nodular ones, may suggest those of systemic candidiasis, a diagnosis that may seem to be supported by the presence of budding yeasts on Gram-stained material from unroofed lesions. Unlike *Candida, M. furfur* requires lipid-supplemented media for primary isolation.

A rare pruritic dermatosis, eosinophilic pustular folliculitis, characterized by recurrent crops of follicular papules and pustules with eosinophilic infiltration of perifollicular dermis, resembles bacterial or mycotic folliculitis but is a sterile process.[26]

Local measures (saline compresses and topical antibacterials or antifungals such as clotrimazole) are usually sufficient to control the infection.

Furuncles and Carbuncles

Definition and Pathologic Characteristics. A furuncle is a deep inflammatory nodule, usually developing from a preceding folliculitis. A carbuncle is a more extensive process extending into the subcutaneous fat in areas covered by thick, inelastic skin. In the latter, multiple abscesses develop, separated by connective tissue septae, and drain to the surface along hair follicles. *Staphylococcus aureus* is almost invariably the etiologic agent (see also Ch. 173).

Clinical Findings. Furuncles occur in skin areas subject to friction and perspiration and containing hair follicles (neck, face, axillae, buttocks). Predisposing factors include obesity, blood dyscrasias, treatment with corticosteroids, defects in neutrophil function, and probably diabetes mellitus. A furuncle begins as a firm, tender, red nodule that soon becomes painful and fluctuant. Spontaneous drainage of pus commonly occurs, and the lesion subsides. A carbuncle is a larger, deeper, indurated, more serious lesion, usually located at the nape of the neck, on the back, or on the thighs. Fever and malaise are frequent, and some patients are acutely ill. As the lesion progresses, drainage occurs externally along the course of multiple hair follicles. A leukocytosis occurs, particularly when the lesion contains a large amount of undrained pus or when there is a complicating cellulitis or bacteremia.

Blood stream invasion may occur unpredictably (but is sometimes precipitated by manipulation of the lesions), resulting in osteomyelitis, endocarditis, or other metastatic foci. Lesions about the upper lip and nose present the special problem of spread of infection via the facial and angular emissary veins to the cavernous sinus.

Presumptive Therapy. Most furuncles are satisfactorily treated by the application of moist heat, which promotes localization and drainage of the process. A carbuncle or a furuncle with surrounding cellulitis and/or fever, or if located about the midface, should be treated with an antistaphylococcal antibiotic (e.g., cloxacillin, 0.5–1.0 g, or dicloxacillin, 0.125–0.25 g orally every 6 hours for an adult). In the penicillin-allergic adult, clindamycin (150–300 mg orally every 6 hours) or erythromycin (0.25–0.5 g orally every 6 hours) are alternatives. If the lesions are large and fluctuant, surgical drainage is indicated. Antibiotic treatment should be continued until evidences of acute inflammation have subsided.

Management of patients with recurrent furunculosis presents

a troublesome problem. This disease does not appear to be due to specific staphylococcal strains with special biologic properties, and most patients do not have definable underlying defects in host defenses. Prophylaxis of recurrent episodes involves several measures:

1. *Antibiotic treatment.* Systemic antibiotic treatment, as described above, should be administered for the most recent episode. Prolonged treatment (2 months) is no more effective than a 10- to 14-day course in preventing recurrences.[27]
2. *General skin care.* Soap and water should be used to reduce the number of *S. aureus* organisms on the body surface, and careful handwashing should be performed after contact with lesions. A separate towel and washcloth (carefully washed in hot water before reuse) should be reserved for the patient. Chlorhexidine solution (4%), an antimicrobial skin cleanser, or hexachlorophene may be used to decrease staphylococcal skin colonization further.
3. *Care of clothing.* Sheets and underclothing should be laundered at high temperatures and should be changed daily for problem patients.
4. *Care of dressings.* Draining lesions should be covered at all times with sterile dressings to prevent autoinoculation, and the dressings should be wrapped and promptly disposed of after removal.

Further measures, aimed at elimination of nasal carriage and subsequent shedding of *S. aureus* (methicillin susceptible or methicillin resistant) onto the skin, may be warranted in management of refractory cases. Intranasal application of a 2% mupirocin calcium ointment in a white, soft paraffin base for 5 days can eliminate *S. aureus* carriage in healthy persons for up to 90 days[28] (bacitracin or neomycin ointments have been used previously for the same purpose). Similarly, prophylaxis with antibiotic ointment (fusidic acid) in the nares twice daily for every fourth week for the patient (along with a perioral antistaphylococcal antimicrobial for 10–14 days for the patient) and family members who are nasal carriers has been used with some success.[27] Oral antibiotics such as rifampin (600 mg daily for 10 days) have been effective in eradicating coagulase-positive staphylococci from the majority of nasal carriers for periods up to 3 months.[29] Such use of rifampin to eliminate nasal carriage of *S. aureus* and interrupt a continuing cycle of recurrent furunculosis might be considered in the patient for whom other measures have failed. However, such therapy can lead to rapid selection of rifampin-resistant strains. The addition of a second drug (cloxacillin if the *S. aureus* is methicillin susceptible; trimethoprim-sulfamethoxazole, ciprofloxacin, or minocycline if the strain is methicillin resistant) has been used to reduce the emergence of rifampin resistance.[30] In one very limited study, prophylaxis with oral clindamycin alone (150 mg daily for 3 months), without an accompanying intranasal antimicrobial agent, reduced the frequency of recurrent staphylococcal skin infections.[31] Various staphylococcal vaccines have not proven effective in preventing recurrent furunculosis.

Ecthyma

Clinical Findings. The lesions of ecthyma begin in a fashion similar to those of impetigo but penetrate through the epidermis. Group A streptococci either produce the lesions de novo or secondarily infect preexisting superficial lesions (insect bites, excoriations), resulting in the same clinical picture.[32] It is important to note that lesions with the same ultimate appearance can be produced in the course of *Pseudomonas* bacteremia (see below). The lesions most frequently occur on the lower extremities, particularly of children and the elderly. They consist of ''punched-out'' ulcers, covered by greenish yellow crusts, extending deeply into the dermis and surrounded by raised violaceous margins. Treatment is the same as for impetigo. Very extensive involvement with complicating bacteremia has oc-

curred in a patient with the acquired immunodeficiency syndrome (AIDS).[33]

Chancriform Lesions

A variety of infections, often with systemic consequences, are characterized by an initial chancriform lesion (Table 1). Of the nonvenereal infections, anthrax has one of the most prominent chancriform lesions.

Anthrax. See Chapter 186 for a detailed discussion.

PATHOGENESIS. Anthrax is a very rare disease in the United States. Infections are limited to persons working with raw imported wool and other animal products contaminated with highly resistant spores of *Bacillus anthracis*. Routine safety measures for employees in wool plants and so forth virtually have eliminated anthrax from this group; sporadic cases still occur in transient workers in factories (e.g., ventilation repairmen) and in persons directly importing wool for their own weaving. Most infections occur on the face, neck, or arms in an area of a minor abrasion. Rarely, pulmonary infection follows inhalation of *B. anthracis*, or intestinal anthrax results from ingestion of the organism.

CLINICAL FINDINGS. After an incubation period of 1–3 days, a painless papule develops on an exposed area. The lesion enlarges, vesiculates (''malignant pustule''), and is surrounded by a wide zone of brawny, erythematous, gelatinous, nonpitting edema.[34,35] Malaise and low-grade fever are present. As the lesion evolves, the vesicle becomes hemorrhagic, necrotic, and covered by an eschar of variable dimensions (Fig. 2). At all stages the lesion remains painless. Bacteremic dissemination of infection from a skin site may occur, accompanied by high fever and hypotension. Meningitis may complicate either such a bacteremic infection or primary pulmonary anthrax.

The epidemiologic background and the striking appearance of extensive gelatinous edema serve to distinguish anthrax from other types of chancriform lesion. A staphylococcal pustule or carbuncle with a necrotic eschar may be mistaken for early anthrax. However, the former is very painful and tender, and the etiologic agent can usually be demonstrated on a Gram-stained smear of material from the lesion.

PRESUMPTIVE TREATMENT. Incision and débridement should be avoided, since they increase the likelihood of bacteremia. Parenteral penicillin G (1 million units every 4–6 hours) is used. In the penicillin-allergic patient, tetracycline (1.0–2.0 g/day intravenously in the adult) is an alternative.

Erysipelas

Erysipelas is a distinctive type of superficial cellulitis of the skin with prominent lymphatic involvement. It is almost always due

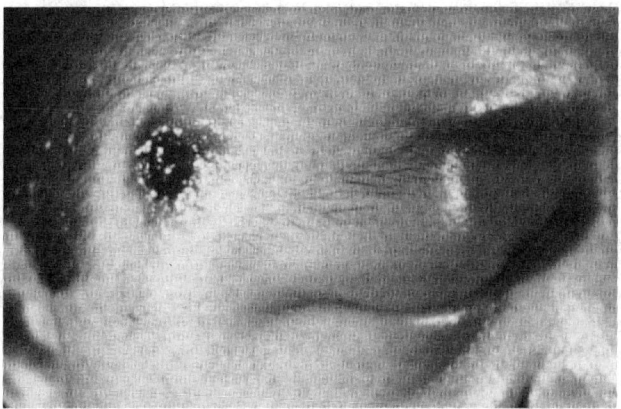

FIG. 2. Chancriform lesion of anthrax on the forehead. There is a prominent surrounding zone of gelatinous edema that is most evident on the eyelids. (Courtesy of Dr. Louis Weinstein, Boston, MA.)

to group A streptococci (uncommonly, group C or G). Group B streptococci have produced erysipelas in the newborn. Evidence of streptococcal infections (groups A, G, and C) was found in 26 of 27 patients with clinical erysipelas, utilizing the combination of direct immunofluorescence and cultures of punch biopsy specimens along with serologic titers.[36] Very rarely, a similar skin lesion is caused by *S. aureus.*

Clinical Findings. Erysipelas is more common in infants, young children, and older adults. Formerly, the face was most commonly involved, and an antecedent streptococcal respiratory tract infection preceded cutaneous involvement in about one-third of patients even though streptococci might not be found on culture at the time the skin lesion became evident. Now the localization of erysipelas has changes: 70–80 percent of the lesions are on the lower extremities and 5–20 percent are on the face.[37] Portals of entry are commonly skin ulcers, local trauma or abrasions, psoriatic or eczematous lesions, or fungal infections; in the neonate, erysipelas may develop from an infection of the umbilical stump. Predisposing factors include venous stasis, paraparesis, diabetes mellitus, and alcohol abuse. Patients with the nephrotic syndrome are particularly susceptible. Erysipelas tends to occur in areas of preexisting lymphatic obstruction or edema (e.g., after a radical mastectomy). Also, because erysipelas itself produces lymphatic obstruction, it tends to recur in an area of earlier infection. Over a 3-year period, the recurrence rate is about 30 percent,[37] predominantly in individuals with venous insufficiency or lymphedema.

Streptococcal bacteremia occurs in about 5 percent of patients with erysipelas; group A, C, or G streptococci can be isolated on throat culture from about 20 percent of cases.[37]

Erysipelas is a painful lesion with a bright red, edematous, indurated (''peau d'orange'') appearance and an advancing, raised border that is sharply demarcated from the adjacent normal skin (Fig. 3). Fever is a feature. A common form of erysipelas involves the bridge of the nose and the cheeks. Uncomplicated erysipelas remains confined primarily to the lymphatics and the dermis. Occasionally, the infection extends more deeply, producing cellulitis, subcutaneous abscess, and necrotizing fasciitis.

A leukocytosis is common with erysipelas. Group A streptococci usually cannot be cultured from the surface of the skin lesion, and only rarely can they be isolated from tissue fluid aspirated from the advancing edge of the lesion. In cases of erysipelas complicating infected ulcers, group A streptococci have been isolated from the ulcerated area in 30 percent of patients.[37]

Differential Diagnosis. The diagnosis is made on the basis of the appearance of the lesion and the clinical setting. Early herpes zoster involving the second division of the fifth cranial nerve may resemble unilateral facial erysipelas but can be distinguished by the pain and hyperesthesia preceding the skin lesions. Occasionally contact dermatitis or giant urticaria may look like erysipelas but can be distinguished by the absence of fever and the presence of pruritus. Lesions closely resembling erysipelas, but apparently not due to streptococcal infection, may occur recurrently in patients with familial Mediterranean fever. Diffuse inflammatory carcinoma of the breast may mimic a low-grade erysipelas. Erythema chronicum migrans, the cutaneous lesion of Lyme disease, resembles erysipelas but is not painful and progresses much more slowly, and the associated fever is less marked. An erysipelaslike skin lesion has occurred in several patients with hypogammaglobulinemia and *Campylobacter jejuni* bacteremia.[39]

Presumptive Therapy. Mild early cases of erysipelas in the adult may be treated with intramuscular procaine penicillin (600,000 units once or twice daily) or with oral penicillin V (250–500 mg every 6 hours). Erythromycin (250–500 mg orally

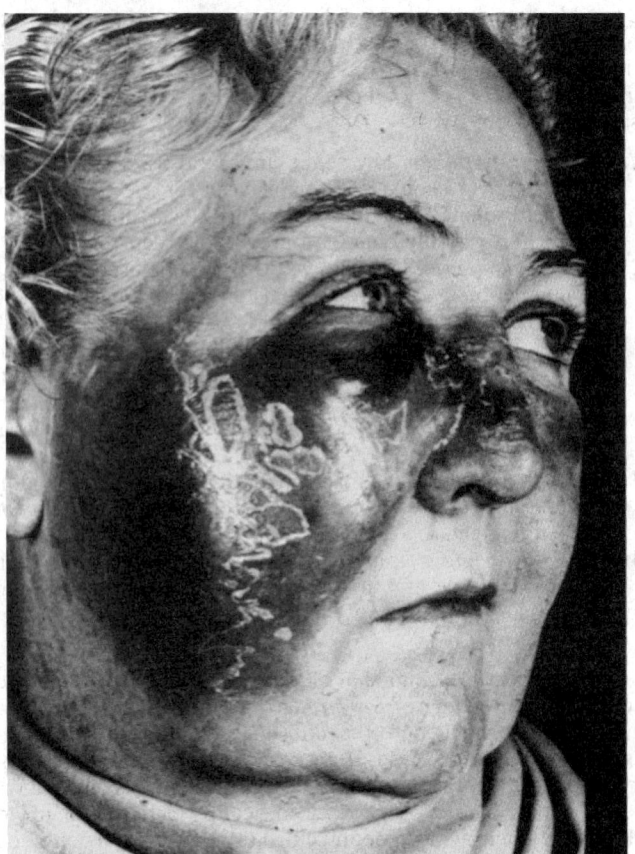

FIG. 3.   Facial erysipelas involving both cheeks and the bridge of the nose. The sharp demarcation between the bright red area of erythema and the normal surrounding skin is evident. (From Fitzpatrick et al.,[38] with permission.)

every 6 hours) is a suitable alternative. For more extensive erysipelas, patients should be hospitalized and receive parenteral aqueous penicillin G (600,000–2,000,000 units every 6 hours).

Cellulitis

Cellulitis is an acute spreading infection of the skin extending deeper than erysipelas to involve the subcutaneous tissues. Group A streptococcus or *S. aureus* is most frequently the etiologic agent.

Clinical Findings. Previous trauma (laceration, puncture wound) or an underlying skin lesion (furuncle, ulcer) predisposes to the development of cellulitis; rarely, the latter may result from blood-borne spread of infection to the skin and subcutaneous tissues. Within several days of the inciting trauma, local tenderness, pain, and erythema develop and rapidly intensify. Malaise, fever, and chills develop. The involved area is often extensive and the lesion is very red, hot, and swollen. In contrast to erysipelas, the borders of an area of cellulitis are not elevated and sharply demarcated. Regional lymphadenopathy is common, and bacteremia can occur. Local abscesses may develop; small patches of overlying skin may subsequently undergo necrosis. Superinfection with gram-negative bacilli may supervene.

Cellulitis due to group A streptococci may occur as a postoperative wound infection. Although uncommon today, it is particularly noteworthy because of the rapidity with which it can spread and invade the blood stream. Such infection may manifest itself within 6–48 hours of surgery (comparable to the short incubation period of postoperative clostridial myonecrosis), earlier than the usual postoperative staphylococcal infection, which is not evident for at least several days after operation. Hypotension, often due to bacteremia, may be the initial sign of infection before significant erythema is evident about the incision. A thin serous discharge may be expressed on compression of the wound margins, and streptococci can be identified on a Gram-stained smear.

Cellulitis is a serious disease because of the propensity of infection to spread via the lymphatics and blood stream. Cellulitis of the lower extremities in older patients may be complicated by thrombophlebitis. In patients with chronic dependent edema, cellulitis may spread extremely rapidly.

A distinctive (by virtue of the clinical setting) form of cellulitis occurs in the lower extremities of patients whose saphenous veins have been removed for coronary artery bypass surgery.[40] Occasionally, an associated lymphangitis is present. In some patients, episodes of cellulitis are recurrent. Systemic manifestations such as chills, high fever, and toxicity are prominent. The area of cellulitis extends along the course of the saphenous venectomy. Edema, erythema, and tenderness are marked. Occasionally, the involved areas are somewhat similar to those of erysipelas ("pseudoerysipelas"). Although the bacterial etiology has not been defined in most cases, the available isolates from involved skin or blood implicate non-group A β-hemolytic streptococci (groups C, G, B) as major etiologies.[41] The portal of entry of the infection is often an associated area of tinea pedis. The combination of compromised lymphatic drainage and minor venous insufficiency secondary to saphenous venectomy may result in lower leg edema, a favorable setting for cellulitis. The inflammation from an initial episode of cellulitis, erysipelas, or lymphangitis obstructs lymphatic drainage, thus enhancing the predisposition to further episodes of infections.

Similar recurrent episodes of cellulitis or pseudoerysipelas due to groups B and G streptococci have occurred in patients with lower extremity lymphedema secondary to radical pelvic surgery, radiation therapy, or neoplastic involvement of pelvic lymph nodes.[42] Typically, the cellulitis involves the vulva, inguinal areas, and both lower extremities. In this setting, recurrent episodes have occurred in association with recent coitus.[33]

An uncommon but distinctive form of cellulitis, perianal streptococcal (group A) cellulitis, occurs principally in children.[44] The clinical features consist of intense perianal erythema, pain on defecation, blood-streaked stools from anal fissures, and chronicity (months) if not treated with penicillin.

A rare but particularly troublesome, chronic, and progressive form of cellulitis, known as *dissecting cellulitis of the scalp* or *perifolliculitis capitis,* is probably similar to hydradenitis suppurativa and acne conglobata in pathogenesis. The clinical features consist of recurrent painful, fluctuant dermal and subcutaneous nodules, purulent drainage from burrowing interconnecting abscesses, scarring, and alopecia. The pathogenesis, as in hydradenitis suppurativa, is probably related to follicular plugging, secondary infection, and deep dissecting inflammation. *Staphylococcus aureus* is most commonly isolated. Effective treatment has involved wide excision and skin grafting.[45]

Lymphatic cutaneous metastases from neoplasms, particularly adenocarcinoma, may produce a localized, edematous, erythematous lesion resembling cellulitis. Inflammatory carcinoma of the breast, carcinoma erysipeloides, involves the skin overlying the site of the primary tumor.

A polymorphonuclear leukocytosis is usually present, regardless of the bacterial etiology.

Etiologic Agents. Group A streptococci and *S. aureus* are responsible for the overwhelming majority of cases of cellulitis, but other organisms may be involved occasionally. Streptococci belonging to other groups (group C, group G, and, in neonates particularly, group B) are sometimes the etiologic agents.

Erysipelothrix rhusiopathiae is the etiologic agent of erysipe-

loid, a cellulitis occurring principally in persons handling saltwater fish, shellfish, poultry, meat, and hides (see Ch. 188). The infection, usually occurring in the summer, is introduced through an abrasion on the hands. A painful violaceous area appears within 1 week of the injury. As the process spreads peripherally with distinct raised borders, the central portion of the lesion clears. Ulceration is not a feature. Occasionally an adjacent joint is involved, and, rarely, bacteremia and endocarditis may follow. The causative organism is generally not observed on Gram-stained drainage from the lesion but may be isolated on culture of a biopsy specimen taken from the advancing margin of the lesion. The development of a typical lesion in a person handling fish or meat products suggests the diagnosis. Other forms of bacterial cellulitis or erysipelas may resemble erysipeloid, particularly when the lesion is on the hand. A somewhat similar lesion of unknown etiology, "seal finger," occurs in aquarium workers and veterinarians secondary to seal bites or trauma sustained in caring for these animals. While penicillin is the antibiotic of choice in the treatment of erysipeloid, it appears that seal finger responds to tetracycline.[46]

Rare cases of pneumococcal cellulitis acquired through the bacteremic route have been reported.[47] Soft tissue infections due to the pneumococcus can bear a striking resemblance to streptococcal erysipelas. A variety of bacteria (*Serratia, Proteus,* and other Enterobacteriaceae) and fungi (*Cryptococcus neoformans*)[48] that are not the cause of cellulitis in normal individuals may produce cellulitis in the immunocompromised or granulocytopenic patient. *Legionella* spp. have very rarely produced cellulitis: *L. pneumophila* in association with pneumonia[49] and *L. micdadei* in a renal transplant recipient.[50] Spontaneous *Escherichia coli* cellulitis occurs in children with the nephrotic syndrome in relapse.[51]

An environmental gram-negative bacillus, *Aeromonas hydrophila,* found particularly in lakes, rivers, and soil, may produce an acute cellulitis after introduction of the organism through a laceration acquired during swimming in fresh water.[52]

Cellulitis, bullous lesions, or necrotic ulcers may complicate infection of a traumatic wound sustained in salt water (or brackish inland waters) or exposed to drippings from raw seafood. Such infections, due to *Vibrio* spp. (primarily *V. vulnificus,* but also, occasionally, *V. alginolyticus,* nonserogroup 01 *V. cholerae,* and *V. parahaemolyticus*) can result in bacteremia and progress to necrosis, requiring extensive surgical débridement.[53,54] A rapidly progressive primary septicemia due to *V. vulnificus* may follow entry of the organism through the gastrointestinal tract (e.g., consumption of raw oysters) rather than through abraded skin. Cellulitis with hemorrhagic skin bullae often rapidly follows the bacteremia. Particularly at risk for the septicemic form of disease are patients with alcoholic cirrhosis, hemochromatosis, and thalassemia—presumably as a result of enhanced growth of *V. vulnificus* mediated by these processes with enhanced iron storage.[55] These vibrios are generally susceptible in vitro to tetracyclines, chloramphenicol, the aminoglycosides, and third-generation cephalosporins. Tetracyclines have been considered the treatment for *V. vulnificus* infections, although use of the combination of a third-generation cephalosporin plus an aminoglycoside has been advocated.[54]

Envenomation following puncture wounds by the spines of a stonefish (indigenous to shallow waters of the South Pacific) produces local edema and erythema that may suggest acute bacterial cellulitis acquired in seawater.[56] This may be accompanied by serious systemic toxicity, including acute pulmonary edema.

Although needle aspiration of the lesion of erysipelas is commonly unsuccessful in providing a bacteriologic diagnosis (by Gram stain or culture), it is sometimes helpful in defining the pathogen in cases of cellulitis. Using aspirates from the advancing edge of cellulitis, skin biopsy, and blood cultures, potential pathogens are isolated in only about 25 percent of patients.[57] Positive cultures can be obtained from 30 percent of closed lesions of cellulitis by use of a fine-needle aspiration technique.[58]

In view of the overall limited yield of pathogens on aspiration of areas of cellulitis, it is reasonable to employ this technique primarily when unusual pathogens are suspected (e.g., in immunocompromised patients), when fluctuant areas are detected, or when initial antimicrobial therapy has been unsuccessful.[59] When a site of origin (abrasion, ulcer) for the infection is present, isolates of potential pathogens (*S. aureus,* group A streptococci) can be obtained in about one-third of cases.

The appearance and clinical features of a noninfectious process, eosinophilic cellulitis, may suggest the appearance of bacterial cellulitis on the extremities or trunk.[60] The involved area is moderately erythematous and edematous. The lesion develops rapidly, is often accompanied by fever, and enlarges over several days. It can be distinguished from the usual bacterial cellulitis by its minimal tenderness, lack of local heat, and its failure to respond to antibiotics. Biopsy of the early lesion shows marked infiltration of the dermis with eosinophils. The lesions resolve in several weeks but frequently recur.

Presumptive Therapy.   If a mild early cellulitis is suspected to be of streptococcal etiology, it may be treated with an initial injection of aqueous penicillin G (600,000 units) followed by intramuscular procaine penicillin (600,000 units every 8–12 hours). When staphylococcal infection is suspected, or when there are no initial clues to the etiology, a penicillinase-resistant penicillin (e.g., cloxacillin, 0.5–1.0 g, or dicloxacillin, 0.25–0.5 g, orally every 6 hours) should be used. In adults allergic to penicillin, erythromycin (0.5 g orally every 6 hours) is an alternative. For more severe infections where both streptococcal and staphylococcal etiologies are considered, parenteral administration of a penicillinase-resistant penicillin (e.g., nafcillin, 1.0–1.5 g intravenously every 4 hours) should be used. Vancomycin (1.0–1.5 g/day intravenously) is an alternative for the highly penicillin-allergic patient. If the clinical setting suggests a gram-negative bacillus as a possible etiology of a serious cellulitis, an aminoglycoside such as gentamicin may be added to the semisynthetic penicillin initially while awaiting definitive bacteriologic results. In the setting of diabetes mellitus and a diabetic leg ulcer, the development of cellulitis may warrant broader initial antimicrobial coverage such as with a parenteral cephalosporin (cefazolin or cefoxitin) plus an aminoglycoside, or with a combination of clindamycin and an aminoglycoside. Gentamicin, along with a penicillinase-resistant penicillin, is probably indicated in the initial treatment of a rapidly progressive cellulitis developing after a freshwater injury. *Aeromonas hydrophila* is usually susceptible to gentamicin, chloramphenicol, trimethoprim-sulfamethoxazole, ciprofloxacin, and aztreonam (tetracycline to a slightly lesser degree).

Initial local care of cellulitis includes immobilization and elevation of the involved limb to reduce swelling and cool sterile saline dressing to decrease local pain. Subsequently, application of moist heat may aid in localization of the infection in those cases in which suggestive signs of fluctuation develop, indicating early abscess formation.

Patients with cellulitis at the saphenous site after coronary bypass surgery who have fungal infection in the interdigital spaces should be treated topically for the latter with miconazole or clotrimazole. The initial antibiotic (penicillin or nafcillin) should be given in high dosage by the intravenous route for 6–7 days to ensure prompt resolution before switching to other routes of therapy. Attention to the problem of tinea pedis before bypass surgery can prevent this form of cellulitis. Similar prompt attention to pedal epidermophytosis in patients who have had one such episode of cellulitis can obviate subsequent episodes.

Recurrent episodes of cellulitis usually occur in patients with peripheral edema. The use of support stockings and good skin hygiene can reduce its frequency or eliminate recurrences. In the occasional patient who continues to have frequent episodes of cellulitis or erysipelas despite such measures, prophylactic penicillin G (250–500 mg orally twice daily) or erythromycin (250 mg orally once or twice daily) if penicillin allergic, may be indicated.[61]

Membranous Ulcers

Infected ulcers of varied or mixed bacterial etiology may be covered at their base by a layer of necrotic debris resembling a membrane. The latter usually is not strongly adherent and can be removed without much difficulty. In addition, such a lesion has abundant purulent drainage attributable to infection with pyogenic bacteria. Membrane-covered lesions (both superficial and deep ulcers) also are produced by cutaneous infection with *Corynebacterium diphtheriae.*

Cutaneous Diphtheria.   Cutaneous diphtheria (see Ch. 183) is uncommon in developed countries; most cases occur in unimmunized persons in overcrowded, underdeveloped parts of the world, particularly in tropical areas, and are associated with skin trauma and poor hygiene. Recent increases in cutaneous diphtheria have been noted in the Pacific Northwest and the South.

CLINICAL FINDINGS.   Three types of cutaneous lesions have been described in cutaneous diphtheria: *(1) Wound diphtheria*—secondary infection with *C. diphtheriae* of a preexisting wound, which becomes partially covered by a membrane and encircled by a zone of erythema; *(2) primary cutaneous diphtheria*—a disease of the tropics, which begins as a single or several pustules, usually on a lower extremity, and progresses to form a punched-out ulcer covered by a gray-brown membrane; and *(3) superinfection of exzematized skin lesions*—a superficial membranous infection; *C. diphtheriae* also have been isolated from lesions resembling impetigo, ecthyma, and infected insect bites, where they may represent true infections or merely a cutaneous carrier state.[62] Cutaneous diphtheria may be as contagious as the respiratory form of the disease among school children.

Occasionally, membranous pharyngitis may accompany cutaneous diphtheria. However, 20–40 percent of the patients with cutaneous diphtheria carry *C. diphtheriae* in their upper respiratory tract.[62,63] Myocarditis is extremely rare as a complication of cutaneous diphtheria, but cranial nerve palsies and Guillain-Barré syndrome occur in 3–5 percent of the patients with membranous diphtheritic skin ulcers.

LABORATORY FINDINGS.   Characteristic beaded, metachromatically staining bacilli can be found in methylene blue-stained smears of the edge of the membrane. However, the diagnosis can be established only by isolation of *C. diphtheriae* from a suggestive skin lesion. Selective media (Loeffler's or tellurite agar) are necessary for isolation in order to inhibit other bacteria in skin ulcers. In addition to isolation of the organism, toxigenicity should be demonstrated by an Elek plate (agar diffusion precipitin reaction) or by guinea pig inoculation (dermonecrosis).

DIFFERENTIAL DIAGNOSIS.   Pyogenic infection of ulcerated traumatic lesions is usually purulent, and the lesions are not covered by a membrane. Cutaneous fungal infections have more proliferative and irregular margins. The early stages of primary cutaneous diphtheria and of secondary infection of insect bites and abrasions with *C. diphtheriae* may closely resemble impetigo.

PRESUMPTIVE THERAPY.   If a presumptive diagnosis of ulcerative cutaneous diphtheria is made on clinical grounds and on the basis of preliminary bacteriologic findings, antitoxin is administered (20,000–40,000 units intramuscularly or intravenously) after testing for sensitivity to horse serum. Antibiotic administration (erythromycin, 2.0 g/day orally, or procaine penicillin, 1.2–2.4 million units/day intramuscularly in the adult for 7–10 days) also assists elimination of the convalescent carrier state. Removal of necrotic debris aids in healing of the lesions.

Infectious Gangrene (Gangrenous Cellulitis)

Infectious gangrene is a cellulitis that has rapidly progressed, with extensive necrosis of subcutaneous tissues and overlying skin. Several different clinically distinguishable pictures may be produced, depending to varying extents on the specific causative organism, the anatomic location of the infection, and the predisposing conditions. Such clinical entities include *(1)* necrotizing fasciitis (streptococcal gangrene), *(2)* gas gangrene (clostridial myonecrosis) and anaerobic cellulitis, *(3)* progressive bacterial synergistic gangrene, *(4)* synergistic necrotizing cellulitis (perineal phlegmon) and gangrenous balanitis, *(5)* gangrenous cellulitis in the immunosuppressed patient, and *(6)* very localized areas of skin necrosis complicating conventional cellulitis.

Pathologic Characteristics and Pathogenesis. The pathologic changes of gangrenous cellulitis are those of necrosis and some hemorrhage in skin and subcutaneous tissues. In most types of gangrenous cellulitis an abundant polymorphonuclear leukocytic exudate is present, but in clostridial myonecrosis the exudate is thin, consisting of fluid, fibrin, and gas, but with few leukocytes. In most types of gangrenous cellulitis (particularly streptococcal gangrene), fibrin thrombi are present in small arteries and veins of the dermis and subcutaneous fat.[64] In most instances, gangrenous cellulitis has developed secondary to introduction of the infecting organism at the infected site. It also may result from extension of infection from a deeper site to involve the subcutaneous tissues and skin (as in clostridial myonecrosis after intestinal surgery or in perineal phlegmon after dissection of infection from a perirectal abscess). Occasionally, gangrenous cellulitis may begin at a site of metastatic infection in the course of a bacteremia (clostridial myonecrosis due to *Clostridium septicum* at a peripheral site secondary to spread from an associated colonic neoplasm; *Pseudomonas* gangrenous cellulitis).

Clinical Findings. STREPTOCOCCAL GANGRENE. This is a rare form of gangrene, due to group A (or C or G) streptococci, which usually develops at a site of trauma on an extremity but may occur in the absence of an obvious portal of entry. The lesion begins as a local painful area of erythema and edema. Over the next 1–3 days the skin becomes dusky. Bullae containing yellowish to red-black fluid develop and rupture.[65] The lesion evolves into a sharply demarcated area covered by a necrotic eschar and surrounded by a border of erythema. The process at this point resembles a third-degree burn, for which it could be mistaken if a history were not available. Lymphangitis is rarely evident. Extensive necrotic sloughs can result because of deep penetration of the infection along fascial planes. Bacteremia, metastatic abscesses, and death may result from this life-threatening illness if appropriate antibiotic therapy is not initiated promptly. Secondary thrombophlebitis may be a complication when the lower extremities are involved. Streptococci can usually be cultured from the early bullous lesions and frequently from the blood.

PROGRESSIVE BACTERIAL SYNERGISTIC GANGRENE. This distinctive lesion usually follows infection at an abdominal operative wound site (frequently when wire sutures have been used), about an ileostomy or colostomy, at the exit of a fistulous tract, or in proximity to a chronic ulceration on an extremity.[66,67] It begins as a local tender area of swelling and erythema that subsequently ulcerates. The painful, shaggy ulcer gradually enlarges and is characteristically encircled by a margin of gangrenous skin (Fig. 4). Surrounding the latter is a violaceous zone that fades into an outer pink edematous border area. If untreated, the process extends slowly but relentlessly, ultimately producing an enormous ulceration. A related lesion, Meleney's ulcer, is essentially bacterial synergistic gangrene with the additional feature of burrowing necrotic tracts through tissue planes emerging at distant skin sites.

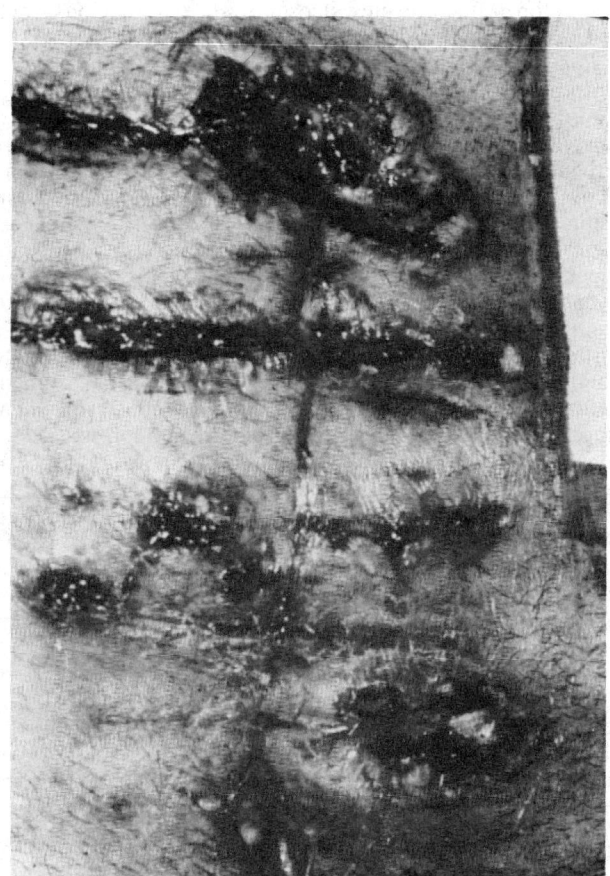

FIG. 4. Progressive bacterial synergistic gangrene of the abdominal wall. Ulcerated areas had developed about wire stay sutures that have since been removed. (From Bornstein et al.,[105] with permission.)

Microaerophilic or anaerobic streptococci can be recovered from aspirates of the advancing margin of the lesion, and *S. aureus* (or occasionally *Proteus* or other gram-negative bacilli) are present in the ulcerated area. Meleney has reproduced the same type of lesions by injecting both microaerophilic streptococci and *S. aureus* (but not either alone) into the skin of experimental animals. The similarity between the appearance of Meleney's progressive bacterial synergistic gangrene and amebic *(Entamoeba histolytica)* skin gangrene, as well as the usual occurrence of both processes at abdominal or thoracic operative wound sites, has led to the suggestion that *E. histolytica* is the principal cause of Meleney's gangrene.[68] However, the development of the latter following gynecologic surgery and its occurrence in countries where amebic infections are rare argue against this concept of pathogenesis. Nonetheless, the capacity of amebic infection to involve the skin of the abdominal wall in a gangrenous process following abdominal surgery should not be overlooked[69]; and appropriate measures (stool examination for amebae, serologic tests, periodic acid-Schiff stain of scrapings, or biopsy of the lesion) should be undertaken to exclude this diagnosis.

GAS GANGRENE, ANAEROBIC CELLULITIS, AND OTHER FORMS OF CREPITANT CELLULITIS. See Chapters 73 and 224.

GANGRENOUS CELLULITIS IN THE PREDISPOSED HOST. The etiologic considerations in cellulitis occurring in the compromised host include agents that produce such infections in healthy persons, as well as a variety of other organisms not ordinarily regarded as causes of cellulitis. Mucormycotic gangrenous cellulitis may be engrafted on an extensive burn wound, or it may develop rarely in patients with diabetes mellitus or in those who are receiving immunosuppressive therapy. Local factors (open fracture sites, ileostomy stomas, fistulous tracts) also play a predisposing role in this type of infection. Spores of *Rhizopus* spp. (members of the Mucoraceae) contaminating Elastoplast tape used for occlusive dressings have resulted in progressive local and disseminated infection in immunosuppressed patients.[70] The infection may exhibit an indolent course with minimal fever and a slowly enlarging black ulcer, or it may follow a rapidly progressive febrile course. The characteristic lesion consists of a central anesthetic black necrotic area with a surrounding raised zone of violaceous cellulitis and edema.[71] Superficial vesicles may occur in the gangrenous area. Hematogenous dissemination is not ordinarily demonstrable, and the skin infection usually does not result from an initial pulmonary or rhinocerebral focus. Cultures of the necrotic skin or aspirates from the advancing margin usually do not reveal the fungus. Definition of the etiology is best obtained on biopsy specimens: fungal wet mount on a crushed tissue preparation, tissue sections stained with hematoxylin and eosin (showing tissue and vascular invasion by characteristic broad hyphae), and culture.

Pseudomonas bacteremia may also produce a gangrenous cellulitis (see the section on "Cutaneous Involvement in Systemic Bacterial and Mycotic Infections" later in this chapter) in immunocompromised hosts, patients with thermal burns, and so forth. In similar settings, gangrenous skin lesions may occur with disseminated aspergillosis.

Prominent necrosis of skin and subcutaneous fat occurs rarely in patients who have chronic renal failure (with secondary hyperparathyroidism), are on chronic dialysis, have extensive calcification of small arteries of subcutaneous tissue, and in whom the calcium-phosphate product is markedly elevated.[72] The process that results in acute local calcification has been termed *calciphylaxis*.[73] Precipitating factors for development of calci-

phylaxis are poorly defined but include local trauma and systemic infection. The skin lesions begin as dark red irregular areas, resembling livido reticularis. They become plaque-like or nodular, are painful, and rapidly increase in size but remain well demarcated. They progress to gangrenous necrosis with eschar formation. Secondary infection of the necrotic areas may follow. Histologically, involved areas show extensive vascular calcification, calcinosis cutis, and ischemic skin necrosis. Bacteremia, originating elsewhere, may contribute to the local ischemic process through further lesional thromboses mediated by DIC. These necrotic skin ulcers in patients with chronic renal failure resemble those of infective gangrenous cellulitis, particularly if they become secondarily infected.

Differential Diagnosis. See Table 2. The bite of the brown recluse house spider can produce a necrotizing skin lesion that resembles infectious gangrenous cellulitis. The occurrence of fever and chills 24–48 hours after the bite enhances the mimicry.

Presumptive Therapy. Treatment of streptococcal gangrene consists of immediate surgical drainage with longitudinal incisions extending through the deep fascia and beyond the involved gangrenous and undermined areas.[65] Initial resuscitation measures with intravenous fluids are essential in the presence of hypotension due to accompanying streptococcal bacteremia or the streptococcal toxic shock-like syndrome.[74] Areas of cutaneous necrosis are excised and nonviable fascia is débrided. Reexploration is commonly performed within 24 hours. Antibiotic therapy consists of parenteral aqueous penicillin G (600,000–2,000,000 units every 4–6 hours). If there is any question as to the etiologic agent (e.g., possibly *S. aureus* rather than group A streptococcus), then nafcillin (1.5–2.0 g intravenously

TABLE 2. Differential Diagnosis of Infectious Gangrene and Gangrenous Cellulitis

	Progressive Bacterial Synergistic Gangrene	Synergistic Necrotizing Cellulitis	Streptococcal Gangrene	Clostridial Myonecrosis (Gas Gangrene)	Necrotizing Cutaneous Mucormycosis	Bacteremic Pseudomonas Gangrenous Cellulitis	Pyoderma Gangrenosum
Predisposing conditions	Surgery; draining sinus	Diabetes common	Occasionally diabetes or myxedema; after abdominal surgery	Local trauma	Diabetes; corticosteroid therapy	Burns, immunosuppression	Ulcerative colitis; rheumatoid arthritis
Pain	Prominent	Prominent	Prominent	Prominent	Minimal	Mild	Moderate
Systemic toxicity	Minimal	Marked	Marked	Very marked	Variable	Marked	Minimal
Course	Slow	Rapid	Very rapid	Extremely rapid	Rapid	Rapid	Slow
Fever	Minimal or absent	Moderate	High	Moderate or high	Low grade	High	Low grade
Anesthesia of lesion	–	–	±	–	+	±	–
Crepitus	–	Often present	–	+	–	–	–
Appearance of the involved area	Central shaggy, necrotic ulcer surrounded by dusky margin and erythematous periphery	Crepitant cellulitis; thick, copious, foul-smelling "dishwater" drainage from scattered areas of skin necrosis	Necrosis of subcutaneous tissue and fascia; black necrotic "burned" appearance of overlying skin	Marked swelling; yellow-bronzed discoloration of skin; brown bullae; green-black patches of necrosis; serosanguineous discharge	Usually a central black necrotic area with purple raised margin; also may present as just a black ulcer	A sharply demarcated necrotic area with black eschar and surrounding erythema, resembling a decubitus ulcer; may evolve from initial hemorrhagic bulla	Begin as bullae, pustules, or erythematous nodules that ulcerate deeply; often multiple, large and coalesce; usually on lower extremities or abdomen
Etiology	Microaerophilic streptococcus plus *S. aureus* (or *Proteus* sometimes)	Usually a mixture of organisms (e.g., *Bacteroides*, peptostreptococci, *E. coli*, etc.)	Primarily group A streptococci; when develops secondary to abdominal surgery, enteric bacteria also involved	*C. perfringens* (occasionally other clostridia)	*Rhizopus*, *Mucor*, *Absidia*	*P. aeruginosa*	Not an infection primarily; may be confused with such due to secondary colonization by Enterobacteriaceae, microaerophilic streptococci, *P. aeruginosa*, *S. aureus*

(Modified from Wilson et al.,[71] with permission.)

every 4–6 hours) should be used. The etiology of necrotizing fasciitis due to mixed anaerobes and facultative organisms (synergistic necrotizing cellulitis) can usually be suspected at the outset from the foul odor and the appearance of the exudate on a Gram-stained smear. After surgery the wound is treated with elevation and moist dressings. Skin grafting is usually required later.

Progressive bacterial synergistic gangrene is very difficult to treat. Local irrigations with bacitracin and systemic therapy with parenteral penicillin (4–6 million units/day intravenously) and a second drug (based on antibiotic susceptibility testing of bacteria other than microaerophilic streptococci isolated from the lesion) is sometimes helpful. However, wide excision of all necrotic tissue (extending well into normal tissue) combined with antibiotic treatment usually is required.

Erythrasma

Clinical Findings.   Erythrasma is a common superficial bacterial infection of the skin characterized by slowly spreading, pruritic, reddish-brown macular patches, usually located in the genitocrural area.[75] The lesions are finely scaled and finely wrinkled, and they are more common in men and in obese individuals with diabetes mellitus. The disease may be asymptomatic or may undergo periodic exacerbations. The etiology appears to be bacterial: *Corynebacterium minutissimum*, a species that can be grown aerobically. Gram-stained imprints of the skin surface show large numbers of small gram-positive bacilli. Examination of the lesions under a Wood's lamp reveals a distinctive coral red fluorescence.

The principal superficial skin infections to be considered in the differential diagnosis are tinea versicolor lesions on the trunk and tinea cruris (a deeper, more inflammatory, and more rapidly progressive process).

Treatment with oral erythromycin (1.0 g/day orally for 5–7 days) is usually efficacious, clearing the lesions within several weeks. Topical treatment with an aqueous solution of 2% clindamycin hydrochloride can also be effective.[76]

SECONDARY BACTERIAL INFECTIONS COMPLICATING PRE-EXISTING SKIN LESIONS

A variety of skin lesions (burns, eczematous dermatitides, traumatic lesions, and so on) may become secondarily infected (Table 1). Such infected lesions usually do not exhibit distinctive morphologic characteristics based on the infecting organism; rather, the appearance of the lesions is determined to a large measure by the nature of the preexisting injury or dermatosis, such as dermatophytosis and acne conglabata, which are often treated primarily by dermatologists. Several of the other secondarily infected dermatoses have some distinctive clinical and bacteriologic features and merit brief consideration here.

Diabetic Foot and Other Chronic Superficial Skin Ulcers

A variety of aerobic and facultative organisms (*Pseudomonas, Proteus,* enterococci, and so on) colonize and secondarily infect decubitus ulcers. Only in recent years has the prominent role of anaerobic bacteria in such infections been recognized.[77] The character of the ulcers (extensive undermining and necrosis of tissue) and their location, frequently in proximity to the anus, provide the opportunity for invasion by anaerobes. *Bacteroides fragilis* and other Bacteroidaceae and *Clostridium perfringens* have commonly been isolated from infected decubitus ulcers. Such lesions have been the sources of symptomatic bacteremias caused by *B. fragilis, Peptostreptococcus* spp., *S. aureus, Enterococcus,* various streptococci, and a variety of facultative gram-negative bacilli.[77,78]

Chronic foot infections in patients with diabetes mellitus are common and difficult problems. They usually begin after minor trauma in patients with peripheral neuropathy and arterial vascular insufficiency and take the form of cellulitis, soft tissue necrosis, or osteomyelitis with a draining sinus. For convenience, foot infections in diabetic patients are classified into two categories[79]: *non-limb-threatening infections* (superficial, lack systemic toxicity, minimal cellulitis extending less than 2 cm from portal of entry, ulceration [if present] not extending fully through the skin, lacking significant ischemia); and *limb-threatening infections* (more extensive cellulitis, lymphangitis, ulcers penetrating through skin into subcutaneous tissues, prominent ischemia). *S. aureus* is the major pathogen in the former. Facultative streptococci are isolated in about one-third of patients. Facultative gram-negative bacilli and anaerobes are uncommonly isolated. In the limb-threatening category, in contrast, infection is commonly polymicrobial.[79–81] *Staphylococcus aureus,* group B streptococci, *Enterococcus,* and facultative gram-negative bacilli are major pathogens in this situation, along with anaerobic gram-positive cocci and *Bacteroides* species.

Deep tissue cultures provide the most reliable bacteriologic information in diabetic foot infections. When these are not available, cultures and gram-stained smears of material obtained from curettage of the base of the ulcer or from a purulent exudate may provide the needed information to guide antimicrobial therapy. When gas is present in surrounding tissues on radiologic examination, it may represent air introduced through the ulcer or gas generated in the soft tissues by the infecting anaerobic or coliform organisms.

Antibiotic treatment of infected diabetic foot ulcers is based on bacteriologic data if available and meaningful. Initial antimicrobial treatment in a previously untreated patient with a non-limb-threatening infection is focused primarily on staphylococci and streptococci. For mild infections that can be treated at home, oral clindamycin or cephalexin for 2 weeks has been satisfactory.[79] Similarly, cloxacillin or dicloxacillin might be effective. When superficial ulcers are complicated by cellulitis warranting parenteral antibiotics, cefazolin intravenously is effective.[79] Initial antimicrobial treatment of limb-threatening infections involves use of broad-spectrum antibiotics aimed at its polymicrobial nature (group B streptococci, other streptococci, Enterobacteriaceae, anaerobic gram-positive cocci, and *Bacteroides* spp. including *B. fragilis*). In the past, the combination of clindamycin and an aminoglycoside have often been used. Cefoxitin or ceftizoxime have also been employed. Although ciprofloxacin has been used successfully as monotherapy, potential problems are presented by the possible role of *Bacteroides* spp. in these infections and by the emerging resistance to this drug among *S. aureus* strains. Currently, a variety of regimens are advocated for initial empiric therapy of limb-threatening infections[79]: ampicillin-sulbactam, clindamycin plus a third-generation cephalosporin; ticarcillin-clavulanate; clindamycin plus ciprofloxacin.

Initial surgical management includes unroofing of encrusted areas and probing the wound to determine the extent of tissue destruction and possible bone involvement. Edema should be reduced by bed rest, elevation, and diuretic therapy as indicated. Control of diabetes is of considerable importance. Open ulcers should be gently packed three times daily with sterile gauze moistened with normal saline or one-quarter strength betadine. Surgical débridement and drainage should be carried out promptly for patients with deep ulcers extending to subcutaneous tissues or where deep tissue necrosis or suppuration is present.[79]

Occupationally related contaminated traumatic wounds often involve loss of skin and subcutaneous tissues, with ensuing cellulitis and deeper infections. Comparison of the bacteriology of initial wounds sustained in factories with those on farms (associated with corn-harvesting machinery) indicates that gram-negative bacilli (particularly *Enterobacter* spp. and *Pseudomonas maltophilia*) are 10 times more common in the latter.[82]

Sport fishing in freshwater may result in puncture wounds or lacerations incurred from venomous spines of catfish.[83] Such wounds may rapidly become secondarily infected, particularly by gram-negative bacilli found in ponds and lakes (e.g., *Aeromonas hydrophila, Klebsiella, E. coli*).

Post-Traumatic Opportunistic Skin Infections in Immunocompromised Patients

A variety of unusual pathogens may invade the skin of immunocompromised patients after some local, often minor laceration or abrasion. Such pathogens include fungi, *(Paecilomyces, Penicillium, Trichosporon, Fusarium, Alternaria)*, mycobacteria *(M. marinum)*, and even algae *(Prototheca wickerhamii)*.[70] The lesions are usually ulcerative or nodular[84] but, in the case of *M. marinum*, may take the form of a nodular lymphangitis extending from the original focus. A typical dermatophyte, *Trichophyton rubrum*, which ordinarily produces only superficial skin infections, may invade the deeper subcutaneous tissues of immunosuppressed hosts and produce multiple nodular or fluctuant masses.[85] Primary cutaneous *Bacillus cereus* infection can occur in neutropenic patients. The lesions are vesicular or pustular and usually occur on the hand or an extremity during warm weather. Bacteremia is not a feature. Intravenous vancomycin is the preferred treatment.[86]

Rarely, scattered papular and nodular lesions in patients with AIDS show on biopsy an abscess containing a granule consisting of basophilic-staining cocci surrounded by eosinophilic material (Splendore-Hoeppli phenomenon). This superficially resembles a "sulfur granule" of actinomycosis or a mycetoma, but is the lesion of botryomycosis due to *S. aureus*.[87] Botryomycosis also occurs in immunocompetent patients; a foreign body may play a role in initiating or perpetuating the lesion, which has the gross appearance of a small infected sebaceous cyst or may resemble prurigo nodularis. Several cases of botryomycosis have occurred in patients with the hyperimmunoglobulin E syndrome associated in patients with the hyperimmunoglobulin E syndrome associated with recurrent staphylococcal infections.

Bacillary Angiomatosis in Patients with AIDS

Bacillary angiomatosis (epitheloid angiomatosis) is an infection that involves primarily the skin but also visceral organs in patients with AIDS. The lesions begin as tiny red papules that enlarge to become exophytic or pedunculated nodules, occasionally reaching several centimeters in diameter.[88] They often are dome-shaped vascular lesions with a collarette of scale.[89] Deeper nodules that may occur in the dermis or subcutaneous tissue are flesh colored, somewhat rubbery to firm in consistency, and may be movable or fixed to underlying structures. The lesions bleed readily if incised. There may be only a few, or they may number in the hundreds, covering the body. Oral, nasal, conjunctival, genital, and anal mucosal lesions occur. Visceral involvement takes the form of bacillary peliosis hepatis with hypodense lesions of liver and spleen demonstrable on abdominal computed tomographic scans.

The lesions of bacillary angiomatosis resemble grossly those of Kaposi sarcoma, pyogenic granuloma, hemangioma, subcutaneous tumors, or verruga peruana (eruptive phase of bartonellosis in Peru and Ecuador). Histologically, bacillary angiomatosis consists of a circumscribed lobular proliferation of capillaries lined with prominent large endothelial cells, an inflammatory infiltrate with neutrophils, and, characteristically, aggregates of bacillary bodies that are demonstrable on Warthin-Starry stain.

The initially uncultivatable etiologic agent of bacillary angiomatosis was first defined in tissue samples as a rickettsia-like organism closely related to *Bartonella (Rochalimaea) quintana* by utilizing techniques for analysis of phylogenetic relatedness of eubacterial 16S ribosomal gene fragments.[90] A newly described species of *Bartonella, B. henselae*, a fastidious gram-negative organism, has been isolated in blood cultures of immunocompromised and nonimmunocompromised patients with an abrupt febrile illness as well as from cutaneous and osseous lesions of patients with bacillary angiomatosis.[89] *Bartonella quintana* has been cultured from other patients with bacillary angiomatosis.

Based on results of a recently developed IFA assay for antibody to *B. henselae* and on the isolation of this organism from the lymph nodes of several nonimmunosuppressed patients with clinical cat-scratch disease, *B. henselae* (or a closely related organism) rather than *Afipia felis* appears to be the causative agent in most cases of cat-scratch disease. It is of interest that many patients with bacillary angiomatosis have a history of cat contact or cat scratches.

The diagnosis of bacillary angiomatosis is made by clinical appearance of the lesions in an HIV-infected patient and confirmed on biopsy (Warthin-Starry stain). Since the skin lesions are often extensive and since systemic manifestations (fever, peliosis hepatis) can be features, antimicrobial treatment is indicated. Erythromycin (0.5 g orally four times daily for 2–8 weeks) is the drug of choice. Some patients have responded to doxycycline, and azithromycin (1.0 g orally once daily) has been used successfully in a patient with skin lesions, fever, and bacillary peliosis hepatis.

Hidradenitis Suppurativa

Hidradenitis suppurativa is an extremely troublesome, chronic, suppurative, ciccatricial disease of apocrine glands in the axillary, genital, and perianal areas. The primary lesion appears to be an unexplained keratinous plugging of the ducts of the apocrine glands resulting in dilation and eventual rupture of the gland and surrounding tissue inflammation. The initial lesions are reddish-purple nodules that slowly become fluctuant and drain. Irregular sinus tracts are formed with repeated crops of lesions; reparative processes are only partially successful. Ultimately the involved areas show a mixture of burrowing, draining tracts, and ciccatricial scarring. In some patients, hidradenitis suppurativa is associated with acne conglobata or dissecting cellulitis of the scalp. In such patients, a distinctive spondyloarthropathy may occur.[91]

Although not initially infected, the lesions frequently become so secondarily. Staphylococci, nonhemolytic streptococci, *E. coli, Proteus*, and *Pseudomonas* are often isolated from draining lesions. Anaerobic organisms (*Bacteroides*, anaerobic gram-positive cocci) also have been reported from such lesions. The foul odor of the discharge from such lesions would suggest the presence of anaerobes.

Treatment of hidradenitis suppurativa is difficult, particularly when the process is chronic and extensive, because of the multiple deep-seated sites of secondary infection that are inaccessible to antibiotics. Antimicrobial therapy (based on Gram-stained smears and culture results) and local moist heat to establish drainage are helpful in the treatment of the initial phases of infection. Surgical drainage is required in the management of large abscesses. In very severe, resistant cases exhibiting chronicity and scarring, radical excision of most of the involved area followed by skin grafting may become necessary.

Infected Epidermal Cysts

Epidermal cysts are closed sacs lined with proliferating epidermal cells located about the head, trunk, extremities, and vulvovaginal and scrotal areas. Lacking communication with the skin surface, they can become infected with resultant abscess formation. *Staphylococcus aureus* (frequently present as the sole aerobic organism) and various streptococci are the principal aerobic/facultative isolates from these abscesses.

Peptostreptococcus and *Bacteroides* spp. are the primary anaerobic isolates, often present in polymicrobial mixtures in cyst abscesses about the head, perineum, and vulvovaginal area.[92] Treatment consists principally of surgical drainage; and initial antimicrobial therapy (clindamycin, cefoxitin, or amoxicillin–clavulanate), if needed, is aimed at *S. aureus* and the likely anaerobes, pending results of gram-stained smears and cultures.

Self-Induced Skin Infections

Rarely, persisting unexplained skin ulcers are self-induced. Their colonization with a variety of gram-negative and gram-positive bacteria is inevitable. However, the continuing ulceration is the result of repeated, self-induced trauma rather than of bacterial infection per se. Very rarely, unexplained continuing or recurrent polymicrobial (oral or intestinal flora) cellulitis or a subcutaneous abscess is the result of injection of foreign material containing saliva or contaminated fluids into subcutaneous tissue. Examination of biopsy specimens from the involved area by polarizing microscopy may reveal the presence of birefringent foreign bodies, suggesting the true diagnosis.

CUTANEOUS INVOLVEMENT IN SYSTEMIC BACTERIAL AND MYCOTIC INFECTIONS

Cutaneous manifestations may be a feature of a variety of bacteremias, fungemias, and systemic bacterial infections (Table 1).[93] In leptospirosis, rat-bite fever, and listeriosis cutaneous manifestations are a small part of the total clinical picture and are considered elsewhere in chapters dealing with the responsible organisms. In some systemic infections cutaneous manifestations are noninfectious complications of the illness (erythema nodosum, purpura fulminans).

Bacteremias

Staphylococcus Aureus. The occurrence of skin lesions (pustules, subcutaneous abscesses, purulent purpura) in the course of bacteremia or endocarditis due to *S. aureus* can provide a clue to the nature of the infecting organism. The most distinctive of these lesions is that of purulent purpura. This is a small area of purpura with a white, purulent center. Aspiration of the contents of the central portion reveals staphylococci and polymorphonuclear leukocytes. Rarely, scattered tender subcutaneous nodules may develop during *S. aureus* bacteremia.

Pseudomonas Aeruginosa. Four types of skin lesion have been described in the course of *Pseudomonas* septicemia:

1. *Vesicles and bullae.* These occur as isolated bullae, or occasionally in small clusters, anywhere on the skin surface. They rapidly become hemorrhagic and have a narrow encircling zone of dusky erythema. Occasionally, in infants, the lesions are surrounded by large, erythematous halos resembling insect bites or erythema multiforme.
2. *Ecthyma gangrenosum.* This is a round, indurated, ulcerated, painless area with a central gray-black eschar and a surrounding narrow zone of erythema. The lesions may develop de novo or may evolve from an initial bullous lesion.
3. *Gangrenous cellulitis.* This is either a superficial, sharply demarcated necrotic area that may resemble a decubitus ulcer or an area of cellulitis with edema and some necrosis of the overlying skin.
4. *Macular or maculopapular lesions.* These are small, oval, erythematous macules, located predominantly over the trunk, resembling the "rose spots" of typhoid fever. Such lesions have been reported, particularly in the tropics, in association with fever and diarrhea, the syndrome described as *Shanghai fever.*

The foregoing types of metastatic lesion contain numerous gram-negative bacilli but relatively few polymorphonuclear leukocytes. The development of such lesions in a febrile patient with leukemia undergoing induction chemotherapy or on uninvolved skin areas of a patient with extensive thermal burns should strongly suggest the presence of *Pseudomonas* bacteremia. Presumptive antibiotic management should be aimed at *P. aeruginosa* and includes a combination of ceftazidime or ticarcillin with tobramycin. Rarely, ecthyma gangrenosum occurs in the course of bacteremia due to other gram-negative bacilli or in disseminated candidiasis; or it may occur in the absence of bacteremia as progression of *Pseudomonas* folliculitis in an immunocompromised patient.[94]

Neisseria Meningitidis. The skin lesion of acute meningococcemia consist of erythematous macules (initially), petechiae, purpura, and ecchymoses located on the extremities and trunk. Extensive gun-metal gray, hemorrhagic, necrotic patches can develop by confluence of petechial and purpuric lesions in fulminant meningococcemia. Symmetric peripheral gangrene and purpura fulminans occur with prominent disseminated intravascular coagulation. Occasionally, gram-negative diplococci can be observed on smears of serum obtained from the skin lesions of acute meningococcemia.

Skin lesions are an important feature of the unusual syndrome of chronic meningococcemia, characterized by recurrent cycles of fever, arthralgias, and rash over a period of 2–3 months.[95] The rash appears in crops, each consisting of a small number of individual lesions during febrile episodes. The lesions are generally located on the extremities, particularly about joints. They may consist of erythematous maculopapules, petechiae, petechiae with vesiculopustular centers, petechiae with small areolas of pale erythema, suggilations, or tender erythema nodosum-like nodules. Biopsy specimens of the lesions reveal the histologic picture of leukocytoclastic angiitis, a finding that may erroneously direct attention toward a diagnosis of a small vessel hypersensitivity vasculitis and away from that of vasculitis secondary to systemic infection.

Neisseria Gonorrhoeae. The skin lesions of gonococcemia consist of pustules surrounded by a thin zone of purpura, macules, papules, purpuric vesicles and bullae, and/or purpuric infarcts. The lesions are few, scattered over the distal extremities particularly, and frequently painful. They are part of the gonococcemic dermatitis-arthritis syndrome.[96] *Neisseria gonorrhoeae* are isolated from fewer than 5 percent of skin lesions, but, in one study, gonococcal antigens have been identified by immunofluorescent staining procedures in the majority of lesions. In addition to arthralgias and frank arthritis, tenosynovitis may be a conspicuous feature.

Salmonella Typhi. "Rose spots" frequently appear 7–10 days into the febrile course of untreated typhoid fever. The lesions are slightly raised, small (1–3 mm), pink papules that tend to occur in crops of 10–20 lesions. They are found most commonly on the upper abdomen, lower chest, and back. Rose spots are less frequently found in enteric fevers due to *Salmonella* spp. other than *S. typhi*. Early treatment with ampicillin or chloramphenicol will prevent the appearance of these skin lesions. *Salmonella typhi* can sometimes be found on Gram-stained preparations from the papules and isolated on culture.

Haemophilus Influenzae. Cellulitis involving the face, neck, or upper extremities occasionally occurs with bacteremic *Haemophilus influenzae* type b infections in children, particularly under the age of 3 years. Although commonly described as having a peculiar purple-red or blue-red hue, the lesion most often is erythematous, indurated, and indistinguishable from cellulitis due to streptococci or staphylococci. The site of primary infection is in the pharynx, the middle ear, or elsewhere in the upper respiratory tract. Direct invasion across traumatized buccal mucous membranes by *H. influenzae* type b colonizing the respiratory tract has been suggested as the pathogenesis of most cases of buccal cellulitis in children.[97] This is a life-threatening acute infection, since bacteremia (sometimes complicated by meningitis) occurs in about 80 percent of cases.[98] Until recently, this uncommon lesion had been described only in pediatric practice, but now a few cases have been reported in adults with epiglottitis and other forms of upper respiratory disease due to *H. influenzae*.[99] Although almost all cases of *H. influenzae* cellulitis in adults have involved cervical or thoracic areas, one case of bacteremic *H. influenzae* type b cellulitis has occurred on the foot of an otherwise well octogenarian.[100] In view of the increasing incidence of ampicillin resistance in clinical strains of *H. influenzae* type b, provisional antibiotic therapy should use a third-generation cephalosporin or chloramphenicol (either alone or in combination with ampicillin) until the isolate can be tested for β-lactamase activity.

Infective Endocarditis

The cutaneous lesions of subacute bacterial endocarditis consist of petechiae, subungual "splinter" hemorrhages, Osler's nodes, and Janeway's lesions. Petechiae tend to occur in small crops, particularly in the conjunctivae, on the palate, and on the upper chest and extremities. These are the most common skin lesions of endocarditis. Rarely, petechiae are extremely numerous, particularly on the lower extremities, and suggest a primary vasculitis. Osler's nodes are split-pea-sized, erythematous, tender nodules located principally on the pads of the fingers and toes. They are few at any given time and occur in about 15 percent of the patients with subacute bacterial endocarditis. The lesions are usually transient, clearing in 1–2 days. Similar lesions may also occur in acute endocarditis (e.g., due to *S. aureus*). Histologic examination of such lesions in several cases of acute endocarditis has suggested septic embolization in their pathogenesis.[101] The genesis of Osler's nodes in subacute bacterial endocarditis may have a different basis, perhaps sterile embolization or an allergic vasculitis. Janeway's lesions are painless, small, erythematous macules or minimally nodular hemorrhages in the palms or soles occurring in either acute or subacute endocarditis (more commonly in the former, particularly when *S. aureus* is the etiology). Histologic findings in a case *S. aureus* endocarditis indicate that Janeway's lesions are caused by septic microembolization.[102]

Fungemias: Candida albicans

Systemic candidiasis developing in the setting of leukemia, immunosuppression, extensive antibiotic therapy, hyperalimentation, heroin addiction, cardiac surgery, and so on may be difficult to diagnose clinically until the organism is isolated from routine blood cultures—often not until 5–7 days of incubation (more rapidly with lysis-centrifugation culture methods). The portal for disseminated candidiasis (or aspergillosis) may be an area of skin injured in the course of intravenous therapy (or trauma induced by adhesive tape or extravasation of intravenous fluid).[70] Examination of the optic fundi (for evidence of candidal ophthalmitis) and the search for *Candida* pseudohyphae and yeast forms on a smear of buffy coat of venous blood are sometimes helpful in making an early diagnosis of candidal fungemia while awaiting isolation of the organism from blood cultures. In occasional patients, the appearance of multiple discrete (2–5 mm) pink maculopapules (sometimes with pale centers) on the trunk or extremities can suggest the diagnosis.[103] In some of these patients severe diffuse muscle tenderness has been present, and muscle biopsy specimens have shown necrosis with yeast and pseudohyphal forms.[104] Occasionally, subcutaneous abscesses due to *Candida* may develop in the course of fungemia. Aspiration of such abscesses reveals the etiology

on stained smear. Punch biopsy specimens of the maculopapular lesions provide a more accurate diagnosis than simple culture, since histologic sections can reveal *Candida* emboli in blood vessels and pseudohyphae in adjacent soft tissues. The isolation of *Candida* from an unroofed lesion may only represent surface colonization or may be consistent with *Candida* folliculitis rather than disseminated candidiasis.

SUBCUTANEOUS TISSUE INFECTIONS AND ABSCESSES

Exact categorization of some bacterial infections of the soft tissues (skin, subcutaneous tissues, fascia, and skeletal muscle) may be difficult. While the differences between a superficial pyoderma and a necrotizing myositis[105] like gas gangrene are readily apparent, distinctions between many other types of soft tissue infection are sometimes blurred. Classification is usually based on features such as the anatomic structure involved, the infecting organism(s), and the clinical picture. Unfortunately for convenience in categorization, some infections may involve several components of the soft tissues, and multiple bacterial species may produce infections with the same clinical appearance.

To compound the problem of classification further, a variety of designations have been given to closely related or virtually identical processes. For example, *streptococcal gangrene* has also been referred to as *necrotizing fasciitis*. Subsequent to the initial descriptions of this condition, it became apparent that it was sometimes caused by bacteria other than group A streptococci.[106] Thus, streptococcal gangrene can be considered the major subset of necrotizing fasciitis. For convenience, because a major feature of its manifestation is cutaneous gangrene, streptococcal gangrene has been considered in the preceding chapter with cellulitis and infectious cutaneous gangrene. Necrotizing fasciitis is reconsidered in this chapter on subcutaneous tissue infections, particularly in relation to its nonstreptococcal etiologies. Another example of the problems in nomenclature is that presented by infections that involve multiple soft tissue strata and that can be caused by a variety of bacterial species. Thus, the condition known as *synergistic necrotizing cellulitis* has also been described as *gram-negative anaerobic cutaneous gangrene* and *synergistic nonclostridial anaerobic myonecrosis*.[107,108] Because of the prominence of subcutaneous tissue involvement in this condition, it is considered primarily in this part of the chapter, although it could be considered almost as readily in the first part (Cellulitis and Superficial Infections) or in the chapter on myositis (Ch. 73).

CLOSTRIDIAL ANAEROBIC CELLULITIS

Clostridial anaerobic cellulitis is a necrotizing clostridial infection of devitalized subcutaneous tissues. Deep fascia is not appreciably involved, and ordinarily there is no associated myositis. Gas formation is common and often extensive. Anaerobic cellulitis is several times more common than gas gangrene in war wounds.

Pathogenesis and Pathologic Characteristics

Clostridial species, usually *Clostridium perfringens,* are introduced into subcutaneous tissues through a dirty or inadequately débrided traumatic wound, through contamination at operation, or from a preexisting localized infection. The last is frequently located in the perineum, abdominal wall, buttocks, and lower extremities, areas that are readily contaminated with fecal flora. The presence of foreign debris and necrotic tissue in the depths of a wound provides a suitable anaerobic milieu for clostridial proliferation. Very rarely, clostridial anaerobic cellulitis develops, not following primary cutaneous injury, but rather as a consequence of *C. septicum* bacteremia in the setting of leukemia and granulocytopenia.[109] Intestinal erosions are the presumed initial portals of entry. This type of *C. septicum* cellulitis should be distinguished from the even more life-threatening bacteremic *C. septicum* myonecrosis, which is often associated with a cryptic underlying colonic neoplasm (see Ch. 73).

Clinical Findings

The incubation period is several days, longer than the 1–2 days for clostridial myonecrosis. The onset is gradual, but the process subsequently may spread rapidly.[110] Local pain, tissue swelling, and systemic toxicity are not prominent features, and the relative mildness of the process helps to distinguish it from true gas gangrene. The dark blebs and bronzing of the skin seen in gas gangrene are not usually features of clostridial cellulitis. A thin, dark, sometimes foul-smelling drainage (often containing fat globules) from the wound is characteristic, as is extensive tissue gas formation, more prominent than that observed in clostridial myonecrosis. Frank crepitus is present in the involved area and may extent very widely, even beyond the limits of the active infection.

Gram-stained smears of the drainage show numerous bluntended, thick, gram-positive bacilli and variable numbers of polymorphonuclear leukocytes. Soft tissue x-ray films show abundant gas, but usually not in the feathery linear pattern in muscles observed in clostridial myonecrosis.

Etiologic Agents

Clostridium perfringens is the most common clostridial species responsible for this infection, but *C. septicum* and other species have been isolated. Sometimes, the clostridia are present in mixed culture with facultative organisms.

Differential Diagnosis

When crepitus is observed with a wound, a variety of possibilities must be considered in the differential diagnosis (Table 3). The first is clostridial myonecrosis (gas gangrene) because of the fulminant nature of the infection and the requirement for emergency surgery. At the same time, distinguishing between clostridial gas gangrene and anaerobic cellulitis is essential to avoid performing unnecessarily extensive surgery. Ultimately, the two processes are differentiated in the operating room when the wound is laid open and the viability and appearance of the muscle are observed. The muscle is normal (pink) in clostridial cellulitis but distinctly abnormal (discolored, fails to contract on stimulation, does not bleed from cut surface) in clostridial myonecrosis (see Ch. 73).

Presumptive Therapy

Surgical exploration is essential to determine the presence of any muscle involvement. If no myonecrosis is found, treatment should be limited to débridement of necrotic tissue and drainage of pus after the wound is opened widely. Initial antimicrobial management of clostridial cellulitis involves the use of several antibiotics, because, until surgical exploration has been carried out to distinguish between clostridial myonecrosis and anaerobic cellulitis and until Gram-stained smears of material from the lesion have been evaluated, gas gangrene or a potentially polymicrobial infection are important considerations. Intravenous penicillin (1–2 million units q3h) or ampicillin (1–1.5 g q3–4h) plus intravenous clindamycin (0.6 g q6–8h) or metronidazole (1 g loading dose followed by 0.5 g q6h) provide a two-drug combination for treating anaerobic organisms likely to be involved. Use of an additional antimicrobial (an aminoglycoside, ciprofloxacin, or a third-generation cephalosporin) aimed

at aerobic gram-negative bacilli would be based on evaluation of Gram-stained smears of exudate and tissue. Definitive antimicrobial selection is subsequently based on results of cultures and antimicrobial susceptibility tests.

NONCLOSTRIDIAL ANAEROBIC CELLULITIS

A clinical picture very similar that of clostridial anaerobic cellulitis can be produced by infection with a variety of nonsporeforming anaerobic bacteria (various *Bacteroides* spp., peptostreptococci, peptococci—either alone or as mixed infections).[108] The anaerobic bacteria may be present along with facultative species (coliform bacilli, various streptococci, staphylococci) in a mixed infection. Gas-forming soft tissue infections have been produced by *Escherichia coli, Klebsiella, Aeromonas,* and perhaps other facultative bacteria.[111,112]

Since the clinical presentation and setting is very similar to that of clostridial anaerobic cellulitis, the same initial antimicrobial therapy (vide supra) would be appropriate to cover the mixed bacterial nature of the infection. In the past, the combination of penicillin or ampicillin (aimed at *Peptostreptococcus* spp., *Peptococcus* spp., *Clostridium* spp., and various streptococcal species) plus chloramphenicol (directed at *Bacteroides* spp. and facultative gram-negative bacilli) has been used as preliminary therapy and is still favored by some. Ampicillin-sulbactam can also be used as initial therapy. Evaluation of Gram-stained smears of exudate aspirated from the lesion supplies a more focused basis for initial antimicrobial therapy. Subsequent results of cultures and susceptibility testing of aspirates or tissue removed at surgical exploration provide the needed information for narrowing (or extending) antimicrobial therapy. The surgical approach used is the same as in the treatment of clostridial anaerobic cellulitis.

NECROTIZING FASCIITIS

The term *necrotizing fasciitis* encompasses two bacteriologic entities[113,114]: *Type I* is the first entity, in which at least one anaerobic species (most commonly *Bacteroides* and *Peptostreptococcus* spp.) is isolated in combination with one or more facultative anaerobic species such as streptococci (other than group A) and members of the Enterobacteriaceae (e.g., *E. coli, Enterobacter, Klebsiella, Proteus*). An obligate aerobe such as *Pseudomonas aeruginosa* is only rarely a component of such a mixed infection. Cases in which only anaerobes are present appear to be rare.[114]

Type II is the second entity (corresponding to the entity known also as *hemolytic streptococcal gangrene*) in which group A streptococci, either alone or in combination with other species, *Staphylococcus aureus* most commonly, are isolated. Streptococcal gangrene has been considered in the first part of this chapter as a form of gangrenous cellulitis. At this point specific comments about streptococcal gangrene will be limited to the expanded setting in which the disease can appear and the changes in clinical features noted with the very recent apparent increase in bacteremic and severe invasive group A streptococcal infections and their association with the *streptococcal toxic shocklike syndrome* (TSLS).[115,116] Hemolytic streptococcal gangrene occurs not only following minor trauma, stab wounds, or surgery, particularly in the background of diabetes and peripheral vascular disease, but cirrhosis and corticosteroid therapy as well have been predisposing factors.[117] In one study of an outbreak of streptococcal TSLS, fever (or profound hypothermia and shock), confusion, tachycardia, hypotension, multiorgan failure and, in 80 percent of patients, evidence of soft-tissue infection (localized swelling, erythema) were presenting manifestations.[115] Leukocytosis, thrombocytopenia, azotemia, and increased serum levels of creatine phosphokinase (CPK) were commonly present. Rising CPK levels may serve as an indication of progression of streptococcal cellulitis to necrotizing fas-

TABLE 3. Differential Diagnosis of Crepitant Soft Tissue Wounds[a]

	Clostridial Cellulitis	Nonclostridial Anaerobic Cellulitis	Clostridial Myonecrosis (Gas Gangrene)	Anaerobic Streptococcal Myositis	Necrotizing Fasciitis[b]	Infected Vascular Gangrene	Synergistic Necrotizing Cellulitis[c]	Noninfectious Causes of Gas in Tissues
Predisposing conditions	Local trauma or surgery	Diabetes mellitus; preexisting localized infection	Local trauma or surgery	Local trauma	Diabetes mellitus; abdominal surgery; perineal infection	Peripheral arterial insufficiency	Diabetes mellitus; cardiorenal disease; obesity; perirectal infection	Mechanical effects of penetrating trauma; injuries involving use of compressed air; entrapment of air under loosely sutured wounds or under ulcers; irrigation of wounds with hydrogen peroxide; intravenous catheter placement; dissection of air from tracheostomy or spontaneous mediastinal emphysema
Incubation period	Usually over 3 days	Several days	1–2 days	3–4 days	1–4 days	>5 days	3–14 days	Less than an hour
Onset	Gradual	Gradual or rapid	Acute	Not as rapid as gas gangrene	Acute	Gradual	Acute	Usually present immediately after trauma or manipulation; may not be recognized until examined several hours later
Pain	Mild	Mild	Marked	Occurs late; marked	Moderate or severe	Variable	Severe	Mild
Swelling	Moderate	Moderate	Marked	Moderate	Marked	Moderate or marked	Moderate or marked	Slight or absent
Skin appearance	Minimal discoloration	Minimal discoloration	Yellow-bronze; dark bullae; green-black patches of necrosis	Erythema	Erythematous cellulitis; areas of skin necrosis	Discolored or black	Scattered areas of skin necrosis	Only those due to initiating trauma
Exudate	Thin, dark	Dark pus	Serosanguinous	Abundant seropurulent	Seropurulent	0	"Dishwater" pus	0
Gas	++++	++++	++	±	++	+++	++	Variable but present; does not extend
Odor	Sometimes foul	Foul	Variable; slightly foul or peculiar sweet	Slight; "sour"	Foul	Foul	Foul	0
Systemic toxicity	Minimal	Moderate	Marked	Only late in course	Moderate or marked	Minimal	Marked	0
Muscle involvement	0	0	++++	+++	0	Dead	++	0

Key: ±: rarely present; ++: present to mild extent; +++: present to moderate extent; ++++: extensive.

[a] In addition to the causes of crepitant infections listed in this table, *Aeromonas hydrophila* myositis may be associated with gas in soft tissues.

[b] The term *necrotizing faciitis* is employed here to designate forms of this syndrome of streptococcal gangrene.

[c] Synergistic necrotizing cellulitis is essentially the same process as type I necrotizing fasciitis. Since the former occasionally tends to involve muscle it is given a separate designation here; however, the two processes are clinically indistinguishable in most instances.

(Modified from Finegold SM,[142] with permission.)

ciitis and myositis. Unlike many earlier studies of hemolytic streptococcal gangrene, which affected older individuals with underlying diseases, this recent outbreak of streptococcal TSLS occurred primarily in young, previously healthy adults following minor trauma. In 70 percent of the patients, soft-tissue findings progressed to hemolytic streptococcal gangrene with development of vesicles, violaceous bullae, and necrosis of subcutaneous tissues, typical of necrotizing fasciitis (or myositis) and requiring surgical débridement.[115] The mortality rate was about 30 percent.

In a study in Ontario, Canada, in the late 1980s, a primary site of infection could be defined in 38 of 50 (75 percent) cases of severe, invasive group A streptococcal infections.[118] Of these, skin and soft tissue infections numbered 26 (68 percent), and necrotizing fasciitis was present in 15 (57 percent) of these cases. The most common group A streptococci in recent outbreaks have been M1/T1 or M12/T12 types containing pyrogenic exotoxin A (spe A) or C (spe C) genes,[118] and M1 or M3 types producing pyrogenic exotoxins A or B.[115] Recent examination of types M1 and M3 isolates from cases of streptococcal TSLS suggests their possible clonal origin.[119] The finding of a characteristic restriction enzyme fragment profile of streptococcal

DNA (hybridized with a spe A probe) from patients with serious streptococcal disease (mainly TSLS) of several different serotypes suggests further that the invasive strains are not serotype specific, but that a strain of a given serotype can acquire a new gene (toxin gene) and, with it, enhanced virulence.[120] The more general features of necrotizing fasciitis will now be considered here.

Clinical Findings

Necrotizing fasciitis is an uncommon severe infection involving the subcutaneous soft tissues, particularly the superficial (and often the deep) fascia. It usually is an acute process but rarely may follow a subacute progressive course. It can affect any part of the body but is most common on the extremities, particularly the legs. Other sites of predilection are the abdominal wall, perianal and groin areas, and postoperative wounds.[121] The portal of entry is usually a site of trauma (laceration, abrasion, burn, insect bite), a laparotomy performed in the presence of peritoneal soiling (penetrating abdominal trauma or perforated viscus) or other surgical procedure (e.g., hemorrhoidectomy or vasectomy), perirectal abscess, decubitus ulcer, or an intestinal perforation. The last may be secondary to occult diverticulitis,[122,123] rectosigmoid neoplasm, or a foreign body such as chicken bone or toothpick. Necrotizing fasciitis from such intestinal sources may occur in the lower extremity (extension along the psoas muscle), as well as in the groin or abdominal wall (via a colocutaneous fistula). Particular clinical settings in which necrotizing fasciitis may develop include diabetes mellitus, alcoholism, and parenteral drug abuse.[124]

In the newborn necrotizing fasciitis can be a serious complication of omphalitis. Initial swelling and erythema about the umbilicus can progress over several hours to several days, resulting in purplish discoloration and periumbilical necrosis.[125] Involvement of the anterior abdominal wall frequently extends to the flanks and even onto the chest wall.

The affected area initially is erythematous, swollen, without sharp margins, hot, shiny, exquisitely tender, and painful.[126] Lymphangitis and lymphadenitis are infrequent. The process progresses rapidly over several days, with sequential skin color changes from red-purple to patches of blue-gray. Within 3–5 days of onset, skin breakdown with bullae (containing thick pink or purple fluid) and frank cutaneous gangrene (resembling a thermal burn) occurs. By this time, the involved area is no longer tender but has become anesthetic secondary to thrombosis of small blood vessels and destruction of superficial nerves located in the necrotic undermined subcutaneous tissues. The development of anesthesia may antedate the appearance of skin necrosis, and this may provide a clue that the process is necrotizing fasciitis and not a simple cellulitis. Subcutaneous gas is often present in the polymicrobial form of necrotizing fasciitis, particularly in patients with diabetes mellitus. Systemic toxicity is prominent, and the temperature is elevated in the 102–105°F range. On probing of the lesion with a hemostat through a limited incision, easy passage of the instrument along a plane just superficial to the deep fascia occurs. This would not occur with ordinary cellulitis.

A leukocytosis is commonly present. Gram-stained smears of the exudate usually reveal a mixture of organisms or, in the case of streptococcal gangrene, chains of gram-positive cocci. In one instance, we observed numerous long gram-positive bacilli with subterminal spores (along with gram-negative bacilli) in the foul-smelling, purulent exudate of a patient with crepitant necrotizing fasciitis after a lower leg amputation for peripheral vascular disease. The presence of numerous spores in the wound exudate indicated that the gram-positive bacilli were unlikely to be *C. perfringens*. Before surgery the patient had had *Clostridium difficile* enterocolitis, and *C. difficile* was isolated, along with several members of the Enterobacteriaceae, from the wound drainage.

Blood cultures are frequently positive. Hypocalcemia (without tetany) may occur when necrosis of subcutaneous fat is extensive.

Fournier's Gangrene.   A form of necrotizing fasciitis occurring about the male genitals is known as *Fournier's gangrene*[108] *(idiopathic gangrene of the scrotum, streptococcal scrotal gangrene, perineal phlegmon)*. It may be confined to the scrotum or may extend to involve the perineum, penis, and abdominal wall. Predisposing factors include diabetes mellitus, local trauma, paraphimosis, periurethral extravasation of urine, perirectal or perianal infections,[127] and surgery in the area (circumcision, herniorrhaphy). In cases originating in the genitalia, the infecting bacteria probably pass through Buck's fascia of the penis and spread along the dartos fascia of the scrotum and penis, Colles' fascia of the perineum, and Scarpa's fascia of the anterior abdominal wall. In view of the typical foul odor associated with this form of necrotizing fasciitis, a major role for anaerobic bacteria is likely. Mixed cultures containing facultative organisms (*E. coli, Klebsiella,* enterococci), along with anaerobes (*Bacteroides, Fusobacterium, Clostridium,* anaerobic or microaerophilic streptococci), have been obtained from the lesions in the limited number of cases studied. Group A streptococcal gangrene can, on rare occasions, also involve the male genital area, evolving from a streptococcal balanitis.

The infection commonly starts as cellulitis adjacent to the portal of entry. Early on, the involved area is swollen, erythematous, and tender as the infection begins to involve the deep fascia. Pain is prominent; fever and systemic toxicity are marked.[128] The swelling and crepitus of the scrotum quickly increase, and dark purple areas develop and progress to extensive scrotal gangrene. If the abdominal wall becomes involved in an obese patient with diabetes, the process can spread like wildfire.

Other Special Anatomic Forms of Necrotizing Fasciitis.   Necrotizing fasciitis of the face and eyelids,[129] of the neck,[130] and of the lip[131] are uncommon but life-threatening forms of this disease. Although most often due to group A streptococcus, alone or with *S. aureus* and representing streptococcal gangrene, they occasionally represent mixed infections of group A streptococcus with *Enterobacteriaceae* or oral *Bacteroides* spp. In mixed infections, crepitus may be a feature as well as necrosis of epidermis and superficial fascia. Trauma is the usual precipitating cause of necrotizing fasciitis of periorbital areas and face; dental, oral, or pharyngeal infections predispose to cervical necrotizing fasciitis. Differentiation of the latter from cervical soft tissue infection of odontogenic origin may be difficult, but rapid spread of infection to other areas of the neck, severe pain, and systemic symptoms along with subcutaneous crepitus suggest the diagnosis of necrotizing fasciitis. When crepitus is not palpable, soft tissue radiographs may help in the diagnosis by demonstrating subcutaneous gas.

Differential Diagnosis

See Table 3.

Presumptive Therapy

Prompt diagnosis is of paramount importance because of the rapidity with which the process can progress. The mortality rate of necrotizing fasciitis ranges from 20 to 47 percent overall (13 and 22 percent for Fournier's gangrene).[127,138] Among patients (including those with either type I or type II necrotizing fasciitis) in whom the diagnosis is made within 4 days of appearance of the initial symptoms, the mortality rate is reduced to 12 percent.[132] Early clinical differentiation of necrotizing fasciitis from cellulitis may be difficult, since the initial signs, including pain, edema, and erythema, are not distinctive. However, the presence of marked systemic toxicity out of proportion to the local findings should alert the physician. Frozen section examination of biopsy specimens (including dermis, infected subcutaneous tissue, fascia, and underlying muscle) has been found to be helpful for early diagnosis.[132] Once the diagnosis is made, immediate surgical débridement is essential. In the patient in whom the diagnosis is clearly suspected on clinical grounds—deep pain with patchy areas of surface hypesthesia, or crepitation, or bullae and skin necrosis—direct operative intervention is indicated. Extensive incisions should be made through the skin and subcutaneous tissues, going beyond the area of involvement until normal fascia is found. Necrotic fat and fascia should be excised, and the wound should be left open. A second-look procedure is frequently necessary 24 hours later to ensure the adequacy of the initial débridement.[126] In the case of Fournier's gangrene, orchiectomy is almost never required, since the testes have their own blood supply independent of the compromised fascial and cutaneous circulation of the scrotum. Initial antimicrobial therapy is based on the evidence for prominent roles for anaerobic bacteria, Enterobacteriaceae, and various streptococci in this process and on the specific findings on Gram-stained smears. Antibiotics employed before obtaining bacteriologic data include combinations of ampicillin, gentamicin, and clindamycin; or ampicillin, gentamicin, and metronidazole; or ampicillin-sulbactam and gentamicin.

SYNERGISTIC NECROTIZING CELLULITIS

Clinical Findings

Synergistic necrotizing cellulitis (gram-negative anaerobic cutaneous gangrene, necrotizing cutaneous myositis, synergistic nonclostridial anaerobic myonecrosis) is a variant of necrotizing fasciitis, one in which there is prominent involvement of skin *and muscle* as well as of subcutaneous tissue and fascia. Some cases of Fournier's gangrene extending onto the abdominal wall represent this condition. Predisposing factors include diabetes mellitus, obesity, advanced age, and cardiorenal disease. Most infections are located on the lower extremities or near the perineum (e.g., originating in a perirectal abscess).[107]

The lesion may first manifest with small skin ulcers draining foul-smelling reddish-brown ("dishwater") pus. Circumscribed areas of blue-gray gangrene surround these draining sites, but the intervening skin appears normal despite necrosis of underlying subcutaneous tissues, fascia, and muscle. Local pain and tenderness are marked. Tissue gas is noted in about a quarter of the patients. Systemic toxicity is a feature; about half the patients have bacteremia.

Etiologic Agents

Cultures consistently show mixtures of anaerobic (anaerobic streptococci and/or *Bacteroides*) and facultative bacteria (*Klebsiella-Enterobacter, E. coli, Proteus*).[107] *Bacteroides* has been reported as the major pathogen on occasion.[133]

Presumptive Therapy

Initial surgery involves incision and drainage, but radical débridement is often necessary because of extensive involvement of deep fascia and muscle.[107,133] Amputation may be required. Antibiotic management initially is based on the results of Gram-stained smears of wound exudates, but it should include an antimicrobial effective against *Bacteroides* (see "Presumptive Therapy," above, for type I necrotizing fasciitis).

MISCELLANEOUS INFECTIONS SECONDARY TO TRAUMA

Bite Infections

See Chapter 299.

Burn Infections

See Chapter 298.

Injection Site Abscesses

Subcutaneous and intramuscular abscesses infrequently occur after therapeutic injections. *Staphylococcus aureus*, facultative gram-negative bacilli, and anaerobic bacteria are usually implicated. Hematomas may be the site of delayed infections. Gas gangrene has followed various injections, particularly epinephrine in oil.[111] Subcutaneous and intramuscular abscesses due to a variety of oral anaerobes and streptococci have occurred after "skin popping" or attempted intravenous injections by narcotic addicts.[108] In the case of subcutaneous abscesses secondary to intravenous drug abuse, appropriate débridement and drainage should include excision of involved veins, which often contain pus or an infected thrombus.[134]

Factitial Disease (Self-Induced Abscesses)

Occasionally, subcutaneous abscesses and cellulitis are produced when a patient deliberately injects or inserts into the skin contaminated substances.[135,136] Such abscesses often are recurrent and may be of mono- or polymicrobial etiology (often consisting of oral or fecal flora). Sterile abscesses may be induced by introduction of foreign material without bacterial contamination. Such foreign material may be identified by examination of biopsy specimens with polarizing microscopy.

SUBCUTANEOUS INFECTIONS ORIGINATING IN CONTIGUOUS FOCI

Osteomyelitis

In an occasional patient, most commonly a child, acute hematogenous osteomyelitis may manifest as a subcutaneous abscess. Under these circumstances, a subperiosteal abscess has ruptured through intervening tissues into the subcutaneous tissues. *Staphylococcus aureus* is the most common etiologic agent in such infections. It is important to recognize the nature of the process because of the different therapeutic programs required for osteomyelitis in contrast to a subcutaneous abscess of cutaneous origin. Involvement of subcutaneous tissues as a consequence of osteomyelitis may also occur in the form of a draining sinus associated with chronic osteomyelitis and sequestrum formation. Multiple draining sinuses may occur as a result of multiple foci of osteomyelitis in disseminated blastomycosis.

Actinomycosis

Subcutaneous abscesses frequently develop in the course of cervical, thoracic, or sometimes abdominal actinomycosis. Draining sinuses ultimately result (see Ch. 235).

Primary Pyodermas

On occasion, more superficial skin infections, beginning as folliculitis, furunculosis, or cellulitis, may progress into the deeper subcutaneous tissues and form a subcutaneous (sometimes "cold") abscess. *Staphylococcus aureus* is commonly the etiology. Such progression repeatedly might suggest certain underlying phagocytic cell defects such as chronic granulomatous disease of childhood or hyperimmunoglobulin E syndrome (Job syndrome).[137,138]

In a cataloguing of the bacteriology of a large number of cutaneous abscesses (unspecified as to individual predisposing causes), *S. aureus* is the single most common aerobic/facultative isolate, followed in frequency by streptococci, groupable (A, B, C, D) and nongroupable.[139] Among anaerobic isolates, *Bacteroides* spp. (most commonly *B. fragilis* group) is the most frequent, followed by *Peptostreptococcus* spp. and *Clostridium* spp. These abscesses are commonly polymicrobial (mixed aerobic-anaerobic). As might be predicted, *S. aureus* is the principal isolate in infections (both abscesses and wounds) of the extremities and trunk, whereas anaerobes are more numerous than aerobic/facultative species in such infections in the genital, perirectal, inguinal, and head and neck areas.

SUBCUTANEOUS ABSCESSES IN THE COURSE OF BACTEREMIC INFECTIONS

Metastatic pyogenic infections can occur during the course of bacteremias or endocarditis due to various common invasive organisms (e.g., *S. aureus*) in subcutaneous tissues as well as a variety of other organs and tissues. These abscesses are tender and fluctuant. Rarely, multiple, firm, nodular subcutaneous lesions, clinically resembling those of Weber-Christian disease, occur in the course of a staphylococcal bacteremia. If promptly identified and treated, the process may be aborted before frank abscess formation occurs.

Less common bacterial pathogens, infrequently responsible for bacteremia (e.g., *Nocardia* spp.,[140] *Corynebacterium* (*jeikeium*[141]) may also occasionally produce metastatic cutaneous abscesses in immunocompromised or debilitated individuals.

MYCETOMA

See Chapter 242.

REFERENCES

1. Ferrieri P, Dajani AS, Wannamaker LW, et al. Natural history of impetigo. I. Site sequence of acquisition and familial patterns of spread of cutaneous streptococci. J Clin Invest. 1972;51:2851.
2. Demidovich CW, Wittler RR, Ruff ME, et al. Impetigo. Current etiology and comparison of penicillin, erythromycin, and cephalexin therapies. Am J Dis Child. 1990;144:1313.
3. Britton JW, Fajardo JE, Krafte-Jacobs B. Comparison of mupirocin and erythromycin in the treatment of impetigo. J Pediatr. 1990;117:827.
4. Dagan R, Bar-David Y. Double-blind study comparing erythromycin and mupirocin for treatment of impetigo in children: Implications of a high prevalence of erythromycin-resistant *Staphylococcus aureus* strains. Antimicrob Agents Chemother. 1992;36:287.
5. Esterly NB, Nelson DB, Dunne WM Jr. Impetigo. Am J Dis Child. 1991;145:125.
6. Dajani AS, Wannamaker LW. Experimental infection of the skin in the hamster simulating human impetigo. III. Interaction between staphylococci and group A streptocci. J Exp Med. 1971;134:588.
7. Dajani AS, Ferrieri P, Wannamaker LW. Natural history of impetigo. II. Etiologic agents and bacterial interactions. J Clin Invest. 1972;51:2863.
8. Dillon HC. Impetigo contagiosa: Suppurative and non-suppurative complications. I. Clinical bacteriologic, and epidemiologic characteristics of impetigo. Am J Dis Child. 1968;115:530.
9. Dillon HC. Post-streptococcal glomerulonephritis following pyoderma. Rev Infect Dis. 1979;1:935.
10. Baltimore RS. Treatment of impetigo: A review. Pediatr Infect Dis. 1985;4:597.
11. Feder HM Jr, Abrahamian LM, Grant-Kels JM. Is penicillin still the drug of choice for non-bullous impetigo? Lancet. 1991;2:803.
12. Jackson MP, Iandolo JJ. Sequence of the exfoliative toxin B gene of *Staphylococcus* aureus. J Bacteriol. 1986;167:726.
13. Dancer SJ, Garratt R, Saldanha J, et al. The epidermolytic toxins are serine proteases. FEBS Lett. 1990;268:129.
14. Dajani AS. The scalded-skin syndrome: Relation to phage group II staphylococci. J Infect Dis. 1972;125:548.
15. Melish ME, Glascow LA, Turner MD, et al. The staphylococcal epidermolytic toxin: Its isolation, characterization, and site of action. Ann NY Acad Sci. 1974;236:317.
16. Elias PM, Fritsch P, Epstein EH Jr. Staphylococcal scalded skin syndrome:

Clinical features, pathogenesis, and recent microbiological and biochemical developments. Arch Dermatol. 1977;113:207.
17. Curran JP, Al-Salihi FL. Neonatal staphylococcal scalded skin syndrome: Massive outbreak due to an unusual phage type. Pediatrics. 1980;66:285.
18. Shands KN, Schmid GP, Dan BB, et al. Toxic-shock syndrome in menstruating women: Its association with tampon use and *Staphylococcus aureus* and the clinical features in 52 cases. N Engl J Med. 1980;303:1436.
19. Institute of Medicine, National Academy of Science: Conference on the Toxic Shock Syndrome. Ann Intern Med. 1978;96:835.
20. Todd JT, Fishaut M, Kapral F, et al. Toxic shock syndrome associated with phage-group-I staphylococci. Lancet. 1978;2:1116.
21. Gustafson LT, Band JD, Hutcheson RH, et al. *Pseudomonas* folliculitis: An outbreak and review. Rev Infect Dis. 1983;5:1.
22. El Baze P, Thyss A, Caldini C, et al. *Pseudomonas aeruginosa* 0-11 folliculitis: Development into ecthyma gangrenosum in immunosuppressed patients. Arch Dermatol. 1985;121:873.
23. Blankenship MI. Gram negative folliculitis. Arch Dermatol. 1984;120:1301.
24. Klotz SA, Drutz DJ, Huppert M, et al. *Pityrosporum* folliculitis. Its potential for confusion with skin lesions of systemic candidiasis. Arch Intern Med. 1982;142:2126.
25. Bufill JA, Lum LG, Caya JG, et al. Pityrosporum folliculitis after bone marrow transplantation. Ann Intern Med. 1988;108:560.
26. Buchness MR, Lim HW, Hatcher VA, et al. Eosinophilic pustular folliculitis in the acquired immunodeficiency syndrome. N Engl J Med. 1988;318:1183.
27. Hedstrom SA. Treatment and prevention of recurrent staphylococcal furunculosis: Clinical and bacteriologic follow-up. Scand J Infect Dis. 1985;17:55.
28. Reagan DR, Doebbeling BN, Pfaller AM, et al. Elimination of coincident *Staphylococcus aureus* nasal and hand carriage with intranasal application of mupirocin calcium ointment. Ann Intern Med. 1991;114:101.
29. Wheat LJ, Kohler RB, Luft FC, et al. Long-term studies of the effect of rifampin on nasal carriage of coagulase-positive staphylococci. Rev Infect Dis. 1983;5:459S.
30. Darouiche R, Wright C, Hamill R, et al. Eradication of colonization by methicillin-resistant *Staphylococcus aureus* using oral minocycline–rifampin and topical mupirocin. Antimicrob Agents Chemother. 1991;35:1612.
31. Klempner MS, Styrt B. Prevention of recurrent staphylococcal skin infections with low-dose oral clindamycin therapy. JAMA. 1988;260:2682.
32. Allen AM, Taplin D, Twigg L. Cutaneous streptococcal infections in Vietnam. Arch Dermatol. 1971;104:271.
33. Hewitt WD, Farrar WE. Case report: Bacteremia and ecthyma caused by *Streptococcus pyogenes* in a patient with acquired immunodeficiency syndrome. Am J Med Sci. 1988;295:52.
34. Gold H. Anthrax: A report of 117 cases. Arch Intern Med. 1955;96:387.
35. Aksaray N, Cinaz P, Coskun U, et al. Cutaneous anthrax. Trop Geogr Med. 1990;42:168.
36. Bernard P, Bedame C, Mounier M, et al. Streptococcal cause of erysipelas and cellulitis in adults. Arch Dermatol. 1989;125:779.
37. Jorup-Ronstrom C. Epidemiological, bacteriological and complicating features of erysipelas. Scand J Infect Dis. 1986;18:519.
38. Fitzpatrick TB, Eisen AZ, Wolff K, et al, eds. Dermatology in General Medicine. New York: McGraw-Hill; 1971.
39. Kerstens PJ, Endtz HP, Meis JF, et al. Erysipelas-like lesions associated with *Campylobacter jejuni* septicemia in patients with hypogammaglobulinemia. Eur J Clin Microbiol Infect Dis. 1992;11:842.
40. Baddour LM, Bisno AL. Recurrent cellulitis after saphenous venectomy for coronary bypass surgery. Ann Intern Med. 1982;97:493.
41. Baddour LM, Bisno AL. Non-group A beta-hemolytic streptococcal cellulitis. Association with venous and lymphatic compromise. Am J Med. 1985;79:155.
42. Chmel H, Hamdy M. Recurrent streptococcal cellulitis complicating radical hysterectomy and radiation therapy. Obstet Gynecol. 1984;63:862.
43. Ellison RT III, McGregor JA. Recurrent postcoital lower extremity streptococcal erythroderma in women. Streptococcal-sex syndrome. JAMA. 1987;257:3260.
44. Spear RM, Rothbaum RJ, Keating JP, et al. Perianal streptococcal cellulitis. J Pediatr. 1985;107:557.
45. Williams CN, Cohen M, Ronan SG, et al. Dissecting cellulitis of the scalp. Plast Reconstr Surg. 1986;77:378.
46. Markham RB, Polk BF. Seal finger. Rev Infect Dis. 1979;1:567.
47. Miyais S, Uwaydah M. Pneumococcal cellulitis. Infection. 1983;11:173.
48. Anderson DJ, Schmidt C, Goodman J, et al. Cryptococcal disease presenting as cellulitis. Clin Infect Dis. 1992;14:666.
49. Waldor MK, Wilson B, Swartz M. Cellulitis caused by *Legionella* pneumophila. Clin Infect Dis. 1993;16:51.
50. Kilborn JA, Manz LA, O'Brien M, et al. Necrotizing cellulitis caused by *Legionella micdadei*. Am J Med. 1992;92:104.
51. Asmar BI, Bashour BN, Fleischmann LE. *Escherichia coli* cellulitis in children with idiopathic nephrotic syndrome. Clin Pediatr. 1987;26:592.
52. Gold WL, Salit IE. *Aeromonas hydrophila* infections of skin and soft tissue: report of 11 cases and review. Clin Infect Dis. 1993;16:69.
53. Bonner JR, Coker AS, Berryman CR, et al. Spectrum of *Vibrio* infections in a gulf coast community. Ann Intern Med. 1983;99:464.
54. Chuang Y-C, Yuan C-Y, Liu C-Y, et al. *Vibrio vulnificus* infection in Taiwan: Report of 28 cases and review of clinical manifestations and treatment. Clin Infect Dis. 1992;15:271.
55. Arnold M, Woo M-L, French GL. *Vibrio vulnificus* septicemia presenting

as spontaneous necrotizing cellulitis in a woman with hepatic cirrhosis. Scand J Infect Dis. 1989;21:727.

56. Lehman DF, Hardy JC. Stonefish envenomation. N Engl J Med. 1993;329:510.

57. Hook EW III, Hooton TM, Horton CA, et al. Microbiologic evaluation of cutaneous cellulitis in adults. Arch Intern Med. 1986;146:295.

58. Sigurdsson AF, Gundmundsson S. The etiology of bacterial cellulitis as determined by fine-needle aspiration. Scand J Infect Dis. 1989;21:537.

59. Sachs MK. The optimum use of needle aspiration in the bacteriologic diagnosis for cellulitis in adults. Arch Intern Med. 1990;150:1907.

60. Saulsbury FT, Cooper PH, Bracikowski A, et al. Eosinophilic cellulitis in a child. J Pediatr. 1983;102:266.

61. Kremer M, Zuckerman R, Avraham Z, et al. Long-term antimicrobial therapy in the prevention of recurrent soft-tissue infections. J Infect. 1991;22:37.

62. Belsey MA, Sinclair M, Roder MR, et al. *Corynebacterium diphtheriae* skin infections in Alabama and Louisiana. A factor in the epidemiology of diphtheria. N Engl J Med. 1969;280:135.

63. Koopman JS, Campbell J. The role of cutaneous diphtheria infections in a diphtheria epidemic. J Infect Dis. 1975;131:239.

64. Barker FG, Leppard BJ, Seal DV. Streptococcal necrotizing fasciitis: Comparison between histological and clinical features. J Clin Pathol. 1987;40:335.

65. Strasberg SM, Silver MS. Hemolytic streptococcus gangrene. An uncommon but frequently fatal infection in the antibiotic era. Am J Surg. 1968;115:763.

66. Meleney FL. Bacterial synergism in disease processes with a confirmation of the synergistic bacterial etiology of a certain type of progressive gangrene of the abdominal wall. Ann Surg. 1931;94:961.

67. Husseinzadeh N, Nahas WA, Manders EK, et al. Spontaneous occurrence of synergistic bacterial gangrene following external pelvic irradiation. Obstet Gynecol. 1984;63:859.

68. Davson J, Jones DM, Turner L. Diagnosis of Meleney's synergistic gangrene. Br J Surg. 1988;75:267.

69. Turner L, Jones DM, Davson J. Cutaneous amoebiasis: Case report. Br Med J. 1985;291:635.

70. Wolfson JS, Sober AJ, Rubin RH. Dermatologic manifestations in the compromised host. Annu Rev Med. 1983;14:205.

71. Wilson CB, Siber GR, O'Brien TF, et al. Phycomycotic gangrenous cellulitis. Arch Surg. 1976;111:532.

72. Richardson JA, Herron G, Reitz R, et al. Ischemic ulcerations of skin and necrosis of muscle in azotemic hyperparathyroidism. Ann Intern Med. 1969;71:129.

73. Khafif RA, DeLima C, Silverberg A, et al. Calciphylaxis and systemic calcinosis. Arch Intern Med. 1990;150:956.

74. Cone LA, Woodward DA, Schlievert PM, et al. Clinical and bacteriologic observations of a toxic-shock–like syndrome due to *Streptococcus pyogenes*. N Engl J Med. 1987;317:146.

75. Sarkany I, Taplin D, Blank H. The etiology and treatment of erythrasma. J Invest Dermatol. 1961;37:283.

76. Sindhuphak W, MacDonald E, Smith EB. Erythrasma: Overlooked or misdiagnosed. Int J Dermatol. 1985;24:95.

77. George WL. Other infections of skin, soft tissue, and muscle. In: Finegold SM, George WL, eds. Anaerobic Infections in Humans. New York: Academic Press; 1989:491.

78. Allman RM. Pressure ulcers among the elderly. N Engl J Med. 1989;320:850.

79. Karchmer AW, Gibbons GW. Foot infections in diabetes: Evaluation and management. In: Remington JS, Swartz MN, eds. Current Clinical Topics in Infectious Diseases. v. 14. Boston: Blackwell Scientific; 1994;7–10.

80. Sapico FL, Witte JL, Canawati HN, et al. The infected foot of the diabetic patient: Quantitative microbiology and analysis of clinical features. Rev Infect Dis. 1984;6(Suppl 1):S171.

81. Wheat LJ, Allen SD, Henry M, et al. Diabetic foot infections: Bacteriologic analysis. Arch Intern Med. 1986;146:1935.

82. Agger WA, Cogbill TH, Busch H Jr, et al. Wounds caused by corn-harvesting machines: An unusual source of infection due to gram-negative bacilli. Rev Infect Dis. 1986;8:927.

83. Baack BR, Kucan JO, Zook EG, et al. Hand infections secondary to catfish spines: Case reports and literature review. J Trauma. 1991;31:1432.

84. Benedict LM, Kusne S, Torre-Cisneros J, et al. Primary cutaneous fungal infection after solid-organ transplantation: Report of five cases and review. Clin Infect Dis. 1992;15:17.

85. Novick NL, Tapia L, Bottone EJ. Invasive *Trichophyton rubrum* infection in an immunocompromised host. Am J Med. 1987;82:321.

86. Henrickson KJ, Flynn PM, Shenep JL, et al. Primary cutaneous *Bacillus cereus* infection in neutropenic children. Lancet. 1989;1:601.

87. Patterson JW, Kitces EN, Neafie RC. Cutaneous botryomycosis in a patient with acquired immunodeficiency syndrome. J Am Acad Dermatol. 1987;16:238.

88. Cockerell CJ, LeBoit PE. Bacillary angiomatosis: A newly characterized, pseudoneoplastic, infectious, cutaneous vascular disorder. J Am Acad Dermatol. 1990;22:501.

89. Schwartzman WA. Infections due to *Rochalimaea*: The expanding clinical spectrum. Clin Infect Dis. 1992;15:893.

90. Relman DA, Loutit JS, Schmidt TM, et al. The agent of bacillary angiomatosis. An approach to the identification of uncultured pathogens. N Engl J Med. 1990;323:1573.

91. Olafsson S, Khan MA. Musculoskeletal features of acne, hidradenitis suppurativa, and dissecting cellulitis of the scalp. Rheum Dis Clin North Am. 1992;18:215.

92. Brook I. Microbiology of infected epidermal cysts. Arch Dermatol. 1989;125:1658.

93. Kingston ME, Mackey D. Skin clues in the diagnosis of life-threatening infections. Rev Infect Dis. 1986;8:1.

94. Huminer D, Siegman-Igra Y, Morduchowicz G, et al. Ecthyma gangrenosum without bacteremia: Report of six cases and review of the literature. Arch Intern Med. 1987;147:299.

95. Benoit FL. Chronic meningococcemia. Am J Med. 1963;35:103.

96. O'Brien JP, Goldenberg DL, Rice PA. Disseminated gonococcal infection: A prospective analysis of 49 patients and a review of pathophysiology and immune mechanisms. Medicine. 1983;62:395.

97. Chartrand SA, Harrison CJ. Buccal cellulitis reevaluated. Am J Dis Child. 1986;140:891.

98. Walker JS, Corcoran KJ. Buccal cellulitis. Am J Emerg Med. 1990;8:542.

99. Drapkin MS, Wilson ME, Shrager SM, et al. Bacteremid *Hemophilus influenzae* type B cellulitis in the adult. Am J Med. 1977;63:449.

100. Bernard P, Mounier M, Acouturier P, et al. *Haemophilus* influenzae type B cellulitis of the lower extremity in a non-immunosuppressed elderly patient. Acta Dermatol Venereol (Stockh). 1990;70:359.

101. Alpert JS, Krous HF, Dalen JE. Pathogenesis of Osler's nodes. Ann Intern Med. 1976;85:471.

102. Cardullo AC, Silvers DN, Grossman ME. Janeway lesions and Osler's nodes: A review of histopathologic findings. J Am Acad Dermatol. 1990;22:1088.

103. Balandral L, Rothschild H, Pugh N, et al. A cutaneous manifestation of systemic candidiasis. Ann Intern Med. 1973;78:400.

104. Jarowski CI, Fialk MA, Murray HW, et al. Fever, rash, and muscle tenderness. A distinctive clinical presentation of disseminated candidiasis. Arch Intern Med. 1978;138:544.

105. Bornstein DL, Weinberg AN, Swartz MN, et al. Anaerobic infections. Review of current experience. Medicine. 1964;43:207.

106. Wilson HD, Haltalin KC. Acute necrotizing fasciitis in childhood. Am J Dis Child. 1973;125:591.

107. Stone HH, Martin JJ Jr. Synergistic necrotizing cellulitis. Ann Surg. 1972;175:702.

108. George WL. Other infections of skin, soft tissue, and muscle. In: Finegold SM, George WL, eds. Anaerobic Infections in Humans. New York: Academic Press; 1989;492–504.

109. Moses AE, Hardan I, Simhon A, et al. *Clostridium septicum* bacteremia and diffuse spreading cellulitis of the head and neck in a leukemic patient. Rev Infect Dis. 1991;15:525.

110. MacLennan JD. The histotoxic clostridial infections of man. Bacteriol Rev. 1962;26:177.

111. Bornstein DL, Weinberg AN, Swartz MN, et al. Anaerobic infections: A review of current experience. Medicine. 1964;43:207.

112. Bessman AN, Wagner W. Nonclostridial gas gangrene. JAMA 1975;233:958.

113. Rea WJ, Wyrick WJ Jr. Necrotizing fasciitis. Ann Surg. 1970;172:957.

114. Giuliano A, Lewis F Jr, Hadley K, et al. Bacteriology of necrotizing fasciitis. Am J Surg. 1977;134:52.

115. Stevens DL, Tanner MH, Winship J, et al. Severe group A streptococcal infections associated with a toxic shock-like syndrome and a scarlet fever toxin A. N Engl J Med. 1989;321:1.

116. Stevens SL. Invasive group A streptococcus infections. Clin Infect Dis. 1992;14:2.

117. Aitken DR, Mackett MC, Smith LL. The changing pattern of hemolytic streptococcal gangrene. Arch Surg. 1982;117:561.

118. Demers B, Simor AE, Vellend H, et al. Severe invasive group A streptococcal infections in Ontario, Canada: 1987–1991. Clin Infect Dis. 1993;16:792.

119. Musser JM, Hauser AR, Kim MH, et al. *Streptococcus pyogenes* causing toxic-shock-like syndrome and other invasive diseases: Clonal diversity and pyrogenic exotoxin expression. Proc Natl Acad Sci USA. 1991;88:2668.

120. Cleary PP, Kaplan EL, Handley JP, et al. Clonal basis for resurgence of serious *Streptococcus pyogenes* disease in the 1980s. Lancet. 1992;339:518.

121. Casali RE, Tucker WE, Petrino RA, et al. Postoperative necrotizing fasciitis of the abdominal wall. Am J Surg. 1980;140:787.

122. Galbut DL, Gerber DL, Belgraier AH. Spontaneous necrotizing fasciitis. Occurrence secondary to occult diverticulitis. JAMA. 1977;238:2302.

123. Barza MJ, Proppe KH. Case records of the Massachusetts General Hospital. N Engl J Med. 1979;301:370.

124. Schecter W, Meyer A, Schecter G, et al. Necrotizing fasciitis of the upper extremity. J Hand Surg. 1982;7:15.

125. Lally KP, Atkinson JB, Woolley MM, et al. Necrotizing fasciitis: A serious sequela of omphalitis in the newborn. Ann Surg. 1984;199:101.

126. Sudarsky LA, Laschinger JC, Coppa GF, et al. Improved results from a standardized approach in treating patients with necrotizing fasciitis. Ann Surg. 1987;206:661.

127. Iorianni P, Oliver GC. Synergistic soft tissue infections of the perineum. Dis Colon Rectum. 1992;35:640.

128. Nickel JC, Morales A. Necrotizing fasciitis of the male genitalia (Fournier's gangrene). Can Med Assoc J. 1983;129:445.

129. Kronish JW, McLeish WM. Eyelid necrosis and periorbital necrotizing fasciitis. Report of a case and review of the literature. Ophthalmology. 1991;98:92.

130. Rapoport Y, Himelfarb MZ, Zikk D, et al. Cervical necrotizing fasciitis of odontogenic origin. Oral Surg Oral Med Oral Pathol. 1991;72:15.

131. Margolis RD, Cohen KR, Loftus MJ, et al. Nonodontogenic β-hemolytic necrotizing fasciitis of the face. J Oral Maxillofac Surg. 1989;47:1098.
132. Stamenkovic I, Lew PD. Early recognition of potentially fatal necrotizing fasciitis: Use of frozen-section biopsy. N Engl J Med. 1984;310:1689.
133. Baxter CR. Surgical management of soft tissue infections. Surg Clin North Am. 1972;52:1483.
134. Biderman P, Hiatt JR. Management of soft-tissue infections of the upper extremity in parenteral drug abusers. Am J Surg. 1987;154:526.
135. Aduan RP, Fauci AS, Dale DC, et al. Factitious fever and self-induced infection: A report of 32 cases and review of the literature. Ann Intern Med. 1979; 90:230.
136. Reich P, Gottfried LA. Factitious disorders in a teaching hospital. Ann Intern Med. 1983;99:240.
137. Dreskin SC, Gallin JI. Evolution of the hyperimmunoglobulin E and recurrent infection (HIE, Job's) syndrome in a young girl. J Allergy Clin Immunol. 1987;80:746.
138. Curnutte JT, Boxer LA. Clinically significant phagocytic cell defects. In: Remington JS, Swartz MN, eds. Current Clinical Topics in Infectious Diseases. v. 6. New York: McGraw-Hill; 1985:103–56.
139. Brook I, Frazier EH. Aerobic and anaerobic bacteriology of wounds and cutaneous abscesses. Arch Surg. 1990;125:1990.
140. Curley RK, Hayward T, Holden CA. Cutaneous abscesses due to systemic nocardiosis. Clin Exp Dermatol. 1990;15:459.
141. Dan M, Somer I, Knobel B, et al. Cutaneous manifestations of infection with Corynebacterium group JK. Rev Infect Dis. 1988;10:1204.
142. Finegold SM. Anaerobic Bacteria in Human Disease. New York: Academic Press; 1977.

73. MYOSITIS

MORTON N. SWARTZ

Infection of skeletal muscle (infectious myositis) is uncommon. When it occurs, a wide range of organisms may be responsible: bacteria, mycobacteria, fungi, viruses, and parasitic agents. Bacteria invade muscle either from contiguous sites of infection (skin and subcutaneous abscesses, penetrating wounds, decubitus ulcers, osteomyelitis) or by hematogenous spread from a distant focus. It is helpful to categorize infectious myositis on the basis of clinical manifestations. These may be very distinctive, as in clostridial gas gangrene, and suggest the specific etiologic agent; or they may be very nonspecific, as in the myalgias of viral infections and infective endocarditis (Table 1). In certain instances (e.g., psoas abscess), it is the anatomic location rather than the morphologic characteristics of the lesion or the nature of the infecting agent that distinguishes the particular type of muscle infection.

PYOMYOSITIS

Pyomyositis is an acute bacterial infection of skeletal muscle usually due to *Staphylococcus aureus*. The accumulation of pus is always intramuscular initially. Clinically, it is characterized by localized muscle pain, swelling, and tenderness.

Pathogenesis and Pathologic Characteristics

Bacterial infections of muscle usually occur after a penetrating wound, prolonged vascular insufficiency in an extremity, or a contiguous infection. Bacteremic spread of infection to skeletal muscle is extremely uncommon. Of fatal cases of staphylococcal septicemia, abscesses in skeletal muscle are found in less than 1 percent.[1] Pyomyositis (primary muscle abscess) is a bacterial infection of muscle occurring in the absence of a predisposing site of infection. *Staphylococcus aureus* is the most common etiology.[2] Blood cultures are positive in 5–35 percent of the cases at the time of clinical manifestation; metastatic infections in tissue other than muscle are rare.

Most cases of pyomyositis occur in the tropics, hence the term *tropical pyomyositis*. It accounts for 1–4 percent of hospital admissions in some tropical areas.[2,3] In the United States pyomyositis is very uncommon (only ~100 cases reported over the past 20 years in North America), occurring both in persons who have recently immigrated from the tropics and in those who have always resided in a temperate climate.[4,5] It occurs at all ages, in the tropics more frequently among children, but in North America more often in adults. As yet, no convincing evidence to relate pyomyositis causally to predisposing circumstances peculiar to the tropics (malaria, filariasis, arbovirus infection) has been developed. Migration of the guinea worm, *Dracunculus medinensis,* in the deep connective tissues of the lower extremities may be complicated by staphylococcal abscesses. However, these are located between muscle groups and are not the intramuscular abscesses typical of pyomyositis. About 40 percent of cases in temperate climates lack any relevant underlying diseases, but the remainder have possible predisposing conditions: diabetes mellitus, alcoholic liver disease, corticosteroid therapy, and immunosuppressive illnesses such as leukemia, lymphoma, or other hematologic processes (Felty syndrome, myelodysplasia, sickle cell disease), and human im-

TABLE 1. Classification of Infectious Myositis

Type of Process	Clinical Pattern	Principal Specific Etiologies
Pyogenic and predominantly localized (spreading by contiguity)	Pyomyositis	S. aureus; group A streptococcus (rarely); gram-negative bacilli (very rarely)
	Gas gangrene	C. perfringens; occasionally other histotoxic clostridial species
	Nonclostridial (crepitant) myositis	
	Anaerobic streptococcal gangrene	Peptostreptococcus (plus group A streptococci or S. aureus)
	Group A streptococcal necrotizing myositis	Group A streptococcus
	Synergistic nonclostridial anaerobic myonecrosis	Mixed infections: Bacteroides and other anaerobic non-spore-forming gram-negative bacilli; Peptostreptococcus and various streptococci; E. coli; Klebsiella; Enterobacter
	Infected vascular gangrene	Same as for synergistic nonclostridial anaerobic myonecrosis
	Aeromonas hydrophila myonecrosis	Aeromonas hydrophila
	Psoas abscess	Gram-negative bacilli; S. aureus; mixed infections; M. tuberculosis
Nonpyogenic and predominantly generalized	Myalgias	Viral infections (e.g., influenza, dengue); infective endocarditis; bacteremias (e.g., meningococcemia); rickettsioses (e.g., Rocky Mountain spotted fever); toxoplasmosis
	Pleurodynia	Coxsackievirus B
	Myalgias with eosinophilia	
	Trichinosis	Trichinella spiralis
	Cysticercosis (also subcutaneous nodules)	Taenia solium
	Muscle degeneration and destruction associated with infections elsewhere	
	Acute rhabdomyolysis	Viral influenza, echovirus, coxsackie and Epstein-Barr viruses, Legionella

munodeficiency virus (HIV) infection.[5] Pyomyositis has been reported in 22 patients with HIV infection, with or without acquired immunodeficiency syndrome (AIDS) (including one neonate); and in all except one, due to *S. aureus*.[5-7] The predisposition to pyomyositis in patients with AIDS likely stems from the combination of defective bactericidal activity of neutrophils,[8] the underlying cell-mediated immunodeficiency, and the potential for muscle injury (HIV myopathy, zidovudine-associated mitochondrial myopathy, myositis from parasitic disease, *Mycobacterium avium-intracellulare* infection) associated with this disease.

The presumed pathogenesis of pyomyositis involves a prior bacteremia, commonly asymptomatic and transient. Since traumatizing muscle is necessary in order to produce pyomyositis in experimental animals following intravenous injection of *S. aureus*,[9] a role for local mechanical injury has been hypothesized.

Clinical Findings

In 20–50 percent of cases, there has been recent blunt trauma to or vigorous exercise of the involved area. The clinical picture often involves three stages. In the first or *invasive* stage, the onset is subacute with variable fever, local swelling with or without erythema, mild pain, and minimal tenderness. The area is indurated or has a wooden consistency. This stage is often overlooked. Since the initial swelling is firm and since pain is not striking, attention is directed away from an infectious etiology. Aspiration, if attempted, yields no pus. The second or *suppurative* stage occurs 10–21 or more days later, and this is the time when most patients are seen and diagnosed. Distinct muscle tenderness and swelling are present, and the patient is febrile. At this point, pus can be aspirated from the involved muscle. In the third stage, systemic manifestations of sepsis and local findings of erythema, exquisite tenderness, and fluctuance are striking. If untreated the infection can progress to metastatic abscesses, shock, and renal failure.

In an occasional patient the onset is acute rather than subacute with malaise, chills, and high fever. In a rare patient, the clinical picture is combined with that of toxic shock syndrome.[10] Since the muscle abscesses are contained by the overlying fascia, local erythema and heat may be minimal until the process extends through to the subcutaneous tissues some days or weeks later. Regional lymphadenitis is not a feature. Only a single muscle group is usually involved, but multiple muscle abscesses occur in up to 40 percent of the patients. The most frequent sites of involvement are the large muscles of the lower extremities (e.g., quadriceps femoris, gluteus group) and the trunk muscles. Involvement of the abdominal muscles is uncommon but noteworthy, since it may mimic an "acute abdomen."

A leukocytosis occurs. Eosinophilia is common in patients (even in the presence of a prominent leukocytosis) with tropical pyomyositis and appears to reflect the prevalence of parasitic infestation. Serum muscle enzyme levels may be elevated but frequently are normal despite gross muscle destruction. However, marked rhabdomyolysis with myoglobinuria and acute renal failure have developed in a patient with pyomyositis.[12]

Etiologic Agents

Staphylococcus aureus is responsible for 95 percent of the cases in tropical areas. In North America, *S. aureus* is the cause of 75 percent of cases.[5] Group A streptococci account for 1–5 percent of the cases. Other gram-positive organisms uncommonly implicated in pyomyositis include various streptococci (groups B, C, and G), *Streptococcus pneumoniae*, and *Streptococcus anginosus*. Other very rare causes include Enterobacteriaceae (*Escherichia coli, Klebsiella oxytoca, Serratia marcescens, Citrobacter freundii*), *Yersinia enterocolitica, Neisseria gonor-*

rhoeae, Haemophilus influenzae, and *Aeromonas hydrophila*.[5,13] Anaerobes (*Fusobacterium nucleatum, Clostridium septicum*) have been the etiology in several cases. *Pseudomonas mallei* and *Pseudomonas pseudomallei* in the past have very rarely caused abscesses in muscle in the septicemic or chronic suppurative forms of the diseases they produce, glanders and melioidosis, respectively. *Aspergillus fumigatus* has caused localized myositis in a patient with myelodysplasia. Other causes of fungal myositis include disseminated cryptococcal and candidal infections.

Differential Diagnosis

Early in the course of pyomyositis, other diagnoses may be suspected, particularly in nontropical areas: fever of obscure origin (in the early phase when localizing findings may be minimal or absent), osteomyelitis, septic arthritis, appendicitis or diverticulitis, muscle hematoma, muscle rupture, and thrombophlebitis. The presence of a slowly enlarging painful mass in an extremity of a patient with only low-grade fever may suggest the diagnosis of sarcoma. Pyomyositis of the pectoral muscle may present a particular problem in diagnosis and must be distinguished not only from muscle rupture, hematoma and sarcoma but also from cryptic abscessed subpectoral nodes, developing via lymphatic extension of an initiating infection on the thumb or index finger of the ipsilateral hand. Streptococcal necrotizing fasciitis, like gangrenous streptococcal myositis, produces localized swelling, tenderness, and erythema, but it is less common and produces necrosis of fascia and skin. In the patient with multiple sites of muscle involvement and eosinophilia (from incidental parasitic infestation), the picture may suggest trichinosis. This resemblance ends when localized swellings become prominent and markedly tender. Rupture of the muscle abscess through the fascia into subcutaneous tissues may suggest the diagnosis of cellulitis. Radionuclide (^{67}Ga) scanning shows diffuse uptake in the involved area but does not distinguish an intramuscular abscess from necrotizing myositis or necrotizing fasciitis. It may be helpful when several areas of pyomyositis are present, or it may be helpful in the patient with diffuse myalgias in the early phase of the disease. Computed tomography can reveal low-density areas with loss of muscle planes and a surrounding rim of contrast enhancement characteristic of pyomyositis. Enlargement of the involved muscle is usually evident. Sonography may reveal an increase in muscle mass and a hypoechoic collection with internal echoes,[15] but is less useful than computed tomographic (CT) scanning or magnetic resonance imaging (MRI) for early diagnosis. Magnetic resonance scanning can demonstrate enlargement of involved muscles and areas of signal attenuation suggestive of fluid collections.[16] Sonography or CT scanning can guide aspiration which provides specific diagnosis of pyomyositis.

Presumptive Therapy

Surgical (open or ultrasound-guided percutaneous) drainage of all abscesses is essential. Initial antibiotic therapy should consist of intravenous administration of a β-lactamase-resistant penicillin because of the preponderance of penicillin-resistant *S. aureus* isolates from such abscesses. If a group A streptococcus is isolated, treatment should be changed to penicillin G. Early modification of initial antimicrobial therapy is based on interpretation of Gram-stained smear of pus and subsequent results of cultures and susceptibility testing. Continued fever after surgical drainage of a muscle abscess while the patient is receiving appropriate antimicrobial therapy should suggest the presence of other undrained suppurative foci.

GROUP A STREPTOCOCCAL NECROTIZING MYOSITIS

In addition to producing an occasional case of typical pyomyositis with abscess formation, on rare occasions group A streptococci cause a fulminant form of myositis (peracute streptococcal pyomyositis, streptococcal necrotizing myositis, or spontaneous streptococcal gangrenous myositis).[17,18] A recent report of one case of myositis and of three cases of myositis with necrotizing fasciitis among 20 patients with invasive group A streptococcal infections associated with a toxic shock-like syndrome in a recent outbreak suggests that this form of infection may be currently more frequent than in the past.[19] The entire clinical course may be telescoped to 2–3 days. The clinical features are usually intense pain, boardlike swelling of the affected muscle, and fever. The overlying skin may be uninvolved or become erythematous and contain petechiae and vesicles.[20] Most cases involve the extremities and appear to develop spontaneously without antecedent pharyngitis or tonsillitis. Bacteremia and toxemia are prominent features and contribute to the very high mortality (80–100 percent).[19] The rapid spread of infection in a closed compartment of muscles can markedly raise intramuscular pressure, resulting in further necrosis of muscle.[20,21] However, both processes may be simultaneously present in the same area. Laboratory findings include a leukocytosis and elevated serum creatine phosphokinase levels.

This disease is a medical emergency requiring prompt clinical diagnosis with verification at surgery. Distinguishing group A streptococcal necrotizing myositis from spontaneous clostridial myonecrosis may be difficult clinically, but gas in the tissue would suggest the latter. Sonography, CT, or MRI scanning will usually reveal muscle swelling and fluid collection in muscle compartments. Early aggressive surgical intervention with fasciotomy and débridement of necrotic tissue are indicated; in some instances amputation is required. Antibiotic therapy involves high doses of penicillin G (2 million units IV q3–4h) along with clindamycin[23] (600 mg IV q6–8h, based on the gram-stained smear).

GAS GANGRENE (CLOSTRIDIAL MYONECROSIS)

Gas gangrene is a rapidly progressive, life-threatening, toxemic infection of skeletal muscle due to clostridia (principally *Clostridium perfringens*). It usually follows muscle injury and contamination, as in a dirty traumatic wound, or sometimes surgery.

Pathogenesis and Pathologic Characteristics

Gas gangrene occurs in settings having in common muscle injury and contamination with soil or other foreign material containing spores of *C. perfringens* or other histotoxic clostridial species: *(1)* accidental traumatic civilian injuries such as compound fractures[24]; *(2)* penetrating war wounds[25]; *(3)* surgical wounds, particularly after bowel or biliary tract surgery[26]; and *(4)* arterial insufficiency in an extremity.[26] Rare cases of gas gangrene have occurred after parenteral injection of medication, particularly epinephrine in oil. A fulminant case has been described beginning at the site of a simple venipuncture in a granulocytopenic patient.[26] *Clostridium perfringens* are usually present in large numbers as normal flora in human feces and thus can endogenously contaminate skin surfaces. Despite a high frequency (up to 88 percent) of clostridial contamination of major traumatic, open wounds, the incidence of gas gangrene in this setting is only 1–2 percent,[27] emphasizing the importance of devitalized tissue and the presence of foreign bodies in the pathogenesis of gas gangrene. The minimal dose of *C. perfringens* needed to produce fatal gas gangrene in the experimental animal is reduced by a factor of 10^6 when injected into devitalized muscle contaminated with sterile dirt rather than into normal muscle. The policy of prompt, thorough débridement and of leaving wounds open has decreased the incidence of gas gangrene in wartime injuries; only 22 cases among 139,000 combat casualties in Vietnam have been reported.[28]

Gas gangrene may occasionally develop in the absence of an obvious external wound. This form of clostridial myonecrosis is designated *spontaneous, nontraumatic gas gangrene*. Its principal cause is *Clostridium septicum,* a relatively aerotolerant species, which is spread by the bacteremic route and is apparently more capable of establishing infection without significant antecedent tissue injury than other clostridia. Intestinal tract abnormalities (colon cancer, diverticulitis, bowel infarction, necrotizing enterocolitis, volvulus) are the major predisposing conditions.[29] Colon cancer, often cryptic, is the most common of these, occurring in up to 88 percent of patients with *C. septicum* bacteremia. Other predisposing disorders include leukemia, other causes of neutropenia, and diabetes mellitus. The primary source of the organism is probably mucosal ulceration or perforation of the intestinal tract. The spread by the bacteremic route probably accounts for the occasional bilateral (but separated) involvement observed in a few patients with spontaneous gas gangrene. However, it may manifest in the buttocks or flanks as the consequence of an intra-abdominal catastrophe, with rapid extension of infection along the iliopsoas or other deep muscle groups. The progression of *C. septicum* spontaneous gas gangrene may be even more fulminant than that of traumatic *C. perfringens* gas gangrene; the mortality of the former is 67–100 percent, with the majority dying within 24 hours of onset.[29]

The involved muscle undergoes rapid disintegration. Initially, it may exhibit only pallor, edema, and loss of elasticity. When examined in the operating room, it fails to contract on stimulation and does not bleed from a cut surface. Later it becomes discolored (reddish purple, then greenish purple and gangrenous) and friable. Histologically, the muscle fibers show coagulation necrosis, contain cavities due to gas production, and have a destroyed supporting connective tissue; numerous gram-positive bacilli are present. Few if any inflammatory cells are present.

Clinical Findings

The usual incubation period between injury and the development of clostridial myonecrosis is 2–3 days, but it may be as short as 6 hours. The onset is acute. Pain is the earliest and most important symptom, although a sense of heaviness may be the only initial symptom occasionally. It rapidly increases in intensity, is more severe than the pain that is generally associated with the preceding injury or surgical procedure, and may become excruciating. The patient soon appears severely ill, pale, and sweaty. The pulse is rapid, the blood pressure falls, and shock and renal failure follow. The patient may be apathetic or may be apprehensive and restless but mentally clear. Delirium, stupor, and unconsciousness may supervene. Fever is frequently present, but often with temperature elevations of less than 38.3°C (101°F). Hypothermia is a poor prognostic sign and is usually associated with shock. Jaundice may become evident. The process may rapidly progress over a period of hours, with a fatal outcome if not properly treated.

Very early, tense edema and local tenderness may be the only findings of local lesions. If an open wound is present, swollen muscle may herniate through. A serosanguineous, dirty-appearing discharge, containing numerous organisms but few leukocytes, escapes from the wound. The wound has a peculiar foul odor. Gas bubbles may be visible in the discharge. Crepitus is usually present but not prominent; sometimes it is completely obscured by very marked edema. The skin adjacent to the wound is initially swollen and white, but rapidly takes on a yellowish or bronze discoloration (Fig. 1). Tense blebs containing thin serosanguineous or dark fluid develop in the overlying skin, and areas of green-black cutaneous necrosis appear. In fulminant cases, progression of the changes occurs over 2–4 hours, as indicated by the advance of the area of edema and crepitation.

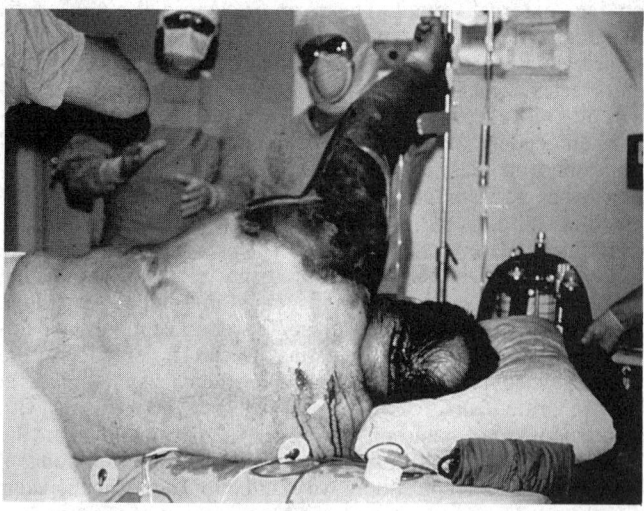

FIG. 1. Clostridial gas gangrene of the left upper extremity. There is prominent characteristic bronze discoloration of the skin extending over the shoulder. Crepitus could be palpated beyond the area of discoloration onto the back.

Laboratory Findings

The hematocrit level is usually reduced. *Clostridium perfringens* bacteremia occurs in about 15 percent of the patients with gas gangrene.[30] Intense bacteremia (with associated intravascular hemolysis) is more likely to occur as a complication of uterine infection.[31] A leukocytosis is common.

Gram-stained smear of the wound exudate or of an aspirate from one of the blebs reveals many large, gram-positive bacilli with blunt ends but few polymorphonuclear leukocytes (see Ch. 224). In almost all cases, spores are not evident. The presence of spores (subterminal) might suggest *C. septicum.*[32] Not infrequently, scattered gram-negative bacilli are also present, particularly in grossly contaminated wounds. The growth of *C. perfringens* in culture can be extraordinarily rapid (generation time of as little as 8 minutes), paralleling the rapidity of advance of the infection in devitalized tissue. Examination of liquid anaerobic cultures for gas production (and subsequent Gram-stain examination) as little as 6 hours after inoculation may provide an early presumptive diagnosis of the infecting species.

X-ray films of the involved areas show extensive and progressive gaseous dissection of muscle and fascial planes.

Etiologic Agents

Clostridium perfringens is most commonly isolated from the lesions of gas gangrene (80–95 percent of the cases).[24,28] *Clostridium novyi* is involved in 10–40 percent of the cases and *C. septicum* in 5–20 percent. Other clostridial species (*C. bifermentans, C. histolyticum, C. fallax*) have been implicated on rare occasions. In addition to clostridia, other organisms (*E. coli, Enterobacter,* enterococci, and so forth) are sometimes isolated from the lesions of gas gangrene, reflecting the contaminated character of the initiating trauma or lesion.[30]

Differential Diagnosis

The major considerations in differential diagnosis are gas-forming infections of the soft tissues (clostridial anaerobic cellulitis, nonclostridial crepitant myositis, nonclostridial crepitant cellulitis). Clostridial anaerobic cellulitis (see Ch. 72) is more gradual in onset and progression, and the systemic manifestations of illness are much milder than in gas gangrene. Local pain is relatively mild, and the skin lesions of gas gangrene (bronzing, dark blebs) do not develop. Gas formation is often much more exten-sive in clostridial cellulitis than in gas gangrene. Clinically, it is often difficult to distinguish between early clostridial cellulitis and myonecrosis. Definitive evaluation requires examination in the operating room for the characteristic changes of myonecrosis described earlier. The clinical picture of nonclostridial crepitant cellulitis is very similar to that of clostridial cellulitis. Although contamination of an operative or traumatic wound may be the source of infection in both types of cellulitis, nonclostridial crepitant cellulitis frequently develops in the setting of vascular insufficiency or perirectal infection. Bacteria isolated from nonclostridial crepitant cellulitis include facultative species (*E. coli, Klebsiella,* various streptococci) and anaerobic bacteria (*Bacteroides, Peptostreptococcus,* and so forth). Commonly, these are present in mixed culture and can be seen on Gram-stained smear of a wound aspirate.

Presumptive Therapy

Treatment includes emergency surgical exploration both to define the nature of the process (gas gangrene vs. crepitant cellulitis) by direct examination of muscles at the site of infection and to carry out appropriate débridement. Prompt and extensive surgery is the principal element in the treatment of gas gangrene. This includes excision of involved muscles (or amputation when necessary) and fasciotomies to decompress and to drain the swollen fascial compartments. Antibiotic therapy is an important adjunct to surgical management. Penicillin G has been the antibiotic of choice in the past and is administered intravenously in a dosage for the adult of 1–2 million units every 2–3 hours. Currently, the combination of penicillin with clindamycin (600 mg IV q6h) is widely used in treatment. The addition of clindamycin is based on results of experimental studies of fulminant clostridial myonecrosis in mice, where clindamycin, metronidazole, and tetracycline were each more effective than penicillin.[33] In vitro, the addition of penicillin to metronidazole antagonizes the activity of the latter; in contrast, the combination of penicillin with clindamycin provides slightly greater efficacy than clindamycin alone, but significantly enhanced efficacy over that of penicillin alone.[34]

An additional antimicrobial (e.g., chloramphenicol, third-generation cephalosporin, ciprofloxacin) may be employed initially when Gram-stained smears of the wound exudate show gramnegative bacilli as well as the predominant gram-positive bacilli. Chloramphenicol is also a good alternative drug in the highly penicillin-allergic patient; it is preferable to tetracycline in view of the resistance of some clostridia to the latter. Although the majority of *C. perfringens* isolates are susceptible in vitro to first-, second-, and third-generation cephalosporins, the minimum inhibitory concentrations for at least 10 percent of isolates are above levels readily achievable in vivo.[35] The demonstration of plasmids mediating transferable drug resistance (tetracycline and chloramphenicol; perhaps erythromycin and clindamycin) in *C. perfringens*[36] suggests the need for periodic monitoring of antibiotic susceptibilities of clinical isolates. Some strains of this organism may be showing somewhat less susceptibility in vitro to penicillin than was formerly the case.[35] *Clostridium perfringens* are susceptible in vitro to metronidazole, but experience with the clinical use of this drug in clostridial myonecrosis is lacking.

The role of hyperbaric oxygen therapy is still under debate. Its use should never delay immediate surgical débridement when possible. Its most appropriate role at present would appear to be in the management of patients with extensive involvement of the trunk in whom surgical excision would be impossible (paraspinal sites) or mutilating.[37] Initial hyperbaric oxygen therapy may reduce the extent of débridement necessary under these circumstances. The efficacy of intravenously administered polyvalent gas gangrene antitoxin has never been established clinically. It is no longer available. Ancillary therapy is essential in the management of gas gangrene. This includes attention to fluid and electrolyte replacement and maintenance of adequate hematocrit levels by transfusions.

NONCLOSTRIDIAL (CREPITANT) MYOSITIS

Nonclostridial (crepitant) myositis includes four relatively distinct entities, differing from gas gangrene in their clinical picture and bacteriologic characteristics: *(1)* anaerobic streptococcal myonecrosis, *(2)* synergistic nonclostridial anaerobic myonecrosis, *(3)* infected vascular gangrene, and *(4) Aeromonas hydrophila* myonecrosis.

Anaerobic Streptococcal Myonecrosis

Anaerobic streptococcal myonecrosis is an acute interstitial myositis that clinically resembles subacute clostridial gas gangrene. The initial manifestations are swelling and a copious seropurulent exudate occurring 3–4 days after injury. Pain develops subsequently, unlike the early occurrence of pain in gas gangrene. Tissue gas is present in muscle and fascial planes but is not extensive. The wound has an unpleasant sour odor. The involved muscles are discolored but do react to stimulation. In contrast to gas gangrene, early cutaneous erythema is prominent. If not adequately treated, the infection progresses, with the development of toxemia, frank gangrene, and shock.

Numerous streptococci and polymorphonuclear leukocytes are present in the exudate. The infection is usually mixed (anaerobic streptococci with group A streptococci or *Staphylococcus aureus*). A mixed infection of muscle with both peptostreptococci and *Bacillus subtilis* has been observed on several occasions in the setting of vascular injury. The clinical picture, along with the appearance of the Gram-stained smear, initially might suggest the diagnosis of clostridial myonecrosis.[38] Treatment involves the use of large doses of penicillin (and an antistaphylococcal agent, if indicated) and surgical débridement.

Synergistic Nonclostridial Anaerobic Myonecrosis

Synergistic nonclostridial anaerobic myonecrosis is a severe infection and is also known as *synergistic necrotizing cellulitis* (see Ch. 72); it involves skin, subcutaneous tissue, fascia, and muscle. The most extensive involvement is in the subcutaneous tissues and fascia; changes in the overlying skin and underlying muscle are usually secondary.

Very rarely crepitant myonecrosis may be caused by *Klebsiella pneumoniae*, unaccompanied by other organisms (aerobic or anaerobic), in a patient with diabetes mellitus.[39] The clinical course is rapidly progressive, with a fatal outcome.

Infected Vascular Gangrene

Infected vascular gangrene is a mixed infection developing in a group of muscles or in a limb devitalized as a result of arterial insufficiency, particularly in patients with diabetes mellitus. *Proteus, Bacteroides,* and anaerobic streptococci are among the bacteria found in such lesions. Gas formation and foul-smelling pus are prominent. The infection does not extend beyond the area of vascular gangrene to involve healthy muscle. *Bacillus cereus* infection has been associated with myonecrosis with slight crepitance after thrombosis of arterial grafts.[41]

Aeromonas Hydrophila Myonecrosis

Rapidly progressive myonecrosis due to *Aeromonas hydrophila*, a facultatively anaerobic, gram-negative bacillus, may follow penetrating trauma either in a freshwater environment or associated with fish or other aquatic animals.[42,43] In a few instances, myonecrosis has been accompanied by gas spreading extensively in soft tissue planes. The rapid onset (24–48 hours) and rapid progression after trauma resemble those of clostridial gas gangrene. The prominence of pain, marked edema, serosanguineous bullae, and toxicity, as well as the presence of gas in fascial planes, adds to the similarity of these conditions. Bacteremia is frequently present. Treatment consists of extensive surgical débridement and prompt initiation of antimicrobial therapy. Most isolates of *Aeromonas* are susceptible in vitro to gentamicin, tobramycin, trimethoprim-sulfamethoxazole, chloramphenicol, and ciprofloxacin.[44] Third-generation cephalosporins and aztreonam also appear to be active.

PSOAS ABSCESS

Infection of the psoas muscle takes the form of either an abscess or a phlegmon. It is usually the consequence of spread of infection from an adjacent structure. Rarely, it develops by the hematogenous route[45]; in children particularly, there may be no prior inciting event such as trauma or preceding infection, and *S. aureus* is the most common etiology in this setting. Psoas abscess usually is confined within the psoas fascia, but occasionally, due to anatomic relations, infection extends to the buttock, hip, or upper thigh. Psoas abscess may complicate pyogenic or tuberculous vertebral osteomyelitis. The latter was formerly the principal cause of a psoas abscess; now psoas abscesses most commonly result from direct extension of intra-abdominal infections (diverticulitis, appendicitis, Crohn's disease, and so on).[45] Occasionally, a psoas abscess results from extension of a perinephric abscess or from secondary infection of a retroperitoneal hematoma. The organisms involved in spread of infection from an intestinal site are usually members of the aerobic and anaerobic bowel flora. *Staphylococcus aureus* is the most common cause of psoas abscess secondary to vertebral osteomyelitis.

The iliacus muscle, applied to the ilium in the iliac fossa, forms a conjoined tendon with the lower portion of the psoas muscle. Osteomyelitis of the ilium or septic arthritis of the sacroiliac joint can penetrate the sheaths of either or both muscles in this location, producing an iliacus or psoas abscess.[47]

Clinical manifestations of a psoas abscess include fever, lower abdominal or back pain, or pain referred to the hip or knee. A limp may be evident, and flexion deformity of the hip may develop from reflex spasm, suggesting septic arthritis of the hip. The psoas sign is evident. Often a tender mass can be palpated in the groin.

Roentgenograms may show a bulge produced by a psoas muscle abscess or the presence of gas within the psoas sheath. Calcification in a psoas abscess strongly suggests a tuberculous etiology.

Of the five noninvasive techniques currently available for visualization of the psoas (and iliacus) muscles, CT scanning is the most rapid and sensitive. Ultrasound is less reliable for detecting small lesions or a phlegmon. Gallium scanning does not provide as sharp a localization and takes up to 72 hours; indium-labeled white blood cell scanning may be preferable to the latter. Computed tomography scanning may show diffuse enlargement of the psoas (phlegmon) or sharply circumscribed, low-density fluid collections (abscess) within the muscle, or may demonstrate the presence of gas within the muscle (indicative of abscess).[48] Magnetic resonance scanning of the pelvis can show enlarged psoas and iliacus muscles displaying grossly abnormal signal intensities.

Pyogenic psoas abscesses are treated by surgical drainage and provisional initial antibiotic therapy based on knowledge of the origin of the infection. Computed tomography scanning may be of considerable value for guidance of direct needle aspiration of an abscess for culture or for drainage when the direct surgical approach is not preferable or warranted. When the process appears to be a phlegmon, repeated CT scanning during the course of antibiotic therapy can confirm resolution of the anatomic changes.

MYALGIAS

Myalgias are prominent features of a variety of infections such as dengue, influenza, and Rocky Mountain spotted fever. Little information is available on the presence of specific histologic findings indicative of myositis.

Influenza

Muscle aches are common early in the course of influenza. Occasionally, severe bilateral muscle pains in the lower limbs may develop in the recovery phase, particularly in young children.[49,50] Muscle tenderness, principally in the gastrocnemius and soleus muscles, is demonstrable, and calf swelling may be present. Deep tendon reflexes and muscle strength are normal, but there is considerable difficulty in walking. The leg pains and muscle tenderness subside in less than a week. Mild elevations of serum levels of aldolase and creatine phosphokinase occur. The few biopsies performed have shown either nonspecific degenerative changes or muscle necrosis with polymorphonuclear leukocytic infiltration. Whether this "myositis" is due to direct viral invasion or to some immunologic or other response is unknown. However, influenza A virus has been isolated from the muscle biopsy specimen of an adult with generalized muscle weakness occurring during an influenza A outbreak.[51]

Infective Endocarditis

Prominent myalgias occur in about 15 percent of patients with infective endocarditis.[52] They may be either diffuse or localized. The pathogenesis is not known, but in one instance muscle biopsy specimens showed a small focus of muscle fiber destruction and leukocytic infiltration consistent with embolization to a small artery.[52]

Toxoplasmosis

The major features of acute acquired disseminated toxoplasmosis are those of meningoencephalitis, myocarditis, pneumonitis, skin rash, and occasionally hepatitis (see Ch. 257). In rare instances, polymyositis may be a prominent clinical manifestation. Marked myalgias, muscle weakness and swelling, and fasciculations occur in such patients. Muscle biopsy specimens show interstitial myositis with destruction of muscle fibers, and pseudocysts of *Toxoplasma gondii* can be found in areas of muscle free of inflammatory reaction. In several cases *Toxoplasma* have been isolated by animal inoculation.[53,54]

Other Etiologies

Occasionally, the only clinical manifestations of initial infection with HIV-1 are those of polymyositis (myalgias, muscle weakness, and increased serum levels of muscle enzymes). HIV-1 viral antigens can be found in CD4 cells in areas of muscle fiber inflammation and necrosis.[55] During the subsequent course of HIV-1 infection various forms of muscular involvement may develop: generalized or localized myalgias, HIV myopathy (polymyositis),[56] muscle atrophy secondary to the anorexia and cachexia of the "wasting syndrome" of AIDS,[57] and the mitochondrial myopathy related to prolonged zidovudine therapy.[58] The clinical presentation of HIV-1 myopathy (inflammatory polymyositis) is that of progressive proximal muscle weakness. Elevated serum creatine phosphokinase levels and electromyographic changes assist in diagnosis. Muscle biopsy material shows either of two histologic patterns alone or in combination: *(1)* an inflammatory myopathy with lymphocytic infiltration and muscle fiber necrosis or *(2)* abundant nemaline rod bodies and muscle fiber necrosis. In patients receiving prolonged zidovudine therapy in whom myopathy develops, muscle biopsy material shows a combination of endomyosial inflammatory infiltrate (CD8 cells and macrophages) and a mitochondrial myopathy characterized by proliferation of large numbers of abnormal mitochondria ("ragged-red fibers") in the subsarcolemmal spaces.[59] The mitochondrial changes appear to represent toxic changes associated with zidovudine therapy, and clinical improvement in some patients may follow discontinuance of the drug. The inflammatory myopathy may represent primarily an HIV-associated autoimmune process and may respond clinically to prednisone.

Inflammatory myositis with a lymphoplasmacytic cellular response was the major feature in a case of Lyme disease.[60] Spirochetes morphologically similar to *Borrelia burgdorferi* were present on Dieterle silver stain of biopsied muscle. Rarely, *Sarcocystis* (an intracellular sporozoan parasite) infection has been observed in histologic sections of muscle of individuals, mainly from abroad, with muscle pain or weakness.[61] Microsporidia myositis has occurred in a patient with AIDS.[62]

PLEURODYNIA SYNDROMES

Epidemic pleurodynia is an acute, febrile disease due to group B coxsackieviruses and is characterized by the sudden onset of sharp chest pain over the lower ribs or sternum (see Ch. 149). Paroxysms of knifelike pain are precipitated by voluntary or respiratory movements. Muscle tenderness may be present. Abdominal pain may also be present in some patients; in others abdominal pain may be the sole manifestation, simulating intraperitoneal processes.

Group B coxsackieviruses produce visceral lesions and also some focal myositis in experimental animals. Myositis has not been demonstrated as a feature pathologically either in the fatal cases of severe neonatal coxsackievirus B infection or in the few biopsy specimens obtained from affected muscles of patients with epidemic pleurodynia.[63,64]

MYALGIAS WITH EOSINOPHILIA (PARASITIC MYOSITIS)

Trichinosis

The prominent clinical manifestations of trichinosis include fever, myositis, periorbital edema, and eosinophilia. An initial intestinal phase during the first week after infection is followed during the second week by larval invasion of skeletal muscle (see Ch. 267). Serious complications in the form of myocarditis, meningoencephalitis, and pneumonitis can occur.[65] Myalgias, frequently accompanied by muscle swelling and weakness and occasionally associated with fasciculations, are present in most patients with the disease. Muscles commonly involved include the extraocular muscles, flexor muscles of the extremities, back muscles, and the muscles used in chewing and swallowing. Periorbital edema, chemosis, and conjunctival hemorrhages are related to larval invasion of extraocular muscles. The inflammatory response in muscle produces an elevation of serum levels of muscle enzymes.

Muscle biopsy specimens reveal encysted larval trichinae in necrotic muscle fibers surrounded by inflammatory cells (predominantly eosinophils and neutrophils, but also lymphocytes). Severe skeletal muscle involvement has been reported in a case of trichinosis in an immunosuppressed patient.[66] Although granulomatous reactions have been observed in the heart and lungs of fatal cases, larval encystment does not take place in organs other than skeletal muscle.

Trichinosis should be distinguished from the eosinophilia-myalgia syndrome resulting from the ingestion of certain tryptophan products and characterized by prominent myalgias, fatigue, and eosinophilia, followed, in some instances, by development of neurologic and sclerodermalike skin changes.[67]

Cysticercosis (Cysticercus Cellulosal Myositis)

Human cysticercosis is rare in the United States but is common in Latin America and Asia. It results from the ingestion and subsequent hatching of viable eggs of *Taenia solium* into the larval form of the parasite *Cysticercus cellulosae* (see Ch. 269). Eggs reach the upper intestinal tract from food contaminated by feces from a person parasitized by the adult worm. Autoinfection can occur through the fecal-oral route and possibly when reverse peristalsis introduces egg-laden proglottids back into the duodenum or stomach where they hatch. From there they are distributed widely (skeletal muscle, subcutaneous tissues, heart, eye).

Symptomatic involvement of muscle is uncommon. Occasionally, the stage of invasion is characterized by fever, muscle tenderness, and eosinophilia. More characteristically, asymptomatic calcified cysts ("puffed rice" appearance) are detected in muscles on soft tissue x-ray films of patients with neurologic manifestations.

MUSCLE DEGENERATION ASSOCIATED WITH INFECTIONS AT OTHER SITES

Acute Rhabdomyolysis

Myoglobinuria occasionally follows an acute illness with symptoms suggesting an upper respiratory tract infection. Scattered cases in recent years have been shown to follow documented influenza A virus infections in children and adults,[68] legionnaires' disease, leptospirosis (Weil's disease),[69] pneumococcal sepsis,[70] echovirus infections,[71] and infections due to coxsackievirus, Epstein-Barr virus, and adenovirus.[72] Diffuse muscle pains (especially in the extremities), weakness, swelling, and tenderness are prominent features, along with myoglobinuria. Rhabdomyolysis has occurred in patients who have had no previous episodes and no family history of this condition. Like the myositis after influenza occurring in children, it develops when respiratory symptoms are resolving.

Muscle Proteolysis and Mediators of Fever in Patients with Sepsis

Muscle involvement, in the form of myalgias and weakness, is common in the course of systemic infections. Accelerated catabolism of skeletal muscle contributes to the marked weakness and muscle wasting that can be observed in systemic infections. This appears to be part of a protective "acute phase" host response to sepsis and trauma. Important roles are played by interleukin-1 (IL-1), tumor necrosis factor, interferon-α, and IL-6. A polypeptide (possibly a breakdown product of IL-1) that produces a rapid increase in protein degradation in rat or human muscle preparations[73] has been observed in the plasma of patients with sepsis. Similar changes are produced by IL-1 itself.[74] This accelerated proteolysis is effected through increased synthesis in muscle of prostaglandin E_2, which in turn activates proteases in muscle-cell lysosomes. This catabolic activity is accompanied by IL-1-stimulated hepatic protein synthesis (using the newly generated source of amino acids) and other elements of the acute phase response and by fever (also generated by IL-1 and mediated by prostaglandin E_2). The important role of prostaglandin E_2 in the generation of the muscle aches and fever of infection is consistent with the amelioration of these symptoms produced by prostaglandin synthesis inhibitors such as aspirin.

REFERENCES

1. Smith IM, Vickers AB. Natural history of 338 treated and untreated patients with staphylococcal septicaemia. Lancet. 1960;1:1318.
2. Levin MJ, Gardner P, Waldvogel FA. "Tropical" pyomyositis. An unusual infection due to *Staphylococcus aureus*. N Engl J Med. 1971;284:196.
3. Horn CV, Master S. Pyomyositis tropicans in Uganda. E Afr Med J. 1968; 45:463.
4. Gibson RK, Rosenthal SJ, Lukert BP. Pyomyositis: Increasing recognition in temperate climates. Am J Med. 1984;77:768.
5. Christin L, Sarosi GA. Pyomyositis in North America: Case reports and review. CID. 1992;15:668.
6. Gardiner JS, Zauk AM, Minnefor AB, et al. Pyomyositis in an HIV-positive premature infant: Case report and review of the literature. J Pediatr Orthop 1990;10:791.
7. Rodgers WB, Yodlowski ML, Mintzer CM. Pyomyositis in patients who have the human immunodeficiency virus. Case report and review of the literature. J Bone Joint Surg (A) 1993;75:588.
8. Murphy PM, Lane HC, Fauci AS, et al. Impairment of neutrophil bactericidal capacity in patients with AIDS. J Infect Dis. 1988;158:627.
9. Miyake H. Beitrag zur Kenntniss des sogenannten Myositis infectiosa. Mitt Grenzgeb Med Chir. 1904;13:155.
10. Immerman RP, Greenman RL. Toxic shock syndrome associated with pyomyositis caused by a strain of *Staphylococcus aureus* that does not produce toxic-shock-syndrome toxin—1. J Infect Dis. 1987;156:505.
11. Kennedy CA, Mathisen G, Goetz MB. Tropical pyomyositis of the abdominal wall musculature mimicking acute abdomen. West J Med. 1990;152:296.
12. Armstrong JH. Tropical pyomyositis and myoglobinuria. Arch Intern Med. 1978;138:1145.
13. Sarubbi FA, Gafford GD, Bishop DR. Gram-negative bacterial pyomyositis: Unique case and review. Rev Infect Dis. 1989;11:789.
14. Schiff RG, Silver L. Tropical pyomyositis. Demonstration of extent and distribution of disease by gallium scintigraphy. Clin Nucl Med. 1990;15:542.
15. Quillin SP, McAlister WH. Rapidly progressive pyomyositis. Diagnosis by repeat sonography. J Ultrasound Med. 1991;10:181.
16. Back SA, O'Neill T, Fishbein G, et al. A case of group B streptococcal pyomyositis. Rev Infect Dis. 1990;12:784.
17. Svane S. Peracute spontaneous streptococcal myositis. Acta Chir Scand. 1971;137:155.
18. Moore DL, Delage G, Labelle H, et al. Peracute streptococcal pyomyositis: Report of two cases and review of the literature. J Pediatr Orthop. 1986;6: 232.
19. Stevens DL, Tanner MH, Winship J, et al. Severe group A streptococcal infections associated with a toxic shock-like syndrome and scarlet fever toxin A. N Engl J Med. 1989;321:1.
20. Johnson L, Berggren L, Björsell-Östling E, et al. Streptococcal myositis. Scand J Infect Dis. 1992;24:661.
21. Nather A, Wong FY, Balasubramaniam P, et al. Streptococcal necrotizing myositis: A rare entity. Clin Orthop Rel Res. 1987;215:206.
22. Yoder EL, Mendez J, Khatib R. Spontaneous gangrenous myositis induced by *Streptococcus pyogenes:* Case report and review of the literature. Rev Infect Dis. 1987;9:382.
23. Stevens DL, Gibbons AE, Bergstrom R, et al. The Eagle effect revisited: Efficacy of clindamycin, erythromycin, and penicillin in the treatment of streptococcal myositis. J Infect Dis. 1988;158:23.
24. Altemeier WA, Fullen WD. Prevention and treatment of gas gangrene. JAMA. 1971;217:806.
25. MacLennan JD. The histotoxic clostridial infections of man. Bacteriol Rev. 1962;26:177.
26. Bornstein DL, Weinberg AN, Swartz MN, et al. Anaerobic infections: Review of current experience. Medicine. 1964;43:207.
27. Altemeier WA, Furste WL. Gas gangrene. Surg Gynecol Obstet. 1947;84: 507.
28. Finegold SM. Anaerobic Bacteria in Human Disease. New York: Academic Press; 1977:424.
29. Stevens DL, Musher DM, Watson DA, et al. Spontaneous, nontraumatic gangrene due to *Clostridium septicum*. Rev Infect Dis. 1990;12:286.
30. Caplan ES, Kluge RM. Gas gangrene: Review of 34 cases. Arch Intern Med. 1976;136:788.
31. Dyelewski J, Wiesenfeld H, Latour A. Postpartum uterine infection with *Clostridium perfringens*. Rev Infect Dis. 1989;11:470.
32. Case Records of the Massachusetts General Hospital. N Engl J Med. 1993; 328:340.
33. Stevens DL, Maier KA, Laine BM, et al. Comparison of clindamycin, rifampin, tetracycline, metronidazole, and penicillin for efficacy in prevention of experimental gas gangrene due to *Clostridium perfringens*. J Infect Dis. 1987; 155:220.
34. Stevens DL, Laine BM, Mitten JE. Comparison of single and combination antimicrobial agents for prevention of experimental gas gangrene caused by *Clostridium perfringens*. Antimicrob Agents Chemother. 1987;31:312.
35. Marrie TJ, Haldane EV, Swantee CA, et al. Susceptibility of anaerobic bacteria to nine antimicrobial agents and demonstration of decreased susceptibility of *Clostridium perfringens* to penicillin. Antimicrob Agents Chemother. 1981; 19:51.
36. Brefort G, Magot M, Ionesco H, et al. Characterization and transferability of *Clostridium perfringens* plasmids. Plasmid. 1977;1:52.
37. Shupak A, Halpern P, Ziser A, et al. Hyperbaric oxygen therapy for

gas gangrene casualties in the Lebanon War, 1982. Isr J Med Sci. 1984;20:323.

38. Chambers CH, Bond GF, Morris JH. Synergistic necrotizing myositis complicating vascular injury. J Trauma. 1974;14:980.

39. Bruno-Murtha LA, Sedghivaziri MA, Arbeit RD. Crepitant myonecrosis caused by *Klebsiella pneumoniae* in an immunocompromised diabetic patient. J Infect Dis. 1990;162:1416.

40. George WL. Other infections of skin, soft tissue, and muscle. In: Finegold SM, George WL, eds. Anaerobic Infections in Humans. New York: Academic Press; 1989:504.

41. Johnson DA, Aulicino PL, Newby JG. *Bacillus cereus*–induced myonecrosis. J Trauma. 1984;24:267.

42. Davis WA, Kane JG, Garagusi VF. Human *Aeromonas* infections: A review of the literature and case report of endocarditis. Medicine. 1978;57:267.

43. Heckerling PS, Stine TM, Pottage JC, et al. *Aeromonas hydrophila* myonecrosis and gas gangrene in a nonimmunocompromised host. Arch Intern Med. 1983;143:2005.

44. San Joaquin VH, Scribner RK, Picket DA, et al. Antimicrobial susceptibility of *Aeromonas species* isolated from patients with diarrhea. Antimicrob Agents Chemother. 1986;30:794.

45. Steiner JL, Septimus EJ, Vartian CV. Infection of the psoas muscle secondary to *Streptococcus pneumoniae* infection. CID. 1992;15:1047.

46. Kyle J. Psoas abscess in Crohn's disease. Gastroenterology. 1971;61:149.

47. Simons GW, Sty JR, Starshak RJ, et al. Retroperitoneal and retrofascial abscesses. J Bone Joint Surg. 1983;65-A:1041.

48. Gordin F, Stamler C, Mills J. Pyogenic psoas abscesses: Noninvasive diagnostic techniques and review of the literature. Rev Infect Dis. 1983;5:1003.

49. Middleton PJ, Alexander RM, Szymanski MT. Severe myositis during recovery from influenza. Lancet. 1970;2:533.

50. Mejlszenkier JD, Safran AP, Healy JJ, et al. The myositis of influenza. Arch Neurol. 1973;29:441.

51. Kessler HA, Trenholme GM, Harris AA, et al. Acute myopathy associated with influenza A/Texas/1/77 infection. JAMA. 1980;243:461.

52. Churchill MA, Geraci JE, Hunder GG. Musculoskeletal manifestations of bacterial endocarditis. Ann Intern Med. 1977;87:754.

53. Greenlee JE, Johnson WD, Campa JF, et al. Adult toxoplasmosis presenting as polymyositis and cerebral ataxia. Ann Intern Med. 1975;82:367.

54. Kass EH, Andrus SB, Adams RD, et al. Toxoplasmosis in the human adult. Arch Intern Med. 1952;89:759.

55. Dalakas MC, Pezeshkpour GH, Gravell M, et al. Polymyositis associated with AIDS retrovirus. JAMA. 1986;256:2381.

56. Simpson DM, Bender AN. Human immunodeficiency virus-associated myopathy: Analysis of 11 patients. Ann Neurol. 1988;24:79.

57. Grunfeld C, Feingold KR. Metabolic disturbances and wasting in the acquired immunodeficiency syndrome. N Engl J Med. 1992;327:329.

58. Till M, MacDonell KB. Myopathy with human immunodeficiency virus type 1 (HIV-1) infection: HIV-1 or zidovudine? Ann Intern Med. 1990;113:492.

59. Dalakas MC, Illa I, Pezeshkpour GH, et al. Mitochondrial myopathy caused by long-term zidovudine therapy. N Engl J Med. 1990;322:1098.

60. Atlas E, Novak SN, Duray P, et al. Lyme myositis: Muscle invasion by *Borrelia burgdorferi*. Ann Intern Med. 1988;109:245.

61. Beaver PC, Gadgil RK, Morera P. Sarcocystis: A review and report of five cases. Am J Trop Med Hyg. 1979;28:819.

62. Ledford DK, Overman MD, Gonzalvo A, et al. Microsporidiosis myositis in a patient with the acquired immunodeficiency syndrome. Ann Intern Med. 1985;102:628.

63. Adams RD. Diseases of Muscle. A Study in Pathology, Hagerstown, MD: Harper and Row; 1975:318.

64. Cherry JD. Enteroviruses. In: Remington JS, Klein JO, eds. Infectious Diseases of the Fetus and Newborn Infant. Philadelphia: WB Saunders; 1976:397.

65. Most H. Trichinosis: Preventable but still with us. N Engl J Med. 1978;298:1178.

66. Jacobson ES, Jacobson HG. Trichinosis in an immunosuppressed human host. Am J Clin Pathol. 1977;68:791.

67. Culpepper RC, Williams RG, Mease PJ, et al. Natural history of the eosinophilia-myalgia syndrome. Ann Intern Med. 1991;115:437.

68. Minow RA, Gorbach S, Johnson BL, et al. Myoglobinuria associated with influenza A infection. Ann Intern Med. 1974;80:359.

69. Solbrig MV, Sher JH, Kula RW. Rhabdomyolysis in leptospirosis (Weil's disease). J Infect Dis. 1987;156:692.

70. Naschitz JE, Yeshurun D, Shagrawi I. Rhabdomyolysis in pneumococcal sepsis. Am J Med. 1989;87:479.

71. Josselson J, Pula T, Sadler JH. Acute rhabdomyolysis associated with an echovirus 9 infection. Arch Intern Med. 1980;140:1671.

72. Meshkinpour H, Vaziri ND. Acute rhabdomyolysis associated with adenovirus infection. J Infect Dis. 1981;143:133.

73. Clowes GHA Jr, George BC, Villee CA Jr, et al. Muscle proteolysis induced by a circulating peptide in patients with sepsis or trauma. N Engl J Med. 1983;308:545.

74. Baracos V, Rodemann HP, Dinarello CA, et al. Stimulation of muscle protein degradation and prostaglandin E_2 release by leukocytic pyrogen (interleukin-1). A mechanism for the increased degradation of muscle proteins during fever. N Engl J Med. 1983;308:553.

74. LYMPHADENITIS AND LYMPHANGITIS

MORTON N. SWARTZ

LYMPHADENITIS

Lymphadenitis is an acute or chronic inflammation of lymph nodes. It may be restricted to a solitary node or to a localized group of nodes draining an anatomic area (regional lymphadenitis), or the involvement can be generalized during a systemic infection. The gross features may be those of nonsuppurative, suppurative, or caseous inflammation, depending on the nature of the infecting microorganism.

Pathogenesis and Pathologic Changes

Acute Lymphadenitis. Lymph nodes serve as filters, removing infectious agents from lymphatics draining areas of acute inflammation. The initial histologic response consists of swelling and hyperplasia of sinusoidal lining cells and the infiltration of leukocytes. Depending on the nature of the infecting organism, host defenses, and antimicrobial therapy, the process may or may not progress to abscess formation. With some microorganisms, more distinctive pathologic pictures may be seen—caseation necrosis with infections due to *Mycobacterium tuberculosis, Histoplasma capsulatum, Coccidioides immitis,* and various atypical mycobacteria; stellate abscesses surrounded by palisading epithelioid cells (''granulomatous abscess'') with lymphogranuloma venereum and cat scratch disease; reactive follicular hyperplasia with scattered clusters of epithelioid histiocytes, located in cortical and paracortical zones and characteristically blurring the margins of germinal centers, along with focal distension of subcapsular and trabecular sinuses by monocytoid cells (monocytoid B cells) in toxoplasmosis.[1] The necrotizing granulomatous lymphadenitis that occurs in tularemia can resemble that occurring in cat scratch disease but often exhibits more granulomatous inflammation. Yersinia (*Y. pseudotuberculosis* or *Y. enterocolitica*) infection in mesenteric lymph nodes can also cause a necrotizing lymphadenitis. Necrotizing nongranulomatous lymphadenitis may be a feature of processes to which an infectious etiology has not yet been ascribed: Kikuchi's necrotizing lymphadenitis, Kawasaki syndrome, and systemic lupus erythematosus.[2]

Chronic Lymphadenitis. Histologically, the response is proliferative with hyperplasia of reticuloendothelial cells, prominent germinal centers, and dilated lymph sinuses filled with mononuclear cells. This picture is nonspecific, can be seen with a variety of infections, and may be observed initially on biopsy in a patient subsequently proven to have a lymphoproliferative disorder.

Dermatophathic lymphadenitis is a distinctive form of chronic lymphadenitis involving lymph nodes draining sites of chronic pruritic dermatitides. Histologically, the enlarged nodes show hyperplasia of reticulum cells in the germinal follicles and of sinusoidal lining cells, as well as the accumulation of lipid and melanin in macrophages (released from the inflammatory process in the skin). The latter feature is the basis for the pathologic designation *lipomelanotic reticuloendotheliosis*. The hyperplastic appearance of such nodes may be so prominent as to suggest erroneously the diagnosis of a lymphoproliferative disorder.

Clinical Findings

Acute Regional Lymphadenitis Due to Pyogenic Bacteria. Palpable lymph nodes do not always indicate serious or ongoing disease. Some degree of inguinal lymphadenopathy is relatively common, reflecting prior episodes of infection on the lower extremities (e.g., interdigital web infections secondary to epidermophytosis); similarly, minor enlargement of cervical nodes may be the residual from previous pharyngeal or dental infections. Lymphadenopathy in certain anatomic areas (preauricular, posterior auricular, supraclavicular, deltoidopectoral, and pectoral) should be viewed with greater suspicion because they are not frequently enlarged as a result of local subclinical infections or minor trauma. Enlargement of superficial lymph nodes along the external jugular vein, as well as of nodes that drain the earlobe and the floor of the external acoustic meatus, is very infrequent but may be associated with superficial infection accompanying recent initial earring insertion. Rarely, a firm mass in the tail or lateral aspect of the breast, suggestive of carcinoma, proves to be an enlarged lymph node in an unusual location due to toxoplasmosis.[1]

Acute suppurative lymphadenitis is more common in children than in adults. In the past three decades, *Staphylococcus aureus* has superseded group A streptococci as the most frequent etiology. The most common sites of involvement are, in order, submandibular (submaxillary), anterior and posterior cervical, inguinal, and axillary lymph nodes. The portal of entry for infection is frequently difficult to determine in children when cervical lymph nodes are involved.

On examination the involved area is swollen and the node(s) is usually at least 3 cm in diameter and tender. Fever is commonly present. The node(s) may be very firm or frankly fluctuant. The overlying skin is warm and often erythematous and edematous.

Syndromes Due to Suppurative Lymphadenitis at Specific Anatomic Sites. CERVICAL LYMPHADENITIS. Acute unilateral adenitis of pyogenic origin occurs most often in pre-school-aged children. The temperature is usually elevated (100–101°F), and local swelling may have been present for some days before the patient is seen by a physician. In only a minority of the cases is there a history of sore throat. However, in the past, group A streptococci have been implicated in about 75 percent of the cases of untreated suppurative cervical lymphadenitis in children.[3,4] *Staphylococcus aureus,* or a combination of *S. aureus* and group A streptococci, is often the etiology of suppurative cervical lymphadenitis associated with pyodermas of the face and scalp. Acute torticollis may result from cervical lymphadenitis, due to either bacterial or viral (e.g., infectious mononucleosis) etiologies, and may be the initial symptom that brings the child to the physician.[5]

On examination, there is prominent swelling of the neck or face due to the enlargement usually of a single node, which is often walnut sized. The node is exquisitely tender and firm but may be fluctuant. The swelling may be sufficiently marked to interfere with opening of the mouth. A leukocytosis of 12,000–25,000 white blood cells per cubic millimeter is commonly present.

Acute bilateral cervical adenitis usually involves multiple nodes that are enlarged and somewhat tender in association with viral pharyngitis, infectious mononucleosis, streptococcal pharyngitis, or periodontal infections. Such lymphadenopathy does not ordinarily go on to suppuration unless the symptomatic streptococcal pharyngitis or periodontal infections are ignored.

ACUTE AXILLARY LYMPHADENITIS. This process, when due to *S. pyogenes,* is characterized by an abrupt onset with chills, fever, marked axillary pain, and prominent edema of the shoulder, arm, axilla, supraclavicular fossa, and pectoral areas.[6] The initiating infection is usually a pustule or traumatic lesion on the hand or arm. The involved area, although edematous, does not have features of cellulitis, lymphangitis, or erysipelas. Ipsilateral pleural effusion may develop due to blockage of lymphatic vessels draining the parietal pleura into involved lymph nodes at the junction of the internal jugular and subclavian veins. Thrombosis of the axillary and subclavian veins may be a complication.

SUBPECTORAL LYMPHADENITIS. An unusual course may be taken occasionally by infection (usually streptococcal but sometimes staphylococcal) of the thumb or of the interdigital web between the thumb and index finger. Lymphatics from this area do not pass through the epitrochlear nodes but drain directly into the axillary nodes, which in turn communicate with the subpectoral nodes. If infection is not contained in the axillary nodes, subpectoral lymphadenitis develops.[7] Suppuration of these subpectoral nodes can follow. Infection in this area may dissect downward and manifest as cellulitis over the lower chest and upper abdomen, suggesting an intra-abdominal infection. Occasionally, large subpectoral abscesses may suggest a tumor because the overlying pectoralis major obscures the local warmth and erythema commonly associated with infection. Rarely, contraction of the pectoral muscle (as on elevating the arm) causes cephalad movement of the pectoral area swelling, suggesting avulsion of the inferior attachments of this muscle to sternum, sixth costal cartilage, and the aponeurosis of the external abdominal oblique muscle. The suppurating nodes may drain onto the chest wall. A pleural effusion may develop on the involved side.

ACUTE SUPPURATIVE EPITROCHLEAR LYMPHADENITIS. The epitrochlear nodes receive lymphatic drainage from the middle, ring, and little fingers and from the medial portion of the hand and the ulnar aspect of the forearm. Acute suppurative epitrochlear lymphadenitis is uncommon. The predisposing infection in most patients is a primary pyoderma or secondarily infected skin lesions. Unilateral tender swelling, erythema, and induration of the epitrochlear area develop and may subsequently spread along the medial aspect of the arm and forearm. Pain on movement of the elbow is evident. There is often a moderate fever and leukocytosis. The diagnosis is apparent when a discrete, tender nodular swelling can be palpated; but when the area is diffusely swollen and movement at the elbow is limited, the picture may suggest septic arthritis or osteomyelitis.[8] Group A streptococci and *S. aureus* are implicated most commonly.

SUPPURATIVE ILIAC LYMPHADENITIS. The iliac lymph nodes are located along the external and common iliac arteries in the anterior retroperitoneal space. They receive deep lymphatic drainage from the lower abdominal wall and afferents from the superficial and deep inguinal nodes. Iliac lymphadenitis may develop secondary to infection of the lower extremities, lower abdominal wall, perineum, and so forth, or rarely it may result from hematogenous infection. After infection develops, it appears to break through fascial compartments in the iliac fossa and abscess formation ensues. Formerly, most cases occurred in children and young adults, but more recently there appears to be no age predilection. The suppurative lymphadenitis progresses to abscess formation in the space between the posterior peritoneum and the psoas and iliacus fascia.[9] An unexplained limp may be the initial symptom; the acute onset with fever may not occur for some days or weeks. Back and hip pain becomes prominent; extension of the thigh is very painful, but abduction and adduction of the hip evoke minimal discomfort. The symptomatology and clinical findings direct attention to the diagnoses of septic arthritis and osteomyelitis. Only after some days or weeks does lower abdominal pain develop, and the patient becomes acutely ill with high fever and marked leukocytosis. Examination at this point reveals a tightly flexed hip, rectus muscle spasm on the affected aide, possibly a tender posterolateral pelvic mass, or a tender inguinal mass suggesting an incarcerated inguinal hernia. By this stage, the abscess may be sizable and may produce elevation and medial displacement of the sigmoid colon and medial displacement of the lower one-third of the ureter. When the symptoms are on the right side, the diagnosis of *retrocecal* appendicitis with abscess may be suggested, but the antecedent limp is an important clinical clue. Other diagnoses that may be suggested by the clinical manifestations include tuberculosis of the spine with psoas abscess formation, pelvic inflammatory disease, and tumor of the thigh.[10] Body computed tomography (CT) scanning can be very helpful in defining an inflammatory collection abutting the psoas and iliacus muscles. *Staphylococcus aureus* is the microorganism most commonly implicated, followed in frequency by streptococci.

Acute Regional Lymphadenitis Due to Infecting Agents Other Than Pyogenic Bacteria. A variety of organisms other than the common pyogens may produce localized lymphadenitis (in some cases, going on to abscess and sinus tract formation). These infections resemble pyogenic lymphadenitis but are distinguishable by a prolonged and indolent course, the atypical anatomic areas involved, the lack of prior pyogenic infection, and clues in the history (scratch by a cat, previous tuberculosis, recent sexual exposure, and so forth). Occasionally, the nature of the clinical setting broadens the spectrum of microorganisms to be considered in causing firm or fluctuant lymphadenitis. Mycotic (*Candida albicans, aspergillus* spp.) cervical lymphadenitis has occurred after oral mucositis in neutropenic children with leukemia.[11] In patients with suppurative lymphadenitis complicating chronic granulomatous disease, the microbial etiology is usually a catalase-positive pathogen. In addition to the commonly involved *S. aureus*, these include Enterobactericeae (*Klebsiella, Serratia, Salmonella*), *Pseudomonas* (often *cepacia*), *Aspergillus, Nocardia,* Calmette-Guérin bacillus (BCG), and *Chromobacterium violaceum*.[12–14]

SPECIFIC TYPES OF NONPYOGENIC REGIONAL LYMPHADENITIS. *Scrofula (Tuberculous Cervical Lymphadenitis).* Tuberculous cervical adenitis, formerly a common disease in children and young adults, has become infrequent. It is still occasionally seen in older adults who many years earlier had immigrated to this country from endemic areas (British Isles, Europe, and the Far East) or who lived in rural areas in this country. In this setting it represents breakdown of prior cervical node tuberculosis, acquired either by ingestion of infected milk (bovine tuberculosis) or by lymphohematogenous spread of infection from an initial pulmonary focus to this group of lymph nodes. *Mycobacterium tuberculosis* is seen in this country as the etiology of cervical adenitis also in adults of particular ethnic groups: Native Americans, Hispanics, and recent immigrants from Haiti and Asia. In this country mycobacterial cervical lymphadenitis (scrofula) is four to five times more frequently due to atypical mycobacteria, commonly *Mycobacterium scrofulaceum* in children,[15] than to *M. tuberculosis.* In certain areas of the United States, *M. avium-intracellulare* complex is the principal etiology,[16] particularly in adults. *Mycobacterium tuberculosis* infections, including cervical lymphadenitis, are frequent in the human immunodeficiency virus (HIV)-infected population. *Mycobacterium tuberculosis* lymphadenitis in the HIV-infected patient differs in several respects from the infection in HIV-negative patients: higher frequency of fever, often negative PPD skin test, and higher frequency of positive smears for acid-fast bacilli (and greater numbers of organisms) on fine-needle aspirates of involved lymph nodes.[17] In parts of the world where BCG vaccination of infants is commonly practiced, subcutaneous abscesses and regional lymphadenitis are not uncommon complications, occurring 2–8 weeks after vaccination, but usually heal spontaneously. Occasionally, the regional (axillary, supraclavicular, or cervical) lymphadenitis progressively enlarges and goes on to caseating suppuration.[18]

The onset of scrofula is insidious, and fever and other systemic manifestations are absent. Several nodes are enlarged and matted together; the mass so formed may develop a swollen fluctuant area, and this brings the patient to medical attention. The process is usually painless. In most cases, clinical evidence of tuberculosis elsewhere is absent. Spontaneous drainage of caseous material onto the skin surface (scrofuloderma) may eventually occur.

Definition of the mycobacterial species involved is important. The atypical mycobacteria causing cervical lymphadenitis are frequently resistant to the usual antituberculous chemotherapy, and surgical excision of the involved fluctuant node(s) is indicated. Antituberculous therapy is usually not needed for BCG nonsuppurative lymphadenitis, but if suppurative lymphadenitis develops, complete excision[19] and antituberculous chemotherapy are indicated.

Granulomatous Lymphadenitis Caused by Nondiphtheria Corynebacteria. Subacute or chronic relapsing lymphadenitis has been reported occasionally to be due to *Corynebacterium pseudotuberculosis (C. ovis).*[20] Most patients have had extensive contact with animals, particularly sheep. The histologic picture is that of a suppurative or necrotizing granulomatous process. Treatment consists of prolonged antibiotic (erythromycin or penicillin) therapy combined with surgical drainage or excision of the involved nodes.

Oculoglandular (Parinaud) Syndrome. Preauricular lymphadenopathy can occur secondary to granulomatous nodular conjunctival infection caused by the introduction of certain pathogens onto the external eye. Oculoglandular syndromes occur occasionally in tularemia, cat scratch disease,[21] listeriosis, sporotrichosis, and lymphogranuloma venereum. Epidemic keratoconjunctivitis due to adenoviruses is often associated with an enlarged preauricular lymph node.

Cat Scratch Disease.[21] Cat scratch disease is a slowly progressive and sometimes chronic form of regional lymphadenitis (see Ch. 108). In the past, the clinical diagnosis was made on the basis of meeting three of the following four criteria: *(1)* appropriate cat contact with evidence of a scratch, a primary dermal lesion or conjunctivitis; *(2)* regional lymphadenopathy with failure to isolate a known etiologic agent from aspirated pus or with normal results from laboratory tests for other causes of lymphadenopathy; *(3)* a bimorphic histologic picture consisting of stellate abscesses with necrotic centers and of granulomas with epitheloid cells; and *(4)* a positive intradermal skin test of a known preparation of cat scratch skin test antigen (derived from pus from a suppurative node of a patient with cat scratch disease). In view of the possibility of spread of viral hepatitis or of HIV infection from such a human source of the antigenic preparation, such skin testing is no longer performed. Although cat scratch disease is usually a benign and ultimately self-limited process, it may be complicated by acute encephalitis, hepatitis, osteolysis, neuroretinitis, arthritis, pleuritis, atypical pneumonia, hilar adenopathy, and thrombocytopenia.

In 1983, small bacilli were demonstrated for the first time by use of the Warthin-Starry silver impregnation stain to be present in walls of capillaries, in macrophages lining sinuses near germinal centers, and in necrotic areas of involved lymph nodes of patients with cat scratch disease.[22] A hitherto undescribed pleomorphic, fastidious gram-negative bacillus was subsequently isolated from lymph nodes of a small number of patients with cat scratch disease, and several of the patients had fourfold or greater rises in indirect fluorescent antibody titers against this organism,[23] now a designated *Afipia felis.*[24] However, in most patients with cat scratch disease, *A. felis* is not isolated on culture nor is there an antibody response to this organism. In almost 90 percent of individuals with cat scratch disease, moreover, antibodies appear to *Bartonella (Rochalimaea) henselae,*[25,26] the causative agent of bacillary angiomatosis and peliosis hepatitis in patients with HIV infection.[27,28] Further support for the role of *B. henselae* in cat scratch disease comes from *(1)* the detection by polymerase chain reaction (PCR) of sequences of 16S rRNA from *B. henselae* and not from any other organism, including *A. felis,* in a cat scratch disease skin test antigen preparation[29] and from *(2)* the isolation of *B. henselae* from the blood of a sick cat.[30] Current evidence suggests that *B. henselae* is the causative agent of most cases of cat scratch disease but whether *A. felis* is responsible for a small number of cases remains controversial. Recently, *B. henselae* has been isolated from infected lymph nodes of two immuno-competent patients with cat scratch disease.[31] The organisms are small, pleomorphic, curved gram-negative rods that are oxidase-negative, catalase-negative, and X-factor dependent. *B. henselae* are slow growing, requiring 2–6 weeks' incubation in a moist environment (e.g., in a sealed, gas-permeable plastic bag) under 5% CO_2 for growth on blood agar plates (human blood preferable to sheep or horse blood) (see Ch. 170).[31]

Cat scratch disease sometimes occurs in patients with HIV infection. In this setting the disease may have prominent systemic manifestations and high fever, involve multiple skin sites, be prolonged, and frequently recur.[32] Bacillary angiomatosis rarely has involved lymph nodes in immunosuppressed patients and may simulate, histologically, vascular neoplasms such as Kaposi sarcoma, angiosarcoma, and hemangioendothelioma.[33] Because *B. henselae* (or a closely related organism) is the etiology of cat scratch disease in the immunocompetent patient and bacillary angiomatosis in the immunocompromised patient with acquired immunodeficiency syndrome (AIDS), the pathophysiologic basis for the differing clinical pictures is unclear (possible *B. henselae* strain differences; differences in state of cellular immune function).

About 90 percent of patients with cat scratch disease give a history of contact with cats (most often kittens), and most have been scratched. A primary lesion (small papule or vesicle resembling an insect bite) develops at the site of the scratch 7–14 days after contact with the cat. This primary lesion lasts for several weeks to months and may be helpful in diagnosis. Lymphadenopathy develops within 1–2 weeks of the appearance of the skin papule.[34] There is no lymphangitis. The lymphadenopathy progresses to suppuration in 10–50 percent of cases, but the course is slower than that of suppurative lymphadenitis due to pyogenic bacteria, and most patients are only mildly ill. Regional lymphadenitis is the sole manifestation of cat scratch disease in half of the cases. Almost any peripheral lymph nodes may be involved, but the axillary nodes are most commonly affected. The nodes are tender, acutely so when there is frank suppuration. Fever is present in only about one-third of patients and is low grade. About 10–15 percent of patients suffer features of a more systemic illness: anorexia, headache, weight loss, and splenomegaly. Unusual clinical presentations include Parinaud's oculoglandular syndrome (conjunctivitis from ocular inoculation associated with ipsilateral preauricular lymphadenopathy) in 4 percent of patients and acute encephalitis/encephalopathy occurring in a rare patient, usually with a sudden seizure as the initial neurologic manifestation, several weeks after the first symptoms of cat scratch disease.

Inguinal Buboes of Venereal Origin.   Inguinal lymphadenopathy due to pyogenic infections or cat scratch disease is usually unilateral. Prominent bilateral (or unilateral) adenopathy, particularly in the adult man, is suggestive of several venereal diseases. The genital chancre of primary syphilis is usually accompanied by one or several discrete, firm, nonsuppurative, painless, enlarged nodes in one or both inguinal areas. Constitutional signs are lacking. The overlying skin is uninflamed. In secondary syphilis the lymphadenopathy is generalized, painless, and usually precedes the cutaneous eruption.

In lymphogranuloma venereum (LGV), the primary genital lesion (painless papule, vesicle, or erosion) is usually transient and asymptomatic. The initial manifestation of the disease is usually the characteristic inguinal bubo, occurring 10–30 days after sexual exposure and 1–2 weeks after the primary lesion. The adenopathy is more commonly unilateral. Initially the node is tender, discrete, hard, and movable, but subsequently the inflammatory process involves multiple nodes in the area. Chills, fever, and constitutional symptoms are common at this stage. As a result of periadenitis, the nodes become fixed and matted into an oval or lobulated mass. The latter is adherent to the overlying skin that is purplish in color. Foci of suppuration develop with multiple fistulous tracts. A central lengthwise linear depression (so-called groove sign of LGV) is produced by involvement of nodes above and below the inguinal ligament. Although characteristic of LGV, the groove sign may rarely be produced by suppurative bacterial lymphadenitis or by lymphomatous involvement of inguinal nodes.

Chancroid is usually accompanied by painful, tender inguinal adenopathy. The primary lesion is a papule or pustule that progresses to form an extremely painful and tender but nonindurated ulceration with undermined edges, quite in contrast to a syphilitic chancre. Autoinoculation is common with lesions on opposing or contiguous areas of the skin. The adenopathy of chancroid develops about 1 week after the primary lesion appears and, unlike LGV, is present while the ulcer is still active. Systemic symptoms accompany chancroid only rarely. The chancroidal bubo is typically unilateral, made up of fused inguinal nodes, and is more painful than that of LGV. Unilocular suppuration may develop. However, in most patients, the lymphadenitis subsides without suppuration.

Primary genital herpetic infection in men and women is often associated with tender inguinal adenopathy. Histologically, the nodes show paracortical hyperplasia (with a prominent admixture of immunoblasts, plasma cells, and macrophages), along with sinus histiocytosis, discrete foci of necrosis, and intranuclear inclusions within scattered mononuclear and giant cells. Similar, histologically proven, recurrent, localized, as well as generalized, herpetic lymphadenitis can occur in immunocompromised patients in the absence of overt mucocutaneous lesions.[35,36] The "pseudobuboes" of granuloma inguinale are produced by subcutaneous granulomatous infection rather than by suppurative lymphadenitis.

Suppurative inguinal lymphadenitis due to group A streptococci has been superimposed on chronic lymphadenopathy in homosexual males.[37]

Inguinal Buboes of Nonvenereal Origin.   Inguinal or femoral buboes occur in bubonic plague, since the flea bite initiating the infection is commonly on a lower extremity.[38] However, involvement of most other peripheral nodes can occur. The disease begins with fever, malaise, headache, and tender regional adenopathy after an incubation period of 2–6 days. Only rarely is a lesion (papule, pustule) at the site of the insect bite evident at the onset of clinical illness. A large, matted collection of lymph nodes with surrounding edema quickly develops and may go on to suppuration and spontaneous drainage. If not treated promptly, the infection rapidly progresses to a septicemic phase. The diagnosis should be suspected in a febrile, acutely ill patient with a large cluster of extremely tender lymph nodes and a history of exposure to fleas, rodents, or rabbits in the western United States. (Tularemia may mimic the epidemiologic and clinical features of bubonic plague but is more likely to produce an *ulceroglandular syndrome* [Table 1], with a primary lesion at the site of inoculation.[39]) Diagnostic procedures include blood cultures (uniformly positive in the septicemic phase of plague), as well as cultures and stained smears (see Ch. 208) of carefully obtained bubo aspirates. Appropriate treatment (see below) should be instituted immediately while awaiting results of cultures if bubonic plague is suspected.

GENERALIZED LYMPHADENITIS ASSOCIATED WITH SYSTEMIC INFECTIONS.   Widespread lymphadenitis is a feature of a variety of infections disseminated by the blood stream. In most instances, suppuration of the involved nodes does not occur. Generalized lymphadenopathy is a feature, for example, of secondary syphilis, HIV infection, infectious mononucleosis, leptospirosis, and miliary tuberculosis. Generalized lymphadenopathy associated with infections is commonly due to the presence

TABLE 1. Clinical Patterns and Microbial Etiologies of Infectious Lymphadenitis

Disease	Infecting Organism	Regional	Regional with Suppuration (or Caseation)	Inguinal Bubo Formation	Ulceroglandular	Oculoglandular	Generalized
Bacterial							
Pyogenic	Group A strep; S. aureus	+	+				
Scarlet fever	Group A strep.	+	+				+
Diphtheria	C. diphtheriae	+					
Fusospirochetal angina	P. melaninogenica; peptostreptococci, etc.	+					
Scrofula	M. tuberculosis	+	+				
	M. scrofulaceum; M. avium-intracellulare	+	+				
Miliary tuberculosis	M. tuberculosis						+
Brucellosis	Brucella						+
Leptospirosis	Leptospira						+
Syphilis	T. pallidum	+					+
Chancroid	H. ducreyi			+			
Plague	Y. pestis	+	+	+			
Tularemia	F. tularensis		+		+	+	
Rat-bite fever	Streptobaccillus moniliformis; Spirillum minus	+			+		
Anthrax	B. anthracis	+			+		
Listeriosis	L. monocytogenes					+	
Melioidosis	P. pseudomallei	+	+				+
Glanders	P. mallei	+	+				+
Cat scratch	B. henselae	+	+		±	+	
Typhoid fever	S. typhi						+
Mycotic							
Histoplasmosis	H. capsulatum						+
	H. capsulatum var. duboisii	+					
Coccidioidomycosis	Coccidioides immitis	+					
Paracoccidioidomycosis	P. brasiliensis	+					
Cryptococcosis	C. neoformans						+
Rickettsial							
Boutonneuse fever, etc.	R. conori				+		
Scrub typhus	R. tsutsugamushi	+					+
Rickettsialpox	R. akari	+					
Chlamydial							
Lymphogranuloma venereum	C. trachomatis			+		+	+
Viral							
Measles	Measles virus						+
Rubella	Rubella virus						+
Infectious mononucleosis	EB virus						+
CMV mononucleosis	CMV virus						+
Dengue fever	Dengue virus						+
West Nile fever	West Nile virus						+
Lassa fever	Lassa virus						+
Genital herpes infection	HSV type 2	+					
Pharyngoconjunctival fever	Adenovirus (types 3 and 7)					+	
Epidemic keratoconjunctivitis	Adenovirus (types 8 and 19)					+	
AIDS; AIDS-related complex	HIV						+
Protozoan							
Kala azar	Leishmania donovani						+
African trypanosomiasis	Trypanosoma brucei	+					+
Chagas disease	T. cruzi					+	+
Toxoplasmosis	Toxoplasma gondii						+
Helminthic							
Filariasis	Wucheria bancrofti						+
	Brugia malayi						+
Loiasis	Loa loa			+			
Oncocerciasis	Oncocerca volvulus			+			

Abbreviations: CMV, cytomegalovirus; HSV, herpes simplex virus; AIDS, acquired immunodeficiency syndrome; HIV, human immunodeficiency virus.

of the invading microorganism in the nodes. Generalized lymph node enlargement is a feature of a variety of infectious diseases due to bacterial, rickettsial, chlamydial, spirochetal, viral, protozoal, and helminthic agents (Table 1).

Etiologic Agents and Differential Diagnosis

It is helpful for purposes of the differential diagnosis to consider infective lymphadenitis in several categories (Table 1): (1) regional lymphadenopathy, (2) regional lymphadenopathy with breakdown of nodes, (3) inguinal bubo formation, (4) ulceroglandular syndrome, (5) oculoglandular syndrome, and (6) generalized lymphadenopathy.

In distinguishing among the causes of fluctuant cervical lymphadenitis, the history may suggest a streptococcal (preceding tonsillitis), staphylococcal (recent facial or neck infection), tuberculous (prior exposure to tuberculosis), or cat scratch disease (exposure to cat) etiology. In a study of suppurative cervical adenitis S. aureus was the etiology more frequently than group A streptococci (36 percent vs. 26 percent), and in another one-quarter of the cases a bacteriologic diagnosis could not be made.[40] A subacute clinical course with little fever and a normal leukocyte count would be more consistent with cat scratch disease or tuberculous involvement. Sinus tract formation suggests infection due to M. tuberculosis or an atypical mycobacterium. Gram-stained and Ziehl-Neelsen smears and culture (including cultures for mycobacteria) of material aspirated or drained from suppurating nodes provides a diagnosis in about two-thirds of such cases of cervical lymphadenitis. Further information may be provided by skin tests (purified protein derivative), serologic tests (antistreptolysin O antibody titer), and histologic examination (caseation necrosis suggesting mycobacterial infection; bimorphic appearance suggesting cat scratch disease) of an excised node when culture of aspirated material is unrevealing. A variety of noninfectious processes may resemble unilateral cervical lymphadenitis. Lymphoma may be suggested by the indolent course of cat scratch disease. Acute febrile mucocutaneous lymph node syndrome (Kawasaki syndrome), a disease of infants and young children of unknown etiology, is characterized by nonsuppurative cervical lymphadenopathy.[41] The age of the patient, febrile course, conjunctival injection, erythematous rash, and subsequent desquamation suggest the diagnosis. A recently described benign disorder of lymph nodes, histiocytic necrotizing lymphadenitis or Kikuchi's disease, was first recognized in Japan and now has been observed in the United States.[42] Clinically, its features consist of localized, sometimes tender, cervical lymphadenopathy, often with an upper respiratory prodrome and associated in some patients with fever. Most cases occur in women, commonly under 30 years of age. Occasional patients present with generalized lymphadenopathy, and rarely hepatosplenomegaly occurs.[43] Less frequent symptoms include nausea, vomiting, weight loss, and night sweats, suggesting the diagnosis of lymphoma. Mild leukopenia and lymphocytosis may suggest infectious mononucleosis. The illness does not respond to antibiotics, but it usually resolves spontaneously within 1 or 2 months. Histologically, biopsy specimens may be erroneously interpreted as lymphoma, but the principal findings are those of focal reticulum cell hyperplasia combined with patchy areas of coagulative necrosis. Although a viral etiology is suspected on the basis of the clinical features, serologic and ultrastructural studies have failed to identify a specific agent.

Bronchial cleft cysts and cystic hygromas may be mistaken for cervical lymphadenitis, particularly if infected; thyroglossal duct cysts may suggest infected submental nodes. Submaxillary sialadenitis or salivary gland tumors may mimic submandibular lymphadenitis. Bimanual (intraoral and submandibular) palpation can be helpful in distinguishing between these processes.

Isolated inguinal lymphadenitis or bubo formation in the adult suggests venereal disease (syphilis, LGV, chancroid). Distinctive associated primary lesions are usually features of syphilis and chancroid but not of LGV. The inguinal adenopathy of primary syphilis consists of painless, firm, discrete, movable nodes without erythema of the overlying skin. The nodes do not suppurate, whereas spontaneous rupture of the buboes of LGV and chancroid may occur. The groove sign is suggestive of LGV. The buboes of chancroid are characteristically painful. Axillary, cervical, and inguinal buboes may occur with plague and tularemia. In plague, an inguinal location is common. The geographic locale and a history of animal exposure are important clues to the diagnosis. Inguinal and femoral nodes can be involved in cat scratch disease, although much less frequently than axillary or cervical nodes.

Generalized lymphadenopathy is frequently a manifestation of disseminated infection (Table 1). Clues may be provided by the age of the patient and the presence of a characteristic rash (childhood exanthems, secondary syphilis), geographic factors (dengue, filariasis, localized leishmania lymphadenitis,[44] histoplasmosis), occupation and/or dietary history (brucellosis, toxoplasmosis), exposure to animals (leptospirosis), and the presence of atypical lymphocytes (infectious mononucleosis, cytomegalovirus infection). Diagnosis of toxoplasmic lymphadenitis in the immunocompetent patient is based primarily on serologic testing, although sometimes a node biopsy is performed because of initial concern for lymphoma. A negative result in the Sabin-Feldman dye test or in a comparable test

for toxoplasma IgG antibody (indirect immunofluorescent [IIF], passive hemagglutination [PHA], or enzyme-linked immunosorbent assay [ELISA]) practically excludes the diagnosis. Acute infection is likely if a high IgM antibody titer is present with a high IgG antibody titer (dye test or IIF test titers of >1:1000) in a single serum specimen. Laboratory diagnosis of acute toxoplasmic lymphadenitis can also be made by seroconversion from a negative to a positive IgG antibody test or by demonstration of a fourfold titer rise over 3 weeks. In endemic areas, generalized nonsuppurative (and very rarely, suppurative) lymphadenopathy occurs in typhoid fever.[45]

Widespread suppurative infections of lymph nodes occur as a result of the microbicidal defect characteristic of neutrophils and monocytes of patients with chronic granulomatous disease. Recurrent infections (skin, bones, lungs, and liver, as well as lymph nodes) beginning in childhood and due to *S. aureus* and certain gram-negative bacilli (*Escherichia coli,* salmonella, *Serratia marcescens*) suggest the diagnosis.

Widespread lymphadenopathy may be a feature of many noninfectious diseases, particularly infiltrative processes such as lymphoma and reticuloendothelioses. Prominent peripheral lymphadenopathy may be a feature of rheumatoid arthritis. Lymphadenopathy may occur as an adverse effect of prolonged use of phenytoin. Widespread lymphadenopathy is a feature of the syndrome of immunoblastic lymphadenopathy, which is often accompanied by skin rash, polyclonal hypergammaglobulinemia, and immunosuppression. This disorder of immune regulation often eventuates in B-cell or T-cell lymphomas.[46]

Sinus histiocytosis with massive lymphadenopathy (Rosai-Dorfman disease) is another benign process that produce extensive, painless lymphadenopathy in the cervical areas in children and adolescents.[47] It is often accompanied by fever, neutrophilic leukocytosis, and polyclonal hypergammaglobulinemia. Histologically there is extensive proliferation of histiocytelike cells within the sinuses of the involved lymph nodes.[48] The etiology is unknown, and the prognosis is favorable. A very rare form of regional lymphadenopathy, showing sinus histiocytosis (containing metal granules) histologically, can be the result of wear-induced debris from an adjacent metallic prosthesis.[49] Similarly, enlarged regional lymph nodes (showing noncaseating granulomas containing silicone) have been described draining areas in which a silicone mammary prosthesis or a silastic joint prosthesis[50] had been inserted previously.

Generalized Lymphadenopathy with AIDS or with the AIDS-Related Complex.   Patients with AIDS may have generalized lymphadenopathy in which involvement with opportunistic infection or neoplastic disease (particularly Kaposi sarcoma) is evident on histologic examination. The infections have included those due to cytomegalovirus and *M. avium-intracellulare*.[51] The latter usually show a few poorly formed or no granulomas and a prominent histiocytic reaction. Large clusters ("globi") of acid-fast bacilli are present within the cytoplasm of histiocytes. Kaposi sarcoma in patients with AIDS often follows the pattern of generalized lymph node involvement and a fulminant course with mucosal and visceral lesions.[52] In AIDS other neoplasms can involve lymph nodes. These are primarily of the B-cell type and include B-cell immunoblastic sarcomas, small noncleaved, Burkitt-like lymphoma, and plasmacytoid lymphocytic lymphoma.[53] Patients with AIDS surviving for up to 3 years on antiretroviral therapy have a relatively high probability of a supervening non-Hodgkin's lymphoma.[54]

Lymphadenopathy occurs in 50–75 percent of patients at risk for AIDs who develop an acute illness approximately 3–6 weeks after initial exposure to HIV.[55,56] It often is one feature of a mononucleosislike syndrome consisting of fever, malaise, myalgias, headaches, sore throat, diarrhea, leukopenia, thrombocytopenia, and a maculopapular rash. After the acute clinical illness subsides, lymphadenopathy may remain as persistent generalized lymphadenopathy (PGL), involving at least several extrainguinal sites, of at least 3 months' duration. This progressive lymphadenopathy early in the course of this infection may be the result of an active immune response against HIV in the affected lymph nodes[57] (see Ch. 101). PGL may also occur in male homosexuals, intravenous drug abusers, and other individuals in high-risk groups without any history of prior clinically apparent initial HIV infection. The nodes are discrete and nontender; suppuration does not occur. HIV replication takes place in such lymph nodes,[58] which histologically show follicular hyperplasia or mixed follicular and interfollicular hyperplasia.[59] With progression to AIDS, lymphocyte depletion supervenes. PGL is frequently one of the manifestations of what has been termed the *AIDS-related complex,* a group of clinical manifestations (including fever, weight loss, diarrhea, fatigue, and night sweats) occurring in individuals at risk for developing AIDS but not as yet having any definable underlying infectious or neoplastic cause for the symptoms. Laboratory findings in this clinical syndrome include two or more of the following: *(1)* lymphopenia, *(2)* decreased numbers of helper T cells, *(3)* depressed helper/suppressor cell ratio, *(4)* increased levels of serum globulins, *(5)* decreased blastogenesis in response to mitogens, and *(6)* anergy to skin test antigens. A sizable number of patients with such chronic generalized lymphadenopathy go on eventually to develop AIDS, with its complicating opportunistic infections and Kaposi sarcoma[57] (see Ch. 102). Regression of the lymphadenopathy may occur after 8–19 months in some patients.

During the intense viremia of primary HIV infection, seeding of multiple lymph nodes occurs producing detectable or subclinical lymphadenopathy. Nodal accumulation of activated CD4 T cells ensues. Thereafter, throughout the period of clinical latency, the HIV burden in lymphoid tissue is greater than in peripheral blood. This is thought to be related to the follicular hyperplasia and expansion of the meshwork of follicular dendritic cells in the lymph nodes and the trapping therein of HIV (either in T cells that cannot recirculate or as extracellular virus). In the later stages of HIV disease, nodal architecture, including the network of follicular dendritic cells, is extensively disrupted, ablating the trapping mechanisms for HIV particles. The return of prominent viremia in the late stages of infection probably represents the consequence of loss of capacity of lymph node entrapment, as well as the progressive loss of other anti-HIV host defenses.[57]

Presumptive Treatment

Initial treatment of infective lymphadenitis requires some narrowing of the diagnostic possibilities (Table 1). Localized pyogenic lymphadenitis responds well to early antibiotic treatment. When cervical lymphadenitis has developed from a pharyngeal or periodontal portal, initial treatment with penicillin is appropriate (procaine penicillin G, 300,000–600,000 units intramuscularly every 12–24 hours initially to ensure receipt of therapy when the patient may be nauseated; subsequently 250–500 mg of penicillin V may be administered orally every 6 hours for at least 20 days for older children and adults). In patients who are more acutely ill, larger doses of aqueous penicillin G parenterally are indicated. Erythromycin (20–40 mg/kg/day orally in divided doses every 6 hours) is an alternative for patients allergic to penicillin.

Pyogenic lymphadenitis complicating skin infections may be staphylococcal or streptococcal in etiology, and a penicillinase-resistant penicillin is the drug of choice (e.g., dicloxacillin, 0.25–0.5 g orally every 6 hours for the older child or an adult). In the more acutely ill patient, intravenous administration of a semisynthetic penicillinase-resistant penicillin (e.g., nafcillin) or a first-generation cephalosporin should be employed. Failure to show improvement, or progression to suppuration, is an indication for percutaneous needle aspiration (for bacteriologic diagnosis and treatment) or surgical drainage.

For cat scratch disease, usually a self-limited process resolving in 2–4 months, treatment is principally symptomatic. If the nodes become fluctuant, aspiration is appropriate both for relief of pain and for bacteriologic diagnosis. The few strains of *R. henselae* from cat scratch disease that have been studied show in vitro susceptibility to a variety of antimicrobial agents, with the notable exception of first-generation cephalosporins.[31] In a retrospective review of antimicrobial treatment of several hundred patients with cat scratch disease, clinical efficacy (58–87 percent) was attributed to four drugs (in increasing order): trimethoprim-sulfamethoxazole, gentamicin, ciprofloxacin, and rifampin.[60] Antimicrobial therapy may be reasonable in patients with more severe or extranodal cat scratch disease. Bacillary angiomatosis and bacillary peliosis hepatitis, infections in patients with AIDS and due to *B. henselae* or a closely related *Bartonellaceae* sp., appear to respond to prolonged antimicrobial therapy with either erythromycin, doxycycline, or rifampin.[28]

If the diagnosis of bubonic plague is suspected, antibiotic treatment should be instituted promptly. Streptomycin (1.0 g intramuscularly every 12 hours in adults) or tetracycline (0.5 g orally every 6 hours in adults) are the preferred drugs, and treatment is continued for 10 days.

LYMPHANGITIS

Lymphangitis is an inflammation of lymphatic channels, usually in the subcutaneous tissues. It occurs either as an acute process of bacterial origin or as a chronic process of mycotic, mycobacterial, or filarial etiology.

Pathologic Changes and Pathogenesis

The visible red streaking in acute lymphangitis stems from the inflammatory process in the walls (and surrounding tissue spaces) of dilated lymphatic channels. Lymphatic obstruction often occurs on healing, resulting sometimes in persistent lymphedema. Cutaneous lymphatic sporotrichosis, a form of chronic lymphangitis, produces a combined suppurative and granulomatous response.

Clinical Findings

Acute Lymphangitis. Acute lymphangitis develops when an infection, commonly on an extremity, is not contained locally but spreads along lymphatic channels. Such infections are most often due to group A streptococci (occasionally streptococci of other groups; very rarely *S. aureus*). Systemic manifestations may develop rapidly before evidence of infection becomes apparent at the site of inoculation of organisms, and they may be more prominent than might be anticipated on the basis of local pain and erythema. Red linear streaks, a few millimeters to several centimeters in width, extend from the initial site of infection toward the regional lymph nodes, which are enlarged and tender. Peripheral edema of the involved extremity often occurs. The time course of this type of infection can be accelerated from initial lesion to lymphangitis to complicating bacteremia in 24–48 hours. Occasionally, recurrent episodes of lymphangitis occur, with the initial episode causing some degree of chronic lymphedema, in turn predisposing to another episode. Rarely, elephantiasis nostras, a temperate zone (nonfilarial) form of progressive lymphatic obstruction of a lower limb, can follow recurrent episodes of streptococcal lymphangitis. With each episode, further localized edema occurs, eventuating in grotesque enlargement of the extremity due to permanent solid edema, fibrosis of dermis and subcutaneous tissues, and verrucous pachydermia.[61]

The peripheral white blood cell count is commonly elevated. The etiologic agent often can be identified on gram-stained smears and cultures obtained from the initial lesion. Blood cultures also may reveal the causative organism.

Acute lymphangitis and/or lymphadenitis, usually involving the lower extremities, is a feature of filariasis due to *Wuchereria bancrofti* (and sometimes to *Brugia malayi*).[62] These mosquito-borne diseases are endemic to Africa, Southeast Asia and the Pacific, and tropical South America. The acute form of disease is characterized by recurrent episodes of headache, backache, lymphangitis, lymphadenitis, epididymitis, and orchitis. Bancroftian lymphangitis may involve the breast, suggesting clinically the appearance of carcinoma.[63] Fever is uncommon. The adult filariae reside in lymphatics and lymph nodes and discharge microfilariae into the blood stream. With prolonged exposure in an endemic area, chronic lymphatic obstruction can develop with elephantiasis of the skin and scrotum. In this setting, recurrent episodes of lymphangitis may be the result of both the parasitic infestation and superimposed streptococcal infections (to which the chronic lymphedema predisposes). Serologic tests for filariasis may be helpful in diagnosis if microfilariae are not found, but they are positive in many other filarial infections. Lymph node or lymphatic vessel biopsy may be necessary for diagnosis.

Chronic Granulomatous Lymphangitis.   Unlike acute lymphangitis, this is an indolent process with little pain or systemic evidences of infection. Sporotrichosis is most commonly the underlying disease.[64] This infection frequently is introduced by minor trauma (e.g., from a thorn of a barberry or rose bush) into the skin of a gardener. An erythematous subcutaneous nodule (often becoming fluctuant) or a chancriform ulcer subsequently develops at the site of inoculation of *Sporothrix schenckii* (present on some plants and in sphagnum moss used in gardening) on the hand or finger.[65] The lesion does not respond to local treatment or to administration of the common antibacterial agents. Slowly, multiple subcutaneous nodules appear and extend proximally along the course of regional lymphatics, which become thickened. Other infections producing a "sporotrichoid" pattern are characterized as nodular lymphangitis.[66]

Cutaneous infection ("swimming pool granuloma") with *Mycobacterium marinum*, an atypical mycobacterium that grows optimally at 25–32°C and is found in swimming pools and fish tanks, produces a chronic nodular, verrucous or ulcerative lesion at the site of an abrasion, usually about the knees or elbows. The lesion is usually solitary, but in an occasional patient new lesions develop proximally, as in sporotrichosis. Multiple sporotrichoid lesions have occurred in occasional infections due to *Nocardia brasiliensis*[67] and in rare infections due to *Mycobacterium kansasii, M. chelonae, and N. asteroides.* Even rarer causes of nodular lymphangitis include American leishmaniasis, staphylococcal botryomycosis, and tularemia (reported earlier this century but not in the past 40 years).[66]

Etiologic Agents

In the United States acute lymphangitis is most commonly due to group A streptococci, and chronic lymphangitis is usually caused by *S. schenckii.* Other infectious agents occasionally produce lymphangitis (Table 2).

Differential Diagnosis

The combination of a peripheral infection or traumatic lesion and the acute onset of fever with proximal red linear streaks directed toward regional lymph nodes is diagnostic of acute lymphangitis. In the legs, thrombophlebitis may produce linear areas of tender erythema, but the absence of an initiating lesion and of tender regional adenopathy is helpful in distinguishing it from lymphangitis. A history of rat bite and the subsequent development of lymphangitis suggest *Spirillum minus* infection. Filariasis is a consideration when an appropriate geographic his-

TABLE 2. Causes of Lymphangitis

Clinical Form	Etiologic Agent	Relative Frequency as Etiology of Lymphangitis
Acute	Group A streptococcus	Common
	S. aureus	Occasional
	Pasteurella multocida	Occasional
	Spirillum minus (rat-bite fever)	Rare
	W. bancrofti; B. malayi (filariasis)	Rare (only in immigrants from endemic areas)
Chronic	*Sporothrix schenckii* (sporotrichosis)	Occasional
	M. marinum (swimming pool granuloma)	Occasional
	M. kansasii	Rare
	Nocardia brasiliensis	Rare
	W. bancrofti; B. malayi	Rare (only in immigrants from endemic areas)
	N. asteroides	Very rare
	M. chelonae	Very rare
	S. aureus (botryomycosis)	Very rare
	Leishmania brasiliensis or *mexicana*	Very rare
	Francisella tularensis	Very rare

tory is obtained. Sporotrichosis is considered when chronic ulcerative lymphangitis develops in someone working with plants, soil, or timbers. *Mycobacterium marinum* is suggested as the etiology when sporotrichoid lesions develop in a person who has been around swimming pools and fish tanks.

Presumptive Therapy

Penicillin is the initial treatment of acute lymphangitis. In a mildly ill adult, 600,000 units of procaine penicillin G once or twice daily is administered initially, with supplementary oral penicillin V. More acutely ill patients in whom bacteremia may have developed should be hospitalized and treated with parenteral aqueous penicillin G (600,000–2,000,000 units every 4–6 hours). If a staphylococcal etiology is suspected, a penicillinase-resistant penicillin is used.

The initial treatment of presumptive lymphocutaneous sporotrichosis is saturated solution of potassium iodide, and itraconazole is also effective[66] (see Ch. 240). If sporotrichoid *M. marinum* infection is suspected, the diagnosis should be confirmed by demonstration of acid-fast bacilli and by isolation of the organism at 30°C on appropriate media. Localized swimming pool granulomas are often treated by surgical excision. Chemotherapy is reserved for more extensive and sporotrichoid forms of infection. On the basis of limited data, the combination of choice would appear to be rifampin and ethambutol[66,68] (see Ch. 233). Prolonged tetracycline or minocycline therapy has also been reported as successful in a small number of cases,[66,69] but in vitro resistance to and treatment failure with doxycycline have been reported.[70] Trimethoprim-sulfamethoxazole has been reported as effective in several studies. However, in vitro activity requires drug concentrations greater than those usually achieved in serum and tissues.[71]

REFERENCES

1. McCabe RE, Brooks RG, Dorfman RF, et al. Clinical spectrum in 107 cases of toxoplasmic lymphadenopathy. Rev Infect Dis. 1987;9:754.
2. Strickler JG, Warnke RA, Weiss LM. Necrosis in lymph nodes. Pathol Annu. 1987;2:253.
3. Scobie WG. Acute suppurative adenitis in children. Scot Med J. 1969;14:352.
4. Dajani AS, Garcia RE, Wolinski E. Etiology of cervical lymphadenitis in children. N Engl J Med. 1963;268:1329.
5. Bredenkamp JK, Maceri DR. Inflammatory torticillis in children. Arch Otolaryngol Head Neck Surg. 1990;116:310.
6. Boyce JM. Severe streptococcal lymphadenitis. N Engl J Med. 1990;323:655.
7. Amren DP. Unusual forms of streptococcal disease. In: Wannamaker LW, Matsen JM, eds. Streptococci and Streptococcal Disease. New York: Academic Press; 1972:545.
8. Currarino G. Acute epitrochlear lymphadenitis. Pediatr Radiol. 1977;6:160.

9. Maull KI, Sachatello CII. Retroperitoneal iliac fossa abscess. A complication of suppurative iliac lymphadenitis. Am J Surg. 1974;127:270.

10. Oliff M, Chuang VP. Retroperitoneal iliac fossa pyogenic abscess. Radiology. 1978;126:647.

11. Shenep JL, Kalwinsky DK, Feldman S, et al. Mycotic cervical lymphadenitis following oral mucositis in children with leukemia. J Pediatr. 1985;106:243.

12. Curnutte JT, Boxer LA. Clinically significant phagocytic cell defects. In: Remington JS, Swartz MN, eds. Current Clinical Topics in Infectious Diseases. v. 4. New York: McGraw-Hill; 1985:103–55.

13. Sorensen RU, Jacobs MR, Shurin SB. *Chromobacterium violaceum* adenitis acquired in the northern United States as a complication of chronic granulomatous disease. Pediatr Infect Dis. 1985;4:701.

14. Kobayashi Y, Komazawa Y, Kobayashi M, et al. Presumed BCG infection in a boy with chronic granulomatous disease. A report of a case and review of the literature. Clin Pediatr. 1984;23:586.

15. Lincoln EM, Gilbert LA. Disease in children due to mycobacteria other than *Mycobacterium tuberculosis*. Am Rev Respir Dis. 1972;105:683.

16. Spark RP, Fried ML, Bean CK, et al. Nontuberculous mycobacterial adenitis of childhood. The ten-year experience at a community hospital. Am J Dis Child. 1988;142:106.

17. Shriner KA, Mathisen GE, Goetz MB. Comparison of mycobacterial lymphadenitis among persons infected with human immunodeficiency virus and seronegative controls. Clin Infect Dis. 1992;15:601.

18. Victoria MS, Shah BR. Bacillus Calmette-Guérin lymphadenitis: A case report and review of the literature. Pediatr Infect Dis. 1985;4:295.

19. Oguz F, Mujgan S, Alper G, et al. Treatment of Bacillus Calmette-Guérin-associated lymphadenitis. Pediatr Infect Dis. J. 1992;11:887.

20. Lipsky BA, Goldberger AC, Tompkins LS, et al. Infections caused by nondiphtheria corynebacteria. Rev Infect Dis. 1982;4:1220.

21. Carithers HA, Carithers CM, Edwards RO Jr. Cat-scratch disease. Its natural history. JAMA. 1969;207:312.

22. Wear DJ, Margileth AM, Hadfield TL, et al. Cat-scratch disease. A bacterial infection. Science. 1983;221:1403.

23. English CK, Wear DJ, Margileth AM, et al. Cat-scratch disease. Isolation and culture of the bacterial agent. JAMA. 1988;259:1347.

24. Brenner DJ, Hollis DG, Moss CW, et al. Proposal of *Afipia* gen. nov., with *Afipia felis* sp. nov. (formerly the cat scratch disease bacillus), *Afipia clevelandensis* sp. nov. (formerly the Cleveland Clinic Foundation strain), *Afipia broomeae* sp. nov., and three unnamed genospecies. J Clin Microbial. 1991; 29:2450.

25. Regnery RL, Olson JG, Perkins BA, et al. Serological response to "*Rochalimaea henselae*" antigen in suspected cat-scratch disease. Lancet. 1992;339: 1443.

26. Zangwill KM, Hamilton DH, Perkins BA, et al. Cat scratch disease in Connecticut. Epidemiology, risk factors, and evaluation of a new diagnostic test. N Engl J Med. 1992;329:8.

27. Relman DA, Loutit JS, Schmidt TM, et al. The agent of bacillary angiomatosis. An approach to the identification of uncultured pathogens. N Engl J Med. 1990;323:1573.

28. Koehler JE, Quinn FD, Berger TG. Isolation of *Rochalimaea* species from cutaneous and osseous lesions of bacillary angiomatosis. N Engl J Med. 1992; 327:1625.

29. Anderson B, Kelly C, Threlkel R, et al. Detection of *Rochalimaea henselae* in cat-scratch disease skin test antigens. J Infect Dis. 1993;168:1034.

30. Regnery R, Martin M, Olson J. Naturally occurring "*Rochalimaea henselae*" infection in domestic cat. Lancet. 1992;340:557.

31. Dolan MJ, Wong MT, Regnery RL, et al. Syndrome of *Rochalimaea henselae* adenitis suggesting cat scratch disease. Ann Intern Med. 1993;118:331.

32. Marasco WA, Lester S, Parsonnet J. Unusual presentation of cat scratch disease in a patient positive for antibody to the human immunodeficiency virus. Rev Infect Dis. 1989;11:793.

33. Chan JK, Lewin KJ, Lombard CM, et al. Histopathology of bacillary angiomatosis of lymph node. Am J Surg Pathol. 1991;15:430.

34. Carithers HA. Cat-scratch disease. An overview based on a study of 1,200 patients. Am J Dis Child. 1985;139:1124.

35. Epstein JI, Ambinder RF, Kuhajda, et al. Localized herpes simplex lymphadenitis. Am J Clin Pathol. 1986;86:444.

36. Miliauskas JR, Leong AS. Localized herpes simplex lymphadenitis: Report of three cases and review of the literature. Histopathology. 1991;19:355.

37. Ho DD, Murata GH. Streptococcal lymphadenitis in homosexual men with chronic lymphadenopathy. Am J Med. 1984;77:151.

38. Reed WB, Palmer DL, Williams RC, et al. Bubonic plague in southwestern United States. Medicine. 1970;49:465.

39. Young LS, Bicknell DS, Archer BG, et al. Tularemia epidemic: Vermont 1968. Forty-seven cases linked to contact with muskrats. N Engl J Med. 1969; 280:1253.

40. Barton LL, Feigin RD. Childhood cervical lymphadenitis: A reappraisal. J Pediatr. 1974;84:846.

41. Feigin RD, Schleien CI. Kawasaki's disease. In: Remington J, Swartz MN,

eds. Current Clinical Topics in Infectious Disease, v. 4. New York: McGraw-Hill; 1983;30.

42. Unger PD, Rappaport KM, Strauchen JA. Necrotizing lymphadenitis (Kikuchi's disease). Arch Pathol Lab Med. 1987;111:1031.

43. Dorfman RF. Histiocytic necrotizing lymphadenitis of Kikuchi and Fujimoto. Arch Pathol Lab Med. 1987;111:1026.

44. Garcia-González R, Sanz I, Saus C, et al. Localized lymphadenitis due to leishmania. Diagnosis by fine needle aspiration cytology. Postgrad Med J. 1990;66:326.

45. Naqvi SH, Thobani S, Moazam F, et al. Generalized suppurative lymphadenitis with typhoidal salmonellosis. Pediatr Infect Dis J. 1988;7:882.

46. Abruzzo LV, Schmidt K, Weiss LM, et al. B-cell lymphoma after angioimmunoblastic lymphadenopathy: A case with oligoclonal gene rearrangements associated with Epstein-Barr virus. Blood. 1993;82:241.

47. Rosai J, Dorfman RF. Sinus histiocytosis with massive lymphadenopathy a pseudolymphomatous benign disorder: Analysis of 34 cases. Cancer. 1972; 30:1174.

48. Paulli M, Locatelli F, Kindl S, et al. Sinus histiocytosis with massive lymphadenopathy (Rosai-Dorfman disease). Clinico-pathological analysis of a paediatric case. Eur J Pediatr. 1992;151:672.

49. Shinto Y, Uchida A, Yoshikawa H, et al. Inguinal lymphadenopathy due to metal release from a prosthesis. J Bone Joint Surg. 1993;75B:266.

50. Rogers LA, Longtine JA, Garnick MB, et al. Silicone lymphadenopathy in a long distance runner: Complication of a silastic prosthesis. Hum Pathol. 1988; 19:1237.

51. Fauci AS, Macher AM, Longo DL, et al. Acquired immunodeficiency syndrome: Epidemiologic, clinical, immunologic, and therapeutic considerations. Ann Intern Med. 1984;100:92.

52. Gottlieb MS, Groopman JE, Weinstein WM, et al. The acquired immunodeficiency syndrome. Ann Intern Med. 1983;99:208.

53. Levine AM, Meyer PR, Begandy MK, et al. Development of B-cell lymphoma in homosexual men: Clinical and immunological findings. Ann Intern Med. 1984;100:7.

54. Pluda JM, Yarchoan R, Jaffe ES, et al. Development of non-Hodgkin lymphoma in a cohort of patients with severe human immunodeficiency virus (HIV) infection on long-term antiretroviral therapy. Ann Intern Med. 1990; 113:276.

55. Kinloch-de Loës S, deSaussure P, Saurat J-H, et al. Symptomatic primary infection due to human immunodeficiency virus type 1: Review of 31 cases. Clin Infect Dis. 1993;17:59.

56. Clark SJ, Saag MS, Decker WD, et al. High titers of cytopathic virus in plasma of patients with symptomatic primary HIV-1 infection. N Engl J Med. 1991; 324:954.

57. Pantaleo G, Graziosi C, Fauci AS. The immunopathogenesis of human immunodeficiency virus infection. N Engl J Med. 1993;328:327.

58. Biberfeld P, Chayt KJ, Marselle LM, et al. HTLV-III expression in infected lymph nodes and relevance to pathogenesis of lymphadenopathy. Am J Pathol. 1986;125:436.

59. Baroni CD, Uccini S. The lymphadenopathy of HIV infection. Am J Clin Pathol. 1993;99:397.

60. Margileth AM. Antibiotic therapy for cat-scratch disease: Clinical study of therapeutic outcome in 268 patients and a review of the literature. Pediatr Infect Dis J. 1992;11:474.

61. Sanders LJ, Slomsky JM, Burger-Caplan C. Elephantiasis nostras: An eight year observation of progressive nonfilarial elephantiasis of the lower extremity. Cutis. 1988;42:406.

62. Grove DI, Warren KS, Mahmoud AAF. Algorithms in the diagnosis and management of exotic diseases. VI. The filariases. J Infect Dis. 1975;132:340.

63. Jungmann P, Figueredo-Silva J, Dreyer G. Bancroftian lymphangitis in northeastern Brazil: A histopathological study of 17 cases. J Trop Med Hyg. 1992; 95:114.

64. Orr ER, Riley HD Jr. Sporotrichosis in childhood: Report of ten cases. J Pediatr. 1971;78:951.

65. Duran RJ, Coventry MB, Weed LA, et al. Sporotrichosis: A report of twenty-three cases in the upper extremity. J Bone Joint Surg. 1957;39(A):1330.

66. Heller HM, Swartz MN. Nodular lymphangitis: Clinical features, differential diagnosis and management. In: Remington JS, Swartz MN, eds. Current Clinical Topics in Infectious Diseases. v. 14. Boston: Blackwell Scientific; 1994; 142–58.

67. Smego RA Jr, Gallis HA. The clinical spectrum of *Nocardia brasiliensis* infection in the United States. Rev Infect Dis. 1984;6:164.

68. Van Dyke JJ, Lake KB. Chemotherapy for aquarium granuloma. JAMA. 1975; 233:1380.

69. Izumi AK, Hanke W, Higaki M. *Mycobacterium marinum* infections treated with tetracycline. Arch Dermatol. 1977;1313:1067.

70. Ljungberg B, Christensson B, Grubb R. Failure of doxycycline treatment in aquarium-associated *Mycobacterium marinum* infections. Scand J Infect Dis. 1987;19:539.

71. Sanders WJ, Wolinsky E. In vitro susceptibility of *Mycobacterium marinum* to eight antimicrobial agents. Antimicrob Agents Chemother. 1980;18:529.

SECTION J. GASTROINTESTINAL INFECTIONS AND FOOD POISONING

75. PRINCIPLES AND SYNDROMES OF ENTERIC INFECTION

RICHARD L. GUERRANT

Gastrointestinal infections encompass a wide variety of symptom complexes and recognized infectious agents. With the exception of recently recognized *Helicobacter pylori* gastritis, the term *gastroenteritis* is applied to syndromes of diarrhea or vomiting that tend to involve noninflammatory infection in the upper small bowel or inflammatory infection in the colon. Other enteric infections and infestations cause predominantly systemic symptoms. Infections of the gastrointestinal tract, especially infectious diarrhea, are among the most common debilitating infectious diseases, afflicting people of all ages around the world. In many heavily populated areas, deaths from diarrheal illnesses exceed those from any other single cause.

In the absence of demonstrable causal forces, many descriptive terms have arisen through the years. Names such as "Montezuma's revenge," "Delhi belly," "Aden gut," "gyppi tummy," "Aztec two-step," "Greek gallop," "Rome runs," "Hong Kong dog," "Turkey trots," "La turista," "Basra belly," and "back door sprint" illustrate its widespread occurrence. Although an etiologic agent is not found in many cases, the infectious nature of most acute diarrheal diseases is suggested by their epidemiologic behavior showing case clustering, spread in families and other groups, and occurrence among travelers. In the last two decades, much has been learned about bacterial and viral agents capable of causing acute gastrointestinal illnesses. These include *Escherichia coli* that produce enterotoxins, which cause fluid secretion, other *E. coli* capable of causing tissue destruction and inflammation, and pathogens such as *Yersinia, Campylobacter, Clostridium, Cryptosporidium, Cyclospora,* rotaviruses, and Norwalk-like viruses. With the development of new tools for diagnosis, important information has been gained in our understanding of the etiologies, pathogenesis, epidemiology, and control of acute gastrointestinal infections.

OCCURRENCE AND SCOPE OF GASTROINTESTINAL INFECTIONS

On a global scale, diarrheal diseases are second only to cardiovascular diseases as a cause of death[1]; they are the leading cause of childhood death, and, in some populous, developing areas, they are responsible for more years of potential life loss than all other causes combined.[2] Estimates are that 4,600,000–6,000,000 children die each year (>12,600/day) in Asia, Africa, and Latin America[3–6] and that over 10,000 die from diarrhea each year in the United States.[7,8] Over 13 percent of the children born in certain parts of Latin America die before their fifth birthday. In more than half, diarrhea is the major or associated cause of death.[2] Although the global mortality is decreasing (especially with oral rehydration therapy),[9] some transitional areas have a worsening diarrhea mortality,[10] and prolonged diarrhea is

emerging as the major cause of death.[11] Even greater than the mortality is the serious morbidity from diarrheal diseases, especially in association with malabsorption and malnutrition in tropical, developing areas. In areas such as Bangladesh, India, Guatemala, and Brazil, the attack rates often reach 7–19 cases per person per year among children under 2 years of age.[12–17] The attack rate is highest at the time of weaning.[15–18]

Over 60 percent of the children dying with diarrhea in Latin America also had nutritional deficiencies as associated causes of death, suggesting that diarrhea may precipitate malnutrition.[2] Acute infectious diarrhea exacerbates nutritional deficiencies in several ways. As with any acute infection, caloric demands are increased, and often catabolic steroids, glucagon, and adrenergic amines cause increased breakdown of structural proteins.[18] Through vicious cycles of transient malabsorption and anorexia, repeated bouts of acute diarrhea are major contributors to malnutrition.[19–25] The converse is also true; undernutrition appears to reduce resistance to acute infectious diarrhea. Increased attack rates and increased mortality from acute infectious diarrheal illnesses occur with progressive severity of malnutrition.[25–28] As a specific example, shigellae are shed longer and there is an increased relapse rate in children if they are malnourished.[26] In addition, malnutrition appears to predispose to more prolonged diarrheal illnesses.[28,29]

Military history indicates that acute diarrheal illnesses have played decisive roles in numerous campaigns. Diarrheal diseases and enteric infections comprised the major nontraumatic cause of hospitalization among U.S. troops in Vietnam and in Saudi Arabia and approached the number of hospitalizations resulting from injuries due to hostile action.[30–32] Overall rates of gastrointestinal illness in the United States range from 1.5 to 5 illnesses per person per year from studies done in communities and day care centers, respectively.[5,33–35] Rates are highest in young children, but may sometimes increase during young adulthood (as with *Campylobacter jejuni* in the second weaning)[36] or in the elderly (as with *Clostridium difficile* and *Salmonella*).[5,7,37] Diarrhea remains the third most frequent syndrome seen in general practice.[31] In studies of community illness among urban and suburban families in Cleveland, Dingle et al.[33] identified "infectious gastroenteritis" as the second most common class of illnesses after common respiratory diseases. In this community, 1.5 bouts of gastroenteritis occurred per person each year and accounted for 16 percent of all illnesses.

EPIDEMIOLOGIC AND ENVIRONMENTAL FACTORS

The frequency, type, and severity of enteric infections are determined by *who* you are, *where* you are, and *when* you are there.

Who is at risk of acquiring a gastrointestinal infection varies greatly with age, living conditions, personal and cultural habits, and group exposures. Although the infant who is being breast-fed is relatively protected from contaminated food and water and probably to some degree by maternal colostral antibodies and lactoferrin, at weaning there is a great increase in the risk of diarrheal illness. Adults, particularly if living for many years in the same environment, may become asymptomatic reservoirs of microorganisms that cause diarrhea in the immunologically untutored child or visitor. Living conditions often reflect socioeconomic conditions; type of housing, population density, sanitation facilities, and water sources are major determinants of environmental exposure to enteric pathogens. The quantity of water available for hygienic and sanitation purposes is often as important as the quality of the water supply.[38] Personal hygienic habits determine how many organisms are ingested. Although the infectious dose varies with the organisms, relatively small inocula of certain organisms may result in disease. Shigellae are acquired with an unusually low infectious dose and are often spread by direct contact among children in day care centers. Conversely, *Clostridium difficile* colitis occurs with increasing frequency with age. The majority of nonspecific diarrheal illnesses acquired in communities occur in family clusters, often with small children having the first illness. Of great importance whenever a patient has an enteric illness is a careful history of other illnesses in the family or community. Multiple illnesses and common exposure may be clues to a food-borne outbreak or to the causative agent.

The second epidemiologic determinant of risk for enteric infection is *where* one is. The pattern of illnesses and the etiologic agents vary greatly with climate. For example, *E. coli* that produce heat-labile (LT) or heat-stable (ST) enterotoxins cause disease primarily in the tropics, where the heaviest burden of parasites also occurs. Viral causes of common enteric illnesses have been found among young children in temperate and tropical climates. Despite their clustering, however, many community cases of diarrhea remain unexplained.

Finally, the third determinant of risk is *when* you are there. The majority of enteric illnesses in temperate climates occur during winter months. The opposite is true in tropical countries, where distinct summer peaks of illnesses are common. The role of rainfall is uncertain, as some adjacent areas with similar monsoon climates have opposite seasons of major diarrheal illnesses, as illustrated by the peak seasons for cholera in different parts of Bengal. In Dhaka, endemic cholera occurs during the winter dry months, whereas less than 200 miles away, the peak cholera season in Calcutta occurs during the summer monsoon.

HOST FACTORS

Considering the ubiquity of potential enteric pathogens, it is surprising that enteric infections are not even more common. After exposure to infectious agents, several host factors determine who becomes ill. Several enteric host defenses provide substantial protection against many intestinal pathogens (Table 1).

Host Species, Genotype, and Age

Host species, genotype, and age are complex but major determinants of susceptibility to colonization and disease with enteric pathogens. While a broad spectrum of animal hosts are infected with pathogens such as *Salmonella enteritidis* and *Campylobacter jejuni*, only primates or humans are characteristically infected with *Salmonella typhi* or *Shigella* spp. In addition, the intestinal cell receptors for the K88, K99, and colonization factor (CF) attachment traits of enterotoxigenic *E. coli* are largely species specific.[39,40] Interspecies variation and host genotype are also important. Individuals with blood group O appear to be more susceptible to cholera, possibly others with type A to giardiasis.[41,42] Furthermore, Rutter et al.[43] have bred a strain of piglets that do not have the single-locus dominant allele for the intestinal receptor for *E. coli* K88 adherence antigen and are consequently resistant to diarrhea caused by these organisms. Such species or even genotype specificities play tremendously important roles in determining the host susceptibility as well as the epidemiology of these infections.

The role of age in determining host susceptibility is complex. In animals a narrow "age window" of susceptibility to specific enteric infections is well recognized. In humans, the tendency of rotaviral and enteropathogenic *E. coli* (EPEC) infections to affect young children is impressive. The explanations likely re-

TABLE 1. Enteric Host Defenses

Host species, genotype, and age
Personal hygiene
Gastric acidity and other physical barriers
Intestinal motility
Enteric microflora
Specific immunity
   Phagocytic
   Humoral
   Cell mediated
Nonspecific protective factors and human milk
Intestinal receptors

side in age-related changes in gut mucus, cell surface factors, microbial flora, environmental exposure, and specific immune factors. In addition, specific receptors for microbial adhesins or toxins may be developmentally regulated, such as that for *Shigella*, *Shiga*-like, cholera, *E. coli*, and *Clostridium difficile* enterotoxins.[44,47]

Specific receptor components or antagonists such as monosaccharides like N-acetylneuraminic acid (NANA) can be added exogenously and compete with intestinal binding sites for *E. coli*.[40,48] Conversely, lectin-like substances that bind to the intestinal cell receptors may compete with the bacterial attachment factors. Positive chemotaxis of *V. cholerae*, *E. coli*, and *S. typhimurium* has been shown toward rabbit ileal mucosa and a role of negative chemotactic factors have been postulated as new types of host defense.[49]

Personal Hygiene

Whether we acquire an enteric infection depends first on the number of pathogens ingested. Nearly all agents of concern are acquired by the oral route. The majority of identified enteric pathogens have come from other mammalian intestinal tracts; often a human fecal–oral route can be traced. A plentiful, conveniently located supply of uncontaminated water, in conjunction with improved sanitary facilities, is critically important in reducing this mode of spread.[38,50] Studies of presumptive viral agents that have not yet been defined strongly implicate the human fecal–oral route of infection.[51,52] In the cases of bacterial infections, a large number (100,000–100,000,000) of organisms must usually be ingested to overcome host defenses and to cause disease[53] (Table 2). Such numbers may require growth in food that is allowed to stand unrefrigerated for several hours after the initial contaminating inoculum. Exceptions to the large number of organisms usually required for an infecting dose are *Shigella* and cysts of certain parasites, which can be reproducibly transmitted with only 10–100 organisms. This small inoculum can be readily transmitted directly by person-to-person contact (as in day care centers). This is an unusual route of spread for other bacterial enteric pathogens in all but hosts with impaired defenses or newborn infants.

Gastric Acidity and Other Physical Barriers

The majority of bacterial pathogens ingested never reach the intestinal tract because of the normal gastric acid barrier. When this barrier is neutralized with antacids, both the susceptibility

TABLE 2. Infectious Doses of Enteric Pathogens

Shigella	10^{1-2}
Campylobacter jejuni	10^{2-6}
Salmonella	10^5
Escherichia coli	10^8
Vibrio cholerae	10^8
Giardia lamblia	10^{1-2} cysts
Entamoeba histolytica	10^{1-2} cysts

and severity of several enteric bacterial and parasitic infections is increased. At the normal gastric pH (<4), over 99.9 percent of the ingested coliform bacteria are killed within 30 minutes. There is no reduction of an experimental bacterial inoculum in achlorhydric stomachs for 1 hour. Not surprisingly, then, the gastric coliform flora in fasting subjects (normally fewer than 10/ml) exceed 10,000/ml in the majority of achlorhydric patients.[54] Excessive numbers of normal bacterial flora in the upper small bowel may contribute to malabsorption and diarrheal syndromes.[55,56]

The inoculum of *V. cholerae* required to cause disease can be reduced 10,000-fold (from 10^8 to 10^4 organisms) by neutralizing gastric acid with 2 g of sodium bicarbonate.[57] In an outbreak of cholera in Israel, 25 percent of the patients had had previous gastric resection, whereas none of a comparable control group had had gastric surgery.[58] The similar association of previous gastric surgery or achlorhydria with increased frequency and severity of *Salmonella* infections has also been noted in several studies.[59] Likewise, the frequency of enteric multiplication of a vaccine strain of *Shigella flexneri* increases threefold with sodium bicarbonate neutralization of gastric acid. With *Campylobacter jejuni*, a substantial range in infectious doses has been documented with different strains.[60] Although gastric acidity may enhance the process of excystation and infection by some parasites after ingestion of the ova, it may provide protection against other parasites. The fragile trophozoite of *Giardia lamblia* (requiring a pH of 6.4–7.1) causes more severe symptoms in association with hypochlorhydria or achlorhydria, perhaps by increased survival of trophozoites refluxed to the stomach and proximal duodenum. The association of achlorhydria and hypochlorhydria with symptomatic strongyloidiasis has also been noted. Some have suggested that vitamin B_{12} deficiency occurs more often in association with fish tapeworm (*Diphyllobothrium latum*) in patients who are achlorhydric and who have high jejunal infestations. Finally, certain parasitic, viral, or bacterial processes such as *Helicobacter pylori* infections may in themselves alter gastric acidity and thus increase host susceptibility to other enteric pathogens.[61] The further importance of gastric acidity in preventing gastric, pharyngeal, and tracheal colonization by gram-negative bacilli and even nosocomial pneumonia has been shown by the increased risk of patients taking antacids or H2 blockers compared to sucralfate, which preserves gastric acidity.[62]

Other physical barriers such as mucus and mucosal tissue integrity are important resistance factors in healthy hosts and work in concert with gastric acidity and intestinal motility to clear many bacteria from the upper small bowel.[63] Continuous removal and renewal of gastrointestinal mucus may bind organisms and toxins and further aid in protecting the intact mucosa from enzymatic and microbial attack.[64]

Intestinal Motility

Intestinal motility plays the following important roles in normal intestinal physiology: *(1)* in the fluid absorptive process, *(2)* in maintaining the appropriate distribution of indigenous enteric microflora, and *(3)* in ridding the host of pathogenic microorganisms. The role of motility in aiding fluid absorption has been demonstrated in a study done on human volunteers by Higgens et al.[65] Using methantheline bromide (Banthine), they showed that inhibition of normal intestinal motility resulted in impaired absorption of radiolabeled water and sodium. Whereas over 90 percent of a labeled saline bolus was normally absorbed in less than 10 minutes, less than 70 percent was absorbed over a half hour after methantheline bromide administration. Intraluminal distribution of a barium bolus in small bowel before and after methantheline bromide suggested that a reasonable explanation for this impaired absorption was a reduction in the absorptive surface area exposed to the intralumenal fluid. In contrast to the distribution within 2–3 minutes of the bolus of barium

throughout the small bowel of healthy persons, methantheline bromide caused a puddling of barium near the injection site in the upper small bowel, which often persisted for over 60 minutes.

Motility also helps to maintain normal distribution and flow of microflora. The risk of bowel stasis is evident in the bacterial overgrowth syndromes in the small bowel and in the added risk of "toxic megacolon" in inflammatory bowel disease after antimotility drugs are administered.

In addition, intestinal motility appears to play a role in providing protection from enteric pathogens. Experimental animals are much more easily infected with enteric pathogens after the inhibition of gut motility with opiates.[66] *Salmonella* bacteremia may develop in patients after opiates are taken for relatively mild gastroenteritis.[67] A controlled study of adults with shigellosis treated with diphenoxylate hydrochloride with atropine (Lomotil) revealed that the antimotility drug abolished antibiotic effectiveness in reducing diarrhea and positive cultures and was associated with prolonged fever and shedding of the *Shigella* organisms.[68] Gut motility and diarrhea that help rid the host of offending pathogens may therefore be analogous to the cough in pulmonary infections as a mechanism to expel pathogens.

Normal Enteric Microflora

In recent years, there have been several developments in our understanding of the composition of intestinal microflora. With improved culture techniques,[69] we now recognize that 99.9 percent of the normal enteric bacterial flora are anaerobes (approximately 10^{11} organisms/g of normal feces). These organisms (*Bacteroides,* clostridia, peptostreptococci, peptococci, and others) far exceed the number of aerobes. The gram-negative aerobic coliform rods are *E. coli,* 10^8/g; *Klebsiella, Proteus,* enterococci, and other species, approximately $10^{5–7}$/g. We are only beginning to appreciate the role of normal flora as an extremely important and often overlooked host defense. In several situations normal bacterial flora can be shown to be highly effective in resisting colonization by potentially pathogenic invaders. The loss of normal flora or a shift in their balance by antibiotics is often attended with their replacement by organisms such as *Pseudomonas, Klebsiella, Clostridium,* and *Candida.* When these organisms take up residence, there is a risk of their causing serious systemic infections, especially in a nosocomial setting. There are numerous examples of the increased susceptibility to infection of patients with reduced bacterial flora.[70,71] Several enteric infections, such as infant botulism, nosocomial salmonellosis, and enteropathogenic *E. coli,* occur with increased frequency in newborn infants who have not acquired a normal enteric flora. Diarrhea associated with the use of antibiotics is common and, in many cases, is likely related to an alteration in the balance of normal enteric microflora.

The basis for the resistance provided by normal bacterial flora in the intestinal tract has been elucidated in an elegant series of studies by Bohnhoff et al.[72] In experimental mice, the protective effect of normal flora is eradicated by a single injection of streptomycin. They showed that an infecting dose of *Salmonella typhimurium* was reduced over 100,000-fold by the administration of a single dose of streptomycin. This reduced resistance correlated with the reduction in the normal colonic flora and their toxic acidic products. Resistance was restored with the return of enteric flora (especially *Bacteroides*), either by inoculation or naturally. The importance of a reduced pH and volatile fatty acids from the anaerobic flora in colonization resistance has been further shown by Van der Waaj et al.[73] and by Que et al.[74] It has been shown that indigenous microbes such as *Lactobacillus, Bacteroides,* and *Clostridium* spp. attach to the intestinal epithelial surface and act synergistically with host immunity to interfere with experimental *S. typhimurium* challenge.[75] Enteric bacteria including *Proteus, Enterobacter,* and *E. coli* also act synergistically in mice with vibriocidal immunity from vaccination to antagonize *V. cholerae*.[76] The protective role of normal enteric bacterial flora in humans has been documented by the increased frequency of *Salmonella* infections among Swedish tourists who took a prophylactic antibiotic compared with those who took no antimicrobial agent.[71] In a huge outbreak of antimicrobial-resistant *S. typhimurium* enteritis involving nearly 200,000 people in Illinois in the spring of 1985, there was a significant association of illness with having taken antimicrobials the month before the illness. There was a fivefold increase (from 6 percent of well controls to 30 percent) of persons having taken antibiotics to which the outbreak strain was resistant.[77] Others have reported an increased risk of antimicrobial-sensitive *Salmonella* infections following antimicrobial exposure.[78] Some have even used normal colonic or other competing bacterial flora in treating refractory *Clostridium difficile* colitis.[79,80] In addition, cytotoxic chemotherapy with agents such as methotrexate, cyclophosphamide, or fluorouracil may also suppress normal flora and predispose to *C. difficile* colitis.[80-84]

Intestinal Immunity

Enteric immunity is composed of phagocytic, humoral, and cell-mediated elements. Each component has specific contributions to host resistance to enteric infections. The normal intestinal mucosa demonstrates a state of "physiologic inflammation" in the lamina propria with numerous neutrophils, macrophages, plasma cells, and lymphocytes that suggest a constant battle of the host with luminal challenges to maintain the integrity of the mucosa. The importance of intact phagocytic immunity becomes evident when neutrophils are absent in hosts, who then become particularly susceptible to gram-negative rod infections that often originate in the gastrointestinal tract.[85] In addition, neutropenic patients may develop stomatitis or necrotizing typhlitis (with fever, abdominal pain, cecal necrosis and edema, and sometimes bloody diarrhea).[86-89] The importance of immunity is also demonstrated by the potentially severe adenoviral, rotaviral, coxsackieviral, and *Clostridium difficile* infections in bone marrow transplant patients.[90]

Diarrhea in patients with the acquired immunodeficiency syndrome (AIDS) is becoming increasingly common and raises a special set of diagnostic and therapeutic questions. The growing range of severe, recurring enteric infections in immunocompromised patients,[89] especially those with AIDS, demonstrates the critical role of immunity in resisting a broad range of viral, bacterial, parasitic, and fungal enteric infections. The majority of AIDS patients with diarrhea have a documentable infectious etiology such as cytomegalovirus, *Entamoeba histolytica*, *Cryptosporidium*, *Microsporidia*, *Salmonella*, *Giardia*, *Campylobacter jejuni*, *Shigella*, *Mycobacterium* or herpes simplex virus.[91,92] In Haiti and Africa, up to 95 percent of AIDS patients initially present with diarrhea; up to 50 percent may have *Cryptosporidium* infections, followed by 15 percent with *Isospora belli*.[93-95] Still other patients may have the human immunodeficiency virus, which may infect cells in the bowel mucosa.[96]

The gut-associated lymphoid tissue (GALT) is comprised of Peyer's patches, lamina propria lymphocytes, and intraepithelial lymphocytes.[6,97] Microfold (M) cells take up antigen and microbes such as *Yersinia*, *Shigella*, and *Cryptosporidium*.[98-100] Specific active humoral intestinal immunity (coproantibody) arises either from a leakage of serum immunoglobulin (predominantly IgG or IgM) or from the formation of IgA by plasma cells located predominantly in the lamina propria. Secretory IgA (an 11S dimer [MW 390,000] with a secretory piece [MW 60,000] from the mucosal epithelial cells) is found in the lumen.[101-103] Selective deficiency of secretory component has been associated with intestinal candidiasis.[103] Certain mucosal pathogens produce an IgA protease or degrade IgA.[104,105] Both serum and secretory antibody responses have been demonstrated in response to parenteral and intraluminal challenge with cholera toxoid.[106] Secretory IgA is resistant to intraluminal degradation by enzymatic proteolysis and sulfhydryl reduction. The dynamics of local intestinal immunity have been elucidated in several experimental models. The most efficient method of eliciting a local antibody response is with a parenteral priming challenge followed by an intestinal booster antigen challenge. Studies of cholera toxoid immunity in rats suggest that the parenteral priming toxoid prepares a wide-spread distribution of precursor lymphocytes in areas like the Peyer's patches.[107] These cells are then capable of responding to a booster challenge to produce many large IgA-bearing lymphocytes that appear in the thoracic duct before "homing" back to the lamina propria as specific IgA-secreting plasma cells at or distal to this site of booster toxoid. Passively acquired IgA probably accounts for part of the protection against enteric infections in infants who are breast fed. Colostral antibody against rotaviruses and the enterotoxins of *V. cholerae* and *E. coli* have been demonstrated in breast milk.[108,109]

Intestinal antibodies may be directed at any of a number of different bacterial antigens such as endotoxin, capsular material, or exotoxins and may have bactericidal, opsonic, or neutralizing effects. Although IgA can have hemagglutinating, precipitating, or virus-neutralizing properties, it does not appear capable of fixing complement in order to have the direct bactericidal effect that IgG and IgM may have. Selective IgA deficiency is often associated with a compensatory increase in IgM levels. Hereditary telangiectasia with IgA deficiency is associated with recurrent rhinopulmonary infection but is rarely associated with intestinal infection or dysfunction.[101] Although debated by others,[110] Zinneman and Kaplan[111] and Ament et al.[112] have suggested that patients with giardiasis have lower IgA levels and that hypogammaglobulinemic patients have more malabsorption and diarrhea with giardiasis. Patients with type 2 combined IgA and IgM deficiency and small intestinal lymphoid hyperplasia with a sparsity of plasma cells may have diarrhea, malabsorption, and giardiasis.[113] Crabbe and Heremans[114] have described three patients with another type of selective IgA deficiency with spruelike intestinal symptoms and histopathologic changes. The role of cell-mediated immune processes in the intestine is suggested by adjuvant enhancement of vaccine efficacy against intracellular infections such as *S. typhi*.[115]

Other Protective Factors in Human Milk and Serum

The protection afforded by breast-feeding likely relates to several passively transmitted factors, as well as to reduced exposure to a contaminated environment.[15-18,116,117] In addition to antibody, these include lactoferrin, lysozyme, phagocytes, high lactose, low protein, low phosphate, low pH (in part from bifidobacteria) and oligosaccharide fractions.[116-122] The role of lactoferrin in human milk is suggested by the abolition of milk's bacteriostatic properties against *V. cholerae* and enteropathogenic *E. coli* by saturation with iron.[121] In addition, patients with chronic iron excess from hemolytic processes such as malaria, sickle cell anemia, and Oroya fever are at increased risk of infection with organisms such as *Salmonella*. Some of the bacteriostatic properties of normal serum were abolished when iron-binding proteins were saturated with iron.[121]

MICROBIAL FACTORS

A number of bacterial virulence traits determine the pathogenic mechanisms responsible for diarrhea. This entire range of traits is demonstrated by the various types of *E. coli*, as summarized in Table 3. This versatile species may represent the predominant normal colonic flora or may be a urinary or enteric pathogen. Depending largely on the transmissible virulence traits encoded on plasmids or phage, *E. coli* may produce one of three families of enterotoxins (LT, STa, or STb), may be invasive (EIEC), may cause hemorrhagic colitis (EHEC), or may exhibit three

TABLE 3. Different Pathogenic Mechanisms of *Escherichia coli* Diarrhea[a]

	Mechanism	Model	Gene Code	Predominant Serogroups
I. Enterotoxigenic *E. coli* (ETEC)	(ETEC first adhere via CFA)	Hemagglutination (for most)	Plasmid	—
LT *E. coli* (LTEC)	Adenylate cyclase-like choleratoxin	Rabbit loops (18h) CHO, Y1 cell immunoassay	Plasmid	LT: O groups 1, 6, 7, 8, 9, 128. LT + ST: O groups 11, 15, 20, 25, 27, 60, 63, 75, 80, 85, 88, 89, 99, 101, 109, 114, 139, 153
STa *E. coli* (STaEC)	Guanylate cyclase	Suckling mice	Plasmid	ST:O groups 12, 78, 115, 148, 149, 153, 159, 166, 167
STb *E. coli* (STbEC)	Noncyclic nucleotide-dependent bicarbonate secretion	Piglet loops	Plasmid	—
II. Enterohemorrhagic *E. coli* (EHEC)	Shiga-like (Vero) toxin 1 or 2 inhibits protein synthesis	HeLa cell cytotoxicity	Phage	Predominantly O157:H7, O26:H11; O103:H2; O111:H⁻; O113:H21 + some 50 others
III. Enteroinvasive *E. coli* (EIEC)	Local mucosal invasion	Sereny test	Plasmid	O groups 11, 28ac, 29, 112ac, 115, 124, 136, 143, 144, 147, 152, 164, 167, 173
IV. Enteropathogenic *E. coli* (EPEC)				
Locally adherent (LA)	Adhere focally	Localized HEp-2 cell adherence	Plasmid (60 M DA, pMAR2, with EAF and bfpA)	O18:H⁻, 7, 14; O26:H⁻, 11; O44:H18, 44; O55:H⁻, 6, 7; O86:H34; O88;
Attaching and effacing *E. coli*	Attach to and efface brush border epithelium, tyrosine kinase–dependent cytoskeletal rearrangement	Fluorescent Actin Staining (FAS)	Chromosome (eaeA → 94 kD intimin; cfm)	O111:H⁻, 2, 12, 21; O114:H2; O119:H⁻, 6; O125ac:H⁻, 21; O126:H⁻, 27; O127:H⁻, 6[b]; O128ab:H2, 7; O142:H6; O145; O157:H8; O158:H23
V. Enteroaggregative *E. coli* (EAggEC)	Aggregative adherence to HEp-2 cells ? EAST-1 ? EALT	Aggregative pattern of HEp-2 cell adherence	Plasmid	O3:H2; O44; O78:H33; O15:H11; O77:H18; O51:H11, among others (O78, 86, 91, 92)
VI. Diffusely adherent *E. coli* (DAEC)	Diffuse adherence	Diffuse adherence to HEp-2 cells	Chromosomal	(Strain F1845, 189, 57-1)
Normal enteric flora	? Adherence traits	—	—	O groups 1, 2, 4, 6, 7, 25, 45, 75, 81
Genitourinary, blood stream, or meningeal pathogens	? Capsular polysaccharide ± adherence pili	Several animals (mice, rabbits)	—	O groups 1, 2, 4, 6, 7, 11, 18, 22, 25, 45, 62, 75, 81 (K antigens 1, 2, 3, 5, 13)

[a] In addition, nontoxigenic *E. coli* with recognized or new colonization factor fimbriae can cause diarrhea, as documented in experimental animals and in human volunteers; several reviews comment on O and H serotypes.[374–378]

[b] O127:H6 is the focally HEp-2 cell adherent strain (E2348) from which the plasmid pMAR-2 was isolated.

or four distinct types of adherence (class I and II EPEC, with or without the plasmid-encoded focal HEp-2 cell enteroadherence factor (EAF); enteroaggregative *E. coli*, EAggEC; and *E. coli* with one of the recognized or new colonization traits, CFAI, CFAII, E8775, 260-1, and O159:H4). Study of *E. coli* with these varied pathogenic traits have greatly helped to unravel the way that enteric pathogens alter normal intestinal absorptive function to cause diarrheal diseases.[123,124]

Toxins

Toxic microbial components or products are implicated in the disease-producing capacity of several enteric pathogens. Culture filtrates of toxigenic microorganisms are capable of altering gastrointestinal structure or function in the absence of the organisms themselves. Toxins produced by enteric pathogens can be classified as *neurotoxins*, *enterotoxins*, or *cytotoxins* (Table 4). Neurotoxins are usually ingested as preformed toxins that often cause enteric symptoms. These include staphylococcal, *Bacillus cereus*, and botulinal toxins. Although staphylococcal food poisoning is an abrupt upper gastrointestinal syndrome attributed to staphylococcal enterotoxin, the effect appears to be due to the action of this toxin on the central autonomic nervous system rather than to destruction or fluid secretion in the intestine per se.[125,126] An exotoxin related to enterotoxin A may cause fluid

TABLE 4. Enteric Bacterial Toxins

Neurotoxin group
  Clostridium botulinum
  Staphylococcus aureus (enterotoxin b)
  Bacillus cereus (emetic toxin)
Secretory enterotoxin group
  Vibrio cholerae (cAMP)
  Noncholera vibrios
  Escherichia coli—LT (cAMP)
  E. coli—STa (cGMP)
  E. coli—STb
  Salmonella
  Klebsiella
  Clostridium perfringens (A)
  Shigella dysenteriae
  B. cereus
Possible Enterotoxins
  E. coli: EIET, EAST, EALT
  V. cholerae: Ace, Zot

Cytotoxin group:
  Shigella
  C. perfringens (A)
  Vibrio parahemolyticus
  S. aureus
  Clostridium difficile (A and B)
  E. coli (EHEC) (certain O groups: 26, 39, 128, 157); *C. jejuni; H. pylori*

accumulation in rabbit ileal loops directly.[127,128] A different staphylococcal α-toxin elicits hyperperistalsis. Certain strains of *B. cereus* isolated from patients with acute food poisoning also produce a highly heat-stable emetic toxin (especially when cultured with rice) that is a small (Mr <5000), nonantigenic polypeptide capable of causing vomiting in monkeys, much like staphylococcal enterotoxin.[129,130] Botulinal toxin has a primary effect on the neuromuscular junction to prevent the release of acetylcholine from the presynaptic vesicle.[126]

True *enterotoxins* are defined as having a direct effect on the intestinal mucosa to elicit net fluid secretion. The classic enterotoxin, choleratoxin, has been extensively studied and causes fluid secretion after the ganglioside-binding subunit releases the A2 toxin subunit, which activates basolateral epithelial adenylate cyclase via ADP-ribosylation of Gsα to increase intestinal cyclic AMP (cAMP) concentrations.[131,132] In addition, prostaglandins, platelet-activating factor (PAF), and possibly neurohumoral mediators like serotonin may be involved in the secretory or tissue culture responses to choleratoxin.[133–137] Similar toxins both antigenically and mechanistically have been described for other closely related vibrios[138,139] and *E. coli*.[140,141] Because there are no reliable markers such as serotype or biotype for enterotoxigenicity, demonstration of the toxin itself is necessary to identify which *E. coli* are enterotoxigenic. The genetic codes for enterotoxigenicity reside on transmissible plasmids that can be lost or transferred to other *E. coli* by conjugation[142,143] or by phage transduction.[144] To recognize which *E. coli* are enterotoxigenic, we must identify enterotoxin activity in culture filtrates of the organisms in question. This had once required inoculation into a ligated rabbit ileal segment[145] or into rabbit skin to test for toxin associated "permeability factor."[146] The ability of the heat-labile enterotoxin of *E. coli* to activate adenylate cyclase has been used in the development of tissue culture bioassays.[147,148] Its similar antigenicity to cholera toxin has provided immunoassay techniques as well.[149–151] Oligonucleotide gene probes for LT and STa are now available with nonradioactive enzyme markers and provide a simple, sensitive, and highly specific detection method for these enterotoxins.[152] The LT-producing *E. coli* are associated with watery diarrhea among adults in Asia,[153,154] travelers to Central America,[155–157] and children in a number of areas.[158–160] In addition, *Klebsiella, Citrobacter, Salmonella,* and *Campylobacter jejuni* produce choleralike heat-labile toxins that also activate adenylate cyclase, bind to ganglioside, and share some immunogenicity with *E. coli* LT.[161–167]

Another plasmid-mediated but smaller, less antigenic, heat-stable toxin may be produced by *E. coli*. The ST-producing *E. coli*, first described as a cause of diarrhea in piglets and calves,[39,168] are capable of causing diarrhea in human volunteers as well.[169] It appears to be significantly associated with diarrhea among tourists to Central America,[170] occasional newborn nursery outbreaks in this country,[171] and among adults with noninflammatory diarrhea on a Navajo reservation[172] or in Brazil.[16,173] The mechanism of action of ST involves the specific activation of intestinal guanylate cyclase.[174–176] Like cyclic AMP, cyclic GMP analogs (such as 8 Br-cyclic GMP) can mimic the secretory effect of the enterotoxin.[174] *Yersinia*, non-O1 *V. cholerae,* and *Citrobacter freundii* also produce cross-reacting homologous ST of 17–19 amino acids with conservation of six cysteines (with three disulfide bonds) and a central asp-pro-ala region that is required for ST-binding and activation of enterocyte guanylate cyclase.[177–181] Furthermore, endogenous ST-like compounds are now being isolated from mammalian cells that may play key roles in normal intestinal and renal physiology.[182–184]

Other bacterial products that induce intestinal secretion include *C. difficile* toxin A,[185] *C. perfringens* type A, *Staphylococcus aureus* (and coagulase-negative staphylococci),[186,187] *B. cereus,* and *B. fragilis.* In addition electrogenic responses in Ussing chambers are induced by a chromosomally mediated 68–80 kD secretory toxin produced in iron-deprived conditions by enteroinvasive *E. coli,* EIET,[188] and by a 2–5 kD heat-stable, plasmid-encoded STa-like loop negative toxin produced by enteroaggregative *E. coli* (EAST).[189] *Clostridium difficile* toxin A disrupts microfilaments and tight junctions and causes striking intestinal inflammation and secretion, the latter blocked by PAF antagonists or by pertussis toxin.[190–193] Because of its different receptor specificity, *C. difficile* toxin B is usually the cytotoxin detected in tissue culture. Enterotoxic and cytotoxic products of certain *Bacteroides fragilis* isolates from children and adults with diarrhea in Arizona and Montana have also been described.[194–197] A protein neuroenterotoxin isolated from *S. dysenteriae* I (that may be responsible for the headache, meningismus, and seizures) also causes fluid secretion in rabbit ileal loops.[198] Although experimental findings have been contradictory, the activation of adenylate cyclase by this *Shigella* enterotoxin has been demonstrated in rabbit ileal loops.[199] Noninflammatory secretion also occurs in the small bowel of experimental monkeys infected with *S. flexneri* 2A,[200] and 80 percent of the patients infected with *S. flexneri* or *Shigella sonnei* develop neutralizing antibodies to the toxin.[201] However, the toxin alone does not appear to be sufficient to cause *Shigella* diarrhea, because toxigenic, noninvasive opaque colonial mutants of virulent *Shigella* are totally avirulent.[202,203] Certain strains of *B. cereus* have also been reported to produce a heat-labile, adenylate-cyclase–activating rabbit ileal loop-positive, dermonecrotic, and intestinonecrotic enterotoxin.[129,130,204,205]

Certain strains of *S. typhimurium* may cause severe watery cholera-like diarrhea[206,207] that can be prevented in experimental models by indomethacin. As noted in Chapter 83, the products of an inflammatory response could act to cause mucosal secretion.[208,209] Sandefur and Peterson[164] have described a heat-labile enterotoxinlike effect in rabbit skin and Chinese hamster ovary cell models after separation from an inhibitor. Others have described a heat-stable enterotoxin from *Salmonella.*[210] Other enteric organisms with which enterotoxin-like activity has been reported include *Klebsiella, Citrobacter, Aeromonas,* and *Enterobacter* spp.[162,163,211–213] Both heat-labile and heat-stable toxins have been reported. Although these enterotoxigenic organisms appear to be infrequent at the present time, much needs to be learned about the occurrence and the mechanism of action of enterotoxins from these organisms other than *E. coli.*

Cytotoxic products of several enteric pathogens are responsible for the mucosal destruction that often results in inflammatory colitis. Bacillary dysentery is a colonic mucosal destructive process in which a cytotoxin isolated from *S. dysenteriae* type 1 may play a role.[203,214] Whether this cytotoxin is a component or a digestive product of the larger neuroenterotoxin mentioned above is unknown.

Enterohemorrhagic *E. coli* that cause hemorrhagic colitis or the hemolytic uremic syndrome (O groups 26, 39, 111, 113, 121, 128, and 157) produce one or two *Shiga*-like Vero cell cytotoxins.[215–219] Two groups have recorded the transfer of Vero toxin production to recipient *E. coli* or its association with a large plasmid,[217,219] whereas others have associated the production of *Shiga*-like toxins I and II with bacteriophages in *E. coli* O157: H7.[220] The heat-labile Verocytotoxin, initially found in *E. coli* O26:H11, O128, and O39, has a slight secretory effect in 18-hour ligated rabbit ileal loops.[216] The multistate outbreak of hemorrhagic colitis with *E. coli* O157:H7 in 1982[218] was followed by studies showing the near identity (one amino acid difference) of Verocytotoxin to Shigatoxin (hence the term *Shiga-like toxin* [*SLT*] and the increasing association of these enterohemorrhagic *E. coli* (EHEC) with numerous outbreaks and sporadic cases of hemorrhagic colitis or childhood hemolytic uremic syndrome in schools, day care centers, nursing homes and communities, including over 500 documented cases and 4 deaths in four western states associated with a single hamburger chain in 1993.[218,221–225] Like Shigatoxin, *E. coli* SLT has binding and active subunits, is neutralized by anti-Shigatoxin antibody, binds to globotriaosylceramide (Gb3) via its B subunit and the active A subunit (analogous to that of the plant toxin, ricin) enzymatically cleaves the N-glycoside bond of adenine at position 4324 in the 28SrRNA of the 60S ribosomal subunit, to prevent elongation factor 1-dependent aminoacyl tRNA binding to the ribosome and thereby halt protein synthesis.[198,221,226–230] Subtle differences in the B subunit specificities for Gb4 or Gb5 (globotetraosyl or globopentaosyl ceramide, respectively) as well as Gb3 may help explain differences in cell culture effects as well as in the disease manifestations of SLT-I and SLT-II, SLT-IIvh, and SLT-IIvp (to cause bloody diarrhea or hemolytic uremic syndrome in patients or edema diseases in swine).[229–231] Shigatoxin causes limb paralysis and death in mice and rabbits, and axonal transport of toxin with vagal sensory neuron damage has been described.[232–235] Examination of histopathologic sections, however, suggests that neuronal damage may be indirect, via endothelial cell damage.[232,233] In addition, a 110-kD heat- and trypsin-labile cytotoxin that is distinct from Shigatoxin has recently been implicated in patients with seizures or encephalopathy with shigellosis.[236]

Clostridium perfringens enterotoxin also produces cytotoxicity similar to that of *S. dysenteriae* toxin in HeLa cell and in animal models.[237] More recent studies have used Vero cells to detect cytotoxicity in fecal filtrates that is neutralized by specific antiserum or toxin fragments.[238–240] These methods have enabled studies to be done that implicate enterocytotoxigenic *C. perfringens* in geriatric institutions and with antibiotic-associated diarrhea.[241–243] *Clostridium perfringens* type C produces a trypsin-sensitive β-toxin.[244] Another enteric pathogen for which a cytotoxin has been described is *Vibrio parahemolyticus*. Although some have reported the presence of a true enterotoxin with this organism,[245] others have described a cytotoxin;[246] still others note the tendency of *V. parahemolyticus* to penetrate and cause bacteremia in animal models[247] or an invasive colitis in patients.[248] *Vibrio parahemolyticus* typically causes explosive watery diarrhea in food-borne outbreaks in coastal areas of the United States.[249] *Staphylococcus aureus* produce a nonantigenic Δ-toxin that impairs water absorption and causes cytotoxic disruption of intestinal mucosa or cells in tissue culture.[250] The clindamycin-resistant *C. difficile* isolated from patients with antibiotic-associated pseudomembranous enterocolitis produces a potent cytotoxin capable of causing cytotoxicity in tissue culture and lethality in a hamster model,[251–253] as well as an enterotoxic product that causes hemorrhagic fluid secretion in rabbit ileal loops.[190,253] Finally, the pathogenesis of *Campylobacter jejuni*, *Helicobacter pylori*, and possibly even *V. cholerae* may also involve cytotoxic products.[254–262]

Attachment

The ability of many enteric pathogens to cause disease depends not only on the organisms's ability to penetrate the mucosa or to produce enterotoxin or cytotoxin but also on their ability to adhere to and colonize the mucosa. This adherence capacity has been well described with enterotoxigenic *E. coli*, which, in order to cause disease, must not only produce an enterotoxin but also must first adhere to and colonize in the upper small bowel of humans or animals. This adherence capacity for *E. coli* is variously called *K88, K99,* or *colonization factor antigen* (*CFA*) for piglet, calf, and human strains, respectively. As with enterotoxigenicity, the production of these adherence antigens also appears to be genetically encoded by transmissible plasmids. These fimbriate bacterial surface adhesins are distinct from type 1 pili and from recognized urinary tract adhesins[263–265] and usually cause hemagglutination that is mannose resistant.[266,267] Although these adhesins hold great promise for immunization against colonization, there are now at least five different types of CFA among human enterotoxigenic *E. coli*: CFAI, CFAII, E8775, 260-1, and O159:H4.[260,266–270]

Analogous to ETEC adhesins, fimbriate or fibrillar adhesins

may also aid in the initial colonization of EHEC O157, EPEC, and enteroaggregative *E. coli* (EAggEC). The enterohemorrhagic, Shigatoxin-producing *E. coli* (EHEC) O26 has been shown to adhere to the mucosa of human fetal small intestinal tissue *in vitro* in a mannose-resistant fashion, a trait that is transmissible by a colicinogenic conjugative plasmid.[271] In addition, EHEC strain O157:H7 has been shown to have a 60-mD plasmid that encodes a new type of fimbria that appear to mediate attachment to Henle 407 cells in tissue culture.[272]

Classic enteropathogenic *E. coli* (EPEC) exhibit a qualitatively different localized and attaching and effacing adherence and F-actin polymerization in intestinal brush border and in HEp-2 cells.[273–279] This localized EPEC adherence involves a complex array of plasmid-mediated adherence,[280] followed by chromosomally mediated effacement, protein phosphorylation, and actin condensation in the host cell.[281–284] The 50–60 mDa plasmid in EPEC encodes inducible, bundle-forming pili that share amino-terminal sequence homology with the toxin coregulated pili (TCP) in *V. cholerae* and are responsible for efficient adherence to HEp-2 cells in "localized" colonies.[285–287] This may be followed by tyrosine phosphorylation of a 90-kD host protein (HP 90) and then by host cytoskeletal assembly by a 94-kD "intimin" to result in actin accumulation and effacement encoded by EPEC chromosomal cfm (class four mutant) and eae (*E. coli* attachment and effacement), respectively,[281] with the role of intracellular calcium-induced protein phosphorylation by a heat-labile product by EPEC being unclear at present.[283,284]

Distinct from the localized adherence of EPEC to HEp-2 cells are the "aggregative" and "diffuse" adherence (AA and DA) patterns, for which gene probes have been developed that detect some, but not all, *E. coli* with these phenotypes.[288–292] EAgg *E. coli* have been associated with persistent diarrhea in studies in India and Brazil,[295–297] while DAEC have been variably seen in association with diarrhea and controls.[298,299] The roles of novel EAST or a distinct 12-kD heat labile "toxin" that is antigenically related to the carboxy-terminal region of the *E. coli* hemolysin and induces host cell calcium-dependent protein phosphorylation (distinct from dantrolene-inhibitable, calcium-dependent phosphorylation seen with EPEC) released by the organism in causing diarrhea remains unclear.[300] The diffusely adherent *E. coli* (DAEC) represent several serotypes as identified by gene probes for strain 1845[293] and for a 100-kb plasmid-encoded 100-kD protein adhesin (AIDA-I) from strain 2787 (O126:H27).[301]

Finally, *E. coli* with the colonization traits mentioned above, but without enterotoxin production, like an engineered colonizing multiply toxin-deleted *V. cholerae* vaccine strain (lacking ctxA, zot, ace, or hly) are capable of causing diarrhea in animals[302–307] and in human volunteers fed *E. coli* with the colonization trait as a potential vaccine.[308] Whether such colonizing *E. coli* are responsible, alone or in part, for naturally occurring acute or prolonged diarrhea remains to be determined.

Invasiveness

The capacity of organisms such as *Shigella* and certain invasive strains of *E. coli* to invade and destroy epithelial cells is responsible for the inflammatory or dysenteric diarrhea they cause. This capacity is demonstrated in the laboratory by the guinea pig conjunctivitis (Sereny) test.[309] There is cell destruction and superficial inflammatory invasion of the cornea similar to that noted in colonic mucosa. Modifications in the specific components of the O side chain of the cell wall lipopolysaccharide alter this invasive property in *Shigella*.[310,311] There is also evidence that the invasiveness of certain *E. coli* may be reflected in their O antigens or serotype.[312,313] Recent evidence has associated invasiveness with large 120–140-mD plasmids in *S. sonnei*,[199] *S. flexneri*,[314] and invasive *E. coli*.[315] HeLa cell, rabbit loop, and Sereny test invasiveness can be genetically constructed by the sequential transfer of defined chromosomal and plasmid genes for *Shigella flexneri* to *E. coli* K12.[316]

Cell invasion, unlike superficial colonization, may involve attachment to transmembrane glycoproteins (instead of carbohydrates and glycolipids) such as *integrin* bound by *Yersinia invasin*.[317] The expression of ''invasiveness'' is complex. In *Shigella* and enteroinvasive *E. coli*, it appears to involve a series of plasmid-encoded invasion and adhesin proteins (ipa A-D) that are regulated by key chromosomal codons (such as kcpA).[316–318] In *Salmonella*, both adherence and invasion appear closely linked and may require bacterial proteins that are induced by trypsin and neuraminidase-sensitive structures present on the epithelial cell surface.[319] The capacity of *Entamoeba histolytica* to adhere and ''invade'' relates, at least in part, to a GalNAc-inhibitable amebic lectin that leads to contact-dependent cytolysis of host cells, particularly attracted neutrophils.[320–322] As discussed above, cytotoxic exotoxins may well play roles in the invasive and destructive properties of certain shigellae, *V. parahemolyticus*, staphylococci, and clostridia.

Other Virulence Factors

In addition to enterotoxin production and adherence, an orchestrated set of additional virulence traits appear to be critical to the ability of pathogens such as *V. cholerae* to succeed in colonizing the intestinal mucosa. These include motility,[323,324] chemotaxis,[49,327] and mucinase production,[325,326] any one of which can be missing and lead to reduced virulence. The virulence of certain enteric pathogens such as *S. typhi* appears to be related to the Vi antigen[327] and to the polysaccharide composition of the O side chain of its lipopolysaccharide cell wall content,[328,329] both of which have been used in vaccine production.[308,330,331] The virulence factors that enable enteric pathogens such as *Yersinia enterocolitica* to cause an enteric feverlike illness or mesenteric adenitis are less clear.

Another potential enteric pathogen that is increasingly recognized with improved culture techniques is *Campylobacter*. *Campylobacter jejuni* tends to cause more diarrhea than *C. fetus;* some *C. jejuni* have been reported to produce an LT-like enterotoxin,[332] or a cytotoxin,[256] and *C. fetus* causes more febrile systemic illness with bacteremia, perhaps related to the LPS and greater serum resistance of the organism.[333,334] The mechanisms by which *Campylobacter* cause disease still remain unclear.[333]

Still another way that organisms may cause diarrhea involves the selective destruction of absorptive cells (villus tip cells) in the mucosa, leaving secretory cells (crypt cells) intact.[334,335] Thus it is not surprising that both the rotaviruses and the Norwalk-like viruses, which selectively infect and disrupt the villus tip cells, alter the normal absorptive fluid balance as well as reduce the brush border digestive enzymes present during active infection.[334,336–338] Such an imbalanced disruption of the specialized absorptive surface may also be involved in other small bowel infections that are often associated with villus tip flattening or microvillus destruction, including bacterial overgrowth syndromes, EPEC infections, giardiasis, strongyloidiasis, and cryptosporidiosis.

MAJOR SYNDROMES OF DERANGED GASTROINTESTINAL PHYSIOLOGY

The elements of net fluid balance in the healthy adult intestinal tract are shown diagrammatically in Figure 1. With a daily oral intake of 1.5 liters, salivary, gastric, biliary, and pancreatic secretions contribute a total of approximately 8.5 liters of fluid that enters the upper gastrointestinal tract each day. However, daily fecal fluid excretion is normally less than 150 ml, indicating a net absorption in excess of 8 liters each day by the intestinal tract. Over 90 percent of this net absorption occurs in the small bowel, where there is a massive bidirectional flux that probably

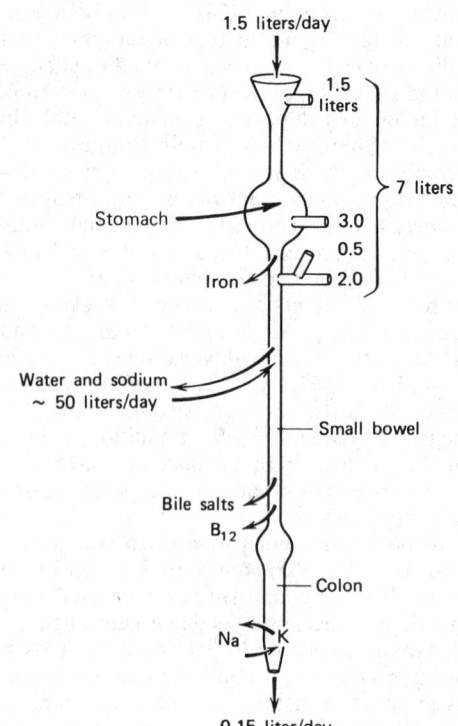

FIG. 1.   Diagram of fluid balance in the healthy adult gastrointestinal tract.

exceeds 50 liters a day. We can readily see how a relatively slight shift in the bidirectional flux can result in substantial overload of the colonic absorptive capacity that rarely exceeds 2–3 liters a day. As in the kidney, there are analogous hormonal, physical, and osmotic factors active in the intestinal tract. Aldosterone, for example, enhances intestinal sodium absorption at the expense of potassium.[339,340] Excessive fluid volume results in a ''third factor'' effect that may elicit or prolong diarrhea,[341] and osmotic laxatives are as familiar as osmotic diuretics.

Enteric disease can be produced by the microbe–host interaction that alters normal gastrointestinal physiology in one or more of these three ways: *(1)* a shift in the delicate balance of bidirectional water and electrolyte fluxes in the upper small bowel by intraluminal processes such as enterotoxin action, *(2)* inflammatory destruction of the ileal or colonic mucosa, or *(3)* penetration through an intact mucosa to the reticuloendothelial system. These three types of enteric infections are outlined in Table 5.

They can often be distinguished by a quick, simple examination. Mucus from a fresh stool specimen is mixed with a drop of methylene blue on a slide and examined for the presence of fecal leukocytes.[342,343] In the majority of cases, no leukocytes will be noted. This suggests a noninflammatory process in which diarrhea usually arises from the upper small bowel by the action of a true enterotoxin or by agents such as *Giardia* or viruses. The secretory effects of certain enterotoxins share similar mechanisms with noninfectious endocrine causes of diarrhea such as non-β-cell islet tumors, medullary carcinoma of the thyroid, carcinoid tumors, and other benign or malignant neoplasms that are associated with increased serum prostaglandins, vasoactive intestinal polypeptide, or changes in cyclic nucleotide concentrations.[344] Impaired small bowel absorption is important in tropical sprue, enzyme deficiencies, and solute loads. Enhanced colonic secretion without an inflammatory response characteristic of microbial or ulcerative colitis may result from excessive bile salts or fatty acids or from malignancies such as villous adenomas.

The presence of numerous polymorphonuclear leukocytes documents an inflammatory or invasive process that usually

TABLE 5. Three Types of Enteric Infection

	I	II	III
Mechanism	Noninflammatory (enterotoxin)	Inflammatory (invasion ?cytotoxin)	Penetrating
Location	Proximal small bowel	Colon	Distal small bowel
Illness	Watery diarrhea	Dysentery	Enteric fever
Stool examination	No fecal leukocytes	Fecal polymorphonuclear leukocytes	Fecal mononuclear leukocytes
Examples	*Vibrio cholerae*	*Shigella*	*Salmonella typhi*
	Escherichia coli (LT)	Invasive *E. coli*	*Yersinia enterocolitica*
	E. coli (ST)	*Salmonella enteritidis*	*?Campylobacter fetus*
	Clostridium perfringens	*V. parahemolyticus*	
	Bacillus cereus	*?Clostridium difficile*	
	Staphylococcus aureus	*?Campylobacter jejuni*	
	?Salmonella	*Entamoeba histolytica*[a]	
	?Vibrio parahemolyticus		
	Giardia lamblia		
	Rotavirus		
	Norwalk-like viruses		
	Cryptosporidium		

[a] Although amebic dysentery involves tissue inflammation, the leukocytes are characteristically pyknotic or absent, having been destroyed by the virulent amebae.[345]

arises from the colon or distal small bowel. Amebic colitis can often be distinguished from bacterial dysenteries by microscopic fecal examination. In addition to the amebic trophozoites or cysts, fecal neutrophils are usually pyknotic or absent with amebiasis, probably because of the cytopathic effect of virulent amebae on mammalian cells, including neutrophils.[345,346] Impaired colonic absorption may contribute to the diarrhea in inflammatory colitis due to shigellosis, pseudomembranous enterocolitis, amebic colitis, or idiopathic ulcerative colitis. In addition, recent evidence suggests that the products of the lipoxygenase and other pathways in neutrophils may also contribute to a secretory process.[208,209] Agents that cause an inflammatory colitis may require specific antimicrobial intervention, as well as supportive fluid therapy.[343]

The third type of enteric infection is caused by organisms that penetrate the intact intestinal mucosa, often in the distal small bowel, to multiply in the lymphatic or reticuloendothelial cells. This usually results in a febrile systemic illness with or without diarrhea. If diarrhea is present, mononuclear leukocytes may be found in the stools of these patients.[342] Cultural documentation of the pathogen is important, since a bacteremia that necessitates specific antimicrobial therapy may result in this setting.

DIAGNOSTIC APPROACH TO ENTERIC INFECTIONS

The appropriate diagnostic approach to diarrheal illness is determined by the patient's age, severity of illness, duration of illness, type of illness, and the available facilities. Of greatest importance in patients with diarrhea are a careful history, physical examination, and examination of a fresh stool specimen for fecal leukocytes. A *history* of recent antibiotic use, weight loss, underlying diseases, other illnesses in the family or in other contacts, or of travel outside the United States, to the seacoast, or to rural mountainous areas should elicit a more careful investigation of specific etiologic agents. A prompt evaluation of *physical* signs of fever, toxicity, or severe dehydration may result in lifesaving supportive fluid therapy. Particularly worrisome signs of severe dehydration, especially in children, include lethargy, postural hypotension and tachycardia, sunken fontanelles, and dry skin (with decreased turgor), dry eyes, or dry mucous membranes. As noted in Figure 2, if the history of physical findings indicate anything more than a mild, isolated, afebrile illness, examination of a fresh *stool* specimen, preferably collected in a cup, is particularly valuable. First, it provides the physician with an objective determination of the patient's subjective complaints. Second, a gross description of the stool as either watery, mucoid, or bloody will provide important clues about its cause and appropriate management. Third, a microscopic examination for fecal leukocytes, as described above, may reveal heavy parasitic intestinal infestations or maldigested

fat or meat fibers, suggesting pancreatic insufficiency, or lipid droplets suggesting malabsorption with steatorrhea. If fever or fecal neutrophils are present, the physician should selectively take a culture for the most commonly recognized invasive pathogens—*Campylobacter jejuni, Salmonella,* and *Shigella.*[343] Cup specimens, when promptly examined for leukocytes, provide a highly sensitive screen for invasive processes such as shigellosis or *C. jejuni* enteritis.[347,348] Swab or diaper specimens appear to be less sensitive.[348] A new, simple test for fecal lactoferrin provides a rapid, sensitive marker for fecal leukocytes that is effective, even with swab or refrigerated samples.[349] The history of recent antibiotic use, weight loss, and chronic diarrhea (>10 days), seacoast or other exposures, or immunocompromised states should prompt the physician to consider other agents as noted.

Other diagnostic studies that can be made on fecal specimens include special stains for fat or muscle and determinations of pH and reducing substances. A Sudan stain may reveal many large (10–75 μm) orange-stained globules of fat suggesting malabsorption or smaller (1–4 μm) globules or needlelike crystals of fatty acid that may be normal. Numerous undigested muscle fibers may be seen with an aqueous 2% eosin stain that suggest pancreatic insufficiency and maldigestion.

An acidic stool pH may be helpful in the identification of lactose intolerance, especially in children with diarrhea. Although breast-fed infants have a fecal pH ranging from 4.7 to 5.1, stool pH usually exceeds 7.0 if the infant is on a regular milk-containing diet. On a regular diet, a fecal pH less than 5.0 suggests the presence of lactic acid from the action of colonic bacterial flora on unabsorbed lactose. Stool-reducing substances may also be helpful in the detection of carbohydrate malabsorption. A simple test uses copper sulfate (Clinitest) tablets. Mix 1 ml stool with 2 ml water, add 15 drops of this mixture to a test tube, and then add one copper sulfate tablet. A reduction positive for "sugar" indicates reducing substances. Positive tests for blood may suggest an invasive process such as amebiasis or shigellosis. Although this is usually evident from a gross examination of the stool, tests for occult blood are much more sensitive but less specific. Tests for hemoglobin peroxidase use orthotolidine, benzidine, or guaiac reagents in descending order of sensitivity. Some are so sensitive that they may be positive with ingested meat myoglobin. Twenty-four-hour determinations for fecal fat (normal <7.2 g/day fecal fat or <150–200 g/day total stool weight) may also be of value.

For culture of enteric pathogens, the specimen should be inoculated onto culture plates as promptly as possible.[350] The media used are selective and often contain indicator substances that aid in initial identification. Routine techniques must now include selective culture for *C. jejuni*, one of the most common causes of inflammatory diarrhea throughout the world.[351] For optimal

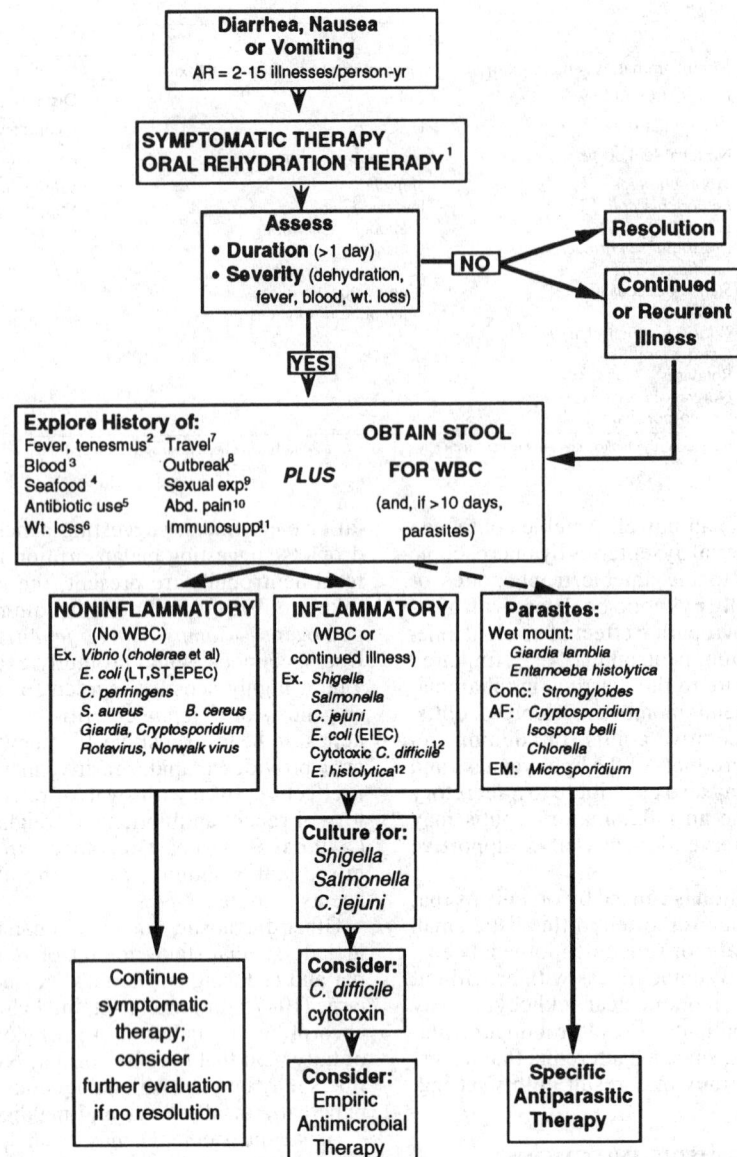

FIG. 2. Approach to diagnosis and management of infectious diarrhea. Key to superscripts: *1.* ORS can be prepared by adding 3.5 g NaCl, 2.5 g NaHCO3 (or 2.9 g Na citrate), 1.5 g KCl and 20 g glucose *or* glucose polymer (ex. 40 g sucrose *or* 4 tablespoons sugar *or* 50–60 g cereal flour such as rice, maize, sorghum, millet, wheat, or potato) per liter (1.05 qt.) of clean water. This makes approximately Na 90, K 20, Cl 80, HCO3 30, glucose 111 mmol/liter. One level teaspoon table salt and 8 level teaspoons table sugar per liter makes about 86 mmol Na and 30 g sucrose/liter to which one could add 1 cup orange juice or two bananas for potassium. *2.* Fever or tenesmus suggest an inflammatory proctocolitis. *3.* Diarrhea with blood, especially without fecal leukocytes, suggests enterohemorrhagic (Shiga-like toxin-producing) *E. coli* O157 or amebiasis (in which leukocytes are destroyed by the parasite). *4.* Ingestion of inadequately cooked seafood should prompt consideration of infections with *Vibrio* or Norwalk-like viruses. *5.* Antibiotics should be stopped if possible and cytotoxigenic *Clostridium difficile* considered. Antibiotics may also predispose to other infections such as salmonellosis. *6.* Persistence (>10 days) with weight loss should prompt consideration of giardiasis or cryptosporidiosis. *7.* Travel to tropical areas increases the chance of developing enterotoxigenic *E. coli*, as well as viral (Norwalk-like or rotaviral), parasitic (*Giardia, Entamoeba, Strongyloides, Cryptosporidium*), and, if fecal leukocytes are present, invasive bacterial infections as noted in the algorithm. *8.* Outbreaks should prompt consideration of *S. aureus, B. cereus*, anisakiasis (incubation period <6 hours), *Campylobacter perfringens*, ETEC, *Vibrio, Salmonella, Campylobacter, Shigella*, or EIEC infection. Consider saving *E. coli* for LT, ST, invasiveness, adherence testing, serotyping, and stool for rotavirus, and stool plus paired sera for Norwalk-like virus or toxin testing. *9.* Sigmoidoscopy in symptomatic homosexual men should distinguish proctitis in the distal 15 cm only (caused by herpesvirus, gonococcal, chlamydial, or syphilitic infection) from colitis (*Campylobacter, Shigella, Clostridium difficile*, or chlamydial [LGV serotypes] infections) or noninflammatory diarrhea (due to giardiasis). *10.* If unexplained abdominal pain and fever persist or suggest an appendicitis-like syndrome, culture for *Y. enterocolitica* with cold enrichment. *11.* In immunocompromised hosts, a wide range of viral (cytomegalovirus, herpes simplex virus, coxsackievirus, rotavirus), bacterial (*Salmonella, M. avium-intracellulare*), and parasitic (*Cryptosporidium, Isospora, Strongyloides, Entamoeba,* and *Giardia*) agents should be considered. *12.* Some inflammatory, colonic pathogens, such as, cytotoxigenic *Clostridium difficile* or *Entamoeba histolytica* may destroy fecal leukocyte morphology, so a reliable leukocyte marker would provide a better screening test. (Adapted from Guerrant and Bobak[6] with permission.)

results, this requires a highly selective atmosphere of reduced oxygen (4–6 percent) and increased carbon dioxide (6–10 percent) and an increased incubator temperature (42°C). Selective media and means to obtain the proper atmosphere are now available.[351–354] When culturing stool from homosexual men with diarrhea, it should be kept in mind that *Helicobacter cinaedi* and *Campylobacter fenelliae* will not grow at 42°C. Routine stool culture also includes a medium, such as MacConkey's or eosin methylene blue (EMB) agar, that inhibits gram-positive organisms and selects predominantly for aerobic gram-negative rods. In addition more selective media (such as xylose-lysine-deoxycholate [XLD] or *Salmonella–Shigella* [SS] agar) and enrichment broth (such as gram-negative [GN], selenite, or tetrathionate) that inhibit most organisms except *Salmonella* and *Shigella* should be used. However, since highly selective media are also more inhibitory, we should also examine the less selective MacConkey's and EMB agar for nonlactose-fermenting (colorless) colonies that may be salmonellae or shigellae. Even the best techniques with fresh specimens may miss fragile organisms such as shigella.[350,353] Fecal cultures failed to yield shigellae in 40 percent of volunteers with inflammatory diarrhea from experimental *Shigella* infection.[342] When immediate culture of specimen is impossible, specimens may be transported to a laboratory in a non-nutrient-holding medium, such as Cary-Blair soft agar, which prevents drying and overgrowth of normal flora.

Culture of vibrios (*V. cholerae, V. parahemolyticus,* and others), which should be suspected after any exposure to coastal areas or seafood, requires the highly selective thiosulfate citrate bile salt sucrose (TCBS) agar.[6,354] Selective culture for *Clostridium difficile* and examination for fecal cytotoxin[248,249,355] may be indicated in patients with refractory antibiotic-associated diarrhea or colitis. Culture of *Y. enterocolitica* may require the selective process of "cold enrichment" on sheep blood agar or phosphate buffered saline for 2–3 weeks.[356]

Escherichia coli that grow readily as dry lactose-fermenting (purple) colonies on EMB or MacConkey's agar are major aerobic constituents of normal fecal flora but should also be considered as potential pathogens. Certain serotypes have been associated with inflammatory diarrhea,[308] recently with bloody diarrhea,[215–220] with outbreaks of diarrhea in newborn nurseries, and even with some enterotoxigenic *E. coli.*[357] However, detection of enterotoxigenicity depends not on serotypes but on detection of the toxin itself. Therefore, routine serotyping of *E. coli* in sporadic cases is of limited value at present and should be considered a special tool for investigating epidemic diarrhea in settings such as nurseries for newborns or unexplained dysentery. Special tests for the cholera-like, heat-labile, adenylate-cyclase–activating enterotoxin may use rabbit ileal loop,[145] rabbit skin permeability,[146] Chinese hamster ovary cell,[147] Y-1 adrenal cell,[148] immunoassay,[149–151] or direct assay for the enterotoxin genome.[152,358] The heat-stable enterotoxin acts through a different mechanism and currently requires the suckling mouse assay for its detection.[359,360] Invasive *E. coli* may be identified by inoculation into the conjunctival sac of guinea pigs (Sereny test).[308] Particularly important with the increasing problem of enterohemorrhagic *E. coli* (EHEC) infections is that stools from patients with bloody diarrhea should be cultured on sorbitol-MacConkey agar to screen for sorbitol-negative enterohemorrhagic *E. coli* O157:H7, which may then be selected for further serotyping.[361–363]

When diarrhea persists unexplained, especially with blood or weight loss, examinations for *Entamoeba, Giardia,* or *Strongyloides* parasites are indicated, using concentration or special staining techniques.[364,365] In immunosuppressed patients with persisting unexplained diarrhea, sugar flotation or modified Kinyoun's acid-fast stains should be done for cryptosporidiosis.[366]

Proctoscopic examination may be very helpful in the differential diagnosis, especially when inflammatory colitis is present. Although necrotic ulcers may be seen in acute shigellosis, discrete ulcers are more suggestive of amebiasis or Crohn's disease. Mucosal friability is more suggestive of inflammatory bowel disease such as ulcerative colitis. The appearance of raised, plaque-like pseudomembranes is diagnostic of pseudomembranous colitis that may be associated with staphylococci or antibiotics such as clindamycin. Large amounts of mucus may be present in "mucous colitis" or with a villous adenoma; melanosis coli may suggest laxative abuse.

Rectal mucosal biopsy specimens, especially when ulcers are present, may be of great help in the identification of the parasite *Entameba histolytica,* granulomata, amyloidosis (with Congo red stain), or Whipple's disease (with periodic acid-Schiff [PAS] stain). Small bowel biopsy specimens may also be diagnostic in Whipple's disease, giardiasis, amyloidosis, a β-lipoproteinemia, lymphoma, coccidiosis, or mast cell disease. Characteristic but not necessarily diagnostic histopathologic changes may be seen in celiac disease, tropical sprue, eosinophilic gastroenteritis, dermatitis herpetiformis, and dysgammaglobulinemia. However, several conditions, including Crohn's disease, bacterial overgrowth syndrome, and pancreatic or bile salt insufficiency, may be associated with normal small bowel histologic findings or with nonspecific changes.

Radiologic studies of the intestinal tract may reveal toxic megacolon, pancreatic calcifications, or nodular adrenal calcifications suggestive of tuberculosis or histoplasmosis. Colonic mucosal edema with a "thumbprint" appearance has been reported on barium enema studies of patients with bloody diarrhea and *E. coli* O157 infection.[218] Although barium studies may reveal nonspecific changes in the small bowel (giardiasis) or colon (inflammatory colitis), they are less useful in diagnosing microbial diarrheas. Indeed, the barium contrast material renders a microscopic examination of stool virtually useless.

Bacterial overgrowth syndrome may result in deconjugation of bile salts that can be tested with a ^{14}C-glycocholic acid breath test. Carbon-14–labeled carbon dioxide in the breath represents the degradation product of bacterial deconjugation of bile salts.

APPROACH TO PREVENTION, CONTROL, AND THERAPY

The public health measures of improved water supply and sanitation facilities are most important for the control of the majority of enteric infections. Another important area for intervention in the spread of enteric infection lies in the quality control of commercial products such as bottled water and beverages. These may be responsible for outbreaks of significant enteric infections such as those of cholera in Portugal[367] or typhoid fever in Mexico.[368]

Nonspecific host factors should be appreciated to minimize their violation. Examples include careful personal hygiene and limited judicious use of antacids, antimotility drugs, or antimicrobial agents.

Vaccines may be used to boost specific immune processes that may be directed against bacteria themselves, adherence appendages, cytotoxins, or enterotoxins. Perhaps the most useful at present are the newly developed live gal-epimerase mutant typhoid vaccine,[328] and the new Vi polysaccharide capsule vaccine against typhoid fever.[329,330] Several additional live and killed bacterial vaccines are currently under study,[307] and new rotavirus vaccines are being studied.[337] To date, there are no effective vaccines against a parasitic enteric infection, and much new work is required to improve the understanding of host defenses against enteric parasitic processes.

New possibilities for pharmacologic antagonists to microbial adherence or to toxin action are now on the horizon. New types of "antibiotics" may work by blocking the formation of bacterial adherence factors, binding bacterial adherence appendages, or lectin-like competitors for the host cell receptors that enable microorganisms to colonize the gastrointestinal tract.[369] Finally, specific competitors for either the binding or the action of enterotoxins hold promise. For example, monosialoganglioside

(G_{m1}) successfully binds cholera toxin or the heat-labile enterotoxin of *E. coli* in vitro and in animal experiments. Pharmacologic reversal of the cyclic nucleotide-associated secretory process may also be possible. Such a mechanism has been suggested for bismuth subsalicylate (Pepto-Bismol).[370]

Specific antimicrobial chemotherapy may be indicated, especially in inflammatory processes such as shigellosis or in parasitic diseases such as giardiasis or amebiasis.

Of greatest importance in the treatment of microbial diarrhea, regardless of the cause or category, is fluid replacement. The degree of volume depletion must be first assessed by examining the turgor of the skin and mucous membranes, by noting the amount of lacrimation, and by obtaining a history of urinary output. Postural light-headedness with changes in pulse and blood pressure are helpful objective parameters in volume depletion. Recent observations have documented that, despite the severest form of secretory derangement in cholera, glucose absorption and its coupled sodium and water absorption remain intact in the upper small bowel. Thus, many patients can be completely rehydrated and maintained by a simple oral-glucose–containing electrolyte solution. A controlled study of patients with cholera and other noninflammatory watery diarrhea in Dacca, Bangladesh, documents the efficacy of sucrose (table sugar) as well as glucose in the oral therapy solution.[371] Electrolyte losses in severe watery diarrhea are similar to the electrolyte composition of serum, and fluid replacement should contain approximately these concentrations of electrolytes. A standard oral fluid regimen contains 3.5 g NaCl, 2.5 g NaHCO$_3$, 1.5 g KCl, and 20 g glucose per liter of boiled water. This corresponds to sodium 90, potassium 20, bicarbonate 30, chloride 80, and glucose 110 mM/liter.[372] A similar solution may be prepared with 3 level tablespoons of sugar, 3/4 teaspoon salt, 1/2 teaspoon sodium bicarbonate in 1 cup of orange juice to make up 1 liter (1.05 qt) in water. If there is concern about hypertonicity, particularly in children, the salt can be reduced in cases of milder diarrhea, and the solution should be given with ad libitum water. Still an additional alternative is 1 level teaspoon of salt and 8 level teaspoons of sugar per liter (or quart) of water, which makes approximately 86 mmol sodium and 30 g sucrose per liter, to which one could add one cup of orange juice or two bananas for potassium. A still further improvement can be made by substituting 40–50 g cereal flour (rice, maize, sorghum, millet, wheat, or potato) for glucose.[373] The electrolyte contents of commonly available soft drinks are quite variable, although solutions of similar electrolyte composition to the ideal as described above can be made in dilute solutions of bouillon or gelatin water. New developments in oral rehydration therapy under study include the use of rice powder or other glucose polymers and the use of amino acids such as glycine, alanine, and glutamine, which enhance sodium absorption independently of glucose.

REFERENCES

1. World Health Organization. Tropical disease 1990. ASM News. 1990;56: 358–9.
2. Guerrant RL, McAuliffe JF. Special problems in developing countries. In: Gorbach SL, ed. Infectious Diarrhea. Boston: Blackwell Scientific, 1986: 287–307.
3. Snyder JD, Merson MH. The magnitude of the global problem of acute diarrhoeal disease: A review of active surveillance data. Bull WHO. 1982;60: 604–13.
4. Warren KS. Tropical medicine or tropical health: The Heath Clark Lectures, 1988. Rev Infect Dis. 1990;12:142–56.
5. Guerrant RL, Hughes JM, Lima NL, et al. Diarrhea in developed and developing countries: Magnitude, special settings, and etiologies. Rev Infect Dis. 1990;12(Suppl 1):S41–50.
6. Guerrant RL, Bobak DA. Bacterial and protozoal gastroenteritis. N Engl J Med. 1991;325:327–40.
7. Cohen ML. The epidemiology of diarrheal disease in the United States. Infect Dis Clin North Am. 1988;2:557–70.
8. Ho M-S, Glass RI, Pinsky PR, et al. Diarrheal deaths in American children—Are they preventable? JAMA. 1988;260:3281–5.
9. Impact of oral rehydration therapy on hospital admission and case-fatality rates for diarrhoeal disease: Results from 11 countries. WHO Weekly Epidemiol Rec No. 8. 1988;49–52.
10. Yunes J. Evaluation of infant mortality and proportional infant mortality in Brazil. World Health Stats Q. 1981;34:200–19.
11. McAuliffe JF, Shields DS, de Souza MA, et al. Prolonged and recurring diarrhea in the northeast of Brazil: Examination of cases from a community-based study. J Pediatr Gastroenterol Nutr. 1986;5:902–6.
12. Schorling JB, Wanke CA, Schorling SK, et al. A prospective study of persistent diarrhea among children in an urban Brazilian slum. Am J Epidemiol. 1990;132:144–56.
13. Bhatnagar S, Dosajh U. Diarrhoeal disease morbidity in children below 5 years in urban slums of Delhi. Indian J Med Res. 1986;84:53–8.
14. Black RE, Brown KH, Becker S, et al. Longitudinal studies of infectious diseases and physical growth of children in rural Bangladesh. Am J Epidemiol. 1982;115:315–24.
15. Mata LJ. The Children of Santa Maria Cauque: A Prospective Field Study of Health and Growth. Cambridge, MA: MIT Press; 1978.
16. Guerrant RL, Kirchhoff LV, Shields DS, et al. Prospective study of diarrheal illness in northeastern Brazil: Patterns of disease, nutritional impact, etiologies and risk factors. J Infect Dis. 1983;148:986.
17. Guerrant RL, Moore RA, Kirschfeld PM, et al. Role of toxigenic and invasive bacteria in acute diarrhea of childhood. N Engl J Med. 1975;293: 567–73.
18. Gordon JE, Chitkara ID, Wyon JB. Weanling diarrhea. Am J Med Sci. 1963; 245:345.
19. Gordon JE, Scrimshaw NS. Infectious disease in the malnourished. Med Clin North Am. 1970;54:1495.
20. Lindenbaum J. Malabsorption during and after recovery from acute intestinal infection. Br Med J. 1965;2:326.
21. Hirschhorn N, Molla A. Reversible jejunal disaccharidase deficiency in cholera and other acute diarrheal diseases. J Hopkins Med J. 1969;125:291.
22. Lindenbaum J, Kent TH, Sprinz H. Malabsorption and jejunitis in American Peace Corps volunteers in Pakistan. Ann Intern Med. 1966;65:1201.
23. Chen LC, Scrimshaw NS, eds. Diarrhea and Malnutrition: Interactions, Mechanisms and Interventions. New York: Plenum Press; 1983.
24. Schorling JB, Guerrant RL. Diarrhea and catch-up growth. Lancet 1990;335: 599–600.
25. Guerrant RL, Schorling JB, McAuliffe JF, et al. Diarrhea as a cause and effect of malnutrition: Diarrhea prevents catch-up growth and malnutrition increases diarrhea frequency and duration. Am J Trop Med Hyg. 1992;47: 28–35.
26. Gordon JE, Guzman MA, Ascoli W, et al. Acute diarrhoeal disease in less developed countries. 2. Patterns of epidemiological behaviour in rural Guatemalan villages. Bull WHO. 1964;31:9.
27. Bowie MD. Malnutrition and diarrhea. S Afr Med J. 1960;34:344.
28. Schorling JB, McAuliffe JF, de Souza MA, et al. Malnutrition is associated with increased diarrhoea incidence and duration among children in an urban Brazilian slum. Int J Epidemiol. 1990;19:728–35.
29. Black RE, Brown RH, Becker S. Malnutrition is determining factor in diarrheal duration, but not incidence, among young children in a longitudinal study in rural Bangladesh. Am J Clin Nutr. 1984;37:87–94.
30. Sheehy TW. Digestive diseases as a national problem. VI. Enteric disease among United States troops in Vietnam. Gastroenterology. 1968;55:105.
31. Hodgkin K. Towards Earlier Diagnosis. A Family Doctor's Approach. Baltimore: Williams & Wilkins; 1963.
32. Hyams KC, Malone JD, Kapikian AZ, et al. Norwalk virus infection among Desert Storm troops. J Infect Dis. 1993;167:986–7.
33. Dingle JH, Badger GF, Jordan WS Jr. Illnesses in the Home, A Study of 25,000 Illnesses in a Group of Cleveland Families. Cleveland: The Press of Western Reserve University; 1964.
34. Bartlett AV, Moore M, Gary GW, et al. Diarrheal illness among infants and toddlers in daycare centers. II. Comparison with daycare home and households. J Pediatr. 1985;107:503–9.
35. Guerrant RL, Lohr JA, Williams EK. Acute infectious diarrhea. I. Epidemiology, etiology, and pathogenesis. Pediatr Infect Dis J 1986;5:353–9.
36. Tauxe RV, Deming MS, Blake PA. *Campylobacter jejuni* infections on college campuses: A national survey. Am J Public Health. 1985;75:659–60.
37. Bartlett JG. *Clostridium difficile:* Clinical considerations. Rev Infect Dis. 1990;12(Suppl 2):S243–51.
38. Hollister AC, Beck MD, Gittelsohn AM, et al. Influence of water availability on shigella prevalence in childre of farm labor families. Am J Public Health. 1955;45:354.
39. Smith HW, Linggood MA. Observations of the pathogenic properties of the K88, Hly and Ent plasmids of *Escherichia coli* with particular reference to porcine diarrhea. J Med Microbiol. 1971;4:467.
40. Evans DG, Silver RP, Evans DJ, et al. Plasmid-controlled colonization factor associated with virulence in *Escherichia coli* enterotoxigenic for humans. Infect Immun. 1975;12:656.
41. Levine MM, Nalin DR, Rennels MB, et al. Genetic susceptibility to cholera. Ann Hum Biol. 1979;6:369–74.
42. Zisman M. Blood group A and giardiasis. Lancet. 1977;2:1285.
43. Rutter JM, Burrows MR, Sellwood R, et al. A genetic basis for resistance to enteric disease caused by *E. coli*. Nature. 1975;257:135.
44. Mobassaleh M, Koul O, Mishra K, et al. The developmental pattern of the regulatory enzymes involved in the synthesis and breakdown of the Shiga toxin receptor in rabbit small intestine. Gastroenterology. 1992;102:A567.

45. Chu SW, Walker WA. Bacterial toxin interaction with the developing intestine: A possible explanation for toxigenic diarrhea of infancy. Gastroenterology. 1993;104:916–25.
46. Cohen MB, Giannella RA. Jejunal toxin inactivation regulates susceptibility of the immature rat to STa. Gastroenterology. 1992;102:1988–96.
47. Eglow R, Pothoulakis C, Itzkowitz S, et al. Diminished *Clostridium difficile* toxin A sensitivity in newborn rabbit ileum is associated with decreased toxin A receptor. J Clin Invest. 1992;90:822–9.
48. Bergman MJ, Evans DG, Sullivan JA, et al. Attachment of *E. coli* to human intestinal epithelial cells: A functional in vitro test for intestinal colonization factor. Trans Assoc Am Physicians. 1978;91:80.
49. Allweiss B, Dostal J, Carey KE, et al. The role of chemotaxis in the ecology of bacterial pathogens of mucosal surfaces. Nature. 1977;266:448.
50. Briscoe J. A role for water supply and sanitation in the child survival revolution. PAHO Bull. 1987;21:93–105.
51. Dolin R, Treanor JJ, Madore HP. Novel agents of viral enteritis in humans. J Infect Dis. 1987;55:365–75.
52. Blackow NR, Greenberg HB. Viral gastroenteritis. N Engl J Med. 1991;325:252–64.
53. Blacklow NR, Dolin R, Fedson DS, et al. Acute infectious nonbacterial gastroenteritis: Etiology and pathogenesis. Ann Intern Med. 1972;76:993.
54. Giannella RA, Broitman SA, Zamcheck N. Gastric acid barrier to ingested microorganisms in man: Studies in vivo and in vitro. Gut. 1972;13:251.
55. Gorbach SL. Progress in gastroenterology: Intestinal microflora. Gastroenterology. 1971;60:1110.
56. Roberts SH, James O, Jarvis EH. Bacterial overgrowth syndrome without "blind loop": A cause for malnutrition in the elderly. Lancet. 1977;2:1193.
57. Hornick RB, Musik SI, Wenzel R, et al. The Broad Street pump revisited: Response to volunteers to ingested cholera vibrios. Bull NY Acad Med. 1971;47:1181.
58. Gitelson S. Gastrectomy, achlorhydria and cholera. Isr J Med Sci. 1971;7:663.
59. Giannella RA, Broitman SA, Zamcheck N. Influence of gastric acidity on bacterial and parasitic enteric infections: A perspective. Ann Intern Med. 1973;78:271.
60. Black RE, Levine MM, Clements ML, et al. Experimental *Campylobacter jejuni* infection in humans. J Infect Dis. 1988;157:472–9.
61. Nurko SS, Garcia-Aranda JA, Consuelo A, et al. Is *Helicobacter pylori* a significant risk factor for persistent diarrhea in Mexican children? (Abstract). Gastroenterology. 1993;104:A160.
62. Driks MR, Craven DE, Celli BR, et al. Nosocomial pneumonia in intubated patients given sucralfate as compared with antacids or histamine type 2 blockers. The role of gastric colonization. N Engl J Med. 1987;317:1376.
63. Dixon JMS. The fate of bacteria in the small intestine. J Pathol Bacteriol. 1960;79:131.
64. Schrager J. The chemical composition and function of gastrointestinal mucus. Gut. 1970;11:450.
65. Higgens JA, Code CF, Orvis AL. The influence of motility on the rate of absorption of sodium and water from the small intestine of healthy persons. Gastroenterology. 1956;31:708.
66. Formal SB, Abrams GD, Schneider H, et al. Experimental *Shigella* infections. VI. Role of the small intestine in an experimental infection in guinea pigs. J Bacteriol. 1963;85:119.
67. Sprinz H. Pathogenesis of intestinal infections. Arch Pathol. 1969;87:556.
68. DuPont HL, Hornick RB. Adverse effect of Lomotil therapy in shigellosis. JAMA. 1973;226:1525.
69. Holdeman LV, Cato EP, Moore WEC, eds. Anaerobe Laboratory Manual. Blacksburg, VA: Virginia Polytechnic and State University Anaerobe Laboratory; 1977.
70. Price DJE, Sleigh JD. Control of infection due to *Klebsiella* aerogenes in a neurosurgical unit by withdrawal of all antibiotics. Lancet. 1970;2:1213.
71. Mentzing LO, Ringertz O. *Salmonella* infection in tourists. 2. Prophylaxis against salmonellosis. Acta Pathol Microbiol Scand. 1968;74:405.
72. Bohnhoff M, Miller CP, Martin WR. Resistance of the mouse's intestinal track to experimental *Salmonella* infections. J Exp Med. 1964;120:805.
73. Van der Waaj D, Berguis JM, Lekkerkerk JEC. Colonization resistance of the digestive tract of mice during systemic antibiotic treatment. J Hyg. 1972;70:605–10.
74. Que JU, Casey SW, Hentges DJ. Factors responsible for increased susceptibility of mice to intestinal colonization after treatment with streptomycin. Infect Immun. 1986;53:116–23.
75. Tannock GW, Savage DC. Indigenous microorganisms prevent reduction in fecal size induced by *Salmonella typhimurium* in vaccinated gnotobiotic mice. Infect Immun. 1976;13:172.
76. Schrank GD, Verwey WF. Distribution of cholera organisms in experimental *Vibrio cholerae* infections: Proposed mechanisms of pathogenesis and antibacterial immunity. Infect Immun. 1976;13:195.
77. Ryan CA, Nickels MK, Hargrett-Bean NT, et al. Massive outbreak of antimicrobial-resistant salmonellosis traced to pasteurized milk. JAMA. 1987;258:3269–74.
78. Pavia AT, Shipman LD, Wells JG, et al. Epidemiologic evidence that prior antimicrobial exposure decreases resistance to infection by antimicrobial-sensitive *Salmonella*. J Infect Dis. 1990;161:255–60.
79. Gorbach SL, Chang T-W, Goldin B. Successful treatment of relapsing *Clostridium difficile* colitis with lactobacillus GG. Lancet. 1987;2:1519.
80. Tvede M, Rask-Madsen J. Bacteriotherapy for chronic relapsing *Clostridium difficile* diarrhoea in six patients. Lancet. 1989;1:1156–60.
81. Cuzzolin L, Zambreri D, Donini M, et al. Influence of radiotherapy on intestinal microflora in cancer patients. J Chemother. 1992;4:176–9.
82. Cudmore MA, Silva J Jr, Fekety R, et al. *Clostridium difficile* colitis associated with cancer chemotherapy. Arch Intern Med. 1982;142:333–5.
83. Silva J, Fekety R, Werk C, et al. Inciting and etiologic agents of colitis. Rev Infect Dis. 1984;6:S214.
84. Milligan DW, Kelly JK. Pseudomembranous colitis in a leukemia unit: Report of five fatal cases. J Clin Pathol. 1979;32:1237–43.
85. Bodey GP, Buckley M, Sathe YS, et al. Quantitative relationships between circulating leukocytes and infection in patients with acute leukemia. Ann Intern Med. 1966;64:328.
86. Gandy W, Greenberg BR. Successful medical management of neutropenic enterocolitis. Cancer. 1983;51:1551–5.
87. Dosik GM, Luna M, Valdivieso M, et al. Necrotizing colitis in patients with cancer. Am J Med. 1979;67:646–56.
88. Hopkins DG, Kushner JP. Clostridial species in the pathogenesis of necrotizing enterocolitis in patients with neutropenia. Am J Hematol. 1983;14:289–95.
89. Bodey GD, Fainstein V, Guerrant RL. Infections of the gastrointestinal tract in the immunocompromised patient. Annu Rev Med. 1986;37:271–81.
90. Yolken RH, Bishop CA, Townsend TR, et al. Infectious gastroenteritis in bone-marrow-transplant recipients. N Engl J Med. 1982;306:1009.
91. Smith PD, Lane C, Gill VJ, et al. Intestinal infections in patients with the acquired immunodeficiency syndrome (AIDS). Ann Intern Med. 1988;108:328–33.
92. Sperber SJ, Schlenpner CJ. Salmonellosis during infection with human immunodeficiency virus. Rev Infect Dis. 1987;9:925–34.
93. Soave R, Johnson WD. *Cryptosporidium* and *Isospora belli* infections. J Infect Dis. 1988;157:225–9.
94. Colebunders R, Franastt, Mann J, et al. Persistent diarrhea, strongly associated with HIV infection in Kinshasa, Zaire. Am J Gastroenterol. 1987;82:859–64.
95. Sewankambo N, Mugerwa RD, Goodgame R, et al. Enteropathic AIDS in Uganda. An endoscopic, histological and microbiological study. AIDS. 1987;1:9–13.
96. Nelson JA, Reynolds-Kohler C, Margaretten W, et al. Human immunodeficiency virus detected in bowel epithelium from patients with gastrointestinal symptoms. Lancet. 1988;1:259–62.
97. Brandtzaeg P, Halstensen TS, Kett K, et al. Immunobiology and immunopathology of human gut mucosa: Humoral immunity and intraepithelial lymphocytes. Gastroenterology. 1989;97:1562–84.
98. Grutzkau A, Hanski C, Hahn H, et al. Involvement of M cells in the bacterial invasion of Peyer's patches: A common mechanism shared by *Yersinia enterocolitica* and other enteroinvasive bacteria. Gut. 1990;31:1011–5.
99. Wassef JS, Keren DF, Mailloux JL. Role of M cells in initial antigen uptake and in ulcer formation in the rabbit intestinal loop model of shigellosis. Infect Immun. 1989;57:858–63.
100. Marcial MM, Madara JL. *Cryptosporidium:* Cellular localization, structural analysis of absorptive cell-parasite membrane—membrane interactions in guinea pigs, and suggestion of protozoan transport by M cells. Gastroenterology. 1986;90:583–94.
101. Bull DM, Tomasi TB. Deficiency of immunoglobulin A in intestinal disease. Gastroenterology. 1968;54:313.
102. Hirschowitz B, Streeton D, Pollard M, et al. Role of gastric secretions in activation of peptic ulcers by corticotrophin (ACTA). JAMA. 1955;158:27–32.
103. Strober W, Krakauer R, Klaeveman HL, et al. Secretory component deficiency: A disorder of the IgA immune system. N Engl J Med. 1976;294:351–6.
104. Plaut AG. The IgAI proteases of pathogenic bacteria. Annu Rev Microbiol. 1983;37:603–22.
105. Kelsall BL, Ravdin JI. Degradation of human immunoglobulin by *Entamoeba histolytica*. Nov. 4–8. 39th Meeting of the American Society for Microbiology 1990; Abstract No. 284:197.
106. Pierce NF, Reynolds HY: Immunity to experimental cholera. II. Secretory and humoral antitoxin response to local and systemic toxoid administration. J Infect Dis. 1975;131:383.
107. Pierce NF, Gowans JL. Cellular kinetics of the intestinal immune responses to cholera toxoid in rats. J Exp Med. 1975;142:1550.
108. Stoliar OA, Pelley RP, Kaniecki-Green E, et al. Secretory IgA against enterotoxins in breast-milk. Lancet. 1976;1:1258.
109. Brown SE III, Sauer KT, Nations-Shields M, et al. Comparison of paired whole milk and dried filter paper samples for antienterotoxin and anti-rotavirus activities. J Clin Microbiol. 1982;16:103.
110. Jones EG, Brown WR. Serum and intestinal fluid immunoglobulins in patients with giardiasis. Am J Dig Dis. 1974;19:791.
111. Zinneman HH, Kaplan AP. The associate of giardiasis with reduced intestinal secretory immunoglobulin A. Am J Dig Dis. 1972;17:793.
112. Ament ME, Ochs HD, Davis SD. Structure and function of the gastrointestinal tract in primary immunodeficiency syndromes: A study of 39 patients. Medicine. 1973;52:227.
113. Hermans PE, Huizenga KA, Hoffman HN, et al. Dysgammaglobulinemia associated with nodular lymphoid hyperplasia of the small intestine. Am J Med. 1966;40:78.
114. Crabbe PA, Heremans JF. Lack of gamma A-immunoglobulin in serum of patients with steatorrhea. Gut. 1966;7:119.

115. Collins FM, Carter PB. Cellular immunity in enteric disease. Am J Clin Nutr. 1974;27:1424.
116. Welsh JK, May JT. Anti-infective properties of breast milk. J Pediatr. 1979; 94:1.
117. McClelland DBL, McGrath J, Samson RR. Antimicrobial factors in human milk: Studies of concentration and transfer to the infant during the early stages of lactation. Acta Paediatr Scand. 1978;27(Suppl):1.
118. Arnold RR, Cole MF, McGhee JR. A bactericidal effect for human lactoferrin. Science. 1977;197:263.
119. Griffiths E, Humphreys J. Bacteriostatic effect of human milk and bovine colostrum on *Escherichia coli:* Importance of bicarbonate. Infect Immun. 1977;15:396.
120. Bullen JJ, Rogers HJ, Leight L. Iron-binding proteins in milk and resistance to *Escherichia coli* infection in infants. Br Med J. 1975;1:69.
121. Hanson LA, Winberg J. Breast milk and defence against infection in the newborn. Arch Dis Child. 1972;47:845.
122. Cravioto A, Tello A, Villafán H, et al. Inhibition of localized adhesion of enteropathogenic *Escherichia coli* to HEp-2 cells by immunoglobulin and oligosaccharide fractions of human colostrum and breast milk. J Infect Dis. 1991;163:1247–55.
123. Levine MM. *Escherichia coli* that cause diarrhea: Enterotoxigenic enteropathogenic, enteroinvasive, enterohemorrhagic, and enteroadherent. J Infect Dis. 1987;155:377–88.
124. Schlager TA, Guerrant RL. Seven possible pathogenic mechanisms for *Escherichia coli* diarrhea. Infect Dis Clin North Am. 1988;2:1–18.
125. Bobak DA, Guerrant RL. New developments in enteric bacterial toxins. Adv Pharmacol. 1992;23:85–108.
126. Lamanna C, Carr CJ. The botulinal, tetanal, and enterostaphylococcal toxins: A review. Clin Pharmacol Ther. 1967;8:286.
127. Koupal A, Deibel RH. Rabbit intestinal fluid accumulation by an enterotoxigenic factor of *Staphylococcus aureus*. Infect Immun. 1977;18:298–303.
128. Freer JH, Arbuthnott JP. Toxins of *Staphylococcus aureus*. In: Dorner F, Drews J, eds. Pharmacology of Bacterial Toxins. Oxford: Pergamon Press; 1986:581–633.
129. Terranova W, Blake PA. *Bacillus cereus* food poisoning. N Engl J Med. 1978;298:143.
130. Turnbull PCB. *Bacillus cereus* toxins. In: Dorner F, Drews J, eds. Pharmacology of Bacterial Toxins. Oxford: Pergamon Press; 1986:397–448.
131. Chen LC, Rohde JE, Sharp GWG. Intestinal adenyl-cyclase activity in human cholera. Lancet. 1971;1:939.
132. Guerrant RL, Chen LC, Sharp GWG. Intestinal adenyl-cyclase activity in canine cholera: Correlation with fluid accumulation. J Infect Dis. 1972;125: 377.
133. Peterson JW, Ochoa G. Role of prostaglandins and cAMP in the secretory effects of cholera toxin. Science. 1989;245:857–9.
134. Peterson JW, Chopra AK, Prasad R. Fine mapping of the rrnE, purHD, and hydGH operons on the *Escherichia coli* chromosome. J Bacteriol. 1991;173: 3274–3275.
135. Fang GD, Fonteles MC, Barrett LJ, et al. Inhibition by platelet activating factor (PAF) antagonists of the effects of choleratoxin on intestinal secretion and cytoskeleton of Chinese hamster ovary (CHO) cells (Abstract). Clin Res. 1993;41:222A.
136. Cassuto J, Jodal M, Tuttle R, et al. On the role of intramural nerves in the pathogenesis of cholera toxin-induced intestinal secretion. Scand J Gastroenterol. 1981;16:377–84.
137. Beubler E, Horina G. 5-HT₂ and 5-HT₃ receptor subtypes mediate cholera toxin-induced intestinal fluid secretion in the rat. Gastroenterology. 1990; 99:1–7.
138. Honda T, Shimizu M, Takeda Y, et al. Isolation of a factor causing morphological changes of Chinese hamster ovary cells from the culture filtrates of *Vibrio parahemolyticus*. Infect Immun. 1976;14:1028.
139. Blake PA, Weaver RE, Hollis DG. Diseases of humans (other than cholera) caused by vibrios. Annu Rev Microbiol. 1980;34:341.
140. Evans DJ Jr., Chen LC, Curlin GT. Stimulation of adenyl cyclase by *Escherichia coli* enterotoxin. Nature [New Biol]. 1972;236:137.
141. Guerrant RL, Ganguly U, Casper AGT, et al. Effect of *Escherichia coli* on fluid transport across canine small bowel: Mechanism and time-course with enterotoxin and whole bacterial cell. J Clin Invest. 1973;52:1707.
142. Skerman FJ, Formal SB, Falkow S. Plasmid-associated enterotoxin production in a strain of *Escherichia coli* isolated from humans. Infect Immun. 1972; 5:622.
143. Lathe R, Hirth P. Cell-free synthesis of enterotoxin of *E. coli* from a cloned gene. Nature. 1980;284:473.
144. Takeda Y, Murphy J. Bacteriophage conversion of heat-labile enterotoxin in *Escherichia coli*. J Bacteriol. 1978;133:172.
145. Evans DG, Evans DJ Jr, Pierce NF. Differences in the response of rabbit small intestine to heat-labile and heat-stable enterotoxins of *Escherichia coli*. Infect Immun. 1973;7:873.
146. Craig JP. A permeability factor (toxin) found in cholera stools and culture filtrates and its neutralization by convalescent cholera sera. Nature. 1965; 207:614.
147. Guerrant RL, Brunton LL, Schnaitman TC, et al. Cyclic adenosine monophosphate and alteration of Chinese hamster ovary cell morphology: A rapid, sensitive in vitro assay for the enterotoxins of *Vibrio cholerae* and *Escherichia coli*. Infect Immun. 1974;10:320.
148. Donta ST, Moon HW, Whipp SC. Detection of heat-labile *Escherichia coli* enterotoxins with the use of adrenal cells in tissue culture. Science. 1974; 183:334.
149. Greenberg HB, Sack DA, Rodriguez W, et al. A microtiter solid-phase radioimmunoassay for detection of *Escherichia coli* heat-labile enterotoxin. Infect Immun. 1977;17:541.
150. Yoiken RH, Greenberg HB, Merson MH, et al. Enzyme-linked immunosorbent assay for detection of *Escherichia coli* heat-labile enterotoxin. J Clin Microbiol. 1977;6:439.
151. Honda T, Tage S, Takeda Y, et al. Modified Elek test for detection of heat-labile enterotoxin of enterotoxigenic *E. coli*. J Clin Microbiol. 1981;13:1.
152. Sommerfelt H, Svennerholm AM, Kalland KH, et al. Comparative study of colony hybridizations with synthetic oligonucleotide probes and enzyme-linked immunosorbent assay for identification of *Escherichia coli*. J Clin Microbiol. 1988;26:530–4.
153. Gorbach SL, Banwell JG, Chatterjee BD, et al. Acute undifferentiated human diarrhea in the tropics. I. Alterations in intestinal microflora. J Clin Invest. 1971;50:881.
154. Ryder RW, Sack DA, Kapikian AZ, et al. Enterotoxigenic *Escherichia coli* and reovirus-like agent in rural Bangladesh. Lancet. 1976;1:659.
155. Gorbach SL, Kean BH, Evans DG: Traveler's diarrhea and toxigenic *Escherichia coli*. N Engl J Med. 1975;292:933.
156. Merson MH, Morris GK, Sack DA, et al. Travelers' diarrhea in Mexico: A prospective study. Abstract 149 presented at the 15th Interscience Conference on Antimicrobial Agents and Chemotherapy; September 1975.
157. Guerrant RL, Rouse JD, Hughes JM. Turista among members of the Yale Glee Club in Latin America. Am J Trop Med Hyg. 1980;29:895.
158. Gorbach SL, Khurana CM. Toxigenic *Escherichia coli:* A cause of infantile diarrhea in Chicago. N Engl J Med. 1972;287:791.
159. Sack RB, Hirschhorn N, Brownlee I, et al. Enterotoxigenic *Escherichia coli*–associated diarrheal disease in Apache children. N Engl J Med. 1975; 292:1041.
160. Guerrant RL, Moore RA, Kirschenfeld PM, et al. Role of toxigenic and invasive bacteria in acute diarrhea of childhood. N Engl J Med. 1975;293: 567.
161. Guerrant RL, Dickens MD, Wenzel RP, et al. Toxigenic bacterial diarrhea: Nursery outbreak involving multiple bacterial strains. J Pediatr. 1976;89: 885–91.
162. Wachsmuth K, Wells J, Shipley P. Heat-labile enterotoxin production in isolates from a shipboard outbreak of human diarrheal illness. Infect Immun. 1979;24:793–7.
163. Honda T, Shimizu M, Takeda Y, et al. Isolation of a factor causing morphological changes of Chinese hamster ovary cells from the culture filtrates of *Vibrio parahemolyticus*. Infect Immun. 1976;14:1028–33.
164. Sandefur PD, Peterson JW. Neutralization of *Salmonella* toxin-induced elongation of Chinese hamster ovary cells by cholera antitoxin. Infect Immun. 1977;15:988–92.
165. Ruiz-Palacios GM, Torres J, Torres NI, et al. Cholera-like enterotoxin produced by *Campylobacter jejuni:* Characterization and clinical significance. Lancet. 1983;2:250–3.
166. Ruiz-Palacios GM, Lopez-Vidal Y, Torres J, et al. Serum antibodies to heat-labile enterotoxin of *Campylobacter jejuni*. J Infect Dis. 1985;152:413–6.
167. Daikoku T, Kawaguchi M, Takama K, et al. Partial purification and characterization of the enterotoxin produced by *Campylobacter jejuni*. Infect Immun. 1990;58:2414–9.
168. Gyles CL. Heat-labile and heat-stable forms of the enterotoxin from *E. coli* strains enteropathogenic for pigs. Ann NY Acad Sci. 1971;176:315.
169. Levine MM, Caplan ES, Waterman D, et al. Diarrhea caused by *Escherichia coli* that produce only heat-stable enterotoxins. Infect Immun. 1977;17:78.
170. Sack DA, Wells JG, Merson MH. Diarrhoea associated with heat-stable enterotoxin-producing strains of *Escherichia coli*. Lancet. 1975;2:239.
171. Ryder RW, Wachsmuth IK, Buxton AE, et al. Infantile diarrhea produced by heat-stable enterotoxin *Escherichia coli*. N Engl J Med. 1976;295:849.
172. Hughes JM, Rouse JD, Barada FA, et al. Etiology of summer diarrhea among the Navajo. Am J Trop Med Hyg. 1980;29:613.
173. Korzeniowski OM, Dantas W, Trabulsi LR, et al. A controlled study of endemic sporadic diarrhoea among adult residents of southern Brazil. Trans R Soc Trop Med Hyg. 1984;78:363–9.
174. Hughes JM, Murad F, Chang B, et al. Role of cyclic GMP in the action of heat-stable enterotoxin of *Escherichia coli*. Nature. 1978;271:755.
175. Field M, Graf LH Jr, Laird WJ, et al. Heat stable enterotoxin of *E. coli*. In vitro effects on guanylate cyclase activity, cyclic GMP concentration, and ion transportin small small intestine. Proc Natl Acad Sci USA. 1978;75:2800.
176. Guerrant RL, Hughes JM, Chang B, et al. Activation of intestinal guanylate cyclase by heat-stable enterotoxin of *E. coli:* Studies of tissue specificity, potential receptors and intermediates. J Infect Dis. 1980;142:220.
177. Aimoto S, Takao T, Shimonishi Y, et al. Amino-acid sequence of a heat stable enterotoxin produced by human enterotoxigenic *Escherichia coli*. Eur J Biochem. 1982;129:257–263.
178. Takao T, Hitouji T, Aimoto S, et al. Amino-acid sequence of a heat-stable enterotoxin isolated from enterotoxigenic *Escherichia coli* strain 18D. FEBS Lett. 1983;152:1–5.
179. Guarino A, Giannella R, Thompson MR. *Citrobacter freundii* produces an 18-amino-acid heat-stable enterotoxin identical to the 18-amino-acid *Escherichia coli* heat-stable enterotoxin (ST Ia). Infect Immun. 1989;57:649–52.
180. Takeda T, Balakrish Nair G, et al. Production of a monoclonal antibody to *Vibrio cholerae* Non-01 heat-stable enterotoxin (ST) which is cross-reactive with *Yersinia enterocolitica* ST. Infect Immun. 1990;58:2755–2759.

181. Guerrant RL, Fang G, Lima AAM, et al. Pathophysiology of enterotoxic diarrheas. 28th Joint Conference US-Japan Cooperative Medical Science Program on Cholera and Related Diarrheal Diseases Panel, Tokyo 1992; July 20:31–36.

182. Fonteles MC, Lima AAM, Fang G, et al. Effect of STa and cholera toxin on renal electrolyte transport: Possible roles of an endogenous ST-like compound in the isolated kidney. 27th U S Japan Cholera Meeting, Charlottesville, VA 1991;100–105.

183. Currie MG, Fok KF, Kato J, et al. Guanylin: An endogenous activator of intestinal guanylate cyclase. Proc Natl Acad Sci USA. 1992;89:947–51.

184. Fonteles MC, Villar-Palasi C, Fang G, et al. Partial characterization of an ANF/urodilatin-like substance released from perfused rabbit kidney under hypoxia. Brazilian J Med Biol Res. 1993;26:75–9.

185. Lyerly DM, Krivan HC, Wilkins TD. *Clostridium difficile:* Its disease and toxins. J Clin Microbiol. 1988;1:1–18.

186. Kapral FA. *Staphylococcus aureus* delta toxin as an enterotoxin. Ciba Found Symp. 1985;112:215–29.

187. Scheifele DW. Role of bacterial toxins in neonatal necrotizing enterocolitis. J Pediatr. 1990;117(No 1, Part 2):S45–6.

188. Fasano A, Kay BA, Russell RG, et al. Enterotoxin and cytotoxin production by enteroinvasive *Escherichia coli.* Infect Immun. 1990;58:3717–23.

189. Savarino SJ, Fasano A, Robertson DC, et al. Enteroaggregative *Escherichia coli* elaborate a heat-stable enterotoxin demonstrable in an *in vitro* rabbit intestinal model. J Clin Invest. 1991;87:1450–5.

190. Lima AAM, Lyerly DM, Wilkins TD, et al. Effects of *Clostridium difficile* toxins A and B in rabbit small and large intestine *in vivo* and on cultured cells *in vitro.* Infect Immun. 1988;56:582–8.

191. Lima AAM, Innes DJ, Chadee K, et al. *Clostridium difficile* toxin A: Early sequential histopathologic effects in rabbit small intestine. Lab Invest. 1989; 61:419–25.

192. Guerrant RL, Fang G, Lima AAM, et al. PAF antagonists, inhibitors of phospholipase A_2 and cyclooxygenase block the secretory and cytoskeletal effects of *C. difficile* toxin A. 1992. Presented in Utah at the Fourth International Congress on PAF and Related Lipid Mediators.

193. Fang GD, Yotseff P, Lyerly DM, et al. Pertussis toxin (PT) inhibits the secretory effect of *C. difficile* toxin A (Abstract). Clin Res. 1993;41:175A.

194. Moore R, Pothoulakis C, LaMont JT, et al. *C. difficile* toxin A increases intestinal permeability and induces Cl⁻ secretion. Am Physiol Soc. 1990; G165–72.

195. Myers LL, Shoop DS, Stackhouse LL, et al. Isolation of enterotoxigenic *Bacteroides fragilis* from humans with diarrhea. J Clin Microbiol. 1987;25: 2330–3.

196. Myers LL, Shoop DS, Collins JE. Rabbit model to evaluate enterovirulence of *Bacteroides fragilis.* J Clin Microbiol. 1990;28:1658–60.

197. Weikel CS, Grieco FD, Reuben J, et al. Human colonic epithelial cells, HT29/C₁, treated with crude *Bacteroides fragilis* enterotoxin dramatically alter their morphology. Infect Immun. 1992;60:321–7.

198. Keusch GT, Grady GF, Mata LJ, et al. The pathogenesis of *Shigella* diarrhea. I. Enterotoxin production by *Shigella dysenteriae* 1. J Clin Invest. 1972;51: 1212.

199. Charney AN, Gots RE, Formal SB, et al. Activation of intestinal mucosal adenylate cyclase by *Shigella dysenteriae* I enterotoxin. Gastroenterology. 1976;70:1085.

200. Rout WR, Formal SB, Giannella RA, et al. Pathophysiology of *Shigella* diarrhea in the rhesus monkey: Intestinal transport, morphological and bacteriological studies. Gastroenterology. 1975;68:270.

201. Keusch FT, Jacewicz M. Serum enterotoxin neutralizing antibody in human shigellosis. Nature [New Biol]. 1973;241:31.

202. Kopecko DJ, Washington O, Formal SB. Genetic and physical evidence for plasmid control of *Shigella sonnei* form I cell surface antigen. Infect Immun. 1980;29:207.

203. Keusch GT. Invasive bacterial diarrhea. In: LC Chen, NS Scrimshaw, eds. Diarrhea and Malnutrition. New York: Plenum Press; 1983:45.

204. Turnbull PCB: Studies on the production of enterotoxins by *Bacillus cereus.* J Clin Pathol. 1976;29:941–9.

205. Gilbert RJ, Kramer JM. *Bacillus ceseus* enterotoxins: Present status. Biochem Soc Trans. 1984;12:198–200.

206. Giannella RA, Formal SB, Dammin GJ, et al. Pathogenesis of salmonellosis. Studies of fluid secretion, mucosal invasion, and morphologic reaction in the rabbit ileum. J Clin Invest. 1973;52:441.

207. Giannella RA, Gots RE, Charney AN, et al. Pathogenesis of *Salmonella*-mediated intestinal fluid secretion: Activation of adenylate cyclase and inhibition by indomethacin. Gastroenterology. 1975;69:1238.

208. Musch MW, Miller RJ, Field M, et al. Stimulation of colonic secretion by lipoxygenase metabolites of arachidonic acid. Science. 1982;217:1255.

209. Madara JL, Patapoff TW, Gillece-Castro B, et al. 5'-Adenosine monophosphate is the neutrophil-derived paracrine factor that elicits chloride secretion from T-84 intestinal epithelial cell monolayers. J Clin Invest. 1993;91:2320–5.

210. Koupal LR, Deibel RH. Assay, characterization and localization of an enterotoxin produced by *Salmonella.* Infect Immun. 1975;11:14.

211. Klipstein FA, Holdeman LV, Corcino JJ. Enterotoxigenic intestinal bacteria in tropical sprue. Ann Intern Med. 1973;79:632.

212. Wasdtrom T, Aust-Kettis A, Habte D, et al. Enterotoxin-producing bacteria and parasites in stools of Ethiopian children with diarrhoeal disease. Arch Dis Child. 1976;51:865.

213. Ljungh A, Popoff M, Wadstrom T. *Aeromonas hydrophila* in acute diarrhea

disease: Detection of enterotoxin and biotyping of strains. J Clin Microbiol. 1977;6:96.

214. Keusch GT, Jacewicz M. The pathogenesis of *Shigella* diarrhea. V. Relationship of Shiga enterotoxin, neurotoxin and cytotoxin. J Infect Dis. 1975;131S: S33.

215. Konowalchuk J, Speirs JI, Stavric S. Vero response to a cytotoxin of *Escherichia coli.* Infect Immun. 1977;18:775.

216. Konowalchuk J, Dickie N, Stavric S, et al. Properties of an *Escherichia coli* cytotoxin. Infect Immun. 1978;10:575.

217. Scotland SM, Day NP, Willshaw GA, et al. Cytotoxic enteropathogenic *Escherichia coli.* Lancet. 1980;1:90.

218. Riley LW, Remia RS, Helgerson SD, et al. Outbreaks of hemorrhagic colitis associated with a rare *Escherichia coli* serotype. N Engl J Med. 1983;308: 681.

219. Johnson WM, Lior H, Bezanson GS. Cytotoxic *Escherichia coli* O157:H7 associated with hemorrhagic colitis in Canada. Lancet. 1983;1:76.

220. Strockbine NA, Marques LRM, Newland JW, et al. Two toxin-converting phages from *E. coli* O157:H7 strains 933 encode antigenically distinct toxins with similar biologic activities. Infect Immun. 1986;53:135–40.

221. Karmali MA, Petric M, Lim C, et al. The association between idiopathic hemolytic uremic syndrome and infection by verotoxin producing *E. coli.* J Infect Dis. 1985;151:775–82.

222. Pai CH, Gordon R, Sims HU, et al. Sporadic cases of hemorrhagic colitis associated with *E. coli* O157:H7. Ann Intern Med. 1984;101:738–42.

223. Carter AO, Borczyk AA, Carlson AK, et al. A severe outbreak of *E. coli* O157:H7 associated hemorrhagic colitis in a nursing home. N Engl J Med. 1987;317:1496–500.

224. Griffin PM, Tauxe RV. The epidemiology of infections caused by *Escherichia coli* O157:H7, other enterohemorrhagic E. coli, and the associated hemolytic uremic syndrome. Epidemiol Rev. 1991;13:60–98.

225. Centers for Disease Control and Prevention. Update: Multistate outbreak of *E. coli* O157:H7 infections from hamburgers—W. U.S., 1992–1993. MMWR 1993;42:258–63.

226. O'Brien AD, Holmes RK. Shiga and shiga-like toxins. Microbiol Rev. 1987; 51:206–20.

227. Obrig TG, Moran RP, Colinas RJ. Ribonuclease activity associated with the 60-S ribosome inactivating proteins Ricin A, phytolacin and shiga toxin. Biochem Biophys Res Commun. 1985;1300:8790–840.

228. Reisbig R, Olsnes S, Eiklid K. The cytotoxic activity of *Shigella* toxin: Evidence for catalytic inactivation of the 60-S ribosomal subunit. J Biol Chem. 1981;2560:8739–44.

229. Jackson MP. Structure–function analysis of Shiga toxin and the Shiga-like toxins. Microbial Pathogenesis. 1990;8:235–42.

230. Karmall MA. Infection by verocytotoxin-producing *Escherichia coli.* Clin Microbiol Rev. 1989;2:15–38.

231. Samuel JE, Perera LP, Ward S, et al. Comparison of the glycolipid receptor specificities of Shiga-like toxin type II and Shiga-like toxin type II variants. Infect Immun. 1990;58:611–8.

232. Bridgewater FAJ, Morgan RS, Rowson KEK, et al. The neurotoxin of *Shigella shigae.* Morphological and functional lesions produced in the central nervous system of rabbits. Br J Exp Pathol. 1955;36:447–53.

233. Cavanagh JB, Howard JG, Whitby JL. The neurotoxin of *Shigella shigae:* A comparative study of the effects produced in various laboratory animals. Br J Exp Med. 1956;370:272–8.

234. Howard JG. Observations on the intoxication produced in mice and rabbits by the neurotoxin of *Shigella shigae.* Br J Exp Pathol. 1955;36:439–46.

235. Wiley RG, Donohue-Rolfe A, Keusch GT. Axonally transported *Shigella* cytotoxin is neurotoxic? J Neuropathol Exp Neurol. 1985;440:496–506.

236. Ashkenazi A, Cleary KR, Pickering LK, et al. The association of Shiga toxin and other cytotoxins with the neurologic manifestations of shigellosis. J Infect Dis. 1990;161:961–5.

237. McDonel JL, Duncan CL. Histopathological effect of *Clostridium perfringens* enterotoxin in the rabbit ileum. Infect Immun. 1975;12:1214.

238. Bartholomew BA, Stringer MF. Observations on the purification of *Clostridium perfringens* type A enterotoxin and the production of a specific antiserum. Fems Microbiol Lett. 1983;18:43–8.

239. Bartholomew BA, Stringer MF. *Clostridium perfringens* enterotoxin: A brief review. Biochem Soc Trans. 1984;12:195–7.

240. Horiguchi Y, Akai T, Sakaguchi G. Isolation and function of a *Clostridium perfringens* enterotoxin fragment. Infect Immun. 1987;55:2912–5.

241. Borriello SP, Barclay F, Welch AR, et al. Epidemiology of diarrhea caused by enterotoxigenic *Clostridium perfringens.* J Med Microbiol. 1985;20: 363–72.

242. Borriello SP, Welch AR, Larson HE, et al. Enterotoxigenic *Clostridium perfringens:* A possible cause of antibiotic associated diarrhea. Lancet. 1984; 1:305–7.

243. Larson HE, Borriello SP. Infectious diarrhea due to *Clostridium perfringens.* J Infect Dis. 1988;157:390–2.

244. Lawrence GW, Lehmann D, Anian G, et al. Impact of active immunization against enteritis necroticans in Papua, New Guinea. Lancet. 1990:336.

245. Bhattacharya S, Bose AK, Ghosh AK: Permeability and enterotoxic factors of nonagglutinable vibrios V. *alcaligenes* and V. *parahaemolyticus.* Appl Microbiol. 1971;22:1159.

246. Carruthers MM. Cytotoxicity of *Vibrio parahemolyticus* in HeLa cell culture. J Infect Dis. 1975;132:555.

247. Calia FM, Johnson DE. Bacteremia in suckling rabbits after oral challenge with *Vibrio parahemolyticus.* Infect Immun. 1975;11:1222.

248. Bolen JL, Zamiska SA, Grennough WB III. Clinical features in enteritis due to *Vibrio parahemolyticus*. Am J Med. 1974;57:638.
249. Barker WH, MacKowiak PA, Fishbein M, et al. *Vibrio parahaemolyticus* gastroenteritis outbreak in Covington, Louisiana in August 1972. Am J Epidemiol. 1974;100:316.
250. Kapral FA, O'Brien AD, Ruff PD, et al. Inhibition of water absorption in the intestine by *Staphylococcal aureus* delta toxin. Infect Immun. 1976;13:140.
251. Bartlett JG, Chang TW, Gurwith M, et al. Antibiotic-associated pseudomembranous colitis due to toxin-producing clostridia. N Engl J Med. 1978;298:531.
252. Rifkin GD, Fekety FR, Silva J Jr, et al. Antibiotic-induced colitis: Implication of a toxin neutralized by *Clostridium sordelli* antitoxin. Lancet. 1977;2:1103.
253. Taylor NS, Thorne GM, Bartlett JG. Comparison of two toxins produced by *Clostridium difficile*. Infect Immun. 1981;34:1036.
254. Johnson WM, Lior H. Toxins produced by *Campylobacter jejuni* and *Campylobacter coli*. Lancet. 1984;1:229–30.
255. Yeen WP, Pothocheary SD, Pang T. Demonstration of a cytotoxin from *Campylobacter jejuni*. J Clin Pathol. 1983;36:1237–40.
256. Guerrant RL, Wanke CA, Pennie RA, et al. Production of a unique cytotoxin by *Campylobacter jejuni*. Infect Immun. 1987;55:2526–30.
257. Perez-Perez GL, Cohn DL, Guerrant RL, et al. Clinical and immunologic significance of cholera-like toxin and cytotoxin production by *Campylobacter* species in patients with acute inflammatory diarrhea in the USA. J Infect Dis. 1989;160:460–7.
258. Leunk RD, Johnson PT, David BC, et al. Cytotoxic activity in broth-culture filtrates of *Campylobacter pylori*. J Med Microbiol. 1988;26:93–9.
259. Leunk RD, Ferguson MA, Morgan DR, et al. Antibody to cytotoxin in infection by *Helicobacter pylori*. J Clin Microbiol. 1990;28:1181–4.
260. Guerrant RL, Lingwood CA. Glycoconjugate receptors for adhesins and toxins. In: Marshall BJ, McCallum RW, Guerrant RL, eds. *Helicobacter pylori* in Peptic Ulceration and Gastritis. Boston: Blackwell Scientific Publication, Inc.; 1991:66–80.
261. Smoot DT, Mobley HLT, Chippendale GR, et al. *Helicobacter pylori* urease activity is toxic to human gastric epithelial cells. Infect Immun. 1990;58:1992–4.
262. Fasano A, Baudry B, Pumplin DW, et al. *Vibrio cholerae* produces a second enterotoxin which affects intestinal tight junctions. Proc Natl Acad Sci USA. 1991;88:5242–6.
263. Salit IE, Gostchlich EC. Type I *Escherichia coli* pili: Characterization of binding to monkey kidney cells. J Exp Med. 1977;146:1182.
264. Silverblatt FJ. Host parasitic in the rat renal pelvis: A possible role for pili in the pathogenesis of pyelonephritis. J Exp Med. 1974;140:1696.
265. Eden CS, Hausson S, Jodal U, et al. Host–parasite interaction in the urinary tract. J Infect Dis. 1988;157:421–6.
266. Evans DG, Satterwhite TK, Evans DJ Jr, et al. Differences in serological responses and excretion patterns of volunteers challenged with enterotoxigenic *Escherichia coli* with and without the colonization factor antigen. Infect Immun. 1978;19:883.
267. Bergman MJ, Updike WS, Wood SJ, et al. Attachment factors among enterotoxigenic *Escherichia coli* from patients with acute diarrhea from diverse geographic areas. Infect Immun. 1981;32:881.
268. Thomas LV, Cravioto A, Scotland SM, et al. New fimbrial antigenic type E8775 that may represent a colonization factor in enterotoxigenic *E. coli* in humans. Infect Immun. 1982;35:1119–24.
269. Honda T, Arita M, Miwatani T: Characterization of new hydrophobic pili of human enterotoxigenic *Escherichia coli*: A possible new colonization. Infect Immun. 1984;43:959–65.
270. Tacket CO, Maneval DR, Levine MM. Purification, morphology, and genetics of a new fimbrial putative colonization factor of enterotoxigenic *Escherichia coli* O159:H4. Infect Immun. 1987;55:1063–9.
271. Williams PH, Sedgwick MI, Evans N, et al. Adherence of an enteropathogenic strain of *Escherichia coli* is mediated by a colicinogenic conjugative plasmid. Infect Immun. 1978;22:393.
272. Karch H, Heesemann J, Laufs R, et al. A plasmid of enterohemorrhagic *Escherichia coli* O157:H7 is required for expression of a new fimbrial antigen and for adhesion to epithelial cells. Infect Immun. 1987;55:455–61.
273. Levine MM, Nalin DR, Hornick RB, et al. *Escherichia coli* strains that cause diarrhea but do not produce heat-labile or heat-stable enterotoxins and are noninvasive. Lancet. 1978;1:1119.
274. Ulshen MH, Rollo JL. Pathogenesis of *Escherichia coli* gastroenteritis in man: Another mechanism. N Engl J Med. 1980;302:99.
275. Polotsky YE, Dragunskaya EM, Seliverstova VG, et al. Pathogenic effect of enterotoxigenic *Escherichia coli* and *Escherichia coli* causing infantile diarrhoea. Acta Microbiol Acad Sci Hung. 1977;24:221.
276. Guerrant RL. Yet another pathogenic mechanism for *Escherichia coli* diarrhea? N Engl J Med. 1980;302:113.
277. Rothbaum R, McAdams AJ, Giannella R, et al. A clinicopathologic study of enterocyte-adherent *Escherichia coli*: A cause of protracted diarrhea in infants. Gastroenterology. 1982;83:441.
278. Cravioto A, Gross RJ, Scotland S, et al. An adhesive factor found in strains of *Escherichia coli* belonging to the traditional infantile enteropathogenic serotypes. Curr Microbiol. 1979;3:95–9.
279. Knutton S, Baldwin T, Williams PH, et al. Actin accumulation at sites of bacterial adhesion to tissue culture cells: Basis of a new diagnostic test for enteropathogenic and enterohemorrhagic *Escherichia coli*. Infect Immun. 1989;57:1290–8.
280. Baldini MM, Kaper JB, Levine MM, et al. Plasmid mediated adhesion of enteropathogentic *Escherichia coli*. J Pediatr Gastroenterol Nutr. 1983;2:534–8.
281. Rosenshine I, Donnenberg MS, Kaper JB, et al. Signal transduction between enteropathogenic *Escherichia coli* (EPEC) and epithelial cells: EPEC induces tyrosine phosphorylation of host cell proteins to initiate cytoskeletal rearrangement and bacterial uptake. EMBO J. 1992;11:3551–60.
282. Jerse AE, Martin WC, Galen JE, et al. Oligonucleotide probe for detection of the enteropathogenic *Escherichia coli* (EPEC) adherence factor of localized adherent EPEC. J Clin Microbiol. 1990;28:2842–4.
283. Baldwin TJ, Brooks SF, Knutton S, et al. Protein phosphorylation by protein kinase C in HEp-2 cells infected with enteropathogenic *Escherichia coli*. Infect Immun. 1990;58:761–5.
284. Baldwin TJ, Ward W, Aitken A, et al. Elevation of intracellular free calcium levels in HEp-2 cells infected with enteropathogenic *Escherichia coli*. Infect Immun. 1991;59:1599–604.
285. Francis CL, Jerse AE, Kaper JB, et al. Characterization of interactions of enteropathogenic *Escherichia coli* O127:H6 with mammalian cells *in vitro*. J Infect Dis. 1991;164:693–703.
286. Vuopio-Varkila J, Schoolnik GK. Localized adherence by enteropathogenic *Escherichia coli* is an inducible phenotype associated with the expression of new outer membrane proteins. J Exp Med. 1991;174:1167–77.
287. Girón JA, Ho ASY, Schoolnik GK. An inducible bundle-forming pilus of enteropathogenic *Escherichia coli*. Science. 1992;254:710.
288. Nataro JP, Kaper JB, Robins-Browne R, et al. Patterns of adherence of diarrheagenic *Escherichia coli* to HEp-2 cells. Pediatr Infect Dis J. 1987;6:829–31.
289. Mathewson JJ, Johnson PC, Dupont HL, et al. Pathogenicity of enteroadherent *Escherichia coli* in adult volunteers. J Infect Dis. 1986;154:524–7.
290. Scaletsky ICA, Silva MLM, Toledo MRF, et al. Correlation between adherence to HeLa cells and serogroups, serotypes, and bioserotypes of *Escherichia coli*. Infect Immun. 1985;49:528–32.
291. Mathewson JJ, Cravioto A. HEp-2 cell adherence as an assay for virulence among diarrrheagenic *Escherichia coli*. J Infect Dis. 1989;159:1057–60.
292. Baudry B, Savarino SJ, Vial P, et al. A sensitive and specific DNA probe to identify enteroaggregative *Escherichia coli*, a recently discovered diarrheal pathogen. J Infect Dis. 1990;161:1249–51.
293. Bilge SS, Clausen CR, Lau W, et al. Molecular characterization of a fimbrial adhesin, F1845, mediating diffuse adherence of diarrhea-associated *Escherichia coli* to HEp-2 cells. J Bacteriol. 1989;171:4281–9.
294. Vial P, Robins-Browne R, Lior H, et al. Characterization of enteroadherent-aggregative *Escherichia coli*, a putative agent of diarrheal disease. J Infect Dis. 1988;158:70–9.
295. Bhan MK, Raj P, Levine MM, et al. Enteroaggregative *Escherichia coli* associated with persistent diarrhea in a cohort of rural children in India. J Infect Dis. 1989;159:1061–4.
296. Bhan MK, Khoshoo V, Sommerfelt H, et al. Enteroaggregative *Escherichia coli* and *Salmonella* associated with nondysenteric persistent diarrhea. Pediatr Infect Dis J. 1989;8:499–502.
297. Wanke CA, Schorling JB, Barrett LJ, et al. Adherence traits of *Escherichia coli*, alone and in association with other stool pathogens: Potential role in pathogenesis of persistent diarrhea in an urban Brazilian slum. Pediatr J Infect Dis. 1991;10:746–51.
298. Girón JA, Fry J, Frankel G, et al. Diffuse-adhering *Escherichia coli* (DAEC) as a putative cause of diarrhea in Mayan children in Mexico. J Infect Dis. 1991;163:507–13.
299. Baqui AH, Sack RB, Black RE, et al. Enteropathogens associated with acute and persistent diarrhea in Bangladeshi children <5 years of age. J Infect Dis. 1992;166:792–6.
300. Baldwin TJ, Knutton S, Sellers L, et al. Enteroaggregative *Escherichia coli* strains secrete a heat-labile toxin antigenically related to *E. coli* hemolysin. Infect Immun. 1992;60:2092–5.
301. Benz I, Schmidt MA. Isolation and serologic characterization of AIDA-I, the adhesin mediating the diffuse adherence phenotype of the diarrhea-associated *Escherichia coli* strain 2787 (O126:H27). Infect Immun. 1992;60:13–8.
302. Wanke C, Guerrant RL. Small-bowel colonization alone is a cause of diarrhea. Infect Immun. 1987;55:1924–6.
303. Schlager TA, Wanke CA, Guerrant RL. Net fluid secretion and impaired villous function induced by colonization of the small intestine by nontoxigenic colonizing *Escherichia coli*. Infect Immun. 1990;58:1337–43.
304. Tacket CO, Losonsky G, Nataro JP, et al. Safety, immunogenicity and transmissibility of live oral cholera vaccine candidate CVD110, a delta CTXA delta ZOT delta ace derivative of El Tor Ogawa *Vibrio cholerae*. J Infect Dis. 1993;168:1536–40.
305. Trucksis M, Galen JE, Michalski J, et al. Accessory cholera enterotoxin (Ace) the third member of a *Vibrio cholerae* virulence cassette. Proc Natl Acad Sci. 1993. In press.
306. Madden JM, McCardell MBA, Shah DB. Cytotoxin production by members of genus *Vibrio*. Lancet. 1990;1:1217–8.
307. Kandel G, Donohue-Rolfe A, Donowitz M, et al. Pathogenesis of *Shigella* diarrhea. XVI. Selective targeting of shigatoxin to villous cells of rabbit jejunum explains the effect of toxin on intestinal electrolyte transport. J Clin Invest. 1989;84:1509–17.
308. Levine MM, Kaper JB, Black RE, et al. New knowledge on pathogenesis of bacterial enteric infections as applied to vaccine development. Microbiol Rev. 1983;47:510–50.

309. Sereny B. Experimental *Shigella* keratoconjunctivitis: A preliminary report. Acta Microbiol Acad Sci Hung. 1955;2:293.

310. Gemski P Jr, Sheahan DG, Washington O, et al. Virulence of *Shigella flexneri* hybrids expressing *Escherichia coli* somatic antigens. Infect Immun. 1972; 6:104.

311. Keusch GT. *Shigella* infections. Clin Gastroenterol. 1979;8:645.

312. Trabulsi LR, Fernandes MFR. *Escherichia coli* serogroup 0115 isolated from patients with enteritis: Biochemical characteristics and experimental pathogenicity. Rev Inst Med Trop Sao Paulo. 1969;11:358.

313. DuPont HL, Formal SB, Hornick RB, et al. Pathogenesis of *Escherichia coli* diarrhea. N Engl J Med. 1971;285:1.

314. Sansonetti PJ, Kopecko DJ, Formal SB. Involvement of an plasmid in the invasive ability of *Shigella flexneri*. Infect Immun. 1982;35:852.

315. Harris JR, Wachsmuth IK, Davis BR, et al. High-molecular-weight plasmid correlates with *Escherichia coli* invasiveness. Infect Immun. 1982;37:1295.

316. Sansonetti PJ, Hale TL, Oaks EV. Genetics of virulence in enteroinvasive *Escherichia coli*. Microbiology. 1985;74–7.

317. Isberg RR. Discrimination between intracellular uptake and surface adhesion of bacterial pathogens. Science. 1991;252:934–8.

318. Maurelli AT, Sansonetti P. Identification of a chromosomal gene controlling temperature-regulated expression of *Shigella* virulence. Proc Natl Acad Sci USA. 1988;85:2820–4.

319. Finlay BB, Heffron F, Falkow S. Epithelial cell surfaces induce *Salmonella* proteins required for bacterial adherence and invasion. Science. 1989;243: 940–3.

320. Ravdin JI, Guerrant RL. Role of adherence in cytopathogenic mechanisms of *Entamoeba histolytica*. J Clin Invest. 1981;68:1305–13.

321. Guerrant RL, Brush JE, Ravdin JI, et al. Interaction between *Entamoeba histolytica* and human polymorphonuclear leukocytes. J Infect Dis. 1981; 143:83–93.

322. Petri WA Jr, Chapman MD, Snodgrass T, et al. Subunit structure of the galactose and *N*-acetyl-D-galactosamine-inhibitable adherence lectin of *Entamoeba histolytica*. J Biol Chem. 1989;264:3007–12.

323. Guentzel MN, Berry LJ. Motility as a virulence factor for *Vibrio cholerae*. Infect Immun. 1975;2:890–7.

324. Freter R, Allweiss B, O'Brien PCM, et al. Role of chemotaxis in the association of motile bacteria with intestinal mucosa: In vitro studies. Infect Immun. 1981;34:241–9.

325. Schneider DR, Parker CD. Isolation and characterization of protease-deficient mutants of *Vibrio cholerae*. J Infect Dis. 1978;138:143–51.

326. Schneider DR, Parker CD. Purification and characterization of the mucinase of *Vibrio cholerae*. J Infect Dis. 1982;145:474–82.

327. Hornick RB, Greisman SE, Woodward TE, et al. Typhoid fever: Pathogenesis and immunologic control. N Engl J Med. 1970;283:686.

328. Robbins PW, Uchida T. Determinants of specificity in *Salmonella*: Changes in antigenic structure mediated by bacteriophage. Immunochemistry. 1962; 21:702.

329. Germanier R, Furer E. Isolation and characterization of Gal E Mutant Ty 21a of *Salmonella typhi*: A candidate strain for a live, oral typhoid vaccine. J Infect Dis. 1975;131:553.

330. Acharva IL, Lowe CU, Thapa R, et al. Prevention of typhoid fever in nepal with the Vi capsular polysaccharide of *Salmonella typhi*. N Engl J Med. 1987;317:1102–4.

331. Klugman KP, Koornhof H, Schneerson R, et al. Protective activity of Vi capsular polysaccharide vaccine against typhoid fever. Lancet. 1987;2: 1165–7.

332. Ruiz-Palacios GM, Torres J, Torres NI, et al. Cholera-like enterotoxin produced by *Campylobacter jejuni*. Characterization and clinical significance. Lancet. 1983;2:250.

333. Guerrant RL, Lahita RG, Winn WC Jr, et al. Campylobacteriosis in man: Pathogenic mechanisms and review of 91 bloodstream infections. Am J Med. 1878;65:584.

334. Perez-Perez GI, Hopkins JA, Blaser MJ. Antigenic heterogeneity of lipopolysaccharides from *Campylobacter jejuni* and *Campylobacter fetus*. Infect Immun. 1985;48:528–33.

335. Field M. Cholera toxin, adenylate cyclase, and the process of active secretion in the small intestine. The pathogenesis of diarrhea in cholera. In: Andreoli TE, Hoffman JF, Fauestil DD, eds. Physiology of Membrane Disorder. New York: Plenum Press; 1978.

336. Davidson GP, Barnes GL. Structural and functional abnormalities of the small intestine in infants and young children with rotavirus enteritis. Acta Paediatr Scand. 1979;68:181.

337. Hamilton JR. Viral enteritis. Pediatr Clin North Am. 1988;35:89–102.

338. Agus SG, Dolin R, Wyatt RG, et al. Acute infectious nonbacterial gastroenteritis: Intestinal histopathology, histologic and enzymatic alterations during illness produced by Norwalk agent in man. Ann Intern Med. 1973;79:18.

339. Levitan R, Ingelfinger FJ. Effect of *d*-aldosterone on salt and water absorption from the intact human colon. J Clin Invest. 1965;44:801.

340. Guerrant RL, Chen LC, Rohde JE. Effect of spironolactone on stool electrolyte losses during human cholera. Gut. 1972;13:197.

341. Guerrant RL, Carpenter CCJ. Diarrheagenic effect of volume expansion: Intestinal fluid secretion without mucosal adenyl cyclase stimulation. Johns Hopkins Med J. 1975;136:209.

342. Harris JC, DuPont HL, Hornick RB. Fecal leukocytes in diarrheal illness. Ann Intern Med. 1972;76:697.

343. Guerrant RL, Shields DS, Thorson SM, et al. Evaluation and diagnosis of acute infectious diarrhea. Am J Med. 1985;78:91–8.

344. Said SI, Faloona GR. Elevated plasma and tissue levels of vasoactive intestinal polypeptide in the watery-diarrhea syndrome due to pancreatic, bronchogenic and other tumors. N Engl J Med. 1975;293:155.

345. Guerrant RL, Brush JE, Ravdin JI, et al. The interaction between *Entamoeba histolytica* and human polymorphonuclear leukocytes. J Infect Dis. 1981; 143:83.

346. Ravdin JI, Guerrant RL. A review of the parasite cellular mechanisms involved in the pathogenesis of amebiasis. Rev Infect Dis. 1982;4:1185.

347. Guerrant RL. *Campylobacter* enteritis. In: Wyngaarden JB, Smith LH Jr, eds. Cecil Textbook of Medicine. Philadelphia: Saunders; 1988:1648–51.

348. Korzeniowski OM, Basada FA, Rouse JD, et al. Value of examination for fecal leukocytes in the early diagnosis of shigellosis. Am J Trop Med Hyg. 1979;28:1031–5.

349. Guerrant RL, Araujo V, Soares E, et al. Measurement of fecal lactoferrin as a marker of fecal leukocytes. J Clin Microbiol. 1992;30:1238–42.

350. Rahaman MM, Huq I, Dey CR: Superiority of MacConkey's agar over *Salmonella–Shigella* agar for isolation of *Shigella dysenteria* type 1. J Infect Dis. 1975;131:700.

351. Blaser MJ, Reller LB. Campylobacter enteritis. N Engl J Med. 1981;305: 1444.

352. Kaplan RL, Barrett JE: Monograph: *Campylobacter*. Kansas City, MO: Marion Scientific; 1981.

353. Rahaman MM, Khan MM, Azi KMS, et al. An outbreak of dysentery caused by *Shigella dysenteriae* type I on a coral island in the Bay of Bengal. J Infect Dis. 1975;132:15.

354. Feeley JC, Balows A. *Vibrio*. In: Lennette EH, Spaulding EH, Truant JP, eds. Manual of Clinical Microbiology. Washington, DC: American Society for Microbiology; 1974:238.

355. Ryan RW, Kwasnik I, Tilton RC. Rapid detection of *Clostridium difficile* in human feces. J Clin Microbiol. 1980;12:776.

356. Morris GK, Feeley JC, Martin WT, et al. Isolation and identification of *Yersinia enterocolitica*. Public Health Lab. 1977;35:217.

357. Merson MH, Black RE, Gross RJ, et al. Use of antisera for identification of enterotoxigenic *E. coli*. Lancet. 1980;2:222.

358. Moseley SL, Escheverria P, Seriwatana J, et al. Identification of enterotoxigenic *E. coli* by colony hybridization using three enterotoxin fene probes. J Infect Dis. 1982;145:863.

359. Dean AG, Ching Y-C, Williams RG, et al. Test for *Escherichia coli* using infant mice: Application in a study of diarrhea in children in Honolulu. J Infect Dis. 1972;125:407.

360. Giannella RA. Suckling mouse model for detection of heat-stable *Escherichia coli* enterotoxin: Characteristic of the model. Infect Immun. 1976;14:95.

361. March SB, Ratnam S. Latex agglutination test for detection of *Escherichia coli* serotype O157:H7. J Clin Microbiol. 1989;27:1675–7.

362. Chapman PA, Siddons CA, Zadik PM, et al. An improved selective medium for the isolation of *Escherichia coli* O157. J Med Microbiol. 1991;35:107–10.

363. Bitzan M, Karch H. Indirect hemagglutination assay for diagnosis of *Escherichia coli* O157 infection in patients with hemolytic-uremic syndrome. J Clin Microbiol. 1992;30:1174–8.

364. Brown HW, Neva FA. Basic Clinical Parasitology. Norwalk, CT: Appleton-Century-Crofts; 1983.

365. Lima JP, Delgado PG. Diagnosis of stronygloidiasis: Importance of Baermann's method. Am J Dig Dis. 1961;6:899.

366. Current WL, Reese NC, Ernst JV, et al. Human cryptosporidiosis in immunocompetent and immunodeficient persons: Studies of an outbreak and experimental transmission. N Engl J Med. 1983;21:1252.

367. Blake PA, Rosenberg ML, Florencia J, et al. Cholera in Portugal, 1974. Am J Epidemiol. 1977;105:344.

368. Lee JA, Kean BH. International Conference on the Diarrhea of Travelers. New Directions in Research: A summary. J Infect Dis. 1978;137:360.

369. Costerton JW, Geesey GG, Cheng K-J. How bacteria stick. Sci Am. 1977; 1:86.

370. Ericsson CD, Evans DG, DuPont HL, et al. Bismuth subsalicylate inhibits activity of crude toxins of *Escherichia coli* and *Vibrio cholerae*. J Infect Dis. 1977;136:693.

371. Palmer DL, Koster FT, Islam AFRM, et al. A comparison of sucrose and glucose in oral electrolyte treatment of cholera and other severe diarrheas. N Engl J Med. 1977;297:1107.

372. Oral glucose/electrolyte therapy for acute diarrhea (Editorial). Lancet. 1975; 1:79.

373. Molla AM, Molla A, Nath SK, et al. Food-based oral rehydration salt solutions for acute childhood diarrhoea. Lancet. 1989;2:429–31.

374. Robbins-Browne RM. Traditional enteropathogenic *Escherichia coli* of infantile diarrhea. Rev Infect Dis. 1987;9:28–53.

375. Echeverria P, Orskov F, Orskov I, et al. Attaching and effacing enteropathogenic *Escherichia coli* as a caujse of infantile diarrhea in Bangkok. J Infect Dis. 1991;164:550–4.

376. Levine MM, Edelman R. Enteropathogenic *Escherichia coli* of classic serotypes associated with infant diarrhea: Epidemiol Rev. 1984;6:31–51.

377. Whittam TS, Wolfe ML, Wachsmuth IK, et al. Clonal relationships among *Escherichia coli* strains that cause hemorrhagic colitis and infantile diarrhea. Infect Immun. 1993;61:1619–29.

378. Scotland SM, Willshaw GA, Cheasty T, et al. Strains of *Escherichia coli* O157:H8 from human diarrhoea belong to attaching and effacing class of *E. coli*. J Clin Pathol. 1992;45:1075–8.

379. Molla AM, Molla A, Nath SK, et al. Food-based oral rehydration salt solution for acute childhood diarrhoea. Lancet. 1989;2:429–31.

TABLE 2. Underlying Conditions Predisposing to Esophageal Candidiasis

Systemic
Acute HIV-1
Acquired immunodeficiency syndrome due to HIV-1
Diabetes mellitus
Broad-spectrum antibacterial therapy
Certain antineoplastic or immunosuppressive drugs, including supraphysiologic doses of adrenal corticosteroids
Chronic mucocutaneous candidiasis
Local
Peptic (reflux) esophagitis, with or without hiatal hernia; Barrett's esophagus; esophageal stenosis; webs or rings
Disordered esophageal motility due to achalasia, scleroderma
Herpes simplex

76. ESOPHAGITIS

MICHAEL A. POLIS

For the purposes of this chapter, *esophagitis* refers to infections of the esophageal mucosa that may or may not extend into the submucosa. Mediastinal infections that begin by perforation of the esophageal mucosa as a result of endoscopy, transesophageal echocardiography, ingestion of fish bones, or other trauma are not included. Nor will infections extending into the esophagus from the mediastinal lymph nodes, such as histoplasmosis, be discussed.

SYMPTOMS

Symptoms most suggestive of esophagitis are odynophagia, a substernal, anterior cervical, or epigastric burning pain on swallowing, or dysphagia, a dull sense of obstruction low in the throat or substernally on swallowing. Odynophagia may be worse on ingesting fruit juice or acid liquids. Both odynophagia and dysphagia tend to be worse on ingesting large, firm objects, such as meat, rather than liquids. Esophageal pain may be present intermittently, unrelated to swallowing, or exacerbated by eructation. Concomitant disease of the oropharynx or stomach may increase pharyngeal or epigastric symptoms. Concomitant gastritis may cause nausea. Endoscopy done for gastrointestinal symptoms has found that esophagitis may be present and even extensive in the absence of symptoms.

ETIOLOGY

Both noninfectious and infectious causes of esophagitis are listed in Table 1. Multiple etiologies are common. For example, the esophagus of a single patient receiving chemotherapy for acute leukemia may have mucositis from antineoplastic therapy, herpes simplex ulcerations, and *Candida* invading the submucosa of the herpetic ulcerations. Presence of multiple etiologies must be kept in mind when therapeutic response is not optimal.

Candida

Patients with esophageal candidiasis usually have local or systemic underlying diseases that must be recognized and, if possible, treated in order to obtain a therapeutic response to antifungal therapy (Table 2). Mucositis from antineoplastic drugs, such as methotrexate or 5-fluorouracil, can mimic or predispose to candidiasis. Reflux esophagitis commonly coexists with esophageal candidiasis and complicates therapy in that absorption of ketoconazole and itraconazole is impaired by drugs that block gastric acid production. This includes agents that block H_2 receptors (e.g., ranitidine), as well as agents that block the gastric proton pump (e.g., omeprazole) (see Ch. 31). HIV-1 infections predispose to esophageal disease late in the course, usually after the CD4 count has begun to fall, for which reason esophageal candidiasis has been part of the definition of acquired immunodeficiency syndrome (AIDS). However, esophageal candidiasis may also occur in the acute human immunodeficiency virus type 1 (HIV-1) syndrome.[9] Oropharyngeal candiasis usually accompanies esophageal candidiasis in AIDS.[10] In patients with hematologic malignancies, oropharyngeal candidiasis is not a reliable herald for esophageal candidiasis. In patients with AIDS or receiving substantial immunosuppressive drugs, concomitant esophagitis due to *Candida* plus either herpes simplex virus or cytomegalovirus is quite common.[11] Diagnostic and management strategies must generally include these diseases along with candidiasis.

Chronic mucocutaneous candidiasis is a syndrome that often begins in childhood and may be accompanied by hypoparathyroidism, hypothyroidism, or Addison's disease (see Ch. 237). Esophageal candidiasis is frequently present and, though asymptomatic, over the years may lead to severe esophageal stenosis.

Endoscopy has permitted classification of esophageal candidiasis into four stages. Each stage tends to be accompanied by manifestations of the less severe stages: I, Diffuse mucosal hyperemia with or without edema; II, discrete white mucosal patches on the mucosa, consisting of desquamated squamous cells, *Candida*, leukocytes, and necrotic debris (Fig. 1; brushing one of these patches may lift up an edge of the lesion, revealing a rough, red base); III, mucosal ulceration, typically with a gray necrotic base (the ulceration may be due to *Candida*, or *Candida* may secondarily invade ulcerations due to herpes simplex virus, cytomegalovirus, or other causes); and IV, bleeding or esophageal perforation.[12] Diagnosis may be suspected when typical white plaques are present but is confirmed by the demonstration of *Candida* pseudohyphae and yeasts in biopsies or smears of brushings (Table 3). With *Candida glabrata*, only yeasts are seen, with no pseudohyphae. Severity of disease as seen on endoscopy correlates poorly with severity of symptoms.[13] Even extensive disease may be asymptomatic.

Esophagram is normal in many patients with esophageal candidiasis and is never diagnostic. Spasm may be appreciated on fluoroscopy and, particularly with air contrast, mucosal irregularities may be seen (Fig. 2).[14] On either esophagram or endoscopy, lesions are most commonly located in the distal third of the esophagus.

TABLE 1. Etiology of Esophagitis

More Common Causes	Less Common Causes
Infectious	
Candidiasis	Cryptococcosis[1]
Herpes simplex	Histoplasmosis[2]
Cytomegalovirus	Tuberculosis[3]
HIV infection, acute[5] or late	Cryptosporidiosis[4]
stage	Pneumocystosis[6]
Noninfectious	
Peptic esophagitis	Local mucositis from tablets or capsules[7]
Mucositis from antineoplastic therapy, zalcitabine, x-irradiation	(e.g., doxycycline, zidovudine[8])
	Ingestion of corrosive substances such as lye
Aphthous ulcers (AIDS patients)	Sclerotherapy for esophageal varices

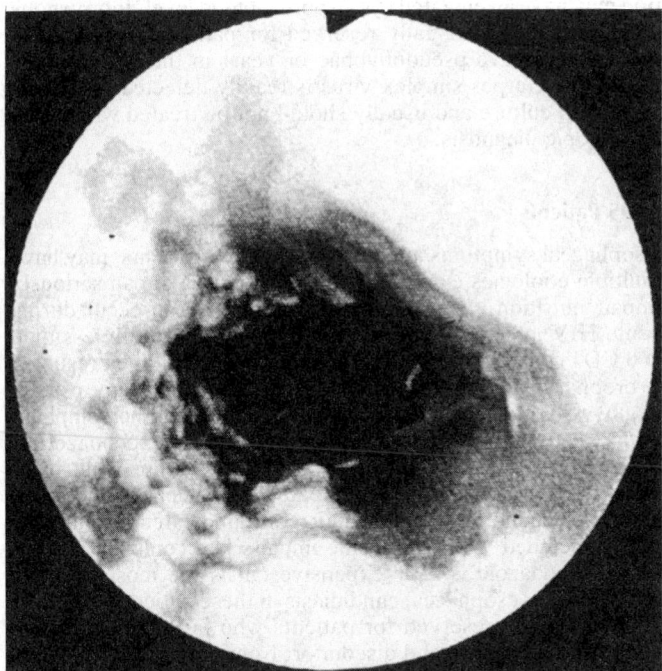

FIG. 1. Endoscopic appearance showing the characteristic raised white plaques of *Candida* opposite an esophageal ulcer due to cytomegalovirus in a patient with acquired immunodeficiency infection and esophagitis due to both *Candida* and cytomegalovirus. (Courtesy of Dr. Douglas T. Dieterich, New York, NY.)

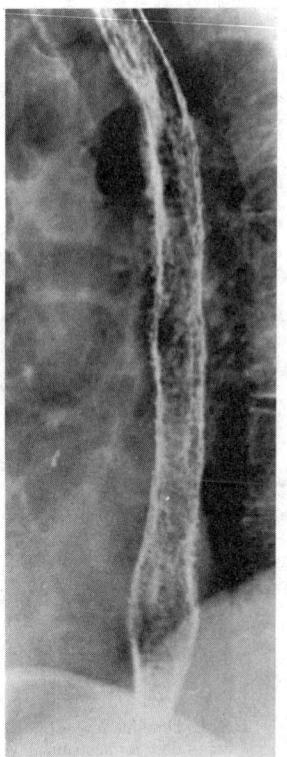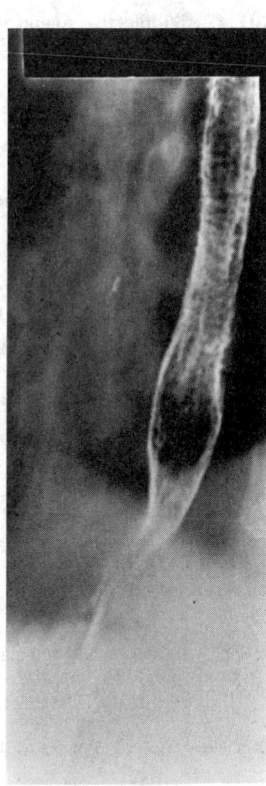

FIG. 2. **(A & B)** Barium contrast esophagrams of *Candida* esophagitis showing a markedly irregular esophagus due to multiple plaques in a patient with AIDS and severe odynophagia.

TABLE 3. Endoscopy for Esophagitis

Specimen	Procedure
Brushings	Send either brush (in nonbacteristatic saline) or smears of brushing on clean glass slides for the following: wet mount or calcifluor white stain or Gram stain for *Candida*; consider direct fluorescent stain or immunochemical stains for HSV and CMV
Biopsy tissue	Send several biopsies specimens of lesions and edges of ulcers in sterile, nonbacteriostatic saline for fungal, HSV, and CMV (shell vial) culture. Histopathology is useful for identifying Kaposi sarcoma, lymphoma, other malignancies, *Preumocystis carinii*, histoplasmosis, and cryptococcosis

Herpes Simplex Virus

Herpes simplex esophagitis occurs in patients who have other serious illnesses. In one representative series of 23 patients, 12 (52 percent) had hematologic malignancies, 8 (35 percent) were receiving immunosuppressive therapy for nonmalignant conditions, 2 (9 percent) had AIDS, and only 1 was previously normal.[15] Other conditions predisposing to herpetic esophagitis include severe burns, nonhematologic malignancies, esophageal x-irradiation, and surgery.[16] Esophageal herpes simplex is less often asymptomatic than candidiasis and is also less frequently accompanied by lesions of the oropharynx. Discrete ulcerations of the mucosa are seen on endoscopy, particularly in the distal third, and, when severe, herpes simplex virus (HSV) lesions may ooze blood. However, endoscopic appearance is variable. In one series, HSV was not suspected by the appearance in 30 percent of cases, heightening the interest in routine cultures for HSV.[15] Diagnosis is best made by culture of brushing or biopsies (Table 3). Direct fluorescent antibody staining for HSV-1 is less sensitive and less specific but more rapid than culture. On biopsy, epithelial cells show ballooning degeneration. In the submucosa, giant cells and cells with intranuclear inclusions typical of herpesviruses may be seen (Cowdry type A inclusion), but cells with inclusions are usually sparse. Esophagram may show mucosal irregularities that are suggestive of herpes simplex.

Cytomegalovirus

Esophageal disease due to cytomegalovirus (CMV) has been difficult to diagnose by culture because CMV from saliva or blood may contaminate the specimen. Cytomegalovirus viremia is common in the late stages of AIDS. In addition, the facilities to culture for CMV are not routinely available in many medical centers, and the virus may be difficult to recover in culture. Typical large cells with large, dense intranuclear inclusions and small, dense intracytoplasmic inclusions are diagnostic but occur infrequently in the submucosa. They are easier to find in autopsy specimens because more tissue is available for study. Response to empiric therapy with ganciclovir or foscarnet is not easy to interpret because success has not been uniform in well-documented CMV cases and the drugs are also active against HSV. Most cases of CMV esophagitis have been recognized in patients with AIDS or severe immunosuppression.[17] Symptoms of CMV esophagitis cannot be distinguished from those due to herpes simplex or *Candida*.[18,19] Extensive large, shallow ulcers of the distal esophagus appear to be the hallmark of CMV esophagitis.[11,18] Diagnosis is certain if the typical cells are seen in biopsy material. Immunohistochemical and direct fluorescent stains for CMV are also available. Culture of CMV supports but does not establish the diagnosis.

APPROACH TO THE PATIENT WITH ESOPHAGEAL SYMPTOMS

Chemotherapy Patients

Patients with severe mucositis due to cancer chemotherapy often have severe throat pain even on swallowing saliva. When pain is also substernal, concern about superimposed esophageal herpes simplex or candidiasis is heightened. An esophageal portal for disseminated candidiasis is a serious concern for the patient with less than 100 neutrophils per cubic millimeter, al-

TABLE 4. Anti-Infective Agents for Esophagitis

Drug	Adult Dose	Comments
Antifungal		
Nystatin suspension (100,000 U/ml)	5 ml PO qid	Inexpensive, efficacy poor, bitter taste
Clotrimazole (10 mg troche)	10 mg 5×/day	Taste variably accepted; compliance often poor
Ketoconazole (200 mg tablet)	400 mg PO qd	Absorption requires gastric acid; rifampin drops ketoconazole levels and other drug interactions exist; rare hepatotoxicity; occasional nausea or rash
Itraconazole (100 mg capsule)	200 mg PO qd	Same as ketoconazole but more expensive, less studied. Less nausea and hepatotoxicity than with ketoconazole
Fluconazole (50, 100, 200 mg tablets)	100–200 mg PO or IV qd	Absorbed well, expensive, (IV very expensive), rash. Drug interactions exist
Amphotericin B, IV	See text	Toxic
Antiviral		
Acyclovir (200 mg capsules) or IV	200–400 mg PO 5×/day 5 mg/kg q8h (HSV dose)	Occasional nausea, headache Adjust dose for azotemia
Ganciclovir, IV	5 mg/kg q12h	Toxic to bone marrow, CNS; adjust dose for azotemia
Foscarnet, IV	60 mg/kg/q8h (CMV dose) 40 mg/kg q8h (HSV dose)	Toxic to kidneys; adjust dose for azotemia

though HSV rarely disseminates in those patients. Prophylactic or empiric oral therapy for *Candida* or HSV is taken irregularly or not at all because of pain on swallowing. The decision to perform endoscopy is difficult because of the patient's oropharyngeal pain and an esophageal mucosa that is friable and bleeds readily. Concern about the necessity of anesthesia and the complications of bleeding, esophageal perforation, or bacteremia from esophagoscopy usually leads to empiric parenteral therapy until such time as endoscopy is less risky. If the patient is febrile and markedly neutropenic, amphotericin B is usually given in doses that would be adequate for disseminated as well as esophageal candidiasis (i.e., 0.5–1 mg/kg daily; see Ch. 289). Patients who are afebrile and not suspected of having disseminated candidiasis might receive intravenous fluconazole (Table 4) or lower doses of amphotericin B, such as 0.3–0.5 mg/kg daily. Patients with severe symptoms or who do not respond to antifungal therapy may be given intravenous acyclovir. Response of esophageal symptoms to antifungal or antiviral therapy generally awaits resolution of the mucositis.

Transplant Recipients

Solid organ transplant recipients are susceptible to esophagitis due to *Candida*, HSV, and CMV. Empiric therapy of esophageal symptoms may be begun with clotrimazole, which is not absorbed systemically, because of the absence of both systemic toxicity and drug interactions. In contrast, patients receiving cyclosporine may develop elevated, nephrotoxic cyclosporine blood concentrations when given ketoconazole, itraconazole, or fluconazole, although any one of these agents is effective treatment for *Candida* esophagitis in this population. Although patients with normal renal function will not usually experience a drug interaction between cyclosporine and 200 mg daily doses of fluconazole, patients who take higher fluconazole doses or who have high fluconazole levels due to decreased renal func-

tion may have an elevated cyclosporine blood level. Intravenous amphotericin B is usually reserved for patients who fail oral therapy and have pseudohyphae or yeast in their endoscopic brushings. Herpes simplex virus is readily detected on endoscopy with culture and usually should not be treated without an endoscopic diagnosis.

AIDS Patients

Esophageal symptoms are frequent in AIDS patients, may have multiple etiologies even in the same patient, and can seriously impair nutrition.[11,19] Esophageal candidiasis can occur during acute HIV infection[9] and is common in patients with less than 200 CD4 cells/mm[3]. Esophageal extension should be presumed if oropharyngeal candidiasis is seen. Empiric therapy usually begins with clotrimazole if the patient is likely to be compliant with at least three of the five doses per day. Ketoconazole is useful if gastric acid is not suppressed, interactions with rifampin or other drugs are not anticipated, and hepatic function is stable. Concomitant didanosine is contraindicated because the buffer included with didanosine impairs ketoconazole absorption. Fluconazole is very expensive but is the most effective oral agent for esophageal candidiasis in these patients.[21] Endoscopy is usually reserved for patients who fail fluconazole because of the expense and discomfort from the procedure. Blind esophageal brushing through a tube has been advocated but not widely used.[22] Empiric therapy for HSV is usually not indicated because HSV is not commonly the only pathogen. In one series of 110 patients with AIDS and esophagitis, only 6 had HSV esophagitis and another 4 had HSV plus *Candida*, CMV, or both.[11] Empiric acyclovir could be considered if endoscopy is not available and the patient fails fluconazole. Ganciclovir should be used for patients who have a positive biopsy for CMV.[23] Patients who have documented HSV but fail acyclovir due to drug resistance will usually not respond to ganciclovir and should be given foscarnet 40 mg/kg IV q8h. Similarly, patients with CMV who fail ganciclovir may respond to foscarnet 60 mg/kg q8h. Low doses of intravenous amphotericin B, about 0.3 mg/kg daily, or double that dose on alternate days, are useful in *Candida* esophagitis that has become resistant to fluconazole.

Patients in the late stages of HIV-1 infection may have aphthous ulcerations of the oropharynx or esophagus. Whether these ulcerations are due to HIV-1 itself is unclear, but some patients have improved within 48 hours of starting prednisone 40 mg per day.[24] Anecdotal responses to thalidomide have also been reported.[25] Such therapy could be considered for patients with endoscopically proven esophageal ulcers and no evidence of an etiology, including negative cultures for *Candida*, HSV, and CMV.

With fungal, viral, or aphthous esophagitis, relapse of esophageal symptoms after an initial response is usual. Long-term prophylaxis for *Candida* esophagitis with once weekly fluconazole is being used[26] but is not recommended because drug resistance to azoles, including clotrimazole, ketoconazole, itraconazole, and fluconazole, has arisen. Susceptibility testing is not helpful in identifying such patients, but patients with well-documented *Candida* esophagitis, no other esophageal disease, and no response to fluconazole 400 mg per day can be assumed to have azole-resistant *Candida*. This problem is no longer rare.

REFERENCES

1. Jacobs DH, et al. Esophageal cryptococcosis in a patient with the hyperimmunoglobulin E-recurrent infection (Job's) syndrome. Gastroenterology. 1984; 87:201–3.
2. Forsmark CE, Wilcox CM, Darragh TM, et al. Disseminated histoplasmosis in AIDS: An unusual case of esophageal involvement and gastrointestinal bleeding. Gastrointest Endosc. 1990;36:604–5.
3. Rosario MT, Raso CL, Comer GM. Esophageal tuberculosis. Dig Dis Sci. 1989;34:1281–4.
4. Kazlow PG, Shah K, Benkov KJ, et al. Esophageal cryptosporidiosis in a

child with acquired immune deficiency syndrome. Gastroenterology. 1986;91:1301–3.

5. Rabeneck L, Popovic M, Gartner S, et al. Acute HIV infection presenting with painful swallowing and esophageal ulcers. JAMA. 1990;263:2318–22.
6. Grimes MM, LaPook JD, Bar MH, et al. Disseminated *Pneumocystis carinii* infection in a patient with acquired immunodeficiency syndrome. Hum Pathol. 1987;18:307.
7. Kikendall JW, Friedman AC, Oyewole MA, et al. Pill-induced oesophageal injury. Case reports and review of the medical literature. Dig Dis Sci. 1983;28:174–82.
8. Edwards P, Turner J, Gold J, et al. Esophageal ulceration induced by zidovudine. Ann Intern Med. 1990;112:65–6.
9. Peña JM, Martínez-López MA, Arnalich F, et al. Esophageal candidiasis associated with acute infection due to human immunodeficiency virus: Case report and review. Rev Infect Dis. 1991;13:872–5.
10. Tavitian A, Raufman JP, Rosenthal LE. Oral candidiasis as a marker for esophageal candidiasis in the acquired immunodeficiency syndrome. Ann Intern Med. 1986;104:54–5.
11. Bonacini M, Young T, Laine L. The causes of esophageal symptoms in human immunodeficiency virus infection. A prospective study of 110 patients. Arch Intern Med. 1991;151:1567–72.
12. Sehhat S, Hazeghi K, Bajoghli M, et al. Oesophageal moniliasis causing fistula formation and lung abscess. Thorax. 1976;31:361–4.
13. Jones JM. Necrotizing *Candida* esophagitis. Failure of symptoms and roentgenographic findings to reflect severity. JAMA. 1980;244:2190–1.
14. Levine MS, Macones AJ, Laufer I. *Candida* esophagitis: Accuracy of radiographic diagnosis. Radiology. 1985;154:581–7.
15. McBane RD, Gross JB. Herpes esophagitis: Clinical syndrome, endoscopic appearance and diagnosis in 23 patients. Gastrointest Endosc. 1991;37:600–3.
16. Nash G, Ross JS. Herpetic esophagitis. A common cause of esophageal ulceration. Hum Pathol. 1974;5:339–345.
17. Laine L, Bonacini M, Sattler F, et al. Cytomegalovirus and *Candida* esophagitis in patients with AIDS. J AIDS. 1992;5:605–9.
18. Wilcox CM, Diehl DL, Cello JP, et al. Cytomegalovirus esophagitis in patients with AIDS. A clinical, endoscopic, and pathologic correlation. Ann Intern Med. 1990;113:589–93.
19. Wilcox CM. Esophageal disease in the acquired immunodeficiency syndrome: Etiology, diagnosis, and management. Am J Med. 1992;92:412–21.
20. Lalor E, Rabeneck L. Esophageal candidiasis in AIDS. Digest Dis Sci. 1991;36:279–281.
21. Laine L, Dretler RH, Conteas CN, et al. Fluconazole compared with ketoconazole for the treatment of *Candida* esophagitis in AIDS. A randomized trail. Ann Intern Med. 1992;117:655–60.
22. Bonacini M, Laine L, Gal AA, et al. Prospective evaluation of blind brushing of the esophagus for *Candida* esophagitis in patients with human immunodeficiency virus infection. Am J Gastroenterol. 1990;85:385–9.
23. Gallant JE, Moore RD, Richman DD, et al. Incidence and natural history of cytomegalovirus disease in patients with advanced human immunodeficiency virus disease treated with zidovudine. J Infect Dis. 1992;166:1223–7.
24. Bach MC, Howell DA, Valenti AJ, et al. Aphthous ulceration of the gastrointestinal tract in patients with the acquired immunodeficiency syndrome (AIDS). Ann Intern Med. 1990;112:465–7.
25. Youle M, Clarbour J, Farthing C, et al. Treatment of resistant aphthous ulceration with thalidomide in patients positive for HIV antibody. Br Med J. 1989;298:432.
26. Leen CLS, Dunbar EM, Ellis ME, et al. Once-weekly fluconazole to prevent recurrence of oropharyngeal cnadidiasis in patients with AIDS and AIDS-related complex: a double-blind placebo-controlled study. J Infect. 1990;21:55–60.

77. NAUSEA, VOMITING, AND NONINFLAMMATORY DIARRHEA

RICHARD L. GUERRANT
DAVID A. BOBAK

The vast majority of acute gastrointestinal illnesses do not involve a recognizable inflammatory process.[1–3] Although there is considerable inflammatory enteritis during summer months in warm areas with poor sanitation, most cases of diarrhea in these areas are noninflammatory, which suggests an enterotoxic bacterial, viral, or noninvasive parasitic process.[4–9]

EPIDEMIC DIARRHEA IN NEWBORN NURSERIES

Epidemic infantile diarrhea has long been recognized as a potentially serious problem that occurs in newborn nurseries. Its mortality has been as high as 24–50 percent.[10,11] Epidemic diarrhea among hospitalized newborns has been associated with certain "enteropathogenic" serotypes of *Escherichia coli* (EPEC). Enteropathogenic *E. coli* serotypes have been associated with diarrhea in hospitalized infants under 4 months of age.

The unusual susceptibility of newborns may be explained by their unique host status; they have not yet acquired a normal intestinal flora or specific immunity. Infants in special care nurseries have this situation compounded by severe underlying diseases such as prematurity or congenital cardiac or pulmonary disease. The consequences of diarrhea in the newborn are unusually severe because of poorly developed homeostatic mechanisms and limited water and electrolyte reserves. Nosocomial transmission may occur since the newborn nurseries may be crowded with susceptible infants.[12] A nursery outbreak can go unrecognized since infants may develop diarrhea after being discharged.

The onset is insidious, with the development of listlessness, irritability, and poor feeding over a period of 3–6 days.[11,13,14] Vomiting and fever are infrequent, and the stools tend to be watery, yellow-green, and usually without mucus, pus, or blood. Early signs such as failure to gain weight or a slight weight loss and abdominal distension may be subtle. The disease may progress to more severe signs of dehydration and shock with depressed sensorium, drowsiness, coma, sunken eyes, circumoral cyanosis, and grayish discoloration of the skin. Shock without hyperpnea often occurs in this setting despite the development of severe acidosis. Poorly nourished infants with decreased protein and potassium reserves may have severe hypokalemia, hyponatremic dehydration, and paradoxical edema. The illness usually lasts 5–15 days but may persist or relapse over the course of several weeks. Complications may include intercurrent otitis media, pneumonia, bacteremia, peritonitis, and renal vein or cerebral sinus thrombosis. Dissemination of EPEC to the lungs has been demonstrated by immunofluorescent staining of tissue at autopsy.[15] While the mortality may be quite high, as noted above, South[16] and Kaslow et al.[17] have reported a milder illness with lower morbidity and mortality in recent years. However, in many areas such as South Africa and southern Brazil, EPEC remain among the most common causes of diarrhea in infants and young children, especially during the summer months.[18–20] Endemic childhood diarrheal illness in areas like England and Canada also remain associated with EPEC in 6–18 percent of cases.[18,19]

Several potentially life-threatening processes may mimic this infantile diarrhea syndrome. So-called parenteral diarrhea is the well-recognized, but poorly understood tendency for systemic or localized infections elsewhere (such as otitis or meningitis) to be manifested clinically with diarrhea. Likewise, a strangulated hernia, intussusception, or torsion of an ovary or testis may be manifested by abdominal pain or diarrhea.

Appropriate antibiotic therapy must be tailored to the specific sensitivity pattern of the organism isolated.[16] If systemic infection is suspected, parenteral therapy should be started and should be tailored to the antibiotic sensitivity pattern of the organism isolated. Appropriate preventive measures include cohorting of nursery admissions, avoidance of overcrowding in nurseries, utilization of individual units and equipment, careful formula preparation, isolation of infants with diarrhea, and careful hand washing by hospital personnel.

The association of a certain strain of *E. coli* with infantile diarrhea was first demonstrated by slide agglutination by Bray and Beavan[21] in 1945 and reported in further detail in 1948. They identified serologically homogeneous *E. coli* in most infants with summer diarrhea (87.5 vs. 4 percent of the controls), half of which was hospital acquired. Varela et al.[22] and Olarte and Varela[23] subsequently found this strain (called *E. coli*-"gomez" by Varela) in cases of infantile diarrhea in Mexico. A second serotype, initially designated as *beta* to distinguish it from the earlier serotype called *alpha*, was described by Giles and Sangster[24] as the cause of an outbreak of infantile gastroenteritis in Aberdeen.

Escherichia coli strains are classified into a large number of serotypes on the basis of three major types of antigens: the "O" or heat-stable somatic antigen (lipopolysaccharide endotoxin), which forms the basis for 169 serogroups; an outer, heat-labile "capsular" antigen called "K" that may inhibit O agglutination; and, for motile organisms, the "H" or flagellar antigen, which is also heat labile. Three different kinds of "K" antigens have been identified: L, A, and B, the latter being of importance in the identification of EPEC serotypes. The original α- and β-serotypes of *E. coli* were subsequently associated with several outbreaks of infantile epidemic gastroenteritis and were classified as serotypes of O111:B4 and O55:B5, respectively, by Kaufmann and Dupont.[25] As shown in Table 1, exclusive of certain invasive serotypes (see Table 2 in Ch. 79), there are some 14 classically recognized EPEC *E. coli* serotypes, beginning with O111:K58 (α), O55:K59 (β), O127:K63, O128:K67, O26:B6, O86:K61, O119:K69, O125:K70, O126:K71, O20:B7, and O44:K74. Additional serotypes recently recognized as causes of epidemic infantile diarrhea include O114,[10,29,30] O142,[12,27] and O158.[28] *E. coli* O157:H7 associated with hemorrhagic diarrhea and hemolytic uremic syndrome (HUS) in several outbreaks as well as sporadic cases, provides yet another mechanism of pathogenesis and serotype.[31-33] It now appears likely that EPEC strains are more related to each other than to other O-antigen–bearing *E. coli*.[34] Furthermore, some investigators have described disease-producing EPEC strains which differ from the previously described EPEC serotypes.[34]

The evidence that EPEC serotypes are responsible for infantile diarrhea has been outlined.[11,18] There is a strong association for these organisms with cases of epidemic infantile diarrhea, and these organisms are infrequently encountered in healthy infants, children, or adults not exposed to cases of diarrhea. The mechanism by which most EPEC organisms cause disease is a topic of intense investigation and involves a complex set of attachment and effacement traits, as detailed in Chapter 79. Although most are not invasive and do not produce conventionally recognized heat-labile or heat-stable enterotoxins, these organisms are capable of causing diarrheal disease in human volunteers, from whom the organism can be reisolated and in whom

TABLE 1. Enteropathogenic and Enterohemorrhagic *E. coli* Serotypes Classically Recognized in Infantile Diarrhea Outbreaks[a]

Serotype	Difco Serogroup and References
Class I (EAF-positive) EPEC	
O55:K59(B5):H⁻/6/7	A (24–26)
O111ab:K58(B4):H⁻/5/12	A (21–23, 25, 26)
O127a:K63(B8):H6	A (26)
O119:K69(B14)	B (26)
O125ac:K70(B15):H21	B (26)
O126:K71(B10):H⁻/H2	B (26)
O128ab:K67(B12)	B (26)
O142	(12, 26, 27)
O158	(26, 28)
Class II (EAF-negative) EPEC	
O44:K74	C (26)
O114	(10, 26, 29, 30)
O86a:K61(B7)	B (26)
Enterohemorrhagic *E. coli* (EHEC)	
O157:H7	(31–33)
O26:B6	A (26)

Abbreviation: EAF: enteroadherence factor probe for focal HEp-2 cell adherence plasmid pMAR2.
[a] See also Table 3, Chapter 75.

TABLE 2. Serotypes of *E. coli* That Appear with Increased Frequency among Enterotoxigenic Isolates

LT *E. coli*
O6:K15:H16
O8:K40:H9, O8:K25:H9
LT + ST *E. coli*
O11:H27
O15:H22
O20:H⁻, O20:H11
O25:K7:H42, O25:K98:H⁻
O27:H7
O63:H12
O80, O85, O139
ST *E. coli*
O78:H11, O78:H12
O115:H40
O128:H7
O148:H28
O149:H10
O153
O159:H20
O166, O167

an antibody response can be documented.[13,35] As noted in Table 3 in Chapter 75, these EPEC serotypes differ from those *E. coli* isolated from patients with nonenteric infections.[36]

Epidemic infantile diarrhea may also be caused by enterotoxigenic organisms that are not limited to certain serotypes of *E. coli*. An outbreak has been described in which multiple serotypes of different organisms (*E. coli*, *Klebsiella*, and *Citrobacter*) that were demonstrated to be transiently enterotoxigenic were isolated,[37] which suggests the transmission of enterotoxigenicity among etiologic strains by plasmids[38] or by bacteriophages.[39] A subsequent outbreak of diarrhea on a cruise ship also documented the association of enterotoxigenic *Klebsiella* and *Citrobacter* as well as *E. coli* with watery diarrhea.[40] Another report of sporadic diarrhea among infants and children in Africa has shown that enteric organisms other than *E. coli* may produce an enterotoxin.[6] Enterotoxigenicity is not limited to specific serotypes, and most EPEC serotypes do not produce recognizable enterotoxins.[5-7,41] There do, however, tend to be a number of serotypes of *E. coli* that are more often enterotoxigenic, as shown in Table 2.[26,42] Whether these organisms are better recipients for enterotoxin plasmids or whether they are simply better adapted to maintaining these plasmids is not known.

A 9-month-long outbreak of diarrhea in the special care nurseries of a pediatric hospital has been reported in association with a multiple drug-resistant *E. coli* O78 that produced only the heat-stable type of enterotoxin.[43] Another outbreak of diarrhea lasting 3 months in a newborn nursery is Scotland was related to ST-producing *E. coli* O159.[44]

Shigellosis[45] and epidemic salmonellosis[46,47] may readily spread in the newborn nursery setting. Echoviruses,[48] coxsackieviruses,[49] adenoviruses,[50] and rotaviruses[51-53] are potential viral causes of epidemic infantile diarrhea. Echovirus 18 was isolated from 10 of 12 infants who had watery noninflammatory diarrhea in a 21-patient premature nursery. The virus was also isolated from two nurses, one of whom was implicated in the spread of the agent to five other babies in another ward.[48] While there are conflicting interpretations of the significance of isolation of enteroviruses and adenoviruses among controls as well as patients, some have suspected that they may cause summer or winter gastroenteritis, respectively. Hospital acquisition of rotaviruses may be common among newborns; some suggest that mild diarrhea develops relatively infrequently.[54] However, rotaviruses have been clearly implicated in epidemic neonatal diarrhea,[51-53] as well as in sporadic infantile diarrhea after the neonatal period.

WEANLING DIARRHEA

Weanling diarrhea usually occurs in the second year of life in areas where sanitation is poor. In contrast to cases of diarrhea where EPEC are still found in many areas,[18–21] EPEC were not found in the relatively infrequent cases of diarrhea among breast-fed neonates studied in rural Guatemala.[55] The greatest attack rate of diarrhea in the community occurs at the time of weaning, usually between 6 and 24 months of age.[9,11,12,56] As noted in the previous chapter, weanling diarrhea is a major cause of mortality around the world. The increased susceptibility of a recently weaned infant relates to several factors.[57] In areas with poor sanitation the infant ingests large numbers of many new organisms at the time of weaning. In developing countries, weaning foods prepared under conditions of poor hygiene are frequently found to be contaminated with large numbers of potential pathogens.[58,59] A second contributing factor is the deteriorating nutritional status that may occur with weaning in many parts of the world.[60,61] Finally there are cellular and humoral factors passively transferred in human breast milk that convey resistance to agents that commonly cause diarrhea in this age group.[62–66] Weanling diarrhea is manifested clinically as an acute, sporadic, watery diarrheal illness that occurs with increased frequency, especially in the summer months, in areas with poor sanitation. In the well-nourished infant, the disease is usually short lived and resolves within 2–3 days with adequate hydration. A low-grade fever may be present, and vomiting is common.[5,56] Diarrhea in the malnourished child tends to persist or to recur and is often much more severe.

Weanling diarrhea is usually an acute, noninflammatory process. Acute diarrhea in children 6–24 months of age has been commonly associated with rotaviruses[2–4] and with enterotoxigenic *E. coli.*[5–7] Shigellosis may also occur in this setting. From 16 to 83 percent of acute diarrheal illnesses among infants and young children have been associated with enterotoxigenic *E. coli.*[5–7,67] Most of these reports involve studies of the summer peak of diarrhea in areas with poor sanitation. The presence of antibody to the heat-labile enterotoxin (LT) of *E. coli* in colostrum[62,63] may provide some protection against LT-producing *E. coli* diarrhea among breast-fed infants exposed to unsanitary conditions. The recent demonstration of passive protection against experimental enterotoxigenic *E. coli* infections in human volunteers with immune bovine colostrum further documents the potential protective role of passive antibody in colostrum or milk.[68] The role of enterotoxigenic *E. coli* in causing infantile diarrhea in temperate climates is less clear. Enterotoxigenic *E. coli* serotypes are uncommon among children with diarrhea in Massachusetts and Virginia.[69–71]

The ability of enteric organisms other than *E. coli* to produce enterotoxins has been suggested, but these organisms appear to be considerably less common than enterotoxigenic *E. coli.* Studies from Ethiopia suggested that young children with sporadic diarrhea may have *Klebsiella, Citrobacter, Aeromonas,* or *E. coli* that produce an LT-like toxin.[6] However, in Brazil enterotoxigenic *Klebsiella* organisms were found in only 2 of 40 patients, both of whom also had enterotoxigenic *E. coli.*[5] Diarrhea produced by LT shares the adenylate cyclase–activating mechanism with cholera toxin,[72–76] while the heat–stable toxin (STa) activates intestinal guanylate cyclase.[77–79]

The major nonbacterial causes of weanling diarrhea are rotaviruses. While most adults have demonstrable antibody to rotaviruses that may protect against symptomatic disease, children less than 2 years of age throughout temperate and tropical climates appear to be highly susceptible to rotavirus diarrhea, which occurs most frequently in the winter or cooler, dry months[2,4,69,80–87] and occasionally in the summer months.[88] Rotavirus diarrhea appears to be associated with low humidity and possibly indoor crowding to a greater extent than with temperature or inadequate sanitation.[89–91] The illness tends to have a more insidious onset and to last slightly longer than bacterial diarrheas do, is slightly more common in males than in females, is usually mild and without fever, and is often associated with vomiting.[2,4,92] Rotaviruses probably account for most cases of "pseudocholera infantum" or hakuri ("white stool diarrhea")

in Japan.[83] They have been associated with initial bouts of weanling diarrhea in aboriginal communities,[93] and antirotavirus antibody has been demonstrated in human colostrum among patients in Costa Rica and Brazil.[63,66] There is a high frequency of rotavirus shedding or seroconversion among parents and other household contacts of cases of rotavirus-associated diarrhea.[2,94,95] Up to 40 percent of these infected adult contacts may develop mild abdominal cramps or diarrhea.[96]

The human rotaviruses demonstrate antigenic cross reaction with several animal strains, including the Nebraska calf diarrhea virus (NCDV), the agent of epizootic diarrhea of infant mice (EDIM), simian rotavirus (SA-11), and the "O" agent of monkeys.[2,97] However, there are three to five different antigenic types of rotaviruses,[98–101] so multiple attacks may occur.[102]

The laboratory diagnosis of rotavirus diarrhea may be made by examining the stool directly for viruses or the rotaviral RNA genome or by testing for an antibody titer increase in serum. Rotaviruses can be detected in fecal material by direct electron microscopy or by using immunologic techniques such as the enzyme-linked immunosorbent assay (ELISA),[103] radioimmunoassay,[104] counterimmunoelectrophoresis,[105] or fluorescent antibody staining of stool or biopsy specimens.[106,107] Immunoassays for rotaviral antigen are available, with ELISA being the most sensitive. Simple rapid latex agglutination assays with 86 percent sensitivity and 95 percent specificity have been developed.[108] Detection of rotaviral genomic RNA in stools by using "dot" hybridization with labeled RNA probes appears to be sensitive, specific, and convenient.[109] Methods for detecting serum antibody titers to rotaviruses use their cross-reactivity with NCDV, SA-11, or O agents of animals that can be cultivated in bovine embryonic kidney or in African green monkey kidney cells in tissue culture. Serum antibody has been measured by using immunoelectron microscopy,[82,110] complement fixation,[2,82] and immunofluorescence[69] with one of the substitute antigens.

In vitro studies were initially difficult because rotaviruses do not grow in most widely used tissue culture systems. Human rotaviruses incorporate into human embryonic gut monolayers,[111] guinea pig intestinal monolayers,[112] and human embryonic kidney cells in tissue culture.[113] Gnotobiotic piglets[114] and colostrum-deprived newborn rhesus monkeys[115] also acquire diarrhea after experimental infection with human rotaviruses. After the initial adaptation of human rotavirus type 2 in African green monkey kidney cell cultures after 11 passages through gnotobiotic newborn piglets,[116] several reports demonstrate the primary isolation of two human rotaviral types in MA104 cells in tissue culture with demonstrable cytopathic effects and without requiring animal passage.[117–119]

Much has been learned about the pathogenesis and the pathologic characteristics of intestinal rotavirus infections. Biopsy specimens from confirmed cases have shown transient, patchy, irregular inflammatory responses in the lamina propria and immature, cuboidal epithelium with 70–90-nm rotavirus particles in the distended cisternae of the endoplasmic reticulum.[80] Normal columnar epithelium at the villus tips was replaced by irregular cuboidal cryptlike cells. As would be expected from the destruction of villous type epithelial cells, a transient brush border disaccharidase deficiency in the duodenal and upper jejunal mucosa and, despite the efficacy of oral therapy with glucose–electrolyte solutions, increased fecal-reducing substances have been noted in children with rotavirus diarrhea.[120–122] The degree of microvillus damage parallels the severity of diarrhea and dehydration.[124] As with transmissible gastroenteritis in piglets, experimental rotaviral infections in animals confirm the shortened villi, reduced sucrase activity, increased thymidine kinase activity, no change in cyclic AMP concentrations, and blunted glucose-induced sodium absorption.[125–126] As noted in Chapter 75, this loss of absorptive villus tip cells may be responsible for the fluid imbalance and nutritional impact of rotaviral infections.

The availability, convenience, and cost-effectiveness of enzyme immunoassays or latex agglutination tests for rotavirus infections may enable improved diagnosis and epidemiologic control.[108] Therapy should be directed first at the immediate restoration of fluid balance by intravenous or oral glucose–electrolyte therapy and then at restoring the nutritional state to normal. Although several candidate live oral rotavirus vaccines (including bovine, rhesus monkey, and reassortant rotaviruses) show promise, questions remain about their efficacy in infants (<1 year old), especially in developing countries, and about the optimal means of delivery, age, and serotype to provide protection with minimal side effects.[127,128] Reasonable preventive measures include the provision of improved sanitation facilities and safe water supplies, as well as efforts to develop protective antibacterial, antitoxic, or antiviral immunity.

ACUTE NAUSEA AND VOMITING (WINTER VOMITING DISEASE)

The syndrome of acute nausea and vomiting, "intestinal flu," or "viral gastroenteritis" commonly occurs in winter months in temperate climates. While there is some overlap of this syndrome with rotavirus-associated infantile gastroenteritis, rotaviruses appear to be relatively uncommon causes of winter vomiting disease in older children and adults. The Cleveland family studies of Dingle et al.[1] showed that enteritis was second only to upper respiratory infection as a cause of illness in homes. Gastrointestinal illnesses were most common between the ages of 1 and 10 years, when approximately two illnesses occurred per person per year. The peak season of these gastrointestinal illnesses was November through February, with June being the lowest point of the year over this continuous study period. Most illnesses were of less than 1–3 days' duration; 20 percent occurred with respiratory symptoms, and 20 percent involved only diarrhea.

Illnesses tended to occur in one of two patterns: (1) mild afebrile illness with watery diarrhea or (2) a more severe febrile illness with vomiting, headache, and constitutional symptoms. Although etiologic agents were rarely identified, these two patterns of illness subsequently developed among volunteers who ingested filtrates prepared from the feces of ill patients.[129–131] Studies done in 1975–1977 in Charlottesville, Virginia, confirmed this pattern of winter illnesses, with clustering in families, highest attack rates in children, and the absence of identifiable etiologic agents in most cases despite the application of techniques for virologic and enterotoxin studies.[70,71]

Although there has been little consistent documentation of enteroviruses in association with febrile winter vomiting disease, echovirus type II has been demonstrated in association with a small laboratory outbreak of febrile vomiting disease.[132] Abdominal pain and vomiting have been described with influenza B infections in children between the ages of 4 and 10 years.[133]

Careful evaluation of specimens from an outbreak of winter vomiting disease in an elementary school revealed a 27-nm parvovirus-like agent.[134–136] Typical winter vomiting disease, first described in 1929 by Zahorsky,[137] occurred over a 2-day period in late October 1968 in Norwalk, Ohio. Fifty percent of 232 students and teachers in an elementary school developed a mild illness characterized by nausea, vomiting, and abdominal cramps that usually lasted only 12–24 hours. Diarrhea occurred in fewer than half, and a low-grade fever occurred in approximately one-third. A remarkable 32 percent secondary attack rate in family contacts occurred approximately 48 hours later. A bacteria-free fecal suspension from a secondary case from the Norwalk outbreak caused an illness with low-grade fever and diarrhea in two of three volunteers. A second passage in volunteers produced either a febrile vomiting disease or an afebrile diarrheal disease, and illness was also produced in one of four volunteers who ingested an inoculum after three passages

in human fetal intestinal organ culture.[135] From the stool of a second human passage in these volunteers, Kapikian and his colleagues[136] used convalescent serum to identify a 27-nm agent by immunoelectron microscopy. Antibody in the convalescent serum of other volunteers and in three of five patients with naturally acquired illness was shown to coat and to aggregate these particles. Biopsy specimens revealed an intact small intestinal mucosa but blunted villi, shortened microvilli, and dilatation of the endoplasmic reticulum with intracellular multivesiculate bodies. Dilated mitochondria and intercellular spaces were observed.[138] There was a transient decrease in the activities of the brush border enzymes, alkaline phosphatase, sucrase, and trehalase. All changes had returned to normal by 2 weeks after the illness. The colon is relatively spared, and fecal leukocytes are absent in this noninflammatory type of diarrhea.

The pathophysiologic features of winter vomiting disease caused by Norwalk-like agents may be parallel in some respects to that mentioned in the previous section for rotaviruses. Both cause mucosal villus disruption and transient brush border enzyme deficiencies in the upper portion of the small bowel without any alteration in adenylate cyclase activity.[100,139,140] The roles of transient enzyme deficiency, malabsorption of xylose and lactose, and the slight increase in the number of bacteria present during the Norwalk illness remain unclear.[139,141]

Similar outbreaks of vomiting disease have occurred elsewhere with either documented or suspected Norwalk-like agents. In March 1971, all four members of a household in Honolulu, Hawaii, developed a vomiting illness over a 4-day period with an apparent 44- to 48-hour incubation period, and in June 1971 another family of four in Montgomery County, Maryland, developed illnesses at 24- to 48-hour intervals that were characterized by vomiting, diarrhea, and occasional myalgias.[142] Fecal specimens from these patients revealed 27-nm Norwalk-like particles, and subsequent cross-challenge volunteer studies suggested that the Norwalk and Montgomery County agents were antigenically similar and conferred cross-immunity, while the Hawaii agent appeared to be antigenically different and failed to confer cross-immunity to the other agents.[142] Other Norwalk-like agents include the Snow Mountain and Taunton agents.[143] Clarke and associates[144] reported an outbreak from a boys' boarding school in Britain. The illness was transmitted to volunteers with filtered extracts of feces from one ill boy (W agent). Another outbreak in a primary school in Ditchling, England, in October 1975 revealed 26-nm particles that aggregated in convalescent serum and appeared to be antigenically similar to the W agent but different from the Hawaii and Norwalk agents.[145] Another 27-nm Norwalk-like agent was associated with an outbreak of gastroenteritis in a winter resort camp in Colorado.[146] From a convalescent hospital in Marin County, California, and a social gathering nearby, outbreaks of acute gastroenteritis have been associated with yet another viral agent capable of causing gastroenteritis, the Marin County agent.[147]

Several small (ranging from 20 to 35 nm in diameter), round (variably structured) viral agents of gastroenteritis have been grouped into four categories.[143,148] The first three categories have a better-defined surface morphology: (1) Norwalk-like viruses (including Norwalk or Montgomery County agent, Hawaii, Snow Mountain, and Tauton agents); (2) caliciviruses, with characteristic "chalicelike" surface hollows (including agents described in the United Kingdom [UK1-4] and Japan); (3) astroviruses, with five- or six-pointed starlike surface structure (including Marin County, UK1-5, and Japan agents; and (4) other less-well-defined, small round viruses (including Wollan, Wor Ditchling agent, Cockle, Paramatta, and other agents). Except for certain astrovirus and calicivirus strains, these have not yet been cultivated in vitro, and the lack of a convenient animal model has restricted their study. The roles of other viral agents, including enteroviruses (especially echovirus types 11, 14, and 18), enteric adenoviruses (said to cause up to 9 percent of pediatric impatient diarrhea[149]), human coronaviruses (reported from infants with gastroenteritis[150,151]), and the recently reported pestiviruses[152] are beyond the scope of this chapter. Over one-third of outbreaks of nonbacterial gastroenteritis in the United States have been associated with the Norwalk virus.[153,154] Astroviruses have been found to be among the most common causes of viral gastroenteritis in the pediatric age group.[155–158] Infection with astrovirus occasionally occurs in association with other enteric pathogens; in these cases the illness is more severe and protracted.[157] In a review of electron microscopy results from 10 centers in the United States and Canada over 6 years, a viral agent was seen in 16 percent, including rotavirus, adenovirus, small round virus (SRV), astroviruses and caliciviruses, the latter three being associated with nosocomial diarrhea.[158]

Identification of Norwalk-like agents capable of causing winter vomiting disease requires immune electron microscopy[136] or radioimmunoassay for demonstration of a serologic response.[159] In vitro expression of the Norwalk virus capsid protein results in the production of capsid structures resembling clinical isolates of this agent.[160] These recombinant particles may facilitate generation of clinically useful diagnostic tests for Norwalk virus (see Ch. 153). It is clear that there are multiple antigenic types of these agents that are capable of causing similar disease and that resistance may relate to individual (genetic) differences rather than to lasting protective immunity after symptomatic infection.[160,161] The detection of other viral causes of gastroenteritis includes monoclonal antibody-based enzyme immunoassay,[152,162] tissue culture,[163] or gene probes.[164]

ACUTE NONINFLAMMATORY DIARRHEA IN ADULTS

In temperate climates, acute noninflammatory diarrhea in adults may be caused by rotaviruses[165,166] or by Norwalk-like viruses.[96,100,135,165] The association of rotaviruses as well as adenoviruses, coxsackieviruses, and toxigenic *Clostridium difficile* with diarrhea, abdominal cramps, and a higher mortality among adult bone marrow transplant recipients has also been noted.[167] Additionally, several agents of food poisoning such as *Clostridium perfringens*, *Bacillus cereus*, or *Staphylococcus aureus* commonly cause noninflammatory diarrheal syndromes in adults (see Ch. 81).

In adults living in areas with poor sanitation, several other agents commonly cause sporadic noninflammatory diarrhea. In certain areas in South Asia, cholera is an endemic cause of severe watery diarrhea. With the increased infection-to-case ratio of El Tor cholera, the seventh pandemic has swept most of the continents of the Eastern Hemisphere, including Asia, Africa, and the Mediterranean portions of Europe.[168] Isolated cases have also occurred in the United States.[169,170] Outbreaks have been related to contaminated mineral water[171] and to undercooked shellfish.[172,173] Beginning in Madras, India, in late 1992 and rapidly spreading to Calcutta and Bangladesh in 1993, a new strain of non-O1 *Vibrio cholerae*, O139, "Bengal" is causing epidemic cholera gravis and may represent the beginning of an eighth pandemic.[174–178] One should suspect cholera in any patient who has severe dehydration and watery diarrhea, especially if the patient has a history of recent travel to a cholera-endemic area. The disease can be so fulminant as to cause hypovolemic shock and death from the outpouring of fluid into the upper portion of the small bowel before the first diarrheal stool occurs.[179] As discussed in detail in Chapter 192, the entire dehydrating syndrome of cholera appears to be related to the activation of intestinal adenylate cyclase by the potent cholera enterotoxin.[72,73] To make the diagnosis of cholera bacteriologically, one should culture stool specimens onto thiosulfate citrate bile salts sucrose agar. Of prime importance in therapy is fluid replacement either intravenously with isotonic fluids or orally with glucose electrolyte solutions.

Patients from whom *V. cholerae* cannot be isolated may also have a cholera-like syndrome. In 1956, De et al.[180] demonstrated

that *E. coli* isolated from adults and children with this syndrome caused fluid accumulation similar to that seen with *V. cholerae* in ligated rabbit ileal loops. In the early 1960s Trabulsi,[181] working in São Paulo, reported a similar finding with "toxigenic" *E. coli*. Subsequently studies by Taylor et al.[182,183] demonstrated that enterotoxigenicity correlated poorly with classic serotypes and that viable organisms were not required. Smith and Halls[184] identified several enterotoxigenic strains in association with animal diarrhea. Other workers showed that several adult cases of "acute undifferentiated diarrhea" in tropical Bengal were due to enterotoxigenic *E. coli* strains that were usually not of the classically recognized pathogenic serotypes.[185–188] These strains were transiently present during acute illness and elicited a net jejunal fluid secretion. The toxic material present in the culture filtrate of these *E. coli* strains was demonstrated to be heat labile and nondialyzable and was precipitated in 40% ammonium sulfate. Subsequent studies have demonstrated that two types of enterotoxin are produced by *E. coli*, a heat-labile enterotoxin (LT) and a heat-stable enterotoxin (ST).[189] Like cholera toxin, the *E. coli* LT activates mucosal adenylate cyclase.[61–63] LT is larger, inactivated by heating at 60°C for 30 minutes, and antigenically and mechanistically similar to cholera toxin with a lag period before the activation of adenylate cyclase. LT is detected by several bioassay systems that use the adenylate cyclase activating property of this toxin[190–192] or by immunoassay methods.[193] In contrast, STa activates guanylate cyclase,[77–79] has an earlier onset of action,[189] has greater tissue specificity,[79] and has a much lower molecular weight than LT does.[194] It is assayed in suckling mice.[195] The role of yet a different type of enterotoxin, STb, that causes secretion in piglets without altering intestinal cyclic AMP or cyclic GMP remains unclear in humans at present.[196–198]

Methods for demonstrating enterotoxigenic *E. coli* are limited by the lack of a selective culture process (as routinely used, for example, to identify salmonellae or shigellae) and the necessity to pick a few random colonies of *E. coli* for enterotoxin testing. Data from a common-source outbreak of enterotoxigenic *E. coli* diarrhea in Crater Lake National Park in Oregon demonstrate the insensitivity of nonselective culture methods.[199] Fourteen patients in this outbreak had enterotoxigenic *E. coli* diarrhea by epidemiologic and clinical criteria, and each had multiple, random *E. coli* stool isolates tested for enterotoxin as well as paired sera examined for antitoxic immunity. Only 43 percent had enterotoxigenic *E. coli* identified, 36 percent had significant serum antitoxic antibody titer increases, and only 64 percent had either one or the other. Thirty-six percent of the cases could not be confirmed by current, nonselective methods. The lack of a serum antibody response in many patients with this intraluminal toxinosis is not surprising.

Other studies have shown that, in addition to the association with diarrhea in children, LT-only, ST-only, and LT-plus-ST–producing strains are associated with adult diarrhea.[3] Adults living in areas of poor sanitation may often carry LT-producing *E. coli* asymptomatically.[200,201] In contrast, ST-producing *E. coli* strains are significantly associated with diarrheal disease and are less frequently present in asymptomatic control patients living in areas with poor sanitation. However, studies suggest that enterotoxigenic *E. coli* serotypes are uncommonly associated with diarrhea in the United States.[69,70]

A cause of acute, noninflammatory, self-limited diarrhea among those exposed to infected animals and patients is cryptosporidiosis.[202–204] This tiny coccidian protozoan parasite causes more severe, watery, prolonged diarrhea in immunocompromised hosts.

Treatment of diarrhea in adults consists primarily of rehydration. If glucose or sucrose accompany the isotonic fluid taken orally, the coupled absorption of sodium and water are often sufficient to replace fluid loss.[205] Pepto-Bismol may reduce enterotoxin action,[206] and if there is no significant febrile or inflammatory process, low doses of antimotility agents may offer some relief with minimum risk if cramping is severe.

DIARRHEA IN AIDS PATIENTS

Patients with the acquired immunodeficiency syndrome (AIDS) often develop or present with diarrhea. Among AIDS patients in the United States, 50–60 percent present with diarrhea,[207,208] a number that reaches 95 percent in tropical developing areas such as Africa or Haiti.[208] In many of these patients, diarrhea becomes prolonged and life-threatening and may present major difficulties in management. Although some have reported an enteropathy without identifiable pathogens[209,210] or with primary human immunodeficiency virus (HIV) infection of enterochromaffin cells in the bowel mucosal crypts and lamina propria,[211] others report one or more enteric pathogens in 55–85 percent of patients with AIDS and diarrhea.[212,213] Sexually promiscuous homosexual males often become infected with *Giardia lamblia, Entamoeba histolytica, Campylobacter jejuni, Shigella, Chlamydia trachomatis, Clostridium difficile,* or (with proctitis) *Neisseria gonorrheae,* herpes simplex virus, or *Treponema pallidum.*[214] As shown in Table 3, the leading agents found in AIDS patients with diarrhea are cytomegalovirus, *Cryptosporidium, Microsporidium, Entamoeba histolytica, Giardia lamblia, Salmonella, Campylobacter, Shingella, Clostridium difficile, Vibrio parahaemolyticus,* and *Mycobacterium* spp.[212,213,215–217] Even *Pneumoncystis carinii* can occasionally involve the intestinal tract in this setting.[218] Although eradicative treatment may be difficult, most of these patients respond to specific antimicrobial or antiparasitic therapy, thus emphasizing the need to diagnose specifically the etiologies of these infections whenever possible. The antiviral agent ganciclovir can transiently reverse intestinal cytomegalovirus infection,[219] and most bacterial and parasitic agents can be treated with some improvement. *Cryptosporidium,* which infects 3–21 percent of AIDS patients in the United States, can be found in as many as 50 percent of patients in Africa and Haiti with AIDS and diarrhea.[208] *Cryptosporidium* may also extend into the biliary tract as well in this setting. The same acid-fast stain that detects *Cryptosporidium* or *Mycobacterium* in fecal specimens may also reveal *Isosora belli* in 2–15 percent of AIDS patients with diarrhea in the United States and Africa, respectively.[208] *Cryptosporidium* and microsporidial infections are associated with vil-

lus atrophy, crypt hyperplasia, increased intraepithelial lymphocytes, and D-xylose malabsorption.[215] An increased yield for pathogens may be found when there is a 5–10 kg weight loss or an abnormal Schilling test.[216] Nontyphoidal *Salmonella* infections occur with an estimated 20-fold increase in frequency as well as increased severity in AIDS patients.[220–223] Enteric viruses have also emerged as significant potential pathogens seen with diarrhea in HIV-infected individuals. In one study, astrovirus, picobirnavirus, calicivirus, and adenovirus were found in 6–12 percent of HIV-positive patients with diarrhea.[224] Nevertheless, these infections, as those with *Campylobacter jejuni* and other species, are treatable. Other common enteric infections include esophagitis or stomatitis with *Candida* or herpes simplex virus.

DIARRHEA IN INSTITUTIONS

Institutions provide special host and environmental settings for the acquisition of certain enteric pathogens. As with diarrhea in AIDS patients and travelers' diarrhea, most cases are still noninflammatory; however, an increased frequency of certain causes of inflammatory diarrhea should prompt a careful search for fecal leukocytes in sporadic or clustered cases in hospitals, chronic care facilities, or day care centers.[225]

Hospitals

Nosocomial diarrhea is among the most common of reported nosocomial outbreaks to the Centers for Disease Control and Prevention (CDC) and accounts for 21 percent of all 223 nosocomial outbreaks reported from 1956 to 1979.[226] However, its frequency is often overlooked, and it has been suggested to be the most common nosocomial infection in some areas.[227] Furthermore, nosocomial diarrhea appears to be a significant predisposing factor to other nosocomial infections such as urinary tract infections.[228] Overall rates range from 2.3 to 4.1 illnesses per 100 admissions on pediatric wards[227,229] and from 7.7 per 100 admissions to 41 percent of adults hospitalized in intensive care units.[227,230] From limited available data, *Clostridium difficile* appears to be associated with most cases with a recognized etiology (45 percent), followed by *Salmonella* (12 percent).[231] *Salmonella* is the most common cause among reported outbreaks of nosocomial gastroenteritis.[226] In young children and in immunocompromised hosts, viral agents (rotaviruses, adenoviruses, coxsackieviruses, and others) are often found as well.[229,232]

Chronic Care Facilities

Diarrheal illnesses are also significant problems in extended care facilities for the elderly. Conservative estimates based on passively reported illness rates are that one-third of patients in chronic care facilities experience diarrhea each year.[233,234] About one-fourth of these patients have *Clostridium difficile* cytotoxin, one-third of whom are symptomatic with diarrhea.[235] Over 20 percent have fecal cytotoxin on admission, and a comparable number acquire cytotoxigenic *C. difficile* in the institution.[235] When those with diarrhea are studied, 18–53 percent have cytotoxin or *C. difficile,* respectively.[236] The frequency of potentially transmissible enteric pathogens emphasizes the importance of careful hand washing in situations in which hygiene is often difficult. Similar problems have been long recognized in mental institutions where hepatitis, *Strongyloides,* and amebiasis are readily acquired.

Day Care Centers

Another special institutional setting in which hygiene is difficult and enteric infections are increasingly appreciated is in day care centers. Numerous outbreaks have been reported in association with viruses, bacteria, or parasites. Most common in infants

TABLE 3. Possible Enteric Pathogens in AIDS Patients

Pathogen	Diarrhea (n = 181)	No Diarrhea (n = 28)
Cytomegalovirus	12–45%	15%
Cryptosporidium	14–26	0
Microsporidium	7.5–33	0
Entamoeba histolytica	0–15	0
Giardia lamblia	2–15	5
Salmonella spp.	0–15	0
Campylobacter spp.	2–11	8
Shigella spp.	5–10	0
Clostridium difficile toxin	6–7	0
Vibrio parahaemolyticus	4	0
Mycobacterium spp.	2–25	0
Isospora belli	2–6	0
Blastocystis hominis	2–15	16
Candida albicans	6–53	24
Herpes simplex	5–18	40
Chlamydia trachomatis	11	13
Strongyloides	0–6	0
Intestinal spirochetes	11	11
One or more pathogens	55–86	39

(Data from refs. 212, 213, 215, 216.)

and children less than 2 years old are rotaviruses, while older toddlers are more likely to acquire *Giardia lamblia*.[237] An identical clinical syndrome of prolonged noninflammatory diarrhea may be seen with *Cryptosporidium* in day care centers.[238–240] Outbreaks of inflammatory diarrhea in the day care center setting include those due to *Shigella, Campylobacter jejuni,* and *Clostridium difficile*.[241,242]

THE DIARRHEA OF TRAVELERS (TURISTA)

Whether it "arouses one from bed with a start at 4 A.M. for a record-breaking race to th bathroom to begin a staccato ballet"[243] or it produces the poetry of the Psalmist, "I am poured out like water . . . my heart like wax is melted in the midst of my bowels,"[244] travelers' diarrhea has a major impact each year on the 300 million international travelers and probably on the distribution of $100 billion in international tourism receipts.[245] Sixteen million people (8 million from the United States) travel from industrialized to developing countries. It is by far the most common and among the most feared illnesses that threaten the traveler. Many studies have focused on North Americans and northern Europeans, who appear to be the groups at greatest risk when they travel to Latin America, Southern Europe, Africa, or Asia.[246–249] Travelers' diarrhea, which may be severe and incapacitating (albeit rarely if ever fatal), is by far the most common health problem encountered with travel to developing countries.[250] The global nature of the problem and some suggested causal forces are illustrated by its more euphemistic names: "Delhi belly," "Gyppi tummy," "GIs," "Rome runs," "Greek gallop," "Turkey trots," "Montezuma's revenge," "Aztec two-step," "Aden gut," "San Franciscitis," "Basra belly," "La turista," "backdoor sprint," "summer complaint," "coeliac flux," "Canary disease," "passion," "Hong Kong dog," "Poona poohs," "Casablanca crud," "tourist trots," "Malta dog," and many more.

The onset of the vast majority of travelers' diarrhea is usually between 5 and 15 days after arrival, with a range from 3 to 31 days in several reported series.[243,251–257] The illness is typically manifested by malaise, anorexia, and abdominal cramps, followed by the sudden onset of watery diarrhea. Nausea and vomiting may accompany 10–25 percent of the illnesses. The diarrhea is usually noninflammatory, without blood or pus. A low-grade fever may be present in approximately one-third of the cases. The duration is usually 1–5 days, but a significant number of people (19–50 percent) have an illness that continues beyond 5–10 days.

The attack rate ranges from 7 percent after 2 weeks in Aden[252] to 54 percent after 8 days in Mexico[246] and was 4–51 percent over a 14-day period among 17,280 Swiss tourists, depending on where they went.[249] One report of British tourists notes an attack rate ranging from 26 percent in Africa to 7.7 percent in North America. In descending order of risk after Africa in this study were the Middle East, southern Europe, Central Europe, Asia (including India and Pakistan), South America, Australia, and North America.[257] In general, it appears that one approaches a 50 percent risk of acquiring turista during travel to a tropical country from a temperate climate for 2 weeks or more. The attack rate also appears to decrease with age after 25 years, an observation that may reflect different habits and exposures rather than inherent susceptibility.[243,249]

For many years, the etiology of turista was an enigma; only infrequently have parasites or bacteria such as amebas, *Giardia, Salmonella,* or *Shigella* been identified. Likewise viral studies have failed to elucidate significant viral etiologies of travelers' diarrhea. The first suggestion that an infectious bacterial process was likely came from the effective reduction in the attack rate by the use of prophylactic antimicrobial agents.[198,204,251,257] Studies by Kean[243] suggested that *E. coli* of certain enteropathogenic serotypes might be involved in up to one-third of the cases. The involvement of *E. coli* was further confirmed in an outbreak

of travelers' diarrhea among the British troops in Aden, where *E. coli* O148 was identified among 54 percent of British troops with diarrhea.[252]

Subsequent studies have demonstrated ETEC in approximately 50 percent (range, 20–75 percent) of cases of travelers' diarrhea in Latin America, Africa, and Asia (Table 4).[241,242] The attack rate ranged from 20 to 100 percent (median, 52–54 percent) in 26 studies reviewed (Table 4).[258,259] Enterotoxigenic *E. coli* organisms were almost never present before the travel; they were acquired by only 14 of 111 (12.6 percent) fellow travelers who did not become ill.[254–256] The type of enterotoxin produced by *E. coli* associated with travelers' diarrhea may be the heat-labile type (LT), the heat-stable type (ST), or both LT and ST (Table 5). In contrast to adults who live in tropical areas and may often carry enterotoxigenic *E. coli* asymptomatically, the traveler appears to be susceptible to illness caused by enterotoxin-producing *E. coli*. Salmonellae, shigellae, or vibrios are present in only 1–16 percent of the patients with travelers' diarrhea. Rotavirus infections have been described in 0–36 percent of cases of travelers' diarrhea, often in association with bacterial or parasitic pathogens.[260] In a study of Panamanian tourists to Mexico, rotavirus or Norwalk virus was found in 41 percent, *Campylobacter* in 11 percent, and ETEC in only one case of diarrhea.[261] Cholera is rarely a problem for U.S. travelers.[249,262]

In contrast to the frequent identification of potential etiologic agents among travelers to tropical areas who develop diarrhea, careful studies of a group of marines who developed diarrhea upon arrival in temperate South Korea (21 percent in 3 weeks) failed to reveal any evidence of bacterial, parasitic, or rotaviral pathogens.[263] Travelers to certain areas such as Russia and national parks in the United States may be especially prone to the more insidious watery diarrhea seen with giardiasis or cryptosporidiosis.[264–267] Strongyloidiasis may also be acquired in tropical areas and may cause noninflammatory diarrhea, abdominal pain, and eosinophilia.[268]

Several other potentially serious infections may be acquired by travelers whose major complaint is diarrhea or abdominal pain. Malaria may be manifested initially as "gastroenteritis" with nausea, vomiting, diarrhea, or abdominal pain in 30–50 percent of the cases.[269] The physician caring for world travelers should also remember to consider typhoid fever and other infections that may be manifested with a "typhoidal pattern" including plague, meloidosis, typhus, and arboviral hemorrhagic fevers.[269,270]

The desire to control the bothersome problem of diarrhea in travelers has led to extreme and sometimes irrational attempts.[243] Some travelers persist in using iodochlorhydroxquin (Entero-Vioform, clioquinol), which has been shown not only to be ineffective for travelers' diarrhea[246,271] but also to carry a risk of severe subacute myelo-optic atrophy.[272] Other commonly used remedies such as diphenoxylate-atropine (Lomotil) and kaolin-pectin suspension were of no value in treating children with acute diarrhea in Guatemala.[273] The former and other antimotility agents may actually worsen the illness with inflam-

TABLE 4. Etiologies of Travelers' Diarrhea

Characteristics	Latin America (15 Studies)	Africa (3 Studies)	Asia (8 Studies)
Duration of stay (days)	21 (2–42)[a]	28 (28–35)	(28–42)
Attack rate (%)	52 (21–100)	54 (36–62)	(39–57)
Percentage with			
Enterotoxigenic *E. coli*	46 (28–72)	36 (31–75)	(20–34)
Shigella	0 (0–30)	0 (0–15)	(4–7)
Salmonella		0 (0–0)	(11–15)
C. jejuni	—	—	(2–15)
V. parahaemolyticus	—	—	(1–13)
Rotavirus	23 (0–36)	0 (0–0)	—

[a] Median (range) from 26 studies.[258,259]

TABLE 5. Frequency of Enterotoxigenic *E. coli* in Association with Travelers' Diarrhea in Latin America, Africa, and Asia

	Study				
Feature	Gastroenterologists in Mexico[149]	Peace Corps Volunteers in Kenya[150]	Yale Glee Club in Latin America[151]	Japanese Travelers Returning to Tokyo from India, Southeast Asia, Orient[259]	Total
Illness attack rate (%)	49% in 16 days	69% in 5 wk	74% in 1 mo	—	
Type of enterotoxin					
LT only (%)	16%	33%	25%	4.8%	21%
LT and ST (%)	16%	15%	12.5%	11.8%	38%
ST only (%)	9.8%	2%	19%	13.6%	41%
Total	21/51 cases	14/27 cases	9/16 cases	226/749 cases	270/843 cases
(Percentage of illness with ETEC)	(41%)	(52%)	(56%)	(30.2%)	(32%)

Abbreviations: LT: heat-labile; ST: heat-stable.

matory processes such as shigellosis.[274] Bismuth subsalicylate (Pepto-Bismol) has been shown to inhibit enterotoxin activity in experimental animal models[206] and has been recommended for symptomatic therapy and, in doses as low as 1.05 g/day (2 tablets bid), for prophylaxis.[274,275] The mainstay of therapy, as with any diarrheal illness, is adequate hydration with an oral glucose—or sucrose—electrolyte solution.

Prevention of travelers' diarrhea should be directed toward reducing the consumption of infectious agents in food and water. Salads, raw vegetables, and untreated water (or ice) are high-risk foods.[277] Bottled, noncarbonated water cannot be considered safe since outbreaks of cholera[171] and typhoid fever[278,279] have been traced to bottled water and beverages, respectively. It has been suggested that even brief, 10-minute heating to 50–55°C (the temperature of some hot tap water, "too hot for the hand to tolerate") may kill many enteric bacterial and parasitic pathogens.[280] Care in eating and drinking may reduce one's risk even in highly endemic areas to less than 15 percent.[277,281]

The efficacy of prophylactic antimicrobial agents has been documented in several studies.[251,257,282] However, multiple drug-resistant enterotoxigenic *E. coli* occur and have demonstrated cotransfer of enterotoxigenicity and drug resistance.[283,284] The increased risk of acquiring a more severe infection such as salmonellosis,[285] the risk of drug side effects (such as photosensitivity in the tropics), and the emergence of drug-resistant organisms should preclude the widespread use of antibiotic prophylaxis at this time. Because treatment regimens combining loperamide with antibiotic are rapidly effective in controlling travelers' diarrhea (<10 hours), most experts consider prophylactic therapy only in travelers with special considerations (e.g., high risk of infection, importance to remain disease-free during the trip).[286,287] Until more widespread resistance develops,[288,289] treatment of travelers' diarrhea with trimethoprim, trimethoprim–sulfamethoxazole, bicozamycin, or ciprofloxacin may reduce a 3- to 4-day illness to 1–1.5 days.[290–292] In 1993, trimethoprim–sulfamethoxazole was effective for treatment in those traveling to inland Mexico.[287,293] Because of bacterial resistance patterns, travelers to other developing countries should be given a fluoroquinolone such as ciprofloxacin or ofloxacin to use if needed.[287] Fluoroquinolone drugs are contraindicated in pregnant women (a nonsorbable agent such as attapulgite can be tried[287–294]) and children under the age of 16 years (combination therapy with trimethoprim–sulfamethoxazole and erythromycin has been suggested[287,294]).

DIFFERENTIAL DIAGNOSIS OF ACUTE NONINFLAMMATORY DIARRHEA

Acute noninflammatory diarrhea may also be the consequence of several noninfectious processes. As with agents that effect an osmotic diuresis, nonabsorbable agents such as sorbitol may cause diarrhea if consumed in excess. Ipecac fluid extract used by mistake instead of ipecac syrup may cause watery diarrhea instead of vomiting. Heavy metal poisoning (As, Sn, Fe, Cd,

Hg, Pb) is often associated with diarrhea, probably as a result of toxic effects on the rapidly growing mucosal epithelium. Endocrine causes of diarrhea that may share the adenylate cyclase–activating mechanism with enterotoxins include non-β-islet cell tumors, medullary carcinoma of the thyroid, carcinoid tumors, and others that are associated with increased serum prostaglandins or vasoactive intestinal polypeptide (VIP).[295] Patients with thyrotoxicosis and adrenal or parathyroid insufficiency may also have diarrhea. Congenital and acquired enzyme deficiencies include lactase deficiency and pancreatic or biliary insufficiency with which inadequately degraded or absorbed nutrients may promote an osmotic diarrhea. A child with diarrhea as well as with edema, hypertension, or petechiae should be suspected of having HUS with or without enterohemorrhagic *E. coli* O157:H7. Patients with dermatitis herpetiformis may also have diarrhea that may respond to sulfone or sulfapyridine therapy or to a gluten-free diet.

CHRONIC NONINFLAMMATORY DIARRHEA

Syndrome of chronic noninflammatory diarrhea of infectious etiology include giardiasis, tropical spruelike syndromes, syndromes of bacterial "overgrowth," and *Cryptosporidium* or *Isospora belli* infection (especially in immunocompromised hosts).[202,203,208,226,296]

The patient with weight loss, malaise, and watery or fatty stools should be suspected of having giardiasis or some other cause of a malabsorption syndrome. This syndrome may also be associated with hypocalcemia, with iron or folate deficiency anemia, or with vitamin D, vitamin K, or protein deficiency.

Giardiasis may go undiagnosed for weeks. While it is endemic throughout most of the United States and much of the world, giardiasis received attention when acquired in Rocky Mountain ski resorts and in Leningrad.[224,225] Effective management requires a high index of suspicion followed by a careful search by a competent experienced person for the trophozoite or cyst of *G. lamblia* in multiple stool specimens or in a small bowel aspirate or "string" (Enterotest; Hedeco, Palo Alto, CA) sample. Recommended therapy is quinacrine (Atabrine), 100 mg tid for 5–7 days, with a reported 95 percent cure rate, or metronidazole (Flagyl), 250 mg tid for 7–10 days, with a reported 70 percent cure rate.[296] Higher doses of metronidazole may be more effective. Furazolidone, which is available in liquid form for pediatric use, divided into three daily doses with meals (total, 8 mg/kg/day) for 10 days is often used in children.[297]

The diagnosis of *Cryptosporidium* or *Isospora belli* infection is best made by phase microscopic or modified Kinyoun acid-fast stain examination of fecal specimens with or without sugar flotation.[202,208,298]

BACTERIAL OVERGROWTH SYNDROMES

Many syndromes have been described in which impaired absorption was attributed to abnormal bacterial colonization in the upper segment of the small bowel.[299] Whether these organisms are virulent pathogens or simply normal colonic flora abnormally distributed is currently unclear.

Normally, the upper portion of the small bowel is relatively sparsely populated with fewer than 10^5 organisms/ml that are predominantly facultative gram-positive organisms (diptheroids, streptococci, and lactobacilli).[300] The organisms most often incriminated in bacterial overgrowth syndromes in the small bowel are aerobic enteric coliforms (Enterobacteriaceae) and anaerobic gram-negative fecal flora (*Bacteroides* and other genera). Other organisms such as *Plesiomonas shigelloides* may occasionally be responsible.[301] Bacterial colonization in the upper part of the small bowel may be associated with malabsorption or chronic diarrhea in the absence of significant histopathologic changes. Small bowel overgrowth is usually associated with a predisposing bowel abnormality such as achlorhydria (from gastritis, pernicious anemia, or gastric surgery), blind-loop syndromes, cholangitis, impaired motility (scleroderma, diabetic neuropathy, vagotomy), surgery, strictures, diverticula, or radiation damage.[302,303] Malnutrition, especially with protein, folate, or B_{12} deficiency, may also render the bowel more susceptible to microbial colonization and injury.[300,304] An episode of acute infectious diarrhea may also provide the initiating event in the establishment of small bowel colonization and chronic diarrhea.[300,305,306] Lindenbaum et al.[307] described spruelike morphologic changes in the upper portion of the small bowel in association with increased numbers of bacteria and malabsorption among Peace Corps volunteers living in Pakistan.

The mechanism by which fecal flora in the small bowel cause malabsorption may involve bacterial binding or utilization of nutrients (such as vitamin B_{12} or carbohydrates, respectively), deconjugation of bile salts by bacteria such as enterococci and anaerobes,[308] or the toxic effects of bacterial products such as fatty acids or amines.[300] Indeed, colonizing *E. coli* without other recognized virulence traits have been shown to cause prolonged diarrhea in a rabbit model,[309] with an associated impairment in water and electrolyte absorption as well as disaccharidase activity.[310]

The approach to the patient suspected of having bacterial "overgrowth" as a cause of malabsorption or chronic diarrhea should include quantitative aerobic and anaerobic cultures of the upper small bowel contents obtained by intubation or "string" passage. Since the critical number of organisms appears to be approximately 10^5 organisms/ml, semiquantitative estimates from a Gram stain analogous to the urine Gram stain may also prove to be of value. Roberts et al.[305] have suggested that unexplained malnutrition in the elderly may be due to clinically inapparent bacterial overgrowth that can be detected by the ^{14}C-glycocholic acid breath test for bacterial deconjugation of bile salts. Tests for urinary indican (from bacterial conversion of tryptophan) have proved to be insensitive and nonspecific for bacterial overgrowth syndromes.[311]

Patients with diarrhea or malabsorption and bacterial overgrowth should be considered for antibiotic therapy, especially if predisposing conditions like achlorhydria, scleroderma, or diabetes are present. Depending on results of quantitative cultures of upper small bowel aspirates, therapy may need to be directed against anaerobes as well as aerobic coliform organisms.[300,305] While small amounts of antibiotics have been used to improve the nutritional status of animals and poultry and even of malnourished children,[312] the potential risks of widespread antibiotic use[313] must be weighed against potential benefits.

Noninfectious causes of chronic noninflammatory diarrhea should also be considered in the differential diagnosis. These include congenital deficiency syndromes and food allergies, certain neoplastic and endocrine processes, and less-well-understood functional disorders. In the first categories one may consider milk allergies, disaccharidase deficiencies, gluten enteropathy, acrodermatitis enteropathica, β-lipoprotein deficiency, familial hyperchloremic alkalosis (congenital "chlo-

ridorrhea"), Leiner's disease, and Wiskott-Aldrich syndrome. Neoplastic and endocrine causes of diarrhea include carcinoid, Werner syndrome (multiple endocrine adenomatosis), Zollinger-Ellison syndrome (gastrinoma), "pancreatic cholera" syndromes, medullary carcinoma of the thyroid, and thyrotoxicosis. Patients with partial mechanical bowel obstruction or pellagra may also have chronic diarrhea. Finally, frequent small stools may suggest an irritable bowel syndrome of presumed functional etiology. However, a search for the treatable infectious agents reviewed in this chapter should always precede the latter diagnosis.

REFERENCES

1. Dingle JH, Badger GF, Jordan WS Jr. Illnesses in the Home: A Study of 25,000 Illnesses in a Group of Cleveland Families. Cleveland: Press of Western Reserve University; 1964.
2. Kapikian AZ, Kim H-W, Wyatt RG, et al. Human reovirus-like agent as the pathogen associated with "winter" gastroenteritis in hospitalized infants and young children. N Engl J Med. 1976;294:965.
3. Black RE, Merson MH, Huq I, et al. Incidence and severity of rotavirus and E. coli diarrhea in rural Bangladesh. Lancet. 1981;1:141.
4. Ryder TW, Sack DA, Kapikian AZ, et al. Enterotoxigenic *Escherichia coli* and reovirus-like agent in rural Bangladesh. Lancet. 1976;1:659.
5. Guerrant RL, Moore RA, Kirschenfeld PM, et al. Role of toxigenic and invasive bacteria in acute diarrhea of childhood. N Engl J Med. 1975;293:567.
6. Wadstrom T, Aust-Kettis A, Habte D, et al. Enterotoxin-producing bacteria and parasites in stools of Ethiopian children with diarrhoeal disease. Arch Dis Child. 1976;51:865.
7. Sack RB, Hirschhorn N, Brownlee I, et al. Enterotoxigenic *Escherichia coli*–associated diarrheal disease in Apache children. N Engl J Med. 1975; 292:1041.
8. Black RE, Brown KH, Becker S, et al. Longitudinal studies of infectious diseases and physical growth of children in rural Bangladesh. I. Patterns of morbidity. Am J Epidemiol. 1982;115:305.
9. Guerrant RL, Kirchoff LV, Shields DS, et al. Prospective study of diarrheal illnesses in Northeastern Brazil: Patterns of disease, nutritional impact and risk factors. J Infect Dis. 1983;148:986.
10. Jacobs SI, Holzel A, Wolman B, et al. Outbreak of infantile gastroenteritis caused by Escherichia coli O114. Arch Dis Child. 1970;45:656.
11. Neter E. Enteritis due to enteropathogenic *Escherichia coli:* Present-day status and unsolved problems. J Pediatr. 1959;55:223.
12. Hone R, Fitzpatrick S, Keane C, et al. Infantile enteritis in Dublin caused by Escherichia coli O142. Med Microbiol. 1973;6:505.
13. Levine MM, Nalin DR, Hornick RB, et al. *Escherichia coli* strains that cause diarrhea but do not produce heat-labile or heat-stable enterotoxins and are noninvasive. Lancet. 1978;1:1119.
14. Nelson JD, Haltalin KC. Accuracy of diagnosis of bacterial diarrheal disease by clinical features. J Pediatr. 1971;78:519.
15. Drucker MM, Polliack A, Yeivin R, et al. Immunofluorescent demonstration of enteropathogenic Escherichia coli in tissues of infants dying with enteritis. Pediatrics. 1970;46:855.
16. South MA: Enteropathogenic *Escherichia coli* disease: New developments and perspectives. J Pediatr. 1971;79:1.
17. Kaslow RA, Taylor A, Dweck HS, et al. Enteropathogenic *Escherichia coli* infection in a newborn nursery. Am J Dis Child. 1974;128:797.
18. Levine MM, Edelman R. Enteropathogenic *Escherichia coli* of classic serotypes associated with infant diarrhea: Epidemiology and pathogenesis. Epidemiol Rev. 1984;6:31–51.
19. Gurwith M, Hinde D, Gross R, et al. A prospective study of enteropathogenic E. coli in endemic diarrheal disease. J Infect Dis. 1978;137:292.
20. Toledo MRF, Alvariza MCB, Murahovschi J, et al. Enteropathogenic *Escherichia coli* serotypes and endemic diarrhea in infants. Infect Immun. 1983; 39:586–9.
21. Bray J, Beavan TED. Slide agglutination of *Bacterium coli* var. *Neopolitanum* in summer diarrhea. J Pathol Bacteriol. 1948;60:395.
22. Varela G, Aguirre A, Grillo J. *Escherichia coli*-gomez, nueva especie aislada de un caso mortal de diarrea. Bol Med Hosp Infantil Mexico. 1946;3:3.
23. Olarte J, Varela G. A complete somatic antigen common to *Salmonella adelaide, Escherichia coli*-gomez and *Escherichia coli* O111:B4. J Lab Clin Med. 1952;40:252.
24. Giles C, Sangster G. An outbreak of infantile gastro-enteritis in Aberdeen. J Hyg (Camb) 1948;46:1.
25. Kaufmann F, Dupont A. *Escherichia* strains from infantile epidemic gastroenteritis. Acta Pathol Microbiol Scand. 1950;27:552.
26. Ørskov I, Ørskov F, Jann B, et al. Serology, chemistry and genetics of O and K antigens of *Escherichia coli*. Bacteriol Rev. 1977;41:667.
27. Rowe B, Gion RJ. *Escherichia coli* O142 and infantile enteritis in Scotland. Lancet. 1971;1:649.
28. Rowe B, Gross J, Lindop R, et al. A new *E. coli* O group O158 associated with an outbreak of infantile enteritis. J Clin Pathol. 1974;27:832.
29. Rogers KB, Cracknell VM. Epidemic infantile gastro-enteritis due to *Escherichia coli* type O114. J Pathol Bacteriol. 1956;72:27.

30. Charter RE. *Escherichia coli* type O114 isolated from infantile diarrhea and calf scours. J Pathol Bacteriol. 1956;72:33.
31. Riley LW, Remis RS, Helgerson SD, et al. Outbreaks of hemorrhagic colitis associated with a rare *Escherichia coli* serotype. N Engl J Med. 1983;308:681.
32. Johnson WM, Lior H, Bezanson GS. Cytotoxic *Escherichia coli* O157:H7 associated with hemorrhagic colitis in Canada. Lancet. 1983;1:76.
33. Outbreak of hemorrhagic colitis—Ottawa, Canada. MMWR. 1983;32:133.
34. Donnenberg MS, Kaper JB. Enteropathogenic *Escherichia coli*. Infect Immun. 1992;60:3953–61.
35. Neter E, Shumway CN: *E. coli* serotype D433: Occurrence in intestinal and respiratory tracts, cultural characteristics, pathogenicity, sensitivity to antibiotics. Proc Soc Exp Biol Med. 1950;74:504.
36. Ørskov F. Virulence factors of the bacterial cell surface. J Infect Dis. 1978;137:630.
37. Guerrant RL, Dickens MD, Wenzel RP, et al. Toxigenic bacterial diarrhea: Nursery outbreak involving multiple bacterial strains. J Pediatr. 1976;89:885.
38. Skerman FJ, Formal SB, Falkow S. Plasmid-associated enterotoxin production in a strain of *Escherichia coli* isolated from humans. Infect Immun. 1972;5:622.
39. Takeda Y, Murphy J. Bacteriophage conversion of heat labile enterotoxin in *Escherichia coli*. J Bacteriol. 1978;133:172.
40. Wachsmith K, Wells J, Shipley P, et al. Heat-labile enterotoxin production in isolates from a shipboard outbreak of human diarrheal illness. Infect Immun. 1979;24:793–7.
41. Sack RB. Human diarrheal disease caused by enterotoxigenic *Escherichia coli*. Annu Rev Microbiol. 1975;29:333.
42. Merson MH, Black RE, Gross RJ, et al. Use of antisera for identification of enterotoxigenic *E. coli*. Lancet. 1980;2:222.
43. Ryder RW, Wachsmuth IK, Buxton AE, et al. Infantile diarrhea produced by heat-stable enterotoxigenic *Escherichia coli*. N Engl J Med. 1976;295:849.
44. Gross RJ, Rowe B, Henderson A, et al. A new *Escherichia coli* O-group, O159, associated with outbreaks of enteritis in infants. Scand J Infect Dis. 1976;8:195.
45. Haltalin KC. Neonatal shigellosis. Am J Dis Child. 1967;114:603.
46. Schroeder SA, Aserkoff B, Brachman PS. Epidemic salmonellosis in hospitals and institutions. N Engl J Med. 1968;279:674.
47. Rice PA, Craven PC, Wells JG: *Salmonella heidelberg* enteritis and bacteremia. An epidemic on two pediatric wards. Am J Med. 1976;60:509.
48. Eichenwald HF, Ababio A, Arky AM, et al. Epidemic diarrhea in premature and older infants caused by echo virus type 18. JAMA. 1958;166:1563.
49. Yow MD, Melnick JL, Blattner RJ, et al. The association of viruses and bacteria with infantile diarrhea. Am J Epidemiol. 1970;92:33.
50. Moffet HL, Shulenberger HK, Burkholder ER. Epidemiology and etiology of severe infantile diarrhea. J Pediatr. 1968;72:1.
51. Murphy AM, Albrey MB, Crew EB. Rotavirus infections of neonates. Lancet. 1977;2:1149.
52. Cameron DJS, Bishop RF, Davidson GP, et al. New virus associated with diarrhea in neonates. Med J Aust. 1976;1:85.
53. Bishop RF, Hewstone AS, Davidson GP, et al. An epidemic of diarrhea in human neonates involving a reoviruslike agent and "enteropathogenic" serotypes of *Escherichia coli*. J Clin Pathol. 1976;29:46.
54. Chrystie IL, Totterdell BM, Banatvala JE. Asymptomatic endemic rotavirus infections in the newborn. Lancet. 1978;1:1176.
55. Mata LJ, Urrutia JJ. Intestinal colonization of breast-fed children in a rural area of low socioeconomic level. Ann NY Acad Sci. 1971;176:93.
56. Gordon JE, Chitkara ID, Wyon JB. Weanling diarrhea. Am J Med Sci. 1963;245:345.
57. Welsh JK, May JT. Anti-infective properties of breast-milk. J Pediatr. 1979;94:1.
58. Motarjemi Y, Kaferstein F, Moy G, Quevedo F. Contaminated weaning food: A major risk factor for diarrhoea and associated malnutrition. Bull WHO. 1993;71:79–92.
59. King J, Ashworth A. Contemporary feeding practices in infancy and early childhood in developing countries. In: King J, Ashworth A, ed. Infant and child nutrition, worldwide-issues and perspectives. Boca Raton, FL: CRC Press; 1991:141–74.
60. Gordon JE, Guzman MA, Ascoli W, et al. Acute diarrhoeal disease in less developed countries. Bull WHO. 1964;31:9.
61. Reddy V, Rashuramulu N, Bhaskaram C. Secretory IgA in protein-calorie malnutrition. Arch Dis Child. 1976;51:871.
62. Stollar OA, Kaniecki-Green E, Pelley RP, et al. Secretory IgA against enterotoxins in breast milk. Lancet. 1976;1:1258.
63. Brown SE III, Sauer KT, Nations MK, et al. Comparison of paired whole milk and dried filter paper samples for anti-enterotoxin and antirotavirus activities. J Clin Microbiol. 1982;16:103.
64. Bullen CL, Willis AT. Resistance of the breast-fed infant to gastroenteritis. Br Med J. 1971;3:338.
65. Bullen JJ, Rogers HJ, Leigh L. Iron-binding proteins in milk and resistance of *Escherichia coli* infection in infants. Br Med J. 1972;1:69.
66. Simhon A, Mata LJ. Anti-rotavirus antibody in human colostrum. Lancet. 1978;1:39.
67. Gorbach SL, Khurana CM. Toxigenic *Escherichia coli*: A cause of infantile diarrhea in Chicago. N Engl J Med. 1972;287:791.
68. Tacket CO, Losonsky G, Link H, et al. Protection by milk immunoglobulin concentrate against oral challenge with enterotoxigenic *Escherichia coli*. N Engl J Med. 1988;318:1240–3.
69. Echeverria P, Blacklow NR, Smith DH. Role of heat-labile toxigenic *Escherichia coli* and reovirus-like agent in diarrhea in Boston children. Lancet. 1975;2:1113.
70. Hughes JM, Gwaltney JM, Hughes DH, et al. Acute gastrointestinal illness in Charlottesville: A prospective family study (Abstract). Clin Res. 1978;26:24.
71. Guerrant RL, Hughes JM, Lima NL, et al. Microbiology of diarrhea in developed and developing countries. Rev Inf Dis. 1990;12:S41–50.
72. Chen LC, Rohde JE, Sharp GWG. Intestinal adenyl-cyclase activity in human cholera. Lancet. 1971;1:939.
73. Guerrant RL, Chen LC, Sharp GWG. Intestinal adenyl-cyclase activity in canine cholera: Correlation with fluid accumulation. J Infect Dis. 1972;125:377.
74. Evans DJ Jr, Chen LC, Curlin GT, et al. Stimulation of adenyl cyclase by *Escherichia coli* enterotoxin. Nature. 1972;236:137.
75. Guerrant RL, Ganguly U, Casper AGT, et al. Effect of *Escherichia coli* on fluid transport across canine small bowel: Mechanism and time course—with enterotoxin and whole bacterial cells. J Clin Invest. 1973;52:1707.
76. Kantor HS, Tao P, Gorbach SL. Stimulation of intestinal adenyl cyclase by *Escherichia coli* enterotoxin: Comparison of strains from an infant and an adult with diarrhea. J Infect Dis. 1974;129:1.
77. Hughes JM, Murad F, Chang B, et al. Role of cyclic GMP in the action of heat stable enterotoxin of *Escherichia coli*. Nature. 1978;271:755.
78. Field M, Graf LH Jr, Laird WJ, et al. Heat-stable enterotoxin of *Escherichia coli*: In vitro effects on guanylate cyclase activity, cyclic GMP concentration, and ion transport in small intestine. Proc Natl Acad Sci USA. 1978;75:2800.
79. Guerrant RL, Hughes JM, Chang B, et al. Activation of intestinal guanylate cyclase by heat stable enterotoxin of *E. coli*: Studies of tissue specificity, potential receptors, and intermediates. J Infect Dis. 1980;142:220.
80. Bishop RF, Davidson GP, Holmes IH, et al. Virus particles in epithelial cells of duodenal mucosa from children with acute non-bacterial gastroenteritis. Lancet. 1973;2:1281.
81. Flewett TH, Bryden AS, Davies H. Virus particles in gastroenteritis. Lancet. 1973;2:1497.
82. Kapikian AZ, Kim HW, Wyatt RG, et al. Reoviruslike agent in stools: Association with infantile diarrhea and development of serologic tests. Science. 1974;185:1049.
83. Kanno T, Suzuki H, Ishida N. Reovirus-like agent in Japanese infants with gastroenteritis. Lancet. 1975;1:918.
84. Virus of infantile gastroenteritis (Editorial). Br Med J. 1975;3:555.
85. Rotaviruses of man and animals (Editorial). Lancet. 1975;1:257.
86. Mata L, Simhon A, Padilla R, et al. Diarrhea associated with rotaviruses, enterotoxigenic *E. coli*, *Campylobacter*, and other agents in Costa Rican children, 1976–1981. Am J Trop Med Hyg. 1983;32:146.
87. Black RE, Merson MH, Rahman ASMM, et al. A two-year study of bacterial, viral, and parasitic agents associated with diarrhea in rural Bangladesh. J Infect Dis. 1980;142:660.
88. Echeverria P, Ho MT, Blacklow NR, et al. Relative importance of viruses and bacteria in the etiology of pediatric diarrhea in Taiwan. J Infect Dis. 1977;136:383.
89. Paul MO, Erinle EA. Influence of humidity on rotavirus prevalence among Nigerian infants and young children with gastroenteritis. J Clin Microbiol. 1982;15:212.
90. Brandt CD, Kim HW, Rodriguez WJ. Rotavirus gastroenteritis and weather. J Clin Microbiol. 1982;16:478.
91. Gurwith M, Wenman W, Gurwith D, et al. Diarrhea among infants and young children in Canada: A longitudinal study in three Northern communities. J Infect Dis. 1983;147:685.
92. Shepherd RW, Truslow S, Walker-Smith JA. Infantile gastroenteritis: A clinical study of reovirus-like agent infection. Lancet. 1975;2:1082.
93. Sexton M, Davidson GP, Bishop RF, et al. Viruses in gastroenteritis. Lancet. 1974;2:355.
94. Tallett S, MacKenzie C, Middleton P, et al. Clinical, laboratory, and epidemiologic features of a viral gastroenteritis in infants and children. Pediatrics. 1977;60:217.
95. Kim HW, Brandt CD, Kapikian AZ, et al. Human reoviruslike agent infection. Occurrence in adult contacts of pediatric patients with gastroenteritis. JAMA. 1977;238:404.
96. Wenman WM, Hinde D, Feltham S, et al. Rotavirus infection in adults: Results of a prospective family study. N Engl J Med. 1979;301:303.
97. Kapikian AZ, Dienstag JL, Purcell RH. Immune electron microscopy as a method for the detection, identification, and characterization of agents not cultivable in an in vitro system. In: Rose NR, Friedman H, eds: Manual of Clinical Immunology. Washington, DC: American Society for Microbiology; 1976.
98. Zissis G, Lambert JP. Different serotypes of human rotaviruses. Lancet. 1978;1:38.
99. Beards GM, Pilford JN, Thouless ME, et al. Rotavirus serotypes by serum neutralization. J Med Virol. 1980;5:231.

100. Blacklow NR, Cukor G. Viral gastroenteritis. N Engl J Med. 1981;304:397.
101. Urasawa S, Urasawa T, Taniguchi K. Three human rotavirus serotypes demonstrated by plaque neutralization of isolated strains. Infect Immun. 1982; 38:781.
102. Fonteyne J, Zissis G, Lambert JP. Recurrent rotavirus gastroenteritis. Lancet. 1978;1:983.
103. Yolken R, Kim HW, Clem T, et al. Enzyme immunoassay (ELISA) for the detection of human reovirus-like agent in human stools. Lancet. 1977;2:263.
104. Kalica AR, Purcell RH, Sereno NM, et al. Microtiter solid phase radioimmunoassay for detection of the human reovirus-like agent in stools. J Immunol. 1977;118:1275.
105. Middleton PJ, Petrie M, Hewitt CM, et al. Counter-immunoelectroosmophoresis for the detection of infantile gastroenteritis virus (orbi group) antigen and antibody. J Clin Pathol. 1976;29:191.
106. Middleton PJ, Szymanski MT, Abbott GD, et al. Orbivirus acute gastroenteritis of infancy. Lancet. 1974;1:1241.
107. Davidson GP, Goller I, Bishop RF, et al. Immunofluorescence in duodenal mucosa of children with acute enteritis due to a new virus. J Clin Pathol. 1975;28:263.
108. Thomas EE, Puterman ML, Kawano E, et al. Evaluation of seven immunoassays for detection of rotavirus in pediatric stool samples. J Clin Microbiol. 1988;26:1189–93.
109. Flores J, Purcell RH, Perez I, et al. A dot hybridization assay for detection of rotavirus. Lancet. 1983;1:555.
110. Flewett TH, Bryden AS, Davies H, et al. Relation between viruses from acute gastroenteritis of children and newborn calves. Lancet. 1974;2:61.
111. Purdham DR, Purdham PA, Evans N, et al. Isolation of human rotavirus using human embryonic gut monolayers. Lancet. 1975;2:977.
112. Banatvala JE, Totterdell B, Chrystie IL, et al. In vitro detection of human rotaviruses. Lancet. 1975;2:821.
113. Wyatt RG, Gill VW, Sereno MM, et al. Probable in vitro cultivation of human reovirus-like agent of infantile diarrhea. Lancet. 1976;1:98.
114. Middleton PJ, Petric M, Szymanski MT. Propagation of infantile gastroenteritis virus (orbi-group) in conventional and germfree piglets. Infect Immun. 1975;12:1276.
115. Wyatt RG, Sly DL, London WT, et al. Induction of diarrhea in colostrum deprived newborn rhesus monkeys with human reovirus-like agent of infantile gastroenteritis. Arch Virol. 1976;50:17.
116. Wyatt RG, James SD, Bohl EH, et al. Human rotavirus type 2: Cultivation in vitro. Science. 1980;207:189.
117. Sato K, Inaba Y, Shinozuka T, et al. Isolation of human rotavirus in cell cultures. Arch Virol. 1981;69:155.
118. Urasawa T, Urasawa S, Taniguchi K. Sequential passages of human rotavirus in MA-104 cells. Microbiol Immunol. 1981;25:1025.
119. Kutsuzawa T, Konno T, Suzuki H, et al. Isolation of human rotavirus subgroups 1 and 2 in cell culture. J Clin Microbiol. 1982;16:727.
120. Guerrant RL. Pathophysiology of the enterotoxic and viral diarrhea. In: Chen LC, Scrimshaw NS, eds. Diarrhea and Malnutrition: Interactions, Mechanisms and Interventions. New York: Plenum; 1983;23–43.
121. Middleton PJ, Szymanski MT, Abbott GD, et al. Orbivirus acute gastroenteritis of infancy. Lancet. 1974;1:1241.
122. Davidson GP, Goller I, Bishop RF, et al. Immunofluorescence in duodenal mucosa of children with acute enteritis due to a new virus. J Clin Pathol. 1974;28:263.
123. Sack DA, Chowdhury AMAK, Eusof A, et al. Oral hydration in rotavirus diarrhea: A double blind comparison of sucrose with glucose electrolyte solution. Lancet. 1978;2:280.
124. Davidson GP, Barnes GL. Structural and functional abnormalities of the small intestine in infants and young children with rotavirus enteritis. Acta Paediatr Scand. 1979;68:181.
125. Shepherd RW, Butler DG, Cutz E, et al. The mucosal lesion in viral enteritis: Extent and dynamics of the epithelial response to virus invasion in transmissible gastroenteritis of piglets. Gastroenterology. 1979;76:770.
126. Davidson GP, Gall DG, Petric M, et al. Human rotavirus enteritis induced in conventional piglets: Intestinal structure and transport. J Clin Invest. 1977; 60:1402.
127. Vesikari T, Isolauri E, D'Hondt E, et al. Protection of infants against rotavirus diarrhea: R1T 4237 attenuated bovine rotavirus vaccine. Lancet. 1984; 1:977–80.
128. Edelman R. Perspective on the development and deployment of rotavirus vaccines. Pediatr Infect Dis. 1987;6:704.
129. Gordon I, Ingraham HS, Korns RF. Transmission of epidemic gastroenteritis to human volunteers by oral administration of fecal filtrates. J Exp Med. 1947;86:409.
130. Jordan WS, Gordon I, Dorrance WR. A study of illness in a group of Cleveland families. VII. Transmission of acute nonbacterial gastroenteritis to volunteers: Evidence for two different etiologic agents. J Exp Med. 1953;98: 461.
131. Kojima S, Fukumi H, Kusama H, et al. Studies on the causative agent of the infectious diarrhea; records of the experiments on human volunteers. Jpn Med J. 1948;1:467.
132. Klein JO, Lerner AM, Finland M. Acute gastroenteritis associated with echo virus, type II. Am J Med Sci. 1950;240:749.
133. Kerr AA, McQuillin J, Downham MAPS, et al. Gastric "flu" influenza B causing abdominal symptoms in children. Lancet. 1975;1:291.
134. Adler JL, Zickl R. Winter vomiting disease. J Infect Dis. 1969;119:668.
135. Dolin R, Blacklow NR, DuPont H, et al. Transmission of acute infectious nonbacterial gastroenteritis to volunteers by oral administration of stool filtrates. J Infect Dis. 1971;123:307.
136. Kapikian AZ, Wyatt RG, Dolin R, et al. Visualization by immune electron microscopy of a 27-nm particle associated with acute infectious nonbacterial gastroenteritis. J Virol. 1972;10:1075.
137. Zahorsky J. Hyperemesis heimis or the winter vomiting disease. Arch Pediatr. 1929;46:391.
138. Agus SG, Dolin R, Wyatt RG, et al. Acute infectious nonbacterial gastroenteritis. Intestinal histopathology. Ann Intern Med. 1973;79:18.
139. Schreiber DS, Trier JS, Blacklow NR. Recent advances in viral gastroenteritis. Gastroenterology. 1977;73:174.
140. Levy AG, Widerlite L, Schwartz CJ, et al. Jejunal adenylate cyclase activity in human subjects during viral gastroenteritis. Gastroenterology. 1976;70: 321.
141. Blacklow NR, Dolin R, Fedson DS, et al. Acute infectious nonbacterial gastroenteritis: Etiology and pathogenesis. Ann Intern Med. 1972;76:993.
142. Wyatt RG, Dolin R, Blacklow NR, et al. Comparison of three agents of acute infectious nonbacterial gastroenteritis by cross-challenge in volunteers. J Infect Dis. 1974;129:709.
143. Dolin R, Treanor JJ, Madore HP. Novel agents of viral enteritis in humans. J Infect Dis. 1987;155:365–76.
144. Clarke SKR, Cook GT, Egglestone SI, et al. A virus from epidemic vomiting disease. Br Med J. 1972;3:86.
145. Appleton H, Buckley M, Thom BT, et al. Virus-like particles in winter vomiting disease. Lancet. 1977;1:409.
146. Morens DM, Zweighaft RM, Vernon TM. A waterborne outbreak of gastroenteritis with secondary person-to-person spread. Lancet. 1979;1:964.
147. Oshiro LS, Haley CE, Roberto RR, et al. A 27-nm virus isolated during an outbreak of acute infectious nonbacterial gastroenteritis in a convalescent hospital: A possible new serotype. J Infect Dis. 1981;143:791.
148. Caul EO, Appleton H. The electron microscopical and physical characteristics of small round human fecal viruses: An interim scheme for classification. J Med Virol. 1982;9:257–65.
149. Brandt CD, Kim HW, Rodriguez WJ, et al. Adenoviruses and pediatric gastroenteritis. J Infect Dis. 1985;151:437–43.
150. Gerna G, Passarani N, Battaglia M, et al. Human enteric coronaviruses: Antigenic relatedness to human coronavirus OC43 and possible etiologic role in viral gastroenteritis. J Infect Dis. 1985;151:796–802.
151. Battaglia M, Passarani N, DiMatteo A, et al. Human enteric coronaviruses: Further characterization and immunoblotting of viral proteins. J Infect Dis. 1987;144:140–3.
152. Yolken R, Santosham M, Reid R, et al. Pestiviruses: Major etiological agents of gastroenteritis in human infants and children (Abstract). Clin Res. 1988; 36:780.
153. Greenberg HB, Valdesuso J, Yolken RH, et al. Role of Norwalk virus in outbreaks of nonbacterial gastroenteritis. J Infect Dis. 1979;139:564.
154. Kaplan JE, Gary GW Jr, Baron RC, et al. Epidemiology of Norwalk gastroenteritis and the role of the Norwalk virus in outbreaks of nonbacterial gastroenteritis. Ann Intern Med. 1982;96:756.
155. Moe CL, Monroe SS, Gary HE Jr, et al. Detection of astrovirus in pediatric stool samples by immunoassay and RNA probe. J Clin Microbiol. 1991;29: 2390–6.
156. Lew JF, Moe CL, Monroe SS, et al. Astrovirus and adenovirus associated with diarrhea in children in day care settings. J Infect Dis. 1991;164:673–8.
157. Cruz JR, Bartlett AV, Herrmann JE, et al. Astrovirus-associated diarrhea among Guatemalan ambulatory, rural children. J Clin Microbiol. 1992;30: 1140–4.
158. Lew JF, Glass RI, Petric M, et al. Six-year retrospective surveillance of gastroenteritis virus identified at ten electron microscopy centers in the United States and Canada. Pediatr Infect Dis. 1990;9:709–14.
159. Greenberg HB, Wyatt RG, Valdesuso J, et al. Solid-phase microtiter radioimmunoassay for detection of the Norwalk strain of acute nonbacterial, epidemic gastroenteritis virus and its antibodies. J Med Virol. 1978;2:97.
160. Jiang X, Wang M, Graham DY, et al. Expression, self-assembly, and antigenicity of the Norwalk virus capsid protein. J Virol. 1992;66:6527–32.
161. Parrino TA, Schreiber DS, Trier JS, et al. Clinical immunity in acute gastroenteritis caused by Norwalk agent. N Engl J Med. 297:86–89, 1977;297: 86–9.
162. Herrmann JE, Perron-Henry DM, Blacklow NR. Antigen detection with monoclonal antibodies for the diagnosis of adenovirus gastroenteritis. J Infect Dis. 1987;155:1167–71.
163. Shinozaki T, Araki K, Ushijima H, et al. Use of Graham 293 cells in suspension for isolating enteric adenoviruses from the stools of patients with acute gastroenteritis. J Infect Dis. 1987;156:246.
164. Neil C, Gomes SA, Leite JPG, et al. Direct detection and differentiation of fastidious and nonfastidious adenoviruses in stools by using a specific nonradioactive probe. J Clin Microbiol. 1986;24:785–9.
165. von Bonsdorff CH, Hovi T, Makela P, et al. Rotavirus associated with acute gastroenteritis in adults. Lancet. 1976;2:423.

166. Wenman WM, Hinde D, Feltham S, et al. Rotavirus infection in adults. Results of a prospective study. N Engl J Med. 1979;301:306.

167. Yolken RH, Bishop CA, Townsend TR, et al. Infectious gastroenteritis in bone-marrow transplant recipients. N Engl J Med. 1982;306:1099.

168. Goodgame RW, Greenough WBIII. Cholera in Africa: A message for the west. Ann Intern Med. 1975;82:101.

169. Weissman JB, DeWitt WE, Thompson J, et al. A case of cholera in Texas, 1973. Am J Epidemiol. 1975;100:487.

170. Blake PA, Allegra DT, Snyder JD, et al. Cholera: A possible endemic focus in the United States. N Engl J Med. 1980;302:305.

171. Blake PA, Rosenberg ML, Florencia J, et al. Cholera in Portugal, 1974. II. Transmission by bottled mineral water. Am J Epidemiol. 1977;105:344.

172. Baine WB, Mazzotti M, Greco D, et al. Epidemiology of cholera in Italy in 1973. Lancet. 1974;2:1370.

173. Gitelson S. Gastrectomy, achlorhydria and cholera. Isr J Med Sci. 1971;7:663.

174. Ramamurthy T, Garg S, Sharma R, et al. Emergence of novel strain of *Vibrio cholerae* with epidemic potential in southern and eastern India (Letter). Lancet. 1993;341:703–4.

175. Albert MJ, Siddique AK, Islam MS, et al. Large outbreak of clinical cholera due to *Vibrio cholerae* non-O1 in Bangladesh (Letter). Lancet. 1993;341:704.

176. Bhattacharya MK, Bhattacharya SK, Garg S, et al. Outbreak of *Vibrio cholerae* non-O1 in India and Bangladesh (Letter). Lancet. 1993;341:1346–7.

177. Shimada T, Nair GB, Deb BC, et al. Outbreak of *Vibrio cholerae* non-O1 in India and Bangladesh (Letter). Lancet. 1993;341:1347.

178. Centers for Disease Control and Prevention. Emerging infectious diseases: Imported cholera associated with a newly described toxigenic *Vibrio cholerae* O139 strain—California, 1993. MMWR. 1993;42:501–3.

179. Snow J. On the Mode of Communication of Cholera. 2nd ed. London: Churchill; 1855.

180. De SN, Bhattacharya K, Sarkar JK. A study of the pathogenicity of strains of *Bacterium coli* from acute and chronic enteritis. J Pathol Bacteriol. 1956;71:201.

181. Trabulsi LR. Revelação de colibacilos associados as diarreias infantis pelo metodo da infeção experimental da alca ligade do intestino do coelho. Rev Inst Med Trop Sao Paulo. 1964;6:197.

182. Taylor J, Wilkins MP, Payne JM. Relation of rabbit gut reaction to enteropathogenic *Escherichia coli*. Br J Exp Pathol. 1961;42:43.

183. Taylor J, Bettleheim KA. The action of chloroform-killed suspensions of enteropathegenic *Escherichia coli* on ligated rabbit-gut segments. J Gen Microbiol. 1966;42:309.

184. Smith HW, Halls S. Studies on *Escherichia coli* enterotoxin. J Pathol Bacteriol. 1967;93:531.

185. Gorbach SL, Banwell JG, Chatterjee BD, et al. Acute undifferentiated human diarrhea in the tropics. I. Alterations in intestinal microflora. J Clin Invest. 1971;50:881.

186. Banwell JG, Gorbach SL, Pierce NF, et al. Acute undifferentiated human diarrhea in the tropics. II. Alterations in intestinal fluid and electrolyte movements. J Clin Invest. 1971;50:890.

187. Sack RB, Gorbach SL, Banwell JG, et al. Enterotoxigenic *Escherichia coli* isolated from patients with severe cholera-like disease. J Infect Dis. 1971;123:378.

188. DuPont HL, Formal SB, Hornick RB, et al. Pathogenesis of *Escherichia coli* diarrhea. N Engl J Med. 1971;285:1.

189. Evans DG, Evans DJ Jr, Pierce NF. Differences in the response of rabbit small intestine to heat-labile and heat-stable enterotoxins of *Escherichia coli*. Infect Immun. 1973;7:873.

190. Guerrant RL, Brunton LL, Schnaitman TC, et al. Cyclic adenosine monophosphate and alteration of Chinese hamster ovary cell morphology: A rapid, sensitive in vitro assay for the enterotoxins of *Vibrio cholerae* ane *Escherichia coli*. Infect Immun. 1974;10:320.

191. Donta ST, Moon HW, Whipp SC. Detection of heat-labile *Escherichia coli* enterotoxin with the use of adrenal cells in tissue culture. Science. 1974;183:334.

192. Guerrant RL, Brunton LL. Characterization of the Chinese hamster ovary cell assy for the enterotoxins of *Vibrio cholerae* and *Escherichia coli* and for antitoxin: Differential inhibition by gangliosides, specific antisera, and toxoid. J Infect Dis. 1977;135:720.

193. Honda T, Arita M, Takeda Y, et al. Further evaluation of the Biken test (modified Elek test) for detection of enterotoxigenic *E. coli* producing heat-labile enterotoxin and application of the test to sampling of heat-stable enterotoxin. J Clin Microbiol. 1982;16:60.

194. Alderete JF, Robertson DC. Purification and chemical characterization of the heat-stable enterotoxin produced by porcine strains of enterotoxigenic *Escherichia coli*. Infect Immun. 1978;19:1021.

195. Dean AG, Ching YC, Williams RG, et al. Test for *Escherichia coli* enterotoxin using infant mice: Application in a study of diarrhea in children in Honolulu. J Infect Dis. 1972;125:407.

196. Gyles CL. Limitation of the infant mouse test for *E. coli* heat-stable enterotoxin. Can J Comp Med. 1979;43:371–9.

197. Kennedy DJ, Greenberg RN, Dunn JA, et al. Effects of *Escherichia coli* heat stable enterotoxin STb on intestines of mice, rats, rabbits and piglets. Infect Immun. 1984;46:639–43.

198. Weikel CS, Mellans HN, Guerrant RL. In vivo and in vitro effects of a novel enterotoxin, STb, produced by *Escherichia coli*. J Infect Dis. 1986;153:893–901.

199. Rosenberg ML, Koplan JP, Wachsmuth IK, et al. Epidemic diarrhea at Crater Lake from enterotoxigenic *Escherichia coli*. A large, waterborne outbreak. Ann Intern Med. 1977;86:714.

200. Korzeniowski OM, Dantas W, Trabulsi LR, et al. A controlled study of endemic sporadic diarrhea among adult residents of southern Brazil. Trans R Soc Trop Med Hyg. 1984;78:363–9.

201. Hughes JM, Rouse JD, Barada FA, et al. Etiology of summer diarrhea among the Navajo. Am J Trop Med Hyg. 1980;29:613.

202. Current WL, Reese NC, Ernst JV, et al. Human cryptosporidiosis in immunocompetent and immunodeficient persons. N Engl J Med. 1983;308:1252.

203. Tzipori S. Cryptosporidiosis in animals and humans. Microbiol Rev. 1983;47:84.

204. Wolfson JS, Richter JM, Waldron MA, et al. Cryptosporidiosis in immunocompetent patients. N Engl J Med. 1985;312:1278–82.

205. Palmer DL, Koster FT, Islam AFMR, et al. A comparison of sucrose and glucose in oral electrolyte therapy of cholera and other severe diarrheas. N Engl J Med. 1977;297:1107.

206. Ericsson CD, Evans DG, DuPont HL, et al. Bismuth subsalicylate inhibits activity of crude toxins of *Escherichia coli* and *Vibrio cholerae*. J Infect Dis. 1977;136:693.

207. Gelb A, Miller S. AIDS and gastroenterology. Am J Gastroenterol. 1986;81:619–22.

208. Soave R, Johnson WD. *Crytposporidium* and *Isospora belli* infections. J Infect Dis. 1988;157:225–9.

209. Kotler DP, Goetz HP, Lange M, et al. Enteropathy associated with the acquired immunodeficiency syndrome. Ann Intern Med. 1984;101:421–8.

210. Gillin JS, Shike M, Alcock N, et al. Malabsorption and mucosal abnormalities of the small intestine in the acquired immunodeficiency syndrome. Ann Intern Med. 1985;102:619–22.

211. Nelson JA, Reynolds-Kohler G, Margaretten W, et al. Human immunodeficiency virus detected in bowel eptiehlium from patients with gastro-intestinal symptoms. Lancet. 1988;1:259–62.

212. Smith PD, Lance C, Gill VJ, et al. Intestinal infections in patients with the acquired immunodeficiency syndrome (AIDS). Ann Intern Med. 1988;108:328–33.

213. Laughon BE, Druckman DA, Vernon A, et al. Prevalence of enteric pathogens in homosexual men with and without acquired immunodeficiency syndrome. Gastroenterology. 1988;94:984.

214. Quinn TC, Stamm WE, Goodell SE, et al. The polymicrobial origin of intestinal infections in homosexual men. N Engl J Med. 1983;309:576–82.

215. Kotler DP, Francisco A, Clayton F, et al. Small intestinal injury and parasitic diseases in AIDS. Ann Intern Med. 1990;113:444–9.

216. Connolly GM, Forbes A, Gazzard BG. Investigation of seemingly pathogen-negative diarrhoea in patients infected with HIV1. Gut 1990;31:886–9.

217. Guerrant RL, Bobak DA. Bacterial and protozoal gastroenteritis. N Engl J Med 1991;325:327–40.

218. Carter TR, Cooper PH, Petri WA Jr, et al. *Pneumocystis carinii* infection of the small intestine in a patient with acquired immune deficiency syndrome. Am J Clin Pathol. 1988;89:679–83.

219. Chachoua A, Dieterich D, Krasinski K, et al. 9-(1,3-Dihydroxy-2-propoxymethyl) guanine (ganciclovir) in the treatment of cytomegalovirus gastrointestinal disease with the acquired immunodeficiency syndrome. Ann Intern Med. 1987;107:133–7.

220. Celum CL, Chaisson RE, Rutherford GW, et al. Incidence of salmonellosis in patients with AIDS. J Infect Dis. 1987;156:998–1002.

221. Jacobs JL, Gold JWM, Murray HW, et al. *Salmonella* infections in patients with the acquired immunodeficiency syndrome. Ann Intern Med. 1985;102:186–8.

222. Glaser JB, Morton-Kute L, Berger SR, et al. Recurrent *Salmonella typhimurium* bacteremia associated with the acquired immunodeficiency syndrome. Ann Intern Med. 1985;102:189–93.

223. Sperber SJ, Schleupner CJ: Salmonellosis during infection with human immunodeficiency virus. Rev Infect Dis. 1987;9:925–34.

224. Grohman GS, Glass RI, Pereira HG, et al. Enteric viruses and diarrhea in HIV-infected patients. N Engl J Med 1993;329:14–20.

225. Guerrant RL, Hughes JM, Lima NL, et al. Microbiology of diarrhea in developed and developing countries. Rev Infect Dis. 1990;12:S41–50.

226. Stamm WE, Weinstein RA, Dixon RE. Comparison of endemic and epidemic nosocomial infections. Am J Med. 1981;70:393–7.

227. Lima N, Searcy M, Guerrant RL. Nosocomial diarrhea rates exceed those of other nosocomial infections on ICU and pediatric wards (Abstract 1050). In: Proceedings of the 26th Interscience Conference on Antimicrobial Agents and Chemotherapy, New Orleans, 1986.

228. Lima NL, Guerrant RL, Kaiser DL, et al. Nosocomial diarrhea: A possible risk factor for nosocomial infections (Abstract). Clin Res. 1988;36:580.

229. Welliver RC, McLaughlin S. Unique epidemiology of nosocomial infection in a children's hospital. Am J Dis Child. 1984;138:131–5.

230. Kelly WJ, Patrick MR, Hilman KM. Study of diarrhea in critically ill patients. Crit Care Med. 1983;1:7–9.

231. Hughes JM, Jarvis WR. Nosocomial gastrointestinal infections. In: Wenzel RP, ed. Prevention and Control of Nosocomial Infections. Boston: Williams & Wilkins; 1987.

232. Yolken RJ, Bishop CA, Towsend R, et al. Infectious gastroenteritis in bone marrow transplant recipients. N Engl J Med. 1982;306:1009–12.

233. Farber BF, Brennen JC, Puntereri AJ, et al. A prospective study of nosocomial infections in a chronic care facility. J Am Geriatr Soc. 1984;32:499.

234. Nicolle LE, McIntyre M, Zacharias H, et al. Twelve-month surveillance of infections in institutionalized elderly men. J Am Geriatr Soc. 1984;32:513.

235. Bender BS, Laughon BE, Gaydos C, et al. Is Clostridum difficile endemic in chronic-care facilities? Lancet. 1986;2:1279.

236. Treolar AJ, Kalra L. Mortality and Clostridium difficile diarrhoea in the elderly. Lancet. 1987;2:1279.

237. Pickering LK, Evans DG, Dupont HL, et al. Diarrhea caused by Shigella, rotavirus and Giardia in day care centers: Prospective study. J Pediatr. 1981; 99:51–6.

238. Centers for Disease Control and Prevention. Cryptosporidiosis among children attending day-care centers: Georgia, Pennsylvania, Michigan, California, New Mexico. MMWR. 1984;33:599.

239. Alpert G, Bell LM, Kirkpatrick CE, et al. Crystosporidiosis in a day-care center. N Engl J Med. 1984;311:860–1.

240. Taylor JP, Perdue JN, Dingley D, et al. Cryptosporidiosis outbreak in a day-care center. Am J Dis Child. 1985;139:1023–5.

241. Bartlett AV, Moore M, Gary GW, et al. Diarrheal illness among infants and toddlers in daycare centers. I. Epidemiology and pathogens. J Pediatr. 1985; 107:495–502.

242. Guerrant RL, Lohr JA, Williams EK. Acute infectious diarrhea. I. Epidemiology, etiology, and pathogenesis. Pediatr Infect Dis. 1986;5:353–9.

243. Kean BH. The diarrhea of travelers to Mexico. Summary of five-year study. Ann Intern Med. 1963;59:605.

244. Psalms 22:14.

245. Consensus development conference statement on travelers' diarrhea. Rev Infect Dis. 1986;8(Suppl):227–33.

246. Lowenstein MS, Balows A, Gangarosa EJ. Turista at an international congress in Mexico. Lancet. 1973;1:529.

247. Editorial. The diarrhea of travelers: Turista. JAMA. 1962;180:402.

248. Higgens AR. Observations on the health of United States personnel living in Cairo, Egypt. Am J Trop Med Hyg. 1955;4:970.

249. Steffen R. Epidemiologic studies of travelers' diarrhea, severe gastrointestinal infections, and cholera. Rev Infect Dis. 1986;8(Suppl 2):122–30.

250. Steffen R, Rickernbach M, Wilhelm U, et al. Health problems after travel to developing countries. J Infect Dis. 1987;156:84–91.

251. Kean BH, Schaffner W, Brennan RW. The diarrhea of travelers. V. Prophylaxis with phthalylsulfathiazole and neomycin sulphate. JAMA. 1962;180: 367–71.

252. Rowe B, Taylor J, Bettelheim KA. An investigation of travelers' diarrhea. Lancet. 1970;1:1.

253. Gorbach SL, Kean BH, Evans DG, et al. Travelers' diarrhea and toxigenic Escherichia coli. N Engl J Med. 1975;292:933.

254. Merson MH, Morris GK, Sack DA, et al. Travelers' diarrhea in Mexico, a prospective study of physicians and family members attending a congress. N Engl J Med. 1976;294:1299.

255. Sack DA, Kaminsky DC, Sack RB, et al. Enterotoxigenic Escherichia coli diarrhea of travelers: A prospective study of American Peace Corps volunteers. Johns Hopkins Med J. 1977;141:63.

256. Guerrant RL, Rouse JD, Hughes JM. Turista among members of the Yale Glee Club in Latin America. Am J Trop Med Hyg. 1980;29:895.

257. Turner AC. Travelers' diarrhoea: A survey of symptoms, occurrence, and possible prophylaxis. Br Med. J. 1967;4:453–4.

258. Black RE. Pathogens that cause travelers' diarrhea in Latin America and Africa. Rev Infect Dis. 1986;8(Suppl 2):131–5.

259. Taylor DN, Echeverria P. Etiology and epidemiology of travelers' diarrhea in Asia. Rev Infect Dis. 1986;8(Suppl 2):136–41.

260. Bolivar R, Conklin RH, Vollet JJ, et al. Rotavirus in travelers' diarrhea: Study of an adult student population in Mexico. J Infect Dis. 1978;137:324.

261. Ryder RW, Oquist CA, Greenberg H, et al. Travelers' diarrhea in Panamanian tourists in Mexico. J Infect Dis. 1981;144:442.

262. Snyder JD, Blake PA. Is cholera a problem for US travelers? JAMA. 1982; 247:2268.

263. Echeverria P, Hodge FA, Blacklow NR, et al. Travelers' diarrhea among United States marines in South Korea. Am J Epidemiol. 1978;108:68.

264. Wolfe MS. Current concepts in parasitology. Giardiasis. N Engl J Med. 1978; 298:319.

265. Brodsky RE, Spencer HC Jr, Schultz MG. Giardiasis in American travelers to the Soviet Union. J Infect Dis. 1974;130:319.

266. Soave R, Armstrong D. Cryptosporidium and cryptosporidiosis. Rev Infect Dis. 1986;8:1012–23.

267. Jokipii L, Pohjola S, Jokipii AMM. Cryptosporidium: A frequent finding in patients with gastrointestinal symptoms. Lancet. 1983;2:358–60.

268. Kean BH, Reilly PC. Malaria—The mime. Recent lessons from a group of civilian travelers. Am J Med. 1976;61:159.

269. Pearson RD, Hewlett EL, Guerrant RL. Tropical diseases in North America. DM. 1984;30:1–68.

270. Hill DR, Pearson RD. Health advice for international travel. Ann Intern Med. 1988;108:839–52.

271. Kean BH, Waters SR. Diarrhea of travelers. III. Drug prophylaxis in Mexico. N Engl J Med. 1959;261:71.

272. Oakley GP. The neurotoxicity of the halogenated hydroxyquinolines. JAMA. 1973;225:395.

273. Portnoy BL, DuPont HL, Pruitt D, et al. Antidiarrheal agents in the treatment of acute diarrhea in children. JAMA. 1976;236:844.

274. DuPont HL, Hornick RB. Adverse effect of Lomotil therapy in shigellosis. JAMA. 1973;226:1525.

275. DuPont HL, Sullivan P, Pickering LK, et al. Symptomatic treatment of diarrhea with bismuth subsalicylate among students attending a Mexican university. Gastroenterology. 1977;73:715.

276. Steffen R, Heusser R, DuPont HL. Prevention of travelers' diarrhea by non-antibiotic drugs. Rev Infect Dis. 1986;8:(Suppl 2):151–9.

277. Blaser MJ. Environmental interventions for the prevention of travelers' diarrhea. Rev Infect Dis. 1986;8(Suppl 2):142–50.

278. Gonzales-Cortez A, Gangarosa EJ, Parrilla C, et al. Bottled beverages and typhoid fever: The Mexican epidemic of 1972–3. Am J Public Health. 1982; 72:844.

279. Harris JR. Are bottled beverages safe for travelers? Am J Public Health. 1982;72:787.

280. Neumann HH. Travellers' diarrhea. Lancet. 1970;1:420.

281. Tjoa W, DuPont HL, Sullivan P, et al. Location of food consumption and travelers' diarrhea. Am J Epidemiol. 1977;106:61.

282. Sack DA, Kaminsky DC, Sack RB, et al. Prophylactic doxycycline for travelers' diarrhea, results of a prospective double-blind study of Peace Corps volunteers in Kenya. N Engl J Med. 1978;298:758.

283. Echeverria P, Verhaert L, Ulyangco CV, et al. Antimicrobial resistance and enterotoxin production among isolates of Escherichia coli in the Far East. Lancet. 1978;2:589.

284. Murray BE. Resistance of Shigella, Salmonella and other selected enteric pathogens. Rev Infect Dis. 1986;8(Suppl 2):172–81.

285. Mentzing LO, Ringertz O. Salmonella infection in tourists. 2. Prophylaxis against salmonellosis. Acta Pathol Microbiol Scand. 1968;74:405.

286. Ericsson CD, DuPont HL, Matthewson JJ et al. Treatment of travelers' diarrhea with sulfamethoxazole and trimethoprim and loperamide. JAMA. 1990;263:257–61.

287. DuPont HL, Ericsson CD. Prevention and treatment of travelers' diarrhea. N Engl J Med. 1993;328:1821–6.

288. Murray BE, Rensimer ER, DuPont HL. Emergence of high level trimethoprim resistance in fecal E. coli during oral administration of trimethoprim or trimethoprim/sulfamethoxazole. N Engl J Med. 1982;306:130.

289. Tiemens KM, Shipley PL, Correia RA, et al. Sulfamethoxazole–trimethoprim resistant Shigella flexneri in northeastern Brazil. Antimicrob Agents Chemother. 1984;25:653–4.

290. DuPont HL, Reves RR, Galindo E, et al. Treatment of travelers' diarrhea with trimethoprim/sulfamethoxazole and with trimethoprim alone. N Engl J Med. 1983;307:841–4.

291. Ericsson CD, DuPont HL, Sullivan P, et al. Bicozamycin, a poorly absorbable antibiotic, effectively treats travelers' diarrhea. Ann Intern Med. 1983; 98:20.

292. Ericsson CD, Johnson PC, DuPont HL, et al. Ciprofloxacin or trimethoprim–sulfamethoxazole as initial therapy for travelers' diarrhea. Ann Intern Med. 1987;106:216–20.

293. Bandres JC, Mathewson JJ, Ericsson CD, et al. Trimethoprim/sulfamethoxazole remains active against enterotoxigenic Escherichia coli and Shigella species in Guadalajara, Mexico. Am J Med Sci. 1992;303:289–91.

294. Gough A, Barsoum NJ, Mitchell L, et al. Juvenile canine drug-induced arthropathy. Toxicol Appl Pharmacol. 1979;51:177–87.

295. Said SI, Faloona GR. Elevated plasma and tissue levels of vasoactive intestinal polypeptide in the watery diarrhea syndrome due to pancreatic, bronchogenic, and other tumors. N Engl J Med. 1975;293:155.

296. Wolff MS, Giardiasis. JAMA. 1975;233:1362.

297. Murphy TV, Nelson JD. Five vs ten days' therapy with furazolidone for giardiasis. Am J Dis Child. 1983;137:267.

298. Ma P, Soave R. Three-step stool examination for cryptosporidiosis in 10 homosexual men with protracted watery diarrhea. J Infect Dis. 1983;147: 824.

299. Donaldson RM Jr. Small bowel bacterial overgrowth. Adv Intern Med. 1970; 16:191.

300. Gorbach SL. Intestinal microflora. Gastroenterology. 1971;60:1110.

301. Penn RG, Giger DK, Knoop FC, et al. Plesiomonas shigelloides overgrowth in the small intestine. J Clin Microbiol. 1982;15:869.

302. Scott AJ, Khan GA. Partial biliary obstruction with cholangitis producing a blind loop syndrome. Gut. 1968;9:187.

303. Vantrappen G, Janssens J, Hellemans J, et al. Interdigestive motor complex of normal subjects and patients with bacterial overgrowth of the small intestine. J Clin Invest. 1977;59:1158.

304. Heyworth B, Brown J. Jejunal microflora in malnourished Gambian children. Arch Dis Child. 1975;50:27.

305. Roberts SH, James O, Jarvis EH. Bacterial overgrowth syndrome without "blind loop": A cause for malnutrition in the elderly. Lancet. 1977;2:1193.

306. Ruiz-Palacios GM, DuPont HL. Bacterial overgrowth syndrome after acute nonspecific diarrhoea. Lancet. 1978;1:337.

307. Lindenbaum J, Kent TH, Sprinz H. Malabsorption and jejunitis in American Peace Corps Volunteers in Pakistan. Ann Intern Med. 1955;65:1201.

308. Shimada K, Bricknell KS, Finegold SM. Deconjugation of bile acids by intes-

tinal bacteria: Review of literature and additional studies. J Infect Dis. 1969; 119:273.

309. Wanke CA, Guerrant RL. Small bowel colonization alone is a cause of diarrhea. Infect Immun. 1987;55:1924–6.

310. Schlager TA, Guerrant RL. Net fluid secretion and impaired villous function induced by small intestinal colonization by non-toxigenic, colonizing E. coli. Abst. No. 1133, 28th Intersci Conf Antimicrob Agents Chemother. 1988;310.

311. Hamilton JD, Dyer NH, Dawson AM, et al. Assessment and significance of bacterial overgrowth in the small bowel. Q J Med. 1970;39:265.

312. MacDougall LG. The effect of aueromycin on undernourished African children. J Trop Pediatr. 1957;3:74.

313. Levy SB, FitzGerald GB, Macone AB. Changes in intestinal flora of farm personnel after introduction of a tetracycline-supplemented feed on a farm. N Engl J Med. 1976;295:583.

78. ANTIBIOTIC-ASSOCIATED COLITIS

ROBERT FEKETY

Antibiotics are the most important precipitating causes of pseudomembranous colitis, but it is noteworthy that this disease was recognized in the preantibiotic era.[1] Many other factors such as abdominal surgery and antineoplastic chemotherapy are also important in pathogenesis. Cases diagnosed in the 1950s were attributed to *Staphylococcus aureus* and treated with oral vancomycin, but in retrospect some investigators believe that this association was coincidental. Pseudomembranous colitis was rarely recognized from 1960 to 1970, but thereafter it was often diagnosed in patients treated with lincomycin, clindamycin, or broad-spectrum β-lactam antibiotics. In these patients, staphylococci could not be implicated, and many patients died because no effective antibiotic therapy was known. At the University of Michigan Hospitals in 1976, 19 (8 percent) of 242 patients receiving ampicillin or clindamycin developed diarrhea.[2] Only 3 (16 percent) of those 19 patients had pseudomembranous colitis, while the rest had a benign diarrhea of unknown cause that was believed to be related to still poorly defined changes in the bowel flora. We now know that this type of diarrhea is very much more common than pseudomembranous colitis in patients treated with antibiotics.

To better understand the causation of pseudomembranous colitis in the 1970s, investigators administered antibiotics to various species of animals in the hope of producing a model of the human disease. They found that Golden Syrian hamsters were highly susceptible to diarrhea and fatal enterocolitis after being given any one of many antibiotics either orally or parenterally.[3,4] After a cytotoxin neutralizable by *Clostridium sordellii* antitoxin was detected in the feces of these hamsters,[5] cultural studies revealed large numbers of *Clostridium difficile* in their feces and also that this organism produced a cytotoxin that was neutralizable by *C. sordellii* antitoxin.[1] An identical toxin neutralizable with *C. sordellii* antitoxin was then found in the diarrheal stools of a female patient with pseudomembranous colitis who responded to treatment with oral vancomycin.[6] Her stools were subsequently found to be culture positive for *C. difficile* (R Fekety, J Silva, GD Rifkin, VR Dowell, unpublished observations, 1977), and the toxin was neutralizable with *C. difficile* antitoxin. Hamsters inoculated with cell-free filtrates (containing toxin) of broth cultures of *C. difficile* developed enterocolitis,[1] and hamsters passively immunized with *C. sordellii* antitoxin did not develop colitis after being given antibiotics.[7] After *C. difficile* isolates were shown to be uniformly susceptible to vancomycin, antibiotic-treated hamsters were given vancomycin prophylactically per os, and colitis was prevented,[8,9] at least until the

vancomycin was discontinued. When humans with pseudomembranous colitis were studied, it was found that *C. difficile* and/or its cytotoxin were almost always present in stools (R Fekety, J Silva, GD Rifkin, VR Dowell, unpublished observations, 1977).[1,10] It was also learned that many patients with *C. difficile* antibiotic-associated colitis (AAC) did not have grossly visible pseudomembranes and that both pseudomembranous colitis and AAC could be treated successfully by the oral administration of vancomycin or metronidazole. However, most patients with antibiotic-associated diarrhea had neither colitis nor *C. difficile* or its toxin in their stools. This more common and benign type of diarrhea was found to be treatable simply by discontinuing antibiotic therapy and replacing fluid and electrolyte losses.

As a result of these studies, *C. difficile* has become recognized as the most frequent cause of AAC and pseudomembranous colitis. Antibiotics operate in pathogenesis primarily by inhibiting the growth of other species of organisms in the gastrointestinal tract that inhibit the growth and/or toxin production of *C. difficile*. Two comprehensive reviews and a book on *C. difficile* and its role in intestinal disease have been published.[11–13]

PATHOLOGY

The most important characteristic of the disease is acute inflammation of the colonic mucosa. Pseudomembranes may be either extensive or absent; they consist of small, discrete yellow-white plaques or nodules that are easily dislodged (Fig. 1). The pseudomembranes and plaques consist of fibrin, mucus, necrotic epithelial cells, and leukocytes adherent to the underlying inflamed mucosa.[14] Usually only the epithelium and superficial lamina propria are affected, but in severe cases deeper tissues are involved. In some cases, colitis and/or pseudomembranes may not be visible to the naked eye but are detectable microscopically if a biopsy specimen is obtained. The latter patients are often categorized as having nonspecific or acute simple colitis unless *C. difficile* and its toxins are detected in their stools. Pseudomembranes occur throughout the colon, but are usually most prominent in the rectosigmoid area; the ileum is rarely involved unless the patient has a colostomy or ileostomy. Anti-

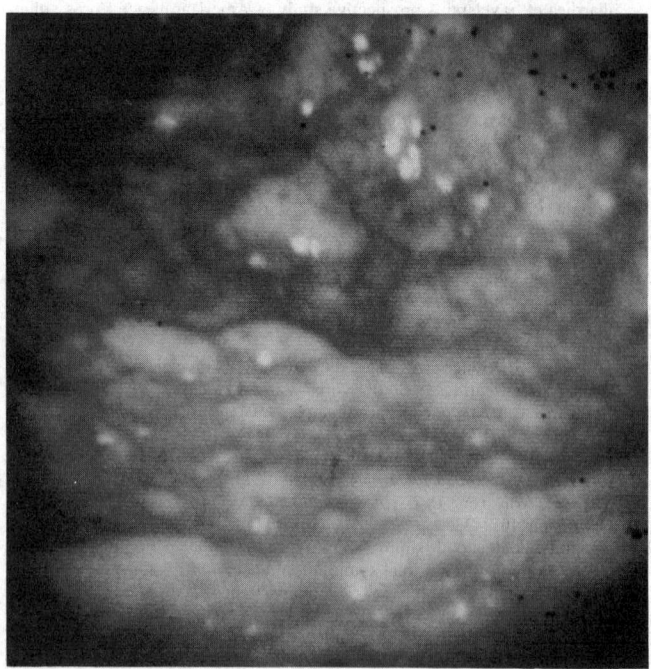

FIG. 1. Proctoscopic view of pseudomembranous colitis in a patient who received clindamycin. Note the 4–8 mm raised white plaques overlying an erythematous mucosa. (From Tedesco et al.,[14] with permission).

biotic-associated colitis is uncommon in infants, who commonly harbor the organism in their stools, but cases have been recognized.[15] Some infants with chronic diarrhea, failure to thrive, and stools positive for *C. difficile* and its toxin have undergone rectal biopsies that revealed cryptitis, and some of them became well after treatment with oral vancomycin.[16]

MICROBIOLOGY, EPIDEMIOLOGY, AND PATHOGENESIS

Clostridium difficile is a spore-forming, gram-positive, obligate anaerobic bacillus that is part of the normal fecal flora of about 3 percent of healthy adults. Colonization rates may be much higher than that (10 to 30 percent or more) in hospitalized persons and in newborns (60–70 percent); often the organism is acquired as a result of cross-infection. We found small numbers of *C. difficile* in the stools of 15 percent of medical patients without diarrhea in our hospital, and stools from 71 percent of asymptomatic infants were positive on a pediatric ward for infants where there was a patient with AAC.[17] The organism has been isolated from healthy dogs, cats, waterfowl, horses, camels, donkeys, seals, hamsters, and guinea pigs,[18] but animals are not considered important in transmission of the organism to humans. Because the organism is not easily distinguished from *C. sporogenes* and several other organisms commonly found in stools, it was difficult initially to detect with ordinary cultural techniques and was overlooked as a cause of pseudomembranous colitis until 1977.[1] In 1979, George and his associates[19] reported that a selective medium containing cycloserine, cefoxitin, and fructose in agar was helpful in isolation of *C. difficile* from stools. The addition of 0.2% highly purified sodium taurocholate to CCFA further increased its ability to detect small numbers of spores in stools or on surfaces.[20] *Clostridium difficile* can be detected in cultures because of its production of *p*-cresol from *p*-hydroxyphenylacetic acid.[21] Alcohol or heat shock techniques also facilitate isolation of the organism from stools.[22]

Staphylococcus aureus is now a very uncommon cause of AAC, and many doubt that it can cause the disease, although our experience suggests that it can.[23] As observed in earlier times, staphylococcal enterocolitis involved the ileum and cecum more often than it did the colon and rectum and usually followed the use of tetracyclines or chloramphenicol, antibiotics that are now rarely associated with colitis. *Clostridium perfringens* type C and salmonellae have also been implicated in rare cases of pseudomembranous colitis.[24,25]

Clostridium difficile colitis occurs at all ages but is most frequent in middle-aged or elderly adults and debilitated patients. Other groups at higher risk include women, patients with cancer or burns, and patients undergoing surgery (especially abdominal surgery) or who are in intensive care units.[17] Even a short course of antibiotic therapy given for prophylaxis or treatment of minor infections may permit spores of the organism to germinate, overgrow, produce toxins, and cause colitis. AAC may follow the oral, intramuscular, intravenous, or topical administration of antibiotics. The list of inciting antimicrobials is extensive and includes penicillin G, ampicillin, amoxicillin, carbenicillin, ticarcillin, cephalothin, cefazolin, cephalexin, cefamandole, cefoxitin, cefotaxime, moxalactam, cefoperazone, ceftizoxime, ceftazidime, ceftriaxone, cefpodoxime, cefixime, imipenemcilastatin, ciprofloxacin, clindamycin, lincomycin, metronidazole, vancomycin, tetracycline, erythromycin, trimethoprimsulfamethoxazole, chloramphenicol, and rifampin. A few cases have been related to the oral administration of aminoglycosides.[1,17] It is probably justified to believe that any antimicrobial agent that can get into the intestinal lumen, even in small amounts, can induce the disease.

The relative risks of various antimicrobials in inducing AAC are not known with precision because antibiotic-specific attack rates in well-controlled studies of well-matched patient groups have not been reported. The incidence of AAC in adults treated with clindamycin has ranged from 1 in 10,000 to as high as 1 in 10 in various reports[2]; perhaps some of this variation is related not only to variations in the prevalence of the organism but also to the variable susceptibility of the organism and/or its suppressors within the intestines to antimicrobials. The high rates reported from some hospitals suggest that the disease can be transmitted nosocomially, either via the hands of personnel or (less likely) by direct contact with patients or contaminated surfaces or objects.[17] Most cases of AAC reported in th 1970s were related to clindamycin or lincomycin (to which *C. difficile* is often resistant), to ampicillin (to which it is usually susceptible), or to cephalosporins (to which susceptibility varies).[8] This paradox is not completely understood, but β-lactamase production by intestinal bacteria seems important in the pathogenesis of cases associated with ampicillin.

Since alterations of the intestinal flora that permit overgrowth by *C. difficile* and production of its toxins are so important in the pathogenesis of AAC, it is not surprising that almost every antibiotic used in treating humans has been implicated in its production. The components of the normal intestinal flora that suppress colonization, overgrowth, or toxin production by *C. difficile* are not completely identified or understood, but the suspects include *Escherichia coli,* enterococci, lactobacilli, *Bacteroides,* and *Clostridial* spp. Factors predisposing to colitis presumably inhibit or eliminate these competing organisms and thus enhance growth of *C. difficile;* certain antibiotics may also stimulate toxin production by *C. difficile.* Hamsters inoculated orally with large numbers of *C. difficile* remain well, while antibiotic-treated hamsters given only two colony-forming units of *C. difficile* developed lethal enterocolitis.[10] The effects of antibiotics on the stool flora may persist for long periods, and the acquisition and overgrowth of *C. difficile* with production of colitis may begin as late at 6 weeks after discontinuation of antibiotic therapy. Many reported patients with pseudomembranous colitis had received no antibiotics; these cases suggest that dietary changes, anesthesia, uremia, and various nonantibiotic medications (such as methotrexate or gold salts) may precipitate the disease.[26]

Clostridium difficile has been isolated from the hands of hospital personnel caring for colonized patients. The spores of *C. difficile* can persist on fomites and surfaces for several months. They have been found in abundance in the environment of patients with AAC.[17] While vegetative forms of the organism are oxygen sensitive and easily killed, spores are very resistant to adverse conditions and to most of the disinfectants used in hospitals. When instruments and tubes inserted into the gastrointestinal tract need to be cleaned and disinfected before use on other patients, alkaline glutaraldehyde and sodium hypochlorite and possibly iodine disinfectants are most effective against spores. Enteric isolation precautions, use of vinyl gloves, and careful handwashing after contact with patients with AAC are also recommended for prevention of cross-infection.

Clostridium difficile rarely invades the colonic tissues, but it may do so in infants or neutropenic patients. Colitis results from production of toxins by the organism within the intestinal lumen. Isolates from patients with colitis usually produce at least two and possibly more exotoxins.[27,28] About 25 percent of isolates obtained from humans lack genes for production of toxins A and B and are nontoxigenic; these never cause diarrhea or colitis. The two best-characterized toxins are toxin A (enterotoxin) and toxin B (cytotoxin). Isolates producing toxin A also produce toxin B and vice versa, with rare exceptions. Because it has been somewhat difficult to purify these toxins in a stable form, their characteristics and mechanisms of action are not yet completely understood. The reported molecular weights of toxins A and B have ranged widely (50,000–600,000). These toxins attack the membranes or microfilaments of cells and produce contraction, hemorrhage, necrosis, inflammation and leakage of protein into the intestinal lumen.[29,30] Other toxins produced by some isolates increase intestinal myoelectric responses and peristalsis[31] and may induce secretion of fluid and electrolytes by purely biochemical mechanisms. Diarrhea associated with *C. difficile* toxins in humans who have undergone colonoscopy to detect colitis has almost always been associated with inflammatory mucosal lesions, but biopsy of minor lesions may be necessary to find the inflammation. Toxin A is lethal for certain rodents, causes intestinal hemorrhage and fluid secretion, and is cytotoxic for certain cell lines in culture. Toxin B is detectable by its cytotoxic or actinomorphic effects on many different cell culture monolayers, but the amount of toxin required to produce cytotoxic effects varies widely between some cell lines.

Newborn infants colonized with toxigenic *C. difficile* organisms usually remain well despite the presence of large amounts of toxins A and B in their stools. Colonization rates as high as 50–60 percent have been reported in newborns.[16,32] In one study, the nursery environment appeared to be the main source of the organism[34]; in another, hand transmission of the organism from infant to infant by nursery personnel seemed responsible[34] for spread within the nursery. A glycoprotein found in milk (fetulin) or a subunit of it may interfere with the action of these toxins on the cecum.[35] In addition, the toxins do not bind well to the intestinal mucosa of newborns.[36] However, pseudomembranous colitis *has* been reported in infants.[5] As newborn infants acquire their normal intestinal flora, the rate of isolation of *C. difficile* and its toxins from their stools declines toward the rates of older children and adults.

Hamsters immunized with toxoids prepared from both toxins A and B (but less often from those immunized with either one alone) were protected against AAC.[37] The toxins are poor immunogens, but immunization with toxin A appears more protective than with toxin B. Toxoid vaccines for use in humans are not available, but would be very helpful. Neutralizing or other types of serum antibodies to the toxins of *C. difficile* have been detected in adults,[38–40] but their protective function in humans is unknown. Colostral or IgA antibodies may be protective against the disease. In one report, antibodies against *C. difficile* antigens were found much less often in sera from elderly than from young adults[37]; this may be an important observation, as AAC is more common in elderly patients.

CLINICAL MANIFESTATIONS

The range of severity of the symptoms associated with *C. difficile* colitis is wide.[1,41–44] Early reports in the preantibiotic era consisted mostly of severe cases documented at the time of surgery, often because of an illness requiring colectomy, or at autopsy. Now that there is a high index of suspicion of AAC and noninvasive tests are available to aid in diagnosis, mild cases of AAC not only have been documented but have been shown to be commonplace and much more frequent than severe cases.

Typically, profuse watery or mucoid green, foul-smelling diarrhea begins, along with cramping abdominal pain, 4–9 days after starting antibiotics. It may begin as early as 24 hours after starting antimicrobials. In as many as 20 percent of patients, diarrhea does not begin until up to 6 weeks after antibiotic treatment has been discontinued. Sometimes the diarrhea is heme positive or bloody, especially if the patient has a coagulopathy. Hypoproteinemia and edema can develop with profuse diarrhea. *Clostridium difficile* is not reliably identifiable on gram-stained smears of stools, and leukocytes are found in smears from only 30–50 percent of patients with AAC. Measurement of fecal lactoferrin as a marker of fecal leukocytes, which may be destroyed by the toxins or during transport of the fecal specimen, can be used as a screening test and as an adjunct to other tests for the presence of clostridial toxins.[45] High fever (temperatures of 103–105°F), marked abdominal tenderness, a peripheral blood leukocyte count as high as 35,000/mm³, and hypoalbuminemia are common and point strongly to the diagnosis of colitis rather than benign diarrhea. Peripheral leukocyte counts as high as

50,000–100,000/mm³ are occasionally seen. Sometimes patients with AAC have little or no diarrhea but present instead with an acute abdominal syndrome with toxic megacolon, colonic perforation, or peritonitis.[46] Such patients may require surgery or emergency colonoscopy with decompression, along with appropriate antibiotic therapy. Acute arthritis resembling Reiter syndrome has complicated the illness.[47]

The pseudomembranous nodules or plaques of *C. difficile* colitis are usually most numerous in the distal colon, sigmoid, or rectum and are easily detected at sigmoidoscopy (Fig. 1). In about 10 percent of cases, lesions are present only in the cecum or transverse colon; this form of the illness may present as an acute abdominal syndrome without diarrhea and is difficult to detect without performing colonoscopy or computerized tomography[48,49]; it should be suspected when patients with diarrhea and toxin-positive stools have no visible lesions at proctosigmoidoscopy.[50] Diarrhea caused by *C. difficile* without colitis has been postulated but has not been proven to occur.[51] This mechanism probably depends on a purely secretory diarrhea or a diarrhea caused by a motility-altering factor.[30,52] Some patients with leukemia or granulocytopenia or who are receiving antineoplastic chemotherapy may develop neutropenic ileocecitis or enterocolitis (typhlitis), which is similar to the disease seen in hamsters.[53,54] Sometimes the diarrhea attributed to the effects of cancer chemotherapeutic agents on the intestinal mucosa may be due to *C. difficile* colitis.[55,56] If *C. difficile* colitis goes unrecognized and untreated, the outcome may be fatal. Death rates of 10–20 percent are reported in untreated elderly or chronically debilitated patients. Hypovolemic shock, toxic megacolon, cecal perforation, secondary sepsis, and hemorrhage are the most serious complications that can result in death.

Clostridium difficile colitis can cause symptoms that may be erroneously interpreted as an exacerbation of an underlying chronic inflammatory bowel disease. This presentation usually occurs during or within a month of treatment of such patients with antibiotics.[57]

LABORATORY DIAGNOSIS

The laboratory tests most useful in confirmation of the diagnosis of AAC include stool cultures for *C. difficile* and tests for the presence of its toxins in stools. A selective medium containing cycloserine, cefoxitin, and fructose in agar (CCFA) is useful for isolation of the organism.[19] *Clostridium difficile* has a characteristic chartreuse fluorescence and gross appearance on CCFA. CCFA can detect as few as 100 cfu of *C. difficile* per gram of stool.[20] Patients with AAC usually have many more organisms than that (typically 10^4–10^6/g), while asymptomatic carriers may have only a few organisms per gram. Almost all untreated patients with AAC are culture positive if the culture is processed properly. A negative culture should suggest the possibility of another etiologic organism, such as staphylococci, unless antimicrobials such as vancomycin, metronidazole, or others to which *C. difficile* is susceptible have been administered. Use of CCFA containing sodium taurocholate or use of alcohol shock or heat shock prior to inoculating cultures may increase sensitivity. These are especially useful when searching for asymptomatic carriers.[58,59] Vegetative forms of the organism are easily killed on exposure to air or other adverse conditions; spores are hardy but less numerous and harder to detect. Anaerobe jars or bags incubated at 35–37°C provide adequate cultural conditions. When using CCFA, it is possible to isolate and presumptively identify *C. difficile* in just a few days. Confirmation is not difficult using biochemical reactions, gas-liquid chromatography to detect the production of characteristic fatty acids, or tests of toxin production.[60,61] Only a few other species of fecal organisms that resemble *C. difficile* can grow on CCFA. *Clostridium sporogenes* is similar but does not produce a cytotoxin.[60] While not all isolates of *C. difficile* are toxigenic, those that are not have not caused colitis or diarrhea.[62]

The isolation of *C. difficile* from diarrheal stools does not in itself prove that the patient has colitis caused by this organism. As mentioned previously, 60–70 percent of healthy newborns can carry it in their stools for a few weeks or months, and 3 percent or more of healthy adults are asymptomatic carriers. In some hospitals where AAC is frequent, 20–30 percent or more of asymptomatic patients may harbor the organism.[17] Nevertheless, a positive culture may be useful in making therapeutic decisions. In our hospital, about 85 percent of adults with antibiotic-associated diarrhea and positive stool cultures have had colitis, and more than 95 percent with toxin B in their stools have had colitis. Since the toxin B (cytotoxin) produced by the organism is the basis for a commonly used laboratory test and is heat and acid labile, stools from patients with AAC may be culture positive but toxin negative because of inactivation of the toxin during transport, or for other reasons. Cultures are used in the detection of post-treatment carriers of the organism, who appear to be at an increased risk of relapse, but since there is as yet no effective way to eradicate the carrier state, post-treatment cultures are of little value and need not be performed routinely.

Tests to detect the cytotoxic effects of *C. difficile* toxin B usually employ monolayer cultures of fibroblasts or other cell lines.[5,60,61] Vero cells appear to be the most sensitive cell line of those used in the United States. All are difficult to maintain, and most are not available in many U.S. hospitals. However, demonstration of cytotoxin in stools is very helpful to the clinician. Toxin B can be detected by counterelectrophoresis, but this method is much less sensitive than the cytotoxin assay.[63] In our hospital, more than 95 percent of adults with antibiotic-associated diarrhea and *C. difficile* cytotoxin-positive stools have had documentable colitis. When proctosigmoidoscopy performed on patients with toxin titers of greater than 1:10 on undiluted stools reveals a normal mucosa, it is likely that they have colitis demonstrable only by colonoscopy or by biopsy and microscopic examination. Isolated cecitis (typhlitis) is more common in patients treated with ampicillin or penicillin G or who have leukemia or granulocytopenia.[54] Colonoscopy, radionuclide scans using gallium or indium, or computerized tomography may be helpful in detecting and localizing colitis in these patients.[48–50]

With tests for cytotoxin B, a cytopathic effect may be seen within 4–6 hours but usually is not definite until 18–24 hours. Nonspecific (false-positive) toxicity can occur, especially with concentrated specimens, but these are not neutralizable by antitoxin. Thus, it is necessary to confirm all positive results by demonstrating neutralization of cytotoxicity by incubation with *C. difficile* or *C. sordellii* antitoxin (these reagents are equivalent). Patients with AAC usually have large amounts of toxin in their stool filtrates and have positive titers at dilutions of 10^{-3}–10^{-5} or more. The amount of toxin B in individual patients does not correlate well with the severity of the illness.[43,64] This discrepancy may be either artifactual or indicative of the greater importance of toxin A in determining the severity of the disease. More than one exotoxin (or more than one aggregate of toxin subunits) produced by *C. difficile* can be found in stools of patients with AAC.[27,28,65] However, usually both toxins A and B are present when either one is present in stools of patient with colitis.

Toxin A is a so-called enterotoxin that causes inflammation and the accumulation of hemorrhagic fluid in inoculated rabbit ileal loops. It is cytotoxic for certain cell lines not used for routine testing for the presence of toxin B.[66] Toxin A is thought by many to be the cause of the symptoms of the disease in most patients,[67] while toxin B may attach to colonic tissues and cause severe disease only after toxin A has exerted its effects. Toxigenic strains usually produce both toxins, and a test for the presence of either one is useful in diagnosis. A latex agglutination test kit for presumed detection of toxin A in stools actually demonstrates instead a glutamate dehydrogenase of *C. difficile*.[68] Other organisms found in stools can produce an immuno-

logically cross-reactive protein; therefore, a positive latex test suggests only that *C. difficile* is probably present,[69] and its value is similar to that of a positive culture. Nontoxigenic isolates are positive using the latex agglutination test.

Several new enzyme immunoassays for the presence of toxin A or B or both have become available recently. They have the advantages of relative ease and speed of performance without the need for expensive equipment. Most have been evaluated using clinical criteria and/or culture and toxin B cytotoxicity assays as the "gold standard." None has been adequately evaluated using the results of colonoscopy and biopsy, as well as highly sensitive toxin B test results, as the standard. The main problem with all the newer tests for toxin A is their relative insensitivity when used alone as a diagnostic test; this is especially evident if indeterminate results have been excluded during evaluation of these tests in clinical trials. Their sensitivity has ranged from 63 to 88 percent,[70] but specificity is usually better. Many early, mild cases are not detected using the EIA test for toxin A. False-positive tests also occur, especially if the endpoint used is chosen to maximize sensitivity.

Now that the genes of toxin A and toxin B have been identified and characterized, novel tests for detecting their presence in the stools of patients with antibiotic-associated diarrhea are being developed. Hybridization probe or polymerase chain reaction (PCR) tests for toxin A have been developed that appear sensitive and specific enough for further use.[71,72] More recently, PCR has been used to identify strains of *C. Difficile* that are positive for toxin B DNA or its 16S RNA in the stools of humans with diarrhea.[72–74] These appear highly sensitive, specific, clinically applicable, and relatively rapid. Continued research along these lines probably will result in the wider availability of a satisfactory clinical test.

Further details of the laboratory aspects of diagnosis of *C. difficile* disease have recently been expertly reviewed.[63,67,70]

Staphylococcal toxins can produce cytopathic effects in Walker rat carcinoma cell culture monolayers (as do *C. difficile* toxins), but not in the fibroblast monolayers used to detect *C. difficile* toxins.[23] This difference may be useful in the diagnosis of staphylococcal enterocolitis.

CLINICAL DIAGNOSIS

When patients with antibiotic-associated diarrhea have high fever, severe abdominal pain and tenderness, bloody stools, or large numbers of leukocytes in their stools, benign diarrhea is ruled out, and colitis is probably present. If they develop diarrhea while in the hospital for treatment of a different condition, the colitis is probably caused by *C. difficile*. The diagnosis of AAC is most rapidly and certainly established by endoscopy, which detects evidence of inflammation (colitis) and/or pseudomembranous lesions. Colonoscopy may be required to detect isolated proximal colonic lesions,[50] which occur in almost ten percent of cases. Colonic biopsy is not needed when typical gross findings are seen, but may aid in the diagnosis of clostridial colitis when so-called nonspecific colitis is visualized, because biopsies may reveal pseudomembranes too small to be seen grossly. When colonoscopy is contraindicated, computerized tomography or abdominal x-ray studies may be helpful in diagnosis. Air-contrast barium enema radiologic studies may show signs of pseudomembranous colitis, but these signs are not specific and are often absent early in the illness. In severe colitis, barium studies may precipitate toxic megacolon, perforation, or other complications, and they are not recommended.

In patients with nonspecific colitis associated with antibiotic usage, it is important also to consider Crohn's disease, idiopathic ulcerative colitis, and ischemic colitis. Infection with other intestinal pathogens such as *Salmonella*, *Edwardsiella*, *Shigella*, invasive *E. coli* (especially the 0157:H7 serotype if the colitis is hemorrhagic), *Entamoeba histolytica*, *Staphylococcus aureus*, *Campylobacter*, *Yersinia*, and *Strongyloides* should be considered. Enterotoxin-producing organisms that can cause diarrhea without colitis include *E. coli, Bacillus cereus, Aeromonas, Vibrio,* and possibly other Enterobacteriaceae, pseudomonads, and staphylococci. Colitis has been reported following gold therapy or use of nonsteroidal anti-inflammatory drugs and in some cases may present with pseudomembranes.[75,76]

TREATMENT

Antibiotics

Clostridium difficile isolates are very susceptible to vancomycin and metronidazole, and most isolates are susceptible to bacitracin and rifampin. The minimal inhibitory concentrations with vancomycin or metronidazole are usually about 5 mg/liter or less. Since resistance to rifampin can develop rapidly, this antimicrobial should not be used alone in the treatment of AAC. Isolates resistant to metronidazole have been reported (they number about 3 percent in our hospital). Vancomycin-resistant isolates have not been documented. *Clostridium difficile* is often susceptible to tetracycline, erythromycin, ampicillin, cefamandole, cefazolin, and various other antibiotics[8,64]; however, all of these except bacitracin have induced AAC, and more importantly they have not been very useful for treating the disease.

Not all patients with AAC need to be treated with antimicrobials. When patients have mild or moderate symptoms, it is sufficient in about 25 percent of instances to discontinue treatment with the precipitating antibiotic and to give supportive therapy with fluids and electrolytes. If such patients improve within 48 hours, supportive therapy can be continued, and the diarrhea usually subsides within 7–10 days or less. If treatment with the inducing antibiotic must be continued, specific antimicrobial treatment for *C. difficile* should be begun promptly, even if symptoms are mild. Patients with high fever, leukocytosis, marked abdominal pain, and signs of peritoneal inflammation should be treated promptly with specific antibiotics, as should patients who are elderly, toxic, debilitated, or unresponsive to supportive therapy or cholestyramine.

Discontinuation of treatment with the inducing antibiotic, although desirable, is probably not essential if specific therapy for AAC is given. For example, the antibacterial effects of vancomycin on *C. difficile* in vitro are not antagonized by clindamycin, and the continuation of clindamycin therapy in patients (and hamsters) treated with oral vancomycin has not been harmful. Furthermore, many of the antibiotics that might be chosen as alternative therapy are themselves capable of inducing AAC. An algorithm for the management of *C. difficile* colitis has been published recently.[12]

Vancomycin. Vancomycin given orally is expensive but still the therapy of choice for severe AAC.[41,42,64,77] Metronidazole[78] and bacitracin[79] are less expensive alternatives for treating mild or moderately severely ill patients or when vancomycin is unavailable. The efficacy of vancomycin has been so well documented in different parts of the world that it must be considered the most reliable treatment of AAC. *Clostridium difficile* is usually susceptible to vancomycin at concentrations of less than 5 mg/liter, and no isolate has been identified that required more than 16 mg/liter. Since vancomycin is poorly absorbed from the gastrointestinal tract when given orally, it is rarely toxic when given in this way, and concentrations far exceeding 16 mg/liter are easily achieved in stools. When 500 mg is given orally four times daily, stool concentrations average 2000 mg/liter or more. When the usual dose of 125 mg is given four times daily, concentrations reach 300–1000 mg/liter. Even patients with profuse diarrhea achieve adequate therapeutic concentrations in stools with these regimens. Vancomycin has been detected in the urine of patients treated orally, but only in low concentrations. Vancomycin is usually undetectable in serum, but concentrations of 5–30 mg/liter were detectable in a few patients with renal

failure. Systemic toxic reactions (except for rare rashes) have been very rare with oral vancomycin, even in patients with an inflamed colonic mucosa.[42,64,77]

Oral vancomycin was evaluated in a controlled study and was found to be significantly better than placebo in the treatment of *C. difficile* toxin-positive postoperative diarrheal syndromes.[77] The dose was 125 mg every 6 hours for 5 days or more. Vancomycin-treated patients who had *C. difficile*–negative antibiotic-associated diarrhea fared no better than did placebo-treated patients. In controlled studies many patients with *C. difficile* colitis have been treated with oral vancomycin. The clinical response almost invariably has been excellent unless the disease was far advanced when treatment was begun or when oral therapy was not possible. It is important to stress that antibacterial activity within colonic tissues does not appear necessary; cessation of toxin production within the lumen of the bowel or at the mucosal surface seems sufficient and indeed essential. Since parenterally administered vancomycin does not reliably yield adequate fecal concentrations, it should not be used in this way unless oral therapy is not possible.

Patients treated with oral vancomycin usually show improvement in fever, diarrhea, abdominal cramps, and malaise within 48 hours, but it may take more than a week for cessation of diarrhea. Toxin titers in stools usually decline within a few days after treatment is begun. Some investigators believe that treatment should continue until stools no longer contain toxin, but it is an unnecessary expense to repeat these tests in a patient who is doing well. Treatment should continue for at least 5–10 days, but is rarely needed for more than 14 days. Longer therapeutic courses given when the illness has subsided are unnecessary and may delay the return of the normal fecal flora and other inhibitors of *C. difficile*.

The major disadvantages to the use of vancomycin are its expense ($16–$25 or more per day), its short supply in some parts of the world, and its bitter taste. In addition, this therapy may result in resistant bacterial strains (e.g., enterococci). A less expensive capsule form of vancomycin for oral use has been made available in the United States and many other parts of the world. Rare patients have not responded to therapy with the capsule form, but have done so subsequently after vancomycin powder (for parenteral or oral use) has been dissolved and given orally, presumably because the capsules did not dissolve rapidly enough in patients with severe diarrhea and rapid intestinal transit.

In about 50 patients entered into a randomized study of treatment of pseudomembranous colitis with vancomycin, there were no significant differences in the overall clinical or bacteriologic responses of those treated with oral vancomycin every 6 hours in dosages of either 125 or 500 mg four times per day,[80] although diarrhea in very ill patients ceased slightly sooner with the higher dose. The 500 mg/day regimen is less expensive and is therefore preferable except for extremely ill patients. For the oral treatment of infants and children with AAC, a dose of 500 mg/1.73 m² every 6 hours or 40 mg/kg in three or four divided doses has been recommended.[15,16]

Vancomycin is also the drug of choice for the treatment of staphylococcal pseudomembranous colitis, which may be suspected when gram-stained smears and cultures of stools show very little except gram-positive cocci or when stool cultures grow large numbers of staphylococci and *C. difficile* and its toxins are not present.

Patients who are unable to take vancomycin orally can be given it via a nasogastric tube instead, but patients with adynamic ileus may still not achieve adequate concentrations within the colonic lumen, where it is needed to stop toxin production. These patients pose a formidable therapeutic problem since they are usually seriously ill and there is no parenteral regimen for treatment of AAC that is of proven reliability. When healthy adults were given intravenous vancomycin, their stools concentrations ranged from 0 to 100 mg/liter.[81] Thus, some patients with colitis treated intravenously might not achieve adequate concentrations within the bowel lumen. A few patients with colitis appear to have responded to intravenous vancomycin,[82] but other seriously ill patients have failed to respond. Evidence suggests that metronidazole given intravenously may also reach therapeutic concentrations in the colonic lumen in some patients.[46] However, reliance on either intravenous metronidazole or vancomycin for the treatment of AAC, to the exclusion of oral therapy, is *not* recommended.

When parenteral therapy is essential (as in patients with adynamic ileus), treatment with both intravenous vancomycin and metronidazole (see below) supplemented by vancomycin given via nasogastric tube (500 mg four times per day for adults), or into ileostomies and colostomies, or by enema is recommended. Oral metronidazole plays *no* role in this setting, since, if small amounts of the drug pass down the gastrointestinal tract, they are likely to be absorbed from the small intestine and little or none will reach the colon. When vancomycin is given both orally and parenterally, serum concentrations should be monitored.

Metronidazole. Metronidazole is very active against almost all isolates of *C. difficile,* and it has been effective in the treatment of patients with AAC.[78,83,84] It is inactive against staphylococci and has no value in treatment of staphylococcal enterocolitis. In a randomized comparative study of the treatment of *C. difficile* diarrhea, oral metronidazole was associated with a cure rate of 95 percent within 7 days, while the rate was 100 percent with vancomycin (the difference was not statistically significant).[84] Metronidazole was well tolerated, significantly less expensive than vancomycin, and associated with about the same rate of post-treatment carriage and relapse as vancomycin. The usual oral dose of metronidazole is 500–750 mg three times daily or 250–500 mg four times daily. The drug is so well absorbed from the small intestine that concerns have been raised about whether the concentrations achieved within the colonic lumen will be adequate in all patients, especially those who are seriously ill. Seriously ill patients may fail to respond to metronidazole[54] and then respond to oral vancomycin. We reserve metronidazole for mildly or moderately ill patients with AAC. Metronidazole has a number of side effects, some serious, and is not recommended for use in pregnant women or children. About 3 percent of isolates are resistant to metronidazole. Furthermore, one case of colitis with a metronidazole-resistant organism has been reported.[85] Recent reports have encouraged the use of intravenous metronidazole for treatment of patients with AAC who are too sick to be treated via the oral route.[46,86–88] The usual intravenous dose was 500 mg every 6–8 hours. Metronidazole given parenterally was detected with a chemical assay in stools of patients and in rat intestinal tissues.[88] However, adequate bioactivity within the colonic lumen of patients treated parenterally has not been documented. Furthermore, it is possible that the biliary excretion of metronidazole was responsible for the clinical improvement noted in patients treated in this way, most of whom did not have decreased intestinal motility. Since no form of parenteral therapy has been proved to be reliably effective in AAC, metronidazole given parenterally should be used only when oral therapy is not possible.

In patients unable to be treated by the oral route, both metronidazole and vancomycin may be given intravenously. Vancomycin (500 mg four times per day for adults) should also be given via nasogastric tube with intermittent clamping, or by enema, or by direct instillation through an ileostomy or colostomy, or via a colonoscopically introduced catheter.[89] A solution containing 200–500 mg vancomycin/liter can be used for infusion into the colonic lumen. A high proportion of these patients ultimately require an emergent colectomy as a life-saving measure. If vancomycin is given both orally and intravenously, serum concentrations should be monitored, especially if the patient has renal impairment.

Bacitracin. Several investigators[80,90–92] reported patients whose pseudomembranous colitis improved with treatment with oral bacitracin. The dosage was 25,000 units (about 500 mg) four times per day for 7–19 days. One patient relapsed after this therapy and then was treated successfully with vancomycin. Bacitracin has a very bitter taste and is nauseating if not given in capsule form (which requires special preparation). Although bacitracin is a useful alternative to vancomycin and metronidazole, the response to bacitracin is slower and less reliable than with vancomycin; furthermore, carrier rates and stool toxin titers decline less rapidly than with vancomycin.[93,94] Most isolates of *C. difficile* are susceptible to bacitracin, but some require more than 20 units/ml (about 1000 mg/liter) for inhibition, which may indicate resistance, since these concentrations may not be achieved in the stools of some patients with diarrhea. Some absorption of the drug occurs when it is given orally. The systemic absorption and safety of bacitracin in patients with an inflamed intestinal mucosa, as well as the frequency of relapse after treatment with this drug, need better documentation. Bacitracin is often unavailable and is only slightly less expensive than vancomycin. Bacitracin is also active against staphylococci and is an alternative therapy when staphylococcal enterocolitis is suspected.

Other Antibiotics. Fusidic acid is highly active against *C. difficile* and has been used successfully for the oral treatment of 15 patients with AAC.[93] It is also active against staphylococci. Tetracycline and erythromycin have been used occasionally in the treatment of AAC of unknown cause, but many isolates of *C. difficile* are resistant to these antibiotics, and their use is not recommended. Teicoplanin (100 mg twice daily per os) was as effective as vancomycin in one study.[94a]

Cholestyramine and Colestipol

Cholestyramine and colestipol, anion-exchange resins, were used in the treatment of pseudomembranous colitis before the cause of the disease was known. Their early use was based on speculation that secretory bile acids might be responsible for antibiotic-associated diarrhea or colitis.[94] However, studies in hamsters suggested that secretory bile acids were unlikely to be the cause of antibiotic-associated diarrhea.[95] Cholestyramine binds *C. difficile* toxin B (and probably also toxin A), which is its presumed mechanism of action in this condition. It may also bind vancomycin, so their simultaneous use should be avoided.[96] Since many patients with AAC respond slowly or not at all to cholestyramine or colestipol and require a change to treatment with antibiotics, they are usually reserved for mild illness. The usual oral dose of cholestyramine for adults in 4 g three or four times per day. Obstipation is the most serious side effect.

Antidiarrheal Agents

Opiates and other antiperistaltic agents should be avoided in patients with AAC. They are especially dangerous in infants. While they often provide symptomatic relief, they probably decrease diarrhea primarily by causing pooling of fluid within the lumen of the intestines; at the same time they may promote more severe damage to the colon because of toxin retention. Some patients have become worse when given these drugs.[97]

Adrenal Steroids

Adrenal steroids are not of proven value in this disease. Reported mortality is higher in patients who received steroids, although such patients have tended to be sicker than others being treated without corticosteroids.

Evaluation of New Therapies of Colitis

Guidelines for the evaluation of new anti-infective agents for treatment of AAC have recently been published.[98] They have been endorsed by the U.S. Food and Drug Administration (FDA) and by the Infectious Diseases Society of America. Such trials should be based on a firm diagnosis and should be placebo controlled for mild disease or with an active drug for severe disease. A randomized, double-blind study design is preferred. Outcome should be assessed by monitoring the degree of inflammation of the bowel mucosa, the intensity and severity of diarrhea, the duration of illness, the eradication of *C. difficile* or its toxins from stools, and the overall outcome.

Relapse or Recurrence of Colitis

More than one episode of colitis has been observed in 10–20 percent or more of patients treated with vancomycin, metronidazole, or bacitracin.[42,80,99–102] Recurrences respond promptly to retreatment with vancomycin or, if the organism is susceptible, to metronidazole or bacitracin, unless treatment is delayed until the patient is critically ill. Recurrences may be caused either by germination of persistent spores or by reinfection from environmental or human contacts; persistence appears to be the more common mechanism on the basis of typing isolates. Persistence results in relapse; acquisition of a new strain results in reinfection. The distinction is probably academic. Not all patients who remain fecal carriers of the organism after successful treatment experience recurrence of the disease; in fact, most do not. Unfortunately, the carrier state cannot be reliably eradicated with antimicrobials or any other regimen.[102] Long-term suppression of the organism with oral vancomycin or oral metronidazole until the carrier leaves an outbreak environment may be helpful. Most relapses are spontaneous and occur within a few weeks or months of the first episode.

Little is known about local, humoral, or cellular immunity to either toxin A or B, to the organism, or to the disease. Serum antibodies to the toxins have been detected in most healthy adults but in a minority of patients who recovered from the disease.[38,40,103] Toxin A–specific IgG was found in higher titers in convalescent sera from patients with *C. difficile* diarrhea than in acute sera or in controls or asymptomatic carriers. Toxin A–specific serum and intestinal IgA levels were similar to those of serum IgG. Neutralization of toxin A was demonstrated with sera of 5 of 14 convalescent patients but with only 1 of 13 acute patients. The presence of neutralizing activity did not appear to alter the subsequent clinical course.[104] One patient developed neutralizing antibodies to toxin B in serum after eight episodes of colitis.[105] He suffered no further recurrences. Children with chronic relapsing *C. difficile* colitis had lower IgG antitoxin A levels than did a group of normal children and adults. Five of these children were treated with 400 mg γ-globulin/kg administered intravenously every 3 weeks and had significant increases in their IgG but not IgA antitoxin levels. They had clinical resolution of their symptoms as well as clearing of cytotoxin B from their stools. This interesting approach deserves further study.[106]

Patients who relapse may be treated initially with oral vancomycin, metronidazole, or bacitracin for 7–14 days or until their diarrhea ceases. Longer courses do not eradicate the carrier state and do not appear more efficacious in preventing recurrences. Indeed, shorter courses of antibiotics may permit more rapid restoration of the normal fecal flora, which in some way inhibits *C. difficile*. Although most patients have only a single recurrence, some unfortunate persons have multiple recurrences. Patients with more than one recurrence tend to have a high rate of subsequent recurrences. No reliable way to manage this problem is yet available, but anecdotal experiences suggest they may respond to long courses (4–6 weeks) of oral vancomycin or metronidazole followed by a gradual tapering of the dose[107]; or to intermittent short periods (days) of treatment alternating with periods of no treatment; or to postantibiotic therapy with cholestyramine to suppress symptoms by binding toxin while the normal flora is being reestablished; or to recolonization of the intestines by administration of oral lactobacillus preparations after antibiotic therapy; or even to enemas with feces from healthy persons.[108,109] Oral vancomycin plus rifampin has seemed useful in the treatment of a few cases in an uncontrolled study.[105] Since recent evidence suggests lactobacilli, enterococci, *Saccharomyces boulardii* and nontoxigenic *C. difficile* isolates are important inhibitors of *C. difficile* or its toxins within the gut, interest in their use for treatment of patients who relapse is growing.[110–117] Administration of a nontoxigenic strain of *C. difficile* orally has been used in two patients with relapsing disease in an uncontrolled study.[113]

Saccharomyces boulardii is a novel living nonpathogenic biotherapeutic agent that has been used in France for the treatment of diarrhea since the 1950s. A lyophilized form was marketed in France in 1962 and used mainly for treatment of antibiotic-associated diarrhea. Widely available in Europe, South America, and Africa, it is an investigational new drug in the United States and is currently undergoing FDA-approved clinical trials.[118] It has been shown to prevent clindamycin-induced mortality in hamsters,[119] *C. difficile*–induced experimental pseudomembranous colitis in mice (along with a reduction in the amounts of toxins A and B but not the number of *C. difficile* in the digestive tracts),[120] to suppress the overgrowth of *C. difficile* and production of toxin B after cessation of vancomycin therapy of hamsters,[121] and to significantly reduce the frequency of antibiotic-associated diarrhea in a prospective double-blind controlled study in a hospital in the United States.[122] In uncontrolled open studies in humans, its oral administration (500 mg twice per day for 30 days) was followed by the apparent prevention of further recurrences in 85 percent of patients.[123] A study of 19 infants who presented with enteral symptoms consisting of persistent or protracted diarrhea, malabsorption, failure to grow, or repeated attacks of colic or emesis without diarrhea, along with *C. difficile*–positive stools with positive toxin B assays (without evidence of colitis), and who were given live *S. boulardii* orally for 15 days demonstrated resolution of enteral symptoms and physical findings, a marked decrease in the number of stools or episodes of colic, and clearing of toxin B in 85 percent or more of cases. Eradication of *C. difficile* from stools was complete after a month in 14 (73 percent) of the 19 patients.[124] These studies suggest that *C. difficile* may cause chronic enteropathies without colitis in infants and that they may be helped by treatment with *S. boulardii*. Finally, in a double-blind placebo-controlled clinical trial in the United States of 51 patients with recurrent *C. difficile* disease who were given live *S. boulardii* orally for 30 days, with a least 4 days overlap with oral antibiotic therapy, it was found that 19 of 28 (68 percent) patients on placebo had a further recurrence, while only 9 of 23 (39 percent) patients on *S. boulardii* had a further recurrence ($p < 0.04$).[118] There were no significant adverse reactions to *S. boulardii* in this study. Further controlled studies with this interesting biotherapeutic agent for the treatment or prevention of gastrointestinal diseases associated with *C. difficile* are indicated and underway.

Surgical Measures

Before specific antibiotic therapy was available for AAC, diversion of the fecal stream or resection of the diseased bowel was often necessary to end the illness. These drastic measures are now rarely performed except in life-threatening situations, such as with toxic megacolon or cecal perforation. However, a colostomy or ileostomy may be needed to facilitate instillation of vancomycin or metronidazole into the colonic lumen of patients with pseudomembranous colitis and ileus.[101]

PREVENTION

Treatment of fecal carriers of *C. difficile* with oral vancomycin until discharge or transfer from a hospital unit where there is a high rate of the disease may be useful in terminating outbreaks. The use of sodium hypochlorite diluted 1:500 to disinfect contaminated surfaces and prevent reinfection has been recommended for control of nosocomial outbreaks.[125] Use of vinyl gloves and careful hand washing by staff after contact with cases or carriers is urged.[126]

Eventually it may be possible to immunize patients against the toxins or other virulence factors of *C. difficile*, but this is not yet possible. Passive immunization of hamsters with *C. sordellii* antitoxin, which cross-reacts with toxin B of *C. difficile*, protected them against clindamycin-induced colitis.[7] However, it has been difficult to purify the toxins and to prepare potent toxoids. Ordinary immune serum globulin does not appear useful in primary prophylaxis, but has been of apparent value in treatment of possibly immunodeficient children with relapsing *C. difficile* colitis.[106] Prophylaxis with antibiotics such as vancomycin or metronidazole in patients who are carriers of *C. difficile* or at high risk of AAC is *not* of proven value in eradicating asymptomatic carriage of the organism,[126] and it is expensive and theoretically undesirable as it may encourage the development of antibiotic resistance by organisms in the gastrointestinal tract and should not be given. Bacteriophage and bacteriocin typing systems as well as immunologic and antibiogram systems for typing *C. difficile* have recently become available, and their use in epidemiologic studies may lead to new or better preventive measures.[127,128]

REFERENCES

1. Bartlett JG. Antibiotic-associated pseudomembranous colitis. Rev Infect Dis. 1979;1:530–9.
2. Lusk RH, Fekety FR, Silva J, et al. Gastrointestinal side effects of clindamycin and ampicillin therapy. J Infect Dis. 1977;135(Suppl):111–9.
3. Lusk RH, Fekety FR, Silva J, et al. Clindamycin-induced enterocolitis in hamsters. J Infect Dis. 1978;137:464–75.
4. Rifkin GD, Silva J, Fekety R. Gastrointestinal and systemic toxicity of fecal extracts from hamsters with clindamycin-induced colitis. Gastroenterology. 1978;74:52–7.
5. Rifkin GD, Fekety R, Silva J. Neutralization by *Clostridium sordellii* antitoxin of toxins implicated in clindamycin-induced colitis in the hamster. Gastroenterology. 1978;75:422–4.
6. Rifkin GD, Fekety FR, Silva J, et al. Antibiotic-induced colitis: Implication of a toxin neutralized by *Clostridium sordellii* antitoxin. Lancet. 1977;2:1103–6.
7. Allo M, Silva J, Fekety FR, et al. Prevention of clindamycin-induced colitis in hamsters by *Clostridium sordellii* antitoxin. Gastroenterology. 1979;76:351–5.
8. Fekety R, Silva J, Toshniwal R, et al. Antibiotic-associated colitis: Effects of antibiotics upon *Clostridium difficile* and the disease in hamsters. Rev Infect Dis. 1979;1:386–97.
9. Borriello SP, Barclay FE. An in vitro model of colonization resistance to *Clostridium difficile* infection. Med Microbiol 1986;21:299–309.
10. Larson HE, Price AB, Honour P, et al. *Clostridium difficile* and the aetiology of pseudomembranous colitis. Lancet. 1978;1:1063–6.
11. Lyerly DM, Korwan HC, Wilkins TD. *Clostridium difficile:* Its disease and toxins. Clin Microbiol Rev. 1988;1:1–18.
12. Fekety R, Shah AB. Diagnosis and treatment of *C. difficile* colitis. JAMA. 1993;269:71–5.
13. Rolfe RD, Finegold SM, eds. *Clostridium difficile:* Its Role in Intestinal Disease. San Diego: Academic Press; 1988:408.
14. Tedesco FJ, et al. Clindamycin-associated colitis: A prospective study. Ann Intern Med. 1974;81:429–433.
15. Scapa E. Pseudomembranous colitis in a 5 week old infant. Br Med J. 1982;284:824.
16. Batts DH, Martin D, Holmes R, et al. Treatment of antibiotic-associated *Clostridium difficile* diarrhea with oral vancomycin. J Pediatr. 1980;97:151–3.
17. Fekety R, Kim K-H, Brown D, et al. Epidemiology of antibiotic-associated colitis. Isolation of *Clostridium difficile* from the hospital environment. Am J Med. 1981;70:906–8.
18. Borriello SP, Honour P, Turner T, et al. Household pets as a potential reservoir for *Clostridium difficile* infection. J Clin Pathol. 1983;36:84–7.
19. George WL, Sutter VL, Citron D, et al. Selective and differential medium for isolation of *Clostridium difficile*. J Clin Microbiol. 1979;9:214–9.
20. Wilson KH, Kennedy MJ, Fekety FR. Use of sodium taurocholate to enhance spore recovery on a medium selective for *Clostridium difficile*. J Clin Microbiol. 1982;15:443–6.
21. Phillips KD, Rogers PA. Rapid detection and presumptive identification of *Clostridium difficile* by p-cresol production on a selective medium. J Clin Pathol. 1981;36:642–4.
22. Borriello SP, Honour P. Simplified procedure for the routine isolation of *Clostridium difficile* from faeces. J Clin Pathol. 1981;34:1124–7.
23. Batts DH, Silva J, Fekety R. Staphylococcal enterocolitis. In: Nelson JD, Grassi C, eds. Current Chemotherapy for Infectious Disease. v. 2. Washington, DC: American Society for Microbiology; 1980:944.
24. Schwartz JN, Hamilton JP, Fekety R, et al. Ampicillin-induced enterocolitis: Implication of toxigenic *Clostridium difficile* type C. J Pediatr. 1980;97:661–3.
25. Hovius SER, Rietra PJ. *Salmonella* colitis clinically presenting as a pseudomembranous colitis. Neth J Surg. 1982;34:81–2.
26. Peikin SR, Galdibini J, Bartlett JG. Role of *Clostridium difficile* in a case of nonantibiotic-associated pseudomembranous colitis. Gastroenterology. 1980;79:948–51.
27. Banno Y, Kobayashi T, Watanabe K, et al. Two toxins (D-1 and D-2) of *Clostridium difficile* causing antibiotic-associated colitis: Purification and some characterization. Biochem Int. 1981;2:629.
28. Taylor NS, Thorne GM, Bartlett JG. Comparison of two toxins produced by *Clostridium difficile*. Infect Immun. 1981;34:1036–43.
29. Thelestam M, Bronnegard M. Interaction of cytopathogenic toxin from *Clostridium difficile* with cells in tissue culture. Scand J Infect Dis. 1980;22(Suppl):16–29.
30. Lima AA, Lyerly DM, Wilkins TD, et al. Effect of *Clostridium difficile* toxins A and B in rabbit small and large intestines in vivo and on cultured cells in vitro. Infect Immun. 1988;56:582–8.
31. Justus PG, Martin JI, Golberg DA, et al. Myoelectric effects of *Clostridium difficile:* Motility-altering factors distinct from its cytotoxin and enterotoxin in rabbits. Gastroenterology. 1982;83:836–43.
32. Welch DF, Marks MI. Is *Clostridium difficile* pathogenic in infants? J Pediatr. 1982;100:393–5.
33. Delmee M, Verellen G, Avesani V, et al. *Clostridium difficile* in neonates: Serogrouping and epidemiology. Eur J Pediatr. 1988;147:36–40.
34. Bacon AE, Fekety R, Schaberg DRS, et al. Epidemiology of *C. difficile* colonization in newborns: Results using a bacteriophage and bacteriolin typing system. J Infect Dis. 1988;158:349–54.
35. Griffin GE, Heath J, Knox P. The action of *Clostridium difficile* cytotoxin is inhibited by specific glycoproteins (Abstract 596). Proceedings of the 22nd Interscience Conference on Antimicrobial Agents and Chemotherapy. Washington, DC: American Society for Microbiology; 1982.
36. Chang TW, Sullivan NM, Wilkins TD. Insusceptibility of fetal intestinal mucosa and fetal cells to *Clostridium difficile* toxins. Acta Pharmacol Sin [Chung Kuo Yao Li Hsueh Pao]. 1967;7:448–53.
37. Libby JM, Wilkins TD. Production of antitoxins to two toxins of *Clostridium difficile* and immunological comparison of the toxins by cross-neutralization studies. Infect Immun. 1982;35:374–6.
38. Nakamura S, Mikawa M, Nakashio S, et al. Identification of *Clostridium difficile* from the feces and the antibody in sera of young and elderly adults. Microbiol Immunol. 1981;25:345–51.
39. Viscidi R, Yolken R, Laughon B, et al. Serum antibody response to toxins A and B of *Clostridium difficile* (Abstract 595). Proceedings of the 22nd Interscience Conference on Antimicrobial Agents and Chemotherapy. Washington, DC: American Society for Microbiology; 1982.
40. Lishman AH, Al-Jumaili IJ, Record CO. Antitoxin production in antibiotic-associated colitis? J Clin Pathol. 1981;34:414–5.
41. Fekety R, Silva J, Armstrong J, et al. Treatment of antibiotic-associated enterocolitis with vancomycin. Rev Infect Dis. 1981;3(Suppl):273–81.
42. Silva J, Batts DH, Fekety R. Treatment of *Clostridium difficile* colitis and diarrhea with vancomycin. Am J Med. 1981;71:815–22.
43. Burdon DW, George RH, Mogg G, et al. Faecal toxin and severity of antibiotic-associated pseudomembranous colitis. J Clin Pathol. 1981;34:548–51.
44. Thompson Jr CM, Gilligan PH, Fisher MC, et al. *Clostridium difficile* cytotoxin in a pediatric population. Am J Dis Child. 1983;137:271–4.
45. Guerrant RL, Araiys V, Soares E, et al. Measurement of fecal lactoferrin as a marker of fecal leukocytes. J Clin Microbiol. 1992;30:1238–42.
46. Triadofilopoulas G, Hallstone AE. Acute abdomen as the first presentation of pseudomembranous colitis. Gastroenterology. 1991;101:685–91.
47. Puddey IB. Reiter's syndrome following antibiotic-associated colitis. Aust NZ J Med. 1982;12:292.
48. Megibow AJ, Strieter ML, Balthazar EJ, et al. Pseudomembranous colitis: Diagnosis by computed tomography. J Comput Assist Tomogr. 1984;8:281–3.
49. Yankes JR, Baker ME, Cooper C, et al. CT appearance of fecal pseudomembranous colitis. J Comput Assist Tomogr. 1988;12:394–6.
50. Tedesco FJ. Antibiotic-associated pseudomembranous colitis with negative proctosigmoidoscopy examination. Gastroenterology. 1979;77:295–7.
51. Gerding DN, Olson MM, Peterson LR, et al. *Clostridium difficile*–associated diarrhea and colitis in adults. A prospective case-controlled epidemiologic study. Arch Intern Med. 1986;146:95–100.
52. Lashner BA, Todorczvk J, Sahm DF, et al. *Clostridium difficile* culture-positive toxin-negative diarrhea. Am J Gastroenterol. 1986;81:940–3.
53. Ikard RW: Neutropenic typhilitis in adults. Arch Surg. 1981;116:943–5.
54. Rampling A, Warren RE, Berry PJ, et al. Atypical *Clostridium difficile* colitis in neutropenic patients. Lancet. 1982;2:162–3.
55. Cudmore MA, Silva J, Fekety R, et al. *Clostridium difficile* colitis associated with cancer chemotherapy. Arch Intern Med. 1982;142:333–5.

56. Fainstein V, Bodey GP, Fekety R. *Clostridium difficile* colonization in cancer patients admitted to laminar air-flow units (Abstract). Clin Res. 1982;30:365.

57. Trnka YM, LaMont JT. Associations of *Clostridium difficile* toxin with symptomatic relapse of chronic inflammatory bowel disease. Gastroenterology. 1981;80:693–6.

58. Clabots CR, Gerding SJ, Olson MM, et al. Detection of asymptomatic *Clostridium difficile* carriage by an alcohol shock procedure. J Clin Microbiol. 1989;27:2386–7.

59. Hanff PA, Zaleznik DF, Kent KC, et al. Use of heat shock for culturing *Clostridium difficile* from rectal swabs. Clin Infect Dis. 1993;16(Suppl. 4): S245–S247.

60. Larson L, Holst E, Gemmell CG, et al. Characterization of *Clostridium difficile* and its differentiation from *Clostridium sporogenes* by automatic headspace gas chromatography. Scand J Infect Dis. 1980;22(Suppl):37.

61. Chang TW, Lauermann M, Bartlett JG. Cytotoxicity assay in antibiotic-associated colitis. J Infect Dis. 1979;140:765–70.

62. Chang TW. *Clostridium difficile* toxin and antimicrobial agent-induced diarrhea. J Infect Dis. 1978;137:854–5.

63. Gerding A, Brazier JS. Optimal methods for indentifying *C. difficile* infections. Clin Infect Dis. 1993;16(Suppl 4):S439–42.

64. Tedesco F, Markham R, Gurwith M, et al. Oral vancomycin for antibiotic-associated pseudomembranous colitis. Lancet. 1978;2:226–8.

65. Aronsson B, Granstrom M, Molby R, et al. Toxin A (enterotoxin) from *Clostridium difficile* in antibiotic-associated colitis. Lancet. 1982;2:1279.

66. Tucker KD, Carrig PE, Wilkins TD. Toxin A of *Clostridium difficile* is a potent cytotoxin. J Clin Microbiol. 1990;28:869–71.

67. Brazier JS. Role of the laboratory in investigation of *Clostridium difficile* diarrhea. Clin Infect Dis. 1993;16(Suppl 4):S228–33.

68. Lyerly DM, Barroso LA, Wilkins TD. Identification of the latex test-reactive protein of *Clostridium difficile* as glutamate dehydrogenase. J Clin Microbiol. 1988;29:2639–42.

69. Lyerly DM, Barraso LA, Wilkins TD. Characterization of cross-reactive proteins detected by Culturette Brand Rapid Latex Test for *Clostridium difficile*. J Clin Microbiol. 1988;29:397–400.

70. Peterson LC, Kelly PJ. The role of the clinical microbiology laboratory in the management of *C. difficile*–associated diarrhea. Infect Dis Clin North Am. 1993;7:277–93.

71. Wren BW, Clayton CL, Castledine NB, et al. Identification of toxigenic *C. difficile* strains by using a toxin A gene-specific proble. J Clin Microbiol. 1990;28:1808–12.

72. Katon, Ou C-Y, Kato H, et al. Identification of toxigenic *C. difficile* by the polymerase chain reaction. J Clin Microbiol. 1991;29:33–7.

73. Gumerlock PH, Tang YJ, Weiss JB, et al. Specific detection of toxigenic strains of *C. difficile* in stools. J Clin Microbiol. 1993;31:507–11.

74. Kuhl SJ, Tang YJ, Navarro L, et al. Diagnosis and monitoring *C. difficile* infections with the polymerase chain reaction. Clin Infect Dis. 1993;16(Suppl 4):S234–8.

75. Gibson GR, Whitacre EB, Ricotti CA. Colitis induced by nonsteroidal antiinflammatory drugs: Report of four cases and review of the literature. Arch Intern Med. 1992;152:625–32.

76. Gentric A, Pennec YL. Diclofenac-induced pseudomembranous colitis. Lancet. 1992;340:126–7.

77. Keighley MRB, Burdon DW, Arabi Y, et al. Randomized controlled trial of vancomycin for pseudomembranous colitis and postoperative diarrhea. Br Med J. 1978;2:1667.

78. Pashby NL, Bolton RP, Sherriff RJ. Oral metronidazole in *Clostridium difficile* colitis. Br Med J. 1979;1:1605–6.

79. Chang T-W, Gorbach SL, Bartlett JG, et al. Bacitracin treatment of antibiotic-associated colitis and diarrhea caused by *Clostridium difficile* toxin. Gastroenterology. 1980;78:1584–6.

80. Fekety R, Silva J, Kauffman C, et al. Treatment of *Clostridium difficile* antibiotic-associated colitis with oral vancomycin: Comparison of two dosage regimens. Am J Med. 1989;86:15–9.

81. Geraci JE, Heilman FR, Nichols DR, et al. Some laboratory and clinical experiences with a new antibiotic, vancomycin. Proc Staff Meet Mayo Clin. 1956;31:564.

82. Donta ST, Lamps GM, Summers KW, et al. Cephalosporin-associated colitis and *Clostridium difficile*. Arch Intern Med. 1980;140:574–7.

83. Cherry RD, Portnoy D, Jabbari M, et al. Metronidazole: An alternate therapy for antibiotic-associated colitis. Gastroenterology. 1982;82:849–51.

84. Teasley DG, Gerding DN, Olson MN, et al. Prospective randomized trial of metronidazole versus vancomycin for the treatment of *Clostridium difficile* associated diarrhea and colitis. Lancet. 1983;2:1043–6.

85. Saginur R, Hawley CR, Bartlett JG. Colitis associated with metronidazole therapy. J Infect Dis. 1980;141:772–4.

86. Bolton RF, Culshaw MA. Faecal metronidazole concentrations during oral and intravenous therapy for antibiotic-associated colitis due to *Clostridium difficile*. Gut. 1986;27:1169–72.

87. Kleinfeld DI, Sharpe RJ, Donta ST. Parenteral therapy for antibiotic-associated pseudomembranous colitis. J Infect Dis. 1988;157:389.

88. Bergan T, Solhaug JH, Soreide O, et al. Comparative pharmacokinetics of metronidazole and tinidazole and their tissue penetration. Scand J Gastroenterol. 1985;20:945–50.

89. Pasic M, Jost R, Carell T, et al. Intracolonic vancomycin for pseudomembranous colitis. N Engl J Med. 1993;329:583.

90. Tedesco FJ. Bacitracin therapy in antibiotic-associated pseudomembranous colitis. Dig Dis Sci. 1980;25:783–4.

91. Young GP, Ward PB, Bayley N, et al. Antibiotic-associated colitis due to *Clostridium difficile*: Double-blind comparison of vancomycin with bacitracin. Gastroenterology. 1985;89:1038–45.

92. Dudley MN, McLaughlin JC, Carrington G, et al. Oral bacitracin vs vancomycin therapy for *Clostridium difficile*–induced diarrhea. A randomized double-blind trial. Arch Intern Med. 1986;146:1101–4.

93. Cronberg S, Castor B, Thoren A. Fusidic acid for the treatment of antibiotic-associated colitis induced by *Clostridium difficile*. Infection. 1984;12:276–9.

94. Kreutzer EW, Milligan FD. Treatment of antibiotic-associated pseudomembranous colitis with cholestyramine resin. Johns Hopkins Med J. 1978;143: 67–72.

94a. de Lalla F, Nicolin R, Rinaldi E, et al. Prospective study of oral teicoplanin versus oral vancomycin for therapy of pseudomembranous colitis and *Clostridium difficile*-associated diarrhea. Antimicrob Agents Chemother. 1992; 36:2192–6.

95. Fekety R, Browne RA, Silva J, et al. Fecal bile acids and cholestyramine in hamsters with clindamycin-associated colitis (Abstract 129). Proceedings of the 18th Interscience Conference on Antimicrobial Agents and Chemotherapy. Atlanta: American Society for Microbiology; 1978.

96. King CY, Barriere SL. Analysis of the in vitro interaction between vancomycin and cholestyramine. Antimicrob Agents Chemother. 1981;19:326–7.

97. Novak E, Lee JG, Seckman E, et al. Unfavorable effect of atropine-diphenoxylate (Lomotil) therapy in lincomycin-caused diarrhea. JAMA. 1976;235: 1451–4.

98. DuPont H, Cooperstock M, Corrado ML, et al. Evaluation of new anti-infective agents for the treatment of antibiotic-associated colitis. Clin Infect Dis. 1992;15(Suppl 1):S263–7.

99. George WL, Volpicelli NA, Stiner DB, et al. Relapse of pseudomembranous colitis after vancomycin therapy. N Engl J Med. 1979;301:414–5.

100. Bartlett JG, Tedesco FJ, Shull S, et al. Symptomatic relapse after oral vancomycin therapy of antibiotic-associated pseudomembranous colitis. Gastroenterology. 1980;78:431–4.

101. George WL, Rolfe RD, Finegold SM. Treatment and prevention of antimicrobial agent-induced colitis and diarrhea. Gastroenterology. 1980;79:366–72.

102. Walters BAJ, Roberts R, Stafford R, et al. Relapse of antibiotic-associated colitis: Endogenous persistence of *Clostridium difficile* during vancomycin therapy. Gut. 1983;24:206–12.

103. Silva J, Lusk R, Fekety R, et al. Immune responses of hamsters and humans with antibiotic-associated colitis. In: Lambe DW Jr, Genco RJ, Mayberry-Carson KJ, eds. Anaerobic Bacteria: Selected Topics. New York: Plenum; 1980:295.

104. Johnson G, Gerding DN, Janoff EN. Systemic and mucosal antibody responses to toxin A in patients infected with *C. difficile*. J Infect Dis. 1992; 166:1287–94.

105. Buggy BP, Fekety R, Silva J. Therapy of relapsing *Clostridium difficile*–associated diarrhea and colitis with the combination of vancomycin and rifampin. J Clin Gastroenterol. 1987;9:155–9.

106. Leving DYM, Kelly CP, Boguniewicz M, et al. Treatment with intravenously administered gamma globulin of relapsing colitis induced by *C. difficile* toxin. J Pediatr. 1991;118:633–7.

107. Tedesco FJ. Treatment of recurrent antibiotic-associated pseudomembranous colitis. Am J Gastroenterol. 1982;77:220–1.

108. Schwan A, Sjolin S, Trottestan U. Relapsing *Clostridium difficile* enterocolitis cured by rectal infusion of homologous faeces. Lancet. 1983;2:845.

109. Schwan A, Sjolin S, Trottesam U, et al. Relapsing *Clostridium difficile* enterocolitis cured by rectal infusion of normal faeces. Scand J Infect Dis 1984; 16:211–5.

110. Wilson KH, Sheagren JH, Freter R, et al. Gnotobiotic models for study of the microbiol ecology of *Clostridium difficile* and *Escherichia coli*. J Infect Dis. 1986;153:547–51.

111. Borriello SP, Barclay FP. An in vitro model of colonisation resistance to *Clostridium difficile* infection. J Med Microbiol. 1986;21:299–309.

112. Elmer G, McFarland LV. Suppression by *Saccharomyces boulardii* of toxigenic *Clostridium difficile* overgrowth after vancomycin treatment of hamsters. Antimicrob Agents Chemother. 1987;31:129–31.

113. Seal D, Borriello SP, Barclay FE, et al. Treatment of relapsing *Clostridium difficile* diarrhoeae by administration of a non-toxigenic strain. Eur J Clin Microbiol. 1987;6:51–3.

114. Wilson KH, Silva J, Fekety FR. Suppression of *Clostridium difficile* by normal hamster cecal flora and prevention of antibiotic-associated cecitis. Infect Immun. 1981;34:626–8.

115. Wilson KH, Sheagren JN. Antagonism of toxigenic *Clostridium difficile* by nontoxigenic *C. difficile*. J Infect Dis. 1983;147:733–6.

116. Rolfe RD, Helebian S, Finegold SM. Bacterial interference between *Clostridium difficile* and normal fecal flora. J Infect Dis. 1981;143:470–5.

117. Malamoa-Lodas H, Tabaqchali S. Inhibition of *Clostridium difficile* by fecal streptococci. J Med Microbiol. 1982;15:569–74.

118. McFarland LV, Bernasconi P. *Saccharomyces boulardii*: A review of an innovative biotherapeutic agent. Microb Etiol Health Dis. 1993;6:157–171.

119. Toothaker RD, Elmer GW. Prevention of clindamycin-induced mortality in hamsters by *Saccharomyces boulardii*. Antimicrob Agents Chemother. 1984; 26:552–6.

120. Castex F, Corthier G, Jowert S, et al. Prevention of *Clostridium difficile*–induced experimental pseudomembranous colitis by *Saccharomyces boulardii*: A scanning electron microscopic and microbiologic study. J Gen Microbiol. 1990;136:1085–9.

121. Elmer G, McFarland LV. Suppression by *S. boulardii* of toxigenic *C. difficile*

overgrowth after vancomycin treatment of hamsters. Antimicrob Agents Chemother. 1987;31:129–31.

122. Surawicz CM, Elmer GW, Speelman P, et al. Prevention of antibiotic-associated diarrhea by *S. boulardii:* A prospective study. Gastroenterology. 1989; 96:991–8.

123. Surawicz CM, McFarland LV, Elmer G, et al. Treatment of recurrent *C. difficile* colitis with vancomycin and *S. boulardii.* Am J Gastroenterol. 1989; 84:1285–7.

124. Buts JP, Corthier G, Delmar M. *S. boulardii* for *C. difficile*–associated enteropathies in infants. J Pediatr Gastroenterol Nutr. 1993;16:419–25.

125. Johnson S, Gerding DN, Olson M, et al. Prospective, controlled study of vinyl glove use to interrupt *Clostridium difficile.* J Infect Dis. 1992;166: 1287–94.

126. Johnson S, Homann SR, Bettin KM, et al. Treatment of asymptomatic *Clostridium difficile* carriers (fecal excretors) with vancomycin or metronidazole. A randomized, placebo-controlled trial. Ann Intern Med. 1992;117:297–302.

127. Wust J, Sullivan NM, Hardegger U, et al. Investigation of an outbreak of antibiotic-associated colitis by various typing methods. J Clin Microbiol. 1982;16:1096–101.

128. Sell TL, Schaberg DR, Fekety FR. Bacteriophage and bacteriocin typing scheme for *Clostridium difficile.* J Clin Microbiol. 1983;17:1148–52.

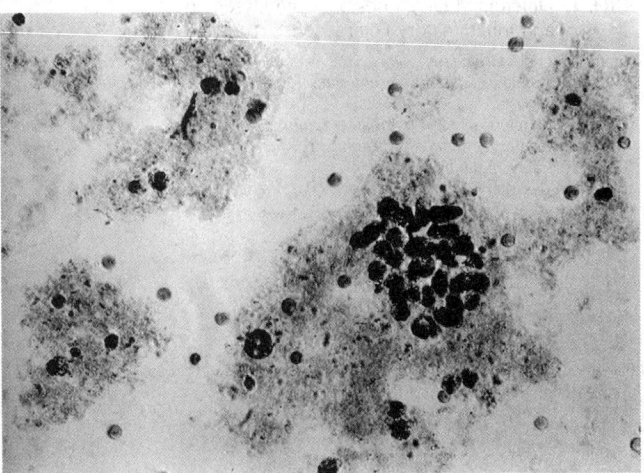

FIG. 1. Methylene blue stain of fecal leukocytes found in colitis. This exudative response may be seen in shigellosis, salmonellosis, *Campylobacter* infection, and colitis due to invasive *E. coli.*

79. INFLAMMATORY ENTERITIDES

RICHARD L. GUERRANT

The acute inflammatory enteritides include several specific distal small bowel and colonic infections such as campylobacteriosis salmonellosis, shigellosis, and amebiasis, as well as the syndromes of necrotizing enteritis and antibiotic-associated pseudomembranous enterocolitis. Several other infectious agents cause chronic enteric inflammatory processes that may result in syndromes of abdominal pain, weight loss, diarrhea, or malabsorption. These include such processes as gastrointestinal mycoses, mycobacterioses, bacterial infections, and certain parasitic infections such as coccidiosis.

ACUTE DYSENTERY: HISTORY, EPIDEMIOLOGY, AND DIAGNOSIS

Syndromes of acute dysentery with fecal blood and pus have been well recognized since the days of Hippocrates. Dysentery implies frequent, small bowel movements accompanied by blood and mucus with tenesmus or pain on defecation. This syndrome implies an inflammatory invasion of the colonic mucosa resulting from bacterial, cytotoxic, or parasitic destruction.

The pathologic changes of inflammatory colitis range from a superficial intense exudative inflammatory process involving the colonic mucosa by shigellae or invasive *Escherichia coli* to deeper, penetrating, ''flask-shaped'' ulcers with undermined edges as seen in amebic dysentery. The pathogenesis of the inflammatory colitides may involve cytotoxic products of shigellae,[1] certain *E. coli*,[2] clostridia, or other organisms.

The epidemiologic patterns of acute dysenteric syndromes are influenced by the unusually low inoculum required by organisms such as shigellae or amebae for infection. As few as 10^2 shigellae or as few as 10 cysts of enteric parasites such as *Entamoeba coli* or *Giardia lamblia* may cause infection in adult volunteers.[3,4] Consequently, there is a substantial risk of person-to-person spread in day care centers,[5] institutions, or other areas where nonhygienic conditions may allow direct fecal–oral spread. The cysts of parasites such as *Entamoeba histolytica* or *Balantidium coli* often resist chlorination and therefore may cause waterborne outbreaks of dysenteric illnesses. Saltwater or seafood exposure should lead one to consider *Vibrio parahaemolyticus* as a cause of inflammatory colitis, and farm or domestic animal exposure might lead one to consider nontyphoid *Salmonella* spp., *Campylobacter jejuni,* or *Yersina enterocolitica.* In addition, when typhoid fever is present with diarrhea in an endemic area, the diarrhea is often inflammatory, with many fecal polymorphonuclear leukocytes seen on microscopic examination.[6] Travel to areas of poor sanitation might implicate any of the aforementioned pathogens. Finally, venereal exposure, particularly among male homosexuals, might implicate *Gonococcus,* herpes simplex virus, *Chlamydia trachomatis,* or *Treponema pallidum* as causes of proctitis or *Campylobacter, Shigella, Chlamydia trachomatis* (lymphogranuloma venereum serotypes), *E. histolytica,* or *Clostridium difficile* as causes of colitis.[7]

Examination for fecal leukocytes often reveals sheets of polymorphonuclear leukocytes in clumps of mucus even in the absence of gross blood in the stool specimen (Fig. 1).[8,9] Fewer pyknotic leukocytes are reported in amebic dysentery[10–12]; this may be attributable to the deeper, undermining ulcers characteristic of intestinal amebiasis or to a contact-dependent cytolytic effect of the ameba on leukocytes. A prompt culture of fresh specimens onto appropriate enteric culture media is very important in the isolation of shigellae.[13] Specialized techniques are required to isolate *Vibrio* (thiosulfate citrate bile salt agar),[14] *Yersinia* (cold enrichment),[15] or *C. jejuni.*[16] The identification of toxigenic *C. difficile* colitis is done by immunoassay or cell culture cytotoxicity assay for *C. difficile* toxin A or B, respectively.[17–19] Leukocytosis or even a leukemoid reaction has been described. Sigmoidoscopic examination, especially with biopsy, may be useful in the diagnosis of a pseudomembranous enterocolitis or in the identification of parasites such as *En. histolytica* (with special PAS stain) or *Balantidium coli.* Amebic colitis is associated with discrete small ulcerations with undermined edges amid relatively normal mucosa. Acute shigellosis causes more widespread, shallow, 3- to 7-mm ulcers with a more intense inflammatory exudate. Barium studies are unnecessary and are relatively contradicted in toxic patients with acute colitis. Therapy consists of careful supportive fluid management with specific antimicrobial therapy directed at a specific pathogen if suspected by the epidemiologic setting or culture results.

The potential etiologies of acute dysentery are listed in Table 1.

Bacillary Dysentery (Shigellosis and Enteroinvasive E. coli)

It is estimated that *Shigella* spp. infect over 200 million people and cause 650,000 deaths each year worldwide.[20] *Shigella* spp.

TABLE 1. Differential Diagnoses of Acute Dysentery and Inflammatory Enterocolitis

Specific infectious processes
  Bacillary dysentery (*Shigella dysenteriae, flexneri, sonnei, boydii;* invasive *E. coli*)
    Campylobacteriosis (*Campylobacter jejuni*)
  Amebic dysentery (*Entamoeba histolytica*)
  Ciliar dysentery (*Balantidium coli*)
  Bilharzial dysentery (*Schistosma japonicum, mansoni*)
  Other parasites (*Trichinella spiralis*)
  Vibriosis (*Vibrio parahaemolyticus*)
  Salmonellosis (*Salmonella typhimurium*)
  Typhoid fever (*Salmonella typhi*)
  Enteric fever (*Salmonella choleraesuis, paratyphi*)
  Yersiniosis (*Yersinia enterocolitica*)
  Spirillar dysentery (*Spirillum* sp.)
Proctitis
  Gonococcal (*Neisseria gonorrhoeae*)
  Herpetic (herpes simplex virus)
  Chlamydial (*Chlamydia trachomatis*)
  Syphilitic (*Treponema pallidum*)
Other syndromes
  Necrotizing enterocolitis of the newborn
  Enteritis necroticans
  Pseudomembraneous enterocolitis (*Clostridium difficile*)
  Diverticulitis
  Typhlitis
Syndromes without known infectious etiology
  Idiopathic ulcerative colitis
  Crohn's disease
  Radiation enteritis
  Ischemic colitis
  Allergic enteritis

TABLE 2. Enteroinvasive *E. coli* Serotypes

Serotype	Difco Serogroup	References
O28 ac	C	31, 34
O29		35
O112 a,c	C	34
O124	B	31, 34, 36
O136	C (Trabulsi's 193-T-64)	34, 36
O143		34
O144		34, 36
O152	(Trabulsi's 185-T-64)	34, 36
O164		34
O167		35
O173		51

(types A–D: *dysenteriae, flexneri, sonnei,* and *boydii*) may cause acute bloody dysentery with high fever and systemic manifestations of malaise, headache, and abdominal pain. The incubation period ranges from 6 hours to 9 days but is usually less than 72 hours. This syndrome may be particularly severe in poorly nourished children. As noted previously, this organism may be spread with relatively small inocula by direct contact as well as in food or water.

Despite the intense superficial destructive process in the colonic epithelium that typifies acute shigellosis, bacteremia and disseminated infection are relatively rare.[21] *Shigella* infection (especially with *Sh. dysenteriae* type 1) is associated with enteric protein loss that improves after appropriate antimicrobial therapy.[22] This may contribute to increased susceptibility to secondary infections or growth stunting.[23,24] A complication of severe shigellosis in childhood is a hemolytic-uremic syndrome that may be associated with a leukemoid reaction, pseudomembranous colitis, circulating immune complexes, and circulating endotoxin, usually in the absence of demonstrable bacteremia.[25]

Intestinal obstruction, which occurs in about 3 percent of patients, is a poor prognostic sign, not infrequently associated with death or the development of hemolytic uremic syndrome.[26] Other less common extraintestinal manifestations of shigellosis include headache, meningismus, and even seizures, especially in children.[27] These findings may be attributable to a neurotoxin that has been demonstrated with *S. dysenteriae* type I.[1,28] A serious arthritis similar to that seen in Reiter's syndrome has been described in up to 10 percent of the patients 2–5 weeks after the dysenteric illness that characteristically occurs in patients with histocompatibility antigen HLA B27.[29,30] Culture-positive conjunctivitis during acute shigellosis has also been described and may represent autoinoculation of the conjunctiva analogous to that induced in the guinea pigs in the Sereny test.[31] Arthritis syndromes have also been described after inflammatory colitis with *Y. enterocolitica, S. enteritidis,* or C. difficile again in association with HLA B27.[32,33]

Certain *E. coli* strains may produce an identical syndrome to that seen with acute shigellosis. The incubation period is usually 2–3 days after ingestion. Although invasive *E. coli* organisms

appear to be limited to certain serotypes (Table 2),[31,34] to identify invasive *E. coli* one should demonstrate their invasive potential in the guinea pig conjunctivitis (Sereny) test,[37] in Hela cells,[38] or identify the 120–140 megadalton plasmid that is associated with invasiveness in *Shigella* and invasive *E. coli*.[39–41] Invasive *E. coli* organisms were responsible for a single widespread outbreak of dysentery associated with imported French Camembert cheese.[36,42] While they have been identified as occasional causes of diarrhea in Brazil,[31] invasive *E. coli* do not appear to be frequent causes of sporadic diarrhea in the United States. Because they are often slow to ferment lactose in the laboratory, invasive *E. coli* may be initially mistaken for shigellae,[31,36,43] to which they are closely related. Invasive *E. coli* are also usually lysine negative and often nonmotile[44] and are antigenitically related to *Shigella*.[45]

Enterohemorrhagic E. coli Diarrhea

Although the frequency with which it causes inflammatory diarrhea is not clear, a significant cause of bloody diarrhea and potentially fatal hemolytic uremic syndrome (HUS) is now recognized to be enterhemorrhagic *E. coli* (EHEC) that produce relatively large amounts of Shiga-like (Vero) cytotoxin (SLT I and/or II).[2,46] These organisms have attracted particular attention with recent widespread outbreaks in popular hamburger chain restaurants.[47–49] While they account for only 0.8–3.0 percent of all diarrhea in the United States and Canada, EHEC (of serotype O157) are estimated to account for 15–36 percent of cases of bloody diarrhea.[2,50] The majority of recognized EHEC are of serotype O157; others include O26:K60:H11; O103:H2; O91:H2; O145:H–; O111:K58:H–; O38:H21; O6:H–;O5: H–O128; O139; O113:K75; O121; and O172.[2,35,50,51] EHEC were the most commonly recognized cause of diarrhea (3 percent) among 5415 patients studied in Calgary, Canada, where they showed a summer seasonal peak.[50] In addition to causing 15–36 percent of all cases of bloody diarrhea, including outbreaks of hemorrhagic colitis, EHEC are associated with 75–90 percent of cases of hemolytic-uremic syndrome in North America, a complication that develops in 8 percent of EHEC infections.[2] After binding to a globotrisylceramide receptor, the Shiga-like toxin cleaves adenosine from an *N*-glycoside bond at nucleotide residue 4324 on the 60 S ribosomal RNA to block protein synthesis by inhibiting EF1-dependent aminoacyl t-RNA binding.[2,52,53] The diagnosis is suspected on clinical grounds and confirmed by serotyping sorbitol-negative *E. coli* insolates or by using tissue culture or gene probes to detect the cytotoxin.

Campylobacter Enteritis

Campylobacter jejuni (formerly *C. fetus* or "*Vibrio fetus*") systemic infections have been recognized for many years. While the majority of *Campylobacter* blood stream infections in humans are with *C. fetus* (old subspecies, *intestinalis*),[54] *C. jejuni* commonly causes an enteric infection in all ages. This organism was recognized many years ago as a cause of swine dysentery.[55] Commercially available techniques of fecal culture have enabled the culture of *C. jejuni* on highly selective media at 42°C from fecal specimens of patients with diarrhea.[16,56] These techniques have revealed a syndrome of severe abdominal pain, fever, and acute inflammatory enteritis that may result in dysentery with blood and pus in the stools.[56–58] Reports from Belgium, England, and central Africa reveal that 5–14 percent of unselected cases of diarrhea have *C. jejuni*,[57–59] and outbreaks of *Campylobacter* enteritis have been associated with ingestion of contaminated water, raw milk, or uncooked meat or poultry. The roles of toxins, adhesins, and lipopolysaccharides in the pathogenesis of *Campylobacter* enteritis remains uncertain.[60]

Amebic Dysentery

Entamoeba histolytica cysts are ingested, pass through the gastric acidity, and have the capsule digested in the small bowel. Trophozoites then invade the colonic mucosa and produce shallow, flasklike undermining ulcers. The capacity of this parasite to invade tissue has been attributed to histolytic enzymes, but likely also involves contact-dependent cytolysis of target cells, especially polymorphonuclear leukocytes that then discharge their cytolytic contents.[61–67] After their invasion in the intestine, amebae may then seed the liver via the portal vein, from which extension may occur to the skin, diaphragm, lung, or pericardium. While extraintestinal amebiasis occurs with less than one-tenth the frequency of symptomatic intestinal amebic dysentery, dissemination is reportedly more common in states of undernutrition, cytotoxic or steroid medication, late pregnancy, carcinoma, or other overwhelming systemic diseases. Asymptomatic cyst carriage occurs in 1–5 percent of the population in the southern United States. The frequency of amebiasis is greater in rural and lower socioeconomic groups and in institutions where fecal–oral spread of this human parasite may occur.[68] The role of amebic infections that are highly prevalent among promiscuous male homosexuals in producing symptoms or invasive disease remain unclear.[69,70]

Ciliar Dysentery

Balantidium coli is the only ciliate parasite that is pathogenic for humans. The most common reservoir is swine. Like *E. histolytica*, this parasite excysts in the small bowel, invades the terminal ileum and colon, and may cause appendicitis or a dysenteric syndrome with rectosigmoid ulceration (with heaped-up 1.5- to 3-cm ulcers) and secondary bacteremia. However, there is no extraintestinal extension of *B. coli* as one may see with amebiasis. The diagnosis is made by scraping the margin of the ulcer and examining microscopically for the ciliate trophozoite. Mucosal invasion is usually limited to the rectal vault. Symptoms may last for 1–4 weeks and may recur several times a year if the diagnosis is not suspected. Treatment is usually successful with tetracycline.

Bilharzial Dysentery

Schistosomiasis may cause acute bloody diarrhea, abdominal pain, and weight loss when the adult schistosomes (usually *S. japonicum* or *S. mansoni*) migrate to the intestinal tract where they begin egg deposition. This occurs 3–8 weeks after initial skin exposure to the cercariae and may last for several weeks. Fecal examination reveals blood, pus, and numerous ova. Fever, leukocytosis, and increasing eosinophilia may be associated with this illness, and hepatosplenic disease may follow. *S. mansoni* may also cause chronic blood or protein loss via inflammatory "polyps."

Other Parasites

Another potential parasitic cause of inflammatory enteritis is acute trichinosis. Approximately 24 hours after the ingestion of infested pork, the larvae excyst and invade the intestinal mucosa, often resulting in nausea, vomiting, diarrhea, and abdominal pain. This precedes the systemic manifestation of periorbital edema, fever, myositis, and eosinophilis by 1–2 weeks.

Vibriosis

In addition to classic and El Tor *Vibrio cholerae* O1, non-O1 *V. cholerae* and several halophilic *Vibrio* species are now recognized to cause diarrhea and occasional wound or blood stream infection.[71,72] The most common and best characterized is *V. parahaemolyticus*. *Vibrio parahaemolyticus* has been recognized since 1950 in Japan and was identified as a *Vibrio* in 1963. *Vibrio parahaemolyticus* is a cause of seafood poisoning 9–25 hours after the ingestion of inadequately cooked fish or shellfish. This has been reported throughout the coastal areas of the United States and on cruise ships and is the most common cause of food poisoning in Japan, where raw seafood is commonly eaten.[73] Diarrhea may be explosive and watery or may be characterized by full-blown dysentery with blood and pus and superficial ulceration on proctoscopic examination.[74,75] The latter syndrome may be associated with cramps, nausea, vomiting, headache, and fever. The illness usually is self-limited within 3–4 days. The pathogenic Kanagawa-positive strains from patients produce β-hemolysis on special (Wagatsuma) medium—in contrast to environmental isolates—and are best isolated as blue-green colonies (alkaline) on thiosulfate citrate bile salt sucrose (TCBS) agar.[14]

Other halophilic vibrios include *V. alginolyticus, fluvialis, hollisase, damsella,* and *vulnificus,* which have been associated with enteric, wound, or systemic infections in humans.[71,72] *Vibrio vulnificus* has been associated with life-threatening septicemia within 24 hours of ingesting raw oysters.[72,76]

Salmonellosis

Salmonella enterocolitis is characterized by fever, cramping, abdominal pain, and diarrhea that begins 8–48 hours after ingestion of an infection dose, usually with food, and usually lasts 3–5 days. The diarrheal stools of patients with salmonellosis often contain a moderate number of polymorphonuclear leukocytes, usually fewer than is typical of shigellosis.

While salmonella enteritis predominantly involves the lamina propria in the small bowel, several reports have noted colitis due to *S. typhimurium,* with crypt abscesses and erosion and ulcerations of the colonic mucosa resulting in blood and pus in the stool.[77–81] Certain other strains of salmonella (*S. choleraesuis* and *S. paratyphi*), like *S. typhi,* tend to elicit a mononuclear response and cause a bacteremia characteristic of enteric fever.

Typhoid Fever

Typhoid fever may lead to an erosion of the blood vessels in Peyer's patches that, if untreated, may result in gross blood in the feces in 10–20 percent of the patients. Severe intestinal hemorrhage may complicate approximately 2 percent of the cases late in the course of untreated typhoid fever. Such intestinal bleeding may precede perforation, another complication of typhoid fever.[82]

Yersiniosis

Yersinia enterocolitica is another increasingly recognized enteric pathogen that may be responsible for an enteric feverlike illness, mesenteric adenitis (that may mimic acute appendicitis), or an inflammatory ileitis or ulcerative colitis syndrome with fecal neutrophils and mononuclear cells.[83-85] *Yersinia* may also be associated with migratory polyarthritis, Reiter syndrome, or erythema nodosum. A syndrome with acute diarrhea and vomiting is especially common in young children.[86] The organism may cause disseminated abscesses in the liver and spleen[87] or an inflammatory colitis.[88] The causative agent, a gram-negative member of the family Enterobacteriaceae, is in the same genus as the plague bacillus *Y. pestis* and is sometimes mistaken for *Proteus* on initial culture plates. Cultivation may require "cold enrichment."[15]

Gonococcal Proctitis

Neisseria gonorrhoeae may be the cause of ulcerative proctitis, usually acquired by venereal exposure.[7] The resultant purulent proctitis appears with an erythematous friable mucous membrane in the rectal vault and occasional abscess or fistula formation. While copious purulent discharge, tenesmus, and burning rectal pain may be noted, two-thirds of the culture-positive patients with anorectal gonococcal infection are asymptomatic.[89,90] Also in the differential diagnosis of venereally acquired proctitis are syphylitic, herpetic, and chlamydial proctitis.[91]

Spirillar Dysentery

"Spirillar" or "spirochetal" dysentery has been reported to occur in southern France and has been attributed to *Spirillum* spp.[92] While severe mucoid diarrhea or dysentery has been associated with intestinal spirochetes, their frequency and role in causing enteric disease is unclear.[93] A DNA probe for the 16 S rRNA of the cause of swine dysentery, *Treponema hyodysenteriae* has been developed and may open new approaches to the recognition of similar infections in humans.[94]

Other unusual or emerging causes of colitis include brucellosis[95] and adenovirus infections.[96,97]

Approach to Diagnosis and Treatment of Acute Dysentery

Any of the aforementioned microorganisms may cause an acute dysentery syndrome with blood and pus in the stool; examination for leukocytes or for indirect evidence such as fecal lactoferrin[98] may suggest one of the above etiologies even if blood is not present in the stool on gross examination. Other diagnoses to be considered in the differential diagnosis of inflammatory colitis are pseudomembranous enterocolitis, which may be associated with antibiotic use, and the potentially rapidly progressive necrotizing enterocolitis syndromes, which are discussed in the subsequent sections. These diagnoses are suspected by clinical course, history, and radiologic and proctoscopic examinations. Noninfectious syndromes that may be manifested with acute inflammatory enterocolitis include idiopathic ulcerative colitis and Crohn's disease.

Presumptive therapy for the inflammatory colitides varies greatly with the suspected etiology (see "Algorithm" in Ch. 75). For example, an acute febrile dysenteric illness in a young child with day care exposure or in an area where shigellosis is common should be treated with an appropriate absorbable antimicrobial agent such as ampicillin or sulfamethoxazole-trimethoprim. If the *Shigella* organism is sensitive, prompt therapy can successfully reduce the diarrhea, systemic symptoms, and shedding of the organisms in the feces.[99-101] Nonabsorbable antibiotics such as colistin or aminoglycosides are ineffective, possibly because they do not prevent the spread of shigellae to adjacent epithelial cells.[102] Because shigellae are increasingly antibiotic resistant,[103,104] one must be familiar with the local resistance pattern of shigellae to appropriate treat acute shigellosis when it is first suspected. The quinolone antibiotics offer a considerable advance in treating inflammatory diarrhea. Not only are they effective in treating otherwise resistant shigellosis, but they re-

duce fecal shedding and the duration of illness with *C. jejuni* and, although they do not necessarily eradicate the organism, may shorten symptoms even with *Salmonella* infections.[105-107]

Amebic dysentery is usually diagnosed by direct examination of wet mounts of fresh fecal or proctoscopic specimens, which reveal *E. histolytica* trophozoites or cysts in 60–80 percent of the cases. The cysts and trophozoites are characterized by four or fewer delicate nuclei with central karyosomes. Additional patients may be diagnosed by biopsy, where PAS-positive trophozoites or cysts may be found in the undermining ulcer in the lamina propria, or by a serum indirect hemagglutinating antibody (IHA) test, which is positive in approximately 90 percent of the patients with intestinal amebiasis.[108] While the systemic amebacide metronidazole is effective in eradicating hepatic amebiasis and may eradicate intestinal disease, the lumenocide diiodohydroxyquin may be required to eradicate intestinal infection. The therapy for balantidiasis is tetracycline or diiodohydroxyquin. Praziquantel is used for significant schistosomal infections. The optimal therapies for *V. parahaemolyticus*, *Y. enterocolitica*, and *C. jejuni* infections are not well established and should be tailored to the specific sensitivity pattern of the organism isolated. Gonococcal proctitis may be difficult to eradicate but should be treated (ceftriaxone, 250 mg im).

As with all diarrheas, the therapy for *Salmonella* gastroenteritis is supportive fluid management. With the apparent exception of ciprofloxacin,[105] oral antibiotics are of no benefit and may actually prolong shedding of the organism and even be associated with increased risk of relapse in children.[109,110]

NECROTIZING ENTEROCOLITIS IN THE NEWBORN

The syndrome of diffuse fulminating necrotizing colitis has been increasingly recognized among infants since reports by Waldhausen et al.[111] in 1963 and Mizrahi and colleagues[112] in 1965. This syndrome probably represents the same entity described as "spontaneous" intestinal perforation and peritonitis as early as 1838.[113-115] While milder forms of the syndrome doubtless exist, the syndrome of necrotizing enterocolitis (NEC) is defined by air in the wall of the intestine, portal venous system, or peritoneal cavity or by necrosis of the bowel wall with mucosal sloughing. This fulminant syndrome often leads to intestinal perforation, peritonitis, and bacteremia. It is a major cause of mortality in low-birth-weight infants (<1500 g) after the first week of life.[116] The diffuse necrotic changes that characterize this syndrome most often occur in the terminal ileum but may be seen in the colon or in the proximal portion of the gastrointestinal tract.

The pathogenesis of NEC appears to involve mucosal injury that is most often ischemic from hypoxemic or hypotensive episodes that may occur in premature infants or infants with complicating features such as an umbilical vein exchange transfusion. Ischemia may also result from the effects of endotoxemia followed by the effects of epinephrine, to which the vessels supplying the terminal ileum may be especially sensitive. Other predisposing factors to mucosal ischemia include asphyxia in association with hyaline membrane disease in premature infants or cyanotic heart disease. Increased intraluminal pressures may contribute to ischemia and pneumatosis, a process that may also play a role in previously normal infants who develop necrotizing colitis after protracted periods of diarrhea.[117] Others have suggested a localized Schwarzman reaction to endotoxemia or gram-negative bacteria.[118] The absence of lysozyme (normally present in human breast milk) may allow overgrowth of gram-negative bacilli. McKay and Wahle[119] have reported the association of "enteropathogenic" *E. coli* serotype 0111:B4 with NEC. Because of the association with umbilical vein polyvinylchloride catheters and feeding tubes, the toxic effect of plasticizers leached from the polyvinylchloride materials has been suggested.[120] Reports of outbreaks of NEC in newborn intensive care units[121-124] have led to a careful search for infectious agents including viral, fungal, or bacterial pathogens.[125–127] Among bacteria, *Pseudomonas*, *Klebsiella*,[125,126] certain *E. coli*,[119,128,129] *Salmonella*,[130] and *Clostridium butyricum*[123] have been implicated. The roles of both ischemia and bacteria have been suggested by Barlow et al.[131] with work in an experimental rat model of NEC in which breast milk was also shown to be protective. Based on acidic intraluminal pH (<5.0) and organic acids in human neonates with NEC,[132] increased lactose fermenting *Klebsiella* have been postulated to play a role in the pathogenesis.[133] Others have suggested a role for platelet-activating factor (PAF),[134] and protection by superoxide dismutase or by endogenous nitric oxide.[134–136]

Clinical features of this serious condition in newborn infants include apneic spells, vomiting, abdominal distension, and occasionally bloody diarrhea. Most infants are less than 1 week of age, and there is an association with prematurity, maternal infections during delivery (such as amnionitis with prolonged ruptured membranes), and exchange transfusion via the umbilical vein. There is no sexual or seasonal predilection. The disease often progresses rapidly to intestinal perforation, shock, septicemia, and pneumatosis intestinalis. Air may also be evident in the portal venous system or biliary tract on plain roentgenograms. This syndrome is associated with mortality rate that is often in excess of 70 percent.

The diagnosis of NEC should be considered in any premature infant with altered gastrointestinal function, abdominal distension, or apneic spells. It may be further suspected by examination of the stool for occult blood and for the presence of reducing substances.[137] Plain abdominal roentgenograms may reveal air in the bowel wall, peritoneal cavity, or portal venous system, and there may be bloody diarrhea late in the course of the disease. Management must be initiated early and aggressively for any infant suspected of having NEC. Umbilical catheters should be removed, oral feeding should be stopped, and nasogastric aspiration should be initiated. Intravenous fluid therapy is of paramount importance. Laparotomy and excision of the necrotic bowel is often necessary and should be done aggressively if there is any evidence of peritonitis or obstruction.[138]

Prevention of NEC includes avoidance of risk factors and careful infection control measures in newborn intensive care units. Hypertonic elemental formulas have been implicated and should be avoided in high-risk patients.[139] Necrotizing enterocolitis rarely occurs in breast-fed infants. Explanations of the advantage of human breast milk include the presence of lysozyme, antibodies, and cellular elements that may play a protective role against potential infectious agents. While oral prophylactic nonabsorbable antibiotics have been suggested,[140] serious questions remain about the use of prophylactic antibiotics, even in high-risk newborn infants weighing less than 1500 g.[141]

DARMBRAND, PIG-BEL, NECROTIZING ENTERITIS IN ADULTS (ENTERITIS NECROTICANS)

First described as "Darmbrand" (meaning "fire bowels") in epidemics of enteritis necroticans in northern Germany in the immediate postwar period in the mid-1940s,[142] a severe necrotizing jejunitis has also been recognized in both epidemic and sporadic forms after pork feasting in the highlands of New Guinea.[143] "Pig-bel" was the name given to the syndrome of abdominal discomfort that followed a large pork meal, commonly eaten after a large "pig kill," which takes place every 3–10 years among the highland Melanesians of New Guinea. Sporadic cases have been reported from other parts of the world, including the United States.[144,145]

The pathologic findings involved are acute patchy, necrotizing disease of the small bowel in previously healthy people that may proceed rapidly to segmental gangrene with small amounts of gas in the mucosa, mesentery, or nodes.

Several theories of pathogenesis have been suggested, most of which involve the toxic products of *C. perfringens* type C,

including α- and β-toxins. Sporadic cases of NEC have been noted in association with nutritional disorders, alcoholism, and malabsorption and after pancreatic or gastric resection.[146,147] After gastric surgery, increased numbers of *C. perfringens* and α-toxin have been noted in the upper small bowel and stomach.[148] Whether α- or β-toxins are capable of causing the necrotizing enteritis alone or whether they initiate the invasion of the mucosa by other organisms such as gram-negative rods is currently nuclear. An attractive hypothesis has been suggested by Lawrence and Walker[147] that could explain the association of necrotizing enteritis with poor nutrition and episodic dietetic overindulgence. The low-protein diet of New Guinea highlanders is associated with low levels of digestive proteases in the intestinal lumen that can be shown to inactivate the β-toxin. The proteases can be further blocked by the oral intake of trypsin inhibitors, which are found in such dietary staples as sweet potatoes. Proteases return with improved diet,[149] as occurred in postwar Germany. This hypothesis has been confirmed in an animal model that required protease inhibitors for symptomatic infection.[150]

The clinical syndromes of necrotizing enteritis range from anorexia, vomiting, severe abdominal pain, and bloody diarrhea to fulminant toxemia and shock. Acute complications that require emergency surgery include paralytic ileus, strangulation, and bowel perforation with peritonitis. These complications are common in the first 2 weeks of illness. Later complications that may also require surgery include scarring that may lead to stenosis, obstruction, malabsorption, or fistulas. Necrotizing enteritis occurs with greater frequency and greater severity in children under 10 years of age. In contrast to European controls, 70 percent of the healthy adults in New Guinea have demonstrable antibody to clostridial β-toxin.[143,147]

The syndrome is defined pathologically but must be suspected in patients who develop severe abdominal pain, bloody diarrhea, ileus, and toxemia. The course is often too fulminant for detection of air in the bowel wall radiologically to be of any diagnostic value.

Etiologic agents held responsible for necrotizing enteritis include *C. perfringens* type C, once designated as type F in the older classification of *Clostridium welchii*. The majority of surgically resected bowel samples with necrotizing enteritis contain *C. perfringens*, over half of which are type C. Furthermore, 12 of 21 cases described had a significant change in serum β-antitoxin titer after illness with pig-bel in New Guinea.[143] While polyvalent gas gangrene antiserum was ineffective, administration of type C antiserum resulted in a 30 percent decrease in the need for surgery and a reduced mortality from 43 to 19 percent.[143] Furthermore, active immunization against the β-toxin has also proved effective in preventing pig-bel.[151,152]

Others have suggested that type A *C. perfringens*, staphylococci, or even hepatitis virus may be responsible for necrotizing enteritis.[153] The syndrome of "enteritis gravis" has been described in association with infectious hepatitis, although no viral etiology has been documented.

The differential diagnosis of necrotizing enteritis include acute shigellosis, acute food poisoning syndromes, antibiotic-associated pseudomembranous colitis, and acute ulcerative colitis. The absence of colonic involvement, the epidemiologic setting, especially in poorly nourished patients, and the rapid progression to toxemia and shock are strongly suggestive of necrotizing enteritis.

Therapy for necrotizing enteritis includes careful supportive care and bowel decompression. Fluid requirements may be substantially greater than what is indicated by fecal output. Resection of the involved bowel must be considered if there is a persistence of paralytic ileus, a rapid increase in signs of toxemia, localized or diffuse signs of peritonitis, persistent pain, or a palpable mass lesion. If subacute obstruction or malabsorption is suspected on the basis of weight loss, elective surgery may be required up to 6 months after the acute illness. Raw peanut or soybean diets should be avoided since they contain trypsin inhibitors. *Clostridium perfringens* type C antiserum containing β-antitoxin or the active β-toxin vaccine should be available and should be used in areas where necrotizing enteritis may be expected to occur.

PSEUDOMEMBRANOUS ENTEROCOLITIS (C. DIFFICILE COLITIS)

First reported by Coats[154] in 1883 and described by Finney[155] as postoperative diphtheritic enteritis in 1893, the syndrome of pseudomembranous enterocolitis has received increasing attention in recent years as different host and etiologic factors have been unraveled. Pettet and colleagues[156] characterized pseudomembranous enterocolitis as occurring typically 4–5 days after abdominal surgery, often for colonic obstruction due to a carcinoma. The association of pseudomembranous enterocolitis with antibiotics was first noted by Reiner et al.[157] in 1952. While this disease occurred in the pre-antibiotic era in association with intestinal obstruction, surgery, uremia, pneumonia, myocardial infarction, and sepsis,[158,159] most reports in the last decade have identified an association with the administration of antimicrobial agents, especially those with a broad antianaerobic spectrum. Diarrhea constitutes a major side effect of many antibiotics. From 4 to 50 percent of the patients taking tetracycline, chloramphenicol, penicillin, ampicillin, lincomycin, and clindamycin will develop diarrhea. Furthermore, each of these antibiotics has also been associated with the potentially life-threatening pseudomembranous enterocolitis.

Pseudomembranous enterocolitis is defined by the protoscopic appearance of small 1- to 5-mm raised whitish yellow plaques of "pseudomembrane" that may become confluent and overlie an erythematous, minimally friable, colonic mucosa (Fig. 2).[160] It is often necessary to remove a thick layer of mucus to identify the characteristic "pseudomembrane." Ulcers and erosions as seen in amebic, bacillary, or ulcerative colitis are usually absent in pseudomembranous enterocolitis. The "pseudomembrane" is composed microscopically of epithelial debris,

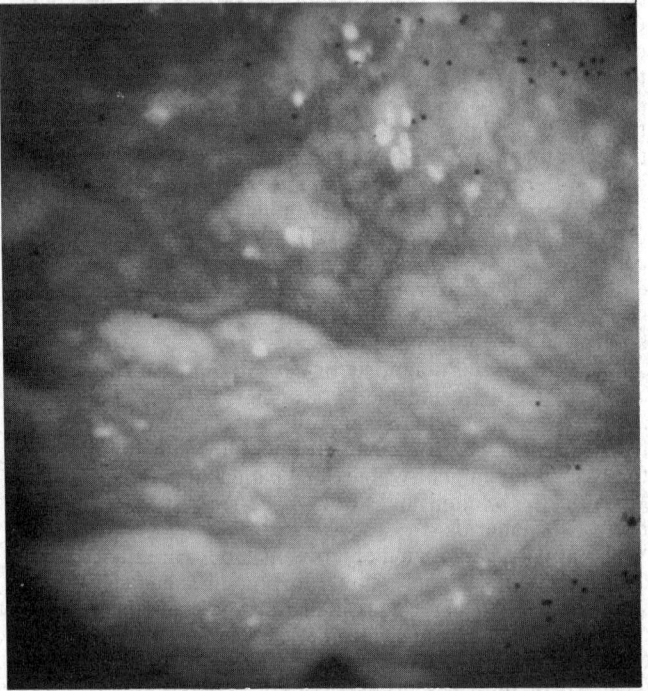

FIG. 2. Proctoscopic view of pseudomembranous colitis in a patient who received clindamycin. Note the 4–8-mm raised, white plaques overlying an erythematous mucosa. (From Tedesco et al.,[160] with permission.)

fibrin, and polymorphonuclear leukocytes and may be found on biopsy if the whole plaque is obtained.[161] The appearance of filling defects or "thumb printing" on plain and barium roentgenograms is inconstant and not reliable for diagnosis.

The pathogenesis of pseudomembranous enterocolitis associated with surgery, intestinal obstruction, debilitating diseases, or antibiotics undoubtedly involves multiple factors. Theories have ranged from circulatory failure with intravascular coagulation[162] and localized Schwartzman reaction or lumenal obstruction to toxic substances that are ingested or produced in the intestinal tract by microorganisms locally on the bowel mucosa. However, the pathologic changes are quite distinct from the hemorrhagic lesions of ischemic colitis or vasculitic processes. Some antibiotics such as neomycin have direct effects on binding bowel salts that may result in diarrhea.[163] Other antibiotics that inhibit protein synthesis may have direct effects on mammalian cells as well. Antibiotics may also induce toxin production by bacteria. Lincomycin enhances enterotoxin production by *V. cholerae* and enterotoxigenic *E. coli*.[164] Still others have described the appearance of viral particles in the intestinal mucosa of patients with antibiotic-associated colitis.[165] However, the majority of cases involve the alteration of normal bowel flora, especially of anaerobes, which allows the emergence of resistant organisms such as *C. difficile* that are capable of producing cytotoxic substances that alter mucosal function and integrity. While *Candida* often appears in the stools of patients taking broad-spectrum antibiotics and may be associated with diarrhea,[166] a double-blind, controlled trial of antifungal therapy failed to reduce the high frequency of gastrointestinal symptoms with oral tetracycline.[167] Pseudomembranous colitis in humans and animals has been associated with overgrowth of staphylococci in the stool.[168,169] While there is debate about their role in causing colitis,[170] staphylococci are capable of producing a cytotoxic Δ-toxin that causes tissue destruction and cell damage and elicits a net secretory response in animal models.[171]

Most cases of antibiotic-associated pseudomembranous colitis are now associated with cytotoxigenic *C. difficile* (see Ch. 78). Larson et al.[172] reported a nondialyzable heat-labile cytotoxin in the stools of five of six patients with antibiotic-associated pseudomembranous colitis that produced a cytopathic effect. Using a hamster model described by Small[173] in 1968, investigators obtained a heat-labile cytotoxic material from patients with clindamycin-associated pseudomembranous colitis that caused cecal damage and death in hamsters similar to that resulting from administering clindamycin to the animals.[174,175] This effect is neutralized by pentavalent clostridial antiserum, by the human immune serum globulin, and by *Cl. difficile* or *Cl. sordellii* antiserum but not by specific antisera against *Cl. perfringens (welchii), septicum, novyi,* or *histolyticum.* Bartlett and colleagues[176] and George et al.[177] have further demonstrated such cytotoxic activity in the broth culture filtrates of strains of *Cl. difficile* isolated from patients with antibiotic-associated colitis. This organism was described and noted to be pathogenic for guinea pigs and rabbits by Hall and O'Toole[178] in 1935, who found the organism in 4 of 10 newborn infants. Snyder[179] had noted in 1937 that certain strains of this organism produced a thermolabile toxin that was lethal for guinea pigs and that the guinea pigs could be protected with specific antiserum.

The association of pseudomembranous enterocolitis with several antibiotics is well documented.[180,181] Pseudomembranous colitis is said to occur in 0.1–10 percent of the patients given clindamycin irrespective of dose.[182,183] While it occurs more frequently with oral than with parenteral antibiotic, there are several cases in which it has followed intravenous or intramuscular drug administration. There is a slight predominance of females over males and of adults over children in most series. However, children have been reported with the syndrome as well.[184] In one series, clindamycin-associated diarrhea was reported to occur in 46 percent of the patients 60 years old or older.[185] The discrepant incidence figures for pseudomembranous colitis with clindamycin may have their explanation in the apparent clustering of cases in several reports.[186,187] Case clusters suggest and molecular marker studies demonstrate that the agent responsible for pseudomembranous colitis may be transmitted in the nosocomial setting.[188]

The onset of clinical illness is usually abrupt, often with fever and abdominal pain. While most patients develop symptoms after receiving antibiotics for 4–9 days, several cases have been reported to begin 2–4 weeks after the discontinuation of clindamycin therapy. Early diagnosis and discontinuation of treatment usually result in resolution of symptoms within 1 week. However, the continuation of the drug or the occurrence of colitis after a full course of antibiotic may lead to diarrhea of 6–10 weeks' duration that may cause severe electrolyte abnormalities and protein loss with significant mortality.

The etiologies of antibiotic-associated diarrhea and of the syndrome pseudomembranous colitis may involve direct effects of antimicrobial agents on gastrointestinal function, effects of antimicrobial agents on microorganisms, or indirect effects of surgery, debilitating disease, or antimicrobial agents on intestinal flora that allows an overgrowth of abnormal, sometimes cytotoxigenic organisms such as staphylococci or clostridia. *Clostridium difficile* colitis is increasingly recognized in patients receiving chemotherapy and in day care centers or institutions for the elderly.[189]

Any patient who develops diarrhea while taking antibiotics should stop taking the antibiotic immediately if at all possible. If symptoms are severe or persistent or if an inflammatory process is noted by fecal leukocyte examination, one should perform a proctoscopic examination to make the diagnosis of pseudomembranous colitis.

Therapy, after discontinuing treatment with the antibiotic, is mainly supportive. Most patients will improve within 1 week. The potential risk of *increased* diarrheal symptoms when antimotility drugs are used has been documented with lincomycin-associated colitis.[190] Oral vancomycin or the less expensive metronidazole are used for treating pseudomembranous enterocolitis.[177,191,192] Although vancomycin protects Syrian hamsters against lethal clindamycin-associated enterocolitis,[193] symptoms may recur after vancomycin therapy, and vancomycin itself can cause colitis in experimental animals[194] and should be used only when symptoms persist or worsen. The emergence of vancomycin-resistant enterococci also poses potential risks of excessive vancomycin use.[195] (See Ch. 79 for a complete discussion of diagnosis and therapy.)

CHRONIC INFLAMMATORY PROCESSES

Chronic inflammatory enteritides are often indolent, slowly progressive infections. Often there is a history of weeks or months of fever, abdominal pain, weight loss, or other systemic manifestations. Recurring or relapsing symptoms may be seen with *C. jejuni* or *Salmonella* gastroenteritis. In addition, 16 percent of cases of shigellosis may become prolonged for 3 weeks or longer.[196] Any diarrheal illness that extends beyond 2 weeks identifies a high-risk child for severe diarrhea and nutritional morbidity in tropical, developing areas.[197–200]

Chronic E. coli Diarrhea

"Enteropathogenic" *E. coli* organisms that cause acute diarrhea in infants by largely unknown mechanisms may rarely be associated with an insidious persistent or relapsing diarrheal illness.[201] *Escherichia coli* in O groups 1, 2, 4, 7, and 75 that produce hemolysin and necrotoxin have been isolated from patients with ulcerative colitis. These toxic organisms were not present in healthy people or in patients with acute diarrheal syndromes.[202] In addition, enteroaggregative *E. coli* are increasingly recognized as a cause of persistent diarrhea in India, Brazil, and Mexico.[203–205]

Gastrointestinal Tuberculosis

Intestinal tuberculosis, once considered common, had become a relatively rare disease, but is now reemerging with the advent of AIDS and with multidrug-resistant tuberculosis.[206] Intestinal involvement with tuberculosis may be either *primary,* from ingestion of the organism or from spread of miliary tuberculosis, or *secondary,* usually from a pulmonary source.

Primary infected tuberculosis without pulmonary disease often results in hypertrophic mucosal changes. Sixty-four percent of the cases of acute miliary tuberculosis may also have gastrointestinal involvement.[207] Primary intestinal tuberculosis may present with abdominal pain, fever, and a tender, fixed palpable mass in the ileocecal area.[208] Primary hypertrophic intestinal tuberculosis continues to occur in the Near East[209] and in India[210] where infection is most often due to the human strain *Mycobacterium tuberculosis.*[211]

Intestinal involvement secondary to pulmonary tuberculosis may result from swallowing infected sputum or from biliary excretion of the organism from an infected liver. The frequency of secondary intestinal tuberculosis increases to 25–80 percent with far-advanced pulmonary disease.[212] Hippocrates stated: "diarrhea attacking a person with phthisis is a mortal symptom."[213]

Tuberculosis may involve any part of the gastrointestinal tract, but most ulcerative and hypertrophic types occur in the ileocecal region where there is a predominance of submucosal lymphatic tissue.[214] The most common features are fever and abdominal pain that is often relieved by defecation or vomiting. Weight loss is more common in secondary intestinal tuberculosis. Only one-third of the patients with gastrointestinal tuberculosis have diarrhea. Diarrhea may be related to exacerbations of abdominal pain and occasionally occurs with extensive involvement of the small intestine that may cause steatorrhea and a malabsorption syndrome. While ulceration and mucous diarrhea are relatively common with secondary intestinal tuberculosis, hemorrhage and the presence of gross blood in the stool are distinctly uncommon, perhaps because of the obliterative endarteritis.

The diagnosis of gastrointestinal tuberculosis may be very difficult radiologically and even histologically. It must be distinguished from regional enteritis, sarcoidosis, actinomycosis, ameboma, carcinoma, and periappendiceal abscess. In contrast to Crohn's disease, gastrointestinal tuberculosis rarely causes anal lesions, fistulas, or perforation; is often associated with miliary nodules on the serosa, rarely causes strictures longer than 3 cm, and may cause circumferential transverse ulcers. Tuberculosis may also cause fibrosis of the muscularis mucosa, pyloric metaplasia, and epithelial regeneration.[215] There may be minimal or no radiologic changes in the bowel mucosa. Small mucosal ulcerations may result in tiny calcified nodules in the mucosa in association with calcified mesenteric lymph nodes analogous to the pulmonary Ghon complex. The ileocecal region often reveals radiologic evidence of irritability and hypermotility, with hypersegmentation of the mucosal folds or poor filling of the ileocecal region detected by barium enema. Occasionally, frank ulcerations can be noted on contrast studies, and late in the course there is scarring. The diagnosis requires a careful examination of involved tissue for acid-fast bacilli by special stain and culture. Caseous necrosis is more frequently found in the mesenteric nodes than in intestinal tissue itself. Complications of intestinal tuberculosis include perforation, peritonitis, and obstruction from either hypertrophy, scarring, or tuberculoma.

Candidiasis

Candida albicans can cause ulcerations in any part of the gastrointestinal tract.[216] Although shallow invasion of gastric or duodenal ulcers may have no obvious clinical consequence in the nonimmunosuppressed patient,[217] ulcerations anywhere from the distal third of the esophagus to the rectum may be deeply invaded and numerous in the neutropenic patient, constituting an important entry site for hematogenously disseminated candidiasis. Patients infected with HIV-1 are prone to esophageal candidiasis, but dissemination from that site is rare.[218] Several reports have implicated *Candida* species as a cause of diarrhea.[219–221] Although *Candida* may reach high concentrations in the stool of patients receiving antimicrobial agents, it has no established role in causing diarrhea.

South American Blastomycosis

While gastrointestinal involvement with the North American blastomycosis is quite rare, South American blastomycosis (*Paracoccidioides brasiliensis*) often presents as lesions of the skin, oral mucosa, or intestinal tract where it causes granulomatous or ulcerative disease.[222] The most common intestinal sites of involvement are the appendix, cecum, and anorectal areas. There is often abscess formation and lymphatic spread to regional nodes and to the spleen, liver, or even the lungs. The major symptoms are abdominal pain and ulcerative, granulomatous lesions, especially in the oropharynx. Palpable, tender abdominal masses in the ileocecal region may be noted on physical examination. Peritoneal signs are often absent. Diagnosis is made by biopsy, stain, and culture of the ulcerative lesion.

Phycomycosis

Other fungi usually involve the intestinal tract only as one feature of disseminated granulomatous disease, some of which may be acquired through a gastrointestinal portal of entry. Phycomycosis (*Absidia, Rhizopus,* and *Mucor* spp.) may invade the predisposed host via the gastrointestinal tract[223] or may involve the gastrointestinal tract by hematogenous spread and cause abdominal pain, diarrhea, gastrointestinal bleeding, and peritonitis.[224]

Histoplasmosis

Histoplasmosis may also involve the intestinal tract as a part of disseminated infection. In the gastrointestinal tract, histoplasmosis presents as ulceration, bleeding, obstruction, or, rarely, protein-losing enteropathy.[225–227] Lesions tend to be single and may be considered initially to be neoplastic.

Syphilis

Syphilis can also involve the gastrointestinal tract, usually in the upper part of the small bowel or stomach. An acute erosive and infiltrative gastritis with motile spirochetes and positive specific treponemal immunofluorescence test response has been reported in late secondary syphilis.[228] The initial complaints are upper abdominal pain, vomiting, and weight loss. More classic are the late gastrointestinal manifestations of lues with pyloric obstruction, "hourglass" constriction, or linitis plastica of the stomach. Less commonly, gumma may be seen in the small bowel or colon.

Parasites

Parasitic enteritides that should be considered among causes of chronic inflammatory bowel processes include coccidiosis, chronic or recurrent amebiasis, and the rare invasive, inflammatory form of giardiasis.

Human coccidiosis is an upper small bowel inflammatory process caused by *Isospora belli* that should be considered in patients with obscure chronic diarrhea and eosinophilia,[229,230] especially in AIDS patients.[219,231] Weight loss, fever, headache, and colicky abdominal pain may also be present with steatorrhea

and malabsorption. This infection is common in Chile and has occurred in nontraveling U.S. residents. It is likely that it often is unrecognized. This unicellular sporazoan parasite undergoes asexual schizogony in the intestinal epithelial cells from which merozoites are released. Like malarial plasmodia, the merozoite may then invade other cells and repeat the asexual schizogony cycle or may mature into sexual gametocytes and form a zygote and then a sporulated oocyst that ruptures to yield sporozoites that restart the enterocyte cycle. Sporulated oocysts are the infective form and have caused laboratory-acquired infections. The diagnosis is made by careful examination of multiple serial sections of intestinal biopsy specimens for any stage of the parasite or by examining small bowel contents for oocysts. Stool oocysts may be seen with a modified acid-fast stain as for *Cryptosporidium*[231] or may rarely be demonstrated with some difficulty by incubating a specimen at room temperature for 1–2 days to permit their maturation before examining using a concentration technique such as zinc sulfate flotation. While many therapeutic agents have been used unsuccessfully (including quinacrine, nitrofuranotin, tetracycline, and metronadizole), sulfamethoxazole-trimethoprim or pyramethamine and sulfadiazine in combination have been effective even in AIDS patients, in whom multiple courses or suppressive therapy may be required.[230–232]

The related protozoan parasite *Cryptosporidium* is a cause of severe chronic diarrhea in immunosuppressed hosts.[231,233,234] It may also cause diarrhea that is self-limited in normal hosts.[234] Unlike *Isospora,* cryptosporidia usually infect only the surface of the mucosal epithelium, and the process is usually noninflammatory. The organism may be identified by sugar floatation or modified acid-fast stains of fecal specimens.[231,235] A newly recognized sporozoon parasite, *Cyclospora* (also called *cynobacterium-like bodies*) has also now been associated with persistent diarrhea in travelers, those living in tropical areas, health care workers, and AIDS patients.[236–238]

Invasive syndromes may occur over a long period of time or in a recurring pattern with intestinal amebiasis. This syndrome may even extend into an entity called *ulcerative postdysenteric colitis* that may no longer respond to antiamebic therapy.[239]

Inflammatory small bowel disease may occur with unusually severe *Giardia lamblia* infection. This may result in severe villus atrophy, with dense plasma cell infiltration and acute inflammation in the lamina propria.[240]

The differential diagnosis of chronic inflammatory diarrhea includes several syndromes of noninfectious or unknown etiology. Idiopathic inflammatory bowel disease including regional enteritis, granulomatous colitis, and ulcerative colitis may be difficult to distinguish from infectious enteritides. Other processes that often require biopsy and culture to exclude infectious processes are intestinal involvement with sarcoidosis, lymphoma, or carcinoma. Radiation enterocolitis, ischemic colitis, and diverticulitis may also be manifested with chronic inflammatory diarrhea.

Few generalizations can be made about the management of infectious chronic inflammatory enteritides. The causes are so varied that the diagnosis often requires a careful search outside the gastrointestinal tract or surgical biopsy of the involved bowel. Only after the diagnosis is made can specific, effective therapy be instituted.

REFERENCES

1. Keusch GT, Jacewicz M. The pathogenesis of *Shigella* diarrhea. V. Relationship of Shiga enterotoxin, neurotoxin and cytotoxin. J Infect Dis. 1975; 131(Suppl):33.
2. Edelman R, Karmali MA, Fleming PA. Summary of the International Symposium and Workshop on Infections due to Verocytotoxin (Shiga-like toxin)-Producing *Escherichia coli*. J Infect Dis. 1988;157:1102–4.
3. Blacklow NR, Dolin R, Fedson DS, et al. Acute infectious nonbacterial gastroenteritis: Etiology and pathogensis. Ann Intern Med. 1972;76:993.
4. Rendtorff RC. The experimental transmission of human intestinal protozoan parasites. Am J Hyg. 1954;59:196.

5. Weissman JB, Schmerler A, Gangarosa EJ, et al. Shigellosis in day-care centres. Lancet. 1975;1:88.
6. Roy SK, Speelman P, Butler T, et al. Diarrhea associated with typhoid fever. J Infect Dis. 1985;151:1138–43.
7. Quinn TC, Stamm WE, Goodell SE, et al. The polymicrobial origin of intestinal infections in homosexual men. N Engl J Med. 1983;309:576.
8. Korzeniowski OM, Barada FA, Rouse JD, et al. Value of examination for fecal leukocytes in the early diagnosis of shigellosis. Am J Trop Med Hyg. 1979;28:1031.
9. Pickering LK, DuPont HL, Olarte J, et al. Fecal leukocytes in enteric infections. Am J Clin Pathol. 1977;68:562–5.
10. Haugwout FG. The microscopic diagnosis of the dysenteries at their onset. JAMA. 1924;83:1156.
11. Guerrant RL, Brush JE, Ravdin JI, et al. Interaction between *Entamoeba histolytica* and human polymorphonuclear neutrophils. J Infect Dis. 1981;143:83–93.
12. Speelman P, McGlaughlin R, Kabir I, et al. Differential clinical features and stool findings in shigellosis and amebic dysentery. Trans R Soc Trop Med Hyg. 1987;81:549–51.
13. Rahaman MM, Khan MM, Azi KMS, et al. An outbreak of dysentery caused by *Shigella dysenteriae* type I on a coral island in the Bay of Bengal. J Infect Dis. 1975;132:15
14. Feeley JC, Balows A. *Vibrio.* In: Lennette EH, Spaulding EH, Truant JP, eds. Manual of Clinical Microbiology. Washington, DC: American Society for Microbiology; 1974:238–45.
15. Morris GK, Feeley JC, Martin WT, et al. Isolation and identification of *Yersinia enterocolitica.* Public Health Lab. 1977;35:217.
16. Skirrow MB. *Campylobacter enteritis:* A "new" disease. Br Med J 1972;2:9.
17. Lyerly DM, Krivan HC, Wilkins TD. *Clostridium difficile:* Its disease and toxins. J Clin Microbiol. 1988;1:1–18.
18. Doern GV, Coughlin RT, Wu L. Laboratory diagnosis of *Clostridium difficile*–associated gastrointestinal disease: Comparison of a monoclonal antibody enzyme immunoassay for toxins A and B with a monoclonal antibody enzyme immunoassay for toxin A only and two cytotoxicity assays. J Clin Microbiol. 1992;30;2042–6.
19. Lima AAM, Lyerly DM, Wilkins TD, et al. Effects of *Clostridium difficile* toxins A and B in rabbit small and large intestine *in vivo* and on cultured cells *in vitro.* Infect Immun. 1988;56:582–8.
20. Lindberg AA, Pal T. Strategies for develpoment of potential candidate *Shigella* vaccines. Vaccine. 1993;11:168–79.
21. Struelens MJ, Mondal G, Roberts M, et al. Role of bacterial and host factors in the pathogenesis of *Shigella* septicemia. Eur J Clin Microbiol Infect Dis 1990;9:337–44.
22. Bennish ML, Salam MA, Wahed MA. Enteric protein loss during shigellosis. Am J Gastroenterol 1993;88:53–7.
23. Black RE, Brown KH, Becker S. Effects of diarrhea associated with specific enteropathogens on the growth of children in rural Bangladesh. Pediatrics. 1984;73:799–805.
24. Henry FJ, Alam N, Aziz KMS, et al. Dysentery, not watery diarrhea, is associated with stunting in Bangladeshi children. Hum Nutr Clin Nutr. 1987;41C:243–9.
25. Koster F, Levin J, Walker L, et al. Hemolytic uremic syndrome after shigellosis. Relation to endotoxemia and circulating immune complexes. N Engl J Med. 1978;298:927.
26. Bennish ML, Azad AK, Yousefzadeh D. Intestinal obstruction during shigellosis: incidence, clinical features, risk factors, and outcome. Gastroenterology. 1991;101:626–34.
27. Barrett-Connor E, Connor JD. Extraintestinal manifestations of shigellosis. Am J Gastroenterol. 1970;53:234.
28. Keusch GT, Grady GF, Mata LJ, et al. The pathogenesis of *Shigella* diarrhea. I. Enterotoxin production by *Shigella dysenteriae* 1. J Clin Invest. 1972;51:1212.
29. Calin A, Fries JF. An "experimental" epidemic of Reiter's syndrome revisited. Follow-up evidence on genetic and environmental factors. Ann Intern Med. 1976;84:564.
30. Aho K, Ahvonen P, Alkio P, et al. HLA-27 in reactive arthritis following infection. Ann Rheum Dis. 1975;34(Suppl):29.
31. Trabulsi LR, Fernandes MFR, Zuliani ME. Noval bacterias pathogenicas para o intestino do homn. Rev Inst Med Trop Sao Paulo. 1967;9:31.
32. Hayward RS, Wensel RH, Kibsey P. Relapsing *Clostridium difficile*, colitis and Reiter's syndrome. Am J Gastroenterol. 1990;85:752–6.
33. Mermel LA, Osborn TG. *Clostridium difficile* associated reactive arthritis in an HLA-B27 positive female: Report and literature review. J Rheumatol. 1989;16:133–5.
34. Ørskov F. Virulence factors of the bacterial cell surface. J Infect Dis. 1978;137:630.
35. Levine MM. *Escherichia coli* that cause diarrhea: Enterotoxigenic, enteropathogenic, enteroinvasive, enterohemorrhagic, and enteroadherent. J Infect Dis. 1987;155:377–89.
36. Tulloch EF Jr, Ryan KJ, Formal SB, et al. Invasive enteropathic *Escherichia coli* dysentery. An outbreak in 28 adults. Ann Intern Med. 1973;79:13.
37. Sereny B. Experimental shigella keratoconjunctivitis: A preliminary report. Acta Microbiol Acad Sci Hung. 1955;2:293.
38. DuPont HL, Formal SB, Hornick R. Pathogenesis of *E. coli* diarrhea. N Engl J Med. 1971;285:1–9.

39. Harris JR, Wachsmuth IK, Davis BF, et al. High molecular weight plasmid correlates with *E. coli* enteroinvasiveness. Infect Immun. 1982;37:1295–8.
40. Sansonetti PS, d'Hauteville H, Ecobiochon C. Moleculare comparison of virulence in *Shigella* and enteroinvasive *E. coli* (Abstract). Ann Microbiol (Paris). 1983;134:295–318.
41. Silva RM, Toledo MRF, Trabulsi LR. Correlations of invasiveness with plasmids in enteroinvasive strains of *E. coli.* J Infect Dis. 1982;146:706.
42. Marier R, Wells JG, Swanson RC, et al. An outbreak of enteropathogenic *Escherichia coli* foodborne disease traced to imported French cheese. Lancet. 1973;2:1376.
43. DuPont HL, Formal SB, Hornick RB, et al. Pathogenesis of *Escherichia coli* diarrhea. N Engl J Med 1971;285:1.
44. Silva RM, Toledo MRF, Trabulsi LF. Biochemical and cultural characteristics of invasive *Escherichia coli.* J Clin Microbiol 1980;11:441.
45. Pal T, Pasca S, Emody L, et al. Antigenic relationship among virulent enteroinvasive *E. coli, Shigella flexneri* and *Shigella sonnei* detected by ELISA. Lancet. 1983;2:102.
46. O'Brien AD, Newland JW, Miller SF, et al. Shiga-like toxin-converting phages from *Escherichia coli* strains that cause hemorrhagic colitis or infantile diarrhea. Science. 1984;226:694–6.
47. Riley LW, Remis RS, Helgerson SD, et al. Outbreak of hemorrhagic colitis associated with a rare *E. coli* serotype. N Engl J Med. 1983;308:681–5.
48. Griffin PM, Tauxe RV. The epidemiology of infections caused by *Escherichia coli* O157:H7, other enterohemmorhagic *E. coli,* and the associated hemolytic uremic syndrome. Epidemiol. Rev. 1991;13:60–98.
49. Centers for Disease Control and Prevention. Preliminary Report: Foodborne outbreak of *Escherichia coli* O157:H7 infections from hamburgers—Western United States, 1993. MMWR. 1993;42:85–6.
50. Pai CH, Ahmed N, Lior H, et al. Epidemiology of sporadic diarrhea due to Verocytotoxin-producing *Escherichia coli:* A two-year prospective study. J Infect Dis. 1988;157:1054–7.
51. Orskov I, Wachsmuth IK, Taylor DN, et al. Two new *Escherichia coli* O groups: 0172 from "Shiga-like" toxin II-producing strains (EHEC) and 0173 from enteroinvasive E. coli (EIEC). Acta Patho Microbiol Immunol Scand. 1991;99:30–2.
52. Obrig TG, Moran TP, Brown JE. The mode of action of shigatoxin on peptide elongation of eukaryotic protein synthesis. Biochem J. 1987;244:287–94.
53. Takeda Y, Yutsudo T, Igarashi K, et al. Mode of action of Vero toxins (VT1 and VT2) from *Escherichia coli* and of Shiga toxin. Williamsburg, VA: Twenty-third US–Japan Joint Conference on Cholera; 1987:104.
54. Guerrant RL, Lahita RG, Winn WC, et al. Campylobacteriosis in man: Pathogenic mechanisms and review of 91 bloodstream infections. Am J Med. 1978;65:584.
55. Doyle LP. A vibrio associated with swine dysentery. Am J Vet Res. 1944;5:3.
56. Dekeyser P, Gossuin-Detrain M, Butzler JP, et al. Acute enteritis due to related *Vibrio:* First positive stool cultures. J Infect Dis. 1972;125:390.
57. Butzler JP, Dekeyser P, Detrain M, et al. Related vibrio in stools. J Pediatr. 1973;82:493.
58. Blaser MJ, Reller LB, Campylobacter enteritis. N Engl J Med. 1981;305:1444.
59. DeMol P, Bosmans E. Campylobacter enteritis in Central Africa. Lancet. 1978;1:604.
60. Perez-Perez GL, Cohn DL, Guerrant RL, et al. Clinical and immunologic significance of choleralike toxin and cytotoxin production by *Campylobacter* species in patients with acute inflammatory diarrhea in the USA. J Infect Dis. 1989;160:460–7.
61. Ravdin JI, Croft BY, Guerrant RL. Cytopathologic mechanisms of *Entamoeba histolytica.* J Exp Med. 1980;152:377.
62. Lynch EC, Rosenberg IM, Gitler C. An ion-channel forming protein produced by *Entamoeba histolytica. EMBO J.* 1982;1:801.
63. Young JDE, Young TM, Lu LP, et al. Characterization of a membrane pore-forming protein from Entamoeba histolytica. J Exp Med. 1982;156:1677.
64. Ravdin JI, Guerrant RL. A review of the parasite cellular mechanisms involved in the pathogenesis of amebiasis. Rev Infect Dis. 1982;4:1185–207.
65. Wittner M, Rosenbaum RM, Role of bacteria in modifying virulence of *Entamoeba histolytica:* Studies of amebae from axenic cultures. Am J Trop Med Hyg. 1970;19:755.
66. Bracha R, Mirelman D. Virulence of *Entamoeba histolytica* trophozoites. Effects of bacteria, microaerobic conditions and metronidazole. J Exp Med. 1984;160:353.
67. Petri WA Jr, Chapman MD, Snodgrass T, et al. Subunit structure of the galacotse and *N*-acetyl-D-galactosamine-inhibitable adherence lectin of *Entamoeba histolytica.* J Biol Chem. 1989;264:3007–12.
68. Krogstad DJ, Spencer HC Jr, Healy GR, et al. Amebiasis: Epidemiologic studies in the United States, 1971–1974. Ann Intern Med. 1978;88:89.
69. Kean BH, Venereal amoebiasis. NY State J Med. 1967;76:930.
70. Keystone JS, Keystone DL, Proctor LM. Intestinal parasitic infections in homosexual men: Prevalence, symptoms, and factors in transmissions. Can Med Assoc J. 1980;123:512.
71. Blake PA. Disease of humans (other than cholera) caused by vibrios. Annu Rev Microbiol. 1980;34:341.
72. Morris JG, Black RE. Colera and other vibrioses in the United States. N Engl J Med. 1985;312:343.
73. Hughes JM, Boyce JM, Aleen ARMA, et al. *Vibrio parahemoliticus* enterocolitis in Bangladesh: Report of an outbreak. Am J Trop Med Hyg. 1978;27:106.

74. Bolen JL, Zamiska SA, Greenough WB III. Clinical features in enteritis due to *Vibrio parahemolyticus*. Am J Med. 1974;57:638.
75. Barker WH. *Vibrio parahemolyticus* outbreaks in the United States. Lancet. 1974;1:551.
76. Blake PA, Merson MH, Weaver RE, et al. Disease caused by a marine vibrio: Clinical characteristics and epidemiology. N Engl J Med. 1979;300:1.
77. Mandal BK, Mani V. Colonic involvement in salmonellosis. Lancet. 1976; 1:887.
78. Thomas M, Tillett H. Colonic involvement in salmonellosis. Lancet. 1976; 1:1129.
79. Boyd JF. Colonic involvement in salmonellosis. Lancet. 1976;1:1415.
80. Appelbaum PC, Scragg J, Schonland MM. Colonic involvement in salmonellosis. Lancet. 1976;2:102.
81. Radsel-Medvescek A, Zargi R, Acko M, et al. Colonic involvement in salmonellosis. Lancet. 1977;1:601.
82. Rowland HAK. The complications of typhoid fever. J Trop Med Hyg. 1961; 64:143.
83. Sonnenwirth AC, Weaver RE. *Yersinia enterocolitica*. N Engl J Med. 1970; 283:1468.
84. Black RE, Jackson RJ, Tsai T, et al. Epidemic *Yersinia enterocolitica* infection due to contaminated chocolate milk. N Engl J Med. 1978;298:76.
85. Leino R, Kalliomaki JL. Yersiniosis as an internal disease. Ann Intern Med. 1974;81:458.
86. Ahvonen P. Human yersiniosis in Finland. II. Clinical features. Ann Clin Res. 1972;4:39.
87. Rabson AR, Hallett AF, Koornhof HJ, Generalized *Yersinia enterocolitica* infection. J Infect Dis. 1975;131:447.
88. Bradford WD, Noce PS, Gutman LT. Pathologic features of enteric infection with *Yersinia enterocolitica*. Arch Pathol. 1974;98:7.
89. Kilpatrick AM. Medical intelligence—Current concepts: Gonorrheal proctitis. N Engl J Med. 1972;287:967.
90. Klein EJ, Fisher LS, Chow AW. Anorectal gonococcal infection. Ann Intern Med. 1977;86:340.
91. Quinn TC, Stamm WE, Gardell SE. The polymicrobial etiology of intestinal infections in homosexual men. N Engl J Med. 1983;309:576–82.
92. Dantec LE. Dysenterie spirillaire. CR Soc Biol. 1903;55:617.
93. Lee FD, Kraszewski A, Gordon J, et al. Intestinal spirochaetosis. Gut. 1971; 12:126.
94. Jensen NS, Casey TA, Stanton TB. Detection and identification of *Treponema hyodysenteriae* by using oligodeoxynucleotide probes complementary to 16S rRNA. J Clin Microbiol. 1990;28:2717–21.
95. Stermer E, Levy N, Potasman I, et al. Brucellosis as a cause of severe colitis. Am J Gastroenterol. 1991;86:917–9.
96. Krajden M, Brown M, Petrasek A, et al. Clinical features of adenovirus enteritis: A review of 127 cases. Pediatr Infect Dis J. 1990;9:636–41.
97. Janoff EN, Orenstein JM, Manischewitz JF, et al. Adenovirus colitis in the acquired immunodeficiency syndrome. Gastroenterology 1991;100:976–9.
98. Guerrant RL, Araujo V, Cooper WH, et al. Measurement of fecal lactoferrin as a marker of fecal leukocytes and inflammatory enteritis. J Clin Microbiol. 1992;30:1238–42.
99. Haltalin KC, Nelson JD, Ring R III, et al. Double-blind treatment study of shigellosis comparing ampicillin, sulfadiazine, and placebo. J Pediatr. 1967; 70:970.
100. Tong MJ, Martin DG, Cunningham JJ, et al. Clinical and bacteriological elevation of antibiotic treatment in shigellosis. JAMA. 1970;214:1841.
101. Barada FA, Guerrant RL. Sulfamethoxazole-trimethoprim versus ampicillin in treatment of acute invasive diarrhea in adults. Antimicrob Agents Chemother. 1980;17:961.
102. Osada Y, Une T, Ogawa H. Inhibition of cell to cell transfer of *Shigella* by treatment with some antibiotics. Jpn Microbiol. 1973;17:233.
103. Farrar WE Jr, Eidson M: Antibiotic resistance to *Shigella* mediated by R factors. J Infect Dis. 1971;123:477.
104. Ross S, Controni G, Khan W. Resistance of shigellae to ampicillin and other antibiotics. Its clinical and epidemiological implications. JAMA. 1972;221: 45.
105. Pichler HET, Diridl G, Sticklerk, et al. Clinical efficacy of ciprofloxacin compared with placebo in bacterial diarrhea. Am J Med. 1987;82(Suppl 4A): 329–32.
106. DuPont HL, Ericsson CD, Robinson A, et al. Current problems in antimicrobial therapy for bacterial enteric infection. Am J Med. 1987;82(Suppl 4A): 324–8.
107. Neill MA, Opal SM, Heelan J, et al. Failure of ciprofloxacin to eradicate convalescent fecal excretion after acute Salmonellosis: Experience during and outbreak in health care workers. Ann Intern Med. 1991;114:195–9.
108. Healy GR. Laboratory diagnosis of amebiasis. Bull NY Acad Med. 1971;47: 478.
109. Aserkoff B, Bennett JV. Effect of antibiotic therapy in acute salmonellosis on the fecal excretion of salmonellae. N Engl J Med. 1969;281:636.
110. Nelson JD, Jusmiesz H, Jackson LH, et al. Treatment of *Salmonella* gastroenteritis with ampicillin, amoxicillin or placebo. Pediatrics. 1980;65:1125.
111. Waldhausen JA, Herendeen T, King H. Necrotizing colitis of the newborn: Common cause of perforation of the colon. Surgery. 1963;54:365.
112. Mizrahi A, Barlow O, Berdon W, et al. Necrotizing enterocolitis in premature infants. J Pediatr. 1965;66:697.
113. Simpson JY. Peritonitis in the fetus in uterus. Edinb Med Surg J. 1838;15: 390.
114. Genersich A. Bauchfellentzondung beim Neugeboreneh in Folg von Perforation des Ileums. Arch Pathol Anat. 1891;126:485.
115. Thelander HE. Perforation of the gastrointestinal tract of the newborn infant. Am Dis J Child. 1939;58:371.
116. Wilson R, Kanto WP, McCarthy BJ, et al. Epidemiologic characteristics of necrotizing enterocolitis: A population-based study. Am J Epidemiol. 1981; 114:880.
117. Fairborn RA. Etiology of necrotizing enterocolitis. Lancet. 1977;1:956.
118. Hermann RE. Perforation of the colon from necrotizing colitis in the neborn: Report of a survival and new etiologic concept. Surgery. 1965;58:436.
119. McKay DG, Wahle GH. Epidemic gastroenteritis due to *Escherichia coli* 0111B4. Arch Pathol. 1955;60:679.
120. Rogers AF, Dunn PM. Intestinal perforation, exchange transfusion and P.V.C. Lancet. 1969;2:1246.
121. Virnig NL, Reynolds JW. Epidemiological aspects of neonatal necrotizing enterocolitis. Am J Dis Child. 1974;128:186.
122. Book LS, Overall JC, Herbst JJ, et al. Clustering of necrotizing enterocolitis. Interruption by infection-control measures. N Engl J Med. 1977;297:984.
123. Howard FM, Flynn DM, Bradley JM, et al. Outbreak of necrotizing enterocolitis caused by *Clostridium butyricum*. Lancet 1977;2:1099.
124. Ryder RW, Buxton AE, Wachsmuth IK. Heat-stable enterotoxigenic *Escherichia coli* and necrotizing enterocolitis: Lack of an association. J Pediatr. 1977;91:302.
125. Olarte J, Ferguson WW, Henderson NI, et al. *Klebsiella* strains isolated from diarrheal infants. Am J Dis Child. 1961;101:763.
126. Frantz ID, L'Heureux P, Engel RR, et al. Necrotizing enterocolitis. J Pediatr. 1975;86:259.
127. Levin SE, Isaacson C. Spontaneous perforation of the colon in the newborn infant. Arch Dis Child. 1960;35:378.
128. Speer ME, Taber LH, Yow MD, et al. Fulminant neonatal sepsis and necrotizing enterocolitis associated with a "nonenteropathogenic" strain of *Escherhichia coli*. J Pediatr. 1976;89:91.
129. Drucker MM, Polliack A, Yeivin R, et al. Immunofluorescent demonstration of enteropathogenic *Escherichia coli* in tissue of infants dying with enteritis. Pediatrics. 1970;46:855.
130. Stein H, Beck J, Solomon A, et al. Gastroenteritis with necrotizing enterocolitis in premature babies. Br Med J. 1972;2:616.
131. Barlow B, Santulli TV, Heird WC, et al. An experimental study of acute neonatal enterocolitis—The importance of breast milk. J Pediatr Surg. 1974; 9:587.
132. Clark DA, Thompson JE, Weiner LB, et al. Necrotizing enterocolitis: Intraluminal biochemistry in human neonates and a rabbit model. Pediatr Res. 1985;19:919–21.
133. Carbonaro CA, Clark DA, Elseviers D. A bacterial pathogenicity determinant associated with necrotizing enterocolitis. Microb Pathogen. 1988;5: 427–36.
134. Miller MJ, McNeill H, Mullane KM. SOD prevents damage and attenuates eicosanoid release in a rabbit model of necrotizing enterocolitis. Am J Physiol. 1988;255:G556–65.
135. Clark DA, Fornabaio DM, McNeill H, et al. Contribution of oxygen-derived free radicals to experimenatl necrotizing enterocolitis. Am J Pathol. 1988; 130:537–42.
136. MacKendrick W, Caplan M, Hsueh W. Endogenous nitric oxide protects against platelet-activating factor-induced bowel injury in the rat. Pediatr Res. 1993;34:222–8.
137. Book LS, Herbst JJ. Jung AL: Carbohydrate malabsorption in necrotizing enterocolitis. Pdiatrics, 1975;57:201.
138. Stevenson JK, Oliver TK, Graham CB, et al. Aggressive treatment of neonatal necrotizing enterocolitis: Thirty-eight patients with 25 survivors. J Pediatr Surg. 1971;6:28.
139. Book LS, Herbst JJ, Atherton SO, et al. Necrotizing enterocolitis in low-birth-weight infants fed on elemental formula. J Pediatr. 1975;87:602.
140. Egan EA, Mantilla G, Nelson RM, et al. A prospective controlled trial of oral kanamycin in the prevention of neonatal necrotizing enterocolitis. J Pediatr. 1976;89:467.
141. Nelson JD. Commentary. J Pediatr. 1976;89:471.
142. Hansen K, Jeckeln E, Jochims J, et al. Darmbrand-Enteritis Necroticanss. Stuttgart: Georg Thiem Verlag; 1949.
143. Murrell TGC, Roth L, Egerton J, et al. Pig-bel: Enteritis necroticans. Lancet. 1966;1:217.
144. Patterson M, Rosenbaum HD. Enteritis necroticans. Gastroenterology. 1952; 21:110.
145. Fick KA, Wolken AP. Necrotic jejunitis. Lancet. 1949;1:519.
146. Williams MR, Pullan JM. Necrotising enteritis following gastric surgery. Lancet. 1953;2:1013.
147. Lawrence G, Walker PD. Pathogenesis of enteritis necroticans in Papua, New Guinea. Lancet. 1976;1:125.
148. Howie JW, Duncan IBR, Mackie LM. Growth of *Clostridium welchii* in the stomach after partial gastrectomy. Lancet. 1953;2:1018.
149. Kumar R, Banks PA, George PK, et al. Early recovery of exocrine pancreatic function in adult protein-calorie malnutrition. Gastroenterology. 1975;68: 1593.
150. Lawrence G, Coake R. Experimental pigbel: The production and pathology of necrotizing enteritis due to *Clostridium welchii* type C in the guinea pig. Br J Exp Pathol. 1980;61:261–71.
151. Lawrence G, Shann F, Frestone DS, et al. Prevention of necrotising enteritis in Papua New Guinea by active immunization. Lancet. 1979;1:227–30.
152. Lawrence GW, Lehmann D, Anian G, et al. Impact of active immunization against enteritis necroticans in Papua New Guinea. Lancet. 1990;336:1165–7.
153. Kravetz RE, Brazenas NV. Viral hepatitis associated with enteritis gravis. Arch Intern Med. 1963;112:179.
154. Coats J. A Manual of Pathology. Philadelphia: Henry C Lea's Sons; 1883: 567.

155. Finney JMT. Gastroenterostomy for cicatrizing ulcer of the pylorus. Bull John Hopkins Hosp. 1893;4:53.
156. Pettet JD, Baggenstoss AH, Dearing WH, et al. Postoperative pseudomembranous enterocolitis. Surg Gynecol Obstet. 1954;98:546.
157. Reiner L, Schlesinger MJ, Miller GM. Pseudomembranous colitis following aureomycin and chloramphenicol. Arch Pathol. 1952;54:39.
158. Hardaway RM, McKay DG. Pseudomembranous enterocolitis. Are antibiotics wholly responsible? Arch Surg. 1959;78:446.
159. Goulston SJM, McGovern VJ. Pseudo-membranous colitis. Gut. 1965;6:207.
160. Tedesco FJ, Barton RW, Alpers DH. Clindamycin-associated colitis. Ann Intern Med. 1974;81:429.
161. Sumner HW, Tedesco FJ. Rectal biopsy in clindamycin-associated colitis. Arch Pathol. 1975;99:237.
162. McKay DG, Hardaway RM, Whale GH, et al. Experimental pseudomembranous enterocolitis. Arch Intern Med. 1955;95:779.
163. Antibiotic diarrhea (Editorial). Br Med J. 1975;4:243.
164. Levner M, Wiener FP, Rubin BA. Introduction of Escherichia coli and Vibrio cholerae enterotoxins by an inhibition of protein synthesis. Infect Immun. 1977;15:132.
165. Steer HW. The pseudomembranous colitis associated with clindamycin therapy—A viral colitis. Gut. 1975;16:695.
166. Kane JG, Chretien JH, Garagusi VF. Diarrhoea caused by Candida. Lancet. 1976;1:335.
167. Comparison of side-effects of tetracycline and tetracyline plus nystatin. Report of the Research Committe of the British Tuberculosis Association by the Clinical Trials Subcommittee. Br Med J. 1968;4:411.
168. Dearing WH, Baggenstoss AH, Weed LA. Studies on the relationship of Staphylococcus aureus to pseudomembranous enteritis and to postantibiotic enteritis. Gastroenterology. 1960;38:441.
169. Bennett IL, Wood JS Jr, Yardley JH. Staphylococcal pseudomembraneous enterocolitis in chinchillas: A clinico-pathologic study. Trans Assoc Am Physicians. 1956;69:116.
170. Bartlett JG, Chang TW, Taylor NS, et al. Colitis induced by Clostridium difficile. Rev Infect Dis. 1979;1:370.
171. Kapral FA, O'Brien AD, Ruff PD, et al. Inhibition of water absorption in the intestine by Staphylococcus aureus delta toxin. Infect Immun. 1976;13:140.
172. Larson HE, Parry JV, Price AB, et al. Undescribed toxin in pseudomembranous colitis. Br Med J 1977;1:1246.
173. Small JD. Fatal enterocolitis in hamsters given lincomycin hydrochloride. Lab Anim Care. 1968;18:411.
174. Bartlett JG, Gorbach SL. Pseudomembranous enterocolitis (antibiotic-related colitis). Adv Intern Med. 1977;22:455.
175. Rifkin GD, Fekety FR, Silva J, et al. Antibiotic-induced colitis: Implications of a toxin neutralized by Clostridium sordellii antitoxin. Lancet. 1977;2:1103.
176. Bartlett JG, Chang TW, Gurwith M, et al. Antibiotic-associated pseudomembranous colitis due to toxin-producing clostridia. N Engl J Med. 1978;298:531.
177. George RH, Symonds JM, Dimock F, et al. Identification of Clostridium difficile as a cause of pseusomembranous colitis. Br Med J. 1978;1:695.
178. Hall IC, O'Toole E. Intestinal flora in new-born infants with a description of a new pathogenic anaerobe, Bacillus difficilis. Am J Dis Child. 1935;49:390.
179. Snyder ML: Further studies on Bacillus difficillis. J Infect Dis. 1937;60:223.
180. Silva J, Fekety R, Werk C, et al. Inciting and etiologic agents of colitis. Rev Infect Dis. 1984;6(Suppl):214–21.
181. Aronsson B, Mollby R, Nord CE. Antimicrobial agents and Clostridium difficile in acute enteric disease: Epidemiological data from Sweden, 1980–1982. J Infect Dis. 1985;151:476–81.
182. Colitis associated with clindamycin. Med Lett. 1974;16:73.
183. Tedesco FJ, Stanley RJ, Alpers DH. Diagnostic features of clindamycin-associated pseudomembranous colitis. N Engl J Med. 1974;290:841.
184. Buts J-P, Weber AM, Roy CC, et al. Pseudomembranous enterocolitis in childhood. Gastroenterology. 1977;73:823.
185. Tedesco FJ. Clindamycin-associated colitis—Review of the clinical spectrum of 47 cases. Am J Dig Dis. 1976;21:26.
186. Kabins SA. Outbreak of clindamycin-associated colitis. Ann Intern Med. 1975;83:830.
187. Keefe EB, Katon RM, Chan TT, et al. Pseudomembranous enterocolitis. Resurgence related to newer antibiotic therapy. West J Med. 1974;121:462.
188. Getchell-White SI, Barrett JA, Barton BA, et al. Nosocomial significance of Clostridium difficile: An epidemiological study using molecular markers. Med Microbiol Lett. 1992;1:49–55.
189. Guerrant RL, Hughes JM, Lima NL, et al. Microbiology of diarrhea in developed and developing countries. Rev Infect Dis. 1990;12:S41–50.
190. Novak E, Lee JG, Seckman CE, et al. Unfavorable effect of atropine-diphenoxylate (Lomotil) therapy in lincomycin caused diarrhea. JAMA. 1976;235:1451.
191. Khan MY, Hall WH. Staphyloccoccal enterocolitis—Treatment with oral vancomycin. Ann Intern Med. 1966;65:1.
192. Keighley MRB, Burdon DW, Arabi Y, et al. Randomised controlled trial of vancomycin for pseudomembranous colitis and postoperative diarrhoea. Br Med J. 1978;2:1667.
193. Bartlett JG, Onderdonk AB, Cisneros RL. Clindamycin-associated colitis in hamsters: Protection with vancomycin. Gastroenterology. 1977;73:772.
194. Browne RA, Fekety Jr, Silva J Jr, et al. The protective effect of vancomycin on clindamycin-induced colitis in hamsters. Johns Hopkins Med J. 1977;141:183.
195. Frieden TR, Munsiff SS, Low DE, et al. Emergence of vancomycin-resistant enterococci in New York City. Lancet. 1993;342:76–9.
196. Black RE, Merson MH, Rahaman SMM, et al. Prospective study of bacterial, viral, and parasitic agents associated with diarrhea in rural Bangladesh. J Infect Dis. 1980;142:660.
197. McAuliffe JF, Shields DS, de Souza MA, et al. Prolonged and recurring diarrhea in the northeast of Brazil: Examination of cases from a community-based study. J Pediatr Gastroenterol Nutr. 1986;5:902–6.
198. McAuliffe JF, Shields DS, de Souza MA, et al. Prolonged and recurring diarrhea in the Northeast of Brazil: Examination of cases from a community-based study. J Pediatr Gastroenterol Nutr. 1986;5:902–6.
199. Schorling JB, Wanke CA, Schorling SK, et al. A prospective study of persistent diarrhea among children in an urban Brazilian slum. Am J Epidemiol. 1990;132:144–56.
200. Guerrant RL, Schorling JB, McAuliffe JF, et al. Diarrhea as a cause and effect of malnutrition: Diarrhea prevents catch-up growth and malnutrition increases diarrhea frequency and duration. Am J Trop Med Hyg. 1992;47:28–35.
201. Nelson JD, Haltalin KC. Accuracy of diagnosis of bacterial diarrheal disease by clinical features. J Pediatr. 1971;78:519.
202. Cooke EM. Properties of strains of Escherichia coli isolated from the feces of patients with ulcerative colitis, patients with acute diarrhea and normal persons. J Pathol Bacteriol. 1968;95:101.
203. Bhan MK, Raj P, Levine MM, et al. Enteroaggregative Escherichia coli associated with persistent diarrhea in a cohort of rural children in India. J Infect Dis 1989;159:1061–4.
204. Wanke CA, Schorling JB, Barrett LJ, et al. Adherence traits of Escherichia coli, alone and in association with other stool pathogens: Potential role in pathogenesis of persistent diarrhea in an urban Brazilian slum. Pediatr J Infect Dis. 1991;10:746–51.
205. Cravioto A, Tello A, Navarro A, et al. Association of Escherichia coli Hep-2 adherence patterns with type and duration of diarrhoea. Lancet. 1991;337:262–4.
206. Fischl MA, Daikos GL, Uttamchandani RB, et al. Clinical presentation and outcome of patients with HIV infection and tuberculosis caused by multiple-drug-resistant bacilli. Ann Intern Med. 1992;117:184–90.
207. Cullen JH. Intestinal tuberculosis—A clinic pathologic study. Q Bull Sea View Hosp. 1940;5:143.
208. Davis AA. Hypertrophic intestinal tuberculosis. Surg Gynecol Obstet. 1933;56:907.
209. Hamandi WJ, Thamer MA. Tuberculosis of the bowel in Iraq: A study of 86 cases. Dis Colon Rectum. 1965;8:158.
210. Anand SS. Hypertrophic ileo-cecal tuberculosis in India with a record of fifty hemicolectomies. Ann R Coll Surg Engl. 1956;19:205.
211. Blacklock JWS. Tuberculous diseases in children. Medical Research Council, Spec Rep Ser 1972. London: His Majesty's Stationery Office; 1932.
212. Blumberg A. Pathology of intestinal tuberculosis. J Lab Clin Med. 1928;13:405.
213. Walsh J. Diagnosis of intestinal tuberculosis. Trans Natl Assoc Prev Tuberc Lond. 1909;5:217.
214. Paustian FF, Monto GL. Tuberculosis of the intestines. In: Bockus HL, ed. Gastroenterology. v. 2. Philadelphia: WB Saunders; 1976:750–77.
215. Tandon HD, Prakach A. Pathology of intestinal tuberculosis and its distinction from Crohn's disease. Gut. 1972;13:260.
216. Eras P, Goldstein MJ, Sherlock P. Candida infection of the gastrointestinal tract. Medicine (Baltimore). 1972;51:367.
217. Bensaude A, Breging E. Examen anorecto-sigmoidien au cours des colopathies a Candida albicans. Ann Gastroenterol Hepatol. 1972;8:199.
218. Smith PD, Lane C, Gill VJ, et al. Intestinal infections in patients with the acquired immunodeficiency syndrome (AIDS): Etiology and response to therapy. Ann Intern Med. 1988;108:328–33.
219. Gupta TP, Ehrinpreis MN. Candida associated diarrhea in hospitalized patients. Gastroenterology. 1990;98:780–5.
220. Margolis BD, Tsang TK, Kuo D. Persistent diarrhea secondary to Candida overgrowth (Letter). Am J Gastroenterol. 1990;85:329–30.
221. Zaidi M, Ponce de Leon S, Ortiz RM, et al. Hospital-acquired diarrhea in adults: A prospective case-controlled study in Mexico. Infection Control Hosp Epidemiol. 1991;12:349–355.
222. Restrepo A, Robledo M, Gutierrey F, et al. Paracoccidioidomycosis (South American blastomycosis). Am J Trop Med Hyg. 1970;19:68.
223. Satir AA, Alla MD, Mahgoub S, et al. Systemic phycomycosis. Br Med J. 1971;1:440.
224. Smith JMB. Mycoses of the alimentary tract. Gut. 1969;10:1035.
225. Bank S, Trey C, Gans I, et al. Histoplasmosis of the small bowel with "giant" intestinal villi and secondary protein-losing enteropathy. Am J Med. 1965;39:492.
226. Shull HJ. Human histoplasmosis. Disease with protean manifestations, often with digestive system involvement. Gastroenterology. 1953;25:582.
227. Kirk ME, Lough J, Warner HA. Histoplasma colitis: An electron microscopic study. Gastroenterology. 1971;61:46.
228. Sachar DB, Klein RS, Swerdlow F, Erosive syphilitic gastritis: Dark-field and immunofluorescent diagnosis from biopsy specimen. Ann Intern Med. 1974;80:512.
229. Brandborg LL, Goldberg SB, Breidenbach WC. Human coccidiosis—A possible cause of malabsorption. The life cycle in small-bowel mucosal biopsies as a diagnostic feature. N Engl J Med. 1970;24:1306.
230. Trier JS, Moxey PC, Schimmel EM, et al. Chronic intestinal coccidiosis in man: Intestinal morphology and response to treatment. Gastroenterology. 1974;66:923.
231. Soave R, Johnson WD Jr. Cryptosporidium and Isospora belli infections. J Infect Dis. 1988;157:225.
232. Pape JW, Verdier R, Johnson WD. Treatment and prophylaxis of Isospora

belli infection in patients with the acquired immunodeficiency syndrome. N Engl J Med. 1989;320:1044–7.

233. Tzipori S. Cryptosporidiosis in animals and humans. Microbiol Rev. 1983; 47:84.
234. Current WL, Reese NC, Ernst JV, et al. Human cryptosporidiosis in immunocompetent and immunodeficient persons. N Engl J Med. 1983;308:1252.
235. Ma P, Soave R. Three-step stool examination for cryptosporidiosis in homosexual men with protracted watery diarrhea. J Infect Dis. 1983;147:824.
236. Soave R, Dubey JP, Ramos LJ, et al. A new intestinal pathogen? Clin Res. 1986;34:533A.
237. Long EG, Ebrahimzadeh A, White EH, et al. Alga associated with diarrhea in patients with acquired immunodeficiency syndrome and in travelers. J Clin Microbiol. 1990;28:1101–4.
238. Ortega YR, Sterling CR, Gilman RH, et al. *Cyclospora* sp—A new protozoan pathogen of humans. N Engl J Med. 1993;328:1308–12.
239. Powell SJ, Wilmot AJ. Ulcerative post-dysenteric colitis. Gut. 1966;7:438.
240. Blenkinsopp WK, Gibson JA, Haffenden GP. Giardiasis and severe jejunal abnormality. Lancet. 1978;1:994.

80. ENTERIC FEVER AND OTHER CAUSES OF ABDOMINAL SYMPTOMS WITH FEVER

RICHARD D. PEARSON
RICHARD L. GUERRANT

Several enteric infections are characterized by clinical syndromes of abdominal pain and fever distinct from acute gastroenteritis. The portal of entry of the responsible infectious agents is usually the gastrointestinal tract, but several other infections and some noninfectious conditions may mimic enteric fever. After a systemic phase, these infections may subsequently involve intestinal tissue and are then manifest as one of three clinical syndromes. *(1)* Enteric fever, characterized by sustained fever, headache, abdominal pain, splenomegaly, bacteremia, and occasionally skin rash, is the most serious of these syndromes and may result from infection by several bacteria. A range of systemic bacterial, rickettsial, viral, fungal, and parasitic infections may mimic enteric fever, and these are discussed later in the chapter. *(2)* Mesenteric adenitis, a syndrome that may mimic acute appendicitis, may be caused by several bacteria. *(3)* Eosinophilia, associated with abdominal cramps or diarrhea often accompanied by fever, may be caused by a number of parasites, usually helminths, several diseases of unknown cause, and intestinal lymphomas.

We focus on the differential diagnosis of these syndromes. Important clinical and epidemiologic features, appropriate diagnostic approaches, and antimicrobial therapeutic considerations are discussed.

ENTERIC FEVER

The classic syndrome of enteric fever is an acute illness, the first typical manifestations of which are fever, headache, abdominal pain, relative bradycardia, splenomegaly, and leukopenia.[1] The prototype of the syndrome is typhoid fever caused by *Salmonella typhi* (see Ch. 200), in which fever is present in 75–100 percent of cases[2,3] and is often initially of the remittent type, rising in a stepwise fashion during the first week of illness, after which it becomes sustained.[4,5] Annually, 300–500 cases of typhoid fever are reported in the United States, over half of which are imported, often from Mexico or India.[6,7] In addition, outbreaks continue to occur in the United States.[8]

Pathogenesis

Organisms that cause the enteric fever syndrome must be ingested and must survive exposure to gastric acid before gaining access to the small bowel, where they penetrate the intestinal epithelium possibly via microfold (M) cells over Peyer's patches and then multiply in intestinal lymphoid tissue before systemic dissemination via the lymphatic or hematogenous route. Organisms causing enteric fever grow intracellularly, primarily in reticuloendothelial cells in lymph nodes, liver, and spleen. Animal models for this syndrome in which mice are infected orally with *Salmonella enteritidis* or *Yersinia enterocolitica* have been developed.[9] After multiplication in ileal and distal mesenteric lymphoid tissue, organisms disseminate with the production of microabscesses in the liver and spleen.

Clinical Features

The organism classically responsible for the enteric fever syndrome is *S. typhi*. Other salmonellae (especially *Salmonella paratyphi* A and B, *S. choleraesuis,* and other *Salmonella* serotypes) may cause a similar clinical syndrome (Table 1). Other diseases that may mimic enteric fever early in their course and that must be included in the differential diagnosis of enteric fever are also summarized in Table 1; important clinical and epidemiologic clues to these specific diagnoses are indicated.

Symptoms. Classic "typhoidal" fever begins with a remittent fever pattern that becomes sustained over the first few days of illness. The frequencies of reported symptoms from several series of patients infected by *S. typhi* and *S. paratyphi* A and B are summarized in Table 2. Most patients report fever and headache. Although reports from the preantibiotic era suggest that constipation occurs more frequently than diarrhea (79 vs. 43 percent),[5] more recent reports suggest that these symptoms occur with approximately equal frequency.[2,10] or that diarrhea may be more common.[11–14] Extraintestinal symptoms reported by patients include cough and conjunctivitis. Although enteric fever caused by salmonellae other than *S. typhi* is usually less severe and of shorter duration than typhoid fever,[15] the syndromes are not sufficiently different to permit clinical separation of the individual case.[10–14]

Physical Findings. In evaluating patients with possible enteric fever syndrome, the physical examination should focus on characteristics of the fever curve and accompanying pulse, skin, eyes, oral cavity and oropharynx, chest, abdomen, and lymph nodes. The frequencies of commonly reported physical findings are summarized in Table 2. Fever is present in most series in over 90 percent of the cases. However, bacteriologic confirmation of typhoid fever has been obtained in patients who were afebrile when the culture was obtained.[11,12] Classically, the fever is remittent during the first week, rising in a stepwise fashion in both naturally acquired infection[5] and volunteer studies[4,16]; after the first week, the fever usually becomes sustained. Deviations from this classic pattern frequently occur, particularly in endemic areas. In two studies from India, fever was remittent in 30 and 60 percent of the cases, sustained in 22–25 percent, and intermittent in 15–46 percent.[3,13] Relative bradycardia suggests the diagnosis of enteric fever. The presence of rose spots, although not pathognomonic, is extremely helpful in confirming the impression of enteric fever;[17] however, they are observed in less than half of the patients and are even less common in dark-skinned people.[5] Rose spots may be observed more frequently in infection caused by *S. typhi* than in other forms of enteric fever.[9,14,18] Conjunctivitis is reported in up to 44 percent of the patients with enteric fever,[10] but it is usually less common.[5] Pharyngitis is infrequent and is usually not a prominent feature of the illness. Rales or other auscultatory abnormalities in the chest may be present. Abdominal tender-

TABLE 1. Clinical, Epidemiologic, and Laboratory Clues to the Causes of Enteric Fever and Conditions That May Mimic Enteric Fever

Etiologic Agent or Disease	Clinical Clues	Epidemiologic Clues	Laboratory Clues
Causes of enteric fever			
Salmonella typhi	Relative bradycardia, splenomegaly, rose spots, conjunctivitis	Young adults, travel, especially to India, Mexico, and other tropical areas,[a] exposure to known carrier	Cultures (B, BM, U, F), leukopenia
Salmonella paratyphi A, B			
Salmonella choleraesuis			
Yersinia enterocolitica	Chronic liver or other underlying disease, arthritis, erythema nodosum	Older adults ± pet exposure	Cultures (B, F, J), serology
Yersinia pseudotuberculosis			
Campylobacter fetus	Stigmata or chronic liver disease, phlebitis	Older adults, ± farm or small animal contact	Cultures (B, F), serology
Brucellosis (Brucella spp.)	Paucity of physical findings	Occupation (abattoir employee, butcher), animal contact (goats, sheep, cattle), diet (unpasteurized cheese)	Cultures (B, BM), serology, leukopenia
Typhoidal tularemia	Severe prostration, splenomegaly	Animal contact (especially rabbits), vector exposure (ticks)	Serology
Conditions that may mimic enteric fever			
Bacterial infections			
Septicemic plague (Yersinia pestis)	Severe prostration	Rodent contact, vector exposure (fleas), travel	Cultures (B), serology
Intestinal anthrax (Bacillus anthracis)	Severe prostration	Travel,[a] diet (undercooked meat)	Cultures (B, F)
Septicemia melioidosis (Pseudomonas pseudomallei)	Severe prostration, pustular skin lesions	Travel,[a] especially Southeast Asia	Cultures (B), serology, chest x-ray (C)
Acute bartonellosis (Bartonella bacilliformis)	Severe prostration, hemolysis, renal failure	Travel to Andean valleys in Peru, Ecuador and Columbia,[a] vector exposure (sandfly)	Cultures (B), blood smear, acute hemolysis
Leptospirosis (Leptospira spp.)	Relative bradycardia, conjunctival suffusion	Occupation (farmers, abattoir and sewer workers, veterinarians), animal contact (especially cattle, dogs), swimming[b]	Cultures (B, CSF, U), serology, hepatorenal dysfunction
Relapsing fever (Borrelia spp.)	Fever pattern, conjunctival suffusion, splenomegaly, skin rash	Travel, especially to Southeast Asia, Far East, Ethiopia, and the western United States),[a] vector exposure (louse, tick)	Blood smear
Legionellosis (Legionella spp.)	Pneumonia, CNS symptoms	Normal or compromised host	Chest radiogram, purulent sputum, DFA of sputum
Intestinal tuberculosis (Mycobacterium tuberculosis, Mycobacterium avium-intracellulare)	Stigmata of tuberculosis or AIDS	Exposure to known case, ± travel[a] ± diet (unpasteurized milk and milk products), malnourished children, HIV infection	Cultures (S, G, BM, L), x-ray (UGI, SBFT)
Abdominal actinomycosis (Actinomyces spp.)	Abdominal mass, fistula	Adult males	Culture (FD, A), radiograph (UGI, SBFT)
Intra-abdominal abscess	Spiking daily fever, reduced diaphragmatic excursion, intraabdominal or diaphragmatic pain	Previous surgery, bowel or biliary tract disease	Leukocytosis, computed tomography, gallium scan, sonography, fluoroscopy
Rat bite fever Streptobacillus moniliformis	Headache, nausea, vomiting, rash, myalgia, polyarthritis	Rat bite or foot-borne outbreak	Culture (B, J), serology
Spirillum minus	Headache, nausea, adenopathy, roseolar-urticarial rash	Rat bite	Serology
Mycoplasma pneumoniae	Cough, headache, bullous myringitis	Children and adolescents	Serology
Chlamydia psittaci	Headache, nausea, vomiting, arthralgias, cough	Exposure to parrots, parakeets, related birds	Serology
Bacterial pneumonia (Streptococcus pneumoniae, Legionella spp.)	Cough, sputum, rales headache, delirium, pulmonary infiltrates	Older adults, underlying diseases	Sputum Gram stain, culture (S, B)
Viral infections			
Hepatitis	Jaundice, arthritis (with hepatitis B)	Exposure to known case, drug abuse, travel[a]	Liver dysfunction, antibody and/or antigen detection
Dengue	Relative bradycardia, myalgia, conjunctival suffusion, rash	Travel,[a] vector exposure (mosquito)	Culture (B), serology, leukopenia
Infectious mononucleosis	Pharyngitis, lymphadenopathy, splenomegaly, rash	Young adults	Serology, lymphocyte morphology
Rickettsial infections			
Epidemic typhus	Conjunctival suffusion, rash, severe prostration	Travel,[a] vector exposure (louse)	Serology
Brill-Zinsser disease	Rash	Older adults, remote travel[a] history	Serology
Endemic typhus	Conjunctival suffusion, rash, splenomegaly	Rat contact, vector exposure (flea)	Serology
Scrub typhus	Conjunctival suffusion, rash, lymphadenopathy	Travel,[a] vector exposure (mites)	Serology
Q fever	Pneumonia, hepatitis	Animal contact (especially livestock), ± travel, ± diet (especially unpasteurized milk)	Serology, chest radiograph, liver dysfunction

(Continued)

TABLE 1. (Continued)

Etiologic Agent or Disease	Clinical Clues	Epidemiologic Clues	Laboratory Clues
Mycotic infections			
Disseminated histoplasmosis	Mucocutaneous lesions, adrenal insufficiency	Travel,[a] animal contact (chicken, birds, bats), hobby (cave exploration)	Culture (B, BM, L, MM), biopsy (BM, L, MM), chest radiograph
Parasitic infections			
Malaria	Fever pattern, splenomegaly	Travel,[a] vector exposure (mosquito)	Blood smear
Amebiasis	Colitis, liver abscess	Travel[a]	Stool examination, serology, liver scan, sonography, computed tomography, colon biopsy
Babesiosis	Paucity of physical findings	Travel,[a] vector exposure (tick)	Blood smear, serology
Toxoplasmosis	Lymphadenopathy	Animal contact (cat); diet (undercooked pork)	Serology, biopsy (lymph node), lymphocyte morphology
Trichinosis	Periorbital edema, muscle tenderness	Diet (undercooked pork or bear meat)	Serology, eosinophilia, biopsy (muscle)
Katayama fever (acute schistosomiasis)	Urticaria, lymphadenopathy	Travel,[a] swimming	Eosinophilia
Visceral larva migrans	Hepatosplenomegaly, rash, bronchospasm, ocular lesions	Young children with history of pica, animal contact (dog, cat)	Serology, biopsy (L), eosinophilia
Noninfectious causes			
Malignancy			
Hematologic, intra-abdominal	Adenopathy, anergy, weight loss	Family history or prior malignancy	Sonography, computed tomography, gallium scan, biopsy
Vasculitic or granulomatous disease (e.g., sarcoidosis, granulomatous hepatitis, Crohn's disease, Still's disease)	Skin lesions, arthritis, serositis	Family history	Biopsy of involved tissue, serology (ANA, C'), exclusion of other causes

Abbreviations for cultures: B: blood; BM: bone marrow; U: urine; F: feces; J: joint fluid; S: sputum; CSF: cerebrospinal fluid; G: gastric aspirate; L: liver; FD: fistula drainage; A: abscess; T: throat; N: nasal; MM: mucous membrane.
Abbreviations for x-rays: UGI, SBFT: upper gastrointestinal tract with small bowel follow-through.
Abbreviations for serology: ANA: antinuclear antibody; C': complement; DFA: direct fluorescent antibody test.
[a] Travel to endemic areas, either domestic or foreign.
[b] Swimming in contaminated surface water.

TABLE 2. Frequency of Symptoms and Physical Findings in Patients with Enteric Fever

	Typhoid Fever[a] (%)	Paratyphoid A and B[b] (%)
Symptoms		
Fever	39–100	92–100
Headache	43–90	60–100
Nausea	23–36	33–58
Vomiting	24–35	22–45
Abdominal cramps	8–52	29–92
Diarrhea	30–57	17–68
Constipation	10–79	2–29
Cough	11–86	10–68
Physical findings		
Fever	98–100	100
Abdominal tenderness	33–84	6–29
Splenomegaly	23–65	0–74
Hepatomegaly	15–52	16–32
Relative bradycardia	17–50	11–100
Rose spots	2–46	0–3
Rales or rhonchi	4–84	2–87
Epistaxis	1–21	2–13
Meningismus	1–12	0–3

[a] Data from refs. 2, 3, 5, 10–13.
[b] Data from refs. 10, 14, 18.

ness may be diffuse or localized, most often in the right lower quadrant. Splenomegaly is noted more frequently than hepatomegaly. Two physical findings that may be useful in suggesting alternative diagnoses because they are rarely reported in patients with enteric fever are lymphadenopathy and herpes simplex labialis.

Laboratory Findings. The definitive diagnosis of enteric fever is made by isolating *S. typhi* or another *Salmonella* from blood, bone marrow, stool, or urine. Multiple cultures of blood as well as stool and urine should be obtained from every patient with a syndrome compatible with enteric fever before the initiation of antimicrobial therapy. If multiple blood cultures are obtained, 73–97 percent[5,10] of the cases can be confirmed. Culture of the blood clot after the serum is removed may yield more positive results.[2,10,19] Bone marrow cultures may be positive when blood cultures are negative.[14,20,21] Stool cultures are positive in less than half the patients,[5,20] and urine cultures are even less frequently positive.[5,20] If patients have received antimicrobial therapy, blood cultures may be positive in only 40 percent of the cases. In that instance, cultures of biopsy specimens of rose spots may be useful. These cultures are reported to be positive in nearly two-thirds of the patients, including some who have received previous antimicrobial therapy.[20] Counterimmunoelectrophoresis of serum may reveal circulating *S. typhi* antigen in patients who have received prior antimicrobial therapy.[22,23] Antigens can also be detected in urine, but specificity may be a problem.[24] Finally, polymerase chain reaction (PCR) is now being applied to *S. typhi* as well as to many other organisms.[25]

The role of serologic testing (Widal's reaction) in the diagnosis of typhoid fever is controversial. The minimum positive titer must be determined in individual geographic areas and is higher in endemic regions.[11] Cross-reactions occur with both non-*S. typhi* group D salmonellae[26] and salmonellae from other groups.[27] Antibody titers to the O antigen, especially if paired sera demonstrate a fourfold or greater increase, are generally more useful than antibodies to the H antigen, which are often elevated after vaccination.[26,28] However, in at least one outbreak, antibody titers to the H antigen were more helpful.

Widal's reactions have been reported positive in 46–94 percent of cases of typhoid fever.[3,28,30] The test is most reliable in areas in which data on Widal's titer results in control groups of patients without enteric fever are available; the sensitivity of the test can be improved when diseases such as rheumatoid arthritis, which are associated with false-positive reactions, are identified.[28] Although single elevated titers (O ≥ 1:40 and H ≥

1:80) may suggest the diagnosis of typhoid fever in unvaccinated people in nonendemic areas or in children under 10 years of age in endemic areas,[31] it is not diagnostic. The consensus is that the diagnostic role of Widal's reaction is limited.[32]

Widal's reaction is not helpful in the diagnosis of enteric fever caused by organisms other than *S. typhi*. The roles of the enzyme-linked immunoabsorbent assay (ELISA) using a cell envelope antigen or lipopolysaccharide (LPS) of *S. typhi*[32-34] or a purified Vi antigen[35,36] and radial counterimmunoelectrophoresis[37] in the serodiagnosis of acute typhoid fever need to be defined.

Additional laboratory tests that may be of value include the white blood cell count and differential, liver function tests, urinalysis, and chest radiograph. Leukopenia is reported in 16–46 percent of the cases.[11,12] In two series, two-thirds of patients had no eosinophils on peripheral smear,[3,10] a finding that may be helpful in areas in which helminthic diseases are prevalent and eosinophilia is common. Liver function tests may reveal a mildly elevated bilirubin[10] and a slight to threefold elevation in alkaline phosphatase and transaminase levels in from one-third to two-thirds of the patients[10,12]; on occasion, hepatic manifestations may be prominent.[38] Urinalysis frequently reveals proteinura, pyuria, and casts[5,10]; immune complex glomerulonephritis with red blood cell casts occasionally occurs.[39] Coagulation abnormalities compatible with mild disseminated intravascular coagulation are common, but the syndrome is rarely clinically apparent.[40] Chest radiographic films reveal infiltrates in 2–11 percent of the cases.[2,5] In patients with diarrhea, a methylene blue stain of a fresh stool specimen for fecal leukocytes may reveal mononuclear cells.[41]

Epidemiology

Certain epidemiologic data may be of value in the diagnosis of enteric fever. Typhoid fever is most common in children and young adults both in the United States[6] and abroad.[10,11] In the United States, cases occur throughout the year. Since humans are the only reservoir for *S. typhi*, history of contact abroad in settings where sanitation is poor or with a known typhoid case or carrier may be extremely useful, but a specific contact is identified in the minority of cases.[6,7] Over the past 10 years, the proportion of the cases in the United States that were acquired abroad has increased dramatically; during 1975–1984, 62 percent of the cases were acquired abroad, most frequently in Mexico and India.[7] The attack rates were highest for travelers to Pakistan and India.[7] Patients who acquired infection abroad were older than those who acquired disease in the United States.[6] The importance of the microbiology laboratory as a source of domestic *S. typhi* infection has also been recognized.[42,43] In most laboratory-acquired cases, *S. typhi* had been used for proficiency testing or research.[42] Most patients with enteric fever caused by *S. paratyphi* A or B acquire their infection abroad; *S. paratyphi* B is only occasionally and *S. paratyphi* A is rarely isolated in the United States.

Differential Diagnosis

Enteric Feverlike Syndromes Caused by Other Bacteria. *Yersinia enterocolitica, Yersinia pseudotuberculosis,* and *Campylobacter fetus* can each produce an enteric feverlike illness characterized by fever, headache, and abdominal pain that may be clinically indistinguishable from enteric fever caused by *S. typhi* or other salmonellae (see Table 1). However, certain features of these infections may serve to differentiate them from true enteric fever. Acute diarrhea is often a prominent feature of enteric feverlike illnesses caused by *Y. enterocolitica*[44,45] and occasionally *Y. pseudotuberculosis*.[46] Diarrhea is less frequent in enteric feverlike illness caused by *C. fetus;* the acute gastrointestinal symptoms of nausea, vomiting, abdominal cramps, and diarrhea were present in only 27 percent of bacteremic illnesses

caused by *C. fetus*.[47] A clue to the diagnosis of *Campylobacter* infection is associated phlebitis.[47-49]

The enteric feverlike syndromes caused by *Y. enterocolitica, Y. pseudotuberculosis,* and *C. fetus* more frequently occur in patients with significant underlying disease. Of 31 patients with *Y. enterocolitica* bacteremia for whom information was available, 12 had cirrhosis of the liver; 4 others had thalassemia and 1 had kwashiorkor.[45] Only 5 were known to be free of underlying disease. In another series, five of seven patients with the acute septicemic or typhoidal form of *Y. enterocolitica* infection had evidence of liver disease; in addition all six patients with the subacute, localized form of the disease characterized by hepatic and splenic abscesses had cirrhosis of the liver.[44] Of 20 patients with the enteric feverlike syndrome caused by *Y. pseudotuberculosis,* 11 had evidence of significant underlying disease; the liver was involved in 10 of these patients.[46] This syndrome has also been reported in a patient with amyloidosis and *Y. pseudotuberculosis* bacteremia.[50] In a series of patients with bacteremic *C. fetus* illness, 73 percent had a significant underlying disease, frequently involving the liver.[47]

Epidemiologic clues in differentiating true enteric fever from these enteric feverlike syndromes include the patient's age, residence, and recent travel history. Patients with *Salmonella*-induced enteric fever are most often less than 30 years of age,[6] whereas the vast majority of patients with non-*Salmonella* enteric feverlike syndromes are over 40.[44-47,51] As with typhoid fever, men are more frequently affected than women. Patients with *Salmonella*-induced enteric fever frequently have a history of recent foreign travel, most often to developing countries. Diseases caused by *Y. enterocolitica* and *Y. pseudotuberculosis* appear to be common in Europe, particularly in Scandinavia,[52,53] and in South Africa[42] and are not frequently reported from developing countries. Infections due to both *Y. enterocolitica* and *Y. pseudotuberculosis* may be acquired in the United States as well.[46,54-56] Although bacteremic *C. fetus* infection is relatively rarely documented, the majority of cases have been reported from the United States, and foreign travel has not appeared to be a significant predisposing factor.[47,51]

A pulse–temperature deficit similar to that observed in typhoid fever has been reported in enteric feverlike illness caused by *Y. enterocolitica*[45,56-58] and *Y. pseudotuberculosis*[46,52] but not with *C. fetus*.[47] An additional clue may be provided by the fever pattern. In contrast to *Salmonella*-induced enteric fevers in which sustained fever is common, intermittent fever throughout the illness caused by *Y. enterocolitica* has been reported.[59] Because of the increased frequency of chronic liver disease in patients with these enteric feverlike syndromes, physical examination is more likely to reveal stigmata of chronic liver disease such as spider angiomata, gynecomastia, ascites, and testicular atrophy. In addition, hepatomegaly is frequent and may be more pronounced than in patients with typhoid fever.[45] Both erythema nodosum and polyarthritis may occur in patients with illnesses caused by *Y. enterocolitica* and *Y. pseudotuberculosis;* in one series 55 percent of the patients with yersiniosis had arthritis, and 88 percent of these had multiple joint involvement.[52] Nonsuppurative arthritis is more common in infections caused by *Y. enterocolitica* (43 percent) than in those caused by *Y. pseudotuberculosis* (10 percent).[60] Patients with bacteremic infection caused by *Y. enterocolitica* and *C. fetus* may also have acute septic arthritis,[45,51,56,58] a condition that is infrequently found in patients with classic enteric fever. Erythema nodosum has been reported in 15–24 percent of patients with *Yersinia* and may be slightly more common with *Y. pseudotuberculosis* infection than with *Y. enterocolitica* infection.[52,60] Thrombophlebitis has been reported in patients with *C. fetus* bacteremia and may be an additional diagnostic clue.[61]

As in the *Salmonella*-induced enteric fevers, blood cultures are the key to the diagnosis. Each of the three organisms is more frequently isolated from blood than from other specimens.[44-47,51] The isolation rate from stool cultures may be improved if cold-enrichment techniques are used for *Yersinia*[62] and if special selective media are used for *Campylobacter*.[63,64] However, because of its sensitivity to cephalosporins, *C. fetus* cannot be cultured from stool on commonly used *C. jejuni* selective agars if they contain cephalosporins. In addition, serologic tests are available for documenting infection with *Y. enterocolitica* and *Y. pseudotuberculosis* and appear to be more sensitive and more specific than those for *Salmonella* infection.[53,65] Leukopenia is infrequent in patients with enteric feverlike syndromes; its presence suggests that *Salmonella* are responsible. Findings on abdominal computed tomography (CT) scan or ultrasound suggestive of hepatic or splenic abscesses favor the diagnosis of yersiniosis.[44,66] Glomerulitis complicating both typhoid fever and *Y. enterocolitica* has been reported; therefore, the presence of protein, red blood cells, and red blood cell casts in the urine is compatible with either of these syndromes.[39,67]

Patients with typhoidal tularemia may be clinically indistinguishable from those with enteric fever. The epidemiologic history may be of value. A history of rabbit or tick exposure within 7 days before the onset of illness supports the diagnosis of tularemia.[68] Although potentially dangerous, *Francisella tularensis* may be isolated from blood if the appropriate medium is used. More often serologic tests are used to confirm the diagnosis of tularemia.

Acute brucellosis may manifest with fever, myalgias, and splenomegaly.[69] As in typhoid fever, white blood cell counts are frequently normal or low. Skin lesions are uncommon in brucellosis. Blood and bone marrow cultures and serologic testing should permit separation of these entities.

Systemic Infections That May Mimic Enteric Fever. A number of other potentially fatal infections may be initially confused with enteric fever. These are particularly important because several are potentially fatal illnesses if not promptly recognized and specifically treated. Among the most common serious febrile illnesses following travel to tropical areas is malaria, which should be sought even in individuals who claim to have been careful about insect repellents and antimalarial prophylaxis. Intestinal and extraintestinal amebiases may present as acute or subacute febrile illnesses. The symptoms of dengue fever may begin up to 7 days after exposure in an endemic area. Other less common infectious etiologies of fever and enteric symptoms are discussed below. Some are endemic in North America, and others are not. In addition common extraintestinal infections such as otitis or pneumococcal, *Legionella,* or *Mycoplasma* pneumonia may present with enteric symptoms on occasion.

Septicemic plague may mimic enteric fever. The diagnosis of plague may be suggested by the sudden onset and rapid progression of the illness. Epidemiologic history may again provide a clue to the differentiation of these entities; plague is endemic in wild rodents in the southwestern United States, and a history of travel to that area with rodent exposure during the previous 2 weeks supports the diagnosis of plague.[70] In addition, a history of recent foreign travel to countries in which plague is endemic may suggest the diagnosis. Blood cultures, methylene blue stains of peripheral blood,[71] and serologic testing aid in the identification of this entity.

Intestinal anthrax may be characterized by fever and severe abdominal pain. However, intestinal anthrax is acute in onset and rapid in progression, and patients usually die during the first few days of their illness. A history of ingestion of raw or undercooked meat in an area in which anthrax is endemic should suggest the diagnosis.[72]

Acute septicemic melioidosis may be confused clinically with enteric fever; this disease is endemic in Southeast Asia. Physical findings that may support the diagnosis of septicemic melioidosis include pustular skin lesions.[73] In melioidosis, the chest radiographic film may reveal nodular pulmonary densities. Blood cultures and serologic studies again permit differentiation of these syndromes.

Acute bartonellosis (Oroya fever) may manifest with fever, headache, and abdominal pain. Since this disease occurs only in certain valleys in the Andes in Peru, Ecuador, and Columbia, a lack of travel in the preceding month is helpful in excluding this possibility.[74] Evidence of acute hemolysis suggests the diagnosis. The causative organisms are frequently seen on the stained peripheral blood smear. Since Oroya fever predisposes to *Salmonella*-induced bacteremia, both infections may be encountered simultaneously.[75]

Rat-bite fever caused by *Streptobacillus moniliformis* may mimic enteric fever when the rat puncture site is not clinically evident or when the infection is food borne.[76] This illness may also mimic enteric feverlike syndromes. History of a recent rat bite suggests the diagnosis.[76] Cultures of blood and joint fluid may confirm this diagnosis; serologic tests may also be helpful. The other cause of rat-bite fever, *Spirillum minus,* causes subacute fever, headache, nausea, and vomiting, often with an urticarial rash (soduku) 1–4 weeks after an initial rat-bite injury that heals with residual regional adenopathy.[77,78] Spirillary fever causes a false-positive serologic test for syphilis in the majority of cases; *Spirillum minus* requires mouse inoculation for its isolation or demonstration of the 2- to 5-μm twisted gram-negative rod in tissue or blood for diagnosis. Like syphilis and relapsing fever, spirillary fever is often associated with a Herxheimer's reaction when treatment is started with penicillin G.

Leptospirosis frequently manifests with fever and headache and is most prevalent in young adults. Abdominal pain occurs in approximately 30 percent of cases.[79] Diarrhea and constipation are less frequent. Muscle pain and tenderness occur in nearly 70 percent of the cases, more frequently than in enteric fever. Additional differentiating features are the fever curve and clinical course; leptospirosis is characteristically a biphasic illness.[80] Evidence of liver dysfunction is present in approximately 50 percent of the patients with leptospirosis.[79] Although conjunctival suffusion is characteristic of leptospirosis and is reported in one-third of patients, conjunctivitis occurs in enteric fever as well. Two findings that would favor the diagnosis of leptospirosis are azotemia (26 percent of cases) and cerebrospinal fluid pleocytosis (47 percent of cases).[79] Serologic tests are of value in confirming the diagnosis of leptospirosis.

Relapsing fever due to *Borrelia recurrentis* may simulate enteric fever. The history of travel during the previous 3 weeks to an area where louse-borne relapsing fever is endemic (Ethiopia, South America, Far East) raises the possibility of this diagnosis. However, tick-borne relapsing fever may be acquired in the western United States.[81] Conjunctivitis, rash, and hepatosplenomegaly are common. However, in contrast to patients with enteric fever, those with tick-borne relapsing fever resolve their fever in a crisis during the first week of their illness.[82] Giemsa or Wright stain of the spirochetes in peripheral blood during a febrile episode may confirm the diagnosis of relapsing fever.

Patients with intestinal tuberculosis may present with fever and findings referable to the gastrointestinal tract. In addition, radiologic studies of the terminal ileum may show evidence of a terminal ileitis that can be confused with the terminal ileitis sometimes associated with typhoid fever or *Y. enterocolitica* infection.[83] This disease is currently rare in the United States, but it may be on the increase with the reemergence of tuberculosis, especially multidrug-resistant disease with AIDS.[84,85] Abdominal tuberculosis remains an important, treatable disease in developing areas, especially in malnourished children.[86] Evidence of active pulmonary or extrapulmonary tuberculosis or of delayed hypersensitivity to tuberculin, provided the person is not anergic, suggests the diagnosis.

Abdominal actinomycosis may also mimic enteric fever. Physical examination may reveal an abdominal mass; the presence of a draining sinus tract strongly favors this diagnosis.[87]

Intra-abdominal pyogenic abscesses pose difficult diagnostic challenges and remain high on the list of undiagnosed causes of fever.[88] They should be suspected when fever persists or recurs and may be detected by sonography, CT, gallium scans, or magnetic resonance imaging (MRI).

Patients with *Mycoplasma pneumoniae* infection may rarely be confused clinically with those with enteric fever. Fever and headache may be prominent. The presence of tracheobronchitis with severe, nonproductive cough or pneumonia determined by physical examination or on the chest radiographic film suggests this diagnosis, although infiltrates may also occur in patients with enteric fever due to *S. typhi*. The presence of bullous myringitis suggests *M. pneumoniae* infection.[89] The appearance of upper or lower respiratory illness in other members of the patient's family also favors this diagnosis. Serologic studies may be helpful in confirmation of *M. pneumoniae* infection.

Patients with psittacosis frequently have an illness characterized by fever, headache, myalgia, abdominal pain, vomiting, and diarrhea. On physical examination a faint macular rash may be noted; splenomgaly occurs in some patients.[90] A history of exposure to birds suggests the diagnosis, and serologic testing is helpful in confirmation.

Several rickettsial infections, especially epidemic typhus, Brill-Zinsser disease, endemic typhus, Rocky Mountain spotted fever, scrub typhus, and Q fever are characterized by fever, headache, myalgia, and, except in Q fever, skin rash. Of these, Rocky Mountain spotted fever and endemic typhus are most likely to be encountered in the United States.[91,92] The gastrointestinal manifestations of Rocky Mountain spotted fever include abdominal pain, diarrhea, vomiting and upper gastrointestinal tract bleeding, and an initial diagnosis of appendicitis, cholecystitis, or gastroenteritis is often considered.[93–95] History of recent tick exposure suggests the diagnosis. Although failure of the characteristic rash to develop may lead to a fatal delay in diagnosis and treatment,[96] once the characteristic rashes associated with these illnesses appear, the diagnostic confusion is lessened. Serologic testing may provide documentation of rickettsial infection. In addition, fluorescent antibody techniques may be used to demonstrate the etiologic agent of Rocky Mountain spotted fever in biopsy specimens of involved skin.[97] Q fever is associated with cattle exposure or ingestion of unpasteurized milk.[98] Sporadic cases of epidemic typhus associated with flying squirrels have been reported in the United States since 1976.[99,100] The majority of these have occurred in the southeastern states during the winter months.

Legionella infections in normal or compromised hosts may present with gastrointestinal symptoms of abdominal pain, nausea, vomiting, or diarrhea (usually watery, noninflammatory) in up to 47 percent of patients.[101–103] Patients with disseminated histoplasmosis may have fever, abdominal pain, nausea, vomiting, and diarrhea.[104] The diagnosis may be suggested by the presence of mucous membrane lesions or adrenal insufficiency. Biopsy specimens and cultures of liver, blood, urine, and bone marrow may be useful in confirming the diagnosis.

Several acute viral infections have gastrointestinal manifestations. Abdominal pain, nausea, and vomiting are frequent symptoms in patients with hepatitis. However, the severity of jaundice and the extent of transaminase elevations are much greater than those observed in enteric fever. Influenza (particularly type B) may manifest with fever, headache, and abdominal pain. Nasopharyngeal and serologic studies may distinguish these illnesses. In dengue, headache, severe myalgias, and leukopenia are common. The maculopapular skin rash that characteristically appears on the trunk on the third to fifth day of illness and subsequently spreads peripherally, the biphasic clinical course, and a history of recent travel (within the previous 7 days) to areas in which dengue is endemic may suggest the diagnosis. Infectious mononucleosis may mimic enteric fever, particularly when acute pharyngitis is not a prominent part of the syndrome. Examination of a peripheral blood smear and a heterophil antibody determination are helpful in differentiating this illness from enteric fever.

A number of protozoan and helminthic infections may mimic the enteric fever syndrome. Malaria is endemic in many areas of the world in which enteric fever also occurs. Both may present with fever, headache, abdominal pain, and other gastrointestinal symptoms. Two-thirds of 25 cases of malaria in one series presented with prominent gastrointestinal symptoms (nausea, vomiting, abdominal pain, or diarrhea) that might have misled one from an early diagnosis of malaria.[105] The intermittent fever in malaria is a useful diagnostic clue, but it is often not present early in infection in nonimmune individuals. Peripheral blood smear confirms the diagnosis of malaria when positive. Fever, chills and hemolytic anemia in an area with the soft tick (nymphal stage of *Ixodes scapularis [dammini]*, the same vector as for Lyme disease) and white-foot mice *(Peromyscus)* or white-tailed deer *(Odocoileus virginianus)* may represent infection with the malaria-like sporozoan *Babesia microti*, especially in an asplenic patient.[106,107] Either intestinal or hepatic amebiasis may mimic acute enteric fever. In patients with hepatic abscesses, documentation of a single abscess cavity somewhat favors the diagnosis of amebiasis.[108] The diagnosis may be confirmed either by demonstration of *Entamoeba histolytica* in stool or colonic mucosal biopsy or by means of the indirect hemagglutination assay.

Patients with trichinosis may have fever, headache, myalgias, abdominal pain, and diarrhea; however, the presence of eosinophilia rather than the eosinopenia frequently noted in enteric fever should suggest the diagnosis, which can be confirmed eventually by serology. The history of recent ingestion of raw or undercooked pork suggests the diagnosis. Patients with acute schistosomiasis (Katayama fever) may be thought to have an enteric fever syndrome. Eosinophilia is helpful in separating these possibilities. The history of swimming in fresh water during the previous month in areas in which schistosomiasis is endemic also favors this diagnosis. Patients with visceral leishmaniasis frequently present with fever, malaise, and hepatosplenomegaly and may be confused with those with enteric fever. Patients with visceral lava migrans may also have fever and hepatomegaly; in more severe infections, splenomegaly, rashes, and pneumonitis may also occur. In contrast to enteric fever, visceral larva migrans is most common in children less than 5 years of age. The diagnosis is suggested by a history of pica. Serologic tests may confirm the diagnosis of visceral larva migrans.

Noninfectious causes of fever and abdominal pain, such as eosinophilic gastroenteritis, hematologic and other malignancies involving abdominal lymph nodes or organs, and vasculitic and granulomatous diseases, must also be considered. Diagnosis often requires biopsy of involved tissues, scans, serologic tests, or exclusion of other processes.[88] Also, see Chapter 37 for a discussion of the differential diagnosis of fever of unknown origin.

Therapy of Enteric Fever

In many patients with the enteric fever syndrome, antimicrobial therapy must be initiated before the diagnosis is documented by culture. Until recently chloramphenicol was the drug of choice for the treatment of *S. typhi*–induced enteric fever,[109] but multiple-drug-resistant isolates unresponsive to chloramphenicol, ampicillin, and trimethoprim–sulfamethoxazole are becoming increasingly prevalent.[110–114] Third-generation cephalosporins, such as ceftriaxone, or quinolones, such as ciprofloxacin, are now used in most areas.[115–120] Ciprofloxacin has the advantage of being available in both oral and parenteral formulations. For chloramphenicol-sensitive *S. typhi*, chloramphenicol remains effective. Strains may occasionally acquire resistance during therapy.[121] While chloramphenicol can be used for the empiric therapy of rickettsial diseases, other pathogens such as *Pseudomonas pseudomallei* or *Francisella tularensis* require different antimicrobial agents. A patient's recent travel history should be considered before initial empiric antimicrobial therapy is selected.

MESENTERIC ADENITIS

Patients with mesenteric adenitis typically have a history of fever and abdominal pain, frequently with localization in the right lower quadrant. The illness closely mimics acute appendicitis. Few data on the incidence of this syndrome are available. In the preantibiotic era, mesenteric adenitis was present in 43 of 2140 patients (2 percent) undergoing appendectomy.[122] In a report from the antibiotic era, 20 of 93 (22 percent) of patients undergoing appendectomy for suspected appendicitis had mesenteric adenitis.[123]

Etiologic Agents and Pathogenesis

At present, the most frequently reported etiologic agents in the syndrome of mesenteric adenitis are *Y. enterocolitica* and *Y. pseudotuberculosis*. Among 2861 consecutive patients undergoing appendectomy for suspected appendicitis in a Belgium hospital, *Y. enterocolitica* was isolated from the appendix or stool in 3.6 percent. Of those with histologically confirmed mesenteric adenitis and/or terminal ileitis without appendicitis, *Y. enterocolitica* was cultured in 75 percent.[124] In another report, five of eight patients (63 percent) who had mesenteric adenitis confirmed at surgery also had serologic evidence of recent *Y. enterocolitica* infection.[125] Again, few valid data on incidence are available. Of the 20 patients with mesenteric adenitis reported by Mair et al.,[123] 17 were adequately studied; 3 (18 percent) had evidence of infection with *Y. pseudotuberculosis*. In a school-related outbreak of *Y. pseudotuberculosis* among 34 children in Finland, 3 children went to surgery for suspected appendicitis and were found to have mesenteric lymphadenitis.[126]

In a mouse model, following intragastric administration of *Y. enterocolitica*, polymorphonuclear leukocytes appear in Peyer's patches within 24 hours. The infection then spreads to the mesenteric lymph nodes, where abscesses develop.[127] The invasive potential of pathogenic strains of *Y. enterocolitica* has also been demonstrated in HeLa cells in tissue culture[128,129] and in the guinea pig conjunctival (Sereny) test.[129,130] Invasiveness is plasmid mediated,[131,132] but the correlation of this and other plasmid-mediated traits with the production of human disease remains unclear.

In the preantibiotic era, hemolytic streptococci were frequently reported as etiologic agents in this syndrome; in one study, 19 of 36 patients (53 percent) with mesenteric adenitis in whom cultures were obtained grew hemolytic streptococci; 4 (11 percent) grew *E. coli*. Of interest is the fact that 37 of 39 patients (97 percent) had throat cultures positive for hemolytic streptococci, and 35 of these had a history of a recent sore throat.[122] In another report from the preantibiotic era, of two patients with mesenteric abscess secondary to suppurative mesenteric adenitis, one had enterococci and an unidentified hemolytic bacillus isolated from the abscess, whereas the other had both *Bacteroides* and *Clostridium* spp. isolated; in both cases the appendix was normal.[133] Hemolytic streptococci appear to be responsible for a few cases of mesenteric adenitis in the antibiotic era as well. Asch et al.[134] reported on one patient from whom β-hemolytic streptococci were isolated from an inflamed mesenteric node and in whom subsequent studies revealed an elevated ASO titer. In another case, both a β-hemolytic streptococcus and a coagulase-positive staphylococcus were isolated from an inflamed mesenteric node in an infant.[134] Of two 9-year-old children, β-hemolytic streptococci were isolated from one and *S. aureus* from the other.[135] A viral cause has also been suspected for this syndrome; however, 17 well-studied patients in one series had no evidence of viral infection.[123]

Clinical Features

Symptoms. *Yersinia enterocolitica* produces a spectrum of disease, including acute enterocolitis, terminal ileitis, and mesenteric adenitis. *Yersinia pseudotuberculosis*, which commonly infects animals, is a less frequent cause of human disease. When it infects humans, it usually produces mesenteric adenitis, especially in older children and adults. Patients with mesenteric adenitis have an illness clinically indistinguishable from acute appendicitis.[136] Symptoms reported by ill people in four common-source outbreaks are summarized in Table 3.[137–139] Fever, abdominal pain, vomiting, and diarrhea are frequent. In a series of 37 sporadic cases of *Yersinia*-induced enteritis reported from Belgium, 84 percent of the patients had abdominal pain, 78 percent had diarrhea, 43 percent had fever, and 22 percent reported anorexia; only 13 percent had nausea and 8 percent vomited.[140] Patients with sporadic cases of mesenteric adenitis caused by *Yersinia* may have a history of biphasic illness[141] or experience of similar illnesses in the remote past.[123] Consumption of raw pork in the 2 weeks before illness has been strikingly associated with *Y. enterocolitica* infection in the most highly endemic country, Belgium.[142]

Physical Examination. Regardless of cause, the clinical syndrome of mesenteric adenitis typically includes fever, right-lower-quadrant tenderness, and rebound tenderness.[60,139] In the setting of a common-source outbreak, rectal tenderness was present in nearly one-third of people examined.[139] In contrast to the enteric fever syndromes, a pulse–temperature deficit is not reported.

Laboratory Findings. Leukocytosis is usually present in patients with mesenteric adenitis[141–146]; white blood cell counts typically are between 10,000 and 15,000/mm^3. A methlene blue examination of fresh feces may reveal polymorphonuclear leukocytes.[147] Blood cultures are rarely positive in this syndrome; however, both *Y. enterocolitica* and *Y. pseudotuberculosis* have been isolated from stool cultures. Frequency of isolation is improved by use of cold enrichment techniques.[62,148] Stool cultures were positive in 56 percent of the hospitalized patients with the syndrome in a recent common-source outbreak[139]; isolation of *Y. pseudotuberculosis* from feces may be less frequent but has been reported.[149] Serologic testing may help in the diagnosis, although agglutinins are rarely present during the first week of illness,[53,140] and cross-reactions can occur with *Brucella* and *Vibrio* spp. and some Enterobacteriaceae. Serologic confirmation was made in 84 percent of the hospitalized patients in one outbreak.[139] The isolation of *Y. enterocolitica* from a stool culture should be considered significant; the organism was isolated from only 1 out of 974 controls in one study and from none of 545 controls in another.[150,151]

Sonographic or radiologic contrast studies of the small bowel may provide a clue to the diagnosis, particularly if ileitis is associated with the mesenteric adenitis. Sonography, using graded compression, may help distinguish appendicitis from mesenteric

TABLE 3. Symptoms in Four Outbreaks of Mesenteric Adenitis Caused by *Y. enterocolitica*

Location	Japan (131)	Japan (132)	Japan (132)	United States (133)
Serotype	03	03	03	08
Number ill	198	188	544	38
Percentage with				
Abdominal pain	76	86	64	97
Fever	61	76	50	100
Diarrhea	36	60	32	47
Vomiting	12	4	11	
Percentage undergoing appendectomy		2		42

adenitis. Of 170 patients presenting with a clinical syndrome suggesting acute appendicitis, 14 had only enlarged mesenteric nodes with mural thickening of the terminal ileum (without visualization of the appendix); none of the 14 had appendicitis; and 8 (of 9 cultured) had *Y. enterocolitica* in the stool.[152] In a series of 37 adult patients with documented *Y. enterocolitica* infection, 40 percent of whom had symptoms compatible with appendicitis, 21 of the 24 patients studied had a radiologic abnormality of the terminal ileum consisting of coarse mucosal folds in 67 percent, nodularity in 45 percent, and ulceration in 45 percent.[140] Although radiologic studies of the colon were normal in these patients, sigmoidoscopic or colonoscopic examination in 13 revealed evidence of colitis in 6 and aphthoid ulceration in 2, indicating that colonic involvement may occur.[140] In another series of 25 patients with *Yersinia* infection with the clinical diagnosis of acute appendicitis who underwent appendectomy, acute terminal ileitis was confirmed at surgery. When these patients were examined within 1 week of surgery by a barium contrast study of the small bowel, abnormalities were confined to the distal 20 cm of the ileum. The lesions evolved from an initial nodular pattern to an edematous pattern before resolution within 10 weeks in all cases.[153]

At surgery, patients with mesenteric adenitis may also have evidence of acute appendicitis, but the organ is rarely severely inflamed or ruptured. Patients may also have evidence of acute terminal ileitis.[125,136,143,144,146,153] Culture of the terminal ileum at surgery may yield the organism.[145]

Histopathologic examination of resected mesenteric lymph nodes in cases of *Y. enterocolitica* infection frequently reveals histiocytic infiltration and the presence of large pyroninophilic cells; abscesses are typically absent.[154,155] In contrast, although reticulum cell hyperplasia is frequently seen in nodes infected with *Y. pseudotuberculosis*, granulomas, polymorphonuclear leukocyte infiltration, and abscess formation are more frequent.[123,145,154,156] In both infections, tissue Gram stain may reveal the responsible organisms. Two fatal cases occurred in a *Y. enterocolitica* outbreak among four families in North Carolina.[157] Postmortem examination revealed extensive ulceration and necrosis extending from the stomach or small bowel to the colon. Mesenteric lymph nodes were necrotic in one case, and the sinusoids were filled with leukocytes and mononuclear cells. In the second case, the lymph nodes were large, firm, and edematous. There was reticuloendothelial hyperplasia with abundant histiocytes and plasma cells within the sinusoids.[147]

Epidemiology

Mesenteric adenitis caused by *Y. enterocolitica* or *Y. pseudotuberculosis* is a syndrome of children and young adults,[123] is most frequent in people between 5 and 14 years of age,[60] is more common in boys,[123,150] and is most often encountered during the winter and spring. This seasonal pattern is reported from both the preantibiotic[122] and antibiotic eras.[143,158]

The mode of transmission of *Y. enterocolitica* and *Y. pseudotuberculosis* has not been well defined; outbreaks involving several members of several families[157] or from the same school have been reported. In these and other episodes of *Yersinia* infection, simultaneous documentation of infection in family pets has been obtained[159]; whether these animals were the source of the human infection or merely acquired the infection simultaneously is unknown. Person-to-person spread to family members does occur.[151] Large common-source outbreaks of mesenteric adenitis have also been reported[137–139,160,161]; in one of these, chocolate milk was the vehicle of transmission.[139] *Yersinia enterocolitica* has been isolated from drinking water,[162,163] but water-borne transmission of these organisms has not been well documented. Results of one study in Wisconsin suggested that *Y. enterocolitica* infection was more common in rural areas.[164]

Differential Diagnosis

The major consideration in the differential diagnosis of mesenteric adenitis is acute appendicitis. Other inflammatory diseases characteristically involving the terminal ileum and/or mesenteric lymph nodes, such as tuberculosis, *Mycobacterium avium-intracellulare,* in patients with AIDS,[165] or actinomycosis, should also be considered. Parvovirus B19 has been associated with pseudoappendicitis,[166] and infectious mononucleosis can cause mesenteric lymphadenopathy.[167] *Angiostrongylus costaricensis* can also produce an appendicitislike syndrome, but usually is associated with eosinophilia as described below.[168]

Therapy

Mesenteric adenitis is a self-limited illness in the vast majority of cases. Specific antimicrobial therapy is often not required. In patients with the syndrome who are severely ill, the selection of an antimicrobial agent should be based, if possible, on the results of antimicrobial sensitivity tests. When these data are not available, therapeutic agents to be considered include tetracycline, chloramphenicol, trimethoprim–sulfamethoxazole, third-generation cephalosporins, ciprofloxacin, and other quinolones.[169,170] The trimethoprim–sulfamethoxazole combination has been shown to be synergistic against 100 percent of 23 human *Y. enterocolitica* isolates.[169] Although *Y. enterocolitica* isolates may also be sensitive in vitro to aminoglycosides,[171] these drugs should probably not be the initial choice for treatment of this syndrome because of their toxicity and their reported failure to eradicate systemic infection caused by these organisms.[44] *Y. pseudotuberculosis* is usually sensitive to tetracycline, chloramphenicol, cephalosporins, and aminoglycosides. Persons with septicemic disease should receive antibiotic therapy because of the high mortality.

THE SYNDROME OF ABDOMINAL PAIN AND/OR DIARRHEA WITH EOSINOPHILIA

The differential diagnosis and etiologic considerations for the syndrome of abdominal pain, diarrhea, and eosinophilia as well as useful diagnostic tests are summarized in Table 4. Most cases are caused by helminths. Additional diagnostic considerations include eosinophilic gastroenteritis, dermatitis herpetiformis, periarteritis nodosa, regional enteritis, and ulcerative colitis. In addition, lymphomas and some solid tumors may manifest with abdominal pain and eosinophilia. Epidemiologic data, particularly dietary and travel histories, may provide important clues to the diagnosis in patients with this syndrome. Valuable laboratory tests in these patients include examination of stool and small bowel contents for ova and parasites, specific serologic tests, and, in some cases, tissue biopsy and radiologic studies.

Differential Diagnosis

Strongyloides stercoralis is unique among intestinal nematodes in its ability to persist for many years through autoinfection and to produce life-threatening hyperinfection in immunocompromised hosts.[172] It infects people in areas where sanitation is poor. Patients with strongyloidiasis frequently have abdominal pain, diarrhea, or bloating with eosinophilia. In a study of 100 hospitalized adult men, abdominal pain was reported by 79 percent and diarrhea by 36 percent.[173] Pain was most often epigastric, although some patients reported pain in the right-upper and right-lower quadrants and in the periumbilical region. Ninety percent of these patients had eosinophilia. More than 30 cases of severe strongyloidiasis hyperinfection after renal transplantation or in association with Hodgkin's disease or cimetidine use have been reported.[174–176] Hyperinfection is often associated with secondary bacteremia, meningitis, urinary tract infection, or pneumonia due to enteric bacteria.

TABLE 4. Etiologic Agents and Useful Laboratory Studies in the Differential Diagnosis of Infectious Causes of the Syndrome of Abdominal Pain and/or Diarrhea with Eosinophilia

Etiologic Agents or Disease	Stool Examination	Small Bowel Fluid Examination or Biopsy	Tissue Biopsy	Serology	Radiologic and Other Studies
Nematodes					
Strongyloides stercoralis	+	+	−	+	−
Ascaris lumbricoides	+	+	−	−	± (Small bowel)
Visceral larva migrans (Toxocara canis, T. cati, and others)	−	−	+ (Liver)	+	−
Trichinella spiralis	−	−	+ (Muscle)	+	−
Anisakiasis (Anisakis spp. and other genera)	−	+	−	−	+ (Endoscopy)
Capillaria philippinensis	+	+	−	−	−
Angiostrongylus costaricensis	−	−	+ (Ileum, colon)	−	+ (UGI series; small bowel)
Trematodes					
Schistosoma spp.	+	−	+ (Rectum)	+	−
Fasciola hepatica	+	−	−	−	+ (Ultrasound, liver CT scan)
Fasciolopsis buski	+	−	−	−	−
Clonorchis sinensis	+	−	−	−	± (Biliary tract abnormalities)
Opisthorchis spp.	+	−	−	−	± (Biliary tract abnormalities)
Cestodes					
Echinococcosis	−	−	−	+	+ (Chest radiograph, abdominal ultrasound or CT scan)
Protozoa					
Isospora belli	+	+	−	−	−
Dientamoeba fragilis	+	−	−	−	−
Diseases of unknown etiology					
Eosinophilic gastroenteritis	−	+	−	−	+ (UGI series; small bowel CT scan)
Periarteritis nodosa and other forms of vasculitis	−	−	+ (Skin, muscle, kidney)	−	+ (Angiography)
Inflammatory bowel disease	−	−	+ (Colon)	−	+ (Small bowel, colonoscopy)
Malignancies	−	±	+ (Lymph nodes, liver, bone marrow)	−	+ (UGI Series, barium enema, CT scan, ultrasound)

Key: +: feature present; −: feature absent.

In the United States, strongyloidiasis is most often found in residents of the southeast, immigrants, or veterans who served in endemic areas. Prolonged infections have been demonstrated in troops and former prisoners of World War II who served in Southeast Asia.[177–180] A prospective study in rural Tennessee documented S. stercoralis in 6.1 percent of patients at a Veterans Administration hospital and in 2.6 percent of their household contacts.[181] The diagnosis of strongyloidiasis is made by demonstration of larvae in fresh concentrated stool specimens, which may require the Baermann funnel gauze test,[182,183] or in duodenal contents.[184] Although improved immunofluorescence and ELISA serologic tests are under study, they have not been fully tested.[185–187] Eosinophilia is often not present in immunocompromised patients, particularly those taking corticosteroids.[174,175]

Most patients infected with Ascaris lumbricoides are asymptomatic. Although ascariasis is not usually associated with diarrhea, severe abdominal pain may occur when patients with heavy worm burdens develop intestinal obstruction or adult worms occlude the biliary or pancreatic ducts. These complications are most frequent in young children.[188,189] It is estimated that acute intestinal obstruction due to Ascaris occurs in 1 in 1000 persons in endemic areas.[190] Ascariasis is most common in areas where sanitation is poor; the eggs may be ingested in contaminated food or water or, by children, in dirt. In the United States, this infection was once common in the southeastern states,[188] but symptomatic infections are now rare. The diagnosis is made by demonstration of the typical eggs in stool specimens. Eosinophilia may or may not be present. Since a single worm produces large numbers of eggs, concentration of feces is not necessary. In patients with intestinal or biliary tract obstruction, radiologic studies and liver or pancreatic enzyme elevations may provide a clue to the diagnosis.

Patients with toxocariasis (visceral larva migrans) caused by animal nematodes such as Toxocara canis or Toxocara cati may have abdominal pain and eosinophilia. In temperate climates, T. canis is the more important etiologic agent.[191] The abdominal pain may be associated with the presence of tender hepatomegaly. Clinical clues to the diagnosis include the simultaneous occurrence of splenomegaly or pneumonitis with bronchospasm.[192–194] Patients may have pruritic rashes on the trunk or lower extremities. The presence of a granuloma in the ocular fundus or other evidence of ocular inflammation, high titers of isoagglutinins, and hypergammaglobulinemia provide additional diagnostic clues. The total white count is often elevated, and eosinophils may exceed 50 percent. Patients are usually young children; additional epidemiologic clues are a history of pica or close contact with dogs or cats. As many as 10–30 percent of the soil samples in public playgrounds and parks in the United States have been found to be contaminated with Toxocara eggs.[191] Serologic tests are available; an ELISA seems to be the most sensitive and specific.[192–194] On rare occasions, larvae are identified in biopsies of hepatic granulomas.

Infection with Trichinella spiralis may be characterized initially by diarrhea, which occurs in approximately 40 percent of the cases; abdominal pain, which occurs in approximately 20 percent; or even by constipation.[195,196] The intestinal symptoms are attributed to the presence of adult worms or invading larvae in the intestinal tract, occur during the first week of illness, and may precede the appearance of eosinophilia. Approximately 100 cases are reported annually in the United States.[197] Infection occurs by the ingestion of raw or undercooked pork or pork products such as sausage, bear meat, and horse meat, and occasionally by other vehicles such as ground beef contaminated during processing with pork.[196–200] Prolonged diarrhea has been the dominant symptom among Inuit inhabitants of northern Canada who acquired *Trichinella nativa* from contaminated, uncooked walrus meat. Myalgia and muscle weakness were less prominent complaints.[201] This unusual presentation is felt to be the result of second infections in previously infected individuals.[202] The presence of myalgias, periorbital edema, muscle tenderness, splinter hemorrhages, and evidence of myocarditis or central nervous system involvement may suggest the diagnosis. The diagnosis is usually made on clinical grounds and confirmed serologically with either the bentonite flocculation or immunofluorescence test; they typically do not become positive until several weeks into infection.[203] Definitive diagnosis may be made by demonstration of larvae in specimens from a muscle biopsy, but biopsy is seldom necessary.

Patients with anisakiasis caused by nematodes of the family Anisakidae, ascarid parasites of marine animals, may have an acute illness characterized by epigastric pain, nausea, and vomiting or a chronic illness characterized by abdominal pain and fever. The disease is caused by larvae that penetrate the gastrointestinal tract. The stomach, small bowel, or colon may be involved. Necrotizing eosinophilic granulomatous inflammation with peripheral eosinophilia occur at the sites where larvae attempt to invade.[204-206] The pathologic and radiologic manifestations may resemble regional enteritis[207]; mass lesions resembling malignancies may also occur.[208] The disease is rarely reported in the United States. It is most common in the Netherlands and Japan. The infection is acquired by the ingestion of raw or undercooked marine fish such as cod, salmon, and herring. In Japan, raw or pickled marine fish are common vehicles; in the Netherlands, raw or slightly salted herring is the most common source of infection.[206] Therefore, a travel or a dietary history may suggest the diagnosis. Confirmation is obtained by identification of the larvae by endoscopy or in tissue specimens.

Patients infected with *Capillaria philippinesis* typically give a history of vague abdominal pain and voluminous watery diarrhea.[209] The illness is characterized by a protein-losing enteropathy and malabsorption. Electrolyte abnormalities and hypoproteinemia are common. Weight loss, muscle wasting, weakness, hyporeflexia, and edema occur.[210,211] The worms are found in the small bowel, especially in the jejunum, and the adults are partially embedded in the mucosa.[212] The intestinal villi are flattened in focal areas.[212] The disease is most common in the Philippines; a few cases have also been reported from Thailand and other sites in Southeast Asia. Freshwater fish eaten raw or poorly cooked appear to be the vehicle of transmission.[213] The diagnosis is made by demonstration of the eggs of *Capillaria philippinensis* in fecal specimens. The finding of eggs, adult worms, and larvae in the small bowel contents suggests that autoinfection may occur.[214,215] Travel and dietary histories may provide a clue to the diagnosis. Eustrongyliasis is another helminthic infection associated with abdominal pain, diarrhea, and eosinophilia following ingestion of *Eustrongylides* in uncooked fish or minnows.[216]

Angiostrongylus costaricensis lives in the lumen of mesenteric arteries of the ileocecal region of rodents and occasionally involves the same site in humans. Eggs form emboli to terminal branches of the mesenteric arteries. Disease, usually encountered in children, may present as an acute abdominal infection with fever, nausea, vomiting, pain, and sometimes a right-lower-quadrant mass. Leukocytosis and eosinophilia (11–82 percent) are usually present. It may be impossible to distinguish infection with *A. costaricensis* from acute appendicitis.[215] Humans are thought to become infected by ingesting material contaminated by infected slugs or snails, which are intermediate hosts. *Angiostrongylus costaricensis* is found in areas of Central and South America. Two cases have been reported that were acquired in the United States.[217] The diagnosis is suggested by the clinical syndrome, occasionally filling defects in the colon on barium enema, and a positive latex test or ELISA.[216] It is confirmed at the time of surgical exploration and resection by identifying adult worms and eggs in tissue.

Patients with trematode infection may occasionally have a syndrome characterized by abdominal pain and/or diarrhea and eosinophilia. Katayama fever, a clinical syndrome characterized by fever, headache, diarrhea, hepatosplenomegaly, generalized lymphadenopathy, urticaria, and eosinophilia, may occur within 4–8 weeks after primary exposure to schistosomes. This syndrome is most common in the presence of heavy infections and occurs most frequently with *Schistosoma japonicum* infection, less frequently with *Schistosoma mansoni* infection, and rarely with *Schistosoma haematobium* infection.[218] The acute manifestations of schistosomiasis are usually self-limited, although deaths may occur. The diagnosis should be suspected in patients with a serum sickness-like illness accompanied by eosinophilia who have had exposure during the previous 4–8 weeks through swimming or bathing in fresh water in an area where schistosomiasis is endemic.[219,220] As *S. japonicum* is found mainly in China, Japan, and Southeast Asia,[219] a history of recent exposure in those areas would suggest the diagnosis. The diagnosis is made by demonstration of the characteristic ova in feces[218] or a rectal biopsy specimen. Serologic tests provide suggestive evidence of infection.

Acute infection with the liver fluke *Fasciola hepatica,* which is found in many sheep-raising areas of the world, is characterized by fever and pain in the right upper quadrant, hepatomegaly, and often marked eosinophilia.[221-223] Human infections are acquired by ingestion of encysted metacercariae on aquatic plants such as wild watercress. Infections have been reported from South America, Africa, Europe, China, and Australia. The laboratory diagnosis is based on identification of characteristic ova in the feces or bile. Concentration techniques increase the likelihood of finding ova.

Another trematode that may be associated with abdominal pain or diarrhea and eosinophilia is the intestinal fluke *Fasciolopsis buski.* Although infection with *F. buski* is usually asymptomatic, patients with heavy infections may have both abdominal pain and diarrhea.[224,225] The diagnosis is suggested by a history of exposure in the Far East and Southeast Asia, where the disease is endemic.[225] Infection is acquired through the ingestion of water chestnuts or the peeling of other freshwater plants with the teeth before ingestion. Diagnosis is made by demonstration of *F. buski* eggs in feces and usually requires a concentration technique.[225] A similar syndrome may be observed with other intestinal flukes. *Heterophyes heterophyes* and *Metagonimus yokogawi* are acquired through ingestion of raw or undercooked infested freshwater fish.[226,227] *Echinostoma* species are ingested in raw, infected snails, amphibians, or fish.[228]

Acute infections with the liver flukes *Clonorchis sinensis* and *Opisthorchis* spp. may be associated with fever, abdominal pain, diarrhea, hepatomegaly, and eosinophilia. Although at increased risk of ascending cholangitis and cholangiocarcinoma, persons with established infection are usually free of specific symptoms and eosinophilia.[229,230]

Abdominal pain and/or diarrhea and eosinophilia are very uncommon in cestode (tapeworm) infections.[231] Eosinophilia may occur in conjunction with abdominal pain in patients with echinococcosis when cysts leak. Ultrasound or CT studies may show a cystic lesion(s) in the liver or other organs. The diagnosis should be suspected in patients who have lived in or traveled to areas where the disease is endemic. In the United States, endemic areas include California, Utah, and Alaska. Other endemic areas include sheep- and cattle-raising areas of Australia, South America, South Africa, the Soviet Union, and Mediterranean countries.[232] The diagnosis is usually made on the basis of radiologic or ultrasound findings and a positive serologic test.[233]

Patients with protozoal infections (e.g., *Entamoeba histolytica*) typically do not have eosinophilia. *Isospora belli* is an important exception.[234,235] It can cause abdominal pain, watery diarrhea, and malabsorption in association with eosinophilia. The disease occurs throughout the world, but it is most prevalent in the tropics where sanitation is poor. In healthy adults, *Isospora belli* produces a self-limited disease. The diagnosis may be suggested by an appropriate history of travel. *Isospora belli* is an important cause of severe, chronic diarrhea and weight loss in Haitians with AIDS.[236] Infection has been documented in a few patients with AIDS in the United States.

The diagnosis of *Isospora belli* is established by the demonstration of oocysts in feces[236]; concentration techniques and acid-fast staining may be helpful.[237,238] Examination of duodenal contents or small bowel biopsy specimens are more sensitive diagnostic techniques. Mucosal abnormalities are frequently seen on small bowel biopsy specimens and include blunted villus tips, shortened villi, hypertrophied crypts, and eosinophilic infiltration of the lamina propria.[234] *Dientamoeba fragilis* is another protozoan that can cause diarrhea and abdominal discomfort and has been associated with pinworm infection and eosinophilia.[239,240]

Eosinophilic gastroenteritis is a disease of adults with clinical manifestations that may include abdominal pain, diarrhea, gastrointestinal bleeding, protein-losing enteropathy, a malabsorption syndrome, or gastric outlet obstruction.[241] Manifestations depend both on the portion of bowel involved (stomach, duodenum, jejunum, or ileum) and on the layer involved (mucosa, muscular layer, or submucosa). The stomach and small intestine are the most common sites, but eosinophilic ileocolitis has also been reported.[242] Patients frequently have a history compatible with an allergic diathesis.[243] The sedimentation rate is usually normal or mildly elevated. Additional clues to the diagnosis include peripheral blood eosinophilia and the presence of Charcot-Leyden crystals in stools.[243,244] Radiologic studies may reveal polyploid gastric or duodenal mucosal folds and rigid dilated loops of jejunum with a sawtooth muscosal pattern.[245] Diagnosis may be made by perioral or endoscopic biopsy. Histologic examination of involved tissue reveals eosinophilia in the absence of both granulomas and vasculitis.[243] Since the involvement may be patchy, multiple biopsies are usually required. All biopsies may be negative if the disease involves only the muscular or subserosal layers. In the latter case, the presence of eosinophils in ascitic fluid may suggest the diagnosis.[243] The disease is chronic and occasionally fatal,[246] but most patients respond to corticosteroid therapy.[241,243]

Gastrointestinal involvement with eosinophilia may occur as manifestations of vasculitis.[247–249] Up to 25 percent of the patients with periarteritis nodosa have involvement of the gastrointestinal tract. It is the initial manifestation of disease in 15 percent of patients.[242,248,249] Abdominal pain is a prominent symptom, and eosinophilia is frequent. The clue to the diagnosis, which may be confirmed by biopsy or angiography, is provided by the systemic nature of the disease with frequent involvement of the kidneys, heart, musculoskeletal, and nervous systems. In allergic angiitis and granulomatosis of the Churg-Strauss syndrome type, lung involvement is pronounced, patients manifest prominent eosinophilia, and there is a strong allergic diathesis, often with asthma.[247] Some of the patients with this syndrome also have abdominal involvement and have been classified as having a polyangiitis overlap syndrome.[250,251]

Abdominal pain and diarrhea accompanied by eosinophilia may occur in patients with regional enteritis, Whipple's disease, or ulcerative colitis.[252] In one series, 32 percent of the patients with radiologically or surgically proven regional enteritis had eosinophilia on more than one occasion.[253] The average elevated eosinophil count was 6.2 percent; the range was from 4 to 22 percent.[253] On occasion the extraintestinal manifestations of inflammatory bowel diseases provide clues to their diagnosis.[254]

Patients with solid tumors and lymphomas may also have abdominal pain, diarrhea, and eosinophilia.[252] Eosinophilia is most commonly associated with solid tumors after metastasis has occurred.[255,256] Among those solid tumors, frequently implicated malignancies are gastric, colonic, lung, pancreatic, and uterine carcinomas.[255,257] A history of weight loss and the presence of

melena or guaiac-positive stools and anemia may suggest the diagnosis, which may be confirmed by appropriate radiographic, endoscopic, or cytologic studies. Both Hodgkin's disease and non-Hodgkin's lymphomas may also be associated with eosinophilia, diarrhea, and abdominal pain when the bowel or abdominal or retroperitoneal nodes are involved.

REFERENCES

1. Christie AB. Typhoid and paratyphoid fevers. In: Infectious Diseases: Epidemiology and Clinical Practice, 2nd ed. Churchill Livingstone; New York: 1974:55–130.
2. Walker W, ed. The Aberdeen typhoid outbreak of 1964. Scott Med J. 1965; 10:466–79.
3. Gulati PD, Saxena SN, Gupta PS, et al. Changing pattern of typhoid fever. Am J Med. 1968;45:544–8.
4. Hornick RB, Greisman SE, Woodward TE, et al. Typhoid fever: Pathogenesis and immunologic control. N Engl J Med. 1970;283:686–91.
5. Stuart BM, Pullen RL: Typhoid: Clinical analysis of three hundred and sixty cases. Arch Intern Med. 1946;78:629–61.
6. Rice PA, Baine WB, Gangarosa EJ. *Salmonella typhi* infections in the United States, 1967–1972: Increasing importance of international travelers. Am J Epidemiol. 1977;106:160–6.
7. Ryan CA, Hargrett-Bean NT, Blake PA. *Salmonella typhi* infections in the United States, 1975–1984: Increasing role of foreign travel. Rev Infect Dis. 1989;11:1–8.
8. Birkhead GS, Morse DL, Levine WC, et al. Typhoid fever at a resort hotel in New York: A large outbreak with an unusual vehicle. J Infect Dis. 1993; 167:1228–32.
9. Carter PB, Collins FM. The route of enteric infection in normal mice. J Exp Med. 1974;139:1189–203.
10. Kamat SA, Herzog C. Typhoid: Clinical picture and response to chloramphenicol: Prospective study in Bombay (1972). Infection. 1977;5:85–91.
11. Wicks ACB, Holmes GS, Davidson L. Endemic typhoid fever: A diagnostic pitfall. Q J Med. 1971;40:341–54.
12. Hoffman TA, Ruiz CJ, Counts GW, et al. Waterborne typhoid fever in Dade County, Florida: Clinical and therapeutic evaluation of 105 bacteremic patients. Am J Med. 1975;59:481–7.
13. Samantray SK, Johnson SC, Chakrabarti AK. Enteric fever: An analysis of 500 cases. Practitioner. 1977;218:400–8.
14. Wahab MFA, Robertson RP, Raasch FO. Paratyphoid A fever, Cairo, Egypt. Ann Intern Med. 1969;70:913–7.
15. Black PH, Kunz LJ, Swartz MN. Salmonellosis: A review of some unusual aspects. N Engl J Med. 1960;262:811–7.
16. Sprinz H, Gangarosa EJ, Williams M, et al. Histopathology of the upper small intestines in typhoid fever: Biopsy study of experimental disease in man. Am J Dig Dis. 1966;11:615–24.
17. Litwack KD, Hoke AW, Borchardt KA. Rose spots in typhoid fever. Arch Dermatol. 1972;105:252–5.
18. Meals RA. Paratyphoid fever: A report of 62 cases with several unusual findings and a review of the literature. Arch Intern Med. 1976;136:1422–8.
19. Watson KC. Laboratory and clinical investigation of recovery of *Salmonella typhi* from blood. J Clin Microbiol. 1978;7:122–6.
20. Gilman RH, Terminel M, Levine MM, et al. Relative efficacy of blood, urine, rectal swab, bone-marrow, and rose-spot cultures for recovery of *Salmonella typhi* in typhoid fever. Lancet. 1975;1:1211–3.
21. Guerra-Caceres JG, Gotuzzo-Herencia E, Crosby-Dagnino E, et al. Diagnostic value of bone marrow culture in typhoid fever. Trans R Soc Trop Med Hyg. 1979;73:680–3.
22. Tsang RSW, Chau PY. Serological diagnosis of typhoid fever by counter-immunoelectrophoresis. Br Med J. 1981;282:1505–7.
23. Sundararaj T, Ilango B, Subramanian S. A study on the usefulness of counter immuno-electrophoresis for the detection of *Salmonella typhi* antigen in the sera of suspected cases of enteric fever. Trans R Soc Trop Med Hyg. 1983; 77:194–7.
24. Taylor DN, Harris JR, Barrett TJ, et al. Detection of urinary Vi antigen as a diagnostic test for typhoid fever. J Clin Microbiol. 1983;18:872–6.
25. Song JH, Cho H, Park MY, et al. Detection of *Salmonella typhi* in the blood of patients with typhoid fever by polymerase chain reaction. J Clin Microbiol. 1993;31:1439–43.
26. Schroeder SA. Interpretation of serologic tests for typhoid fever. JAMA. 1968;206:839–40.
27. Reynolds DW, Carpenter RL, Simon WH. Diagnostic specificity of Widal's reaction for typhoid fever. JAMA. 1970;214:2192–3.
28. Senewiratne B, Chir B. Senewiratne K. Reassessment of the Widal test in the diagnosis of typhoid. Gastroenterology. 1977;73:233–6.
29. Brodie J: Antibodies and the Aberdeen typhoid outbreak of 1964: I. The Widal reaction. J Hyg. 1977;79:161–80.
30. Buck RL, Escamilla J, Sangalang RP, et al. Diagnostic value of a single, pretreatment Widal test in suspected enteric fever cases in the Philippines. Trans R Soc Trop Med Hyg. 1987;81:871–3.
31. Levine MM, Grados O, Gilman RH, et al. Diagnostic value of the Widal test in areas endemic for typhoid fever. Am J Trop Med Hyg. 1978;27:795–800.
32. Editorial: Typhoid and its serology. Br Med J. 1978;1:389.
33. Beasley WJ, Joseph SW, Weiss E: Improved serodiagnosis of *Salmonella*

enteric fevers by an enzyme-linked immunosorbent assay. J Clin Microbiol. 1981;13:106–14.

34. Petchclai B, Ausavarungnirun R, Manatsathit S. Passive hemagglutination test for enteric fever. J Clin Microbiol. 1987;25:138–41.

35. Nolan CM, Feeley JC, White PC Jr, et al. Evaluation of a new assay for Vi antibody in chronic carriers of *Salmonella typhi*. J Clin Microbiol. 1980;12:22–6.

36. Barrett TJ, Blake PA, Brown SL, et al. Enzyme-linked immunosorbent assay for detection of human antibodies to *Salmonella typhi* Vi antigen. J Clin Microbiol. 1983;17:625–7.

37. Gupta AK, Rao KM. Radial counter-immunoelectrophoresis for rapid serodiagnosis of typhoid fever. J Immunol Methods. 1981;40:373–6.

38. Ramachandran S, Godfrey JJ, Perera MVF. Typhoid hepatitis. JAMA. 1974;230:236–42.

39. Sitprija V, Pipatanagul V, Boonpucknavig V, et al. Glomerulitis in typhoid fever. Ann Intern Med. 1974;81:210–3.

40. Butler W, Bell WR, Levin J, et al. Typhoid fever: Studies of blood coagulation, bacteremia, and endotoxemia. Arch Intern Med. 1978;138:407–10.

41. Harris JC, DuPont HL, Hornick RB. Fecal leukocytes in diarrheal illness. Ann Intern Med. 1972;76:697–703.

42. Blaser MJ, Hickman FW, Farmer JJ III, et al. *Salmonella typhi:* The laboratory as a reservoir of infection. J Infect Dis. 1980;142:934–8.

43. Blaser MJ, Lofgren JP. Fatal salmonellosis originating in a clinical microbiology laboratory. J Clin Microbiol. 1981;13:855–8.

44. Rabson AR, Hallett AF, Koornhof JH. Generalized *Yersinia enterocolitica* infection. J Infect Dis. 1975;131:447–51.

45. Spira TJ, Kabins SA. *Yersinia enterocolitica* septicemia with septic arthritis. Arch Intern Med. 1976;136:1305–8.

46. Marlon A, Gentry L, Merigan TC. Septicemia with *Pasteurella pseudotuberculosis* and liver disease. Arch Intern Med. 1971;127:947–9.

47. Guerrant RL, Lahita RG, Winn WC Jr, et al. Campylobacteriosis in man: Pathogenic mechanisms and review of 91 bloodstream infections. Am J Med. 1978;65:584–92.

48. Schmidt U, Chmel H, Kaminski Z, et al. The clinical spectrum of *Campylobacter fetus* infection: Report of 5 cases and review of the literature. Q J Med. 1980;49:431–42.

49. Carbone KM, Heinrich MC, Quinn TC. Thrombophlebitis and cellulitis due to *Campylobacter fetus* spp *fetus*. Medicine. 1984;64:244–50.

50. Bevanger L. *Yersinia pseudotuberculosis* as the cause of septicemia in a patient with amyloidosis. Acta Pathol Microbiol Scand [B]. 1976;84:461–2.

51. Bokkenheuser V. *Vibrio fetus* infection in man: I. Ten new cases and some epidemiologic observations. Am J Epidemiol. 1970;91:400–9.

52. Leino R, Kalliomäki JL. Yersiniosis as an internal disease. Ann Intern Med. 1974;81:458–61.

53. Ahvonen P. Human yersiniosis in Finland: I. Bacteriology and serology. Ann Clin Res. 1972;4:30–8.

54. Hubbert WT, Petenyi CW, Glasgow LA, et al. *Yersinia pseudotuberculosis* infection in the United States: Septicemia, appendicitis, and mesenteric lymphadenitis. Am J Trop Med Hyg. 1971;20:679–84.

55. Yamashiro KM, Goldman RH, Harris D, et al. *Pasteurella pseudotuberculosis:* Acute sepsis with survival. Arch Intern Med. 1971;128:605–8.

56. Keet EE. *Yersinia enterocolitica* septicemia: Source of infection and incubation period identified. NY State J Med. 1974;74:2226–30.

57. Sonnenwirth AC. Bacteremia with and without meningitis due to *Yersinia enterocolitica, Edwardsiella tarda, Comamonas terrigena,* and *Pseudomonas maltophilia*. Ann NY Acad Sci. 1970;174:488–502.

58. Taykor BG, Zafarzai MZ, Humphreys DW, et al. Nodular pulmonary infiltrates and septic arthritis associated with *Yersinia enterocolitica* bacteremia. Am Rev Respir Dis. 1977;116:525–9.

59. Bliddal J, Kaliszan S. Prolonged monosymptomatic fever due to *Yersinia enterocolitica*. Acta Med Scand. 1977;201:387–9.

60. Ahvonen P. Human yersiniosis in Finland: II. Clinical features. Ann Clin Res. 1972;4:39–48.

61. Franklin B, Ulmer DD. Human infection with *Vibrio fetus*. West J Med. 1974;120:200–4.

62. Greenwood JR, Flanigan SW, Pickett MJ, et al. Clinical isolation of *Yersinia enterocolitica:* Cold temperature enrichment. J Clin Microbiol. 1975;2:559–60.

63. Skirrow MB. *Campylobacter* enteritis: A "new" disease. Br Med J. 1977;2:9–11.

64. Lauwers S, DeBoeck M, Butzler JP. *Campylobacter* enteritis in Brussels. Lancet. 1978;1:604–5.

65. Bokkenheuser V. *Vibrio fetus* infection in man: A serological test. Infect Immun. 1972;5:222–226.

66. Reinicke V, Korner B. Case report: Fulminant septicemia caused by *Yersinia enterocolitica*. Scand J Infect Dis. 1977;9:249–51.

67. Forrström J, Viander M, Lehtonen A, et al. Case report: *Yersinia enterocolitica* infection complicated by glomerulonephritis. Scand J Infect Dis. 1977;9:253–6.

68. Guerrant RL, Humphries MK Jr, Butler JE, et al. Tickborne oculoglandular tularemia. Arch Intern Med. 1976;136:811–3.

69. Buchanan TM, Faber LC, Feldman RA. Brucellosis in the United States, 1960–1972: An abattoir-associated disease: I. Clinical features and therapy. Medicine. 1974;53:403–13.

70. Reed WP, Palmer DL, Williams RC Jr, et al. Bubonic plague in the southwestern United States: A review of recent experience. Medicine. 1970;49:465–86.

71. Cantey JR. Plague in Vietnam: Clinical observations and treatment with kanamycin. Arch Intern Med. 1974;133:280–3.

72. Nalin DR, Sultana B, Sahunja R, et al. Survival of a patient with intestinal anthrax. Am J Med. 1977;62:130–2.

73. Brundage WG, Thuss CJ Jr, Walden DG. Four fatal cases of melioidosis in U.S. soldiers in Vietnam: Bacteriologic and pathologic characteristics. Am J Trop Med Hyg. 1968;17:183–91.

74. Schultz MG. A history of bartonellosis (Carrión's disease). Am J Trop Med Hyg. 1968;17:503–15.

75. Cuadra M. Salmonellosis complication in human bartonellosis. Tex Rep Biol Med. 1956;14:97–113.

76. Cole JS, Stoll RW, Bulger RJ. Rat-bite fever: Report of three cases. Ann Intern Med. 1969;71:979–81.

77. Kowal J. Spirillum fever: Report of a case and review of the literature. N Engl J Med. 1961;264:123–8.

78. Anderson LC, Leary SL, Manning PJ. Rat bite fever in animal research laboratory personnel. Lab Anim Sci. 1983;33:292–4.

79. Heath CW Jr, Alexander AD, Galton MM. Leptospirosis in the United States: Analysis of 483 cases in man, 1949–1961. N Engl J Med. 1965;273:857–64.

80. Edwards GA, Domm BM. Human leptospirosis. Medicine. 1960;39:117–56.

81. Boyer KM, Munford RS, Maupin GO, et al. Tick-borne relapsing fever: An interstate outbreak originating at Grand Canyon National Park. Am J Epidemiol. 1977;105:469–79.

82. Southern PM Jr, Sanford JP. Relapsing fever: A clinical and microbiological review. Medicine. 1969;48:129–49.

83. Lewis EA, Kolawole RM. Tuberculous ileo-colitis in Ibadan: A clinico-radiological review. Gut. 1972;13:646–53.

84. Johnson CAC, Hill ID, Bowie MD. Abdominal tuberculosis in children: A survey of cases at the Red Cross War Memorial Children's Hospital. 1976–1985. S Afr Med J. 1987;72:20–2.

85. Fischl MA, Daikos GL, Uttamchandani RB, et al. Clinical presentation and outcome of patients with HIV infection and tuberculosis caused by multiple-drug–resistant bacilli. Ann Intern Med. 1992;117:184–90.

86 Dooley SW, Jarvis WR, Martone WJ, et al. Multidrug-resistant tuberculosis (Editoral; Comment). Ann Intern Med. 1992;117:257–9.

87. Weese WC, Smith IM. A study of 57 cases of actinomycosis over a 36-year period: A diagnostic "failure" with good prognosis after treatment. Arch Intern Med. 1975;135:1562–8.

88. Larson EB, Featherstone HJ, Petersdorf RG. Fever of undetermined origin: Diagnosis and follow-up of 105 cases, 1970–1980. Medicine. 1982;61:269–92.

89. Murray HW, Masur H, Senterfit LB, et al. The protean manifestations of *Mycoplasma pneumoniae* infection in adults. Am J Med. 1975;58:229–42.

90. Schaffner W, Drutz DJ, Duncan GW, et al. The clinical spectrum of endemic psittacosis. Arch Intern Med. 1967;119:433–43.

91. Hattwick MAW, O'Brien RJ, Hanson BF. Rocky Mountain spotted fever: Epidemiology of an increasing problem. Ann Intern Med. 1976;84:732–9.

92. Woodward TE. A historical account of the rickettsial diseases with a discussion of unsolved problems. J Infect Dis. 1973;127:583–94.

93. Walker DH. Gastroenterology of Rocky Mountain spotted fever. Practical Gastroenterol. 1986;10:25–39.

94. Jiminez J, Byrne WJ, Seibert JJ, et al. Gastrointestinal symptoms in Rocky Mountain spotted fever: Histopathologic finding of ulcerative enteritis with vasculitis. Clin Pediatr. 1982;21:581–4.

95. Middleton DB. Rocky Mountain spotted fever: Gastrointestinal and laboratory manifestations. South Med J. 1978;71:629–32.

96. Westerman EL. Rocky Mountain spotted fever: A dilemma for the clinician. Arch Intern Med. 1982;142:1106–7.

97. Woodward TE, Pedersen CE Jr, Oster CN, et al. Prompt confirmation of Rocky Mountain spotted fever: Identification of rickettsiae in skin tissues. J Infect Dis. 1976;134:297–301.

98. Marrie TJ, Schlech WF III, Williams JC, et al. Q fever pneumonia associated with exposure to wild rabbits. Lancet 1986;1:427–9.

99. Duma RJ, Sonenshine DE, Bozeman FM, et al. Epidemic typhus in the United States associated with flying squirrels. JAMA. 1981;245:2318–23.

100. Centers for Disease Control and Prevention. Epidemic typhus associated with flying squirrels: United States. MMWR. 1982;31:555–61.

101. Yu VL, Kroboth FJ, Shonnard J, et al. Legionnaires' disease: New clinical perspecive from a prospective pneumonia study. Am J Med. 1982;73:357–61.

102. Kirby BD, Snyder KM, Meyer RD, et al. Legionnaires' disease: Report of 65 nosocomially acquired cases and a review of the literature. Medicine. 1980;59:188–205.

103. Chow JW, Lu VL. New perspectives on *Legionella* pneumonia: Dignosis, management and prevention. J Crit Illness. 1988;3:17–27.

104. Sturim HS, Kouchonkos NT, Ahlvin RC. Gastrointestinal manifestations of disseminated histoplasmosis. Am J Surg. 1965;110:435–40.

105. Gordon S, Brennessel DJ, Goldstein JA, et al. Malaria: A city hospital experience. Arch Intern Med. 1988;148:1569–71.

106. Steketee RW, Eckman MR, Burgess EC, et al. Babesiosis in Wisconsin: A new focus of disease transmission. JAMA. 1985;253:2675–8.

107. Ruebush TK II, Cassaday PB, Marsh HJ, et al. Human babesiosis on Nantucket Island: Clinical features. Ann Intern Med. 1977;86:6–9.

108. May RP, Lehmann JD, Sanford JP. Difficulties in differentiating amebic from pyogenic liver abscess. Arch Intern Med. 1967;119:69–74.

109. Robertson RP, Wahab MFA, Raasch FO. Evaluation of chloramphenicol and ampicillin in salmonella enteric fever. N Engl J Med. 1968;278:171–6.

110. Baine WB, Farmer JJ III, Gangarosa EJ. Typhoid fever in the United States associated with the 1972–1973 epidemic in Mexico. J Infect Dis. 1977;135:649–53.

111. Butler T, Arnold K, Linh NN, et al. Chloramphenicol-resistant typhoid fever in Vietnam associated with R factor. Lancet. 1973;2:983–91.

112. Brown JD, Mo DH, Rhoades ER. Chloramphenicol-resistant *Salmonella typhi* in Saigon. JAMA. 1975;231:162–6.

113. Olarte J, Galindo E. *Salmonella typhi* resistant to chloramphenicol, ampicillin and other antimicrobial agents: Strains isolated during an extensive typhoid fever epidemic in Mexico. Antimicrob Agents Chemother. 1973;4:597–603.

114. Bhutta ZA, Naqvi SH, Razzaq RA, et al. Multidrug-resistant typhoid in children. Presentation and clinical features. Rev Infect Dis. 1991;13:832–6.

115. Lasserre R, Sangalang RP, Santiago L. Three-day treatment of typhoid fever with two different doses of ceftriaxone, compared to 14-day therapy with chloramphenicol: A randomized trial. J Antimicrob Chemother 1991;28:765–72.

116. Bryan JP, Rocha H, Scheld WM. Problems in salmonellosis: Rationale for clinical trials with newer beta-lactam agents and quinolones. Rev Infect Dis. 1986;8:189–207.

117. Soe GB, Overturf GD. Treatment of typhoid fever and other systemic salmonellosis with cefotaxime, ceftriaxone, cefoperazone and other newer cephalosporins. Rev Infect Dis. 1987;9:719–36.

118. Chew SK, Monteiro EH, Lim YS, et al. A 7-day course of ciprofloxacin for enteric fever. J Infect. 1992;25:267–71.

119. Uwaydah AK, al Soub H, Matar I. Randomized prospective study comparing two dosage regimens of ciprofloxacin for the treatment of typhoid fever. J Antimicrob Chemother. 1992;30:707–11.

120. Dutta P, Rasaily R, Saha MR, et al. Ciprofloxacin for treatment of severe typhoid fever in children. Antimicrob Agents Chemother. 1993;37:1197–9.

121. Datta N, Richards H, Datta C. *Salmonella typhi* in vivo acquires resistance to both chloramphenicol and co-trimoxazole. Lancet. 1981;1:1181–3.

122. Collins DC. Mesenteric lymphadenitis in adolescents simulating appendicitis. Can Med Assoc J. 1936;34:402–5.

123. Mair NS, Mair HJ, Stirk EM, et al. Three cases of acute mesenteric lymphadenitis due to *Pasteurella pseudotuberculosis*. J Clin Pathol. 1960;13:432–9.

124. Van Noyen R, Selderslaghs R, Bekaert J, et al. Causative role of *Yersinia* and other enteric pathogens in the appendicular syndrome. Eur J Clin Microbiol Infect Dis. 1991;10:735–41.

125. Winblad S, Nilehn B, Sternby NJ. *Yersinia enterocolitica* (Pasteurella X) in human enteric infections. Br Med J. 1966;2:1363–6.

126. Tertti R, Vuento R, Mikkola P, et al. Clinical manifestations of *Yersinia pseudotuberculosis* infection in children. Eur J Clin Microbiol Infect Dis. 1989;8:587–91.

127. Carter PB. Pathogenicity of *Yersinia enterocolitica* for mice. Infect Immun. 1975;11:164–70.

128. Une T. Studies on the pathogenicity of *Yersinia enterocolitica*: II. Interaction with cultured cells in vitro. Microbiol Immunol. 1977;21:365–77.

129. Kay BA, Wachsmuth K, Gemski P, et al. Virulence and phenotypic characterization of *Yersinia enterocolitica* isolated from humans in the United States. J Clin Microbiol. 1983;17:128–38.

130. Feeley JC, Wells JG, Tsai TF, et al. Detection of enterotoxigenic and invasive strains of *Yersinia enterocolitica*. Contrib Microbiol Immunol. 1979;5:329–34.

131. Zink DL, Feeley JC, Wells JG, et al. Plasmid-mediated tissue invasiveness in *Yersinia enterocolitica*. Nature. 1980;283:224–6.

132. Kay BA, Wachsmuth K, Gemski P. New virulence-associated plasmid in *Yersinia enterocolitica*. J Clin Microbiol. 1982;15:1161–3.

133. Dudley HAF, MacLaren IF. Primary mesenteric abscess. Lancet. 1956;2:1182–4.

134. Asch MJ, Amoury RA, Touloukian RJ, et al. Suppurative mesenteric lymphadenitis: A report of two cases and review of the literature. Am J Surg. 1968;115:570–3.

135. Constantinides CG, Davies MRQ, Cywes S. Suppurative mesenteric lymphadenitis in children: Case reports. S Afr Med J. 1981;60:629–31.

136. Jepsen OB, Korner B, Lauritsen KB, et al. *Yersinia enterocolitica* infection in patients with acute surgical abdominal disease: A prospective study. Scand J Infect Dis. 1976;8:189–94.

137. Zen-Yoji H, Maruyama T, Sakai S, et al. An outbreak of enteritis due to *Yersinia enterocolitica* occurring at a junior high school. Jpn J Microbiol. 1973;17:220.

138. Asakawa Y, Akahane S, Kagata N, et al. Two community outbreaks of human infection with *Yersinia enterocolitica*. J Hyg (Camb). 1973;71:715–23.

139. Black RE, Jackson RJ, Tsai T, et al. Epidemic *Yersinia enterocolitica* infection due to contaminated chocolate milk. N Engl J Med. 1978;298:76–9.

140. Vantrappen G, Agg HO, Ponette E, et al. *Yersinia* enteritis and enterocolitis: Gastroenterological aspects. Gastroenterology. 1977;72:220–7.

141. Jansson E, Wallgren GR, Ahvonen P. *Yersinia enterocolitica* as a cause of acute mesenteric lymphadenitis. Acta Paediatr Scand. 1968;57:448–50.

142. Tauxe RV, Vandepitte J, Wauters G, et al. *Yersinia enterocolitica* infections and pork: The missing link. Lancet. 1987;1:1129–32.

143. Knapp W. Mesenteric adenitis due to *Pasteurella pseudotuberculosis* in young people. N Engl J Med. 1958;259:776–8.

144. Randall KJ, Mair NS. Family outbreak of *Pasteurella pseudotuberculosis* infection. Lancet. 162;1:1042–3.

145. Weber J, Finlayson NB, Mark JBD. Mesenteric lymphadenitis and terminal ileitis due to *Yersinia pseudotuberculosis*. N Engl J Med. 1970;283:172–4.

146. Saari TN, Triplett DA. *Yersinia pseudotuberculosis* mesenteric adenitis. J Pediatr. 1974;85:656–9.

147. Bradford WD, Noce PS, Gutman LT. Pathologic features of enteric infection with *Yersinia enterocolitica*. Arch Pathol. 1974;98:17–22.

148. Weissfeld AS, Sonnenwirth AC. *Yersinia enterocolitica* in adults with gastrointestinal disturbances: Need for cold enrichment. J Clin Microbiol. 1980;11:196–7.

149. Daniëls JJHM. Enteral infection with *Pasteurella pseudotuberculosis*: Isolation of the oganism from human feces. Br Med J. 1961;2:997.

150. Niléhn B, Sjöström B. Studies on *Yersinia enterocolitica*. Acta Pathol Microbiol Scand. 1967;71:12–28.

151. Marks MI, Pai CH, Lafleur L, et al. *Yersinia enterocolitica* gastroenteritis: A prospective study of clinical, bacteriologic, and epidemiologic features. J Pediatr. 1980;96:26–31.

152. Puylaert JB. Mesenteric adenitis and acute terminal ileitis: Ultrasound evaluation using graded compression. Radiol. 1986;161:691–5.

153. Ekberg O, Sjöström B, Brahme F. Radiological findings in *Yersinia* ileitis. Radiology. 1977;123:15–9.

154. Ahlqvist J, Ahvonen P, Räsänen JA, et al. Enteric infection with *Yersinia enterocolitica*: Large pyroninophilic cell reproduction in mesenteric lymph nodes associated with early production of specific antibodies. Acta Pathol Microbiol Scand [A]. 1971;79:109–22.

155. Braunstein H, Tucker EB, Gibson BC. Mesenteric lymphadenitis due to *Yersinia enterocolitica*: Report of a case. Am J Clin Pathol. 1971;55:506–10.

156. El-Maraghi NRH, Mair NS. The histopathology of enteric infecton with *Yersinia pseudotuberculosis*. Am J Clin Pathol. 1979;71:631–9.

157. Gutman LT, Ottesen EA, Quan TJ, et al. An inter-familial outbreak of *Yersinia enterocolitica* enteritis. N Engl J Med. 1973;288:1372–7.

158. Arvastson B, Damgaard K, Winblad S. Clinical symptoms of infection with *Yersinia enterocolitica*. Scand J Infect Dis. 1971;3:37–40.

159. Wilson HD, McCormick JB, Feeley JC. *Yersinia enterocolitica* infection in a 4-month-old infant associated with infection in household dogs. J Pediatr. 1976;89:767–8.

160. Tacket CO, Narain JP, Sattin R, et al. A multistate outbreak of infections caused by *Yersinia enterocolitica* transmitted by pasteurized milk. JAMA. 1984;251:483–6.

161. Nolan C, Harris N, Ballard J, et al. Outbreak of *Yersinia enterocolitica*: Washington State. MMWR. 1982;31:562.

162. Laasen J. *Yersinia enterocolitica* in drinking-water. Scand J Infect Dis. 1972;4:125–7.

163. Highsmith AK, Feeley JC, Skaliy P, et al. Isolation of *Yersinia enterocolitica* from well water and growth in distilled water. Appl Environ Microbiol. 1977;34:745–50.

164. Snyder JD, Christenson E, Feldman RA. Human *Yersinia enterocolitica* infections in Wisconsin. Am J Med. 1982;72:768–74.

165. Berkowitz FE, Nesheim S. Chylous ascites caused by *Mycobacterium avium* complex and mesenteric lymphadenitis in a child with the acquired immunodeficiency syndrome. Pediatr Infect Dis J. 1993;12:99–101.

166. Morinet F, Monsuez JJ, Roger P, et al. Parvovirus B19 associated with pseudoappendicitis [Letter]. Lancet. 1987;2:1466.

167. Chen CM, Chao K, Su IJ. Acute primary Epstein-Barr virus infection presenting as acute abdomen. Peditr Infect Dis J. 1991;10:471–3.

168. Loría-Cortés R, Lobo-Sanahuja JF. Clinical abdominal angiostrongylosis: A study of 116 children with intestinal eosinophilic granuloma caused by *Angiostrongylus costaricensis*. Am J Trop Med Hyg. 1980;29:538–44.

169. Gutman LT, Wilfert CM, Quan T. Susceptibility of *Yersinia enterocolitica* to trimethoprim–sulfamethoxazole. J Infect Dis. 1973;128(Suppl):S538.

170. Hornstein MJ, Jupeau AM, Scavizzi MR, et al. In vitro susceptibilities of 126 clinical isolates of *Yersinia enterocolitica* to 21 β-lactam antibiotics. Antimicrob Agents Chemother. 1985;27:806–11.

171. Hammerberg S, Sorger S, Marks MI. Antimicrobial susceptibilities of *Yersinia enterocolitica* biotype 4, serotype O:3. Antimicrob Agents Chemother. 1977;11:566–8.

172. Grove DI, Warren KS, Mahmoud AAF. Algorithms in the diagnosis and management of exotic diseases: III. Strongyloidiasis. J Infect Dis. 1975;131:755–8.

173. Jones CA. Clinical studies in human strongyloidiasis: I. Semeiology. Gastroenterology. 1950;16:743–56.

174. Purtilo DT, Meyers WM, Connor DH. Fatal strongyloidiasis in immunosuppressed patients. Am J Med. 1974;56:488–93.

175. Morgan JS, Schaffner W, Stone WJ. Opportunistic strongyloidiasis in renal transplant recipients. Transplantation. 1986;42:518–24.

176. Cadranel JF, Eugene C. Another example of *Strongyloides stercoralis* infec-

tion associated with cimetidine in an immunosuppressed patient. Gut. 1986; 27:1229.

177. Pelletier LL Jr, Baker CB, Gam AA, et al. Diagnosis and evaluation of treatment of chronic strongyloidiasis in ex-prisoners of war. J Infect Dis. 1988;157:573–6.

178. Gill GV, Bell DR. *Strongyloides stercoralis* infection in former Far East prisoners of war. Br Med J [Clin Res]. 1979;2:572–4.

179. Grove DI. Strongyloidiasis in Allied ex-prisoners of war in south-east Asia. Br Med J [Clin Res]. 1980;280:598–601.

180. Pelletier LL Jr. Chronic strongyloidiasis in World War II Far East ex-prisoners of war. Am J Trop Med Hyg. 1984;33:55–61.

181. Berk SL, Verghese A, Alvarez S, et al. Clinical and epidemiologic features of strongyloidiasis: A prospective study in rural Tennessee. Arch Intern Med. 1987;147:1257–61.

182. Lima JP, Delgado PG. Dignosis of strongyloidiasis: Importance of Baermann's method. Am J Diagn Dis. 1961;6:899.

183. de Kaminsky RG. Evaluation of three methods for laboratory diagnosis of *Strongyloides stercoralis* infection. J Parasitol. 1993;79:277–80.

184. Beal CB, Viens P, Grant RGL, et al. A new technique for sampling duodenal contents: Demonstration of upper small bowel pathogens. Am J Trop Med Hyg. 1970;19:399–52.

185. Grove DI, Blair AJ. Dignosis of human strongyloidiasis by immunofluorescence using *Strongyloides ratti* and *S. stercoralis* larvae. Am J Trop Med Hyg. 1981;30:344–9.

186. Kagen IG, Maddison SE. Parasitic immunodiagnosis. In Strickland GT (ed): Hunter's Tropical Medicine, 7th ed. Philadelphia: WB Saunders; 1991: 1090–5.

187. Gam AA, Neva FA, Krotoski WA. Comparative sensitivity and specificity of ELISA and IHA for serodiagnosis of strongyloidiasis with larval antigens. Am J Trop Med Hyg. 1987;37:157–61.

188. Blumenthal DS, Schultz MG. Incidence of intestinal obstruction in children infected with *Ascaris lumbricoides*. Am J Trop Med Hyg. 1975;24:801–5.

189. Krige JEJ, Lewis G, Bornman PC. Recurrent pancreatitis caused by a calcified ascaris in the duct of Wirsung. Am J Gastroenterol. 1987;82:256–7.

190. Blumenthal DS, Schultz MG. Incidence of intestinal obstruction in children infected with *Ascaris lumbricoides*. Am J Trop Med Hyg. 1975;24:801–5.

191. Schantz PM, Glickman LT. Toxocaral visceral larva migrans. N Engl J Med. 1978;298:436–9.

192. Taylor MRH, Keane CT, O'Connor P, et al. The expanded spectrum of toxocaral disease. Lancet. 1988;1:692–5.

193. Thompson DE, Bundy DAP, Cooper ES, et al. Epidemiological characteristics of *Toxocara canis* zoonotic infection of children in a Caribbean community. Bull WHO. 1986;64:283–90.

194. Glickman LT, Magnaval J-F, Domanski LM, et al. Visceral larva migrans in French adutls: A new disease syndrome. Am J Epidemiol. 1987;125:1019–34.

195. Grove DI, Warren KS, Mahmoud AAF. Algorithms in the diagnosis and management of exotic diseases: VII. Trichinosis. J Infect Dis. 1975;132: 485–8.

196. Campbell WC. Trichinella and Trichinosis. New York: Plenum Press; 1983.

197. Stehr-Green JK, Schantz PM, Chisolm EM. Trichinosis surveillance, 1984. MMWR. 1985;35:11–15SS.

198. Singal M, Schantz PM, Werner SB. Trichinosis acquired at sea: Report of an outbreak. Am J Trop Med Hyg. 1976;25:675–81.

199. Petri WA Jr, Holsinger JR, Pearson RD. Common-source outbreak of trichinosis associated with eating raw home-butchered pork. South Med J. 1988; 81:1056–8.

200. Trichinosis outbreaks associated with horsemeat. Parasitol Today. 1986;2: 295.

201. Viallet J, MacLean JD, Goresky CA, et al. Arctic trichinosis presenting as prolonged diarrhea. Gastroenterology. 1986;91:938–46.

202. MacLean JD, Poirier L, Gyorkos TW, et al. Epidemiologic and serologic definition of primary and secondary trichinosis in the Arctic. J Infect Dis. 1992;165:908–12.

203. Kagan IG. Serodiagnosis of trichinosis. In: Cohen S, Sadun EH, eds. Immunology of Parasitic Infections. Oxfod: Blackwell Scientific; 1976:143–51.

204. Kwee HG, Sautter RL. Anisakiasis. Am Fam Physician. 1987;36:137–40.

205. Smith JW, Wooten R. Anisakis and anisakiasis. Adv Parasitol. 1978;16: 93–163.

206. Pinkus GS, Coolidge C. Intestinal anisakiasis: First case report from North America. Am J Med. 1975;59:114–20.

207. Richman RH, Lewicki AM. Right ileocolitis secondary to anisakiasis. Am J Roentgen Rad Ther Nucl Med. 1973;119:329–31.

208. Yokogawa M, Yoshimura H. Clinicopathologic studies on larval anisakiasis in Japan. Am J Trop Med Hyg. 1967;16:723–34.

209. Cross JH. Intestinal capillariasis. Clin Microbiol Rev. 1992;5:120.

210. Whalen GE, Strickland GT, Cross JH, et al. Intestinal capillariasis: A new disease in man. Lancet. 1969;1:13–6.

211. Watten RH, Beckner WM, Cross JH, et al. Clinical studies of capillariasis philippinensis. Trans R Soc Trop Med Hyg. 1972;66:828–34.

212. Fresh JW, Cross JH, Reyes V, et al. Necropsy findings in intestinal capillariasis. Am J Trop Med Hyg. 1972;21:169–73.

213. Cross JH, Banzon T, Clarke MD, et al. Studies on the experimental transmission of *Capillaria philippinensis* in monkeys. Trans R Soc Trop Med Hyg. 1972;66:819–27.

214. Whittner M, Turner JW, Jacquette G, et al. Eustrongylidiasis—A parasitic infection acquired by eating sushi. N Engl J Med. 1989;320:1124–6.

215. Morera P, Perez F, Mora F, et al. Visceral larva migrans-like syndrome caused by *Angiostrongylus costaricensis*. Am J Trop Med Hyg. 1982;31: 67–70.

216. Morera P. Abdominal angiostrongyliasis. Clin Trop Med Commun Dis. 1987; 2:747–54.

217. Hulbert TV, Larsen RA, Chandrasoma PT. Abdominal angiostrongyliasis mimicking acute appendicitis and Meckel's diverticulum: Report of a case in the United States and review. Clin Infect Dis. 1992;14:836–40.

218. Mahmoud AA. Schistosomiasis. N Engl J Med. 1977;297:1329–31.

219. Warren KS. Schistosomiasis japonicum. In: Marsden PD, ed. Clinics in Gastroenterology. v. 17. no. 1: Intestinal Parasites. London: WB Saunders; 1978: 77–85.

220. Farid Z, Trabolsi B, Hafez A. Acute schistosomiasis mansoni (Katayama syndrome). Ann Trop Med Parasitol. 1986;80:563–4.

221. Hardman EW, Jones RL, Davies AH. Fascioliasis—A large outbreak. Br Med J. 1970;3:502–5.

222. Stork MG, Venables GS, Jennings SMF, et al. An investigation of endemic fascioliasis in Peruvian village children. J Trop Med Hyg. 1973;76:231–5.

223. Jones EA, Kay JM, Milligan HP, et al. Masive infection with *Fasciola hepatica* in man. Am J Med. 1977;63:836–42.

224. Plaut AG, Kampanart-Sanyakorn C, Manning GS. A clinical study of *Fasciolopsis buski* infection in Thailand. Trans R Soc Trop Med Hyg. 1969;63: 470–8.

225. Warren KS, Mahmoud AAF. Algorithms in the diagnosis and management of exotic diseases. XXI. Liver, intestinal and lung flukes. J Infect Dis. 1977; 135:692–6.

226. Adams KO, Jungkind DL, Bergquist EJ, et al. Intestinal fluke infection as a result of eating sushi. Am J Clin Pathol. 1986;86:688–9.

227. Goldsmith RS. Chronic diarrhea in returning travelers: Intestinal parasite infection with the fluke *Metagonimus yokogawi*. South Med J. 1978;71: 1513–5.

228. Huffman JE, Fried B. *Echinostoma* and echinostomiasis. Adv Parasitol. 1990;29:215–69.

229. Lin AC, Chapman SW, Turner HR, et al. Clonorchiasis: An update. South Med J. 1987;80:919–22.

230. Brockelman WY, Upatham ES, Viyanant V, et al. Measurement of incidence of the human liver fluke, *Opisthorchis viverrini*, in northeast Thailand. Trans R Soc Trop Med Hyg. 1987;81:327–35.

231. Warren KS, Mahmoud AAF. Algorithms in the diagnosis and management of exotic diseases: XIV. Tapeworms. J Infect Dis. 1976;134:108–12.

232. Grove DI, Warren KS, Mahmoud AAF. Algorithms in the diagnosis and management of exotic diseases. X. Echinococcosis. J Infect Dis. 1976;133: 354–8.

233. Kagan IG. Current status of serologic testing for parasitic diseases. Hosp Pract. 1974;9:157–63.

234. Trier JS, Moxey PC, Schimmel EM, et al. Chronic intestinal coccidiosis in man: Intestinal morphology and response to treatment. Gastroenterology. 1974;66:923–35.

235. Liebman WM, Thaler MM, DeLorimier A, et al. Intractable diarrhea of infancy due to intestinal coccidiosis. Gastroenterology. 1980;78:579–84.

236. DeHovitz JA, Page JW, Boncy M, et al. Clinical manifestations and therapy of *Isospora belli* infection in patients with the acquired immunodeficiency syndrome. N Engl J Med. 1986;315:87–90.

237. Guerrant RL, Bobak DA. Bacterial and protozoal gastroenteritis. N Engl J Med. 1991;325:327–40.

238. Pape JW, Verdier R, Johnson WD. Treatment and prophylaxis of *Isospora belli* infection in patients with the acquired immunodeficiency syndrome. N Engl J Med. 1989;320:1044–7.

239. Spencer MJ, Garcia LS, Chapin MR. *Dientamoeba fragilis*: An intestinal pathogen in children? Am J Dis Child. 1979;133:390–3.

240. Yang J, Scholten TH. *Dientamoeba fragilis*: A review with notes on its epidemiology, pathogenicity, mode of transmission, and diagnosis. Am J Trop Med Hyg. 1977;26:16–22.

241. Blackshaw AJ, Levison DA. Eosinophilic infiltrates of the gastrointestinal tract. J Clin Pathol. 1986;39:1–7.

242. Tedesco FJ, Huckaby CB, Hamby-Allen M, et al. Eosinophilic ileocolitis: Expanding spectrum of eosinophilic gastroenteritis. Dig Dis Sci. 1981;26: 943–8.

243. Klein NC, Hargrove L, Sleisenger MH, et al. Eosinophilic gastroenteritis. Medicine. 1970;49:299–319.

244. Leinbach GE, Rubin CE. Eosinophilic gastroenteritis: A simple reaction to food allergens? Gastroenterology. 1970;59:874–89.

245. Goldberg HI, O'Kieffe D, Jenis EH, et al. Diffuse eosinophilic gastroenteritis. Am J Roentgen Rad Therapy Nucl Med. 1973;119:342–51.

246. Tytgat GN, Grijm R, Dekker W, et al. Fatal eosinophilic enteritis. Gastroenterology. 1976;71:479–83.

247. Cupps TR, Fauci AS. The Vasculitides. Philadelphia: WB Saunders; 1981.

248. Mowrey FH, Lundberg EA. The clinical manifestations of essential polyangiitis (periarteritis nodosa), with emphasis on the hepatic manifestations. Ann Intern Med. 1954;40:1145–64.

249. Nightingale EJ. The gastroenterological aspects of periarteritis nodosa. Am J Gastroenterol. 1959;31:152–65.

250. Leavitt RY, Fauci AS. Polyangiitis overlap syndrome. Am J Med. 1986;81: 79–85.

251. Churg J, Strauss L. Allergic granulomatosis, allergic angiitis and periarteritis nodosa. Am J Pathol. 1951;27:277–301.

252. Finch SC. Granulocytosis. In: Williams WJ, Beutler E, Erslev AJ, et al., eds. Hematology. New York: McGraw-Hill; 1977:746–55.

253. Haeberle MG, Griffen WO Jr. Eosinophiia and regional enteritis: A possible diagnostic aid. Am J Dig Dis. 1972;17:200–4.

254. Glotzer DJ, Gardner RC, Goldman H, et al. Comparative features and course of ulcerative and granulomatous colitis. N Engl J Med. 1970;282:582–7.

255. Isaacson NJ, Rapoport P. Eosinophilia in malignant tumors: Its significance. Ann Intern Med. 1946;25:893–902.

256. Banerjee RN, Narang RM. Haematological changes in malignancy. Br J Haematol. 1967;13:829–43.

257. Beeson P. Cancer and eosinophilia. N Engl J Med. 1983;309:792–3.

81. FOOD-BORNE DISEASE

ROBERT V. TAUXE
JAMES M. HUGHES

Food-borne disease syndromes result from ingestion of a wide variety of foods contaminated with pathogenic microorganisms, microbial toxins, or chemicals. From 1973 to 1987, a mean of 500 outbreaks of food-borne disease affecting 16,000 persons in the United States were reported annually to the Centers for Disease Control and Prevention (CDC).[1] These figures certainly underestimate the magnitude of the problem. The actual incidence of food-borne disease is unknown, but estimates range from 6,500,000 to 81,000,000 illnesses annually.[2,3]

Although a wide variety of microorganisms and toxins can cause food-borne disease, this discussion focuses on food-borne disease syndromes that are acute (onset of symptoms usually within 72 hours of ingestion) and whose clinical features include gastrointestinal manifestations. The diseases to be discussed and the frequency with which outbreaks were reported to the CDC from 1973 to 1987 are indicated in Table 1.

The spectrum of food-borne diseases has expanded in recent years.[4] New food-borne agents causing severe disease have emerged, such as *Escherichia coli* O157:H7 and domoic acid.[5] Important food sources have been defined for other established pathogens, such as *Vibrio cholerae* O1 and *Listeria monocytogenes*. Postinfectious syndromes have been recognized as important sequelae of food-borne infections, including hemolytic uremic syndrome after infections with *E. coli* O157:H7,[6] Reiter syndrome after salmonellosis,[7] and Guillain-Barré syndrome after campylobacteriosis.[8] The emergence of epidemic cholera in Latin America in 1991 has caused cholera in travelers and their families exposed to contaminated foods from Latin America.[9] The growing population of persons with immunosuppressive conditions or treatments and the increasing number of institutionalized elderly mean that more of the population is exquisitely susceptible to microbial contamination of food.[10]

PATHOGENESIS AND CLINICAL FEATURES

Food-borne disease can appear as an isolated sporadic case or, less frequently, as an outbreak of illnesses following a common food exposure. The diagnosis of food-borne disease should be considered when an acute illness with gastrointestinal or neurologic manifestations affects two or more persons who have shared a meal during the previous 72 hours. Important clues to the etiologic agent are provided by both the symptoms and the incubation period.

TABLE 1. Food-Borne Disease Outbreaks and Outbreak-Associated Cases of Known Etiology Reported to the CDC, 1973–1987

Etiologic Agent	Outbreaks		Cases	
	No.	%	No.	%
Bacterial				
Bacillus cereus	58	2	1123	1
Campylobacter	53	2	1547	1
Clostridium botulinum	231	8	494	0
Clostridium perfringens	190	7	12,234	10
Escherichia coli	10	0	1187	1
Salmonella	790	28	55,864	45
Shigella	104	4	14,399	12
Staphylococcus aureus	367	13	17,248	14
Vibrio cholerae O1	6	0	916	1
Vibrio cholerae non-O1	2	0	11	0
Vibrio parahaemolyticus	23	1	535	0
Yersinia enterocolitica	5	0	767	1
Other bacterial	30	1	2581	2
Chemical				
Ciguatera	234	8	1052	1
Heavy metals	46	2	753	1
Histamine fish poisoning	202	7	1046	1
Monosodium glutamate	18	1	58	0
Mushrooms	61	2	169	0
Paralytic shellfish poisoning (PSP)	21	1	160	0
Other chemical	115	4	1046	1
Parasitic				
Giardia	5	0	131	0
Trichinella spiralis	128	5	843	1
Other parasitic	7	0	30	0
Viral				
Hepatitis A	110	4	3133	3
Norwalk virus	15	1	6474	5
Other viral	10	0	1023	1
Total	2841	100	124,824	100

TABLE 2. Pathogenic Mechanisms in Bacterial Food-Borne Disease

Preformed Toxin	Toxin Production In Vivo	Tissue Invasion	Toxin Production and/or Tissue Invasion
S. aureus	C. perfringens	C. jejuni	V. parahaemolyticus
B. cereus (short incubation)	B. cereus (long incubation)	Salmonella	Y. enterocolitica
C. botulinum	C. botulinum (infant botulism)	Shigella	
	Enterotoxigenic E. coli	Invasive E. coli	
	V. cholerae O1		
	V. cholerae non-O1		
	Verotoxigenic E. coli		

Food-Borne Disease Due to Microbial Agents or Their Toxins (Table 2)

Nausea and Vomiting Within 1–6 Hours. The major etiologic considerations are *Staphylococcus aureus* and *Bacillus cereus*. The relatively short incubation period reflects the fact that these diseases are caused by a preformed enterotoxin. Staphylococcal food poisoning is characterized by vomiting (76 percent of the cases) and diarrhea (77 percent); fever is relatively uncommon (23 percent).[11] Staphylococci responsible for episodes of food poisoning produce one or more enterotoxins; five immunologically distinct heat-stable proteins (A, B, C, D, and E) with molecular weights ranging from 28,000 to 35,000 daltons have been identified.[12] Another staphylococcal protein, enterotoxin F, is produced by the majority of *S. aureus* strains causing toxic shock syndrome[13] but has not been reported to cause food-borne disease. Although the mechanism of action of these enterotoxins in humans has not been clarified, studies in monkeys and cats suggest that the enterotoxin produces its emetic action after interaction with abdominal viscera.[14,15] The sensory stimulus is carried to the vomiting center in the brain by the vagus and sympathetic nerves.[14] Other studies suggest that diarrhea may result from inhibition of water and sodium absorption in the small intestine by enterotoxin.[16]

Enterotoxigenic staphylococci isolated from implicated foods in outbreaks are most often lysed by group III phages; less commonly, they are lysed by both group I and group III phages or by group I phages alone.[17] Over 99 percent of enterotoxigenic staphylococci associated with food poisoning are coagulase positive; occasionally, an outbreak caused by enterotoxigenic *Staphylococcus epidermidis* is reported.[18] In the past, strains producing type A enterotoxin alone accounted for 44–69 percent of the reported outbreaks of staphylococcal food poisoning in the United States and England.[19,20] Strains producing type D enterotoxin, either alone or in combination with type A, were the next most frequently implicated. Strains producing enterotoxins B, C, or E alone accounted for fewer than 10 percent of the outbreaks. During 1979–1981, all reported staphylococcal food-borne outbreaks in the United States of known toxin type were caused by strains producing type A enterotoxin alone.[21]

Bacillus cereus strains can cause two types of food poisoning syndromes: one characterized primarily by nausea and vomiting with an incubation period of 1–6 hours (short-incubation "emetic" syndrome) and a second manifested primarily by abdominal cramps and diarrhea with an incubation period of 8–16 hours (long-incubation "diarrhea" syndrome).[22,23] Recent evidence suggests that the short-incubation syndrome, which is characterized by vomiting (100 percent of the cases), abdominal cramps (100 percent), and, less frequently, diarrhea (33 percent),[24] may be caused by a heat-stable toxin produced by some *B. cereus* strains and capable of causing vomiting when fed to monkeys.[25] The mechanism and site of action of this toxin, which has a molecular weight of less than 5000, are unknown.[26]

Another clue to the cause of both staphylococcal and short-incubation *B. cereus* outbreaks is provided by the fact that the illnesses are of short duration, usually lasting less than 12 hours.[11,24]

Abdominal Cramps and Diarrhea within 8–16 Hours. The major etiologic considerations for this syndrome, which is also enterotoxin mediated, are *Clostridium perfringens* and *B. cereus*. In contrast to staphylococcal food poisoning and the short-incubation *B. cereus* disease, which are caused by ingestion of preformed enterotoxins in food, *C. perfringens* and long-incubation *B. cereus* food poisoning are caused by toxins produced in vivo, accounting for the longer incubation period. In *C. perfringens* food poisoning, the most common symptoms are diarrhea and abdominal cramps. Although nausea may occur, vomiting and fever are uncommon, occurring in less than 10 percent of the patients.[27,28] Only *C. perfringens* type A strains have been associated with this food poisoning syndrome.[28,29] *Clostridium perfringens* enterotoxin is a heat-labile protein with a molecular weight of approximately 35,000 daltons[30] synthesized during sporulation of the vegetative cells of *C. perfringens* in the gastrointestinal tract; the enterotoxin is released during lysis of the sporangium.[31] Studies in rabbits and rats indicate that the enterotoxin is active throughout the small intestine, with greatest activity in the ileum, in which net secretion of sodium and fluid and inhibition of chloride and glucose absorption occur.[32,33] The enterotoxin damages brush borders of epithelial cells at villus tips.[33]

Bacillus cereus strains, which cause a similar syndrome characterized by diarrhea (96 percent) and abdominal cramps (75 percent), sometimes vomiting (33 percent), and rarely fever,[24] elaborate a heat-labile enterotoxin with a molecular weight of

approximately 50,000 Da[26] that activates intestinal adenylate cyclase and results in intestinal fluid secretion.[34] This enterotoxin appears also to have cytotoxic properties in rabbit small intestine and guinea pig skin.[26,34]

Although nausea occurs in many patients with *C. perfringens* and long-incubation *B. cereus* food poisoning, vomiting occurs infrequently. In fact, occurrence of vomiting in greater than one-third of affected people suggests that these organisms are not involved. Although these illnesses last longer than staphylococcal and short-incubation *B. cereus* food poisoning, symptoms usually resolve within 24 hours.[24,35] However, in one large long-incubation *B. cereus* outbreak involving elderly patients in a chronic disease hospital, the mean duration of illness was 2.3 days, and one patient was ill for 10 days.[36]

Fever, Abdominal Cramps, and Diarrhea within 16–48 Hours. The major etiologic considerations for this syndrome are salmonellae, shigellae, *Campylobacter jejuni*, *Vibrio parahaemolyticus*, and invasive *E. coli*. These organisms cause this syndrome after tissue invasion.[37–42] Vomiting occurs in 35–80 percent of the patients.[43–46] These illnesses usually resolve within 2–7 days.

Campylobacter jejuni is the most common food-borne bacterial pathogen.[47,48] The frequency of fecal blood and polymorphonuclear leukocytes[49] and colitis[50] suggests that this organism also causes this syndrome after tissue invasion. In contrast to the illnesses caused by other organisms in this group, *C. jejuni* food poisoning is characterized by vomiting in only 15–25 percent of cases[49,51,52] and a longer incubation period of 1–7 days.[47] The duration of illness is usually less than 1 week, but relapses may occur in untreated patients.[53]

The diarrhea experienced by patients with *Vibrio cholerae* non-O1 infection is sometimes bloody, and fever may be present.[54–56]

Abdominal Cramps and Watery Diarrhea within 16–72 Hours. The major etiologic considerations in this syndrome are enterotoxigenic strains of *E. coli*, *V. parahaemolyticus*, *V. cholerae* non-O1, and, in endemic areas, *V. cholerae* O1; *C. jejuni*, salmonellae, and shigellae may also cause this syndrome. Enterotoxins synthesized in vivo are responsible for the syndrome caused by *V. cholerae* O1.[57] *Vibrio cholerae* non-O1,[58,59] and enterotoxigenic strains of *E. coli*[60]; enterotoxigenic and/or cytotoxic substances may also play a role in the pathogenesis of this syndrome when caused by salmonellae,[61,62] shigellae,[63–65] and *V. parahaemolyticus*.[66,67]

Severe cholera presents as a profuse watery diarrhea accompanied by vomiting and muscular cramps. Among the other infections, fever and vomiting occur in a minority of cases.[68–71] With the exception of cholera, which may last for 5 days, and disease due to *V. cholerae* non-O1, which may last for 2–12 days, these illnesses usually resolve within 72–96 hours. However, in one documented enterotoxigenic *E. coli* outbreak, the median duration of illness was 7 days.[72]

Food-borne transmission of the Norwalk agent, and related 27-nm viruses may be common.[73–76] In contrast to the illness produced by bacterial agents causing this syndrome, vomiting and headache are prominent features or Norwalk agent gastroenteritis and occur in the majority of cases.[73] The duration of illness is usually 24–48 hours. The occurrence of secondary cases in close contacts not exposed to the suspected food is an important clue to the possibility of a Norwalk agent etiology. A Norwalk-like virus (Snow Mountain agent) has been reported to be transmitted by food.[77] The importance of food in transmission of other similar viral agents (e.g., Hawaii, Ditchling, and Marin County agents) remains to be determined.[78]

Fever and Abdominal Cramps within 16–48 Hours. *Yersinia enterocolitica* has been incriminated as a cause of food-borne outbreaks in the United States and is a more common cause of food-borne disease in Northern Europe and Canada.[79–82] Although some strains of this organism have been reported to produce a heat-stable enterotoxin,[83,84] the frequent occurrence of fever and mesenteric adenitis suggests that this organism causes disease as a result of tissue invasion. In other children and adults, the clinical illness may be prolonged, and one syndrome may closely resemble acute appendicitis; nausea and vomiting are relatively uncommon, occurring in less than 25–40 percent of the cases.[79,85] Diarrhea is the most common symptom in infants.[86] Duration of the illness may range from 24 hours to 4 weeks.[81,85]

Bloody Diarrhea without Fever within 72–120 Hours. The distinctive syndrome of hemorrhagic colitis has been linked to verotoxigenic strains of *E. coli*, most often serotype O157:H7.[6,87,88] These strains produce cytotoxins for Vero cells, which are neutralized by antiserum to Shiga toxin.[89,90] These strains produce cytotoxins that affect Vero kidney cell cultures, are neutralized by antiserum to Shiga toxin, and have been called Shiga-like toxins or verotoxins.[89,90] The bacteria are noninvasive. The toxins are absorbed from the gut and damage vascular endothelial cells in target organs such as the gut and kidney.[91] The illness is characterized by severe abdominal cramps and diarrhea, which is initially watery but subsequently grossly bloody.[91] Patients with uncomplicated infection usually remain afebrile. The mean incubation period in outbreaks is 4–8 days. The duration of uncomplicated illness ranges from 1 to 12 days. The development of fever and leukocytosis may herald complications, which include hemolytic uremic syndrome, thrombotic thrombocytopenic purpura, and death.[88,93–95] Hemolytic uremic syndrome can occur in 2–7 percent of infections, with onset 5–10 days after the beginning of the diarrheal illness.[6] The case-fatality rate in outbreaks has been 2 percent, with rates as high as 16–35 percent in nursing homes.[6,88,93] Other *E. coli* serotypes that produce verotoxins can also cause hemorrhagic colitis and hemolytic uremic syndrome, but have not yet caused outbreaks.[6]

Nausea, Vomiting, Diarrhea, and Paralysis within 18–36 Hours. The occurrence of acute gastrointestinal symptoms simultaneously with or just before the onset of descending weakness or paralysis strongly suggests the diagnosis of food-borne botulism. Constipation is common once the neurologic syndrome is well established, but nausea and vomiting occur at onset in 50 percent of the patients, and diarrhea occurs in approximately 20–25 percent.[96–98] The pathogenesis of the acute gastrointestinal symptoms is not understood; the botulinal toxins, which inhibit acetylcholine release from nerve endings,[99,100] do not appear to be responsible. The disease in humans is usually caused by one of three immunologically distinct heat-labile protein neurotoxins designated A, B, and E,[101] which are produced after germination of *Clostridium botulinum* spores in inadequately processed foods. The disease in older children and adults results from ingestion of performed toxin. The syndrome of infant botulism appears to result from ingestion of spores with subsequent toxin production in vivo.[102–104] Both illnesses last from several weeks to several months. Clinical suspicion is critical if the disease is to be correctly diagnosed.[105]

Guillain-Barré syndrome (GBS) has been associated with serologic evidence of recent infection with *Campylobacter jejuni*.[8] In one reported series, approximately 20 percent of GBS patients had evidence of recent campylobacteriosis. When preceding diarrheal illness is reported, it typically occurs 1–3 weeks before the onset of neurologic symptoms.[8] In contrast to botulism, GBS is usually an ascending paralysis, accompanied by sensory findings and abnormal nerve conduction velocity.

Food-borne Disease due to Chemicals of Nonmicrobial Origin

Nausea, Vomiting, and Abdominal Cramps within 1 Hour. The major etiologic considerations for this syndrome are heavy metals; copper, zinc, tin, and cadmium have caused food-borne outbreaks.[106–110] Incubation periods most often range from 5 to 15 minutes. Nausea, vomiting, and abdominal cramps result from irritation of the gastric mucosa and usually resolve within 2–3 hours after removal of the offending agent during emesis.

Paresthesias within 1 Hour. When patients have this symptom, fish poisoning, shellfish poisoning (Table 3), the "Chinese restaurant syndrome," and niacin poisoning are the major possibilities. Histamine fish poisoning (scombroid) is characterized by symptoms resembling those of a histamine reaction. Burning of the mouth and throat, flushing, headache, and dizziness are common; abdominal cramps, nausea, vomiting, and diarrhea also occur in a majority of the cases.[111] In severe cases, urticaria and bronchospasm may also occur. Symptoms are thought to result from histamine and inhibitors of histamine degradation produced in fish flesh by the enzymatic decarboxylation of histidine by certain marine bacteria.[112–115] In an outbreak traced to tuna sashimi,[116] a strain of *Klebsiella pneumoniae* capable of producing large quantities of histamine was implicated.[117] Symptoms usually resolve in a few hours.

Three types of shellfish poisoning should be considered: paralytic (PSP), neurotoxic (NSP), and amnesic (ASP).[118,119] PSP is characterized by paresthesias of the mouth, lips, face, and extremities.[120–123] In severe cases, dyspnea, dysphagia, muscle weakness or frank paralysis, ataxia, and respiratory insufficiency may occur.[122,123] Respiratory failure may occur during the first 12 hours of the illness.[122] Some patients also have nausea, vomiting, and diarrhea.[118] The disease is caused by neurotoxic substances in dinoflagellates, one of which is known as *saxitoxin*. Bivalve molusks feed on these dinoflagellates; the toxins are concentrated in their flesh but do not affect the mollusks.[120] Saxitoxin appears to be the only neurotoxin produced by *Gonyaulax catenella*, whereas *Gonyaulax tamarensis* produces saxitoxin and several additional neurotoxic substances.[124–126] The structure of saxitoxin has been determined[127]; it is heat stable and blocks the propagation of nerve and muscle action potentials by interfering with the increase in sodium permeability by acting at a metal cation-binding site in the sodium channels or nerve membranes.[128–130] The mechanism of action of the other neurotoxins is unknown. Duration of the illness ranges from a few hours to a few days.[118]

Although many patients with PSP experience the onset of symptoms within 1 hour of ingestion, the incubation period is often inversely related to the amount of toxin ingested. A European outbreak involved 120 cases after the ingestion of contaminated mussels; the median incubation period in this outbreak was 3.5 hours, with a range of 1–10 hours.[121]

The clinical features of NSP are similar to those of PSP, but paralysis does not occur.[118,120] Several poorly characterized neurotoxins responsible for this illness are found in *Gymnodinium breve*, the responsible dinoflagellate.[131,132] One of these neurotoxins stimulates postganglionic cholinergic nerve fibers.[133] Duration of the illness ranges from a few hours to a few days.[118]

The clinical features of ASP are initially nonspecific, including vomiting, abdominal cramps, and diarrhea. Confusion, amnesia, coma, and cardiovascular instability follow within hours in severe cases, which tend to occur in older persons and in those with underlying renal disease. The hallmark of the disease is antegrade amnesia, which was reported in 25 percent of affected persons in a large Canadian outbreak.[119] The disease is caused by domoic acid, a toxin produced by the dinoflagellate *Nitzchia pungens* and concentrated in the flesh of mollusks. Amnesia can be permanent and is the result of bilateral destruction of the hippocampi by the toxin.[134]

The Chinese restaurant syndrome is characterized by a burning sensation in the neck, chest, abdomen, or arms and by a sensation of tightness over the face and chest.[135] Headache, flushing, diaphoresis, lacrimation, weakness, nausea, abdomi-

TABLE 3. Fish and Shellfish Poisoning Syndromes

Syndrome	Incubation Period	Duration	Geographic Location[a]	Season
Histamine fish poisoning (scombroid)	5 min–1 hr	Few hours	Primarily coastal areas (Hawaii, California)	Year round
Ciguatera	1–6 hr	Few days–few months	35°N–35°S latitude (Hawaii, Florida)	Feb.–Sept.
Paralytic shellfish poisoning	5 min–4 hr	Few hours–few days	Above 30°N and below 30°S latitude (New England, West Coast)	May–Nov.
Neurotoxic shellfish poisoning	5 min–4 hr	Few hours–few days	Gulf and Atlantic coasts of Florida (Florida)	Spring, fall
Amnesic shellfish poisoning	15 min–6 hr	Few days–permanent	Coastal areas?	Uncertain

[a] Location of U.S. outbreaks in parentheses.

TABLE 4. Mushroom Poisoning Syndromes

Syndrome	Mushroom Species	Toxins
Short incubation		
Delirium	Amanita muscaria A. pantherina	Ibotenic acid, muscimol
Parasympathetic hyperactivity	Inocybe spp. Clitocybe spp.	Muscarine
Hallucinations	Psilocybe spp. Panaeolus spp.	Psilocybin, psilocin
Disulfiram reaction	Coprinus atramentarius	Disulfiram-like substance
Gastroenteritis	Many	?
Long incubation		
Gastroenteritis, hepatorenal failure	Amanita phalloides A. virosa A. verna Galerina autumnalis G. marginata G. venenata	Amatoxins, phallotoxins
Gastroenteritis, hepatic failure	Gyromitra spp.	Gyromitrin

nal cramps, and thirst frequently occur.[135,136] Symptoms appear to be caused by excessive amounts of monosodium L-glutamate in foods, although other undefined substances may also play a role.[135,136] The illness usually resolves within several hours.

Niacin poisoning produces a burning facial erythema within 20 minutes of ingestion, which rapidly resolves.[137]

Paresthesias within 1–6 Hours. The major diagnostic considerations for this syndrome are PSP and ciguatera fish poisoning (Table 3), which is often characterized by the onset of abdominal cramps, nausea, vomiting, and diarrhea preceded or followed by numbness and paresthesias of the lips, tongue, and throat.[138–140] Malaise, headache, pruritus, dry mouth, metallic taste, myalgias, arthralgias, blurred vision, photophobia, and transient blindness have also been reported.[141–143] Sharp shooting pains in the legs and a sensation of looseness and pain in the teeth are characteristic.[139] In severe cases, reversal of hot and cold temperature sensations, sinus bradycardia, hypotension, cranial nerve palsies, and respiratory paralysis may occur.[140,141,144] The illness is caused by ciguatoxin, a poorly characterized lipid-soluble, relatively heat-stable compound,[145] which is acquired by fish through the food chain.[146] The dinoflagellate *Gambierdiscus toxicus* has been identified as the source of the toxin in the food chain.[147] Ciguatoxin inhibits red blood cell cholinesterase activity,[148] increases membrane sodium permeability,[149] and changes the electrical potential of cells through its action on sodium channels.[150,151] Duration of the acute illness ranges from a few days to a few months; pain in the extremities has been reported to occur intermittently for years after an episode of ciguatera.

Miscellaneous Mushroom Poisoning Syndromes within 2 Hours. At least five clinical syndromes may occur within 2 hours of ingestion of toxic mushrooms (Table 4).[152–155] Species containing ibotenic acid and muscimol cause an illness mimicking acute alcoholic intoxication characterized by confusion, restlessness, and visual disturbances followed by lethargy; symptoms resolve within 24 hours. Species containing muscarine cause an illness characterized by evidence of parasympathetic hyperactivity, for example, salivation, lacrimation, diaphoresis, blurred vision, abdominal cramps, and diarrhea. Some patients experience miosis, bradycardia, and bronchospasm. Symptoms usually resolve within 24 hours. Species containing the toxic substances psilocybin and psilocin cause an acute psychotic reaction manifested by hallucinations and inappropriate behavior, which usually resolves within 12 hours. The mushroom *Coprinus atramentarius* contains a disulfiramlike substance that can result in headache, flushing, paresthesias, nausea, vomiting, and tachycardia if alcohol is consumed during the 48-hour period after ingestion. The fifth clinical syndrome is characterized by nausea, vomiting, abdominal cramps, and diarrhea after the ingestion of mushrooms containing gastrointestinal irritants that are not well characterized.

Abdominal Cramps and Diarrhea within 6–24 Hours Followed by Hepatorenal Failure. Species of poisonous mushrooms containing amatoxins and phallotoxins.[152,153,155] are responsible for this syndrome (Table 4).[152,153,155] The most common implicated species are *Amanita phalloides, A. virosa,* and *A. verna.*[156,157] The illness is typically biphasic; the abdominal cramps and diarrhea, which may be quite severe, usually resolve within 24 hours. The patient then remains well for 1–2 days before evidence of hepatic and renal failure supervenes. A mortality of 30–50 percent has been reported.[158,159]

A similar clinical syndrome follows the ingestion of mushrooms of the *Gyromitra* genus, which contain the toxic substance gyromitrin. However, this toxin does not cause acute renal failure.[160]

Chronic Diarrhea within 1–3 Weeks. A food-borne disease, chronic watery diarrhea, also known as Brainerd diarrhea, has been described among persons drinking raw milk.[161] After a mean incubation period of 15 days, affected persons developed acute watery diarrhea with marked urgency and abdominal cramps. Diarrhea persisted for a mean period of 2 years. No etiologic agent was identified. A second restaurant-associated outbreak of a similar illness suggests that food vehicles other than raw milk may also be involved.[162]

Water-Borne Disease. The evaluation of a suspected food-borne outbreak may reveal that water was the vehicle. Pathogens incriminated in water-borne outbreaks are different from those most often responsible for food-borne disease; the responsible etiologic agents for water-borne outbreaks reported to the CDC from 1972 through 1990 are shown in Table 5.[163–176] *Giardia lamblia* is the single most frequently recognized pathogen in the United States and has been responsible for several large outbreaks traced to a municipal water supply.[177–179] This illness is characterized by abdominal pain, bloating, flatulence, and occasionally malabsorption. The incubation period is typically 1–4 weeks, and duration of the illness may be several weeks. Large water-borne outbreaks caused by *E. coli* O157:H7,[179] shigellae,[180] hepatitis A,[181] *Salmonella typhi,*[182] nontyphoid salmonellae,[183] enterotoxigenic *E. coli,*[184] *C. jejuni,*[185,186] Brainerd

TABLE 5. Water-Borne Disease Outbreaks of Known Etiology Reported to the CDC, 1972–1990

Etiologic Agent	Outbreaks	
	No.	%
Giardia lamblia	100	39.5
Shigella	29	11.5
Hepatitis A	20	7.9
Norwalk-like agents	16	6.3
Campylobacter jejuni	12	4.7
Nontyphoid salmonella	12	4.7
Salmonella typhi	5	2.0
Enterotoxigenic Escherichia coli	1	0.4
Escherichia coli O157:H7	1	0.4
Vibrio cholerae O1	1	0.4
Yersinia enterocolitica	1	0.4
Rotavirus	1	0.4
Cryptosporidium	2	0.8
Entamoeba histolytica	1	0.4
Miscellaneous chemicals	51	20.2
Total	253	100

diarrhea,[187] the Norwalk agent,[188,189] and a Norwalk-like virus, the Snow Mountain agent,[190] have been reported. The majority of water-borne outbreaks are of unknown etiology.

Miscellaneous Food-Borne Infections. This discussion has focused on diseases often transmitted by foods and manifested primarily by gastrointestinal or neurologic symptoms and signs. Some food-borne diseases present largely as invasive infections in immunocompromised patients. Listeriosis typically affects pregnant women, fetuses and persons with compromised cellular immunity, who present with fever, myalgias, and primary bacteremia or meningitis. Identified sources are most often food borne, including cole slaw, dairy products, and cold processed meats. The incubation period if prolonged, ranging from 2 to 6 weeks, and the case-fatality rate is 23 percent.[191] Vibrio vulnificus infections present as fulminant myonecrosis or primary bacteremia following ingestion of raw oysters. This severe syndrome is almost exclusively seen in patients with underlying liver disease, especially those associated with iron-overload states.[192]

Other infectious diseases with primary symptoms outside the gastrointestinal and neurologic systems, which are occasionally or usually transmitted by foods and their most common vehicles of transmission, include group A β-hemolytic streptococci (potato and egg salads), brucellosis (goat's milk cheese), anthrax (meat), tularemia (water), tuberculosis (milk), Q fever (milk), hepatitis A (shellfish, salads), trichinosis (pork), toxoplasmosis (beef), anisakiasis (fish), and tapeworms (beef, pork, fish).

EPIDEMIOLOGY

In addition to the clinical syndrome and incubation period, additional clues to the cause of an outbreak of food-borne disease may be provided by the type of food responsible and the setting in which it is eaten (Table 6).[193]

Foods

Outbreaks of staphylococcal food poisoning are associated with foods of high protein content, such as ham, poultry, potato and egg salads, and cream-filled pastries, which are thought to be contaminated during preparation by a food handler. Although in the classic staphylococcal food-borne outbreak a food handler has a purulent skin lesion on his or her hand, in actuality this is true in only a minority of outbreaks. In contrast, outbreaks of B. cereus food poisoning of the short-incubation type are

most often associated with fried rice that has been cooked and held warm for extended periods. The growth of B. cereus under similar experimental conditions in rice has been well documented.[194] The vehicle in a recently reported outbreak was macaroni and cheese that was mishandled after preparation; investigation revealed that powdered milk was the source of the organism.[195]

Clostridium perfringens outbreaks usually follow the ingestion of meat (especially beef and poultry) and gravies; organisms have been isolated from 16–85 percent of raw meat, poultry, and fish specimens.[196–198] Outbreaks are more likely to occur when these items are prepared in large quantities for banquets or in institutional settings when food is prepared well in advance without adequate final reheating.[199] Long-incubation B. cereus food poisoning is also frequently associated with meat or vegetable dishes. In addition to the frequent contamination of raw meats, vegetables, and milk products with B. cereus, the organism has been isolated from 25 percent of dried foods such as seasoning mixes, spices, and dried potatoes[200] and from over 50 percent of dried beans and cereals.[201] A long-incubation B. cereus outbreak has also been traced to a "meals-on-wheels" operation in which food was held at and above room temperature for an extended period.[202] E. coli O157:H7 outbreaks have typically followed consumption of undercooked beef or, occasionally, raw milk.[6]

Salmonella food-borne outbreaks most frequently follow the ingestion of poultry, beef, egg, or dairy products. Internally contaminated shell eggs cause many outbreaks of infections with Salmonella enteritidis.[203] Foods made with raw or undercooked shell eggs are now a dominant source of outbreaks and sporadic cases of salmonellosis in the United States.[204,205] The role of raw milk in the transmission of Salmonella infections persists.[206,207] Two large international outbreaks have been caused by contaminated chocolate candy.[208,209] Shigella outbreaks are most often associated with cool, moist foods such as potato and egg salads that require much handling after cooking. In an outbreak caused by Shigella dysenteriae type 2, the vehicle was raw vegetables served at a salad bar.[210] Campylobacter jejuni outbreaks most often follow the ingestion of raw milk and poultry.[47] Vibrio parahaemolyticus outbreaks in the United States are associated with the ingestion of bivalve mollusks and crustaceans[211,212]; in Japan, these outbreaks are more often associated with the ingestion of a variety of saltwater fish.[213] Vibrio cholerae O1 and non-O1 outbreaks have been traced to contaminated shellfish eaten raw or inadequately cooked.[214,215] Crabs, shrimp, and raw oysters have been implicated as the vehicles of transmission of a unique epidemic strain of V. cholerae in Louisiana.[216–219] Crabs brought in travelers' luggage from Latin America have recently caused outbreaks of cholera in the United States.[220] Sporadic cases of diarrhea associated with V. cholerae non-O1 strains in the United States have also been linked to shellfish ingestion.[54,55] Food-borne outbreaks in the United States due to Y. enterocolitica were caused by contaminated milk[79,80] and tofu.[81] In Europe, this illness is associated with eating raw pork.[82] A food-borne outbreak caused by invasive E. coli followed the ingestion of cheese.[46] Travelers' diarrhea caused by enterotoxigenic E. coli has been associated with consumption of salads in Mexico,[221] a food-borne outbreak of enterotoxigenic E. coli followed the ingestion of imported cheese,[222] and enterotoxigenic isolates have been obtained from a variety of foods including hamburger, sausage, seafood, and cheese in the United States.[223] Botulism outbreaks are most often associated with the ingestion of low-acid (pH ≥ 4.4) home-canned vegetables, fruits, and fish. Recent outbreaks of botulism followed ingestion of unusual vehicles including baked potatoes, sauteed onions, and chopped garlic.[105,224] Honey was the source of C. botulinum in some cases of infant botulism.[225] In Norwalk agent outbreaks, shellfish[74,75,226,227] and salads[278] have been implicated. In a recent large outbreak, cake and frosting were implicated.[229] Contamination of food by an ill food handler has been docu-

TABLE 6. Etiology of Food-Borne Disease Outbreaks by Food, Season, and Geographic Predilection

Etiology	Foods	Season	Geographic Predilection
Bacterial			
Salmonella	Beef, poultry, eggs, dairy products	Summer	None
S. aureus	Ham, poultry, egg salads, pastries	Summer	None
C. jejuni	Poultry, raw milk	Spring, summer	None
C. botulinum	Vegetables, fruits, fish, honey (infants)	Summer, fall	West, Northeast
C. perfringens	Beef, poultry, gravy, Mexican food	Fall, winter, spring	None
Shigella	Egg salads, lettuce	Summer	None
V. parahaemolyticus	Crabs	Spring, summer, fall	Coastal states
B. cereus	Fried rice, meats, vegetables	Year round	None
Y. enterocolitica	Milk, tofu, pork	Winter	Unknown
V. cholerae O1	Shellfish	Variable	Tropical, Gulf Coast, Latin America
V. cholerae non-O1	Shellfish	Unknown	Tropical, Gulf Coast
Verotoxigenic E. coli	Beef, raw milk	Summer, fall	Unknown
Viral			
Norwalk agent	Shellfish, salads	Year round	Northeast
Chemical			
Ciguatera	Barracuda, snapper, amberjack, grouper	Spring, summer (in Florida)	Tropical
Histamine fish poisoning (scombroid)	Tuna, mackerel, bonito, skipjack, mahi-mahi	Year round	Coastal
Mushroom poisoning	Mushrooms	Spring, fall	Temperate
Heavy metals	Acidic beverages	Year round	None
Monosodium-L-glutamate	Chinese food	Year round	None
Paralytic shellfish poisoning	Shellfish	Summer, fall	Temperate
Neurotoxic shellfish poisoning	Shellfish	Spring, fall	Subtropical

mented.[230] Food-borne transmission of the Snow Mountain agent has been associated with clams.[77]

Outbreaks of heavy metal poisoning are most often associated with acidic beverages such as lemonade, fruit punch, and carbonated drinks that have been stored in corroded metallic containers such as punch bowls[108] or that have been in contact with metallic tubing (e.g., in vending machines)[231] for periods of time sufficient to leach the metallic ions from the container. Histamine fish poisoning outbreaks are associated with scombroid fish, the most common of which are tuna, mackerel, bonito, and skipjack. In addition, the nonscombroid fish mahi-mahi has caused outbreaks of scombroidlike fish poisoning. Ciguatera fish poisoning has been associated with over 400 species of fish. Barracuda, red snapper, amberjack, and grouper are most commonly implicated. The disease is more often associated with large fish; in one study, 69 percent of red snappers weighing 2.8 kg or more were toxic, compared with only 18 percent of smaller fish.[232] PSP, NSP, and ASP follow the ingestion of bivalve mollusks, most often oysters, clams, and mussels. The most common Chinese food item associated with the Chinese restaurant syndrome is soup, which is frequently the first item ingested at a meal; the absorption of monosodium L-glutamate is most rapid when the stomach is empty.[135]

Seasonality

The time of year may also provide a clue to the cause of a food-borne outbreak. Outbreaks caused by the bacterial pathogens S. aureus, Salmonella, and Shigella, are most common during the summer months. Campylobacter jejuni outbreaks are more common during the spring and fall, Clostridium perfringens outbreaks occur throughout the year but least often during the summer months, and botulism outbreaks are more common during the summer and fall. Shellfish-associated Vibrio infections are largely limited to late summer and early fall.

In general, chemical food poisoning occurs throughout the year. Exceptions are PSP, which often occurs in association with a red tide[233] and is most common in the summer and fall; ciguatera, which is most common in the spring and summer in

Florida[234]; and mushroom poisoning, which is most common in the spring, late summer, and fall.

Geographic Location

The geographic setting may also provide a clue to the cause of food-borne disease. Vibrio parahaemolyticus outbreaks are most frequently reported from coastal states. The initial 13 outbreaks reported in the United States all occurred in coastal states.[211] An outbreak of cholera and sporadic cases of V. cholerae O1 and non-O1 infection have been reported from the Gulf Coast of the United States.[217] Type A botulism outbreaks are most common west of the Mississippi River, whereas type B outbreaks are most common in the East, and type E outbreaks are most common in the Great Lakes Region and Alaska.[101]

Ciguatera outbreaks occur in tropical and subtropical regions between 35°N and 35°S latitudes. Over 90 percent of outbreaks in the United States have been reported from Florida and Hawaii.[118] Ciguatera is common in the West Indies,[236] and travelers who return with the characteristic syndrome should be questioned regarding fish consumption. PSP and NSP outbreaks occur in coastal areas.

Epidemiologic Assessment

For a food to provide a clue to the cause of a food-borne outbreak, it must be identified. Once a common meal is identified through interviews with ill people, food-specific attack rates should be determined for all foods and beverages served at the meal (see example in Table 7). People who were present at the same meal but did not become ill must also be interviewed to serve as controls. Food-specific attack rates may identify the responsible vehicle of transmission. To be adequately incriminated, a food must have a significantly higher attack rate for those who ate it than for those who did not, and most of those who became ill must have eaten the food. On occasion, more than one food item may be incriminated. On these occasions, simple cross-table analysis may indicate whether both items were contaminated by the etiologic agent or whether both were eaten by most people at the meal (e.g., meat and gravy) (Table 7). For example, if meat loaf and gravy were both incriminated, subsequent analysis may indicate that attack rates were equally high for those who ate meat loaf, regardless of whether they ate gravy, and were similarly low for those who did not eat meat loaf, regardless of whether they ate gravy, indicating that the meat loaf alone was responsible for the outbreak.

LABORATORY DIAGNOSIS

Appropriate specimens for laboratory confirmation vary with the etiologic agents but include feces, vomitus, serum, and blood (Table 8). In addition, cultures of the leftover food, the food preparation environment, and food handlers may be indicated. The laboratory should be alerted to suspected causes so that special techniques can be used for isolation of *Clostridium perfringens,* vibrios, *Campylobacter jejuni, E. coli* O157:H7, and *Y. enterocolitica* and so that organisms considered part of the normal flora (other *E. coli, B. cereus*) are not overlooked.

Outbreaks of staphylococcal food poisoning may be confirmed by the isolation of *S. aureus* of the same phage type from vomitus or feces of ill people and from the incriminated food or skin lesion or hand of a food handler, by the isolation of more than 10^5 *S. aureus* organisms per gram of incriminated food, or by the demonstration of staphylococcal enterotoxin in the food by gel diffusion, radioimmunoassay (RIA), or the enzyme-linked immunosorbent assay (ELISA), which have sensitivities of 0.1–3 ng/g of food.[237–241] *Bacillus cereus* outbreaks may be documented by the isolation of organisms from the feces of ill people who shared the same meal or by the isolation of 10^5 or more *B. cereus* per gram of incriminated food. Serotyping, if available, may be of value in confirming that isolates were derived from a common source, since 14 percent of healthy adults have been reported to have transient gastrointestinal colonization with *B. cereus.*[242] Plasmid analysis may also be useful.[243]

The laboratory confirmation of *Clostridium perfringens* outbreaks is more difficult. Since both heat-sensitive and heat-resistant strains of *C. perfringens* type A have been implicated as causes of food poisoning, selective isolation procedures involving heat treatment of food and fecal specimens should not be used. Because *C. perfringens* organisms are variably reported as normal flora in 42–100 percent of healthy people,[244,245] organisms of the same serotype[246–248] or bacteriocin type[249] should be demonstrated in stools of ill people and the incriminated food or in stools of ill people and not in those of people who ate the same meal but did not become ill, or median counts of 10^6 or more *C. perfringens* spores per gram of feces obtained within 48 hours after onset of illness should be demonstrated.[246,250] Alternatively, counts of 10^5 or more organisms per gram of food provide etiologic confirmation. Demonstration of *C. perfringens* enterotoxin in stools of ill people and not in control subjects is possible with ELISA or latex agglutination.[251–253] For serotyping, approximately 90 *C. perfringens* antisera, including the original 13 Hobbs serotypes, are available, but many isolates cannot

TABLE 7. Example of Use of Food-Specific Attack Rates and Cross-Table Analysis To Identify Food Vehicle in a Food-Borne Outbreak

	Food-Specific Attack Rates					
	No. of People Eating Food			No. of People Not Eating Food		
Food	Total	Ill	Percent Ill	Total	Ill	Percent Ill
Meat loaf	100	88	88[a]	10	2	20[a]
Gravy	80	80	100[b]	30	10	33[b]
Potatoes	95	78	82	15	12	80
Salad	90	74	82	20	16	80
Water	70	58	82	40	32	80
	Cross-Table Analysis					
	No. of People Eating Meat Loaf			No. of People Not Eating Meat Loaf		
	Total	Ill	Percent Ill	Total	Ill	Percent Ill
No. eating gravy	75	67	89[c]	5	1	20[d]
No. not eating gravy	25	21	84[c]	5	1	20[d]

[a] p < .05 (Fisher's exact test).
[b] p < .05 (Chi-square analysis).
[c] p > .05 (Chi-square analysis).
[d] p > .05 (Fisher's exact test).

TABLE 8. Appropriate Laboratory Specimens for Documentation of Etiology of a Food-Borne Outbreak

	Patient			Food Handler				Food-Preparation Environment
	Stools	Vomitus	Blood	Stools	Nose	Hands	Food	
Bacterial								
Salmonella	C		C	C			C	C
S. aureus	C	C			C	C	C, T	
C. jejuni	C			C			C	C
C. botulinum	C, T	C, T	T				C, T	
C. perfringens	C, T						C	
Shigella	C			C			C	
V. parahaemolyticus	C						C	C
B. cereus	C	C					C	
Y. enterocolitica	C		S	C			C	C
V. cholerae O1 and non-O1	C		S	C			C	C
Verotoxigenic E. coli	C, T						C	
Viral								
Norwalk agent	I		S					
Chemical								
Ciguatera							T	
Histamine fish poisoning (scombroid)							T	
Mushroom	T	T	T				T	
Heavy metals							T	
Monosodium-L-glutamate							T	
Paralytic shellfish poisoning							T	
Neurotoxic shellfish poisoning							T	

Abbreviations: C: culture; T: toxin testing; S: serology; I: immune electron microscopy.

be typed. In the United Kingdom, serotyping implicates a specific serotype in nearly two-thirds of outbreaks,[247] whereas in the United States serotyping is helpful in only approximately 20 percent of outbreaks.[254]

Salmonella, Shigella, Campylobacter jejuni, V. cholerae O1 and non-O1, *V. parahaemolyticus,* and *Y. enterocolitica* outbreaks may be confirmed by the isolation and serotyping of the organisms from the feces of ill people. In *Salmonella* outbreaks in which it is uncertain whether a common vehicle is responsible, plasmid profiling or determination of phage type may be necessary.[255–257] Strains of *V. parahaemolyticus* isolated from patients are hemolytic on special blood agar medium (Kanagawa-positive strains). Isolation and serotyping of salmonellae, shigellae, *C. jejuni,* vibrios, and *Y. enterocolitica* from the incriminated food may also be confirmatory. Molecular characterization of *V. cholerae* O1 may help to define the geographic origins of the infecting organism.[258] Because *V. parahaemolyticus* in low numbers are a frequent contaminant of shellfish, counts of 10^5 or more organisms per gram are required for confirmation; food isolates are usually Kanagawa negative. Serologic testing of acute and convalescent sera may be helpful in confirming the diagnosis in patients in *Y. enterocolitica,* cholera, and typhoid fever outbreaks but currently plays no important role in the investigation of nontyphoid *Salmonella, Shigella, C. jejuni,* and *V. parahaemolyticus* outbreaks.

Infection with *E. coli* O157:H7 can be diagnosed by isolating sorbitol-negative *E. coli* from stools of ill persons on sorbitol-MacConkey medium and confirming the serotype.[259] Infection with other verotoxigenic *E. coli* can be diagnosed by demonstrating free verotoxin in stools, or by isolating other verotoxigenic strains from stools from ill individuals.[95] Enterotoxigenic *E. coli* can be identified by gene probe for the toxin gene[260] or by detecting the toxins themselves: heat-labile enterotoxin (LT) in tissue culture assays,[261] ELISA,[262] or the Biken test[263] and heat-stable enterotoxin (ST) in the suckling mouse assay[264] in ill people and not in control subjects. Invasive strains may be identified by gene probe,[265] or by using the Sereny test.[266] Since *E. coli* serotypes have been shown to cause diarrhea in volunteers in the absence of detectable enterotoxin production or invasiveness, use of the EAF gene probe for the enteropathogenic *E. coli,*[267] and serotyping of *E. coli* isolates from both patients and controls may also be useful in outbreak settings if cases are found to have a serotype absent from controls.

Botulism outbreaks may be confirmed by the demonstration of botulinal toxin in the serum or stool of ill people or in incriminated food by the mouse neutralization test or by the isolation of *Clostridium botulinum* from the feces of ill people or from the incriminated food.[268,269] Laboratory confirmation by testing of clinical specimens can be obtained in approximately 70–75 percent of the cases of botulism.[268,269] Norwalk agent outbreaks may be confirmed by the demonstration of viral particles in stools of ill people by immunoelectron microscopy[270] or of a serologic response by a biotin-avidin immunoassay procedure.[271]

Outbreaks caused by heavy metals may be documented by the demonstration of the metallic ion in the incriminated food. Histamine fish poisoning may be confirmed by the demonstration of histamine in the fish; concentrations of 100 mg in 100 g of fish flesh correlate with toxicity. The diagnosis of ciguatera is based on the clinical picture.[272] However, ciguatera outbreaks may be documented by the demonstration of ciguatoxin in the incriminated fish using a bioassay in the mongoose, rat, or cat; RIA and ELISA techniques have been developed but are not generally available.[273] Shellfish poisoning may be confirmed either by demonstrating the toxin in mollusks by the mouse bioassay technique or by finding elevated numbers of the responsible dinoflagellate in the water from which the mollusks were obtained. Outbreaks of Chinese restaurant syndrome may be confirmed by the demonstration of elevated monosodium L-glutamate levels in the food. Mushroom poisoning may be

confirmed either by the identification of the responsible toxin in gastric contents, blood, urine, or fecal specimens by thin-layer chromatography or RIA or by the identification of the mushroom by a mycologist.

An additional diagnostic tool that may be of value in food-borne disease outbreaks characterized by diarrhea is the fecal leukocyte examination.[274] The presence of leukocytes implies that the responsible organism has invaded the intestinal tract, suggesting that salmonellae, shigellae, *Campylobacter jejuni,* invasive *E. coli, V. parahaemolyticus,* or *Y. enterocolitica* are responsible for the illness.

Over 50 percent of the reported food-borne disease outbreaks in the United States are of unknown cause. In some cases, appropriate diagnostic procedures are not conducted. In others, no agent is identified, raising the possibility that other etiologic agents are responsible. Possibilities include *Aeromonas hydrophila, Plesiomonas shigelloides,* rotaviruses, and Norwalk-like agents. In several outbreaks in England traced to cockles, 25–26-nm viral particles similar to Norwalk-like agents have been seen in stool specimens.[275] Although enterococci and gram-negative rods (*Klebsiella, Enterobacter, Proteus, Citrobacter,* and *Pseudomonas* spp.) have been reported as causes of food-borne outbreaks on rare occasions, their role in the cause of food-borne outbreaks has not been well documented. Because these latter organisms may be part of the normal fecal flora, documentation of their presence in ill people and their absence from well people will be required to confirm their role in food-borne outbreaks. That the gram-negative organisms might be responsible for some outbreaks is suggested by reports of the production of LT[276,277] and ST enterotoxins[278,279] by some of these organisms.

THERAPY

Supportive measures are the mainstay of therapy in most cases of food poisoning. The majority of these illnesses are self-limited; exceptions are botulism, long-incubation mushroom poisoning, and PSP, which may be fatal in previously healthy people; listeriosis, which is often fatal in neonates and immunocompromised persons; cholera; and *Vibrio vulnificus* infection, which is often fatal in persons with underlying liver disease. In addition, fatalities occasionally occur due to staphylococcal and *Clostridium perfringens* food poisoning, salmonellosis, verotoxigenic *E. coli* infections, and shigellosis in infants, the elderly, and debilitated people (Table 9).

Adequate treatment of cholera requires vigorous volume replacement with appropriate fluids. In any diarrheal illness, gastrointestinal fluid losses should be replaced either orally or parenterally. Antimicrobial agents may be used in the therapy for shigellosis, cholera, and typhoid fever but should be avoided in uncomplicated gastrointestinal infection caused by nontyphoid salmonellae. Tetracycline shortens both the duration of clinical cholera and the excretion of *V. cholerae* O1. Erythromycin eradicates carriage of *Campylobacter jejuni* and can shorten the duration of illness if given early in the disease.[280] The role of antimicrobial gents in the management of food poisoning due to *V. parahaemolyticus,* enterotoxigenic, verotoxigenic, and invasive *E. coli,* and *Y. enterocolitica* is unsettled but probably minimal. Antimicrobial agents are of no value in the management of staphylococcal, *Clostridium perfringens,* or *B. cereus* food-poisoning. Antiperistaltic agents appear to be of little if any benefit in controlling diarrhea and are contraindicated in patients with fever or fecal leukocytes, which suggest a syndrome associated with an invasive pathogen. Patients with botulism present several additional therapeutic problems, which are discussed in Chapter 223.

Patients with PSP and occasional patients with ciguatera may require ventilatory support; in these illnesses, this support is usually required for only a few days. Recent reports suggest that intravenous mannitol may ameliorate the acute neurologic

TABLE 9. Number of Deaths in Death-to-Case Ratios in Food-Borne Disease Outbreaks Reported to the CDC, 1973–1987

Etiologic Agent	No. Deaths	Death-to-Case Ratio[a]
Bacterial		
Bacillus cereus	0	0
Campylobacter	2	2
Clostridium botulinum	47	192
Clostridium perfringens	12	1
Escherichia coli	4	3
Listeria monocytogenes	70	317
Salmonella	88	2
Shigella	4	1
Staphylococcus aureus	4	<1
Vibrio cholerae O1	12	13
Vibrio cholerae non-O1	0	0
Yersinia enterocolitica	0	0
Other bacterial	4	2
Chemical		
Mushrooms	8	49
Paralytic shellfish poisoning (PSP)	1	6
Other chemical	12	3
Parasitic		
Trichinella spiralis	5	8
Other parasitic	0	0
Viral	2	<1
Unknown	26	<1

[a] Per 1000 cases.

symptoms of severe ciguatera and that tocainide may improve persistent dysesthesias.[281,282] Therapy is otherwise supportive; no antitoxins are available. If not contraindicated by the presence of ileus, enemas or cathartics may be administered to these patients in an effort to remove unabsorbed toxin from the intestinal tract. Because of the severe dysesthesias associated with ciguatera, analgesics may also be required. Symptoms of histamine fish poisoning may be relieved by antihistamines. In severe cases with bronchospasm, epinephrine or aminophylline may be required.

Therapy for short-incubation types of mushroom poisoning is primarily supportive.[283] Patients who have ingested species containing pharmacologically active amounts of muscarine and who manifest evidence of parasympathetic hyperactivity may be treated with atropine. Patents who are severely ill after ingestion of species containing ibotenic acid and muscimol may be treated with physostigmine. Therapy for the long-incubation illness includes cathartics and enemas in an effort to remove unabsorbed toxin, as well as a number of specific and supportive measures.[283] Since hypoglycemia often occurs, intravenous glucose may be required. Thioctic acid is an experimental drug that appears to be an effective antidote in these patients[153]; the drug may be obtained from Burton M. Berkson, M.D., Ph.D., in Las Cruces, New Mexico (505-678-2321 or 505-521-1609). Pyridoxine is indicated in the management of patients poisoned with *Gyromitra* spp.

Therapy for acute heavy metal poisoning is supportive. Emesis should be induced if it does not occur spontaneously. Antiemetics are contraindicated, since retention of the toxic ions in the gut with subsequent systemic absorption may result. In severe cases with systemic manifestations of heavy metal toxicity, use of specific antidotes may be considered but is rarely necessary in these outbreaks.

PREVENTION

Food-borne disease prevention requires efforts at many levels. Contamination of raw animal products can be reduced by better animal production and slaughter practices This is important be-

cause raw animal products, including meat, milk, eggs, and shellfish, are common sources of contamination leading to food-borne diseases. Monitoring the safety of industrial food processing is increasingly important as the nation's food supply becomes more centralized and precooked for the convenience of the consumer. In large kitchens and in homes, careful cooking and storage are necessary to kill pathogens and to prevent their growth following recontamination of food after cooking. Because they serve high-risk populations, the kitchens of hospitals and nursing homes must pay particular attention to food safety; for example, routine use of pasteurized eggs instead of shell eggs will prevent many nosocomial outbreaks of food-borne salmonellosis. The role of the clinician goes beyond that of diagnosis and treatment and includes warning high-risk patients of the hazards of raw oysters, raw eggs, and unpasteurized milk and detecting outbreaks and reporting them to public health authorities.[284]

Food-borne disease can be prevented if food is selected, prepared, and stored properly. In outbreaks reported to the CDC, the most common error is storage of food at inappropriate temperatures; this error is most often identified in staphylococcal, short- and long-incubation *B. cereus, Clostridium perfringens,* and *Salmonella* outbreaks. Bacterial pathogens grow in food at temperatures ranging from 40 to 140°F; growth may be prevented if cold food is adequately refrigerated and if hot food is held at temperatures above 140°F before serving.

The usual source of contamination for *Salmonella, Campylobacter, Clostridium perfringens,* vibrios, and *Y. enterocolitica* and other zoonoses is raw foods of animal origin, not infected food handlers.[285] However, poor personal hygiene by food handlers frequently contributes to *Staphylococcus, Shigella,* hepatitis A, and some Norwalk-like agent outbreaks. Although thorough cooking of food just before consumption will eliminate the risk of many illnesses, protection against staphylococcal food poisoning is not provided, since the staphylococcal enterotoxins are heat stable. Inadequate heat processing may lead to botulism, and the use of contaminated equipment such as knives and meat slicers may result in nontyphoid salmonellosis.[286] Particular care in handling and cooking raw poultry, raw beef, raw pork, raw shellfish, and raw eggs is important in preventing many food-borne diseases. Avoiding consumption of raw milk is important in preventing *Salmonella, E. coli* O157:H7, and *Campylobacter jejuni* outbreaks.[6,287,288]

Food-handling errors resulting in chemical intoxication are different from those leading to bacterial outbreaks. Heavy metal poisoning occurs when acidic beverages are stored in defective metallic containers or when valves in vending machines malfunction. Ciguatera and shellfish poisoning occur when fish or shellfish are obtained from unsafe sources. Items contaminated with these toxins appear and taste normal; in addition, cooking of these items does not provide protection, since the toxins are heat stable.

Public health surveillance of food-borne infections and outbreaks is important to understand the magnitude and complexity of the problem and to guide targeted prevention efforts. Food-borne disease outbreaks should be reported to public health authorities. Reporting is essential if investigations are to be conducted to identify the source of the outbreak so that it can be corrected. Prompt reporting may also lead to the prevention of additional cases; there are well-documented outbreaks of botulism,[105,289] salmonellosis,[290] and *E. coli* O157:H7[291] in which recognition and reporting of the initial illness could have prevented many subsequent cases. Reporting illnesses with the potential for intrafamilial spread (e.g., shigellosis or *E. coli* O157:H7 infection) can prevent secondary transmission. Reporting is critical to stimulate concerted action to control major new hazards, such as *Salmonella enteritidis* in eggs, or *E. coli* O157:H7 in beef. Finally, reporting is vital to detect and intervene in outbreaks caused by commercially distributed foods before large numbers of people become ill.

REFERENCES

1. Bean NH, Griffin PM. Foodborne disease outbreaks in the United States, 1973–1987: Pathogens, vehicles and trends. J Food Protection. 1990;53:804–17.
2. Bennett JV, Holmberg SD, Rogers MF, et al. Infectious and parasitic diseases. In: Amler RW, Dull HB, eds. Closing the Gap: The Burden of Unnecessary Illness. New York: Oxford University Press; 1987:102–14.
3. Archer DL, Kvenberg JE. Incidence and cost of foodborne diarrheal disease in the United States. J Food Protection. 1985;48:887–94.
4. Waites WM, Arbuthnott JP. Foodborne illness: An overview. Lancet. 1990;336:722–5.
5. Lederberg J, Shope RE, Oaks SC Jr, eds. Emerging infections: Microbial threats to health in the United States. Washington, DC: National Academy Press; 1992.
6. Griffin PM, Tauxe RV. The epidemiology of infections caused by *Escherichia coli* O157:H7, other enterohemorrhagic *E. coli*, and the associated hemolytic uremic syndrome. Epidemiol Rev. 1991;13:60–98.
7. Swerdlow DL, Lee LA, Tauxe RV, et al. Reactive arthropathy following a multisate outbreak of *Salmonella typhimurium* infections (Abstract 916). 30th Interscience Conference on Antimicrobial Agents and Chemotherapy. Atlanta, October 21–24, 1990.
8. Mishu B, Ilyas AA, Kosli CL, et al. Serologic evidence of previous *Campylobacter jejuni* infections in patients with the Guillain-Barré syndrome. Ann Intern Med. 1993;118:947–53.
9. Tauxe RV, Blake PA. Epidemic cholera in Latin America. JAMA. 1992;267:1388–90.
10. Levine WC, Smart JF, Archer DL, et al. Foodborne disease outbreaks in nursing homes, 1973 through 1987. JAMA. 1991;266:2105–9.
11. Feig M. Staphylococcal food poisoning. A report of two related outbreaks, and a discussion of the data presented. Am J Public Health. 1950;40:279.
12. Bergdoll MS. The enterotoxins. In: Cohen JO, ed. The Staphylococci. New York: Wiley; 1972:301.
13. Bergdoll MS, Crass BA, Reiser RF, et al. A new staphylococcal enterotoxin, enterotoxin F, associated with toxic-shock-syndrome *Staphylococcus aureus* isolates. Lancet. 1981;1:1017.
14. Sugiyama H, Hayama T. Abdominal viscera as site of emetic action for staphylococcal enterotoxin in the monkey. J Infect Dis. 1965;115:330.
15. Clark WG, Vanderhooft GF, Borison HL. Emetic effect of purified staphylococcal enterotoxin in cats. Proc Soc Exp Biol Med. 1962;111:205.
16. Elias J, Shields R. Influence of staphylococal enterotoxin on water and electrolyte transport in the small intestine. Gut. 1976;17:527.
17. Gilbert RJ. Staphylococcal food poisoning and botulism. Postgrad Med J. 1974;50:603.
18. Breckinridge JC, Bergdoll MS. Outbreak of foodborne gastroenteritis due to a coagulase-negative enterotoxin-producing staphylococcus. N Engl J Med. 1971;284:541.
19. Merson MH. The epidemiology of staphylococcal foodborne disease. Proc Staph Foods Conf. University Park, PA: Pennsylvania State University; 1973:20.
20. Šimkovičova M, Gilbert RJ. Serological detection of enterotoxin from food-poisoning strains of *Staphylococcus aureus*. J Med Microbiol. 1971;4:19.
21. Holmberg SD, Blake PA. Staphylococcal food poisoning in the United States: New facts and old misconceptions. JAMA. 1984;251:487.
22. Mortimer PR, McCann G. Food-poisoning episodes associated with *Bacillus cereus* in fried rice. Lancet. 1974;1:1043.
23. Midura T, Gerber M, Wood R, et al. Outbreak of food poisoning caused by *Bacillus cereus*. Public Health Rep. 1970;85:45.
24. Terranova W, Blake PA. *Bacillus cereus* food poisoning. N Engl J Med. 1978;298:143.
25. Melling J, Capel BJ, Turnbull PCB, et al. Identification of a novel enterotoxigenic activity associated with *Bacillus cereus*. J Clin Pathol. 1976;29:938.
26. Turnbull PCB, Kramer JM, Jorgensen K. Properties and production characteristics of vomiting, diarrheal, and necrotizing toxins of *Bacillus cereus*. Am J Clin Nutr. 1979;32:219.
27. Hobbs BC, Smith ME, Oakley CL, et al. *Clostridium welchii* food poisoning. J Hyg. 1953;51:75.
28. Shandera WX, Tacket CO, Blake PA. Food poisoning due to *Clostridium perfringens* in the United States. J Infect Dis. 1983;147:167.
29. Smith LDS. *Clostridium perfringens*. The Pathoenic Anaerobic Bacteria. Springfield, IL: Charles C Thomas; 1975:115.
30. Stark RL, Duncan CL. Purification and biochemical properties of *Clostridium perfringens* type A enterotoxin. Infect Immun. 1972;6:662.
31. Duncan CL. Time of enterotoxin formation and release during sporulation of *Clostridium perfringens* type A. J Bacteriol. 1973;113:932.
32. McDonel JL, Duncan CL. Regional localization of activity of *Clostridium perfringens* type A enterotoxin in the rabbit ileum, jejunum, and duodenum. J Infect Dis. 1977;136:661.
33. McDonel JL. The molecular mode of action of *Clostridium perfringens* enterotoxin. Am J Clin Nutr. 1979;32:210.
34. Turnbull PCB. Studies on the production of enterotoxins by *Bacillus cereus*. J Clin Pathol. 1976;29:941.
35. Loewenstein MS. Epidemiology of *Clostridium perfringens* food poisoning. N Engl J Med. 1972;286:1026.
36. Giannella RA, Brasile L: A hospital food-borne outbreak of diarrhea caused by *Bacillus cereus*. Cinical, epidemiologic, and microbiologic studies. J Infect Dis. 1979;139:366.
37. Giannella RA, Formal SB, Dammin GJ, et al. Pathogenesis of salmonellosis: Studies of fluid secretion, mucosal invasion, and morphologic reaction in the rabbit ileum. J Clin Invest. 1973;52:441.
38. Rout WR, Formal SB, Giannella RA, et al. Pathophysiology of shigella diarrhea in the rhesus monkey: Intestinal transport, morphological, and bacteriological studies. Gastroenterology. 1975;68:270.
39. Bolen JL, Zamiska SA, Greenough WB III. Clinical features in enteritis due to *Vibrio parahaemolyticus*. Am J Med. 1974;57:638.
40. Hughes JM, Boyce JM, Aloem ARMA, et al. *Vibrio parahaemolyticus* enterocolitis in Bangladesh: Report of an outbreak. Am J Trop Med Hyg. 1978;27:106.
41. Boutin BK, Townsend SF, Scarpino PV, et al: Demonstration of invasiveness of *Vibrio parahaemolyticus* in adult rabbits by immunofluorescence. Appl Environ Microbiol. 1979;37:647.
42. Tulloch EF, Ryan KJ, Formal SB, et al. Invasive enteropathic *Escherichia coli* dysentery: An outbreak in 28 adults. Ann Intern Med. 1973;79:13.
43. Horwitz MA, Pollard RA, Merson MH, et al. A large outbreak of foodborne salmonellosis on the Navaho Nation Indian Reservation: Epidemiology and secondary transmission. Am J Pubic Health. 1977;67:1071.
44. Weissman JB, Williams SV, Hinman AR, et al. Foodborne shigellosis at a country fair. Am J Epidemiol. 1974;100:178.
45. Chatterjee BD, Neogy KN, Gorbach SL. Studies of *Vibrio parahaemolyticus* from cases of diarrhea in Calcutta. Indian J Med Res. 1970;58:234.
46. Marier R, Wells JG, Swanson RC, et al. An outbreak of enteropathogenic *Escherichia coli* foodborne disease traced to imported French cheese. Lancet. 1973;2:1376.
47. Tauxe RV. Epidemiology of *Campylobacter jejuni* infections in the United States and other industrialized nations. In: Nachamkin I, Blaser ML, Tompkins L, eds. *Campylobacter jejuni*: Current status and future trends. Washington, DC: American Society of Microbiology; 1992:9–19.
48. Tauxe RV, Bean NH, Patton CH. *Campylobacter* isolates in the United States, 1982–1986. CDC surveillance summaries. MMWR. 1988;37(No. SS-2):1–13.
49. Blaser MJ, Wells JG, Feldman RA. *Campylobacter* enteritis in the United States: A multicenter study. Ann Intern Med. 1983;98:360.
50. Lambert ME, Schofield PF, Ironside AG, et al. *Campylobacter* colitis. Br Med J. 1979;1:857.
51. Taylor DN, Porter BW, Williams CA, et al. *Campylobacter* enteritis: A large outbreak traced to commercial raw milk. West J Med. 1982;137:365.
52. Blaser MJ, Checko P, Bopp C, et al. *Campylobacter* enteritis associated with foodborne transmission. Am J Epidemiol. 1982;116:886.
53. Blaser MJ, Berkowitz ID, LaForce FM, et al. *Campylobacter* enteritis: Clinical and epidemiologic features. Ann Intrn Med. 1979;91:179.
54. Hughes JM, Hollis DG, Gangarosa E, et al. Non-*cholera vibrio* infections in the United States: Clinical, epidemiologic, and laboratory features. Ann Intern Med. 1978;88:602–6.
55. Morris JG Jr, Wilson R, Davis BR, et al. Non-O group 1 *Vibrio cholerae* gastroeneritis in the United States: Clinical, epidemiologic, and laboratory characteristics of sporadic cases. Ann Intern Med. 1981;94:656.
56. Wilson R, Lieb S, Roberts A, et al. Non-O group 1 *Vibrio cholerae* gastroenteritis associated with eating raw oysters. Am J Epidemiol. 1981;114:293.
57. Carpenter CCJ Jr. Cholera enterotoxin: Recent investigations yield insights into transport processes. Am J Med. 1971;50:1.
58. Zinnaka Y, Carpenter CCJ Jr. An enterotoxin produced by noncholera vibrios. Johns Hopkins Med J. 1972;131:403.
59. Craig JP, Yamamoto K, Takeda Y, et al. Production of cholera-like enterotoxin by a *Vibrio cholerae* non-O1 strain isolated from the environment. Infect Immun. 1981;34:90.
60. Sack RB. Human diarrheal disease caused by enterotoxigenic *Escherichia coli*. Annu Rev Microbiol. 1975;29:333.
61. Sandefur PD, Peterson JW. Neutralization of *Salmonella* toxin-induced elongation of Chinese hamster ovary cells by cholera antitoxin. Infect Immun. 1977;15:988.
62. Sedlock DM, Deibel RH. Detection of *Salmonella* enterotoxin using rabbit ileal loops. Can J Microbiol. 1978;24:268.
63. Keusch GT, Donta ST. Classification of enterotoxins on the basis of activity in cell culture. J Infect Dis. 1975;131:58.
64. Keusch GT, Jacewicz M. The pathogenesis of *Shigella* diarrhea. IV. Toxin and antitoxin in *Shigella flexneri* and *Shigella sonnei* infections in humans. J Infect Dis. 1977;135:552.
65. O'Brien AD, Gentry MK, Thompson MR, et al. Shigellosis and *Escherichia coli* diarrhea: Relative importance of invasive and toxigenic mechanisms. Am J Clin Nutr. 1979;32:229.
66. Honda T, Shimizu M, Takeda Y, et al. Isolation of a factor causing morphological changes in Chinese hamster ovary cells from the culture filtrate of *Vibrio parahaemolyticus*. Infect Immun. 1976;14:1028.
67. Carruthers MM. Cytotoxicity of *Vibrio parahaemolyticus* in HeLa cell culture. J Infect Dis. 1975;132:555.
68. Banwell JG, Gorbach SL, Pierce NF, et al. Acute undifferentiated human diarrhea in the tropics. II. Alterations in instestinal fluid and electrolye movements. J Clin Invest. 1971;50:890.
69. Barker WH Jr, Mackowiak PA, Fishbein M, et al. *Vibrio parahaemolyticus* gastroenteritis outbreak in Covington, Louisiana, in August 1972. Am J Epidemiol. 1974;100:316.
70. Aldova E, Lázničková K, Stěpankova E, et al. Isolation of nonagglutinable vibrios from an enteritis outbreak in Czechoslovakia. J Infect Dis. 1968;118:25.

71. Carpenter CCJ Jr, Mitra PP, Sack RB. Clinical studies in Asiatic cholera. I. Preliminary observations, November 1962–March 1963. Bull Johns Hopkins Hosp. 1966;118:165.

72. Taylor WR, Schell WL, Wells JG, et al. A foodborne outbreak of enterotoxigenic Escherichia coli diarrhea. N Engl J Med. 1982;306:1093.

73. Kaplan JE, Gary GW, Baron RC, et al. Epidemiology of Norwalk gastroenteritis and the role of Norwalk virus in outbreaks of acute nonbacterial gastroenteritis. Ann Intern Med. 1982;96:756.

74. Murphy AM, Grohmann GS, Christopher PJ, et al. An Australia-wide outbreak of gastroenteritis from oysters caused by Norwalk virus. Med J Aust. 1979;2:329.

75. Morse DL, Guzewich JJ, Hanrahan JP, et al. Widespread outbreaks of clam- and oyster-associated gastroenteritis: Role of Norwalk virus. N Engl J Med. 1986;314:678–32.

76. Kaplan JE, Feldman R, Campbell DS, et al. The frequency of a Norwalk-like pattern of illness in outbreaks of acute gastroenteritis. Am J Public Health. 1982;72:1329–32.

77. Truman BI, Madore HP, Menegus MA, et al. Snow Mountain Agent gastroenteritis from clams. Am J Epidemiol. 1987;126:516–25.

78. Dolin R, Treanor JJ, Madore HP. Novel agents of viral enteritis in humans. J Infect Dis. 1987;155:365–76.

79. Black RE, Jackson RJ, Tsai T, et al. Epidemic Yersinia enterocolitica infection due to contaminated chocolate milk. N Engl J Med. 1978;298:76.

80. Tacket CO, Narain JP, Sattin R, et al. A multistate outbreak of infections caused by Yersinia enterocolitica transmitted by pasteurized milk. JAMA. 1984;251:483.

81. Ostroff SM, Kapperud G, Lassen J, et al. Clinical features of sporadic Yersinia enterocolitica infections in Norway. J Infect Dis. 1992;166:812–7.

82. Tauxe RV, Vandepitte J, Wauters G, et al. Yersinia enterocolitica infections and pork: The missing link. Lancet. 1987;1:1129–32.

83. Pai CH, Mors V. Production of enterotoxin by Yersinia enterocolitica. Infect Immun. 1978;19:908.

84. Boyce JM, Doyle DJ Jr, Evans DG, et al. Production of heat-stable, methanol-soluble enterotoxin by Yersinia enterocolitica. Infect Immun. 1979;25:532.

85. Asakawa Y, Akahane S, Kagata N, et al. Two community outbreaks of human infection with Yersinia enterocolitica. J Hyg (Camb). 1973;71:715.

86. Arvastson B, Damgaard K, Winblad S. Clinical symptoms of infection with Yersinia enterocolitica. Scand J Infect Dis. 1971;3:37.

87. Riley LW, Remis RS, Helgerson SD, et al. Hemorrhagic colitis associated with a rare Escherichia coli serotype. N Engl J Med. 1983;308:681.

88. Ryan CA, Tauxe RV, Hosek GW, et al. Escherichia coli O157:H7 diarrhea in a nursing home: Clinical, epidemiological, and pathological findings. J Infect Dis. 1986;154:631–8.

89. Johnson WM, Lior H, Bezanson GS. Cytotoxic Escherichia coli O157:H7 associated with haemorrhagic colitis in Canada. Lancet. 1983;1:76.

90. O'Brien AD, Lively TA, Chen ME, et al. Escherichia coli O157:H7 strains associated with haemorrhagic colitis in the United States produce a Shigella dysenteriae 1 (shiga) like cytotoxin. Lancet. 1983;1:702.

91. Boyd B, Lingwood C. Verotoxin receptor glycolipid in human renal tissue. Nephron. 1989;51:207–10.

92. Griffin PM, Ostroff SM, Tauxe RV, et al. Illnesses associated with Escherichia coli O157:H7 infections: A broad clinical spectrum. Ann Intern Med. 1988;109:705–12.

93. Carter AO, Borczyk AA, Carlson JAK, et al. A severe outbreak of Escherichia coli O157:H7-associated hemorrhagic colitis in a nursing home. N Engl J Med. 1987;317:1496–1500.

94. Centers for Disease Control and Prevention. Thrombotic thrombocytopenic purpura associated with Escherichia coli O157:H7–Washington. MMWR. 1986;35:549–51.

95. Pavia AT, Nichols CR, Green DP, et al. Hemolytic-uremic syndrome during an outbreak of Escherichia coli O157:H7 infections in institutions for mentally retarded persons: Clinical and epidemiologic observations. J Pediatr. 1990;116:544–51.

96. Koenig MG, Spickard A, Cardella MA, et al. Clinical and laboratory observations of type E botulism in man. Medicine. 1964;43:517.

97. Barker WH Jr, Weissman JB, Dowell VR Jr, et al. Type B botulism outbreak caused by a commercial food product. JAMA. 1977;237:456.

98. Hughes JM, Blumenthal JR, Merson MH, et al. Clinical features of types A and B food-borne botulism. Ann Intern Med. 1981;95:442.

99. Kao I, Drachman DB, Price DL. Botulinum toxin: Mechanism of presynaptic blockade. Science. 1976;193:1256.

100. Simpson LL. The origin, structure, and pharmacological activity of botulinum toxin. Pharmacol Rev. 1981;33:155.

101. Horwitz MA, Hughes JM, Merson MH, et al. Food-borne botulism in the United States, 1970–1975. J Infect Dis. 1977;136:153.

102. Midura TF, Arnon SS. Infant botulism: Identification of Clostridium botulinum and its toxins in feces. Lancet. 1976;2:934.

103. Arnon SS, Midura TF, Clay SA, et al. Infant botulism: Epidemiological, clinical, and laboratory aspects. JAMA. 1977;237:1946.

104. Sugiyama H, Mills DC. Intraintestinal toxin in infant mice challenged intragastrically with Clostridium botulinum spores. Infect Immun. 1978;21:59.

105. St Louis ME, Shaun HS, Peck MB, et al. Botulism from chopped garlic: Delayed recognition of a major outbreak. Ann Intern Med. 1988;108:363–8.

106. Semple AB, Parry WH, Phillips DE. Acute copper poisoning: An outbreak traced to contaminated water from a corroded geyser. Lancet 1960;2:700.

107. Brown MA, Thom JV, Orth GL, et al. Food poisoning involving zinc contamination. Arch Environ Health. 1964;8:657.

108. Centers for Disease Control and Prevention. Illness associated with elevated levels of zinc in fruit punch: New Mexico. MMWR. 1983;32:257.

109. Barker WH Jr, Runte V. Tomato juice–associated gastroenteritis, Washington and Oregon, 1969. Am J Epidemiol. 1972;96:219.

110. Baker TD, Hafner WG. Cadmium poisoning from a refrigerator shelf used as an improvised barbecue grill. Public Health Rep. 1961;76:543.

111. Merson MH, Baine WB, Gangarosa EJ, et al. Scombroid fish poisoning: Outbreak traced to commercially canned tuna fish. JAMA. 1974;228:1268.

112. Kawabata T, Ishizaka K, Miura T. Studies on the allergy-like food poisoning associated with putrefaction of marine products. III. Physiological and pharmacological action of "saurine," a vagus stimulant of unknown structure recently isolated by the authors, and its characteristics in developing allergy-like symptoms. Jpn J Med Sci Biol. 1955;8:521.

113. Foo LY. Scombroid poisoning: Recapitulation on the role of histamine. NZ Med J. 1977;85:425.

114. Geiger E, Courtney G, Schnakenberg G. The content and formation of histamine in fish muscle. Arch Biochem. 1944;3:311.

115. Taylor SL. Histamine food poisoning: Toxicology and clinical aspects. CRC Crit Rev Toxicol. 1986;17:91–128.

116. Lerke PA, Werner SB, Taylor SL, et al. Scombroid poisoning: Report of an outbreak. West J Med. 1978;129:381.

117. Taylor SL, Guthertz LS, Leatherwood M, et al. Histamine production by Klebsiella pneumoniae and an incident of scombroid fish poisoning. Appl Environ Microbiol. 1979;37:274.

118. Hughes JM, Merson MH. Fish and shellfish poisoning. N Engl J Med. 1976;295:1117.

119. Perl TM, Bedard L, Kosatsky T, et al. An outbreak of toxic encephalopathy caused by eating mussels contaminated with domoic acid. New Engl J Med. 1990;322:1775–80.

120. Halstead BW, Courville DA. Poisonous and Venomous Marine Animals of the World. v. 1. Invertebrates. Washington, DC: Government Printing Office; 1965:157.

121. Zwahlen A, Blanc MH, Robert M. Epidémie d'intoxication par les moules ("Paralytic Shellfish Poisoning"). Schweiz Med Wochenschr. 1977;107:226.

122. Acres J, Gray J. Paralytic shellfish poisoning. Can Med Assoc J. 1978;119:1195.

123. Rodriguez DC, Etzel RA, Hall S, et al. Lethal paralytic shellfish poisoning in Guatemala. Am J Trop Med Hyg. 1990;42:267–71.

124. Proctor NH, Chan SL, Trevor AJ: Production of saxitoxin by cultures of Gonyaulax catenella. Toxicon 1975;13:1.

125. Ghazarossian VE, Schantz EJ, Schnoes HK, et al. Identification of a poison in toxic scallops from a Gonyaulax tamarensis red tide. Biochem Biophys Res Comm. 1974;59:1219.

126. Shimizu Y, Buckley LJ, Alam M, et al. Structures of gonyautoxin II and III from the East Coast toxic dinoflagellate Gonyaulax tamarensis. J Am Chem Soc. 1976;98:5414.

127. Schantz EJ, Ghazarossian VE, Schnoes HK, et al. The structure of saxitoxin. J Am Chem Soc. 1975;97:1238.

128. Henderson R, Ritchie JM, Strichartz GR. The binding of labelled saxitoxin to the sodium channels in nerve membranes. J Physiol. 1973;235:783.

129. Henderson R, Ritchie JM, Strichartz GR. Evidence that tetrodotoxin and saxitoxin act at a metal cation binding site in the sodium channels of nerve membrane. Proc Natl Acad Sci USA. 1974;71:3936.

130. Catterall WA. Neurotoxins that act on voltage-sensitive sodium channels in excitable membranes. Annu Rev Pharmacol Toxicol. 1980;20:15.

131. Spiegelstein MY, Paster Z, Abbott BC. Purification and biological activity of Gymnodinium breve toxins. 1973;11:85.

132. Kim YS, Padilla GM. Purification of the ichthyotoxic component of Gymnodinium breve (red tide dinoflagellate) toxin by high pressure liquid chromatography. Toxicon. 1976;14:379.

133. Grunfeld Y, Spiegelstein MY. Effects of Gymnodinium breve toxin on the smooth muscle preparation of guinea-pig ileum. Br J Pharmacol. 1974;51:67.

134. Teitlebaum JS, Zatorre RJ, Carpenter S, et al. Neurologic sequelae of domoic acid intoxication due to the ingestion of contaminated mussels. N Engl J Med. 1990;322:1781–7.

135. Schaumburg HH, Byck R, Gerstl R, et al. Monosodium L-glutamate: Its pharmacology and role in the Chinese restaurant syndrome. Science. 1969;163:826.

136. Reif-Lehrer L. A questionnaire study of the prevalence of Chinese restaurant syndrome. Fed Proc. 1977;36:1617.

137. Hudson PJ, Vogt RL. A foodborne outbreak traced to niacin overenrichment. J Food Protection. 1985;48:249–51.

138. Barkin RM. Ciguatera poisoning: A common source outbreak. South Med J. 1974;67:13.

139. Halstead BW. Fish poisoning: The diagnosis, pharmacology and treatment. Clin Pharmacol Ther. 1964;5:615.

140. Russell FE. Ciguatera poisoning: A report of 35 cases. Toxicon. 1975;13:383.

141. Halstead BW, Courville DA. Poisonous and Venomous Marine Animals of the World. v. 1. Vertebrates. Washington, DC: Government Printing Office; 1967:63.

142. Engleberg NC, Morris JG Jr, Lewis J, et al. Ciguatera fish poisoning: A major common-source outbreak in the U.S. Virgin Islands. Ann Intern Med. 1983;98:336.

143. Bagnis R, Kuberski T, Laugier S. Cinical observations on 3,009 cases of

ciguatera (fish poisoning) in the South Pacific. Am J Trop Med Hyg. 1979; 28:1067.

144. Morris JG Jr, Lewin P, Hargrett NT, et al. Clinical features of ciguatera fish poisoning: A study of the disease in the U.S. Virgin Islands. Arch Intern Med. 1982;142:1090.

145. Scheuer PJ, Takahashi W, Tsutsumi J, et al. Ciguatoxin: Isolation and chemical nature. Science. 1967;155:1267.

146. Helfrich P, Banner AH. Experimental induction of ciguatera: Toxicity in fish through diet. Nature. 1963;197:1025.

147. Bagnis R, Chanteau S, Chungue E, et al. Origins of ciguatera fish poisoning: A new dinoflagellate, *Gambierdiscus toxicus* Adachi and Fukuyo, definitively involved as a causal agent. Toxicon. 1980;18:199.

148. Li K-M. Ciguatera fish poison: A cholinesterase inhibitor. Science. 1965; 147:1580.

149. Halstead BW. Current status of marine biotoxicology: An overview. Clin Toxicol. 1981;18:1.

150. Le Grand AM, Galonnier M, Bagnis R. Studies on the mode of action of ciguateric toxins. Toxicon. 1982;20:311–5.

151. Bidard JN, Vijverberg HPM, Frelin C, et al. Ciguatoxin is a novel type of Na$^+$ channel toxin. J Biol Chem. 1984;259:8353–7.

152. Lampe KF. Current concepts of therapy in mushroom intoxication. Clin Toxicol. 1974;7:115.

153. Becker CE, Tong TG, Boerner U, et al. Diagnosis and treatment of *Amanita phalloides*–type mushroom poisoning: Use of thioctic acid. West J Med. 1976;125:100.

154. McCormick DJ, Avbel AJ, Gibbons RB. Nonlethal mushroom poisoning. Ann Intern Med. 1979;90:332.

155. Lampe KF. Toxic fungi. Annu Rev Pharmacol Toxicol. 1979;19:85.

156. Paaso B, Harrison DC. A new look at an old problem: Mushroom poisoning. Am J Med. 1975;58:505.

157. Hughes JM, Horwitz MA, Merson MH, et al. Foodborne disease outbreaks of chemical etiology in the United States, 1970–1974. Am J Epidemiol. 1977; 105:233.

158. Editorial: Death-cap poisoning. Lancet. 1972;1:1320.

159. Centers for Disease Control and Prevention: Mushroom poisoning among Laotian refugees: 1981. MMWR. 1982;31:287.

160. Wieland T, Wieland O. The toxic peptides of *Amanita* species. In: Kadis S, Ciegler A, Aji SJ, eds. Microbiol Toxins. v. 8. Fungal Toxins. New York: Academic Press; 1972:249.

161. Osterholm MT, MacDonald KL, White KE, et al. An outbreak of a newly recognized chronic diarrhea syndrome associated with raw milk consumption. JAMA. 1986;256:484–90.

162. Martin DL, Hoberman LJ. A point source outbreak of chronic diarrhea in Texas: No known exposure to raw milk. JAMA. 1986;256:469.

163. Merson MH, Barker WH Jr, Craun GF, et al. Outbreaks of waterborne disease in the United States, 1971–1972. J Infect Dis. 1974;129:614.

164. Hughes JM, Merson MH, Craun GF, et al. Outbreaks of waterborne disease in the United States, 1973. J Infect Dis. 1975;132:336.

165. Horwitz MA, Hughes JM, Craun GF. Outbreaks of waterborne disease in the United States, 1974. J Infect Dis. 1976;133:588.

166. Black RE, Horwitz MA, Craun GF. Outbreaks of waterborne disease in the United States, 1975. J Infect Dis. 1978;137:370.

167. Centers for Disease Control and Prevention. Foodborne and Waterborne Disease Outbreaks Annual Summary 1976. October 1977.

168. Centers for Disease Control and Prevention. Foodborne and Waterborne Disease Surveillance Annual Summary 1977. August 1979.

169. Centers for Disease Control and Prevention. Water-Related Disease Outbreaks Surveillance Annual Summary 1978. May 1980.

170. Centers for Disease Control and Prevention. Water-Related Disease Outbreaks Surveillance Annual Summary 1979. September 1981.

171. Centers for Disease Control and Prevention. Water-Related Disease Outbreaks Surveillance Annual Summary 1980. February 1982.

172. Centers for Disease Control and Prevention. Water-Related Disease Outbreaks Surveillance Annual Summary 1981. September 1982.

173. Centers for Disease Control and Prevention. Water-Related Disease Outbreaks Surveillance Annual Summary 1982. Centers for Disease Control. 1983;1–15.

174. Centers for Disease Control and Prevention. Water-Related Disease Outbreaks Surveillance Annual Summary 1983. 1984;1–15.

175. Centers for Disease Control and Prevention. Water-Related Disease Outbreaks Surveillance Annual Summary 1984. 1985;1–15.

176. St Louis ME. Water-Related Disease Outbreaks, 1985. CDC surveillance summaries. MMWR. 1986;37(No. SS-2):15–24.

177. Levine WC, Stephenson WT, Craun GF. Waterborne disease outbreaks, 1986–1988. Centers for Disease Control Surveillance Summaries, March 1990. MMWR. 1990;39(No. SS-1):1–13.

178. Herwaldt BL, Craun GF, Stokes SL, et al. Waterborne disease outbreaks, 1989–1990. Centers for Disease Control Surveillance Summaries, December 1991. MMWR. 1991;40(No. SS-3):1–21.

179. Swerdlow DL, Woodruff BA, Brady RC, et al. A waterborne outbreak in Missouri of *Escherichia coli* O157:H7 associated with bloody diarrhea and death. Ann Intern Med. 1992;117:812–9.

180. Weissman JB, Craun GF, Lawrence DN, et al. An epidemic of gastroenteritis traced to a contaminated public water supply. Am J Epidemiol. 1976;103: 391.

181. Mosley JW. Water-borne infectious hepatitis. N Engl J Med. 1959;261:703.

182. Feldman RE, Baine WB, Nitzkin JL, et al. Epidemiology of *Salmonella typhi*

183. A collaborative report. A waterborne epidemic of salmonellosis in Riverside, California, 1965: Epidemiologic aspects. Am J Epidemiol. 1971;93:33.

184. Rosenberg ML, Koplan JP, Wachsmuth IK, et al. Epidemic diarrhea at Crater Lake from enterotoxigenic *Escherichia coli*. A large waterborne outbreak. Ann Intern Med. 1977;86:714.

185. Vogt RL, Sours HE, Barrett T, et al. *Campylobacter* enteritis associated with contaminated water. Ann Intern Med. 1982;96:292.

186. Palmer SR, Gully PR, White JM, et al. Water-borne outbreak of *Campylobacter* gastroenteritis. Lancet. 1983;1:287.

187. Parsonnet J, Trock SC, Bopp CA, et al. Chronic diarrhea associated with drinking untreated water. Ann Intern Med. 1989;110:985–91.

188. Wilson R, Anderson LJ, Holman RC, et al. Waterborne gastroenteritis due to the Norwalk agent: Clinical and epidemiologic investigation. Am J Public Health. 1982;72:72.

189. Kaplan JE, Goodman RA, Schonberger LB, et al. Gastroenteritis due to Norwalk virus: An outbreak associated with a municipal water system. J Infect Dis. 1982;146:190.

190. Morens DM, Zweighaft RM, Vernon TM, et al. A waterborne outbreak of gastroenteritis with secondary person-to-person spread. Lancet. 1979;1:964.

191. Jackson LA, Wenger JD. Listeriosis: A foodborne disease. Infections Med. 1993;10:61–6.

192. Blake PA, Merson MH, Weaver RE, et al. Disease caused by a marine *Vibrio*: Clinical characteristics and epidemiology. N Engl J Med. 1979;300: 1–5.

193. Horwitz A. Specific diagnosis of foodborne disease. Gastroenterology. 1977; 73:375.

194. Gilbert RJ, Stringer MF, Peace TC. The survival and growth of *Bacillus cereus* in boiled and fried rice in relation to outbreaks of food poisoning. J Hyg (Camb). 1974;73:433.

195. Holmes JR, Plunkett T, Pate P, et al. Emetic food poisoning caused by *Bacillus cereus*. Arch Intern Med. 1981;141:766.

196. Strong DH, Canada JC, Griffiths BB. Incidence of *Clostridium perfringens* in American foods. Appl Microbiol. 1963;11:42.

197. Hall HE, Angelotti R. *Closridium perfringens* in meat and meat products. Appl Microbiol. 1965;13:352.

198. Smart JL, Roberts TA, Stringer MF, et al. The incidence and serotypes of *Clostridium perfringens* on beef, pork and lamb carcasses. J Appl Bacteriol. 1979;46:377.

199. Petersen LR, Mshar R, Cooper GH Jr, et al. A large *Clostridium perfringens* foodborne outbreak with an unusual attack rate pattern. Am J Epidemiol. 1988;127:605–11.

200. Kim HU, Goepfert JM. Enumeration and identification of *Bacillus cereus* in foods. I. 24-hour presumptive test medium. Appl Microbiol. 1971;22:581.

201. Blakey LJ, Priest FG. The occurrence of *Bacillus cereus* in some dried foods including pulses and cereals. J Appl Bacteriol. 1980;48:297.

202. Jephcott AE, Barton BW, Gilbert RJ, et al. An unusual outbreak of food-poisoning associated with meals-on-wheels. Lancet. 1977;2:129.

203. St Louis ME, Morse DL, Potter ME, et al. The emergence of grade A eggs as a major source of *Salmonella enteritidis* infections. JAMA. 1988;259:2103–7.

204. Centers for Disease Control and Prevention. Outbreak of *Salmonella enteritidis* infection associated with consumption of raw shell eggs, 1991. MMWR. 1992;41:369–72.

205. Hedberg CW, David MJ, White KE, et al. Role of egg consumption in sporadic *Salmonella enteritidis* and *Salmonella typhimurium* infections in Minnesota. J Infect Dis. 1993;167:107–11.

206. Werner SB, Humphrey GL, Kamel I. Association between raw milk and human *Salmonella dublin* infection. Br Med J. 1979;2:238.

207. Galbraith NS, Forbes P, Clifford C. Communicable disease associated with milk and dairy products in England and Wales 1951–80. Br Med J. 1982;284: 1761.

208. Gill ON, Bartlett CLR, Sockett PN, et al. Outbreak of *Salmonella napoli* infection caused by contaminated chocolate bars. Lancet. 1983;1:574.

209. Craven PC, Baine WB, Mackel DC, et al. International outbreak of *Salmonella eastbourne* infection traced to contaminated chocolate. Lancet. 1975; 1:788.

210. Centers for Disease Control and Prevention. Hospital-associated outbreak of *Shigella dysenteriae* type 2: Maryland. MMWR. 1983;32:250.

211. Barker WH Jr. *Vibrio parahaemolyticus* outbreaks in the United States. Lancet. 1974;1:551.

212. Lawrence DN, Blake PA, Yashuk JC, et al. *Vibrio parahaemolyticus* gastroenteritis outbreaks aboard two cruise ships. Am J Epidemiol. 1979;109: 71.

213. Kudoh Y, Sakai S, Zen-Yoji H, et al. Epidemiology of food poisoning due to *Vibrio parahaemolyticus* occurring in Tokyo during the last decade. In: Fujino T, Sakaguchi G, Sakazaki R, et al., eds. International Symposium on *Vibrio parahaemolyticus*. Tokyo: Saikon; 1974:9.

214. Baine WB, Zampieri A, Mazzotti M, et al. Epidemiology of cholera in Italy in 1973. Lancet. 1974;2:1370.

215. Blake PA, Rosenberg ML, Costa JB, et al. Cholera in Portugal, 1974: I. Modes of transmission. Am J Epidemiol. 1977;105:337–43.

216. Barrett TJ, Blake PA. Epidemiological usefulness of changes in hemolytic activity of *Vibrio cholerae* biotype El Tor during the seventh pandemic. J Clin Microbiol. 1981;13:126.

217. Blake PA, Allegra DT, Snyder JD, et al. Cholera: A possible endemic focus in the United States. N Engl J Med. 1980;302:305.

infection in a migrant labor camp in Dade County, Florida. J Infect Dis. 1974;130:334.

218. Pavia AT, Campbell JF, Blake PA, et al. Cholera from raw oysters shipped interstate. JAMA. 1987;258:2374.
219. Lowry PW, Pavia AT, McFarland LM, et al. Cholera in Louisiana: Widening spectrum of seafood vehicles. Arch Intern Med. 1989;149:2079–84.
220. Finelli L, Swerdlow D, Mertz K, et al. Outbreak of cholera associated with crab brought from an area with epidemic disease. J Infect Dis. 1992;166:1433–5.
221. Merson MH, Morris GH, Sack DA, et al. Travelers' diarrhea in Mexico. N Engl J Med. 1976;294:1299.
222. MacDonald KL, Eidson M, Strohmeyer C, et al. A multistate outbreak of gastrointestinal illness caused by enterotoxigenic Escherichia coli in imported semisoft cheese. J Infect Dis. 1985;151:716–20.
223. Sack RB, Sack DA, Mehlman IF, et al. Enterotoxigenic Escherichia coli isolated from food. J Infect Dis. 1977;135:313.
224. MacDonald KL, Cohen ML, Blake PA. The changing epidemiology of adult botulism in the United States. Am J Epidemiol. 1986;124:794–9.
225. Spika JS, Shaffer N, Hargrett-Bean N. Risk factors for infant botulism in the United States. Am J Dis Child. 1989;143:828–32.
226. Linco SJ, Grohmann GS. The Darwin outbreak of oyster-associated viral gastroenteritis. Med J Aust. 1980;1:211.
227. Gunn RA, Janowski HT, Lieb S, et al. Norwalk virus gastroenteritis following raw oyster consumption. Am J Epidemiol. 1982;115:348.
228. Griffin MR, Surowiec JJ, McCloskey DI, et al. Foodborne Norwalk virus. Am J Epidemiol. 1982;115:178.
229. Kuritsky JN, Osterholm MT, Greenberg HB, et al. Norwalk gastroenteritis: A community outbreak associated with bakery product consumption. Ann Intern Med. 1984;100:519.
230. Reid JA, Caul EO, White OG, et al. Role of infected food handler in hotel outbreak of Norwalk-like viral gastroenteritis: Implications for control. Lancet. 1988;2:321–3.
231. Hopper SH, Adams HS. Copper poisoning from vending machines. Public Health Rep. 1958;73:910.
232. Hesse IDW, Halstead BW, Peckham NH. Marine biotoxins. I. Ciguatera poison: Some biological and chemical aspects. Ann NY Acad Sci. 1960;90:788–97.
233. Collins JC, Bicknell WJ. The red tide: A pubic-health emergency. N Engl J Med. 1974;288:1126.
234. Lawrence DN, Enriquez MB, Lumish RM, et al. Ciguatera fish poisoning in Miami. JAMA. 1980;244:254.
235. Kelly MT, Peterson JW, Sarles HE Jr, et al. Cholera on the Texas Gulf Coast. JAMA. 1982;247:1598.
236. Morris JG Jr, Lewin P, Smith CW, et al. Ciguatera fish poisoning: Epidemiology of the disease on St. Thomas, U.S. Virgin Islands. Am J Trop Med Hyg. 1982;31:574.
237. Casman EP, Bennett RW. Detection of staphylococcal enterotoxin in food. Appl Microbiol. 1965;13:181.
238. Pober Z, Silverman GJ. Modified radioimmunoassay determination for staphylococcal enterotoxin B in foods. Appl Environ Microbiol. 1977;33:620.
239. Saunders GC, Bartlett ML. Double-antibody solid-phase enzyme immunoassay for the detection of staphylococcal enterotoxin. A. Appl Environ Microbiol. 1977;34:518.
240. Stiffler-Rosenberg G, Fey H. Simple assay for staphylococcal enterotoxins A, B, and C: Modification of enzyme-linked immunosorbent assay. J Clin Microbiol. 1978;8:473.
241. Freed RC, Evenson ML, Reiser RF, et al. Enzyme-linked immunosorbent assay for detection of staphylcoocal enterotoxins in foods. Appl Environ Microbiol. 1982;44:1349.
242. Ghosh AC. Prevalence of Bacillus cereus in the faeces of healthy adults. J Hyg (Lond). 1978;80:233.
243. De Buono BA, Brondum J, Kramer JM, et al. Plasmid, serotypic, and enterotoxin analysis of Bacillus cereus in an outbreak setting. J Clin Microbiol. 1988;26:1571–4.
244. Mansson I, Colldahl H. The intestinal flora in patients with bronchial asthma and rheumatoid arthritis: With special reference to Clostridium perfringens. Acta Allergy. 1965;20:94.
245. Akama K, Otani S. Clostridium perfringens as the flora in the intestine of healthy persons. Jpn J Med Sci Biol. 1970;23:161.
246. Hauschild AHW. Criteria and procedures for implicating Clostridium perfringens in food-borne outbreaks. Can J Public Health. 1975;66:388.
247. Stringer MF, Turnbull PCB, Gilbert RJ. Application of serological typing to the investigation of outbreaks of Clostridium perfringens food poisoning, 1970–1978. J Hyg (Lond). 1980;84:443.
248. Harmon SM, Kautter DA, Hatheway CL. Enumeration and characterization of Clostridium perfringens spores in the feces of food poisoning patients and normal controls. J Food Protection. 1986;49:23–8.
249. Watson GN, Stringer MF, Gilbert RJ, et al. The potential of bacteriocin typing in the study of Clostridium perfringens food poisoning. J Clin Pathol. 1982;35:1361.
250. Schiemann DA. Laboratory confirmation of an outbreak of Clostridium perfringens food poisoning. Health Lab Sci. 1977;14:35–8.
251. Harmon SM, Kautter DA. Evaluation of a reversed passive latex agglutination test kit for Clostridium perfringens enterotoxin. J Food Protection. 1986;49:523–5.
252. McClane BA, Strouse RJ. Rapid detection of Clostridium perfringens type A enterotoxin by enzyme-linked immunosorbent assay. J Clin Microbiol. 1984;19:112–5.
253. Birkhead G, Vogt RL, Heun EM, et al. Characterization of an outbreak of Clostridium perfringens food poisoning by quantitative fecal culture and fecal enterotoxin measurement. J Clin Microbiol. 1988;26:471–4.
254. Hatheway CL, Whaley DN, Dowell VR Jr. Epidemiological aspects of Clostridium perfringens foodborne illness. Food Technol. 1980;34:77.
255. Taylor DN, Wachsmuth IK, Shangkuan YH. Salmonellosis associated with marijuana: A multistate outbreak traced by plasmid fingerprinting. N Engl J Med. 1982;306:1249.
256. Riley LW, Cohen ML. Plasmid profiles and Salmonella epidemiology. Lancet. 1982;1:573.
257. Rodriguez DC, Cameron DN, Puhr ND, et al. Comparison of plasmid profiles, phage types, and antimicrobial resistance patterns of Salmonella enteritidis isolates in the United States. J Clin Microbiol. 1992;30:854–7.
258. Wachsmuth IK, Evins GM, Fields PI, et al. The molecular epidemiology of cholera in Latin America. J Infect Dis. 1993;167:621–6.
259. March SB, Ratnam S. Latex agglutination test for detection of Escherichia coli serotype O157:H7. J Clin Microbiol. 1989;27:1675–7.
260. Murray B, Mathewson J, Dupont H, et al. Utility of oligodeoxyribonucleotide probes for detecting enterotoxigenic Escherichia coli. J Infect Dis. 1987;155:809–11.
261. Guerrant RL, Brunton LL, Schnaitman TC, et al. Cyclic adenosine monophosphate and alteration of Chinese hamster ovary cell morphology: A rapid, sensitive in vitro assay for the enterotoxins of Vibrio cholerae and Escherichia coli. Infect Immun. 1974;10:320.
262. Svennerholm AM, Wiklund G. Rapid GMl-enzyme-linked immunosorbent assay with visual reading for identification of Escherichia coli heat-labile enterotoxin. J Clin Microbiol. 1983;17:596.
263. Honda T, Arita M, Takeda Y, et al. Further evaluation of the Biken test (modified Elek test) for detection of enterotoxigenic Escherichia coli producing heat-labile enterotoxin and application of the test to sampling of heat-stable enterotoxin. J Clin Microbiol. 1982;16:60.
264. Giannella RA. Suckling mouse model for detection of heat-stable Escherichia coli enterotoxin: Characteirstics of the model. Infect Immun. 1976;14:95.
265. Venkatesen M, Buysse J, Vandendries E, et al. Development and testing of invasion-associated DNA probes for detection of Shigella spp and enteroinvasive Escherichia coli. J Clin Microbiol. 1988;26:261–6.
266. Sereny B. Experimental Shigella keratoconjunctivitis: A preliminary report. Acta Microbiol Acad Sci Hung. 1955;2:293.
267. Jerse A, Martin W, Galen J, et al. Oligonucleotide probe for the detection of enteropathogenic Escherichia coli (EPEC) adherence factor of localized adherent EPEC. J Clin Microbiol. 1990;28:2842–4.
268. Dowell VR Jr, McCroskey LM, Hatheway CL, et al. Coproexamination for botulinal toxin and Clostridium botulinum. JAMA. 1977;238:1829.
269. Mann JM, Hatheway CL, Gardiner TM. Laboratory diagnosis in a large outbreak of type A botulism. Am J Epidemiol. 1982;115:598.
270. Kapikian AZ, Wyatt RG, Dolin R et al. Visualization by immune electron microscopy of a 27-nm particle associated with acute infectious nonbacterial gastroenteritis. J Virol. 1972;10:1075.
271. Gary GW Jr, Kaplan JE, Stine SE, et al. Detection of Norwalk virus antibodies and antigen with a biotin-avidin immunoassay. J Clin Microbiol. 1985;22:274–8.
272. Morris JG Jr. Ciguatera fish poisoning. JAMA. 1980;244:73.
273. Hokama Y, Abad MA, Kimura LH. A rapid enzyme-immunoassay for the detection of ciguatoxin in contaminated fish tissues. Toxicon. 1983;21:817–24.
274. Harris JC, DuPont HL, Hornick RB. Fecal leukocytes in diarrheal illness. Ann Intern Med. 1972;76:697.
275. Appleton H, Pereira MS. A possible virus etiology in outbreaks of foodpoisoning from cockles. Lancet. 1977;1:780.
276. Guerrant RL, Dickens MD, Wenzel RP, et al. Toxigenic bacterial diarrhea: Nursery outbreak involving multiple bacterial strains. J Pediatr. 1976;89:885.
277. Wadström T, Aust-Kettis A, Habte D, et al. Enterotoxin-producing bacteria and parasites in stools of Ethiopian children with diarrhoeal disease. Arch Dis Child. 1976;51:865.
278. Klipstein FA, Engert RF. Purification and properties of Klebsiella pneumoniae heat-stable enterotoxin. Infect Immun. 1976;13:373.
279. Klipstein FA, Engert RF. Partial purification and properties of Enterobacter cloacae heat-stable enterotoxin. Infect Immun. 1976;13:1307.
280. Salazar-Lindo E, Sack RB, Chea-Woo E, et al. Early treatment with erythromycin of Campylobacter jejuni–associated dysentery in children. J Pediatr. 1986;109:355–60.
281. Swift AEB, Swift TR. Ciguatera. Clin Toxicol. 1993;31:1–29.
282. Lange WR, Kreider SD, Hatwick M, et al. Potential benefit of tocainide in the treatment of ciguatera: Report of three cases. Am J Med. 1988;84:1087–8.
283. Mitchel DH. Amanita mushroom poisoning. Ann Rev Med. 1980;31:51.
284. Dupont HL. How safe is the food we eat? JAMA. 1992;268:3240.
285. Cruickshank JG, Humphrey TJ. The carrier food-handler and non-typhoid salmonellosis. Epidemiol Infect. 1987;98:223–30.
286. Jordan MC, Powell KE, Corothers TE, et al. Salmonellosis among restaurant patrons: The incisive role of a meat slicer. Am J Public Health. 1973;63:982.
287. Chin J. Raw milk: A continuing vehicle for the transmission of infectious disease agents in the United States. J Infect Dis. 1982;146:440.
288. Potter ME, Kauffman AF, Blake PA, et al. Unpasteurized milk: The hazards of a health fetish. JAMA. 1984;252:2048–52.
289. Horwitz MA, Marr JS, Merson MH, et al. A continuing common-source outbreak of botulism in a family. Lancet. 1975;2:861.
290. Payne DJH, Scudamore JM. Outbreaks of salmonella food poisoning over a period of eight years from a common source. Lancet. 1977;1:1249.
291. Centers for Disease Control and Prevention. Update: Multistate outbreak of Escherichia coli O157:H7 infections from hamburgers—Western United States, 1992–1993. MMWR. 1993;42:258–63.

82. TROPICAL SPRUE

CHRISTINE A. WANKE
RICHARD L. GUERRANT

Tropical sprue, also called *postinfectious tropical malabsorption,* is a syndrome of enigmatic etiology that is characterized by a prolonged diarrheal illness and malabsorption of two or more substances in individuals in the tropics who have no other obvious reason to malabsorb. Tropical sprue has been recognized since the second or third century AD, when Aretaeus of Cappadocchia reported on "The Coeliac Affection." The first mention of sprue in the modern medical literature was in 1747, when Dr. William Hillary emigrated from England to Barbados and published his observations on a prolonged tropical diarrheal disease in native islanders. The English term *sprue* is an adaptation from the Dutch *sprouw,* which was originally used to refer to persistent diarrheal disease in Holland, which was probably coeliac disease. The term *sprue* was first used in 1880 by Manson for the persistent wasting diarrhea that occurred in tropical countries.[1] Knowledge about the etiology or pathogenesis of sprue did not advance significantly until investigations were begun after recognized outbreaks during the World War II. The distinction between coeliac sprue and tropical sprue was not truly clear until the early 1970s.

EPIDEMIOLOGY

While sprue is considered a disease of tropical locales, there are distinct geographic areas of risk within the tropics. Tropical sprue has been most readily identified in Asia and the Caribbean islands, and there are isolated areas of particular risk within both hemispheres. Sprue is relatively common among the indigenous populations of Puerto Rico, Haiti, the Dominican Republic, and Cuba, but it is not seen in the rest of the Caribbean islands and is no longer recognized in Barbados.[2,3] It is seen in northern South America, in Venezuela and Columbia, but rarely in Central America or Mexico. It is common on the Indian subcontinent, from the Himalayas to the south; it has been recognized in Mayanmar and the Philippines.[4–6] Surprisingly, little tropical sprue had been documented in Africa until the 1970s; at present, cases have been recognized in Rhodesia and South Africa, and tropical sprue has developed in expatriates living in Nigeria.[7] There may be endemic foci of tropical sprue in the Middle East as well, with a spruelike illness recognized in Turkey.

Unlike other endemic diarrheal illnesses in the tropical world, tropical sprue is a disease mainly of adults. Children have been thought to be relatively spared, although clearly disease has been documented in all age groups. Very young children have not developed tropical sprue; this may be due to beneficial effects of breast-feeding. In studies of family outbreaks of tropical sprue in South India, even older children developed disease at a significantly lower rate than adults.[8] The reason for this is not clear. Certainly persistent diarrhea develops in children more commonly in the less developed parts of the world. Tropical sprue may be one of the etiologies of prolonged diarrhea and wasting in this age group as well, but etiologic studies such as small bowel intubation and cultures or biopsy have been hampered by the difficulty in obtaining adequate control specimens for comparison.

Some patterns of disease expression are of particular interest in tropical sprue. There are clear epidemics of tropical sprue, which have been best documented in families and villages in South India.[8] There have been descriptions of sprue houses, in which successive tenants have developed disease, and an outbreak was described in which over half of the exposed individuals in an isolated extended family developed tropical sprue within 3 months of the onset of disease in the index case. Well-documented outbreaks of sprue affecting entire villages have also been reported, mostly from the Indian subcontinent. Such an epidemic pattern suggests an underlying infectious etiology.

There has been a seasonal variation in outbreaks of tropical sprue as well. An increased rate of mild tropical sprue in the setting of an increased rate of diarrheal disease was seen more often in the period from March to July than at other times of the year for at least 4 years at an American military base in the Philippines.[6] In these outbreaks, sprue occurred among American military personnel and their dependents, who were eating a well-balanced Western style diet. A seasonal variation has also been documented in the rate of occurrence of tropical sprue in the indigenous population of Puerto Rico.[3] Such a seasonal variation also lends credence to the possibility of an underlying infectious etiology.

As suggested by the above-mentioned outbreaks in American military personnel, tropical sprue develops in expatriates living in endemic areas.[9] Tropical sprue was originally recognized in expatriates and British colonists in India in the early nineteenth century and subsequently in the Dutch in Java, the French in Indochina, and Americans in the Philippines, Vietnam, and Puerto Rico. Tropical sprue or malabsorption with jejunitis ("tropical enteropathy") has been described in Peace Corps volunteers and has occurred sporadically in travelers.[10] Generally tropical sprue develops in an expatriate who has lived for a prolonged time, 6 months to 1 year, in an endemic area. Rare cases have been described in short-term travelers as well.[11] Tropical sprue is also recognized in immigrants who leave endemic areas, although they may not complain of gastrointestinal symptoms until they have been out of the endemic area for prolonged periods.[12,13] These exposure data also suggest an infectious etiology for tropical sprue.

ETIOLOGY

There is a strong presumption that tropical sprue is caused by an enteric infection. The facts lending support to this theory include *(1)* often the prolonged episode of tropical sprue is initiated by an episode of acute diarrheal disease; *(2)* there is an epidemic and seasonal nature to the epidemiology of the disease, as discussed above; and *(3)* the disease responds most often to treatment with antibiotics. The precise nature of the infection that leads to development of tropical sprue is less clear.

Multiple studies in Asia and the Caribbean have demonstrated small bowel bacterial overgrowth in patients with tropical sprue.[10,14,15] While some bacteria normally live in the upper small bowel of healthy individuals, the organisms isolated from this region of the gut in healthy asymptomatic individuals are most often gram positive. Streptococci, staphylococci and lactobacilli are among the common isolates, and these are present in small numbers. In the distal small bowel, the cecum, and colon, anaerobes and gram-negative organisms predominate in normal individuals. Small bowel cultures done in travelers with tropical sprue have demonstrated increased numbers of gram-negative rods, including Alcaligenes, *Enterobacter aerogenes,* and *Hafnia* spp. in the small bowel. In small bowel cultures done in individuals with tropical sprue native to India, Haiti, or Puerto Rico, *Klebsiella, E. coli,* and *Enterobacter cloacae* were the most common organisms. However, carefully done studies in South Africa and India have also documented similar organisms in similar concentrations in the small bowel of asymptomatic control patients as well as patients with tropical sprue, suggesting that environmental contamination may predispose to increased small bowel flora. In another series of patients from India, the numbers of organisms found in the small bowel of tropical sprue patients was the same as that found in the small bowel of healthy controls, but the type of organisms isolated varied.[14] Other organisms, especially *Enterobacter* and *Veillonella* were isolated more frequently from the small bowels of patients with tropical sprue than from healthy controls.[16] Gram-negative organisms isolated from the small bowels of tropical sprue patients in Haiti were found to have a secretory effect, presumably by toxin production, in rabbit ileal loops and rat perfusion studies.[17,18] These supposedly enterotoxigenic organisms have not been studied for the presence of any of the recognized secretory toxins by currently available methodology such as DNA probes or ELISA; nor have these organisms been studied for the presence of colonizing factors, such as pili or the hydophobic surface proteins that are found in many enteric pathogens. *Escherichia coli* and *Klebsiella* isolated from Indian patients with tropical sprue were not found to produce heat-stable or heat-labile enterotoxins when they were tested.[19] Other in vivo data have suggested that small bowel overgrowth by nonpathogenic, nontoxigenic *E. coli* can produce a secretory diarrheal syndrome if the level of colonization by these organisms reaches a high enough concentration within the small bowel.[20,21]

The presence of bacteria in the small bowel may potentiate the symptoms caused by the small bowel parasite *Giardia lamblia,* and the interaction of small bowel bacteria and parasites has been considered as a possible etiology for tropical sprue.[22] Infections with hookworm or *Strongyloides stercoralis* have also been discussed as a possible etiology for tropical sprue. Reports of tropical sprue occurring in the setting of the presence of orthomyxovirus or corona virus particles in the stool have also appeared in the literature. Cases of tropical sprue have been reported after an intestinal infection with either fungus or the blue green algae prototheca,[23,24] but the present definition of tropical sprue excludes those patients with diarrhea on the basis of recognized pathogens.

That small bowel overgrowth, as it occurs spontaneously in a certain segment of the population in the less developed countries or after an acute enteric infection, may precipitate a series of intestinal insults that proceed to full-blown tropical sprue in susceptible individuals is at present the most likely etiologic explanation for tropical sprue. The predisposition for progression from intestinal insult to tropical sprue is less easy to explain. Malnutrition may be a predisposing factor, but is neither necessary nor sufficient as demonstrated by the occurrence of tropical sprue in well-nourished military personnel and their dependents. Small bowel overgrowth may alter intestinal transit time and promote further overgrowth and intestinal stasis, but cannot explain the initial colonization that induces the episode. In vitro data suggest that small bowel colonization by *Escherichia coli* may be increased by low levels of cytokines, as might be expected in chronic parasitic infections in the developing world, but this does not explain the occurrence of sprue in the traveler or uninfested expatriate.[25] There has been no genetic predisposition noted for tropical sprue as there has been for coeliac sprue.

The processes that control the normal colonization of the small bowel are not well understood; therefore, the forces that may disrupt these normal processes to permit abnormal colonization are even less well understood. However, some of the factors that may affect the normal small bowel colonization process include gastric acidity, which controls the entry of viable organisms into the small bowel; and intestinal mucin glycoprotein, which contains receptors for and specifically binds a variety of bacteria within the small bowel lumen.[26] *Helicobacter pylori,* for example, may impair gastric acidity and thereby predispose to small bowel colonization or persistent diarrhea.[27,28] Bacterial binding to mucin is presumed to promote clearance of pathogenic organisms to protect the small bowel, but may promote colonization by nonpathogenic organisms or may promote small bowel colonization by pathogens when the mucin is damaged by malnutrition, an inflammatory process, or bacterial proteases or mucinases. Some loss of the protective mucin layer in tropical sprue is suggested by data from biopsy specimens obtained from patients with tropical sprue that demonstrate that the bacteria visualized are often tightly associated within the mucosa rather than being free within the lumen of the gut.[1] Damage to the protective mucin layer may also permit epithelial cell damage by food or other small bowel antigens. The presence of free bile acids within the upper small bowel can alter intestinal bacterial growth rates and colonization, but bile acid concentrations have not been abnormal in patients with tropical sprue, and the bacterial organisms that have been cultured from patients with tropical sprue are not those that classically alter bile salt metabolism.[19]

Intestinal immunologic dysfunction has been suggested as a factor that might predispose to abnormal bacterial colonization in tropical sprue. Patients with deficiencies of secretory IgA are subject to more frequent and severe bouts of enteric infections. In addition to secretory IgA there is lymphoid tissue present throughout the small bowel focally in Peyer's patches and diffusely as mucosal lymphocytes. When small bowel lymphocytes were characterized in patients with tropical sprue and in control patients with irritable bowel syndrome in southern India, there was no difference in the number of IgA-, IgG-, or IgM-producing lymphocytes between the two groups.[29,30] Patients with sprue were noted to have increased numbers of lymphocytes in the crypt epithelium, with a higher percentage of immunoblasts and a higher mitotic index.[31] These data can be interpreted as evidence that lymphoid activation does occur in tropical sprue but that it is likely secondary to whatever primary process institutes tropical sprue rather than being an inciting process itself.

It has also been postulated that dietary fat might play a role in the etiology of tropical sprue. Similar to the permissive effect of protein ingestion in the pathogenesis of pig bel, the intake of long chain fatty acids has been studied as a potential etiologic factor for tropical sprue.[32] The seasonal epidemic occurrence of tropical sprue in Puerto Rico immediately follows a traditional holiday feast of pork, which is rich in long chain fatty acids.[33] There are several mechanisms by which these long chain fatty acids might contribute to the production of clinical tropical sprue. Long chain fatty acids can alter intestinal motility and delay intestinal transit time. Plasma levels of enteroglucagon and motilin are significantly elevated in patients with tropical sprue; motilin slows gastric emptying and enteroglucagon slows intestinal transit.[34] Intubation studies have demonstrated that intestinal infusions of fat increase plasma enteroglucagon levels and decrease intestinal motor activity. Fat within the gut lumen also inhibits both the mucosal sodium-potassium and magnesium ATPases, which can contribute to malabsorption of water and electrolytes in the intestine as well as raise the pH of the mucosal microenvironment.[32,35] The elevated mucosal pH produced by intestinal fats has also been associated with increased growth of gram-negative bacteria in the lumen of the small bowel.[11,36]

The elevation of mucosal pH and the presence of fatty acids within the lumen of the gut may also impair the ability of the intestine to absorb folate; folate deficiency may then potentiate the intestinal dysfunction that precedes it.[37] Folate deficiency leads to a decreased number of gut epithelial cells, as assessed by DNA concentrations, and to villus atrophy. Additional structural alterations are seen in the intestine with folate deficiency; these include crypt hypertrophy, villus blunting, and megaloblastic changes in the epithelial cells. These changes are somewhat nonspecific and are similar to those seen with vitamin B_{12} deficiency as well as those seen with tropical sprue. Functionally the folate deficient gut is less efficient in absorbing water, electrolytes, and carbohydrates than the normal small bowel.[38] It is likely that whatever the initial insult to the gut may be in tropical sprue, the resulting folate malabsorption and deficiency contributes to the further pathogenesis of disease (Fig. 1).

CLINICAL MANIFESTATIONS

The classic clinical features of tropical sprue are nonspecific and simply reflect the symptoms of malabsorption. These symptoms

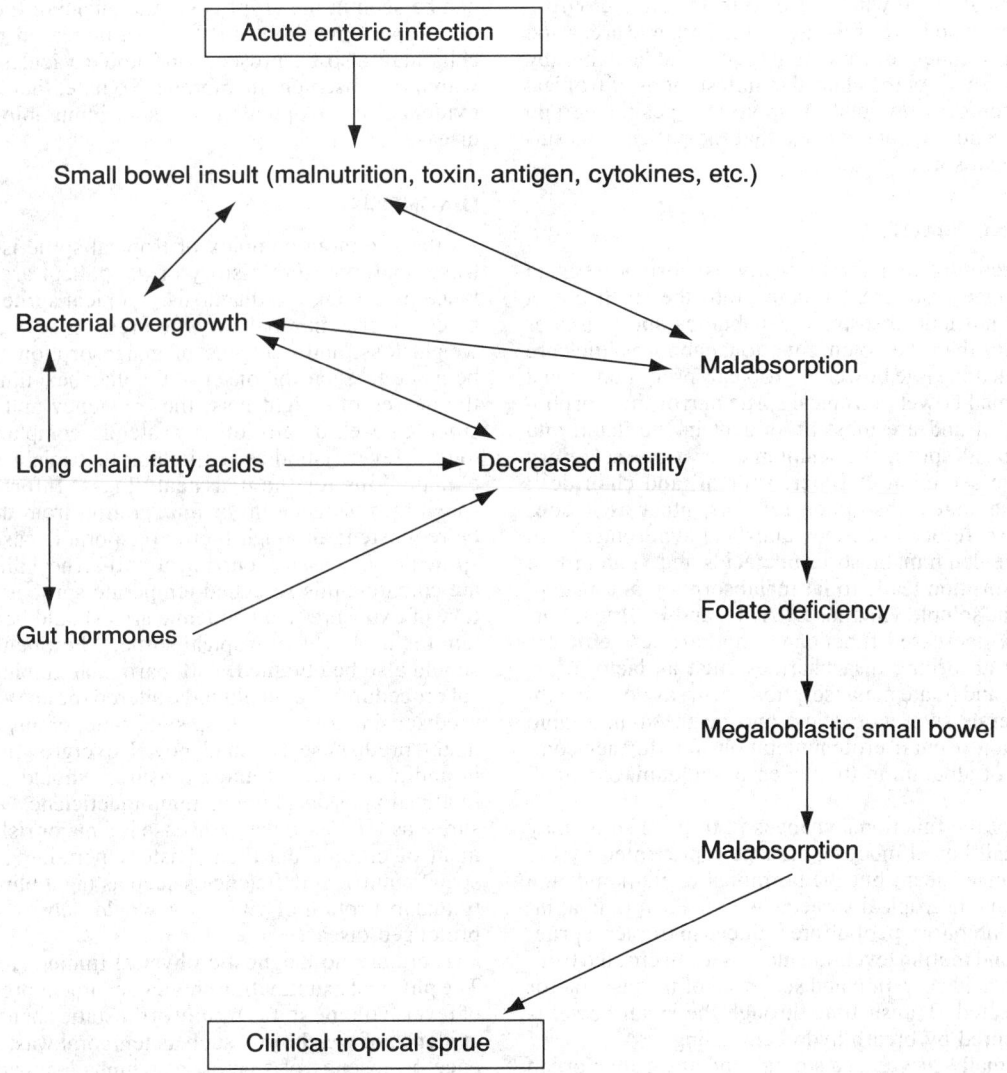

FIG. 1. Proposed pathogenesis of tropical sprue. The complex vicious cycle of small bowel insult that may result in bacterial overgrowth and malabsorption and further small bowel damage by luminal long chain fatty acids and dysregulation of intestinal hormones is likely the mechanism that promotes disease in susceptible individuals with an acute enteric infection.

include prolonged diarrhea, abdominal cramping, and anorexia, with or without nausea and secondary weight loss. Other associated although less common symptoms also related to the malabsorption of nutrients and subsequent malnutrition include peripheral edema, glossitis, stomatitis, and dermatitis.[11,12] Fever may occur at the onset of diarrhea (especially in Asia), and, although the presence of fever has been suggested as a means to distinguish Caribbean from Asian sprue, this distinction has not been consistently observed. Fever rarely persists for the course of disease, which may span months to years. Signs and symptoms related to anemia may also occur; pallor and weakness are most common early in disease. Later in the course of tropical sprue, peripheral neuropathy, confusion, and, if the anemia is severe enough, congestive symptoms reflecting high output failure may occur.

Many individuals can pinpoint the onset of disease; tropical sprue rarely has an insidious onset and is far more often associated with an obvious acute episode of diarrhea that then becomes prolonged. Individuals with tropical sprue may recall other people with similar acute illnesses or being exposed to someone with an acute illness just prior to developing disease themselves. As the operative definition of tropical sprue implies that the function of the gut was normal prior to the development of tropical sprue, ideally the alteration of bowel habits from a

normal pattern by the inciting episode of acute diarrheal disease should be notable. In practice, especially in the developing world, the distinction between normal and abnormal bowel habits may not be so clear.

Patients describe crampy abdominal pain, multiple soft or loose stools daily often with mucus, and the exacerbation of symptoms with food consumption. Patients may also complain of nausea and bloating, which lead to decreased appetite and decreased oral intake. The precise presentation of a patient with tropical sprue depends on the duration of illness and the extent of malabsorption.

Malabsorption of specific nutrients may lead to other symptoms and syndromes.[39] Lactose intolerance often develops early in the course of tropical sprue. The anemia of tropical sprue is most often macrocytic and related to vitamin B_{12} and folate malabsorption. Iron deficiency may also occur, again related to malabsorption and turn a macrocytic anemia into a normocytic anemia. Impaired absorption of calcium, vitamin D, and magnesium may occur, with resulting osteopenia.[40] Patients with tropical sprue also malabsorb fats and, depending on the severity of fat malabsorption, may complain of bulky, floating, or foul smelling stools.

Spontaneous recovery may occur, but this is not inevitable. Spontaneous recovery is more common in travelers to areas endemic for tropical sprue who return to their native environments. Individuals who have emigrated from endemic areas and individuals living in endemic areas often require medical therapy to alleviate symptoms. As the clinical manifestations of tropical sprue are nonspecific, symptomatic response to specific therapy can be considered additional evidence that the patient was suffering from tropical sprue.

INTESTINAL ABNORMALITIES

Although the secretory and malabsorptive syndrome seen in tropical sprue suggest preferential damage to the small bowel that has greater nutrient absorptive capabilities and a greater secretory capacity than the colon, functional abnormalities are seen in both small and large bowels in tropical sprue. Functional changes in the small bowel in tropical sprue mirror the morphologic changes seen and are most prominent in the ileum and jejunum. In tropical sprue, the jejunum is in a net secretory state, with active secretion of water, sodium, and chloride[41]; however, glucose-linked absorption remains intact as it does for many other secretory infectious diarrheal syndromes.[42] In tropical sprue the ileum malabsorbs bile acids and vitamin B_{12}. Bile acid malabsorption leads to fat malabsorption and malabsorption of the fat-soluble vitamins D, A, K, and E. Brush border enzymes are decreased functionally and are less efficient in digesting and absorbing disaccharides such as lactose.[43,44] Xylose, glucose, and folate malabsorption occur, as does malabsorption of minerals such as calcium and magnesium. Amino acid malabsorption occurs; protein metabolism is further complicated by loss of albumin in the lumen of the damaged small bowel.[45]

The majority of the functional changes in tropical sprue may be related to small bowel mucosal damage represented by the morphologic changes seen, but the hormonal regulation of the gut is dysfunctional in tropical sprue as well.[46] Postprandial insulin and gastric inhibitory peptide are reduced in tropical sprue; enteroglucagon and motilin levels are increased. In chronic tropical sprue gastric acid secretion and secretion of intrinsic factor may also be affected. Transit time through the small bowel is slowed, as measured by breath hydrogen testing.[47,48]

The colon normally serves as a storage and absorptive organ and normally absorbs 4–7 liters of water and 100–160 mmol of carbohydrate per day. In the few studies of colonic function that have been done in tropical sprue, the ability of the colon to absorb water is decreased in patients with tropical sprue as compared to controls. There is speculation that the dysfunction of colonic cells may be related to damage by excess fatty acids in the gut lumen or bacterial toxins or infection. While there is physiologic confirmation of the ability of fatty acids to disturb the absorptive function of colonocytes as well as small bowel enterocytes, data suggesting that colonic infections are of importance in the pathogenesis of tropical sprue are lacking.

MORPHOLOGY

Partial villus atrophy is the hallmark histologic change seen in the small bowel in tropical sprue, as opposed to the flattened mucosa that is characteristic of coeliac sprue.[49] The villi in tropical sprue progressively shorten and thicken, forming fused leaves after about 4 months of illness. These histologic changes are seen in the jejunum and the ileum, where the changes in absorption are localized as well. These histologic changes are not specific for tropical sprue, but might also be present in severe folate deficiency or with bacterial overgrowth.

Microscopically, the mucosa is thin, with an infiltrate of chronic inflammatory cells, consisting of plasma cells, histiocytes, lymphocytes, and eosinophils. As mentioned previously, these lymphocytes have been characterized, and IgA, IgG, and IgM lymphocytes are present in numbers equal to those of asymptomatic control patients.[29,30] An increased mitotic index

can be seen in the crypt cells; the nuclei of the crypt cells may also appear megaloblastic.[45,50] An increased number of goblet cells may also be present, and lipoid vacules have been seen within the basement membrane. To date, there is no convincing evidence that tropical sprue is an immunologically mediated disease.

DIAGNOSIS

As the symptom complex of tropical sprue is nonspecific, the travel and exposure history of the patient are of prime importance in making the diagnosis. Tropical sprue should certainly be considered in a patient who presents with chronic diarrhea, weight loss, and evidence of malabsorption. Attempts should be made to elicit the onset of the diarrheal illness, its duration, the degree of weight loss, the frequency and character of the stool, as well as any other systemic complaints such as prolonged fever, jaundice, or itching that might suggest alternate explanations for the diarrheal illness. Information regarding travel to, residence in, or immigration from the tropics should be requested; although there are sporadic case reports of mild sprue like illnesses occurring after diarrheal illnesses in temperate climates, this so-called temperate sprue is rare and the history of exposure to an endemic area should be present to entertain the diagnosis of tropical sprue.[33] Pertinent medical history should also be obtained, with particular emphasis on any surgical procedures that might have altered the anatomy of the bowel, predisposing to a blind loop syndrome, or any medications that might predispose to small bowel overgrowth. Social history, in addition to travel and exposures, should include questions relating to possible human immunodeficiency virus (HIV) exposures, as HIV-associated disease is a major risk for the development of chronic diarrhea. History pertaining to symptoms of specific nutrient deficiencies such as night blindness secondary to malabsorption of vitamin A would only be expected in very prolonged disease.

There are no diagnostic physical findings for tropical sprue. The physical examination should document presence or absence of fever, volume status by any orthostatic changes, body weight, evidence of weight loss such as temporal wasting, and the presence or absence of significant lymphadenopathy or abdominal masses. Hyperactive bowel sounds may be the only pertinent abdominal finding. Signs of anemia, such as pallor, are notoriously nonspecific, but can be looked for. Signs of specific nutrient deficiencies may also be present on physical examination: cheilosis, stomatitis, glossitis, rashes, dermatitis, koilonychia, muscle pain or weakness, peripheral neuropathy, or edema can suggest deficiencies of iron, zinc, vitamin B_{12}, folate, vitamins D and E, or protein. Deficiencies of any of these nutrients could be present in tropical sprue because of malabsorption by the damaged small bowel.

Laboratory evaluation of the patient suspected to have tropical sprue can be minimal or extensive, depending on the degree of suspicion and the urgency for diagnosis. A simple CBC demonstrating a macrocytic anemia in a high-risk patient in the appropriate clinical setting could be sufficient to proceed with other more confirmatory diagnostic tests such as a small bowel biopsy. A more complete laboratory evaluation would include serum vitamin B_{12} level and red blood cell folate levels, a serum carotene, or, preferably, a 72-hour fecal fat determination. Stool examination to exclude *Giardia* is very useful; stool culture looking for bacterial pathogens is less likely to be helpful in chronic diarrhea.

Ultimately, a small bowel series with small bowel followthrough showing flattened mucosal folds, luminal dilatation, or flocculation of the barium meal can be suggestive of tropical sprue.[51] An upper endoscopy with duodenal aspirate for parasites, biopsy, and quantitative small bowel culture, if available, can be diagnostic of tropical sprue in the appropriate clinical setting. Documentation of abnormal transit time by small bowel follow-through or breath hydrogen testing, which can also imply bacterial overgrowth, can be suggestive but not diagnostic of tropical sprue. The differential diagnosis that must be considered in a patient with chronic diarrhea, weight loss, and malabsorption, even in a clinical setting consistent with tropical sprue, should include giardiasis, cryptosporidiosis, coccidiosis (*Isosospora belli*), capillariasis, strongybidiasis coeliac sprue (gluten enteropathy), lymphoma, intestinal tuberculosis, the blind loop syndrome, pancreatic tumors, Whipple's disease, and microsporidia associated with HIV or HIV enteropathy.

TREATMENT

The treatment of tropical sprue with folate alone improves the symptoms of tropical sprue but does not cure the diarrhea. Combination therapy with tetracycline and folate seems to be most effective in symptom resolution and cure of diarrhea with promotion of weight gain.[52,53] Treatment with 250 mg of tetracycline four times a day and 5 mg of folate daily for 1 month has been effective in travelers with tropical sprue, but therapy must be prolonged for 6 months or more for residents of the tropics who have had long-term disease. Even with prolonged therapy, relapses have been seen in this population, although it is not possible to exclude the possibility that there has been reexposure to an infecting organism and recurrent rather than relapsing disease (54). Reports have suggested that tropical sprue in the Caribbean has been more amenable to therapy than has sprue in India, but these studies are difficult to compare.[51] Poorly absorbed sulfa drugs are an acceptable alternative to tetracycline in children or pregnant women.[55] A favorable symptomatic response to therapy with folate and antibiotics can provide additional evidence that tropical sprue was the etiology of chronic diarrhea and malabsorption in a patient; however, even this is not specific, as bacterial overgrowth in a blind loop syndrome would also be expected to respond.

REFERENCES

1. Bartholomew C. William Hillary and sprue in the Caribbean: 230 years later. Gut Festschr. 1989;17–21.
2. Klipstein FA, Samloff IM, Smarth G, Schenk EA. Treatment of overt and subclinical malabsorption in Haiti. Gut. 1969;10:315–22.
3. Klipstein FA, Corcino JJ. Seasonal occurrence of overt and subclinical tropical malabsorption in Puerto Rico. Am J Trop Med Hyg. 1974;23:1189–96.
4. Gorbach SL, Banwell JG, Jacobs B, Chatterjee BD. Tropical Sprue and malnutrition in West Bengal. Am J Clin Nutr. 1970;23:1515–58.
5. Mathan VI, Baker SJ. Epidemic tropical Sprue and other epidemics of diarrhea in South Indian villages. Am J Clin Nutr. 1968;21:1077–87.
6. Jones TC, Dean AG, Parker GW. Seasonal gastroenteritis and malabsorption at an American military base in the Phillipines. Am J Epdemiol. 1973;95:128–39.
7. Thomas G, Clain DJ, Wicks CB. Tropical enteropathy in Rhodesia. Gut. 1976;17:888:894.
8. Mathan VI, Ignatius M, Baker SJ. A household epidemic of tropical sprue. Gut. 1966;7:490.
9. Klipstein FA. Tropical Sprue in travelers and expatriates living abroad. Gastroenterology. 1981;80:590.
10. Lindenbaum J, Kent TH, Sprine H. Malabsorption and jejunitis in American Peace Corps volunteers in Pakistan. Ann Intern Med. 1966;65:1201.
11. Davis JS, Klipstein FA. Tropical sprue in visitor to Mexico. Lancet. 1985;454.
12. Klipstein FA, Falaiye JM. Tropical sprue in expatriates from the tropics living in the continental United States. Medicine. 1969;48:475.
13. Montgomery RD, Beale DJ, Sammons HG, Schneider R. Postinfective malabsorption: a sprue syndrome. Br Med J. 1973;2:265–8.
14. Appelbaum PC, Moshal MG, Hift W, Chatterton SA. Intestinal bacteria in patients with tropical sprue. S Afr Med J. 1980;57:1081.
15. Bhat P, Shantakumari S, Rajan D, et al. Bacterial flora of the gastrointestinal tract in southern Indian control subjects and patients with tropical sprue. Gastroenterology. 1972;62:11.
16. Tomkins AM, Drasbar BS, James WPT. Bacterial colonisation of jejunal mucosa in acute tropical sprue. Lancet. 1975;59.
17. Klipstein FA, Engert RF, Short HB. Enterotoxigenicity of colonising coliform bacteria in tropical sprue and blind-loop syndrome. Lancet. 1978;342.
18. Klipstein FA, Holdeman LV, Corcino JJ. Enterotoxigenic intestinal bacteria in tropical sprue. Ann Intern Med. 1973;79:632–41.
19. Ramakrishna BS, Mathan VI. Role of bacterial toxins, bile acids, and free fatty acids in colonic water malabsorption in tropical sprue. Dig Dis Sci. 1987;32:500–5.
20. Wanke CA, Guerrant RL. Small-bowel colonization alone is a cause of diarrhea. Infect Immun. 1987;55:1924–6.
21. Schlager TA, Wanke CA, Guerrant RL. Net fluid secretion and impaired villous function induced by colonization of the small intestine by non-toxigenic, colonizing E. coli. Infect Immun. 1990;58:1337–1343.
22. Tomkins AM, Wright SG, Drasbar BS, James WPT. Bacterial colonisation of jejunal mucosa in giardiasis. Trans R Soc Trop Med Hyg. 1978;72:33.
23. Klipstein FA, Schneider R. Prototheca and sprue. Gastroenterology. 1975;69:1372.
24. Swanson VL, Haley LD, Wheby MS. Mycological study of jejunal biopsy specimens from patients with tropical sprue. Am J Trop Med Hyg. 1965;14:1066.
25. Wanke CA, Cronan S, Bistrian B. Recombinant tumor necrosis factor alters the avidity of bacterial binding to small bowel mucin and the HT29 intestinal cell line (Abstract). In: Abstracts of the 31st Interscience Conference on Antimicrobial Agents and Chemotherapy, Chicago, IL, 1991; Abstract No. 40.
26. Wanke CA, Cronan S, Goss C, et al. Characterization of binding of Escherichia coli strains which are enteropathogens to small-bowel mucin. Infect Immun. 1990;58:794–800.
27. Graham D, Alpert L, Smith J, et al. Iatrogenic Campylobacter pylori infection is a cause of epidemic achlorhydria. Am J Gastroenterol. 1988;83:974.
28. Nurko SS, García-Aranda JA, Consuelo A, et al. Is Helicobacter pylori a significant risk factor for persistent diarrhea in Mexican children? Gastroenterology. 1993;104:A160.
29. Malik AK, Mehta SK, Chandrashekhar Y, et al. Quantitation of immunoglobin-containing cells in the jejunal lamina propria in tropical sprue. J Clin Gasterol. 1992;14:163–6.
30. Marsh MN. Functional and structural aspects of the epithelial lymphocyte, with implications for coeliac disease and tropical sprue. Scand J Gastroenterol. 1985;115:55–75.
31. Marsh MN, Mathan M, Mathan VI. Studies of intestinal lymphoid tissue. VII. The secondary nature of lymphoid cell "Activation" in the jejunal lesion of tropical sprue. Am J Pathol. 1983;112:302–12.
32. Tiruppathi C, Balasubramanian KA, Hill PG, Mathan VI. Faecal free fatty acids in tropical sprue and their possible role in the production of diarrhoea by inhibition of ATPases. Gut. 1983;24:300–5.
33. Glynn J. Tropical sprue—its aetiology and pathogenesis. J R Soc Med. 1986;79:599.
34. Cook GC. Aetiology and pathogenesis of postinfective tropical malabsorption (tropical sprue). Lancet. 1984;721.
35. Ramakrishna BS, Mathan VI. Absorption of water and sodium and activity of adenosine triphosphatases in the rectal mucusoa in tropical sprue. Gut. 1988;29:665–8.
36. Lucas ML, Mathan VI. Jejunal surface pH measurements in tropical sprue. Trans R Soc Trop Med Hyg. 1989;83:138–42.
37. Kesavan V, Noronha JM. An ATPase dependent, radio sensitive, acidic microclimate essential for folate absorption. J Physiol. 1978;280:1–7.
38. Davidson GP, Townley RRW. Structural and functional abnormalities of the small bowel due to nutritional folate deficiency in infancy. J Pediatr. 1977;90:590–4.
39. Chacko A, Begum A, Mathan VI. Absorption of nutrient energy in southern Indian control subjects and patients with tropical sprue. Am J Clin Nutr. 1984;40:771–5.
40. Haddock L, Vazquez MDC, Rivera R, Corcino J. The kinetics of D3–3H metabolism in tropical sprue. PR Health Sci J. 1985;4:47.
41. Tompkins A. Tropical malabsorption: recent concepts in pathogenesis and nutritional significance. Clin Sci. 1981;60:131–7.
42. Rolston DDK, Mathan VI. Jejunal and ileal glucose-stimulated water and sodium absorption in tropical enteropathy: implications for oral rehydration therapy. Digestion. 1990;46:55–60.
43. Batt RM, Bush BM, Peters TJ. Subcellular biochemical studies of a naturally occurring enteropathy in the dog resembling chronic tropical sprue in human beings. Am J Vet Res. 1993;44:1492.
44. Cook GC, Menzies IS. Intestinal absorption and unmediated permeation of sugars in post-infective tropical malabsorption (tropical sprue). Digestion. 1986;33:109–16.
45. Westergaard H. Southwestern Internal Medicine Conference: The sprue syndromes. Am J Med Sci. 1985;290:249–62.
46. Besterman HS, Cook GC, Sarson DL, et al. Gut hormones in tropical malabsorption. Br Med J. 1979;1252–5.
47. Cook GC. Delayed small-intestinal transit in tropical malabsorption. Br Med J. 1978;2:238–40.
48. Jayanthi V, Chacko A, Gani IK, Mathan VI. Intestinal transit in healthy southern Indian subjects and in patients with tropical sprue. Gut. 1989;30:35–8.
49. Tawil SC, Brandt LJ, Bernstein LH. Scalloping of the valvulae conniventes and mosaic mucosa in tropical sprue. Gastroenterology. 1991;37:365.
50. Mathan MM, Ponniah J, Mathan VI. Epithelial cell renewal and turnover and relationship to morphologic abnormalities in jejunal mucosa in tropical sprue. Dig Dis Sci. 1986;31:586–92.
51. Scully RE, Mark EJ, McNeely WF, McNeely BU. Weekly clinicopathologic exercises: Case 15–1990. N Engl J Med. 1990;322:1067–75.
52. Guerra R, Wheby MS, Bayless TM. Long-term antibiotic therapy in tropical sprue. Ann Intern Med. 1965;63:619.

53. Rickles FR, Klipstein FA, Tomasini J, Corcino JJ. Long-term follow-up of antibiotic-treated tropical sprue. Ann Intern Med. 1972;76:203–10.
54. Gerson CD, Kent TH, Saha JR, et al. Recovery of small-intestinal structure and function after residence in the tropics. II. Studies in Indians and Pakistanis living in New York City. Ann Intern Med. 1971;75:41–8.
55. Maldonado N, Horta E, Guerra R, Perez-Santiago H: Poorly absorbed sulfonamides in the treatment of tropical sprue. Gastroenterology. 1969;57:559.

83. WHIPPLE'S DISEASE

WILLIAM O. DOBBINS III

Whipple's disease, first described in 1907,[1] is a systemic bacterial illness affecting primarily middle-aged, white men. It is characterized morphologically by an infiltrate of macrophages that are intensely stained by the periodic acid–Schiff (PAS) stain in virtually all organ systems. There may be a subtle cell-mediated immune deficit that predisposes to the infection. Whipple organisms have all the structural characteristics of bacteria.[2–4] The organism has a unique 1321-base rRNA sequence and according to phylogenetic analysis is a gram-positive actinomycete not closely related to any known genus.[5] Its proposed name is *Tropheryma whippelii*.[5,6] This microorganism has not yet been cultured in vitro, and the disease has not been reproduced in animals. Most patients respond to treatment with antibiotics.

PATHOGENESIS AND PATHOLOGIC CHARACTERISTICS

Sieracki and Fine[7] first emphasized the presence of systemic involvement when they found characteristic PAS-positive macrophages in body tissues. The PAS reaction has a strong affinity for glycoproteins, and electron microscopic studies have shown that the rod-shaped masses found within macrophages are actually masses of intact and degenerating bacteria, the walls of which are apparently in part composed of glycoproteins.[3,4] Greatest involvement occurs in the lamina propria of the small intestine and its lymphatic drainage, in the heart (with valvular lesions being particularly prominent), and in the central nervous system (CNS).

Electron microscopic studies from many laboratories have documented the presence of bacilli in involved tissues,[3] both intracellularly and extracellularly. These bacilli have been remarkably uniform in appearance and are approximately 0.2 μm wide by 1.5–2.5 μm long (Fig. 1). The organism possesses a trilaminar plasma membrane that is surrounded by a homogeneous cell wall approximately 20 nm thick. The cell wall itself is enclosed within an outer trilaminar "membrane."[3] This latter feature is more characteristic of gram-negative bacilli. Tubules and vesicles are located centrally within the bacilli and resemble the mesosomes that are characteristic of gram-positive bacteria. Nucleoids can often be identified within the core of the bacilli. Binary fission is often present. The Whipple bacillus is present within a variety of cells, including macrophages, intestinal epithelial cells, lymphatic and capillary endothelial cells, smooth muscle cells, polymorphonuclear leukocytes, plasma cells, mast cells, and even intraepithelial lymphocytes.[8] The intracellular bacilli are often intact in structure, which suggests that these organisms may be intracellular pathogens.[4] Immunofluorescence studies have shown that the material found within macrophages has a strong antigenic similarity to material found within streptococci groups B and G.

Because the disease has not been reproduced in laboratory animals and because the organism has not been convincingly cultured in vitro, the only sure method to detect Whipple's dis-

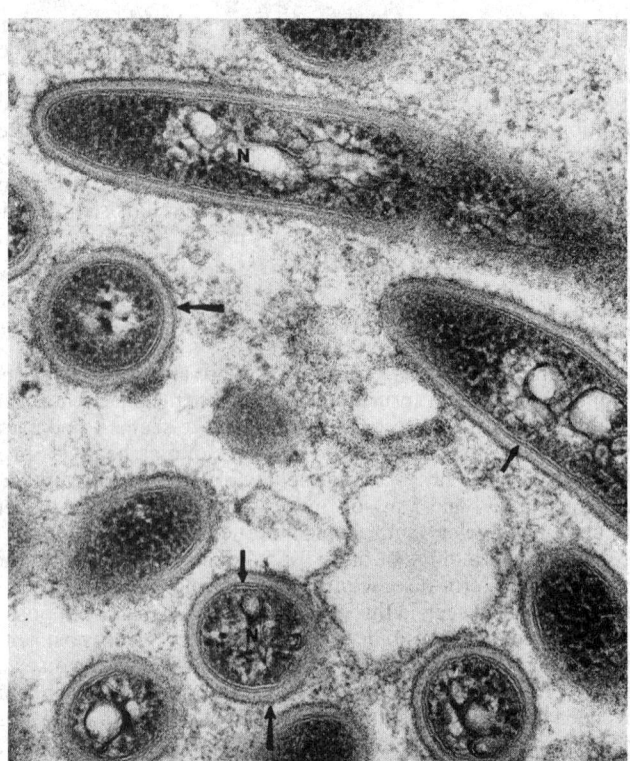

FIG. 1. Electron micrograph showing the characteristic appearance of the Whipple bacilli, many of which have been cut obliquely. These bacilli are up to 0.25 μm wide and, when sectioned lengthwise, up to 2.5 μm long. The nucleoid (N) is enclosed within a typical trilaminar plasma membrane (small arrows). A homogeneous cell wall about 20 nm thick surrounds the plasma membrane, and the cell wall itself is surrounded by a less well characterized "membrane," which has a trilaminar appearance (large arrows). The bacilli have electron microscopic characteristics, therefore, of both gram-positive and gram-negative bacilli. (× 100,000)

ease is the structural characteristic of the organism as seen by electron microscopy and possibly its antigenic structure as defined by immunofluorescence staining. Now its molecular genetic structure can be detected by polymerase chain reaction,[6,9] and this can be used for diagnosis.

Microscopic pathology in the proximal small intestine shows the presence of typical club-shaped villi containing PAS-positive macrophages. The macrophages are found chiefly in the gastrointestinal tract, the mesenteric and retroperitoneal nodes, the heart, and the CNS. Occasional involvement has been found in the lungs, spleen, pancreas, and peripheral lymph nodes. Minimal changes have been noted in the genitourinary tract, adrenals, joints, skin, bone marrow, and skeletal muscle.

There is evidence supporting the presence of cell-mediated immune deficiency in patients with Whipple's disease. Even after successful treatment, the cutaneous response to antigens and the responsiveness of lymphocytes to nonspecific mitogens, although improved, are subnormal. There may be an increased association with HLA-B27 (28 percent of Whipple's patients and 10 percent of healthy people).[10]

CLINICAL AND LABORATORY FINDINGS

The patient is typically a middle-aged white man with a history of intermittent arthralgia involving multiple joints over a period of years.[11] The actual illness develops gradually, with diarrhea followed by the development of steatorrhea, weight loss, and finally a progressive downhill course. Rarely, there is no diarrhea, and the illness is characterized by nondescript abdominal pain and low-grade fever. Arthralgias may appear 10–30 years before the development of gastrointestinal symptoms and are usually migratory. Usually the large joints are most prominently involved.

Evidence of weight loss is usual. The abdomen is often distended and tender to palpation, and abdominal nodes may be palpable. Hypotension is often present, and hyperpigmentation of the skin is found in 50 percent of patients. Fever is usually low grade, but on occasion spiking temperatures to 103°F are present. Peripheral lymphadenopathy is often present. Cardiac murmurs (often with marantic endocarditis) have been noted in 25 percent of patients. Ascites is uncommon, and splenomegaly and hepatomegaly occur in less than 5 percent of patients. All of the manifestations of advanced malabsorption may be present in those patients diagnosed late in their clinical course. Neurologic abnormalities are often present and include ophthalmoplegia, dementia, ataxia, myoclonus, hyperreflexia, paresis, and sensory changes such as hearing loss and visual disturbances. The patient may present with neurologic and personality changes as the initial manifestation in the absence of significant gastrointestinal signs or symptoms.[12–14] Exceedingly rarely, Whipple's disease of the CNS has been reported in the absence of involvement of the gastrointestinal tract.

Laboratory findings include a normocytic, normochromic anemia in 90 percent of the patients. Occasional patients have iron deficiency. Megaloblastic anemia is rare. The white blood cell count is usually not elevated, and the differential count is usually normal. Hypoalbuminenia, hypocholesterolemia, hypokalemia, and prolonged prothrombin times are usually present. Steatorrhea is present in 93 percent and decreased D-xylose absorption in 78 percent of patients, whereas decreased vitamin B_{12} absorption is found in only 15 percent of patients.[11]

DIAGNOSIS

Whipple's disease should be suspected in people with the four most prominent symptoms—weight loss, diarrhea, arthralgia, and abdominal pain.[11] If the arthralgias precede the other symptoms, the diagnosis deserves very serious consideration. Histologically, the most severe and consistent changes are seen in the proximal small intestine. Thus, small bowel biopsy is the diagnostic procedure of choice. Rarely, the intestinal mucosa will contain numerous macrophages in patients with diffuse histoplasmosis and in patients with acquired immune deficiency syndrome (AIDS). Macrophages found in these diseases are distinguished from those found in Whipple's disease by using special stains for *Histoplasma capsulatum* in histoplasmosis and for intracellular *Mycobacterium avium* in AIDS.

PAS-positive macrophages can also be found in most tissues from healthy subjects. This is particularly true in the rectal and colonic mucosa. PAS-positive macrophages in the small intestinal mucosa but not in other tissues are unique and may be considered diagnostic. It is helpful to have electron microscopic confirmation of the presence of the characteristic Whipple bacilli, although these bacilli can be seen by light microscopy in properly prepared specimens.[15]

Occasionally, biopsy specimens of a lymph node or other tissue may permit the diagnosis, but this requires electron microscopic or polymerase chain reaction confirmation.[6,16] Brain biopsy specimens have been used to establish the diagnosis in the rare person with CNS Whipple's disease in the absence of intestinal involvement.[13]

TREATMENT

Antibiotics are the treatment of choice, and good responses to a variety of antibiotics have been reported.[17–19] The appropriate duration of therapy is unclear, but, because occasional patients have had a relapse after several weeks to a few months of treatment, antibiotics should be given for 1 year.[11,17–19]

Initial treatment should consist of one double-strength tablet of trimethoprimsulfamethoxazole (TMP/SMX) given twice daily for 1 year. TMP/SMX penetrates the blood-brain barrier well. Indeed, two patients who presented with CNS Whipple's disease have responded to treatment with TMP/SMX.[17,18] If the patient is severely ill, the double-strength tablet may be given three times per day for 2 weeks and then given twice daily for 1 year. Folic acid deficiency is a potential complication of such therapy, especially in a malnourished individual. Folinic acid in a dose of 3 mg twice weekly should prevent this complication and should be administered routinely during the 2-week period that patients are given three double-strength tablets on a daily basis.

In the patient allergic to or unable to tolerate sulfonamides, treatment with oral penicillin (penicillin V, 250 mg four times per day) for 1 year is recommended. Reed et al.[19] elected to treat their patient initially with high doses (20 million units per 24 hours) of penicillin for 30 days because of the suspicion of subclinical cerebral involvement. Because patients with Whipple's disease may be severely malnourished, folate, vitamin B_{12}, vitamin K, iron, and other dietary supplements may be beneficial.

The duration of therapy should not be determined by the presence or absence of PAS-positive macrophages within the intestinal lamina propria. The macrophages may persist within the lamina propria for many years after successful treatment, whereas free bacilli clear very rapidly and have never been reported to persist longer than 9 weeks after the initiation of treatment. Routine follow-up intestinal biopsies are thus not necessary. However, it is becoming apparent that many successfully treated patients will develop a clinical relapse years after treatment, with or without intestinal symptoms.[18] Thus, all treated patients should be followed up by careful clinical evaluation on a yearly basis. If a relapse is suspected, then intestinal biopsy specimens should be obtained and the presence or absence of free bacilli determined. An empirical trial of antibiotics may still be appropriate.

Treatment for relapse is the same as that outlined for initial therapy. If a patient with CNS relapse fails to respond to oral TMP/SMX, treatment with oral chloramphenicol, 1 g/day (250 mg qid) for 6–12 months, is indicated. Chloramphenicol, like TMP/SMX, results in a relatively high CNS concentration of the drug. One patient with a CNS relapse responded partially to treatment for 30 days with intravenous ceftriaxone, 2 g twice a day.[20] Failure of the patient with non-CNS relapse to respond to TMP/SMX may require trials of oral penicillin (penicillin V, 250 mg four times per day) or oral tetracycline (250 mg four times per day).

REFERENCES

1. Whipple GH. A hitherto undescribed disease characterized anatomically by deposits of fat and fatty acids in the intestinal and mesenteric lymphatic tissues. Johns Hopkins Hosp Bull. 1907;18:382.
2. Dobbins WO III. Whipple's Disease. Springfield, IL: Charles C Thomas; 1987.
3. Silva MT, Macedo PM, Moura Nunes JF. Ultrastructure of bacilli and the bacillary origin of the macrophage inclusions in Whipple's disease. J Gen Microbiol. 1985;131:1001.
4. Dobbins WO III, Kawanishi H. Bacillary characteristics in Whipple's disease: An electron microscopic study. Gastroenterology. 1981;80:1468.
5. Relman DA, Schmidt TM, MacDermott RP, Falkow S. Identification of the uncultured bacillus of Whipple's disease. N Engl J Med. 1992;327:293.
6. Donaldson RM Jr. Whipple's disease—Rare malady with uncommon potential. N Engl J Med. 1992;327:346.
7. Sieracki JC, Fine G. Whipple's disease: Observation on systemic involvement. I. Gross and histologic observation. Arch Pathol. 1959;67:81.
8. Austin LL, Dobbins WO III. Intraepithelial leucocytes of the intestinal mucosa in normal man and in Whipple's disease: A light and electron microscopic study. Dig Dis Sci. 1982;27:311.
9. Relman DA, Falkow S, Dobbins WO III, et al. *Tropheryma whippelii* gen. nov. sp. nov., the causative agent of Whipple's disease. 1994. Submitted for publication.
10. Dobbins WO III. HLA antigens in Whipple's disease. Arthritis Rheum. 1987; 30:102.
11. Maizel H, Ruffin JM, Dobbins WO III. Whipple's disease. A review of 19

patients from one hospital and review of the literature since 1950. Medicine (Baltimore) 1970;49:175.

12. Finelli PF, McEntee WJ, Lessel S, et al. Whipple's disease with predominantly neuroophthalmic manifestations. Ann Neurol. 1977;1:247.

13. Johnson L, Diamond I. Cerebral Whipple's disease: Diagnosis by brain biopsy. Am J Clin Pathol. 1979;74:486.

14. Schmitt BP, Richardson H, Smith E, et al. Encephalopathy complicating Whipple's disease. Ann Intern Med. 1981;94:51.

15. Trier JS, Phelps PC, Eidelman S, et al. Whipple's disease: Light and electron microscope correlation of jejunal mucosal histology with antibiotic treatment and clinical status. Gastroenterology 1965;48:684.

16. Mansbach CM II, Shelburne FA, Stevens RD, et al. Lymph node bacilliform bodies resembling those of Whipple's disease in a patient without intestinal involvement. Ann Intern Med. 1978;89:64.

17. Keinath RD, Merrell DE, Vlietstra R, et al. Antibiotic treatment and relapse in Whipple's disease: Long-term follow up of 88 patients. Gastroenterology. 1985;88:1867.

18. Ryser RJ, Locksley RM, Eng SC, et al. Reversal of dementia associated with Whipple's disease by trimethoprim-sulfamethoxazole, drugs that cross the blood-brain barrier. Gastroenterology. 1984;86:745.

19. Reed JI, Sipe JD, Wohlgethan JR, et al. Response of the acute phase reactants to antibiotic treatment of Whipple's disease. Arthritis Rheum. 1985;28:352.

20. Adler CH, Galetta SL. Oculo-facial-skeletal myorhythmia in Whipple's disease: Treatment with ceftriaxone. Ann Intern Med. 1990;112:467.

SECTION K. BONE AND JOINT INFECTIONS

84. INFECTIOUS ARTHRITIS

JAMES W. SMITH
ELIZABETH ANNE PIERCY

An inflammatory reaction in the joint space (arthritis) follows infection with many different microorganisms. Bacterial invasion of the joint generally leads to a suppurative arthritis, principally of one joint (monarticular). Certain bacteria may produce symptoms in multiple joints during bacteremia, and some, such as *Neisseria gonorrhoeae*, may induce inflammation in the neighboring tendon sheaths. Viral infections frequently involve multiple joints and demonstrate inflammation without suppuration. A chronic granulomatous monarticular arthritis due to either mycobacteria or fungi must be differentiated from other causes of chronic monarticular arthritis. A sterile arthritis may occur early in the infection, as with hepatitis B, or later, as with a postinfectious arthritis. Infectious arthritis has a low case fatality rate but can leave residual symptoms if not recognized and treated promptly. Any person with an inflamed joint must have infection included as a diagnostic possibility.

PATHOGENESIS AND PREDISPOSING FACTORS

Infectious arthritis usually follows hematogenous inoculation of pathogenic organisms,[1-3] except in infants. Under 1 year of age, capillaries perforate the epiphyseal growth plate, providing a conduit from bone to joint space. After 1 year of age the capillaries recede, and infection is usually limited to the joint since the growth plate contains the infection.[4] Patients with rheumatoid arthritis and osteoarthritis are predisposed to infectious arthritis, especially those with more debilitating arthritis who require intra-articular injection.[5,6] Many patients with bacterial arthritis give a history of trauma (Table 1).[1,7] Intra-articular injection

or trauma may lead to infection because capillary integrity is interrupted so that microbial seeding takes place during bacteremia.[2] Other systemic conditions predisposing to infectious arthritis include immunosuppressive therapy and chronic debilitating illnesses such as diabetes mellitus or malignancies.[1,8] Extra-articular infections are found in both adults and children with bacterial arthritis (Table 1).

Synovial tissue is highly vascular and lacks a basement membrane and thus is susceptible to hematogenous seeding by bacteria.[8] The most common pathogen, *Staphylococcus aureus*, has been demonstrated in vitro to bind to bone sialoprotein, a glycoprotein found in joints.[9] Endocrine factors appear to be important in the genesis of the disseminated gonococcal syndrome and viral arthritis.[10,11] Gonococcal infections tend to occur in women during pregnancy and during menstruation,[10] when endocervical shedding of *N. gonorrhoeae* is maximal and access to the blood stream is greatest. Rubella arthritis principally occurs in postpubertal women, whereas mumps arthritis is seen exclusively in postpubertal men.[11]

Immunologic response accounts for clinical expression of arthritis with hepatitis B, meningococci, and lymphocytic choriomeningitis virus.[12-14] Arthritis in patients with hepatitis B infection relates to the transient appearance of complement-fixing complexes in patients with arthritis.[12] As the arthritis disappears with the onset of jaundice, complement components can no longer be demonstrated in the immune complexes. Postinfectious arthritis can also develop in persons after sexually transmitted diseases or after enteric infections with *Shigella, Salmonella, Campylobacter,* and *Yersinia*.[15,16] The presence of the specific histocompatibility antigen HLA-B27 increases the likelihood of postinfectious arthritis 50-fold and has been reported to predispose to more severe diseases.[15]

CLINICAL FEATURES

Children and adults with bacterial arthritis present with fever in 60–80 percent of cases and monarticular involvement in 90 percent.[4,17,18] Most have mild temperature elevation, with only 30–40 percent having a temperature exceeding 39°C.[1,8,17] Joint motion is limited, and swelling representing synovial effusion is visible in peripheral joints. Joint tenderness may vary from minimal to severe. The knee is the most commonly affected joint in both children and adults with bacterial arthritis, as well as infections with *Mycobacterium tuberculosis* (Table 2).[19] The hip is the next most commonly involved joint, but correct diagnosis of bacterial infection of the hip and shoulder joints is frequently delayed since effusions may be difficult to demon-

TABLE 1. Predisposing Factors in Bacterial Arthritis

Factor	In Adult[a] (%)	In Children (%)
Preexisting arthritis	46	—
Trauma	32	28
Other diseases	23	3
Other infection	9 +	26
None	8	43

[a] More than one predisposing factor existed in some patients.

(Data from Cooper et al.[1] and Nelson et al.[7])

TABLE 2. Frequency (Percentages) of Joint Involvement in Infectious Arthritis[a]

Joint	Bacterial (Suppurative)		Mycobacterial	Viral
	Children	Adults		
Knee	41	54	24	60
Hip	23	16	20	4
Ankle	14	7	12	30
Elbow	12	3	8	20
Wrist	4	7	20	55
Shoulder	4	8	4	5
Interphalangeal and metacarpal	1.4	4	12	75
Sternoclavicular	0.4	<1	0	0
Sacroiliac	0.4	<1	0	0

[a] More than one joint may be involved, so the percentages exceed 100 percent.

(Data from refs. 1, 4, 11, 17–20).

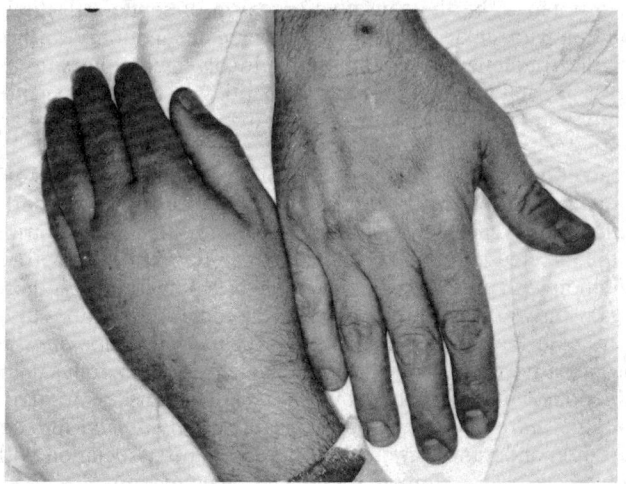

FIG. 1. Patient with chromic gonococcemia with swollen hand and skin lesions over dorsal surface of wrist. (Courtesy of *Current Prescribing*, April, 1979.)

strate.[1,21] Children tend to have infection more commonly of the ankle and elbow,[4] whereas adults tend to have more involvement of the shoulder and wrist.[17,21] Interphalangeal joints of the hand are infrequently involved with bacterial arthritis except for *N. gonorrhoeae* and *M. tuberculosis* and following human and animal bites. Infection of the sacroiliac and sternoclavicular joint is infrequent except when parenteral drug abuse is a predisposing factor.[8,22] Most patients with bacterial arthritis have an acute presentation, but a prolonged duration of symptoms has been reported with neisserial infections.[13] Infections with mycobacteria and certain fungi such as *Sporothrix schenckii* have such an insidious onset that a diagnosis of infection may not be considered.[23]

Multiple joint involvement is observed in 10 percent of patients, especially those with rheumatoid arthritis.[6] Infectious arthritis of viral etiology (e.g., rubella) tends to involve multiple joints, with most having symptoms in the interphalangeal joints of the hands, the wrist, as well as the knees, ankles, and elbows[11,20] (Table 2). Inflammation of multiple tendon sheaths (tenosynovitis) occurs commonly with the disseminated gonococcal syndrome (Fig. 1).[10] Tenosynovitis also may be seen with other infections such as *Moraxella*, rubella, nontuberculous mycobacteria, and sporotrichosis. Carpal tunnel syndrome (paresthesias of the hands), with or without joint symptoms, occurs with rubella, nontuberculous mycobacteria, sporotrichosis, and histoplasmosis.

Septic bursitis is usually due to *S. aureus* and commonly fol-

lows local trauma.[24] Bursitis also may be the first manifestation of infectious arthritis in patients with rheumatoid arthritis. The olecranon and prepatellar bursae are the usual sites. Occasionally, organisms of low pathogenicity cause chronic olecranon bursitis, such as nontuberculous *Mycobacterium*, *Prototheca*, and *Phialophora*.

LABORATORY FINDINGS

Patients with infectious arthritis, whether bacterial, viral, or mycobacterial, usually have an elevated erythrocyte sedimentation rate (ESR). The ESR is higher in those with bacterial infection and can be helpful in the assessment of patients with rheumatoid arthritis.[6] Anemia may be noted, particularly in those with chronic infections or in those who develop infectious arthritis secondary to underlying joint disease such as rheumatoid arthritis. Children tend to have elevated white blood cell counts with a predominance of polymorphonuclear leukocytes, whereas many adults have minimal or no elevation of the peripheral blood leukocyte count.[1,7]

Examination of synovial fluid from inflamed joints is essential to distinguish infectious from noninfectious arthritis. Joint fluid from monarticular bacterial arthritis generally appears turbid or purulent, although 10–20 percent have serosanguineous fluid. The synovial leukocyte count usually exceeds 50,000/mm³, and most have a differential count of more than 75 percent polymorphonuclear leukocytes.[1,25] However, this finding is not specific for bacterial arthritis, since synovial fluid in rheumatoid arthritis and crystalline joint disease also shows a preponderance of polymorphonuclear leukocytes; furthermore, bacterial infections in patients who have malignancy, are on corticosteroids, or who are intravenous drug abusers do not elicit as high a synovial fluid leukocyte count (half below 28,000 cells/mm³), although their percentage of segmented neutrophils exceeds 90 percent.[26] Protein levels are generally elevated, but this has little specificity for joint infection. A low synovial fluid glucose level is neither sensitive nor specific for bacterial arthritis.[17,25] Viral arthritis may be associated with a modest elevation of the synovial fluid leukocyte count.[11] In most instances, the preponderant cell is mononuclear, although some cases with proven rubella arthritis have had a majority of polymorphonuclear leukocytes.[20] Leukocyte counts exceeding 1000/mm³ are characteristic of staphylococcal bursitis.[24]

Smears of joint fluid stained for bacteria from persons with bacterial arthritis show the organisms in one-third of the cases.[4] The Gram stain can give false-positive results (positive test results not confirmed by a positive cultures). Both blood and joint fluid should be cultured aerobically and anaerobically. In addition, other sites should be cultured, if appropriate, such as spinal fluid in a patient with central nervous system manifestations. Pharyngeal, rectal, and cervical or urethral cultures should be plated on gonococcal media if the disseminated gonococcal syndrome is considered.[15,17] Blood cultures have been positive in 10–60 percent of adults and in 29 percent of children with bacterial arthritis.[1,4,17] Joint cultures are positive in up to 90 percent of those in whom a diagnosis of bacterial arthritis has been established and in 79 percent of those with tuberculosis.[8,17,19] Cultures of synovial tissue produce higher yields for mycobacterial and fungal infection than synovial fluid.[19,23]

RADIOLOGIC AND IMAGING EVALUATION

Imaging studies do not play as crucial a role in the diagnosis of joint infection as they do in osteomyelitis. However, radiographic or arthrographic studies may be helpful to assess the extent of soft tissue and osseous involvement or to monitor percutaneous aspiration and biopsy.[27] The most frequent radiographic abnormality in bacterial arthritis is distension of the joint capsule, soft tissue swelling, or fat pad edema.[28] Destructive changes are rarely noted in bacterial infections except in those who are seen late (more than 2 weeks into the course of infection).[6] Erosion of the central articular surface is seen in adults, whereas in children displacement of the ossific nucleus or destruction of cartilage can be seen.[27] If the infection complicates rheumatoid arthritis, then rapid articular destruction and asymmetry of involvement has been useful in distinguishing infection from rheumatoid arthritis.[28] Radiographs of the joint in those with mycobacterial infection show joint space narrowing, erosions, and cyst formation.[19] Viral infections rarely produce radiographic changes unless significant quantities of fluid are present and result in distension of the joint capsule.

Sonography, computed tomography (CT), and magnetic resonance imaging (MRI) are more sensitive than radiographs for detecting joint effusions.[29] CT can detect abnormalities present in cases of arthritis with osteomyelitis, and MRI is helpful for cases with extra-articular spread of infections, especially in those with sinus tract formation. Injection of contrast (arthrography) into joint spaces can be a valuable supplement to plain radiographs for identifying spaces that require direct puncture, such as the hip and shoulder, and for identifying rotator cuff tears.[6,21,27]

Radionuclide imaging with the three-phase bone scan is also helpful in evaluating joint infection in the setting of suspected osteomyelitis or in detecting bacterial sacroiliitis.[22] Although bone and gallium scans are frequently positive with asymmetrical uptake in patients with septic arthritis, these scans were of little use in distinguishing rheumatoid from septic synovitis.[29] Radionuclide scans can be used to confirm arthritis when involvement of muscle is the predominant physical abnormality.

PATHOLOGIC CHANGES

In experimental arthritis produced by the intra-articular injection of *Staphylococcus aureus*, this organism is destructive to cartilage due to the production of chondrocyte proteases.[30] In rabbits, early pathologic changes were noted on the surface and in the matrix of the superficial zone of the articular surface by electron microscopy within 24 hours.[31] At this time, the joint cavity showed polymorphonuclear leukocytes, and lysosomal bodies were present in the synovial cells. By 3 days, the destruction of articular cartilage was more extensive and was even visible with light microscopy. The matrix appeared loose in the superficial zones, and degeneration of chondrocytes was noted in deeper zones. In chronic arthritis due to mycobacteria or fungi, histologic evidence of a granulomatous inflammation occurs with dense mononuclear inflammatory infiltrates consisting of lymphocytes.[19]

SYNDROMES OF INFECTIOUS ARTHRITIS

Acute Bacterial Arthritis

The frequencies of the etiologic agents that induce bacterial arthritis vary with age (Table 3). *Haemophilus influenzae* type b is the preponderant causative organism in children under 2 years of age. Arthritis or meningitis due to this causative organism has been seen infrequently in the past 3 years since introduction of the conjugate vaccine. In infants under 1 month of age, group B streptococci, gram-negative bacilli, and *S. aureus* are causative organisms. *Staphylococcus aureus* is the most frequent organism causing bacterial arthritis in children over 2 years of age[4] and is the causative organism in the vast majority of cases of suppurative arthritis in adults.[1,17,18] *Neisseria gonorrhoeae* is the preponderant cause of bacterial arthritis in adults under 30 years.[17] The frequency of streptococcal infections as a cause of bacterial arthritis is relatively constant from childhood through the adult years (13–27 percent). The most frequently isolated type in both children and adults is group A β-hemolytic streptococci; however, group B (in the neonate and adult diabetic), viridans streptococci, and microaerophilic and anaerobic streptococci have been isolated. *Streptococcus pneumoniae* is rarely encountered now as a cause of suppurative arthritis, but has been noted to be the causative organism of septic arthritis in children with sickle disease.[32] The course of suppurative arthritis, the frequency of multiple joint involvement, the sites of infection, and the laboratory abnormalities do not differ significantly with any of these major causative agents of bacterial arthritis.[17]

Infectious arthritis due to gram-negative bacilli is seen in 9–17 percent of cases of infectious arthritis.[1,17] Most were elderly with either a chronic debilitating disease or a chronic arthritis in the infected joint, and some had an intercurrent urinary tract infection with gram-negative bacteremia.[33] Infection with these organisms was associated with good outcome. Intravenous drug users who develop septic arthritis may have *Pseudomonas* as the causative organism with sternoclavicular and sacroiliac joint infections, but in non-drug abusers such infections are primarily due to *S. aureus*.[8,22] Septic arthritis due to *Salmonella* spp. occurs preponderantly in children but bears no association with sickle cell disease, unlike *Salmonella* osteomyelitis.

Gonococcal arthritis, one of the more commonly recognized features of disseminated gonococcal infections, is caused by organisms with protein 1-A serotype, which are also resistant to serum.[10,34] The syndrome exists in either of two forms. In one form, patients have systemic symptoms with fever, shaking chills, skin lesions, and a polyarticular syndrome. Blood cultures are frequently positive, particularly within 2 days of the onset of symptoms, whereas synovial fluid cultures are rarely positive. *Neisseria gonorrhoeae* can be recovered from cultures of genital, rectal, and pharyngeal areas. The skin lesions begin as tiny erythematous papules, frequently petechiae, and may evolve to become vesicles or pustules (Fig. 1). These lesions are fairly transient and last 3–4 days. An occasional patient who fails to come to medical attention may have recurrent episodes of skin lesions and polyarthralgias for periods up to 3 months (as in the case in Fig. 1). The organism is occasionally recovered from scrapings of the skin lesion, although more frequently organisms are recovered from blood. Other microorganisms to be considered in the differential diagnosis of patients with skin rash and arthritis include *H. influenzae*, *Moraxella osloenis*, *Streptobacillus moniliformis*, and *Neisseria meningitidis*.

In the other form of gonococcal infection, patients have a monarticular suppurative infection with recovery of the organism from joint fluid.[10] These patients may give a history of having had transient polyarthralgias before the monarticular arthritis developed and may even have a history of skin lesions; however, skin lesions are rarely present in those with a monarticular arthritis. Infection with *N. meningitidis* may mimic the disseminated gonococcemia syndrome; patients with greater than 100 skin lesions have a high probability of meningococcal

TABLE 3. Etiologic Agents as Causes of Bacterial (Suppurative) Arthritis (Percentages)

Agent	Children <5 Yr	Children >5 Yr	Adults
Staphylococcus aureus	11	33	55
Haemophilus influenzae, type b	31	1	<1
Streptococcus spp.[a]	12	13	27
Gram-negative bacilli	5	6	14
Anaerobes	0	1	<1
Neisseria	5	8	—[b]
Other	2	5	0
Unknown	35	34	3

[a] Includes *Streptococcus pneumoniae*, groups A and B streptococci, viridans group streptococci, and microaerophilic and anaerobic streptococci.
[b] Excluded from most series of adult suppurative arthritis.

(Data from refs. 1, 4, 17, 18.)

TABLE 4. Historical or Physical Features of Importance in Patients with Bacterial Arthritis

Organism	Arthritis-Associated Condition
Neisseria gonorrhoeae	Female during menstrual cycle or pregnancy; multiple skin lesions[10]
Neisseria meningitidis	Greater than 100 skin lesions[35]
Organisms from oral flora (Eikenella corrodens, Fusobacterium nucleatum)	Human bite[36]
Pasteurella multocida	Cat or dog bite[37]
Streptobacillus moniliformis	Rat bite[38]
Borrelia burgdorferi (Lyme disease)	Tick exposure[39]

TABLE 5. Infectious Causes of Chronic Monarticular Arthritis

Bacterial
    Brucella spp.
Mycobacteria and Nocardia
    Mycobacterium tuberculosis
    M. kansasii
    M. marinum
    M. intracellulare
    M. fortuitum
    M. leprae
    Nocardia asteroides
Fungi
    Sporothrix schenckii
    Coccidioides immitis
    Blastomyces dermatitidis
    Candida albicans
    Pseudallescheria boydii

infection (Table 4).[35] In addition, patients with meningococcemia may develop joint effusions 5–10 days after the onset of the infection. Sterile effusions are found in multiple joints and resolve rather rapidly. An uncommon variety of meningococcal infection is chronic meningococcemia in which symptoms are present for more than 1 week without meningeal involvement.[13] These patients have low-grade fever; a rash that may be macular, papular, or petechial; joint involvement; and headache. Two-thirds of the patients have polyarthralgias, and one-third have arthritis with joint effusions.

Septic arthritis of the metacarpophalangeal joint following human bites can be caused by oral microbes or, after cat or dog bites, by *Pasteurella multocida* (Table 4).[36,37] Infections with *S. moniliformis* occur 2–3 days after rat bites with the onset of chills, a macular rash of the palms and soles, and arthralgias in large joints.[38] The organism, a pleomorphic gram-negative bacillus, can be grown in blood cultures but not from joint fluid. The arthritis of Lyme disease is characterized by intermittent attacks of a migratory polyarticular arthritis lasting weeks to months, usually in large joints, that occur late in the course of the disease.[39] This spirochetal infection transmitted by tick bite (see Ch. 219) also rarely can result in a long-standing chronic arthritis of the knee joint.[39] Brucella arthritis most commonly affects the sacroiliac joint, then the knee, hip, and others less often.[40] The diagnosis is most frequently made by serologic tests.

Obligate anaerobic bacteria, principally gram-positive cocci, are rarely the causative agents in bacterial arthritis, even when anaerobic cultures are performed routinely on joint fluid.[8] *Bacteroides* species are rarely encountered. The most frequent anaerobic pathogen in arthritis of children is due to *Clostridium* spp.[4]

Chronic Monarticular Arthritis

Chronic monarticular arthritis with a granulomatous reaction on pathologic examination may be caused by a variety of organisms (Table 5). Mycobacterial infections of the joint are chronic, slowly progressive monarticular infections that may also involve the tendon sheaths, particularly the carpal tunnel area of the wrist.[19] A granulomatous reaction of the synovium is seen pathologically in young adults with tuberculosis, although only 60 percent of elderly patients had granulomas histologically.[19] Patients less than 60 years of age with tuberculous infections principally presented with arthritis of a single weight-bearing joint such as the knee and few systemic symptoms, whereas those over 60 had systemic symptoms, other foci of tuberculosis, and arthritis of nonweight-bearing joints such as the shoulder.[19]

Nontuberculous mycobacteria also produce infections of the joints (Table 5). *Mycobacterium kansasii* was the most common cause of monarticular synovitis seen in Dallas, Texas.[41] This organism has a propensity to involve the wrist and hands and to cause flexor tenosynovitis, carpal tunnel syndrome, and, rarely, olecranon bursitis.[41] *Mycobacterium kansasii* may localize to a

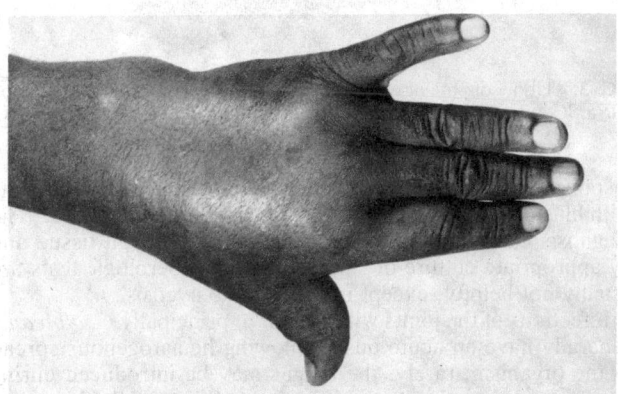

FIG. 2. Wrist of patient who had sporotrichosis of wrist and olecranon bursa. (Courtesy of *Current Prescribing*, April, 1979.)

joint after trauma or spread from a pulmonary focus. These patients do not usually have extra-articular infection. *Mycobacterium marinum* would be suspected in a patient with arthritis who develops the infection after exposure to tropical fish aquariums or marine life.

Synovial tissue from a patient with a chronic monarticular arthritis should be cultured for mycobacteria, inspected at a few days (to recognize *M. fortuitum*, a rapid grower), and incubated at 30°C (*M. marinum* grows better at this temperature than at 37°C). Patients with lepromatous leprosy may have a symmetrical polyarthritis of wrist, metacarpal, and small joints of the hands, especially patients with erythema nodosum leprosum.[42] Juxtaarticular erosions are seen in the carpal bones.

Fungal arthritis can be caused by a number of fungi with some variation based on geographic localization. *Sporothrix schenckii* causes infections of the joints world-wide in warm, moist environments; the majority of patients have contact with moist soil but rarely have penetrating joint trauma.[43] The most commonly affected joint is the knee, followed by the wrist and the elbow. The infection occasionally involves the wrist and the small joints of the hand with a chronic tenosynovitis (Figs. 2 and 3). Radiologic findings are nonspecific. The course is progressive over months and years, usually without fever. With time, infection appears in contiguous bursae or bones as well as in distant joints. Diagnosis is by culture of fluid or tissue; fungal elements of *Sporothrix* may be infrequent in tissue and difficult to find in pathologic specimens.

A chronic monarticular arthritis is seen with *Coccidioides immitis* in non-white immunocompromised men from endemic areas.[44] The knee is the most frequently involved joint. The joint fluid may show either a polymorphonuclear or a lymphocytic cellular response, but smears and cultures are often negative. Radiographs show variable evidence of bony destruction even after many months of illness. Diagnosis is made by culture of synovium. Patients' sera also have positive complement fixation

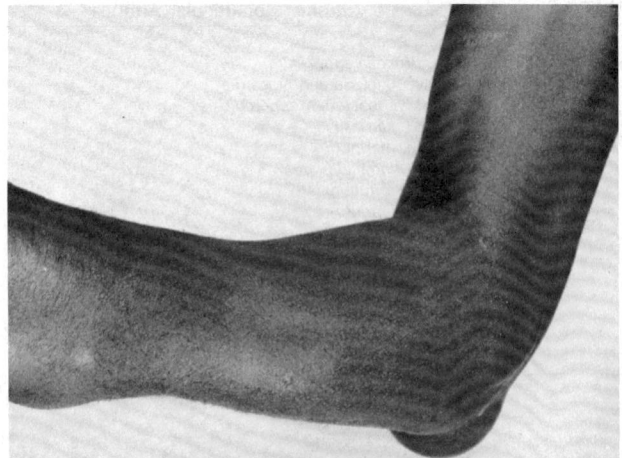

FIG. 3. Elbow of patient who had sporotrichosis of wrist and olecranon bursa. (Courtesy of *Current Prescribing*, April, 1979.)

responses with *Coccidioides* antigen. Joint infection in patients with blastomycosis primarily spreads from osteomyelitis.[23] The diagnosis can be made by examination of synovial tissue and by appropriate culture of surgical material. Serologic tests are usually not helpful, except in coccidioidomycosis.

Infections of the joints with *Candida*, principally *C. albicans*, generally have an acute onset following hematogenous spread of the organism; rarely, the fungus may be introduced during intra-articular corticosteroid injection.[23] Synovial fluid shows a polymorphonuclear leukocytic response. Any peripheral joint can be involved, but multiple joint infection is observed in up to 37 percent.[23] Migratory polyarthritis, usually in association with skin lesions or erythema nodosum and erythema multiforme, has been seen with acute histoplasmosis.[23] Arthritis is rare with cryptococcosis and aspergillosis and usually extends from osteomyelitis.[23] Carpal tunnel syndrome has also been noted in patients with disseminated histoplasmosis. *Pseudallescheria (Petriellidium) boydii* arthritis has occurred in men living in rural areas with a history of penetrating trauma of the knee.[23] Penetrating trauma precedes infection with *Scedosporium inflatum*.[45] Dematiaceous fungi such as *Exophiala jeanselmei* can cause a chronic bursitis following penetrating trauma.

Viral Arthritis

Viral agents associated with symptoms and signs of arthritis are listed in Table 6. Arthritis is a reasonably frequent event of infection with rubella and mumps, whereas it is an atypical manifestation of infection with varicella, adenovirus, echovirus, and rubeola.[11] A polyarthritis due to rubella occurs principally in adult women (Table 7).[46] The onset of joint symptoms occurs either with the rash or within 3 days after the eruption in 52 percent of females.[46] The small joints of the hand are most frequently involved, with knees, wrists, and ankles less commonly affected. Synovial fluid shows a predominance of mononuclear cells, and virus is rarely isolated from the joint fluid. The course is self-limited in most people, although some have recurrent episodes of joint symptoms up to 6 months after infection.[46] Rubella vaccine induces joint symptoms in 41 percent of susceptible postpubertal women.[46] The vaccine virus most frequently associated with symptoms replicates better in human joint cell cultures; the strains less likely to cause symptoms replicate less well in organ cultures.[47]

Up to 20 percent of patients with hepatitis B have been noted to develop arthritis, frequently in association with urticaria 2 days to 6 weeks before the onset of jaundice.[12] In the great majority, the symptoms disappear with the onset of the jaundice.[12] The arthritis is symmetrical with predilection for the

TABLE 6. Viral Agents Associated with Arthritis

Group	Virus
DNA viruses	
Poxvirus	Smallpox
	Vaccinia[a]
Adenovirus	Adenovirus[a]
Herpesvirus	Varicella[a]
	Epstein-Barr (infectious mononucleosis)[a]
Parvovirus B19	Erythema infectiosum
Hepadnavirus	Hepatitis B
RNA viruses	
Paramyxoviruses	Mumps
	Rubeola[a]
Orthomyxoviruses	Influenza[a]
Picornavirus	Echovirus[a]
Togavirus	
Alphavirus	Chikungunya
	O'nyong-nyong
	Sindbis
	Ockelbo disease
	Ross River virus
Rubivirus	Rubella
Arenavirus	Lymphocytic choriomeningitis virus
Lentivirus	
Retrovirus	HTLV-1
	HIV-1

[a] Unusual manifestation of infection.

TABLE 7. Clinical or Epidemiologic Characteristics of Viral Agents Causing Arthritis

Virus	Characteristic
Rubella	Adult females
Hepatitis B	Preicteric phase
Mumps	Adult males
Lymphocytic choriomeningitis virus	Adults with aseptic meningitis
Parvovirus B19	Adult females with erythema infectiosum
Site of arthropod-borne alphavirus infection	
Chikungunya	East Africa, India
O'nyong-Nyong	East Africa
Ockelbo agent	Sweden
Ross River agent	Australia
Barmah Forest virus	Australia

hands followed by knees and ankles; joint effusions are scanty when present and reveal predominantly mononuclear cells. Arthritis occurs in association with mumps with a frequency of 0.44 percent and is seen more commonly in men.[48] The arthritis begins from 1 day before to 15 days after the onset of parotitis, with multiple large and small joints affected. Effusions are infrequent. Symptoms subside within 2 weeks, although arthritis may persist for up to 3 months.[48]

A number of alphaviruses of the togavirus family, which are arthropod-borne, have arthritis as a frequent manifestation of the illness they cause. *Chikungunya* derives its name from its characteristic clinical finding (that which bends up). This disease is characterized by an abrupt onset of fever, chills, and severe incapacitating pain in the large joints, although hot, swollen joints are infrequently seen.[11] Maculopapular eruption occurred over the trunk and extensor surfaces of the extremities in 80 percent of those with the disease. A similar illness in Uganda in 1959 was given the name *O'nyong-nyong* fever (weakening of the joints).[11] The onset of O'nyong-nyong fever was also abrupt, with symmetric involvement of most of the large joints with excruciating pain. All eventually made a full recovery. Sindbis virus and Sindbis-related diseases such as Ockelbo disease in Sweden have been noted to have arthritis as a prominent manifestation of the illness.[49] In Australia, epidemics of polyarthritis with rash have been observed that are due to two different alphaviruses, the Ross River agent and the Barmah Forest virus.[50,51]

Lymphocytic choriomeningitis, caused by an arenavirus, was associated with arthritis in one outbreak among laboratory personnel.[14] The development of a severe influenza-like disease with headache and arthritis may be due to lymphocytic chorio-meningitis virus rather than influenza, a disease in which arthritis is an uncommon complication. In late winter and spring, outbreaks of epidemic erythema infectiosum, an infection caused by parvovirus B19, are associated with a symmetric arthritis in adults, particularly in women.[52]

Patients with human T-lymphotropic virus type 1 (HTLV-1) have a chronic persistent oligoarthritis. This is a proliferative synovitis involving large joints with atypical lymphocytes in synovial fluid and proviral DNA within tissue cells.[53] Human immunodeficiency virus type 1 (HIV-1) infection has been associated with arthralgias of multiple joints, rarely a monarticular arthritis, and a propensity to have septic arthritis.[54]

PARASITES

Joint manifestations are not a feature of any of the commonly recognized parasitic infections. However, in the Sepik district of Papua, New Guinea, arthritis in association with filarial infections was the most frequent cause of arthritis.[55] The knee was the most frequently involved joint and showed warmth, tenderness, and limitation of motion. Joint effusions were present in slightly less than one-half of the cases, and the fluid aspirated was creamy yellow. Radiograms showed no articular destruction, only soft tissue swelling. Microfilariae were present in the blood. A reactive polyarthropathy is seen with schistosomiasis characterized by high IgE levels, an inflammatory exudate, and low complement in synovial fluid.[56]

APPROACH TO THE PATIENT

Differential Considerations

Bacterial infection should be suspected in any patient with acute monarticular arthritis, even in the absence of fever. However, a number of noninfectious conditions may involve single joints, including acute rheumatoid arthritis, gout, and chondrocalcinosis (pseudogout). As stated earlier, all of these illnesses can cause an inflammatory arthritis with more than 75 percent polymorphonuclear leukocytes.[25] Hence, the ultimate diagnosis must be based on Gram stain and culture of joint fluid and blood. Synovial fluid from any adult with monarticular arthritis should be examined for negatively birefringent (uric acid) and positively birefringent (calcium pyrophosphate) crystals. Simultaneous bacterial infection and crystalline joint disease has been reported.[57] Serologic studies including rheumatoid factor, antinuclear antibody tests, and acute and convalescent studies for antistreptolysin O (ASO) should be performed if more than one joint is affected. Any hot, tender joints with a fluid collection in a rheumatoid patient should be aspirated and the fluid be submitted for smear and culture. Gonococcal arthritis, Reiter syndrome, or acute rheumatic fever should be suspected in any adult having fever and multiple joint involvement; characteristic skin lesions and tenosynovitis suggest the disseminated gonococcal syndrome. The other features of the triad of Reiter syndrome, conjunctivitis and urethritis, may not be apparent initially. Frequently, the only way to distinguish between gonococcal infection and Reiter syndrome is to observe response to treatment with antibiotics appropriate for *N. gonorrhoeae*: if a new joint develops after the second day of therapy, then Reiter syndrome is the more likely diagnosis. HLA-B27 testing is not helpful in individual cases of Reiter syndrome.

When a monarticular arthritis has a chronic course, an infectious etiology should also be considered uppermost in the differential diagnosis. The leading infectious cause has been infection with nontuberculous mycobacteria, followed closely by *S. schenckii*. Infection with *M. tuberculosis* in some countries predominates,[19] and the increase in tuberculosis in association with HIV could presage a rise in tuberculous arthritis.[19,54] Synovial fluid cultures for acid-fast bacteria and fungi should be consid-

ered for any patient who is immunocompromised, on immunosuppressive therapy, or who has a persistent effusion. A synovial biopsy culture should be done for fungus and acid-fast organisms in any person with a chronic monarticular involvement whose synovial fluid cultures are negative or with tenosynovitis as a prominent feature. In addition, Lyme arthritis should be considered if the patient is from an endemic area.[39] In Lyme arthritis, the infectious agent can be demonstrated by Dieterle silver stain in 25 percent of cases, but all should have a diagnostic titer in a serum indirect immunofluorescent assay of 1:256 or greater.[39] A diagnosis of viral arthritis should be considered if a person presents with multiple joint involvement and systemic manifestations consistent with a viral infection. It is frequently not possible to isolate virus from the joint fluid, so serologic confirmation of the infection is necessary using acute and convalescent sera. In general, the course is the major determinant in distinguishing between viral arthritis and rheumatic disorders such as adult Still's disease, since the former has a self-limited course with no residual joint abnormalities.

Antimicrobial Therapy

Empiric antimicrobial therapy for presumed bacterial arthritis would be given after obtaining blood culture and withdrawing synovial fluid for culture, Gram stain, leukocyte count, and chemistries. The choice of drug will depend on the Gram stain result and the patient's age and sexual activity.

In children under 5 years of age, cefuroxime, 100 mg/kg/day divided into q8h doses; cefotaxime; or ceftriaxone would be reasonable initial therapy pending culture results. For children over 5 years of age and adults, if clusters of gram-positive organisms suggestive of *S. aureus* are seen on Gram stain, then one would use an intravenous penicillinase-resistant penicillin such as nafcillin, 150 mg/kg/day divided into q4–6h doses, or oxacillin. If gram-positive organisms in chains consistent with streptococci are seen on Gram stain, then penicillin G would be indicated. If the Gram stain is negative, then a second-generation cephalosporin or intravenous nafcillin (adult dose, 1.5 g q4h iv) would be appropriate. Ceftriaxone is a reasonable initial drug in sexually active adults, particularly when the gonococcus is suggested by organisms on Gram stain or by the presence of skin lesions or tenosynovitis. Recommendations for treatment of infections in prosthetic joints are given in Chapter 87. When culture and susceptibility results are available, therapy can be changed to the optimal and perhaps less expensive agent.

The usual course of therapy for suppurative arthritis is 2 weeks for *H. influenza,* streptococci, or gram-negative cocci and 3 weeks for staphylococci or gram-negative bacilli.[58] Intra-articular injections of drugs used to treat suppurative bacterial arthritis are unnecessary. Most agents used to treat suppurative arthritis reach sufficient levels in the joint when given intravenously.[59,60] Inclusion of antibiotics in solutions used to irrigate the joint is not indicated. The reader is referred to the relevant chapters of this text for treatment of other specific organisms such as fungi, mycobacteria, and Lyme borreliosis.

Other Therapeutic Modalities

Most people with suppurative arthritis respond adequately to appropriate antimicrobial agents after an initial joint aspiration for diagnosis. Early treatment in experimental infectious arthritis prevented reduction in loss of collagen and erosion of articular surface and therefore should minimize the need for ancillary treatment.[61] Repeated needle aspiration for recurrent joint effusions has been used with success during the first 5–7 days of treatment.[8,62] If the volume of synovial fluid, the cell count, and the percentage of polymorphonuclear leukocytes decrease with each aspiration, then the combination of antimicrobial therapy and aspiration as needed is probably adequate. Persistence of effusion beyond 7 days is evidence that surgical drainage is re-

TABLE 8. Predictors of Poor Outcome with Bacterial Arthritis

Age over 60 years
Infection in hip and shoulder
Duration of symptoms before treatment of greater than 1 week
≥Four joints
Persistently positive culture after 7 days of appropriate therapy

(Data from refs. 1, 18, 21, 63.)

quired.[8,62] Suppurative arthritis of the hip and shoulder[1,21] frequently requires aspiration under radiologic imaging or surgical drainage. In some medical centers, surgical drainage is generally preferred for adults with infections of weight-bearing joints and infections due to *S. aureus* or gram-negative bacilli. If open surgical drainage is performed, continued irrigation of the joint after drainage is of little value. Treatment with systemic antimicrobial agents should be continued for up to 1 week after open drainage and the wound be allowed to close by secondary closure.

In the usual case of septic arthritis, immobilization of the infected joint is not necessary, although weight bearing should be avoided until signs of inflammation and pain have disappeared. The joint should be maintained in the functional position, and passive motion may be instituted early, once the symptoms of pain have subsided. As the inflammation diminishes, active exercises may be instituted, and weight bearing may be permitted when all signs of inflammation have disappeared and no evidence of effusion is present.[8]

Course of the Illness

Although some persons with bacterial arthritis recover without long-term residual abnormalities, certain persons have a poor long-term response (Table 8). The elderly do poorly, especially with infections of the hip and with underlying joint disease.[64,65] The frequency of sequelae in children was shown to be 27 percent,[66] including slight limitation of movement, impairment of ambulation, and shortening of the extremity. These residua were more common with hip and ankle infection. In adults, up to 50 percent had limitation of motion or persistence of pain.[17] Most with septic arthritis immediately following arthroscopy did well with few sequelae.[67] Infectious causes of chronic monarticular arthritis are occasionally associated with substantial residua even after maximal therapy.[23,41] Synovectomy has been combined with chemotherapy to achieve an inactive joint infection.[44]

REFERENCES

1. Cooper C, Cawley MID. Bacterial arthritis in an English health district: A 10 year review. Ann Rheum Dis. 1986;45:458–63.
2. McCarty DJ. Joint sepsis: A chance for cure. JAMA. 1982;247:835.
3. Smith JW. Infectious arthritis. Infect Dis Clin North Am. 1990;4:523–38.
4. Jackson MA, Nelson JD. Etiology and medical management of acute suppurative bone and joint infections in pediatric patients. J Pediatr Orthop. 1982;2:313–23.
5. Ostenssan A, Geborek P. Septic arthritis as a non-surgical complication in rheumatoid arthritis: Relation to disease severity and therapy. Br Rheum. 1991;30:35–8.
6. Gardner GC, Weisman MH. Pyarthrosis in patients with rheumatoid arthritis: A report of 13 cases and a review of the literature from the past 40 years. Am J Med. 1990;88:503–511.
7. Nelson JD, Koontz WC. Septic arthritis in infants and children: A review of 117 cases. Pediatrics. 1966;38:966–71.
8. Goldenberg DL, Reed JI. Bacterial arthritis. N Engl J Med. 1985;312:764–71.
9. Bremell T, Lange S, Yacoub A, et al. Experimental *Staphylococcus aureus* arthritis in mice. Infect Immun. 1991;59:2615–23.
10. O'Brien JPP, Goldenberg DL, Rice PA. Disseminated gonococcal infection: A prospective analysis of 49 patients and a review of pathophysiology and immune mechanisms. Medicine. 1983;62:395–406.
11. Smith JW, Sanford JP. Viral arthritis. Ann Intern Med. 1967;67:651–9.
12. Inman RD. Rheumatic manifestations of hepatitis B virus infection. Semin Arthritis Rheum. 1982;11:406–20.
13. Kidd BL, Hart HH, Grigor RR. Clinical features of meningococcal arthritis: A report of four cases. Ann Rheum Dis. 1985;44:790–2.
14. Baum SG, Lewis AM Jr, Rowe WP, et al. Epidemic nonmeningitis lymphocytic–choriomeningitis–virus infection. N Engl J Med. 1966;274:934–6.
15. Keat A. Sexually transmitted arthritis syndromes. Med Clin North Am. 1990;74:1617–1631.
16. Fryden A, Bengtsson A, Foberg U, et al. Early antibiotic treatment of reactive arthritis associated with enteric infections: Clinical and serological study. Br Med J. 1990;301:1299–302.
17. Sharp JT, Lidsky MD, Duffy J, et al. Infectious arthritis. Arch Intern Med. 1979;139:1125–30.
18. Ho G Jr, Su EY. Therapy for septic arthritis. JAMA. 1982;247:797–800.
19. Garrido G, Gomez-Reino J, Fernandez-Dapica P, et al. A review of peripheral tuberculous arthritis. Semin Arthritis Rheum. 1988;18:142–149.
20. Medical Staff Conference: Arthritis caused by viruses. Calif Med. 1973;119:38–44.
21. Leslie BM, Harris III JM, Driscoll D. Septic arthritis of the shoulder in adults. J Bone Joint Surg. 1989;71A:1516–22.
22. Vyskocil JJ, McIlroy MA, Brennan TA, et al. Pyogenic infection of the sacroiliac joint. Case reports and review of the literature. Medicine. 1991;70:188–97.
23. Cuellar ML, Silveira LH, Espinoza LR. Fungal arthritis. Ann Rheum Dis. 1992;51:690–7.
24. Ho Jr G, Mikolich DJ. Bacterial infection of the superficial subcutaneous bursae. Clin Rheum Dis. 1986;12:437–57.
25. Shemerling RH, Delbanco TL, Tosetson ANA, et al. Synovial fluid tests. JAMA. 1990;264:1009–14.
26. McCutchan HJ, Fisher RC. Synovial leukocytosis in infectious arthritis. Clin Orthop. 1990;257:226–30.
27. Goldman AB. Arthrography for rheumatic disease: When, why, and for whom. Rheum Dis Clin North Am. 1991;17:505–42.
28. Gelman MI, Ward JR. Septic arthritis: A complication of rheumatoid arthritis. Radiology. 1975;122:17–24.
29. Kim EE, Haynie PP. Radionuclide imaging in the evaluation of osteomyelitis and septic arthritis. Crit Rev Diagn Imaging. 1989;29:257–305.
30. Williams III RJ, Smith RL, Schurman DJ. Septic arthritis: staphylococcal induction of chondrocyte proteolytic activity. Arthritis Rheum. 1990;33:533–41.
31. Roy S, Bhawan J. Ultrastructure of articular cartilage in pyogenic arthritis. Arch Pathol. 1975;99:44–7.
32. Syrogiannopoulos GA, McCracken GH Jr, Nelson JD. Osteoarticular infections in children with sickle cell disease. Pediatrics. 1986;78:1090–6.
33. Newman ED, Davis DE, Harrington TM. Septic arthritis due to gram negative bacilli: Older patients with good outcome. J Rheum. 1988;15:659–62.
34. Hook EW. Septic arthritis: Gonococcal arthritis is much more common in the USA than in the UK. Br J Rheum. 1990;29:283.
35. Rompalo AM, Hook EW, Roberts PL, et al. The acute arthritis-dermatitis syndrome. The changing importance of *Neisseria gonorrhoeae* and *Neisseria meningitidis*. Arch Intern Med. 1987;147:281–3.
36. Resnick D, Pineda CJ, Weisman MH, et al. Osteomyelitis and septic arthritis of the hand following human bites. Skeletal Radiol. 1985;14:263–6.
37. Ewing R, Fainstein V, Musher DM, Lidsky M, Clarridge J. Articular and skeletal infections caused by *Pasteurella multocida*. South Med J. 1980;73:1349–52.
38. Holroyd KJ, Reiner AP, Dick JD. *Streptobacillus moniliformis* polyarthritis mimicking rheumatoid arthritis: An urban case of rat bite fever. Am J Med. 1988;85:711–4.
39. Goldings EA, Jericho J. Lyme disease. Clin Rheum Dis. 1986;12:343–67.
40. Khateeb MI, Araj GF, Majeed SA, Lulu AR. Brucella arthritis: A study of 96 cases in Kuwait. Ann Rhem Dis. 1990;49:994–8.
41. Sutker WL, Lankford LL, Tompsett R. Granulomatous synovitis: The role of atypical mycobacteria. Rev Infect Dis. 1979;1:729–35.
42. Atkin SL, El-Ghobarey A, Kamel M, Owen JP, Dick WC. Clinical and laboratory studies of arthritis in leprosy. Br Med J. 1989;298:1423–5.
43. Bayer AS, Scott VJ, Guze LB. Fungal arthritis. III. Sporotrichal arthritis. Semin Arthritis Rheum. 1979;9:66–74.
44. Bayer AS, Guze LB. Fungal arthritis. II. Coccidioidal synovitis: clinical diagnostic, therapeutic, and prognostic considerations. Semin Arthritis Rheum. 1979;8:200–11.
45. Wilson CM, O'Rourke EJ, McGinnis MR, Salkin IF. *Scedosporium inflatum*: Clinical spectrum of a newly recognized pathogen. J Infect Dis. 1990;161:102–7.
46. Tingle AJ, Allen M, Petty RE, Kettyls GD, Chantler JK. Rubella-associated arthritis I. Comparative study of joint manifestations associated with natural rubella infection and RA 27/3 rubella immunization. Ann Rheum Dis. 1986;45:110–4.
47. Miki NPH, Chantler JK. Differential ability of wild-type and vaccine strains of rubella virus to replicate and persist in human joint tissue. Clin Exp Rheum. 1992;10:3–12.
48. Gordon SC, Lauter CB. Mumps arthritis: A review of the literature. Rev Infect Dis. 1984;6:388–44.
49. Niklasson B, Espmark A, Lundstrom J. Occurrence of arthralgia and specific IgM antibodies three to four years after Ockelbo disease. J Infect Dis. 1988;157:832–5.
50. Fraser JRE. Epidemic polyarthritis and Ross River virus disease. Clin Rheum Dis. 1986;12:369–88.
51. Phillips DA, Murray JR, Aaskov JG, et al. Clinical and subclinical Barmah Forest virus infection in Queensland. Med J Aust. 1990;152:463–6.
52. Reid DM, Brown T, Reid TMS, et al. Human parvovirus-associated arthritis: A clinical and laboratory description. Lancet. 1985;1:422–5.
53. Sato K, Maruyama I, Maruyama Y, et al. Arthritis in patients infected with

human T lymphotropic virus type I. Clinical and immunopathologic features. Arthritis Rheum. 1991;34:714–21.

54. Monteagudo I, Rivera J, Lopez-Longo J, et al. AIDS and rheumatic manifestations in patients addicted to drugs. An analysis of 106 cases. J Rheum. 1991; 18:1038–41.
55. Salfield S. Filarial arthritis in the Sepik District of Papua New Guinea. Med J Aust. 1975;1:264–7.
56. Kamal M, Safwat E, Eltayeb S. Bilharzial arthropathy. Scand J Rheum. 1989; 18:315–9.
57. Baer PA, Tenenbaum J, Fam AG, et al. Coexistent septic and crystal arthritis. Report of four cases and literature review. J Rheumatol. 1986;13:604–7.
58. Syrogiannopoulos GA, Nelson JD. Duration of antimicrobial therapy for acute suppurative osteoarticular infections. Lancet. 1988;1:37–40.
59. Nelson JD. Antibiotic concentration in septic joint effusions. N Engl J Med. 1971;284:349–53.
60. Sattar MA, Barrett SP, Cawley MID. Concentrations of some antibiotics in synovial fluid after oral administration, with special reference to antistaphylococcal activity. Ann Rheum Dis. 1983;42:67–74.
61. Smith RL, Schurman DJ, Kajiyama G, et al. The effect of antibiotics on the destruction of cartilage in experimental infectious arthritis. J Bone Joint Surg. 1987;69A:1063–8.
62. Rosenthal J, Giles GB, Robinson WD. Acute nongonococcal infectious arthritis. Evaluation of risk factors, therapy, and outcome. Arthritis and Rheum. 1980;23:889–97.
63. Yu LP, Bradley JD, Hugenberg ST, Brandt KD. Predictors of mortality in non-post-operative patients with septic arthritis. Scand J Rheumatol. 1992; 21:142–4.
64. Cooper C, Cawley MID. Bacterial arthritis in the elderly. Gerontology. 1986; 32:222–227.
65. McGuire NM, Kauffman CA. Septic arthritis in the elderly. J Am Geriatr Soc. 1985;33:170–4.
66. Howard JG, Highgenboten CL, Nelson JD. Residual effects of septic arthritis in infancy and childhood. JAMA. 1976;236:932–5.
67. Armstrong RW, Bolding F, Joseph R. Septic arthritis following arthroscopy: Clinical syndrome and analysis of risk factors. J Arthrosc. 1992;8:213–23.

85. OSTEOMYELITIS

JON T. MADER
JASON CALHOUN

GENERAL CONCEPT OF OSTEOMYELITIS

Bone infections are currently classified by the Waldvogel et al.[1,2] system as either hematogenous osteomyelitis or osteomyelitis secondary to a contiguous focus of infection. Contiguous focus osteomyelitis has been further subdivided into osteomyelitis with or without vascular insufficiency. Hematogenous and contiguous focus osteomyelitis have been further divided into acute or chronic disease. Acute disease presents as a suppurative infection accompanied by edema, vascular congestion, and small vessel thrombosis. In early acute disease the vascular supply to the bone is compromised by infection extending into the surrounding soft tissue. When both the medullary and periosteal blood supplies are compromised, large areas of dead bone (sequestra) may be formed. Within this necrotic and ischemic tissue, the bacteria may be difficult to eradicate even after an intense host response, surgery, and/or antibiotic therapy. Clinically, acute osteomyelitis evolves into chronic disease. The hallmarks of chronic disease are a nidus of infected dead bone or scar tissue, an ischemic soft tissue envelope, and a refractory clinical course.[3]

The term *cure* is not used in osteomyelitis, since the bone infection may recur years after apparent successful treatment of the disease. If the patient suffers trauma in the involved area and/or the host response to the infection is suppressed, the organism(s) may again proliferate and lead to an exacerbation of the infection. Therefore, in osteomyelitis treatment the infection is said to be "arrested" rather than "cured."

An alternative classification system has been developed by Cierny and Mader.[4] This classification takes into consideration

the quality of host, the anatomic nature of the disease, treatment factors, and prognosis factors (Table 1). This staging system combines four anatomic disease types (Fig. 1) and three physiologic host categories to define 12 discrete clinical stages of osteomyelitis.

Stage 1, or medullary, osteomyelitis, equates with early hematogenous osteomyelitis where the primary lesion is endosteal. Pediatric stage 1 usually can be treated with antibiotics alone. Adult stage 1 osteomyelitis is usually treated with cortical unroofing and intramedullary reaming. An infected intramedullary rod in a stable bone is another example of stage 1 osteomyelitis. In this case the infected intramedullary rod must be removed, followed by intramedullary reaming.

In stage 2, or superficial, osteomyelitis, the bone infection results from an adjacent soft tissue infection and represents a true contiguous focus lesion. An exposed, infected necrotic outer surface of the bone lies at the base of a soft tissue wound. Stage 2 osteomyelitis requires superficial débridement and coverage with a local or microvascular flap.

Stage 3, or localized, osteomyelitis is characterized by full thickness cortical sequestration that can be surgically removed without compromising stability of the infected bone. Stage 3 osteomyelitis requires débridement, saucerization, and possibly a bone graft to improve stability.

Stage 4, or diffuse, osteomyelitis, represents a through and through section of the bone and usually requires segmental resection of the bone. The stage 4 patient may also have bone infection on both sides of a nonunion or major joint. Diffuse osteomyelitis includes those infections with a loss of bony stability either before or after débridement surgery. Stage 4 osteomyelitis requires débridement, dead space management, and stabilization.

In this system, patients are classified as A, B, or C hosts. A hosts are those patients with normal physiologic, metabolic, and immunologic capabilities. B hosts (Table 1) are patients who are locally compromised, systemically compromised, or both. It is important to improve the factors and diseases that made the patient a B host. The goal of host modification is to make a B host as much like an A host as possible. The final category, or C host, represents the patient for whom the treatment of the bone infection is worse than the osteomyelitis itself.

TABLE 1. Cierny and Mader Classification System

Anatomic type
  Stage 1, medullary osteomyelitis
  Stage 2, superficial osteomyelitis
  Stage 3, localized osteomyelitis
  Stage 4, diffuse osteomyelitis

Physiologic class
A host, Normal host
B host, Systemic compromise (Bs)
     Local compromise (Bl)
C host, Treatment worse than the disease

Systemic or Local Factors that Affect Immune Surveillance, Metabolism, and Local Vascularity
Systemic (Bs)
  Malnutrition
  Renal, liver failure
  Diabetes mellitus
  Chronic hypoxia
  Immune disease
  Malignancy
  Extremes of age
  Immunosuppression or immune deficiency
  Tobacco abuse

Local (Bl)
  Chronic lymphedema
  Venous stasis
  Major vessel compromise
  Arteritis
  Extensive scarring
  Radiation fibrosis
  Small vessel disease
  Complete loss of local sensation

Stage I (Medullary Osteomyelitis)

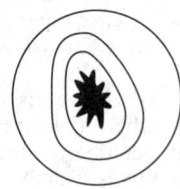

Necrosis limited to medullary contents and endosteal surfaces.
Etiology: Hematogenous
Treatment:
Early: Antibiotics/ Host alteration
Late: Unroofing, intramedullary reaming

Stage II (Superficial Osteomyelitis)

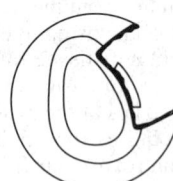

Necrosis limited to exposed surfaces.
Etiology: Contiguous soft tissue infection
Treatment:
Early: Antibiotics/ Host alteration
Late: Superficial debridement/ Coverage
        Possible ablation

Stage III (Localized Osteomyelitis)

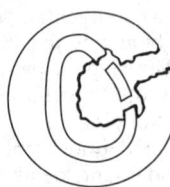

Well marginated and stable before and after debridement.
Etiology: Trauma, evolving stages I and II, Iatrogenic
Treatment:
Antibiotics/ Host alteration
Debridement, Dead space management
Temporary stabilization, Bone graft optional

Stage IV (Diffuse Osteomyelitis)

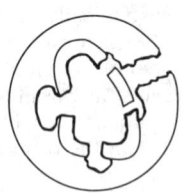

Circumferential and/or permeative.
Unstable prior to or after debridement
Etiology: Trauma, evolving stages I and II and III, Iatrogenic
Treatment:
Antibiotics/ Host alteration
Stabilization - ORIF, External fixation (Ilizarov)
Debridement, Dead space management
Possible ablation

FIG. 1. Anatomic classification of adult long bone osteomyelitis, etiology, and treatment. ORIF, orthopaedic rod internal fixation.

This staging system has been used to determine optimal treatment protocols, and prognoses and to compare therapy results between institutions. The stages are dynamic and may be altered by therapy outcome or change in host status. The traditional Waldvogel classification system will be used throughout this chapter, but reference to the Cierny-Mader classification will be made when appropriate.

HEMATOGENOUS OSTEOMYELITIS

Hematogenous osteomyelitis occurs mainly in infants and children. The metaphyses of the long bones (tibia, femur) are most frequently involved (Fig. 2). The anatomy of the metaphyseal region seems to explain this clinical localization.[5] Nonanastomosing capillary ends of the nutrient artery make sharp loops under the growth plate and enter a system of large venous sinusoids where the blood flow becomes slow and turbulent. These capillary loops are essentially "end-artery" branches of the nutrient artery. Any end capillary obstruction can lead to an area of avascular necrosis. The metaphyseal capillaries lack phagocytic lining cells, and sinusoidal veins contain functionally inactive phagocytic cells.[6] The infant or child is predisposed to infection by minor trauma that produces a small hematoma, vascular obstruction, and subsequent bone necrosis. The area is then susceptible to inoculation from a transient bacteremia.[7] The acute infection initially produces a local cellulitis that results in a infiltration with leukocytes, increased bone pressure, decreased pH, and decreased oxygen tension. The cumulative effects of these physiologic factors further compromise the medullary circulation and enhance the spread of infection. The infection may proceed laterally through the Haversian and Volkmann canal systems, perforate the bony cortex, and lift the periosteum from the surface of the bone. When this occurs in the presence of medullary extension, both the periosteal and endosteal circulations are lost, and large segments of dead cortical and cancellous bone are formed. In the infant, medullary infection may spread to the epiphysis and joint surfaces through capillaries that cross the growth plate. In the child over 1 year of age, since the growth plate is avascular the infection is confined to the metaphysis and diaphysis. The joint is spared unless the metaphysis is intracapsular. Thus, cortical perforation at the proximal radius, humerus, or femur infects the elbow, shoulder, or hip joint, respectively, regardless of the age of the patient.

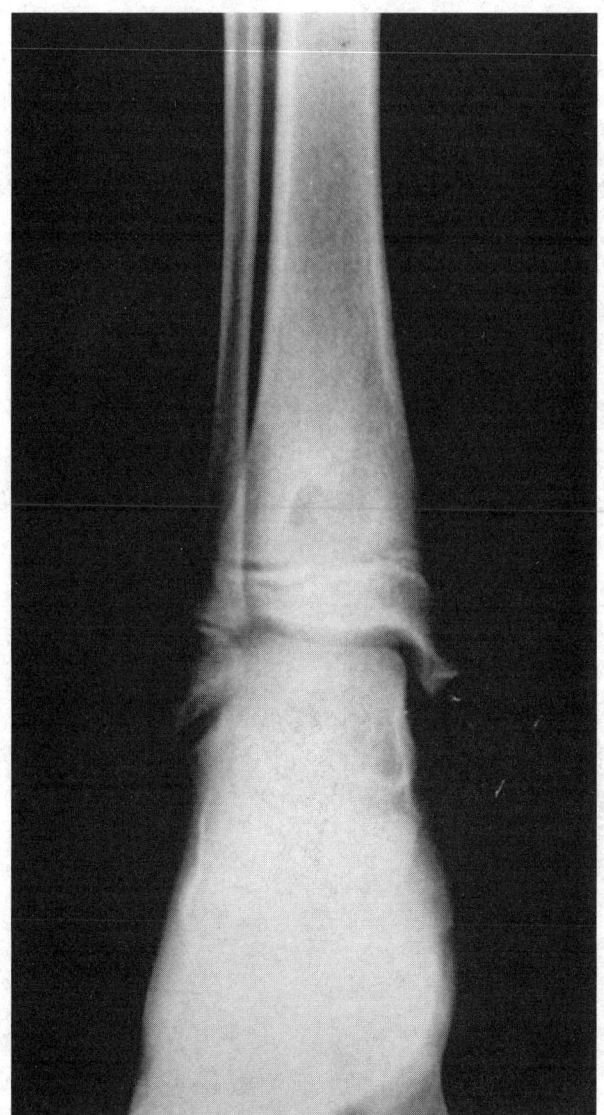

FIG. 2. Hematogenous osteomyelitis in a child. There is bony involvement with lytic changes in the metaphysis of the distal tibia.

Hematogenous osteomyelitis is also found in the adult population. The infection usually begins in the diaphysis but may spread to involve the entire medullary canal (Fig. 3). Extension into the joint may occur since the growth plate has matured and once again shares vessels with the metaphysis. As the periosteum is firmly adherent to the bone, cortical penetration usually leads to a soft tissue abscess. In time sinus tracts connecting the sequestered nidus of infection to the skin via soft tissue extension may form.

A single pathogenic organism is almost always recovered from the bone. In infants, *Staphylococcus aureus, Streptococcus agalactiae,* and *Escherichia coli* are most frequently isolated from blood or bones, whereas in children over 1 year of age *S. aureus, Streptococcus pyogenes,* and *Haemophilus influenzae* are most commonly isolated. The incidence of *H. influenzae* infection decreases after age 4 years. In adults, *S. aureus* is the most common organism isolated.

Neonatal osteomyelitis is characterized by a paucity of systemic and local findings.[8] Local findings include edema and decreased motion of a limb. A joint effusion adjacent to the bone infection is present in approximately 60 percent of the cases. Children with hematogenous osteomyelitis may present with abrupt fever, irritability, lethargy, and local signs of inflamma-

tion 3 weeks or less in duration.[9] However, 50 percent of children present with vague complaints, including pain of the involved limb of 1–3 months in duration and minimal if any temperature elevation. Infants and children with hematogenous osteomyelitis usually have normal soft tissue enveloping the infected bone and are capable of a very efficient metabolic response to infection. Therefore, children have the potential to resorb large sequestra and generate a significant periosteal response to the infection. This latter feature leads to substantial formation of bone formed at the margin of the infection (involucrum). The involucrum affords skeletal continuity and maintenance of function during the healing phase. If antimicrobial therapy directed at the responsible pathogen is begun prior to extensive bone necrosis, the patient has an excellent probability of disease arrest.

Adults usually present with vague complaints consisting of nonspecific pain and few constitutional symptoms of 1–3 months in duration. However, acute clinical presentations with fever, chills, swelling, and erythema over the involved bone(s) are occasionally seen.

VERTEBRAL OSTEOMYELITIS

Pyogenic vertebral osteomyelitis is usually hematogenous in origin. An arterial route rather than Batson's venous plexus is believed to be the most likely route of infection.[10] The segmental arteries supplying the vertebrae usually bifurcate to supply two adjacent bony segments.[11,12] Therefore, the disease usually involves two adjacent vertebrae and the intervertebral disc. In the normal host, *S. aureus* remains the most commonly isolated organism.[13] However, in intravenous drug users, *Pseudomonas aeruginosa* is the most commonly isolated organism.[14,15] Other sources of infection include the genitourinary tract, skin and soft tissue, respiratory tract, infected IV sites, endocarditis, dental infection, or unknown sources.[16–18]

Localized pain and tenderness of the involved bone segments is present in at least 90 percent of the cases. The pain is usually insidious and slowly progresses over 3 weeks to 3 months.

Fever and peripheral leukocytosis are absent in approximately 50 percent of the cases. The erythrocyte sedimentation rate is usually elevated and may be used as a prognostic guide during treatment. Posterior extension of the infection may lead to epidural and subdural abscesses or even to meningitis. Extension anteriorly or laterally may lead to paravertebral, retropharyngeal, mediastinal, subphrenic, or retroperitoneal abscesses. Motor and sensory neurologic defects can be detected in 6–15 percent of cases.[13] The lumbar region is affected in at least 45 percent of cases of hematogenous vertebral osteomyelitis, followed by the thoracic spine (35 percent) and the cervical spine (20 percent).[10]

CONTIGUOUS FOCUS OSTEOMYELITIS WITHOUT GENERALIZED VASCULAR INSUFFICIENCY

In contiguous focus osteomyelitis, the organisms may be directly inoculated into the bone at the time of trauma, spread by nosocomial contamination during perioperative or intraoperative procedures, or extend from an adjacent soft tissue infection (Fig. 4). Common predisposing factors include surgical reduction and internal fixation of fractures, prosthetic devices, open fractures, and chronic soft tissue infections. In contrast to hematogenous osteomyelitis, multiple organisms are usually isolated from the infected bone. *Staphylococcus aureus* remains the most commonly isolated pathogen. However, gram-negative bacilli and anaerobic organisms are frequently isolated.

The infection usually occurs within 1 month after inoculation of the organism from trauma, surgery, or a soft tissue infection. The patient presents with low-grade fever, pain, and drainage. Loss of bone stability, bone necrosis, and soft tissue damage

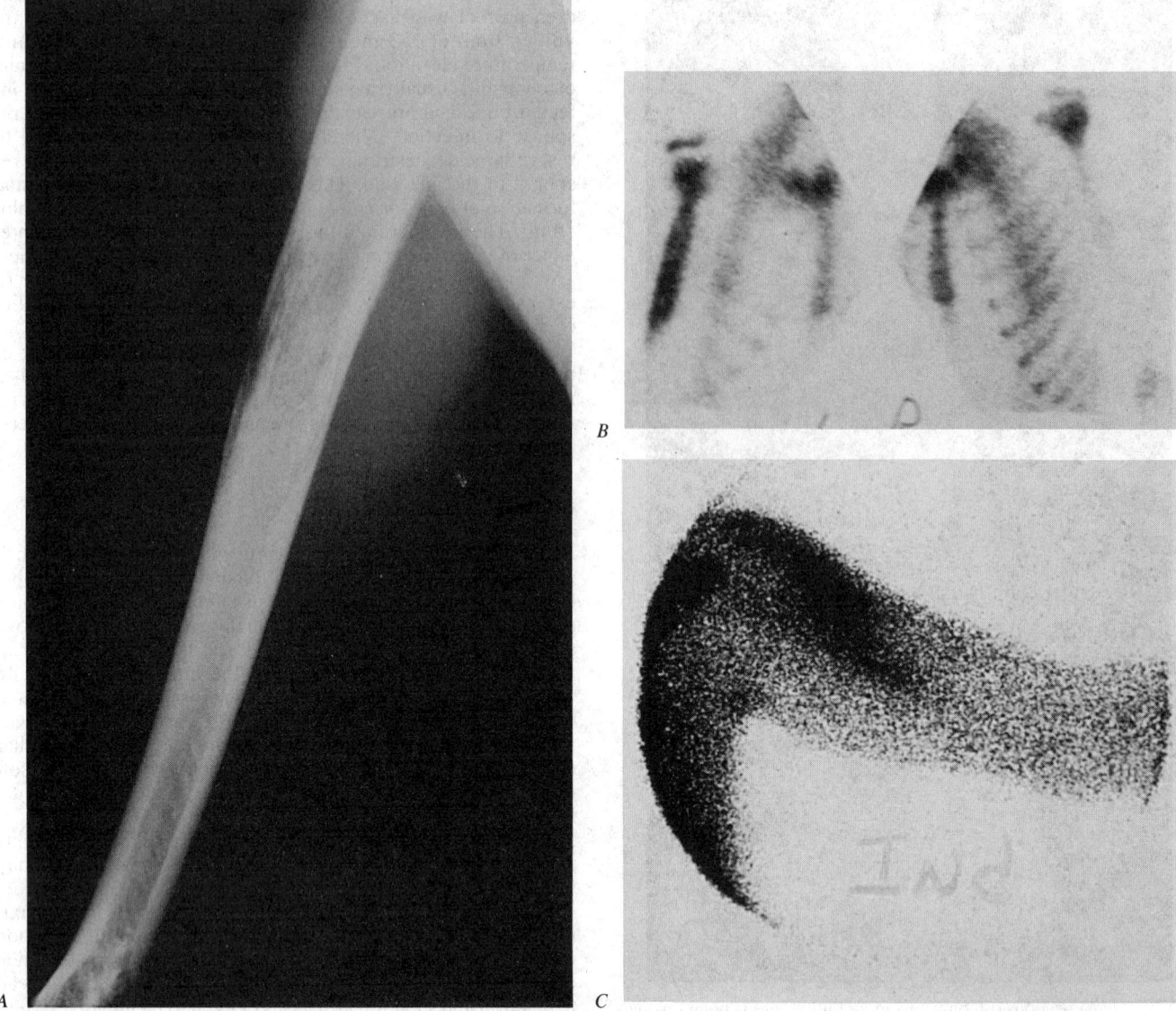

FIG. 3.   (A) Hematogenous osteomyelitis in the diaphysis of the humerus of a 28-year-old man. There is involvement of the intramedullary canal with cortical extension to the periosteum and soft tissue. (B) ^{99m}Technetium polyphosphate scan showing involvement of the humerus. In our experience the technetium scan tends to show more bony involvement than is surgically present. Minor trauma may also cause a positive technetium scan. (C) Indium chloride scan showing involvement of the intramedullary canal of the humerus with extension to the adjacent soft tissue.

frequently occur, making this form of osteomyelitis difficult to treat.

CONTIGUOUS FOCUS OSTEOMYELITIS WITH GENERALIZED VASCULAR INSUFFICIENCY

The majority of the patients in this category of osteomyelitis have diabetes mellitus. The small bones of the feet are commonly involved in this type of infection (Fig. 5). Blunting of the local tissue response due to inadequate tissue perfusion predisposes the patient to infection. Commonly, the infection is initiated by minor trauma of the feet. Multiple organisms are usually isolated from the infected bone. The most common organisms are coagulase-positive and -negative staphylococci, *Streptococcus* spp., *Enterococcus* spp., gram-negative bacilli, and anaerobes. Aerobic gram-negative bacilli are usually a part of a mixed infection.

Osteomyelitis in vascularly compromised patients can be difficult to diagnose. The patient may present with an ingrown toenail, a perforating foot ulcer, cellulitis, or a deep space infection. Concurrent peripheral neuropathy mutes the patient's perception of pain. Fever and systemic toxicity are often absent. Examination shows decreased dorsal pedis and posterior tibial pulses, poor capillary refill, and decreased sensation.

Although arrest of the infection is desirable, a more attainable treatment goal is to suppress the infection and maintain the functional integrity of the involved limb. Recurrent or new bone infections occur in the majority of the patients even after appropriate treatment. Resection of the infected area is almost always necessary.

CHRONIC OSTEOMYELITIS

Both hematogenous and contiguous focus osteomyelitis can progress to a chronic condition. Local bone loss, persistent drainage, and/or sinus tracts are common.[19] The nidus of the persistent contamination must be removed before the infection will start to regress. Antibiotic therapy alone is usually unsuc-

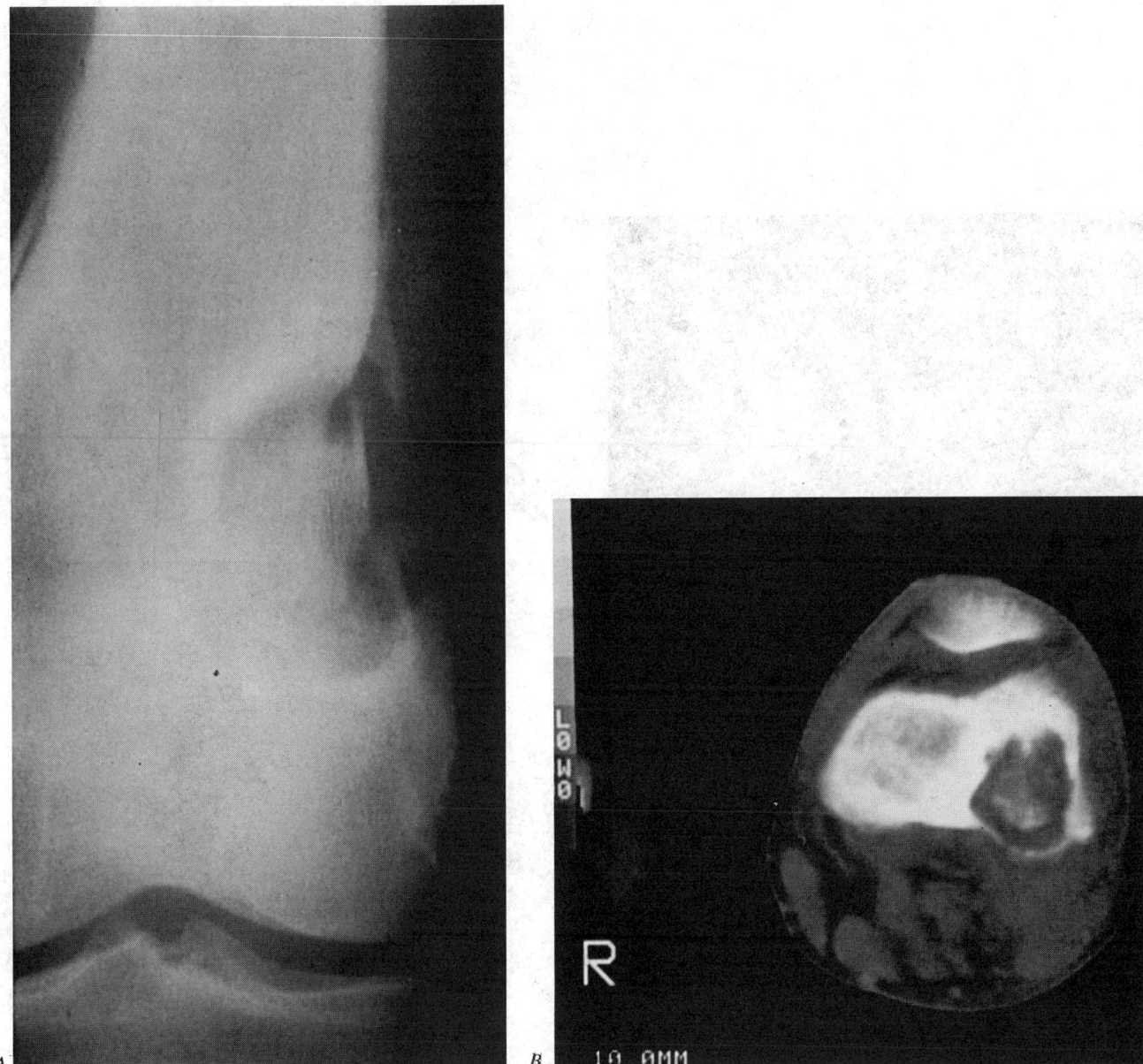

FIG. 4. **(A)** Contiguous focus osteomyelitis in a 20-year-old man. The radiograph shows a large sequestrum in the distal femur. **(B)** CT scan showing the large sequestrum in the distal femur. The femur was saucerized, and the resulting defect was bone grafted.

cessful in the treatment of chronic osteomyelitis. Prospects of arresting the infection are reduced when the integrity of surrounding soft tissue is poor or the bone is unstable secondary to an infected nonunion or an adjacent septic joint.

The patient usually presents with chronic pain and drainage. If present, fever is low grade. The sedimentation rate is usually elevated, reflecting chronic inflammation, but the leukocyte count is usually normal. The chronic disease is usually nonprogressive or slowly progressive. If a sinus tract becomes obstructed, the patient may present with a localized abscess and/or a soft tissue infection. Squamous cell carcinoma at the site of tissue drainage and amyloidosis are rare complications of chronic osteomyelitis.

DIAGNOSIS OF OSTEOMYELITIS

The diagnosis of long bone osteomyelitis rests on the obligatory isolation of the pathogen from the bone lesion or blood culture. In hematogenous osteomyelitis, positive blood cultures can

often obviate the need for a bone biopsy when there is radiographic or radionuclide scan evidence of osteomyelitis.

Sinus tract cultures are not reliable for predicting gram-negative organisms causing osteomyelitis.[20] In most cases, antibiotic treatment of osteomyelitis should be based on meticulous cultures taken at débridement surgery or from deep bone biopsies and antibiotic susceptibilities.[21]

Sedimentation rates and leukocyte counts are frequently elevated prior to therapy in the acute disease, but the leukocyte count rarely exceeds $15,000/mm^3$, and it is usually normal in patients with chronic osteomyelitis. Elevated sedimentation rates and leukocyte counts may fall with appropriate therapy. However, both values may elevate acutely around each débridement surgery. A sedimentation rate that returns to normal during the course of therapy is a favorable prognostic sign. However, in the compromised host this laboratory determination is not reliable since these patients are constantly challenged by minor illnesses and peripheral lesions that may elevate this index.

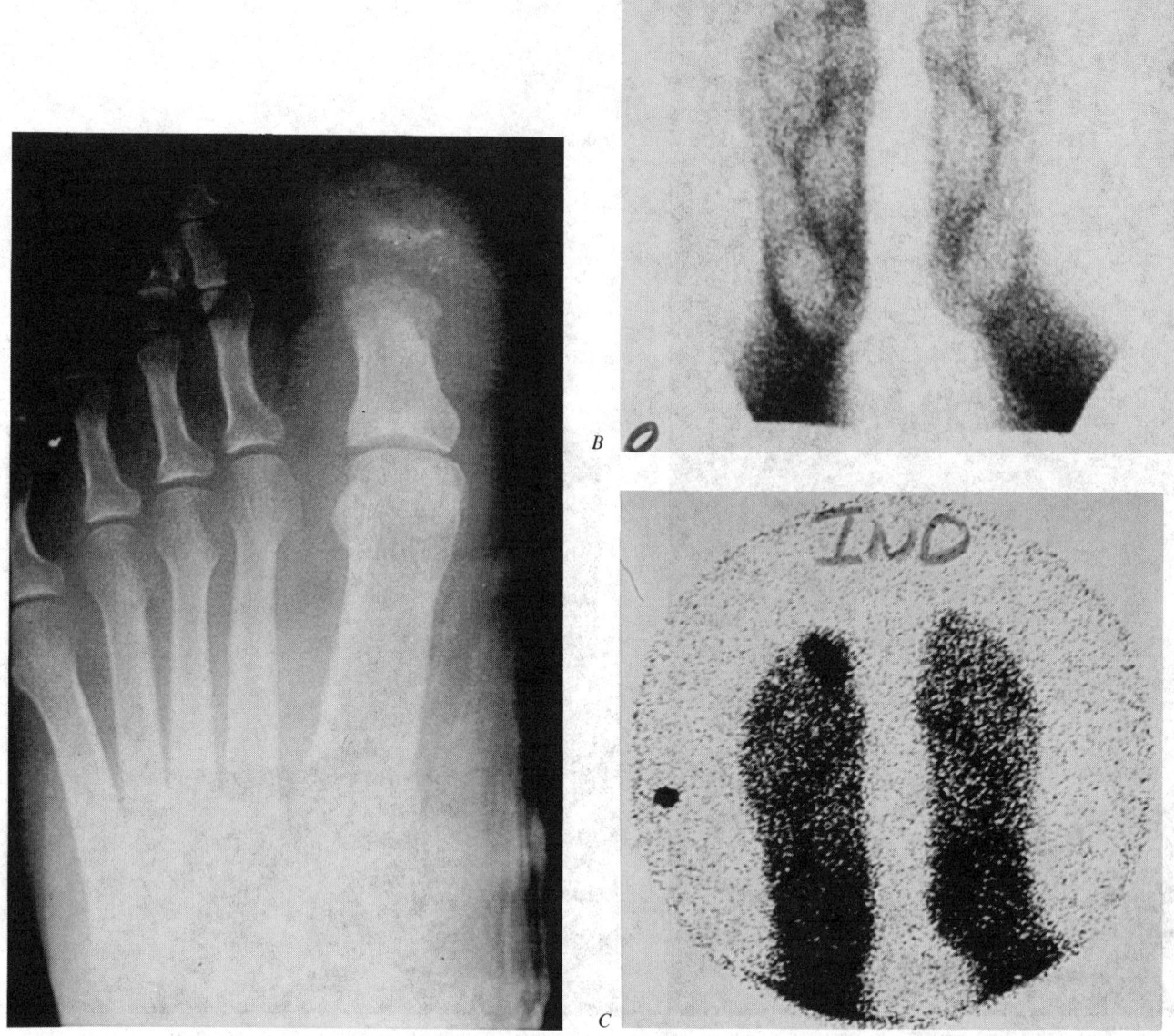

FIG. 5. **(A)** Contiguous focus osteomyelitis in a 40-year-old man with diabetes mellitus. The proximal and distal phalanges of the first toe around the proximal interphalangeal joint show bony destruction. **(B)** A 3-minute ^{99m}Tc polyphosphate scan (venous pool) of the first toe showing increased uptake consistent with osteomyelitis. **(C)** Indium chloride scan showing increased uptake in the bones of the first toe. The indium scan is consistent with (inflammation) osteomyelitis of the first toe. Comparison of the technetium and indium scans supports osteomyelitis of the first toe. A more diffuse pattern on both scans would suggest a soft tissue process.

Diagnosis of Long Bone Osteomyelitis

Radiograph Studies. In acute hematogenous osteomyelitis, radiographic changes accurately reflect the destructive process, but lag at least 2 weeks behind the evolution of infection. The earliest changes are swelling of the soft tissue, periosteal thickening and/or elevation, and focal osteopenia (Figs. 2 and 3A). At least 50–75 percent of the bone matrix must be destroyed before radiographs show lytic changes. The more diagnostic lytic changes are delayed and often associated with an indolent infection of several months duration. Radiographic improvement may lag behind clinical recovery, even when the patient is receiving appropriate antimicrobial therapy.[22] In contiguous focus and chronic osteomyelitis, the radiographic changes are subtle, often found in association with other nonspecific radiographic findings, and require a careful clinical correlation to achieve diagnostic significance (Fig. 4A and 5A).

Radionuclide Studies. An earlier diagnosis of osteomyelitis may be achieved with radionuclide imaging. However, the actual mechanism of bone labeling with radiopharmaceuticals is still unclear. The technetium polyphosphate ^{99m}Tc scan demonstrates increased isotope accumulation in areas of increased blood flow and reactive new bone formation (Figs. 3B and 5B).[23] In biopsy-confirmed cases of hematogenous osteomyelitis, it is usually positive as early as 48 hours following the initiation of the bone infection.[24] Negative ^{99m}Tc scans in documented cases of osteomyelitis may reflect impaired blood supply to the infected area.[25]

A second class of radiopharmaceuticals used for the evaluation of osteomyelitis includes gallium citrate and indium chloride. Gallium and indium attach to transferrin, which leaks from the blood stream into areas of inflammation. Gallium and indium scans also show increased isotope uptake in areas concentrating polymorphonuclear leukocytes, macrophages, and malignant tumors.[26,27] Since these scans do not show bone detail well, it is often difficult to distinguish between bone and soft tissue inflammation; a comparison with a [99mTc] scan helps to resolve this problem (Figs. 3B and 5B).[28] In contrast to gallium citrate, indium chloride is more heavily concentrated by hematopoietic tissue and is not found to accumulate in areas of reactive bone.[26]

Indium-labeled leukocyte scans are less useful in the evaluation of osteomyelitis. Indium leukocyte scans are positive in approximately 40 percent of patients with acute osteomyelitis and 60 percent of patients with septic arthritis.[29] Patients who have chronic osteomyelitis, bony metastases, and degenerative arthritis often have negative scans.

Computed Tomography. Computed axial tomography (CT) may play a role in the diagnosis of osteomyelitis. Increased marrow density occurs early in the infection,[30] and intramedullary gas has been reported in patients with hematogenous osteomyelitis.[31] The CT scan can also help to identify areas of necrotic bone and to assess the involvement of the surrounding soft tissues (Fig. 4b). In a recalcitrant infection, the CT scan may assist in identifying the surgical approach and augment débridement.[30,32] One disadvantage of this study is the scatter phenomenon, which occurs when metal is present in or near the area of bone infection. This scatter results in a significant loss of image resolution.

Magnetic Resonance Imaging. Magnetic resonance imaging (MRI) has been recognized as a useful modality for diagnosing the presence and scope of musculoskeletal sepsis.[33–35] The spatial resolution of MRI makes it useful in differentiating between bone and soft tissue infection, often a problem with radionuclide studies.[36] Unlike the radionuclide studies, MRI is not useful for whole-body examinations. Metallic implants in the region of interest may produce focal artifacts, thereby decreasing the utility of the image.[37] Initial MRI screening usually consists of a T1-weighted and a T2-weighted spin-echo pulse sequence. In a T1-weighted study, edema is dark and fat is bright. In a T2-weighted study, the reverse is true. The typical appearance of osteomyelitis is a localized area of abnormal marrow with decreased signal intensity on T1-weighted images and increased signal intensity on T2-weighted images. On occasion there may be decreased signal intensity on T2-weighted images.[37] Posttraumatic or surgical scarring of the marrow is seen as a region of decreased signal intensity on T1-weighted images with no change of the T2-weighted image. Sinus tracts are seen as areas of high signal intensity on the T2-weighted image extending from the marrow and bone through the soft tissues and out of the skin. Cellulitis is seen as diffuse areas of intermediate signal in the T1-weighted images of the soft tissues, with increased signal on the T2-weighted images of the same area. Since differentiation of infection from neoplasm on the basis of the MRI may be difficult, clinical and radiographic confirmation is necessary.[37]

Vertebral Osteomyelitis

Anteroposterior and lateral radiographic views of the spine will reveal intervertebral disc space narrowing, with destruction and new bone formation at the anterior edge of the vertebral disc (Fig. 6A). A CT or MRI scan that can demonstrate evidence of osteomyelitis before radiographic changes occur shows early evidence of paravertebral soft tissue swelling and bone destruction (Fig. 6B, 6C).[38–40]

The technetium polyphosphate [99mTc] scan also can detect spinal abnormalities in the early stages of infection, even before radiographic changes are seen.[41] Gallium/indium scans are difficult to interpret due to the high concentration of hematopoietic tissue in vertebral bodies.

A definitive diagnosis of vertebral osteomyelitis rests on the isolation of the organism from bone. A bone biopsy is generally required, since blood cultures are usually sterile. The biopsy should be performed under fluoroscopy or CT scan for guidance into the infected areas. In addition to aerobic and anaerobic bacterial cultures, the specimens should be sent for fungal and mycobacterial stains and cultures, as well as histology. If the original cultures are negative, an open surgical biopsy should be performed before starting empiric antibiotic therapy.

TREATMENT

The components of osteomyelitis treatment include patient evaluation, staging assessment, identification and sensitivity of microorganism(s), administration of antibiotics, débridement surgery, dead space management, and, if necessary, stabilization.[3,42] Reconstruction is considered at the first surgery.

Acute Hematogenous Osteomyelitis

In children, acute hematogenous osteomyelitis is primarily a medical disease. In the adult, débridement surgery, bone unroofing, intramedullary reaming, and/or incision and drainage of soft tissue abscesses are often required. Identification of the causative pathogen is essential. The infection is usually susceptible to specific antimicrobial therapy. Mismanagement with inappropriate antibiotic(s) encourages disease extension, necrosis, and sequestra formation. Surgical intervention is indicated if the patient has not responded to specific antimicrobial therapy within 48 hours, has evidence of a persistent soft tissue abscess, or diagnosed or suspected joint sepsis. A bone biopsy for culture is necessary unless the patient has positive blood cultures along with radiographic or bone scan findings consistent with osteomyelitis. After cultures are obtained, a parenteral antimicrobial regimen is begun to cover the clinically suspected pathogens. Once the organism is identified, the antibiotic regimen may be continued or changed on the basis of sensitivity results.[43] The patient is treated for 4–6 weeks with appropriate parenteral antimicrobial therapy, dated from the initiation of therapy or after the last major débridement surgery. If the initial medical management fails and the patient is clinically compromised by a recurrent infection, medullary and/or soft tissue débridement will be necessary in conjunction with another 4–6 weeks course of antibiotics.

Oral antibiotic therapy can be utilized for treatment of childhood osteomyelitis. However, it is recommended that the patient initially receive 2 weeks of parenteral antibiotic therapy prior to changing to an oral regimen.[44,45] In addition, the patient must be compliant and have close outpatient follow-up. Absorption and activity of the orally administered antibiotic should be monitored. Pediatric patients should not be given oral antimicrobial therapy with quinolones.[46,47]

Vertebral Osteomyelitis

Biopsy and débridement cultures dictate the choice of antibiotic(s). The antibiotics are given for 4–6 weeks and are dated from the initiation of therapy or from the last major débridement surgery. Surgical therapy is usually not necessary, except in cases in which the patient develops an extension of the infection, such as paravertebral or epidural abscesses, when medical management fails or when instability is pending. The neurologic status of the patient must be closely monitored. Surgical fusion of the involved vertebrae is usually not required, as spontaneous bony fusion occurs in 1–12 months following appropriate antibiotic therapy. The success of patients treated with bedrest alone is not substantially different from those who are ambulatory and stabilized with a cast, a corset, or a brace.

Osteomyelitis Secondary to Contiguous Focus Infection or Chronic Osteomyelitis

In contiguous focus and chronic osteomyelitis, the primary problem is infected necrotic bone having a poorly perfused sur-

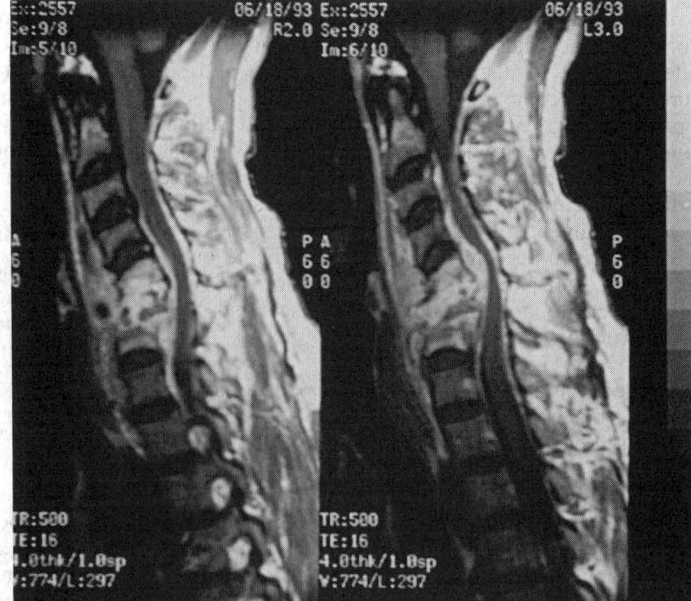

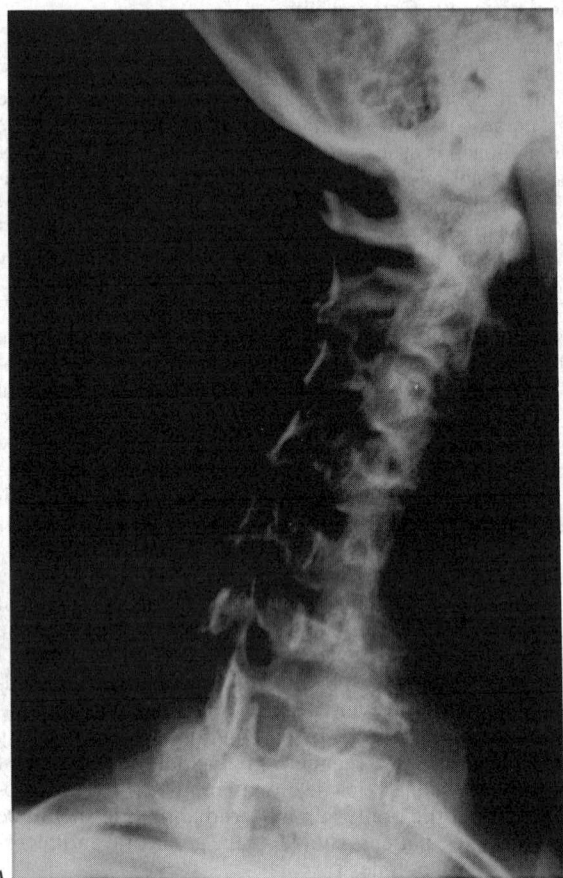

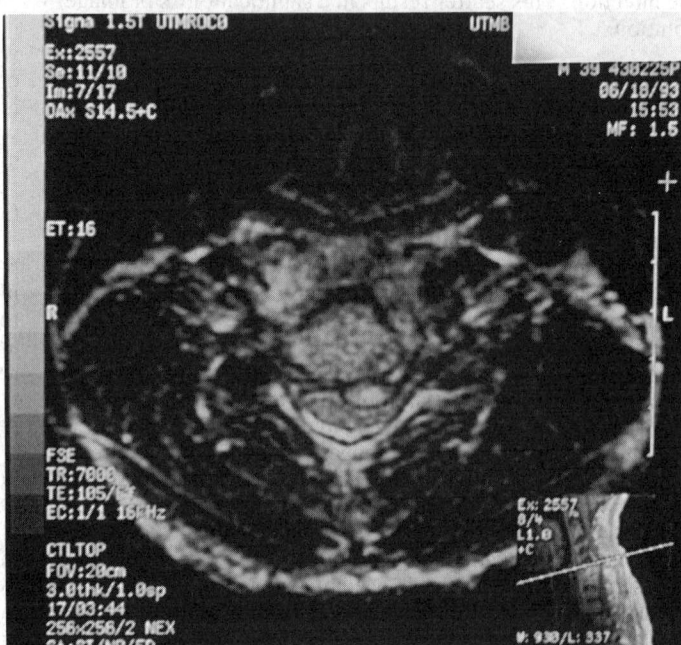

FIG. 6. **(A)** Cervical spine film showing involvement of the C5–6, C6–7 cervical vertebral disc spaces. There is destructive involvement of the body of C6. **(B)** MRI showing involvement of C5–6 and C6–7 disc spaces. There is destruction of the body of C6. There is an associated extension of the infection into the prevertebral and epidural areas. **(C)** MRI cross section at C6. There is osteomyelitis of the body of C6 and epidural extension of the infection.

rounding soft tissue envelope. The infection cannot be arrested until the nidus for the persistent contamination is removed. Adequate drainage, thorough débridement, obliteration of dead space, hardware removal, wound protection, and specific antimicrobial therapy are the mainstays of treatment.[48]

If possible, antibiotics should not be initiated until the results of the bone bacterial culture and sensitivities are known. However, if immediate débridement surgery is required, empiric broad-spectrum antibiotics can be started. The antibiotics may be modified, if necessary, when results of the débridement cultures and sensitivities are available. Surgical exposure is direct, atraumatic, and designed to avoid unnecessary devitalization of bone and soft tissue. The wound is débrided until all nonviable tissue and superfluous hardware have been removed. To ensure

antibiotic perfusion and avoid continued sequestration, the cancellous and cortical bone remaining in the wound after débridement must bleed uniformly.

Since it takes 3–4 weeks for bone to revascularize following débridement surgery, antibiotics are used to treat live infected bone and to protect bone undergoing revascularization. The patient is treated with 4–6 weeks of parenteral antimicrobial therapy dated from the last major débridement surgery.[42] Outpatient intravenous therapy with long-term intravenous access catheters such as Hickman or Groshong catheters makes outpatient intravenous antibiotic treatment possible.[49–51] Outpatient intramuscular antibiotic administration is also feasible. Oral therapy using quinolones for gram-negative organisms is currently being utilized in adult patients with osteomyelitis.[52,53] The current quinolones have poor activity against *Streptococcus* spp., *Enterococcus* spp., and anaerobic bacteria.[54] The quinolones also have variable *S. aureus* and *S. epidermidis* coverage, and resistance is increasing.[55] Coverage of aerobic gram-positive organisms should be obtained with other oral antibiotics such as clindamycin or amoxicillin-clavulanate. Before changing to an oral regimen, it is recommended that the patient initially receive 2 weeks of parenteral antibiotic therapy. The patient must be compliant and have close outpatient follow-up.

A combination of parenteral and oral antibiotics has been used in some situations. Methicillin-sensitive *S. aureus* osteomyelitis has been successfully treated with a semisynthetic penicillin and rifamipin.[56]

In general, it is not necessary to follow antibiotic levels,[57] because most treatment failures are due to a lack of adequate surgical débridement rather than antibiotic efficacy.[42] It may be necessary to follow serum levels in cases of relatively resistant organisms or when combination antibiotic therapy is necessary.

Appropriate management of any dead space created by débridement surgery is mandatory to arrest the disease and to maintain the integrity of the skeletal part (Fig. 7). The goal of dead space management is to replace dead bone and scar tissue with durable vascularized tissue.[42] Secondary intention healing is discouraged, since the scar tissue that fills the defect may later become avascular. Suction irrigation systems are not recommended because of the high incidence of associated nosocomial infections and the unreliability of these setups.[58,59] Complete wound closure should be attained whenever possible. Local tissue flaps or free flaps may be used to fill dead space.[60–62] An alternative technique is to place cancellous bone grafts beneath local or transferred tissues where structural augmentation is necessary. Careful preoperative planning is critical to the conservation of the patient's limited cancellous bone reserves. Open cancellous grafts without soft tissue coverage are useful when a free tissue transfer is not a treatment option and local tissue flaps are inadequate.[63] Antibiotic-impregnated acrylic beads may be used to sterilize and temporarily maintain dead space (Fig. 8). The beads are usually removed within 2–4 weeks and replaced with a cancellous bone graft.[42,64–69] Antibiotics (clindamycin, amikacin) have also been delivered directly into dead space with an implantable pump.[70]

If movement is present at the site of infection, measures must be taken to achieve permanent stability of the skeletal unit. Stability may be achieved with plates, screws, rods, and/or an external fixator. A new type of external fixator allows bone reconstruction of segmental defects and difficult infected nonunions.[71] The Ilizarov external fixation method uses distraction or compression histogenesis, a process of bone regeneration to fill bone defects or to compress nonunions and correct malunion. In one clinical series,[72] 92 percent of patients with chronic osteomyelitis with segmental defects, ranging from simple nonunions to 8 cm gaps, were successfully reconstructed. The technique is labor intensive and requires an extended period of treatment averaging 8.5 months in the device. The Ilizarov pins usually become infected, and the device is painful.

Osteomyelitis Secondary to Contiguous Focus Infection with Vascular Diseases

Because of the relative inability of the host to participate in the eradication of the infectious process, this type of osteomyelitis

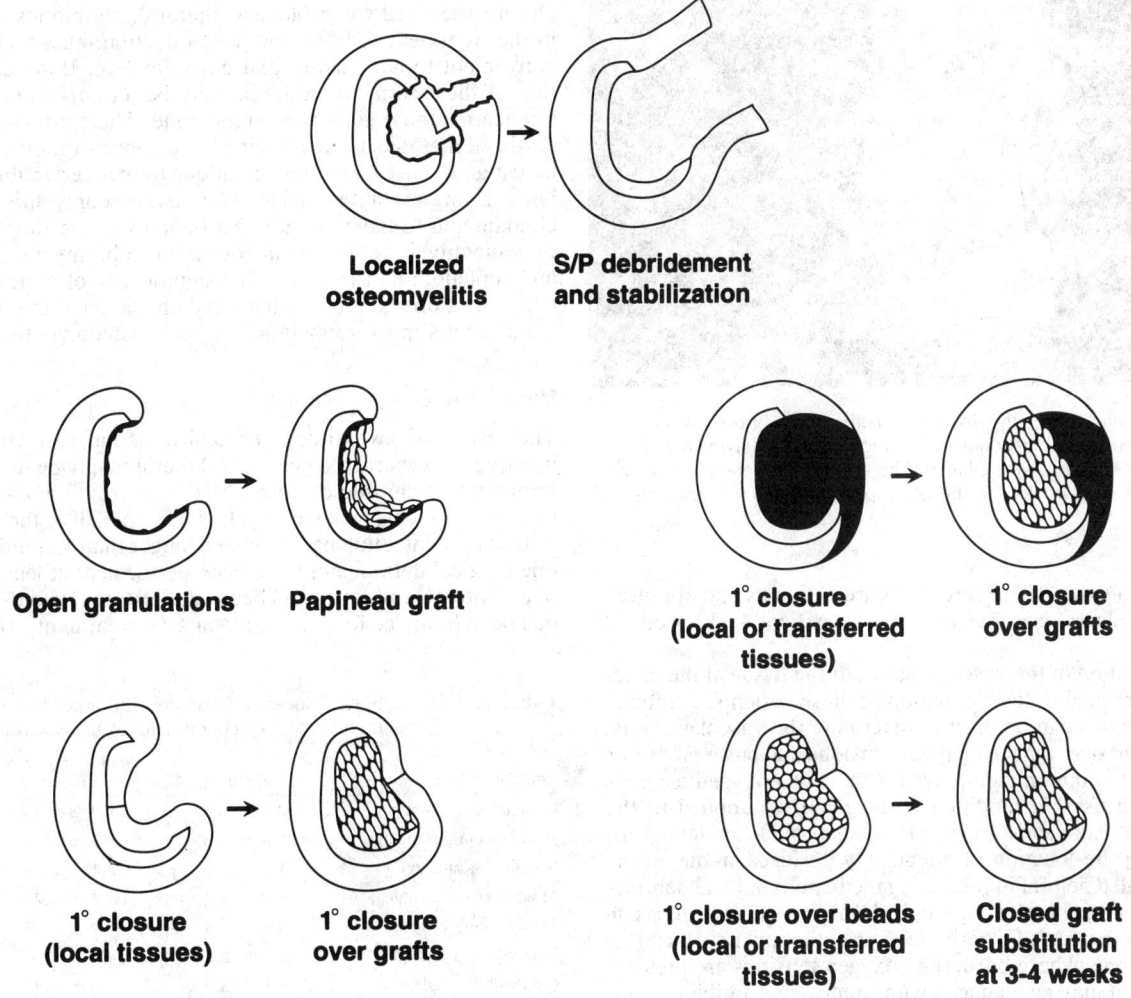

Localized osteomyelitis   S/P debridement and stabilization

Open granulations   Papineau graft

1° closure (local or transferred tissues)   1° closure over grafts

1° closure (local tissues)   1° closure over grafts

1° closure over beads (local or transferred tissues)   Closed graft substitution at 3-4 weeks

FIG. 7. Dead space management of long bone osteomyelitis.

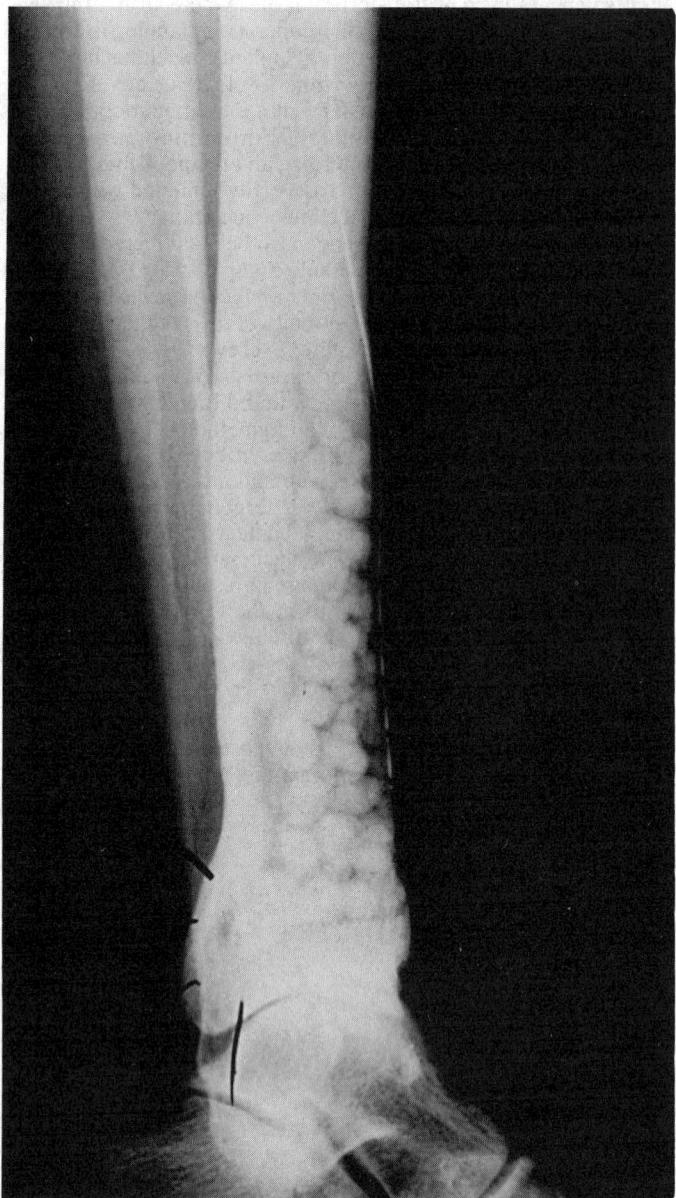

FIG. 8. Osteomyelitis of the distal tibia. Following débridement surgery, antibiotic-impregnated (vancomycin and tobramycin) polymethylmethacrylate (PMMA) beads were placed. The antibiotic-impregnated beads were removed at 3 weeks and the dead space replaced with cancellous bone graft.

is difficult to treat. These infections are insidious and are often beyond simple salvage by the time the patient seeks medical therapy.

Determination of the vascular status of the tissue at the infection site is crucial in the evaluation of these patients. Although several methods can be used to determine the vascular status, measurement of cutaneous oxygen tensions and pulse pressures are the most commonly employed. Cutaneous oxygen tensions are obtained using a modified Clark electrode applied to the skin surface. Cutaneous oxygen tensions provide guidelines for determining the location of adequately perfused tissue.[73] The values are also helpful in predicting the benefit of local débridement surgery and in selecting surgical margins where healing can be expected to occur. Hyperbaric oxygen therapy may facilitate healing in areas where borderline oxygen tensions are present.

The patient may be managed with suppressive antibiotic therapy, local débridement surgery, or ablative surgery. The deci-

sion regarding treatment options used is based on tissue oxygen perfusion at the infection site, extent of the osteomyelitis, and patient preference.[74,75]

The patient can be offered long-term suppressive antibiotic therapy when a definitive surgical procedure would lead to unacceptable patient morbidity or disability or in cases in which the patient refuses local débridement or ablative surgery. Even with suppressive antibiotic therapy, in time most of these patients will require an amputation of the involved bone.

Local débridement surgery and a 4 week course of antibiotics may be employed in the patient who has localized osteomyelitis and good tissue oxygen perfusion. Unless good oxygen tensions are present, the wound will fail to heal and ultimately require an ablative procedure.

The patient with extensive osteomyelitis and poor tissue oxygen perfusion usually requires some type of ablative surgery. Digital and ray resections, transmetatarsal amputations, midfoot disarticulations, and Syme amputations (amputation of the foot with retention of the heel pad) permit the patient to ambulate without a prosthesis. The amputation level is determined by the vascularity of the tissues proximal to the site of infection and the requirements of a thorough débridement. The patient is given 4 weeks of antibiotics when infected bone is surgically transected. Two weeks of antibiotics are given when the infected bone is completely excised, but some residual soft tissue infection remains. When the amputation is performed proximal to the bone and soft tissue infection, the patient is given 1–3 days of antibiotic therapy.

Bone Concentrations

Due to the need for prolonged therapy, antibiotics employed in the treatment of bone and joint infection must be nontoxic, convenient to administer, and cost effective. Bone concentration of the treatment antibiotic may be an important factor in eradicating the organism from the bone. There are still no standardized methods for measuring bone concentrations, but most investigators use an elution technique to recover antibiotic from bone. Using a rabbit model for *S. aureus* osteomyelitis we found clindamycin to have the greatest bone-to-serum ratio followed by vancomycin, nafcillin, moxalactam, tobramycin, cefazolin, and cephalothin (Table 2).[76] The significance of bone antibiotic concentrations is unclear, but clindamycin gave the best treatment results in experimental *S. aureus* osteomyelitis.[77]

Hyperbaric Oxygen Therapy

The results of several open clinical trials have shown that adjunctive hyperbaric oxygen (HBO) therapy may be useful in the treatment of chronic osteomyelitis.[78] Morrey[79] reported on 40 patients with chronic osteomyelitis who met all of the following criteria: the infection had persisted longer than 1 month; at least one surgical débridement had been performed; at least 2 weeks of parenteral antibiotics had been administered; and the patients had been followed for at least 1 year after treatment. All patients

TABLE 2. Infected Bone Concentrations after Antibiotic Administration in Experimental Staphylococcus Aureus Osteomyelitis

Antibiotic	Serum μg/ml	Infected Bone μg/g	Serum (%)
Clindamycin (70 mg/kg)	12.1 ± 0.6	11.9 ± 1.9	98.3
Vancomycin (30 mg/kg)	36.4 ± 4.6	05.3 ± 0.8	14.5
Nafcillin (40 mg/kg)	21.8 ± 4.6	02.1 ± 0.3	09.6
Moxalactam (40 mg/kg)	65.2 ± 5.2	06.2 ± 0.7	09.5
Tobramycin (5 mg/kg)	14.3 ± 1.3	01.3 ± 0.1	09.1
Cefazolin (15 mg/kg)	67.2 ± 2.6	04.1 ± 0.7	06.1
Cefazolin (5 mg/kg)	45.6 ± 3.2	02.6 ± 0.2	05.7
Cephalothin (40 mg/kg)	34.8 ± 2.8	01.3 ± 0.2	03.7

had chronic refractory osteomyelitis with a recurrence of this infection despite previous aggressive antibiotics and surgical treatment. After HBO therapy, appropriate surgery, and treatment with antibiotics, 34 patients (85 percent) remained clinically free of disease, and six experienced recurrences of their osteomyelitis. Using the same criteria, Davis[80] evaluated 38 patients who were treated with adjunctive HBO. Of these 38 patients, 34 remained free of clinical signs of osteomyelitis. While the results of these clinical trials are encouraging, the adjunctive role of HBO in the treatment of osteomyelitis is difficult to assess because of the multiple patient, surgical, organism, bone, and antibiotic variables.

Animal studies performed in an experimental *S. aureus* osteomyelitis model have shown that hyperbaric oxygen administered under standard treatment conditions was as effective as cephalothin in eradicating *S. aureus* from infected bone.[81] Osteomyelitic bone in this experimental model has decreased blood flow and greatly decreased partial pressure of oxygen. Hyperoxia did not directly affect this strain of *S. aureus*. HBO was found to restore intramedullary oxygen tensions to physiologic or supraphysiologic tensions, but did not acutely increase blood flow in osteomyelitic bone. HBO was effective in *S. aureus* osteomyelitis because it increased intramedullary oxygen to tensions at which phagocytic killing may proceed more efficiently.[82] In a *P. aeruginosa* osteomyelitis model, HBO potentiated the aminoglycoside tobramycin.[83-85]

Wound healing is a dynamic process that requires an adequate oxygen tension to proceed.[86,87] In the ischemic or infected wound, HBO provides oxygen to promote collagen production, angiogenesis, and ultimately wound healing.

OTHER CLINICAL SITUATIONS

Osteomyelitis in Hemodialysis Patients

Osteomyelitis sometimes occurs as a complication of hemodialysis. Since *S. aureus* and *S. epidermidis* are common blood isolates in hemodialysis patients in whom indwelling cannulae allow portals for bacterial entry, bone infections are probably hematogenous in origin. The ribs and the thoracic vertebral column are the most common sites of involvement. The diagnosis of osteomyelitis is usually made 12–72 months after the initiation of hemodialysis. Surgical intervention and antibiotic treatment can result in an arrest of the infection. The infection may not be recognized as the clinical signs and radiographs may mimic those of renal osteodystrophy.

Osteomyelitis in Patients with Sickle Cell Disease

One large series reviewing sickle cell disease and osteomyelitis reported that 20 of 70 patients with complete hemoglobin defects had at least one hospitalization for the treatment of osteomyelitis during a 10-year period.[88] In essentially all cases, the infecting organisms were gram-negative rods. *Salmonella* spp. accounted for approximately 80 percent of the gram-negative organisms. In the same hospital series, one out of 117 patients with normal hemoglobin levels who had osteomyelitis exhibited a *Salmonella* sp. infection of the bone. In a second series of osteomyelitis patients with sickle cell disease, *S. aureus* was the most common pathogen followed by *Salmonella* sp. and *Proteus mirabilis*.[89]

It is often difficult to differentiate thrombotic marrow crisis from osteomyelitis in patients with sickle cell disease. Often a history of bone pain and fever followed in 1–2 weeks by the onset of spiking fever, chills, and leukocytosis is suggestive of osteomyelitis after a crisis. Patients with sickle cell disease may present with multiple sites of bone infection. Since the presenting symptoms are often insidious and mimic those of marrow crisis, early cultures of blood and stool offer clues to the correct diagnosis. Presumptive antibiotic therapy in patients suspected

of having osteomyelitis should include antibiotics effective against *Salmonella* spp. Radiographs of appropriately treated patients will usually show complete healing of the bone.

Osteomyelitis in Heroin Addicts

Osteomyelitis is a complication of intravenous drug addiction.[90-92] Clinical symptoms and signs of infection may be subtle and include localized pain. Fever is often absent. The infection is commonly found in the vertebrae, pubis, and clavicles, but may occur in any bone. *S. aureus*, *S. epidermidis*, gram-negative rods, and *Candida* spp. are the most commonly isolated pathogens. Since the initial films are often normal, serial radiographs of the involved area may be necessary. Unless blood cultures are positive along with radiographs or scan evidence of osteomyelitis, surgical exploration is mandatory to make a bacteriologic diagnosis.

Brodie's Abscess

Brodie's abscess is the name given to a chronic localized bone abscess. Subacute cases may present with fever, pain, and periosteal elevation, while chronic cases are often afebrile and present with long-standing dull pain. The most common site of involvement is the distal part of the tibia. The lesion is typically single and located near the metaphysis. Seventy-five percent of the patients are less than 25 years of age. Surgical débridement and culture-directed antibiotics are often curative.[93,94]

Gaucher's Disease

Patients, particularly children with Gaucher's disease, have noninfectious bone crises that mimic the signs and symptoms of acute bacterial osteomyelitis.[95,96] Patients with bone crises present with acute pain, usually over the tibia. The overlying area is tender to palpation, and the skin may be warm. The process is accompanied by high fever, leukocytosis, and an elevated sedimentation rate. Radionuclide scans may be compatible with osteomyelitis. A bone biopsy specimen shows bone necrosis, but no organisms are isolated.

Skeletal Tuberculosis

Skeletal tuberculosis is the result of hematogenous spread of *M. tuberculosis* early in the course of a primary infection. Rarely, skeletal tuberculosis may be a contiguous infection from an adjacent caseating lymph node. If the primary bone infection is not initially arrested, or a quiescent primary bone infection is reactivated, an inflammatory reaction is produced, followed by the development of granulation tissue. The granulation tissue erodes and destroys the cartilage and cancellous bone. Eventually the infection causes bone demineralization and necrosis. Proteolytic enzymes that can destroy cartilage are not produced in skeletal tuberculosis. Cartilage is destroyed slowly by granulation tissue, preserving the joint or disc space for considerable periods of time. Healing of the infection involves deposition of fibrous tissue. Pain is the most frequent clinical complaint.

Any bone may be involved in skeletal tuberculosis, but the infection usually involves one site. In children or adolescents the metaphysis of the long bones are most frequently infected. In the adult, the axial skeleton followed by the proximal femur, knee, and small bones of the hands and feet are most often involved. In the axial skeleton, the thoracic vertebral bodies are most frequently infected, followed by the lumbar and cervical vertebral bodies. Vertebral infection usually begins in the anterior portion of a vertebral body and is adjacent to an intervertebral disc. The infection produces destruction of the nearby bone and the intervertebral disc. Adjacent vertebral bodies may become involved, and a paravertebral abscess may develop. Generally, pyogenic osteomyelitis involves the disc early on and produces rapid sclerosis by 3–4 months. Tuberculosis spondylitis progresses slowly, over a period of years. Sixty percent of the patients with skeletal tuberculosis have evidence of extraosseous tuberculosis.[97]

Tissue for culture and histology is almost always required for the diagnosis of skeletal tuberculosis. Cultures for *M. tuberculosis* are positive in approximately 60 percent of the cases. But since 6 weeks may be required for growth and identification of the organism,[98,99] histology showing granulomatous tissue compatible with tuberculosis and a positive tuberculosis skin test are sufficient to begin therapy. However, a negative skin test does not rule out skeletal tuberculosis.[100] Therapy for skeletal tuberculosis involves prolonged chemotherapy, and in some cases surgical débridement.

Nontuberculous Mycobacterial Infections

Osteoarticular infections with nontuberculous mycobacteria fall into three distinct types: tenosynovitis, synovitis, and osteomyelitis. Multiple diverse species including *M. marinum, M. avium-intracellulare, M. fortuitum,* and *M. gordonae* have all been associated with infection. Many of these infections seem to respond well to surgery alone. The role of antituberculous therapy, particularly with organisms like *M. avium-intracellulare,* is not clear.[101]

Fungal Osteomyelitis

Bone infections may be caused by a variety of fungal organisms, including coccidioidomycosis, blastomycosis, cryptococcosis, candidiasis, and sporotrichosis. The most common presentation is a cold abscess overlying an osteolytic lesion. Joint space extension may occur in coccidioidomycosis and blastomycosis. Therapy for fungal osteomyelitis involves surgical débridement and antifungal chemotherapy.[102]

ACKNOWLEDGMENTS

We thank Joan Mader, M.S.N., Diane Staebler, Donna Gobert, and Mark Wade, M.D., for manuscript research and preparation.

REFERENCES

1. Waldvogel FA, Medoff G, Swartz MN. Osteomyelitis: A review of clinical features, therapeutic considerations, and unusual aspect. N Engl J Med. 1970;282:198–206,260–6,316–22.
2. Waldvogel FA, Vasey H. Osteomyelitis: The past decade. N Engl J Med. 1980;303:360–70.
3. Cierny G, Mader JT. Adult chronic osteomyelitis. Orthopedics 1984;7:1557–64.
4. Cierny G, Mader JT, Pennick H. A clinical staging system of adult osteomyelitis. Contemp Orthop. 1985;10:17–37.
5. Trueta J, Morgan JD. The vascular contribution to osteogenesis. I. Studies by the injection method. J Bone Joint Surg. 1960;42B:97–109.
6. Hobo T, Zur pathogenese de akuten haematogenen Osteomyelitis, mit Berucksichtigung der Vitalfarbungslehre. Acta Sch Med Univ Imp Kioto. 1922;4:1–29.
7. Morrissy RT, Haynes DW. Acute Hematogenous Osteomyelitis: A Model With Trauma as an Etiologic Agent (Abstract). Kappa Delta Paper 2. American Academy of Orthopaedic Surgeons 51st Annual Meeting, Atlanta, GA, 1984.
8. Ish-Horowicz MR, McIntyre P, Nade S. Bone and joint infections caused by multiply resistant *Staphylococcus aureus* in a neonatal intensive care unit. Pediatr Infect Dis J. 1992;11:82–7.
9. Morrey BF, Peterson HA. Hematogenous pyogenic osteomyelitis in children. Orthop Clin North Am. 1975;6:935–51.
10. Batson OV. The function of the vertebral veins and their role in the spread of metastases. Ann Surg. 1940;112:138–40.
11. Wiley AM, Trueta J. The vascular anatomy of the spine and its relationship to pyogenic vertebral osteomyelitis. J Bone Joint Surg. 1959;41B:796–804.
12. Croke HV, Goldwasser M. Anatomic studies of the circulation in the region of the vertebral end-plate in adult greyhound dogs. Spine. 1984;9:702–6.
13. Sapico FL, Montgomerie JZ. Pyogenic vertebral osteomyelitis: Report of nine cases and review of the literature. Rev Infect Dis. 1979;1:754–76.
14. Holzman RS, Bishko F. Osteomyelitis in heroin addicts. Ann Intern Med. 1971;75:693–6.
15. Sapico FL, Montgomerie JZ. Vertebral osteomyelitis in intravenous drug abusers: Report of three cases and review of the literature. Rev Infect Dis. 1980;2:196–206.
16. Lee YH, Kerstein MD. Osteomyelitis and septic arthritis: A complication of subclavian venous catheterization. N Engl J Med. 1971;285:1179–80.
17. Leonard A, Comty CM, Shapiro FL, et al. Osteomyelitis in hemodialysis patients. Ann Intern Med. 1973;78:651–8.
18. Watanakunakorn C. Vertebral osteomyelitis as a complicatioon of *P. aeruginosa* pneumonia. South Med J. 1975;68:173–6.
19. Gruber HE. Bone and the immune system. Proc Soc Exp Biol Med. 1991;197:219–25.
20. Mackowiak PA, Jones SR, Smith JW. Diagnostic value of sinus tract cultures in chronic osteomyelitis. JAMA. 1978;239:2772–5.
21. Perry CR, Pearson RL, Miller GA. Accuracy of cultures of material from swabbing of the superficial aspect of the wound and needle biopsy in the preoperative assessment of osteomyelitis. J Bone Joint Surg. 1991;73(A):745–9.
22. Butt WP. The radiology of infection. Clin Orthop. 1973;96:20–30.
23. Jones AG, Francis MD, Davis MA. Bone scanning: Radionuclide reaction mechanisms. Semin Nucl Med. 1976;6:3–18.
24. Treves S, Khettry J, Broker FH, et al. Osteomyelitis: Early scintigraphic detection in children. Pediatrics. 1976;57:173–86.
25. Russin LD, Staab EV. Unusual bone-scan findings in acute osteomyelitis: Case report. J Nucle Med. 1976;17:617–9.
26. Deysine M, Rafkin H, Teicher I, et al. Diagnosis of chronic and postoperative osteomyelitis with gallium 67 citrate scans. Am J Surg. 1975;129:632–5.
27. Sayle B, Cierny G, Mader JT. Indium-111 chloride imaging in the detection of osteomyelitis. J Nucle Med. 1983;24:72.
28. Lisbona R, Rosenthall L. Observations of the sequential use of ⁹⁹ᵐTc phosphate complex and ⁶⁷Ga imaging in osteomyelitis, cellulitis, and septic arthritis. Radiology. 1977;123:123–9.
29. Propst-Proctor SL, Dillingham MF, McDougall IR, et al. The white blood cell scan in orthopedics. Clin Orthop. 1982;168:157–65.
30. Kuhn JP, Berger PE. Computed tomographic diagnosis of osteomyelitis: Radiology. 1979;130:503–6.
31. Ram PC, Martinez S, Korobkin M, et al. CT detection of intraosseous gas: A new sign of osteomyelitis. Am J Roentgenol. 1981;137:721–3.
32. Seltzer SE. Value of computed tomography in planning medical and surgical treatment of chronic osteomyelitis. J Comput Assist Tomogr. 1984;8:482–7.
33. Mason MD, Zlatkin MB, Esterhai JL, et al. Chronic complicated osteomyelitis of the lower extremity: Evaluation with MR imaging. Radiology 1989;173:355.
34. Erdman WA, Tamburro F, Jayson HT, et al. Osteomyelitis: Characteristics and pitfalls of diagnosis with MR imaging. Radiology. 1991;180:533–9.
35. Tehranzadeh J, Wang F, Mesgarzadeh M. Magnetic resonance imaging of osteomyelitis. Crit Rev Diagn Imaging. 1992;33:495–534.
36. Unger E, Moldofsky P, Gatenby R, et al. Diagnosis of osteomyelitis by MR imaging. Am J Roentgenol. 1988;150:605–10.
37. Modic MT, Pflanze W, Feiglin DHI, et al. Magnetic resonance imaging of musculoskeletal infections. Radiol Clin North Am. 1986;24:247–58.
38. Golimbu C, Firooznia H, Rafii M. CT of osteomyelitis of the spine. Am J Roentgenol. 1984;142:159–63.
39. Post MJ, Quencer RM, Montalvo BM, et al. Spinal infection: Evaluation with MR imaging and intraoperative US. Radiology. 1988;169:765–71.
40. Post MJ, Sze G, Quencer RM, et al. Gadolinium-enhanced MR in spinal infection. J Comput Assist Tomogr. 1990;14:721–9.
41. Adatepe MH, Powell OM, Isaacs GH, et al. Hematogenous pyogenic vertebral osteomyelitis: Diagnostic value of radionuclide bone imaging. J Nucle Med. 1986;27:1680–5.
42. Cierny G, Mader JT. The surgical treatment of adult osteomyelitis. In: Evarts CMC, ed. Surgery of the Musculoskeletal System. New York: Churchill Livingstone; 1983;10, 15–35.
43. Ericcson HM, Sherris JC. Antibiotic sensitivity testing: Report of an international collaborative study. Acta Pathol Microbiol Scand. 1971;227(Suppl B):1–90.
44. Tetzloff TR, McCracken GH, Nelson FD. Oral antibiotic therapy for skeletal infections in children. II. Therapy of osteomyelitis and suppurative arthritis. J Pediatr. 1978;92:485–90.
45. Nelson JD. A critical review of the role of oral antibiotics in the management of hematogenous osteomyelitis. In: Remington RS, Swartz MN, eds. Current Clinical Topics in Infectious Diseases. v 4. New York: McGraw-Hill; 1983:64–74.
46. Christ W, Lehnert T, Ulbrich. Specific toxicologic aspects of the quinolones. Rev Infect Dis. 1988;10(Suppl 1):141–6.
47. Mayer DG. Overview of toxicological studies. Drugs 1987;34(Suppl 1):150–3.
48. Anthony JP, Mathes SJ. Update on chronic osteomyelitis. Clin Plast Surg. 1991;18:515–23.
49. Hickman RO, Buckner CD, Clift RA, et al. A modified right atrial catheter for

access to the venous system in marrow transplant recipients. Surg Gynecol Obstet. 1979;148:871–5.

50. Couch L, Cierny G, Mader JT. Inpatient and outpatient use of the Hickman catheter for adults with osteomyelitis. Clin Orthop. 1987;219:226–35.

51. Graham DR, Keldermans MM, Klemm LW, et al. Infectious complications among patients receiving home intravenous therapy with peripheral, central, or peripherally placed central venous catheters. Am J Med. 1991;91: 95S–100S.

52. Mader JT. Fluoroquinolones in bone and joint infections. In: Sanders WE Jr, Sanders CC, eds. Fluoroquinolones in the Treatment of Infectious Diseases. Glenview, IL; Physicians & Scientists; 1990:71–86.

53. Mader JT, Cantrell JS, Calhoun JH. Oral ciprofloxacin compared with standard parenteral antibiotic therapy for chronic osteomyelitis in adults. J Bone Joint Surg. 1990;72(A):104–10.

54. Schamberg DR, Dillon WI, Terpenning MS, et al. Increasing resistance of enterococci to ciprofloxacin. Antimicrob Agents Chemother. 1992;36: 2533–5.

55. Blumberg HM, Rimland D, Carroll DJ, et al. Rapid development of ciprofloxacin resistance in methicillin-susceptible and -resistant *Staphylococcus aureus*. J Infect Dis. 1991;163:1279–85.

56. Norden CW, Bryant R, Palmer D, et al. Chronic osteomyelitis caused by *Staphylococcus aureus*: Controlled clinical trial of nafcillin therapy and nafcillin-rifampin therapy. South Med J. 1986;79:947–51.

57. Reller LB, Stratton CW. Serum dilution test for bactericidal activity. II. Standardization and correlation with antimicrobial assays and susceptibility tests. J Infect Dis. 1977;136:196–204.

58. Clawson DK, Davis FJ, Hansen ST. Treatment of chronic osteomyelitis with emphasis on closed suction-irrigation technique. Clin Orthop. 1973;96:88–97.

59. Letts RM, Wong E. Treatment of acute osteomyelitis in children by closed-tube irrigation: A reassessment. Can J Surg. 1975;18:60–3.

60. Ruttle PE, Kelley PJ, Arnold PG, et al. Chronic osteomyelitis treated with a muscle flap. Orthop Clin North Am. 1984;15:451–9.

61. May JW Jr, Jupiter JB, Gallico GG 3d, et al. Treatment of chronic traumatic bone wounds. Microvascular free tissue transfer: A 13-year experience in 96 patients. Ann Surg. 1991;214:241–50.

62. Anthony JP, Mathes SJ, Alpert BS. The muscle flap in the treatment of chronic lower extremity osteomyelitis: Results in patients over 5 years after treatment. Plast Reconstr Surg. 1991;88:311–8.

63. Papineau LJ, Alfageme A, Dalcourt JP, et al. Osteomyelite chronique: Excision et greffe de spongieux a l'air libre apres mises a plat extensives. Int Orthop. 1979;3:165–76.

64. Scott DM, Rotschafer JC, Behrens F. Use of vancomycin and tobramycin polymethylmethacrylate impregnated beads in the management of chronic osteomyelitis. Drug Intell Clin Pharmacol. 1988;22:480–3.

65. Wilson KJ, Cierny G, Adams KR, et al. Comparative evaluation of the diffusion of tobramycin and cefotaxime out of antibiotic-impregnated polymethylmethacrylate beads. J Orthop Res. 1988;6:279–86.

66. Adams K, Couch MSL, Cierny G, et al. In vitro and in vivo evaluation of antibiotic diffusion from antibiotic-impregnated polymethylmethacrylate (PMMA) beads. Clin Orthop. 1992;276:244–52.

67. Calhoun JH, Mader JT. Antibiotic beads in the management of surgical infection. Am J Surg. 1989;157:443–9.

68. Henry SL, Seligson D, Mangino P, et al. Antibiotic-impregnated beads. Part I: Bead implantation versus systemic therapy. Orthop Rev. 1991;20:242–7.

69. Popham GJ, Mangino P, Seligson D, et al. Antibiotic-impregnated beads. Part II: Factors in antibiotic selection. Orthop Rev. 1991;20:331–7.

70. Perry CR, Davenport K, Vossen MK. Local delivery of antibiotics via an implantable pump in the treatment of osteomyelitis. Clin Orthop. 1988;226: 222–30.

71. Green SA. Osteomyelitis. The Ilizarov perspective. Orthop Clin North Am. 1991;22:515–21.

72. Calhoun JH, Anger DM, Mader JT. The Ilizarov technique in the treatment of osteomyelitis. Texas Med. 1991;87:56–9.

73. Matsen FA, Wyss CR, Pedegana LR, et al. Transcutaneous oxygen tension measurement in peripheral vascular disease. Surg Gynecol Obstet. 1980;150: 525–8.

74. Calhoun JH, Cantrell J, Lacy J, et al. Treatment of diabetic foot infection. Wagner classification, and outcome. Foot Ankle. 1988;9:101–6.

75. Calhoun JH, Mader JT. Osteomyelitis of the diabetic foot. In: Frykberg SRG, ed. The High Risk Foot in Diabetes Mellitus. New York: Churchill Livingstone; 1991:213–39.

76. Mader JT, Adams KR. Experimental osteomyelitis. In: Schlossberg D, ed. Orthopedic Infection. New York: Springer/Verlag; 1988:39–48.

77. Mader JT, Adams KR, Morrison L. Comparative evaluation of cefazolin and clindamycin in the treatment of experimental *Staphylococcus aureus* osteomyelitis in rabbits. Antimicrob Agent Chemother. 1989;33:1760–4.

78. Mader JT, Adams KR, Sutton TE. Infectious diseases: Pathophysiology and mechanisms of hyperbaric oxygen. J Hyperbaric Med. 1987;2:133–40.

79. Morrey BF, Dunn JM, Heimbach RD, et al. Hyperbaric oxygen and chronic osteomyelitis. Clin Orthopp. 1979;144:121–7.

80. Davis JC, Heckman JD, DeLee JC, et al. Chronic non-hematogenous osteomyelitis treated with adjuvant hyperbaric oxygen. J Bone Joint Surg. 1986; 68A:1210–7.

81. Mader JT, Guckian JC, Glass DL, et al. Therapy with hyperbaric oxygen for experimental osteomyelitis due to *Staphylococcus aureus* in rabbits. J Infect Dis. 1978;138:312–8.

82. Mader JT, Brown GL, Guckian JC, et al. A mechanism for the amelioration by hyperbaric oxygen of experimental staphylococcal osteomyelitis in rabbits. J Infect Dis. 1980;142:915–22.

83. Verklin RM, Mandell GL. Alteration of effectiveness of antibiotics by anaerobiosis. J Lab Clin Med. 1977;89:65–71.

84. Reynolds AV, Hamilton-Miller JMT, Brumfittt W. Diminished effect of gentamicin under anaerobic and hypercapnic conditions. Lancet 1976;1:447–9.

85. Mader JT, Adams KR, Couch LA, et al. Potentiation of tobramycin by hyperbaric oxygen in experimental *Pseudomonas aeruginosa* osteomyelitis (Abstract 1331). Abstracts of the 27th Interscience Conference on Antimicrobial Agents and Chemotherapy. American Society for Microbiology, Washington, DC, 1987.

86. Hunt TK, Pai MP. The effect of varying ambient oxygen tensions on wound metabolism and collagen synthesis. Surg Gynecol Obstet. 1972;135:756–8.

87. Hunt TK, Zederfeldt B, Goldstick TK. Oxygen and healing. Am J Surg. 1969;118:521–5.

88. Engh C, Hughes J, Abrams R, et al. Osteomyelitis in the patient with sickle cell disease. J Bone Joint Surg. 1971;53A:1–15.

89. Epps CH Jr, Bryant DD 3d, Coles MJ, et al. Osteomyelitis in patients who have sickle-cell disease: Diagnosis and management. J Bone Joint surg. 1991; 73(A):1281–94.

90. Gifford DB, Patzakis M, Ivler D, et al. Septic arthritis due to *Pseudomonas* in heroin addicts. J Bone Joint Surg. 1975;57A:631–5.

91. Roca RPP, Yoshikawa TT. Primary skeletal infections in heroin users: A clinical characterization, diagnosis, and therapy. Clin Orthop. 1979;144: 238–48.

92. Chandrasekar PH, Narula AP. Bone and joint infections in intravenous drug abusers. Rev Infect Dis. 1986;8:904–11.

93. Miller W, Murphy W, Gilula L. Brodie abscess: Reappraisal. Radiology 1979; 132:15–23.

94. Dunn EC, Singer L. Operative treatment of Brodie's abscess. J Foot Surg. 1991;30:443–5.

95. Beighton P, Goldblatt J, Sacks S. Bone involvement in Gaucher disease. In: Desnick RJ, Gatt S, Grabowski GA, eds. Gaucher Disease: A Century of Delineation and Research. New York: Alan R. Liss; 1982:107–9.

96. Noyes FR, Smith WS. Bone crises and chronic osteomyelitis in Gaucher's disease. Clin Ortho. 1971;79:132–40.

97. Falk A. Results of long-term chemotherapy in spinal tuberculosis. XVII. A follow-up study of 235 patients. Am Rev Respir Dis. 1967;95:1–5.

98. Wallace R, Cohen AS. Tuberculosis arthritis: A report of two cases with review of biopsy and synovial fluid findings. Am J Med. 1976;61:277–82.

99. Gorse GJ, Pais MJ, Kusske JA, et al. Tuberculosis spondylitis: A report of six cases and a review of the literature. Medicine. 1983;62:178–93.

100. Davidson PT, Horowitz I. Skeletal tuberculosis: A review with patient presentations and discussion. Am J Med. 1970;48:77–84.

101. Marchevsky A, Damsker B, Green S, et al. The clinicopathological spectrum of non-tuberculous mycobacterial osteoarticular infection. J Bone Joint Surg. 1985;67A:925–9.

102. Gathe J Jr, Harris R, Garland B, et al. *Candida* osteomyelitis: Report of 5 cases and review of the literature. Am J Med. 1987;82:927–37.

86. INFECTIONS WITH PROSTHESES IN BONES AND JOINTS

BARRY D. BRAUSE

Over the past 25 years joint replacement surgery has become commonplace due to the magnificent success of these procedures in restoring function to disabled arthritic individuals. Initially, total prosthetic hip implantation techniques were devised. Subsequently, total knee replacement, total shoulder replacement, and total elbow replacement procedures using many of the same orthopedic principles became available. Patients receiving total joint replacements number in the hundreds of thousands each year worldwide, and virtually millions of people have indwelling prosthetic articulations. One to five percent of indwelling prostheses become infected; this is a calamity for the patient and is associated with significant morbidity and occasionally death. Prosthesis removal, which usually is necessary to treat these infections, produces large skeletal defects, shortening of the extremity, and severe functional impairment. The health care cost of treating septic prosthetic articulations has been estimated conservatively at 40–80 million dollars per year in the United States alone.[1] The patient faces protracted hospitalization, sizable financial expense, and potentially renewed disability.

PATHOGENESIS

Certain patient populations have been identified as predisposed toward infection of their prosthetic joints, including those with prior surgery at the site of the prosthesis, rheumatoid arthritis, corticosteroid therapy, diabetes mellitus, poor nutritional status, obesity, and extremely advanced age.[2,3] Infection usually occurs in osseous tissue adjacent to the foreign body. Since most prostheses are cemented in place with polymethylmethacrylate, infection develops at the bone–cement interface. Sepsis involving cementless prostheses develops in the bone contiguous with the metallic alloy.

Prosthetic joints become infected by two different pathogenetic routes: locally introduced and hematogenous types of osteomyelitis. The locally introduced form of infection is the result of wound sepsis contiguous to the prosthesis or operative contamination. Any factor or event that delays wound healing increases the risk of infection. Ischemic necrosis, infected wound hematomas, wound infection (with or without identifiable cellulitis), and suture abscesses are common preceding events for joint replacement sepsis. During the early postimplantation period, when these superficial infections develop, the fascial layers have not yet healed, and the deep, periprosthesis tissue is not protected by the usual physical barriers. Generally these infections are caused by a single pathogen, but polymicrobial sepsis with as many as five different organisms is also observed. Coagulase-negative staphylococci are the most common etiologic agents in this clinical setting. Infrequently, latent foci of chronic, quiescent osteomyelitis are reactivated by the disruption of tissue associated with implantation surgery. Although bone cultures at the time of the joint replacement operation are sterile, old *Staphylococcus aureus* and *Mycobacterium tuberculosis* infections can recrudesce postoperatively.[3]

Any bacteremia can induce infection of a total joint replacement by the hematogenous route.[4–6] Dentogingival infections and manipulations are known causes of viridans streptococcal and anaerobic (*Peptococcus, Peptostreptococcus*) infections in prostheses. Pyogenic skin processes can cause staphylococcal (*S. aureus, S. epidermidis*) and streptococcal (groups A, B, C, and G streptococci) infections of joint replacements. Genitourinary and gastrointestinal tract procedures or infections are associated with gram-negative bacillary, enterococcal, and anaerobic infections of prostheses. Twenty to forty percent of prosthetic joint infections arise by the hematogenous route, the remainder being of the locally introduced type.

The frequency of specific microorganisms etiologic in prosthetic joint sepsis varies among the published studies, but a general view of the spectrum of this bacteriology, as well as the prominence of certain microbial groups, is given in Table 1. Staphylococci (coagulase-negative staphylococci and *S. aureus*) are the principal causative agents, aerobic streptococci and gram-negative bacilli are each responsible for approximately 20 percent, and anaerobes represent 5–10 percent of these infections. The spectrum of microbial agents capable of causing

TABLE 1. Bacteriology of Prosthetic Joint Infection

Pathogens	Frequency (%)
Staphylococci	53
Coagulase-negative	28
S. aureus	25
Streptococci	20
β-Hemolytic streptococci	12
Viridans streptococci	8
Gram-negative aerobic bacilli	20
Anaerobes	7

prosthetic joint infection is unlimited and includes organisms ordinarily considered "contaminants" of cultures such as corynebacteria, propionibacteria, and *Bacillus* spp. Rarely have infections with fungi (particularly *Candida*) and mycobacteria been described.[3]

As foreign bodies, the indwelling metallic prosthesis and the polymethylmethacrylate cement, which binds the metal alloy to adjacent bone, predispose both joint space and osseous tissue to septic processes. Foreign substances contribute to local sepsis experimentally by decreasing the quantity of bacteria necessary to establish infection and by permitting pathogens to persist on their avascular surface, sequestered from circulating immunologic defenses (leukocytes, antibodies, and complement) as well as systemic antibiotics.[3,7] Polymethylmethacrylate cement appears to predispose toward infection to an extent beyond that of other inert foreign substances. The cement in unpolymerized form has been shown to inhibit phagocytic, lymphocytic, and complement function in vitro.[8,9] The polymerization process itself appears to enhance the risk of infection, possibly due to the substantial heat generated by this in vivo reaction.[8] In an effort to provide total joint replacement without polymethylmethacrylate, cementless prostheses have been designed. These devices have textured surfaces to provide fixation by the growth of adjacent bone into the "porous" interface of the prosthesis. The performance and durability of this new form of arthroplasty is uncertain.

Host responses to methylmethacrylate also may play a role in the pathogenesis of infection. Fibronectin, a connective tissue and plasma glycoprotein, appears to enhance *S. aureus* adherence to polymethylmethacrylate in vivo and thus may contribute to the occurrence of sepsis.[10] Microbial products may assist the development and persistence of infection in association with foreign substances. In the presence of prosthetic devices, many bacteria elaborate a fibrous exopolysaccharide material called *glycocalyx*. Organisms can grow within this matrix and form thick biofilms that are protected at least in part from host defense mechanisms (see Ch. 2)[2,11]. Bacteria adherent to biomaterials demonstrate decreased quantitative susceptibility to antibiotics both in vitro and in vivo.[12,13]

CLINICAL PRESENTATION

Prosthetic joint sepsis produces the cardinal symptoms of inflammation with a wide spectrum of severity. Most patients present with a long indolent course characterized by a progressive increase in joint pain and occasionally the formation of cutaneous draining sinuses but no fever, soft tissue swelling, or systemic toxicity. Others present with an acute, fulminant illness with high fever, severe joint pain, local swelling, and erythema. The frequencies of these presenting symptoms are listed in Table 2.[14]

The pattern of clinical presentation is determined largely by three factors: *(1)* the virulence of the infecting pathogen, *(2)* the nature of the host tissue in which the microorganism grows, and *(3)* the route of infection. *Staphylococcus aureus* is a particu-

TABLE 2. Presenting Symptoms of Prosthetic Joint Infection

Symptom	Frequency (%)
Joint pain	95
Fever	43
Periarticular swelling	38
Wound or cutaneous sinus drainage	32

larly virulent pathogen in this setting and usually produces a fulminant infection (occasionally with septic shock). β-Hemolytic streptococci and aerobic gram-negative bacilli are also capable of causing this clinical picture. Alternatively, the relatively avirulent but tenacious coagulase-negative staphylococci are consistently associated with an indolent course. Characteristics of the involved tissue can influence the type of presentation on the basis of their support of microbial growth. Wound hematomas (as well as seromas and hemarthroses), fresh operative wounds, ischemic wounds, and tissues in diabetic and steroid-treated patients all enhance the ability of bacteria to multiply rapidly in expansive tissue planes. These factors promote the development of a more fulminant infection when a large inoculum of bacteria is allowed access to deep tissue compartments during surgery or in a slowly healing wound postoperatively. The hematogenous route of infection theoretically seeds the bone–cement interface with a relatively small number of organisms. When a blood-borne infection arises in a prosthetic joint several months or years after implantation surgery, the fully healed connective tissue often is capable of restricting the septic process to a relatively small but critical focus at the bone–cement interface. Joint pain is the principal symptom of deep tissue infection irrespective of the mode of presentation and suggests either acute inflammation of periarticular tissue or loosening of the prosthesis due to subacute erosion of bone at the bone–cement interface.

DIAGNOSIS

The clinical manifestations previously described (i.e., joint pain, swelling, erythema, and warmth) all reflect an underlying inflammatory process in the surrounding tissues but are not specific for infection. When a painful prosthesis is accompanied by a fever or purulent drainage from overlying cutaneous sinuses, infection may be presumed, pending further confirmatory tests. However, in the vast preponderance of cases, infection must be differentiated from aseptic and mechanical problems (e.g., hemarthrosis, gout, bland loosening, and dislocation), which are more common causes of pain and inflammatory symptoms in these patients.

Constant joint pain is suggestive of infection, whereas mechanical loosening commonly causes pain only with motion and weight bearing.[2] Plain radiographs can reveal (1) abnormal lucencies greater than 2 mm in width at the bone–cement interface, (2) changes in the position of prosthetic components, (3) cement fractures, (4) periosteal reaction, or (5) motion of components on stress views. In addition, the intra-articular injection of dye (arthrography) may reveal abnormal communications between the joint space and multiple defects in the bone–cement interface. These radiologic abnormalities (Fig. 1) are found in 50 percent of septic prostheses. They are generally related to the duration of infection since it may require 3–6 months to manifest such changes. When both distal and proximal components of a prosthetic joint demonstrate radiographic pathology, sepsis is more likely than is simple mechanical loosening. However, these changes seen on radiographs are not specific for infection because they are also seen frequently with aseptic processes.

Radioisotopic scans with technetium diphosphonate demonstrate increased uptake in areas of bone with enhanced blood supply or increased metabolic activity. Increased technetium uptake is seen routinely around normal prostheses for 6 months

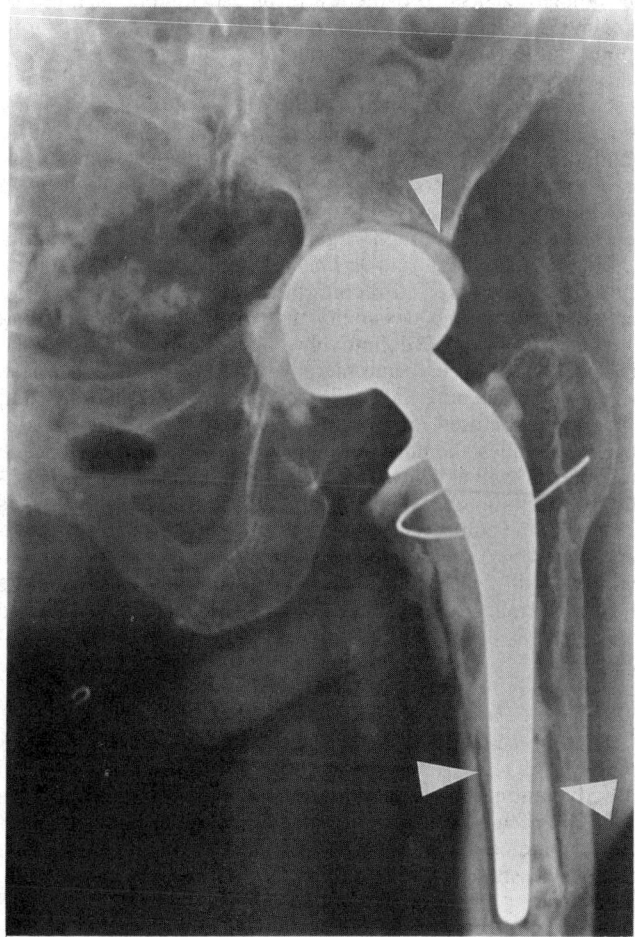

FIG. 1. A plain radiograph of an infected total hip prosthesis demonstrates lucencies at the bone–cement interface of both femoral and acetabular components (arrowheads).

after arthroplasty. Positive scan findings after this period are abnormal and reflect inflammation and possible loosening but not specifically infection of the implant. Sequential technetium-gallium bone scanning is also nondiagnostic due to unacceptable sensitivity (66 percent) and specificity (81 percent).[15] Indium-labeled leukocyte scanning, although very sensitive, also provides only nonspecific results.[16] Therefore, normal or negative technetium or indium leukocyte scan findings can be considered strong evidence against the presence of infection, but they are not definitive in establishing the diagnosis. Elevated peripheral white blood cell counts and erythrocyte sedimentation rates, although suggestive, also are inadequate in diagnosing sepsis in this clinical setting.

The specific diagnosis of joint replacement infection is dependent, in large part, upon isolation of the pathogen by aspiration of joint fluid or by culture of tissue obtained at arthrotomy.[17] Analysis of joint fluid often reveals a high leukocyte count (mainly polymorphonuclear cells), a high protein content, and a low glucose concentration. However, the changes are only variably present and are neither prerequisites for making the diagnosis of joint replacement infection nor specific for this entity. Histopathologic examination of periprosthetic tissue frequently reveals an infiltration of polymorphonuclear leukocytes indicative of an acute inflammatory reaction, but this parameter is positive in only 55 percent of infected patients and also may not be sufficiently specific. Therefore, the single observation that delineates the presence of implant infection is isolation of the pathogen by arthrocentesis or surgical débridement.

Since fastidious microorganisms, including anaerobes, may

be etiologic agents in prosthetic arthroplasty infections, multiple specimens should be obtained and rapidly cultured in appropriate media. Arthrocentesis demonstrates the pathogen in 85–98 percent of cases.[17,18] Gram stain is positive in 32 percent. Fluoroscopic guidance and arthrography are useful in documenting accurate needle placement. When difficulty is encountered in obtaining intra-articular fluid, irrigation with sterile normal saline (without antiseptic preservative additives) can be used to provide the necessary fluid for culture. When initial cultures reveal a relatively avirulent organism (*S. epidermidis*, corynebacteria, propionibacteria, or *Bacillus* spp.), a second aspirate should be considered to reconfirm the bacteriologic diagnosis and to eliminate the possibility that the isolate is artifactual. Operative cultures are definitively diagnostic; therefore, the patient should not receive antimicrobial therapy for several weeks before the procedure. Multiple specimens of tissue and fluid should be submitted for culture. The results of these microbiologic techniques should confirm the presence and nature of the infection as well as allow for optimal treatment. In the uncommon circumstance when the clinical suggestion of sepsis is strong but the cultures are sterile, fastidious organisms (particularly anaerobes) should be suspected. To design the most efficacious and the least toxic antimicrobial therapy, the patient's infecting strain of bacteria must first be available for in vitro evaluation as described later in this chapter.

THERAPY

Successful treatment of a total joint arthroplasty infection depends on extensive and meticulous surgical débridement and effective antimicrobial therapy. Simple surgical drainage (with retention of the prosthesis in situ) followed by a nonstandardized, finite course of antibiotic therapy has been only 20 percent successful.[19] In response to this 80 percent failure rate, two different approaches to more effective treatment of prosthetic joint infection have evolved over the past decade. Complete removal of all foreign materials (metallic prosthesis and cement) is an essential component of both regimens.

The most successful protocol incorporates standardized antimicrobial therapy with a two-stage surgical procedure. Removal of the prosthesis and cement is followed by a 6-week course of bactericidal antibiotic therapy chosen on the basis of in vitro susceptibility studies. Reimplantation is performed at the conclusion of the 6-week antibiotic course. With this protocol a 90 percent success rate has been achieved in total hip replacement infections, and a 97 percent success rate has been obtained in total knee replacement infections.[20–22] The success of this regimen relies on thorough débridement techniques and effective antimicrobial therapy. In this manner, both gram-positive bacteria (including multidrug-resistant staphylococci and enterococci) as well as gram-negative bacteria (including *Pseudomonas aeruginosa*) can be eliminated if the specific sensitivity of each isolate allows eradication. The empirical selection of a 6-week duration of antibiotic therapy may be critical for efficacy. Others have employed a similar approach to therapy but only a 2-week course of antibiotic treatment before reinsertion of the prosthesis.[23] With this protocol the pathogen was eradicated in only 79 percent of the cases, and only 35 percent of the patients obtained good function in the new prosthesis.

The alternative method of treatment involves metallic joint and cement extraction with immediate reimplantation of a new prosthesis in a one-stage surgical procedure (exchange operation) accompanied by nonstandardized antimicrobial therapy. Methylmethacrylate cement impregnated with an antibiotic (usually gentamicin or tobramycin) is employed during reimplantation. The antimicrobial agent leaches out from the hardened plastic to produce variable but high initial release, as well as protracted diffusion, of antibiotic into surrounding tissues at the bone–cement interface.[24] The protocol is effective in 70–80 percent of cases.[25–27] When using repeated exchange operations

(in the 20–30 percent failure group) incorporating antibiotic-laden cement, the success rate is increased to 90 percent.[26] It has been suggested that this mode of therapy is applicable only to infections with the less virulent microorganisms, since high failure rates are observed when *S. aureus* or gram-negative bacilli are the pathogens.[28] Systemic antibiotics are administered rarely and without standardization in this regimen. Moreover, the selection of an aminoglycoside as a component in the recementing phase of these operations may not have reflected the susceptibility of the pathogen being treated.

Future therapeutic approaches will likely include the most efficacious parts of these two protocols: combining the specific, standardized 6-week antibiotic regimen and two-stage prosthesis removal-reimplantation surgery with the incorporation of antibiotic-impregnated cement during arthroplasty reinsertion.[29] In those clinical situations in which adequate antimicrobial potency cannot be achieved, arthrodesis or resection arthroplasty is recommended rather than attempting prosthesis reimplantation. However, with the advent of antibiotic-impregnated cement even these difficult cases may be candidates for another total joint arthroplasty.

SUPPRESSIVE ANTIBIOTIC THERAPY

Although removal of the implanted prosthesis is necessary to eradicate deep infection associated with these devices, this therapeutic approach is not always available. Occasionally surgical excision is contraindicated due to medical and surgical conditions or patient refusal. Since it is likely that the pathogen will be able to persist at the undébrided bone–cement interface despite high-dose, finite systemic antimicrobial therapy, lifelong oral antibiotic treatment can be considered to suppress the infection and retain the usefulness of the total joint replacement. In selected cases in which (1) prosthesis removal is not possible, (2) the pathogen is relatively avirulent, (3) the pathogen is exquisitely sensitive to an orally absorbed antibiotic, (4) the patient can tolerate an appropriate oral antibiotic, and (5) the prosthesis is not loose, suppressive oral antimicrobial therapy may be of value. Successful retention of the functioning hip arthroplasty has been seen in 63 percent of patients when all of these five criteria are fulfilled.[30] However, when similar therapy is employed in total knee replacements infected with a variety of microorganisms (both virulent and relatively avirulent), successful joint function is maintained in only 23 percent.[31] The suppressive approach is not without risk. Serial radiographs are needed over the course of treatment to monitor for progressive bone resorption at the bone–cement interface that could reduce the success of any future revision surgery. Despite continual antibiotic therapy the localized septic process could extend into adjacent tissue compartments or become a systemic infection. Moreover, the patient would be subjected to the potential side effects of chronic antibiotic administration.

PREVENTION OF JOINT PROSTHESIS INFECTION

In view of the catastrophic effects of prosthetic arthroplasty infection, prevention of these septic processes is of prime importance. In anticipation of elective total joint replacement surgery, the patient should be evaluated for the presence of pyogenic dentogingival pathology, obstructive uropathy, and dermatologic conditions that might predispose to infection and bacteremia. Strong consideration should be given to reducing the risks represented by these factors (i.e., dental extraction, prostatic resection, control of dermatitis) before insertion of the prosthesis. Perioperative antibiotic prophylaxis has been shown to reduce deep wound infection effectively in total joint replacement surgery.[32] Oxacillin or cefazolin are commonly administered as antistaphylococcal agents immediately before the operation and for 1–2 days thereafter. Filtered laminar airflow systems in the operating room further reduce infection rates, especially when whole-body, exhaust-ventilated suits are worn by the operating team.[33,34]

For patients with indwelling joint prostheses, early recognition and prompt therapy for infection in any location is critical to reduce the risk of seeding the joint implant hematogenously. Situations likely to cause bacteremia should be avoided. The use of prophylactic antibiotics in anticipation of bacteremic events (i.e., dental surgery, cystoscopy, colonoscopic biopsy, surgical procedures on infected or contaminated tissues) has been suggested on the same empirical basis upon which endocarditis prophylaxis is recommended.[3,5] This approach to prevention is controversial at the present time, and no data are available with which to determine the adequacy or the cost-effectiveness of such measures. Clinical decisions regarding prophylactic antibiotics for expected bacteremias in patients with prosthetic joints should be made on an individual basis.

REFERENCES

1. Salvati EA, Small RD, Brause BD, et al. Infections associated with orthopedic devices. In: Sugarman B, Young EJ, eds. Infections Associated with Prosthetic Devices. Boca Raton, FL: CRC Press; 1984:181–218.
2. Gristina AG, Kolkin J. Total joint replacement and sepsis. J Bone Joint Surg [Am] 1983;65:128–34.
3. Brause BD. Prosthetic joint infections. Curr Opin Rheumatol. 1989;1:194–8.
4. Ahlberg A, Carlsson AS, Lindberg L. Hematogenous infection in total joint replacement. Clin Orthop. 1978;137:69–75.
5. Maderazo EG, Judson S, Pasternak H. Late infections of total joint prostheses: A review and recommendations for prevention. Clin Orthop. 1988; 229:131–42.
6. Lindqvist C, Slatis P. Dental bacteremia—A neglected cause of arthroplasty infections? Acta Orthop Scand. 1985;56:506–8.
7. Petty W, Spanier S, Shuster JJ, et al. The influence of skeletal implants on incidence of infection. J Bone Joint Surg [Am]. 1985;67:1236–44.
8. Petty W. The effect of methylmethacrylate on bacterial inhibiting properties of normal human serum. Clin Orthop. 1978;132:266–77.
9. Petty W. The effect of methylmethacrylate on bacterial phagocytosis and killing by human polymorphonuclear leukocytes. J Bone Joint Surg [Am]. 1978; 60:752–7.
10. Vaudaux P, Suzuki R, Waldvogel FA, et al. Foreign-body infection: Role of fibronectin as a ligand for the adherence of *Staphylococcus aureus*. J Infect Dis. 1984;150:546–53.
11. Costerton JW, Irvin RT, Cheng K-J. The bacterial glycocalyx in nature and disease. Annu Rev Microbiol 1981;35:299–324.
12. Gristina AG, Jennings RA, Naylor PT, et al. Comparative in vitro antibiotic resistance of surface-colonizing coagulase-negative staphylococci. Antimicrob Agents Chemother. 1989;33:813–6.
13. Widmer AF, Frei R, Rajacic Z, et al. Correlation between in vivo and in vitro efficacy of antimicrobial agents against foreign body infections. J Infect Dis. 1990;162:96–102.
14. Inman JN, Gallegos KV, Brause BD, et al. Clinical and microbial features of prosthetic joint infection. Am J Med. 1984;77:47–53.
15. Merkel KD, Brown ML, Fitzgerald RH. Sequential technetium-99m HMDP-gallium-67 citrate imaging for the evaluation of infection in the painful prosthesis. J Nucl Med. 1986;27:1413–7.
16. Pring DJ, Henderson RG, Rivett AG, et al. Autologous granulocyte scanning of painful prosthetic joints. J Bone Joint Surg [Br]. 1986;68:647–52.
17. O'Neill DA, Harris WH. Failed total hip replacement: Assessment by plain radiographs, arthrograms and aspiration of the hip joint. J Bone Joint Surg [Am]. 1984;66:540–6.
18. Eftehar NS. Wound infection complicating total hip joint arthroplasty. Orthop Rev. 1979;8:49–64.
19. Fitzgerald RH, Nolan DR, Ilstrup DM, et al. Deep wound sepsis following total hip replacement. J Bone Joint Surg [Am]. 1977;59:847–55.
20. Callaghan JJ, Salvati EA, Brause BD, et al. Reimplantation for salvage of the infected hip. In: The Hip: Proceedings of the 14th Open Scientific Meeting of The Hip Society. St Louis: CV Mosby; 1986:65–94.
21. Windsor RE, Insall JN, Urs WK, et al. Two-stage reimplantation for the salvage of total knee arthroplasty complicated by infection. J Bone Joint Surg [Am]. 1990;72:272–8.
22. Salvati EA, Chekofsky KM, Brause BD, et al. Reimplantation in infection. Clin Orthop. 1982;170:62–75.
23. Rand JA, Bryan RS. Reimplantation for the salvage of an infected total knee arthroplasty. J Bone Joint Surg [Am]. 1983;65:1081–6.
24. Trippel SB. Antibiotic-impregnated cement in total joint arthroplasty. J Bone Joint Surg [Am]. 1986;68:1297–302.
25. Buchholz HW, Elson RA, Lodenkamper H. The infected joint implant. In: McKibbin B, ed. Recent Advances in Orthopedics. Edinburgh: Churchill Livingstone; 1979:139–61.
26. Buchholz HW, Elson R, Engelbrecht E. Management of deep infection of total hip replacement. J Bone Joint Surg [Br]. 1981;63:342–53.
27. Carlsson AS, Josefsson G, Lindberg L. Revision with gentamicin-impregnated cement for deep infection in total hip arthroplasties. J Bone Joint Surg [Am]. 1978;60:1059–64.
28. Fitzgerald RH, Jones DR. Hip implant infection. Am J Med. 1986;78(Suppl 6B):225–8.
29. Garvin KL, Salvati EA, Brause BD. Role of gentamicin-impregnated cement in total joint arthroplasty. Orthop Clin North Am. 1988;19:605–10.
30. Goulet JA, Pellicci PM, Brause BD, et al. Prolonged suppression of infection in total hip arthroplasty. J Arthroplasty. 1988;3:109–16.
31. Schoifet SD, Morrey BF. Treatment of infection after total knee arthroplasty by débridement with retention of the components. J Bone Joint Surg [Am]. 1990;72:1383–90.
32. Norden C. A critical review of antibiotic prophylaxis in orthopedic surgery. Rev Infect Dis. 1983;5:928–32.
33. Lidwell O, Lowbury E, Whyte E. Effect of ultraclean air in operating rooms on deep sepsis in the joint after total hip or total knee replacement. Br Med J. 1982;285:10–4.
34. Salvati EA, Robinson RP, Zeno SM, et al. Infection rates after 3175 total hip and total knee replacements performed with and without a horizontal unidirectional filtered air-flow system. J Bone Joint Surg [Am]. 1982;64: 525–35.

SECTION L. DISEASES OF THE REPRODUCTIVE ORGANS AND SEXUALLY TRANSMITTED DISEASES

---

87. GENITAL SKIN AND MUCOUS MEMBRANE LESIONS

MICHAEL F. REIN

The skin of the genital area is subject to many of the same diseases that affect other anatomic sites. Nonvenereal and noninfectious conditions can involve the genital epithelium alone or as part of a more generalized disease process.[1–4] Among adults, sexually transmitted diseases (STD) are a frequent cause of genital lesions, and a sexual history and diligent search for confirmatory manifestations of STD should be a part of the initial work-up.

HISTORY

Age

Candida albicans or herpes simplex virus can infect the neonatal genitalia, and herpetic vulvitis occurs occasionally in young children as the initial manifestation of exposure to the virus. Molluscum contagiosum is a common pediatric infection that only occasionally involves the genitalia, probably by autoinfection. The presence of sexually transmitted lesions such as herpes genitalis in an older child,[5] condylomata accuminata,[6–8] or exclusively genital molluscum contagiosum[9] in a child should prompt an evaluation for, but does not prove the existence of, sexual abuse.[10,11]

Sexual History

Exposure to multiple partners increases the risk of sexually acquired infection. Orogenital contact can inoculate sexually transmitted pathogens into the oral or pharyngeal mucosa.[12–15] Receptive anal intercourse predisposes to perianal, anal, and rectal infection.[13–17] A history of genital symptoms in, or recent treatment of, a sexual partner may be helpful diagnostically. Specific sexual practices such as particularly vigorous coitus or masturbation[18] or a history of being bitten by a sexual partner should be sought.

Incubation Period

We can sometimes estimate the incubation period of a sexually transmitted infection by obtaining the history of a single sexual contact or exposure to a new partner. Genital lesions developing within hours of sexual exposure suggest trauma, chemical irritation, or hypersensitivity.[1,18–20] Localized penile edema occurring within hours of vigorous coitus has been reported.[18] The swelling decreased spontaneously, and no specific therapy was required. Incubation periods of less than 24 hours are occasionally observed in chancroid.[21,22] Some patients experience reactivation of herpes genitalis within 12 hours after coitus.[13,14,23]

Somewhat longer incubation periods of 2–5 days are usually seen with chancroid[21,22] or herpes genitalis,[13,14,23] although the mean incubation period for primary genital herpes is actually about 6 days.[13,14,23] Clinical manifestations may follow infection by as much as 2–3 weeks for either of these diseases. An incubation period of 1–3 weeks is usually seen with syphilis,[15] although this may rarely extend up to 12 weeks. An incubation period of 4–12 weeks usually precedes the development of genital warts,[17] and the symptoms of pubic lice[24] and scabies generally follow infection by about 4 weeks (see Chs. 272 and 273). The incubation period for molluscum contagiosum is not well documented and apparently ranges from 2 to 26 weeks.[25,26] The incubation period for donovanosis is also poorly defined[21] but appears to average around 2 weeks.[27,28]

Residence and Travel

Lymphogranuloma venereum is considerably more common in Africa and the Far East than in the United States. Chancroid was diagnosed in 40 to 90 percent of patients with genital ulcerations in some African and Indian series.[29–36] Donovanosis is endemic in India, New Guinea, the West Indies, and some parts of Africa and South America.[21,27,28,37] Dual or multiple infections, in which some combination of *Treponema pallidum, Haemophilus ducreyi, Calymmatobacterium granulomatis,* and herpes simplex virus is isolated from a single lesion, are frequently reported in the developing world and may result in partial responses to therapy aimed only at a single agent. Whereas lymphogranuloma venereum and donovanosis are distinctly rare in the United States, chancroid has recently become far more common in major metropolitan areas,[38–41] where it often presents as localized epidemics.

Use of Antimicrobials

Antimicrobials and other drugs have been reported to cause fixed drug eruptions (FDE) that occasionally involve the genita-

lia.[1,42–45] The tetracyclines, commonly used in the treatment of sexually transmitted diseases, are incriminated with particular frequency as a cause of genital FDE.[43] Such lesions may take several forms but frequently manifest yellow ulcerations. Antimicrobials may predispose to the development of candidiasis and may alter or completely eliminate the lesions of syphilis,[46] chancroid, or lymphogranuloma venereum.

Underlying Diseases

Immunodeficiency states predispose to a variety of genital lesions. Balanitis due to *Candida*[47] or gram-negative bacteria[48] has been reported in neutropenic patients wearing condom catheters. The acquired immunodeficiency syndrome (AIDS) is associated with chronic necrotizing and recurrent genital[49] and perianal[59] herpes simplex virus infections, and recalcitrant genital candidiasis as well.[51]

Mode of Onset and Course

Because lesions often change over time, a history of the initial manifestation may be helpful in making the diagnosis. Thus, the patient with genital ulcerations who can state with surety that the lesions began as vesicles has helped to make a diagnosis of herpes genitalis. Vesicles often rupture quickly so that this stage of the lesions can go unnoticed by women.[23] A prodrome of local paresthesia preceding the appearance of lesions is reported by 50–90 percent of patients with recurrent genital herpes.[13,14,52,53] Venereal warts and molluscum contagiosum may remain relatively static for long periods of time after their initial appearance. The lesions of syphilis often last for many weeks and then heal without antibiotic intervention.[15] Pearly penile papules, appearing in single or multiple rows around the penile corona at puberty, are a completely benign condition.[54]

A recurrence of the lesions at intervals strongly suggests genital herpes. The rate of recurrence varies strikingly among individuals, but the average rate of recurrence among patients genitally infected with herpes simplex virus type 2 is 0.33 per month, whereas genital infections with herpes simplex virus type 1 recur at an average rate of but 0.02 per month.[55] Indeed, whereas 90 percent of patients with type 2 genital infections report a recurrence within 1 year, recurrences are experienced by only 25 percent of the patients genitally infected with herpes simplex virus type 1.

Pain

Although the syphilitic chancre is usually described as nontender, up to 30 percent of the patients with primary syphilis experience either pain or tenderness of the lesions.[46] The relative indolence of the lesions of donovanosis[21,37,56] sometimes results in long delays before the patient seeks medical attention. Pain usually accompanies the lesions of chancroid,[21,57] herpes genitalis,[13,14,23] tularemia,[58,59] and amebiasis.[60–62]

Pruritis

Itching is associated with herpes genitalis and is described by 50–90 percent of patients with recurrent disease,[13,14,23,52] particularly in the prodromal period. Pruritus accompanies 90 percent of infestations with pubic lice,[24] and severe itching, increased by warming the skin, either in bed or when taking a bath, suggests scabies. Although *severe* pruritis is uncommon in secondary syphilis,[15] 42 percent of patients describe at least mild itching.[63] Pruritis also characterizes candidal balanitis, which is observed occasionally in male sexual partners of women with vulvovaginal candidiasis.[64,65]

Vaginal Discharge

Several infectious vaginitides are associated with vulvar lesions. The vulvovaginitis syndrome is discussed in Chapter 89.

Fever

Fever occurs in 5–8 percent of the patients with secondary syphilis[15,63] and in many patients with disseminated gonococcal infection.[66,67] Fever accompanies primary herpes genitalis in 70 percent of women and 40 percent of men but is uncommon in recurrent disease.[13,14,23,52]

Other Features

Sacral root neurologic symptoms suggest herpes,[13,14,23] and a urethral discharge suggests gonorrhea or, less commonly, Reiter syndrome (see Ch. 88). Inguinal adenopathy accompanies syphilis, chancroid, herpes genitalis, and lymphogranuloma venereum when lesions involve the vulva, distal two-thirds of the vagina, shaft of the penis, or scrotum. The cervix and proximal third of the vagina and the glans penis drain to the iliac rather than the inguinal nodes, and lesions in these regions are not associated with palpable adenopathy. The adenopathy of herpes genitalis or chancroid is usually tender, whereas the adenopathy of syphilis in characteristically indolent.

MORPHOLOGIC CHARACTERISTICS OF GENITAL LESIONS

Careful examination of the entire genital area is essential and will be facilitated by a good light source and a hand lens. A differential diagnosis can often be made on the basis of the morphologic characteristics of genital lesions, but variations from the typical appearance and clinical overlap among the various diseases are unfortunately common.[46,68–70a] A clinical differential diagnosis of genital ulcers is perhaps the greatest challenge,[26,68–71] with the most common error involving the overdiagnosis of chancroid.[30] Nonetheless, the morphologic characteristics of genital lesions often supply the first and most important clue to their cause. Table 1 provides a classification of genital lesions but can serve only as a rough guide.

The absence of lesions does not rule out active disease. From 1 to 8 percent of asymptomatic individuals attending STD clinics are shedding herpes simplex virus.[72] About 60 percent of infected individuals give no prior history of genital lesions,[73,74] although with instruction some 50 percent of these women subsequently recognize symptomatic outbreaks in the future.[75] Subclinical carriage of human papillomavirus (HPV) is common and greatly exceeds the prevalence of visible warts.[76,77] Colposcopy has become a standard diagnostic approach to subclinical lesions in women, and the same technique is being applied with increasing enthusiasm to men.[78–80] Subclinical HPV lesions will stain white when 5% acetic acid is applied for several minutes. The etiology of such "acetowhite" lesions must be confirmed by biopsy, because several other inflammatory conditions produce the same reaction.[79,80]

Vesicles or Bullae

The classic initial lesion of genital herpes is grouped vesicles on an erythematous base.[13,14] Umbilications are sometimes observed.[13,14] The vesicles have often ruptured by the time the patient seeks medical attention, and only ulcers are observed. Scabies occasionally manifests vesicular or bullous lesions.[81]

Genital Ulcers

As noted earlier, the causes of genital ulcers vary markedly in different parts of the world. Chancroid is becoming far more

TABLE 1. Morphologic Classification of Genital Lesions

Ulcers
  Herpes genitalis
  Syphilis
  Trauma
  Chancroid
  Fixed drug eruption
  Lymphogranuloma venereum
  Tularemia
  Behçet syndrome
  Malignancy
  Donovanosis (granuloma inguinale)
  Candidiasis
  Histoplasmosis
  Mycobacterioses
  Amebiasis
  Gonorrhea
  Trichomoniasis
Papules
  Venereal warts
  Scabies
  Molluscum contagiosum
  Candidiasis
  Syphilis
Vesicles and bullae
  Scabies
  Herpes genitalis
Diffuse erythema
  Candidiasis
  Trauma
  Contact dermatitis
  Fixed drug eruption
Crusts
  Herpes genitalis
  Scabies
Miscellaneous findings
  Linear tracks: scabies
  Reddish flecks: crab louse excreta
  Maculae ceruleae (sky blue spots): crab lice
  Nits: crab lice
  Hypertrophic: donovanosis

common in major metropolitan areas of the United States,[38–41] and we can no longer regard a clinical diagnosis of chancroid with suspicion.[68] Tuberculosis,[82–85] histoplasmosis, and amebiasis[60–62] are rare causes of destructive penile ulcerations. Genital ulcers have assumed a particularly ominous importance, for it appears that they can serve as a portal of entry for human immunodeficiency virus.[36,86]

Number. The classic chancre of primary syphilis is a single lesion (Figs. 1 and 2)[15,87]; however, in some series, almost half of the patients with proven primary syphilis had more than one penile ulcer.[31,46,87] Chancroid is usually said to be present as multiple ulcerations, yet in some series 40–70 percent of the affected men had but a single lesion.[57,88] The genital lesion of tick-borne tularemia is single.[58] Herpes genitalis characteristically produces multiple ulcerations in groups surrounded by an erythematous border (Fig. 3).[13,14,23,52] The vagina per se is involved in only 4 percent of cases.[13,14,46] Although the multiple lesions of syphilis and herpes are generally of uniform size, the lesions of chancroid may vary in an individual patient.[21] A rare cause of recurrent, multiple genital ulcerations in the United States is Behçet syndrome,[89] an inflammatory disease of unknown cause that usually also involves the oral, conjunctival, and synovial membranes. Behçet's ulcers involve the scrotum and vulva more frequently than they do the penis, anus, or vagina, and scars from previous episodes may be present.[89] Ulcers are occasionally observed in vulvovaginal or penile candidiasis. Intravaginal ulcers may follow tampon use,[90] but infectious and neoplastic causes must be ruled out in these cases.

Tenderness. Tenderness on palpation may be extreme with herpes genitalis,[13,14,23] and chancroid[21,57] is present in 30 percent of syphilitic chancres[46] and characterizes tularemia.[58] Even massive, ulcerated lesions of donovanosis are nontender.[21,37]

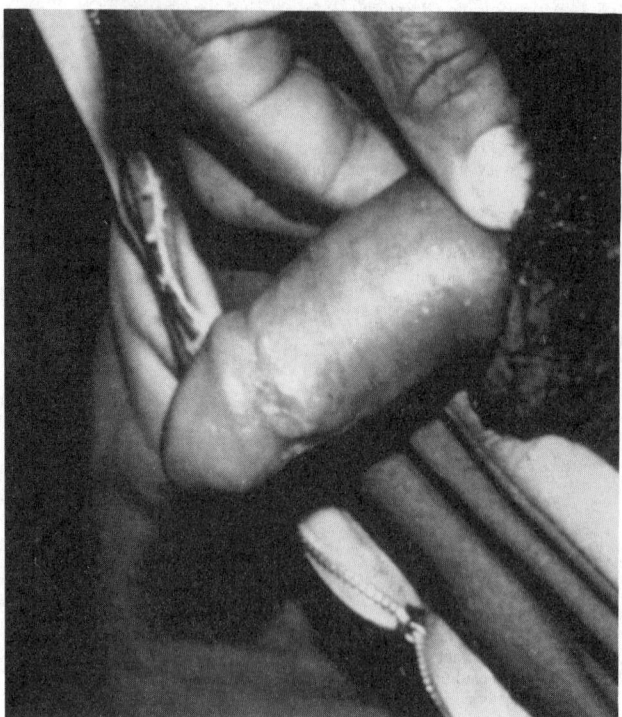

FIG. 1. Primary syphilitic chancre of the penis.

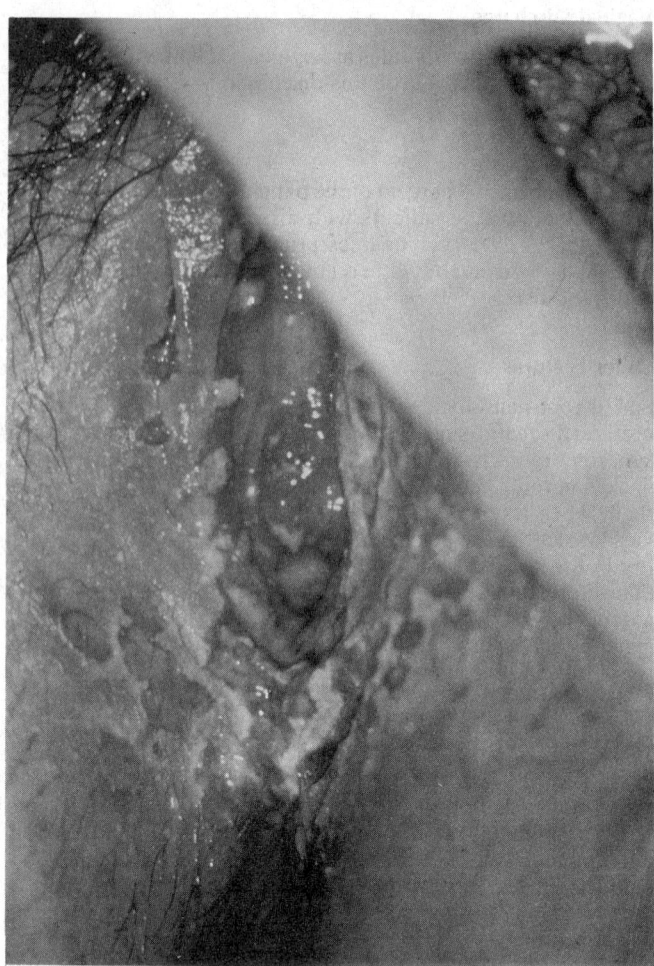

FIG. 3. Herpes (HSV-2) of the vulva.

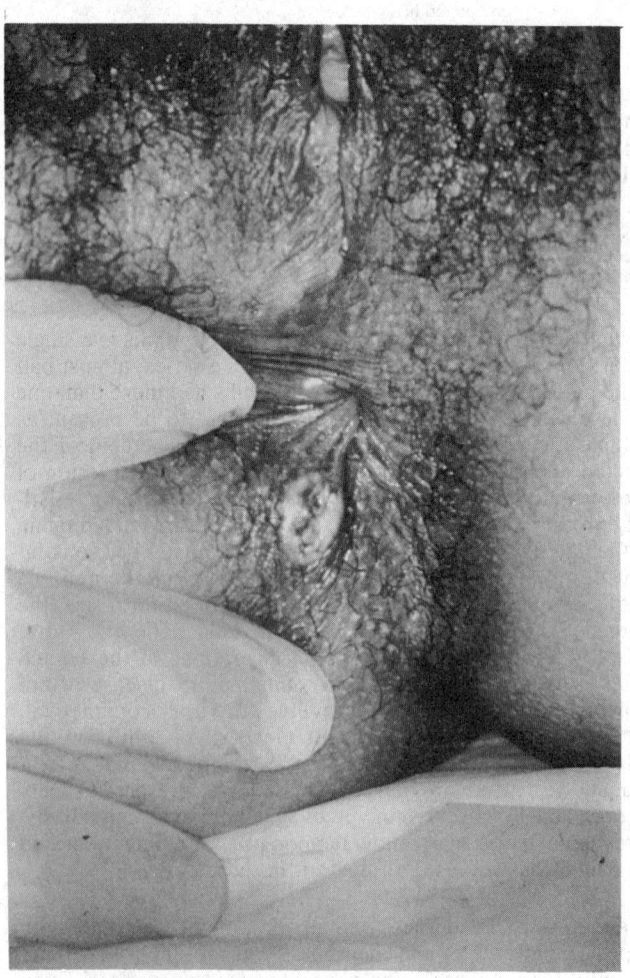

FIG. 2. Primary syphilitic chancre of the perineum.

Ulcer Base. The lesions of chancroid are usually ragged and have a necrotic base.[21,32,57] On the other hand, syphilitic and herpetic ulcers are relatively clean (Figs. 1–3). The ulcers of Behçet syndrome often have a yellow, necrotic base.[89] Donovanosis results in ulcers with granulation tissue at the base yielding beefy red lesions that often become exuberantly hypertrophic and produce large, friable, ulcerated masses projecting above the skin.[21,37]

Ulcer Edge. The ulcers of chancroid are characteristically undermined, but the edge is not indurated,[21,22,57,91] giving rise to the informal name "soft chancre." An indurated lesion is highly suggestive of syphilis[15,31,87] and occurs in 92 percent of the infected patients.[46] An erythematous border is seen both with herpes[13,14,23] and with chancroid.[21,57] The border of the lesion in donovanosis is often a stark white, which is characteristic of no other genital infection.[56] Lesions of donovanosis also often manifest a thickening of the edge that yields a rolled appearance.[37] Serpiginous lesions, progressing in one area as they heal in another, are characteristic of donovanosis[21,37] and less so of chancroid.[21]

Genital Papules

Careful examination of the papules with the aid of a hand lens often suggests a specific etiologic diagnosis. Papules may be the transient, initial state of a variety of genital infections, including syphilis,[46] scabies,[92] lymphogranuloma venereum,[93] chancroid,[21] and herpes.[13,14,23] Early condylomata acuminata usually appear as simple papules that can be identified when the hand lens reveals the beginning of a verrucous cap or tiny blood vessels at the base. Papular or papulosquamous lesions are seen on the external genitalia in most patients with secondary syphilis.[15,63,69,87]

Pearly penile papules are normal and occur in 8–25 percent of men.[54] They are found more commonly in uncircumcised men and present as one or more rows of grayish white or pink papules along the corona or in the coronal sulcus. They usually appear at puberty and are of no pathologic significance. Patients concerned about venereal disease will occasionally notice the lesions and will seek medical attention. Although the histologic appearance is characteristic, biopsy is rarely warranted because the diagnosis can be made clinically.

Umbilication. The hand lens will reveal tiny umbilications at the vertex of the lesions of molluscum contagiosum (see Ch. 113).[25,26] The umbilications often appear to contain keratin plugs. These 1–5 mm papules occur singly or in small clusters on the penile shaft, glans, labia majora, thighs, and buttocks. The lesions may be particularly abundant and disseminated in patients with AIDS,[94] but almost identical lesions are also seen in disseminated cryptococcosis in the same population.[95] In children, the disease is nonvenereally acquired and usually affects the trunk and extremities. The lesions are nonpruritic and may coalesce to form larger masses.[25,26] Squeezing expresses caseous material from the umbilication. Curettage easily removes the entire lesion and leaves a shallow, slightly hemorrhagic ulceration that heals without scarring. If the diagnosis is in doubt, a papule may be removed and crushed between two microscope slides. Wright or Giemsa stain reveals cells distended by intracytoplasmic inclusions (see Ch. 113).

Verrucous Lesions. Verrucous papules suggest a diagnosis of condylomata acuminata (venereal warts). The lesions are usually multiple and may show a satelliting phenomenon wherein a larger wart is surrounded by smaller lesions. Stalked or sessile, the warts can be found anywhere on the external genitalia and in the vagina or on the cervix. Perianal warts in women may occur as a result of the spread from a genital focus. Perianal condylomas in men are associated with receptive anal intercourse,[16,17,96] and such men should be evaluated for intra-anal warts[25] and other anorectal infections as well.[97] Perianal warts in men should prompt the clinician vigorously to recommend serologic testing for human immunodeficiency virus.

In moist areas, warts may become relatively elongated. The major source of diagnostic difficulty is differentiating these from the moist lesions of secondary syphilis, condylomata lata. The syphilitic lesions tend to be flatter and more grayish than are condylomata acuminata.[15] A differential diagnosis is best made by carefully abrading the lesions and performing a darkfield examination; condylomata lata are teeming with spirochetes. Unfortunately, anaerobic spirochetes occasionally superinfect condylomata acuminata and may give an initial appearance of darkfield positivity. Venereal warts, particularly flat warts of the cervix, are strongly associated with cervical intraepithelial neoplasia and cancer (see Ch. 122),[98] and culposcopy or biopsy may be indicated for suspicious lesions.

Although acetic acid applications have long been used to identify subclinical HPV infections of the cervix and vagina, the technique is now also employed to detect otherwise invisible lesions in men.[78–80,99–103] Acetic acid, 3–5%, is applied to the penis for 3–5 minutes, and the skin is examined with the colposcope. Flat white lesions are revealed in 40–80 percent of the male partners of women with warts, and 60–80 percent of such lesions are identified as HPV by biopsy.[78–80,99–103] Thus the mere presence of acetowhite lesions does not confirm the presence of HPV; other inflammatory conditions also yield a similar reaction with acetic acid.

Candidal balanitis occurs uncommonly in men who are the sexual partners of women with candidal vulvovaginitis[64,65,104] and is sometimes manifested as pruritic plaques of the glans, foreskin, or shaft of the penis surrounded by small, discrete papules (satellite lesions), which are helpful diagnostically. Similar papular or papulopustular lesions accompany candidal infection of the groin, scrotum, and vulva.

Crusted Lesions. Herpetic ulcers heal by crusting over. Crusts are also characteristic of scabies (see Ch. 273) and may be accompanied by moist papules[47] and burrows. These thread-like lesions, often stippled, are 1–10 mm long and are specific for scabies. They may be dramatically demonstrated by covering a papule with ink (as from a fountain pen) and the wiping it off with an alcohol swab. In about two-thirds of cases the burrow, now filled with ink, is readily visualized.[105]

Diffuse Erythematous Lesions

Superficial infection with tinea or candida may cause diffusely erythematous, intensely pruritic lesions of the genitalia and groin. Candidal lesions are often more intensely erythematous, whereas lesions caused by tinea are usually somewhat brown and may show central clearing. Involvement of the scrotum or the appearance of small papules or pustules beyond the main border of the lesion suggests candidal infection. Group A[106] and group B[104,106,107] streptococci have caused balanitis. *Gardnerella vaginalis* and *Trichomonas vaginalis* are also felt to cause some cases of balanitis in uncircumcised men.[108,109] Either infection responds to metronidazole. Human papillomavirus should be considered as a cause of recurrent or intractable, patchy balanitis[110]; the diagnosis is confirmed histologically. Atopic dermatitis and reaction to soaps have also been implicated.[111]

Pubic Hair

Crab lice are usually present in very small numbers, an average infestation consisting of fewer than 10.[112] Some lice are, however, observed in 97 percent of infested patients who have not treated themselves before seeking medical attention.[24] Examination of the pubic hair with a hand lens reveals the lice as gray-brown creatures climbing along the shafts or partially buried at the bases. They are found in perianal hair in about 50 percent of patients and in abdominal hair in about 17 percent.[24] If the organisms themselves are not observed, the diagnosis can still be made in 80 percent of patients by recognizing the eggs or nits, 0.5-mm ovoids adherent to the hair shafts, and a careful examination will reveal tiny reddish spots of louse excreta at the base of the hair in about 15 percent of patients.[24] Crab lice bites sometimes result in round to oval, 0.5–1.5-mm, bluish red macules called *maculae ceruleae* or *sky blue spots*.[24,113]

EXTRAGENITAL DERMATOLOGIC MANIFESTATIONS OF SEXUALLY TRANSMITTED DISEASES

Patients should be questioned about orogenital and receptive anal practices, since these may result in direct inoculation of sexually transmitted pathogens into extragenital sites. Additionally, sexually transmitted infections sometimes disseminate, producing secondary, extragenital manifestations.

Mouth

Direct inoculation of sexually transmitted viruses can cause oral lesions. Intraoral condyloma acuminata[23] and molluscum contagiosum[114] are reported, and lesions resemble those of the genital area. Herpes simplex has been transmitted from the genital tract to the mouth and vice versa.[13,14,23,55] Genital lesions produced by herpes simplex virus type 1 are indistinguishable from those produced by type 2. Likewise, oral inoculation can result in fever blisters, a primary gingivostomatitis, or a herpanginalike picture, with clusters of vesicles and ulcers on the hard palate.[13,14,23,115]

Although the oral mucosa is generally resistant to gonococcal infection, occasional cases of gonococcal stomatitis, presumably resulting from the direct inoculation, have been reported.[116] Syphilitic chancres of the lip, buccal mucous membranes, gingiva, and tonsils are becoming relatively more common. They are usually painless and may be difficult to diagnose because normal oral spirochetes confound the darkfield examination.[15,87]

Disseminated infections may also affect the mouth. Mucous patches occur in about 20 percent of patients with secondary syphilis and appear on the oral mucous membranes and the tongue as painless, relatively clean, shallow ulcerations, often with a yellow or gray base and a small amount of surrounding erythema.[9,63,87] Atypical presentations are described in patients with AIDS.[117] Palatal petechiae may accompany gonococcal bacteremia. Recurrent oral and genital ulcers suggest Behçet syndrome.[87]

Anorectum

A similar spectrum of diseases affects the rectal mucosa.[97] Perianal warts[16,17,96] and herpetic lesions[50,118] are seen in homosexual men who practice receptive anal intercourse. Both processes can involve women in the same manner, but in women they may also have extended to the anus from a primary genital focus. Among patients with AIDS, herpetic proctitis may be chronic and relentlessly destructive.[50] Necrotizing perianal lesions occasionally result from amebiasis in endemic areas.[43]

Other Skin

The generalized rash of secondary syphilis frequently involves the genitalia. In fact, a generalized eruption sparing the genital area and the oral mucous membranes is unlikely to be syphilis.[15] The rash is highly variable, and the differential diagnosis is challenging.[15,63,69,87] One should consider secondary syphilis in the differential diagnosis of any generalized, relatively indolent eruption, particularly if the palms and soles are involved, if there is accompanying generalized lymphadenopathy (70–86 percent), or if there is a patchy hair loss.[15,63] The lesions are usually macular, maculopapular (70 percent), or papulosquamous, and symmetrically distributed.[15,63] Markedly pruritic or vesicular lesions in an adult are unlikely to be syphilis.

About 33–50 percent of the patients with disseminated gonococcal infections will have small numbers of skin lesions, usually found on the distal portions of the extremities and occasionally involving the palms and the soles. Some cases with very large numbers of lesions have also been reported, but in these settings meningococcemia must also be considered.[119] Lesions are relatively pleomorphic and may be macular, maculopapular, petechial, vesicular, pustular, or necrotic.[67] The typical lesion is an erythematous or hemorrhagic spot, 2–5 mm in diameter, that is surmounted by a gray pustule, sometimes displaying a small eschar in its center.[66] The lesions of subacute meningococcemia may be similar and represent an important differential diagnosis.[119]

The interdigital webs, wrists, and ankles are often involved in scabies.[120] Secondary papular lesions, thought to represent a hypersensitivity phenomenon, may occur on the abdomen or the pelvic girdle area. Burrows, described above, are pathognomonic of scabies.[105] Maculae ceruleae (see above) are occasionally observed on the anterior and lateral portions of the abdomen and thorax of patients with crab lice.[113]

Herpes genitalis involves the thigh or buttock in some 15 percent of infected women.[121–123] Many of these women simultaneously shed virus from genital sites.[123] Patients with AIDS demonstrate a variety of skin lesions, including Kaposi sarcoma, at some distance from sexual orifices (see Ch. 102).

LABORATORY EXAMINATIONS

Sufficiently accurate etiologic diagnoses can often be made on the basis of clinical examination when genital lesions are classical. In many situations, particularly in the etiologic diagnosis of genital ulcers, laboratory examination is required.

Direct Microscopic Examinations

Any ulcerated genital lesion or hypertrophic lesion in a moist area may be examined by darkfield microscopy (see Ch. 215). The diagnosis of chancroid is sometimes confirmed by cleaning the lesion with gauze and swabbing material from the undermined edge. Gram staining of this material may reveal chains of streptobacilli suggestive of *H. ducreyi*,[57] but the smear technique has a low sensitivity and specificity and is not useful in a clinical setting.[33,34,88,124] Direct fluorescent antibody staining is under investigation.[125]

A smear of material from the base of a freshly ruptured vesicle may be stained with Wright or Giemsa stain and examined for the multinucleated giant cells that are diagnostic of herpetic infection.[13,14,23] This Tzanck test is not generally helpful, however, because the presence of vesicles is essentially diagnostic of herpetic infection, and the test is insensitive on genital ulcers, being positive in fewer than 40 percent of culture-proven cases.[126] Monoclonal antibodies will detect herpes viral antigens in material from 75 percent of herpetic lesions by direct examination with fluorescence microscopy,[127,128] and the technique also differentiates type 1 virus from type 2.

Bits of tissue from a hypertrophic lesion may be crushed between microscope slides, treated with Wright or Giemsa stain, and examined for the characteristic intracytoplasmic bacterial inclusions of donovanosis.[21,27,28,37] Papular lesions may be scraped, crushed, stained with a variety of agents, and examined for the balloonlike cells of molluscum contagiosum.[26] Heating such scrapings with 10% potassium hydroxide will destroy the squamous elements and may reveal tinea, candida, or the mites or larvae of scabies.[92] Mixing scrapings with mineral oil rather than potassium hydroxide may give an advantage in the diagnosis of scabies, for, unlike potassium hydroxide, mineral oil preserves mite fecal pellets and motility.[129] Scrapings or aspirations of the peripheral lesions of disseminated gonococcal infection reveal the organisms only infrequently by Gram stain but may be subjected to immunofluorescence microscopy, which will be diagnostic in about half the cases.[67,130]

Antigen and Genome Detection

Because of the cost of viral culture, there has been considerable interest in alternative methods for identifying the presence of herpes simplex virus. Commercially available ELISA tests are as sensitive as culture in early lesions and almost twice as sensitive in crusted lesions.[131,132] Culture remains more sensitive when applied to cervical swabs.[132] DNA hybridization with radiolabeled probes and DNA polymerase chain reaction are under investigation.[133–136]

Detection of HPV infection by DNA hybridization has become a valuable diagnostic tool.[53,76,80,137,137a] Polymerase chain reaction is more sensitive and is under investigation as well.[137,138] Polymerase chain reaction for *H. ducreyi* is also under development.[139]

Serologic Tests

Serologic tests are occasionally misleading in the diagnosis of syphilis. From 20 to 30 percent of the patients with a chancre, particularly if the lesion has just appeared, will have nonreactive

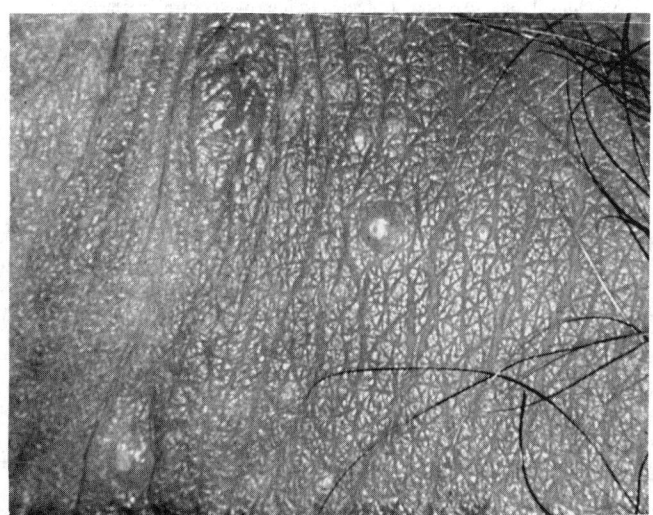

FIG. 4. Molluscum contagiosum: penile lesions displaying characteristic keratin-plugged umbilications.

nontreponemal results for syphilis.[140–142] About 10–17 percent of the patients may have a reactive fluorescent treponemal antibody absorption (FTA-ABS) test even if the nontreponemal tests (e.g., Venereal Disease Research Laboratory [VDRL], rapid plasma reagin [RPR], automated reagin test [ART]) (see Ch. 215) are nonreactive.[140–142] The clinician may therefore wish to obtain an FTA-ABS test from patients with suspicious genital lesions, even if the nontreponemal test result is negative. In many areas, the microhemagglutination test for *Treponema pallidum* antibodies (MHA-TP) has replaced the more demanding FTA-ABS as the confirmatory treponemal test. The tests are not entirely equivalent, since the MHA-TP is only about 89 percent sensitive in primary syphilis and will therefore miss about 10 percent of cases that would be detected by the FTA-ABS.[142] The vast majority of patients will have positive nontreponemal test findings within the week after the appearance of the chancre, and repeated serologic testing and a darkfield examination may be necessary to make the diagnosis. The sensitivities of nontreponemal and treponemal tests are almost 100 percent in secondary syphilis. Thus, a negative serologic examination essentially rules out this diagnosis.[140,142]

Commercially available serologic tests have almost no current role in the routine clinical diagnosis of genital herpes simplex virus infection because of their low sensitivity in primary infection and cross-reactions resulting from highly prevalent herpes simplex type 1 infections.[143–146] Research tests capable of differentiating antibodies directed against types 1 and 2 infections avoid this confusion but still suffer from a lack of sensitivity in primary infection.[73,147] The finding of serum antibody only to type 1 in a patient without symptoms or with recurrent genital lesions does not rule out genital herpes, since genital infection may be caused by either herpes simplex type. Serologic tests may, however, be the only way to establish a diagnosis in the 60 percent of patients with genital herpes who give no history of lesions.[73]

A serologic test for donovanosis is being studied.[148] The serodiagnosis of chancroid is experimental and, not surprisingly in face of the short incubation period, is plagued by insensitivity in acute disease and lack of specificity for current infection in populations with high endemicity.[149] The infrequency of a carrier state in chancroid further reduces the likely clinical utility of serodiagnosis.

Culture

Tissue culture for herpes simplex identifies the agent in 70–80 percent of first episode infections.[73] Once the lesions have

crusted over, however, sensitivity of the culture is reduced to about 30 percent.[130,150] The sensitivity is lower in recurrent disease, dropping to 30 percent in ulcers and to less than 20 percent in crusted lesions.[128] Patients with asymptomatic infections shed virus only rarely (perhaps only 1 percent of the time), and even repeated negative viral cultures cannot rule out infection in an asymptomatic patient.

The edge of a clean lesion may be cultured for *H. ducreyi*.[151,152] The medium employed dramatically affects sensitivity,[151–154] which is, even under the best circumstances, probably no higher than 80 percent.[32,35,88,151–154] Material from the lesion suspected of being molluscum contagiosum may be inoculated into tissue culture, and a cytopathic effect may be observed (see Chapter 113). Culture for the agent of donovanosis is unreliable and not generally available.[37]

REFERENCES

1. Wilson JF. The nonvenereal diseases of the genitals: Their differentiation from venereal lesions. Med Clin North Am. 1964;48:787.
2. Hillman RJ, Wladron S, Walker MM, et al. Granuloma annulare of the penis. Genitourin Med. 1992;68:47–9.
3. Hillman RJ, Walker MM, Harris JRW, et al. Penile dermatoses: A clinical and histopathological study. Genitourin Med. 1992;68:166–9.
4. Shen RN, Cybulska RA, Thin RN, et al. Vulval Crohn's disease mimicking genital herpes. Intern J STD AIDS. 1993;4:54–5.
5. Hibbard RA. Herpetic vulvovaginitis and child abuse. Am J Dis Child. 1985;139:542–5.
6. Gutman LT, Herman-Giddens ME, Phelps WC. Transmission of human genital papillomavirus disease: Comparison of data from adults and children. Pediatrics. 1993;91:31–8.
7. Amschler DH. Condylomata accuminata in children: Is sexual abuse implicated? J School Health. 1992;62:191–3.
8. Derksen DJ. Children and condylomata accuminata. J Fam Pract. 1992;34:419–23.
9. Bargman H, Schachner L, Hankim D. Is genital molluscum contagiousum a cutaneous manifestation of sexual abuse in children? J Am Acad Dermatol. 1986;14:847–9.
10. Ross JD, Scott GR, Busuttil A. Condylomata accuminata in pre-pubertal children. Med Sci Law. 1993;33:78–82.
11. Cohen BA, Honig P, Androphy E. Anogenital warts in children. Clinical and virological evidence for sexual abuse. Arch Dermatol. 1990;126:1575–80.
12. Choukass NC, Toto PD. Condyloma accuminatum of the oral cavity. Oral Surg. 1982;54:480.
13. Corey L, Adams HG, Brown ZA, et al. Genital herpes simplex infection: Clinical manifestations, course, and complications. Ann Intern Med. 1983;98:958.
14. Mertz GJ. Genital herpes simplex virus infections. Med Clin North Amer. 1990;74:1433–54.
15. Stokes HJ, Beerman H, Ingraham NR. Modern Clinical Syphilology. 3rd ed. Philadelphia: WB Saunders; 1944.
16. Carr G, William DC. Anal warts in a population of gay men in New York City. Sex Transm Dis. 1977;4:56.
17. Oriel JD. Genital warts. Sex Transm Dis. 1981;8:326.
18. Wilde H, Canby JP. Penile venereal edema. Arch Dermatol. 1973;108:263.
19. Fried FA. Glans penis dermatitis after treatment of wife's vaginitis. JAMA. 1981;245:2532.
20. Gochfeld M, Burger J. Sexual transmission of nickel and poison oak contact dermatitis. Lancet. 1983;1:589.
21. Hart G. Chancroid, Donovanosis, Lymphogranuloma Venereum. DHEW publication (CDC) 75-8302. Atlanta, GA: Centers for Disease Control and Prevention; 1975.
22. Fiumara NJ. A guide to lesions of the penis. Hosp Med. March 1970.
23. Pazin GJ. Management of oral and genital herpes simplex virus infections: Diagnosis and treatment. DM 1986;32:725–824.
24. Chapel TA, Katta T, Kuszmar T, et al. Pediculosis pubis in a clinic for sexually transmitted diseases. Sex Transm Dis. 1979;6:257.
25. Margolis S. Genital warts and molluscum contagiosum. Urol Clin North Am. 1984;11:163–70.
26. Brown ST, Nalley JF, Kraus SJ. Molluscum contagiosum. Sex Transm Dis. 1981;8:227.
27. Sehgal VN, Shyam Prasad AL. Donovanosis: Current concepts. Int J Dermatol. 1986;25:8–16.
28. Rosen T, Tschen JA, Ramsdell W, et al. Granuloma inguinale. J Am Acad Dermatol. 1984;433–7.
29. Meheus A, Van Dyck E, Ursi JP, et al. Etiology of genital ulcers in Swaziland. Sex Transm Dis. 1983;10:33.
30. Sturm AW, Stoltung GJ, Cormane RH, et al. Clinical and microbiological evaluation of 46 episodes of genital ulceration. Genitourin Med. 1987;63:98, 101.

31. Diaz-Mitoma F, Benninger G, Slutchuk M, et al. Etiology of nonvesicular genital ulcers in Winnipeg. Sex Transm Dis. 1987;14:33–6.
32. Nsanze H, Fast MV, D'Costa LJ. Genital ulcers in Kenya: Clinical and laboratory study. Br J Vener Dis. 1981;57:378.
33. Coovadia YM, Kharsany A, Hoosen A. The microbiol etiology of genital ulcers in black men in Durban, South Africa. Genitourin Med. 1985;61:266–9.
34. Plummer FA, D'Costa LJ, Nsanze H, et al. Clinical and microbiologic studies of genital ulcers in Kenyan women. Sex Transm Dis. 1985;12:193–7.
35. Fast MV, D'Costa LJ, Nsanze H, et al. The clinical diagnosis of genital ulcer disease in men in the tropics. Sex Transm Dis. 1984;11:72–6.
36. Bogearts J, Ricart CA, Van Dyck E, et al. The etiology of genital ulceration in Rwanda. Sex Transm Dis. 1989;16:123–6.
37. Kuberski T. Granuloma inguinale (donovanosis). Sex Transm Dis. 1980;7:29.
38. Flood JM, Sarafian SK, Bolan GA, et al. Multistrain outbreak of chancroid in San Francisco. J Infect Dis. 1993;167:1106–11.
39. Schulte JM, Martich FA, Schmid GP. Chancroid in the United States, 1981–1990: Evidence for underreporting of cases. MMWR. 1992;41:57–61.
40. Farris JR, Hutcheson D, Cartwright G, et al. Chancroid in Dallas: New lessons from an old disease. Texas Med 1991;87:78–81.
41. Blackmore CA, Kimpakarnjanarat K, Rigau-Perez JG, et al. An outbreak of chancroid in Orange County, California: Descriptive epidemiology and disease control measures. J Infect Dis. 1985;151:840–4.
42. Talbot MD. Fixed genital drug eruption. Practitioner. 1980;224:823.
43. Dodds PR, Chi T-N. Balanitis as a fixed drug eruption to tetracycline. J Urol. 1981;133:1044–5.
44. Cohen HA, Ashkenazi A, Nussinovitch M, et al. Fixed drug eruption of the scrotum due to methylphenidate. Ann Pharmacother. 1992;26:1378.
45. Lacey HB, Ness A, Mandal BK. Vulval ulceration associated with foscarnet. Genitourin Med. 1992;68:182.
46. Chapel TA. The variability of syphilitic chancres. Sex Transm Dis. 1978;5:68.
47. Morrissey R, Xavier A, Nguyen N, et al. Invasive candidal balanitis due to a condom catheter in a neutropenic patient. South Med J. 1985;78:1247–9.
48. Manian FA, Alford RH. Nosocomial infectious balanoposthitis in neutropenic patients. South Med J. 1987;80:909–11.
49. Maier JA, Bergman A, Ross MG. Acquired immunodeficiency syndrome manifested by chronic primary genital herpes. Am J Obstet Gynecol. 1986;155:756–8.
50. Siegal FP, Lopez C, Hammer GS, et al. Severe acquired immunodeficiency in male homosexuals manifested by chronic perianal herpes simplex lesions. N Engl J Med. 1981;305:1439–44.
51. Imam N, Carpenter CCJ, Mayer KH, et al. Hierarchical pattern of mucosal *Candida* infections with HIV seropositive women. Am J Med. 1990;89:142.
52. Guinan ME, MacCalman J, Kern ER, et al. The course of untreated recurrent genital herpes simplex infection in 27 women. N Engl J Med. 1981;304:759.
53. Brookes JL, Haywood S, Green J. Prodromal symptoms in genital herpes simplex infection. Genitourin Med. 1992;68:347–8.
54. Rehbein HM. Pearly penile papules: Incidence. Cutis. 1977;19:54.
55. Lafferty WE, Coombs RW, Benedetti J, et al. Recurrences after oral and genital herpes simplex virus infection. Influence of site of infection and viral type. N Engl J Med. 1987;316:1444–9.
56. D'Aunoy R, Von Hamm E. Granuloma inguinale. Am J Trop Med. 1937;17:747.
57. Asm J. Chancroid: A report of 1402 cases. Am J Syph Gonorr Vener Dis. 1952;36:483.
58. Dienst FT. Tularemia: A perusal of 339 cases. J LA State Med Soc. 1963;115:114.
59. Evans ME, Gregory DW, Schaffner W, et al. Tularemia: A 30 year experience with 88 cases. Medicine. 1985;64:251–69.
60. Parkash S, Ramakrishnan K, Ananthakrishnan N, et al. Amoebic ulcer of the penis. Postgrad Med J. 1982;58:375.
61. Veliath AJ, Bansal R, Sankaran V, et al. Genital amebiasis. Int J Gynaecol Obstet. 1987;25:249–56.
62. O'Leary RK, Posen J. Amoebiasis of the penis. S Afr Med J. 1984;65:113–6.
63. Chapel TA. The signs and symptoms of secondary syphilis. Sex Transm Dis. 1980;7:161.
64. Oriel JD, Partridge BM, Denny MJ, et al. Genital yeast infections. Br Med J. 1972;4:761.
65. Diddle AW. Oral contraceptive medication and vulvovaginal candidiasis. Obstet Gynecol. 1969;34:373.
66. Holmes KK, Counts GW, Beaty HN. Disseminated gonococcal infection. Ann Intern Med. 1971;74:979.
67. Masi AT, Eisenstein BI. Disseminated gonococcal infection (DGI) and gonococcal arthritis (GCA): II. Clinical manifestations, diagnosis, complications, treatment, and prevention. Semin Arthritis Rheum. 1981;10:173.
68. Chapel TA, Brown WJ, Jeffries C, et al. How reliable is the morphologic diagnosis of penile ulcerations? Sex Transm Dis. 1977;4:150.
69. Chapel TA. Physician recognition of the signs and symptoms of secondary syphilis. JAMA. 1981;246:250.
70. Dangor Y, Ballard RC, Exposto FDL, et al. Accuracy of clinical diagnosis of genital ulcer disease. Sex Transm Dis. 1990;17:184–9.
70a. O'Farrell N, Hoosen AA, Coetzee KD, et al. Genital ulcer disease: Accuracy of clinical diagnosis and strategies to improve control in Durban, South Africa. Genitourin Med. 1994;70:7–11.
71. Verdich J. *Haemophilus ducreyi* infection resembling granuloma inguinale. Acta Dermatol Venereol. 1984;64:452–5.
72. Guinan ME, Wolinsky SM, Reichman RC. Epidemiology of genital herpes simplex virus infection. Epidemiol Rev. 1985;7:127–46.
73. Koutsky LA, Stevens CE, Holmes KK, et al. Underdiagnosis of genital herpes by current clinical and viral-isolation procedures. N Engl J Med. 1992;326:1533–9.
74. Koutsky LA, Ashley RL, Holmes KK, et al. The frequency of unrecognized type 2 herpes simplex virus infection among women. Implications for the control of genital herpes. Sex Transm Dis. 1990;17:90–4.
75. Langenberg A, Benedetti J, Jenkins J, et al. Development of clinically recognizable genital lesions among women previously identified as having "asymptomatic" herpes simplex virus type 2 infection. Ann Intern Med. 1989;110:882–7.
76. Horn JE, McQuillan GM, Shah KV, et al. Genital human papillomavirus infection in patients attending an inner-city STD clinic. Sex Transm Dis. 1991;18:183–7.
77. Kiviat NB, Koutsky LA, Paavonen JA, et al. Prevalence of genital papillomavirus infection among women attending a college student health clinic or a sexually transmitted disease clinic. J Infect Dis. 1989;159:293–302.
78. Laurikka J, Ala-Opas M, Kivinen S. Genital human papillomavirus infections in the male partners of 45 female patients with papillomavirus infection. Ann Chir Gynaecol. 1990;79:54–7.
79. Wikstrom A, Hedblad M-A, Johansson B, et al. The acetic acid test in evaluation of subclinical genital papillomavirus infection: A comparative study on penoscopy, histopathology, virology and scanning electron microscopy findings. Genitourin Med. 1992;68:90–9.
80. Hippeläinen MI, Syrjänen, Hippeläinen MJ, et al. Diagnosis of genital human papillomavirus (HPV) lesions in the male: correlation of penoscopy, histology, and in situ hybridisation. Genitourin Med. 1993;69:346–51.
81. Bhawan J, Milstone MD, Malhotra R, et al. Scabies presenting as bullous pemphigoid-like eruption. J Am Acad Dermatol. 1991;24:179–81.
82. Vekataramaiah NR, van Raate JA, Dutta SN. Tuberculous ulcer of the penis. Postgrad Med J. 1982;58:59.
83. Nishigori C, Taniguchi S, Hayakawa M, et al. Penis tuberculosis: Papulonecrotic tuberculosis on the glans penis. Dermatologica. 1986;172:93–7.
84. Kumar B, Skarma VK. Papulonecrotic tuberculids on glans penis. Dermatologica. 1987;174:151–3.
85. Carroll PR, Cattokica EV, Turzan CW, et al. Necrotizing soft-tissue infections of the perineum and genitalia. Etiology and early reconstruction. West J Med. 1986;144:174–8.
86. Cameron DW, Simonsen JN, D'Costa LJ, et al. Female to male transmission of human immunodeficiency virus type 1: Risk factors for seroconversion in men. Lancet. 1989;2:403–7.
87. Hutchinson CVM, Hook EW 3d. Syphilis in adults. Med Clin North Am. 1990;74:1389–416.
88. D'Costa LJ, Bowmer I, Nsanze H, et al. Advances in the diagnosis and management of chancroid. Sex Transm Dis. 1986;13:189–91.
89. Shmmizu T, Ehrlich GE, Inaba G, et al. Behçet disease (Behçet syndrome). Semin Arthritis Rheum. 1979;8:223.
90. Weissberg SM, Dodson MG. Recurrent vaginal and cervical ulcers associated with tampon use. JAMA. 1983;250:1430.
91. Kraus SJ. Evaluation and management of acute genital ulcers in sexually active patients. Urol Clin North Am. 1984;11:155–62.
92. Shelley WB, Wood MG. Larval papule as a sign of scabies. JAMA. 1976;236:1144.
93. Schachter J, Dawson CR. Human Chlamydial Infection. Littleton, MA: PSG Publishing; 1978:45.
94. Schwartz JJ, Myskowski PI. Molluscum contagiosum in patients with human immunodeficiency virus infection. A review of twenty-seven patients. J Am Acad Dermatol. 1992;27:583–8.
95. Ghigliotti G, Carrega G, Farris A, et al. Cutaneous cryptococcosis resembling molluscum contagiosum in a homosexual man with AIDS. Report of a case and review of the literature. Acta Dermato-Venereol. 1992;72:182–4.
96. Oriel JD. Genital warts. Sex Transm Dis. 1977;4:153.
97. Quinn TC, Stamm WE, Goodell SE, et al. The polymicrobial origin of intestinal infections in homosexual men. N Engl J Med. 1983;309:576.
98. Koutsky LA, Holmes KK, Critchlow CW, et al. A cohort study of the risk of cervical intraepithelial neoplasia grade 2 or 3 in relation to papillomavirus infection. N Engl J Med. 1992;327:1272–8.
99. Rosenberg SK. Subclinical papilloma viral infection of male genitalia. Urology. 1985;26:554–7.
100. Sand PK, Baven LW, Blischke PA, et al. Evaluation of male consorts of women with genital human papilloma virus infections. Obstet Gynecol. 1986;68:679–81.
101. Schultz RE, Skelton HG. Value of acetic acid screening for flat genital condylomata in men. J Urol. 1988;139:777–975.
102. Krebs H-B, Schneider V. Human papillomavirus–associated lesions of the penis: Colposcopy, cytology, and histology. Obstet Gynecol. 1987;70:299–304.
103. Sedlack TV, Cunnane M, Carpiniello V. Colposcopy in the diagnosis of penile condyloma. Am J Obstet Gynecol. 1986;154:494–6.

104. Abdullah AN, Drake SM, Wade AA, Walzman M. Balanitis (balanoposthitis) in patients attending a department of genitourinary medicine. Internat J STD AIDS. 1992;3:128–9.

105. Woodley D, Saurat JH. The burrow ink test and the scabies mite. J Am Acad Dermatol. 1981;4:715.

106. Kyriazi NC, Costenbader CL. Group A beta-hemolytic streptococcal balanitis: It may be more common than you think. Pediatrics. 1991;88:154–6.

107. Lucks DA, Venezio FR, Lakin CM. Balanitis caused by group B streptococcus. J Urol. 1986;135:1015.

108. Burdge DR, Bowie WR, Chow A. Gardnerella vaginalis–associated balanoposthitis. Sex Transm Dis. 1986;13:159–62.

109. Krieger JN. Epidemiology and clinical manifestations of urogenital trichomoniasis in men. In: Honigberg BM, ed. Trichomonads Parasitic in Humans. New York: Springer-Verlag; 1990:235–45.

110. Arumainayagam JT, Sumathipala AH, Smallman LA, et al. Flat condylomata of the penis presenting as patchy balanoposthitis. Genitourin Med. 1990;66:251–3.

111. Birley HDL, Walker MM, Luzzi GA, et al. Clinical features and management of recurrent balanitis. Association with atopy and genital washing. Genitourin Med. 1993;69:400–3.

112. Ackerman A. Crabs: The resurgence of Phthirus pubis. N Engl J Med. 1968;278:950.

113. Miller RA. Maculae ceruleae. Int J Dermatol. 1986;25:383–4.

114. Whitaker SB, Wiegand SE, Budnick SD. Intraoral molluscum contagiosum. Oral Surg Oral Med Oral Pathol. 1991;72:334–6.

115. Chang TW. Herpetic angina following orogenital exposure. J Am Vener Dis. 1975;1:163.

116. Jamsky RJ, Christen AG. Oral gonococcal infections. Oral Surg. 1982;53:358.

117. Ficarra G, Zaragoza AM, Stendardi L, et al. Early oral presentation of lues maligna in a patient with HIV infection. Oral Surg Oral Med Oral Pathol. 1993;75:728–32.

118. Goodell SE, Quinn TC, Mkrtichian PA-C, et al. Herpes simplex virus proctitis in homosexual men. Clinical, sigmoidoscopic and histopathological features. N Engl J Med. 1983;308:868.

119. Rompalo AM, Hook EW 3rd, Roberts PL, et al. The acute arthritis dermatitis syndrome. The changing importance of Neisseria gonorrhoeae and Neisseria meningitidis. Arch Intern Med. 1987;147:281–3.

120. Burkhart CG. Scabies: An epidemiologic reassessment. Ann Intern Med. 1983;98:498.

121. Weisman K, Secher L, Hjorth N. Recurrent genital herpes on the buttocks: "Herpes disciformis." Cutis. 1987;40:166–8.

122. Wickett WH, Miller RD. Sites of multiple lesions in recurrent genital herpes. Am Fam Physician. 1985;32:145–52.

123. Mead PB, Amstey MS, Gail SA, et al. Report on asymptomatic genital excretion of herpes simplex virus (HSV) in 21.9% of 41 women with clinical buttock herpes. J Reprod Med. 1991;36:831–4.

124. Nsanze H, Fast MV, D'Costa LJ, et al. Genital ulcers in Kenya: Clinical and laboratory study. Br J Vener Dis. 1981;57:378.

125. Karim QN, Finn GY, Easmon CS, et al. Rapid detection of Haemophilus ducreyi in clinical and experimental infections using monoclonal antibody: A preliminary evaluation. Genitourin Med. 1989;65:361–5.

126. Brown ST, Jaffe HW, Zaidi A, et al. Sensitivity and specificity of diagnostic tests for genital infection with Herpesvirus hominis. Sex Transm Dis. 1979;6:10.

127. Goldstein LC, Corey L, McDougall JK, et al. Monoclonal antibodies to herpes simplex virus: Use in antigenic typing and rapid diagnosis. J Infect Dis. 1983;47:829.

128. Lafferty WF, Kron S, Remington M, et al. Diagnosis of herpes simplex virus by direct immunofluorescence and viral isolation from samples of external genital lesions in a high prevalence population. J Clin Microbiol. 1987;25:323–6.

129. Austin VH, Topham EB. Mineral oil versus KOH for Sarcoptes. J Am Acad Dermatol. 1982;7:555.

130. Tronca E, Handsfield HH, Wiesner PJ, et al. Demonstration of Neisseria gonorrhoeae with fluorescent antibody in patients with disseminated gonococcal infection. J Infect Dis. 1974;129:583.

131. Cone RW, Swenson PD, Hobson AC, et al. Herpes simplex virus detection from genital lesions: A comparative study using antigen detection (Herp-Chek) and culture. J Clin Microbiol. 1993;31:1774–6.

132. Kudesia G, Van Hegam A, Wake S, et al. Comparison of cell culture with an amplified enzyme immunoassay for diagnosing genital herpes simplex infection. J Clin Pathol. 1991;44:778–80.

133. Redfield DC, Richman DD, Albanil S, et al. Detection of herpes simplex virus in clinical specimens by DNA hybridization. Diagn Microbiol Infect Dis. 1983;1:117.

134. Corey L. Laboratory diagnosis of herpes simplex virus infections. Principles guiding the development of rapid diagnostic tests. Diagn Microbiol Infect Dis. 1986;4(Suppl):III-9.

135. Seal LA, Toyama PS, Fleet KM, et al. Comparison of standard culture methods, a shell vial assay, and a DNA probe for the detection of herpes simplex virus. J Clin Microbiol. 1991;29:650–2.

136. Rogers BB, Josephson SL, Mak SK, et al. Polymerase chain reaction amplifi-

cation of herpes simplex virus DNA from clinical samples. Obstet Gynecol. 1992;79:464–9.

137. Gjoen K, Siebke JC, Flikke M, et al. Genital human papillomavirus infection in Oslo studied by dot blot DNA hybridization and the polymerase chain reaction. J Med Virol. 1991;34:159–64.

137a. Felix JC, Wright TC. Analysis of lower genital tract lesions clinically suspicious for condylomata using in situ hybridization and the polymerase chain reaction for the detection of human papillomavirus. Arch Pathol Lab Med. 1994;118:39–43.

138. Tabrizi SN, Tan J, Quinn M, et al. Detection of human papillomaviruses (HPV) DNA by PCR and other conventional hybridization techniques in male partners of women with abnormal Papanicolaou smears. Genitourin Med. 1992;68:370–3.

139. Chui L, Albritton W, Paster B, et al. Development of the polymerase chain reaction for the diagnosis of chancroid. J Clin Microbiol. 1993;31:659–64.

140. Deacon WE, Lucas JB, Price EV. Fluorescent treponemal antibody absorption (FTA-ABS) test for syphilis. JAMA. 1966;198:624.

141. Duncan W, Knox J, Wende R. The FTA-ABS test in darkfield positive primary syphilis. JAMA. 1974;228:859.

142. Larsen SA, Hambie EA, Pettit DE, et al. Specificity, sensitivity, and reproducibility among the fluorescent treponemal antibody absorption test, the hemagglutination assay for Treponemal pallidum antibodies, and the hemagglutination treponemal test for syphilis. J Clin Microbiol. 1981;14:441.

143. Ashley RL. Laboratory techniques in the diagnosis of herpes simplex infection. Genitourin Med. 1993;69:174–83.

144. Ashley R, Cent A, Maggs V, et al. Inability of enzyme immunoassays to discriminate between infections with herpes simplex virus types 1 and 2. Ann Intern Med. 1991;115:520–6.

145. Field PR, Ho DWT, Irving WL, et al. The reliability of serological tests for the diagnosis of genital herpes: A critique. Pathology. 1993;25:175–9.

146. Field PR, Ho DW, Cunningham AL. The diagnosis of recent herpes simplex virus type 2 genital infections by the simplex-2 test. Pathology. 1992;24:302–6.

147. Ho DW, Field PR, Sjogren-Jansson E, et al. Indirect ELISA for the detection of HSV-2 specific IgG and IgM antibodies with glycoprotein G (gG-2). J Virol Methods. 1992;36:249–64.

148. Freinkel AL, Dangor Y, Koornhof HJ, et al. A serologic test for granuloma inguinale. Genitourin Med. 1992;68:269–72.

149. Alfa MJ, Olson N, Degangke P, et al. Use of an adsorbtion enzyme immunoassay to evaluate the Hemophilus ducreyi: Specific and cross-reactive humoral immune response of humans. Sex Transm Dis. 1992;19:309–14.

150. Moseley RC, Corey L, Benjamin D, et al. Comparison of viral isolation, direct immunofluorescence, and indirect immunoperoxidase techniques for detection of genital herpes simplex virus infection. J Clin Microbiol. 1981;13:913–8.

151. Nsanze H, Plummer FA, Maggwa AB, et al. Comparison of media for the primary isolation of Haemophilus ducreyi. Sex Transm Dis. 1984;11:6–9.

152. Jones CC, Rosen T. Cultural diagnosis of chancroid. Arch Dermatol. 1991;127:1823–7.

153. Dangor Y, Miller SD, Koornhof HJ, et al. A simple medium for the primary isolation of Haemophilus ducreyi. Eur J Clin Microbiol Infect Dis. 1992;11:930–4.

154. Macdonald K, Cameron DW, Irungu G, et al. Comparison of Sheffield media with the standard media for the isolation of Haemophilus ducreyi. Sex Transm Dis. 1989;16:88–90.

88. URETHRITIS

WILLIAM M. McCORMACK
MICHAEL F. REIN

Urethritis affects an estimated 4 million American men each year.[1] The symptoms range from the trivial and often overlooked to the disabling. Urethral discharge is more frequently recognized by men than by women. It may be apparent at all times during the day and may be present in sufficient quantity to stain undergarments, or it may be so scanty that it is noted only on arising as a small bead of moisture or crust at the meatus. It may be completely clear, mucopurulent, or frankly purulent, and it may be white, yellow, green, or brown. Some patients complain only of a deviation of the first morning urine stream. Occasionally, urethral discharge comes to the attention of the patient through the observation of mucous strands in the urine specimen.

The urine stream transiently eliminates most inflammatory discharges; thus, scanty discharges are best observed on arising before the passage of any urine. Micturition immediately preceding urethral examination may completely eliminate signs of infection.

The discomfort of urethritis can take several forms. Dysuria is common, and men variously localize it to the meatus, the distal portion of the penis, or anywhere along the shaft. Discomfort is sometimes increased by the acidity or solute content of the urine and therefore may be most marked during the passage of a concentrated first morning urine. Dysuria may be increased in the presence of irritants such as alcohol, which is an observation that sometimes leads the patient to attribute his disease to the ingestion of specific foods or fluids. Discomfort may persist between micturitions and is perceived as pain, itching, frequency, urgency, or a feeling of heaviness in the genitals. Women may complain of dysuria, but urethral pain between micturitions is uncommon.

Discomfort only during ejaculation, deep pelvic pain, or pain radiating to the back is infrequent in uncomplicated urethritis and suggests prostatitis or inflammation involving other portions of the urogenital tract such as the epididymis. Hematuria, particularly if painless, or blood in the ejaculate are uncommon in urethritis.[2] The persistence of hematuria after cure of urethritis demands a thorough urologic evaluation.[2]

EXAMINATION OF THE URETHRA

Men should stand before the seated examiner so that the external genitalia are approximately eye level. Alternatively, the genitalia can be examined while the patient is supine. A good light source is essential. The patient should lower his pants and underwear so the entire genital area may be observed. The underwear may reveal stains of dried discharge, which suggest that it is being produced in large amounts. This observation is particularly useful if the patient has recently urinated.

The patient is preferably examined at least 2 hours after his last micturition. If advised to restrict his fluids during the day preceding the examination, he may be able to present for evaluation before passing his first urine of the day, which sometimes permits the recovery of very small amounts of discharge.[3]

The entire genital area should be carefully examined since other sexually transmitted infections are relatively common in patients with urethritis. Inguinal adenopathy should be sought, and tenderness should be noted. The skin of the entire pubic area, scrotum, groin, and penis should be examined for lesions, and the hair should be examined for nits. The testes and the spermatic cords should be palpated for masses or tenderness. The foreskin should be completely retracted and the glans examined. The urethral meatus should be examined for dried crusts, redness, and spontaneous discharge. If no discharge is present, the urethra should be gently stripped by placing the gloved thumb along the ventral surface of the base of the penis and the forefinger on the dorsum and then applying gentle pressure. The examiner's hand is moved slowly toward the meatus. This will frequently expel a discharge that may be collected on a swab for examination as described below.

If no discharge is delivered by this maneuver, the third and fourth fingers should be used to grip the penis lightly from above, just behind the glans. The thumb and forefinger can then spread open the meatus to examine for urethral redness or the presence of small amounts of discharge. Unless the patient has recently urinated or has been in a state of sexual arousal, virtually no fluid should be expressible from the urethra or observed by spreading the meatus.

If expressed material cannot be collected at the meatus, a specimen must be recovered from inside the urethra. This is best accomplished with a calcium alginate urethral or nasopha-

ryngeal swab.[4] The swab should be inserted gently at least 2 cm into the urethra while taking care not to attempt to force the tip past an obstruction. The patient should be warned that the examination is uncomfortable; also, the insertion and removal of the swab should be accomplished as quickly as possible. Patients may tolerate the examination better if they are supine. If additional specimens are required for multiple examinations or cultures, separate swabs should be used while taking care to insert each at least 1 cm deeper than that preceding it.

Regular cotton swabs should not be used for urethral examination, because their larger diameter makes insertion extremely uncomfortable and because of the possibility that the cotton or the wooden shaft may be toxic to some fastidious pathogens. A small platinum loop is effective, but it must be sterilized in a flame and carefully cooled between uses.

A woman's urethra is best examined when she is in the lithotomy position. The entire genital area should be examined for lesions, and the vagina should be examined as described in Chapter 89. The urethral meatus may be directly visualized, and the urethra may be stripped by placing the gloved finger inside the vagina and gently moving it along the urethra. A calcium alginate swab may be inserted a short distance within the meatus to obtain a urethral specimen.

EXAMINATION OF THE URETHRAL SPECIMEN

A swab that contains material from the urethra should be rolled across a clean microscope slide. Rolling rather than streaking the swab brings all its surfaces into contact with the slide and better preserves cellular morphologic characteristics. The material may be air dried and fixed by gentle heating or by rinsing with methanol. Gram staining of urethral material is particularly useful in the work-up of urethritis, and the specimen should be examined by using the oil-immersion objective. Specimens obtained from within the urethra generally reveal urethral epithelial cells. When recovered from near the meatus, these are typical squamous cells with a very large cytoplasmic/nuclear ratio, or when obtained from further within the urethra they are cuboidal epithelial cells, which are smaller and have relatively larger, less dense nuclei.

Urethral material from patients with acute urethritis will contain polymorphonuclear neutrophils (PMN). The area of the smear that contains most PMN should be sought. More than four PMN per oil-immersion microscopic field is always abnormal and is seen in 60–90 percent of all patients with acute symptomatic urethritis.[4-6] However, 16–50 percent of all men with documented urethral infection will not show four PMN in maximally dense oil-immersion fields.[7-12] The number of PMN in the smear is reduced by recent micturition[13]; also, there often is considerable observer variation in the number of PMN detected in a single specimen.[14] Thus, although purulent discharges may reveal sheets of PMN, the minimal number of these cells that indicates disease is not known. In general, the presence of even rare PMN suggests infection, particularly in the patient who has urethral symptoms or who is found to have a small amount of discharge on examination.

The distal centimeter of the urethra is colonized by normal skin or introital flora. One usually will observe a variety of gram-positive and gram-negative organisms that have no particular significance. Of great diagnostic value, however, is the presence of typical gram-negative, "intracellular" diplococci (Fig. 1). These organisms are not randomly distributed among the cells but are seen in large numbers in a few PMN. They will be observed in more than 95 percent of all symptomatic patients with gonococcal urethritis and in fewer than 2 percent of all symptomatic men who cannot be shown to have gonorrhea by culture.[15-17] Some strains of *Neisseria gonorrhoeae* are inhibited by the concentrations of vancomycin that usually are employed in selective isolation media; these organisms will not be recovered by standard culture techniques.[18] Extracellular diplo-

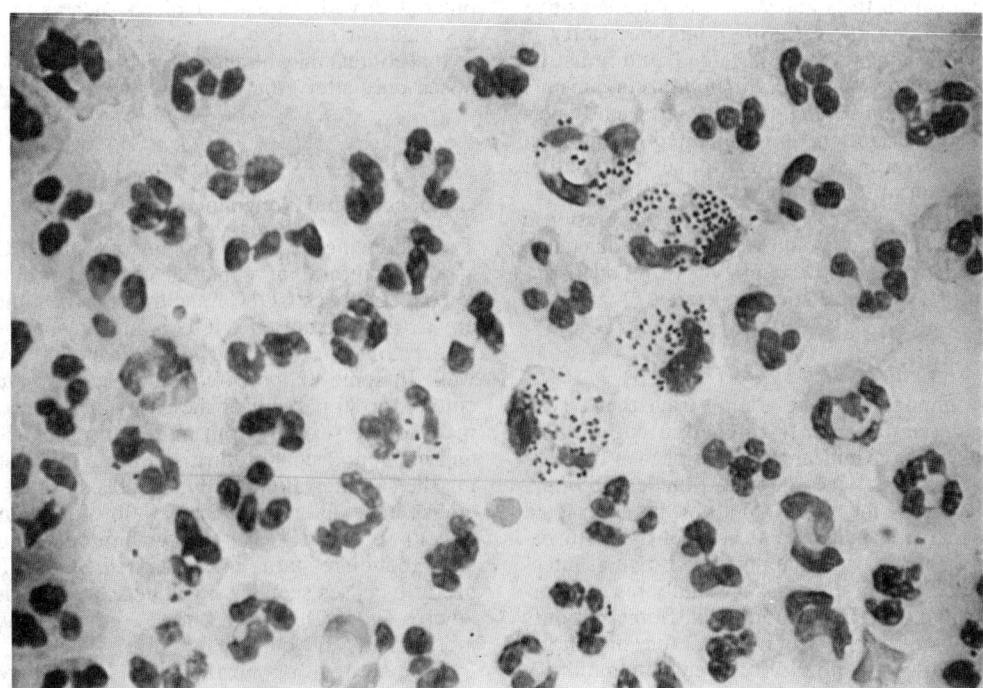

FIG. 1. Gram stain of urethral exudate from a man with gonorrhea. Several neutrophils contain many gram-negative cell-associated diplococci.

cocci indicate gonorrhea in only 10–29 percent of all cases, and this predictive value is even further reduced in populations with a low prevalence of gonorrhea.[17] A shortcoming of the gram-stained smear is that it cannot diagnose coincidental nongonococcal urethritis (NGU) in the presence of gonorrhea. Although a smear containing PMN that does not reveal gram-negative intracellular diplococci strongly suggests NGU, a smear revealing these organisms does not rule out NGU.

In men with adequate amounts of urethral discharge, one can test for the presence of gonococcal oxidase. Experience with the technique is limited; however, preliminary data suggest a sensitivity of 96 percent but a specificity of only 85 percent.[19] *Limulus* lysate assays for gonococcal endotoxin, although greater than 95 percent sensitive and specific,[20] are of limited clinical utility because many patients have inadequate amounts of discharge.[21]

Candida may be recognized as gram-positive or beaded, oval bodies about 3 × 6 μm. Observing small numbers of yeast cells does not prove a candidial etiology for the urethritis, since *Candida* may be recovered from normal patients, particularly if they are uncircumcised.

Trichomonads are very difficult to identify on gram-stained smears. Urethral material may be mixed with a small amount of saline and observed as a wet mount with the substage condenser racked down or the substage diaphragm partially closed. Motile trichomonads occasionally are observed but are rarely seen unless the examination is carried out before the first voiding. A positive wet mount diagnoses trichomoniasis, but the wet mount is often negative in infected men. Endourethral cultures or cultures of first-void urine sediment in media such as modified Diamond's medium is the preferred method for diagnosis of trichomoniasis in men.[22,23]

After the patient's urethra has been carefully examined, he may be asked to provide a divided urine specimen. The patient delivers the first 10 ml of urine into one container and the remainder of the urine specimen into a second. Mucous strands in the first fraction that clear in the second portion suggest urethritis. Equal aliquots of the fractions may be centrifuged and the sediments examined as wet mounts. Observing more white

blood cells in the initial than in the second fraction suggests urethritis, while observing equal numbers of white cells in both fractions suggests cystitis or infection higher in the urinary tract.[3] A total of more than 15 white blood cells in five ×400 microscopic fields of the sediment from the initial fraction strongly suggests urethritis,[4,7,10] but the minimum significant number of white blood cells is unknown. More than 10 PMN per high-power field have been observed in 90 percent of all men with chlamydial urethritis.[7]

White blood cells in the initial urine fraction provide no clue to the etiology of the urethritis. Such a finding, however, may allow an objective diagnosis of urethritis to be made in a man whose gram-stained smear does not contain PMN.

Many men who are infected with *N. gonorrhoeae* or *Chlamydia trachomatis* have no symptoms. Such men often have pyuria that can be detected by examination of the first 10 ml urine sample either by microscopy or a leukocyte-esterase "dip stick." This approach provides a noninvasive, inexpensive method for screening men for urethral infection. Screened men who have pyuria are candidates for further examination, including examination of endourethral specimens for gonococci and chlamydia.[24]

If the urine specimen is a first morning micturition, motile trichomonads may be observed in the sediment. In one study, *Trichomonas vaginalis* organisms were recovered by culture of urethral swabs in 80 percent and first-void urine in 68 percent of infected patients. When combined, these two cultures detected 49 (98 percent) of 50 infected men.[22] Trichomonads are recovered less frequently from patients who have already voided during the day.

Material recovered from the urethra can be cultured with appropriate media for *N. gonorrhoeae*. Culture systems for *C. trachomatis* are becoming more generally available and less costly. Nonculture tests such as enzyme-linked immunosorbent assay (ELISA) and gene-amplification techniques such as polymerase chain reaction for identifying *C. trachomatis* in genital specimens have been developed (see Ch. 157) and are changing our approach to these infections. Although ELISA, DNA probes, and immunofluorescence tests are less sensitive than cultures, gene-amplification tests appear to be more sensitive than chlamydial cultures while retaining high specificity.[25] Gene-amplification techniques may replace cell culture as the "gold standard" for identification of *C. trachomatis* organisms.

Cultures for *Ureaplasma urealyticum* are less frequently performed; also, their interpretation is complicated by the high prevalence of colonization in asymptomatic, sexually active people. Although present in the distal urethra, normal skin organisms (such as *Staphylococcus epidermidis,* α-hemolytic streptococci, and propionibacteria) and vaginal organisms (such as *Candida albicans,* lactobacilli, *Escherichia coli,* and *Gardnerella vaginalis*) are of no diagnostic significance.[26,27]

NONINFECTIOUS URETHRITIS

So psychologically important is the genital tract that trivial symptoms often receive patients' frightened attention. The "worried well" make up a significant fraction of men who are seen in venereal disease clinics and in private practices. Sympathetic questioning as to why the patient thinks he has contracted a genital infection may reveal guilt over an act such as masturbation, which does not put the patient at significant risk of infection. The urethral specimen in these cases usually reveals normal epithelial cells and no white blood cells. Some patients confuse dried remnants of semen with inflammatory discharge. Microscopic examination again fails to reveal inflammatory cells, but spermatozoa may be recognized on the Gram stain as gram-positive ovoids whose coloration fades gradually toward the acrosomal cap or may be recognized on the wet mount. However, the physician must remember that symptoms and signs of true urethritis can be trivial and that microscopic examination may miss minimal inflammation, particularly if the patient has recently voided. Symptomatic patients with negative examinations should have urethral specimens examined for gonococci and chlamydiae and be asked to return in several days, by which time the symptoms may have resolved or examination may provide a diagnosis. Antimicrobial treatment of symptomatic men who have neither objective evidence of urethritis nor positive cultures for urethral pathogens is inadvisable and may serve to reinforce psychosomatic contributions to their symptoms.[28] An occasional patient who complains of a discharge is really suffering from urinary incontinence.

Chronic irritation of the urethra can elicit a clear, mucoid discharge. Occasional patients, concerned that they may have contracted a venereal disease, vigorously strip the urethra looking for a discharge. After several days of this, a clear discharge obligingly appears that may contain a few white blood cells. A history of vigorous urethral stripping is helpful diagnostically. Patients treated for other forms of urethritis should be cautioned not to examine themselves too vigorously for fear that such a traumatic discharge may confuse the clinical picture. Very rarely, patients will insert foreign bodies into the urethra and produce a mechanical urethritis.[29] This sort of self-abuse should be considered in retarded or psychotic individuals.

A heavy precipitation of crystals in the urine can suggest a discharge, and the presence of large amounts of crystalline material or calculous gravel may produce urinary discomfort. The intermittent nature of pain associated with the passage of gravel or the obvious presence of crystals on microscopic examination of the urine sediment usually confirms this diagnosis. White blood cells may be present.

Urethritis may accompany noninfectious systemic diseases such as Stevens-Johnson syndrome or Wegener's granulomatosis.

Chemicals may irritate the urethra, and alcohol has long been known to produce mild dysuria. The ingestion of alcohol during the treatment for gonorrhea was at one time thought to be responsible for the syndrome of postgonococcal urethritis, discussed later, although it is now known to have an infectious etiology. An occasional patient may develop urethral symptoms on contact with vaginal chemicals such as spermicides used by a sexual partner. The history of discomfort immediately after sexual contact may be suggestive. This condition should be diagnosed only after other etiologies have been excluded.

INFECTIOUS URETHRITIS

Gonococcal and Nongonococcal Urethritis

The major single specific etiology of acute urethritis is *N. gonorrhoeae*. Urethral inflammation of all other etiologies is referred to collectively as NGU. As with gonorrhea, most cases of NGU are sexually acquired. NGU is more common than gonorrhea in the United States and in much of the developed world as well. In some underdeveloped areas, however, gonorrhea accounts for 80 percent of the cases of acute urethritis. As with many other sexually transmitted diseases (STD), gonococcal and nongonococcal urethritis have an increased incidence during the summer months, presumably because of a seasonal increase in sexual activity. The ratio of nongonococcal to gonococcal urethritis is greater among groups of higher socioeconomic status in the United States. Thus, most of the urethritis cases seen among college students is nongonococcal, whereas gonorrhea is the most common cause of urethritis in most urban STD clinics.[30–33]

Compared with gonorrhea, NGU is relatively less prevalent among homosexual than among heterosexual men with urethritis. Examining consecutive men attending an STD clinic, Stamm and colleagues[9] recovered gonococci from 12 percent of heterosexual and 25 percent of homosexual men, whereas they recovered chlamydiae from 14 percent of heterosexual but only 5 percent of homosexual men.

Historically, there has been considerable interest in the possible contribution of circumcision to the epidemiology of STD. Such studies are difficult to interpret, because certain behavioral factors are associated with circumcision.[34] The presence of a foreskin may mask a urethral discharge and delay patients from presenting for evaluation, but other roles remain speculative.[34]

The clinical spectrum of gonorrhea differs from that of NGU, but there is sufficient overlap so that an accurate differential diagnosis must be based on examination of the urethral specimen. Seventy-five percent of men acquiring urethral gonorrhea develop symptoms within 4 days[3] and 80–90 percent within 2 weeks.[30,35,36] The incubation period for NGU is much more variable and is often longer, usually between 7 and 14 days, but incubation periods ranging from 2 to 35 days have been described,[30,33,35] and almost 50 percent of the men with NGU developed urethral symptoms within 4 days.[3,30,35] Thus, an incubation period of less than 1 week is not a reliable factor in the differential diagnosis.[3,30,35,37] The incubation period of either infection can be prolonged by the ingestion of subcurative doses of antibiotics.[38]

The urethral discharge is described as frankly purulent in three-fourths of the patients with gonorrhea but in only 11–33 percent of the patients with NGU.[15,33,39] A purulent discharge issuing from the meatus without stripping the urethra correlates strongly with the diagnosis of gonorrhea but is also seen in 4 percent of patients with NGU.[15,39] Mucopurulent discharge, consisting of thin cloudy fluid or mucoid fluid with purulent flecks, is seen in about 50 percent of the patients with NGU but in only 25 percent of the patients with symptomatic gonorrhea.[15,39] The discharge is completely clear and moderately viscid in 10–50 percent of the patients with NGU, principally those who are minimally symptomatic, but in only 4 percent of symptomatic patients with gonorrhea.[15,39,40] A differential diagnosis on the basis of the clinical characteristics of the urethral discharge is unreliable and yields a correct diagnosis in only 73 percent of all cases, even under optimal circumstances.[39] Microscopic examination always should be part of the initial evaluation.

Dysuria has been described in 53–75 percent of the patients with NGU and in 73–88 percent of the patients with symptomatic gonorrhea.[15,41] Only about 10 percent of the patients complaining of dysuria without discharge have gonorrhea; the remainder suffer from NGU.[15] A combination of dysuria and discharge is seen in 71 percent of the patients with gonococcal urethritis but in only 38 percent of the patients with NGU. Thus, the combination of discharge and dysuria is associated with gonorrhea, while the appearance of one without the other is more frequently seen with NGU. The association is insufficiently specific for differential diagnosis. Urethral discomfort may mimic cystitis in men and women and result in urinary frequency and urgency.

Symptoms of gonorrhea often begin abruptly, and the patient may remember the specific time of day when they were first noted. Nongonococcal urethritis usually has a less acute onset, with symptoms increasing over several days. A urethral discharge may appear days in advance of dysuria; the symptoms may wax and wane, even to the point of transiently disappearing before the patient seeks therapy. The mildness and variability of the symptoms may erroneously convince the patient with NGU that he does not have a significant disease; such patients often delay seeking medical attention.[15,41]

The symptoms of infectious urethritis will, in most cases, resolve even if the patient remains untreated. Ninety-five percent of untreated patients with acute gonococcal urethritis will be free of symptoms 6 months after contracting the disease,[36] and the symptoms of NGU gradually subside over a period of 1–3 months in 30–70 percent of the patients.[42] How many of these asymptomatic patients remain infected and potentially infectious is unknown. Untreated gonococcal urethritis may subside to a chronic state characterized by little or no urethral discomfort and a small amount of mucoid discharge called *gleet*. This discharge contains small numbers of gonococci and PMN.

So great are the clinical overlaps between nongonococcal and gonococcal urethritis that a differential diagnosis should not be made on clinical grounds alone. A Gram stain of urethral discharge material will reveal typical, gram-negative, "intracellular" diplococci in about 95 percent of the cases of gonococcal urethritis and will be negative in about 97 percent of the patients with NGU.[15–17] Thus, in a population in which about 50 percent of the acute urethritis is gonococcal, a positive Gram stain suggests gonorrhea, and a negative Gram stain suggests NGU with 98 percent accuracy.[15,17] The observation of typically shaped extracellular diplococci diagnoses gonorrhea with an accuracy of 10–30 percent.[17] This is known as an *equivocal* Gram stain and is found in about 15 percent of patients with symptomatic urethritis.[15] Other techniques for diagnosing gonococcal urethritis are described above.[19–21]

The sensitivity of the culture for *N. gonorrhoeae* is less than 100 percent, partly because some gonococci are inhibited by the vancomycin concentrations used in selective media. The chances of isolating the organism are further reduced if the patient has recently taken antibiotics or if there is a delay in processing the culture. Thus, it seems likely that most of the few patients with positive Gram stains and negative cultures actually have gonorrhea. In most cases of acute symptomatic urethritis it is unnecessary to confirm culturally a Gram stain diagnostic of gonorrhea. It must be remembered that the Gram stain will be negative in as many as 5 percent of such patients who have gonorrhea, so a Gram stain suggestive of NGU should be confirmed with a culture for gonococci, although therapy need not be delayed until the results are known. The Gram stain cannot be used to make a diagnosis of simultaneous NGU in the presence of gonorrhea. Because of the frequency with which trichomonads may be missed with direct microscopic techniques, patients in whom trichomonal urethritis is suspected should be evaluated by culture of urethral and/or first-void urine specimens as well as by wet mount.[22]

There is no doubt that urethritis is sexually transmitted. It occurs most frequently during the ages of peak sexual activity and in groups with a high prevalence of other STDs. It is found with increased frequency in persons with a history of other sexually transmitted genital infections.[30,33] It frequently follows sexual exposure to a new partner and is almost never seen in virgins except as a part of some systemic conditions. As the etiologic agents of urethritis have been defined, they have been isolated with high frequency from the female and homosexual male sexual partners of infected men by whom, however, they usually are carried asymptomatically.

Recognizing urethritis as an STD is important for several practical reasons. It allows one to define a population at very high risk for carrying the agents, namely, the sexual partners of infected patients. The prevalence of infection with these agents is sufficiently high among sexual partners to justify their treatment on epidemiologic grounds, even if they are asymptomatic. Many episodes of recurrent NGU are terminated only by the treatment of an asymptomatic sexual partner of the infected patient. Since persons with one STD are at increased risk for others, it is important to screen patients with urethritis for other STDs.

Etiology of NGU

The organism most clearly associated with nongonococcal urethritis, *C. trachomatis,* is discussed in detail in Chapter 157. This obligate intracellular parasite causes 30–50 percent of the cases of NGU.[7,26,31,43,44] *Chlamydia trachomatis* is susceptible to several antimicrobial agents, including the tetracyclines, sulfonamides, and erythromycin. Significantly, it is not reliably eradicated by penicillins, cephalosporins, fluoroquinolones, or spectinomycin in the single doses used to treat uncomplicated gonorrhea.

Chlamydiae are not recovered from at least 50 percent of men with NGU. Although the clinical features of *Chlamydia*-negative NGU are very similar to those of *Chlamydia*-positive NGU,[30,45] some workers have suggested that less discharge is produced in patients who are positive for *Chlamydia* than in those who are not, and the mean incubation period may be slightly shorter.[30,45]

The agents responsible for *Chlamydia*-negative NGU remain, to some extent, unidentified. *Ureaplasma urealyticum,* formerly known as the *T-strain mycoplasma,* has been recovered from 81 percent of the men with *Chlamydia*-negative NGU, which is significantly higher than the 60 percent isolation rate from asymptomatic controls.[26,46] Furthermore, *U. urealyticum* can be recovered in larger numbers from men with *Chlamydia*-negative NGU than from control subjects.[46,48] Supporting the hypothesis that these agents (see Ch. 162) cause some cases of NGU is the observation that sulfonamides or rifampin, to which the organisms are insensitive, fail to cure most patients with *Chlamydia*-negative NGU.[49,50] Conversely, spectinomycin, which is active against ureaplasmas but inactive against *Chlamydia,* cures patients with NGU from whom only *U. urealyticum* has been isolated.[49] Additional support comes from experiments in which two investigators inoculated themselves with ureaplasmas; both developed NGU.[51] Furthermore, some patients with NGU show rises in IgM and IgG antibody titers against *U. urealyticum.*[52] Thus, the weight of evidence favors an etiologic role for *U. urealyticum* organisms in NGU. Accurate assessment of the relative contribution of ureaplasmas is hindered by the ubiquity of the organisms that can be recovered from urethral cultures from many sexually experienced men who have no evidence of urethritis.[53,54] *Mycoplasma hominis* is not a cause of NGU,[53,54] whereas *Mycoplasma genitalium* has been recovered from a few patients with NGU[55] and been shown to cause inflammation in the urethras of experimental animals.[56,57] *Mycoplasma genitalium* does not, however, appear to be an important cause of urethritis in humans.

As with *Chlamydia,* the ureaplasmas are susceptible to erythromycin and, usually, tetracyclines—the agents that have been most successful in treating NGU. Some patients, however, are infected with tetracycline-resistant *U. urealyticum*[5,58-61]; such patients may not be cured by tetracycline therapy. A significant minority of men with NGU do not carry either *C. trachomatis* or *U. urealyticum*,[49,50,62,63] and it would not be surprising if other agents were in the future identified as causes of NGU. Patients with nonchlamydial, nonureaplasmal NGU have a higher recurrence rate after therapy than do men with chlamydial urethritis.[50,62,63]

Uncommon Causes of Nongonococcal Urethritis

Dysuria is described by 83 percent of women and 44 percent of men with primary herpes simplex genital infection. Some men notice a clear, mucoid discharge that seems disproportionately mild when compared with the amount of dysuria that they experience. Herpes simplex virus (HSV) is recovered from the urethras of about 80 percent of women and 30 percent of men with primary infection, and HSV must be regarded as a cause of some cases of NGU. In most such instances, however, the diagnosis of HSV is obvious because of genital lesions. Urethral involvement is less common in recurrent disease, and dysuria is described by only 27 percent of women and 9 percent of men.[64]

Trichomonas vaginalis has been isolated from patients with NGU,[22,23,27] and it causes a small percentage of the cases. The syndrome is not clinically distinguishable from NGU of other etiologies, although the discharge often is so scant that it may be noticed only as a small bead at the meatus on arising in the morning.

Preexisting urethral stricture, particularly in the presence of other infectious agents, may (it is said) produce a urethritis-like syndrome. Urethral infection with gram-negative bacilli can be seen in men with diabetes or who practice insertive anal intercourse and may occur in patients with phimosis or with urethral trauma after instrumentation or indwelling catheterization.[65] Periurethral abscesses may occur in this setting. Somewhat fewer than 3 percent of the cases of urethritis are due to infection higher up in the urinary tract. Syphilis, with an endourethral chancre, and intraurethral condylomata acuminata occasionally cause a urethral discharge. *Neisseria meningitidis* organisms have been isolated from some patients who had urethritis.[66]

A few investigators have attributed some cases of NGU to *Clostridium difficile, Branhamella catarrhalis, Haemophilus influenzae*, corynebacteria, *Gardnerella vaginalis, Bacteroides ureolyticus*,[67] adenoviruses,[68] and schistosomes. Most of these observations, however, are uncontrolled for the presence of such important pathogens as *C. trachomatis* and *U. urealyticum*, and the role of these organisms must be considered unproven. Indeed, other studies have recovered corynebacteria, *G. vaginalis*, and anaerobes less frequently from patients with NGU than from asymptomatic controls.[26,46,69]

POSTGONOCOCCAL URETHRITIS

Some patients who receive single dose treatment for acute gonococcal urethritis experience prompt resolution followed in a few days by a recurrence of symptoms—usually a mucoid or mucopurulent discharge and sometimes mild dysuria. Other patients may note that their symptoms have never entirely disappeared and, after initial rapid improvement, stabilized at a low level. This syndrome is referred to as *postgonococcal urethritis* (PGU) and should be suspected if signs, symptoms, or laboratory evidence of urethritis is found 4–7 days after single-dose treatment for gonorrhea.[70,71] It is a manifestation of dual urethral infection. The gonococci and the agents of NGU are extremely prevalent in sexually active populations, and they are carried simultaneously and asymptomatically by many swomen. Male sexual partners of these women may acquire both agents during the same sexual exposure. In the presence of gonorrhea, coincident NGU

cannot be diagnosed by Gram stain. Single-dose treatment of gonorrhea with cephalosporins, quinolones, or spectinomycin eradicates the gonococci (eliminating the symptoms of gonorrhea), but it usually spares the agents of NGU. When the incubation period of NGU is exceeded, the patient experiences a recurrence or persistence of milder symptoms that is consistent with the latter infection.

Although PGU was originally thought to result from the consumption of alcohol or other irritants during therapy for gonorrhea, dual infection is now well established as the explanation for PGU. *Chlamydia trachomatis* has been recovered from 11–50 percent of men with gonorrhea[43]; 75–100 percent of patients with gonorrhea who are also culture positive for *Chlamydia* will develop PGU if their gonorrhea is treated with an agent that does not eradicate *Chlamydia*.[70-74] *Chlamydia trachomatis* can be recovered from almost 50 percent of the patients with PGU, which is similar to the recovery rate in NGU. Postgonococcal urethritis, however, also develops in 20–50 percent of the patients with gonorrhea from whom chlamydiae are not recovered[70,71,73]; some of these cases appear to be associated with ureaplasmal infection.[71] As one might expect, if gonorrhea is treated with a regimen active against the agents of NGU, the incidence of PGU is lower.[74-76] Accordingly, current treatment schedules for gonorrhea include a second agent such as doxycycline.

Patients suffering persistence or recurrence of urethral symptoms after therapy for acute gonococcal urethritis may indeed have PGU, but the physician also should remember the possibilities of gonococcal reinfection or frank treatment failure. The patient who is having recurrent urethritis must be evaluated as a new patient to differentiate gonococcal from nongonococcal infection.

ASYMPTOMATIC URETHRAL INFECTION

Many patients without specific complaints that are referable to the urethra will be found to have signs of urethritis on physical examination; sexually transmitted pathogens can be recovered from some patients who have neither symptoms nor signs of urethritis. Infected adolescents are less likely to complain of urethral symptoms than are adults.[77]

The importance of asymptomatic urethral gonococcal infection in men is well recognized.[78] Prolonged asymptomatic urethral carriage of gonococci occurs in about 2–3 percent of newly infected men[78]; however, since these men do not seek treatment, the prevalence of asymptomatic urethral gonococcal infections is distinctly higher than 3 percent and may have considerable epidemiologic significance. Random screening of asymptomatic populations is unrewarding[78] except in high-risk populations.[79] Most cases of asymptomatic urethral infection are detected when gonorrhea is diagnosed in female sexual partners or if complications subsequently develop in the infected man. Asymptomatic urethral infection therefore is particularly prevalent among the male sexual partners of women who develop symptomatic complications of gonorrhea or when gonorrhea is detected by screening.[78] Up to 40 percent of the asymptomatic sexual partners of women with disseminated gonococcal infection or pelvic inflammatory disease are found to be infected[78]; 60 percent of the infected men may be asymptomatic. Asymptomatic urethral infection also is prevalent among men with gonococcal dermatitis-arthritis syndrome.[78] Asymptomatic gonorrhea may be diagnosed by a Gram stain of urethral material collected on a swab with a sensitivity of about 70 percent.[78]

Part of the controversy over the etiologic role of *U. urealyticum* is its recovery from 59 percent of sexually active, asymptomatic men attending venereal disease clinics.[26,46] *Chlamydia trachomatis* is recovered from about 3 percent of such men.[26,46] Many men harboring trichomonads are asymptomatic[23] and represent an important vector of infection.

Asymptomatic urethritis in many cases can be rapidly detected by observing PMN in material recovered from the urethra with a swab or loop. About 25 percent of asymptomatic men with four or more PMN per oil-immersion microscopic field were found to carry *C. trachomatis* in their urethras.[80] Endourethral sampling, however, is uncomfortable and is poorly accepted by asymptomatic men. Examination of first-void urine for leukocyte esterase[24] or for evidence of gonococcal or chlamydial infection with nucleic acid amplification techniques[25] may provide an acceptable means of examining men for asymptomatic urethral infection.

Because of the frequency of asymptomatic, sexually transmitted urethral infections in men, asymptomatic sexual partners of infected women or homosexual men should always be evaluated. Since immediate diagnostic techniques are of relatively low sensitivity, such men should be treated at the time of their initial presentation (epidemiologic treatment).

URETHRAL SYNDROME AND RELATED DISEASES OF WOMEN

Dysuria, frequency, urgency, and nocturia are frequent symptoms of bacterial cystitis in women. A similar syndrome occurs in women who do not have classic bacterial infection of the lower urinary tract. Such women are said to have the acute urethral syndrome.[81] The usual work-up for bacterial urinary tract infection is unrewarding because fewer than 10^5 organisms are recovered from each milliliter of urine. If the urine sediment contains PMN, the symptoms frequently respond to antimicrobial therapy. Some of these patients appear to suffer from bacterial cystitis, although bacteria are recovered from the urine in smaller than traditional numbers.[81,82] Other patients' symptoms, however, appear to be related to urethritis rather than to cystitis. *Escherichia coli* sometimes apparently causes urethritis in the absence of cystitis.[83] When ordinary bacterial pathogens associated with urinary tract infections are not isolated (even in small numbers), the condition is often due to sexually transmitted agents.[81,82] If pyuria is absent, cultures for enteric bacteria and agents of STD are less likely to be positive, and antimicrobial treatment is less likely to be effective; a noninfectious explanation for urethral symptoms should be sought in such patients.

Neisseria gonorrhoeae can affect the urethra in women as it does in men, and it occasionally causes the urethral syndrome.[84] Gently stripping the urethra may deliver a purulent discharge that with a Gram stain will reveal typical gram-negative, cell-associated diplococci. The gram-stained smear from the female urethra has a sensitivity of about 50 percent for gonorrhea.[85] About three-fourths of these women also will have gonococci recoverable from the endocervix.[84] The syndrome responds to standard therapy for uncomplicated anogenital gonorrhea (see Ch. 19).

Chlamydia trachomatis is frequently recovered from women with dysuria, frequency, and pyuria.[81,82] Indeed, urinary tract symptoms are described by 53 percent of women from whom *C. trachomatis* is isolated from the urethra.[86,87] This association suggests that in some cases the urethral syndrome is the clinical counterpart of NGU in women. If such patients are initially treated with antimicrobial agents that are active against chlamydiae (e.g., tetracyclines, amoxicillin, fluoroquinolones, sulfonamides, and sulfamethoxazole-trimethoprim [SMX-TMP]), their symptoms are likely to respond. Relapses, however, are frequent and may reflect reinfection from an asymptomatic male sexual partner. In most studies, *U. urealyticum* has not been statistically associated with the urethral syndrome,[81,82,86–88] although one group found an association with $>10^3$ organisms per milliliter and pyuria.[89] The acute urethral syndrome, which is associated with pyuria, must be differentiated from the chronic urethral syndrome. The latter is not associated with pyuria and responds poorly to antimicrobial therapy.[90–93]

Dysuria is a common complaint of women with trichomoniasis. The parasite is recovered from the urethra and periurethral

glands of over 90 percent of women with the infection (see Ch. 260) and is associated with pyuria.[94] Dysuria also may result from vulvar irritation such as that accompanying vaginal candidiasis. It is far less common in patients with bacterial vaginosis.

The urethral syndrome has been treated with steroids[82] or with urethral dilatation and other types of instrumentation. Among sexually active women, however, gonococcal, chlamydial, and trichomonal infection should be ruled out before other therapies are tried.

TREATMENT OF SEXUAL PARTNERS OF MEN WITH NGU

Chlamydia trachomatis can be recovered from the endocervix of 45–90 percent of the sexual partners of infected men[31,42,95–97] and from the urethra alone in about 15–25 percent of these women.[86,94,98,99] Although infected women usually are asymptomatic, the organism is far from benign (see Ch. 157). Chlamydial infection can be documented in as many as 50 percent of the women with mucopurulent cervicitis who are attending an STD clinic. Indeed, cervical abnormalities, often mild, may be seen in many women from whom *C. trachomatis* is recovered. *Chlamydia trachomatis* is a cause of acute salpingitis and bartholinitis. In addition, babies born to infected women may develop chlamydial ophthalmia neonatorum or pneumonia, and asymptomatic women undoubtedly are a reservoir for recurrent NGU. The carriage of ureaplasmas has been linked to infertility,[100] although the causal nature of the relationship is controversial.[53,54] These considerations support the routine treatment of female sexual partners of men with NGU.

COMPLICATIONS OF URETHRITIS

Both *N. gonorrhoeae* and *C. trachomatis* have been identified as causes of acute epididymitis among sexually active men.[101,102] In 20–30 percent of the men with NGU, prostatic involvement is documented; however, it is usually asymptomatic[5,103] and responds to standard treatments. The role of chlamydia in the development of chronic nonbacterial prostatitis remains unproven. The organism has been recovered from some men with chronic nonbacterial prostatitis,[104–106] and in some patients the condition appeared to respond to treatment with tetracyclines. The role of *U. urealyticum* is even more controversial. The organism has been associated with prostatitis in some series but not in others.[53,54] An association with infertility and abnormal semen specimens has been described,[100,107] but it also is regarded as controversial.[54] Stricture may follow gonococcal or nongonococcal urethritis. *Chlamydia trachomatis* can infect the conjunctiva. Also, an oculogenital syndrome consisting of NGU and conjunctivitis may be seen in about 4 percent of the patients with NGU[108,109]; it responds to standard therapy with tetracyclines and must be differentiated from Reiter syndrome.

THERAPY

Specific forms of urethritis including chlamydial and ureaplasmal infections, gonorrhea, trichomoniasis, and syphilis should be treated as discussed in the appropriate chapters in Part III. As a syndrome, NGU has been treated with a variety of regimens, but a tetracycline (to which *C. trachomatis* and most *U. urealyticum* strains are sensitive) is the drug of choice. Treatment for 7 days will cure 65–94 percent of the patients.[8,9,44,49, 50,62,70,100–113] Although longer treatment for 14–21 days has been tried, there is little convincing evidence that full-dose regimens exceeding 7 days have any additional benefits.[42,63,111]

Tetracycline hydrochloride may be administered in doses of 500 mg four times a day,[8,9,44,49,50,62,70,110–113] which appears to be superior to 250 mg four times a day.[111–113] The patient should be instructed to take the drug on an empty stomach and not accompanied by milk or antacids. Alternatively, doxycycline can be administered in a dose of 100 mg orally twice daily for 7 days.[114] This drug is highly effective, well tolerated by patients, and can be taken with food. Twice daily administration and fewer side effects are probably associated with better compliance.[115] Since inexpensive generic preparations are now available, doxycycline is the tetracycline of choice for treatment of NGU. Administration of doxycycline may be associated with photosensitivity reactions. Minocycline has no apparent advantages over doxycycline, and it produces dizziness in many patients.[63]

Azithromycin is an azalide antimicrobial agent with a prolonged half-life that is active against *C. trachomatis* and *U. urealyticum*. A single 1.0 g oral dose is effective against chlamydial infections[116] and in syndromic NGU.[117]

Erythromycin is as effective as tetracycline in chlamydial infections[8] and is active against tetracycline-resistant ureaplasmas.[5,61] Erythromycin has the additional theoretic advantage of producing higher prostatic levels than tetracycline hydrochloride does, and it may be of use in the retreatment of patients whose symptoms are relieved by tetracycline but return after therapy is completed. Such patients may have a prostatic focus of infection that is not cured by tetracycline.[8,118] Gastrointestinal discomfort is an unfortunately common adverse effect of erythromycin therapy. Patients who cannot tolerate a dose of 500 mg four times daily for 7 days can be treated with 250 mg four times daily for 14 days, a regimen that is almost as effective in NGU.[8]

Fluoroquinolone antimicrobial agents have been evaluated in chlamydial urethritis and in syndromic NGU. Ciprofloxacin was ineffective,[119] whereas ofloxacin (300 mg twice daily for 7 days) was effective.[120] Sulfonamides including sulfisoxazole and SMX-TMP can be used to treat chlamydial NGU, but are less effective in *Chlamydia*-negative NGU.[49,121]

Even if untreated, the symptoms of NGU will resolve within 2 weeks in 14–30 percent of the patients;[110] up to 70 percent of the patients will have a complete resolution of symptoms within 6 months.[42] Resolution of symptoms does not, of course, mean that the infection is cured. Such asymptomatic patients may remain infected and infectious. Conversely, the inflammatory response accompanying NGU may take some time to resolve, even after the pathogens have been eliminated.[51]

During treatment, the symptoms of NGU frequently resolve before the patient has completed the therapy. Patients should be cautioned to complete the entire course of antibiotics, since a relapse is considerably more common if therapy is aborted. To differentiate reliably a relapse from reinfection and to protect sexual partners, patients undergoing treatment for urethritis should refrain from coitus or use condoms until both partners have completed their medication and their symptoms have resolved.

Because coincident chlamydial infection is very common in men with gonorrhea, the Centers for Disease Control and Prevention have suggested that uncomplicated gonococcal urethritis should be treated with a combined regimen consisting of a single dose of a suitable cephalosporin or fluoroquinolone antibiotic followed by 7 days of doxycycline (100 mg orally twice daily), or erythromycin (500 mg orally four times daily). This regimen has the advantage of providing effective single-dose therapy for gonorrhea and effective therapy for coincident, undiagnosed NGU.[122] Its disadvantages include increased cost and the potential for adverse reactions. It is also prudent to use one of these combined regimens to treat urethritis of undetermined etiology.

Patients who are being treated for urethritis should be examined for other STDs and should be tested serologically for syphilis at the initial visit. An initial work-up for trichomoniasis probably is not indicated in most routine settings since the infection accounts for a small proportion of cases.[23] Additionally, direct microscopic examination of a urethral specimen for trichomo-

nads usually is unrewarding unless the patient can be seen before first morning micturition. If the patient's urethritis has not been cured by previous antibacterial therapy or if symptoms or signs in the sexual partner suggest trichomonal infection, the patient's first-void urine sediment can be examined as a wet mount or can be cultured on suitable media.[22] Empiric treatment for trichomoniasis with oral metronidazole may be warranted in some patients.

Men whose symptoms do not resolve or recur following appropriate treatment for urethritis should have urethral Gram stains or first-void urine sediments examined to establish the existence of persistent urethritis. Symptoms may persist in the absense of objective evidence of urethritis. Antimicrobial treatment of symptomatic men who do not have objective evidence of urethritis is of questionable value.[28]

Patients initially treated for NGU whose urethritis is not eliminated by doxycycline should be suspected of having infection with *Trichomonas* or doxycycline-resistant *Ureaplasma*.[5,58,59,61] Because these infections may be impossible to differentiate clinically, such patients may be empirically treated with a single 2-g dose of metronidazole followed by erythromycin, 500 mg orally four times daily for 7 days. It is, of course, important that their sexual partners be treated with the same regimen.

Some men report that their urethral symptoms disappeared while they were taking a tetracycline but reappeared days to weeks after completing therapy. Such recurrences with objective evidence of urethritis are seen in about 20 percent of patients with chlamydial NGU and in about 40 percent of patients with nonchlamydial infection. Among NGU patients from whom neither chlamydiae nor ureaplasmas are isolated, the recurrence rate is greater than 50 percent.[50,62,63] Eighty percent of recurrent NGU occurs in patients in whom neither organism is initially recovered,[63] and 70–80 percent of men with recurrent NGU are culture negative for both organisms at the time of recurrence.[85]

Men with recurrent urethritis should be questioned closely about the possibility of reexposure, and attention should be given to ensuring simultaneous treatment of all sexual partners. If reexposure is likely, the patient may be retreated with the initial doxycycline regimen. If the patient has not been reexposed, a recurrence of urethritis suggests the possibility that some pathogens remained in a relatively antibiotic protected site. Prostatic involvement is common in NGU. It is possible that some men may have a prostatic focus of infection. Men with repeated relapses occasionally are successfully treated with a 3-week course of erythromycin.[123] Patients whose relapses are not eliminated by these maneuvers should be referred for urologic evaluation to rule out anatomic abnormalities.[118] Such men most likely are not infected with *Chlamydia* or *Ureaplasma*. About one-fourth will be found to have a partial obstruction to urine flow, and about half of these will have urethral strictures.[118] They and their sexual partners do not appear to be at significant risk for infectious complications.[124] Long-term antimicrobial suppression is useful in this setting.[124]

Sexual partners of patients with sexually transmitted urethritis should be treated simultaneously. A woman who has been the sexual partner of a man with urethritis of undetermined etiology should be treated with a regimen that is effective against gonococci, chlamydiae, and ureaplasmas. A regimen combining a cephalosporin or a fluoroquinolone with doxycycline as described above is suitable in nonpregnant women. Erythromycin, amoxicillin,[125] or clindamycin[126] may be substituted for doxycycline in pregnancy. Asymptomatic male sexual partners of women known to have gonorrhea, chlamydial infection, or trichomoniasis should be treated even if direct microscopic examinations are negative.

REITER SYNDROME

Some cases of nongonococcal urethritis appear as one element of Reiter syndrome, which also includes arthritis, uveitis, and, often, lesions of the skin and mucous membranes. The syndrome complicates 1–2 percent of the cases of NGU[127,128] and is felt to be the most common peripheral inflammatory arthritis in young men.[129] Its pathogenesis is unclear, but it probably represents an abnormal host response to any of a number of infections.[130] The idiosyncratic nature of the host's response is supported by a strong correlation between the development of Reiter syndrome and the presence of the HLA-B27 histocompatibility antigen. This antigen has been found in 60–96 percent of the patients with Reiter syndrome,[128,129,131,132] and it also has been related to uveitis and sacroiliitis.[128] Although possibly providing a clue to pathogenesis, it is not diagnostic.[133]

The inciting infection is of two types. Reiter syndrome may follow sexually transmitted urethritis, and most cases in North America and Europe seem to occur in sexually active young people.[134,135] Many cases occur after contact with a new partner, and some cases have been epidemiologically linked.[128,136] In one series, 9 percent of cases followed gonococcal urethritis, although 50 percent of these patients subsequently developed PGU.[137] *Chlamydia trachomatis* has been implicated in the pathogenesis of Reiter syndrome[138] since it has been recovered from the urethras of 16–44 percent of the patients with Reiter syndrome and from 69 percent of those men who had signs of urogenital inflammation at the time of examination.[135,139,140] In addition, antibodies to *Chlamydia* have been detected in 46–67 percent and cell-mediated immunity in 72 percent of patients with Reiter syndrome.[130,140,141] Chlamydial RNA has been identified in synovial membranes,[142] and chlamydial elementary bodies have been observed in joint fluid[143] in a few patients. The significance of these observations is not yet defined, but the failure of antichlamydial therapy to influence the course of disease argues against a direct cause and effect relationship.

Reiter syndrome also follows bacterial gastroenteritis and has been described after infection with *Salmonella, Shigella, Yersinia,* and *Campylobacter*[127–129,131,137,144–148] and after antibiotic-associated colitis.[149] Postdysenteric Reiter syndrome has been reported in 0.24–1.50 percent of patients after epidemics of gastrointestinal infection[145,147]; it is considerably more common among patients who are HLA-B27-positive. Antibodies reacting with *Yersinia* proteins occur in the sera of many patients with Reiter syndrome.[150]

Clinically, Reiter syndrome after genital infection is indistinguishable from that following bacterial gastroenteritis; indeed, 12–80 percent of the patients with postdysenteric Reiter syndrome have genital symptoms.[128,151] The age- and sex-specific attack rates, however, are different; 94–99 percent of the cases of Reiter syndrome after sexually transmitted infections occur in men. However, a much larger fraction—up to 10 percent—of the cases of postdysenteric Reiter syndrome occur in women.[134,147,152,153] It also is reported in sexually inactive children.[134,146]

Clinical Features

Nongonococcal urethritis is the initial manifestation in 80 percent of the patients.[128,129] As with other forms of NGU, it usually occurs 7–14 days after sexual exposure.[128] The urethritis may be mild and may be unnoticed by the patient,[127] and it may be detectable only by physical examination performed before the first micturition. Gonococcal urethritis sometimes precedes Reiter syndrome.[137] The discharge may be purulent or mucopurulent, and patients may or may not complain of dysuria. Accompanying prostatitis has been described by some authors.[127,129,151,153] If present, it is usually asymptomatic. Cystitis without urethritis has also been reported and may be a manifestation, particularly in women.[151] Cervicitis is associated with Reiter syndrome[154] and may represent female genital infection with the inciting microorganism.

The other features of Reiter syndrome develop 1–5 weeks after the onset of urethritis.[151] Arthritis begins within 4 weeks

of the onset of urethritis in four-fifths of patients,[127,128] but it precedes urethritis in about 15 percent.[134] The knees are the most frequently involved area, followed by the ankles and small joints of the feet. Sacroiliitis, either symmetric[151] or, more frequently, asymmetric,[134,146,153] may develop in up to two-thirds of patients.[151] It is more frequent in patients with the HLA-B27 antigen.[146] Ankylosing spondylitis, which occurs in only about 1 percent of the general population, complicates a significant minority of cases of Reiter syndrome[128,132,146,155]; also, back pain is reported by 60 percent of all patients.[129] Many patients with the HLA-B27 antigen who develop Reiter syndrome develop ankylosing spondylitis,[155,156] which is rare in patients without the antigen.[156] Spurring of the calcaneus may be seen in up to one-fourth of the patients with Reiter syndrome[134,153] and may produce heel pain. A dactylitis resulting in sausage-shaped swelling of the digits is also characteristic.[134] Arthritis is the most persistent feature of the syndrome and may last for months to years after other manifestations have disappeared.[134,151]

Mild bilateral conjunctivitis, iritis, or uveitis is sometimes present but often lasts for only a few days.[127,151,153,157] It is occasionally accompanied by a purulent discharge or frank keratitis.[151,157] Unlike the conjunctivitis caused by direct infection with *C. trachomatis,* the inflamed conjunctivae in Reiter syndrome do not manifest follicular hypertrophy.

Dermatologic manifestations occur in up to 50 percent of the patients.[127–129] The initial lesions are waxy papules, which often display a central yellow spot and occur most frequently on the soles and palms[151] and with decreasing frequency on the nails, scrotum, scalp, and trunk.[127] The papules epithelialize and thicken to produce keratoderma blenorrhagicum in about 10–25 percent of the patients.[129,154] Circinate balanitis is usually painless and occurs in about 25–40 percent of all patients.[128,129,151] Circinate and ulcerative vulvitis also are described.[158] Painless erosions on the dorsum of the tongue and fauces occur most commonly with the initial episode and less frequently with recurrences.[153,154] Incomplete Reiter syndrome consisting of urethritis and arthritis or arthritis alone has been reported.[129,144,159]

The initial episode of Reiter syndrome usually lasts for 2–6 months, but episodes lasting for 1 year have been described.[129,151,153] Most patients feel completely well after the attack subsides, but the disease recurs in many of them[128,129,134,143,155] at a rate of about 15 percent in each 5-year period after the initial attack.[160] During recurrences, the genital symptoms are usually less marked and may be entirely absent.[161,162] Over half of the patients will have active disease 15–20 years after the initial episode,[129,132,155,160] with the risk of residuals being somewhat higher among patients with the HLA-B27 antigen.[163] Almost 50 percent of the affected patients develop some degree of permanent disability.[132,155]

Rare complications of Reiter syndrome include pericarditis,[154] myocarditis,[151] first-degree atrioventricular block,[153,164] and aortic insufficiency.[132,153] Thrombophlebitis, radiculitis,[154] and myelopathy[165] are occasionally described.

Laboratory Features

Anemia is common,[129] and the erythrocyte sedimentation rate is elevated in about 50 percent of the patients.[134,154] Fluid recovered at the same time from different joints may be different.[151] Synovial fluid may contain 1000–200,000 white blood cells, more than two-thirds of which are PMN.[151] The glucose level is low in about 50 percent of the joints.[151] Synovial biopsy specimens reveal nonspecific inflammatory changes.[154]

Therapy

Treatment of Reiter syndrome is quite controversial. Because of the possibility that the inciting infection may be sexually transmitted NGU, treatment with doxycycline for 7 days is recommended[127,154] and has been said by some to reduce or eliminate the urethritis.[166] Others, however, have seen no effect on the arthritis or on the overall course of the disease.[154,161] The relative safety of oral doxycycline and the frequency with which chlamydiae are isolated from patients with Reiter syndrome make a course of doxycycline reasonable. Among a population in Greenland with a high prevalence of HLA-B27, treatment of patients who had urethritis or cervicitis with tetracycline or erythromycin was associated with a lower incidence of subsequent arthritis than was treatment with penicillin or no treatment at all.[167]

Nonsteroidal anti-inflammatory drugs (NSAID) are the most effective treatment.[129] Indomethacin or tolmetin are favored by some workers,[168] and all of these agents are superior to salicylates or corticosteroids. Sulfasalazine may be beneficial for patients whose symptoms do not respond to NSAID. Cytotoxic agents such as methotrexate may be of value in recalcitrant cases.[168]

REFERENCES

1. Braun P, Sherman H, Komaroff AL. Urethritis in men: Benefits, risks, and costs of alternative strategies of management. Sex Transm Dis. 1982;9: 188–99.
2. Amarasuriya KL. Haematuria presenting in outpatients attending a department of genitourinary medicine. Br J Vener Dis. 1979;55:214–7.
3. Swartz SL. Diagnosis of nongonococcal urethritis. In: Hobson D, Holmes KK, eds. Nongonococcal Urethritis and Related Infections. Washington, DC: American Society for Microbiology; 1977:15–8.
4. Bowie WR. Comparison of Gram stain and first-voided urine sediment in the diagnosis of urethritis. Sex Transm Dis. 1978;5:39–42.
5. Root TE, Edwards LD, Spengler PJ. Nongonococcal urethritis: A survey of clinical and laboratory features. Sex Transm Dis. 1980;7:59–65.
6. Swartz SL, Kraus SJ, Herrmann KL, et al. Diagnosis and etiology of nongonococcal urethritis. J Infect Dis. 1978;138:445–54.
7. Desai K, Robson HG. Comparison of the gram-stained urethral smear and first-voided urine sediment in the diagnosis of nongonococcal urethritis. Sex Transm Dis. 1982;9:21–5.
8. Scheibel JH, Kristensen JK, Hentzer B, et al. Treatment of chlamydial urethritis in men and Chlamydia trachomatis–positive female partners: Comparison of erythromycin and tetracycline in treatment courses of one week. Sex Transm Dis. 1982;9:128–31.
9. Stamm WE, Koutsky LA, Benedetti JK, et al. Chlamydia trachomatis urethral infections in men. Prevalence, risk factors, and clinical manifestations. Ann Intern Med. 1984;100:47–51.
10. Perera SAB. Use of Kova-Slide II with grid and uncentrifuged segmented urine specimens in the diagnosis of nongonococcal urethritis: A quantitative technique. Sex Transm Dis. 1985;12:14–8.
11. Veeravahu M, Smyth RW, Clay JC. Detection of leukocyte esterase in urine: A new screening test for nongonococcal urethritis compared with two microscopic methods. Sex Transm Dis. 1987;14:180–4.
12. Perera SAB, Jones C, Srikantha V, et al. Leukocyte esterase test as rapid screen for non-gonococcal urethritis. Genitourin Med. 1987;63:380–3.
13. Simmons PD. Evaluation of the early morning smear investigation. Br J Vener Dis. 1978;54:128–9.
14. Willcox JR, Adler MW, Belsey EM. Observer variation in the interpretation of gram-stained urethral smears. Br J Vener Dis. 1981;57:134–6.
15. Jacobs NF Jr, Kraus SJ. Gonococcal and nongonococcal urethritis in men. Clinical and laboratory differentiation. Ann Intern Med. 1975;82:7–12.
16. Kraus SJ. Semiquantitation of urethral polymorphonuclear leukocytes as objective evidence of nongonococcal urethritis. Sex Transm Dis. 1982;9: 52–5.
17. Goodhart ME, Ogden J, Zaidi AA, Kraus SJ. Factors affecting the performance of smear and culture tests for the detection of Neisseria gonorrhoeae. Sex Transm Dis. 1982;9:63–9.
18. Haberberger RL Jr, Mikhail IA, Fox E, et al. Predominance of vancomycin-sensitive strains of Neisseria gonorrhoeae in Djibouti. Lancet 1989;2:683.
19. Janda WM, Jackson T. Evaluation of Gonodecten for the presumptive diagnosis of gonococcal urethritis in men. J Clin Microbiol. 1985;21:143–5.
20. Prior RB, Spagna VA. Improved utility of Gonoscreen, a Limulus amoebocyte lysate assay, in the evaluation of urethral discharges in men. J Clin Microbiol. 1985;22:141–4.
21. Judson FN, Werness BA, Shahan MR. Lack of utility of a Limulus amoebocyte lysate assay in the diagnosis of urethral discharges in men. J Clin Microbiol. 1985;21:152–4.
22. Krieger JN, Verdon M, Siegel N, et al. Risk assessment and laboratory diagnosis of trichomoniasis in men. J Infect Dis. 1992;166:1362–6.
23. Krieger JN, Jenny C, Verdon M, et al. Clinical manifestations of trichomoniasis in men. Ann Intern Med. 1993;118:844–9.
24. Shafer M-A, Schachter J, Moscicki AB, et al. Urinary leukocyte esterase screening test for asymptomatic chlamydial and gonococcal infections in males. JAMA. 1989;262:2562–6.
25. Jaschek G, Gaydos CA, Welsh LE, et al. Direct detection of Chlamydia trachomatis in urine specimens from symptomatic and asymptomatic men by using a rapid polymerase chain reaction assay. J Clin Microbiol. 1993;31: 1209–12.
26. Bowie WR, Pollock HM, Forsyth PS, et al. Bacteriology of the urethra in normal men and men with nongonococcal urethritis. J Clin Microbiol. 1977; 6:482–8.
27. Wong JL, Hines PA, Brasher MD, et al. The etiology of nongonococcal urethritis in men attending a venereal disease clinic. Sex Transm Dis. 1977; 4:4–8.
28. Augenbraun MH, Cummings M, McCormack WM. Management of chronic urethral symptoms in men. Clin Infect Dis. 1992;15:714–5.
29. Pec J, Straka S, Novomesky F, et al. Mechanical urethritis and ascendent genitourinary infections due to sexual stimulation of the urethra by inserted foreign bodies. Genitourin Med. 1992;68:399–400.
30. McCutchan JA. Epidemiology of venereal urethritis: Comparison of gonorrhea and nongonococcal urethritis. Rev Infect Dis. 1984;6:669–88.
31. Judson FN. Epidemiology and control of nongonococcal urethritis and genital chlamydial infections: A review. Sex Transm Dis. 1981;8:117–26.
32. Wright RA, Judson FN. Relative and seasonal incidences of the sexually transmitted diseases. A two-year statistical review. Br J Vener Dis. 1978; 54:433–40.
33. McChesney JA, Zedd A, King H, et al. Acute urethritis in male college students. JAMA. 1973;226:37–9.
34. Smith GL, Greenup R, Takafuji ET. Circumcision as a risk factor for urethritis in racial groups. Am J Public Health. 1987;77:452–4.
35. Boyd JT, Csonka GW, Oates JK. Epidemiology of non-specific urethritis. Br J Vener Dis. 1958;34:40–3.
36. Holmes KK. Gonococcal infection. Clinical, epidemiologic and laboratory perspectives. Adv Intern Med. 1974;19:259–85.
37. Schofield CBS. Some factors affecting the incubation period and duration of symptoms of urethritis in men. Br J Vener Dis. 1982;58:184–7.
38. Harrison WO, Hooper RR, Wiesner PJ, et al. A trial of minocycline given after exposure to prevent gonorrhea. N Engl J Med. 1979;300:1074–80.
39. Rothenberg R, Judson FN. The clinical diagnosis of urethral discharge. Sex Transm Dis. 1983;10:24–8.
40. Lee Y-H, Rosner B, Alpert S, et al. Clinical and microbiological investigation of men with urethritis. J Infect Dis. 1978;138:798–803.
41. Volk J, Kraus SJ. Nongonococcal urethritis. A venereal disease as prevalent as epidemic gonorrhea. Arch Intern Med. 1974;134:511–4.
42. Oriel JD. Treatment of nongonococcal urethritis. In: Hobson D, Holmes KK, eds. Nongonococcal Urethritis and Related Infections. Washington, DC: American Society for Microbiology; 1977:38–42.
43. Johannisson G, Lowhagen G-B, Nilsson S. Chlamydia trachomatis and urethritis in men. Scand J Infect Dis 1982;32(Suppl):87–92.
44. Handsfield HH, Alexander ER, Wang SP, Pedersen AHB, Holmes KK. Differences in the therapeutic response of chlamydia-positive and chlamydia-negative forms of nongonococcal urethritis. J Am Vener Dis Assoc. 1976;2: 5–9.
45. Jacobs NF Jr, Arum ES, Kraus SJ. Nongonococcal urethritis: The role of Chlamydia trachomatis. Ann Intern Med. 1977;86:313–4.
46. Bowie WR, Wang S-P, Alexander ER, et al. Etiology of nongonococcal urethritis. Evidence for Chlamydia trachomatis and Ureaplasma urealyticum. J Clin Invest. 1977;59:735–42.
47. Viarengo J, Hebrant F, Piot P. Ureaplasma urealyticum in the urethra of healthy men. Br J Vener Dis. 1980;56:169–72.
48. Hunter JM, Smith IW, Peutherer JF, et al. Chlamydia trachomatis and Ureaplasma urealyticum in men attending a sexually transmitted diseases clinic. Br J Vener Dis. 1981;57:130–3.
49. Bowie WR, Floyd JF, Miller Y, et al. Differential response of chlamydial and ureaplasma-associated urethritis to sulphafurazole (sulfisoxazole) and aminocyclitols. Lancet. 1976;2:1276–8.
50. Coufalik ED, Taylor-Robinson D, Csonka GW. Treatment of nongonococcal urethritis with rifampicin as a means of defining the role of Ureaplasma urealyticum. Br J Vener Dis. 1979;55:36–43.
51. Taylor-Robinson D, Csonka GW, Prentice MJ. Human intraurethral inoculation of ureaplasmas. Q J Med. 1977;46:309–26.
52. Brown MB, Cassell GH, Taylor-Robinson D, et al. Measurement of antibody to Ureaplasma urealyticum by an enzyme-linked immunosorbent assay and detection of antibody responses in patients with nongonococcal urethritis. J Clin Microbiol. 1983;17:288–95.
53. Cassell GH, Cole BC. Mycoplasmas as agents of human disease. N Engl J Med. 1981;304:80–9.
54. Taylor-Robinson D, McCormack WM. The genital mycoplasmas. N Engl J Med. 1980;302:1003–10, 1063–7.
55. Tully JG, Cole RM, Taylor-Robinson D, et al. A newly discovered mycoplasma in the human urogenital tract. Lancet. 1981;1:1288–91.
56. Taylor-Robinson D, Furr PM, Hetherington CM. The pathogenicity of a newly discovered human mycoplasma (strain G37) for the genital tract of marmosets. J Hyg. 1982;89:449–55.
57. Taylor-Robinson D, Tully JG, Barile MF. Urethral infection in male chimpanzees produced experimentally by Mycoplasma genitalium. Br J Exp Pathol. 1985;66:95–101.
58. Magalhaes M. Persistent nongonococcal urethritis associated with a minocycline-resistant strain of Ureaplasma urealyticum: A case report. Sex Transm Dis. 1983;10:151–2.

59. Arya OP, Pratt BC. Persistent urethritis due to *Ureaplasma urealyticum* in conjungal or stable partnerships. Genitourin Med. 1986;62:329–32.

60. Magalhaes M, Veras A. Minocycline resistance among clinical isolates of *Ureaplasma urealyticum*. J Infect Dis. 1984;149:117.

61. Stimson JB, Hale J, Bowie WR, Holmes KK. Tetracycline-resistant *Ureaplasma urealyticum*: A cause of persistent nongonococcal urethritis. Ann Intern Med. 1981;94:192–4.

62. Bowie WR. Urethritis and infections of the lower urogenital tract. Urol Clin North Am. 1980;7:17–28.

63. Bowie WR, Alexander ER, Stimson JB, et al. Therapy for nongonococcal urethritis. Double-blind, randomized comparison of two doses and two durations of minocycline. Ann Intern Med. 1981;95:306–11.

64. Corey L, Adams HG, Brown ZA, et al. Genital herpes simplex virus infection: Clinical manifestations, course, and complications. Ann Intern Med. 1983;98:958–72.

65. Nacey JN, Tulloch AGS, Ferguson AF. Catheter-induced urethritis: A comparison between latex and silicone catheters in a prospective clinical trial. Br J Urol. 1985;57:325–8.

66. Conde-Glez CJ, Calderon E. Urogenital infection due to meningococcus in men and women. Sex Transm Dis. 1991;18:72–5.

67. Fontaine EAR, Bryant TN, Taylor-Robinson D, et al. A numerical taxonomic study of anaerobic gram-negative bacilli classified as *Bacteroides ureolyticus* isolated from patients with non-gonococcal urethritis. J Gen Microbiol. 1986; 132:3137–46.

68. Harnett GB, Phillips PA, Gollow MM. Association of genital adenovirus infection with urethritis in med. Med J Aust. 1984;141:337–8.

69. Woolley PD, Kinghorn GR, Talbot MD, Duerden BI. Microbiological flora in men with non-gonococcal urethritis with particular reference to anaerobic bacteria. Int J STD AIDS. 1990;1:122–5.

70. Arya OP, Mallinson H, Pareek SS, et al. Post-gonococcal cervicitis and post-gonococcal urethritis. A study of their epidemiological correlation and the role of *Chlamydia trachomatis* in their aetiology. Br J Vener Dis. 1981;57: 395–9.

71. Bowie WR, Alexander ER, Holmes KK. Etiologies of postgonococcal urethritis in homosexual and heterosexual men: Roles of *Chlamydia trachomatis* and *Ureaplasma urealyticum*. Sex Transm Dis. 1978;5:151–4.

72. Terho P. *Chlamydia trachomatis* in gonococcal and postgonococcal urethritis. Br J Vener Dis. 1978;54:326–9.

73. Oriel JD, Ridgway GL, Reeve P, et al. The lack of effect of ampicillin plus probenecid given for genital infections with *Neisseria gonorrhoeae* on associated infections with *Chlamydia trachomatis*. J Infect Dis. 1976;133:568–71.

74. Stamm WE, Guinan ME, Johnson C, et al. Effect of treatment regimens for *Neisseria gonorrhoeae* on simultaneous infection with *Chlamydia trachomatis*. N Engl J Med. 1984;310:545–9.

75. Patrone P, Negosanti M, Ghetti P, et al. A combined treatment in prevention of postgonococcal urethritis. Dermatologica. 1984;168:300–2.

76. Holmes KK, Johnson DW, Floyd TM, et al. Studies of venereal disease. II. Observations on the incidence, etiology, and treatment of the postgonococcal urethritis syndrome. JAMA. 1967;202:467–73.

77. Chambers CV, Shafer M-A, Adger H, et al. Microflora of the urethra in adolescent boys: Relationships to sexual activity and nongonococcal urethritis. J Pediatr. 1987;110:314–21.

78. Handsfield HH, Lipman TO, Harnisch JP, et al. Asymptomatic gonorrhea in men. Diagnosis, natural course, prevalence and significance. N Engl J Med. 1974;290:117–23.

79. Smith JA, Linder CW, Jay MS, et al. Isolation of *Neisseria gonorrhoeae* from the urethra of asymptomatic adolescent males. Clin Pediatr (Phila). 1986;25:566–8.

80. Swartz SL, Kraus SJ. Persistent urethral leukocytosis and asymptomatic chlamydial urethritis. J Infect Dis. 1979;140:614–7.

81. Stamm WE. Etiology and management of the acute urethral syndrome. Sex Transm Dis. 1981;8:235–8.

82. Stamm WE, Wagner KF, Amsel R, et al. Causes of the acute urethral syndrome in women. N Engl J Med. 1980;303:409–14.

83. Fihn SD, Johnson C, Stamm WE. *Escherichia coli* urethritis in women with symptoms of acute urinary tract infection. J Infect Dis. 1988;157:196–9.

84. Curran JW. Gonorrhea and the urethral syndrome. Sex Transm Dis. 1977; 4:119–21.

85. Goh BT, Varia KB, Ayliffe PF, et al. Diagnosis of gonorrhea by gram-stained smears and cultures in men and women: Role of the urethral smear. Sex Transm Dis. 1985;12:135–9.

86. Paavonen J. *Chlamydia trachomatis*–induced urethritis in female partners of men with nongonococcal urethritis. Sex Transm Dis. 1979;6:69–71.

87. Paavonen J, Vesterinen E. *Chlamydia trachomatis* in cervicitis and urethritis in women. Scand J Infect Dis. 1982;32(Suppl):45–54.

88. Hunter JM, Young H, Harris AB. Genitourinary infection with *Ureaplasma urealyticum* in women attending a sexually transmitted diseases clinic. Br J Vener Dis. 1981;57:338–42.

89. Stamm WE, Running K, Hale J, et al. Etiologic role of *Mycoplasma hominis* and *Ureaplasma urealyticum* in women with the acute urethral syndrome. Sex Transm Dis. 1983;10:318–22.

90. Fihn SD, Stamm WE. The urethral syndrome. Semin Urol. 1983;1:121–9.

91. Latham RH, Stamm WE. Urethral syndrome in women. Urol Clin North Am. 1984;11:95–101.

92. Scotti RJ, Ostergard DR. The urethral syndrome. Clin Obstet Gynecol. 1984; 27:515–29.

93. Bump RC, Copeland WE Jr. Urethral isolation of the genital mycoplasmas and *Chlamydia trachomatis* in women with chronic urologic complaints. Am J Obstet Gynecol. 1985;152:38–41.

94. Feldman RG, Johnson AL, Schober PC, et al. Aetiology of urinary symptoms in sexually active women. Genitourin Med. 1986;62:333–41.

95. Ghadirian FD, Robson HG. *Chlamydia trachomatis* genital infections. Br J Vener Dis. 1979;55:415–8.

96. Paavonen J, Kousa M, Saikku P, et al. Examination of men with nongonococcal urethritis and their sexual partners for *Chlamydia trachomatis* and *Ureaplasma urealyticum*. Sex Transm Dis. 1978;5:93–6.

97. Thelin I, Mardh P-A. Contact tracing in genital chlamydial infection. Scand J Infect Dis. 1982;32(Suppl):163–6.

98. Johannison G, Lowhagen G-B, Lycke E. Genital *Chlamydia trachomatis* infection in women. Obstet Gynecol. 1980;56:671–5.

99. Wallin JE, Thompson SE, Zaidi A, et al. Urethritis in women attending an STD clinic. Br J Vener Dis. 1981;57:50–4.

100. Toth A, Lesser ML, Brooks C, et al. Subsequent pregnancies among 161 couples treated for T-mycoplasma genital-tract infection. N Engl J Med. 1983;308:505–7.

101. Berger RE. Acute epididymitis. Sex Transm Dis. 1981;8:286–9.

102. Berger RE, Alexander ER, Harnisch JP, et al. Etiology, manifestations and therapy of acute epididymitis: Prospective study of 50 cases. J Urol. 1979; 121:750–4.

103. Holmes KK, Hansfield HH, Wang SP, et al. Etiology of nongonococcal urethritis. N Engl Med. 1975;292:1199–205.

104. Bruce AW, Chadwick P, Willett WS, O'Shaughnessy M. The role of chlamydiae in genitourinary disease. J Urol. 1981;126:625–9.

105. Mardh P-A, Ripa KT, Colleen S, et al. Role of *Chlamydia trachomatis* in non-acute prostatitis. Br J Vener Dis. 1978;54:330–4.

106. Nilsson S, Johannisson G, Lycke E. Isolation of *Chlamydia trachomatis* from the urethra and from prostatic fluid in men with signs and symptoms of acute urethritis. Acta Dermatol Venereol (Stockh). 1981;61:456–9.

107. Cassell GH, Younger JB, Brown MB, et al. Microbiologic study of infertile women at the time of diagnostic laparoscopy. Association of *Ureaplasma urealyticum* with a defined subpopulation. N Engl J Med. 1983;308:502–5.

108. Mordhorst CH. Clinical epidemiology of oculogenital *Chlamydia* infection. In: Hobson D, Holmes KK, eds. Nongonococcal Urethritis and Related Infections. Washington, DC: American Society for Microbiology; 1977:126–34.

109. Ronnerstam R, Persson K. Chlamydial eye infection in adults. Scand J Infect Dis. 1982;32(Suppl):111–5.

110. Holmes KK, Johnson DW, Floyd TM. Studies of venereal disease. III. Double-blind comparison of tetracycline hydrochloride and placebo in treatment of nongonococcal urethritis. JAMA. 1967;202:474–6.

111. Arya OP, Alergant CD, Annels EH, et al. Management of non-specific urethritis in men. Evaluation of six treatment regimens and effect of other factors including alcohol and sexual intercourse. Br J Vener Dis. 1978;54:414–21.

112. Thambar IV, Simmons PD, Thin RN, et al. Double-blind comparison of two regimens in the treatment of nongonococcal urethritis. Seven-day vs 21-day courses of triple tetracycline (Deteclo). Br J Vener Dis. 1979;55:284–8.

113. Bowie WR, Yu JS, Fawcett A, et al. Tetracycline in nongonococcal urethritis. Comparison of 2 g and 1 g daily for seven days. Br J Vener Dis. 1980; 56:332–6.

114. Juvakoski T, Lauharanta J, Kanerva L, et al. One-week treatment of chlamydia-positive urethritis with doxycycline and tetracycline chloride in males. Acta Dermatol Venereol (Stockh). 1981;61:273–5.

115. Jordan WC. Doxycycline vs. tetracycline in the treatment of men with gonorrhea: The compliance factor. Sex Transm Dis. 1981;8:105–9.

116. Martin DH, Mroczkowski TF, Dalu ZA, et al. A controlled trial of a single dose of azithromycin for the treatment of chlamydial urethritis and cervicitis. N Engl J Med. 1992;327:921–5.

117. Whatley JD, Thin RN, Mumtaz G, et al. Azithromycin vs doxycycline in the treatment of non-gonococcal urethritis. Int J STD AIDS. 1991;2:248–51.

118. Krieger JN, Hooton TM, Brust PJ, et al. Evaluation of chronic urethritis. Defining the role for endoscopic procedures. Arch Intern Med. 1988;148: 703–7.

119. Hooton TM, Rogers ME, Medina TG, et al. Ciprofloxacin compared with doxycycline for nongonococcal urethritis. Ineffectiveness against *Chlamydia trachomatis* due to relapsing infection. JAMA. 1990;264:1418–21.

120. Mogabgab WJ, Holmes B, Murray M, et al. Randomized comparison of ofloxacin and doxycycline for chlamydia and ureaplasma urethritis and cervicitis. Chemotherapy. 1990;36:70–6.

121. Willcox RR, Sparrow RW. Cortrimoxazole in the treatment of non-gonococcal urethritis. Acta Dermatol Venereol (Stockh). 1974;54:317–20.

122. Centers for Disease Control and Prevention. Sexually transmitted diseases treatment guidelines, 1993. MMWR. 1993;42(RR-14):75–81.

123. Hooton TM, Wong ES, Barnes RC, et al. Erythromycin for persistent or recurrent nongonococcal urethritis. A randomized placebo-controlled trial. Ann Intern Med. 1990;113:21–6.

124. Berger RE. Recurrent nongonococcal urethritis. JAMA. 1983;249:409.

125. Crombleholme WR, Schachter J, Grossman M, et al. Amoxicillin therapy for *Chlamydia trachomatis* in pregnancy. Obstet Gynecol. 1990;75:752–6.

126. Campbell WR, Dodson MG. Clindamycin therapy for *Chlamydia trachomatis* in women. Am J Obstet Gynecol. 1990;162:343–7.

127. Morton RS. Reiter's disease. Practitioner. 1972;209:631–8.

128. Keat A. Reiter's syndrome and reactive arthritis in perspective. N Engl J Med. 1983;309:1606–15.

129. Arnett FC Jr. Reiter's syndrome. Johns Hopkins Med J. 1982;150:39–44.

130. Ford DK, deRoza DM, Schulzer M. The specificity of synovial mononuclear cell responses to microbiological antigens in Reiter's syndrome. J Rheumatol. 1982;9:561–7.

131. Lehman DH. Postdysenteric Reiter's syndrome. West J Med. 1977;126:405–7.

132. Sairanen E, Paronen I, Mahonen H. Reiter's syndrome: A follow-up study. Acta Med Scand. 1969;185:57–63.

133. Kahn MA, Kahn MK. Diagnostic value of HLA-B27 testing in ankylosing spondylitis and Reiter's syndrome. Ann Intern Med. 1982;96:70–6.

134. Hawkes JG. Clinical and diagnostic features of Reiter's disease: A follow-up study of 39 patients. NZ Med J. 1973;78:347–53.

135. Kousa M, Saikku P, Richmond S, et al. Frequent association of chlamydial infection with Reiter's syndrome. Sex Transm Dis. 1978;5:57–61.

136. Rustin MHA, Wedzicha JA, Keat AC, et al. Sexually transmitted arthritis? Two informative cases. J Rheumatol. 1982;9:646.

137. Leirisalo M, Skylv G, Kousa M, et al. Followup study on patients with Reiter's disease and reactive arthritis, with special reference to HLA-B27. Arthritis Rheum. 1982;25:249–59.

138. Editorial. Is Reiter's syndrome caused by chlamydia? Lancet. 1985;1:317–9.

139. Keat AC, Thomas BJ, Taylor-Robinson D, et al. Evidence of *Chlamydia trachomatis* infection in sexually acquired reactive arthritis. Ann Rheum Dis. 1980;39:431–7.

140. Kousa M. Evidence of chlamydial involvement in the development of arthritis. Scand J Infect Dis 1982;32(Suppl):116–21.

141. Inman RD, Johnston MEA, Chiu B, et al. Immunochemical analysis of immune response to *Chlamydia trachomatis* in Reiter's syndrome and nonspecific urethritis. Clin Exp Immunol. 1987;69:246–54.

142. Rahman MU, Cheema MA, Schumacher HR, et al. Molecular evidence for the presence of *Chlamydia* in the synovium of patients with Reiter's syndrome. Arthritis Rheum. 1992;35:521–9.

143. Keat A, Dixey J, Sonnex C, et al. *Chlamydia trachomatis* and reactive arthritis: The missing link. Lancet. 1987;1:72–5.

144. Jones RAK. Reiter's disease after *Salmonella typhimurium* enteritis. Br Med J. 1977;1:1391.

145. Noer HR. An "experimental" epidemic of Reiter's syndrome. JAMA. 1966;198:693–8.

146. Calin A. Reiter's syndrome. Med Clin North Am. 1977;61:365–76.

147. Paronon I. Reiter's disease. A study of 344 cases observed in Finland. Acta Med Scand. 1948;131(suppl 212):1–112.

148. Urman JD, Zurier RB, Rothfield NF. Reiter's syndrome associated with *Campylobacter fetus* infection. Ann Intern Med. 1977;86:444–4.

149. Hayward RS, Wensel RH, Kibsey P. Relapsing *Clostridium difficile* colitis and Reiter's syndrome. Am J Gastroenterol. 1990;85:752–6.

150. Kobayashi S, Ogasawara M, Maeda K, et al. Antibodies against *Yersinia enterocolitica* in patients with Reiter's syndrome. J Lab Clin Med. 1985;105:380–9.

151. Weinberger HW, Ropes MW, Kulka JP, et al. Reiter's syndrome, clinical and pathologic observations. A long term study of 16 cases. Medicine (Baltimore). 1962;41:35–91.

152. Smith DL, Bennett RM, Regan MG. Reiter's disease in women. Arthritis Rheum. 1980;23:335–40.

153. Good AE. Reiter's disease. Postgrad Med. 1977;61:153–8.

154. Catterall RD. Reiter's disease. In: Danielsson D, Juhlin L, Mardh P-A, eds. Genital Infections and Their Complications. Stockholm: Almquist & Wildsell; 1975:205–9.

155. Marks JS, Holt PJL. The natural history of Reiter's disease—21 years of observations. Q J Med. 1986;60:685–97.

156. Morris R, Metzger AL, Bluestone R, et al. HL-A W27-A clue to the diagnosis and pathogenesis of Reiter's syndrome. N Engl J Med. 1974;290:554–6.

157. Mark DB, McCulley JB. Reiter's keratitis. Arch Ophthalmol. 1982;100:781–4.

158. Daunt SON, Kotowski KE, O'Reilly AP, et al. Ulcerative vulvitis in Reiter's syndrome. A case report. Br J Vener Dis. 1982;58:405–7.

159. Arnett FC, McClusky OE, Schacter BZ, et al. Incomplete Reiter's syndrome: Discriminating features and HL-A W27 in diagnosis. Ann Intern Med. 1976;84:8–12.

160. Csonka GW. Recurrent attacks in Reiter's disease. Arthritis Rheum. 1960;3:164–9.

161. Catterall RD. The role of microbial infection in Reiter's syndrome. In: Dumont DC, ed. Infection and Immunology in the Rheumatic Diseases. Oxford: Blackwell Scientific Publications; 1976:147–50.

162. Butler MJ, Russell AS, Percy JS, et al. A follow-up study of 48 patients with Reiter's syndrome. Am J Med. 1979;67:808–10.

163. Calin A, Fried JF. An "experimental" epidemic of Reiter's syndrome revisited. Ann Intern Med. 1976;84:564–6.

164. Ruppert GB, Lindsay J, Barth WF. Cardiac conduction abnormalities in Reiter's syndrome. Am J Med. 1982;73:335–40.

165. Montanaro A, Bennett RM. Myelopathy in Reiter's disease. J Rheumatol. 1984;11:540–1.

166. Ford DK. Reiter's syndrome: Current concepts of etiology and pathogenesis. In: Hobson D, Holmes KK, eds. Nongonococcal Urethritis and Related Infections. Washington, DC: American Society for Microbiology; 1977:64–6.

167. Bardin T, Enel C, Cornelis F, et al. Antibiotic treatment of venereal disease and Reiter's syndrome in a Greenland population. Arthritis Rheum. 1992;35:190–4.

168. Editorial. Treating Reiter's syndrome. Lancet. 1987;2:1125–6.

89. VULVOVAGINITIS AND CERVICITIS

MICHAEL F. REIN

THE NORMAL VAGINA

Under the influence of estrogens, the vaginal epithelium becomes cornified and supports a prodigious microbial flora. This adult microenvironment were may develop transiently in neonates because of transplacentally acquired maternal estrogens[1] but resolves within several weeks as they are metabolized. The prepubescent vagina supports a flora rich in anaerobic bacteria, in particular, more *Bacteroides* species than are commonly found in the adult.[2] *Staphylococcus epidermidis* is frequently recovered,[2] and yeasts and *Gardnerella vaginalis* are isolated from 10 percent of girls.[2,3] The vagina again matures in the immediate premenarchal period.

In its mature state the vagina is colonized by a variety of bacteria,[4–8] primarily obligate and facultative anaerobes. More than 10^5 lactobacilli per milliliter of vaginal material are recovered from three-fourths of women. These are usually of the *Lactobacillus acidophilus* group.[9] Viridans streptococci and *S. epidermidis* are isolated from almost one-half of asymptomatic women of childbearing age. Surprisingly, 10^5 *Bacteroides* and *Prevotella* species were recovered from only one-sixth of these women[4,5,7,8] and *G. vaginalis* from 30–90 percent.[10,11] *Staphylococcus aureus* is recovered from the vaginas of only about 5 percent of healthy women.[12] Pregnancy has little effect on the distribution of most of the bacteria,[6,7,13] although the flora varies slightly during the menstrual cycle. Yeasts are carried by about 15–20 percent of healthy women.[14] With the onset of sexual activity, statistically significant increases are observed in the prevalence of *G. vaginalis,* lactobacilli, mycoplasmas, and ureaplasmas, but the prevalences of group B streptococci, *S. aureus,* and yeasts are not significantly altered.[15] It is of interest that ureaplasmas and *G. vaginalis* are recovered from 20–25 percent of young women who have not commenced sexual activity.[15]

Although our descriptive knowledge of vaginal microbiology has increased, our understanding of the factors controlling the flora remains primitive.[13,16] Changes in the level of gestational hormones influence the relative numbers of organisms of various species.[13] Specific and nonspecific vaginal host defenses have been cataloged, but again, their precise significance is unclear.[17,18] The metabolic products of some bacteria, for example, the hydrogen peroxide produced by some lactobacilli, may suppress other organisms such as anaerobes.[18] The vaginal microflora remains remarkably stable even through repeated douching.[13]

Mucoid endocervical secretions combine with sloughed vaginal epithelial cells and normal bacteria to form a physiologic vaginal discharge. This material is usually unnoticed but may produce symptomatic "leukorrhea." It is often increased during pregnancy or with the use of oral contraceptives.

VULVOVAGINITIS

Vulvovaginitis is a common clinical syndrome and is diagnosed in more than one-fourth of women attending sexually transmitted disease clinics.[19] Its incidence appears to be increasing.[20,21] Treatment should be based on a specific etiologic diagnosis that can usually be made at the time of the initial evaluation (Table 1).[22] Symptoms alone are inadequate for differential diagnosis,[23] and the use of over-the-counter antifungal therapy is therefore slightly treacherous.[23a] Multiple infections are not rare.[24]

Candidiasis

The archaic term *moniliasis* should be discarded.[25] *Candida albicans* is isolated from about 80–90 percent of cases of vulvovaginal candidiasis, and other species of *Candida* account for about 15 percent of cases.[20,26] *Candida tropicalis* is isolated from about 5 percent[27] and may be associated with a higher rate of recurrence after standard treatments.[28] *Candida (Torulopsis) glabrata* accounts for about 10 percent of vaginal yeast isolates.[10,20,26,29] Symptomatic vaginitis caused by this organism is not clinically distinguishable from that caused by other *Candida* species, but the organism may be harder to eradicate with standard therapies.[29] The relative incidence of vaginitis caused by fungi other than *C. albicans* appears to be increasing in some populations,[21] but not in others,[30] and it is thought that the widespread use of topical antifungals, especially in short courses, may contribute to selection for non-*albicans* yeasts, which are less susceptible to these agents than is *C. albicans*.[27] Cases of vaginitis caused by *Saccharomyces cerevisiae* have been reported.[31]

Vulvovaginal candidiasis (VC) accounts for about one-third of the vaginitis cases seen in private practice.[32] Some workers have estimated that 75 percent of adult women suffer at least one episode of VC during their lifetimes.[14] Yeast carried vaginally in small numbers and producing no symptoms may be considered part of the normal vaginal flora. VC may result if conditions in the vagina change so as to give the yeast an advantage over competing normal vaginal bacteria and induce an inflammatory response. Inhibition of normal bacterial flora by broad-spectrum antibiotics favors the growth of yeasts.[30] Thus yeasts were isolated from about 10 percent of women before but from 30 percent of women after 2- to 3-week courses of various tetracyclines.[10] Vulvovaginal candidiasis is said to follow 6–8 percent

of single doses and 26 percent of 1-week courses of metronidazole[33] and about 6–11 percent of courses of vaginal antimicrobials used to treat bacterial vaginosis.

Overgrowth of yeasts is apparently favored by high estrogen levels, although such levels also promote the growth of lactobacilli.[13] Vulvovaginal candidiasis is more common in pregnancy; it occurs in 10 percent of first-trimester women and 36–55 percent of women in their third trimesters.[10] Symptomatic disease has eventually developed in 60–90 percent of pregnant carriers, and old inoculation studies confirm the increased susceptibility of pregnant women.[10] Some nonpregnant women note recurrent or increasing symptoms preceding each menstrual period. The prevalence of vaginal carriage of *Candida* is higher among users of oral contraceptives than among women using other methods of birth control, but regimens based on lower estrogen doses are associated with a lower incidence of disease.[20,30] Small series and anecdotal reports suggest that some patients with recurrent VC can be cured only when oral contraceptives are discontinued.[10,30] The mechanism of estrogenic predisposition is unclear, although some investigators have suggested that increased vaginal glycogen stores may play a role[10] or that estrogens influence vaginal pH in a way that makes the milieu more hospitable to the fungi.[14] Estrogens induce changes in vaginal epithelial cells that increase the adherence of yeasts, and an estrogen receptor in the cytosol of *C. albicans* suggests a possible direct effect of gestational hormones on the organism.[20,34] The mechanism of increased glycogen stores has also been adduced to explain the association of VC with poorly controlled diabetes mellitus, but testing for diabetes in women with recurrent VC is not cost effective.[30]

It has been suggested that tight, insulating clothing predisposes to VC by increasing vulvar warmth and moisture. In prospective studies, a higher prevalence of candidal carriage and higher concentrations of organisms were found among women who wore tight rather than loose clothing.[35–37] Impairment of phagocytic cells or cell-mediated immunity (e.g., transplantation, chemotherapy) also predisposes to VC, and severe, refractory disease plagues women with the acquired immunodeficiency syndrome (AIDS).[38,39]

The mechanism by which *Candida* produces disease is not well defined. Although it is postulated that differences in virulence must exist,[30] strains isolated from symptomatic women are not demonstrably different than are isolates from asymptomatic carriers.[40] Filamentous forms (hyphae and pseudohyphae) are associated with active disease.[25] Pseudohyphae have been observed to penetrate the vaginal epithelial cells[41] and are more adherent to cells than are blastospores.[42]

TABLE 1. Typical Features of the Common Infectious Vaginitides

	Physiologic	Trichomonal	Candidal	Bacterial Vaginosis
Symptoms				
Vulvar irritation	—	+ +	+ +	− to +
Dysuria	—	20%	+	—
Odor	—	− to +	—	+ +
Signs				
Labial erythema	—	− to +	− to +	—
Satellite lesions	—	—	+	—
Discharge				
Consistency	Floccular	Frothy 25%	± Curdy	Homogeneous, ± Frothy
Color	White	Yellow-green 25%	White	Gray, white
Adherence to vaginal walls	—	—	+	+
pH	≤4.5	± ≥4.7	≤4.5	≥4.7
Microscopy				
Epithelial cells	Normal	Normal	Normal	Clue cells
PMN per epithelial cells	≤1	≥1	Variable	≤1
Bacteria	Gram + rods	Gram + rods	Gram + rods	Gram-variable coccobacilli
Pathogens	—	Trichomonads 70%	Yeasts and pseudohyphae 50%	Coccobacilli and motile rods
Bimanual examination				
Vaginal tenderness	—	+	+	—
Rugal hypertrophy	—	+	− to +	—
Adnexal tenderness	—	Occasionally	—	—

Adherence appears to be an important pathogenic feature of *Candida* species,[43] and sublethal concentrations of antifungals may ameliorate disease by reducing adherence.[44]

The severity of symptoms in VC is not directly related to the number of yeasts present.[10] Indeed, very small numbers of yeasts may be present in vaginal material recovered from highly symptomatic women.[10,45] An immunologic reaction has been suggested as the mechanism for symptomatic disease in such women.[20] A small series suggests that desensitization may decrease the frequency of symptomatic episodes.[46]

Clinical Features.   Patients with candidal vulvovaginitis generally complain of perivaginal pruritus, often with little or no discharge. Dysuria is occasionally noted and is likely to be perceived as vulvar rather than urethral. The labia may be pale or erythematous, and excoriation is often present. Shallow, linear ulcerations, especially on the posterior portion of the introitus, are common. Tiny satellite papules or papulopustules just beyond the main area of erythema are helpful diagnostically. The vaginal walls may be erythematous. Candidal discharge is classically thick and adherent and contains curds. It may, however, be thin and loose and thus resemble the discharge of other vaginitides.

Diagnosis.   The vaginal pH is generally normal (approximately 4.5) in women with VC[47–49] in contrast to trichomoniasis or bacterial vaginosis, in which it is characteristically elevated. Thus, demonstrating a normal pH (Table 1) in a woman with signs and symptoms of vaginitis suggests that she has candidiasis rather than one of the other infections. The addition of 10% potassium hydroxide (KOH) to vaginal discharge on a slide or in the speculum (Table 1) fails to elicit a fishy odor in most women with VC. Such an odor (a positive "whiff" test) suggests trichomoniasis or bacterial vaginosis.

An attempt should be made to demonstrate the organism on a wet mount of vaginal discharge. Adding 10–20% KOH to the specimen destroys the cellular elements and facilitates recognizing the fungi. Although classic descriptions and most textbook pictures suggest that one sees extensive tangles of filamentous forms, many patients in fact carry only small numbers of yeasts. Indeed, direct microscopic examination fails to reveal fungi in 30–50 percent of infected women,[14,50,51] and a presumptive diagnosis must be made on the basis of clinical features, pH, whiff test, and microscopy negative for other pathogens. A commercially available latex agglutination test has a limited sensitivity of about 60 percent.[52–54] The discharge usually contains relatively few polymorphonuclear neutrophils.

Treatment.   Currently available regimens are listed in Table 2.

Topical Therapy.   Vulvovaginal candidiasis is usually treated with the topical application of an antifungal agent. The striking variety of available drugs and regimens attests to the size of the market and the lack of a clear superiority of one product over another.

Commercially available preparations are characterized by high patient acceptability and safety in pregnancy. Most of the commercially available drugs are imidazoles (e.g., clotrimazole, miconazole, butoconozole, tioconazole, and econazole) or triazoles (terconazole). They are available in a variety of forms, including creams, tablets, and coated tampons.[49] Nystatin is the only polyene antifungal currently available for vaginal use in the United States. It is difficult to compare therapies directly because of the variety of protocols used in various studies. Odds[55] reviewed studies published through 1975 and concluded that imidazoles cured about 90 percent of patients and were superior to polyenes, which cured about 80 percent. There are no significant differences among currently available topical

TABLE 2. Regimens for the Treatment of Vulvovaginal Candidiasis

Duration	Drug	Regimen
Single dose	Miconazole	1200-mg suppository
	Clotrimazole	500-mg suppository
		10% cream, 5 g
	Tioconazole	6.5% cream, 4.6 g
3 Day	Miconazole	200-mg suppository qhs
	Clotrimazole	200-mg suppository qhs
	Butoconazole	2% cream, 5 g qhs
	Tioconazole	2% cream, 5 g qhs
	Econzole	150-mg suppository qhs
	Terconazole	0.8% cream, 5 g qhs
		80-mg suppository qhs
7 days	Miconazole	2% cream, 5 g qhs
		100-mg suppository qhs
	Clotrimazole	100-mg suppository qhs
		1% cream, 5 g qhs
	Terconazole	0.4% cream, 5 g qhs
	Fenticonazole	2% cream, 5 g qhs[a]
14 Day	Nystatin	100,000 U suppository qhs
Oral	Ketoconazole	200-mg po bid × 3–5 days[b]
		200-mg po × 3 days[b,c]
	Fluconazole	150-mg po × 1[b]
	Itraconazole	200-mg po bid × 1 day[b,c]
		200-mg po qd × 3[b,c]

[a] Not currently available in the United States.
[b] Not FDA approved for this use.
[c] Clinical data are limited.

preparations or between delivery systems consisting of creams or vaginal tablets.[56]

Current interest centers on shorter courses of therapy. Seven days of treatment with an imidazole yields cure rates ranging from 80 to 94 percent.[10] Newer, 3-day regimens produce approximately equivalent cure rates,[57–63] although some reviews suggest marginally better results with 7 days of therapy.[57] Because patients' compliance is likely to be better, it seems reasonable to recommend a 3-day regimen.[64]

A few studies have examined the efficacy of single-dose treatments with larger amounts of imidazoles such as 500 mg of clotrimazole.[58,59,65,66] Such regimens may be preferred for the sake of convenience in the treatment of mild infections. Cure rates obtained in some of these studies have not quite matched those obtained with longer courses. Treatment in pregnancy is more often unsuccessful, and the longer course regimens may be preferred in this setting.

Nystatin is a polyene that has been used in the United States for many years in a regimen consisting of one 100,000 unit tablet inserted intravaginally daily for 14 days. Although older series suggested a cure rate of about 80 percent,[55] more recent studies have yielded cure rates in excess of 90 percent, approximately equivalent to those obtained with the imidazoles.[10] It must be remembered, however, that treatment with nystatin requires 2 weeks as compared with shorter course regimens now recommended for the imidazoles.

Oral Therapy.   Several orally administered and well-absorbed imidazoles and triazoles are of great value in treating systemic mycoses. Several regimens of ketoconazole have been found effective in the treatment of VC (Table 2).[10,67–69] A number of studies strongly support the efficacy of a single oral dose of 150 mg of fluconazole for VC.[70–76] Preliminary experience also supports the use of oral itraconazole in a single- or 3-day regimen.[77–82] Results do not appear to be substantially superior to those obtained with topical regimens, and the clinician must carefully consider the need for systemic therapy for VC in view of the potential toxicities and possible teratogenicity of the drugs (see Ch. 31).

Other Therapies.   Gentian violet, a classic treatment, has suffered from low patient acceptability because it stains clothing. Newer delivery systems, such as impregnated tampons, may be easier to use.[83] Povidone-iodine cures about 65 percent of patients.[84] It should probably be avoided in pregnancy because absorption of iodine might suppress fetal thyroid development.[85] Treatment with 600 mg of boric acid powder in gelatin capsules intravaginally each evening or as vaginal suppositories used twice daily for 14 days cured 85–92 percent of women.[83,86] The regimens may have some role in the treatment of infection with species of yeast other than *C. albicans,* which are resistant to the topical imidazoles[9,29] but should be used with caution because experience is limited, and toxicity may well result from chronic use. Treatment of VC with various topical and oral *Lactobacillus* preparations has long been recommended in published anecdotes and in the lay press.[87] Theoretically acting by restoring a normal bacterial flora that can successfully compete with yeasts, these regimens have not been evaluated in well-controlled trials.

Recurrent Infection. When patients treated for VC are recultured 3–6 weeks after the completion of therapy, a sizable proportion are found once again to harbor the yeasts. Results from many studies[10,65,77,88] suggest a late recolonization rate of 21 ± 12 percent (mean ± SD), which is largely independent of the regimen used and often precedes symptomatic recurrence by 1–2 months.[30,67] Recurrent symptomatic infection is a major problem. The mechanisms of recurrence remain obscure, but what is known has been analyzed by Sobel and others.[14,30,89] Recurrence does not appear to result from the development of resistance to antifungals.[14,20,26,30]

Techniques for subspeciating *Candida* will increase our understanding of recurrence.[14,30] Such analyses suggest that about 40 percent of women with recurrent disease are demonstrably infected with new strains of *Candida*.[10,14,30] Obviously, women whose recurrence is associated with reappearance of the same strain might have suffered either recurrence or reinfection. The source of putative reinfection is poorly defined. Sexual transmission may be implicated in some cases, but its overall contribution to recurrent disease is unclear and probably low.[20,30] About 15 percent of women associate recurrences with sexual contact.[14,30] Yeasts are carried by 5–26 percent of male partners,[14,26] and 80 percent of the female partners of infected men are vaginally colonized.[14,30] Conjugal partners usually carry the same strain.[14,90] Simultaneous treatment of male partners, however, does not delay symptomatic recurrence,[91] and the effect on vaginal recolonization is minimal.[67,77] Reinfection from contaminated douche equipment has also been proposed.[14] Contaminated underwear appears to play no role.[89]

Vaginal reinfection from a persistent rectal focus has been alleged, but support for this contention is weak. Admittedly, 40–70 percent of women with VC have positive rectal cultures, and 80 percent of doubly colonized women carry the same strain in rectal and vaginal sites,[14,26,30,92] but simultaneous treatment of a rectal focus with oral nystatin or systemic ketoconazole[67–69] does not significantly lower recolonization or recurrence rates over vaginal therapy alone. One large study does suggest a benefit of adding oral nystatin to topical therapy, showing decreased colonization and symptomatic relapse rates. The study suffers from a relatively short, 3–7 week, follow-up period and a poorly defined subject population.[95] Care must therefore be taken in interpreting these results. Whether selected women might benefit from coincident gastrointestinal therapy is unclear.

Endogenous vaginal relapse from small numbers of yeasts that survive chemotherapy has also been suggested.[12,27,30] This contention is supported by the rapidity with which vaginal cultures return to positive after treatment and the frequency with which recurring strains are the same as those causing the previous infection.[30] Intracellular residence may protect some fungal cells from antimycotic agents.[14,26,30] Small numbers of yeasts would certainly be invisible on wet mount and even by culture,[14] so early post-treatment evaluation might erroneously suggest a cure. As Lossick[96] has remarked, the frequency with which

Candida is carried asymptomatically suggests that mere reintroduction of yeasts into the vagina is not an adequate cause of symptomatic recurrence; host susceptibility must also play a role.[30] In addition to the risk factors described above, some women with recurrent VC appear to be mildly zinc deficient[97] or have defective cell-mediated immunity to yeasts.[98,99] The significance of these findings is unclear. Tolerance may be induced by chronic infection rather than serving as its cause.[14,30]

If our lack of understanding of recurrence is dispiriting, our lack of effective therapy is intensely frustrating to patients and clinicians. One should attempt to reduce or eliminate the aforementioned risk factors. Short courses of topical antifungal therapy administered on the days 5–11 of the menstrual cycle[100] or immediately preceding[67,68] or following[101,102] menses reduce but by no means eliminate symptomatic recurrences. Likewise, 200 mg of itraconazole orally on days 5 and 6 of the menstrual cycle suppresses symptoms for the duration of therapy.[103] Such treatment is obviously not curative and rapidly becomes oppressively expensive. Simultaneous treatment of a rectal focus with oral nystatin or systemic treatment with ketoconazole does not significantly reduce the relapse rate.[69,93,94] Continuous daily treatment with ketoconazole,[68] or fluconazole[30] prevents recurrences but only for the duration of treatment. In some cases of frequently recurrent VC, a switch to lower dose oral contraceptives or even a discontinuance of oral contraceptives may be indicated. Oral glucose tolerance tests in such women have very low yield and are not routinely recommended.[14,30] Rarely, examination of sexual partners may reveal candidal balanitis, which could conceivably be a source of exogenous reinfection.

A recent, prospective, much publicized study[104] reported that daily ingestion of yogurt containing live *Lactobacillus acidophilus* decreased the rate of vaginal recolonization and symptomatic relapse in women with frequently recurrent disease. The study is flawed by small sample size, lack of suitable design (i.e., double blinding) and controls (i.e., yogurt lacking live organisms), and possible biases.[105] Although oral administration of lactobacilli does increase the lactobacillary content of the intestine,[9] its value in preventing VC remains highly speculative.

Disease in Men. The contribution of sexual transmission to vaginal candidiasis is apparently considerably smaller than for other forms of vaginitis. Balanitis, however, has been reported in 3–10 percent of the male sexual partners of women with candidal vulvovaginitis, and this condition is clearly sexually transmitted.[14,47,106,107] It responds to antifungal creams or ointments and treatment of the involved women. Some men develop pruritus within minutes of sexual contact. Symptoms usually resolve by the following day, and this syndrome may result from hypersensitivity to a partner's vaginal yeast.[14]

Trichomoniasis

Estimates based on the amount of metronidazole sold in this country suggest that 3 million Americans are infected with *Trichomonas vaginalis* each year. The disease is almost always sexually acquired and usually produces a combination of vaginal discharge and vulvovaginal irritation. About 25 percent of the women carrying trichomonads are asymptomatic, and the parasite has been recovered from up to 5 percent of sexually active asymptomatic women in Great Britain. The infection is discussed in detail in Chapter 260, to which the reader is referred.

Bacterial Vaginosis

Most women presenting to their physicians with vaginal symptoms have a specific condition first described by Gardner and Dukes in 1955.[108] This condition is now usually referred to, perhaps unfortunately from a linguistic standpoint,[109] as *bacterial vaginosis* (BV).[110,111] Inflammation and perivaginal irritation are considerably milder than in trichomoniasis or candidiasis. Dysuria and dyspareunia are correspondingly rare. Affected women are usually sexually active and often complain predominantly of vaginal odor. This odor is described as "fishy" in the textbooks more frequently than by the patients. About 90 percent of patients also notice a mild to moderate discharge. Abdominal discomfort is occasionally present, but it is usually mild and should prompt evaluation for coincident infections, including salpingitis.

Discharge is often present at the introitus and visible on the labia minora. The labia and vulva are generally not erythematous or edematous. On speculum examination, the vaginal walls usually appear uninflamed. The vagina often contains a grayish, thin, homogeneous discharge manifesting small bubbles. This discharge differs from normal, physiologic discharge in that the latter has a floccular appearance, and bubbles are absent. Although the discharge may be heavy enough to pool in the posterior fornix, it is usually present in smaller amounts. In some patients, the discharge may be so slight that it does not conspicuously pool. Because it is relatively thin but adherent to the vaginal walls, it is often apparent only as an increased light reflex, giving rise to the impression that the vaginal walls are too wet. A distinct, pungent odor may be noted by the examiner.

The endocervix is unaffected by the process, and cervical discharge should be physiologic and therefore mucoid. The presence of a purulent cervical discharge or frank cervicitis is not rare but results from coincident gonococcal, chlamydial, or herpetic infection.[112] Abnormalities on bimanual examination are unusual in uncomplicated BV and should prompt a search for other pathologic processes. There is an increased risk of salpingitis among women with BV.[113]

Other vaginal infections may closely resemble BV; an accurate differential diagnosis depends on laboratory examination of the genital specimen. The pH of vaginal discharge is elevated above the normal of 4.5 in about 90 percent of women with BV.[108,114,115] Although the pH may also be elevated in trichomoniasis, it is usually normal in VC. A vaginal pH of 5 or higher strongly suggests infection.[116] If 10–20% KOH is added to vaginal discharge samples either in the speculum blade or on a microscope slide, a distinctively pungent, fishy odor is generated.[9,10,114,117–119] This positive "whiff test" has been used as part of the case definition of BV by some workers and has been found to be positive in about 70 percent of cases in other series.[114,118] The accuracy of this test appears to improve with experience,[119] but the test is also positive in some patients with trichomoniasis, and its predictive value is therefore limited in populations with a high prevalence of the protozoal infection.

Bacterial vaginosis is perhaps most easily differentiated from trichomoniasis on the basis of direct microscopic examination of vaginal discharge. A wet mount of the discharge from patients with BV reveals clue cells, which are vaginal epithelial cells studded with tiny coccobacilli. These organisms are best appreciated at the edges of the cell (Fig. 1) but may be dense enough to obscure the nucleus partially. Not all cells in the specimen are clue cells, but some clue cells are seen in over 90 percent of patients with BV.[119,120] Predominant bacterial flora can also be assessed on a wet mount slide. In healthy women, the predominant morphotype is a large rod (presumably *Lactobacillus* species). In the discharge from a patient with BV, these rods have been completely supplanted by clumps of coccobacilli. Similar discrimination can be made on the basis of a Gram stain of the vaginal discharge[10,111,121–123] or on cervical cytology.[124] Discharge in BV contains few polymorphonuclear neutrophils (PMN). This may in part explain the absence of the green or yellow color that frequently characterizes the discharge in trichomoniasis. Up to about one PMN per epithelial cell is considered normal in a vaginal wet mount. Finding increased numbers of PMN in a patient with BV suggests the presence of a second inflammatory process, often coincidental cervicitis.[112]

Culture for *G. vaginalis* is easily accomplished on a variety

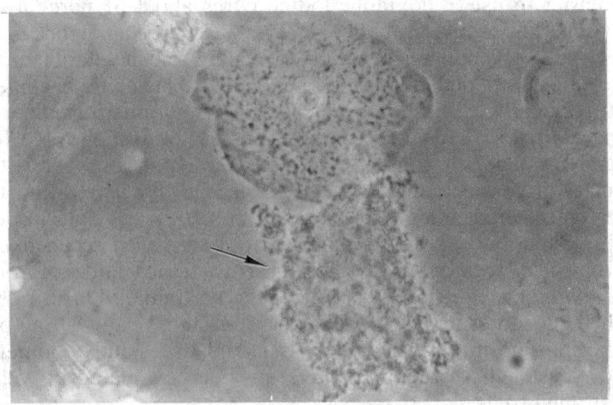

FIG. 1. A wet mount of vaginal discharge from a patient with bacterial vaginosis shows epithelial cells, neutrophils, and trichomonads (arrows). (Phase microscopy, ×400)

of media (see Ch. 204). The organism is isolated from 92–98 percent of women with BV,[10,111,119,125] but it is also recovered in smaller numbers from up to 70 percent of some populations of asymptomatic women,[2,3,10,15,111,125–127] and its presence does not therefore prove that the patient has BV or suggest a need for treatment. Thin-layer chromatography, gas-liquid chromatography, and enzyme assays can be used to diagnose BV by identifying specific bacterial products.[10,111,115,128–130] These techniques are not routinely performed, but they provide insight into the pathophysiology of BV.

Amsel et al.[119] have suggested that the clinician look for a pH greater than 4.5; homogeneous, white, adherent vaginal discharge; a positive whiff test; and clue cells. Finding any three of these four signs strongly supports the diagnosis of BV, although an abnormal discharge, an elevated pH, and a positive whiff test often accompany trichomoniasis as well. These criteria have become somewhat standardized in the literature, but several reasonable modifications have been suggested, and studies confirm that the finding of clue cells is the most specific of the criteria.[111,131] Rather than rigidly adhering to statistical criteria, however, the clinician should base the final diagnosis and decision to treat on a complete evaluation of the patient. Speigel[111] provides a recent, excellent review of the topic.

Epidemiology. Bacterial vaginosis was initially described in sexually active women and is common in populations with a high prevalence of sexually transmitted diseases. The precise contribution of sexual transmission to the overall epidemiology of the condition remains controversial. Support of a significant role for sexual transmission includes the following observations: *(1)* BV is more prevalent among women with greater numbers of recent and lifetime sexual partners[132–134] and in populations with a higher prevalence of other STD[21]; *(2)* symptoms first develop in many women shortly after they become sexually active[108]; *(3)* vaginal recolonization with *G. vaginalis* is far more common in women reexposed to untreated male partners than to those who are not[114]; and *(4) G. vaginalis* is recovered from the urethras of more than 80 percent of the male sexual partners of infected women,[108,114] and they are almost always of the same biotype.[111]

Several observations argue against exclusively sexual transmission: *(1) G. vaginalis* can be isolated from prepubescent girls[2,3] and sexually inactive women[10,11]; *(2)* the syndrome of bacterial vaginosis has been recognized in virgins[135]; *(3)* recurrences are observed in the absence of sexual reexposure; *(4)* initial, simultaneous treatment of sexual partners cannot be shown to reduce recurrence rates[136–138]; *(5)* the age and racial distribution of BV differs from that of gonorrhea, being relatively more likely to occur in older, white women[21]; and *(6)* the organisms associated with BV can be cultured from the rectum, from which site, it is speculated, they might colonize the vagina.[139]

The association of bacterial vaginosis with sexual transmission is sufficiently well established that clinicians diagnosing bacterial vaginosis should screen affected women for other sexually transmitted diseases, such as gonococcal or chlamydial infections, which may be clinically silent but of greater eventual medical significance. It is not demonstrably necessary to treat male sexual partners of women with an initial diagnosis of BV. Some women suffering from frequently recurring BV can be cured, however, only if sexual partners are treated as well. Still, the factors leading to recurrence are not completely understood, and recurrence should not be considered diagnostic of reinfection. The possible contribution of sexual contact to recurrent disease in an individual case may be difficult to determine, but the need for treating sexual partners might be supported by a history of symptoms recurring only after contact with a particular partner.

Pathophysiology. Microscopic examination of vaginal discharge in BV characteristically reveals a predominant flora of coccobacilli. On the basis of its morphology, this organism was originally called *Haemophilus vaginalis*.[108] It has now been given to its own genus and is called *Gardnerella vaginalis* in honor of Dr. Gardner's initial observations (see Ch. 204).[140] Several observations suggest a less than straightforward relationship between *G. vaginalis* and BV. Although Gardner and Dukes regularly produced BV by inoculating fresh vaginal discharge from patients into the vaginas of healthy recipients, inoculation of a pure culture of *G. vaginalis* was far less likely to produce disease.[108] In addition, *G. vaginalis* is isolated from 30–40 percent of asymptomatic women,[2,3,10,11,15,119,125–127] and only 50 percent of women with heavy vaginal colonization by *G. vaginalis* actually have BV.[127] Finally, the in vitro sensitivity of *G. vaginalis* to antimicrobial agents does not match the effectiveness of these agents in clinical disease. Metronidazole is highly effective therapy for BV[114,117,138,141–145] despite the fact that *G. vaginalis* is relatively resistant to the drug in vitro.[114,142,146]

An explanation for all these observations is that *G. vaginalis* is not the single cause of BV. There is considerable experimental support for the hypothesis that BV is actually a synergistic infection involving not only *G. vaginalis* but certain anaerobic bacteria as well.[8,10,18,111,114,115,118,130,145,147] The total number of such organisms is dramatically increased in the vaginas of women with BV. Various *Bacteroides* and *Prevotella* species other than *B. fragilis* and various peptococci are principally involved. Asymptomatic carriers of *G. vaginalis* might lack the anaerobic synergants. Pure cultures of *G. vaginalis* would not be able to produce clinical disease in patients lacking the other necessary bacteria, but the vaginal discharge from symptomatic women would be expected to contain all the necessary bacterial components. Drugs relatively inactive against *G. vaginalis* might still cure the disease if they acted against the other bacteria, and metronidazole is highly active against most strict anaerobes. The characteristic odor of BV is due to various aromatic amines such as triethylamine, putrescine, and cadaverine, which are produced by anaerobes but not by *G. vaginalis*.[115] These aromatic diamines are volatilized at basic pH, which explains the positive whiff test associated with the infection.

Most cases of BV are also associated with motile, curved anaerobic rods that are gram negative or gram variable.[111,139,148–155] These organisms, classified in the new genus *Mobiluncus*,[156] are sensitive to ampicillin, but some species are relatively resistant to metronidazole.[151,154] The precise pathogenic role of these organisms remains to be elucidated.

Mycoplasma hominis is isolated from the vaginas of many women with BV.[15,16,125,157,158] A role in the production of BV has not been established.

Hydrogen peroxide–producing lactobacilli appear to play a major role in limiting *Gardnerella* and the anaerobic flora of the vagina.[113,125,159,160] These lactobacilli are present in the vaginas of 60 percent of normal women but in only 5 percent of women with BV.[125,159,160]

Treatment. Applicable regimens are summarized in Table 3. Many studies[114,117,136,141–145,161,162] have shown that BV is successfully treated with metronidazole, 500 mg orally twice daily or 250 mg orally three times daily for 7 days. Cure rates of 80–90 percent are reported. Several good studies suggest that single doses of metronidazole are inadequate,[10,129,136,137,142–144,161,162] but a recent meta-analysis supports the value of a single 2 g dose.[138] Clindamycin is active against anaerobes and *G. vaginalis* in vitro, and 300 mg orally twice daily for 7 days is effective therapy for BV.[163] Ampicillin is highly active in vitro against *G. vaginalis*, with a minimum inhibitory concentration (MIC) of less than 2 μg/ml for most strains.[10,145,161] Although a few small studies have suggested a high cure rate for BV with ampicillin or amoxicillin,[120,145] larger experience reveals inadequate efficacy.[114,141,144,145] The inferiority of ampicillin to metronidazole probably derives in part from its inactivation by penicillinase elaborated by *Bacteroides* or *Prevotella* species in the vagina[114,145]; however, the combination of amoxicillin with clavulanic acid is still inferior to metronidazole.[144] Ampicillin, amoxicillin, and probably clindamycin block recolonization of the vagina by normal lactobacilli, whereas metronidazole does not.[145] Recolonization with lactobacilli may be part of the process of recovery from BV.

The value of oral cephalosporins for BV remains somewhat controversial. Gardner and Dukes praised them anecdotally,[108,164] as do other workers. Indeed, cephalexin, 500 mg taken four times daily for 1 week, has cured some women whose disease relapsed after repeated treatments with metronidazole. Limited data also suggest a role for cefadroxil, 500 mg twice daily for 7 days.[165] Oral therapy with tetracyclines, erythromycin, or the fluoroquinolones has been disappointing.[10,166]

Recently released topical therapies have proven effective and are of use in women who prefer not to take oral medications. Clindamycin 2% cream used in an intravaginal regimen of 5 g nightly for seven doses yields cure rates of about 75–95 percent, results that are not significantly different from those obtained with oral metronidazole in the same studies.[167–171] Metronidazole 0.75 percent vaginal gel is applied as 5 g twice daily for 5 days. Data on this regimen suggest cure rates of about 80–90 percent, again comparable to the results obtained with oral metronidazole.[172–174] Vulvovaginal candidiasis occurred in some women receiving topical treatments, but other toxicities were rare. Absorption of metronidazole from the vagina produces serum levels approximately 4 percent of those following a single 500-mg oral dose, and steady-state levels after multiple doses are about 275 ng/ml.[175] The cost of the topicals is currently considerably higher than that of oral metronidazole.

Sulfanilamide-aminacrine-allantoin cream is no longer available. Povidone-iodine has an unacceptably low cure rate.[10] Triple sulfa preparations have been used topically for some de-

TABLE 3. Regimens for the Treatment of Bacterial Vaginosis

Oral regimens
  Metronidazole, 500 mg po bid for 7 days
  Metronidazole, 250 mg po tid for 7 days
  Metronidazole, 2 g po as a single dose[a]
  Clindamycin, 300 mg po bid for 7 days[b]
  Cephalexin, 250 mg po qid for 7 days[c]
  Cefadroxil, 500 mg po bid for 7 days[b]
Vaginal regimens
  Clindamycin 2% vaginal cream, 5 g vaginally qhs for 7 days
  Metronidazole 0.75% vaginal gel, 5 g vaginally bid for 5 days

[a] The equivalence of this regimen to the week courses remains somewhat controversial.
[b] Limited clinical data.
[c] Principally anecdotal data.

cades, but small series suggest that the compounds are ineffective.[114,176] Topical therapy with acetic acid has no value.[177,178] On the other hand, preliminary European experience supports the value of a topical lactate gel.[179,180] Topical treatment with yogurt, in an effort to reinstitute a lactobacillary flora, has yielded inconsistent results in very small studies. One study shows little effect,[181] whereas another describes a cure in 28 out of 32 women at a 2-month follow-up.[178] The difference might have resulted from the presence of live hydrogen peroxide–producing lactobacilli in one yogurt preparation but not the other. Further study is required before such treatment can be recommended. A trial of a commercially available, Danish, topical *Lactobacillus* product showed no benefit among women evaluated 20–40 days following treatment.[182] Several other commercially available topical *Lactobacillus*-containing products have not been subject to clinical trial and may not be microbiologically suitable because they are likely to contain inappropriate *Lactobacillus* species, which do not produce hydrogen peroxide, and they are frequently contaminated with other bacteria.[183]

There are no data supporting the need to treat asymptomatic male sexual partners initially.[10,138] Some women, however, suffer from frequently relapsing disease that can be controlled only by the simultaneous treatment of male sexual partners. The drug of choice for the treatment of such partners has not been defined; metronidazole, clindamycin, or even amoxicillin each has advocates. Vaginal carriage of *G. vaginalis* in the absence of signs or symptoms of BV is common and need not be treated. The treatment of asymptomatic women with BV diagnosed on examination remains controversial[184] but should be undertaken in women about to undergo instrumentation of the upper genital tract[129,184] or prior to delivery (see below).

Complications of Bacterial Vaginosis. The reader is referred to Chapter 204 for a description of other infections caused by *Gardnerella vaginalis*. The organism is recovered from the urethras of asymptomatic men; it does not cause urethritis.

Bacterial vaginosis cannot be considered a totally benign condition. Among women with BV there is a significantly increased risk of salpingitis,[113] particularly following abortion,[185,186] and of vaginal cuff and wound infection after hysterectomy.[113,187,188] BV is associated with postpartum fever, endometritis, and salpingitis.[167,185,189–194] Premature labor and delivery occur more frequently in women with BV than in other women.[191,195–199] A true pathogenic role for BV in these settings is supported by the recovery of microorganisms associated with BV from amniotic fluid, wound infections, and blood. These observations give added impetus to the treatment of BV in pregnancy and before instrumentation.

Other Vaginal Infections

Staphylococci. *Staphylococcus aureus* is recovered from the vaginas of only about 5 percent of healthy women.[11] The organism is isolated, however, from most women with catamenial toxic shock syndrome (see Ch. 173).[200,201] A history of vaginitis is associated with an increased incidence of toxic shock syndrome.[202] The disease is usually characterized by vulvar edema and vulvar and vaginal erythema.[210] A vaginal discharge, purulent but often scanty, is observed in about one-fourth to one-third of these patients,[200,201] and vaginal ulceration was noted in about 7 percent.[201] The pathogenesis of the vaginitis is not entirely understood. Toxic shock syndrome is manifested as a polymucositis, and vaginitis is also reported in about one-third of women who have nonmenstrual toxic shock syndrome, sometimes with the staphylococcal source at sites other than the vagina. Thus, the vaginitis may reflect direct infection or may be a secondary effect of staphylococcal toxin. The ulcerations sometimes observed may result from tampon use, with which toxic shock syndrome is associated.

Foreign Body Vaginitis. Secondary anaerobic infections may be associated with foreign bodies in the vagina. In adults, the most common of these are the forgotten vaginal tampon and various contraceptive devices such as the diaphragm, cervical cap, or a condom that has slipped off during coitus. Objects apparently used in masturbation are occasionally implicated.[203] In children and the mentally incompetent, a variety of objects may be found.[1] These infections often produce an intensely foul odor, and the discharge is usually scanty and contains small amounts of blood. Therapy often requires only the removal of the offending object, but oral metronidazole may speed recovery.

Tampon use affects the vaginal mucosa.[204–207] Extended tampon use, particularly of superabsorbent tampons, may produce local drying and peeling of the vaginal mucosa and result in frank ulceration of the vaginal wall and endocervix. Tampon fibers have been observed within ulcerations.[206] Microscopic ulcers have been noted in up to one-fifth of women using tampons,[123] and larger lesions are occasionally observed.[205,207] Ulceration may be associated with vaginal bleeding and pain on insertion of the tampons. Because of possible confusion with other ulcerating vaginal diseases, including malignancy, a thorough work-up is essential.[207]

Herpes Simplex Virus. The adult vaginal epithelium is relatively resistant to herpetic infection. Vaginal lesions have been observed in only about 4 percent of infected women.[208,209] Fourteen percent of women with primary genital herpes developed vulvovaginal candidiasis during the second week of infection.[208,209] Treatment of these secondary infections, however, must be done carefully, because the topical antifungal miconazole cream appears to be associated with delayed healing of genital herpetic lesions.[210] Indeed, the application of any occlusive preparation to herpetic lesions should probably be avoided,[208,209] and therapy of accompanying VC with an oral imidazole or triazole would be preferred in this setting.

Human Papillomavirus. Genital warts inside the vagina often assume a more filiform shape than do those on the vulva. Micropapillomatosis manifests as sheets of tiny warts (see Ch. 122).

Less Common Infections. True vaginal infections with other specific agents such as *Mycobacterium tuberculosis,* salmonellae, Enterobacteriaceae, actinomycetes, and schistosomes are rare and usually occur in patients with underlying diseases or who are systemically ill. Group A streptococcal vaginitis has been described in children aged 3–5 years old. It presents with a blood-tinged discharge, "firey red" vaginal mucosae, and dysuria. A Gram stain is usually negative, and the disease responds promptly to penicillin G.[211]

Preexisting lesions due to other diseases may become secondarily infected with a mixed anaerobic flora of fusobacteria and spirochetes. Such "fusospirochetal" infections can progress rapidly. Metronidazole, 250 mg orally three times daily, is recommended therapy.

Pinworms are an occasional cause of perivaginal itching, especially in children.[1] Perianal pruritus that becomes worse at night may suggest this diagnosis. True vaginal infestation has been described.[212]

Neisseria gonorrhoeae and *C. trachomatis* can cause frank vaginitis in prepubescent girls.[213]

"Doderlein cytolysis" or "cytolytic vaginosis," a condition characterized by irritative symptoms exacerbated in the premenstrual interval and theoretically caused by microbially induced hyperacidity, is poorly substantiated. It is said to result from an overgrowth of lactobacilli and to be diagnosed by finding abnormally large numbers of rods, "bare or naked intermediate [cell] nuclei," and relatively few PMN on a vaginal wet mount. The vaginal pH is reportedly below 4.5. The condition is said to respond to akalinizing douches.[214]

Noninfectious Vulvovaginitis

Genital neoplasm may result in an abnormal vaginal discharge. Such conditions are more common in older women and are usually manifested by the gradual onset of a thin, often foul-smelling discharge that may be blood tinged. In postmenopausal women, the absence of estrogen stimulation results in atrophy of the vaginal epithelium, which may lead to an atrophic vaginitis. The vaginal walls become secondarily infected with a number of different organisms, but treatment of the primary disease often requires estrogenic supplementation.

Occasional cases of vulvovaginal inflammation from chemicals,[215] including deodorant sprays[216] and allergic reactions to semen[217] and nickel,[218] have been reported. Fixed drug eruptions frequently involve the genitalia, particularly in association with oral tetracyclines or sulfonamides. Lesions usually consist of dusky red to purple plaques that may be surmounted by ulcers. Patients with episodic genital lesions should be carefully questioned about recent oral medications.

Desquamative or purulent vaginitis is characterized by a vaginal discharge containing large numbers of PMN. The etiology and therapy of the condition are unknown, but lichen planus should be considered in the differential diagnosis.[219–221] Treatment is not well defined, but anecdotal experience supports the use of topical steroids[221] or clindamycin.

Related Considerations and Conditions

Physiologic or normal vaginal discharge is sometimes referred to as *leukorrhea* and generally consists of cervical mucus combined with desquamated vaginal epithelial cells. This material passes through the vaginal introitus, where it is perceived by the patient as a vaginal discharge. Neonates may have a transient physiologic discharge until transplacentally acquired maternal estrogens are metabolized. In the adult, the output of the endocervical glands is highly responsive to hormonal levels and sometimes increases at the time of ovulation or in the immediate premenstrual period. Oral contraceptives may increase the cervical component, and women sometimes note a new discharge when they start to use these agents. This leukorrhea may cause considerable concern since it often begins coincidentally with first sexual exposures, thus raising the specter of venereal disease. Physiologic discharge accounted for 10 percent of women attending a private practice with vaginal complaints.[32] It may be heavy enough to stain underwear and may dry to a brown residue, which patients sometimes associate with infectious vaginitis. Unlike most infections, it is usually not associated with perineal burning or pruritus, dyspareunia, or dysuria, but an odor is sometimes described.[222] Abdominal pain does not occur unless another process is present. Microscopic examination reveals normal vaginal flora and few PMN. More than one PMN per epithelial cell is unusual in physiologic vaginal discharge.

Infectious cervicitis due to any of several different organisms may result in an inflammatory cervical discharge that passes through the vagina. This condition is discussed in a later section of this chapter. A variety of inflammatory diseases confined to the perineum may produce symptoms suggesting vaginitis to the patient. The lesions of herpes genitalis or chancroid produce considerable perineal discomfort. Intertrigo may result in burning, an unpleasant odor, and staining of underwear. Infections of Bartholin's glands and Skene's glands sometimes produce perineal discomfort and a discharge and are discussed in a later section of this chapter. Inflammatory diseases of the rectum occasionally result in a discharge that suggests vaginitis to the patient. Dysuria may be a symptom of urinary tract infection.

Of particular interest is a condition referred to as *vulvar vestibulitis, focal vulvitis,* or *vestibular adenitis* and that may be more common than previously suspected.[223–226] Affected women suffer vulvar pain and significant dyspareunia. They are sometimes unable to sit comfortably or wear tight clothing. These women frequently undergo repeated treatments for vulvovaginal candidiasis, and they are often thought to be neurotic. Physical examination reveals rather subtle but exquisitely tender, erythematous patches, usually along the posterior portion of the introital ring. Biopsy demonstrates nonspecific inflammation of vestibular glands.[224,227] The condition may be associated with interstitial cystitis.[228] Current therapy is surgical excision[229,230] or laser ablation[230] of the affected areas, with relief of discomfort obtained in about two-thirds of cases. An infectious etiology has not been convincingly demonstrated for all cases, but some infections with human papillomavirus (HPV) present with diffuse involvement of the labia minora yielding clinically similar pain.[231–233] When associated with HPV infection, vulvar vestibulitis appears to respond to intradermal interferon.[234] Biopsy and DNA probe may be required to differentiate between the conditions.

Vaginitis emphysematosa is an uncommon condition in which the vaginal walls contain submucosal, gas-filled cysts.[235–237] The endocervix too may be involved.[238] This benign condition is frequently associated with trichomoniasis or with bacterial vaginosis and resolves after treatment of the accompanying infection.

Obstruction of the pelvic nodes is a rare cause of lymphatic weeping of the vagina. Massive lymphedema of the lower extremities usually accompanies this finding, and the diagnosis is not difficult to make.

There are small numbers of women who complain of vaginal discharge, discomfort, or odor without any objective findings.[239] Such women may be motivated by a neurotic fear of uncleanliness, guilt concerning sexual activities (or a desire to avoid them), or anxiety about venereal disease, whether or not sexual exposure has actually taken place. These patients have often sought advice from numerous physicians and have symptoms that have failed to respond to a variety of standard therapies. They require careful and complete medical evaluation. The diagnosis of "worried well" must not be made without a thorough examination for physical disease. Women with psychosomatic complaints may respond to a careful and sympathetic explanation of the results of the examination and to psychotherapy.[239]

Scabies, pediculosis, or enterobiasis may produce intense perivaginal itching and soreness.

APPROACH TO THE PATIENT WITH VAGINAL COMPLAINTS

History

The etiologic diagnosis of vaginitis depends on a careful evaluation of the history, physical examination, and immediate laboratory tests. Historical features are relatively nonspecific,[10,23] but they may direct clinical suspicion toward certain causes.

Age. Neonates can acquire trichomonal or candidal vulvovaginitis during passage through an infected birth canal, an argument for treating these infections in pregnant women before term. Neonatal vaginal thrush responds promptly to topical antifungal medications.[1] Neonatal trichomoniasis often does not require specific therapy and disappears when the estrogens are metabolized.[240] After the neonatal period, any vaginal discharge is abnormal and should prompt a vigorous search for disease. Sexual abuse may also be a consideration. Prepubescent vaginal epithelium is not cornified, and the entire vagina is susceptible to infection with *N. gonorrhoeae* or *C. trachomatis.* Gonococcal vulvovaginitis often causes profuse vaginal discharge, and the rectum is almost always involved. Vaginal candidiasis is extremely rare in prepubescent girls.[241] Immediately before menarche, physiologic discharge reappears. A diagnosis of sexually transmitted disease in a young girl should raise the suspicion of child abuse, although some agents have been transmitted to children in the absence of frank sexual contact.

Patients in the sexually active years are more likely to have a sexually transmitted disease. Genital neoplasia is more common among older women, and postmenopausal women are more likely to have atrophic vaginitis.

Mode of Onset. An abrupt and identifiable time of onset of symptoms suggests infection. Vaginal discharge associated with neoplasia, estrogen depletion, or a foreign body often has a subacute onset, with symptoms progressing over a period of weeks. Symptoms beginning during or immediately after the menstrual period are somewhat suggestive of trichomoniasis, and a premenstrual onset more frequently accompanies candidiasis.

Quantity of Discharge. The amount of discharge is highly variable in all conditions. Patients with candidiasis often have scanty discharge or note no discharge at all. Atrophic or neoplastic discharges are commonly scanty unless infection has supervened.

Perineal Irritation. Physiologic discharge is rarely associated with perineal discomfort. Pruritus with a scanty or absent discharge is frequently seen in candidiasis and less commonly with trichomoniasis. Perineal discomfort is an infrequent complaint in BV. Severe episodic perineal pain sometimes preventing urination is strongly suggestive of herpes genitalis, which affects the labia but usually spares the vagina per se.[35,36] Chronic discomfort, often interfering with sexual activity, should prompt consideration of vulvar vestibulitis.

Odor. An unpleasant odor accompanies many vaginal infections and sometimes physiologic discharge as well.[222] Vaginal odor in the absence of other symptoms is the initial complaint in many cases of BV. A feculent odor may accompany anaerobic superinfection of genital lesions or may be noted in the presence of a foreign body.

Abdominal Pain. Abdominal discomfort is rare in uncomplicated vulvovaginitis except for occasional cases of trichomoniasis. Women complaining of abdominal pain should be examined carefully for evidence of coincidental infections, including cystitis and pelvic inflammatory disease.

Sexual History. Exposure to a new sexual partner increases the likelihood of sexually transmitted disease. A history of genital symptoms in a sexual partner is helpful diagnostically. The commencement of oral contraceptive use may be associated with increased physiologic discharge. The use of tampons, particularly the prolonged use of superabsorbent tampons, may be associated with ulcerative vaginitis.[204–207]

Other Diseases. Diabetes, AIDS, malignancy and the treatment thereof, and possibly hypoparathyroidism increase the risk of candidal vaginitis. Diseases known to impair host defenses may predispose to otherwise rare infections. Other diseases may be treated with drugs that predispose to vaginal infection.

Medication. Systemic or local medication influences the spectrum of vaginal infection. Antibiotics, particularly tetracyclines and ampicillin, are active against much of the normal bacterial flora of the vagina, and their use predisposes to candidal vaginitis. Metronidazole is active against vaginal anaerobes and also predisposes to candidal infection, but less frequently than with many other antimicrobials. Low doses of many antibiotics can interfere with the isolation of *N. gonorrhoeae* and possibly *C. trachomatis*. Low-dose antibiotics may result in the development of atypical syphilitic chancres or may entirely eliminate the primary stage of syphilis. Patients taking corticosteroids or oral contraceptives are at increased risk for developing vulvovaginal candidiasis. Oral contraceptive use may also be associated with the development of a physiologic vaginal discharge. Local medication including vaginal douches rarely produce a chemical vaginitis, but douching immediately before examination makes etiologic diagnosis difficult.

Examination of the Female Genitalia

With the patient supine on the examining table, the pubic hair should be examined for the presence of crab lice or nits. The inguinofemoral areas are palpated for adenopathy. Suprapubic and lower abdominal tenderness or masses are sought by palpation. With the patient in the lithotomy position, the labia and the perineum should be examined for erythema, lichenification, excoriation, or discrete lesions. Diffuse perineal erythema may accompany trichomoniasis or candidiasis. Diffuse reddening with small satellite lesions, usually papular or papulopustular, suggests candidiasis. The degree of perineal irritation is quite variable with all infections, but severe perivaginal irritation is uncommon with BV. Labial edema may accompany severe irritation.

Careful examination of all the extravaginal surfaces may reveal lesions of herpes genitalis, syphilis, condyloma accuminata, molluscum contagiosum, scabies (which are discussed in Ch. 87), or vulvar vestibulitis. Even though the patient's chief complaint may strongly suggest a true vaginitis, examination of the external genitalia for coincident infections is very important because multiple, coexistent sexually transmitted diseases are common.

Applying a 3–5% solution of acetic acid to the vulva may reveal white areas where no lesions were grossly visible. Such acetowhite staining suggests the possibility of human papillomavirus infection. Several other conditions, such as lichen planus, psoriasis, acute inflammation, or healing tissue, may also stain acetowhite. Diagnosis must be based on the histologic appearance[242] of a biopsy specimen. Acetic acid staining is not indicated as part of the routine gynecologic examination but may be a useful adjunct in evaluating the patient with vulvar symptoms or known HPV infection.

By spreading the labia with the gloved hand, the urethral meatus is examined. The urethra may be gently stripped with the finger placed inside the introitus. Urethral discharge is not a common finding, but, if delivered, such material should be examined microscopically and cultured. The introitus and the internal surfaces of the labia minora should be examined for lesions. Vaginal discharge is sometimes observed on the labia or actually running out onto the perineum. Such copious discharge is usually associated with trichomoniasis but may accompany other infections.

If the patient has had a hysterectomy, a calcium alginate urethral swab should be inserted gently into the urethra and the recovered material inoculated for gonococcal culture. Urethral culture is unnecessary if the cervix is present since gonococci are more often recovered from the cervix than from the urethra. The urethra is in 25 percent of cases the only site from which *C. trachomatis* can be recovered.

A vaginal speculum moistened with warm water is gently inserted. In the presence of severe herpes genitalis or, occasionally, trichomoniasis, insertion of the speculum may be impossible because of the patient's discomfort. In such a case, a primary diagnosis is sometimes made from material recovered on a cotton swab gently inserted into the vagina. After the speculum has been inserted, the vaginal walls are examined. Candidal or trichomonal vaginitis is often accompanied by erythema of the vaginal walls. The degree of erythema, however, is often very difficult to assess in an individual patient. Punctate hemorrhages of the vaginal walls strongly suggest trichomoniasis. A diffuse sheen, manifested by an increased light reflex, may be caused by thin discharge adhering to the walls. This is seen most frequently with BV but may accompany other infections. Fingerlike projections within the vagina may be condylomata accuminata, but these must be differentiated from hymenal tags. The latter are normal but are usually found only near the introitus.

The surface of the cervix may be inflamed. Punctate hemorrhages are only rarely observed with the naked eye in patients with severe trichomoniasis (colpitis macularis, strawberry cervix), although they are revealed by colposcopy in almost 50 percent of cases.[243] Cervical ulcerations may be present in herpes genitalis. Mucoid material is normally observed at the cervical os and is present in increased amounts in women taking oral contraceptives. A normal cervical discharge may be clear or white, but purulent or mucopurulent discharge is associated with infectious cervicitis, primarily chlamydial, gonococcal, or herpetic.

Acetic acid staining of the vagina and cervix is useful as an adjunct to colposcopy but is not indicated during the routine genital examination.

Bimanual examination for adnexal tenderness and masses should be a part of the evaluation. Adnexal tenderness is sufficiently uncommon with local vaginal infections that its presence suggests salpingitis.

Other Bedside Evaluation. After the speculum is withdrawn, the pH of vaginal secretions can be determined by inserting a strip of indicator paper into the material collected in the lower lip of the speculum. We have found nitrazine paper with a pH range of 4.5–7.0 to be useful. A normal pH of 4.5 is seen in most patients with vulvovaginal candidiasis, whereas a pH elevated to 5.0 or above is associated with BV and trichomoniasis. Several drops of 10% KOH are then added to the material on the speculum. A resultant pungent, fishy, aminelike odor, constitutes a positive "whiff test." The whiff test is positive in more than 90 percent of patients with BV and in many patients with trichomoniasis. It is negative in women with vulvovaginal candidiasis. The whiff test may also be evaluated on a slide that has been prepared for KOH microscopic examination.

Laboratory Examination

A wet mount is of greatest value in the differential diagnosis of a vaginal discharge, and the specimen may be prepared in several ways. A swab of vaginal discharge may be agitated in a tube containing about 0.5 ml of normal saline. One drop of the resulting suspension is put on a microscope slide, and a coverslip is applied. Alternatively, the examiner may place a drop of saline on the slide and mix in a loop full of vaginal material, after which a coverslip is applied. The slide is examined initially under low power (×100) and then under high power (×400) on a brightfield microscope with the substage condenser racked down and with the substage diaphragm closed down to increase the contrast. Phase-contrast microscopy is becoming more widely available in clinical settings and provides an excellent means of evaluating vaginal wet mounts. The relative numbers of epithelial cells and PMN should be noted. PMN are present in physiologic endocervical discharge[243] that collects in the vagina, so small numbers of PMN may be observed in the vaginal material recovered from healthy women. Finding more than one PMN per epithelial cell should raise the examiner's suspicion of cervical or vaginal inflammation. Observing relatively few PMN, however, does not rule out vaginal infection. Vaginal candidiasis often produces a discharge containing only small numbers of PMN.[48] The relative absence of PMN is characteristic of the discharge of BV.[10] In fact, finding many PMN in the vaginal discharge of a patient with BV should prompt the examiner to search for simultaneous infection such as trichomoniasis, gonorrhea, or chlamydial cervicitis. Large clumps of pseudohyphae suggest vaginal candidiasis, but the examiner often sees only moderate or even very small numbers of yeasts in this condition. Indeed, some patients

with VC have organisms identified only by culture. The wet preparation should be scanned for motile trichomonads.

Normal squamous epithelial cells have transparent cytoplasm and small nuclei. Epithelial cells covered with tiny coccobacillary forms (Fig. 1) are called *clue cells* and are associated with BV. Clue cells are best recognized by observing the edges of epithelial cells, which may be obscured by the adherent coccobacilli. Some cells are so heavily encrusted that the nuclei are obscured. Trichomonads (Fig. 2) are best be recognized by their characteristic twitching motility. The flagella and undulating membrane may be observed by carefully focusing the microscope and adjusting the light source. Trichomonad motility is improved by gently warming the preparation. Unfortunately, the wet mount is negative in about 30 percent of the women with trichomoniasis (see Ch. 260), and a negative wet mount does not rule out this infection, particularly in relatively asymptomatic women. A negative wet mount should be confirmed with a culture. Small numbers of yeasts are frequently observed and do not necessarily indicate that the patient's vaginitis is of fungal etiology.

The bacterial flora can be assessed on the wet mount. Normal vaginal flora consists primarily of rods. In BV, the predominant flora is tiny coccobacilli. Spermatozoa may be observed as long as 10 days after the last coitus, but motile sperm suggest sexual contact within the preceding 24 hours.[244]

Combining a drop of 10% or 20% KOH with the vaginal material on a microscope slide, applying a coverslip, and gently heating will destroy cellular elements but leave the bacteria and fungi unscathed. The KOH preparation cannot be used for a microscopic diagnosis of trichomoniasis or BV, but elaboration of a fishy odor from the slide suggests either of these infections.

A Gram stain of vaginal material is somewhat less useful for differential diagnosis than is the wet mount, because, although *G. vaginalis* and *Candida* species are readily recognized on the Gram-stained smear, trichomonads are very difficult to identify. Normal vaginal flora consists primarily of gram-positive rods, which are presumably lactobacilli. In BV the normal flora is replaced by sheets of gram-variable coccobacilli, which often overly the surface of epithelial cells. Small numbers of yeasts are occasionally observed as dense, gram-positive or beaded ovoids, and women with active vaginal candidiasis sometimes have large numbers of budding yeasts and pseudohyphae recognizable as thick gram-positive or beaded tubes. Unfortunately, the Gram stain is positive in fewer than one-third of the women from whom *Candida* can be cultured.[50] The Gram stain of vaginal material should not be used for the diagnosis of gonorrhea, as gonorrhea is a cervicitis rather than a vaginitis in the adult.

Material recovered from the endocervix can be Gram stained. Cervical discharge always contains moderate numbers of PMN,

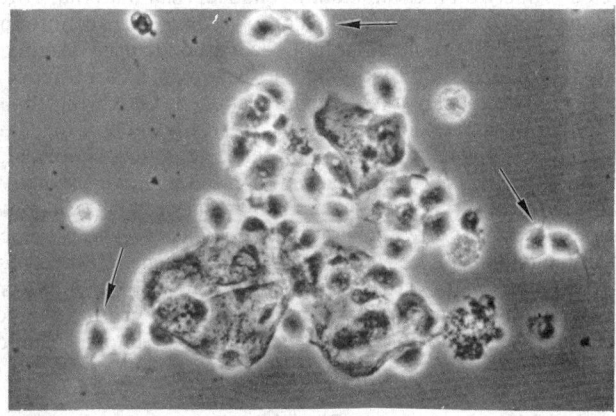

FIG. 2. A wet mount of vaginal discharge from a patient with trichomonal vaginitis shows epithelial cells, neutrophils, and trichomonads (arrows). (Phase microscopy, ×400)

and their presence is not necessarily an indication of specific inflammation.[243] Large numbers of PMN indicate cervicitis. Gram-negative, intracellular diplococci accurately diagnose gonorrhea (see Ch. 190), but extracellular diplococci are of no significance, since nonpathogenic *Neisseria* is part of the normal flora of the female genital tract. Unfortunately, the cervical Gram stain is positive in only about one-half of the women with cervical gonorrhea, and a negative Gram stain does not rule out the infection.[50] Trichomonads are only infrequently found in the endocervix, and cervical material should not be used to examine for trichomoniasis. Cervical material recovered from women at risk should be cultured for *N. gonorrhoeae* and evaluated for *C. trachomatis*. The Papanicolaou smear may reveal *T. vaginalis* or clue cells, but neither of these findings is sufficiently sensitive for a negative result to rule out infection. Direct staining of cervical specimens using the Giemsa or Papanicolaou methods is insufficiently sensitive for the diagnosis of chlamydial cervicitis (see Ch. 157).

CERVICITIS

Under the influence of estrogens, the normal vaginal epithelium cornifies and becomes relatively resistant to infection with a number of pathogens. The endocervix, however, is lined with columnar epithelium, which remains susceptible to many of these infections. Therefore, the examiner frequently finds infectious cervicitis in the absence of vaginitis and vice versa. Studies of the etiology of cervicitis have been hampered by the lack of a reliable definition of the syndrome.[110,245,246] Erythema around the cervical os may indicate infection or may merely represent cervical ectropion (previously called *erosion* or *eversion*), a term indicating migration of endocervical epithelium over the surface of the cervix. This lesion is usually symmetric about the os and is not particularly friable. It is accompanied by a mucoid cervical discharge. Ectropion is more common in women taking oral contraceptives, and the increased amount of exposed columnar epithelium may contribute to the greater risk of chlamydial infection among women taking oral contraceptives. It is often impossible on clinical grounds alone to differentiate ectropion from true infection. *Hypertrophic cervicitis,* on the other hand, is manifested as an intensely erythematous, raised, irregular lesion that bleeds easily.[112,245-247] This lesion is often associated with chlamydial infection.[112,245-247]

Normal cervical discharge is clear and mucoid. Purulent or mucopurulent discharge is associated with gonococcal or chlamydial infection.[112,248-250] The nature of the cervical discharge can be assessed by obtaining endocervical material on a swab and comparing its consistency and color against a well-illuminated sheet of white paper or cloth.

Polymorphonuclear neutrophils are normally present in the endocervix,[243] but abnormally increased numbers can be detected crudely on a Gram stain of endocervical material. After the endocervix has been cleaned off, a swab is inserted into the cervix and gently rotated, and the recovered material is applied to a microscope slide by rolling the swab over an area about 1 × 2 cm. The specimen is then Gram stained. Observing 10–30 PMN per oil-immersion field in the densest portion of the slide correlates statistically with the presence of gonococci or chlamydiae,[112,249,251-254] but the sensitivity and positive predictive value of the observation (both 25–45 percent in a high risk population) are far too low for a definitive diagnosis. The presence of inflammation on cervical cytology may suggest a need for further investigation, but only about 25 percent of high-risk women with inflammation on cervical cytology will have infection with *N. gonorrhoeae, C. trachomatis,* or human papillomavirus.[255-257]

Specific Etiologies of Acute Cervicitis

The clinical features of specific cervical infections overlap too much to permit an accurate etiologic diagnosis without labora-

tory assistance.[112,245,258] Multiple infections are common[258] and may be missed if the diagnosis is attempted on clinical grounds alone.

Acute gonococcal cervicitis has been known for hundreds of years. The endocervix is the site from which gonococci are most frequently isolated in women with uncomplicated gonococcal infections. In typical cases, the cervical os is reddened and productive of a purulent discharge.[259] A Gram stain of this material reveals typical gram-negative cell-associated diplococci in only about 50–75 percent of the infected women (Fig. 3),[50,253] and a negative Gram stain must never be used as an argument against treating women for uncomplicated gonorrhea. Examination for gonococcal cervicitis must include an appropriate culture. The sensitivity of the endocervical culture is disputed but is generally held to be on the order of 90 percent. Most women with uncomplicated gonococcal cervicitis are asymptomatic, but about one-third note vaginal discharge.[243,259] *Chlamydia trachomatis* can be recovered from the endocervix of 60–90 percent of the sexual partners of men with chlamydial urethritis.[243,245-247,260,261] Cervical abnormalities, often subtle, have been observed in 80–90 percent of chlamydia-positive women,[243,245-247,260,261] but about one-third note a discharge from the vagina[243] that actually originates in the inflamed cervix. Chlamydiae have been isolated from 50–90 percent of sexually active patients with hypertrophic cervicitis.[243] Only 19–32 percent of women with chlamydial cervical infection manifest hypertrophic cervicitis, and only about 30 percent have a mucopurulent or purulent cervical discharge.[243,245,246,248,262] On examination 20–70 percent[248,262] of infected women have a completely normal cervix. Therefore, physical examination never adequately excludes chlamydial infection, similar to the situation with gonococcal cervicitis. Female partners of men with nongonococcal urethritis should be epidemiologically treated even before the diagnosis of chlamydial infection is confirmed by laboratory techniques.

Chlamydiae can be identified in cervical specimens from 75 to 95 percent of infected women by using immunofluorescence microscopy.[250,262-265] Enzyme immunoassays are also 65–95 percent sensitive in women.[264-269] DNA probes detect chlamydial infection with a sensitivity of about 80 percent.[270,271] The lower cost of these culture-independent tests has made selective screening for chlamydiae advisable in certain populations.[272] Cervical cytology is not useful for screening because of its low sensitivity.[248,262,273] Colposcopy has revealed a typical follicular appearance in most cases and may be useful diagnostically.[274,275]

Herpes simplex virus is isolated from the cervix in 88 percent

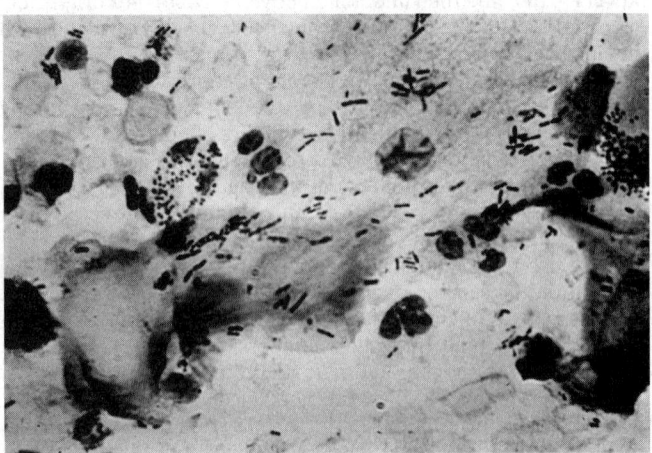

FIG. 3. Gram stain of cervical exudate from a woman with gonorrhea. A neutrophil contains many gram-negative diplococci. Other bacteria are normal vaginal flora. (×1000)

of women with primary infection but only from 12 percent of women with recurrent herpetic infection.[208,209] Herpetic cervicitis may be present without external lesions. Cervicitis is seen on physical examination in about 90 percent of women whose cervical culture are positive for herpes simplex virus.[208,209] The cervix usually displays diffuse friability and, less frequently, frank ulcers or necrosis.[208] Cervical discharge is usually mucoid, but it is occasionally mucopurulent, and in one series herpetic cervical infection caused 8 percent of cases of mucopurulent cervicitis.[112] Affected patients may have lower abdominal pain, but inguinal adenopathy is rare unless the disease is accompanied by lesions of the external genitalia[276] because lymphatic drainage of the cervix involves the external iliac rather than the inguinofemoral nodes. The diagnosis of herpetic cervicitis may be made cytologically by observing multinucleated giant cells, often with intranuclear inclusions.[277] In the presence of severe necrosis, however, cellular architecture is so distorted that cytologic examination becomes insensitive, and the diagnosis is best made by recovering the virus in tissue culture or by immunofluorescent staining.[278]

Human papillomavirus, particularly certain subtypes, frequently infects the cervix.[279] It has been observed since 1837 that cancer of the cervix behaves epidemiologically as if it were a sexually transmitted disease. The strongest infectious association with cancer of the cervix has been established for some types of human papillomavirus (see Ch. 122).[279,281,282]

Other organisms occasionally considered causes of cervicitis include adenovirus,[283] measles virus,[284] cytomegalovirus,[285] *Enterobius vermicularis*,[286] amoebae,[287] *Mycobacterium tuberculosis*,[288] group B streptococci,[289] *Neisseria meningitidis*,[290] and actinomycetes,[291] the last usually in association with the use of intrauterine contraceptive devices.

Therapeutic Approach to Cervicitis

Specifically diagnosed gonococcal cervicitis should be treated as recommended in Chapter 190. Because 30–60 percent of women with gonococcal cervicitis also have chlamydial infection, simultaneous treatment for both infections is advised when gonorrhea is diagnosed.[292,293] Cervicitis in patients who are the sexual partners of men with nongonococcal urethritis should be treated with doxycycline, 100 mg orally twice daily for 7 days; erythromycin, 500 mg orally four times daily for 7 days; or azithromycin, 1 g orally as a single dose (see Ch. 157). Because none of these regimens reliably cures gonorrhea, cervicitis of unknown etiology should probably be treated with one of the aforementioned regimens plus effective antigonococcal therapy. Management of cervicitis due to herpes simplex is discussed in Chapter 115.

INFECTIONS OF BARTHOLIN'S AND SKENE'S GLANDS

Bartholinitis

In the adult, Bartholin's gland is a 1 cm structure on each side of the vagina near the base of the labia minora. The healthy gland is not palpable and nontender. A 2 cm long duct lined with columnar epithelium opens on the inner surface of the labia minora at the junction of the posterior and middle thirds. Inflammation of the duct can produce blockage resulting in the development of a sterile cyst, and infection of the duct is said to be more common than infection of the gland itself.[294,295] Infection of the gland behind a blocked duct can result in the development of a Bartholin's gland abscess.

The frequency with which specific organisms infect Bartholin's glands is incompletely defined. Anaerobic and polymicrobic infections are common.[296] Early writers felt that clinically significant bartholinitis accompanied 2–50 percent of gonococcal infections.[294,295,297] Rees[295] recovered gonococci from the

glands of 28 percent of women with gonorrhea, most of whom were asymptomatic, but later workers recovered gonococci from only 5–12 percent of a series of patients with Bartholin's gland abscess.[298,299] Gonococcal bartholinitis is usually asymptomatic, but about 1 in 5 women has a palpable enlargement or tenderness of the glands, and 1 in 20 has edema.[295] The examiner should attempt to palpate the glands during the pelvic examination. If material can be expressed from the duct opening, it should be examined with the Gram stain, and it should be cultured.

Chlamydia trachomatis causes occasional cases of bartholinitis,[300] although its incidence is apparently low. Infection with normal genital flora is also significant. Single or mixed species of anaerobes have been recovered from up to 90 percent of the infected glands.[296,298,301-303] *Escherichia coli* and *Proteus mirabilis* are also frequently recovered.[298,301,303,304] *Staphylococcus aureus* is apparently a rare cause of abscess, but streptococci are frequently isolated.[298,301,305,306] *Haempohilus influenzae* has been recovered.[307]

Lee et al.[298] recovered *Ureaplasma urealyticum* from two-thirds of Bartholin's gland abscesses. Occasionally, herpes genitalis involves the duct and produces a transient but recurrent swelling of the gland.

Bartholinitis accompanying gonococcal infection can be treated like acute gonorrhea,[295] although some workers have recommended repeating the treatment daily for 3 days.[294] The optimal initial therapy for bartholinitis of uncertain etiology is not known. A combination of ofloxacin, in doses adequate for chlamydial infection, with clindamycin might be considered. Doxycycline alone has been used traditionally with good anecdotal results. A failure of bartholinitis to respond to antibiotic therapy suggests the need for surgical drainage of the abscess.[308,309] Complications of bartholinitis include toxic shock,[306] septic shock,[310] and necrotizing fasciitis.[311]

Skenitis

Skene's glands are small structures that empty into the urethra. Dysuria is the usual complaint of patients with infection of these glands, and sometimes a bead of pus can be expressed. The gonococcus is felt to produce some cases of skenitis,[294] but the role of other potential pathogens has not been determined. Empirical therapy should resemble that for bartholinitis.

REFERENCES

1. Lang WR. Pediatric vaginitis. N Engl J Med. 1955;253:1153.
2. Hammerschlag MR, Alpert S, Onderdonk AB, et al. Anaerobic microflora of the vagina in children. Am J Obstet Gynecol. 1978;131:853–60.
3. Hammerschlag MR, Alpert S, Rosner I, et al. Microbiology of the vagina in children: Normal and potentially pathogenic organisms. Pediatrics. 1978;62: 57–62.
4. Levison ME, Corman LC, Carrington ER, et al. Quantitative microflora of the vagina. Am J Obstet Gynecol. 1977;127:80.
5. Tashijan JH, Coulam CB, Washington JA. Vaginal flora in asymptomatic women. Mayo Clin Proc. 1976;51:557.
6. Brown WJ. Variations in the bacterial flora: A preliminary report. Ann Intern Med. 1982;96:131.
7. Larsen B, Galask RP. Vaginal microbial flora: Composition and influences of host physiology. Ann Intern Med. 1982;96(Suppl 6):926.
8. Spiegel CA, Amsel R, Eschenbach D, et al. Anaerobic bacteria in nonspecific vaginitis. N Engl J Med. 1980;303:601.
9. Lidbeck A, Nord CE. Lactobacilli and the normal human anaerobic microflora. Clin Infect Dis. 1993;16(Suppl 4):S181–7.
10. Rein MF, Holmes KK. "Nonspecific vaginitis," vulvovaginal candidiasis, and trichomoniasis. In: Remington JS, Swartz MN, eds. Current Clinical Topics in Infectious Diseases. v. 4. New York: McGraw-Hill; 1983:281.
11. Easmon CSF, Ison CA. *Gardnerella vaginalis*. Lancet. 1983;2:343.
12. Guinan ME, Dan BB, Guidotti RJ, et al. Vaginal colonization with *Staphylococcus aureus* in healthy women: A review of four studies. Ann Intern Med. 1982;94:944.
13. Larsen B. Vaginal flora in health and disease. Clin Obstet Gynecol 1993;36: 107–21.
14. Sobel JD. Epidemiology and pathogenesis of recurrent vulvovaginal candidiasis. Am J Obstet Gynecol. 1985;1523:924–35.

15. Shafer MA, Sweet FL, Ohm-Smith MJ, et al. Microbiology of the lower genital tract in postmenarchal adolescents girls: Differences in sexual activity, contraception, and presence of nonspecific vaginitis. J Pediatr. 1985;107: 974–81.

16. Hill GB, Eschenbach DA, Holmes KK. Bacteriology of the vagina. Scand J Urol Nephrol. 1984;18:(Suppl 86):23–30.

17. Cohen MS, Black JR, Proctor RA, et al. Host defenses and the vaginal mucosa: A reevaluation. Scand J Urol Nephrol. 1984;(Suppl 86):13–22.

18. Eschenbach DA, Davick PR, Williams BL, et al. Prevalence of hydrogen peroxide–producing *Lactobacillus* species in normal women and women with bacterial vaginosis. J Clin Microbiol. 1989;27:251.

19. Centers for Disease Control and Prevention. Nonreported sexually transmitted diseases. MMWR. 1979;28:61.

20. Sobel JD. Candidal vulvovaginitis. Clin Obstet Gynecol. 1993;36:153–65.

21. Kent HL. Epidemiology of vaginitis. Am J Obstet Gynecol. 1991;165: 1168–76.

22. Sweet RL. Importance of differential diagnosis in acute vaginitis. Am J Obstet Gynecol. 1985;152:921–3.

23. Schaaf VM, Perez-Stable EJ, Borchardt K. The limited value of symptoms and signs in the diagnosis of vaginal infections. Arch Intern Med. 1990;150: 1929–33.

23a. Taylor CA, Lipsky MS. Physicians' perceptions of the impact of the reclassification of vaginal antifungal agents. J Fam Pract. 1994;38:157–60.

24. Redondo-Lopez V, Meriwether C, Schmitt C, et al. Vulvovaginal candidiasis complicating recurrent bacterial vaginosis. Sex Transm Dis 1990;17:51–3.

25. Odds FC. *Candida* and Candidosis. Baltimore: University Park Press; 1979: 4.

26. O'Connor MI, Sobel JD. Epidemiology of recurrent vulvovaginal candidiasis: Identification and strain differentiation of *Candida albicans*. J Infect Dis. 1986;154:358–63.

27. Horowitz BJ. Mycotic vulvovaginitis: A broad overview. Am J Obstet Gynecol. 1991;165:1188–92.

28. Horowitz BJ, Edelstein SW, Lippman L. *Candida tropicalis* vulvovaginitis. Obstet Gynecol. 1985;66:229–32.

29. Redondo-Lopez V, Lynch M, Schmitt CA, et al. *Torulopsis glabrata* vaginitis: Clinical aspects and susceptibility to antifungal agents. Obstet Gynecol. 1990;76:651.

30. Sobel JD. Pathogenesis and treatment of recurrent vulvovaginal candidiasis. Clin Infect Dis. 1992;14(Suppl 1):S148–53.

31. Sobel JD, Vazquez J, Lynch M, et al. Vaginitis due to *Saccharomyces cerevisiae*: Epidemiology, clinical aspects, and therapy. Clin Infect Dis. 1993; 16:93–9.

32. Fleury FJ. Adult vaginitis. Clin Obstet Gynecol. 1981;24:407.

33. Heary FL. Recurrent *Candida* vulvovaginitis. Chemotherapy. 1982;28(Suppl 1):48–50.

34. Powell BL, Frey CL, Drutz DJ. Estrogen receptor in *Candida albicans*. A possible explanation for hormonal influences in vaginal candidiasis (Abstract 751). In: Proceedings of the 23rd ICAAC. Las Vegas, 1983.

35. Elgebe IA, Botu M. A preliminary study on dressing patterns and incidence of candidiasis. Am J Public Health. 1982;72:176.

36. Elgebe IA, Elgebe I. Quantitative relationships of *Candida albicans* infections and dressing patterns in Nigerian women. Am J Public Health. 1983; 73:450–2.

37. Heidrich FE, Berg AO, Bergman JJ. Clothing factors and vaginitis. J Family Pract. 1984;19:491–4.

38. Rhoads JL, Wright DC, Redfield RR, et al. Chronic vaginal candidiasis in women with human immunodeficiency virus infection. JAMA. 1987;257: 3105–9.

39. Imam N, Carpenter CCJ, Mayer KH, et al. Hierarchical pattern of mucosal *Candida* infections with HIV seropositive women. Am J Med. 1990;89:142.

40. Odds FC. Genital candidosis. Clin Exp Dermatol. 1982;7:345–54.

41. Garcia-Tamayo J, Castillo G, Martinez AJ. Human genital candidiasis: Histochemistry, scanning and transmission electron microscopy. Acta Cytol (Baltimore). 1982;26:7.

42. Kimura LH, Pearsal NH. Relationship between germination of *Candida albicans* and increased adherence to human buccal epithelial cells. Infect Immun. 1980;28:464.

43. King RD, Lee JC, Morris AL. Adherence of *Candida albicans* and other *Candida* species to mucosal epithelial cells. Infect Immun. 1980;27:667.

44. Sobel JD, Muller G. Ketoconazole in the prevention of experimental candidal vaginitis. Antimicrob Agents Chemother. 1984;25:281–2.

45. Oriel JD, Partridge BM, Denny MJ, et al. Genital yeast infections. Br Med J. 1972;4:761.

46. Rigg D, Miller MM, Motzger WJ. Recurrent allergic vulvovaginitis treatment with *Candida albicans* allergen immunotherapy. Am J Obstet Gynecol. 1990; 162:232.

47. Drake SM, Evans BA, Gerken A. Vaginal pH and microflora related to yeast infections and treatment. Br J Vener Dis. 1980;56:107.

48. Peeters F, Snauwaert R, Segers J, et al. Observations on candidal vaginitis: Vaginal pH, microbiology. Am J Obstet Gynecol. 1972;112:80.

49. Baldson MJ. Comparison of miconazole-coated tampons with clotrimazole vaginal tablets in the treatment of vaginal candidosis. Br J Vener Dis. 1981; 57:275.

50. Rothenberg RB, Simm R, Chipperfield E, et al. Efficacy of selected diagnostic tests for sexually transmitted diseases. JAMA. 1976;235:49.

51. Pattman RS. Evaluation of a culture in the diagnosis of vaginal candidiasis. Br J Vener Dis. 1981;57:67.

52. Rajakumar R, Lacey CJN, Evans EGV, et al. Use of a slide latex agglutination test for rapid diagnosis of vaginal candidosis. Genitourin Med. 1987;63: 192–5.

53. Sobel JD, Schmitt C, Meriwether C. A new slide agglutination test for the diagnosis of acute *Candida* vaginitis. Am J Clin Pathol. 1990;94:323–5.

54. Reed BD, Pierson CL. Evaluation of a latex agglutination test for identification of *Candida* species in vaginal discharge. J Am Board Fam Pract. 1992; 5:375–80.

55. Odds FC. Cure and relapse with antifungal therapy. Proc R Soc Med. 1977; 70(Suppl 4):24.

56. Doering PL, Santiago TM. Drugs for treatment of vulvovaginal candidiasis: Comparative efficacy of agents and regimens. DICP. 1990;24:1078–83.

57. Weisberg M. Treatment of vaginal candidiasis in pregnant women. Clin Ther. 1986;8:563–7.

58. Lebherz T, Guess E, Wolfson N. Efficacy of single-versus multiple-dose clotrimazole therapy in the management of vulvovaginal candidiasis. Am J Obstet Gynecol. 1985;152:965–7.

59. Heary F, Hughes D, Floyd R. Therapeutic results obtained in vaginal mycoses after single-dose treatment with 500 mg clotrimazole vaginal tablets. Am J Obstet Gynecol. 1985;152:968–70.

60. Anonymous. Butoconazole for vulvovaginal candidiasis. Med Lett Drugs Ther. 1986;28:68.

61. Loendersloot EW, Goormans E, Wieshann E, et al. Efficacy and tolerability of single-dose versus six-day treatment of candidal vulvovaginitis with vaginal tablets of clotrimazole. Am J Obstet Gynecol. 1985;152:953–5.

62. Bradbeer CS, Mayhew SR, Barlow D. Butoconazole and miconazole in treating vaginal candidiasis. Genitourin Med. 1985;61:270–2.

63. Droegemuller W, Adamson DG, Brown D, et al. Three-day treatment with butoconazole nitrate for vulvovaginal candidiasis. Obstet Gynecol. 1984;64: 530–4.

64. Nixon SA. Vulvovaginitis: The role of patient compliance in treatment success. Am J Obstet Gynecol. 1991;165:1207–9.

65. Cohen L. Single dose treatment of vaginal candidosis: Comparison of clotrimazole and isoconazole. Br J Vener Dis. 1984;60:40–2.

66. Milson I, Forssman L. Treatment of vaginal candidosis with a single 500 mg clotrimazole pessary. Br J Vener Dis. 1982;58:124.

67. Sobel JD. Management of recurrent vulvovaginal candidiasis with intermittent ketoconazole prophylaxis. Obstet Gynecol. 1985;65:435–40.

68. Sobel JD. Recurrent vulvovaginal candidiasis. A prospective study of the efficacy of maintenance ketoconazole therapy. N Engl J Med. 1986;315: 1455–8.

69. Eschenbach DA, Hummel D, Gravett MG. Recurrent and persistent vulvovaginal candidiasis: Treatment with ketoconazole. Obstet Gynecol. 1985;66: 248–54.

70. Houang ET, Chappatte O, Byrne D, et al. Fluconazole levels in plasma and vaginal secretions of patients after a 150-milligram single oral dose and rate of eradication of infection in vaginal candidiasis. Antimicrob Agents Chemother. 1990;34:909–10.

71. van Heusden AM, Merkus HMWM, Corbeij RSACM, et al. Single-dose oral fluconazole versus single-dose topical miconazole for the treatment of acute vulvovaginal candidosis. Acta Obstet Gynecol Scand. 1990;69:417–22.

72. Boag FC, Houang ET, Westrom R, et al. Comparison of vaginal flora after treatment with a clotrimazole 500 mg pessary or a fluconazole 150 mg capsule for vaginal candidosis. Genitourin Med. 1991;67:232–4.

73. Salem HT, Salah M, Farid A, et al. Oral versus local treatment of vaginal candidosis. Int J Gynaecol Obstet. 1989;30:57–62.

74. Osser S, Haglund A, Westrom L. Treatment of candidal vaginitis: A prospective randomized investigator-blind multicenter study comparing topically applied econazole with oral fluconazole. Acta Obstet Gynecol Scand. 1991;70: 73–8.

75. Brammer KW, et al. A comparison of single dose oral fluconazole with 3-day intravaginal clotrimazole in the treatment of vaginal candidiasis. Report of an international multicenter trial. Br J Obstet Gynecol. 1989;96:226–32.

76. Phillips RJ, Watson SA, McKay FF. An open multicentre study of the efficacy and safety of a single dose of fluconazole 150 mg in the treatment of vaginal candidiasis in a general practice. Br J Clin Pract. 1990;44:219–22.

77. Calderon-Marquez JJ. Itraconazole in the treatment of vaginal candidosis and the effect of treatment of the sexual partner. Rev Infect Dis. 1987;9(Suppl 1):143–5.

78. Tobin JM, Loo P, Granger SE: Treatment of vaginal candidosis: A comparative study of the efficacy and acceptability of itraconazole and clotrimazole. Genitourin Med. 1992;68:36–8.

79. Stein GE, Mummaw N: Placebo-controlled trial of itraconazole for treatment of acute vaginal candidiasis. Antimicrob Agents Chemother. 1992;37:89–92.

80. Silva-Cruz A, Andrade L, Sobral L, et al. Itraconazole versus placebo in the management of vaginal candidiasis. Int J Gynecol Obstet. 1991;36:229–32.

81. Roongpisuthipong A, Sentrakul P, Bhiraleus P, et al. Itraconazole in the treatment of acute vaginal candidiasis. J Med Assoc Thailand. 1992;75:30–4.

82. Wesel S. Itraconazole: A single-day oral treatment for acute vulvovaginal candidosis. Br J Clin Pract (Symp Suppl). 1990;71:S77–80.

83. Jovanovic R, Congema E, Nguyen HT. Antifungal agents vs. boric acid for treating chronic mycotic vulvovaginitis. J Reprod Med. 1991;36:593–7.

84. Clayton YM. Antifungal drugs in current use. A review. Proc R Soc Med. 1977;70(Suppl 4):15.

85. Vorherr H, Vorherr UF, Mehta P, et al. Vaginal absorption of povidone-iodine. JAMA. 1980;244:2628.

86. van Slyke KK, Michel VP, Rein MF. Treatment of vulvovaginal candidiasis with boric acid powder. Am J Obstet Gynecol. 1981;141:145–8.
87. Podolsky S, Tauber AI. Yogurt for candidal vaginitis. Ann Intern Med. 1992;117:345–6.
88. Cohen L. Is more than one application of an antifungal necessary in the treatment of acute vaginal candidiasis. Am J Obstet Gynecol. 1985;152:961–4.
89. Rashid S, Collins M, Kennedy RJ. A study of candidosis: the role of fomites. Genitourin Med. 1991;67:137–42.
90. Schmidt J, Rotman M, Reed B, et al. Genetic similarity of *Candida albicans* strains from vaginitis patients and their partners. J Clin Microbiol. 1993;31:39–46.
91. Fong IW. The value of treating the sexual partners of women with recurrent vaginal candidiasis with ketoconazole. Genitourin Med. 1992;68:147–6.
92. Hill LVH, Embil JA. Vaginitis: Current microbiological and clinical concepts. Can Med Assoc J. 1986;134:3221–31.
93. Milne JD, Warnock DW. Effect of simultaneous oral and vaginal treatment on the rate of cure and relapse in vaginal candidosis. Br J Vener Dis. 1979;55:362.
94. Velupillai S, Thin RN. Treatment of vulvovaginal yeast infection with nystatin. Practitioner. 1977;219:897.
95. Nystatin Multicenter Study Group. Therapy of candidal vaginitis: The effect of eliminating intestinal Candida. Am J Obstet Gynecol. 1986;155:651–5.
96. Lossick JG. Sexually transmitted vaginitis. Semin Adolesc Med. 1985;2:131–42.
97. Edman J, Sobel JD, Taylor ML. Zinc status in women with recurrent vulvovaginal candidiasis. Am J Obstet Gynecol. 1986;155:1082–5.
98. Witkin SS, Yu IR, Ledger WJ. Inhibition of *Candida albicans*–induced lymphocyte proliferation by lymphocytes and sera from women with recurrent vaginitis. Am J Obstet Gynecol. 1983;147:809–11.
99. Witkin SS, Hirsch J, Ledger WJ. A macrophage defect in women with recurrent *Candida* vaginitis and its reversal by prostaglandin inhibitors. Am J Obstet Gynecol. 1986;155:790–5.
100. Davidson F, Mould RF. Recurrent genital candidosis in women and the effect of intermittent prophylactic treatment. Br J Vener Dis. 1978;54:176.
101. Roth AC, Milson I, Forssman L, et al. Intermittent prophylactic treatment of recurrent vaginal candidiasis by postmenstrual application of a 500 mg clotrimazole tablet. Genitourin Med. 1990;66:357–60.
102. Sobel JD, Schmitt C, Meriwether C. Clotrimazole treatment of recurrent and chronic *Candida* vulvovaginitis. Obstet Gynecol. 1989;73:330–4.
103. van Heusden AM, Merkus JM. Chronic recurrent vaginal candidiasis: Easy to treat, difficult to cure. Results of treatment with a new oral antifungal. Eur J Obstet Gynecol Reprod Biol. 1990;35:75–83.
104. Hilton E, Isenberg HD, Alperstein P, et al. Ingestion of yogurt containing *Lactobacillus acidophilus* as prophylaxis for candidal vaginitis. Ann Intern Med. 1992;116:353–7.
105. Drutz DJ. *Lactobacillus* prophylaxis for *Candida* vaginitis. Ann Intern Med. 1992;116:419–20.
106. Waugh MA. Clinical presentation of candidal balanitis—Its differential diagnosis and treatment. Chemotherapy. 1982;28(Suppl 1):56–60.
107. Oriel JD, Partridge BM, Denny MJ, et al. Genital yeast infections. Br Med J. 1972;4:761.
108. Gardner HL, Dukes CD. *Haemophilus vaginalis* vaginitis: A newly defined specific infection previously classified "non-specific" vaginitis. Am J Obstet Gynecol. 1955;69:962.
109. Huth EJ. Style note: Bacterial vaginosis of vaginal bacteriosis. Ann Intern Med. 1989;111:553–4.
110. Mardh PA, Taylor-Robinson D, eds. Bacterial vaginosis. Scand J Urol Nephrol. 1984;18(Suppl 86):1–270.
111. Speigel CA. Bacterial vaginosis. Clin Microbiol Rev. 1991;4:485–502.
112. Brunham RC, Pavonen J, Stevens CE, et al. Mucopurulent cervicitis—The ignored counterpart in women of urethritis in men. N Engl J Med. 1984;311:1–6.
113. Eschenbach DA. Bacterial vaginosis and anaerobes in obstetric-gynecologic infections. Clin Infect Dis. 1993;16(Suppl 4):S282–7.
114. Pheifer TA, Forsyth PS, Durfee MA, et al. Nonspecific vaginitis: Role of *Haemophilus vaginalis* and treatment with metronidazole. N Engl J Med. 1978;298:1429.
115. Chen KCS, Forsyth PS, Buchman TM, et al. Amine content of vaginal fluid from untreated and treated patients with nonspecific vaginitis. J Clin Invest. 1979;63:828.
116. Hanna NF, Taylor-Robinson D, Kalodiki-Karammanoki M, et al. The relation between vaginal pH and the microbiological status in vaginitis. Br J Obstet Gynaecol. 1985;92:1267–71.
117. Baldson MJ, Taylor GE, Pead L, et al. *Corynebacterium vaginale* and vaginitis: A controlled trial of treatment. Lancet. 1980;1:501.
118. Vontver LA, Eschenbach DA. The role of *Gardnerella vaginalis* in nonspecific vaginitis. Clin Obstet Gynecol. 1981;24:439.
119. Amsel R, Totten PA, Spiegel CA, et al. Nonspecific vaginitis: Diagnostic criteria and microbial and epidemiological associations. Am J Med. 1983;74:14.
120. Bhattycharyya MN, Jones BM. *Haemophilus vaginalis* infection: Diagnosis and treatment. J Reprod Med. 1980;24:71.
121. Spiegel CA, Amsel R, Holmes KK. Diagnosis of bacterial vaginosis by direct Gram stain of vaginal fluid. J Clin Microbiol. 1983;18:170–7.
122. Thomasen JL, Andersen RJ, Gelbart SM, et al. Simplified Gram stain interpretative methods for diagnosis of bacterial vaginosis. Am J Obstet Gynecol. 1992;167:16–9.
123. Nugent RP, Krohn MA, Hillier SI. Reliability of diagnosing bacterial vaginosis is improved by a standardized method of Gram stain interpretation. J Clin Microbiol. 1991;29:297–301.
124. Platz-Christensen JJ, Larsson PG, Sundstrom E, et al. Detection of bacterial vaginosis in Papanicolaou smears. Am J Obstet Gynecol. 1998;158:953–9.
125. Hillier SL, Krohn MA, Rabe LK, et al. The normal vaginal flora, H₂O₂-producing lactobacilli to bacterial vaginosis in pregnant women. Clin Infect Dis 1993;16(Suppl 4)S273–81.
126. Ratnam S, Fitzgerald BL. Semiquantitative culture of *Gardnerella vaginalis* in laboratory determination of nonspecific vaginitis. J Clin Microbiol. 1983;18:344.
127. Totten PA, Amsel R, Hale J, et al. Selective differential human blood bilayer media for isolation of *Gardnerella* (*Haemophilus*) *vaginalis*. J Clin Microbiol. 1982;15:141–7.
128. Schoonmaker JN, Lunt BD, Lawellin DW, et al. A new proline aminopeptidase assay for the diagnosis of bacterial vaginosis. Am J Obstet Gynecol. 1991;165:737–42.
129. Biswas MK. Bacterial vaginosis. Clin Obstet Gynecol 1993;36:166–76.
130. Chen KCS, Amsel R, Eschenbach DA, et al. Biochemical diagnosis of vaginitis: Determination of diamines in vaginal fluid. J Infect Dis. 1982;145:337.
131. Thomason JL, Gelbart SM, Andersen RJ, et al. Statistical evaluation of diagnostic criteria for bacterial vaginosis. Am J Obstet Gynecol 1990;102:155–60.
132. Larsson PG, Platz-Christensen JJ, Sundstrom E. Is bacterial vaginosis a sexually transmitted disease? Int J STD AIDS. 1991;2:362–4.
133. Barbone F, Austin H, Louv WC, et al. A follow-up study of methods of contraception, sexual activity, and rates of trichomoniasis, candidiasis, and bacterial vaginosis. Am J Obstet Gynecol. 1990;163:510–4.
134. Avonts D, Sercu M, Heyetick P, et al. Incidence of uncomplicated genital infections in women using oral contraception or an intrauterine device: A prospective study. Sex Transm Dis. 1990;17:23–9.
135. Bump RC, Buesching WJ III. Bacterial vaginosis in virginal and sexually active adolescent females: Evidence against exclusive sexual transmission. Am J Obstet Gynecol 1988;158:935–9.
136. Swedberg J, Steiner JF, Deiss F, et al. Comparison of single-dose vs one-week course of metronidazole for symptomatic bacterial vaginosis. JAMA. 1985;254:1046–9.
137. Jones BM, Geary I, Alawattegama AB, et al. In vitro and in vivo activity of metronidazole against *Gardnerella vaginalis*, *Bacteroides* spp. and *Mobiluncus* spp. in bacterial vaginosis. J Antimicrob Chemother. 1985;16:189–97.
138. Lugo-Miro VI, Green M, Mazur L. Comparison of different metronidazole regimens for bacterial vaginosis. JAMA. 1992;268:92–5.
139. Holst E. Reservoir of four organisms associated with bacterial vaginosis suggests lack of sexual transmission. J Clin Microbiol 1990;28:2035–9.
140. Greenwood JR, Picket MJ. Transfer of *Haemophilus vaginalis* to a new genus, *Gardnerella*: G. *vaginalis* (Gardner and Dukes) com. nov. Int J Syst Bacteriol. 1980;30:170.
141. Malouf M, Fortier M, Morin G, et al. Treatment of *Hemophilus vaginalis* vaginitis. Obstet Gynecol. 1980;57:711.
142. Monhanty KC, Deighton R. Comparison of 2 g single dose of metronidazole, nimorazole and tinidazole in the treatment of vaginitis associated with *Gardnerella vaginalis*. J Antimicrob Chemother. 1987;19:393–9.
143. Monhanty KC, Deighton R. Comparison of two different metronidazole regimens in the treatment of *Gardnerella vaginalis* infection with or without trichomoniasis. J Antimicrob Chemother. 1985;16:799–803.
144. van der Meijden WI, Piot P, Loriaux SM, et al. Amoxycillin, amoxycillin-clavulanic acid and metronidazole in the treatment of clue cell positive discharge. A comparative clinical and laboratory study. J Antimicrob Chemother. 1987;20:735–42.
145. Amsel R, Critchlow CW, Spiegel CA, et al. Comparison of metronidaozle, ampicillin, and amoxicillin for treatment of bacterial vaginosis (nonspecific vaginitis): Possible explanation for the greater efficacy of metronidazole. In: Finegold S, ed. *United States Metronidazole Conference. Proceedings from a Symposium*, Tarpon Springs, Florida, February 18–20, 1982. New York: Biomedical Information Corp. 1982;225.
146. Shander S, Munro R. Sensitivity of *Gardnerella vaginalis* to metabolites of metronidazole and tinidazole. Lancet. 1982;1:167.
147. Taylor E, Blackwell AL, Barlow D, et al. *Gardnerella vaginalis*, anaerobes, and vaginal discharge. Lancet. 1982;1:1376.
148. Hillier SL, Critchlow CW, Stevens CE, et al. Microbiological, epidemiological and clinical correlates of vaginal colonization by *Mobiluncus* species. Genitourin Med 1991;67:26–31.
149. Darieux R, Dublanchet A. Les "vibrions" anaerobics des leucorrhees. I: Technique d'osolement et sensibilite aux antibitiques. Med Mal Infect. 1980;10:109.
150. Sprott MS, Pattman RS, Ingham HR, et al. Anaerobic curved rods in vaginitis. Lancet. 1982;1:54.
151. Hjelm E, Hallen A, Forsum U, et al. Motile anaerobic curved rods in nonspecific vaginitis. Lancet 1982;1:9.
152. Spiegel CA, Eschenbach DA, Amsel R, et al. Curved anaerobic bacteria in bacterial vaginosis and their response to antimicrobial therapy. J Infect Dis. 1983;148:817.
153. Thomason JL, Schreckenberger PC, Spellacy WN, et al. Clinical and microbiological characterization of patients with nonspecific vaginosis associated with motile, curved anaerobic rods. J Infect Dis. 1984;149:801–9.

154. Spiegel CA. New developments in the etiology and pathogenesis of bacterial vaginosis. Adv Exp Med Biol. 1987;224:127–34.

155. Thomason JL and the Working Group. Diagnosis of infection with anaerobic cervical rods. Scan J Urol Nephrol. 1984;18(Suppl 86):261–2.

156. Spiegel CA, Roberts M. *Mobiluncus* gen nov, *Mobiluncus curtisii* subspecies *curtisii* sp. nov., *Mobiluncus curtisii* subspecies *holmesii* subsp. nov., and *Mobiluncus mulieris* sp. nov., curved rods from the human vagina. Int J Syst Bacteriol. 1984;34:177–84.

157. Eschenbach DA, Gravett MG, Chen KCS, et al. Bacterial vaginosis during pregnancy: An association with prematurity and postpartum complications. Scand J Urol Nephrol. 1984;18(Suppl 86):213–22.

158. Paavonen J, Miettinen A, Stevens CE, et al. *Mycoplasma hominis* in nonspecific vaginitis. Sex Transm Dis. 1983;10:271–5.

159. Hillier SL, Krohn MA, Klebanoff SJ, et al. The relationship of hydrogen-peroxide–producing lactobacilli to bacterial vaginosis and genital microflora in pregnant women. Obstet Gynecol 1992;79:369–73.

160. Eschenbach DA, Davick PR, Williams BL, et al. Prevalence of hydrogen peroxide–producing *Lactobacillus* species in normal women and women with bacterial vaginosis. J Clin Microbiol. 1989;27:251–6.

161. Alawattengama AB, Jones BM, Kinghorn GR, et al. Single-dose versus seven-day metronidazole in *Gardnerella vaginalis* associated with nonspecific vaginitis. Lancet. 1984;1355–7.

162. Eschenbach DA, Critchlow CW, Watkins H, et al. A dose-duration study of metronidazole for the treatment of nonspecific vaginosis. Scand J Infect Dis. 1983;(Suppl)40:73–80.

163. Greaves WL, Chungfung J, Morris B, et al. Clindamycin versus metronidazole in the treatment of bacterial vaginosis. Obstet Gynecol. 1988;72:799–802.

164. Gardner H. *Hemophilus vaginalis* vaginitis after twenty-five years. Am J Obstet Gynecol. 1980;137:385–92.

165. Wathne B, Hovelius B, Holst E. Cefadroxil as an alternative to metronidazole in the treatment of bacterial vaginosis. Scand J Infect Dis. 1989;21:585–6.

166. Nayagam AT, Smith MD, Ridgeway GL, et al. Comparison of ofloxacin and metronidazole for the treatment of bacterial vaginosis. Int J STD AIDS. 1992;3:204–7.

167. Hillier S, Krohn MA, Watts P, et al. Microbiological efficacy of intravaginal clindamycin cream for the treatment of bacterial vaginosis. Obstet Gynecol 1990;76:407–13.

168. Livengood CH, Thomason JL, Hill GB. Bacterial vaginosis: Treatment with topical intravaginal clindamycin phosphate. Obstet Gynecol. 1990;76:118–23.

169. Schmitt C, Sobel JD, Meriwether C. Bacterial vaginosis: Treatment with clindamycin cream *versus* oral metronidazole. Obstet Gynecol. 1992;79:1020–3.

170. Livengood CH, III, Thomason JL, Hill GB. Bacterial vaginosis: diagnostic and pathologic findings during topical clindamycin therapy. Am J Obstet Gynecol 1990;163:515–20.

171. Andres FJ, Parker R, Hosein I, et al. Clindamycin cream versus oral metronidazole in the treatment of bacterial vaginosis: A prospective, double-blind clinical trial. South Med J. 1992;85:1077–80.

172. Galask RP, Bowdler N. Open label evaluation of 0.75% metronidazole gel in the treatment of bacterial vaginosis. Annual Meeting of the Infectious Disease Society for Obstetrics and Gynecology, August 6–8, 1992, San Diego.

173. McGregor JA, Livengood C, III, French JI, et al. Intravaginal metronidazole gel (0.75%) for bacterial vaginosis: Results of a double-blinded, randomized, placebo-controlled trial. Annual Meeting of the Infectious Disease Society for Obstetrics and Gynecology, August 6–8, 1992, San Diego.

174. Hillier SL, Lipinski C, Briselden AM, et al. Efficacy of intravaginal 0.75% metronidazole gel for the treatment of bacterial vaginosis. Obstet Gynecol. 1993;81:963–7.

175. Curatek Pharmaceuticals. MetroGel-Vaginal Clinical Monograph. Elk Grove Village, IL: Curatek; 1992;13–14.

176. Piot P, Van Dyck E, Godts P, et al. A placebo-controlled, double-blind comparison of tinidazole and triple sulfonamide cream for the treatment of non-specific vaginitis. Am J Obstet Gynecol 1983;147:85–9.

177. Fredricsson B, Englund K, Weintraub L, et al. Bacterial vaginosis is not a simple ecological disorder. Gynecol Obstet Invest. 1989;28:156–60.

178. Neri A, Sabah G, Samra Z. Bacterial vaginosis in pregnancy treated with yoghurt. Acta Obstet Gynecol Scand. 1993;72:17–19.

179. Holst E, Brandberg A. Treatment of bacterial vaginosis in pregnancy with a lactate gel. Scand J Infect Dis. 1990;22:625–6.

180. Andersch B, Lindell D, Dahlen I, et al. Bacterial vaginosis and the effect of intermittent treatment with an acid lactate gel. Gynecol Obstet Invest. 1990;30:114–9.

181. Fredricsson B, Englund K, Weintraub L, et al. Ecological treatment of bacterial vaginosis. Lancet. 1987;1:276.

182. Hallen A, Jarstrand C, Pahlson C. Treatment of bacterial vaginosis with lactobacilli. Sex Transm Dis. 1992;19:146–8.

183. Hughes VL, Hillier SL. Microbiologic characteristics of *Lactobacillus* products used for colonization of the vagina. Obstet Gynecol. 1990;75:244–8.

184. Thomason JL, Gelbart SM, Scaglione NJ. Bacterial vaginosis: Current review with indications for asymptomatic therapy. Am J Obstet Gynecol. 1991;165:1210–7.

185. Larsson P-G, Platz Christensen J-J, Thejls H, et al. Incidence of pelvic inflammatory disease after first-trimester legal abortion in women with bacte-

rial vaginosis after treatment with metronidazole: A double-blind, randomized study. Am J Obstet Gynecol. 1992;166:100–3.

186. Larsson P-G, Bergman B, Forsum U, et al. *Mobiluncus* and clue cells as predictors of PID after first trimester abortion. Acta Obstet Gynecol Scand. 1989;68:217–20.

187. Soper DE, Bump RC, Hurt WG. Bacterial vaginosis and trichomoniasis vaginitis are risk factors for cuff cellulitis after abdominal hysterectomy. Am J Obstet Gynecol. 1990;163:1016–23.

188. Larsson P-G, Platz-Christensen J-J, Forsum U, et al. Clue cells in predicting infections after abdominal hysterectomy. Obstet Gynecol. 1991;77:450.

189. Rosene K, Eschenbach DA, Tompkins LS, et al. Polymicrobial early postpartum endometritis with facultative and anaerobic bacteria, genital mycoplasma, and *Chlamydia trachomatis:* Treatment with piperacillin or cefoxtin. J Infect Dis. 1986;153:1028–37.

190. Lamey JR, Eschenbach DA, Mitchell SH, et al. Isolation of mycoplasmas and bacteria from the blood of postpartum women. Am J Obstet Gynecol. 1982;143:104–12.

191. Gravett MG, Hummel DH, Eschenbach DA, et al. Preterm labor associated with subclinical amniotic fluid infection and with bacterial vaginosis. Obstet Gynecol. 1986;67:229–37.

192. Venkataramani TK, Rathbun HK. *Corynebacterium vaginale (Hemophilus vaginalis)* bacteremia: Clinical study of 29 cases. Johns Hopkins Med J. 1976;139:93.

193. Reimer LG, Reller LB. *Gardnerella vaginalis* bacteremia: A review of 30 cases. Obstet Gynecol. 1984;65:180–2.

194. Watts DH, Krohn MA, Hillier SL, et al. Bacterial vaginosis as a risk factor for postcesarian endometritis. Obstet Gynecol. 1990;75:52–8.

195. Gravett MG, Nelson HP, DeRouen T, et al. Independent association of bacterial vaginosis and *Chlamydia trachomatis* infection with adverse pregnancy outcome. JAMA 1986;256:1899–903.

196. McGregor JA, French JI, Richter R, et al. Antenatal microbiologic and maternal risk factors associated with prematurity. Am J Obstet Gynecol. 1990;163:1465–73.

197. Martius J, Krohn MA, Hillier SL, et al. Relationships of vaginal *Lactobacillus* species, cervical *Chlamydia trachomatis,* and bacterial vaginosis to preterm birth. Obstet Gynecol 1988;71:89–95.

198. Krohn MA, Hillier SL, Lee ML, et al. Vaginal *Bacteroides* species are associated with an increased risk of preterm delivery among women in preterm labor. J Infect Dis. 1991;164:88–93.

199. Kurki T, Sivonen A, Renkonen OV, et al. Bacterial vaginosis in early pregnancy and pregnancy outcome. Obstet Gynecol 1992;80:173–7.

200. Shands KN, Schmid GP, Dan BB, et al. Toxic shock syndrome in menstruating women. Association with tampon use and *Staphylococcus aureus* and clinical features in 52 cases. N Engl J Med. 1980;303:1436.

201. Tofte RW, Williams DN. Clinical and laboratory manifestations of toxic shock syndrome. Ann Intern Med. 1982;96:843.

202. Lanes SF, Poole C, Dreyer NA. Toxic shock syndrome, contraceptive methods, and vaginitis. Am J Obstet Gynecol. 1986;154:989–91.

203. Zaaijman JD, deBeer J. An unusual vaginal foreign body. S Afr Med J. 1982;61:33.

204. Friedrich EG, Siegesmund KA. Tampon associated vaginal ulcerations. Obstet Gynecol. 1980;55:149.

205. Friedrich EG. Tampon effects on vaginal health. Clin Obstet Gynecol. 1981;24:295.

206. Jimerson SD, Becker JD. Vaginal ulcers associated with tampon usage. Obstet Gynecol. 1980;56:97.

207. Weissberg SM, Dodson MG. Recurrent vaginal and cervical ulcers associated with tampon use. JAMA. 1983;250:1430.

208. Corey L, Adams HG, Brown AZ, et al. Genital herpes simplex virus infections. Clinical manifestations, course, and complications. Ann Intern Med. 1983;98:958.

209. Pazin GH. Management of oral and genital herpes simplex viral infections: Diagnosis and treatment. DM. 2986;32:725–84.

210. Corey L, Holmes KK. The use of 2-deoxy-D-glucose for genital herpes. JAMA. 1980;243:29.

211. Ginsburg CM. Group A streptococcal vaginitis in children. Pediatr Infect Dis. 1982;1:36.

212. Symmers WstC. Pathology of oxyuriasis. Arch Pathol. 1950;50:475.

213. Dump RC. *Chlamydia trachomatis* as a cause of prepubertal vaginitis. Obstet Gynecol. 1985;65:384–8.

214. Cibley LJ, Cibley LJ. Cytolytic vaginosis. Am J Obstet Gynecol 1991;165:1245–9.

215. Sharp HC. Vulvovaginal conditions mimicking vaginitis. Clin Obstet Gynecol. 1993;36:129–36.

216. Fisher AA. Allergic reactions to feminine hygiene sprays. Arch Dermatol. 1973;108:801.

217. Chang T. Familial allergic seminal vulvovaginitis. Am J Obstet Gynecol. 1976;126:442.

218. Gochfeld M, Burger J. Sexual transmission of nickel and poison oak contact dermatitis. Lancet. 1983;1:589.

219. Gardner HL. Desquamative inflammatory vaginitis: A newly defined entity. Am J Obstet Gynecol. 1968;102:1102–5.

220. Edwards L, Friedrich EG. Desquamative inflammatory vaginitis: Lichen planus in disguise. Obstet Gynecol. 1988;71:832–6.

221. Oates JK, Rowen D. Desquamative inflammatory vaginitis. A review. Genitourin Med 1990;66:274–9.

222. Huggins GR, Preti G. Vaginal odors and secretions. Clin Obstet Gynecol. 1981;24:355.
223. Friedrich EG. The vulvar vestibule. J Reprod Med. 1983;28:773–7.
224. Peckham BM, Maki DG, Patterson JJ, et al. Focal vulvitis: A characteristic syndrome and cause of dyspareunia. Features, natural history, and management. Am J Obstet Gynecol. 1986;154:855–64.
225. Goetsch MF. Vulvar vestibulitis: Prevalence and historic features in a general gynecologic practice population. Am J Obstet Gynecol 1991;164:1609–14.
226. Marinoff SC, Turner ML. Vulvar vestibulitis syndrome. Dermatol Clin 1992; 10:435–44.
227. Pyka RE, Wilkinson EJ, Friedrich EG, et al. The histopathology of vulvar vestibulitis syndrome. Int J Gynecol Pathol. 1988;7:249.
228. McCormack WM. Two urogenital sinus syndromes: Interstitial cystitis and focal vulvitis. J Reprod Med. 1990;35:873–6.
229. Mann MS, Kaufman RH, Brown DJ, et al. Vulvar vestibulitis: Significant clinical variables and treatment outcome. Obstet Gynecol. 1992;79:122–5.
230. Micklewitz H, Kennison RD, Turksoy RN, et al. Vulvar vestibulitis: Subgroup with Bartholin gland duct inflammation. Obstet Gynecol. 1989;73:410–3.
231. Reid R, Greenberg MD, Daoud MA. Colposcopic findings in women with vulvar pain syndromes: A preliminary report. J Reprod Med. 1988;33:523.
232. Potkul RK, Lancaster WD, Kurman RJ, et al. Vulvar condylomas and squamous vestibular micropapilloma: differences in appearance and response to treatment. J Reprod Med. 1990;35:1019–22.
233. Umpierre SA, Kaufman RH, Adam E, et al. Human papillomavirus DNA in tissue biopsy specimens of vulvar vestibulitis patients treated with interferon. Obstet Gynecol 1991;78:693–5.
234. Horowitz BJ. Interferon therapy for condylomatous vulvitis. Obstet Gynecol 1989;73:446–8.
235. Gardner HL, Fernet P. Etiology of vaginitis emphysematosa: Report of ten cases and review of the literature. Am J Obstet Gynecol 1946;88:680–94.
236. Kramer K, Jobon H. Vaginitis emphysematosa. Arch Pathol Lab Med. 1987; 111:746–11.
237. Josey WE, Campbell WG. Vaginitis emphysematosa: Report of four cases. J Reprod Med. 1990;35:974–7.
238. McCallion JS, Parkin DE. Emphysematous vaginitis masquerading as carcinoma of the cervix. Case report. Br J Obstet Gynaecol. 1988;95:309–11.
239. Dodson MG, Friedrich EG. Psychosomatic vulvovaginitis. Obstet Gynecol. 1978;51(Suppl):23.
240. Al-Saliki FL, Curran JP, Wong JS. Neonatal *Trichomonas vaginalis:* Report of three cases and review of the literature. Pediatrics. 1974;53:196.
241. Paradise JE, Campos JM, Friedman HM, et al. Vulvovaginitis in premenarchal girls. Clinical features and diagnostic evaluation. Pediatrics. 1982;70:193.
241a. Nuovo GJ. Human papillomavirus DNA in genital tract lesions histologically negative for condylomata: Analysis by in situ, Southern blot hybridization and polymerase chain reaction. Am J Surg Pathol. 1990;14:643–51.
242. Wolner-Hanssen P, Krieger JN, Stevens CE, et al. Clinical manifestations of vaginal trichomoniasis: Implications for strategies for diagnosis and control of the infection. JAMA 1989;261:571–6.
243. Rees E, Tait IA, Hobson D, et al. *Chlamydia* in relation to cervical infection and pelvic inflammatory disease. In: Hobson D, Holmes KK, eds. *Nongonococcal Urethritis and Related Infections.* Lake Placid, NY: American Society for Microbiology; 1976;67–76.
244. Silverman EM, Silverman AG. Persistence of spermatozoa in the lower genital tracts of women. JAMA. 1978;240:1875.
245. Tait IA, Rees E, Hobson D, et al. Chlamydial infection of the cervix in contacts of men with nongonococcal urethritis. Br J Vener Dis. 1980;56:37.
246. Mardh PA, Moller BR, Paavonen J. Chlamydial infection of the female genital tract with emphasis on pelvic inflammatory disease. A review of Scandinavian studies. Sex Transm Dis. 1981;8:140.
247. Paavonen J, Vesterinen E. *Chlamydia trachomatis* in cervicitis and urethritis in women. Scand J Infect Dis. 1982;32(Suppl):45.
248. Spence MR, Barbacci M, Kappus E, et al. A correlative study of Papanicolaou smear, fluorescent antibody, and culture for the diagnosis of *Chlamydia trachomatis.* Obstet Gynecol. 1986;68:691–5.
249. Paavonen J, Critchlow CW, DeRouen T, et al. Etiology of cervical inflammation. Am J Obstet Gynecol. 1986;154:556–64.
250. Harrison HR, Costin M, Meder JB, et al. Cervical *Chlamydia trachomatis* infection in university women: Relationship to history, contraceptives, ectopy, and cervicitis. Am J Obstet Gynecol. 1985;153:224–51.
251. Moscicki B, Shafer MA, Millstein SG, et al. The use and limitations of endocervical Gram stain and mucopurulent cervicitis as predictors for *Chlamydia trachomatis* in female adolescents. Am J Obstet Gynecol. 1987;157:65–71.
252. Nugent RP, Hillier SL. Mucopurulent cervicitis as a predictor of chlamydial infection and adverse pregnancy outcome. Sex Transm Dis. 1992;19:198–202.
253. Knud-Hansen CR, Dallabetta GA, Reichart C, et al. Surrogate methods to diagnose gonococcal and chlamydial cervicitis: Comparison of leukocyte esterase dipstick, endocervical Gram stain, and culture. Sex Transm Dis. 1991;18:211–6.
254. Katz BP, Caine VA, Jones RB. Diagnosis of mucopurulent cervicitis among women at risk for *Chlamydia trachomatis* infection. Sex Transm Dis. 1989;16:103–6.
255. Dimian C, Nayagam M, Bradbeer C. The association between sexually transmitted diseases and inflammatory cervical cytology. Genitourin Med. 1992;68:305–6.
256. Bertolino JG, Rangel JE, Blake RL Jr, et al. Inflammation on the cervical Papanicolaou smear: The predictive value for infection in asymptomatic women. Fam Med 1992;241:447–52.
257. Lowley TB, Lee RB, Kapela R. The significance of moderate and severe inflammation on class I Papanicolaou smear. Obstet Gynecol. 1990;76:997–9.
258. Wentworth BB, Bonin P, Holmes KK, et al. Isolation of viruses, bacteria and other organisms from venereal disease clinic patients: Methodology and problems associated with multiple isolations. Health Lab Sci. 1973;10:75.
259. Curran JW, Rendtorff RC, Chandler RW, et al. Female gonorrhea: Its relationship to abnormal uterine bleeding, urinary tract symptoms and cervicitis. Obstet Gynecol. 1975;45:195.
260. Hilton AL, Richmond SJ, Milne JD, et al. Chlamydia A in the female genital tract. Br J Vener Dis. 1974;50:1.
261. Oriel JD, Powis PA, Reeve P, et al. Chlamydial infection of the cervix. Br J Vener Dis. 1974;50:11.
262. Quinn TC, Gupta PK, Burkman RT. Detection of *Chlamydia trachomatis* cervical infections: A comparison of Papanicolaou and immunofluorescent staining with cell cultures. Am J Obstet Gynecol. 1987;157:394–9.
263. Stamm WE, Harrison HR, Alexander ET, et al. Diagnosis of *Chlamydia trachomatis* infections by direct immunofluorescence staining of genital secretions: A multicenter trial. Ann Intern Med. 1984;101:638–42.
264. Hipp SS, Han V, Murphy D. Assessment of enzyme immunoassay and immunofluorescence tests for detection of *Chlamydia trachomatis.* J Clin Microbiol. 1987;25:1938–43.
265. LeBar W, Schubiner H, Jemal C, et al. Comparison of the Kallstead Pathfinder EIA, cytocentrifuged direct fluorescent antibody, and culture for the diagnosis of *Chlamydia trachomatis.* Diagn Microbiol Infect Dis. 1991;14:17–20.
266. Coleman P, Varitek V, Mushahwar IK, et al. TestPack Chlamydia, a new rapid assay for the direct detection of *Chlamydia trachomatis.* J Clin Microbiol. 1989;27:2811–4.
267. Ferris DG, Martin WH. A comparison of three rapid chlamydial tests in pregnant and nonpregnant women. J Fam Pract. 1992;34:593–7.
268. Skulnick M, Small GW, Simor AE, et al. Comparison of the Clearview Chlamydia test, Chlamydiazyme, and cell culture for the detection of *Chlamydia trachomatis* in women with a low prevalence of infection. J Clin Microbiol. 1991;29:2056–8.
269. Moncada J, Schachter J, Bolan G, et al. Confirmatory assay increases specificity of the Chlamydiazyme test for *Chlamydia trachomatis* infections. J Clin Microbiol 1990;28:1770–3.
270. Nohara M, Sugase M, Kawana T. Evaluation of DNA probe for chlamydial and gonococcal infections of the uterine cervix. Acta Obstet Gynecol Jpn. 1991;43:459–64.
271. Mercer LJ, Robinson DC, Sahon DF, et al. Comparison of chemiluminescent DNA probe to cell culture for the screening of *Chlamydia trachomatis* in a gynecology clinic population. Obstet Gynecol. 1990;76:114–7.
272. Phillps RS, Aronson MD, Taylor WC, et al. Should tests for *Chlamydia trachomatis* cervical infection be done during routine gynecological visits? An analysis of the costs of alternative strategies. Ann Intern Med. 1987;107:188–94.
273. Purola E, Paavonen J. Routine cytology as a diagnostic aid in chlamydial cervicitis. Scand J Infect Dis. 1982;32(Suppl):55.
274. Hare MJ, Toone E, Taylor-Robinson D, et al. Follicular cervicitis: Colposcopic appearances and association with *Chlamydia trachomatis.* Br J Obstet Gynecol. 1981;88:174.
275. Paavonen J, Vesterinen E, Meyer B, et al. Colposcopic and histological findings in cervical chlamydial infection. Obstet Gynecol. 1982;59:712.
276. Willcox RR. Necrotic cervicitis due to primary infection with the virus of herpes simplex. Br Med J. 1968;1:610.
277. Morse AR, Coleman DV, Gardner SD. An evaluation of cytology in the diagnosis of herpes simplex virus infection and cytomegalovirus infection of the cervix uteri. J Obstet Gynecol Br Common. 1974;81:393.
278. Corey L. Laboratory diagnosis of herpes simplex virus infections. Principles guiding the development of rapid diagnostic tests. Diagn Microbiol Infect Dis. 1986;4(Suppl):111S–9S.
279. Reid R, Greenberg M, Jensen AB, et al. Sexually transmitted papillomavirus infections. I. The anatomic distribution and pathologic grade of neoplastic lesions associated with different viral types. Am J Obstet Gynecol 1987;156:212–22.
280. Waugh MA. History of clinical developments in sexually transmitted diseases. In: Holmes KK, Mardh P-A, Sparling PF, et al (eds): *Sexually Transmitted Diseases.* 2nd ed. New York: McGraw Hill; 1990:3–16.
281. Pfister H. Relationship of papillomaviruses to anogenital cancer. Obstet Gynecol Clin North Am. 1987;14:349–62.
282. Koutsky LA, Holmes KK, Critchlow CW, et al. A cohort study of the risk of cervical intrepithelial neoplasia grade 2 or 3 in relation to papillomavirus infection. N Engl J Med. 1992;327:1272–8.
283. Laverty CR, Russell P, Black J, et al. Adenovirus infection of the cervix. Acta Cytol 1977;21:114.
284. Heimann A, Scanlon R, Gentile J, et al. Measles cervicitis. Report of a case with cytologic and molecular biologic analysis. Acta Cytol 1992;36:727–30.

285. Deppisch LM. Cytomegalovirus inclusion body endocervicitis: Significance of CMV inclusions in endocervical biopsies. Mt Sinai J Med. 1981;48:418.

286. Wong JV, Becker SN. *Enterobius vermicularis* ova in routine cervicovaginal smears. Light scanning electron microscopic observations. Acta Cytol. 1982; 26:484.

287. Arroyo G, Elgueta R. Squamous cell carcinoma associated with amoebic cervicitis. Acta Cytol. 1989;33:301–4.

288. Tang LCH. Postmenopausal tuberculous cervicitis. Acta Obstet Gynecol Scand. 1986;65:279–81.

289. Buttigieg G. Cervicitis and urethritis caused by group B streptococcus: Case report. Genitourin Med. 1985;61:343–4.

290. Conde-Glez CJ, Calderon E. Urogenital infection due to meningococcus in men and women. Sex Transm Dis. 1991;18:72–5.

291. Mao K, Guillebaud J. Influence of removal of intrauterine contraceptive devices on colonization of the cervix by *Actinomyces*-like organisms. Contraception. 1984;30:535–44.

292. Washington AE, Browner WS, Korenbrot CC. Cost effectiveness of combined treatment for endocervical gonorrhea. Considering coinfection with *Chlamydia trachomatis*. JAMA. 1987;257:2056–60.

293. Centers for Disease Control and Prevention. 1993 sexually transmitted disease treatment guidelines. MMWR 1993;42(RR-14):49.

294. Morton RS. *Gonorrhea*. London: WB Saunders; 1977:108.

295. Rees E. Gonococcal bartholinitis. Br J Vener Dis. 1967;43:150.

296. Brook I. Aerobic and anaerobic microbiology of Bartholin's abscess. Surg Gynecol Obstet. 1989;169:32–4.

297. Norris CC. Gonorrhea in Women. Philadelphia: WB Saunders; 1913:202.

298. Lee Y-H, Rankin JS, Alpert S, et al. Microbiological investigation of Bartholin's gland abscesses and cysts. Am J Obstet Gynecol. 1977;129–150.

299. Blecker OP, Smalbraak DJ, Schutte MF. Bartholin's abscess: The role of *Chlamydia trachomatis*. Genitourin Med 1990;66:24–5.

300. Davies JA, Rees E, Hobson D, et al. Isolation of *Chlamydia trachomatis* from Bartholin's duct. Br J Vener Dis. 1978;54:409.

301. Swensen RM. Anaerobic bacteria in infections of the female genital tract. In: Balows A, DeHaan RM, Dowell VR, et al (eds). *Anaerobic Bacteria: Role in Disease*. Springfield, IL: Charles C. Thomas, 1974.

302. Swenson RM, Michaelson TC, Dayl MJ, et al. Anaerobic bacterial infections of the female genital tract. Obstet Gynecol. 1973;42:538.

303. Kubitz R, Hoffman K. Bartholin's gland abscess in an infant. A case report. J Reprod Med. 1986;31:67–9.

304. Carson GD, Smith LP. *Escherichia coli* endotoxic shock complicating Bartholin's gland abscess. Can Med Assoc J. 1980;122:1397.

305. Morton BD, McCarthy LR. Bartholinitis: An unusual etiologic agent. Obstet Gynecol. 1980;55:(Suppl):97.

306. Shearin RS, Boehlke J, Karanth S. Toxic shock-like syndrome associated with Bartholin's gland abscess: Case report. Am J Obstet Gynecol 1989;160: 1073–4.

307. van Bosterhaut B, Buts R, Veys A, et al. *Haemophilus influenzae* bartholinitis. Eur J Clin Microbiol Infect Dis. 1990;9:442.

308. Azzan BB. Bartholin's cyst and abscess: A review of treatment of 53 cases. Br J Clin Pract. 1978;32:101.

309. Anderson PG, Christensen S, Detlefsen GU, et al. Treatment of Bartholin's abscess. Marsupializtion versus incision, curettage and suture under antibiotic cover. A randomized study with six months' follow up. Acta Obstet Gynecol Scand. 1992;71:59–62.

310. Lopez-Zeno JA, Ross E, O'Grady JP. Septic shock complicating drainage of a Bartholin gland abscess. Obstet Gynecol 1990;76:915–6.

311. Frolich EP, Schein M. Necrotizing fasciitis arising from Bartholin's abscess. Case report and review of the literature. Isr J Med Sci. 1989;25:644–7.

90. INFECTIONS OF THE FEMALE PELVIS

PHILIP B. MEAD

Infections of the female pelvis constitute a diverse group of both community- and hospital-acquired infections. They are conveniently considered in three categories: infections related to pregnancy; infections following gynecologic surgery; and sexually transmitted pelvic inflammatory disease.

INTRAPARTUM, POSTPARTUM, AND POSTABORTAL INFECTIONS

Intra-Amniotic Infection Syndrome

Intra-amniotic infection syndrome (IAIS), known also as *chorioamnionitis*, is a clinically detectable infection of the uterus and

its contents during pregnancy.[1] IAIS occurs in 1–2 percent of term patients and in up to 25 percent of women with preterm labor. Most cases of IAIS are ascending in origin, occurring after prolonged rupture of the membranes or labor in patients with multiple vaginal examinations. A few cases, most notably those caused by *Listeria monocytogenes,* result from transplacental hematogenous spread in mothers with bacteremia.[2] Rare cases have been reported following diagnostic amniocentesis, intrauterine transfusions, or percutaneous umbilical blood sampling. Intrauterine infection also follows the placement of a cervical cerclage in 1–2 percent of patients, and this risk may be as high as 25 percent if the cerclage is carried out after prolapse of the membranes into the vagina. Risk factors for IAIS include prolonged duration of labor or rupture of membranes, multiple vaginal examinations, young age, low socioeconomic class, nulliparity, and preexisting bacterial vaginosis.

The most common organisms isolated from amniotic fluid in cases of IAIS are anaerobes, genital mycoplasmas, group B streptococci, and *Escherichia coli*. The latter two are found most commonly in maternal or neonatal bacteremia complicating intra-amniotic infection. Two constellations of organisms have been noted. In one, presumed to be from a vaginal source, *Gardnerella vaginalis, Mycoplasma hominis,* and anaerobes are associated. In the other, enterococci, *E. coli,* and other aerobic gram-negative bacilli are associated, suggesting an intestinal source.[3]

Maternal manifestations of IAIS are fever, tachycardia, and uterine tenderness. Foul-smelling or grossly purulent amniotic fluid is an uncommon finding. Fetal heart rate abnormalities, primarily tachycardia and decreased variability, are important markers of intrauterine infection. Approximately 5–10 percent of women with preterm labor and intact membranes have symptomatic chorioamnionitis, while another 10 percent have subclinical infection. In patients with preterm premature rupture of the membranes, the frequency of subclinical infection at the time of admission may be as high as 25 percent. In term patients, chorioamnionitis typically causes dysfunctional labor. About 75 percent of infected women require augmentation of labor with oxytocin, and about 40 percent require cesarean delivery, usually for arrest of progress in labor.

Although diagnosis is based largely on clinical findings, amniotic fluid Gram stain, leukocyte esterase activity, and glucose concentration have been shown to be useful in supporting the clinical impression.[4,5]

Management of IAIS is based on the principles that antibiotic therapy should be started as soon as the diagnosis is made and that delivery is essential to cure. Antibiotic administration seeks to reduce the frequency of neonatal pneumonia and bacteremia and to cure the maternal infection. Because group B streptococci and *E. coli* are the most frequent isolates from infected newborns, a combination of ampicillin plus gentamicin is a reasonable initial regimen for IAIS. In patients who deliver vaginally, this is usually sufficient to treat the mother as well. If cesarean delivery is required, however, 20–30 percent of operative patients given only ampicillin and gentamicin will experience treatment failure. These patients probably require better anaerobic coverage, and accordingly a drug such as clindamycin should be added to the treatment regimen. Other broad-spectrum regimens may be equally effective. Gibbs et al.[6] have documented improved neonatal and maternal outcome when antibiotic therapy is begun as soon as the diagnosis of IAIS is made rather than immediately postpartum. This is currently the standard of care.

Although delivery is essential to cure, no critical diagnosis-to-delivery interval beyond which the frequency of neonatal complications escalates dramatically has been identified. Accordingly, labor must be managed actively, but cesarean delivery should be performed only for accepted obstetric indications.

Postpartum Endometritis

Postpartum infection of the uterus, the most common cause of puerperal fever, is designated *endometritis, endomyometritis,* or *endoparametritis* depending on the extent of disease. Cesarean delivery, particularly following labor or rupture of the membranes of any duration, is the dominant predictor of postpartum endometritis (PPE).[7] Following vaginal delivery, reported incidence ranges from 0.9–3.9 percent, while the incidence of PPE following cesarean section ranges from 10 percent or less in most private services to 50 percent or more in large teaching services caring for indigent patients. Postulated secondary predictors of postcesarean endometritis include duration of labor or rupture of membranes, presence of bacterial vaginosis, number of vaginal examinations, and use of internal fetal monitoring.[8–10]

Although prolonged membrane rupture, midforceps delivery, anemia, and maternal soft tissue trauma are commonly mentioned as factors predisposing to endometritis following vaginal delivery, these events are not identified in the vast majority of patients who develop such infections and are probably relative risk factors. Indigent patients are at substantially higher risk of developing PPE following either vaginal or abdominal delivery, although the reasons for this have never been fully delineated.

Postpartum endometritis is a polymicrobial infection caused by a wide variety of bacteria. Group B streptococci, enterococci, other aerobic streptococci, *G. vaginalis, E. coli, Prevotella bivia,* other *Bacteroides* spp., and peptostreptococci are the most common endometrial isolates, with group B streptococci and *G. vaginalis* the most common isolates from blood.[11–13]

The isolation of *Ureaplasma urealyticum* and *M. hominis* from endometrium and blood suggests that these organisms can cause PPE, although good clinical responses have been obtained in patients with mycoplasmas cultured from blood who were treated with antibiotics not active against these organisms.

Chlamydia trachomatis has been associated with a late form of PPE occurring more than 2 days to 6 weeks postpartum among women who deliver vaginally.[14] Group A β-hemolytic streptococcal endometritis is rare, epidemiologically unique because its source is exogenous infection (usually in a caregiver), and characterized by early onset and rapid progression with poor localization.

The diagnosis of PPE is suggested by the development of fever, usually on the first or second postpartum day. Significant fever is defined as an oral temperature of 38.5°C or higher in the first 24 hours after delivery or 38°C or higher for at least 4 consecutive hours 24 or more hours after delivery. Other consistently associated findings are lower abdominal pain, uterine tenderness and leukocytosis.

Patients suspected of having PPE should undergo a bimanual pelvic examination to determine uterine size, consistency, and tenderness. The presence of an adnexal mass can also be ascertained at this time.

The value of transvaginally obtained uterine cultures, and the optimal method of obtaining such cultures, are currently matters of controversy. While cultures obtained transvaginally are often difficult to interpret because of contaminants, they may be useful in those patients failing initial therapy.[15] It is important to obtain blood cultures because 10–20 percent of patients will have a documentable bacteremia. Bacteremia does not predict the severity of clinical illness or a prolonged recovery, however. Cultures or rapid antigen detection tests for *Chlamydia* should be obtained from patients with late-onset PPE or those with PPE at high risk for chlamydial infection (e.g., teenage pregnancy). *Mycoplasma* cultures are presently a research tool only.

Based on findings of general systemic toxicity, patterns of pulse and fever, and clinical course, some patients will be classified as having severe PPE. Clindamycin plus gentamicin has proved to be an effective regimen for these patients, especially if they developed PPE following cesarean section. PPE of mild to moderate severity is typically treated with one of the extended-spectrum penicillins or second-generation cephalosporins (e.g., cefotetan, cefoxitin, ampicillin/sulbactam, ticarcillin/clavulanic acid). Parenteral therapy should be continued until the patient's temperature has remained lower than 37.5°C for 24 hours, she is pain free, and the white blood cell count is normal. The use of oral antibiotics after discharge has been shown to be unnecessary. Women with positive cultures for *Chlamydia* should receive erythromycin or doxycycline therapy for a full 10 days even if they have had an initial clinical response to one of the above regimens.

Failure of antimicrobial therapy usually results from either enterococcal superinfection or inadequate coverage of a multiresistant anaerobe. Enterococcal superinfection is suggested when patients fail to respond or relapse on regimens that are not effective against enterococci (e.g., cephalosporins; clindamycin plus gentamicin), particularly when this organism is isolated in pure culture or heavy growth from an endometrial specimen. If enterococcal superinfection is suspected, one of the following regimens should be employed: clindamycin or metronidazole plus ampicillin plus gentamicin; ampicillin/sulbactam; cefoxitin or cefotetan plus ampicillin; ticarcillin/clavulanic acid; piperacillin; or mezlocillin. Antimicrobial failure due to lack of coverage of a multiresistant anaerobe often responds to a regimen containing either metronidazole or clindamycin.

If fever persists despite apparently appropriate antimicrobial therapy, the differential diagnosis includes a wound or pelvic abscess, puerperal ovarian vein thrombosis, or noninfectious fever (e.g., drug fever or breast engorgement).

Prophylactic antimicrobial agents can be expected to decrease the postcesarean endometritis rate in a given institution by 50 percent,[16,17] and are currently the standard of care for any patient who requires a cesarean section after labor or rupture of the membranes of any duration.[10] About 15 percent of women undergoing nonelective cesarean section develop PPE despite receiving antimicrobial prophylaxis,[9] possibly because of unrecognized subclinical infection at the time of cesarean delivery.[18]

PPE caused by group A β-hemolytic streptococci has special epidemiologic significance.[19–21] If group A β-hemolytic streptococci are isolated from more than one patient over a brief time span, the following measures should be initiated: notify local public health authorities; employ contact isolation of all infected patients for 24 hours after the start of effective antimicrobial therapy; institute a cohort nursery system; culture all involved professional and support staff and relieve from duty any who are colonized; culture all newborns for group A streptococci; stress rigid adherence to aseptic technique and handwashing; consider stringent reduction of visitors; and save all positive group A streptococcal isolates for typing.

Puerperal Ovarian Vein Thrombophlebitis

Puerperal ovarian vein thrombophlebitis (POVT) is a syndrome resulting from the acute thrombosis of one or both ovarian veins in the postpartum period. It can follow either cesarean or vaginal delivery and is rare, with a reported incidence of 1 per 2000 deliveries or 1–2 per 100 patients with postpartum infection. Puerperal ovarian vein thrombophlebitis is usually associated with postcesarean endometritis, but may occur in the absence of infection. Onset is variable but most often occurs 2–4 days postpartum.

Clinical symptoms have an acute onset, and patients appear ill. Most have a moderate temperature elevation and complain of lower abdominal pain, usually on the right side. Many patients will have previously been diagnosed with PPE but failed to respond to appropriate antibiotics.

The pulse rate usually is elevated, often disproportionately compared with the temperature. Temperature elevations persist, often accompanied by shaking chills. On physical examination a tender, sausage-shaped or ropelike abdominal mass can be palpated in one-half to two-thirds of patients. The mass usually originates centrally near the right uterine cornua and extends laterally and cephalad toward the upper abdomen. An ileus is frequently present. Tachypnea, stridor, and other signs of respiratory distress may be present if pulmonary embolization has occurred.[22]

In the absence of a thrombosed vessel palpable abdominally, the diagnosis is one of exclusion based on the clinical history. Computed tomography, duplex Doppler ultrasonography, and magnetic resonance imaging have all been used to confirm the presence of POVT.[23,24]

Therapy consists of broad-spectrum antibiotics, effective against the common pelvic pathogens, and continuous intravenous heparin anticoagulation. The optimal duration of anticoagulation is unknown, but, in the absence of pulmonary embolization, most clinicians have utilized a course of 7–10 days, concurrent with antibiotic administration. Even though blood cultures are usually sterile in women with POVT, evidence for an infection-related etiology is convincing since resected thrombi usually contain microorganisms, a hectic fever course is common, and not all patients treated with heparin alone respond.[23]

Episiotomy Infections

Infection of the episiotomy site is an uncommon occurrence. Overall only 0.1 percent of episiotomies become infected, although this rate increases to 1–2 percent of episiotomies complicated by third- or fourth-degree extensions.

Shy and Eschenbach[25] have classified episiotomy infections into four categories, depending on the depth of infection (see Fig. 1). The *simple episiotomy infection* is a local infection that is limited to the skin and superficial fascia along the episiotomy incision. In contrast to deeper infection, the associated skin changes of edema and erythema only occur adjacent to the episiotomy. The simple episiotomy infection should be opened, explored, and débrided under adequate anesthesia to exclude a hematoma or previously unrecognized rectovaginal communication. If the superficial fascial layer is extensively infected, antibiotic administration is appropriate to inhibit streptococci, staphylococci, Enterobacteriaceae, and anaerobes, including *Bacteroides fragilis*.

Two infections of the two layers of the superficial fascia may occur. The more common is *superficial fascia infection without necrosis*, the clinical presentation of which is neither striking nor distinctive. The skin may be erythematous and edematous, but severe systemic manifestations do not occur. If response to broad-spectrum antibiotic therapy does not occur in 24–48 hours, or if the clinical condition worsens during antibiotic therapy, then the episiotomy should be surgically explored.

Infection of the superficial fascia with necrosis, most commonly referred to as *necrotizing fasciitis*, is an infection of the subcutaneous tissues (i.e., the superficial fascia) that spreads in the fascial clefts overlying the deep fascia. The deep fascia usually, but not always, is spared; skin involvement results only secondarily after the nutrient vessels to the skin thrombose. Because the skin is not primarily involved, the episiotomy wound may appear normal, making early recognition difficult and causing fatal delay in treatment. Despite the minimal local findings, patients may appear severely ill, with marked local pain, high fever, and prominent systemic manifestations. Most patients are diabetic. Definitive diagnosis is made at surgery when the operator discovers extensive undermining of surrounding tissues and lack of resistance in the superficial fascial plane to probing with a blunt instrument. Treatment includes

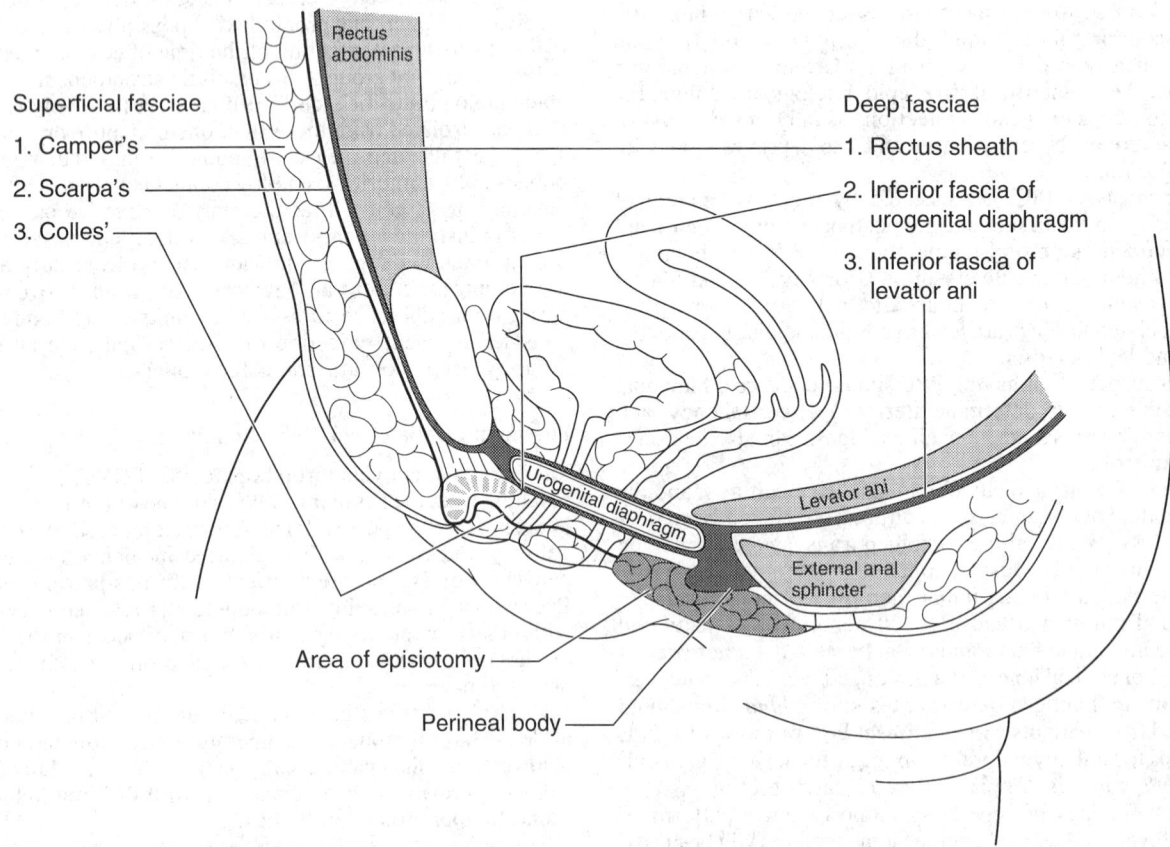

FIG. 1. Diagrammatic representation of the fascial layers of the lower abdomen and perineum in paramedian sagittal section. (From Shy and Eschenbach,[25] with permission.)

broad-spectrum antibiotics (e.g., clindamycin plus ampicillin plus gentamicin) and radical débridement to include removal of all necrotic and pale tissue.

In the extremely rare event of infection beneath the deep fascia, muscle may be involved, resulting in the fourth type of episiotomy infection, *myonecrosis.* Myonecrosis is most commonly caused by *Clostridium perfringens,* although it can occur from a neglected necrotizing fasciitis infection that invades deep fascia. Myonecrosis of the subgluteal muscles surrounding the hip joint or the psoas muscles can also occur from bacteria introduced into this deep space by a paracervical or pudendal needle. These patients experience severe hip pain associated with marked limitation of motion.[26]

Both myonecrosis and clostridial infection should be treated with surgical resection and antibiotic therapy. For clostridial infection, high-dose penicillin is the therapy of choice. Radical wide excision may be necessary. Hyperbaric oxygen therapy is at best an adjunctive measure to surgical débridement. Polyvalent gas gangrene antitoxin is probably ineffective (see Ch. 225).

Soper[27] has reported an unusually severe form of clostridial myonecrosis arising from an episiotomy due to *Clostridium sordelli.* The patient had a distinctive course characterized by sudden onset of severe and unrelenting hypotension associated with marked, generalized tissue edema and third spacing, with increased hematocrit, marked leukemoid reaction, absence of rash or fever, and a rapid fatal course. This syndrome has subsequently been reported in association with retention of a vaginal pack, degeneration of a cervical myoma, and postpartum endometritis.[28,29]

Postabortion Infection

Infection after abortion is an ascending process and occurs more commonly in the presence of retained products of conception or operative trauma. Risk factors include greater duration of pregnancy, technical difficulties, and the presence of unsuspected sexually transmitted pathogens.

Symptoms include fever, chills, abdominal pain, and vaginal bleeding, often with the passage of placental tissue. Postabortal infection typically has its onset within 4 days of the procedure.

Physical findings include an elevated temperature, tachycardia, tachypnea, and abdominal tenderness. In the presence of bacteremia, hypotension or frank shock may occur, and the patient may be agitated or disoriented. Pelvic examination reveals a sanguinopurulent discharge and uterine tenderness, with or without adnexal and parametrial tenderness. It is important to look for cervical or vaginal lacerations, especially in a suspected illegal abortion.

Septic abortion due to *C. perfringens* infection has a characteristic clinical presentation. In severe cases, massive intravascular hemolysis produces jaundice, mahogany-colored urine, and severe anemia.

Laboratory evaluation for patients with more than early uncomplicated postabortal endometritis should include complete blood count, urinalysis, culture, and Gram stain of cervical material, blood cultures, anteroposterior radiographs of the abdomen and pelvis and upright chest roentgenograms.

Simple endometritis, defined as low-grade fever associated with mild uterine tenderness after uncomplicated elective abortion, can be treated with oral doxycycline. Persistent bleeding or signs of infection require curettage.

Patients with more serious infection require early curettage and broad-spectrum parenteral antibiotic therapy. For the patient with septic shock, clindamycin plus ampicillin plus either gentamicin or aztreonam is advisable. If *C. perfringens* infection is suspected, the regimen should include high-dose penicillin.

Surgical removal of infected tissue is essential in all but the mildest of postabortal infections.[30] Pelvic ultrasound can be employed to confirm the presence of retained tissue. In most cases, prompt curettage will control the infection. When the uterus is too large to allow suction curettage, oxytocin administration is often successful. Prostaglandin suppositories are contraindicated in the presence of acute pelvic infection. Concurrent laparoscopy may be needed when curetting a uterus perforated at the time of abortion.

Indications for laparotomy and hysterectomy include failure to respond to curettage and appropriate medical therapy, perforation and infection with suspected bowel injury, pelvic and adnexal abscess, and clostridial necrotizing myometritis (gas gangrene). Isolation of *C. perfringens* does not mandate hysterectomy. Initial treatment should be with high-dose penicillin, curettage, supportive therapy, and intensive cardiovascular monitoring. Laparotomy is indicated if there is deterioration or no response.

Avoidance of unwanted pregnancies by making contraceptives available is the most important preventive measure. Screening for sexually transmitted diseases prior to performing elective abortion is optimal but often impractical. Prophylactic antibiotics may be effective in reducing infection morbidity when used routinely for first-trimester elective suction curettage abortion.[31]

INFECTION FOLLOWING GYNECOLOGIC SURGERY

Pathogens

The normal vaginal flora consists of lactobacilli, various species of streptococci, *G. vaginalis,* strains of Enterobacteriaceae, and anaerobes. Anaerobes predominate numerically, with a ratio of 10:1.[32] The normal flora mirrors the major pathogens in nonvenereal infections of the female pelvis (Table 1), supporting an endogenous route of infection as postulated by Schottmueller[33] more than 80 years ago. Unexplained exceptions to this association are *Fusobacteria* and *B. fragilis,* both infrequent members of the normal vaginal flora.

Many factors alter the vaginal flora and may indirectly predispose to postoperative infection. Ohm and Galask[34,35] have shown that, after abdominal or vaginal hysterectomy, *E. coli, Klebsiella, Proteus, Enterobacter, B. fragilis,* and enterococci are more common in 5-day postoperative vaginal cultures than in preoperative cultures from the same patients. Although several studies have documented increased enterococcal colonization after perioperative cephalosporin prophylaxis, other factors must be involved since placebo groups show increased enterococcal colonization as well. Hospitalization appears to exert a profound effect on the vaginal flora, regardless of surgery or antibiotic prophylaxis, and this change tends to be in the direction of more virulent organisms, including enterococci, *B. fragilis,* and resistant Enterobacteriaceae.

Other factors that affect the vaginal flora include use of non-

TABLE 1. Endogenous Pathogens Commonly Isolated from Postoperative Pevic Infections

Aerobic gram-positive cocci
  Viridans and nongroup A, B, and D streptococci
  Group B streptococci
  Enterococcus faecalis
  Staphylococcus aureus
  Staphylococcus epidermidis
Aerobic gram-negative bacilli
  Escherichia coli
  Klebsiella species
  Proteus mirabilis
  Gardnerella vaginalis
Anaerobic organisms
  Peptostreptococcus species
  Bacteroides fragilis group
  Prevotella bivia (Bacteroides bivius)
  Prevotella disiens (Bacteroides disiens)
  Fusobacterium species
Mycoplasmas
  Mycoplasma hominis
  Ureaplasma urealyticum

oxynol-9-containing vaginal contraceptive preparations,[36,37] douching,[38] use of the female condom,[39] and the phase of the menstrual cycle. The significance of these factors in relation to infection after gynecologic surgery is presently unknown.

The animal model of intra-abdominal infection devised by Weinstein and colleagues[40,41] has clarified the distinctive roles played by different bacteria in the natural history of pelvic infection. These investigators documented a biphasic response to infection consisting of an early-onset phase with high rates of sepsis and death in which gram-negative aerobic bacteria predominate (peritonitis stage) and a late-onset phase with abscess formation in which anaerobes predominate (abscess stage).

Risk Factors

Several factors, many beyond the surgeon's control, influence the likelihood of developing a postoperative infection. Febrile morbidity is more common following abdominal than vaginal hysterectomy.[42] The incidence of postoperative infection is higher in patients of lower socioeconomic status, irrespective of the surgical approach. Age has inconsistently been shown to be a risk factor after hysterectomy, with premenopausal women shown to be at increased risk in some studies, especially after vaginal hysterectomy. It is not known whether this increased risk in younger women is due to estrogen-mediated influences on vaginal flora and host response[43] or to greater difficulty in obtaining hemostasis. Duration of surgery is directly correlated with postoperative infection rates. For infections of the operative site (i.e., "deep" as opposed to incisional infections) duration of surgery probably reflects the degree of technical difficulty of a procedure, the skill of the surgeon, or both.

Bacterial vaginosis has been associated with an increased risk of infection following abdominal hysterectomy.[44,45] Patients scheduled for elective hysterectomy should be screened for bacterial vaginosis 1 month before the planned procedure. Those found to have bacterial vaginosis should be treated and allowed several weeks to reestablish a normal lactobacillus-dominant flora prior to surgery.

Pelvic Cellulitis

The most common infection after hysterectomy is pelvic cellulitis. Patients complain of increasing lower abdominal and pelvic pain that is usually more severe on one side. Symptoms typically develop on the second or third postoperative day, and the temperature is greater than 38.5°C. Direct tenderness over the parametrial area is elicited by abdominal and confirmed by bimanual examinations.

The value of obtaining a culture from the vaginal cuff is controversial. Some believe cultures can identify the responsible pathogens, especially when an infection has not responded to the initial antimicrobial regimen. Others argue that the inevitable contamination with vaginal flora renders such cultures uninterpretable.

Women with pelvic cellulitis usually respond promptly to single-agent parenteral antibiotic therapy. Successful regimens include cefotetan, cefoxitin, ampicillin/sulbactam, or ticarcillin/clavulanic acid. Patients with true allergy to β-lactam antibiotics, or those who fail initial therapy, can be treated with a regimen of clindamycin plus gentamicin. Parenteral therapy is continued until the patient has been afebrile for 24–36 hours. Hager et al.[46] have shown that oral outpatient antibiotic therapy after successful parenteral therapy is unnecessary.

It should be emphasized that not all patients who are febrile following hysterectomy are infected. Hemsell[47] has observed that 17 percent of women undergoing vaginal hysterectomy and 35 percent undergoing abdominal hysterectomy have recurrent temperature elevations on the second or third postoperative day, but have normal abdominal and pelvic examinations and no pain. These patients become afebrile without therapy.[47]

Cuff Cellulitis

An inflammatory response at the margins of the vaginal cuff incision is a normal part of the healing process in the early postoperative period. Host defense mechanisms quickly resolve this cellulitis in most patients without need for antibiotic administration. In a small number of cases, however, cuff cellulitis after hysterectomy will require antibiotic therapy. These cases usually occur in the 10-day period following discharge from the hospital. Patients complain of increasing central lower abdominal or pelvic pain, increased vaginal discharge, and low-grade temperature elevation. Abdominal examination is normal or elicits only slight suprapubic tenderness to deep palpation. On bimanual examination only the vaginal surgical margin is tender, and no masses are palpable. Women with cuff cellulitis have been treated successfully as outpatients with oral antibiotics such as amoxicillin/clavulanic acid. Patients should monitor their temperatures at home, and clinical reevaluation must be carried out at 72 hours.

Cuff Abscess

A few patients will develop a well-localized collection just above the vaginal cuff. They usually become febrile on the second or third postoperative day and may complain of a sense of fullness in the lower abdomen. Drainage facilitates cure and may be accomplished in a treatment room. Any purulent material recovered should be cultured for aerobic and anaerobic pathogens. Parenteral antibiotics should be given until the patient has been afebrile for 24–36 hours.[48]

Pelvic Abscess

The most serious late postoperative complication is an adnexal abscess. These infections are rare, occur almost exclusively in premenopausal women, occur despite the use of prophylactic antibiotics, and often have a latent period of many weeks between surgery and onset of symptoms.[49,50]

Patients may have had no apparent infection during their initial hospitalization, or, alternatively, they may have appeared to respond rapidly to the initial selection of antibiotics for presumed pelvic cellulitis, only to relapse after discharge. Typically the fever curve is characterized by a high spike late in the afternoon or early evening. The white blood cell count is often in the 20,000/mm³ range, and the erythrocyte sedimentation rate is markedly elevated. Patients with postoperative adnexal abscesses often have a palpable mass high in the pelvis. Ultrasonography and computed tomography (CT) scans both confirm the presence of the mass as well as help determine if it is loculated, related to an intraperitoneal structure, or drainable percutaneously.

Identification of a postoperative pelvic abscess does not mandate immediate drainage if it is inaccessible, as antibiotic therapy alone is often successful in the treatment of this complication. The frequent isolation of *B. fragilis* from these abscesses warrants the use of clindamycin, metronidazole, or other agents effective against gram-negative anaerobes. A regimen of clindamycin plus gentamicin is frequently employed. In patients who fail to respond to appropriate antibiotic therapy, drainage is necessary. Ledger et al.[51] have shown that most such antibiotic failures are due not to antimicrobial resistance but to the unique environment of the abscess, which inhibits antibiotic effectiveness.

If the abscess is located in the posterior cul-de-sac, colpotomy drainage can be attempted under ultrasound guidance.[52] The abscess cavity should be completely evacuated and a drain placed to prevent reaccumulation of fluid. Abscesses not located in the cul-de-sac may be drained percutaneously if located adjacent to the abdominal wall or determined to be accessible by CT scan. A pigtail or equivalent catheter should remain in place until drainage ceases, usually 4–8 days.[53–57] Patients with suspected postoperative pelvic abscess who fail to respond to antibiotic therapy, and whose abscess is not able to be drained by one of the above techniques, will require laparotomy. The least extensive operation compatible with cure should be used. If the abscess is amenable to extraperitoneal drainage, this alone should suffice. If not, as in a postoperative adnexal abscess, extirpation may be necessary.

Purulent material obtained at drainage procedures should be submitted for culture in an anaerobic transport vial. Fluid should be inoculated through the rubber diaphragm, and tissue, such as a specimen of abscess wall, may be placed into the vial after the cap has been briefly removed. Introduction of oxygen into the vial is not a problem if tissue or pus is being cultured. Material placed in an anaerobic transport vial is adequate for every type of culture, including aerobes, anaerobes, fungi, and mycobacteria. For most purposes several milliliters of pus or a 0.5-cm cube of tissue is adequate.

Parenteral antibiotics should be administered until the patient remains afebrile for 48–72 hours, the white blood cell count is normal, and signs and symptoms have resolved. Controversy exists as to the need for postdischarge oral antibiotics for patients with pelvic abscesses that have responded to parenteral therapy and where the abscess was neither excised nor drained. Some clinicians choose to treat these patients for 7 days after discharge with oral agents such as amoxicillin/clavulanic acid or metronidazole. Regardless of whether they receive such therapy, all patients should be reexamined 2 weeks after discharge to ensure recurrence or reaccumulation of the abscess has not occurred. Sauer and Paulson[58] have recently reported the unusual case of a pelvic abscess complicating transcervical embryo transfer.

Septic Pelvic Thrombophlebitis

Pelvic vein thrombophlebitis may present as the so-called enigmatic fever syndrome, a rare cause of obscure postoperative fever.[22,59] This condition is almost always associated with a diagnosed operative site infection and typically has a gradual onset 4–8 days after surgery. Patients are begun on antibiotic therapy, and, unlike the patients with POVT, (see above), usually experience definite improvement in all clinical parameters except temperature. They do not appear to be acutely ill, and positive physical findings are usually limited to recurrent temperature elevations, often as high as 39.4–40.0°C, and tachycardia proportional to the fever. Pain, tenderness, palpable mass, and adynamic ileus are usually not present. Because there is no obvious source for the recurrent temperature elevations, this syndrome is aptly described as "enigmatic fever." The diagnosis of septic pelvic thrombophlebitis should be suspected in any patient with a recent soft tissue pelvic infection and recurrent temperature elevations that persist despite appropriate broad-spectrum antibiotic therapy. Differential diagnoses include drug fever, viral illness, collagen-vascular disease, and pelvic or incisional abscess. The diagnosis of septic pelvic thrombophlebitis is almost invariably one of exclusion and is verified by observing defervesence following therapeutic anticoagulation with heparin.[60]

Osteomyelitis Pubis

Osteomyelitis of the pubis is a rare infection that results from either bacteremic seeding or extension of a contiguous focus of infection. Most cases in women occur after urethral suspension, radical vulvectomy, or pelvic exenteration. In the study conducted by Hoyme and colleagues,[61] symptoms, consisting of pubic bone pain and tenderness, avoidance of ambulation, and pain on abduction, did not appear until more than 8 weeks after the initial operation. Wound drainage, low-grade fever, moderate leukocytosis, and an elevated erythrocyte sedimentation

rate or alkaline phosphatase level may be present. Blood and bone biopsy specimens or aspirated material should be cultured.

The radiograph or CT scan of the pubic bone often shows rarefaction, erosion, osteolytic lesions, or irregularities of the bone margins with separation of the symphysis. Later in the course of disease there is evidence of bone repair, with new bone formation or sclerosis of the symphysis. Radioactive scanning techniques may show increased activity.

Antimicrobial therapy must be prolonged and capable of covering both *Staphylococcus aureus* and aerobic gram-negative bacteria, the usual pathogens, unless a specific organism is isolated. Surgical débridement may be necessary as well.[61]

PELVIC INFLAMMATORY DISEASE

Acute pelvic inflammatory disease (PID) refers to the clinical syndrome, unrelated to pregnancy or surgery, that results when cervical microorganisms ascend to the endometrium, fallopian tubes, and contiguous pelvic structures producing one or more of the following inflammatory conditions: endometritis, salpingitis, pelvic peritonitis, or tuboovarian abscess. Each year approximately 1 million women in the United States experience an episode of symptomatic PID. Many women with PID have minimal or no symptoms.

PID results from direct canalicular spread of organisms from the endocervix to the endometrial and fallopian tube mucosa. Both *N. gonorrhoeae* and *C. trachomatis* commonly cause endocervicitis, and 10–40 percent of women with these infections who do not receive adequate treatment develop clinical symptoms of acute PID.[62] In addition to *N. gonorrhoeae* and *C. trachomatis,* a wide variety of bacteria have been isolated from the upper genital tracts of women with acute PID, including anaerobes, gram-negative rods, streptococci, and mycoplasmas. Barham et al.[63] have recently reported a rare case of acute salpingitis due to group A β-hemolytic streptococci following endometrial biopsy.

Risk Factors

Age is inversely related to PID rates, with sexually experienced teenagers three times more likely to be diagnosed with PID than are 25- to 29-year-old women. A history of multiple sexual partners, an increased rate of acquiring new partners within the previous 30 days,[64] and frequent intercourse with a single partner[65] are all associated with an increased risk of PID. Contraceptive choice modifies PID risk in a complex manner (i.e., mechanical and chemical barriers decrease risk; oral contraceptives have a variable effect; and intrauterine devices confer a slightly increased risk of nonsexually transmitted PID in the first months after insertion). Other suggested associations with PID include bacterial vaginosis,[66] douching,[67] menses, cigarette smoking,[68] and substance abuse.

Although an association between the use of an intrauterine contraceptive device (IUD) and increased risk of PID has been documented for many years, recent studies suggest that the magnitude of this association has been overestimated.[69,70] Contamination of the endometrial cavity at insertion apparently results in a slightly increased risk of acute PID that is limited to the first 4 months of use. Infections occurring after 4 months are believed to be the result of acquired sexually transmitted pathogens, not of the IUD itself.

A unique role for *Actinomyces* organisms in IUD PID has been suggested, but this relationship remains unclear. Although as many as 4–8 percent of IUD users may have *Actinomyces*-like organisms identified on a Pap smear, this presence has not been equated with pelvic actinomycosis, nor has the risk of subsequent pelvic infection been quantified.[71]

Diagnosis

Classic clinical criteria for acute PID include direct lower quadrant tenderness, cervical motion tenderness, and adnexal tenderness, plus one or more of the following: mucopurulent cervicitis, culture or nonculture evidence of cervical infection with *N. gonorrhoeae* or *C. trachomatis*, temperature greater than 38°C, leukocytosis, elevated erythrocyte sedimentation rate or C-reactive protein, pelvic abscess or inflammatory complex on bimanual examination or by sonography, and purulent material from peritoneal cavity by culdocentesis or laparoscopy.[72]

Unfortunately, asymptomatic PID may be a common occurrence. Gump et al.[73] found that two-thirds of patients with evidence of old PID on laparoscopy or hysterosalpingography could not recall a history of PID and yet had sufficient residual disease to impair fertility. Walters and colleagues[74] have reported that only 18 percent of women with ectopic pregnancies and detectable antichlamydial antibody or inflammatory tubal damage report a history of PID.

Endometrial biopsy and ultrasonography have been used to support a clinical diagnosis of PID. The finding of plasma cell endometritis on endometrial biopsy has a sensitivity of 89 percent and specificity of 67 percent compared with laparoscopically detected salpingitis.[75] Transvaginal sonograms showing thickened, fluid-filled tubes correlate well with plasma cell endometritis and may improve the accuracy of diagnosing PID.[76]

Clinical diagnosis and grading of PID has poor specificity.[77] Patients with atypical clinical presentations, those with other suspected diagnoses, and those who fail empiric therapy should undergo laparoscopy for definitive diagnosis.

Although rare, acute salpingitis can occur in the proximal stump of patients who have undergone surgical sterilization.[78-80]

Management of Acute Pelvic Inflammatory Disease

There is no consensus on the need to carry out treatment in the hospital. The Centers for Disease Control and Prevention (CDC) recommends hospitalization of patients with acute PID in the following situations: the diagnosis is uncertain; surgical emergencies such as appendicitis and ectopic pregnancy cannot be excluded; a pelvic abscess is suspected; the patient is pregnant; the patient is an adolescent; severe illness precludes outpatient management; the patient is unable to tolerate an outpatient regimen; the patient has failed to respond to outpatient therapy; and clinical follow-up within 72 hours of starting antibiotic treatment cannot be arranged. Many authorities recommend that all patients with acute PID be hospitalized so that treatment with parenteral antibiotics can be initiated.[64]

Treatment consists of bedrest, pelvic rest, and antibiotics. The antimicrobial regimen of choice has not been established by randomized clinical trials. No single agent is active against the entire spectrum of potential pathogens. A variety of combination antimicrobial regimens are highly effective in producing clinical and microbiologic cures. Uncertainties regarding the effectiveness of antimicrobial therapy in preventing late sequelae, and the appropriateness of ambulatory treatment further complicate therapeutic decisions. The CDC has published antibiotic treatment guidelines for acute PID (Table 2).[64,64a,81,82]

All patients treated as outpatients should be clinically reevaluated within 72 hours. Those not responding favorably should be hospitalized. All male sex partners of women with acute PID should be evaluated for sexually transmitted diseases and empirically treated with regimens effective against *C. trachomatis* and *N. gonorrhoeae* infections.

Management of Suspected Tuboovarian Abscess

Patients suspected of having a tuboovarian abscess (TOA) should be hospitalized and begun on broad-spectrum antimicrobials that include adequate coverage for gram-negative anaer-

TABLE 2. Treatment Regimens for Acute Pelvic Inflammatory Disease

1. Inpatient Treatment
One of the following:
  Recommended regimen A
    Cefoxitin, 2 g iv every 6 hours, or cefotetan,[a] 2g iv every 12 hours
                    plus
    Doxycycline, 100 mg orally or iv every 12 hours
The above regimen is given for at least 48 hours after the patient clinically improves. After discharge from hospital, doxycycline, 100 mg orally two times a day, should be continued for a total of 10–14 days.

  Recommended regimen B
    Clindamycin, 900 mg iv every 8 hours
                    plus
    Gentamicin, loading dose iv or im (2 mg/kg of body weight) followed by a maintenance dose (1.5 mg/kg) every 8 hours
The above regimen is given for at least 48 hours after the patient improves. After discharge from hospital, doxycycline, 100 mg orally two times a day, should be continued for 14 days total. Continuation of clindamycin, 450 mg orally four times a day for 14 days, may be considered as an alternative.

2. Outpatient Management
  Recommended regimen A
    Cefoxitin, 2 g im, *plus* probenecid, 1 g orally, concurrently *or* ceftriaxone, 250 mg im, *or* equivalent cephalosporin
                    plus
    Doxycycline, 100 mg orally two times a day for 14 days
  Recommended regimen B
    Ofloxacin, 400 mg orally 2 times a day for 14 days
                    plus
    Either clindamycin, 450 mg orally 4 times a day, or metronidazole, 500 mg orally 2 times a day for 14 days

[a] Other cephalosporins such as ceftizoxime, cefotaxime, and ceftriaxone, which provide adequate gonococcal, other gram-negative aerobic, and anaerobic coverage, may be utilized in appropriate doses.

(From Centers for Disease Control and Prevention.[64,64a])

obes.[83] Failure of response to medical therapy is suggested by failure to defervesce in 72 hours or increase in the size of the mass. Eighty-five percent of abscesses with a diameter of 4–6 cm respond to antibiotics alone, while only 40 percent of those 10 cm or larger respond.[84]

Surgical intervention for TOAs failing to respond to antimicrobial therapy can be carried out laparoscopically,[85,86] percutaneously,[53-55,57,87] transvaginally,[52,56,88] or by laparotomy. Patients with a suspected leaking or ruptured abscess should undergo immediate laparotomy after rapid stabilization and institution of broad-spectrum antibiotics.

Prognosis

After one episode of PID a woman's risk of ectopic pregnancy increases sevenfold. Approximately 13 percent of women are infertile after a single episode of PID, 25–35 percent after two episodes, and 50–75 percent after three or more episodes.[64,89] If a true TOA is present, only 7–14 percent will conceive subsequent to treatment. Following treatment for a tuboovarian complex, a less restrictive diagnostic category than TOA, approximately two-thirds of women attempting pregnancy will be unable to conceive.[90] Other sequelae associated with PID include dyspareunia, pelvic adhesions, and chronic pelvic pain.[91]

REFERENCES

1. Gibbs RS, Duff P. Progress in pathogenesis and management of clinical intra-amniotic infection. Am J Obstet Gynecol. 1991;164:1317–26.
2. Liner RI. Intrauterine *Listeria* infection: Prenatal diagnosis by biophysical assessment and amniocentesis. Am J Obstet Gynecol. 1990;163:1596–7.
3. Silver HM, Sperling RS, St. Clair PJ, Gibbs RS. Evidence relating bacterial vaginosis to intraamniotic infection. Am J Obstet Gynecol. 1989;161:808–12.
4. Gauthier DW, Meyer WJ. Comparison of Gram stain, leukocyte esterase activity, and amniotic fluid glucose concentration in predicting amniotic fluid culture results in preterm premature rupture of membranes. Am J Obstet Gynecol. 1992;167:1092–5.
5. Coultrip LL, Grossman JH. Evaluation of rapid diagnostic tests in the detection of microbial invasion of the amniotic cavity. Am J Obstet Gynecol. 1992;167:1231–42.
6. Gibbs RS, Dinsmoor MJ, Newton ER, Ramamurthy RS. A randomized trial of intrapartum versus immediate postpartum treatment of women with intra-amniotic infection. Obstet Gynecol. 1988;72:823–8.

7. Newton ER, Prihoda TJ, Gibbs RS. A clinical and microbiologic analysis of risk factors for puerperal endometritis. Obstet Gynecol. 1990;75:402–6.
8. Watts DH, Krohn MA, Hillier SL, Eschenbach DA. Bacterial vaginosis as a risk factor for post-cesarean endometritis. Obstet Gynecol. 1990;75:52–8.
9. Chang PL, Newton ER. Predictors of antibiotic prophylactic failure in post-cesarean endometritis. Obstet Gynecol. 1992;80:117–22.
10. Hemsell DL. Prophylactic antibiotics in gynecologic and obstetric surgery. Rev Infect Dis. 1991;13(10):S821–41.
11. Watts DH, Eschenbach DA, Kenny GE. Early postpartum endometritis: The role of bacteria, genital mycoplasmas, and *Chlamydia trachomatis*. Obstet Gynecol. 1989;73:52–60.
12. Eschenbach DA, Rosene K, Tompkins LS, et al. Endometrial cultures obtained by a triple-lumen method from afebrile and febrile postpartum women. J Infect Dis. 1986;153:1038–45.
13. Watts DH, Hillier SL, Eschenbach DA. Upper genital tract isolates at delivery as predictors of post-cesarean infection among women receiving antibiotic prophylaxis. Obstet Gynecol. 1991;77:287–92.
14. Hoyme UB, Kiviat N, Eschenbach DA. The microbiology and treatment of late postpartum endometritis. Obstet Gynecol. 1986;68:226–32.
15. Martens MG, Faro S, Hammil HA, et al. Transcervical uterine cultures with a new endometrial suction curette: A comparison of three sampling methods in postpartum endometritis. Obstet Gynecol. 1989;74:273–6.
16. Faro S, Martens MG, Hammill HA, et al. Antibiotic prophylaxis: Is there a difference? Am J Obstet Gynecol. 1990;162:900–9.
17. Polk BF. Antimicrobial prophylaxis to prevent mixed bacterial infection. J Antimicrob Chemother. 1981;8(D):115–29.
18. Gonik B, Shannon RL, Shawar R, et al. Why patients fail antibiotic prophylaxis at cesarean delivery: Histologic evidence for incipient infection. Obstet Gynecol. 1992;79:179–84.
19. Ledger WJ, Headington JT. Group A beta-hemolytic *Streptococcus*. Obstet Gynecol. 1972;39:474–82.
20. Mead PB, Ribble JC, Dillon TF. Group A streptococcal puerperal infection: Report of an epidemic. Obstet Gynecol. 1968;32:460–4.
21. Stevens DL, Tanner MH, Winship J, et al. Severe group A streptococcal infections associated with a toxic shock-like syndrome and scarlet fever toxin A. N Engl J Med. 1989;321:1–7.
22. Duff P, Gibbs RS. Pelvic vein thrombophlebitis: Diagnostic dilemma and therapeutic challenge. Obstet Gynecol Surv. 1983;38:365–73.
23. Brown CEL, Lowe TW, Cunningham FG, Weinreb JC. Puerperal pelvic thrombophlebitis: Impact on diagnosis and treatment using x-ray computed tomography and magnetic resonance imaging. Obstet Gynecol. 1986;68:789–94.
24. Baka JJ, Lev-Toaff AS, Friedman AC, et al. Ovarian vein thrombosis with atypical presentation: Role of sonography and duplex Doppler. Obstet Gynecol. 1989;73:887–9.
25. Shy KK, Eschenbach DA. Fatal perineal cellulitis from an episiotomy site. Obstet Gynecol. 1979;54:292–8.
26. Hibbard LT, Snyder EN, McVann RM. Subgluteal and retroposal infection in obstetric practice. Obstet Gynecol. 1972;39:137–50.
27. Soper DE. Clostridial myonecrosis arising from an episiotomy. Obstet Gynecol. 1986;68:26S–8S.
28. McGregor JA, Soper DE, Lovell G, Todd JK. Maternal deaths associated with *Clostridium sordelli* infection. Am J Obstet Gynecol. 1989;161:987–95.
29. Spera RV, Kaplan MH, Allen SL. *Clostridium sordelli* bacteremia: Case report and review. Clinical Infect Dis. 1992;15:950–4.
30. Chow AW, Marshall JR, Guze LB. A double-blind comparison of clindamycin with penicillin plus chloramphenicol in treatment of septic abortion. J Infect Dis. 1977;135:S35–9.
31. Levallois P, Rioux JE. Prophylactic antibiotics for suction curettage abortion: Results of a controlled clinical trial. Am J Obstet Gynecol. 1985;158:100–5.
32. Bartlett JG, Moon NE, Goldstein PR, et al. Cervical and vaginal bacterial flora: Ecologic niches in the female lower genital tract. Am J Obstet Gynecol. 1978;130:658–61.
33. Schottmueller H. Significance of several anaerobes in pathology, especially in puerperal illnesses. Mitt Grenzt Med Chir. 1910;21:450.
34. Ohm MJ, Galask RP. The effect of antibiotic prophylaxis on patients undergoing vaginal operations. Am J Obstet Gynecol. 1975;123:597–604.
35. Ohm MJ, Galask RP. The effect of antibiotic prophylaxis on patients undergoing total abdominal hysterectomy. Am J Obstet Gynecol. 1976;125:448–54.
36. McGroarty JA, Tomeczek L, Pond DG, et al. Hydrogen peroxide production by *Lactobacillus* species: Correlation with susceptibility to the spermicidal compound nonoxynol-9. J Infect Dis. 1992;165:1142–4.
37. Klebanoff SJ. Effects of the spermicidal agent nonoxynol-9 on vaginal microbial flora. J Infect Dis. 1992;165:19–25.
38. Onderdonk AB, Delaney ML, Hinkson PL, DuBois AM. Quantitative and qualitative effects of douche preparations on vaginal microflora. Obstet Gynecol. 1992;80:333–8.
39. Soper DE, Brockwell NJ, Dalton HP. Evaluation of the effects of a female condom on the female lower genital tract. Contraception. 1991;44:21–9.
40. Weinstein WM, Onderdonk AB, Bartlett JG, Gorbach SI. Experimental intra-abdominal abscesses in rats. Development of an experimental model. Infect Immun. 1974;10:1250–5.
41. Bartlett JG, Onderdonk AB, Louie T, et al. Lessons from an animal model of intraabdominal sepsis. Arch Surg. 1978;113:853–7.
42. Dicker RC, Greenspan JR, Strauss LT, et al. Complications of abdominal and vaginal hysterectomy among women of reproductive age in the United States. Am J Obstet Gynecol. 1982;144:841–8.
43. Styrt B, Sugarman B. Estrogens and infection. Rev Infect Dis. 1991;13:1139–50.
44. Soper DE, Bump RC, Hurt WG. Bacterial vaginosis and trichomoniasis are

45. Larsson P-G, Platz-Christensen J-J, Forsum U, Pahlson C. Clue cells in predicting infections after abdominal hysterectomy. Obstet Gynecol. 1991;77:450–2.
46. Hager WD, Pascuzzi M, Vernon M. Efficacy of oral antibiotics following parenteral antibiotics for serious infections in obstetrics and gynecology. Obstet Gynecol. 1989;73:326–9.
47. Hemsell DL. Posthysterectomy cuff and pelvic cellulitis. In: Mead PB, Hager WD, eds. Infection Protocols for Obstetrics and Gynecology. Montvale, NJ: Medical Economics Publishing; 1992:283–7.
48. Hemsell DL, Nobles B, Heard MC. Recognition and treatment of post-hysterectomy pelvic infections. Infect Surg. 1988;7:47–68.
49. Livengood CH, Addison WA. Adnexal abscess as a delayed complication of vaginal hysterectomy. Am J Obstet Gynecol. 1982;143:596–7.
50. Ledger WJ, Campbell C, Wilson JR. Postoperative adnexal infection. Obstet Gynecol. 1968;31:83–9.
51. Ledger WJ, Moore DE, Lowensohn RI, Gee CL. A fever index evaluation of chloramphenicol or clindamycin in patients with serious pelvic infections. Obstet Gynecol. 1977;50:523–30.
52. Rubenstein PR, Mishell DR, Ledger WJ. Colpotomy drainage of pelvic abscess. Obstet Gynecol. 1976;48:142–5.
53. Tyrrel RT, Murphy FB, Bernardino ME. Tubo-ovarian abscesses: CT-guided percutaneous drainage. Radiology. 1990;175:87–9.
54. Mueller PR, Van Sonnenberg E. Interventional radiology in the chest and abdomen. N Engl J Med. 1990;322:1364–74.
55. Martin EC, Karlson KB, Fankuchen EI, et al. Percutaneous drainage of postoperative intra-abdominal abscesses. Am J Roentgenol. 1982;138:13–5.
56. Loy RA, Gallup DG, Hill JA, et al. Pelvic abscesses. Examination and transvaginal drainage guided by real-time ultrasonography. South Med J. 1989;82:788–90.
57. Casola G, Van Sonnenberg E, D'Agostino HB, et al. Percutaneous drainage of tuboovarian abscesses. Radiology. 1992;182:399–402.
58. Sauer MV, Paulson RJ. Pelvic abscess complicating transcervical embryo transfer. Am J Obstet Gynecol. 1992;166:148–9.
59. Dunn LJ, Van Voorhis LW. Enigmatic fever and pelvic thrombophlebitis. N Engl J Med. 1967;276:265–8.
60. Josey WE, Staggers SR. Heparin therapy in septic pelvic vein thrombophlebitis: A study of 46 cases. Am J Obstet Gynecol. 1974;120:228–33.
61. Hoyme UB, Tamimi HK, Eschenbach DA, et al. Osteomyelitis pubis after radical gynecologic operations. Obstet Gynecol. 1984;63:47S–53S.
62. Stamm WE, Guinan ME, Johnson C, et al. Effect of treatment regimens for *Neiserria gonorrhoeae* on simultaneous infection with *Chlamydia trachomatis*. N Engl J Med. 1984;310:545–9.
63. Barham WB, Haberberger RL, Decker CF. Group A streptococcal sepsis secondary to acute salpingitis. Clin Infect Dis. 1993;16:444–5.
64. Centers for Disease Control and Prevention. Pelvic inflammatory disease: Guidelines for prevention and management. MMWR 1991;40:1–25.
64a.Centers for Disease Control and Prevention. 1993 sexually transmitted diseases treatment guidelines. MMWR. 1993;42:75–81.
65. Lee NC, Rubin GL, Grimes DA. Measures of sexual behavior and the risk of pelvic inflammatory disease. Obstet Gynecol. 1991;77:425–30.
66. Eschenbach DA, Hillier S, Critchlow C, et al. Diagnosis and clinical manifestations of bacterial vaginosis. Am J Obstet Gynecol. 1988;158:819–28.
67. Wolner-Hanssen P, Eschenbach DA, Paavonen J, et al. Association between vaginal douching and acute pelvic inflammatory disease. JAMA. 1990;263:1936–41.
68. Scholes D, Daling JR, Stergachis AS. Cigarette smoking and risk of pelvic inflammatory disease. Am J Epidemiol. 1990;132:759.
69. Kessel E. Pelvic inflammatory disease with intrauterine device use: A reassessment. Fertil Steril. 1989;51:1–11.
70. Lee NC, Rubin GL, Borucki R. The intrauterine device and pelvic inflammatory disease revisited: New results from the Women's Health Study. Obstet Gynecol. 1988;72:1–6.
71. Scully RE, Mark EJ, McNeely WF, McNeely BU. Case records of the Massachusetts General Hospital: Case 10–1992. N Engl J Med. 1992;326:692–9.
72. Hager WD, Eschenbach DA, Spence MR, Sweet RL. Criteria for diagnosis and grading of salpingitis. Obstet Gynecol. 1983;61:113–4.
73. Gump DW, Gibson M, Ashikaga T. Evidence of prior pelvic inflammatory disease and its relationship to *Chlamydia trachomatis* antibody and intrauterine contraceptive device use in infertile women. Am J Obstet Gynecol. 1983;146:153–9.
74. Walters MD, Eddy CA, Gibbs RS, et al. Antibodies to *Chlamydia trachomatis* and risk for tubal pregnancy. Am J Obstet Gynecol. 1988;159:942–6.
75. Paavonen J, Aine T, Teisala K, et al. Comparison of endometrial biopsy and peritoneal fluid cytologic testing with laparoscopy in the diagnosis of acute pelvic inflammatory disease. Am J Obstet Gynecol. 1985;151:645–50.
76. Cacciatore B, Leminen A, Ingman-Friberg S, et al. Transvaginal sonographic findings in ambulatory patients with suspected pelvic inflammatory disease. Obstet Gynecol. 1992;80:912–6.
77. Livengood CH, Hill GB, Addison WA. Pelvic inflammatory disease: Findings during inpatient treatment of clinically severe, laparoscopy-documented disease. Am J Obstet Gynecol. 1992;166:519–24.
78. Fletcher V. Proximal stump salpingitis. Am J Obstet Gynecol. 1986;155:496–500.
79. Vermesh M, Confino E, Boler LR, et al. Acute salpingitis in sterilized women. Obstet Gynecol. 1987;69:245–9.
80. Green MM, Vicario SJ, Sanfilippo JS, Lochhead SA. Acute pelvic inflammatory disease after surgical sterilization. Ann Emerg Med. 1991;20:344–7.

81. Peterson HB, Walker CK, Kahn JG, et al. Pelvic inflammatory disease. JAMA. 1991;266:2605–11.
82. Landers DV, Wolner-Hanssen P, Paavonen J, et al. Combination antimicrobial therapy in the treatment of acute pelvic inflammatory disease. Am J Obstet Gynecol. 1991;164:849–58.
83. Reed SD, Landers DV, Sweet RL. Antibiotic treatment of tuboovarian abscess. Am J Obstet Gynecol. 1991;164:1556–61.
84. Amstey MS, Sweet RL. Definition of pelvic abscess (Letter). Am J Obstet Gynecol. 1993;168:740–1.
85. Henry-Suchet J, Soler A, Loffredo V. Laparoscopic treatment of tuboovarian abscesses. J Reprod Med. 1984;29:579–82.
86. Reich H. Role of laparoscopy in treating TOA and pelvic abscess. Contemp OB/GYN 1989;34(June):91–102.
87. Shulman A, Maymon R, Shapiro A, Bahary C. Percutaneous catheter drainage of tubo-ovarian abscesses. Obstet Gynecol. 1992;80:555–7.
88. Teisala K, Heinonen PK, Punnonen R. Transvaginal ultrasound in the diagnosis and treatment of tubo-ovarian abscess. Br J Obstet Gynaecol. 1990;97:178–80.
89. Westrom L. Effect of acute pelvic inflammatory disease on fertility. Am J Obstet Gynecol. 1975;121:707–13.
90. Brumsted JR, Clifford PM, Nakajima ST, Gibson M. Reproductive outcome after medical management of complicated pelvic inflammatory disease. Fertil Steril. 1988;50:667–9.
91. Safrin S, Schachter J, Dahrouge D, Sweet RL. Long-term sequelae of acute pelvic inflammatory disease. Am J Obstet Gynecol. 1992;166:1300–5.

91. PROSTATITIS, EPIDIDYMITIS, AND ORCHITIS

JOHN N. KRIEGER

ANATOMY AND PHYSIOLOGY OF THE TESTES AND MALE ACCESSORY SEX ORGANS

The testicle has two functional components, seminiferous tubules and interstitial cells. Sperm production is the primary function of the seminiferous tubules. Interstitial cells, located between the seminiferous tubules, are primarily responsible for hormone production. After spermatogenesis spermatozoa are transported from the testis into the epididymis (Fig. 1). Sperm

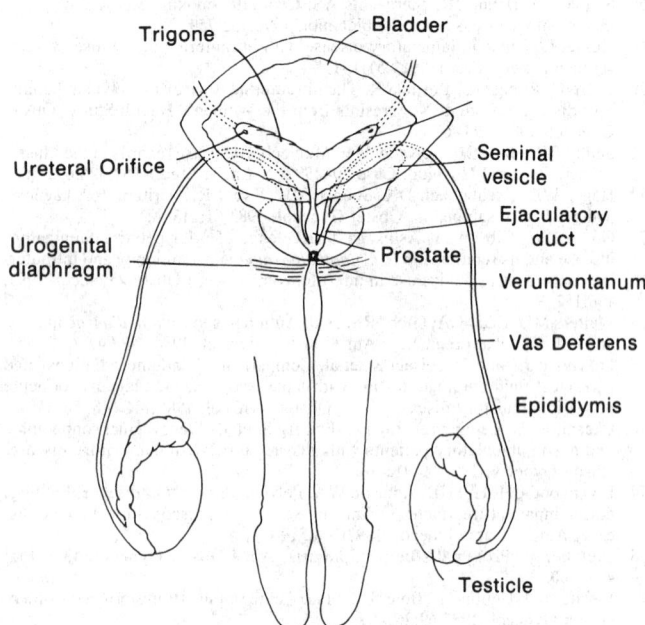

Trigone
Bladder
Ureteral Orifice
Seminal vesicle
Ejaculatory duct
Urogenital diaphragm
Prostate
Verumontanum
Vas Deferens
Epididymis
Testicle

FIG. 1. Anatomy of the male sex organs and lower urinary tract.

then move into the vas deferens, a muscular tube approximately 12 inches long that is easily palpable in the scrotum. Fructose from the seminal vesicles is the major energy source for ejaculated sperm. In addition, the seminal vesicles provide a number of proteins that cause coagulation of the ejaculate. Liquification of the semen occurs within 5–30 minutes after ejaculation as a result of proteolytic enzymes from the prostate.[1]

HOST DEFENSES OF THE MALE LOWER UROGENITAL TRACT

Organisms ascend via the urethra to cause most infections of the urogenital ducts and accessory sex organs.[2] Thus, mechanical factors such as the flushing action of micturition and ejaculation should provide some protection against infection, although the relative significance of such defenses is unclear.

A zinc-containing polypeptide known as the *prostatic antibacterial factor* is the most important antimicrobial substance secreted by the prostate.[2,3] Men with well-documented chronic bacterial prostatitis have significantly lower levels of zinc in their prostatic fluid than do healthy men, but their serum zinc levels are within normal limits.[3] Other findings indicating that bacterial prostatitis is associated with generalized secretory dysfunction include increased pH of prostatic fluid; reduced calcium, citric acid, and spermine concentrations; and changes in prostatic fluid enzymes.[4] It is unclear whether reduced zinc concentrations precede the development of prostatic infection or represent a secretory dysfunction resulting from such infections. Prostatic secretions of patients with bacterial prostatitis contain high concentrations of immunoglobulins.[5,6] Several studies have demonstrated antigen-specific antibody coating of bacteria isolated from the lower urinary tracts of patients with prostatitis syndromes. The antigen-specific antibody response in prostatic secretions (predominately secretory IgA) is significantly greater than is the serologic response.[6]

The presence of leukocytes is characteristic of many conditions of the male lower urinary tract, including prostatitis.[7] Phagocytosis of abnormal sperm by leukocytes in some infertile men with pyosemina has been observed.

PROSTATITIS

Classification of Prostatitis

The term *prostatitis* is employed clinically to describe a large group of adult men with a variety of complaints referable to the lower urogenital tract and perineum.[2,8] It has been estimated that 50 percent of men will experience symptoms of prostatitis at some time in their lives.[2] It is of critical importance to distinguish patients with lower urinary tract complaints associated with bacteriuria, such as patients who may have bacterial prostatitis, from the larger number of patients without bacteriuria. Further classification of patients with prostatitis depends on careful bacteriologic assessment of the lower urinary tract that is based on sequential urine cultures obtained during micturition (Table 1).[8,9] On the basis of results of lower urinary tract locali-

TABLE 1. Lower Urinary Tract Localization Using Segmented Urine Cultures[a]

Specimen	Symbol	Description
Voided bladder 1	VB_1	Initial 5–10 ml of urinary stream
Voided bladder 2	VB_2	Midstream specimen
Expressed prostatic secretions	EPS	Secretions expressed from prostate by digital massage after midstream specimen
Voided bladder 3	VB_3	First 5–10 ml of urinary stream immediately after prostatic massage

[a] Unequivocal diagnosis of bacterial prostatitis requires that the colony count in the VB_3 specimen greatly exceed the count in the VB_1 specimen, preferably by at least 10-fold.[2,9] Many patients who have chronic bacterial prostatitis, however, harbor only small numbers of bacteria in their prostates. In such patients, direct culture of the prostatic secretions is particularly useful. Microscopic examination of the EPS is useful for identifying white blood cells and "oval fat bodies," large lipid-laden macrophages characteristic of the prostatic inflammatory response.[2,8]

TABLE 2. Classification of Prostatitis Syndromes on the Basis of Lower Urinary Tract Localization Studies

Condition	Bacteriuria[a]	Infection Localized to Prostate[b]	Inflammatory Response in EPS[c]	Abnormal Rectal Examination of Prostate[d]	Systemic Illness[e]
Acute bacterial prostatitis	+	+	+	+	+
Chronic bacterial prostatitis	+	+	+	−	−
"Nonbacterial" prostatitis	−	−	+	−	−
Prostatodynia	−	−	−	−	−

[a] Documented with an identical organism that is shown to localize to a prostatic focus when the midstream urine culture is negative.
[b] Refer to the text for diagnostic criteria.
[c] Prostatic secretions containing ≥12 WBC/HPF in a patient with no objective evidence of urethritis.
[d] Abnormal findings include exquisite tenderness and swelling that may be associated with signs of lower urinary tract obstruction.
[e] Systemic findings frequently include fever and rigors and may include signs of bacteremia.

zation, men with prostatitis syndromes may be classified into four major groups: acute bacterial prostatitis, chronic bacterial prostatitis, nonbacterial prostatitis, and prostatodynia (Table 2).[8] In addition, rare patients develop granulomatous prostatitis.

Bacterial prostatitis is a frequent diagnosis in general clinical practice, but well-documented bacterial infections of the prostate, whether acute or chronic, are uncommon.[2,6] The great majority of patients with a diagnosis of prostatitis are adult men with perineal, lower back, or lower abdominal pain; urinary discomfort; or ejaculatory complaints. Most of these patients have no history of bacteriuria, and there is little objective evidence of bacterial infection of the prostate. Thus, most patients with prostatitis may be classified in the groups of nonbacterial prostatitis or prostatodynia, conditions about which there are few firm data to base therapeutic decisions.

Acute Bacterial Prostatitis. Acute bacterial prostatitis is usually not a subtle or difficult diagnosis. Patients complain of symptoms associated with lower urinary tract infection such as urinary frequency and dysuria. Patients may also experience lower urinary tract obstruction due to acute edema of the prostate. Signs of systemic toxicity are common. On physical examination patients may have a high temperature and lower abdominal or suprapubic discomfort due to bladder infection. The rectal examination is frequently impressive, with an exquisitely tender, tense prostate on palpation. Urinalysis is abnormal, with evidence of pyuria, and cultures are positive. Bacteremia may be present spontaneously or may result from overly vigorous rectal examinations.

Results of antimicrobial therapy for acute bacterial prostatitis are often dramatic. Many drugs that do not penetrate into the prostate under normal conditions are effective in acute bacterial prostatitis.[2] Thus, drugs that would be appropriate in patients with bacteremia caused by Enterobacteriaceae, pseudomonads, and enterococci should be administered once specimens have been obtained for urine and blood cultures. Urinary retention is best managed with a suprapubic cystostomy, rather than a transurethral catheter, to avoid obstructing drainage of infected prostatic secretions into the urethra. General measures, including hydration, analgesics, and bed rest, are also indicated. The most important complications of acute bacterial prostatitis include prostatic abscess, prostatic infarction, chronic bacterial prostatitis, and granulomatous prostatitis.

Chronic Bacterial Prostatitis. Chronic bacterial prostatitis is an important cause of bacterial persistence in the male lower urinary tract. Patients characteristically experience recurrent bacterial urinary tract infections caused by the same organism.[2] Patients are generally asymptomatic between episodes of bladder bacteriuria. The prostate gland is usually normal on either rectal or endoscopic evaluation. Thus, careful lower urinary tract localization studies are the cornerstone on which to base a diagnosis of chronic bacterial prostatitis (Tables 1 and 2).[9] Diagnosis of chronic bacterial prostatitis based solely on symptoms, the number of leukocytes in expressed prostatic secretions, or the use of prostate biopsy specimens is inadequate.

Gram-negative rods (Enterobacteriaceae or pseudomonads) are by far the most important pathogens in chronic bacterial prostatitis. Gram-positive cocci such as *Enterococcus faecalis* or, perhaps, *Staphylococcus saprophyticus* may be the etiologic organisms in a few cases. Reports implicating many other organisms are generally difficult to evaluate due to methodologic problems with case definition or a lack of documentation of bacteriuria by the alleged pathogen.

Medical management is effective in curing or suppressing bacterial infections of the prostate. Trimethoprim has two useful characteristics: it achieves good levels in the prostatic parenchyma and is effective against most of the common bacterial pathogens.[2] Available studies have most commonly employed the combination of trimethoprim and sulfamethoxazole for the treatment of patients with well-documented chronic bacterial prostatitis. Long treatment courses result in symptomatic and bacteriologic cure in approximately one-third of patients, symptomatic improvement while receiving therapy in approximately one-third of patients who relapse after the drug therapy is stopped, and no improvement in the remaining patients.[10] The newer quinolones are promising alternative agents for treatment of bacterial prostatitis.[11–14]

Bacteria isolated from patients with chronic bacterial prostatitis, even after multiple episodes of symptomatic bacteriuria and prolonged courses of antibiotics, are generally antibiotic-sensitive strains.[2,10] Several findings may explain the disappointing results of antibiotic therapy, including poor diffusion of many drugs into the prostatic parenchyma, changes in prostatic fluid pH level that are associated with infection, and infected calculi that may serve as persistent foci for bacteria.[10,15]

Patients with chronic bacterial prostatitis who are not cured may be rendered asymptomatic by long-term, suppressive treatment. Since patients are usually asymptomatic between episodes of bacteriuria, the goal of suppressive therapy is to prevent symptomatic episodes despite the persistence of bacteria in the prostate. Very low doses of agents such as penicillin, tetracycline, nitrofurantoin, nalidixic acid, trimethoprim sulfamethoxazole, or newer guinolones are remarkably effective in preventing episodes of symptomatic bladder infection in patients with chronic bacterial prostatitis.[2,12]

Nonbacterial Prostatitis and Prostatodynia. Patients with nonbacterial prostatitis and prostatodynia have no history of bacteriuria and lack objective evidence of bacterial infection of their prostatic secretions on careful lower urinary tract localization studies (Table 2).[8] Such patients may complain of a variety of perineal and pelvic symptoms. Pain or vague discomfort is common and may be suprapubic, infrapubic, scrotal, or inguinal in location. The discomfort may be described as either continuous or spasmodic and is commonly described as a "dull ache." Occasional patients complain of increased urinary frequency or dysuria, and ejaculatory complaints are not infrequent. Systemic symptoms or signs are absent. Physical examination is generally unremarkable.

Nonbacterial prostatitis and prostatodynia are distinguished by microscopic examination of the expressed prostatic secretions. Patients with nonbacterial prostatitis have objective evidence of an inflammatory response in their prostatic secretions, while patients with prostatodynia have no evidence of inflammation.

The etiologies of nonbacterial prostatitis and prostatodynia remain uncertain. Mardh and Colleen[16] and Mardh et al.[17] found no evidence for an etiologic role for *Neisseria gonorrhoeae, Trichomonas vaginalis, Ureaplasma urealyticum, Mycoplasma hominis, Candida albicans,* anaerobic bacteria, *Chlamydia trachomatis,* or viruses in these syndromes. However, other researchers have reported that many patients with "subacute or chronic prostatitis" are infected with *C. trachomatis*[18-20] or *U. urealyticum.*[21,22] The techniques, control groups, and findings in these later studies have been questioned by other workers.[2,23-25] Some workers have proposed that nonbacterial prostatitis is not an infectious disease.[26,27] In poorly controlled studies, prostaglandins, autoimmunity, psychological abnormalities, neuromuscular dysfunction of the bladder neck or urogenital diaphragm, and allergy to environmental agents have all been suggested as etiologic factors.

Current therapy for symptomatic patients with nonbacterial prostatitis is unsatisfactory. There is little objective evidence that patients with nonbacterial prostatitis or prostatodynia benefit from empirical antimicrobial therapy.

Granulomatous Prostatitis. Granulomatous prostatitis is a characteristic histologic reaction of the prostate to a variety of insults, with granulomas containing lipid-laden histiocytes, plasma cells, and scattered giant cells. In most cases granulomatous prostatitis follows an episode of acute bacterial prostatitis.[28,29] There are also a number of specific infectious causes of granulomatous reaction by the prostate. Tuberculous prostatitis is usually secondary to tuberculosis elsewhere in the genital tract.[30,31] Most patients have no symptoms referable to prostatic infection. On biopsy the granulomas may contain typical Langhans giant cells and may be associated with caseous necrosis. Such infections are most often caused by *Mycobacterium tuberculosis* but have also been reported to be caused by nontuberculous mycobacteria.[32] Iatrogenic mycobacterial prostatitis may develop in patients treated with intravesicular Calmette-Guérin bacillus for transitional cell carcinoma of the bladder.[33,34] Prostatitis may be secondary to systemic involvement with many of the deep mycoses.[35] Most cases of mycotic prostatitis reported have been associated with blastomycosis,[35] coccidioidomycosis,[36] and cryptococcosis.[37] The prostate may be a focus of persistent cryptococcosis in patients with acquired immunodeficiency syndrome (AIDS).[38] Rarely, prostatic histoplasmosis occurs in this population.[39]

Granulomatous prostatitis is most important in the differential diagnosis of an indurated, firm, or nodular prostate. The rectal examination of such patients raises the suspicion of prostatic carcinoma. Biopsy is usually necessary for diagnosis, and it is important that appropriate stains be used for the detection of specific etiologic agents.

Prostatic Abscess

Prostatic abscess is a rare complication in patients who receive appropriate treatment for acute bacterial prostatitis.[40] Most prostatic abscesses occur in patients with diabetes, in immunocompromised patients, and in patients who have not received appropriate therapy for acute prostatitis. The presence of a foreign body or urinary tract obstruction are other predisposing factors. In the past, *N. gonorrhoeae* was a common pathogen, but most cases are now caused by the common uropathogens. Infection generally occurs by the ascending route.[41] On occasion, *Staphylococcus aureus* is the pathogen, which suggests the possibility of hematogenous infection. Patients are usually febrile with irritative voiding symptoms, and they may have signs of urosepsis. Thus, the clinical presentation closely resembles that of acute bacterial prostatitis. Classically, the abscess presents as a fluctuant area in the prostate that can be palpated during rectal examination. However, the presentation may be more subtle. The use of ultrasonography,[42] computed tomography,[43] or magnetic resonance imaging of the pelvis is helpful for confirming the diagnosis or in patients with equivocal clinical findings. Treatment includes draining the abscess, via either a perineal or transurethral route, in addition to appropriate antimicrobial therapy.

EPIDIDYMITIS

Epididymitis is an inflammatory reaction of the epididymis to a variety of infectious agents or to local trauma. Epididymitis is common, accounting for over 600,000 visits to physicians per year in the United States. Acute epididymitis is responsible for more days lost from military service than any other disease and is responsible for 20 percent of urologic admissions in military populations.[44]

Patients with epididymitis usually complain of painful swelling of the scrotum. The onset may be acute over 1 or 2 days or more gradual and is often associated with dysuria or irritative lower urinary tract symptoms. Many patients have a urethral discharge.[45] Specific attention should be directed to eliciting a past history of genitourinary tract disease or sexual exposure. Some patients may have only a nonspecific finding of fever or other signs of infection. This is particularly frequent in hospitalized patients who have recent urinary tract manipulation and may be obtunded by medication.

Tender swelling, frequently accompanied by erythema, generally unilateral, may be noted primarily in the posterior aspect of the scrotum. If the patient is examined early in the course of the disease, the swelling may be localized to one portion of the epididymitis. Later, involvement of the ipsilateral testis is frequent, producing an epididymo-orchitis, and it may be difficult to distinguish the testicle from the epididymis within the inflammatory mass. Scrotal examination commonly reveals the presence of a hydrocele caused by the secretion of inflammatory fluid between the layers of the tunica vaginalis. Urethral discharge may be apparent on inspection or stripping of the urethra.

There are two common types of epididymitis, nonspecific bacterial epididymitis and sexually transmitted epididymitis. In addition, epididymitis may occur rarely after genital trauma or with disseminated infections.

Nonspecific Bacterial Epididymitis

The most common cause of epididymitis in men over 35 years old is infection with coliform or *Pseudomonas* species.[45,46] In most series, gram-negative aerobic rods caused over two-thirds of the cases of bacterial epididymitis.[45-47] However, gram-positive cocci are also important pathogens and were the most common organisms in some reports.[48]

Many patients who develop bacterial epididymitis have underlying urologic pathology or have a history of recent genitourinary tract manipulation.[44,45] The development of epididymitis after surgery or urethral catheterization may occur weeks or rarely months after the manipulation. Epididymitis is particularly likely in patients who undergo urinary tract surgery or instrumentation while they are bacteriuric. Acute and chronic bacterial prostatitis are other important predisposing conditions for the development of bacterial epididymitis.

Bacterial epididymitis may be an important focus of organisms causing bacteremia and local morbidity in patients with indwelling transurethral catheters. Genitourinary tract complications of acute bacterial epididymitis include testicular infarction, scrotal abscess, pyocele, a chronic draining scrotal sinus, chronic epididymitis, and infertility.[49,50]

Tuberculous epididymitis is the most common manifestation of male genital tuberculosis, with orchitis and prostatitis being less common. The usual symptom is heaviness or swelling. There is characteristic scrotal swelling with "beadlike" enlargement of the vas deferens. Chronic draining scrotal sinuses may be present. The systemic mycoses may rarely cause epididymitis; blastomycosis is the most common pathogen and may also cause a draining sinus through the scrotal wall.

Medical management is appropriate for most patients with bacterial epididymitis. Initial empirical treatment with agents appropriate for both gram-negative rods and gram-positive cocci should be initiated pending urine culture and sensitivity results. Nonspecific measures such as bed rest, scrotal elevation analgesics, and local ice packs are helpful. Surgery may be necessary for complications of acute epididymal infections but has no role in tuberculous or fungal epididymitis.

Sexually Transmitted Epididymitis

Sexually transmitted epididymitis is the most common type of epididymitis in young men. *Chlamydia trachomatis* and *N. gonorrhoeae* are the major pathogens in this population. Chlamydiae have been identified as the most common cause of epididymitis in younger, sexually active populations.[51,52] Such patients were formerly considered to have "idiopathic," nonspecific epididymitis. Berger et al.[45] documented infections with *C. trachomatis* in 17 of 34 cases of epididymitis in patients less than 35 years old and only 1 of 16 cases of epididymitis in patients older than 35. Patients with chlamydial epididymitis frequently did not complain of urethral discharge. However, 11 of 17 patients with epididymitis caused by chlamydiae had demonstrable discharge, usually the scant, watery discharge characteristic of nonspecific urethritis. The median interval from the last sexual exposure was 10 days and ranged from 1 to 45 days. Thus, patients may carry chlamydiae for long periods before the development of overt epididymitis.

Before the availability of penicillin, it was estimated that epididymitis occurred in 10–30 percent of men with gonococcal urethritis. In more recent studies, *N. gonorrhoeae* was identified as the cause of acute epididymitis in 16 percent of cases in military populations[53] and in 21 percent of cases of epididymitis in civilians less than 35 years old.[45] Many patients with gonococcal epididymitis do not have a history of urethral discharge, and a discharge may be demonstrable in only 50 percent of such patients.

Underlying genitourinary tract abnormalities are uncommon in this population. Diagnosis depends on a high index of clinical suspicion, evaluation for presence of urethritis (which may be asymptomatic), and appropriate cultures. Specific antibiotic therapy, generally employing drugs appropriate for both chlamydiae and gonococci (i.e., tetracycline, 500 mg po four times daily for at least 10 days), is the most important aspect of treatment.[50,54] Patients should be evaluated for other sexually transmitted pathogens, and treatment of sexual partners is important. In general, a complete urologic work-up is not indicated for patients with uncomplicated sexually transmitted epididymitis. Complications of sexually transmitted epididymitis include abscess formation, testicular infarction, chronic epididymitis, and infertility. Ultrasonography, particularly color-flow Doppler ultrasonography, is useful for the differential diagnosis of complicated cases of epididymitis.[55,56]

ORCHITIS

Orchitis is significantly less common than is either prostatitis or epididymitis. Orchitis differs from infections of the male accessory sex glands in two important respects: blood-borne dissemination is the major route of infection, and viruses are clearly implicated as important pathogens.

Viral Orchitis

Viral infections, particularly mumps, are associated with most cases of orchitis. Although mumps rarely causes orchitis in pre-pubertal boys, orchitis occurs in approximately 20 percent of postpubertal patients with mumps.[57] Testicular pain and swelling usually begin 4–6 days after the onset of parotitis but may occur without parotid involvement. Orchitis is unilateral in approximately 70 percent of cases. Contralateral testicular swelling may occur 1–9 days after involvement of the first side. The clinical course is variable and ranges from mild testicular discomfort and swelling to severe testicular pain and marked swelling accompanied by nausea, vomiting, prostration, high fever, and constitutional symptoms. Epididymitis and inflammation of the spermatic cord may be noted on physical examination. Resolution of mild cases may occur in 4–5 days. More severe cases usually resolve in 3–4 weeks. Approximately one-half of the involved testes undergo some degree of atrophy. In older series, sterility was reported in 25 percent of patients with bilateral disease. However, more recent studies have found that mumps orchitis seldom results in infertility.[57] Coxsackie B virus produces a disease that clinically and histologically resembles mumps orchitis.

Bacterial Orchitis

With the exception of viral diseases, acute genitourinary tract infections involving only the testis are distinctly unusual. Pyogenic bacterial orchitis usually occurs as a consequence of the contiguous spread from an inflammatory process in the epididymis to cause an epididymo-orchitis. Thus, most cases of pyogenic orchitis are caused by *Escherichia coli, Klebsiella pneumoniae, Pseudomonas aeruginosa,* staphylococci, or streptococci. Occasionally, acute orchitis may be caused by other organisms as a result of metastatic seeding.

The patient with pyogenic orchitis appears acutely ill with a high fever and marked discomfort and swelling of the involved testicle. Generally the pain is described as radiating to the inguinal canal and is frequently accompanied by nausea and vomiting. On examination, there is usually an acute hydrocele, and the testis is swollen and exquisitely tender. The overlying scrotal skin is generally erythematous and edematous. Complications of pyogenic bacterial orchitis include testicular infarction, abscess formation, and pyocele of the scrotum.[50] Surgery is usually required for treatment of these conditions. Orchitis can be caused by tuberculosis and blastomycosis, but by extension from the epididymis. Involvement of the testicle without palpable abnormality in the adjacent epididymis has rarely been observed with these agents.

PROSTATITIS, EPIDIDYMITIS, AND ORCHITIS IN MEN WITH HIV-1 INFECTION

One study of 80 autopsied AIDS patients found that 2 of 11 cases with systemic toxoplasmosis involved the testes, 4 of 48 cases of systemic cytomegalovirus infection involved the prostate and 1 involved the testes, and 1 of 27 cases of systemic candidiasis involved the prostate.[58] Other opportunistic infections involving the male genital tract include *Mycobacterium avium* complex,[59] cryptococcosis,[60] toxoplasmosis,[61] *Haemophilus parainfluenzae,*[62] and candidiasis.[63] The testes characteristically exhibit azospermia, marked spermatogenic arrest, germ cell degeneration, peritubular fibrosis, and Leydig cell depletion. These nonspecific findings most likely reflect the severe systemic disease in these patients. Focal accumulations of leukocytes in the connective tissue stroma of the testes and epididymedes may represent a portal of entry for HIV-1 into the semen.[64]

Urologic Manifestations

Other urologic manifestations in patients with AIDS and HIV-1 infections reflect involvement of related organ systems. For example, bladder dysfunction may occur in patients with HIV-

1–associated neurologic disorders. Such bladder dysfunction increases the risk of urinary tract infection. Urinary tract infections were diagnosed in 14–20 percent of HIV-1–seropositive in patients.[65,66] In another study, bacterial prostatitis was diagnosed in 17 (8 percent) of 209 men hospitalized for treatment of HIV-1 infections.[67] The most common presentation of prostatitis was fever plus irritative lower tract symptoms associated with bacteriuria.

Semen

Epidemiologic studies suggest that direct contact with semen is the most important route for sexual transmission of HIV-1.[59,64] HIV-1 was first isolated by cocultivation of seminal cells and donor lymphocytes.[68,69] Shedding of HIV-1 in semen was associated with no significant changes in semen parameters that assess fertility in one study of 50 semen specimens from asymptomatic or minimally symptomatic HIV-1–seropositive men.[70] In contrast, three men with AIDS all had pyosemia and grossly abnormal sperm.

The effects of the clinical stage of HIV infection and nucleoside therapy on shedding of HIV were evaluated by at least three groups. The first report described cultivation of HIV from semen in only 11 (32 percent) of 34 men, including 3 of 6 studied sequentially over time. HIV-1 was isolated from 6 (32 percent) of 19 semen specimens from 14 asymptomatic or minimally symptomatic persons (Centers for Disease Control and Prevention [CDC] class II or III) and from 10 (28 percent) of 36 semen specimens from 20 symptomatic patients (CDC class IV).[71] In this study, isolation of HIV-1 from semen did not correlate with CD4+ T-lymphocyte count or zidovudine therapy. The second study cultured HIV-1 from the semen of 9 (9 percent) of 95 men.[72] Factors associated with shedding of HIV-1 in semen were peripheral CD4+ cell counts of 200/ul or less, symptomatic (CDC class IV) disease, and lack of zidovudine therapy. The third study used polymerase chain reaction–based methods to detect HIV-1 in 45 (87 percent) of 52 semen specimens from 29 (81 percent) of 36 men. Seventeen (77 percent) of 22 stage II or III subjects and 12 (86 percent) of 14 stage IV subjects had positive specimens. Similar to the initial report, CD4+ lymphocyte count was not significantly different comparing subjects with positive and negative semen. Moreover, 6 (67 percent) of 9 untreated men had positive specimens compared with 23 (85 percent) of 27 men treated with zidovudine, 2′,3′-dideoxyinosine, or both. Thus, the detection of HIV-1 in semen was independent of both stage of infection and treatment.[73] All three studies support current recommendations for safe sexual practices by all persons infected with HIV-1 regardless of the stage of infection or concurrent antiviral chemotherapy.

REFERENCES

1. Jenkins AD, Turner TT, Howards SS. Physiology of the male reproductive system. Urol Clin North Am. 1978;5:437.
2. Stamey TA: Pathogenesis and Treatment of Urinary Tract Infections. Baltimore: Williams & Wilkins; 1980;1, 342.
3. Fair WR, Couch J, Wehner N. Prostatic antibacterial factor: Identity and significance. Urology. 1976;7:169.
4. Meares EM Jr. Prostatitis syndromes: New perspectives about old woes. J Urol. 1980;123:141.
5. Shortliffe LMD, Wehner N, Stamey TA. Use of solid-phase radioimmunoassay and formalin-fixed whole bacterial antigen in the detection of antigen-specific immunoglobulin in prostatic fluid. J Clin Invest. 1981;67:780.
6. Fowler JE Jr, Mariano M. Immunologic response of the prostate to bacteriuria and bacterial prostatitis: II. Antigen specific immunoglobulin in prostatic fluid. J Urol. 1982;128:165.
7. Schaeffer AJ, Wendel EF, Dunn JK, et al. Prevalence and significance of prostatic inflammation. J Urol. 1981;125:215.
8. Drach GW, Meares EM, Fair WR, et al. Classification of benign diseases associated with prostatic pain: Prostatitis or prostatodynia? J Urol. 1978;120:266.
9. Meares EM, Stamey TA. Bacteriologic localization patterns in bacterial prostatitis and urethritis. Invest Urol. 1968;5:492.
10. Fair WR, Crane DB, Schiller N, et al. Re-appraisal of treatment in chronic bacterial prostatitis. J Urol. 1979;121:437.
11. Malinverni R, Glausser MP. Comparative studies of fluoroquinolones in the treatment of urinary tract infections. Rev Infect Dis. 1988;10(Suppl 1):153.
12. Naber KG: Use of quinolones in urinary tract infections and prostatitis. Rev Infect Dis. 1989:11(Suppl 5):S1321.
13. Weidner W, Schiefer HG, Brahler E: Refractory chronic bacterial prostatitis: A re-evaluation of ciprofloxacin treatment after a median followup of 30 months. J Urol. 146:350.
14. Corrado ML: Worldwide clinical experience with ofloxacin in urologic cases. Urology. 1991;37(Suppl):28.
15. Eykyn S, Bultitude MI, Mayo ME, et al. Prostatitic calculi as a source of recurrent bacteriuria in the male. Br J Urol. 1974;46:527.
16. Mardh PA, Colleen S. Search for uro-genital tract infections in patients with symptoms of prostatitis. Scand J Urol Nephrol. 1975;9:8.
17. Mardh PA, Ripa KT, Colleen S, et al. Role of Chlamydia trachomatis in non-acute prostatitis. Br J Vener Dis. 1978;54:330.
18. Weidner W, Arens M, Krauss H, et al. Chlamydia trachomatis in "abacterial" prostatitis: Microbiological, cytological, and serological studies. Urol Int. 1983;38:146.
19. Poletti F, Medici MC, Alinovi A, et al. Isolation of Chlamydia trachomatis from the prostatic cells in patients affected by nonacute abacterial prostatitis. J Urol. 1985;134:691.
20. Bruce AW, Chadwick P, Willet WS, O'Shaughnesey M. The role of chlamydiae in genitourinary disease. J Urol. 1981;126:625.
21. Weidner W, Brunner H, Krause W. Quantitative culture of Ureaplasma urealyticum in patients with chronic prostatitis or prostatosis. J Urol. 1980;124:622.
22. Brunner H, Weidner W, Schiefer H-G. Studies on the role of Ureaplasma urealyticum and Mycoplasma hominis in prostatitis. J Infect Dis. 1983;147:807.
23. Schacter J. Is Chlamydia trachomatis a cause of prostatitis? J Urol. 1985;134:711.
24. Taylor-Robinson D. The role of chlamydiae in genitourinary disease (Letter). J Urol. 1982;128:156.
25. Doble A, Walker TMM, Harris JRW, et al. The role of Chlamydia trachomatis in chronic abacterial prostatitis: A study using ultrasound guided biopsy. J Urol. 1989;141:332.
26. Segura JW, Opitz JL, Green L. Prostatosis prostatitis or pelvic floor tension myalgia? J Urol. 1979;122:168.
27. Nilsson JK, Colleen S, Mardh PA. Relationship between psychological and laboratory findings in patients with symptoms of non-acute prostatitis. In: Danielsson D, Juhlin L, Mardh PA, eds. Genital Infections and Their Complications. Stockholm: Almquist and Wiksell; 1975:133.
28. Krieger, JN. Prostatitis syndromes: Pathophysiology, differential diagnosis and treatment. Sex Transm Dis. 1984;11:100.
29. Stillwell TJ, Engen DE, Farrow GM. The clinical spectrum of granulomatous prostatitis: A report of 200 cases. J Urol. 1987;138:320.
30. Venema RJ, Lattimer, JK. Genital tuberculosis in the male. J Urol. 1957;78:65.
31. Simon HB. Genitourinary tuberculosis: Clinical features in a general hospital population. Am J Med. 1977;63:410.
32. Brooker WJ, Aufderheide AC. Genitourinary tract infections due to atypical mycobacteria. J Urol. 1980;124:242.
33. Oates RD, Stilmant MM, Freedlund MC, Siroky MB. Granulomatous prostatitis following Bacillus Calmette-Guérin immunotherapy for bladder cancer. J Urol. 1988;140:751.
34. Miyashita H, Troncoso P, Babaian RJ. BCG-induced granulomatous prostatitis: A comparative ultrasound and pathologic study. Urology. 1992;39:364.
35. Inoshita T, Youngberg GA, Boelen LJ, Langston J. Blastomycosis presenting with prostatic involvement: Report of 2 cases and review of the literature. J Urol. 1983;130:160–216.
36. Price MJ, Lewis EL, Carmalt JE. Coccidioidomycosis of prostate gland. Urology. 1982;19:653.
37. Hinchley WW, Someren A. Cryptococcal prostatitis. Am J Clin Pathol. 1981;75:257.
38. Bozzette SA, Larsen RA, Chiu J, et al. Fluconazole treatment of persistent Cryptococcus neoformans prostatic infection in AIDS. Ann Intern Med. 1991;115:285–286.
39. Zighelboim J, Goldfarb RA, Mody D, et al. Prostatic abscess due to Histoplasma capsulatum in a patient with the acquired immunodeficiency syndrome. J Urol. 1992;147:166.
40. Meares EM Jr. Prostatic Abscess. J Urol. 1986;136:1281.
41. Weinberger M, Cytron S, Servadio C, et al. Prostatic abscess in the antibiotic era. Rev Infect Dis. 1988;10:239.
42. Suago H, Takiuchi H, Sakurai T. Transrectal longitudinal ultrasonography of prostatic abscess. J Urol. 1986;136:1316.
43. Vaccaro JA, Belville WD, Kiesling VJ Jr, et al. Prostatic abscesses: Computerized tomography scanning as an aid to diagnosis and treatment. J Urol. 1986;136:1318.
44. Bormel P. Current concepts on the etiology and treatment of epididymitis. Med Bull US Army Europe. 1963;20:332.
45. Berger RE, Alexander ER, Harnisch JP, et al. Etiology, manifestations and therapy of acute epididymitis: Prospective study of 50 cases. J Urol. 1979;121:750.
46. Berger RE, Alexander ER, Monda GD, et al. Chlamydia trachomatis as a cause of acute "idiopathic" epididymitis. N Engl J Med. 1978;298:301.

47. Mittemeyer BT, Lennox KW, Borski AA. Epididymitis—a review of 610 cases. J Urol. 1966;95:390.
48. Nilsson S, Obrant KD, Persson PS. Changes in the testes parenchyma caused by acute nonspecific epididymitis. Fertil Steril. 1968;19:748.
49. Witherington R, Harper WM IV. The surgical management of acute bacterial epididymitis with emphasis on epididymotomy. J Urol. 1982;128:722.
50. Krieger JN. Epididymitis, orchitis, and related conditions. Sex Transm Dis. 1984;11:173.
51. Shapiro FR, Breschi LC. Acute epididymitis in Viet Nam. Review of 52 cases. Milit Med. 1973;138:643.
52. Harnisch JP, Berger RE, Alexander ER, et al. Aetiology of acute epididymitis. Lancet. 1977;1:819.
53. Watson RA. Gonorrhea and acute epididymitis. Milit Med. 1979;144:785.
54. Drotman PD. Epidemiology and treatment of epididymitis. Rev Infect Dis. 1982;4(Suppl):788.
55. Krieger JN, Wang K, Mack L. Preliminary evaluation of color Doppler imaging for investigation of intrascrotal pathology. J Urol. 1990;140:904.
56. Erden MI, Ozbeck SS, et al. Color-Doppler imaging in acute scrotal disorders. Urol Int. 1993;50:39.
57. Beard CM, Benson RC, Kelalis PP, et al. The incidence and outcome of mumps orchitis in Rochester, Minn. Mayo, 1935–1974. Mayo Clin Proc. 1977;52:3.
58. Shevchuk M, de Silza M, Armenakas N, et al. The male genital tract in AIDS. J Urol. 141:354, 1989.
59. Mikolich DJ, Mates SM. Granulomatous prostatitis due to *Mycobacterium avium* complex. Clin Infect Dis. 1992;14:589.
60. Adams JRJ, Mata JA, Culkin DJ, et al. Acquired immunodeficiency syndrome manifesting as prostate nodule secondary to cryptococcal infection. Urology. 1992;39:289.
61. Haskell L, Fusco MJ, Ares L. Disseminated toxoplasmosis presenting as symptomatic orchitis and nephrotic syndrome. Am J Med Sci. 1989;298:185.
62. Clairmont GJ, Zon LI, Groopman JE. *Hemophilus parainfluenzae* prostatitis in a homosexual man with chronic lymphadenopathy syndrome and HTLV-III infection. Am J Med. 1987;82:175.
63. Swartz DA, Harrington P, Wilcox R. Candidal epididymitis treated with ketoconazole. N Engl J Med 1988;319:1485.
64. Pudney J, Anderson D. Orchitis and human immunodeficiency virus type 1 infected cells in reproductive tissues from men with the acquired immune deficiency syndrome. Am J Pathol. 1991;139:149.
65. Miles BJ, Melser M, Farah R, et al. The urological manifestations of the acquired immunodeficiency syndrome. J Urol. 1989;142:771.
66. Kaplan MS, Wechsler M, Benson MC. Urologic manifestations of AIDS. Urology. 30:1987.
67. Leport C, Rousseau F, Perronne C, et al. Bacterial prostatitis in patients infected with the human immunodeficiency virus. J Urol. 1989;141:334.
68. Ho DD, Schooley R, Rota T, et al. HTLV-III in the semen and blood of a healthy homosexual man. Science. 1984;226:451.
69. Zagury D, et al. Evidence for HTLV-III in T-cells from semen of AIDS patients. Cancer Res. 1985;45(S):4595.
70. Krieger JN, Coombs RW, Collier AC, et al. Fertility parameters in men infected with human immunodeficiency virus. J Infect Dis. 1991;164:464.
71. Krieger JN, Coombs RW, Collier AC, et al. Recovery of human immunodeficiency virus type 1 from semen: Minimal impact of stage of infection and current antiviral chemotherapy. J Infect Dis. 1991;163:386.
72. Anderson DJ, O'Brien TR, Politch JA, et al. Effects of disease stage and zidovudine therapy on the detection of human immunodeficiency virus type 1 in semen. JAMA. 1992;267:2769.
73. Hamed KA, Winters MA, Holodniy M, et al. Detection of human immunodeficiency virus type 1 in semen: Effects of disease stage and nucleoside therapy. J Infect Dis. 1993;167:798.

SECTION M. EYE INFECTIONS

92. CONJUNCTIVITIS

TERRENCE P. O'BRIEN
W. RICHARD GREEN

Conjunctivitis is the most common ocular inflammation; it involves all ages and occurs worldwide. The principal causes of acute conjunctivitis are infections, allergens, and irritative toxins. Accurate diagnosis and management of conjunctivitis requires distinguishing between an acute or chronic pace of inflammation, identification of any precipitating event(s), consideration of the role of any antecedent medication, and utilization of the principal ocular signs with identification of the key distinctive conjunctival signs. The principal ocular signs in external diseases of the eye include skin and mucous membrane involvement, orbital involvement, regional lymphadenopathy, type and amount of conjunctival discharge, morphologic pattern of conjunctival inflammation, and the type of corneal epithelial abnormality. Infectious conjunctivitis may cause significant morbidity, depending in part on the type of invading organism and local ocular defense mechanisms. The normal flora of the conjunctiva, various sources of infection in conjunctivitis, and factors important in the resistance of the conjunctiva to infections have been well described.[1–15]

ETIOLOGIC AGENTS

The numerous agents that may cause conjunctivitis are listed in Table 1.

CLINICAL MANIFESTATIONS

The clinical findings and the course of infection are influenced by the pathogenic features of the exogenous microorganisms. The most obvious clinical manifestation of conjunctivitis is hyperemia of the conjunctiva. The dilatation and congestion of the vessels are greater near the periphery of the bulbar conjunctiva and become less marked as the corneal margin (limbus) is approached.

The presence of secretion is almost always a feature of conjunctivitis. This is due to an exudation of inflammatory cells and a fibrin-rich edematous fluid from the blood, and the exudate is combined with denuded epithelial cells and mucus. The secretion may be purulent, mucopurulent, fibrinous, or serosanguineous, depending on the cause and severity of the disease. When the exudate dries, the eyelids may stick together. Conjunctival edema (chemosis) may be present in parts of the conjunctiva that are freely movable over the globe and lids. The normal transparency of the conjunctiva may be lost, and it may appear thickened due to the infiltration of the tissues with leukocytes. If there is diffuse leukocytic infiltration of the conjunctival stroma, with hyperplasia of the overlying epithelium, papillae may form. A papilla contains a central blood vessel in its core. This vessel branches on the surface of the papilla. Papillae usually occur in the tarsal conjunctiva. The conjunctiva may have a velvety appearance from numerous small papillae. When large, the papillae have the appearance of cobblestone excrescences. This is unusual in acute infectious conjunctivitis but more common in allergic and chronic conjunctivitis. Papillae are nonspecific conjunctival signs, but are most commonly observed with bacterial infection and allergy.

The conjunctiva contains lymphatic tissue that may be stimulated by various microbial antigens to form a follicle. Normal

TABLE 1. Etiologic Agents of Conjunctivitis

Bacteria
  Streptococcus pneumoniae
  Streptococcus pyogenes
  Streptococci of the viridans group
  Staphylococcus aureus
  Haemophilus influenzae (includes *H. aegyptius*)
  Neisseria gonorrhoeae
  Haemophilus ducreyi
  Neisseria meningitidis
  Proteus vulgaris
  Moraxella lacunata
  Corynebacterium diphtheriae
  Mycobacterium tuberculosis
  Francisella tularensis
  Treponema pallidum
  Moraxella catarrhalis
  Shigella flexneri
  Yersinia enterocolitica
  Staphylococcus epidermidis
  Acinetobacter species
  Aeromonas hydrophila
  Peptostreptococcus
  Bartonella (Rochalimaea) henselae (cat scratch bacillus)
Viruses
  Adenoviruses
  Poxviruses (variola, vaccinia, molluscum contagiosum)
  Herpesviruses (herpes simplex, varicella-zoster, Epstein-Barr virus)
  Papillomaviruses
  Influenza A and B viruses
  Paramyxoviruses (measles, mumps, Newcastle disease virus)
  Picornaviruses (echovirus, enterovirus, coxsackievirus, and poliovirus)
Chlamydia trachomatis
Fungi
  Candida spp.
  Sporothrix schenckii
  Rhinosporidium seeberi
Parasites
  Onchocerca volvulus
  Loa loa
  Wuchereria bancrofti
  Oestrus ovis (myiasis)
  Microsporidiosis
    Nosema spp.
    Encephalitozoon spp.
  Toxocara canis

conjunctiva has an occasional follicle in its substantia propria, especially in the fornices. In certain forms of conjunctivitis, especially viral, chlamydial, or toxic, a follicular reaction may predominate. Follicles and papillae are differentiated clinically by appearance with follicles resembling smooth, glistening bumps, whereas papillae are smaller (<1 mm) and red with a central vascular core.

Membrane formation is also seen in some cases of conjunctivitis, especially with viral and some bacterial causes. This membrane consists of a superficial fibrinous layer connected to subconjunctival granulation tissue. When this membrane is excised, a raw, bleeding surface is exposed.

Corneal involvement may occur in conjunctivitis, especially viral, due to the close proximity of the corneal epithelium to the inflamed tarsal and limbal conjunctivae. Symptoms of corneal involvement include a gritty foreign body sensation, photophobia, diminished vision, and pain. The various forms of conjunctivitis have many of the aforementioned signs and symptoms in common. Awareness of the principal ocular signs with selection of the most distinctive conjunctival sign can narrow the differential diagnosis.

BACTERIAL CONJUNCTIVITIS

Bacterial conjunctivitis is among the most common type of ocular infection. Typically, pathogenesis involves exogenous routes of infection with airborne fomites, contact with upper respiratory tract infections, hand to eye contact, and possible relationship with genital tract infections. Less frequently, endogenous routes of infection with spread from adjacent structures such as

the face and eyelids, lacrimal drainage apparatus, and paranasal sinuses occurs. Hematogenous routes of infection in acute bacterial conjunctivitis are rare.

The principle causes of acute conjunctivitis in the normal host include *Staphylococcus aureus*, *Streptococcus pneumoniae*, *Neisseria gonorrhoeae*, and *Haemophilus influenzae*. Age-related factors are important determinants of causative organisms. In neonates, there is a notorious invalidity of clinical signs due to the immature immunologic system. There is a frequency of neisserial and chlamydial infections in the newborn.[16] In children, there is an opportunity for severe conjunctivitis caused by *H. influenzae*.[17–19] *Streptococcus pneumoniae* and occasionally *Staphylococcus aureus* may also cause acute conjunctivitis in children.[20–22] In young adults, there may be a higher frequency of neisserial and chlamydial infections.[23]

In adults, the most common bacterial isolates from an acute conjunctivitis are *Streptococcus pneumoniae*, *Staphylococcus aureus*, and *Staphylococcus epidermidis*. The role of the latter two organisms in causation is, however, disputed.[24–26] Although leptospirosis commonly causes conjunctival suffusion, this infection is a rare cause of conjunctivitis.

The bacterial etiology of chronic bacterial conjunctivitis is less well defined.[27]

Anaerobic bacteria have been isolated from conjunctivitis in association with aerobic organisms thought to be the cause of the conjunctivitis.[20,25] The same organisms have been isolated from immunodeficient patients, in whom acute and chronic conjunctivitis are more common than in normal patients.[28] Table 1 lists the bacteria that have been noted to cause conjunctivitis.

The clinical significance of certain organisms isolated in studies of bacterial cultures during conjunctivitis remains incompletely determined. However, early in the course of infection, bacterial and viral conjunctivitis may not have distinctive clinical signs to differentiate the conditions.[24]

Investigations into the cause of epidemics of bacterial conjunctivitis have improved to better establish, for example, *Streptococcus pneumoniae*,[29] *Pseudomonas aeruginosa*,[30] and *Moraxella* spp.[31] as significant pathogens.

In acute bacterial conjunctivitis, it is helpful to assess the severity of inflammation based on the rate of evolution of certain distinctive signs, including corneal involvement.

In nonsevere bacterial conjunctivitis, there is minimal to no lid edema, scant purulent discharge with mild to moderate conjunctival hyperemia, and a normal cornea. In contrast, severe conjunctivitis is characterized often by marked lid edema with copious purulent discharge, marked conjunctival hyperemia, chemosis, membrane formation, and suppurative or nonsuppurative keratitis.

The principle causes of nonsevere bacterial conjunctivitis are *Staphylococcus aureus*, *Streptococcus pneumoniae*, *Haemophilus* spp., especially after age 5 years, and *Moraxella* spp.

Severe bacterial conjunctivitis is most often caused by *Neisseria* spp., *H. influenzae* in children, *Streptococcus pyogenes*, and *Staphylococcus aureus*.

Severe conjunctivitis caused by *Neisseria gonorrhoeae* or *N. meningitidis* deserves special recognition. Infection with *Neisseria* may result in markedly swollen eyelids, extreme hyperemia and chemosis, and a profuse purulent discharge.[32] The massively swollen conjunctiva infiltrated with polymorphonuclear neutrophils may become draped over the peripheral cornea at the limbus. The action of lytic enzymes from the neutrophils may cause serious complications in untreated gonococcal conjunctivitis, including corneal ulceration with subsequent perforation. Occasionally, gonococcal conjunctivitis may have a prolonged asymptomatic course, in a manner similar to some of the genital infections.[33] Gonococcal conjunctivitis can occur without sexual transmission, though a healthy suspicion for possible sexual abuse should be maintained in prepubertal children.[35]

Neisseria meningitidis is an uncommon cause of acute bacterial conjunctivitis. In 84 cases of primary meningococcal conjunctivitis, the male to female ratio was 1.76:1, with 9 neonates, 55 children, and 20 adults.[34] Systemic meningococcal disease develops in 17.8 percent of the patients, and the overall mortality was 13.3 percent. Other *Neisseria* spp., including *N. cinerea*, may cause acute purulent conjunctivitis.[36]

Membrane formation may be seen in any severe infection of the conjunctiva, but it is typically present in infections with streptococci and *Corynebacterium diphtheriae* or with adenovirus. These membranes may lead to a spectrum of changes from fine corneal scarring to obliteration of the fornices and permanent dry eye states. In contrast to most other types of conjunctivitis, pain is a common symptom with *C. diphtheriae* infection. Diphtheritic conjunctivitis does not occur as the sole manifestation of diphtheria, and so other manifestations of the disease should be sought. Widespread immunization programs have made diphtheritic conjunctivitis extremely rare.[37]

Moraxella lacunata produces a localized "angular" conjunctivitis associated with fissuring and dermatitis of the external canthi and a scanty conjunctival discharge. *Moraxella* conjunctival infection may be incorrectly diagnosed as chlamydial, epidemic keratoconjunctivitis, and herpes simplex infections. Although *Moraxella* conjunctivitis is associated with adolescent girls, 13 of 27 female patients with culture-proven *Moraxella* infection (48 percent) were 20 years or older.[38] *Moraxella* conjunctivitis can occur in epidemics from sharing contaminated eye makeup.[31]

Certain nonpyogenic organisms (*Mycobacterium tuberculosis, Francisella tularensis, Treponema pallidum*) produce an atypical clinical picture characterized by unilateral conjunctival nodules that tend to ulcerate. Moderate localized conjunctival injection, minimal discharge, and a palpable preauricular lymph node on the affected side are present. Nonsyphilitic spirochetal infection with *Borrelia burgdorferi* has reportedly caused conjunctivitis in association with Lyme disease.[39,40]

The cat scratch disease bacillus *Bartonella (Rochalimeae) henselae*[41–43] produces a unilateral follicular conjunctivitis associated with prominent enlargement of the ipsilateral preauricular lymph node[44] (see Ch. 108). *Yersinia* infection has been implicated[45] in a syndrome similar to Reiter syndrome and consisting of a self-limited conjunctivitis, acute myalgia, fever, gastrointestinal symptoms, and a prolonged anterior uveitis, polyarthritis, sacroiliitis, and HLA-B27 association. Similar syndrome complexes were seen within family groups. *Yersinia enterocolitica* has also been associated with an isolated conjunctivitis.[46]

Haemophilus ducreyi,[47] *Pasteurella multocida,*[48] *Francisella tularensis,*[49] *Neisseria meningitidis,*[50] *Streptococcus* spp.,[51] *Acinetobacter* spp.,[52] and *Aeromonas hydrophila*[53] have caused isolated cases of acute conjunctivitis.

FUNGAL CONJUNCTIVITIS

Primary fungal conjunctivitis is infrequently encountered clinically, though *Candida* spp. and others (Table 1) may be isolated from the conjunctiva. Blastomycosis involving the eyelid may cause a granulomatous conjunctivitis.[54] Lid or conjunctival nodules are the usual form of ocular involvement with *Sporothrix schenckii*. *Rhinosporidium seeberi* may cause a characteristic granulomatous inflammatory mass in the conjunctiva, which may become pedunculated.[55] Other fungi are also occasionally recovered from cultures in immunocompromised individuals.

VIRAL CONJUNCTIVITIS

Viral conjunctivitis is common, causing 20 percent of nonepidemic cases of conjunctivitis in one study in children[21] and 14 percent of adult patients in another study.[24] The morphology of associated corneal changes, the time course, systemic involvement, and epidemic characteristics will usually permit presumptive clinical diagnosis of viral conjunctivitis. The actual causative virus usually cannot be determined by ocular morphologic

characteristics alone, and definitive diagnosis requires cultures and serologic studies. Most viral conjunctivitides are self-limited but highly contagious, with potential for causing considerable morbidity. The discharge is usually serous rather than mucoid or purulent. A generalized conjunctival hyperemia, moderate tearing, and mild itching are present. Follicle formation stimulated by viral antigen may be prominent. Regional lymphadenopathy with preauricular and submandibular node enlargement is common, and occasionally the conjunctivitis is associated with an upper respiratory tract infection. The preauricular node is usually exquisitely tender to palpation.

Adenoviruses are responsible for the most frequent epidemics of viral conjunctivitis in the United States and are a major occupational hazard for eye care professionals.

Serotypes of adenoviruses typically associated with pharyngoconjunctival fever are 3 and 7, with occasional involvement by types 1, 2, 4, 5, 6, 8, and 14. The clinical complex of pharyngitis, fever, and conjunctivitis, inferior forniceal follicles, and, rarely, keratitis may help to identify this conjunctivitis. Spontaneous resolution within 1–2 weeks is the rule.[56] Outbreaks among children may occur after swimming pool inoculation or hand to eye contact.[57]

Epidemic keratoconjunctivitis has most commonly resulted from infection with serotype 8, but types 2, 3, 4, 7, 9, 10, 11, 14, 16, 19, and 29 have been reported.[58–65] The clinical picture includes pharyngitis, preauricular lymphadenopathy, and follicular conjunctivitis, and there is a 7- to 10-day incubation period with a 5- to 12-day interval before characteristic (but inconsistent) corneal subepithelial infiltrates develop. These epidemics are sometimes propagated by eye health care personnel. Despite a wide spectrum of symptoms ranging from severe photophobia to mild irritation only, this disease is usually self-limited and is rarely associated with visual loss from corneal changes.[66,67] Occasional reports have described raised intraocular pressure[68] and chronic keratitis and Stevens-Johnson syndrome[69] as a result of epidemic keratoconjunctivitis. Chronic adenovirus conjunctivitis has also been reported.[70,71]

Reports of epidemics in Florida have emphasized the emergence of an enterovirus as a cause of epidemic hemorrhagic conjunctivitis in the United States. Previous reports have been mainly from Africa.[72,73] Enterovirus type 70, coxsackievirus A24, and adenovirus 11 have all resulted in a similar clinical picture (Fig. 1).[74–80] This consists of bilateral follicular conjunctivitis of sudden onset, with (rarely) corneal changes and systemic symptoms, a short (4–5 day) symptomatic course, and bulbar conjunctival hemorrhages.[81,82] Spontaneous resolution with low morbidity is the usual course, although occasional re-

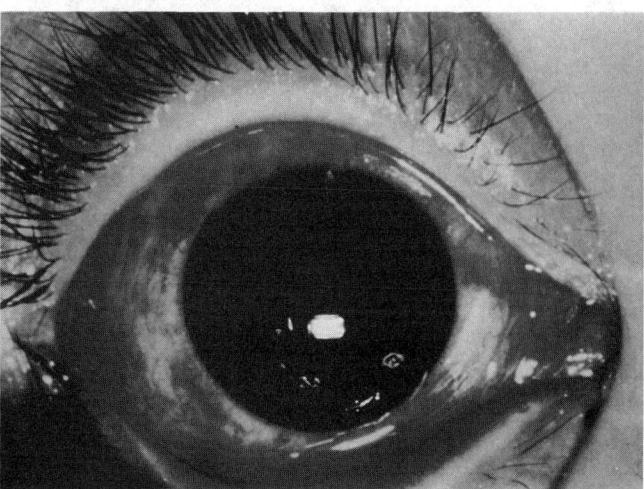

FIG. 1. Acute hemorrhagic conjunctivitis due to enterovirus 70. (From Kono et al.,[78] with permission.)

ports have described Bell's palsy, radiculomyelitis, cranial nerve palsies, and other types of central nervous system involvement.[83–86]

Ocular infection with vaccinia virus occurs when the virus is accidentally transferred from the site of medical inoculation to the eye. Vesicles appear on the lid margin,[87] and a conjunctivitis may follow. Conjunctivitis without lid lesions has also been reported.[88]

Molluscum contagiosum virus produces small, waxy, elevated lid-margin nodules with umbilicated centers that are associated with a chronic follicular conjunctivitis caused by the toxic effect of incomplete virions that are shed.[89]

Herpes simplex virus types 1 and 2, varicella-zoster virus, and Epstein-Barr virus can cause conjunctivitis.[90,91] Primary herpes simplex is responsible for the majority of cases of nonepidemic follicular conjunctivitis in young children.[92] Vesicular lid lesions, preauricular lymphadenopathy, and transient keratitis may be noted. The conjunctivitis is self-limited and is rarely associated with significant morbidity.

In patients with chickenpox, papules may develop on the lids and conjunctiva and at the limbus during the infection. These papules may become pustules and ulcerate. Vesicles may be found on the conjunctiva, particularly on the semilunar fold. Four percent of patients with chickenpox have conjunctival and corneal manifestations.[93] In herpes zoster ophthalmicus, a follicular conjunctivitis with regional adenopathy rarely occurs. In less than 5 percent of patients with infectious mononucleosis, a mild conjunctivitis is present.[94,95]

Human papillomavirus may produce lesions on the tarsal and bulbar conjunctivae and on the lid margin. A catarrhal conjunctivitis may result, and the cornea may show multiple punctate erosions. The presence of viral antigen and DNA sequences in some dysplastic epithelial lesions of the conjunctiva has raised concern that the virus may have a role in the development of conjunctival epithelial malignancies similar to its suspected role in the female genital tract.[96]

Congenital rubella is associated with numerous ocular abnormalities.[97,98] Epidemic rubella in young children has produced a follicular conjunctivitis associated with occasional corneal epithelial changes.

Influenza viruses often cause catarrhal conjunctivitis and occasionally an acute follicular conjunctivitis. This ocular manifestation of influenza has been reported in both 48 percent and 60 percent of patients in two studies.

Infections due to measles (rubeola) virus may be associated with mild paralimbal conjunctival epithelial erosion; the epithelia contain measles antigens that develop during the prodrome before the skin rash.[101] An epithelial keratitis with photophobia may occur after the skin rash occurs. Koplik's spots may be found on the semilunar fold.[102]

Conjunctivitis occurs rarely with mumps.[103] Newcastle disease virus (which causes a fatal pneumoencephalitis in fowl) may produce a self-limited, unilateral follicular conjunctivitis in humans.[104] Echovirus 11[105] and poliovirus[106] have occasionally been described as a cause of follicular conjunctivitis.

Parinaud's oculoglandular syndrome is a clinical complex of conjunctivitis, prominent preauricular lymphadenopathy, and a febrile illness with various possible causes, including infectious mononucleosis,[107] cat-scratch disease,[108] syphilis, tuberculosis, and sarcoidosis.

CHLAMYDIAL CONJUNCTIVITIS

Trachoma, one of the leading causes of blindness in the world,[109,110] is caused by a *Chlamydia trachomatis*. In the United States, the disease is largely confined to certain Native American populations that are characterized by poverty and poor communal hygiene. Repeated infections appear necessary to establish clinical trachoma. The conjunctivitis is characterized by a follicular reaction in the superior tarsal conjunctiva that is often associated with a concurrent papillary response. As follicles resolve, they appear to be replaced with fine subconjunctival scars. The degree of scarring seems to be related to the intensity of the follicular response and also to the presence of secondary bacterial infection. The subconjunctival scarring may in time lead to distortion of the tarsal plate and result in trichiasis. *Chlamydia trachomatis* serotypes A, B, Ba, and C have been most commonly found in hyperendemic areas of trachoma.

Also associated with trachoma is the development of a superior limbic pannus with opacification of the corneal stroma and neovascularization. Follicles may occur in the limbus, and when these resolve a clear depression persists (Herbert's pit).

Inclusion conjunctivitis is a fairly common infection caused by *Chlamydia trachomatis* that is most often sexually transmitted.[111,112] Since an infant may acquire the organism during passage through the birth canal, it is one of the causes of ophthalmia neonatorum. Because the conjunctiva in the newborn does not form follicles, the injected appearance of this conjunctivitis in newborns is nonspecific. In adults, numerous papillae and follicles form on the tarsal conjunctiva and are more pronounced on the lower. Bulbar conjunctival follicles may appear, and their presence is highly suggestive of chlamydial infection. The disease is usually bilateral, and the discharge is often profuse. Inclusion conjunctivitis is differentiated from trachoma by two important features: *(1)* corneal scarring rarely occurs in inclusion conjunctivitis; and *(2)* in trachoma the upper tarsal conjunctiva is more involved than the lower, although occasionally inclusion conjunctivitis may take on the characteristics of trachoma and various corneal changes have been described in inclusion conjunctivitis. In adults with *C. trachomatis* conjunctivitis, infection is sexually acquired, acute, and accompanied by copious mucopurulent conjunctival discharge. Chlamydial urethritis or cervicitis is commonly present.[113]

Conjunctivitis is a rare manifestation of systemic lymphogranuloma venereum that is caused by certain immunotypes (L-1, L-2, L-3) of *C. trachomatis*. Moderate unilateral conjunctival injection, slight conjunctival discharge, and extreme edema of the upper and lower lids are present. In addition, ipsilateral preauricular, parotid, and submaxillary lymphadenopathy is present.[114] *Lymphogranuloma venereum* conjunctivitis has caused marginal keratitis with corneal perforation in an HIV-positive individual.[115]

PARASITIC CONJUNCTIVITIS

A number of ocular parasites may cause conjunctivitis. Blepharoconjunctivitis due to *Leishmania donovani* in association with nodules of post-kala azar dermal leishmaniasis can infect the conjunctiva by spread from contaminated fingers.[116] Parasites are being recovered in increasing frequency from the conjunctiva of individuals with the acquired immunodeficiency syndrome (AIDS). Microsporidiosis, most often due to Encephalitozoon species, are small ubiquitous obligate intracellular parasites that usually cause infections in animals and rarely in humans. Encephalitozoon species may cause a mild conjunctivitis with punctate keratopathy in patients with AIDS.[117] The symptoms may mimic those of blepharitis or dry eye, and a high index of suspicion should be maintained to diagnose this parasitic keratoconjunctivitis in immunodeficient individuals. Cryptosporidial enteritis has also been complicated by conjunctivitis.[118] Conjunctival involvement with fly larvae,[119] nematodes,[120] and trematodes[121,122] has been described.

OPHTHALMIA NEONATORUM

The incidence of acute conjunctivitis of the newborn (ophthalmia neonatorum) is reported to be as high as 12 percent of all newborns.[123] It has been most commonly the result of mild chemical irritation after ocular silver nitrate prophylaxis. This self-limited conjunctivitis appears within the first 24 hours, and it lasts 1–2 days. However, chlamydial conjunctivitis is becoming much more common, with an incidence of approximately 2.8 percent of all births at one clinic and occurring in more than 35 percent of the infants who are born to mothers with proven chlamydial cervicitis.[124] This has been substantiated by other studies.[125,126] The onset generally occurs within 5–19 days of delivery, with no pathologic features except for an association with other systemic chlamydial infections such as pneumonia and otitis media.[127,128] It has been suggested that the organism in these cases gains entry to the neonate through the conjunctival mucosa. There have been reports of occasional cases of chlamydial conjunctivitis in infants delivered by cesarean section.[129]

Bacterial conjunctivitis is most often the result of *Staphylococcus aureus* infection, with *Streptococcus pneumoniae* and *H. influenzae* the next most common.[130,131] There are no pathognomonic features of these infections, and they may occur as early as 24 hours after birth. Streptococcal infections may be associated with acute dacryocystitis of the newborn, and *Pseudomonas* spp. have been reported as an occasional cause.[132] Cases of staphylococcal "scalded skin" syndrome have been attributed to primary staphylococcal conjunctivitis.[133] *Haemophilus influenzae* conjunctivitis has been implicated in neonatal meningitis. *Shigella flexneri* has caused ethmoiditis and conjunctivitis.[134] *Moraxella catarrhalis* conjunctivitis is being more frequently diagnosed[135–137] and has been confused with true gonococcal ophthalmia neonatorum.

The prevailing incidence of gonococcal ophthalmia neonatorum is not known, but it is usually seen 1–2 days after birth and is characterized by a florid course and the threat of corneal ulceration and perforation. Cases of penicillin-resistant strains[138,139] and occasional cases with a deceptively mild course have made diagnosis and management more difficult.[140]

Infants born to mothers with herpes simplex virus cervicitis may develop a conjunctivitis within a few days of birth. The conjunctivitis is usually self-limited but may be associated with corneal epithelial changes and, rarely, stromal keratitis.

NONINFECTIOUS CONJUNCTIVITIS

Conjunctival inflammation (chemosis, injection, and discharge) is seen as a result of many noninfectious conditions, but particularly as an allergic mucosal response. The agents responsible include drugs and devices such as hard and soft contact lenses.[141,142] contact lens sterilizing solutions (usually the preservative thiomerosol),[143,144] and prostheses,[145,146] which can cause giant papillary conjunctivitis. Other agents implicated include topical timolol,[147] atropine, antiviral agents, and other drugs,[148–152] cosmetics,[153] and external allergens that cause vernal keratoconjunctivitis.[154] Conjunctivitis may occur as a response to toxic agents such as gentian violet,[155] latex,[156] and ultraviolet irradiation.[157–159] Phlyctenular keratoconjunctivitis has occurred in patients with increased tuberculin sensitivity[160] and staphylococcal hypersensitivity.[161]

The precise mechanisms eliciting conjunctivitis in numerous other conditions with fairly specific clinical features have not been conclusively identified. These include keratoconjunctivitis sicca, superior limbic keratoconjunctivitis, ligneous conjunctivitis, mucocutaneous lymph node syndrome, and Reiter syndrome. Immune-mediated conjunctivitis has been implicated in mucous membrane pemphigoid[162] and in the conjunctivitis associated with graft-vs-host disease in bone marrow transplant patients.[163]

DIFFERENTIAL DIAGNOSIS

Other serious, sight-threatening conditions that present as "red eye" may superficially resemble a conjunctivitis. The points of

TABLE 2. Comparison of Conjunctivitis and Other Conditions

Characteristics	Conjunctivitis	Uveitis	Acute Angle Closure Glaucoma
Prominent symptoms	Discharge, irritation	Photophobia, visual loss	Pain, visual loss
Vision	Usually normal	Normal and occasionally decreased	Markedly reduced
Ocular injection	Conjunctival injection generalized	Paralimbal injection	Paralimbal injection
Cornea	Usually clear	Usually clear	Edematous and cloudy
Pupil	Normal	May be normal or small	Usually mid-dilated, irregular, and immobile
Intraocular pressure	Normal	Normal or elevated	Markedly elevated

difference are highlighted in Table 2. Chronic, unilateral conjunctivitis in which a specific diagnosis is not made should alert the physician to the possibility of a meibomian gland carcinoma.[164]

LABORATORY INVESTIGATIONS

Mild, nonsevere conjunctivitis is not routinely investigated and is often treated empirically without benefit of knowledge from microbial culture. Reports differ on the value of culturing suspected bacterial conjunctivitis.[165–167] In nonsevere conjunctivitis, a calcium alginate swab dipped in trypticase soy broth may be used to obtain material from the conjunctival sacs. Cultures should be obtained from both eyes and plated on chocolate agar. In severe conjunctivitis scrapings of the superior and inferior tarsal conjunctiva should be taken after the administration of topical proparacaine HCl, 0.5% for diagnostic smears, as well as microbial culture in a manner similar to that described in Chapter 93. Cultures are occasionally taken separately from both lids in suspected conjunctivitis, though the value of this practice is less certain. Chlamydial cultures are usually taken with a dry calcium alginate swab, which is then placed in special *Chlamydia* transport medium prior to processing for cell culture.

All cases of suspected ophthalmia neonatorum should have cultures and smears performed for bacteria, *Chlamydia,* and herpes simplex virus. Acute and convalescent serologic tests for adenovirus and some enteroviruses may help in diagnosing epidemic conjunctivitis, but these are generally not required because of the self-limited nature of the infection, the nonspecific treatment available, and the diagnostic characteristics of the epidemic features. Serodiagnostic testing of tears and serum by using microimmunofluorescent tests has been described for patients with *Chlamydia trachomatis* inclusion conjunctivitis.[168] Serologic testing for SS-A and SS-B autoantibodies has assisted in the early diagnosis of keratoconjunctivitis sicca that is a prodrome of Sjögren syndrome.[169]

In a conjunctival scraping from a normal healthy eye, epithelial cells and occasional goblet cells are present. In acute bacterial infection, the scraping shows large numbers of neutrophils. Bacteria may be present within or outside leukocytes. In chronic bacterial infections, there is a decrease in neutrophils and an increase in lymphocytes and large mononuclear cells. In viral conjunctivitis, lymphocytes and monocytes are predominant. In herpes simplex infections, multinucleated epithelial cells may be seen. In chlamydial infections, a mixed inflammatory cell population (polymorphonuclear leukocytes and lymphocytes) is present, and basophilic intracytoplasmic inclusion bodies may be seen in epithelial cells; the latter finding is common in children and less common in adults. Immunofluorescent techniques provide more sensitivity in identification.[170] Topically applied fluorescein does not appear to have an effect on fluorescent monoclonal antibodies in the diagnosis of chlamydial conjunctivitis. In allergic conjunctivitis, scrapings characteristically reveal eosinophils.[171] They are found in greatest abundance in vernal conjunctivitis. Between attacks of vernal conjunctivitis, mast cells and no eosinophils are seen.

Scrapings from patients with keratoconjunctivitis sicca and superior limbic keratoconjunctivitis reveal keratinized epithelial cells or condensed chromatin patterns when using the Papanicolaou staining technique.[172]

Impression cytology may offer an alternative to the conjunctival scraping method.[173] Immunoelectron microscopy and immunofluorescent techniques may aid in diagnosing viral conjunctivitis.[174,175]

TREATMENT

Most types of mild bacterial conjunctivitis and most types of viral conjunctivitis are usually self-limited, benign conditions that perhaps require no treatment. Topical gentamicin or tobramycin[176] for gram-negative rod infections; and erythromycin, bacitracin, polymixin B/trimethoprim, or neomycin/polymixin for gram-positive infections, given every 2–4 hours for 7–10 days, are usually effective.[26,166] Topical fluoroquinolone solutions should probably be reserved for severe conjunctivitis and keratitis. Often an organism reported to be resistant to a specific antibiotic in the laboratory based on achievable serum levels will respond to that antibiotic clinically because of the high concentrations achievable in the tear film by topical application.

Gonococcal conjunctivitis requires urgent therapy with parenteral ceftriaxone and frequent instillations of normal saline for lavage. A single intramuscular dose of 125 mg of ceftriaxone has resulted in a 100 percent cure rate for gonococcal ophthalmia neonatorum without the need for concomitant topical therapy.[177]

Herpes simplex virus conjunctivitis may be treated with topical trifluridine every 2 hours for 7 days, although this condition is usually benign and self-limited.

Adult inclusion conjunctivitis requires a 1-week course of either doxycycline 100 mg twice daily, or, in pregnant or lactating women, erythromycin or sulfamethoxazole may be substituted orally. Adjunctive topical tetracycline ointment or erythromycin drops may also be prescribed. A similar therapy is effective in treating trachoma, but prevention of reinfection and bacterial superinfection are equally important. Macrolide antibiotics having long serum half-lives and favorable tissue penetration (e.g., azithromycin, clarithromycin, and roxithromycin) are under investigation for a potential role in therapy of trachoma in developing nations.

Since interferon and interferon inducers have been shown to be largely ineffective in therapy of viral conjunctivitis, the search continues for an effective broad-spectrum antiviral preparation for ocular use.

Allergic and immune-mediated conjunctivitis responds best to topical corticosteroids. The long-term use of topical steroids may be associated with glaucoma and cataracts, whereas short-term use may aggravate herpes simplex epithelial keratitis. Nonsteroidal anti-inflammatory agents such as aspirin[178] and cromolyn sodium[179,180] ketorolac tromethamine and others are useful adjunctive measures.

PROPHYLAXIS OF OPHTHALMIA NEONATORUM

There is considerable debate over the relative efficacy of 1% silver nitrate vs. topical antibiotics such as 0.5% erythromycin or 1% tetracyclines. Silver nitrate is still extremely effective, particularly against gonococcal infection, but it has little impact on the increasing incidence of chlamydial infections. Topical erythromycin seems the most effective agent in preventing this infection.[181] In infants born to mothers with known genital chlamydial infection, the routine use of erythromycin ointment will eliminate chlamydial conjunctivitis, but systemic erythromycin estolate is preferred to prevent nasopharyngeal colonization.[182,183]

REFERENCES

1. Allansmith MR, Ostler HB, Butterworth M. Concomitance of bacteria in various areas of the eye. Arch Ophthalmol. 1969;82:37.
2. Lucic H. Bacteriology of the normal conjunctiva. Am J Ophthalmol. 1927:10:829.
3. Khorazo D, Thompson R. The bacterial flora of the normal conjunctiva. Am J Ophthalmol. 1935;18:1114.
4. Gowen GH. Source of staphylococci on normal conjunctiva of human eye. Am J Ophthalmol. 1934;17:36.
5. Locatcher-Khorazo D, Benham RW, Silva-Hunter M. Incidence of fungi from clinically healthy eyes of 508 young people 10–18 years of age and in 1347 adults 19–80 years of age. In: Locatcher-Khorazo D, Seegal BC, eds. Microbiology of the Eye. St. Louis, CV Mosby; 1972:213.
6. Hammeke JC, Ellis PP. Mycotic flora of the conjunctiva. Am J Ophthalmol. 1960;49:1174.
7. Williamson J, Gordon AM, Wood R, et al. Fungal flora of the conjunctival sac in health and disease: Influence of topical and systemic steroids. Br J Ophthalmol. 1968;52:127.
8. Nema HV, Ahuja OP, Bal A, et al. Mycotic flora of the conjunctiva. Am J Ophthalmol. 1966;62:968.
9. Locatcher-Khorazo D, Guiterrez E. Eye infections following cataract extraction, with special reference to the role of Staphylococcus aureus. Am J Ophthalmol. 1956;41:981.
10. Allen HF, Mangiaracine AB. Bacterial endophthalmitis after cataract extraction. II. Incidence in 36,000 Consecutive operations, with special reference to preoperative topical antibiotics. Trans Am Acad Ophthalmol Otolaryngol. 1973;77:581.
11. McMeel JW, Wapner JM. Infections and retina surgery. I. Bacteriologic contamination during scleral buckling surgery. Arch Ophthalmol. 1965;74:42.
12. Howard HJ. Role of the epithelial cell in conjunctival and corneal infections. Am J Ophthalmol. 1924;7:909.
13. Halbert SP, Locatcher-Khorazo D, Sonn-Kazar C, et al. Further studies on the incidence of antibiotic-producing microorganisms of the ocular flora. Arch Ophthalmol. 1957;58:66.
14. Halbert SP, Swick LS. Antibiotic-producing bacteria of the ocular flora. Am J Ophthalmol. 1952;35(5 Pt 2):73.
15. Halbert SP, Swick LS, Sonn C, et al. Ocular antibiotic-producing bacteria in normal eyes and in conjunctivitis. Arch Ophthalmol. 1954;51:7.
16. deToledo AR, Chandler JW. Conjunctivitis of the newborn. Infect Dis Clin North Am. 1992;6:807–13.
17. Trottier S, Stenberg K, VonRosen IA, et al. Haemophilus influenzae causing conjunctivitis in day-care children. Pediatr Infect Dis J. 1991;10:578–84.
18. Roberts MC, Bell TA, Sandstrom KI, et al. Characterization of Haemophilus species isolated from infant conjunctivitis. J Med Microbiol. 1986;21:219–24.
19. Weiss A, Brinser JH, Nazar-Stewart V. Acute conjunctivitis in childhood. J Pediatr. 1993;122:10–14.
20. Brook I. Anaerobic and aerobic bacterial flora of acute conjunctivitis in children. Arch Ophthalmol. 1980;98:833.
21. Gigliotti F, Williams WT, Hayden FG, et al. Etiology of acute conjunctivitis in children. J Pediatr. 1981;98:531.
22. Levin RM, Ticknor W, Jordan C, et al. Etiology of conjunctivitis. J Pediatr. 1981;99:831.
23. Olafsen LD, Storvold, Melby K. A microbiological study of conjunctivitis, with emphasis on Chlamydia trachomatis, in Northern Norway. Acta Ophthalmol. 1986;64:463–70.
24. Leibowitz HM, Pratt MV, Flagstad IJ, et al. Human conjunctivitis. A diagnostic evaluation. Arch Ophthalmol. 1976;94:1747.
25. Brook I, Pettit TH, Martin WJ, et al. Anaerobic and aerobic bacteriology of acute conjunctivitis. Ann Ophthalmol. 1979;11:389.
26. Seal DV, Barrett SP, McGill JI. Aetiology and treatment of acute bacterial infection of the external eye. Br J Ophthalmol. 1982;66:357.
27. Syed MA, Hyndiuk RA. Infectious conjunctivitis. Infect Dis Clin North Am. 1992;6:789–805.
28. Friedlaender MH, Masi RJ, Osumoto M, et al. Ocular microbial flora in immunodeficient patients. Arch Ophthalmol. 1980;98:1211.
29. Shayegani M, Parsons LM, Gibbons WE Jr, et al. Characterization of nontypeable Streptococcus pneumoniae-like organisms isolated from outbreaks of conjunctivitis. J Clin Microbiol. 1982;16:8.
30. King S, Devi SP, Mindroff C, et al. Nosocomial Pseudomonas aeruginosa conjunctivitis in a pediatric hospital. Infection Control Hosp Epidemiol. 1988;9:77–80.
31. Schwartz B, Harrison LH, Motter JS, et al. Investigation of an outbreak of Moraxella conjunctivitis at a Navajo boarding school. Am J Ophthalmol. 1988;107:341–7.
32. Valenton MJ, Abendanio R. Gonorrhea conjunctivitis. Can J Ophthalmol. 1973;8:421.
33. Tight RR. Gonococcal conjunctivitis. J Am Med Assoc. 1982;247:2499.
34. Barquet N, Gasser I, Domingo P, et al. Primary meningococcal conjunctivitis: Report of 21 patients and review. Rev Infect Dis. 1990;12:838–47.
35. Lewis LS, Glauser TA, Joffe E. Gonococcal conjunctivitis in pre-pubertal children. Am J Dis Child. 1990;144:546–8.

36. Au YK, Reynolds MD, Rambin ED, et al. *Neisseria cinerea* acute purulent conjunctivitis. Am J Ophthalmol. 1990;109:96–7.
37. Boralkar AN. Diphtheritic conjunctivitis. A rare case report in Indian literature. Ind J Ophthalmol. 1989;37:49–50.
38. Kowalski RP, Hardwick JC. Incidence of *Moraxella* conjunctivial infection. Am J Ophthalmol. 1986;101:437–40.
39. Flach AJ, Lavoie PE. Episcleritis, conjunctivitis and keratitis as ocular manifestations of Lyme disease. Ophthalmology. 1990;97:973–5.
40. Mombaerts IM, Maudgal P, Knockaert DC. Bilateral follicular conjunctivitis as a manifestation of lyme disease. Am J Ophthalmol. 1991;112:96–7.
41. English CK, Wear DJ, Margileth AM, et al. Cat-scratch disease, isolation and culture of the bacterial agent. JAMA. 1988;259:1347–52.
42. Tappero JW, Mohle-Boetani J, Koehler JE, et al. The epidemiology of bacillary angiomatosis and bacillary peliosis. JAMA. 1993;269:770–5.
43. Koehler JE, Quinn FD, Berger TG, et al. Isolation of *Rochalimae* species from cutaneous and osseous lesions of bacillary angiomatosis. N Engl J Med. 1992;327:1625–31.
44. Wear DJ, Malaty RH, Zimmerman LE, et al. Cat-scratch disease bacilli in the conjunctiva of patients with Parinaud's oculoglandular syndrome. Ophthalmology. 1985;92:1282–7.
45. Saari KM, Laitinen O, Leirisalo M, et al. Ocular inflammation associated with *Yersinia* infection. Am J Ophthalmol. 1980;89:84.
46. Crichton EP. Suppurative conjunctivitis caused by *Yersinia enterocolitica*. Can Med J. 1978;118:22.
47. Gregory JE, Henderson RW, Smith R. Conjunctivitis due to *Haemophilus ducreyi* infection. Br J Vener Dis. 1980;56:414.
48. Eschete ML, Rambin ED, West BC. *Clostridium pseudotetanicum* bacteremia in a patient with *Pasteurella multocida* conjunctivitis. J Clin Microbiol. 1978;8:509.
49. Guerrant RL, Humphries MK, Butler JE, et al. Tickborne oculoglandular tularemia. Case report and review of seasonal and vectorial associations in 106 cases. Arch Intern Med. 1976;136:811.
50. Brook I, Bateman JB, Pettit TH. Meningococcal conjunctivitis. Arch Ophthalmol. 1979;97:890.
51. Cohn H, Mondino BJ, Brown SI, et al. Marginal corneal ulcers with acute beta streptococcal conjunctivitis and chronic dacryocystitis. Am J Ophthalmol. 1979;87:541.
52. Abel R, Shulman J, Boyle GL, et al. *Herellea vaginicola* and ocular infections. Ann Ophthalmol. 1975;7:1485.
53. Smith JA. Ocular *Aeromonas hydrophila*. Am J Ophthalmol. 1980;89:449.
54. Slack JW, Hyndiuk RA, Harris GJ, et al. Blastomycosis of the eyelid and conjunctiva. Ophthalmol Plast Reconstructr Surg. 1992;8:143–149.
55. Arnold R, Whiddin J. Rhinosporidiosis of the conjunctiva. Am J Ophthalmol. 1942;25:1227–30.
56. Bell JA, Rowe WP, Engler JI, et al. Pharyngoconjunctival fever: Epidemiological studies of a recently recognized disease entity. JAMA. 1955;175:1083.
57. Outbreak of pharyngoconjunctival fever at a summer camp. North Carolina, 1991. Infection Control Hosp Epidemiol. 1992;13:499–500.
58. O'Day DM, Guyer B, Hierholzer JC, et al. Clinical and laboratory evaluation of epidemic keratoconjunctivitis due to adenovirus type 8 and 19. Am J Ophthalmol. 1976;81:207.
59. Aoki K, Kato M, Ohtsuka H, et al. Clinical and aetiological study of adenoviral conjunctivitis, with special reference to adenovirus types 4 and 19 infections. Br J Ophthalmol. 1982;66:776.
60. Tullo AB, Higgins PG. An outbreak of adenovirus type 14 conjunctivitis. Br J Ophthalmol. 1980;64:489.
61. D'Angelo LJ, Hierholzer JC, Holman RC, et al. Epidemic keratoconjunctivitis caused by adenovirus type 8: Epidemiologic and laboratory aspects of a large outbreak. Am J Epidemiol. 1981;113:44.
62. Darougar S, Pearce R, Gibson JA, et al. Adenovirus type 21 keratoconjunctivitis. Br J Ophthalmol. 1978;62:836.
63. Taylor JW, Chandler JW, Cooney MK. Conjunctivitis due to adenovirus type 19. J Clin Microbiol. 1978;8:209.
64. Schaap GJP, deJong JC, van Bijsterveld OP, et al. A new intermediate adenovirus type causing conjunctivitis. Arch Ophthalmol. 1979;97:2336.
65. Newland JC, Cooney MK. Characteristics of an adenovirus type 19 conjunctivitis isolate and evidence for a subgroup associated with epidemic conjunctivitis. Infect Immun. 1978;21:303.
66. Beale AJ, Doane F, Ornsby HL. Studies on adenovirus infections of the eye in Toronto. Am J Ophthalmol. 1957;43:26.
67. Boniuk M, Phillips CA, Hines MJ. Adenovirus infections of the conjunctiva. Trans Am Acad Ophthalmol Otolaryngol. 1966;70:1016.
68. Hara J, Ishibashi T, Fujimoto F, et al. Adenovirus type 10 keratoconjunctivitis with increased intraocular pressure. Am J Ophthalmol. 1980;90:481.
69. Kiernan JP, Schanzlin DJ, Leveille AS. Stevens-Johnson syndrome associated with adenovirus conjunctivitis. Am J Ophthalmol. 1981;92:543.
70. Pettit TH, Holland GN. Chronic keratoconjunctivitis associated with ocular adenovirus infection. Am J Ophthalmol. 1979;88:748.
71. Darougar S, Quinlan MP, Gibson JA, et al. Epidemic keratoconjunctivitis and chronic papillary conjunctivitis in London due to adenovirus type 19. Br J Ophthalmol. 1977;61:76.
72. Epidemiology: Acute haemorrhagic conjunctivitis. Br Med J. 1982;284:833.
73. Hoffman M. Acute haemorrhagic conjunctivitis. S Afr Med J. 1982;62:311.
74. Christopher S, Theogaraj S, Godbole S, et al. An epidemic of acute hemorrhagic conjunctivitis due to Coxsackievirus A24. J Infect Dis. 1982;146:16.
75. Langford MP, Stanton GJ, Barber JC, et al. Early-appearing antiviral activity in human tears during a case of picornavirus epidemic conjunctivitis. J Infect Dis. 1979;139:653.
76. Goh KT, Doraisingham S, Yin-Murphy M. An epidemic of acute conjunctivitis caused by enterovirus-70 in Singapore in 1980. Southeast Asian J Trop Med Public Health. 1981;12:473.
77. Hatch MH, Malison MD, Palmer EL. Isolation of enterovirus 70 from patients with acute hemorrhagic conjunctivitis in Key West, Florida. N Engl J Med. 1981;305:1648.
78. Kono R, Miyamura K, Yamazaki S, et al. Seroepidemiologic studies of acute hemorrhagic conjunctivitis virus (enterovirus type 70) in West Africa. II. Studies with human sera collected in West African countries other than Ghana. Am J Epidemiol. 1981;114:274.
79. Bernard KW, Hierholzer JC, Dugan JB, et al. Acute hemorrhagic conjunctivitis in Southeast Asian refugees arriving in the United States: Isolation of enterovirus 70. Am J Trop Med Hyg. 1982;31:541.
80. Minami K, Otatsume S, Mingle JAA, et al. Seroepidemiologic studies of acute hemorrhagic conjunctivitis virus (enterovirus type 70) in West Africa. I. Studies with human sera from Ghana collected eight years after the first outbreak. Am J Epidemiol. 1981;114:267.
81. Kono R, Uchida Y. Acute hemorrhagic conjunctivitis. Ophthalmol Dig. 1977;39:14.
82. Wolken SH. Acute hemorrhagic conjunctivitis. Surv Ophthalmol. 1974;19:71.
83. Wadia NH, Wadia PN, Katrak SM, et al. Neurological manifestations of acute hemorrhagic conjunctivitis. Lancet. 1981;2:528.
84. Thakur LC. Cranial nerve paralyses associated with acute haemorrhagic conjunctivitis. Lancet. 1981;2:584.
85. Katiyar BC, Surendra M, Singh RB, et al. Neurological syndromes after acute epidemic conjunctivitis. Lancet. 1981;2:866.
86. John TJ, Christopher S, Abraham J. Neurological manifestation of acute haemorrhagic conjunctivitis due to enterovirus 70. Lancet. 1981;2:1283.
87. Bybee JD, Phillips CA, Ory EM, et al. Vaccinia of the eyelid. J Am Med Assoc. 1967;199:126.
88. Croffead GW, Harrison SW. Vaccinia conjunctivitis. Am J Ophthalmol. 1962;53:531.
89. Denis J, Chauvaud D, Savoldelli M, et al. Fine structure of palpebral molluscum contagiosum and its secondary conjunctival lesions. Graefes Arch Ophthalmol. 1978;208:207.
90. North RD. Presumptive viral keratoconjunctivitis, mononucleosis, and the oncogenic viruses. Int Ophthalmol Clin. 1975;15:211.
91. Darougar S, Hunter PA, Viswalingham M, et al. Acute follicular conjunctivitis and keratoconjunctivitis due to herpes simplex virus in London. Br J Ophthalmol. 1978;62:843.
92. Jones BR. The management of ocular herpes. Trans Ophthalmol Soc UK. 1959;79:425.
93. Stucchi CA, Bianchi G. Complications oculaires graves postvaricelleuses chez l'adulte. Ophthalmologica. 1970;161:108.
94. Carter RL, Penman HG. Infectious Mononucleosis. Oxford: Blackwell Scientific Publications; 1969.
95. Wilhelmus KR. Ocular involvement in infectious mononucleosis. Am J Ophthalmol. 1981;91:117.
96. McDonnell JM, McDonnell PK, Green WR, et al. Demonstration of Papillomavirus capsid antigen in human conjunctival neoplasia. Arch Ophthalmol. 1986;104:1801.
97. Roy FH, Hiatt RL, Korones SB, et al. Ocular manifestations of congenital rubella syndrome. Arch Ophthalmol. 1966;75:601.
98. Hara J, Fujimoto F, Ishibashi T, et al. Ocular manifestations of the 1976 rubella epidemic in Japan. Am J Ophthalmol. 1979;87:642.
99. Holland WW. A clinical study of influenza in the Royal Air Force. Lancet. 1957;2:840.
100. Jordan WS Jr, Denny FW Jr, Badger GF, et al. A study of illness in a group of Cleveland families. Am J Hyg. 1958;68:190.
101. Nommensen FE, Dekkers NWHM. Detection of measles antigen in conjunctival epithelial lesions staining by lissamine green during measles virus infection. J Med Virol. 1981;7:157.
102. Deckard PS, Bergstrom TJ. Rubeola keratitis. Ophthalmol. 1981;88:810.
103. Riffenburgh RS. Ocular manifestations of mumps. Arch Ophthalmol. 1961;66:739.
104. Lippman O. Human conjunctivitis due to the Newcastle-disease virus of fowls. Am J Ophthalmol. 1952;35:1021.
105. Spalton DJ, Palmer S, Logan LC. Echo 11 conjunctivitis. Br J Ophthalmol. 1980;64:487.
106. Kasova V, John J, Koza J, et al. Poliovirus type 3 keratoconjunctivitis. J Infect Dis. 1980;42:292.
107. Meisler DM, Bosworth DE, Krachmer JH. Ocular infectious mononucleosis manifested as Parinaud's oculoglandular syndrome. Am J Ophthalmol. 1981;92:722.
108. Loftus MJ, Sweeney G, Goldberg MH. Parinaud oculoglandular syndrome and cat-scratch fever. J Oral Surg. 1980;38:218.
109. Schacter J, Dawson CR. Human Chlamydial Infections. Littleton, MA: PSG Publishing; 1978.
110. Schacter J. Chlamydial ocular infection. J Antimicrob Chemother. 1981;8:350.
111. Schacter J. Chlamydial infections. N Engl J Med. 1978;298:428.
112. Holmes KK. The *Chlamydia* epidemic. J Am Med Assoc. 1981;245:1718.
113. Stenson S. Adult inclusion conjunctivitis. Clinical characteristics and corneal changes. Arch Ophthalmol. 1981;99:605.
114. Macnie JP. Ocular lymphogranuloma venereum. Arch Ophthalmol. 1941;25:255.
115. Buus DR, Pflugfelder SC, Schachter J, et al. Lymphogranuloma venereum conjunctivitis with a marginal corneal perforation. Ophthalmology. 1988;95:799–802.

116. Nandy A, Addy M, Chowdhury AB. Leishmanial blepharoconjunctivitis. Trop Geog Med. 1991;43:303–6.
117. Friedberg TN, Stenson SM, Orenstein JM, et al. Microsporidian keratoconjunctivitis in acquired immunodeficiency syndrome. Arch Ophthalmol. 1990; 108:504–8.
118. Green ST, Scott V, McMenamin J, et al. Cryptosporidial enteritis complicated by conjunctivitis. Ann Rheum Dis. 1991;50:526.
119. Wong D. External ophthalmomyiasis caused by the sheep bot *Oestrus ovis*. Br J Ophthalmol. 1982;66:786.
120. Ashton N, Cook C. Allergic granulomatous nodules of the eyelid and conjunctiva. The XXXV Edward Jackson Memorial Lecture. Am J Ophthalmol. 1979;87:1.
121. Mimori T, Hirai H, Kifune T, et al. *Philophthalmus sp. (trematoda)* in a human eye. Am J Trop Med Hyg. 1982;31:859.
122. Gutierrez Y, Grossniklaus HE, Annabelle WL. Human conjunctivitis caused by the bird parasite *Philophthalmus*. Am J Ophthalmol. 1987;104:417–9.
123. Pierce JM, Ward ME, Seal DV. Ophthalmia neonatorum in the 1980's: Incidence, aetiology and treatment. Br J Ophthalmol. 1982;66:728.
124. Schachter J, Holt J, Goodner E, et al. Prospective study of chlamydial infection in neonates. Lancet. 1979;2:377.
125. Heggie AD, Lumicao GG, Stuart LA, et al. *Chlamydia trachomatis* infection in mothers and infants. A prospective study. Am J Dis Child. 1981;135:507.
126. Persson K, Ronnerstam R, Svanberg L, et al. Maternal and infantile infection with chlamydia in a swedish population. Acta Paediatr Scand. 1981;70:101.
127. Schachter J, Lum L, Goodnig CA, et al. Pneumonitis following inclusion blennorrhea. J Pediatr. 1975;87:779.
128. Beem MO, Saxon EM. Respiratory-tract colonization and a distinctive pneumonia syndrome in infants infected with *Chlamydia trachomatis*. N Engl J Med. 1977;296:306.
129. Givner LB, Rennels MB, Woodward CL, et al. Chlamydia trachomatis infection in infant delivered by cesarean section. Pediatrics. 1981;68:420.
130. Stenson S, Newman R, Fedukowicz H. Conjunctivitis in the newborn: Observations on incidence, cause, and prophylaxis. Ann Ophthalmol. 1981;13: 329.
131. Cohen KL, McCarthy LR. *Haemophilus influenzae* ophthalmia neonatorum. Arch Ophthalmol. 1980;98:1214.
132. Cole GF, Davies DP, Austin DJ. *Pseudomonas* ophthalmia neonatorum: A cause of blindness. Br Med J. 1980;281:440.
133. Fox KR, Golomb HS. Staphylococcal ophthalmia neonatorum and the staphylococcal scalded skin syndrome. Am J Ophthalmol. 1979;88:1052.
134. Overton ME, Heath JD, Stapleton FB. Conjunctivitis and ethmoiditis due to *Shigella flexneri* in an infant. Clin Pediatr (Phila). 1981;20:231.
135. Garvey RJP, Reed TAG. Ophthalmia neonatorum due to *Branhamella (Neisseria) catarrhalis*. Case reports. Br J Vener Dis. 1981;57:346.
136. Spark RP, Dahlberg PW, LaBelle JW. Pseudogonococcal ophthalmia neonatorum. *Branhamella (Neisseria) catarrhalis* conjunctivitis. Am J Clin Pathol. 1979;72:471.
137. Leu YA, Simms DH, Ubriani R, et al. Ophthalmia neonatorum caused by penicillin-resistant *Branhamella catarrhalis*. NY State J Med. 1981;81:1775.
138. Pang R, Teh LB, Rajan VS. Gonococcal ophthalmia neonatorum caused by beta-lactamase–producing *Neisseria gonorrhoeae*. Br Med J. 1979;280:380.
139. Dunlop EMC, Rodin P, Seth AD, et al. Ophthalmia neonatorum due to beta-lactamase–producing gonococci. Br Med J. 1980;281:483.
140. Podgore JK, Holmes KK. Ocular gonococcal infection with minimal or no inflammatory response. J Am Med Assoc. 1981;246:242.
141. Stenson S. Superior limbic keratoconjunctivitis associated with soft contact lens wear. Arch Ophthalmol. 1983;101:402.
142. Allansmith MR, Baird RS, Greiner JV. Vernal conjunctivitis and contact lens-associated giant papillary conjunctivitis compared and contrasted. Am J Ophthalmol. 1979;87:544.
143. Binder PS, Rasmussen RM, Gordon M. Keratoconjunctivitis and soft contact lens solutions. Arch Ophthalmol. 1981;99:87.
144. Wright P, Mackie I. Preservative-related problems in soft contact lens wearers. Trans Ophthalmol Soc UK. 1982;102:3.
145. Srinivasan RB, Jakobiet FA, Iwamoto T, et al. Giant papillary conjunctivitis with ocular prostheses. Arch Ophthalmol. 1979;97:892.
146. Meisler DM, Krachmer JH, Goeken JA. An immunopathologic study of giant papillary conjunctivitis associated with an ocular prosthesis. Am J Ophthalmol. 1981;92:368.
147. Baldone JA, Hankin JS, Zimmerman TJ. Allergic conjunctivitis associated with timolol therapy in an adult. Ann Ophthalmol. 1982;14:364.
148. Vizel M, Oster MW. Ocular side effects of cancer chemotherapy. Cancer. 1982;49:1999.
149. Ostler HB. Acute chemotic reaction to cromolyn. Arch Ophthalmol. 1982; 100:412.
150. Umez-Eronini EM. Conjunctivitis due to ketoprofen. Lancet. 1978;2:737.
151. Flach AJ, Peterson JS, Mathias CGT. Photosensitivity to topically applied sulfisoxazole ointment. Evidence for a phototoxic reaction. Arch Ophthalmol. 1982;100:1286.
152. Wilson FM II. Adverse external ocular effects of topical ophthalmic medications. Surv. Ophthalmol. 1979;24:57.
153. Jacobson JH. Blepharitis and secondary conjunctivitis. Am J Ophthalmol. 1980;89:609.
154. Neumann E, Gutman MJ, Blumenkrantz N, et al. A review of 400 cases of vernal conjunctivitis. Am J Ophthalmol. 1959;47:166.
155. Parker WT, Binder PS. Gentian violet keratoconjunctivitis. Am J Ophthalmol. 1979;87:340.
156. Biedner BZ, Sachs U, Witztum A. *Euphorbia paplus* latex keratoconjunctivitis. Ann Ophthalmol. 1981;13:739.
157. Backman HA. The effects of PUVA on the eye. Am J Optom Physiol Opt. 1982;59:86.
158. Halperin W, Altman R, Black K, et al. Conjunctivitis and skin erythema. Outbreak caused by a damaged high-intensity lamp. JAMA. 1978;240:1980.
159. Rose RC, Parker RL. Erythema and conjunctivitis. Outbreak caused by inadvertent exposure to ultraviolet light. JAMA. 1979;242:1155.
160. Philip RN. Comstock GW, Shelton JH. Phlyctenular keratoconjunctivitis among eskimos in southern Alaska: I. Epidemiologic characteristics. Am Rev Respir Dis. 1965;91:171.
161. Ostler HB, Lanier JD. Phlyctenular keratoconjunctivitis with special reference to the staphylococcal type. Trans Pacific Coast Otoophthalmol Soc Annu Meet. 1974;55:237.
162. Mondino BJ, Brown SI, Lempert S, et al. The acute manifestations of ocular cicatricial pemphigoid: Diagnosis and treatment. Ophthalmology. 1979;86: 543.
163. Hirst LW, Jabs DA, Tutschka PJ, et al. The eye in bone marrow transplantation. I. Clinical study. Arch Ophthalmol. 1983;101:580.
164. Perlman E, McMahon RT. Sebaceous gland carcinoma of the eyelid. Am J Ophthalmol. 1978;86:699.
165. Stenson S, Newman R, Fedukowicz H. Laboratory studies in acute conjunctivitis. Arch Ophthalmol. 1982;100:1275.
166. Leibowitz HM, Pratt MV, Flagstad IJ, et al. Human conjunctivitis. II. treatment. Arch Ophthalmol. 1976;94:1752.
167. Jones DB, Liesegang TJ, Robinson NM. Laboratory diagnosis of ocular infections. Cumitech. 1980;13:1.
168. Darougar S, Treharne JD, Minassian D, et al. Rapid serological test for diagnosis of chlamydial ocular infections. Br J Ophthalmol. 1978;62:503.
169. Forstot SL, Forstot JZ, Peebles CL, et al. Serologic studies in patients with keratoconjunctivitis sicca. Arch Ophthalmol. 1981;99:888.
170. Sheppard JD, Kowalski RP, Meyer MP, et al. Immunodiagnosis of adult chlamydial conjunctivitis. Ophthalmology. 1988;95:434–442.
171. Abelson MB, Madiwale N, Weston JH. Conjunctival eosinophils in allergic ocular disease. Arch Ophthalmol. 1983;101:555.
172. Wander AH, Masukawa T. Unusual appearance of condensed chromatin in conjunctival cells in superior limbic keratoconjunctivitis. Lancet. 1981;2:42.
173. Hershenfeld S, Kazdan JJ, Mancer K, et al. Impression cytology in conjunctivitis. Can J Ophthalmol. 1981;16:76.
174. Rodrigues MR, Leennette DA, Arentsen JJ, et al. Methods for rapid detection of human ocular viral infections. Ophthalmology. 1979;86:452.
175. Van Rij G, Klepper L, Peperkamp E, et al. Immune electron microscopy and a cultural test in the diagnosis of adenovirus ocular infection. Br J Ophthalmol. 1982;66:317.
176. Liebowitz HM, Hyndiuk RA, Smolin GR, et al. Tobramycin in external eye disease. A double-masked study vs. Gentamicin. Curr Eye Res. 1981;1:259.
177. Laga M, Naamara W, Brunham RC, et al. Single-dose therapy of gonococcal ophthalmia neonatorum with ceftriaxone. N Engl J Med. 1986;315:1382.
178. Abelson MB, Butrus SI, Weston JH. Aspirin therapy in vernal conjunctivitis. Am J Ophthalmol. 1983;95:502.
179. Foster CS, Duncan J. Randomized clinical trial of topically administered cromolyn sodium for vernal conjunctivitis. Am J Ophthalmol. 1980;90:175.
180. Friday GA, Biglan AW, Hiles DA, et al. Treatment of ragweed allergic conjunctivitis with cromolyn sodium 4% ophthalmic solution. Am J Ophthalmol. 1983;95:169.
181. Hammerschlag MR, Chandler JW, Alexander ER, et al. Erythromycin ointment for ocular prophylaxis of neonatal chlamydial infection. JAMA. 1980; 244:2291.
182. Patamasucon P, Rettig PJ, Faust KL, et al. Oral versus topical erythromycin therapies for chlamydial conjunctivitis. Am J Dis Child. 1982;136:817.
183. Rees E, Tait A, Hobson D, et al. Persistence of chlamydial infection after treatment for neonatal conjunctivitis. Arch Dis Child. 1981;56:193.

93. KERATITIS

TERRENCE P. O'BRIEN
W. RICHARD GREEN

Keratitis, or inflammation of the cornea, may be produced by infectious organisms or by noninfectious stimuli. Microbial keratitis is a common, potentially site-threatening ocular infection that may be caused by bacteria, fungi, viruses, or parasites. The challenge for the clinician is to distinguish microbial keratitis from other noninfectious inflammatory conditions of the cornea resulting from trauma, hypersensitivity, and other immune-mediated reactions. There are no absolutely specific clinical signs that confirm infection, yet the clinician should assess and define distinctive corneal signs based on the status of the epithelium (intact or ulcerated), type of stromal inflammation (nonsuppurative or suppurative), and site of stromal inflammation (focal, diffuse, multifocal, or marginal). If infection is considered likely or possible, laboratory investigations are performed, in all cases utilizing appropriate special stains and media, depending on which organisms are suspected. Based on clinical suspicion, the results of initial laboratory studies and a knowledge of potentially etiologic organisms, appropriate antimicrobial therapy is initiated. Initial therapy is subsequently modified based on the clinical response, results of in vitro susceptibility determination, and tolerance of the antimicrobial agents. With careful clinical monitoring, antimicrobial therapy is then terminated and any residual structural alterations corrected. With advanced corneal infection or severe host-inflammatory response, permanent structural alterations such as thinning, perforation, or scleral extension can occur and require surgical intervention.

Since the corneal epithelium and conjunctival epithelium are continuous, forming the ocular surface, agents causing conjunctival disease may also affect the cornea. Before most infectious agents and some mediators of the immune reaction can invade the corneal stroma, a defect in the ocular surface must usually be present. This defect can be caused by various kinds of external trauma, including trauma from contact lenses, trichiasis, entropion, or abnormal lid margins. Surface defects may also result from chronic problems in severe dry eyes, exposure, or neurogenic corneal anesthesia. Systemic diseases such as diabetes mellitus or immunodeficiency states decrease the corneal host resistance when the ocular surface has been broached by one of the above mechanisms.

Any corneal inflammation should be considered potentially sight threatening and require prompt management. Corneal perforation and loss of the eye can occur rapidly after a severe inflammatory episode or infection with virulent organisms. Even minor corneal ulcerations occurring in the central visual axis can disrupt visual acuity.

ETIOLOGIC AGENTS

The various agents known to cause keratitis are listed in Table 1. The organisms most commonly identified in microbial keratitis vary geographically depending on the climate, soil, and individual patient factors. Under the appropriate opportunistic conditions, any organism can cause keratitis.

CLINICAL MANIFESTATIONS

Because of the rich innervation of the cornea, the most common symptom of inflammatory lesions of the cornea is pain. The movement of the eyelids over the ulcerated corneal epithelium increases the pain. Examination of patients with microbial keratitis is greatly facilitated by first instilling a drop of topical anesthetic.

Unlike conjunctival infections, keratitis is usually accompanied by a variable decrease in vision. Discharge, which is a distinctive feature of conjunctivitis, is generally absent in patients with keratitis unless a purulent bacterial keratitis is present. Reflex tearing, photophobia, and blepharospasm are common.

Since the cornea is normally a clear, avascular tissue, the clinical appearance of an inflammatory reaction is different from that observed in other tissues. After a noxious agent enters the cornea, inflammatory cells migrate into the cornea from dilated limbal vessels and from the preocular tear film. An early sign of keratitis is therefore a subtle loss of corneal transparency, localized or generalized and frequently a focal epithelial defect that is best observed with a Cobalt blue light after instillation of fluorescein using a sterile strip. Signs distinctive for microbial keratitis include an ulceration of the epithelium with suppurative stromal inflammation that is either focal or diffuse. Multifocal suppurative keratitis is suggestive of mixed infection (polymicrobial keratitis). Microbial keratitis occasionally may present

TABLE 1. Some Infectious Agents That Cause Keratitis

Bacteria
  Gram-postive cocci
    Staphylococcus aureus
    Staphylococcus epidermidis
    Streptococcus pneumoniae
    Streptococci of the viridans group
    Streptococcus pyogenes (group A)
    Enterococcus (Streptococcus) faecalis
    Peptostreptococcus spp.
  Gram-negative bacilli
    Pseudomonas aeruginosa, P. mallei, P. fluorescens, P. pseudomallei, P. stutzeri
    Comamonas (Pseudomonas) acidovorans
    Proteus mirabilis
    Morganella moragnii
    Klebsiella pneumoniae
    Serratia marcescens
    Escherichia coli
    Aeromonas hydrophila
    Cat-scratch bacillus
  Gram-negative coccobacilli
    Moraxella lacunata, M. nonliquefaciens
    Acinetobacter calcoaceticus
    Pasteurella multocida
    Neisseria gonorrhoeae
    Moraxella (Branhamella) catarrhalis
  Gram-positive bacilli
    Bacillus coagulans, B. laterosporus, B. cereus, B. licheniformis, B. brevis
    Corynebacterium diphtheriae
    Clostridium perfringens, C. tetani
  Spirochetes
    Treponema pallidum
    Borrelia burgdorferi
  Mycobacteria
    Mycobacterium tuberculosis, M. fortuitum, M. chelonae, M. gordonae, M. avium-intracellulare
  Actinomycetes
    Nocardia spp.
Chlamydia
  Chlamydia trachomatis
Viruses
  Herpes simplex virus
  Adenovirus
  Varicella-zoster virus
  Epstein-Barr virus
  Poxviruses (vaccinia, molluscum contagiosum)
  Rubeola (measles)
Fungi
  Acremonium spp.
  Fusarium spp.
  Bipolaris spp.
  Candida spp.
  Aspergillus spp.
  Pseudallescheria boydii
  Penicillium spp.
  Paecilomyces spp.
  Neurospora spp.
  Phialophora spp.
  Curvularia spp.
Parasites
  Onchocerca volvulus
  Acanthamoeba polyphaga, A. castellani
  Leishmania brasiliensis
  Trypanosoma spp.
  Microsporidia
    Nosema spp.
    Encephalitozoon spp.

with an intact epithelium and nonsuppurative multifocal stromal inflammation. Perhaps the most important result of the inflammatory reaction with invasion by microbial pathogens is loss of corneal substance (keratolysis), which may rapidly lead to perforation if untreated or sometimes to a corneal scar (leukoma) even if successful therapy is promptly initiated.

In severe keratitis, there is frequently an invasion of the cornea by blood vessels (neovascularization). After the inflammation subsides, residual microscopic empty blood channels (ghost vessels) may be the only evidence of a previous inflammatory condition.

Some degree of corneal edema accompanies almost all inflammatory conditions of the cornea, leading to a loss of corneal transparency and a resultant decrease in vision. Edema fluid

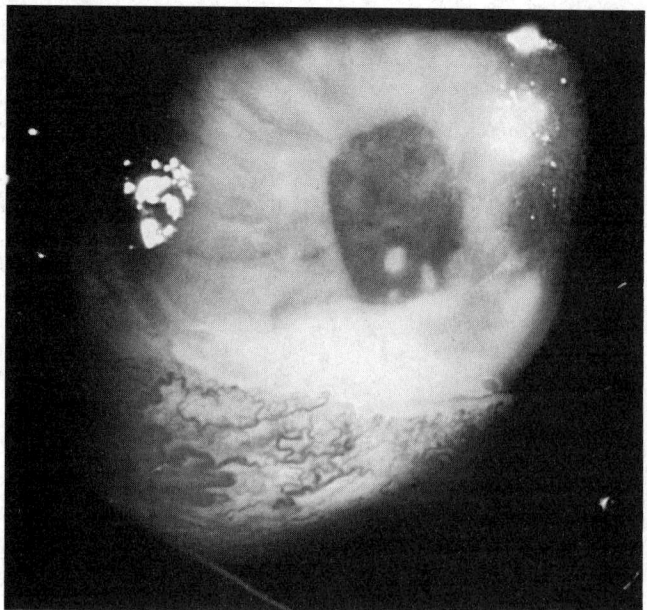

FIG. 1. Hypopyon, corneal clouding, and conjunctival hyperemia due to *Capnocytophaga canimosus* keratitis.

may also accumulate under the corneal epithelium and form bullae that cause severe "foreign body" pain and rupture and predispose to microbial invasion.

An associated intraocular inflammation is common. Early inflammatory changes may only be discernible by careful slit-lamp biomicroscopic examination (flare and cells). Severe inflammation may lead to layering of fibrin and white blood cells in the inferior portion of the anterior chamber (hypopyon) by gravity (Fig. 1). There may also be hyphema, extensive synechiae, and glaucoma. The aqueous and vitreous humors remain sterile in most microbial keratitis until a late stage when infective endophthalmitis may occur.

BACTERIAL KERATITIS

Bacterial keratitis accounts for approximately 65–90 percent of all microbial corneal infections.[1-4] Four principle groups of bacterial pathogens responsible for the majority of infective keratitis include the micrococcaceae (*Staphylococcus, Micrococcus*), the *Streptococcus* species, the *Pseudomonas* species, and the Enterobacteriaceae (*Citrobacter, Klebsiella, Enterobacter, Serratia, Proteus*). Eighty-seven percent of cases of bacterial keratitis are caused by organisms in these four groups.[1] The prevalence of organisms incriminated in bacterial keratitis have shifted somewhat over the past several decades. Previously, pneumococci were the most commonly isolated organisms from corneal infections. Opportunistic commensals are now frequently isolated, and in some series *Pseudomonas* is the most common bacterial isolate. In addition, anaerobes and protozoa have been reported with increasing frequency. Any apparent changes that have occurred result from improved isolation techniques from the cornea, an increase in the population of patients who are systemically immunosuppressed, an increase in topical steroid administration, and an increase in the use of soft contact lenses,[4-6] especially for extended wear.[7,8] There have been occasional cases of bacterial keratitis as a result of organ-cultured and MK medium–stored corneal buttons used for corneal transplantation.[9]

A geographic variation in causes of microbial keratitis has also been noted. *Pneumococcus (Streptococcus pneumoniae)* was the predominant cause of microbial keratitis in the past, often in association with chronic dacryocystitis. In most large series, gram-positive organisms continue to be the predominant cause of microbial keratitis. *Staphylococcus aureus* is now the most commonly isolated agent in microbial keratitis, especially in the Northern and Northeastern United States and Canada. In a reported series from New York City,[2] *Staph. aureus* was the most common organism, followed by *Moraxella, P. aeruginosa,* and *Strep. pneumoniae.* In London,[10] the most common organisms are *Staph. aureus, Strep. pneumoniae, Pseudomonas,* and *Moraxella.* Streptococcal species are still commonly isolated causative organisms in eastern and western United States.

Pseudomonas aeruginosa is an increasingly frequent organism encountered in infectious keratitis, especially among contact lens wearers. *P. aeruginosa* is more common in the South than *Staph. aureus.*[3,11] *Pseudomonas* and *Streptococcus* are the main pathogens in previously healthy eyes in the southern United States. In a series from South Florida, there were 238 bacterial corneal infections among 663 patients with suspected microbial keratitis.[3] *Pseudomonas aeruginosa* was the single most common organism (31 percent) and was frequently observed in association with hard or soft contact lens wear. *Staphylococcus aureus* and *Strep. pneumoniae* combined caused 22 percent of the total bacterial keratitis cases.

The pathogenesis of bacterial keratitis involves several routes of inoculation. Direct penetration of intact corneal epithelium occurs only by organisms releasing special toxins, enzymes, and other virulent factors (*Neisseria gonorrhoeae, N. meningitidis, Corynebacterium diphtheriae, Listeria,* and *Shigella* spp.). More commonly any organism may be introduced through a corneal epithelial defect or a gap in epithelial bridges occurring by mechanical thermal, or chemical injury or by epithelial erosion secondary to ocular conditions, including eyelid abnormalities, tear dysfunction states, corneal anesthesia, or decreased adherence of the corneal epithelium as in bullous keratopathy or epithelial basement membrane and other dystrophies. The inoculation of organisms into the corneal stroma may occur via obvious exogenous penetrating trauma (cat-scratch bacillus)[12] or more often via inapparent minor corneal epithelial abrasions such as from contaminated mascara.[13,14]

Strains of staphylococci causing extensive corneal ulcerations are the same ones that are found as inhabitants in other noninfected parts of the body.[15,16] Marginal keratitis with or without corneal epithelial ulceration found in association with conjunctival cultures that are positive for staphylococci have been thought to be due to toxins or hypersensitivity reactions to the α-riboteichoic acid moieties in these bacterial cell walls. *Staphylococcus epidermidis* and streptococci can cause corneal ulceration, usually in immunocompromised hosts and occasionally in association with chronic dacryocystitis,[17] in which a peripheral corneal ulcer may occur that is similar in appearance of the staphylococcal hypersensitivity ulcer described above.[18] A toxic factor (pneumolysin) having exopeptidase activity has been implicated in the pathogenesis of corneal ulceration caused by *Strep. pneumoniae.*[19]

Pseudomonas aeruginosa is recognized for its particular swift suppurative course to perforation because of its proteolytic enzyme production,[20-23] which degrades the corneal stroma. Endotoxin may produce characteristic inflammatory rings consisting of polymorphonuclear leukocytes within the corneal stroma that are attracted through activation of the alternative complement pathway.[24,25] Similar stromal ring infiltrates may be observed in fungal, viral, and Acanthamoeba keratitis. Host-derived enzymes also contribute in the pathogenesis of *Pseudomonas* corneal infection.[26] Following invasion, there is stimulation release of chemotactic substances that initiate polymorphonuclear leukocyte migration from the limbus.[27] Polymorphonuclear leukocytes are important in host defenses, including phagocytosis, but are also implicated in the destruction of the corneal collagen matrix in ground substance. The extent of visual impairment is directly related to severity of inflammatory cell infiltration, phagocytic activity, cell death, release of proteolytic enzymes, and damage to corneal endothelium.

In comatose patients with corneal exposure and tracheostomies colonized by *P. aeruginosa*, the danger of corneal infection is greatly increased.[28] Unusual extension of the keratitis into the sclera has been reported.[29,30] Other related species such as *Comamonas (Pseudomonas) acidovorans* and *P. stutzeri* have caused bacterial keratitis with less malignant course.[31] Infectious keratitis due to *Morganella morganii* may be clinically indistinguishable from *Pseudomonas* ulcerative keratitis. *Serratia marcescens* corneal ulcerations have been associated with contact lens wear[32] and contaminated eyedrops.[33] *Moraxella* keratitis has been described in debilitated alcoholic patients in whom the organism is also frequently a nasopharyngeal commensual[34] and in otherwise well patients when chronic ocular surface disease is present.[35] The infrequency of isolation of this bacteria may perhaps be explained by its fastidious nature and culture and the inhibitory topical anesthetic agent instilled prior to obtaining corneal scrapings for microbial cultures.

Neisseria gonorrhoeae may cause a keratitis during an episode of untreated or inadequately treated conjunctivitis. It is one of the few organisms that can penetrate an intact corneal epithelium. *Neisseria* spp. can produce marked conjunctival chemosis and infiltration of the conjunctiva with polymorphonuclear neutrophils. The edematous, infiltrated conjunctiva may drape over the peripheral cornea with resultant exposure to lytic enzymes capable of producing epithelial ulceration. It is essential that the presence of the gonococcus be verified by culture because *Acinetobacter*, which is morphologically identical to the gonococcus, can also cause corneal perforation.

Gram-positive aerobic bacilli are widespread in nature and are of low virulence. They produce infections of the cornea when host resistance is lowered.[36] *Bacillus cereus* is a large, aerobic, gram-positive rod that may produce an extremely virulent course following introduction after foreign body injury.[37] *Corynebacterium diphtheriae* may also penetrate intact corneal epithelium to produce keratitis.[38] Studies of the cell wall of the organism indicate that *Actinomyces* and *Nocardia* more closely resemble bacteria than fungi, despite their filamentous character. These bacteria are gram positive and replicate by fragmentation of filaments. *Nocardia* is weakly acid fast. Corneal infections by these organisms are infrequent.

Primary tuberculous keratitis is now extremely rare. Nontubeculous mycobacteria *(Mycobacterium fortuitum* and *M. chelonae)* are known to cause keratitis, especially after injury with a foreign body or following office surgical procedures.[39–43] The nontuberculous mycobacteria cause chronic indolent corneal ulcerations with frequent resistance to conventional antituberculous medications. Other nontuberculous mycobacterial species including *M. gordonae* and *M. avium-intracellulare* are also capable of causing ulcerative keratitis.

The incidence of ocular lesions of leprosy varies from about 15 percent of patients with tuberculoid leprosy to about 100 percent of the patients with long-standing lepromatous leprosy.[44–46]

Organisms less frequently causing bacterial keratitis include *Azotobacter*,[47] *Moraxella catarrhalis*,[48] *Aeromonas hydrophilia*,[49] *Pasteurella multocida*,[50] *Clostridium perfringens*,[51] *Bacillus licheniformis*,[52] *B. thuringiensis*,[53] and anaerobic streptococci including *Peptostreptococcus* and *Peptococcus*.[54] Other nonsporaforming anaerobic bacteria causing keratitis include *Propionibacterium* spp. Polymicrobial keratitis was seen in about 78 percent of one series of bacterial and fungal keratitis and is associated with the use of therapeutic soft "bandage" contact lenses in diseased corneas.

FUNGAL KERATITIS

In one series of culture-positive ulcerative keratitis,[3] approximately 35 percent were of fungal origin, whereas another study found 20 percent to have a fungal etiology.[1] Over 70 genera of filamentous fungi and yeast forms have been identified in fungal keratitis.[3,55] The septate filamentous fungi are the most common causes of fungal keratitis, with a variable geographic distribution generally occurring in the southern and southwestern United States. *Fusarium solani* is the most common etiologic organism and has been isolated in up to 65 percent of cases.[56–58] *Aspergillus*,[59] *Curvularia*, *Paecilomyces*, *Phialophora*, *Blastomyces*, *Sporothrix*, *Exophiala*, *Pseudallescheria*, an many fungi can cause keratitis. Nonseptate filamentous fungi such as Mucoraceae rarely are responsible. The most common predisposing factor to fungal keratitis with filamentous organisms is corneal injury, usually by tree branches or vegetative material. Filamentous fungi can infect the cornea of patients with soft contact lenses, especially when the lens is used therapeutically as a "bandage" for a diseased cornea.

Distinctive signs of fungal keratitis in early nonsevere infection include either an intact or an ulcerated epithelium with nonsuppurative stromal inflammation, often with fine feathery infiltrates. Inflammation early in the course may be minimal and either focal or multifocal with "satellite" stromal infiltrates. In advanced severe fungal keratitis, the epithelium may be ulcerated with diffuse suppurative stromal inflammation.

Candida and other yeasts are more commonly isolated in cooler climates from patients with previous existent disease. Risk factors for *Candida* keratitis include protracted epithelial ulceration, topical corticosteroid therapy, keratoplasty treated with topical corticosteroids, and therapeutic soft contact lens wear. In patients with local ocular surface abnormalities such as dry eyes, exposure keratitis, and previous herpes simplex keratitis or with systemic immunosuppression, infection with *Candida* is more common. In contrast to filamentous keratitis, *Candida* keratitis typically causes a small oval ulceration of the corneal epithelium with an expanding, discrete, sharply demarcated, dense yellow-white stromal suppuration lacking the delicate features observed with filamentous organisms. Indeed, *Candida* keratitis may closely mimic a gram-positive bacterial keratitis, such as that caused by *Staph. aureus* or *Strep. pneumoniae*. The inflammatory reaction in *Candida* keratitis is somewhat less marked than in bacterial keratitis, often sparing the periphery of the cornea and less often associated with hypopyon.

Nocardia[60] and *Corynebacterium (Bacterionema) matruchotii*[61] are rare causes of infective keratitis, and the lesions are indistinguishable from those of a fungal origin. Rare causes of fungal keratitis include *Pullularia*,[62] *Helminthosporium*,[63] *Rhodotorula*,[64] *Scedosporium*,[65] *Phialophora bubakii*,[66] and *Tritirachium roseum*.[67] Because these agents can also be isolated from the environment, it is often difficult to be sure of their role when isolated from an infected cornea.

PARASITIC KERATITIS

Parasitic keratitis is a major cause of blindness in some tropical areas. Sclerosing keratitis and stromal opacification occur from invasion of the corneal stroma by microfilariae of *Onchocerca volvulus*.[68–70] Black fly vectors are found in Africa and in scattered areas of Central and South America. The gravid female fly deposits her eggs on rocks and vegetation in rivers and streams, hence the common term *river blindness*. Onchocerciasis is one of the leading causes of blindness worldwide.[71] The ocular lesions in onchocerciasis are the direct result of microfilarial invasion of the anterior segment of the eye. Excessive tearing, conjunctival hyperemia, and photophobia are early symptoms of infection. Living microfilaria are well tolerated by the host and are often seen floating in the anterior chamber or traversing slowly through the cornea near Bowman's layer.[72] Once the intracorneal microfilariae dies, a severe inflammatory reaction ensues.[73] Sclerosing keratitis is the blinding complication that usually occurs following a high-intensity infection of several years duration.

Leishmania may produce a keratitis quite similar to that observed in onchocerciasis.[74] *Leishmania* are obligate intracellular parasites transmitted by the bites of infected sand flies. Depending on the parasite species, human infection can result in cutaneous, mucocutaneous, or visceral disease. Infection of the eyelids and conjunctiva may result in edema, ulceration, and scarring. Corneal involvement begins with superficial phlyctenules that may progress to abscess formation and ultimately result in corneal perforation.

Acanthamoeba is now a worldwide infectious agent being recognized more frequently as the cause of painful, recalcitrant keratitis, frequently leading to loss of vision or even loss of the eye.[75] These free-living amoebae may be isolated from fresh water, well water, and brackish water, soil, and even air. There many different species, of which at least seven have been associated with human keratitis. *Acanthamoeba* exist in nature and tissue in two forms. The trophozoite form is a uninucleated, motile stage that reproduces by conventional mitosis. The cystic form is double walled with a wrinkled outer wall (ectocyst) and a stellate, polygonal inner wall (endocyst). The ability of the trophozoite to encyst under adverse conditions renders *Acanthamoeba* highly resistant to freezing, desiccation, standard chlorination of water supplies, and a variety of antimicrobial agents.

Risk factors for *Acanthamoeba* keratitis include contact lens wear, especially extended or daily wear soft contact lenses.[76,77] Contaminated home-made saline solutions, failure of cold contact lens sterilization, and a predilection for substrate of gram-negative organisms are additional risk factors. *Acanthamoeba* keratitis may follow corneal trauma, especially with contaminated water.

The clinical features of *Acanthamoeba* keratitis early in the course may be nonspecific with patchy corneal epithelial irregularity or focal and multifocal, pleomorphic epithelial ulceration. Early in the course of infection, the epithelial abnormality may mimic dendritic ulceration, as seen with herpes simplex keratitis. Established infection typically develops a ring-shaped corneal stromal infiltrate that may be partial or complete. The patient typically complains of severe pain, and there may be a nodular, diffuse, or posterior scleritis associated. Presence of risk factors and intense pain should suggest the diagnosis. Although a stromal ring infiltrate is diagnostically helpful, it may not be seen early in the course. *Acanthamoeba* can be seen in smear and cultured by appropriate techniques.

Microsporidia are ubiquitous small obligate intracellular parasites that have rarely caused human infection. The two main genuses causing keratitis are *Nosema* and *Encephalitozoon*. Corneal nosematosis has been observed in a 26-year-old woman in Africa,[78] in an 11-year-old boy with ulceration in India,[79] and in a 9-year-old boy in Japan with granulomatous meningoencephalitis, chorioretinitis, and meningitis.[80] Patients with acquired immunodeficiency syndrome (AIDS) may develop mild conjunctivitis with punctate keratitis due to *Encephalitozoon* spp.[81] Symptoms may be subtle and mimic dry eye syndromes or blepharitis. A high index of suspicion in any patient with AIDS is necessary to make the clinical diagnosis of microsporidial corneal infection.

African trypanosomiasis, or African sleeping sickness, is caused by hemoflagellates that are transmitted to humans via the bite of tse tse flys of the genus *Glossina*. Unilateral conjunctivitis, periorbital edema, and preauricular lymph adenopathy may be observed. Interstitial keratitis similar to that observed in syphilitic keratitis with iritis and conjunctival hyperemia have been observed.[82]

OTHER CAUSES OF KERATITIS

Corneal changes secondary to trachoma conjunctivitis are major causes of worldwide blindness.[83] Trachoma affects approxi-

mately 500 million people in the world and represents a major health problem in both developing and highly industrialized countries. The major clinical eye diseases caused by *Chlamydia trachomatis* include trachoma, adult inclusion conjunctivitis, and neonatal inclusion conjunctivitis. In developed countries, sexually transmitted *C. trachomatis* infection rarely mimics the morphology of true trachoma, which requires chronicity. Trachoma begins as an acute follicular conjunctivitis, which may progress to a chronic phase. The cicatricial phase of the disease causes conjunctival and lid reformation (entropion and trichiasis), which ultimately leads to corneal ulceration and opacification often long after active infection has subsided. The disease is often characterized by repeated reinfection. Bacterial superinfection may prolong and exacerbate inflammation.

Perhaps the most common cause of keratitis results from a hypersensitivity reaction to the exotoxin of *Staphylococcus*. Typically, inferior punctate corneal epithelial defects, marginal corneal stromal infiltrates, and ulcers are clinical manifestations of this allergy. Histologically, lymphocytes and plasma cells are present in the peripheral cornea, but the cornea is free of infectious organisms. Marginal keratitis associated with inflammation of the lid margin from staphylococcal blepharitis has two principal forms. *(1)* Marginal infiltrative and/or ulcerative keratitis is presumably caused by hypersensitivity reaction (type III, immune complex mediated) to staphylococcal exotoxins or other antigens. *(2)* Phlyctenular keratitis is presumably caused by hypersensitivity reaction (type IV, cell mediated) to staphylococci and other organisms.

Ring ulcerations of the cornea may give the appearance of coalesced marginal ulcerative keratitis. These ulcers may progress to total corneal destruction. The precise etiology is uncertain, but these ulcerations are sometimes associated with acute systemic diseases such as influenza, bacillary dysentery, brucellosis, gonococcal arthritis, dengue, herpes zoster ophthalmicus, diabetes mellitus, and hook-worm. The ring ulcerations may also be associated with a number of autoimmune connective tissue diseases such as periarteritis nodosa, rheumatoid arthritis,[84] Wegener's granulomatosis,[85] systemic lupus erythematosus, and giant cell arteritis.[86]

The two major types of interstitial keratitis encountered clinically are due to syphilis and tuberculosis. About 90 percent of all cases of interstitial keratitis are caused by congenital syphilis. Mycobacteria other than *M. tuberculosis* rarely cause a similar keratitis. The best explanation for the occurrence of interstitial keratitis in these two main conditions is as a host-immune response rather than an active microbial infection.

Ocular involvement with syphilis may be acquired or congenital. The chancre of acquired primary syphilis has been reported to have occurred in the conjunctiva.[87] Among patients with acquired secondary syphilis, the incidence of ocular complications is 4.5 percent.[88] These include papulosquamous lesions of the skin of the lids, temporary loss of the eyebrows, diffuse papillary conjunctivitis, scleroconjunctivitis, interstitial keratitis, iritis, chorioretinitis,[89,90] and optic[91] and retrobulbar[92] neuritis. The most common eye lesion in secondary syphilis is iridocyclitis, which accounts for about 75 percent of all eye lesions of the early acquired disease.[93] In almost all cases of iridocyclitis, there are other manifestations of early syphilis. Iridocyclitis can also be a late manifestation of acquired syphilis.[94]

Interstitial keratitis is a rare complication of acquired primary or secondary syphilis. Fewer than 3 percent of all cases of interstitial keratitis are due to acquired syphilis. Interstitial keratitis is also rare in early congenital syphilis. However, it is the most common lesion of late congenital syphilis and occurs in about 52 percent of untreated patients. It typically occurs in the early teens, with most of the cases occurring in patients between the ages of 5 and 20 years. In the acute stage, patients have decreased visual acuity, photophobia, pain, blepharospasm, and lacrimation. The corneal stroma becomes hazy within a few days and has a ground-glass appearance with marked reduction in vision. A severe iridocyclitis is present in the early stages. Over a period of months, new vessels grow into the corneal stroma from the limbus at all levels. When the vessels meet in the center of the cornea, there is a dramatic regression of the disease; the corneal infiltrates are resorbed, and the vessels are partially obliterated. The final visual prognosis in some of these patients is surprisingly good. Seventy percent have 20/20 to 20/100 acuity, and only 10 percent have poorer than 20/200 acuity. Nonsyphilitic spirochetal infection of the cornea may occur in Lyme disease. An interstitial keratitis similar to that observed in syphilis may be caused by the spirochete *Borrelia burgdorferi*.[95]

A syndrome of acute stromal keratitis and vestibuloauditory dysfunction affecting young adults following a hypersensitivity response to upper respiratory tract infection has been described. Besides stromal keratitis, other infrequent eye findings include episcleritis, scleritis, uveitis, and optic disc edema. Ocular involvement in Cogan syndrome[96] must be differentiated from that occurring in congenital and acquired syphilis, chlamydial infection, mumps, herpes zoster, herpes simplex, and rubeola.

A deep, nonsuppurative stromal keratitis of uncertain pathogenesis may simulate herpes simplex stromal keratitis and may follow penetrating keratoplasty and is caused by complex, gram-negative bacilli including *Methylobacterium (Pseudomonas) mesophilica, Capnocytophaga* spp., and *Alcaligenes xylosooxidans* subsp. *denitrificans*.

A severe liquefactive keratitis may develop secondarily to decreased tear production, which may be idiopathic[97,98] or due to decreased corneal sensation after local corneal disease (e.g., herpes zoster infection), to neurologic lesions of the ophthalmic division of the trigeminal nerve, or to medullary infarction. This problem is greatly compounded when associated with inadequate lid closure.

VIRAL KERATITIS

About 20 percent of infants born with herpes simplex virus types 1 or 2 infection have ocular changes.[99] Seven percent will have keratitis with either punctate keratopathy, dendritic ulcers, or disciform keratitis. Of these, 30 percent are infected by herpes simplex type 1. Keratouveitis may occasionally be present at the time of birth. Prophylactic silver nitrate use is not uniformly successful in preventing ocular disease in neonates born to mothers with genital herpes simplex. Atypically, the primary keratitis may present as subepithelial dendritic opacities.[100] Morphologically the lesions of herpes simplex types 1 and 2 are identical.

Ocular herpes simplex acquired during childhood usually presents as a follicular conjunctivitis and is frequently undiagnosed. Transient epithelial lesions are common. However, very similar changes to those described below in adults may also be encountered.[101]

In adults with documented previous corneal herpetic infection, the recurrence rates are approximately 25 percent within 12 months of the last attack and 33 percent within 24 months.[102] Another study suggested a 40 percent recurrence rate for all cases of corneal epithelial herpes and a 25 percent recurrence rate in the form of stromal disease or keratouveitis.[103] Six percent develop visual loss secondary to stromal scarring. The clinical forms of herpes simplex epithelial keratitis include a punctate (nondendritiform) that may occur with or without conjunctivitis. The more classic form of herpes simplex virus epithelial keratitis is the linear, dendritic figure. There also may be geographic, macroulceration of the epithelium. In the nonlinear and dendritic forms, active viral replication in the ulcer margin has been documented in the epithelium. The geographic type is notable for a prolonged course. Dendritic and geographic epithelial keratitis are known to heal spontaneously within 10–14 days in 80 percent of the cases. Stromal involvement is usually seen in recurrent attacks, and the cornea has not been conclusively shown to harbor active viral particles. Herpes simplex

virus stromal involvement (disciform keratitis) is an immune-mediated reaction. The process frequently results in some stromal scarring commonly with thinning and occasionally with perforation. An associated uveitis is common. Recurrent ocular herpes simplex is thought to result from reactivation of latent herpes in the trigeminal ganglion and centripetal spread to the eye.[104,105] Herpes simplex viral DNA has been detected using the polymerase chain reaction. Corneal hypesthesia,[106] which worsens with repeated attacks, is common.

The pattern of disease is different in immunosuppressed patients.[107,108] They may have bilateral corneal involvement, which is seen in only 5 percent of other patients and may also have extensive and multiple lesions on the cornea and conjunctiva. These lesions tend to persist or recur with topical antiviral therapy until immunosuppressive therapy is reduced.

The precise mechanisms for viral reactivation are incompletely understood, yet some of the factors that may precipitate recurrent episodes are exposure to sunlight, menstruation, psychiatric disturbances, fever, and other acute stresses.[109] Acute illnesses may temporarily suppress the immune mechanisms, and the most common cause of a unilateral red eye in a hospitalized patient is herpes simplex keratitis. Topical and systemic steroids and immunosuppressive agents may provoke recurrences in corneal epithelium, and they enhance replication in established lesions.[110]

The subepithelial corneal opacities occurring in epidemic keratoconjunctivitis caused by adenovirus probably represent an immune phenomenon. These opacities tend to appear approximately 10–14 days after the symptoms commence. The natural course of the corneal lesions is resolution over 2–3 weeks, although patients may be very photophobic during this period. The lesions tend to clear dramatically with the use of topical corticosteroids, with occasional reappearance when the steroid therapy is discontinued.[110]

In about 10 percent of the patients with herpes zoster infections, the ophthalmic division of the trigeminal nerve is involved. The various ocular manifestations include vesicles on the lid and conjunctiva, iridocyclitis, secondary glaucoma, ophthalmoplegia, neuroretinitis, optic neuritis, and retinal vascular occlusion.[111,112] Corneal findings include decreased corneal sensation, epithelial and subepithelial punctate keratitis, dendritic figures, disciform keratitis, segmental keratitis, and corneal vascularization. The corneal disease may occur after the skin eruption has healed, and it can be prolonged.[113] Visual loss may result from peripheral and central stromal involvement.[114]

In varicella infections (chickenpox), ocular involvement is usually limited to the appearance of vesicles on the lids, conjunctiva, and limbus. Superficial punctate keratitis, interstitial and disciform keratitis, and uveitis have also been reported.[115] Epithelial dendritic figures that are identical to those seen in herpes zoster keratitis may occur immediately or up to several months after the skin eruption.[116] A scleritis may also accompany varicella disciform keratitis.[117] Vaccinia infections of the eye occur from accidental autoinoculation.[118] Corneal complications occur in one-third of the patients with ocular vaccinia and may consist of superficial punctate keratitis, epithelial ulcers, and rarely disciform keratitis. The epithelial ulcers may superficially resemble herpetic keratitis.[119,120]

The keratitis that is occasionally associated with measles (rubeola) infections causes punctate or dendritic epithelial defects in the cornea.[121] In one adult population study, all rubeola patients had epithelial keratitis that followed a benign course.[122] The changing immune status of the population after vaccination programs is changing the pattern of clinical disease—from a childhood illness to an adult disease and perhaps a different ocular expression of measles infection. In developing countries, vitamin A deficiency and malnutrition sometimes make measles keratitis a binding disease with secondary bacterial infection and perforation of the globe.

Epstein-Barr virus infections may cause a spectrum of ocular involvement, including dacryoadenitis, oculoglandular syndrome, follicular conjunctivitis, punctate and dendritic epithelial keratitis, and stromal keratitis. Cranial nerve palsies, papilledema, and optic neuritis may also be observed. The stromal keratitis may involve the subepithelial region,[123] the anterior and midstroma, or the deep stroma.[124]

There have been occasional reported cases of Jacob-Kreutzfeldt disease[125] and rabies transmission[126] by the use of infected donor tissue in corneal transplantation. Human immunodeficiency virus (HIV) has been demonstrated to be present within the corneal epithelium.[127] All potential donors of corneas considered for transplantation are screened for possible HIV infection and the hepatitis viruses.

LABORATORY INVESTIGATIONS FOR DIAGNOSIS

Since the morphologic features of infectious and noninfectious keratitis are sometimes indistinguishable, diagnostic laboratory evaluation of corneal scrapings is imperative if there is a suspicion of microbial keratitis. One of the basic principals of laboratory investigation is to follow a standard set plan for all suspected cases of microbial keratitis. The ophthalmologist and clinical microbiology laboratory should establish a routine method for obtaining diagnostic material and maintaining standard materials for collection, transport, and culture.[128] Other basic principles include maintaining complete patient control to ensure adequate sampling of the area of corneal suppuration. This can be achieved through administration of local anesthetic to achieve akinesia in noncooperative adults or general anesthesia in children if necessary. Multiple samples from areas of suppuration should be obtained for *each* stain and media. The smears of corneal scrapings on glass slides should be fixed promptly in methyl alcohol. Material from corneal scrapings should also be inoculated directly to fresh culture media, which has been warmed to room temperature. Special stains and media should be utilized if directed by clinical signs or results of prior studies. Methods for obtaining material and techniques for culture vary considerably. Proparacaine hydrochloride (0.5%) is less antiseptic than other topical anesthetics and is the preferred topical anesthetic for performing corneal scrapings. Corneal scraping can be achieved using a blunt platinum (Kimura) spatula, sterile surgical blade (Bard-Parker), or calcium alginate swab dipped in trypticase soy broth. The calcium alginate swab dipped in trypticase soy broth may adhere corneal pathogens better than the platinum spatula, thereby increasing the yield of diagnostic corneal scrapings. Superficial keratectomy may be helpful in dry nonsuppurative infections and is aided by the use of sharp sterile blade or scissors and forceps. Corneal biopsy[129] may assist in diagnosis in dry, nonsuppurative infections if the surface of the cornea is spared. A corneal shave biopsy can be completed with a sterile surgical blade, or adequate corneal biopsy may be performed with a 1.5- or 2.0-mm trephine and unguarded diamond blade. Corneal biopsy can usually be performed at the slit-lamp biomicroscope, though some patients may require the operating room and adjunctive anesthesia for controlled biopsy. Lamellar keratoplasty is typically unnecessary for diagnostic purposes. A penetrating therapeutic keratoplasty may be required for diagnosis and therapy of progressive, destructive keratitis if the etiology is not determined by other methods.

Corneal scrapings are transferred to clean glass slides for Gram, Giemsa, acid-fast and calcofluor white, or methenamine silver stains. Multiple inoculations of the corneal scraping with the spatula or calcium alginate swab are completed on blood agar, chocolate agar, thioglycolate or Schaedler broth, brain–heart infusion or Sabouraud's agar, and blood agar incubated anaerobically. Special methods are required to recover *Chlamydia* or *Acanthamoeba*. For mycobacteria, Lowenstein-Jensen agar at 35°C, Petragnani's agar, Middlebrook 7H10 or 7H11, or commercial radiometric broth (Bactec) medium is ap-

propriate. In many cases, concomitant cultures of the conjunctiva and lid on the involved and uninvolved eye are obtained to ascertain the persons' flora and to assist in assessing the significance of positive corneal cultures taken from the area of ulceration. The type and number of positive cultures needed to support a microbial diagnosis are still unsettled.[130,131] Negative cultures obtained from corneal scrapings in the face of a suspicious ulcerative keratitis should lead to a superficial keratectomy or corneal biopsy. These investigations may prove positive when superficial scrapings were previously negative since fungi and *Acanthamoeba* are characteristically deep in corneal parenchyma and conspicuously absent on the surface.[128,129] Viral keratitis does not often require culture, and the diagnosis is sustained by the morphology of the lesions. Careful débridement of the corneal epithelium and transfer to viral transport media will usually suffice to grow herpes simplex virus types 1 and 2 and adenovirus. Herpes zoster virus is rarely isolated from corneal lesions. In doubtful cases, transmission electron microscopy may occasionally be helpful in establishing the viral etiology.[129,132]

The majority of aerobic bacteria causing keratitis grow on the standard media within 48 hours, and sometimes a pathogen may be recognized in 12–15 hours. Some criteria suggested for confirming an infectious corneal process include growth of an organism in two or more media; confluent growth of a known ocular pathogen in one solid medium; or growth in one medium of an organism identified on routine stain.

Once a corneal pathogen has been identified from the appropriate media, antimicrobial susceptibility testing should proceed according to the usual laboratory techniques. Laboratory antifungal sensitivity testing currently lacks optimal standardization and reproducibility.

TREATMENT

Because of the rapid evolution to perforation in keratitis due to virulent pathogens and visual loss secondary to central scarring, many patients with bacterial keratitis with significant ulceration need to be hospitalized. The high frequency and intense dosage scheduling of antimicrobial therapy often requires the assistance of trained nursing personnel.

In infectious keratitis, aggressive antibiotic therapy is the mainstay, and there are several routes of administration, including topical antibiotic drops and ointments, continuous lavage, antibiotic-soaked collagen corneal shields or therapeutic soft contact lenses, iontophoresis, subconjunctival injection, and parenteral administration.

The objective of therapy in bacterial keratitis is to eliminate the infective organism in a rapid fashion, reduce the inflammatory response, prevent structural damage to the cornea, and promote healing of the epithelial surface. With suspected infectious keratitis, the clinician has the option of initiating specific directed or broad-spectrum antimicrobial therapy or deferring treatment pending the results of laboratory investigation, or monitoring the clinical signs. In general, because of the potential rapid destruction of corneal tissue that may accompany bacterial keratitis, if there is a clinical suspicion suggestive of a bacterial pathogen, the patient should be treated appropriately for bacterial keratitis until a definitive diagnosis is substantiated.

A basic plan for therapy of severe suppurative keratitis depends on the results of Gram stains on smears from diagnostic corneal scrapings. If a single type of bacterium is observed with microscopic analysis of smears and the patient has not been on antecedent therapy, a single specific antibacterial agent is selected. If two or more bacteria are present on Gram stain, combined specific antibacterial therapy is recommended. If a single bacterium is observed on Gram stain, however, and the patient has received prior therapy, a broad-spectrum antibacterial therapeutic regimen is recommended.

The decision to base initial antibiotic therapy on the results of Gram stain requires high technical proficiency of the Microbiology Laboratory. With optimal conditions, the Microbiology Laboratory can identify the pathogen on Gram stain in 75 percent of monobacterial keratitis cases and 37 percent of polybacterial keratitis. If the Gram stain is equivocal or there is uncertainty in interpretation of diagnostic smears, broad-spectrum antibiotic coverage should be initiated in the initial treatment of all cases of severe suppurative microbial keratitis since the consequences of inappropriate or inadequate therapy can be devastating.[133]

The design for drug administration in severe suppurative keratitis includes antibiotics administered frequently. Topical antibiotics in solution are preferred over ointments because concentrated antibiotic solutions can penetrate into ocular tissues to achieve higher concentration in ocular tissues than with ointment preparations. Hospital pharmacies can readily prepare highly concentrated (fortified) solutions by using commercially available ocular lubricants and parenteral antibiotic formulations.[134]

Subconjunctival administration of antibiotics, although painful, provides a transient peak concentration of drug within the corneal stroma, yet equivalent drug levels may be attained with highly concentrated antibiotic solutions administered at great frequency.[135]

Continuous lavage of the cornea with antibiotic solutions has been described.[136] The advantages of this method include potentially increased drug levels obtained within the aqueous humor,[137] as well as a lack of dependence on nursing personnel for frequent drop instillations.

Soft hydrophilic contact lenses have been used as drug delivery systems to achieve higher intraocular drug concentrations than can be obtained with frequent topical administration.[138,139] Collagen corneal shields soaked in antibiotic solutions have also been shown to increase antibiotic penetration compared with therapeutic soft contact lenses.[140,141] Use of collagen corneal shields as adjuncts in the therapy of bacterial keratitis has been experimentally documented.[142] No controlled clinical trials documenting efficacy and safety have been completed. Polymer inserts have also been designed to prolong the presence of drug in the tear film. Liposomal systems have been designed to improve the interaction of drugs with the corneal surface.[143,144] Transcorneal iontophoresis of antibiotics has also been employed to increase attainable drug concentrations and increase efficacy of antibacterial therapy.[145] Other strategies to improve drug delivery to the cornea include placement of temporary punctal occlusion plugs to maintain more antibiotic in the preocular tear film.

Parenteral (intramuscular or intravenous) administration of antibiotic compounds is reserved for severe suppurative keratitis with impending perforation. Intravenous antibiotic administration is also recommended for contiguous spread of infection to involve the sclera (sclerokeratitis).

Factors that frequently guide the choice of appropriate antibiotic for systemic infection are not necessarily applicable to the topical therapy of ocular infections. The minimal inhibitory concentration determinations in antimicrobial susceptibility testing are based on achievable serum levels and do not directly apply to topical therapy of infective keratitis. Other factors important in therapy of systemic infections such as distribution space, mode of excretion, influence of renal or hepatic failure, and absorption characteristics are also not directly applicable to ocular infections. The antimicrobial agent selected for initial therapy should have bactericidal activity against common corneal pathogens, low rates of acquired resistance, favorable solubility characteristics to enhance penetration, and minimal toxicity to ocular tissues. Initial broad-spectrum therapy for suspected bacterial keratitis has traditionally been with a topical first-generation cephalosporin (e.g., cefazolin) and an aminoglycoside (gentamicin, tobramycin, or amikacin). Second- and third-generation cephalosporins have also been utilized for therapy

of bacterial keratitis, though the stability of the β-lactam ring in solution in these compounds and sustained efficacy have not been well studied.

Many classes of antibiotic compounds have been used for the directed specific therapy of bacterial keratitis. Gram-positive keratitis, especially from staphylococcal species, is most often treated with topical cephalosporin antibiotics. If there is suspected resistance of the staphylococcal species to cephalosporins or semisynthetic penicillins, topical vancomycin should be considered. Penicillin G is the therapy of choice for pneumococcal keratitis.

Gentamicin has been the therapy of choice for gram-negative keratitis and can be administered by topical, subconjunctival, and parenteral routes. Tobramycin is similar. The aminoglycosides may be synergistic with ticarcillin or piperacillin against *Pseudomonas* and *Proteus* spp., but they may be inactivated if mixed in the same solution.

Fluoroquinolone antibiotics have been developed for topical ocular use and are especially effective in the therapy of *Pseudomonas* and other gram-negative keratitis.[146] Topical fluoroquinolones have some activity against gram-positive corneal pathogens, though clinical treatment failures have occurred in keratitis due to streptococci and enterococci. Sulfonamides have been replaced by more effective antibiotics in the treatment of bacterial keratitis, but they remain indicated for corneal infections caused by *Nocardia*.[60]

Supportive therapy in the treatment of infectious keratitis consists of topical cycloplegics to reduce photophobia, enzyme inhibitors, metalloproteinase inhibitors, therapeutic soft contact lenses, collagen corneal shields, and topical corticosteroids. Since severe anterior chamber inflammatory reaction may occur with bacterial keratitis, cycloplegics should be administered to prevent the formation of synechiae and to relieve the discomfort of ciliary spasm.

If corneal ulceration is marked, the temporary use of a therapeutic soft contact lens or "bandage" lens may facilitate stromal repair and promote reepithelialization by protecting the corneal surface from mechanical trauma of lid movement. Topical medication may be continued after the contact lens insertion, and drug delivery to the cornea may also be enhanced.

The use of topical corticosteroids in the management of bacterial keratitis is somewhat controversial. It has been suggested that steroids in conjunction with specific antibacterial therapy minimize the inflammatory sequelae of bacterial keratitis. A number of experimental studies have concluded that corticosteroid therapy does not adversely affect results of antibiotic therapy in bacterial keratitis.[147–149] *Pseudomonas* keratitis requires long-term high-dose antibiotic therapy prior to cautious introduction of corticosteroid therapy.

Signs of clinical improvement are based on frequent slit-lamp examination. Clinical changes may be difficult to appreciate in the early course of therapy due to the effects of diagnostic corneal scraping and frequent topical antibiotic therapy. After the first 48 hours, frequency of antibiotic administration can usually be gradually decreased. Highly concentrated antibiotic solutions may be converted to commercial-strength drops after several days. The therapeutic endpoint in ulcerative keratitis is epithelial healing, yet concentrated antibiotics may retard reepithelialization.

The research and development of effective antifungal compounds for ocular mycotic infections has lagged behind that for antibacterial agents.[150] Therapy of fungal keratitis generally requires prolonged use of topical antifungal agents and occasionally adjunctive parenteral therapy. Topical natamycin (Pimaricin) has sometimes been available in the United States as a 5% suspension. If hyphal fragments are observed on diagnostic smears from corneal scrapings, natamycin should be administered hourly for the initial 24–48 hours. Natamycin, if available, is the therapy of choice for keratitis due to filamentous fungi. Amphotericin B desoxycholate (Fungizone) can be prepared in the pharmacy in sterile water as 1.5 mg/ml. Amphotericin B is active against fungi, particularly *Candida,* though the desoxycholate formulation is toxic to the corneal epithelium. Ketoconazole[151] and particularly itraconazole have been used orally for fungal keratitis, but experience is meager. Fluconazole is available as a sterile solution for intravenous use and might be considered for topical therapy of *Candida* keratitis. Caution must be exercised when adding topical corticosteroid to therapy when a response to the antifungal agent has been observed to help reduce corneal destruction caused by host response. In severe cases of fungal keratitis, corneal transplantation, keratoplasty, or conjunctival flaps may be needed to stabilize the eye. Penetrating keratoplasty and conjunctival flaps were the main defense against fungal keratitis prior to antifungal chemotherapy.

Medical therapy for *Acanthamoeba* keratitis remains challenging. The ability of the amoeba to transform from the relatively susceptible trophozoite form to the highly recalcitrant cystic form makes eradication difficult. In vitro susceptibility determinations suggest that trophozoites may be killed by certain antibacterial compounds (paromomycin, neomycin), antifungals (imidazoles and triazoles), and antiparasitic agents (propamidine isethionate, hydroxystilbamidine). The principles in management of *Acanthamoeba* keratitis have most often employed a combined therapeutic approach with multiple agents. Polyhexamethylene biguanide, a polymeric biguanide and environmental biocide, has been shown to have clinical efficacy in the therapy of keratitis.[152] Many cases of *Acanthamoeba* keratitis require medical therapy and therapeutic keratoplasty to eradicate the cyst effectively from the corneal tissue.

Diethylcarbamazine (DEC) has been previously used both topically and systemically to kill the microfilariae in onchocerciasis, but is ineffective in killing the adult worm. Both the microfilariae and adult worm can be killed by suramin, but therapy is highly toxic. Patients may exhibit marked inflammatory reactions to multiple dead microfilariae and should be given corticosteroids to reduce this response. Topical levamisole and mebendazole have also been recommended. Ivermectin is highly effective and less toxic with fewer ocular complications than DEC[153] and has evolved as the preferred therapy for onchocerciasis. Since syphilitic interstitial keratitis is a manifestation of an immune phenomenon, specific antitreponemal therapy does not greatly affect the course of the acute inflammation. However, therapy reduces the chances of recurrence from 27 percent in untreated cases to 3.6 percent in treated cases. Treatment also reduces the likelihood of bilateral ocular involvement. Topical steroids are used during the acute stages of the keratitis to avoid severe postinflammatory sequelae. Since Lyme keratitis is a manifestation of a systemic infection having potentially protean manifestations, including neurologic, cardiologic, rheumatologic, and dermatologic complications, a course of systemic parenteral therapy with intravenous ceftriaxone is indicated. Topical corticosteroids to reduce interstitial inflammation should be applied and may require a prolonged taper.

The treatment of epithelial keratitis in herpes simplex viral infections consists of minimal wiping débridement of the epithelium[154] and use of a topical antiviral agent; this is effective in most cases of corneal dendritic ulcerations. Extensive involvement, central lesions, geographic macroulcerations, or resistent lesions are usually treated with a 10-day course of topical antiviral agents. Trifluridine and acyclovir are the agents used topically because of their lower corneal toxicity. The use of corticosteroids is contraindicated in isolated herpes simplex epithelial keratitis. Active epithelial keratitis generally resolves within 5–10 days, and judgment of activity is aided clinically by the use of Rose Bengal solution, which also has antiviral activity. Concurrent prophylactic antibacterial antibiotics are generally not indicated, as they may enhance drug toxicity. Herpes simplex viral nonnecrotizing (disciform) stromal keratitis or necrotizing (suppurative) stromal keratitis may occur sequential to epithelial keratitis or as isolated inflammations. Corticosteroids are the only effective therapeutic measure, and their use and dosage is determined by the severity of the stromal inflammation, presence of or interval since active epithelial keratitis, and antecedent corticosteroid use. Use of concurrent topical antiviral agent as a prophylaxis against recurrent epithelial keratitis is recommended when corticosteroid therapy is administered greater than once daily. The role of oral acyclovir in combination with topical steroid has not been shown to be beneficial in control of stromal keratitis, and the efficacy of long-term oral acyclovir in suppressing recurrence has not been established. Other methods of therapy for herpes simplex corneal infection such as topical interferon[155] and cryotherapy have been used. Uncontrolled herpetic stromal keratitis and secondary stromal scarring may require corneal transplantation.[156,157]

Stromal keratitis caused by herpes zoster frequently requires corticosteroids to reduce the inflammatory response and resultant corneal destruction, including neovascularization and lipid deposition along with permanent endothelial dysfunction.

Oral acyclovir or topical antiviral agents are not indicated for therapy of herpes zoster stromal keratitis even with concomitant corticosteroid administration. Oral corticosteroids may be required for concurrent scleritis.[158,159]

Epidemic keratoconjunctivitis from adenovirus rarely requires more therapy than supportive measures such as artificial tears and mild cycloplegics. Severe photophobia, incapacitating irritation, and decreased vision during acute episodes may be relieved with topical corticosteroids. It is unclear whether their use prolongs the course of the disease. Ocular involvement in infectious mononucleosis also typically only requires the use of ocular lubricants or mild corticosteroids to control the stromal keratitis.

REFERENCES

1. Jones DB. Polymicrobial keratitis. Trans Am Ophthalmol Soc. 1981;79:153.
2. Asbell P, Stenson S. Ulcerative keratitis. Survey of 30 years laboratory experience. Arch Ophthalmol. 1982;100:77.
3. Liesegang TJ, Forster RK. Spectrum of microbial keratitis in South Florida. Am J Ophthalmol. 1980;90:38.
4. Eichenbaum JW, Feldstein M, Podos SM. Extended-wear aphakic soft contact lenses in corneal ulcers. Br J Ophthalmol. 1982;66:663.
5. Wilson LA, Schlitzer RL, Ahearn DG. Pseudomonas corneal ulcers associated with soft contact lens wear. Am J Ophthalmol. 1981;92:546.
6. Krachmer JH, Purcell JJ. Bacterial corneal ulcers in cosmetic soft contact lens wearers. Arch Ophthalmol. 1978;96:57.
7. Schein OD, Poggio EC, Seddon JM, et al. The incidence of ulcerative keratitis among extended contact lens wearers. N Engl J Med. 1989;321:773.
8. Glynn RJ, Schein OD, Seddon JM, et al. The incidence of ulcerative keratitis among aphakic contact lens wearers in New England. Arch Ophthalmol. 1991;109:104–7.
9. Escapini H Jr, Olson RJ, Kaufman HE. Donor cornea contamination with McCarey-Kaufman medium preservation. Am J Ophthalmol. 1979;88:59.
10. Coster DJ, Wilhelmus KR, Peacock J, et al. Suppurative keratitis in London. In: Trevor-Roper T, ed. European Society of Ophthalmology. The Cornea, Health, and Disease. London: Academic Press; 1981:395.
11. Ostler HB, Okumoto M, Wilkey C. The changing pattern of the etiology of central bacterial corneal (hypopyon) ulcer. Trans Pacific Coast Oto-Ophthalmol Soc. 1976;57:235.
12. Udell IJ, Kelly CG, Woolf TC, et al. Cat scratch keratitis. Ophthalmology. 1987;94(Suppl)124.
13. Wilson LA, Ahearn DG. *Pseudomonas* induced corneal ulcers associated with contaminated eye mascaras. Am J Ophthalmol. 1977;84:112.
14. Reid PR, Wood TO. *Pseudomonas* corneal ulcer. The causative role of contaminated eye cosmetics. Arch Ophthalmol. 1979;97:1640.
15. Locatcher-Khorazo D, Gutierrez E. Bacteria typing of *Staphylococcus aureus.* A study of normal, infected eyes in environment. Arch Ophthalmol. 1960;63:774.
16. Locatcher-Khorazo D, Sullivan N, Gutierrez E. *Staphylococcus aureus* isolated from normal and infected eyes. Stage types and sensitivity to antibacterial agents. Arch Ophthalmol. 1967;77:370.
17. Kim HB, Ostler HB. Marginal corneal ulcer due to beta-*Streptococcus.* Arch Ophthalmol. 1977;95:454.
18. Cohn H, Mondino BJ, Brown SI, et al. Marginal corneal ulcers with acute beta-streptococcal conjunctivitis in chronic dacryocystitis. Am J Ophthalmol. 1979;87:541.
19. Johnson MK, Allen JH. Ocular toxin of the *Pneumococcus.* Am J Ophthalmol. 1971;72:175.

20. Brown SI, Bloomfield SE, Wai-Fong IC. The cornea-destroying enzyme of *Pseudomonas aeruginosa*. Invest Ophthalmol. 1974;13:174.

21. Kreger AS, Griffin OK. Physiochemical fractionation of extracellular cornea-damaging proteases of *Pseudomonas aeruginosa*. Infect Immun. 1974;9:829.

22. Liu PV. Extracellular toxins of *Pseudomonas aeruginosa*. J Infect Dis. 1974; 130(Suppl):94.

23. Ohman DR, Burns RP, Iglewski BH. Corneal infections in mice with toxin-A and elastase mutants of *Pseudomonas aeruginosa*. J Infect Dis. 1980; 142:547.

24. Mondino BJ, Rabin BS, Kessler E, et al. Corneal rings with gram-negative bacteria. Arch Ophthalmol. 1977;95:2222.

25. Belmont JB, Ostler HB, Chandler RD, et al. Non-infectious ring-shaped keratitis associated with *Pseudomonas aeruginosa*. Am J Ophthalmol. 1982; 93:338.

26. Kessler E, Mondino BJ, Brown SI. The corneal response to *Pseudomonas aeruginosa*: Histopathological and enzymatic characterization. Invest Ophthalmol Vis Sci. 1977;16:116.

27. Chusid MJ, Davis SD. Polymorphonuclear leukocyte kinetics in experimentally induced keratitis. Arch Ophthalmol. 1985;103:270.

28. Hutton WL, Sexton RR. Atypical *Pseudomonas* corneal ulcers in semi-comatose patients. Am J Ophthalmol. 1972;73:37.

29. Codere F, Brownstein S, Jackson WB. *Pseudomonas aeruginosa* scleritis. Am J Ophthalmol. 1981;91:706.

30. Raber IM, Laibson PR, Kurz GH, et al. *Pseudomonas* corneoscleral ulcers. Am J Ophthalmol. 1981;92:353.

31. Brinser JH, Torczynski E. Unusual *Pseudomonas* corneal ulcers. Am J Ophthalmol. 1977;84:462.

32. Lass JH, Haaf J, Foster CS, et al. Visual outcome in eight cases of *Serratia marcescens* keratitis. Am J Ophthalmol. 1981;92:384.

33. Templeton WC, Eiferman RA, Snyder JW, et al. *Serratia* keratitis transmitted by contaminated eyedroppers. Am J Ophthalmol. 1982;93:723.

34. Baum J, Fedukowicz HB, Jordan A. A Survey of *Moraxella* corneal ulcers in a derelict population. Am J Ophthalmol. 1980;90:476.

35. Cobo LM, Coster DJ, Peacock J. *Moraxella* keratitis in a nonalcoholic population. Br J Ophthalmol. 1981;65:683.

36. vanBusterveld OP, Richards RD. Bacillus infection of the cornea. Arch Ophthalmol. 1965;74:91.

37. O'Day DM, Ho PC, Andrews JS, et al. Mechanism of tissue destruction in ocular *Bacillus cereus* infections. In: Trevor-Roper T, ed. European Society of Ophthalmology. The Cornea, Health, and Disease. London: Academic Press; 1981:403.

38. Chandler JW, Milam DF. Diphtheria corneal ulcers. Arch Ophthalmol. 1978;96:53.

39. Turner L, Stinson I. *Mycobacterium fortuitum* as a cause of corneal ulcer. Am J Ophthalmol. 1965;60:329.

40. Meisler DM, Friedlaender MH, Okumoto M. *Mycobacterium chelonei* keratitis. Am J Ophthalmol. 1982;94:398.

41. Gangadharam PRJ, Lanier JD, Jones DB. Keratitis due to *Mycobacterium chelonei*. Tubercle. 1978;59:55.

42. Lazar M, Nemet P, Bracha R, et al. *Mycobacterium fortuitum* keratitis. Am J Ophthalmol. 1974;78:530.

43. Newman PE, Goodman RA, Waring GA, et al. A cluster of cases of *Mycobacterium chelonei* keratitis associated with outpatient office procedures. Am J Ophthalmol. 1984;97:344.

44. Allen JH, Byers JL. The pathology of ocular leprosy. I. Cornea. Arch Ophthalmol. 1960;64:216.

45. Elliott DC. An Interpretation of the ocular manifestations of leprosy. Ann NY Acad Sci. 1951;54:84.

46. Pillat A. Leprosy bacilli in the scraping from the diseased cornea in a leper and comments on keratitis punctata superficialis leprosa. Arch Ophthalmol. 1930;3:306.

47. Liesegang TJ, Jones DB, Robinson NN. Azotobacter keratitis. Arch Ophthalmol. 1981;99:1587.

48. Wilhelmus KR, Peacock J, Coster BJ. *Branhamella* keratitis. Br J Ophthalmol. 1980;64:892.

49. Feaster FT, Nisbet RN, Barber JC. *Aeromonas hydrophilia* corneal ulcer. Am J Ophthalmol. 1978;85:114.

50. Purcell JJ, Krachmer JH. Corneal ulcer caused by *Pasteurella multocida*. Am J Ophthalmol. 1977;83:540.

51. Stern GA, Hodes BL, Stock EL. *Clostridium perfringens* corneal ulcer. Arch Ophthalmol. 1979;97:661.

52. Tabbara KF, Taraba VN. *Bacillus licheniformis* corneal ulcer. Am J Ophthalmol. 1979;87:717.

53. Samples JR, Buettner H. Corneal ulcer caused by a biologic insecticide (*B. thuringiensis*). Am J Ophthalmol. 1983;95:258.

54. Ostler HB, Okumoto M. Anaerobic streptococcal corneal ulcer. Am J Ophthalmol. 1976;81:518.

55. Jones DB. Opportunistic fungal infections in ophthalmology. Fungal keratitis. In: Chic ED, Balows A, Furcolow ML, eds. Opportunistic Fungal Infections. Springfield, IL: Charles C. Thomas; 1975:103.

56. Jones BR, Richards HB, Morgan G. Direct fungal infection of the eye in Britain. Trans Ophthalmol Soc UK. 1969;89:727.

57. DeVoe AG, Silva-Hunter M. Fungal infections of the eye. In: Locatcher-Khorazo D, Seegal BC, eds. Microbiology of the Eye. St. Louis: CV Mosby; 1972:208.

58. Jones DB, Forster RK, Rebell G. *Fusarium solani* keratitis treated with natamycin (Pimaricin): 18 consecutive cases. Arch Ophthalmol. 1972;88:147.

59. Searl SS, Udell IJ, Sadun A, et al. *Aspergillus* keratitis with intraocular invasion. Ophthalmology. 1981;88:1244.

60. Hirst LW, Harrison GK, Merz EG, et al. *Nocardia asteroides* keratitis. Br J Ophthalmol. 1979;63:449.

61. Wilhelmus KR, Robinson NN, Jones DB. *Bacterionema matruchotii* ocular infections. Am J Ophthalmol. 1979;87:143.

62. Jones BR, Christensen GR. *Pullularia* corneal ulcer. Arch Ophthalmol. 1974; 92:529.

63. Krachmer JH, Anderson RL, Binder PS, et al. *Helminthosporium* corneal ulcers. Am J Ophthalmol. 1978;85:66.

64. Francois J, Rijsselae RE. Corneal infections by *Rhodotorula*. Ophthalmologica. 1979;178:241.

65. Zapater RC, Albesi EJ. Corneal monosporiosis. A review and report of one case. Ophthalmologica 1979;178:142.

66. Eiferman RA, Snyder JW, Barbee JV Jr. Corneal chromomycosis. Am J Ophthalmol. 1982;95:255.

67. Rodrigues MM, Laibson P, Kaplan W. Exogenous corneal ulcer caused by *Tritirachium roseum*. Am J Ophthalmol. 1979;80:804.

68. Taylor HR. Treatment of onchocerciasis in the 1980's. Onchocerciasis is one of the Leading Causes of Blindness Worldwide. Postgrad Doctor AFR. 1983; 5:74.

69. Buck AA, ed. Onchocerciasis: Symptomatology, pathology, diagnosis. Geneva: World Health Organization; 1974.

70. Gibson DW, Heggie C, Connor DA. Clinical and pathologic aspects of onchocerciasis. Pathol Ann. 1980;15:195.

71. Thylefors B. Ocular onchocerciasis. Bull WHO. 1978;56:63.

72. Fuglsang JA. Living microfilariae of *Onchocerca volvulus* in the cornea. Br J Ophthalmol. 1983;57:712.

73. Rodger FC, Chir M. The pathogenesis and pathology of ocular onchocerciasis. Am J Ophthalmol. 1960;49:104.

74. Roizenblatt J. Interstitial keratitis caused by American (mucocutaneous) leishmaniasis. Am J Ophthalmol. 1979;87:175.

75. Jones DB, Visvesvara GS, Robinson NM. *Acanthamoeba polyphaga* keratitis and *Acanthamoeba uveitis* associated with fatal meningoencephalitis. Trans Ophthalmol Soc UK. 1975;95:221.

76. Ma P, Willaert E, Juechter KB, et al. A case of keratitis due to *Acanthamoeba* in New York, New York and features of ten cases. J Infect Dis. 1981; 143:662.

77. Mannis NJ, Tamaro R, Roth AM, et al. *Acanthamoeba* scleral keratitis. Determining diagnostic criteria. Arch Ophthalmol. 1986;104:1313–17.

78. Pinnolis M, Egbert PR, Font RL, et al. Nosematosis of the cornea. Arch Ophthalmol. 1981;99:1044.

79. Ashton N, Wirasinha P. Encephalitozoonosis (nosematosis) of the cornea. Br J Ophthalmol. 1973;57:669.

80. Matsubayashi H, Koike T, Mikata I, et al. A case of eencephalitozoon-like body infection in man. Arch Pathol. 1959;67:181.

81. Friedberg DN, Stenson SM, Orenstein JM, et al. Microsporidial keratoconjunctivitis in acquired immunodeficiency syndrome. Arch Ophthalmol. 1990; 108:504–8.

82. Neame H. Parenchymatous keratitis in trypanosomiasis in cattle and in dogs and in man. Br J Ophthalmol. 1927;11:209.

83. Dawson CR, Jones BR, Tarizzo ML. Guide to Trachoma Control in Programs for the Prevention of Blindness. Geneva: World Health Organization; 1981.

84. Eiferman RA, Carothers DJ, Yangeelow JA. Peripheral rheumatoid ulceration and evidence for conjunctival collagenase production. Am J Ophthalmol. 1979;87:703.

85. Austin P, Green WR, Sallyer DC, et al. Peripheral corneal degeneration and occlusive vasculitis in Wegener's granulomatosis. Am J Ophthalmol. 1978; 85:311.

86. Gerstle CC, Friedman AH. Marginal corneal ulceration (limbal guttering) as a presenting sign of temporal arteritis. Ophthalmology. 1980;87:1173.

87. Duke-Elder S. System of Ophthalmology. v. 8. Diseases of the Outer Eye. St. Louis: CV Mosby; 1965;237, 259, 539, 828, 829, 1032.

88. Woods AC. Syphilis of the eye. Am J Syph Gonor Vener Dis. 1943;27:133.

89. Ballantyne AJ, Michaelson IC. Textbook of the Fundus of the Eye. Baltimore: Williams & Wilkins; 1962;564.

90. Knapp A. Bilateral circumpapullary chorioretinitis with detachment of the retina in syphilis. Trans Am Acad Ophthalmol Otolaryngol. 1920;25:132.

91. Stokes JH, Beerman H, Ingraham NR. Modern Clinical Syphilology. Philadelphia: WB Saunders; 1949:59.

92. Carrol FD. Retrobulbar neuritis. Arch Ophthalmol. 1940;24:44.

93. Hogan MJ, Zimmerman LE, et al. Ophthalmic Pathology, 3rd ed. Philadelphia: WB Saunders; 1968:397.

94. Moore JE. Syphilitic iritis. Am J Ophthalmol. 1931;14:110.

95. Baum J, Bavza M, Weinstein P, et al. Bilateral keratitis as a manifestation of Lyme disease. Am J Ophthalmol. 1988;105:75.

96. Vollerstein RS, McDonald TJ, Younge BR, et al. Coagan's syndrome: 18 cases and a review of the literature. Mayo Clin Proc. 1986;61:344–361.

97. Krachmer JH, Laibson PR. Corneal Thinning and Perforation in Sjögren's syndrome. Am J Ophthalmol. 1974;78:917.

98. Pfister RR, Murphy GE. Corneal ulceration and perforation associated with Sjögren's syndrome. Arch Ophthalmol. 1980;98:89.

99. Nahmias AJ, Visintine AM, Caldwell DR, et al. Eye infections with herpes simplex viruses in neonates. Surv Ophthalmol. 1976;21:100.

100. Stern DA, Zam ZS, Gutgesell VJ. Primary herpes simplex subepithelial dendritic keratitis. Am J Ophthalmol. 1981;91:496.

101. Poirier RH. Herpetic ocular infections of childhood. Arch Ophthalmol. 1980; 98:704.

102. Shuster JJ, Kaufman HE, Nesburn AB. Statistical analysis of the rate of recurrence of herpes virus ocular epithelial disease. Am J Ophthalmol. 1981; 91:328.

103. Wilhelmus KR, Coster DJ, Donovan HC, et al. Prognostic indicators of herpetic keratitis. Analysis of a five year observation after corneal ulceration. Arch Ophthalmol. 981;99:1578.

104. Stevens JG, Nesburn AB, Cook M. Latent herpes simplex virus recovered from trigeminal ganglia of rabbits with recurrent eye infections. Nature. 1972; 235:216.

105. Baringer J, Swoveland P. Recovery of herpes simplex virus from human trigeminal ganglions. N Engl J Med. 1973;288:648.

106. Norn MS. Dendritic (herpetic keratitis). IV. Follow-up examination of corneal sensitivity. Acta Ophthalmol. 1970;48:383.

107. Bloomfield SE, Lopez C. Herpes infections in the immunosuppressed host. Ophthalmology. 1980;87:1226.

108. Howcroft MJ, Breslin CW. Herpes simplex keratitis in renal transplant recipients. Can Med Assoc J. 1981;124:292.

109. Cleobury JF, Skinner GRB, Thouless ME, et al. Association between psychopathic disorder in serum antibody to herpes simplex virus (type I). Br Med J. 1971;261:438.

110. Patterson A, Jones BR. Management of ocular herpes. Trans Ophthalmol Soc UK. 1967;87:59.

111. Womack LW, Liesegang TJ. Complications of herpes zoster ophthalmicus. Arch Ophthalmol. 1983;101:42.

112. Hedges TR III, Elbert DM. The progression of ocular abnormalities of herpes zoster. Histopathologic observations of nine cases. Ophthalmology. 1982; 89:165.

113. Edgerton AE. Herpes zoster ophthalmicus: Report of cases and review of literature. Arch Ophthalmol. 1945;34:40.

114. Mondino BJ, Brown SI, Mondzelewski JP. Peripheral corneal ulcers with herpes zoster ophthalmicus. Am J Ophthalmol. 1978;86:611.

115. Strachman J. Uveitis associated with chicken pox. J Pediatr. 1955;46:327.

116. Uchida Y, Kaneko M, Hyashi K. Varicella dendritic keratitis. Am J Ophthalmol. 1980;89:259.

117. Threlkeld AB, Elliot D, O'Brien TP. Scleritis in varicella-zoster disciform keratitis. Am J Ophthalmol. 1992;113:721.

118. Frampton G, Smith C. Primary vaccinia of the eyelid. Br J Ophthalmol. 1952; 36:214.

119. Bedell AJ. Multiple vaccination of the eyelids. Trans Am Ophthalmol Soc. 1919;17:273.

120. Darrell RW, Vrabec F. Vaccinia virus infection of the rabbit cornea. Arch Ophthalmol. 1971;86:568.

121. Sachs U, Marcus M. Bilateral herpetic keratitis during measles. Am J Ophthalmol. 1981;91:796.

122. Deckard PS, Bergstrom TJ. Rubeola keratitis. Ophthalmology. 1981;88:810.

123. Pinnolis M, McCulley JP, Urman JD. Nummular keratitis associated with infectious mononucleosis. Am J Ophthalmol. 1980;89:791.

124. Matoba AY, Wilhelmus KR, Jones DB. Epstein-Barr viral stromal keratitis. Ophthalmology. 1986;93:746–51.

125. Manuelidis EE, Angelo JN, Gorgacz EJ, et al. Experimental Kreutzfeldt-Jacob disease transmitted via the eye with infected cornea. N Engl J Med. 1977;296:1334.

126. Houff SA, Burton RC, Wilson RW, et al. Human to human transmission of rabies virus by corneal transplant. N Engl J Med. 1979;300:603.

127. Salahuddin SZ, Palestine AG, Heck E, et al. Isolation of the human T-cell leukemia/lymphotropic virus type III from the cornea. Am J Ophthalmol. 1986;101:149–52.

128. Jones DB, Liesegang TJ, Robinson NM. Cumitech 13, laboratory diagnosis of ocular infections. In: Washington JA II,. Brewer NS, eds. Laboratory Procedures in Clinical Microbiology. Washington, DC: American Society for Microbiology; 1981;1–27.

129. Lee P, Green WR. Corneal biopsy: Indications, techniques and a report of 87 cases. Ophthalmology. 1990;97:718–21.

130. Forster RK, Rebell G. The diagnosis and management of keratomycoses II. Medical and surgical management. Arch Ophthalmol. 1975;93:1134.

131. Jones DB. Decision making in the management of microbial keratitis. Ophthalmology. 1981;88:814.

132. Boerner CF, Lee FK, Wichliffe CL, et al. Electron microscopy for the diagnosis of ocular viral infections. Ophthalmology. 1981;88:1377.

133. Baum JL. Initial therapy of suspected microbial corneal ulcers. I. Broad antibiotic therapy based on prevalence of organisms. Surv Ophthalmol. 1979; 24:97.

134. Chaudhuri PR, Godfrey B. Treatment of bacterial corneal ulcers with concentrated antibiotic eyedrops. Trans Ophthalmol Soc UK. 1982;102:11.

135. Baum JL, Barza M. Topical versus subconjunctival treatment of bacterial corneal ulcers. Ophthalmology. 1983;90:162.

136. Hessburg PC. Treatment of *Pseudomonas* keratitis in humans. Am J Ophthalmol. 1966;61:896.

137. Golden B, Fingerman LH, Allen HF. *Pseudomonas* corneal ulcers in contact lens wearers. Arch Ophthalmol. 1971;85:543.

138. Waltman SR, Kaufman HE. Use of hydrophilic contact lenses to increase ocular penetration of topical drugs. Invest Ophthalmol. 1970;9:250–5.

139. Matoba AI, McCulley JP. The effect of therapeutic soft contact lenses on antibiotic delivery to the cornea. Ophthalmology. 1985;92:97–9.

140. O'Brien TP, Sawusch MR, Dick JD, et al. Use of collagen corneal shields versus soft contact lenses to enhance penetration of topical tobramycin. J Cataract Refract Surg. 1988;14:505–7.

141. Unterman SR, Rootman DS, Hill JM, et al. Collagen shield drug delivery: Therapeutic concentrations of tobramycin in the rabbit cornea and aqueous humor. J Cataract Refract Surg. 1988;14:500–3.

142. Sawusch MR, O'Brien TP, Dick JD, et al. Use of collagen corneal shields in the treatment of bacterial keratitis. Am J Ophthalmol. 1988;106:279–81.

143. Smolin G, Okumoto M, Feiler S, et al. Idoxuridine-liposome therapy for herpes simplex keratitis. Am J Ophthalmol. 1981;91:220–5.

144. Schaeffer HE, Krohn DL. Liposomes in topical drug delivery. Invest Ophthalmol Vis Sci. 1982;22:220–7.

145. Rootman DS, Hobden JA, Jantzen JA, et al. Iontophoresis of tobramycin for the treatment of experimental *Pseudomonas* keratitis in the rabbit. Arch Ophthalmol. 1988;106:262–5.

146. O'Brien TP, Sawusch MR, Dick JD, et al. Topical ciprofloxacin in the treatment of aminoglycoside resistant *Pseudomonas aeruginosa* keratitis in rabbits. Arch Ophthalmol. 1988;106:1444–6.

147. Davis SD, Sarff LD, Hyndiuk RA. Corticosteroid in experimentally induced *Pseudomonas* keratitis: Failure of prednisolone to impair the efficacy of tobramycin and carbenicillin therapy. Arch Ophthalmol. 1978;96:126–8.

148. Leibowitz HM, Kupferman A. Topically administered corticosteroids: Effect on antibiotic-treated bacterial keratitis. Arch Ophthalmol. 1980;98:1287–90.

149. Badenoch PR, Hay GJ, McDonald PJ, et al. A rat model of bacterial keratitis: Effect of antibiotics and corticosteroids. Arch Ophthalmol. 1985;103:718–22.

150. Jones BR. Antifungal drugs for oculomycoses I: Selection of possible useful substances. Trans Ophthalmol Soc UK. 1969;89:819.

151. Ishibashi Y. Oral ketoconazole therapy for keratomycosis. Am J Ophthalmol. 1983;95:342.

152. Larkin DFP, Kilingman S, Dart JKG. Treatment of *Acanthamoeba* keratitis with polyhexamethylene biguanide. Ophthalmology. 1992;99:185–91.

153. White AT, Newland HS, Taylor HR, et al. Controlled trial and dose-finding study of ivermectin for treatment of onchocerciasis. J Infect Dis. 1987;156: 463–70.

154. LaLau C, Oosterhuis A, Versteeg J, et al. Acyclovir and trifluorothymidine in herpetic keratitis; A multicentre trial. Br J Ophthalmol. 1982;66:506.

155. Cobo LN, Coster DJ, Rice NSC, et al. Prognosis and management of corneal transplantation for herpetic keratitis. Arch Ophthalmol. 1980;98:1755.

156. Foster CS, Duncan J. Penetrating keratoplasty for herpes simplex keratitis. Am J Ophthalmol. 1981;92:336.

157. Liesegang TJ. Corneal complications from herpes zoster ophthalmicus. Ophthalmology. 1985;92:316.

158. Bergaust B, Westby RK. Zoster ophthalmicus: Local treatment with cortisone. Acta Ophthalmol. 1967;45:787.

94. ENDOPHTHALMITIS

TERRENCE P. O'BRIEN
W. RICHARD GREEN

Endophthalmitis is an inflammatory process involving the ocular cavity and adjacent structures. Based on the clinical setting in which the disease occurs, endophthalmitis can be classified according to the type of etiologic agent, the mode of entry, and the location within the eye. Infectious etiologic agents include bacteria, fungi, viruses, protozoa, and parasites (Table 1). Infectious microorganisms may be introduced directly into the eye as in cases of surgical and nonsurgical trauma, or may reach the eye via hematogenous spread from a distant site of infection. Noninfectious stimuli causing endophthalmitis include retained lens material after cataract surgery, foreign materials introduced at the time of surgery, intraocular blood, and neoplasms. The inflammatory process may be localized to specific tissues within the eye or may involve the intraocular contents in a generalized fashion. Inflammation involving all ocular tissue layers, including the episclera, is termed *panophthalmitis*. Pain with movement of the eye is a prominent feature of panophthalmitis.

TABLE 1. Infectious Agents That Cause Endophthalmitis

Bacteria	Fungi
Aerobic	Acremonium (Cephalosporium)
Gram-positive cocci	spp.
Staphylococcus aureus, S. epidermidis	Aspergillus spp.
Streptococcus pneumoniae, other	Blastomyces dermatitidis
Streptococcus and Enterococcus	Candida spp., including
spp.	C. (Torulopsis) glabrata
Gram-positive bacilli	Cladosporium spp.
Bacillus cereus, B. subtilis, and other	Coccidioides immitis
Bacillus spp.	Cryptococcus neoformans
Corynebacterium	Exophiala jeanselmei
pseudodiphtheriticum	Fusarium spp.
(C. hofmannii)	Graphium spp.
Corynebacterium spp.	Histoplasma capsulatum
Listeria monocytogenes	Mucor spp.
Gram-negative cocci	Neurospora sitophila
Neisseria meningitidis	Rhizopus spp.
Gram-negative bacilli	Paecilomyces spp.
Acinetobacter spp.	Penicillium spp.
Alcaligenes faecalis	Pseudallescheria (Petriellidium)
Enterobacter spp.	boydii (Scedosporium
Escherichia coli	apiospermum)
Flavobacterium meningosepticum	Sporothrix schenckii
Haemophilus influenzae	Trichosporon beigelii
Klebsiella spp.	(cutaneum)
Moraxella spp.	Volutella spp.
Proteus spp.	Virus
Pseudomonas aeruginosa	Herpes simplex virus
Salmonella typhimurium	Herpes zoster virus
Serratia marcescens	Cytomegalovirus
Anaerobic	Rubella
Clostridium spp.	Rubeola
Propionibacterium acnes	Parasites
Never grown in vitro	Onchocerca volvulus
Whipples' disease bacillus	Taenia solium (cysticercosis)
("Tropherema whippelii")	Toxocara canis and T. cati
Spirochetes	Toxoplasma gondii
Treponema pallidum	Pneumocystis carinii
Higher bacteria	
Actinomyces israelii	
Mycobacterium tuberculosis,	
M. leprae, and other nontuberculous	
mycobacteria	

BACTERIAL ENDOPHTHALMITIS

Bacteria are the most common causative infectious agents of endophthalmitis. The typical clinical course of bacterial endophthalmitis develops suddenly with rapid progression.[1] Symptoms and signs of ocular inflammation manifest in the first 24–48 hours following surgical or nonsurgical trauma. Development of increasing pain with progressive blurred vision in the early postoperative period accompanied by exaggerated conjunctival hyperemia, chemosis, lid edema, corneal edema, with anterior chamber and vitreous inflammatory cell reaction, is highly suggestive of bacterial endophthalmitis. Careful slit-lamp biomicroscopic examination and direct or indirect ophthalmoscopy are necessary to detect the earliest signs of endophthalmitis.

Most cases of bacterial endophthalmitis develop after intraocular surgery. Since cataract surgery with placement of intraocular lenses has evolved as the most common intraocular operative procedure, bacterial endophthalmitis is encountered most frequently after cataract surgery. The usefulness of prophylactic antiseptics and antibiotics applied topically or subconjunctivally before, during, or after surgery remains unproven, although preoperative topical antibiotics are widely used.[2–5] The ocular surface microflora are responsible for the majority of infections and probably gain access to the eye during surgery. The techniques of molecular epidemiology implicate the patient's external ocular tissue as the source of the infecting organism in a majority of cases of acute postoperative endophthalmitis.[6] Conjunctival preparation with povidone-iodine appears to reduce the incidence of postoperative endophthalmitis.[7]

Virtually any bacterial microorganism, including those previously considered saprophytic, may cause endophthalmitis[8–26] (Table 1). Staphylococcus aureus is responsible for 50 percent

of the cases of endophthalmitis after cataract extraction.[4] Infections due to S. aureus and Pseudomonas are usually manifested in a fulminating fashion in the early postoperative period.

The incidence of endophthalmitis after cataract extraction varies from 0.078 percent[4,27] to 0.496 percent[5] and 0.53 percent.[28] Postoperative endophthalmitis occurs in 0.2 percent of cases after penetrating keratoplasties.[29,30] Contamination of intraocular lenses has produced isolated endophthalmitis.[31–33] Short-term storage of corneal buttons in McCarey-Kaufman media[34] has resulted in endophthalmitis.

Bacterial endophthalmitis may follow surgical procedures for glaucoma,[35–37] retinal detachment,[38] strabismus,[39] pterygia,[40] myopia,[41] and corneal transplantation.[34,42] Postoperative complications such as wound leaks,[43] unplanned filtering blebs,[44,45] vitreous wick syndrome,[46] epithelial ingrowth, and retained lens material[47] may predispose to bacterial endophthalmitis. An incidence of 1.2–9.0 percent has been reported for late endophthalmitis in patients who have had glaucoma procedures.[48] The use of contact lenses in patients with inadvertent postoperative blebs may lead to endophthalmitis.[44] Recently, persistent low-grade infections with organisms of low virulence such as Propionibacterium acnes have been recognized to cause chronic inflammation after cataract extraction.[49]

Bacterial endophthalmitis is surprisingly rare after penetrating nonsurgical trauma.[50–52] Bacillus species are the most commonly isolated organisms following penetrating trauma.[53] The development of tetanus has been reported after penetrating ocular trauma.[54,55]

Sudden onset of endophthalmitis in an unoperated nontraumatized eye suggests hematogenous spread from a distant focus of infection.[56–62] The clinical picture of endogenous endophthalmitis is similar to that seen in postoperative bacterial endophthalmitis except that the posterior segment of the eye is usually involved and the patients are usually extremely ill and often immunologically compromised.[59,63–65] Dental procedures have occasionally preceded the development of bacterial endophthalmitis.[66,67] Neonates and women in the puerperal period may also occasionally develop endogenous endophthalmitis.[68–70]

Common clinical features of endogenous endophthalmitis include decreased visual acuity, pain, hypopyon, or severe anterior uveitis and conjunctival hyperemia. Often a focal chorioretinitis may develop within hours of metastatic seeding. Vitreous infection and finally an acute panophthalmitis may follow. Endophthalmitis may also rarely occur as a result of progressive severe bacterial corneal ulceration.

In hematogenous bacterial disease, a septic focus may be apparent prior to the onset of endophthalmitis. Meningitis, abdominal infection, endocarditis, pneumonia, otitis media, breast abscess, paronychia, pharyngitis, or lymphangitis may be the origin of septic foci.

Since the etiologic agents are usually of low virulence in subacute bacterial endocarditis, ocular findings may be minimal. Conjunctival and retinal hemorrhages are the most frequent findings. Retinal hemorrhages having white centers, called Roth spots, may represent septic retinitis. These lesions are characteristic but not pathognomonic of subacute bacterial endocarditis, since most hemorrhages with white centers are due to the accumulation of platelets and fibrin. Rapidly progressive bacterial endophthalmitis due to Bacillus cereus may occur after trauma, following transfusion with contaminated blood, and after intravenous heroin injection.[71] Various agents, including Haemophilus influenzae, Streptococcus, and Neisseria meningitidis have been implicated in unilateral and bilateral endophthalmitis associated with meningitis.[60,61,72]

In miliary tuberculosis, small elevated yellow-white choroidal nodules with indistinct borders may be observed.[73] Tuberculous retinitis and endophthalmitis have been observed.[74]

In congenital syphilis, a severe chorioretinitis leads to extensive chorioretinal scarring with a variety of patterns.[74]

In secondary and late acquired syphilis, iridocyclitis is the most frequent ocular finding.[75] Other inflammatory features include retinal vasculitis, phlebitis, periarteritis, panuveitis, "posterior uveitis," multifocal choroiditis ("salt and pepper fundus"), chorioretinitis, papillitis, and neuroretinitis.[74]

Nocardiosis may cause hematogenous endophthalmitis by dissemination from the lung, usually in immunosuppressed patients. There have been 11 reported cases of hematogenous intraocular involvement and three cases after trauma or surgery.[74] With ocular involvement, the patients complain of blurred vision and pain. Ophthalmoscopic examination discloses central or paracentral foci of necrotizing chorioretinitis.[76,77] Discrete detachments of the retinal pigment epithelium may occur in early cases. A vitreous abscess may ensue.

Endogenous bacterial endophthalmitis may occur in Whipple's disease, and macrophages with phagocytosed bacilli in varying stages of breakdown have been observed in the vitreous cavity and retina.[78]

Delayed-onset postcataract extraction endophthalmitis in pseudophakic patients can have a chronic course with recurrent low-grade inflammation. The spectrum of organisms include most notably *Propionibacterium acnes,* as well as coagulase-negative staphylococci, nontuberculous mycobacteria, and *Corynebacterium* spp.[79]

FUNGAL ENDOPHTHALMITIS

The incidence of systemic fungal infections has increased over the past several decades, perhaps in part due to the widespread use of antibiotics, corticosteroids, chemotherapy, and immunosuppressive therapy; to increased intravenous narcotic abuse[80–85]; and to hyperalimentation.[86–88]

Fungi generally considered to be saprophytes can cause endophthalmitis. Over 20 different fungal organisms have been isolated from cases of intraocular mycoses.[89]

Fungal endophthalmitis may occur after exogenous or endogenous routes of organism entry. Exogenous sources include extension of a fungal keratitis with or without perforation and following surgical or nonsurgical trauma,[90] including outbreaks of fungal endophthalmitis due to contaminated ophthalmic irrigation solution.[91] The principal clinical difference between bacterial and fungal endophthalmitis after trauma or surgery is the time of onset of symptoms and signs. Typically, in a fungal endophthalmitis the onset of symptoms and signs is delayed in comparison with bacterial endophthalmitis. After intraocular surgery, there may be a lapse of several weeks before the development of ocular pain, ciliary injection, and signs of a nonspecific uveitis. On slit-lamp examination, a localized gray-white area may be seen in the anterior vitreous adjacent to the pupillary border. A transient hypopyon may occur, and additional satellite lesions occur in the anterior vitreous. In rare instances, the site of infection and abscess formation may occur in the anterior chamber usually near the chamber angle.

The incidence of fungal endophthalmitis after cataract surgery is very low. In one series of 36,000 cataract extractions, only 2 cases of fungal infection were reported.[92] However, an outbreak of fungal endophthalmitis has occurred after implantation of contaminated intraocular lenses[93,94] and in isolated cases after retinal reattachment surgery.[95] Fungal endophthalmitis has also occurred after penetrating keratoplasty using cryopreserved or organ-cultured tissue.[96,97] Fungi isolated postoperatively have included *Volutella* spp.,[98] *Neurospora sitophila,*[99] *Scedosporium apiospermum,*[100] *Candida parapsilosis,*[101] *Trichosporon beigelii (cutaneum),*[102] *Paecilomyces lilacinus,*[92,103] *Acremonium (cephalosporium),*[97] and *Candida (Torulopsis) glabrata* (Table 1).[96]

After penetrating nonsurgical trauma, signs of fungal endophthalmitis may develop in an indolent fashion many weeks later.[104–106] Extension of fungal ulcerative keratitis may also lead to endophthalmitis.[107,108] In endogenous fungal endophthalmitis from hematogenous dissemination, the ocular involvement

may be the first or only manifestation. Evidence of nonocular foci of metastatic fungal disease may not be present. In one series of 133 patients who died with a deep mycosis, 14 (10.5 percent) were found to have ocular involvement (11 with *Candida,* 2 with *Aspergillus,* and 1 with *Cryptococcus*).[109] Reduction of vision is the usual initial symptom. At first, only a slight preretinal vitreous haze may be seen. Within a few days, fluffy white exudates in the anterior vitreous occur. The degree of inflammation may vary from a localized abscess to a diffuse vitritis and total endophthalmitis. Chorioretinal or vitreoretinal scarring may result in a severe reduction of vision or even loss of the eye.

Candida albicans is the most frequently reported cause of endogenous fungal endophthalmitis (see Ch. 237).[110–116] Intraocular infection by *Candida* spp. has increased impressively over the past three to four decades, partly accounted for by increased clinical suspicion.

Candida is a common colonizing organism of the human mouth, vagina, and colon. Colonization is enhanced by administration of broad-spectrum antibiotics. The fungus can gain access to the body from these sites or from skin contamination when integumentary barriers are broken by intravenous catheters and either trauma or surgery on the gastrointestinal tract. Host defenses may be weakened by corticosteroid or other immunosuppressive therapy, diabetes mellitus, and the extremes of age. In a review of 100 cases of endophthalmitis due to *Candida,* 85 percent of patients previously received broad-spectrum antibiotics and 17 percent received systemic corticosteroids.[117] Approximately one-half of the patients treated with corticosteroids were concurrently on systemic antibiotics. Other associations included abdominal, thoracic, or cardiac surgery performed a short time before development of candidiasis (53 patients), diabetes mellitus (9 patients), and chronic alcoholism with cirrhosis (6 patients). In this series, *Candida* was commonly isolated from the blood, urine, or tip of intravenous catheters and sometimes from more than one of these sites.

Candida endophthalmitis may occur in otherwise healthy persons following intravenous injection of a contaminated anesthetic,[118] although the majority of cases originate with catheter-acquired candidemia. The ocular symptoms generally become manifest following a latent period of many days after *Candida* is recovered from the blood, although retinal lesions are generally visible much earlier.[117] Symptoms include blurred vision, pain, and redness of the eyes. Frequently, the patient does not report early symptoms because of concomitant grave illness, endotracheal intubation, or depressed mentation. Fluffy yellow-white retinal, chorioretinal, or vitreoretinal lesions are seen. Although the border of the lesions eventually may become cloudy because of vitreous extension, early lesions resemble the cotton wool spots of diabetes mellitus, retinal lesions of HIV-1 infection, a Roth spot of subacute bacterial endocarditis, or the cytoid body of systemic lupus erythematosus. Gradual enlargement over a few days aids in distinguishing *Candida* endophthalmitis, although *Candida* lesions may regress spontaneously. Ocular lesions are unilateral in one-half of the cases. Spread of retinal infection into the vitreous leads to a vitreous abscess, which is later obscured by diffuse inflammation and clouding of the vitreous. Vitritis may provide an early clue that the lesion is not due to cytomegalovirus or toxoplasmosis. Occasionally patients present with an abscess of the iris or ciliary body. More commonly, extension of *Candida* endophthalmitis into the anterior chamber is a late finding.[119] Prognosis for the return of normal visual acuity in an eye with a *Candida* vitreous abscess is guarded despite appropriate therapy.[110–112] Recognition of an early ophthalmoscopic lesion may not only preserve vision, but may provide useful evidence of disseminated candidiasis. In one autopsy series of 15 cases with *Candida* endophthalmitis, 13 had *Candida* in other organs.[111] Periodic ophthalmoscopic examinations are indicated in patients with known or suspected candidemia.

In reported cases of endophthalmitis due to *Aspergillus*[74,117] a high percentage of patients had underlying systemic debilitating conditions. Antibiotics, corticosteroids, and immunosuppressive therapy alone or in combination were used in about one-half of patients before the onset of infection. Intravenous injection of illicit drugs is another cause of *Aspergillus* endophthalmitis.[80,84] The most common sign is an iridocyclitis or a vitritis with associated yellow-white retinal lesions. Retinal hemorrhages, hypopyon, scleritis, and panophthalmitis are also seen. Endophthalmitis due to *Aspergillus* has also been observed after accidental and surgical trauma.[120]

Cryptococcosis may occur in previously normal patients but more commonly occurs in patients immunocompromised by adrenal corticosteroid therapy or advanced HIV-1 infection.[124] Although the presumed portal is always the lung, most patients present with symptoms of meningitis. Diagnosis is made by isolating *Cryptococcus neoformans* from cerebrospinal fluid (CSF), blood, or other sites. Detection of the capsular polysaccharide antigen in serum or CSF or visualizing the organism in biopsy or India ink smear of CSF provides presumptive diagnosis. Infection is already extensive when cryptococcosis is first detected because of the paucity of inflammatory response elicited by the fungus.[121,122]

Ocular manifestations sometimes accompanying intracranial involvement include papilledema, nystagmus, extraocular muscle paresis, and blindness.[123] Intraocular involvement may occur as a complication of disseminated cryptococcosis or as the sole manifestation. The most common ocular symptom is blurred vision. Intraocular signs include uveitis, papilledema, retinal hemorrhages, exudates, optic atrophy, and detachment. Discrete yellow choroidal or chorioretinal lesions may be seen.

Acute or chronic pneumonia is the most common manifestation of coccidioidomycosis (see ch. 246). Hematogenous spread results in lesions elsewhere, especially in the bone and the skin. Dissemination from the lung is more likely in black and immunocompromised patients, particularly those receiving adrenal corticosteroids or with advanced HIV-1 infection. Ocular coccidioidomycosis is generally part of a widespread infection but may be the only evidence of disseminated disease. Ocular symptoms include blurred vision, pain, and photophobia. Multiple yellow-white chorioretinal lesions that are 0.1–0.5 optic disc diameter in size are present, often with pigmented borders. Juxtapapillary chorioretinal lesions, retinal exudates,[125] recurrent uveitis,[126,127] secondary glaucoma, perivascular sheathing, and serous retinal detachment overlying the lesion in the macular area have been reported.[128,129] A combination of diffuse pulmonary disease and widespread dissemination may occur in AIDS.[130]

The usual form of ocular involvement with *Sporothrix schenckii* is a lid or conjunctival nodule. In the rare case of intraocular sporotrichosis, the most common presenting sign has been anterior uveitis.[117,126] Of 22 reported cases of sporotrichosis,[74] a lid or conjunctival lesion was present in 4 patients.

Lid lesions are the most common ocular manifestation of North American blastomycosis. In the rare patient with intraocular involvement, blurred vision and pain may occur. An anterior uveitis and secondary glaucoma can be present.[131] Yellow nodules on the iris and yellow-white posterior fundus lesions may also be seen. Of the six cases of intraocular blastomycosis reported, endophthalmitis was observed in three, an iritis or iridocyclitis in two, and bilateral choroiditis in one. A mixed acute and chronic granulomatous inflammatory response is characteristic of North American blastomycosis.

In mucormycosis, the orbit is involved by direct extension from infection of the sinuses. No cases of hematogenous endophthalmitis due to mucormycosis have been reported.[117] In craniofacial mucormycosis, however, eyes examined histopathologically have shown changes varying from normal to panophthalmitis with ophthalmic artery and central retinal artery occlusion or thrombosis.[132]

A clinically distinctive form of uveitis has been termed the *presumed ocular histoplasmosis syndrome*. Although the relationship to histoplasmosis remains conjectural, multifocal choroiditis is found to be scattered throughout the fundus, in the peripapillary area, and sometimes in the macular area.[74] The lesions heal with variable chorioretinal scarring. This pattern of chorioretinal scars is the principle basis on which the diagnosis of the presumed ocular histoplasmosis syndrome is made. Even after years of quiescence, macular and, sometimes, lesions at other sites may become "active." Such activity is due to leakage and hemorrhage from choroidal neovascularization tissue that extends to the scar. This sequence of change may threaten vision. The mechanism by which the macular lesion develops neovascularization and its sequelae are unknown. Recurrent low-grade inflammation, presumably related to residual *Histoplasma* antigen, may play a role. Argon laser photocoagulation of vision-threatening macular lesions can significantly reduce the risk of visual loss.[133] Patients do not have active infection due to *Histoplasma capsulatum* in the eye or other sites, and antifungal treatment is not effective. The relationship to histoplasmosis has been predicated on a positive histoplasmin skin test and, rarely, by pulmonary calcifications suggestive of healed histoplasmosis. *Histoplasma* spp. have been identified with varying degrees of certainty in the eyes of six patients with the funduscopic findings of the presumed ocular histoplasmosis syndrome.[134] In eight additional cases in which the fungus has been seen in the eye, the patients had disseminated histoplasmosis and a different fundoscopic picture.

There have been reports of 17 cases of ophthalmic infections by *Pseudallescheria boydii*, of which 7 were endophthalmitis.[135] Predisposing factors in these cases were trauma (3 cases) and immunosuppression (3 cases), but in one patient there were no predisposing factors.

Pneumocystis carinii has not been cultivated in vitro but is likely closer to fungi than to protozoa, based on sequence homology of the small unit ribosomal RNA.[136,137] *Pneumocystis carinii* most commonly presents as pneumonia in patients who are immunocompromised, particularly those receiving adrenal corticosteroid or with advanced HIV-1 infection (AIDS). Extrapulmonary pneumocystosis remains rare but has been seen more commonly in AIDS patients receiving inhalation pentamidine for prophylaxis than in those taking prophylactic oral trimethoprim-sulfamethoxazole. *Pneumocystis carinii* causes choroiditis in patients with AIDS.[138–140] Clinically, the choroidal lesions are pale and oval with minimal evidence of inflammation.

VIRAL INFECTIONS

Herpes Simplex

In herpes simplex keratitis, generally from herpes simplex virus type 1, intraocular inflammation in the form of a persistent, nongranulomatous iridocyclitis may be present. Occasionally, an iridocyclitis is seen in the absence of keratitis. In a few cases, herpes simplex virus has been isolated from the aqueous humor.[141]

The intraocular inflammation from herpes simplex is usually located in the anterior segment of the eye. However, posterior involvement has been documented,[142–145] especially in the newborn,[146–148] usually as a result of herpes simplex virus type 2 infection. Large patches of yellow-white retinal exudates accompanying perivascular and vitreous inflammatory infiltrates are present. The posterior pole of the fundus is usually more extensively involved than is the periphery. When the lesions heal, sharply circumscribed punched-out chorioretinal scars that may be confused with toxoplasmic scars are seen.

Histopathologically, areas of retinal necrosis are present.[149] Inflammatory cells are noted in the vitreous and choroid adjacent to these areas of necrosis. By electron microscopy, viral particles consistent with herpes simplex virus are present in the retinal pigment epithelium,[150] retinal ganglion cell, and inner nuclear layers.[143]

Varicella-Zoster Virus

Herpes zoster keratitis is commonly followed by iridocyclitis. A diffuse choroiditis may occur. The characteristic histopathologic feature of ocular herpes zoster infection is a chronic, nongranulomatous infiltration around posterior ciliary nerves and vessels.[74] Occlusive vasculitis may lead to iris and ciliary body necrosis and to anterior chamber hemorrhage. A perivasculitis and vasculitis of retinal vessels may lead to hemorrhagic retinopathy. Viral inclusions have been described in the necrotizing retinopathy of herpes zoster ophthalmicus.[153] An optic neuritis may occur secondary to periarteritis.[152] Varicella-zoster virus is at least one cause of the acute retinal necrosis syndrome.[78,153]

In varicella infections, uveitis may develop either during the acutely infectious stage, or during convalescence.

Cytomegalovirus

Congenital cytomegalovirus infection is a well-recognized cause of chorioretinitis[154] and occurs in 23–29 percent of the neonates with the disease.[155] Iritis, cataracts, and optic atrophy may also accompany congenital infections.

Cytomegalovirus (CMV) retinitis in adults was uncommon prior to the AIDS epidemic.[156–158] It occurs in patients receiving chemotherapy for acute leukemia and malignant lymphomas.[159] However, CMV retinitis most frequently occurs in patients who have advanced HIV-1 infection and CD4 counts below $100/mm^3$. Less often, retinitis occurs in solid organ and bone marrow transplant recipients.[160–165] Patients usually complain of blurred vision and scotomas. Initially, this visual impairment is mild; but, with progression of the disease, severe and permanent visual loss occurs. Ocular pain is usually not present. Ophthalmoscopic examination discloses retinal edema, scattered intraretinal hemorrhages, yellow-white exudates, vessel attenuation, and sheathing.[78] The picture of a branch retinal vein occlusion or a necrotizing vasculitis may be simulated.[156] As the initial lesions heal, retinal and pigment epithelial atrophy occurs. Adjacent areas of active infection may be seen to progress through the same exudative, hemorrhagic, and atrophic stages. The appearance of the fundus and the maintenance of a clear vitreous humor is quite distinctive and usually is the only clinical sign of CMV infection other than fever.[157] Regular ophthalmoscopic examinations should be performed in all patients with advanced HIV-1 infection or organ transplantation.[166]

Rubeola and Rubella

Measles (rubeola) retinopathy occurs 6–12 days after the skin rash and is clinically manifested by acute blindness due to macular involvement. It may or may not accompany measles encephalitis. In the early stages, retinal edema, attenuated vessels, and a stellate macular figure are seen in the fundus.[78] In the later stages of the disease, there is frequently a return of useful vision and the occurrence of a secondary pigmentary retinopathy that may have a "salt-and-pepper" appearance.[167]

Subacute sclerosing panencephalitis is a progressive, invariably fatal disease of childhood caused by measles virus, and it appears years after the attack of clinical measles. Chorioretinitis is a common ocular complication occurring in about 30 percent of the cases.[168] Optic atrophy, papilledema, and cortical blindness may also occur.[169]

The ocular complications of rubella virus infection include congenital cataracts, glaucoma, and a pigmentary retinopathy.[170]

PARASITIC ENDOPHTHALMITIS

Toxoplasma gondii is a protozoan that causes retinochoroiditis.[78] Since *Toxoplasma* are found primarily in an area of coagulative necrosis of the retina, with a secondary granulomatous

choroiditis, the term *retinochoroiditis* is applied to the ocular lesion. Ocular involvement is present in both the congenital and acquired forms of the disease. A retinochoroiditis usually affecting the macula is present in 80 percent of the patients with congenital toxoplasmosis. The eye is rarely affected in the acquired form of the disease, and it has been suggested that almost all cases of ocular toxoplasmosis are congenital.[171]

In the active stage, the fundus lesion is yellow-white, with indistinct borders and an overlying hazy vitreous. In recurrent disease, an active focus of inflammation is present at the border of an area of an inactive healed scar of retinochoroiditis. An iridocyclitis is usually present, and posterior vitreous detachment with vitreous precipitates on its detached surface is common. As the activity of the retinochoroiditis subsides, its color changes from yellow-white to gray and the vitreous haze recedes. Glaucoma, cataract, vitreous hemorrhage, and retinal detachment are possible complications.

Toxoplasma retinochoroiditis in the immunodeficient individual has more extensive tissue destruction, may be more difficult to diagnose and treat, may have single or multifocal lesions in one or both eye, or diffuse retinal necrosis. The disease responds to conventional antiparasitic therapy, but continued treatment is probably necessary to prevent reactivation.[172,173]

The nematode *Toxocara* is the most common parasitic cause of endophthalmitis.[174,175] The second-stage larva of this nematode is responsible for endophthalmitis with or without visceral larva migrans. The average age of the patients affected is 7.5 years, with a range of 2–31 years. Children become infected by the ingestion of ova present in soil contaminated with the excrement of dogs or cats. Nematode endophthalmitis has been diagnosed in 2 percent of 1000 eyes enucleated in children under 15 years of age[176] and is thought to be responsible for 10 percent of the cases of uveitis in children.[177]

Infection may present as a diffuse chronic endophthalmitis, as a posterior-pole granuloma, or as a peripheral granuloma in a quiet eye.[178] A cloudy vitreous, cyclitic membrane, and posterior synechiae may be present. A *Toxocara* granuloma is typically white with a diameter roughly equal to or larger than the optic disc (1.5 mm). It is primarily located in the retina. It may be present at the macula or at the periphery of the fundus. Other ocular manifestations of *Toxocara* infestation include a localized vitreous abscess, papillitis,[179] pars planitis, and iridocyclitis. In the presence of systemic visceral larva migrans, ocular involvement is rare. Nematode granulomas in the eye may be confused with retinoblastoma and the differential diagnosis is critical.

Diffuse unilateral neuroretinitis is a syndrome characterized by a loss of vision, vitritis, papillitis, and recurrent crops of gray-white retinal lesions; the syndrome progresses to optic atrophy, retinal vessel narrowing, and diffuse pigmentary changes. Diffuse unilateral neuroretinitis may be caused by at least two different nematodes.[180]

Ocular infestation with *Cysticercus cellulosae* may occur in 13 percent[181] of patients with cysticercosis (see Ch. 267). The parasite may be found in the vitreous cavity, anterior chamber, or subretinal space.[182] Ocular inflammation and characteristic retinal tracks may be seen with fly larvae *(Myiasis)*.[183] Onchocerciasis (river blindness) is usually manifested in the eye as keratitis, but iridocyclitis, glaucoma, and choroiditis also may occur (see Ch. 267).

NONINFECTIOUS ENDOPHTHALMITIS

Other intraocular inflammatory syndromes such as sympathetic ophthalmia, idiopathic uveitis, and pars planitis may be confused with the previously described infectious diseases. Sterile endophthalmitis has resulted from surgical contamination of the intraocular contents by starch particles[184] and from probable ethylene oxide/polymer byproducts of the intraocular lens sterilization process.[185] Infection of an implanted intraocular lens by

Propionibacterium acnes may be difficult to distinguish from a reaction to the lens.

Retained lens fragments following nuclear dislocation in complicated phacoemulsification cataract surgery may result in vitreous and aqueous inflammation. In the immediate postoperative period, such sterile inflammation may be confused with the aforementioned infectious endophthalmitides.

LABORATORY FINDINGS

Early recognition of distinctive clinical signs and prompt and accurate microbiologic investigation utilizing the microbiology laboratory to assist with rapid diagnosis of the etiologic agent is essential if functional vision is to be salvaged in acute bacterial endophthalmitis. Although initial selection of antimicrobial therapy is generally not dependent on microbiologic results, subsequent modification and specification of treatment require proper identification of the microbial pathogen and antimicrobial susceptibility pattern. The vitreous humor is the intraocular site from which microbial isolation has the highest yield. Conjunctival cultures are inadequate and often misleading in bacterial endophthalmitis. The anterior chamber, vitreous cavity, wound abscesses, and wound dehiscences are all potential sites from which material should be obtained for culture on appropriate media.[186-188]

In cases of suspected infectious endophthalmitis following trauma or after surgical intervention, both aqueous and vitreous aspiration for microbial culture and smear should be performed. In a study of 140 cases of endophthalmitis, a microbial agent was isolated by vitreous and aqueous paracentesis in 78 cases. In 27 of these, the organism was isolated from the vitreous alone with a negative aqueous culture.[186] The vitreous specimen should be specially prepared for cytology,[189] and centrifugal cytology may be helpful.[190]

Smears of material from each site should be separately stained with Gram, Giemsa, and periodic acid-Schiff (PAS) and cultured for aerobic and anaerobic bacteria, mycobacteria, and fungi.[191] Vitreous irrigation material from vitrectomy fluid can be centrifuged and smeared or passed through a millipore filter that can then be stained and cultured. Care must be taken to exclude contamination by airborne fungi, because they could be suspected of causing endophthalmitis. For the same reason, slides should be cleaned with alcohol to remove organisms before smears are made. Calcofluor white staining for fungi and fluorochrome staining for mycobacteria aid in detecting small numbers of those organisms. *Bacillus* spp., infrequent in pseudophakic and bleb-associated endophthalmitis, is the most common organism isolated after trauma and overall occurs in approximately one of five infected traumatic endophthalmitis patients.[26] The *Limulus* lysate test on aqueous and vitreous material has been suggested to assist rapid detection of gram-negative endophthalmitis.[192] In patients with leukocoria and suspected nematode endophthalmitis, microscopic cytologic examination of aqueous humor disclosing eosinophils and normal lactate dehydrogenase levels[193] may prevent enucleation as a result of a misdiagnosis of retinoblastoma. Enzyme-linked immunosorbent assay testing of aqueous humor material may also aid in the diagnosis.[194,195]

TREATMENT

Successful outcome of management of endophthalmitis requires a low threshold of clinical suspicion for diagnosing infectious endophthalmitis. Acute bacterial endophthalmitis represents a true ophthalmologic emergency, and effective therapy requires early diagnostic aspirates, immediate initial broad-spectrum antimicrobial coverage, followed by appropriate therapy to reduce the host immune and anti-inflammatory response, and, finally, modification of the antibiotic therapy based on results of microbial culture organism(s) identification and susceptibility testing,

plus clinical response to therapy.[186,187,196,197] Surgical removal (pars plana vitrectomy) of vitreous infected by certain organisms may facilitate diagnosis and cure.

Animal and human studies demonstrate that the visual outcome is greatly influenced by the virulence of the infectious etiologic agent. *Staphylococcus epidermidis* endophthalmitis, which appears to be increasing in frequency, responds well to relatively conservative therapy with vancomycin, with or without corticosteroids.[187,198]

Unfortunately, reliable and rapid diagnosis of the etiologic organism can sometimes be challenging. Destruction of the eye by virulent pathogens such as *Pseudomonas aeruginosa, Bacillus cereus,* and *Staphylococcus aureus* may occur within 24 hours, so aggressive therapy appears warranted if these organisms are suspected. Improvements in understanding of the role of the vitreous humor and pathogenesis of acute bacterial endophthalmitis have resulted in an evolving preference toward early mechanical vitrectomy with intravitreal administration of broad-spectrum antibiotics. There is currently no consensus, however, on what constitutes appropriately aggressive therapy. It may include early mechanical vitrectomy[199-202]; intravitreal antibiotics[203]; early systemic, topical, and perhaps intravitreal corticosteroids[187]; and intravenous broad-spectrum antibiotics most commonly including a third-generation cephalosporin. Selection of the optimal agent for intravitreal administration includes consideration of maximum efficacy against the suspected pathogen(s) and potential toxicity of the intravitreal antibiotic preparation. Because of the potential extreme toxicity of aminoglycoside antibiotics to the retina,[204] there has been a trend toward utilization of third-generation cephalosporins having activity against gram-negative pathogens.[205] In cases of oxacillin-resistant *Staphylococcus aureus* intravitreal vancomycin may be the agent of choice. In cases of post-traumatic endophthalmitis, intravitreal and systemic clindamycin therapy should be considered because of the risk of *Bacillus cereus* endophthalmitis.[206]

Effective management of *Propionibacterium acnes* infection may require adjunctive surgical removal of all residual lens material and capsule when the organism is sequestered in the lens capsule.[207] Intravitreal, as well as systemic, antibiotic therapy may be necessary. The organism is susceptible to a wide variety of agents, including penicillins and cephalosporins.

The rationale for the use of early corticosteroids as an addition to antimicrobial therapy is based on the recognition of the visually destructive secondary processes that can occur from host inflammatory and immune response to the causative organism. Unlike various extraocular infections, effective elimination of the organism is not the only criteria of successful treatment of endophthalmitis. If vision is to be retained, control of the inflammatory and immune response, in addition to elimination of the organism, is crucial.

Therapy for suspected fungal endophthalmitis remains challenging due to delays in diagnosis and less information available on pharmacokinetics and sensitivity testing of preferred antifungal agents. Natamycin is the only FDA-approved agent for topical therapy of ocular fungal infections but is no longer commercially available in the United States. Oral imidazoles, newer triazole agents, flucytosine, intravenous amphotericin B, and possibly intraocular amphotericin B have been the therapies recommended.[208] This should be combined with mechanical vitrectomy if any intravitreal abscess is present. The use of corticosteroids, either orally or intravitreally, together with antifungal agents remains controversial.

Candida endophthalmitis appears to be best treated with intravenous amphotericin B.[117] Use of systemic fluconazole for hematogenous endophthalmitis due to *Candida albicans* may offer less toxicity than treatment with amphotericin B, though comparative efficacy is unknown. As *Candida* endophthalmitis resolves with therapy, scarring is a common occurrence. Once vitreous invasion is present, significant intraocular morbidity occurs despite appropriate antifungal therapy. Vitreous organization and vitreous traction leading to retinal detachment may occur.[112]

Candida infection not involving the vitreous may sometimes resolve spontaneously without antifungal treatment.[86] Presumably, these patients have relatively intact immunologic systems. Once extension to the vitreous or anterior chamber occurs, progression to blindness is anticipated in the absence of appropriate therapy.

Combined therapy with amphotericin B and flucytosine appears to provide a synergistic effect in vitro. This combination has been reported to the successful in the treatment of endogenous and postsurgical *Candida* endophthalmitis.[208,209] Pars plana vitrectomy is both a diagnostic and a therapeutic modality that may be used in the management of *Candida* endophthalmitis. It facilitates diagnosis by making tissue available for culture and microscopic evaluation.[188,189] It plays a therapeutic role by removing replicating fungi in the vitreous body, by improving the diffusion of systematically administered antifungal agents into the vitreous cavity, and by preventing future vitreoretinal traction.[210] Because of potential toxicity, the place of intravitreal amphotericin B is unclear.[211-213] However, 5–10 μg of amphotericin B have been injected into the vitreous with reported success.[211]

High-dose intravenous amphotericin B is the treatment of choice for *Aspergillus* endophthalmitis, although the prognosis remains grave.[214] Successful treatment of endogenous *Aspergillus* endophthalmitis usually requires combined surgical removal of infected vitreous combined with aggressive administration of intravenous amphotericin B.[78,80] High-dose oral itraconazole may have some role late in the course of treatment, after the infection has become more indolent.

Of five patients who received amphotericin B for cryptococcal endophthalmitis, two were successfully treated.[215,216] Of 12 patients with endophthalmitis secondary to *Coccidiodes immitis*[117,209] treated with amphotericin B, there was dramatic improvement in both systemic and ocular disease manifestations in two. In the ocular histoplasmosis syndrome, systemic steroids have been reported to be of some value in treating the early stage of serous and/or hemorrhagic detachment of the retina and/or retinal pigment epithelium that occurs in an old macular scar. Corticosteroids do not activate any latent histoplasmosis in such patients. In almost all instances, there is no evidence of actively replicating *Histoplasma* in the lesions. Photocoagulation of macular lesions not involving the fovea has proved to reduce the risk of visual loss.[133] Surgical excision of the submacular fibrovascular membrane offers some hope for treatment of such lesions.[217]

Topical corticosteroids and cycloplegics are used to reduce the inflammation and accompanying photophobia in herpetic keratouveitis. A topical antiviral prophylactic "umbrella" to reduce the chance recurrence of epithelial herpetic disease is usually coadministered. Systemic acyclovir has been shown to be effective in the treatment of retinitis associated with varicella-zoster virus.[153,218] Herpetic retinitis may also be treated with short courses of systemic corticosteroids.[141]

Herpes zoster iridocyclitis is best treated with topical corticosteroids and cycloplegia. The role of acyclovir in the management of this iridocyclitis remains unclear.

In the treatment of CMV infection in adults, early reduction or discontinuation of immunosuppressive therapy, if possible, should help in limiting the progression of the ocular and systemic infection.[219] Ganciclovir is effective therapy for AIDS patients with CMV retinitis. Ganciclovir should be given in a maintenance dose to delay relapse in AIDS patients, but those who do not die from other causes will have recurrent CMV retinitis.[220] A randomized comparative treatment trial for CMV retinitis with ganciclovir and foscarnet demonstrated improved survival for those individuals randomized to treatment with foscarnet, but this may have been due to the lack of concomitant antiretroviral

therapy in the ganciclovir group.[221] Both ganciclovir and foscarnet had similar efficacy in controlling the CMV retinitis. Intraocular delivery devices for sustained release application of ganciclovir are under investigation.

In the treatment of ocular toxoplasmosis, mydriatics, topical corticosteroids, systemic and/or periocular depot administration of corticosteroids, and pyrimethamine with sulfonamides have been recommended.[222] Some authorities recommend treatment of cases only with extensive involvement or those in which the macula is threatened with involvement. Clindamycin has been combined with pyrimethamine to treat intracerebral toxoplasmosis and might be considered for treatment of ocular toxoplasmosis in patients allergic to sulfonamides (see Ch. 257).[223]

To avoid ocular toxocariasis, children should be instructed not to eat dirt that may be contaminated with dog feces. Handwashing after handling young dogs that have not been dewormed can prevent ingestion of infectious dog feces. Thiabendazole is effective in the treatment of visceral larva migrans. However, intraocular inflammation develops when the *Toxocara* larvae die within the eye. Therefore, systemic or periocular injection of corticosteroids is the usual therapy of choice.[175,224] Removal of the encysted larvae, lysis of traction bands, and removal of epiretinal membranes can be helpful.[224-228] Diethylcarbamazine treatment of onchocerciasis may cause intense ocular inflammation due to the death of microfilariae. Ocular corticosteroids are often administered to ameliorate the inflammatory response. Ivermectin has become the treatment of choice for onchocerciasis because of the slower mechanism of action and less ocular inflammation.[229]

In cases in which no infectious organism(s) are recovered, intensive topical and systemic corticosteroids most effectively treat the sterile endophthalmitis. Mechanical vitrectomy may be necessary to remove retained lens fragments along with adjunctive steroid therapy.

REFERENCES

1. Forster RK. Etiology and diagnosis of bacterial postoperative endophthalmitis. Ophthalmology. 1978;85:320.
2. Allen HF. Prevention of postoperative endophthalmitis. Ophthalmology. 1978;85:386.
3. Binder PS, Abel R Jr, Bellows R. Postoperative bacterial endophthalmitis. Section II. Ann Ophthalmol. 1976;6:1129.
4. Allen HF, Mangiaracine AB. Bacterial endophthalmitis after cataract extraction. II. Incidence in 36,000 consecutive operations with special reference to preoperative topical antibiotics. Arch Ophthalmol. 1974;91:3.
5. Christy NE, Lall P. Postoperative endophthalmitis following cataract surgery. Effects of subconjunctival antibiotics and other factors. Arch Ophthalmol. 1973;90:361.
6. Speaker MG, Milch FA, Shah MK, et al. Role of external bacterial flora in the pathogenesis of acute postoperative endophthalmitis. Ophthalmology. 1991;98:639–50.
7. Speaker MG, Menikoff JA. Prophylaxis of endophthalmitis with topical povidone-iodine. Ophthalmology. 1991;98:1769–75.
8. Brisner JH, Hess JB. Meningococcal endophthalmitis without meningitis. Can J Ophthalmol. 1981;16:100.
9. Wasserman HE. Avian tuberculosis endophthalmitis. Arch Ophthalmol. 1973;89:321.
10. Ebright JR, Lentino JR, Juni E. Endophthalmitis caused by *Moraxella non-liquefaciens*. Am J Clin Pathol. 1982;77:362.
11. Salceda SR, Lapuz J, Vizconde R. *Serratia marcescens* endophthalmitis. Arch Ophthalmol. 1973;89:163.
12. Bigger JF, Miltzer G, Mandell A, et al. *Serratia marcescens* endophthalmitis. Am J Ophthalmol. 1971;72:1102.
13. Oesterle CS, Kronenberg HA, Peyman GA. Endophthalmitis caused by an *Erwinia* species. Arch Ophthalmol. 1977;95:824.
14. Peyman GA, Vastine BW, Diamond JG. Vitrectomy and intraocular gentamicin management of *Herellea* endophthalmitis after incomplete phacoemulsification. Am J Ophthalmol. 1975;80:764.
15. Wahl JW. *Vibrio* endophthalmitis. Arch Ophthalmol 1974;91:423.
16. Smolin G. *Proteus* endophthalmitis. Arch Ophthalmol 1974;91:419.
17. Tabbara KF, Juffali F, Matossian RM. *Bacillus laterosporus* endophthalmitis. Arch Ophthalmol. 1977;95:2187.
18. Snead JW, Stern WH, Whitcher JP, et al. *Listeria monocytogenes* endophthalmitis. Am J Ophthalmol 1977;84:337.
19. Abbott RL, Forster RK, Rebell G. *Listeria monocytogenes* endophthalmitis with a black-hypopyon. Am J Ophthalmol. 1978;86:715.

20. Ballen PH, Loffredo FR, Painter B. *Listeria* endophthalmitis. Arch Ophthalmol. 1979;97:101.
21. Eliott D, O'Brien TP, Green WR, et al. Elevated intraocular pressure, pigment dispersion and dark hypopyon in endogenous endophthalmitis from *Listeria monocytogenes*. Surv Ophthalmol. 1992;37:117–24.
22. Bagnarello AG, Berlin AJ, Weinstein AJ, et al. *Listeria monocytogenes* endophthalmitis. Arch Ophthalmol. 1977;95:1004.
23. Friedman E, Peyman GA, May DR. Endophthalmitis caused by *Propionibacterium acnes*. Can J Ophthalmol. 1978;13:50.
24. Hanscom T, Maxwell WA. *Corynebacterium* endophthalmitis. Laboratory studies and report of a case treated by vitrectomy. Arch Ophthalmol. 1979;97:500.
25. Cooperman EW, Friedman AH. Exogenous *Moraxella liquefaciens* endophthalmitis. Ophthalmologica. 1975;171:177.
26. O'Day DM, Smith RS, Gregg CR, et al. The problem of *Bacillus* species infection, with special emphasis on the virulence of *Bacillus cereus*. Ophthalmology 1981;88:833.
27. Allen HF. Symposium: Postoperative endophthalmitis. Introduction: Incidence and etiology. Ophthalmology. 1978;85:317.
28. Fahmy JA. Endophthalmitis following cataract extraction. A study of 24 cases in 4,498 operations. Acta Ophthalmol. 1975;53:522.
29. Leveille AS, McMullan D, Cavanagh HD. Endophthalmitis following penetrating keratoplasty. Ophthalmology. 1983;90;38–39.
30. Cameron JA, Antonios SR, Cotter JB, et al. Endophthalmitis from contaminated donor corneas following penetrating keratoplasty. Arch Ophthalmol. 1991;109:54–59.
31. Zaidman GW, Mondino BJ. Postoperative pseudophakic bacterial endophthalmitis. Am J Ophthalmol. 1982;93:218.
32. Schanzlian DJ, Goldberg DB, Brown SI. *Staphylococcus epidermidis* endophthalmitis following intraocular lens implantation. Br J Ophthalmol. 1980;64:684.
33. Gerding DN, Poley BJ, Hal WH, et al. Treatment of *Pseudomonas* endophthalmitis associated with prosthetic intraocular lens implantation. Am J Ophthalmol. 1979;88:902.
34. Shaw BL, Aquavella JV. *Pneumococcal* endophthalmitis following grafting of corneal tissue from a (cadaver) kidney donor. Ann Ophthalmol. 1977;9:435.
35. Hattenhauer JM, Lipsich MP. Late endophthalmitis after filtering surgery. Am J Ophthalmol. 1971;72:1097.
36. Kanski JJ. Treatment of late endophthalmitis associated with filtering blebs. Arch Ophthalmol. 1974;91:339.
37. Freedman J, Gupta M, Bunke A. Endophthalmitis after trabeculectomy. Arch Ophthalmol. 1978;96:1017.
38. Pusin SM, Green WR, Tasman W, et al. Simultaneous bacterial endophthalmitis and sympathetic uveitis after retinal detachment surgery. Am J Ophthalmol. 1976;81:57.
39. Salamon SM, Friberg TR, Luxenberg MN. Endophthalmitis after strabismus surgery. Am J Ophthalmol. 1982;93:39.
40. Tarr KH, Constable IJ. *Pseudomonas* endophthalmitis associated with scleral necrosis. Br J Ophthalmol. 1980;64:676.
41. Gelender H, Flynn HW, Mandelbaum SH. Bacterial endophthalmitis resulting from radial keratotomy. Am J Ophthalmol. 1982;93:323.
42. LeFrancois M, Baum JL, *Flavobacterium* endophthalmitis following keratoplasty. Use of a tissue culture medium-stored cornea. Arch Ophthalmol. 1976;94:1907.
43. Gelender H. Bacterial endophthalmitis following cutting of sutures after cataract surgery. Am J Ophthalmol. 1982;94:528.
44. Bellows AR, McCulley JP. Endophthalmitis in aphakic patients with unplanned filtering blebs wearing contact lenses. Ophthalmology. 1981;88:839.
45. Swan KC, Campbell L. Unintentional filtration following cataract surgery. Arch Ophthalmol. 1964;71:43.
46. Ruiz RS, Teeters VW. The vitreous wick syndrome. A late complication following cataract extraction. Am J Ophthalmol. 1970;70:483.
47. Allen HF. Recent advances in aseptic surgical technique. Trans Am Acad Ophthalmol Otolaryngol. 1960;64:493.
48. Sugar HS, Zekman T. Late infection of filtering conjunctival scar. Am J Ophthalmol. 1971;72:1097.
49. Meisler DM, Palestine AG, Vastine DW, et al. Chronic *Propionibacterium* endophthalmitis after extracapsular cataract extraction and intraocular lens implantation. Am J Ophthalmol. 1986;102:733.
50. Mason GI, Peyman GA, Jampol LM, et al. Peptostreptococcal endophthalmitis with a relapsing course. Arch Ophthalmol. 1978;96:1813.
51. Mason GI, Bottone EJ, Podos SN. Traumatic endophthalmitis caused by an *Erwinia* species. Am J Ophthalmol. 1976;82:709.
52. Lass JH, Thoft RA, Bellows AR, et al. Exogenous *Nocardia asteroides* endophthalmitis associated with malignant glaucoma. Ann Ophthalmol. 1981;13:317.
53. Affeldt JC, Flynn HW, Forster RK, et al. Microbial endophthalmitis resulting from ocular trauma. Ophthalmology. 1987;94:407.
54. Wetzel JO. Tetanus following eye injury. Report of a case: Review of the literature. Am J Ophthalmol. 1942;25:933.
55. Muddappa TM, Rao RNS. Ocular tetanus. Ind J Ophthalmol. 1982;30:163.
56. Burns CL. Bilateral endophthalmitis in acute bacterial endocarditis. Am J Ophthalmol. 1979;88:809.
57. Jensen AD, Naidoff NA. Bilateral meningococcal endophthalmitis. Arch Ophthalmol. 1973;90:396.
58. Shammas HF. Endogenous *E. coli* endophthalmitis. Surv Ophthalmol. 1977;21:429.
59. Weinstein JM, Elliott J, Tilford RH. Metastatic endophthalmitis due to *Salmonella typhimurium*. Arch Ophthalmol. 1982;100:293.
60. Taylor JRW, Cibis GW, Hantil LW, Endophthalmitis complicating *Hemophilus influenzae* type b meningitis. Arch Ophthalmol 1980;98:324.
61. Hull DS, Patipa M, Cox F. Metastatic endophthalmitis: A complication of meningococcal meningitis. Ann Ophthalmol. 1982;14:29.
62. Gamel JW, Allansmith MR. Metastatic staphylococcal endophthalmitis presenting as chronic iridocyclitis. Am J Ophthalmol. 1974;77:454.
63. Rogers SJ, Johnson BL. Endogenous *Nocardia* endophthalmitis: Report of a case in a patient treated for lymphocytic lymphoma. Ann Ophthalmol. 1977;9:1123.
64. Nigrin J, Tyrrell DU, Jackson FL, et al. *Listeria monocytogenes* endophthalmitis in an immune suppressed host. Can Med Assoc J. 1977;116:1378.
65. Blumfield SE, David DS, Cheigh JS, et al. Endophthalmitis following staphylococcal sepsis in renal failure patients. Arch Intern Med. 1978;138:706.
66. Folk JC, Lobes LA Jr. Bacterial endophthalmitis and traumatic hyphema resulting from ocular injuries during dental procedures. Can J Ophthalmol. 1981;16:151.
67. May DR, Peyman GA, Raichand M, et al. Metastatic *Peptostreptococcus intermedius* endophthalmitis after a dental procedure. Am J Ophthalmol. 1978;85:662.
68. Weintraub MI, Otto RN. Pneumococcal meningitis and endophthalmitis in a newborn. JAMA. 1972;219:1763.
69. Berger BB. Endophthalmitis complicating neonatal group b streptococcal septicemia. Am J Ophthalmol. 1981;92:681.
70. Jain MR, Sharma HR. Puerperal sepsis leading to bilateral fulminating purulent endophthalmitis with tenonitis. Br J Ophthalmol. 1973;57:698.
71. Kerkenezov N. Panophthalmitis after a blood transfusion. Responsible organism *Bacillus cereus*. Br J Ophthalmol. 1953;37:632.
72. McLendon BF, Bron AJ, Mitchell CJ. *Streptotoccus suis* type II (group r) as a cause of endophthalmitis. Br J Ophthalmol. 1978;62:729.
73. Massaro D, Katz S, Sachs M. Choroidal tubercles. A clue to hematogenous tubercles. Ann Intern Med. 1964;60:231.
74. Green WR. Uvea. In: Spencer WH, ed. Ophthalmic Pathology. An Atlas and Textbook. v. 5. Philadelphia: WB Saunders; 1985;1352–2071.
75. Moore JE. Syphilitic iritis: A study of 249 patients. Am J Ophthalmol. 1931;14:110.
76. Jampol LM, Strauch BS, Albert BM. Intraocular nocardiosis. Am J Ophthalmol. 1973;76:568.
77. Meyer SL, Font RL, Shaver RP. Intraocular nocardiosis: Report of 3 cases. Arch Ophthalmol. 1970;83:536.
78. Green WR. Retina. In: Spencer WH, ed. Ophthalmic Pathology. An Atlas and Textbook. v. 2. Philadelphia: WB Saunders; 1985;589:1291.
79. Fox GM, Joondeph BC, Flynn HW Jr, et al. Delayed-onset pseudophakic endophthalmitis. Am J Ophthalmol. 1991;111:163–73.
80. Doft BH, Clarkson JG, Febell G, et al. Endogenous *Aspergillus* endophthalmitis in drug abusers. Arch Ophthalmol. 1980;98:859.
81. Elliott JH, O'Day DM, Gutow GS, et al. Mycotic endophthalmitis in drug abusers. Am J Ophthalmol. 1979;98:66.
82. Getnick RA, Rodrigues MM. Endogenous fungal endophthalmitis in a drug addict. Am J Ophthalmol. 1974;77:680.
83. Aguilar GL, Blumenkrantz MS, Egbert PR, et al. *Candida* endophthalmitis after intravenous drug abuse. Arch Ophthalmol. 1979;97:96.
84. Sugar HS, Mandell GH, Shalev J. Metastatic endophthalmitis associated with injection of addictive drugs. Am J Ophthalmol. 1971;71:1055.
85. Michelson JB, Freedman SD, Boyden BG. *Aspergillus* endophthalmitis in a drug abuser. Ann Ophthalmol. 1982;14:1051.
86. Dellon AL, Stark WJ, Chretien PB. Spontaneous resolution of endogenous *Candida* endophthalmitis complicating intravenous hyperalimentation. Am J Ophthalmol. 1978;79:648.
87. Henderson DK, Edwards JE, Montgomerie JZ. Hematogenous *Candida* endophthalmitis in patients receiving parenteral hyperalimentation fluids. J Infect Dis. 1981;143:655.
88. Freeman JB, Davis PL, MacLean LD. *Candida* endophthalmitis associated with intravenous hyperalimentation. Arch Surg. 1974;108:237.
89. François J, Rysselaere M. Oculomycoses. Springfield, MA: Charles C. Thomas; 1972.
90. Fine BS, Zimmerman LE. Exogenous intraocular fungus infections: With particular reference to complications of intraocular surgery. Am J Ophthalmol. 1959;48:151.
91. McCray E, Rampell N, Solomon SL, et al. Outbreak of *Candida parapsilosis* endophthalmitis after cataract extraction and intraocular lens implantation. J Clin Microbiol. 1986;24:625.
92. Allen HF. Amphotericin-B and exogenous mycotic endophthalmitis after cataract extraction. Arch Ophthalmol. 1972;88:640.
93. Pettit TH, Olsen RJ, Foos RY, et al. Fungal endophthalmitis following intraocular lens implantation. Arch Ophthalmol. 1980;98:1025.
94. O'Day DN. Fungal endophthalmitis caused by *Paecilomyces lilacinus* after intraocular lens implantation. Am J Ophthalmol. 1977;83:130.
95. Landott E, Zuccoli A. Mycotic endophthalmitis after retinal surgery. Ophthalmologica. 1970;161:237.
96. Larsen PA, Lindstrom RL, Doughman BJ. *Torulopsis glabrata* endophthalmitis after keratoplasty with an organ-cultured cornea. Arch Ophthalmol. 1978;96:1019.

97. Rao GN, Aquavella JV. Cephalosporium endophthalmitis following penetrating keratoplasty. Ophthalmic Surg. 1979;10:34.

98. Foster JBL, Almeda E, Liltman ML, et al. Some intraocular and conjunctival effects of amphotericin-b in man and the rabbit. Arch Ophthalmol. 1958;60: 555.

99. Theodore FH, Littman ML, Almeda E. Endophthalmitis following cataract extraction: Due to *Neurospora sitophila*, a so-called nonpathogenic fungus. Am J Ophthalmol. 1962;53:35.

100. Glassman MI, Henkind P, Alture-Werker E. *Monosporium apiospernum* endophthalmitis. Am J Ophthamol. 1973;76:821.

101. Rosen R, Friedman AH. Successfully treated postoperative *Candida parakrusei* endophthalmitis. Am J Ophthalmol. 1973;76:574.

102. Sheikh HA, Mahgoub S, Badi K. Postoperative endophthalmitis due to *Trichosporum cutaneum*. Br J Ophthalmol. 1974;58:591.

103. Miller GR, Rebell G, Magoon RC, et al. Intravitreal antimycotic therapy and the cure of mycotic endophthalmitis caused by a *Paecilomyces lilacinus* as contaminated pseudophakos. Ophthalmic Surg. 1978;9:54.

104. Searl SS, Udell IJ, Sadun A, et al. *Aspergillus* keratitis with intraocular invasion. Ophthalmology. 1981;88:1244.

105. Rodrigues MM, MacLeod D. Exogenous fungal endophthalmitis caused by *Paecilomyces*. Am J Ophthalmol. 1975;79:687.

106. Elliott IB, Halde C, Shapiro J. Keratitis and endophthalmitis caused by *Petriellidium boydii*. Am J Ophthalmol. 1977;83:16.

107. Rowsey JJ, Acers TE, Smith BL, et al. *Fusarium oxysporum* endophthalmitis. Arch Ophthalmol. 1979;97:103.

108. Apostol JG, Meyer SL. Graphium endophthalmitis. Am J Ophthalmol. 1972; 73:566.

109. McDonnell PJ, McDonnell JM, Brown RH, et al. Ocular involvement in patients with fungal infections. Ophthalmology. 1985;92:706.

110. Fishman LS, Griffin JR, Sapico FL, et al. Hematogenous *Candida* endophthalmitis: A complication of candidemia. N Engl J Med. 1972;286:675.

111. Griffin JR, Pettit TH, Fishman LS, et al. Blood borne *Candida* endophthalmitis: A clinical and pathologic study of 21 cases. Arch Ophthalmol. 1973; 88:450.

112. Michelson PE, Stark WJ, Reeser F, et al. Endogenous *Candida* endophthalmitis: Report of 13 cases of 16 from the literature. In: Smith ME, ed. International Ophthalmology Clinics: Ocular Pathology. v. 2. Boston: Little, Brown; 1971:125.

113. Edwards JE Jr, Foos RY, Montgomerie JF, et al. Ocular manifestations of Candida septicemia: Review of 76 cases of hematogenous *Candida* endophthalmitis. Medicine (Baltimore). 1974;53:47.

114. Michelson PE, Rupp R, Efthimiadis B. Endogenous *Candida* endophthalmitis leading to bilateral corneal perforation. Am J Ophthalmol. 1975;80:800.

115. Cantrill HL, Rodman WP, Ramsay RC, et al. Postpartum *Candida* endophthalmitis. JAMA. 1980;243:1163.

116. Baley JE, Annabeele WL, Kleigman RM. *Candida* endophthalmitis in the premature infant. J Pediatr. 1981;98:458.

117. Brod RD, Clarkson JG, Flynn HW Jr, et al. Endogenous fungal endophthalmitis. In: Duane's Clinical Ophthalmology. v. 3. Hagerstown, MD: Harper & Row, 1976;1–39.

118. Daily MJ, Dickey JB, Packo KH. Endogenous *Candida* endophthalmitis after intravenous anesthesia with propofol. Arch Ophthalmol. 1991;109:1081–4.

119. Meyers BR, Lieberman TW, Ferry AP. *Candida* endophthalmitis complicating candidemia. Ann Intern Med. 1973;79:647.

120. Roney P, Barr CC, Chun CH, et al. Exogenous *Aspergillus* endophthalmitis. Rev Infect Dis. 1986;8:955.

121. Grosse G, Mishra SK, Staib F. Selective involvement of the brain in experimental murine *Cryptococcus*. II. Histopathological observations. Zentralbl Bakteriol. 1975;233:106–22.

122. Macher A, Bennett J, Gadek J, et al. Complement depletion in cryptococcal sepsis. J Immunol. 1978;120:1686–90.

123. Rex JR, Larsen RA, Dismukes WE, et al. Catastrophic visual loss due to *Cryptococcus neoformans* meningitis. Medicine. 1993;72:207–24.

124. Kovacs JA, Kovacs AA, Polis M, et al. Cryptococcosis in the acquired immunodeficiency syndrome. Ann Intern Med. 1985;103:533.

125. Blumenkranz NS, Stevens DS. Endogenous coccidiodal endophthalmitis. Ophthalmology. 1980;87:974.

126. Bell R, Font RL. Granulomatous anterior uveitis caused by *Coccidioides immitis*. Am J Ophthalmol. 1972;74:93.

127. Cutler JE, Binder PS, Paul TO, et al. Metastatic coccidioidal endophthalmitis. Arch Ophthalmol. 1978;96:689.

128. Rainin EA, Little HL. Ocular coccoidal mycosis: A clinical pathological case report. Trans Am Acad Ophthalmol Otolaryngol. 1972;76:645.

129. Glasgow BJ, Brown HH, Foos RV. Miliary retinitis in coccidiomycoses. Am J Ophthalmol. 1987;104:24.

130. Bronnimann BA, Adam RB, Galgiani JN, et al. Coccidiomycosis in the acquired immunodeficiency syndrome. Ann Intern Med. 1987;106:372–9.

131. Font RL, Spaulding AB, Green WR. Endogenous mycotic panophthalmitis caused by *Blastomyces dermatidis*. Arch Ophthalmol. 1967;77:217.

132. Straatsma BR, Zimmerman LE, Gass JDM. Phycomycosis: A clinical pathologic study of 51 cases. Lab Invest. 1962;2:963.

133. Macular Photocoagulation Study Group. Argon laser photocoagulation for ocular histoplasmosis: Results of a randomized clinical trial. Arch Ophthalmol. 1983;101:1347.

134. Scholz R, Green WR, Kutys R, et al. *Histoplasma capsulatum* in the eye. Ophthalmology. 1984;91:1100.

135. McGuire TW, Bullock JD, Bullock JD Jr, et al. Fungal endophthalmitis. An experimental study with a review of 17 human ocular cases. Arch Ophthalmol. 1991;109:1289–96.

136. Edman JC, Kovacs JA, Masur H, et al. Ribosomal RNA sequence shows *Pneumocystis carinii* to be a member of the fungi. Nature. 1988;334:519–22.

137. Pixley FJ, Wakefield AE, Banerji S, et al. Mitochondrial gene sequences show fungal homology for *Pneumocystis carinii*. Mol Microbiol J. 1991;5: 1347–51.

138. Dugel PU, Rao NA, Forster DJ, et al. *Pneumocystis carinii* choroiditis after long-term aerosolized pentamidine therapy. Am J Ophthalmol. 1990;110: 113–7.

139. Freeman WR, Gross JG, Labelle J, et al. *Pneumocystis carinii* choroidopathy: A new clinical entity. Arch Ophthalmol. 1989;107:863–7.

140. Macher AM, Bardenstein DS, Zimmerman LE, et al. *Pneumocystis carinii* choroiditis in a male homosexual with AIDS and disseminated pulmonary and extrapulmonary *P. carinii* infection. N Engl J Med. 1987;316:1092.

141. Pavan Langston D, Brockhurst RJ. Herpes simplex panuveitis. Arch Ophthalmol. 1969;81:783.

142. Bloom JN, Katz JI, Kaufman HE. Herpes simplex retinitis and encephalitis in an adult. Arch Ophthalmol. 1964;95:1798.

143. Cibis GW, Flynn JT, David EB. Herpes simplex retinitis. Arch Ophthalmol. 1978;96:299.

144. Partamian LG, Morse PH, Klein HZ. Herpes simplex type I retinitis in an adult with systemic herpes zoster. Am J Ophthalmol. 1982;92:215.

145. Uninsky E, Jampol LM, Kaufman S, et al. Disseminated herpes simplex infection with retinitis in a renal allograft recipient. Ophthalmology. 1983; 90:175.

146. Nahmias AJ, Hagler WS. Ocular manifestations of herpes simplex in the newborn (neonatal ocular herpes). In: Boniuk M, ed. Rubella and Other Intraocular Viral Diseases in Infancy. International Ophthalmology Clinics. v. 12. Boston: Little, Brown; 1972:191.

147. Cibis A, Burde RM. Herpes simplex virus–induced congenital cataracts. Arch Ophthalmol. 1971;85:220.

148. Yanoff M, Allman FI, Fine BS. Congenital herpes simplex virus, type II, bacterial endophthalmitis. Trans Am Ophthalmol Soc. 1977;75:325.

149. Green WR. Retina. In: Spencer WH, ed. Ophthalmic Pathology. An Atlas and Textbook. v. 2. Philadelphia: WB Saunders; 1985:589–1291.

150. Minckler DS, McLean EB, Shaw CM, et al. Herpes virus hominis encephalitis and retinitis. Arch Ophthalmol. 1976;94:89.

151. Schwartz JN, Cashwell F, Hawkins HK, et al. Necrotizing retinopathy with herpes zoster ophthalmicus: A light and electron microscopic study. Arch Pathol Lab Med. 1976;100:386.

152. Bartlett RE, Mumma CS, Irvine AR. Herpes zoster ophthalmicus with bilateral hemorrhagic retinopathy. Am J Ophthalmol. 1951;34:485.

153. Culbertson WW, Blumenkranz MS, Pepose JS, et al. Varicella-zoster virus is a cause of the acute retinal necrosis syndrome. Ophthalmology. 1986;93: 559.

154. Boniuk I. The cytomegaloviruses in the eye. Int Ophthalmol Clin. 1979;12: 169.

155. Lonn LI. Neonatal cytomegalic inclusion disease chorioretinitis. Arch Ophthalmol. 1972;88:434.

156. DeVenecia G, Zu Rhein GM, Pratt MV, et al. Cytomegalovirus retinitis in adults: A clinical, histopathologic, and ultrastructural study. Arch Ophthalmol. 1971;86:44.

157. Murray HW, Knox DL, Green WR, et al. Cytomegalovirus retinitis in adults: A manifestation of disseminated viral infection. Am J Ophthalmol. 1977;63: 574.

158. Egbert PR, Pollard RB, Gallagher JG, et al. Cytomegalovirus retinitis in immunosuppressed hosts. II. Ocular manifestations. Ann Intern Med. 1980; 93:664.

159. Smith ME. Retinal involvement in adult cytomegalic inclusion disease. Arch Ophthalmol. 1964;72:44.

160. Aaberg TM, Cesarz TJ, Rytel MW. Correlation of virology and clinical course of cytomegalovirus retinitis. Am J Ophthalmol. 1972;74:407.

161. Porter R. Acute necrotizing retinitis in a patient receiving immunosuppressive therapy. Br J Ophthalmol. 1972;36:555.

162. Wyhinny GJ, Apple DJ, Guastella FR, et al. Adult cytomegalic inclusion retinitis. Am J Ophthalmol. 1973;76:773.

163. Newman NN, Mandel MR, Gullett J, et al. Clinical and histologic findings in opportunistic ocular infections. Arch Ophthalmol. 1983;101:396.

164. Holland GN, Gottlieb MS, Yee RD, et al. Ocular disorders associated with a new severe acquired cellular immunodeficiency syndrome. Am J Ophthalmol. 1982;93:393.

165. Astle JN, Ellis PP. Ocular complications in renal transplant patients. Ann Ophthalmol. 1974;6:1269.

166. Porter R, Crombie AL, Gardner PS, et al. Incidence of ocular complications in patients undergoing renal transplantation. Br Med J. 1972;3:133.

167. Scheie HJ, Morse PH. Rubeola retinopathy. Arch Ophthalmol. 1972;88:341.

168. Robb RM, Walters GV. Ophthalmic manifestations of subacute sclerosing panencephalitis. Arch Ophthalmol. 1970;83:426.

169. Lapiana FG, Tso MOM, Jenis EH. The retinal lesions of subacute sclerosing panencephalitis. Ann Ophthalmol. 1974;6:603.

170. Krill AE. Retinal disease of rubella. Arch Ophthalmol. 1967;77:445.

171. Perkins ES. Ocular toxoplasmosis. Br J Ophthalmol. 1973;57:1.

172. Holland GN, Engstrom RE, Glasgow BJ. Ocular toxoplasmosis in patients

with the acquired immunodeficiency syndrome. Am J Ophthalmol. 1988;106:653–7.

173. Heineman MH, Gold JMW, Maisel JM. Bilateral *Toxoplasma* retinochoroiditis in a patient with the acquired immunodeficiency syndrome. Retina. 1986;6:224–6.
174. Molk R. Ocular toxocariasis: A review of the literature. Ann Ophthalmol. 1983;15:216.
175. Shields JA. Ocular toxocariasis. A review. Surv Ophthalmol. 1984;28:361.
176. Leopold IH. Is the dog really man's best friend? Am J Ophthalmol. 1965;59:717.
177. Perkins ES. Pattern of uveitis in children. Br J Ophthalmol. 1966;50:169.
178. Wilkinson CP, Welch RB. Intraocular toxocara. Am J Ophthalmol. 1971;71:921.
179. Bird AC, Smith JL, Curtin VT. Nematode optic neuritis. Am J Ophthalmol. 1970;69:72.
180. Gass JDM, Braunstein RA. Further observations concerning the diffuse unilateral subacute neuroretinitis syndrome. Arch Ophthalmol. 1983;101:1689.
181. Malik SRK, Gupta AK, Chounhry S. Ocular cysticerosis. Am J Ophthalmol. 1968;66:1168.
182. Topilow HW, Yimoyines DJ, Freeman HM, et al. Bilateral multifocal intraocular cysticercosis. Ophthalmology. 1981;88:1166.
183. Rapoza PA, Michels RG, Semeraro RJ, et al. Vitrectomy for excision of intraocular larva (*Hypoderma* species). Retina. 1986;6:99–104.
184. Aronson SV. Starch endophthalmitis. Am J Ophthalmol. 1972;73:570.
185. Stark WJ, Rosenblum P, Maumenee AE, et al. Postoperative inflammatory reactions to intraocular lens sterilized with ethylene-oxide. Ophthalmology. 1980;87:385.
186. Forster RK, Zachary IG, Cottingham AJ, Jr, et al. Further observations on the diagnosis, cause, and treatment of endophthalmitis. Am J Ophthalmol. 1976;81:52.
187. Forster RK, Abbott RL, Gelender H. Management of infectious endophthalmitis. Ophthalmology. 1980;87:313.
188. Engel HM, Green WR, Michels RG, et al. Diagnostic vitrectomy. Retina. 1981;1:121.
189. Engel HM, DelaCruz ZC, Jimenes-Abalahin LD, et al. Cytoprepatory techniques for eye fluid specimens obtained by vitrectomy. Acta Cytol (Baltimore). 1982;26:551.
190. Stulting RD, Leif RC, Clarkson JG, et al. Centrifugal cytology of ocular fluids. Arch Ophthalmol. 1982;100:822.
191. Jones DB, Liesegang TJ, Robinson NM. Laboratory diagnosis of ocular infections. Cumitech. 1981;13:16.
192. Ellison AC. The *Limulus* lysate test. A rapid test for diagnosis of *pseudomonas* keratitis or endophthalmitis. Arch Ophthalmol. 1978;96:1268.
193. Shields JA, Lerner HA, Felberg NT. Aqueous cytology and enzymes in nematode endophthalmitis. Am J Ophthalmol. 1977;84:319.
194. Felberg NT, Shields JA, Federman JL. Antibody *Toxocara canis* in the aqueous humor. Arch Ophthalmol. 1981;99:1563.
195. Searl SS, Moazed K, Albert DM, et al. Ocular toxocariasis presenting as leukocoria in a patient with low ELISA titer to *Toxocara canis*. Ophthalmology. 1981;88:1302.
196. Forster RK. Endophthalmitis. Diagnostic cultures and visual results. Arch Ophthalmol. 1974;92:387.
197. Baum JL. The treatment of bacterial endophthalmitis. Ophthalmology. 1978;83:350.
198. O'Day DM, Jones DB, Patrinely J, et al. *Staphylococcus epidermidis* endophthalmitis. Visual outcome following noninvasive therapy. Ophthalmology. 1982;89:354.
199. Eichenbaum DM, Jaffe NS, Clayman HN, et al. Pars plana vitrectomy as a primary treatment for acute bacterial endophthalmitis. Am J Ophthalmol. 1978;86:167.
200. Diamond JG. Intraocular management of endophthalmitis. A systematic approach. Arch Ophthalmol. 1981;99:96.
201. Algvere P, Alanko H, Dickhoff K, et al. Pars plana vitrectomy in the management of intraocular inflammation. Acta Ophthalmol. 1981;59:727.
202. Peyman GA, Raichand M, Bennett T. Management of endophthalmitis with pars plana vitrectomy. Br J Ophthalmol. 1980;64:474.
203. Baum J, Peyman GA, Barza M. Intravitreal administration of antibiotics in the treatment of bacterial endophthalmitis III. Consensus. Surv Ophthalmol. 1982;26:204.
204. Campochiaro PA, Conway BP. Aminoglycoside toxicity—A survey of retinal specialists: Implications for ocular use. Arch Ophthalmol. 199;109:946–50.
205. Campochiaro PA, Green WR. Toxicity of intravenous ceftazidime in primate retina. Arch Ophthalmol. 1992;110:1625–9.
206. Schemmer GD, Drickee WJ. Post-traumatic *Bacillus cereus* endophthalmitis. Arch Ophthalmol. 1987;105:342.
207. Sawusch MR, Michels RG, Stark WJ, et al. Endophthalmitis due to *Propionibacterium acnes* sequestered between IOL optic and posterior capsule. Ophthalmic Surg. 1989;20:90–2.
208. Jones DB. Therapy of post-surgical fungal endophthalmitis. Ophthalmology. 1978;85:357.
209. Glumenkranz MS, Stevens DA. Therapy of endogenous fungal endophthalmitis. Miconazole or amphotericin-b for coccidiodal and candidal infection. Arch Ophthalmol. 1980;98:1216.
210. Snip RC, Michels RG. Pars plana vitrectomy in the management of endogenous *Candida* endophthalmitis. Am J Ophthalmol. 1976;82:699.
211. Perraut LE Jr, Perraut LE, Bleiman B, et al. Successful treatment of *Candida albicans* endophthalmitis with intravitreal amphotericin b. Arch Ophthalmol. 1981;99:1565.
212. Axelrod AJ, Peyman GA, Apple DJ. Toxicity of intravitreal injection of amphotericin B. Am J Ophthalmol. 1973;76:578.
213. Souri EN, Green WR. Intravitreal amphotericin-b toxicity. Am J Ophthalmol. 1974;78:77.
214. Naidoff NA, Green WR. Endogenous *Aspergillus* endophthalmitis occurring after kidney transplant. Am J Ophthalmol. 1975;79:502.
215. Grieco MH, Freilich DB, Louria BV. Diagnosis of cryptococcal uveitis with hypertonic media. Am J Ophthalmol. 1971;72:171.
216. Cameron ME, Harrison A. Ocular cryptococcosis in australia: With a report of two further cases. Med J Aust. 1970;1:935.
217. Thomas MA, Kaplan JH. Surgical removal of subfoveal neovascularization in the presumed ocular histoplasmosis syndrome. Am J Ophthalmol. 1991;11:1–7.
218. Jabs DA, Schachat AP, Liss R, et al. Presumed varicella-zoster retinitis in immunocompromised patients. Retina. 1987;7:9.
219. Dorfman LJ. Cytomegalovirus encephalitis in adults. Neurology (Minn). 1973;23:136.
220. Henderly DE, Freeman WR, Causey DM, et al. Cytomegalovirus retinitis in response to therapy with ganciclovir. Ophthalmology. 1987;94:425.
221. Studies of ocular complications of AIDS research group. Mortality in patients with the acquired immunodeficiency syndrome treated with either foscarnet or ganciclovir for cytomegalovirus retinitis. N Engl J Med. 1992;326:213–20.
222. Schlaegel TF Jr. Toxoplasmosis. In: Duane TD, ed. Clinical Ophthalmology. v. 4. Hagerstown, MD: Harper & Row; 1976:12.
223. Tabbara KF, O'Connor GR. Treatment of ocular toxoplasmosis with clindamycin and sulfadiazine. Ophthalmology. 1980;87:129.
224. Byers B, Kimura SJ. Uveitis after death of a larvae in the vitreous cavity. Am J Ophthalmol. 1974;77:63.
225. Belmont JV, Irvine A, Benson W, et al. Vitrectomy in ocular toxocariasis. Arch Ophthalmol. 1982;100:1912.
226. Grand MG, Roper-Hall G. Pars plana vitrectomy for ocular toxocariasis. Retina. 1981;1:258.
227. Maguire AM, Green WR, Michels RG, et al. Recovery of intraocular *Toxocara canis* by pars plana vitrectomy. Ophthalmology. 1990;97:675–80.
228. Green WR. Diagnostic cytopathology of ocular fluid specimens. Ophthalmology. 1984;91:726–749.
229. White AT, Newland HS, Taylor HR, et al. Controlled trial and dose-finding study of ivermectin for treatment of onchocerciasis. J Infect Dis. 1987;156:463.

95. PERIOCULAR INFECTIONS

TERRENCE P. O'BRIEN
W. RICHARD GREEN

Serious ocular and systemic complications may result from microbial infections of the orbit and ocular adnexa. Prevention of complications requires early recognition of distinctive clinical features, prompt microbiologic investigation, aggressive antimicrobial therapy, and proper adjunctive surgery.

The principal periocular structures susceptible to microbial infection include the eyelids, the components of the lacrimal apparatus, the orbit, and the paranasal and cavernous sinuses.

EYELIDS

Inflammation of the eyelids is a common condition that may be due to several causes, including infection with excess oil production. The eyelids display signs of inflammation quite readily due to the overlying thin skin and a subcutaneous layer composed of loose strands of connective tissue without fat. Bacteria are the principle pathogens responsible for most infections of the eyelids, with *Staphylococcus* spp. being the most common cause.[1] The term *blepharitis* connotes inflammation of the lid margins, which is typically chronic and bilateral. There are two main types: anterior (staphylococcal) and posterior (meibomian gland dysfunction). Both forms have similar symptoms, including chronic irritation, a burning sensation, mild redness, and occasional itching of the lid margins.

Staphylococcal blepharitis may be acute and ulcerative due to infection of the skin of the eyelids, ciliofollicles, or accessory glandular structures by *Staphylococcus aureus*. Chronic blepharitis and blepharoconjunctivitis involving the anterior lid margin is most commonly caused by infection with *Staphylococcus aureus* and *Staphylococcus epidermidis*. Chronic infection is often manifested by hyperemia with small ulcerations along the lid margins, crusted exudate in the form of dry scales around the base of the lashes, and even loss of the lashes (madarosis). Exotoxins elaborated by the staphylococcal species may cause nonspecific conjunctivitis, inferior punctate epithelial keratitis, and peripheral corneal infiltrates.[2] Corneal involvement occurs with two principal forms: a marginal infiltrative and/or ulcerative keratitis presumably caused by hypersensitivity reaction (type III, immune- complex-mediated) to staphylococcal exotoxins or other antigens; or a phlyctenular keratitis presumably caused by hypersensitivity reaction (type IV, cell-mediated) to staphylococci and other organisms.

Other bacteria less frequently implicated in anterior blepharitis include *Pseudomonas* spp.,[3] *Proteus mirabalis*,[4] and *Moraxella*.[5] Anterior blepharitis may be secondary to contact allergies caused by agents such as cosmetics.[6] Mascara use has been implicated in some cases of blepharitis.[7]

Molluscum contagiosum may cause unilateral red, irritated eyes with an associated waxy dome-shaped nodule that becomes umbilicated. These nodules may be hidden between the eyelashes and contribute to a toxic conjunctivitis often with diffuse fine punctate epithelial keratitis. Hair follicle mites *Demodex folliculorum* and *D. brevis* have been associated with anterior blepharitis, though their precise role in pathogenesis is unclear.[8-10]

Infestation of the anterior lid margins (*Phthiriasis palpebrarum*) by the pubic or "crab" louse (*Phthirus pubis*) causes itching and red swollen lid margins. Nits (0.5–1 mm) and adult lice (3 mm) may be observed on and between the lashes with red or rust-colored flecks on the lid margin (lice excreta). An irritating bloody blepharitis is sometimes experienced. Phthiriasis palpebrarum is most commonly a sexually transmitted disease.[11]

Posterior lid margin disease (meibomian gland dysfunction) is caused by a complex abnormality of meibomian secretion with alterations of meibomian ductal epithelium and surrounding tissues. The posterior inflammation is probably not due to direct infection, though bacterial flora lipases may play a role in breaking down meibum into irritating free fatty acids. The role of fungi (*Malassezia furfur*) is not well established.

A chalazion is a nontender, sterile, chronic lipogranulomatous inflammation of the meibomian gland that has a tendency to recur. It presents as a lid nodule and may begin with inflammation and tenderness. Once fully developed, the chalazion is characterized by an absence of acute inflammatory signs. If a chalazion becomes secondarily infected, signs of acute inflammation are evident. The majority of these lesions point toward the conjunctival surface of the lid, and they may be large enough to press on the globe and distort vision. Since sebaceous gland carcinoma of the lid may be confused clinically with a chalazion, any recurrent chalazion should be examined histopathologically. The main histopathologic feature of a chalazion is a chronic granulomatous inflammatory reaction centered around clear spaces. These spaces represent areas of lipid material that are dissolved out during tissue processing.

If a chalazion ruptures through the tarsal conjunctiva, there may be an outgrowth of granulation tissue that results in a rapidly enlarging, painless polypoid mass called a *granuloma pyogenicum*. Histopathologically it is composed of capillaries in a radiating pattern and is separated by a loose connective tissue with an acute and chronic inflammatory cell infiltrate.

The skin around the eyelids is thin and may become inflamed (dermatoblepharitis). Dermatoblepharitis may be due to infection, allergy, connective tissue disease, or other dermatologic disease.

Infectious dermatoblepharitis may be caused by primary or secondary infection with herpes simplex virus (type 1 or 2).[12] Herpes simplex virus dermatoblepharitis is more commonly seen in children under age 6, but may occur in adolescents or adults. Primary infection may be associated with symptoms of upper respiratory infection. Ocular signs include ipsilateral preauricular lymphadenopathy, follicular conjunctivitis, and pleomorphic epithelial keratitis.

Varicella-zoster virus may cause dermatoblepharitis in a characteristic dermatomal distribution involving ophthalmic division of the trigeminal nerve. Usually all three branches (frontal, lacrimal, nasociliary) are involved, but isolated branch involvement may occur. Nasociliary involvement does not necessarily predict ocular involvement. Laboratory diagnosis is often not necessary unless there is a question of immune compromise of the host, dissemination, or atypical features. Human immunodeficiency virus testing is recommended in young patients with any potential risk factors.

Dermatoblepharitis of bacterial etiology (impetigo) results from skin infection caused by *Staphylococcus aureus* or occasionally *Streptococcus pyogenes*. Impetigo is most common in children under age 6 years and may complicate preexisting skin lesions in varicella, herpes simplex virus infection, or eczema.

Erysipelas is acute cellulitis caused by *Streptococcus pyogenes*, less commonly other streptococci and *Staphylococcus aureus*. Erysipelas presumably occurs by invasion of the organism into the subcutaneous tissue through an abrasion or inflammatory ulceration and is often accompanied by marked lymphatic involvement. Clinical features include an elevated, erythematous skin plaque with a brawny indurated appearance that progresses to sharply demarcated, bright-red, or crimson erythema with marked edema of the eyelids. A high temperature (103–104°F), leukocytosis, chills, and malaise may occur.

A hordeolum is a common acute purulent infection of the glands of the eyelids and is usually caused by *Staphylococcus*. Depending on the glands affected, a hordeolum can be classified into two types, internal and external.

A internal hordeolum is an infection of the meibomian glands. Hordeola may be associated with diffuse lid swelling, erythema, and tenderness. They may point toward the skin, or the conjunctival surface of the lid.

An external hordeolum (or sty) is an infection of the glands of Zeis, which are small sebaceous glands connected with the follicles of the eyelashes and the glands of Moll, which are apocrine sweat glands near the lid margin. External hordeola are smaller and more superficial than internal hordeola. They are discrete, elevated, erythematous, tender pustules and point toward the skin surface of the lid, usually near the margin. Warm compresses may provide localized hyperthermia to promote drainage, and systemic or topical antibiotics are rarely indicated.

LACRIMAL APPARATUS

The lacrimal apparatus has two major functions. The main lacrimal gland (located anteriorly in the superotemporal quadrant of the orbit) and the accessory lacrimal glands of Krause and Wolfring (located in the conjunctiva) produce the aqueous component of the tear film. The lacrimal puncta, the superior and inferior canaliculi, the common canaliculus, the lacrimal sac, and the nasolacrimal duct are concerned with the drainage of tears from the conjunctival sac and tear lake to the nasal cavity. Pathologic processes affecting the main and accessory lacrimal glands result in diminished tear production, whereas those affecting the lacrimal drainage apparatus cause obstruction resulting in excessive tearing (epiphora).

Canaliculitis is a low-grade chronic inflammation in the canaliculi that is usually due to infection from the anaerobic, gram-positive filamentous organisms *Propionibacterium propionicus* and species of *Actinomyces*.[13] Other organisms less frequently causing canaliculitis include *Pityrosporum pachydermatis*,[14] *Fusobacterium*,[15] *Enterobacter cloacae*,[16] *Nocardia asteroides*, *Candida albicans*, and *Aspergillus niger*.[17] Viruses implicated in canaliculitis include herpes simplex,[18–20] herpes zoster,[18,19] and vaccinia.[19] Inflammation leads to obstruction of the lumen of the canaliculus,[21] which results in epiphora, chronic conjunctivitis, and a tender swollen nasal lid margin that may go undiagnosed for years. Typically, the punctum has a slightly distended appearance. In cases due to *P. propionicus*, a gritty sensation is felt when the canaliculus is probed. Trachoma and medications (antivirals, silver nitrate, miotics, and thiotepa) may contribute to canalicular scarring that can predispose to infection.

Dacryocystitis is inflammation of the lacrimal sac. It is clinically useful to divide dacryocystitis into chronic and acute forms. Chronic dacryocystitis is usually caused by a single site of partial or complete obstruction within the lacrimal sac or within the nasolacrimal duct. The infection is usually the result and not the cause of the obstruction.

There are many causes of obstruction. In about 5 percent of all newborns the distal end of the nasolacrimal duct is not patent at birth, but in most cases there is spontaneous opening of the duct during the first few days or weeks of life.[22,23]

Trauma causing fractures in the nasoethmoid region may obstruct the drainage system at the junction of the lacrimal sac and the nasolacrimal duct. Infection of the lacrimal sac by *Aspergillus*, *Candida albicans*, or *Actinomyces* may occur. With partial or complete obstruction of the nasolacrimal duct, a laminated concretion (dacryolith) may develop in the lacrimal sac and often has associated bacteria and fungi present.[24] Benign and malignant tumors of the lacrimal sac may cause obstruction of the outflow system. Obstruction in the area of the sac-duct junction from a silicone implant used for an orbital floor fracture repair has been reported; a chronic dacryocystitis developed.[25] Foreign bodies such as wood or cilia are rare causes of obstruction of the drainage apparatus.

Streptococcus pneumoniae is most commonly isolated from cases of chronic dacryocystitis. However, a mixed infection with *Staphylococcus*, *Streptococcus*, and *Pseudomonas aeruginosa* can occur. Sarcoidosis[26,27] and *Chlamydia trachomatis*[28] may cause a chronic recurrent dacryocystitis.

Epiphora may be the only clinical finding in patients with chronic dacryocystitis. On palpation of the tear sac area, a mucoid discharge may be expressed through the lacrimal puncta.

Acute dacryocystitis occurs when both the proximal and distal ends of the drainage system become partially or totally obstructed. The obstruction may be due to trauma, dacryoliths acting as ball valves, or flare-up of a chronic dacryocystitis or lacrimal sac sarcoidosis. The major symptom in patients with acute dacryocystitis is pain in the tear sac area. On palpation, tenderness in the lacrimal sac area is present, and purulent material can be expressed in a retrograde fashion through the lacrimal puncta. Localized cellulitis may progress to dacryocystopyocele and orbital abscess. A serious complication of acute dacryocystitis is orbital cellulitis (see below).[29,30] This occurs if the inflammation process involving the lacrimal sac spreads posterior through the orbital septum; this is more likely in older patients with attenuated septa.[31] Marginal corneal ulcers have been described in streptococcal dacryocystitis.[32]

The common pathogens in acute dacryocystitis are *Staphylococcus aureus*, *Streptococcus* spp., and *Haemophilus influenzae* in children.[29]

Histopathologic study of bone from the area adjacent to the lacrimal sac showed normal bone in approximately one-half of patients undergoing dacryocystorhinostomy for acute or chronic dacryocystitis. The other half of the bone samples revealed evidence of bone remodeling or woven bone, but no inflammation. The periosteum of the lacrimal fossa may help to prevent bony changes in dacryocystitis.[31]

Dacryoadenitis refers to inflammation of the main lacrimal gland. Acute dacryoadenitis is characterized by localized tenderness and swelling of the outer half of the upper eyelid, producing S-curved deformity of the lid margin. There may be associated conjunctivitis and periorbital edema. Acute bacterial infections of the gland are uncommon. Infections may occur from an exogenous site on the skin or the gland may be seeded during a bacteremia. Local trauma is a predisposing factor. The palpebral lobe of the gland is more frequently involved than is the orbital lobe.[33] Pyogenic bacteria such as *Staphylococcus aureus* and streptococci are the bacteria most often implicated as causes. Rarely, gonococcal bacteremia may result in an acute dacryoadenitis. Dacryocystitis due to *Cysticercus cellulosae* has been reported.[34] Viral infections of the lacrimal gland cause acute inflammation and usually occur in children. The two viral diseases that most often involve the gland are mumps[35] and infectious mononucleosis.[36] Clinically inapparent infection of the lacrimal gland may occur with cytomegalovirus, coxsackievirus A, echoviruses, or varicella-zoster virus infections.[37] Patients with acute dacryoadenitis complain of severe pain in the lacrimal gland region, and signs of inflammation including erythema of overlying skin, swelling, and tenderness on palpation of the region are noted. Ocular motility defects such as combined abduction and elevation deficiency or isolated abduction deficiency may be seen.[33,38] In some cases (particularly in children), fever and leukocytosis occur.[37]

Chronic infections of the lacrimal gland may be bilateral with minimal eyelid edema. Infectious etiologies include tuberculosis,[39] syphilis, leprosy, cysticercosis, and schistosomiasis.[40] Clinically, painless enlargement of one or both lacrimal glands may occur, and signs of acute inflammation are not present. Similar clinical features may be present in noninfectious causes, including sarcoidosis.[41] Fungal infections involving the lacrimal gland are rare, but include blastomycosis, histoplasmosis, nocardiosis, and sporotrichosis.[39]

Chronic dacryoadenitis of unknown etiology is a nonspecific inflammatory condition, occurring mainly in males over 40, that is characterized by mild tenderness, bulbar conjunctival stasis, and chemosis.[42,43] There is slight exophthalmos and good visual acuity. The cause, although presumed to be an immune disorder, remains unknown.

ORBIT AND CAVERNOUS SINUS

Preseptal cellulitis is infection confined anterior to the orbital septum. Distinctive features include hyperemia of the skin of the eyelids, distension of the soft tissue, and absence of signs of orbital congestion. Postseptal (orbital) cellulitis is an acute infection of the orbital contents. It is most commonly caused by bacteria, although it may be caused by fungi in debilitated patients. It is a serious infection because of the risk of visual loss and the possibility of posterior spread to involve the cavernous sinus, which may lead to thrombosis and death.

There are many causes of orbital cellulitis. Most cases occur by spread from contiguous structures such as the paranasal sinuses. The potentially serious nature of this condition is frequently underestimated.[44] Any of the sinuses may be involved. The lamina papyracea separating the ethmoid air cells from the orbit is thin and may permit the spread of infection. Congenital or traumatic breaks may further compromise this barrier. Additionally, the anterior and posterior ethmoidal foramina allow communication between the sinus and orbit. The bones separating the frontal and maxillary sinuses from the orbit are also thin. In children, since the ethmoid sinuses are the first to pneumatize, ethmoiditis is the most common source.[45,46] In one large series, 84 percent of the children with orbital cellulitis had roentgenographic evidence of sinusitis. This sinusitis was bilateral in almost half the cases.[47] In adults, a frontal sinusitis is a common cause.

Direct inoculation of organisms may occur after puncture wounds to the orbit when they perforate the orbital septum. Retained orbital foreign bodies are another source of infection.[48] Orbital cellulitis may occur as a complication of orbital fractures, even in the absence of adjacent sinusitis.[49] Certain surgical procedures can rarely cause orbital infections. These include exploration for orbital tumors, retinal reattachment procedures, and strabismus operations.[50,51] Foreign materials such as sutures, encircling ocular bands, and sponges may serve as the nidus in postoperative orbital infections, and such materials must be removed to eliminate the infection. Acute dacryocystitis[29,49,52] or posterior perforation of the lacrimal sac during therapeutic probing may result in orbital cellulitis. Rare cases from bites by house pets and rats have been reported.[53] Dental and intracranial infections may extend into the orbit and produce an orbital cellulitis.

In adults, infection of the orbit by blood-borne bacterial metastases from a distant site is extremely rare. In children, however, orbital cellulitis may develop secondarily to a bacteremia caused by *Haemophilus influenzae*.[45] *Enterococcus faecalis* causing a bacteremia with the subsequent development of orbital cellulitis has also been reported.[54] Systemic diseases that may result in orbital infection include influenza, subacute bacterial endocarditis, scarlet fever, vaccinia, herpes simplex, and herpes zoster.[55] In newborns, intrauterine infections have been implicated in the causation of orbital cellulitis.[56] Anaerobes are frequently present in cases of chronic sinusitis and should be suspected in orbital cellulitis associated with long-standing sinus disease. Multiple anaerobic strains may be found.[57,58] Trauma with resultant inoculation of earthen material is a cause of orbital cellulitis due to *Clostridium perfringens*.[59]

The bacteria most commonly causing orbital cellulitis are *Staphylococcus aureus, Streptococcus pyogenes,* and *Streptococcus pneumoniae*.[45,46] Of these, *Staphylococcus aureus* is the most common etiologic agent. However, given the variability of organisms found on the skin and conjunctiva and from foreign bodies, a mixed infection is usual. In children under 5 years of age, *H. influenzae* is the most common cause.[60] Anaerobic organisms found in infected paranasal sinuses can also cause orbital cellulitis.[57,58,61] If crepitation is present, the possibility of cellulitis secondary to clostridial organisms should be considered.[59,62] In patients receiving immunosuppressive drugs, nontuberculous mycobacteria may rarely cause orbital cellulitis.[63]

Regardless of the source of the infection, many of the symptoms and signs of orbital cellulitis are distinctive. However, in some cases it may be difficult to establish an early diagnosis. For example, after severe injuries, hemorrhage and edema in the lids and orbit may prevent early recognition of the signs of infection. Likewise, nonseptic inflammation after intraorbital surgical procedures often mimics bacterial cellulitis by the presence of lid edema, chemosis, orbital edema, and restricted ocular motion. These factors may contribute to a delay in diagnosis. Therefore, it is imperative that the clinician maintain a high index of suspicion of the possibility of infection in such cases. After trauma, symptoms and signs of orbital cellulitis usually begin within 48–72 hours. However, occasionally a retained intraorbital foreign body may reveal signs of infection only several months later.

Fever, lid edema, and rhinorrhea are the most frequent early signs. They are followed by orbital pain, tenderness on palpation of the lids, and headache. Vision is usually normal during the early stages. As the infection progresses, the lids acquire a dark red discoloration and increased warmth. Conjunctival hyperemia, chemosis, and proptosis follow. The direction of proptosis may help to indicate the primary site of involvement in the orbit. There is limitation of ocular motility, with pain on attempted motion and increased resistance to retropulsion of the globe.

Increased orbital pressure, reduced corneal sensation, congestion of retinal veins, and chorioretinal striae may be present later in the course of the infection. In severe cases of orbital cellulitis, gangrene and sloughing of the lids have been reported.[64] Acute infarction of the choroid and retina from involvement of the posterior ciliary vessels and ophthalmic artery may rarely occur.[65] A leukocytosis with a white blood cell count greater than 15,000/mm^3 is usually present.

A different clinical course is seen in "posterior" orbital cellulitis.[66] These patients manifest an orbital apex syndrome in which profound visual loss and ophthalmoplegia develop with minimal external inflammatory signs.[67–69] This condition occurs as a result of contiguous spread into the orbit from an adjacent sphenoidal and/or ethmoidal sinusitis. The cause of visual loss in posterior orbital cellulitis is probably vascular compromise, but vasculitis of the optic nerve vasculature may also be of etiologic importance.[65,66] In the few cases reported, the visual loss has been almost uniformly irreversible. Posterior orbital cellulitis is less common than is orbital cellulitis.[66]

Preseptal and postseptal (orbital) cellulitis secondary to paranasal sinusitis may be classified into five clinical stages.[69] In the first stage (preseptal cellulitis), bacteria are not present within the orbit, but inflammatory orbital edema produced by the proximity of a suppurative sinusitis is present. During the second stage there is a direct extension through bone, with infiltration of the orbital contents by bacteria and inflammatory cells. The third stage occurs after the infection has extended beneath bone, thereby leading to formation of a subperiosteal abscess. The fourth stage is reached when the infection within the orbit consolidates as an abscess. This may be clinically verifiable by the subcutaneous induration of the lids, as mentioned above, and by fluctuance in the orbit that is detectable on retropulsion of the globe. This is quite unlike the usual loss of resiliency and the difficulty in retropulsion that accompanies orbital cellulitis without abscess formation. Occasionally, the abscess may rupture through the orbital septum and present beneath the skin of the lid.[70] The fifth stage is the uncommon late complication of cavernous sinus thrombosis.

Before antibiotics became available, about 19 percent of the patients with orbital cellulitis died of intracranial complications. About 20 percent of the patients were blinded in the involved eye, and an additional 13 percent suffered some visual loss from the infection.[71] Additional complications include osteomyelitis, strabismus, an afferent pupillary defect, a chronic draining sinus, and a scarred upper eyelid.[72] With antibiotic therapy, the prognosis in cases of orbital cellulitis has markedly improved.

Tuberculous involvement of the orbit is very rare, occurs by a hematogenous route, and is unassociated with miliary tuberculosis.[73] The patients are apparently healthy, without pulmonary disease or other signs of systemic tuberculosis.

Syphilitic gummas in the orbit are rare. They may occur in the extraocular muscles, the orbital nerves, and the optic nerve.[74]

The two most common fungal infections causing orbital infection are mucormycosis (see Ch. 239) and aspergillosis (see Ch. 238). Conditions predisposing to orbital mucormycosis and the clinical and pathologic features of the infection have been well described.[75–80]

Aspergillus is an opportunistic mold that is common in the air. The infection begins in a sinus and may extend from the ethmoid sinus to the orbit.[81,82] Chronic sinus aspergillosis usually occurs in persons who have a chronically obstructed sinus due to allergic diathesis, often with nasal polyps. There may be a geographic factor related to humidity.[83] A similar syndrome (phaeohyphomycosis of the paranasal sinus) is produced by *Exserohilum, Bipolaris, Curvularia,* and other species of dematiaceous (dark-walled) molds. Orbital infection with these fungi in the normal host progresses over many months to years. Painless unilateral proptosis is the usual presenting manifestation, but dull pain or decreased vision may be present. Patients with an allergic background have a mass of expanding mucopus containing eosinophils, Charcot-Leiden crystals, and occasional hyphae. Other previously normal patients will have a firm, pyogranulomatous inflammatory mass extending into the orbit suggestive of neoplasm. Other signs of inflammation—such as lid edema, chemosis, fever, and leukocytosis—are usually absent.

Aspergillosis in the sinus of an immunosuppressed patient is typically an acute infection resembling mucormycosis.[82] As a third clinical manifestation, *Aspergillus* may form a fungus ball in a chronically obstructed maxillary sinus without invading the sinus lining.[83] These patients do not have orbital extension. Orbital infections caused by other fungi[84–87] and parasites[75,88–95] are rare.

Craniofacial mucormycosis most often occurs in patients with poorly controlled diabetes mellitus but patients with prolonged, profound neutropenia and those receiving immunosuppressive drugs or deferoxamine are also at risk. Mucormycosis is usually not considered until orbital extension occurs but is preceded by fever and dull sinus pain. Proptosis and chemosis are rapidly followed by external ophthalmoplegia and decreasing visual acuity. Extension into the facial skin or hard palate with infarction and necrosis may also suggest the diagnosis.

The nematode *Trichinella spiralis* may invade the extraocular muscles and result in periorbital edema and pain on movement of the eyes.[91]

Orbital inflammation may be due to a wide variety of noninfectious causes. The differential diagnosis of orbital inflammation has been well reviewed.[96]

Cavernous sinus thrombosis may be difficult to distinguish from mucormycosis and orbital cellulitis. Most often, cavernous sinus thrombosis results from blood-borne infection from the face, nasal cavity, paranasal sinuses, and ear.[97,98] It may also occur as a rare complication of orbital cellulitis.[99,100] Evidence of orbital infection was found in all six cases of cavernous sinus thrombosis that came to autopsy at one series.[101] This suggests that although orbital cellulitis often occurs without involvement of the cavernous sinus, most cases of cavernous sinus thrombosis will have coinvolvement of the orbit.[102] Aseptic thrombosis of the sinus is uncommon, and it usually follows surgical and/or nonsurgical trauma.[103]

The symptoms and signs of cavernous sinus thrombosis are graver than those or orbital cellulitis. The early onset of internal and external ophthalmoplegia is a suggestive feature. Decreased sensation about the eye, indicating involvement of the trigeminal nerve, and signs of bilaterality with paretic muscles in the contralateral eye are strong evidence of cavernous sinus thrombosis. Altered consciousness and other signs of meningitis indicate the seriousness of this clinical entity.

LABORATORY FEATURES

Patients with blepharitis may often be more symptomatic than the clinical findings seem to warrant. In such cases, bacteriologic culture of the lid margins may reveal a dense population of *Staphylococcus*.

In canaliculitis from *Propionibacterium propionicus (Arachnia propionica)* the recovery of concretions is diagnostic. Branching filamentous organisms may be seen with Gram and periodic acid-Schiff stains. Fluorescein-labeled antisera may aid in diagnosis.[13] Anaerobic cultures should be obtained for confirmation, but the organisms may be difficult to isolate.[13]

When obstruction of the lacrimal drainage system is suspected, several procedures are available to evaluate its patency. When the drainage apparatus is fully patent, 2% fluorescein dye instilled in the conjunctival sac may usually be collected on a nasal applicator passed beneath the inferior turbinate (Jones I test). If no dye is recovered, the fornices are irrigated to remove residual fluorescein. The nasolacrimal sac is then cannulated and irrigated with saline (Jones II test). If dye is recovered with the Jones II test when none could be recovered with the Jones I

test, a partial nasolacrimal duct obstruction is probably present. Probing of the lacrimal passages may provide information regarding the site of the obstruction.

Several other techniques have been devised to assess the patency and status of the lacrimal drainage system. Thermography, a process by which body surface temperatures are recorded in the form of thermal images, has been used to study lacrimal system obstructions and inflammations.[104,105] Inflammation induces hyperthermia, and canaliculitis and acute dacryocystitis may be demonstrated by comparisons to a normal contralateral side. Radiographic studies that have been used to evaluate the patency of the drainage system include plain film dacryocystography with contrast injection (distension dacryocystography), macrodacryocystography, scintillography, and tomography (including computed tomography).[106–108] Computed tomography of the outflow system after topical instillation of a contrast agent is useful as a physiologic test with good anatomic resolution.[109]

In cases of orbital cellulitis, the isolation of the causative agent is often difficult because external drainage is often absent, aspiration of fluid from the orbit is contraindicated (unless an abscess is present), and results of efforts to isolate organisms in periorbital and orbital cellulitis are variable. The assistance of otolaryngologist is essential in the management of this infection, because infectious sinusitis is commonly associated with orbital cellulitis. Careful clinical examination of the sinuses with microbiologic investigation of purulent material obtained from the nasopharynx, nasal mucosa, and conjunctiva is important. Blood cultures are essential and are more likely to be positive in children under 5 years of age with periorbital cellulitis associated with an upper respiratory tract infection.[46] Microbiologic investigation should consist of Gram and PAS stains and inoculation of blood agar, chocolate agar, Sabouraud agar and thioglycollate broth, and reduced blood agar in an anaerobic environment.

Ultrasonography is useful in the diagnosis of orbital cellulitis and orbital abscess. B-scan ultrasound may indicate fingerlike clear areas in the retrobulbar space in cases of cellulitis, and an abscess may be manifested as an area of low or medium reflectivity.[55] Plain orbital and sinus films are helpful in these cases and may show sinus opacification, air-fluid levels, bony abnormalities, or foreign bodies.

Computed tomography (CT) and magnetic resonance imaging (MRI) are the preferred techniques for imaging patients with suspected orbital cellulitis.[55,109] Closely spaced sections, with and without intravenous contrast, are helpful. A correlation of CT findings with the clinical stages of orbital cellulitis mentioned previously has been proposed.[109] In stage II disease (orbital cellulitis without abscess), a low-density fluid collection is present between the periosteum and the adjacent rectus muscle. In stage III (subperiosteal abscess), the periosteum is elevated and the rectus muscle displaced by an abscess defined by an enhancing periosteal border. An orbital abscess (stage IV) is manifested by a homogeneous, heterogeneous, or ringlike mass within the orbital space.[110] Computed tomography will also delineate sinus and bony abnormalities and most orbital foreign bodies. Magnetic resonance imaging is excellent for visualizing orbital and sinus inflammation but gives less resolution of bony structures. Orbital venography may show attenuation of the superior ophthalmic vein from increased orbital pressure, which is compatible with cellulitis.

In cases of suspected cavernous sinus thrombosis, MRI is the imaging modality of choice. Carotid arteriography is of diagnostic usefulness, but is potentially dangerous. Orbital venography is effective in the region of the cavernous sinus, and modification of this technique by digital subtraction has also been used to diagnose thrombosis.[111] Contrast-enhanced CT has been beneficial in some cases of cavernous sinus thrombosis[102,112,113] but is inferior to MRI.[114] The cerebrospinal fluid will often show pleocytosis with an abundance of polymorphonuclear cells and an increased protein level, although this is of little diagnostic utility.[102] Cultures of the cerebrospinal fluid are almost always negative in cases of cavernous sinus thrombosis. Blood cultures may be positive.[115]

Paranasal sinus aspergillosis with orbital extension is best diagnosed by tissue removed from the paranasal sinus. Fungal cultures of sinus tissue alone are not diagnostic because the molds also can be airborne contaminants. Septated hyphae can be readily visualized in resected tissue if Gomori methenamine silver or periodic acid-Schiff stain is done. In cases of mucormycosis, positive cultures are often difficult to obtain, and the diagnosis is usually made by histologic examination of excised tissue. Otolaryngologic consultation is necessary, and a biopsy and scraping samples from any necrotic area of the nasal mucosa or palate are essential. On tissue sections, nonseptate branching hyphae that are large (6–20 μm wide) with an irregular diameter are found.

TREATMENT

In staphylococcal blepharitis, the use of a topical antibiotic (bacitracin, erythromycin, or sulfacetamide) or antibiotics/steroid combination ointment and lid scrubs with or without diluted shampoo applied to the lid margins may decrease lid inflammation.[116] Resistant cases or those associated with acne rosacea may benefit from the long-term, low-dose use of oral tetracyclines. Topical corticosteroid drops are occasionally briefly used to decrease ocular surface inflammation. Caution must be exercised to avoid complications from chronic steroid use, including cataract formation and possible glaucoma.

Any internal or external hordeolum should be treated with warm compresses until the inflammation subsides. The use of topical and systemic antibiotics are rarely indicated, and surgical drainage is seldom required.

Because most chalazia infrequently subside spontaneously, typically having chronic or subacute inflammation, surgical curettage and excision may be performed. However, simple observation is reasonable because chalazia tend to decrease in size with time. The use of intralesional long-acting corticosteroids (e.g., triamcinolone acetate) has been suggested. *Phthirus pubis* may be treated by manual epilation of involved lashes together with the use of gamma benzene hexachloride shampoo on the body hair of the patient and that of other family members and sexual contacts. In more widely involved cases, the application of a pediculocide—such as yellow mercuric oxide twice a day for a week, 0.25% physostigmine ointment twice a day for 10 days, or 20% fluorescein topically—may be used.[117]

The value of topical antiviral ointment to treat ulcerative herpes simplex blepharitis is unclear, although a short course of topical trifluridine is reasonable in an effort to prevent inoculation of the ocular surface with herpes simplex virus.

Antibiotic irrigation of the canaliculi combined with topical antibiotic eyedrops is useful in the treatment of canaliculitis. Penicillin G (160,000 units/ml as an irrigant, 60,000 units/ml as drops) is used for *Propionibacterium propionicus* and *Actinomyces* spp.; amphotericin B (1–5 mg/ml) is used against *Candida* and *Aspergillus* spp.[17] Systemic penicillin, erythromycin, or cephalosporins should be part of the treatment regimen in cases due to *Propionibacterium propionicus*.[17,118] When concretions are present, they should be removed by canaliculotomy and curettage. The canaliculus should then be reconstructed; silicone intubation may be needed.[119] Cases of canicular obstruction associated with herpes simplex virus infection may require surgical intervention more frequently than in cases caused by bacteria. A possible explanation is that, in the situation with herpes, the epithelial lining of the canaliculi is damaged with resultant adherence of the subepithelial layers with scar formation. In the cases of bacterial infection, however, the epithelium remains intact, and the obstruction is due to edema, which is more reversible.[20]

Parents of infants with nasolacrimal duct obstruction should be taught to massage the lacrimal sac area firmly several times daily. Topical antibiotic eyedrops may be used for lid mattering. If symptoms persist for 6–8 months, the lacrimal drainage apparatus should be irrigated and possibly probed. Probing is more successful in cases of lacrimal duct obstruction due to membranous obstruction than in cases due to narrowing of the duct. If probing is unsuccessful, repeat probing is done a few months later. Silicone intubation of the drainage apparatus is performed if the repeat probing also fails to succeed.[23]

In adults with acute dacryocystitis, treatment with warm compresses and systemic antibiotics should be given. If *Streptococcus pyogenes* is isolated or suspected, oral penicillin is used.[17] Staphylococci are best treated with a penicillinase-resistant penicillin.[17,29] After the acute infection is controlled, the patient should be taught to perform digital massage of the lacrimal sac, and topical antibiotic drops should be used. If epiphora persists, a dacryocystorhinostomy is performed in most cases to obtain adequate tear drainage.

Bacterial dacryoadenitis is treated with systemic antibiotics. If an orbital abscess forms, surgical drainage is necessary.

Management of post-traumatic preseptal cellulitis includes clinical assessment of degree and evolution of conjunctival injection and chemosis, presence or absence of proptosis, limitation of or pain on extraocular movement, visual acuity, and pupillary reaction. A CT scan or MRI of the orbit should be performed if there is any question of orbital involvement.

In post-traumatic preseptal cellulitis wound sites should be cultured on appropriate media and antibiotic selection based on Gram stain morphology. If gram-positive cocci are observed on diagnostic smears, intravenous nafcillin or oxacillin and, in milder cases, oral cloxacillin or dicloxacillin are recommended. Intravenous cefazolin or oral cephalexin may be administered to nonanaphylactic penicillin-allergic patients. If there is a history of anaphylactic penicillin allergy, intravenous vancomycin is recommended. If gram-negative rods are observed on diagnostic smears, an intravenous third-generation cephalosporin or oral ciprofloxacin depending on severity may be administered. If anaerobic bacteria are isolated with culture, clindamycin is often the therapy of choice. For preseptal cellulitis in children, intravenous cephalosporins that are effective against *H. influenzae, Streptococcus pneumoniae,* other streptococci, and *Staphylococcus aureus* (e.g., cefuroxime or ceftriaxone) are recommended until clinical improvement is obvious and the child is afebrile for 24 hours prior to switching to oral antibiotic therapy (e.g., amoxicillin-clavulanate or trimethoprim-sulfamethoxazole).

In treating orbital cellulitis, appropriate intravenous antibiotics are urgently required, as well as surgical consultation for possible drainage of the paranasal sinuses. The bacterial agents most commonly responsible for this infection were mentioned above. In adults, nafcillin or oxacillin (1.5 g) every 4 hours should be the initial therapy. In cases of penicillin allergy, vancomycin may be used.[72,120] Because *H. influenzae* is a common cause of orbital cellulitis in children, cefotaxime or ceftriaxone is the drug of choice until culture and susceptibility results are available.[69,120,121] If the infection progresses and the clinical situation deteriorates despite adequate intravenous antibiotic therapy, it is probably due to the development of a subperiosteal or orbital abscess, and surgical drainage is imperative.[45–47] Material obtained from such drainage should have the complete microbiologic evaluation mentioned previously. In cases of radiographically suspected subperiosteal abscess that seem to be responding to conservative measures, surgery may be deferred, but inflammatory signs may persist much longer than in those patients treated by drainage.[109,122–124]

If the management of patients with orbital mucormycosis is to be successful, the combined efforts of internists, mycologists, otolaryngologists, and ophthalmologists are essential. The underlying disease, for example, diabetic ketoacidosis, should be treated. Intravenous amphotericin B is of value if begun early in the disease.[125–127] Surgical débridement of devitalized tissue is extremely important. Frequently the involved eye may need to be sacrificed to obtain adequate orbital débridement.

In the treatment of chronic orbital aspergillosis or phaeohyphomycosis, surgical excision appears to be the best method. Amphotericin B is only of ancillary help.

Cavernous sinus thrombosis is treated with high-dose intravenous antibiotics. Adjunctive corticosteroids have been recommended in this entity.[102,128] The role of anticoagulants is still unclear.[97,129,130]

REFERENCES

1. Smolin G, Okumoto M. Staphylococcal blepharitis. Arch Ophthalmol. 1977; 95:812.
2. Valenton MJ, Okumoto M. Toxin-producing strains of *Staphylococcus epidermidis (albus)*. Isolates from patients with staphylococcic blepharoconjunctivitis. Arch Ophthalmol. 1973;89:186.
3. Rosenoff SH, Wolfe ML, Chabner BA. *Pseudomonas* blepharoconjunctivitis. A complication of combination chemotherapy. Arch Ophthalmol. 1974; 90:490.
4. Parunovic A. *Proteus mirabilis* causing necrotic inflammation of the eyelid. Am J Ophthalmol. 1973;76:543.
5. Van Bijsterveld OP. The incidence of *Moraxella* on mucous membranes in the skin. Am J Ophthalmol. 1972;74:72.
6. Van Ketel WG, Liem DH. Eyelid dermatitis from nickel contaminated cosmetics. Contact Dermatitis. 1981;4:217.
7. Wilson LA, Julian AJ, Ahearn DG. The survival and growth of microorganisms in mascara during use. Am J Ophthalmol. 1975;79:596.
8. Rufli T, Mumcuoglu Y. The hair follicle mites *Demodex folliculorum* and *Demodex brevis:* Biology and medical importance. A review. Dermatologica. 1981;162:1.
9. Roth AM. Demodex folliculorum in hair follicles of eyelid skin. Ann Ophthalmol. 1979;11:37.
10. Jutgesell VJ, Stern GA, Hood CI. Histopathology of meibomian gland dysfunction. Am J Ophthalmol. 1982;94:383.
11. Couch JM, Green WR, Hirst LW, et al. Diagnosing and treating phthirus pubis palpebrarum. Surv Ophthalmol. 1982;26:219.
12. Egerer I, Stary A. Erosive-ulcerative herpes simplex blepharitis. Arch Ophthalmol. 1980;98:1760.
13. Hirst LW, Merz WB, Kaufmann CS, et al. *Actinomyces/Arachnia* lacrimal canaliculitis. Cornea. 1982;1:259.
14. Romano A, Segal E, Blumenthal M. Canaliculitis with isolation of *Pityrosporum pachydermatis*. Brit J Ophthalmol. 1978;62:732.
15. Weinberg RJ, Sartoris MJ, Buerger GF Jr, et al. *Fusobacterium* in presumed *Actinomyces* canaliculitis. Am J Ophthalmol. 1977;84:371.
16. Chumble LC. Canaliculitis caused by *Enterobacter cloacae:* Report of a case. Br J Ophthalmol. 1984;68:564–6.
17. Starr MB. Lacrimal drainage system infections. In: Smith BC, Della Rocca RC, Nesi FA, et al, eds. Ophthalmic Plastic and Reconstructive Surgery. St. Louis: CV Mosby; 1987;947–5.
18. Bouzas AG. Canalicular inflammation in ophthalmic cases of herpes zoster and herpes simplex. Am J Ophthalmol. 1965;60:713–6.
19. Bouzas AG. Virus etiology aetiology of certain cases of lacrimal obstruction. Br J Ophthalmol. 1973;57:849–51.
20. Harris GJ, Hyndiuk RA, Fox MJ, et al. Herpetic canicular obstruction. Arch Ophthalmol. 1981;99:282–3.
21. Wolter JR. *Pityrosporum* species associated with dacryoliths in obstructive dacryocystitis. Am J Ophthalmol. 1977;84:806.
22. Corchmaros I, Szalay E. Canula-probing combined with nasal procedure for dacryocystitis neonaturum. Acta Ophthalmol. 1978;56:357.
23. Kushner BJ. Congenital nasolacrimal system obstruction. Arch Ophthalmol. 1982;100:597.
24. Berlin AJ, Ruth R, Rich L. Lacrimal system dacryoliths. Ophthalmic Surg. 1980;11:435.
25. Mauriello JA, Fiore PM, Kotch M. Dacryocystitis—Late complications of orbital floor fracture repaired with implant. Ophthalmology. 1987;94:248–50.
26. Harris GJ, Williams GA, Clarke GP. Sarcoidosis of the lacrimal sac. Arch Ophthalmol. 1981;99:1198.
27. Coleman SL, Brull S, Green WR. Sarcoid of the lacrimal sac and surrounding area. Arch Ophthalmol. 1972;88:645.
28. Bahnasawi SA, Abdalla MI, Ghaly AF, et al. Trachoma of the lacrimal sac. Bull Ophthalmol Soc Egypt. 1976;69:619.
29. Hurwitz JJ, Rodgers KJA. Management of acquired dacryocystitis. Can J Ophthalmol. 1983;18:213–6.
30. Ahrens-Palumbo MJ, Ballen PH. Primary dacryocystitis causing orbital cellulitis. Ann Ophthalmol. 1982;14:600.
31. Hinton P, Hurwitz JJ, Cruickshank B. Nasolacrimal bone changes and diseases of the lacrimal drainage sytsem. Ophthalmic Surg. 1984;15:516–21.
32. Cohn H, Mondino BJ, Brown SI, et al. Marginal corneal ulcers with acute beta-streptococcal conjunctivitis and chronic dacryocystitis. Am J Ophthalmol. 1979;87:541.
33. Ulman S, Sergott R. Abduction deficit secondary to presumed bacterial dacryocystitis. Arch Ophthalmol. 1986;104:1127–8.
34. Sen DK. Acute suppurative dacryocystitis caused by a cysticercus cellulosae. J Pediatr Ophthalmol Strabismus. 1982;19:100.
35. Riffenburgh RS. Ocular manifestations of mumps. Arch Ophthalmol. 1961; 56:739.
36. Jones BR. Lacrimal diseases associated with infectious mononucleosis. Trans Ophthalmol Soc UK. 1955;75:101.
37. Jakobiec FA, Jones IS. Orbital inflammations. In: Duan CD, ed. Clinical Ophthalmology. v. 2. Philadelphia: Harper & Row; 1987:65.
38. Duke-Elder S. The ocular adnexa. In: Duke-Elder S, ed. System of Ophthalmology. v. 13. St. Louis: CV Mosby; 1974:601.
39. Baghdassarian SA, Zakharia H, Asdourian KK. Report of a case of bilateral caseous tuberculous dacryocystitis. Am J Ophthalmol. 1972;74:744.
40. Jakobiec FA, Gess L, Zimmerman LE. Granulomatous dacryoadenitis caused by *Schistosoma haematobium*. Arch Ophthalmol. 1977;95:278.
41. Obernauf CD, Shaw HE, Sydnor CJ, et al. Sarcoidosis and its ophthalmic manifestations. Am J Ophthalmol. 1978;86:8648.
42. Amemiya T, Mori H, Koizumi K. Clinical and histocytopathological study of chronic dacryoadenitis. Graefes Arch Clin Exp Ophthalmol. 1983;220: 229–32.
43. Mcnally L, Jakobiec FA, Knowles DM. Clinical, morphologic, immunophenotypic, and molecular genetic analysis of bilateral ocular adnexal lymphoid neoplasms in 17 patients. Am J Ophthalmol. 1987;103:555.
44. Check WA. Many misjudge severity of orbital cellulitis. JAMA. 1982;247: 1236.
45. Brook I, Friedman EM, Rodriguez WJ, et al. Complications of sinusitis in children. Pediatrics. 1980;66:568.
46. Noel LP, Clark WN, Peacocke TA. Periorbital and orbital cellulitis in children. Can J Ophthalmol. 1981;16:178.
47. Weiss A, Friendly D, Eglin K, et al. Bacterial periorbital and orbital cellulitis in children. Ophthalmology. 1983;90:195.
48. Ferguson EC III. Deep wooden foreign bodies of the orbit: A report of two cases. Trans Am Acad Ophthalmol Otolaryngol. 1970;74:778.
49. Goldfarb MS, Hoffman DS, Rosenberg S. Orbital cellulitis and orbital fractures. Ann Ophthalmol. 1987;19:97–9.
50. Von Noorden GK. Orbital cellulitis following extraocular muscle surgery. Am J Ophthalmol. 1972;74:627.
51. Wilson ME, Paul TO. Orbital cellulitis following strabismus surgery. Ophthalmic Surg. 1987;18:92–4.
52. Allen MV, Cohen KL, Grimson BS. Orbital cellulitis secondary to dacryocystitis following blepharoplasty. Ann Ophthalmol. 1985;17:498–9.
53. Diwan R, Sen DK, Sood GC. Rat bite orbital cellulitis. Br J Ophthalmol. 1970;54:211.
54. Biedner BZ, Marmur U, Yassur Y. *Streptococcus faecalis* orbital cellulitis. Ann Ophthalmol. 1986;18:194–5.
55. Hornblass A, Herschorn BJ, Stern RK, et al. Orbital abscess. Surv Ophthalmol. 1984;29:169–78.
56. Appalanarasayya K, Murthy ASR, Viswanath CK, et al. Proptosis in a newborn due to orbital infection: Case report. Int Surg. 1971;55:149.
57. Frederick J, Braude AL. Anaerobic infection of the paranasal sinuses. N Engl J Med. 1974;290:135.
58. Partamian LG, Jay WM, Fritz KL. Anaerobic orbital cellulitis. Ann Ophthalmol. 1983;15:123–6.
59. Crock GW, Heriot WJ, Janakiraman P, et al. Gas gangrene infection of the eyes and orbits. Br J Ophthalmol. 1985;69:143–8.
60. Londer L, Nelson DL. Orbital cellulitis due to *Haemophilus influenzae*. Arch Ophthalmol. 1974;91:89.
61. Gorbach SL, Bartlett JG. Anaerobic infections. Part I. N Engl J Med. 1974; 290:1177.
62. Sevel D, Tobias B, Sellars SL, et al. Gas in the orbit associated with orbital cellulitis and paranasal sinusitis. Br J Ophthalmol. 1973;57:133.
63. Levine RA. Infection of the orbit by an atypical mycobacterium. Arch Ophthalmol. 1969;82:608.
64. Ross J, Kohlhepp PA. Gangrene of the eyelids. Ann Ophthalmol. 1973;5:84.
65. El-Shewy TM. Acute infarction of the choroid and retina: A complication of orbital cellulitis. Br J Ophthalmol. 1973;57:204.
66. Slavin ML, Glaser JS. Acute severe irreversible visual loss with sphenoethmoiditis—''Posterior'' orbital cellulitis. Arch Ophthalmol. 1987;105:345–8.
67. Kjoer I. A case of orbital apex syndrome in collateral pansinusitis. Acta Ophthalmol. 1945;23:357–66.
68. Jarrett WH, Gutman FA. Ocular complications of infection in the paranasal sinuses. Arch Ophthalmol. 1969;81:683–86.
69. Chandler JR, Langenbrunner DJ, Stevens ER. The pathogenesis of orbital complications in acute sinusitis. Laryngoscope. 1970;80:1414–28.
70. Sen D. Surgical treatment of ''collar-stud'' orbital abscess. Int Surg. 1970; 54:379.
71. Birch-Hirshfield, cited by Duke-Elder S. The ocular abscess. In: Textbook of Ophthalmology. v. 5. St. Louis: CV Mosby; 1952;5420–44.
72. Bergin DJ, Wright JE. Orbital cellulitis. Br J Ophthalmol. 1986;70:174–8.
73. Mortada A. Tuberculoma of the orbit and lacrimal gland. Br J Ophthalmol. 1971;55:565.
74. Whitfield R, Wirotsko E. Ocular syphilis. In: Locatcher-Khorazo D, Seegal BC, eds. Microbiology of the Eye. St. Louis: CV Mosby; 1972:322.
75. Jakobiec FA. Orbital infections. In: Spencer WH, ed. Ophthalmic Pathology: An Atlas and Textbook. 3rd ed. Philadelphia: WB Saunders; 1986:2812–31.
76. Gass JDM. Ocular manifestations of acute mucormycosis. Arch Ophthalmol. 1961;65:226.
77. Baum JL. Rhino-orbital mucormycosis occurring in an otherwise apparently healthy individual. Am J Ophthalmol. 1967;63:335.

78. Hale LM. Orbital-cerebral phycomycosis: Report of a case and a review of the disease in infants. Arch Ophthalmol. 1971;86:39.

79. Blodi FC, Hannah FT, Wadsworth JAC. Lethal orbitocerebral phycomycosis in otherwise healthy children. Am J Ophthalmol. 1969;67:698.

80. Straatsma BR, Zimmerman LE, Gass JDM. Phycomycosis: A clinico-pathologic study of fifty-one cases. Lab Invest. 1962;11:963.

81. Green WR, Font RL, Zimmerman LE. Aspergillosis of the orbit: Report of ten cases and review of the literature. Arch Ophthalmol. 1969;82:302.

82. Houle TV, Ellis PP. Aspergillosis of the orbit with immunosuppressive therapy. Surv Ophthalmol. 1975;20:35.

83. Miloshev B, Davidson CM, Gentles JC, et al. Aspergilloma of the paranasal sinuses and orbit in northern sudanese. Lancet. 1966;1:746.

84. Morris FH Jr, Spock A. Intracranial aneurysm secondary to mycotic orbital and sinus infection: Report of a case implicating *Penicillium* as an opportunistic fungus. Am J Ophthalmol. 1969;68:14.

85. Olurin O, Lucas AO, Oyediran ABO. Orbital histoplasmosis due to *Histoplasma duboisii*. Am J Ophthalmol. 1969;68:14.

86. Vida L, Moel SA. Systemic North American blastomycosis with orbital involvement. Am J Ophthalmol. 1974;77:240.

87. Streeten BW, Rabuzzi DD, Jones DB. Sporotrichosis of the orbital margin. Am J Ophthalmol. 1974;77:750.

88. Baghdassarian SA, Zekheria H. Report of three cases of hydatid cyst of the orbit. Am J Ophthalmol. 1971;71:1081.

89. Mehra KS, Banerjee C, Somani PN, et al. Hydatid cyst in orbit. Acta Ophthalmol. 1965;43:761.

90. Talib H. Orbital hydatid cyst in Iraq. Br J Surg. 1972;59:391.

91. Kagan IG. Trichinosis: A review of biologic, serologic and immunologic aspects. J Infect Dis. 1960;107:65.

92. Hamed HH. Orbital affection with cysticercus cellulosae. Bull Ophthalmol Soc Egypt. 1968;61:253.

93. Jones BR. Inflammatory pseudotumors of the orbit: A probable case of microfilarial granuloma of the orbit. Trans Ophthalmol Soc UK. 1970;90:299.

94. Mathur SP, Makhija JM. Invasion of the orbit by maggots. Br J Ophthalmol. 1967;51:406.

95. Wood TR, Slight JR. Bilateral orbital myiasis. Arch Ophthalmol. 1970;84:692.

96. Blodi FC. Orbital inflammations. Symposiun on diseases and surgery of the lids, lacrimal apparatus, and orbit. Trans N Orleans Acad Ophthalmol. 1982;1–17.

97. Clune JP. Septic thrombosis within the cavernous chamber: Review of the literature with recent advances in diagnosis and treatment. Am J Ophthalmol. 1963;56:33.

98. Yarington CR Jr. The prognosis and treatment of cavernous sinus thrombosis: A review of 878 cases in the literature. Ann Otol Rhinol Layngol. 1961;70:263.

99. Price CD, Hameroff SB, Richards RD. Cavernous sinus thrombosis and orbital cellulitis. South Med J. 1971;64:1243.

100. Bell RW. Orbital cellulitis and cavernous sinus thrombosis caused by rhabdomyosarcoma of the middle ear. Ann Ophthalmol. 1972;4:1090.

101. Walsh FB. Ocular signs of thrombosis of the intracranial sinuses. Arch Ophthalmol. 1937;17:46.

102. Clifford-Jones RE, Ellis CJK, Stevens JM, et al. Cavernous sinus thrombosis. J Neurol Neurosurg Psychiatry. 1982;45:1092.

103. Geggel HS, Isenberg SJ. Cavernous sinus thrombosis as a cause of unilateral blindness. Ann Ophthalmol. 1982;14:569.

104. Raflo GT, Chart P, Hurwitz JJ. Thermographic evaluation of the human lacrimal drainage system. Ophthalmic Surg. 1982;13:119–24.

105. Rosenstock T, Chart P, Hurwitz JJ. Inflammation of the lacrimal drainage system—assessment by thermography. Ophthalmic Surg. 1983;14:229–37.

106. Galloway JE, Kavic TA, Raflo GT. Digital subtraction macrodacryocystography: A new method of lacrimal system imaging. Ophthalmology. 1984;91:956.

107. Rossomondo RM, Carlton WH, Trueblood JH, et al. A new method of evaluating lacrimal drainage. Arch Ophthalmol. 1972;88:523.

108. Freeman LN, Zinreich SJ, Iliff NT. Radiography of the lacrimal system using topical CT dacryocystography (abstract). Ophthalmology. 1987;94:142.

109. Eustis HS, Amstrong DC, Buncie JR, et al. Staging of orbital cellulitis in children: Computed tomography characteristics and treatment guidelines. J Pediatr Ophthalmol Strabismus. 1986;23:246–51.

110. Harr DL, Quencer RM, Abrams GW. Computed tomography and ultrasound in the evaluation of orbital infection and pseudotumor. Radiology. 1982;152:395.

111. Fiandaca MS, Spector RH, Hartmann TM, et al. Unilateral septic cavernous sinus thrombosis—a case report with digital orbital venograhpic documentation. J Clin Neuro-Ophthalmol. 1986;6:35–8.

112. Kline LB, Acker JD, Post MJD, et al. The cavernous sinus: A computed tomographic study. Am J Neurol Radiol. 1981;2:299.

113. Lew D, Southwick FS, Montgomery WW, et al. Sphenoid sinusitis: a review of 30 cases. N Engl J Med. 1983;309:1149.

114. Savino PJ, Grossman RI, Schatz NJ, et al. High-field magnetic resonance imaging in the diagnosis of cavernous sinus thrombosis. Arch Neurol. 1986;43:1081–2.

115. Taylor PJ. Cavernous sinus thrombophlebitis. Br J Ophthalmol. 1957;41:228–37.

116. Aragones JV. The treatment of blepharitis: A controlled double blind study of combination therapy. Ann Ophthalmol. 1973;5:49.

117. Mathew M, D'Souza P, Mehta DK. A new treatment of pthiriasis palpebrarum. Ann Ophthalmol. 1982;14:439.

118. Seal DV, McGill J, Flanagan D. Lacrimal canaliculitis due to *Arachnia (Actinomyces) propionica*. Br J Ophthalmol. 1981;65:10–3.

119. Campbell CB, Flanagan JC, Schaefer AJ. Acquired lacrimal disorders. In: Smith BC, Della Rocca RC, Nesi FA, eds. Ophthalmic Plastic and Reconstructive Surgery. St. Louis: CV Mosby; 1987:956.

120. Krohel G. Orbital cellulitis and abscess. In: Fraunfelder F, Roy H, eds. Current Ocular Therapy. 2nd ed. Philadelphia: WB Saunders; 1985:451.

121. Gutman L. Appropriate antibiotics in orbital cellulitis. Arch Ophthalmol. 1977;95:170.

122. Tannenbaum M, Tenzel J, Byrne SF, et al. Medical management of orbital abscess. Surv Ophthalmol. 1985;30:211–2.

123. Gold SC, Arrigg PG, Hedges TR. Computed tomography in the management of acute orbital cellulitis. Ophthalmic Surg. 1987;18:753–6.

124. Harris GJ. Subperiosteal inflammation of the orbit: A bacteriological analysis of 17 cases. Arch Ophthalmol. 1988;106:947–52.

125. Best M, Obstbaum SA, Friedman B, et al. Survival in orbital phycomycosis. Am J Ophthalmol. 1971;71:1078.

126. Bullock JD, Jampol LM, Fezza AJ. Two cases of orbital phycomycosis with recovery. Am J Ophthalmol. 1974;78:811.

127. Jones DB. Microbial preseptal and orbital cellulitis. In: Duane TD, ed. Clinical Ophthalmology. v. 4. Hagerstown, MD: Harper & Row; 1976:17.

128. Solomon OD, Moses L, Volk M. Steroid therapy in cavernous sinus thrombosis. Am J Ophthalmol. 1962;54:1122–5.

129. Parsons M. Intracranial venous thrombosis. Postgrad Med J. 1967;43:409–14.

130. Lyons C. Treatment of staphylococcal cavernous sinus thrombophlebitis with heparin and chemotherapy. Ann Surg. 1941;113:113–7.

SECTION N. HEPATITIS

96. ACUTE VIRAL HEPATITIS

HENRY H. HSU
STEPHEN M. FEINSTONE
JAY H. HOOFNAGLE

Acute viral hepatitis is a common and sometimes serious viral infection of the liver leading to inflammation and necrosis. This disease was traditionally separated into two types based on its clinical and epidemiologic characteristics: type A or "infectious" hepatitis caused by the hepatitis A virus (HAV) and type B or "serum" hepatitis caused by the hepatitis B virus (HBV).[1-4] In the last 25 years, it has become clear that there are at least five distinct viral agents that cause acute viral hepatitis: HAV[5]; HBV[6,7]; hepatitis delta virus or hepatitis D virus (HDV)[8-11]; hepatitis C virus (HCV), the cause of parenterally transmitted, non-A, non-B hepatitis as well as community acquired non-A, non-B hepatitis[12-14]; and hepatitis E virus (HEV), an enterically transmitted, epidemic non-A, non-B hepatitis agent.[15-17] Acute hepatitis caused by any of these agents is clinically very similar. Therefore, etiologic diagnosis now depends on serologic assays specific for each of the different viruses.

These five recognized hepatitis viruses infect primarily the liver and result in hepatic inflammation and hepatocellular necrosis without major pathologic involvement of other organs. Many other known viral agents can also infect the liver and induce a viral hepatitislike syndrome, but they do so in the context of a more widespread disease. For instance, yellow fever virus (YFV) frequently causes severe hepatic necrosis, but it is a systemic viral infection with widespread pathology affecting multiple organs. Other common viruses that cause hepatitis in the United States are Epstein-Barr virus (EBV) and cytomegalovirus (CMV). Liver disease can also occur with infections with herpes simplex viruses, varicella-zoster virus, as well as measles, rubella, rubeola, coxsackie B viruses, and adenoviruses. While these agents produce some degree of liver inflammation and dysfunction and deserve diagnostic consideration, they are not major causes of acute or chronic viral hepatitis.

A minority of patients remain in a category of a viral hepatitislike syndrome without serologic evidence for infection by any of the recognized agents. These patients may have disease caused by one of the five known viral agents but have levels of antigen or antibody that are undetectable by any of the specific serologic tests, or they may be infected by other yet-to-be-identified viruses; alternatively, they may have a noninfectious etiology for their illness.

Acute viral hepatitis is a common disease. Yearly estimates from the Centers for Disease Control and Prevention (CDC) suggest that the incidence of acute viral hepatitis has been rising slowly over the last 20 years.[18] During 1985, there were approximately 60,000 cases of viral hepatitis reported, among which an estimated 29 percent were due to hepatitis A, 44 percent to hepatitis B, and 27 percent to non-A, non-B hepatitis.[19–21] Thus, the annual incidence of acute viral hepatitis in the United States is calculated to be about 0.25 per 1000 population. This is clearly an underestimate. Attempts to quantify the degree of underreporting of viral hepatitis[22] have suggested that the true incidence is five to eight times that reported each year (thus 1–2 per 1000 population). Indeed, use of serologic markers for evidence of previous HAV and HBV infections reveal that by age 50 years, 70 percent of middle-class white Americans have had HAV infection, and 7 percent have had HBV infection.[23] The prevalence of antibody markers is higher among lower socioeconomic groups and among foreign-born U.S. citizens.

Acute viral hepatitis can be a serious disease. The overall mortality rate for icteric viral hepatitis is approximately 1 percent, and it is age dependent. The mortality rate is higher in older persons, and some of the reported variation in mortality rates relates to the age of the affected patients. The frequency of fulminant hepatitis is also dependent on the etiology of the hepatitis. Fulminant disease occurs more commonly in hepatitis B and D than in the other forms of acute viral hepatitis. In various outbreaks of delta hepatitis, the mortality rate has been between 2 and 20 percent.[9,24] A striking characteristic of type E hepatitis is an increased incidence of fulminant disease and a high mortality rate (~10 percent) in pregnant women, especially during the third trimester.[17]

In addition to morbidity and mortality from the acute disease, the progression of viral hepatitis B, C, and D from an acute to a chronic state can also lead to serious sequelae (see Ch. 97), including chronic liver disease, cirrhosis, and hepatocellular carcinoma; in addition, polyarteritis nodosa, cryoglobulinemia, glomerulonephritis, and aplastic anemia have been associated with either acute or chronic infection.[25–27] In the United States and Western Europe, chronic viral hepatitis is probably the second most frequent cause of cirrhosis, second only to alcohol abuse. The chronic forms of hepatitis B, delta hepatitis, and hepatitis C are frequent causes of terminal liver disease for which hepatic transplantation is performed. On a worldwide scale, chronic hepatitis B infection is the most important cause

of cirrhosis and is a major cause of cancer mortality. It is estimated that 5 percent of the world's population has chronic HBV infection (the chronic carrier state), and hepatocellular carcinoma resulting from such chronic infections is among the most common malignancies worldwide.[28] Chronic infection by HCV is also associated with a greatly increased risk of liver cancer.[29–32]

Major advances during the past 25 years have been made in definition of the agents of viral hepatitis; this has translated into means of detection and prevention of these infections. Less progress has been made in the realm of specific treatment to prevent complications, such as chronic infections. A safe, highly effective hepatitis B vaccine made from hepatitis B surface antigen (HBsAg) purified from the plasma of chronic carriers has been available since 1982, and safe and effective vaccines prepared from bioengineered recombinant yeast expressing HBsAg have been available since 1986.[33] Recently, both killed and live attenuated vaccines against hepatitis A have been developed. A formalin-inactivated hepatitis A vaccine has been demonstrated to be highly effective in preventing clinically apparent infection.[34–38]

CLINICAL MANIFESTATIONS

Symptoms

The clinical presentation of acute viral hepatitis ranges from asymptomatic subclinical illness to fulminant hepatic failure with its attendant high mortality rate. There are no clinical features that unequivocally distinguish the individual types of hepatitis, although certain epidemiologic patterns of transmission may suggest a particular etiology. Acute viral hepatitis is conveniently separated into four clinical stages: incubation period, preicteric phase, icteric phase, and convalescence. The timing of the symptoms in relation to the laboratory, serologic, and virologic findings during each of these stages of a generalized case of acute viral hepatitis is shown diagrammatically in Figure 1.

The incubation period of acute viral hepatitis varies from as short as a few weeks to as long as 6 months, depending on the particular infecting virus. The incubation period of hepatitis A averages about 21 days (range, 15–45 days), type B hepatitis about 70 days (range, 30–180 days), type C hepatitis (classic non-A, non-B hepatitis) 50 days (range, 15–150 days), and type E hepatitis (epidemic non-A, non-B hepatitis) about 40 days (range, 15–60 days). The incubation period of delta hepatitis has not been well documented. Because delta hepatitis invariably occurs in conjunction with hepatitis B, its incubation period probably is similar to that of hepatitis B. Because there is considerable overlap in the incubation periods of each of the viruses, one cannot reliably ascertain the etiologic agent based on such information. During the incubation period, the patient is asymptomatic and feels well.

The initial symptoms of acute hepatitis are nonspecific; typically, the patient develops malaise and weakness, followed shortly by anorexia, nausea, vomiting, and a vague, dull, right upper quadrant pain. These symptoms of the preicteric phase usually last 3–10 days. The onset of jaundice and/or dark urine then ushers in the icteric phase. It is these symptoms that usually bring the patient to the doctor. The patient may begin to feel better even while jaundice persists.

While this may represent the typical case, one must stress that there is considerable variation in the clinical presentation. Clinically evident icteric cases account for only 20–50 percent of hepatitis virus infections. The remainder pass unnoticed, without symptoms or with such mild symptoms that they are dismissed as inconsequential ("indigestion" or "the flu"). The spectrum of clinical disease ranges from inapparent to anicteric (but symptomatic) to icteric to fulminant.

The onset of viral hepatitis can be either sudden (most typical

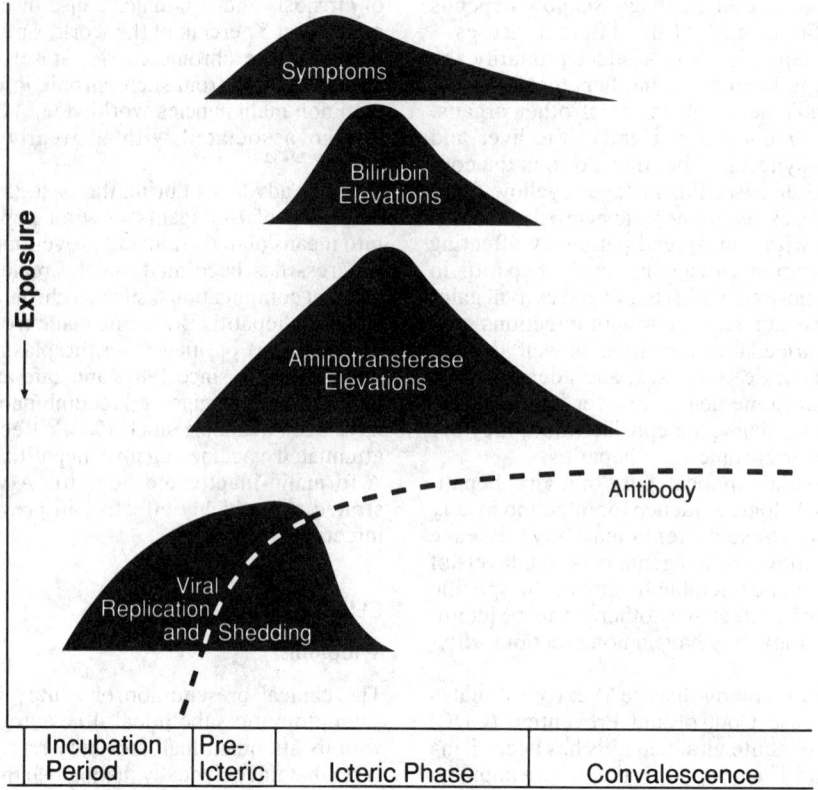

FIG. 1.   The course of acute viral hepatitis. The timing of the clinical symptoms related to laboratory findings, virologic events, and development of serum antibodies is shown.

of hepatitis A) or insidious (more typical of type B or C). At least 25 percent of the patients with viral hepatitis describe the onset of their disease as an "influenzalike" illness with weakness, headaches, myalgias, chills, and fever. This type of onset is most common with hepatitis A. Symptoms of an upper respiratory infection such as a sore throat and cough may be present. These symptoms are short-lived (1–3 days) and are replaced by the more typical symptoms of anorexia, nausea, and then jaundice. Fever, in particular, rarely persists into the icteric phase. Jaundice with high fever is *not* characteristic of viral hepatitis.

Malaise is the earliest and most common (~95 percent) symptom of this disease. It usually is the first symptom to appear and the last to leave. *Anorexia* is frequently present in symptomatic viral hepatitis, but it typically is one of the first symptoms to abate. There may be a change in taste and smell with a concomitant aversion to food and often to cigarettes. This dysgeusia is not specific for viral hepatitis and may be seen with any form of acute hepatitis. *Nausea* and vomiting occur in about 80 percent of patients with symptomatic viral hepatitis. The nausea is typically intermittent and rarely intractable. Nausea, as with malaise, may be absent early in the day and then appear and worsen as the day progresses. Mild weight loss is common during viral hepatitis. Abdominal *pain* can accompany acute viral hepatitis (~60 percent), and it usually consists of a mild, dull, right upper quadrant, aching discomfort and is unaffected by meals, antacids, stool patterns, or position.

A minority of patients with acute hepatitis (5–15 percent) experience a "serum sicknesslike syndrome" at the onset of their illness.[39,40] This consists of a triad of symptoms: fever, rash, and arthritis. It is a manifestation of immune complex (virus/antibody) deposition. This syndrome occurs during the preicteric phase and almost invariably will resolve dramatically with

the onset of jaundice. *Fever* is usual but not invariable. The *rash* is typically urticarial, with pruritic hives appearing and disappearing in a largely peripheral distribution. More exanthemlike macular-papular lesions can also occur as well as fleeting irregular patches of erythema. The *arthritis* is mild to moderate, nondeforming, polyarticular, and migratory. Major joints involved are the elbows, wrists, knees, and small joints of the hands. Arthralgias probably are more common than frank arthritis. This syndrome is most common with hepatitis B, but it also has been reported with hepatitis A. In children with hepatitis B, a condition perhaps related to this syndrome has been described—papular acrodermatitis (Gianotti's disease)—which is characterized by skin eruptions, lymphadenopathy and lymphadenitis, and mild, usually anicteric, acute viral hepatitis.[41]

Jaundice and dark urine are the most distinctive symptoms of acute hepatitis, but they can be unreliable. Scleral icterus may go unnoticed, even with a serum bilirubin level as high as 10 mg/dl. *Dark urine* often is more noticeable than scleral icterus. Dark urine also is helpful in indicating that the jaundice is accompanied by conjugated (direct) hyperbilirubinemia (not found with jaundice due to hemolysis or Gilbert syndrome). While jaundice and dark urine usually occur after a 4- to 10-day preicteric phase, some patients have jaundice only and deny any prodrome of malaise, anorexia, or nausea. Light-colored stools also can occur with the jaundice of viral hepatitis, reflecting the lack of bile pigments being added to the intestinal contents. The lightening of stool color in viral hepatitis, however, usually is not as great as in obstructive jaundice, and white or chalky stools are uncommon. Persons with prominent jaundice will also often complain of *pruritus*. Approximately 40 percent of jaundiced patients will complain of itching at the peak of icterus or sometime into convalescence.

In addition to a serum sicknesslike syndrome, there are other immune complex–mediated diseases that have been described in association with acute (and chronic) viral hepatitis. Polyarteritis nodosa, associated with hepatitis B virus infection, leads to a small, medium, and large vessel arteritis that affects multiple organs. Symptoms include fever, abdominal pain, arthralgias, mononeuritis, renal disease, hypertension, central nervous system abnormalities, and skin rashes. Recent studies show that up to 69 percent of patients with established polyarteritis nodosa are HBsAg positive.[42] Both hepatitis B and C have been associated with glomerulonephritis thought to be due to immune complex deposition of viral antigen and/or antibody within the glomerular basement membrane, which can lead to membranous and membranoproliferative glomerulonephritis.[43–45] Not infrequently, the severity of the renal disease overshadows the hepatitis. Mixed cryoglobulinemia, due to the production of antibodies with altered physical characteristics such that they form a precipitate when subjected to lower temperatures, has been associated with hepatitis B and, more recently, hepatitis C viral infection.[46,47] The rare occurrence of other manifestations such as Raynaud's phenomenon, bullous formation, and erythema nodosa also have been described in acute hepatitis.

Fulminant viral hepatitis is defined as the development of severe acute liver failure with hepatic encephalopathy within 8 weeks of the onset of symptoms with jaundice.[48,49] Late-onset hepatic failure is defined as severe acute liver failure from 8 to 12 weeks after the onset of symptoms with jaundice. Approximately 75 percent of cases of fulminant hepatic failure are due to viral hepatitis with hepatitis B being responsible for 30–60 percent of all cases. Up to 30–40 percent of patients with fulminant hepatic failure caused by hepatitis B also test positive for the delta virus and are presumably coinfected. Hepatitis A is an uncommon cause of hepatic failure, with less than 0.1 percent of cases progressing to hepatic failure. Hepatitis C virus has not been implicated in causing acute fulminant hepatic failure by itself, although it may act as a cofactor in causing fulminant hepatitis among patients who are coinfected with another virus, such as hepatitis B. Fulminant hepatic failure can occur at any time—early or late—during the course of the disease. The first symptoms usually are lethargy, somnolence, and a change in personality. Patients may be excited, euphoric, and unruly. These symptoms are followed in more severe cases by stupor and then coma.

Physical Findings

The physical findings in acute viral hepatitis are few. Vital signs are normal, although bradycardia can occur when significant hyperbilirubinemia is present. Icterus can be detected if the bilirubin level exceeds 2.5–3.0 mg/dl. It is seen most easily in the sclera or under the tongue. In light-skinned people, the skin may have a yellowish hue. Palpation of the abdomen often demonstrates a slightly enlarged and tender liver. A spleen tip is felt in 5–25 percent of patients. Signs of portal hypertension are not seen in acute hepatitis except in late, severe disease (as with subacute hepatic necrosis). Adenopathy, if present, is not prominent.

There are several skin findings in acute viral hepatitis. Vascular spiders often are found in light-skinned persons, but they are few and small. Severe pruritus may lead to excoriations. One should search for forearm venipuncture marks suggesting drug addiction, a common source of hepatitis virus infection. Patients with the serum sicknesslike syndrome will have urticaria or a mild, fleeting erythematous rash and (occasionally) red, warm, and tender joints. Finally, acne-prone persons may exhibit an exacerbation of this condition with acute hepatitis.

When fulminant hepatitis supervenes, signs of hepatic encephalopathy appear. These consist of lethargy, somnolence, untidiness, confusion, forgetfulness, and then stupor and full coma. Typical of hepatic encephalopathy is asterixis—the asynchronous irregular flapping of the forcibly dorsiflexed, outstretched hands. In stage I coma, mild mental changes are present, but asterixis is minimal or absent. Stage II coma is marked by worsening of mental changes and definite asterixis. In stage III coma, the patient develops stupor and semicoma but can still be aroused. With stage IV coma, the patient no longer is arousable, and there may or may not be a response to deep pain stimuli. Patients with hepatic failure may demonstrate other neurologic signs—flapping of the tongue, involuntary movements, long-tract signs, and decerebrate posturing. They also may demonstrate the distinctive sweetish smell of fetor hepaticus.

Laboratory Findings

While the symptoms and signs of acute viral hepatitis are frequently nonspecific or vague, laboratory findings are quite characteristic. The ranges of serum enzyme and bilirubin levels in acute viral hepatitis and other common liver diseases are shown in Figure 2. Most distinctive of viral hepatitis are the dramatic elevations in the aminotransferases—aspartate aminotransferase (AST) and alanine aminotransferase (ALT). In acute viral hepatitis, concentrations of both of the aminotransferases are elevated to levels usually greater than eight times normal at the time of the appearance of jaundice. The AST to ALT ratio is usually less than 1 in viral hepatitis while it usually exceeds 1.5 in alcoholic liver disease.[50–52] The alkaline phosphatase and other serum enzyme levels that denote biliary obstruction or cholestasis (γ-glutamyl-transferase, 5′-nucleotidase) are only mildly elevated (one to three times normal). The lactic dehydrogenase (LDH) concentration usually is mildly elevated in acute viral hepatitis (one to three times normal). Indeed, the dramatic elevation of both AST and ALT levels with only mild elevation in alkaline phosphatase and LDH levels is virtually diagnostic of "acute hepatitis" or "acute necroinflammatory disease of the liver." Given this enzyme pattern, one need then only to resolve whether this acute hepatitis is due to a hepatitis virus, a hepatotoxic drug, a toxin, or a nonspecific liver injury (e.g., anoxia, shock, or severe heart failure).

The AST and ALT levels become abnormal during the late incubation period of this disease. They are invariably abnormal once symptoms occur, usually rise during the preicteric phase, and peak early in the icteric phase. With recovery, the aminotransferase levels quickly fall but almost always remain slightly abnormal for several weeks after the jaundice and symptoms have abated.

The bilirubin level is variably elevated in icteric viral hepatitis. This elevation involves both the direct and indirect fractions, with the ratio being approximately equal. Disproportionate elevations in direct bilirubin concentration suggest cholestasis, whereas the preponderance of indirect bilirubin (>80 percent) suggests hemolysis. Persons with underlying hemolytic states (glucose-6-phosphate dehydrogenase [G6PD] deficiency or sickle cell disease) may suffer accelerated hemolysis with many viral infections and especially viral hepatitis.[53] These persons may become markedly jaundiced and yet have relatively mild symptoms and aminotransferase level elevations.

The prothrombin time generally is normal in typical acute viral hepatitis and when prolonged should raise the suspicion of more severe liver necrosis that may progress to fulminant hepatic failure. Any elevation should be regarded as a serious sign. When the prothrombin time is greater than 100 seconds, or greater than 50 seconds in association with a bilirubin greater than 17.6 mg/dl in a patient who is less than 11 or greater than 40 years of age, the probability that spontaneous recovery will occur is low, and the patient should be promptly considered for liver transplantation.[54] The partial thromboplastin time is not as sensitive or reliable a measure as the prothrombin time.

Other laboratory test results rarely are abnormal. The serum albumin and globulin levels usually are normal in acute viral hepatitis as are hemoglobin values. A white blood cell count is

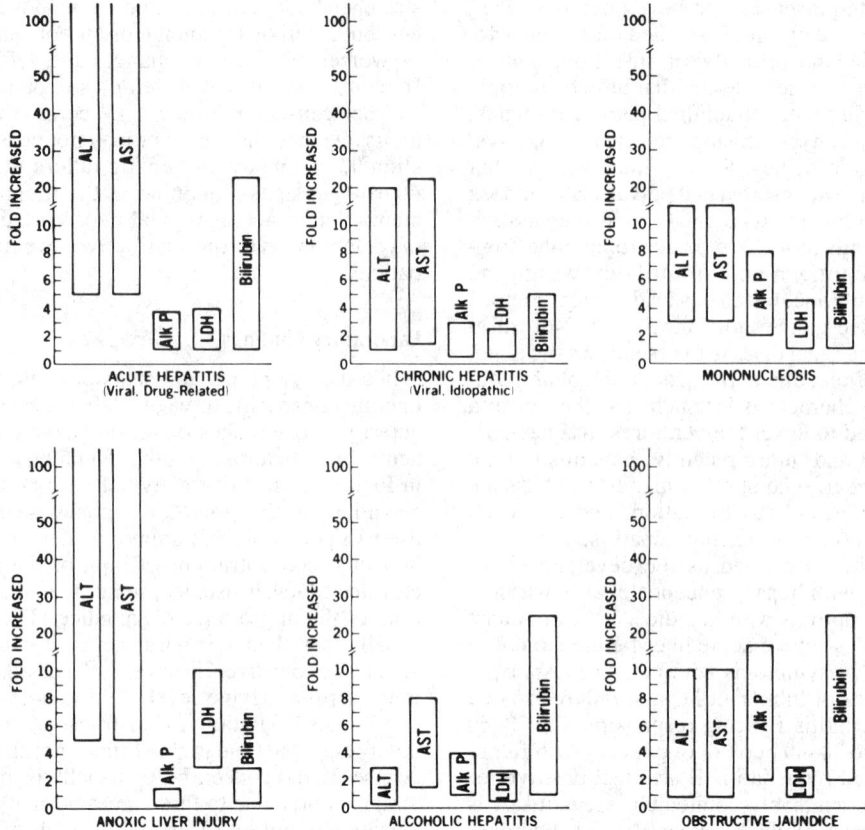

FIG. 2. The range of elevation of key serum enzyme levels in acute viral hepatitis and other common liver diseases. ALT: alanine aminotransferase; AST: aspartate aminotransferase; Alk P: alkaline phosphate; LDH: lactic dehydrogenase.

either normal or slightly low. A mild lymphocytosis can occur. The platelet count remains normal except with fulminant hepatitis, in which case disseminated intravascular coagulation can supervene. Patients with acute viral hepatitis often develop low levels of anti-DNA and smooth muscle antibodies (SMA). Biologic false-positive VDRL test reactions are rare. The sedimentation rate is normal or minimally elevated. Serum immunoglobulin levels usually are normal except in hepatitis A, in which case the serum IgM level may double during the course of the disease.

Pathologic Findings

The clinical history, pattern of serum enzyme levels, and serologic findings in acute viral hepatitis are sufficiently characteristic that a percutaneous liver biopsy specimen is rarely indicated for diagnosis. However, when several possible causes of acute liver disease are present or when therapy is a consideration, a liver biopsy can be helpful. The typical liver biopsy findings of acute viral hepatitis are the following: *(1)* lobular disarray, *(2)* ballooning and eosinophilic degeneration, *(3)* liver cell necrosis, *(4)* mononuclear cell infiltration of the parenchyma and portal tracts, and *(5)* variable degrees of cholestasis.[55] These changes are diffuse and generalized; therefore, sampling error from needle biopsy usually is not a problem. *Lobular disarray* refers to a loss of the orderly pattern of hepatic sinusoidal cords, which results from widespread anisocytosis, liver cell degeneration, regeneration, or death (Fig. 3). Liver cells demonstrate two forms of degeneration: ballooning degeneration (in which there is swelling of the liver cell and rarefaction of the cytoplasm) and eosinophilic degeneration (in which the cell shrinks and becomes a deeper red and more angular). The end result of eosinophilic degeneration is the free hyaline body (Fig. 4). There also may be "smudging" of hepatocytes with indistinctness of cell

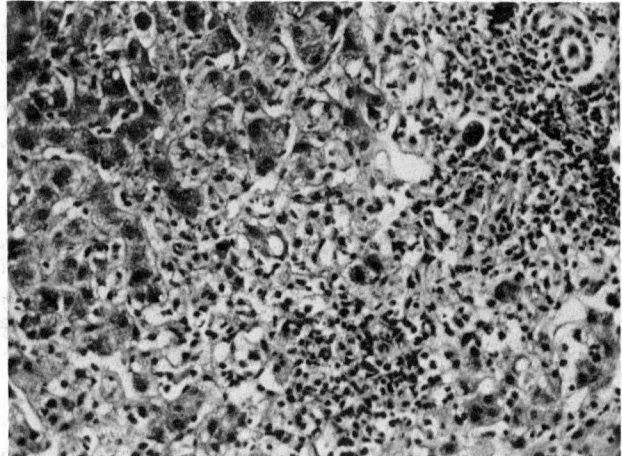

FIG. 3. Liver biopsy specimen from a patient with acute viral hepatitis. Note the lobular disarray, the occurrence of eosinophilic degeneration, free hyaline bodies, and spotty hepatocellular necrosis and the prominent mononuclear cell infiltrates in the portal zone and areas of parenchyma. (H&E, × 240) (Photomicrograph courtesy of Dr. Kamal Ishak, Washington, DC.)

outline as well as cell "dropout"—with or without associated inflammatory cell reaction. Kupffer cells appear to be more numerous and enlarged. Areas of lymphocytic infiltration are common both in the parenchyma and in portal tracts. Polymorphonuclear leukocytes are not numerous. A few plasma cells and eosinophils may be found, but a prominence of portal tract plasma cells suggests chronic hepatitis; also, unusual numbers of eosinophils suggest drug addiction or a drug-related hepatitis.

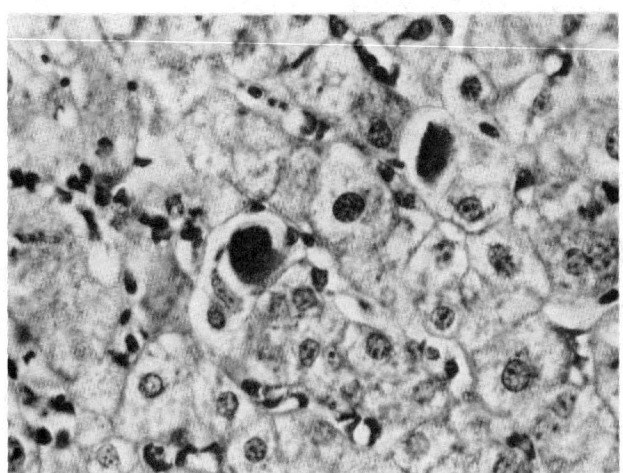

FIG. 4. The free hyaline body and eosinophilic degeneration typical of acute viral hepatitis. (H&E, ×660) (Photomicrograph courtesy of Dr. Kamal Ishak, Washington, DC.)

Cholestasis (bile staining of liver cells and bile "plugs") may be seen on liver biopsy specimens and generally corresponds in degree to the height of the serum bilirubin level. The portal bile ducts, however, usually appear to be normal. In typical viral hepatitis, cell necrosis is spotty and focal. More severe hepatitis may be accompanied by coalescent or bridging necrosis (between portal zones or from portal zones to central veins), multilobular necrosis, or massive necrosis.[55–58] Bridging necrosis found during acute viral hepatitis indicates a serious lesion that can progress to postnecrotic cirrhosis. Multilobular or massive necrosis is seen in severe and fulminant disease.

DIFFERENTIAL DIAGNOSIS

The specific etiologic diagnosis of acute viral hepatitis depends primarily on serologic testing once it has been demonstrated that acute necroinflammatory disease (acute hepatitis) is present. The latter is based largely on the pattern of serum enzyme concentrations—dramatic elevations in aminotransferase levels with mild elevations in the alkaline phosphatase level. One should always keep in mind that the differential diagnosis of acute hepatitis includes other infectious diseases as well as noninfectious forms of liver disease. These include bacterial infections (pneumococcal pneumonia, leptospirosis), various drugs (acetaminophen, isoniazid), toxins (alcohol, carbon tetrachloride), and nonspecific injury (shock, ischemia). These types of acute hepatitis usually can be excluded by a careful history and physical examination with some support from laboratory data. In addition to identification of the responsible viral agent using serologies, one should attempt to identify the source of infection. Most cases of acute viral hepatitis are caused by one of five agents: HAV, HBV, HCV, HDV, or HEV. While these agents are virologically distinct, the diseases that they cause are quite similar. They overlap so much in symptoms and severity that they cannot be reliably distinguished on clinical grounds, by biochemical tests, or even by liver biopsy findings. Specific serologic assays can usually determine which of the five types of viral hepatitis is present, but in some circumstances diagnostic uncertainties remain. A flow diagram for the specific diagnosis of acute viral hepatitis is shown in Figure 5.

Hepatitis A

Hepatitis A is an acute self-limited disease that only rarely causes death (see Ch. 150). Hepatitis A characteristically has an acute, sudden, influenza-like onset with a prominence of my-

algia, headache, fever, and malaise.[1,59–61] The ratio of anicteric to icteric hepatitis is high, particularly in children. Hepatitis A usually is not as severe or as long-lasting as hepatitis B. However, a transient relapsing course has been reported,[62] and a prolonged cholestasis appearing late in the acute phase and lasting for several months may be seen.[63,64] Both of these unusual forms of hepatitis A are usually benign; the mortality rate of hepatitis A is low (~2/1000 icteric cases),[60,65] and the disease ultimately resolves. Hepatitis A never leads to a chronic hepatitis or a carrier state.[66]

Epidemiologic features can be helpful in distinguishing hepatitis A from other forms of viral hepatitis.[18,67] Hepatitis A is spread predominantly by the fecal-oral route. It is highly contagious and spreads rapidly to close contacts. Hepatitis A can occur in outbreaks that may have an identifiable point source (often a person in the incubation period of acute disease). Hepatitis A has been shown to be spread by (1) contaminated water, milk, or food[68]; (2) after breakdown in usual sanitary conditions or after floods or natural disasters[69]; (3) by ingestion of raw or undercooked shellfish (oysters, clams, and mussels) from contaminated waters[69]; (4) during travel to areas of the world with poor hygienic conditions where hepatitis A is endemic[70]; (5) in institutionalized children and adults[1]; and (6) after exposure to recently imported chimpanzees or apes.[71]

Three other epidemiologic sources have recently been shown to be important in spread of hepatitis A: exposure to children in day care centers,[67,72] male homosexuality,[73] and intravenous drug addiction.[18,67] Day care centers can serve as sources of outbreaks of hepatitis A, especially when there are children who are still not toilet trained in the centers. Male homosexuals may have a high incidence of hepatitis A that probably is related to sexual practices. Some cases occur without any known point-source of infection. Blood transfusion is a very rare mode of transmission of hepatitis A.[18]

The clinical and laboratory findings during the course of a typical case of hepatitis A are shown in Figure 6. Fecal shedding of HAV is found during both the incubation period and the early symptomatic phase of illness, but may no longer be detectable at the time of onset of jaundice. Antibody to HAV (anti-HAV) is detectable in serum by the onset of disease. Initially, the anti-HAV consists of both IgG and IgM class antibodies. After 3–12 months, IgM anti-HAV disappears, whereas IgG anti-HAV persists in high titer, which confers life-long immunity. Thus, the diagnosis of acute hepatitis A is made by the finding of IgM anti-HAV in a patient with either clinical symptoms or biochemical evidence of acute hepatitis.[74] Immunoassays are now available for IgM anti-HAV and for total anti-HAV. These assays allow for diagnosis (IgM anti-HAV) and for assessment of immunity (total anti-HAV) to hepatitis A. For the purposes of the diagnosis of acute hepatitis A, only the IgM anti-HAV is necessary.

Hepatitis B

Hepatitis B appears to be a more serious disease than hepatitis A, and it has a definite propensity to chronicity (see Ch. 124). It usually has a more insidious onset and a more prolonged course than hepatitis A. In the individual case, however, hepatitis B cannot be distinguished from hepatitis A or from hepatitis C on clinical grounds alone. The occurrence of the serum sicknesslike syndrome of fever, rash, and polyarthritis during the preicteric phase favors the diagnosis of hepatitis B.

Epidemiologic features can suggest HBV infection. This disease has a long incubation period (30–180 days) and is more likely to occur as sporadic rather than epidemic hepatitis.[1] Whether apparent or not, HBV is spread predominantly by the parenteral route. On a worldwide basis, the most common forms of spread are from mother to child during or soon after birth and by sexual contact. In the United States, hepatitis B often occurred in persons with exposure to blood or blood products (multiply transfused patients, hemophiliacs, renal dialysis, and

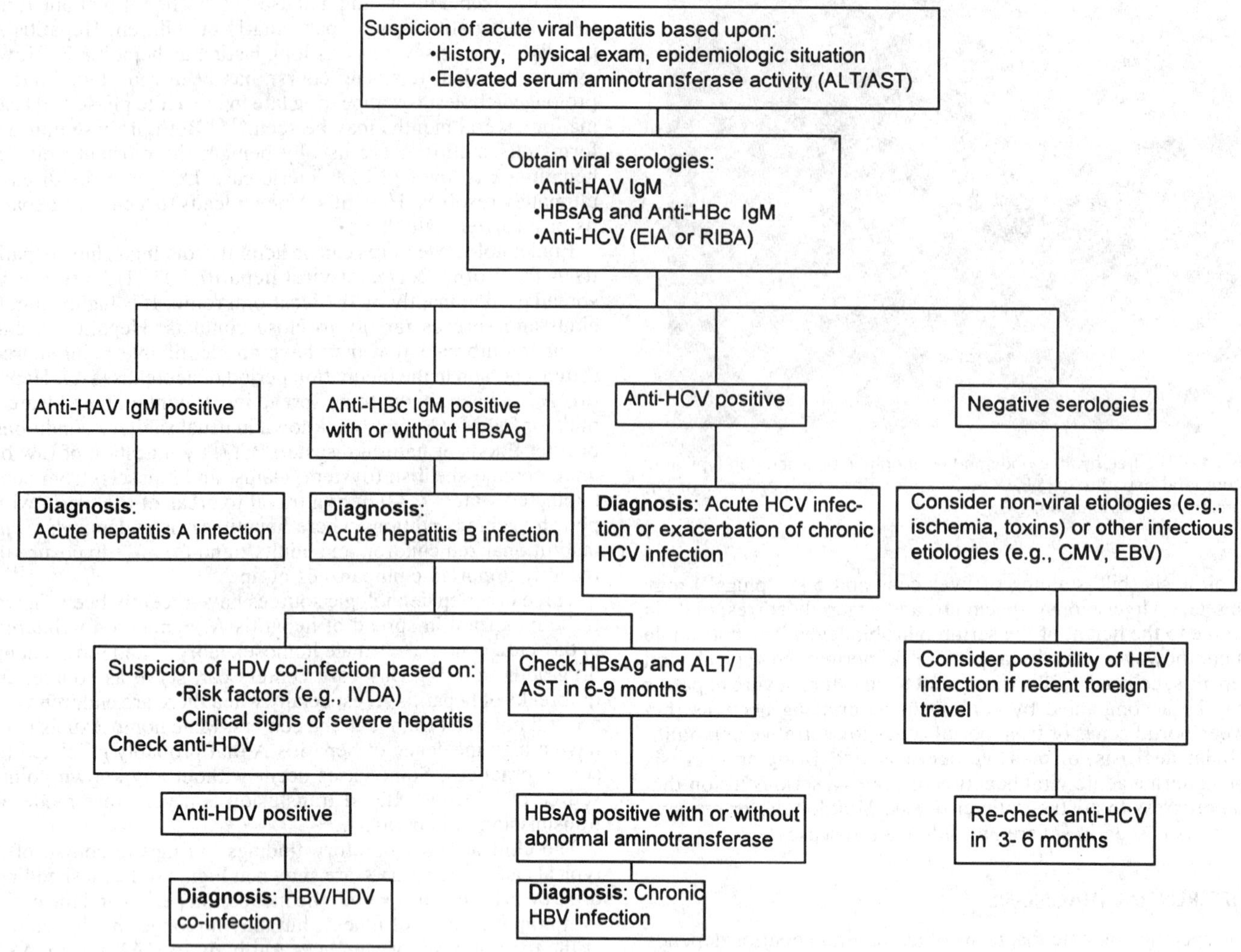

Suspicion of acute viral hepatitis based upon:
•History, physical exam, epidemiologic situation
•Elevated serum aminotransferase activity (ALT/AST)

Obtain viral serologies:
•Anti-HAV IgM
•HBsAg and Anti-HBc IgM
•Anti-HCV (EIA or RIBA)

Anti-HAV IgM positive

Anti-HBc IgM positive with or without HBsAg

Anti-HCV positive

Negative serologies

Diagnosis: Acute hepatitis A infection

Diagnosis: Acute hepatitis B infection

Diagnosis: Acute HCV infection or exacerbation of chronic HCV infection

Consider non-viral etiologies (e.g., ischemia, toxins) or other infectious etiologies (e.g., CMV, EBV)

Suspicion of HDV co-infection based on:
•Risk factors (e.g., IVDA)
•Clinical signs of severe hepatitis
Check anti-HDV

Check HBsAg and ALT/AST in 6-9 months

Consider possibility of HEV infection if recent foreign travel

Anti-HDV positive

HBsAg positive with or without abnormal aminotransferase

Re-check anti-HCV in 3- 6 months

Diagnosis: HBV/HDV co-infection

Diagnosis: Chronic HBV infection

FIG. 5. A flow diagram showing the use of specific serologic tests for the diagnosis of acute viral hepatitis in relation to the clinical and epidemiologic setting. Coinfections and superinfections of chronic hepatitis B or C patients should always be considered in cases that do not fit well with the clinical or serologic picture.

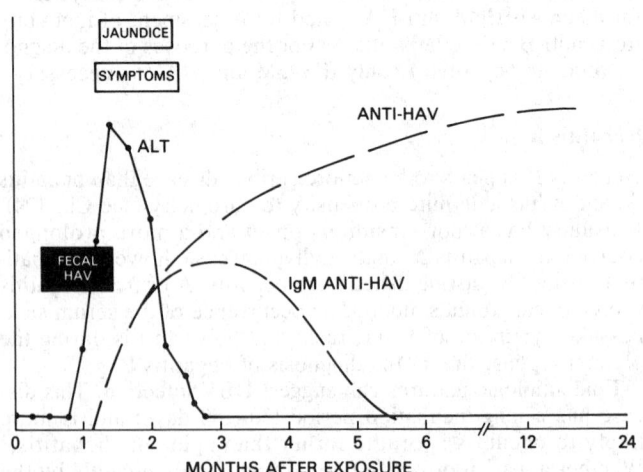

FIG. 6. The clinical, virologic, and serologic courses of a typical case of hepatitis A. HAV: hepatitis A virus; ANTI-HAV: antibody to hepatitis A virus; ALT: alanine aminotransferase.

oncology ward patients), with exposure to contaminated needles and syringes (medical personnel with accidental needlesticks, drug addicts), with multiple sexual contacts (homosexuals, prostitutes, the sexually active),[75] and with exposure to saliva or other potentially infectious excreta (children in institutions for the mentally retarded).[1] However, the same epidemiologic features also can be found in cases of non-A, non-B hepatitis (hepatitis C) and (occasionally) in hepatitis A. In at least 50 percent of acute hepatitis B cases, no history of parenteral exposure is uncovered. Whether these cases were acquired by ''nonparenteral'' routes or by inapparent parenteral routes is not known. At the present time, with screening of all blood donors for high-risk behavior and the testing of all donated blood and source plasma for HBsAg and anti-HBc, as well as specific viral inactivation of most plasma-derived products, the transmission of HBV by blood or blood products is now rare.

The diagnosis of hepatitis B should rest on specific serologic testing, with the finding of hepatitis B surface antigen (HBsAg) in the serum during the acute disease, which is shown diagrammatically in Figure 7. HBsAg appears in the serum during the incubation period 2–7 weeks before the onset of symptoms. It usually persists in the blood throughout the illness and disappears with convalescence.[76,77] The majority (95 percent) will be HBsAg positive at the onset of symptoms and jaundice. In some patients, however, HBsAg is cleared rapidly and may be absent by the time the patient is tested. In this situation, tests for anti-

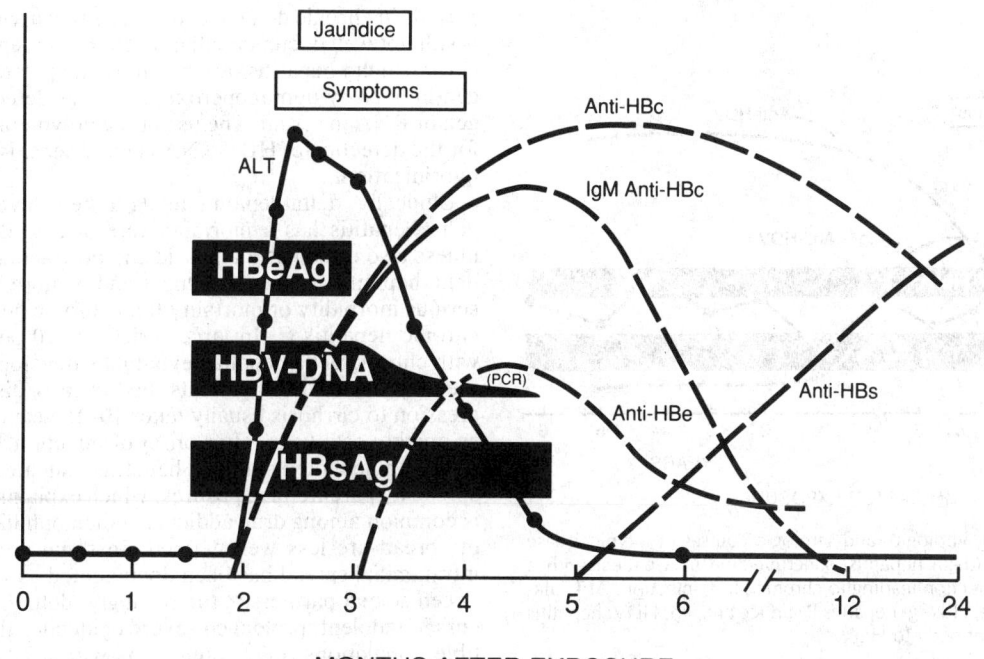

FIG. 7. The clinical, virologic, and serologic courses of a typical case of acute hepatitis B. HBsAg: hepatitis B surface antigen; HBeAg: hepatitis B e antigen; DNA-p: hepatitis B DNA polymerase activity; HBV-DNA: hepatitis B DNA; Anti-HBc: antibody to hepatitis B core antigen; anti-HBe: antibody to hepatitis B e antigen; anti-HBs: antibody to hepatitis B surface antigen.

body must be used to make this diagnosis. Antibody to HBsAg (anti-HBs) usually arises during convalescence from hepatitis B and, indeed, may not be detectable for some time into the recovery phase. Antibody to hepatitis B core antigen (anti-HBc) is a more reliable marker of HBV infection and usually appears at or about the time of onset of symptoms. Sensitive and specific immunoassays are now available for assaying both anti-HBs and anti-HBc. However, neither of these assays are definitive in the serodiagnosis of acute hepatitis B, since both anti-HBs and anti-HBc are long-lived. The finding of either of these antibodies in the serum of a patient with acute hepatitis does not prove that the disease is due to HBV infection, since infection with another virus might have occurred in a patient previously infected with hepatitis B. However, immunoassays for IgM anti-HBc have been developed that are very useful in the diagnosis of hepatitis B. IgM anti-HBc arises early in the illness of patients with acute hepatitis B, but it rapidly decreases in titer and no longer may be detectable 6–24 months after the illness.[43] Both false-positive and false-negative results can occur with the IgM anti-HBc test, but they are rare.

Patients with acute hepatitis B also develop hepatitis B e antigen (HBeAg) as well as direct markers for the presence of HBV in serum such as HBV DNA (as detected by molecular hybridization or polymerase chain reaction) and DNA polymerase (the endogenous polymerase of this virus). These are markers of active viral replication and are detected early in the course of acute hepatitis. By the peak of clinical illness and jaundice, levels of HBV in serum usually are decreasing or absent. Indeed, the seroconversion from HBeAg to antibody to HBeAg (anti-HBe) may be a favorable serologic sign indicating that the height of the viral replication has passed and that the infection is on the wane.[9]

From 5 to 10 percent of patients with HBV infection do not clear HBsAg but become HBsAg carriers.[1,77,78] These people typically have mild, often anicteric and asymptomatic disease, which may explain why most chronic HBsAg carriers do not give a history of acute hepatitis. As many as 0.2–1.0 percent of adults in the United States are chronic HBsAg carriers. The prevalence of the carrier state is even higher in "high-risk"

populations such as male homosexuals (6 percent), IV drug abusers (7 percent), hemophiliacs (7 percent), and renal dialysis patients (2–15 percent).[77] Most chronic HBsAg carriers are asymptomatic of their infection and have minimal or no accompanying liver injury.

The development of the chronic HBsAg carrier state as a result of symptomatic acute viral hepatitis occurs less commonly than with asymptomatic disease. Progression to a chronic carrier state should be suspected if the patient remains HBeAg positive or if HBsAg persists beyond 6 months after acute infection.[76]

The presence of the chronic HBsAg carrier state also can create diagnostic confusion in the serodiagnosis of acute viral hepatitis. A patient with acute viral hepatitis who is HBsAg positive does not necessarily have acute hepatitis B; the patient may be a chronic HBsAg carrier and have a superimposed and unrelated form of acute liver injury. This possibility is not as unlikely as it may seem. People who are at high risk for developing hepatitis B and, therefore, may have the chronic HBsAg carrier state often are at high risk for developing other forms of acute viral hepatitis. Indeed, delta hepatitis represents this phenomenon: an acute viral hepatitis superimposed on the chronic HBsAg carrier state.[9] In this situation, testing for IgM anti-HBc can be helpful. This marker of acute type B hepatitis should be absent if the patient is a chronic HBsAg carrier and has another form of acute hepatocellular injury.[79]

Hepatitis D (Delta)

Delta hepatitis is unusual in that it absolutely requires coinfection with hepatitis B virus (see Ch. 124). It is a defective RNA virus that utilizes HBsAg for its structural protein shell.[9,80] HDV infection occurs only in patients who also have HBsAg in serum and thus have either acute or chronic HBV infection. In the United States and Western Europe, delta hepatitis occurs most commonly in persons who have multiple parenteral exposures such as IV drug addicts, hemophiliacs, and persons who have multiple transfusions.[80] HDV infection is uncommon in medical care workers and male homosexuals. There are several areas

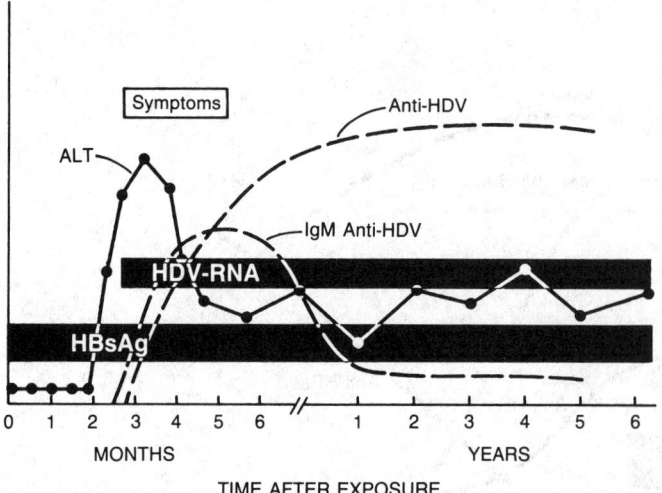

FIG. 8. The clinical, virologic, and serologic courses of a typical case of acute hepatitis D (delta hepatitis) superinfection in a patient with a chronic hepatitis B infection leading to chronic HDV infection. ALT: alanine aminotransferase; HBsAg: hepatitis B surface antigen; HDV: hepatitis D virus; anti-HDV: antibody to HDV.

of the world with a high prevalence of HDV infection among HBV carriers, including the Amazon basin in South America, Central Africa, Southern Italy, and Middle Eastern countries. Why HDV infection became established among HBsAg carriers in those particular areas of the world and not in others such as China and Southeast Asia (where hepatitis B is very common) is not known. Acute delta infection occurs in two forms, depending on the state of the underlying HBV infection: *(1)* as coinfection in which acute delta hepatitis occurs simultaneously with acute hepatitis B; and *(2)* more commonly, as superinfection in which acute delta hepatitis is superimposed on an chronic hepatitis B (Fig. 8).[81] Delta antigen can sometimes be detected in the serum during the early phase of acute delta hepatitis; with disappearance of antigen, anti-HDV arises.[82] However, the appearance of anti-HDV may be delayed, short lived, and low in titer. Thus, many patients with acute delta hepatitis will test negative for anti-HDV during the acute illness and will only become positive in convalescence and then only in low titer. A radioimmunoassay for anti-HDV is commercially available,[83] but anti-HDV tests are not always reliable for diagnosis of acute HDV infection.

Most patients with acute delta coinfection recover; as the hepatitis B resolves and HBsAg is cleared from the serum, the HDV infection also resolves. Less than 5 percent of cases of acute delta coinfection result in chronic delta hepatitis. In contrast, most patients with delta superinfection are left with chronic delta hepatitis; because HBsAg persists, the HDV infection can persist. More than 70 percent of cases of delta superinfection result in chronic hepatitis.[82] The diagnosis of chronic HDV infection is easier than that of acute type D hepatitis; high titers of anti-HDV (>1:100 by commercial radioimmunoassay) indicate ongoing delta infection. Furthermore, patients with chronic delta hepatitis have HDV antigen detectable by immunohistochemical techniques in the liver and persistence of IgM anti-HDV in serum.[82]

Two research assays have provided information regarding the natural history and biology of HDV infection: tests of HDV antigen in serum and liver using immunoblotting[84] and tests for HDV RNA in serum and liver using molecular hybridization technology with probes made from cloned cDNA or RNA.[85] The finding of HDV antigen or RNA in serum is a direct demonstration of the presence of virus and indicates active viral replication. HDV antigen and RNA are typically present transiently during the early phases of acute delta hepatitis and for prolonged periods in chronic delta hepatitis. The sensitivity of these assays is still not well documented; only 50–80 percent of patients with chronic delta hepatitis (as shown by the presence of delta antigen in liver by immunoperoxidase) have detectable HDV antigen or RNA in serum. The use of the polymerase chain reaction for the detection of HDV RNA is more sensitive than molecular hybridization.

Clinically, delta hepatitis tends to be a severe illness. Acute delta hepatitis has a mortality rate of 2 to 20 percent.[80] The illness also often has a biphasic and protracted course. Chronic delta hepatitis is a severe illness and is more likely to result in serious morbidity or mortality than chronic hepatitis B alone or chronic hepatitis C. In large series, 60–70 percent of patients with chronic delta hepatitis eventually developed cirrhosis, and the majority of these patients died of liver disease.[86] The progression to cirrhosis usually takes 10–15 years, but it can occur as quickly as 2 years after onset of infection.[80]

The epidemiology of delta hepatitis indicates that it is usually spread by parenteral exposures, which explains why this disease is common among drug addicts and hemophiliacs. Other modes of spread are less well defined. In some areas of the world, intrafamilial spread has been documented as well as spread between sexual partners.[87] Interestingly, delta hepatitis often occurs in indolent, prolonged severe epidemics that strike susceptible populations (i.e., populations with a high HBsAg carrier rate).[24] Epidemics of delta virus have been described in the Amazon Basin, Central Africa, as well as among communities of drug addicts and institutionalized, mentally handicapped children.[80]

The diagnosis of delta hepatitis should be suspected in any HBsAg-positive patient with acute or chronic hepatitis, especially if the disease is severe or if the patient is a drug addict or has had multiple parenteral exposures. The diagnosis can be made by the finding of HBsAg and anti-HDV in serum: rising titers of antibody indicate acute infection, and sustained high titers indicate chronic infection. Confirmation of the diagnosis rests in finding HDV antigen or RNA in serum or liver.

Hepatitis C

Hepatitis C is the designation for what had been referred to as parenterally transmitted or "classic" non-A, non-B hepatitis until the causative agent of this disease was identified (see Ch. 132). Although acute hepatitis caused by HCV obviously occurs, HCV infection presents much more frequently as a chronic hepatitis diagnosed on the basis of blood chemistry testing. Indeed, the singular feature that distinguishes disease caused by hepatitis C in comparison to the other hepatotropic viral infections is the propensity toward the development of chronic infection. The original description of the existence of a non-A, non-B form of viral hepatitis was made in 1974 and 1975, when Prince and colleagues[12a] studied a group of patients who had non-B post-transfusion hepatitis in which the incubation periods clearly exceeded the range accepted for hepatitis A infections. Feinstone and colleagues[12] showed that non-B transfusion-associated hepatitis was serologically unrelated to infection by HAV, and the term *non-A, non-B hepatitis* was introduced. Attempts to identify the non-A, non-B hepatitis agent were undertaken by many investigators during the following 15 years without convincing success until 1989, when Choo and coworkers,[13] using advanced molecular biology techniques, identified the etiologic agent of non-A, non-B hepatitis and named it the *hepatitis C virus*. The molecular cloning, sequencing, and analysis of the HCV genome has enabled characterization and classification of the virus.[88,89] The expression and synthesis of specific viral proteins using recombinant technology has led to the development of clinically useful diagnostic tests based on the detection of serum antibody to these viral antigens.[14]

Hepatitis C virus is the most common cause of post-transfusion hepatitis, accounting for 70–95 percent of post-transfusion hepatitis. With the implementation of universal donor testing by the new assays for antibody to HCV, HCV infection, like HBV, is rapidly becoming a rare event following blood transfusion. However, the majority of HCV infections occur in individuals without previous transfusions, and it appears that parenteral exposure due to illicit drug use and needle sharing constitutes the major means of transmission in the United States. A large proportion of such sporadically acquired infections are also unassociated with obvious risk factors such as parenteral exposure, and there may be means of transmission that have not been fully defined. In recent American surveys, HCV was considered to be the cause of 65–90 percent of cases of sporadic acute viral hepatitis.[20,67,91–95] Surveys of the seroprevalence of antibodies to HCV indicate that between 0.2 and 0.6 percent of volunteer blood donors in the United States are infected. However, much higher prevalence rates have been found among high-risk populations; for example, 18 percent of all patients seen in a major inner city emergency room in Baltimore were seropositive.[96] In part because hepatitis C is associated with a high rate of chronicity, there is a very large reservoir of infected and infectious persons among the general population.

Approximately 25 percent of cases of acute hepatitis C are icteric, and the mortality rate during acute infection is less than 1 percent.[90] There is a high rate of subclinical acute infection, since the majority of individuals with sporadically acquired chronic infections do not recall any previous history suggestive of acute hepatitis. On average, hepatitis C has a more indolent and prolonged course than hepatitis B (Fig. 9). Serum aminotransferases often fluctuate widely and peak at levels (10–20 times normal) somewhat lower than those in hepatitis B (20–50 times normal). The onset also tends to be more insidious than hepatitis B.

In prospective studies, 50–70 percent of persons with acute hepatitis C have persistent abnormalities in liver enzymes indicative of progression to chronic hepatitis.[90,97] Liver biopsy specimens show evidence of chronic hepatitis that may progress to chronic active disease, fibrosis, and cirrhosis. The chronicity rate tends to be just as high after sporadic as after transfusion-related infections.[95] Chronic hepatitis C is frequently indolent and often silent. However, long-term follow-up studies of patients with this disease have shown that 20–25 percent ultimately develop cirrhosis of the liver.[97] It is often with the development of end-stage liver disease that symptoms first appear in patients infected by HCV. Chronic hepatitis C is one of the major causes of cirrhosis in the United States and is one of the most common

indications for liver transplantation in adults. Chronic HCV infections may also be a major cause of hepatocellular carcinoma worldwide.

Antibodies to HCV (anti-HCV) can be detected by immunoassays that utilize recombinant or synthesized antigens based on the deduced genomic sequence of the virus. The commercially available diagnostic tests for HCV detect antibodies to recombinant viral antigens and are most useful to screen blood donors who are chronic HCV carriers as well as to diagnose chronic infection. Since seroconversion may not occur early in acute infection, the antibody tests cannot be relied on for diagnosis of acute hepatitis C infection. However, the anti-HCV almost invariably becomes positive later in the course of the disease. Thus, a patient with an initially seronegative sample during acute disease should be retested in 3–6 months. In addition, a positive antibody test does not distinguish between an acute infection and a chronic infection, and antibody may persist in the minority of patients who have cleared the infection.

Hepatitis E

In certain developing countries of the world, both large outbreaks and sporadic cases of non-B hepatitis have occurred in individuals already immune to HAV.[99] These outbreaks did not fit the epidemiologic picture of what we now call hepatitis C and were therefore thought to represent a second form of non-A, non-B hepatitis that had been termed enterically transmitted non-A, non-B hepatitis. The causative agent was originally identified in much the same way as HAV was—by use of immunoelectron microscopy on stool samples of an infected individual. In this case, the individual was the investigator who ingested a stool filtrate that he had collected during his investigations of an outbreak.[15] The genome of this virus has now been molecularly cloned and has organizational features similar to those of caliciviruses. It has been named hepatitis E virus (see Ch. 152).[16]

Epidemiologically, hepatitis E resembles hepatitis A: both are transmitted by the fecal-oral route, and disease tends to occur both in epidemics and as sporadic cases. Outbreaks of hepatitis E have been described from India, Pakistan, Russia, China, Central and Northern Africa, Peru, and Mexico.[17] Most outbreaks have been linked to fecal contamination of the water supply. The outbreaks were distinctive in that they largely affected young adults and had unusually high mortality rates in pregnant women.[99–101] Secondary cases in families were uncommon, and the outbreaks were generally self-limited. No outbreaks of this disease have been described in the United States or Western Europe, but cases have occurred in travelers returning from endemic areas.

Clinically, hepatitis E is characterized as an acute self-limited disease that is often cholestatic. Serum aminotransferase levels tend to be lower in this disease than in other forms of acute viral hepatitis, but serum alkaline phosphatase tends to be somewhat higher.[99] Prolonged jaundice can occur. As is the case with hepatitis A, this disease does not lead to chronic hepatitis or to a carrier state.

HEV is a small RNA virus that is found in the stools of patients during the incubation period and early acute phase of illness.[15,101] The amount of HEV shedding in stool is generally not as great as the amount of virus found in the stools of patients with hepatitis A. HEV may also be more labile in the environment than HAV. These features may explain the low levels of secondary spread of HEV infections.

Antibody to HEV (anti-HEV) can be detected by immunoelectron microscopy, by inhibition of immunofluorescence detection of HEV antigen in hepatocyte cytoplasm[101,102] and recently by enzyme immunoassays using antigen expressed in recombinant DNA systems. These techniques have shown that antibody develops early during the course of illness. Cases of hepatitis associated with large-scale epidemics of enterically transmitted non-A, non-B hepatitis have invariably demon-

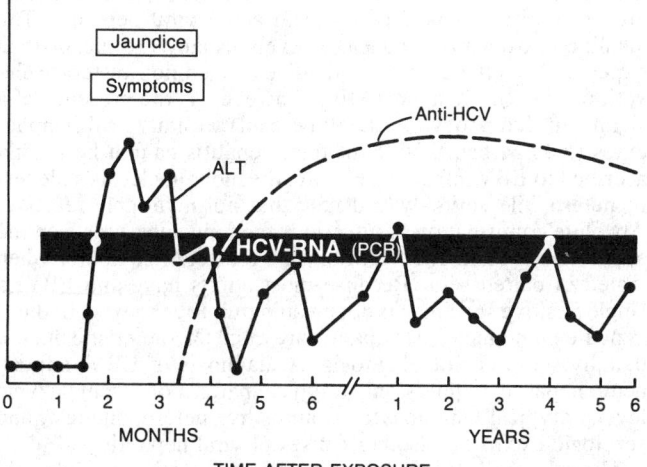

FIG. 9. The clinical, virologic, and serologic courses of a typical case of acute hepatitis C. ALT: alanine aminotransferase; HCV-RNA: hepatitis C virus RNA as determined by polymerase chain reaction; anti-HCV: antibody to HCV.

strated the development of anti-HEV. In contrast, none of a large number of cases of sporadic non-A, non-B hepatitis from the United States have demonstrated anti-HEV reactivity. These preliminary results suggest that HEV may be a common cause of jaundice and acute hepatitis in the developing world, but is still a very rare cause of hepatitis in the United States.

Serodiagnosis of Acute Viral Hepatitis

A guide to the serodiagnosis of acute viral hepatitis is given in Figure 5. Patients in whom acute hepatitis is suspected based on history, physical examination, and elevated serum aminotransferase activity should be tested for IgM anti-HAV, HBsAg, IgM anti-HBc, and anti-HCV. The presence of IgM anti-HAV establishes the diagnosis of acute hepatitis A. The presence of HBsAg suggests the diagnosis of hepatitis B, but does not differentiate between acute versus chronic disease. The presence of IgM anti-HBc confirms the diagnosis of *acute* hepatitis B; its absence suggests that the patient is actually a chronic carrier of HBsAg and that the acute hepatitis is either due to an exacerbation of the underlying chronic hepatitis B or due to superinfection with another hepatitis agent. Patients with chronic hepatitis B may have low levels of IgM anti-HBc as long as viral replication persists; however, the commercial assays for IgM anti-HBc detect this antibody only when present in high titer.[78]

Anti-HDV should be sought only when evidence of HBV infection is found, since delta hepatitis can occur only in the presence of hepatitis B. The presence of anti-HDV suggests the diagnosis of delta hepatitis coinfection, although it is not conclusive and does not indicate whether the delta infection is resolved, ongoing, acute, or chronic. The titer of anti-HDV can help to separate acute (low or rising titers) from chronic delta hepatitis (sustained high titers >1:100).

Hepatitis C can be diagnosed on the basis of finding anti-HCV antibodies in serum, although the presence of such antibodies does not distinguish between acute and chronic HCV infections. Indeed, because of the fluctuating nature of the transaminase elevations seen in association with chronic hepatitis C, it may be difficult to determine clinically whether the patient is acutely infected or his having a flare of chronic disease unless a source of infection is found (such as contaminated blood) or previous chemistries indicate ongoing liver inflammation. Antibody is not always detectable early in the course of the acute infection, and assays to detect IgM anti-HCV are not clinically available. The first-generation HCV immunodetection assays were insensitive in diagnosing acute infection and frequently did not detect antibodies until as long as 6–12 months after infection occurred; however, current second-generation assays have shortened the window period to about 8–12 weeks. Patients can be antibody negative during early acute infection, and one should retest such individuals 3–6 months later if there is a suspicion of hepatitis C infection. Because of the high incidence of chronicity associated with hepatitis C, acutely infected patients should always be followed for 6–12 months to determine whether chronic hepatitis C has developed. Mixed infections of hepatitis C with any of the other viruses are always a possibility and should be considered. Many research centers use the polymerase chain reaction to obtain direct evidence for the presence of HCV. At present this is the only technology available with the sensitivity required to detect HCV (as opposed to antibodies) in clinical samples. Unfortunately, it has been very difficult to bring polymerase chain reaction technology to the clinical diagnostic laboratory, and it remains a research tool.

Anti-HEV testing is rarely necessary in the United States or Western Europe, as the only cases of HEV infections in these areas to date have been in travelers returning from endemic areas. Immunoassays to detect anti-HEV antibody are not currently commercially available in the United States. Nevertheless, this situation may change, and diagnostic tests could be made available based on present technology.

Chronic Hepatitis

Chronic hepatitis with an acute exacerbation can mimic acute viral hepatitis and can represent a significant problem in the differential diagnosis. This is best demonstrated for HBsAg-positive chronic hepatitis. These patients occasionally can be asymptomatic, except for recurrent bouts of jaundice and symptoms of hepatitis that can occur with almost seasonal regularity. Several features should suggest the presence of chronic hepatitis. These include previous bouts of hepatitis or jaundice, a prolonged and indolent preicteric phase of disease, protracted and only mild-to-moderate elevations in aminotransferase and serum bilirubin levels, and increased globulin and decreased serum albumin levels. In most instances the presence of HBsAg with absence of IgM anti-HBc confirms the diagnosis of chronic infection. In the final analysis, however, differentiation requires the test of time. The persistence of symptoms or abnormal serum enzyme levels for more than 6 months indicates chronic hepatitis. A liver biopsy specimen usually can be helpful if it demonstrates chronic hepatitis with fibrosis, piecemeal necrosis, or ground-glass cells; it can also be helpful in determining the severity and aggressiveness of the hepatic inflammatory process. However, it may not clearly differentiate acute from chronic hepatitis at the height of an acute exacerbation. Other features of chronic hepatitis are discussed in Chapter 97.

Acute Hepatitis Due to Other Viruses

Several other common viral infections can secondarily affect the liver and can cause an acute hepatitislike picture. The liver disease associated with these infections usually is mild, self-limited, subclinical, and overshadowed by the other symptoms in these diseases.

Of prime importance as a secondary cause of viral hepatitis is EBV, the agent of heterophile-positive infectious mononucleosis. Mild elevations in serum aminotransferase levels (two to five times normal) in the absence of symptoms suggestive of liver disease are very common in acute mononucleosis. This syndrome generally does not present a diagnostic confusion with acute viral hepatitis; the liver disease is mild and subclinical. However, on rare occasions, EBV infection can be manifested as acute icteric hepatitis without the usual symptoms of mononucleosis.[50] Physical examination may reveal little or no evidence of pharyngitis or lymphadenopathy. Several features of the hepatitis should suggest that it is due to EBV infection. First, if fever (which is low grade in acute viral hepatitis) is prominent and persistent into the icteric phase, this is suggestive of mononucleosis. Second, the serum enzyme levels in mononucleosis are not entirely typical of those in acute viral hepatitis. The alkaline phosphatase and LDH levels usually are higher than expected from the degree of jaundice and aminotransferase elevation (Fig. 2). Most suggestive, however, is the presence of a significant lymphocytosis (>50 percent) with atypical lymphocytes (>20 percent). Without this, hepatitis cannot be readily ascribed to EBV infection. Finally, the mononucleosis slide test or heterophile antibody is usually but not invariably reactive. Absolute confirmation of infectious mononucleosis rests on the appearance of anti-EBV IgM or on a fourfold rise in titer when tested in paired sera. Because most adults have anti-EBV, a single positive specimen is not meaningful. Liver biopsy findings in acute mononucleosis hepatitis are quite characteristic but not usually required for diagnosis. A diagnosis of EBV-induced acute hepatitis requires only a typical pattern of serum enzyme levels, atypical lymphocytosis, a positive heterophile test, and serologic exclusion of other causes of viral hepatitis.

The role of CMV infection in causing a hepatitis in adults still is subject to debate, especially as it relates to post-transfusion hepatitis.[97,103–105] The problem centers on relating changes in anti-CMV titers and/or excretion of the virus to an episode of hepatitis. Such changes can occur in totally asymptomatic patients and are frequent after blood transfusions (regardless of the occurrence of hepatitis).[103] There is no doubt that primary CMV infection can cause a heterophile-negative mononucleosis syndrome that frequently is accompanied by hepatosplenomegaly and minor elevations of serum aminotransferase levels.[103-105] Whether CMV can induce a purely hepatitislike syndrome is unclear. If it can, it probably is rare in adults. The diagnosis rests on the finding of atypical lymphocytosis with acute liver injury or the absence of heterophile antibody along with laboratory evidence of acute CMV infection, such as serum anti-CMV IgM, a seroconversion or rise in anti-CMV IgG titers, or excretion of virus in blood, urine, or oropharyngeal secretions.

Several other common human viruses (including rubella, rubeola, mumps viruses, and coxsackie B viruses) can induce mild abnormalities in liver enzymes.[106] These changes are not common and rarely are accompanied by jaundice. In the immunosuppressed host, however, several usually benign viruses can cause a disseminated infection, part of which may be hepatic involvement. Chief among these are herpes simplex virus, CMV, and varicella-zoster virus.[103-107] Hepatic necrosis, marked elevations in the serum aminotransferase levels, icterus, and even death from hepatic failure have been described. In the immunosuppressed host with fulminant hepatic failure, a search for these viruses should be made. Liver biopsy specimens may demonstrate inclusion bodies and/or intranuclear herpesvirus particles. These viruses, however, are not common causes of sporadic acute hepatitis in the otherwise healthy host.

Though yellow fever has not been reported in the United States for over 40 years, it is still enzootic in Central America, South America, and central Africa, and the mosquito vector does exist in the United States. Yellow fever is marked by a short incubation period (3–7 days), severe hepatitis with high aminotransferase level elevations, and a high mortality rate (approximately 20 percent).[108] It need be considered only in the recent traveler to enzootic areas who has not received adequate immunization. The diagnosis is made by isolation of virus from blood, by finding a significant rise in antibody titers or by characteristic pathologic findings in the liver.

Hepatitis Due To Nonviral Infectious Diseases

Elevations in serum enzyme levels and liver dysfunction can occur with many nonviral infectious diseases due to bacteria, mycobacteria, rickettsia, and fungi. Thus, jaundice with mild elevations in aminotransferase and alkaline phosphatase levels (two to five times normal) can be seen with sepsis as well as with pneumococcal pneumonia.[50,109] Furthermore, minor elevations in liver enzyme levels without jaundice are often seen with many severe infections that usually do not primarily involve the liver, including pulmonary and miliary tuberculosis,[110-114] brucellosis, tularemia, plague, bacterial sepsis, and legionnaires' disease. Liver biopsy specimens usually show nonspecific changes and focal areas of necrosis. However, at times (as in miliary tuberculosis), a liver biopsy specimen can be very helpful in establishing the primary diagnosis.

Three nonviral infectious agents that can produce an acute hepatitislike syndrome deserve special note: syphilis, leptospirosis, and Q fever. Early syphilis, either primary or early secondary, can be accompanied by significant serum aminotransferase level elevations (three to eight times normal).[115] Jaundice, however, is rare, and the chancre of primary syphilis or the rash of secondary syphilis should be present. The liver enzyme tests, as in mononucleosis hepatitis, show atypically high elevations of alkaline phosphatase levels (four to eight times normal) when compared with the extent of aminotransferase abnormalities. Diagnosis is established by the finding of a reactive VDRL and fluorescent treponemal antibody, as well as by the typical clinical setting and response to treatment.

Leptospirosis is an unusual cause of jaundice and hepatitis in the United States. The disease is caused by at least 15 serotypes of *Leptospira interrogans*.[116] The serotypes that are responsible for most of the infections in this country are (1) icterohemorrhagiae (30–40 percent), which is enzootic in rats; (2) canicola (30 percent), enzootic in dogs; and (3) pomona (10–20 percent), enzootic in cattle and swine. The history usually points to exposure to these animals or their urine (lake water, swimming holes). The clinical manifestations include malaise, fever, chills, severe myalgias, and headache.[116] Later symptoms of cough, sputum production, prostration, and hepatic and renal involvement appear. Hepatic involvement is most common with the serotype icterohemorrhagiae. Evaluation may demonstrate fever, prostration, severe muscle tenderness, hepatosplenomegaly, and pneumonitis. Laboratory abnormalities include leukocytosis and a left shift in the differential count. The urinalysis may show albuminuria, casts, and white and red blood cells. In severe cases, the urine output falls, and the blood urea nitrogen level rises; central nervous system manifestations and pneumonitis may also appear. Liver function tests reveal jaundice that is often out of proportion to the degree of serum enzyme level elevations. As with the jaundice of pneumococcal pneumonia,[109] the jaundice in leptospirosis appears to be a result of a defect in bilirubin excretion rather than the result of hepatic necrosis.[116] The diagnosis is made by finding a high titer or a significant rise in leptospiral agglutinins. Due to the variable course of this disease, the value of antibiotic therapy has been difficult to demonstrate. Nevertheless, a 1 week course of intravenous penicillin or ampicillin in moderate or severe cases or oral doxycycline, ampicillin, or amoxicillin in milder cases is recommended and should commence as early in the disease as possible.

Q fever is the third nonviral infectious disease that may be mistaken for acute viral hepatitis. This disease is caused by the rickettsial agent *Coxiella burnetii* and is uncommon in the United States. In this disease, as in leptospirosis, constitutional symptoms are prominent with fever, chills, and pneumonitis. Overt jaundice occurs in only about 5 percent of the cases, although subclinical hepatic involvement is quite common. In rare cases, hepatitis without pneumonitis occurs, and a differentiation from acute viral hepatitis may be difficult.[117] Epidemiologic features should reveal exposure to farm or wild animals (cows, goats, sheep). Clinically, persistent fever, pneumonitis, and prostration are more prominent than in viral hepatitis. Liver function tests reveal jaundice with only mild elevations in aminotransferase levels (two to five times normal) and sometimes marked elevations in the alkaline phosphatase concentration. The diagnosis is made by demonstration of a rise in agglutination titers against *C. burnetii* in paired sera. The diagnosis and treatment of Q fever are discussed in Chapter 166.

Drug-Related Acute Hepatitis

The major differential diagnosis in acute hepatitis is often between viral and drug-related hepatitis. Every patient with hepatitis should be questioned carefully about all medications taken, and should be specifically asked about over-the-counter products. Drug-related acute liver injury is not nearly as common as acute viral hepatitis, but it often is much more serious and is a prominent cause of fulminant hepatic failure.[118] Drug-related acute liver injury may act synergistically with acute viral hepatitis to increase the severity of liver necrosis. Many drugs and toxins have been shown to induce hepatic injury, but few have actually been repeatedly implicated as causing an acute hepatitislike syndrome. The major common medications available in the United States that are associated with significant hepatotoxicity are listed in Table 1 by the type of injury usually seen and with an approximate incidence. This is not an exhaustive list. Any patient who develops hepatitis while taking a drug that is a known or potential hepatotoxin should have treatment with the medication stopped until the full clinical picture can be eval-

TABLE 1. Common Causes of Drug-Related Liver Injury

Agent Class	Agent	Frequency of Occurrence[a]	Type of Injury
Analgesic	Acetaminophen	Dose-related	Hepatitis
	Aspirin	Dose-related	Hepatitis
Anesthetic	Halothane	Rare	Hepatitis
	Methoxyflurane	(0.01–0.1%) Rare	Hepatitis
Antiarthritic	Allopurinol	Rare	Granuloma/hepatitis
	Indomethacin	Very rare	Hepatitis
	Phenylbutazone	Rare	Granuloma/mixed
Antibacterial	Carbenicillin	Low[b]	Hepatitis
	Erythromycin estolate	Low	Cholestasis
	Nitrofurantoin	Rare	Mixed
	Oxacillin	Rare	Hepatitis
	Sulfonadmides/sulfones	Rare	Hepatitis
	Tetracycline	Dose-related	Steatosis/necrosis
Antifungal	Ketoconazole	Rare	Hepatitis
Antineoplastic	Azathioprine	Rare[b]	Cholestasis
	6-Mercaptopurine	Common[b]	Hepatitis
	Methotrexate	(10–35%)	Fibrosis
	Mithromycin	Dose-related Rare[b]	Necrosis
Antituberculosis	Isoniazid	Low (1%)	Hepatitis
	Para-aminosalicylic acid	Low (0.1–1%)	Hepatitis
	Rifampin	Low	Hepatitis
Cardiovascular	Methyldopa	Low	Hepatitis
	Quinidine	Rare	Granuloma/hepatitis
	Thiazides	Very rare	
	Amiodarone	Low (1–3%)	Mixed Steatosis/necrosis
Endocrinologic	17-Alkylated androgens	Dose-related	Cholestasis
	Chlorpropamide	Rare	Cholestasis
	Oral contraceptives	Rare	Cholestasis
	Propylthiouracil	Rare	Hepatitis
	Tolbutamine	Very rare	Cholestasis
	Dantrolene	Low (1–2%)	Hepatitis
Neuro- and psychopharmacologic	Monoamine oxidase inhibitors	Low	Hepatitis
	Phenothiazines	Low (1–2%)	Cholestasis
	Phenytoin	Rare	Hepatitis
	Valproic acid	Low (1–2%)	Steatosis/necrosis

[a] The frequency of occurrence is an estimate from the literature[118]: common = >2 percent, low = 0.1–2 percent, rare = <0.1 percent; very rare = isolated case reports only.
[b] Dose-related to some degree.

uated. The most serious mistake that can be made in caring for patients with acute hepatic injury is to underestimate the role of drugs and to continue administering them in the face of acute hepatitis. The suspicion of drug-induced liver injury should be the greatest when epidemiologic features are not absolutely typical of acute viral hepatitis (e.g., in the elderly, in patients with underlying diseases, and in patients who develop fulminant hepatitis). However, even when epidemiologic features are appropriate for acute viral hepatitis, the role of drugs should not be dismissed: the renal dialysis patient taking methyldopa or the drug addict receiving isoniazid who develops acute hepatitis should have treatment with these medications stopped until adequate evaluation dismisses their role.

Some of the most commonly encountered causes of drug-related acute hepatitis are aspirin, acetaminophen, isoniazid, rifampin, phenytoin, and the anesthetic halothane. Aspirin (acetylsalicylic acid) can cause moderate elevations in serum enzyme levels (two to five times normal), but it rarely causes jaundice. Aspirin hepatotoxicity seems to occur only with a high maintenance dosage, usually with serum salicylate levels of 20 mg/dl or greater. Characteristically, the biochemical abnormalities subside rapidly on withdrawing the drug. Acetaminophen

overdose, both purposeful and accidental, has become a major cause of fulminant hepatic failure.[119–121] The liver disease appears 2–5 days after the overdose. Every patient with evidence of severe hepatic injury should be carefully questioned regarding acetaminophen use, since the liver injury can be averted if the patient is treated within 10 hours of the overdose with large doses of N-acetyl cysteine (mucomyst). Liver injury from the chronic use of acetaminophen in high doses also has been described.[119] Both isoniazid and rifampin have been implicated in causing an acute hepatitislike syndrome; both have been associated with fulminant hepatic failure. Rifampin hepatic injury usually has its onset within the first weeks of therapy, whereas isoniazid hepatotoxicity is most common after 1–2 months of therapy. The incidence of isoniazid hepatotoxicity is approximately 1 percent, but it is definitely higher in older age groups and approaches 10 percent in patients over the age of 40. Treatment with these drugs should be discontinued if symptoms of hepatitis or jaundice appear or if aminotransferase levels are persistently elevated more than five times normal. Phenytoin can cause an acute hepatitis, usually within 1–6 weeks of starting the medication, and is associated with other manifestations of hypersensitivity such as fever, rash, lymphadenopathy, and eosinophilia. It has a mortality of approximately 10 percent. A cooperative study on halothane-induced hepatitis suggested that approximately 1/10,000 patients given this anesthetic for the first time and 1/1000 given it more than once develop fulminant hepatic necrosis.[122–125] Clinically, halothane-related jaundice appears within 3–14 days of its use and resembles an acute, severe viral hepatitis. Fever is very characteristic early in the course, and many patients have an accompanying leukocytosis and eosinophilia. Halothane-induced hepatitis usually is not confused with post-transfusion hepatitis because of its early onset after surgery and anesthesia.

Anoxic Liver Injury

A syndrome resembling acute viral hepatitis can occur after anoxic injury to the liver due to a period of hypotension, severe left- or right-sided heart failure, or cardiopulmonary arrest.[126] An inciting event is frequently obvious; however, in some cases, no clear history of an anoxic episode is obtained, or the patient is brought to the hospital comatose and unable to give an adequate history. In these situations, a diagnosis usually can be made on the basis of serum enzymes. Within hours of an anoxic episode, there are marked elevations of aminotransferase levels into the range seen with acute viral hepatitis (Fig. 2). The LDH level is dramatically elevated (as is the creatinine phosphokinase level), and it may be most helpful in suggesting this diagnosis. Most typical of anoxic liver injury, however, is the rapid resolution of these enzyme abnormalities. The aminotransferase levels can fall from 50–100 times elevated to normal within 1 week. Jaundice is uncommon and mild. In some cases, aminotransferase levels remain elevated to two to five times normal for 5–14 days after the injury, in which case differentiation from acute viral hepatitis may be difficult and may require a liver biopsy procedure (which will show a bland centrozonal necrosis). While a liver biopsy specimen is diagnostic, it generally is not needed for the diagnosis when the clinical history and pattern of enzyme levels are typical.

Alcoholic Liver Disease

Alcohol abuse is the most common cause of serious liver disease in the United States. Acute alcoholic hepatitis may be confused with viral hepatitis. These patients have the gradual and imprecisely dated onset of malaise, anorexia, weight loss, nausea and vomiting, fever chills, abdominal swelling, and jaundice or dark urine. The history of alcohol intake should suggest the diagnosis, but many patients conceal or underestimate the amount of alcohol they consume. The lower limit of alcohol intake said to lead to alcoholic liver disease is 80 g/day; the equivalent of a half-pint of 86 proof whiskey, four conventional cocktails, five to six cans of beer, or 1 quart of wine each day.[118,127] Alcoholic liver disease is rarely manifested until after 10 or more years of excessive drinking.

Clinically, the patient usually appears chronically ill. Fever and tachycardia are common. Examination may reveal evidence of chronic liver disease and alcohol abuse that is not seen with acute viral hepatitis—wasting, parotid enlargement, palmar erythema, vascular spiders, gynecomastia, testicular atrophy, significant hepatomegaly, and signs of portal hypertension. The laboratory data may be helpful.[50] The white blood cell count is usually elevated with a left shift. The hematocrit may be slightly decreased, and the red blood cell indices reveal macrocytosis (with or without folate deficiency). Liver function tests reveal hyperbilirubinemia and typically a low albumin level and a prolonged prothrombin time. The aminotransferase values are most characteristic (Fig. 2) in that the AST level is elevated out of proportion to the ALT level (which can be slightly elevated, normal, or even low), while in viral hepatitis the ALT and AST are comparably elevated.

Cholestatic Liver Disease

Cholestatic liver disease refers to a host of diseases marked by bile retention. Cholestasis can be due either to extrahepatic biliary obstruction (from gallstones, stricture, pancreatitis, or tumor) or to intrahepatic causes (from primary biliary cirrhosis, several childhood cholestatic syndromes, and drug-induced cholestasis from phenothiazines or methyltestosterone). These patients have the nonspecific symptoms of acute liver disease with jaundice, but the signs and symptoms of cholestasis are prominent—the degree of jaundice, lightening of stools, and itching overshadow the amount of anorexia or malaise. Laboratory data are confirmatory and show modest abnormalities in aminotransferase levels but marked elevations in alkaline phosphatase levels (Fig. 2).

Other Liver Diseases

Few other causes of jaundice pose a problem in the differential diagnosis of acute hepatitis. Rare causes of an acute hepatitislike syndrome include Wilson's disease,[128] sickle cell crisis,[129] acute Budd-Chiari syndrome or veno-occlusive disease,[130] and massive replacement of the liver by tumor.[131] These causes usually are associated with a fulminant or severe hepatitis. Patients with hemolytic anemia may have vague nonspecific symptoms and jaundice, but the urine will have no bilirubin, and the aminotransferase levels will be normal. Patients with congenital disorders of bilirubin metabolism (Gilbert and Dubin-Johnson syndromes) may become notably jaundiced, especially during intercurrent viral illnesses, but serum enzyme levels should be normal.

MANAGEMENT

Supportive Care

There is limited specific therapy for acute viral hepatitis. Good management consists of supportive measures, relief of symptoms, and avoidance of further injury. An important role of the physician is to identify and carefully follow the rare patient who develops fulminant hepatic failure; early consultation and referral to a liver transplant center is essential in such cases.

Hospitalization. Most patients with acute viral hepatitis do not require hospitalization. Little can be done for most patients in the hospital that is not available at home. Hospitalization is advisable for any patient who is in danger from dehydration due to poor oral intake, whose prothrombin time shows prolonga-

tion, who has a rising bilirubin level (>15–20 mg/dl), or who has any clinical evidence of hepatic failure. The duration of hospitalization, of course, will vary with the severity of illness. Once symptoms have abated, the patient usually can be discharged to continue convalescence at home. There is no need to continue hospitalization until laboratory test values return to normal.

Rest. Bed rest should be prescribed for patients with acute viral hepatitis during the period of symptoms. However, the bed rest should not be absolute; use of the bathroom and periods of being up each day should be encouraged. Traditionally, it has been recommended that bed rest be continued until recovery is complete and liver function test values have returned to normal. While most patients are willing to remain at bed rest for the duration of the symptoms, most—and especially the young—will be anxious to return to normal activity once the symptoms abate. Indeed, controlled studies have shown that after the symptoms have cleared normal activity and even strenuous exercise does not slow recovery, induce relapses, or predispose to chronic liver disease.[132] It is unnecessarily restrictive to insist on bed rest until the aminotransferase levels return to normal or until HBsAg is negative. A gradual return to activity with monitoring of liver function test values is warranted once the symptoms have abated. Relapses of symptoms should be treated with a return to bed rest.

Alcohol. Alcohol should be avoided during the acute illness. However, there are no data to suggest that moderate alcohol intake after recovery leads to a worsening of acute hepatitis or predisposes to chronic hepatitis. While it is prudent to advise abstinence during the acute symptomatic phase of viral hepatitis, the recommendation of total abstinence for 6–12 months after viral hepatitis is unnecessarily strict.

Diet. There is little evidence that any dietary regimen has any effect on the course of acute hepatitis. A generally nutritious diet should be encouraged. During the symptomatic phase, patients frequently are anorexic and may have distinct likes and dislikes. The person with anorexia cannot be forced to eat; however, some encouragement can come from the use of frequent small feedings and a diet low in fat but high in carbohydrates. Forced or nasogastric tube feedings should be avoided.

Drugs. Most medications are best avoided during acute hepatitis. In particular, sedatives should not be given, since their elimination is altered in patients with hepatic disease. Antibiotics are not indicated. Immune serum globulin has no effect. Symptomatic therapy for nausea, pain, or sleeplessness may be needed at times. Antiemetics can be helpful, but chlorpromazine (because of its potential to cause intrahepatic cholestasis) should be avoided. Among analgesics, acetaminophen is preferable to aspirin (because of its reduced effects on platelet function and the gastric mucosa) and to codeine or morphine derivatives (because of their sedative effects). Previous data have suggested that estrogens might worsen the course of typical acute viral hepatitis; however, prospective studies of women with acute viral hepatitis who were taking oral contraceptives have failed to support this.[133] Nevertheless, it is advisable that treatment with all but the most necessary medications be discontinued during the acute phase of viral hepatitis. Vitamins often are given but have not been shown to be beneficial in patients with acute hepatitis. If the prothrombin time is prolonged, a trial of vitamin K (1–5 mg IM) can be given. The administration of vitamin K, however, will have little or no effect on the prothrombin time in typical viral hepatitis unless there has been prolonged cholestasis.

Treatment

There are no well accepted specific therapies for acute viral hepatitis. Corticosteroids have not been shown to shorten the course or to aid in healing of acute viral hepatitis.[134,135] Indeed, some studies have indicated that corticosteroids may predispose to more prolonged illness, more relapses, and more chronic liver disease.[135] Therefore corticosteroids are definitely not indicated for the typical uncomplicated case of acute viral hepatitis.

Corticosteroids have sometimes been recommended for two situations in acute viral hepatitis: cholestatic hepatitis and fulminant hepatic failure. In prolonged cholestasis after acute viral hepatitis, corticosteroids can decrease serum bilirubin levels and ameliorate symptoms of fatigue and itching. Use of corticosteroids in this situation, however, should be limited to cases of hepatitis A, in which there is no possibility of transition to chronic hepatitis. In fulminant hepatitis, corticosteroids are often used, frequently because no other options are available. However, controlled clinical trials have failed to demonstrate any benefit of corticosteroids in acute viral hepatitis, and some have indicated that the adverse side effects of high doses of corticosteroids outweigh their potential benefit.[135]

Interferon-α has been demonstrated to be efficacious as therapy in certain settings of chronic hepatitis B and C.[136-141] It may also hold promise as therapy of acute disease. However, the only studies of antiviral treatment in severe acute viral hepatitis have been in small number of patients. In a study from Israel,[142] five patients with fulminant hepatitis were treated with interferon-α and three survived, which led the authors to suggest that antiviral therapy might be helpful in a subset of patients with severe or fulminant hepatitis. However, in a later study from Spain, only 2 of 12 patients with fulminant hepatitis B or hepatitis B plus delta who were treated with high doses of parenteral interferon-α survived, indicating that this medication is unlikely to be of benefit in reversing fulminant viral hepatitis.[143] The absence of a beneficial effect of therapy in fulminant hepatitis does not necessarily indicate that the therapy will have no effect in patients with less advanced or severe hepatic injury. Indeed, there is preliminary evidence in a limited number of patients with acute hepatitis C that treatment with natural interferon-β can prevent the development of chronic hepatitis C.[144] It has not been determined whether treatment with recombinant interferon-α may be associated with similarly positive results.

Monitoring

Monitoring during acute viral hepatitis should be regular and specific. If hospitalization is necessary, a once or twice daily check on major symptoms is important. The patient should be examined for the degree of icterus, liver size, and the presence of asterixis or other evidence of hepatic encephalopathy. The ALT, AST, alkaline phosphatase, and bilirubin levels and the prothrombin time should be monitored once or twice a week during hospitalization and every 1–2 weeks thereafter until they return to normal. Initially, the patient should be tested for HBsAg. If positive, the test is best repeated every 1–2 months until HBsAg disappears. The continued presence of HBsAg 4–6 months after acute viral hepatitis indicates the establishment of the chronic HBsAg carrier state. If all initial serologies are negative, antibodies to hepatitis C should be re-checked in 6 months, and, if positive, the patient should be further followed for the probable development of chronic hepatitis C.

A percutaneous liver biopsy specimen in acute viral hepatitis may establish the diagnosis, but generally it is not necessary. However, liver biopsy is indicated in several situations: when the diagnosis is in doubt and diagnostic confusion remains despite clinical, biochemical, and serologic data; if more than one explanation of acute liver injury exists; if drug-related acute hepatitis is a possibility; and when specific therapy is being considered.

Fulminant Viral Hepatitis

The management of fulminant viral hepatitis should begin with its early recognition. The initial signs and symptoms of hepatic encephalopathy may be subtle (nightmares, slight changes in personality, restlessness) or dramatic (unexpected aggressive physical or sexual activity). It is important to recognize these signs for what they are and not to use sedatives or physical restraints injudiciously.

At the first sign of encephalopathy, vigorous management should be started.[48,49,145-147] This should include bed rest, a low-protein diet (20–30 g/day), the administration of enemas to cleanse the bowel, and the use of oral neomycin (1.0–1.5 g every 6 hours) or lactulose (30–60 cc in sorbitol every 2–6 hours until loose stools are achieved). Treatment with all sedatives is contraindicated. With deepening coma, the patient should be monitored in an intensive care unit and may require intravenous fluids, a central venous pressure line, a nasogastric tube, and a urinary bladder catheter. Coagulation defects may require correction with the use of fresh frozen plasma (the coagulation factor concentrates such as fibrinogen and prothrombin complex should not be used). The patient should be carefully monitored for gastrointestinal bleeding. Cimetidine (300–500 mg IV every 6 hours) or vigorous antacid therapy may be begun to help prevent upper gastrointestinal bleeding. Most important is careful attention to all the details of "routine" medical management (fluid and electrolyte balance, acid-base balance, pulmonary toilet, IV and bladder catheter care, skin care, and monitoring for signs of blood loss or superinfection). More aggressive experimental approaches such as exchange transfusions, "total body washout," charcoal hemoperfusion, cross-circulation with a human or baboon liver, and immunotherapy with antibody to HBsAg each have had their advocates, but none has been repeatedly shown to be more effective than "conventional" medical management.

The most promising new therapy for fulminant hepatic failure is emergency hepatic transplantation.[145-148] Since the introduction of cyclosporin A as an immunosuppressive agent in the early 1980s, liver transplantation has become a successful and well-accepted approach to severe liver disease. At present more than 2500 liver transplants are done yearly in the United States in 40–50 different medical centers. Approximately 7 percent of patients undergo liver transplantation for fulminant or subacute hepatic failure. The 1–2 year survival rates have ranged between 60 and 90 percent.[147]

The major reason to avoid liver transplantation in fulminant hepatic failure is the possibility of spontaneous recovery. The survival rate of patients with fulminant hepatitis in stages III to IV coma averages 20–30 percent. Features that predict a poor outcome include age (either less than 11 or greater than 40 years), medications as a cause of the liver injury, a prothrombin time greater than 50 seconds in conjunction with a bilirubin greater than 17.6 mg/dl, or a prothrombin time alone greater than 100 seconds.[54,149] The decision for transplantation needs to be made before severe complications supervene, in particular, severe intracranial hypertension with decerebration, after which recovery is unlikely even with transplantation. Interestingly, fulminant hepatitis does not recur in the transplanted liver, although reinfection by the virus may occur.[150,151] Thus, at the first sign of hepatic failure, the physician should refer the patient with acute viral hepatitis to a liver transplant center. The criteria for transplantation in fulminant hepatitis are evolving, and the decision for transplant should be made by a team of physicians with experience in treating fulminant hepatic failure.

PREVENTION

Specifics of prevention in viral hepatitis will be presented in later chapters. Management of needle stick injuries in hospital employees is discussed in Chapters 284 and 285. Certain nonspecific measures regarding the patient with acute hepatitis should be stressed here. If the patient is hospitalized, he should be placed in enteric isolation to prevent the spread of type A hepatitis. Even with lax precautions, such spread is very rare; most patients with hepatitis A are no longer excreting virus once they have become symptomatic. Nevertheless, there are exceptions, and isolation is prudent. Health care personnel should use universal blood and secretion precautions when handling specimens. Labeling of blood specimens to indicate an infectious source is a common practice. It should be stressed, however, that all blood from any patient should be handled as if potentially infectious.

If at home, the patient should be advised about care in personal hygiene—use of a private bathroom, if possible, and careful hand washing. Attention should also be paid to the handling of cuts and lacerations.

Recommendations regarding the prevention of acute hepatitis are governed by the type of viral hepatitis that is being considered. In the case of acute hepatitis A, all family members and close personal contacts should receive immune serum globulin, 0.02–0.06 ml/kg IM, as soon as possible after exposure. Office, factory, and school contacts do not need to be treated. Immune serum globulin can be given for up to 4 weeks after exposure, but it probably is only effective if given within 7–14 days. In the case of acute hepatitis B, prophylaxis only needs to be provided for "regular" sexual contacts. Combined passive-active immunization is considered the preferable method of prophylaxis. Hepatitis B immune globulin (HBIG), 0.06 ml/kg IM as soon as possible and again 1 month later, has been the conventional recommendation in this situation. However, the efficacy of HBIG in preventing the sexual spread of acute hepatitis B has not been well proved.[152,153] In addition, there is now evidence that postexposure immunization with HBV vaccine can attenuate or prevent acute hepatitis B.[154–157] In view of this, the combined approach dictates that vaccine should be given at the recommended dose as soon as possible and then 1 month and 6 months later. In the case of acute delta hepatitis, no specific immunoprophylaxis is available and efforts should be directed toward the prevention of hepatitis B. In the case of non-A, non-B hepatitis (hepatitis C), there is little or no information concerning the efficacy of any mode of prevention. One can administer immunoglobulin (0.06 ml/kg) as soon as possible after percutaneous exposure, but there are no data demonstrating that this approach is efficacious. Similarly, there are no data on the efficacy of immunoglobulin prophylaxis of sexual or household contacts of patients with hepatitis C; however, in view of epidemiologic studies showing that there is a very low rate of transmission of hepatitis C to household or even regular sexual contacts of chronically infected patients, it is unlikely that passive prophylaxis will greatly affect the already low rate of transmission.

There is often a delay between the diagnosis of acute viral hepatitis and the identification of whether the disease is due to hepatitis A, B, C, or D. The recommendations given above require that the prophylaxis of family and intimate contacts of patients be postponed until the results of serologic testing are known. A simplified approach to prophylaxis is to administer immune serum globulin immediately to all family, household, and intimate contacts and to begin HBV vaccination of the sexual contact(s) if the disease is subsequently shown to be type B (or delta) hepatitis. This schema could be modified if the hepatitis is obviously not due to HAV (e.g., post-transfusion hepatitis). This approach is appealing because of its simplicity and also because the titers of anti-HBs (the protective antibody in hepatitis B) in standard preparations of immune serum globulin have been increasing over the past 10–15 years.[152,155] Thus, immune serum globulin that is currently being produced may be partially effective in preventing hepatitis B.

Finally, it should be stressed that viral hepatitis is a reportable disease. Once the diagnosis is verified and serologic testing data are available, they should be reported to the local or state department of health.

REFERENCES

1. Krugman S, Giles JP. Viral hepatitis. New light on an old disease. JAMA. 1970;212:1019.
2. Carey WD, Patel G. Viral hepatitis in the 1990s, part I: Current principles of management. Cleve Clin J Med. 1992;59:317–25.
3. Carey WD, Patel G. Viral hepatitis in the 1990s, part II: Hepatitis B and delta virus. Cleve Clin J Med. 1992;59:393–401.
4. Carey WD, Patel G. Viral hepatitis in the 1990s, part III: Hepatitis C, hepatitis E, and other viruses. Cleve Clin J Med. 1992;59:595–601.
5. Feinstone SM, Kapikian AZ, Purcell RH. Hepatitis A: Detection by immune electron microscopy of a virus-like antigen associated with acute illness. Science. 1973;182:1026.
6. Blumberg BS, Alter HJ, Visnich S. A "new" antigen in leukemia sera. JAMA. 1965;191:541.
7. Tiollais P, Pourcel C, Dejean A. The hepatitis B virus. Nature. 1985;317:489.
8. Rizzetto M, Canese MG, Arico S, et al. Immunofluorescence detection of a new antigen-antibody system (delta/anti-delta) associated with hepatitis B virus in liver and serum of HBsAg carriers. Gut. 1977;18:997.
9. Rizzetto M. The delta agent. Hepatology. 1983;3:729.
10. Thomas HC, Karayiannis P, Monjardino J, et al. Hepatitis delta virus and the host response: Current status and future perspectives. Prog Clin Biol Res. 1993;382:431–5.
11. Karayiannis P, Saldanha J, Monjardino J, et al. Prevention and treatment of hepatitis delta virus infection. Prog Clin Biol Res. 1991;364:377–83.
12. Feinstone SM, Kapikian AZ, Purcell RH, et al. Transfusion-associated hepatitis not due to viral hepatitis type A or B. N Engl J Med. 1975;292:767.
12a. Prince AM, Brotman B, Grady GF, et al. Long-incubation post-transfusion hepatitis without serological evidence of exposure to hepatitis B virus. Lancet. 1974;2:241–6.
13. Choo Q-L, Kuo G, Weiner AJ, et al. Isolation of a cDNA clone from a blood-borne non-A non-B viral hepatitis genome. Science. 1989;244:329–2.
14. Kuo G, Choo Q-L, Alter HJ, et al. An assay for circulating antibodies to a major etiologic virus of human non-A, non-B hepatitis. Science. 1989;244:262–4.
15. Balayan MS, Andjaparidze AG, Savinskaya SS, et al. Evidence for a virus in non-A/non-B hepatitis transmitted via the fecal oral route. Intervirology. 1983;20:23.
16. Reyes GR, Purdy MA, Kim JP. Isolation of cDNA from the virus responsible for enterically transmitted non-A, non-B hepatitis. Science. 1990;247:1335–9.
17. Gust ED, Purcell RH. Waterborne non-A, non-B hepatitis. J Infect Dis. 1987;156:630.
18. Centers for Disease Control and Prevention. Hepatitis surveillance report. No 51:13, 1987.
19. Alter MJ, Hadler SC, Margolis HS, et al. The changing epidemiology of hepatitis B in the United States: Need for alternative vaccination strategies. JAMA. 1990;263:1218–22.
20. Alter MJ, Hadler SC, Judson FN, et al. Risk factors for acute non-A, non-B hepatitis in the United States and association with hepatitis C virus infection. JAMA. 1990;264:2231–5.
21. Margolis HS, Alter MJ, Hadler SC. Hepatitis B: Evolving epidemiology and implications for control. Semin Liver Dis. 1992;11:84–92.
22. Koff RS, Chalmers TC, Culhane PO, et al. Underreporting of viral hepatitis. Gastroenterology. 1973;64:1194.
23. Szmuness W, Dienstag JL, Purcell RH, et al. Distribution of antibody to hepatitis A antigen in urban adult populations. N Engl J Med. 1976;295:755.
24. Hadler SC, de Monzon M, Ponzetto A, et al. An epidemic of severe hepatitis due to delta virus infection in Yucpa Indians of Venezuela. Ann Intern Med. 1984;100:339.
25. Hoofnagle JH, Shafritz DA, Popper H. Chronic hepatitis B and the "healthy" HBsAg carrier state. Hepatology. 1987;7:758.
26. Zeldis JB, Dienstag JL, Gale RP. Aplastic anemia and non-A, non-B hepatitis. Am J Med. 1983;74:64.
27. Beasley RP, Hwang LY, Lin CC, et al. Hepatocellular carcinoma and hepatitis B virus. A prospective study of 22,707 men in Taiwan. Lancet. 1981;2:1129.
28. Beasley RP. Hepatitis B virus as the etiologic agent in hepatocellular carcinoma—Epidemiologic considerations. Hepatology. 1982;2(Suppl):21.
29. Saito I, Miyamura T, Ohbayashi A, et al. Hepatitis C virus infection is associated with the development of hepatocellular carcinoma. Proc Natl Acad Sci USA. 1990;87:6547–9.
30. Nishioka K, Watanabe J, Furuta S. A high prevalence of antibody to hepatitis C virus in patients with hepatocellular carcinoma in Japan. Cancer. 1991;67:429–33.
31. Kaklamani E, Trichopoulos D, Tzonou A. Hepatitis B and C viruses and their interaction in the origin of hepatocellular carcinoma. JAMA. 1991;265:1974–6.
32. Simonetti RG, Camma C, Fiorello F. Hepatitis C virus infection as a risk factor for hepatocellular carcinoma in patients with cirrhosis: A case-controlled study. Ann Intern Med. 1992;115:97–102.
33. Stevens CE, Taylor PE. Hepatitis B vaccine: Issues, recommendations, and new developments. Semin Liver Dis. 1986;6:23.
34. Werzberg A, Mensch B, Kuter B, et al. A controlled trial of a formalin-

inactivated hepatitis A vaccine in healthy children. N Engl J Med. 1992;327: 453–7.

35. Kane MA. Perspectives on the control of hepatitis A by vaccination. Vaccine. 1992;10(Suppl 1):S93–6.
36. Margolis HS. Prevention of acute and chronic liver disease through immunization: Hepatitis B and beyond. J Infect Dis. 1993;168:9–14.
37. Steffen R. Hepatitis A and hepatitis B: Risks compared with other vaccine preventable diseases and immunization recommendations. Vaccine. 1993; 11:518–20.
38. Gardner P, Schaffner W. Immunization of adults. N Engl J Med. 1993;328: 1252–8.
39. Alpert E, Isselbacher KJ, Schur PH. The pathogenesis of arthritis associated with viral hepatitis. N Engl J Med. 1971;285:185.
40. Heermann KH, Gerlich WH. Immunology of hepatitis B virus infections. Rheumatol Int. 1989;9:167–73.
41. Gianotti F. Hepatitis B antigen in papular acrodermatitis of children. Br Med J. 1974;3:169.
42. Michalak T. Immune complexes of hepatitis B surface antigen in the pathogenesis of periarteritis nodosa. Am J Pathol. 1978;90:619.
43. Eknoyan G, Gyorkey F, Dicheso C, et al. Renal morphological and immunological changes associated with acute viral hepatitis. Kidney Int. 1972;1:413.
44. Kneiser MR, Jhenis EH, Lowenthal DT, et al. Pathogenesis of renal disease associated with viral hepatitis. Arch Pathol. 1974;97:193.
45. Johnson RJ, Gretch DR, Yamabe H, et al. Membranoproliferative glomerulonephritis associated with hepatitis C virus infection. N Engl J Med. 1993; 328:465–70.
46. Levo Y, Gorevic PD, Kassab, et al. Liver involvement in the syndrome of mixed cryoglobulinemia. N Engl J Med. 1977;296:1501.
47. Agnello V, Chung RT, Kaplan LM. A role for hepatitis C virus infection in type II cryoglobulinemia. N Engl J Med. 1992;327:1490–5.
48. Bernuau J, Rueff B, Benhamou JP. Fulminant and subfulminant liver failure: Definition and causes. Semin Liver Dis. 1985;6:97–106.
49. Katelaris PH, Jones DB. Fulminant hepatic failure. Med Clin North Am. 1989;73:955–70.
50. Zimmerman HG. The differential diagnosis of jaundice. Med Clin North Am. 1968;52:1417.
51. Frank BB. Clinical evaluation of jaundice. A guideline of the Patient Care Committee of the American Gastroenterological Association. JAMA. 1989; 262:3031–4.
52. Elias E. Clinical and biochemical diagnosis of jaundice. Baillieres Clin Gastroenterol. 1989;3:357–85.
53. Salen G, Goldstein F, Haurani F, et al. Acute hemolytic anemia complicating viral hepatitis in patients with glucose-6-phosphate dehydrogenase deficiency. Ann Intern Med. 1966;65:1210.
54. O'Grady JG, Alexander GJ, Hayllar KM, et al. Early indicators of prognosis in fulminant hepatic failure. Gastroenterology. 1989;97:439–45.
55. Ishak KG. Light microscopic morphology of viral hepatitis. Am J Clin Pathol. 1976;65:787.
56. Boyer JL, Klatskin G. Pattern of necrosis in acute viral hepatitis. Prognostic value of bridging (subacute hepatic necrosis). N Engl J Med. 1970;283:1063.
57. Lefkowitch JH, Schiff ER, Davis GL, et al. Pathological diagnosis of chronic hepatitis C: A multicenter comparative study with chronic hepatitis B. The Hepatitis Interventional Therapy Group. Gastroenterology. 1993;104: 595–603.
58. Mathiesen LR, Fauerholt L, Moller AM, et al. Immunofluorescence studies for hepatitis A virus and hepatitis B surface and core antigen in liver biopsies from patients with acute viral hepatitis. Gastroenterology. 1979;77:623.
59. Boggs JD, Melnick JL, Conrad ME, et al. Viral hepatitis, clinical and tissue culture studies. JAMA. 1970;214:1041.
60. Lemon S. Type A viral hepatitis. New developments in an old disease. N Engl J Med. 1985;313:1059.
61. Koff RS. Clinical manifestations and diagnosis of hepatitis A virus infection. Vaccine. 1992;10:S15–7.
62. Sjogren MH, Tanno H, Fay O, et al. Hepatitis A virus in stool dunng clinical relapse. Ann Intern Med. 1987;106:221.
63. Gordon SC, Reddy KR, Schiff L, et al. Prolonged intrahepatic cholestasis secondary to acute hepatitis A. Ann Intern Med. 1984;101:635.
64. Schiff ER. Atypical clinical manifestations of hepatitis A. Vaccine. 1992;10: S18–20.
65. O'Grady J. Management of acute and fulminant hepatitis A. Vaccine. 1992; 10:S21–3.
66. Rakela A, Radeker AF, Edwards VM, et al. Hepatitis A virus infection in fulminant hepatitis and chronic active hepatitis. Gastroenterology. 1978;74: 879.
67. Francis DP, Hadler SC, Prendergast TJ, et al. Occurrence of hepatitis A, B, and non-A, non-B hepatitis in the United States—CDC Sentinel County hepatitis study I. Am J Med. 1984;76:69.
68. Dienstag JL, Routenberg JA, Purcell RH, et al. Foodhandler-associated outbreak of hepatitis type A. An immune electron microscopic study. Ann Intern Med. 1975;83:647.
69. Mackowiak PA, Caraway CT, Portnoy EL. Oyster-associated hepatitis. Lessons from the Louisiana experience. Am J Epidemiol. 1976;103:181.
70. Woodson RD, Clinton JJ. Hepatitis prophylaxis abroad. Effectiveness of immune serum globulin in protecting Peace Corps volunteers. JAMA. 1968; 109:1053.
71. Pattison CP, Maynard JE, Bryan JS. Subhuman primate-associated hepatitis. J Infect Dis. 1975;132:478.
72. Hadler SC, Erben JJ, Francis DP, et al. Risk factors for hepatitis A in daycare centers. J Infect Dis. 1982;145:255.

73. Corey L, Holmes KK. Sexual transmission of hepatitis A in homosexual men. Incidence and mechanism. N Engl J Med. 1980;302:435.
74. Decker RH, Kosakowski SM, Vanderbilt AS, et al. Diagnosis of acute hepatitis A by HAVab-M, a direct radioimmunoassay for IgM anti-HAV. Am J Clin Pathol. 1981;76:140.
75. Szmuness W, Much ML, Prince AM, et al. On the role of sexual behavior in the spread of hepatitis B infection. Ann Intern Med. 1975;83:489.
76. Krugman S, Overby LR, Mushahwar IK, et al. Viral hepatitis type B. Studies on the natural history and prevention reexamined. N Engl J Med. 1979;300: 101.
77. Hoofnagle JH, Seeff LB, Bales ZB, et al. Serologic responses in hepatitis B. In: Vyas GN, Cohen SN, Schmid R, eds. Viral Hepatitis. Philadelphia: Franklin Institute Press; 1978:219–44.
78. Hoofnagle JH, Di Bisceglie AM. Serologic diagnosis of acute and chronic viral hepatitis. Semin Liver Dis. 1991;11:73–83.
79. Chau KH, Hargie MP, Decker RH, et al. Serodiagnosis of recent hepatitis B infection by IgM class anti-HBc. Hepatology. 1983;3:142.
80. Rizzetto M, Gerin JL, Purcell RH, eds. Hepatitis Delta Virus and Its Infection. New York: Alan R Liss; 1987.
81. Hoofnagle JH. Type D hepatitis. JAMA. 1989;261:1321.
82. Farci P, Gerin JL, Aragona M, et al. Diagnostic and prognostic significance of the IgM antibody to the hepatitis delta virus. JAMA. 1986;255:1443.
83. Mushawar IK, Decker RH. Prevalence of delta antigen and anti-delta detected by immunoassays in various HBsAg positive populations. In: Vyas GN, Dienstag JL, Hoofnagle JH, eds. Viral Hepatitis and Liver Disease. Orlando, FL: Grune & Stratton; 1984:617.
84. Bergmann KF, Gerin JL. Antigens of hepatitis delta virus in the serum of humans and animals. J Infect Dis. 1986;514:702.
85. Smedile A, Baroudy BM, Bergman KF, et al. Clinical significance of HDV RNA in HDV disease. In: Rizzetto M, Gerin JL, Purcell RH, eds. Hepatitis Delta Virus and Its Infection. New York: Alan R. Liss; 1987:31–4.
86. Rizzetto M, Verme G, Recchia S, et al. Chronic HBsAg hepatitis with intrahepatic expression of delta antigen. An active and progressive disease unresponsive to immunosuppressive treatment. Ann Intern Med. 1983;98:437.
87. Rocca G, Poli G, Gerardo P, et al. Familial clustering of delta infection. In: Verme G, Bonino F, Rizzetto M, eds. Viral Hepatitis and Delta Infection. New York: Alan R Liss; 1984:133–7.
88. Dienstag JL. Non-A, non-B hepatitis. 1. Recognition, epidemiology, and clinical features. Gastroenterology. 1983;85:439.
89. Dienstag JL. Non-A, non-B hepatitis. 11. Experimental transmission, putative virus agents and markers, and prevention. Gastroenterology. 1983;85: 743.
90. Esteban JI, Genesca J, Alter JH. Hepatitis C: Molecular biology, pathogenesis, epidemiology, clinical features, and prevention. Prog Liver Dis. 1992; 10:253–82.
91. Houghton M, Weiner A, Han J, et al. Molecular biology of the hepatitis C viruses: Implications for diagnosis, development and control of viral disease. Hepatology. 1991;14:381–8.
92. Hsia PC, Seeff LB. Non-A, non-B hepatitis: Impact of the emergence of the hepatitis C virus. Adv Int Med. 1992;37:197–222.
93. Alter MJ, Margolis HS, Krawczynski K, et al. The natural history of community-acquired hepatitis C in the United States. The Sentinel Counties Chronic non-A, non-B Hepatitis Study Team. N Engl J Med. 1992;327:1899–905.
94. Seeff LB, Buskell-Bales Z, Wright EC, et al. Long-term mortality after transfusion-associated non-A, non-B hepatitis. The National Heart, Lung, and Blood Institute Study Group. N Engl J Med. 1992;327:1906–11.
95. Alter MJ, Gerety RJ, Smallwood LA, et al. Sporadic non-A, non-B hepatitis: Frequency and epidemiology in an urban U.S. population. J Infect Dis. 1982; 145:886.
96. Kelen GD, Green GB, Purcell RH. Hepatitis B and hepatitis C in emergency department patients. N Engl J Med. 1992;326:1399–404.
97. Alter HJ, Hoofnagle JH. Non-A, non-B. Observations on the first decade. In: Vyas GN, Dienstag JL, Hoofnagle JH, eds. Viral Hepatitis and Liver Disease. Orlando, FL: Grune & Stratton; 1984:345–55.
98. Wong DC, Purcell RH, Sreenivasan MA, et al. Epidemic and endemic hepatitis in India: Evidence for non-A/non-B hepatitis virus etiology. Lancet. 1980; 2:876.
99. Khuroo SM. Study of an epidemic of non-A, non-B hepatitis. Possibility of another human hepatitis virus distinct from post-transfusion non-A, non-B type. Am J Med. 1980;68:818.
100. Krawczynski K. Hepatitis E. Hepatology. 1993;17:932–41.
101. Kane MA, Bradley DW, Shrestha SM, et al. Epidemic non-A, non-B hepatitis in Nepal: Recovery of a possible etiologic agent and transmission studies in marmoset. JAMA. 1984;252:3140.
102. Kraczynski K, Bradley DW, Kane MA. Virus associated antigen of epidemic non-A, non-B hepatitis and specific antibodies in outbreaks and in sporadic cases of NANB hepatitis. Hepatology. 1988;8:1223.
103. Purcell RH, Walsh IH, Holland PV, et al. Seroepidemiological studies of transfusion-associated hepatitis. J Infect Dis. 1981;123:406.
104. Lamb B, Stern H. Cytomegalovirus hepatitis. Lancet. 1966;2:1003.
105. Laskus T, Lupa E, Cianciara J, et al. Cytomegalovirus infection presenting as hepatitis. Digestion. 1990;47:167–71.
106. Gabish D, Kleinman Y, Morag A, et al. Hepatitis and jaundice associated with measles in young adults. Arch Intern Med. 1983;143:674.
107. Shalev-Zimels H, Weizman Z, Lotan C, et al. Extent of measles hepatitis in various ages. Hepatology. 1988;8:1138.
108. Francis TL, Moore DL, Edington GM, et al. A clinicopathological study of human yellow fever. Bull WHO. 1972;46:659.
109. Zimmerman HG, Fang M, Utili R, et al. Jaundice due to bacterial infection. Gastroenterology. 1979;77:362.

110. Bowry S, Chan CH, Weiss H, et al. Hepatic involvement in pulmonary tuberculosis. Histologic and functional characteristics. Am Rev Respir Dis. 1970;101:941.
111. Godwin JE, Coleman AA, Sahn SA. Military tuberculosis presenting as hepatic and renal failure. Chest. 1991;99:752–4.
112. Kielhofner MA, Hamill RJ. Focal hepatic tuberculosis in a patient with acquired immunodeficiency syndrome. South Med J. 1991;84:401–4.
113. Asada Y, Hayashi T, Sumiyoshi A, et al. Military tuberculosis presenting as fever and jaundice with hepatic failure. Hum Pathol. 1991;22:92–4.
114. Oliva A, Duarte B, Jonasson O, et al. The nodular form of local hepatic tuberculosis. A review. J Clin Gastroenterol 1990;12:166–73.
115. Lee RV, Thornton GF, Conn HO. Liver disease associated with secondary syphilis. N Engl J Med. 1971;284:1423.
116. Heath CW Jr, Alexander AD, Galton MM. Leptospirosis in the United States. Analysis of 483 cases in man, 1949–1961. N Engl J Med. 1965;273:857.
117. Bernstein M, Edmondson HA, Barhour BH. The liver lesion in Q fever. Clinical and pathologic features. Arch Intern Med. 1965;116:491.
118. Zimmerman HJ. Hepatotoxicity. The Adverse Effects of Drugs and Other Chemicals on the Liver. New York: Appleton-Century-Crofts; 1978.
119. Johnson GK, Tolman KG. Chronic liver disease and acetaminophen. Ann Intern Med. 1977;87:302.
120. Janes J, Routledge PA. Recent developments in the management of paracetamol (acetaminophen) poisoning. Drug Safety. 1992;7:170–7.
121. Nelson SD. Molecular mechanisms of the hepatotoxicity caused by acetaminophen. Semin Liver Dis. 1990;10:267–78.
122. Subcommittee on the National Halothane Study of the Committee on Anesthesia. Possible association between halothane anesthesia and postoperative hepatic necrosis. JAMA. 1966;197:775.
123. Ray DC, Drummond GB. Halothane hepatitis. Br J Anaesth 1991;67:84–99.
124. Kenna JG. The molecular basis of halothane-induced hepatitis. Biochem Soc Trans. 1991;19:191–5.
125. Neuberger JM. Halothane and hepatitis. Incidence, predisposing factors and exposure guidelines. Drug Safety. 1990;5:28–38.
126. Bynum TE, Boinoit JK, Maddrey WC. Ischemic hepatitis. Am J Dig Dis. 1979;24:129.
127. Lieber CS. Biochemical and molecular basis of alcohol-induced injury to the liver and other tissues. N Engl J Med. 1988;319:1639.
128. Roche-Sicot J, Benhamou JP. Acute intravascular hemolysis and acute liver failure associated as a first manifestation of Wilson's disease. Ann Intern Med. 1977;86:301.
129. Rosenblate HJ, Eisenstein R, Halmes AW. The liver in sickle cell anemia. Arch Pathol Lab Med. 1970;90:235.
130. Parker RGF. Occlusion of the hepatic veins in man. Medicine (Baltimore). 1959;38:369.
131. Harrison HB, Middleton HM, Crosby JH, et al. Fulminant hepatic failure. An unusual presentation of metastatic liver disease. Gastroenterology. 1981;80:820.
132. Repsher LH, Freebern RK. Effects of early and vigorous exercise on recovery from infectious hepatitis. N Engl J Med. 1969;281:1393.
133. Schweitzer IL, Weiner JM, McPeak CM, et al. Oral contraceptives in acute viral hepatitis. JAMA. 1975;233:979.
134. Blum AL, Stutz R, Haemmerli UP, et al. A fortuitously controlled study of steroid therapy in acute viral hepatitis. I. Acute disease. Am J Med. 1969;47:82.
135. Gregory PB, Knauer CM, Miller R, et al. Steroid therapy in severe viral hepatitis. N Engl J Med. 1976;294:681.
136. Sherlock S, Thomas HC. Treatment of chronic hepatitis due to hepatitis B virus. Lancet. 1985;2:1343.
137. Hoofnagle JH, Mullen KD, Jones DB, et al. Treatment of chronic non-A, non-B hepatitis with recombinant human alpha interferon. N Engl J Med. 1986;315:1575.
138. Perrillo RP, Schiff ER, Davis GL, et al. A randomized, controlled trial of interferon alfa-2b alone and after prednisone withdrawal for the treatment of chronic hepatitis B. The Hepatitis Interventional Therapy Group. N Engl J Med. 1990;323:295–301.
139. Davis GL, Balart LA, Schiff ER, et al. Treatment of chronic hepatitis C with recombinant interferon alpha. A multicenter randomized, controlled trial. Hepatitis Interventional Therapy Group. N Engl J Med. 1989;321:1501–6.
140. Davis GL. Recombinant alpha-interferon treatment of non-A, and non-B (type C) hepatitis: Review of studies and recommendations for treatment. J Hepatol. 1990;11:S72–7.
141. Hoofnagle JH, Di Bisceglie AM. Treatment of chronic type C hepatitis with alpha interferon. Semin Liver Dis. 1989;9:259–63.
142. Levin S, Hahn T. Interferon system in acute viral hepatitis. Lancet. 1982;1:592.
143. Sanchez-Tapias JM, Mas A, Costa J, et al. Recombinant alpha 2c interferon therapy in fulminant viral hepatitis. J Hepatol. 1987;5:205.
144. Omata M, Yokosuka O, Takano S, et al. Resolution of acute hepatitis C after therapy with natural beta interferon. Lancet. 1991;338:914–5.
145. Peleman RR, Gavaler JS, Van Thiel DH, et al. Liver transplantation for acute and subacute hepatic failure. Hepatology. 1985;5:1045.
146. Mutimer DJ, Elias E. Liver transplantation for fulminant hepatic failure. Prog Liver Dis. 1992;10:349–67.
147. Lidofsky SD. Liver transplantation for fulminant hepatic failure. Gastroenterol Clin North Am. 1993;22:257–69.
148. Vickers C, Neuberger J, Buckels J, et al. Transplantation of the liver in adults and children with fulminant hepatic failure. J Hepatol. 1988;7:143.
149. Bernuau J, Gordeau A, Poynard T, et al. Multivariate analysis of prognostic factors in fulminant hepatitis. Hepatology. 1986;6:648.
150. Auslander MO, Gitnick GL. Vigorous medical management of acute fulminant hepatitis. Arch Intern Med. 1977;137:599.
151. Katelaris PH, Jones DB. Fulminant hepatic failure. Med Clin North Am. 1989;73:955–70.
152. Seeff LB, Hoofnagle JH. Immunoprophylaxis of viral hepatitis. Gastroenterology. 1979;77:161.
153. Margolis HS. Prevention of acute and chronic liver disease through immunization: Hepatitis B and beyond. J Infect Dis. 1993;168:9–14.
154. Centers for Disease Control and Prevention. Post-exposure prophylaxis of hepatitis B. Ann Intern Med. 1984;101:351.
155. Catterall AP, Murray-Lyon IM. Strategies for hepatitis B immunisation. Gut. 1992;33:576–9.
156. Hadler SC, Margolis HS. Hepatitis B immunization: Vaccine types, efficacy, and indications for immunization. Curr Clin Top Infect Dis. 1992;12:282–308.
157. Beasley RP, Hwang LY, Lee GC, et al. Prevention of perinatally transmitted hepatitis B virus infections with hepatitis B immune globulin and hepatitis B vaccine. Lancet. 1983;2:1099.

97. CHRONIC HEPATITIS

EDWARD L. KRAWITT

Although it is now recognized that five hepatitis viruses cause acute hepatitis, only three, hepatitis B (HBV), hepatitis C (HCV), and hepatitis delta (HDV), are known to result in chronic viral hepatitis, a heterogeneous disorder defined by duration and histologic appearance, which may eventuate in cirrhosis and hepatocellular carcinoma (Table 1). In general, persistence of viral hepatitis for more than 6 months is considered adequate to satisfy the criterion for duration, but on occasion a slowly resolving acute viral hepatitis may exceed 6 months before achieving complete resolution. However, because of the variable clinical presentations of chronic hepatitis, it may be difficult to determine precisely the onset of disease. A history of exposure and/or a typical clinical history with serologic identification may help, but these data may not be available to help establish duration. The histologic features of chronic viral hepatitis are rather characteristic, but are not specific for any agent and cannot be distinguished from the chronic necroinflammatory changes seen in autoimmune hepatitis, the other major type of chronic hepatitis that must be considered in the differential diagnosis of chronic viral hepatitis.

The presentations of chronic hepatitis span a wide clinical spectrum. They range from the asymptomatic patient, who may be discovered when abnormal laboratory values are obtained during a screening examination, to patients with an insidious presentation characterized by mild nonspecific symptomatology, to patients who present with new onset or reactivation with a severe and sometimes fulminant picture. On occasion, patients with chronic hepatitis may present with extrahepatic manifestations such as polyarteritis nodosa, glomerulonephritis, cryoglobulinemia, or porphyria cutanea tarda as the major problem

TABLE 1. Consequences of Viral Hepatitis Infection

| | Hepatitis | | | | Hepatocellular |
Agent	Acute	Fulminant	Chronic	Cirrhosis	Carcinoma
A	+	+	0	0	0
B	+	+	5–10%[a]	+	+
C	+	?[b]	~50%	+	+
Delta	+	+	co, <5%; super, ~50%[c]	+	+
E	+	+	0	0	0

[a] Adults (infants and children, 20–50%).
[b] Conflicting data.
[c] Coinfection, <5%; superinfection, ~50%.

TABLE 2. Extrahepatic Manifestations of Chronic Hepatitis

Condition	Hepatitis B	Hepatitis C
Polyarteritis nodosa	+	+
Glomerulonephritis	+	+
Essential mixed cryoglobulinemia	+	+
Porphyria cutanea tarda	?[a]	+

[a] Not known.

(Table 2). Physicians may also be confronted by a patient whose liver biopsy specimen obtained at the time of abdominal surgery for another condition reveals chronic hepatitis in whom identification of the etiology may be required. Usually, however, a biopsy is performed only after having obtained pertinent subjective and objective information in patients seen for jaundice or other signs of liver disease, evidence of abnormal laboratory values, or extrahepatic manifestations of disease.

Findings on physical examination are rarely helpful in patients with chronic hepatitis unless jaundice is present or the disease is already accompanied by cirrhosis, in which case signs of chronic liver disease such as spider angiomata, hepatomegaly, splenomegaly, or ascites may be obvious to the examiner. The presence of tatoos, scars of acupuncture, intravenous drug use, or major surgery may alert the physician to evidence of exposure to blood products, wherein a hepatitis virus may have been transmitted.

Major clues to the etiology of chronic hepatitis are to be found in historical and serologic data. Whenever the etiology of abnormal liver function tests is unclear, chronic hepatitis should be considered. Circulating hepatitis B surface antigen (HBsAg) and antibodies to the hepatitis core antigen (anti-HBc) and hepatitis B surface antigen (anti-HBs), as well as antibodies to the hepatitis C antigen (anti-HC), should be determined. Where appropriate, hepatitis B e antigen (HBeAg) and antibodies to the hepatitis B e antigen (anti-HBe), hepatitis delta antigen (HDAg) and antibodies to the hepatitis delta antigen (anti-HD), and hepatitis B virus DNA and hepatitis C virus RNA should be measured.

Histologic confirmation is necessary to eliminate other causes for abnormalities encountered and to document the presence and severity of disease. The histopathologic changes in chronic hepatitis also cover a wide spectrum. In the mildest of cases, minimal inflammatory changes are present in the portal and/or lobular areas, but in general, changes are those of a progressive necroinflammatory disorder characterized by portal and periportal infiltrates of mononuclear cells that invade the hepatocytes surrounding the portal triad (limiting plate) and percolate into the surrounding lobule. The term *chronic persistent hepatitis* was introduced to designate changes that for the most part were confined to the portal area without significant extension beyond the limiting plate or significant fibrosis as opposed to *chronic active hepatitis* (or chronic aggressive hepatitis), which indicated invasion into the surrounding lobule. These descriptions do have some prognostic implications, although many pathologists now use the term *chronic hepatitis* and describe specific findings rather than use the terms *chronic persistent* and *chronic active*.[1-3] With more advanced disease, damage becomes extensive and results in bridging inflammation between portal/central areas, fibrosis, and eventual cirrhosis. There is no absolute correlation between the clinical presentation and the pathologic appearance. Thus, although patients with severe clinical presentations often have more advanced histopathologic findings, the asymptomatic patient may also be discovered to have cirrhosis when biopsied.

Histologic severity of disease appears to be the most important prognosticator in chronic hepatitis.[4] Survival over a period of 5–10 years is in the range of 90 percent for patients whose histologic picture includes chronic hepatitis without fibrosis. Patients with a histologic picture that includes fibrosis or cirrhosis have a significantly shortened survival. These prognostic implications have become much more important in this modern era when treatment options are available but involve the risk of serious side effects.

DIFFERENTIAL DIAGNOSIS IN CHRONIC HEPATITIS

A variety of diseases other than chronic viral hepatitis and autoimmune hepatitis must be considered as causes of a histologic picture characterized by portal, periportal, and lobular inflammation, fibrosis, and/or cirrhosis. α_1-Antitrypsin deficiency is a disorder in which there is abnormal polymerization of this globulin in hepatocytes such that it is not secreted into the plasma, resulting in a "storage/transport" disease that progresses to cirrhosis. Wilson's disease is a copper storage disease marked by decreased levels of circulating ceruloplasmin. Other autoimmune liver diseases, namely, primary biliary cirrhosis and primary sclerosing cholangitis, the latter seen frequently as a complication of inflammatory bowel disease (Crohn's disease and ulcerative colitis), must be considered. AIDS cholangiopathy, granulomatous hepatitis, systemic lupus erythematosus, graft-versus-host disease, and drug-induced chronic hepatitis are to be included in the differential diagnosis. Oxyphenisatin (no longer available in the United States), methyldopa, nitrofurantoin, and dantrolene are drugs that cause chronic hepatitis most frequently. Isoniazid, halothane, papaverine, sulfonamides, propylthiouracil, ticrynafen (no longer available in the United States), etretinate, and acetaminophen have also been implicated. On occasion, alcoholic liver disease presents with a picture of chronic hepatitis. An inflammatory component may be seen in patients with genetic hemochromatosis, an iron storage disease that progresses to cirrhosis if untreated.

CHRONIC HEPATITIS B

Although it is estimated that there are about 400 million patients with chronic hepatitis B,[5] most are in the developing world. In the United States, the disease is seen primarily in special high-risk groups and is not compounded by the high percentages of vertical transmission and frequent childhood acquisition that occur in the developing world. These high-risk groups include Alaskan natives; immigrants from China, Southeast Asia, and other areas where prevalence is high; male homosexuals; promiscuous heterosexuals; intravenous drug users; recipients of blood products; and healthcare workers. Nevertheless, there is a significant percentage of patients in whom no risk factor can be identified. With the introduction of screening for hepatitis markers and transaminase elevations in American blood banks, and the advent of hepatitis B vaccination programs, the incidence of hepatitis B in the United States should continue to lessen. It is estimated that chronicity occurs in 5–10 percent of adults with acute hepatitis B, although chronicity rates are considerably higher in those acquiring disease at birth or during childhood (Table 1). Susceptibility to chronicity may also be increased in immunosuppressed individuals, which is of importance in terms of the common risk factors for acquisition of HIV and hepatitis viruses in some groups. Coincidental infection with HCV or HDV may affect hepatitis B chronicity.

Patients with chronic hepatitis B may exist as asymptomatic carriers (i.e., they have circulating HBsAg without evidence of abnormal liver function tests). In general, carriers also have anti-HBc present. Patients considered to be in a replicative viral stage are HBeAg positive and anti-HBe negative. Patients in a nonreplicative viral state are in general HBeAg negative and anti-HBe positive, although it has recently been established that some patients who are infected by a mutant HBV do not express HBe activity.[6] Circulating HBV DNA is present in patients in the replicative stage.

Occasionally, patients with chronic hepatitis B present with an isolated anti-HBc. Although an isolated anti-HBc frequently represents a false-positive result, it may occur in the presence of a low level of HBsAg that is undetectable by present methods. In those patients in whom the assay is so insensitive as to be negative for HBsAg, serum HBV DNA testing will reveal the presence of replicating virus. In one group of Chinese patients who were exclusively positive for anti-HBc, over one-third were found to be HBV DNA positive and therefore carriers.[7] The primary type of response to hepatitis B immunization seen in patients with isolated anti-HBc indicates, however, that in many of these patients the result is simply a false positive.[8] Although the presence of circulating anti-HBs in the absence of HBsAg has been presumed to signify resolution of hepatitis B infection and to be incompatible with chronic infection, a recent study also found HBV DNA in serum in HBsAg negative, anti-HBs positive patients, suggesting that our presently accepted standards of chronicity may be less accurate than heretofore thought.[9] On occasion, an isolated anti-HBc indicates resolved infection with a level of anti-HBs too low to be detected by standard techniques.

It has been over 20 years since it was recognized that chronic hepatitis B may appear as a variety of extrahepatic syndromes (Table 2)[10–12] such as periarteritis nodosa, glomerulonephritis, and cryoglobulinemia. There are few data to implicate HBV as a cause of acquired porphyria cutanea tarda. Polyarthritis is not uncommon in hepatitis.[13]

The distinction between the HBsAg carrier state and chronic hepatitis ultimately depends on the histologically confirmed presence of a chronic necroinflammatory disease in the liver. Although an elevated serum transaminase level in the presence of circulating HBsAg is presumptive evidence of chronic hepatitis, elevated transaminase levels may occur independent of HBsAg infection, and one cannot assume that the levels do not reflect another condition such as chronic hepatitis C infection, alcohol-induced liver disease, drug-induced changes, nonalcoholic fatty liver, and so forth.

The histologic changes in chronic hepatitis B may be accompanied by characteristic ground-glass cells, which may indicate the presence of HBsAg in the cytoplasm. With the availability of immunohistochemical techniques that demonstrate HBsAg and HBcAg in hepatocytes, confirmation of chronic hepatitis B is generally accomplished through immunohistochemical staining. The risk of developing cirrhosis is greater in patients with a severe chronic active hepatitis, but progression to cirrhosis does occur in patients with only moderate chronic active hepatitis or chronic persistent hepatitis, although it is less frequent.[14,15] Other predictors of mortality include age, serum bilirubin levels, and complications of cirrhosis. Survival of patients with established cirrhosis *and* symptoms is poor. In one study it was only 14–15 percent.[15] Calculating survival in patients with hepatitis B in the presence of HIV infection presents another facet of this problem.[16]

The course of chronic hepatitis B appears to involve the replicative phase followed by a nonreplicative phase. The replicative phase is characterized by inflammatory activity in the liver, circulating HBV DNA, and generally HBeAg positivity. During the latter stages of the replicative phase, inflammatory activity and HBV DNA levels decrease until the nonreplicative phase begins, where there is no inflammation present, HBeAg is absent, and anti-HBe is present. In this phase, circulating HBV DNA is presumably absent, but polymerase chain reaction (PCR) determinations of circulating HBV DNA have indicated that even in patients in the so-called nonreplicative phase with anti-HBe, HBV DNA detection indicates viral replication may be still present.[17,18]

There has been increased insight into the immunopathogenesis of chronic hepatitis B infection, vis-à-vis decreases in interferon production and viral cytopathic effects and immunological damage, perhaps mediated by a cellular cytolytic mechanism directed against nucleocapsid antigens in the context of HLA antigens. However, attempts at effective treatment have been disappointing. Based on the data obtained in clinical trials,[19–22] a common treatment regimen in the United States for patients in the replicative stage is interferon-α administered subcutaneously at a dosage of 5 million units a day for a 4-month course. Therapy is aimed at eliminating or decreasing viral replication, mitigating the necroinflammatory process, and/or halting progression of disease, and effectiveness is determined by measurement of serum transaminase levels, serologic markers of HBV replication, and histologic resolution. The results of many trials have differed, in part because of the criteria used to define responses, the different regimens used, and the different populations treated. Thus, evaluation of results must take into consideration the characteristics of the population (replicative phase, gender, sexual orientation, HIV status, duration of infection, possibly race, histologic stage) and status of hepatic compensation. The phenomenon of coinfection or superinfection with HDV, HIV, or HCV also may confound interpretation of treatment results. Response rates after 4–6 months of therapy have been in the range of 25–50 percent measured by markers of viral replication, which in general are accompanied by a decrease in transaminase levels and improved histology. Long-term remission rates are estimated at 20–30 percent.[22,23] However, it should be noted that HBV DNA as detected by PCR may be present in liver tissue long after the disappearance of circulating HBsAg and HBV DNA.[24] Studies in native-born Asians indicate less seroconversion in both children and adults, which may reflect duration of disease, immunologic tolerance in individuals who acquire the disease in the neonatal or early childhood periods, or immunogenetic differences. Geographic differences may also reflect different mutations in viruses, although conclusive data demonstrating this are not yet available.

Patients who are HIV negative and those with higher transaminase levels and lower levels of HBV DNA are more likely to respond to interferon treatment. Development of neutralizing interferon antibodies during treatment may have an effect on treatment results.[25] Individuals with recent infection and women appear to have better response rates.[26] Interferon treatment regimens using alternate forms and schedules of interferons as well as the use of other viral and/or immunomodulatory agents are currently under study.

Despite the obvious need for orthotopic liver transplantation in patients with advanced chronic hepatitis B and end-stage liver disease, continuing infection after transplantation, sometimes in a particularly aggressive fashion, has tempered enthusiasm for this approach. Studies directed toward improving results after orthotopic liver transplantation for HBsAg-positive patients are also under way.

CHRONIC DELTA HEPATITIS

Chronic delta hepatitis occurs only in the presence of hepatitis B. HDV is a cytopathic single-stranded circular RNA virus, which requires HBV for production of its surface protein and which is dependent on HBV for membrane attachment and entry to cells, although not for intracellular replication. The diagnosis is established on the basis of titers of anti-HDV and/or the persistence of HDV antigen in the liver, and, when available, serum HDV RNA levels. HDV infection can occur simultaneously with HBV infection (coinfection) or superimposed on an underlying HBV infection (superinfection). The incidence of chronicity is less than 5 percent with coinfection and approximately 50 percent with superinfection. "Healthy" delta carriers (i.e., those without evidence of liver disease), similar to HBV carriers, are also seen in patients with chronic delta infections. Although it is estimated that 15 million people in the world are infected with HDV, it is rare in the United States, where it is seen most often in patients with a history of intravenous drug use. HDV infection has also been observed in hemophiliacs, nonintravenous drug-using male homosexuals, female prostitutes, and individuals in institutions for the mentally retarded.[27,28]

Therapeutic trials have not uncovered an effective treatment for chronic delta hepatitis. Interferon-α is not very promising, as decreases in necroinflammatory changes have occurred in only a minority of patients. Attempts have been made to improve the response rate by different regimens. A 12-month course of interferon-α studied in Italy, an area of high endemicity, demonstrated no antiviral effects; and, although biochemical and histologic improvement was observed, patients relapsed after discontinuation of therapy.[29] Reactivation of disease in chronic delta hepatitis patients is more likely to be secondary to HDV activity than to HBV activity.[30] Because of the high incidence of HDV infection in intravenous drug users, interrelationships between HBV, HDV, HCV, and HIV may complicate the clinical picture.[30] Persistence of infection after orthotopic liver transplantation is also a problem for patients with chronic delta hepatitis.[31]

CHRONIC HEPATITIS C

Chronic hepatitis C represents a major health problem in the United States and in the world at large. It is estimated that the annual incidence of HCV infection in the United States is approximately half that of HBV, but, considering that approximately 50% of patients with acute HCV go on to develop a chronic form of hepatitis C, the problem of chronic hepatitis C surpasses that of chronic hepatitis B. The epidemiology of chronic hepatitis C is currently being elucidated due in large part to the availability of more sensitive and specific tests of HCV infection, which can now determine the role of HCV in what was formerly referred to as *non-A, non-B chronic hepatitis*. The discovery of a variety of hepatitis C genotypes defined by nucleotide heterogeneity should also be important in defining the epidemiology of chronic hepatitis C and may also help in explaining variations in disease severity, chronicity, response to therapy, and case identification.

The sequelae of acute hepatitis C are the same as those for HBV and HDV infections. Chronicity may be manifested as a carrier state without apparent liver disease or as mild or severe chronic hepatitis, which may progress to cirrhosis and primary hepatocellular carcinoma.[32-35] Although the immunopathogenesis has not been fully elucidated, it would appear that direct viral cytopathic effects as well as host-directed immunologic events mediate injury, although cytopathic effects appear to be more important in chronic hepatitis C than in chronic hepatitis B. Frequently, asymptomatic patients are discovered only at the time of screening examinations or when their blood is refused for donation because of abnormalities found during biochemical or serologic testing. Patients may present with insidious symptoms, the most prominent being easy fatiguability. On occasion, patients present with signs and symptoms of end-stage liver disease or evidence of unsuspected advanced liver disease at the time of laparotomy for another condition. Patients with chronic hepatitis C may report risk factors for infection such as blood product transfusion, intravenous drug use, acupuncture, tatoos, occupational exposure, or intimate contact with others who have these risk factors, suggesting apparent or inapparent parenteral infection. With widespread screening of potential blood donors for evidence of HIV, HBV, and HCV infection, the incidence of post-transfusion hepatitis C has decreased.[36] However, risk factors are often not uncovered, and between one-third and one-half of patients with chronic hepatitis C are presently categorized as having community-acquired disease.[34] Whether community-acquired disease represents inapparent parenteral infection or nonparenteral infection is not clear.

Although there are conflicting data regarding vertical transmission, it is clear that anti-HC may be passively transferred from mother to child. Vertical transmission of HCV appears to be uncommon at least in the absence of concurrent HIV infection.[37-40] Although there is an increase in incidence in some populations of homosexual and heterosexual partners and household members, it similarly is unclear whether this represents inapparent parenteral infection of blood or actual transmission through body fluids other than blood.[41-45] Some of the increased incidence in sexual partners is due to the occurrence of similar risk factors. The results of detection of HCV in serum and saliva are contradictory[46-50] and not readily explained at this time. Differences may depend on methodology and viral load and/or may relate to variations in HCV genotypes encountered in different populations.

As was noted for hepatitis B, the presenting signs and symptoms of chronic hepatitis C in some cases may be manifested as extrahepatic manifestations (Table 2).[51-56] Essential mixed cryoglobulinemia presenting with vascular purpura, arthralgia, systemic vasculitis, neuropathy, and glomerulonephritis, as well as polyarteritis and acquired porphyria cutanea tarda, have been reported.

It should also be noted that circulating antibodies to a variety of unrelated proteins may be seen in patients with chronic hepatitis, including antibodies to nuclei, smooth muscle, and microsomes. An autoantibody to a protein termed GOR has also been described in patients with chronic hepatitis C.[57-59] Approximately 5 percent of patients with chronic hepatitis C have circulating antinuclear or antismooth muscle antibodies with titers of $\geq 1:100$ (E. L. Krawitt, K. R. Reddy, and J.-C. Homberg, unpublished data.) Antibodies to liver/kidney microsomes have been observed in European patients but have not been seen in a group of patients from the United States (E. L. Krawitt, K. R. Reddy, and J.-C. Homberg, unpublished data.) The presence of these autoantibodies may provide diagnostic difficulties for clinicians in determining whether patients have chronic hepatitis C or a form of autoimmune hepatitis (see Autoimmune Hepatitis, below).[59]

The serologic diagnosis of hepatitis C evolved quickly from a first-generation enzyme-linked immunosorbent assay (ELISA) for anti-HCV, to a second-generation ELISA, and confirmatory recombinant immunoblotting assays (RIBA).[60] A high correlation of positivity with the presence of HCV by PCR exists when second-generation tests are positive in the presence of abnormal transaminases and risk factors. Properly performed PCR techniques, in carefully prepared samples, are now required for confirmation of the existence of HCV RNA,[61,62] but new assays including a quantitative branched-signal amplification assay may enter the diagnostic armamentarium soon. When immunohistochemical identification is readily available, it will aid in the diagnosis of patients with chronic hepatitis C. As noted, the histologic appearance of chronic hepatitis C cannot be differentiated from that of chronic hepatitis B or of autoimmune hepatitis,[1-3] although lymphoid aggregates in the portal areas, steatosis, and destruction of small intrahepatic bile ducts are more characteristic of chronic hepatitis C.[2,3]

Treatment of chronic hepatitis C is also directed at eliminating or decreasing viral replication, mitigating the necroinflammatory process, and halting the progression of disease. Based on the results of a number of controlled trials,[63-66] interferon-α has become the drug of choice. Unfortunately, the results of these initial trials, which have been confirmed by additional trials and by experience in practice, indicate that responses, as measured by transaminase diminution, are generally short-lived. Responses may occur in more than 50 percent of patients, but when interferon is stopped and patients are evaluated 6 months later, only 10–25 percent will have maintained a response. Histologic improvement is less striking than biochemical improvement. Viral replication as measured by HCV RNA determinations in serum and in the liver parallel transaminase data.[67,68] Whether patients with specific genotypes have more frequent complete and sustained resolution rates remains to be determined. Oral ribavirin in pilot studies has reduced transaminase and HCV levels, but the effects were not sustained after discontinuation of treatment.[69,70]

In general, the initial regimen used in the United States has been 3 million units 3 times a week subcutaneously for 6 months. It appears that if a response is to be achieved with this regimen, it will be seen within 3 months. Studies are in progress to see if response rates may be improved by higher dosage, prolongation of treatment, dose escalation regimens, retreatment regimens after relapse, low dosage maintenance regimens, intermittent administration, and use of other forms of interferon-α and other antiviral and immunomodulatory agents. Decisions regarding treatment of chronic hepatitis C must be made anticipating the likelihood of response, the side effects of medication, and the severity of the underlying disease. The dilemma for the patient with mild disease is that this form of disease is less likely to progress, but is also more likely to respond to treatment. If long-term follow-up is available for a patient who was infected with HCV in the distant past, clinicians may be better able to assess the likelihood of progression of disease in that patient. Treatment may be more appropriate for patients who seem to have more severe disease as measured by AST elevations and histologic appearance. The correlation between symptoms and severity of disease is not very strong, however, and symptoms are difficult to use as a reliable indicator for treatment. Patients with chronic hepatitis C with cirrhosis may still be asymptomatic while patients with milder disease may complain of fatiguability. If treatment is undertaken in patients with far-advanced disease and in those with some evidence of hepatic decompensation, low doses of interferon should be used, and frequent monitoring of clinical status and of side effects of medication should be carried out.

For those patients with progressive disease who do not respond to treatment, orthotopic liver transplantation is the only option. Unfortunately, hepatitis C may infect the graft, but the problem does not appear to be as severe as that seen with transplantation in chronic hepatitis B patients. The presence of viremia post-transplantation does not necessarily mean the development of hepatitis.[71]

AUTOIMMUNE HEPATITIS

Autoimmune hepatitis is of unknown etiology, devoid of evidence of antecedent viral infection, and characterized by immunologic and autoimmunologic features, including the presence of circulating autoantibodies, high serum globulin, and a therapeutic response to glucocorticosteroid therapy.[72] The distinction between autoimmune hepatitis and other autoimmune liver diseases (i.e., primary biliary cirrhosis and primary sclerosing cholangitis) has been based primarily on the histologic appearance and characteristic clinical and immunologic features of these disorders. Overlap, however, may occur that obscures the classic boundaries among these autoimmune disorders. Moreover, as noted, the presence of autoantibodies in chronic viral hepatitis (and drug-induced hepatitis), in which histopathologic features may be identical with those in autoimmune hepatitis, further blurs distinctions between disorders of known and unknown etiologies.

Genetic factors appear to play a major role in autoimmune hepatitis, perhaps by predisposing to cirrhosis-producing immunopathogenic processes, although the genetic basis for this remains largely undefined. Although many investigations have been undertaken, the basis for immunopathogenesis is not well understood. Different viruses, including hepatitis A,[73] chemicals, and host proteins have been suggested as triggering agents.

Histologically, autoimmune hepatitis is also characterized by a portal/periportal infiltrate of mononuclear cells.[1] It may be accompanied by more extensive inflammatory changes with resulting bridging inflammation and fibrosis between portal/central areas (severe chronic active hepatitis) and eventuate in cirrhosis. As with chronic viral hepatitis, there is no absolute

TABLE 3. Classification of Autoimmune Hepatitis

Type 1 (classic)
Anti-nuclear antibody
Anti-smooth muscle antibody, anti-actin antibody
Soluble liver antigen antibodies
Anti-liver/pancrease antibody
Anti-lamins A and C antibody
Type 2
Anti-liver/kidney microsome-1 antibody
Anti-liver cytosol-1 antibody
Overlap syndrome
Anti-mitochondrial antibody
Immune cholangiopathy
Anti-nuclear antibody
Anti-smooth muscle antibody

correlation between the clinical presentation and the histopathologic appearance. Thus, although patients with severe clinical presentation often have more advanced histopathologic findings, the asymptomatic patient may also be discovered to have cirrhosis. The histologic picture in patients with a spontaneous or a pharmacologically induced remission may revert to that of strictly portal inflammation or, if cirrhosis has already ensued, to that of an inactive cirrhosis.

Classification (Table 3) is based on the presence of circulating autoantibodies, although it is not known what role, if any, these antibodies play in pathogenesis of disease. The form of autoimmune hepatitis presently identified as type 1 or classical was originally known as *active chronic hepatitis*. Subsequently, it was known as *lupoid hepatitis* because of the presence of the lupus erythematosus cell phenomenon and has most frequently been referred to as *autoimmune chronic active hepatitis*. It is characterized by circulating antibodies to nuclei (ANA) and/or to smooth muscle (ASMA), the latter thought to be reflective of the more specific antibodies to actin (AAA). Antibodies to a liver-pancreas protein and to nuclear envelope proteins (lamins A + C), a variety of anti-cytoskeleton antibodies and soluble liver antigens (SLA) (cytokeratins 8 and 18) have also been described in patients with type 1 autoimmune hepatitis.

A second type of autoimmune hepatitis often seen in children and characterized by the presence of antibodies to cytochrome P-450 IID6—antiliver/kidney microsomal antibodies (ALKM-1)—is now referred to as *type 2 or ALKM-1*.[74] These patients frequently possess antiliver cytosol antibodies (ALC-1). On occasion, type 2 may be marked exclusively by antibodies to ALC-1. ALKM-2 antibodies, which are seen in ticrynafen-induced hepatitis, and ALKM-3 antibodies, which are seen in chronic delta hepatitis, are not thought to be characteristic of type 2.

In addition to type 1 and type 2 autoimmune hepatitis, there are two conditions in which features of both autoimmune hepatitis and primary biliary cirrhosis (PBC) occur. In the so-called overlap syndrome, serologic findings are those of primary biliary cirrhosis, characterized by antimitochondrial antibodies directed toward enzymes in the 2-oxo-acid dehydrogenase family but whose histologic picture is that of a chronic active hepatitis.[75] These patients generally respond to glucocorticosteroid therapy. Immunocholangitis or immune cholangiothopathy, on the other hand, has the histopathologic features of PBC but circulating ANA and ASMA and also responds to glucocorticosteroid treatment.[76]

The heterogeneity of autoimmune hepatitis is illustrated by histologic findings, circulating autoantibody patterns, immunogenetic status, and a variable clinical picture. Presentation of the classic type extends from the asymptomatic patient to those patients who present with an acute or even fulminant picture. Although more prevalent in women, the female preponderance in autoimmune hepatitis is not nearly as great as that seen in primary biliary cirrhosis. It commonly affects girls and premenopausal women, but is also seen in postmenopausal women and in males. Type 2 is predominantly a disease of girls or young women.

One laboratory feature of autoimmune hepatitis that seems rather consistent is hyperglobulinemia. Although not specific, marked elevations of serum globulins, in particular of the IgG type, are characteristic and more striking in general than those seen in chronic viral hepatitis. This nonspecific response may also manifest itself in the presence of circulating antibodies to a variety of viruses and to nonorgan-specific cellular constituents, a feature that may provide diagnostic uncertainties for clinicians trying to distinguish autoimmune from viral hepatitis. Antibodies to HCV determined by ELISA in patients with classic autoimmune hepatitis probably represent nonspecific responses that in general disappear after drug-induced remission of disease.[77,78] Anti-HC determined by RIBA or the presence of HCV RNA in ALKM-1–positive hepatitis patients more likely represents hepatitis C with coincidental circulating autoantibodies. In general, those patients with HCV infection and ALKM-1 antibodies are older and have lower ALKM-1 titers and anti-GOR antibodies in comparison to patients with type 2 autoimmune hepatitis.[59]

Although some patients present with clinically advanced cirrhosis with characteristic circulating autoantibodies, others may present with cirrhosis *without* evidence of circulating autoantibodies and no evidence of HBV or HCV infection and are labeled as cryptogeneic cirrhosis. In those cases, a therapeutic response to glucocorticosteroid therapy may be the only indication that AH is the underlying disease. Autoimmune hepatitis may also present in conjunction with other diseases in which immune or autoimmune features appear to play a role, such as ulcerative colitis, hemolytic anemia, or thyroiditis, with or without the presence of circulating autoantibodies.

In terms of immunogenetic heterogeneity, type 1 and also probably type 2 are examples of autoimmune disorders found in white people in association with the class I HLA-B8 and class II HLA-DR3 phenotypes, although the frequency of those phenotypes in the general population makes them of little use in establishing the diagnosis in given patient.[79] In Japanese patients, a primary association exists with HLA-DR4. A secondary association with this phenotype has also been observed in white patients with classic AH who did not possess HLA-B8,DR3.[80] Classic autoimmune hepatitis patients who are characterized by HLA-B8,DR3 are predominantly female, develop the disease earlier in life, and are less likely to have a lasting response to anti-inflammatory treatment.

Despite its striking heterogeneity and our incomplete understanding of its pathogenesis, autoimmune hepatitis is in general, a "steroid-responsive" condition.[72,81] The response rate is probably better than that reported in early controlled trials that involved, for the most part, patients with severe disease and antedated our ability to test for hepatitis B and C markers. The remission rate induced by initial therapy (prednisone or a combination of prednisone and azathioprine) is in the range of 60–80 percent. In general, the prognosis is inversely correlated with the histologic severity of disease. Although some patients will remain in remission after initial suppression by anti-inflammatory therapy, the large majority requires long-term maintenance therapy. Patients whose initial biopsy indicates chronic active hepatitis with cirrhosis rarely stay in remission when treatment is withdrawn and almost always require maintenance therapy. In general, steroid response is marked by a decrease in transaminase and globulin levels within 1–3 months of initiation of treatment, although remission has been reported in a small percentage of patients only after treatment for 2–4 years.

Despite anti-inflammatory therapy, treatment failures and drug intolerance occur. Sustained disease activity results in the development or worsening of cirrhosis with eventual complications and death if patients are not treated with orthotopic liver transplantation.[81] It is not established whether autoimmune hepatitis recurs in the graft in these patients, all of whom receive immunosuppressive therapy after transplantation.

REFERENCES

1. Batts KP, Ludwig J. Histopathology of autoimmune chronic active hepatitis, primary biliary cirrhosis, and primary sclerosing cholangitis. In: Krawitt EL, Wiesner RH, eds. Autoimmune Liver Diseases. New York: Raven Press; 1991:75–92.
2. Scheuer PJ, Ashrafzadeh P, Sherlock S, Brown D, Dusheiko GM. The pathology of hepatitis C. Hepatology. 1992;15:567–71.
3. Bach N, Thung SN, Schaffner F. The histological features of chronic hepatitis C and autoimmune chronic hepatitis: A comparative analysis. Hepatology. 1992;15:572–7.
4. Lashner BA, Jonas RB, Tang H-S, Evans AA, Ozeran SE, Baker AL. Chronic hepatitis: Disease factors at diagnosis predictive of mortality. Am J Med. 1988;85:609–13.
5. Ndumbe PM. Control of hepatitis B. Lancet. 1991;338:1136.
6. Carman WF, Thomas HC. Genetic variation in hepatitis B virus. Gastroenterology. 1992;102:711–9.
7. Luo K-X, Zhou R, He C, Liang Z-S, Jiang S. Hepatitis B virus DNA in sera of virus carriers positive exclusively for antibodies to the hepatitis B core antigen. J Med Virol. 1991;35:55–9.
8. McMahon BJ, Parkinson AJ, Helminiak C, et al. Response to hepatitis B vaccine of persons positive for antibody to hepatitis B core antigen. Gastroenterology. 1992;103:590–4.
9. Zhang Y-Y, Hansson BG, Kuo LS, Widell A, Nordenfelt E. Hepatitis B virus DNA in serum and liver is commonly found in Chinese patients with chronic liver disease despite the presence of antibodies to HBsAg. Hepatology. 1993; 17:538–44.
10. Koff RS. Immunologically mediated extrahepatic manifestations of viral hepatitis. In: Krawitt EL, Wiesner RH, eds. Autoimmune Liver Diseases. New York: Raven Press; 1991:233–45.
11. Venkataseshan VS, Lieberman K, Kim DU, et al. Hepatitis-B–associated glomerulonephritis: Pathology, pathogenesis, and clinical course. Medicine. 1990;69:200–16.
12. Lai KN, Li PKT, Lui SF, et al. Membranous nephropathy related to hepatitis B virus in adults. N Engl J Med. 1991;324:1457–63.
13. Scully LJ, Karayiannis P, Thomas HC. Interferon therapy is effective in treatment of hepatitis B–induced polyarthritis. Dig Dis Sci. 1992;37:1757–60.
14. Fattovich G, Brollo L, Giustina G, et al. Natural history and prognostic factors for chronic hepatitis type B. Gut. 1991;32:294–8.
15. De Johngh FE, Janssen HLA, De Man RA, Jop WCJ, Schalm SW, Van Blankenstein M. Survival and prognostic indicators in hepatitis B surface antigen-positive cirrhosis of the liver. Gastroenterology. 1992;103:1630–5.
16. Scharschmidt BF, Held MJ, Hollander HH, et al. Hepatitis B in patients with HIV infection: Relationship to AIDS and patient survival. Ann Intern Med. 1992;117:837–8.
17. Moraleda G, Bartolome J, Molina J, Castillo I, Carreno V. Analysis of hepatitis B virus DNA, liver disease and influence of antibody to hepatitis C virus in anti-HBe chronic carriers. Liver. 1991;11:352–7.
18. Loriot M-A, Marcellin P, Bismuth E, et al. Demonstration of hepatitis B virus DNA by polymerase chain reaction in the serum and the liver after spontaneous or therapeutically induced HBeAG to anti-HBe or HBsAg to anti-HBs seroconversion in patients with chronic hepatitis B. Hepatology. 1992;15:32–6.
19. Brook MG, McDonald JA, Karayiannis P, et al. Randomised controlled trial of interferon alfa 2A (rbe) (Roferon-A) for the treatment of chronic hepatitis B virus (HBV) infection: Factors that influence response. Gut. 1989;30:1116–22.
20. Perrillo RP, Schiff ER, Davis GL, et al. A randomized, controlled trial of interferon alfa-2b alone and after prednisone withdrawal for the treatment of chronic hepatitis B. N Engl J Med. 1990;323:295–301.
21. Lok AS, Wu P-C, Lai C-L, et al. A controlled trial of interferon with or without prednisone priming for chronic hepatitis B. Gastroenterology. 1992; 102:2091–7.
22. Korenman J, Baker B, Waggoner J, Everhart JE, Di Bisceglie AM, and Hoofnagle JH. Long-term remission of chronic hepatitis B after alpha-interferon therapy. Ann Intern Med. 1991;114:629–34.
23. Carreno V, Castillo I, Molina J, Porres JC, Bartolome J. Long-term follow-up of hepatitis B chronic carriers who responded to interferon therapy. J Hepatol. 1992;15:102–6.
24. Kuhns M, McNamara A, Mason A, Campbell C, Perrillo R. Serum and liver hepatitis B virus DNA in chronic hepatitis B after sustained loss of surface antigen. Gastroenterology. 1992;103:1649–56.
25. Lok AS-F, Lai C-L, Leung EK-Y. Interferon antibodies may negate the antiviral effects of recombinant α-interferon treatment in patients with chronic hepatitis B virus infection. Hepatology. 1990;12:1266–70.
26. Brook MG, Karayiannis P, Thomas HC. Which patients with chronic hepatitis B virus infection will respond to α-interferon therapy? A statistical analysis of predictive factors. Hepatology. 1989;10:761–3.
27. Rosenblum L, Darrow W, Witte J, et al. Sexual practices in the transmission of hepatitis B virus and prevalence of hepatitis delta virus infection in female prostitutes in the United States. JAMA. 1992;267:2477–81.
28. Hershow RC, Chomel BB, Graham DR, et al. Hepatitis D virus infection in Illinois state facilities for the developmentally disabled. Ann Intern Med. 1989; 110:779–85.
29. Rosina F, Pintus C, Meschievitz C, Rizzetto M. A randomized controlled trial of a 12-month course of recombinant human interferon-α in chronic delta (type D) hepatitis: A multicenter Italian study. Hepatology. 1991;13:1052–6.
30. Ackerman Z, Valinluck B, McHutchison JG, Redeker AG, Govindarajan S.

Spontaneous exacerbation of disease activity in patients with chronic delta hepatitis infection: The role of hepatitis B, C or D? Hepatology. 1992;16:625–9.

31. Ottobrelli A, Marzano A, Smedile A, et al. Patterns of hepatitis delta virus reinfection and disease in liver transplantation. Gastroenterology. 1991;101:1649–55.
32. Brillanti S, Foli M, Gaiani S, Masci C, Miglioli M, Barbara L. Persistent hepatitis C viraemia without liver disease. Lancet. 1993;1:464–5.
33. Seeff LB, Buskell-Bales Z, Wright EC, et al. Long-term mortality after transfusion-associated non-A, non-B hepatitis. N Engl J Med. 1992;327:1906–11.
34. Alter MJ, Margolis HS, Krawczynski K, et al. The natural history of community-acquired hepatitis C in the United States. N Engl J Med. 1992;327:1899–905.
35. Bukh J, Miller RH, Kew MC, Purcell RH. Hepatitis C virus RNA in southern African blacks with hepatocellular carcinoma. Proc Natl Acad Sci USA. 1993;90:1848–51.
36. Donahue JG, Muñoz A, Ness PM, et al. The declining risk of post-transfusion hepatitis C virus infection. N Engl J Med. 1992;327:369–73.
37. Thaler MM, Park C-K, Landers DV, et al. Vertical transmission of hepatitis C virus. Lancet. 1991;1:17–18.
38. Reinus JF, Leikin EL, Alter HJ, et al. Failure to detect vertical transmission of hepatitis C virus. Ann Intern Med. 1992;117:881–6.
39. Wejstål R, Widell A, Månsson A-S, Hermodsson S, Norkrans G. Mother-to-infant transmission of hepatitis C virus. Ann Intern Med. 1992;117:887–90.
40. Roudet-Thormawal F, Paulotsky J-M, Thiers V, et al. Lack of mother-to-infant transmission of hepatitis C virus in human immunodeficiency virus-seronegative women: A prospective study with hepatitis C virus RNA testing. Hepatology. 1993;17:772–7.
41. Tedder RS, Gilson RJC, Briggs M, et al. Hepatitis C virus: Evidence for sexual transmission. Br Med J. 1991;302:1299–302.
42. Melbye M, Biggar RJ, Wantzin P, Krogsgaard K, Ebbesen P, Becker NG. Sexual transmission of hepatitis C virus: Cohort study (1981–9) among European homosexual Men. Br Med J. 1990;301:210–12.
43. Osmond DH, Padian NS, Sheppard HW, Glass S, Shiboski SC, Reingold A. Risk factors for hepatitis C virus seropositivity in heterosexual couples. JAMA. 1993;269:361–5.
44. van Doornum GJJ, Hooykaas C, Cuypers MT, van der Linden MMD, Coutinho RA. Prevalence of hepatitis C virus infections among heterosexuals with multiple partners. J Med Virol. 1991;35:22–7.
45. Gordon SC, Patel AH, Kulesza GW, Barnes RE, Silverman AL. Lack of evidence for the heterosexual transmission of hepatitis C. Am J Gastroenterol. 1992;87:1849–51.
46. Kotwal GJ, Rustgi VK, Baroudy BM. Detection of hepatitis C virus–specific antigens in semen from non-A, non-B hepatitis patients. Dig Dis Sci. 1992;37:641–4.
47. Fried MW, Shindo M, Fong T-L, Fox PC, Hoofnagle JH, Di Bisceglie AM. Absence of hepatitis C viral RNA from saliva and semen of patients with chronic hepatitis C. Gastroenterology. 1992;102:1306–8.
48. Hsu HH, Wright TL, Luba D, Martin M, Feinstone SM, Garcia G, Greenberg HB. Failure to detect hepatitis C virus genome in human secretions with the polymerase chain reaction. Hepatology. 1991;14:763–7.
49. Wange J-T, Wange T-H, Sheu J-C, Lin J-T, Chen D-S. Hepatitis C virus RNA in saliva of patients with posttransfusion hepatitis and low efficiency of transmission among spouses. J Med Virol. 1992;36:28–31.
50. Liou T-C, Chang T-T, Young K-C, Lin X-Z, Lin C-Y, Wu H-L. Detection of HCV RNA in saliva, urine, seminal fluid, and ascites. J Med Virol. 1992;37:197–202.
51. Marcellin P, Descamps V, Martinot-Peignoux M, et al. Cryoglobulinemia with vasculitis associated with hepatitis C infection. Gastroenterology. 1992;103:272–7.
52. Dammacco F, Sansonno D. Antibodies to hepatitis C virus in essential mixed cryoglobulinaemia. Clin Exp Immunol. 1992;87:352–6.
53. Agnello V, Chung RT, Kaplan LM. A role for hepatitis C virus infection in type II cryoglobulinemia. N Engl J Med. 1992;327:1490–5.
54. Johnson RJ, Gretch DR, Yamabe H, et al. Membranoproliferative glomerulonephritis associated with hepatitis C virus infection. N Engl J Med. 1993;328:465–70.
55. Fargion S, Piperno A, Cappellini MD, et al. Hepatitis C virus and porphyria cutanea tarda: Evidence of a strong association. Hepatology. 1992;16:1322–6.
56. Herrero C, Vicenter A, Bruguera M, et al. Is hepatitis C virus infection a trigger or porphyria cutanea tarda? Lancet. 1993;341:788–90.
57. Mishiro S, Hoshi Y, Takeda K, et al. Non-A, non-B hepatitis specific antibodies directed at host-derived epitope: Implication for an autoimmune process. Lancet. 1990;336:1400–3.
58. Mehta SU, Mishiro S, Sekiguchi K, et al. Immune response to GOR, a marker for non-A, non-B hepatitis and its correlation with hepatitis C virus infection. J Clin Immunol. 1992;12:178–84.
59. Michel G, Ritter A, Gerken G, Meyer zum Buschenfelde K-H, Decker R, and Manns MF. Anti-GOR and hepatitis C virus in autoimmune liver diseases. Lancet. 1992;339:267–9.
60. Alter HJ. New kit on the block: Evaluation of second-generation assays for detection of antibody to the hepatitis C virus. Hepatology. 1992;15:350–3.
61. Hagiwara H, Hayashi N, Mita E, et al. Detection of hepatitis C virus RNA in chronic non-A, non-B liver disease. Gastroenterology. 1992;102:692–4.
62. Lok ASF, Cheung R, Chan R, Liu V. Hepatitis C viremia in patients with hepatitis C virus infection. Hepatology. 1992;15:1007–12.
63. Davis GL, Balart LA, Schiff ER, et al. Treatment of chronic hepatitis C with recombinant interferon alfa. A multicenter randomized, controlled trial. N Engl J Med. 1989;321:1501–6.
64. Di Bisceglie AM, Martin P, Kassianides C, et al. Recombinant interferon alfa therapy for chronic hepatitis C. A randomized, double-blind, placebo-controlled trial. N Engl J Med. 1989;321:1506–10.
65. Causse X, Godinot H, Chevallier M, et al. Comparison of 1 or 3 MU of interferon alfa-2b and placebo in patients with chronic non-A, non-B hepatitis. Gastroenterology. 1991;101:497–502.
66. Marcellin P, Boyer N, Giostra E, et al. Recombinant human α-interferon in patients with chronic non-A, non-B hepatitis: A multicenter randomized controlled trial from France. Hepatology. 1991;13:393–7.
67. Shindo M, Di Bisceglie AM, Cheung L, Shih JW-K, Cristiano K, Feinstone SM, Hoofnagle JH. Decrease in serum hepatitis C viral RNA during alpha-interferon therapy for chronic hepatitis C. Ann Intern Med. 1991;115:700–4.
68. Chayama K, Saitoh S, Arase Y, et al. Effect of interferon administration on serum hepatitis C virus RNA in patients with chronic hepatitis C. Hepatology. 1991;13:1040–3.
69. Reichard O, Andersson J, Schvarcz R, Weiland O. Ribavirin treatment for chronic hepatitis C. Lancet 1991;337:1058–61.
70. Di Bisceglie AM, Shindo M, Fong T-L, et al. A pilot study of ribavirin therapy for chronic hepatitis C. Hepatology. 1992;16:649–54.
71. Wright TL, Donegan E, Hsu HH, et al. Recurrent and acquired hepatitis C viral infection in liver transplant recipients. Gastroenterology. 1992;103:317–322.
72. Czaja AJ. Diagnosis, prognosis and treatment of classical autoimmune chronic active hepatitis. In: Krawitt EL, Wiesner RH, eds. Autoimmune Liver Diseases. New York: Raven Press; 1991:143–66.
73. Vento S, Garofano T, Di Perri G, Dolci L, Concia E, Bassetti D. Identification of hepatitis A virus as a trigger for autoimmune chronic hepatitis type 1 in susceptible individuals. Lancet. 1991;337:1183–7.
74. Homberg J-C, Nisen A, Bernard O, et al. Chronic active hepatitis associated with antiliver/kidney microsome antibody type 1: A second type of "autoimmune" hepatitis. Hepatology. 1987;7:1333–9.
75. Davis PA, Leung P, Manns M, et al. M4 and M9 antibodies in the overlap syndrome of primary biliary cirrhosis and chronic active hepatitis: Epitopes of epiphenomena? Hepatology. 1992;16:1128–36.
76. Carrougher JG, Shaffer RT, Canales LI, Goodman ZD. Diagnostic problems in clinical hepatology: A 33-year-old woman with an autoimmune syndrome. Semin Liver Dis. 1991;11:256–62.
77. McFarlane IG, Smith HM, Johnson PJ, Bray GP, Vergani D, Williams R. Hepatitis C virus antibodies in chronic active hepatitis: Pathogenic factor or false-positive result? Lancet. 1990;335:754–7.
78. Nishiguchi S, Kuroki T, Ueda T, et al. Detection of hepatitis C virus antibody in the absence of viral RNA in patients with autoimmune hepatitis. Ann Intern Med. 1992;116:21–5.
79. Krawitt EL, Albertini RJ. Immunogenetic studies of autoimmune liver disease. In: Krawitt EL, Wiesner RH, eds. Autoimmune Liver Diseases. New York: Raven Press; 1991:63–73.
80. Donaldson PT, Doherty DG, Hayllar KM, McFarlane IG, Johnson PJ, and Williams R. Susceptibility to autoimmune chronic active hepatitis: Human leukocyte antigens DR4 and A1-B8-DR3 are independent risk factors. Hepatology. 1991;13:701–6.
81. Sanchez-Urdazpal L, Czaja AJ, Van Hoek B, Krom RAF, Wiesner RJ. Prognostic features and role of liver transplantation in severe corticosteroid-treated autoimmune chronic active hepatitis. Hepatology. 1992;15:215–21.

98. GRANULOMATOUS HEPATITIS

ANTHONY S. FAUCI
GARY S. HOFFMAN

Granulomas in the liver are histopathologic manifestations of a broad range of disease processes that may be of diverse etiologies, both infectious and noninfectious. They do not represent a distinct disease; also, in and of themselves, they rarely are diagnostic of a particular disease entity since their etiology is seldom determined purely on histologic criteria.[1] Most often (74 percent), they reflect a systemic granulomatous disease. Less frequently (21 percent), they represent a process that primarily is neither a systemic granulomatous nor a hepatic disease; only rarely (4 percent) do they represent an isolated hepatic disease.[1] However, the relative frequency of isolated, idiopathic granulomatous hepatic disease may be considerably greater among patients who are referred to a tertiary care center and who have likely undergone an extensive work-up for causes of granulomatous liver disease. In one series of such patients, the frequency of idiopathic granulomatous hepatitis was 50 percent.[2]

The demonstration of hepatic granulomas may serve to confirm documented underlying disease, or it may present a diagnostic challenge requiring an organized and directed approach in determining its underlying etiology. Since the histopathologic features of granulomas resulting from infectious and noninfectious etiologies may be identical and since the treatment regimens (particularly corticosteroids) used in diseases with hepatic granulomata of noninfectious etiologies are directly contraindicated in most disorders of infectious etiologies, it is imperative to appreciate the intricacies of this clinicopathologic process.

PATHOPHYSIOLOGIC MECHANISMS OF GRANULOMA FORMATION

Granulomas form by a stepwise series of events that include the migration of monocyte–macrophages into an area of inflammatory or immunologic reactivity and the transformation of these cells into epithelioid cells, which may remain as such or may fuse to form the characteristic multinucleated giant cells.[3–6] The morphologic changes that impart an epithelial-like appearance to the macrophage are accompanied by functional changes. The macrophage–phagocyte becomes a nonphagocytic epithelioid cell having increased organelles for enzyme and other protein synthesis and secretion.[7,8] The persistence of incompletely degraded foreign matter in tissues represents one type of stimulus for such cellular transformation. An example is found in tuberculosis, the clinically most common microbial cause of granulomata. It has been demonstrated that mycobacterial lipids persist within the macrophage and trigger its transformation.[9] Although this is an excellent example of persistence of microbial intracellular antigen-enhancing granuloma formation, persistent extracellular stimuli such as schistosome eggs lead to similar responses.[8] In addition, nonmicrobial particles may also stimulate granuloma formation (e.g., silica, metal salts). In these last examples, nonimmunologic mechanisms appear to activate macrophages.

Undegraded materials are not the only stimuli of epithelioid cell transformation and granuloma formation, since antigen persistence cannot adequately explain many of the granulomatous responses of hypersensitivity etiology.[4] Pure foreign body granulomas in which antigen persistence triggers the reaction fall on one end of the spectrum, and pure hypersensitivity responses in which it is highly unlikely that antigen persists form the other end of the spectrum.[10] In the latter circumstance, sensitized lymphocytes on exposure to antigen (which, in many cases, is soluble) amplify the immune response by release of mediators. Monocyte–macrophages accumulate, most likely in response to mediators, and subsequently undergo transformation as described above. In experimental animals, cyclosporine A has been demonstrated to reduce markedly the granulomatous response induced with a variety of mycobacterial agents.[7] This observation suggests that, at least in this setting, granuloma formation is highly dependent upon T-lymphocyte mediators that may inhibit migration and cause activation of macrophages (e.g., interferon-γ).[11,12]

Most infectious diseases in which granulomas occur constitute an overlap of mechanisms since microbes can serve both as a foreign body and as an antigen for an immunologic response. In addition, immune complexes made up of host antibody and microbial or nonmicrobial antigen may, under certain circumstances, stimulate granuloma formation. Finally, certain T-lymphocyte neoplasms may secrete soluble factors that activate macrophages,[13] an alternative mechanism for granuloma formation in diseases such as lymphomatoid granulomatosis.[14]

The liver serves as a particularly susceptible target organ for

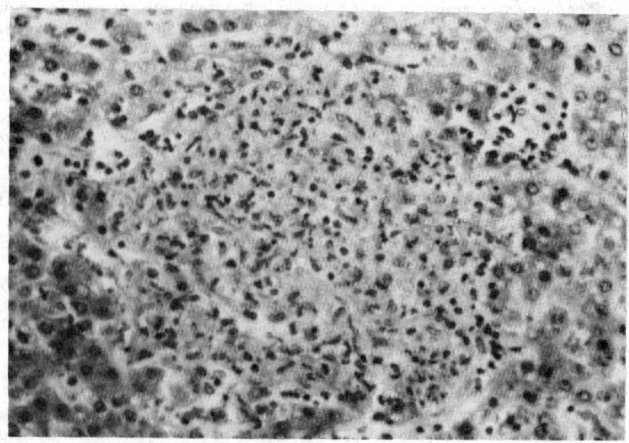

FIG. 1   Liver biopsy specimen from a patient with disseminated histoplasmosis. A typical granuloma is shown with epithelioid cells and mononuclear cell infiltration. (H&E, ×220)

granuloma formation. It is an extremely large organ rich in reticuloendothelial cells. In addition to their phagocytic ability, certain of these cells possess receptors such as those for the Fc portion of immunoglobulin,[15] thus allowing for nonspecific (as well as a degree of immunologically specific) clearance of circulating antigens, unopsonized and opsonized microorganisms, and immune complexes. It is clear then why hepatic granulomas are found in such a high proportion of diseases with systemic granulomatous responses and why a liver biopsy specimen provides such a high-yield source of diagnostic tissue in such diseases (Fig. 1).

Histopathologically, hepatic granulomas are characterized by the presence of generally discrete nodular infiltrates of epithelioid cells interspersed with greater or lesser degrees of mononuclear cells. The epithelioid cells usually are compactly arranged and may merge to form typical multinucleated giant cells. However, the presence of these giant cells is not necessary to make the diagnosis of a granulomatous reaction. This histopathologic picture of hepatic granulomas is clearly distinguishable from portal triaditis, which is more commonly seen in a number of inflammatory conditions and which is characterized by the infiltration of mononuclear cells as well as granulocytes around the portal tract areas. Thus, it is not strictly correct to term granulomatous hepatitis a true *hepatitis* since classic inflammatory responses are rarely seen, and, as will be discussed below, significant hepatocellular dysfunction is rare.[16,17]

DISEASES CHARACTERIZED BY HEPATIC GRANULOMAS

Infectious Diseases

Infectious diseases clearly are the most common underlying causes of granulomas in general and of hepatic granulomas in particular.[18–20] Table 1 lists some of the various types of infectious diseases that may be associated with granulomas in the liver. Tuberculosis continues to lead the list as the most common infectious disease cause of hepatic granulomas.[18–20] Even when one considers all causes of hepatic granulomas (infectious and noninfectious), tuberculosis still ranks very high in incidence. In Klatskin's series[1] of 433 patients with documented granulomatous diseases in other organs, tuberculosis ranked second to sarcoidosis in the incidence of demonstrable hepatic granulomas. Of 164 tuberculous patients, 70 had granulomas on liver biopsy specimens. Caseating granulomas are the classic findings in tuberculosis. However, noncaseating granulomas also are quite common in tuberculous hepatic involvement. In one series reporting noncaseating granulomas of infectious and noninfec-

TABLE 1. Infectious Disease Causes of Granulomatous Hepatitis

Bacterial
  Mycobacteriosis
    Tuberculous
    Nontuberculous
    BCG vaccination or immunotherapy
  Lepromatous leprosy
  Brucellosis (*Brucella abortus*)
  Tularemia
  Granuloma inguinale
  Melioidosis
  Listeriosis
  Cat-scratch disease
Fungal
  Histoplasmosis
  Coccidioidomycosis
  Candidiasis
Viral
  Cytomegalovirus
  Epstein-Barr virus
  Viral hepatitis
Parasitic
  Schistosomiasis (*Schistosoma mansoni*)
  Visceral larva migrans (*Toxocara canis* or *catis*)
  Fascioliasis (*Fasciola hepatica*)
  Capillaria hepatica
Rickettsial
  Q fever (*Coxiella burnetii*)
Spirochetal
  Syphilis

tious etiology in 50 liver biopsy specimens, tuberculosis again ranked second to sarcoidosis and accounted for 10 percent of the total.[21] In other studies of hepatic granulomas unrestricted with regard to the presence or absence of caseous changes, fewer than 15 percent of patients found to have tuberculosis had caseous necrosis in the liver.[22,23] Certain consistent findings emerge from various series on the diagnostic import of liver biopsy specimens in patients who ultimately are proved to have tuberculosis. Thirty-one percent of the patients with "isolated" active pulmonary tuberculosis were shown to have hepatic granulomas.[1] In series of patients with documented pulmonary and extrapulmonary tuberculosis (exclusive of miliary involvement), 70–80 percent had hepatic granulomas.[1,24] In cases of miliary tuberculosis, greater than 90 percent of the patients will have hepatic granulomas.[1,25] There is no question that *Mycobacterium tuberculosis* can be demonstrated by appropriate staining techniques as well as by culture from liver biopsy specimens.[24–27] Yet, when one looks at all cases of hepatic granulomas associated with tuberculosis of any extent, this demonstration is rather uncommon.[28,29] However, in a series of 23 liver biopsies in documented miliary tuberculosis, 43 percent either had a positive culture or smear.[25]

Other mycobacterial infections that may cause hepatic granulomas are disseminated mycobacteriosis other than tuberculosis,[30] lepromatous leprosy,[31] and BCG-osis after Calmette-Guérin bacillus (BCG) vaccination, immunotherapy for neoplasms, or intravesical therapy in the treatment of bladder cancer.[32–34] It is noteworthy that, in the hepatic granulomas associated with lepromatous leprosy, organisms are plentiful and can be easily demonstrated within Kupffer cells.[31] It is of interest that granulomatous tissue reactions rarely are found and if present, they are poorly formed in the *Mycobacterium avium-intracellulare* and *M. tuberculosis* infections that are commonly seen in patients with acquired immunodeficiency syndrome (AIDS).[35] This is likely due to the fact that these patients have markedly suppressed inducer–helper T-lymphocyte numbers and function,[36] which are required for the immunologic component of the granulomatous response to mycobacteria. Although less common, AIDS patients may also develop hepatic granulomas in association with cryptococcosis, histoplasmosis, cytomegalovirus, hepatitis virus infection, and Kaposi's sarcoma.[37]

Brucellosis is quite commonly associated with hepatic granulomas.[36] In infections with *Brucella abortus*, the granulomas

are well formed and discrete. Infections with *Brucella suis* and *Brucella melitensis* result in less distinct changes in the liver, which may be manifested merely as isolated areas of necrosis.[29,38]

Although tularemia often is cited as one of the bacterial diseases that can lead to hepatic granulomas, classic well-formed granulomas with multinucleated giant cells are seldom seen in this disease. The most common finding is scattered necrotic nodules with neutrophil infiltration.[39]

Other uncommon bacterial causes of hepatic granulomas are granuloma inguinale,[40] melioidosis,[41] cat scratch disease,[42] and disseminated infection with *Listeria monocytogenes*, particularly in a rare syndrome in neonates called *miliary granulomatosis* or *granulomatosis infantisepticum*.[43]

Fungi are another common cause of hepatic granulomas. Depending on the reported series and geographic location, they may be the most common infectious disease cause, surpassing even tuberculosis in some individual reports.[21] In the United States, disseminated histoplasmosis is the most common of the fungal etiologies of hepatic granulomas. A hepatic biopsy specimen is a more fruitful source of diagnostic tissue in histoplasmosis as compared with tuberculosis.[44] In a prospective study of 26 patients with disseminated histoplasmosis at the National Institutes of Health, 21 of 26 patients had liver function abnormalities; in the 8 in whom liver biopsy specimens were obtained, 5 had granulomas.[45] Furthermore, *Histoplasma* was cultured from four of the eight biopsy specimens and was demonstrated by staining techniques in three of the four cultured specimens.

Other disseminated mycotic infections such as coccidioidomycosis, candidiasis, and aspergillosis rarely may cause hepatic granulomas. However, the other organ system manifestations of these diseases in their disseminated form overshadow the hepatic granulomas when present. For the most part, the finding of hepatic granulomas in this setting adds little to an already obvious clinical diagnosis.

It is now well established that viral infections may cause hepatic granulomas. Cytomegalovirus and infectious mononucleosis,[1] in particular, have been associated with granulomatous hepatitis. In addition, in a large biopsy series of hepatitis of various causes, granulomas were demonstrated in the liver biopsy specimens of 2 percent of the patients with acute viral hepatitis and in 12 percent of the patients with chronic active hepatitis.[1]

It is uncertain whether influenza virus may cause granulomatous hepatitis. There has been an association of influenza B infection and granulomatous hepatitis,[46] but the two may have been unrelated.[18]

Several parasites encountered throughout the world may cause hepatic granulomas.[18,47] Of particular importance are schistosomiasis (resulting from *Schistosoma mansoni*) and visceral larva migrans (caused by *Toxocara canis* or *Toxocara cati*). Granuloma formation in these disorders most likely results from a deposition of eggs in the liver, with a subsequent combination foreign body reaction to the eggs themselves and a cell-mediated or delayed hypersensitivity reaction to antigenic determinants of the parasite. Another potential cause of parasite-related granulomatous reaction in the liver is fascioliasis caused by the liver fluke *Fasciola hepatica*.

Of the rickettsioses, *Coxiella burnettii*, which causes Q fever, most often is associated with granulomatous hepatitis.[48,49] Q fever is not associated with an exanthem (characteristic of the other rickettsioses); in some cases, it may present with a clinical syndrome identical to viral hepatitis. Thus, the finding of granulomas on a liver biopsy specimen in such a clinical setting should suggest Q fever as part of the differential diagnosis.

The liver may be involved in secondary and tertiary syphilis. During the era when late syphilis was much more common than it is at present, variable degrees of hepatic involvement were frequently seen. Hepatic gummas and hepar lobatum are the typical changes of late syphilitic liver involvement, and interstitial hepatitis is the typical finding in congenital syphilis.[50] Well-formed granulomas are not characteristic but may be found in some cases.

Noninfectious Diseases

Among diseases in which a diagnosis is ultimately made, sarcoidosis is the most common noninfectious disease cause of hepatic granulomas[1,18]; in addition, it is the most common cause—infectious and noninfectious—of noncaseating hepatic granulomas.[21] It is the histopathologic prototype of the classic noncaseating granuloma. Most authorities accept the working definition of sarcoidosis to be a multisystem granulomatous disorder of unknown etiology. Although typical patients present with bilateral hilar lymphadenopathy, skin or eye lesions, these features are not considered essential.[2,21]

Other noninfectious disease causes of granulomatous hepatitis are listed in Table 2 and have been reviewed in detail elsewhere.[49-52] Of particular interest in this group, with regard to infectious diseases, are erythema nodosum and chronic granulomatous disease (CGD) of childhood.

Erythema nodosum is a hypersensitivity manifestation of several different clinical entities that is characterized predominantly by tender subcutaneous nodules over the anterior surface of the lower extremities beneath the knees and (occasionally) elsewhere.[53] It can be associated with granulomatous hepatitis as part of the syndrome complex itself. In addition, some of the infectious disease entities with which it is associated (e.g., tuberculosis, coccidioidomycosis, histoplasmosis, and lepromatous leprosy), in and of themselves, can cause hepatic granulomas; this makes the diagnostic approach even more complex when hepatic granulomas are found in erythema nodosum.

In up to 29 percent of patients with hepatic granulomas, medications have been suspected causes. Granulomas are said to always be noncaseating and often contain large numbers of eosinophils (>5–10 per granuloma), a finding that would be very unusual in tuberculosis or sarcoidosis. In a minority of cases, drug-induced granulomas may be found in extrahepatic sites such as lymph nodes and bone marrow. Eosinophilic granulomas may also occur in schistosomiasis, visceral larva migrans, Hodgkin's disease, and histoplasmosis. In the absence of these disorders, the question of drug-induced disease should be considered.[2,54-56] The terms *probable* and *possible* have been applied to drug-suspected cases when the withdrawal of a drug has been associated with resolution of symptoms, normalization of liver function test results (if these had been abnormal), and diminution or absence of granulomas in a repeat liver biopsy specimen. A "definite" diagnosis of drug-induced disease would require the demonstration of recurrent abnormalities after reinstitution of the suspected agent. However, rechallenge of patients with the suspected medication should not be carried out unless the medication is essential and an appropriate alternative is not available. Since it is conceivable that many different medications may play a role in granuloma formation, treatment with nonessential drugs should be discontinued and the patient's clinical course be followed subsequently. A repeat liver biopsy can be considered approximately 8 weeks after the drug has been stopped, to assess the effect of discontinuation of the drug on liver histopathology.

Patients with the host defense defect of CGD frequently have disseminated granulomas with a predominance of liver involvement.[57] It is felt that the mechanism of granuloma formation in this disease is an intracellular persistence of microorganisms or their products that is related to the well-established microbial killing defect. This triggers the epithelioid cell transformation with subsequent granuloma formation as described above. Granulomas persist in these patients, and it is difficult to recover microorganisms from liver tissue. The granulomatous reaction results from an inability to handle a variety of microorganisms normally.

Hodgkin's disease and other lymphomas are recognized as the most common malignancies associated with hepatic granulomas. Although other tumors (renal cell, rectal, nasopharyngeal, and primary hepatocellular carcinoma) have also been noted to share this association, those examples are not as well documented.[23,52,54] Further confusion is added by the observation that malignancies related to hepatic granulomas may not become apparent until months or even several years after the initial evaluation. Preliminary data suggest that individuals with hepatic granulomas who are later (4–40 months) demonstrated to have lymphomas are more likely to have at initial presentation: (1) prolonged (>4 weeks) unexplained fevers; (2) liver or (3) spleen size extending more than 4 cm below the costal margins; and (4) eosinophilia of greater than 4 percent of the peripheral white blood cell count. The presence of any two of these features had a specificity of 80 percent and a sensitivity of 100 percent for lymphoma as a cause of the hepatic granulomas.[58]

Another interesting and perplexing category of granulomatous hepatitis is that group of patients in whom the etiology of the granulomatous reaction remains unknown despite extensive diagnostic investigation.[59] In various series, this group of idiopathic granulomatous hepatitis ranged from 4 to 50 percent of the cases with documented hepatic granulomas.[1,2,18,20,28,31] In addition, in a group of 72 patients with hepatic granulomas whose underlying disease did not appear to be hepatic or granulomatous in nature, 37 of these remained undiagnosed.[1] These patients do not have extra-abdominal granulomas, and other criteria for sarcoidosis are absent. This group probably represents hypersensitivity states that are clinically and histopathologically reflected primarily in the liver, with the responsible antigen remaining unidentified.

GRANULOMATOUS HEPATITIS AND FEVER

Fever is a major manifestation in most cases of granulomatous hepatitis. In one large series, over 40 percent of the patients with hepatic granulomas had fevers of unknown origin.[18] The liver is rich in phagocytic Kupffer cells, which are highly efficient producers of interleukin-1 and other endogenous pyrogens.[60] Triggering of these cells by antigens, immune complexes, or microorganisms in the pathogenesis of granuloma formation can lead to the release of pyrogen. On the one hand, an infectious agent that may be the underlying cause of the hepatic granulomas can cause fever; conversely, the hepatic granulomas, whether resulting from infectious or noninfectious causes, can themselves be the sources of fever. Interleukin-1 is secreted by monocyte–macrophages and is critically involved in the activation of T lymphocytes,[61] which further indicates the complex relationship among immunologic reactions, granuloma formation, and febrile responses.

TABLE 2. Noninfectious Disease Causes of Granulomatous Hepatitis

Sarcoidosis
Hypersensitivity diseases
  Erythema nodosum
  Berylliosis
  Hypersenitivity drug reactions
Primary liver disease
  Primary biliary cirrhosis
  Rarely, others such as Laennec's cirrhosis, postnecrotic cirrhosis, alcoholic hepatitis, or chronic active hepatitis
Neoplasms
  Hodgkin's disease and, rarely, other lymphomas and solid tumors
Host defense defects
  Chronic granulomatous disease of childhood
  Immune deficiencies (hypogammaglobulinemia)
Others
  Temporal artertis—polymyalgia rheumatica syndrome
  Allergic granulomatosis
  Idiopathic granulomatous hepatitis
  Ulcerative colitis
  Crohn's disease

DIAGNOSTIC APPROACH TO HEPATIC GRANULOMAS

Hepatic granulomas are quite common and may be found in up to 10 percent of specimens from liver biopsies performed in general hospitals.[18] Although a liver biopsy specimen obtained by laparotomy may offer the highest yield, a percutaneous needle biopsy is a relatively safe and efficient procedure for obtaining tissue for diagnosis, assessment of extent of disease, follow-up, and evaluation of therapy. Its value in the diagnostic approach to fevers of unknown origin is well established.[62] Once hepatic granulomas have been demonstrated histologically and the underlying diagnosis is still not established, a stepwise diagnostic approach should be undertaken. Because infectious diseases are the leading causes of all types of hepatic granulomas, bacterial, fungal, and mycobacterial cultures should be obtained. In addition, special stains, including silver impregnation stains for cat scratch microbes[42] and spirochetes,[50] should be applied to histologic sections, and appropriate skin tests and diagnostic serologic tests should be used. Also, viruses such as cytomegalovirus (CMV) and Epstein-Barr virus (EBV) may infrequently cause granulomatous hepatitis (Table 1). The diagnosis of CMV or EBV infection can be suspected on clinical grounds and is usually established by serologic tests.

If infectious disease causes have been ruled out and the diagnosis is still unknown, an orderly diagnostic approach that includes clinical, histopathologic, serologic, and radiologic parameters should be used to exclude noninfectious disease causes (Table 2). Medications instituted within the last 6 months should be suspected as a possible cause, and treatment with nonessential medications should be stopped. If after this one is still left with a diagnosis of granulomatous hepatitis of unknown etiology, careful follow-up, subsequent reevaluation, and, in some cases, empirical therapy are indicated, as discussed below.

There may be specific laboratory abnormalities associated with various diseases in which granulomatous hepatitis can be present.[14,21,59] However, laboratory abnormalities usually associated with hepatic granulomas are generally nonspecific. The erythrocyte sedimentation rate is variably elevated (40–80 percent).[2,53] Increased serum levels of alkaline phosphatase and transaminases are frequently abnormal. Hyperbilirubinemia is most unusual except in cases of primary biliary cirrhosis. Mild hyperglobulinemia may be found, and prothrombin elevations are unusual.

TREATMENT OF GRANULOMATOUS HEPATITIS

When the underlying cause of the granulomatous hepatitis is known, treatment should be directed toward the specific etiology, whether it be infectious or noninfectious. The disappearance of granulomas usually parallels the therapeutic response of the underlying disease. After successful therapy for the underlying disease, little if any histopathologic residue of the granulomas remain.[51,59]

In the clinical setting where infectious and other causes of granulomatous hepatitis have been excluded in so far as possible, and where the diagnosis of idiopathic granulomatous hepatitis remains, corticosteroids often lead to clinical and histopathologic improvement.[59,63] Because of the risk of administration of corticosteroids to a patient with an underlying, but undetected infection (particularly tuberculosis), empirical antituberculous therapy should be considered. Cases of granulomatous hepatitis in which tuberculosis could not be demonstrated have responded to antituberculous drugs. Conversely, patients who lacked evidence for tuberculosis and were treated with steroids for idiopathic granulomatous hepatitis have died of disseminated tuberculosis.[23] Because of these observations, it is recommended that all patients with granulomatous hepatitis in whom an etiology cannot be established be given an empirical trial of two-drug antituberculous therapy. If a clinical response is seen,

the drugs are continued for the usual recommended course. If no clinical response is seen after 2 months, anti-tuberculous drugs are stopped once corticosteroids are added. If the patient is tuberculin skin test–positive, a single drug (isoniazid) should be continued with the corticosteroid. If symptoms are modest and tolerable, treatment may be deferred and the patient carefully followed. In one recent study of fever of unknown origin and idiopathic granulomatous hepatitis, 41 percent of 17 patients had self-limiting disease, 18 percent of patients experienced disease resolution within 3 months of corticosteroid or indomethacin therapy, and 41 percent of patients required long-term low-dose corticosteroid therapy.[63] Therapeutic responses should be monitored by clinical and laboratory parameters as well as by repeat liver biopsies every 6–12 months. If corticosteroid therapy has been instituted it is highly recommended to convert the therapeutic regimen to alternate-day corticosteroids once clinical improvement has occurred, since granulomatous hepatitis can be adequately controlled in many patients with alternate-day low-dose (e.g. prednisone, 10 mg) corticosteroid regimens.[59]

REFERENCES

1. Klatskin G. Hepatic granulomata: Problems in interpretation. Ann NY Acad Sci. 1976;278:427.
2. Sartin JS, Walker RD. Granulomatous hepatitis: A retrospective review of 88 cases at the Mayo Clinic. Mayo Clin Proc. 1991;66:914–8.
3. Silverman L, Shorter RG. Histogenesis of the multinucleated giant cell. Lab Invest. 1963;12:985.
4. Epstein WL. Granulomatous hypersensitivity. Prog Allergy. 1967;11:36.
5. Epstein WL, Krasnobrod H. The origin of epithelioid cells in experimental granulomas of man. Lab Invest. 1968;18:190.
6. Gillman T, Wright LJ. Probable in vivo origin of multinucleated giant cells from circulating mononuclears. Nature. 1963;209:263.
7. Muller-Hermelink HK, Kaiserling E, Sonntag HG. Modulation of epithelioid cell granuloma formation to apathogenic mycobacteria by cyclosporin A. Pathol Res Pract. 1982;175:80.
8. Williams GT, Williams WJ. Granulomatous inflammation—A review. J Clin Pathol. 1983;36:723.
9. Rich AR. The Pathogenesis of Tuberculosis. Springfield, IL: Charles C Thomas; 1951:13.
10. Warren KS. Granulomatous inflammation. In: Lepow IH, Ward PW, eds. Inflammation: Mechanisms and Control. New York: Academic Press; 1972; 203.
11. Weinberg JB, Hobbs MM, Misukonis MA. Recombinant human γ-interferon induces human monocyte polykaryon formation. Proc Natl Acad Sci USA 1984;81:4554.
12. Block CM, Catterall JR, Remington JS. In vivo and in vitro activation of alveolar macrophages by recombinant interferon-γ. J Immunol. 1987;138:491.
13. Simrell CR, Crabtree GR, Cossman J, et al. Stimulation of phagocytosis by a T cell lymphoma derived lymphokine. In: Vitetta E, Fox CF, eds. B and T Cell Tumors: Biological and Clinical Aspects. UCLA Symposia on Molecular and Cellular Biology. v. 24. New York: Academic Press; 1982:247.
14. Fauci AS, Haynes BF, Costa J, et al. Lymphomatoid granulomatosis. Prospective clinical and therapeutic experience over 10 years. N Engl J Med. 1982;306:68.
15. Atkinson JP, Frank MM. Studies on the in vivo antibody and complement in the immune clearance and destruction of erythrocytes in man. J Clin Invest. 1974;54:339.
16. Sherlock S. Hepatic granulomas. In: Sherlock S, ed. Diseases of the Liver and Biliary System. 5th ed. Oxford: Blackwell Scientific Publications; 1975: 598.
17. Harrington PT, Gutierrez JJ, Ramirez-Ronda CH, et al. Granulomatous hepatitis. Rev Infect Dis. 1982;4:638.
18. Guckian JC, Perry JE. Granulomatous hepatitis. An analysis of 63 cases and review of the literature. Ann Intern Med. 1969;65:1081.
19. Gold J, Wigderson A, Leiman E, et al. Report of a case with review of the literature. Gastroenterology. 1957;33:113.
20. Bowry S, Chan CH, Weiss H, et al. Hepatic involvement in pulmonary tuberculosis. Histologic and functional characteristics. Am Rev Respir Dis. 1970; 101:941.
21. Mir-Madjlessi SH, Farmer RG, Hawk WA. Granulomatous hepatitis. A review of 50 cases. Am J Gastroenterol. 1973;60:122.
22. Irani SK, Dobbins WO III. Hepatic granulomas: A review of 73 patients from one hospital and survey of the literature. J Clin Gastroenterol. 1979;1:131.
23. Cunningham D, Mills PR, Quigley EMM, et al. Hepatic granulomas: Experience over a 10-year period in West of Scotland. Q J Med. 1982;51:162.
24. Korn RJ, Kellow WF, Heller P, et al. Hepatic involvement in extrapulmonary tuberculosis. Histologic and functional characteristics. Am J Med. 1959;27: 60.
25. Cucin RL, Coleman M, Eckardt JJ, et al. The diagnosis of miliary tuberculosis:

Utility of peripheral blood abnormalities, bone marrow and liver needle biopsy. J Chronic Dis. 1973;26:355.

26. Healey RJ, Leff AH, Rosenak BD. Needle biopsy in tuberculosis of the liver, with culture of acid-fast bacilli. Am J Dig Dis. 1959;4:638.

27. Rumball JM, Baum GL. Liver biopsy culture in the diagnosis of miliary tuberculosis: A case report. Gastroenterology. 1952;22:124.

28. Wagoner GP, Anton AT, Gall EA, et al. Needle biopsy of the liver. VII. Experiences with hepatic granulomas. Gastroenterology. 1953;25:487.

29. Rubin E. Interpretation of the liver biopsy. Diagnostic criteria. Gastroenterology. 1963;45:400.

30. Koenig MG, Collins RD, Heyssel RM. Disseminated mycobacteriosis caused by Battey type mycobacteria. Ann Intern Med. 1966;64:145.

31. Browne SG. The liver in leprosy: A review. W Afr Med J. 1964;13:35.

32. Marans HY, Bekirov HM. Granulomatous hepatitis following intravesical bacillus Calmette-Guerin therapy for bladder carcinoma. J Urol. 1987;137:111.

33. Hunt JS, Silverstein MJ, Spark FC, et al. Granulomatous hepatitis: A complication of BCG immunotherapy. Lancet. 1973;2:820.

34. Bodurtha A, Kim YH, Laucius JF, et al. Hepatic granulomas and other hepatic lesions associated with BCG immunotherapy for cancer. Am J Clin Pathol. 1974;61:714.

35. Greene JB, Sidhu GS, Lewin S, et al. *Mycobacterium avium-intracellulare:* A cause of disseminated life-threatening infection in homosexuals and drug abusers. Ann Intern Med. 1982;97:539.

36. Fauci AS. The syndrome of Kaposi's sarcoma-opportunistic infections: An epidemiologically restricted disorder of immunoregulation. Ann Intern Med. 1982;96:777.

37. Jonas MM, Roldan EO, Lyons HJ, et al. Histopathologic features of the liver in pediatric acquired immune deficiency syndrome. J Pediatr Gastroenterol Nutr. 1989;9:73–81.

38. Spink WW, Hoffbauer FW, Walher WW, et al. Histopathology of the liver in human brucellosis. J Lab Clin Med. 1949;34:40.

39. Foshay L. Tularemia: A summary of certain aspects of the disease including methods for early diagnosis and the results of serum treatment in 600 patients. Medicine (Baltimore). 1940;19:1.

40. Lyford J III, Johnson RW Jr, Blackman S, et al. Pathologic findings in a fatal case of disseminated granuloma inguinale with miliary bone and joint involvement. Bull Johns Hopkins Hosp. 1946;79:349.

41. Borchardt KA, Stansifer P, Albano PM. Osteomyelitis due to *Pseudomonas pseudomallei.* JAMA. 1966;196:660.

42. Delahoussaye PM, Osborne BM: Cat-scratch disease presenting as abdominal visceral granulomas. J Infect Dis. 1990;161:71–8.

43. Ray CJ, Wedgewood RJ. Neonatal listeriosis: Six case reports and a review of the literature. Pediatrics. 1964;34:378.

44. Schiff L. The clinical value of needle biopsy of the liver. Ann Intern Med. 1951;34:948.

45. Smith JW, Utz JP. Progressive disseminated histoplasmosis. A prospective study of 26 patients. Ann Intern Med. 1972;76:557.

46. Klatskin G, Yesner R. Hepatic manifestations of sarcoidosis and other granulomatous diseases. Yale J Biol Med. 1950;23:207.

47. Marcial Rojas RA. Helminthic diseases. In: Schiff L, ed. Diseases of the Liver. 2nd ed. Philadelphia: JB Lippincott; 1963:800.

48. Dupont HL, Hornick RB, Levin HS, et al. Q fever hepatitis. Ann Intern Med. 1971;74:198.

49. Travis LB, Travis WD, Li C-Y, et al. Q fever: A clinicopathologic study of five cases. Arch Pathol Lab Med 1986;110:1017.

50. Murray FE, O'Loughlin S, Dervan P, et al. Granulomatous hepatitis in secondary syphilis. Irish J Med Sci 1990;159:53–4.

51. Fauci AS, Wolff SM. Granulomatous hepatitis. In: Popper H, Schaffner F, eds. Progress in Liver Diseases. v. 5. New York: Grune & Stratton; 1976: 609.

52. Anderson CS, Nicholls J, Rowland R, et al. Hepatic granulomas: A 15-year experience in the Royal Adelaide Hospital. Med J Aust. 1988;148:71.

53. Epstein WL. Erythema nodosum. In: Samter M, ed. Immunological Diseases. v. 2. Boston: Little, Brown; 1971:944.

54. McMaster KR III, Hennigar GR. Drug-induced granulomatous hepatitis. Lab Invest. 1981;44:61.

55. Stricker BHC, Blok APR, Babany G, et al. Fibrin ring granulomas and allopurinol. Gastroenterology. 1989;96:1199–203.

56. Larrey D, Vial T, Micaleff A, et al. Hepatitis associated with amoxycillin-clavulanic acid combination: Report of 15 cases. Gut 1992;33:368–71.

57. Good RA, Quie PG, Windhorst DB, et al. Fatal (chronic) granulomatous disease of childhood: A hereditary defect of leukocyte function. Semin Hematol. 1968;5:215.

58. Aderka D, Kraus M, Weinberger A, et al. Parameters which can differentiate patients with "idiopathic" from patients with lymphoma-induced liver granulomas. Am J Gastroenterol. 1985;80:1004.

59. Simon HB, Wolff SM. Granulomatous hepatitis and prolonged fever of unknown origin: A study of 13 patients. Medicine (Baltimore). 1973;52:1.

60. Dinarello CA, Wolff SM. Exogenous and endogenous pyrogen. In: Brazier MAB, Coceani F, eds. Brain Dysfunction in Infantile Febrile Convulsions. v. 2. New York: Raven Press; 1976:117.

61. Oppenheim JJ, Gery I. Interleukin 1 is more than an interleukin. Immunol Today. 1982;3:113.

62. Wolff SM, Simon HB. Granulomatous hepatitis and prolonged fever of unknown origin. Trans Am Clin Climatol Assoc. 1973;84:149.

63. Zoutman DE, Ralph ED, Frei JV: Granulomatous hepatitis and fever of unknown origin. An 11 year experience of 23 cases with three years follow-up. J Clin Gastroenterol 1991;13:69–75.

SECTION O. ACQUIRED IMMUNODEFICIENCY SYNDROME (AIDS)

99. GLOBAL PERSPECTIVES ON HIV INFECTION AND AIDS

PETER PIOT
MICHAEL H. MERSON

More than a decade after the recognition of acquired immunodeficiency syndrome (AIDS) in the United States, the global epidemiologic pattern of human immunodeficiency virus (HIV) infection has changed dramatically. Whereas the disease was originally confined primarily to North America, Western Europe, and parts of sub-Saharan Africa, HIV has now spread throughout the world, with major epidemic foci in all continents. In addition, on a world-wide scale, the epidemic is now evolving into a mainly heterosexually transmitted disease of the developing world, and increasingly, of underprivileged populations in the industrialized world. In this aspect, HIV infection now resembles the "classic" infectious diseases, disproportionately affecting the most socially and economically vulnerable.

This chapter discusses specific features of the epidemiology and impact of HIV infection and AIDS in the developing world, as well as the response to the epidemic. Whereas two serotypes of HIV are currently recognized, namely, HIV-1 and HIV-2, *HIV* will be used in the text to designate HIV-1, which is the major virus.

THE SIZE OF THE PROBLEM

As of June 30, 1993, a cumulative total of 718,894 cases of AIDS have been reported to the World Health Organization (WHO).[1] However, especially in the developing world, these reported cases represent only a small proportion of the actual number of cases. Thus, WHO estimates that a total of a little over 2.5 million AIDS cases in adults and children have occurred by mid-1993, with over 80 percent originating from the Third World.[2]

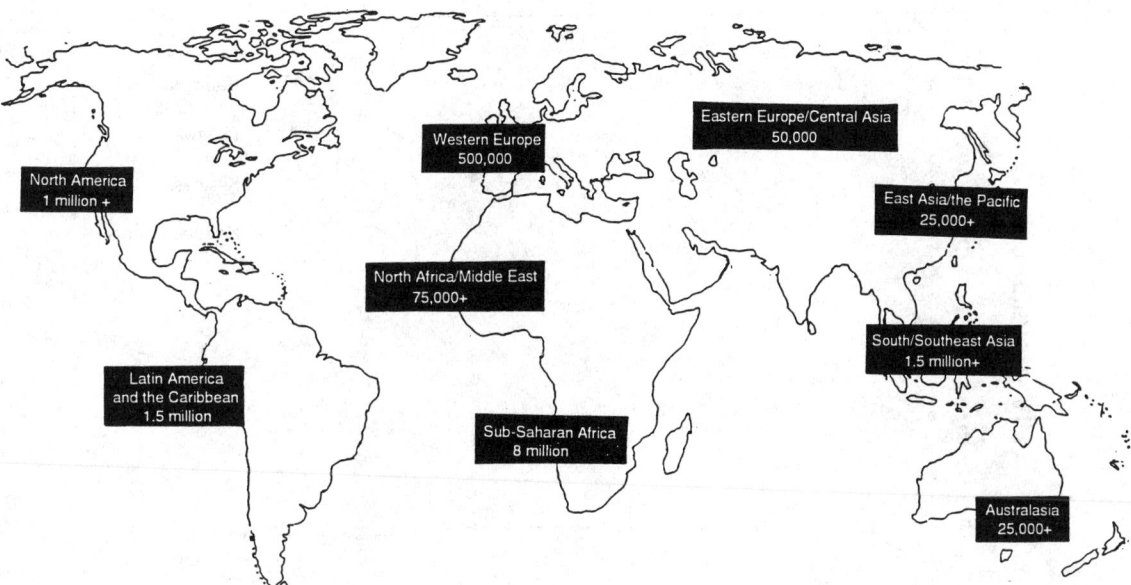

FIG. 1. Estimated distribution of cumulative HIV infections in adults, by continent or region: mid-1993. Global total: 13 million +. (Data from World Health Organization.)

A more complete picture of the extent of the epidemic is given by the number of persons with HIV infection, conservatively estimated for mid-1993 by the WHO at approximately 14 million individuals, including 1 million children. The regional distribution of cumulative HIV infections in adults in the world is shown in Figure 1, illustrating that over 70 percent of cases have occurred in Africa. These cumulative incidence figures keep increasing at a staggering rate. Thus, in 1992 alone, it has been estimated that nearly 2 million people became infected, with a majority of these new infections occurring in sub-Saharan Africa, South Asia, and Southeast Asia.

The ultimate global dimensions of the epidemic are uncertain, but a conservative estimate is that by the year 2000 there will have occurred a cumulative total of 30–40 million cases of HIV infection and close to 10 million cases of AIDS. Over 90 percent of HIV infections will likely have occurred in the developing world.[2,3]

Industrialized Countries

The epidemiology of HIV/AIDS in North America is extensively discussed in Chapter 100, and the present chapter deals mainly with the situation in the developing world. By March 31, 1993, a cumulative total of 83,973 AIDS cases had been reported in the 12 countries of the European Community. In general, in the industrialized countries of Europe, Australia, and New Zealand, there has been a marked fall in HIV incidence among homosexual and bisexual men. Heterosexual transmission is rising, however, in part because of rising infection rates among drug users, who also have sex with noninjectors. In some Scottish cities, up to one-third of new infections now occur through heterosexual intercourse, and among women attending antenatal clinics in London in 1992, HIV prevalence ranged between 1 and 5 per 1000.

In 1993, over half of all new cases of AIDS in Europe occurred in injecting drug users. These contribute particularly to the epidemic in Spain, Italy, and France, which contain 71 percent of all cases reported in the European Community.[4] However, homosexual and bisexual men still represent the largest number of AIDS cases in Europe, including 41 percent of adult cases in 1991–1993, which reflects the high incidence of infection in those populations a decade ago.

In Eastern Europe, HIV incidence is believed still to be relatively low, though conflict, displacement, and slow economic development are undermining health preventive and care services and encouraging high risk behavior. These are key elements for an uncontrolled epidemic to emerge in future.

Sub-Saharan Africa

Sub-Saharan Africa remains by far the worst affected region. In cities such as Kigali, Rwanda, and Kampala, Uganda, as many as one-third of all sexually active adults are infected. However, the HIV prevalence rate is still well below 1 percent in many rural areas or in a country such as Madagascar.[5,6]

In most parts of Africa, the epidemic is still expanding. Figure 2 shows the evolution of HIV prevalence among pregnant women in various African cities. In general, prevalence of HIV infection is highest in eastern and southern Africa, though in Côte d'Ivoire and surrounding countries in West Africa it is now rapidly increasing. Prevalence rates are generally highest among the sexually most active parts of the population, as illustrated by the age distribution of HIV infections, which peak between the ages of 20 and 40 years, by very high infection rates among men with a sexually transmitted disease (STD), and by high rates among prostitutes. Even in areas where HIV infection is still relatively uncommon in the population as a whole, prevalence rates well over 10 percent can be found in these higher risk populations (Table 1). It is now increasingly common in Africa to find HIV prevalence rates exceeding 80 percent in prostitutes and 50 percent in STD patients, particularly when the latter have genital ulcers. However, studies in antenatal clinics in Rwanda, Kenya, and Malawi demonstrate that the HIV epidemic is not limited any longer to people with high-risk sexual behavior.[7–9] They also show that sexual behavior of the partner may be an important risk factor of being infected with HIV.

HIV continues to spread in all populations in Africa, as illustrated by annual HIV incidence rates of 0.3 percent to as high as 5 percent in cohorts thought to be representative of the general population.[5] Among highly exposed female prostitutes such incidence rates may be as high as 12–50 percent per year.[10,11] In contrast, the prevalence of HIV seems to have stabilized around 5–10 percent in some Zairian populations,[6] suggesting that the incidence of HIV has peaked at least in some parts of Africa. However, it should be kept in mind that "stable" prevalence still implies active spread of HIV, but at a rate more or less

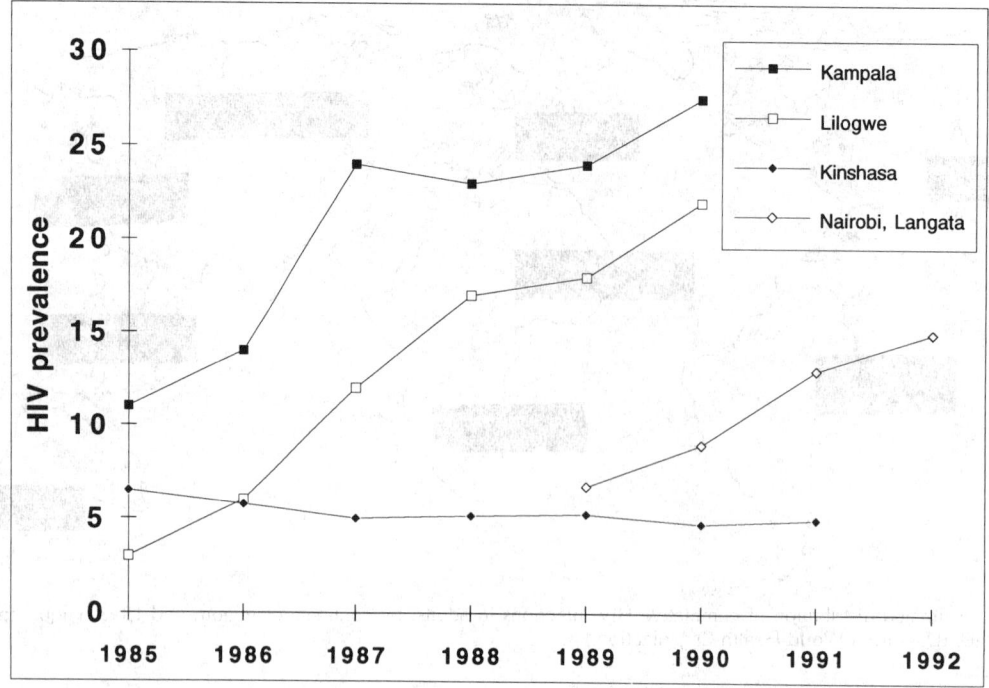

FIG. 2. Evolution of HIV-1 prevalence among pregnant women in four African cities. (Adapted from World Health Organization,[2] with permission.)

TABLE 1. HIV Antibody Prevalence Rates in Pregnant Women Attending Antenatal Clinics, Men with a Sexually Transmitted Disease, and Prostitutes in Selected African Cities, 1989–1991

City, Country	% with HIV Antibody		
	Pregnant Women	Men with STD	Prostitutes
Bobo Dioulas, Burkina Fasso	7.8	18.2	NA
Yaounde, Cameroon	1.1	2.9	9.3
Abidjan, Côte d'Ivoire	12.2	22.0	91.8
Addis Ababa, Ethiopia	2.1	17.1	22.0
Nairobi, Kenya	5.8–15.8	44.7	85.9
Various towns, Malawi	22.0–23.1	62.4	NA
Kigali, Rwanda	26.2	69.0	NA
Dakar, Senegal	0.6*	2.7*	33.4*
Dar-es-Salaam, Tanzania	8.9	19.8	45.0
Kampala, Uganda	29.5	45.0	NA
Kinshasa, Zaire	4.8	NA	35.0
Lusaka, Zambia	25.0	54.0	NA

[a] Includes HIV-2.
Abbreviation: STD, sexually transmitted disease; NA, data not available.

(Data from U.S. Bureau of the Census, 1992.)

equalling the mortality from AIDS in that population.[12] Overall, about equal numbers of men and women are infected. However, there is significant geographic variation in the male-to-female ratio, with ratios of 1:1.2 in Zaire and Uganda but of 2:1 in Côte d'Ivoire.

The disease burden of HIV infection in sub-Saharan Africa is high and will grow considerably higher. WHO estimates that as of June 1993 over 1.5 million AIDS cases had occurred in this region, constituting over two-thirds of the global total.[2] In addition, approximately a half million children have developed AIDS. The enormous impact of AIDS on health services, individuals, and communities is discussed below.

A second human immunodeficiency virus, HIV-2, is found in West Africa and, to a much lesser extent, in Angola and Mozambique.[13] The highest HIV-2 prevalence rates are found in Guinea-Bissau, with nearly 10 percent of the sexually active population being infected.[14] In the other countries where HIV-2 infection is found, prevalence rates are usually below 2 percent among pregnant women.[13]

HIV-2 seems to spread slower, and the average age of infection appears to be higher than that of HIV-1 infection in the same population. On the other hand, STD patients and prostitutes have the highest risk of HIV-2 infection, indicating that transmission is also mainly sexual. However, mother-to-child transmission and HIV-2 infection in infants and children are unusual.[15] Overall, the risk of transmission of HIV-2 appears to be significantly less than that of HIV-1.

Dually reactive sera for both HIV-1 and HIV-2 antibodies occur frequently in HIV-2–prevalent populations. One-third to one-half of such cases are due to concomitant infection with both viruses.[16,17] The epidemiology and natural history of double reactivity is under study.

Asia

In recent years HIV has been spreading considerably in South and Southeast Asia, where more than 1.5 million people were infected by mid-1993.[2] At the same time, less than 4000 cases of AIDS were reported from Asia, though the actual number is probably over 30,000.

The extent of the spread of HIV in Asia is critical for the future of the pandemic, as over half of the world's population lives on this continent. In addition, the full consequences of HIV infection in Asia will only begin to be seen after the year 2000, when many of the currently HIV-infected individuals will have progressed to AIDS.

HIV-1 spread was first detected in Asia among injecting drug users. The virus has spread fulminantly among drug users in selected areas of Thailand, Myanmar, Northeast India, and Malaysia, where HIV seroprevalence levels around 50 percent are not uncommon in such populations.[6,18–22] The situation is similar in some parts of Yunnan province in Southern China,[23] Malaysia, and Viet Nam.

In a simultaneously occurring epidemic, the virus has also

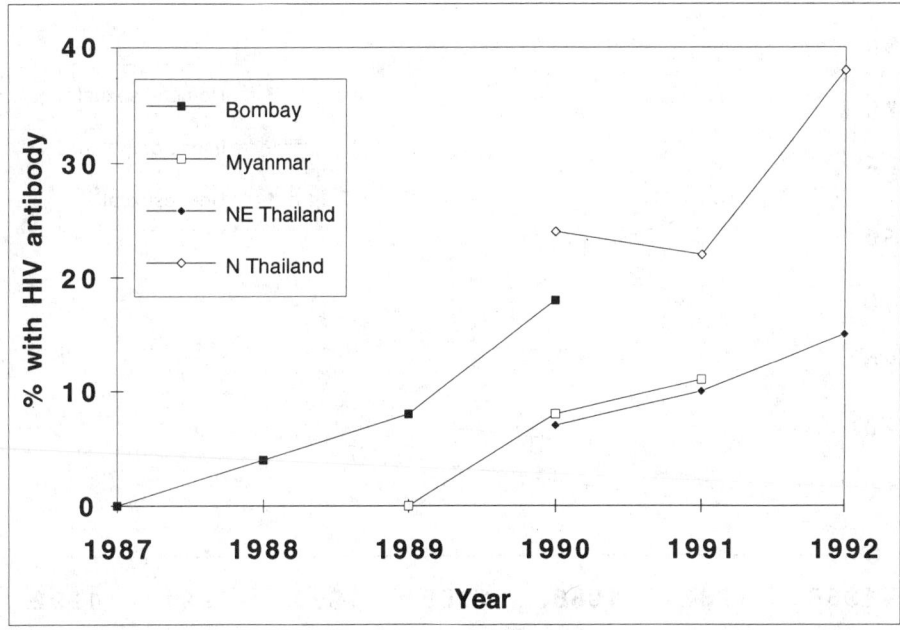

FIG. 3. Evolution of HIV prevalence among female prostitutes in Bombay, India, and Thailand. (Adapted from World Health Organization,[2] with permission.)

been spreading heterosexually, which is now the main mode of transmission of HIV in Asia. As in Africa, it was initially among female prostitutes that HIV infection rates increased most dramatically (Fig. 3). In Bombay, India, HIV seroprevalence among prostitutes appears to have increased from zero in 1987 to 20 percent in 1990. In Thailand, prostitutes from all regions of the country are not equally affected, but rapidly rising rates of HIV prevalence are common (Fig. 3). Molecular and serologic techniques support the separate introduction of a different HIV virus subtype among prostitutes and injecting drug users.[25,26] In contrast, as of early 1993, HIV had not spread as yet or spread only to a very limited extent among prostitutes in countries such as Korea, the Philippines, and Taiwan.[6]

In Thailand, HIV has now spread well beyond the most vulnerable groups, as illustrated by a nearly 6 percent HIV antibody prevalence rate among military recruits in the Thai Army in mid-1992, up from 0.5 percent in 1989.[27] Among young recruits from the northern part of the country, the prevalence rate was as high as 20 percent. These figures illustrate the depth of HIV spread into the general adult population of Thailand.

In India, heterosexual intercourse is now also the main mode of spread of HIV, with infections now reported from every state. HIV-2 infection has been documented in the Bombay area.

In most other Asian countries, HIV infection and AIDS are still uncommon, but the conditions for an imminent spread of HIV are present. The current epidemiologic trends suggest that Asia is experiencing the initial phases of the epidemic reminiscent of that in sub-Saharan Africa 10 years ago. High-risk and vulnerable environments are not confined to Thailand and India, and significant spread of HIV is likely elsewhere in the region.

Latin America and the Caribbean

Spread of HIV in the Caribbean and Latin America probably started around the same time as in the United States. By mid-1993, approximately 250,000 cases of AIDS had occurred in this region, with a cumulative number of 1.5 million adults infected with HIV.[2] Some islands in the Caribbean have now among the highest cumulative incidence rates of AIDS in the world.

Epidemiologic patterns in the region have been diverse and are changing over time. In general, homosexual and bisexual activity has been the main mode of spread since the beginning of the epidemic, but heterosexual intercourse and injecting drug use have become increasingly the main routes of transmission since the late 1980s in many countries.[28–31] For instance, in Brazil the proportion of AIDS cases attributable to homosexual or bisexual transmission decreased from approximately 79 percent in 1980–1986 to below 35 percent in 1992 (Fig. 4). If current trends are confirmed, heterosexuals and injecting drug users will become the major transmission groups among AIDS cases during the second half of the 1990s.[30]

As in most industrialized countries women are increasingly infected with HIV, as reflected by increasing prevalence rates in pregnant women and by a declining male-to-female ratio among AIDS cases. Bisexual behavior of their male partners is an important source of HIV infection for women in several Latin American countries.[32]

HIV infection in the Caribbean is a true mosaic of different epidemiologic patterns determined by the local interaction of various risk determinants of HIV transmission.[33] Male homosexual transmission predominates in Trinidad, Tobago, Barbados, and Guyana.[34] Injecting drug use and sex for drugs (mainly cocaine/crack) are major risk factors in the Bahamas, Bermuda, Puerto Rico, and Trinidad.[35] Finally, heterosexual transmission is predominant in Haiti and in the neighboring Dominican Republic.[28,36,37] In fact, Haiti was one of the first countries where a sustained AIDS epidemic in a heterosexual population was documented[38]; around 10 percent of pregnant women in urban areas in Haiti are now infected. Other nearby countries may rapidly catch up as suggested by data from San Pedro Sula, Honduras, where an HIV prevalence rate of 4 percent was documented in 1991 among pregnant women.

North Africa and the Middle East

The few studies that are available regarding North Africa and the Middle East suggest that the extensive spread of HIV began in some parts of this region in the late 1980s. As of mid-1993, WHO estimates that more than 75,000 cumulative adult HIV infections have occurred in North Africa and the Middle East. An HIV prevalence as high as 40 percent has been found among female sex workers in southern Sudan and Djibouti, both of

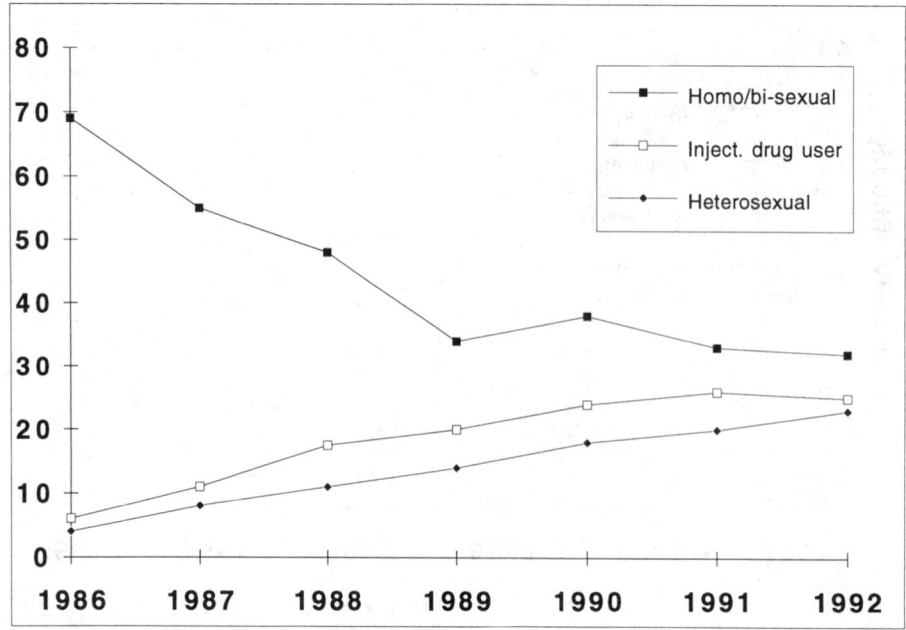

FIG. 4. Changing transmission group among AIDS patients in Brazil. (From Boletim Epidemiológico AIDS 1992,[30] with permission.)

which are in fact part of the HIV/AIDS epidemic in sub-Saharan Africa.[2]

Only limited and indirect information is available regarding the extent of high-risk behaviors in North Africa and the Middle East. For example, reports have suggested substantial numbers of STD among the employees of some oil companies. Substantial trade in drugs such as heroin also appears to occur in some parts of the region. An HIV prevalence of about 14 percent was reported among injecting drug users known to police authorities in one Gulf state in 1989.

Of the approximately 1500 HIV infections among resident and immigrant expatriates reported over the past 7 years in another Gulf state, one-third were believed to have occurred during 1992 alone, indicating the rapid evolution of the epidemic in the region.

THE DYNAMICS OF HIV SPREAD

There is no difference between the modes of transmission of HIV in the developing world and the industrialized countries. We review briefly selected aspects of HIV transmission in the developing world, as well as other determinants of HIV spread.

Modes of Transmission

World-wide HIV infection is basically a sexually transmitted infection. However, unprotected heterosexual intercourse accounts for the large majority of cases of HIV infection in the developing world, in contrast to the situation in North America and Western Europe, though the situation in the regions is gradually changing with increasing heterosexual transmission.

The low efficiency of penile–vaginal intercourse for the transmission of HIV has now been well documented,[39,40] especially from women to men. A sustained and fulminant heterosexual epidemic can only be explained by a common occurrence of factors amplifying heterosexual transmission, possibly in addition to high-risk sexual behavior patterns.

Factors that may enhance the efficiency of heterosexual transmission of HIV include higher viremia or more advanced immunodeficiency in the infecting partner, receptive anal intercourse, sex during menses, and the presence of other STD. Other factors

that may increase the risk of heterosexual transmission but are less well documented include lack of circumcision in men, the use of various desiccating vaginal agents, and cervical ectopy.[41,44]

Conventional STD have attracted the most attention as a risk factor since many are curable with relatively inexpensive antibiotics, leading to public health interventions for HIV prevention. There is now convincing evidence from prospective studies that particularly genital ulcers such as chancroid, syphilis, and genital herpes, but also the more common nonulcerative STD such as gonorrhea and chlamydial infection, enhance the sexual transmission of HIV.[45] This has been extensively documented in Africa, mainly in Kenya and Zaire.[10,46,47]

Cohort studies in Nairobi found adjusted relative risks of 3 to 8 of genital ulcers, mainly chancroid, for HIV transmission, but it is plausible that these increase the risk of HIV transmission during a single sexual act by a factor between 10 and 100. In addition, people with HIV infection with declining immunity have more genital ulcers, probably increasing their infectiousness during sexual intercourse, as HIV can often be detected in ulcer material obtained from such individuals.[48,49]

The relative risks of gonorrhea and chlamydial infection for HIV acquisition in women are smaller than those of genital ulcers.[10] However, as these STD are far more common in most populations than genital ulcers, their contribution to the heterosexual spread of HIV may also be greater.[46] The increased risks can probably be attributed to the presence of HIV in the white blood cells accompanying the infection.

Globally, mother-to-child transmission during pregnancy, delivery, or breast-feeding is a second major mode of spread of HIV. Most of the over 1 million African children with HIV were infected by this route.

Studies on mother-to-child transmission of HIV have consistently found higher rates of transmission in Africa than in North America or Europe (approximately 30–40 percent vs. 15–20 percent, respectively).[49]

At least three factors may play a role in this higher risk of transmission in Africa. The first is breast-feeding, which is much more common than in the industrialized world.[49,50] Studies in Rwanda showed that the risk of transmission through breast-feeding may be as high as 50 percent when the mother becomes infected during late pregnancy or after delivery.[49] This is probably due to high levels of virus production in the blood stream shortly after infection.[50] A second factor is the more common occurrence of advanced immunodeficiency among women in Africa, as HIV has been spreading for a longer time among heterosexuals on this continent resulting in more infected women with immunodeficiency. Thus, HIV transmission was associated with maternal P24 antigenemia, low CD4+ lymphocyte counts, and elevated CD8+ lymphocyte counts. Again, this is probably an indicator of a higher viral load. Finally, placental membrane inflammation may be more common as a result of genital infections and was associated with an increased risk for mother-to-child transmission in two studies in Kinshasa, Zaire.[51,52]

The impact of maternal HIV infection on pregnancy outcome is unclear.[53] In several studies in Kenya and Zaire, maternal HIV infection was associated with adverse pregnancy outcome, including stillbirth, premature delivery, and low birth weight.[52,54] However, this was not the case in studies in Congo and Rwanda.[55,56]

As mentioned earlier, HIV has spread considerably among injecting drug users in parts of Asia, Latin America, and the Caribbean; this has sometimes occurred where in several populations injecting has been replacing smoking and inhaling as a way of administering drugs.[19] Sharing injection equipment and imprisonment were the strongest predictors of HIV infection in Thailand.[57]

Transfusion with HIV-contaminated blood continues to be a source of HIV infection in some parts of the developing world, particularly in sub-Saharan Africa.[58,59] This illustrates tragically that mere availability of technology (i.e., serologic tests for HIV antibody) is not sufficient to solve a public health problem. It was estimated that in 1989 in Zaire, less than half of all blood donations were tested for HIV antibody.[60]

Nosocomial transmission of HIV via injection with nonsterile syringes and needles occurs, but its contribution to the spread of HIV in the developing world is not well documented, though it is probably very low.[61,62] However, outbreaks of injection-associated nosocomial HIV infection in the former Soviet Union and in Romania show that injections for medical purposes may be a source of HIV infection in the community.[63,64]

Factors Influencing the Spread of HIV

The HIV/AIDS epidemic is still in a dynamic phase in most parts of the world, with continuing geographic spread and changing epidemiologic patterns. Moreover, there is substantial heterogeneity in the epidemiology of HIV throughout the world.[65,66]

A multitude of variables may influence the spread of HIV (Table 2). It is the complex mix and interaction of these direct (i.e., behavioral) and indirect (i.e., demographic) risk factors that determine how and when HIV spreads in the population.

Sexual Behavior

HIV infection is foremost a sexually transmitted disease, and sexual behavior is undoubtedly the most important determinant of HIV spread. Such behavior is very heterogeneous among and within populations. Recent surveys on sexual behavior in sub-Saharan Africa have documented this heterogeneity in terms of the number of partners, age of sexual debut, and rate of casual and commercial sex.[67] In addition, these studies found that men have generally more partners than women and that in some societies higher socioeconomic status is associated with a higher number of partners. However, according to mathematical models, sexual mixing patterns are equally important in determining the spread of HIV, particularly in the early stages of the epidemic.[68,69] The "core group" concept postulates that a relatively small proportion of the population is contributing to the maintenance of the epidemic. This concept was first described in the 1970s with respect to the epidemiology of gonorrhea in the United States.[70]

TABLE 2. Variables That May Influence the Spread of HIV Infection in a Population

Behavioral variables	Demographic variables
Rate of partner change	Size of the population in the sexually most active age groups
Sexual mixing patterns	
Size and rate of contact with "core" groups	Male-to-female ratio
	Rate and growth of urbanization
Sexual practices (anal intercourse, intercourse during menses)	Migration patterns
Level of condom use	
Behavior and infection rate of partners	
Prevalence of injecting drug use	
Biologic variables	**Economic and political factors**
Level of viremia	Response to the epidemic
Infectivity and virulence of HIV strains (strain variation)	Performance of the health care system
	Poverty, deprivation, lack of education
Prevalence of other sexually transmitted diseases	War and social disturbance
	Women's status
Lack of male circumcision	Attitudes towards sex
Use of certain vaginal products	

(From Piot et al.,[66] with permission.)

The behavior of one's partner is as relevant for the risk of HIV infection as one's own. This seems particularly the case for women, who often become infected by their stable male partner. Recent data suggest that an increasing proportion of women with HIV infection in Rwanda, Kenya, and Zaire have their husbands as the only sexual contact.[5,6,71]

Sexual practices, in particular the frequency of anal intercourse, which is the most efficient mode of sexual transmission of HIV, may also vary among populations. Thus, heterosexuality anal intercourse appear to be more frequent in some Latin American countries, as well as male bisexual behavior.[32]

Last, but not least, the rate of condom use plays a major role in the extent of HIV spread. Despite much early skepticism, condoms have become increasingly popular in many parts of the developing world, particularly where social marketing programs are active.[72] The use of condoms has played a role in the significant reduction of HIV incidence in discordant couples in Zaire, as well as in female prostitutes in Thailand, Kenya, and Zaire (Fig. 5).[71,73–75] These "success stories" demonstrate that effective HIV prevention is possible, even under the difficult conditions of the developing world.

Demography

One of the most striking differences between the industrialized and the developing world is the age structure of the population, with a much higher proportion belonging to the sexually most active age group. This by itself often results in higher incidence rates of sexually transmitted infections such as HIV infection.

Traditionally, migration and rapid urbanization have also been associated with higher rates of STD. Both rural-to-urban and international migrations occur basically all over the developing world.[76]

An imbalance in numbers or accessibility between the sexes may be an important determinant of HIV epidemiology, as cities with such an imbalance appear to experience a more rapid spread of HIV.[12,77] Migration of male labor into the cities of the developing world may create such a situation, but also social constraints on sexual behavior, such as disapproval of premarital and extramarital sex among women, and late marriage by men for economic reasons may be contributing factors. These demographic and social patterns in general are associated with a higher rate of prostitute contacts by men.

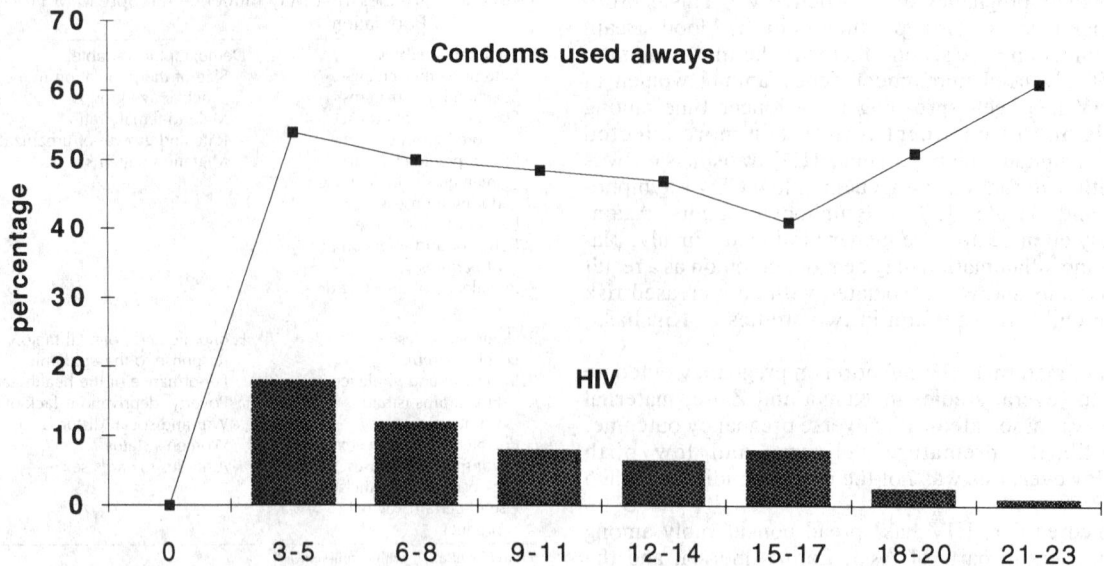

FIG. 5. Increase in condom use and decrease in new infections among female prostitutes in Kinshasa, Zaire. *n* = 1266. (Adapted from Laga et al.,[75] with permission.)

Biologic Variables

As mentioned earlier, several studies have documented a higher efficiency of heterosexual transmission of HIV in the presence of more advanced immunodeficiency in the index case.[46,78] This is probably due to higher levels of viremia and virus excretion in patients with symptomatic HIV infection, than in asymptomatically infected individuals.[79] In populations that have experienced an HIV epidemic for a longer time, this may imply an increased overall efficiency of heterosexual and perinatal transmission of HIV. Such higher rates of transmission have been observed in Africa.

African HIV isolates exhibit a higher degree of genetic variability than American or European isolates.[78,79] It is not known whether such viral variation has implications for the epidemiology of HIV, through strain differences in infectivity and cell tropism, or in capacity to reach higher levels of viremia. However, it is likely that differences in these features play a role in the different epidemiology of HIV-1 and HIV-2 infection.

As STD enhance the efficiency of sexual transmission of HIV, their prevalence in a population partly determines its vulnerability for the spread of HIV. Prevalence rates of various STD vary widely among populations, but are generally higher in the developing world, particularly in urban Africa.[45,46] They are particularly high in so-called core groups for STD and HIV infection, which in the developing world may include prostitutes and their clients, truck drivers, fishermen, and the military.[82] Most importantly, high levels of STD are not only a result of unsafe sexual behavior, but also of inadequate care for patients with an STD. Lack of circumcision in men, if confirmed as a risk factor for HIV transmission, may also play a role in the differential spread of HIV, since male circumcision is practiced to a varying degree throughout the world.

Economic and Political Factors

The effectiveness of national responses to the AIDS pandemic will ultimately determine how extensive HIV will spread. This requires, in the first place, political commitment to AIDS/HIV prevention, which is insufficient in many countries. In addition, the developing world needs about 5–10 times more financial resources than presently available to control the AIDS epidemic.

In many developing countries, public health care systems have deteriorated during the past two decades, and the introduction of user fees has resulted in declining access to health services and in poorer management of people with STD. Thus, in Nairobi, Kenya, after introduction of user fees at the main STD clinic, the attendance of men decreased significantly to 40 percent of that before fees were levied.[84]

Lastly, poverty is not only a consequence of epidemics, but also one of the major driving forces. It is associated with prostitution, homeless adults and street children, low rates of literacy, migration and separated families, and low status of women, all of which provide a fertile ground for an HIV epidemic.

CLINICAL EXPRESSION

The clinical manifestations and opportunistic diseases associated with HIV infection differ from one geographic area to another. First, there are indications that the progression to disease among individuals with HIV infection may be more rapid in Africa.[84,86] In a rural cohort in Uganda, the rate of disease progression was as high as 12.4 percent per year.[86] If confirmed, this may be explained by a lack of medical care and prophylaxis for opportunistic infections (particularly for tuberculosis), as well as by a higher occurrence of other endemic diseases such as parasitoses and tuberculosis, which depress the immune response. A study in Haiti found that chemoprophylaxis with isoniazid in patients infected with both HIV and *Mycobacterium tuberculosis* considerably extended the life expectancy of these individuals, supporting both hypotheses.[87]

However, the most striking difference in the natural history of HIV infection in adults is the short survival time of AIDS patients in Africa compared with the industrialized world.[88,89] This is obviously a consequence of inadequate medical care for most patients in Africa.

Though all opportunistic diseases may occur in AIDS patients throughout the world, the relative importance of specific diseases may be different. For instance, major opportunistic diseases in North America such as *Pneumocystis carinii* pneumonia and Kaposi sarcoma are less frequent in African AIDS patients than elsewhere.[89–91] In contrast, tuberculosis, chronic diarrhea, and bacteremia due to pathogens such as *Salmonella typhimurium* and *Streptococcus pneumoniae* are all very common.[92,96] In Southeast Asia, systemic infection with *Penicillium marneffei* is a common opportunistic mycosis in patients with HIV infection. Thus, in Chiang Mai, Northern Thailand, penicil-

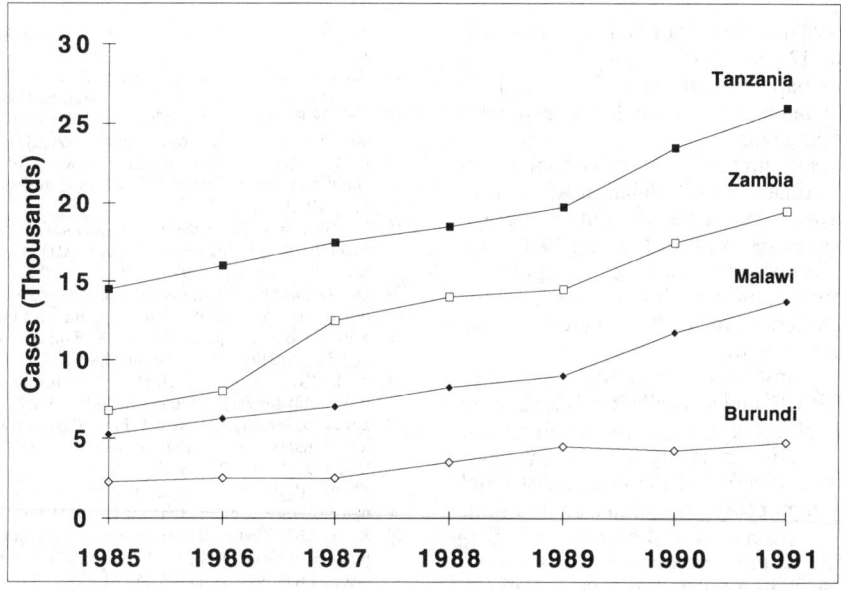

FIG. 6. Annual tuberculosis notification in selected African countries. (Data from World Health Organization.)

TABLE 3. HIV Seroprevalence Among Patients with Tuberculosis

Country	Years	No. Patients Studied	% HIV Positive
Africa			
Burundi	1985–86	328	55
Ivory Coast	1989–90	2043	40
Kenya	1990	NA	27
Zaire	1990	1011	20
Zambia	1988–90	346	60
Asia			
Hong Kong	1985–1991	1548	0
Tamil Nadu, India	1991–92	278	1
Latin America/Caribbean			
Brazil	1991	1398	3
Haiti	1990	NA	57
Mexico	1991	NA	5

Abbreviation: NA: data not available.

(Data from U.S. Bureau of the Census, 1992.)

linosis was diagnosed in 140 (35 percent) of 400 consecutive AIDS cases.[97] A nearly pathognomonic generalized papular pruritic skin eruption, mainly on the extremities, is observed in around 20 percent of African patients with HIV infection, but rarely in patients from other continents.[98] Its etiology is unknown.

Tuberculosis is not only the leading opportunistic infection among adult AIDS patients in Africa, but is itself greatly affected by the HIV epidemic, with rising incidence rates wherever HIV has become endemic (Fig. 6).[92,99,100] Thus, in several African countries with a reasonably well functioning tuberculosis control program, the annual incidence of tuberculosis doubled between 1985 and 1990.[92,100,101] This rise in incidence is probably entirely attributable to the spread of HIV infection in populations where 50–80 percent of all adults are infected with *M. tuberculosis*. A new tuberculosis epidemic is now accompanying the AIDS epidemic in many countries, and is one of the major public health consequences of HIV infection in the developing world.

In Africa and Haiti, around 30–50 percent of tuberculosis patients are now infected with HIV (Table 3). In other developing countries, the HIV prevalence is still low among tuberculosis patients, but is usually higher than in the general population. However, as pulmonary tuberculosis may develop across a broad spectrum of HIV-associated immunodeficiency in tuber-

culosis endemic populations, it is of limited use as an AIDS-defining illness.[102]

Additional consequences of dual HIV–*M. tuberculosis* infection include a high mortality among tuberculosis patients with HIV infection (mostly due to HIV-related illness), a growing rate of multidrug resistance of *M. tuberculosis*, and an up to 10-fold increase in severe skin reactions, including Stevens-Johnson syndrome, during antituberculous therapy in HIV-positive patients.[92,100]

The cause of death in patients with HIV infection in the developing world is not well studied.[88] In a large study of a representative sample of patients who died during hospitalization in Abidjan, Côte d'Ivoire, tuberculosis, bacteremia due to gram-negative rods, and cerebral toxoplasmosis caused 53 percent of deaths.[97] Tuberculosis was found in half of the cadavers with an AIDS-defining pathology as compared with only 4 percent for *P. carinii* pneumonia. Interestingly, in this population, where both HIV-1 and HIV-2 occur, patients with HIV-2 infection more often had severe cytomegalovirus infection and HIV-associated encephalitis than did patients with HIV-1 infection, which is compatible with the more prolonged course of disease associated with HIV-2 infection.

IMPACT OF THE HIV/AIDS EPIDEMIC

The impact of the AIDS epidemic on many parts of the developing world is already severe, but will undoubtedly become worse as the number of people with AIDS and HIV-related illness continue to increase over the next decades. AIDS not only affects infected individuals and their relatives and friends, but also communities at large, with a long-term impact on households, on the health sector, on demography, and on the economic and social systems.[103]

Perhaps the most visible aspect of the burden of AIDS are the large numbers of men and women with AIDS in the hospitals of many African countries. In cities such as Abidjan, Kampala, Lusaka, and Kinshasa, they now make up at least 50 percent of all patients. AIDS has also become the major cause of death among hospitalized patients.[104,105] By the end of the 1990s, many Asian and Latin American cities will probably face the same problem as Africa today.

With a growing number of individuals with HIV infection developing AIDS, the demand for health services will expand rapidly. In a country such as Rwanda, the cost of hospital-based AIDS care increased from 2.1 to 9.7 percent of the national hospital budget between 1988 and 1993.[106] In Thailand, it is estimated that by the year 2000 12 percent of all hospital bed days will be required to care for patients with AIDS.[107] Absorbing this growing burden of patients is a major challenge for health care systems in the developing world.

The long-term demographic impact of AIDS is controversial.[108–110] A conservative estimate for sub-Saharan Africa predicts that the population growth will decrease from an average of 3 percent to less than 2 percent per year by the year 2000, with the most affected areas possibly approaching zero population growth.[108,109] Where the population growth is slower, such as in Southeast Asia or Latin America, an equally severe epidemic may even reverse population growth.

AIDS is now the leading cause of death in adults in a city such as Abidjan in West Africa,[104] and in Thailand it is estimated that by the year 2000 nearly 30 percent of all deaths will be due to AIDS.[111] AIDS is also affecting mortality in children under five years of age, leading to a reversal of the benefits of child survival initiatives in many high-prevalence areas. In addition, the number of orphans from parents who died from AIDS is growing at a staggering rate in the worse affected countries, with over 1 million AIDS orphans expected in 1998 in Uganda alone, and 5–10 million expected world wide by the year 2000.[112]

In economic terms, AIDS is now among the top five causes of healthy life lost in urban sub-Saharan Africa, accounting for 15 percent of the total disease burden.[82] Because HIV infection occurs mostly in adults in their most productive years, it profoundly affects various economic and social sectors. The gross domestic product (GDP) of severely affected countries will decline because of loss of productivity in agriculture, industry, and services. Thus, in Tanzania it is estimated that the real GDP growth rate will decline by 15–28 percent as a result of AIDS between 1995 and 2010.[113]

To paraphrase the World Development Report 1993: "Historians will look back on the latter half of this century as having had one great medical triumph, the eradication of smallpox, and one great medical tragedy, AIDS."[103]

REFERENCES

1. World Health Organization. AIDS. The current global situation of the HIV/AIDS pandemic. Weekly Epidemiol Rec 1993;68:193–6.
2. World Health Organization. The HIV/AIDS pandemic. 1993 Overview. Geneva: World Health Organization; 1993.
3. Mann JM, Tarantola DM, Netter TW, eds. AIDS in the World. Cambridge, MA; Harvard University Press; 1992.
4. European Centre for the Epidemiological Monitoring of AIDS. AIDS Surveillance in the European Community and Cost countries. Quarterly Report, March 1993, Paris.
5. Nkowane BM. Prevalence and incidence of HIV infection in Africa: A review of data published in 1990. AIDS. 1991;5(Suppl 1):S7–15.
6. United States Bureau of the Census, Center for International Research. AIDS/HIV Surveillance Database. Washington, DC: Bureau of the Census; 1989.
7. Allen S, Lindan C, Serufila A, et al. Human immunodeficiency virus infection in urban Rwanda: Demographic and behavioural correlates in a representative sample of child bearing women. JAMA. 1991;226:1657–63.
8. Temmerman M, Mohammed Ali F, Ndinya-Achola JO, et al. Rapid increase of both HIV-1 infection and syphilis among pregnant women in Nairobi, Kenya. AIDS. 1992;6:1181–5.
9. Dallabetta GA, Miotti PG, Chiphangur JD, et al. High socio-economic status is a risk factor for human immunodeficiency virus type 1 (HIV-1) infection but not for sexually transmitted diseases in women in Malawi: Implications for HIV-1 control. J Infect Dis. 1993;167:36–42.
10. Laga M, Manoka A, Kivuvu M, et al. Non-ulcerative sexually transmitted diseases as risk factors for HIV-1 transmission in women: Results from a cohort study. AIDS. 1993;7:95–102.
11. Ngugi EN, Plummer FA, Simonsen JN, et al. Prevention of HIV transmission in Africa: The effectiveness of condom promotion and health education among high-risk prostitutes. Lancet. 1988;2:887–90.
12. Anderson RM, May RM, Boily MC, et al. The spread of HIV-1 in Africa: Sexual contact patterns and the predicted demographic impact of AIDS. Nature. 1991;352:581–9.
13. De Cock KM, Brun-Vézinet F, Soro B. HIV-1 and HIV-2 infections and AIDS in West Africa. AIDS. 1991;5(Suppl 1):S21–28.
14. Poulsen AG, Krinesdal B, Aaby P, et al. Prevalence of and mortality from human immunodeficiency virus type 2 in Bissau, West Africa. Lancet. 1989; 1:827–31.
15. Andreasson PA, Dias F, Nauclér A, et al. A prospective study of vertical transmission of HIV-2 in Bissau, Guinea-Bissau. AIDS. 1993;7:989–94.
16. George R, Ou C-Y, Parekh B, et al. Prevalence of HIV/1 and HIV/2 mixed infections in Côte d'Ivoire. Lancet. 1992;1:338–9.
17. Peeters M, Gershy-Damet GM, Fransen K, et al. Virological and polymerase chain reaction studies of HIV-1/HIV-2 dual infection in Côte d'Ivoire. Lancet. 1992;1:339–40.
18. Li PCK, Yeoh EK. Current epidemiological trends of HIV infection in Asia. In Volberding P, Jacobson MA, eds. AIDS Clinical Review 1992. New York: Marcel Dekker Inc.; 1992:1–24.
19. Des Jarlais DC, Friedman SR, Choopanyq K, et al. International epidemiology of HIV and AIDS among injecting drug users. AIDS. 1992;6:1053–68.
20. Weinger BG, Limpakarnjanarat K, Ungchusok K, et al. The epidemiology of HIV infection and AIDS in Thailand. AIDS 1991;5(Suppl 2):S71–85.
21. Naik TN, Sarkar S, Singh HL, et al. Intravenous drug users—A new high risk group for HIV infection in India. AIDS. 1991;5:117–8.
22. Sarkat S, Mokerjee P, Roy A, et al. Descriptive epidemiology of intravenous heroin users—A new risk group for transmission of HIV in India. J Infect Dis. 1991;23:201–7.
23. Zhang JP. An epidemiological study on HIV infection in Ruili county, Yennan Province. Chung Hua Liu Hsing Hsueh Tsa Chih. 1991;12:9–12.
24. Bhave GG, Wagle UD, Tripathy SP. HIV sero-surveillance in promiscuous females of Bombay, India. VI International Conference on AIDS, San Francisco, June 1991, Abstract FC 612.
25. Ou C-Y, Auwanet W, Pan C-P, et al. Wide distribution of two subtypes of HIV-1 in Thailand. AIDS Res Hum Retroviruses. 1992;8:1471–2.
26. Pau C-P, Lee-Thomas S, Auwanit W, et al. Highly specific V3 peptide enzyme immunoassay for serotyping HIV-1 specimens from Thailand. AIDS. 1993;7:337–40.
27. Sirisopana N, Torugsok, McNeil J, et al. The temporal trend of HIV seroprevalence among young men entering the Royal Thai Army: 1989–91. 8th International Conference on AIDS, Amsterdam, The Netherlands, July 1992. Abstract POC 4084.
28. Hospedales J, White F, Gayle C, et al. Epidemiology of HIV/AIDS in the Caribbean. In: Lamptey P, White F, Figueroa JP, et al., eds. The Handbook for AIDS Prevention in the Caribbean. Research Triangle Park, NC: Family Health International; 1992:1–23.
29. Basset D, Narain J. Changing pattern of HIV transmission in the Caribbean. In: AIDS: Profile of an Epidemic. PAHO Sci Pub. No. 514, 1988:200–204.
30. Boletim Epidemiológico AIDS 1992. Brasilia: Programo Nacional de Doencas Sexualmente Transmissiveis/AIDS; 1992.
31. Pan American Health Organization/WHO 1990 AIDS/HIV/STD Annual Surveillance Report. Washington DC, 1991.
32. Parker RG, Tawil O. Bisexual behavior and HIV transmission in Latin America. In: Tielman R, Carballo M, Hendriks A, eds. Bisexuality and HIV/AIDS. New York: Prometheus Press; 1991;59–63.
33. Piot P, Laga M. Epidemiology of AIDS in the developing world. In: Textbook of AIDS Medicine. Baltimore: Williams & Wilkins; 1993;109–32.
34. Bartholomew C, Sayinger C, Clard J, et al. Transmission of HTLV-1 and HIV among homosexual men in Trinidad. JAMA. 1987;257:2604–8.
35. Lewis P, Hospedales J, Francis M, et al. HIV seroprevalence among cocaine addicts in Trinidad. West Ind Med J. 1989;4(Suppl).
36. Pape JW, Johnson WD Jr. Epidemiology of AIDS in the Caribbean. In: Piot P, Mann JM, eds. AIDS and HIV Infection in the Tropics. London: Baillière Tindall; 1988:31–42.
37. Garris I, Rodriguez E, de Moya E, et al. AIDS heterosexual predominance in the Dominican Republic. J AIDS. 1991;4:1173–8.
38. Pape J, Liautaud B, Thomas F, et al. Characteristics of the acquired immunodeficiency syndrome (AIDS) in Haiti. N Engl J Med. 1983;309:945–50.
39. Johnson AM, Laga M. Heterosexual transmission of HIV. AIDS. 1988; 2(Suppl 1):S49–56.
40. Holmberg SD, Horsburgh CR Jr, Ward JW, et al. Biological factors in the sexual transmission of human immunodeficiency virus. J Infect Dis. 1989; 160:116–125.
41. Bongaarts J, Reining P, Way P, et al. The relationship between male circumcision and HIV infection in African populations. AIDS. 1989;3:373–7.
42. Moses S, Bradley JE, Nagelkerke NJD, et al. Geographical patterns of male circumcision practices in Africa: Association with HIV seroprevalence. Int J Epidemiol. 1990;19:693–7.
43. Dallabetta GA, Miotti PG, Chiphangui JD, et al. Traditional vaginal agents: Prevalence of use and association with HIV-1 infection in Malawian women. Submitted for publication.
44. Clemetson DBA, Moss GB, Willerford DM, et al. Detection of HIV DNA in cervical and vaginal secretions. Prevalence and correlates among women in Nairobi, Kenya. JAMA. 1993;269:2860–4.
45. Wasserheit JN. Epidemiological synergy: Interrelationships between HIV infection and other STDs. Sex Transm Dis. 1992;19:61–77.
46. Laga M, Nzila N, Goeman J. The interrelationship of sexually transmitted diseases and HIV infection: Implications for the control of both epidemics in Africa. AIDS 1991;5(Suppl 1):S55–64.
47. Cameron DW, Simonsen JN, D'Costa LJ, et al. Female to male transmission

of human immunodeficiency virus type 1: Risk factors for seroconversion in man. Lancet 1989;2:401–7.

48. Ghys P, Diallo MO, Traore-Ettiegne V, et al. Genital ulcer disease in HIV positive female prostitutes in Abidjan: Association with low CD4 + counts and low CD4 + /CD8 + ratios. IXth International Conference on AIDS, Berlin, June 1993.

49. Dunn DT, Newell ML, Ades AE, et al. Risk of human immunodeficiency virus type 1 transmission through breast feeding. Lancet. 1992;1:585–8.

50. Van de Perre P, Simonon A, Msellati P, et al. Postnatal transmission of human immunodeficiency virus in infants born to seropositive mothers. N Engl J Med. 1991;325:593–9.

51. St Louis ME, Kamenga M, Brown C, et al. Risk for perinatal HIV-1 transmission according to maternal immunologic, virologic and placental factors. JAMA. 1993;269:2853–9.

52. Ryder RW, Nsa W, Hassig SE, et al. Perinatal transmission of the human immunodeficiency virus type 1 to infants of seropositive women in Zaire. N Engl J Med. 1989;302:1637–42.

53. Newell ML, Peckham CS, Lepage P. HIV infection in pregnancy: Implications for women and children. AIDS. 1990;4(Suppl):S111–7.

54. Temmerman M, Plummer F, Mirza NB, et al. Infection with HIV as a risk factor for adverse obstetrical outcome. AIDS 1990;4:1087–93.

55. Lepage P, Msellati P, Van de Perre P, et al. Newborn characteristics and HIV-1 infection in Rwanda. AIDS. 1992;6:882–3.

56. Lallemant M, Lallemant-Lecoeur S, Cheynier D, et al. Mother–child transmission of HIV-1 and infant survival in Brazzaville, Congo. AIDS. 1989;3:643–6.

57. Choopanya K, Vanichseni S, Des Jarlais DC, et al. Risk factors and HIV seropositivity among injecting drug users in Bangkok. AIDS. 1991;5:1509–13.

58. Jäger H, Jersild C, Emmanuel JC. Safe blood transfusions in Africa. AIDS. 1991;5:(Suppl 1):S163–8.

59. Colebunders R, Ryder R, Francis H, et al. Seroconversion rate, mortality and clinical manifestations associated with the receipt of a human immunodeficiency virus infected blood transfusion. J Infect Dis. 1991;164:450–6.

60. Jäger H, N'galy B, Perriëns J, et al. Prevention of transfusion-associated HIV transmission in Kinshasa, Zaire: HIV screening is not enough. AIDS. 1990;4:571–4.

61. Berkeley S. Parenteral transmission of HIV in Africa. AIDS. 1991;5(Suppl 1):S163–8.

62. Lepage P, Van de Perre P. Nosocomial transmission of HIV in Africa: What tribute is paid to contaminated blood transfusions and medical injections? Infect Control Hosp Epidemiol. 1989;9:200–3.

63. Pokrovsky VV, Eramone EV. Nosocomial outbreak of HIV infection in Elista, USSR. Vth International Conference on AIDS, Montreal, June 1989, Abstract WA 05.

64. Hersh BS, Popovici F, Apetrei RC, et al. Acquired immunodeficiency syndrome in Romania. Lancet. 1991;1:645&9.

65. Piot P, Plummer FA, Mhalu FS, et al. AIDS: An international perspective. Science. 1988;239:573–9.

66. Piot P, Laga M, Ryder RW, et al. The global epidemiology of HIV infection: Continuity, heterogeneity, and change. J AIDS. 1990;3:403–12.

67. Carael M, Cleland J, Adeokun L. Overview and selected findings of sexual behaviour surveys. AIDS. 1991;5(Suppl 1):S65–74.

68. Anderson RM, May RM. Transmission dynamics of HIV infection. Nature. 1987;26:137–42.

69. Boily MC, Anderson RM. Sexual contact patterns between men and women and the spread of HIV-1 in urban centres in Africa. IMAJ Math Appl Med Biol. 1991;8:221–47.

70. Yorke JA, Heathcote HW, Nold A. Dynamics and control of the transmission of gonorrhoea. Sex Transm Dis. 1978;5:31–7.

71. Kamenga M, Ryder RW, Jingu M, et al. Evidence of marked sexual behaviour change associated with low HIV-1 seroconversion in 149 married couples with discordant HIV-1 status: Experiences at an HIV counseling center in Zaire. AIDS. 1991;5:61–7.

72. Lamptey P, Goodridge GAW. Condom issues in AIDS prevention in Africa. AIDS. 1991;5(Suppl 1):S183–91.

73. World Health Organization. Effective approaches to AIDS prevention. Report of the meeting, Geneva 26/29 May 1992.

74. Moses S, Plummer FA, Ngugi E, et al. Controlling HIV in Africa: Effectiveness and cost of an intervention in a high-frequency STD transmitter core group. AIDS. 1991;5:407–11.

75. Laga M, Alary M, Nzila N, et al. Condom promotion and STD treatment leading to a declining incidence of HIV-1 infection in a cohort of high risk women. Submitted for publication.

76. Hunt CW. Migrant labor and sexually transmitted disease: AIDS Africa J Health Soc Beh. 1991:353–73.

77. Larson A. Social context of HIV transmission in Africa: historical and cultural bases of East and Central African sexual relations. Rev Infect Dis. 1989;11:71–3.

78. Goedert JJ, Eyster ME, Giggar RJ. Heterosexual transmission of human immunodeficiency virus infection: association with severe depletion of T-helper cells in men with hemophilia. AIDS Res Hum Retroviruses. 1987;4:335–61.

79. Weiss RA. How does HIV cause AIDS? Science 1993;260:1273–8.

80. Meyers G, Rabson AB, Smith TF, et al., eds. Human Retroviruses and AIDS. Los Alamos: Los Alamos National Laboratory; 1992.

81. Louwagie J, McCutchan FE, Peeters M, et al. Comparison of *gag* genes from sixty one international HIV-1 isolates provides evidence for multiple genetic subgroups. AIDS. 1993;7:769–80.

82. Over M, Piot P. HIV infection and sexually transmitted diseases. In: Jamison DT, Mosley WH, eds. Disease Control Priorities in Developing Countries. Washington, DC: The World Bank, 1993.

83. Moses S, Manji F, Bradley JE, et al. Impact of user fees on attendance at a referral centre for sexually transmitted diseases in Kenya. Lancet. 1992; 340:463–6.

84. N'Galy B, Ryder RW, Kapita B, et al. Human immunodeficiency virus infection among employees in an African hospital. N Engl J Med. 1988;319:1123–7.

85. Anzala A, Wambugu P, Plummer FA, et al. Incubation time to symptomatic disease and AIDS in women with known duration of infection. VII International Conference on AIDS, Florence, June 1991. Abstract TUC 103.

86. Mulder D, Kamali A, Nakyinge J, et al. HIV-1 associated mortality in a rural Ugandian cohort: results of a two year follow-up (14,913 person years). IX International Conference on AIDS, Berlin, June 1993. Abstract WS-CO3–6.

87. Pape JW, Ho J, Haffner A, Johnson WD. Effect of isoniazid on the natural history of HIV infection in Haiti. VIII International Conference on AIDS, Amsterdam, July 1992. Abstract PoB 3091.

88. Mbaga JM, Pallangyo KJ, Bakari M, et al. Survival time of patients with acquired immunodeficiency syndrome: experience with 274 patients in Dar es Salaam. East Afr Med J. 1990;3:55–61.

89. Colebunders RL, Latif AS. Natural history and clinical presentation of HIV-1 infection in adults. AIDS. 1991;5(Suppl 1):S103–12.

90. Lucas SB, Odida M, Wabinga H. The pathology of severe morbidity and mortality due to HIV infection in Africa. AIDS. 1991;5(Suppl 1):S143–8.

91. Desmond-Hellmann SD, Katongole-Mbidde E. Kaposi's sarcoma: Recent developments. AIDS. 1991;5(Suppl 1):S135–42.

92. Perriëns JH, Mukadi Y, Nunn NP. Tuberculosis and HIV infection: implications for Africa. AIDS. 1991;5(Suppl 1):S127–33.

93. Gilks CF, Ojoo SA, Brindle RJ. Non-opportunistic bacterial infections in HIV-1 seropositive adults in Nairobi, Kenya. AIDS. 1991;5(Suppl 1):S113–6.

94. Colebunders R, Frances H, Mann JM, et al. Persistent diarrhoea, strongly associated with HIV in Kinshasa, Zaire. Am J Gastroentorol. 1987;82:859–64.

95. Gilks CF, Brindle RJ, Otieno LS, et al. Life-threatening bacteremia in HIV-1 seropositive adults admitted to hospital in Nairobi, Kenya. Lancet. 1990; 336:545–9.

96. Taelman H, Bogaerts J, Batungwanayo J, et al. Community acquired bacteraemia, fungaemia and parasitaemia in febrile adults infected with HIV in Central Africa. V International Conference on AIDS in Africa; Kinshasa, October 1990. Abstract FOD1.

97. Sirisanthana F. Mycotic infections in patients infected with HIV. IX International Conference on AIDS, Berlin, June 1993, Abstract PS-07-2.

98. Colebunders R, Mann JM, Francis H, et al. Generalized popular prunitic eruption in African patients with human immunodeficiency virus infection. AIDS. 1987;1:117–21.

99. Lucas SB, Hounnou A, Peacock C, et al. The mortality and pathology of HIV infection in a West African city. AIDS. 1993;7;1569–79.

100. De Cock KM, Soro B, Koulibaly IM, et al. Tuberculosis and HIV infection in sub-Saharan Africa. JAMA. 1992;268:1581–7.

101. Murray CJL, Styblo K, Rouillon A. Tuberculosis in developing countries: Burden, intervention and cost. Bull Int Union Tuber Lung Dis. 1990;65:6–24.

102. Mukadi Y, Perriëns JH, St Louis ME, et al. Spectrum of immunodeficiency in HIV-1 infected patients with pulmonary tuberculosis in Zaire. Lancet. 1993;342:143–6.

103. The World Bank. World Development Report 1993. Investing in Health. New York: Oxford University Press; 1993.

104. De Cock KM, Barrere B, Diaby L, et al. AIDS: The leading cause of adult death in the West African city of Abidjan, Ivory Coast. Science. 1990;249:793–6.

105. Hassig SE, Perriens J, Baende E, et al. An analysis of the economic impact of HIV infection among patients at Mama Yemo Hospital, Kinshasa, Zaire. AIDS. 1990;4:883–7.

106. Cameron C, Shepard J. The cost of AIDS care and prevention. In Mann J, Tarantola DJM, Netter TW, eds. AIDS in the World. Cambridge, MA: Harvard University Press; 1992:477–535.

107. Viravoidya M, Obremsky S, Myers C. The Economic Impact of AIDS on Thailand. Cambridge, MA: Harvard School of Public Health, Department of Population and International Health; Working Paper No. 4, March 1992.

108. Bongaarts J. A model of the spread of HIV infection and the demographic impact of AIDS. Statist Med. 1989;8:103–20.

109. Stanley EA, Seity ST, Way PO, et al. The iwg AIDS model for the heterosexual spread of HIV and the demographic impact of the AIDS epidemic in Proceedings of the UN/WHO Workshop on Modeling the Demographic Impact of the AIDS Epidemic in Pattern II Countries, December 13–15, 1989. United Nations and World Health Organization; 1989.

110. Anderson RM, May R, McLean AR. Possible demographic consequences of AIDS in developing countries. Nature. 1988;332:228–34.

111. Sittitrai W, Brown T, Obremskey S, et al. Projection of HIV/AIDS in Thailand and social and demographic impacts. Paper presented at the Workshop on Population Programme Policies: New directions Chiang Mai, September 11, 1992. National Economic and Social Development Board, Thailand.

112. Barnett T, Blaikie P. AIDS in Africa: Its Present and Future Impact. London: Bellhaven Press; 1992.

113. The World Bank. Tanzania. AIDS assessment and planning study. Washington, DC: The World Bank; 1992.

100. EPIDEMIOLOGY AND PREVENTION OF AIDS AND HIV INFECTION

MARY E. CHAMBERLAND
JOHN W. WARD
JAMES W. CURRAN

Acquired immunodeficiency syndrome (AIDS) is the most severe manifestation of a clinical spectrum of illness following infection with the retrovirus human immunodeficiency virus (HIV). The syndrome is defined by the development of serious opportunistic infections, neoplasms, or other life-threatening manifestations resulting from progressive HIV-induced immunosuppression. AIDS was first recognized in mid-1981, when unusual clusters of *Pneumocystis carinii* pneumonia and Kaposi sarcoma were reported in young, previously healthy homosexual men in New York City, Los Angeles, and San Francisco.[1,2] The subsequent documentation of cases among persons with hemophilia, blood transfusion recipients, and heterosexual injecting drug users and their sex partners suggested that a transmissible agent was the primary cause of the immunologic defects characteristic of AIDS. In 1983, 2 years after the first reports of AIDS, a cytopathic retrovirus was isolated from persons with AIDS and with associated conditions such as chronic lymphadenopathy. By 1985, serologic tests to detect evidence of infection with HIV had been developed and licensed.

In the decade since the initial recognition of the epidemic, there have been important changes in the epidemiology of HIV infection. Most significantly, HIV infection has become a pandemic affecting every region of the world and a major cause of morbidity and mortality, particularly among young adults. HIV is spread primarily through heterosexual contact; women account for 5 of every 11 new HIV infections in adults.[3] Even in many developed countries where transmission through male homosexual contact predominated for the first decade, the number of persons infected through heterosexual contact and injecting drug use is increasing. In contrast, transmission through transfusion of blood and blood products has been virtually eliminated in countries that have systematically instituted HIV-antibody screening of donated blood and plasma and heat treatment of clotting factors. The epidemiology of AIDS has been affected by the increasing use of antiretroviral therapies such as zidovudine and other treatment strategies that have delayed the development of certain opportunistic conditions, such as *P. carinii* pneumonia, in infected persons. In comparison, the HIV epidemic has contributed to a marked and alarming increase in tuberculosis infection in the United States and other countries, which has been further complicated by the development of multidrug-resistant strains of *Mycobacterium tuberculosis*.

Now more than ever, the control and prevention of HIV infection, whether on a global or an individual scale, must be grounded in an understanding of HIV's changing epidemiology.

HIV AND AIDS SURVEILLANCE IN THE UNITED STATES

All 50 states, the District of Columbia, and all U.S. territories require reporting of AIDS cases to local health authorities.

TABLE 1. Conditions Included in the 1993 AIDS Surveillance Case Definition

Bacterial infections, multiple or recurrent[a]
Candidiasis of bronchi, trachea, or lungs
Candidiasis, esophageal
Cervical cancer, invasive[b]
Coccidioidomycosis, disseminated or extrapulmonary
Cryptococcosis, extrapulmonary
Cryptosporidiosis, chronic intestinal (>1 month duration)
Cytomegalovirus disease (other than liver, spleen, or nodes)
Cytomegalovirus retinitis (with loss of vision)
Encephalopathy, HIV-related
Herpes simplex, chronic ulcer(s) (>1 month duration); or bronchitis, pneumonitis, or esophagitis
Histoplasmosis, disseminated or extrapulmonary
Isosporiasis, chronic intestinal (>1 month duration)
Kaposi sarcoma
Lymphoid interstitial pneumonia and/or pulmonary lymphoid hyperplasia[a]
Lymphoma, Burkitt's (or equivalent term)
Lymphoma, immunoblastic (or equivalent term)
Lymphoma, primary, of brain
Mycobacterium avium-intracellulare complex or *M. kansasii*, disseminated or extrapulmonary
Mycobacterium tuberculosis, any site (pulmonary[b] or extrapulmonary)
Mycobacterium, other species or unidentified species, disseminated or extrapulmonary
Pneumocystis carinii pneumonia
Pneumonia, recurrent[b]
Progressive multifocal leukoencephalopathy
Salmonella septicemia, recurrent
Toxoplasmosis of brain
Wasting syndrome due to HIV

[a] Children less than 13 years old.
[b] Added in the 1993 expansion of the AIDS surveillance case definition for adolescents and adults.

AIDS surveillance is based on a standard case definition comprising the opportunistic illnesses and laboratory markers indicative of severe HIV-related immunosuppression and disease (Table 1). Health department staff actively survey case reports submitted from physicians, hospitals, and other medical care facilities and from record systems such as death certificates and tumor registries. Along with HIV serologic surveys and HIV infection reporting, the AIDS surveillance system serves as a major resource to monitor and anticipate trends in HIV morbidity.

The initial AIDS surveillance case definition was established soon after the first reports of unexplained illnesses associated with cellular immunodeficiency in homosexual/bisexual men, and formally listed the opportunistic infections and neoplasms indicative of underlying immunosuppression.[4] In the absence of previously described causes of immunosuppression, a diagnosis of one of these conditions was defined as AIDS. The definition did not include the less severe manifestations of HIV infection and was designed to be highly specific and to provide a standard means to monitor trends of severe immunodeficiency caused by what was then an unknown agent.

One of the initial uses of AIDS surveillance was to search medical records and death certificates retrospectively for previously unrecognized or unreported cases of similar immunodeficiency. This review identified only 125 cases of AIDS diagnosed between 1977 and 1981 and provided evidence that the condition was a new disease in the United States. Although a few isolated cases compatible with AIDS have been retrospectively diagnosed from the 1950s and 1960s, the AIDS epidemic in the United States essentially began in the late 1970s.[5,6]

The AIDS surveillance case definition was modified in 1985, in 1987, and again in 1993.[7-9] These revisions were made to reflect the development of serologic tests to detect HIV in 1985, the recognition of additional clinical illnesses associated with or directly caused by HIV infection, and changes in the clinical management of HIV-infected persons. Each revision to the AIDS surveillance case definition has subsequently resulted in a higher proportion of HIV-infected persons being defined as having AIDS.

The 1985 and 1987 revisions added several new diseases to the

AIDS surveillance definition for persons with diagnosed HIV infection. The 1985 revision included disseminated histoplasmosis, chronic isosporiasis, and certain non-Hodgkin's lymphomas. Following this revision, the reported number of AIDS cases increased by an estimated 3–4 percent.[10] The 1987 revision incorporated HIV encephalopathy, wasting syndrome, and other AIDS-indicator diseases that are diagnosed presumptively (i.e., without definitive laboratory evidence). As a result of this revision, an estimated additional 10–15 percent of HIV-infected persons became reportable as having AIDS, and AIDS cases increased by as much as 28 percent in some areas.[11,12] The increase in AIDS case reporting resulting from these revisions was greatest for women, blacks, Hispanics, and injecting drug users.[11,12]

In 1993, the AIDS surveillance definition was expanded to include HIV-infected adolescents and adults with severe immunosuppression (<200 $CD4^+$ T lymphocytes/μl, or a CD4+ T-lymphocyte percentage of total lymphocytes of <14), pulmonary tuberculosis, recurrent (i.e., two or more episodes in a 12-month period) pneumonia, and invasive cervical cancer. Measures of CD4+ T lymphocytes are a recommended guide for the clinical and therapeutic management of HIV-infected persons. Considerations of antiretroviral therapy is recommended for persons with CD4+ T-lymphocyte counts of less than 500 cells/μl, and prophylaxis against *P. carinii* pneumonia is recommended for all persons with CD4+ T-lymphocyte counts of less than 200 cells/μl.[13–15a] These clinical interventions have delayed or prevented the development of previous AIDS-defining opportunistic illnesses in many HIV-infected patients, which in turn has directly affected the timeliness and representativeness of AIDS case reporting.[16] The inclusion of these immunologic criteria allow for more accurate representation of the number of persons with severe HIV-related immunosuppression and should also simplify the reporting process, particularly for physicians and other outpatient reporting sources.

The clinical conditions added to the 1993 surveillance case definition have documented their potential importance for the health of HIV-infected persons. Persons coinfected with HIV and *M. tuberculosis* have a much greater likelihood of developing clinical tuberculosis and may be more difficult to diagnose and treat than non-HIV-infected persons.[17,18] Other than the conditions in the 1987 surveillance definition, pneumonia is the leading cause of serious illness, hospitalizations, and death for HIV-infected persons.[19–21] Cervical dysplasia, a precursor lesion that may progress to cervical cancer, is common among HIV-infected women and increases in severity as immunosuppression worsens.[22–24] The addition of invasive cervical cancer to the definition emphasizes the importance of gynecologic care for HIV-infected women and will allow for assessment of trends in the diagnosis of this condition as the number of HIV-infected women increases.

Evaluation studies have shown that AIDS surveillance provides complete and timely information. A national multicenter study utilizing computerized medical records in six areas determined that 92 percent of persons with AIDS-defining conditions were reported to local health departments.[25] Of these previously reported cases, 67 percent were reported to local health departments within 2 months of the date of diagnosis. Studies of state and local death certificate information and national vital statistics found that completeness of reporting of persons with AIDS ranged from 80 to 96 percent and that 70–90 percent of HIV-related deaths were reported to AIDS surveillance groups.[19,20,26] Completeness of reporting for AIDS is comparable with or higher than that for other disease surveillance systems.[27,28]

Twenty-five states require confidential reporting by name of persons who test positive for HIV antibody.[29] HIV infection reporting is often a useful adjunct to AIDS case surveillance and may assist efforts to plan, implement, and evaluate HIV prevention and medical intervention programs.[29–31] HIV infection reporting provides a minimum estimate of the number of

TABLE 2. 1993 Revised Classification System for HIV Infection and Expanded AIDS Surveillance Case Definition for Adolescents and Adults[a]

CD4+ T-Cell Categories	Clinical Categories		
	A — Asymptomatic, Acute (Primary) HIV, or PGL	B — Symptomatic, Not A or C Conditions	C[b] — AIDS-Indicator Conditions
1. $\geq$500/μl	A1	B1	C1
2. 200–499/μl	A2	B2	C2
3. $<$200/μl AIDS-indicator T-cell count[a]	A3	B3	C3

Abbreviation: PGL, persistent generalized lymphadenopathy.
[a] Shading indicates conditions included in the 1993 AIDS surveillance case definition for adolescents and adults.
[b] Clinical conditions in category C are listed in Table 1.

(From Centers for Disease Control and Prevention.[9])

persons known to be infected in a given area and also provides information regarding more recently infected persons than those reported with AIDS.[30] In states where HIV infection is a reportable condition, the number of persons reported with HIV infection is on average twice that of persons reported with AIDS. In addition, persons reported with HIV infection are more likely than those reported with AIDS to be women, adolescents, and racial/ethnic minorities, reflecting more recent trends in HIV transmission.[30]

Concurrent with the revision of the AIDS surveillance case definition in 1993, the Centers for Disease Control and Prevention (CDC) implemented a revised classification system for HIV-infected adolescents and adults.[9] The system reflects both the evolving knowledge about the spectrum and progression of HIV infection and current standards of medical care for infected persons. The system is based on a combination of three ranges of CD4+ T-lymphocyte counts and three clinical categories (Table 2). Dividing the continuum of HIV infection into mutually exclusive and descriptive categories serves many useful purposes, including increased awareness of the spectrum of clinical manifestations of HIV infection; facilitation of surveillance and reporting for AIDS and HIV infections; provision of information for designing, standardizing, and evaluating drug and vaccine trials and epidemiologic and natural history studies and for formulating health policy and strategy; and facilitation of scientific communication.[32–34] The public health orientation of the CDC's classification system is complemented by other proposed systems for classifying the natural history of HIV infection, including prognostic staging systems,[34–36] prognostic scoring indices,[37] and systems that can be adapted to settings that lack testing for sophisticated laboratory markers.[33]

HIV INFECTION AND AIDS IN ADULTS

Incidence and Prevalence of AIDS in the United States

As of December 31, 1992, 249,199 adolescents and adults were reported with AIDS in the United States.[38] Since 1981, when the first cases were reported,[1,2] the number of persons with AIDS has increased rapidly. As a result of this rapid growth, the first 100,000 AIDS cases were reported during an 8-year period (1981–89), whereas the second 100,000 cases were reported in just over 2 years (1989–91).[39]

In the early 1990s, the number of persons reported with AIDS in the United States is likely to increase further, although at a much slower rate than during the earlier years of the epidemic. However, an aberration in the temporal trends will result from the expansion in the surveillance definition for AIDS[9] primarily due to the inclusion of markers of severe HIV-related immunosuppression. As a result of this expansion, the number of reported AIDS cases is expected to increase by more than 100 percent in 1993[39a] and by 15–20 percent in 1994. In 1994, 160,000–200,000 persons are expected to be living with AIDS in the United States.

Serologic Monitoring of the HIV Epidemic

Because of the long period between infection with HIV and the development of AIDS, surveillance systems for HIV infection are needed to supplement the information available through AIDS case surveillance. Estimates of the prevalence and incidence of HIV infection have been developed periodically over the course of the epidemic using various methods. The U.S. Public Health Service has estimated that approximately 1 million U.S. residents are infected with HIV, with at least 40,000 new infections occurring annually.[40]

HIV seroprevalence surveys describe patterns of current HIV infection. These surveys have been conducted on (1) specimens not linked to personal identifiers and collected for other purposes; (2) name-identified specimens; and (3) specimens collected among populations subject to routine or mandatory HIV screening such as blood donors or military personnel. In general, the patterns of HIV transmission observed in these studies in the United States are similar to those observed through AIDS case surveillance—higher rates of HIV infection are found among men than women, among blacks and Hispanics than whites, and among persons 20–45 years of age then persons in other age groups.

Homosexual and bisexual men remain a major population with an increased prevalence of HIV infection. Of surveys conducted primarily in sexually transmitted disease clinics in the early to mid-1980s, HIV seroprevalence rates in homosexual and bisexual men ranged from 10 to as high 70 percent, with most rates falling between 20 and 50 percent.[41] Although the highest rates were found in New York City and San Francisco, areas of high-to-moderate HIV seroprevalence are dispersed throughout the country.[41,42] In 1991–92, a subsequent study of unlinked serologic specimens collected from homosexual/bisexual men attending sexually transmitted disease clinics in 36 cities had a median seroprevalence rate of 26 percent, with a range of 4–47 percent (Fig. 1).[43] The HIV seroprevalence rate in this population is lower than that found in earlier surveys in the same clinics and suggests a decrease in HIV infection incidence.[44] The incidence of HIV infection among homosexual/bisexual men in some cohort studies dropped in the mid- to late-1980s.[41,45,46] However, the prevalence of HIV infection remains high, and new infections continue to occur since not all men in this population have adopted or sustained safer sexual practices.[47,48] Adolescent and young adult homosexual/bisexual men appear to be at particular risk for acquiring HIV.[48]

In contrast to the epidemic among homosexual/bisexual men, the epidemic among injecting drug users has been more concentrated geographically within the United States. Among injecting drug users, the initial HIV seroprevalence studies demonstrated very high rates of HIV infection in the northeastern United States and very low rates on the western coast and in cities in other areas.[41,49,50] Although the highest rates of HIV infection continue to be observed among cities in the Northeast, the rate of HIV infection among drug users in other cities has increased. Studies conducted in the late 1980s in Atlanta, Chicago, and Baltimore have shown HIV seroprevalence rates greater than 12 percent.[51–53] In 1991–92, surveys in 35 cities observed a me-

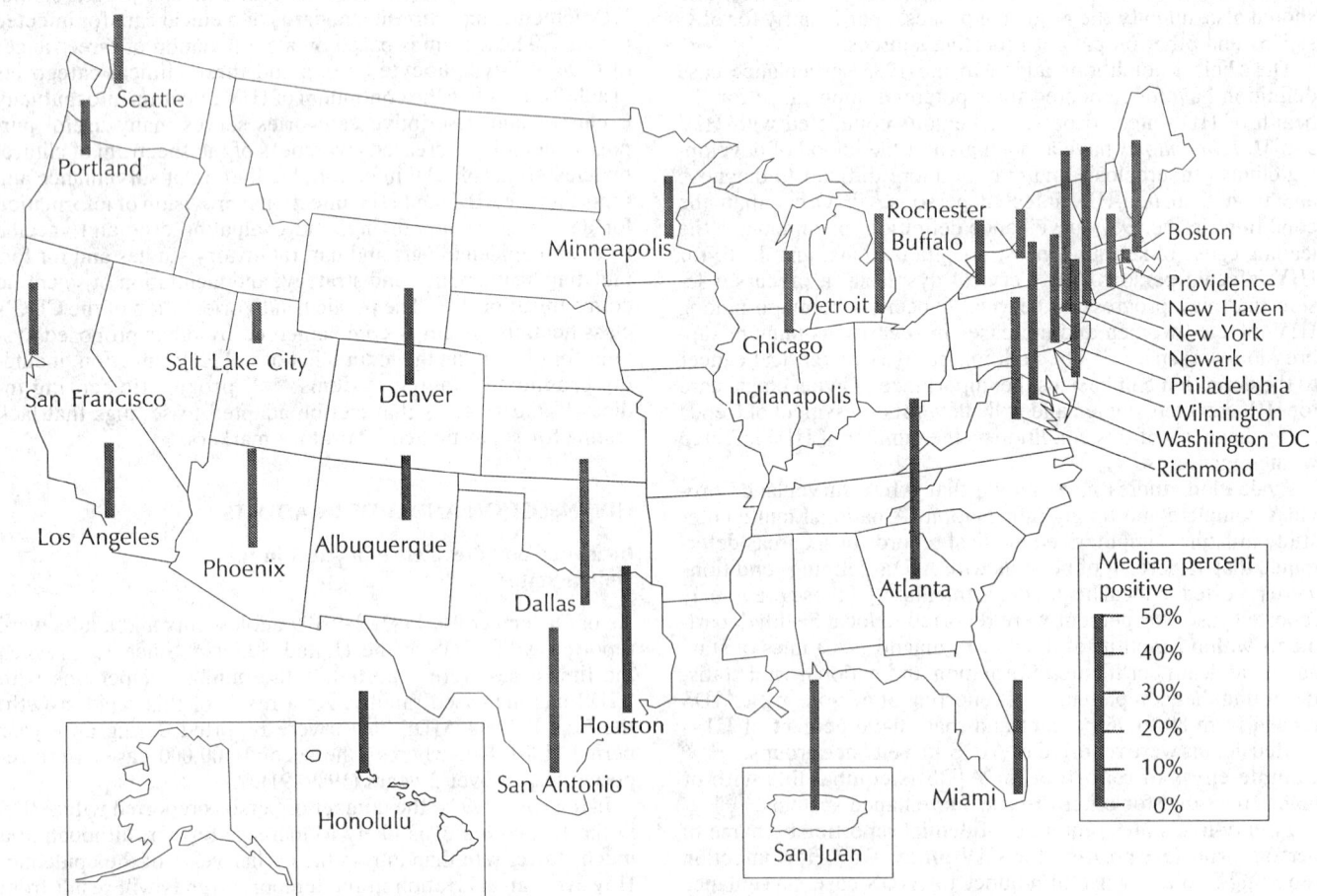

FIG. 1. HIV seroprevalence in men having sex with men, sexually transmitted disease clinic surveys, 1991–1992. (From Centers for Disease Control and Prevention.[43])

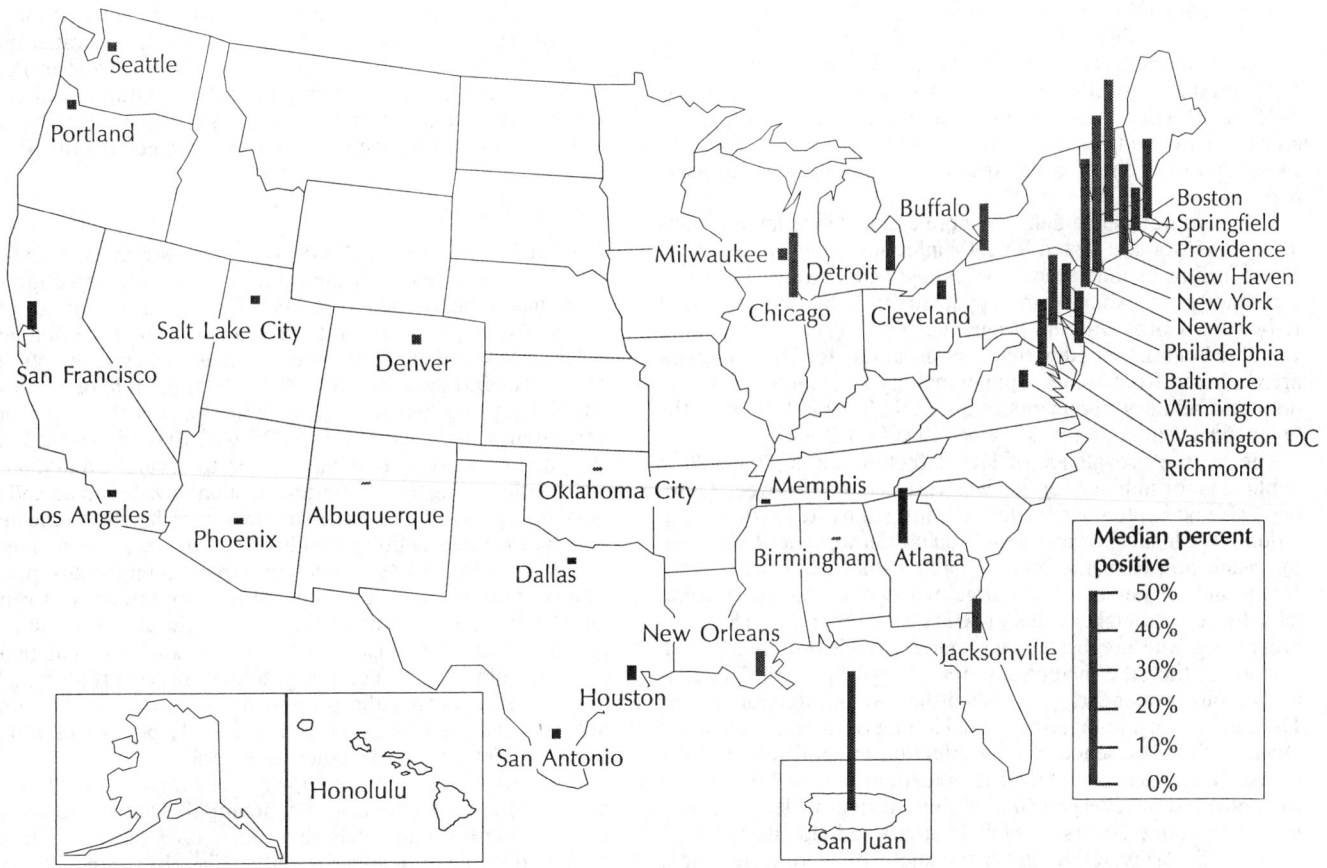

FIG. 2. HIV seroprevalence in injecting drug users, drug treatment center surveys, 1991–1992. (From Centers for Disease Control and Prevention.[43])

dian HIV seroprevalence rate of 7.5 percent (range 1–53 percent) among injecting drug users entering drug treatment programs (Fig. 2).[43,53] The rate of infection was higher in the Atlantic coast states than the rest of the country. Studies in sexually transmitted disease clinics have also shown elevated rates of HIV infection among heterosexual injecting drug users compared with other heterosexual men and women.[43,44] Although heroin injection is typically associated with the parenteral transmission of HIV, injectors of cocaine and other drugs also have increased rates of HIV infection.[53–55]

Some populations of heterosexual men and women who do not inject drugs may also have appreciable rates of HIV infection. In 1988–89, studies in sexually transmitted disease clinics of heterosexual persons who do not inject drugs but who have other sexually transmitted diseases found a median seroprevalence of 2.3 percent, with a range of 0–14 percent.[44] Although men in these clinics typically had higher rates than women, in some areas adolescent women had higher rates of HIV infection than adolescent men. Nearly one-third of persons infected heterosexually are estimated to have been infected as adolescents.[56]

Of persons infected heterosexually, sexual contact with an injecting drug user is the most frequently reported risk. Accordingly, the geographic distribution of HIV rates among persons who acquired their infection through heterosexual contact and among injecting drug users is similar.[57] In addition, persons who use smokable forms of cocaine and other noninjected illicit drugs have elevated risks for HIV infection as a result of exchanging sex for drugs or money and the presence of other sexually transmitted diseases.[58–61] Some persons infected through heterosexual contact may not report a risk of HIV infection because they are unaware of the serostatus of their heterosexual partners.[38,44,61]

Female commercial sex workers (prostitutes) are at increased risk for HIV infection because of injecting drug use and multiple sex partners. In a 1987 multicenter study of prostitutes in various settings in selected cities, 65 (10 percent) of 670 women tested positive for HIV antibody.[62] Seroprevalence rates for HIV infection ranged from 0 percent for prescreened prostitutes in Nevada to 69 percent for prostitutes being treated for drug addiction in New Jersey. Among prostitutes who were studied, the major risk factor was injecting drug use. In a study in south Florida in 1987, 37 (41 percent) of 90 inner-city sex workers were HIV-antibody positive, including 29 (46 percent) of 63 women who reported drug use and 8 (30 percent) of 27 women who denied using drugs.[63] From 1987 to 1991, the prevalence of HIV infection among female sex workers in south Florida remained relatively stable at approximately 24 percent. However, the incidence of HIV infection among female sex workers in this area who received multiple HIV tests increased from 0.3 percent per 100 person years in 1987 to 15 percent in 1991.[64]

Surveys conducted in some clinical settings indicate that the HIV infection rate is higher than in a more representative sample of the general population.[65,66] In 1989–91, a survey of persons admitted to 20 hospitals observed an HIV-seroprevalence of 4.7 percent (range 0.2–14.2 percent); in one hospital, 24 percent of men 15–54 years of age were HIV infected.[65] Using data from this survey, an estimated 225,000 HIV-infected persons were hospitalized in 1990; 72 percent of these persons were admitted for conditions other than HIV infection or AIDS.

In many areas, persons with tuberculosis have high rates of HIV infection. Among 20 tuberculosis treatment clinics surveyed in 1988–89, HIV seroprevalence ranged from 0 to 46 percent, with a median rate of 3.4 percent.[66] The highest rates were found in the Northeast and Atlantic Coast areas and among persons with extrapulmonary disease.

Studies of HIV seroprevalence among entrants to correctional facilities have indicated a wide range of rates, with the highest in areas with moderate-to-high AIDS incidence.[67] From 1991 to 1992, the median HIV seroprevalence was 2.9 percent (range 0–15 percent) in 35 correctional facilities in 17 metropolitan areas.[43] Rates ranged from 1 to 12.5 percent for men and 0 to 24 percent for women, reflecting high rates of drug use in these persons.

HIV seroprevalence data are more available for large groups of persons who are tested for HIV infection on a routine basis. These groups include blood donors, applicants for military service, military personnel, and applicants to U.S. Department of Labor Job Corps training programs.[43,68–75] These surveys are valuable but are limited in that persons at risk for HIV infection are excluded from some populations (e.g., potential blood donors and military applicants). Among U.S. blood donors, the level of HIV infection was 1.4 per 10,000 to 1992.[68]

The overall prevalence of HIV infection among 2.3 million applicants for military service was 1.31 per 1000 between October 1985 and September 1989.[69] HIV infection rates in this population were higher for men (1.42/1000) than women (0.66/1000), for black non-Hispanic men (3.7/1000) than white men (0.61/1000), and for persons from large metropolitan areas, particularly those with higher rates of AIDS case reporting. The seroprevalence rate among teenage military applicants (0.34/1000) was lower than the median rate for all applicants; the male-to-female ratio was nearly 1 to 1 and the rate of infection among 17- and 18-year-old females exceeded that of same-age males.[70] Overall, the prevalence of HIV infection in applicants has decreased from approximately 0.15 percent in 1985 to 0.06 percent (one positive for every 1640 applicants tested) in 1991–92, due in part to active efforts to exclude at-risk individuals.[43]

For U.S. Army active-duty personnel who were tested more than once; the HIV-seroconversion rate was 0.39 per 1000 person years.[74] The rate of seroconversion decreased from 0.49 per 1000 person years in 1985–87 to 0.29 per 1000 person years in 1988–89. However, a reduction in the seroconversion rate was not observed for black soldiers, suggesting a higher rate of continued transmission in this population.

Students who enter Job Corps training programs tend to be economically disadvantaged school-aged youths drawn from racial and ethnic minority communities in both rural and urban areas. For students aged 16–21 years who entered training from October 1987 through 1992, 3.0 per 1000 were infected with HIV—a rate almost 10 times that seen among applicants for military service.[43,75] The infection rate increased with age. For 21-year-old students, the infection rate was 4.8 per 1000 for men and 7.0 per 1000 for women. HIV seroprevalence rates have decreased among men, while rates have increased among women. The highest rates were observed in students from large Northeast urban centers and also among students from rural and smaller urban centers in the South.

Another type of broad population survey is the survey of childbearing women, which provides unbiased population-based estimates of HIV infection in women giving birth in the United States. HIV antibody prevalence for childbearing women has been ascertained by blinded surveys conducted on residual blood samples collected on filter paper from newborns for routine metabolic screening such as that for phenylketonuria.[76] Based on data from 35 states, there were approximately 7000 annual births to HIV-infected women during 1991–92, for an estimated annual national HIV infection prevalence of 1.7 per 1000 childbearing women.[77] Assuming a perinatal transmission rate of 20–30 percent, an estimated 1400–2100 infants born in the United States in 1992 were HIV-infected. By state, New York, Florida, and New Jersey had the highest HIV seroprevalence rates; infection rates were also higher in metropolitan areas than nonmetropolitan areas, and among black women than women of other race/ethnicities. In the South, from 1989 to 1992, the rate among women increased from 1.7 to 2.1 per 1000.[77] The

findings of seroprevalence studies of women seeking reproductive care services have also shown the highest HIV rates among clinics located among the Atlantic Coast area and in Puerto Rico.[43,78] If HIV seroprevalence rates among childbearing women are similar for all women of reproductive age, 80,000 or more women in this age group could be infected with HIV.

Exposure Categories

Since the first cases of AIDS were reported in 1981, cases in men who have sex with men and heterosexual injecting drug users have consistently represented the largest number of reported AIDS cases. The rate of growth in the total number of AIDS cases and in these two exposure categories was most rapid through 1986 (Fig. 3a).[79,80] In 1987, the rate of increase in AIDS reporting began to slow for homosexual/bisexual men, particularly in cities where AIDS was first recognized. This slowing in case reporting was related to several events, including the increasing use of therapies, such as zidovudine and prophylaxis against *P. carinii* pneumonia, which delayed the development of AIDS-defining conditions; a decrease in the number of new HIV infections, reflecting in part the impact of prevention programs; and a decline in the completeness of reporting.[40,45,81,82] As a result of this slowing in case reporting, the proportion of AIDS cases among homosexual/bisexual men decreased from 65 to 52 percent of total cases reported from 1987 to 1992. In contrast, the proportion of cases reported among heterosexual drug users increased from 17 percent of all cases to 25 percent during the same time period.

Cases of AIDS among recipients of blood or blood components and among persons with hemophilia increased dramatically during the mid-1980s, but since 1987 the numbers have remained stable or declined slightly (Fig. 3b).[80] Since the initiation of HIV antibody screening of donated blood and plasma and heat treatment of clotting factors, transmission of HIV through blood and blood products has been reported only rarely.[83] Additional cases with these modes of transmission continue to be diagnosed as a consequence of infections that occurred before screening and treatment practices were initiated and because of the long period between infection with HIV and AIDS.

Heterosexual contact cases comprise persons who report heterosexual exposure to a person with, or at increased risk for, HIV infection (e.g., an injecting drug user) or persons born in countries were heterosexual transmission is the major route of HIV infection (e.g., areas of sub-Saharan Africa and some Caribbean countries). AIDS cases associated with heterosexual contact have been increasing steadily and in 1992 represented 9 percent of all reported cases. Since 1986 the annual percent increase in this group has been higher than that of any other exposure category and has been most striking for women (Fig. 3C). In 1992, the number of cases diagnosed among women infected through heterosexual contact exceeded those infected through injecting drug use for the first time.[84]

For AIDS cases reported in 1992, most of the source partners for persons with heterosexually acquired AIDS were injecting drug users (49 percent) or persons born in countries where heterosexual contact is the major transmission mode (11 percent). The risk of the partner was not specified for 34 percent. Persons with sex partners of unknown HIV infection or risk status are classified in the undetermined category (see below). Selected follow-up and investigation of heterosexual contact cases has identified other sources of exposure to HIV infection for some persons, especially men.[85] Nonetheless, it is unlikely that such misclassification bias has significantly influenced national trends.[79]

Of the 46,335 adults and adolescents with AIDS reported in 1992, 11 percent had two or more reported risk factors for infection. The largest overlaps occurred in men who reported both having sex with men and injecting drugs (5 percent of all cases) and among heterosexual persons who reported both injecting

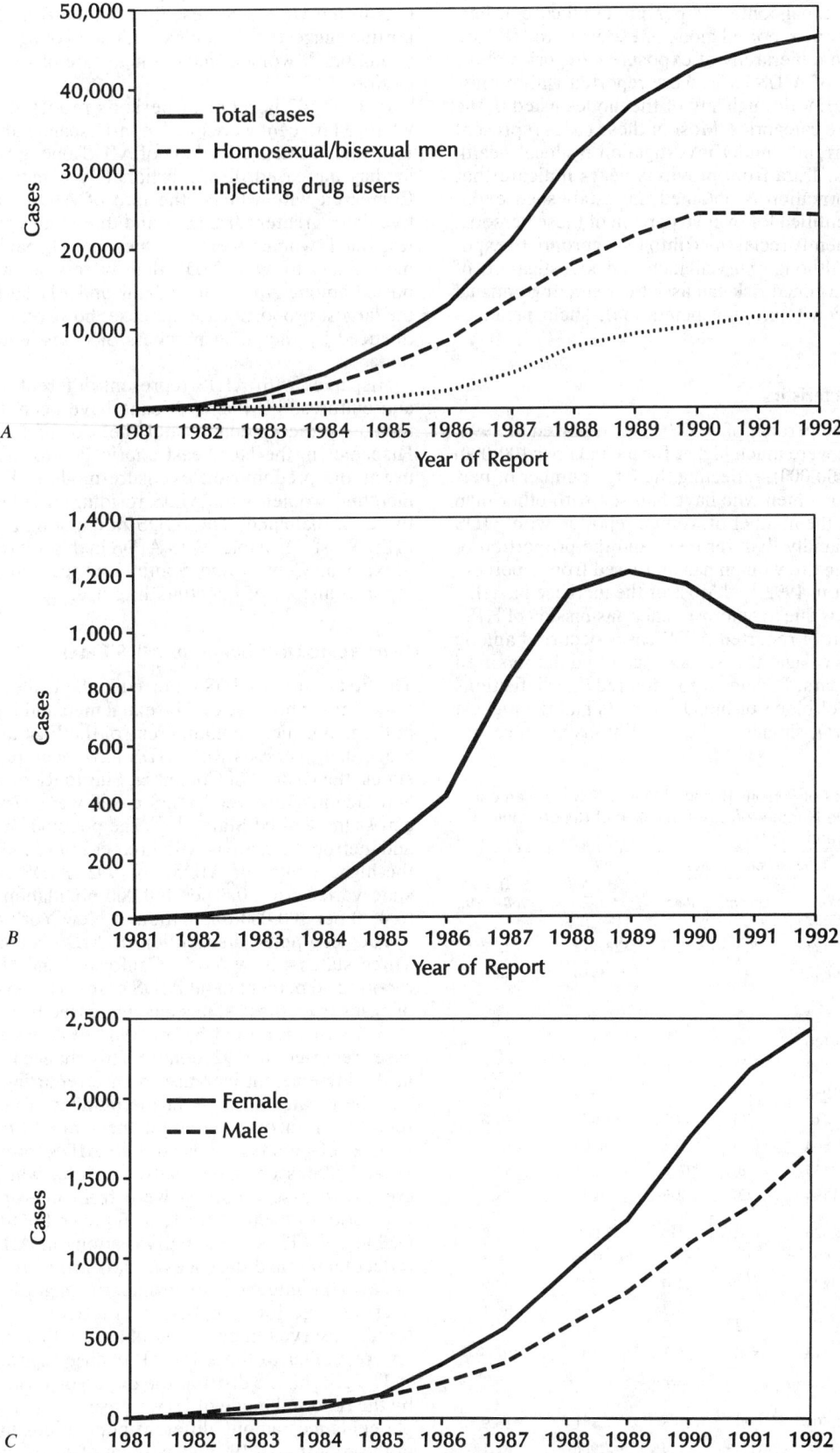

FIG. 3. (A) Total reported AIDS cases, cases among homosexual/bisexual men (excluding injecting drug users), and cases among women and heterosexual men reporting injecting drug use, United States, by year of report. (B) AIDS case attributed to receipt of HIV-infected blood and blood products. (C) AIDS cases reported among men and women infected through heterosexual contact. Data include persons born in countries where heterosexual transmission is the predominant mode of transmission.

drug use and heterosexual contact (4 percent of all cases). Persons with more than one reported mode of exposure to HIV are counted only once in a hierarchy of exposure categories.[38]

In 1992, 7 percent of AIDS cases were reported with no history of exposure to HIV through any of the modes listed in the hierarchy of exposure categories. Most of these cases represent persons who are currently under investigation by local health department officials. Data from previous years indicate that when follow-up information is obtained, an established exposure mode can be identified for over 90 percent of these persons, and they are subsequently reclassified into the appropriate exposure category.[59,86] Although surveillance and investigation of cases with an undetermined risk can assist in detecting unusual modes of transmission (e.g., transplantation), such instances remain rare.[87]

Demographic Characteristics

Men accounted for 86 percent of AIDS cases reported in 1992, and AIDS case rates were much higher for men (33 per 100,000) than women (5 per 100,000), reflecting the large number of persons with AIDS among men who have had sex with other men (Table 3). However, the number of women reported with AIDS is increasing more rapidly than for men, and the proportion of total AIDS cases who are women has increased from 8 percent in 1988 to 14 percent in 1992.[10,84] Most of the increase in AIDS cases among women is due to heterosexual transmission of HIV.

In 1992, 62 percent of reported AIDS cases occurred among persons 20–39 years of age; the average age of adults reported with AIDS was 38 years. Persons who acquired their infections through transfusion of blood or blood products had the highest average age (53 years), similar to that of all transfusion recipi-

ents in the United States. Information from HIV infection reporting suggests that adolescents and young adults, particularly young black women, have a high rate of recently acquired infection.[30]

In 1992, 47 percent of persons reported with AIDS were white, 34 percent were black non-Hispanic, and 18 percent were Hispanic (Table 3). The rate of AIDS among blacks and Hispanics has increased disproportionately compared with whites.[10] Compared with whites, the rate of AIDS was approximately five times greater for blacks and three times greater for Hispanics. Black women were 17 times and Hispanic women 8 times more likely to have AIDS than were white women. Cases reported among American Indians and Alaska Natives have had the largest proportionate increase; however, this increase is influenced by the small numbers of cases among these populations.

Hispanics with AIDS represent different countries of origin and cultures.[89,90] Puerto Ricans have been disportionately affected by the epidemic, and the rate of AIDS is highest for Hispanics in the Northeast and in Puerto Rico. Injecting drug use is the predominant exposure mode in Puerto Rican–born men and women with AIDS residing in either Puerto Rico or the U.S. mainland. The AIDS rate among Hispanics is lowest in the West. Hispanics with AIDS in this area are primarily from Mexico or Central and South America and are less likely to report a history of injecting drug use.

Geographic Distribution of AIDS Cases

The first cases of AIDS reported in the United States were clustered among homosexual/bisexual men and injecting drug users in the major metropolitan areas of the East and West coasts.[1,2] Since then, persons with AIDS have been reported from all 50 states, the District of Columbia, Puerto Rico, the Virgin Islands, and Guam. However, AIDS cases were distributed unevenly across the United States.[38,79] The populous northeastern states and metropolitan areas with greater than 1 million persons have the highest rates of AIDS. In 1992, AIDS incidence rates by state varied from 0.8 per 100,000 population in North Dakota to 46.0 per 100,000 population in New York (Fig. 4).

The geographic distribution of AIDS is changing over time. Three states—New York, California, and New Jersey—have reported 46 percent of all AIDS cases. However, the proportion of cases from these states has decreased from 54 percent of the 50,316 cases reported before 1988 to 40 percent of the 47,106 cases reported in 1992 alone.[10] This change reflects the slowing in the incremental increase in case reporting from these areas and the greater increase in the number of persons with AIDS reported from other areas of the United States. In 1992, the number of persons reported with AIDS from the northeastern United States changed relatively little, while the greatest increases in case reporting were from metropolitan areas with populations of 500,000 or less and from the South and Midwest (Table 3).[84] These regional variations in AIDS case reporting reflect temporal differences in the introduction of HIV, the rate of new HIV infections over time, the migration of HIV-infected persons, and local reporting practices.[81,90] The geographic trends observed in population-based HIV seroprevalence studies are similar to those for AIDS case reporting.[69,73–76]

The geographic distribution of persons with AIDS also varies by the reported mode of HIV transmission, reflecting the multiple epidemics among different populations in different regions of the country. In 1992, 46 percent of cases among homosexual/bisexual men were reported from California, Florida, and New York. However, men with AIDS who report sexual contact with other men are increasingly distributed throughout all regions of the United States.[91] Since 1987, the incidence of AIDS among homosexual/bisexual men in New York City, Los Angeles, and San Francisco has increased much less rapidly than in earlier years. In contrast, in 1991 and 1992, the South had the largest

TABLE 3. Characteristics of Persons Reported With AIDS and Percent Change in the Number of Cases, by Year of Report, United States, 1988 and 1992

Category	1992 Reported Cases			1988 Reported Cases	% Change 1988–1992
	No.	Percent	Rate[a]		
Sex					
Male	40,453	(86)	32.6	28,449	42.2
Female	6642	(14)	5.1	3516	88.9
Age (years)					
0–4	624	(1)	3.2	464	34.5
5–12	146	(<1)	0.5	131	11.5
13–19	159	(<1)	0.6	120	32.5
20–29	7982	(17)	19.5	6574	21.4
30–39	21,212	(45)	49.1	14,671	44.6
40–49	11,963	(25)	36.7	6762	76.9
50–59	3515	(8)	16.0	2201	59.7
≥60	1494	(3)	3.5	1042	43.4
Race/ethnicity[b]					
White	22,328	(47)	11.8	17,068	30.8
Black	15,890	(34)	53.7	9118	74.3
Hispanic	8282	(18)	31.0	5501	50.6
Asian/Pacific Islander	314	(1)	4.3	189	66.1
American Indian/ Alaskan Native	113	(<1)	6.1	38	197.4[c]
Region					
Northeast	13,507	(29)	26.5	11,551	16.9
Midwest	5296	(11)	8.9	2908	82.1
South	15,788	(34)	18.3	9022	75.0
West	10,881	(23)	20.2	7,238	50.3
U.S. territories	1623	(4)	45.6	1246	30.3

[a] Per 100,000 population. 1992 population counts were estimated from 1990 U.S. Census Bureau data. For categories of sex, race/ethnicity, and HIV exposure, denominator was population in 50 states and Puerto Rico (excluding other U.S. territories).
[b] Excludes persons with unspecified race/ethnicity (168 [0.4%] in 1992, 57 [0.2%] in 1988).
[c] Percentage change reflects small number of cases among this population.

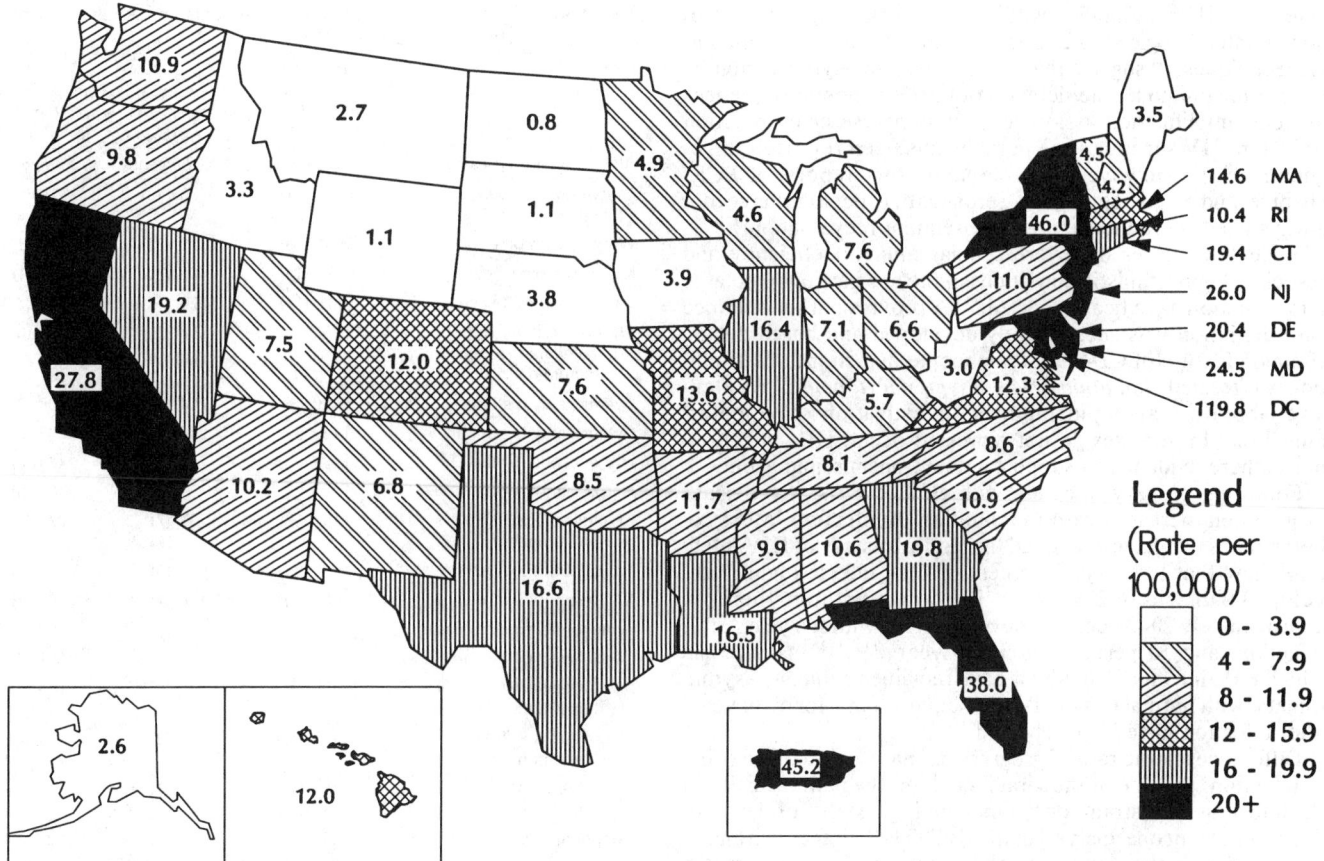

FIG. 4. AIDS annual rates per 100,000 population for cases reported in the United States, 1992. (From Centers for Disease Control and Prevention.[38])

increase in the number of cases reported among homosexual/bisexual men.

Injecting drug users with AIDS are clustered in states along the Atlantic coast of the United States. In 1992, approximately half of the AIDS cases among heterosexual injecting drug users and among persons infected through heterosexual contact (many of whom had contact with injecting drug users) were reported from New York, New Jersey, and Florida. However, the southern and midwestern United States had the greatest rise in the number of cases reported among injecting drug users.[84,92]

All areas of the country have had an increase in the number of men and women with AIDS reportedly infected through heterosexual contact; the largest increase in the number of these cases occurred in the South. This trend is associated with a 30 percent increase in the South in the number of births to HIV-seropositive women from 1989 to 1992, representing the largest increase of any region of the United States.[77]

AIDS cases reported among persons infected with HIV through the receipt of blood or blood products are also clustered in areas of high AIDS incidence. However, these cases are distributed throughout the United States, reflecting the distribution of collected blood and the migration patterns of persons who require medical care involving transfusions.

Clinical Manifestations of HIV Infection

Spectrum and Progression of HIV Infection. The spectrum of HIV infection ranges from an asymptomatic state to severe immunodeficiency and associated serious secondary infections, neoplasms, and other conditions.[21,93] Initial or primary infection with HIV can be followed by an acute mononucleosis-like illness. Features of this acute illness associated with seroconver-

sion include fever, lymphadenopathy, sweats, myalgia, arthralgia, rash, malaise, lethargy, sore throat, anorexia, nausea, vomiting, diarrhea, headache, photophobia, and mucocutaneous ulcers.[94,95] Less common manifestations have also been reported, including a variety of neurologic conditions (e.g., myelopathy, radiculopathy, peripheral neuropathy, and Guillain-Barré syndrome)[96] and *Candida* esophagitis,[97] which responds well to treatment in contrast to the esophagitis associated with advanced infection.[95]

The relative frequency of symptomatic primary HIV infection has been difficult to determine because symptoms tend to be nonspecific, may cause little discomfort, pass largely unnoticed by the patient, and are often assessed retrospectively. However, more recent studies indicate that between 50 and 70 percent of persons with primary HIV infection develop an acute retroviral illness, reflecting in part an increased recognition of this symptom complex by both physicians and patients.[95,98,99] In a comprehensive review of primary HIV infection, the interval between exposure and symptomatic illness was reported to range on average between 2 and 4 weeks, with the duration of illness lasting from 1 to 2 weeks.[95]

Laboratory evaluation of some persons with primary, symptomatic HIV infection has found transient high levels of p24 antigen in plasma and cytopathic HIV in peripheral blood mononuclear cells.[100,101] It has been suggested that the intensity and/or resolution of symptomatic primary HIV infection may be related to the level of viremia, which declines precipitously soon after initial infection, coincident with increasing levels of antiviral antibodies[100–102] and a high level of antiviral activity mediated by CD8+ T lymphocytes.[103] Studies of homosexual men,[104,105] persons with hemophilia,[104,106] and intravenous drug users,[107] consistently have demonstrated the development of detectable HIV antibodies within 3–12 weeks following infection. Epidemiologic studies and case reports, as well as modeling techniques,[104] suggest that seroconversion beyond 6 months is very uncommon. The detection of HIV genomic sequences by gene amplification assays (e.g., polymerase chain reaction [PCR] in HIV seronegative persons has been reported infrequently.[108,109] However, isolated laboratory reports of PCR-positive and persistently HIV-seronegative persons have not always been reproducible upon subsequent reevaluation.[110]

Since 1989, cases of severe cellular immunodeficiency and associated opportunistic conditions in the absence of detectable HIV infection have been reported.[111] A provisional surveillance case definition was subsequently developed and based on the common feature of CD4+ T-lymphocyte depletion; this condition was termed *idiopathic CD4+ T lymphocytopenia*.[112] Extensive laboratory and epidemiologic investigations have determined that these cases do not represent occult HIV infection, nor is there evidence to support a new transmissible agent.[113]

Following primary infection with HIV, the risk for disease progression increases with the duration of infection. Most cohort studies that have evaluated the natural history of HIV infection show that less than 5 percent of HIV-infected adults develop AIDS within 2 years of infection; without therapy, approximately 20–25 percent develop AIDS within 6 years after infection, and 50 percent within 10 years.[114–117] Instances in which HIV-infected individuals have remained clinically asymptomatic with normal CD4+ T-lymphocyte counts for 5–10 years after infection have been reported.[118,119]

Differences in the rate of progression may be due to the route of infection, the size of the viral inoculum, the pathogenicity of the infecting viral strain, or the immunologic status of the host. For example, in one analysis of nearly 700 HIV-infected transfusion recipients, the estimated risk for the development of AIDS was 33 percent for persons within 5 years of infection and 49 percent within 7 years of infection.[120] Among recipients infected for similar periods of time, AIDS developed more rapidly in those who received blood from donors who progressed to AIDS soon after donation (50 percent), in comparison to those who received blood from other HIV-infected donors (26 percent). In the same study, recipients who developed AIDS received significantly more units of blood at the time of infection than recipients without AIDS, raising the possibility that underlying clinical status, particularly the degree of immunosuppression, or exposure to other viral cofactors, may also have affected disease progression.

The role of exogenous biologic and behavioral cofactors in the progression to AIDS remains uncertain. Coinfection with other viruses, use of tobacco, and injecting or recreational drug use have not been consistently associated with acceleration of HIV disease.[121–124] Several studies have suggested that the risk of developing AIDS increases significantly with age.[115,124,125] Pregnancy has not been shown to affect the progression of HIV infection.[126]

Because the natural history of HIV infection can vary considerably from person to person, clinical and laboratory predictors of progression are helpful. Oral candidiasis,[127] oral hairy leukoplakia,[128] and severe, recurrent herpes zoster[129] have been associated with an increased likelihood of developing AIDS. Measures of CD4+ T lymphocytes are the most specific laboratory markers of HIV-related immunosuppression and are strongly predictive of disease progression; such testing is also widely available.[130,131] Other immunologic markers, including serum neopterin, β_2-microglobulin, soluble interleukin-2 receptors, and immunoglobulin A may be useful adjuncts in assessing the clinical prognosis of individuals with HIV infection.[131]

AIDS Indicator Diseases. The relative frequency of individual AIDS-indicator diseases is most representative for those diseases diagnosed at the time of the initial case report to national

TABLE 4. AIDS-Indicator Diseases in Adolescents and Adults Reported in 1992, United States[a]

AIDS-Indicator Diseases	Men Who Have Sex With Men[b] (N = 23,936) No. (Percent)	Heterosexual Men[c] (N = 10,997) No. (Percent)	Heterosexual Women (N = 6,255) No. (Percent)
Pneumocystis carinii pneumonia	9842 (41)	4700 (43)	2716 (43)
Wasting syndrome	4374 (18)	2388 (22)	1324 (21)
Kaposi sarcoma	3695 (15)	306 (3)	74 (1)
Candidiasis, esophageal	3081 (13)	1873 (17)	1319 (21)
Mycobacterium avium-intracellulare complex, extrapulmonary	1986 (8)	556 (5)	344 (6)
Cytomegalovirus disease	1490 (6)	211 (2)	208 (3)
Cytomegalovirus, retinitis	1468 (6)	270 (3)	205 (3)
HIV encephalopathy	1437 (6)	760 (7)	383 (6)
Herpes simplex disease	1201 (5)	371 (3)	382 (6)
Cryptococcosis, extrapulmonary	1191 (5)	734 (7)	270 (4)
Toxoplasmosis of brain	1078 (5)	656 (6)	372 (6)
Cryptosporidiosis, chronic	680 (3)	126 (1)	85 (1)
Lymphoma, immunoblastic	595 (2)	157 (1)	68 (1)
Candidiasis, pulmonary	394 (2)	209 (2)	151 (2)
Mycobacterium tuberculosis, extrapulmonary	380 (2)	445 (4)	184 (3)
Mycobacterial disease, extrapulmonary	371 (1)	214 (2)	93 (2)
Histoplasmosis, extrapulmonary	265 (1)	76 (1)	38 (1)
Lymphoma, Burkitt's	259 (1)	50 (1)	20 (<1)
Progressive multifocal leukoencephalopathy	247 (1)	80 (1)	40 (1)
Lymphoma, brain, primary	193 (1)	57 (1)	27 (<1)
Isosporiasis, chronic	100 (<1)	22 (<1)	3 (<1)
Coccidioidomycosis, extrapulmonary	69 (<1)	25 (<1)	9 (<1)
Salmonella, septicemia	31 (<1)	48 (<1)	16 (<1)

[a] Percentages exceed 100 percent because some persons were reported with more than one AIDS-indicator disease.
[b] Excludes men who have sex with men and use injecting drugs.
[c] Excludes men with an undetermined risk.

AIDS surveillance because subsequent diagnoses are much less completely reported.

Three clinical conditions accounted for more than three-fourths of all initial AIDS-indicator conditions reported in 1992: *P. carinii* pneumonia (42 percent); HIV wasting syndrome (20 percent); and candidiasis of the esophagus (15 percent). The prevalences of several AIDS-indicator diseases were higher for men who have sex with men compared with either heterosexual men or women (Table 4). In general, the reported frequency of AIDS-indicator diseases is similar for men and women with similar modes of exposure to HIV. However, among injecting drug users, esophageal candidiasis, cytomegalovirus disease and retinitis, and *Herpes simplex* virus disease have been reported more frequently for women than men.[132]

Since most AIDS-indicator infections result from the endogenous reactivation of previously acquired pathogens, the frequency of reported opportunistic infections likely reflects, in part, geographic-specific prevalences of endemic infections. For example, African and Haitian patients are more likely to develop toxoplasmosis and cryptococcosis.[133] Similarly, the risk of extrapulmonary tuberculosis among foreign-born persons with AIDS in the United States is highest among persons from Haiti, the Philippines, Central America, and Africa.[134] Among U.S.-born persons, those at increased risk for extrapulmonary tuberculosis include residents of the South and Northeast, blacks and Hispanics, and injecting drug users.[134]

Changes in incidence and prevalence trends of some AIDS-defining diseases may be related to the increasing use of antiretroviral therapy and prophylaxis against *P. carinii* pneumonia. For example, among adults and adolescents with a single AIDS-defining disease reported through 1992, the proportion with *P. carinii* pneumonia decreased from 50 percent in 1988 to 38 percent in 1992. Although declines were seen in all persons with AIDS during this period, it was most striking for homosexual/bisexual men and persons with hemophilia or a coagulation disorder. During 1988–92, *P. carinii* pneumonia decreased from 53 to 37 percent and from 47 to 29 percent among homosexual/bisexual men and persons with hemophilia and coagulation disorders, respectively. More modest declines were reported among injecting drug users (45–40 percent) and women (48–40 percent), which may reflect differences in access to and/or use of early medical interventions. A similar pattern of decreasing incidence of *P. carinii* pneumonia and corresponding increases in other AIDS-defining conditions has been observed in well-studied cohorts of homosexual and bisexual men.[135]

Esophageal candidiasis and disseminated *Mycobacterium avium-intracellulare* complex have increased proportionately over time. Among adults and adolescents with a single AIDS-defining disease diagnosed from 1988 through 1992, esophageal candidiasis increased from 6 to 9 percent and *M. avium-intracellulare* increased from 2 to 4 percent. Because disseminated *M. avium-intracellulare* infection usually is diagnosed after the development of AIDS, national surveillance data significantly underestimate its true incidence. In a study of 1006 HIV-infected patients followed over a 3-year period with monthly blood cultures, the incidences of *M. avium-intracellulare* bacteremia were 21 percent at 12 months after AIDS diagnosis, 41 percent at 24 months, and 50 percent at 827 days.[136]

Kaposi sarcoma is another opportunistic condition whose reported frequency has changed dramatically over time. In 1981, the proportion of persons with AIDS who presented with Kaposi sarcoma as their initial manifestation of AIDS was 28 percent nationwide and 59 percent in San Francisco.[137] By 1987, this percentage decreased dramatically to 11 percent overall in the United States and to 19 percent in San Francisco.[137] Although this decline was steepest among homosexual/bisexual men, it was observed among persons in all risk groups.[138] In subsequent years, the proportion of all persons presenting with Kaposi sarcoma has declined only slightly from 8 percent in 1988 to 7 percent in 1992. The reason for this proportional decrease in new cases of AIDS manifesting as Kaposi sarcoma is not completely understood. Studies in San Francisco suggest that the decline is not secondary to diagnostic bias or selective underreporting.[137] The possibility of a concomitant decrease in exposure to an infectious or environmental cofactor necessary for the development of Kaposi sarcoma has been suggested, but remains unproven.[138] Interestingly, in a prospective follow-up study of homosexual and bisexual men, the incidence rate of Kaposi sarcoma as the initial AIDS-defining diagnosis declined from 1.7 per 100 person-years in 1985 to 1.3 in 1987, but then increased to 2.1 in 1991.[135] The authors hypothesized that the more recent increase in Kaposi sarcoma in this cohort might be explained by progressive immunosuppression associated with longer survival. Similarly, the risk of other clinical conditions such as non-Hodgkin's lymphomas may be increased for HIV-infected persons who survive for prolonged periods of time with advanced immunodeficiency.[139]

Several studies have shown that persons with HIV-related immunosuppression are at increased risk of bacterial pneumonia,[21,140] which can result in significant morbidity and mortality.[19,20] One study among injecting drug users found that the annual incidence rate of bacterial pneumonia was five times higher for those who were HIV-infected than for those who are seronegative injecting drug users.[140] *Streptococcus pneumoniae* is the most commonly isolated bacterial pathogen and has been reported to precede the onset of AIDS in 57–81 percent of persons with HIV-infection.[141] In a population-based survey in San Francisco, the rate of pneumococcal bacteremia (89 percent of HIV-infected patients with bacteremia had pneumonia as a major clinical syndrome) among persons with AIDS was nearly 100 times higher than rates reported before the HIV epidemic.[142] The risk of pneumonia in HIV-infected patients is inversely related to their CD4+ T-lymphocyte counts.[21]

Precursor lesions to invasive cervical cancer such as cervical dysplasia-neoplasia and genital papillomavirus infection are more commonly diagnosed in HIV-infected women than in other women.[22,143] In a prospective clinic-based study of more than 500 women, HIV-infected women were nearly three times more likely to have colposcopy- or biopsy-confirmed cervical intraepithelial neoplasia (CIN) than HIV-seronegative women.[144] This risk was independent of other potentially confounding factors such as sexual behavior. In this same study, although HIV-infected women had an increased prevalence (52 percent) of human papillomavirus (HPV) compared with uninfected women (22 percent), HPV infection was strongly associated with CIN in both groups of women.[144,145] The increased risk for HPV and the development of CIN in HIV-infected women was related to the degree of HIV-related immunosuppression.[22,145] Whether the increased frequency of these precursor conditions will translate into a significantly increased frequency of invasive cervical cancer is the subject of current study.

HIV Infection and Tuberculosis. After several decades of declining incidence, the number of new cases of tuberculosis in the United States has increased annually since 1986.[146] This increase is inextricably linked to the HIV epidemic. More than 100,000 persons in the United States are estimated to be coinfected with HIV and *M. tuberculosis*.[147] In a survey of tuberculosis clinics in 14 U.S. cities, HIV seroprevalence was highest in clinics in New York City (46 percent), Newark, NJ (34 percent), Boston (27 percent), and Miami (24 percent).[66] Both tuberculosis and HIV infection disproportionately affect racial/ethnic minorities and the urban poor.[146] In one analysis, black and Hispanic adults who died with AIDS were nearly three times more likely than whites also to have tuberculosis.[148]

HIV infection is a strong risk factor for the development of active tuberculosis in persons with latent *M. tuberculosis* infection. In a prospective study of injecting drug users with documented positive tuberculin skin tests, the observed incidence of active tuberculosis was 7.9 per 100 person-years for 49 HIV-infected persons compared with no cases among 62 HIV seronegative persons.[17] The risk of active tuberculosis in HIV-seropositive persons in this study—14 percent over 2 years[17]—contrasts strikingly with the estimated 10 percent lifetime risk in HIV-negative persons with latent tuberculosis infection.[149] In addition, HIV-infected persons are at greatly increased risk of developing active, symptomatic tuberculosis after their initial exposure and subsequent infection with *M. tuberculosis*.[150]

Recently, there has been a notable rise in drug-resistant tuberculosis in the United States.[151] For example, in New York City, the proportion of isolates resistant to one or more antituberculosis drugs increased from 10 percent in 1982–84 to 23 percent in 1991.[152] Persons with or at risk for HIV infection (especially injecting drug users) appear to be at increased risk for active infection with drug-resistant strains of *M. tuberculosis*.[152] This is due, in part, to their susceptibility to develop active disease rapidly after infection. Outbreaks of multidrug-resistant tuberculosis (e.g., resistant to both isoniazid and rifampin and/or other drugs) have been characterized by (1) a high prevalence of HIV infection among the outbreak cases (range 20–100 percent); (2) a high mortality rate among persons infected with resistant strains (range 72–89 percent); (3) a short median interval between diagnosis and death (range 4–16 weeks); and (4) nosocomial transmission to health care and other workers.[151] There have been at least 20 health care workers who developed multidrug-resistant tuberculosis in association with these outbreaks (CDC, unpublished data).[151,153-155] Many, but not all, of these reports were from health care facilities in urban areas with high rates of HIV infection in the population.

Mortality of Persons with HIV Infection and AIDS

Through December 31, 1992, 68 percent of the 249,199 adolescents and adults diagnosed with AIDS in the United States were reported to have died.[38] Reported fatalities increase as time from the diagnosis of AIDS increases, with 43 percent reported to have died within 1 year of diagnosis and 62 and 75 percent reported to have died 2 and 3 years, respectively, after diagnosis. Of 1622 HIV-infected persons who received medical care for their infection and who died in 10 U.S. cities from January 1990 through August 1992, 1578 (97 percent) were diagnosed with an AIDS-defining condition before death.[156]

In 1990, for all ages, HIV infection was the tenth leading cause of death for persons in the United States and caused the largest increase (13 percent) in mortality among the 15 leading causes of death.[42] The impact of HIV-related mortality is greatest among young adults.[157] Approximately three-fourths of the HIV-related deaths occurred among persons 25–44 years of age. For this age group, in 1990, HIV infection was the second leading cause of death for men and the sixth leading cause of death for women, causing 17 percent of deaths in men and 5 percent of deaths in women of this age group.[157] HIV-related death rates in this age group were highest for black males (105.0 per 100,000 population) followed by white males (31.4), black females (24.4), and white females (1.5). Provisional data for 1992 indicate that HIV infection became the leading cause of death for men 25 to 44 years of age and the fourth leading cause of death among women in this age group.[157a]

In 1990, HIV infection was the leading cause of death for persons 25–44 years of age in many metropolitan areas of the United States.[42] For young men, HIV infection was the leading cause of death in 64 cities in 27 states and caused 16–61 percent of deaths in these cities (Fig. 5A). For young women, HIV infection was the leading cause of death in nine cities in five states on the East Coast, where the proportion of deaths due to HIV ranged from 15 to 43 percent (Fig. 5B). Subsequent analysis of mortality data for 1991 has shown that the number of cities where HIV infection is the leading cause of death increased.[157b]

One measure of premature mortality is the years of potential life lost (YPLL) before the age of 65.[158] From 1989 to 1990, YPLL before the age of 65 years attributed to AIDS and HIV infection increased by 13 percent. When final mortality data are analyzed for 1991, HIV/AIDS is projected to be the fifth leading cause of YPLL before the age of 65 years.

The survival of persons diagnosed with AIDS-defining conditions has increased over time. Studies of persons diagnosed from 1980 through 1987 estimated a median length of survival from diagnosis of an AIDS-defining condition to death of 10.0–12.5 months and a survival rate 3 years after diagnosis of an AIDS-defining condition of 9–22 percent.[159-163] These studies found that the type and number of opportunistic illnesses, older age at the time of AIDS diagnosis, black race and Hispanic ethnicity, and female sex were associated with shortened survival. Persons diagnosed in the more recent years had longer survival, most likely reflecting earlier diagnosis of HIV infection and related illnesses due to the availability of serologic tests to diagnose HIV infection. Longer survival was associated with the diagnosis of Kaposi sarcoma, particularly when it occurred at an earlier stage of illness as measured by immunologic parameters.[159-166] However, this difference in survival has decreased over time. From 1983 to 1987 in San Francisco, the median survival of persons with *P. carinii* pneumonia increased from 10 to 18 months, while the survival for those with Kaposi sarcoma alone decreased from 20 to 18 months, and the survival of persons with other opportunistic illnesses increased slightly from 9 to 10 months.[161] The decrease in survival for persons

with Kaposi sarcoma may be due in part to the occurrence of this disease later in the course of HIV infection.

Observational studies have indicated that the use of antiretroviral therapy and the use of prophylactic therapy to prevent *P. carinii* pneumonia are associated with improved survival of persons with AIDS.[161,163,167-173] For HIV-infected persons receiving zidovudine, those with CD4+ T-lymphocyte counts of less than 50 cells/μl are at the greatest risk of death.[174,175] The time in the course of HIV disease during which zidovudine therapy should be initiated for maximum therapeutic benefit has not yet been determined (see Ch. 104).[167,172,176]

AIDS IN CHILDREN

Through December 31, 1992, a total of 4249 cases of AIDS in children less than 13 years of age were reported in the United States. Pediatric cases of AIDS include children who have one of a broad range of "indicator" diseases (Table 1).[9] Although the spectrum of AIDS-defining opportunistic infections and malignancies in children overlaps considerably with those that are included in the surveillance case definition for adults and adolescents, there are some differences. Three important exceptions for children younger than 13 years of age are the inclusion of lymphoid interstitial pneumonia and/or pulmonary lymphoid hyperplasia (LIP/PLH complex) and recurrent bacterial infections, and the exclusion of a threshold CD4+ T-lymphocyte count (e.g., <200 CD4+ T lymphocytes/μl). Longitudinal evaluations of lymphocyte subsets in both HIV-infected and uninfected children have been conducted recently and suggest some measure of prognostic value.[177,178] However, because normal newborns and young infants have a prominent lymphocytosis,[179] moderate declines in CD4+ T lymphocytes by adult standards can represent significant impairment in young children.[177,180]

Pediatric cases are ordered into a hierarchy of mutually exclusive exposure categories.[38] Of the 1463 children reported in 1991–92, 3 percent had hemophilia or another coagulation disorder; 90 percent were born to mothers either with or at risk for HIV infection; 4 percent received a transfusion of blood, blood components, or tissue; and 3 percent had an undetermined risk. Similar to adults, when follow-up information is available, most children who are initially reported with an undetermined risk are reclassified. In one study, half of those children who were reclassified had mothers who used injecting drugs or were partners of men who used injecting drugs.[181] Of the 1311 children born to mothers with, or at risk for, HIV infection, 56 percent had mothers who reported injecting drugs or having sex with an injecting drug user. The remaining mothers acquired their infection through heterosexual contact with infected men other than injecting drug users (17 percent); received a transfusion of blood or blood components (3 percent); or had an undetermined risk for HIV infection (24 percent).

Temporal trends for individual pediatric exposure categories vary. Similar to adults, the incidence of AIDS in children who received blood and blood products (including children with hemophilia) began to decline in 1989 (Fig. 6). Children with perinatally acquired HIV infection have accounted for the largest number of pediatric AIDS cases throughout the epidemic. However, with the number of reported cases in blood and blood product recipients declining over time, there has been a corresponding increase in the proportion of cases attributable to perinatal transmission. In 1982, perinatally acquired cases accounted for 62 percent of all AIDS cases in children; this has steadily increased to 90 percent of cases reported in 1992. The rate of AIDS cases associated with perinatal HIV transmission increased most rapidly in the mid-1980s, but appears to have slowed beginning in 1990 (Fig. 6). This most likely reflects changes in reporting practices or delay in onset of AIDS secondary to antiretrovirals and other therapeutic agents, and not a stabilization of HIV seroprevalence in childbearing women.[79,92,182] Extrapolating from the national HIV serosurvey

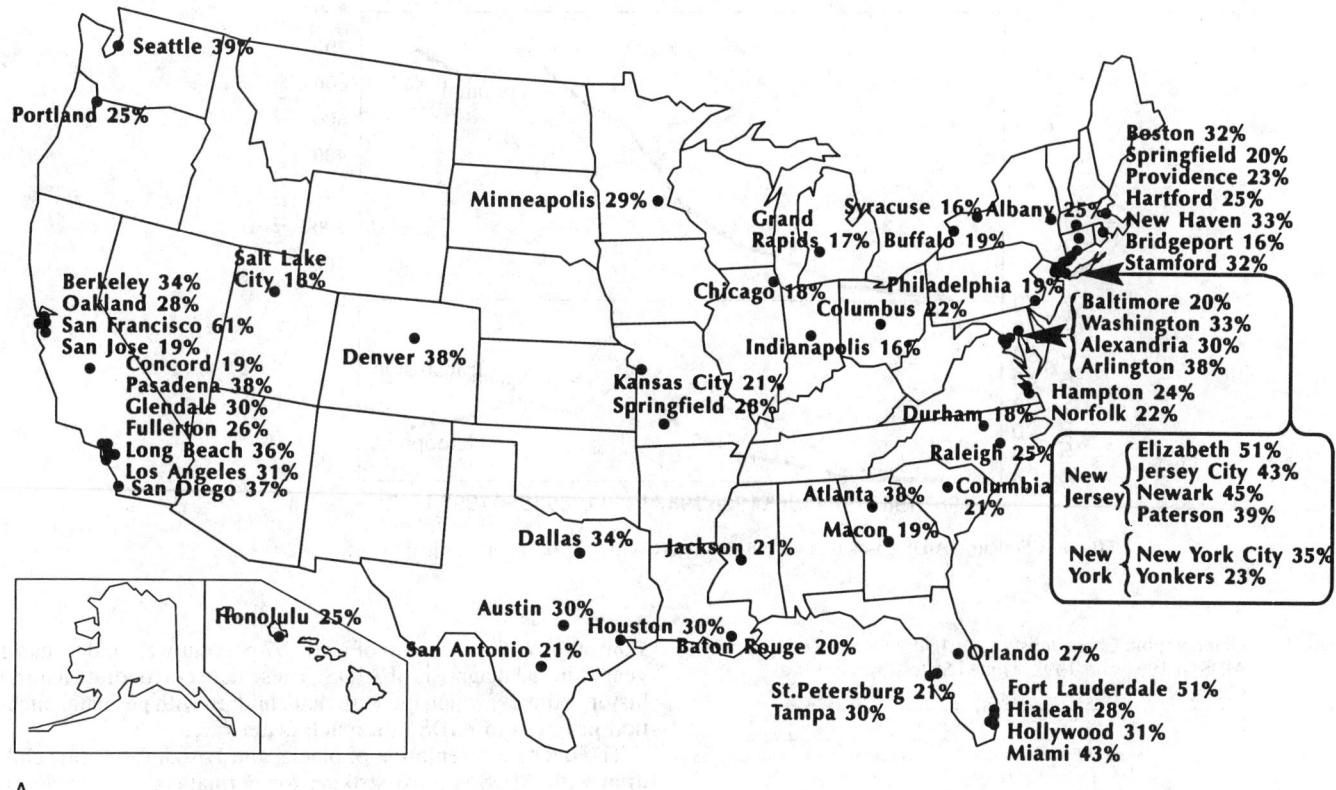

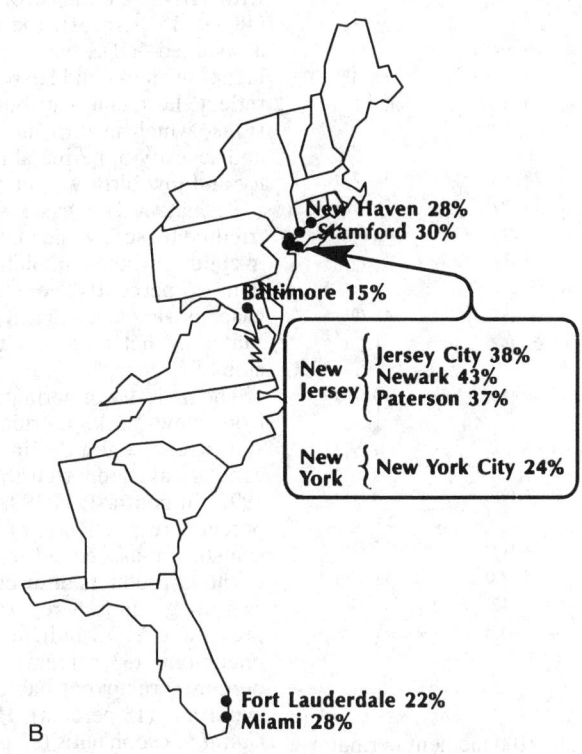

FIG. 5. The proportion of deaths caused by HIV infection in 1990 among **(A)** young men (aged 25–44 years) and **(B)** young women (aged 24–44 years) in selected U.S. cities of at least 100,000 population in which HIV was the leading cause of deaths in young men and for which the denominator was at least 25 deaths from all causes. (From Selik et al.[42])

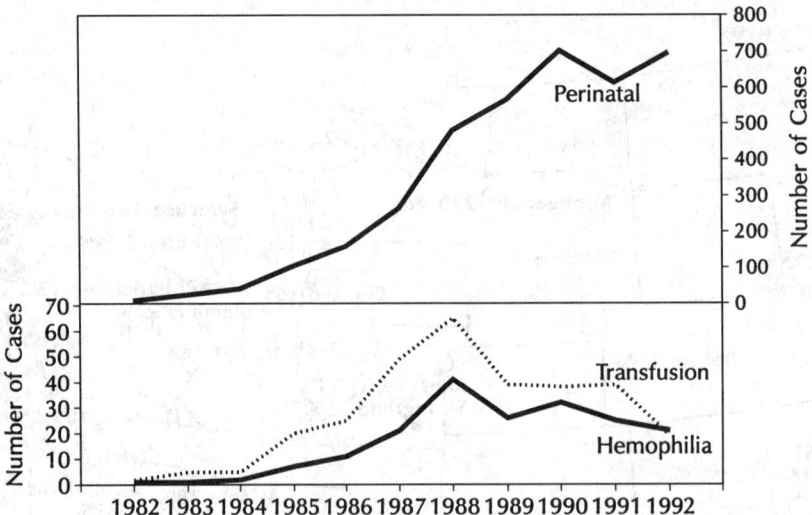

FIG. 6. Pediatric AIDS cases by exposure category and year of report, United States, 1982–1992.

TABLE 5. Demographic Characteristics of Children Reported With AIDS in 1991 and 1992, United States, by Exposure Category

	Exposure Category		
	Perinatal (N = 1311)	Transfusion (N = 58)	Hemophilia (N = 46)
Characteristic	No. (Percent)	No. (Percent)	No. (Percent)
Age at diagnosis			
0–6 months	376 (29)	2 (3)	1 (2)
7–12 months	186 (14)	1 (2)	0 (0)
13 months–4 years	546 (42)	9 (16)	1 (2)
5–10 years	184 (14)	36 (62)	21 (46)
>10 years	17 (1)	10 (17)	22 (48)
Mean/median age at diagnosis (years)	2.4/1.4	7.6/8.1	10.3/11.0
Race			
White	201 (15)	28 (48)	33 (72)
Black	820 (63)	13 (22)	6 (13)
Hispanic	278 (21)	14 (24)	6 (13)
Other/unknown	12 (1)	3 (6)	1 (2)
Sex			
Male	654 (50)	33 (57)	45 (98)
Female	657 (50)	25 (43)	1 (2)
AIDS-indicator diseases[a]			
Pneumocystis carinii pneumonia	430 (33)	9 (16)	10 (22)
Lymphoid interstitial pneumonitis	282 (22)	9 (16)	3 (7)
HIV encephalopathy	203 (16)	5 (9)	6 (13)
Recurrent bacterial infections	198 (15)	12 (21)	7 (15)
Wasting syndrome	188 (14)	13 (22)	11 (24)
Candida esophagitis	158 (12)	7 (12)	14 (30)

[a] Percentages exceed 100 percent because some children were reported with more than one AIDS-indicator disease.

of childbearing women,[76] approximately 2100 incident perinatal infections occurred in the United States in 1991.[77]

Examination of the demographic and clinical characteristics of children with AIDS reveals considerable variation depending on their mode of exposure (Table 5). While 43 percent of children who acquired their HIV infection perinatally are initially diagnosed at 1 year of age or less, children with AIDS who received contaminated blood or blood products are usually older at the time of initial diagnosis. Of children who received transfu-

sions at or within 1 month of birth, 97 percent were older than 1 year at initial diagnosis of AIDS. These data corroborate natural history studies, which indicate that children with perinatal infection progress to AIDS at a much faster rate.

The over-representation of blacks and Hispanics among children with AIDS is most striking for perinatal cases (Table 5), reflecting the racial/ethnic distribution of women with HIV infection. Although children with transfusion-associated AIDS reported in 1991–92 were more likely to be white than children with AIDS resulting from perinatally acquired HIV infection (48 vs. 15 percent), the cumulative incidence of transfusion-associated AIDS has been reported to be two to three times higher in blacks and Hispanics than whites.[183] This may, in part, reflect the racial distribution of children who receive transfusions, which in turn may reflect differences in the frequency and severity of perinatal medical problems related to prematurity and low birth weight.[183]

Perinatal AIDS cases reported in 1991–92 were equally distributed by sex, while males accounted for the majority of cases in children with hemophilia (98 percent) and in transfusion recipients (57 percent). The sex distribution of transfusion-associated cases is similar to that for all transfused infants in the United States in that more male than female infants receive transfusions.[183]

The majority of perinatal AIDS cases continue to be reported from New York, Florida, New Jersey, and Texas, but these states represent a declining proportion of cases—from 83 percent of cases reported through 1984 to 55 percent reported in 1992. In contrast, in 1992 these four states reported 33 and 47 percent, respectively, of cases in children with hemophilia or transfusion-associated infection due in part to the distribution of blood products after collection.

Among children reported with AIDS in 1991–92, the most prevalent AIDS indicator diseases reported were *P. carinii* pneumonia (33 percent), lymphoid interstitial pneumonitis (21 percent), recurrent bacterial infections (15 percent), wasting syndrome (15 percent), HIV encephalopathy (15 percent), and *Candida* esophagitis (12 percent). The proportional distribution of these opportunistic conditions varied by exposure category (Table 5). The reported frequency of each of these opportunistic diseases represents a minimum estimate of their actual incidence among children with AIDS, since there is underreporting of opportunistic diseases diagnosed after the initial case report to CDC. For example, disseminated nontuberculous mycobacterial disease was reported to the CDC for 6 percent of 3472 children with AIDS through 1991; in comparison, 11 percent of 739 children enrolled in an active HIV infection surveillance project had disseminated nontuberculous mycobacterial disease.[184]

The relative frequency of certain AIDS-indicator diseases appears to vary with age. For example, lymphoid interstitial pneumonitis is more common in older children. Of children reported with AIDS in 1991–92 who were diagnosed before or at 12 months of age, 7 percent had lymphoid interstitial pneumonitis compared with 36 percent of children diagnosed at ages 1–4 years. In contrast, of children diagnosed before or at 12 months of age, 58 percent had *P. carinii* compared with 14 percent of those aged 1–4 years. This early age at onset, as well as the high mortality rate associated with *P. carinii* pneumonia in infants and children, reinforces recommendations that HIV-infected infants should be diagnosed as soon as possible after birth so that prophylaxis can be promptly initiated when indicated.[185]

Disease presentation and progression in children with perinatally acquired HIV infection have been characterized as fitting into a "biomodal" pattern.[186,187] In general, one group of children develops HIV-related symptoms that can include AIDS-defining, life-threatening opportunistic conditions at an early age (i.e., between 4 and 8 months) and has a rapid and poor rate of survival; other children develop less severe HIV-related symptoms, often at a later age, and consequently have a much better survival experience.

Overall, 53 percent of children with AIDS reported through national surveillance are reported to have died. Survival in HIV-infected children is closely related to age at initial diagnosis of AIDS and to the specific AIDS-defining condition. Case-fatality rates derived from national surveillance data indicate that 65 percent of infants aged 1 year or younger at diagnosis have died compared with 44 percent of children between 13 months and 4 years. The shortest durations of survival, ranging from 1 to 9 months, have been reported for children with an initial AIDS diagnosis of *P. carinii* pneumonia.[188–190] In contrast, longer median survival times ranging from 65 to 72 months have been reported for LIP.[188,189] In a longitudinal evaluation of 789 children enrolled in the New York State Medicaid Programs, the proportion of children younger than 6 months of age who survived 1 year after being diagnosed with AIDS (40–54 percent) was substantially less than children older than 6 months (70–85 percent), irrespective of the AIDS-indicator disease.[189] Similar to adults, it is likely that early and effective treatment for children, such as zidovudine, *P. carinii* prophylaxis, and intravenous immunoglobulin, will impact positively on survival by delaying disease progression. Recent declines in the proportion of reported perinatal AIDS cases with *P. carinii* pneumonia are modest compared with the decrease in *P. carinii* pneumonia among adults with AIDS.[190] This emphasizes the need for early diagnosis of HIV infection among children at risk for perinatally acquired HIV infection and frequent and careful clinical monitoring subsequently.

MODES OF TRANSMISSION

More than a decade after the initial studies were conducted to determine the ways in which HIV is transmitted, surveillance and epidemiologic data throughout the world continue to support strongly three primary modes of transmission: sexual contact; exposure to blood, largely through injecting drug use and transfusion; and perinatal transmission from infected mothers to their infants.

Sexual Transmission

Sexual contact is the predominant mode of HIV transmission throughout the world. However, the geographic distribution of cases attributable to homosexual and heterosexual transmission varies markedly.[191] Whereas heterosexual transmission is the major mode of spread of HIV infection in Africa, most of South America, and the Caribbean, it accounts for a smaller, albeit

growing, proportion of AIDS cases in North America and Europe, where male-to-male sexual transmission continues to account for most reported cases of AIDS.[192]

The likelihood of acquiring or transmitting HIV infection through a single sexual contact is directly related to certain correlates of exposure, such as the number of partners and the prevalence of HIV infection in the population. Sexual transmission of HIV occurs with variable efficiency and is affected by overlapping factors related both to the infectiousness of the source partner, including properties of the infecting virus, and the susceptibility of the recipient partner.[193] None of these factors can account entirely for differences in transmission efficiency, nor are they absolute. Nonetheless, they can serve as a useful point of reference in attempting to understand the observed differences in the epidemiology of HIV through sexual contact, whether on a global scale or between individuals of the same or different sex.

Infectiousness of the Source Partner. Variability in the infectiousness of the source partner has been suggested by observations that some persons appear to be highly efficient transmitters of HIV through sexual contact. Such efficiency is manifested by the infection of a high proportion of an individual's sexual partners,[193,194] often after only a single contact.[195,196]

Multiple lines of evidence point to an association of increased infectiousness of the source partner with the development of severe immunodeficiency. This association was first suggested in a prospective study of infected hemophilic men and their female sex partners.[197] Subsequent epidemiologic studies have supported the correlation of advanced disease stage, as measured by diseases indicative of AIDS or decreased numbers of peripheral CD4+ T lymphocytes, with an increased likelihood of transmission to sexual partners.[198–201] Furthermore, this association has been observed for male-to-male, male-to-female, and female-to-male transmission. A more recent study found an inverse dose-response relationship between the absolute number of CD4+ T lymphocytes in the source partner and the infection rate among sexual partners, with increasing rates of HIV infection observed in recipient partners as the number of CD4+ T lymphocytes in the source partner decreased.[200] These observations correlate well with laboratory studies demonstrating that both the ability to isolate HIV from semen as well as the concentration of virus in plasma are inversely proportional to the number of CD4+ T-lymphocyte cells.[202–204] In another study, HIV was isolated more frequently from the cervicovaginal secretions of women with AIDS than from those of women in earlier stages of disease.[205] In addition to a low CD4+ T-lymphocyte count, other indicators of increased viral titer in the blood and probable concomitantly increased excretion of HIV include the presence of HIV antigen, the absence of HIV antibody, and elevated CD8+ T lymphocytes.[193] At least one study has suggested that men with higher numbers of suppressor cells are more likely to transmit HIV to their male partners than are men with fewer suppressor cells.[206] These findings notwithstanding, all infected persons must be presumed to be capable of sexually transmitting HIV, regardless of their stage of infection.

Antiretroviral therapy may influence infectivity and the subsequent risk of transmission through sexual contact. First, treatment with zidovudine has been associated with decreased detection of HIV in semen.[203] In addition, at least two epidemiologic studies have demonstrated that antiretroviral therapy was associated with a reduced risk of HIV transmission among discordant heterosexual couples.[207,208] Further studies are needed to evaluate the influence of antiviral drugs on HIV transmission. However, any protective effect exerted by zidovudine or other antiviral drugs is likely to be partial and not render an individual completely noninfectious.[209]

The presence of antibodies to certain HIV-1 antigens may influence the probability of transmission of HIV through sexual contact. For example, neutralizing antibodies to the V3 loop region of the viral gp120 envelope protein inhibit virus infectivity.[210] Limited epidemiologic data suggest that the presence of V3 antibodies may be associated with a reduced rate of heterosexual transmission.[211]

Because HIV is present in both blood cells and cervicovaginal secretions, sexual contact with an HIV-infected woman during menses has been postulated to increase the risk of female-to-male HIV transmission. However, information about such an association has been inconsistent. While cross-sectional surveys have not found such an association,[212,213] one large longitudinal study of heterosexual couples found that the risk of HIV transmission was increased for men who reported sexual contact during their partner's menses.[198] However, such contact was not an absolute requirement, as 8 of 19 infected men in this study had never had intercourse during their partner's menses. Nonmenstrual vaginal and penile bleeding have also been reported to be associated with HIV transmission.[214,215]

The probability of saliva from HIV-infected persons transmitting HIV through oral-oral or oral-genital sexual contact is very low. HIV is found in very low concentrations in the saliva of infected persons.[216,217] Moreover, when sex practices result in the mixing of saliva with genital secretions, the precise mechanism of transmission cannot be determined with certainty.

Epidemiologic and laboratory data indicate that genital ulcer disease in the source partner is an important factor facilitating HIV transmission. The higher rates of heterosexual transmission in Africa may be explained in part by the higher prevalences of genital ulcer disease in many developing countries, including those in Africa, than in countries in North America and Europe.[218] Genital ulcers likely increase the infectiousness of both male and female source partners.[219,220] In a prospective study of over 400 men who acquired a sexually transmitted disease (including HIV infection) from a group of prostitutes in Nairobi, Kenya, seroconversion to HIV was independently associated with the concurrent acquisition of genital ulcer disease.[221] Genital ulcer disease may have augmented the women's infectiousness by increasing viral shedding in the female genital tract through a local inflammatory response mediated by the recruitment and activation of HIV-infected macrophages and lymphocytes to the disrupted mucosal surface.[221,222] The recovery of HIV from genital ulcers in HIV-infected women supports this hypothesis.[223]

Nonulcerative sexually transmitted diseases may also enhance sexual transmission of HIV. In a longitudinal study of female prostitutes in Kinshasa, Zaire, incident gonorrhea, chlamydial infections, and trichomoniasis were associated with an elevated rate of HIV seroconversion in these women, independent of number of partners and frequency of condom use.[224] However, because the prevalences of neither HIV infection nor these sexually transmitted diseases were measured directly among the male source partners, it is possible that men with these sexually transmitted diseases may simply have had a higher prevalence of HIV than men without them. Another study has shown that gonococcal or chlamydial infection in the male source partner can result in an increased number of T lymphocytes, monocytes, and macrophages in the male genital tract,[225] which could increase the man's infectiousness. Thus, as with genital ulcer disease, additional studies will be needed to determine if nonulcerative sexually transmitted diseases facilitate HIV transmission by increasing the infectiousness of the source partner, increasing the susceptibility of the recipient partner, or augmenting both processes concurrently.[224]

Rates of heterosexual transmission of HIV have been reported to vary depending on the mode by which the source partner presumably acquired HIV. In some studies, rates of HIV infection among partners of hemophilic men and transfusion recipients have been lower than those among partners of injecting drug users.[195,197,214,226,227] However, these observed rates may not reflect a truly higher risk because most of these studies have been cross sectional and retrospective in design

and did not control for factors such as duration of the relationship, frequency of sexual contact, use of condoms, and presence of other risk factors for HIV infection.[228,229] Differences in the rates of transmission to partners may instead reflect biologic factors, such as stage of disease and varying levels of infectivity, the presence of other sexually transmitted diseases (in either the source partner or the recipient partner), and behavioral factors, such as unreported drug use by the recipient partner.

Similar factors must be considered when examining the comparative efficiency of male-to-female and female-to-male transmission.[228] Although findings from multiple "partner studies" suggest that male-to-female transmission is more efficient,[214,230] behavioral and biologic variables that might interact with HIV transmission need to be carefully controlled.[200] For example, in a large prospective study of heterosexual couples, men and women in advanced stages of HIV infection had similar rates of transmission; however, asymptomatic men were five times more efficient transmitters than asymptomatic women.[198] These findings suggest that, as the HIV epidemic matures in the United States and Europe and more women develop symptomatic HIV infection, increased female-to-male transmission may be observed.[191,212]

Susceptibility of the Recipient Partner. Genital and anorectal ulceration or mucosal disruption due to infection has emerged as one of the most consistent and biologically plausible factors affecting the acquisition of HIV infection through sexual transmission. While ulcerations that disrupt the genital epithelium can serve simply as a portal of entry for HIV-infected genital secretions, ulcerations may have a more complex role in HIV transmission. Genital ulcerations cause an inflammatory response that in turn may increase the number of stimulated T lymphocytes at the surface of the ulceration.[222] In vitro, stimulated T lymphocytes are more susceptible to infection with HIV than are unstimulated cells.[231]

A number of epidemiologic studies have demonstrated that a history of genital ulcer disease in the recipient partner is a risk factor for acquiring HIV in both heterosexual and homosexual men[222,232] and women.[220,232] While this association may not be surprising, two seroepidemiologic studies of homosexual men have convincingly demonstrated that genital ulcer disease is not simply a marker for increased sexual activity.[222,233] Rather, infection with HIV was independently associated with serologic evidence of prior syphilis or infection with herpes simplex virus type 2, the two most common causes of genital ulcers among homosexual men in the United States. In another study among female prostitutes in Nairobi, 60 percent of seroconverting women experienced one or more episodes of genital ulcers before seroconverting.[220] As in other studies,[224] this association may be confounded by an increased seroprevalence of HIV infection among male partners with sexually transmitted diseases.

Nonulcerative sexually transmitted diseases such as gonorrhea and chlamydial infection may also facilitate acquisition of HIV infection by causing mucosal disruption of the genital tract.[220,224] Other nonulcerative sexually transmitted diseases (e.g., urethritis, cervicitis, balanitis, vaginosis, and genital warts) and their associated inflammatory responses may increase the risk of acquiring HIV infection.[224,234] The higher frequency of balanitis in uncircumcised men has been postulated as a partial explanation for the increased risk of HIV observed among uncircumcised men in developing countries.[221,234,235] Alternatively, the intact foreskin may be more susceptible to traumatic injury during sexual contact.[221,234]

Noninfectious causes of ulcerations of the genital tract may also pose a risk for sexual transmission of HIV. For example, frequent use of the nonoxynol 9 contraceptive sponge by female prostitutes in Nairobi was associated with increased rates of genital ulcers, vulvitis, and HIV seroconversion in one study.[236] The increased risk for HIV acquisition may be attributable to chemical irritation from the spermicide or to mechanical trauma, both of which can result in inflammation and ulceration.[237] The prevention or prompt identification and treatment of both infectious and noninfectious causes of genital ulcerations should be useful adjuncts in reducing sexual transmission of HIV.

Certain traumatic sexual practices that result in rectal mucosal disruption and lesions have been associated with HIV infection. Early epidemiologic studies of homosexual men found that receptive anal intercourse, "fisting," and douching increased the risk of HIV transmission.[238–240] Subsequent studies have both supported these findings and extended the association of receptive anal intercourse to heterosexual transmission of HIV.[198,199,206,215]

Although cases of AIDS have been reported among lesbian and bisexual women, most were infected through injecting drug use practices.[241] Female-to-female transmission of HIV appears to be very rare.[242] Only two such instances have been reported, and both were associated with traumatic sex practices.[243,244]

No consistent association between oral contraceptive use by women and acquisition of HIV infection has been found. In one study, women who reported taking oral contraceptives had a reduced risk of HIV infection.[199] However, in a longitudinal cohort study of Nairobi prostitutes and a cross-sectional study of sex partners at a sexually transmitted disease clinic in Nairobi, oral contraceptive use was an independent risk factor for HIV seroconversion and for prevalent infection, respectively.[213,220] In contrast, a study of prostitutes in Zaire[232] and a study of pregnant women in a rural U.S. community with a high prevalence of HIV infection[59] found no association between HIV infection and the use of oral contraceptives. The presence of cervical ectopy has been associated with an increased risk of HIV seropositivity among long-term female partners of HIV positive men in Nairobi.[213] Because oral contraceptives are associated with higher rates of ectopy, the relationship, if any, between oral contraceptives and HIV requires further study.

While anal and vaginal intercourse are the two sex practices associated with the greatest risk of transmission, other sexual activities involving exposure to semen or blood also carry a potential risk of transmission. For example, seroconversion for HIV antibody after multiple episodes of receptive oral intercourse with ejaculation has been documented.[245]

Finally, underlying immune function may affect the recipient partner's susceptibility to infection. Studies of HIV seronegative homosexual men and persons with hemophilia have demonstrated that impaired functional cellular immunity, as measured by abnormal skin testing responses, is predictive of HIV seroconversion following exposure to the virus.[246,247]

Transmission Through Injecting Drug Use

Among injecting drug users, HIV is transmitted by parenteral exposure to HIV-infected blood through use of contaminated needles and other injection equipment. Specific factors that have been associated with HIV infection among injecting drug users include duration of injecting drug use since 1977, frequency of needle sharing, number of needle-sharing partners, number of injections, median number of injections in "shooting galleries," and prevalence of HIV infection in area of residence.[41,50,248,249] The rate of HIV infection among injecting drug users varies widely among different geographic areas. In the United States, the rate of HIV infection has been highest in the Northeast.[49,250]

Most studies have found higher rates of HIV infection associated with cocaine and heroin injection than with heroin injection alone, probably due to the greater frequency of cocaine injections.[54,251,252] Among injecting drug users, poor socioeconomic conditions, homelessness, and minority race/ethnicity are associated with an increased frequency of risk behaviors and higher rates of HIV infection.[52,55,253,254] Among injecting drug users enrolled in a study in Baltimore from 1988 to 1989, the 703 HIV-infected users were more likely to have a history of syphilis

(16.8 percent) than were the 2218 uninfected injecting drug users (11.3 percent).[255] The higher rates of sexually transmitted diseases among HIV-infected injecting drug users than among uninfected users suggests that some infections are transmitted through unsafe sexual practices.[255,256]

Many injecting drug users have changed their drug-use behaviors to reduce their risk of HIV infection.[257–259] The rate of needle sharing has decreased in some areas, and the use of bleach to clean needles and other drug-use paraphernalia between uses has increased. Drug-abuse treatment, street outreach programs, needle and syringe exchange programs, AIDS educational efforts, and HIV counseling and testing programs have all been shown to be effective in reducing, but not eliminating, the risk of HIV transmission.

Transmission by Blood and Other Tissues

Recipients of unscreened blood or blood products from HIV-infected donors are at high risk for HIV infection. HIV has been transmitted through receipt of whole blood, blood cellular components, plasma, and clotting factors.[260,261] The likelihood of a person becoming infected with HIV after receiving a single-donor blood product documented to be HIV-positive approaches 100 percent.[262,263] Other blood or plasma products, such as hepatitis B immune globulin, immune serum globulin, Rh(D) immune globulin, and hepatitis B vaccine, are prepared by using one of several fractionation processes that inactivate HIV; use of these products has not been associated with transmission.[264,265]

Before serologic testing for HIV was begun in 1985, 0.04 percent of 1,200,000 donations in the United States were estimated to be HIV positive.[266] During this time an estimated 29,000 blood or blood-product recipients were exposed to HIV; since many died of underlying conditions, 12,000 of these persons were estimated to survive long enough to develop AIDS.[267] Since screening was instituted, the risk of HIV transmission through transfusion of blood screened as HIV negative has been estimated to be 1 in 36,000 to 1 to 225,000 per unit transfused.[268–270] Such rare transmissions are due to donations from recently infected donors who have not developed detectable antibody.[83,268] This "window period" is estimated to last an average of 1.5–2.1 months, with 95 percent of persons developing detectable antibody within 6 months.[104]

The risk of HIV infection for patients with hemophilia who received concentrated clotting factors composed of blood components from potentially thousands of donors was substantial before 1984–85.[271,272] Episodes of HIV transmission by transplantation of liver, heart, kidney, pancreas, bone, and possibly skin have been reported.[87,273,274] Relatively avascular tissues such as corneas and processed tissues have not been associated with transmission.[87,275]

Perinatal Transmission

Vertical transmission of HIV from an infected woman to her infant can occur during intrauterine gestation, delivery, or the postpartum period through breastfeeding. Progress has been made in elucidating risk factors that influence transmission during these three periods and in detecting infection in the newborn earlier and more reliably. However, the relative efficiency and the precise mechanisms of transmission during each period and the role of viral and other biologic cofactors remain incompletely understood.

The occurrence of intrauterine infection is supported by the detection of HIV both in fetal tissue as early as 8 weeks gestation[276] and in placental tissue infected in vivo and in vitro.[277] In addition, the 30–50 percent of infected infants who test positive by PCR or HIV culture at birth[278–280] probably reflect transmission during early or midgestational periods. Transmission to the infant early in pregnancy would presumably allow for viral replication to reach a level sufficient for detection by these tests.[281] In contrast, HIV-infected infants who test negative by PCR or HIV culture at birth may have become infected late in pregnancy or during the intrapartum period. Similarly, differences in the onset and progression of clinical disease and attendant immunodeficiency in children with prepartum- or intrapartum-acquired HIV infection may be explained in part by differences in the timing of their infection.[180,186]

Accumulating information suggests that a sizable proportion of vertical transmission may occur during the intrapartum period.[282,283] Both vaginal and cesarean delivery present frequent and varied opportunities for the infant to be exposed to infected maternal blood and/or cervicovaginal fluids. Although many studies have found statistically similar rates of transmission for vaginal and cesarean section delivery,[284–286] some have suggested that cesarean section delivery may offer a slight protective effect.[283,287] However, no randomized control trials have been conducted. Moreover, the only one of these studies[283] that evaluated elective vs. emergency cesarean sections did not find a significant difference between the two. A recent meta-analysis of available epidemiologic studies found that the overall weighted risk of perinatal HIV infection was lower for cesarean delivery (14.0 percent) than for vaginal delivery (20.2 percent).[288] Controlled trials comparing elective cesarean section delivery prior to rupture of membranes with vaginal delivery will be required to evaluate fully whether the route of delivery can influence the probability of HIV transmission.

The isolation of HIV from breast milk,[289] as well as reports of breast-feeding mothers who infected their infants after they had acquired HIV infection through postpartum blood transfusions, provided initial evidence for postnatal HIV transmission.[290] Subsequent evaluation has focused on estimating the added, or attributable, risk of perinatal transmission conveyed by breast-feeding. Several prospective cohort studies that compared breast-fed and bottle-fed infants have detected higher rates of HIV infection in breast-fed children.[283–285,291] A comprehensive analysis of available data estimated that the attributable risk of transmission through breast-feeding ranged from 14 to 29 percent.[292] Mothers who themselves acquired HIV infection in the postpartum period were more efficient transmitters, presumably because of the increased viral burden associated with primary HIV infection.[293] Epidemiologic studies[291] and mathematical models[294] have evaluated the competing risks of acquiring HIV infection by breast-feeding and the increased morbidity and mortality associated with alternatives to breast-feeding. Both approaches have found that, for children in many developing countries, the benefits from breast-feeding outweigh the risk of HIV transmission through breast-feeding.

Prospective studies of infants born to women with HIV infection have found rates of transmission ranging from 13 to 40 percent.[283–286,295] Recent comprehensive reviews have highlighted the geographic variability of observed vertical transmission rates.[180,296] The European Collaborative Study followed more than 700 infants born to HIV-infected mothers for a minimum of 18 months and found 14 percent to be infected.[283] Collaborative studies undertaken in France, Italy, and the United States have found rates of infection between 24 and 30 percent.[284–286] The highest rates of perinatally acquired HIV infection, which approach 40 percent, have been reported from Africa.[295] The disparity in these rates most likely reflects differences in the severity of maternal disease stage, nutritional status, rates of breast-feeding, study design, completeness and length of follow-up, and use of different diagnostic criteria.[180,296] The relative contribution of differences in viral strains and genetic factors is unknown.

The risk of perinatal transmission appears to vary by the disease stage of the mother. Mothers at both extremes of the clinical spectrum of HIV infection with either acute, primary infection[293] or advanced, symptomatic disease[283,295] have been reported to be more likely to transmit HIV to their infants than

asymptomatic seropositive women. Cellular markers of maternal immune status associated with an increased likelihood of perinatal transmission include high CD8 + T lymphocytes[297] and low CD4 + T lymphocytes.[283,295,297] Reports assessing the predictive value of maternal HIV p24 antigenemia for perinatal transmission have been conflicting.[283,298] Although some early studies found a correlation between maternal antibodies to specific epitopes within one of the variable regions (V3 loop) of the HIV envelope protein and lower rates of mother-to-infant transmission,[299,300] subsequent evaluations have not confirmed these findings.[301,302]

In addition to maternal risk factors, placental factors that disrupt the maternal-fetal barrier can increase perinatal transmission. In one study conducted among Zairean women, the presence of histologic chorioamnionitis and funisitis was associated with an overall twofold increase in transmission risk.[297] Placental inflammation posed a fourfold increased risk for infants born to HIV-infected women with normal CD8 + and CD4 + T lymphocytes.

Epidemiologic studies to assess the risk of perinatal transmission and to identify risk factors have been greatly aided by significant advancements in the development of laboratory tests to detect HIV infection in infants by 6 months of age. Infants born to HIV-infected mothers have passively acquired maternal antibody to HIV that persists for 12–18 months. For infants 0–6 months of age, PCR and virus culture offer the greatest sensitivity and specificity for detecting HIV-infection.[303] Nonetheless, these tests can detect only one-half or fewer of the perinatally infected infants, reflecting a very low viral burden, sequestration of the virus in other tissues, or recent transmission to the infant either late in the third trimester or at the time of delivery.[304] Other options for diagnosing HIV infection in infants include HIV-specific IgA assays and an in vitro antibody production assay, such as the ELISPOT.[281] However, the overall sensitivity and specificity of these tests are less than those of PCR and viral culture, especially for infants less than 3 months of age.[281]

Transmission of HIV in Health Care Settings

Percutaneous, mucous membrane, and cutaneous exposures to blood-contaminated body fluids can occur frequently in the health care setting.[305–307] Such exposures have resulted in occupationally acquired HIV infection in health care workers.[308–311] Data from several prospective surveillance projects among health care workers indicate that the average risk of seroconversion after a needlestick injury with HIV-infected blood is approximately 0.3 percent.[308,309] Transmission of HIV after mucous membrane and cutaneous exposures to blood has been reported, although too few seroconversions have occurred in prospective studies to quantify risk precisely. Data from 21 studies worldwide include one seroconversion (0.09 percent) among 1107 mucous membrane exposures.[310]

Because health care workers are more likely than patients to have contact with blood in the health care setting, the risk of HIV transmission from patient to health care worker clearly exceeds that of health care worker to patient.[312] Transmission of HIV from a health care worker to patients has been documented in only one instance, in a dental practice in Florida.[313,314] The precise events that resulted in the dentist transmitting HIV to 6 of approximately 1100 patients tested for HIV in this practice remain unknown. However, the six patients had no other confirmed exposures to HIV other than receiving treatment from the dentist, and each was infected with a viral strain that was very similar to that of the dentist but dissimilar to those from other HIV-infected persons in the local area.[313,315] The very small risk of a health care worker transmitting HIV to a patient probably depends on several factors, including the type of procedure; the technique, skill, and medical condition of the health care worker; and the titer of circulating virus.[312,316]

Two patients undergoing nuclear medicine procedures have been reported to have been infected through inadvertent intravenous injections of blood or other material from HIV-infected patients.[317] Also, transmission of HIV through percutaneous or mucocutaneous exposures to blood or other body substances has occurred in homes in which health care has been provided.[318,318a] Transmission of HIV from patient to patient through improper sterilization or reuse of contaminated needles and syringes has been reported in Romania and the former Soviet Union.[319,320] Similarly, preliminary results of an investigation in Australia suggest that a breach in infection control precautions caused HIV to be transmitted from one patient to four other patients during minor surgical procedures performed on the same day by an HIV-negative surgeon.[320a] A more detailed review of transmission in the health care setting can be found in Chapter 285.

Other Modes of Transmission

Although HIV has been isolated from a variety of body fluids,[203–205,216,217,289,321–323] only contacts with blood, semen, other genital secretions, and breast milk have been implicated as sources of infection. HIV infection is acquired through exposure to blood principally through injecting drug use and receipt of contaminated blood, blood products, organs, and tissues. Exposure of nonintact skin to blood after a motor vehicle accident and a sports injury have been reported to result in HIV infection, but these are rare occurrences.[324,325]

Vaginal and anal intercourse are the predominant ways in which persons are exposed to HIV-infected semen and cervicovaginal fluids. However, transmission of HIV through intravaginal insemination with unprocessed donor semen[326,327] and through intrauterine insemination with processed semen[328] have both been reported. Although data regarding the magnitude of the risk are conflicting,[326–328] there is no evidence that any procedure can reliably eliminate HIV from semen.[328]

Laboratory and epidemiologic studies indicate that the infectivity of saliva from HIV-infected persons through human bites or occupational contact is extremely low. Furthermore, definitive attribution of HIV transmission to contact with saliva is difficult because saliva is often commingled with blood in these settings. The low risk of saliva-mediated HIV transmission is likely attributable to the very low concentrations of HIV in the saliva of infected persons,[216,217] as well as to the presence of HIV inhibitory activity in saliva.[329] One case report of two siblings infected with HIV suggested a bite as the route of transmission for the previously uninfected child.[330] However, because the bite did not break the skin or result in bleeding, the precise mode of transmission remains uncertain. Multiple epidemiologic studies, including occupational and household contact studies, have found no evidence of transmission via a human bite.[331] Similarly, studies of health care workers followed prospectively after percutaneous, mucous membrane (e.g., during the administration of cardiopulmonary resuscitation), or nonintact skin exposure to saliva from HIV-infected patients have not detected any instances of seroconversion to HIV antibody.[309,332]

To examine the risk of HIV transmission through causal contact, studies have evaluated more than 1000 nonsexual household contacts of both adults and children with HIV infection.[331,333–335] In these households, transmission of HIV was found only among sex partners, children born to infected mothers, and persons who themselves had risk factors for HIV infection. However, there have been 8 case reports of household transmission of HIV not associated with sexual contact, injecting drug use, or breast feeding. Five of the 8 reports were associated with documented or probable blood contact.[318a,335a–c] Two reports involved nursing care of terminally ill persons with AIDS in which a blood exposure might have occurred, but was not documented; in both reports, skin contact with other secretions and excretions occurred.[318a,335d] In the last report, a bite

was suggested but not documented to have resulted in transmission.[330]

Laboratory and epidemiologic studies have produced no evidence of replication of HIV within insects, in vitro mechanical transmission of HIV, or transmission through biting or bloodsucking insects.[336–338] The potential role of insect-mediated HIV infection was evaluated in a study of residents in a southern Florida community with a high rate of HIV infection.[339] HIV seropositivity was not associated with either epidemiologic or laboratory evidence of exposure to mosquitoes, as measured by the presence of antibodies to five arboviruses. Additional studies in Africa failed to establish an association between the presence of malaria antibodies and HIV.[340]

HIV INFECTION AND AIDS OUTSIDE THE UNITED STATES

HIV infection is a pandemic affecting almost all countries. Through June 1993, the World Health Organization (WHO) had received reports of 718,894 persons with AIDS.[341] In mid-1993, WHO estimated that as many as 2.5 million persons had developed AIDS and that 13 million persons had been infected with HIV.[341] While similar modes of transmission exist worldwide, the relative importance of the different transmission modes varies considerably by geographic area. In western Europe, North America, and Australia, as well as some parts of South America and the Caribbean, homosexual/bisexual men and injecting drug users remain the predominantly affected groups.[342] In northern Europe the majority of AIDS cases have occurred among homosexual and bisexual men, while in southern Europe more than 60 percent of persons with AIDS are injecting drug users.[343] The sex partners of injecting drug users have been particularly affected by heterosexual transmission of HIV. The proportion of infections attributed to heterosexual transmission has increased over time, particularly in Brazil and other countries in South America, where infection rates among injecting drug users are relatively high.[344,345]

In sub-Saharan Africa and some areas of the Caribbean, heterosexual contact is the most common mode of transmission.[341,346–352] High rates of HIV infection among pregnant women have resulted in a substantial number of children with perinatally acquired HIV.[342,352] The highest rates of HIV infection in Africa and some Caribbean countries are found among female prostitutes and persons treated for other sexually transmitted diseases.[224,351,352–357] Injecting drug use in less common in developing countries than in some areas of the United States. In contrast, receipt of contaminated blood products remains a major source of HIV transmission in many developing countries, and medical injections using contaminated medical devices continue to result in some HIV infections.[340,342]

HIV was introduced later (middle to late 1980s) in Asia, the Middle East, North Africa, and eastern Europe than in other regions. The HIV seroprevalence rates in these areas are variable and the major modes of transmission diverse. The explosive increase in HIV infection among injecting drug users, prostitutes, and other populations of young adults in Southeast Asia, India, Malaysia, and southeast is of particular concern.[358–366] Korea and Japan continue to have low rates of HIV infection among their populations at risk.[367,368]

In eastern Europe, rates of HIV infection are, as yet, lower than in other European countries. In Poland and Yugoslavia, HIV transmission is most commonly associated with injecting drug use, and the prevalence of HIV among persons who inject drugs is growing. In the Czech Republic, Estonia, and Bulgaria, HIV infections are typically due to sexual transmission. In the former Soviet Union and Romania, outbreaks of HIV have been related to contaminated blood products and medical equipment. In 1990, several thousand Romanian children were infected after receiving multiple injections with improperly cleaned needles and syringes and transfusions of unscreened blood.[319] In Russia, a nosocomial outbreak of HIV infection among 152 hospitalized children was associated with the multiple use of unsterilized syringes.[320]

The HIV epidemic is expected to continue to grow in the coming years, with an increasing proportion of infected persons residing in developing countries. From 1992 to 1995, 5.6 million persons are expected to become infected with HIV; 3.6 million of these infections are expected to occur in sub-Saharan Africa alone.[369] Estimates indicate that, by 1995, 17.4 million persons will be infected with HIV, and 6.4 million of these persons will have developed AIDS, with the developing world having approximately 84 percent of all infected persons.[369] A more extensive discussion of AIDS in the developing world is presented in Chapter 99.

HIV-2

A second retrovirus, HIV-2, can result in severe immunosuppression and the development of serious opportunistic diseases that are clinically indistinguishable from those caused by HIV-1. Infection with HIV-2 was first reported in West Africa in 1986.[370] Although cases of HIV-2 infection have since been reported in other parts of Africa, several European countries, Canada, the United States, Brazil, and India,[371] the virus continues to be found mostly among heterosexual persons in West Africa.[371a] Differences in the geographic distribution of HIV-1 and HIV-2 may reflect differences in viral load, which in turn can affect transmissibility and duration of infectiousness.[371a] Data from surveillance and serologic surveys indicate that the prevalence of HIV-2 infection in the United States is extremely low.[371,372] Serologic testing of more than 24 million blood donations found no HIV-2 infected persons.[372] Similarly, surveys conducted among persons presumably at increased risk of infection with retroviruses through sexual contact and injecting drug use have found very low rates of HIV-2 infection.[371,372] In a survey performed during 1988–1990, of 31,533 persons at high risk for HIV infection in the United States 10 percent were found to be infected with HIV-1, but only two persons (0.006 percent) were seropositive for HIV-2.[373]

Accumulating information suggests that the modes of transmission for HIV-1 and HIV-2 are similar. Worldwide, HIV-2 infections have been diagnosed predominantly in men and women infected through heterosexual contact and, to a lesser extent, in homosexual men, injecting drug users, transfusion recipients, and persons with hemophilia.[371,374] In general, the patterns of HIV-1 and HIV-2 transmissions within a country are similar. Although perinatal transmissions of HIV-2 has been reported, preliminary data suggest that HIV-2 is transmitted less efficiently than HIV-1 from mother to child.[374–376] The natural histories of HIV-1 and HIV-2 infections appear similar in that both are characterized by a broad spectrum of disease. However, preliminary observations indicate that the incubation period from the time of initial infection to the eventual development of AIDS may be longer for HIV-2.[374,377,378]

HIV-1 and HIV-2 are genetically and immunologically distinct. However, nucleotide sequence analyses indicate that HIV-1 and HIV-2 share a similar genomic organization, suggesting a common evolutionary origin.[379] Overall, the nucleotide sequence homology for HIV-1 and HIV-2 is approximately 40 percent; the *gag* and *pol* genes for the two viruses are approximately 60 percent homologous.[379] These genetic similarities can result in frequent serologic cross reactions between HIV-1 and HIV-2. HIV-1 antibody tests using whole virus lysate EIA will detect 41–91 percent of HIV-2–infected persons.[380] Similarly, because the *gag* and *pol* proteins of HIV-1 and HIV-2 are antigenically cross reactive, HIV-2–infected persons may have an indeterminate HIV-1 Western blot.[381] Available HIV-2 EIA tests have a reported sensitivity of greater than 99 percent.[371] However, a licensed supplemental confirmatory test, similar to the Western blot for HIV-1, is not currently available for HIV-

2.[371] While dual infection with both HIV-1 and HIV-2 has been reported, in one study among persons in Cote d'Ivoire with antibodies to both retroviruses, PCR and viral isolation results suggested that more than half were likely infected with HIV-1 alone.[382]

Currently, blood donations in the United States are tested for evidence of both HIV-1 and HIV-2 antibodies. The very low prevalence of HIV-2 infection in the United States does not warrant routine testing for HIV-2 in settings other than blood centers. The CDC has recommended that tests for both HIV-1 and HIV-2 be performed in two HIV-testing situations: *(1)* if demographic or behavioral information suggests that HIV-2 infection might be present (e.g., sexual or blood contact with a person from a country where HIV-2 is endemic or with a person known to be infected with HIV-2; or *(2)* when clinical evidence suggests HIV disease in the absence of a positive test for antibodies to HIV-1 or in the presence of an HIV-1 Western blot with only *gag* and *pol* bands.[371] Detailed HIV-2 testing and counseling algorithms have been developed.[371] In general, preventive counseling and medical management for persons infected with HIV-2 are similar to those for persons diagnosed with HIV-1 infection.

PREVENTION OF HIV INFECTION IN THE COMMUNITY

Prevention of HIV infection must be based on strategies that interrupt sexual, blood-borne, and perinatal transmission of the virus. Such strategies must be grounded in an understanding of the epidemiology of HIV infection and knowledge of the science of human behavior. These science-based strategies are the foundation for the design, implementation, and evaluation of prevention efforts.

Prevention of Sexual Transmission

The risk of sexual transmission of HIV can be completely eliminated by avoiding sexual activity with infected partners. However, many sexually active persons do not know the HIV infection status of their partners, while others knowingly choose to have sexual contact with an infected partner. Multiple epidemiologic studies of heterosexual couples in which one partner is HIV positive and the other is HIV negative indicate that the correct and consistent use of condoms can significantly reduce transmission of HIV and other sexually transmitted diseases.[383,384]

In one prospective study of 342 HIV-seronegative women who had no exposure to HIV other than participation in a stable, monogamous relationship with an infected man, 19 seroconversions were detected, for an incidence rate of 3.6 per 100 person-years.[385] The risk of acquiring HIV infection was sixfold greater for women whose partners were inconsistent (i.e., never or not always) condom users than for women who reported that their partners always used condoms. A second longitudinal study of heterosexual HIV serodiscordant couples reported similar findings: no seroconversions occurred among 123 partners who always used condoms, while 12 of 122 partners who were irregular condom users seroconverted, for an incidence rate of 5.0/100 person-years.[386] Deriving precise and consistent estimates of condom efficacy is often hindered by the inability to control for potentially important confounders that may significantly affect transmission; these include the presence of other concurrent sexually transmitted diseases, the frequency of sex, the duration of the partnership, anal intercourse, and the source partner's degree of immunosuppression.[384] Two large prospective studies of serodiscordant couples have demonstrated that, among partners who do not use condoms regularly, the risk of seroconversion is further increased if the partner has symptomatic HIV infection.[385,386] Such information reinforces the need for ongoing counseling of persons involved in long-term partnerships with infected partners whose clinical condition will deteriorate over time.

The effectiveness of condoms in reducing the risk of HIV transmission can potentially be affected by condom breakage, leakage, and slippage. While condom breakage can occur, it appears uncommon, particularly in developed countries where studies have found breakage rates of 2 percent or less for vaginal or anal intercourse.[383,383a] Similarly, low rates of slippage (i.e., less than 1 percent) have been reported.[387] In vitro testing of intact latex condoms to detect leakage of HIV-sized particles suggests that condoms, when properly used, can act as an effective physical barrier and substantially reduce contact with fluid containing HIV-sized particles, even if leakage were to occur.[388]

Intravaginal pouches ("female condoms"), advocated as a "female-controlled" barrier prevention method, also require correct and consistent use.[383,389] While the female condom may act as an effective physical barrier to viruses, data regarding measurement of the efficacy of this type of condom in preventing HIV transmission are not yet available. The female condom's contraceptive failure rate has ranged from 11 to 26 percent, depending on the consistency and correctness of usage.[390] However, a condom's contraceptive failure rate may not accurately reflect its effectiveness in reducing heterosexual HIV transmission.[384]

Whether data on the protective effect of spermicides against a variety of sexually transmitted diseases apply to HIV as well has not been determined.[383,391] The irritative effects of spermicides on the vaginal epithelium may in fact facilitate, rather than reduce, HIV transmission.[237,391] In a randomized trial among prostitutes in Kenya, the use of a vaginal sponge containing a high dose of nonoxynol-9 was associated with an increased risk of HIV transmission.[236]

Despite the demonstrated benefits of condom use, multiple studies have found relatively low rates of consistent condom use among sexually active homosexual men and heterosexual men and women. Factors that influence condom use are complex.[392] Concern about decreased sexual pleasure or a partner's noncooperation, inadequate communication skills, the temporal effects of drugs or alcohol, use of other methods for contraception, and cultural influences have been correlated with low rates of condom use.[392–395]

Among homosexual and bisexual men, significant reductions in certain high-risk behaviors, such as sex with nonsteady partners and insertive anal intercourse, have been reported; importantly, reductions in incident HIV infections have been observed.[45,396] However, coincident with these observation in selected populations is accumulating evidence that such risk reduction behaviors have not been universally adopted and are difficult to maintain over extended periods of time. In cross-sectional studies of homosexual and bisexual men, younger men aged 18–25 years,[397] blacks,[394] and men from cities with low AIDS prevalence[398] reported the highest rates of unprotected anal intercourse. Two longitudinal studies of men who adopted safer sexual practices found that 12 percent of participants in San Francisco[399] and 47 percent in Chicago[400] acknowledged relapsing to unprotected receptive anal intercourse. One study of men who engaged in receptive anal intercourse found that heavy alcohol ingestion, moderate to heavy drug use, and younger age were associated with subsequent seroconversion.[401] Collectively, these studies highlight the diversity among men who have sex with men, the challenges in preventing new HIV infections, and the need for continued commitment to the development, implementation, and targeting of intervention and education programs suitable for different age, racial/ethnic, socioeconomic, and geographic populations.[402]

Available data suggest that changes in sexual behavior by heterosexual men and women at risk for HIV infection have been limited. In the United States, the HIV epidemic among heterosexual men and women has its roots in injecting drug use, crack cocaine use, and the exchange of sex for drugs.[57,58,403]

Prevention of heterosexually acquired HIV will require efforts to prevent HIV transmission associated with drug use, especially injecting drug use, as well as the prevention and treatment of other sexually transmitted diseases that facilitate HIV transmission.[255,403,404]

Partner notification is another mechanism to assist in the prevention of sexual transmission of HIV. Many infected persons inform their sex partners, while others do not[405,406]; the effectiveness of contact tracing and partner notification has been hotly debated.[407] The prioritization of partner notification as a public health intervention strategy is likely to depend on geographic considerations related to HIV prevalence, predominant modes of transmission, and available resources.[408] The efficacy of contact tracing for preventing incident HIV infection or reducing high risk behavior by both the infected person and his or her partners has not been evaluated extensively,[409,409a] but it must be carefully weighed against other activities and be conducted with special attention to confidentiality concerns.

Prevention of Transmission by Injecting Drug Use

Prevention and treatment of injecting drug use is critical for reducing HIV transmission among injecting drug users.[410] However, an estimated 80 percent of active drug users are not in treatment because of either choice or the unavailability of treatment.[411] This has necessitated the development of a creative blend of educational and alternative therapeutic approaches, including the removal of restrictions on the purchase of needles and syringes,[412] needle and syringe exchange programs,[413] proper use of bleach for disinfection of drug injection equipment,[414] and interim methadone maintenance programs.[415] Improvement in selected drug use behaviors, including a decrease in sharing of drug-injecting equipment and an increase in the use of bleach for cleaning equipment, has been reported,[257,416] although the duration of such behaviors has not been studied extensively. Recent reviews of needle exchange programs have found that most programs did not appear to increase drug injection use[413] and that many were strongly associated with decreases in needle-sharing and other drug behaviors known to transmit HIV infection.[417]

Prevention of Transmission Through Blood and Other Tissues

The first report of transfusion-associated AIDS was in 1982. In 1983, blood banks initiated the voluntary self-exclusion of donors with risks for HIV infection. In 1985, the first serologic assays for HIV antibody became available, and the use of these HIV serologic tests to screen blood donations dramatically decreased the risk of transfusion-associated HIV transmission.[266,267] The serologic identification of repeat donors with HIV infection, the screening of blood for non-A/non-B (C) hepatitis and human T-lymphotrophic virus types I and II and reductions in the number of transfusions used have also lowered transmission risks.[418–420] In addition to HIV antibody testing of plasma donors and deferral procedures for donors with risks for HIV infection, the implementation of viral inactivation procedures such as heat and solvent/detergent treatments and purification with monoclonal antibody have virtually eliminated the risk of HIV transmission through pooled plasma products for persons with hemophilia. In 1993, a recombinant Factor VIII product obtained from hamster cells containing the gene for human Factor VIII became available as an alternative therapy to pooled human plasma products. Organ and tissue donors should be evaluated and serologically screened in a manner similar to blood donors.[421,422] In addition, donations of semen and bone from a living donor may be quarantined until subsequent testing has definitively ruled out the possibility of delayed seroconversion in the donor.

Prevention of Transmission in the Health Care Setting

Effective prevention of HIV transmission in the health care setting requires a multifaceted approach to reduce the frequency of occupational blood exposure among health care workers. Such a strategy includes engineering controls that do not rely on worker compliance (e.g., self-sheathing needles), safe work practices and techniques, personal protective equipment, and training.[423] In particular, the reduction of percutaneous injuries will require the development of puncture-resistant gloves and/or the redesign of needles and other sharp instruments. The CDC has recommended that the principles of "universal precautions" be incorporated in programs for infection control.[424] Under universal precautions, blood and certain other body fluids from *all* patients are considered to be potentially infective. Universal precautions includes the appropriate use of handwashing and protective barriers, care in the use and disposal of needles and other sharp instruments, and appropriate disinfection and sterilization of reusable equipment. A detailed discussion of the prevention of transmission of HIV in the health care setting, including the use of zidovudine after occupational exposure,[425] is presented in Chapter 285.

Prevention of Perinatal Infection

Primary prevention of perinatally acquired HIV infection must center on routine, voluntary counseling and HIV antibody testing and on the availability of reproductive health services for women of reproductive age.[426,427] Because a substantial proportion of women may not initially acknowledge high-risk behavior or know the infection status of their partners, routine HIV testing and counseling must be considered a standard of care, especially in areas of high prevalence,[428] and not be reserved for those women with self-reported risk histories. Preliminary results from a randomized, double-blinded clinical trial found that zidovudine therapy administered to HIV-infected pregnant women who had a CD4+ T-lymphocyte count of greater than $200/\mu l$ and their infants was associated with a 67.5 percent reduction in the risk of perinatal HIV transmission.[428a] The Public Health Service has recommended that HIV-infected pregnant women who meet the protocol eligibility criteria should be informed of the potential benefits and potential risks of zidovudine therapy. Additional recommendations are pending. In the United States and some other developed countries, the effective treatment of injecting drug use remains an essential adjunct to preventing perinatal transmission, because mothers of most children with perinatally acquired HIV infection either inject drugs themselves or have partners who do.

Prevention of postnatal transmission of HIV infection through breast-feeding must take into account the likelihood of competing risks for morbidity and mortality associated with feeding alternatives in developing countries. In 1985, after the first case report implicating HIV transmission from breast milk and the isolation of HIV from breast milk, the CDC recommended that HIV-seropositive women should not breast-feed their infants.[429] This recommendation was intended for mothers in the United States, where alternative, safe, and nutritious substitute feeding methods are readily available.[290] In 1992, the WHO and UNICEF developed a consensus statement on HIV transmission related to breast-feeding, stating[430]:

> In settings where the primary causes of infant deaths are infectious diseases and malnutrition, breast-feeding should remain the standard advice to pregnant women, including those who are HIV-infected . . . . In settings where infectious diseases are not the primary causes of death during infancy, pregnant women known to be infected with HIV should be advised not to breast-feed but to use a safe feeding alternative.

COUNSELING AND HIV ANTIBODY TESTING

Early recognition of HIV infection through HIV antibody testing is one of the primary objectives of HIV prevention efforts. The major benefits of HIV testing programs are *(1)* the referral of HIV-seropositive persons for medical evaluation and treatment and other social services and *(2)* counseling to promote the behavior change necessary to reduce HIV transmission. Physicians have an essential role in this public health effort. As the principal providers of primary health care, they are most frequently named by the general public as the desired source for HIV testing.[431] It is likely that an increasing number of physicians will be requested to provide HIV testing services.

Indications for HIV Testing

Knowledge of the behaviors that place persons at risk for HIV infection, the clinical conditions associated with HIV infection, and the estimated rate of HIV infection in the community served by the health care facility or practitioner is necessary to target effectively HIV counseling and testing. Specific populations or clinical settings in which testing is recommended include the following[426,432,433]:

1. *Persons with behavioral risks for HIV infection.* Persons at risk for HIV infection include men who have had sex with other men, persons who have injected drugs, male and female prostitutes, sex partners of persons with or at increased risk for HIV infection, and other persons who consider themselves at risk. To identify risks associated with HIV transmission, physicians should interview patients regarding their sexual and drug-use practices.

   Injecting drug users are at increased risk of HIV infection through contact with contaminated needles or syringes. HIV counseling can provide these persons with information on safer sexual and needle-sharing practices that can reduce further HIV transmissions, as well as with referrals for substance abuse treatment and preventive services.

2. *Persons with clinical conditions associated with HIV infection.* The HIV antibody test is a useful diagnostic tool for evaluating persons with generalized lymphadenopathy; unexplained weight loss, fever, diarrhea, or dementia; diseases such as tuberculosis, generalized herpes, and chronic candidiasis; and other conditions suggestive of HIV infection.[9]

3. *Persons who received blood or blood products between 1978 and 1985.* Persons who received transfusions of blood or blood components from 1978 to 1985 are at increased risk of transfusion-associated HIV transmission. The risk of transfusion-associated transmission is greatest for persons who received relatively large numbers of units in geographic areas with high rates of AIDS and HIV infection.[434] Because clotting factor concentrates are derived from many donors nationwide, all persons with hemophilia who received clotting factor concentrate during this time are considered to be at risk for HIV infection.

4. *Persons with other sexually transmitted disease.* HIV testing should be considered for persons with other sexually transmitted diseases, because many of these persons have likely practiced behaviors that place them at risk for HIV infection.

5. *Selected women of reproductive age.* Women at risk for HIV infection include those with the behavioral risks outlined above and all women living in communities or born in countries where the prevalence of HIV infection among women is known or suspected to be high. Offering HIV testing to all women in these areas is particularly important, because many people may neither recognize nor report a risk on interview.[428]

6. *Children born to mothers with HIV infection or at increased risk.* Children born to infected mothers should be evaluated as early as possible after delivery for laboratory and clinical evidence of HIV infection so that appropriate prophylactic and therapeutic interventions can begin. Infected infants often have life-threatening complications of HIV infection in the first few months of life.

7. *Patients aged 15–54 years in acute health care settings with high rates of unsuspected HIV infection.* High rates of unrecognized HIV infection have been found among patients at some U.S. hospitals and associated clinics.[65,306] In anonymous unlinked serologic surveys, 0.2–8.9 percent of persons receiving care in emergency departments and 0.1–7.8 percent of persons admitted to hospitals were HIV-antibody positive. In two studies that collected data on previous HIV testing, a number of persons were unaware of their HIV infection before hospital admission.[65] Thus, testing persons on the basis of acknowledged risk behaviors or clinical signs and symptoms will recognize only a minority of HIV-infected persons. To address this shortcoming, routine, voluntary HIV counseling and testing programs are recommended for hospitals and associated clinics with a high rate of HIV infection. A high rate of HIV infection is defined as an estimated HIV seroprevalence rate of at least 1 percent or an AIDS diagnosis rate greater than or equal to 1.0 per 1000 discharges. The AIDS diagnosis rate is the annual number of AIDS patients diagnosed and reported to the health department divided by the annual number of discharges times 1000. Acute care facilities and other health-care institutions, such as mental health facilities or private medical practitioners' offices with high rates of HIV infection, should strongly consider routinely offering HIV counseling and testing to all patients aged 15–54 years.

8. *Persons who sustain occupational exposures that may place them at risk of HIV infection.* Occupational exposures that may place a worker at risk of HIV infection include percutaneous injuries and contact of mucous membranes or skin (especially when the skin is chapped, abraded, or afflicted with dermatitis or the contact is prolonged or involves an extensive area) with blood and other body fluids to which universal precautions apply.[424] After such an exposure, if the source individual has AIDS, is known to be HIV seropositive, or refuses testing, the worker should be evaluated clinically and serologically for evidence of HIV infection as soon as possible after the exposure (baseline) and, if seronegative, should be retested periodically for a minimum of 6 months after exposure (e.g., 6 weeks, 12 weeks, and 6 months after exposure) to determine whether HIV infection has occurred.[425] If the source individual is HIV seronegative and has no other clinical manifestations of AIDS or HIV infection, no further HIV follow-up of the exposed worker is necessary unless epidemiologic evidence suggests that the source individual may have recently been exposed to HIV or if testing is desired by the worker or recommended by the health care provider.[425]

9. *Health care workers who perform exposure-prone procedures.* Health care workers who perform invasive procedures that are considered exposure prone (e.g., procedures that include digital palpation of a needle tip in a body cavity or the simultaneous presence of the health care worker's fingers and a needle or other sharp object in a poorly visualized or highly confined anatomic site) should know their HIV antibody status. Mandatory testing of health care workers for HIV antibody is not recommended.[435]

Guidelines for HIV Counseling and Testing

Testing for HIV infection should be voluntary, with informed consent obtained in accordance with local laws.[433] Confidentiality and the avoidance of discrimination toward persons who test positive must be ensured. Mandatory testing is not recommended except in the limited setting of tissue and organ donation. HIV testing for purposes other than immediate medical care should be deferred until a later time for persons who are too severely ill to give informed consent. Testing patients to reduce the risk of HIV transmission within health care settings has not been shown to be effective and is not a substitute for universal precautions.[305,436]

Although study results have differed, HIV counseling and testing may reduce high-risk behaviors in persons tested and can be a cost-effective prevention strategy when properly conducted and linked to follow-up prevention and medical services.[437–440] Counseling should be performed in accordance with existing CDC recommendations by health care providers knowledgeable about HIV infection.[426,433] HIV testing should be preceded by information about the testing policies of the physician or institution, the medical implications of the test, an assessment of risk, and the opportunity to receive additional information. Following testing, HIV-seronegative persons should be informed that continued high-risk sexual or drug-use behaviors could result in HIV infection. Seronegative persons concerned about a recent exposure should be advised to seek repeated testing at least 6 months after the exposure.

The counseling of HIV-seropositive persons should be tailored for each individual and include an interpretation of the test results and a discussion of the medical, social, and psychological implications of a positive test result. HIV-infected persons should also be instructed how to notify sex or needle-sharing partners and to refer them for HIV counseling and testing. If HIV-infected persons are reluctant to inform their partners directly, physicians may offer to inform partners or to seek local health department assistance. Confidentiality is very important to protect individuals and not discourage persons from seeking HIV testing.

Persons found to be HIV seropositive require a medical evaluation, including immunologic monitoring, screening for other sexually transmitted diseases, prophylaxis against certain opportunistic illnesses, vaccinations, antiretroviral therapy, and other preventive and therapeutic services.[433,441] Physicians who offer HIV testing should be able to provide these services or have an effective referral mechanism.

REFERENCES

1. Centers for Disease Control and Prevention. *Pneumocystis* pneumonia—Los Angeles. MMWR. 1981;30:250–2.
2. Centers for Disease Control and Prevention. Kaposi's sarcoma and *Pneumocystis* pneumonia among homosexual men—New York City and California. MMWR. 1981;30:305–8.
3. Merson MH. The HIV pandemic: Global spread and global response (Abstract PS-01-1). In: Abstracts of the IX International Conference on AIDS/IVth STD World Congress. v. I. Berlin, Germany, June 6–11, 1993:9.
4. Centers for Disease Control and Prevention: Update on acquired immune deficiency syndrome (AIDS)—United States. MMWR. 1982;31:507–8, 513–4.
5. Garry RF, Witte MH, Gottlieb AA, et al. Documentation of an AIDS virus infection in the United States in 1968. JAMA. 1988;260:2085–7.
6. Huminer D, Rosenfeld JB, Pitlik SD. AIDS in the pre-AIDS era. Rev Infect Dis. 1987;9:1102–8.
7. Centers for Disease Control and Prevention: Revision of the case definition of acquired immunodeficiency syndrome for national reporting—United States. MMWR. 1985;34:373–5.
8. Centers for Disease Control and Prevention: Revision of the CDC surveillance case definition for acquired immunodeficiency syndrome. MMWR. 1987;36(Suppl):1S–15S.
9. Centers for Disease Control and Prevention: 1993 Revised classification system for HIV infection and expanded surveillance case definition for AIDS among adolescents and adults. MMWR. 1992;41(No. RR-17):1–19.
10. Centers for Disease Control and Prevention: Update: Acquired immunodeficiensy syndrome—United States, 1981–1988. MMWR. 1989;38:229–36.
11. Selik RM, Buehler JW, Karon JM, et al. Impact of the 1987 revision of the case definition of the acquired immunodeficiency syndrome in the United States. J Acquir Immune Defic Syndr. 1990;3:73–82.
12. Payne SF, Rutherford GW, Lemp GF, et al. Effect of the revised AIDS case definition on AIDS reporting in San Francisco: Evidence of increased reporting in intravenous drug users. AIDS. 1990;4:335–9.
13. National Institutes of Health. State-of-the-art conference on azidothymidine therapy for early HIV infection. Am J Med. 1990;89:335–44.
14. Volberding PA, Lagakos SW, Koch MA, et al. Zidovudine in asymptomatic human immunodeficiency virus infection: A controlled trial in persons with fewer than 500 CD4-positive cells per cubic millimeter. N Engl J Med. 1990;322:941.
15. Centers for Disease Control and Prevention: Recommendations for prophy-

laxis against *Pneumocystis carinii* pneumonia for adults and adolescents infected with human immunodeficiency virus. MMWR. 1992;41(RR-4):1–11.

15a. El Sadr W, Oleshe JM, Agins BD, et al. Evaluation and management of early HIV infection. In: Clinical Practice Guideline No. 7, Publication No. 94-0572. Rockville, MD: Agency for Health Care Policy and Research, Public Health Service, U.S. Department of Health and Human Services, January 1994;28.

16. Brookmeyer R. Reconstruction and future trends of the AIDS epidemic in the United States. Science. 1991;253:37–42.

17. Selwyn PA, Hartel D, Lewis VA, et al. A prosective study of the risk of tuberculosis among intravenous drug users with human immunodeficiency virus infection. N Engl J Med. 1989;320:545–50.

18. Selwyn PA, Sckell BM, Alcabes P, et al. High risk of active tuberculosis in HIV infected drug users with cutaneous anergy. JAMA. 1992;268:504–9.

19. Buehler JW, Devine OJ, Berkelman RL, et al. Impact of the human immunodeficiency virus epidemic on mortality trends in young men, United States. Am J Public Health. 1990;80:1080–6.

20. Chu SY, Buehler JW, Berkelman RL. Impact of the human immunodeficiency virus epidemic on mortality in women of reproductive age, United States. JAMA. 1990;264:225–9.

21. Farizo KM, Buehler JW, Chamberland ME, et al. Spectrum of disease in persons with human immunodeficiency virus infection in the United States. JAMA. 1992;267:1798–805.

22. Schafer A, Friedmann W, Mielke M, et al. The increased frequency of cervical dysplasia-neoplasia in women infected with the human immunodeficiency virus is related to the degree of immunosuppression. Am J Obstet Gynecol. 1991;164:593–9.

23. Feingold AR, Vermund SH, Burk RD, et al. Cervical cytologic abnormalities and papillomavirus in women infected with human immunodeficiency virus. J Acquir Immune Defic Syndr. 1990;3:896–903.

24. Maiman M, Fruchter RG, Serur E, et al. Human immunodeficiency virus infection and cervical neoplasia. Gynecol Oncol. 1990;38:377–82.

25. Rosenblum LS, Buehler JW, Morgan MW, et al. The completeness of AIDS case reporting, 1988: A multisite collaborative surveillance project. Am J Public Health. 1992;82:1495–9.

26. Buehler JW, Berkelman RL, Stehr-Green JK. The completeness of AIDS surveillance. J Acquir Immune Defic Syndr. 1992;5:257–64.

27. Thacker SB, Choi K, Brachman PS. The surveillance of infectious disease. JAMA. 1983;249:1181–5.

28. Vogt RL, Clark SW, Kappel S. Evaluation of the state surveillance system using hospital discharge diagnoses, 1982–83. Am J Epidemiol. 1986;123:197–8.

29. Centers for Disease Control and Prevention: Update: Public health surveillance for HIV infection—United States, 1989 and 1990. MMWR. 1990;39:853, 859–61.

30. Fleming PL, Ward JW, Morgan MW, et al. Mandatory HIV reporting: Characteristics of adults reported with HIV compared to AIDS in the United States (Abstract WS-C17-2). In: Abstracts of the IXth International Conference on AIDS/IVth STD World Congress (v.I). Berlin, Germany, June 6–11, 1993;98.

31. Centers for Disease Control and Prevention: Public health uses of HIV-infection reports—South Carolina, 1986–1991. MMWR. 1992;41:245–9.

32. Solomon SL, Curran JW. Public health applications of a classification system for human immunodeficiency virus infection (Editorial). Ann Intern Med. 1987;106:319–21.

33. World Health Organization. Interim proposal for a WHO staging system for HIV infection and diseases. Weekly Epidemiol Rec. 1990;65:221–4.

34. Royce RA, Luckmann RS, Fusaro RE, et al. The natural history of HIV-1 infection: Staging classifications of disease. AIDS. 1991;5:355–64.

35. Redfield RR, Wright DC, Tramont EC. The Walter Reed staging classification for HTLV-III/LAV infection. N Engl J Med. 1986;314:131–2.

36. Zolla-Pazner S, DesJarlais DC, Friedman SR, et al. Nonrandom development of immunologic abnormalities after infection with human immunodeficiency virus: Implications for immunologic classification of the disease. Proc Natl Acad Sci USA. 1987;84:5404–8.

37. Justice AC, Feinstein AR, Wells CK. A new prognostic staging system for the acquired immunodeficiency syndrome. N Engl J Med. 1989;320:1388–93.

38. Centers for Disease Control and Prevention. HIV/AIDS Surveillance Report, February 1993:1–23.

39. Centers for Disease Control and Prevention. The second 100,000 cases of acquired immunodeficiency syndrome—United States, June 1981–December 1991. MMWR. 1992;41:28–9.

39a. Centers for Disease Control and Prevention. Update: Impact of the expanded AIDS surveillance case distribution for adolescents and adults on case reporting—United States, 1993. MMWR. 1994;43:160–1;167–70.

40. Centers for Disease Control and Prevention. HIV prevalence estimates and AIDS case projections for the United States: Report based upon a workshop. MMWR. 1990;39(No. RR-16):1–31.

41. Centers for Disease Control and Prevention. Human immunodeficiency virus infection in the United States: A review of current knowledge. MMWR. 1987;36(No. S6):1S–48S.

42. Selik RM, Chu SY, Buehler JW. Human immunodeficiency virus (HIV) infection as a leading cause of death among young adults in U.S. cities and states. JAMA. 1993;269:2991–4.

43. Centers for Disease Control and Prevention (CDC). National HIV serosurveillance summary—results through 1992. Atlanta, GA: U.S. Department of Health and Human Services, Public Health Service, 1993, Publication No. HIV/NCID/11-93/036.

44. McCray E, Onorato IM, the Field Services Branch. Sentinel surveillance of human immunodeficiency virus infection in sexually transmitted disease clinics in the United States. Sex Transm Dis. 1992;19:235–41.

45. Winkelstein W Jr, Wiley JA, Padian NS, et al. The San Francisco Men's Health Study: Continued decline in HIV seroconversion rates among homosexual/bisexual men. Am J Public Health. 1988;78:1472–4.

46. Kingsley LA, Bacellar H, Zhou S, et al. Temporal trends in HIV seroconversion: A report from the multicenter AIDS cohort study (MACS) [Abstract F.C.550]. In: Final Program and Abstracts of the VIth International Conference on AIDS. v. 2. San Francisco, CA, June 20–24, 1990:218.

47. Nieri GN, Lemp GF, Watson RP, et al. HIV-1 seroprevalence and risk behaviors among young gay and bisexual men in San Francisco (Abstract PoC 4092). In: Poster Abstracts of the VIIIth International Conference on AIDS/III STD World Congress. v. 2. Amsterdam, The Netherlands. July 19–24, 1992:C260.

48. Hernandez SR, Kellogg TA, Wilson MJ, et al. Prevalnce of HIV-1 among homosexual and bisexual men in the San Francisco Bay area: Evidence of infection among young gay men (Abstract W.C.3010). In: Abstracts of the VIIth International Conference on AIDS. v. 2. Florence, Italy, June 16–21, 1991:298.

49. Hahn RA, Onorato IM, Jones TS, et al. Prevalence of HIV infection among intravenous drug users in the United States. JAMA. 1989;261:2677–84.

50. Des Jarlais DC, Friedman SR, Novick DM, et al. HIV-1 infection among intravenous drug users in Manhattan, New York City, from 1977 through 1987. JAMA. 1989;261:1008–12.

51. Weibel W, Lampinen T, Chene D, et al. HIV-1 seroconversion in a cohort of street intravenous drug users in Chicago (Abstract F.C.556). In: Final Program and Abstracts of the VIth International Conference on AIDS. v. 2. San Francisco, CA, June 20–24, 1990:220.

52. National HIV Serosurveillance Summary. v. 2. Results through 1990. Atlanta, GA: U.S. Department of Health and Human Services, Public Health Service, 1991; Publication No. HIV/NCID/11-91/011.

53. Allen DM, Onorato IM, Green TA, et al. HIV infection in intravenous drug users entering drug treatment, United States, 1988 to 1989. Am J Public Health. 1992;82:541–6.

54. Chaisson RE, Bacchetti P, Osmond D, et al. Cocaine use and HIV infection in intravenous drug users in San Francisco. JAMA. 1989;261:561–5.

55. Chaisson RE, Moss AR, Onishi R, et al. Human immunodeficiency virus infection in heterosexual intravenous drug users in San Francisco. Am J Public Health. 1987;77:169–72.

56. Byers RH, Lindegren ML, Hanson IC, et al. AIDS patients infected during adolescence, United States (Abstract 284). In: Program and Abstracts of the 32nd Interscience Conference on Antimicrobial Agents and Chemotherapy. Anaheim, CA, October 11–14, 1992:158.

57. Dondero TJ, Allen DM, McCray D, et al. Injected drug use: The driving force for much of the U.S. epidemic (Abstract WC 3356). In: Abstracts of the VIIth International Conference on AIDS. v. 2. Florence, Italy, June 16–21, 1991:385.

58. Chaisson MA, Stoneburner RL, Hildebrandt DS, et al. Heterosexual transmission of HIV-1 associated with the use of smokable freebase cocaine (crack). AIDS. 19912;5:1121–6.

59. Ellerbrock TV, Lieb S, Harrington PE, et al. Heterosexually transmitted human immunodeficiency virus infection among pregnant women in a rural Florida community. N Engl J Med. 1992;327:1704–9.

60. Kim MY, Marmor M, Dubin N, et al. HIV risk-related sexual behaviors among heterosexuals in New York City: Associations with race, sex, and intravenous drug use. AIDS. 1993;7:409–14.

61. Stoneburner RL, Chaisson MA, Weisfuse IB, et al. The epidemic of AIDS and HIV-1 infection among heterosexuals in New York City. AIDS. 1990;4:99–106.

62. Darrow WW, Cohen JB, French J, et al. Multicenter study of HIV antibody in U.S. prostitutes (Abstract W.2.1). In: Abstracts of the III International Conference on AIDS. Washington, DC, June 1–5, 1987:105.

63. Fischl MA, Dickinson GM, Flanagan S, et al. Human immunodeficiency virus (HIV) among female prostitutes in south Florida (Abstract W.2.2). In: Proceedings of the Third International Conference on AIDS. Washington, D.C., June 1–5, 1987:105.

64. Onorato IM, Klaskala W, Morgan M. High and rising HIV incidence in female sex workers in Miami, Florida, despite stable HIV prevalence over time (Abstract 285). In: Program and Abstracts of the 32nd Interscience Conference on Antimicrobial Agents and Chemotherapy. Anaheim, CA, October 11–14, 1992:158.

65. Janssen RS, St. Louis ME, Satten GA, et al. HIV infection among patients in U.S. acute care hospitals: Strategies for the counseling and testing of hospital patients. N Engl J Med. 1992;327:445–52.

66. Onorato IM, McCray E, the Field Services Branch. Prevalence of human immunodeficiency virus infection among patients attending tuberculosis clinics in the United States. J Infect Dis. 1992;165:86–92.

67. Withum DG, Guerena-Burgueno F, Gwinn M, et al. High HIV prevalence among female and male prisoners in the United States, 1989–1992: Implications for prevention and treatment strategies (Abstract PO-C21-3115). In: Abstracts of the IX International Conference on AIDS/STD World Congress. v. II. Berlin, Germany, 1993:736.

68. Kennedy M, Petersen L, Doll L, et al. Five year trends in HIV seroprevalence and risk behaviors among U.S. blood donors: A multicenter study

[Abstract P]-C21-3118]. In: Abstracts of the IXth International Conference on AIDS/STD World Congress. v. II. Berlin, Germany, 1993:737.

69. Brundage JF, Burke DS, Gardner LI, et al. Tracking the spread of the HIV infection epidemic among young adults in the United States: Results of the first four years of screening among civilian applicants for U.S. military service. J Acquir Immune Defic Syndr. 1990;3:1168–80.

70. Burke DS, Brundage JF, Goldenbaum M, et al. Human immunodeficiency virus infections in teenagers. JAMA. 1990;263:2074–7.

71. Withers BG, Kelley PW, McNeil JG. A brief review of the epidemiology of HIV in the U.S. Army. Milit Med. 1992;157:80–4.

72. Cowan DN, Pomerantz RS, Wann ZF, et al. Human immunodeficiency virus infection among members of the reserve components of the U.S. Army: Prevalence, incidence, and demographic characteristics. J Infect. Dis. 1990; 162:827–36.

73. Kelley PW, Miller RN, Pomerantz R, et al. Human immunodeficiency virus seropositivity among members of the active duty U.S. Army 1985–89. Am J Public Health. 1990;80:405–10.

74. McNeil JG, Brundage JF, Gardner LI, et al. Trends of HIV seroconversion among young adults in the U.S. Army, 1985 to 1989. JAMA. 1991;265:1709–14.

75. St. Louis ME, Conway GA, Hayman CR, et al. Human immunodeficiency virus infection in disadvantaged adolescents. JAMA. 1991;266:2387–91.

76. Gwinn M, Pappaioanou M, George JR, et al. Prevalence of HIV infection in childbearing women in the United States. JAMA. 1991;265:1704–8.

77. Davis S, Gwinn M, Wasser S, et al. HIV prevalence among U.S. childbearing women, 1989–1992 (Abstract 27). In: Program and Abstracts of the First National Conference on Human Retroviruses and Related Infections. Washington, D.C., December 12–16, 1993:60.

78. Sweeney PA, Onorato IM, Allen DM, et al. Sentinel surveillance of human immunodeficiency virus infection in women seeking reproductive health services in the United States, 1988–1989. Obstet Gynecol. 1992;79:503–10.

79. Green TA, Karon JM, Nwanyanwu OC. Changes in AIDS incidence trends in the United States. J Acquir Immune Defic Syndr. 1992;5:547–55.

80. Centers for Disease Control and Prevention: Update: Acquired immunodeficiency syndrome—United States, 1981–1990. MMWR. 1991;40:358–63, 369.

81. Berkelman R, Karon J, Thomas P, et al. Are AIDS cases among homosexual men leveling (Abstract W.A.O.13). In: Abstracts of the V International Conference on AIDS. Montreal, Canada, June 4–9, 1989:66.

82. Gail MH, Rosenberg PS, Goedert JJ. Therapy may explain recent deficits in AIDS incidence. J Acquire Immune Defic Syndr. 1990;3:296–306.

83. Conley LJ, Holmberg SD. Transmission of AIDS from blood screened negative for antibody to the human immunodeficiency virus (Letter). N Engl J Med. 1992;326:1499–500.

84. Centers for Disease Control and Prevention: Update: Acquired immunodeficiency syndrome—United States, 1992. MMWR. 1993;42:547–51, 557.

85. Nwanyanwu OC, Conti LA, Ciesielski CA, et al. Increasing frequency of heterosexually transmitted AIDS in southern Florida: Artifact or reality? Am J Public Health. 1993;83:571–3.

86. Castro KG, Lifson AR, White CR, et al. Investigations of AIDS patients with no previously identified risk factors. JAMA. 1988;259:1338–42.

87. Simonds RJ, Holmberg SD, Hurwitz RL, et al. Transmission of human immunodeficiency virus type 1 from a seronegative organ and tissue donor. N Engl J Med. 1992;326:726–32.

88. Selik RM, Castro KG, Pappaioanou M. Racial/ethnic differences in the risk of AIDS in the United States. Am J Public Health. 1988;78:1539–45.

89. Diaz T, Buehler JW, Castro KG, et al. AIDS trends among Hispanics in the United States. Am J Public Health. 1993;83:504–9.

90. Thomas PA, Hindin R, Greenberg A, et al. Decreased incidence of reported AIDS cases, New York City (Abstract Th.C.707). In: Abstracts of the VIth International Conference on AIDS. v. 1. San Francisco, CA, June 20–24, 1990:301.

91. Karon J, Berkelman RL. The geographic and ethnic diversity of AIDS incidence trends in homosexual/bisexual men in the United States. J Acquir Immune Defic Syndr. 1991;4:1179–89.

92. Centers for Disease Control and Prevention: Update: Acquired immunodeficiency syndrome—United States, 1991. MMWR. 1992;41:463–8.

93. Greenberg AE, Thomas PA, Landesman SH, et al. The spectrum of HIV-1–related disease among outpatients in New York City. AIDS. 1992;6:849–59.

94. Kinloch-de Loes, de Saussure P, Saurat J-H, et al. Symptomatic primary infection due to human immunodeficiency virus type 1: Review of 31 cases. Clin Infect Dis. 1993;17:59–65.

95. Tindall B, Cooper DA. Primary HIV infection: Host responses and intervention strategies. AIDS. 1991;5:1–14.

96. Hardy WD, Daar ES, Sokolov RT Jr, et al. Acute neurologic deterioration in a young man. Rev Infect Dis. 1991;13:745–50.

97. Pena JM, Martinez-Lopez MA, Arnalich F, et al. Esophageal candidiasis associated with acute infection due to human immunodeficiency virus: Case report and review. Rev Infect Dis. 1991;13:872–5.

98. Fox R, Eldred LJ, Fuchs EJ, et al. Clinical manifestations of acute infection with human immunodeficiency virus in a cohort of gay men. AIDS. 1987;1:35–8.

99. Pedersen C, Lindhardt BO, Jensen BL, et al. Clinical course of primary HIV infection: Consequences for subsequent course of infection. Br Med J. 1989;299:154–7.

100. Clark SJ, Saag MS, Decker WD, et al. High titers of cytopathic virus in plasma of patients with symptomatic primary HIV-1 infection. N Engl J Med. 1991;324:954–60.

101. Daar ES, Moudgil T, Meyer RD, et al. Transient high levels of viremia in patients with primary immunodeficiency virus type 1 infection. N Engl J Med. 1991;324:961–4.

102. Busch MP, Amad ZE, Sheppard HW, et al. Primary HIV-1 infection (Letter). N Engl J Med. 1991;325:733.

103. Levy JA, Mackewicz CE, Walker CM. Primary HIV-1 infection (Letter). N Engl J Med. 1991;325:734.

104. Horsburgh CR Jr, Ou C-Y, Jason J, et al. Duration of human immunodeficiency virus infection before detection of antibody. Lancet. 1989;2:637–40.

105. Pan L-Z, Sheppard HW, Winkelstein W, et al. Lack of detection of human immunodeficiency virus in persistently seronegative homosexual men with high or medium risks for infection. J Infect Dis. 1991;164:962–4.

106. Simmonds P, Lainson FAL, Cuthbert R, et al. HIV antigen and antibody detection: Variable responses to infection in the Edinburgh haemophiliac cohort. Br Med J. 1988;296:593–8.

107. Yerly S, Chamot E, Deglon J-J, et al. Absence of chronic human immunodeficiency virus infection without seroconversion in intravenous drug users: A prospective and retrospective study. J Infect Dis. 1991;164:965–8.

108. Imagawa DT, Lee MH, Wolinsky SM, et al. Human immunodeficiency virus type 1 infection in homosexual men who remain seronegative for prolonged periods. N Engl J Med. 1989;320:1458–62.

109. Wolinsky SM, Rinaldo CR, Kwok S, et al. Human immunodeficiency virus type 1 (HIV-1) infection a median of 18 months before a diagnostic western blot: Evidence from a cohort of homosexual men. Ann Intern Med. 1989; 111:961–72.

110. Imagawa D, Detels R. HIV-1 in seronegative homosexual men (Letter). N Engl J Med. 1991;325:1250–1.

111. Laurence J, Siegal FP, Schattner E, et al. Acquired immunodeficiency syndrome without evidence of infection with human immunodeficiency virus types 1 and 2. Lancet. 1992;340:273–4.

112. Centers for Disease Control and Prevention: Unexplained CD4+ T-lymphocyte depletion in persons without evident HIV infection—United States. MMWR. 1992;41:541–5.

113. Smith DK, Neal JJ, Holmberg SD, et al. Unexplained opportunistic infections and CD4+ T-lymphocytopenia without HIV infection. An investigation of cases in the United States. N Engl J Med. 1993;328:373–9.

114. Centers for Disease Control and Prevention: Projections of the number of persons diagnosed with AIDS and the number of immunosuppressed HIV-infected persons—United States, 1992–1994. MMWR. 1992;41(No.RR-18):1–29.

115. Ragni MV, Kingsley LA. Cumulative risk for AIDS and other HIV outcomes in a cohort of hemophiliacs in western Pennsylvania. J Acquir Immune Defic Syndr. 1990;3:708–13.

116. Kuo J-M, Taylor JMG, Detels R. Estimating the AIDS incubation period from a prevalent cohort. Am J Epidemiol. 1991;133:1050–7.

117. Rutherford GW, Lifson AR, Hessol NA, et al. Course of HIV-1 infection in a cohort of homosexual and bisexual men: An 11 year follow up study. Br Med J. 1990;301:1183–8.

118. Lifson AR, Buchbinder SP, Sheppard HW, et al. Long-term human immunodeficiency virus infection in asymptomatic homosexual and bisexual men with normal CD4+ lymphocyte counts: Immunologic and virologic characteristics. J Infect Dis. 1991;163:959–65.

119. Learmont J, Tindall B, Evans L, et al. Long-term symptomless HIV-1 infection in recipients of blood products from a single donor. Lancet. 1992;340:863–7.

120. Ward JW, Bush TJ, Perkins HA, et al. The natural history of transfusion-associated infection with human immunodeficiency virus. N Engl J Med. 1989;321:947–52.

121. Selwyn PA, Alcabes P, Hartel D, et al. Clinical manifestations and predictors of disease progression in drug users with human immunodeficiency virus infection. N Engl J Med. 1992;327:1697–703.

122. Coates RA, Farwell VT, Raboud J, et al. Cofactors of progression to acquired immunodeficiency syndrome in a cohort of male sexual contacts of men with human immunodeficiency virus disease. Am J Epidemiol. 1990;132:717–22.

123. Kaslow RA, Blackwelder WC, Ostrow DG, et al. No evidence for a role of alcohol or other psychoactive drugs in accelerating immunodeficiency in HIV-1 positive individuals. A report from the Multicenter AIDS Cohort Study. JAMA. 1989;261:3424–9.

124. Goedert JJ, Kessler CM, Aledort LM, et al. A prospective study of human immunodeficiency virus type 1 infection and the development of AIDS in subjects with hemophilia. N Engl J Med. 1989;321:1141–8.

125. Mariotto AB, Mariotti S, Pezzotti P, et al. Estimation of the acquired immunodeficiency syndrome incubation period in intravenous drug users: A comparison with male homosexuals. Am J Epidemiol. 1992;135:428–37.

126. Vermund SH, Galbraith MA, Ebner SC, et al. Human immunodeficiency virus/acquired immunodeficiency syndrome in pregnant women. Ann Epidemiol. 1992;2:773–803.

127. Klein RS, Harris CA, Small CB, et al. Oral candidiasis in high-risk patients as the initial manifestation of the acquired immunodeficiency syndrome. N Engl J Med. 1984;311:354–8.

128. Greenspan D, Greenspan JS, Hearst NG, et al. Relation of oral hairy leukoplakia to infection with the human immunodeficiency virus and the risk of developing AIDS. J Infect Dis. 1987;155:475–81.

129. Melbye M, Grossman RJ, Goedert JJ, et al. Risk of AIDS after herpes zoster. Lancet. 1987;1:728–31.

130. Stein DS, Korvick JA, Vermund SH. CD4+ lymphocyte cell enumeration for prediction of clinical course of human immunodeficiency virus disease: A review. J Infect Dis. 1992;165:352–63.

131. Fahey JL, Taylor JMG, Detels R, et al. The prognostic value of cellular and serologic markers in infection with human immunodeficiency virus type 1. N Engl J Med. 1990;322:166–72.

132. Fleming PL, Ciesielski CA, Byers RH, et al. Gender differences in reported AIDS-indicative diagnoses. J Infect Dis. 1993;168:61–7.

133. Kreiss JK, Castro KG. Special considerations for managing suspected human immunodeficiency virus infection and AIDS in patients from developing countries. J Infect Dis. 1990;162:955–60.

134. Slutsker L, Castro KG, Ward JW, et al. Epidemiology of extrapulmonary tuberculosis among persons with AIDS in the United States. Clin Infect Dis. 1993;16:513–8.

135. Munoz A, Schrager LK, Bacellar H, et al. Trends in the incidence of outcomes defining acquired immunodeficiency syndrome (AIDS) in the Multicenter AIDS Cohort Study: 1985–1991. Am J Epidemiol. 1993;137:423–38.

136. Nightingale SD, Byrd LT, Southern PM, et al. Incidence of *Mycobacterium avium-intracellulare* complex bacteremia in human immunodeficiency virus-positive patients. J Infect Dis. 1992;165:1082–5.

137. Rutherford GW, Schwarcz SK, Lemp GF, et al. The epidemiology of AIDS-related Kaposi's sarcoma in San Francisco. J Infect Dis. 1989;159:569–72.

138. Beral V, Peterman TA, Berkelman RL, et al. Kaposi's sarcoma among persons with AIDS: A sexually transmitted infection? Lancet. 1990;335:123–8.

139. Moore RD, Kessler H, Richman DD, et al. Non-Hodgkin's lymphoma in patients with advanced HIV infection treated with zidovudine. JAMA. 1991; 265:2208–11.

140. Selwyn PA, Feingold AR, Hartel D, et al. Increased risk of bacterial pneumonia in HIV-infected intravenous drug users without AIDS. AIDS. 1988;2: 167–72.

141. Janoff EN, Breiman RF, Daley CL, et al. Pneumococcal disease during HIV infection. Epidemiologic, clinical, and immunologic perspectives. Ann Intern Med. 1992;117:314–24.

142. Redd SC, Rutherford GW III, Sande MA, et al. The role of human immunodeficiency virus infection in pneumococcal bacteremia in San Francisco residents. J Infect Dis. 1990;162:1012–7.

143. Laga M, Icenogle JP, Marsella R, et al. Genital papillomavirus infection and cervical dysplasia—opportunistic complications of HIV infection. Int J Cancer. 1992;50:45–8.

144. Ellerbrock T, Wright TC, Chiasson MA, et al. Strong independent association between HIV infection and cervical intraepithelial neoplasia (CIN) (Abstract WS-B07-5). In: Abstracts of the IX International Conference on AIDS/IVth STD World Congress. v. I. Berlin, Germany, June 6–11, 1993:50.

145. Wright T, Sun X, Ellerbrock T, et al. Human papillomavirus infections in HIV+ and HIV− women: Prevalence, association with cervical intraepithelial neoplasia, and impact of CD4+ count (Abstract WS-B17-2). In: Abstracts of the IX International Conference on AIDS/IVth STD World Congress. v. I. Berlin, Germany, June 6–11, 1993:60.

146. Barnes PF, Bloch AB, Davidson PT, et al. Tuberculosis in patients with human immunodeficiency virus infection. N Engl J Med. 1991;324:1644–50.

147. Raviglione MC, Narain JP, Kochi A. HIV-associated tuberculosis in developing countries: Clinical features, diagnosis, and treatment. Bull WHO. 1992; 70:515–26.

148. Braun MM, Cote TR, Rabkin CS. Trends in death with tuberculosis during the AIDS era. JAMA. 1993;269:2865–8.

149. Rieder HL, Snider DE Jr. Tuberculosis and the acquired immunodeficiency syndrome (Editorial). Chest. 1986;90:469–70.

150. Castro KG, Curran JW. Overview of the tuberculosis and human immunodeficiency virus epidemics. J Law Med Ethics. In press.

151. Centers for Disease Control and Prevention: Initial therapy for tuberculosis in the era of multidrug resistance. Recommendations of the Advisory Council for the Elimination of Tuberculosis. MMWR. 1993;42(No.RR-7):1–8.

152. Frieden TR, Sterling T, Pablos-Mendez A, et al. The emergence of drug-resistant tuberculosis in New York City. N Engl J Med. 1993;328:521–6.

153. Edlin BR, Tokars JI, Grieco MH, et al. An outbreak of multidrug-resistant buerculosis among hospitalized patients with the acquired immunodeficiency syndrome. N Engl J Med. 1992;326:1514–21.

154. Pearson ML, Jereb JA, Frieden TR, et al. Nosocomial transmission of multidrug-resistant *Mycobacterium tuberculosis*. A risk to patients and health care workers. Ann Intern Med. 1992;117:191–6.

155. Beck-Sague C, Dooley SW, Hutton MD, et al. Hospital outbreak of multidrug-resistant *Mycobacterium tuberculosis* infections. Factors in transmission to staff and HIV-infected patients. JAMA. 1992;268:1280–6.

156. Chu SY, Farizo K, Hanson D, et al. Capturing HIV-related mortality—effect of the 1993 expanded AIDS surveillance case definition (Abstract WS-C01-5). In: Abstracts of the IXth International Conference on AIDS/IVth STD World Congress. v. I. Berlin, Germany, June 6–11, 1993:82.

157. Centers for Disease Control and Prevention: Update: Mortality attributable to HIV infection/AIDS among persons aged 25–44 years—United States, 1990 and 1991. MMWR. 1993;42:481–6.

157a.Centers for Disease Control and Prevention. Update: Mortality attributable to HIV infection among persons aged 25–44 years—United States, 1991 and 1992. MMWR. 1993;42:869–70.

157b.Selik RM, Chu SY. HIV infection as the leading cause of death among young adults in U.S. cities and states: 1991. JAMA. 1994;271:903.

158. Centers for Disease Control and Prevention: Years of potential life lost before age 65—United States, 1990 and 1991. MMWR. 1993;42:251–2.

159. Rothenberg R, Woelfel M, Stoneburner R, et al. Survival with the acquired immunodeficiency syndrome. N Engl J Med. 1987;317:1297–302.

160. Bacchetti P, Osmond D, Chaisson RE, et al. Survival patterns of the first 500 patients with AIDS in San Francisco. J Infect Dis. 1988;157:1044–7.

161. Lemp GF, Payne SF, Neal D, et al. Survival trends for patients with AIDS. JAMA. 1990;263:402–6.

162. Moore RD, Hidalgo J, Sugland BW, et al. Zidovudine and the natural history of the acquired immunodeficiency syndrome. N Engl J Med. 1991;324: 1412–6.

163. Swanson CE, Cooper DA. Factors influencing outcome of treatment with zidovudine of patients with AIDS in Australia. AIDS. 1990;4:749–57.

164. Hardy AM, Long-term Survivor Collaborative Study Group. Characterization of long-term survivors of acquired immunodeficiency syndrome. J Acquir Immune Defic Syndr. 1991;4:386–91.

165. Moss AR, McCallum G, Volberding PA, et al. Mortality associated with mode of presentation in the acquired immune deficiency syndrome. J Natl Cancer Int. 1984;73:1281–4.

166. Vadhan-Raj S, Wong G, Gnecco C, et al. Immunological variables as predictors of prognosis in patients with Kaposi's sarcoma and the acquired immunodeficiency syndrome. Cancer Res. 1986;46:417–25.

167. Ragni MV, Kingsley LA, Zhou SJ. The effect of antiviral therapy on the natural history of human immunodeficiency virus infection in a cohort of hemophiliacs. J Acquir Immune Defic Syndr. 1992;5:120–6.

168. Drabick JJ, Williams WJ, Tang DB, et al. CD4 lymphocyte decline and survival in human immunodeficiency virus infection. AIDS Res Hum Restroviruses. 1992;8:2039–47.

169. Vella S, Giuliano M, Pezzotti P, et al. Survival of zidovudine-treated patients with AIDS compared with that of contemporary untreated patients. JAMA. 1992;267:1232–6.

170. Buira E, Gatell JM, Miro JM, et al. Influence of treatment with zidovudine (ZDV) on the long-term survival of AIDS patients. J Acquir Immune Defic Syndr. 1992;5:737–42.

171. Creagh-Kirk T, Doi P, Andrews E, et al. Survival experience among patients with AIDS receiving zidovudine. JAMA. 1989;260:3009–15.

172. Graham NM, Zeger SL, Park LP. The effects on survival of early treatment of human immunodeficiency virus infection. N Engl J Med. 1992; 326:1037–42.

173. Chaisson RE, Keruly J, Richman DD, et al. Pneumocystis prophylaxis and survival in patients with advanced human immunodeficiency virus infection treated with zidovudine. Arch Intern Med. 1992;152:2009–13.

174. Yarchoan R, Venzon DJ, Pluda JM, et al. CD4 count and the risk for death in patients infected with HIV receiving antiretroviral therapy. Ann Intern Med. 1991;115:184–9.

175. Williams WJ, Drabick JJ, Tang DB. CD4 cell counts and the risk of death in HIV infection (Letter). Ann Intern Med. 1992;116:168.

176. Hamilton JD, Hartigan PM, Simberkoff MS, et al. A controlled trial of early versus late treatment with zidovudine in symptomatic human immunodeficiency virus infection. N Engl J Med. 1992;326:437–43.

177. Duliege A-M, Messiah A, Blanche S, et al. Natural history of human immunodeficiency virus type 1 infection in children: Prognostic value of laboratory tests on the biomodal progression of the disease. Pediatr Infect Dis J. 1992; 11:630–5.

178. McKinney RE Jr, Wilfert CM. Lymphocyte subsets in children younger than 2 years old: Normal values in a population at risk for human immunodeficiency virus infection and diagnostic and prognostic application to infected children. Pediatr Infect Dis J. 1992;11:639–44.

179. Waecker NJ Jr, Ascher DP, Robb ML, et al. Age-adjusted CD4+ lymphocyte parameters in healthy children at risk for infection with human immunodeficiency virus. Clin Infect Dis. 1993;17:123–5.

180. Quinn TC, Ruff A, Modlin J. HIV infection and AIDS in children. Annu Rev Public Health. 1992;13:1–30.

181. Lifson AR, Rogers MF, White C, et al. Unrecognized modes of transmission of HIV: Acquired immunodeficiency syndrome in children reported without risk factors. Pediatr Infect Dis. 1987;6:292–3.

182. Lindegren ML, Simonds RJ, Gwinn M, et al. Why are perinatal AIDS cases in the United States (US) not increasing (Abstract PO-C16-2988)? In: Abstracts of the IX International Conference on AIDS/IVth STD World Congress. v. II. Berlin, Germany, June 6–11, 1993:715.

183. Jones DS, Byers RH, Bush TJ, et al. Epidemiology of transfusion-associated acquired immunodeficiency syndrome in children in the United States, 1981 through 1989. Pediatrics. 1992;89:123–7.

184. Horsburgh CR Jr, Caldwell MB, Simonds RJ. Epidemiology of disseminated nontuberculous mycobacterial disease in children with acquired immunodeficiency syndrome. Pediatr Infect Dis J. 1993;12:219–22.

185. Centers for Disease Control and Prevention: Guidelines for prophylaxis against *Pneumocystis carinii* pneumonia for children infected with human immunodeficiency virus. MMWR. 1991;40(RR-2):1–13.

186. Blanche S, Tardieu M, Duliege A-M, et al. Longitudinal study of 94 symptomatic infants with perinatally acquired human immunodeficiency virus infection. Evidence for a bimodal expression of clinical and biological symptoms. Am J Dis Child. 1990;144:1210–5.

187. Byers B, Caldwell B, Oxtoby M, et al. Survival of children with perinatal HIV-infection: Evidence for two distinct populations (Abstract WS-C10-6). In: Abstracts of the IX International Conference on AIDS/IVth STD World Congress. v. I. Berlin, Germany, June 6–11, 1993:91.

188. Scott GB, Hutto C, Makuch RW, et al. Survival in children with perinatally

acquired human immunodeficiency virus type 1 infection. N Engl J Med. 1989;321:1791–6.

189. Turner BJ, Denison M, Eppes SC, et al. Survial experience of 789 children with the acquired immunodeficiency syndrome. Pediatr Infect Dis J. 1993; 12:310–20.

190. Simonds RJ, Oxtoby MJ, Caldwell MB, et al. *Pneumocystis carinii* pneumonia among U.S. children with perinatally acquired HIV infection. JAMA. 1993;270:470–3.

191. Padian NS. Heterosexual transmission of acquired immunodeficiency syndrome: International perspectives and national projections. Rev Infect Dis. 1987;9:947–60.

192. Chin J, Sato PA, Mann JM. Projections of HIV infections and AIDS cases to the year 2000. Bull WHO. 1990;68:1–11.

193. Holmberg SD, Horsburgh CR Jr, Ward JW, et al. Biologic factors in the sexual transmission of human immunodeficiency virus. J Infect Dis. 1989; 160:116–25.

194. Clumeck N, Taelman H, Hermans P, et al. A cluster of HIV infection among heterosexual people without apparent risk factors. N Engl J Med. 1989;321: 1460–2.

195. Peterman TA, Stoneburner RL, Allen JR, et al. Risk of human immunodeficiency virus transmission from heterosexual adults with transfusion-associated infections. JAMA. 1988;59:55–8.

196. Johnson AM, Petherick A, Davidson SJ, et al. Transmission of HIV to heterosexual partners of infected men and women. AIDS. 1989;3:367–72.

197. Goedert JJ, Eyster ME, Bigger RJ, et al. Heterosexual transmission of human immunodeficiency virus: Association with severe depletion of T-helper lymphocytes in men with hemophilia. AIDS Res Hum Retroviruses. 1987;3: 355–61.

198. European Study Group on Heterosexual Transmission of HIV. Comparison of female to male and male to female transmission of HIV in 563 stable couples. Br Med J. 1992;304:809–13.

199. Lazzarin A, Saracco A, Musicco M, et al. Man-to-woman sexual transmission of the human immunodeficiency virus. Risk factors related to sexual behavior, man's infectiousness, and woman's susceptibility. Arch Intern Med. 1991;151:2411–6.

200. Laga M, Taelman H, Van der Stuyft P, et al. Advanced immunodeficiency as a risk factor for heterosexual transmission of HIV. AIDS. 1989;3:361–6.

201. Seage GR III, Mayer KH, Horsburgh CR Jr. Risk of human immunodeficiency virus infection from unprotected receptive anal intercourse increases with decline in immunologic status of infected partners. Am J Epidemiol. 1993;137:899–908.

202. Anderson DJ, Hill JA. CD4 (T4+) lymphocytes in semen of healthy heterosexual men: Implications for the transmission of AIDS (Letter). Fertil Steril. 1987;48:703–4.

203. Anderson DJ, O'Brien TR, Politch JA, et al. Effects of disease stage and zodivudine therapy on the detection of human immunodeficiency virus type 1 in semen. JAMA. 1992;267:2769–74.

204. Ho DD, Moudgil T, Alam M. Quantitation of human immunodeficiency virus type 1 in the blood of infected persons. N Engl J Med. 1989;321:1621–5.

205. Henin Y, Porrot F, Montagnier L, et al. Prevalence of HIV in the cervicovaginal secretions of women seropositive for HIV: Correlation with the clinical status and implications for heterosexual transmission (Abstract Th.C. 554). In: Abstracts of the VIth International Conference on AIDS. v. 1. San Francisco, CA, June 20–24, 1990:263.

206. Seage GR III, Horsburgh CR Jr, Hardy AM, et al. Increased suppressor T cells in probable transmitters of human immunodeficiency virus infection. Am J Public Health. 1989;79:1638–42.

207. Massimo M, Angarano G, Saracco A, et al. Antiretroviral therapy reduces the rate of sexual transmission of HIV-1 from man to women (Abstract WeC 1088). In: Abstracts of the VIII International Conference on AIDS/III STD World Congress. v. 1. Amsterdam, the Netherlands, July 19–24, 1992:We61.

208. Chirianni A, Perna E, Liuzzi G, et al. Absence of anti-HIV seroconversion in heterosexual partners of HIV patients treated with zidovudine (Abstract PoC 4530). In: Poster Abstracts of the VIII International Conference on AIDS/III STD World Congress. v. 2. Amsterdam, the Netherlands, July 19–24, 1992:C333.

209. Routy JP, Blanc AP, Allegre T, et al. HIV-1 transmission by a heterosexual man treated with zidovudine (Letter). J Acquir Immune Defic Syndr. 1991; 4:1166–7.

210. Ivanoff LA, Dubay JW, Morris JF, et al. V3 loop region of the HIV-1 gp 120 envelope protein is essential for virus infectivity. Virology. 1992;187: 423–32.

211. Fiore JR, Jansson M, Scarlatti G, et al. Correlation between seroreactivity to HIV-1 V3 loop peptides and male-to-female heterosexual transmission. AIDS. 1993;7:29–31.

212. Padian NS, Shiboski SC, Jewell NP. Female-to-male transmission of HIV (Letter). JAMA. 1992;268:1856–7.

213. Moss GB, Clemetson D, D'Costa L, et al. Association of cervical ectopy with heterosexual transmission of human immunodeficiency virus: Results of a study of couples in Nairobi, Kenya. J Infect Dis. 1991;164:588–91.

214. Padian NS, Shiboski SC, Jewell NP. Female-to-male transmission of human immunodeficiency virus. JAMA. 1991;266:1664–7.

215. Padian NS, Shiboski SC, Jewell NP. The effect of number of exposures on the risk of heterosexual HIV transmission. J Infect Dis. 1990;161:883–7.

216. Goto Y, Yeh C-K, Notkins AL, et al. Detection of proviral sequences in saliva of patients infected with human immunodeficiency virus type 1. AIDS Res Hum Retroviruses. 1991;7:343–7.

217. Levy JA, Greenspan D. HIV in saliva (Letter). Lancet. 1988;2:1248.

218. Piot P, Plummer PA. Genital ulcer adenopathy syndrome. In: Holmes KK, Mardh PA, Sparling PF, eds. Sexually Transmitted Diseases. 2nd ed. New York: McGraw-Hill; 1990:711–6.

219. Piot P, Laga M. Genital ulcers, other sexually transmitted diseases, and the sexual transmission of HIV. The first two may be important risk factors for the third. Br Med J. 1989;298:623–4.

220. Plummer FA, Simonsen JN, Cameron DW, et al. Cofactors in male-female sexual transmission of human immunodeficiency virus type 1. J Infect Dis. 1991;163:233–9.

221. Cameron DW, Simonsen JN, D'Costa LJ, et al. Female to male transmission of human immunodeficiency virus type 1: Risk factors for seroconversion in men. Lancet. 1989;2:403–7.

222. Stamm WE, Handsfield HH, Rompalo AM, et al. The association between genital ulcer disease and acquisition of HIV infection in homosexual men. JAMA. 1988;260:1429–33.

223. Kreiss KJ, Coombs R, Plummer F, et al. Isolation of human immunodeficiency virus from genital ulcers in Nairobi prostitutes. J Infect Dis. 1989; 160:380–4.

224. Laga M, Manoka A, Kivuvu M, et al. Non-ulcerative sexually transmitted diseases as risk factors for HIV-1 transmission in women: Results from a cohort study. AIDS. 1993;7:95–102.

225. Wolff H, Anderson DJ. Male genital tract inflammation associated with increased numbers of potential human immunodeficiency virus host cells in semen. Andrologia. 1988;20:404–10.

226. Fischl MA, Dickinson GM, Scott GB, et al. Evaluation of heterosexual partners, children, and household contacts of adults with AIDS. JAMA. 1987; 257:640–4.

227. Padian N, Marquis L, Francis DP, et al. Male-to-female transmission of human immunodeficiency virus. JAMA. 1987;258:788–90.

228. Kim MY, Lagakos SW. Estimating the infectivity of HIV from partner studies. Ann Epidemiol. 1990;1:117–28.

229. Feldblum PJ. Results from prospective studies of HIV-discordant couples (Letter). AIDS. 1991;5:1265–6.

230. Haverkos HW, Battjes RJ. Female-to-male transmission of HIV (Letter). JAMA. 1992;268:1855.

231. Popovic M, Sarngadharan MG, Reed E, et al. Detection, isolation, and continuous production of cytopathic retroviruses (HTLV-III) from patients with AIDS and pre-AIDS. Science. 1984;224:497–500.

232. Greenblatt RM, Lukehart SA, Plummer FA, et al. Genital ulceration as a risk factor for human immunodeficiency virus infection. AIDS. 1988;2:47–50.

233. Holmberg SD, Stewart JA, Gerber AR, et al. Prior herpes simplex virus type 2 infection as a risk factor for HIV infection. JAMA. 1988;259:1048–50.

234. Hira SK, Kamanga J, Macuacua R, et al. Genital ulcers and male circumcision as risk factors for acquiring HIV-1 in Zambia (Letter). J Infect Dis. 1990;161:584–5.

235. Jessamine PG, Plummer FA, Achola JON, et al. Human immunodeficiency virus, genital ulcers and the male foreskin: Synergism in HIV-1 transmission. Scand J Infect Dis. 1990;69(Suppl):181–6.

236. Kreiss J, Ngugi E, Holmes K, et al. Efficacy of nonoxynol 9 contraceptive sponge in preventing heterosexual acquisition of HIV in Nairobi prostitutes. JAMA. 1992;268:477–82.

237. Stone KM, Peterson HB. Spermicides, HIV, and the vaginal sponge (Editorial). JAMA. 1992;268:521–3.

238. Darrow WW, Echenberg DF, Jaffe HW, et al. Risk factors for human immunodeficiency virus (HIV) infections in homosexual men. Am J Public Health. 1987;77:479–83.

239. Winkelstein W, Lyman DM, Padian N, et al. Sexual practices and risk of infection by the human immunodeficiency virus. The San Francisco Men's Health Study. JAMA. 1987;257:321–5.

240. Kingsley LA, Detels R, Kaslow R, et al. Risk factors for seroconversion to human immunodeficiency virus among male homosexuals. Results from the Multicenter AIDS Cohort Study. Lancet. 1987;1:345–9.

241. Chu SY, Buehler JW, Fleming PL, et al. Epidemiology of reported cases of AIDS in lesbians, United States 1980–89. Am J Public Health. 1990;80: 1380–1.

242. Petersen LR, Doll L, White C, et al. No evidence for female-to-female HIV transmission among 960,000 female blood donors. J Acquir Immune Defic Syndr. 1992;5:853–5.

243. Marmor M, Weiss LR, Lyden M, et al. Possible female-to-female transmission of human immunodeficiency virus (Letter). Ann Intern Med. 1986;105: 969.

244. Monzon OT, Capellan JMB. Female-to-female transmission of HIV (Letter). Lancet. 1987;2:40–1.

245. Lifson AR, O'Malley PM, Hessol NA, et al. HIV seroconversion in two homosexual men after receptive oral intercourse with ejaculation: Implications for counseling concerning safe sexual practices. Am J Public Health. 1990;80:1509–11.

246. Marion SA, Schechter MT, Weaver MS, et al. Evidence that prior immune dysfunction predisposes to human immunodeficiency virus infection in homosexual men. J Acquir Immune Defic Syndr. 1989;2:178–86.

247. Madhok R, Gracie A, Lowe GDO, et al. Impaired cell mediated immunity in haemophilia in the absence of infection with human immunodeficiency virus. Br Med J. 1986;293:978–80.

248. Schoenbaum EE, Hartel D, Selwyn PA, et al. Risk factors for human immunodeficiency virus infection in intravenous drug users. N Engl J Med. 1989; 321:874–9.

249. Lange WR, Synder FR, Lozovsky D, et al. The geographic distribution of human immunodeficiency virus markers in parenteral drug abusers. Am J Public Health. 1988;78:443–6.

250. Allen DM, Onorato IM, Sweeney PA, et al. Seroprevalence of HIV infection in intravenous drug users (IVDUs) in the United States (U.S.) (Abstract F.C.551). In: Final program and Abstracts of the VIth International Conference on AIDS. v. 2. San Francisco, CA, June 20–24, 1990:218.

251. Anthony JC, Vlahov D, Nelson KE, et al. New evidence on intravenous cocaine use and the risk of infection with human immunodeficiency virus type 1. Am J Epidemiol. 1991;134:1175–89.

252. Koblin BA, McCusker J, Lewis BF, et al. Racial/ethnic differences in HIV-1 seroprevalence and risky behaviors among intravenous drug users in a multisite study. Am J Epidemiol. 1990;132:837–46.

253. Selik RM, Castro KG, Pappaioanou M, et al. Birthplace and the risk of AIDS among Hispanics in the United States. Am J Public Health. 1989;79:836–9.

254. McCusker J, Koblin B, Lewis BF, et al. Demographic characteristics, risk behaviors, and HIV seroprevalence among intravenous drug users by site of contact: Results from a community-wide HIV surveillance project. Am J Public Health. 1990;80:1062–7.

255. Nelson KE, Vlahov D, Cohn S, et al. Sexually transmitted diseases in a population of intravenous drug users: Association with seropositivity to the human immunodeficiency virus (HIV). J Infect Dis. 1991;164:457–63.

256. Rolfs RT, Goldberg M, Sharrar RG. Risk factors for syphilis: Cocaine use and prostitution. Am J Public Health. 1990;80:853–7.

257. Magura S, Grossman JI, Lipton DS, et al. Determinants of needle sharing among intravenous drug users. Am J Public Health. 1989;79:459–62.

258. Guydish JR, Abramowitz A, Woods W, et al. Changes in needle sharing behavior among intravenous drug users: San Francisco, 1986–88. Am J Public Health. 1990;80:995–7.

259. Neaigus A, Sufian M, Friedman SR, et al. Effects of outreach intervention on risk reduction among intravenous drug users. AIDS Educ Prev. 1990;2: 253–71.

260. Curran JW, Lawrence DN, Jaffe H, et al. Acquired immunodeficiency syndrome (AIDS) associated with transfusions. N Engl J Med. 1984;310:69–75.

261. Evatt BL, Ramsey RB, Lawrence DN, et al. The acquired immunodeficiency syndrome in patients with hemophilia. Ann Intern Med. 1984;100:499–504.

262. Donegan E, Stuart M, Niland JC, et al. Infection with human immunodeficiency virus type 1 (HIV-1) among recipients of antibody-positive blood donations. Ann Intern Med. 1990;113:733–9.

263. Ward JW, Deppe DA, Samson S, et al. Risk of human immunodeficiency virus infection from blood donors who later developed the acquired immunodeficiency syndrome. Ann Intern Med. 1987;106:61–2.

264. Centers for Disease Control and Prevention: Safety of therapeutic immune globulin preparations with respect to transmission of human T-lymphocytropic virus type III/lymphadenopathy-associated virus infection. MMWR. 1986;35:231–3.

265. Wells MA, Wittek AE, Epstein JS, et al. Inactivation and partition of human T-cell lymphotrophic virus, type III, during ethanol fractionation of plasma. Transfusion. 1986;26:210–3.

266. Ward JW, Grindon AJ, Feorino PM, et al. Laboratory and epidemiologic evalaution of an enzyme immunoassay for antibodies to HTLV-III. JAMA. 1986;256:357–61.

267. Peterman TA, Lui K-J, Lawrence DN, et al. Estimating the risks of transfusion-associated acquired immune deficiency syndrome and human immunodeficiency virus infection. Transfusion. 1987;27:371–4.

268. Ward JW, Holmberg SD, Allen JR, et al. Transmission of human immunodeficiency virus (HIV) by blood transfusions screened as negative for HIV antibody. N Engl J Med. 1988;318:473–8.

269. Nelson KE, Donahue JG, Munoz A, et al. Transmission of retroviruses from seronegative donors by transfusion during cardiac surgery. Ann Intern Med. 1992;117:554–9.

270. Cumming PD, Wallace EL, Schorr JB, et al. Exposure of transfused patients to human immunodeficiency virus through the transfusion of blood components that test antibody negative. N Engl J Med. 1989;321:917–24.

271. Stehr-Green JK, Jason JM, Evatt BL, et al. Geographic variability of hemophilia-associated AIDS in the United States: Effect of population characteristics. Am J Hematol. 1989;32:178–83.

272. Eyster ME, Gail MH, Ballard ID, et al. Natural history of human immunodeficiency virus infection in hemophiliacs: Effects of t-cell subsets, platelet counts and age. Ann Intern Med. 1987;107:1–6.

273. Erice A, Rhame FS, Heussner RC, et al. Human immunodeficiency virus infection in patients with solid-organ transplants: Report of five cases and review. Rev Infect Dis. 1991;13:537–47.

274. Clarke JA. HIV transmission and skin grafts. Lancet. 1987;1:983.

275. Pepose JS, McRae S, Quinn TC, et al. Serologic markers after the transplantation of corneas from donors infected with human immunodeficiency virus. Am J Ophthalmol. 1987;103:798–801.

276. Lewis SH, Reynolds-Kohler C, Fox HE, et al. HIV-1 in trophoblastic and villous Hofbauer cells, and haematological precursors in eight-week fetuses. Lancet. 1990;335:565–8.

277. Douglas GC, King BF. Maternal-fetal transmission of human immunodeficiency virus: A review of possible routes and cellular mechanisms of infection. Clin Infect Dis. 1992;15:678–91.

278. Krivine A, Firtion G, Cao L, et al. HIV replication during the first weeks of life. Lancet. 1992;339:1187–9.

279. Rogers MF, Ou C-Y, Rayfield M, et al. Use of the polymerase chain reaction for early detection of the proviral sequences of human immunodeficiency virus in infants born to seropositive mothers. N Engl J Med. 1989;320: 1649–54.

280. Burgard M, Mayaux M-J, Blanche S, et al. The use of viral culture and p24 antigen testing to diagnose human immunodeficiency virus infection in neonates. N Engl J Med. 1992;327:1192–7.

281. Rogers MF, Schochetman G, Hoff R. Advances in diagnosis of HIV infection in infants. In: Pizzo PA, Wilfert CM, eds. Pediatric AIDS: The Challenge of HIV Infection in Infants, Children and Adolescents. 2nd ed. Baltimore: Williams & Wilkins; 1994:219–38.

282. Ehrnst A, Lindgren S, Dictor M, et al. HIV in pregnant women and their offspring: Evidence for late transmission. Lancet. 1991;338:203–7.

283. Euorpean Collaborative Study. Risk factors for mother-to-child transmission of HIV-1. Lancet. 1992;339:1007–12.

284. Gabiano C, Tovo P-A, de Martino M, et al. Mother-to-child tranmission of human immunodeficiency virus type 1: Risk of infection and correlates of transmission. Pediatrics. 1992;90:369–74.

285. Blanche S, Rouzioux C, Moscato M-LG, et al. A prospective study of infants born to women seropositive for human immunodeficiency virus type 1. N Engl J Med. 1989;320:1643–8.

286. Hutto C, Parks WP, Lai S, et al. A hospital-based prospective study of perinatal infection with human immunodeficiency virus type 1. J Pediatr. 1991;118:347–53.

287. Goedert JJ, Duliege A-M, Amos CI, et al. High risk of HIV-1 infection for first-born twins. Lancet. 1991;338:1471–5.

288. Villari P, Spino C, Chalmers TC, et al. Cesarean section to reduce perinatal transmission of human immunodeficiency virus. A metaanalysis [Serial online]. Online J Curr Clin Trials. Jul 8, 1993 (Doc No. 74).

289. Thiry L, Sprecher-Goldberger S, Jonchkheer T, et al. Isolation of AIDS virus from cell-free breast milk of three heatlhy virus carriers (Letter). Lancet. 1985;2:891–2.

290. Oxtoby MJ. Human immunodeficiency virus and other viruses in human milk: Placing the issues in broader perspective. Pediatr Infect Dis. J. 1988; 7:825–35.

291. Ryder RW, Manzila T, Baende E, et al. Evidence from Zaire that breast-feeding by HIV-1 seropositive mothers is not a major route for perinatal HIV-1 transmission but does decrease morbidity. AIDS. 1991;5:709–14.

292. Dunn DT, Newell ML, Ades AE, et al. Risk of human immunodeficiency virus type 1 transmission through breastfeeding. Lancet. 1992;340:585–8.

293. Van de Perre P, Simonon A, Msellati P, et al. Postnatal transmission of human immunodeficiency virus type 1 from mother to infant. A prospective cohort study in Kigali, Rwanda. N Engl J Med. 1991;325:593–8.

294. Hu DJ, Heyward WL, Byers RH Jr, et al. HIV infection and breast-feeding: Policy implications through a decision analysis model. AIDS. 1992;6: 1505–13.

295. Ryder RW, Nsa W, Hassig SE, et al. Perinatal transmission of the human immunodeficiency virus type 1 to infants of seropsoitive women in Zaire. N Engl J Med. 1989;320:1637–42.

296. Mofenson LM. Preventing mother to infant HIV transmission: What we know so far. The AIDS Reader. 1992;March/April 42–51.

297. St. Louis ME, Kamenga M, Brown C, et al. Risk for perinatal HIV-1 transmission according to maternal immunologic, virologic, and placental factors. JAMA. 1993;269:2853–9.

298. Papaevangelou V, Moore T, Nagaraj V, et al. Lack of predictive value of maternal human immunodeficiency virus p24 antigen for transmission of infection to their children. Pediatr Infect Dis. J. 1992;11:851–5.

299. Goedert JJ, Mendez H, Drummond JE, et al. Mother-to-infant transmission of human immunodeficiency virus type 1: Association with prematurity or low anti-gp120. Lancet. 1989;2:1351–4.

300. Devash Y, Calvelli TA, Wood DG, et al. Vertical transmission of human immunodeficiency virus is correlated with the absence of high-affinity/avidity maternal antibodies to the gp120 principal neutralizing domain. Proc Natl Acad Sci USA. 1990;87:3445–9.

301. Parekh BS, Shaffer N, Pau C-P, et al. Lack of correlation between maternal antibodies to V3 loop peptides of gp120 and perinatal HIV-1 transmission. AIDS. 1991;5:1179–84.

302. Robertson CA, Mok JYQ, Froebel KS, et al. Maternal antibodies to gp120 V3 sequence do not correlate with protection against vertical transmission of human immunodeficiency virus. J Infect Dis. 1992;166:704–9.

303. Borkowsky W, Krasinski K, Pollack H, et al. Early diagnosis of human immunodeficiency virus infection in children <6 months of age: Comparison of polymerase chain reaction, culture, and plasma antigen capture techniques. J Infect Dis. 1992;166:616–9.

304. Report of a Consensus Workshop, Siena, Italy, January 17–18, 1992. Early diagnosis of HIV infection in infants. J Acquir Immun Defic Syndr. 1992;5: 1169–78.

305. Tokars JI, Bell DM, Culver DH, et al. Percutaneous injuries during surgical procedures. JAMA. 1992;267:2899–904.

306. Marcus R, Culver DH, Bell DM, et al. Risk of human immunodeficiency virus infection among emergency department workers. Am J Med. 1993;94: 363–70.

307. Wong ES, Stotka JL, Chinchilli VM, et al. Are universal precautions effective in reducing the number of occupational exposures among health care workers? A prospective study of physicians on a medical service. JAMA. 1991;265:1123–8.

308. Tokars JI, Marcus R, Culver DH, et al. Survillance of HIV infection and zidovudine use among health care workers after occupational exposure to HIV-infected blood. Ann Intern Med. 1993;118:913–9.

309. Henderson DK, Fahey BJ, Willy M, et al. Risk for occupational transmission of human immunodeficiency virus type 1 (HIV-1) associated with clinical exposures. A prospective evaluation. Ann Intern Med. 1990;113:740–6.

310. Ippolito G, Puro V, De Carli G. The risk of occupational human immunodeficiency virus infection in health care workers. Italian multicenter study. Arch Intern Med. 1993;153:1451–8.

311. Chamberland ME, Conley LJ, Bush TJ, et al. Health care workers with AIDS. National surveillance update. JAMA. 1991;266:3459–62.

312. Chamberland ME, Bell DM. HIV transmission from health care worker to patient: What is the risk (Editorial). Ann Intern Med. 1992;116:871–3.

313. Ciesielski C, Marianos D, Ou C-Y, et al. Transmission of human immunodeficiency virus in a dental practice. Ann Intern Med. 1992;116:798–805.

314. Centers for Disease Control and Prevention: Update: Investigations of patients who have been treated by HIV-infected health-care workers—United States. MMWR. 1993;42:329–31, 337.

315. Ou C-Y, Ciesielski CA, Myers G, et al. Molecular epidemiology of HIV transmission in a dental practice. Science. 1992;256:1165–71.

316. Bell DM, Shapiro CN, Gooch BF. Preventing HIV transmission to patients during invasive procedures. J Public Health Dent. 1993;53:170–3.

317. Centers for Disease Control and Prevention: Patient exposures to HIV during nuclear medicine procedures. MMWR. 1992;41:575–8.

318. Centers for Disease Control and Prevention: HIV infection in two brothers receiving intravenous therapy for hemophilia. MMWR. 1992;41:228–31.

318a. Centers for Disease Control and Prevention: Human immunodeficiency virus transmission in household settings—United States. MMWR. 1994;43:347; 353–6.

319. Hersh BS, Popovici F, Apetrei RC, et al. Acquired immunodeficiency syndrome in Romania. Lancet. 1991;338:645–9.

320. Pokrovsky VV, Eramova EU. Nosocomial outbreak of HIV infection in Elista, USSR (Abstract W.A.O.5). In: Abstracts of the V International Conference on AIDS. Montreal, Canada, June 4–9, 1989:63.

320a. Chant K, Lowe D, Rubin G, et al. Patient-to-patient transmission of HIV in private surgical consulting rooms (Letter). Lancet. 1993;342:1548–9.

321. Fujikawa LS, Salahuddin SZ, Palestine AG, et al. Isolation of human T-lymphotropic virus type III from the tears of a patient with the acquired immunodeficiency syndrome. Lancet. 1985;2:529–30.

322. Ho DD, Rota TR, Schooley RT, et al. Isolation of HTLV-III from cerebrospinal fluid and neural tissues of patients with neurologic syndromes related to the acquired immunodeficiency syndrome. N Engl J Med. 1985;313:1493–7.

323. Mundy DC, Schinazi RF, Gerber AR, et al. Human immunodeficiency virus isolated from amniotic fluid (Letter). Lancet. 1987;2:459–60.

324. Hill DR. HIV infection following motor vehicle trauma in central Africa. JAMA. 1989;261:3282–3.

325. Torre D, Sampietro C, Ferraro G, et al. Transmission of HIV-1 infection via sports injury (Letter). Lancet. 1990;335:1105.

326. Stewart GJ, Tyler JPP, Cunningham AL, et al. Transmission of human T-cell lymphotropic virus type III (HTLV-III) by artificial insemination by donor. Lancet. 1985;2:581–5.

327. Chiasson MA, Stoneburner RL, Joseph SC. Human immunodeficiency virus transmission through artificial insemination. J Acquir Immune Defic Syndr. 1990;3:69–72.

328. Centers for Disease Control and Prevention: HIV-1 infection and artificial insemination with processed semen. MMWR. 1990;39:249,255–6.

329. Yeh C-K, Handelman B, Fox PC, et al. Further studies of salivary inhibition of HIV-1 infectivity. J Acquir Immun Defic Syndr. 1992;5:898–903.

330. Wahn V, Kramer HH, Voit T, et al. Horizontal transmission of HIV infection between two siblings (Letter). Lancet. 1986;2:694.

331. Rogers MF, White CR, Sanders R, et al. Lack of transmission of human immunodeficiency virus from infected children to their household contacts. Pediatrics. 1990;85:210–4.

332. Saviteer SM, White GC, Cohen MS, et al. HTLV-III exposure during cardiopulmonary resuscitation (Letter). N Engl J Med. 1985;313:1606–7.

333. Lifson AR. Do alternate modes for transmission of human immunodeficiency virus exist? A review. JAMA. 1988;259:1353–6.

334. Gershon RRM, Vlahov D, Nelson KE. The risk of transmission of HIV-1 through non-percutaneous, non-sexual modes—A review. AIDS. 1990;4:645–50.

335. Lusher JM, Operskalski EA, Aledort LM, et al. Risk of human immunodeficiency virus type 1 infection among sexual and nonsexual household contacts of persons with congenital clotting disorders. Pediatrics. 1991;88:242–9.

335a. Centers for Disease Control and Prevention: Apparent transmission of human T-lymphotrophic virus type III/lymphadenopathy-associated virus from a child to a mother providing health care. MMWR. 1986;35:76–9.

335b. Centers for Disease Control and Prevention: HIV transmission between two adolescent brothers with hemophilia. MMWR. 1993;42:948–51.

335c. Fitzgibbon JE, Gaur S, Frenkel LD, et al. Transmission from one child to another of human immunodeficiency virus type 1 with a zidovudine-resistance mutation. N Engl J Med. 1993;329:1835–41.

335d. Grint P, McEvoy M. Two associated cases of the acquired immunodeficiency syndrome (AIDS). Communicable Disease Report. 1985;42:4.

336. Srinivasan A, York D, Bohan C. Lack of HIV replication in arthropod cells (Letter). Lancet. 1987;1:1094–5.

337. Miike L. Do Insects Transmit AIDS? Washington, D.C.: Health Program, Office of Technology Assessment, U.S. Congress. 1987:1–43.

338. Webb PA, Happ CM, Maupin GO, et al. Potential for insect transmission of HIV: Experimental exposure of *Cimex hemipterus* and *Toxorhynchites amboinensis* to human immunodeficiency virus. J Infect Dis. 1989;160:970–7.

339. Castro KG, Lieb S, Jaffe HW, et al. Transmission of HIV in Belle Glade, Florida: Lessons for other communities in the United States. Science. 1988; 239:193–7.

340. Greenberg AE, Nguyen-Dinh P, Mann JM, et al. The association between malaria, blood transfusions, and HIV seropositivity in a pediatric population in Kinshasa, Zaire. JAMA. 1988;259:545–9.

341. World Health Organization. The current global situation of the HIV/AIDS pandemic. Global Programme on AIDS. July 1, 1993.

342. Chin J, Mann JM. The global patterns and prevalence of AIDS and HIV infection. AIDS 1988;2(Suppl 1):S247–52.

343. World Health Organization. Global programme on AIDS: Current and future dimensions of the HIV/AIDS pandemic—A capsule summary. Geneva: World Health Organization, April 1991.

344. Mann JM, Tarantola DJM, Netter TW, eds. Global AIDS Policy Coalition. AIDS in the World: A Global Report. Cambridge MA: Harvard University Press, 1992:88.

345. Cortes E, Detels R, Aboulafia D, et al. HIV-1, HIV-2, and HTLV-1 infection in high risk groups in Brazil. N Engl J Med. 1989;320:953–8.

346. Torrey BB, Way PO. Seroprevalence of HIV in Africa: Winter 1990. CIR staff paper No. 55, May 1990. Washington, DC: Center for International Research, U.S. Bureau of the Census.

347. Rwandan HIV Seroprevalence Study Group. Nationwide community based serological survey of HIV-1 and other human retroviruses infections in a central African country. Lancet. 1989;1:941–3.

348. Serwadda D, Wawer MJ, Musgrave SD, et al. HIV risk factors in three geographic strata of rural Rakai District, Uganda. AIDS. 1992;6:983–9.

349. Miotti PG, Dallabetta GA, Ndovi E, et al. HIV-1 and pregnant women: Associated factors, prevalence, estimate of incidence and role in fetal wastage in Central Africa. AIDS. 1990;4:733–6.

350. Allen S, Lindan C, Serufilira A, et al. Human immunodeficiency virus infection in urban Rwanda: Demographic and behavioral correlates in a representative sample of childbearing women. JAMA. 1991;226:1657–63.

351. N'Galy B, Ryder RW. Epidemiology of HIV infection in Africa. J Acquir Immune Defic Syndr. 1988;1:551–8.

352. Dallabetta GA, Miotti PG, Chiphangwi JD, et al. High socioeconomic status is a risk factor for human immunodeficiency virus type 1 (HIV-1) infection but not for sexually transmitted diseases in women in Malawi: Implications for HIV-1 control. J Infect Dis. 1993;167:36–42.

353. Piot P, Plummer FA, Rey M-A, et al. Retrospective seroepidemiology of AIDS virus infections in Nairobi populations. J Infect Dis. 1987;155:1108–12.

354. Simonsen JN, Plummer FA, Ngugi EN, et al. HIV infection among lower socioeconomic strata prostitutes in Nairobi. AIDS. 1990;4:139–44.

355. Simonsen JN, Cameron W, Gakinya MN, et al. Human immunodeficiency virus infection among men with sexually transmitted diseases. N Engl J Med. 1988;319:274–8.

356. Pape JW, Stanback ME, Pamphile M, et al. Prevalence of HIV infection and high-risk activities in Haiti. J Acquire Immune Defic Syndr. 1990;3:995–1001.

357. Diallo MO, Ackah AN, Lafontaine M-F, et al. HIV-1 and HIV-2 infections in men attending sexually transmitted disease clinics in Abidjan, Cote D'Ivoire. AIDS. 1992;6:581–5.

358. Weniger BG, Limpakarnjanarat K, Ungchusak K, et al. The epidemiology of HIV infection and AIDS in Thailand. AIDS. 1991;5(Suppl 2):S71–85.

359. Ou C-Y, Takebe Y, Weniger BG, et al. Independent introduction of two major HIV-1 genotypes into distinct high-risk populations in Thailand. Lancet. 1993;341:1171–4.

360. Sirisopana N, Torugsa K, Carr J, et al. Prevalence of HIV-1 infection in young men entering the Royal Thai Army (Abstract PO-C08-2778). In: Abstracts of the IXth International Conference on AIDS/IVth STD World Congress. v. II. Berlin, Germany, June 6–11, 1993:680.

361. Brajachand SN, Ibotoma SY, Naik TN, et al. Spread of HIV infection in Manipur, a border state of India (Abstract PO-C08-2763). In: Abstracts of the IXth International Conference on AIDS/IVth STD World Congress. v. II. Berlin, Germany, June 6–11, 1993:677.

362. Tripathy S, Banerjee K, Rodriques J, et al. Increasing HIV infection in western India (Abstract PO-CO8-2764). In: Abstracts of the IXth International Conference on AIDS/IVth STD World Congress. v. II. Berlin, Germany, June 6–11, 1993:678.

363. Singh YN, Malaviya AN, Tripathy SP, et al. HIV serosurveillance among prostitutes and patients from a sexually transmitted diseases clinic in Delhi, India. J Acquire Immune Defic Syndr. 1990;3:287–9.

364. Singh S, Crofts N, Gertig D. HIV infection among IDU's in northeast Malaysia (Abstract PO-C08-2777). In: Abstracts of the IXth International Conference on AIDS/IVth STD World Congress. v. II. Berlin, Germany, June 6–11, 1993:680.

365. Zheng X, Thian C, Zhang J, et al. Rapid spread of HIV among drug users and their wives in southwest China (Abstract PO-CO8-2766). In: Abstracts of the IXth International Conference on AIDS/IVth STD World Congress. v. II. Berlin, Germany, June 6–11, 1993:678.

366. Bhave GG, Wagle UD, Tripathi SP, et al. HIV serosurveillance in promiscuous females of Bombay, India (Abstract FC.612). In: Final Program and Abstracts of the VIth International Conference on AIDS. v. 2. San Francisco, CA, June 20–24, 1990:234.

367. Oh M-d, Choe K, Shin Y, et al. Current status of HIV/AIDS epidemic in South Korea (Abstract PO-C08-2769). In: Abstracts of the IXth International Conference on AIDS/IVth STD World Congress. v. II. Berlin, Germany, June 6–11, 1993:678.

368. Soda K, Fukutomi K, Hashimoto S, et al. Temporal trend and projections

of HIV/AIDS epidemic in Japan (Abstract PO-CO8-2779). In: Abstracts of the IXth International Conference on AIDS/IVth STD World Congress. v. II. Berlin, Germany, June 6–11, 1993:680.

369. Mann JM, Tarantola DJM, Netter TW, eds. Global AIDS Policy Coalition. AIDS in the World: A Global Report. Cambridge MA: Harvard University Press; 1992:105–6, 127–8.

370. Clavel F, Guetard D, Brun-Vezinet F, et al. Isolation of a new human retrovirus from West African patients with AIDS. Science. 1986;233:343–6.

371. Centers for Disease Control and Prevention: Testing for antibodies to human immunodeficiency virus type 2 in the United States. MMWR. 1992; 41(No.RR-12):1–9.

371a.DeCock KM, Adjorlolo G, Ekpini E, et al. Epidemiology and transmission of HIV-2: Why there is no HIV-2 pandemic. JAMA. 1993;270:2083–6.

372. O'Brien TR, George JR, Holmberg SD. Human immunodeficiency virus type 2 infection in the United States: Epidemiology, diagnosis, and public health implications. JAMA. 1992;267:2775–9.

373. Onorato IM, O'Brien TR, Schable CA, et al. Sentinel surveillance for HIV-2 infection in high-risk US populations. Am J Public Health. 1993;83:515–9.

374. Markovitz DM. Infection with the human immunodeficiency virus type 2. Ann Intern Med. 1993;118:211–8.

375. Poulsen A-G, Kvinesdal BB, Aaby P, et al. Lack of evidence of vertical transmission of human immunodeficiency virus type 2 in a sample of the general population in Bissau. J Acquir Immun Dis Syndr. 1992;5:25–30.

376. Del Mistro A, Chotard J, Hall AJ, et al. HIV-1 and HIV-2 seroprevalence rates in mother-child pairs living in The Gambia (West Africa). J Acquir Immun Defic Syndr. 1992;5:19–24.

377. Dufoort G, Courouce A-M, Ancelle-Park R, et al. No clinical signs 14 years after HIV-2 transmission via blood transfusion (Letter). Lancet. 1988;2:510.

378. Pepin J, Morgan G, Dunn D, et al. HIV-2-induced immunosuppression among asymptomatic West African prostitutes: Evidence that HIV-2 is pathogenic, but less so than HIV-1. AIDS. 1991;5:1165–72.

379. Guyader M, Emerman M, Sonigo P, et al. Genome organization and trans-activation of the human immunodeficiency virus type 2. Nature. 1987;326: 662–9.

380. George JR, Rayfield MA, Phillips S, et al. Efficacies of US Food and Drug Administration-licensed HIV-1-screening enzyme immunoassays for detecting antibodies to HIV-2. AIDS. 1990;4:321–6.

381. Myers RA, Patel JD, Joseph JM. Identifying HIV-2 seropositive individuals by reevaluating HIV-1 indeterminate sera. J Acquir Immun Defic Syndr. 1992;5:417–23.

382. Peeters M, Gershy-Damet G-M, Fransen K, et al. Virological and polymerase chain reaction studies of HIV-1/HIV-2 dual infection in Cote d'Ivoire. Lancet. 1992;340:339–40.

383. Cates W Jr, Stone KM. Family planning, sexually transmitted diseases and contraceptive choice: A literature update-part I. Fam Plan Perspect 1992;24: 75–84.

383a.Thompson JL, Yager TJ, Martin JL. Estimated condom failure and frequency of condom use among gay men. Am J Public Health. 1993;83:1409–13.

384. Weller SC. A meta-analysis of condom effectiveness in reducing sexually transmitted HIV. Soc Sci Med. 1993;36:1635–44.

385. Saracco A, Musicco M, Nicolosi A, et al. Man-to-women sexual transmission of HIV: Longitudinal study of 343 steady partners of infected men. J Acquir Immune Defic Syndr. 1993;6:497–502.

386. De Vincenzi I for the European Communities Study Group on Heterosexual Transmission of HIV. Heterosexual transmission of HIV in a European cohort of couples (Abstract WS-C02-1). In: Abstracts of the IX International Conference on AIDS/IVth STD World Congress. v. I. Berlin, Germany, June 6–11, 1993:83.

387. Trussell J, Warner DL, Hatcher R. Condom performance during vaginal intercourse: Comparison of Trojan-Enz™ and Tactylon™ condoms. Contraception. 1992;45:11–9.

388. Carey RF, Herman WA, Retta SM, et al. Effectiveness of latex condoms as a barrier to human immunodeficiency virus-sized particles under conditions of simulated use. Sex Transm Dis. 1992;19:230–4.

389. Rosenberg MJ, Gollub EL. Commentary: Methods women can use that may prevent sexually transmitted disease, including HIV. Am J Public Health. 1992;82:1473–8.

390. Centers for Disease Control and Prevention: Update: Barrier protection against HIV infection and other sexually transmitted disease. MMWR. 1993; 42:589–91, 597.

391. Cates W Jr, Stewart FH, Trussell J. Commentary: The quest for women's prophylactic methods—hopes vs science. Am J Public Health. 1992;82: 1479–82.

392. Roper WL, Peterson HB, Curran JW. Commentary: Condoms and HIV/STD prevention—Clarifying the message. Am J Public Health. 1993;83:501–3.

393. Centers for Disease Control and Prevention: Heterosexual behaviors and factors that influence condom use among patients attending a sexually transmitted disease clinic—San Francisco. MMWR. 1990;39:685–9.

394. Peterson JL, Coates TJ, Catania JA, et al. High-risk sexual behavior and condom use among gay and bisexual African-American men. Am J Public Health. 1992;82:1490–4.

395. Catania JA, Coates TJ, Kegeles S, et al. Condom use in multi-ethnic neighborhoods of San Francisco: The population-based AMEN (AIDS in multi-ethnic neighborhoods) study. Am J Public Health. 1991;81:284–7.

396. Martin JL. The impact of AIDS on gay male sexual behavior patterns in New York City. Am J Public Health. 1987;77:578–81.

397. Hays RB, Kegeles SM, Coates TJ. High HIV risk-taking among young gay men. AIDS. 1990;4:901–7.

398. St. Lawrence JS, Hood HV, Brasfield T, et al. Differences in gay men's AIDS risk knowledge and behavior patterns in high and low AIDS prevalence cities. Public Health Rep. 1989;104:391–5.

399. Ekstrand ML, Coates TJ. Maintenance of safer sexual behaviors and predictors of risky sex: The San Francisco Men's Health Study. Am J Public Health. 1990;80:973–7.

400. Adib SM, Joseph JG, Ostrow DG, et al. Relapse in sexual behavior among homosexual men: A 2-year follow-up from the Chicago MACS/CCS. AIDS. 1991;5:757–60.

401. Penkower L, Dew MA, Kingsley L, et al. Behavioral, health and psychosocial factors and risk for HIV infection among sexually active homosexual men: The Multicenter AIDS Cohort Study. Am J Public Health. 1991;81: 194–6.

402. Lifson AR. Men who have sex with men: Continued challenges for preventing HIV infection and AIDS (Editorial). Am J Public Health. 1992;82:166–7.

403. Chirgwin K, DeHovitz JA, Dillon S, et al. HIV infection, genital ulcer disease, and crack cocaine uses among patients attending a clinic for sexually transmitted diseases. Am J Public Health. 1992;81:1576–9.

404. Centers for Disease Control and Prevention: Condom use among male injecting-drug users—New York City, 1987–1990. MMWR. 1992;41:617–20.

405. Marks G, Richardson JL, Maldonado N. Self-disclosure of HIV infection to sexual partners. Am J Public Health. 1991;81:1321–3.

406. Landis SE, Schoenbach VJ, Weber DJ, et al. Results of a randomized trial of partner notification in cases of HIV infection in North Carolina. N Engl J Med. 1992;326:101–6.

407. Bayer R, Toomey KE. HIV prevention and the two faces of partner notification. Am Public Health. 1992;82:1158–64.

408. Rutherford GW, Woo JM. Contact tracing to control the spread of HIV (Letter). JAMA. 1988;260:3275.

409. Wykoff RF, Heath CW Jr, Hollis SL, et al. Contact tracing to identify human immunodeficiency virus infection in a rural community. JAMA. 1988;259: 3563–6.

409a.Pavia AT, Benyo M, Niler L, et al. Partner notification for control of HIV: Results after 2 years of a statewide program in Utah. Am J Public Health. 1993;83:1418–24.

410. The Twin Epidemics of Substance Use and HIV. Washington, D.C.: National Commission on AIDS; 1991.

411. Centers for Disease Control and Prevention: Update: Reducing HIV transmission in intravenous-drug users not in drug treatment—United States. MMWR. 1990;39:97–101.

412. Groseclose SL, Weinstein B, Jones S, et al. Legal purchase of clean needles and syringes in Connecticut: Do they make a difference (Abstract PO-D27-4185)? In: Abstracts of the IX International Conference on AIDS/IVth STD World Congress. v. II. Berlin, Germany, June 6–11, 1993:915.

413. U.S. General Accounting Office. Needle exchange programs: Research suggests promise as an AIDS prevention strategy. Washington, D.C.: USGAO, Human Resources Division; 1993. Report to the Chairman, Select Committee on Narcotics Abuse and Control, House of Representatives.

414. Centers for Disease Control and Prevention: Use of bleach for disinfection of drug injection equipment. MMWR. 1993;42:418–9.

415. Yancovitz SR, Des Jarlais DC, Peyser NP, et al. A randomized trial of an interim methadone maintenance clinic. Am J Public Health. 1991;81:1185–91.

416. Stephens RC, Feucht TE, Roman SW. Effects of an intervention program on AIDS-related drug and needle behavior among intravenous drug users. Am J Public Health. 1991;81:568–71.

417. The Public Health Impact of Needle Exchange Programs in the United States and Abroad. Summary, Conclusions, and Recommendations. Report prepared for the Centers for Disease Control and Prevention: September 1993.

418. Carson JL, Russell LB, Taragin MI, et al. The risks of blood transfusion: The relative influence of acquired immunodeficiency syndrome and non-A, non-B hepatitis. Am J Med. 1992;92:45–52.

419. Surgenor DM, Wallace EL, Hao SHS, et al. Collection and transfusion of blood in the United States, 1982–1988. N Engl J Med. 1990;322:1646–51.

420. Ward JW, Kleinman SH, Douglas KD, et al. Epidemiologic characteristics of blood donors with antibody to human immunodeficiency virus. Transfusion. 1988;28:298–301.

421. Semen banking, organ and tissue transplantation, and HIV antibody testing. MMWR. 1988;37:57–8, 63.

422. Centers for Disease Control and Prevention: Transmission of HIV through bone transplantation: Case report and public health recommendations. MMWR. 1988;37:597–9.

423. Bell DM. Human immunodeficiency virus transmission in health care settings: Risk and risk reduction. Am J Med. 1991;91(Suppl 3B):3B-294S–300S.

424. Centers for Disease Control and Prevention: Recommendations for prevention of HIV transmission in health-care settings. MMWR. 1987;36(Suppl No.2S):1S–18S.

425. Centers for Disease Control and Prevention: Public Health Service statement on management of occupational exposure to human immunodeficiency virus, including considerations regarding zidovudine postexposure use. MMWR. 1990;39(No.RR-1):1–14.

426. Centers for Disease Control and Prevention: Public Health Service guidelines for counseling and antibody testing to prevent HIV infection and AIDS. MMWR. 1987;36:509–15.

427. Working Group on HIV Testing of Pregnant Women and Newborns. HIV infection, pregnant women, and newborns. JAMA. 1990;264:2416–20.

428. Lindsay MK, Peterson HB, Feng TI, et al. Routine antepartum human immunodeficiency virus infection screening in an inner-city population. Obstet Gynecol. 1989;74:289–94.

428a. Centers for Disease Control and Prevention: Zidovudine for the prevention of HIV transmission from mother to infant. MMWR. 1994;43:285–7.

429. Centers for Disease Control and Prevention: Recommendations for assisting in the prevention of perinatal transmission of human T-lymphotrophic type III/lymphadenopathy-associated virus. MMWR. 1985;34:721–6, 731–2.

430. World Health Organization. Consensus statement from the WHO/UNICEF consultation on HIV transmission and breast-feeding. Wkly Epidemiol Rec. 1992;67:177–9.

431. Valdiserri RO, Holtgrave DR, Brackbill RM. American adults' knowledge of HIV testing availability. Am J Public Health. 1993;83:525–8.

432. Ward J. Testing for retroviral infections: medical indications and ethical considerations. In: Schochetman G, George JR, eds. AIDS testing. Methodology and Management Issues. New York: Springer-Verlag; 1992:6–17.

433. Centers for Disease Control and Prevention: Recommendations for HIV testing services for inpatients and outpatients in acute-care hospital settings. MMWR. 1993;42(No.RR-2):1–17.

434. Centers for Disease Control and Prevention: Human immunodeficiency virus infection in transfusion recipients and their family members. MMWR. 1987; 36:137–40.

435. Centers for Disease Control and Prevention: Recommendations for preventing transmission of human immunodeficiency virus and hepatitis B virus to patients during exposure-prone invasive procedures. MMWR. 1991; 40(No.RR-8):1–9.

436. Gerberding JL, Littell C, Tarkington A, et al. Risk of exposure of surgical personnel to patients' blood during surgery at San Francisco General Hospital. N Engl J Med. 1990;322:1788–93.

437. Higgins DL, Galavotti C, O'Reilly KR, et al. Evidence for the effects of HIV antibody counseling and testing on risk behaviors. JAMA. 1991;266:2419–29.

438. Otten MW, Zaidi AA, Wroten JE, et al. Changes in sexually transmitted disease rates after HIV testing and posttest counseling, Miami 1988 to 1989. Am J Public Health. 1993;83:529–33.

439. Zenilman JM, Erickson B, Fox R, et al. Effect of HIV posttest counseling on STD incidence. JAMA. 1992;267:843–5.

440. Holtgrave DR, Valdiserri RO, Gerber AR, et al. Human immunodeficiency virus counseling, testing, referral, and partner notification services: A cost-benefit analysis. Arch Intern Med. 1993;153:1225–30.

441. Jewett JF, Hecht FM. Preventive health care for adults with HIV infection. JAMA. 1993;269:1144–53.

101. IMMUNOLOGY OF AIDS AND HIV INFECTION

SHARILYN K. STANLEY
ANTHONY S. FAUCI

Since the initial identification of the human immunodeficiency virus (HIV) in 1983[1,2] much has been learned about the organism, its transmission, and its pathogenic mechanisms. HIV is transmitted through sexual contact, injection drug use with contaminated needles, blood and blood product transfusion, and maternal to fetal and infant transfer. Although an acute mononucleosislike illness may occur just before or at the time of seroconversion, infection is characteristically followed by a prolonged period of clinical latency[3] with the median period of latency estimated to be approximately 10 years. It is now clear that during this clinically quiescent period viral replication continues and is associated with a gradual erosion of immune competence. Subsequently, as the patient becomes progressively immunosuppressed, opportunistic infections and malignancies develop that are responsible for most of the morbidity and mortality of this disease.

Although much is known about the genomic structure of HIV, its life cycle, and the regulation of viral replication (reviewed in ref. 4), the study of pathogenesis of disease and the immune response to the virus are still rapidly evolving fields. For example, although individuals can be shown to develop a vigorous antibody and cytotoxic T-cell (CTL) response after infection with HIV, these responses wane over time and the factors that

contribute to long-term protective immunity remain unknown. Additionally, concepts of pathogenesis are being revised in response to recent observations regarding the role of lymphoid tissue in disease,[5] and new clinical parameters for following disease progression may need to be identified.

This chapter examines the immunologic features of HIV infection and the mechanisms whereby the virus contributes to the deterioration of the immune system. The immune response to infection and the role of particular tissues, such as brain, bone marrow, and lymph nodes in pathogenesis are discussed.

VIROLOGY OF HIV

The molecular virology and life cycle of HIV is discussed in detail in Chapter 146, and will be reviewed briefly below. HIV is an RNA virus in the lentivirus subfamily of retroviruses and is closely related to two other human retroviruses, human T-lymphotropic virus (HTLV) type I and II.[2,6] HIV is primarily a cytopathic virus whereas the HTLV I and II viruses are notable for their ability to transform infected cells. Two predominant forms of HIV have been identified, with HIV-1 being much more common than HIV-2 in most parts of the world (reviewed in ref. 7). HIV-2 was first identified in prostitutes from western Africa and has remained the predominant virus in West African countries such as Guinea Bissau, Ivory Coast, and Senegal; however, it has also been reported in other parts of the world. HIV-2 differs from HIV-1 in that it appears to cause less aggressive disease, is not transmitted as readily from mother to infant, and there are differences in the regulation of the virus at the genetic level (reviewed in ref. 7). Finally, the HIV-2 genome is only 40–50 percent similar to the HIV-1 genome whereas it is highly homologous (75 percent) to the simian immunodeficiency virus (SIV); certain investigators have suggested that, because sequence data from a given isolate cannot distinguish between SIV and HIV-2, the two viruses are identical.[8]

Genomic Organization

The HIV genome is approximately 10 kilobases long and contains the genes common to all retroviruses; these encode for structural proteins (*gag*), polymerase enzymes (*pol*), and envelope proteins (*env*).[9,10] As with other retroviruses, regulation of expression of these genes occurs through the binding of regulatory proteins to promoter and enhancer sequences found in the long terminal repeat (LTR) regions that flank the gene coding sequences on both the 5′ and 3′ ends of the genome. Although potential binding sites exist in the HIV-LTR for multiple human cellular transcription factors, of particular note is the fact that the LTR contains sequences that bind the human regulatory factors SP-1 (LTR contains three binding sites) and NF-κB (LTR contains two binding sites), and these appear to be important regulators of constitutive and inducible HIV expression (discussed further below). HIV differs from other retroviruses in that, in addition to these three major groups of proteins, the genome also encodes for several regulatory proteins. The best studied of these include *tat*, which is the viral transactivator of the LTR leading to increased transcription; *rev*, which favors the expression or translation of unspliced or partially spliced structural over multiply spliced regulatory mRNAs, possibly by enhancing rapid transport of mRNAs out of the nucleus before completion of slicing; and *nef*, initially defined as a negative viral regulator that has subsequently been shown to upregulate virus expression in certain circumstances. Three other regulatory genes encoded in the HIV genome include *vif*, a virion infectivity factor that may be necessary for productive infection; *vpu* (viral protein U), which appears to facilitate envelope processing and viral budding; and *vpr* (viral protein R) whose function remains unknown. Additionally, HIV-2, which lacks a coding region for *vpu*, contains an open-reading frame termed *vpx* (viral protein X), which appears to be necessary for efficient

TABLE 1. Life Cycle of the Human Immunodeficiency Virus[a]

Process	Factors Involved	
	Viral	Cellular
Viral binding to cell	gp120	CD4
Internalization of virus/fusion with cell membrane	gp41	Cell membrane; "human factor"
Uncoating of virion core	Protease enzyme	?
Reverse transcription of full-length viral RNA	RT enzyme	nucleotides
Degradation of viral RNA and synthesis of second DNA strand	Ribonuclease H and RT enzymes	?
Translocation of ds DNA (provirus) to nucleus and integration	Integrase enzyme	?
Activation of transcription from integrated provirus	—	Cellular activation signals (e.g., antigen, cytokines), nuclear transcription factors
Production of early regulatory messages	tat; ?nef, vpr	Transcriptional and translational machinery
Production of spliced and unspliced structural gene products	rev	Transcriptional and translational machinery
Translation of mRNA into proteins	?rev	Translational machinery
Viral assembly (full-length RNA, pol enzymes, gag, and env proteins)	?vpu, vif	?
Viral budding from cell surface	Protease, other pol enzymes, vpu	Cell membrane

[a] Also see Chapter 146.
(From Green,[9] with permission.)

viral replication.[7] The complexity of the HIV genome endows this virus with a versatility lacking in most other retroviruses, as demonstrated, for example, by the variety of means by which expression of the integrated provirus can be regulated (discussed below).

Viral Life Cycle

The critical step in infection with HIV is the binding of the viral envelope protein, gp120, to the cellular CD4 molecule[11,12] (Table 1). This binding is both specific and highly efficient, in that the affinity of gp120 for the CD4 molecule is greater than the affinity for CD4 of its natural ligand, the class II major histocompatibility (MHC) molecule.[13] In vitro infection of cells with HIV can be blocked by incubating the cells with antibodies to the CD4 molecule, the T4A epitope being especially critical in this binding reaction. Conversely, incubating the viral preparation with soluble CD4 also blocks infectivity by competitively binding to the viral gp120 surface proteins and preventing their interaction with cell-associated CD4.[14] Thus, CD4 acts as the primary receptor for HIV, targeting the infection primarily to cells that express this protein.

After binding, the virus fuses with the cell membrane and is internalized in an incompletely understood reaction that appears to involve the viral gp41 protein. The fact that CD4-gp120 binding alone is not sufficient for entry of the virus into the cell was clearly demonstrated in experiments in which the human CD4 gene was transfected into mouse cells or human HELA cells, which were then shown to express CD4 on their surface.[15] Upon subsequent exposure to HIV, the CD4-transfected HELA cells became infected, whereas the CD4 transfected mouse cells bound virus efficiently but remained uninfected. This lack of detectable infection did not result from an inability of the mouse

cells to support HIV replication because experiments in which HIV was directly transfected into the cells resulted in the production of infectious virions by the mouse cells. Taken together, these data implicate some yet undefined human factor in the initial internalization step of infection.

After internalization and uncoating of the virus, the viral reverse transcriptase (RT) enzyme transcribes viral RNA into double-stranded DNA, which then may circularize and either persist in the unintegrated form or, through the actions of the viral integrase protein, is integrated as a provirus into cellular DNA[9] (Table 1). At this point the virus may enter a quiescent or latent phase. When the infected cell is subsequently activated, transcription of the proviral DNA is initiated with resultant RNA production, protein synthesis and processing, viral assembly, and budding from the cell[9] (Table 1).

Cellular activation plays a critical role in the expression of HIV. During the course of an immune response an HIV-infected T cell may become activated and concomitantly initiate expression of latent provirus, resulting in spreading of infection. A variety of activating signals, including antigens, heterologous viruses, and cytokines are capable of enhancing virus expression from chronically infected cells in vitro (reviewed in ref. 16 and discussed under "Co-factors" below). The mechanisms of this viral activation are becoming increasingly clear. Stimulation of T cells results in the activation of several transcription factors, including the cellular transcription factor NF-κB, which then induce transcription of specific genes involved in T-cell responses. Because the HIV-LTR contains regulatory sequences that bind NF-κB, much of the upregulation of virus expression that occurs with activation signals appears to be mediated by this cellular factor.

A second manner in which cellular activation may accelerate or facilitate the course of HIV disease involves the initial process of infection. Although resting cells can support viral entry, uncoating, and partial reverse transcription, reverse transcription of full-length DNA and integration occur only in cells that are activated.[17,18] Indeed, initial attempts to isolate HIV required the activation of target cells so that viral propagation became detectable.[2] Subsequent studies have shown that infection of resting cells with HIV results in the appearance of partially reverse-transcribed DNA products that are the result of a block in the reverse transcription process.[18] Although these partial transcripts can support productive infection of the quiescent cell if the cell receives a stimulus as late as 2 days after infection, the efficiency of infection is markedly reduced because these partial transcripts are labile and disappear with a half-life of 1 day.[19] Thus, because immune activation clearly can result in both spread of infection, by increasing transcription of latent provirus, as well as increased susceptibility of individual cells to infection with HIV, consideration is now being given to a potential role for the cautious application of therapies that block cellular activation early in the course of disease.

Cellular Targets of Infection

Because the primary receptor for HIV is the CD4 molecule, any cell that expresses this protein becomes a target for infection with the virus. In this regard, the CD4+ T lymphocyte is extraordinarily susceptible to infection and is the predominant cell type targeted by HIV, but cells of the monocyte/macrophage (M/M) lineage also express CD4 and are capable of being infected. As discussed below, the course of infection in these two cell types is very different and they probably play distinct roles in the pathogenesis of HIV disease. HIV has also been detected in a wide variety of cell types that express variable amounts of CD4 or even lack detectable CD4 expression. These cells include megakaryocytes, peripheral blood dendritic cells, follicular dendritic cells, epidermal Langerhans cells, astrocytes, oligodendroglia and microglia, CD8+ cells, cervical cells, rectal mucosal cells, trophoblastic cells, renal epithelial cells, cardiac myocytes, and retinal cells. Although infection of many of these cell types has been accomplished in vitro, this may not be a reflection of what actually occurs in vivo. As an example, although epidermal Langerhans cells are easily infectable in vitro and support active viral replication, there are conflicting reports regarding the presence and/or prevalence of infected Langerhans cells in vivo (reviewed in ref. 20). In addition, many cell types thought to be CD4− but infectable with HIV have, in fact, been subsequently found to express CD4. As an example, immature bone marrow CD34+ precursor cells as well as immature thymocyte precursors, both of which were thought to lack CD4 expression, have been shown to be infectable with HIV.[21,22] The fact that HIV infection of these two cell types can be blocked by monoclonal antibodies to CD4 suggests that infection is due to extremely low levels of surface CD4 that is undetectable by currently available assays. However, because some cells are truly CD4− and are infectable with HIV in a CD4-independent manner, the existence of a second receptor for HIV has been postulated; both Fc receptors and galactosyl ceramide have been suggested as possible mediators of viral entry in certain cell types.[23]

HIV Variation and Potential Cell Tropism

Because of the infidelity of the reverse transcriptase enzyme, genomic mutation occurs and HIV variants arise during the course of viral replication (reviewed in ref. 24). It is thought that most individuals are infected with a relatively homogeneous strain of virus that diverges over time into heterogeneous quasispecies. Most of these mutations occur in the envelope gene and it has been shown that these differences in envelope protein can result in a differential cytopathic capability of the virus. Additionally, differences in the ability of the variant HIV strains to infect primary T cells or M/M in vitro appear to be due to changes in the envelope region (reviewed in ref. 24). In this regard, during the early clinically latent period of infection, viral isolates from most individuals replicate slowly in culture, cause minimal cytopathicity, and are preferentially grown in macrophages.[25] Later in the course of disease, more cytopathic HIV variants are detected that grow well in T cells, and it has been postulated that these isolates that are identified in vitro as the more cytotoxic "syncytia inducing" (SI) strains are responsible for the accelerated decline in CD4+ T cells often observed clinically in late-stage disease.[26] In addition to the increase in cytopathic potential that appears to develop with in vivo viral mutation over time, the generation of antigenic variants that results from these mutations may allow the virus to evade immune surveillance. Although cytotoxicity and escape from an immune response may be important sequelae of viral variation in vivo, the significance of the in vitro tropism for T cells or M/M is unclear, because viruses that grow in T cells in vivo can infect M/M in vitro.[27]

IMMUNOPATHOGENIC MECHANISMS OF HIV INFECTION

Although the hallmark of infection with HIV is progressive depletion of CD4+ T cells, a broad array of defects in the immune function of a variety of cell types also occurs. In some instances these cellular defects are due to direct infection of the cell (as, for example, with T cells and M/M), whereas other effects on function are indirect (as is the case with natural killer [NK] and B cells as well as with uninfected T cells and M/M).

T-Cell Abnormalities

Mechanisms of CD4+ T-cell Depletion. The mechanism of the severe depletion of CD4+ T cells that occurs with disease progression is currently an area of intense investigation. Early after infection, total CD4+ T cells drop, sometimes precipitously, and often associated with a burst of viremia and signs and symptoms of an acute viral syndrome (Fig. 1). As viremia

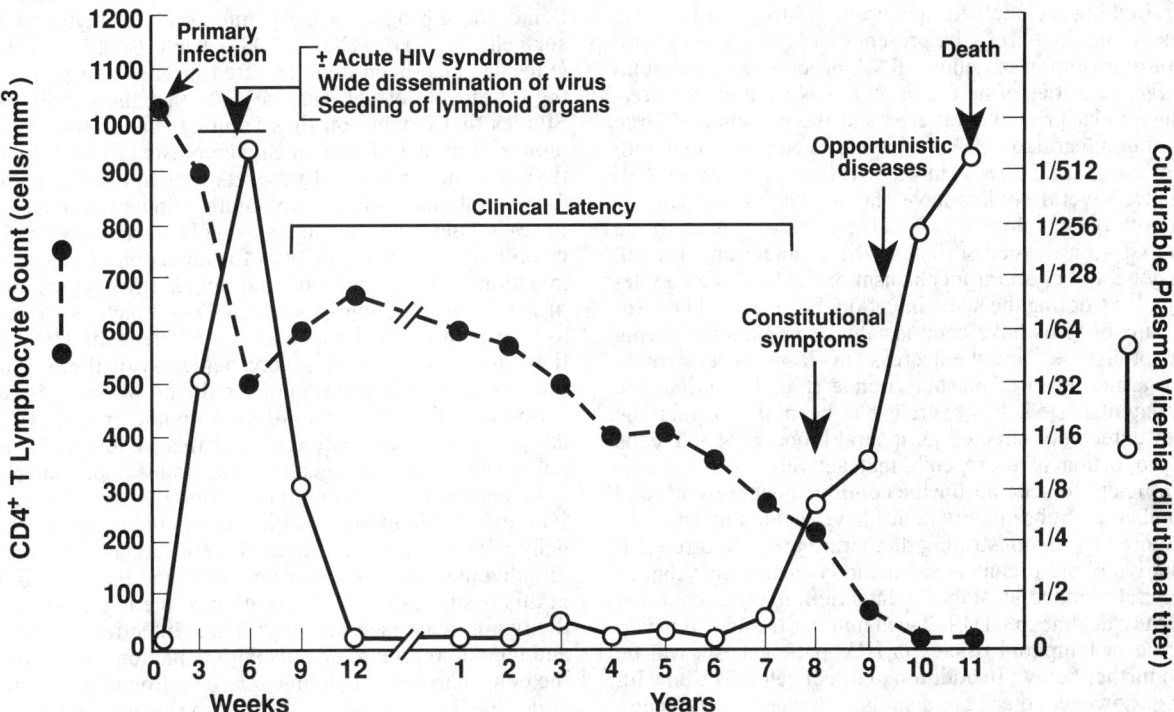

FIG. 1. Typical course of HIV infection. Widespread dissemination of virus occurs early during the primary infection and is associated with an abrupt decline in peripheral blood CD4+ T-cell number. The ensuing immune response is accompanied by a decrease in culturable plasma viremia and a lengthy period of clinical latency. However, the CD4+ T-cell count continues to decline during this period until a critical level is reached where the risk of opportunistic infections is markedly increased. (Adapted from Pantaleo et al.,[5] with permission.)

TABLE 2. Potential Mechanisms of CD4+ T-Cell Depletion in HIV Infection

Direct infection with cytopathicity
  Membrane effects
  Accumulation of viral or heterodisperse RNA
  Interruption of cellular RNA and protein processing
  Unintegrated DNA
Bystander killing
  Syncytia
  Soluble gp120 binding to CD4+ cells with subsequent apoptosis or cell killing by ADCC or CTL
Inability to regenerate mature T cells
  Bone marrow infection, altered hematopoiesis
  Thymus infection, destruction of microenvironment
Autoimmunity
  Homology of HIV to MHC class I and II
  Homology of HIV to other cell surface proteins
Apoptosis due to gp120 cross-linking of CD4
Superantigen effects of HIV or opportunistic pathogens

Abbreviations: ADCC, antibody-dependent cellular cytotoxicity; CTL, cytotoxic T cell; MHC, major histocompatibility.

resolves, total CD4+ T cells may rise to near normal levels.[28,29] Over the ensuing clinically latent period, often lasting more than 10 years, CD4+ T-cell levels decline at rates that vary between individuals; in general, the secondary complications of opportunistic infections and neoplasms develop at levels below 200 cells/mm³. It is currently felt that monitoring of the total CD4+ T-cell count is the best way to follow disease progression because these levels correlate with the severity of immune suppression. Indeed, the case definition for AIDS was recently modified to include patients with a total CD4+ T-cell count below 200/mm³ even in the absence of symptoms or any other AIDS-defining illnesses.[30]

A variety of mechanisms have been postulated to account for this CD4+ T-cell depletion (Table 2). Direct infection of the cells with subsequent cytotoxicity, particularly due to virulent strains arising during the course of infection, is the most obvious explanation for loss of CD4+ T cells. Potential mechanisms of direct viral killing include cell membrane destruction by large quantities of budding virus; the presence of high levels of viral RNA with interruption of cellular RNA processing, accumulation of large quantities of heterodisperse RNAs, and the interruption of cellular protein synthesis; and the presence of large amounts of unintegrated DNA, which has been associated with significant cytopathic effects in other retroviral diseases.[31,32] Additionally, several studies have shown that cytotoxicity is linked to both the envelope region of the virus as well as to the amount of CD4 on the cell surface.[33] Direct infection with cell killing may be an important mechanism of CD4+ T-cell depletion particularly during the acute infection, because highly cytopathic strains of virus have been isolated from patients during this phase of disease[34] and the decrease in CD4+ T cells correlates with a high level of plasma viremia (Fig. 1). During the clinically latent period, however, it has been shown that the number of detectably infected peripheral blood CD4+ T cells and the proportion of those cells that actively express virus seem insufficient to account for the continued decrease in total T-cell numbers.[35] Subsequent studies have yielded insight into this dichotomy by demonstrating that viral burden and replication in the lymphoid organs is significantly higher than that in the peripheral blood at all stages of infection, likely accounting for the steady decline in CD4+ T-cell number (reviewed in ref. 5). The role of lymphoid tissues in HIV pathogenesis will be discussed further below. In addition to direct cell infection with cell killing, however, there are also data to suggest that many other mechanisms may contribute to CD4+ T-cell depletion; these include indirect killing, stem cell infection or failure, autoimmunity, apoptosis, and superantigen effects. Indirect killing of bystander T cells has been postulated to occur through the formation of syncytia when infected cells expressing gp120 on the surface bind to and fuse with uninfected CD4+ T cells.[36] Although syncytia occur in vitro and are responsible for some degree of cytopathicity in culture, and multinucleated thymocytes with morphology suggestive of syncytia have been observed in infected human thymic tissues in the SCID-hu mouse (S. Stanley and A. S. Fauci, unpublished observations), the role of cell fusion in in vivo CD4+ T-cell toxicity is unknown. An additional bystander mechanism of cytotoxicity involves the binding of soluble gp120, thought to be shed from infected cells, to the surface CD4 molecules on uninfected cells. These cells subsequently become targets for anti-gp120 directed antibody-dependent cellular cytotoxicity (ADCC) and cytotoxic T-cell (CTL) killing.[37] In this regard, cells from infected individuals have demonstrated both CTL and NK cell mediated ADCC against uninfected cells coated with HIV antigens in vitro.[38,39]

The progressive decline in CD4+ T-cell numbers in the face of effective antiretroviral therapy that suppresses viral replication suggests that the ability to regenerate CD4+ cells may be defective. Indeed, infection or dysfunction of both myeloid and lymphoid progenitor cells has been demonstrated by numerous groups. Decreased myeloid, erythroid, granulocyte, and megakaryocyte colony formation and bone marrow suppression manifested as thrombocytopenia, granulocytopenia, anemia, and lymphopenia occur in HIV-infected individuals (reviewed in ref. 40). Pathologically, the bone marrow in acquired immunodeficiency syndrome (AIDS) is abnormal and displays an increased plasmacytosis, fibrosis, and dysmyelopoiesis[41]; loss of circulating peripheral blood progenitor cells has also been noted. These effects have been postulated to be related to the abnormal production of suppressive cytokines or soluble factors by infected T cells or macrophages in the bone marrow, or to the presence of serum antibodies against HIV mediating a direct or indirect inhibition of progenitor cells. Additionally, infection of the CD34+ myeloid precursor cell has been shown to occur both in vitro and in vivo,[21,42] and the presence of these infected cells has been shown to correlate in North American patients with advanced disease as indicated by very low CD4+ T-cell counts (<50/mm³). It is not yet known whether infection leads to depletion of these progenitor cells. Infection of the lymphoid precursor cell, the CD3−CD4−CD8− triple negative (TN) thymocyte, has also been demonstrated in vitro and is mediated by the low levels of cell surface CD4 that these cells express.[22] Studies that expand on these findings have used the SCID-hu mouse, a model of human thymopoiesis in which human fetal thymic tissue grows and supports normal human thymopoiesis for several months after implantation under the renal capsule of the SCID mouse.[43] In studies using DNA and RNA polymerase chain reaction (PCR) analysis for detection of productive HIV infection, it has been found that human thymocytes at all levels of maturation (double-positive, CD4+ single-positive, as well as CD8+ single-positive cells) are infected with HIV.[44] In addition, infection leads to severe depletion of these lymphocyte precursors.[44–46] Disruption of the thymic stroma with internalization of HIV within the stromal thymic epithelial (TE) cells has also been demonstrated, and this undoubtedly interrupts normal thymopoietic mechanisms. Indeed, pathologic studies have demonstrated premature atrophy of the thymus gland in HIV-infected individuals with thymocyte loss and fibrosis.[47] Finally, HIV is present and actively replicating in the lymph nodes of individuals at all stages of disease, and the high viral burden in this tissue results in destruction of the microenvironment of the lymph node (see below).[48] Thus, infection of both myeloid and lymphoid precursor cells with depletion and dysfunction of the bone marrow, the thymic microenvironment, and the lymph node, has been demonstrated. In the face of peripheral T-cell destruction, this organ damage likely contributes to the failure of regeneration of mature hematolymphoid cells, which compounds the CD4+ T-cell depletion as well as the other cytopenias that are observed in HIV-infected individuals.

Autoimmunity has also been postulated to contribute to

CD4+ T-cell depletion and indeed a spectrum of autoimmune responses has been observed in HIV-infected individuals. There is homology between the gp120 molecule and the β chains of MHC class II molecules, the natural ligand for CD4.[49] Additionally, gp41 shares homology with regions of class II molecules, and homology exists between envelope proteins and interleukin (IL)-2 as well as MHC class I proteins[50] (reviewed in ref. 16). Immune responses targeted to these HIV proteins may therefore cross react with self MHC or IL-2 proteins and lead to the destruction of uninfected cells expressing these molecules on their surface. In this regard, sera of infected individuals have been shown to contain antilymphocyte antibodies reacting with MHC class II molecules. Additional antiself antibodies have been found in HIV-infected patients and include antibodies reacting with normal platelets, neutrophils, CD4 molecules, CD43 molecules, and IL-2 (reviewed in ref. 51). These antibodies may mediate ADCC killing of uninfected cells; in fact, there are reports of autologous antibodies bound to T cells in HIV-infected individuals.[52]

The contribution of apoptosis of mature peripheral blood T cells to cell depletion in HIV-infected individuals is currently an area of intense discussion and research. Apoptosis, a form of programmed cell death, is characterized by a rise in intracellular calcium levels with activation of a specific endogenous nuclease that cuts the nuclear DNA into oligonucleotide fragments detected as a ladder pattern on Southern blot analysis.[53] Apoptosis occurs naturally intrathymically in the process of negative selection of T cells resulting in the elimination of autoreactive thymocytes, and it has been shown to be initiated in mature mouse T cells by cross liking of the CD4 receptor followed by signaling through the T-cell receptor (TCR).[54] Cross linking of the CD4 receptor on cells in HIV-infected individuals could occur through the binding of gp120 with or without anti-gp120 antibodies, and subsequent antigen recognition through the TCR could theoretically result in apoptotic death of the cell. Many lines of evidence support a role for apoptosis in HIV infection, including the detection of gp120/anti-gp120 complexes on peripheral blood mononuclear cells (PBMCs) from AIDS patients,[55] the occurrence of apoptosis in vitro with acute infection of activated PBMCs,[56] and the presence of autoantibodies to double-stranded DNA and histones in HIV-infected individuals.[57] Poke week mitogen (PWM) or superantigen stimulated CD4+ T cells from HIV-infected individuals have been shown by one group of investigators to undergo apoptosis in vitro,[58] whereas others

have found that CD8+ as well as CD4+ T cells from infected individuals undergo spontaneous apoptosis in vitro without the addition of exogenous stimuli[59] (reviewed in ref. 60). It is clear that further investigation is needed to delineate the possible contribution of apoptosis to the T-cell depletion observed in HIV-infected individuals.

Finally, a potential role of superantigens in T-cell depletion in HIV-infected individuals has recently been postulated (reviewed in ref. 61). The normal binding of antigen to the TCR requires that the variable (V), diversity (D), and joining (J) regions of both the α and β chains cooperate to form a specific antigen binding domain to which antigen bound within the groove of the MHC class II molecule is presented (Fig. 2A). In humans there are 100 variable regions of the α (Vα) chain and 60 variable regions of the β (Vβ) chain that are subdivided into 29 and 24 families, respectively.[62] Thus, most antigens requiring interaction with both Vα and Vβ chains will activate only a small number of T cells that possess the appropriate combination of α and β chains. Superantigens recognize the TCR differently in that only the Vβ chain of the receptor is required for recognition and binding (Fig. 2B).[63] Additionally, because superantigens bind MHC class II molecules outside of the normal antigen binding groove, they are MHC dependent but not MHC restricted in the classic sense. As such, then, superantigens can recognize and activate a large number of T cells that use one of a limited number of Vβ chains in their TCR. This superantigen activation leads to an initial expansion of T cells bearing these specific Vβ chains followed ultimately by deletion or anergy of the expanded clones. Both bacterial cell proteins (e.g., staphylococcal enterotoxins) and mouse exogenous and endogenous viral gene products, particularly those of mouse mammary tumor virus (MMTV), have demonstrated superantigen effects.[64] Infection of mice with exogenous MMTV, or genetic engineering to induce expression of the exogenous MMTV transmembrane glycoprotein on mouse cells leads to the depletion of specific Vβ subsets of T cells. The defective mouse leukemia virus that causes mouse acquired immunodeficiency syndrome (MAIDS) also encodes a superantigenlike protein that stimulates the expansion of specific Vβ-bearing T-cell subsets.[65] Because MAIDS and AIDS share many features, and because CD4+ T-cell anergy and depletion are characteristic of HIV infection, it has been postulated that HIV encodes a protein that functions as a superantigen.[66] In this regard, the Vβ T-cell repertoire in HIV-infected individuals was examined in one study and expan-

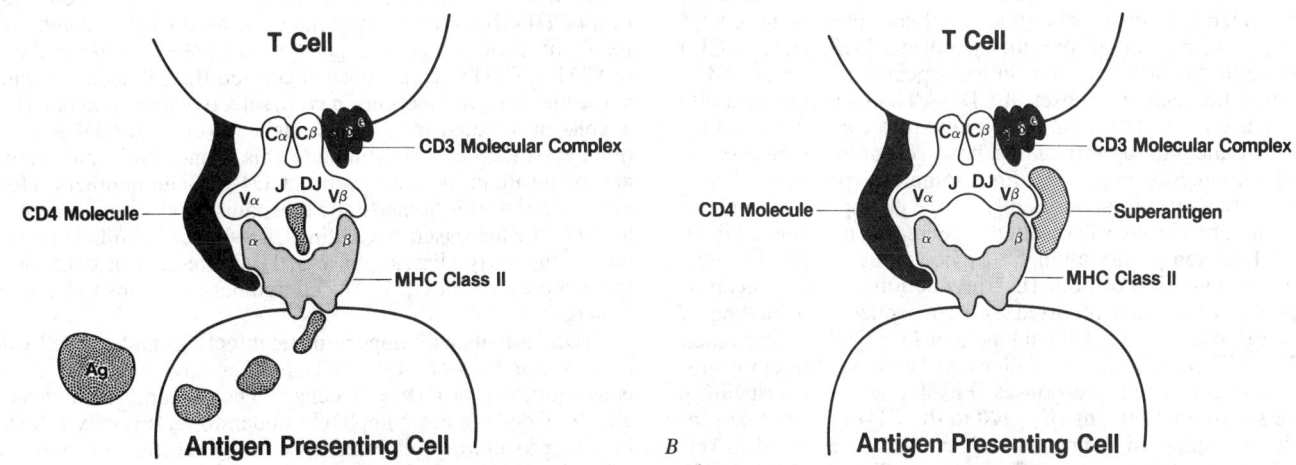

FIG. 2. Interactions of conventional antigens and superantigens with CD4+ T cells **(A)** Conventional antigens are bound within the groove of a particular MHC class II molecule and require the interaction of all of the variable regions of the α- and β-chains of the T-cell antigen receptor for recognition by the T cell. **(B)** Superantigens bind to a variety of MHC molecules outside of the normal antigen binding groove and require predominantly the variable region of the β-chain of the T-cell antigen receptor for T-cell recognition. Ag denotes antigen; V, D, and J denote variable, diversity, and joining, respectively. (Adapted from Pantaleo et al.,[5] with permission.)

sion or deletion of certain subsets was observed.[67] However, other explanations may exist for these findings, such as the encoding of a superantigen by an opportunistic pathogen present in some patients or the different genetic backgrounds, a factor known to influence Vβ utilization, which exist between unrelated infected individuals. Recently, studies of monozygotic twins discordant for HIV infection as well as HIV-infected mothers with their infected or uninfected offspring have indicated perturbations of Vβ subsets consistent with the presence of a superantigen.[67a] Other evidence comes from a study showing that HIV replicates up to 100-fold more efficiently in T-cell lines bearing specific Vβ chains and that T cells from HIV-infected individuals bearing these same Vβ chains preferentially expressed HIV proteins.[68] Thus a major role for superantigen in HIV disease may be the stimulation of specific Vβ-bearing T-cell subsets resulting in enhanced infectability, replication, and cytopathicity.

Functional Impairment of CD4 + T Cells. Even before significant CD4 + T-cell depletion, functional abnormalities of CD4 + T cells are detected (reviewed in ref. 16). Autologous mixed lymphocyte reactions (MLR), T-cell colony formation, expression of IL-2 receptors, and production of IL-2 have all been reported to be abnormal in HIV-infected individuals. Early during the clinically asymptomatic stage of disease, the ability of T cells to proliferate in response to recall antigens such as tetanus toxoid or influenza is markedly diminished in a substantial proportion of patients (reviewed in ref. 69). Indeed, asymptomatic HIV-seropositive individuals are often found to be anergic on skin testing for delayed hypersensitivity. In some studies, the diminished proliferative responses were independent of antigen presenting cells (APCs) in that proliferation could not be restored even when APCs from uninfected identical twins were used.[69] Conversely, other groups have found that the decreased proliferative responses of T cells appeared to be secondary to abnormal APC function.[70] Recently, it has been shown that loss of in vitro proliferative responses of PBMC to recall antigen, alloantigen, and mitogen occur in a predictable sequential fashion[71]; proliferation to recall antigens is lost first (−/+/+ phenotype), followed by loss of in vitro proliferation to alloantigens (−/−/+ phenotype), and finally to mitogens (−/−/− phenotype). These progressive defects in T-cell proliferation correlate with progressive immune dysfunction so that most AIDS patients express the −/−/− phenotype of T-cell proliferation.

Functional impairment of T-cell responses may be due to direct infection of these cells and subsequent downmodulation of CD4 expression, as has been shown in vitro.[72] This downregulation, which is probably due to intracellular complexing of CD4 with gp120, may interfere with the normal MHC class II-CD4 binding that is necessary for antigen-specific responses. Additionally, the memory subset of CD4 + T cells is preferentially infected and could account for a failure to recognize recall antigens.[73] Functional abnormalities, however, occur in the absence of direct infection of T cells. For example, exposure of T cells to noninfectious virus, purified envelope glycoproteins, and purified *tat* protein have all resulted in decreased mitogen, antigen, or TCR-driven proliferation[74,75] (reviewed in ref. 16). Furthermore, suppression of both IL-2 production and IL-2 receptor expression has been reported as a consequence of binding of HIV gp120 to CD4. Gp120 binding to surface CD4 can also block CD4-MHC class II mediated adhesion[76] and may therefore suppress antigen specific responses. Finally, several investigators have shown that binding of gp120 to the CD4 molecule can inhibit subsequent signaling through the TCR (reviewed in ref. 16). In this regard, exposure of primary T cells to gp120 results in increased activity of the cellular CD4-associated p56[lck] tyrosine phosphorylase enzyme.[77] The resultant pattern of proteins phosphorylated in response to this stimulus are different than those phosphorylated in response to p56[lck] activation via CD4 binding by MHC class II molecules or by TCR-mediated activation. This

suggests that gp120 delivers a negative signal to the cell through an as yet unidentified protein phosphorylated in response to gp120-mediated activation of p56[lck], and may explain certain of the functional abnormalities present in uninfected CD4 + T cells.

An additional functional disturbance of T cells has been proposed that involves an imbalance between two types of T-helper cells and the cytokines they produce. Two distinct and mutually exclusive subsets of T-helper cells, called T-helper (Th)-1 and Th-2, have been clearly demonstrated in the mouse. These two subsets appear to contribute to activation of the cellular and humoral arms of the immune system, respectively (reviewed in ref. 78). Th-1 cells produce predominantly IL-2 and interferon (IFN)-γ whereas Th-2 cells produce primarily IL-4, IL-5, IL-6, and IL-10, and cross-regulation between these subsets occurs.[79] In addition, there is a subset of T cells termed Th-0 cells that display a more generalized pattern of cytokine secretion and is now felt to represent the precursor cell to both Th-1 and Th-2 cells. It has been postulated that there is an imbalance between the functioning of these two subsets in HIV-infected individuals with Th-2 effects becoming dominant as disease progresses (reviewed in ref. 80). It is unclear whether such an imbalance does indeed exist and what effect this would have on the ability of the immune system to effectively respond to HIV.

Abnormalities in CD8 + T cells. Similar to CD4 + T cells, CD8 + T cells are decreased during the acute syndrome of HIV infection. Within 3–4 weeks, however, CD8 + T-cell numbers return to normal and even exceed normal levels.[28,81] During the clinically asymptomatic period of infection CD8 + T-cell numbers often remain higher than normal. This increase in CD8 + T cells has been postulated to reflect the presence of an expanded population of circulating CTLs against HIV. An alternative postulate relates to the mechanism whereby the body regulates T-cell homeostasis (ref. 82 and references therein). According to this theory, supported indirectly by clinical data obtained through the multicenter AIDS cohort study (MACS), the immune system does not recognize a specific depletion of CD4 + or CD8 + T cells, but rather regulates T-cell homeostasis by recognizing alterations in the total CD3 + T-cell number. Thus, a response to either selective CD4 + or CD8 + T-cell depletion results in an increase in total CD3 + T cells consisting of both CD3 + CD4 + and CD3 + CD8 + T cells. In the face of a balanced loss of T cells, such as that which occurs with blood loss, this strategy would lead to the replacement of both CD4 + and CD8 + cells in a normal ratio. However, when one T-cell subset is selectively lost, as occurs with the CD4 + T-cell depletion of HIV infection, replacement of total CD3 + T cells will result in a progressive accumulation of CD8 + T cells in relation to CD4 + T cells. It has been suggested that, if such a homeostatic mechanism functions in vivo, selective depletion of CD8 + T cells in infected individuals might lower total CD3 + T-cell number sufficiently to stimulate this homeostatic mechanism and result in an increase in total CD4 + T-cell numbers. However, whether this homeostatic mechanism exists and is contributory to the increased circulating CD8 + T-cell numbers present during the early clinical phase of HIV infection or contributes to a suppression of CD4 + T-cell numbers, remains to be determined.

AIDS patients with opportunistic infections and markedly decreased numbers of CD4 + T cells often have markedly diminished numbers of CD8 + T cells.[83] The reason for this loss of CD8 + T cells is not completely understood, but may reflect a loss of progenitor cell capacity for regeneration of mature T cells. In this regard, the finding that the human thymus in the SCID-hu mouse is highly susceptible to infection with HIV and that infection is seen within both the CD4 and CD8 single-positive thymocyte populations is of interest.[44] Whether this CD8 + thymocyte infection results in a loss of immature thymocytes with failure to generate sufficient mature T-cell numbers is not currently known. Alternatively, the loss of CD8+ T cells could reflect a complete breakdown in he body's normal T-cell homeostatic mechanisms with failure to respond to decreased numbers of T cells.

Abnormalities in CD8+ T-cell function have been noted at all stages of infection. A deficiency in MHC-restricted CTLs against influenza and cytomegalovirus (CMV) has been observed, and loss of HIV CTL activity also occurs with disease progression.[84,85] Later in the course of disease circulating CD8+ T cells display an impaired clonogenic potential.[86] These nonclonogenic cells are HLA-DR positive but CD25 (IL-2 receptor) negative, and appear to constitute the anti-HIV specific CTLs. The loss of clonogenic potential may explain the disappearance of HIV CTLs observed late in the course of disease.

Abnormalities in Monocyte/Macrophages

Infection with HIV. Because M/M express the CD4 molecule on their surface, they are targets for infection with HIV. There are several distinguishing features between HIV infection of M/M and CD4+ T cells that are likely important in the overall pathogenesis of HIV infection (reviewed in ref. 87). First, contrary to what is observed with infection of the CD4+ T-cell, HIV infection of M/M does not result in significant cell killing. Second, as opposed to virus budding strictly from the cell surface membrane in T cells, virus production and budding from the infected M/M can occur both at the cell membrane and intracellularly into organelles. This intracellular budding of virus may allow the infected M/M to escape detection by the immune system. Third, infection of macrophages can occur efficiently in nonproliferating populations, whereas activation and proliferation are required for efficient HIV infection of T cells.[88] Finally, although infected monocytes are rarely detected in the circulation, HIV-infected macrophages are readily observed in multiple tissues. These features of M/M infection suggest that these cells may serve as an important reservoir for HIV; long-lived noncytopathically infected cells escape immune surveillance and are present in many tissues. These cells may be able to subsequently infect CD4+ T cells that migrate through tissues in response to inflammation. Because cytokines would be present in such areas of inflammation, and because the production of HIV from infected macrophages is upregulated by a number of these cytokines (reviewed in ref. 89 and discussed below), T cells that migrate to a tissue location might be exposed to a high localized concentration of infectious virions.

Functional Abnormalities of the M/M. Multiple abnormalities in M/M function occur after either in vivo or in vitro infection or exposure of these cells to HIV (reviewed in ref. 16). Most frequently these cells exhibit abnormal chemotaxis, possibly due to a downregulation of expression of receptors for chemotactic ligands, an event that occurs in vitro after exposure of M/M to HIV proteins.[90] Additionally, Fc receptor mediated function, C3 receptor mediated clearance, certain monocyte dependent T-cell proliferative responses, and the oxidative burst are impaired to some degree in HIV-infected patients. In vitro infection of M/M results in impaired ADCC activity and decreased killing of intracellular microbes[91] as well as decreased IFN-α secretion.[92] In vitro exposure to viral antigens without infection of the cells results not only in defective chemotactic function, as mentioned above, but also in a decreased respiratory burst.[93] The relevance of some of these in vivo findings remains to be determined because certain of these functions, such as ADCC,[94] antimicrobial activity, and phagocytosis[95] appear to remain intact in the infected individual. Although cytokine production by M/M appears to be intact with the exception of IFN-α secretion, exposure of M/M to HIV proteins in vitro results in the production of inhibitors of IL-1 activity, and some studies suggest that these inhibitors may be present in the circulation of HIV-infected individuals.[96] Additionally, the production of IL-12, a macrophage product that upregulates T-cell production of IFN-γ and appears to be important in establishing a Th-1-like immune response, is decreased in HIV-infected individuals.[97] Thus, analogous to the multiple direct and indirect effects that HIV exerts on the functions of the CD4+ T cell, multiple functional abnormalities are observed in in vivo or in vitro HIV-infected M/M as well as in M/M exposed to HIV proteins in the absence of direct infection.

Pathogenic Effects Related to Infection of M/M. Forty to sixty percent of AIDS patients develop neurologic dysfunction and up to 90 percent have neuropathologic changes at autopsy.[98] HIV itself can cause brain disease manifested as meningoencephalitis, mild cognitive dysfunction, or frank dementia. It is felt that the pathogenesis of this neurologic damage is related to the presence of infected tissue macrophages that may release viral proteins or cytokines that result in brain dysfunction, inflammation, and tissue destruction (reviewed in ref. 99). In this regard, studies of brain tissue from AIDS patients have shown that the predominant cell type infected with HIV is the M/M.[100] Infected M/M may release factors resulting in reactive glial cell growth, and, because glial cells have been shown to be infectable with HIV in vitro,[101] infected brain M/M may provide a source of infectious HIV to these glial cells. The HIV envelope protein can inhibit neuronal growth in vitro; this may be due to competition between neuroleukin and gp120 for binding to the neuroleukin receptor, because there is partial sequence homology between these two proteins.[102] It is possible, but not yet demonstrated, that infected M/M in the brain may release large quantities of gp120 resulting in the inhibition of neuronal growth.

A wide variety of hematologic abnormalities occur in HIV-infected individuals including pancytopenia and myelodysplasia (reviewed in ref. 40). Although the etiology of these multiple abnormalities has not been completely delineated, it has been shown that the CD34+ bone marrow myeloid progenitor cell can be infected with HIV in vitro with the resultant production of large amounts of predominantly intracellular virus and minimal cytopathic effects.[21] More recently, CD34+ cells isolated from the bone marrow of some infected individuals have been shown to be infected with HIV.[42] Whether these precursor cells produce large amounts of virus in the bone marrow in vivo and the potential contribution of these cells to the hematologic abnormalities observed are currently unknown. Infected macrophages within the bone marrow have been reported to produce factors, presumably cytokines, which appear to suppress hematopoiesis through their effects on the CD34+ precursor cell (reviewed in ref. 40). Whether bone marrow macrophages are an important reservoir of HIV has not been definitively determined.

Finally, cells of the monocytic lineage that populate other organs are susceptible to infection with HIV and may contribute to pathogenesis of disease at these sites (reviewed in ref. 89). Specifically, lung alveolar macrophages, Küpffer cells of the liver, and peritoneal macrophages are infectable in vitro with HIV, and alveolar macrophages from HIV-infected individuals are clearly infected in vivo. It is currently unknown whether these cells contribute to tissue-specific disease, such as the diffuse pulmonary fibrosis that occurs frequently in pediatric AIDS patients.

B-Cell Abnormalities

Activation and Impaired Specific Antibody Responses. Pronounced B-cell activation occurs consistently in AIDS patients,[103] manifested as an elevated number of B cells proliferating spontaneously in vitro and producing large amounts of antibody as detected in vivo by elevated serum IgG, IgA, and IgD. A significant proportion of these in vivo activated B cells produce antibodies against HIV, predominantly reactive against envelope antigens.[104] Although they spontaneously proliferate and produce antibody, these B cells are refractory to further activation signals[103] (reviewed in ref. 16), and fail to produce specific antibody or proliferate after antigen or PWM stimulation even in some patients infected for less than 1 year.[105] In vivo responses to primary and secondary immunizations are poor in AIDS patients; specific antibody production against both protein and polysaccharide antigens are decreased. This inability to mount an adequate humoral response results in an increased susceptibility to bacterial infections in many HIV-infected adults; however, it is probably even more significant in infants and children with HIV, who have limited previous exposure to pathogens and must rely on a primary humoral response to control infections.[106] Decreases in circulating B-cell numbers occur early in the course of HIV infection and may increase with increasing severity of disease.[107]

The mechanism of this B-cell activation is probably multifactorial. HIV itself may have a direct B-cell stimulating effect. Although there is currently no evidence that HIV infects B cells either in vivo or in vitro, may of the functional abnormalities of B cells from HIV-infected patients can be observed on exposure of B cells to intact or disrupted virus[108] (reviewed in ref. 16). Additionally, the carboxyl terminus of gp41 has been shown in one study to have polyclonal B-cell activating capability.[109] Infection with Epstein-Barr virus (EBV) or CMV, well-established polyclonal B-cell stimulators, is common in HIV-infected individuals and these may contribute to the B-cell activation.[110] Finally, the loss of appropriate CD4+ T-helper cell function must certainly contribute to abnormal humoral responses.

Lymphomas in HIV Infection. AIDS patients have a significantly increased incidence of lymphomas, most of which are B cell in origin. Although EBV infection is present in many HIV-infected individuals and HIV has been shown in vitro to infect EBV-transformed B cells, there is currently no evidence to suggest that HIV infection of B cells occurs or results in the formation of lymphomas.[111] EBV has been suggested as playing a role in the development of central nervous system (CNS) lymphomas in AIDS patients (see Ch. 146). Spontaneous transformation of B cells from AIDS patients by EBV occurs in vitro[112] and is felt to be due to deficient T-cell and NK-cell immune surveillance. Hence, the occurrence of lymphomas in these immunocompromised patients probably does not reflect a dysfunction of B cells as much as it indicates a lack of adequate tumor surveillance.

Cytokine Production. Cytokines play an important role in HIV pathogenesis and can increase and decrease the production of virus from acutely and chronically infected cells. Because B cells from HIV-infected individuals are activated in vivo, investigators have examined the ability of these cells to produce cytokines that might influence the course of HIV infection. After exposure to HIV or gp120, B cells from HIV-infected individuals, but not normal controls, secrete increased levels of cytokines in vitro.[113,114] Furthermore, B cells from HIV-infected individuals but not uninfected controls secrete both tumor necrosis factor (TNF)-α and IL-6 constitutively.[115] These cytokines were active in that either co-culture of B cells with or transfer of the B cell supernatants onto chronically infected T and promonocytic cell lines resulted in an upregulation of HIV production. Finally, activation of virus expression was also noted upon co-culture of B cells with autologous T cells from HIV-infected individuals. Thus, it is apparent that B cells from HIV-infected individuals produce cytokines both spontaneously and after exposure to HIV that can enhance the production of HIV from infected cells. This may be particularly significant in the environment of the lymph node, where infected CD4+ T cells migrating through the node likely encounter a permissive cytokines milieu that supports active viral replication (discussed further below).

Natural Killer Cells

NK cells are a group of phenotypically distinct cell types that have the functional property of killing tumor cells, allogeneic cells, and virally infected cells. Most of the cells are large granular lymphocytes (LGL) that bear the CD16 antigen on their surface, and a smaller population of these cells also bear the γδ T-cell receptor.[116] These cells are thought to play a critical role in the normal immune surveillance mechanisms that detect and kill virally infected cells and spontaneously arising tumor cells. Although most investigators have reported that the number of circulating NK cells is not altered in HIV-infected individuals, more recent studies suggest that these cells are depleted early in the course of infection.[117] Whether present in normal numbers or not, NK cell function is significantly impaired in HIV-infected individuals (reviewed in ref. 16). NK cells from HIV-seropositive individuals bind normally to target cells but cytotoxicity is decreased. This does not reflect a defect in the lytic machinery of the cell in that these cells can still mediate normal ADCC in vitro.[118] Activation of NK cells does not increase their in vitro cytotoxicity, whereas the addition of IL-2 to cultures results in an increase of this activity,[119] suggesting that IL-2 specifically triggers the production or release of the cytotoxic factor that results in cytolysis. Although a deficiency in IL-2 may contribute to decreased NK cell function, HIV may directly depress NK function. In this regard, in vitro exposure of NK cells to peptides homologous to HIV gp41 results in significant suppression of NK cell function.[120] Finally, the addition of IL-12 to cultures of PBMCs from HIV-infected individuals augments in vitro NK function,[121] and, because IL-12 secretion is defective in these patients,[97] depressed NK cell cytotoxicity may reflect an in vivo deficiency of this cytokine.

Dendritic Cells

Over the past several years the role of the peripheral blood dendritic cell in HIV infection and pathogenesis has been explored. These cells, first described by Steinmann and colleagues in 1974, are now recognized to be potent APCs that not only activate T cells in a secondary response to recall antigens but also, unlike other known APCs, initiate a primary immune response to viruses and other antigens (reviewed in ref. 122). Dendritic cells are bone marrow derived cells that express high levels of HLA-DR but lack surface molecules of the T, B, NK, or M/M lineage. Additionally, they have a distinct morphology and can be readily identified on electron microscopy (EM) examination by their convoluted cell membrane with its multiple and extensive dendritic processes that give them a "veiled" appearance. These cells are felt to belong to a single family of bone marrow derived cells, including the skin Langerhans cells, afferent lymph veiled cells, and interdigitating dendritic cells in the T-dependent area of the lymph node. The function of these cells is to carry antigen acquired in the periphery via blood or lymphatics to T cells in the lymph node, thereby initiating a primary immune response. Because patients infected with HIV have impaired T-cell responses, it has been of considerable interest to determine whether this may reflect a dysfunction of this class of potent antigen presenting cells.

To date, conflicting results have been obtained by several groups of investigators studying dendritic cells. One group of investigators has found that some proportion of dendritic cells are infected in vivo in HIV-infected individuals and that these cells are deficient in their ability to stimulate T-cell responses.[123] Additionally, this group finds that the number of HLA-DR expressing dendritic cells is decreased in HIV infection. Both this group and one other have also found that dendritic cells from normal donors can be infected with HIV in vitro and support high titers of virus replication (ref. 123 and references therein). In contrast, others have found that there is no preferential loss of dendritic cells in HIV-infected individuals; that these cells are probably not infected either in vivo or infectable in vitro with HIV; and that dendritic cells from HIV-infected people maintain normal function in stimulating T cells, as measured by the mixed leukocyte reaction (MLR).[124] Indeed, highly purified (>95 percent) dendritic cells from normal donors retain their potent APC activity after in vitro exposure to HIV in that they present HIV efficiently to autologous CD4+ T cells that become infected, whereas the dendritic cells themselves remain uninfected with HIV (D. Weissman and A. S. Fauci, unpublished observation).

The explanation for these widely divergent findings may lie in the methodology employed by the separate groups in isolating dendritic cells. Indeed, because there is currently no specific surface marker that identifies these cells and morphology remains the sine qua non for identification, most investigators are generally studying populations of cells that are not purified but rather enriched for dendritic cells, with the enriched population of cells usually containing only 20–50 percent dendritic cells. Because the contaminating populations of cells may be very different depending on the isolation techniques employed, variant results are possible. In addition, Patterson et al. have proposed that there are several stages of maturation of peripheral blood dendritic cells, identified morphologically, and that susceptibility to HIV infection may differ with developmental stage.[123]

Co-factors in Pathogenesis

Cytokine Regulation of HIV Expression. Whereas viral replication occurs in vivo throughout the course of infection with HIV[125] it is clear that individual cells may be latently infected and express virus only after immunologic activation. Regulation of expression of the latent provirus has been studied in detail, and it is now apparent that cytokines play an important role in this process (reviewed in ref. 126). In this regard, a number of endogenous cytokines have been shown to upregulate virus expression from both acutely and chronically HIV-infected cells, whereas other cytokines can suppress viral expression and still others exert bimodal effects depending on the conditions of the assay.

Among those cytokines which can upregulate virus expression, TNF-α has been the most extensively studied. TNF-α has been shown to upregulate virus expression from acutely and chronically infected cell lines of both T and monocytic lineage, as well as primary macrophages.[127–129] TNF-α induces HIV expression by increasing the binding of cellular NF-κB to the enhancer sequences in the integrated proviral LTR with subsequent initiation of transcription.[130] IL-1 also induces HIV expression from chronically infected monocyte and T-cell lines as well as primary monocyte-derived macrophages through both transcriptional and post-transcriptional mechanisms (reviewed in ref. 126). This is in contrast to the mechanism of induction of virus expression by two other upregulatory cytokines, namely IL-6 and granulocyte-macrophage colony-stimulating factor (GM-CSF)[131] (reviewed in ref. 126). These cytokines induce virus expression in both chronically infected promonocytic cell lines and, in the case of GM-CSF, in primary PBMC. Both of these cytokines, when acting alone, appear to induce HIV expression primarily through an as yet unidentified post-transcriptional mechanism. However, both of these cytokines can also synergize with TNF-α in the induction of HIV from chronically infected monocytic cells, and, at least in the case of IL-6, the mechanism of this synergy includes both transcriptional and post-transcriptional inductive effects. Finally, IL-3, IL-4, and macrophage colony-stimulating factor (M-CSF) can upregulate HIV expression in certain cells (reviewed in ref. 126), and IL-10, which alone has no effect on HIV expression, can synergize with a variety of cytokines in upregulating HIV expression from monocytic cell lines (D. Weissman and A. S. Fauci, unpublished observations).

A number of studies have demonstrated that exposure of cells to HIV with or without infection can lead to the increased expression of cytokines. In this regard, in vitro infection of cells results in increased production of TNF-α,[129] IL-6,[132] and IL-1.[133,134] Productive infection of cells is not necessary for the induction of cytokines, because exposure of cells to HIV gp120 results in an increased expression of TNF-α, IL-6, IL-1, and GM-CSF.[116,135,136] Additionally, memory and naive CD4+ T cells from HIV-infected individuals display abnormal secretion of both IL-6 and IFN-γ.[137] The ability of HIV to induce the cellular production of cytokines that are positive modulators of its own expression establishes an autocrine mechanism for cytokine-induced enhancement of viral expression. This has been most clearly demonstrated for TNF-α.[129]

Further evidence for the role of cytokines in HIV pathogenesis is the fact that HIV-infected patients demonstrate abnormal plasma levels of certain cytokines. Specifically, plasma levels of TNF-α, IL-6, and IFN-γ are increased in certain individuals,[138,139] and PBMC from infected individuals secrete, both spontaneously and in response to various stimuli, increased amounts of TNF-α, IL-6, and IL-1[133,139,140]; pulmonary alveolar macrophages from HIV-infected individuals also secrete significantly higher amounts of TNF-α than those from uninfected individuals.[141] Additionally, as discussed previously, B cells from HIV-infected individuals secrete TNF-α and IL-6 both spontaneously and after exposure to HIV.[113–115] Indeed, multiple cytokines are present at abnormal levels, either increased or decreased, in the microenvironment of the lymph node, where these cytokines may be playing an important role in modulating the expression of HIV from infected lymphoid cells (C. Graziosi and A. S. Fauci, unpublished observations). Thus, it appears that HIV has insinuated itself into the very regulatory mechanisms of the host immune system, causing perturbations in cytokine secretion and using these cytokines to enhance its own replication and spread.

There are, however, certain cytokines that can negatively regulate HIV expression. These include IFN-α and β, which can suppress HIV replication in both acutely and chronically infected PBMC, M/M, and cell lines[142,143] (reviewed in ref. 126), and transforming growth factor (TGF)-β, which inhibits the PMA or IL-6 stimulated expression of HIV from chronically infected promonocytic cell lines[144] as well as acute infection of primary M/M.[145] Although the mechanism of suppression by TGF-β remains unclear, IFN-α and IFN-β decrease virus production by inhibiting viral protein production from acutely infected mitogen stimulated PBMCs and M/M and suppress virion release from the cell membrane of chronically infected cells. Because HIV-infected individuals have elevated plasma levels of acid-labile IFN-α,[145] and elevated levels of TGF-β have been demonstrated in brain tissue of infected individuals,[146] these cytokines may play a role in downregulating virus expression in vivo.

Finally, there are several cytokines that appear to have bimodal effects on HIV expression, depending on the conditions of the assay. IFN-γ can stimulate viral expression from both T cells and monocytes[147,148] and appears to function in a manner similar to IL-6 in that, when used as a single agent on a promonocytic cell line it upregulates virus in a post-transcriptional manner but can also synergize with TNF-α in inducing transcription from the viral LTR (reviewed in ref. 126). IFN-γ has also been reported to decrease viral production from chronically infected monocytic cell lines after phorbol ester stimulation, but it has more recently been shown that there is actually not a decrease in virion production but, rather, a redirection of viral budding from the surface into intracellular vacuoles.[149] It has also been reported to have a suppressive effect on viral expression from T cells (reviewed in ref. 126). TGF-β, which suppresses virus expression from chronically infected promonocytic cells, can enhance the acute infection of cell lines and M/M (reviewed in ref. 126). Additionally, IL-4 can suppress or enhance virus expression from cells depending on whether it is added before or after acute infection (reviewed in ref. 126).

In summary, multiple cytokines exert complex effects on the regulation of HIV expression from both T cells and monocytes under experimental conditions, and alterations in cytokine production from PBMCs of infected individuals occurs both in vitro and in vivo. Further understanding of the intricacies of this network may allow manipulation of cytokine production or the use of agents that antagonize cytokine function for the treatment of HIV disease.

Pathogens Other Than HIV as Cofactors in HIV Pathogenesis. Co-infection with pathogens other than HIV has been postulated to modulate HIV disease progression (also see Ch. 146). In this regard, certain investigators have reported an increased incidence of infection with *Mycoplasma fermentans* (incognitus strain) in HIV-infected individuals and have suggested that this organism is responsible for the AIDS-associated nephropathy and in vitro cytotoxicity.[150,151] Others, however, have found no increased incidence of infection with this organism in autopsy studies.[152] Patients co-infected with HTLV-I appear to progress to symptomatic disease more rapidly than those infected with HIV alone[153]; this may be related to the observation that HTLV-I increases the production of HIV from infected cells in vitro by increasing the transactivation of the HIV-LTR.[154] Human herpesvirus type 6 (HHV-6) is present in the PBMCs of up to 83 percent of AIDS patients.[155] HHV-6 can infect cells already infected with HIV,[156] and has been shown to act synergistically with the HIV *tat* protein to transactivate the HIV-LTR.[157] For this reason, it has been postulated that co-infection with this virus may lead to accelerated progression of immunodeficiency in HIV-infected individuals, although there is currently no epidemiologic data to confirm this. Finally, the hepatitis B virus X protein has been shown to transactivate the HIV-LTR,[158] and because this virus is also transmitted both sexually and by blood, co-infection of individuals with HIV and hepatitis B is not uncommon.

Role of Lymphoid Tissue in Pathogenesis

Lymphoid organs play a central role in the pathogenesis of HIV disease. Although HIV infection in human lymph nodes was detected several years ago by a number of investigators[159,160] (reviewed in ref. 5), the extent of viral burden in the nodes and the dichotomy between viral activity in the lymph nodes and blood were not fully recognized. In this regard, Pantaleo and colleagues, using the DNA PCR assay, simultaneously studied lymph node and PBMC from the same HIV-infected individuals; they found that, in all cases, cells from the lymph node contained 5–10 times more viral DNA than equal numbers of cells from peripheral blood.[161] Because the vast majority of lymphoid cells are found in the lymphoid organs as opposed to the peripheral blood, these results indicate that the viral burden reflected in the peripheral blood is not at all representative of total body viral burden. Furthermore, it was demonstrated that, even in an individual with no evidence of active HIV disease in the peripheral blood, viral replication is active and ongoing in the lymph nodes, as detected by RNA PCR techniques[48]; viral replication in the lymph nodes was always greater than that in the peripheral blood at all stages of HIV disease. These findings, together with those from several histopathologic studies that have been performed (reviewed in ref. 162), have led to the formulation of a hypothesis that describes the role of lymphoid organs in HIV disease.[5] The intense viremia that usually accompanies primary infection[34] results in the seeding of multiple lymph nodes with virus. As occurs during the immune response to any pathogen, there is an accompanying antigen-driven expansion of B cells and infiltration of activated CD4+ T cells within the nodes, which, because of the magnitude of the viremia and immune response, may contribute to the initial marked

decline in CD4+ T cells that is observed clinically (Fig. 1). Because these T cells are activated, they are more easily infected with HIV that is trapped as extracellular virions on the processes of the follicular dendritic cells (FDCs) within germinal centers of the node, and viral replication is facilitated by this activated state.[19] In addition, as alluded to previously, cytokines such as TNF-α are released by activated germinal center B cells, and these cytokines further enhance viral replication and spread within the lymph node.

Plasma viremia diminishes markedly and viral replication within PBMC is downregulated as the patient enters the clinically latent period of disease (Fig. 1)[5,29]; this phenomenon is probably reflective of both efficient trapping of virus within the lymph nodes as well as the development of an initial immune response. However, because of the unique environment of the lymph node that brings activated CD4+ T cells and HIV in close proximity and provides an appropriate cytokine milieu for viral replication, virus persists in the lymph nodes and actively replicates within infected cells. The FDC network is important in maintaining this trapping of virus within the node. FDCs, distinct from peripheral blood dendritic cells, are the primary antigen presenting cells for B cells and are capable of trapping antigen/antibody/complement complexes on their extensive processes (reviewed in ref. 163). It has been shown that, as HIV disease worsens, there is progressive destruction of the FDC network within the lymph node and the nodal architecture is effaced.[5,164] At late stages of disease, when FDCs can no longer normally trap antigen and when the HIV-specific immune response diminishes, HIV spills over from the nodes into the circulation and viremia is again detected (Fig. 1).

This hypothesis has several implications in understanding HIV pathogenesis and treatment. It was previously felt that viral replication was minimal during the clinically latent period of disease and the reappearance of viremia in late stages reflected a massive increase in replication and viral burden. It is now clear that there is a significant viral burden in asymptomatic individuals and that viral replication is persistent throughout the course of disease, although it generally increases as disease progresses. This provides the scientific rationale and justification for early and aggressive treatment of HIV infection with antiretroviral agents when effective drugs become available. Second, therapeutic strategies aimed at blocking viral replication as well as those designed to antagonize cytokine effects on HIV will need to consider the concentrations of drug needed to be effective in the lymph node. Finally, the destruction of the lymph node microenvironment, along with the destruction of the thymic microenvironment discussed earlier,[44] implies that reconstitution of the immune system may be more complex than previously imagined if these tissues themselves do not have the capacity to regenerate spontaneously.

IMMUNE RESPONSE TO HIV

Although individuals clearly mount an early vigorous immune response in infection with HIV (Table 3), the fact that the course of HIV infection is chronic and progressive indicates that the immune response is ineffective in completely supressing the

TABLE 3. Immune Responses to HIV

Humoral responses
Neutralizing antibodies
Cytotoxic antibodies (ADCC)
Cellular responses
T-helper cell proliferation to HIV proteins
Cytotoxic T-lymphocyte response, CD8+ and CD4+
Noncytotoxic CD8+ T-cell suppression of HIV
Natural killer (NK) cells
Active in ADCC
Abnormal NK activity
Monocyte-mediated ADCC

virus over a prolonged period of time. It is still not clear which factors constitute an effective response against this particular pathogen, but recent evidence suggests that an effective response can be mounted by certain individuals. In this regard, preliminary data suggest that some individuals, such as health care workers, wives of infected hemophiliacs, and sexual partners of infected individuals, have been exposed to virus, as manifested by a recall proliferative response of their PBMCs in vitro when exposed to HIV peptides. These individuals have successfully avoided established HIV infection, as documented by negative testing by PCR and culture for the presence of HIV.[165] These observations need to be verified by other laboratories, and if confirmed, further study of such individuals may yield important information on the components of the immune response that are effective against HIV.

Humoral Response

The development of an antibody response occurs within 3–6 months in the vast majority of individuals and forms the basis for the diagnostic enzyme-linked immunosorbent assay (ELISA) and Western blot assays to detect HIV infection; however, the production of both neutralizing and cytolytic antibodies can occur as early as 2 weeks after the onset of symptoms of HIV infection.[166] A broad antibody response can occur, with antibodies against the envelope glycoproteins, core antibody, *tat*, *rev*, *nef*, and other regulatory proteins.

Neutralizing Antibody Response.

It is felt that the rapid clearance of plasma viremia after acute infection with HIV is due primarily to the presence of neutralizing antibodies and the formation of antigen/antibody complexes.[167] However, binding antibodies that fix complement may contribute to the clearance of virus from the plasma by enhancing the trapping of virions on the FDCs of the lymph node germinal centers (see above). Variable titers of neutralizing antibodies are detectable throughout the course of infection with HIV.[168] Most responses are against the envelope glycoproteins gp120 and gp41, although neutralizing responses against core proteins have also been detected (reviewed in ref. 16). Antibodies can be either type specific or group specific, depending on whether they neutralize one specific viral isolate or several closely related isolates that share some degree of sequence homology. Many of the antibodies against the gp120 protein recognize sequences within a region termed the V3 loop, and more specifically, a short sequence within this region termed the principle neutralizing determinant (PND).[169,170] Because the PND is highly conserved among various HIV isolates, a response against this region may be broadly reactive.

Despite its role in early clearance of plasma viremia, it is clear that the neutralizing antibody response is ineffective in inhibiting viral replication over the course of infection. Indeed, several studies have found no clear correlation between the clinical course or ability to prevent disease and the in vitro activity of the neutralizing antibodies.[171] This loss of effectiveness over time may be due to viral variants that have been shown to arise in vivo over time. Because HIV replicates with a high mutation rate, HIV strains that are not susceptible to the initial strain specific neutralizing antibody response may arise. Indeed, it has been shown that early serum samples from an individual are unable to neutralize virus isolated at a later time point from the same individual.[167] In addition, in vitro generation of neutralization resistant isolates has been accomplished by passage of susceptible virus in culture in the presence of neutralizing antibodies, and only minor genetic changes (e.g., point mutations) may be responsible for the development of this resistance (reviewed in ref. 16). Thus, it is highly likely that the development of such variants during the prolonged course of HIV disease are responsible in part for the loss of effectiveness of neutralizing antibodies in controlling viral replication.

Antibody-Dependent Cellular Cytotoxicity.

Anti-HIV ADCC activity is directed primarily against the gp120 protein of HIV, although anti-gp41 activity has also been detected (reviewed in refs. 16, 172, and 173). The effector cell for ADCC is generally the CD16+ natural killer cell. This cell is defective in NK activity in HIV-infected individuals (see above); however, it mediates ADCC normally.[118] Monocytes can also mediate anti-HIV ADCC activity in HIV-infected individuals.[174] This antibody-mediated cellular cytolytic activity is non-MHC-restricted and generally involves antibodies that are broadly reactive with numerous strains of HIV-1 (reviewed in ref. 173). Although ADCC activity can be detected at all stages of HIV disease, it is unclear whether this activity declines with disease progression in certain individuals; some reports have found persistently high activity in later stage patients,[175] whereas others have found a decreasing ability to mediate ADCC with disease progression[176] (reviewed in refs. 172 and 173). This loss of ADCC activity did not always correlate with anti-HIV antibody titers and may therefore reflect further suppression of the function of the CD16+ effector cells. In this regard, IL-2 promotes NK cell activity[119] and HIV-infected patients have been shown to have defects in the production of and cellular response to IL-2. Clinical trials are currently underway using IL-2 therapy in an attempt to increase this potentially beneficial ADCC activity in infected individuals (reviewed in ref. 172).

Cell-Mediated Responses

Cytotoxic T-cell Response.

CTL activity can be detected in HIV-infected individuals during the primary acute retroviral syndrome and is present in lymphocytes isolated from peripheral blood, lung, and cerebrospinal fluid (reviewed in refs. 16 and 177). This response is targeted against a variety of both structural and regulatory proteins of HIV, including RT, gp120, gp41, gp160, and *nef* (reviewed in ref. 177). Indeed, the highly conserved regions in gp120, gp41, p24, p17, and *nef* appear to be particularly effective in inducing a CTL response. The CTL response appears early in the course of infection and the early CD8+ T-cell lymphocytosis observed during the acute syndrome[29] has been proposed to reflect this CTL response. This early response may be a major mechanism of clearance of the initial plasma viremia; the appearance of CTLs correlates with the decline in p24 antigenemia and resolution of clinical symptoms.[81] Although the major cell mediating CTL activity is a CD8+ T cell, CD4+ mediated MHC class II-restricted CTLs have been induced after exposure of PBMCs from HIV-infected individuals to gp160 peptides.[178] CD4+ T-cell CTL activity has also been observed in seronegative individuals after vaccination with a recombinant gp160 protein; this response is directed toward a highly conserved region of the gp41 molecule that is recognized in the context of a DP allele prevalent in certain populations.[179] Use of this region in vaccinations might therefore induce effective CTL activity against a number of HIV-1 strains in a significant percentage of vaccines. These findings may be of particular import as it has been shown that cellular immunity alone can provide protection against mouse retroviral infection but this protective effect requires both CD4+ and CD8+ T-cell responses.[180]

HIV-specific CD8+ CTL responses occur early in HIV infection and appear to be effective in controlling HIV replication; however, activity is gradually lost over time as disease progresses. This loss of activity may reflect the emergence of viral variants that escape recognition by CTLs (reviewed in ref. 16). In one instance resistance to cytotoxicity was due to a single amino acid change in the HIV envelope,[181] and loss of recognition by CTLs has also occurred due to genetic alterations within the core antigens.[182] Alternatively, loss of this activity as immunosuppression increases may be due to an absolute decrease in CD8+ T-cell numbers, a loss of CD4+ T cells responsible for inducing or helping the CD8+ T cells, an inability to generate new T cells due to thymic dysfunction, or an inability to initiate or maintain normal CTL activity due to a deficiency of necessary growth factors or cytokines. Because the CTL response appears to be effective in early control of HIV infection, attempts are now being made to expand CD8+ T cells and reinfuse them into infected hosts to potentiate the anti-HIV effects.[183]

Noncytolytic Suppression by CD8+ T Cells. A second mechanism of CD8+ T cell suppression of HIV occurs in a noncytolytic manner.[184] Several years ago it was demonstrated that isolation of HIV from a patient's PBMCs was significantly enhanced by prior removal of the autologous CD8+ T cells. It was subsequently shown by several groups that this is due to a noncytolytic suppression of HIV expression from autologous CD4+ T cells, which involves at least in part the action of an as yet unidentified soluble factor secreted by the CD8+ T cells.[185,186] The presence or effectiveness of this anti-HIV activity differs between infected individuals and correlates with the clinical stage of disease, with more severely immunosuppressed patients lacking this CD8+ T-cell activity.[187] The phenomenon has also been recognized in SIV-infected rhesus monkeys[188] where, although the cell appears to be a CTL, the mechanism of suppression of HIV or SIV expression is not clearly cytolytic. Additionally, CD8+ T cells from asymptomatic HIV-infected individuals can, in an MHC-unrestricted manner, block the replication of HIV in allogeneic CD4+ T cells that are acutely infected with HIV; although a soluble factor was responsible at least in part for this effect, cell co-culture was required for maximum suppression.[189] It remains unclear whether cell contact is required to stimulate the CD8+ T cells to secrete the soluble factor, or whether there are two mechanisms (i.e., contact mediated as well as secreted factor). The disappearance of this function in more clinically advanced patients may be a contributing factor to the progression of disease as well as a result thereof. In any event, it will be of interest to determine the mechanism of this effect that, when present, can be a powerful suppressor of HIV expression and may have important therapeutic implications.

Other Cellular Responses. As mentioned previously, NK cells in HIV-infected individuals are active in mediating ADCC responses to HIV, but generally are deficient in normal NK activity. However, gp120 specific killing by NK-like cells has been observed in some individuals (reviewed in ref. 16). Additionally, helper T lymphocytes from most individuals early in the course of disease display proliferative responses to viral proteins such as gp120, gp41, and p24, although a few cases of T-helper cell anergy to HIV proteins have been described (reviewed in ref. 16). The epitopes responsible for eliciting these proliferative responses are generally distinct from those that are recognized by neutralizing antibodies.

CONCLUSIONS

It has become increasingly clear that the immunopathogenesis of HIV infection is a complex process due to the multiple interactions that occur between the virus and its host throughout the various stages of disease. Resolution of the acute syndrome and the disappearance of plasma viremia would seem to indicate early efficacy of a vigorous immune system in controlling this pathogen. However, the persistence of HIV replication in the tissues, particularly the lymphoid organs, and the insidious erosion of immune competence ultimately result in profound immunosuppression of the host. The ability of HIV to insinuate itself into many different aspects of the immune system, such as intercepting the signals provided by multiple cytokines and interfering with the interaction of cell surface molecules, enables it to disrupt the very system that was designed to control pathogens. Although the relentless destruction of CD4+ T cells is central

to the immune suppression caused by this virus, alterations occur in every component of the immune system, including CD8+ T cells, NK cells, monocytes, and B cells. This widespread disruption of the immune system indicates that therapeutic approaches will need to be comprehensive, such that a broad reconstitution of the immune system must be achieved at the same time as effective and long-lasting viral suppression is accomplished. Recent insights into the pathogenic mechanisms that occur during the acute syndrome, with seeding of peripheral lymphoid organs, have demonstrated that early events are critical to the subsequent course of the disease, and the ongoing viral replication in the lymph nodes throughout the course of HIV disease may be the primary cause for the insidious erosion of the immune system. Continued efforts to broaden our understanding of the pathogenic mechanisms of HIV disease are critical for the design of effective therapeutic strategies.

REFERENCES

1. Barre-Sinoussi F, Chermann JC, Rey F, et al. Isolation of a T-lymphotropic retrovirus from a patient at risk for acquired immunodeficiency syndrome (AIDS). Science. 1983;220:868–71.
2. Gallo RC, Salahuddin SZ, Popovic M, et al. Frequent detection and isolation of cytopathic retroviruses (HTLV-III) from patients with AIDS and at risk for AIDS. Science. 1984;224:500–3.
3. Moss AR, Bacchetti P. Natural history of HIV infection. AIDS. 1989;3:55–61.
4. Cullen BR, Greene WC. Regulatory pathways governing HIV-1 replication. Cell. 1989;58:423–6.
5. Pantaleo G, Graziosi C, Fauci AS. The immunopathogenesis of human immunodeficiency virus infection. N Engl J Med. 1993;328:327–35.
6. Chiu IM, Yaniv A, Dahlberg JE, et al. Nucleotide sequence evidence for relationship of AIDS retrovirus to lentiviruses. Nature. 1985;317:366–68.
7. Markovitz DM. Infection with the human immunodeficiency virus type 2. Ann Intern Med. 1993;118:211–8.
8. Fultz PN, McClure HM, Anderson DC, et al. Isolation of a T-lymphotropic retrovirus from naturally infected sooty mangabey monkeys (Cercocebus atys). Proc Natl Acad Sci USA. 1986;83:5286–90.
9. Greene WC. The molecular biology of human immunodeficiency virus type 1 infection. N Engl J Med. 1991;324:308–18.
10. Gaynor R. Cellular factors involved in regulating HIV gene expression. In: Haseltine WA, Wong-Staal F, eds. Genetic structure and regulation of HIV. New York: Raven Press; 1991:107–34.
11. Fauci AS. The human immunodeficiency virus: Infectivity and mechanisms of pathogenesis. Science. 1988;239:617–22.
12. Dalgleish AG, Beverly CL, Clapham PR, et al. The CD4 (T4) antigen is an essential component of the receptor for the AIDS retrovirus. Nature. 1984;312:763–7.
13. Klatzmann D, Champagne E, Charmaret S, et al. T-lymphocyte T4 molecule behaves as the receptor for human retrovirus LAV. Nature. 1984;312:767–8.
14. Sattentau QJ, Dalgleish AG, Weiss RA, et al. Epitopes of the CD4 antigen and HIV infection. Science. 1986;234:1120.
15. Maddon PJ, Dagleish AG, McDougal JS, et al. The T4 gene encodes the AIDS virus receptor and is expressed in the immune system and the brain. Cell. 1986;47:333–8.
16. Rosenberg ZF, Fauci AS. The immunopathogenesis of HIV infection. Adv Immunol. 1989;47:356–431.
17. Gowda SD, Stein BS, Mohagheghpour N, et al. Evidence that T cell activation is required for HIV-1 entry in CD4+ lymphocytes. J Immunol. 1989;142:773–80.
18. Zack JA, Arrigo SJ, Weitsman SR, et al. HIV-1 entry into quiescent primary lymphocytes: Molecular analysis reveals a labile, latent viral structure. Cell. 1990;61:213–22.
19. Zack JA, Haislip AM, Krogstad P, et al. Incompletely reverse-transcribed human immunodeficiency virus type 1 genomes in quiescent cells can function as intermediates in the retroviral life cycle. J Virol. 1992;66:1717–25.
20. Connor RI, Ho DD. Etiology of AIDS: Biology of human retroviruses. In: DeVita VT Jr, Ho DD, Rosenberg SA, eds. AIDS: Etiology, Diagnosis, Treatment and Prevention. Philadelphia: JB Lippincott; 1992:13–38.
21. Folks TM, Kessler SW, Orenstein JM, et al. Infection and replication of HIV-1 in purified progenitor cells of normal human bone marrow. Science. 1988;242:919–22.
22. Schnittman SM, Denning SM, Greenhouse JJ, et al. Evidence for susceptibility of intrathymic T-cell precursors and their progeny carrying T-cell antigen receptor phenotypes TCR alpha beta + and TCR gamma delta + to human immunodeficiency virus infection: A mechanism for CD4+ (T4) lymphocyte depletion. Proc Natl Acad Sci USA. 1990;87:7727–31.
23. McKeating JA, Griffiths PD, Weiss RA. HIV susceptibility conferred to human fibroblasts by cytomegalovirus-induced Fc receptor. Nature. 1990;343:659–61.
24. Rosenberg ZF, Fauci AS. Immunopathogenesis of HIV infection. In: DeVita VT Jr, Hellman S, Rosenberg SA, eds. AIDS: Etiology, Diagnosis, Treatment and Prevention. Philadelphia: JB Lippincott; 1992:61–76.

25. Schuitemaker H, Kootstra NA, de Goede RE, et al. Monocytotropic human immunodeficiency virus type 1 (HIV-1) variants detectable in all stages of HIV-1 infection lack T-cell line tropism and syncytium-inducing ability in primary T-cell culture. J Virol. 1991;65:356–63.

26. Koot M, Keet IPM, Vos AHV, et al. Prognostic value of HIV-1 syncytium-inducing phenotype for rate of CD4 + cell depletion and progression to AIDS. Ann Intern Med. 1993;118:681–8.

27. Massari FE, Poli G, Schnittman SM, et al. *In vivo* T lymphocyte origin of macrophage-tropic strains of HIV. Role of monocytes during *in vitro* isolation and *in vivo* infection. J Immunol. 1990;144:4628–32.

28. Gaines H, von Sydow MA, von Stedingk LV, et al. Immunological changes in primary HIV-1 infecton. AIDS. 1990;4:995–9.

29. Tindall B, Cooper DA. Primary HIV infection: Host responses and intervention strategies. AIDS. 1991;5:1–14.

30. Centers for Disease Control and Prevention. 1993 revised classification system for HIV infection and expanded surveillance case definition for AIDS among adolescents and adults. MMWR. 1992;41(No.RR-17).

31. Rabson AB. The molecular biology of HIV infection: Clues for possible therapy. In: Levy JA, ed. AIDS Pathogenesis and Treatment. New York: Marcel Dekker. 1989;231–256.

32. Somasundaran M, Robinson HL. Unexpectedly high levels of HIV-1 RNA and protein synthesis in a cytocidal infection. Science. 1988;242:1554–7.

33. Koga Y, Sasaki M, Yoshida H, et al. Cytopathic effect determined by the amount of CD4 molecules in human cell lines expressing envelope glycoprotein of HIV. J Immunol. 1990;144:94–102.

34. Clark SJ, Saag MS, Decker WD, et al. High titers of cytopathic virus in plasma of patients with symptomatic primary HIV-1 infection. N Engl J Med. 1991;324:954–60.

35. Schnittman SM, Psallidopoulos MC, Lane HC, et al. The reservoir for HIV-1 in human peripheral blood is a T cell that maintains expression of CD4. Science. 1989;245:305–8.

36. Yoffe B, Lewis DE, Petrie BL, et al. Fusion as a mediator of cytolysis in mixtures of uninfected CD4 + lymphocytes and cells infected by human immunodeficiency virus. Proc Natl Acad Sci USA. 1987;84:1429–33.

37. Weinhold KJ, Lyerly HK, Stanley SD, et al. HIV-1 gp120-mediated immune suppression and lymphocyte destruction in the absence of viral infection. J Immunol. 1989;142:3091–7.

38. Siliciano RF, Lawton T, Knall C, et al. Analaysis of host-virus interactions in AIDS with anti-gp120 T cell clones: Effect of HIV sequence variation and a mechanism for CD4 + cell depletion. Cell. 1988;54:561–75.

39. Katz JD, Nishanian P, Mitsuyasu R, et al. Antibody-dependent cellular cytotoxicity (ADCC)-mediated destructon of human immunodeficiency virus (HIV)-coated CD4 + T lymphocytes by acquired immunodeficiency syndrome (AIDS) effector cells. J Clin Immunol. 1988;8:453–8.

40. Re MC, Zauli G, Furlini G, et al. HIV-1 infection and hematologic picture. Microbiologica. 1991;14:165–76.

41. Sun NCJ, Shapshak P, Lachant NA, et al. Bone marrow examination in patients with AIDS and AIDS-related complex (ARC). Am J Clin Pathol. 1989;92:589–94.

42. Stanley SK, Kessler SW, Justement JS, et al. CD34 + bone marrow cells are infected with HIV in a subset of seropositive individuals. J Immunol. 1992;149:689–97.

43. McCune JM, Namikawa R, Kaneshima H, et al. The SCID-hu mouse: Murine model for the analysis of human hematolymphoid differentiation and function. Science. 1988;241:1632–9.

44. Stanley SK, McCune JM, Kaneshima H, et al. Human immunodeficiency virus (HIV) infection of the human thymus and disruption of the thymic microenvironment in the SCID-hu mouse. J Exp Med. 1993;178:1151–63.

45. Bonyhadi ML, Rabin L, Salimi S, et al. HIV induces thymus depletion *in vivo*. Nature. 1993;363:728–32.

46. Aldrovandi GM, Feuer G, Lianying G, et al. The SCID-hu mouse as a model for HIV-1 infection. Nature. 1993;363:732–6.

47. Seemayer TA, Laroche AC, Russo P, et al. Precocious thymic involution manifest by epithelial injury in the acquired immune deficiency syndrome. Hum Pathol. 1984;15:469–74.

48. Pantaleo G, Graziosi C, Demarest JF, et al. HIV infection is active and progressive in lymphoid tissue during the clinically latent stage of disease. Nature. 1993;362:355–8.

49. Pugliese O, Viora M, Camponeschi B, et al. A gp120 HIV peptide with high similarity to HLA class II beta chains enhances PPD-specific and autoreactive T cell activation. Clin Exp Immunol. 1992;90:170–4.

50. Reiher WE, Blalock JE, Brunck TK. Sequence homology between acquired immunodeficiency syndrome virus envelope protein and interleukin 2. Proc Natl Acad Sci USA. 1986;83:9188–92.

51. Boyd JE, James K. B cell responses to HIV and the development of human monoconal antibodies. Clin Exp Immunol. 1992;88:189–202.

52. Ardman B, Mayer K, Bristol J, et al. Surface immunoglobulin-positive T lymphocytes in HIV-1 infection: Relationship to CD4 + lymphocyte depletion. Clin Immunol Immunopathol. 1990;56:249–58.

53. Cohen JJ, Duke RC. Apoptosis and programmed cell death in immunity. Annu Rev Immunol. 1992;10:267–93.

54. Newell MK, Haughn LJ, Maroun CR, et al. Death of mature T cells by separate ligation of CD4 and TCR for antigen. Nature. 1990;347:286–9.

55. Amadori A, De Silvestro G, Zamarchi R, et al. CD4 epitope masking by gp120/anti-gp120 antibody complexes. A potential mechanism for CD4 + cell function down-regulation in AIDS patients. J Immunol. 1992;148:2709–16.

56. Laurent-Crawford AG, Krust B, Muller S, et al. The cytopathic effect of HIV is associated with apoptosis. Virology. 1991;185:829–39.

57. Muller S, Richalet P, Laurent-Crawford A, et al. Autoantibodies typical of non-organ-specific autoimmune diseases in HIV-seropositive patients. AIDS. 1992;6:933–42.

58. Groux H, Torpier G, Monte D, et al. Activation-induced death by apoptosis in CD4 + T cells from human immunodeficiency virus-infected asymptomatic individuals. J Exp Med. 1992;175:331–40.

59. Meyaard L, Otto SA, Jonker RR, et al. Programmed death of T cells in HIV-1 infection. Science. 1992;257:217–9.

60. Gougeon ML, Laurent-Crawford AG, Hovanessian AG, et al. Direct and indirect mechanisms mediating apoptosis during HIV infection: Contribution to *in vivo* CD4 T cell depletion. Semin Immunol. 1993;5:187–94.

61. Soudeyns H, Rebai N, Pantaleo G, et al. The T cell receptor Vβ repertoire in HIV-1 infection and disease. Semin Immunol. 1993;5:175–85.

62. Wilson RK, Lai E, Concannon P, et al. Structure, organization and polymorphism of murine and human T cell receptor α and β gene families. Immunol Rev. 1988;101:149–72.

63. Kappler J, Kotzin B, Herron L, et al. V beta-specific stimulation of human T cells by staphylococcal toxins. Science. 1989;244:811–3.

64. Marrack P, Kushnir E, Kappler J. A maternally inherited superantigen encoded by a mammary tumor virus. Nature. 1991;349:524–6.

65. Hugin AW, Vacchio MS, Morse HC 3d. A virus-encoded superantigen: In a retrovirus-induced immunodeficiency syndrome of mice. Science. 1991;252:424–7.

66. Janeway C. MIs: Makes a little sense. Nature. 1991;349:459–61.

67. Imberti L, Sottini A, Bettinardi A, et al. Selective depletion in HIV infection of T cells that bear specific T cell receptor V beta sequences. Science. 1991;254:860–2.

67a.Rebai N, Pantaleo G, Demarest JF, et al. Analysis of the T-cell receptor beta-chain variable-region (Vbeta) repertoire in monozygotic twins discordant for human immunodeficiency virus: Evidence for perturbations of specific Vbeta segments in CD4+ T cells of the virus-positive twins. Proc Natl Acad Sci USA. 1994;91:1529–35.

68. Laurence J, Hodtsev AS, Posnett DN. Superantigen implicated in dependence of HIV-1 replication in T cells on TCR VB expression. Nature. 1992;358:255–9.

69. Fauci AS. AIDS: Immunopathogenic mechanisms and research strategies. Clin Res. 1987;35:503–10.

70. Meyaard L, Schuitemaker H, Miedema F. T-cell dysfunction in HIV infection: Anergy due to defective antigen-presenting cell function? Immunol Today. 1993;14:161–4.

71. Clerici M, Stocks NI, Zajac RA, et al. Detection of three distinct patterns of T helper cell dysfunction in asymptomatic, human immunodeficiency virus-seropositive patients. Independence of CD4 + cell numbers and clinical staging. J Clin Invest. 1989;84:1892–99.

72. Kawamura I, Koga Y, Oh-Hori N, et al. Depletion of the surface CD4 molecule by the envelope protein of human immunodeficiency virus expressed in a human CD4 + monocytoid cell line. J Virol. 1989;63:3748–54.

73. Schnittman SM, Lane HC, Greenhouse J, et al. Preferential infection of CD4+ memory T cells in human immunodeficiency virus type 1: Evidence for a role in the selective T-cell functional defects observed in infected individuals. Proc Natl Acad Sci USA. 1990;87:6058–62.

74. Corado J, Mazerolles F, Le Deist F, et al. Inhibition of CD4 + T cell activation and adhesion by peptides derived from the gp160. J Immunol. 1991;147:475–82.

75. Viscidi RP, Mayur K, Lederman HM, et al. Inhibition of antigen-induced lymphocyte proliferation by Tat protein from HIV-1. Science. 1989;246:1606–8.

76. Rosenstein Y, Burakoff SJ, Herrmann SH. HIV-gp120 can block CD4-class II MHC-mediated adhesion. J Immunol. 1990;144:526–31.

77. Hivroz C, Mazerolles F, Soula M, et al. Human immunodeficiency virus gp120 and derived peptides activate protein tyrosine kinase p56[lck] in human CD4 T lymphocytes. Eur J Immunol. 1993;23:600–7.

78. Sher A, Gazzinelli RT, Oswald IP, et al. Role of T-cell derived cytokines in the downregulation of immune responses in parasitic and retroviral infection. Immunol Rev. 1992;127:183–204.

79. Maggi E, Parronchi P, Manetti R, et al. Reciprocal regulatory effects of IFN-γ and IL-4 on the *in vitro* development of human Th1 and Th2 clones. J Immunol. 1992;148:2142–7.

80. Clerici M, Shearer GM. A T$_{H}$1 T$_{H}$2 switch is a critical step in the etiology of HIV infection. Immunol Today. 1993;14:107–11.

81. Cooper DA, Tindall B, Wilson EJ, et al. Characterization of T lymphocyte responses during primary infection with human immunodeficiency virus. J Infect Dis. 1988;157:889–96.

82. Stanley SK, Fauci AS. T cell homeostasis in HIV infection: Part of the solution, or part of the problem? J Acquir Immune Defic Syndr. 1993;6:142–3.

83. Lane HC, Masur H, Gelmann EP, et al. Correlation between immunologic function and clinical subpopulations of patients with the acquired immune deficiency syndrome. Am J Med. 1985;78:417–22.

84. Shearer GM, Salahuddin SZ, Markham PD, et al. Prospective study of cytotoxic T lymphocyte responses to influenza and antibodies to human T lymphotropic virus-III in homosexual men. J Clin Invest. 1985;76:1699–1704.

85. Rook AH, Manischewitz JF, Frederick WR, et al. Deficient, HLA-restricted, cytomegalovirus-specific cytotoxic T cells and natural killer cells in patients

with the acquired immunodeficiency syndrome. J Infect Dis. 1985;152: 627–30.

86. Pantaleo G, Koenig S, Baseler M, et al. Defective clonogenic potential of CD8+ T lymphocytes in patients with AIDS. Expansion *in vivo* of a nonclonogenic CD3+CD8+ DR+CD25- T cell population. J Immunol. 1990;144: 1696–1704.

87. Meltzer MS, Skillman DR, Hoover DL, et al. Macrophages and the human immunodeficiency virus. Immunol Today. 1990;11:247.

88. Weinberg JB, Matthews TJ, Cullen BR, et al. Productive human immunodeficiency virus type 1 (HIV-1) infection of nonproliferating human monocytes. J Exp Med. 1991;174:1477–82.

89. Poli G, Gauci AS. The role of monocyte/marcrophages and cytokines in the pathogenesis of HIV infection. Pathobiology. 1992;60:246–51.

90. Wahl SM, Allen JB, Gartner S, et al. HIV-1 and its envelope glycoprotein down-regulate chemotactic ligand receptors and chemotactic function of peripheral blood monocytes. J Immunol. 1989;142:3553–9.

91. Baldwin GC, Fleischmann J, Chung Y, et al. Human immunodeficiency virus causes mononuclear phagocyte dysfunction. Proc Natl Acad Sci USA. 190; 87:3933–7.

92. Gendelman HE, Friedman RM, Joe S, et al. A selective defect of interferon alpha production in human immunodeficiency virus-infected monocytes. J Exp Med. 1990;172:1433–42.

93. Harrell RA, Cianciolo GJ, Copeland TD, et al. Supression of the respiratory burst of human monocytes by a synthetic peptide homologous to envelope proteins of human and animal retroviruses. J Immunol. 1986;136:3517–20.

94. Poli G, Bottazzi B, Acero R, et al. Monocyte function in intravenous drug abusers with lymphadenopathy syndrome and in patients with acquired immunodeficiency syndrome: Selective impairment of chemotaxis. Clin Exp Immuno. 1985;62:136–42.

95. Washburn RG, Tuazon CU, Bennett JE. Phagocytic and fungicidal activity of monocytes from patients with acquired immunodeficiency syndrome. J Infect Dis. 1985;151:565.

96. Enk C, Gerstoft J, Moller S, et al. Interleukin 1 activity in the acquired immunodeficiency syndrome. Scand J Immunol. 1986;23:491–7.

97. Chehimi J, Trinchieri G, Frank I, et al. IL-12 deficiency in HIV-infected patients (Abstract). In: IX International Conference on AIDS. Berlin, Germany; 1993:WS-A08-4.

98. Price RW, Brew BJ. The AIDS dementia complex. J Infect Dis. 1988;158: 1079.

99. Tardieu M, Hery C, Peudenier S. Neurotoxicity of macrophages infected by HIV-1. Cell Biol Toxicol. 1992;8:117–21.

100. Koenig S, Gendelman HE, Orenstein JM, et al. Detection of AIDS virus in macrophages in brain tissue from AIDS patients with encephalopathy. Science. 1986;233:1089–193.

101. Chiodi F, Fuerstenberg S, Gidlund M, et al. Infection of brain-derived cells with the human immunodeficiency virus. J Virol. 1987;93:1244–7.

102. Lee MR, Ho DD, Gurney ME. Functional interaction and partial homology between human immunodeficiency virus and neuroleukin. Science. 1987;237: 1047–51.

103. Lane HC, Masur H, Edgar LC, et al. Abnormalities of B-cell activation and immunoregulation in patients with the aquired immunodeficiency syndrome. N Engl J Med. 1983;309:453–8.

104. Shirai A, Cosentino M, Leitman-Klinman SF, et al. Human immunodeficiency virus infection induces both polyclonal and virus-specific B cell activation. J Clin Invest. 1992;89:561–6.

105. Terpstra FG, Al BJ, Roos MT, et al. Longitudinal study of leukocyte functions in homosexual men for HIV: Rapid and persistent loss of B cell function after HIV infection. Eur J Immunol. 1989;19:667–73.

106. Ammann AJ, Schiffman G, Abrams D, et al. B-cell immunodeficiency in acquired immune deficiency syndrome. JAMA. 1984;251:1447–9.

107. Reddy MM, Goetz RR, Gorman JM, et al. Human immunodeficiency virus type-1 infection of homosexual men is accompanied by a decrease in circulating B cells. J Acquir Immune Defic Syndr. 1991;4:428–34.

108. Schnittman SM, Lane HC, Higgins SE, et al. Direct polyclonal activation of human B lymphocyts by the acquired immune deficiency syndrome virus. Science. 1986;233:1084–6.

109. Chirmule N, Kalyanaraman VS, Saxinger C, et al. Localization of B-cell stimulatory activity of HIV-1 to the carboxyl terminus of gp41. AIDS Res Hum Retrovirus. 1990;6:299–305.

110. Pahwa S, Pahwa R, Good RA, et al. Stimulatory and inhibitory influences of human immunodeficiency virus on normal B lymphocytes. Proc Natl Acad Sci USA. 1986;83:9124–8.

111. Pelicci PG, Knowles DM, Arlin ZA, et al. Multiple monoclonal B-cell expansions and c-myc oncogene rearrangements in AIDS-related lymphoproliferative disorders: Implications by lymphomagenesis. J Exp Med. 1986;164: 2049–60.

112. Yarchoan R, Redfield RR, Broder S. Mechanisms of B cell activation in patients with acquired immunodeficiency syndrome and related disorders. J Clin Invest. 1985;78:439–47.

113. Rieckmann P, Poli G, Fox CH, et al. Recombinant gp120 specifically enhances tumor necrosis factor-alpha production and Ig secretion in B lymphocytes from HIV-infected individuals but not from seronegative donors. J Immunol. 1991;147:2922–7.

114. Boue F, Wallon C, Goujard C, et al. HIV induces IL-6 production by human B lymphocytes. Role of IL-4. J Immunol. 1992;148:3761–7.

115. Rieckmann P, Poli G, Kehrl JH, et al. Activated B lymphocytes from human

immunodeficiency virus-infected individuals induce virus expression in infected T cells and a promonocytic cell line, U1. J Exp Med. 1991;173:1–5.

116. Borst J, van de Griend RJ, van Oostveen JW, et al. A T-cell receptor γ/CD3 complex found on cloned functional lymphocytes. Nature. 1987;325:683–8.

117. Mansour I, Doinel C, Rouger P. CD16+ NK cells decrease in all stages of HIV infection through a selective depletion of the CD16+CD8+CD3-subset. AIDS Res Hum Retroviruses. 1990;6:1451–7.

118. Katz JD, Mitsuyasu R, Gottlieb MS, et al. Mechanism of defective NK cell activity in patients with acquired immunodeficiency syndrome (AIDS) and AIDS-related complex. II. Normal antibody-dependent cellular cytotoxicity (ADCC) mediated by effector cells defective in natural killer (NK) cytotoxicity. J Immunol. 1987;139:55–60.

119. Reddy MM, Chinoy P, Grieco MH. Differential effects of interferon-alpha 2 and interleukin-2 on natural killer cell activity in patients with acquired immune deficiency syndrome. J Biol Response Modif. 1984;3:379–86.

120. Cauda R, Tumbarello M, Ortona L, et al. Inhibition of normal human natural killer cell activity by human immunodeficiency virus synthetic transmembrane peptides. Cell Immunol. 1988;115:57–65.

121. Chehimi J, Starr SE, Frank I, et al. Natural killer (NK) cell stimulatory factor increases the cytotoxic activity of NK cells from both healthy donors and human immunodeficiency virus-infected patients. J Exp Med. 1992;175: 789–96.

122. Steinman RM. The dendritic cell system and its role in immunogenicity. Annu Rev Immunol. 1991;9:271–96.

123. Patterson S, Gross J, Bedford P, et al. Morphology and phenotype of dendritic cells from peripheral blood and their productive and non-productive infection with human immunodeficiency virus type 1. Immunology. 1991;72: 361–7.

124. Cameron PU, Forsum U, Teppler H, et al. During HIV-1 infection most blood dendritic cells are not productively infected and can induce allogeneic CD4+ T cells clonal expansion. Clin Exp Immunol. 1992;88:226–36.

125. Michael NL, Vahey M, Burke DS, et al. Viral DNA and mRNA expression correlate with the stage of human immunodeficiency virus (HIV) type 1 infection in humans: Evidence for viral replication in all stages of HIV disease. J Virol. 1992;66:310–6.

126. Poli G, Fauci AS. Cytokine modulation of HIV expression. Semin Immunol. 1993;5:165–73.

127. Folks TM, Clouse KA, Justement J, et al. Tumor necrosis factor-alpha induces the expression of the human immunodeficiency virus from a chronically infected T cell clone. Proc Natl Acad Sci USA. 1989;86:2365–8.

128. Mellors JW, Griffith BP, Ortiz MA, et al. Tumor necrosis factor-alpha/ cachectin enhances human immunodeficiency virus type 1 replication in primary macrophages. J Infect Dis. 1991;163:78–82.

129. Poli G, Kinter A, Justement JS, et al. Tumor necrosis factor alpha functions in an autocrine manner in the induction of human immunodeficiency virus expression. Proc Natl Acad Sci USA. 1990;87:782–5.

130. Duh EJ, Maury WJ, Folks TM, et al. Tumor necrosis factor-alpha activates human immunodeficiency virus-1 through induction of nuclear factor binding to the NF-kB sites in the long terminal repeat. Proc Natl Acad Sci USA. 1989;86:5974–8.

131. Poli G, Bressler P, Kinter A, et al. Interleukin 6 induces human immunodeficiency virus expression in monocytic cells alone and in synergy with tumor necrosis factor alpha by transcriptional and post-transcriptional mechanisms. J Exp Med. 1990;172:151–8.

132. Nakajima K, Martinez-Maza O, Hirano T, et al. Induction of IL-6 (B cell stimulatory factor-2/IFN-beta 2) production by HIV. J Immunol. 1989;142: 531–6.

133. Roux-Lombard P, Modoux C, Cruchaud A, et al. Purified blood monocytes from HIV-1 infected patients produce high levels of TNF-α and IL-1. Clin Immunol Immunopathol. 1989;50:374–84.

134. D'Addario M, Roulston A, Wainberg MA, et al. Coordinate enhancement of cytokine gene expression in human immunodeficiency virus type 1-infected promonocytic cells. J Virol. 1990;64:6080–9.

135. Clouse KA, Robbins PB, Fernie B, et al. Viral antigen stimulation of the production of human monokines capable of regulating HIV-1 expressions. J Immunol. 1989;143:470–5.

136. Merrill JE, Koyanagi Y, Chen ISY. Interleukin-1 and tumor necrosis factor α can be induced from mononuclear phagocytes by human immunodeficiency virus type 1 binding to the CD4 receptor. J Virol. 1989;63:4404–8.

137. Cayota A, Vuillier F, Scott-Algara D, et al. Impaired proliferative capacity and abnormal cytokine profile of naive and memory CD4 T cells from HIV-seropositive patients. Clin Exp Immunol. 1992;88:478–83.

138. Lahdevirta J, Maury CP, Teppo AM, et al. Elevated levels of circulating cachectin/tumor necrosis factor in patients with acquired immunodeficiency syndrome. Am J Med. 1988;85:289–91.

139. Breen EC, Rezai AR, Nakajima K, et al. Infection with HIV is associated with elevated IL-6 levels and production. J Immunol. 1990;144:480–4.

140. Wright SC, Jewett A, Mitsuyasu R, et al. Spontaneous cytotoxicity and tumor necrosis factor production by peripheral blood monocytes from AIDS patients. J Immunol. 1988;141:99–104.

141. Millar AB, Miller RF, Foley NM, et al. Production of tumor necrosis factor-alpha by blood and lung mononuclear phagocytes from patients with human immunodeficiency virus-related lung disease. Am J Respir Cell Mol Biol. 1991;5:144–8.

142. Ho DD, Hartshorn KL, Rota TR, et al. Recombinant human interferon alpha-A suppresses HTLV-III replication *in vitro*. Lancet. 1985;1:602–4.

143. Williams GJ, Colby CB. Recombinant human interferon-beta suppresses the

replication of HIV and acts synergistically with AZT. J Interferon Res. 1989; 9:709–18.

144. Poli G, Kinter AL, Justement JS, et al. Transforming growth factor β suppresses human immunodeficiency virus expression and replication in infected cells of the monocyte/macrophage lineage. J Exp Med. 1991;173:589–97.

145. Lazdins JK, Klimkait T, Woods-Cook K, et al. In vitro effect of transforming growth factor-β on progression of HIV-1 infection in primary mononuclear phagocytes. J Immunol. 1991;147:1201–7.

146. Wahl SM, Allen JB, McCartney-Francis N, et al. Macrophage- and astrocyte-derived transforming growth factor beta as a mediator of central nervous system dysfunction in acquired immune deficiency syndrome. J Exp Med. 1991;173:981–91.

147. Hartshorn KL, Neumeyer D, Vogt MW, et al. Activity of interferons alpha, beta, and gamma against human immunodeficiency virus replication in vitro. AIDS Res Hum Retroviruses. 1987;3:125–33.

148. Koyanagi Y, O'Brien WA, Zhao JQ, et al. Cytokines alter production of HIV-1 from primary mononuclear phagocytes. Science. 1988;241:1673–5.

149. Biswas P, Poli G, Kinter AL, et al. Interferon-γ modulates the expression of human immunodeficiency virus in persistently infected promonocytic cells by redirecting the production of virions to intracytoplasmic vacuoles. J Exp Med. 1992;176:739–50.

150. Hawkins RE, Rickman LS, Vermund SH, et al. Association of mycoplasma and human immunodeficiency virus infection: Detection of amplified Mycoplasma fermentans DNA in blood. J Infect Dis. 1992;165:581–5.

151. Lemaitre M, Henin Y, Destouesse F, et al. Role of mycoplasma infection in the cytopathic effect induced by human immunodeficiency virus type 1 in infected cell lines. Infect Immun. 1992;60:742–8.

152. Miller-Catchpole R, Shattuck M, Kandalaft P, et al. The incidence and distribution of Mycoplasma fermenans (incognitus strain) in the Chicago AIDS autopsy series: An immunohistochemical study. Chicago Associated Pathologists. Mod Pathol. 1991;4:481–6.

153. Page JB, Lai SH, Chitwood DD, et al. HTLV-I/II seropositivity and death from AIDS among HIV-1 seropositive intravenous drug users. Lancet. 1990; 335:1439–41.

154. Okamoto T, Akagi T, Shima H, et al. Superinduction of trans-activation accounts for augmented human immunodeficiency virus replication in HTLV-I-transformed cells. Jpn J Cancer Res. 1987;78:1297.

155. Buchbinder A, Josephs SF, Ablashi D, et al. Polymerase chain reaction amplification and in situ hybridization for the detection of human B-lymphotropic virus. J Virol Methods. 1988;21:191–7.

156. Lusso P, Ensoli B, Markham PD, et al. Productive dual infection of human CD4+ T lymphocytes by HIV-1 and HHV-6. Nature. 1989;337:370–3.

157. Geng YQ, Chandran B, Josephs SF, et al. Identification and characterization of a human herpesvirus 6 gene segment that trans activates the human immunodeficiency virus type 1 promoter. J Virol. 1992;66:1564–70.

158. Seto E, Yen TS, Peterlin BM, et al. Trans-activation of the human immunodeficiency virus long terminal repeat by the hepatitis B virus X protein. Proc Natl Acad Sci USA. 1988;85:8286–90.

159. Tenner-Racz K, Racz P, Bofill M, et al. HTLV-III/LAV viral antigens in lymph nodes of homosexual men with persistent generalized lymphadenopathy and AIDS. Am J Pathol. 1986;123:9–15.

160. Biberfeld P, Ost A, Porwit A, et al. Histopathology and immunohistology of HTLV-III/LAV related lymphadenopathy and AIDS. Acta Pathol Microbiol Immunol Scand A. 1987;95:47–65.

161. Pantaleo G, Graziosi C, Butini L, et al. Lymphoid organs function as major reservoirs for human immunodeficiency virus. Proc Natl Acad Sci USA. 1991;88:9838–42.

162. Wood GS. The immunohistology of lymph nodes in HIV infection: A review. In: Rotterdam H, Racz P, Greco MA, et al., eds. Progress in AIDS Pathology. v. 2. New York: Field & Wood; 1991:25–32.

163. Tew JG, Kosco MH, Burton GF, et al. Follicular dendritic cells as accessory cells. Immunol Rev. 1990;117:185–211.

164. Tenner-Racz K, Racz P, Dietrich M, et al. Altered follicular dendritic cells and virus-like particles in AIDS and AIDS-related lymphadenopathy. Lancet. 1985;1:105–6.

165. Clerici M, Giorgi JV, Chou CC, et al. Cell-mediated immune response to human immunodeficiency virus (HIV) type 1 in seronegative homosexual men with recent sexual exposure to HIV-1. J Infect Dis. 1992;165:1012–9.

166. Gaines H, Sonnerbog A, Czajkowski J, et al. Antibody response in primary human immunodeficiency virus infection. Lancet. 1987;1:1249–53.

167. Albert J, Abrahamsson B, Nagy K, et al. Rapid development of isolate-specific neutralizing antibodies after primary HIV-1 infection and consequent emergence of virus variants which resist neutralization by autologous sera. AIDS. 1990;4:107–12.

168. Robert-Guroff M, Brown M, Gallo RC. HTLV-III-neutralizing antibodies in patients with AIDS and AIDS-related complex. Nature. 1985;316:72–4.

169. Javaherian K, Langlois AJ, McDanal C, et al. Principal neutralizing domain of the human immunodeficiency virus type 1 envelope protein. Proc Natl Acad Sci USA. 1989;86:6768–72.

170. Javaherian K, Langlois AJ, LaRosa GJ, et al. Broadly neutralizing antibodies elicited by the hypervariable neutralizing determinant of HIV-1. Science. 1990;250:1590–3.

171. Weiss RA, Clapham PR, Cheingsong-Popov R, et al. Neutralization of human T-lymphotropic virus type III by sera of AIDS and AIDS-risk patients. Nature. 1985;316:69–72.

172. Weinhold KJ. Anti-HIV-1 ADCC: Clinical and therapeutic implications. Biotechnol Ther. 1991;2:147–57.

173. Brenner BG, Gryllis C, Wainberg MA. Role of antibody-dependent cellular cytotoxicity and lymphokine-activated killer cells in AIDS and related diseases. J Leukocyte Biol. 1991;50:628–40.

174. Jewett A, Giorgi JV, Bonavida B. Antibody-dependent cellular cytotoxicity against HIV-coated target cells by peripheral blood monocytes from HIV seropositive asymptomatic patients. J Immunol. 1990;145:4065–71.

175. Ojo-Amaize E, Nishanian PG, Heitjan DF, et al. Serum and effector-cell antibody-dependent cellular cytotoxicity (ADCC) activity remains high during human immunodeficiency virus (HIV) disease progression. J Clin Immunol. 1989;9:454–61.

176. Tyler DS, Stanley SD, Nastala CA, et al. Alterations in antibody-dependent cellular cytotoxicity during the course of HIV-1 infection. Humoral and cellular defects. J Immunol. 199;144:3375–84.

177. Plata F. Implications of HIV-specific cytotoxic T lymphocytes in AIDS. Biotherapy. 1992;5:31–45.

178. Takahashi H, Germain RN, Moss B, et al. An immunodominant class I-restricted cytotoxic T lymphocyte determinant of human immunodeficiency virus type 1 induces CD4 class II-restricted help for itself. J Exp Med. 1990; 171:571–6.

179. Hammond SA, Obah E, Stanhope P, et al. Characterization of a conserved T cell epitope in HIV-1 gp41 recognized by vaccine-induced human cytolytic T cells. J Immunol. 1991;146:1470–7.

180. Hom RC, Finberg RW, Mullaney S, et al. Protective cellular retroviral immunity requires both CD4+ and CD8+ immune T cells. J Virol. 1991;65:220–4.

181. Takahashi H, Merli S, Putney SD, et al. A single amino acid interchange yields reciprocal CTL specificities for HIV-1 gp160. Science. 1989;246: 118–21.

182. Phillips RE, Rowland-Jones S, Nixon DF, et al. Human immunodeficiency virus genetic variation that can escape cytotoxic T cell recognition. Nature. 1991;354:453–9.

183. Herberman RB. Adoptive therapy with purified CD8 cells in HIV infection. Semin Hematol. 1992;29:35–40.

184. Walker CM, Moody DJ, Stites DP, et al. CD8+ lymphocytes can control HIV infection in vitro by suppressing virus replication. Science. 1986;234: 1563–6.

185. Walker CM, Levy JA. A diffusible lymphokine produced by CD8+ T lymphocytes suppresses HIV replication. Immunology. 1989;66:628–30.

186. Brinchmann JE, Gaudernack G, Vartdal F. In vitro replication of HIV-1 in naturally infected CD4+ T cells is inhibited by rIFN alpha 2 and by a soluble factor secreted by activated CD8+ T cells, but not by rIFN beta, rIFN gamma, or recombinant tumor necrosis factor-alpha. J Acquir Immune Defic Syndr. 1991;4:480–8.

187. Mackewicz CE, Ortega HW, Levy JA. CD8+ cell anti-HIV activity correlates with the clinical state of the infected individual. J Clin Invest. 1991;87: 1462–6.

188. Tsubota H, Lord CI, Watkins DI, et al. A cytotoxic T lymphocyte inhibits acquired immunodeficiency syndrome virus replication in peripheral blood lymphocytes. J Exp Med. 1989;169:1421–34.

189. Walker CM, Erickson AL, Hsueh FC, et al. Inhibition of human immunodeficiency virus replication in acutely infected CD4+ cells by CD8+ cells involves a noncytotoxic mechanism. J Virol. 1991;65:5921–7.

102. CLINICAL MANIFESTATIONS OF HIV INFECTION

RICHARD E. CHAISSON
PAUL A. VOLBERDING

Infection with the human immunodeficiency virus (HIV) results in a wide range of clinical consequences from asymptomatic carriage to life-threatening opportunistic infections and malignancies. The disease state called acquired immunodeficiency syndrome (AIDS) is at the advanced stage of this axis when the infected host can no longer control opportunistic organisms or malignancies that rarely cause illness in immunocompetent individuals. In persons infected with HIV, the sequential decline and ablation of cell-mediated immunity result in diverse manifestations of opportunistic disease. Those manifestations may vary according to the individual's age, sex, race, geographic location, treatment status, and behavioral history. This chapter reviews the clinical features of HIV infection from the acquisition of the virus to death with AIDS and discusses the classification and evaluation of HIV-related syndromes.

HISTORY

Disease caused by HIV-induced immunosuppression was first described in late 1980 and early 1981 when physicians in Los Angeles, New York, and San Francisco observed opportunistic infections in homosexual men.[1-4] Simultaneously, an outbreak of Kaposi sarcoma (KS), a previously rare malignancy, was reported in young homosexual men from the same three cities.[5,6] These patients had a selective defect in cell-mediated immunity that was manifested by low numbers of CD4 + T lymphocytes and the development of opportunistic infections.

That opportunistic diseases occurred in homosexual men who had been healthy previously suggested that immunodeficiency developed because of an acquired rather than a congenital trait. In 1982, the Centers for Disease Control and Prevention (CDC) developed a case definition, based on the clinical, immunologic, and epidemiologic features of the first clusters of cases, for what was called the acquired immunodeficiency syndrome (AIDS).[7] AIDS was defined as the occurrence of a reliably diagnosed disease at least moderately indicative of underlying cellular immunodeficiency in a person without a condition known to be associated with an increased incidence of diseases related to cellular immunodeficiency.[6,8] AIDS became a reportable condition in 1983. Soon after the initial case reports of AIDS, additional cases were observed in persons other than homosexual men. In 1981 and 1982, heterosexual intravenous drug users and immigrants from Haiti were reported to have AIDS.[2,9-12] AIDS cases in hemophiliacs, recipients of blood transfusions, and Africans were also soon reported.[13,14]

While the groups of persons at risk for AIDS expanded, clinicians noted an increasing spectrum of clinical manifestations of

TABLE 1. CDC Surveillance Case Definition for AIDS—1987

Diseases diagnosed definitively without confirmation of HIV infection in patients without other causes of immunodeficiency
  Candidiasis of the esophagus, trachea, bronchi, or lungs
  Cryptococcosis, extrapulmonary
  Cryptosporidiosis >1 month duration
  Cytomegalovirus (CMV) infection of any organ except the liver, spleen, or lymph nodes in patients >1 month old
  Herpes simplex infection, mucocutaneous (>1 month duration) or of the bronchi, lungs, or esophagus in patients? 1 month duration
  Kaposi sarcoma in patients <60 yr old
  Primary central nervous system (CNS) lymphoma in patients <60 yr old
  Lymphoid interstitial pneumonitis (LIP) and/or pulmonary lymphoid hyperplasia (PLH) in patients <13 yr old
  Mycobacterium avium complex or *M. kansasii* disseminated
  Pneumocystis carinii pneumonia
  Progressive multifocal leukoencephalopathy
  Toxoplasmosis of the brain in patients >1 month old
Diseases diagnosed definitively with confirmation of HIV infection
  Multiple or recurrent pyogenic bacterial infections in patients <13 yr old
  Coccidioidomycosis, disseminated
  Histoplasmosis, disseminated
  Isosporiasis >1 month duration
  Kaposi sarcoma, any age
  Primary CNS lymphoma, any age
  Non-Hodgkin's lymphoma (small, noncleaved lymphoma; Burkitt or non-Burkitt type; or immunoblastic sarcoma)
  Mycobacterial disease other than *M. tuberculosis*, disseminated
  M. tuberculosis, extrapulmonary
  Salmonella septicemia, recurrent
Diseases diagnosed presumptively with confirmation of HIV infection
  Candidiasis of the esophagus
  CMV retinitis
  Kaposi sarcoma
  LIP/PLH in patients <13 yr old
  Disseminated mycobacterial disease (not cultured)
  Pneumocystis carinii pneumonia
  Toxoplasmosis of the brain in patients >1 month old
  HIV encephalopathy
  HIV wasting syndrome

(From Centers for Disease Control and Prevention.[28])

TABLE 2. World Health Organization Adult Case Definition for AIDS

Major signs[a]
  >10% weight loss
  Diarrhea >1 month duration
  Fever >1 month duration
Minor signs[a]
  Cough >1 month duration
  General pruritic dermatitis
  Recurrent herpes zoster
  Oropharyngeal candidiasis
  Progressive, disseminated herpes simplex
  Generalized lymphadenopathy
Diagnostic of AIDS
  Cryptococcal meningitis
  Disseminated Kaposi sarcoma

[a] The presence of at least two major signs and one minor sign is diagnostic of AIDS.

(From World Health Organization,[30] with permission.)

TABLE 3. 1993 CDC AIDS Surveillance Case Definition and Staging System[a]

CD4 Categories		Clinical Categories		
CD4 Number	CD4 Percent	Asymptomatic or Acute HIV, PGL	Symptomatic, Not A or C	AIDS-Indicator Conditions
>499	>29	A1	B1	C1
200–499	14–28	A2	B2	C2
<200	<14	A3	B3	C3

Abbreviation: PGL, persistent generalized lymphadenopathy.
[a] AIDS-indicator conditions in 1987 are listed in Table 1. New AIDS-indicator conditions are pulmonary tuberculosis, recurrent bacterial pneumonia, and invasive cervical cancer.

(From Centers for Disease Control and Prevention.[31])

AIDS-associated immunodeficiency. Unexplained generalized lymphadenopathy, idiopathic thrombocytopenia, oral candidiasis, herpes zoster, and a constitutional wasting syndrome were observed in persons from AIDS risk groups who had deficits in cellular immunity.[15-19] The term *AIDS-related complex* (ARC) was coined to describe the symptoms of immunodeficiency recognized with increasing frequency in persons at risk for AIDS.[20] In 1982–1983, several investigators postulated an asymptomatic carrier state of the AIDS agent in healthy homosexual men, heterosexual partners of IV drug users, and Haitians who were noted to have laboratory evidence of impaired cellular immunity.[21] After HIV was first described in 1983–1984,[22-24] serologic tests to identify persons infected with HIV were developed that allowed large serologic surveys of risk group members to estimate the number of individuals infected with the virus and to delineate the spectrum of HIV-associated diseases.

Retrospective studies of serum and tissue indicate that the virus was present in Africa in the mid-1960s and that disease associated with HIV occurred in England in 1959 and the United States in 1968.[25-27] The CDC expanded its case definition of AIDS in 1985 and again in 1987 (Table 1) to accommodate the increased number of manifestations of impaired cellular immunity that had become associated with chronic HIV infection.[28,29] The World Health Organization also promulgated a case definition for AIDS for use in developing countries that lacked sophisticated diagnostic resources (Table 2).[30] The AIDS case definition was revised again in 1993 to include individuals with advanced immunodeficiency and with several other clinical manifestations of HIV disease (Table 3).[31]

CLASSIFICATION OF HIV DISEASE

HIV infection causes a variety of specific and nonspecific defects in immune function that result in diverse clinical consequences. Because HIV infection represents an underlying progressive immunodeficiency disease process that is likely to result in serious immunologic and clinical consequences, HIV infection should be considered a disease state. Individuals who are HIV infected but asymptomatic may not be ill, but do have

TABLE 4. Walter Reed Staging System for HIV Disease

Stage	HIV (Antibody/Antigen)	Lymphadenopathy	CD4 + Lymphocytes/mm³	Skin Tests	Thrush	Opportunistic Infection
WR 0	−	−	>400	NL	−	−
WR 1	+	−	>400	NL	−	−
WR 2	+	+	>400	NL	−	−
WR 3	+	±	<400	NL	−	−
WR 4	+	±	<400	Partial anergy	−	−
WR 5	+	±	<400	Complete anergy	+	−
WR 6	+	±	<400	Complete anergy	+	+

Abbreviations: NL, normal.

(From Redfield et al.,[33] with permission.)

a chronic and progressive condition that may result ultimately in significant impairment or death.

Several systems to classify HIV infection and disease have been proposed. The 1986 CDC classification system placed HIV-infected persons into four categories: group I, acute infection; group II, asymptomatic seropositive; group III, persistent generalized lymphadenopathy; and group IV, symptomatic HIV disease.[32] This system had limited prognostic utility and has been supplanted by the 1993 classification system and revised AIDS case definition (Table 3). The 1993 CDC classification system for HIV categorizes HIV-infected individuals according to clinical and CD4 cell level groupings. The clinical categories are group A, asymptomatic, acute HIV infection or persistent generalized lymphadenopathy (PGL); group B, symptomatic HIV disease; and group C, AIDS-indicator illnesses, encompassed by the 1987 case definition and including recurrent bacterial pneumonia, pulmonary tuberculosis, and invasive cervical cancer. The CD4 cell level categories are *(1)* 500/mm³ or greater, *(2)* 200–499/mm³, and *(3)* less than 200/mm³. CD4 cell percentages may be used in place of CD4 cell number, as indicated in Table 3. As noted above, patients in all three clinical categories whose CD4 cell count in less than 200/mm³ or less than 14 percent are now counted as AIDS cases by the CDC surveillance definition.

The 1993 CDC classification system for HIV infection recognizes the prognostic significance of CD4 cell counts in individuals with HIV infection and also is consistent with clinical standards regarding the institution of antiretroviral therapy and prophylaxis against *Pneumocystis carinii* pneumonia. The CD4 categories in the 1993 classification system separate patients into categories with distinctly different probabilities of developing opportunistic illnesses. Thus, this system classifies patients both by their current clinical status and their likelihood of subsequently developing opportunistic complications of advanced HIV disease.

The Walter Reed (WR) staging system for HIV infection (Table 4) classifies patients on the basis of CD4 lymphocyte counts, delayed type hypersensitivity (DTH), and the presence of lymphadenopathy, oral candidiasis, and opportunistic infections.[33] The stages of the WR system are hierarchical, and they roughly parallel the natural history of HIV in infected individuals. However, the CD4 level separating WR stages 1 and 2 from WR stages 3–5, 400/mm³, does not correspond with therapeutic guidelines and is less prognostically precise than the CD4 levels used in the CDC system. The WR system also requires that skin tests be performed routinely—a practice that is often clinically cumbersome and impractical in managing large numbers of patients. As many as 14–70 percent of HIV-seropositive individuals cannot be placed into WR stages because they have greater than 400/mm³ CD4 + cells but are anergic.[34,35] When use of DTH testing is restricted to patients with less than 400/mm³ CD4 cells, the WR system is predictive of disease progression. A recent study also shows that DTH responsiveness is independently associated with disease progression.[35]

Many clinicians classify HIV disease by a more detailed CD4 cell level schema than those used in the CDC or WR systems

TABLE 5. Clinical Stages of HIV Infection

CD4 Cell Count	Stage	Comment
>500	Early	Risk of disease low. Response to routine immunizations and PPD skin testing reliable.
200–500	Middle	Risk of minor signs and symptoms high; risk of opportunistic disease moderate. May benefit from antiretroviral therapy.
50–200	Late	Risk of opportunistic disease high. Benefit from *Pneumocystis* prophylaxis and antiretroviral therapy.
<50	Advanced	Risk of opportunistic disease and death high. Benefit from *Pneumocystis*, *Mycobacterium avium* complex, and fungal prophylaxis. May benefit from antiretroviral therapy.

TABLE 6. Staging of Pediatric HIV Exposure and Infection

Category	
P-0	Infection status indeterminate. Anti-HIV IgG seropositive and <15 months old.
P-1	Confirmed infection, asymptomatic. Anti-HIV IgG seropositive and >15 months old, or HIV antigen positive, culture positive, or polymerase chain reaction positive and <15 months old.
P-2	Symptomatic HIV disease.

(From Centers for Disease Control and Prevention.[36])

(Table 5). This system focuses more on patients with advanced HIV disease than the CDC and WR system. In particular, this approach includes a category of patients (CD4 count <50/mm³) who are at very high risk of death.[35a]

CLASSIFICATION OF PEDIATRIC HIV INFECTION

The diagnosis of perinatally transmitted HIV infection in young children is difficult because of the presence of passive maternal IgG antibodies, and the clinical manifestations of pediatric HIV disease may differ greatly from adult disease. Consequently, a separate system for the classification of pediatric HIV infection has been developed (Table 6.)[36] Children younger than 15 months born to HIV-infected mothers who are anti-HIV IgG seropositive are considered to have indeterminate HIV infection (stage P-0). After 15 months the presence of anti-HIV IgG is considered indicative of HIV infection in the child. Asymptomatic children older than 15 months who are HIV seropositive or younger than 15 months who are HIV antigen positive, viral culture positive, or IgA seropositive are classified as stage P-1, asymptomatic confirmed infection. Children of any age with symptomatic HIV disease, with other illnesses ruled out, are classified as stage P-2, symptomatic HIV infection. The pediatric classification system applies to children up to the age of 12 years, although it is most relevant in the diagnosis and management of younger children.

DIAGNOSIS OF HIV INFECTION

The diagnosis of HIV infection (see also Ch. 103) is best accomplished by detecting specific antibodies against viral antigens

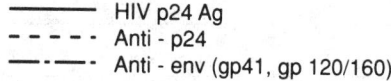

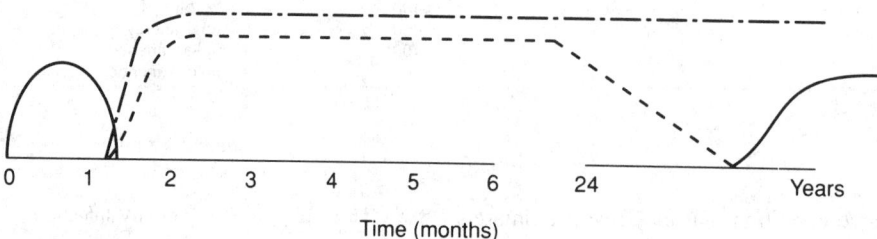

FIG. 1. Serologic response to HIV infection.

serologically. Directly detecting viral antigens and culture of virus in cell culture are also possible; however, the former is relatively insensitive, and the latter is very expensive. Other diagnostic tests have been developed, including the use of polymerase chain reaction assays and other methods to detect genomic DNA or RNA. Use of the enzyme-linked immunosorbent assay (ELISA) for HIV antibodies, however, is the most efficient and practical way to diagnose HIV infection.[37]

Detecting anti-HIV antibodies by ELISA is highly sensitive (>99 percent) and specific (95–99 percent). As with any diagnostic test, the predictive value of a positive test result depends on the prevalence of infected persons in the population being tested. A number of conditions including collagen-vascular diseases, chronic hepatitis, malaria, and certain HLA phenotypes have been associated with false-positive results on ELISA. Serum samples that are reactive by ELISA should be retested; repeatedly positive specimens should then be confirmed with a highly specific test such as an immunofluorescence assay (IFA) or a Western blot (WB). Other specific methods such as radioimmunoprecipitation assay are not practical for routine use in clinical laboratories. When confirmed reactive by IFA or WB, specimens should be considered true positives. Individuals positive by these tests should be informed that they are infected with HIV, counseled about the implications of HIV infection, and advised to eliminate behaviors that might result in transmitting the virus to others. Medical screening and follow-up should be offered to all HIV seropositive individuals.

The serologic response to HIV infection is shown in Figure 1. Shortly after exposure to the virus, a period of viremia and p24 antigenemia occurs. Antigenemia generally occurs within 2 weeks of exposure and lasts for several weeks. Both IgM and IgG antibodies to core (p24) and envelope (gp41, gp120) antigens develop 1–3 months after exposure, although longer periods of seroconversion have been documented. HIV antigen (p24)testing is useful in evaluating patients with suspected acute retroviral syndrome or for newborns and infants.[38,39]

Months to years after seroconversion, a significant proportion of HIV-infected individuals begin to lose antibodies to core antigens, although antibodies to envelope antigens, reverse transcriptase, and regulatory proteins remain. Most such individuals then develop core antigenemia; a minority may have antigen detected in the cerebrospinal fluid (CSF). Developing antigenemia presumably reflects an antigen-excess state, with anti-core antibodies consumed in immune complexes.

NATURAL HISTORY OF HIV INFECTION

The clinical spectrum of HIV infection ranges from acute infection to asymptomatic carriage to advanced immunodeficiency with opportunistic disease. The probability that an infected individual will progress from asymptomatic HIV infection to AIDS,

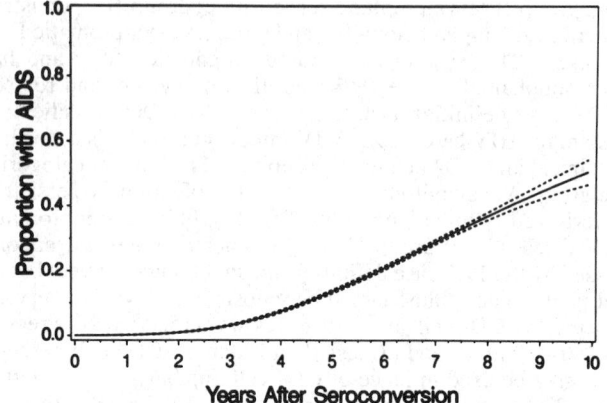

FIG. 2. Probability of progression from HIV seroconversion to diagnosis of AIDS by the 1987 CDC case definition based on estimates from three cohorts of homosexual men in San Francisco. The median time to progression was 9.8 years. (From Bachetti and Moss,[40] with permission.)

and from AIDS to death, has been estimated in a number of studies. Bacchetti and Moss estimated the incubation period from HIV infection to development of AIDS (1987 case definition) in homosexual men in San Francisco (Fig. 2).[40] The median estimated time from seroconversion to AIDS was 9.8 years. Other studies have estimated the period from infection to developing AIDS to range from 6.5 to 13 years with an average of 8–9 years.[41-44] Most studies of the natural history of untreated HIV infection suggest that most infected people will progress to clinical immunodeficiency eventually. Variability in the rate of progression of HIV infection has been attributed to age and the route by which HIV infection was acquired. Transfusion recipients, for example, whose initial inoculum of HIV is undoubtedly larger than individuals infected sexually or by contaminated needles, have a median incubation time of 6 years.[42] Transfusion-related HIV-infected persons tend to be older than those infected sexually, however, which may confound this observation. In addition, the stage of disease in the HIV-infected blood donor is associated with the rate of progression to AIDS in the recipient.

An important study of the natural history of HIV infection is the cohort of homosexual and bisexual men followed by the San Francisco Department of Public Health and the CDC since early in the AIDS epidemic.[45] These subjects were originally enrolled in a study of hepatitis B vaccine in 1978 and have serologic studies and clinical evaluations that date from that time. Of the 489 men for whom the time of HIV seroconversion can be reliably estimated, 13 percent developed AIDS within 5 years, 51 percent within 10 years, and 54 percent at 11 years. In addition, of those who had not developed AIDS within 12 years of sero-

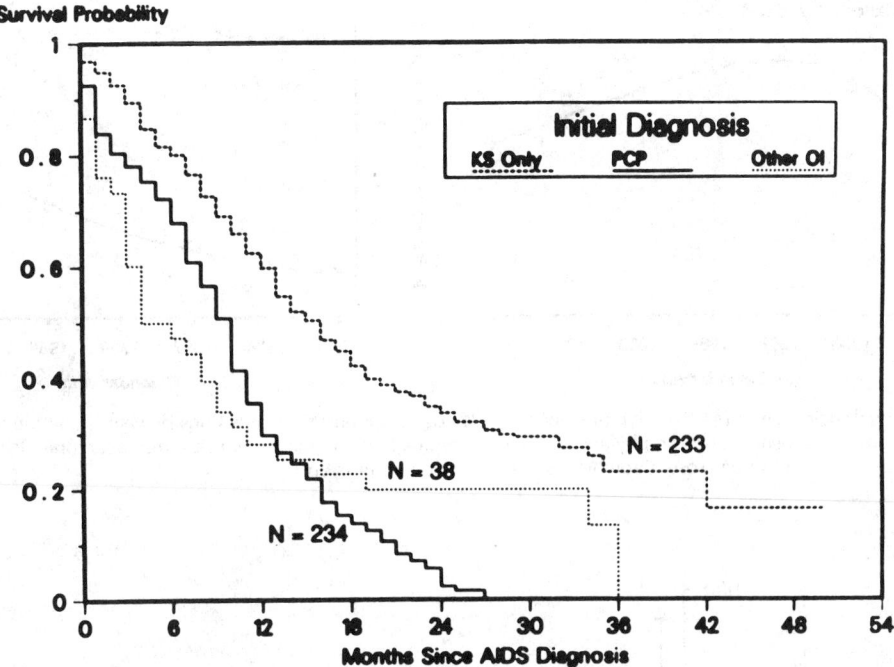

FIG. 3. Probability of surviving from diagnosis of AIDS in 505 patients in San Francisco, by index diagnosis. (Courtesy of P. Bacchetti. Adapted from Bacchetti et al.,[46] with permission.)

conversion, 19 percent had symptomatic HIV disease; 29 percent of individuals infected for more than 11 years without developing AIDS had severe clinical immunodeficiency (CD4 cell count <200/mm³). Thus, after 11 years of follow-up, more than three-quarters of HIV-infected homosexual men had advanced HIV disease, AIDS, or had died.

After the development of AIDS, clinical progression and death ensue rapidly, particularly in the absence of therapy. In a study of survival after diagnosis of AIDS in the first 505 patients with AIDS in San Francisco, Bacchetti et al. found a median survival of 9 months, with most patients dead within 2 years (Fig. 3).[46] Patients diagnosed with an opportunistic infection had the most rapid mortality, whereas survival was significantly longer in patients initially diagnosed with Kaposi sarcoma. Rothenberg and associates found similar results in New York City AIDS patients, although overall survival was slightly longer (median survival 12 months).[47] In New York City patients, women, blacks, and injection drug users had significantly shorter survival than males, whites, and homosexual men. These survival differences may reflect the somewhat different natural history of KS, which occurs predominantly in homosexual men in the United States, as well as differences in access to medical care.

Several studies have confirmed that the advent of antiretroviral therapy and widespread prophylaxis against *P. carinii* pneumonia have substantially altered the natural history of AIDS, with median survival in treated AIDS patients ranging from 2 to 3 years.[48–51] In addition, use of antiretroviral therapy and prophylaxis against opportunistic infections such as *P. carinii* extends the clinical incubation period from infection with HIV to AIDS, as well as overall survival.[52,53] As opportunistic infections such as *P. carinii* are prevented, diseases that occur later in the course of HIV-induced immunodeficiency, such as *Mycobacterium avium* complex bacteremia or cytomegalovirus organ disease may be the first clinical manifestation of HIV disease. Among homosexual men with AIDS in one cohort study, 50 percent of those who received no prophylactic therapy had *P. carinii* pneumonia as an index AIDS diagnosis, compared to 15 percent of those receiving prophylaxis.[54,55] As therapies that inhibit retroviral replication and prevent specific opportun-

istic infections improve, the natural history and clinical spectrum of HIV disease will continue to evolve (Fig. 4).

The probability that an HIV-infected person will develop opportunistic disease is influenced by several factors.[56] First, host immunocompetence is a critical determinant of whether an infected individual can contain a potential pathogen. As discussed below, the CD4 cell count appears to be the most clinically useful measure of host cellular immunocompetence and plays a central role in staging HIV disease. Second, exposure to potential pathogens is required before disease can result. Although some opportunistic pathogens are ubiquitous, resulting in latent infection in a large proportion of HIV-infected persons (e.g., *P. carinii*, cytomegalovirus), others are prevalent in a smaller proportion of individuals and cause disease less often (e.g., *Toxoplasma gondii*, *M. tuberculosis*). Other opportunistic pathogens do not appear to be associated with latent reactivation but rather cause disease when a sufficiently immunocompromised host acquires new infection (e.g., *Cryptococcus neoformans*, *M. avium* complex). Third, the relative virulence of a potential pathogen is a factor determining when disease is likely to occur. For example, more virulent organisms such as *M. tuberculosis* or *Streptococcus pneumoniae* cause clinical illness in patients with less severe immunodeficiency than less virulent organisms such as *P. carinii* or cytomegalovirus.[57–59] Finally, whether a patient is taking chemoprophylactic agents with activity against specific pathogens will influence the risk of disease. Figure 5 shows CD4 cell levels in 222 patients with AIDS-related illnesses evaluated at one center.[60] Although the range of CD4 cell counts for some conditions is broad, most patients with truly opportunistic infections had CD4 counts less than 100/mm³.

The incidence of specific opportunistic diseases has been determined for several large cohorts of HIV-infected individuals. In one study of more than 1000 patients with advanced HIV disease (AIDS or symptomatic HIV with a CD4 cell count <250/mm³) who were starting zidovudine therapy, the 2-year probability of new opportunistic diseases was determined (Fig. 6).[56,61] The most common opportunistic infection was *P. carinii* pneumonia, followed by cytomegalovirus disease and *M. avium* complex disease. The most common opportunistic malignancy in

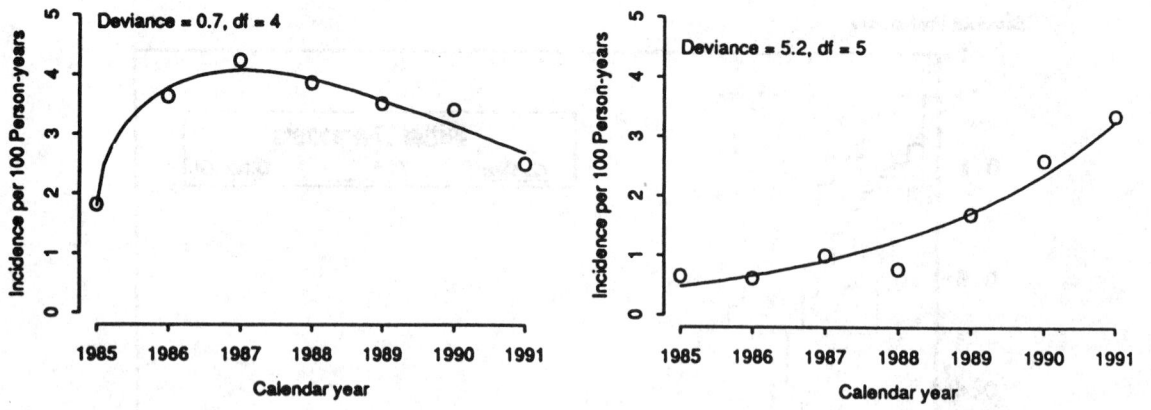

FIG. 4. Annual incidence of **(A)** *P. carinii* pneumonia or **(B)** other opportunistic infections by year in the Multicenter AIDS Cohort Study. As anti-*Pneumocystis* prophylaxis became widespread, the incidence of *P. carinii* pneumonia decreased while the incidence of other infections rose. (From Muñoz et al.,[74] with permission.)

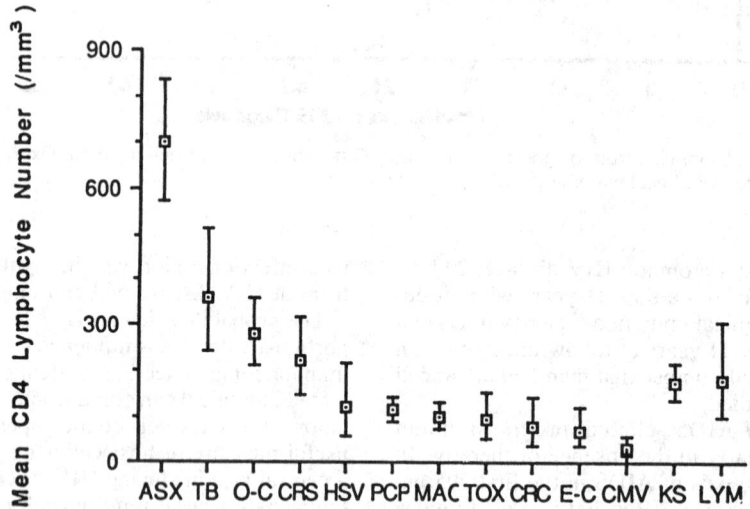

FIG. 5. Mean CD4 cell levels with standard deviations (boxes) and 95 percent confidence intervals (whiskers) in 222 HIV-infected patients with opportunistic diseases and HIV-infected, asymptomatic controls. ASX: asymptomatic; TB: tuberculosis; O-C: oral candidiasis; CRS: cryptosporidiosis; HSV: recurrent herpes simplex virus; PCP: *Pneumocystis carinii* pneumonia; MAC: *Mycobacterium avium* complex; TOX: toxoplasmosis; CRC: cryptococcal meningitis; EC: esophageal candidiasis; CMV: cytomegalovirus retinitis; KS: Kaposi sarcoma; LYM: lymphoma. (From Crowe et al.,[60] with permission.)

this cohort composed largely of homosexual men was KS; the 2-year probability of non-Hodgkin's lymphoma was 2.4 percent.[62] In terms of opportunistic infections, those that appear likely to occur in a large proportion of patients are the ubiquitous organisms *P. carinii*, cytomegalovirus, and *M. avium* complex, whereas organisms such as *M. tuberculosis* and *T. gondii* are far less prevalent. The varying incidences of specific opportunistic infections has implications for prophylactic strategies. Chemoprophylaxis against *P. carinii* and *M. avium* complex is now recommended for all HIV-infected patients with severe enough immunodeficiency to elevate the risk of disease.[63–64] A similar strategy will likely be employed if effective prophylaxis for cytomegalovirus is developed. Conversely, prophylaxis against the less common pathogens *M. tuberculosis* and *T. gondii* is targeted at those individuals known to be latently infected with these organisms (i.e., *T. gondii* IgG seropositive persons or those individuals with a positive tuberculin skin test).

Clinical findings may also predict disease progression in seropositive subjects. Oral candidiasis (thrush), itself an opportunistic infection, is an early clinical marker of immunosuppression and heralds the development of AIDS in many patients.[65] In the Multicenter AIDS Cohort Study, a natural history cohort of homosexual and bisexual men, the presence of oral candidiasis

was associated with an increased risk of subsequent *P. carinii* pneumonia, independent of CD4 cell count.[66] Unexplained fever and diarrhea were also independently associated with development of *P. carinii*. Hairy leukoplakia, an opportunistic infection associated with Epstein-Barr virus (EBV), also predicts the development of AIDS. Greenspan et al. found that a referred population of homosexual men with hairy leukoplakia had an actuarial progression rate to opportunistic infection of 48 percent at 16 months and 83 percent at 31 months.[67] Dermatomal or disseminated outbreaks of herpes zoster appear to be associated with the HIV infection, per se, but not with the progressive development of AIDS.[68–70] Generalized lymphadenopathy is a clinical marker of HIV infection but not a predictor of progression to AIDS. One study found that average CD4 lymphocyte counts were higher in homosexual men with lymphadenopathy than in seropositive individuals without enlarged lymph nodes.[71]

A number of laboratory tests have correlated progressive immunodeficiency and the development of AIDS. CD4 lymphocyte counts, a specific test for HIV-induced immunopathology, have sensitively predicted the development of AIDS and ARC. Goedert et al. found that CD4 cell counts less than 300/mm³ were associated with a progression rate of 18.5 cases/100 person-years in seropositive homosexual men as compared with

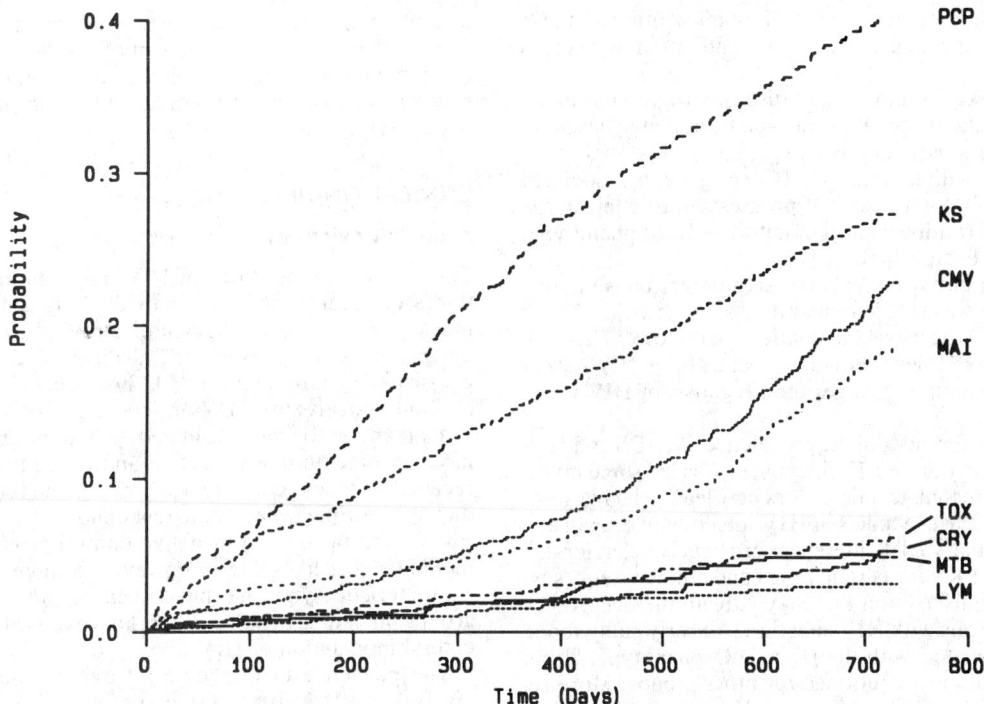

FIG. 6. Probability of developing a new diagnosis of selected AIDS-indicator conditions in a cohort of 1050 patients with advanced symptomatic HIV disease (CD4 count <250/mm³ or AIDS) who were starting zidovudine therapy. PCP: *Pneumocystis carinii* pneumonia; KS: Kaposi sarcoma; CMV: cytomegalovirus; MAI: *Mycobacterium avium* complex; Tox: toxoplasmosis; CRY: cryptococcosis; MTB: tuberculosis; LYM: non-Hodgkin's lymphoma. (Adapted from Gallant et al.[56] and Moore et al.[61] with permission.)

TABLE 7. Predictors of Progression to AIDS in HIV Seropositive Homosexual Men

Variable	Category	3-Year Rate of Progression[a] (%)	Relative Hazard
CD4+ lymphocyte count	<200/mm³	87	13.4
	200–400/mm³	46	3.6
	>400/mm³	16	1.0
CD4+ lymphocyte proportion (of total lymphocytes)	<25%	48	5.1
	≥25%	12	1.0
HIV p24 antigen	Positive	59	4.6
	Negative	16	1.0
Anti-p24 antibody	Negative	43	3.2
	Positive	16	1.0
β₂ Microglobulin	>5 µg/ml	69	16.9
	3.1–5 µg/ml	33	4.5
	≤3 µg/ml	12	1.0
Hemoglobin	<13.5 g/dl	50	4.5
	≥13.5 g/dl	21	1.0

[a] Actuarial progression rate by product-limit method.

(From Moss et al.,[45] with permission.)

1.5 cases/100 person-years for men with greater than 550 CD4 cells/mm³.[72] Polk and associates also showed that the development of AIDS was associated with a CD4 cell count of less than 300/mm³ during a 15-month period of follow-up.[73] Moss and coworkers associated a baseline CD4 cell count of 200/mm³ or less with a 3-year progression rate to AIDS of 87 percent; the rate for those with baseline CD4 counts of 200–400/mm³ was 46 percent, and those with more than 400 cells/mm³ had a 15 percent progression rate (Table 7).[45] Other studies have shown similar findings.[74] Other cell determinations that predict the development of AIDS in a seropositive individual include a total lymphocyte count of less than 1000, a total white blood cell count of less than 4000, a hematocrit of less than 40, and a low proportion of lymphocytes with the CD4 phenotype, regardless of the total CD4 count. Because CD4 percentage has a narrower range of variation in most clinical laboratories than absolute CD4 cell number, many clinicians favor using this measure to stage and monitor patients.[75]

As discussed earlier, the presence of HIV p24 antigen in the serum reflects either recent infection of an antigen-excess state in advanced HIV disease. HIV antigenemia is associated with a high rate of disease progression. Moss et al. compared initially antigenemic subjects with antigen-negative subjects. Of the antigenemic subjects 59 percent developed AIDS, and 30 percent developed ARC in 3 years as compared with 16 and 17 percent, respectively, for antigen-negative subjects.[45] Approximately 7 percent of antigen-negative subjects became antigenemic annually. Allain and coworkers showed that in hemophiliacs HIV antigenemia was a better predictor of progression to disease than was the CD4 cell count.[76] DeWolf and associates also found a higher rate of disease progression in antigenemic homosexual men in Amsterdam.[77] HIV antigenemia is also useful because it responds to effective antiretroviral therapy. However, because a large proportion of patients lack antigenemia, and because quantitation of antigenemia is not predictive of outcome, the clinical utility of this surrogate marker is limited.

Levels of serum β₂-microglobulin, a low-molecular-weight immunoglobulin that forms the light chain of the class I major histocompatibility center (MHC) receptor, are elevated in HIV infection, particularly in subjects with advanced disease. Subjects with a β₂-microglobulin level greater than 5 µg/ml had a 17-fold greater hazard for developing AIDS than did seropositive subjects with normal levels in one study.[45] Serum and urine neopterin concentrations are strongly associated with CD4 cell levels and, when elevated, predictive of disease progression.[78–80] Although β₂-microglobulin declines with antiretroviral therapy, neopterin levels do not appear to be affected by treatment.[81]

Other markers of HIV disease progression that have been described include acid-labile interferon-α (INF-α), soluble CD8, low concentrations of anti-p24 antibodies, and elevated anti-cytomegalovirus antibodies.[73,74,82-84] The clinical utility of these assays in the management of individual patients, however, is very limited.

A virologic marker of more rapid disease progression is the conversion of a patient's viral phenotype from non-syncytium-inducing (NSI) to syncytium-inducing (SI).[85] This phenotype switch, associated with mutations in the *env* gene, is associated with more rapid CD4 cell loss and progression to clinical disease. The value of routine clinical monitoring for SI phenotype, however, has not been established.

Another marker of more rapid disease progression is vitamin A deficiency.[86] Lower serum retinol levels are associated with impaired T-cell blastogenesis, and patients with lower CD4 cell counts tend to have lower retinol concentrations.[87] Whether treatment with vitamin A changes the prognosis of HIV infection is not known.

Striking racial differences in the prevalence of AIDS and HIV infection, particularly among IV drug users, has led some investigators to speculate that genetic factors may lead to higher rates in acquiring the disease. Studies of HIV infection in drug users, however, suggest that racial differences are largely behavioral.[88] The predilection of KS for certain racial and ethnic groups suggests a genetic predisposition that may explain the occurrence of KS in some persons with HIV infection. An early study found that KS was associated with the HLA-DR5 phenotype,[101] but this finding has not been confirmed for other groups. More recent epidemiologic studies suggest that KS may be associated with a sexually transmitted pathogen, although an etiologic agent has not been identified.[89-91]

A number of investigators have examined the potential impact of behaviors on the natural history of HIV infection. To date, there is no compelling evidence that sexual practices, alcohol or drug consumption, lifestyle, or other behavioral characteristics modify the course of HIV infection.[92-95] Other potential cofactors in HIV disease progression that might be related to behaviors have been identified, however. It has been postulated that antigenic stimulation from sexually transmitted diseases, such as herpes simplex virus or syphilis, may upregulate HIV replication and result in a more rapid disease course.[96] Although clinical evidence for this is lacking, several drug trials have demonstrated that acyclovir use is associated with significantly improved survival in patients treated with zidovudine.[97] This effect is unrelated to an impact on cytomegalovirus infections. Although it is prudent to caution HIV-infected persons to avoid contracting new sexually transmitted diseases for the protection of both themselves and their sexual partners, it is unproved that acquiring sexually transmitted diseases has an impact on the natural history of HIV infection. Similarly, although a small study suggested that injection drug users with HIV infection who continued to use intravenous drugs had a more rapid decline in CD4 cell levels,[98] larger cohort studies have failed to detect any association between continued drug use and development of AIDS.[99] Recently, the issue of antigenic stimulation of HIV-infected persons has been raised in relation to the use of influenza vaccine in this patient population. Conflicting results of the impact of influenza vaccine on HIV replication and disease course have been reported.[100] Currently, the evidence that antigen stimulation accelerates HIV disease is limited.

Biologic differences in disease progression do exist. Age is an important factor in the rate at which AIDS develops in seropositive subjects. Eyster et al. reported that disease progression was three- to fivefold higher in adult hemophiliacs with HIV infection when compared with subjects under 21 years old.[102] Moss and associates observed a relative hazard of 2.2 for developing AIDS, independent of the CD4 cell count, in seropositive homosexual men over 36 years old.[45] Bacchetti et al. studied the first 500 AIDS cases in San Francisco and found that patients over the age of 40 had significantly shorter survival than did patients 20–30 years old.[46] This difference was most pronounced for patients with an initial diagnosis of KS. Survival of older

patients with transfusion-related HIV infection is significantly shorter than for younger patients.[42] Although immunocompetence is known to decline with senescence, the striking differences in disease progression and mortality by age are poorly understood.

CLINICAL FINDINGS

Acute Retroviral Syndrome

The initial manifestations of HIV infection in one-half to two-thirds of recently infected individuals is a mononucleosislike illness, referred to as the acute retroviral syndrome. In 1985, Cooper and colleagues in Australia identified an acute mononucleosislike syndrome in 11 of 12 homosexual men who became antibody-positive for HIV antibodies.[103] In a follow-up study, Tindall and associates evaluated 39 homosexual men known to have become antibody-positive and found that 36 (92 percent) recalled an illness consistent with the acute retroviral syndrome during the time when their tests showed seroconversion.[104] Forty percent of a seronegative control group also reported a mononucleosislike illness, however. Similar descriptions of a characteristic syndrome have been reported in all AIDS risk groups, including health care workers exposed to accidental parenteral inoculation of HIV.[106]

The incidence of the acute retroviral syndrome is not precisely known. Retrospective studies of homosexual men infected with HIV find a low prevalence of seroconversion illness.[105,107] A prospective study of homosexual men showed a 55 percent incidence of a mononucleosis-like illness in 22 subjects who became antibody-positive as compared with 21 percent in 44 nonconverting controls.[108] Most health care workers with occupational acquisition of HIV had the acute retroviral syndrome after exposure.[106,109] Overall, this syndrome is probably underreported and underdiagnosed.

The clinical features of the acute retroviral syndrome are nonspecific and variable. The onset of the illness ranges from 1 to 6 weeks after exposure to the virus. Table 8 lists the signs and symptoms of the acute retroviral syndrome reported in 209 cases, reviewed by Niu and coworkers.[110] Fever, sweats, malaise, myalgias, anorexia, nausea, diarrhea, and a nonexudative pharyngitis are prominent symptoms.[110-121] Many patients report headaches, photophobia, and meningismus. Two-thirds of patients may have a truncal exanthem that may be maculopapular, roseola-like, or urticarial. In addition to aseptic meningitis, neurologic symptoms occur in a minority of patients and may include encephalitis, peripheral neuropathy, and an acute, ascending polyneuropathy (Guillain-Barré syndrome). Physical examination frequently reveals cervical, occipital, or axillary lymphadenopathy; rash; and less commonly, hepatosplenomegaly. Oral aphthous ulcerations have been reported in several

TABLE 8. Symptoms and Signs of the Acute Retroviral Syndrome in 209 Patients

Symptom or Sign	No. with Finding	Frequency (%)
Fever	200	96
Adenopathy	154	74
Pharyngitis	146	70
Rash	146	70
Myalgia or arthralgia	112	54
Thrombocytopenia	94	45
Leukopenia	80	38
Diarrhea	67	32
Headache	66	32
Nausea, vomiting	56	27
Elevated transaminases[a]	38	21
Hepatosplenomegaly	30	14
Thrush	24	12
Neuropathy	13	6
Encephalopathy	12	6

[a] Based on 178 subjects.

(Adapted from Niu et al.,[110] with permission.)

cases; these may involve the esophagus. Oral and esophageal candidiasis during the seroconversion illness has been reported. The remainder of the physical examination is usually unremarkable.

Laboratory evaluation of patients with the syndrome reveals a reduced total lymphocyte count, elevated sedimentation rate, negative heterophil-antibody test and elevated transaminase and alkaline phosphatase levels.[110,111] When lymphocyte phenotyping is performed, a characteristic pattern is observed.[122] Initially, the total lymphocyte count, including both CD4 and CD8 T lymphocytes, decreases with a normal ratio of CD4 to CD8 cells. Within several weeks, both the CD4 and CD8 cell populations begin to increase. The rise in CD8 cell numbers is relatively greater than is that in CD4 cells, and the CD4:CD8 ratio is inverted. In the weeks that follow, the CD8 cell population increases rather markedly. The total lymphocyte count also increases, and atypical lymphocytes may be seen on the peripheral smear. The ratio of CD4:CD8 cells usually remains inverted as the acute illness resolves (primarily due to excess numbers of CD8 cells). In patients with neurologic symptoms, CSF may show a lymphocytic pleocytosis with normal levels of protein and glucose.[119,123]

Serologic studies of patients with the acute illness may be useful in making an early diagnosis. HIV core (p24) antigen may be detected in the serum and CSF of patients with primary infection within 2 weeks of exposure, often coincidentally with the onset of symptoms.[123,124] Antigenemia can persist for several weeks or months and generally resolves when antibodies to p24 are produced in sufficient quantity to form complexes with free antigen. High-level viremia is found in patients during the symptomatic state of acute infection, with titers declining in the days to weeks before antibody seroconversion.[111,125,126] The ELISA for HIV antibodies remains negative for an average of 2–3 months despite the appearance of specific antibodies on a Western blot of the patient's serum. Anti-p24 appears on the Western blot shortly before seroconversion is detected by ELISA and by the appearance of antibodies to other antigens.

The differential diagnosis of the acute retroviral syndrome includes a number of other illnesses: infectious mononucleosis; other viral infections such as influenza, measles, rubella, and herpes simplex; and secondary syphilis. Evaluation of patients presenting with an illness consistent with acute retroviral infection should include a careful history to elicit risks for HIV infection, laboratory tests to rule out mononucleosis and syphilis, HIV antibody and antigen tests, and complete blood counts and differential. Sequential HIV antibody tests may need to be performed over several months to confirm the diagnosis.

Persistent Generalized Lymphadenopathy

Infection with HIV is associated with a high prevalence of generalized lymphadenopathy, often beginning with the acute retroviral syndrome. In the early 1980s, PGL was recognized as a prodromal state to the development of AIDS in homosexual men who were otherwise healthy.[15,16] The pathogenesis of generalized lymphadenopathy is related to the rapid infection of CD4 cells in lymph nodes by HIV after initial infection. The syndrome of PGL was defined as the presence of two or more extrainguinal sites of lymphadenopathy for a minimum of 3–6 months for which no other explanation could be found. Biopsy specimens of lymph nodes from such patients usually reveal a follicular hyperplasia without specific pathogens.

After becoming antibody-positive, approximately 50–70 percent of infected individuals develop PGL. The most frequently involved node groups are the posterior and anterior cervical, submandibular, occipital, and axillary chains; epitrochlear and femoral nodes may also be enlarged. Physical examination usually reveals symmetric, mobile, rubbery lymph noes ranging from 0.5 to 2 cm and distributed as previously described. Pain and tenderness are uncommon. Localized (i.e., asymmetric) adenopathy and rapid nodal enlargement are not characteristic and suggest an infectious or malignant process. The remainder of the physical examination is often unremarkable, although other complications of HIV infection may be found such as thrush or hairy leukoplakia. Mediastinal and hilar adenopathy are not characteristic of the syndrome; however, abdominal computed tomography (CT) often reveals enlarged mesenteric and retroperitoneal adenopathy in HIV-infected persons. The natural history of HIV infection in individuals with PGL does not differ significantly from that of HIV infection without PGL.[71,127] Involution of enlarged lymph nodes, with degeneration of follicular germinal centers and loss of hyperplasia, often accompanies progression of HIV infection to advanced disease.

The differential diagnosis of PGL includes HIV infection and a wide variety of other processes that are associated with generalized lymphadenopathy: sarcoid, secondary syphilis, and Hodgkin's disease, for example. In patients with HIV infection, lymphadenopathy may also be caused by mycobacterial infections, KS, and lymphoma.[128] In patients with clinical findings suggesting opportunistic disease, needle aspiration of lymph nodes may help establish a specific diagnosis.[129] Examination of aspirates with cytologic, acid-fast, and Gram stains is valuable in identifying infection or malignancy. If a specific diagnosis is not determined after staining and culture of node aspirates, then lymph node biopsy is indicated. Aspiration of lymph nodes in patients with PGL usually reveals benign cells. Biopsy specimens show follicular hyperplasia, with the normal architecture distorted by greatly expanded germinal centers composed of B lymphocytes. It is now known that active viral replication is occurring in these follicular cells and dendritic cells, although the patient may appear well clinically.[129a]

Most patients with PGL require no invasive evaluation and can be managed expectantly for the occurrence of other AIDS-related manifestations.

Immune Thrombocytopenia and Hematologic Manifestations

A number of hematologic abnormalities have been described in patients with HIV disease.[130] Thrombocytopenia is a relatively common manifestation of HIV infection that may occur throughout the clinical spectrum of disease. HIV-related immune thrombocytopenia may be manifested by easy bruising, petechiae, bleeding gums, and prolonged bleeding from minor cuts and abrasions. Most patients are asymptomatic and are found to have low platelet counts incidentally during routine clinical evaluation. More severe bleeding complications such as gastrointestinal (GI) hemorrhage or cerebrovascular bleeding are very rare. Platelet counts typically remain low for months to years, although platelet counts increase in some patients as HIV disease advances.

The pathophysiology of immune thrombocytopenia has been studied in both homosexual men and drug users, and the primary mechanism of disease has been identified as the peripheral destruction of platelets. Examination of the bone marrow usually shows normal or increased production of megakaryocytes and erythroid hyperplasia. Deposition of immune complexes on platelets has been postulated as one mechanism of destruction.[131] Replication of HIV within megakaryocytes has also been described, and may contribute to thrombocytopenia is some cases.[132]

A limited differential diagnosis of isolated thrombocytopenia in an HIV-infected person includes drug-induced thrombocytopenia, particularly in heroin addicts and alcoholics, consumptive thrombocytopenia, or splenic sequestration. Some patients with thrombocytopenia may also present with leukopenia or anemia. The presence of constitutional symptoms and pancytopenia suggests an opportunistic infection, particularly disseminated mycobacterial or fungal infection, or a lymphoma. Patients with these clinical findings should undergo bone marrow aspiration and biopsy, with appropriate stains and cultures. Isolated immune thrombocytopenia in an HIV-infected person can be managed expectantly by advising the patient to avoid aspirin and drugs that may exacerbate thrombocytopenia. Managing drugs associated with thrombocytopenia depends on the need for the drug and the degree of thrombocytopenia. If the patient does not have significant bleeding and maintains a platelet count above 20,000/mm^3, the medication can be continued with close observation. If an alternative agent can be reasonably substituted, this should be done. Use of zidovudine is associated with increases in platelet counts in most patients, presumably by inhibiting virus, replication within megakaryocytes or elsewhere in the bone marrow.[133]

Thrombotic thrombocytopenic purpura (TTP) has been reported in a small number of persons with HIV disease, and its clinical features appear to be similar to other populations.[134,135] Intravascular hemolysis and thrombocytopenia are pronounced. The prevalence of TTP appears to be extremely low, and it is unclear whether HIV itself or another infectious agent is responsible for TTP in HIV-infected patients.

Anemia is a prominent feature of HIV disease. Most patients with advanced disease, particularly those with opportunistic infections, have a normochromic, normocytic anemia.[130] The anemia is generally mild (hemoglobin content, 11–14 g/dl) and nonprogressive, although patients with a history of multiple opportunistic infections may have a hemoglobin level as low as 8–9 g/dl. Anemia is caused by a number of factors. Nutritional factors, such as deficiencies of vitamin B$_{12}$ or folate, may be a cause of anemia in some patients. HIV may infect erythroid precursors in the bone marrow[136] and inhibit the production of red cells directly. However, AIDS patients with anemia usually show normal erythroid and myeloid precursors and adequate iron stores in the bone marrow. Sequestration of red cells in the spleen and, to a lesser extent, the liver may contribute to the anemia. Concurrent opportunistic infections or malignancies frequently depress the hematocrit value. Suppression of erythropoietin production may also affect red cell production; although serum erythropoietin levels in patients with HIV become elevated with advanced disease, the degree of elevation is often inappropriate for the severity of anemia.[137] In advanced HIV disease, anemia is often a consequence of HIV itself, opportunistic diseases, and drug therapy that causes bone marrow suppression.[138]

Several recent studies have shown that patients with HIV infection and anemia may have persistent B19 parvovirus infection, with a pure red cell aplasia, low reticulocyte counts, and normal leucocyte levels.[139,140]

The differential diagnosis of anemia in a person with HIV disease should include blood loss, infiltration of the bone marrow by opportunistic pathogens (e.g., *M. avium* complex, *Histoplasma capsulatum*), malignancy, and drug toxicity. Depression of all cell lines suggests opportunistic disease, whereas isolated, mild anemia is most often associated with HIV. Bone marrow biopsy is not usually indicated in the latter situation. Although mild HIV-induced anemia generally does not require specific therapy, a low hematocrit predicts disease progression in asymptomatic HIV-seropositive individuals.

A variety of leukocyte disorders have been described in HIV disease. Most prominent is lymphopenia, primarily due to CD4 cell depletion. Dysfunction of neutrophils and monocytes has been reported, although the clinical importance of these findings is unclear.[141] Drug-induced neutropenia or leukopenia is a common finding in advanced HIV disease.[138,142]

Constitutional Disease

Prolonged infection with HIV is often completely asymptomatic; however, a minority of patients complain of nonspecific constitutional symptoms in the months or years after primary infection. Patients commonly complain of being easily fatigued and report the need to reduce their normal activities somewhat. Debilitating fatigue is uncommon in the early years of infection. Low-grade fevers (temperature <38°C), occasional night sweats, and intermittent diarrhea are also reported. The exact incidence of these findings is not known, and attributing them solely to HIV infection may not be accurate. The differential diagnosis of these findings includes intercurrent minor illnesses and psychological or psychiatric disorders. Anxiety and depression are common responses to knowledge or suspicion of HIV infection.[143,144] Many patients infected with HIV may have underlying psychiatric conditions. Intravenous drug users, in particular, have a high prevalence of affective disorders that may result in somatic complaints. Moreover, the physical effects of opiates and withdrawal from stimulants such as cocaine and amphetamines cause fatigue and other constitutional symptoms.

In patients with more advanced HIV disease and severe depletion of CD4+ cells, constitutional disease (fatigue, weight loss, malaise, fever) usually heralds the onset of opportunistic infections or malignancies. In one study of HIV-infected outpatients with fever, a specific etiology could be identified for 83 percent.[145] Common causes of fever in these patients included *P. carinii* pneumonia, *M. avium* complex bacteremia, catheter-related bacteremia, bacterial pneumonia, sinusitis, lymphoma, and drug reactions. Fever of greater than 2 weeks' duration was more often associated with AIDS-defining illnesses.

In African patients with HIV infection, a wasting illness termed "slim disease" has been described.[146] These patients have debilitating fatigue, fevers, sweats, protracted diarrhea, and severe weight loss. Opportunistic or conventional pathogens are not found, but the patients waste away and die of severe malnutrition and terminal secondary infections. This illness has been encountered in developed countries as well, but far less commonly than in Africa—a pattern that suggests underdiagnosis of opportunistic diseases in Africa. One study of African patients with enteropathic slim disease found that most (16 of 22) had enteric pathogens or microsporidia found when a thorough evaluation was performed.[147] In Abidjan, Cote D'Ivoire, 37 percent of patients who died with a diagnosis of slim disease were found at autopsy to have disseminated tuberculosis.[148] The definition of wasting syndrome in the United States is the presence of unexplained constitutional disease for more than 1 month with a temperature greater than 38.3°C, diarrhea, and loss of more than 10 percent of baseline body weight. A thorough evaluation to identify specific pathogens that would explain the symptoms and that might be amenable to treatment is essential before wasting syndrome is diagnosed.

Oral Disease

Abnormalities of the oral cavity occur throughout the course of HIV infection. Primary HIV infection has been associated with severe aphthous stomatitis and with oropharyngeal and esophageal candidiasis. As the infection progresses and immunologic impairment proceeds, numerous oral complications arise. In the late stages of disease, oral manifestations are highly prevalent and frequently severe.[149,150] A number of studies have demonstrated that the occurrence of oral lesions such as candidiasis and hairy leukoplakia is associated with an increased risk of progression to AIDS.[151–153]

Oral Candidiasis. *Candida* infections of the hard and soft palates, buccal mucosa, tongue, pharynx, and hypophyarynx are observed frequently. Contrary to systemic *Candida* infections, which appear to result from defects in phagocyte function and number, mucosal candidal infections result from impaired cellular immunity. The incidence of candidiasis increases with progressive cellular immunodeficiency, particularly as CD4+ lymphocyte counts fall below 200–300/mm^3. Because oral candidiasis itself is an opportunistic infection, it predicts the disease progression and development of other AIDS-related infections.

A variety of manifestations of candidiasis have been described in HIV-infected patients. The most common form is thrush (pseudomembranous candidiasis). Characteristic cottage cheese plaques that can be removed with a tongue blade are seen on the soft palate, tonsils, and buccal mucosa. Less often, thrush involves the lateral and posterior aspects of the tongue, the hard palate, and the hypopharynx. *Candida* infection can produce flat, erythematous plaques distributed in the same way as the pseudomembranous form of the disease, but without the characteristic white exudate. This atrophic form of candidiasis is underdiagnosed because many clinicians are unfamiliar with its appearance. Atrophic candidiasis of the tongue also occurs. *Candida* can cause a nonscrapable white plaque similar to hairy leukoplakia (see below). This hypertrophic form of disease may involve the lateral border of the tongue, the palate, and the buccal mucosa. *Candida* infections of the lateral lip or angular cheilitis, is another common complication. Angular cheilitis can cause pain, fissures, and difficulty opening the mouth. Physical examination, KOH preparation, and the response to antifungal therapy establish the diagnosis.

The diagnosis of candidiasis is frequently made on the basis of physical examination alone. A KOH preparation of scraped material from a plaque is diagnostic and can be performed easily in most clinical settings. Cultures for *Candida* are rarely necessary. Biopsy specimen of oral lesions can distinguish various forms of leukoplakia. A therapeutic trial of antifungal agents can also help to establish a diagnosis. The recent widespread use of oral triazole antifungal agents has been accompanied by the emergence of disease caused by drug-resistant fungi.[154] *Candida glabrata*, *C. krusei*, and *C. albicans* resistant to fluconazole have all been recovered from patients with refractory oropharyngeal or esophageal candidiasis.[155]

Oral Hairy Leukoplakia. Originally described in 1984 by Greenspan et al., oral hairy leukoplakia (OHL) is a raised, white lesion of the oral mucosa that is unique to HIV infection.[156] OHL appears to be caused by the replication of EBV in the epithelium of keratinized cells on the surface of the tongue and buccal mucosa.[157] Other herpesviruses have also been isolated from cultures of biopsied lesions; however, their role in the pathogenesis of OHL is unclear. HIV is not routinely cultured from specimens and is not found with DNA probes. The diagnosis of OHL is established by visual inspection, failure of the lesion to scrape off with a tongue blade, failure to respond to antifungal therapy, and by biopsy material or scrapings in which EBV can be identified. Hairy leukoplakia is usually asymptomatic, although large lesions may impair taste, hinder eating, and cause discomfort.

Gingivitis and Periodontitis. Severe gingivitis and periodontitis have been observed in patients with HIV disease.[158] The onset of symptoms is often insidious but may be abrupt. Pain is often severe; patients may note foul breath, bleeding gums, and loosening of teeth. Physical examination may reveal a bright red marginal line on the gingiva, necrosis and ulceration of interdental papillae, gingival erosion, exfoliation of enamel, and loose teeth. The etiology of gingivitis and periodontitis is unclear. Mixed cultures of aerobic and anaerobic flora have been obtained from gingival biopsy samples. More severe, ulcerating gingivitis can be caused by infections with gram-negative bacilli, particularly *Klebsiella pneumoniae* and *Enterobacter cloacae*. Infections tend to be chronic, but topical antiseptic agents or metronidazole therapy may control some cases.

Oral Ulcers. A number of ulcerative lesions may occur in the oral cavity of patients with HIV infection. Herpes simplex virus types 1 and 2 may cause occasional or recurrent oral ulcers. These lesions generally appear as small, smooth ulcers on an erythematous base without exudate on the lips, buccal mucosa, hard palate, or gums. The ulcers may be single or multi-

ple and are often painful. Cytomegalovirus may rarely cause solitary large ulcers, without involvement of other organ systems. Aphthous stomatitis is manifested by single or multiple painful ulcers, often with exudate or necrosis, that may appear throughout the oral cavity or elsewhere in the GI tract.[159] The etiology of oral ulcers is best determined by biopsy and viral culture, although minor lesions may be observed without specific therapy in many cases. Several drugs have been reported to cause oral and GI ulcers, including zalcitabine, zidovudine, and dapsone.

Genital Tract Disorders

Both men and women with HIV disease have an increased risk of genital tract diseases that occur throughout the course of HIV infection. As noted above, genital herpes virus infections may be chronic or recurrent in HIV-infected individuals, and are associated with increased likelihood of transmission of HIV to sexual partners.[160] Genital warts may also be severe and chronic in HIV-infected persons. Other sexually transmitted diseases may have more atypical and prolonged manifestations in people with HIV infection.

Pelvic inflammatory disease has been reported to be more common, more severe, and require more frequent hospitalization and surgical intervention in HIV-seropositive women than in HIV-seronegative women.[161] Adequate cohort studies and case-control studies have not been conducted, however, to implicate HIV as causing an altered natural history of pelvic inflammatory disease. Nevertheless, several series have suggested that HIV-infected women with pelvic inflammatory disease may have more severe pain, prolonged symptoms, and failure to respond to antimicrobial therapy, which are all potential indications for surgery. The microbiology of pelvic inflammatory disease in women with HIV infection is poorly described.

Vaginal candidiasis also has an increased incidence in HIV-infected women, and recurrent candidiasis is common.[162,163] Vaginal candidiasis presents earlier in the course of HIV disease than oropharyngeal or esophageal candidiasis, often when CD4 cell counts are in the range of 500/mm^3.[163]

Cervical disease is exceedingly common in women with HIV infection, and the prevalence of cervical lesions increases as immunosuppression progresses.[164–166] Human papilloma virus (HPV) co-infection appears to play a major role in the development of cervical atypia and squamous dysplasia (see Ch. 122).[167] The prevalence of both HPV infection and cervical squamous intraepithelial lesions (SIL) increase in more advanced HIV disease, and SIL is strongly associated with HPV co-infection. Although HPV types 16 and 18 have been previously associated with cervical carcinoma, it is not clear that these types are responsible for the squamous dysplasia seen in HIV-seropositive women. The natural history of SIL in women with HIV infection is not currently understood. Women may present with low-grade or high-grade lesions, single or multifocal sites, and recurrent disease after excisional or ablative therapy. Some authorities have recommended that all women with HIV infection undergo cervical examination and Pap smear every 6 months,[168] and that colposcopy be performed for SIL. Others recommend careful observation of low-grade SIL, as spontaneous regression may occur. Invasive cervical carcinoma was added to the AIDS case definition in 1993. As of the end of 1993, fewer than 1 percent of AIDS patients had a diagnosis of cervical cancer.[169] Prospective cohort studies of women are needed to determine whether HIV infection increases the risk of cervical cancer, and what the incidence of this disorder is. Routine gynecologic care and follow-up for HIV-seropositive women are clearly important, however.

The interactions of syphilis and HIV infection are complex and important. Data from a number of studies indicate that syphilis and other genital ulcer diseases are important cofactors in the transmission and acquisition of HIV.[170,171] In addition, the natural history of syphilis appears to be altered by HIV infection.[172–174] Among the features of syphilis described in HIV-infected persons are delayed seroconversion during secondary syphilis,[175] impaired response to penicillin therapy,[176] a serofast state with prolonged elevation of titers of serologic tests for syphilis,[177] and accelerated development of neurologic syphilis (also see Ch. 215).[172,173] The neurologic manifestations of syphilis seen in patients with HIV infection most commonly are meningitis, optic neuritis, and asymptomatic positive CSF Venereal Disease Research Laboratory (VDRL) tests. Whether these findings represent advanced neurosyphilis is controversial. Nonetheless, because the behavior of syphilis in patients with HIV infection is distinctly different than in other populations, more extensive treatment regimens are recommended (see Ch. 215).[178]

Musculoskeletal Complications

Polymyositis complicates HIV infection in a small number of patients.[179] Clinical features include myalgias, weakness of the proximal muscles, muscle tenderness, wasting, and fatigue. Creatinine kinase and other muscle enzyme concentrations are usually elevated, and electrophysiologic studies are consistent with a myopathy.[180] The nucleoside analog antiretroviral agents are associated with myopathy in a small proportion of patients taking these drugs. The mechanism of this toxicity is inhibition of mitochondrial DNA, similar to the situation with neuropathy.[181]

Pyomyositis has been reported in patients with advanced HIV. Skin flora, particularly *Staphylococcus aureus,* are usually recovered from wound cultures, and preexisting skin diseases such as prurigo nodularis are a risk factor.[182]

Although rheumatologic findings in patients with HIV disease are not unusual, the extent to which HIV infection is associated with these disorders is not always clear. Defining a specific arthropathy caused by HIV is difficult because many patients with HIV infection are already at increased risk for inflammatory joint disease. Injection drug users, for example, may develop septic arthritis caused by pyogenic bacteria, particularly *S. aureus*. Homosexual men may have increased risk for gonococcal arthritis or postinfectious reactive arthritis associated with genital or GI tract infections (Reiter syndrome). Immune complex deposition related to hepatitis B infection may also be associated with arthritis in patients with HIV infection. Thus, while some animal retroviruses are clearly associated with arthropathies, the situation with HIV remains somewhat clouded.

In one prospective study of HIV seropositive homosexual men and seronegative controls, the incidence of Reiter syndrome and other arthropathies was similar in both groups.[183] The clinical course of Reiter syndrome in HIV-infected persons may be prolonged and severe, however.[184] Patients with this syndrome are usually HLA-B27-positive and present with an asymmetric oligoarticular arthritis and sacroiliitis with a variety of extra-articular signs and symptoms. Aspiration of synovial fluid is generally unremarkable, and synovial biopsy specimens show mononuclear cell infiltrates. Management is complex, as response to nonsteroidal anti-inflammatory drugs is limited, and the use of steroids will contribute to increased risk of opportunistic infections.

Cutaneous Manifestations

Dermatologic consequences of HIV infection include primary cutaneous opportunistic infections and malignancies (that may also disseminate to the viscera) and systemic, opportunistic diseases with skin involvement.

Viral Infections of the Skin and Mucous Membranes. A wide range of viruses involve the skin in HIV-immunosuppressed patients. Herpes simplex viruses (see Ch. 115) in particular cause frequent morbidity in patients with advanced HIV disease.[185] Serology documents previous infection with HSV-2 in more than 90 percent of homosexual men with HIV infection; it is less prevalent in other groups. Although HSV-2 recurs frequently even in nonimmunosuppressed hosts, it recurs more frequently and for prolonged periods in patients with HIV infection. HSV-2, a common pathogen of the sacral root dermatomes, often causes outbreaks in the buttocks, perineum, scrotum or vulva, and the shaft and glans of the penis. Characteristic lesions of herpes appear first as painful erythematous papules; later they vesiculate and ulcerate, and in superinfection, pustules may form. Chronic ulcers may become granulated and bloody. Herpes proctitis is associated with severe rectal pain, fever, tenesmus, and obstipation. External lesions may be absent, and the diagnosis is established by anoscopic or sigmoidoscopic examination and cultures. Giant perirectal ulcers and lesions at other sites that yield thymidine kinase-resistant strains of HSV-2 have been reported in patients who were previously treated with acyclovir.[187–189] Herpes simplex virus infections are diagnosed by the typical appearance and distribution of the lesions and culture. Tzanck preparations may show giant cells, which suggests HSV infection. Some physicians base their diagnoses on how patients respond to an empirical trial of acyclovir. Orolabial HSV infections in HIV-infected persons may be caused by either HSV-1 or HSV-2. Although primary infections may occur after patients acquire HIV, recurrences are more common. Often, a prodrome of tingling and pain precedes the appearance of painful vesicles and ulcers. Lesions may be found on the lips, buccal mucosa, gingiva, soft palate, uvula, and tongue. Herpes simplex virus disease may recur chronically in patients with advanced immunosuppression.

In persons with HIV infection varicella-zoster virus (shingles) often reactivates[186] (see Ch. 116). Herpes zoster may occur early in the course of HIV infection but the incidence in late HIV disease is 5–10 percent annually.[69,70,190–192] Dermatomal outbreaks are most common, and a substantial proportion of patients may have several dermatomes involved. Shingles is often characterized by radicular pain and itching several days before erythematous papules appear, and vesiculation occurs within several days. Lesions are often extremely pruritic, and excoriation with secondary bacterial infection commonly occurs. Over a period of 4–7 days, lesions form bullae and crusts and begin to heal, although some patients have zoster chronically. Cranial and thoracic dermatomes, followed by lumbar and sacral roots, are most often involved. Outbreaks along the ophthalmic branch of the trigeminal nerve may result in corneal involvement and lead to scarring and opacification that impair vision. Varicella-zoster virus appears to disseminate less often in patients with HIV infection than in other immunosuppressed patients. A substantial proportion of patients may experience post-herpetic scarring and pain. Although considered extremely rare before AIDS, recurrences of herpes zoster have been reported from a number of patients with HIV infection. Chronic or nonremitting herpes zoster has also been observed. In patients with HIV infection who acquire primary varicella (chicken pox), the acute infection may progress to a chronic form in a period of weeks to months.

Molluscum contagiosum, a cutaneous poxvirus infection, is seen more often in HIV-infected persons than in other populations. The agent is transmitted by sexual or other close contact; reactivation of remote infection may cause outbreaks in immunosuppressed hosts. Molluscum lesions are small, firm papules with a pearly white surface distributed on the face, trunk, or genital areas. The lesions are usually painless and can be differentiated from herpetic lesions by the absence of erythema and the smaller size and resolution of lesions without ulcerating or crusting. Molluscum lesions can become superinfected with bacteria if they become excoriated, but otherwise they do not cause complications. Liquid nitrogen is used effectively to treat this condition.

Bacillary Angiomatosis.   A recently described infection, bacillary angiomatosis, is associated with cutaneous and visceral involvement that produces lesions characterized by vascular proliferation, hemorrhage, and necrosis.[193-196] The disease was first described in 1983 in an AIDS patient with subcutaneous nodules with vascular proliferation and evidence of bacterial involvement by electron microscopy.[197] Subsequently, the etiology of bacillary angiomatosis has been attributed to the organisms *Bartonella (Rochalimaea) henselae* and *B. quintana* (see Ch. 170). Identification of *Bartonella (Rochalimaea)* by amplification of 16S RNA by polymerase chain reaction has been accomplished by several groups, and the organisms have been cultured from skin lesions, blood, liver, bone, and other sites.[193-196]

Bacillary angiomatosis usually presents as one or several cutaneous lesions, although disseminated disease is common.[198] The typical skin lesions are nodules or plaques that are erythematous and friable. Lesions may be mistaken for cutaneous KS, skin tags, or basal cell carcinomas. Visceral disease may include hepatitis (bacillary peliosis), osseous lesions, bacillemia, pneumonitis, or, less often, involvement of other organs.[199] Bacillary peliosis is a characteristic illness that presents with fever, right upper quadrant pain, hepatomegaly, and elevation of liver enzymes, particularly alkaline phosphatase. Imaging studies of the liver may reveal echogenic defects; histologically lesions have a cystic appearance, with vascular proliferation, hemorrhage, and necrosis.

The diagnosis of bacillary angiomatosis is best made by biopsy of involved sites. Hematoxylin and eosin stains of biopsies from skin lesions show proliferation of small blood vessels in the dermis or cutis, enlarged endothelial cells with abundant cytoplasm, and necrotic and granulomatous changes. Warthin-Starry stains show perivascular accumulations of bacilli; these findings may be confirmed by electron microscopy, although this is not usually necessary. The diagnosis can also be established by culture of the organism in several special media, or by detection of *Bartonella (Rochalimaea)* DNA by polymerase chain reaction. Serologic assays for anti-*Bartonella* antibodies are available through the Special Pathogens Branch of the CDC. The natural history of the infection in the patient with HIV infection is for disease to relapse in the absence of prolonged therapy with erythromycin or doxycycline.

Other Cutaneous Manifestations.   A variety of other skin disorders have been described in HIV-infected patients. Seborrheic dermatitis, an inflammatory condition of sebaceous glands that may be associated with dermatophytic superinfection, is an early complication. Erythema and scaling of midline areas of the forehead, face, and groin are typical findings. Tinea infections of the scalp, trunk, inguinal and perineal areas, extremities, and feet are also quite common. Onychomycosis, or fungal infections of the fingernails and toenails, are common, although usually asymptomatic, causing only cosmetic difficulty. Bacterial folliculitis may be localized or disseminated in patients with HIV infection, and the condition frequently relapses. Eosinophilic folliculitis is an inflammatory condition associated with raised, pruritic nodules with a pustular head on an erythematous base, similar to bacterial folliculitis. Biopsy specimens of these lesions reveal intense infiltration of eosinophils and an absence of polymorphonuclear cells and organisms. Xerosis and ichthyosis are also very common in patients with more advanced HIV disease, and may be refractory to therapy with emollients and anti-inflammatory agents.

Gastrointestinal Syndromes

As HIV infection progresses, diseases of the GI tract occur with greater frequency. Besides opportunistic disease resulting from HIV-induced immunodeficiency, persons with HIV disease may have more common gastrointestinal problems exacerbated by advanced systemic illness. Therefore, clinicians evaluating gastrointestinal complaints in HIV-infected patients must consider conventional gut pathology.

Esophageal Disease.   Several specific agents cause esophageal pathology in HIV infection. Esophagitis secondary to infections by *Candida*, cytomegalovirus, and herpes simplex viruses are the most common opportunistic manifestations of HIV disease in the upper GI tract.[200-203] *Candida* esophagitis is a more common index to AIDS diagnosis in women in the United States than men, probably as a result of the lower incidence of KS in women.

Esophageal infections most commonly present with dysphagia or odynophagia, often associated with persistent or intermittent retrosternal pain, nausea, anorexia, and weight loss. The duration of symptoms may be brief or prolonged, and other manifestations of immunodeficiency often are present. In particular, the finding of oral candidiasis in a patient with odynophagia strongly suggests esophageal candidiasis.[204] While involvement of another anatomic site by a pathogen (e.g., cytomegalovirus retinitis) may suggest a secondary esophageal process with the same organism, multiple etiologies of diverse organ system disease in AIDS is remarkably common.

Evaluation of patients with symptoms of esophagitis begins with a careful physical examination. The finding of oropharyngeal candidiasis strongly suggests esophageal candidiasis, and physicians may elect a trial of antifungal therapy. If symptoms resolve, the diagnosis can be established empirically. In patients who do not have oral thrush or who fail to respond to empirical antifungal therapy, upper GI contrast radiography may show characteristic abnormalities that suggest a specific diagnosis. *Candida* esophagitis is associated with a classic pattern of diffuse ulcerations and plaques that creates a cobblestone appearance. Cytomegalovirus esophagitis frequently causes numerous, large, shallow ulcerations, although single ulcers are also reported. Herpes simplex infection of the esophagus usually produces multiple, deep ulcers. Patients with dysphagia or odynophagia are most likely to have candidal esophagitis, followed by cytomegalovirus and herpes simplex esophagitis. Other disorders, such as esophageal strictures, esophagotracheal fistulas, or malignancies, are far less common. More than one pathogen may be recovered. Aphthous ulcers and drug-induced ulcers may also be found. Esophageal endoscopy is a highly sensitive procedure to establish a diagnosis in patients with odynophagia or dysphagia and is generally preferred to radiologic studies. Friable cheesy plaques that may be easily removed with biopsy forceps are characteristic in candidal esophagitis, whereas diffuse erythematous ulcers are more common in viral esophagitis. Lesions should be biopsied and tissue sections prepared for histopathologic stains to identify viral inclusion bodies or invasive yeast forms. Cultures for fungi and viruses should also be obtained from biopsy specimens. The yield of endoscopy with biopsy and culture is extremely high; additional diagnostic maneuvers are not usually required. Additional pathology that may be found in evaluating esophageal symptoms in HIV-infected patients includes reflux esophagitis, achalasia, esophageal KS, lymphoma, carcinoma, or peptic ulcer disease.

Disorders of the Stomach, Small Bowel, and Hepatobiliary System.   As with esophageal diseases in HIV-infected patients, gastric disease may be opportunistic or may be unrelated to immunodeficiency. Common complaints include nausea, early satiety, anorexia, vomiting, hematemesis, and abdominal pain. Esophageal pathology may also involve the stomach. Cytomegalovirus gastritis has been described alone or associated with esophageal cytomegalovirus ulcers. Cytomegalovirus gastritis causes an intense inflammatory response, ulceration, enlargement of ruggal folds, and edema. Cytomegalovirus gastritis may appear on a radiograph to be a mass lesion engulfing the entire stomach. Gastric KS is a common complication of cutaneous

KS and is often asymptomatic.[205] The GI tract is the organ system most involved in visceral KS, and gastric lesions may occur in 25 percent of patients who undergo endoscopy. Occasionally, gastrointestinal KS may be associated with nausea, early satiety, severe pain, and gastrointestinal hemorrhage.

Definitive diagnoses of upper GI pathology may be made by endoscopic observation, biopsy, and culture. Kaposi sarcoma typically appears as a violet-blue submucosal mass without mucosal ulceration or bleeding. Biopsy of these lesions results in a histologic diagnosis in only about one-third of the cases—presumably because of the nonmucosal location of the tumor. When other KS lesions are histologically confirmed, observing characteristic lesions on endoscopy is sufficient to make a diagnosis. Gastric lymphomas are diagnosed by endoscopic biopsy with histologic and immunohistochemical stains. Like KS, AIDS-related lymphomas are almost always multifocal, so a biopsy of the most accessible lesion can establish a diagnosis. Gastric ulcers and mass lesions should be sent for viral culture, and standard histologic stains should be performed to identify viral inclusion bodies. *Mycobacterium avium* complex occasionally causes gastric disease in patients with advanced immunodeficiency and disseminated infection. Diagnosis is made by culture and acid-fast tissue stains.

Acalculous cholecystitis has been associated with both *Cryptosporidium* and cytomegalovirus infections.[206,207] The usual presentation is postprandial pain, fever, right upper quadrant pain and tenderness, and an elevated alkaline phosphatase level. Ultrasonography or CT may reveal typical findings of cholecystitis as well as thickened gallbladder wall and obliteration of the bladder lumen. On histologic study, Cryptosporidia have been seen in the gallbladder mucosa, as have cytomegalovirus inclusions.

Papillary stenosis and sclerosing cholangitis occur in AIDS patients who present with right upper quadrant pain and tenderness, fever, and an elevated alkaline phosphatase level.[208,209] Dilatation of intrahepatic and extrahepatic ducts is noted on ultrasonography, and papillary stricture is frequently observed. Schneiderman and coworkers reported that endoscopic retrograde cholangiopancreatography identified cholangitis, ductal sclerosis, isolated papillary stenosis, or a combination of these findings.[209] Papillary stenosis was associated with *Cryptosporidium* or cytomegalovirus in almost one-half of the cases. Jacobson et al. found that 12 of 36 patients with cytomegalovirus end-organ disease had cholestatic liver enzyme abnormalities, and one-third of those undergoing ultrasound had biliary dilatation.[210] A significantly higher proportion of AIDS patients with cytomegalovirus cultured from the blood have elevated liver enzymes than patients with negative blood cultures. Endoscopic sphincterotomy may significantly relieve pain and normalize the alkaline phosphatase level in patients with sclerosing cholangitis.

Enterocolitis. Small and large bowel infections and disease processes may cause symptoms in association with HIV infection. Table 9 lists the principal causes of lower GI tract disease in patients with AIDS. A variety of infectious agents may produce diarrhea, abdominal cramping, and pain, and they may be managed less readily by a host with HIV-induced immunosuppression. Before the AIDS epidemic, both symptomatic and asymptomatic GI infections were found to be prevalent in homosexual men. Asymptomatic carriage of some pathogens has also been observed in patients with HIV infection and AIDS.[211–213] The incidence of gastroenteritis in patients with HIV infection is high, and some specific infections (e.g., *Salmonella, Cryptosporidium, Isospora,* Cytomegalovirus, microsporidia) have been found to occur more frequently in AIDS patients.[214–218]

Small bowel infections generally produce bloating, nausea, cramping, and profuse diarrhea and may be associated with significant weight loss. Colitis and proctitis more often cause lower quadrant cramping and pain, urgency, tenesmus, and smaller, more frequent stools. Distinguishing small bowel infections and colitis clinically may be difficult, however, and some infections may cause a panenteritis. The differential diagnosis of enterocolitis includes bacteria (such as *Salmonella, Shigella, Campylobacter,* mycobacteria) protozoa (such as *Entamoeba histolytica, Giardia lamblia, Cryptosporidium, Isospora*), and viruses, including cytomegalovirus. In addition, *Clostridium difficile*-associated colitis may be more common in patients with HIV disease, particularly in those who have previously received antimicrobial therapy.

A number of studies have attempted to delineate the microbiology of diarrheal disease in patients with HIV infection or AIDS. Studies that include control groups of individuals without diarrhea or without HIV infection indicate that a number of potential pathogens may be recovered from the stools of individuals who are not symptomatic. Whether organisms recovered with similar frequency from asymptomatic and symptomatic patients (e.g., *Blastocystis hominis*) are agents of disease remains controversial.

The common bacterial pathogens associated with enterocolitis in patients with HIV disease are presented in Table 9. These include *Salmonella* spp., *Shigella, Campylobacter jejunii, C. fennellae,* and enterotoxigenic *E. coli. Clostridium difficile*-toxin-associated diarrhea is also common. Small bowel overgrowth has been reported in some patients and appears to be more common in those with hypochlorhydria. Salmonellosis is bacteremic in up to one-half of cases and enteric symptoms may be minimal. Bacteremia with *Shigella* and *Campylobacter* has also been reported.[219,220] Less common bacterial causes of diarrhea include *Aeromonas, Pleisomonas, Yersinia,* and *Vibrio* spp. As noted previously, mycobacterial infection of the small bowel, usually with *M. avium* complex, is more frequent in late-stage HIV disease.

Parasites associated with diarrhea in patients with HIV include *Cryptosporidia, Giardia, Isospora, Entamoeba histolytica,* and the microsporidia. Although *Giardia* and amebic infections may occur throughout the spectrum of HIV infection and are more commonly associated with conventional risk factors for diarrhea (sexual practices, travel), cryptosporidiosis and microsporidiosis are late complications of HIV disease. Several reports of diarrhea associated with cyclospora have also appeared.[221]

The most common viral cause of diarrhea is cytomegalovirus, which causes a painful colitis in late-stage HIV disease. Symptoms include small volume diarrhea, cramping and bloating, pain, fever, and, often, tenesmus. Severe cytomegalovirus colitis may result in perforation of the colon.[222] Cytomegalovirus has also been reported to cause appendicitis in patients with HIV infection.[223] Other viruses that have been implicated as agents of diarrhea include astrovirus, adenovirus, calicivirus, and picobirnavirus.[212]

TABLE 9. Lower Gastrointestinal Tract Disease in Patients with HIV Infection

Causes of enterocolitis	Viruses
Bacteria	Cytomegalovirus
Campylobacter jejunii and other spp.	Adenovirus
Salmonella spp.	Astrovirus
Shigella flexnerii	Calicivirus
Aeromonas hydrophila	Picobirnavirus (?)
Vibrio spp.	HIV (?)
Mycobacterium avium complex	Fungi
M. tuberculosis	*Histoplasma capsulatum*
Clostridium difficile (toxin)	Causes of proctocolitis
Bacterial overgrowth	Bacteria
Enterotoxigenic *E. coli*	*Chlamydia trachomatis*
Parasites	*Neisseria gonorrhoeae*
Cryptosporidium spp.	*Treponema pallidum*
Isospora belli	Viral
Microsporidia	Herpes simplex
Entamoeba histolytica	Cytomegalovirus
Giardia lamblia	

Proctitis in patients with HIV disease may be the result of a conventional or opportunistic infection. Herpes simplex, *Chlamydia trachomatis,* syphilis, and gonorrhea are associated with proctitis in sexually active patients, particularly homosexual men.[224] Chronic and recurrent herpes simplex may cause proctitis in later stages of HIV disease. Cytomegalovirus proctitis is unusual, and is almost always seen in patients with colitis.

The evaluation of patients with HIV infection and diarrhea should be directed toward identifying treatable conditions. A careful assessment of symptoms, medications, travel, and other exposures is important. Initial studies should include stool bacterial cultures, *C. difficile* toxin assay, and several stool examinations for ova and parasites, including modified acid-fast stains for cryptosporidia and chromotrope stains for microsporidia.[224a] If the results of these studies are negative and symptoms persist, endoscopic evaluation with biopsies may prove useful.[225] For patients with predominantly lower GI signs and symptoms, colonoscopy should be performed first and biopsies obtained. The yield of colonoscopy for cytomegalovirus colitis is high (>95 percent). Upper GI endoscopy with duodenal biopsy is performed for patients with symptoms suggesting small bowel disease or those whose previous evaluation is unrevealing. Stains for acid-fast organisms, yeast, and parasites should be performed in addition to standard histologic studies. Electron microscopy is extremely sensitive for identifying microsporidia.

Between 15 and 50 percent of patients with HIV disease and diarrhea will have a negative evaluation. These patients are often considered to have an AIDS-associated enteropathy, the etiology of which is not fully understood. Histologic findings on small bowel biopsy typically reveal an increased ratio of villi to crypts without inflammation or lymphocytic infiltration. As additional agents of disease are identified and diagnostic technology improves, the proportion of patients diagnosed with AIDS enteropathy may decrease.

Renal Disease

A number of renal abnormalities have been described in patients with HIV infection, including a specific HIV-related nephropathy.[226] Ascribing renal dysfunction to HIV infection is problematic, however, because some patients with HIV have a high risk for renal disease from other causes. Intravenous drug use, hepatitis B infection, hypertension, fluid and electrolyte disorders, therapy with nephrotoxic drugs, and concomitant opportunistic infections and malignancies are all associated with renal dysfunction. In 1984, Rao and colleagues reported on 11 AIDS patients who had renal disease.[226] The patients were characterized clinically by proteinuria and mildly elevated serum creatinine levels and pathologically by focal and segmental glomerulosclerosis. Although this entity is similar to heroin-associated nephropathy, only one-half of the patients studied gave a history of iv drug use. In a review of 75 consecutive AIDS patients in Miami, 43 percent of the patients had proteinuria greater than 0.5 g/24 hr; 9 percent had greater than 3 g/24 hr.[227] In 36 autopsied patients, 17 (47 percent) had renal pathology, 5 had focal glomerulosclerosis, and 12 had mesangial proliferation. A subsequent review of the same patient population found that patients with a history of iv drug use had the highest incidence of renal disease; however, other non-drug-using patients, including children, may develop HIV-related nephropathy. In another series of patients, renal disease was observed in 13 of 32 patients and included focal glomerulosclerosis, mesangial proliferation, and glomerulonephritis.[228] HIV-related nephropathy is more commonly reported in blacks than in other racial groups, which suggests a biologic susceptibility to this disorder. Further prospective studies of how HIV-seropositive individuals develop renal disease are needed.

Renal dysfunction in patients with HIV disease is usually diagnosed incidentally when patients present with opportunistic infections and have CD4 cell counts less than 200/mm^3.[229]

Asymptomatic proteinuria, up to 5 g/day, is often the initial finding, and the serum creatinine level is often normal or only mildly elevated. The albumin concentration is almost always low (as is true for most AIDS patients with opportunistic infections), and the blood pressure is usually normal. Renal biopsy most often shows focal and segmental glomerulosclerosis with tubular dilatation and atrophy, fibrosis, and a mononuclear cell infiltrate. Immunofluorescence studies often reveal deposits of IgM and C3, and electron microscopy shows electron-dense mesangial deposits and mesangial hypocellularity.

The clinical course of HIV-related nephropathy progresses quickly, usually because many other opportunistic processes occur simultaneously. Rao et al.[226] originally reported death with renal failure in 8 of 11 patients with HIV-related nephropathy in less than 4 months. Because nephropathy is diagnosed late in the course of HIV disease, it is difficult to determine the effect of renal dysfunction on survival. Some centers have reported that patients with AIDS responded poorly to maintenance by hemodialysis.[230] Activating the cellular immune system through chronic dialysis may accelerate HIV pathology. On the other hand, AIDS patients who have acute renal failure from a reversible insult (such as hypertension or nephrotoxic drugs) respond to conservative measures and the brief use of hemodialysis.

Pulmonary Disease

Opportunistic pulmonary disease remains an important cause of acute illness and death in patients with advanced HIV disease. The clinical spectrum of pulmonary disease is broad, and geographic and temporal variations in the etiology of respiratory illnesses in HIV-infected patients are important. For example, although *P. carinii* pneumonia (PCP) has been the most common AIDS-indicator illness in the United States and other developed countries, accounting for more than 50 percent of all AIDS diagnoses, the disease is much less prevalent in developing countries.[231] In addition, the widespread use of primary prophylaxis for the prevention of PCP in the United States has resulted in a marked decline in the prevalence of this illness in newly diagnosed AIDS patients.[54] Although PCP was reported as the index diagnosis in two-thirds of AIDS patients in the United States in 1985–1988, less than one-half of AIDS patients reported in 1991–1992 had this diagnosis. In the Multicenter AIDS Cohort Study, the incidence of *P. carinii* pneumonia as an initial AIDS diagnosis peaked in 1987 and has declined since then, while other opportunistic infections have become more common (Fig. 4).[74] Bacterial pneumonia has emerged as an important cause of pulmonary morbidity in recent years, as a growing number of patients have risk factors for bacterial infections, including injection drug use and smoking cigarettes and other drugs.[232] As the proportion of HIV-infected people who are also infected with *M. tuberculosis* increases, particularly in developing countries, the incidence of HIV-associated tuberculosis is growing rapidly.[233]

The multiple etiologies of pulmonary disease in patients with HIV infection are listed in Table 10. The differential diagnosis of respiratory complaints in an HIV-seropositive patient is quite extensive. Patients with known or suspected HIV infection who present with pulmonary symptoms should be expeditiously evaluated with reliable diagnostic procedures to achieve a specific diagnosis so that therapy can be initiated as soon as possible. Empirical antimicrobial therapy is often appropriate while the diagnostic evaluation proceeds.

A clinical history is extremely important in evaluating patients who may have AIDS-related pulmonary disease. Information about the patient's CD4 cell level, use of prophylaxis, exposure to tuberculosis, cigarette smoking, and prior respiratory disease should be elicited. Clinical symptoms may also help distinguish etiologic differences between patients. In patients with HIV infection (as opposed to other immunocompromised hosts), PCP

TABLE 10. Pulmonary Complications of HIV Infection

Bacteria	Coccidioides immitis
Mycobacterium tuberculosis	Aspergillus fumigatus
M. kansasii	Penicillium marneffei
M. avium complex	Blastomyces dermatitidis
Streptococcus pneumoniae	(Candida albicans)
Haemophilus influenzae	Protozoa
Group A Streptococcus	Toxoplasma gondii
Staphylococcus aureus	Cryptosporidium spp.
Moraxella catarrhalis	Microsporidia
Pseudomonas aeruginosa	Viruses
Enterobacteriaceae	Cytomegalovirus
Nocardia asteroides	Herpes simplex
Legionella pneumophila	Adenovirus
Rhodococcus equi	HIV (?)
Fungi	Tumors
Pneumocystis carinii	Kaposi sarcoma
Cryptococcus neoformans	Non-Hodgkin's lymphoma
Histoplasma capsulatum	Lymphocytic interstitial pneumonitis (children)

often has an insidious onset.[234] A constitutional prodrome of fevers, night sweats, weight loss, and oral candidiasis for weeks may be followed by increasing respiratory distress—with shortness of breath at first on exertion and finally dyspnea at rest. Approximately 80 percent of patients with PCP note a dry cough, and may report retrosternal irritation on deep breathing. About 5–10 percent of patients with PCP may initially deny respiratory symptoms. These same symptoms may occur in patients with other pulmonary pathogens. Bacterial pneumonias in HIV-seropositive individuals tend to have a more abrupt and severe onset. A productive cough is more likely, although many patients with pyogenic pneumonia do not produce sputum. Seventy percent of patients with bacterial pneumonia report pleuritic chest pain (uncommon in PCP), and most have a fever, a productive cough, and progressive dyspnea. Patients with cryptococcal pneumonitis generally have disseminated disease and may have a paucity of pulmonary complaints.

Tuberculosis in HIV-seropositive patients most often presents as pulmonary disease and often has an accelerated clinical course.[235–240] In patients with advanced immunodeficiency, tuberculosis may be disseminated and may present as a systemic illness with minimal pulmonary symptomatology. Pulmonary Kaposi sarcoma may be a primary lesion but most commonly occurs in patients with extensive disease elsewhere. Respiratory symptoms tend to progress slowly at first, and constitutional symptoms may be minimal. Upper respiratory tract infections are common in AIDS patients and are most often remarkable for pronounced cough without dyspnea.

A variety of upper respiratory tract symptoms and signs may be elicited. Rales are often detected in patients with PCP and other opportunistic infections. Bacterial pneumonias tend to be focal and may result in localized findings of consolidation on auscultation. Pulmonary KS is frequently associated with pleural effusions that are detected by dullness to percussion and diminished breath sounds at the lung bases. Many patients will have normal chest examination findings despite the presence of active pulmonary infection or malignancy. Physical examination may be of limited value to establish a specific diagnosis, and all patients with respiratory symptoms should undergo further diagnostic work-up as outlined below.

Figure 7 shows the diagnostic algorithm employed in the authors' institutions to evaluate patients with suspected AIDS-related pulmonary disease. The protocol has proved to be efficient, cost-effective, and reliable in expeditiously diagnosing both hospitalized and ambulatory patients. A chest radiograph is performed initially and used to guide the work up. Common radiographic patterns associated with diseases in HIV-infected patients are listed in Table 11. When the chest x-ray is normal, noninvasive tests may be used to determine the likelihood of pneumonitis. Among the screening tests with good sensitivity for serious pulmonary pathology (≥90 percent sensitive) are diffusing capacity for carbon monoxide (<80 percent predicted),

gallium lung scanning (any uptake is abnormal), and exercise oximetry (≥5 percent decline in oxygen saturation).[241] When noninvasive tests and the chest film are normal, alternative sources of symptoms should be considered. If these nonspecific tests suggest pneumonitis, however, specific microbiologic studies should be pursued.

Examination of induced sputum is now widely used initially to identify *P. carinii* and other pathogens, including mycobacteria. Specimens should be collected and processed properly, and well-trained laboratory personnel should review stained specimens to identify organisms. A number of reagents may be used to stain *P. carinii*. Modified Giemsa stain (Dif-Quik), silver methenamine, and toluidine blue O, all have sensitivities of 70–80 percent in experienced laboratories. Use of monoclonal antibody-based immunofluorescence assays increases sensitivity to 90 percent.[242,243] Obtaining a second sample of induced sputum increases the yield only slightly. A sample of sputum that is obviously purulent should have a Gram stain and bacterial culture, and antibacterial therapy is appropriate. Acid-fast bacilli (AFB) smears and mycobacterial cultures should be performed on all sputum specimens, even when *P. carinii* has been identified. The sensitivity of AFB smears for tuberculosis is only 50–60 percent, however. When AFB smears are positive, tuberculosis is likely, even in settings where *M. avium* complex is more prevalent than *M. tuberculosis*, as the former only rarely yields AFB smear positive sputum. The utility of fungal and viral cultures from induced sputum is marginal. *Candida* is frequently isolated, but is virtually never a cause of lower respiratory tract disease in HIV-infected patients. Antigen detection tests and blood cultures are more sensitive than sputum cultures for diagnosing pulmonary cryptococcosis or histoplasmosis.[244,245] Cytomegalovirus is frequently isolated from pulmonary specimens but is only very rarely a cause of symptomatic lung disease.[246,247]

Because the negative predictive value of sputum induction is no more than 60 percent, patients who do not have a pathogen identified by this method should undergo a bronchoscopic procedure to establish a diagnosis. Fiber-optic bronchoscopy is an effective, low-morbidity procedure that has a high yield for diagnosing pulmonary pathogens in patients with HIV infection.[248,249] The combination of bronchoalveolar lavage (BAL) and transbronchial biopsy has a diagnostic yield of more than 95 percent for all pathogens in AIDS patients, and its yield is 100 percent for *P. carinii*. Bronchoalveolar lavage alone has a sensitivity of 85–95 percent and can be performed safely in most patients with suspected PCP. When this procedure does not establish a diagnosis, a repeat bronchoscopic examination is performed, and BAL and transbronchial biopsies are done. Six biopsies of the right lower lobe are generally taken—again without fluoroscopic guidance—unless a focal abnormality is present on the chest radiograph. Fresh biopsy material is examined by touch imprints. Formalin-fixed specimens are stained with hematoxylin and eosin (H&E), Giemsa, acid-fast stains, and silver methenamine. Performance of transbronchial biopsy is not recommended for patients who require mechanical ventilation or have an uncorrectable coagulopathy, although BAL may be performed in such instances. Bronchoalveolar lavage can result in hypoxemia transiently after the procedure. A transbronchial biopsy results in pneumothorax in about 10 percent of patients, at least 50 percent of whom require tube thoracostomy for reexpansion.

Open lung biopsy (OLB) is generally restricted to several unusual circumstances in patients with HIV-related pulmonary disease. Rarely, a patient with progressive respiratory impairment will have a nondiagnostic sputum induction and bronchoscopy or will have a coagulopathy that contraindicates transbronchial biopsy. Such patients may benefit from OLB. Nodular or peripheral mass lesions may be successfully biopsied by the transthoracic route.

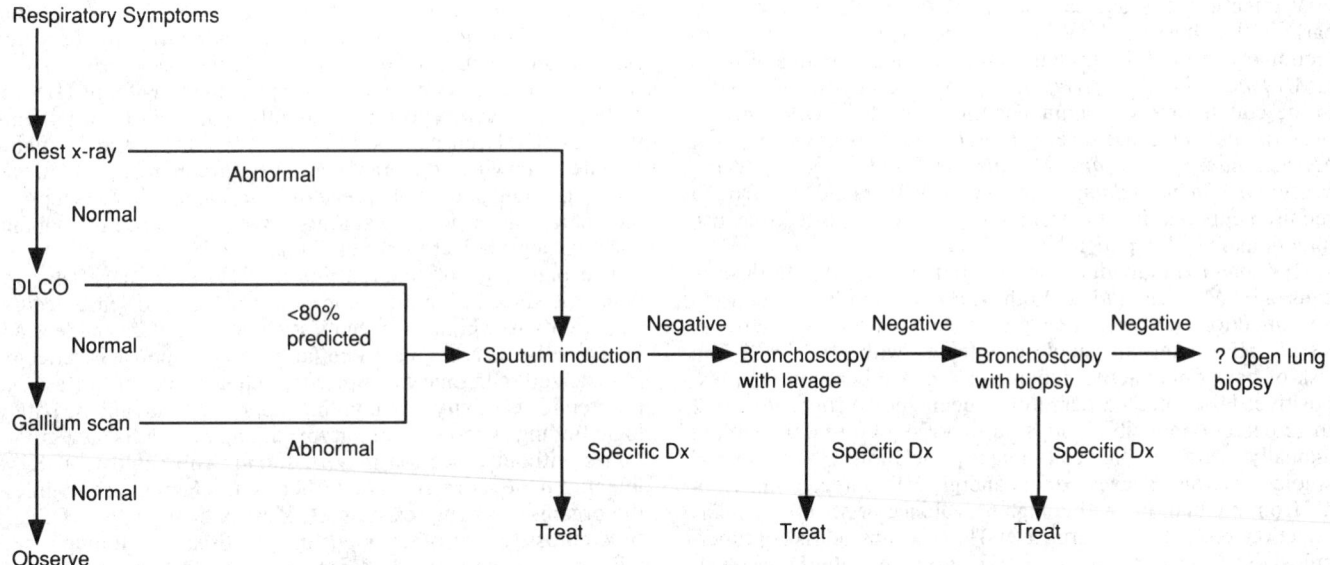

FIG. 7. Algorithm for evaluating pulmonary disease in patients with HIV infection.

TABLE 11. Chest Radiographic Findings in AIDS Patients with Respiratory Disease

CXR Pattern	Illnesses
Normal	No disease *Pneumocystis carinii* pneumonia Disseminated fungal infection
Focal infiltrate	Pyogenic pneumonia Tuberculosis Cryptococcal pneumonia *Pneumocystis carinii* pneumonia
Pleural effusion	Kaposi sarcoma Pyogenic pneumonia Tuberculosis
Mediastinal adenopathy	Tuberculosis/*Mycobacterium avium* complex Lymphoma
Interstitial infiltrate	*Pneumocystis carinii* pneumonitis Tuberculosis Lymphocytic interstitial pneumonia Nonspecific pneumonitis Pyogenic pneumonia

Specific Pathogens. PNEUMOCYSTIS CARINII. Infection with *P. carinii* is common early in life and does not generally result in symptomatic disease in immunocompetent basis (also see Ch. 258). Patients with HIV infection develop disease caused by *P. carinii* very frequently—principally an intra-alveolar pneumonitis. *Pneumocystis carinii* pneumonia often presents as a slowly progressive pneumonitis associated with fever, sweats, weight loss, increasing cough, and dyspnea. Kovacs and colleagues compared patients with AIDS-related PCP with patients with PCP and other types of immunodeficiency.[234] The median duration of symptoms was prolonged in the AIDS group (28 vs. 5 days in non-AIDS patients), and AIDS patients with PCP tended to have less fever, a lower respiratory rate, and a higher arterial PO$_2$. Similar studies by other authors have confirmed the difference between AIDS and non-AIDS PCP. The longer prodrome of PCP in AIDS patients may reflect a different host response to *P. carinii*.

Pathologically, PCP causes air space consolidation because a protein-rich exudate consisting of numerous *P. carinii* trophozoites fills the aveoli and causes intrapulmonary right-to-left shunting and arterial hypoxemia. Alveolar membranes become thickened, and parenchymal inflammation, edema, and fibrosis occur. Patients with advanced PCP may have what physiologically appears to be the adult respiratory distress syndrome. Alveolar capillaries leak solutes into the air spaces, pulmonary fluids increase and worsen the shunting of pulmonary capillary blood flow, and arterial hypoxemia increases. Hughes has proposed a histopathologic staging system for PCP in adults that reflects the natural progression of pneumonitis caused by the organism.[250] In stage 1 (early infection), scattered *P. carinii* cysts can be seen in the alveolar wall, but no inflammatory response is evident. Neither autopsy nor biopsy materials for asymptomatic HIV-infected patients have demonstrated that this stage of the disease is common before patients develop symptomatic PCP. Stage 2 is marked by an increase in the number of *P. carinii* cysts in the alveolar wall, alveolar septal inflammation, and desquamation of alveolar cells into the lumen. In addition, *P. carinii* trophozoites can be seen by electron microscopy. In stage 3, alveolar hypertrophy occurs along with a mononuclear cell infiltration and extensive alveolar desquamation; numerous *P. carinii* cysts and trophozoites are found in pulmonary macrophages. After acute PCP is resolved, *P. carinii* cysts or trophozoites may be found in up to 60 percent of patients, although it is not known whether the organisms are viable. Over time the recovery of *P. carinii* declines. Alveolar hypertrophy, interstitial fibrosis, and nonspecific inflammation may be found on biopsy or at autopsy. Approximately 10–20 percent of patients with an initial episode of PCP die acutely and mortality with subsequent episodes is similar. Early mortality can be predicted by the severity of disease on both clinical grounds and histopathologic findings when the lungs are biopsied.[251] Patients with more extensive edema, fibrosis, and inflammation (stage 3 disease) have a significantly higher mortality rate than do those with less severe disease. Consequently, earlier diagnosis and treatment may improve survival of the first episode of PCP. Patients dying of respiratory failure due to PCP are frequently found to have additional pathogens in the lungs at autopsy (most commonly cytomegalovirus), but how other infections contribute to the morbidity of PCP is not yet known.

Although most patients with disease caused by *P. carinii* appear to have pneumonitis alone, extrapulmonary pneumocystosis occurs occasionally, particularly in patients receiving aerosol pentamidine prophylactic therapy.[252–254] *Pneumocystis carinii* has been identified in specimens obtained from the middle ear, mastoid, retina, liver, lymph nodes, spleen, and bone marrow. More extensive extrapulmonary dissemination has been reported in patients without HIV infection.

MYCOBACTERIA. Both tuberculosis and atypical mycobacterial disease (see Chs. 230, 233) are common manifestations of

HIV infection. Disease caused by *M. tuberculosis* may occur early in the course of HIV-induced immunosuppression.[255] Infections with the less virulent nontuberculous organisms such as *M. kansasii* and *M. avium* complex generally manifest later in the course of severe immunodeficiency.[256–258] Other mycobacteria that can cause disease in AIDS patients are *M. xenopi*, *M. chelonae*, *M. ulcerans*, *M. gordonae*, and *M. bovis*. *Mycobacterium haemophilum*, an organism with fastidious growth requirements that include iron, has also been reported to cause infections in AIDS patients (see Ch. 233).

HIV-infected individuals are uniquely susceptible to disease caused by *M. tuberculosis*. Both reactivation of latent tuberculous infection and accelerated progression of primary tuberculosis are more likely in people co-infected with HIV.[240,259] The risk of developing active tuberculosis in a tuberculin skin test positive, HIV-infected person has been shown to vary from 2 to 12 percent annually, compared to a risk of 0 to 0.02 percent annually for immunologically intact populations.[259–261] Several studies have also suggested that anergic HIV-infected individuals from populations with a high prevalence of *M. tuberculosis* infection (e.g., injection drug users) have an annual risk of tuberculosis of 6–15 percent.[261,262] HIV-infected, tuberculin-negative, nonanergic patients from the same population also have an elevated risk of tuberculosis, albeit lower than anergic persons.

Acceleration of the early natural history of tuberculosis infection with progression to primary disease is a major clinical and public health problem in people with HIV infection. Daley and coworkers showed that 37 percent of HIV-infected injection drug users exposed in a household to an untreated patient with pulmonary tuberculosis developed active pulmonary tuberculosis with an identical organism within 4 months.[240] Other studies of nosocomial transmission of tuberculosis in HIV-infected patients have also documented the rapid progression of primary infection to active disease.[263,264]

The emergence of multidrug resistant (MDR) tuberculosis among patients with HIV infection has been particularly problematic, with epidemic transmission of infection leading to early disease in hospitals, prisons, and drug treatment centers.[265] Although tuberculosis drug resistance is not related to HIV infection, per se, the altered natural history of *M. tuberculosis* infection in persons with HIV infection has resulted in catastrophic consequences when MDR isolates are transmitted.[264–266] Because MDR tuberculosis is often refractory to treatment with second-line and experimental antituberculosis agents,[267] case fatality rates in HIV-infected patients are extremely high with death occurring within several months of diagnosis.[268]

Clinical features of tuberculosis in patients with HIV infection vary with the degree of immunosuppression and how recently *M. tuberculosis* infection was acquired. Most HIV-related tuberculosis is a result of reactivation of latent infection in individuals who become immunosuppressed from HIV infection. These patients may have tuberculosis months to years before the diagnosis of AIDS. The pattern of tuberculosis in these individuals is typical of the reactivation seen in other populations; characteristic pulmonary symptoms and clinical findings are the rule. Most patients (60–80 percent), despite moderately severe CD4 lymphopenia, respond to intradermal tuberculin. Chest radiographs show localized or diffuse lung abnormalities in half of the patients. Tuberculosis most commonly affects the pulmonary system, although 20–60 percent of patients may have extrapulmonary disease concomitantly. Tuberculosis is diagnosed by examining pulmonary specimens with stains for acid-fast organisms and by culture for mycobacteria. Clinicians should employ the diagnostic algorithm for pulmonary disease described above (Fig. 7). In patients with advanced HIV disease, tuberculosis may appear as a late opportunistic complication coinciding with or following other opportunistic diseases. Clinically, this type of tuberculosis often differs from reactivation tuberculosis. Constitutional symptoms are more pronounced; chest radiographic findings are usually atypical, with diffuse infiltrates and intratho-

racic adenopathy predominant; a response to tuberculin testing occurs at a rate of only 30–40 percent; and extrapulmonary dissemination is found in 50–70 percent of the cases. *Mycobacterium tuberculosis* bacteremia, rare in patients without HIV infection, has been reported frequently, particularly in patients with low CD4 cell counts.[269,270] The respiratory tract remains the site from which the organism is most frequently isolated and is an important source of spread of infection to other susceptible individuals, even when respiratory symptoms are minimal and chest radiographs are unremarkable.

The pathology of tuberculosis in HIV-infected persons reflects the stage of immunosuppression at which disease occurs. In patients in whom tuberculosis is reactivated during less advanced HIV disease, a brisk inflammatory response is reflected in localized pulmonary symptoms, radiographic infiltrates, and tuberculin reactivity. As immunosuppression advances, pathologic findings become more atypical, and poorly formed granulomas without caseation may be found. Tuberculosis in HIV-infected patients responds excellently to chemotherapy unless the organism is drug resistant.[237] Most patients with AIDS and tuberculosis die of other opportunistic diseases, although mortality may be as high as 10 percent in the first month of treatment. A recent study suggests that tuberculosis may enhance progression of HIV disease by upregulating viral replication through a tumor necrosis factor (TNF)-β-mediated mechanism.[271] Validation of this hypothesis is required, however.

Atypical or nontuberculous mycobacterial infections are an important complication of HIV-induced immunosuppression. In a study of nontuberculous mycobacterial infections in patients with AIDS reported to the CDC, 97 percent were caused by *M. avium* complex, and 3 percent were due to *M. kansasii*, *M. xenopi*, *M. gordonae*, and others.[272] Nontuberculous mycobacterial disease appears to be equally prevalent in males and females, in all age groups, and in different geographic regions. *Mycobacterium avium* complex, a common environmental saprophyte, may be acquired orally or inhaled. Environmental sources of *M. avium* complex include water, soil, vegetables, unpasteurized milk and milk products and, possibly, aerosols.[273] Because nontuberculous mycobacteria are distributed uniformly among different risk groups, the disease caused by *M. avium* complex is probably a new infection rather than a previous infection reactivated.

The incidence of disseminated *M. avium* complex disease increases as HIV disease progresses. In patients with CD4 cell counts less than 100/mm^3, the incidence of disease is 8–12 percent annually.[257,258] In patients with CD4 cell counts less than 10/mm^3, the 1-year incidence in one study was 39 percent.[258] Colonization of the lung and gut is an insensitive measure of risk in a population as most patients with *M. avium* complex bacteremia do not have detectable colonization.[274] Among those few patients with positive sputum or stool cultures, however, the risk of subsequent dissemination is increased three- to fourfold.

In AIDS patients, *M. avium* complex disease is characterized by continuous bacteremia, with as many as 10^4–10^5 colony-forming units per milliliter of blood. *Mycobacterium avium* complex can infect numerous organs: bone marrow, liver, spleen, gut, lymph nodes, lungs, skin, brain, adrenals, and kidneys. There is little histologic response despite relatively large numbers of organisms. Granulomas, when present, are usually poorly formed. Macrophages may be packed with organisms that have not been killed by antimicrobial therapy.

In patients with PCP, recovery of *M. avium* complex from pulmonary specimens is often an incidental finding, and most patients recover with anti-*Pneumocystis* therapy alone. A minority of patients may have respiratory tract disease caused by *M. avium* complex alone, an infection that results in diffuse pulmonary infiltrates, or nodules, arterial hypoxmia, and progressive respiratory deterioration.[275] Clinicians should evaluate patients carefully for other pulmonary pathogens before ascribing respiratory findings to *M. avium* complex.

Mycobacterium avium complex disease most commonly presents as a systemic illness with fevers, night sweats, fatigue, and weight loss. Gastrointestinal symptoms such as abdominal pain and persistent diarrhea are also often reported. Patients usually appear emaciated and have generalized lymphadenopathy and other findings associated with immunodeficiency (e.g., oral candidiasis). Abdominal examination may show diffuse tenderness and hepatosplenomegaly. Laboratory evaluation is usually nonspecific, although anemia and leukopenia are usually pronounced. Computed tomography scans of the abdomen may show marked hepatosplenomegaly and diffuse lymphadenopathy (often with central attenuation). The bowel wall is often thickened, which is consistent with an inflammatory colitis. Gallium scans may show intense colonic uptake. Biopsy or autopsy specimens of the small bowel and colon show acute and chronic inflammation and numerous AFB in the mucosa and submucosa. Concurrent infections with *Cryptosporidium,* cytomegalovirus, and other pathogens may be found. The small bowel may also be involved and result in a histologic appearance similar to Whipple's disease and the chronic diarrhea syndrome. *Mycobacterium avium* complex has been found in enlarged periportal lymph nodes in patients whose extrahepatic bile ducts were extrinsically obstructed. *Mycobacterium avium* complex has also been found in the adrenals of patients with acute adrenal insufficiency (although cytomegalovirus is most often associated with this clinical entity), in brain abscesses, and in bone biopsies of patients with osteomyelitis.

PYOGENIC BACTERIA. Infections with pyogenic bacteria occur more frequently in patients with HIV disease, particularly in children and IV drug users. The incidence of bacterial pneumonia, for example, is increased greatly in HIV-seropositive IV drug users when compared with seronegative controls.[232] Encapsulated bacteria (particularly *Streptococcus pneumoniae* and *Haemophilus influenzae*) are the most common pathogens. Table 12 lists bacteria that cause serious infections in HIV-infected persons.

In HIV-infected patients, bacterial infections involve primarily the skin, lungs, sinuses, and middle ear. Children appear to have a high prevalence of otitis media and pneumonia caused by *S. pneumoniae* and *H. influenzae*. In adults, pyogenic infections are manifested most commonly as skin and soft tissue infections, sinusitis, and pneumonia. Persistent impetigo, furunculosis, folliculitis, and skin abscesses occur in adults with HIV infection; streptococci and *Staphylococcus aureus* are usually responsible. In patients with HIV infection, sinusitis may be caused by *S. pneumoniae, H. influenzae* or other *Haemophilus* spp., *Moraxella catarrhalis, Pseudomonas aeruginosa,* or other organisms. The clinical presentation is often subacute; congestion, cough, and headache are the most prominent symptoms.[276,277] Sinus tenderness is uncommon, but sinus x-ray films frequently reveal sinus thickening and air-fluid levels within the paranasal sinuses. In more advanced HIV disease, sinusitis is more severe, with involvement of the maxillary, ethmoid, and sphenoid sinuses being more frequent, and relapse after therapy is common. Aspirating the sinus fluids may be both diagnostic and therapeutic.

Bacterial pneumonias (discussed earlier) and bacterial bronchitis present as clinically distinct from PCP. Bacterial pneumonia may occur more frequently in iv drug users, cigarette smokers, and children with HIV infection. Patients with bronchitis usually complain of a chronic cough with scant sputum production and minimal dyspnea. Evaluation reveals rhonchi or wheezes, and chest films are normal. Sputum gram staining may show polymorphonucleocytes (PMNs) and gram-positive diplococci or gram-negative coccobacillary organisms. Although bronchitis is rarely associated with bacteremia, bacterial pneumonias in AIDS patients are often bacteremic. Up to 80 percent of patients with *S. pneumoniae* pneumonia and 25 percent of patients with *H. influenzae* pneumonia have bacteremia. Infection may be more difficult to eradicate in these patients, and relapses after appropriate therapy are common.

Rhodococcus equi is a more unusual bacterial respiratory pathogen in patients with HIV. This pleomorphic gram-positive bacillus causes focal pneumonitis, often with cavitation, and may also cause empyema and bacteremia. Recurrence after therapy is not uncommon. Other bacterial pathogens that are less often associated with pulmonary or disseminated disease in patients with HIV infection include *Nocardia, Legionella,* group A β-hemolytic *Streptococcus,* and *Salmonella.*

Bacteremia occurs more frequently in patients with advanced HIV disease. Risk factors include injection drug use, skin and soft tissue infections, pneumonia, and central venous catheters. Catheter-related sepsis is highly prevalent in AIDS patients, particularly those with central venous lines who are receiving intravenous therapy at home. The organisms responsible for catheter-related sepsis are predominantly *S. aureus* or *epidermidis, P. aeruginosa,* and other gram-negative bacilli. Why the risk of infection increases is not known. AIDS patients may be more likely to employ inadequate hygienic techniques than are other patient groups with indwelling venous catheters, and host mechanisms that control integumental defense may be impaired. Patients with HIV infection who have a central venous catheter should receive careful instructions on how to control infection, adequate nursing supervision, and medical follow-up.

Fungi. Fungi are a less frequent cause of pulmonary disease in patients with HIV infection than in other immunocompromised hosts. In particular, although *C. albicans* is recovered from a high proportion of respiratory secretions in patients with HIV and pulmonary symptoms, pulmonary candidal disease is distinctly uncommon. Pulmonary cryptococcosis complicates cryptococcal meningitis in approximately 20 percent of cases and isolated pneumonitis may occur in up to 5 percent of all cases of disease due to *C. neoformans*.[244] Respiratory symptoms may be mild to severe, and constitutional symptoms are often more pronounced. Radiographic manifestations include focal and diffuse infiltrates, nodules, cavitation, adenopathy, and pleural effusions. The diagnosis is established by identification of the polysaccharide cryptococcal antigen in blood, CSF, or respiratory secretions and isolation of the organism by culture (also see Ch. 243).

Histoplasma capsulatum (see Ch. 244) is an important cause of pulmonary and disseminated disease in patients in endemic areas, including the Ohio River valley and south-central United States, the Caribbean, and Latin America.[245,278] Most patients with HIV infection and histoplasmosis have disseminated disease, although one-half have pulmonary involvement. The most common radiographic presentation of pulmonary histoplasmosis is diffuse interstitial infiltrates, with nodular infiltrates and focal

TABLE 12. Bacteria Causing Serious Infections in Patients with HIV Infection

	Organism	Site(s) of Disease
Gram-positive	*Streptococcus pneumoniae*	Lung, sinuses, blood
	Streptococcus spp.	Lung
	Staphylococcus aureus	Skin, blood, lung, perineum
	Listeria monocytogenes	Meninges, blood
	Nocardia asteroides	Lung, brain
	Rhodococcus equi	Lung, blood
Gram-negative	*Haemophilus influenzae*	Lung, blood
	Haemophilus spp.	Lung
	Moraxella catarrhalis	Lung
	Salmonella spp.	Gut, blood, brain
	Shigella spp.	Gut
	Campylobacter spp.	Gut
	Legionella pneumophila	Lung
	Bartonella (Rochalimaea)	Skin, blood, liver, spleen, bone
Spirochetes	*Treponema pallidum*	Skin, meninges, brain

disease being less frequent. Extrapulmonary histoplasmosis usually presents with severe constitutional symptoms such as fever, night sweats, weight loss, diarrhea, and delirium. In addition to fungemia, patients may have organisms in liver, spleen, bone marrow, gut, and central nervous system. Neurologic involvement occurs in 5–20 percent of patients. Many patients have mucocutaneous ulcers or papular lesions that may be mistaken for molluscum contagiosum or other viral eruptions. Up to 10 percent of patients may have a sepsis syndrome, with fever, hypotension, coagulopathy, and multiorgan system failure. The diagnosis is established by culturing the organisms from blood or other tissue. Histoplasma polysaccharide antigen testing of blood or urine is highly sensitive and specific, although this test is not available in commercial laboratories.[279] Complement fixation or immunodiffusion serologic assays are less sensitive and specific than the antigen assay and are not generally used.

Pulmonary invasive aspergillosis (see Ch. 238) has been described as a late complication of HIV disease in several series of patients.[280,281] Predisposing risk factors such as neutropenia and corticosteroid use appear to be less prevalent in AIDS patients with aspergillosis than in other populations. The clinical presentation may be a chronic, progressive cavitary pneumonitis or obstructive bronchial disease. Pleural-based disease and nodular pulmonary disease have also been described. The diagnosis should be based on histologic findings as well as culture.

Coccidioidomycosis develops in up to 10 percent of HIV-positive individuals in endemic areas for that fungal infection (see Ch. 246). Illness appears to be a mix of new and reactivated infection. Diffuse pulmonary disease and dissemination are common.

Very uncommon fungal causes of pulmonary disease in patients with HIV infection include *Blastomyces dermatitidis* and *Penicillium marneffei*. Blastomycosis is extremely rare, even in endemic areas, but may cause focal pulmonary or disseminated disease. *Penicillium marneffei* has recently been reported as a common cause of disseminated disease in AIDS patients in Thailand.[282] Pulmonary involvement occurs in about one-fourth of patients, with diffuse or focal infiltrates.

Other Organisms. Respiratory disease in patients with HIV infection is occasionally caused by *T. gondii* or *Cryptosporidium*. Cytomegalovirus is frequently isolated from the respiratory secretions of patients with other causes of pneumonitis, and the clinical importance of this finding is controversial.[246,247] Several large studies have shown that the recovery of cytomegalovirus from respiratory specimens of patients with *P. carinii* pneumonia does not influence the subsequent course of illness in the absence of specific therapy for cytomeglovirus. On rare occasions, cytomegalovirus itself can be considered to be a genuine pulmonary pathogen in patients with HIV infection who are severely immunosuppressed, have diffuse pulmonary infiltrates and arterial hypoxemia, and in whom other pathogens cannot be identified. In these circumstances, some authorities recommend anti-cytomegalovirus therapy, although the efficacy of treating cytomegalovirus pneumonitis in patients with HIV disease is unknown (also see Ch. 105).

Neurologic Complications

HIV is a neurotrophic virus with a variety of clinical manifestations in the central (CNS) and peripheral nervous systems. Numerous neurologic opportunistic infections occur in AIDS patients in addition to the direct, immunologic sequelae of HIV infection, so the neurologic complications of HIV infection can best be considered primary and secondary consequences. The

TABLE 13. Neurologic Complications of HIV Infection

Aseptic meningitis
Guillain-Barré syndrome
Chronic inflammatory demyelinating polyneuropathy
Multiple mononeuropathy
Peripheral predominantly sensory neuropathy
HIV encephalopathy
Vascular myelopathy
Opportunistic infections of CNS[a]
Neoplasms of CNS[a]

Abbreviation: CNS, central nervous system.
[a] See Table 14.

spectrum of neurologic complications of HIV infection is shown in Table 13.

Peripheral Neuropathy

In most patients with AIDS, the peripheral nervous system is involved, and 20–40 percent of patients may have symptomatic peripheral nerve disease. Symptoms may occur at any time during the course of HIV infection. The most common peripheral neuropathy, a distal, predominantly sensory polyneuropathy, accounts for most cases and is almost always a late complication of HIV disease.[283] Patients with this neuropathy usually complain of chronic, symmetric, painful dysesthesias in a stocking distribution, particularly in the soles; numbness; and (less often) weakness. Some patients feel pain when lightly touched. Sensory deficits, decreased or absent ankle jerks, and weakness may also be observed on examination, and patellar reflexes may be brisk. Electromyography shows a combined sensory and motor neuropathy consistent with demyelination in the lower extremities. Nerve biopsy may reveal axonal degeneration. Distal, sensory neuropathy is most often found in patients with advanced symptomatic HIV disease. Peripheral neuropathy can also be a consequence of drug therapy; agents associated with peripheral neuropathy include zalcitabine, didanosine, stavudine, and isoniazid. Inhibition of mitochondrial DNA is thought to underly this side effect of the antiretroviral agents, although other mechanisms may also be operative.

Chronic inflammatory demyelinatng polyneuropathy (CIDP), the second most common peripheral neuropathy, tends to occur before other clinical manifestations of HIV develop. Acute, inflammatory, demyelinating polyneuropathy (Guillain-Barré syndrome) is also reported early in the course of HIV disease. Patients report motor weakness that occurs acutely or gradually and have minimal sensory complaints. Weakness and areflexia are often noted on examination; a CSF pleocytosis is often present and the CSF protein level elevated. Nerve biopsy shows mononuclear cell infiltration and demyelination. The clinical course may wax and wane, and some patients recover spontaneously. Inflammatory demyelinating polyneuropathies may be associated with cytomegalovirus infection, although the etiology may be autoimmune.[284]

Other rarer neuropathies include multiple mononeuropathy, possibly associated with vasculitis, herpes simplex virus, cytomegalovirus polyradiculopathies, and neuropathies of vitamin deficiency, particularly vitamin B_{12}.

Aseptic Meningitis. When HIV directly infects the CNS, several distinct clinical syndromes result. In approximately one-quarter to one-third of the cases, an aseptic meningitis characterizes the acute retroviral syndrome (described previously). Although cranial neuropathies have been reported, meningeal signs may be minimal and laboratory evaluation remarkable for only a slight CSF pleocytosis and elevation of the CSF protein. Culture of CSF may reveal HIV, and HIV p24 antigen may be detected. Seroconversion can result in the intrathecal production of anti-HIV antibodies. Patients with this presentation may wax and wane clinically for months. HIV-related meningitis was reported in one series of 14 patients who presented no evidence of recently acquiring HIV.[285] The symptoms that prompted evaluation lasted from 10 days to more than 10 months. Signs of immunodeficiency were found in eight cases (57 percent). A mild CSF pleocytosis was noted in all patients, and both CSF protein levels and opening pressure were elevated in five patients. Eighty percent of patients tested had positive HIV cultures. A CSF pleocytosis, detection of HIV antigen, and positive viral cultures from the CSF can also be found in asymptomatic HIV-seropositive patients, however, so attributing meningitis in HIV-infected persons to HIV itself is problematic.

HIV Encephalopathy. A progressive neurocognitive syndrome (now termed HIV encephalopathy or AIDS-dementia complex) can be caused when HIV infects the brain.[286,286a] HIV encephalopathy is a late complication of HIV infection, occurring in 15–20 percent of individuals with severe immunodeficiency. HIV encephalopathy is rare in HIV-infected adults with CD4 cell counts greater than 200/mm^3. HIV encephalopathy can be divided into two phases, early and late, and each has a distinct clinical presentation. In early HIV encephalopathy, the major symptoms are memory loss, impaired concentration, and mental slowness. Patients also demonstrate affective symptoms, apathy, behavior change, and motor complaints. Patients with early HIV encephalopathy may have hyperreflexia, hypertonia, frontal-release signs, tremor, psychomotor slowing, ataxia, and abnormal results of mental status examination. Laboratory and clinical evaluation is essential to rule out opportunistic infection, depression, tumor, or other causes of mental status changes. Use of neuropsychiatric tests such as trailmaking tests may be helpful, particularly with serial assessments.[286b] In 70–90 percent of patients, cranial imaging studies show generalized atrophy that is usually inconsistent with the patient's age. Magnetic resonance imaging (MRI) shows cerebral atrophy, often with marked abnormalities of the subcortical white matter and an increased T2 signal intensity that is distributed multifically. A slight CSF pleocytosis is found in a minority of individuals, along with normal glucose and elevated CSF protein levels (primarily CSF IgG) in more than half of the patients. Oligoclonal bands are present in one-third of subjects tested but myelin basic protein is normal. HIV isolation and antigen detection assays may be positive, although these tests are both nonspecific and insensitive for predicting and diagnosing HIV encephalopathy. Markers of immune activation such as β-2 microglobulin are usually elevated as is CSF quinolinic acid; these assays are relatively nonspecific, however. Other diagnostic test findings (e.g., electroencephalography [EEG]) may be abnormal but have not been adequately evaluated to be helpful.

Late HIV encephalopathy is a more fulminant process. Patients present with marked cognitive abnormalities, memory loss, behavioral change, and significant psychomotor impairment. Profound weakness, neglect, tremor, seizures, and psychosis may also be noted. Computed tomography and MRI scanning findings are often more severely abnormal; extreme cerebral atrophy and white matter changes are common. Other diagnostic studies are used to rule out opportunistic infections. A clinical diagnosis of HIV encephalopathy is made by excluding other causes of encephalopathy and documenting HIV infection. Characteristic findings on history and examination, suggestive radiographic or imaging findings, and the absence of space-occupying lesions, opportunistic pathogens, or intoxicating drugs all support the diagnosis. Brain biopsy has generally not yielded useful results in this setting. In children infected with HIV, CNS involvement appears very frequently. It can be manifested by a developmental delay, cognitive deficits, abnormalities of muscle tone, and paraparesis. Seizures have been reported occasionally as a late complication in both children and adults.

In the brains of patients with HIV encephalopathy, pathologic findings are varied. Seventy-five percent of patients have cerebral atrophy that is most pronounced in the frontal and temporal lobes. Almost all patients have gliosis and focal necrosis. Microglial nodules of macrophages, lymphocytes, and microglia are reported in up to 70 percent of patients. Demyelination and myelin pallor are common; focal perivascular myelin rarefaction or demyelination and vacuolation are also frequently noted. The basal ganglia are commonly involved. Multinucleated giant cells, produced by direct HIV infection in the brain, can be found scattered throughout the cerebral cortex and white matter. Perivascular and leptomeningeal inflammation may also be found.

Intracranial Mass Lesions. Central nervous system dysfunction from intracranial mass lesions is a late complication of HIV disease. Processes associated with mass lesions of the brain are listed in Table 14. Cerebral toxoplasmosis (Ch. 257) is the most common cause of intracranial masses in patients with AIDS, followed by CNS lymphoma, progressive multifocal leukoencephalopathy (PML), and other infectious agents (e.g., *M. tuberculosis, Cryptococcus, Candida*). As many as 10 percent of biopsied or autopsied intracranial masses have nondiagnostic histopathology. In many cases, neither the clinical presentation nor the neuroradiologic appearance of CNS lesions permits a definitive diagnosis. Patients with opportunistic CNS disease may present with a variety of signs and symptoms. Headache may occur in one-third to three-quarters of patients and altered sensorium in 50–90 percent. Incoordination, ataxia, hemiparesis, and cranial neuropathies are present in fewer than 25 percent of patients with intracranial mass lesions. The radiographic appearance of various CNS lesions may be distinct but not pathognomonic. A diagnosis of CNS disease is challenging without examining tissue. However, given the high frequency of cerebral toxoplasmosis and its rapid response to antimicrobial therapy, patients with intracranial mass lesions consistent with toxoplasmic encephalitis may be given presumptive therapy and followed carefully.[287] A clinical response establishes the diagnosis reliably (see below). Figure 8 presents a diagnostic algorithm for evaluating patients with HIV infection and suspected intracranial mass lesions.

Patients who present with clinical findings suggestive of intracranial pathology should be evaluated with a brain imaging study. Both CT and MRI have been shown to be sensitive for assessing CNS disease in HIV infection, but MRI is generally preferred because of its greater sensitivity. Cranial imaging studies may reveal single or multiple lesions, with or without enhancement. Characteristically, abscesses are enhanced by contrast in toxoplasmosis, tuberculosis, cryptococcosis, nocardiosis, and pyogenic brain abscesses. A lack of enhancement is more often associated with PML and lymphomas, although enhancement can be seen in the latter. Multiple ring-enhancing lesions are the sine qua non of toxoplasmosis; how-

---

TABLE 14. Causes of Intracranial Mass Lesions in AIDS

Infections
   Toxoplasma gondii
   Progressive multifocal leukoencephalopathy (JC virus)
   M. tuberculosis
   Cryptococcus neoformans
   Nocardia asteroides
   Histoplasma capsulatum
   Cytomegalovirus
   Herpes simplex virus
   Human immunodeficiency virus
   Candida albicans
Neoplasms
   Primary CNS lymphoma
   Metastatic lymphoma
   Kaposi sarcoma
Unidentified
   Nonspecific gliosis

Abbreviation: CNS, central nervous system.

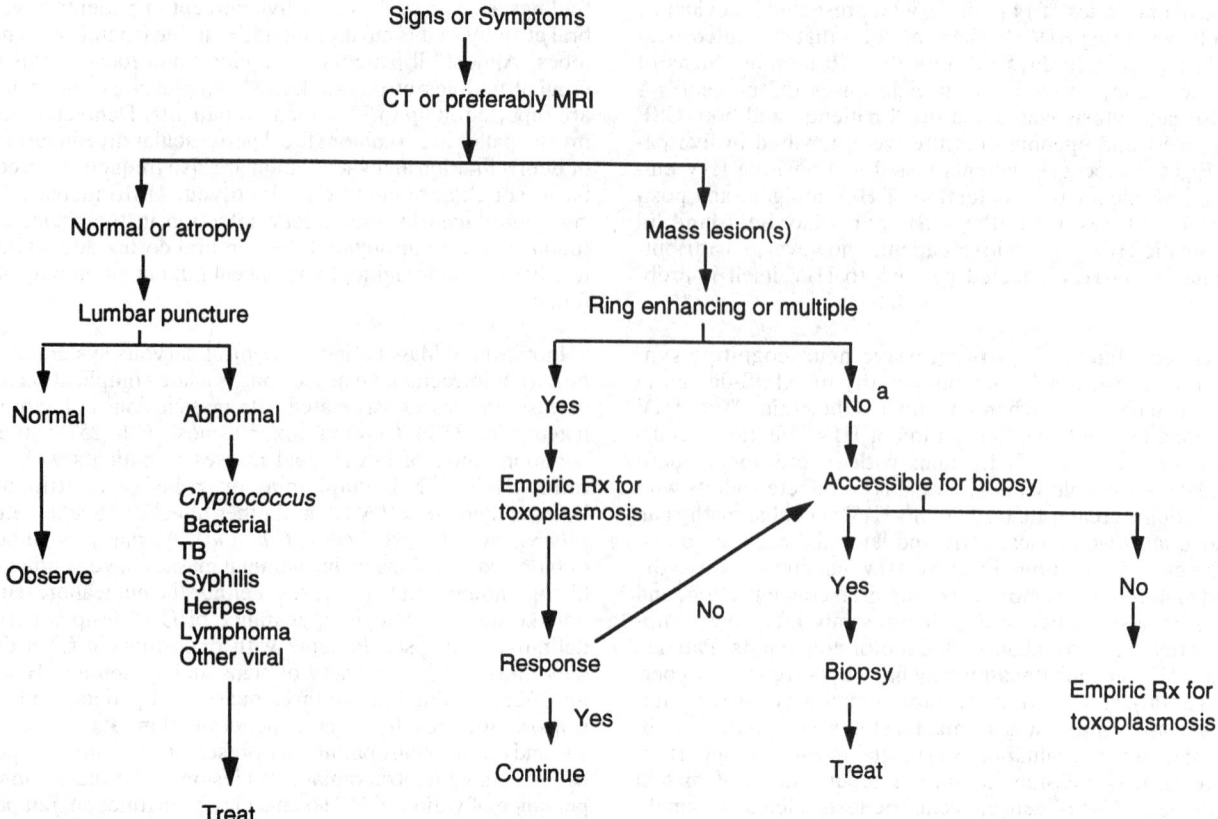

FIG. 8. Algorithm for evaluating neurologic abnormalities in patients with HIV infection. If CT does not show ring-enhancing or multiple lesions, an MRI should be performed (see text).

ever, many toxoplasmic abscesses are not detected by CT scanning. Therefore, the appearance of a single ring-enhancing lesion by CT does not rule out toxoplasmosis. Toxoplasmosis is usually associated with multiple lesions, and most patients have basal ganglia involvement.[288] Lesions are often small (1–3 cm) and hemorrhage rare. Progressive multifocal leukoencephalopathy is a demyelinating disease that results in diffuse, nonenhancing, hemispheric, white matter lesions without edema or mass effect. Primary CNS lymphoma usually produces single, hyperdense lesions that enhance unevenly. Multiple lesions may be found in some patients, particularly in serial studies of untreated individuals. In patients with HIV infection, normal CT scan results do not rule out CNS disease. If clinical findings suggest intracranial mass lesions, a negative CT scan should be followed by an MRI scan. High-field strength, T2-weighted MRI scans are more sensitive than CT scans in detecting cerebral abscesses and other CNS pathology.[289] Magnetic resonance imaging often reveals multiple high-intensity target lesions (which suggest toxoplasmosis) when the CT scan shows only a single ring-enhancing lesion. Magnetic resonance image scanning also reveals lesions in the basal ganglia in virtually all patients with toxoplasmosis. When multiple lesions and basal ganglia lesions are absent in MRI scanning, this finding strongly suggests a diagnosis other than toxoplasmosis. Progressive multifocal leukoencephalopathy characteristically causes hemispheric, white matter lesions; on MRI scans, multiple, high-signal, nonenhancing white matter lesions are found (see Ch. 123). Solitary lesions on MRI scans may be CNS lymphomas, cryptococcomas, tuberculomas, or viral encephalitides.

If the cranial imaging study reveals no mass effect, a lumbar puncture can be performed. Cerebrospinal fluid should be sent for a cell count and differential; protein and glucose determination; cryptococcal antigen assay; bacterial, mycobacterial, viral, and fungal culture; cytology; and VDRL testing. *Tox-*

oplasma serology may be performed, although the sensitivity of serum IgG may be only 80–85 percent in patients with confirmed toxoplasmosis. In patients with advanced immunodeficiency (CD4 count $<100/mm^3$) with clinical and neuroradiologic findings consistent with toxoplasmosis, presumptive therapy is appropriate.

Empirical therapy is less optimal for patients with a single lesion detected by MRI scan; patients with tuberculosis, cryptococcosis, other fungal infection, or malignancy at an anatomic site outside the CNS; or patients allergic to anti-*Toxoplasma* drugs. Early brain biopsy in these instances should be considered. Empirical treatment should be avoided in patients with mass effect who require steroid therapy because the response to steroids alone may confuse the clinical picture and render later biopsy results uninterpretable. These patients and those who have not had a clinical and radiographic response after 10–14 days of empirical antitoxoplasmosis therapy should undergo brain biopsy. Stereotactic needle biopsy is a safe and relatively nonmorbid way to obtain brain tissue for histologic study. In patients with impending herniation, open biopsies should be performed.

Biopsy material obtained from the periphery of an abscess has the highest diagnostic yield, particularly for toxoplasmosis. Fresh tissue may be used for touch preparations and should be cultured for viruses, bacteria, mycobacteria, and fungi. Specimens should be stained with standard cytochemical stains (e.g., hematoxylin and eosin); however, the sensitivity of hematoxylin-eosin staining for *Toxoplasma* may be less than 50 percent. Staining with immunoperoxidase greatly increases the diagnostic yield and should be used routinely to evaluate brain biopsy specimens when standard stains fail to make a specific diagnosis.

The utility of serologic tests for *T. gondii* antibodies is primarily in identifying candidates for chemoprophylaxis. In the

United States 30–50 percent of AIDS patients have previously been infected with *T. gondii* and have demonstrable antibodies.[290] Up to one-third of the IgG-positive patients with HIV will later develop CNS toxoplasmosis. Conversely, IgG-negative patients with biopsy-confirmed CNS toxoplasmosis have been reported.[288] Diagnostic tests that will more reliably distinguish cerebral toxoplasmosis from other CNS mass lesions are needed. Methods under investigation include *T. gondii* antigen detection, polymerase chain reaction, and more sensitive imaging techniques such as single positron emission computed tomography (SPECT) scans.

Specific Etiologies of Opportunistic DNS Disease. TOXO-PLASMOSIS. Toxoplasmosis (see Ch. 257) causes most intracranial mass lesions in AIDS patients. CNS toxoplasmosis is the index diagnosis of AIDS in approximately 2 percent of patients in the United States, and it occurs as a secondary diagnosis in an additional 2–5 percent. In geographic areas where the underlying prevalence of remote infection with *T. gondii* is high (e.g., France, Haiti), cerebral toxoplasmosis among AIDS patients is very prevalent. Of those AIDS patients who have mass lesions revealed by CT head scans, 50–70 percent have toxoplasmosis. The incidence of toxoplasmosis has recently declined as a result of widespread use of trimethoprin-sulfa prophylaxis for *P. carinii*, which is also effective for *T. gondii*.[291]

Central nervous system toxoplasmosis presents as a global encephalitis with altered mental status in up to 75 percent of patients.[288] Fifty percent of patients report headaches, although those headaches are not typically severe. About 50 percent may have focal neurologic signs (i.e., seizure, hemiparesis, or ataxia); fewer than 50 percent may have fever. Symptoms often have a subacute onset—over a period of days to several weeks—with a median of 22 days in one series. Laboratory studies other than cranial imaging scans are generally unhelpful. CD4 cell counts are usually less than 50/mm³. Cerebrospinal fluid findings are often normal. Pathologically, toxoplasmosis results in a diffuse encephalitis with focal areas of intense inflammation and necrosis. Abscesses show acute and chronic inflammation and infiltration by PMNs, lymphocytes, and histiocytes. The abscess centers are necrotic, with scant organisms. On the periphery of an abscess, numerous *T. gondii* tachyzoites may be found, whereas cyst forms can be seen in non-necrotic tissue. In small vessels surrounding abscesses, vasculitis may be present; reactive astrocytosis is seen adjacently.

PROGRESSIVE MULTIFOCAL LEUKOENCEPHALOPATHY. PML (see Ch. 123), a demyelinating disease of cerebral white matter, is characterized by multiple, discrete foci of disease. A papovavirus, JC virus, is consistently identified in oligodendrocytes in affected areas of the syndrome.[291a] In the United States, fewer than 1 percent of patients with AIDS have PML reported to the CDC. The symptoms of PML include headache, ataxia, hemiparesis, confusion, and other mental status changes.[291b] Computed tomography scans most often reveal nonenhancing, low-density lesions of the periventricular white matter. Magnetic resonance imaging scans show high-signal intensity lesions without enhancement. Cerebrospinal fluid studies are usually unrevealing; the diagnosis is established by brain biopsy. JC virus can be identified by typical electron microscopy morphology, by immunofluorescence staining, or by gene amplification techniques. Clinically, patients deteriorate progressively. Death occurs on average in less than 3 months, although spontaneous remission has been reported.

Cryptococcus neoformans. The CDC reports disease caused by *C. neoformans* (see Ch. 243) in up to 10 percent of persons with AIDS. Cryptococcal meningitis occurs in approximately 80 percent of patients with symptomatic cryptococcal disease. Cryptococcosis is more common among IV drug users and ethnic minorities with AIDS and in the south-central United States. No seasonal variation in the occurrence of cryptococcosis has

been reported. A number of other clinical syndromes including pneumonitis, multiple skin lesions resembling molluscum contagiosum, fungemia, and prostatitis may also be seen. Cryptococcal meningitis often presents clinically with nonspecific symptoms. Eighty percent of patients complain only of fever, night sweats, malaise, and a dull headache.[244] Severe headache, photophobia, meningismus, and an altered sensorium occur in 2–20 percent of patients. Focal neurologic complaints such a seizures, cranial nerve abnormalities, or hemiparesis are rare. Many patients may have only low-grade fever. Other symptoms may be elicited retrospectively after cryptococcosis is diagnosed. Clinicians need to be vigilant to detect crytococcal disease early in its course before it disseminates and fulminant disease develops.

The diagnosis of cryptococcal meningitis is made by detecting cryptococcal antigen in blood or CSF and growth of *Cryptococcus* in the CSF. Patients with suspected cryptococcal meningitis should be carefully examined neurologically and ophthalmologically. If no focal neurologic abnormalities are noted and papilledema is absent, a lumbar puncture may be performed with small risk of complication. If neurologic abnormalities or altered sensorium are noted, a CT scan of the head should be obtained before performing a lumbar puncture. In many institutions, clinicians perform CT scanning on all patients before a lumbar puncture. The CSF findings of cryptococcal meningitis in AIDS is usually benign, with a pleocytosis of 5–50 mononuclear cells/mm³, slightly elevated protein levels, and a normal glucose concentration. India ink examination reveals organisms in 50–90 percent of cases, and the cryptococcal antigen is positive in 90–95 percent of patients. The sensitivity of serum cryptococcal antigen was higher in one study (98 percent) than CSF antigen (92 percent) in patients with culture-confirmed meningitis.[244] Cultures of the CSF are invariably positive in primary disease but may be negative in patients who ar relapsing from previously treated cryptococcosis. A rising antigen titer in the CSF strongly suggests relapse in this setting.

Cryptococcal infections are acquired by inhaling the organism into the lungs. The primary pulmonary infection is often asymptomatic, even in immunodeficient hosts; however, cryptococcal pneumonia does occur in patients with advanced HIV infection. The clinical features of cryptococcal pneumonia include the insidious onset of fever, night sweats, malaise, cough, and dyspnea. The radiograph may show focal lobar infiltrates, sometimes with cavitation. Examination of induced sputum (using silver methenamine stain) may show yeast. Bronchoalveolar lavage fluid and transbronchial biopsy specimens may also show yeast, and cultures may yield *C. neoformans*. Cryptococcal antigenemia is present variably, and fungal blood cultures may grow *Cryptococcus*.

Other extraneural sites of disease are common in AIDS patients with cryptococcosis. Fungemia is present in more than 80 percent of patients with cryptococcal meningitis, and the organism has been found in the bone marrow, liver, spleen, kidneys, prostate, skin, and other organs. Prostatic involvement may serve as a source of relapse in patients who do not take suppressive therapy.[292]

Cytomegalovirus. Cytomegalovirus (see Ch. 117) is ubiquitous in patients with HIV infection and causes serious morbidity in AIDS. Cytomegalovirus is transmitted by the same routes as HIV, and almost all patients with sexually acquired HIV infection are also infected with cytomegalovirus. Like other herpesviruses, CMV may infect cells latently and reactivate when host defenses are impaired. Asymptomatic cytomegalovirus viruria and viremia may be found in one-third to one-half of patients with advanced HIV disease. Zurlo and coworkers found that cytomegalovirus viremic patients were 2.5-fold more likely to develop end-organ disease than nonviremic patients, and viruria was associated with a threefold increased risk of cytomegalovirus.[293] However, most patients who developed cytomegalovirus disease in the cohort did not have antecedent viremia or viruria.

Cytomeglovirus has a unique predilection for the retina, with 90 percent of end-organ disease in patients with HIV infection being retinitis.[294] Other involved sites include the colon, esophagus, stomach, adrenals, pancreas, brain, and lungs.

Cytomegalovirus retinitis is the index diagnosis of AIDS in 1–2 percent of patients and occurs subsequently in 4–6 percent. The onset of cytomegalovirus retinitis may be insidious or rapid. Patients complain of painless, progressive visual loss, blurring, and "floaters." Cytomegalovirus retinitis usually presents unilaterally, although it may subsequently progress to the contralateral retina. Funduscopic examination of the involved eye typically reveals coalescing white exudates in a vascular pattern with surrounding hemorrhage and edema.

Often, lesions are peripheral initially, involve the fovea later, and result in visual loss. Retinal detachment may occur as a late complication.

Patients complaining of ocular symptoms should undergo a thorough ophthalmologic examination. The differential diagnosis of retinal lesions includes cotton wool spots, ischemic retinopathy, Roth spots, and toxoplasmic retinitis. Cotton-wool spots are very prevalent in patients with AIDS but do not appear to predict the development of other retinal disease. The cotton-wool spots are distributed in a vascular pattern similar to cytomegalovirus, but do not have the irregular pattern of exudate and hemorrhage that is characteristic of cytomegalovirus retinitis. Similarly, *Toxoplasma* retinitis shows discrete, rounded, pale exudates. Autopsy studies of persons dying with cytomegalovirus retinitis have shown retinal necrosis, hemorrhage, and mononuclear cell infiltration. Cytomegalovirus (but not HIV) DNA and RNA can be detected in affected cells. An ophthalmologist or other highly trained observer can make a premortem diagnosis by visually inspecting the lesions. Cultures of the blood and urine yield cytomegalovirus in 80–100 percent of cases, respectively. At autopsy, one quarter of patients with cytomegalovirus retinitis may also have cytomegalovirus encephalitis.

Other Ocular Diseases. Although cytomegalovirus retinitis is by far the most common serious ocular complication of HIV infection, a number of other ophthalmologic disorders are seen. Varicella-zoster retinitis is a severe, necrotizing retinitis that may occur in patients with higher CD4 cell counts than in patients with cytomegalovirus retinitis.[295] Patients most often note rapid visual loss. Fundoscopic findings include peripheral necrosis, occlusive vasculopathy, optic neuritis, and vitreal and scleral inflammation. The severity of the syndrome has led to its being termed acute retinal necrosis. Varicella-zoster retinitis usually occurs in the absence of zoster at other sites. Ocular toxoplasmosis occurs in patients with advanced immunodeficiency, and many but not all have cerebral toxoplasmosis. Lesions are usually discrete foci of retinal inflammation without hemorrhage or vasculopathy. Vitreal inflammation is common. The diagnosis is made by observation by an experienced ophthalmologist. *Pneumocystis carinii* may cause a choroiditis that may mimic cytomegalovirus retinitis.[296] The lesions are typically posterior, yellow-orange in appearance, and do not cause vitreal inflammation. Choroidal pneumocytosis occurs most often in patients with previous *P. carinii* pneumonia, particularly in those taking aerosolized pentamidine for prophylaxis.

Patients who have had cytomegalovirus retinitis frequently experience acute retinal detachments. Erosion of the retinal border at the site of a necrotic lesions allows the retina to be lifted off underlying tissues. Patients complain of sudden loss of vision "like a curtain falling" in front of the affected eye. Surgical reattachment is often partially successful in restoring vision, although progressive visual loss may ensue.

MALIGNANCIES IN THE HIV-INFECTED PATIENT

Along with opportunistic infections and clinical problems directly attributed to HIV itself, malignant neoplasms are frequent causes of severe morbidity and mortality. The recognition and management of these cancers are key components of comprehensive AIDS care, and research into their etiology and pathogenesis is expected to shed additional light on oncogenesis in non-HIV-infected patients.

Early Reports of AIDS-Related Cancers

Cases of KS in young homosexual men in the early 1980s helped alert the medical community to the AIDS epidemic. Before this, KS had been a rare and relatively indolent cutaneous neoplasm of elderly men in the United States and elsewhere[297] and also an endemic malignancy in parts of central Africa.[298-300] In Africans, KS was more aggressive, particularly in children, where a lymphodenopathic variant was rapidly fatal. In all age groups African KS, before the appearance of HIV, was linked epidemiologically to cytomegalovirus infection. Additionally, KS had been reported as a complication of exogenous corticosteroids taken to prevent organ transplant rejection.[301-307] Although an interesting disease because of these unusual geographic patterns and postulated associations with cytomegalovirus infection[308,309] and iatrogenic immune suppression, KS was not a clinically significant problem in the United States.

In 1980, several cases of KS were diagnosed in homosexual men in New York, and these and similar cases from California were described in a series of reports in 1981 and 1982.[310-312] Several aspects of these cases were distinctly unusual (Table 15). First, they affected a much younger population than prior ("classic") KS in the United States. Second, the tumor was much more aggressive, with early and wide dissemination the rule. Finally, the patients often had the same spectrum of unusual infections being diagnosed simultaneously in other homosexual men but had no known reason for immune deficiency. The combination of these striking findings in similar "risk" populations soon led to the recognition of a common underlying disorder, AIDS.

The second malignancy recognized as part of the AIDS epidemic was non-Hodgkin's lymphoma (NHL). Sporadic cases of NHL of CNS origin in individuals with other manifestations of AIDS resulted in the early inclusion of this cancer in AIDS surveillance definitions.[313-315] Subsequently, NHL of peripheral origin was also reported in association with AIDS.[316-325] Since 1984, NHL in both sites has become increasingly common, and its clinical appearance, biology, and management are important for the clinician to understand.

In addition to KS and NHL, an increasing variety of other cancers have been diagnosed in HIV-infected individuals. Although less common than KS and NHL and less clearly linked causally to HIV infection, these tumors may also offer insight into the relationship between HIV, immune deficiency, and oncogenesis. Although the wide variety of these cancers precludes extensive discussion in this chapter, their diagnosis should be considered when clinically appropriate.

Epidemiology of AIDS-Related Malignancies—Kaposi Sarcoma

Kaposi sarcoma is, by far, the most common neoplasm in HIV-infected patients.[326-328] Overall, 9 percent of all AIDS cases reported to the CDC have been initially diagnosed with KS as compared with less than 1 percent with NHL, the next most common cancer. Many more patients develop KS or lymphoma later in their disease course although no accurate data are collected by the CDC for secondary AIDS-defining opportunistic diseases. Kaposi sarcoma is, in fact, one of the most common clinical manifestations of HIV disease, and as mentioned, its increased incidence was an early indicator of the AIDS epidemic.

Kaposi sarcoma, for reasons still unclear, disproportionately affects HIV-infected male homosexuals.[326–329] In the first several years of the epidemic, for example, 47 percent of newly diagnosed AIDS cases in homosexual and bisexual men had KS as compared with 3.9 percent in intravenous drug users.[330] Kaposi sarcoma is rare in all heterosexuals with HIV disease except black Africans.[331,332] In Africa, KS is more common and clinically more aggressive in the HIV-infected population when compared with reports before the HIV epidemic.[333–337] Although precise incidence figures are not available, KS does seem more common in African AIDS patients than in other groups of heterosexuals.[338,339] Kaposi sarcoma in children with AIDS has been reported but is rare.[340] Recent work suggests that even when adjusted for risk-group category, KS may be more common in whites than blacks.[341]

Adding even more to the interest in KS are studies showing that it is an epidemiologic "moving target." For example, its incidence in homosexual men is clearly decreasing in the United States.[342,343] Compared with initial rates of 36 percent of AIDS cases at diagnosis, more recent work now shows a 6 percent incidence of KS.[344] This decline undoubtedly reflects, in part, the increasing proportion of heterosexuals with AIDS but KS is actually declining in incidence in *each* HIV risk-behavior subgroup.

Not only is the incidence of KS declining, but its mortality rate may also be worsening. In a preliminary study from San Francisco the median duration of survival for a group of KS patients diagnosed in 1982–1983 was 24 months, whereas a cohort diagnosed from 1984 to 1986 had a 14-month median survival.[345] In this study, HIV p24 antigen was more frequently detectable in the more recent group (76 vs. 43 percent, $p = .03$), which suggests that KS had been diagnosed at a later point in the course of the HIV infection.

In several studies, certain sexual practices were found to correlate with KS risk. Particularly significant were behaviors such as oral-anal contact that would result in anal exposure to fecal organisms.

Explanations for the unusual epidemiologic profile of KS in the AIDS epidemic are yet being developed. The relative restriction to homosexuals has been speculated secondary to recreational drug use[346,347] or to a second, as yet unidentified virus or other organism that is enteric and sexually transmitted. Either theory could at least partially explain the change in KS incidence (decreasing exposure to a second "cofactor").

Ideally, information from epidemiology studies could contribute to our knowledge of the pathogenesis of KS, but this is not yet the case. No recreational drug used primarily by homosexual men, including the inhaled nitrites once popular, have been clearly shown to be carcinogenic or particularly immunosuppressive. Similarly, despite some early speculation, no coincident "KS virus" has been found, although investigators are now applying sensitive molecular techniques in this search. Recent work points to cytokines or HIV-induced growth factors such as oncostatin-m as potentially involved in KS formation, but this theory is not yet reconciled with the complex and variable epidemiology of KS in different HIV-infected populations.

Indirect laboratory support for a KS growth factor comes from investigations in which immunodeficient mice were inoculated with cells cultured from human KS tumors. These mice developed vascular tumors that interestingly, were of murine rather than human genetic origin.[348,349]

Clinical Appearance and Pathophysiology of Kaposi Sarcoma in HIV Infection.   Kaposi sarcoma (Table 15) is considered to be an endothelial neoplasm of either capillary or lymphatic origin.[350–353] Histologically, the tumor is typified by a proliferation of vascular structures, often with large malignant-appearing endothelial cells, set against a background of a bland proliferation

TABLE 15. Kaposi Sarcoma (KS) in AIDS—Distinguishing Characteristics

Extent of disease	Unlike "traditional" KS, AIDS/KS is *rarely* limited to a single anatomic region
Site of involvement	The head and neck are common primary sites (including the face, oral cavity)
Visceral involvement	Common, rarely symptomatic except for pulmonary KS, which is *rapidly* fatal
Opportunistic infections	Almost always present during the course of disease; usual cause of death
Social problems	The stigma of AIDS is exacerbated by visible lesions

of spindle-shaped cells and extravasated erythrocytes.[298,353–357] Efforts to establish KS cell lines in culture have made little headway,[348,349] and direct tumor transplants to immunodeficient animals have been unsuccessful. This and the not uncommonly indolent clinical behavior have led to speculation that KS is not a malignancy in the truest sense but is rather a striking benign cellular proliferation[358] in response to some circulating "growth factor."

The clinical pattern of KS is usually not difficult to recognize and can be somewhat predicted from the histologic appearance. Kaposi sarcoma lesions are typically nodular, pigmented, and initially asymptomatic. Size varies from several millimeters to confluent tumor plaques that are 5–10 cm in diameter. Violaceous to red pigmentation is common, but KS in dark-skinned persons may be nearly black, and rarely patients irrespective of race have subcutaneous lesions that are nonpigmented. Nodularity of KS lesions is typical, and even small lesions are usually palpable. Exophytic KS tumors are more common in African-Americans and can cause pain and necrosis. Many areas of the body can be affected by KS, although some are rarely involved. For example, KS is frequently seen on the skin and in the oral cavity, and although the soles are one of the most common KS sites, the tumor rarely affects the palms.[311,359–369]

Kaposi sarcoma is a multicentric tumor, and numerous lesions can appear simultaneously in widely scattered areas of the body. Kaposi sarcoma in the HIV-infected patient, unlike most other KS populations, often involves visceral structures.[370] Kaposi sarcoma in the GI tract is seen in almost 50 percent of cases, most commonly in the stomach, duodenum, and rectum. Another important visceral site of KS is the lung. Both sites will be discussed below.

The lymphatic endothelial origin postulated for KS is often reflected in the gross clinical appearance of the disease. Linearity of lesions after cutaneous lymphatic drainage patterns is particularly common across the chest and back. Lymphedema, often out of proportion to the visible extent of tumor, is seen in some patients and usually affects either the lower extremities or face. In extreme cases, lymphedema of the lower portion of the body to the level of the diaphragm is observed.

Gastrointestinal Kaposi Sarcoma.   The GI tract is the most common visceral site of KS.[371–374] As many as 50 percent of patients with KS have lesions in the GI tract even early in the course of their disease. Gastrointestinal KS is seldom symptomatic and is rarely if ever fatal. In some cases, however, GI KS can cause intestinal obstruction, bleeding, or enteropathy. Essentially, any segment of the GI tract may be involved with KS, although the stomach and duodenum are most commonly affected.[375]

The diagnosis of GI KS is most often made by the endoscopic visualization of typical lesions.[372,376] Endoscopy is not considered mandatory in all KS patients and should be reserved for those with GI symptoms. Radiographic visualization of KS is possible, with contrast studies showing raised, smooth, rounded intraluminal masses. The diagnostic accuracy of these studies, however, is not as high as with endoscopy.[377,378]

On endoscopy, KS lesions are nodular and raised and appear highly vascular. As with cutaneous lesions, they vary in size from several millimeters to several centimeters in diameter. Any number may be present, but confluent tumor masses are unusual. Despite their ready visualization, GI KS lesions are not easily diagnosed by biopsy because the tumor is subcutaneous, beyond the depth of the biopsy forceps in 77 percent of cases.[376] If biopsy confirmation is considered essential for patient management, a high yield may be achieved with loop biopsy technique.

Pulmonary KS. Pulmonary parenchymal involvement by KS is less commonly recognized than GI spread but is more often symptomatic.[379–382] In fact, the general principle that KS, even in the HIV-infected patient, is not directly fatal is not true with symptomatic pulmonary disease where the median duration of survival is approximately 3 months.[380]

The symptoms of pulmonary KS, described in several reviews,[379–381,383] usually consist of dyspnea, a severe but minimally productive cough, chest tightness, and less commonly, fever. These symptoms clearly overlap with those of *P. carinii* and mycobacterial pneumonias, which are the main diseases to be considered in a differential diagnosis. Bronchoconstriction is also common with pulmonary KS.

The diagnosis of pulmonary KS is to some degree one of exclusion, particularly with respect to PCP. The chest x-ray findings in pulmonary KS tend to show a more nodular pattern with less even infiltration than is typical of PCP. Pleural effusions are also more suggestive of pulmonary KS. These effusions are frequently bloody, but cytologic examination is usually nondiagnostic. Pulmonary gallium scans can provide useful information in some cases, generally showing no uptake in patients with pulmonary KS in contrast to those with infectious pneumonias.[383,384]

Bronchoscopy provides the strongest evidence of pulmonary KS. Although the pulmonary parenchyma is the principal site of disease, in most cases endobronchial lesions are easily visualized by an experienced bronchoscopist. Lesions are several millimeters or more in diameter and appear redder and more vascular than cutaneous KS lesions. Biopsy is relatively contraindicated because of possible hemorrhage, but transbronchial biopsy has been used to diagnose KS in some cases. Patients with pulmonary KS almost always have extensive cutaneous KS as well, although primary pulmonary KS has been reported.[379,385] At any rate, the presence of typical pulmonary symptoms and diagnostic tests in the absence of an infectious pneumonia should be considered adequate to warrant management for pulmonary KS.

Diagnosis of Cutaneous Kaposi Sarcoma. A clinician should, with some experience, have no difficulty in recognizing typical cutaneous KS lesions, but biopsy confirmation should be obtained, particularly if this information will be used to make an initial AIDS diagnosis. A punch biopsy (ideally ≥4 mm in diameter) is usually sufficient. The biopsy can be safely performed in an outpatient setting with local anesthesia. Despite the vascular nature of KS, hemorrhage is rarely encountered and healing is unimpaired. Although KS has been diagnosed from fine-needle aspiration cytology specimens, this technique is almost certainly less sensitive and specific, and its use should be limited.

Oral Kaposi Sarcoma. The oral cavity is an extremely common site of KS.[363,386,387] In as many as one-third of patients this represents the first site of disease, whereas it appears later in the course of KS in many others. Intraoral lesions are most common on the hard palate but are not uncommon on the posterior pharyngeal wall or the gingiva.[388] The tongue is an uncommon site of KS, and the buccal mucosa is almost always spared.

The appearance of oral KS is typical and similar to cutaneous disease. Lesions on the hard palate, however, are often not raised and are blue to violet in color. Biopsy (usually by an oral surgeon) can be performed, and this should be done if other, more easily sampled cutaneous lesions are not present.[389,390]

Intraoral KS is initially asymptomatic, but later, with disease progression, the lesions can become bulky, with superficial necrosis leading to pain. bleeding, and occasionally difficulty in swallowing. Gingival KS can additionally contribute to the periodontal disease seen in many AIDS patients.

Staging, Clinical Course, and Management of Kaposi Sarcoma. PROGNOSTIC FACTORS/STAGING   Staging of KS by estimates of tumor burden have been proposed by several groups.[360,391] Usually, KS in these systems is categorized by the number, size, appearance, site of involvement, and the rate of growth. Although most experienced clinicians are convinced that KS patients can be divided into those with "minimal" tumor burden and those with "advanced" KS, no common definitions have been accepted. This is problematic for the individual patient and practitioner who would like more precise information available to better discuss the prognosis and plan therapy, but it is of even more concern for the design and comparison of clinical investigations.

Admitting limitations, some broad staging guidelines of KS extent can be proposed. Patients with "few" lesions (for example, <25) or those without known visceral or intraoral disease, may progress less rapidly than those patients with many lesions or with any extracutaneous involvement. Similarly, patients with a history of minimal increase in lesions size or number over a several month period (not an uncommon observation at the time of biopsy) have a better prognosis than do patients in whom new lesions are rapidly appearing. The prognosis may also be improved when the lesions are geographically confined to one body area, for example, the skin of one extremity. Certainly, the prognosis is worsened if visceral KS is diagnosed. The median duration of survival is less than 3 months, for example, in patients with pulmonary KS. Although the effect of GI and intraoral KS on survival duration is less clear, disease in these sites also carries a worse prognosis.

The symptomatic status of the KS patient is also important in the prognosis. KS patients with chronic systemic ("B") symptoms including unexplained fevers, night sweats, and weight loss have a decrease in median survival duration.[391] Also, this effect is cumulative, and the prognosis is additionally limited in patients with multiple constitutional symptoms.

A final component to staging KS involves laboratory tests grouped into those of general value and those specifically estimating HIV burden and/or immunologic impairment.[360,361, 392,393] Survival duration is decreased in patients with severe anemia or neutropenia or with erythrocyte sedimentation rates above 40 mm/hr.

Probably the strongest laboratory predictors of outcome in KS are likely to be those that are more directly involved in HIV and its immune effects. As is true with HIV-infected patients without KS, prognosis is worse with lower CD4 cell counts, higher HIV p24 antigen levels, and higher markers of immune activation including β-2 microglobulin and neopterin.

Another similar staging system of KS has been proposed by a group of investigators. In this system, patients are also staged by tumor characteristics, their symptomatic status, and laboratory studies. The most favorable groups are those with tumors confined to skin, lymph nodes, or with minimal oral disease, CD4 counts 200/mm³ or greater, and no systemic symptoms.[394]

KS staging is far from being firmly defined and the clinician must take all into account, including that relating to underlying HIV status. Using this information, the clinician can better advise the patient concerning opportunistic infection prophylaxis and the need for specific antineoplastic therapy. The prognostic and staging variables are shown in Table 16.

INITIAL EVALUATION OF THE PATIENT WITH KAPOSI SARCOMA.   The goals of an initial evaluation of a patient with suspected KS vary depending on the patients' prior health status.

TABLE 16. Prognostic Variables in Kaposi Sarcoma (KS)

Predicts Indolent Course	Predicts Aggressive Course
Few lesions (<25)	Many KS lesions
Low rate of growth	Rapid appearance of new lesions
No visceral KS identified	Intraoral or visceral lesions
No fevers, drenching night sweats, or weight loss	One or more constitutional symptoms
No prior opportunistic infection	One prior or concurrent opportunistic infection
Absolute CD4+ count, >400/mm³	CD4+ cell count, <200/mm³
Normal ESR	ESR, >40 mm/hr
HIV p24 antigen not detectable	HIV p24 detectable
Normal β₂-microglobulin	β₂-Microglobulin, >5
Normal blood counts	Leukopenia or anemia present

Abbreviation: ESR, erythrocyte sedimentation rate.

TABLE 17. Guidelines for Kaposi Sarcoma Treatment

Patient Status	Options
Favorable prognostic indicators[a]	Expectant observation
	Alternating single-agent chemotherapy such as vinblastine/vincristine
	Interferon-α with or without zidovudine
	Experimental treatment trials
Unfavorable prognostic indicators[a]	Early initiation of therapy
	Alternating vincristine/vinblastine chemotherapy
	Other single-agent chemotherapy (e.g., doxorubicin)
	Combination chemotherapy (e.g., doxorubicin, bleomycin, vincristine)
Local tumor problems	Radiation therapy
	Topical liquid nitrogen
	Intralesional dilute vinblastine
	Surgical excision

[a] See Table 16.

If KS represents the initial AIDS-defining process, biopsy is essential. If, on the other hand, the patient has had prior opportunistic infections and if the KS is not likely to require treatment either because of poor baseline prognosis or because the extent of KS is still minimal, biopsy may not be required, especially if the lesion sites are on visible skin or are intraoral.

The initial evaluation can, overall, be divided into those tests that would be performed in any new AIDS patient to estimate viral burden and immune damage and to rule out opportunistic infections. The specific application of these tests to the new KS patient is to estimate the prognosis and to plan treatment. To this end, a careful examination of the entire body surface is essential, with recording of the number, size, site, and general appearance of visible KS lesions. Photography of selected areas can be useful for later establishing progression or response to treatment. The examination should include a digital rectal exam to palpate possible KS lesions and a careful examination of the pharynx to identify intraoral KS lesions on the palate, posterior oral pharynx, or gingiva. Routine GI endoscopy is not recommended unless indicated for specific symptomatology.

The initial (and each subsequent) medical history should inquire about the constitutional symptoms discussed previously and about any symptoms potentially related to opportunistic infections. Because these are often the cause of death in patients with KS,[395] their diagnosis, prophylaxis, and treatment must be considered at *all* times by treating physicians.

Laboratory studies in the KS patient should include a complete blood count and a routine chemistry panel. As with all parts of the spectrum of HIV disease, HIV infection must be established with HIV antibody tests, and all patients should be tested for serologic evidence of syphilis and active hepatitis B infection as well as have a PPD applied. HIV status can be additionally evaluated with an HIV p24 antigen and indirectly with β₂-microglobulin determination. Immunologic testing should include T-lymphocyte subset testing with enumeration of CD4+ and CD8+ populations.

As soon as the results of the initial examination are available, the patient should be informed of the results. This discussion should attempt to give the patient a better sense of the disease prognosis to help further decision making.[396] Specific counseling should address the need for considering antiretroviral therapy and the importance of recognizing, treating, and if possible, preventing opportunistic infections. The options for treating the KS directly should also be frankly reviewed. This discussion should, of course, include the possibility of not treating the KS per se if that seems an option and should also address the common concerns about the visible nature of KS and the fear that antineoplastic treatment—particularly chemotherapy and radiation therapy—may cause further immune impairment or may further compromise the ability to tolerate other necessary medications.

Therapy for Kaposi Sarcoma. Although perhaps less dramatic than progress in antiretroviral drug development, research in the treatment of KS has improved overall patient outcome.

Kaposi sarcoma therapy (Table 17) currently reflects the growing realization that the tumor, although not a true malignancy according to some definitions,[359] has a heterogeneous natural history ranging from indolent to rapidly fatal that takes place against a backdrop of progressive HIV-induced immune depletion. Thus, recent reports include both local treatments and increasingly aggressive chemotherapy regimens as well as attempts to combine antineoplastic drugs with agents of antiviral potential such as zidovudine. These approaches are summarized in Table 16, which stresses the individualization of treatment based on the patient's estimated prognosis.

LOCAL THERAPY. Many patients experience more problems from individual lesions than from their overall disease. This is especially common in patients with bulky intraoral KS, those with scattered facial lesions, and those with lesions in areas subjected to recurrent minor trauma (e.g., the ankle). Surgical excision or local radiation therapy remain good options for some of these situations, and increasingly, topical or intralesional treatments are also being evaluated. Radiation therapy rapidly shrinks individual KS lesions but is more frequently administered to somewhat broader areas of the body to control plaques of coalesced lesions or to reduce KS-associated lymphedema.[397–406] Although tumor responses to relatively low doses of radiation therapy (2000–3000 rads) are gratifying, local toxicity remains a problem for some patients. Particularly common are moderate to severe mucositis form radiating large intraoral KS lesions and cutaneous erythema from radiating larger lesions on the feet. These local toxicities are temporary and, in the case of intraoral mucositis, can be reduced by scrupulous attention to oral hygiene and control of minor infections such as with *Candida albicans.*

Intralesional or topical treatments being investigated for KS include some that are not directly antineoplastic in the usual sense such as cryotherapy with liquid nitrogen. This therapy consists of applying liquid nitrogen by a cotton applicator to the lesion until a "halo" of surrounding erythema is observed. A mild inflammation results, and the KS lesion flattens as this resolves. Larger lesions may require repeated applications at approximately 2-week intervals. Small lesions may completely disappear with this therapy; larger ones may leave a residual hemosiderin "tattoo."

A similar result has been reported with injections of small volumes of dilute vinblastine directly into the KS lesions.[407] Here, a 0.2 mg/cc solution of sterile vinblastine is prepared and injected through a fine-gauge needle placed perpendicular to the skin surface in the center of small KS lesions. Larger lesions (>1 cm) may require two or more such injections at separate sites. Sufficient volume is injected into the lesion (usually less than 0.5 cc). Because of the low dose, multiple lesions can be treated simultaneously. As with liquid nitrogen application, a mild inflammatory reaction ensues, but cutaneous ulcerations are not common, and small lesions typically heal without scarring. Therapy can be repeated every 2 weeks if required. This therapy has also been applied to intraoral lesions, but these, if extensive, are probably best treated with radiation therapy.

SYSTEMIC CHEMOTHERAPY. Even early in the AIDS epidemic, recognition of the variable natural history of KS and the many uncertainties of staging led to concern that overly aggressive chemotherapy—particularly the use of combinations of agents—might be inappropriate in some patients. Awareness of the underlying immune deficiency caused fears of the immunologic toxicity resulting from the aggressive use of cytotoxic drugs. Thus, most subsequent efforts were directed at single-agent chemotherapy—giving this more frequently but in lower doses or in alternating regimens with other single-agent therapy. This direction has been of value; single-agent chemotherapy with vinblastine alone at a dose of 4–8 mg weekly or alternated with vincristine[408,409] at 1–2 mg/dose is considered by many as a standard for HIV-related KS, especially if the disease is relatively indolent. Recently, equal or increased activity has been shown for single-agent doxorubicin given in attenuated doses (10–30 mg total dose) intravenously every 1–2 weeks.[410] In a study of the National Institute of Allergy and Infectious Diseases (NIAID)-supported AIDS Clinical Trials Group, for example, doxorubicin therapy administered weekly at a dose of 15 mg/m^2 resulted in a 16 percent partial remission in a group of 32 previously untreated patients. Also, vincristine as a single-drug treatment regimen is used for KS patients who are thrombocytopenic. This regimen has a high response rate—over 50 percent—with acceptable neurotoxicity. A variation of this approach involves the use of liposome encapsulated doxorubicin or daunorubicin, which appears to reduce systemic toxicity.[411]

Although concern about immune toxicity is still appropriate, more information suggests that some combination chemotherapy can be used safely.[412,413] The group of KS patients with rapidly progressing and often fatal disease may, in fact, benefit from these more aggressive chemotherapeutic approaches. Gill et al. have reported that a combination of doxorubicin, bleomycin, and vincristine results in rapid and often complete KS responses with no apparent increase in expected rates of opportunistic infections. Doses of each agent are as follows: doxorubicin, 20 mg/m^2; bleomycin, 10 MG/M^2; vincristine, 1.4 mg/m^2, all given intravenously every other week.[414] Because of the cardiac, pulmonary, and neurologic toxicities of these agents, this regimen should probably be reserved for patients with poor overall prognoses, particularly for those with symptomatic pulmonary KS. Its use should be accompanied by careful monitoring of toxicities.

INTERFERON-α. Systemic recombinant interferon-α has an established level of activity in treating HIV-related KS and is approved by the Food and Drug Administration (FDA) for this indication. Objective response rates of approximately 40 percent can be expected and are even higher in selected patients with a more favorable overall prognosis.[415–419] The doses used have varied widely in reported trials, but daily doses of greater than 10 million units may be required for the optimum antineoplastic effect. The major predictor of poor response in several studies is the presence of chronic constitutional symptoms or a prior AIDS diagnosis when therapy with interferon is initiated. The drawbacks to single-agent interferon-α therapy are the side effects seen with the high doses required and the need for parenteral injection. Toxicities are primarily subjective—fever, malaise, nausea—but neutropenia is not uncommon, and CNS effects including confusion are also seen.

Studies in New York and Miami by the NIAID AIDS Clinical Trials Group show antineoplastic activity with low doses (9–18 million units) of recombinant or lymphoblastoid interferon-α along with low doses (100 mg every 4 hours) of zidovudine.[420–422] Hematologic toxicity was seen in these studies but was considered moderate and usually manageable by the investigators.

Non-Hodgkin's Lymphoma

The second most common HIV-associated malignancy, non-Hodgkin's lymphoma (NHL), bears little epidemiologic resemblance to KS. Non-Hodgkin's lymphoma is less frequent than KS; it is the index AIDS diagnosis in less than 1 percent of cases in the United States, but is not restricted to any specific risk group. Nor does the relative frequency of diagnosed NHL seem to be changing, although the absolute number of cases is increasing with the epidemic.[62,317,322,326,423,424]

The pathogenesis of HIV-associated NHL is unknown but is the subject of active laboratory investigation, although some of the tumor's biologic characteristics are understood.[424,425] Non-Hodgkin's lymphoma in AIDS is a B-lymphocyte neoplasm of unfavorable histologic grade.[321] Most are either large cell, undifferentiated, or immunoblastic types with a clinical presentation and natural history that matches their highly malignant pathologic appearance. No single cytogenetic abnormality has been found, but several different gene rearrangements have been reported. A relationship to EBV has been proposed, and seems probable with NHL in the CNS. Laboratory studies of non-CNS NHL have been inconclusive, with EBV-related DNA sequences found in some, but not all specimens from several tumor sites in a single affected individual.[428]

Non-Hodgkin's lymphoma in HIV can be present in single or multiple sites, and the clinical problems are determined, in part, by areas of involvement, by the rate of tumor growth, and by the presence or absence of underlying or preexisting HIV-related opportunistic infections. Malignant lymphocytes are often found in the peripheral blood of NHL patients with HIV, but it is uncommon for the lymphoma to present without easily identifiable solid tumor masses.

Central Nervous System Non-Hodgkin's Lymphoma. Non-Hodgkin's lymphoma occurring in the CNS in AIDS patients was recognized early in the epidemic, well before the peripheral lymphomas were reported, and thus the early CDC surveillance definitions of AIDS included NHL only of CNS origin.[315,429–433]

Central nervous system lymphomas cause the array of clinical problems expected from space-occupying intracranial masses, but these tumors have been surprisingly difficult to diagnose.[314,434] Diagnosis is often delayed given the other CNS processes that are more common in HIV infection, especially *Toxoplasma* encephalitis. In several autopsy series, CNS lymphomas have been surprisingly frequent, further attesting to the need to consider them in differential diagnoses and obtain a brain biopsy to establish the diagnosis. CNS NHL is a manifestation of very advanced HIV disease. The typical CD4 cell count at diagnosis below 25 cells/mm^3.

Patients with NHL in the CNS may complain of motor deficits, but others present with cranial neuropathies, headache, or seizures, and frequently some combination of these are present. The onset of symptoms is usually rapid, and death can occur quickly in the absence of therapy.

The diagnosis of CNS NHL relies on a combination of suggestive imaging studies and brain biopsy. Either contrast-enhanced CT or MRI head scanning are commonly employed, but MRI is a more sensitive test. In contrast to toxoplasmosis, NHL usually presents with a single mass lesion although the finding of several masses does not exclude the diagnosis. Tumors occurring along the base of the skull can be missed, especially by CT. A brain biopsy must be used to finally establish the NHL diagnosis, especially if an empirical course of therapy for toxoplasmosis fails to rapidly (1–2 weeks) lead to a decrease in mass size. Examination of the CSF is not of significant value and should be deferred until large intracranial mass lesions are excluded by imaging studies.

Peripheral Non-Hodgkin's Lymphoma. The clinical presentation of NHL outside the CNS is highly varied because essentially any organ can be affected. In contrast to NHL in non-HIV-infected patients, extralymphatic disease is extremely common, with 63 percent of patients having stage IV disease.[315,316,321,324,435] Also, NHL in the HIV-infected group presents with disease in sites otherwise rarely seen. These have included primary lymphoma in the liver, common bile duct, rectum, soft tissue, duodenum, and lung.[316,436,437] Peripheral NHL can be seen at essentially any stage of HIV disease with a median CD4 cell count at diagnosis of approximately 200 cells/mm³.

The rapid clinical course and poor prognosis of NHL in the HIV-infected patient is not surprising considering the tumor's aggressive histology. Patients often have fulminant disease progression, even developing the tumor lysis syndrome before initiation of therapy due to rapid tumor cell turnover The prognosis of NHL in HIV infection is extremely grave. In several reports from Los Angeles, New York, and San Francisco, the median survival from diagnosis was less than 12 months.[316,317,438] Markers of prognosis include histologic type and stage as with the non-HIV-infected patient, but the most important factor is whether or not the lymphoma represents the patient's first HIV-induced opportunistic disease. Patients with a prior history of AIDS and a low CD4 cell count have a median survival of 3 months as compared with 12 months for those initially diagnosed with AIDS on the basis of the lymphoma.[316] In fact, some would generally discourage treatment for patients with a prior AIDS diagnosis because of the poor prognosis and limited ability to tolerate the aggressive chemotherapy otherwise essential to control the lymphoma.

The relationship between persistent generalized lymphadenopathy (PGL) and NHL has been widely discussed but is still quite unclear. It is obvious that in some HIV-infected individuals B-cell proliferation results in diffuse and persisting lymph node enlargement. Occasionally, NHL arises in patients with PGL, but it is not certain that the factors responsible for PGL are the same as those causing the malignant proliferation. What is clear is that the usual caveats against biopsying nodes in patients with PGL need revision if one nodal group is rapidly enlarging. Because this is often due to NHL, immediate biopsy is essential.[439,440]

The diagnosis of NHL should ideally be made by histologic examination of tissue obtained by incisional or excisional biopsy. This permits a more accurate assessment of histologic type for special stains and immunologic subtyping. It may be possible, however, to make an adequate diagnosis from needle aspiration cytology, and this may be required if the patient's clinical condition is critical or deteriorating rapidly.[439] Because the disease is so often widespread, the initial clinical evaluation of the NHL patient should include imaging of the head, chest, and abdomen[441,442]; bone marrow aspiration and biopsy; and lumbar puncture. Once staging is completed, therapy, if it is to be recommended, should be initiated promptly and should be coordinated by an oncologist experienced with these extremely complex patients.

Therapy for HIV-Related Non-Hodgkin's Lymphoma. Therapy for HIV-related NHL is still under active investigation. If therapy is to be employed (potentially excluding those with extremely poor prognoses), an aggressive regimen must be used to achieve acceptable complete response rates. However, because patients with HIV infection have a limited bone marrow reserve, the clinician is frequently faced with the dilemma of selecting a regimen and dose of chemotherapy that controls the tumor without precipitating death from secondary infections. For NHL confined to the CNS, these questions are less urgent because primary therapy usually consists of whole brain radiation with intrathecal chemotherapy.[431]

CHEMOTHERAPY FOR NON-HODGKIN'S LYMPHOMA IN HIV-INFECTED PATIENTS. Few definite guidelines are possible for the treatment of HIV-related NHL. As with all aggressive lymphomas, the use of combinations of drugs is essential. In most reports, cyclophosphamide has been the primary agent,[316,321,324,443] however, because of the compromised marrow reserve at least one investigator favors an attenuated dose at the beginning and subsequent dose escalation. Older combinations such as cyclophosphamide, doxorubicin, vincristine, and prednisone (CHOP) are often avoided because their relatively prolonged dosing intervals may allow rapid tumor growth between cycles. Most clinicians favor attenuated doses of aggressive regimens such as M-BACOD (methotrexate, leucovorin rescue, bleomycin, doxorubicin, cyclophosphamide, vincristine, and dexamethasone); methotrexate with leucovorin rescue, doxorubicin, cyclophosphamide, vincristine, prednisone, and bleomycin (MACOP-B); cyclophosphamide, vincristine, prednisone, bleomycin, doxorubicin, and procarbazine (COP-BLAM); or cyclophosphamide, vincristine, methotrexate with leucovorin rescue, and cytarabine (COMLA). Even these general guidelines, however, should not be accepted as established because further clinical trials are clearly needed.

Drug regimens for peripheral NHL must include intrathecal therapy, which can be relatively brief in the absence of identified CNS involvement. Specific guidelines are available in clinical reviews from Los Angeles[323,443] and San Francisco.[316]

Zidovudine, because of its associated myelotoxicity, should, in general, be avoided in the early chemotherapy of HIV-related NHL. If antiretroviral therapy is to be used, nonmyelotoxic drugs such as didanosine or zalcitabine may be used instead.

Other clinical trials are exploring the use of hematopoietic hormones, G-CSF, or Gm-CSF, to support the bone marrow during combination chemotherapy. Such support is clearly able to reduce toxicity and allows higher dosage chemotherapy. Whether this approach is better than chemotherapy with reduced dosages is unclear.

A final area of NHL therapy deserving attention is the prophylaxis of opportunistic infections. Even more than in KS, these are a frequent cause of mortality for patients with NHL.[316] Prophylaxis of PCP should be employed in each NHL patient and all other prophylaxis guidelines should be followed as well.

Other Cancers in HIV Infection

The full spectrum of HIV-induced malignancies has not been fully elucidated but a large number of cancers have been diagnosed in HIV-infected persons[444–447] (Table 18). Some of these may be directly HIV induced but at a much lower rate than seen with KS or B-cell NHL. Others may arise as a secondary consequence of HIV-induced immune dysfunction whereas many may represent nothing more than a chance occurrence of two simultaneous diseases. Regardless of etiology, however, it seems clear that the clinical presentation and course of these rarer cancers is altered in the setting of HIV infection.

Hodgkin's Disease. Hodgkin's lymphoma is relatively common in HIV-infected patients.[448,449] One study finds an increased incidence in HIV,[450] others find no probable etiologic association. When Hodgkin's disease is diagnosed in the HIV-

TABLE 18. Cancers in the HIV Epidemic

Incidence increased:
  Kaposi sarcoma
  CNS non-Hodgkin's lymphoma
  Peripheral non-Hodgkin's lymphoma
Cases reported
  Hodgkin's lymphoma
  Squamous carcinoma
  Small cell carcinoma
  Testicular cancer
  Basal cell cancer
  Melanoma
Anticipated relationship:
  Hepatocellular carcinoma

Abbreviation: CNS, central nervous system.

infected patient it is usually more advanced in stage—often stage IVB—and of mixed cellular histology. Hodgkin's disease responds well to conventional chemotherapy management but a complete regression is less often seen and relapses more common in the HIV-infected patient. Despite this, conventional treatment should be used for HIV-infected Hodgkin's disease patients as durable complete remissions can often be achieved.

Cervical Cancer. Numerous studies document a high frequency of cervical dysplasia in HIV-infected women, which becomes more common and severe in grade with advancing HIV disease.[451] Frank malignancy is less commonly seen although cases of aggressive cervical cancer have occurred. A relationship between cervical changes and human papillomavirus (HPV) is presumed although the relationship between this virus and HIV if any is unknown.

Clinical care of HIV-infected women must recognize the increased risk of cervical disease and routine pelvic examinations with Pap smears included. The optimal frequency of Pap smear is uncertain. Most recommend annual examinations with the frequency increased to every 6 months with CD4 cell counts below 200/mm³. Any abnormalities on Pap smear should be followed by colposcopy.

Anal Squamous Cancer. Similar to cervical cancer in its association with HPV,[452–454] anal cancers are more common in HIV-infected patients and are preceded by a prolonged period of cellular atypia. Invasive cancers are still relatively uncommon but should be considered in the diagnoses of anal disorders.

REFERENCES

1. Gottlieb MS, Schroff R, Schanker HM, et al. *Pneumocystis carinii* pneumonia and mucosal candidiasis in previously healthy homosexual men: Evidence of a new acquired cellular immunodeficiency. N Engl J Med. 1981; 305:1425–31.
2. Masur H, Michelis MA, Greene JB, et al. An outbreak of community-acquired *Pneumocystis carinii* pneumonia: Initial manifestation of cellular immune dysfunction. N Engl J Med. 198;305:1431–8.
3. Siegal FP, Lopez C, Hammer GS, et al. Severe acquired immunodeficiency in male homosexuals manifested by chronic perianal ulcerative herpes simplex lesions. N Engl J Med. 1981;305:1431–8.
4. Follansbee SE, Busch DF, Wofsy CB, et al. An outbreak of *Pneumocystis carinii* pneumonia in homosexual men. Ann Intern Med. 1982;96:705–13.
5. Centers for Disease Control and Prevention. Kaposi's sarcoma and *Pneumocystis* pneumonia among homosexual men—New York City and California. MMWR. 1982;30:305–8.
6. Centers for Disease Control and Prevention. Opportunistic infections and Kaposi's sarcoma among Haitians in the United States. MMWR. 1982;31:353–61.
7. Centers for Disease Control and Prevention. Update on acquired immunodeficiency syndrome (AIDS)—United States. MMWR. 1982;31:507–14.
8. Centers for Disease Control and Prevention. Update: Acquired immunodeficiency syndrome—United States. MMWR. 1985;34:245–8.
9. Centers for Disease Control and Prevention. *Pneumocystis carinii* pneumonia among persons with hemophila A. MMWR. 1982;31:365–7.
10. Centers for Disease Control and Prevention. Update on acquired immune deficiency syndrome (AIDS) among patients with hemophilia A. MMWR. 1982;31:644–6, 652.
11. Pape JW, Liautaud B, Thomas F, et al. Characteristics of the acquired immunodeficiency syndrome (AIDS) in Haiti. N Engl J Med. 1983;309:945–50.
12. Pape JW, Liautaud B, Thomas F, et al. The acquired immunodeficiency syndrome in Haiti. Ann Intern Med. 1985;103:674–8.
13. Malebranche R, Annoux E, Guerin JM, et al. AIDS with severe gastrointestinal manifestations in Haiti. Lancet. 1983;2:873–8.
14. Centers for Disease Control and Prevention. Possible transfusion-associated acquired immune deficiency syndrome AIDS—California. MMWR. 1982;31:652–4.
15. Abrams DI, Lewis BJ, Beckstead JP, et al. Persistent diffuse lymphadenopathy in homosexual men: Endpoint or prodrome? Ann Intern Med. 1984;100:801–8.
16. Metroka CE, Cunningham-Rundles S, Pollack MS, et al. Persistent generalized lymphadenopathy in homosexual men. Ann Intern Med. 1983;99:585.
17. Morris L, Distenfeld A, Amorosi E, et al. Autoimmune thrombocytopenic purpura in homosexual men. Ann Intern Med. 1982;96:714–7.
18. Walsh CM, Nardi MA, Karpatkin S. On the mechanism of thrombocytopenic purpura in sexually active homosexual men. N Engl J Med. 1984;311:635–9.
19. Abrams DI, Volberding PA, Linker CA, et al. Immune thrombocytopenic purpura in homosexual men: Clinical manifestations and treatment results (Abstract). Blood. 1983;62:1082.
20. Abrams DI. AIDS-related conditions. Clinics Immunol Allergy. 1986;6:581.
21. Harris C, Small CB, Klein RS, et al. Immunodeficiency in female sexual patners of men with the acquired immunodeficiency syndrome. N Engl J Med. 1984;308:1181–4.
22. Barre-Sinoussi F, Chermann JC, Rey F, et al. Isolation of a T-lymphotropic retrovirus from a patient at risk for acquired immunodeficiency syndrome (AIDS). Science. 1983;220:868–71.
23. Gallo RC, Salahudin SZ, Popovic M, et al. Frequent detection and isolation of cytopathic retroviruses (HTLV-III) from patients with AIDS and at risk for AIDS. Science. 1984;224:500–3.
24. Levy JA, Hoffman AD, Kramer SD, et al. Isolation of lymphocytopathic retrovirus from San Francisco patients with AIDS. Science. 1984;225:840–2.
25. Nzilambi N, DeCock KM, Forthal DN, et al. The prevalence of infection with human immunodeficiency virus over a 10-year period in rural Zaire. N Engl J Med. 1988;318:276.
26. Corbitt G, Bailey AS, Williams G. HIV infection in Manchester, 1959 (Letter). Lancet. 1990;336:51.
27. Garry RF, Witte MH, Gottlieb AA, et al. Documentation of AIDS virus infection in the United States in 1968. JAMA. 1988;260:2085.
28. Centers for Disease Control and Prevention. Revision of the CDC surveillance case definition for acquired immunodeficiency syndrome. MMWR. 1987;36:1S–15S.
29. Selik RM, Buehler JW, Karon JM, et al. Impact of the 1987 revision of the case definition of acquired immune deficiency syndrome in the United States. J AIDS. 1990;3:73–82.
30. World Health Organization. Interim proposal for a WHO staging system for HIV infection and diseases. Wkly Epidemiol Rec. 1990;65:221–4.
31. Centers for Disease Control and Prevention. 1993 revised classification system for HIV infection and expanded surveillance case definition for AIDS among adolescents and adults. MMWR. 1992;41:1–19.
32. Centers for Disease Control and Prevention. Current trends: Classification system for human T lymphotropic virus type III/lymphadenopathy associated virus infections. MMWR. 1986;35:334–9.
33. Redfield RR, Wright DC, Tramont EC. The Walter Reed staging classification for HTLV-III/LAV infection. N Engl J Med. 1986;314:131–2.
34. MacDonnell KB, Chmiel JS, Goldsmith J, et al. Prognostic usefulness of the Walter Reed Staging classification for HIV infection. JAIDS. 1988;1:367–74.
35. Blatt SP, Hendrix CW, Butzin CA, et al. Delayed-typed hypersensitivity skin testing predicts progression to AIDS in HIV-infected patients. Ann Intern Med. 1993;119:177–84.
35a. Yarchoan R, Venzon DJ, Pluda JM, et al. CD4 count and the risk for death in patients infected with HIV receiving antiretroviral therapy. Ann Intern Med. 1991;115:184–9.
36. Centers for Disease Control and Prevention. Classification system for human immunodeficiency virus (HIV) infection in childen under 13 years of age. MMWR. 1987;36:225–36.
37. Centers for Disease Control and Prevention. Update: Serologic testing for antibody to human immunodeficiency virus. MMWR. 1988;36:833–45.
38. Kessler HA, Blaauw B, Spear J, et al. Diagnosis of human immunodeficiency virus infection in seronegative homosexuals presenting with an acute viral syndrome. JAMA. 1987;258:1196–9.
39. Miles SA, Balden E, Magpantay L, et al. Rapid serologic testing with immune-complex-dissociated HIV p24 antigen for early detection of HIV infection in neonates. N Engl J Med. 1993;328:297–302.
40. Bacchetti P, Moss AR. Incubation period of AIDS in San Francisco. Nature. 1989;338:251–3.
41. Goedert JJ, Biggar RJ, Weiss SH, et al. Three-year incidence of AIDS in five cohorts of HTLV-III-infected risk group members. Science. 1986;231:992–5.
42. Ward JW, Deppe DA, Samson S, et al. Risk of human immunodeficiency virus infection from blood donors who later developed the acquired immunodeficiency syndrome. Ann Intern Med. 1987;106:61–2.
43. Muñoz A, Wang M-C, Bass S, et al. Acquired immunodeficiency syndrome (AIDS)-free time after human immunodeficiency virus type 1 (HIV-1) seroconversion in homosexual men. Am J Epidemiol. 1989;130:530–9.
44. Medley GF, Anderson RM, Cox DR, et al. Estimating the incubation period for AIDS patients. Nature. 1988;333:504–5.
45. Moss AR, Bacchetti P, Osmond D, et al. Seropositivity for HIV and the development of AIDS or AIDS related condition: Three year follow up of the San Francisco General Hospital cohort. Br Med J. 1988;296:745–50.
46. Bacchetti P, Osmond D, Chaisson RE, et al. Patterns of survival in the acquired immunodeficiency syndrome. J Inf Dis. 1988;157:1044–7.
47. Rothenberg R, Woelfel M, Stoneburner R, et al. Survival with the acquired immunodeficiency syndrome: Experience with 5833 cases in New York City. N Engl J Med. 1987;317:1297–302.
48. Lemp GF, Payne SF, Temelso DN, et al. Survival trends for patients with AIDS. JAMA. 1990;263:402–5.
49. Harris JE. Improved short-term survival of AIDS patients initially diagnosed with *Pneumocystis carinii* pneumonia, 1984 through 1987. JAMA. 1990;263:397–405.
50. Moore RD, Hidalgo J, Sugland B, et al. Zidovudine and the natural history of the acquired immunodeficiency syndrome. N Engl J Med. 1991;324:1412–6.
51. Chaisson RE, Keruly J, Richman DD, et al. Pneumocystis prophylaxis and survival in patients with advanced human immunodeficiency virus infection treated with zidovudine. Arch Intern Med. 1992;152:2009–13.

52. Graham NM, Zeger SL, Park LP, et al. Effect of zidovudine and *Pneumocystis carinii* pneumonia prophylaxis on progression of HIV-1 infection to AIDS. Lancet. 1991;338:265–9.

53. Graham NM, Zeger SL, Park LP, et al. The effects on survival of early treatment of human immunodeficiency virus infection. N Engl J Med. 1992; 326:1037–42.

54. Hoover DR, Saah AJ, Bacellar H. Clinical manifesations of AIDS in the era of pneumocystis prophylaxis. N Engl J Med. 1993;329:1922–6.

55. Saah AJ, Munoz A, Kuo V, et al. Predictors of the risk of development of acquired immunodeficiency syndrome within 24 months among gay men seropositive for human immunodeficiency virus type 1: A report from the multicenter AIDS cohort study. Am J Epidemiol. 1992;135:1147–55.

56. Gallant JE, Moore RD, Chaisson RE. Prophylaxis for opportunistic infections in patients with HIV infection. Ann Intern Med. 1994;120:932–43.

57. Masur H, Ognibene FP, Yarchoan R, et al. CD4 counts as predictors of opportunistic pneumonias in human immunodeficiency virus (HIV) infection. Ann Intern Med. 1989;111:223–31.

58. Janoff EN, Breiman RF, Daley CL, et al. Pneumococcal disease during HIV infection. Ann Intern Med. 1992;117:314–24.

59. Theuer CP, Hopewell PC, Elias D, et al. Human immunodeficiency virus infection in tuberculosis patients. J Infect Dis. 1990;162:8–12.

60. Crowe SM, Carlin JB, Stewart KI, et al. Predictive value of CD4 lymphocyte numbers for the development of opportunistic infections and malignancies in HIV-infected persons. J AIDS. 1991;4:770–6.

61. Moore RD, Keruly J, Richman DD, et al. Natural history of advanced HIV disease in patients treated with zidovudine. AIDS. 1992;6:671–7.

62. Moore RD, Kessler H, Richman DD, et al. Non-Hodgkin's lymphoma in patients with advanced HIV infection treated with zidovudine. JAMA. 1991; 265:2208–11.

63. U.S. Public Health Service Task Force on antipneumocystis prophylaxis in patients with human immunodeficiency virus infection. Recommendations for prophylaxis against *Pneumocystis carinii* pneumonia for persons infected with human immunodeficiency virus. J AIDS. 1993;6:46–55.

63a. Centers for Disease Control and Prevention. Recommendations on prophylaxis and therapy for disseminated *Mycobacterium avium* complex for adults and adolescents infected with human immunodeficiency virus. MMWR. 1993;42(RR-9):14–20.

64. Phair J, Muñoz A, Detels R, et al. The risk of *Pneumocystis carinii* pneumonia among men infected with human immunodeficiency virus type 1. N Engl J Med. 1990;322:161–5.

65. Carne CA, Weller IVD, Loveday C, et al. From persistent generalized lymphadenopathy to AIDS: Who will progress? Br Med J. 1987;294:868–9.

66. Polk BF, Fox R, Brookmeyer R, et al. Predictors of the acquired immunodeficiency snydrome developing in a cohort of seropositive homosexual men. N Engl J Med. 1987;316:61–6.

67. Greenspan D, Greenspan JS, Hearst NG, et al. Relation of oral hairy leukoplakia to infection with the human immunodeficiency virus and the risk of developing AIDS. J Infect Dis. 1987;155:475–81.

68. Moss AR: Predicting progression to AIDS. Br Med J. 1988;297:1067–8.

69. Buchbinder SP, Katz MH, Hessol NA, et al. Herpes zoster and human immunodeficiency virus infection. J Infect Dis. 1992;166:1153–6.

70. Glesby MJ, Moore RD, Chaisson RE. Herpes zoster in patients with advanced human immunodeficiency virus infection treated with zidovudine. J Infect Dis. 1993;168:1264–8.

71. Murray HW, Godbold JH, Jurica KB, Roberts RB. Progression to AIDS in patients with lymphadenopathy or AIDS-related complex: Reappraisal of risk and predictive factors. Am J Med. 1989;86:533–8.

72. Goeddert JJ, Biggar RJ, Melbye M, et al. Effect of T4 count and cofactors on the incidence of AIDS in homosexual men infected with human immunodeficiency virus. JAMA. 1987;257:331–4.

73. Polk BF, Fox R, Brookmeyer R, et al. Predictors of the acquired immunodeficiency syndrome developing in a cohort of seropositive homosexual men. N Engl J Med. 1987;316:61–6.

74. Munoz A, Schroger L, Bacellar H, et al. Trends in the incidence of outcomes defining acquired immunodeficiency syndrome (AIDS) in the Multicenter AIDS cohort study: 1985–1991. Am J Epidemiol. 1993;137:423–38.

75. Taylor JM, Fahey JL, Detels R, et al. CD4 percentage, CD4 number, and CD4:CD8 ratio in HIV infection: Which to choose and how to use. J AIDS. 1989;2:114–24.

76. Allain J-P, Laurian Y, Paul DA, et al. Long-term evaluation of HIV antigen and antibodies to p24 and gp41 in patients with hemophilia. N Engl J Med. 1987;317:1114–21.

77. DeWolf F, Goudsmit J, Paul DA, et al. Risk of AIDS-related complex and AIDS in homosexual men with persistent antigenemia. Br Med J. 1987;295: 569–72.

78. Fuchs D, Kramer A, Reibnegger G. Neopterin and B2-microglobulin as prognostic indices in human immunodeficiency virus type 1 infection. Infection. 1991;2:S98–S102.

79. Fahey JL, Taylor J, Detels R, et al. The prognostic value of cellular and serologic markers in infection with human immunodeficiency virus type 1. N Engl J Med. 1990;322:166–72.

80. Chaisson RE, Taylor E, Margolick JB, et al. Immune serum markers and CD4 cell counts in HIV-infected intravenous drug users. J AIDS. 1992;5: 456–60.

81. Jacobson MA, Bacchetti P, Kolokathis A, et al. Surrogate markers for survival in patients with AIDS and AIDS-related complex treated with zidovudine. Br Med J. 1991;302:73–8.

82. Mildvan D, Machado SG, Wilets I, et al. Endogenous interferon and triglyceride concentrations to assess response to zidovudine in AIDS and advanced AIDS-related complex. Lancet. 1992;339:453–6.

83. Osmond DH, Shiboski S, Bacchetti P, et al. Immune activation markers and AIDS prognosis. AIDS. 1991;5:505–11.

84. Burnell R, Jeffries DJ, Pinching AJ, et al. Decline of anti p24 antibody precedes antigenaemia as correlate of prognosis in HIV-1 infection. AIDS. 1987; 1:235–40.

85. Koot M, Keet IP, Vos AH, et al. Prognostic value of HIV-1 syncytium-inducing phenotype for rate of CD4 + cell depletion and progression to AIDS. Ann Intern Med. 1993;118:681–8.

86. Semba RD, Graham NMH, Caiaffa WT, et al. Increased mortality associated with vitamin A deficiency during human immunodeficiency virus type 1 infection. Arch Intern Med. 1993;153:2149–54.

87. Ward BJ, Humphrey JH, Clement L, et al. Vitamin A status in HIV infection. Nutrition Res. 1993;13:157–66.

88. Vlahov D, Muñoz A, Anthony JC, et al. Association of drug injection patterns with antibody to human immunodeficiency virus type 1 among intravenous drug users in Baltimore, Maryland. Am J Epidemiol. 1990;132:847–56.

89. Beral V, Bull D, Darby S, et al. Risk of Kaposi's sarcoma and sexual practices associated with faecal contact in homosexual or bisexual men with AIDS. Lancet. 1992;339:632–5.

90. Hoover DR, Black C, Jacobson LP, et al. Epidemiologic analysis of Kaposi's sarcoma as an early and later AIDS outcome in homosexual men. Am J Epidemiol. 1993;138:266–78.

91. Gallant JE, Moore RD, Richman DD, et al. Risk factors for Kaposi's sarcoma in patients with advanced HIV disease treated with zidovudine. Arch Intern Med.

92. Kaslow RA, Blackwelder WC, Ostrow DG, et al. No evidence for a role of alcohol or psychoactive drugs as cofactors for HIV-1 induced immunodeficiency. JAMA. 1989;261:3424–9.

93. Muñoz A, Vlahov D, Solomon L, et al. Prognostic indicators for development of AIDS among intravenous drug users. J AIDS. 1992;5:694–700.

94. Schecter M'T, Craib KJP, Le TN, et al. Progression to AIDS and predictors of AIDS in seroprevalent and seroincident cohorts of homosexual men. AIDS. 1989;3:347–53.

95. Coates RA, Farewell VT, Raboud J, et al. Cofactors of progression to acquired immunodeficiency syndrome in a cohort of male sexual contacts of men with human immunodeficiency virus disese. Am J Epidemiol. 1990;132: 717–22.

96. Nabael GJ, Rice SA, Knipe DM, et al. Alternative mechanisms for activation of human immunodeficiency virus enhancer in T cells. Science. 1988;239: 1299–302.

97. Cooper DA, Pehson PO, Pedersen C, et al. The efficacy and safety of zidovudine alone or as cotherapy with acyclovir for the treatment of patients with AIDS and AIDS-related complex: A double-blind randomized trial. AIDS. 1993;7:197–207.

98. DesJarlaiś DC, Friedman SR, Marmor M, et al. HTLV-III/LAV-associated disease progression and co-factors in a cohort of IV drug users. AIDS. 1987; 1:105–11.

99. Alcabes P, Schoenbaum EE, Klein RS. Correlates of the rate of decline of CD4 + lymphocytes among injection drug users infected with the human immunodeficiency virus. Am J Epidemiol. 1993;137:989–1000.

100. Nelson KE, Clements ML, Miotti P, et al. The influence of human immunodeficiency virus (HIV) infection on antibody responses to influenza vaccines. Ann Intern Med. 1988;109:383–8.

101. Mann DL, Murray C, Yarchoan R, et al. HLA antigen frequencies in HIV-1 seropositive disease-free individuals and patients with AIDS. J AIDS. 1988; 1:1185–8.

102. Eyster ME, Gail MH, Ballard JO, et al. Natural history of human immunodeficiency virus infections in hemophiliacs: Effects of T-cell subsets, platelet counts and age. Ann Intern Med. 1987;107:1–6.

103. Cooper DA, Gold J, Maclean P, et al. Acute AIDS retrovirus infection: Definition of a clinical illness associated with seroconversion. Lancet. 1985; 1:537–40.

104. Tindall B, Barker S, Donovan B, et al. Characteristics of the acute clinical illness associated with human immunodeficiency virus infection. Arch Intern Med. 1988;148:945–9.

105. Moss AR, Osmond D, Bacchetti P, et al. Risk factors for AIDS and HIV seropositivity in homosexual men. Am J Epidemiol. 1987;125:1035–47.

106. Tokars JI, Marcus R, Culver DH, et al. Surveillance of HIV infection and zidovudine use among health care workers after occupational exposure to HIV-infected blood. Ann Intern Med. 1993;118:913–9.

107. Jaffe HW, Hardy AM, Morgan WM, et al. The acquired immunodeficiency syndrome in gay men. Ann Intern Med. 1985;103:662–4.

108. Fox R, Eldred LJ, Fuchs EJ, et al. Clinical manifestations of acute infection with human immunodeficiency virus in a cohort of gay men. AIDS. 1987;1: 35–8.

109. Anonymous: Needlestick transmission of HTLV-III from a patient infected in Africa. Lancet. 1984;2:1376–7.

110. Niu MT, Stein DS, Schnittman SM. Primary human immunodeficiency virus type 1 infection: Review of pathogenesis and early treatment intervention in humans and animals retrovirus infections. J Infect Dis. 1993;168:1490–501.

111. Clark SJ, Saag MS, Decker WD, et al. High titers of cytopathic virus in plasma of patients with symptomatic primary HIV-1 infection. N Engl J Med. 1991;324:954–60.

112. Niu MT, Jermano JA, Reichelderfer P, et al. Summary of the National Insti-

tutes of Health workshop on primary human immunodeficiency virus type I infection. AIDS Research and Human Retroviruses. 1993;9:913–24.

113. Rustin MHA, Ridely CM, Smith MD, et al. The acute exanthem associated with seroconversion to human T-cell lymphotropic virus III in a homosexual man. J Infect Dis. 1986;12:161–3.

114. Carne CA, Tedder RS, Smith A, et al. Acute encephalopathy coincident with seroconversion for anti-HTLV-III. Lancet. 1985;2:1206–8.

115. Denning DW, Anderson J, Rudge P, et al. Acute myelopathy associated with primary infection with human immunodeficiency virus. Br Med J. 1987;294:143–4.

116. Elder G, Dalakas M, Pezeshkpour G, et al. Ataxic neuropathy due to ganglioneuritis after probable acute human immunodeficiency virus infection. Lancet. 1986;2:1275–6.

117. Farthing C, Gazzard B. Acute illnesses associated with HTLV-III seroconversion. Lancet. 1985;1:935–6.

118. Ho DD, Sarngadharan MG, Resnick L, et al. Primary human T-lymphotropic virus type III infection. Ann Intern Med. 1985;103:880–3.

119. Piette AM, Tusseau F, Vignon D, et al. Acute neuropathy coincident with seroconversion for anti-LAV/HTLV-III. Lancet. 1986;1:852.

120. Podzamczer D, Casanova A, Santa-maria P, et al. Esophageal candidiasis in the diagnosis of HIV-infected patients. JAMA. 1988;259:1328–9.

121. Cooper DA, Imrie AA, Penny R. Antibody response to human immunodeficiency virus after primary infection. J Infect Dis. 1987;155:1113–8.

122. Cooper DA, Tindall B, Wilson E, et al. Characterization of T lymphocyte responses during primary HIV infection. J Infect Dis. 1987;157:889–96.

123. Goudsmit J, De Wolf F, Paul DA, et al. Expression of human immunodeficiency virus antigen (HIV-Ag) in serum and cerebrospinal fluid during acute and chronic infection. Lancet. 1986;2:177–80.

124. Kessler HA, Blaauw B, Spear J, et al. Diagnosis of human immunodeficiency virus infection in seronegative homosexuals presenting with an acute viral syndrome. JAMA. 1987;258:1196–7.

125. Lange JM, Boucher CA, Hollak CE, et al. Failure of zidovudine prophylaxis after accidental exposure to HIV-1. N Engl J Med. 1990;322:1375–7.

126. Daar ES, Mougdil T, Meyer RD, et al. Transient high level of uremia in patients with primary human immunodeficiency virus type 1 infection. N Engl J Med. 1991;324:961–4.

127. Osmond D, Chaisson RE, Moss A, et al. Lymphadenopathy in asymptomatic patients seropositive for HIV. N Engl J Med. 1987;317:246.

128. Bottles K, McPhaul LW, Volberding P. Fine-needle aspiration biopsy of patients with the acquired immunodeficiency syndrome (AIDS): Experience in an outpatient clinic. Ann Intern Med. 1988;108:42–5.

129. Abrams DI. AIDS-related lymphadenopathy: The role of biopsy. J Clin Oncol. 1986;4:126–7.

129a. Pantaleo G, Graziosi C, Demarest JF, et al. HIV infection is active and progressive in lymphoid tissue during the clinically latent stage of disease. Nature. 1993;362:355–8.

130. Hambleton J, Abrams DI. Hematologic manifestations of HIV infection. In: Sande MA, Volberding PA, eds. The Medical Management of AIDS. 3rd ed. Philadelphia: WB Saunders; 1992:234–46.

131. Morris L, Distenfeld A, Amorosi E, et al. Autoimmune thrombocytopenic purpura in homosexual men. Ann Intern Med. 1982;96:714–7.

132. Ballem PJ, Belzberg A, Devine DV, et al. Kinetic studies of the mechanism of thrombocytopenia in patients with human immunodeficiency virus infection. N Engl J Med. 1992;327:1779–84.

133. The Swiss Group for Clinical Studies on AIDS, Luthy R, Chairman. Zidovudine for the treatment of thrombocytopenia associated with human immunodeficiency virus (HIV): A prospective study. Ann Intern Med. 1988;109:718–21.

134. Nair JM, Bellevue R, Bertoni M, et al. Thrombotic thrombocytopenic purpura in patients with the acquired immunodeficiency syndrome (AIDS)-related complex. Ann Intern Med. 1988;109:209–12.

135. Leaf AN, Laubenstein LJ, Raphael B, et al. Thrombotic thrombocytopenic purpura associated with human immunodeficiency virus type 1 (HIV-1) infection. Ann Intern Med. 1988;109:194–7.

136. Folks TM, Kessler SW, Orenstein JM, et al. Infection and replication of HIV-1 in purified progenitor cells of normal human bone marrow. Science. 1988;242:919–22.

137. Spivak JL, Barnes DC, Fuchs E, et al. Serum immunoreactive erythropoietin in HIV-infected patients. JAMA. 1989;261:3104–7.

138. Richman DD, Fischl MA, Grieco MH, et al. The toxicity of azidothymidine (AZT) in the treatment of patients with AIDS and AIDS-related complex. A double-blind, placebo-controlled trial. N Engl J Med. 1987;317:192–7.

139. Frickhofen N, Abkowitz JL, Safford M, et al. Persistent B19 parovirus infection in patients infected with human immunodeficiency virus type 1 (HIV-1): A treatable cause of anemia in AIDS. Ann Intern Med. 1990;113:926–33.

140. Naides SJ, Howard EJ, Swack NS, et al. Parvovirus B19 infection in human immunodeficiency virus type 1-infected persons failing or intolerant to zidovudine therapy. J Infect Dis. 1993;168:101–5.

141. Ellis M, Gupta S, Galant S, et al. Impaired neutrophil function in patients with AIDS or AIDS-related complex: A comprehensive evaluation. J Infect Dis. 1988;158:1268–76.

142. Collaborative DHPG Treatment Study Group. Treatment of serious cytomegalovirus infections with 9-(1,3-dihydroxy-2-propoxymethyl) quanine in patients with AIDS and other immundeficiencies. N Engl J Med. 1986;314:801–5.

143. Miller EN, Selnes OA, McArthur JC, et al. Neuropsychological performance in HIV-1-infected homosexual men. Neurology. 1990;40:197–203.

144. Chuang HT, Devins GM, Hunsley J, et al. Psychosocial distress and well-being among gay and bisexual men with human immunodeficiency virus infection. Am J Psychiatry. 1989;146:876–80.

145. Sepkowitz KA, Telzak EE, Carrow M, et al. Fever among outpatients with advanced human immunodeficiency virus infection. Arch Intern Med. 1993;153:1909–12.

146. Serwadda D, Mugerwa RD, Sewankambo NK, et al. Slim disease: A new disease in Uganda and its association with HTLV-III infection. Lancet. 1985;2:1849.

147. Sewankambo N, Mugerwa R, Goodgame R, et al. Enteropathic AIDS in Uganda: An endoscopic, histologic and microbiologic study. AIDS. 1987;1:9–14.

148. DeCock KM, Soro B, Coulibaly IM, et al. Tuberculosis and HIV infection in sub-Saharan Africa. JAMA. 1992;268:1581–7.

149. Greenspan JS, Greenspan D, Winkler JR. Diagnosis and Management of the Oral Manifestations of HIV Infection and AIDS. In: Sande ME, Volberding PA eds. The Medical Management of AIDS. Philadelphia: WB Saunders; 1988:127–40.

150. Greenspan D, Greenspan JS. Oral manifestations of human immunodeficiency virus infection. Dent Clin North Am. 1993;37:21–32.

151. Royce RA, Luckmann RS, Fusaro RE, et al. The natural history of HIV-1 infection: Staging classifications of disease. AIDS. 1991;5:355–64.

152. Klein RS, Harris CA, Small CB, et al. Oral candidiasis in high-risk patients as the initial manifestation of the acquired immunodeficiency syndrome. N Engl J Med. 1984;311:354–8.

153. Feigal DW, Katz MH, Greenspan D, et al. The prevalence of oral lesions in HIV-infected homosexual and bisexual men: Three San Francisco epidemiological cohorts. AIDS. 1991;5:519–25.

154. Sanguineti A, Carmichael JK, Campbell K. Fluconazole-resistant candida albicans after long-term suppressive therapy. Arch Intern Med. 1993;153:1122–4.

155. Tavitian A, Raufman JP, Rosenthal LE, et al. Ketoconazole-resistant Candida esophatitis in patients with acquired immunodeficiency syndrome. Gastroenterology. 1986;90:443–5.

156. Greenspan D, Greenspan JS, Conant M, et al. Oral "hairy" leukoplakia in male homosexuals: Evidence of association with both papillomavirus and a herpes-group virus. Lancet. 1984;2:831–4.

157. Greenspan JS, Greenspan D, Lennette ET, et al. Replication of Epstein-Barr virus within the epithelial cells of oral "hairy" leukoplakia and AIDS-associated lesion. N Engl J Med. 1985;313:1564–71.

158. Rowland RW, Escobar MR, Friedman RB, et al. Painful gingivitis may be an early sign of infection with the human immunodeficiency virus. Clin Infect Dis. 1993;16:233–6.

159. Bach MC, Howell DA, Valenti AS, et al. Aphthous ulceration of the gastrointesitnal tract in patients with the acquired immunodeficiency syndrome (AIDS). Ann Intern Med. 1990;112:465–7.

160. Hook EW, Cannon RO, Nahmias AJ, et al. Herpes simplex virus infection as a risk factor for human immunodeficiency virus infection in heterosexuals. J Infect Dis. 1992;165:251–5.

161. Hoegsberg B, Abulafia O, Sedis A. Sexually transmitted diseases and human immunodeficiency virus infection among women with pelvic inflammatory disease. Am J Obstet Gynecol. 1990;163:1135–9.

162. Rhoads JL, Wright DC, Redfield RR, et al. Chronic vaginal candidiasis in women with human immunodeficiency virus infection. JAMA. 1987;257:3105–7.

163. Iman N, Carpenter CC, Mayer KH, et al. Hierarchical pattern of mucosal candida infections in HIV-seropositive women. Am J Med. 1990;89:142–6.

164. Maiman M, Fruchter RG, Serur E, et al. Human immunodeficiency virus infection and cervical neoplasia. Gynecol Oncol. 1990;38:377–82.

165. Schafer A, Friedmann W, Mielke M, et al. The increased frequency of cervical dysplasia-neoplasia in women infected with the human immunodeficiency virus is related to the degree of immunosuppression. Am J Obstet Gynecol. 1991;164:593–5.

166. Vermund SH, Kelley KF, Klein RS, et al. High risk of human papillomavirus infection and cervical squamous intraepithelial lesions among women with symptomatic human immunodeficiency virus infection. Am J Obstet Gynecol. 1991;165:392–400.

167. Feingold AR, Vermund SH, Burk RD, et al. Cervical cytologic abnormalities and papillomavirus in women infected with human immunodeficiency virus. J AIDS. 1990;3:896–903.

168. Minkhoff HL, DeHovitz JA. Care of women with human immunodeficiency virus. JAMA. 1991;266:253–8.

169. Centers for Disease Control and Prevention. HIV/AIDS Surveillance Report, February 1994. Atlanta: Centers for Disease Control and Prevention.

170. Stamm WE, Handsfield HH, Rompalo AM, et al. The association between genital ulcer disease and acquisition of HIV infection in homosexual men. JAMA. 1988;260:1429–33.

171. Quinn TC, Cannon RO, Glasser D, et al. The association of syphilis with risk of human immunodeficiency virus infection in patients attending sexually transmitted disease clinics. Arch Intern Med. 1990;150:1297–302.

172. Johns DR, Tierney M, Felsenstein D. Alteration in the natural history of neurosyphilis by concurrent infection with the human immunodeficiency virus. N Engl J Med. 1987;316:1569–72.

173. Berry CD, Hooton TM, Collier AC, et al. Neurologic relapse after benzathine penicillin therapy for secondary syphilis in a patient with HIV infection. N Engl J Med. 1987;316:1587–9.

174. Katz DA, Berger JR, Duncan RC. Neurosyphilis. A comparative study of

the effects of infection with human immunodeficiency virus. Arch Neurol. 1993;50:243–9.

175. Hicks CV, Benson PM, Lupton GP, et al. Seronegative secondary syphilis in a patient infected with the human immunodeficiency virus (HIV) with Kaposi sarcoma. A diagnostic dilemma. Ann Intern Med. 1987;107:492–5.

176. Hook EW, Marra CM. Acquired syphillis in adults. N Engl J Med. 1992; 326:1060–9.

177. Hutchinson CM, Rompalo AM, Reichart CA, et al. Characteristics of patients with syphilis attending Baltimore STD clinics. Multiple high-risk subgroups and interactions with human immunodeficiency virus infection. Arch Intern Med. 1991;151:511–6.

178. Centers for Disease Control and Prevention. Sexually transmitted diseases guidelines. MMWR. 1993;42:(RR-14):1–102.

179. Dalakas MC, Pezeshkpour GH, Gnavall M, et al. Polymyositis associated with AIDS retrovirus. JAMA. 1986;256:2381–3.

180. Dalakas MC, Pezeshkpour GH. Neuromuscular diseases associated with human immunodeficiency virus infection. Ann Neurol. 1988;23:S38–48.

181. Dalakas MC, Illa I, Pezeshkpour GH, et al. Mitochondrial myopathy caused by long-term zidovudine therapy. N Engl J Med. 1990;322:1098–105.

182. Schwartzman WA, Lambertus MW, Kennedy CA, et al. Staphylococcal pyomyositis in patients infected by the human immunodeficiency virus. Am J Med. 1991;90:595–600.

183. Hochberg MC, Fox R, Nelson KE, et al. HIV infection is not associated with Reiter's syndrome: Data from the Johns Hopkins Multicenter AIDS cohort study. AIDS. 1990;4:1149–51.

184. Winchester R, Bernstein DH, Fischer HD, et al. The co-occurrence of Rieter's syndrome and acquired immunodeficiency syndrome. Ann Intern Med. 1987;106:19–26.

185. Quinnan GV, Masur H, Rook AH, et al. Herpesvirus infections in the acquired immune deficiency syndrome. JAMA. 1984;252:72–7.

186. Friedman-Kien AE, Lafleur FL, Gendler E, et al. Herpes zoster: A possible early clinical sign for development of acquired immunodeficiency syndrome in high-risk individuals. J Am Acad Dermatol. 1986;14:1023–8.

187. Safrin S, Crumpacker C, Chatis P, et al. A controlled trial comparing foscarnet with vidarabine for acyclovir-resistant mucocutaneous herpes simplex in the acquired immunodeficiency syndrome. N Engl J Med. 1991;325:551–5.

188. Jacobson MA, Berger TG, Fikrig S, et al. Acyclovir-resistant varicella zoster virus infection after chronic oral acyclovir therapy in patients with the acquired immunodeficiency syndrome (AIDS). Ann Intern Med. 1990;112: 187–91.

189. Erlich KS, Mills J, Chatis P, et al. Acyclovir-resistant herpes simplex virus infections in patients with the acquired immunodeficiency syndrome. N Engl J Med. 1989;320:293–6.

190. Melbye M, Grossman RJ, Goedert JJ, et al. Risk of AIDS after herpes zoster. Lancet. 1987:728–31.

191. Cohen PR, Beltrani VP, Grossman ME. Disseminated herpes zoster in patients with human immunodeficiency virus infection. Am J Med. 1988;84: 1076–80.

192. Grossman MC, Grossman ME. Chronic hyperkeratotic herpes zoster and human immunodeficiency virus infection. J Am Acad Dermatol. 1993;28: 306–8.

193. Tappero JW, Mohle-Boetani J, Koehler JE, et al. The epidemiology of bacillary angiomatosis and bacillary peliosis. JAMA. 1993;269:770–5.

194. Relman DA, Loutit JS, Schmidt TM, et al. The agent of bacillary angiomatosis: An approach to the identification of uncultured pathogens. N Engl J Med. 1990;323:1576–80.

195. Slater LN, Welch DF, Min KW. Rochalimaea hensalae causes bacillary angiomatosis and peliosis hepatis. Arch Intern Med. 1992;152:602–6.

196. Koehler JE, Quinn FD, Berger TG, et al. Isolation of Rochalimaea species from cutaneous and osseous lesions of bacillary angiomatosis. N Engl J Med. 1992;327:1625–31.

197. Stoler MH, Bonfiglio TA, Steigbigel RT, et al. An atypical subcutaneous infection associated with acquired immune deficiency syndrome. Am J Clin Pathol. 1983;80:714–8.

198. Koehler JE, Tappero JW. Bacillary angiomatosis and bacillary peliosis in patients infected with human immunodeficiency virus. Clin Infect Dis. 1993; 17:612–24.

199. Koehler JE, LeBoit PE, Egbert BM, et al. Cutaneous vascular lesions and disseminated cat-scratch disease in patients with the acquired immunodeficiency syndrome (AIDS) and AIDS-related complex. Ann Intern Med. 1988; 109:449–55.

200. Cello J. Gastrointestinal tract manifestations of AIDS. In: Sande MA, Volberding PA, eds. Medical Management of AIDS. 3rd ed. Philadelphia: WB Saunders; 1992:176–92.

201. Wilcox CM, Diehl DL, Cello JP, et al. Cytomegalovirus esophagitis in patients with AIDS: A clinical, endoscopic, and pathologic correlation. Ann Intern Med. 1990;113:589–93.

202. St Onge G, Bezahler GH. Giant esophageal ulcer associated with cytomegalovirus. Gastroenterology. 1983;83:127.

203. Bonacini M, Young T, Laine L. The causes of esophageal symptoms in human immunodeficiency virus infection. A prospective study of 100 patients. Arch Intern Med. 1991;151:1567–72.

204. Tavitian A, Raufman JP, Rosenthal LE. Oral candidiasis as a marker for esophageal candidiasis in the acquired immunodeficiency syndrome. Ann Intern Med. 1986;104:54.

205. Friedman SL, Wright TL, Altman DF. Gastrointestinal Kaposi's sarcoma in patients with acquired immunodeficiency syndrome: Endoscopic and autopsy findings. Gastroenterology. 1985;89:102–8.

206. Blumberg RS, Kelsey P, Perrone T, et al. Cytomegalovirus- and cryptosporidium-associated acalculous gangrenous cholecystitis. Am J Med. 1984;76: 1118.

207. Kavin H, Jonas RB, Chowdhury L, et al. Acalculous cholecystitis and cytomegalovirus infection the acquired immunodeficiency syndrome. Ann Intern Med. 1986;104:53.

208. Margulis SJ, Honig CL, Soave R, et al. Biliary tract obstruction in the acquired immunodeficiency syndrome. Ann Intern Med. 1986;105:207.

209. Schneiderman DJ, Cello JP, Laing FC. Papillary stenosis and sclerosing cholangitis in the acquired immunodeficiency syndrome. Ann Intern Med. 1987; 106:546–9.

210. Jacobson MA, Cello JP, Sande MA. Cholestasis and disseminated cytogalovirus disease in patients with acquired immunodeficiency syndrome. Am J Med. 1987;84:218–24.

211. Laughon BE, Druckman DA, Vernon A, et al. Prevalence of enteric pathogens in homosexual men with and without AIDS. Gastroenterology. 1988; 94:984–93.

212. Grohmann GS, Glass RI, Pereira HG, et al. Enteric viruses and diarrhea in HIV-infected patients. N Engl J Med. 1993;329:14–20.

213. NIH Conference. Gastrointestinal infections in AIDS. Ann Intern Med. 1992; 116:63–77.

214. Celum CL, Chaisson RE, Rutherford GW, et al. Incidence of salmonellosis in patients with the acquired immunodeficiency syndrome. J Infect Dis. 1987; 156:998–1002.

215. Soave R, Johnson WD Jr. Cryptosporidium and Isopora belli infections. J Infect Dis. 1988;157:225–9.

216. DeHovitz JA, Pape JW, Boncy M, et al. Clinical manifestations and therapy of Isospora belli infection in patients with the acquired immunodeficiency syndrome. N Engl J Med. 1986;315:87–90.

217. Orenstein JM, Chiang J, Steinberg W, et al. Intestinal microsporidiosis as a cause of diarrhea in HIV-infected patients: A report of 20 cases. Hum Pathol. 1990;21:475–81.

218. Shadduck JA, Lucas SB, Papadaki L, et al. Human microsporidiosis and AIDS. Rev Infect Dis. 1989;11:203–7.

219. Blaser MJ, Hale TL, Formal SB. Recurrent shigellosis complicating human immunodeficiency virus infection: Failure of pre-existing antibodies to confer protection. Am J Med. 1989;86:105–7.

220. Perlman DM, Ampel NM, Schifman RB, et al. Persistent Campylobacter jejuni infections in patients infected with the human immunodeficiency virus (HIV). Ann Intern Med. 1988;108:540–6.

221. Elder GH, Hunter PR, Codd GA. Hazardous freshwater cyanobacteria (blue-green algae). Lancet. 1993;341:1519–20.

222. Goodgame RW. Gastrointestinal cytomegalovirus disease. Ann Intern Med. 1993;119:924–35.

223. Lin J, Bleiweiss IJ, Mendelson MH, et al. Cytomegalovirus-associated appendicitis in a patient with the acquired immunodeficiency syndrome. Am J Med. 1990;89:377–9.

224. Quinn TC, Goodell SE, Mkrtichian E, et al. Chlamydia trachomatitis proctitis. N Engl J Med. 1981;305:195–200.

224a. Weber R, Bryan RT, Owen RL, et al. Improved light-microscopical detection of microsporidia spores in stool and duodenal aspirates. N Engl J Med. 1992; 326:161–6.

225. Greenson JK, Belitsos PC, Yardley JH, et al. AIDS enteropathy: Occult enteric infections and duodenal mucosal alterations in chronic diarrhea. Ann Intern Med. 1991;114:366–72.

226. Rao TKS, Filippone EJ, Nicastri AD, et al. Associated focal and segmental glomerulosclerosis in the acquired immunodeficiency syndrome. N Engl J Med. 1984;310:669–73.

227. Pardo V, Aldana M, Colton RM, et al. Glomerular lesions in the acquired immunodeficiency syndrome. Ann Intern Med. 1984;101:429–34.

228. Rao TKS, Friedman EA, Nicastri AD. The types of renal disease in the acquired immunodeficiency syndrome. N Engl J Med. 1987;316:1062–8.

229. Carbone L, D'Agati V, Cheng JT, et al. Course and prognosis of human immunodeficiency virus-associated nephropathy. Am J Med. 1989;87: 389–95.

230. Ortiz C, Meneses R, Jaffe D, et al. Outcome of patients with human immunodeficiency virus on maintenance hemodialysis. Kidney Int. 1988;34:248–53.

231. Lucas SB, Hounnou A, Peacock C, et al. The mortality and pathology of HIV infection in a West African city. AIDS. 1993;7:1569–79.

232. Selwyn PA, Feingold AR, Hartel D, et al. Increased risk of bacterial pneumonia in HIV-infected intravenous drug users without AIDS. AIDS. 1988;2: 267–72.

233. Johnson MP, Chaisson RE. Tuberculosis and HIV Disease. In: Volberding PA, Jacobson MA, eds. AIDS Clinical Review 1993/1994. New York: Marcel Dekker; 1994:73–94.

234. Kovacs JA, Hiemenz JW, Macher AM, et al. Pneumocystis carinii pneumonia: A comparison between patients with other immunodeficiencies. Ann Intern Med. 1984;100:663–71.

235. Chaisson RE, Schecter GF, Theuer CP, et al. Tuberculosis in patients with the acquired immunodeficiency syndrome: Clinical features, response to therapy, and survival. Am Rev Respir Dis. 1987;136:570–4.

236. Pitchenik AE, Cole C, Russell BW, et al. Tuberculosis, atypical mycobacteriosis, and the acquired immunodeficiency syndrome among Haitian and non-Haitian patients in south Florida. Ann Intern Med. 1984;101:641–5.

237. Small PM, Schecter GF, Goodman PC, et al. Treatment of tuberculosis in

patients with advanced human immunodeficiency virus infection. N Engl J Med. 1991;324:289–94.

238. Pitchenik AE, Burr J, Suarez M, et al. Human T-cell lymphotropic virus-III (HTLV-III) seropositivity and related disease among 71 consecutive patients in whom tuberculosis was diagnosed. Am Rev Respir Dis. 1987;135:815–9.

239. Louie E, Rice LB, Holzman RS. Tuberculosis in non-Haitian patients with acquired immunodeficiency syndrome. Chest. 1986;90:542–5.

240. Daley CL, Small PM, Schecter GF, et al. An outbreak of tuberculosis with accelerated progression among persons infected with the human immunodeficiency virus—an analysis using restriction-fragment length polymorphisms. N Engl J Med. 1992;326:231–5.

241. Hopewell PC. *Pneumocystis carinii* pneumonia: Current concepts. In: Sande MA, Volberding PA, eds. Medical Management of AIDS. 3rd ed. Philadelphia: WB Saunders. 1992:261–83.

242. Kovacs JA, Ng VL, Masur H, et al. Diagnosis of *Pneumyocystis carinii* pneumonia: Improved detection in sputum with use of monoclonal antibodies. N Engl J Med. 1988;318:589–93.

243. Ng VL, Virani NA, Chaisson RE, et al. Detection of *Pneumocystis carinii* in sputum and bronchoalveolar lavage fluid by direct fluorescent assay using monoclonal antibodies. J Clin Microbiol. 1990;28:2228–33.

244. Chuck SL, Sande MA. Infections with *Cryptococcus neoformans* in the acquired immunodeficiency syndrome. N Engl J Med. 1989;321:794–9.

245. Wheat LJ, Connolly-Stringfield PA, Baker RL, et al. Disseminated histomosis in the acquired immune deficiency syndrome: Clinical findings, diagnosis and treatment, and review of the literature. Medicine. 1990;69:361–74.

246. Millar AB, Patou G, Miller RF, et al. Cytomegalovirus in the lungs of patients with AIDS: Respiratory pathogen or passenger? Am Rev Respir Dis. 1990; 141:1474–7.

247. Jacobson MA, Mills J, Rush J, et al. Morbidity and mortality of patients with AIDS and first-episode *Pneumocystis carinii* pneumonia unaffected by concomitant pulmonary cytomegalovirus infection. Am Rev Respir Dis. 1991;144:6–9.

248. Broaddus C, Dake MD, Stulbarg MS, et al. Bronchoalveolar lavage and transbronchial biopsy for the diagnosis of pulmonary infections in the acquired immunodeficiency syndrome. Ann Intern Med. 1985;102:747–52.

249. Stover DE, White DA, Romano PA, et al. Diagnosis of pulmonary disease in the acquired immunodeficiency syndrome: Roles of bronchoscopy and bronchoalveolar lavage. Am Rev Respir Dis. 1984;131:659.

250. Hughes WT. *Pneumocystis carinii*. Boca Raton, FL: CRC Press; 1987.

251. Brenner M, Ognibene FP, Lack EE, et al. Prognostic factors and life expectancy of acquired immunodeficiency syndrome patients with *Pneumocystis carinii* pneumonia. Am Rev Respir Dis. 1987;136:1199–206.

252. Telzak EE, Cote RJ, Gold JW, et al. Extrapulmonary *Pneumocystis carinii* infections. Rev Infect Dis. 1990;12:380–6.

253. Gherman CR, Ward RR, Basis ML. *Pneumocystis carinii* otitis media and mastoiditis as the initial manifestation of the acquired immunodeficiency syndrome. Am J Med. 1988;85:250–2.

254. Pilon A, Echols RM, Celo JS, et al. Disseminated *Pneumocystis carinii* infection in AIDS. N Engl J Med. 1987;316:1410–1.

255. Theuer CP, Hopewell PC, Elias D, et al. Human immunodeficiency virus infection in tuberculosis patients. J Infect Dis. 1990;162:8–12.

256. Levine B, Chaisson RE. *Mycobacterium kansasii*: A cause of treatable pulmonary disease in patients with advanced human immunodeficiency virus infection. Ann Intern Med. 1991;114:861–8.

257. Chaisson RE, Moore RD, Richman DD, et al. Incidence and natural history of *Mycobacterium avium*-complex infections in patients with advanced HIV disease treated with zidovudine. Am Rev Respir Dis. 1992;146:285–9.

258. Nightingale SD, Byrd LT, Southern PM, et al. Incidence of *Mycobacterium avium*-intracellulare complex bacteremia in human immunodeficiency virus-positive patients. J Infect Dis. 1992;165:1082–5.

259. Selwyn PA, Hartel D, Lewis VA, et al. A prospective study of the risk of tuberculosis among intravenous drug users with human immunodeficiency virus infection. N Engl J Med. 1989;320:545–50.

260. Allen S, Batungwanayo J, Kerlikowske K, et al. Two-year incidence of tuberculosis in cohorts of HIV-infected and uninfected urban Rwandan women. Am Rev Respir Dis. 1992;146:1439–44.

261. Moreno S, Baraia-Etxaburu J, Bouza E, et al. Risk for developing tuberculosis among anergic patients infected with HIV. Ann Intern Med. 1993;119: 194–8.

262. Selwyn PA, Sckell BM, Alcabes P, et al. High risk of active tuberculosis in HIV-infected drug user with cutaneous anergy. JAMA. 1992;268:504–9.

263. DiPerri G, Cruciani M, Danzi MC, et al. Nosocomial epidemic of active tuberculosis among HIV-infected patients. Lancet. 1989;2:1502–4.

264. Edlin BR, Tokars JI, Grieco MH, et al. An outbreak of multidrug-resistant tuberculosis among hospitalized patients with the acquired immunodeficiency syndrome. N Engl J Med. 1992;326:1514–21.

265. Centers for Disease Control and Prevention. Nosocomial transmission of multidrug-resistant tuberculosis among HIV-infected persons—Florida and New York, 1988–1991. MMWR. 1991;40:585–91.

266. Fischl MA, Uttamchandani RB, Daikos GL, et al. An outbreak of tuberculosis caused by multiple-drug-resistant tubercle bacilli among patients with HIV infection. Ann Intern Med. 1992;117:177–83.

267. Goble M, Iseman MD, Madsen LS, et al. Treatment of 171 patients with pulmonary tuberculosis resistant to isoniazid and rifampin. N Engl J Med. 1993;328:527–32.

268. Fischl MA, Daikos GL, Uttamchandani RB, et al. Clinical presentation and

outcome of patient with HIV infection and tuberculosis caused by multiple-drug-resistant bacilli. Ann Intern Med. 1992;117:184–90.

269. Barber TW, Craven DE, McCabe WR. Bacteremia due to mycobacterium tuberculosis in patients with human immunodeficiency virus infection. Medicine. 1990;69:375–83.

270. Jones BE, Young SMM, Antoniskis D, et al. Relationship of the manifestations of tuberculosis to CD4 cell counts in patients with human immunodeficiency virus infection. Am Rev Respir Dis. 1993;148:1292–7.

271. Wallis RS, Vjecha M, Amir-Tahmasseb M, et al. Enhanced cytokine expression and elevated beta-2 microglobulin in HIV-positive tuberculosis. J Infect Dis. 1993;167:43–8.

272. Horsburgh CR Jr, Selik RM. The epidemiology of disseminated nontuberculous mycobacterial infection in the acquired immunodeficiency syndrome (AIDS). Am Rev Respir Dis. 1989;139:4–7.

273. Kirschner RA, Parker BC, Falkinham JO. Epidemiology of infection by nontuberculous mycobacteria. *Mycobacterium avium, Mycobacterium intracellulare*, and *Mycobacterium scrofulaceum* in acid, brown-water swamps of the southwestern United States and their association with environmental variables. Am Rev Respir Dis. 1992;145:271–5.

274. Chin DP, Hopewell PC, Yajko DM, et al. *Mycobacterium avium* complex in the respiratory or gastrointestinal tract and the risk of *M. avium* complex bacteremia in patients with human immunodeficiency virus infection. J Infect Dis. 1994;169:289–95.

275. Packer SJ, Cesario T, Williams JH Jr. *Mycobacterium avium* complex infection presenting as endobronchial lesions in immunosuppressed patients. Ann Intern Med. 1988;109:389–93.

276. Zurlo JJ, Feuerstein IM, Lebovics R, Lane HC. Sinusitis in HIV-1 infection. Am J Med. 1992;93:157–62.

277. Godofsky EW, Zinreich J, Armstrong M, et al. Sinusitis in HIV-infected patients: A clinical and radiographic review. Am J Med. 1992;93:163–70.

278. Johnson PC, Khardori N, Najjar AF, et al. Progressive disseminated histoplasmosis in patients with acquired immunodeficiency syndrome. Am J Med. 1988;85:152–8.

279. Wheat LJ, Connolly-Stringfield P, Kohler RB, et al. *Histoplasma capsulatum* polysaccharide antigen detection in diagnosis and management of disseminated histoplasmosis in patients with acquired immunodeficiency syndrome. Am J Med. 1989;87:396–400.

280. Denning DW, Follansbee SE, Scolaro M, et al. Pulmonary aspergillosis in the acquired immunodeficiency syndrome. N Engl J Med. 1991;324:654–62.

281. Ilortholary O, Meyohas MC, Dupont B, et al. Invasive aspergillosis in patients with acquired immunodeficiency syndrome: Report of 33 cases. Am J Med. 1993;95:177–87.

282. Supparatpinyo K, Chiewchanvit S, Hirursri P, et al. *Penicillium marneffei* infection in patients infected with human immunodeficiency virus. Clin Infect Dis. 1992;14:871–4.

283. Cornblath DR, McArthur JC. Predominantly sensory neuropathy in patients with AIDS and AIDS-related complex. Neurology (NY). 1988;38:794–6.

284. Eidelberg D, Sotrel A, Vogel H, et al. Progressive polyradiculopathy in acquired immune deficiency syndrome. Neurology. 1986;36:912–6.

285. Hollander H, Stringari S. Human immunodeficiency virus-associated meningitis. Am J Med. 1987;83:813–6.

286. McArthur JC, Cohen BA, Selnes OA, et al. Low prevalence of neurological and neuropsychological abnormalities in otherwise healthy HIV-1-infected individuals: results from the Multicenter AIDS Cohort study. Ann Neurol. 1989;26:601–11.

286a. Worley JM, Price RW. Management of neurologic complications of HIV-1 infection and AIDS. In: Sande MA, Volbepding PA, eds. The medical management of AIDS. 3rd ed. Philadelphia: WB Saunders; 1992.

286b. Jones BN, Teng EL, Folstein MF, et al. A new bedside test of cognition for patients with HIV infection. Ann Intern Med. 1993;119:1001–4.

287. Luft BJ, Hafner R, Korzun AH, et al. Toxoplasmic encephalitis in patients with the acquired immunodeficiency syndrome. N Engl J Med. 1993;329: 995–1000.

288. Porter SB, Sande MA. Toxoplasmosis of the central nervous system in the acquired immunodeficiency syndrome. N Engl J Med. 1992;327:1643–8.

289. Levy RM, Mills CM, Posin JP, et al. The efficacy and clinical impact of brain imaging in neurologically symptomatic AIDS patients: A prospective CT/MRI study. J AIDS. 1990;3:461–71.

290. Grant IH, Gold JWM, Rosenblum M, et al. *Toxoplasma gondii* serology in HIV-infected patients: The development of central nervous system toxoplasmosis in AIDS. AIDS. 1990;4:519–21.

291. Carr A, Tindall B, Brew BJ, et al. Low-dose trimethoprim-sulfamethoxazole prophylaxis for toxoplasmic encephalitis in patients with AIDS. Ann Intern Med. 1992;117:106–11.

291a. Chaisson RE, Griffin DE. Progressive multifocal leukoencephalopathy and AIDS. JAMA. 1990;264:79–83.

291b. Berger JR, Kaszovitz B, Post M, et al. Progressive multifocal leukoencephalopathy associated with human immunodeficiency virus: A review of the literature with a report of sixteen cases. Ann Intern Med. 1987;107:78–87.

292. Larsen RA, Bozzette S, McCutchan JA, et al. Persistent *Cryptococcus neoformans* infection of the prostate after successful treatment of meningitis, California Collaborative Treatment Group. Ann Intern Med. 1989;111:125–8.

293. Zurlo JJ, O'Neill D, Pois MA, et al. Lack of clinical utility of cytomegalovirus blood and urine cultures in patients with HIV infection. Ann Intern Med. 1993;118:12–7.

294. Gallant JE, Moore RD, Richman DD, et al. Incidence and natural history of

cytomegalovirus disease in patients with advanced human immunodeficiency virus disease treated with zidovudine. J Infect Dis. 1992;166:1223–7.

295. Margolis TP, Lowder CY, Holland GN, et al. Varicella-zoster virus retinitis in patients with the acquired immunodeficiency syndrome. Am J Ophthalmol. 1991;112:119–31.

296. Wasserman L, Haghighi P. Otic and ophthalmic pneumocystosis in acquired immunodeficiency syndrome. Arch Pathol Lab Med. 1992;116:500–3.

297. Safai B, Good RA. Kaposi's sarcoma: A review and recent developments. Clin Bull. 1980;10:62–8.

298. Templeton AC. Kaposi's sarcoma. Pathol Annu. 1981;16:315–36.

299. Hutt MSR. The epidemiology of Kaposi's sarcoma. Antibiot Chemother. 1981;29:3–8.

300. Taylor JF, Templeton AC, Vogel CL, et al. Kaposi's sarcoma in Uganda: A clinico-pathological study. Int J Cancer. 1971;8:122–35.

301. Zisbrod Z, Haimov M, Schanzer H, et al. Kaposi's sarcoma after kidney transplantation. Transplantation. 1980;30:383–4.

302. Myers BD, Kessler E, Levi J, et al. Kaposi's sarcoma in kidney transplant recipients. Arch Intern Med. 1974;133:307–11.

303. Penn I. Kaposi's sarcoma in immunosuppressed patients. J Clin Lab Immunol. 1983;12:1–10.

304. Little PJ, Al Khader A, Farthing CF, et al. Kaposi's sarcoma in a patient after renal transplantation. Postgrad Med J. 1983;59:325–6.

305. Meyers AM, Rice GC, Kaye S, et al. Kaposi's sarcoma in an immunosuppressed renal allograft recipient. S Afr Med J. 1976;50:1299–300.

306. Stribling J, Weitzner S, Smith GV. Kaposi's sarcoma in renal allograft recipients. Cancer. 1978;42:442–6.

307. Klepp O, Dahi O, Stenwig JT. Association of Kaposi's sarcoma and prior immunosuppressive therapy. Cancer. 1978;42:2626–30.

308. Giraldo G, Beth E, Huang E-S. Kaposi's sarcoma and its relationship to cytomegalovirus (CMV) III. CMV DNA and CMV early antigens in Kaposi's sarcoma. Int J Cancer. 1980;26:23–9.

309. Giraldo G, Beth E, Coeur P, et al. Kaposi's sarcoma: A new model in the search for viruses associated with human malignancies. JNCI. 1972;49:1495–507.

310. Urmacher C, Myskowski P, Ochoa M, et al. Outbreak of Kaposi's sarcoma with cytomegalovirus infection in young homosexual men. Am J Med. 1982;72:569–75.

311. Friedman-Kien AE, Laubenstein LJ, Rubinstein P, et al. Disseminated Kaposi's sarcoma in homosexual men. Ann Intern Med. 1982;96:693–700.

312. Friedman-Kien AE. Kaposi's sarcoma and Pneumocystis pneumonia among homosexual men—New York City and California. MMWR. 1981;30:305–8.

313. Editor. Revision of the case definition of acquired immunodeficiency syndrome for national reporting—United States. N Engl J Med. 1987;34:373–5.

314. Levy RM, Pons VG, Rosenblum ML. Central nervous system mass lesions in the acquired immunodeficiency syndrome (AIDS). J Neurosurg. 1984;61:9–16.

315. Rosenblum ML, Levy RM, Bredesen DE, et al. Primary central nervous system lymphomas in patients with AIDS. Ann Neurol. 1988;23(Suppl):13–6.

316. Kaplan LD. AIDS-associated lymphomas. Infect Dis Clin North Am. 1988;2:525–32.

317. Ioachim HL, Cooper MC, Hellman GC. Lymphomas in men at high risk for acquired immune deficiency syndrome (AIDS). Cancer. 1985;56:2831–42.

318. Hoffken G, Kramer A, Dienemann B, et al. Malignant tumors other than Kaposi's sarcoma in persons at high risk for AIDS (Abstract). Tumor Biol. 1987;286.

319. Monfardini S, Italian Cooperative Group for AIDS-Related tumors. Malignant lymphomas in patients with or at risk for AIDS in Italy. JNCI. 1988;80:855–60.

320. Nasr SA, Brynes RK, Garrison CP, et al. Peripheral T-cell lymphoma in a patient with acquired immune deficiency syndrome. Cancer. 1988;61:947–51.

321. Di Carlo EF, Amberson JB, Metroka CE, et al. Malignant lymphomas and the acquired immunodeficiency syndrome (Abstract). Arch Pathol Lab Med. 1986;110:1012–6.

322. Ziegler JL, Beckstead JA, Volberding PA, et al. Non-Hodgkin's lymphoma in 90 homosexual men. N Engl J Med. 1984;311:565–70.

323. Kreiss JK, Kitchen LW, Prince HE, et al. Antibody to human T-lymphotropic virus type III in wives of hemophiliacs. Ann Intern Med. 1985;102:623–6.

324. Levine AM, Gill PS, Meyer PR, et al. Retrovirus and malignant lymphoma in homosexual men JAMA. 1985;254:1921–5.

325. Ahmed T, Wormser GP, Stahl RE, et al. Malignant lymphomas in a population at risk for acquired immune deficiency syndrome. Cancer. 1987;60:719–23.

326. Levine AM. Non-Hodgkin's lymphomas and other malignancies in the acquired immune deficiency syndrome. Semin Oncol. 1987;14:34–9.

327. Haverkos HW, Drotman DP. Prevalence of Kaposi's sarcoma among patients with AIDS. N Engl J Med. 1985;312:1518.

328. Rogers MF, Morens DM, Stewart JA, et al. National case-control study of Kaposi's sarcoma and Pneumocystis carinii pneumonia in homosexual men: Part 2, laboratory results. Ann Intern Med. 1983;99:151–8.

329. Jaffe HW, Keewhan C, Thomas P, et al. National case-control study of Kaposi's sarcoma and Pneumocystis carinii pneumonia in homosexual men: Part 1, epidemiologic results. Ann Intern Med. 1983;99:145–51.

330. DeJarlais DC, Marmor M, Thomas P, et al. Kaposi's sarcoma among four different AIDS risk groups. Lancet. 1988;1:1119.

331. Jaffe HW, Bregman D, Selik RM. Acquired immune deficiency syndrome in the United States: The first 1,000 cases. J Infect Dis. 1983;148:339–45.

332. Cohn DL, Judson FN. Absence of Kaposi's sarcoma in hemophiliacs with the acquired immunodeficiency syndrome. Ann Intern Med. 1984;101:401.

333. Garrett TJ, Lange M, Ashford A, et al. Kaposi's sarcoma in heterosexual intravenous drug users. Cancer. 1985;55:1146–8.

334. Van de Perre P, Lepage P, Kestelyn P, et al. Acquired immunodeficiency syndrome in Rwanda. Lancet. 1984;2:62–5.

335. Kestens L, Melbye M, Biggar RJ, et al. Endemic African Kaposi's sarcoma is not associated with immunodeficiency. Int J Cancer. 1985;36:49–54.

336. Bayley AC, Cheingsong-Popov R, Dalgleish AG, et al. HTLV-III serology distinguishes atypical and endemic Kaposi's sarcoma in Africa. Lancet. 1985;359–61.

337. Downing RG, Eglin RP, Bayley AC. African Kaposi's sarcoma and AIDS. Lancet. 1984;478–80.

338. Bayley AC. Aggressive Kaposi's sarcoma in Zambia, 1983. Lancet. 1988;1318–22.

339. Montgomery AB, Luce JM, Turner J, et al. Aerosolised pentamidine as sole therapy for Pneumocystis carinii pneumonia in patients with acquired immunodeficiency syndrome. Lancet. 1987;480–3.

340. Buck BE, Scott GB, Valdes-Dapena M, et al. Kaposi's sarcoma in two infants with acquired immune deficiency syndrome. J Pediatr. 1983;103:911–3.

341. Gallant JE, Moore RD, Richman DD, et al. Risk factors for Kaposi's sarcoma in patients with advanced HIV disease treated with zidovudine. Arch Intern Med. 1994;154:566–72.

342. Haverkos HW, Amsel Z, Drotmn DP, et al. Kaposi's sarcoma in homosexual men with AIDS, by race. Lancet. 1988;1075.

343. Drew WL, Mills J, Hauer LB, et al. Declining prevalence of Kaposi's sarcoma in homosexual AIDS patients paralleled by fall in cytomegalovirus transmission. Lancet. 1988;66.

344. Declines in proportion of Kaposi's sarcoma among cases of AIDS in multiple risk groups in New York City. Lancet. 1987;1024.

345. Volberding PA, Kusick P, Feigal DW. HIV antigenemia at diagnosis with Kaposi's sarcoma: Predictors of shortened survival (Abstract). In: Proceedings of the Fourth International Conference on AIDS. 1988:136.

346. Marmor M, Laubenstein LJ, William DC, et al. Risk factors for Kaposi's sarcoma in homosexual men. Lancet. 1982;1083–6.

347. Haverkos HW. Factors associated with the pathogenesis of AIDS. J Infect Dis. 1987;156:251–7.

348. Lesbordes JL, Martin PMV, Ravisse P, et al. Clinical and histopathological aspects of Kaposi's sarcoma in Africa: Relationship with HIV serology. 1988;139:197–203.

349. Nakamura S, Salahuddin SZ, Biberfeld P, et al. Kaposi's sarcoma cells: Long-term culture with growth factor from retrovirus-infected CD4 T cells. Science. 1988;242:426–30.

350. Newell GR, Mansell PWA, Spitz MR, et al. Volatile nitrites use and adverse effects related to the current epidemic of the acquired immune deficiency syndrome. Am J Med. 1985;78:811–6.

351. Hashimoto H, Muller H, Falk S, et al. Histogenesis of Kaposi's sarcoma associated with AIDS: A histologic, immunohistochemical and enzyme histochemical study. Pathol Res Pract. 1987;182:658–68.

352. Nadji M, Morales AR, Ziegles-Weissman J, et al. Kaposi's sarcoma: Immunohistologic evidence for an endothelial origin. Arch Pathol Lab Med. 1981;105:274–5.

353. Beckstead JH, Wood GS, Fletcher V. Evidence for the origin of Kaposi's sarcoma from lymphatic endothelium. Am J Pathol. 1985;119:294–300.

354. Dorfman RF. Kaposi's sarcoma revisited. Hum Pathol. 1984;15:1013–7.

355. McNutt NS, Fletcher V, Conant MA. Early lesions of Kaposi's sarcoma in homosexual men. Am J Pathol. 1983;111:62–77.

356. Jones RR, Spaull J, Spry C, et al. Histogenesis of Kaposi's sarcoma in patients with and without acquired immune deficiency syndrome (AIDS). J Clin Pathol. 1986;39:742–9.

357. Green TL, Beckstead JH, Lozada-Nur F, et al. Histopathologic spectrum of oral Kaposi's sarcoma. Oral Surg. 1984;58:306–14.

358. Salahuddin SZ, Nakamura S, Biberfeld P, et al. Angiogenic properties of Kaposi's sarcoma-derived cells after long-term culture in vitro. Science. 1988;242:430–3.

359. Costa J, Rabson AS. Generalised Kaposi's sarcoma is not a neoplasm. Lancet. 1983;58.

360. Mitsuyasu RT. Clinical variants and staging of Kaposi's sarcoma. Semin Oncol. 1987;14:13–8.

361. Safai B, Sarngadharan MG, Koziner B, et al. Spectrum of Kaposi's sarcoma in the epidemic of AIDS. Cancer Res. 1985;45(Suppl):4646–8.

362. Vadhan-Raj S, Wong G, Gnecco C, et al. Immunological variables as predictors of prognosis in patients with Kaposi's sarcoma and the acquired immunodeficiency syndrome. Cancer Res. 1986;46:417–25.

363. Rawlinson KF, Zubrow AB, Harris MA, et al. Disseminated Kaposi's sarcoma in pregnancy: A manifestation of acquired immune deficiency syndrome. Obstet Gynecol. 1984;63(Suppl):2–6.

364. Patow CA, Steis R, Longo DL, et al. Kaposi's sarcoma of the head and neck in the acquired immune deficiency syndrome. Otolaryngology. 1984;92:255–60.

365. Real FX, Oettgen HF, Krown SE. Kaposi's sarcoma and the acquired immunodeficiency syndrome: Treatment with high and low doses of recombinant leukocyte A interferon. J Clin Oncol. 1986;4:544–51.

366. Hymes KB, Greene JB, Marcus A, et al. Kaposi's sarcoma in homosexual men—a report of eight cases. Lancet. 1981;598–600.

367. Seftel AD, Sadick NS, Waldbaum RS. Kaposi's sarcoma of the penis in a

patient with the acquired immune deficiency syndrome. J Urol. 1986;136: 673–5.

368. Mitsuyasu RT, Taylor J, Glaspy J, et al. Heterogeneity of epidemic Kaposi's sarcoma. Cancer. 1986;57:1657–61.

369. Lumerman H, Freedman PD, Kerpel SM, et al. Oral Kaposi's sarcoma: A clinicopathologic study of 23 homosexual and bisexual men from the New York metropolitan areas. Oral Surg. 1988;65:711–6.

370. Gnepp DR, Chandler W, Hyams V. Primary Kaposi's sarcoma of the head and neck. Ann Intern Med. 1984;100:107–14.

371. Moskowitz LB, Hensley GT, Gould EW, et al. Frequency and anatomic distribution of lymphadenopathic Kaposi's sarcoma in the acquired immunodeficiency syndrome: An autopsy series. Hum Pathol. 1985;16:447–56.

372. Lustbader I, Sherman A. Primary gastrointestinal Kaposi's sarcoma in a patient with acquired immune deficiency syndrome. Am J Gastroenterol. 1987;82:894–5.

373. Rose HS, Balthazar EJ, Megibow AJ, et al. Alimentary tract involvement in Kaposi sarcoma: Radiographic and endoscopic findings in 25 homosexual men. AJR. 1982;139:661–6.

374. Scott LF, Wright TL, Altman DF. Gastrointestinal Kaposi's sarcoma in patients with acquired immunodeficiency syndrome. Gastroenterology. 1988; 89:102–8.

375. Dwordin B, Wormser GP, Rosenthal WS, et al. Gastrointestinal manifestations of the acquired immunodeficiency syndrome: A review of 22 cases. Am J Gastroentrol. 1985;80:774–8.

376. Barrison IG, Foster S, Harris JW, et al. Upper gastrointestinal Kaposi's sarcoma in patients positive for HIV antibody without cutaneous disease. Br Med J. 1988;296:92–3.

377. Friedman SL, Wright TL, Altman DF. Gastrointestinal Kaposi's sarcoma in patients with acquired immunodeficiency syndrome. Gastroenterology. 1985;89:102–8.

378. Federle MP. A radiologist looks at AIDS: Imaging evaluation based on symptom complexes. Radiology. 1988;166:553–62.

379. Frager DH, Frager JD, Brandt LJ, et al. Gastrointestinal complications of AIDS: Radiologic features. Radiology. 1986;158:597–603.

380. Rucker L, Meador J. Kaposi's sarcoma presenting as homogeneous pulmonary infiltrates in a patient with acquired immunodeficiency syndrome. West J Med. 1985;142:831–3.

381. Ognibene FP, Steis RG, Macher AM, et al. Kaposi's sarcoma causing pulmonary infiltrates and respiratory failure in the acquired immunodeficiency syndrome. Ann Intern Med. 1985;102:471–5.

382. Caray SM, Belenko M. Fazzini E, et al. Pulmonary manifestations of Kaposi's sarcoma. Chest. 1987;91:39–43.

383. Meduri GU, Stover D, Lee M, et al. Pulmonary Kaposi's sarcoma in the acquired immune deficiency syndrome. Am J Med. 1986;81:11–8.

384. Kaplan LD, Hopewell PC, Jaffe HW, et al. Kaposi's sarcoma involving the lung in patients with the acquired immunodeficiency syndrome. J AIDS. 1988;1:23–30.

385. Nash G, Fligiel S. Kaposi's sarcoma presenting as pulmonary disease in the acquired immunodeficiency syndrome: Diagnosis by lung biopsy. Hum Pathol. 1984;15:999–1001.

386. Kornfeld H, Axelrod JL. Pulmonary presentation of Kaposi's sarcoma in a homosexual patient. Am Rev Respir Dis. 1983;127:248–9.

387. Keeney K, Abaza NA, Tidwel O, et al. Oral Kaposi's sarcoma in acquired immune deficiency syndrome. J Oral Maxillofac Surg. 1987;45:815–21.

388. Lozada F, Silverman S, Migliorati CA, et al. Oral manifestations of tumor and opportunistic infections in the acquired immunodeficiency syndrome (AIDS): Findings in 53 homosexual men with Kaposi's sarcoma. Oral Surg. 1983;56:491–4.

389. Emery CD, Wall SD, Federle MP, et al. Pharyngeal Kaposi's sarcoma in patients with AIDS. AJR. 1986;147:919–22.

390. Green TL, Beckstead JH, Lozada-Nur F, et al. Histopathologic spectrum of oral Kaposi's sarcoma. Oral Surg. 1984;58:306–14.

391. Krigel RL, Laubenstein LJ, Muggia FM. Kaposi's sarcoma: A new staging classification. Cancer Treat Rep. 1983;67:531–4.

392. Volberding PA. The role of chemotherapy for epidemic Kaposi's sarcoma. Semin Oncol. 1987;16(Suppl 3):23–6.

393. Taylor J, Afrasiabi R, Fahey JL, et al. Prognostically significant classification of immune changes in AIDS with Kaposi's sarcoma. Blood. 1986;67:666–71.

394. Kaplan L, Northfelt DW. Malignancies associated with AIDS. In: Sande MA, Volberding PA, eds. The Medical Management of AIDS. 3rd ed. Philadelphia: WB Saunders; 1992:403.

395. Moss AR. Predicting who will progress to AIDS. Br Med J. 1988;297:1067–8.

396. Moss AR, McCallum G, Volberding PA, et al. Mortality associated with mode of presentation in the acquired immune deficiency syndrome. JNCI. 1984;73:1281–4.

397. El-Akkad S, Bull CA, El-Senoussi MA, et al. Kaposi's sarcoma and its management by radiotherapy. Arch Dermatol. 1986;122:1396–9.

398. Holecek MJ, Harwood AR. Radiotherapy of Kaposi's sarcoma. Cancer. 1978;41:1733–8.

399. Hill DR. The role of radiotherapy for epidemic Kaposi's sarcoma. Semin Oncol. 1987;14:19–22.

400. Groopman JE. AIDS-related Kaposi's sarcoma: Therapeutic modalities. Semin Hematol. 1987;24:5–8.

401. Cooper JS, Fried PR. Treatment of aggressive epidemic Kaposi's sarcoma of the conjunctiva by radiotherapy. Arch Ophthalmol. 1988;106:20–1.

402. Cooper JS, Fried PR, Laubenstein LJ. Initial observations of the effect of radiotherapy on epidemic Kaposi's sarcoma. JAMA. 1984;252:934–5.

403. Volberding PA. Therapy of Kaposi's sarcoma in AIDS. Semin Oncol. 1984; 11:60–7.

404. Harris JW, Reed TA: Kaposi's sarcoma in AIDS: The role of radiation therapy. Front Radiat Ther Oncol. 1985;19:126–32.

405. Nisce LZ, Safai B, Poussin-Rosillo H. Once weekly total and subtotal skin electron beam therapy for Kaposi's sarcoma. Cancer. 1981;47:640–4.

406. Nobler MP, Leddy ME, Huh SH. The impact of palliative irradiation on the management of patients with acquired immune deficiency syndrome. J Clin Oncol. 1987;5:107–12.

407. Kahn J, Kaplan LD, Jaffe HW, et al. Intralesional recombinant tumor necrosis factor for AIDS related Kaposi's sarcoma (Abstract). In: Proceedins of the Fourth International Conference on AIDS. Washington, DC: Bio-Data Publishers; 1988:324.

408. Volberding PA, Abrams DI, Conant MA, et al. Vinblastine therapy for Kaposi's sarcoma in the acquired immunodeficiency syndrome. Ann Intern Med. 1985;103:335–8.

409. Kaplan LD, Abrams DI, Volberding PA. Treatment of Kaposi's sarcoma in acquired immunodeficiency syndrome with an alternating vincristine vinblastine regimen. Cancer Treat Rep. 1986;70:1121–2.

410. Fischl MA, Krown SE, O'Boyle KP, et al. Weekly doxorubicin in the treatment of patients with AIDS-related Kaposi's sarcoma. J AIDS. 1993;6: 259–64.

411. Presant CA, Scolaro M, Kennedy P, et al. Liposomal daunorubicin treatment of HIV-associated Kaposi's sarcoma. Lancet. 1993;341:1242–3.

412. Mintzer DM, Real FX, Jovino L, et al. Treatment of Kaposi's sarcoma and thrombocytopenia with vincristine in patients with the acquired immunodeficiency syndrome. Ann Intern Med. 1985;102:200–2.

413. Laubenstein LJ, Krigel RL, Odajnyk CM, et al. Treatment of epidemic Kaposi's sarcoma with etoposide or a combination of doxorubicin, bleomycin, and vinblastine. J Clin Oncol. 1984;2:1115–20.

414. Gill PS, Krailo MD, Slater L, et al. Results of a randomized trial of ABV (Adriamycin, bleomycin, vincristine) vs an advanced epidemic Kaposi's sarcoma. (Abstract). In: Proceedings of the Fourth International Conference on AIDS. Washington, DC: Bio-Data Publishers; 1988:323.

415. Flepp M, Tauber MG, Luthy R, et al. Kaposi's sarcoma in AIDS patients: Long-term treatment with recombinant interferon alpha-2A and chemotherapy. Klin Wochenschr. 1988;66:437–42.

416. Gelmann EP, Preble OT, Steis R, et al. Human lymphoblastoid interferon treatment of Kaposi's sarcoma in the acquired immune deficiency syndrome. Am J Med. 1985;78:737–41.

417. Krown SE, Real FX, Cunningham-Rundles S, et al. Preliminary observations on the effect of recombinant leukocyte A interferon in homosexual men with Kaposi's sarcoma. N Engl J Med. 1983;308:1071–6.

418. Groopman JE, Scadden DT. Interferon therapy for Kaposi sarcoma associated with the acquired immunodeficiency syndrome. Ann Intern Med. 1989; 110:335–7.

419. Rios A, Mansell PWA, Newell GR, et al. Treatment of acquired immunodeficiency syndrome-related Kaposi's sarcoma with lymphoblastoid interferon. J Clin Oncol. 1985;3:506–12.

420. Krigel RL, Slywotzky CM, Lonberg M, et al. Treatment of epidemic Kaposi's sarcoma with a combination of interferon-alpha 2b and etoposide. J Biol Response Mod. 1988;7:359–64.

421. Krown SE, Bundow D, Tong WP, et al. Interferon-alpha plus azidothymidine (AZT) in AIDS-associated Kaposi's sarcoma (KS). J Interferon Res 1987;7: 688–9.

422. Krown S, Bundow D, Gansbacher B, et al. Interferon-alpha plus zidovudine: A phase I trial in AIDS-associated Kaposi's sarcoma (KS) (Abstract). In: Proceedings of the Fourth International Conference on AIDS. Washington, DC: Bio-Data Publishers; 1988:173.

423. Pluda JM, Yarchoan R, Jaffe ES, et al. Development of non-Hodgkin lymphoma in a cohort of patients with severe human immunodeficiency virus (HIV) infection on long-term antiretroviral therapy. Ann Intern Med. 1990; 113:276–82.

424. Biggar RJ, Horm J, Lubin JH, et al. Cancer trends in a population at risk of acquired immunodeficiency syndrome. JNCI. 1985;74:793–7.

425. Rechavi B, Ben-Bassat B, Berkowicy M, et al. Molecular analysis of Burkitt's leukemia in two hemophilic brothers with AIDS. Blood. 1987;70: 1713–7.

426. Groopman JE, Sullivan JL, Mulder C, et al. Pathogenesis of B cell lymphoma in a patient with AIDS. Blood. 1986;67:612–5.

427. Lippman SM, Volk JR, Spier CM, et al. Clonal ambiguity of human immunodeficiency virus-associated lymphomas. Arch Pathol Lab Med. 1988;122: 128–32.

428. Subar M, Neri A, Inghirami G, et al. Frequent c-*myc* oncogene activation and infrequent presence of Epstein-Barr virus genome in AIDS-associated lymphoma. Blood. 1988;72:667–71.

429. Loeffler JS, Ervin TJ, Mauch P, et al. Primary lymphomas of the central nervous system: Patterns of failure and factors that influence survival. J Clin Oncol. 1985;3:490–4.

430. Elkin CM, Leon E, Grenell SL, et al. Intracranial lesions in the acquired immunodeficiency syndrome. JAMA. 1985;253:393–6.

431. So YT, Beckstead JH, Davis RL. Primary central nervous system lymphoma in acquired immune deficiency syndrome: A clinical and pathological study (Abstract). Ann Neurol. 1986;20:566–72.

432. Galetto G, Levine A. AIDS-associated primary central nervous system lymphoma. JAMA. 1993;269:92–3.

433. Ragni MV, Belle SH, Jaffe RA, et al. Acquired immunodeficiency syndrome-associated non-Hodgkin's lymphomas and other malignancies in patients with hemophilia. Blood. 1993;81:1889–97.

434. Levy RM, Bredesen DE, Rosenblum ML. Neurologic manifestations of the

acquired immunodeficiency syndrome (AIDS): Experience at UCSF and review of the literature. J Neurosurg. 1985;62:475–95.

435. Knowles DM, Chamulak GA, Subar M, et al. Lymphoid neoplasia associated with the acquired immunodeficiency syndrome (AIDS). Ann Intern Med. 1988;108:744–53.

436. Ioachim HL, Weinstein MA, Robbins RD, et al. Primary anorectal lymphoma: A new manifestation of the acquired immune deficiency sndrome (AIDS). Cancer. 1987;60:1449–53.

437. Caccamo D, Pervez NK, Marchevsky A. Primary lymphoma of the liver in the acquired immunodeficiency syndrome. Arch Pathol Lab Med. 1986;110: 553–5.

438. Lowery S, Fallat R, Feigal DW, et al. Changing patterns of *Pneumocystis carinii* pneumonia (PCP) on pentamidine aerosol prophylaxis (Abstract). In: Proceedings of the Fourth International Conference on AIDS. Washington, DC: Bio-Data Publishers; 1988:419.

439. Bottles K, McPhaul LW, Volberding PA. Fine needle aspiration biopsy of patients with acquired immunodeficiency syndrome (AIDS): Experience in an outpatient clinic. Ann Intern Med. 1988;108:42–5.

440. Abrams DI, Kaplan LD, McGrath MS, et al. AIDS-related benign lymphadenopathy and malignant lymphoma: Clinical aspects and virology interactions. AIDS Res. 1986;2:131–40.

441. Jeffrey RB, Nyberg DA, Bottles K, et al. Abdominal CT in acquired immunodeficiency syndrome. AJR. 1986;146:7–13.

442. Nyberg DA, Jeffrey RB, Federle MP, et al. AIDS-related lymphomas: Evaluation by adominal CT. Radiology. 1986;159:59–63.

443. Gill PS, LEvine AM, Krailo MD, et al. AIDS-related malignant lymphoma: Results of prospective treatment trials. J Clin Oncol. 1987;5:1322–8.

444. Maiman M, Fruchter RG, Serur E, et al. Human immunodeficiency virus infection and cervical neoplasia. Gynecol Oncol. 1990;38:377–82.

445. Reynolds P, Saunders LD, Layefsky ME, Lemp GF. The spectrum of acquired immunodeficiency syndrome (AIDS)-associated malignancies in San Francisco, 1980–1987. Am J Epidemiol. 1993;137:19–30.

446. Monfardini S, Vaccher E, Pizzocaro G, et al. Unusual malignant tumours in 49 patients with HIV infection. AIDS. 1989;3:449–52.

447. Johnson JC, Burnett AF, Willet GD, et al. High frequency of latent and clinical human papillomavirus cervical infections in immunocompromised human immunodeficiency virus-infected women. Obstet Gynecol. 1992;79: 321–7.

448. Ames ED, Conjalka MS, Goldberg AF, et al. Hodgkin's disease and AIDS. Hematol/Oncol Clin North Am. 1991;5:343–56.

449. Monfardini S, Tirelli U, Vaccher E, et al. Hodgkin's disease in 63 intravenous drug users infected with human immunodeficiency virus. Anns Oncol. 1991; 2:201–5.

450. Hessol NA, Katz MH, Liu JY, et al. Increased incidence of Hodgkin disease in homosexual men with HIV infection. Ann intern Med. 1992;117:309–11.

451. Byrne MA, Taylor-Robinson D, Munday PE, et al. The common occurrence of human papillomavirus infection and intraepithelial neoplasia in women infected by HIV. AIDS. 1989;3:379–82.

452. Critchlow CW, Holmes KK, Wood R, et al. Association of human immunodeficiency virus and anal human papillomavirus infection among homosexual men. Arch Intern Med. 1992;152:1673–6.

453. Palefsky JM, Holly EA, Gonzales J, et al. Natural history of anal cytologic abnormalities and papillomavirus infection among homosexual men with group IV HIV disease. J AIDS. 1992;5:1258–65.

454. Palefsky JM, Gonzales J, Greenblatt RM, et al. Anal intraepithelial neoplasia and anal papillomavirus infection among homosexual males with group IV HIV disease. JAMA. 1990;263:2911–6.

103. DETECTION OF HIV-1 INFECTION

CHARLES J. SCHLEUPNER

In 1983–1984, as the isolation of human immunodeficiency virus type 1 (HIV-1) was first reported, serologic tests were described that recognized antibodies to HIV-1 in sera of patients with the acquired immunodeficiency syndrome (AIDS).[1–7] The first assay for screening blood became licensed for commercial use on March 2, 1985, when blood centers initiated screening of all donated blood for antibody to HIV-1.[8] The "first generation" of these enzyme immunoassays (EIAs) were adaptations of assays using antigens derived from lysed HIV-1–infected cell cultures.[6] They were designed for sensitivity of detection of HIV-1 infection; the EIA gained specificity only upon repeated testing with positive results and "confirmatory" evaluation with Western

blot (WB). The test was clearly successful at its primary purpose, making the blood supply safer.[8,9]

To prevent individuals in high-risk groups from using blood banks for diagnostic testing (thereby increasing the risk of contamination of the blood supply), alternate test sites were also established where patients in high-risk groups could have EIA evaluations (and WB, if indicated) performed anonymously or confidentially and without charge after appropriate counseling. Therefore, continued self-deferral of high-risk donors was facilitated.[10]

Through counseling, another goal of EIA testing for antibody to HIV-1 evolved (i.e., prevention of infection or spread thereof to others). In December 1985, the Centers for Disease Control and Prevention (CDC) extended its recommendation for EIA testing to pregnant women and women who might become pregnant while being at high risk for HIV-1 infection.[11] In the spring of 1986, serologic testing was additionally recommended for persons attending sexually transmissible disease (STD) clinics and clinics for prostitutes and injectable drug users.[12] Testing was further advised for recipients of transfusions between 1978 and 1985 and for all patients with tuberculosis.[13]

At the same time that the target high-risk populations for diagnostic testing were being extended, the limitations of the "first-generation" EIAs were acknowledged. The rate of false positivity was high (80–90 percent) in low-risk populations, resulting in an unnecessary reduction in the sources of the nation's blood supply and unwarranted emotional stress for individuals receiving such erroneous information.[14–16] With the purpose of increasing the specificity of both screening and confirmatory tests, EIAs using specific HIV-1 synthetic proteins and proteins produced by recombinant technology were developed.[17,18] With the application of these assays, together with the development of an EIA for HIV-1 core antigen,[19–21] the utility of serologic assays has recently been extended to include a better understanding of the pathogenesis of HIV-1 infection, evaluation of the success of therapy, and definition of the strategies for earlier initiation of therapy.[22,23]

SEROLOGIC RESPONSE TO HIV-1 INFECTION

The serologic response to HIV-1 is best understood by an appreciation of the major protein products of the viral genome (see Ch. 146). The temporal course of the appearance of serum HIV-1 antigen and antibodies to several viral proteins as detected by various techniques is shown in Figure 1. After infection, p24 antigen is the first serologic marker to be detected.[24,25] The appearance of antibody to p24 is temporally associated with falling p24 antigen levels and with immune complexes of these reactants.[19,24,26–28] Antibodies to the carboxy-terminal cleavage product (gp41) of gp160 are often detectable before anti-p24 (Fig. 1) by WB, competitive EIA using recombinant antigens (CIA-RA), or radioimmunoprecipitation (RIPA).[24,29] In the peri-

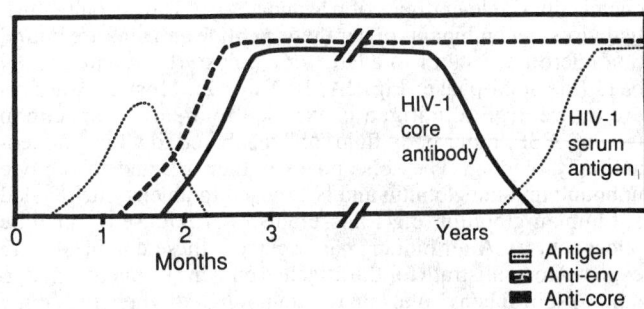

FIG. 1. Chronology of HIV-1 infection defined by presence of core (p24) antigen and antibodies to core protein and envelope (gp41) glycoprotein. (Courtesy of Abbott Diagnostics Division, Abbott Laboratories, North Chicago, IL.)

TABLE 1. Summary of Methodology of Currently Licensed Standard Screening EIAS for Antibody to HIV-1

Manufacturer of Assay	HIV-1 Antigen Source			Cell Line Sourced of Lysate	Solid Phase for Antigen			Enzyme Conjugate
	Viral Lysate	Recombinant Protein	Synthetic Peptide		Latex Bead	Metal Bead	Well	
Abbott	+[a]			H9	+			Antibody[b]
Abbott		+[c]			+			HIV-1 antigen
Genetic Systems	+[d]			CEM-F			+	Antibody
Cambridge Biotech		+[e]					+	Antibody
Ortho	+			H9			+	Antibody
Organon-Technika	+			H9			+	Antibody
Organon-Technika	+			H9		+		Antibody
Cellular Products	+			H9			+	Antibody
United Biomedical, Inc.			+[f]				+	Antibody

[a] Viral lysate with purified antigens.
[b] Antihuman IgG antibody.
[c] Combined HIV-1 (rp24 and rp41) and HIV-2 (rp41) recombinant proteins.
[d] Available as HIV-1 or combined HIV-1/2 viral lysate(s).
[e] rp24, rp41, and gp120 recombinant HIV-1 proteins.
[f] Synthetic, immunodominant epitopes of p24 and gp41.

natally infected infant, IgM antibody to HIV-1 appears by 2–4 weeks after infection and peaks at 3–8 weeks, decreasing slowly thereafter.[30] IgA appears within 3–6 months after infection, paralleling IgG.[31] IgM assays are insensitive due to the lower concentration of IgM–anti-HIV-1 compared with IgA and IgG. Within 6 months of HIV-1 infection, 95% or more of infected persons seroconvert to EIA positivity.[32] Months or years after the development of antibodies to both the core and envelope proteins, the core antigen may reappear (Fig. 1); this is usually coincident with loss of anti-p24 and correlates with the development of AIDS.[20,23,33–39]

HIV-1 ANTIBODY ASSAYS

Enzyme Immunoassays

There are at least nine licensed standard EIAs available for the detection of antibody to HIV-1; most use virus derived from lysed cell cultures, some with partially purified antigens, while two of these assays use protein antigens derived by recombinant technology and one relies upon synthetic peptide antigens ("second generation" assays; Table 1).[18,40–46] All viral lysate kits (first-generation assays) use the human T-cell leukemia/lymphoma virus (HTLV-III) strain of HIV-1, except the Genetic Systems assay, which uses the lymphadenopathy-associated virus (LAV) strain. The cell source of HIV-1 for the viral lysate kits varies according to each manufacturer. The Abbott, Organon-Technika, Cellular Products, and Ortho kits use the H-9 cell line. (The Organon-Technika kit is an improved version of what was formerly the Laden EIA.) Genetic Systems uses the CEM-F line.[42,43,47] The recombinant assays by Abbott and Cambridge Biotech contain p24 and envelope antigens. The United Biomedical kit uses synthetic immunodominant, conserved, and chemically stable epitopes of p24 and gp41.[18] The partially purified virus, recombinant, or synthetic peptide antigens are bound to a microtiter well or to a latex or a polystyrene-coated metal bead (the solid phase; Fig. 2A, B, Table 2). Most EIA assays are indirect; viral antigen is exposed to a patient specimen (serum, CSF, other body fluid) and incubated to allow antigen-antibody binding. The solid phase is then washed to remove unbound immunoglobulin and is exposed to an enzyme-labeled antihuman globulin (e.g., horseradish peroxidase or alkaline phosphatase). After binding has occurred, these complexes are exposed to a substrate for the attached enzyme (o-phenylenediamine, p-nitrophenyl phosphate, amino-di-3-ethybenzthiazoline sulfonate, or tetramethylbenzidine); a calorimetric reaction occurs that is proportional to the amount of bound anti-HIV-1 globulin in the patient specimen. Both strongly and weakly reactive controls, as well as negative controls, are run in parallel on

A. 1st Generation Viral Lysate Assay Format

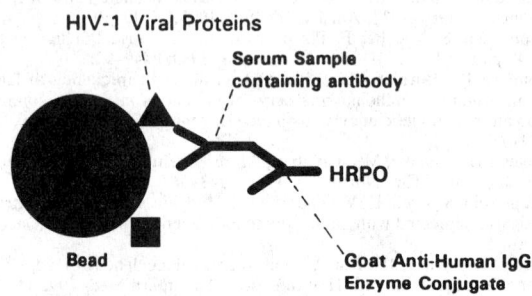

B. 2nd Generation rDNA Assay Format

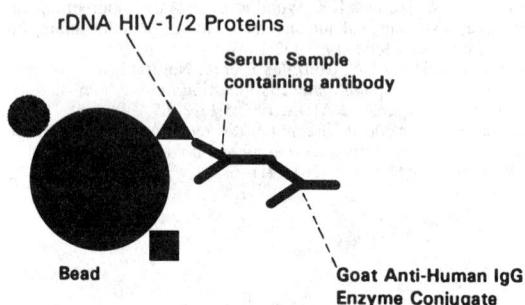

C. 3rd Generation rDNA Assay Format

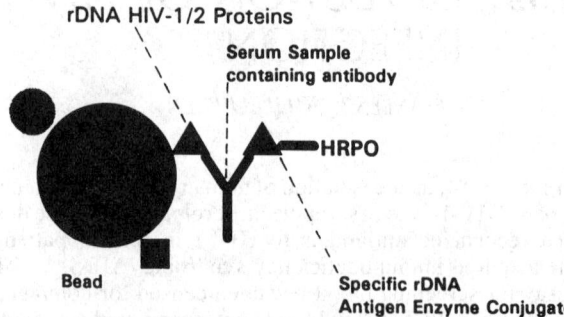

FIG. 2. The three most commonly used formats for the enzyme immunoassay (EIA) to detect antibody against HIV-1 and -2. **(A)** Antibody capture, viral lysate, antibody-enzyme conjugate (indirect sandwich) assay format for HIV-1 antibody assay; **(B)** recombinant DNA (rDNA)-derived HIV-1 antigen "indirect sandwich" assay format for HIV-1 antibody assay; **(C)** rDNA-derived antigen-enzyme conjugate "direct sandwich" format for HIV-1 and -2 antibody assays.

TABLE 2. Example of Problems With the HIV-1 Antibody EIA When Applied to High- and Low-Risk Populations

Assay Result	High-Risk Population	Low-Risk Population
No. tested	10,000	10,000
Percentage positive	10	0.3
Total no. positive	1000	30
No. false positive[a]	27	27
No. true positive	973	3
Positive predictive value	973/1000 (97.3%)	3/30 (10%)

[a] False positive due to intrinsic methodologic inaccuracies, regardless of the population tested.

each occasion when unknown sera are assayed. Some more recent kits use a competitive inhibition enzyme immunoassay. In the latter assay, the color reaction is inversely proportional to the amount of bound anti-HIV-1 globulin in the patient specimen. Abbott has most recently introduced a direct sandwich EIA; in this assay the enzyme is conjugated to HIV-1 (or HIV-2) antigen, which binds to an open binding site of the patients' antibody that is attached to the solid phase (latex bead) bound antigen (Fig. 2C).[48] An EIA assay takes up to 4 hours to perform.

An antibody capture EIA has recently been described, for which microtiter wells are coated with rabbit antihuman IgG, which is then exposed to the patient's serum.[49] After washing, an enzyme-conjugated HIV-1 antigen is added, thereby allowing "captured" human antibody to HIV-1 to bind these antigens. This assay has been readily applied to detection of multiple pathogens (e.g., HIV-1 and HIV-2).

With indirect, direct, competitive, or antibody capture EIA, the optical density (OD) of each unknown (individual or paired) and each control is measured at the optimal wavelength for substrate absorption after undergoing the calorimetric reaction. A cut-off OD is then calculated using negative and/or positive control values (the equation varies with each kit), and a ratio of sample to cut-off OD is calculated. For the indirect or direct ("sandwich") EIA, values of at least 1.0 are considered positive; for the competitive EIA, values less than 1.0 are positive. These EIAs are usually performed with serum, but EIAs using viral lysate and recombinant antigens have been reported to detect HIV-1 antibodies in saliva with a sensitivity equal to that in serum.[50–52] Various EIAs have also been used to assay eluates from dried whole blood impregnated fiber paper disks.[49,53–57] This specimen source has been shown to be as sensitive and specific as serum when performing antibody assays.

Burke et al.[58] have shown that EIA OD readings vary with the intensity of various WB banding patterns. While the first-generation Abbott EIA has greatest sensitivity for antibodies to gp41 and the polymerase gene products, the Dupont and Litton (Organon-Technika) first-generation EIAs were more sensitive for antibodies to the gag (core) proteins.[58] This has relevance to the sensitivity of each EIA for HIV-1 antibody during various stages of infection; for example, during AIDS when anti-p24 has usually disappeared, the latter EIAs were less sensitive for detecting infection due to their greater sensitivity for p24 antibody. Cooper et al.[59] have compared four EIAs for their ability to identify infection during acute HIV-1 illness; the ENI assay (now unavailable) was the most sensitive for early diagnosis, while the Abbott EIA was the least. Weiblin et al.[60] have reported increased sensitivity for early detection of HIV-1 infection with first-generation EIAs after treatment with recombinant protein G to remove IgG antibodies. This allows for easier detection of IgM and IgA antibodies, with the Genetic Systems and Organon/Technika kits performing best. The Abbott antigen-enzyme conjugate direct sandwich assay (third generation; Table 1) also detects infection earlier due to its enhanced IgM sensitivity (Fig. 2C).[48]

If a blood or plasma collection center or a referral laboratory detects HIV-1 antibody by EIA in a plasma or serum sample,

a repeat EIA is performed on a second specimen (Fig. 3). If the repeated assay is positive, a confirmatory test is ordered (usually a WB or immunofluorescence assay) and the donor or patient is notified. If the repeated test is negative, a different EIA should be performed.[8,45,46] In either case the unit of blood or plasma is discarded, and the donor is referred to a private physician, a health department, or an alternate testing site for evaluation and counseling. For specimens indeterminate by WB analysis, a repeat specimen obtained in 2–3 months should be evaluated and/or the specimen can be examined by another confirmatory test method (e.g., immunofluorescence or RIPA).

Because the EIA for anti-HIV-1 has been used for serologic evaluation of high-risk populations in addition to volunteer blood donors,[15,16,42] any discussion of the validity of test results must take into account the population tested and its overall sero-positivity rate. In blood donor populations, initial reports of the performance of the screening first-generation EIA (usually the Abbott test) showed positive predictive values of 3.8–27.3 percent.[9,61] These predictive values varied depending on the EIA OD reactivity, with low positive OD values being associated with greater degrees of false positivity.[61–63] Other early studies compared various EIA tests against the same sera, usually from a group of patients with a spectrum of risk for HIV-1 infection.[64–67] While the Abbott (and the Wellcome Diagnostics) EIAs were usually among the most sensitive, the Abbott assay had the highest false-positive rate among low-risk groups (i.e., blood donors), followed by the Organon, Dupont, and Litton assays. The sensitivity and specificity for most manufacturers' assays were 97.2–100 percent and 99.6–100 percent, respectively, when using sera from patients in high risk groups,[65] except for one report of low specificity for the Abbott test in this population.[68]

Subsequent reports have included evaluations of the Genetic Systems EIA, along with others mentioned previously, using sera from a similar spectrum of patients.[29,62,63,69] The Genetic Systems EIA repeatedly ranked best in these studies in terms of sensitivity, specificity, and reproducibility. The most recent studies, some using EIA assays with more purified disrupted viral antigens, confirm further the excellence of the Genetic Systems and the new, improved Organon-Technika EIAs.[38,60,70–72] A number of studies have pointed out the relevance of the distribution of positive and negative OD values above and below the cut-off to differentiate true-positive from true-negative results.[62,71,72] It is evident that a first-generation EIA with many OD determinations clustered around the OD cut-off will be subject to more false-positive and/or false-negative results (e.g., Litton and Ortho).[62,71,72] A CDC survey of health department and American Red Cross laboratories identified similar problems with specimens having OD results around cut-off values.[73] It was noteworthy that, despite confirmation of higher false-positive rates with the Abbott viral lysate EIA, 80–85 percent of laboratories reported using this assay. Schwartz et al.[74] have discussed arguments for varying the OD cut-off values defining positive and negative specimens. Since a rise in the OD cut-off of the noncompetitive EIA increases specificity at the cost of sensitivity, these authors argued for raising cut-off values when these tests are being used for diagnostic rather than screening purposes. Laboratory experience will determine whether such variations in definition of reactive specimens is warranted.

Variations in specificity and positive predictive value are co-dependent on the prevalence of HIV-1 infection in the population tested, as shown in Table 2. For any laboratory test, methodologic error, regardless of source, occurs with a relatively fixed frequency; therefore, for each population tested, regardless of risk for HIV-1 infection, the number of false positives per 1000 tests will be approximately the same. However, in a low-risk population (with few true positives), the number of false positives will be a much greater percentage of those called positive than for the high-risk population. Therefore, the positive predictive value of such a screening test in a low-risk popu-

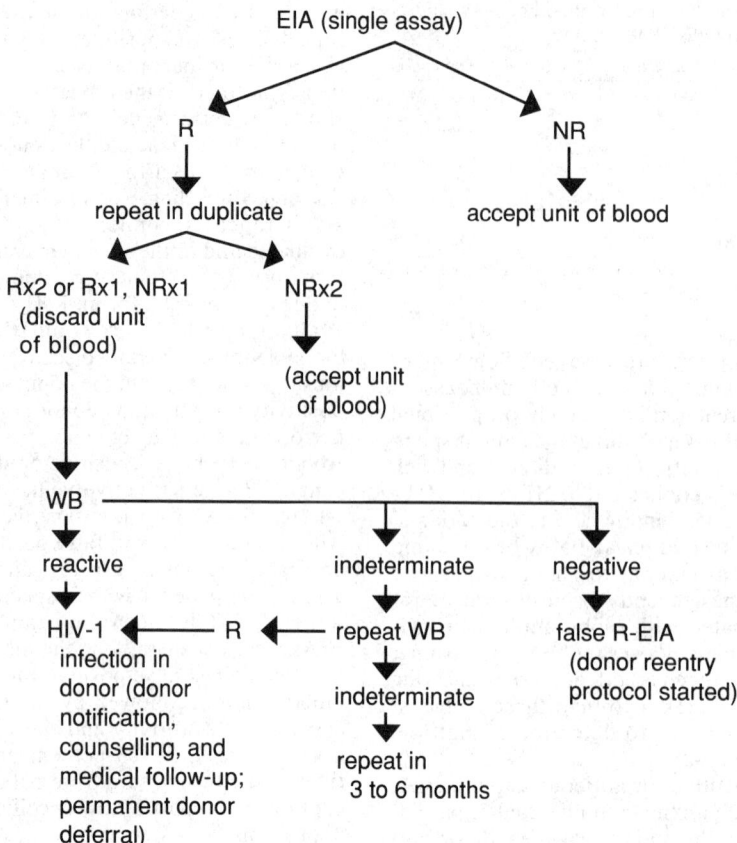

FIG. 3. An algorithm for the management of HIV-1 serologic results. R, reactive; NR, nonreactive.

TABLE 3. Correlation Between EIA and Western Blot Positivity for 2.58 Million American Red Cross Blood Donors

Assay Result	No.	Percent
EIA, initially positive	25,800	1
Repeat EIA positive	6,966	0.27
WB positive	903	0.035
Positive predictive values		
Initial EIA	—	3.5
Repeat EIA	—	13

TABLE 4. Causes of False-Positive Reactions in EIA for Antibody to HIV-1

Antibody against smooth muscle, parietal cell, mitochondrial, nuclear, leukocyte, and T-cell antigens and anti-HAV-IgM, anti-HBc-IgM
Antibodies against class II leukocyte antigens (HLA-DR4, HLA-DQw3) present on H-9 cells (more frequently observed in multiparous women, multiply transfused patients)
Severe alcoholic liver disease, primary biliary cirrhosis, sclerosing cholangitis
Heat inactivation or RPR positivity of serum tested (Abbott unpurified viral lysate EIA only)
Hematologic malignancies, lymphoma
Acute DNA viral infections, HIV-2 infection, influenza immunization
Renal transplantation, chronic renal failure
Stevens-Johnson syndrome
Passively acquired HIV-1 antibody (hepatitis B immunogolbulin)

TABLE 5. Causes of False-Negative Reactions in EIA for Antibody to HIV-1

Incubation period or acute disease before seroconversion (window period)
Malignancy
Intensive or long-term immunosuppressive therapy
Replacement transfusion
Bone marrow transplantation
Kits that detect antibody to p24 primarily
B-cell dysfunction
Rheumatoid factors (with competitive EIA)

lation may only be 10 percent, while it would be as high as 97.3 percent in a high-risk population.[15,16] This was anticipated since these screening viral lysate EIAs were designed for optimum sensitivity at the expense of specificity.[15]

The relevance of these comments about false positivity in a low-risk population are apparent from American Red Cross data (Table 3).[9,47] Among 2.58 million volunteer blood donors, only 3.5 percent of initially positive EIAs and only 13 percent of repeatedly reactive EIAs were reactive by WB.[47] This high prevalence of false positivity in low-risk groups with viral lysate EIAs brings into focus the relatively high cost of identifying one truly infected person in such a population, estimated conservatively by the author to be $35,000 to $40,000 per infected person (e.g., if all hospital admissions underwent mandatory screening annually).

The false-positive and false-negative results obtained with viral lysate EIAs are due to a variety of clinical and technical variables.[75] It has been noted that heat-inactivated sera (treated to enhance laboratory safety) cause false-positive reactions with the former Abbott unpurified viral lysate EIA.[66,76,77] Sera with RPR reactivity have also been reported to cause false-positive EIAs for HIV-1 antibody only with this Abbott kit; the false-positive rate with RPR-positive sera using the most recent viral

lysate Abbott EIA has been reduced to approximately 3 percent.[78] Other factors are also associated with erroneous results, as noted in Tables 4 and 5.[42,61,67,79–90] By far the most important cause of false positivity is cross-reacting antibodies in serum to HLA class II antigens present in HIV-1 preparations harvested from H-9 cells.[61,79–83] The Genetic Systems (and Wellcome) assays avoid this problem by use of CEM-F cells for virus propagation; this cell line lacks such HLA reactivity (Table 1).[71,74] While too insensitive to assay for HIV-2 antibodies, anti-HIV-

1 EIAs, especially competitive EIAs, can be falsely positive due to cross-reacting core antibodies with HIV-2.[43,92] Indeed, some HIV-1 EIAs can serve as screening tests for HIV-2 infection. Due to p24 cross-reactivity, the Genetic Systems and Cellular Products HIV-1 EIAs have a 91 percent sensitivity for HIV-2–seropositive specimens.[43]

Using WB and the Dupont EIA, Tribe et al.[93] have also recognized some sera that are repeatedly reactive by EIA but nonreactive by WB criteria due to their EIA reactivity with gag proteins of HIV-1. These sera react predominantly with p15/p17 and less frequently with p24, while they lack anti-env reactivity. Such individuals must be excluded from blood donation until the reasons for this continued reactivity are clarified (e.g., cross-reactivity with other [retro] viruses or tissue proteins).

Despite the foregoing comments, the probability of a false positive result after the complete testing sequence (Fig. 3) has been estimated to be 1–5 per 100,000 persons screened with viral lysate EIAs.[13,94] Perhaps more important from a clinical perspective, estimates of the false-negative rate of EIAs for HIV-1 antibody range from 1 in 40,000 to 1 in 1 million.[95–97] The causes of such false negativity are presented in Table 5. This problem has been reviewed with regard to transfusion-related transmission of HIV-1.[98]

The most recently developed second-generation EIAs for antibody to HIV-1 use polypeptide antigens of the HIV-1 core and envelope that are synthesized or produced by recombinant DNA technology. Dupont and Cambridge Bioscience (both now merged into Cambridge Biotech) and Smith Kline Bioscience Laboratories have developed similar assays; Abbott produced a competitive enzyme immunoassay (CIA-RA) using recombinant HIV-1 antigens (p24 and gp41) individually and an indirect EIA combining these two proteins (Envacore); each has been evaluated for screening and confirmatory purposes. The initial report with CIA-RAs demonstrated sensitivity superior to both first-generation (viral lysate antigen) EIAs and WB.[23] Subsequent studies confirmed this initial impression and demonstrated greater specificity for CIA-RA.[38,39,68,99]

Other authors reported similarly enhanced sensitivity and specificity for a Cambridge Bioscience assay (recombinant envelope protein only) and another recombinant EIA for HIV-1 antibody.[17,100,101] These studies noted that the enhanced sensitivity of such recombinant-protein assays for antibody were dependent to a significant extent on the presence of envelope patterned peptides, including both gp160 and gp41,[17,39,42,100,101] since antibodies to gp160/120 and gp41 develop before anti-p24 and remain after anti-p24 disappears.[24,39,42]

The newer Cambridge Biotech EIA (with rp24 and rp41) and the Smith Kline EIA (with antigens from the gag, pol, and env genes) are reported to have 99.7–99.9 percent sensitivities and specificities. Both are reported to have fewer indeterminate results (i.e., are better able to distinguish true positives and true negatives; Table 1).[44,45]

Abbott has combined their new third-generation EIA format (antigen–enzyme conjugate, direct sandwich assay) with similar rp24 and rp41 antigens not only to enhance sensitivity and specificity but also to detect infection earlier due to IgM binding (Table 1; Fig. 2C).[48]

Several synthetic peptide antigen EIAs have been developed and studied.[18,46,102] The United Biomedical EIA is the only licensed synthetic antigen assay using conserved, immunogenic portions of p24 and gp41. This assay was found to be as sensitive as the recombinant and viral lysate EIAs (100 percent) and 98.4 percent specific.[46]

Some theoretical limitations of these recombinant and synthetic protein assays include (1) lack of glycosylation of env proteins, which may limit interactions with serum antibodies; and (2) limited cross-reactions with HIV-1 variants (e.g., HIV-2).[17,42] These assays retain the limitations of all antibody assays in that they fail to detect p24 antigen before antibody seroconversion.[17] Their advantages are significant, however, including

safety, reproducibility of antigen content, and lack of contaminating cellular proteins that cause false positivity.[42] Due to their technical ease, assays for antibody to individual recombinant antigens may be useful as (or replace) confirmatory tests such as WB.[42,45,46] It has been suggested that interposition of one of the recombinant assays to confirm screening EIA (viral lysate) could reduce the need for confirmatory WB assays by up to 47 percent.[45,46]

Since March 1985, the American Red Cross blood donor centers have sequentially adopted gradually improving Abbott EIAs. Initially, the purified whole virion lysate antibody assay was introduced, followed, in sequence, by the same lysate assay "spiked" with further purified gp41 (early 1987) and subsequently additionally spiked by further purified p24 antigen (C. Fang, PHD, personal communication, 1989, Director, National Reference Laboratory for Infectious Diseases, American Red Cross, Rockville, MD).

While endemic to west Africa and of low prevalence in the United States, screening for HIV-2 infection was made practicable because of antigenic and genomic characteristics similar to HIV-1. A number of EIA formats (whole virion, recombinant and synthetic peptide antigen, competitive EIA, antigen-enzyme conjugate, and antibody-capture EIAs) have been developed and tested for detection of both HIV-1 and HIV-2.[49,103,104] After reports of high sensitivity, the Genetic system and the Abbott assays were licensed, the former on September 25, 1991, and the latter on February 14, 1992. The Abbott EIA uses a direct sandwich technique with an antigen–enzyme conjugate (third-generation assay; Fig. 2C); the antigens included are the rp24 and rp41 of HIV-1 and the rp41/36 of HIV-2. The Genetic Systems assay uses a viral lysate format. In place of the Abbott purified antigen HIV-1 viral lysate format, the American Red Cross, in March–April 1992, initiated screening all donor blood units with the Abbott recombinant HIV-1/2 EIA, in response to the FDA directive mandating dual screening starting on June 1, 1992.

Western Blot

The WB was developed as a method for separating proteins obtained from HIV-1 harvested from cell lysates and thereby analyzing sera for antibody content to these specific proteins. HIV-1 is allowed to replicate in continuous lymphoid cell lines, usually HUT-78 (H-9) cells. Cells are lysed to release viral and precursor protein yields; virus is then partially purified by centrifugation (Fig. 4).[33,106,107] The viral protein is then placed in multiple, small aliquots at the top of a thin slablike polyacrylamide gel. The viral proteins are then electrophoresed from the negative to positive electrodes attached to each end of the gel slab (the negative electrode is at the site of protein loading at the top of the gel). When completed, the lower molecular weight proteins (p17, p24) have migrated farther in the gel, with the higher molecular weight proteins (gp160/120) remaining near the origin. The proteins are then blotted (or transferred) to nitrocellulose paper electrophoretically by applying a current across the thin slab of gel and nitrocellulose paper (positive on far side of paper). The paper is dried and cut into strips (or lanes) of approximately 5 mm width. The strips are subsequently exposed to a dilution of patient serum, washed, and incubated with anti-human IgG labeled with an enzyme that produces a colored band upon exposure to its substrate. Molecular weight standards, as well as positive and negative control sera, are incorporated into each assay. This reference WB technique is performed according to the method of Towbin et al.[107] Figure 5 depicts test strips developed using the Dupont licensed WB kit, which provides nitrocellulose paper strips with preelectrophoresed disrupted viral proteins blotted onto the strips.

The WB has the advantage over nonrecombinant EIAs that antibodies to individual viral proteins can be assayed. WB is more sensitive for the assay of anti-p24 than anti-gp41, since

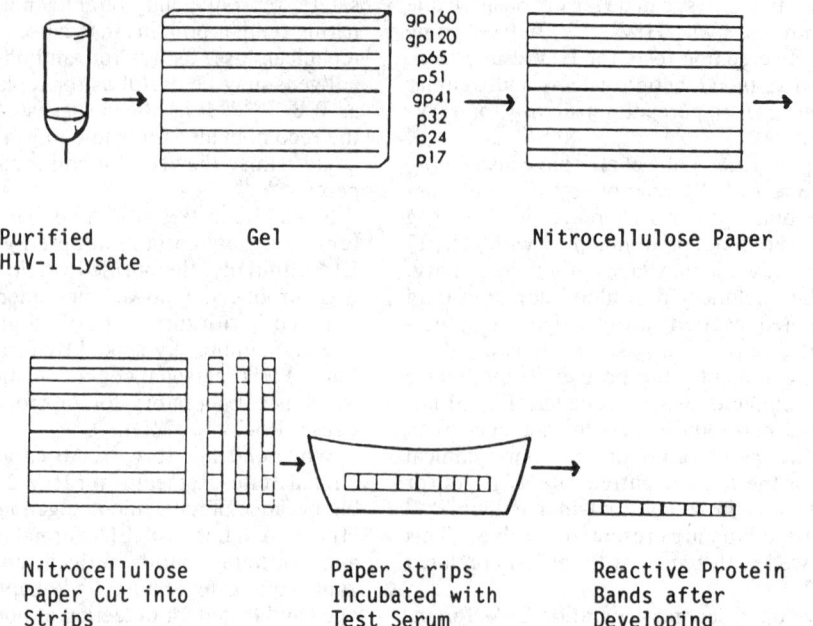

Purified HIV-1 Lysate → Gel → Nitrocellulose Paper →

gp160
gp120
p65
p51
gp41
p32
p24
p17

Nitrocellulose Paper Cut into Strips → Paper Strips Incubated with Test Serum → Reactive Protein Bands after Developing

FIG. 4. Western blot procedure in diagrammatic format. (Modified from Griffith et al.,[106] with permission.)

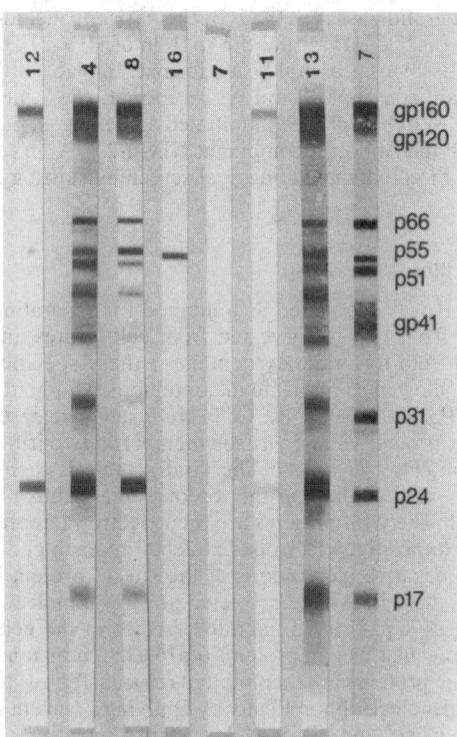

FIG. 5. Typical Western blot result using Dupont immunoblot kit. Number 12 is indeterminate serum; numbers 4, 8, and 13 are positive sera; numbers 7 (middle), 11, and 16 are negative sera; and number 7 (right) is positive control.

the latter glycosylated proteins do not transfer as well to nitrocellulose paper.[24,41,63,69] WB is also less sensitive for the detection of antibody to gp160/120 than other confirmatory assays (e.g., RIPA) because of less resolving power. This is due to clumping of higher molecular weight antigens at the origin.[29,63] During the spectrum of HIV-1 infection, WB is insensitive during early HIV-1 infection (similar to EIA due to lack of anti-

p24 and/or anti-gp41) and in patients with AIDS (due to a loss of anti-p24 late in disease).[29,33,69]

The definition of a positive WB has been in a state of flux for some time. In addition to the cumbersome nature of the assay, which allows for the possibility of multiple technical errors, the test is also subjective in interpretation (reading the presence or absence of faint bands). The CDC has variably called WB with anti-p24 or anti-gp41 bands as positive.[40,41] The licensed Dupont (now Cambridge Biotech) kit requires evidence of antibody against each of the three major gene products (gag, pol, and env) and defines the presence of anti-p24, either anti-gp41 or gp160, and anti-p31 as a positive test[40,41,74,75]; the American Red Cross has used a similar definition,[74] while the U.S. Army accepts the presence of either anti-gp41 or both anti-p24 and anti-p55 bands.[75,108] The Consortium for Retrovirus Serology Standardization recommends at least two antibody bands for positivity; p24 or p31 antibody, plus antibody to gp41 or gp120/160.[109] The Association of State and Territorial Public Health Laboratory Directors (ASTPHLD) published recommended guidelines.[110] A *reactive* WB must contain two of three major bands of diagnostic significance (anti-gp160/120, anti-gp41, anti-p24); a *nonreactive* WB is defined as one without any HIV-1–specific bands, and an *indeterminate* WB contains one or more viral specific bands but insufficient bands to meet their definition of reactive. Such an indeterminate WB should be repeated and, if still indeterminate, followed up with a repeat blot in 2–3 months (Fig. 3). The CDC subsequently adopted the ASTPHLD recommendations.[109] While continuing to use the Dupont (Cambridge Biotech) WB kit, in February 1993 the American Red Cross changed its criteria for a positive WB to those of the ASTPHLD/CDC.

Three different WB techniques, one similar to the Towbin method and two commercially available kits, Bio-RAD and Dupont, have been compared.[111] The Dupont kit had the best sensitivity (dilutional reactivity) and specificity (lack of reaction with cellular and subcellular antisera). It was noted that antibodies to HLA class I cellular antigens tend to cause false-positive anti-gp41 bands, while antibodies to HLA class II antigens primarily caused false-positive anti-p31 bands; a parallel WB of uninfected H-9 cellular proteins was recommended to detect these false-positive reactions. Unexplained occasional anti-HIV-1 gag pro-

TABLE 6. Causes of False-Positive Western Blot Reactions to HIV-1 Antigens (gag, env, and pol Proteins)

Cross-reactions with
  Normal human ribonucleoproteins
  Other human retroviruses
  Antibodies to mitochondrial, nuclear, T-cell, and leukocyte antigens
  Antibodies to HLA antigens (classes I and II)
  Globulins produced during polyclonal gammopathy

TABLE 7. Comparison of IFA and Western Blot: Day of Acute Illness When Initially Positive for Indicated Antibody

| | Day of Illness According to Test | |
Antibody	IFA	WB (8)[a]
IgM	5(5)	—
IgG	11(6)	—
p24/gp41	—	24
p55	—	40
p68	—	57
p34	—	71

[a] The number of patients evaluated are given in parentheses.

(From Cooper et al.,[59] with permission.)

tein bands (falsely positive) were also noted by Blomberg and Klaase[111] and others,[38,108,112,113] as has been noted for EIAs.[93] Overall, false-positive WBs are estimated to occur no more frequently than 1 in 20,000[41]; the potential cross-reacting antibodies are noted in Table 6.[108,112,113] The false positivity of a WB is determined by a negative RIPA or immunofluorescence assay.

False-negative reactions by WB occur usually very early after HIV-1 infection or late after the development of AIDS.[29,33,40,41,69] HIV-1 culture or enzymatic DNA amplification positivity have been noted in WB-negative patients.[41,61,89,114–119] The importance of the use of ongoing quality control (unknown) serum specimens in diagnostic laboratories performing WB assays has been emphasized.[120] In conjunction with serial EIA determinations, the false-negative rate of WB for blood donors is estimated to be 1 in 250,000.[41]

Indeterminate WB (I-WB) reactivity has been recognized as a frequent problem following positive or negative EIAs.[121–123] From 2 to 49 percent of patients assayed may have such reactivity, most commonly caused by cross-reacting antibodies to p24, p55, or p66 bands.[123] In low-risk populations, an I-WB is rarely associated with HIV-1 infection during follow-up testing.[124–133] Even in high-risk patients, an I-WB pattern is variably followed by seroconversion.[131,134] The continued presence of this banding pattern after absorption with recombinant p24 demonstrates a nonspecific cross-reacting antibody to p24 in I-WB assays.[135] To reduce further the incidence of I-WB patterns, the CDC has reinforced its recommendation to all laboratories to adopt the ASTPHLD/CDC criteria for a positive WB.[136]

There are three WB kits commercially available, all using viral lysate antigens. Cambridge Biotech (Dupont) and Ortho distribute the same product, while Biorad and Organon-Technika each have their own licensed viral lysate WB assays. The American Red Cross continues to use the Cambridge Biotech kit, despite their recent adoption of ASTPHLD/CDC criteria.

Indirect Immunofluorescence Assay

The indirect immunofluorescence assay (IFA) is a rapid and reliable supplemental test using uninfected and HIV-1 infected H-9 (or HUT-78) cells in the logarithmic growth phase. The cells are air dried and fixed to a fluorescent glass microscope slide.[41] A small quantity of a 1:10–1:20 test serum dilution is applied to each well, incubated to allow antibody to react with antigen, washed, and air dried. Subsequently, antihuman IgG labeled with fluorescein isothiocyanate is applied to each well, followed again by incubation, washing, drying, and mounting. The use of known positive and negative control sera with both infected and uninfected cells in each assay allows for correction due to nonspecific fluorescence. Specimens are evaluated for fluorescence intensity, percentage of fluorescent cells, and fluorescent pattern; each test serum is determined to be qualitatively positive or negative, but may be quantitatively assayed by use of serial test serum dilutions. Through the use of antihuman globulin specific for IgM, this immunoglobulin response can also be differentiated.

The IgM and IgG antibody responses to acute HIV-1 infection can be detected by IFA earlier than other currently available

antibody assays (Table 7).[59] Sandstrom et al.[137] found excellent overall agreement of IFA results with those of WB for both low- and high-risk populations; IFA was also shown to be more sensitive than EIA. Others have suggested similar sensitivity and specificity for high-risk patients.[33,138–140] However, for a low-risk population, Lennette et al.[140] noted nonspecific staining patterns that could be absorbed by noninfected HUT-78 cell antigens,[140] perhaps accounting for the false positives reported by Carlson et al.[141] when a similar population was screened by IFA in their study. Most authors concur that IFA requires less technical expertise, is quicker to perform (<2 hours), and is less costly than WB, while being equally sensitive and specific.[138–140,142] Infrequently, however, false-negative assays have been identified.[115,137] The sensitivity of IFA may vary according to the cell line in which the virus is grown.[29] Generally, IFA interpretation is subjective and requires an experienced observer, but excellent interlaboratory agreement has been documented.[41,143]

Immunofluorescence can be used to differentiate HIV-1 from HIV-2 infection.[144,145] By using live retrovirus-infected target cells for IFA (instead of acetone-fixed cells), thereby limiting the IFA assay to membrane staining, this differentiation of HIV-1 from HIV-2 is reliable and easier.[145]

Radioimmunoprecipitation Assay

The radioimmunoprecipitation assay is a research technique confined to laboratories capable of propogation of HIV-1 in cell culture. The virus is grown in H-9 cells to logarithmic growth and then exposed to a radiolabeled amino acid or other substance that allows isotopic incorporation in or transfer to viral proteins.[41,146] Cells are subsequently lysed, thereby releasing labeled viral proteins. Cell lysates are exposed to test serum, with resultant HIV-1–specific immune complexes being formed if antibody is present. This reaction mixture is then exposed to Sepharose beads to which protein A is bound, with the exposed Fc receptors of protein A binding the immune complexes. After washing, these immunoprecipitates are then eluted from the beads and separated electrophoretically on polyacrylamide gels, as for WB. The HIV-1 antigen-antibody complexes are detected in the gel by autoradiography (due to isotopic labeling); the bands are similar to those of WB except that the gp160 and gp120 bands are better separated and defined.[29,41,63,69,146]

RIPA is more sensitive than WB for the detection of antibodies to the higher molecular weight proteins of HIV-1; due to this sensitivity, gp 160/120 antibodies may be detected with RIPA before anti-p24 or anti-gp41, thereby potentially allowing for earlier detection of seroconversion.[29,69,146] In contrast, RIPA has been found to be less sensitive than WB at detecting antibodies to p24 in most studies,[29,69] while one group reported greater sensitivity for anti-p24 by RIPA than by WB.[146] Generally RIPA is more sensitive late during HIV-1 infection when WB may revert to negativity.[69] Few false positives have been detected,[29,38] and RIPA is usually negative among blood donors when WB may be falsely reactive with anti-p24 bands.[29,146] There are rare false negatives by RIPA.[69,115] RIPA has also been applied to the detection of salivary antibodies.[147]

Overall, RIPA is slightly more sensitive and specific than WB, and, therefore, can be used to supplement WB assays when results are indeterminate.[29,41] Theoretic reasons for the advantages of this assay include (1) retention of three-dimensional structure by soluble proteins, allowing for more specific antibody binding; (2) greater multivalent binding by antibody in a liquid medium, thereby increasing sensitivity; and (3) formation of more stable antigen-antibody complexes in a soluble phase, thereby detecting low-avidity antibodies.[146] Despite these advantages, whether real or theoretic, RIPA will remain a supplemental test confined to research laboratories due to its being labor intensive, expensive, and requiring the use of HIV-1–infected cell lines and radioisotopes.

Latex Agglutination

For developing countries many of the screening tests described above are not practical due to lack of needed equipment, biohazard containment facilities, sufficient skilled technicians, and/or sufficient financial resources. Furthermore, viral lysate EIAs are recognized to give a high rate of false positivity with African sera,[148] possibly due to cross-reactivity with other retroviruses.[47,92] Riggin et al.[149] have reported development of a rapid latex agglutination (LA) assay using recombinant envelope antigen (CBre3) to detect HIV-1 antibodies. This antigen incorporates the immunodominant regions of gp120 (carboxy-terminal third) and gp41 (amino-terminal half) and has been used by others for a recombinant EIA.[17,100] Riggin et al.[149] showed complete agreement of LA with WB and only one discordant result with EIA among 211 serum specimens (95 positive by WB and EIA); most positive specimens were strongly reactive by LA and easy to interpret. Similar results have been reported by others with this Cambridge Biotech kit when using sera from 300 African patients[70] and 2820 serum specimens from many areas of the globe (the Carribean, Africa, North and South America, and Europe).[150] This assay is now licensed as Recombigen. Van de Perre et al.[70] did note a need to dilute sera for the LA test to avoid a prozone phenomenon causing false-negative results; these authors believed that LA results did not require confirmation. Other studies have also defined disappointing sensitivities of 81 to 86 percent with this assay, despite good specificity.[151,152] Quinn et al.[150] cautioned about the need for positive and negative LA controls and a trained observer due to the subjective determination of reactivity with LA. The need for such training, the limited shelf life of the LA, and need for refrigeration of reagents may unfortunately limit the use of LA in developing countries.[153] The LA does appear to be a good screening (and possibly confirmatory) assay in high-risk populations. However, its applicability to low-risk population screening (e.g., blood donors) requires evaluation, due to anticipated increases in rates of false positivity.

Dot-Blot Immunobinding Assay

A rapid dot immunobinding assay for HIV-1 antibodies has been described recently for screening purposes.[154,155] The lysate of HIV-1–infected cells[155,156] or recombinant HIV-1 polypeptides[154,157] are spotted onto nitrocellulose paper and reacted with test sera; this is followed by typical EIA immunoenzymatic reactions resulting in the development of color. The color intensity is judged as positive or negative by the observer when compared with both positive and negative controls.[158] This assay technique has the advantages of being simple, rapid (30 minutes), stable, and requiring no equipment, but is subject to observer variability. Using recombinant peptides it may detect HIV-1 antibodies to defined viral antigens.[157] The assay is sensitive and at least as specific as the Genetic Systems EIA and

WB. It may have applicability in developing countries but has found recent use in the diagnosis of infection in infants. While the assay for anti-HIV-1 IgM antibodies to diagnose infection in newborns has been disappointing due to both its transiency and its low concentration, its ability to detect IgA antibody to HIV-1 by dot immunoblot is promising.[30,31,159–161] By 6 months of age, 50–93 percent of infected children were detected by this IgA assay before or at the time of viral culture positivity.

A screening second-generation recombinant protein dot immunoblot, HIVCHEK by Dupont, has been extensively tested in the United States and Africa.[151,152,162,163] This assay has been reported to have excellent specificity (97–99 percent) with a sensitivity of 87–99 percent. It is easy to perform and read, as well as quick (5 minutes).[151]

A confirmatory diagnostic technique has been described and marketed, although not licensed for clinical use, that incorporates recombinant HIV-1 antigens with a protein electrophoretic immunoblot technique.[164] In this Chiron immunoblot, recombinant p24, p31, gp41, and gp120 are electrophoresed and blotted onto nitrocellulose sheets, which are cut into strips. Controls include an antibody-negative serum and two sera with high and low levels of antibody. With this kit, the bands are sharp, well separated, and defined; this assay also requires less reaction time with the patient's serum than the WB.[164]

Hofbauer et al.,[165] have reported a similar recombinant envelope (gp41) immunoblot. This recombinant blot was easier to read than was the WB when using viral lysate. This assay detected anti-gp41 before anti-p24 was detected by the conventional WB, lacked any false positives, and was more sensitive than either the conventional WB or IFA. Further studies are needed to define the use of these recombinant antigen immunoblots in the diagnosis of HIV-1 infection.

Other Antibody Tests

Van de Perre et al.[70] have described a dipstick screening test for HIV-1 antibodies (Biotech). An HIV-1–infected H-9 cell lysate is coated to a polystyrene stick, which is then reacted with test serum and immunoenzymatic reagents modified from an EIA. The color reaction is visible to the observer after three 15-minute incubations. This assay was 98 percent sensitive but suffered from false positivity (90 percent specific). Confirmation of results was needed when using the dipstick as a screen. Its low cost and lack of equipment requirements may make this assay applicable as a screening test in developing countries.

The most unique development regarding screening for HIV-1 infection uses the patient's own blood, with autologous red cell agglutination being a positive test.[166] A nonagglutinating murine monoclonal antibody was made to human red blood cells; to this monoclonal antibody was bound a synthetic peptide containing the immunoreactive portion of gp41. The addition of this monoclonal antibody–peptide complex results in binding of the antibody to red blood cells and agglutination if HIV-1 envelope antibodies are present in the patient's blood. This assay can be performed with 0.01 ml of the patient's blood and takes 2 minutes. The sensitivity reported was 98 percent for patients with AIDS; a false-positive rate of 0.1 percent with sera from healthy blood donors was noted, compared with a 0.2 percent rate using the Genetic Systems EIA on the same samples. A similar passive hemagglutination test has proven sensitive and specific on whole blood, serum, and saliva.[167] This assay scheme may have major applications as a screening test in the future, especially considering its simplicity and speed.

The particle agglutination assay has also been utilized with gelatin particles (Serodia)[151,152,162,168] and turkey red blood cells.[151] These rapid gelatin particle assays have sensitivities and specificities greater than 94 percent.

A recently FDA licensed rapid screening EIA is the Murex SUDS (single use diagnostic system). This assay is self-contained, performed manually, read visually, and takes 10 minutes at room temperature. The solid phase is latex particles coated with purified p24 and a recombinant immunodominant peptide of gp41. A positive reaction comprises the development of blue color in the center hole of the microfiltration apparatus. Sensitivity and specificity of 99.9 and 99.6 percent, respectively, have been reported.[163]

A test generating much interest but yet unapproved by the FDA is a saliva-based EIA (Orasure). A test pad is placed between the gingiva and buccal surface for 2 minutes to collect saliva, which subsequently undergoes a standard EIA for HIV-1 antibody. Its ease of collection without venipuncture make it attractive as a mass screening test.[169]

A unique assay method for HIV-1 antibodies has been developed using flow cytometric indirect immunofluorescence. Either HIV-1–infected H9 cells or polystyrene beads of various sizes coated with recombinant HIV-1 proteins according to bead size are exposed to patient serum.[170,171] After washing, the antibody-coated H9 cells or beads are exposed to fluorescent antiglobulin and subjected to flow cytometric assay. These assays are at least as sensitive and specific as current EIAs and WBs. The bead assay is the least cumbersome and most readily applicable.

Another method of antibody detection is demonstration of the presence of antibody-secreting cells in blood. These assays have been developed primarily for detecting HIV-1 infection in newborns. The ELISPOT uses a recombinant gp41 antigen of HIV-1 fixed to nitrocellulose-coated wells of microtiter plates. The wells are exposed overnight to peripheral blood mononuclear cells from patients and treated with an enzyme-conjugated anti-human Ig immunoglobulin.[172] An EIA enzyme substrate is then added. A test for in vitro antibody production (IVAP) assays supernatants from cultures of peripheral blood mononuclear cells for HIV-1 antibody using a WB assay.[173–175] Both of these assays are restricted to research laboratories at present.

Some virologists consider the ability of serum to neutralize the infectivity of a virus to be a reference serologic test. With HIV-1, this is a tedious assay requiring culture in H-9 or other cell culture systems[176,177] and is confined to laboratories with biohazard capabilities. The complexity of the assay for neutralizing antibodies currently limits its application as a diagnostic test for HIV-1 infection.

HIV-1 ANTIGEN DETECTION

The detection of p24 antigen in serum has played an important role in experimental studies of the therapy of HIV-1 infection since the Abbott EIA became available in 1986. Genetic Systems, Cellular Products, Dupont, and Coulter antigen EIAs are also available commercially. The detection of the p24 antigen viral marker differs from antibody detection in two ways: (1) only low antigen concentrations are present and (2) p24 forms immune complexes with its antibody, which are not detected by the antigen assay. The standard EIA for p24 antigen only detects free antigen in excess of antibody. Recently, a modification of the EIA has been described that enhances sensitivity for (free) p24 antigen through pretreatment with HCl or glycine HCl, which dissociates immune complexes by denaturing antibody.[178–180] It is estimated that, using this assay technique, 58.6 percent of sera from HIV-1–infected patients persistently contain p24 as an immune complex, 34.5 percent of sera never contain p24, and 6.9 percent have intermittent antigenemia. Rates generally increase as patients progress to advanced stages of HIV-1 infection.

With this indirect EIA for p24 antigen, the test specimen is incubated overnight with polystyrene beads or in a microtiter well coated with polyclonal HIV-1 antibody. After rinsing, the bead or well is allowed to react with rabbit or goat anti-HIV-1. After rinsing, the bead or well is then exposed to an enzyme-linked antirabbit or antigoat immunoglobulin. The substrate is added to allow the color to develop, after which absorbance is

TABLE 8. Correlation of the Clinical Status of HIV-1 Infection with p24 Antigen Detection

Clinical Status	Percent with p24 Antigenemia
Asymptomatic	4
AIDS-related complex	56
AIDS	70

(From Kenny et al.,[191] with permission.)

measured. The OD is proportional to the amount of antigen present, with the limit of detection for the assay being between 50 and 100 pg/ml.[19,34,181] The entire assay consumes 24–30 hours.[41]

For a specimen that is repeatedly reactive, the specificity of the assay must be confirmed by use of a blocking ("neutralizing") antibody.[41,110] The specimen, as well as positive and negative controls, are incubated with reference human sera with or without antibody to HIV-1 and then reassayed for the presence of detectable p24 antigen. Specificity is confirmed by a concomitant reduction (50 percent or greater) of OD with the specimen exposed to human anti-HIV-1 or by an OD of the non-neutralized specimen equal to or greater than the cut-off value.[41] Including repetition and the blocking assay, confirmation of a positive p24 antigen assay may take 3–4 days.

The major advantages of the antigen assay over viral culture include working with noninfectious HIV-1 antigen and the lack of HLA determinants contaminating the antigen preparation used in the former assay. A major disadvantage is the complexity and duration of the assay itself, especially when coupled with confirmatory tests. Additionally, this assay is not a screening test and must be used in conjunction with an antibody assay.

Suggested uses for the antigen assay are (1) detection of HIV-1 in cell culture, (2) detection of an antiretroviral effect of therapy, and (3) assessment of the HIV-1 infection status of neonates born to seropositive mothers.[110,182,183] Cerebrospinal fluid can also be assayed for p24 to provide evidence for HIV-1 central nervous system involvement.[20] Antigen screening of blood donors, in addition to EIA for antibody, has not been shown to be fruitful due to lack of antigen-positive, antibody-negative donors.[184,185]

During acute infection, p24 antigenemia precedes seroconversion, usually resolves within 2–3 weeks as antibodies to p24 appear,[19,26,28,186–188] but may persist for 6–14 months before seroconversion.[25,26] However, during the early stages of HIV infection, antigen detection is not as sensitive as viral culture.[189] Thus, while detection of p24 antigen has been shown to correlate with virus culture positivity, the antigen assay is an insensitive test for infection due to its usual negativity during asymptomatic illness when patients remain culture positive.[41,190] Its sensitivity improves as HIV-1–related disease develops (Table 8).[191] As the infection progresses clinically with the development of AIDS, p24 antibodies decline and p24 antigen reappears.[20,23,28,34,35,188,190–192] The sensitivity limits of this assay are between 10 and 30 pg/ml.[181] In a diverse group of seropositive males, acid pretreatment increased p24 detection from 12.4 to 50.6 percent.[178] The specificity of p24 antigen positivity by EIA is very good, since Stute[193] found only a 0.43 percent false-positive rate among volunteer blood donors. The p24 antigen assay has been used to detect an initial antiviral effect in patients receiving ZDV and other antivirals active against HIV-1.[21,181,194] Prior to therapy, a high serum antigen concentration correlated with a poor prognosis.[183,194]

In addition to detection of soluble antigen in serum, HIV-1 antigens have also been detected on the surface of peripheral blood lymphocytes from HIV-1–infected patients by direct and indirect immunofluorescence and by flow cytometry.[195,196]

HIV-1 DETECTION
Viral Culture

The in vitro propagation of HIV-1 was initially reported in 1983 and was followed by improvements in culture techniques.[3–5]

The virus was initially identified in cell culture by electron microscopy,[2] but was subsequently detected by assays for reverse transcriptase (RT) activity in cell culture supernatants.[197] Reverse transcriptase activity is not specific for HIV-1, since it is also produced by other retroviruses.[198] More specific indirect assays for the presence of HIV-1 in cell culture have been described, including HIV-1 antigen (p24) detection in culture supernatants by EIA,[22,41,199–201] antigen detection by a dot immunoenzymatic binding assay,[202] and a radioimmunoassay (RIA) designed for antigen detection in cell culture.[200]

Each of these indirect methods of viral detection requires HIV-1 culture, which is cumbersome, costly, and time consuming and exposes personnel to an infectious risk.[41] A typical HIV-1 culture requires (1) separation of peripheral blood mononuclear cells (PBMC) from other blood components, (2) incubation of patient PBMC with PBMC from an HIV-1–seronegative donor for several weeks in the presence of interleukin-2 and phytohemagglutinin (fresh PBMC must be added every 3–5 days), and (3) once or twice weekly assay of supernatants from these cultures for RT activity or p24 antigen.[3–5,41] In culture supernatants, antigen detection is more sensitive and positive earlier than the RT assay for HIV-1[22,41,199,201,203]; 60–94 percent of supernatants are positive by the p24 detection assay at day 10 of culture compared with 20–25 percent by the RT assay. The RIA and EIA are equally sensitive.[200] Technically, however, antigen detection by EIA has numerous advantages over RIA and the RT assay.[41,199–201]

The clinical indications for HIV-1 culture are similar to those for p24 antigen detection, but culture is the more sensitive technique. Sensitivity of HIV-1 culture in infected patients varies from 65 to 100 percent.[204] By viral culture, Ho et al.,[205] established that 1 in 50,000 PBMC in asymptomatic patients and 1 in 400 PBMC in symptomatic patients carry infectious HIV-1. Coombs et al.,[204] found a linear relation of plasma viremia to disease stage, ranging from $10^{1.4}$/ml in asymptomatic patients to $10^{2.5}$/ml in patients with AIDS. By separating monocytes from PBMC for culture, Landay et al.[206] found universal HIV-1 culture positivity regardless of disease stage. Dilution of PBMCs or plasma samples for culture has been used as a method to quantitate virus "load" in peripheral blood. For the diagnosis of neonatal infection with HIV-1, the sensitivity of viral culture at birth (48 percent) and at 3 months of age (75 percent) remains superior to IgA and p24 detection.[207] However, due to the many technical difficulties with HIV-1 culture, it is currently confined to a limited number of laboratories.[41,110]

DNA and RNA Detection

An alternative method for detection of HIV-1 in culture-negative patients is molecular hybridization using DNA probes and peripheral blood nonlymphoid mononuclear cells.[25,41] Attempts at direct detection of the HIV-1 circular proviral genome in the host cell nucleus with hybridization were quite insensitive.[41] To enhance sensitivity, subsequent attempts have relied on amplification of the virus in host cells before hybridization by cocultivation in vitro[208] or by oligonucleotide probes of DNA extracted from mononuclear cells and blotted on nitrocellulose.[41,203] These probes of subgenomic size are made by inserting fragments of the HIV-1 genome into plasmids, by allowing the plasmids to replicate, and then by extracting the subgenomic fragments from the plasmids.[203] These fragments are then isotopically labeled. DNA is extracted from a patient's mononuclear cells and blotted onto nitrocellulose paper. Hybridization is then attempted with the blotted cellular DNA extract and the labeled subgenomic HIV-1 DNA fragments. Blots are subsequently washed, dried, and exposed to film for detection of hybridized, labeled DNA. Such hybridization assays have been shown to be at least as sensitive and specific as HIV-1 culture.[25,203] The method is time consuming and technically diffi-

cult but faster and easier than culture.[203] As few as 1 in 10,000 PBMC may express HIV-1 RNA by hybridization.

Much excitement has been generated by the development of far more sensitive amplification techniques for detection of as little as one genome of nonreplicating HIV-1 in mononuclear cells; these techniques have somewhat downplayed the need for HIV-1 culture.[208] Molecular hybridization without amplification requires an actively replicating HIV-1 infection. The polymerase chain reaction (PCR) involves annealing two oligonucleotide strands (partially analogous to the HIV-1 genome) to the proviral genome after DNA denaturation, one onto each strand of the HIV-1 proviral DNA. This template-directed replication of the HIV-1 genome is initiated by the addition of DNA polymerase; the products of this replication serve as templates for repeated cycles (up to 25) of denaturation, annealing, and replication, until there are sufficient numbers of oligonucleotides to be detected by a complementary, labeled oligonucleotide DNA probe or by incorporation of radiolabeled deoxynucleotides into the amplified product.[209,210] Since the initial description of PCR in 1987, a thermostable DNA polymerase has been substituted for the thermolabile polymerase, allowing the entire procedure to be automated and completed within hours, instead of taking 1 day or more.[209,211] PCR has also been applied to the detection of HIV-1 RNA by a competitive and noncompetitive RT-based amplification system.[212,213] A new modification of PCR is the use of nested primers in a two-step amplification process to enhance sensitivity even further.[214,215] During a second PCR sequence, the nested PCR technique utilizes a second primer that targets an internal portion of the oligonucleotide primer target that was initially amplified.

Applications of PCR include detection and quantitation of HIV-1 proviral DNA in PBMC[216–219] and HIV-1 RNA in serum,[220] identification of all HIV-1–infected blood donors (impractical at present), confirmation of HIV-1 infection (especially when false-positive screening and/or confirmatory tests are suspected), detection of HIV-1 infection in the nonreplicative state in patients who are seronegative,[116–118,221] early diagnosis of infection before seroconversion,[222] confirmation of infection and definition of infection patterns in newborns while maternal antibody persists, and differentiation of HIV-1 and HIV-2 infections.[223–229] PCR is more sensitive than the p24 antigen assay and viral culture for detecting HIV-1 (at least for detecting part of the genome).[216,220,225,226] The sensitivity of PCR is estimated at 92–100 percent.[119,216,222,225,226,230] There are rare false positives due to (1) contamination of a negative sample or the assay vial with HIV-1 genetic material, (2) reagent contamination with the HIV-1 genome or a complimentary oligonucleotide, or (3) experimental "carryover" from a positive sample.[119,229,230] False negatives have usually resulted from compromised analytic technique.[229] PCR has also been used to monitor HIV-1 RNA during therapy, to amplify HIV-1 RNA in cerebrospinal fluid, and to assess virus load.[231–233]

After several authors proposed the concept, based on use of PCR, that some individuals could be infected with HIV-1 and be seronegative,[116–118,221] Imagawa and Detels[234] pointed out a potential fallacy of PCR: that detection is part of the HIV-1 genome with PCR may really reflect incomplete infection rather than latent persistent infection. Others have also questioned the inference that PCR sensitivity always reflects latent (or active) communicable infection.[235,236] While hybridization and PCR technologies are significant advances, they have not currently been applied widely because of cost and potential technical problems, particularly contamination with extraneous nucleic acids.

SURROGATE MARKERS OF HIV-1 INFECTION

During the early part of the HIV-1 epidemic, the value of the percent T-helper (CD4) cells, absolute number of CD4 cells, and the ratio of CD4 to CD8 cells (suppressor T-cells) became evident.[237] A decrease in each of these measures correlates with advancing HIV-1 infection. More recently, other nonspecific markers of HIV-1 infection, once established, were used as correlates of progressive infection. Neopterin (a hydroxypropylpterin metabolite of guanosine triphosphate produced by activated macrophages) and β_2-microglobulin (the light chain common to the three major class I HLA histocompatibility antigens that is increased with monocyte activation) have been found to be progressively elevated during HIV-1 infection.[237–242] Neopterin levels require a high-pressure liquid chromatographic assay, while β_2-microglobulin can be assayed by EIA or radioimmunoassay.[242] Serum β_2-microglobulin may also serve as a surrogate marker for response of HIV-1 to antiretroviral therapy by decreasing during treatment.[243] Soluble interleukin-2 receptors (sIL-2R) have been shown to be elevated nonspecifically during HIV-1 infection. The concentration of sIL-2R has been variably correlated with advancing infection; sIL-2R concentration varies inversely with CD4 count.[244–247]

APPLICATION OF HIV-1 ANTIBODY SCREENING

Since the screening EIA became available in March 1985, much discussion and debate has ensued among the public and among legal and health care professionals as to the appropriateness of broad-based screening programs for HIV-1 antibody. Arguments have been presented for and against premarital and preoperative mandatory screening, as well as employee screening.[248–250] A balanced perspective in this regard has been presented by Bloom and Glied.[251] Issues of ethics, confidentiality, and informed consent have been raised.[252–255] Appropriate hospital policies have been debated.[256,257] Arguments have been presented for universal prenatal testing and for strongly recommending antibody testing for all groups at high risk for HIV-1 infection.[258] Justification has been presented for routine, voluntary testing in clinics and hospital settings of high endemicity.[259–261] It is beyond the scope of this chapter to deal with these issues in detail (see Ch. 100). At present, in the United States, the population groups undergoing mandatory and voluntary screening are defined in Table 9. Current requirements for screening immigrants and international travelers have been questioned.[262] Proposed justifications for mandatory screening are enumerated in Table 10. As the sensitivity and especially the specificity of the current means for diagnosing HIV-1 infection have improved,[74] screening tests for HIV-1 infection have gained broader applicability.

TABLE 9. Population Groups Currently Screened for HIV-1 Antibody

Mandatory in United States
Blood donors
Federal prisoners
Military recruits and active duty personnel
Foreign service officers
Aliens seeking immigration and international travelers
With consent
Patients in STD clinics, prostitutes
Injectable drug users
Women of child-bearing age with a recognized risk for HIV-1 infection
Admissions to hospitals in areas with high HIV-1 infection rates ($\geq$1 per 1000 discharges)
Hospital admissions in high-risk groups

TABLE 10. Considerations for Determining Justification for Mandatory Screening Programs for Antibody to HIV-1

The population selected should have a reservoir of infected persons so that disproportionate numbers of uninfected persons do not have to submit to intrusive testing
The population must pose a significant risk of communication of infection
Knowledge of results should allow for the reduction of transmission
Benefits must outweigh negative effects of testing
No less intrusive/restrictive alternatives are available

(From Gostin et al.,[253] with permission.)

REFERENCES

1. Centers for Disease Control and Prevention. Prevention of acquired immunodeficiency syndrome (AIDS): Report of inter-agency recommendations. MMWR. 1984;32:101–3.
2. Barre-Sinoussi F, Chermann JC, et al. Isolation of a T-lymphotropic retrovirus from a patient at risk for acquired immune deficiency syndrome (AIDS). Science. 1983;20:868–71.
3. Popovic M, Sarngadharan MG, et al. Detection, isolation and continuous production of cytopathic retroviruses (HTLV-III) from patients with AIDS and pre-AIDS. Science. 1984;224:497–500.
4. Gallo RC, Salahuddin SZ, et al. Frequent detection and isolation of cytopathic retroviruses (HTLV-III) from patients with AIDS and at risk for AIDS. Science. 1984;224:500–2.
5. Levy JA, Hoffman AD, et al. Isolation of lymphocytopathic retroviruses from San Francisco patients with AIDS. Science. 1984;225:840–2.
6. Sarngadharan MG, Popovic M, et al. Antibodies reactive with human T-lymphotropic retroviruses (HTLV-III) in serum of patients with AIDS. Science. 1984;224:506–8.
7. Brun-Vezinet F, Barre-Sinoussi F, et al. Detection of IgG antibodies to lymphadenopathy-associated virus in patients with AIDS or lymphadenopathy syndrome. Lancet. 1984;1:1253–6.
8. Centers for Diesase Control and Prevention: Provisional Public Health Service inter-agency recommendations for screening donated blood and plasma for antibody to the virus causing acquired immunodeficiency syndrome. MMWR. 1985;34:1–5.
9. Schorr JB, Berkowitz A, et al. Prevalence of HTLV-III antibody in American blood donors. N Engl J Med. 1985;313:384–5.
10. Centers for Disease Control and Prevention. Human T-lymphotropic virus type III/lymphadenopathy-associated virus antibody testing at alternate sites. MMWR. 1986;35:284–7.
11. Centers for Disease Control and Prevention. Recommendations for assisting in the prevention of perinatal transmission of human T-lymphotropic virus Type III/lymphadenopathy-associated virus and acquired immunodeficiency syndrome. MMWR. 1985;34:721–6, 731–733.
12. Centers for Disease Control and Prevention. Additional recommendations to reduce sexual and drug abuse–related transmission of human T-lymphotropic virus type III/lymphadenopathy-associated virus. MMWR. 1986;35:152–5.
13. Centers for Disease Control and Prevention. Perspectives in disease prevention and health promotion: Public Health Service guidelines for counseling and antibody testing to prevent HIV infection and AIDS. MMWR. 1987;36:509–15.
14. Weiss SH, Goedert JJ, et al. Screening test for HTLV-III (AIDS agent) antibodies: specificity, sensitivity, and applications. JAMA. 1985;253:221–5.
15. Carlson JR, Bryant ML, et al. AIDS serology testing in low and high risk groups. JAMA. 1985;253:3405–8.
16. Sivak SL, Wormser GP. Predictive value of a screening test for antibodies to HTLV-III. Am J Clin Pathol. 1986;85:700–3.
17. Burke DS, Brandt BL, et al. Diagnosis of human immunodeficiency virus infection by immunoassay using a molecularly cloned and expressed virus envelope polypeptide. Comparison to Western blot on 2707 consecutive serum samples. Ann Intern Med. 1987;106:671–6.
18. Wang JJG, Steel S, et al. Detection of antibodies to human T-lymphotropic virus type III by using a synthetic peptide of 21 amino acid residues corresponding to a highly antigenic segment of gp41 envelope protein. Proc Natl Acad Sci USA. 1986;83:6159–63.
19. Goudsmit J, Paul DA, et al. Expression of human immunodeficiency virus antigen (HIV-Ag) in serum and cerebrospinal fluid during acute and chronic infection. Lancet. 1986;2:177–80.
20. Lange JMA, Paul DA, et al. Persistent HIV antigenaemia and decline of HIV core antibodies associated with transition to AIDS. Br Med J. 1986;293:1459–62.
21. Chaisson RE, Allain JP, et al. Significant changes in HIV antigen level in the serum of patients treated with azidothymidine. N Engl J Med. 1986;315:1610–11.
22. Diggs JL. Testing for HIV antigen. Infect Control Hosp Epidermiol. 1988;9:353–4.
23. Allain JP, Laurian Y, et al. Long-term evaluation of HIV antigen and antibodies to p24 and gp41 in patients with hemophilia. N Engl J Med. 1987;317:1114–21.
24. Allain JP, Laurian Y, et al. Serological markers in early stages of human immunodeficiency virus infection in haemophiliacs. Lancet. 1986;2:1233–6.
25. Ranki A, Krohn M, et al. Long latency precedes overt seroconversion in sexually transmitted human-immunodeficiency-virus infection. Lancet. 1987;1:589–93.
26. Simmonds P, Lainson FAL, et al. HIV Antigen and antibody detection: Variable responses to infection in the Edinburgh haemophiliac cohort. Br Med J. 1988;296:593–8.
27. Cooper DA, Tindall B, et al. Characterization of T lymphocyte responses during primary infection with human immunodeficiency virus. J Infect Dis. 1988;157:889–96.
28. Von Sydow M, Gaines H, et al. Antigen detection in primary HIV infection. Br Med J. 1988;296:238–40.
29. Gaines H, Sonnerborg A, et al. Antibody response in primary human immunodeficiency virus infection. Lancet. 1987;1:1249–53.
30. Pyun KH, Ochs HD, et al. Perinatal infection with human immunodeficiency virus. N Engl J Med. 1987;317:611–4.

31. Pizzo PA, Wilfert CM. Perspectives on pediatric human immunodeficiency virus infection. Pediatr Infect Dis J. 1991;10:523–31.

32. Horsburgh CR, Ou CY, et al. Duration of human immunodeficiency virus infection before detection of antibody. Lancet. 1989;2:637–40.

33. Pan LZ, Cheng-Mayer C, et al. Patterns of antibody response in individuals infected with the human immunodeficiency virus. J Infect Dis. 1987;155:626–32.

34. Goudsmit J, Lange JMA, et al. Antigenemia and antibody titers to core and envelope antigens in AIDS, AIDS-related complex, and subclinical human immunodeficiency virus infection. J Infect Dis. 1987;155:558–60.

35. Mayer KH, Falk LA, et al. Correlation of enzyme-linked immunosorbent assays for serum human immunodeficiency virus antigen and antibodies to recombinant viral proteins with subsequent clinical outcomes in a cohort of asymptomatic homosexual men. Am J Med. 1987;83:208–12.

36. Weber JN, Weiss RA, et al. Human immunodeficiency virus infection in two cohorts of homosexual men: Neutralising sera and association of anti-Gag antibody with prognosis. Lancet. 1987;1:119–21.

37. Schupbach J, Haller O, et al. Antibodies to HTLV-III in Swiss patients with AIDS and pre-AIDS and in groups at risk for HIV. N Engl J Med. 1985;312:265–70.

38. Lelie PN, Reesink HW, et al. Evaluation of three second-generation and three confirmatory assays for antibodies to human immunodeficiency virus. Vox Sang. 1988;54:84–91.

39. Dawson GJ, Heller JS, et al. Reliable detection of individuals seropositive for the human immunodeficiency virus (HIV) by competitive immunoassays using *Escherichia coli*–expressed HIV structural proteins. J Infect Dis. 1988;157:149–55.

40. Steckelberg JM, Cockerill FR. Serologic testing for human immunodeficiency virus antibodies. Mayo Clin Proc. 1988;63:373–80.

41. Jackson JB, Balfour HH Jr. Practical diagnostic testing for human immunodeficiency virus. Clin Microbiol Rev. 1988;1:124–38.

42. Allain JP, Hojvat S. Development in HIV Serology. In: de la Maza LM, Peterson EM, eds. Proceedings of the 1987 International Symposium on Medical Virology, Anaheim, CA. Amsterdam: Elsevier Science Publishing; 1987:315–30.

43. George JR, Rayfield MA, et al. Efficacies of US Food and Drug Administration–licensed HIV-1 screening enzyme immunoassays for detecting antibodies to HIV-2. AIDS. 1990;4:321–6.

44. Ng VL, Chiang CS, et al. Reliable confirmation of antibodies to human immunodeficiency virus type 1 (HIV-1) with an enzyme-linked immunoassay using recombinant antigens derived from the HIV-1 gag, pol, and env genes. J Clin Microbiol. 1989;27:977–82.

45. Lepine DG, Neumann PW, et al. Evaluation of a human immunodeficiency virus test algorithm utilizing a recombinant protein enzyme immunoassay. J Clin Microbiol. 1990;28:1169–71.

46. Johnson JE. Detection of human immunodeficiency virus type 1 antibody by using commercially available whole cell viral lysate, synthetic peptide, and recombinant protein enzyme immunoassay systems. J Clin Microbiol. 1992;30:216–8.

47. Houn HY, Pappas AA, et al. Status of current clinical tests for human immunodeficiency virus (HIV): Applications and limitations. Ann Clin Lab Sci. 1987;17:279–85.

48. Gallarda JL, Henrard DR, et al. Early detection of antibody to human immunodeficiency virus type 1 by using an antigen conjugate immunoassay correlates with the presence of immunoglobulin M antibody. J Clin Microbiol. 1992;30:2379–84.

49. Thongcharoen P, Wasi C, et al. Immunoglobulin G antibody capture enzyme-linked immunosorbent assay: A versatile assay for detection of anti-human immunodeficiency virus type 1 and 2 antibodies in body fluids. J Clin Microbiol. 1992;30:3288–9.

50. Parry JV, Perry KR, et al. Sensitive assays for viral antibodies in saliva: An alternative to tests on serum. Lancet. 1987;2:72–5.

51. Major CJ, Read SE, et al. Comparison of saliva and blood for human immunodeficiency virus prevalence testing. J Infect Dis. 1991;163:699–702.

52. Frerichs RR, Htoon MT, et al. Comparison of saliva and serum for HIV surveillance in developing countries. Lancet. 1992;340:1496–9.

53. Lindhardt BO, Bygbjerg IC, et al. Detection of antibodies to human immunodeficiency virus (HIV) in eluates from whole blood impregnated filter paper discs. J Virol Methods. 1987;18:73–7.

54. Varnier ODE, Lillo FB, et al. Whole blood collection on filter paper is an effective means of obtaining samples for human immunodeficiency virus antibody assay. AIDS Res Hum Retrovirus. 1988;4:131–6.

55. Fortes P, Menitove J et al. Evaluation of blood collected on filter paper for detection of antibodies to human immunodeficiency virus type 1. J Clin Microbiol. 1989;27:1380–1.

56. Steger KA, Craven DE, et al. Use of paper-absorbed fingerstick blood samples for studies of antibodies to human immunodeficiency virus type 1 in intravenous drug users. J Infect Dis. 1990;162:964–7.

57. Gwinn M, Redus MA, et al. HIV-1 serologic test results for one million newborn dried-blood specimens: Assay performance and implications for screening. J AIDS. 1992;5:505–12.

58. Burke DS, Redfield RR, et al. Variations in Western blot banding patterns of human T-cell lymphotropic virus type III/lymphadenopathy-associated virus. J Clin Microbiol. 1987;25:81–4.

59. Cooper DA, Imrie AA, et al. Antibody response to human immunodeficiency virus after primary infection. J Infect Dis. 1987;155:1113–8.

60. Weiblen BJ, Schumacher RT, et al. IgA and IgM human immunodeficiency virus antibodies in weakly reactive or false-negative blood donors. Transfusion. 1991;31:397–400.

61. Ward JW, Grindon AJ, et al. Laboratory and epidemiologic evaluation of an enzyme immunoassay for antibodies to HTLV-III. JAMA. 1986;256:357–61.

62. Nishanian P, Taylor JMG, et al. Significance of quantitative enzyme-linked immunosorbent assay (ELISA) results in evaluation of three ELISAs and Western blot tests for detection of antibodies to human immunodeficiency virus in a high risk population. J Clin Microbiol. 1987;25:395–400.

63. Handsfield HH, Wandell M, et al. Screening and diagnostic performance of enzyme immunoassay for antibody to lymphadenopathy-associated virus. J Clin Microbiol. 1987;25:879–84.

64. Voeller B. Evaluation of eight ELISA kits for the detection of anti-LAV/HTLV-III antibodies. Lancet. 1986;1:1152–3.

65. Reesink HW, Huisman JG, et al. Evaluation of six enzyme immunoassays for antibody against human immunodeficiency virus. Lancet. 1986;2:483–6.

66. Evans RP, Shanson DC, et al. Clinical evaluation of Abbott and Wellcome enzyme linked immunosorbent assays for detection of serum antibodies to human immunodeficiency virus (HIV). J Clin Pathol. 1987;40:552–5.

67. Burkhardt U, Mertens TH, et al. Comparison of two commercially available anti-HIV ELISAs: Abbott HTLV-III EIA and Du Pont HTLV-III ELISA. J Med Virol. 1987;23:217–24.

68. Deinhardt F, Eberle J, et al. Sensitivity and specificity of eight commercial and one recombinant anti-HIV ELISA tests. Lancet. 1987;1:40.

69. Saah AJ, Farzadegan H, et al. Detection of early antibodies in human immunodeficiency virus infection by enzyme-linked immunosorbent assay, Western blot, and radioimmunoprecipitation. J Clin Microbiol. 1987;25:1605–10.

70. Van De Perre P, Nzaramba D, et al. Comparison of six serological assays for human immunodeficiency virus antibody detection in developing countries. J Clin Microbiol. 1988;26:552–6.

71. Ozanne G, Fauvel M. Performance and reliability of five commercial enzyme-linked immunosorbent assay kits in screening for anti-human immunodeficiency virus antibody in high-risk subjects. J Clin Microbiol. 1988;26:1496–1500.

72. Engle JC, Schleupner CJ. Performance evaluation of six commercially available enzyme linkd immunosorbent assays kits for antibody to human immunodeficiency virus. In: de la Maza LM, Peterson EM, eds. Proceedings of the 1987 International Symposium on Medical Virology. 1987, Anaheim, CA. Amsterdam: Elsevier Science Publishing; 1987:357.

73. Taylor RN, Przybyszewski VA. Summary of the Centers for Disease Control Human Immunodeficiency Virus (HIV) Performance Evaluation Surveys for 1985 and 1986. Am J Clin Pathol. 1988;89:1–13.

74. Schwartz JS, Dans PE, et al. Human immunodeficiency virus test evaluation, performance, and use. JAMA. 1988;259:2574–9.

75. Centers for Disease Control and Prevention. Update: Serologic testing for antibody to human immunodeficiency virus. MMWR. 1988;36:833–45.

76. Van Den Akker R, Hekker AC, et al. Heat inactivation of serum may interfere with HTLV-III/LAV Serology. Lancet. 1985;2:672.

77. Jungkind DL, DiRenzo SA, et al. Effect of using heat-inactivated serum with the Abbott human T-cell lymphotropic virus type III antibody test. J Clin Microbiol. 1986;23:381–2.

78. Kvinesdal B, Pedersen NS. False-positive HIV antibody tests in RPR-reactive patients. JAMA. 1988;260:923–4.

79. Kuhnl P, Seidl S, et al. HLA DR4 antibodies cause positive HTLV-III antibody ELISA results. Lancet. 1985;1:1222–3.

80. Ameglio F, Dolei A, et al. Antibodies reactive with nonpolymorphic epitopes on HLA molecules interfere in screening tests for the human immunodeficiency virus. J Infect Dis. 1987;156:1034–5.

81. Wartick MG, McCarroll DR, et al. A second discriminator for biological false positive results in enzyme-linked immunosorbent assays for antibodies to human immunodeficiency virus (HTLV-III/LAV). Transfusion. 1987;27:109–11.

82. Blanton M, Balakrishnan K, et al. HLA antibodies in blood donors with reactive screening tests for antibody to the immunodeficiency virus. Transfusion. 1987;27:118–9.

83. Smith DM, Dewhurst S, et al. False-positive enzyme-linked immunosorbent assay reactions for antibody to human immunodeficiency virus in a population of Midwestern patients with congenital bleeding disorders. Transfusion. 1987;127:112.

84. Mendenhall CL, Roselle GA, et al. False positive tests for HTLV-III antibodies in alcoholic patients with hepatitis. N Engl J Med. 1986;314:921–2.

85. Marlink RG, Allain JS, et al. Low sensitivity of ELISA testing in elderly HIV infection. N Engl J Med. 1986;315:1549.

86. Biberfeld G, Bredberg-Raden U, et al. Blood donor sera with false-positive Western blot reactions to human immunodeficiency virus. Lancet. 1986;2:289–91.

87. Albersheim SG, Smyth JA, et al. Passively acquired human immunodeficiency virus seropositivity in a neonate after hepatitis B immunoglobulin. J Pediatr. 1988;112:915–6.

88. Saag MS, Britz J. Asymptomatic blood donor with a false-positive HTLV-III Western blot. N Engl J Med. 1986;314:118.

89. Goetz DW, Hall SE, et al. Pediatric acquired immunodeficiency syndrome with negative human immunodeficiency virus antibody response by enzyme-linked immunosorbent assay and Western Blot. Pediatrics. 1988;81:356–9.

90. MacKenzie WR, Davis JP, et al. Multiple false-positive serologic tests for HIV, HTLV-1, and hepatitis C following influenza vaccination, 1991. JAMA. 1992;268:1015–7.

91. Janvier D, Reviron M, et al. False negative results in a competitive immuno-

assay for anti-HIV-antibodies due to the presence of rheumatoid factors. Vox Sang. 1989;56:237–42.

92. Denis F, Leonard G, et al. Comparison of 10 enzyme immunoassays for detection of antibody to human immunodeficiency virus type 2 in West African sera. J Clin Microbiol. 1988;26:1000–4.

93. Tribe DE, Reed DL, et al. Anibodies reactive with human immunodeficiency virus gag-coded antigens (gag reactive only) are a major cause of enzyme-linked immunosorbent assay reactivity in a blood donor population. J Clin Microbiol. 1988;26:641–7.

94. MacDonald KL, Jackson JB, et al. Performance characteristics of serologic tests for human immunodeficiency virus type 1 (HIV-1) antibody among Minnesota blood donors. Ann Intern Med. 1989;110:617–21.

95. Hickman M, Mortimer JY, et al. Donor screening for HIV: How many false negatives? Lancet. 1988;1:1221.

96. Busch MP, Eble BE, et al. Evaluation of screened blood donations for human immunodeficiency virus type 1 infection by culture and DNA amplication of pooled cells. N Engl J Med. 1991;325:1–5.

97. Lefrere JJ, Mariotti M, et al. No evidence of frequent human immunodeficiency virus type 1 infection in seronegative at-risk individuals. Transfusion. 1991;31:205–11.

98. Ward JW, Holmberg SD, et al. Transmission of human immunodeficiency virus (HIV) by blood transfusions screened as negative for HIV antibody. N Engl J Med. 1988;318:473–8.

99. Navarro MDR, Pineda JA, et al. Recombinant EIA for anti-HIV testing is more specific than conventional EIA. Vox Sang. 1988;54:62–3.

100. Thorn RM, Beltz GA, et al. Enzyme immunoassay using a novel recombinant polypeptide to detect human immunodeficiency virus env antibody. J Clin Microbiol. 1987;25:1207–12.

101. Gnann JW Jr, Schwimmbeck PL, et al. Diagnosis of AIDS by using a 12-amino acid peptide representing an immunodominant epitope of the human immunodeficiency virus. J Infect Dis. 1987;156:261–7.

102. Petrov RV, Khaitov RM, et al. The use of synthetic peptides in the diagnosis of HIV infections. Biomed Sci. 1990;1:239–44.

103. Parry JV, McAlpine L, et al. Sensitivity of six commrecial enzyme immunoassay kits that detect both anti-HIV-1 and anti-HIV-2. AIDS. 1990;4:355–60.

104. Baillou A, Barin F, et al. Competitive enzyme-immunoassays using native viral antigens to discriminate between HIV-1 and HIV-2 infections. J Virol Methods. 1990;29:81–90.

105. Centers for Disease Control and Prevention. Testing for antibodies to human immunodeficiency virus type 2 in the United States. MMWR. 1992;41(RR-12):1–9.

106. Griffith BP, Feguson D, et al. Detection of antibodies to human immunodeficiency virus: Principles, use and interpretation. VA Practitioner. 1988;5:50–61.

107. Towbin H, Staehelin T, et al. Electrophoretic transfer of proteins from polyacrylamide gels to nitrocellulose sheets: Procedure and some applications. Proc Natl Acad Sci USA. 1979;76:4350–4.

108. Burke DC, Redfield RR. False-positive Western blot tests for antibodies to HTLV-III. JAMA. 1986;256:347.

109. Centers for Disease Control and Prevention. Interpretation and use of the Western blot assay for serodiagnosis of human immunodeficiency virus type 1 infections. MMWR. 1989;38(S-7):1–7.

110. Hausler WJ, Jr. Report of the Third Consensus Conference on HIV Testing Sponsored by the Association of State an Territorial Public Health Laboratory Directors. Infect Control Hosp Epidemiol. 9:345–9.

111. Blomberg J, Klasse PJ. Specificities and sensitivities of three systems for determination of antibodies to human immunodeficiency virus by electrophoretic immunoblotting. J Clin Microbiol. 1988;26:106–10.

112. Mathez D, Leibovitch J, et al. LAV/HTLV-III Seroconversion and disease in hemophiliacs treated in France. N Engl J Med. 1986;314:118–9.

113. Courouce AM, Muller JY, et al. False-positive Western blot reactions to human immunodeficiency virus in blood donors. Lancet. 1986;2:921–22.

114. Salahuddin SZ, Groopman JE, et al. HTLV-III in symptom-free seronegative persons. Lancet. 1984;2:1418–20.

115. Groopman JE, Hartzband PI, et al. Antibody seronegative human T-lymphotropic virus type III (HTLV-III)–infected patients with acquired immunodeficiency syndrome or related disorders. Blood. 1985;66:742–4.

116. Farzadegan H, Polis MA, et al. Loss of human immunodeficiency virus type 1 (HIV-1) antibodies with evidence of viral infection in asymptomatic homosexual men. Ann Intern Med. 1988;108:785–90.

117. Imagawa DT, Lee MH, et al. Human immunodeficiency virus type 1 infection in homosexual men who remain seronegative for prolonged periods. N Engl J Med. 1989;320:1458–62.

118. Wolinsky SM, Rinaldo CR, et al. Human immunodeficiency virus type 1 (HIV-1) infection a median of 18 months before a diagnostic western blot. Ann Intern Med. 1989;111:961–72.

119. Lifson AR, Stanley M, et al. Detection of human immunodeficiency virus DNA using the polymerase chain reaction in a well-characterized group of homosexual and bisexual men. J Infect Dis. 1990;161:436–9.

120. Edwards VM, Mosley JW, et al. Reproducibility in quality control of protein (Western) immunoblot assay for antibodies to human immunodeficiency virus. Am J Clin Pathol. 1989;91:75–8.

121. Glassman AB, Sherrill T, et al. Human immunodeficiency virus Western blot tests: Comparisons and considerations. Ann Clin Lab Sci. 1990;20:343–6.

122. Dodd RY, Fang CT. The Western immunoblot procedure for HIV antibodies and its interpretation. Arch Pathol Lab Med. 1990;114:240–5.

123. Midthum K, Garrison L, et al. Frequency of indeterminate Western blot tests in healthy adults at low risk for human immunodeficiency virus infection. J Infect Dis. 1990;162:1379–82.

124. Dock NL, Lamberson HV Jr, et al. Evaluation of atypical human immunodeficiency virus immunoblot reactivity in blood donors. Transfusion. 1988;28:412–8.

125. Kleinman S, Fitzpatrick L, et al. Follow-up testing and notification of anti-HIV Western blot atypical (indeterminant) donors. Transfusion. 1988;28:280–2.

126. van der Poel CL, Lelie PN, et al. Blood donors with indeterminate anti-p24gag reactivity in HIV-1 western blot: Absence of infectivity to transfused patients and in virus culture. Vox Sang. 1989;56:162–7.

127. Josephson SL, Swack NS, et al. Investigation of atypical western blot (immunoblot) reactivity involving core proteins of human immunodeficiency virus type 1. J Clin Microbiol. 1989;27:932–7.

128. Leitman SF, Klein HG, et al. Clinical implications of positive tests for antibodies to human immunodeficiency virus type 1 in asymptomatic blood donors. N Engl J Med. 1989;321:917–24.

129. Genesca J, Shih JW, et al. What do western blot indeterminate patterns for human immunodeficiency virus mean in EIA-negative blood donors? Lancet. 1989;2:1023–5.

130. Jackson JB, MacDonald KL, et al. Absence of HIV infection in blood donors with indeterminate western blot tests for antibody to HIV-1. N Engl J Med. 1990;322:217–22.

131. Celum CL, Coombs RW, et al. Indeterminate human immunodeficiency virus type 1 western blots: Seroconversion risk, specificity of supplemental tests, and an algorithm for evaluation. J Infect Dis. 1991;164:656–64.

132. Dock NL, Kleinman SH, et al. Indeterminate western blot results and HIV infection. Arch Intern Med. 1991;151:525–530.

133. Ramirez E, Uribe P, et al. Reactivity patterns and infection status of serum samples with indeterminate western immunoblot tests for antibody to human immunodeficiency virus type 1. J Clin Microbiol. 1992;30:801–5.

134. Phair J, Hoover D, et al. The significance of western blot assays indeterminate for antibody to HIV in a cohort of homosexual/bisexual men. J AIDS. 1992;5:988–92.

135. Povolotsky J, Gold JWM, et al. Differences in human immunodeficiency virus type 1 (HIV-1) anti-p24 reactivities in serum of HIV-1 infected and uninfected subjects: Analysis of indeterminate western blot reactions. J Infect Dis. 1991;163:247–51.

136. Centers for Disease Control and Prevention. Interpretive criteria used to report western blot results for HIV-1 antibody testing—United States. MMWR. 1991;40:692–5.

137. Sandstrom EG, Schooley RT, et al. Detection of human anti-HTLV-III antibodies by indirect immunofluorescence using fixed cells. Transfusion. 1985;25:308–12.

138. Gallo D, Diggs JL, et al. Comparison of detection of antibody to the acquired immune deficiency syndrome virus by enzyme immunoassay, immunofluorescence, and western blot methods. J Clin Microbiol. 1986;23:1049–51.

139. Hedenskog M, Dewhurst S, et al. Testing for Antibodies to AIDS-associated retrovirus (HTLV-III/LAV) by indirect fixed cell immunofluorescence: Specificity, sensitivity, and applications. J Med Virol. 1986;19:325–34.

140. Lennette ET, Karpatkin S, et al. Indirect Immunofluorescence assay for antibodies to human immunodeficiency virus. J Clin Microbiol. 1987;25:199–202.

141. Carlson JR, Yee J, et al. Comparison of indirect immunofluorescence and Western blot for detection of anti-human immunodeficiency virus antibodies. J Clin Microbiol. 1987;25:494–7.

142. Sullivan MT, Mucke H, et al. Evaluation of an indirect immunofluorescence assay for confirmation of human immunodeficiency virus type 1 in U.S. blood donor sera. J Clin Microbiol. 1992;30:2509–10.

143. Mahony J, Rosenthal K, et al. Agreement study between two laboratories of immunofluorescence as a confirmatory test for human immunodeficiency virus type 1 antibody screening. J Clin Microbiol. 1989;27:1234–7.

144. Kvinesdal BB, Nielsen CM, et al. Immunofluorescence assay for detection of antibodies to human immunodeficiency virus type 2. J Clin Microbiol. 1989;27:2502–4.

145. Gallo D, Hoffman MN, et al. Comparison of indirect immunofluorescence and membrane fluorescence assays for the differentiation of antibodies to human immunodeficiency virus types 1 and 2. J Clin Microbiol. 1992;30:2275–8.

146. Tersmette M, Lelie PN, et al. Confirmation of HIV seropositivity: Comparison of a novel radioimmunoprecipitation assay to immunoblotting and virus culture. J Med Virol. 1988;24:109–16.

147. Archibald DW, Zon LI, et al. Salivary antibodies as a means of detecting human T cell lymphotropic virus type III/lymphadenopathy-associated virus infection. J Clin Microbiol. 1986;24:873–5.

148. Biggar RJ, Gigase PL, et al. ELISA HTLV retrovirus antibody reactivity associated with malaria and immune complexes in healthy Africans. Lancet. 1985;2:520–3.

149. Riggin CH, Beltz GA, et al. Detection of antibodies to human immunodeficiency virus by latex agglutination with recombinant antigen. J Clin Microbiol. 1987;25:1772–3.

150. Quinn TC, Riggin CH, et al. Rapid latex agglutination assay using recombinant envelope polypeptide for the detection of antibody to the HIV. JAMA. 1988;260:510–13.

151. Spielberg F, Kabeya CM, et al. Field testing and comparative evaluation of rapid, visually read screening assays for antibody to human immunodeficiency virus. Lancet. 1989;1:580–4.

152. Constantine NT, Fox E, et al. Diagnostic usefulness of five screening assays for HIV in an east African city where prevalence of infection is low. AIDS. 1989;3:313–7.

153. Heyward WL, Curran JW. Rapid screening tests for HIV infection. JAMA. 1988;260:542.

154. Carlson JR, Yee JL, et al. Rapid, easy, and economical screening test for antibodies to human immunodeficiency virus. Lancet. 1987;1:361–2.

155. Heberling RL, Kalter SS, et al. Dot immunobinding assay compared with enzyme-linked immunosorbent assay for rapid and specific detection of retrovirus antibody induced by human or simian acquired immunodeficiency syndrome. J Clin Microbiol. 1988;26:765–7.

156. Kalter SS, Heberling RL, et al. Detection of antibody to immunodeficiency viruses by dot immunobinding assay. J Clin Microbiol. 1992;30:993–5.

157. Busch MP, Amad ZE, et al. Reliable confirmation and quantitation of human immunodeficiency virus type 1 antibody using a recombinant-antigen immunoblot assay. Transfusion. 1991;31:129–37.

158. Heberling RL, Kalter SS. Rapid dot-immunobinding assay on nitrocellulose for viral antibodies. J Clin Microbiol. 1986;23:190–13.

159. Weiblen BJ, Lee FK, et al. Early diagnosis of HIV infection in infants by detection of IgA HIV antibodies. Lancet. 1990;1:988–90.

160. Martin NL, Levy JA, et al. Detection of infection with human immunodeficiency virus (HIV) type 1 in infants by an anti-HIV immunoglobulin A assay using recombinant proteins. J Pediatr. 1991;118:354–8.

161. Quinn TC, Kline RL, et al. Early diagnosis of perinatal HIV infection by detection of viral-specific IgA antibodies. JAMA. 1991;266:3439–42.

162. Spielberg F, Kabeya CM, et al. Performance and cost-effectiveness of a dual rapid assay system for screening and confirmation of human immunodeficiency virus type 1 seropositivity. J Clin Microbiol. 1990;28:303–6.

163. Malone JD, Smith ES, et al. Comparative evaluation of six rapid serological tests for HIV-1 antibody. J AIDS. 1993;6:115–9.

164. Calarco TL, Polito AJ, et al. Nitrocellulose cellulose strip ELISA for antibodies to human immunodeficiency virus employing recombinant antigens. In: de la Maza LM, Peterson EM, eds. Proceedings of the 1987 International Symposium on Medical Virology, Anaheim, CA. Amsterdam: Elsevier Science Publishing; 1987:293–314.

165. Hofbauer JM, Schulz TF, et al. Comparison of Western blot (immunoblot) based on recombinant-derived p41 with conventional tests for serodiagnosis of human immunodeficiency virus infections. J Clin Microbiol. 1988;26:116–20.

166. Kemp BE, Rylatt DB, et al. Autologous red cell agglutination assay for HIV-1 antibodies: Simplified test with whole blood. Science. 1988;241:1352–4.

167. Vasudevachari MB, Uffelman K, et al. Detection of antibodies to human immunodeficiency virus type 1 in whole blood and saliva by using a passive hemagglutination test. J Clin Microbiol. 1989;27:2384–5.

168. Yoshida T, Matsui T, et al. Evaluation of passive particle agglutination test for antibody to human immunodeficiency virus. J Clin Microbiol. 1987;25:1433–7.

169. Pollner F. Uncertain HIV saliva test approval. ASM News. 1993;59:168–9.

170. Sligh JM, Rodman ST, et al. Flow cytometric indirect immunofluorescence assay with high sensitivity and specificity for detection of antibodies to human immunodeficiency virus (HIV). Am J Clin Pathol. 1989;91:210–4.

171. Scillian JJ, McHugh TM, et al. Early detection of antibodies against rDNA-produced HIV proteins with a flow cytometric assay. Blood. 1989;73:2041–8.

172. Lee FK, Nahmias AJ, et al. ELISPOT: A new approach to studying the dynamics of virus-immune system interaction for diagnosis and monitoring of HIV infection. AIDS Res Hum Retrovirus. 1989;5:517–23.

173. Amadori A, DeRossi A, et al. Diagnosis of human immunodeficiency virus 1 infection in infants: In vitro production of virus-specific antibody in lymphocytes. Peditar Infect Dis J. 1990;9:26–30.

174. Jehuda-Cohen T, Slade BA, et al. Polyclonal B-cell activation reveals antibodies against human immunodeficiency virus type 1 (HIV-1) in HIV-1-seronegative individuals. Proc Natl Acad Sci USA. 1990;87:3972–6.

175. Buseyne F, Blanche S, et al. Detection of HIV-specific cell-mediated cytotoxicity in the peripheral blood from infected children. J Immunol. 1993;150:3569–81.

176. Anderson KC, Gorgone BC, et al. Transfusion-acquired human immunodeficiency virus infection among immunocompromised persons. Ann Intern Med. 1986;105:519–27.

177. Robert-Guroff M, Brown M, et al. HTLV-III–neutralizing antibodies in patients with AIDS and AIDS-related complex. Nature. 1985;316:72–4.

178. Nishanian P, Huskins KR, et al. A simple method for improved assay demonstrates that HIV p24 antigen is present as immune complexes in most sera from HIV-infected individuals. J Infect Dis. 1990;162:21–8.

179. Palomba E, Gay V, et al. Early diagnosis of human immunodeficiency virus infection in infants by detection of free and complexed p24 antigen. J Infect Dis. 1992;165:394–5.

180. Miles SA, Balden E, et al. Rapid serologic testing with immune complex–dissociated HIV p24 antigen for early detection of HIV infection in neonates. N Engl J Med. 1993;328:297–302.

181. Harry DJ, Jennings MB, et al. Antigen detection for human immunodeficiency virus. Clin Microbiol Rev. 1989;2:241–9.

182. Borkowsky W, Paul D, et al. Human-immunodeficiency-virus infections in infants negative for anti-HIV by enzyme-linked immunoassay. Lancet. 1987;1:1168–71.

183. Borkowsky W, Krasinski K, et al. Human immunodeficiency virus type 1 antigenemia in children. J Pediatr. 1989;114:940–5.

184. Alter HJ, Epstein JS, et al. Prevalence of human immunodeficiency virus type 1 p24 antigen in U.S. blood donors—An assessment of the efficacy of testing in donor screening. N Engl J Med. 1990;323:1312–7.

185. Busch MP, Taylor PE, et al. Screening of selected male blood donors for p24 antigen of human immunodeficiency virus type 1. N Engl J Med. 1990;323:1308–12.

186. Kessler HA, Blaauw B, et al. Diagnosis of human immunodeficiency virus infection in seronegative homosexuals presenting with an acute viral syndrome. JAMA. 1987;258:1196–9.

187. Wall RA, Denning DW, et al. HIV antigenaemia in acute HIV infection. Lancet. 1987;1:566.

188. Goudsmit J, Paul DA. Circulation of HIV antigen in blood according to stage of infection, risk group, age and geographic origin. Epidemiol Infect. 1987;99:701–10.

189. Gaines H, Albert J, et al. HIV antigenaemia and virus isolation from plasma during primary HIV infection. Lancet. 1987;1:1317–8.

190. Wittek AE, Phelan MA, et al. Detection of human immunodeficiency virus core protein in plasma by enzyme immunoassay. Ann Intern Med. 1987;107:286–92.

191. Kenny C, Parkin J, et al. HIV antigen testing. Lancet. 1987;1:565–6.

192. Lange J, Goudsmit J. Decline of antibody reactivity to HIV core protein secondary to increased production of HIV antigen. Lancet. 1987;1:488.

193. Stute R. HIV antigen detection in routine blood donor screening. Lancet. 1987;1:566.

194. Jackson GG, Paul DA, et al. Human immunodeficiency virus (HIV) antigenemia (p24) in the acquired immunodeficiency syndrome (AIDS) and the effect of treatment with zidovudine (AZT). Ann Intern Med. 1988;108:175–80.

195. Pekovic DD, Chausseau JP, et al. Detection of HTLV-III/LAV antigens in peripheral blood lymphocytes from patients with AIDs. Arch Virol. 1986;91:11–19.

196. Ohlsson-Wilhelm BM, Cory JM, et al. Circulating human immunodeficiency virus (HIV) p24 antigen-positive lymphocytes: A flow cytometric measure of HIV infection. J Infect Dis. 1990;162:1018–24.

197. Sano K, Lee MH, et al. Antibody that inhibits human immunodeficiency virus reverse transcriptase and association with inability to isolate virus. J Clin Microbiol. 1987;25:2415–7.

198. Poiesz BJ, Ruscetti FW, et al. Detection and isolation of type C retrovirus particles from fresh and cultured lymphocytes of a patient with cutaneous T-cell lymphoma. Proc Natl Acad Sci USA. 1980;77:7415–9.

199. Viscidi R, Farzadegan H, et al. Enzyme immunoassay for detection of human immunodeficiency virus antigens in cell cultures. J Clin Microbiol. 1988;26:453–8.

200. Gupta P, Balachandran R, et al. Detection of human immunodeficiency virus by reverse transcriptase assay, antigen capture assay, and radioimmunoassay. J Clin Microbiol. 1987;25:1122–5.

201. Feorino P, Forrester B, et al. Comparison of antigen assay and reverse transcriptase assay for detecting human immunodeficiency virus in culture. J Clin Microbiol. 1987;25:2344–6.

202. Blumberg RS, Hartshorn KL, et al. Dot immunobinding assay for detection human immunodeficiency virus-associated antigens. J Clin Microbiol. 1987;25:1989–92.

203. Richman DD, McCutchan JA, et al. Detecting human immunodeficiency virus RNA in peripheral blood mononuclear cells by nucleic acid hyridization. J Infect Dis. 1987;156:823–7.

204. Coombs RW, Collier AC, et al. Plasma viremia in human immunodeficiency virus infection. N Engl J Med. 1989;321:1626–31.

205. Ho DD, Moudgil T, et al. Quantitation of human immunodeficiency virus type 1 in the blood of infected persons. N Engl J Med. 1989;321:1621–5.

206. Landay A, Kessler HA, et al. Isolation of HIV-1 from monocytes of individuals negative by conventional culture. J Infect Dis. 1990;161:706–10.

207. Burgard M, Mayaux MJ, et al. The use of viral culture and p24 antigen testing to diagnose human immunodeficiency virus infection in neonates. N Engl J Med. 1992;327:1192–7.

208. Ou CY, Kwok S, et al. DNA amplification for direct detection of HIV-1 in DNA of peripheral blood mononuclear cells. Science. 1988;239:295–7.

209. Guatelli JC, Gingeras TR, et al. Nucleic acid amplification in vitro: Detection of sequences with low copy numbers and application to diagnosis of human immunodeficiency virus type 1 infection. Clin Microbiol Rev. 1989;2:217–26.

210. Carman WF, Williamson C. Detection of enzymatically amplified human immunodeficiency virus DNA by oligonucleotide solution hybridization and by incorporation of radiolabeled deoxynucleotides. J Clin Microbiol. 1989;27:2570–3.

211. Saiki RK, Gelfand DH, et al. Primer-directed enzymatic amplification of DNA with a thermostable DNA polymerase. Science. 1988;239:487–91.

212. Davis GR, Blumeyer K, et al. Detection of human immunodeficiency virus type 1 in AIDS patients using amplification-mediated hyridization analyses: Reproducibility and quantitative limitations. J Infect Dis. 1990;162:13–20.

213. Menzo S, Bagnarelli P, et al. Absolute quantitation of viremia in human immunodeficiency virus infection by competitive reverse transcription and polymerase chain reaction. J Clin Microbiol. 1992;30:1752–7.

214. Zazzi M, Romano L, et al. Nested polymerase chain reaction for detection of human immunodeficiency virus type 1 DNA in clinical specimens. J Med Virol. 1992;38:172–4.

215. Teglbjaerg LLS, Nielsen C, et al. Sensitive non-radioactive detection of HIV-1: Use of nested primers for the amplification of HIV DNA. Mol Cell Probes. 1992;6:175–80.

216. Jackson JB, Kwok SY, et al. Human immunodeficiency virus type 1 detected

in all seropositive symptomatic and asymptomatic individuals. J Clin Microbiol. 1990;28:16–9.

217. Simmonds P, Balfe P, et al. Human immunodeficiency virus–infected individuals contain provirus in small numbers of peripheral mononuclear cells and at low copy numbers. J Virol. 1990;64:864–72.

218. Bagasra O, Hauptman SP, et al. Detection of human immunodeficiency virus type 1 provirus in mononuclear cells by in situ polymerase chain reaction. N Engl J Med. 1992;326:1385–91.

219. Dickover RE, Donovan RM, et al. Quantitation of human immunodeficiency virus DNA by using the polymerase chain reaction. J Clin Microbiol. 1990; 28:2130–3.

220. Holodniy M, Katzenstein DA, et al. Detection and quantification of human immunodeficiency virus RNA in patient serum by use of the polymerase chain reaction. J Infect Dis. 1991;163:862–6.

221. Loche M, Mach B. Identification of HIV-infected seronegative individuals by a direct diagnostic test based on hybridization to amplified viral DNA. Lancet. 1988;2:418–21.

222. Jason J, Ou C, et al. Prevalence of human immunodeficiency virus type 1 DNA in hemophilic men and their sex partners. J Infect Dis. 1989;160: 789–94.

223. Chadwick EG, Yogev R, et al. Enzymatic amplification of the human immunodeficiency virus in peripheral blood mononuclear cells from pediatric patients. J Infect Dis. 1989;160:954–9.

224. Rogers MF, Ou C, et al. Use of the polymerase chain reaction for early detection of the proviral sequences of human immunodeficiency virus in infants born to seropositive mothers. N Engl J Med. 1989;320:1649–54.

225. Krivine A, Yakudima A, et al. A comparative study of virus isolation, polymerase chain reaction, and antigen detection in children of mothers infected with human immunodeficiency virus. J Pediatr. 1990;116:372–6.

226. Petru A, Dunphy MG, et al. Reliability of polymerase chain reaction in the detection of human immunodeficiency virus infection in children. Pediatr Infect Dis J. 1992;11:30–3.

227. Luzuriaga K, McQuilken P, et al. Early viremia and immune responses in vertical human immunodeficiency virus type 1 infection. J Infect Dis. 1993; 167:1008–13.

228. DeRossi A, Amadori A, et al. Polymerase chain reaction and in-vitro antibody production for early diagnosis of paediatric HIV infection. Lancet. 1988;2:278.

229. Schochetman G. Diagnosis of HIV infection. Clin Chim Acta. 1992;211:1–26.

230. Horsburgh CR Jr, Ou C, et al. Concordance of polymerase chain reaction with human immunodeficiency virus antibody detection. J Infect Dis. 1990; 162:542–5.

231. Holodniy M, Katzenstein DA, et al. Reduction in plasma human immunodeficiency virus ribonucleic acid after dideoxynucleoside therapy as determined by the polymerase chain reaction. J Clin Invest. 1991;88:1755–9.

232. Shaunak S, Alright RE, et al. Amplification of HIV-1 provirus from cerebrospinal fluid and its correlation with neurologic disease. J Infect Dis. 1990; 161:1068–72.

233. Yerly S, Chamot E, et al. Quantitation of human immunodeficiency virus provirus and circulating virus: Relationship with immunologic parameters. J Infect Dis. 1992;166:269–76.

234. Imagawa D, Detels R. HIV-1 seronegative homosexual men. N Engl J Med. 1991;325:1250–1.

235. Nielsen C, Teglbjaerg LS, et al. Prevalence of HIV infection in seronegative high-risk individuals examined by virus isolation and PCR. J AIDS. 1991;4: 1107–11.

236. Lee T, El-Amad Z, et al. Absence of HIV-1 DNA in high-risk seronegative individuals using high-input polymerase chain reaction. AIDS. 1991;5: 1201–7.

237. Fahey JL, Taylor JMG, et al. The prognostic value of cellular and serologic markers in infection with human immunodeficiency virus type 1. N Engl J Med. 1990;322:166–72.

238. Fuchs D, Reibnegger G, et al. Neopterin levels correlating with the Walter Reed staging classification in human immunodeficiency virus (HIV) infection. Ann Intern Med. 1987;107:784–5.

239. Reddy MM, Grieco MH. Neopterin and alpha and beta interleukin-1 levels in sera of patients with human immunodeficiency virus infection. J Clin Microbiol. 1989;27:1919–23.

240. Chan MM, Campos JM, et al. β2-Microglobulin and neopterin: Predictive markers for human immunodeficiency virus type 1 infection in children? J Clin Microbiol. 1990;28:2215–19.

241. Anderson RE, Lang W, et al. Use of β2-microglobulin level and CD4 lymphocyte count to predict development of acquired immunodeficiency syndrome in persons with human immunodeficiency virus infection. Arch Intern Med. 1990;150:73–77.

242. Davey RT Jr, Lane HC. Laboratory methods in the diagnosis and prognostic staging of infection with human immunodeficiency virus type 1. Rev Infect Dis. 1990;12:912–30.

243. Jacobson MA, Abrams DI, et al. Serum β2-microglobulin decreases in patients with AIDS or ARC treated with azidothymidine. J Infect Dis. 1989; 159:1029–36.

244. Pizzolo G, Vinante F, et al. Increased levels of soluble interleukin-2 receptor in the serum of patients with human immunodeficiency virus infection. Diagn Clin Immunol. 1987;5:180–3.

245. Prince HE, Kleinman S, et al. Soluble IL-2 receptor levels in serum from blood donors seropositive for HIV. J Immunol. 1988;140:1139–41.

246. Honda M, Kitamura K, et al. Correlation of its serum level with the classifica-

tion of HIV-induced diseases and its characterization. J Immunol. 1989;142: 4248–55.

247. Allen JB, McCartney-Francis N, et al. Expression of interleukin 2 receptors by monocytes from patients with acquired immunodeficiency syndrome and induction of monocyte interleukin 2 receptors by human immunodeficiency virus in vitro. J Clin Invest. 1990;85:192–9.

248. Cleary PD, Barry MJ, et al. Compulsory premarital screening for the human immunodeficiency virus. Techincal and public health considerations. JAMA. 1987;258:1757–62.

249. Hagan MD, Meyer KB, et al. Routine preoperative screening for HIV. Does the risk to the surgeon outweigh the risk to the patient? JAMA. 1988;259: 1357–9.

250. HIV testing in the workplace (Editorial). Lancet. 1988;2:199–200.

251. Bloom DE, Glied S. Benefits and costs of HIV testing. Science. 1991;252: 1798–1804.

252. Bayer R, Levine C, et al. HIV antibody screening: An ethical framework for evaluating proposed programs. JAMA. 1986;256:1768–74.

253. Gostin L, Curran WC. AIDS screening, confidentiality, and the duty to warn. Am J Public Health. 1987;77:361–5.

254. Dixon RE. Sacred secrets: Confidentiality, informed consent, and diagnostic testing in the AIDS era. Infect Control Hosp Epidemiol. 1988;9:187–8.

255. Sherer R. Physician use of the HIV antibody test. The need for consent, counseling, confidentiality, and caution. JAMA. 1988;259:264–5.

256. Eickhoff TC. Hospital policies on HIV antibody testing. JAMA. 1988;259: 1861–62.

257. Henry K, Willenbring K, et al. Human immunodeficiency virus antibody testing: A description of practices and policies at US infectious disease-teaching hospitals and Minnesota hospitals. JAMA. 1988;259:1819–22.

258. Rhame FS, Maki DG. The case for wider use of testing for HIV infection. N Engl J Med. 1989;320:1248–54.

259. Janssen RS, St. Louis ME, et al. HIV infection among patients in U.S. acute care hospitals. N Engl J Med. 1992;327:445–52.

260. Quinn TC. Screening for HIV infection-benefits and costs. N Engl J Med 1992;327:486–8.

261. Centers for Disease Control and Prevention. Recommendations for HIV testing services for inpatients and outpatients in acute-care hospital settings. MMWR. 1993;42:157–8.

262. Gostin LO, Cleary PD, et al. Screening immigrants and international travelers for the human immunodeficiency virus. N Engl J Med. 1990;322:1743–6.

104. THERAPY OF HIV INFECTION

LAWRENCE COREY

During the past decade, extensive efforts have been expended on the development of agents that would be clinically useful in the inhibition of human immunodeficiency viruses (HIV). Several clinical studies have shown the utility of the dideoxynucleoside compounds (ddN) such as zidovudine (ZDV), didanosine (ddI), and zalcitabine (ddC).[1–7] However, the use of these agents remains one of the most controversial areas in the field of anti-infective chemotherapy.[8] Much of this is related to the relative low potency of these agents, the complex life cycle of HIV, and a lack of understanding about both the true mechanism of action of these agents and their effects on the complex immunobiology of HIV.

Figure 1 illustrates the life cycle of HIV. Two phases of the life cycle are of particular relevance to antiviral chemotherapy. The early events of replication include attachment, fusion, reverse transcription, and subsequent integration into the host cell chromosome.[9] These viral functions constitute the *establishment phase* of the HIV life cycle. The later events of replication, or expression phase of infection, start with the transcription and translation of viral proteins from proviral DNA and the subsequent packaging of these proteins into virions that are then released by budding from the cell. The complexity of the HIV life cycle provides many potential targets for attack by chemotherapeutic agents (Fig. 2), but it also provides the virus with a unique opportunity for continued persistence within the

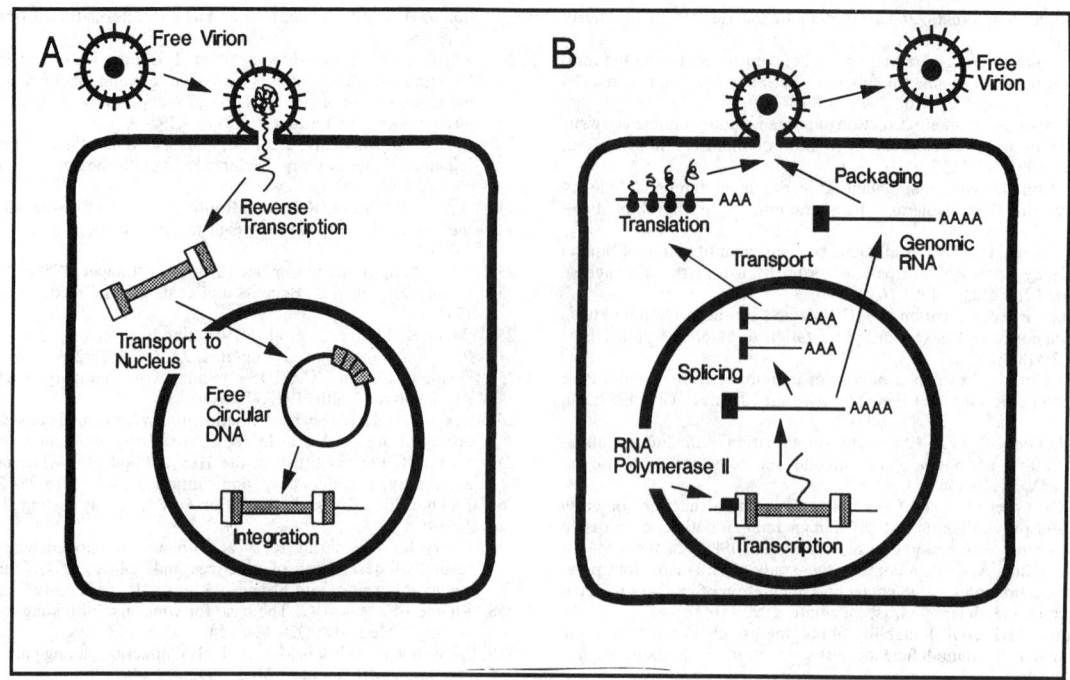

FIG. 1. **(A & B)** Life cycle of retroviruses.

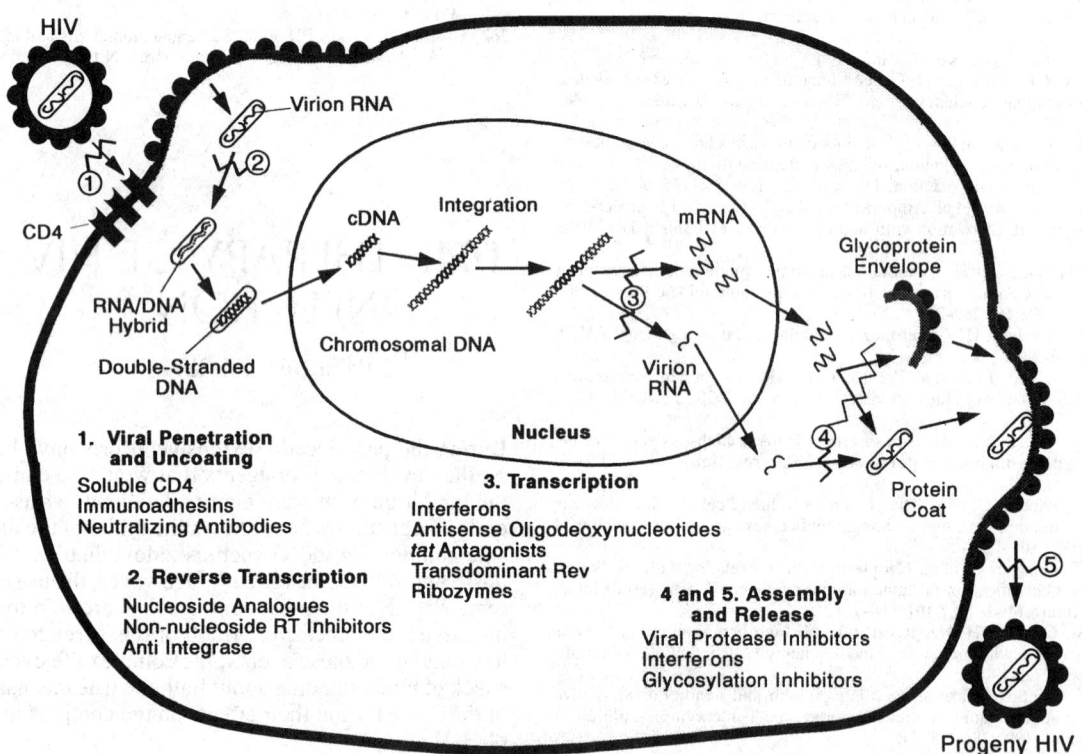

FIG. 2. Stages of HIV replication for which inhibitors have been developed. (Adapted from Fischl,[230] with permission.)

host.[7,10,11] In addition, the rapid mutational variety of HIV has proven a formidable challenge for the development of long-standing antiviral therapy.[12–14]

INTERFERENCE WITH ATTACHMENT

The high affinity between the HIV envelope protein gp120 and the CD4 receptor has made inhibition of attachment an important target for altering the spread of HIV infection.[15] One ap-

proach has been the administration of recombinant soluble CD4 (rsCD4) to attempt to ''flood'' the blood stream with enough CD4 to bind up circulating HIV virions and prevent their subsequent attachment to CD4-bearing cells. Soluble CD4 has been shown to strip gp120 envelope proteins from virions, and in vitro, low doses of soluble CD4 prevent HIV infections at concentrations of less than 1 μm.[16] However, the affinity between CD4 and gp120 varies markedly between clinical and laboratory-based isolates and between isolates from different patients.

Most isolates from HIV-infected individuals require from 100 to 10,000 times more soluble CD4 to inhibit replication in vitro than to inhibit laboratory-adapted strains of HIV-1.[17-21]

Several clinical trials of recombinant soluble CD4 have been conducted.[22-24] Both subcutaneous and intravenous recombinant soluble CD4 have been well tolerated and without significant side effects.[17-21] However, the half-life of rsCD4 is short (½ hour).[22-24] To overcome this, CD4 has been linked to the Fc portion of the immunoglobulin molecule.[23] This hybrid sCD4-IgG molecule has a serum half-life of over 16 hours.[25,26] Although this has favorable pharmacokinetic properties, production costs have limited its use. Current clinical trials of rsCD4 have used dosages of soluble CD4 up to 10 mg/kg/dose.[20,22] These levels are safe, and have resulted in transient binding of virus circulating in plasma. However, prolonged antiviral effects were not apparent, especially when drug levels fell below the ID$_{90}$ of the patient's HIV isolate.[21,22] It appears that the high receptor density of CD4 in HIV-susceptible cells, the density of such cells in lymph nodes where HIV replicates, and the presence of high concentrations of circulating gp120 that may bind up many CD4 molecules may all contribute to the lack of demonstrable clinical efficacy of sCD4.[27,28] However, the transient ability to bind up infectious virus from plasma suggests that rsCD4 may be useful as part of a regimen designed to prevent perinatal transmission or infection after needlestick exposure. As such, preclinical evaluations using newer formulations of CD4 are still under development.

INHIBITION BY IMMUNOGLOBULINS

High titers of immunoglobulin that contain antibodies to HIV have also been used in an attempt to inhibit HIV infection in vivo.[29,30] Such trials have been based on the finding that low levels of neutralizing antibodies to HIV-1 and low titers of antibody to the p24 gag protein are found in persons with long-standing HIV-1 infection.[31-35] Globulin preparations that contain high titers of antibodies to HIV-1 have been made mainly from persons with "early infection."[36] Infectious virus is lost by either heating or in the Cohn fractionation procedure used to prepare immunoglobulin, and the preparations appear safe.[37] Phase I trials have suggested that antibodies to HIV p24 can be increased and circulating levels of HIV in plasma can be reduced.[29,30,37] However, a clinical trial demonstrating the long-term benefit of such preparations has not been reported.

The difficulty of standardizing such immunoglobulin and making it available safely is a formidable task. Approaches that overcome these difficulties are preparation of high-titered globulin from persons immunized with HIV-1 envelope vaccines, or development of humanized monoclonal antibodies to neutralizing epitopes of HIV such as the V3 loop region of the HIV envelope[38-42] (see Ch. 106). Several monoclonals to the V3 loop and CD4 binding domains of HIV have been described and have been shown to neutralize a wide variety of clinical isolates. The use of "cocktails" of monoclonals offers the potential of reducing the spread of HIV. Clinical phase I trials of such preparations are just being initiated.

INHIBITION OF REVERSE TRANSCRIPTION

The reverse transcriptase (RT) enzyme is a unique feature of animal retroviruses. As such, its inhibition offers an attractive target for antiviral drug development.[9,43] The HIV-1 RT uses the two strands of HIV-1 virion RNA as a template to create a first strand DNA copy. The exact mechanism of this process is reviewed in detail in Chapter 146. It appears that an initial short strand of proviral DNA in the long terminal repeat section of the virion is initially transcribed. The enzyme then switches to the second virion RNA template to complete the first (negative strand) DNA copy. RNase H is an intrinsic activity of viral RT and catalyzes the degradation of viral RNA from the RNA-DNA

hybrid. This process is then followed by synthesis of the complementary second strand of DNA. The synthesis of viral DNA (proviral DNA) from virion RNA, by virion RT, takes place in the cell cytoplasm.[44] Transport of double-stranded viral DNA into the nucleus and integration into the host cell genome appears to be a major dividing point in what is a latently infected versus productively infected lymphocyte.[45] Thus, many cells in the body, including most CD4-bearing cells that are infected with HIV, contain HIV-RNA-DNA hybrids that are not fully transcribed by the virion RT.[46,47] This inhibition of the development of double-stranded DNA (proviral DNA) and its integration into the cell nucleus interrupts the ability of HIV to enter the "expressive" phase of its replicative cycle, the phase that in the CD4 lymphocyte leads to cell death and destruction.

At present, two major classes of RT inhibitors exist: competitive inhibitors, which currently are composed of ddN, and noncompetitive inhibitors, which are non-nucleoside RT inhibitors (NNRTI) that allosterically inhibit the HIV RT binding site.[48-51] These latter compounds appear to be very specific for HIV-1 and do not inhibit the HIV-2 RT or the RT of other lentiviruses.

Dideoxynucleoside Analogs

In 1986, a class of nucleoside compounds was first demonstrated to be potent in vitro inhibitors of HIV.[43] They differed from purine and pyramidine deoxynucleotides in that they lacked the 3'-hydroxyl group (Fig. 3). These nucleoside derivatives are essentially prodrugs. They must be metabolically activated to their respective 5'-triphosphates by kinases, nucleotideases, or other cellular phosphorylating enzymes.[43] The exact mechanism by which these nucleotides inhibit HIV-1 RT is unclear. It appears that the 5'-triphosphate competes with the corresponding endogenous 2'-deoxynucleoside-5'-triphosphate (NTP) for binding to the RT and/or acts as an alternative substrate to prevent formation of 3',5'-phosphodiester linkages that lead to premature termination of the elongating viral DNA chain (Fig. 2).[52] The viral RT has a greater affinity for the DNTPs than do host DNA polymerases, a feature that contributes to their selective action. The antiviral activity of the nucleoside analogs is highly dependent on both activating and degrading cellular enzymes whose activity varies among cell types.[54-58] The intracellular concentration of the ddN phosphate derivative as compared with that of the corresponding endogenous deoxynucleoside triphosphate is an important factor in the relative activity of the compound in vitro.[59,60] These interactions appear to account for the differences in the in vivo potency of these compounds on HIV replication. Differences in the intracellular metabolism and affinity for cellular polymerases of the different ddNs also appears to be an important determinant of the clinical toxicities of these agents. Unfortunately, all the current ddNs inhibit HIV-1 replication only partially, and all have significant side effects that complicate their long-term use.[61,62] In addition, in vitro and in vivo resistance have been described for all the drugs and appear to reduce their long-term utility.

Zidovudine

Zidovudine (3'-azido-3'-deoxythymidine or ZDV) was the first antiretroviral compound demonstrated to be effective against HIV in vitro and the first antiretroviral shown to be effective for the treatment of HIV infection.[1-4,62-68] A series of comparative trials with other ddNs have shown zidovudine to be the initial choice for the treatment of HIV infection and currently forms the mainstay of most therapeutic regimens for initial HIV disease. Besides reducing the amount of HIV in peripheral blood mononuclear cells (PBMCs) and plasma, ZDV also appears to enhance certain in vitro and in vivo immune functions of HIV-infected persons.[65]

ZDV is well-absorbed orally. Extensive first-pass glucuronidation through the liver makes the bioavailability of ZDV about

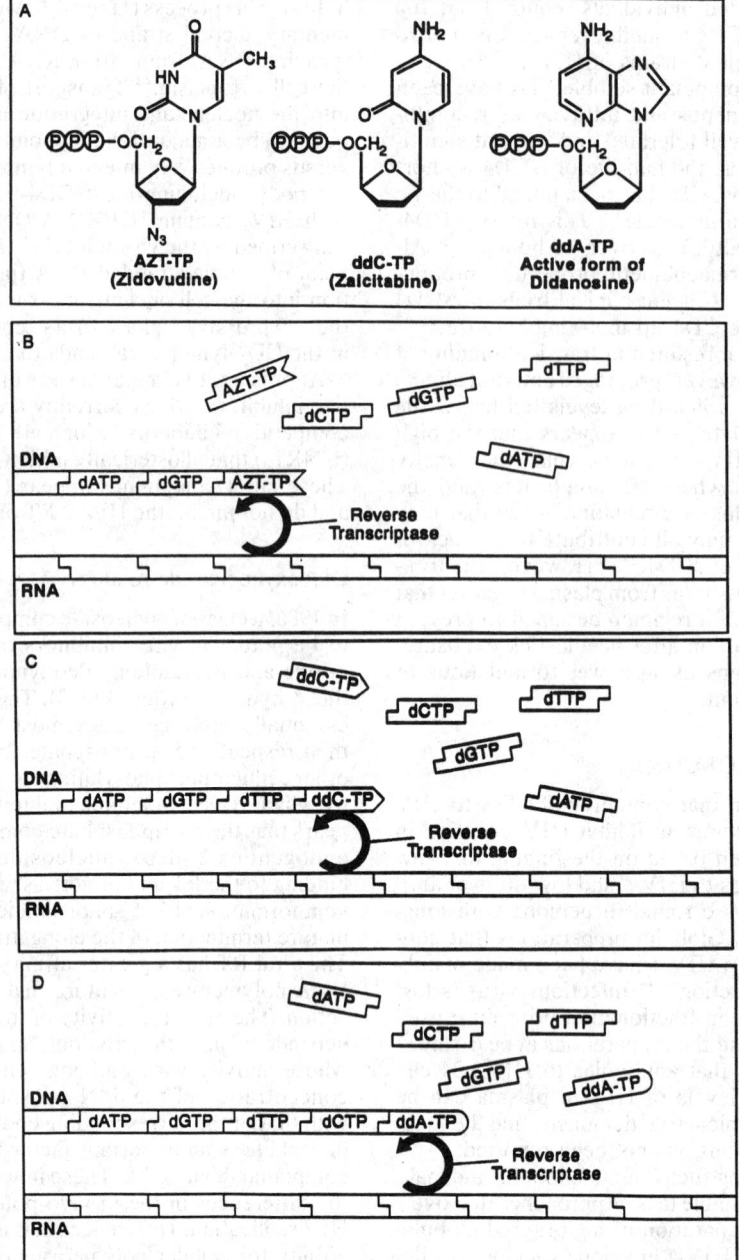

FIG. 3. The nucleoside analogs **(A)** competitively inhibit physiologic deoxynucleoside triphosphates (part of the HIV proviral DNA chain) when incorporated by HIV reverse transcriptase **(B–D)**. Azidothymidine triphosphate (AZT-TP) competes with deoxythymidine triphosphate (dTTP), dideoxycytidine triphosphate (ddC-TP) competes with deoxycytidine triphosphate (dCTP), and dideoxyinosine (ddI) is converted to dideoxyadenosine triphosphate (ddA-TP), which competes with deoxyadenosine triphosphate (dATP). (Adapted from Fischl,[230] with permission.)

60 percent.[69] Metabolic degradation of ZDV involves both glucuronidation and reduction by cytokine p450 activity. Plasma elimination half-life of ZDV is approximately 1 hour, but the intracellular half-life of the active triphosphate is about 3–4 hours.[70-72] As such, most authorities recommend ZDV to be taken on a 3-times-daily regimen.[70] ZDV activation via phosphorylation is mediated by cellular kinases, and in vitro ZDV is most effective in proliferating as compared with quiescent cells.[55,56] Some data suggest that there are large differences among individuals in production of a metabolite of ZDV, adenosine 3'-deoxythymidine (AMT), and concentrations of this metabolite may be associated with ZDV's hematopoietic toxicity.

The major toxicities of ZDV are listed in Table 1 and include neutropenia, anemia, and myopathy.[1-5] Most of these toxicities are dose dependent and are also related to severity of HIV infection, being found much more frequently in persons with more advanced HIV infection.[3,4] ZDV-related anemia can be treated with either transfusion of packed red blood cells or with the administration of recombinant erythropoietin.[73] The responses to erythropoietin in ZDV-treated patients are dependent on endogenous serum erythropoietin level. Patients with erythropoietin levels less than 500 mU/ml should receive erythropoietin at a dose of 100 U/kg 3 times weekly. In such patients, erythropoietin has reduced ZDV-associated transfusion requirements by almost 40 percent. Recombinant erythropoietin is not recommended for HIV-associated anemia due to iron or folate deficiencies, hemolysis, or gastrointestinal losses. ZDV-associated neutropenia is usually reversible by reducing the dose or inter-

TABLE 1. Major Toxicities of Dideoxynucleosides

	ZDV	ddI	ddC	d4T
Anemia	+++	−	−	−
Leukopenia	+++	−	−	−
Neutropenia	+++	−	−	−
Thrombocytopenia	+	−	−	−
Peripheral neuropathy	−	+	++	++
Pancreatitis	−	+++	+	?
Hepatitis	+/−	+/−	+/−	?
Myopathy	++	−	?	?
Mucosal ulcerations	−	−	++	−

TABLE 2. Commonly Used Doses of Antiretrovirals

Zidovudine	200 mg PO tid or 100 mg PO 5 times daily
Didanosine	250 mg PO (sachet) bid
	200-mg tablets PO bid for persons ≥60 kg
	125-mg tablets PO bid for persons <60 kg
Zalcitabine	0.75 mg tid

rupting medication.[61] In selected instances, colony-stimulating factor-granulocyte (CSF-G) and colony-stimulating factor-granulocyte-macrophage (CSF-GM) have been used.[74,75] Myopathy has been associated with prolonged ZDV therapy, an effect that may be related to depletion of muscle cell mitochondrial DNA.[76–79]

ZDV-associated anemia and neutropenia are infrequent in persons with CD4 counts greater than 300 cells/mm³ (e.g., <5 percent per year). In more advanced HIV infections, anemia and neutropenia are seen in 8–20 percent of patients. There are several other toxicities of ZDV that are common and make treatment difficult, especially of patients with subclinical illness. These include nausea, vomiting, diarrhea, fatigue, malaise, myalgias, and headache. The initiation of therapy with lower doses such as 100 mg tid with gradual escalation to standard doses of 200 mg tid or 100 mg 5 times a day can mitigate against these side effects (Table 2). In most patients tachyphylaxis to many of these symptoms will occur. However, in most series, anywhere from 10 to 20 percent of patients initiating ZDV therapy are "intolerant" to medication.[80]

Larder, Richman, and colleagues have described the development of in vitro ZDV resistance during the course of therapy.[81–83] Although nearly all untreated patients have HIV-1 isolates that are susceptible to ZDV, about 20 percent of persons with advanced HIV who have been receiving ZDV for 12–14 months will have isolates that are 50–100-fold less susceptible to ZDV in vitro. In vitro resistance has been shown to be related to the development of several specific point mutations in the RT enzymes[84–86] (Fig. 4). This appears to reduce the ability of ZDV-TP to bind to the RT. Several of these mutations may be present at once. Two in particular, a change from methionine to leucine at amino acid 41, and threonine to tyrosine or phenylalanine at amino acid 215, confer high-grade (50–100-fold) changes in in vitro susceptibility to HIV. Many of these changes appear stable, as ZDV-resistant strains have been transmitted between sexual partners, and from mothers to infants.[87,88] ZDV resistance is a factor in the continued progression of HIV replication that occurs while receiving ZDV monotherapy.[89,90] In vitro resistance to ZDV occurs much sooner in those with AIDS than in those with earlier stages of infection.[7,91,92] However, it is not the sole reason for the clinical failure of ZDV. For example, in a recent study of patients with acquired immunodeficiency syndrome (AIDS) receiving long-term ZDV (mean of 19 months), progression of HIV infection among patients harboring a ZDV-resistant isolate ($IC_{50} > 1.0$ μm) was over twice as common as those harboring a ZDV-sensitive isolate. However, patients with ZDV-resistant strains also possessed syncytium-inducing (SI) isolates of HIV-1, as well as higher quantities of HIV-1 in their plasma and PBMCs.[93] Some data suggest that ZDV can reduce the progression among those with nonsyncy-

tium-inducing (NSI) strains of HIV while not significantly affecting strains that are SI. Because syncytium inhibition is a function associated with the HIV envelope gene, questions have arisen as to whether NSI and SI are markers of other factors associated with HIV replication such as quantity of virus and transcriptional activity. These data indicate that progression of HIV replication on ZDV therapy is a multifactorial process influenced by viral quantity and strain, as well as by a variety of host factors involved in limiting HIV replication.

Didanosine

Didanosine (ddI) is another ddN that has been shown to be of clinical benefit.[5,94–96] The active 5'-triphosphate derivative of ddI is 2',3'-dideoxyadenosine-5'-triphosphate (ddATP).[97–99] ddI is an acid-labile compound and is administered in a buffered solution or in a buffer-containing tablet. Because bioavailability is reduced when ddI is taken with food, the drug should be administered on an empty stomach. Drugs that may be affected by buffering of stomach acids (e.g., ketoconazole, dapsone) should be administered at least 2 hours before ddI. The plasma elimination half-life of ddI is about 1.6 hours; however, the intracellular half-life of ddATP is 8–24 hours, and this is the rationale for use of a twice-daily regimen.[100–101] The major toxicities of ddI are peripheral neuropathy and pancreatitis, and the mechanisms of those toxicities are poorly understood.[94,96,102,103] Neuropathy can be reversed when recognized early by discontinuing treatment. Monitoring of serum amylase levels in patients can reduce the risk of severe pancreatitis, although pancreatitis can occur without premonitory elevations of serum amylase taken as frequently as every 4 weeks.[5,104] Concomitant use of medications that are associated with drug-induced pancreatitis as well as alcohol abuse increase the frequency of ddI-associated pancreatitis.[5,105] Didanosine-associated pancreatitis occurs in about 4–5 percent of patients when used at the currently recommended dose of approximately 250 mg bid of sachet (200 mg bid for the tablet form).[5] The background incidence of pancreatitis among patients with symptomatic HIV appears to be about 3 percent. The lack of overlapping toxicities between ddI and ZDV have allowed the two medications to be used in combination.[106] One of the major inconveniences of ddI therapy is the large tablet size and bitter taste of the current formulations. Use of the sachet preparation or the pediatric formulation may be necessary for some patients who cannot take the tablet. Smaller tablets of ddI and other formulations of the drug are currently under development.

Isolates with decreased sensitivity to ddI have been reported.[107,108] The in vitro change in sensitivity to ddI appears to be a reduction of four-to-fivefold. Isolates that demonstrate a reduced susceptibility to ddI in vitro also show reduced susceptibility to zalcitabine).[109–112] Fortunately, isolates that are resistant to ZDV appear to be sensitive in vitro to ddI.[108,109,112–114] Resistance to ddI has been associated with a change in the RT at amino acid 74 (Fig. 4).

Zalcitabine

Zalcitabine (2',3'-dideoxycytidine or ddC) is another nucleoside analog with anti-HIV activity. ddC is well absorbed and has an oral bioavailability of approximately 80 percent.[115] Food slows absorption and reduces peak plasma concentrations by above 40 percent. The plasma half-life is approximately 1–2 hours, but the intracellular half-life of the triphosphate derivatives is about 2.6 hours. Renal excretion is the primary mode of elimination, and more than 75 percent of the dose is found unchanged in the urine.[116] Dose reductions are recommended when the clearance is 40 ml/min or less. Dosing is generally given on a 3-times-a-day regimen (0.75 mg tid).[117] ddC's major dose-limiting side effect is a painful peripheral neuropathy that is reversible if detected early, but that may be associated with long-term residual effects

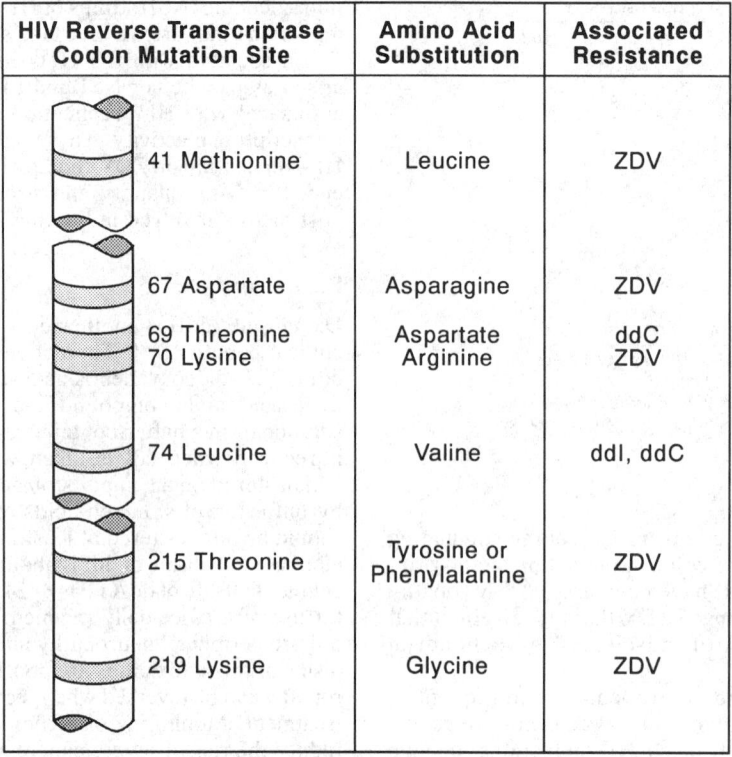

HIV Reverse Transcriptase Codon Mutation Site	Amino Acid Substitution	Associated Resistance
41 Methionine	Leucine	ZDV
67 Aspartate	Asparagine	ZDV
69 Threonine	Aspartate	ddC
70 Lysine	Arginine	ZDV
74 Leucine	Valine	ddl, ddC
215 Threonine	Tyrosine or Phenylalanine	ZDV
219 Lysine	Glycine	ZDV

FIG. 4. Specific mutation sites on the *pol* gene, which codes for reverse transcriptase, have been linked with development of resistance to the nucleoside analogs. Zidovudine resistance is associated with presence of mutations at sites 41, 67, 70, 215, and 219, with 41, 70, and 215 being the most important. Didanosine resistance has been associated with a mutation at site 74 in patients with the zidovudine-resistance mutation at position 215. Resistance to zalcitabine is associated with a mutation at site 69 or 74. (From Fischl,[230] with permission.)

if ddC is continued.[118] Pancreatitis, esophageal and penile ulcerations, and cardiomyopathy are also zalcitabine-associated toxicities.[119–123] Like ddI, ddC exhibits no significant hematologic toxicities, and as such, has been used in combination with ZDV.[124–127] ddC is currently approved by the FDA for use in combination with ZDV for patients with advanced HIV disease.[122] In a head-to-head comparative clinical trial of previously untreated patients with symptomatic HIV, ZDV reduced the development of new opportunistic infections more than ddC.[128]

d4T (Stavudine)

d4T is a thymidine analog whose 5'-triphosphate is also a potent in vitro inhibitor of the HIV RT.[129] d4T is well absorbed with an absolute bioavailability of 90 percent or greater. The plasma half-life is approximately 1 hour, and the intracellular half-life of the triphosphate is approximately 3½ hours.[130,131] Recent clinical trials have indicated that the major dose-limiting toxicity of d4T is, like zalcitabine, painful peripheral neuropathy.[132,133] Hematologic toxicity with d4T is uncommon. At present, d4T is not currently licensed for use as an antiviral in the United States, although an expanded access program for use in patients who are intolerant to other nucleoside analogs is in place. The antiviral activity of d4T appears similar to that of the other ddNs, and a recent product license application for its use in selected patients with HIV-1 infection is under review.[134]

NON-NUCLEOSIDE REVERSE TRANSCRIPTASE INHIBITORS

Several structurally unrelated compounds have recently been demonstrated to be potent and selective inhibitors of HIV-1 replication.[135–139] These drugs noncompetitively inhibit viral RT, presumably by binding to a site other than the nucleoside and template binding sites. This interaction between the NNRTI and the HIV-1 RT produces a conformational change that results in the inactivation of the viral RT. These drugs have great selectivity for the HIV-1 RT.[140–143] They have no antiretroviral activity against HIV-2 or against other animal retroviruses.[141,142] Several have been shown to have potent in vivo antiviral activity, in that marked reductions in p24 antigen and plasma RNA levels have been shown with shot-course therapy.[144] However, the rapid emergence of resistant isolates of HIV-1 has been demonstrated for most of these compounds.[145–147] This has been associated with a marked rise in p24 and plasma RNA levels. For some of these compounds, this increase in susceptibility is more than 100-fold, and may emerge as early as within 2 weeks after initiation of therapy. For others, NNRTI-reduced susceptibility appears to be 10-fold and may take months to develop. As the NNRTIs appear to have an excellent safety profile, very high concentrations of these compounds are being tested both alone and in combination with other nucleoside analogs. Two of these drugs, nevirapine and delaviridine, are described in more detail below.

Nevirapine

Nevirapine is a compound that specifically inhibits HIV-1 RT in nanomolar concentrations.[142] In addition to its ability to block RT, nevirapine also has an inhibitory effect in the HIV RNase activity.[141] Nevirapine has greater than 95 percent bioavailability, and its half-life is 24–48 hours.[148] In vitro synergy has been reported between nevirapine and ddNs such as ZDV and ddI, and the combination of nevirapine, ddI, and ZDV is a potent in vitro inhibitor of HIV-1 replication.[149] Clinical trials of this triple combination therapy are currently in progress in patients with HIV infections at various stages of disease. Early trials of nevirapine at doses less than 400 mg/day showed a rapid emergence of resistance associated with development of mutations at specific amino acid sites of the RT (e.g., 181). This in vitro resistance was associated with a marked reversal of antiviral activity and reversal of the CD4 count elevations seen with initiation of therapy. Use of high concentrations of the compound reduces the frequency of these findings, and concentrations above the ID_{90} of most clinical isolates still appear possible, especially when combined with other retrovirals. Nevirapine at such doses of 400 mg/day appears to be well tolerated. The most common adverse reaction to nevirapine has been rash, occurring most frequently at initiation of treatment.

Delavirdine

Delavirdine is a bisheteroarylpiperazine derivative that is a potent NNRTI.[150,151] In vitro delavirdine inhibits replication in HIV in submicromolar concentrations and both ZDV- and ddI-resistant strains are susceptible to the compound.[152] As with nevirapine, delaviridine and ZDV are synergistic in vitro.[149] Of interest, recent evidence suggests that HIV-1 strains that are resistant to delaviridine are not cross-resistant to other NNRTIs, and mutations at sites that confer delaviridine resistance produce isolates that are more sensitive to nevirapine.[144] If such findings are corroborated in vivo, these findings open up the possibility of using combinations of NNRTIs. Phase III trials to evaluate the clinical utility of delaviridine are under way.

Foscarnet

Foscarnet, a licensed therapy for treatment of cytomegalovirus (CMV) retinitis, has in vitro and in vivo antiretroviral activity.[153,154] In vitro, foscarnet and ZDV are synergistic and foscarnet therapy is associated with a reduction in p24 antigen among persons on ZDV.[155] In a recent study of patients with advanced HIV infection and CMV retinitis, foscarnet therapy prolonged survival.[156] Because the anti-CMV activity of the two agents tested in that study, ganciclovir and foscarnet, appeared similar, the difference in survival in the foscarnet group may have been related to foscarnet's anti-HIV activity. Unfortunately, the high cost, need for parenteral administration, need for preadministration hydration to decrease renal toxicity, and the substantial number of other toxicities associated with foscarnet severely limit its use as an antiretroviral, except for patients with CMV disease.

INTERFERON-α

Parenterally administered interferon-α has been widely used as a therapy for selected patients with AIDS-associated Kaposi sarcoma, and favorable short-term effects on virologic markers such as HIV p24 antigen have been demonstrated among some patients.[157–160] Unfortunately, the toxicities of interferon-α among HIV-infected persons are substantial. In a placebo-controlled study of 34 persons with asymptomatic HIV infection and CD4+ cell counts greater than 400/mm³, 12 weeks of daily interferon-α was associated with a change from positive to negative HIV PBMC cultures, although 35 percent of subjects withdrew because of interferon-associated toxicities.[161–164] An early placebo-controlled study of interferon-α in patients with AIDS showed no differences in outcome among the study groups.[161] The systemic toxicities of parenteral interferon-α (except at very low doses) and need for parenteral administration have limited its widespread use as an antiretroviral agent, particularly in the absence of compelling data about its clinical efficacy.[165,166]

PROTEASE INHIBITORS

The HIV protease protein has been shown to be an essential part of the virion's life cycle and is responsible for cleaving the gag-pol polyprotein into its component parts. Inhibition of the protease results in loss of the gag protein (p24), accumulation of unprocessed full-length gag-pol protein, and the emergence of "defective" particles of HIV.[167–170] The HIV-1 protease belongs to the class of aspartyl proteases, and several inhibitors of this protease have been derived.[171,172] The advantages of such agents is that they are able to inhibit HIV replication in cells that are chronically infected with HIV-1.[173,174] As such, they offer attractive alternatives to RT inhibitors. In addition, in vitro synergism between the two classes of drugs has been readily demonstrated.[175] The major obstacle in the development of the protease inhibitors for HIV therapeutics has been their pharmacokinetic profiles. Many of the initial prototype compounds were peptidometic structures that were insoluble and had extremely poor bioavailability.[176] More recently, several compounds with reasonable (5–20 percent) bioavailability have been described and have entered clinical trials. Limited information suggests these compounds are well tolerated and have in vivo activity (i.e., lower HIV p24 and plasma RNA levels). Again, the development of resistance is of concern as one can readily select out such variants in vitro, albeit not as quickly as with many of the NNRTIs.[177] As of this writing, the role of the protease inhibitors in HIV therapeutics is under intense evaluation, and studies of their clinical utility alone and in combination with ddNs are under way.

OTHER APPROACHES

Because of the desirability to inhibit production of HIV from chronically infected cells, several novel approaches to HIV therapy are undergoing intense preclinical evaluation. These include compounds that inhibit the regulatory genes of HIV such as tat[178,179] or inhibit HIV envelope processing by interfering with glycosylation.[180] Although several of these compounds have entered clinical trials, successful in vivo activity has not been consistently achieved. Other approaches have been to inhibit the spread of HIV using novel strategies such as antisense oligonucleotides that would inhibit HIV transcription and/or translation[181] (also see Ch. 146). Delivery of such compounds to viral-infected cells for an extended time period is an obstacle under intensive study. Another approach under investigation to inhibit HIV is to deliver RNA molecules that are specific to HIV-1 and that can bind and cleave HIV-1 RNA (ribozymes),[16] thus inhibiting subsequent HIV-1 transcription among chronically or even latently infected cells.[182,183]

Another approach for antiviral therapy has been the development of therapies directed at enhancing host responses to HIV-1. Several studies have shown that CD8+ T-cell responses to HIV appear very early in the course of infection (2 weeks) and persist in vitro. CD8+ cytotoxic T-lymphocyte (CTL) activity is reduced as disease progresses.[184–186] As such, "adoptive immunotherapy" with autologous CD8+ CTLs specific to HIV is one approach to inhibit spread of HIV from infected cells. Use of CTLs that are directed at the gag-pol proteins of HIV are underway in phase I trials.[187] Another approach is to replace CD4 cell loss with autologous CD4 cells. Because such cells are likely to be reinfected with HIV-1, introduction of a gene that would prevent HIV-1 replication in these cells is a concept also under investigation.[188,189]

DOES ANTIRETROVIRAL THERAPY PROLONG SURVIVAL?

Studies in patients with AIDS and with advanced constitutional disease (formerly AIDS-related complex) have demonstrated that ZDV delays the development of opportunistic infections and prolongs survival.[4,5,190–193] Observational studies of large cohorts of patients receiving ZDV, often in conjunction with prophylaxis for *Pneumocystis carinii* pneumonia (PCP), have also demonstrated a lengthening of survival, compared with controls who did not receive ZDV. For example, among 1028 persons with AIDS from Maryland, median survival was 770 days among those who received ZDV compared with 190 days among patients who did not receive ZDV ($p < 0.001$).[192] Among 271 Italian patients with AIDS, most of whom had contracted HIV through injection drug use,[194] ZDV prolonged survival (median 21 versus 10 months for those treated and untreated, respectively). In a study of aerosolized pentamidine for prevention of PCP, ZDV recipients lived longer than the non-ZDV-treated patients.[195] Thus, a large body of evidence indicates that among persons with advanced HIV infection, irrespective of risk factors, gender, or race, ZDV prolongs survival, albeit for a limited time span (months).[196,197]

Whether antiretroviral therapy prolongs survival when used in earlier stages of HIV infection has been more difficult to determine. Several large, randomized, double-blind studies using ZDV have demonstrated that treatment of both asymptomatic and symptomatic patients with HIV infection and CD4+ lymphocyte counts less that 500/mm³ delays disease progression. This delay in disease progression results primarily from both a reduction in the frequency of subsequent opportunistic infections and the time to which the peripheral CD4+ cell counts fall to very low levels.[197–201] However, studies have been discontinued by external review boards when therapy was shown to reduce the development of opportunistic infections associated with HIV, an event that may precede death by 1–4 years. In these studies, mortality tended to be lower in treated versus untreated patients, although the differences were not statistically significant. In addition, antiretroviral therapy was often started in placebo recipients after disease progression occurred, and stopped for toxicity in initially treated patients, negating the potential to demonstrate a survival benefit in these studies. Nonetheless, these studies have shown that ZDV therapy reduces the frequency of hospitalization, and reduces the need for medical therapy overall.[202–206] The quality of life appeared to be favorably impacted by ZDV in a study of patients with mildly symptomatic HIV infection.[205] However, a recent study of asymptomatic HIV-infected patients indicated that the beneficial effects of ZDV on quality of life (based on delay in progression of disease) were offset by equivalent negative effects of severe side effects of the drug.[207]

There are, however, two major studies that have not shown a beneficial effect of ZDV on survival.[208,209] A study conducted by the Veteran's Affairs Cooperative Group with 338 HIV-infected, symptomatic patients demonstrated that therapy with ZDV was associated with a reduction in progression to AIDS but not with longer survival in patients with CD4 counts greater than 200 cells/mm³.[208] Unfortunately, the study design was modified in midtrial to allow a crossover from blinded therapy to open-label ZDV when the results of AIDS Clinical Trials Group (ACTG) protocols 016 and 019, which demonstrated that ZDV reduced the time to development of AIDS, became available.[198,200]

More recently a large cooperative study in Europe (Concorde) enrolled 1762 patients with asymptomatic HIV-1 infection and randomized patients into early versus delayed ZDV therapy (early = an entry into the study; delayed = when symptomatic disease developed, or when CD4 counts fell below 500/mm³).[209] This study demonstrated that whereas ZDV again delayed progression to AIDS when given early, no overall difference in long-term mortality was noted in comparison to "delayed" therapy with ZDV. Again, most deaths from HIV were distantly related to the selection of initial therapy. Both of these multicenter trials indicate that progression of HIV-1 infection in adults is an invariable part of ZDV therapy, that is, that ZDV monotherapy has a limited clinical benefit. However, the development of additional antiretrovirals has made the use of long-term monotherapy with ZDV less necessary.[210,211]

WHEN SHOULD ANTIRETROVIRAL THERAPY BE INITIATED?

The above information has created controversy regarding the initial use of ZDV. Should therapy be initiated while patients are asymptomatic with high CD4 counts or should one wait until they develop illnesses or CD4 counts less than 200 cells/mm³? One approach is to use ZDV to increase the duration of time before the development of AIDS. This approach recognizes that alternative therapy will be necessary once the patient progresses on ZDV, and that, at present, alternative therapy also has limited clinical benefit.[210,211] Another management approach is to base therapy on survival benefits. Advocates of this approach generally delay initiation of ZDV until the later stages of infection (AIDS, advanced AIDS-related complex, or CD4 counts <200). I favor discussing the above options with each patient and making an individualized choice. In my experience, among persons who tolerate ZDV, most (>80 percent) prefer earlier rather than delayed therapy.

Although the term "early" intervention is widely used to describe the initiation of ZDV when the CD4 counts approach 500 cells/mm³, this strategy actually delays treatment until years after HIV infection has occurred and after widespread immunologic damage has already been sustained. Ongoing HIV replication is detectable throughout all stages of infection, and the time from infection with HIV-1 until a CD4+ lymphocyte count in peripheral blood is less than 500/mm³ is often 5 years or more.[10,11,212–217] Viral replication causes damage to cells directly, by cell death, by cell fusion and from toxic viral products (e.g., gp 120), and indirectly through widespread immune derangement that results from HIV infection of CD4+ lymphocytes and mononuclear cells, with the resultant cytokine activation (see Ch. 101). RT inhibitors may protect new cells from becoming latently infected, but are ineffective in suppression of replication in chronically infected cells.[210] In theory, the sooner therapy is begun with this class of antiretrovirals, the less spread of HIV and the less damage to the immune system would occur. However, the limited antiviral effects, the potential drug toxicities, and the loss of effectiveness over time of currently available nucleoside analogs have led to a moderation of this view.

One large collaborative trial has demonstrated that ZDV monotherapy in patients with CD4+ cell counts greater than 500/mm³ is beneficial.[218] This European-Australian, collaborative, double-blinded, placebo-controlled trial of 993 HIV-infected patients with CD4 counts greater than 400/mm³ was recently terminated early because the results indicated that ZDV therapy (500 mg bid) significantly reduced the frequency of clinical progression of HIV and frequency with which CD4 counts fell to less than 350 cells/mm³.[218] The median entry CD4 count was almost 600/mm³, and patients were followed for a median of 93 weeks. As in previous placebo-controlled studies of ZDV in patients with lower CD4 cell counts, ZDV therapy reduced progression of HIV disease defined by CD4 cell decreases and/or onset of symptomatic disease in patients who were asymptomatic at study entry. Another large, placebo-controlled trial of ZDV in persons with asymptomatic HIV with CD4+ cell counts greater than 500/mm³ has been under way in the United States for over 5 years. If similar results are found, we will see a greater use of ZDV in patients with CD4 counts greater than 500.

There are limited human data about use of antiretroviral therapies other than ZDV monotherapy as initial treatment in patients with CD4+ cell counts above 300/mm³. However, in two separate trials among persons with CD4 counts less than 300/mm³, ZDV has been noted to be more effective than either didanosine or zalcitabine. One of these trials compared ZDV with ddI in 836 patients, 26 percent of whom had AIDS, 67 percent of whom had symptomatic HIV infection with CD4+ cell counts < 300/mm³, and 7 percent of whom were asymptomatic individuals with CD4+ cell counts less than 200/mm³. Patients were either previously untreated or could have received ZDV alone for up to 16 weeks before entry. In patients who had never received ZDV, ZDV was more effective in delaying disease progression than ddI (rates per 100 years of patient observation were 27 for ZDV versus 32 [500 mg/day] and 37 [750 mg/day] of ddI.[219] Survival was also better in the ZDV-treated subjects who had not had prior ZDV. Fatality rates per 100 years of patient observation were 11.1 for ZDV, and 17.7 and 15.4 for ddI). However, among the subgroup of patients with 8–16 weeks of prior ZDV, switches to ddI therapy appeared better than continuing ZDV in terms of both delay progression of disease and survival.[219] These latter results are consistent with the findings of a companion study (ACTG 116B/117), which showed that "switching" to ddI was beneficial in patients who had received prolonged ddI therapy[5] (see below). Another recently completed study also indicated that "switching" to ddI from ZDV was more effective than remaining on ZDV in patients with advanced disease who were clinically deteriorating on ZDV.[219]

A similar study compared zalcitabine monotherapy with ZDV. Among 635 patients with a median CD4 cell count of 90/mm^3 randomized to ZDV or ddC, survival was better in the ZDV-treated patients (33 deaths versus 59 deaths, $p = 0.007$).[128] Thus, ZDV (at a dose of 500–600 mg daily) is the recommended therapy for the initial treatment of HIV-infected persons. Data from several studies suggest that doses of ZDV as low as 300 mg daily have antiretroviral activity, but that 150 mg daily is less effective than higher doses.[57]

There has been significant interest in enhancing the benefit of ZDV monotherapy among patients by initiating antiretroviral therapy with combinations of ZDV and ddI or ZDV and ddC.[106,220–224] Several studies have shown that among such patients, the combination of either ZDV and ddC or ZDV and ddI is associated with a higher and more prolonged rise of CD4 cells and a greater antiviral effect than ZDV alone.[106,220,221] However, whether the added antiviral effect of combination therapy translates into clinical benefit is currently unclear. As of this writing, I initiate antiretroviral therapy with ZDV alone. In persons with advanced HIV infection (CD4 < 200), addition or substitution of therapy with another antiretroviral such as ddI or ddC soon in the course of infection is often beneficial.

MANAGEMENT OF ZDV FAILURE WITH ddI AND ddC

It is clear that patients with advanced HIV infection eventually "clinically fail" with prolonged ZDV treatment. The rate of progression of disease increases with time on therapy. It appears that among ZDV-treated patients, the time from the development of an opportunistic infection to death is shorter than among comparable patients who have not received previous ZDV.[208] As such, an important management question is whether altering a patient's antiretroviral regimen from ZDV alone can prevent or reverse this clinical deterioration. The answer to this question appears to be—to a limited extent—yes, albeit such "switching" appears to be most beneficial at higher CD4 cell counts (>150 cells/mm^3).

Recently Kahn et al. demonstrated that switching from ZDV to didanosine was beneficial in patients with advanced HIV infection with CD4 counts less than 200/mm^3 or with symptomatic HIV with CD4 counts less than 300/mm^3, who had more than 16 weeks of previous ZDV therapy (ACTG Trial 116B/117).[5] Persons randomized to didanosine (500 mg/day) had a statistically significant delay in time to a clinical endpoint, compared with those assigned to ZDV therapy (1-year rate 28 percent versus 40 percent, $p = 0.008$). Higher dose didanosine (750 mg/day) (1-year rate 34 percent) was not significantly different than ZDV, presumably because of poorer compliance and less actual use of ddI in that group. Of note, the delay in disease progression was seen in the subgroups with asymptomatic or AIDS-related complex (CD4 counts >150), but not among patients with AIDS

(CD4 count <100), suggesting that there may be a point beyond which benefit cannot be gained by a switch from one antiviral to another. No differences in survival were seen between the three treatment groups in this study.[5]

The application of the results of these trials to use of these drugs in clinical practice is not straightforward. The study design for ACTG 116B/117 was based on the assumption that almost all persons with advanced HIV infection who have been on ZDV monotherapy for 6–12 months have HIV isolates with high-grade resistance to ZDV. However, when retrospectively tested, only 20–25 percent of such patients appeared to have isolates with high-grade resistance to ZDV (in vitro susceptibility of ≥1 uM). Although in vitro ZDV resistance was an important factor influencing progression of disease (relative risk of progression of about 2), viral load and phenotype of the virus (SI versus NSI strain) were additional factors influencing progression in such patients.

At present I do not feel it necessary to switch from ZDV therapy of HIV-infected adults at an arbitrary time point. I recommend that any patient on ZDV monotherapy for at least 8 weeks who develops another opportunistic infection, has progressive weight loss or constitutional symptoms, who has a reproducible decrease in CD4+ cells counts, or who doubles serum HIV p24 antigen levels or serum RNA levels on two determinations more than 4 weeks apart, should be offered alternative antiretroviral therapy. One of the central issues for such patients is whether switching to another nucleoside monotherapy or adding a new agent is the best strategy. For didanosine, no data are available. For zalcitabine it appears that adding this drug to ZDV appears preferable, based on the results of a recent study (ACTG 155).[224] This study evaluated the strategy of switching to zalcitabine versus the addition of this agent among persons with advanced HIV infection who had taken ZDV for a prolonged period of time. Little clinical benefit was observed for either strategy among those with CD4 counts less than 150/mm^3. However, among those with CD4 counts between 150 and 300, the addition of ddC or switching to ddC decreased progression to a new opportunistic infection or death by about one-third.[224]

One recently reported trial compared ddC and ddI in late stages of HIV-1 infection.[6] This study enrolled 467 patients (median CD4 count of 73/mm^3), 63 percent who were unable to tolerate ZDV and 37 percent who had failed ZDV, and followed them for a mean of 16 months. After adjustment for factors that might affect disease progression (CD4+ cell counts, presence of AIDS, Karnofsky performance score), both treatments appeared similar in their effects on disease progression, but ddC therapy was associated with prolonged survival compared with ddI (adjusted relative risk of death 0.63 [CI 0.46–0.85], $p = 0.002$). However, overall outcome remained poor, as two-thirds of patients had disease progression and one-third died during the mean 16 months of follow-up.

There are several phase II studies that have used alternating regimens of ZDV and zalcitabine (at 1-monthly intervals). These studies were based on the hope of reducing toxicity to each agent, preserving antiviral activity, and perhaps reducing the time to the development of in vitro resistance to ZDV. It appears that the latter is not achieved, although toxicity can be reduced.[221–223] Whether alternation of two antiretrovirals result in prolonged clinical benefit is unproven.

ANTIRETROVIRAL THERAPY IN PREGNANCY

Recently ZDV has been studied in HIV-infected pregnant women[225,226] and has been shown to reduce the transmission of HIV infection from mother to infant.[227] In a study of over 400 HIV-positive women conducted in the United States and France, the use of ZDV during the second and third trimesters, and during and shortly after parturition reduced the infection rate among infants from 28 percent to 8 percent. At this writing the definitive report of this trial has not been published, but available data indicate that ZDV therapy may be one way to decrease, although not eliminate, transmission of HIV-1 to the infant. The ZDV regimen consisted of antepartum ZDV, 100 mg PO 5 times daily plus intravenous ZDV (IV loading dose of 2 mg/kg followed by continuous infusion 1 mg/kg/day until delivery) plus ZDV treatment of the newborn (syrup, 2 mg/kg every 6 hours for 6 weeks beginning 8–12 hours after birth). Infection rates appeared similar in those starting antepartum therapy between 14 and 26 weeks versus those initiating therapy after 26 weeks' gestation. This is an important advance in the therapy of women with HIV-1.

CURRENT RECOMMENDATIONS

A "state-of-the-art" conference was convened in mid-1993 by the National Institute of Allergy and Infectious Diseases to evaluate current information on the use of nucleoside analog RT inhibitors for the treatment of HIV-1.[228] Table 3 summarizes the consensus recommendations of the conference. As shown, the table suggests that asymptomatic patients with CD4 counts greater than 500 cells/mm³ should not be treated. This recommendation was based on the fact that only one study currently shows benefit of ZDV monotherapy in this patient group. There is a similar study in the United States involving over 1800 patients with high CD4 counts that has been ongoing for over 4 years. If data from the U.S. study are similar to that of the European-Australian study described earlier, then recommen-

dation for using ZDV in such patients may be forthcoming. Review of Table 3 also indicates that it is "acceptable" to withhold ZDV in asymptomatic patients with CD4 counts between 200 and 500. The issues relating to such recommendations have been discussed above and relate to what the provider and patient feel is the primary "goal" of therapy. Is survival of paramount importance? If so, then delaying ZDV to stages where survival benefit has been most clearly demonstrated is an acceptable strategy. However, ZDV has been shown to decrease progression of HIV in asymptomatic persons with CD4 counts below 200 and 500. In addition, the duration of this effect (i.e., delaying the time to AIDS) is nearly twice as long among those with CD4 counts greater than 300 cells/mm³ at initiation of therapy versus those with CD4 counts between 200 and 300 cells/mm³. If one elects to initiate ZDV in persons with CD4 counts of 200 or more, then initiation of alternative therapy with ddI or ddC is suggested if HIV infection progresses.

The consensus panel agreed that among persons with CD4 counts less than 200 cells/mm³, whether symptomatic or asymptomatic, ZDV should be initiated. However, because of the data showing greater CD4 rises and greater antiviral effects with combination therapy, some authorities initiate therapy with combination ZDV and didanosine or ZDV and zalcitabine.

THE NEED TO INDIVIDUALIZE THERAPY

Perhaps the largest single deficiency in our current treatment strategies for HIV-1 infection with antiretrovirals has been our inability to individualize therapy. As shown in Figure 5, at any particular CD4 count, the amount of virus circulating in an HIV-1 infected patient may vary by as much as 10,000-fold. Because ddNs reduce serum HIV-1 concentrations by an average of 5- to 10-fold, the response to therapy among patients with similar CD4 counts is not likely to be the same. Studies of antiretrovirals have used CD4 rather than quantitative measurements of viral load as their initiating and ending points. Analysis of responses to therapy that have used CD4 counts and/or clinical progression of an opportunistic infection as endpoints, rather than direct measurements of the antiviral affects of therapy on HIV, may give imprecise or even misleading results. The difficulty and expense that is entailed in laboratory measurements of HIV-1 has limited the utility of these virologic measurements in patient management. Recently, accurate quantitative assays to measure HIV-1 in plasma and cells have been developed, and technological improvements to allow their use in individual patients are now being devised.[229] Such assays will allow the practitioner to assess the actual antiviral response of an individual to a particular antiviral drug or regimen and to alter therapy

TABLE 3. Antiretroviral Therapy for HIV-Infected Adults: Recommendations From 1993 National Institute of Allergy and Infectious Diseases (NIAID) State-of-the-Art Conference

Clinical Status	CD4+ Range, Cell Count × 10⁹/liter	Recommendation
No Previous Antiretroviral Therapy		
Asymptomatic	>0.50	No therapy
Asymptomatic	0.20–0.50	Zidovudine or no therapy
Symptomatic	0.20–0.50	Zidovudine
Asymptomatic	<0.20	Zidovudine
Symptomatic	<0.20	Zidovudine
Previous Antiretroviral Therapy		
Stable	≥0.30	Continue zidovudine
Stable	<0.30	Continue zidovudine or change to didanosine
Progressing	0.05–0.50	Change to didanosine or zalcitabine
Progressing	<0.05	Change to didanosine or zalcitabine
Intolerant to Zidovudine		
Stable	>0.50	Change to didanosine or zalcitabine

(From Sande et al.,[228] with permission.)

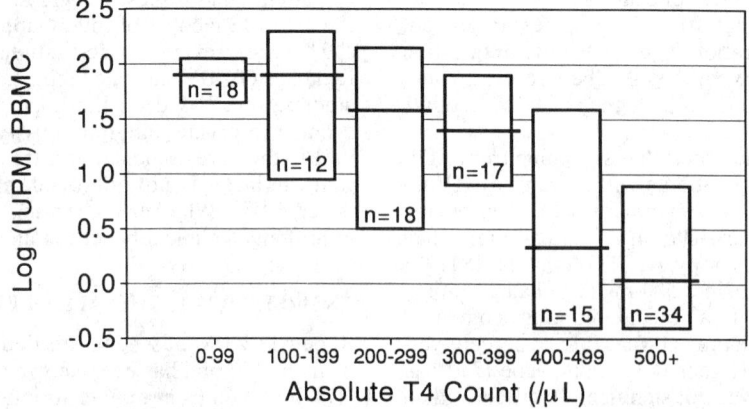

FIG. 5. Relationship between CD4 count and concentration of HIV cultured from PBMCs of 116 patients. The graph illustrates the median (25th to 75th quartile) number of infectious units of HIV per million PMBCs (IUPM). Although the median IUPM is inversely related to CD4 cell count, there is a wide overlap, and many persons with similar CD4 cell counts have infectious titers of HIV that differ by over 3 logs.

based on such assays. These assays should enable the management of HIV infection to follow more closely the paradigm that we use in antimicrobial therapy of other infectious diseases.

REFERENCES

1. Fischl MA, Richman DD, Grieco MH, et al. The efficacy of azidothymidine (AZT) in the treatment of patients with AIDS and AIDS-related complex. A double-blind, placebo-controlled trial. N Engl J Med. 1987;317:185–91.
2. Fischl MA, Richman DD, Hansen N, et al. The safety and efficacy of zidovudine (AZT) in the treatment of subjects with mildly symptomatic human immunodeficiency virus type 1 (HIV) infection: A double-blind, placebo-controlled trial. Ann Intern Med. 1990;112:721–3.
3. Yarchoan R, Klecker RW, Weinhold KJ, et al. Administration of 3'-azido-3'-deoxythymidine, an inhibitor of HTLV-III/LAV replication, to patients with AIDS or AIDS-related complex. Lancet. 1986;7:575–80.
4. Fischl MA, Richman DD, Causey DM, et al. Prolonged zidovudine therapy in patients with AIDS and advanced AIDS-related complex. JAMA. 1989;262:2405–10.
5. Kahn JO, Lagakos SW, Richman DD, et al. A controlled trial comparing continued zidovudine with didanosine in human immunodeficiency virus infection. N Engl J Med. 1992;327:581–7.
6. Abrams DI, Goldman AI, Launer C, et al. A comparative trial of didanosine or zalcitabine after treatment with zidovudine in patients with human immunodeficiency virus infection. N Engl J Med. 1994;330:657–62.
7. Fischl MA, Parker CB, Pettinelli C, et al. A randomized controlled trial of a reduced daily dose of zidovudine in patients with the acquired immunodeficiency syndrome. N Engl J Med. 1990;323:1009–14.
8. Corey L, Fleming TR. Treatment of HIV-1 infection: Progress in perspective (Editorial). N Engl J Med. 1992;326:484–5.
9. Crumpacker CS. Molecular targets of antiviral therapy. N Engl J Med. 1989;321:163–72.
10. Pantaleo G, Graziosi C, Demarest JF, et al. HIV infection is active and progressive in lymphoid tissue during the clinically latent stage of disease. Nature. 1993;362:355–8.
11. Embretson J, Zupancic M, Ribas JL, et al. Massive covert infection of helper T lymphocytes and macrophages by HIV during the incubation period of AIDS. Nature. 1993;362:359–62.
12. Richman DD. Zidovudine resistance of human immunodeficiency virus. Rev Infect Dis. 1990;12(Suppl 5):S507–10.
13. Goodenow M, Huet T, Saurin W, et al. HIV-1 isolates are rapidly evolving quasispecies: Evidence for viral mixtures. J AIDS. 1989;2:344–52.
14. Martin JL, Wilson JE, Haynes RL, et al. Mechanism of resistance of human immunodeficiency virus type 1 to 2',3'-dideoxyinosine. Proc Natl Acad Sci USA. 1993;90:6135–9.
15. Smith DH, Byrn RA, Marsters SA, et al. Blocking of HIV-1 infectivity by a soluble, secreted form of CD4 antigen. Science. 1987;238:1704–7.
16. Moore JP, McKeating JA, Weiss RA, et al. Dissociation of gp120 from HIV-1 virions induced by soluble CD4. Science. 1990;250:1139–42.
17. Daar ES, Li XL, Moudgil T, et al. High concentrations of recombinant soluble CD4 are required to neutralize primary human immunodeficiency virus type 1 isolates. Proc Natl Acad Sci USA. 1990;87:6574–8.
18. Ashkenazi A, Smith DH, Marsters SA, et al. Resistance of primary isolates of human immunodeficiency virus type 1 to soluble CD4 is independent of CD4-rgp120 binding affinity. Proc Natl Acad Sci USA. 1991;88:7056–60; Erratum 1992;89:1517.
19. Brighty DW, Rosenberg M, Chen ISY, et al. Envelope proteins from clinical isolates of human immunodeficiency virus type 1 that are refractory to neutralization by soluble CD4 possess high affinity for the CD4 receptor. Proc Natl Acad Sci USA. 1991;88:7802–5.
20. Moore JP, McKeating JA, Huang YX, et al. Virions of primary human immunodeficiency virus type 1 isolates resistant to soluble CD4 (sCD4) neutralization differs in sCD4 binding and glycoprotein gp120 retention for sCD4-sensitive isolates. J Virol. 1992;66:235–43.
21. Schacker T, Coombs RW, Collier AC, et al. The effects of high-dose recombinant soluble CD4 on human immunodeficiency virus type 1 viremia. J Infect Dis. 1994;169:37–40.
22. Schooley RT, Merigan TC, Gaut P, et al. Recombinant soluble CD4 therapy in patients with the acquired immunodeficiency syndrome (AIDS) and AIDS-related complex. Ann Intern Med. 1990;112:247–53.
23. Schacker T, Collier AC, Coombs R, et al. A phase I study of high dose, intravenous rsCD4 in subjects with advanced HIV-1 infection. J Infect Dis. 1994;169:37–40.
24. Kahn JO, Allan JD, Hodges TL, et al. The safety and pharmacokinetics of recombinant soluble CD4 (rCD4) in subjects with the acquired immunodeficiency syndrome (AIDS) and AIDS-related complex. Ann Intern Med. 1990;112:254–61.
25. Traunecker A, Schneider J, Kiefer H, et al. Highly efficient neutralization of HIV with recombinant CD4-immunoglobulin molecules. Nature. 1989;339:68–70.
26. Hodges TL, Kahn JO, Kaplan LD, et al. Phase I study of recombinant human CD4-immunoglobulin G therapy of patients with AIDS and AIDS-related complex. Antimicrob Agents Chemother. 1991;35:2580–6.
27. Layne SP, Merges MJ, Spouge JL, et al. Blocking of human immunodeficiency virus infection depends on cell density and viral stock age. J Virol. 1991;65:3293–300.
28. Pantaleo G, Grazios C, Butini L, et al. Lymphoid organs function as major reservoirs for human immunodeficiency virus. Proc Natl Acad Sci USA. 1991;88:9838–42.
29. Jackson GG, Perkins JT, Rubenis M, et al. Passive immunoneutralization of human immunodeficiency virus in patients with advanced AIDS. Lancet. 1988;2:647–52.
30. Karpas A, Hill F, Youle M, et al. Effects of passive immunization in patients with advanced immunodeficiency syndrome-related complex and acquired immunodeficiency syndrome. Proc Natl Acad Sci USA. 1988;85:9234–7.
31. Ranki A, Weiss SH, Valle SL, et al. Neutralizing antibodies in HIV (HTLV-III) infection: Correlation with clinical outcome and antibody response against different viral proteins. Clin Exp Immunol. 1987;69:231–9.
32. Steimer K, Puma JP, Power MD, et al. Differential antibody responses of individuals infected with AIDS-associated retroviruses surveyed using the viral core antigen p25 gag expressed in bacteria. Virology. 1986;150:283–90.
33. Biggar RJ, Melbye M, Ebbesen P, et al. Variation in human T lymphotropic virus type III (HTLV-III) antibodies in homosexual men: Decline before onset of illness related to acquired immune deficiency syndrome (AIDS). Br Med J. 1985;291:997–8.
34. Schupbach J, Haller O, Vogt M, et al. Antibodies to HTLV-III in Swiss patients with AIDS and pre-AIDS and in groups at risk for AIDS. N Engl J Med. 1985;312:265–70.
35. Goudsmit J, Lange MA, Paul DA, et al. Antigenemia and antibody titers to core and envelope antigens in AIDS, AIDS-related complex, and subclinical human immunodeficiency virus infection. J Infect Dis. 1987;155:558–60.
36. Vittecoq D, Mattlinger B, Barre-Sinoussi F, et al. Passive immunotherapy in AIDS: A randomized trial of serial human immunodeficiency virus-positive transfusion of plasma rich in p24 antibodies versus transfusions of seronegative plasma. J Infect Dis. 1992;165:364–8.
37. Cummins LM, Weinhold KJ, Matthews TJ, et al. Preparation and characterization of an intravenous solution of IgG from human immunodeficiency virus-seropositive donors. Blood. 1991;77:1111–7.
38. Higgins PJ, Paradis T, Potts BJ, et al. In vitro inhibition of a variety of human immunodeficiency virus isolates by broadly reactive, V3-directed heteroconjugate antibody. J Infect Dis. 1992;166:198–202.
39. LaRosa GJ, Davide JP, Weinhold K, et al. Conserved sequence and structural elements in the HIV-1 principal neutralizing determinant. Science. 1990;249:932–5. [erratum: Science. 1991;251, 811.]
40. Girard M, Kieny MP, Pinter A, et al. Immunization of chimpanzees confers protection against challenge with human immunodeficiency virus. Proc Natl Acad Sci USA. 1991;88:542–6.
41. Javaherian K, Langlois AJ, LaRosa GJ, et al. Broadly neutralizing antibodies elicited by the hypervariable neutralizing determinant of HIV-1. Science. 1990;250:1590–3.
42. Berman PW, Matthews TJ, Riddle L, et al. Neutralization of multiple laboratory and clinical isolates of human immunodeficiency virus type 1 (HIV-1) by antisera raised against gp120 from the MN isolate of HIV-1. J Virol. 1992;66:4464–9.
43. Furman PA, Fyfe JA, St. Clair MH, et al. Phosphorylation of 3'-azido-3'-deoxythymidine and selective interaction of the 5'-triphosphate with human immunodeficiency virus reverse transcriptase. Proc Natl Acad Sci USA. 1986;83:8333–7.
44. Varmus H. Retroviruses. Science. 1988;240:1427–35.
45. Bukrinsky MI, Stanwick TL, Dempsey MP, et al. Quiescent T lymphocytes as an inducible virus reservoir in HIV-1 infection. Science. 1991;254:423–7.
46. Zack JA, Haislip AM, Krogstad P, et al. Incompletely reverse-transcribed human immunodeficiency virus type 1 genomes in quiescent cells can function as intermediates in the retroviral life cycle. J Virol. 1992;66:1717–25.
47. Stevenson M, Haggerty S, Lamonica CA, et al. Integration is not necessary for expression of human immunodeficiency virus type 1 protein products. J Virol. 1990;64:2421–5.
48. Huang P, Farquhar D, Plunkett W. Selective action of 3'-azido-3'-deoxythymidine 5'-triphosphate on viral reverse transcriptases and human DNA polymerases. J Biol Chem. 1990;265:11914–8.
49. Vasudevachari MB, Battista C, Lane HC, et al. Prevention of the spread of HIV-1 infection with nonnucleoside reverse transcriptase inhibitors. Virology. 1992;190:269–77.
50. Yarchoan R, Thomas RV, Grafman J, et al. Long-term administration of 3'-azido-2',3'-dideoxythymidine to patients with AIDS-related neurological disease. Ann Neurol. 1988;23:S82–S87.
51. Merluzzi VJ, Hargrave KD, Labadia M, et al. Inhibition of HIV-1 replication by a nonnucleoside reverse transcriptase inhibitor. Science. 1990;250:1411–3.
52. Yarchoan R, Mitsuya H, Myers CE, et al. Clinical pharmacology of 3'-azido-2',3'-dideoxythymidine (zidovudine) and related dideoxynucleosides. N Engl J Med. 1989;321:725–38.
53. Frick LW, Nelson DJ, St. Clair MH, et al. Effects of 3'-azido-3'-deoxythymidine on the deoxynucleotide triphosphate pools of cultured human cells. Biochem Biophys Res Commun. 1988;154:124–9.
54. Watson AJ, Wilburn LM. Inhibition of HIV infection of resting peripheral blood lymphocytes by nucleosides. AIDS Res Hum Retroviruses. 1992;8:1221–7.
55. Balzarini J, Pauwels R, Baba M, et al. The in vitro and in vivo antiretrovirus activity and intracellular metabolism of 3'-azido-2',3'-dideoxythymidine and 2',3'-dideoxycytidine are highly dependent on the cell species. Biochem Pharmacol. 1988;37:897–903.
56. Tornevik Y, Jacobsson B, Britton S, et al. Intracellular metabolism of 3'-

azidothymidine in isolated human peripheral blood mononuclear cells. AIDS Res Hum Retroviruses. 1991;7:751–9.

57. Collier AC, Bozzette S, Coombs RW, et al. A pilot study of low-dose zidovudine in human immunodeficiency virus infection. N Engl J Med. 1990;323:1015–21.

58. Balzarini J, Herdewijn P, De Clercq E. Differential patterns of intracellular metabolism of 2′,3′-didehydro-2′,3′-dideoxythymidine and 3′-azido-2′,3′-dideoxythymidine, two potent anti-human immunodeficiency virus compounds. J Biol Chem. 1989;264:6127–33.

59. Perno CF, Yarchoan R, Balzarini J, et al. Different pattern of activity of inhibitors of the human immunodeficiency virus in lymphocytes and monocyte/macrophages. Antiviral Res. 1992;17:289–304.

60. Zhu Z, Hitchcock MJM, Sommadossi JP. Metabolism and DNA interaction of 2′,3′-didehydro-2′,3′-dideoxythymidine in human bone marrow cells. Mol Pharmacol. 1991;40:838–45.

61. Richman DD, Fischl MA, Grieco MH, et al. The toxicity of azidothymidine (AZT) in the treatment of patients with AIDS and AIDS-related complex: A double-blind, placebo-controlled trial. N Engl J Med. 1987;317:192–7.

62. Yarchoan R, Brouwers P, Spitzer AR, et al. Response of human-immunodeficiency-virus-associated neurological disease to 3′-azido-3′-deoxythymidine. Lancet. 1987;1:132–6.

63. Berger AR, Arezzo JC, Schaumburg HH, et al. 2′-3′-dideoxycytidine (ddC) toxic neuropathy: A study of 52 patients. Neurology. 1993;43:358–62.

64. Hirsch MS. Azidothymidine. J Infect Dis. 1988;157:427–31.

65. Rinaldo C, Huang XL, Piazza P, et al. Augmentation of cellular immune function during the early phase of zidovudine treatment of AIDS patients. J Infect Dis. 1991;164:638–45.

66. Schmitt FA, Bigley JW, McKinnis R, et al. Neuropsychological outcome of zidovudine (AZT) treatment of patients with AIDS and AIDS-related complex. N Engl J Med. 1988;319:1573–8.

67. Surbone A, Yarchoan R, McAtee N, et al. Treatment of the acquired immunodeficiency syndrome (AIDS) and AIDS-related complex with a regimen of 3′-azido-2′,3′-dideoxythymidine (azidothymidine or zidovudine) and acyclovir. A pilot study. Ann Intern Med. 1988;108:534–40.

68. Cooper DA, Pehrson PO, Pedersen C, et al. The efficacy and safety of zidovudine alone or as cotherapy with acyclovir for the treatment of patients with AIDS and AIDS-related complex: A double-blind, randomized trial. AIDS. 1993;7:197–207.

69. Tadepalli SM, Puckett L, Jeal S, et al. Differential assay of zidovudine and its glucuronide metabolite in serum and urine with a radioimmunoassay kit. Clin Chem. 1990;36:897–900.

70. McLeod GX, Hammer SM. Zidovudine: Five years later. Ann Intern Med. 1992;117:487–501.

71. Henry K, Chinnock BJ, Quinn RP, et al. Concurrent zidovudine levels in semen and serum determined by radioimmunoassay in patients with AIDS or AIDS-related complex. JAMA. 1988;259:3023–6.

72. Kuster H, Vogt M, Joos B, et al. A method for the quantification of intracellular zidovudine nucleotides. J Infect Dis. 1991;164:773–6.

73. Fischl M, Galpin JE, Levine JD, et al. Recombinant human erythropoietin for patients with AIDS treated with zidovudine. N Engl J Med. 1990;322:1488–93.

74. Miles SA, Mitsuyasu RT, Moreno J, et al. Combined therapy with recombinant granulocyte colony-stimulating factor and erythropoietin decreases hematologic toxicity from zidovudine. Blood. 1991;77:2109–17.

75. Mitsuyasu RT. Use of recombinant interferons and hematopoietic growth factors in patients infected with human immunodeficiency virus. Rev Infect Dis. 1991;13:979–84.

76. Mhiri C, Baudrimont M, Bonne G, et al. Zidovudine myopathy: A distinctive disorder associated with mitochondrial dysfunction. Ann Neurol. 1991;29:606–14.

77. Lamperth L, Dalakas MC, Dagani F, et al. Abnormal skeletal and cardiac muscle mitochondria induced by zidovudine (AZT) in human muscle in vitro and in an animal model. Lab Invest. 1991;65:742–51.

78. Dalakas MC, Illa I, Pezeshkpour GH, et al. Mitochondrial myopathy caused by long-term zidovudine therapy. N Engl J Med. 1990;322:1098–105.

79. Arnaudo E, Dalakas M, Shanske S, et al. Depletion of muscle mitochondrial DNA in AIDS patients with zidovudine-induced myopathy. Lancet. 1991;337:508–10.

80. Groopman JE. Zidovudine intolerance. Rev Infect Dis. 1990;12(Suppl 5):S500–6.

81. Larder BA, Darby G, Richman DD. HIV with reduced sensitivity to zidovudine isolated during prolonged therapy. Science. 1989;243:1731–4.

82. Richman DD, Grimes JM, Lagakos SW. Effect of stage of disease and drug dose on zidovudine susceptibilities of isolates of human immunodeficiency virus. J AIDS. 1990;3:743–6.

83. Larder BA, Kemp SD. Multiple mutations in HIV-1 reverse transcriptase confer high-level resistance to zidovudine. Science. 1989;246:1155–9.

84. Kellam PA, Boucher CAB, Larder BA. Fifth mutation in human immunodeficiency virus type 1 reverse transcriptase contributes to the development of high-level resistance to zidovudine. Proc Natl Acad Sci USA. 1992;89:1934–8.

85. Edlin BR, St. Clair MH, Pitha PM, et al. In-vitro resistance to zidovudine and alpha-interferon in HIV-1 isolates from patients: Correlations with treatment duration and response. Ann Intern Med. 1992;117:457–60. [erratum: Ann Intern Med. 1992;117:879.]

86. Larder BA, Kellam P, Kemp SD. Zidovudine resistance predicted by direct detection of mutations in DNA from HIV-infected lymphocytes. AIDS. 1991;5:137–44.

87. Erice A, Mayers DL, Strike DG, et al. Primary infection with zidovudine resistant HIV-type 1. N Engl J Med. 1993;328:110–5.

88. Fitzgibbons JE, Gaur S, Frenkel LD, et al. Transmission from one child to another of HIV type 1 with a zidovudine resistant mutation. N Engl J Med. 1993;329:1835–41.

89. Kozal MJ, Shafer RW, Winters MA, et al. A mutation in human immunodeficiency virus reverse transcriptase and decline in CD4 lymphocyte numbers in long-term zidovudine recipients. J Infect Dis. 1993;167:526–32.

90. Tudor-Williams G, St. Clair MH, McKiney RE, et al. HIV-1 sensitivity to zidovudine and clinical outcome in children. Lancet. 1992;339:15–9.

91. Land S, Treloar G, McPhee D, et al. Decreased in vitro susceptibility to zidovudine of HIV isolates obtained from patients with AIDS. J Infect Dis. 1990;161:326–9.

92. Mayers DL, McCurchan FE, Sanders-Boell EE, et al. Characterization of HIV-1 isolates arising after prolonged zidovudine therapy. J AIDS. 1992;5:749–59.

93. Boucher CAB, Lange JMA, Miedema FF, et al. HIV-1 biological phenotype and the development of zidovudine resistance in relation to disease progression in asymptomatic individuals during treatment. AIDS. 1992;6:1259–64.

94. Lambert JS, Seidlin M, Reichman RC, et al. 2′,3′-Dideoxyinosine (ddI) in patients with the acquired immunodeficiency syndrome or AIDS-related complex. A phase I trial. N Engl J Med. 1990;322:1333–9.

95. Drusano GL, Yuen GJ, Lambert JS, et al. Relationship between dideoxyinosine exposure, CD4 counts, and p24 antigen levels in human immunodeficiency virus infection. Ann Intern Med. 1992;116:562–6.

96. Cooley TP, Kunches LM, Saunders CA, et al. Once-daily administration of 2′,3′-dideoxyinosine (ddI) in patients with the acquired immunodeficiency syndrome or AIDS-related complex. Results of a phase I trial. N Engl J Med. 1990;322:1340–5.

97. Ahluwalia G, Cooney DA, Mitsuya H, et al. Initial studies on the cellular pharmacology of 2′,3′-dideoxyinosine, an inhibitor of HIV infectivity. Biochem Pharmacol. 1987;36:3797–800.

98. Faulds D, Brogden RN. Didanosine. A review of its antiviral activity, pharmacokinetic properties and therapeutic potential in human immunodeficiency virus infection. Drugs. 1992;44:94–116.

99. Yarchoan R, Mitsuya H, Thomas RV, et al. In vivo activity against HIV and favorable toxicity profile of 2′,3′-dideoxyinosine. Science. 1989;245:412–5.

100. Kamali F. Clinical pharmacology of zidovudine and other 2′,3′-dideoxynucleoside analogues. Clin Invest. 1993;71:392–405.

101. Yarchoan R, Mitsuya H, Myers CE, et al. Clinical pharmacology of 3′-azido-2′,3′-dideoxythymidine (zidovudine) and related dideoxynucleosides. N Engl J Med. 1989;321:726–38.

102. Butler KM, Venzon D, Henry N, et al. Pancreatitis in human immunodeficiency virus-infected children receiving dideoxyinosine. Pediatrics. 1993;91:747–51.

103. Kieburtz KD, Seidlin M, Lambert JS, et al. Extended follow-up of peripheral neuropathy in patients with AIDS and AIDS-related complex treated with dideoxyinosine. J Acquir Immune Defic Syndr. 1992;5:60–4.

104. Schwartz MS, Brandt LJ. The spectrum of pancreatic disorders in patients with acquired immunodeficiency syndrome. Am J Gastroenterol. 1989;84:459–62.

105. Mallory A, Kern F Jr. Drug-induced pancreatitis: A critical review. Gastroenterology. 1989;78:813–20.

106. Collier AC, Coombs RW, Fischl MA, et al. Combination therapy with zidovudine and didanosine compared to zidovudine alone in HIV-1 infection. Ann Intern Med. 1993;119:786–93.

107. Martin JL, Wilson JE, Haynes RL, et al. Mechanism of resistance of human immunodeficiency virus type 1 to 2′,3′-dideoxyinosine. Proc Natl Acad Sci USA. 1993;90:6135–9.

108. Eron JJ, Chow YK, Caliendo AM, et al. Pol mutations conferring zidovudine and didanosine resistance with different effects in vitro yield multiply resistant human immunodeficiency virus type 1 isolates in vivo. Antimicrob Agents Chemother. 1993;37:1480–1.

109. St. Clair MH, Martin JL, Tudor-Williams G, et al. Resistance to ddI and sensitivity to AZT induced by a mutation in HIV-1 reverse transcriptase. Science. 1991;253:1557–9.

110. Gu Z, Gao Q, Li X, et al. Novel mutation in the human immunodeficiency virus type 1 reverse transcriptase gene that encodes cross-resistance to 2′,3′-dideoxyinosine and 2′,3′-dideoxycytidine. J Virol. 1992;66:7128–35.

111. Balzarini J, Karlsson A, Perez-Perez MJ, et al. Treatment of human immunodeficiency virus type 1 (HIV-1)-infected cells with combinations of HIV-1-specific inhibitors results in a different resistance pattern than does treatment with single drug therapy. J Virol. 1993;67:5353–9.

112. Shirasaka T, Yarchoan R, O'Brien MC, et al. Changes in drug sensitivity of human immunodeficiency virus type 1 during therapy with azidothymicine, dideoxycytidine, and dideoxyinosine: An in vitro comparative study. Proc Natl Acad Sci USA. 1993;90:562–6.

113. Hitchcock MJ. In vitro antiviral activity of didanosine compared with that of other dideoxynucleoside analogs against laboratory strains and clinical isolates of human immunodeficiency virus. Clin Infect Dis. 1993;(Suppl 1):S16–21.

114. Dimitrov DH, Hollinger FB, Baker CJ, et al. Study of human immunodeficiency virus resistance to 2′-3′-dideoxyinosine and zidovudine in sequential isolates from pediatric patients on long-term therapy. J Infect Dis. 1993;167:818–23.

115. Shelton MJ, O'Donnell AM, Morse GD. Zalcitibine. Ann Pharmacother. 1993;27:480–9.

116. Whittington R, Brogden RN. Zalcitabine. A review of its pharmacology and clinical potential in acquired immunodeficiency syndrome (AIDS). Drugs. 1992;44:656–83.

117. Lipsky JJ. Zalcitabine and didanosine. Lancet. 1993;341:30–2.

118. Fischl MA, Olson RM, Follansbee SE, et al. Zalcitabine compared with

zidovudine in patients with advanced HIV-1 infection who received previous zidovudine therapy. Ann Intern Med. 1993;118:822–3.

119. Yarchoan R, Perno CF, Thomas RV, et al. Phase I studies of 2′,3′-dideoxy-cytidine in severe human immunodeficiency virus infection as a single agent and alternation with zidovudine (AZT). Lancet. 1988;1:76–81.

120. Merigan TC, Skowron G, Bozzette SA, et al. Circulating p24 antigen levels and responses to dideoxycytidine in human immunodeficiency virus (HIV) infections. Ann Intern Med. 1989;110:189–94.

121. Saag MS. Treatment of HIV infection: The antiretroviral nucleoside analogues. Hosp Pract (Off Ed). 1992;(Suppl 2):S26–36.

122. HIVID (zalcitabine) package insert. Roche Laboratories, 340 Kingsland St., Nutley, NJ 07110.

123. Simpson DM, Olney RK. Peripheral neuropathies associated with human immunodeficiency virus infection. Neurol Clin. 1992;10:685–711.

124. Meng TC, Fischl MA, Boota AM, et al. Combination therapy with zidovudine and dideoxycytidine in patients with advanced human immunodeficiency virus infection. A phase I/II study. Ann Intern Med. 1992;116:13–20.

125. Yarchoan R, Pluda JM, Perno CF, et al. Initial clinical experience with dideoxynucleosides as single agents and in combination therapy. Ann NY Acad Sci. 1990;616:328–43.

126. Broder S, Yarchoan R. Dideoxycytidine: Current clinical experience and future prospects. A summary. Am J Med. 1990;88:31S–33S.

127. Pizzo PA, Butler K, Balis F, et al. Dideoxycytidine alone and in an alternating schedule with zidovudine in children with symptomatic human immunodeficiency infection. J Pediatr. 1990;117:799–808.

128. Drew L, Olson R, Pollard R, et al. The efficacy of zalcitabine (ddC, HIVID) versus zidovudine (ZDV) as monotherapy in ZDV naive patients with advanced HIV disease: A randomized, double-blind, comparative trial (ACTG 114:N330) IXth International Conference on AIDS, Berlin, Germany, June 6–11, 1993, Abstract PO-B26-2113.

129. Dudley MN, Graham KK, Kaul S, et al. Pharmacokinetics of stavudine in patients with AIDS or AIDS-related complex. J Infect Dis. 1992;166:480–5.

130. Mansuri MM, Starrett JE, Ghazzouli I, et al. 1-(2,3-dideoxy-B-D-glycero-pent-2-enofuranosyl)thymidine (D4T): A highly potent and selective anti-HIV agent. J Med Chem. 1989;32:461–6.

131. August EM, Marongiu ME, Lin TS, et al. Initial studies on the cellular pharmacology of 3′-deoxythymidin-2′-ene (d4T): A potent and selective inhibitor of human immunodeficiency virus. Biochem Pharmacol. 1988;37:4419–22.

132. Dunkle L, Cross A, Gugliotti R, et al. Dose escalating study of safety and efficacy of dideoxy-didehydrothymidine (d4T) for HIV infection. Antiviral Res. 1990;1(Suppl):116.

133. Browne MJ. Phase I study of 2′,3′-didehydro-2′,3′-dideoxythymidine (D4T) in patients with AIDS or ARC. VI International Conference on AIDS, June 20–23, 1990. Abstract S.B. 456, 1990.

134. Squires KE, Weiss W, Sacks H, et al. Effect of 2′,3′-didehydro-3′-deoxy-thymidine (D4T) on p24 antigenemia in patients with AIDS and ARC. In: VI International Conference on AIDS. Abstract TH.A.241, 180, 1990.

135. Dueweke TJ, Poppe SM, Romero DL, et al. U-90152S, a potent inhibitor of human immunodeficiency virus type 1 replication. Antimicrob Agents Chemother. 1993;37:1127–31.

136. Pauwels R, Andries K, Desmyter J, et al. Potent and selective inhibition of HIV-1 replication by a novel series of TIBO derivatives. Nature (London). 1990;343:470–4.

137. White EL, Buckheit RW, Ross LJ, et al. A TIBO derivative, R82913, is a potent inhibitor of HIV-1 reverse transcriptase with heteropolymer templates. Antiviral Res. 1991;16:257–66.

138. Romero DL, Busso M, Tan CK, et al. Nonnucleoside reverse transcriptase inhibitors that potently and specifically block human immunodeficiency virus type 1 replication. Proc Natl Acad Sci USA. 1991;88:8806–10.

139. Saari WS, Hoffman JM, Wai JS, et al. 2-Pyridinone derivatives: A new class of nonnucleoside HIV-1 specific reverse transcriptase inhibitors. J Med Chem. 1991;34:2922–5.

140. Koup RA, Merluzzi VJ, Hargrave KD, et al. Inhibition of human immunodeficiency virus type 1 (HIV-1) replication by the dipyridodiazepinone BI-RG-587. J Infect Dis. 1991;163:966–70.

141. Starnes MC, Cheng Y-C. Human immunodeficiency virus reverse transcriptase-associated RNase H activity. J Biol Chem. 1989;264:7073–7.

142. Kopp EB, Miglietta JJ, Shrutkowski AG, et al. Steady state kinetics and inhibition of HIV-1 reverse transcriptase by a non-nucleoside dipyridodiazepinone, BI-RG-587, using a heteropolymeric template. Nucleic Acids Res. 1991;19:3035–9.

143. Vasudevachari MB, Battista C, Lane HC, et al. Prevention of the spread of HIV-1 infection with nonnucleoside reverse transcriptase inhibitors. Virology. 1992;190:269–77.

144. Saag MS, Emini EA, Laskin OL, et al. A short clinical evaluation of L-697, 661, a non-nucleoside inhibitor of HIV-1 reverse transcriptase. N Engl J Med. 1993;329:1065–72.

145. Richman D, Shih CK, Lowy I, et al. Human immunodeficiency virus type 1 mutants resistant to nonnucleoside inhibitors of reverse transcriptase arise in tissue culture. Proc Natl Acad Sci USA. 1991;88:11241–5.

146. Dueweke TJ, Pushkarskaya T, Poppe SM, et al. A mutation in reverse transcriptase of bis(heteroaryl)piperazine-resistant human immunodeficiency virus type 1 that confers increased sensitivity to other nonnucleoside inhibitors. Proc Natl Acad Sci USA. 1993;90:4713–7.

147. Nunberg JH, Schleif WA, Boots EJ, et al. Viral resistance to human immunodeficiency virus type 1-specific pyridinone reverse transcriptase inhibitors. J Virol 1991;65:4887–92.

148. Cheeseman SH, Hattox SE, McLaughlin MM, et al. Pharmacokinetics of nevirapine: Initial single-rising dose study in humans. Antimicrob Agents Chemother. 1993;37:178–82.

149. Koup RA, Brewster F, Grob P, et al. Nevirapine synergistically inhibits HIV-1 replication in combination with zidovudine, interferon or CD4 immunoadhesin. AIDS. 1993;7:1181–4.

150. Dueweke TJ, Poppe SM, Romero DL, et al. U-90152S, a potent inhibitor of human immunodeficiency virus type 1 replication. Antimicrob Agents Chemother. 1993;37:1127–31.

151. Romero D, Morge R, Biles C, et al. Discovery, synthesis, and bioactivity of bis(hetero)piperazines: A novel class of non-nucleoside HIV-1 reverse transcriptase inhibitors. J Med Chem. 1994;37:999–1014.

152. Campbell TB, Young RK, Eron JJ, et al. Inhibition of human immunodeficiency virus type 1 replication in vitro by the bis(heteroaryl)piperazine atevirdine (U-87201E) in combination with zidovudine or didanosine. J Infect Dis. 1993;168:318–26.

153. Palestine AG, Polis MA, De Smet MD, et al. A randomized, controlled trial of foscarnet in the treatment of cytomegalovirus retinitis in patients with AIDS. Ann Intern Med. 1991;115:665–73.

154. Jacobson MA, Crowe S, Levy J, et al. Effect of foscarnet therapy on infection with human immunodeficiency virus in patients with AIDS. J Infect Dis. 1988;158:862–5.

155. Jacobson MA, van der Horst C, Causey DM, et al. In vivo additive antiretroviral effect of combined zidovudine and foscarnet for human immunodeficiency virus infection (ACTG Protocol 053). J Infect Dis. 1991;163:1219–22.

156. Studies of Ocular Complications of AIDS Research Group, in collaboration with the AIDS Clinical Trials Group. Mortality in patients with the acquired immunodeficiency syndrome treated with either foscarnet or ganciclovir for cytomegalovirus retinitis. N Engl J Med. 1992;326:213–20.

157. Berglund O, Engman K, Ehrnst A, et al. Combined treatment of symptomatic human immunodeficiency virus type 1 infection with native interferon-alpha and zidovudine. J Infect Dis. 1991;163:710–5.

158. Krown SE, Gold JW, Niedzwiecki D, et al. Interferon-alpha with zidovudine: Safety, tolerance and clinical virologic effects in patients with Kaposi sarcoma associated with the acquired immunodeficiency syndrome (AIDS). Ann Intern Med. 1990;112:812–21. [erratum: Ann Int Med. 1990;1130:334.]

159. Lane HC, Kovacs JA, Feinberg J, et al. Antiretroviral effects of interferon-alpha in AIDS-associated Kaposi's sarcoma. Lancet. 1988;2:1218–22.

160. de Wit R, Schattenkerk JK, Boucher CA, et al. Clinical and virological effects of high-dose recombinant interferon-alpha in disseminated AIDS-related Kaposi's sarcoma. Lancet. 1988;2:1214–7.

161. Interferon Alpha Study Group. A randomized placebo-controlled trial of recombinant human interferon alpha 2a in patients with AIDS. J AIDS. 1988;1:111–8.

162. Lane HC, Davey V, Kovacs JA, et al. Interferon-alpha in patients with asymptomatic human immunodeficiency virus (HIV) infection. Ann Intern Med. 1990;112:805–11.

163. Mildvan D, Bassiakos YD, and the ACTG 068 Collaborative Group. Zidovudine and interferon-alpha 2a: Ongoing assessment of synergy and tolerance in early ARC patients, ACTG 068. Eighth International Conference on AIDS, July 19–24, 1992, Amsterdam, Netherlands, Abstract PoB 3586.

164. Kovacs JA, Deyton L, Davey R, et al. Combined zidovudine and interferon-a therapy in patients with Kaposi sarcoma and the acquired immunodeficiency syndrome (AIDS). Ann Intern Med. 1989;111:280–7.

165. Koech DK, Obel AO, Minowada J, et al. Low dose oral alpha-interferon therapy for patients seropositive for human immunodeficiency virus type-1 (HIV-1). Mol Biother. 1990;2:91–5.

166. Kaiser G, Jaeger H, Birkmann J, et al. Low-dose oral natural human interferon-alpha in 29 patients with HIV-1 infection: A double-blind, randomized, placebo-controlled trial. AIDS. 1992;6:563–9.

167. Navia M, Fitzgerald P, McKeever B, et al. Three-dimensional structure of aspartyl protease from HIV-1. Nature. 1989;337:615–20.

168. Loeb DD, Hutchison CA III, Edgell MH, et al. Mutational analysis of human immunodeficiency virus type 1 protease suggests functional homology with aspartic proteinases. J Virol. 1989;63:111–21.

169. Kohl NE, Emini EA, Schleif WA, et al. Active human immunodeficiency virus protease is required for viral infectivity. Proc Natl Acad Sci USA. 1988;85:4686–90.

170. Peng C, Ho BK, Chang TW, et al. Role of human immunodeficiency virus type 1-specific protease in core protein maturation and viral infectivity. J Virol. 1989;63:2550–6.

171. Robins T, Plattner J. HIV protease inhibitors: Their anti-HIV activity and potential role in treatment. J AIDS. 1993;6:162–70.

172. Roberts NA, Martin JA, Kinchington D, et al. Rational design of peptide-based HIV protease inhibitors. Science. 1990;4:248.

173. Lambert DM, Petteway SJ Jr, McDanal CE, et al. Human immunodeficiency virus type 1 protease inhibitors irreversibly block infectivity of purified virions from chronically infected cells. Antimicrob Agents Chemother. 1992;36:982–8.

174. Perno CF, Bergamini A, Pesce CD, et al. Inhibition of the protease of human immunodeficiency virus blocks replication and infectivity of the virus in chronically infected macrophages. J Infect Dis. 1993;168:1148–56.

175. Kageyama S, Weinstein J, Shirasaka T, et al. In vitro inhibition of HIV-1 replication by C2 symmetry-based HIV protease inhibitors as single agents or in combinations. Antimicrob Agents Chemother. 1992;36:926–33.

176. Kempf DJ, Marsh KC, Paul DA, et al. Antiviral and pharmacokinetic properties of C2 symmetric inhibitors of the human immunodeficiency virus type 1 protease. Antimicrob Agents Chemother. 1991;35:2209–14.

177. Otto MJ, Garber S, Winslow D, et al. In vitro isolation and partial characterization of HIV variants with reduced sensitivity to C2 symmetrical inhibitors of HIV-1 protease. Abstract ThA 1505 presented at the VIIIth International Conference on AIDS, Amsterdam, Netherlands, 1992.

178. Hsu MC, Schutt AD, Holly M, et al. Inhibition of HIV replication in acute

and chronic infection in vitro by a tat antagonist. Science. 1991;254: 1799–802.

179. Potash MJ, Bentsman G, McKinley G, et al. A tat antagonist inhibits HIV-1 induction in naturally infected and experimentally infected T cells. Biochem Biophys Res Commun. 1992;189:250–6.

180. Fischl M, Resnick L, Coombs R, et al. The preliminary efficacy and safety of N-butyl-deoxynojirimycin (SC-48334), an α-glucosidase I inhibitor, in combination with zidovudine (ZDV). IXth International Conference on AIDS, Berlin, Germany, June 6–11, 1993, Abstract PO-B26-2039.

181. Li G, Lisziewicz J, Sun D, et al. Inhibition of rev activity and human immunodeficiency virus type 1 replication by antisense oligodeoxynucleotide phosphorothioate analogs directed against the rev-responsive element. J Virol. 1993;67:6882–8.

182. Sarver N, Cantin EM, Chang PS, et al. Ribozymes as potential anti-HIV-1 therapeutic agents. Science. 191;247:1222–5.

183. Yu M, Ojwang J, Yamada O, et al. A hairpin ribozyme inhibits expression of diverse strains of human immunodeficiency virus type 1. Proc Natl Acad Sci USA. 1993;90:6340–4; Erratum, Proc Natl Acad Sci USA. 1993;90:8303.

184. Plata F, Dadaglio G, Chenciner N, et al. Cytotoxic T lymphocytes in HIV-induced disease: Implications for therapy and vaccination. Immunodef Rev. 1989;1:227–46.

185. Yarchoan R, Mitsuya H, Broder S. The immunology of HIV infection: Implications for therapy. AIDS Res Hum Retrovir. 1992;8:1023–31.

186. Nixon DF, McMichael AJ. Cytotoxic T-cell recognition of HIV proteins and peptides. AIDS. 1991;5:1049–59.

187. Riddell SR, Gilbert MJ, Greenberg PD. CD8+ cytotoxic T cell therapy of cytomegalovirus and HIV infection. Curr Opin Immunol. 1993;5:484–91.

188. Bahner I, Zhou C, Yu XJ, et al. Comparison of transdominant inhibitory mutant human immunodeficiency virus type 1 genes expressed by retroviral vectors in human T lymphocytes. J Virol. 1993;67:3199–207.

189. Bevec D, Dobrovnik M, Hauber J, et al. Inhibition of human immunodeficiency virus type 1 replication in human T cells by retroviral-mediated gene transfer of a dominant-negative rev trans-activator. Proc Natl Acad Sci USA. 1992;89:9870–4.

190. Creagh-Kirk T, Doi P, Andrews E, et al. Survival experience among patients with AIDS receiving zidovudine. JAMA. 1988;260:3009–15.

191. Moore RD, Keruly J, Richman DD, et al. Natural history of advanced HIV disease in patients treated with zidovudine. AIDS. 1992;6:671–7.

192. Moore RD, Hidalgo J, Sugland BW, et al. Zidovudine and the natural history of the acquired immunodeficiency syndrome. N Engl J Med. 1991;324:1412–6.

193. Graham NMH, Zeger SL, Park LP, et al. The effects on survival of early treatment of human immunodeficiency virus infection. N Engl J Med. 1992;326:1037–42.

194. Vella S, Giuliano M, Pezzotti P, et al. Survival of zidovudine-treated patients with AIDS compared with that of contemporary untreated patients. JAMA. 1992;267:1232–6.

195. Leoung GS, Feigal DW, Montgomery AB, et al. Aerosolized pentamidine for prophylaxis against *Pneumocystis carinii* pneumonia. N Engl J Med. 1990;323:769–75.

196. Easterbrook PJ, Keruly JC, Creagh-Kirk T, et al. Racial and ethnic differences in outcome in zidovudine-treated patients with advanced HIV disease. JAMA. 1991;266:2713–8.

197. Lagakos S, Fischl MA, Stein DS, et al. Effects of zidovudine therapy in minority and other subpopulations with early HIV infection. JAMA. 1991;266:2709–12.

198. Volberding P, Lagakos SW, Koch MA, et al. Zidovudine in asymptomatic human immunodeficiency virus infection. A controlled trial in persons with fewer than 500 CD4-positive cells per cubic millimeter. N Engl J Med. 1990;322:941–9.

199. State-of-the-Art Conference on Azidothymidine Therapy for Early HIV Infection. Am J Med. 1990;89:335–44.

200. Fischl MA, Richman DD, Hansen N, et al. The safety and efficacy of zidovudine (AZT) in the treatment of subjects with mildly symptomatic human immunodeficiency virus type 1 (HIV) infection. Ann Intern Med. 1990;112:727–37.

201. Cooper DA, Pedersen C, Aiuti F, et al. The efficacy and safety of zidovudine with or without acyclovir in the treatment of patients with AIDS-related complex. AIDS. 1991;5:933–43.

202. Cosler LE, Lambrinos J. Zidovudine's impact on resource use by patients with symptomatic HIV illness: A large sample analysis. Inquiry. 1992;29:345–55.

203. Hellinger FJ. The lifetime cost of treating a person with HIV. JAMA. 1993;270:474–8.

204. Lynn LA, Schulman KA, Eisenberg JM. The pharmacoeconomics of HIV disease. PharmacoEcon 1992;1:161–74.

205. Gelber RD, Lenderking WR, Cotton DJ, et al. Quality-of-life evaluation in a clinical trial of zidovudine therapy in patients with mildly symptomatic HIV infection. Ann Intern Med. 1992;116:961–6.

206. Schulman KA, Lynn LA, Glick HA, et al. Cost effectiveness of low-dose zidovudine therapy for asymptomatic patients with human immunodeficiency virus (HIV) infection. Ann Intern Med. 1991;114:798–802.

207. Lenderking WR, Gelber RJ, Cotton DJ, et al. Evaluation of the quality of life associated with zidovudine treatment in asymptomatic human immunodeficiency virus infection. N Engl J Med. 1994;330:738–43.

208. Hamilton JD, Hartigan PM, Simberkoff MS, et al. A controlled trial of early versus late treatment with zidovudine in symptomatic human immunodeficiency virus infection. N Engl J Med. 1992;326:437–443.

209. Aboulker J-P, Swart AM. Preliminary analysis of the Concorde trial. Concorde Coordinating Committee (Letter). Lancet 1993;341:889–90.

210. Hirsch MS. Chemotherapy of human immunodeficiency virus infections: current practice and future prospects. J Infect Dis 1990;161:845–57.

211. Broder S, Mitsuya H, Yarchoan R, et al. NIH conference. Antiretroviral therapy in AIDS. Ann Intern Med. 1990;113:604–18.

212. Fauci AS. The human immunodeficiency virus: Infectivity and mechanisms of pathogenesis. Science. 1988;239:617–22.

213. Pantaleo G, Graziosi C, Fauci AS. The immunopathogenesis of human immunodeficiency virus infection. N Engl J Med. 1993;328:327–35.

214. Piatak M, Saag MS, Yang LC, et al. High levels of HIV-1 in plasma during all stages of infection determined by competitive PCR. Science. 1993;259:1749–54.

215. Michael NL, Vahey M, Burke DS, et al. Viral DNA and mRNA expression correlate with the stage of human immunodeficiency virus (HIV) type 1 infection in humans: Evidence for viral replication in all stages of HIV disease. J Virol. 1992;66:310–6.

216. Coombs RW, Collier AC, Allain J-P, et al. Plasma viremia in human immunodeficiency virus infection. N Engl J Med. 1989;321:1626–31.

217. Clark SJ, Saag MS, Decker WD, et al. High titers of cytopathic virus in plasma of patients with symptomatic primary HIV-1 infection. N Engl J Med. 1991;324:954–60.

218. Cooper DA, Gatell JM, Kroon S, et al. Zidovudine in persons with asymptomatic HIV infection and CD4+ cell counts greater than 400 per cubic millimeter. The European-Australian Collaborative Group. N Engl J Med. 1993;329:297–303.

219. Dolin R, Amato DA, Fischl MA. Efficacy of didanosine (ddI) versus zidovudine (ZDV) in patients with no or less than equal to 16 weeks of prior ZDV therapy. Ninth Int Conf AIDS, 1993; Berlin, June 6–11, Abstract No. WS-B24-1.

220. Meng TC, Fischl MA, Boota AM, et al. Combination therapy with zidovudine and dideoxycytidine in patients with advanced human immunodeficiency virus infection. A phase I/II study. Ann Intern Med. 1992;116:13–20.

221. Ragni M, Dafni R, Amato D, et al. Combination zidovudine and dideoxyinosine in asymptomatic HIV(+) patients. Eighth International Conference on AIDS, July 19–24, 1992, Amsterdam, Netherlands, Abstract MoB0055.

222. Yarchoan R, et al. Therapy of AIDS or symptomatic HIV with simultaneous or alternating regimens of AZT and ddI. Eighth International Conference on AIDS, July 19–24, 1992, Amsterdam, Netherlands, Abstract MoB0054.

223. Skowron G, Bozzette SA, Lim L, et al. Alternating and intermittent regimens of zidovudine and dideoxycytidine in patients with AIDS or AIDS-related complex. Ann Intern Med. 1993;118:321–30.

224. Fischl M, Collier A, Stanley K, et al. The safety and efficacy of zidovudine (ZDV) and zalcitabine (DDC) or DDC alone versus ZDV. IXth International Conference on AIDS, Berlin, Germany, June 6–11, 1993, Abstract WS-B25-1.

225. Sperling RS, Stratton P, O'Sullivan MJ, et al. A survey of zidovudine use in pregnant women with human immunodeficiency virus infection. N Engl J Med. 1992;326:857–61.

226. Watts H, Brown ZA, Tartaglione T, et al. Pharmacokinetic disposition of zidovudine during pregnancy. J Infect Dis. 1991;163:226–32.

227. Executive Summary NIAID Bulletin 1994:ACTG-076.

228. Sande MA, Carpenter CCJ, Cobbs CG, et al. for the National Institute of Allergy and Infectious Diseases State of the Art Panel on Anti-Retroviral Therapy for Adult HIV-infected patients. JAMA. 1993;270:2583–9.

229. Katzenstein DA, Holodniy M. Quantitative virological measures of antiretroviral therapy. AIDS Clin Rev. 1992;41–67.

230. Fischl M. Combination antiretroviral therapy for HIV infection. Hosp Pract. 1994;29:43–8.

105. MANAGEMENT OF OPPORTUNISTIC INFECTIONS ASSOCIATED WITH HIV INFECTION

HENRY MASUR

The quality and duration of survival for patients with human immunodeficiency virus (HIV) infection has improved since acquired immunodeficiency syndrome (AIDS) was first recognized in the early 1980s.[1–3] Although much of this improvement is attributable to antiretroviral therapy, a substantial contribution is made by more effective management of the opportunistic processes that complicate immunosuppression caused by HIV.[1]

This increasingly successful management has been due to advances in several convergent areas: understanding unique features of the natural history of HIV-associated opportunistic infections; recognizing when these opportunistic processes occur in the course of immunologic decline; developing new diagnostic techniques; identifying more effective therapies; developing more effective, more comprehensive preventive strategies; and improving education of health care workers and patients.

The range and diversity of new approaches to the management of opportunistic infections in patients with HIV infection present problems as well as opportunities. Many patients have difficulty affording the cost of medical care or cannot take time from work or family responsibilities to obtain optimal management. Most patients find it difficult to comply with highly complex schedules of assessments and medications. Moreover, familiar pathogens such as cytomegalovirus (CMV), *Candida,* and *Mycobacterium tuberculosis* are increasingly resistant to the most widely used agents. In addition, previously unrecognized or seldom recognized pathogens such as *Microsporidia, Mycobacterium haemophilum,* or *Bartonella (Rochalimaea)* are now producing clinical disease as patients live longer and receive preventive management for the more frequently recognized pathogens.

PROSPECTIVE MONITORING

Prospective clinical and laboratory assessment is vital to the effective management of opportunistic infections in patients with HIV infection, just as it is important to determine prognosis and to decide the optimal time for antiretroviral intervention.

The CD4+ T-lymphocyte count is a valuable marker for determining when patients are at increased risk for the development of a specific opportunistic infection[4-9] (also see Ch. 102, Fig. 5). For example, *Pneumocystis carinii* pneumonia (PCP) rarely occurs in patients who have CD4+ T-lymphocyte counts above 200–250 cells/mm^3,[7,8] and disseminated *Mycobacterium avium* complex (MAC) will rarely occur in patients with counts higher than 75–100 cells/mm^3.[10-12] This information is very helpful in a diagnostic evaluation. For example, when a patient with a CD4+ T-lymphocyte count of 700 cells/mm^3 develops cough and fever, the likelihood that this syndrome is caused by PCP is slim. Thus, sputum examination for *Pneumocystis* is generally not necessary and most attention should be directed at common bacterial and viral pathogens when respiratory secretions are processed. In contrast, when the CD4+ T-lymphocyte count is 25 cells/mm^3, identification of *Pneumocystis* in sputum or bronchoalveolar lavage is a very important focus because PCP is so common in this patient population. Sequential CD4+ T-lymphocyte counts in a patient are shown in Figure 1, in Chapter 101, as an example of the chronology of immune dysfunction. There is considerable variability, however, in how quickly immune function deteriorates in individual patients.[4-6,13-16]

Although CD4+ T-lymphocyte counts provide a useful estimate of susceptibility to certain infections, they are not perfect predictive tools. For example, over 90 percent of cases of PCP occur in patients with CD4+ T-lymphocyte counts under 200 cells/mm^3; however, some cases occur in patients with counts reported in the 200–300 cells/mm^3 range, and a few cases occur in patients with counts greater than 300 cells/mm^3.[7,8] Some of these patients have had inaccurate laboratory measurements due to errors such as mislabeled specimens, incorrectly processed specimens, or technical inaccuracies involving the cell count or the fluorescent antibody cell sorter machine. Other patients may have rapidly falling CD4+ T-lymphocyte counts such that a value obtained 2–4 weeks previously is not a true reflection of a patient's current count. However, CD4+ T-lymphocyte counts, even when accurate, provide only a partial assessment of immunologic function. Other assays will likely be developed that will be able to assess immunologic function more precisely and identify clinical susceptibility more accurately.

Currently, clinical findings can be useful predictors of susceptibility to supplement the information derived from CD4+ T-lymphocyte counts. Thus, the development of otherwise unexplained oropharyngeal candidiasis, persistent fever, or previous PCP are good indicators of current susceptibility to PCP and of the need for prophylaxis, independent of the CD4+ T-lymphocyte count.[8,17]

SPECTRUM OF OPPORTUNISTIC PATHOGENS

Patients with HIV infection are highly susceptible to a unique constellation of pathogens (Table 1). The development of an opportunistic infection is related to the degree of immunosuppression as discussed above, and to the exposure of the patient to the pathogen. Most HIV-associated opportunistic infections are thought to be due to reactivation of latent infection, but this concept is based on speculation rather than data. Some episodes of opportunistic infection, such as those that have occurred in outbreaks of multidrug-resistant *M. tuberculosis,* represent either primary infection or exogenous reinfection with new strains of *M. tuberculosis.*[18-21] As techniques to identify strain variants are more widely applied, additional information will be forthcoming about how often multiple episodes of pneumocystis, candida, or CMV disease, for example, represent reinfections rather than relapses.

The infectious manifestations of HIV-induced immunosuppression vary geographically because of different exposure patterns. For example, *Histoplasmosis* is a very common cause of pulmonary infiltrates in the Ohio River Valley[22,23]; *Leishmania chagasi* is frequently recognized as a cause of fever and hepatosplenomegaly in Brazil[24]; *M. tuberculosis* is very common in certain parts of New York City, Miami, Africa, and Haiti[19-21,25,26]; and isosporiasis is common in Haiti.[27] Specific behavior patterns also influence exposure and thus the infectious manifestations of HIV-induced immunosuppression. For example, homosexual males are much more likely to develop Kaposi sarcoma[28] or ulcerative perirectal herpes simplex virus infection than are patients with other behavioral risk factors.

Certain opportunistic infections occur in patients with HIV infection much more frequently than in almost any other patient group. For example, without prophylaxis, PCP will ultimately develop in 60–80 percent of HIV-infected patients in North America.[8,29] The annual attack rate for HIV-infected patients with CD+ T-lymphocyte counts below 100 cells/mm^3 is probably twice that of patients with severe combined immunodeficiency syndromes, and more than 10 times that of patients with

TABLE 1. Therapy for Common Opportunistic Pathogens in HIV-Infected Patients

Pathogens that are common and may respond to therapy
  Pneumocystis carinii
  Toxoplasma gondii
  Leishmania donovani
  Herpes simplex virus
  Varicella-zoster virus
  Cytomegalovirus
  Candida spp.
  Cryptococcus neoformans
  Histoplasma capsulatum
  Coccidioides immitis
  Salmonella spp.
  Campylobacter spp.
  Shigella spp.
  Mycobacterium tuberculosis
  Streptococcus pneumoniae
  Haemophilus influenza
  Mycobacterium avium complex
  Bartonella (*Rochalimaea*)
Pathogens for which no therapy currently appears to be highly effective
  Cryptosporidia
  Epstein-Barr virus
  Microsporidia
  Acanthamoeba

organ transplants, solid tumors, or most hematologic malignancies.[8,30] Disseminated MAC was rarely recognized in humans before the advent of HIV infection, yet disseminated MAC occurs in as many as 30–40 percent of patients with advanced HIV disease.[10–12,31] *Mycobacterium tuberculosis,* cerebral toxoplasmosis, persistent cryptosporidiosis, microsporidiosis, and Kaposi sarcoma are examples of other processes that cause disease much more commonly in patients with HIV infection than with other immunodeficiencies that their presence should strongly suggest that patients be tested for HIV infection.

GENERAL PRINCIPLES OF MANAGEMENT

As indicated in Table 2, most opportunistic pathogens that cause disease in HIV-infected patients can be successfully treated with available anti-infective agents. The opportunistic pathogens commonly seen in HIV-infected patients can be categorized into two groups: *(1)* those that may respond to therapy but have a high likelihood of recurrence or relapse if therapy is discontinued; and *(2)* those for which no therapy currently appears to be effective. The successful management of opportunistic infections depends on *(1)* prompt diagnosis and initiation of therapy before the clinical syndrome is severe; *(2)* recognition that a poor response to therapy may indicate that a pathogen other than the one initially identified may be present, or that the pathogen is resistant to the therapeutic agent employed; and *(3)* recognition that most therapies must be lifelong to prevent relapses or recurrences.

The management of opportunistic infections in HIV-infected patients differs from that in other patient populations because the natural history of specific infections such as PCP[32] or cryptococcal meningitis[33] may be different in AIDS patients. Also, HIV-infected patients may be less tolerant of some therapeutic agents, such as trimethoprim-sulfamethoxazole or flucytosine. Consideration must also be given to interactions between the drug used to treat opportunistic pathogens and the multiplicity of drugs directed against HIV itself, and against other concomitant processes.[34]

An issue that frequently arises is whether to use empirical antimicrobial regimens or to establish a specific diagnosis before therapy, which often requires invasive procedures. For some clinical problem, such as the presence of a central nervous system mass lesion or the presence of active retinitis, empirical therapy is usually reasonable, because clinical features, immune profiles, and noninvasive laboratory tests make establishment of the correct diagnosis very likely. In other situations, such as the presence of pulmonary infiltrates, meningitis, fever and inanition, or diarrhea, the clinical presentation is so nonspecific that a definitive diagnosis should be sought. The costs of embarking on an extensive diagnostic work-up need to be considered, along with the benefits and risks of a trial of antibiotic therapy. For effective therapy of most opportunistic infections patients with HIV infection will usually need lifelong, suppressive therapy. These chronic regimens may also promote the development of microbial resistance and may produce undesirable drug interactions. Thus, the establishment of an accurate diagnosis is particularly important when long, expensive, and often difficult to tolerate therapeutic regimens are to be undertaken.

PNEUMOCYSTIS CARINII

Pneumocystis carinii pneumonia (also see Ch. 102 and 258) continues to be a common complication of HIV infection in North America, although in some areas of the world it is much less common.[35,36] Although prophylaxis has reduced the number of cases, many patients do not recognize that they have HIV infection until they present with PCP. Some patients fail to take prophylaxis, and other patients develop PCP despite prophylaxis.

Thus, PCP continues to be a substantial cause of morbidity and mortality.

Pneumocystis disease most often presents as pulmonary dysfunction in patients with HIV infection. Patients may have chest tightness or exercise intolerance as very early symptoms, before chest radiographs are abnormal and before arterial blood gases reveal hypoxemia.[32,37–39] For therapy to have the highest likelihood of success, patients and clinicians must be trained to initiate diagnostic evaluation at this stage, before pulmonary dysfunction is severe.[37–41] Even with very mild manifestations of disease, organisms can be readily detected in sputum or bronchoalveolar lavage, allowing initiation of therapy on an outpatient basis at a stage when prognosis is excellent.[42–46]

There is no reliable clinical method to distinguish PCP from a variety of other infectious and noninfectious processes, including tuberculosis, histoplasmosis, and nonspecific interstitial pneumonitis.[22,47,48] Thus, it is highly desirable to establish a specific diagnosis to ascertain that the correct pathogen is being treated, and to avoid the toxicities, cost, and inconvenience of unnecessary drugs. Because of the cost of a diagnostic evaluation, it may be appropriate in some settings to treat mild cases of presumptive PCP empirically. If patients do not improve on therapy, the yield of a subsequent diagnostic evaluation for *Pneumocystis* should not be substantially diminished.[42–46,49,50] Evaluation of such patients needs to include screening for tuberculosis, which is very important in many communities for identification of cases early and for reduction of the spread of tuberculosis. The availability of induced sputum examination provides a very sensitive, relatively low-cost method to diagnose PCP, and to search for cases of tuberculosis. Nucleic acid detection systems may prove to be useful for outpatient assessments, but their utility remains to be proven.[51,52]

The likelihood that an AIDS patient will survive an episode of PCP depends on the severity of pulmonary dysfunction at the time therapy is initiated, the patient's ability to tolerate available regimens, the presence of concomitant pathology, and the severity of the patient's immunologic dysfunction. A poor prognosis correlates with an alveolar-arterial gradient greater than 30 mmHg, a severely abnormal chest radiograph, or a high number of organisms detected on lavage or biopsy.[37–39] Thus, drug therapy is more likely to be successful if the therapy is started at a time when pulmonary dysfunction is mild, and if other severe opportunistic infections are absent. Second, third, or subsequent episodes of PCP do not have a worse prognosis than first episodes.[53]

Oral trimethoprim-sulfamethoxazole is the regimen of choice for treatment of PCP because of convenience of administration, high degree of efficacy, and the manageability of associated toxicities. No agent has ever been shown to have a higher efficacy. There is no clear reason to prefer intravenous over oral trimethoprim-sulfamethoxazole in compliant patients with no obvious gastrointestinal dysfunction. Patients usually improve clinically in terms of fever, respiratory rate, arterial-alveolar gradient, and dyspnea within 4–8 days, although there may be an initial worsening during the first 48–72 hours of therapy.[32,37,54–58] Survival for mild episodes treated with trimethoprim–sulfamethoxazole has improved steadily over the past decade. For patients with initial room air PO_2 values over 70 mmHg, survival has improved from 85–90 percent to 95–99 percent in optimal circumstances.[32,37,54,59] Noncompliant patients and patients with significant concomitant disorders will have worse results. This improvement in survival is presumably due to improved understanding of management of the non-life-threatening toxicities associated with trimethoprim-sulfamethoxazole to maintenance of trimethoprim levels in the 5–8 μg/ml range, which appears to improve tolerance, and to the availability of better alternative agents for patients who are truly failing trimethoprim-sulfamethoxazole or who are unable to tolerate the drug.

For trimethoprim-sulfamethoxazole, common adverse reac-

TABLE 2. Therapy of Opportunistic Infections in Patients with HIV Infection

Clinical Disease	Drug	Dose	Route	Interval	Duration
Pneumocystis pneumonia (therapy)	Trimethoprim with sulfamethoxazole	5 mg/kg with 25 mg/kg	PO, IV	q8h	21 days
	OR				
	Trimethoprim	300 mg	PO	q8h	21 days
	plus dapsone	100 mg	PO	qd	
	OR				
	Pentamidine	3–4 mg/kg	IV (IM)	qd	21 days
	OR				
	Atovaquone	750 mg	PO	q8h	21 days
	OR				
	Clindamycin	300–450 mg	PO, IV	q6h	21 days
	plus primaquine	15 mg	PO	qd	
	OR				
	Trimetrexate	45 mg/m^2	IV	q24h	21 days
	plus leucovorin	20 mg/m^2	PO, IV	q6h	
	Prednisone (adjunctive therapy for severe episode)	40 mg	PO	q12h[a]	21 days
Pneumocystis pneumonia (maintenance)	Trimethoprim plus sulfamethoxazole	1 double-strength tablet	PO	q24h	Lifelong
	OR				
	Dapsone	50–100 mg	PO	q24h	Lifelong
Toxoplasmosis	Sulfadiazine	1–2 g	PO	q6h	Lifelong
	plus pyrimethamine	50–100 mg[g]	PO	qd	Lifelong
	plus leucovorin	10–25 mg	PO, IV	qd	Lifelong
	OR				
	Clindamycin	600 mg	PO	q6h	Lifelong
	plus pyrimethamine	50–100 mg[b]	PO	qd	Lifelong
Cryptosporidiosis	None	—	—	—	—
Microsporidiosis	None	—	—	—	—
Isosporiasis	Trimethoprim	160 mg	PO, IV	q6h	7 days
	with sulfamethoxazole	800 mg			
	FOLLOWED BY				
	Trimethoprim	160 mg	PO	qd	Lifelong
	plus sulfamethaxazole	800 mg			
Candidiasis					
Oral	Nystatin	5 × 10^5–1 × 10^6 u	PO	q6h	7–10 days
	OR				
	Fluconazole	100–200 mg	PO, IV	q24h	7–10 days
Esophageal	Fluconazole	100–400 mg	PO, IV	q24h	14–21 days
Coccidioidomycosis	Amphotericin B	0.5–1.0 mg/kg	IV	q24h	≥56 days
	FOLLOWED BY				
	Itraconazole	300 mg	PO	bid	3 days
		then 200 mg	PO	bid	Lifelong
	OR				
	Ketoconazole	400 mg	PO	q24h	Lifelong
Cryptococcus	Amphotericin B	0.3–1.0 mg/kg	IV	q24h	≥14 days
	with or without flucytosine	25 mg/kg	PO	q6h	≥14 days
	OR				
	Fluconazole[c]	400 mg	PO	q24h	≥14 days
	FOLLOWED BY				
	Fluconazole	200 mg	PO	q24h	Lifelong
Histoplasmosis	Amphotericin B	0.5–1.0 mg/kg	IV	q24h	≥28–56 days
	FOLLOWED BY				
	Itraconazole	200 mg	PO	q12h	Lifelong
Herpes simplex virus	Acyclovir	200 mg	PO	5 times/day	≥7 days
Varicella-zoster virus					
Dermatomal	Acyclovir	800 mg	PO	5 times/day	7–10 days
Disseminated	Acyclovir	10–12 mg/kg	IV	q8h	7–14 days
Cytomegalovirus	Ganciclovir	5 mg/kg	IV	q12h	14–21 days
	FOLLOWED BY				
	Ganciclovir	5 mg/kg	IV	q24h	Lifelong
	OR				
	Foscarnet	60 mg/kg	IV	q8h	14–21 days
	FOLLOWED BY				
	Foscarnet	90–120 mg/kg	IV	q24h	Lifelong
Mycobacterium tuberculosis	Isoniazid	300 mg	PO, IM	q24h	At least 9 months
	AND				
	Rifampin	600 mg	PO, IV	q24h	At least 9 months
	AND				
	Ethambutol	15–25 mg/kg	PO	q24h	Depends on sensitivity
	AND				
	Pyrazinamide	15–25 mg/kg	PO	q24h	2 months
Mycobacterium avium complex	Clarithromycin	500 mg	PO	q12h	Lifelong
	AND ONE OR MORE				
	Ethambutol	15 mg/kg	PO	q24h	Lifelong
	Rifabutin	300 mg	PO	q24h	Lifelong
	Clofazimine	100–200 mg	PO	q24h	Lifelong
Bartonella (Rochalimaea) spp.	Erythromycin	500 mg	PO	q6h	≥8–12 weeks
	OR				
	Doxycycline	100 mg	PO	q12h	≥8–12 weeks

[a] Prednisone, 40 mg q12h × 5 days, followed by 20 mg bid × 5 days, followed by 20 mg qd × 11 days.
[b] Following a single loading dose of pyrimethamine, 200 mg. After 3–6 weeks, maintenance doses of pyrimethamine are usually 50–75 mg/day.
[c] Rarely recommended as initial therapy unless very mild episode and favorable prognostic signs.

tions include skin rash, nausea, vomiting, granulocytopenia, transaminase elevations, nephritis, and hyperkalemia.[37,54,55–61] These adverse reactions do not invariably require discontinuation of trimethoprim-sulfamethoxazole therapy. The skin rashes, which commonly occur between the 8th and 12th days of therapy, may be limited in extent and associated with a degree of pruritus that the patient can tolerate for 21 days. It is unclear if they are less frequent in patients with lower CD4+ T-lymphocyte counts, or patients receiving concomitant corticosteroids.[62a,62b,79] Life-threatening desquamating processes such as the Stevens-Johnson syndrome are extraordinarily rare in AIDS patients, although a few fatal cases have been reported. Thus, the development of a rash associated with trimethoprim-sulfamethoxazole therapy is not necessarily an indication to discontinue this drug regimen. Severe febrile, hypotensive episodes that resemble septic shock in terms of hemodynamics have also been reported.[60] Granulocytopenia appears to be a dose-related phenomenon that may resolve partially or completely if the dose of trimethoprim-sulfamethoxazole is reduced by 25 percent.[54] Granulocytopenia only rarely responds to leucovorin administration. Nausea and vomiting can be troublesome complications of trimethoprim-sulfamethoxazole therapy. Severe nausea may be due to very high sulfonamide levels and may improve if the dose is reduced. Transaminase levels may fluctuate until therapy is stopped, and will usually return promptly to baseline values at that time. Overall, adverse reactions have required discontinuation of trimethoprim-sulfamethoxazole therapy in about 25 percent of cases in the past. Although it has not been proved by a prospective study, adverse reactions can probably be reduced without sacrificing efficacy by lowering the recommended dose of trimethoprim-sulfamethoxazole from trimethoprim, 20 mg/kg/day, and sulfamethoxazole, 100 mg/kg/day, to trimethoprim, 15 mg/kg/day, and sulfamethoxazole, 75 mg/kg/day.[54] It is not clear if desensitization is useful, nor is it clear what portion of truly sulfonamide-intolerant individuals can tolerate dapsone for meaningful lengths of time.[63]

Parenteral pentamidine is effective therapy for PCP.[37,54,60,64,65] However, this regimen is inconvenient to administer, and the associated adverse reactions can be life-threatening. Renal dysfunction, hypoglycemia, hyperglycemia, granulocytopenia, cardiac arrhythmias, and hypotension are reported in 10–50 percent of patients.[37,54,64,65] There is growing concern that simultaneous treatment with other drugs that have similar toxicities, such as foscarnet (i.e., nephrotoxicity) or ddI or ddC (i.e., pancreatic toxicity) may greatly increase the likelihood of serious adverse events. For many years, pentamidine was administered intramuscularly because early reports had described fatal hypotension when the drug was given intravenously.[64–66a] Intramuscular administration of pentamidine is no longer recommended except in unusual circumstances, because intramuscular injections are often associated with painful sterile abscesses that can become superinfected. Moreover, the hypotension originally associated with administration of intravenous pentamidine was probably related to the rate of infusion. When pentamidine is administered over at least a 60-minute period in 100–150 ml of dextrose in water, clinically important hypotension is unusual.[66] The renal dysfunction associated with pentamidine can be severe. If the serum creatinine level rises by more than 1.0–2.0 mg/dl, strong consideration should be given to withholding therapy for a few days or switching to an alternative agent. Hypoglycemia can be a life-threatening complication of pentamidine therapy and can occur at any time during therapy or many weeks after therapy has been completed.[67] Hypoglycemia occurs more frequently in patients who have pentamidine-induced renal dysfunction. The unpredictability of the hypoglycemia adds an element of danger to the inpatient or outpatient use of this drug. However, life-threatening hypoglycemia is sufficiently uncommon that this effective agent is still recommended for trimethoprim-sulfamethoxazole-intolerant or trimethoprim-dapsone in-

tolerant patients who have severe disease. Lowering the dose of parenteral pentamidine from 4 to 3 mg/kg/day has been advocated to reduce toxicity; whether this also reduces efficacy is unknown.[68]

Dapsone (100 mg PO qd) plus trimethoprim (5 mg/kg PO q8h or 300 mg PO q8h) appear to be as effective as trimethoprim-sulfamethoxazole but less toxic in a limited, controlled experience.[69] Skin rashes are very common among AIDS patients treated with dapsone, but a 21-day course of therapy can often be completed without interruption. Dapsone alone has some efficacy when 100 mg PO qd is used for 21 days, but there is probably not enough activity to warrant use of this agent as single-drug therapy.[70] Higher doses are not well tolerated.

Atovaquone is a hydroxynaphthoquinone that appears to affect mitochondrial electron transport in microorganisms, and thus has a mechanism of action distinct from trimethoprim-sulfamethoxazole or pentamidine.[59,71,72] Atovaquone is only available as an oral agent. For patients with mild or moderate pneumocystis pneumonia, it has a high degree of efficacy and is extremely well tolerated.[59,72] A large, prospective, double-blind study demonstrated that atovaquone is very effective, and is much better tolerated than trimethoprim-sulfamethoxazole. However, it is associated with more treatment failures than trimethoprim-sulfamethoxazole.[59] A possible explanation for the higher rate of treatment failures and the higher death rate in the atovaquone group is that, unlike trimethoprim-sulfamethoxazole, atovaquone has no antibacterial activity, and therefore patients in the atovaquone groups were more likely to die due to unrecognized, concurrent bacterial processes. Another explanation is that atovaquone absorption can be erratic, especially in patients who cannot consume fatty foods with this medication. In addition, atovaquone is poorly absorbed if diarrhea is present, and should not be used in patients with substantial gastrointestinal dysfunction. The primary toxicity due to atovaquone is skin rash. Atovaquone is a reasonable treatment option for patients with mild or moderate pneumocystis pneumonia who cannot tolerate trimethoprim-sulfamethoxazole and who are good candidates for oral therapy.[30]

Clindamycin plus primaquine is also effective for the therapy of PCP.[73–75] Despite the fact that primaquine can only be given orally, this regimen has been used successfully in patients with mild, moderate, and severe disease. Clindamycin plus primaquine can be associated with considerable toxicity including rash, serum transaminase elevation, diarrhea, and hemolysis. Until a large prospective trial is completed comparing this regimen to standard therapy, the role of clindamycin plus primaquine for the treatment of PCP will remain unclear.

Trimetrexate is a potent inhibitor of dihydrofolate reductase that is effective therapy against PCP when used either alone (45 mg/m² IV qd) or in combination with a sulfonamide.[76–78] Because trimetrexate inhibits the dihydrofolate reductase of human cells as well as the enzyme of *Pneumocystis,* it must be given in conjunction with high-dose leucovorin (20 mg/kg IV or PO q6h), which rescues mammalian cells without diminishing the anti-*Pneumocystis* effect. Trimetrexate is well tolerated when given with leucovorin, and leukopenia is the major adverse effect that is noted. Trimetrexate has a high degree of efficacy, and has the advantage of being available as a parenteral agent. However, a large, multicenter, double-blinded study has demonstrated that trimetrexate therapy is associated with a higher rate of poor response and death than is trimethoprim-sulfamethoxazole.[78] The relapse rate after trimetrexate therapy is high, and 40–60 percent of patients relapse within the first 60 days. This relapse rate is probably much lower if a few days of sulfonamide therapy are given concurrently.

Regardless of which specific therapy is chosen for PCP, adjunctive corticosteroid therapy is indicated for any patient whose initial room air PO₂ is less than 70 mmHg.[79–82] Three prospective trials[79–81] have demonstrated that the frequencies of ventilatory failure and mortality can be reduced substantially by the prompt use of corticosteroids. The precise mechanism by which corticosteroids provide benefit is not well delineated. Adjunctive corticosteroids appear to prevent much of the decline in oxygenation that characteristically occurs during the first 3 days of treatment.[58] This decline may be caused by the inflammatory response elicited by dying organisms. Adjunctive corticosteroids may also provide benefit for patients with an initial room air PO_2 greater than 70 mmHg. There is evidence that shows an improvement in lung function in these patients, but so few patients with mild PCP develop respiratory failure or die that it is difficult to substantiate a survival benefit.

When an AIDS patient with PCP fails to improve while receiving conventional therapy, there are no controlled observations to indicate what modifications in therapy are optimal.[30] The mean time to improvement for AIDS patients treated with conventional therapy is 5–6 days,[32,37,54] so patients should probably not be considered to be therapeutic failures until they have received 7–10 days of therapy. However, clinicians often feel compelled to alter therapy earlier, especially if the patient is deteriorating rapidly. If a patient has not improved after 5–10 days of therapy, a repeat diagnostic procedure should be considered to determine whether another treatable pathogen is present. Bronchoscopy with transbronchial biopsies is the procedure of choice because lung tissue is usually necessary to assess the presence of CMV, and can also be very helpful to establish the presence of fungal or mycobacterial processes, which are major diagnostic considerations. *Pneumocystis* will often be present in lavage or tissue for at least 3–4 weeks after initiating therapy even in patients who respond promptly, so their presence after 7–10 days of therapy does not necessarily imply ineffective therapy.[83] The presence of extensive intra-alveolar exudate or extensive fibrosis after 7–10 days of therapy is probably a more ominous sign. Open lung biopsy should rarely be necessary to establish a diagnosis of PCP, but this procedure is useful for identifying other processes. Kaposi sarcoma of the lung is one treatable process that is difficult or impossible to diagnose reliably from transbronchial biopsy specimens.[28] Nodular lesions on chest computed tomography (CT) scan, extensive intrabronchial lesions, and the presence of a bloody pleural effusion may be helpful clues to the presence of Kaposi sarcoma.

If *Pneumocystis* is the only identifiable cause of the pulmonary dysfunction after 7–10 days of therapy and the patient has failed to improve, there are several therapeutic alternatives: *(1)* switch from trimethoprim-sulfamethoxazole to parenteral pentamidine or vice versa; *(2)* add corticosteroids to conventional therapy if they have not already been added; *(3)* switch to intravenous trimetrexate; *(4)* switch to intravenous clindamycin with oral primaquine; or *(5)* use two specific therapies concurrently (e.g., trimethoprim-sulfamethoxazole plus pentamidine). Each of these approaches has been associated with a successful outcome in some cases. A controlled trial is needed to determine the best approach, but such trials are difficult to perform due to the large size, complexity, and cost for a valid study. Whether AIDS patients with pneumocystis pneumonia should be aggressively supported with intensive care, mechanical ventilation, or other interventions is a controversial issue.[84] The most reasonable approach would appear to be to individualize each management plan in terms of how many days of therapy have been received, what therapeutic alternatives are available, what concomitant processes are present, what the patient's wishes are, and what resources are available. There is published literature to indicate that AIDS patients with PCP can survive intubation and mechanical ventilation and lead independent lives for many months after hospital discharge.[38–41] The best candidates for intensive care and mechanical ventilation would be those patients who have no other serious opportunistic processes, those who have received less than 7 days of therapy, and those who have clearly articulated a desire for aggressive support.

The prevention of PCP is a major priority for the management of patients with HIV infection. Prevention of pneumocystis pneumonia is important because episodes are frequent (at least 60–80 percent of patients in North America will develop an episode at some point during their HIV disease if they do not receive prophylaxis); morbidity and mortality due to PCP can be substantial; low-cost drugs are available that are effective; and the period of high susceptibility can be defined.[29,30,85] Prospective and retrospective studies have shown that most primary episodes of PCP occur in patients with CD4+ T-lymphocyte counts below 200 cells/mm^3, or in those patients, regardless of CD4+ T-lymphocyte count, with otherwise unexplained persistent fever or oropharyngeal candidiasis.[7,8,17] Thus, the presence of those findings are indications for prophylaxis against PCP (primary prophylaxis).[29,30] A few cases of PCP will occur in patients with CD4+ T-lymphocyte counts higher than 200 cells/mm^3 who do not have fever or mucocutaneous candidiasis, and thus some clinicians prefer to initiate prophylaxis at somewhat earlier time points.[7,8] However, such a strategy entails putting a relatively large number of patients on prophylaxis to prevent a relatively small additional number of cases. Secondary prophylaxis (the prevention of second or subsequent episodes of PCP is indicated for any patient who has had a documented case of PCP, because the 1-year rate of subsequent episodes is about 65 percent for patients who receive no prophylaxis.[29]

Trimethoprim-sulfamethoxazole is the preferred prophylactic regimen for any HIV-infected patient who can tolerate the drug[29,85–88] (Table 3). When administered at a daily dose of trimethoprim (160 mg)-sulfamethoxazole (800 mg), that is, one double-strength tablet per day, episodes of PCP are extremely uncommon. Comparative trials have demonstrated that the regimen of trimethoprim-sulfamethoxazole is much more effective than aerosolized pentamidine for either primary or secondary prophylaxis.[86,87] Based on retrospective analyses, trimethoprim-sulfamethoxazole also has the benefit of reducing the frequency of toxoplasmosis, and may have a beneficial effect on the frequency of pneumococcal and *Haemophilus* infections.[86,88] Comparative trials have confirmed that trimethoprim-sulfamethoxazole is not nearly as well tolerated as aerosolized pentamidine.[86,87] About 20–40 percent of patients cannot tolerate trimethoprim-sulfamethoxazole because of rash, pruritus, fever, granulocytopenia, thrombocytopenia, anemia, hepatitis, nephritis, nausea, or vomiting. Reducing the dose of trimethoprim-sulfamethoxazole by 50 percent (i.e., a single-strength tablet daily) or reducing the frequency to two or three times weekly may lower toxicity to a modest degree.[87] Efficacy of these alternative regimens appears to be high although they have not been rigorously studied.[89–91] Aerosolized pentamidine, although not as effective as trimethoprim-sulfamethoxazole, also reduces the frequency of PCP when used for primary or secondary prophylaxis.[92–96] Doses higher than 300 mg monthly (delivered by the Respirgard nebulizer) may have enhanced efficacy as suggested by preliminary trials.[96a] How aerosolized pentamidine is delivered to the patient is a major determinant of efficacy and safety.[97] Different nebulizers deliver different densities of particle sizes, and thus deliver different amounts of drug to the patient. Thus, the dosing regimens for the Respirgard II nebulizer[86,87,96] and the Fisons nebulizer[95] are quite different. Only the Respirgard II jet nebulizer and the Fisons ultrasonic nebulizer have been studied in large, well-controlled trials with clinical endpoints. Aerosolized pentamidine is well tolerated by most patients. Coughing and wheezing can be ameliorated or prevented by nebulized albuterol. A bitter taste is often reported. Cases of pancreatitis and renal dysfunction have been attributed to aerosolized pentamidine, but causality has not been proven. A major concern related to the use of aerosolized pentamidine is the environmental contamination with drug and respiratory secretions that are created when patients cough or become disconnected from the nebulizer. Health care workers and patients may inhale enough pentamidine to develop detectable urine levels of the drug.[98] The clinical importance of this is unknown. More important, should the patient have pulmonary tuberculo-

TABLE 3. Prophylaxis for HIV-Related Opportunistic Infections

Pathogen	Indication for Prophylaxis	First Choice	Alternatives	Comments
Pneumocystis	CD4 + <200/mm³ Persistent unexplained fever Chronic oropharyngeal candidiasis	Trimethoprim-sulfamethoxazole 1 DS qd	Aerosolized pentamidine Dapsone 50 mg qd + pyrimethamine 50 mg per week Dapsone alone (100 mg qd)	Aerosol pentamidine should be delivered by Respirgard or Fisons nebulizer. TMP/SMX can probably be given 2 or 3 days weekly with high efficacy; single-strength tablets may also be effective.
Mycobacterium avium complex	CD+4 <100/mm³	Rifabutin, 300 mg qd	? Clarithromycin ? Azithromycin	Rifabutin increases hepatic metabolism of other drugs.
Toxoplasma	No consensus	Trimethoprim-sulfamethoxazole 1 DS qd	—	Efficacy and safety of pyrimethamine alone is unclear.
Mycobacterium tuberculosis	PPD >5 mm ? High risk	Sensitive: INH 300 mg qd × 12 months Resistant: ?		For resistant strains, two drug regimens using combinations of rifampin, pyrazinamide, or a quinolone can be considered.
Candida	Multiple recurrences	Fluconazole, 200 mg daily	Itraconazole, 100 mg qd	Topical agents such as nystatin or clotrimazole are options.
Herpes simplex	Multiple recurrences	Acyclovir, 200 mg 3–5×/day	—	Some promising new oral agents are currently in clinical trials.
Cytomegalovirus	None	—	—	No convenient and well-tolerated agent available; oral ganciclovir or acyclovir prodrugs are being assessed.
Pneumococcus	All patients	Pneumovax	—	Trimethoprim-sulfamethoxazole appears to prevent some disease.
Haemophilus influenzae	No consensus	Hib vaccine	—	Trimethoprim-sulfamethoxazole appears to prevent some disease.
Influenza	All patients	Influenza vaccine	—	—

sis, the environmental contamination produced by dispersed respiratory particles has considerable potential to spread tuberculosis.[99] Patients need to be carefully screened for pulmonary tuberculosis before aerosolized pentamidine prophylaxis is initiated.

For patients who cannot tolerate trimethoprim-sulfamethoxazole and who either do not tolerate aerosolized pentamidine or who experience multiple breakthroughs, there are several alternatives. Weekly dapsone-pyrimethamine has efficacy comparable to aerosolized pentamidine (i.e., it is not as effective as daily trimethoprim-sulfamethoxazole as prophylaxis for PCP), but it is very effective as prophylaxis against toxoplasmosis.[100] Dapsone-pyrimethamine, like trimethoprim-sulfamethoxazole, is poorly tolerated by a substantial fraction of patients: fever, rash, pruritus, and hemolysis occur. Many patients who cannot tolerate trimethoprim-sulfamethoxazole also cannot tolerate dapsone-containing regimens. Dapsone alone, given daily, is used by many practitioners as a prophylactic regimen, and appears to have anti-*Pneumocystis* potency comparable to that of aerosolized pentamidine.[101,102] Atovaquone and clindamycin-primaquine have been proposed for prophylaxis, but there are no studies substantiating their utility. One reasonable alternative in patients who cannot tolerate any of the above prophylactic regimens and whose episodes of PCP are infrequent, is to use no prophylaxis, but to educate the patient to return immediately when symptoms develop so that each episode is mild and suitable for outpatient therapy.

TOXOPLASMA GONDII

Toxoplasma gondii causes disease in patients with HIV infection by reactivation, rather than by primary infection in most cases[103] (also see Chs. 102 and 257). Thus, patients usually have IgG antibodies against *Toxoplasma*, have fairly advanced disease (CD4+ T-lymphocyte counts below 100 cells/mm³), and have not received trimethoprim-sulfamethoxazole prophylaxis.[86,88,103–105] Because the seroprevalence of toxoplasmosis is much higher in some areas of the world such as western Europe compared to the United States, toxoplasmosis is encountered much more frequently as a complication of HIV infection there.

In patients with HIV infection, toxoplasmosis manifests more often as cerebral disease than any other manifestation. When an HIV-infected patient with a CD4+ lymphocyte count below 100 cells/mm³ presents with a space-occupying cerebral lesion

that involves gray matter, the differential diagnosis primarily consists of toxoplasmosis and lymphoma. Fungal, mycobacterial, and viral processes present as space-occupying lesions infrequently, and progressive multifocal leukoencephalopathy should primarily involve white matter.[106–111]

An empirical approach to diagnosis is reasonable in many instances.[109,110] A definitive diagnostic study (i.e., brain biopsy) has some morbidity associated with it, and the diagnostic yield may only be 50 percent if toxoplasmosis is the etiology.[103,111] The cysts and tachyzoites of *T. gondii* can be very difficult to recognize in fragments of necrotic brain tissue, and even several small needle biopsy samples may miss the area that has abundant organisms. Because toxoplasmosis is the only common etiology for gray matter lesions that clearly benefits from therapy and because needle biopsy has diagnostic limitations, empirical therapy with pyrimethamine (200 mg PO the first day followed by 50–100 mg PO qd) plus sulfadiazine (1–2 g PO q6h) is reasonable.[112,113] Some clinicians use higher doses of both drugs, but there is no clear evidence that higher doses are more effective, and they almost certainly produce more toxicity. If there is not unequivocal improvement by clinical and radiologic criteria within 14–21 days, a biopsy should be performed to establish whether the etiology is an infectious or neoplastic process other than toxoplasmosis.[105,110–113] Corticosteroids to reduce inflammation are sometimes used in patients with substantial or progressive neurologic dysfunction or signs of increased intracranial pressure. The administration of corticosteroids may make evaluation of the clinical and radiologic response to specific therapy difficult because the observed improvement may be solely due to corticosteroid therapy and may be unrelated to the anti-*Toxoplasma* regimen employed. Chronic antiseizure medication may be necessary; although some clinicians institute this prophylactically, most will initiate it only if a seizure occurs. For patients who respond, anti-*Toxoplasma* therapy should be continued for life, because relapses occur in the same sites in which disease presented initially, if therapy is discontinued, even after 8–12 months of treatment.[110–113] Whether the chronic suppressive regimen will be as effective if both pyrimethamine and sulfadiazine are not included at full doses remains to be demonstrated.

Treatment failures are very unusual for patients with toxoplasmosis who are able to tolerate both pyrimethamine and sulfadiazine.[110–113] Radiologically proven failures in patients who are unequivocally taking their drugs should raise the possibility that toxoplasmosis is not the correct or the only diagnosis. Adverse reactions to sulfadiazine (leukopenia, rash, elevated transaminase levels, nausea, nephritis) and to pyrimethamine (leukopenia, thrombocytopenia) are common.[103,110–113] The leukopenia often will not respond to leucovorin therapy, although a short course of leucovorin (10–20 mg PO or IV q6h) should be attempted.

For patients unable to tolerate sulfadiazine, clindamycin plus pyrimethamine is also quite effective.[105,113] Atovaquone plus pyrimethamine[114] or dapsone plus pyrimethamine[115] may also be useful regimens. Pyrimethamine by itself does not appear efficacious,[116] nor does trimetrexate.[117]

Trimethoprim-sulfamethoxazole offers considerable protection as primary prophylaxis, that is, before toxoplasmosis has been manifested clinically.[86,88] Dapsone-pyrimethamine also has substantial efficacy.[110] The efficacy and safety of pyrimethamine alone is controversial.[110a]

HERPES SIMPLEX AND VARICELLA-ZOSTER VIRUS INFECTIONS

Oral acyclovir (200 mg q4h) is very effective therapy for herpes simplex virus perirectal lesions, proctitis, oral lesions, digital lesions, and esophagitis[118] (also see Chs. 102 and 115). Disseminated herpes simplex viral infections are very unusual in HIV-infected patients. Intravenous therapy is rarely necessary unless the patient has a major gastrointestinal disorder that prevents oral absorption. Topical acyclovir has not been demonstrated to be highly effective in patients with HIV infection. The response of acyclovir-sensitive herpes simplex lesions is usually prompt and occurs within 3–10 days. Therapy should continue until the lesions are crusted over or epithelialized. Relapses occur with high frequency. If relapses occur quickly or often, chronic suppression may be necessary. A regimen of oral acyclovir, 200 mg three to five times daily, is often used. Acyclovir-resistant isolates are being recognized.[119,120] Foscarnet is active against herpes simplex, and has been used successfully against acyclovir-resistant strains.[119–120a]

Dermatomal herpes zoster does not always need to be treated in HIV-infected patients, and dissemination of varicella-zoster virus (VZV) is an unusual event (also see Chs. 102 and 116). Local involvement in more than one dermatome can be seen. Even when extensive disseminated cutaneous lesions have been observed, clinically apparent visceral disease is rare. Whether acyclovir therapy has any role in hastening the crusting of lesions, in preventing post-herpetic neuralgia, or in preventing recurrences in HIV-infected patients is not well studied. Patients with persistent or recurrent lesions or zoster ophthalmicus might be logical candidates for high-dose oral acyclovir (800 mg PO five times daily). Corticosteroid therapy to prevent postherpetic neuralgia is not recommended in patients with HIV infection because of the potentially adverse effects of corticosteroids on immune function. Acyclovir-resistant VZV isolates do occur,[120a,121,122] and clinical failures associated with acyclovir-resistant viruses have been successfully treated with foscarnet in some cases.

CYTOMEGALOVIRUS

Cytomegalovirus infection is almost universal among HIV-infected patients as assessed by serology (also see Chs. 102 and 117). HIV-infected patients with fewer than 100 circulating CD4+ T-lymphocyte cells are often viremic and viruric with CMV, but not all of these patients develop specific organ damage.[123] Thus, it is not certain if therapeutic intervention at this point would be useful, although the issue is moot until an oral drug or a long-acting parenteral agent with good activity and safety is available. Retinitis is the most commonly recognized disorder caused by CMV.[124,125] Cytomegalovirus retinitis has the potential to involve the macula and optic disk rapidly and

to cause retinal detachments, which can result in visual impairment and ultimately in blindness.[126–129] Thus, therapy is urgent when disease is recognized unless lesions are small and very peripheral. Cytomegalovirus retinitis responds to either ganciclovir administered at a dose of 5 mg/kg IV q12h or foscarnet (phosphonoformate) at 60 mg/kg IV q8h.[127,130–132] Beginning therapy without a specific histologic or virologic diagnosis is reasonable because the ophthalmologic appearance of CMV retinitis is quite characteristic to an experienced ophthalmologist, and CMV causes almost all the retinitis that occurs in HIV-infected patients. Ganciclovir and foscarnet are equally effective in terms of inducing resolution of retinitis.[130] New lesions or progressive disease may be identified during the first 7 days of therapy and do not necessarily imply a poor response. Considerable improvement in inflammation, edema, and hemorrhage will be recognized in responders before the end of 21 days of therapy. Without maintenance suppressive therapy, relapse at the same site as the initial lesions and at new sites almost invariably occurs within a few weeks or months. The median time to progression when no initial therapy is given is 15–21 days.[131,132] Maintenance regimens using ganciclovir, 5–6 mg/kg IV qd 5–7 days per week, or foscarnet, 90–120 mg/kg IV daily, are often administered, but these regimens seem only to prolong the interval until relapse by several weeks (mean time to progression for patients receiving ganciclovir or foscarnet maintenance regimens is 50–59 days).[130–132] Thus, they do not prevent relapses from occurring. At the time of relapse, patients will usually respond to reinstitution of ganciclovir or foscarnet. Ganciclovir's major toxicity is bone marrow suppression with neutropenia and thrombocytopenia.[127,130] Confusion, nausea, vomiting, transaminase elevation, and inhibition of spermatogenesis also occur. Some AIDS patients are unable to tolerate parenteral ganciclovir therapy. Intravitreal injections and intravitreal implants of ganciclovir have been assessed.[133] These appear to be effective and relatively safe, although retinal detachment and infection resulting from repeated injections is a concern. When patients with sight-threatening CMV lesions become neutropenic due to ganciclovir, other infectious, neoplastic, immunologic, and drug-related causes of the neutropenia should be sought. G-CSF may be useful. Alternatively, another therapy such as intravitreal ganciclovir or parenteral foscarnet may be tried. Foscarnet is nephrotoxic and can cause nausea, vomiting, anorexia, seizures, hypocalcemia, and hypomagnesemia.[130,131,134] Foscarnet generally must be infused over 60 minutes following a 60-minute infusion of normal saline, and thus requires more infusion time than ganciclovir therapy. Foscarnet has in vitro activity against HIV. This feature may be responsible for the apparent survival benefit of foscarnet compared with ganciclovir in a large prospective trial of CMV retinitis.[130,135]

Cytomegalovirus can cause serious and occasional life-threatening infections such as esophagitis, enteritis, colitis, and pneumonitis. For these syndromes, a specific diagnosis should be established by histology because the syndromes are indistinguishable from those caused by other pathogens if clinical criteria alone are used. Culture of CMV from secretions or excretions alone is not sufficient to indicate that CMV is causing disease, and should be correlated with histologic, clinical, and other microbiologic data before concluding that CMV infection warrants specific antiviral therapy (see Ch. 117).

For patients with esophagitis, colitis, or rectal ulcers, improvement in clinical symptoms is usually noted during the first week of therapy.[136–139] Improved performance status and increased weight is often noted, especially if therapy results in less dysphagia or less diarrhea. There is considerably less experience with ganciclovir therapy for CMV pneumonia. There is no consensus about the specific criteria for establishing the diagnosis, however, and some patients who failed ganciclovir therapy had very severe lung damage before ganciclovir treatment was started. Ganciclovir therapy alone has not been reported to be effective in CMV pneumonia in bone marrow transplant recipients unless immune serum globulin or hyperimmune globulin is given concurrently.[140,141] Whether ganciclovir is effective in AIDS patients with CMV pneumonia either alone or in conjunction with immunoglobulin remains to be determined.

Ganciclovir-resistant[142] and foscarnet-resistant[143] isolates are being recognized with increasing frequency. To date, isolates resistant to both ganciclovir and foscarnet have not been isolated from clinical specimens. There is some evidence that ganciclovir in combination with foscarnet may be synergistic.[144,145]

Because CMV frequently causes specific organ damage in patients with HIV infection, and may contribute to the febrile wasting syndromes associated with HIV disease, prevention of CMV disease is a logical goal. There are currently no well-founded guidelines concerning when such prophylaxis might be indicated nor are there effective, well-tolerated, convenient approaches. Acyclovir, oral ganciclovir, oral foscarnet, and CMV immunoglobulin have been considered, but none has yet been shown to be effective.[146–148]

EPSTEIN-BARR VIRUS

Epstein-Barr virus (EBV) can be cultured from the oropharynx and peripheral mononuclear cells of a substantial proportion of AIDS patients (see Ch. 118). This virus has been implicated in the pathogenesis of hairy leukoplakia and may have a role in the pathogenesis of nonspecific pneumonitis, lymphadenopathy, lymphoma, fever, or wasting. There is insufficient evidence to warrant specific therapy for EBV at this point, nor is there a drug that would clearly be effective.

PROGRESSIVE MULTIFOCAL LEUKOENCEPHALOPATHY

Progressive multifocal leukoencephalopathy is caused by JC virus and results in a variety of central nervous system clinical manifestations. Characteristic white matter lesions are seen on magnetic resonance imaging (MRI) of the brain (see Ch. 123). There have been reports that Ara-C and zidovudine may be of benefit, but effective therapy has not been established.[149]

CANDIDA SPECIES

Stomatitis, esophagitis, vaginitis, and proctitis due to *Candida* spp. are common and will often respond to topical therapy (nystatin or clotrimazole), oral therapy (ketoconazole, itraconazole, or fluconazole), or intravenous therapy (fluconazole or amphotericin B) (see Ch. 31). Fluconazole (100–200 mg PO q24h) is the most convenient regimen, and is probably more effective than topical therapy. Single-dose therapy with 400 mg may be adequate,[150] but a variety of daily doses (50–400 mg) and durations of therapy (1–28 days) have been studied, most with reasonable response rates. Ketoconazole is less expensive than fluconazole or itraconazole, but can cause adrenal suppression and is poorly absorbed in the absence of gastric acidity, which is a common occurrence in patients with advanced HIV disease.[151–153] Fluconazole, itraconazole, and ketoconazole all inhibit certain hepatic enzymes of the cytochrome P-450 class, resulting in elevated levels of drugs such as dilantin.

There is usually no urgency to institute antifungal therapy for any of these mucosal disorders: esophagitis is rarely associated with bleeding, perforation, fungemia, or disseminated fungal disease. Stomatitis, esophagitis, and proctitis often recur when therapy is discontinued. Fluconazole administration may have to be continued for life if recurrences are frequent or severe. Occasional patients who do not respond to topical or oral therapy, especially those who are extremely debilitated or immunosuppressed, may respond to amphotericin B. *Candida* spp. that are clinically and microbiologically resistant to fluconazole and/or to amphotericin B are being described with increasing frequency.[154]

Primary prophylaxis with fluconazole appears to be effective compared with topical agents. Whether such prophylaxis is warranted when the benefits are weighed against cost, compliance, and drug interactions is subject to debate.

Disseminated candidiasis is not a common occurrence in AIDS patients unless they are receiving drug therapy that makes them neutropenic (especially cytotoxic antineoplastic therapy) or if they have an infected intravenous catheter. Treatment is similar to that in other patient populations, with particular attention directed at removal of infected intravenous lines or discontinuation of therapies that produce neutropenia.

CRYPTOCOCCUS NEOFORMANS, HISTOPLASMA CAPSULATUM, COCCIDIOIDES IMMITIS

Most experience with therapy of cryptococcal disease in patients with HIV is derived from patients with meningitis. Patients with factors predicting a poor outcome need more aggressive therapy than patients with mild disease. Baseline factors predicting poor therapeutic response include altered mental status (including confusion, lethargy, and obtundation), cerebrospinal fluid (CSF) antigen titer greater than 1:1024, decreased CSF leukocyte count (<20 cells/mm³), age less than 35 years, and perhaps hyponatremia and positive extra central nervous system cultures for cryptococcus[155–157] (also see Ch. 243).

The most potent therapy for cryptococcal meningitis appears to be intravenous amphotericin B with flucytosine.[157–161] A randomized multicenter trial compared fluconazole (200 mg PO qd after a 400-mg loading dose) with amphotericin B (at least 0.3 mg/kg daily). Mortality in the two groups was substantial but comparable (40 and 34 percent, respectively). Amphotericin B was associated with a trend toward fewer deaths during the first 2 weeks, and faster sterilization of CSF.[157] Fluconazole was much better tolerated than amphotericin B. Doses of amphotericin B (0.5–1.0 mg/kg daily) have been associated with survival rates of 70–90 percent in smaller or retrospective series.[156,158,161] The role of flucytosine remains controversial; in the AIDS population there is no unequivocal proof of benefit. Flucytosine can cause granulocytopenia and thrombocytopenia as well as hepatitis and rash. Tolerance may be improved using relatively lower doses of flucytosine (25 mg po q6h), and maintaining serum levels of 50–100 µg/ml.

Some clinicians prefer high-dose amphotericin B therapy (0.5–1.0 mg/kg daily) with or without flucytosine and reserve fluconazole (400 mg po qd) as initial therapy only for patients with extremely mild disease. It is not clear that a central nervous system imaging study such as a CT scan or MRI is necessary for managing uncomplicated cases without focal signs. When there is evidence of increased intracranial pressure or focal neurologic signs, obtaining such a study is prudent to assess the possibility of a mass lesion or obstructive hydrocephalus. If there is evidence of increased intracranial pressure, management with repeated lumbar punctures should be considered. In severe cases, the placement of a CSF drain needs to be considered. The use of corticosteroid therapy in the setting of increased intracranial pressure or cranial nerve dysfunction is controversial. When managing patients with cryptococcal meningitis, many clinicians advocate performing a second lumbar puncture after the course of acute therapy; however, how to modify management on the basis of the subsequent CSF findings is not entirely certain. Chronic suppressive therapy is necessary after acute therapy. Without chronic suppression, the relapse rate is 50–60 percent.[155] After a good clinical response during the initial 2–10 weeks of therapy, chronic suppressive therapy with fluconazole (200 mg PO qd) is well tolerated and is as effective as once-weekly amphotericin B.[159,160] Serial monitoring of serum cryptococcal antigen titers has limited value; cerebrospinal fluid titers are probably more clinically useful than serum antigen levels.[160a] The prostate is one focus of infection that can be especially difficult to eradicate.[162]

Itraconazole has activity against cryptococcus but is not as well studied and appears less promising than fluconazole.[162,163]

Histoplasmosis is the most common life-threatening opportunistic infection in patients with HIV infection in some endemic regions such as the Indianapolis area[22,23] (see Ch. 244). Acute therapy should consist of amphotericin B 0.5–0.6 mg/kg qd with a total dose of about 500 mg.[164] The length of therapy is determined by the clinical response. Itraconazole is given as 300 mg bid for 3 days followed by 200 mg PO bid for 10 weeks in patients with very mild disease. For chronic maintenance therapy, either itraconazole 200 mg PO qd or amphotericin B 0.5–0.8 mg/kg IV weekly is adequate.[165,166] Serum and urine *Histoplasma capsulatum* polysaccharide antigen titers are useful for monitoring chronic suppressive therapy and predicting relapse.[165,166] The role of antigen monitoring during acute therapy is less certain.

Coccidioidomycosis is a common complication of HIV infection in the southwestern United States (see Ch. 246). Therapy usually consists of an initial course of amphotericin B (0.5–1.0 mg/kg/day iv for at least 8 weeks) followed by lifelong suppression with itraconazole (100–200 mg PO bid) or ketoconazole 400 mg PO qd. High-dose fluconazole can also be used for acute therapy (400–800 mg/day) or chronic suppression (400 mg daily), but is not preferred.[167]

MYCOBACTERIUM SPECIES

Mycobacterium Tuberculosis

Therapy for tuberculosis is reviewed in Chapter 230. For patients with HIV infection, initial therapy generally consists of four drugs unless the likelihood of INH resistance is extremely small: INH (300 mg PO qd), rifampin (600 mg PO), pyrazinamide (15–25 mg/kg PO daily) and ethambutol (15–25 mg/kg PO qd).[168–171] If the organism is susceptible to the drugs being used, isoniazid and pyrazinamide and rifampin should be continued to complete an initial 2 months of therapy; isoniazid plus rifampin should then be continued for 7 additional months or 6 months after sputum culture conversion, whichever is longer. Treatment of drug-resistant tuberculosis is discussed in Chapter 230. Drug-resistant strains have been particular problems in primary infections associated with outbreaks at health care facilities or other institutional settings.[172–175] Therapy is based on susceptibility patterns of the organism.

Chemoprophylaxis should be administered to any HIV-infected patient with a tuberculin skin test that is at least 5 mm in diameter who has never received adequate prophylaxis.[170,171] In addition, HIV-infected patients should receive chemoprophylaxis regardless of tuberculin skin test status if they meet the following criteria: a history of a positive tuberculin skin test that was not adequately treated; close contact with a patient with active tuberculosis; a chest radiograph that is consistent with previous untreated tuberculosis.[168–171]

The recommended prophylaxis is isoniazid for 12 months. It is important to recognize that in areas such as Haiti where tuberculosis is endemic, isoniazid prophylaxis can have a major impact on survival.[25] Arguments can be made in favor of lifelong prophylaxis in areas where tuberculosis is endemic. If patients are unable to tolerate isoniazid, or if there is reason to suspect infection with a drug-resistant strain, prophylactic combination regimens should consist of at least two of the following three drugs: rifampin, pyrazinamide, or a quinolone. Precise doses or durations are not well established. The efficacy of such regimens is also unknown.

Mycobacterium Avium Complex

Studies to date have documented that several individual drugs or multiple drug combinations can reduce or eliminate bacteremia with MAC over a period of weeks or months.[176–185] Many of the patients who have favorable microbiologic responses experience improvement in clinical signs and symptoms. Drugs with microbiologic activity include clarithromycin, azithromycin, ethambutol, rifabutin, rifampin, several quinolones, and amikacin.[176–185] After several weeks or months of monotherapy, however, patients again deteriorate clinically in association with rising numbers of circulating organisms.[176–178] These reemerging organisms are often less susceptible to the treatment regimen than the pretreatment isolates. Thus, monotherapy for MAC disease does not seem to be a successful strategy for providing long-term benefit, at least using the agents currently available. It appears logical to employ multiple drug regimens in order to improve the efficacy of the drug regimen and to reduce the likelihood that resistance will develop. As of yet, there is no proof that combination therapy will produce a sustained clinical and microbiologic response. Moreover, there is no consensus regarding the manner in which in vitro susceptibility testings should be performed in order to guide the selection of drugs. Many antimycobacterial drugs are associated with considerable toxicities. Multidrug regimens with these toxic agents often prove intolerable, and patients must modify or terminate them. Some drugs, such as rifabutin, may also alter the pharmacokinetics of other drugs such as clarithromycin or zidovudine.

Because disease caused by MAC is a source of substantial morbidity, and because mycobacterial disease occurs at a predictable time in the natural history of HIV-induced immunosuppression (i.e., at CD4 counts of <100/mm³) prophylaxis is a reasonable consideration.[31] Prophylactic administration of rifabutin can reduce the frequency of MAC bacteremia by 50 percent.[10] How durable this benefit will be is uncertain. Rifabutin prophylaxis is very well tolerated, although as mentioned above, drug interactions are potentially problematic. Clarithromycin, azithromycin, and higher doses of rifabutin are currently being evaluated for prophylaxis against MAC (also see Ch. 232).

ENTERIC PATHOGENS: SALMONELLA SPECIES, SHIGELLA SPECIES, CAMPYLOBACTER SPECIES, ENTAMOEBA HISTOLYTICA, GIARDIA LAMBLIA

Initial therapy for *Salmonella* (Ch. 200), *Shigella* (Ch. 201), *Campylobacter* (Ch. 194), *Entamoeba histolytica* (Ch. 251) and *Giardia lamblia* (Ch. 259) follows standard guidelines. *Salmonella* and perhaps *Shigella* tend to relapse if chronic suppressive therapy is not administered.

CRYPTOSPORIDIA, ISOSPORA, MICROSPORIDIA

Isospora belli (see Ch. 263) responds to trimethoprim-sulfamethoxazole (trimethoprim, 160 mg, plus sulfamethoxazole, 800 mg PO q6h for 7–10 days), but the relapse rate is high and chronic suppression with trimethoprim-sulfamethoxazole is necessary. Pyrimethamine may be an alternative for patients with severe intolerance to trimethoprim-sulfamethoxazole.

Therapy of cryptosporidiosis has been disappointing[186] (see Ch. 262). Paromomycin may offer temporary benefit.[187] Otherwise, therapy consists of supportive measures.

Microsporidia spp. do not respond to most therapies than have been tried (see Ch. 264). High-dose albendazole has been reported to be effective in preliminary reports.[188] As more is learned about species differences among this group of organisms, it is possible that some species may be identified that are more responsive to therapy than others.

TREPONEMA PALLIDUM

Syphilis is often recognized in HIV-infected patients either because characteristic lesions of primary or secondary disease are present or because a screening serology for *T. pallidum* is positive. It is becoming increasingly apparent that in HIV-infected patients with syphilis, central nervous system involvement is relatively common. As many as 40 percent of patients with primary or secondary syphilis will have serologic or microbiologic evidence of *T. pallidum* in their CSF regardless of their HIV status if careful diagnostic studies are employed. It is also becoming increasingly apparent that, in HIV-infected patients with primary, secondary, or latent syphilis, a single dose of 2.4 million units of benzathine penicillin may be inadequate to cure the central nervous system infection or to prevent systemic relapses as measured by subsequent rises in serum Venereal Disease Research Laboratory (VDRL) titers.[189] The optimal treatment for HIV-infected patients with early or latent syphilis is not established: procaine penicillin (2.4 mIU daily plus 1 g probenicid for 10–14 days) may be preferred over serial doses of benzathine penicillin (2.4 mIU every week for 3 or 4 weeks)[189] (also see Ch. 215).

BARTONELLA (ROCHALIMAEA) HENSELAE AND B. QUINTANA

Bartonella (Rochalimea) henselae and *B. quintana* (see Ch. 170) have been described as the cause of a spectrum of clinical syndromes in patients with HIV infection. These syndromes include cutaneous and subcutaneous angiomatosis papules (bacillary angiomatosis) that can be confused with Kaposi sarcoma; peliosis hepatitis; bacteremia; splenic inflammation; cerebral mass lesions; bone lesions; lymphadenitis; and aseptic meningitis. Erythromycin and tetracycline have both been used with success in some patients. At least 2 g daily of erythromycin should be given for at least 8–12 weeks for patients with cutaneous disease. Clinical response may be seen during the first week. Hepatic and osseous disease should be treated initially with intravenous erythromycin, and then therapy should be continued for at least 4–6 months with an oral regimen. Bacteremia alone may respond to 2 months of therapy. A Jarisch-Herxheimer reaction may be seen in response to the first few doses.[190–192] Treatment failures and relapses occur, and more information is needed to establish optimal regimens.

KAPOSI SARCOMA

The presence of Kaposi sarcoma does not necessarily mandate institution of therapy, especially if lesions are few in number and inconspicuous (see Ch. 102 for additional discussions). Local measures include excision, radiation, and intralesional injection with chemotherapy.[28] Kaposi sarcoma lesions tend to recur despite intensive radiation therapy. When lesions in the oropharynx are radiated, mucositis seems to be especially common.

When cutaneous Kaposi sarcoma is extensive, recombinant interferon-α therapy (10–30 million units/m² IM, IV, or SC qd) can be useful, especially for patients with circulating CD4+ T-lymphocyte counts greater than 100–200 cells/mm³.[28] Objective tumor responses can be seen in 4–8 weeks, with maximal responses in 12–24 weeks. Late initial responses after many months of therapy occasionally occur. Tumor response may persist for over 1 year, especially when maintenance interferon-α therapy is given. Because the tumor response is not rapid, interferon-α therapy is not desirable for urgent, life-threatening situations such as laryngeal or extensive pulmonary involvement. Adverse effects of interferon-α include confusion, fatigue, myalgias, leukopenia, thrombocytopenia, hepatitis, and cardiomyopathy.

Kaposi sarcoma can cause life-threatening disease by obstructing a vital structure such as the larynx, bronchus, biliary tract, or bowel. Kaposi sarcoma can occasionally infiltrate a vital organ such as the lung and cause fatal hypoxemia. In these life-threatening situations, either radiation therapy or cytotoxic chemotherapy is necessary to produce a rapid and substantial response. The optimal mode of therapy depends on the location and extent of tumor. In appropriate clinical settings, short-term palliation of life-threatening symptoms rather than long-term survival is the therapeutic goal, and thus the immunosuppres-

sive nature of some therapies is not the overriding concern. A variety of chemotherapeutic regimens have been used with some success, including vinblastine; etoposide; vincristine; vincristine and vinblastine; vinblastine and bleomycin; doxorubicin, bleomycin, and vincristine[28] (see Ch. 102). The optimal drug regimen for specific situations has not been determined.

LYMPHOMA

Lymphomas of the Hodgkin's, non-Hodgkin's, and Burkitt types generally have been associated with short patient survival regardless of the therapeutic modality chosen (see Ch. 102). A variety of cytotoxic regimens and irradiation has been used in order to reduce tumor size or palliate specific syndromes such as neurologic dysfunction caused by central nervous system lesions.[193,194] The response rate has been lower in AIDS patients than in non-AIDS patients, and relapses have been prompt and frequent. Whether any regimen prolongs survival and which regimen is optimal have not yet been determined, although there are some reports that the remission rates and disease-free survival may be improving. Patients die as a direct result of lymphoma, as a result of AIDS-related infections, and as a result of chemotherapy-associated infections.

REFERENCES

1. Osmond D, Charlebois E, Lang W, et al. Changes in AIDS survival time in two San Francisco cohorts of homosexual men, 1983–1993. JAMA. 1994; 271:1083–7.
2. Lafferty WE, Glidden D, Hopkins SG. Survival trends of people with AIDS in Washington state. Am J Public Health. 1991;81:217–9.
3. Moore RD, Hidalgo J, Sugland BW, et al. Zidovudine and the natural history of the acquired immunodeficiency syndrome. N Engl J Med. 1991;324: 1412–6.
4. Goedert JJ, Kessler CM, Aledort M, et al. A prospective study of human immunodeficiency virus type 1 infection and the development of AIDS in subjects with hemophilia. N Engl J Med. 1989;321:1141–8.
5. Moss AR, Bacchetti P, Osmond D, et al. Seropositivity for HIV and the development of AIDS or AIDS related condition: Three year follow up of the San Francisco General Hospital cohort. Br Med J. 1988;296:745–50.
6. Fahey JL, Taylor JMG, Detels R, et al. The prognostic value of cellular and serologic markers in infection with human immunodeficiency virus type 1. N Engl J Med. 1990;322:166–72.
7. Masur H, Ognibene FP, Yarchoan R, et al. CD4 counts as predictors of opportunistic pneumonias in human immunodeficiency virus (HIV) infection. Ann Intern Med. 1989;111:223–31.
8. Phair J, Munoz A, Detels R, et al. The risk of *Pneumocystis carinii* pneumonia among men infected with human immunodeficiency virus type 1. N Engl J Med. 1990;322:161–5.
9. Yarchoan R, Venzon DJ, Pluda JM, et al. CD4 count and the risk for death in patients infected with HIV receiving antiretroviral therapy. Ann Intern Med. 1991;115:184–9.
10. Nightingale SD, Cameron DW, Gordin FM, et al. Two controlled trials of rifabutin prophylaxis against *Mycobacterium avium* complex infection in AIDS. N Engl J Med. 1993;329:828–33.
11. Havlik JA Jr, Horsburgh CR Jr, Metchock B, et al. Disseminated *Mycobacterium avium* complex infection: Clinical identification and epidemiologic trends. J Infect Dis. 1992;165:577–80.
12. Nightingale SD, Byrd LT, Southern PM, et al. Incidence of *Mycobacterium avium* intracellulare complex bacteremia in human immunodeficiency virus-positive patients. J Infect Dis. 1992;165:1082–5.
13. Rutherford GW, Lifson AR, Hessol NA, et al. Course of HIV-1 infection in a cohort of homosexual and bisexual men: An 11 year follow up study. Br Med J. 1990;301:1183–8.
14. Biggar RJ, International Registry of Seroconverters. AIDS incubation in 1891 seroconverters from different exposure groups. AIDS. 1990;4:1059–66.
15. Hessol NA, Byers RH, Lifson AR, et al. Relationship between AIDS latency period and AIDS survival time in homosexual and bisexual men. J AIDS. 1990;3:1078–85.
16. Ward JW, Bush TJ, Perkins HA, et al. The natural history of transfusion-associated infection with human immunodeficiency virus: Factors influencing the rate of progression to disease. N Engl J Med. 1989;321:947–52.
17. Phair J, Munoz A, Saah A, et al. Response to letter to the editor. N Engl J Med. 1990;322:1608.
18. Small PM, Shafer RW, Hopewell PC, et al. Exogenous reinfection with multidrug-resistant *Mycobacterium tuberculosis* in patients with advanced HIV infection. N Engl J Med. 1993;328:1137–44.
19. Centers for Disease Control and Prevention. Nosocomial transmission of multidrug resistant tuberculosis among HIV-infected patients. MMWR. 1991;40:585–91.

20. Daley CL, Small PM, Schecter GF, et al. An outbreak of tuberculosis with accelerated progression among persons infected with human immunodeficiency virus: An analysis using restriction-fragment-length polymorphisms. N Engl J Med. 1992;326:231–5.
21. Pearson ML, Jereb JA, Frieden TR, et al. Nosocomial transmission of multidrug-resistant *Mycobacterium tuberculosis*—a risk to patients and health care workers. Ann Intern Med. 1992;117:191–6.
22. Wheat LJ. Histoplasmosis in Indianapolis. Clin Infect Dis. 1992;14(Suppl 1):S91–S99.
23. Wheat LJ, Connolly-Stringfield PA, Baker RL, et al. Disseminated histoplasmosis in the acquired immunodeficiency syndrome: Clinical findings, diagnosis and treatment, and review of the literature. Medicine (Baltimore). 1990;69:361–74.
24. DeGorgolas M, Castrillo JM, Fernandez Guerrrero AL. Visceral leishmaniasis in patients with AIDS: Report of 3 cases treated with pentavalent antimony and interferon gamma. Clin Infect Dis. 1993;17:56–8.
25. Pape JW, Jean Simone S, Ho JL, et al. Effect of isoniazid prophylaxis on incidence of active tuberculosis and progression in HIV infection. Lancet. 1993;342:268–72.
26. Mukadi Y, Perriens JH, St. Louis ME, et al. Spectrum of immunodeficiency in HIV-1 infected patients with pulmolnary tuberculosis in Zaire. Lancet. 1993;342:143–6.
27. Pape JW, Verdier R, Johnson WD, et al. Treatment and prophylaxis of *Isospora belli* infection. N Engl J Med. 1989;320:1044–7.
28. Kahn JO, Northfelt DW, Miles SA. AIDS associated Kaposi's sarcoma. AIDS Clin Rev. 1992;261–80.
29. Centers for Disease Control and Prevention. Recommendations for prophylaxis against *Pneumocystis carinii* pneumonia for adults and adolescents infected with human immunodeficiency virus. MMWR. 1992;41,RR-4:1–11.
30. Masur H. Prevention and treatment of *Pneumocystis* pneumonia. N Engl J Med. 1992;327:1853–60.
31. Masur H (Chairman) and the U.S. Public Health Service Task Force on Prophylaxis and Therapy for *Mycobacterium avium* Complex. Recommendations on prophylaxis and therapy for disseminated *Mycobacterium avium* complex disease in patients infected with the human immunodeficiency virus. N Engl J Med. 1993;329:898–904.
32. Kovacs JA, Hiemenz JW, Macher AM, et al. Pneumocystis carinii pneumonia: A comparison between patients with the acquired immunodeficiency syndrome and patients with other immunodeficiencies. Ann Intern Med. 1984;100:663–71.
33. Kovacs JA, Kovacs AA, Polis M. Cryptococcosis in the acquired immunodeficiency syndrome. Ann Intern Med. 1985;103:533–8.
34. Lee BL, Safrin S. Interactions and toxicities of drugs used in patients with AIDS. Clin Infect Dis. 1992;14:773–9.
35. Abouya YL, Beaumel A, Lucas A, et al. Pneumocystis pneumonia—an uncommon cause of death in African patients with acquired immunodeficiency syndrome. Am Rev Respir Dis. 1992;145:617–20.
36. Carme B, Mboussa J, Andzin M, et al. *Pneumocystis carinii* is rare in AIDS in Central Africa. Trans R Soc Trop Med Hyg. 1991;85:80.
37. Wharton JM, Coleman DL, Wofsy CB, et al. Adverse reactions to trimethoprim-sulfamethoxazole or pentamidine for *Pneumocystis carinii* pneumonia in the acquired immunodeficiency syndrome. A prospective randomized trial. Ann Intern Med. 1986;195:37–44.
38. Brenner M, Ognibene FP, Lack EE, et al. Prognostic factors and life expectancy of acquired immunodeficiency syndrome patients with *Pneumocystis carinii* pneumonia. Am Rev Respir Dis. 1987;136:1199–206.
39. Garay S, Greene J. Prognostic indicators in the initial presentation of pneumocystis pneumonia. Chest. 1989;95:769–72.
40. Wachter RM, Russi MB, Bloch DA, et al. *Pneumocystis carinii* pneumonia and respiratory failure in AIDS. Am Rev Respir Dis. 1991;143:251–6.
41. el Sadr WM, Simberkoff MS. Survival and prognostic factors in severe *Pneumocystis carinii* pneumonia requiring mechanical ventilation. Am Rev Respir Dis. 1988;137:1264–7.
42. Broaddus C, Dake MD, Stulbarg MS, et al. Bronchoalveolar lavage and transbronchial biopsy for the diagnosis of pulmonary infections in the acquired immunodeficiency syndrome. Ann Intern Med. 1985;102:747–52.
43. Meduri G, Stover DE, Greene RA, et al. Bilateral bronchoalveolar lavage in the diagnosis of opportunistic pulmonary infections. Chest. 1991;100:1272–6.
44. Ognibene FP, Shelhamer J, Gill V, et al. The diagnosis of *Pneumocystis carinii* pneumonia in patients with the acquired immunodeficiency syndrome using subsegmental bronchoalveolar lavage. Am Rev Respir Dis. 1984;129:933–7.
45. Baughman RP, Dohn MN, Shipley R, et al. Increased *Pneumocystis carinii* recovery from the upper lobes in pneumocystis pneumonia—the effect of aerosolized pentamidine prophylaxis. Chest. 1993;103:426–32.
46. Kovacs JA, Ng VL, Leoung G, et al. Diagnosis of pneumocystis pneumonia: Improved detection in sputum with use of monoclonal antibodies. N Engl J Med. 1988;318:589–93.
47. Barnes PF, Steele MA, Young SMM, et al. Tuberculosis in patients with human immunodeficiency virus infection—how often does it mimic *Pneumocystis carinii* pneumonia? Chest. 1992;102:428–32.
48. Ognibene FP, Masur H, Rogers P, et al. Nonspecific interstitial pneumonitis without evidence of *Pneumocystis carinii* in asymptomatic patients infected with human immunodeficiency virus (HIV). Ann Intern Med. 1988;109:874–9.
49. Ng VL, Geaghan SM, Leoung G, et al. Lack of effect of prophylactic aerosolized pentamidine on the detection of *Pneumocystis carinii* in induced sputum

or bronchoalveolar lavage specimens. Arch Pathol Lab Med. 1993;117:493–6.
50. Levine SF, Masur H, Gill VJ, et al. Effect of aerosolized pentamidine prophylaxis on the diagnosis of *Pneumocystis carinii* pneumonia by induced sputum examination in patients infected with HIV. Am Rev Respir Dis. 1991;144:760–4.
51. Wakefield AE, Guiver L, Miller RJ, et al. DNA amplification in induced sputum samples for diagnosis of *Pneumocystis carinii* pneumonia. Lancet. 1991;337:1378.
52. Schluger N, Godwin T, Sepkowitz K, et al. Application of DNA amplification to pneumocystosis: Presence of serum *Pneumocystis carinii* pneumonia. J Exp Med. 1992;176:1327–33.
53. Dohn MN, Baughman RP, Vigdorth EM, et al. Equal survival rates for first, second and third episodes of *Pneumocystis carinii* pneumonia in patients with AIDS. Arch Intern Med. 1992;152:2465–70.
54. Sattler FR, Cowan R, Nielsen DM, et al. Trimethoprim-sulfamethoxazole versus pentamidine for therapy of pneumocystis pneumonia: A prospective noncrossover study in patients with AIDS. Ann Intern Med. 1988;109:280–7.
55. Lee BL, Medina I, Benowitz NL, et al. Dapsone, trimethoprim, and sulfamethoxazole plasma levels during treatment of pneumocystis pneumonia in patients with the acquired immunodeficiency syndrome (AIDS): Evidence of drug interactions. Ann Intern Med. 1989;110:606–11.
56. Lau WK, Young LS. Trimethoprim-sulfamethoxazole treatment of *Pneumocystis carinii* pneumonia in adults. N Engl J Med. 1976;295:716–8.
57. Gordin FM, Simon GL, Wofsy CB, et al. Adverse reactions to trimethoprim-sulfamethoxazole in patients with the acquired immunodeficiency syndrome. Ann Intern Med. 1984;100:495–9.
58. Montaner JSG, Lawson LM, Levitt N, et al. Oral corticosteroids prevent early deterioration in patients with moderately severe AIDS-related *Pneumocystis carinii* pneumonia. Ann Intern Med. 1990;113:14–20.
59. Hughes W, Leoung G, Kramer F, et al. Comparison of atovaquone (566C80) with trimethoprim-sulfamethoxazole to treat *Pneumocystis carinii* pneumonia in patients with AIDS. N Engl J Med. 1993;328:1521–7.
60. Nguyen BY, Landucci DL, Cunnion RE, et al. A case of hyperdynamic shock caused by trimethoprim-sulfamethoxazole in which no tumor necrosis factor or features of anaphylaxis were detected. Clin Infect Dis. 1993;17:885–7.
61. Greenberg S, Reiser JW, Chou SY, et al. Trimethoprim-sulfamethoxazole induces reversible hyperkalemia. Ann Intern Med. 1993;119:291–5.
62. Carr A, Swanson C, Penny R, et al. Clinical and laboratory markers of hypersensitivity to trimethoprim-sulfamethoxazole in patients with pneumocystis pneumonia and AIDS. J Infect Dis. 1993;167:180–5.
62a.Kennedy CA, Pimentel JA, Lewis DE, et al. Crossover of human immunodeficiency virus-infected patients from aerosolized pentamidine to trimethoprim-sulfamethoxazole: Lack of hematologic toxicity and relationships of side effects to CD4+ lymphocyte count. Clin Infect Dis. 1993;168:314–7.
62b.Caumes E, Rodier C, Rogeaux O, et al. Effect of corticosteroids on the incidence of adverse cutaneous reactions to trimethoprim-sulfamethoxazole during treatment of AIDS associated pneumocystis pneumonia. Clin Infect Dis. 1994;18:319–23.
63. Smith RM, Iwamoto GK, Richerson HB, et al. Trimethoprim-sulfamethoxazole desensitization in the acquired immunodeficiency syndrome. Ann Intern Med. 1987;106:335.
64. Pearson RD, Hewlett EL. Pentamidine for the treatment of *Pneumocystis carinii* and other protozoal diseases. Ann Intern Med. 1985;103:782–6.
65. Navin TR, Fontaine RE. Intravenous versus intramuscular administration of pentamidine. N Engl J Med. 1984;311:1701–2.
66. Mallory DL, Parrillo JE, Bailey KR, et al. Cardiovascular effects and safety of intravenous and intramuscular pentamidine isethionate. Crit Care Med. 1987;15:503–5.
66a.Eisenhauer MD, Eliasson AH, Taylor AJ, et al. Incidence of cardiac arrhythmias during intravenous pentamidine therapy in HIV infected patients. Chest. 1994;105:389–94.
67. Waskin H, Stehr-Green JK, Helmick CG, et al. Risk factors for hypoglycemia associated with pentamidine therapy for pneumocystis pneumonia. JAMA. 1988;260:345–7.
68. Conte JE, Chernoff D, Feigal DW, et al. Intravenous or inhaled pentamidine for treating *Pneumocystis carinii* pneumonia in AIDS. Ann Intern Med. 1990;113:203–9.
69. Medina I, Mills J, Leoung G, et al. Oral therapy for *Pneumocystis carinii* pneumonia in the acquired immunodeficiency syndrome—a controlled trial of trimethoprim-sulfamethoxazole versus trimethoprim-dapsone. N Engl J Med. 1990;323:776–82.
70. Mills J, Leoung G, Medina J, et al. Dapsone treatment of *Pneumocystis carinii* pneumonia in the acquired immunodeficiency syndrome. Antimicrob Agents Chemother. 1988;32:1057–60.
71. Hughes WT, Gray VL, Gutteridge WE, et al. Efficacy of a hydroxynaphthoquinone, 566C80, in experimental *Pneumocystis carinii* pneumonitis. Antimicrob Agents Chemother. 1990;34:225–8.
72. Falloon J, Kovacs J, Hughes W, et al. A preliminary evaluation of 566C80 for the treatment of pneumocystis pneumonia in patients with acquired immunodeficiency syndrome. N Engl J Med. 1991;325:1534–8.
73. Toma E, Fournier S, Poisson M, et al. Clindamycin with primaquine for *Pneumocystis carinii* pneumonia. Lancet. 1989;1:1046–8.
74. Ruf B, Pohle HD. Clindamycin/primaquine for *Pneumocystis carinii* pneumonia. Lancet. 1989;2:626–7.
75. Noskin GA, Murphy RL, Black JR, et al. Salvage therapy with clindamycin/

primaquine for *Pneumocystis carinii* pneumonia. Clin Infect Dis. 1992;14: 183–8.

76. Allegra CJ, Chabner BA, Tuazon CU, et al. Trimetrexate for the treatment of *Pneumocystis carinii* pneumonia in patients with the acquired immunodeficiency syndrome. N Engl J Med. 1987;317:978–85.

77. Sattler FR, Allegra CJ, Verdegem TD, et al. Trimetrexate-leucovorin dosage evaluation study for treatment of *Pneumocystis carinii* pneumonia. J Infect Dis. 1990;161:91–6.

78. Sattler FR, Frame P, Davis R, et al. Comparison of trimetrexate with leucovorin versus trimethoprim-sulfamethoxazole for moderate to severe episodes of *Pneumocystis carinii* pneumonia in patients with AIDS. J Infect Dis. 1994 In press.

79. Bozzette SA, Sattler FR, Chiu J, et al. A controlled trial of early adjunctive treatment with corticosteroids for *Pneumocystis carinii* pneumonia in the acquired immunodeficiency syndrome. N Engl J Med. 1990;323:1451–7.

80. Gagnon S, Boota AM, Fischl MA, et al. Corticosteroids as adjunctive therapy for severe *Pneumocystis carinii* pneumonia in the acquired immunodeficiency syndrome—a double-blind, placebo-controlled trial. N Engl J Med. 1990;323:1444–50.

81. Nielsen TL, Schattenkerk JKME, Jensen BN, et al. Adjunctive corticosteroid therapy for *Pneumocystis carinii* pneumonia in AIDS: A randomized European multicenter open label study. J AIDS. 1992;5:726–31.

82. National Institutes of Health–University of California Expert Panel for Corticosteroids as Adjunctive Therapy for Pneumocystis Pneumonia. Consensus statement on the use of corticosteroids as adjunctive therapy for pneumocystis pneumonia in the acquired immunodeficiency syndrome. N Engl J Med. 1990;323:1500–4.

83. Shelhamer JH, Ognibene FP, Macher AM, et al. Persistence of *Pneumocystis carinii* in lung tissue of acquired immunodeficiency syndrome patients treated for pneumocystis pneumonia. Am Rev Respir Dis. 1984;130:1161–5.

84. Wachter RM, Luce JM, Hopewell PC. Critical care of patients with AIDS. JAMA. 1992;267:541–7.

85. Kovacs JA, Masur H. Prophylaxis for *Pneumocystis carinii* pneumonia in patients infected with human immunodeficiency virus. Clin Infect Dis. 1992; 14:1005–9.

86. Hardy WD, Feinberg J, Finkelstein DM, et al. A controlled trial of trimethoprim-sulfamethoxazole or aerosolized pentamidine for secondary prophylaxis of *Pneumocystis carinii* pneumonia in patients with the acquired immunodeficiency syndrome: AIDS Clinical Trials Group protocol 021. N Engl J Med. 1992;327:1842–8.

87. Schneider MME, Hoepelman AIM, Eeftinck Schattenkerk JKM, et al. A controlled trial of aerosolized pentamidine or trimethoprim-sulfamethoxazole as primary prophylaxis against *Pneumocystis carinii* pneumonia in patients with human immunodeficiency virus infection. N Engl J Med. 1992; 327:1836–41.

88. Carr A, Tindall B, Brew BJ, et al. Low-dose trimethoprim-sulfamethoxazole prophylaxis for toxoplasmic encephalitis in patients with AIDS. Ann Intern Med. 1992;117:106–11.

89. Ruskin J, LaRiviere M. Low-dose co-trimoxazole for prevention of *Pneumocystis carinii* pneumonia in human immunodeficiency virus disease. Lancet. 1991;337:468–71.

90. Raviglione M, Nash E, Cortes H, et al. Intermittent co-trimoxazole prophylaxis against *Pneumocystis carinii* pneumonia. Lancet. 1990;336:180.

91. Wormser GP, Horowitz HW, Duncanson FP, et al. Low-dose intermittent trimethoprim-sulfamethoxazole for prevention of *Pneumocystis carinii* pneumonia in patients with human immunodeficiency virus infection. Arch Intern Med. 1991;151:688–92.

92. Leoung GS, Feigal DW Jr, Montgomery AB, et al. Aerosolized pentamidine for prophylaxis against *Pneumocystis carinii* pneumonia—the San Francisco Community Prophylaxis Trial. N Engl J Med. 1990;323:769–75.

93. Murphy RL, Lavelle JP, Allan JD, et al. Aerosol pentamidine prophylaxis following *Pneumocystis carinii* pneumonia in AIDS patients: Results of a blinded dose-comparison study using an ultrasonic nebulizer. Am J Med. 1991;90:418–26.

94. Girard P-M, Landman R, Gaudebout C, et al. Prevention of *Pneumocystis carinii* pneumonia relapse by pentamidine aerosol in zidovudine-treated AIDS patients. Lancet. 1989;1:1348–53.

95. Montaner JSG, Lawson LM, Gervais A, et al. Aerosol pentamidine for secondary prophylaxis of AIDS-related *Pneumocystis carinii* pneumonia: A randomized, placebo-controlled study. Ann Intern Med. 1991;114:948–53.

96. Hirschel B, Lazzarin A, Chopard P, et al. A controlled study of inhaled pentamidine for primary prevention of *Pneumocystis carinii* pneumonia. N Engl J Med. 1991;324:1079–83.

96a. Golden JA, Katz M, Chernoff DN, et al. A randomized comparison of once-monthly or twice-monthly high dose aerosolized pentamidine prophylaxis. Chest. 1993;104:743–52.

97. O'Doherty MJ, Thomas S, Page C, et al. Differences in relative efficacy of nebulizers for pentamidine administration. Lancet. 1988;2:1283–6.

98. O'Riordan TG, Smaldone GC. Exposure of health care workers to aerosolized pentamidine. Chest. 1992;101:1494–9.

99. Centers for Disease Control and Prevention. *Mycobacterium tuberculosis* transmission in a health clinic—Florida, 1988. MMWR. 38:256–8, 263–4.

100. Girard P-M, Landman R, Gaudebout C, et al. Dapsone-pyrimethamine compared with aerosolized pentamidine as primary prophylaxis against *Pneumocystis carinii* pneumonia and toxoplasmosis in HIV infection. N Engl J Med. 1993;328:1514–20.

101. Blum RN, Miller LA, Gaggini LC, et al. Comparative trial of dapsone vs.

trimethoprim-sulfamethoxazole for primary prophylaxis of *Pneumocystis carinii* pneumonia. J AIDS. 1992;15:341–7.

102. Kemper CA, Tucker RM, Lang DS, et al. Low dose dapsone prophylaxis of *Pneumocystis carinii* pneumonia in AIDS and AIDS related complex. AIDS. 1990;4:1145–8.

103. Porter SB, Sande MA. Toxoplasmosis of the central nervous system in the acquired immunodeficiency syndrome. N Engl J Med. 1992;327:1643–8.

104. Israelski DM, Chmiel JS, Poggenser L, et al. Prevalence of toxoplasma infection in a cohort of homosexual men at risk of AIDS and toxoplasmic encephalitis. J AIDS. 1993;6:414–8.

105. Luft BJ, Hafner R, Korzun AH. Toxoplasmic encephalitis in patients with the acquired immunodeficiency syndrome. N Engl J Med. 1993;329: 995–1000.

106. Kupfer MC, Zee CS, Colletti PM, et al. MRI evaluation of AIDS-related encephalopathy: Toxoplasmosis vs. lymphoma. Magn Reson Imag. 1990;8: 51–7.

107. Levy RM, Mills CM, Posin JP, et al. The efficacy and clinical impact of brain imaging in neurologically symptomatic AIDS patients: A prospective CT/MRI study. J AIDS. 1990;3:461–71.

108. Levy RM, Rosenbloom S, Perrett L. Neuroradiologic findings in the acquired immunodeficiency syndrome: A report of 200 cases. Am J Nucl Radiol. 1986; 7:833–9.

109. Cohn JA, McMeeking A, Cohen W, et al. Evaluation of the policy of empiric treatment of suspected toxoplasma encephalitis in patients with the acquired immunodeficiency syndrome. Am J Med. 1989;86:521–7.

110. Luft BJ, Remington JS. Toxoplasmic encephalitis in AIDS. Clin Infect Dis. 1992;15:211–22.

110a. Jacobson MA, Besch CL, Child C, et al. Primary prophylaxis with primethamine for toxoplasmic encephalitis in patients with HIV disease: Results of a randomized trial. J Infect Dis. 1994;165:384–94.

111. Wanke CH, Tuazon CU, Kovacs A, et al. Toxoplasma encephalitis in patients with acquired immune deficiency syndrome. Am J Trop Med Hyg. 1987;36:509–16.

112. Leport C, Raffi F, Matheron S, et al. Treatment of central nervous system toxoplasmosis with pyrimethamine-sulfadiazine combination in 35 AIDS patients: Efficacy of long term continuous therapy. Am J Med. 1988;84:94–100.

113. Dannemann B, McCutchan JA, Israelski D, et al. Treatment of toxoplasmic encephalitis in patients with AIDS: A randomized trial comparing pyrimethamine plus clindamycin to pyrimethamine plus sulfonamides. Ann Intern Med. 1992;116:33–43.

114. Kovacs JA, O'Neill D, Feuerstein I, et al. Efficacy of atovaquone in treatment of toxoplasmosis in patients with AIDS. Lancet. 1992;340:637–8.

115. Derouin F, Piketty C, Chastang C, et al. Antitoxoplasma effects of dapsone alone and combined with pyrimethamine. Antimicrob Agents Chemother. 1991;35:252–5.

116. de Gans J, Portegies P, Reiss P, et al. Pyrimethamine alson as maintenance therapy for central nervous system toxoplasmosis in 38 patients with AIDS. J AIDS. 1992;5:137–42.

117. Masur H, Polis MA, Tuazon CU, et al. Salvage trial of trimetrexate-leucovorin for the treatment of cerebral toxoplasmosis in patients with AIDS. J Infect Dis. 1993;167:1422–6.

118. Kalb RE, Grossman ME. Chronic perianal herpes simplex in immunocompromised hosts. Am J Med. 1986;80:486–90.

119. Hardy WD. Foscarnet treatment of acyclovir-resistant herpes simplex virus infection in patients with AIDS: Preliminary results of a controlled, randomized regimen—comparative trial. Am J Med. 1992;14:305–55.

120. Safrin S, Assay-Keen T, Follansbee S, et al. Foscarnet therapy for acyclovir resistant mucocutaneous herpes simplex virus infection in 26 AIDS patients: Preliminary data. J Infect Dis. 1990;161:1078–84.

120a. Balfour HH, Benson C, Braun J, et al. Management of acyclovir-resistant herpes simplex and varicella-zoster infection. JAIDS. 1994;7:254–260.

121. Safrin S, Berger TG, Gilson I, et al. Foscarnet therapy in five patients with AIDS and acyclovir-resistant varicella zoster virus infection. Ann Intern Med. 1991;115:19–21.

122. Jacobson MA, Berger TG, Fikorg S, et al. Acyclovir-resistant varicella-zoster virus infection after chronic oral acyclovir therapy in patients with AIDS. Ann Intern Med. 1990;112:187–91.

123. Zurlo JJ, O'Neill D, Polis MA, et al. Lack of clinical utility of cytomegalovirus blood and urine cultures in patients with HIV infection. Ann Intern Med. 1993;118:12–7.

124. Jacobson MA, Mills J. Serious cytomegalovirus disease in the acquired immunodeficiency syndrome (AIDS). Ann Intern Med. 1988;108:585–94.

125. Drew WL. Cytomegalovirus infection in patients with AIDS. Clin Infect Dis. 1992;14:608–15.

126. Bloom JN, Palestine AG. The diagnosis of cytomegalovirus retinitis. Ann Intern Med. 1988;109:963–9.

127. Buhles WC, Mastre BJ, Tinker AJ, et al. Ganciclovir treatment of life- or sight-threatening cytomegalovirus infection: Experience in 314 immunocompromised patients. Rev Infect Dis. 1988;10 (Suppl 3):S495–S504.

128. Jabs DA, Enger C, Haller JA, et al. Retinal detachments in patients with cytomegalovirus retinitis. Arch Ophthalmol. 1991;109:794–9.

129. Holland G, Shuler JD. Progression rates of cytomegalovirus retinopathy in ganciclovir-treated and untreated patients. Arch Ophthalmol. 1992;110: 1435–42.

130. Studies of the Ocular Complications of AIDS Research Group, AIDS Clinical Trials Group. Mortality in patients with the acquired immunodeficiency syn-

drome treated with either foscarnet or ganciclovir for cytomegalovirus retinitis. N Engl J Med. 1992;326:213–20.

131. Palestine AG, Polis MA, De Smet MD, et al. A randomized, controlled trial of foscarnet in the treatment of cytomegalovirus retinitis in patients with AIDS. Ann Intern Med. 1991;115:665–73.

132. Spector SA, Barker C, Buhles W, et al. A randomized, controlled study of immediate vs. deferred ganciclovir therapy in AIDS patients with cytomegalovirus peripheral retinitis (Abstract). VII International Conference on AIDS 1991;M.B.86.

133. Cantrill HL, Henry K, Melroe NH, et al. Treatment of cytomegalovirus retinitis with intravitreal ganciclovir: Long-term results. Ophthalmology. 1989;69:367–74.

134. Deray G, Martinez F, Katlama C, et al. Foscarnet nephrotoxicity: Mechanism, incidence, and prevention. Am J Nephrol. 1989;9:316–21.

135. Polis MA, De Smet MD, Baird BF, et al. Increased survival of a cohort of patients with acquired immunodeficiency syndrome and cytomegalovirus retinitis who received sodium phosphonoformate (foscarnet). Am J Med. 1993;94:185–90.

136. Wilcox CM, Diehl DL, Cello JP, et al. Cytomegalovirus esophagitis in patients with AIDS: A clinical, endoscopic, and pathologic correlation. Ann Intern Med. 1990;113:589–93.

137. Wilcox CM. Esophageal disease in the acquired immunodeficiency syndrome: Etiology, diagnosis, and management. Am J Med. 1992;92:412–21.

138. Dieterich DT, Kotler DP, Busch DF, et al. Ganciclovir treatment of cytomegalovirus colitis in AIDS: A randomized, double-blind, placebo-controlled multicenter study. J Infect Dis. 1993;167:278–82.

139. Nelson MR, Connolly GM, Hawkins DA, et al. Foscarnet in the treatment of cytomegalovirus infection of the esophagus and colon in patients with the acquired immune deficiency syndrome. Am J Gastroenterol. 1991;86:876–81.

140. Emanuel D, Cunningham I, Jules-Elysee K, et al. Cytomegalovirus pneumonia after bone-marrow transplantation successfully treated with the combination of ganciclovir and high-dose intravenous immune globulin. Ann Intern Med. 1988;109:777–82.

141. Reed EC, Bowden RA, Dandliker PS, et al. Treatment of cytomegalovirus pneumonia with ganciclovir and intravenous cytomegalovirus immunoglobulin in patients with bone marrow transplants. Ann Intern Med. 1988;109:783–8.

142. Tatarowicz WA, Lurain NS, Thompson KD. A ganciclovir-resistant clinical isolate of human cytomegalovirus exhibiting cross-resistance to other DNA polymerase inhibitors. J Infect Dis. 1992;166:904–7.

143. Sullivan V, Coen DM. Isolation of foscarnet-resistant human cytomegalovirus patterns of resistance and sensitivity to other antiviral drugs. J Infect Dis. 1991;164:781–4.

144. Nelson MR, Barter G, Hawkins D, et al. Simultaneous treatment of cytomegalovirus retinitis with ganciclovir and foscarnet. Lancet. 1991;338:250.

145. Manischewitz JF, Quinnan GV Jr, Lane HC, et al. Synergistic effect of ganciclovir and foscarnet on cytomegalovirus replication *in vitro*. Antimicrob Agents Chemother. 1990;34:373–5.

146. Follansbee S, Busch D, Connor J, et al. Phase I study of the safety and pharmacokinetics of oral ganciclovir (Abstract). VI International Conference on AIDS 1990;F.B.91.

147. Balfour HH Jr, Chace BA, Stapleton JT, et al. A randomized placebo-controlled trial of oral acyclovir for the prevention of cytomegalovirus disease in recipients of renal allografts. N Engl J Med. 1989;320:1381–7.

148. Snydman DR, Werner BC, Heinze-Lacey BH, et al. Use of cytomegalovirus immune globulin to prevent cytomegalovirus disease in renal transplant recipients. N Engl J Med. 1987;317:1049–54.

149. Major EO, Amemiya K, Tornatore CS, et al. Pathogenesis and molecular biology of progressive multifocal leukoencephalopathy, the JC virus-induced demyelinating disease of the human brain. Clin Microbiol Rev. 1992;5:49–73.

150. Chave JP, Francioli P, Hirschel B, et al. Single dose therapy for esophageal candidiasis (Letter). AIDS. 1990;4:1034–5.

151. Lake-Bakaar G, Tom W, Lake-Bakaar D, et al. Gastropathy and ketoconazole in AIDS. Ann Intern Med. 1988;109:471–3.

152. Smith DE, Midgely J, Allen M, et al. Itraconazole vs. ketoconazole in treatment of oral and esophageal candidiasis in patients with HIV. AIDS. 1991;5:1367–71.

153. DeWit S, Weerts D, Goosens H, et al. Comparison of fluconazole and ketoconazole for oropharyngeal candidiasis in AIDS. Lancet. 1989;1:746–7.

154. Fox R, Neal KR, Leen CLS, et al. Fluconazole resistant candida in AIDS. J Infect. 1991;22:201–2.

155. Zuger A, Louis E, Holzman RS, et al. Cryptococcal disease in patients with the acquired immunodeficiency syndrome: Diagnostic features and outcome of treatment. Ann Intern Med. 1986;104:234–40.

156. White M, Cirrincione C, Blevins A, et al. Cryptococcal meningitis: Outcome in patients with AIDS and patients with neoplastic disease. J Infect Dis. 1992;165:960–3.

157. Saag MS, Powderly WG, Clud GA, et al. Comparison of amphotericin B with fluconazole in the treatment of acute AIDS-associated cryptococcal meningitis. The NIAID Mycoses Study Group and the AIDS Clinical Trials Group. N Engl J Med. 1992;326:83–9.

158. Larsen RA, Leal M, Chan L. Fluconazole compared with amphotericin B plus flucytosine for cryptococcal meningitis in AIDS. Ann Intern Med. 1990;113:183–7.

159. Powderly WG, Saag MS, Cloud GA, et al. A controlled trial of fluconazole or amphotericin B to prevent relapse of cryptococcal meningitis in patients with AIDS. N Engl J Med. 1992;326:793–8.

160. Bozzette SA, Larsen R, Chiu J, et al. A controlled trial of maintenance therapy with fluconazole after treatment of cryptococcal meningitis in the acquired immunodeficiency syndrome. N Engl J Med. 1991;324:580–4.

160a. Powderly WG, Cloud GA, Dismutes WE, et al. Measurement of cryptococcal antigen in serum and cerebrospinal fluid: Value in the management of AIDS-associated cryptococcal meningitis. Clin Infect Dis. 1994;18:789–92.

161. Chuck SL, Sande MA. Infections with *Cryptococcus neoformans* in the acquired immunodeficiency syndrome. N Engl J Med. 1989;321:794–9.

162. Larsen RA, Bozzette S, McCutchan JA, et al. Persistent *Cryptococcus neoformans* of the prostate after successful treatment of meningitis. Ann Intern Med. 1989;111:125–8.

163. Denning DW, Tucker RM, Hanson LH, et al. Itraconazole therapy for cryptococcal meningitis and cryptococcosis. Arch Intern Med. 1989;149:2301–8.

164. Wheat LJ, Connolly-Stringfield P, Blair R, et al. Effect of successful treatment with amphotericin B on *Histoplasma capsulatum* variety capsulatum polysaccharide antigen levels in patients with AIDS and histoplasmosis. Am J Med. 1992;92:153–60.

165. Wheat LJ, Hafner R, Wulfsohn M, et al. Prevention of relapse of histoplasmosis with itraconazole in patients with the acquired immunodeficiency syndrome. The National Institute of Allergy and Infectious Diseases Clinical Trials and Mycoses Study Group Collaborators. Ann Intern Med. 1993;118:610–6.

166. Wheat LJ, Connolly-Springfield P, Blair R, et al. Histoplasmosis relapse in patients with AIDS: Detection using *Histoplasma capsulatum* variety capsulatum antigen levels. Ann Intern Med. 1991;115:936–41.

167. Gagliani JN, Catanzaro A, Cloud GA, et al. Fluconazole therapy for coccidioidal meningitis. The NIAID Mycosis Study Group. Ann Intern Med. 1993;119:28–35.

168. Barnes PF, Bloch AB, Davidson PT, et al. Tuberculosis in patients with human immunodeficiency virus infection. N Engl J Med. 1991;324:1644–50.

169. Barnes PF, Barrows SA. Tuberculosis in the 1990s. Ann Intern Med. 1993;119:400–10.

170. Centers for Disease Control and Prevention. Tuberculosis and human immunodeficiency virus infection: Recommendations of the advisory committee for the elimination of tuberculosis. MMWR. 1989;38:236–8.

171. Centers for Disease Control and Prevention. The use of preventive therapy for tuberculosis infection in the United States: Recommendations of the advisory committee for the elimination of tuberculosis. MMWR. 1990;39:9–12.

172. Fischl MA, Daikos GL, Uttamchandani RB, et al. Clinical presentation and outcome of patients with HIV infection and tuberculosis caused by multiple-drug-resistant bacilli. Ann Intern Med. 1992;117:184–90.

173. Pearson ML, Jereb JA, Frieden TR, et al. Nosocomial transmission of multidrug-resistant *Mycobacterium tuberculosis:* A risk to patients and health care workers. Ann Intern Med. 1992;117:191–6.

174. Frieden TR, Sterling T, Pablos-Mendez A, et al. The emergence of drug-resistant tuberculosis in New York City. N Engl J Med. 1993;328:521–6.

175. Iseman MD. Treatment of multidrug-resistant tuberculosis. N Engl J Med. 1993;329:784–91.

176. Chaisson RE, Benson CA, Dube M, et al. Clarithromycin therapy for disseminated *Mycobacterium avium* complex (MAC) in AIDS. Abstract of the 32nd Interscience Conference on Antimicrobial Agents and Chemotherapy, Anaheim, California; 1992:891.

177. Dautzenberg B, Truffot C, Legris S, et al. Activity of clarithromycin against *Mycobacterium avium* infection in patients with the acquired immune deficiency syndrome: A controlled clinical trial. Am Rev Respir Dis. 1992;144:564–9.

178. Young LS, Wiviott L, Wu M, et al. Azithromycin for treatment of *Mycobacterium avium-intracellulare* complex infection in patients with AIDS. Lancet. 1991;338:1107–9.

179. Kemper C, Havlir D, Haghighat D, et al. Effect of ethambutol, rifampin, or clofazimine, given singly, on *Mycobacterium avium* bacteremia in AIDS. VIII International Conference on AIDS; Amsterdam, The Netherlands, July 19–24, 1992;PoB 3087.

180. Kemper CA, Meng TC, Nussenbaum J, et al. Treatment of *Mycobacterium avium* complex bacteremia in AIDS with a four-drug oral regimen: Rifampin, ethambutol, clofazimine and ciprofloxacin. Ann Intern Med. 1992;116:466–72.

181. Agins BD, Berman DS, Spicehandler D, et al. Effect of combined therapy for *Mycobacterium avium* bacteremia in AIDS patients. J Infect Dis. 1990;159:784–7.

182. Hoy J, Mijch A, Sandland M, et al. Quadruple-drug therapy for *Mycobacterium avium* bacteremia in AIDS patients. J Infect Dis. 1990;161:801–5.

183. Horsburgh CR, Havlik JA, Metchock BG, et al. Oral therapy of disseminated *Mycobacterium avium* complex infection in AIDS relieves symptoms and is well tolerated. Am Rev Respir Dis. 1991;143:A115.

184. Chiu J, Nussbaum J, Bozzette S, et al. Treatment of disseminated *Mycobacterium avium* complex infection in AIDS with amikacin, ethambutol, rifampin, and ciprofloxacin. Ann Intern Med. 1990;113:358–61.

185. deLalla F, Maserati R, Scarpellini P, et al. Clarithromycin-ciprofloxacin-amikacin for therapy of *Mycobacterium avium-Mycobacterium intracellulare* bacteremia in patients with AIDS. Antimicrob Agents Chemother. 1992;36:1567–9.

186. Petersen C. Cryptosporidiosis in patients infected with human immunodeficiency virus. Clin Infect Dis. 1992;15:903–9.

187. Fichtenbaum CJ, Ritchie DJ, Powderly WG. Use of paromomycin for treatment of cryptosporidiosis in patients with AIDS. Clin Infect Dis. 1993;16:298–300.

188. Blanshard C, Ellis DS, Tovey DG, et al. Treatment of intestinal microsporidiosis with albendazole in patients with AIDS. AIDS. 1992;6:311–3.
189. Hook EW III, Marra CM. Acquired syphilis in adults. N Engl J Med. 1992; 326:1060–9.
190. Koehler JE, Quinn FD, Berger TG, et al. Isolation of *Rochalimaea* species from cutaneous and osseous lesions of bacillary angiomatosis. N Engl J Med. 1992;327:1625–31.
191. Dolan MJ, Wong MT, Regnery FL, et al. Syndrome of *Rochalimaea henselae* adenitis suggesting cat scratch disease. Ann Intern Med. 1993;118:331–6.
192. Koehler JE, Tappero JW. Bacillary angiomatosis and bacillary peliosis in patients infected with human immunodeficiency virus. Clin Infect Dis. 1993; 17:612–24.
193. von Gunten CF, Von Roenn JH. Clinical aspects of human immunodeficiency virus-related lymphoma. Curr Opin Oncol. 1992;4:894–9.
194. Ragni MV, Belle SH, Jaffe RA, et al. Acquired immunodeficiency syndrome-associated non-Hodgkin's lymphomas and other malignancies in patients with hemophilia. Blood. 1993;81:1889–97.

106. VACCINES FOR HIV-1 INFECTION

RAPHAEL DOLIN
MICHAEL C. KEEFER

Intensive efforts to develop safe and effective vaccines against human immunodeficiency virus (HIV) infection and/or HIV-associated disease are underway in research centers throughout the world. Currently available antiretroviral chemotherapies appear to have relatively modest impact on the progression of disease, and attempts to modify behavior to control the spread of HIV-1 infection have met with limited success. Thus, efforts to develop vaccines are receiving increasing priority as a potential control measure against AIDS. As outlined in Chapter 99, the continued worldwide spread of HIV-1 infection, and particularly the explosive spread of HIV-1 infection in many areas of the developing world, have imparted a sense of particular urgency to these efforts.

The development of HIV-1 vaccines presents formidable scientific, logistic, and social challenges, and these have been the subject of several recent detailed reviews.[1–4] Among the most serious problems is the current lack of understanding of the parameters of immunity that protect against HIV-1 infection and/or disease. Furthermore, the antigenic variation of HIV-1 isolates, particularly in their surface antigens, suggests that vaccines will have to generate broad-based immune responses against antigenically heterologous strains of HIV-1. The development of suitable animal models would greatly facilitate investigations of these questions and are of particular importance to the development of HIV-1 vaccines. While considerable progress has been made in the development of primate animal models of HIV-1 and of related lentivirus infections, there is as yet no fully satisfactory animal model of HIV-associated disease. Nonetheless, important information has emerged from studies carried out in available animal models, as well as from phase I studies of candidate acquired immunodeficiency syndrome (AIDS) vaccines carried out in human volunteers. Information generated from those investigations, as well as from studies of immune responses in patients infected with HIV-1, form the basis for the current approaches to the development of AIDS vaccines.

IMMUNE RESPONSES TO HIV-1

In recent years, extensive knowledge of the molecular virology and antigenic characteristics of HIV-1 has been gained.[5] The structure of the virus, the biochemical events of replication, and the genetic organization of the virus have been studied and described in extraordinary detail (see Chap. 146). Major antigenic components of HIV-1 have been identified, and a variety of epitopes on the major virus proteins have been mapped. The HIV-1 surface proteins have been studied most extensively in this regard. In humans infected with HIV-1, humoral and cell-mediated immune responses directed at a variety of viral antigens have been described.[1–3,6] However, as noted above, the correlation of specific immune responses with protection from infection and/or disease has not yet been accomplished. The specific immune responses that have been described in HIV-1–infected patients are reviewed below.

Neutralizing Antibodies

The level of neutralizing antibodies has been correlated with vaccine efficacy in several viral infections, and protection has been engendered against HIV-1 infection with passive immunization in chimpanzee animal studies (see below). Thus, neutralizing antibodies against HIV-1 have been the object of particular interest in studies of HIV-1 vaccines. Antibodies that neutralize HIV-1 in vitro have been detected against a variety of epitopes on proteins of HIV-1, particularly on the surface glycoproteins (gp120 and gp41),[7–9] but also to some extent on internal proteins, such as p17[10] and p51/p66.[11] A principal neutralizing determinant (PND) has been defined that resides on the third variable region of the HIV-1 gp120 envelope glycoprotein, the "V3 loop" (Fig. 1).[12] Multiple neutralization epitopes have been defined on the loop, using a number of different techniques.[3] The V3 loop contains both variable domains, principally on the sides, and conserved domains, on the crown and base of the loop.[12] The variable domains elicit primarily strain-specific neutralizing antibodies, while the conserved domains induce more broadly cross-reacting neutralizing antibodies. Studies of immunization with envelope glycoproteins or V3 peptides suggest that the dominant neutralizing antibody response is strain specific, although some cross-neutralizing antibodies are also elicited.[9,13] Neutralizing antibodies directed against the transmembrane portion of the envelope glycoprotein of HIV-1, gp41, have also been described.[14] Neutralizing antibodies have been detected against linear epitopes and also against noncontiguous or conformational epitopes on gp120, such as the CD4-binding site.[15–17] Neutralizing antibodies directed at this noncontiguous epitope also have a more broadly directed specificity. Recent observations have indicated that synergy exists between neutralizing antibodies directed against linear regions of the V3 loop and those directed against the conformational gp120–CD4-binding site.[18]

Antibody-Dependent Cellular Cytotoxicity

Antibody-dependent cellular cytotoxicity (ADCC) is a mechanism by which effector cells that contain Fc receptors attach to immunoglobulins that are complexed with virus or virus antigens on cell surfaces.[19] These effector cells can then kill virus-infected target cells that express viral antigen on the cell surface or kill cells that simply may have viral antigen-antibody complexes coating the cell surface. ADCC has been detected in the peripheral blood of individuals with various stages of HIV-1 infection and in some primate models of infection.[20,21] Since it appears likely that transmission of HIV-1 infection can occur by either cell-free or cell-associated virus, ADCC may be particularly relevant to the elimination of virus-infected cells. ADCC may also provide a mechanism by which uninfected CD4+ cells, which have soluble gp120 attached to their surface, may be injured. Epitopes that induce ADCC activity have been identified on gp120, including the V3 loop, and on gp41.[2,20,21]

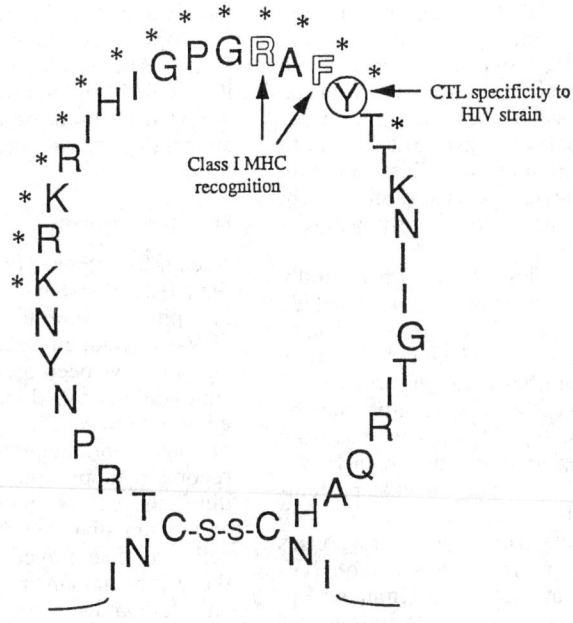

Domains of the V3 Loop

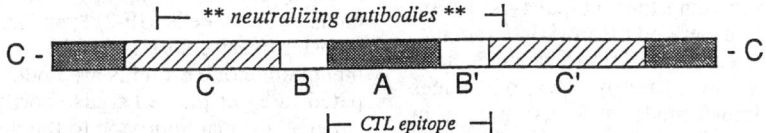

FIG. 1. V3 loop of the envelope glycoprotein (gp120) of an HIV-1 isolate (MN strain). Amino acid sequence is shown with designated linear conserved and variable regions and with regions that elicit neutralizing antibodies and cytotoxic T-cell (CTL) responses. **A,** group specific (conserved); **B,** class specific (semiconserved); **C,** type specific (variable). (Adapted from Broliden et al.,[12] with permission.)

Cell-Mediated Immunity

Cell-mediated immune responses are considered to be important in the restriction of virus replication and in the resolution of infection in a number of viral infections. T-cell cytotoxic activity, mediated by CD8+ T cells in the context of MHC class I restriction, is an important mechanism for elimination of virus-infected host cells. Cytotoxic T-cell (CTL) activity against HIV-1 antigens, including both CD4+ and CD8+ effector cells, has been detected in HIV-1 seropositive individuals[22,23] and appears to wane as HIV-1 disease progresses.[24] Recently, CD4+ and CD8+ CTL activities have also been detected in humans immunized with candidate HIV-1 vaccines (see below). CTL activity has been directed against antigens on a variety of HIV-1 proteins, including envelope glycoproteins, internal structural proteins (p17, p24, p15), as well as against the products of regulatory genes, including *nef* and *vif,* and to *pol* products.[22,25–29] An epitope against which CTL activity is directed has been defined on the V3 loop.[30] In recipients of candidate AIDS vaccines, CD8+ CTL have been detected only after administration of live-virus vector vaccines followed by subunit (protein) boosts.[31,32] The administration of subunit vaccines alone has generated only CD4+ CTL to date.[33,34] Cytotoxic T cells also have the potential to injure uninfected CD4+ cells that have soluble gp120 attached to their cell surface.

Potentially Deleterious Immune Responses

Despite the exceedingly detailed information that has been generated regarding the molecular events of HIV-1 replication, the pathogenesis of T-cell depletion and immunosuppression induced by HIV-1 is incompletely understood (see Ch. 101). As noted above, immunopathology, including T-cell injury or dysfunction, may result from cytotoxic T cells or ADCC. In addition, a number of other potentially deleterious immune responses to HIV infection or immunization have been described. In vitro enhancement of infection by antibodies, by either complement-mediated or Fc-mediated mechanisms, has been reported.[35,36] This apparently occurs by the interaction of virus-antibody complexes, with or without complement, with cells that bear Fc or complement receptors. This interaction may facilitate (enhance) entry of virus into cells that otherwise might not be infected by the virus. Such enhancing antibodies have been detected in vitro in serum specimens from patients with HIV-1 infection, as well as following immunization with recombinant HIV-1 surface glycoproteins.[37,38] However, enhancement of infection has not been observed in vivo, and the biologic significance of enhancing antibodies is not known.

HIV-1, as well as other retroviruses, contains an immunosuppressive peptide in the transmembrane envelope protein (gp41).[39,40] This peptide suppresses stimulation of T-helper-dependent immune responses. It is not known whether antibodies directed against this immunosuppressive protein would be a desirable component of an immune response or conversely whether the absence of an immune response against this immunosuppressive region would be deleterious. Studies of immunization with synthetic HIV-1 peptides in which the immunosuppressive area is deleted may help to clarify this question.

Another potentially deleterious mechanism of the immune response to HIV-1 would be the induction of autoimmunity against CD4-bearing cells. This could occur through the development of antibody to the binding site of HIV-1, which interacts with CD4 receptors and interferes with normal signaling events in CD4+ lymphocytes. It is also possible that anti-idiotype responses to anti-gp160, or to antibodies against gp120 bound to CD4, may also react with CD4-bearing cells and interfere with functions of that subset of lymphocytes. A shared amino acid sequence between CD4 and gp120 has also recently been described.[41]

HIV-1 proteins also have areas of homology with naturally occurring host regulatory and structural proteins. These include areas of homology between gp120 and interleukin-2,[42] neuroluekin,[43] and β-chains of MHC class II molecules[44]; between gp41 and HLA-DR molecules[45]; and between gag protein and thymosin α-1.[46] Recently, induction of anti-HLA antibodies by immunization with HIV-1 envelope (gp160) vaccines has been reported.[47] Thus, it is possible that immunization with HIV-1 vaccines may induce antibodies that react with host proteins and that may have deleterious effects on important host cell functions. While the potential for deleterious immune responses remains an important consideration in the development of HIV-1 vaccines, it should be noted that autoimmunity, immunosuppression, enhancement of infection, or other deleterious effects have not been detected in studies of candidate HIV vaccines in humans or in experimental animals to date (see below).

TYPES OF CANDIDATE HIV-1 VACCINES

Because of the uncertainty regarding the optimal type of immune responses that should be generated by an HIV-1 vaccine, a variety of different types of candidate HIV-1 vaccines have been proposed. Many of these are currently at various stages of preclinical evaluation in animal model systems, and, as of this writing, at least 20 candidate HIV-1 vaccines have reached trials in humans (Table 1). Most of these human trials are phase I studies in HIV-1 seronegative volunteers, but in some cases studies in HIV-1 seropositive asymptomatic individuals are also underway. The major types of candidate vaccines under development or consideration are discussed below.

Whole Virus Vaccines

Traditionally, the initial approach to development of virus vaccines has been to generate an inactivated or "killed" whole virus preparation. This may be particularly advantageous when the parameters of immunity are not defined and, therefore, when the critical antigenic components of a vaccine are difficult to predict. Compared with a subunit preparation, a whole virus vaccine offers inclusion of a larger number of potentially relevant antigens. In HIV-1 vaccine development, this approach has received relatively little emphasis, primarily because of considerations of safety. The chief concern is related to the potential hazard of retained genetic material in such a vaccine (i.e., the potential risk of transmission of infectious HIV-1). Whole virus vaccines can now be prepared by techniques that render any remaining nucleic acid extremely unlikely to be infectious, and such vaccines can be ascertained to be free of nucleic acids by techniques of extraordinarily high sensitivity. However, the lack of an entirely appropriate animal model in which to demonstrate that a vaccine preparation is free of infectious HIV-1 still poses a significant problem.

However, whole inactivated simian immunodeficiency virus (SIV) vaccines have been developed and evaluated in primates and have demonstrated protection from challenge, although the precise mechanism of protection appears to be complex (see below). Salk[48] and coworkers have developed a whole HIV-1 vaccine candidate in which the virus is inactivated by β-propiolactone and γ-irradiation. The inactivation and purification techniques they employed resulted in a vaccine preparation that is largely depleted of gp120 and that has been administered to HIV-1 seropositive individuals without apparent deleterious effects.[49] The developers of this vaccine candidate have targeted its use for "immunotherapy" in HIV-1 infected individuals, in whom it is intended to stimulate cell-mediated immune responses, primarily against internal proteins.

Envelope Proteins

Vaccines composed of HIV-1 envelope proteins have undergone the most extensive study. As noted above, important neutralizing epitopes, as well as T-cell epitopes, have been identified on HIV-1 envelope proteins. Envelope HIV-1 vaccines studied in humans have been generated through recombinant DNA expression systems, which provide an efficient means to prepare large quantities of purified proteins and also bypass concerns about possible contamination with other HIV-1 components. These recombinant proteins have been generated with a number of different vectors and cell systems, including insect,[50] yeast,[51] and mammalian cell cultures.[52,53] Depending on the vector and cell system employed, as well as on the purification procedures, these recombinant proteins can have important differences in structure and in glycosylation compared with their naturally occurring analogs. Envelope protein vaccine candidates that are being evaluated in human trials include an rgp160 generated via a baculovirus vector and produced in insect cells (LAI strain);[38] a fully glycosylated rgp160 made via a vaccinia vector in Vero cells (LAI and MN strains)[54]; a nonglycosylated rgp120 made in yeast cells (SF-2 strain)[55]; an rgp120 generated in Chinese hamster ovary cells (SF-2)[56]; and an rgp120 generated in Chinese hamster ovary cells (LAI and MN).[57] A number of other recombinant envelope proteins are under development and are anticipated to enter phase I trials shortly.

An additional approach to the development of envelope vaccines is the generation of synthetic peptides that include only certain epitopes of the surface proteins rather than the entire gp160 or gp120 proteins themselves. This affords the opportunity to include only those epitopes that are most important for a protective response in the vaccine and to exclude minor or even potentially deleterious epitopes, such as ones that might be associated with enhancement of infection or with immunopathogenesis. On the other hand, a potential disadvantage of this approach is that synthetic peptides may not stimulate immune responses to noncontiguous or highly conformationally dependent epitopes. In addition, synthetic peptides are generally not as immunogenic as whole, or native proteins. However, this problem might be overcome by coupling peptides to certain protein carriers and/or by addition of more potent adjuvants, as discussed below. An example of this approach is a vaccine candidate that consists of synthetically produced peptides from the V3 loops of four strains of HIV-1, which contain epitopes that induce neutralizing antibodies, T-helper cells, and cytotoxic T lymphocytes but that do not contain epitopes for infection-enhancing antibodies.[58] Another example of this approach is a mixture of synthetic peptides from the V3 loop of HIV-1 (MN) attached to a heptalysyl core, which is currently undergoing trials.[59]

Internal or Core Proteins

Vaccine candidates comprised of HIV-1 internal proteins, either entirely or in part, have received relatively less attention. As noted above, it is believed that core proteins are particularly important in the generation of cell-mediated immune responses and especially cytotoxic T cells, although neutralizing antibodies against internal proteins have been reported as well. Examples of vaccine candidates based on internal proteins include a 30 amino acid peptide of p17 of HIV-1 (HGP-30)[60]; a portion of p17/p24 proteins formulated as a viruslike particle by introduc-

TABLE 1. HIV-1 Vaccine Candidates Undergoing Study in HIV-1 Seronegative Volunteers

Vaccine Type	Cell Type/Production Method	HIV-1 Strain	Sponsor	Reference
Envelope proteins				
gp160	Insect (baculovirus)	LAI	MicroGeneSys	38
gp160	Vero (vaccinia)[a]	LAI	Immuno AG	125
gp160	Mammalian	LAI/MN	Pasteur-Merieux-Connaught	4
gp160	Mammalian	LAI	A. Burney, Universite´ Libre de Bruxelles	155, 156
gp120 (Env 2-3)	Yeast	SF-2	Chiron/Biocine	126
gp120	CHO[b]	SF-2	Chiron/Biocine	56, 128
gp120	CHO	LAI/MN	Genentech	57
Envelope peptides				
V3-MAPS	Synthetic, MAPS carrier	MN	United Biomedical Inc.	59
V3	Synthetic	MN	Pasteur-Merieux-Connaught	4
Mixed peptides	Synthetic, KLH carrier	MN, RF, LAI	Yokohama City University, Japan	157
V3	Synthetic, conjugated to PPD	MN	Swiss Serum and Vaccine Institute	4
Core protein/peptides				
HGP-30	Synthetic p17/KLH	LAI	Viral Technologies, Inc.	132, 133
Ty p24 particles	p17/p24 via yeast retrotransposon	LAI	British Biotechnology, Ltd.	134
Live virus vectors				
Vaccinia-gp160	Mammalian	LAI	Oncogen	130, 131
Canarypox-gp160	CEF[c]	MN	Pasteur-Merieux-Connaught	4
Vaccinia-gp160, gag, pol	Mammalian	LAI	Therion Biologics	65[d]
Live vector + subunit boost				
Vaccinia-gp160 + gp160 (baculovirus)	—[e]	LAI	Oncogen/MicroGeneSys	73, 74
Vaccinia-gp160 + gp160 (vaccinia derived)	—	LAI + MN	Oncogen/Immuno AG	McElrath[f]
Vaccinia-gp160 + gp120 (CHO)	—	LAI + SF-2	Oncogen/Chiron	McElrath[f]
Vaccinia-gp160 + gp120 (CHO)	—	LAI + LAI or MN	Oncogen/Genentech	McElrath[f]
Canarypox-gp160 + V3 peptide		MN	Pasteur-Merieux-Connaught	4
Vaccinia-gp160 + gp 160 + envelope peptides		LAI	Institut Jacques Monod, Université Libre de Bruxelles	4

[a] African green monkey kidney cells.
[b] Chinese hamster ovary cells.
[c] Chick embryo fibroblasts.
[d] In future studies.
[e] Individual vaccine candidates produced as noted above.
[f] AIDS vaccine evaluation group protocol OIO (J McElrath, personal communication, 1994).

tion into the yeast retrotransposon Ty (Ty-Gag)[61]; and a p24 protein generated via a baculovirus vector.[62]

Live Vectors

Considerable interest has been focused on the development of a live vector vaccine for HIV-1. Such a vaccine has the potential to present HIV-1 antigens in the context of a replicating microbial system, and, in the case of an obligate intracellular organism such as a virus, the antigens are expressed by host cells. Presentation of antigen to the host in this manner may result in a more efficient immune response, particularly with respect to the generation of MHC class I restricted CD8 + cytotoxic T cells. The development of an efficiently replicating, genetically stable, live vector also offers important advantages for the large-scale production of vaccines. Some live vectors, such as vaccinia virus, are also very resistant to environmental inactivation, which is of practical importance for utilization of vaccines in field conditions in developing countries. However, live vectors need to be selected carefully, since they can contribute morbidity of their own in certain clinical settings (e.g., administration of a vaccinia vector to individuals with eczema or depressed cell-mediated immune defenses). An additional limitation of live vector vaccines is the development of immunity to the vector after initial immunization, so that repeated doses (boosts) with the vector may not be possible, at least over the short term. However, it may be possible to boost with the product of the HIV-1 gene inserted in the vector (e.g., gp160) rather than with the live vector itself, as discussed below.

The most extensively studied live vector HIV-1 vaccine candidate is a vaccinia-gp160 construct in which the *env* gene of HIV-1 (LAI) has been inserted into the thymidine kinase locus of the vaccinia genome.[63] Vaccinia is an extensively studied virus vector with a large DNA genome into which a number of foreign genes have been inserted and successfully expressed. The vaccinia–HIV-1 construct is genetically stable and appears to have biologic properties similar to those of its vaccinia parent. Another live vector vaccine under evaluation is one in which the *env* gene from HIV-1 (MN) has been inserted into the genome of canarypox, a pox virus with an abortive replicative cycle in mammalian cells that does not result in the production of infectious virus.[64] Other virus constructs under development include vaccinia or canarypox vectors in which HIV-1 genes for *gag*, *pol*, and *env* have been inserted.[65] Additional vectors for HIV-1 vaccines that have been proposed and are at various stages of development include adenovirus,[66] poliovirus,[67,68] salmonella,[69] and BCG.[70,71] Administration of live vector followed by a boost with the HIV-1 protein or peptide expressed in the construct (e.g., boosting with gp160, gp120, or V3 peptide) has also been studied. This combination of live vector followed by subunit boost has provided protection from challenge to SIV in the primate model[72] and has shown promise in phase I studies in humans (see below).[73,74]

Live Attenuated Virus Vaccines

The use of live attenuated vaccines has been highly successful in the control of several important viral diseases, such as measles, rubella, and polio. Live attenuated vaccines have the advantage of presenting vaccine antigens in a manner that most closely resembles naturally occurring infection and also stimulate a broad array of humoral and cell-mediated immune responses. With some live attenuated vaccines, immunity may be particularly long-lasting. Depending on the site of immunization, live attenuated viruses (or live vectors) may be highly efficient in stimulation of local (mucosal) immunity, which may be particularly important in prevention of HIV-1 infection transmitted by the sexual route. Boosting by repeated mucosal immunization may also be possible, depending on the intensity and duration of local immune responses stimulated by initial immunization.

Clearly, the major concern in the development of a live attenuated HIV-1 vaccine candidate is safety. The problem of devising adequate safety tests, particularly with the lack of a suitable animal model for HIV-1 disease, has been noted above. The incomplete understanding of the pathogenesis of HIV-1–associated disease, and therefore the difficulty of identification of "virulence" factors, has also inhibited attempts to develop live attenuated viruses. HIV-1 is known to have a number of regulatory genes that affect different points of the virus replicative cycle (see Ch. 146).[5] One approach to the development of a live attenuated vaccine has been to delete one or more regulatory genes, which can result in a mutant virus that has lost pathogenicity. Because such a virus has a genetic deletion, it would be unlikely to revert to its pathogenic parent, at least by reconstruction of the deleted gene. The attenuated mutant virus would nonetheless have to replicate sufficiently well to stimulate humoral and cell-mediated immunity. One such deletion mutant of SIV, in which the *nef* gene has been deleted, has yielded promising results in the rhesus macaque system (see below).[75]

Other Types of Candidate AIDS Vaccines

Candidate AIDS vaccines that do not contain HIV-1 components themselves have also been proposed. These include a recombinant human soluble CD4 preparation, intended to induce antibodies against the HIV-1 binding site to CD4[76]; a vaccine composed of anti-gp120 antibodies, which will induce anti-idiotype antibodies against the CD4 binding site of gp120[77]; and anti-CD4 antibodies to induce anti-idiotype antibodies against the CD4 binding site on gp120.[78] These types of vaccines, since they are either immunoglobulins or soluble proteins, have the advantage that they do not contain HIV-1 components. However, they raise potential safety concerns of their own, related to inhibition or perturbation of CD4 receptors, which are widely distributed in lymphoid cells and in cells of the monocyte macrophage lineage.

Most recently, a novel immunization approach has been reported in which complementary DNA ("naked DNA") is administered, which elicits immune responses to a gene product but does not produce infectious virus.[79] This approach is potentially promising for attempts to develop an HIV-1 vaccine, but additional information regarding safety needs to be obtained.

Adjuvants

An important consideration in the development of HIV-1 vaccines is the availability of well-tolerated and effective adjuvants. It was anticipated that subunit HIV-1 vaccines, particularly glycoproteins and small peptides, would be relatively weak immunogens, and this has been borne out by experience in the phase I trials in humans described below. The only adjuvant currently approved for use with vaccines in the United States is alum (usually as aluminum phosphate or aluminum hydroxide), which has been used with several of the HIV-1 subunit vaccine candidates. Some rgp120 vaccines have utilized a synthetic muramyl tripeptide, linked covalently with dipalmitoyl phosphatidylethanolamine (MTP-PE), which is an analog of muramyl dipeptide (MDP).[80] This is formulated in an oil and water emulsion, MF59, and has undergone phase I trials with herpes simplex virus and influenza virus vaccines, as well as rgp120 vaccines. As noted below, MTP-PE appears to be moderately reactogenic, and its contribution to augmenting immunogenicity above that of the MF59 emulsion is unclear. A squalene-based adjuvant, SAF/2 with MDP, has also been developed and is undergoing evalua-

tion. A variety of other adjuvants have been proposed, including monophosphoryl lipid A (MPL), alum-absorbed liposome-encapsulated MPL, MDP, and QS21, a saponin derived from the soapbark tree *Quillaja saponaria*. Several of these are currently being examined in comparative trials in primate models and in humans. The development of safe and effective adjuvants is clearly an important component of the HIV vaccine development effort.

ANIMAL MODELS

Chimpanzees

The availability of an appropriate and practical animal model would be of great importance to studies of the pathogenesis of HIV-1 disease and to the development of vaccines and chemotherapeutic agents. For the development of vaccines, the availability of an animal model is particularly important, since it offers the opportunity to conduct experimental virus challenges and thus to study the protective effects of candidate vaccines directly, which is otherwise not possible. Despite the fact that considerable progress has been made in this area, there is not as yet an entirely suitable animal model of HIV-1 infection. Chimpanzees are the only animal model system fully established in which experimental infection with HIV-1 can be readily achieved.[81–83] After infection, chimpanzees mount immune responses to HIV-1, and virus can be isolated from peripheral blood mononuclear cells. However, HIV-1–infected chimpanzees do not show consistent evidence of HIV-related disease, and isolation of virus from many animals becomes increasingly difficult as time goes by. In addition, chimpanzees are extraordinarily expensive and in short supply, so that only small numbers are available for experimental studies of candidate vaccines.

Nonetheless, a number of important observations have been made in the study of immunoprophylaxis in the chimpanzee model. Initial studies of passive immunization with anti-HIV-1 immunoglobulin preparations failed to protect chimpanzees against intravenous HIV-1 challenge.[84] The particular immunoglobulin preparation used in those studies had only low levels of neutralizing activity against the HIV-1 IIIB (LAI) challenge virus. In subsequent experiments in which a lower challenge dose of virus was used, protection was achieved with passive administration of this immunoglobulin.[85] Emini and colleagues[86] demonstrated protection with administration of a monoclonal antibody with neutralizing activity directed against the V3 loop, indicating the importance of antibody directed at the principal neutralizing determinant of the envelope glycoprotein. This neutralizing monoclonal antibody provided protection if it was administered within 10–30 minutes after intravenous challenge with HIV-1, but protection was not provided if antibody was administered 1 hour after challenge.

Initial attempts to induce active immunization in chimpanzees were carried out with a variety of candidate vaccines, primarily consisting of HIV-1 envelopes or subunits.[87,88] These preparations generally stimulated low humoral and cellular immune responses and were not successful in inducing protection against subsequent challenge with the homologous HIV-1 (LAI) challenge strain. In an attempt to improve immunogenicity, Girard and colleagues[89] administered combinations of whole killed virus, vaccinia-expressed HIV-1 envelope, subunits of *gag*, envelope peptides, and some nonstructural viral proteins. Although these combinations apparently did not induce high levels of neutralizing activity, a marked increase in neutralizing activity was generated when the animals were boosted with peptides of the principal neutralizing determinant of the envelope. Subsequently, the animals were protected if challenged with homologous HIV-1 (LAI).[89]

Berman and colleagues[90] reported protection against intravenous challenge with HIV-1 virus by administration of a recombinant gp120 (LAI) vaccine produced in Chinese hamster ovary cells, but not with a recombinant gp160 produced in the same cell line. The reason for the failure of rgp160 to protect in this study was not clear, but the rgp160 vaccinated chimpanzees had significantly lower neutralizing antibody titers to the principal neutralizing domain (V3 loop) than did the rgp120 vaccinees. More recently, Fultz and colleagues[91] were able to show that protection was afforded against cell-associated HIV-1 virus challenge after immunization with the combination of HIV proteins and subunits developed by Girard et al.[89] Protection against cell-associated virus challenge persisted for at least 1 year in one chimpanzee, but a second animal challenged with cell-free virus at 1 year after immunization became infected. The neutralizing titer in the chimp protected against cell-associated challenge was significantly higher than in the chimp who was not protected against challenge with cell-free virus.

An initial experiment in which chimpanzees were immunized with a vaccinia-gp160 construct failed to protect against intravenous HIV-1 challenge.[92] Another experiment employed immunization with a vaccinia-gp160 recombinant followed by boosting with recombinant synthetic V3 peptides and demonstrated some protection early, but HIV-1 was isolated from the animal 8 months after challenge.[89]

The above experiments in chimpanzees established that protective immunity could be induced by active immunization. However, correlation of protection with specific parameters of immunity was limited because of the small numbers of animals that have been studied. In some instances at least, protection could be afforded by passive immunization with humoral antibodies with specific neutralizing activity.

Rhesus Macaque Monkeys

Considerable progress has occurred in the development of another primate animal model, the rhesus macaque infected with SIV.[93–95] This model has the advantage that SIV causes disease in macaques, and macaques are much more readily available and less expensive than chimpanzees. After an incubation period that is considerably shorter than that seen in humans, SIV infection results in immunosuppression and in the development of opportunistic infections. Death often results within 3–5 months. A particularly virulent strain, SIV_{pbj}, exists that can cause overwhelming disease in 1–2 weeks after infection.[96] Although differences in the frequency and type of certain opportunistic infections and tumors exist between SIV-induced disease in macaques and HIV-1 disease in humans, overall the disease patterns have many features in common. SIV and HIV-1 are also similar, although some differences exist. The major surface glycoprotein is somewhat smaller in SIV (gp110 in SIV vs. gp120 in HIV-1), and the transmembrane protein is also smaller in SIV (gp31 in SIV vs. gp41 in HIV-1). The SIV external protein also does not contain a loop analogous to the V3 loop in HIV-1.[97,98] Overall, the SIV genome is more closely related to HIV-2 and more distantly related to HIV-1.[97,98]

Beginning in 1989, three groups reported success in providing protection in macaques challenged intravenously with cell-free SIV after immunization with whole inactivated SIV.[99–103] Murphey-Corb et al.[101] also showed that protection was present with an envelope-rich preparation of vaccine but that it was reduced in an envelope-depleted preparation. Studies of protection against intravenous challenge with cell-associated virus in macaques have yielded conflicting results: three groups have reported failure to protect,[87,104] while others reported partial protection.[105] A clear correlation between protection and in vitro parameters of immunity, such as neutralizing antibodies or cell-mediated immunity, has not emerged from the above studies.

The above challenge experiments were usually carried out by intravenous administration of virus. An important question to be addressed was whether protection would be afforded after challenge via the mucosal route, which is the most common route of naturally acquired HIV-1 infection. Initial studies with

whole virus immunization did not show protection when animals were challenged via the mucosal route, but subsequently protection was noted after genital mucosal challenge with SIV.[106]

In 1991, Stott[107] made an observation that confounded interpretation of the above studies. He reported that immunization of macaques with uninfected human cells afforded protection against challenge with SIV strains grown in human cells. Largely for practical considerations, all SIV challenge strains up to that time had been grown in human (xenogeneic) cells. Macaques previously protected against challenge with SIV strains grown in human cells were not protected when challenged with cell-free SIV grown in macaque (allogeneic) cells. The basis for the protection in the xenogeneic system is not fully elucidated at present, but it may be associated with an immune response to a human (xenogeneic) cell antigen rather than to an SIV antigen. However, immunization with xenogeneically grown SIV, followed by an allogeneic *cell-associated* virus challenge, appears to afford some protection, but apparently less efficiently than in the entirely xenogeneic system utilized earlier.[105,108] Experiments are currently being undertaken in which *both* vaccine and challenge SIV strains are allogeneic (i.e., are grown entirely in monkey cells), to elucidate further the basis for protection with whole virus SIV vaccines.

Studies of immunization of macaques with recombinant envelope proteins (subunits) from SIV have failed to show protection.[109,110] One group has reported protection after immunization with a vaccinia vector virus expressing the *env* gene of SIV, and subsequent boosting with a baculovirus produced SIV gp140[72,111]; but other groups have not confirmed this.[112] Most recently, rhesus macaques immunized with canarypox or attenuated vaccinia virus constructs containing *gag*, *pol*, and *env* genes from HIV-2, or with *Salmonella typhimurium* with *gag* and *env* HIV-2 genes, followed by boosting with gp160 subunits, have been reported to be protected against challenge with HIV-2.[113]

The macaque model has also been used to study live attenuated vaccine candidates against SIV. Desrosiers and colleagues have generated several attenuated viruses as potential live vaccine candidates.[75,114] One of these, the SIV_{mac239} Δnef virus, has a deletion of the *nef* gene and produces an infection with a similar serologic response to that seen with the virulent parent strain, but does not produce disease. Virus isolation is uncommon in animals that receive the *nef* deletion mutant, although the monkeys remain positive by polymerase chain reaction (PCR). Recently, macaques vaccinated with Δnef virus were challenged with allogeneically grown SIV some 18 months after immunization.[75] In the Δnef-immunized animals, challenge with either homologous or heterologous SIV resulted in complete protection in three of the four animals; in the other, virus was detected 2 weeks after challenge, but not subsequently. All four animals were subsequently protected from an additional high-dose SIV challenge.

HIV-2 infection of cynomolgous monkeys apparently provides some protection against disease induced by subsequent challenge with SIV_{sm}, although not against infection with the virus.[115,116] Whether HIV-2 can serve as an attenuated vaccine strain in the macaque model is the subject of ongoing investigation.

Passive immunization has been less extensively studied in the macaque model. A report by Putkonen and colleagues[117] indicates that administration of hyperimmune globulin prepared from infected macaques protected macaques from infection with SIV and HIV-2.

Two recent developments offer the potential to provide a direct role for macaques in evaluation of HIV-1 vaccines. One development involves the generation of a chimeric SIV/HIV (SHIV-1) virus in which the HIV-1 envelope gene and the *tat* and *rev* genes have been inserted into the SIV genome.[118–120] This chimeric virus infects macaques and may be useful in examining vaccine candidates comprised of HIV-1 envelope proteins or subunits. The other development relates to the report that a particular strain of macaque, *Macaca nemestrina,* or the pig-tailed macaque, can be infected with HIV-1.[121] The parameters of HIV-1 infection in this system, including the duration and pathogenic effect of infection, are not yet fully elucidated. However, if *M. nemestrina* offers a reproducible model for HIV-1 infection and/or disease, studies of HIV-1 candidate vaccines will be greatly facilitated.

HUMAN TRIALS

The study of candidate HIV-1 vaccines in humans poses several unique problems above and beyond those encountered in studies of other experimental vaccines. Volunteers need to be fully informed of the potential hazards of immunization, including the limitation of our knowledge regarding the pathogenesis of HIV-1–induced immunosuppression. Seronegative volunteers must be aware of the problems of becoming seropositive for HIV-1 by conventional "screening assays" and of the possible difficulties with employment, eligibility for insurance, and immigration that may result. Volunteers must also be counseled not to abandon behaviors to reduce the risk of acquisition of HIV-1 infection because of a false hope that the vaccine under study will provide protection against such infection. A detailed description of the procedures employed in the conduct of phase I studies of HIV-1 candidate vaccines in humans, including measures taken to address the above issues, has been recently published.[38]

The purpose of the initial trials that have been undertaken is to provide information on the immunogenicity and safety (phase I studies) of various vaccine candidates directly in humans, despite the fact that the crucial elements of a protective response have not yet been defined. As noted above, studies in primates have not clearly established the superiority of one vaccine approach over another, and therefore several different types of vaccine candidates are being evaluated (Table 1). The studies directed at the development of preventive vaccines have been carried out in healthy HIV-1 seronegative subjects. In general, these individuals have been determined to be at low risk for acquisition of HIV-1 infection, to avoid the potentially confounding effects of an intercurrent HIV-1 infection in the study. Vaccines intended for immunotherapy have been studied in HIV-1 seropositive subjects as well (Table 2).

Recombinant gp160 Vaccines

Two vaccine candidates consisting of recombinant gp160 proteins derived from the LAI strain of HIV-1 have been studied

in HIV-1 seronegative subjects. The first of these was a baculovirus-generated preparation (MicroGeneSys, Inc., New Haven, CT), which was studied in a dose-escalation trial of doses ranging from 40 to 640 μg, administered intramuscularly in a three-dose schedule (0, 1, and 6 months) followed by a booster dose at 12–18 months.[38,122] The vaccine was generally well-tolerated without evidence of clinical or laboratory toxicity. There was no evidence of immunosuppression by a variety of in vitro tests, nor was any effect noted on delayed-type hypersensitivity as measured by a battery of skin tests. Induction of serum antibody responses required two or three immunizations, and a dose-related effect was noted up to the highest dose (640 μg) administered. After four doses of 640 μg, binding antibodies detected by Western blot and ELISA were seen in most subjects. Neutralizing antibodies against the homologous HIV-1 (LAI) strain developed in approximately 50 percent of subjects, but were of low titer.[38,122] T-cell lymphoproliferative responses to the immunogen also developed, on occasion before humoral antibody responses were noted. Lymphoproliferative responses persisted for as long as 30 months, even among subjects who lost detectable serum antibodies.[123,124] CD4 + MHC class II restricted cytotoxic T lymphocytes directed at gp160 developed in approximately 30 percent of subjects.[33]

The other recombinant gp160 vaccine candidate that has been studied in humans is a fully glycosylated gp160 produced via a vaccinia vector in Vero cells (Immuno AG, Vienna, Austria).[125] This vaccine preparation was administered at a similar dose schedule to that described above and was also generally well tolerated. Binding antibodies as detected by Western blot and ELISA were also generated with high frequency. Neutralizing antibodies against the homologous HIV-1 (LAI) strain developed in a minority of subjects who received doses of 12.5–50 μg, but were more frequent in those who were boosted with a 200-μg dose.[125] Lymphocyte proliferation to gp120 and gp160 proteins was also observed, and CD4 + MHC class II restricted cytotoxic T lymphocytes directed at gp160-bearing target cells developed. Studies of this vaccine candidate with higher doses (200 μg), and with an accelerated dose schedule, as well as with rgp160 derived from the MN strain of HIV-1, are currently under way.

Recombinant gp120 Vaccines

Envelope protein vaccines consisting of gp120 subunits generated by different recombinant DNA techniques have also been

TABLE 2. HIV-1 Candidate Vaccines Undergoing Study in HIV-1–Infected Individuals

Vaccine Type	Cell Type/Production Method	HIV-1 Strain	Sponsor	Reference
Whole virus	Inactivated by β-propiolactone and γ-irradiation	HZ-321	Immune Research Corp.	49
Envelope proteins				
gp160	Insect (baculovirus)	LAI	MicroGeneSys	142
gp160	Vero (vaccinia)[a]	LAI	Immuno AG	158
gp120	CHO[b]	LAI and MN	Genentech	144, 159
gp120 (Env 2-3)	Yeast	SF-2	Biocine/Chiron	151, 160
gp120	CHO	SF-2	Biocine/Chiron	160
Core protein				
p24 + gp160	Ibsect (baculovirus)	LAI	MicroGeneSys	62
Live virus + boost				
Vaccinia-gp160 + gp160 + fixed vaccinia-gp160 infected autologous cells	Vaccinia recombinants, and subunits	LAI	Institut Jacques Monod and Université Libre de Bruxelles	147
Anti-idiotypes				
Anti-gp120 idiotype	Immunoglobulin	—	IDEC	77
Anti-CD4 idiotype (10T4a)	Immunoglobulin	—	Immunotech SA	78
Soluble CD4			Biogen	4

[a] African green monkey kidney cells.
[b] Chinese hamster ovary cells.

studied. One of these is ENV 2–3, which is a yeast-derived, nonglycosylated polypeptide that contains the entire primary sequence of gp120 of HIV-1 (SF-2 strain, Biocine/Chiron, Emeryville, CA). Env 2–3 does not bind to CD4, but does induce strong T-cell proliferative responses in experimental animals. Env 2–3 (30 μg) was combined in an adjuvant preparation consisting of an oil and water emulsion (MF59) with a synthetic lipophilic muramyl tripeptide (MTP-PE) and administered intramuscularly in a three-dose schedule at 0, 1, and 6 months. In studies in HIV-1 seronegative subjects, MTP-PE was associated with significant reactogenicity and did not clearly augment immunogenicity.[126,127] Env 2–3 in MF59 alone was generally well tolerated and induced neutralizing antibodies against the homologous SF-2 strain in approximately 80 percent of subjects after three doses, and in an even higher proportion after four doses. However, little neutralizing activity against heterologous strains was detected. Increasing the dose of Env 2–3 to 100 μg did not appear to increase overall immunogenicity.

A recombinant gp120 from HIV-1 (SF-2 strain) generated in a mammalian cell line, Chinese hamster ovary (CHO) cells (Biocine/Chiron) has also been studied in HIV-1 seronegative subjects, combined with MTP-PE/MF59 as the adjuvant.[56,128] Again, MTP-PE was associated with significant, although self-limited, reactogenicity. After three doses of 15 or 50 μg, neutralizing antibody against SF-2 was seen in 88 percent of subjects, and neutralizing activity against the heterologous LAI strain was seen in 14 percent of subjects in one study. Studies of higher doses of this vaccine candidate (200 μg) in MF-59 alone are currently under way.

Studies of a recombinant gp120 generated from HIV-1 (LAI strain) in CHO cells (Genentech, Inc., South San Francisco, CA) formulated in an alum adjuvant have also been carried out.[57] A three-dose regimen of either 100 or 300 μg of vaccine was administered intramuscularly at 0, 1, and 8 months. This vaccine was also well tolerated, with only mild local reactions. ELISA binding antibody responses developed in all vaccinees and were significantly higher in the 300-μg group. Neutralizing antibody against the homologous strain was detected in 90 percent of subjects who received three 300-μg doses, and heterologous neutralizing antibodies to HIV-1/SF-2 were seen in 67 percent of subjects who received the 300-μg doses.[57] T-cell proliferative responses to gp120 were also observed. Boosting of the vaccine recipients with a heterologous rgp120 (MN strain) appeared to broaden the neutralization antibody responses in some subjects who had previously been immunized with rgp120 from the LAI strain.[129] Similar studies of immunization with recombinant gp120 from the MN strain derived in CHO cells (Genentech), as well as studies of immunization with combined rgp120s from MN and LAI strains, are also under way.

Vaccinia Virus Vector

A vaccinia virus construct in which the *env* gene of HIV-1 (LAI) has been inserted into the thymidine kinase locus of vaccinia (HIVAC-1e, Oncogen, Seattle, WA) has also undergone phase I studies. An initial two-dose study carried out in HIV-1 seronegative individuals, most of whom had had previous smallpox immunization, showed that HIVAC-1e was well tolerated.[130] The reactogenicity was not significantly different from that seen with the standard vaccinia virus that was employed as a control. HIVAC-1e stimulated weak HIV-1 serum antibody responses, particularly in previously vaccinia-immunized subjects. However, in subjects who had never received vaccinia virus previously (vaccinia naive), HIVAC-1e appeared to be more immunogenic, particularly in terms of induction of T-cell proliferative responses.[130,131] However, neutralizing antibody responses were still relatively poor.

Because of the relatively weak immune responses that were observed following administration of HIVAC-1e, even in vaccinia-naive subjects, approaches to augment or boost immune responses have been investigated. It was not possible to boost with additional doses of HIVAC-1e, because subjects had developed immunity to the vaccinia vector after one or two doses. However, administration of a recombinant envelope protein (i.e., the product of the gene inserted into the vaccinia construct) as a booster dose resulted in markedly augmented humoral and cellular immune responses.[73,74] Approximately 50 percent of the recipients of HIVAC-1e who were boosted with an rgp160 protein developed neutralizing antibody against the homologous HIV-1 (LAI) strain. Heterologous neutralizing antibody was also detected, albeit in a minority of subjects. In addition, the regimen of live virus vector followed by a subunit boost generated CD8+ cytotoxic T cells directed against target cells that expressed gp160.[31,32] This was the first time that CD8+ cytotoxic T lymphocytes were detected following immunization with a candidate HIV-1 vaccine in humans. Studies to examine the effects of different schedules of "priming" with a live vector, and boosting with a subunit preparation, as well as boosting with heterologous envelope proteins, are currently under way.

Internal or Core Antigens

Internal or core proteins have been less extensively studied as vaccine candidates in HIV-1 seronegative subjects than have envelope proteins. HGP-30, a 30 amino acid synthetic peptide from p17 coupled to KLH, has been well tolerated in two small phase I trials in HIV-1 seronegative subjects.[132,133] This preparation stimulated serum antibodies to the immunogen p17 and to KLH, but neutralizing antibodies were apparently not detected. T-cell proliferative responses were variably present, and cytotoxic T-lymphocyte responses were noted in some subjects.

A viruslike particle vaccine containing p17/p24 (Ty-Gag) has also been studied in seronegative subjects and appears to be well tolerated.[134] Low titers of binding antibodies have been elicited by this preparation. T-cell proliferative responses to the Ty particles and to p17 were noted, but cytotoxic activity was not seen.

Perinatal Studies

An important potential use of an HIV-1 vaccine would be the interruption of mother-to-child transmission of HIV-1 infection. The risk of such transmission varies from 13 to 65 percent, depending on the cohort, method of diagnosis, and length of follow-up.[135] Risk factors for transmission of HIV-1 infection from mother-to-child include low CD4 count,[136] advanced HIV disease, previous history of delivery of an HIV-infected newborn, serum p24 antigen positivity, and prematurity.[135,137] Transmission can occur in utero, peripartum, and postpartum.[138] Some studies have suggested that the presence of high titers of maternal serum antibodies to the V3 loop are associated with a lower likelihood of transmission of HIV-1 to the newborn,[139,140] although other studies have failed to corroborate this observation.[141] If certain serum antibodies indeed protect against neonatal transmission, then it is possible that passive or active immunization of HIV-1–infected mothers during pregnancy may reduce transmission; and both of these approaches are currently undergoing study. Two separate studies are examining the effects of administration of a recombinant gp120 vaccine (MN strain) or a recombinant gp160 vaccine (LAI strain) to HIV-1–infected pregnant women between weeks 16 and 24 of gestation. Women are to receive up to five monthly injections until delivery and will have the option to receive additional immunizations postpartum. Mother and child are to be followed for 18 months with careful clinical, virologic, and immunologic assessments. The results of these trials will be compared with those of passive immunization with anti-HIV-1 immunoglobulin or administration of zidovudine in this setting.

Studies in HIV-1 Seropositive Persons (Immunotherapy)

The goal of vaccination of HIV-1 seropositive persons (immunotherapy) is to induce an immune response in the host that will retard progression of disease, either through inhibition of virus replication or spread or by other as yet undefined mechanisms. Several HIV-1 vaccine candidates are undergoing study in HIV-1 seropositive individuals (Table 2). These include the inactivated virus preparation of Salk,[48,49] recombinant gp160[142,143] and gp120[144] proteins, and p24 preparations.[62] These candidate vaccines have been studied primarily in asymptomatic individuals with CD4 counts of 400 and above, although some studies in patients with lower CD4 counts have also been carried out. Available results from phase I studies indicate that these vaccines are generally well tolerated and that they induce a variety of humoral and cellular immune responses to the immunogen that were either previously undetectable or present at low levels only.[142,143] These responses have included serum antibody rises to specific epitopes on the immunogen, increased T-cell proliferative responses, and increased cytotoxic T-cell activity.[143-149] In one uncontrolled study, the ability to mount immune responses to the vaccine was associated with stable rather than falling CD4 counts.[142] Preliminary results from two small phase I studies in which HIV-1 subjects received a vaccinia-derived recombinant gp160, a recombinant yeast-derived gp120, or placebo did not show any effect of immunization on CD4 counts or on measures of virus load.[150,151] Larger placebo-controlled, double-blind, randomized trials are under way to determine the efficacy of immunotherapy with HIV-1 vaccine candidates. The measures of efficacy in these trials will be changes in CD4 counts and in HIV-1 virus load, as well as effects on clinical progression of HIV-1 disease.

SUMMARY

In summary, some successes have been achieved in studies of candidate HIV-1 and SIV vaccines in primate models. In the chimpanzee, a relatively limited number of experiments have been carried out in which protection was observed against homologous, intravenously administered cell-free virus and in at least one experiment against cell-associated virus challenge. Although the precise correlates of immunity have not been determined, in some studies protection was associated with levels of neutralizing antibody, particularly directed against the principal neutralizing determinant in the V3 loop. This is also consistent with the demonstration of protection by passive immunization with anti-HIV-1 antibody. Many important questions remain in this system, including duration of protection and ability to protect against mucosal routes of challenge. The critical question of extent of protection, if any, against heterologous HIV-1 strains has not been able to be addressed because of the absence of a heterologous challenge strain for use in chimpanzees. It is anticipated that such strains will become available in the near future to examine this question.

Studies of immunization in macaques have also demonstrated protection against SIV challenges intravenously (and via the mucosal route) with cell-free virus and to a variable degree with cell-associated virus. The largest number of studies that have demonstrated protection employed whole, inactivated virus vaccine preparations, and interpretation of many of these studies is confounded by the xenogeneic challenge system in which protection could be attributed to anti-human cell responses. Nonetheless, some protection has also been demonstrated recently in systems that are not confounded by anti-human cell responses. The experience with subunit vaccines in the macaque SIV system has been disappointing, and experience has been mixed with respect to the protective effects of live vaccinia vector vaccine followed by a subunit boost. A recent notable success has been the use of an SIV deletion mutant as a live attenuated candidate vaccine. Despite the large number of studies that have been carried out, the in vitro correlates of immunity (protection) have not been clearly established.

Considerable experience has been gained in phase I studies of a variety of candidate HIV-1 vaccines in healthy seronegative individuals. With the exception of the acute reactogenicity associated with preparations that contained the MTP-PE adjuvant, vaccine candidates have been generally well tolerated. No significant clinical or laboratory toxicities have been encountered, and evidence of immunosuppression, employing a variety of in vitro assays and skin tests, has not been found. Although the experience with regard to the safety of candidate HIV-1 vaccines is reassuring, it should be acknowledged that subtle forms of immunosuppression or other toxicities have not been excluded, particularly those that may develop after long periods of time. Careful follow-up of subjects for development of such toxicities needs to be maintained.

Studies of the immunogenicity of subunit vaccine candidates that have been carried out thus far in humans indicate that it is likely that at least three doses will be required. Optimal regimens for immunization have not been defined, and will likely vary according to vaccine type. Generation of binding antibodies, as detected by Western blot and EIA, appears to be readily accomplished, but stimulation of neutralizing antibodies is more difficult. To date, the most promising results with respect to neutralizing antibodies have been generated with recombinant gp120 vaccines, in which neutralizing antibody responses develop in most vaccinees after three doses. Administration of a live vaccinia-gp160 construct followed by a subunit boost has also shown promise, and this regimen is the only one in which CD8+ cytotoxic T-lymphocyte activity has been detected to date. As noted earlier, a major problem confronting efforts to develop an HIV-1 vaccine is the antigenic diversity of HIV-1 isolates and the likely need to mount immune responses to heterologous strains for a vaccine to be effective. Studies to date have shown that it is possible to generate some heterologous neutralizing activity with subunit vaccines, and the development of optimal strategies to achieve this is a major goal of studies currently under way. Most recently, questions have been raised regarding possible qualitative differences between neutralizing antibodies stimulated by vaccination and those induced by naturally occurring HIV-1 infection. Vaccine-stimulated antibodies effectively neutralize laboratory-adapted HIV-1 strains, but have been reported to be ineffective in neutralizing primary (nonlaboratory-adapted) HIV-1 isolates, even ones within the same strain designation as the vaccine virus.[152,153] Whether this is merely a laboratory phenomenon related to different in vitro properties of laboratory-adapted and "primary" HIV-1 isolates or whether this indicates that vaccine-induced antibody will be ineffective in neutralizing field isolates of HIV-1 is unknown and is currently under active investigation.

HIV-1 vaccines administered to HIV-1–infected patients (immunotherapy) have also been well tolerated and have elicited humoral and cellular immune responses to the immunogen. Controlled trials are underway to examine the efficacy of this type of immunotherapy in HIV-1–infected individuals.

On the basis of data generated in phase I studies, two candidate HIV-1 vaccines, both produced in CHO cells (rgp 120 [MN] and rgp 120 [SF-2]), are now entering expanded safety and immunogenicity studies in HIV-1 seronegative subjects who are at higher risk for acquisition of HIV-1 infection (phase II studies).[154] These studies are intended to provide additional data on vaccine candidates in populations that are likely to be important targets for the eventual utilization of an HIV-1 vaccine, such as sexually active adolescents, young adults with histories of sexually transmitted diseases, sexual partners of HIV-1–infected individuals, and intravenous drug users. Information from phase II studies is to be used in selection of vaccine(s) to undergo large-scale, placebo-controlled efficacy trials in HIV-1 seronegative subjects (phase III studies). Such trials will require considerable resources, since they necessarily involve large numbers of subjects and prolonged follow-up. The decision to embark on such a trial will depend on multiple factors, including the relative risk-benefit analysis of individual vaccine candidates and the availability of resources to conduct such a trial. Plans are underway to establish the organization and infrastructure with which to carry out efficacy trials at multiple sites within the United States and at one or more sites in Africa, Southeast Asia, and South America.

REFERENCES

1. Berzofsky JA. Approaches and issues in the development of vaccines against HIV. J AIDS. 1991;4:451–9.
2. Kurth R, Binninger D, Ennen J, et al. The quest for an AIDS vaccine: The state of the art and current challenges. AIDS Res Hum Retroviruses. 1991; 7:425–33.
3. Bolognesi DP. Human immunodeficiency virus vaccines. Adv Virus Res. 1993;42:103–48.
4. Fast PE, Walker MC. Human trials of experimental AIDS vaccines. AIDS. 1993;7(Suppl 1):S147–59.
5. Greene WC. The molecular biology of human immunodeficiency virus type 1 infection. N Engl J Med. 1991;324:308–18.
6. Pantaleo G, Graziosi C, Fauci AS. The immunopathogenesis of human immunodeficiency virus infection. N Engl J Med. 1993;328:327–35.
7. Palker TJ, Clark ME, Langlois AJ, et al. Type-specific neutralization of the human immunodeficiency virus with antibodies to env-encoded synthetic peptides. Proc Natl Acad Sci USA. 1988;85:1932–6.
8. Goudsmit J, Debouck C, Meloen RH, et al. Human immunodeficiency virus type 1 neutralization epitope with conserved architecture elicits early type-specific antibodies in experimentally infected chimpanzees. Proc Natl Acad Sci USA. 1988;85:4478–82.
9. Javaherian K, Langlois AJ, McDanal C, et al. Principal neutralizing domain of the human immunodeficiency virus type 1 envelope protein. Proc Natl Acad Sci USA. 1989;86:6768–72.
10. Papsidero LD, Sheu M, Ruscetti FW. Human immunodeficiency virus type-1 neutralizing monoclonal antibodies which react with p17 core protein characterization and epitope mapping. J Virol. 1989;63:267–72.
11. Sano K, Lee MH, Morales F, et al. Antibody that inhibits human immunodeficiency virus reverse transcriptase and association with inability to isolate virus. J Clin Microbiol. 1987;25:2415–7.
12. Broliden PA, Ljunggren K, Hinkula J, et al. A monoclonal antibody to human immunodeficiency virus type 1 which mediates cellular cytotoxicity and neutralization. J Virol. 1990;64:936–40.
13. Javaherian K, Langlois AJ, LaRosa GH, et al. Broadly neutralizing antibodies elicited by the hypervariable neutralizing determinant of HIV-1. Science. 1990;250:1590–3.
14. Veronese FDM, Rahman R, Kalyanaraman VS, et al. Monoclonal antibodies to HTLV-III₄₅₁ gp41: Delineation of an immunoreactive conserved epitope in the transmembrane region of divergent isolates of HIV-1. AIDS Res Hum Retroviruses. 1989;5:479–86.
15. Olshevsky U, Helseth E, Furman C, et al. Identification of individual human immunodeficiency virus type 1 gp120 amino acids important for CD4 receptor binding. J Virol. 1990;64:5701–7.
16. Ho DD, McKeating JA, Li XL, et al. Conformational epitope on gp120 important in CD4 binding and human immunodeficiency virus type 1 neutralization identified by a human monoclonal antibody. J Virol. 1991;65:489–93.
17. Thali M, Olshevsky U, Furman C, et al. Characterization of a discontinuous human immunodeficiency virus type 1 gp120 epitope recognized by a broadly reactive neutralizing human monoclonal antibody. J Virol. 1991;65:6188–93.
18. Montefiori DM, Graham BS, Zhou J, et al, and the NIAID AIDS Clinical Trials Network. V3 specific neutralizing antibodies in sera from HIV-1 gp160-immunized volunteers block virus fusion and act synergistically with human monoclonal antibody to the conformation-dependent CD4 binding site of gp120. J Clin Invest. 1993;92:840–7.
19. Weinhold KJ. Anti-HIV-1 ADCC: Clinical and therapeutic implications. Biotechnol Ther. 1991;2:147–57.
20. Brenner BG, Gryllis C, Wainberg MA. Role of antibody-dependent cellular cytotoxicity and lymphokine-activated killer cells in AIDS and related diseases. J Leukocyte Biol. 1991;50:628–40.
21. Jewett A, Giorgi JV, Bonavida B. Antibody-dependent cellular cytotoxicity against HIV-coated target cells by peripheral blood monocytes from HIV seropositive asymptomatic patients. J Immunol. 1990;145:4065–71.
22. Plata F. Implications of HIV-specific cytotoxic T lymphocytes in AIDS. Biotherapy. 1992;5:31–45.
23. Takahashi H, Germain RN, Moss B, et al. An immunodominant class 1–restricted cytotoxic T lymphocyte determinant of human immunodeficiency virus type 1 induces CD4 class II–restricted help for itself. J Exp Med. 1990; 171:571–6.
24. Rosenberg ZF, Fauci AS. The immunopathogenesis of HIV infection. Adv Immunol. 1989;47:377–431.
25. Langlade-Demoyen P, Michel F, Hoffenbach A, et al. Immune recognition of AIDS virus antigens by human and murine cytotoxic T lymphocytes. J Immunol. 1988;141:1949–1957.

26. Riviere Y, Tanneau-Salvadori F, Regnault A, et al. Human immunodeficiency virus-specific cytotoxic responses of seropositive individuals: Distinct types of effector cells mediate killing of targets expressing gag and env proteins. J Virol. 1989;63:2270–7.
27. Walker BD, Flexner C, Paradis TJ, et al. HIV-1 reverse transcriptase is a target for cytotoxic T lymphocytes in infected individuals. Science. 1988; 240:64–6.
28. Chenciner N, Michel F, Dadaglio G, et al. Multiple subsets of HIV-specific cytotoxic T lymphocytes in humans and in mice. Eur J Immunol. 1989;19: 1537–44.
29. Walker BD, Flexner C, Birch-Limberger K, et al. Long-term culture and fine specificity of human cytotoxic T-lymphocyte clones reactive with human immunodeficiency virus type 1. Proc Natl Acad Sci USA. 1989;86:9514–18.
30. Takahashi H, Merli S, Putney SD, et al. A single amino acid interchange yields reciprocal CTL specificities for HIV-1 gp160. Science. 1989;246: 118–21.
31. Hammond SA, Bollinger RC, Stanhope PE, et al. Comparative clonal analysis of human immunodeficiency virus type 1 (HIV-1) specific CD4+ and CD8+ cytolytic T lymphocytes isolated from seronegative humans immunized with candidate HIV-1 vaccines. J Exp Med. 1992;176:1531–42.
32. El-Daher N, Keefer MC, Reichman RC, et al. Persisting human immunodeficiency virus-1 gp160-specific human T lymphocyte responses including CD8+ cytotoxic activity after receipt of envelope vaccines. J Infect Dis. 1993;168:306–13.
33. Orentas RJ, Hildreth JEK, Obah E. Induction of CD4+ cytolytic T cells specific for HIV-infected cells by a gp160 subunit vaccine. Science. 1990; 248:1234–7.
34. Stanhope PE, Clements ML, Siliciano RF. Human CD4 cytolytic T lymphocyte responses to a human immunodeficiency virus type 1 gp160 subunit vaccine. J Infect Dis. 1993;168:92–100.
35. Robinson WE Jr, Montefiori DC, Mitchell WM. Antibody-dependent enhancement of human immunodeficiency virus type 1 infection. Lancet. 1988; 1:790–794.
36. Takeda A, Tuazon CU, Ennis FA. Antibody-enhanced infection by HIV-1 via Fc receptor-mediated entry. Science. 1988;242:580–3.
37. Montefiori DC, Lefkowitz LB Jr, Keller RE, et al. Absence of a clinical correlation for complement mediated, infection-enhancing antibodies in plasma or sera from HIV-1-infected individuals. AIDS. 1991;5:413–7.
38. Dolin R, Graham B, Greenberg S, et al, and the AIDS Vaccine Clinical Trials Network. Safety and immunogenicity of an HIV-1 recombinant gp160 candidate vaccine in humans. Ann Intern Med. 1991;114:119–27.
39. Cianciolo GJ, Copeland TD, Oroszlan S, et al. Inhibition of lymphocyte proliferation by a synthetic peptide homologous to retroviral envelope proteins. Science. 1985;230:453–5.
40. Ruegg CL, Monell CR, Strand M. Inhibition of lymphoproliferation by a synthetic peptide with sequence identity to gp41 of human immunodeficiency virus type 1. J Virol. 1989;63:3257–60.
41. Zagury JF, Bernard J, Achour A, et al. Identification of CD4 and major histocompatibility complex functional peptide sites and their homology with oligopeptides from human immunodeficiency virus type 1 glycoprotein gp120: Role in AIDS pathogenesis. Proc Natl Acad Sci USA. 1993;90:7573–7.
42. Reiher WE, Blalock JE, Brunek TK. Sequence homology between acquired immunodeficiency syndrome virus envelope protein and interleukin-2. Proc Natl Acad Sci USA. 1986;83:9188–92.
43. Lee MR, Ho DD, Gurney ME. Functional interaction and partial homology between human immunodeficiency virus and neuroleukin. Science. 1987;237: 1047–51.
44. Pugliese O, Viora M, Camponeschi B, et al. A gp120 HIV peptide with high similarity to HLA class II beta chains enhances PPD-specific and autoreactive T cell activation. Clin Exp Immunol. 1992;90:170–4.
45. Golding H, Robey FA, Gates FT, et al. Identification of homologous regions in human immunodeficiency virus 1 gp41 and human MHC class II beta I domain. J Exp Med. 1988;167:914–23.
46. Jarin PS, Sun DK, Thornton AH, et al. Neutralization of HTLV-III/LAV replication by antiserum to thymosin α-1. Science. 1986;232:1135–9.
47. DeSantis C, Robbioni P, Longhi R, et al. Cross-reactive response to HIV-1 gp120 and HLA class I heavy chains induced by receipt of HIV-1 derived envelope vaccines. J Infect Dis. 1993;6:1396–403.
48. Salk J. Prospects for the control of AIDS by immunizing seropositive individuals. Nature. 1987;327:473–6.
49. Levine A, Allen J, Munson K, et al. Initial studies of active immunotherapy in HIV infected patients using a gp120 depleted HIV-1 immunogen: A five year follow up. Abstract WS-B28-2. IXth Int Conf on AIDS/IVth STD World Congress. Berlin, June 1993.
50. Cochran MA, Ericson BL, Knell JD, et al. Use of baculovirus recombinants as a general method for the production of subunit vaccines. In: Ginsberg H, Brown F, Lerner RA, et al., eds. Vaccines 87. Cold Spring Harbor, NY: Cold Spring Harbor Press; 1987:384–8.
51. Steimer KS, van Nest G, Dina D, et al. Genetically engineering human immunodeficiency virus envelope glycoprotein gp120 produced in yeast is the target of neutralizing antibodies. In: Ginsberg H, Brown F, Lerner RA, et al. Vaccines 87. Cold Spring Harbor, NY: Cold Spring Harbor Press; 1987; 236–41.
52. Haigwood NL, Nara PL, Brooks E, et al. Native but not denatured recombinant human immunodeficiency virus type 1 gp120 generates broad-spectrum neutralizing antibodies in baboons. J Virol. 1992;66:172–82.
53. Lasky LA, Groopman JE, Fennie CW, et al. Neutralization of the AIDS

retrovirus by antibodies to a recombinant envelope glycoprotein. Science. 1986;233:209–12.

54. Barrett N, Mitterer A, Mundt W, et al. Large scale production and purification of a vaccinia derived HIV-1 gp160 and analysis of its immunogenicity. AIDS Res Hum Retroviruses. 1989;25:159–71.

55. Dolin R, Corey L, Graham B, et al, and the NIAID AIDS Vaccine Clinical Trials Network and Chiron Corp. Safety and immunogenicity of an HIV vaccine candidate, ENV 2-3, in combination with MTP-PE/MF59 (Abstract PO-A2226). VIIIth International Conference on AIDS/III STD World Congress, Amsterdam, The Netherlands, July 19–24, 1992.

56. Graham B, Keefer M, McElrath MJ, et al, and the NIAID AIDS Vaccine Clinical Trials Network. Phase I trial of native HIV-1 SF-2 rgp120 candidate vaccine (Abstract PO-A29-0692). IXth International Conference on AIDS/IV STD World Congress, Berlin, Germany, June 7–11, 1993.

57. Schwartz D, Gorse G, Clements ML, et al. Induction of HIV-1 neutralizing and syncytium-inhibiting antibodies in seronegative recipients of HIV-1 IIIB rgp120 subunit vaccines. Lancet. 1993;342:69–73.

58. Hart MK, Palker TJ, Matthews TS, et al. Synthetic peptides containing T and B cell epitopes from human immunodeficiency virus envelope gp120 induce anti-HIV proliferative responses and high titers of neutralizing antibodies in rhesus monkeys. J Immunol. 1990;145:2677–85.

59. Wang CY, Looney DJ, Li ML, et al. Long-term high titer neutralizing activity induced by octameric synthetic HIV-1 antigen. Science. 1991;254:285–8.

60. Goldstein AL, Naylor PH, Sarin PS, et al. Progress in the development of a p17-based HIV vaccine: Safety and potential efficacy of the HGP-30 synthetic peptide vaccine in humans (Abstract MA1342). VIIth International Conference on AIDS/IInd STD World Congress, Florence, June 1991.

61. Adams SE, Dawson KM, Gull K, et al. The expression of hybrid HIV: Ty virus-like particles in yeast. Nature. 1987;329:68–70.

62. Blick G, Crook S, Buchanan S, et al. A phase I/II study of the toxicity, immunogenicity and efficacy of recombinant gp160 and p24 vaccines (Vax-Syn) in HIV-infected individuals regardless of CD4+ cell count (Abstract TuB0562). VIIIth International Conference on AIDS/III STD World Congress, Amsterdam, July 1992.

63. Hu SL, Kosowski SG, Dalrymple JM. Expression of AIDS virus envelope in recombinant vaccinia viruses. Nature. 1986;320:537–9.

64. Tartaglia J, Cox WI, Taylor J, et al. Highly attenuated poxvirus vectors. AIDS Res Hum Retroviruses. 1992;8:1445–1447.

65. Hesselton RM, Mazzara GP, Panicali D, et al. HIV-specific immune response in rabbits immunized with HIV-like particles and recombinant vaccinia virus (Abstract MoA0045). VIII International Conference on AIDS/III STD World Congress, Amsterdam, July 1992.

66. Chandra PK, Natuk RJ, Mason BB, et al. High-level expression of the envelope glycoprotein of the human immunodeficiency virus type 1 in presence of rev gene using helper-independent adenovirus type 7 recombinants. Virology. 1990;175:535–47.

67. Evans DJ, McKeating J, Meredith JM, et al. An engineered poliovirus chimaera elicits broadly reactive HIV-1 neutralizing antibodies. Nature. 1989;339:385–8.

68. Burke KL, Almond JW, Evans DJ. Antigen chimeras of poliovirus. Prog Med Virol. 1991;38:56–68.

69. Aggarwal A, Sadoff J, Markham P, et al. Induction of cytotoxic T lymphocytes against HIV-2 in mice immunized with recombinant *Salmonella typhimurium* (Abstract MA1036). VIIth International Conference on AIDS/II STD World Congress, Florence, June 1991.

70. Stover CK, de la Cruz VF, Ruerst TR, et al. New use of BCG for recombinant vaccines. Nature. 1991;351:456–60.

71. Aldovini A, Young RA. Humoral and cell-mediated immune responses to live recombinant BCG-HIV vaccines. Nature. 1991;351:479–82.

72. Hu SL, Abrams K, Barber GN, et al. Protection of macaques against SIV infection by subunit vaccines of SIV envelope glycoprotein gp160. Science. 1992;255:456–9.

73. Cooney EL, McElrath MJ, Corey L, et al. Enhanced immunity to HIV envelope elicited by a combined vaccine regimen consisting of priming with a vaccinia recombinant expressing HIV envelope and boosting with gp160 protein. Proc Natl Acad Sci USA. 1993;90:1882–6.

74. Graham BS, Matthews TJ, Belshe RB, et al, and the NIAID AIDS Vaccine Clinical Trials Network. Augmentation of HIV-1 neutralizing antibody by priming with gp160 recombinant vaccinia and boosting with rgp160. J Infect Dis. 1993;167:533–7.

75. Daniel MD, Kirchoff F, Czajak SC, et al. Protective effects of a live attenuated SIV vaccine with a deletion in the nef gene. Science. 1992;258:1938–41.

76. Letvin N, communicated in Fast PE, Walker MC. Human trials of experimental AIDS vaccines. AIDS. 1993;7:S147–59.

77. Kang CY, Nara P, Chamat S, et al. Anti-idiotype monoclonal antibody elicits broadly neutralizing anti-gp120 antibodies in monkeys. Proc Natl Acad Sci USA. 1992;89:2546–50.

78. Sutor GC, Trussenar J, Jurkiewich E, et al. Anti-CD4 idiotype vaccination of HIV+ volunteers (Abstract POB3042). VIIIth International Conference on AIDS/III STD World Congress, Amsterdam, July 1992.

79. Ulmer JB, Donnelly JJ, Parker SE, et al. Heterologous protection against influenza by infection of DNA encoding a viral protein. Science. 1993;259:1745–9.

80. van Nest GA, Steimer KS, Haigwood NL, et al. Advanced adjuvant formulation for use with recombinant subunit vaccines. In: Brown F, Chanock R, Ginsberg HS, et al., eds. Vaccines. Cold Spring Harbor, NY: Cold Spring Harbor Laboratory Press; 1992:57–62.

81. Gadjusek DC, Amyx HL, Gibbs CJ Jr, et al. Transmission experiments with human T-lymphotropic retroviruses and human AIDS tissue. Lancet. 1984;1:1415–6.

82. Francis DP, Feorino PM, Broderson JR, et al. Infection of chimpanzees with lymphadenopathy associated virus. Lancet. 1984;11:1276–7.

83. Alter JH, Eichberg JW, Masur H, et al. Transmission of HTLV-III infection from human plasma to chimpanzees: An animal model for AIDS. Science. 1984;226:549–52.

84. Prince AM, Horowitz B, Baker L, et al. Failure of a human immunodeficiency virus (HIV) immune globulin to protect chimpanzees against experimental challenge with HIV. Proc Natl Acad Sci USA. 1988;85:6944–8.

85. Prince AM, Reesink H, Pascual D, et al. Prevention of infection by passive immunization with HIV immunoglobulin. AIDS Res Hum Retroviruses. 1991;7:971–3.

86. Emini EA, Schlief WA, Nunberg JH, et al. Prevention of HIV-1 infection in chimpanzees by gp120 V3 domain-specific monoclonal antibody. Nature. 1992;355:728–30.

87. Schultz AM, Hu SL. Primate models for HIV vaccines. AIDS 1993;7(Suppl 1):S161–70.

88. Arthur LO, Bess JW Jr, Waters DJ, et al. Challenge of chimpanzees (*Pan troglodytes*) immunized with human immunodeficiency virus envelope glycoprotein gp120. J Virol. 1989;63:5046–53.

89. Girard M, Kieny MP, Pinter A, et al. Immunization of chimpanzees confers protection against challenge with human immunodeficiency virus. Proc Natl Acad Sci USA. 1991;88:542–6.

90. Berman PW, Gregory TJ, Riddle L, et al. Protection of chimpanzees from infection by HIV-1 after vaccination with recombinant glycoprotein gp120 but not gp160. Nature. 1990;345:622–5.

91. Fultz PN, Nara P, Barre-Sinoussi F, et al. Vaccine protection of chimpanzees against challenge with HIV-1–infected peripheral blood mononuclear cells. Science. 1992;256:1687–90.

92. Hu SL, Fultz PN, McClure HM, et al. Effect of immunization with a vaccinia-HIV env recombinant on HIV infection of chimpanzees. Nature. 1987;328:721–3.

93. Kestler H, Kodama T, Ringler D, et al. Induction of AIDS in rhesus monkeys by molecularly cloned simian immunodeficiency virus. Science. 1990;248:1109–12.

94. Gardner MB, Luciw PA. Animal models of AIDS. FASEB J. 1989;3:2593–606.

95. Daniel MD, Desrosiers RC. Use of simian immunodeficiency virus for evaluation of AIDS vaccine strategies. AIDS. 1989;3:S131–3.

96. Fultz PN, McClure HM, Anderson DC, et al. Identification and biologic characterization of an acutely lethal variant of simian immunodeficiency virus from sooty mangabeys (SIV/SMM). AIDS Res Hum Retroviruses. 1989;5:397–409.

97. Desrosiers RC. The simian immunodeficiency viruses. Annu Rev Immunol. 1990;8:557–76.

98. Kodama T, Wooley DP, Naidu YM, et al. The significance of premature stop codons in env of SIV. J Virol. 1989;63:4709–14.

99. Desrosiers RC, Wyand MS, Kodama T, et al. Vaccine protection against simian immunodeficiency virus infection. Proc Natl Acad Sci USA. 1989;86:6353–7.

100. Murphey-Corb M, Martin LN, Davison-Fairburn B, et al. A formalin-inactivated whole SIV vaccine confers protection in macaques. Science. 1989;246:1293–7.

101. Murphey-Corb M, Montelaro RC, Miller MA, et al. Efficacy of SIV/Delta B670 glycoprotein-enriched and glycoprotein depleted subunit vaccines in protecting against infection and disease in rhesus monkeys. AIDS. 1991;5:655–62.

102. Gardner MB. Vaccination against SIV infection and disease. AIDS Res Hum Retrovirus. 1990;6:835–45.

103. Sutgipto S, Pederien NC, Miller CJ, et al. Inactivated simian immunodeficiency virus vaccine failed to protect *Rhesus macaques* from intravenous or genital mucosal infection but delayed disease in intravenously exposed animals. J Virol. 1990;64:2290–7.

104. Johnson PR, Montefiore DC, Goldstein S, et al. Inactivated whole SIV vaccine in macaques: Evaluation of protective efficacy against challenge with cell-free virus or infected cells. AIDS Res Hum Retroviruses. 1992;8:1501–5.

105. Heeney JL, de Vries P, Dubbes R, et al. Comparison of protection from homologous cell-free versus cell-associated SIV challenge afforded by inactivated whole SIV vaccine. J Med Primatol. 1992;21:126–30.

106. Warren JT, Dolatshai M. First updates and revised survey of worldwide HIV and SIV vaccine challenge studies in nonhuman primates: Progress in first and second order studies. J Med Primatol. 1993;22:203–35.

107. Stott EJ. Anti-cell antibody in macaques (Letter). Nature. 1991;353:393.

108. Osterhalis A, de Vries P, Heeney J. AIDS vaccine developments. Nature. 1992;355:684–5.

109. Planelles V, Giavedoni L, Marthas M, et al. Vaccine studies with SIV$_{mac}$ 1A11 recombinant gp130: Lack of protection from SIV$_{mac251}$ challenge. In: Brown F, Chanock R, Ginsberg H, et al., eds. Vaccines 92. Cold Spring Harbor, NY: Cold Spring Harbor Laboratory Press, 1992:123–129.

110. Mills KHG, Page M, Chal WL, et al. Protection against SIV challenge in macaques. J Med Primatol. 1992;21:50–8.

111. Hu SL, Abrams K, Misher L, et al. Evaluation of protective efficacy of recombinant subunit vaccines against simian immunodeficiency virus infection of macaques. J Med Primatol. 1992;21:119–25.

112. Hoover E, Desrosiers R, Yilma T. Communicated in Fast PE, Walker MC.

Human trials of experimental AIDS vaccines. AIDS. 1993;7(Suppl 1): S147–59.

113. Franchini G, Guroff M, Tartaglia J, et al. Efficacy of canarypox, attenuated vaccinia, and *Salmonella typhimurium* HIV-2 vaccines in rhesus macaques (Abstract WS-B27-5). IXth International Conference on AIDS/IV STD World Congress, Berlin, Germany, June 7–11, 1993.

114. Luciw PA, Shaw KE, Unger RE, et al. Genetic and biological comparisons of pathogenic and non-pathogenic molecular clones of simian immunodeficiency virus (SIV$_{mac}$). AIDS Res Hum Retroviruses. 1992;8:395–402.

115. Putkonen P, Thorstensson R, Biberfeld G, et al. Vaccination against HIV-2 and SIV in cynomolgus monkeys. AIDS Res Hum Retroviruses. 1991;7: 271–7.

116. Putkonen P, Thorstensson R, Albert J, et al. Infection of cynomolgus monkeys with HIV-2 protects against pathogenic consequences of a subsequent simian immunodeficiency virus infection. AIDS. 1990;4:783–9.

117. Putkonen PR, Thorstensson R, Ghavamzadeh J, et al. Prevention of HIV-2 and SIV$_{mac}$ infection by passive immunization in cynomolgus monkeys. Nature. 1991;352:436–8.

118. Shibata R, Kawamura M, Sakaj H, et al. Generation of chimeric human and simian immunodeficiency virus infectious to monkey peripheral blood mononuclear cells. J Virol. 1991;65:3514–20.

119. Li J, Lord CI, Haseltine W, et al. Infection of cynomolgus monkeys with a chimeric HIV-1/SIV$_{mac}$ virus that expresses the HIV-1 envelope glycoproteins. J AIDS. 1992;5:639–46.

120. Sakuragi S, Shibata R, Mukai R, et al. Infection of macaque monkeys with a chimeric human and simian immunodeficiency virus. J Gen Virol. 1992; 73:2983–7.

121. Agy MB, Frumkin LR, Corey L, et al. Infection of *Macaca nemestrina* by human immunodeficiency virus type 1. Science. 1992;257:103–6.

122. Keefer MC, Graham BS, Belshe RB, et al. Studies of high doses of a human immunodeficiency virus type 1 (HIV-1) recombinant gp160 candidate vaccine in HIV-1 seronegative humans. 1994. Submitted.

123. Keefer MC, Bonnez W, Roberts NJ Jr, et al. Human immunodeficiency virus (HIV-1) gp160-specific lymphocyte proliferative responses of mononuclear leukocytes from HIV-1 recombinant gp160 vaccine recipients. J Infect Dis. 1991;163:448–53.

124. Gorse GJ, Belshe RB, Newman FK, et al., and the NIAID AIDS Vaccine Clinical Trials Network. Lymphocyte proliferative responses following immunization with human immunodeficiency virus recombinant gp160. Vaccine. 1992;10:383–8.

125. Belshe R, Clements ML, Dolin R, et al, and the NIAID AIDS Vaccine Clinical Trials Network. Safety and immunogenicity of a fully glycosylated recombinant gp160 HIV-1 vaccine in low risk volunteers. J Infect Dis. 1993;168: 1387–95.

126. Keefer M, Graham B, McElrath MJ, et al, and the AIDS Vaccine Clinical Trials Network. Phase I trial of an HIV-1 candidate vaccine ENV 2-3, in combination with MTP-PE/MF59 (Abstract PO-A29-07083). IXth International Conference on AIDS/IV STD World Congress, Berlin, Germany, June 7–11, 1993.

127. Keefer MC, Graham B, McElrath MJ, et al. Safety and immunogenicity of Env 2-3, a human immunodeficiency virus type-1 candidate vaccine in combination with MTP-PE/MF59 adjuvant. 1994. Submitted.

128. Kahn J, Chernoff D, Sinangil F, et al. A phase I study of HIV-1 gp120 combined with MF59 and with dose escalation of MTP-PE in seronegative adults (Abstract WS-B27-2). IXth International Conference on AIDS/IV STD World Congress, Berlin, Germany, June 7–11, 1993.

129. Schwartz D, Clements ML, Gorse G, et al. Neutralization profile after sequential immunization with IIIB-rgp120 followed by MN-rgp120 (Abstract). Conference on Advances in AIDS Vaccine Development, Sixth Annual Meeting of the National Cooperative Vaccine Development Group, Alexandria, VA, 1993.

130. Cooney EL, Collier AC, Greenberg PD, et al. Safety of and immunological response to a recombinant vaccinia virus vaccine expressing HIV envelope glycoprotein. Lancet. 1991;337:567–72.

131. Graham BS, Belshe RB, Clements ML, et al, and the AIDS Vaccine Clinical Trials Network. Vaccination of vaccinia-naive adults with HIV-1 gp160 recombinant vaccinia (HIVAC-1e) in a blinded, controlled, randomized clinical trial. J Infect Dis. 1992;116:244–52.

132. Kahn J, Coleman R, Stites D, et al. A phase I study of HGP-30, a 30 amino-acid subunit of HIV p17 synthetic peptide analogue subunit vaccine in seronegative subjects (Abstract POB3037). VIIIth International Conference on AIDS/III STD World Congress, Amsterdam, The Netherlands, July 1992.

133. Goldstein AL, Sorin PS, Markham R. Cytotoxic and humoral immune responses to HIV-1 p17 synthetic peptide HGP-30 in human volunteers (Abstract POB27-2139). IXth International Conference on AIDS/IV STD World Congress, Berlin, Germany, June 1993.

134. Martin S, Weber J, Rott I, et al. Recombinant HIV-1 gag p24-Ty virus-like-particles (VLPs) induce HIV-1 p24 specific T helper cells in seronegative subjects vaccinated with these particles (Abstract POA2194). VIIIth International Conference on AIDS/III STD World Congress, Amsterdam, July 1992.

135. Ukwu HN, Graham BS, Lambert JS, et al. Perinatal transmission of human immunodeficiency virus-1 infection and maternal immunization strategies for prevention. Obstet Gynecol. 1992;80:458–68.

136. Ryder RW, Nsa W, Hassig SE, et al. Perinatal transmission of the human immunodeficiency virus type 1 to infants of seropositive women in Zaire. N Engl J Med. 1989;320:1637–42.

137. Goedert JJ, Mendez H, Drummond JE, et al. Mother-to-infant transmission of human immunodeficiency virus type 1: Association with prematurity or low anti-gp120. Lancet. 1989;2:1351–4.

138. Katz SL, Wilfert CM. Human immunodeficiency virus infection of newborns. N Engl J Med. 1989;320:1687–90.

139. Devash Y, Calvelli TA, Wood DG, et al. Vertical transmission of human immunodeficiency virus is correlated with the absence of high-affinity/avidity maternal antibodies to the gp120 principal neutralizing domain. Proc Natl Acad Sci USA. 1990;87:3445–9.

140. Rossi P, Moschese V, Broliden PA, et al. Presence of maternal antibodies of human immunodeficiency virus 1 envelop glycoprotein gp120 epitopes correlates with the uninfected status of children born to seropositive mothers. Proc Natl Acad Sci USA. 1989;86:8055–8.

141. Parekh BS, Shaffer N, Pau CP, et al. Lack of correlation between maternal antibodies to V3 loop peptides of gp120 and perinatal HIV-1 transmission. AIDS 1991;5:1179–84.

142. Redfield R, Birx D, Ketter N, et al. A phase 1 evaluation of the safety and immunogenicity of recombinant gp160 in patients with early human immunodeficiency virus infection. N Engl J Med. 1991;324:1677–84.

143. Redfield R, Birx D, Vahey M, et al. HIV vaccine therapy: phase I safety and immunogenicity using gp160 (Abstract TuB0563). VIIIth International Conference on AIDS/III STD World Congress. Amsterdam, July 1992.

144. Birx D, Johnson S, Amman A, et al. Immunogenicity and safety of rgp120 (LAI) in early-stage HIV-positive patients (Abstract TuB0564). VIIIth International Conference on AIDS/III STD World Congress. Amsterdam, July 1992.

145. Tsoukas C, Sampalis J, Gold P, et al. Specific active immunotherapy in asymptomatic HIV disease using recombinant gp160 (Abstract TuB0560). VIIIth International Conference on AIDS/III STD World Congress. Amsterdam, July 1992.

146. Bratt G, Eriksson L, Sandstrom E, et al. A study of gp160 vaccine in healthy HIV carriers with and without zidovudine (Abstract TuB3036). VIIIth International Conference on AIDS/III STD World Congress. Amsterdam, July 1992.

147. Picard O, Giral P, Defer MC, et al. AIDS vaccine therapy; phase 1 trial. Lancet. 1990;336:179–82.

148. Biselli R, Loomis LD, Del Bono V, et al. Vaccine therapy with gp160; effect on human anti-gp120 antibody spectrotype (Abstract MoA0011). VIIIth International Conference on AIDS/III STD World Congress, Amsterdam, July 1992.

149. Katzenstein D, Valentine F, Kundu SK, et al. Delayed-type hypersensitivity reactions to intradermal gp160 in HIV-infected individuals immunized with gp160 (Abstract POA2192). VIIIth International Conference on AIDS/III STD World Congress. Amsterdam, July 1992.

150. Schwartz D. New immune responses induced by full-length glycosylated IIIB rgp160 vaccine (AVEG-Immuno AG). Sixth Annual Meeting of the National Cooperative Vaccine Development Groups, Alexandria, VA, 1993.

151. Corey L, McElrath MJ, Keefer M, et al. An AVEG phase I randomized, blinded, controlled trial in asymptomatic HIV-infected subjects using Env 2-3 with or without MTP-PE. Sixth Annual Meeting of the National Cooperative Vaccine Development Group, Alexandria, VA, 1993.

152. Mascola J, Weislow O, Snyder S, et al. Neutralizing antibody activity in sera from human immunodeficiency virus type-1 vaccine recipients from the AIDS vaccine clinical trials network. Sixth Annual Meeting of the National Cooperative Vaccine Development Group, Alexandria, VA, 1993.

153. Steimer K, Sinangil F, Kahn J, et al. Primary isolate neutralizing activity of human antibodies directed to recombinant, native HIV-SF-2 GP 120 (rgp120$_{SF-2}$). Sixth Annual Meeting of the National Cooperative Vaccine Development Group, Alexandria, VA, 1993.

154. McElrath MJ, Corey L, Clements ML, et al. Expanded safety and immunogenicity trial of recombinant gp120 vaccines among seronegative volunteers (AVEG Protocol 201). Sixth Annual Meeting of the National Cooperative Vaccine Development Group, Alexandria, VA, 1993.

155. Zagury D, Bernard J, Cheyner R, et al. A group-specific anamnestic reaction against HIV-1 induced by a candidate vaccine against AIDS. Nature. 1988; 332:728–31.

156. Picard O, Achour A, Bernard J, et al. A 2-year follow-up of an anti-HIV immune reaction in HIV gp160-immunized healthy seronegative humans: Evidence for persistent cell-mediated immunity. J AIDS. 1992;6:539–46.

157. Okuda K, Inami S, Kaneko T. Strong synergistic effects of polyvalent vaccine for human immunodeficiency virus (HIV-1) infection (Abstract PoA2425). VIIIth International Conference on AIDS/III STD World Congress, Amsterdam, July 1992.

158. Schwartz D, Clements ML, Belshe R, et al. Interim results of rgp160 vaccine trial in HIV+ volunteers (Abstract PO-A28-0668). IXth International Conference on AIDS/IVth STD World Congress, Berlin, June 1993.

159. Allan JD, Conant M, Lavelle J, et al. Safety and immunogenicity of MN and IIIB rgp120 HIV-1 vaccine in HIV-1 infected subjects with CD4 counts >500 cells/mm³ (Abstract PO-B27-2137). IXth International Conference on AIDS/IVth STD World Congress. Berlin, June 1993.

160. Chernoff D, Lang W, Sinangil F. Comparative safety and immunogenicity of yeast-derived, denatured nonglycosylated SF-2 gp120 (Env 2-3) vs CHO-derived conformationally intact glycosylated gp120 in HIV-1 seropositive subjects. Sixth Annual Meeting of the National Cooperative Vaccine Development Group, Alexandria, VA 1993.

SECTION P. MISCELLANEOUS SYNDROMES

107. CHRONIC FATIGUE SYNDROME

ROBERT T. SCHOOLEY

Over the past decade increasing attention has been paid to a patient population with a clinical syndrome consisting primarily of fatigue and cognitive dysfunction. Despite a number of attempts to define the syndrome on the basis of an etiologic agent, it has become increasingly clear that, despite a somewhat stereotypic presentation, it is unlikely that the majority of patients are suffering from infection with a single etiologic agent. Diagnosis is made primarily by exclusion, and management is largely supportive.

HISTORY

Patients with a syndrome of fatigue and malaise have been recognized in the medical literature for more than two centuries.[1–3] A clinical syndrome consisting of fatigue, palpitations, and breathlessness was further defined by DaCosta[4] in his description of severe exhaustion that often followed an acute bout of gastroenteritis among veterans of the Civil War. The syndrome received much attention in the military medical literature during the first half of the twentieth century before it gradually lost favor in the 1940s with the realization that it was unlikely to represent a discrete clinical entity. Since the demise of DaCosta's syndrome as a discrete clinical entity, a number of authors have described series of patients who are virtually indistinguishable from those described by DaCosta except that the intellectual focus has been on a parade of putative etiologic agents rather than on the clinical features of the syndrome. These authors have described patient populations with overlapping clinical features in which a wide variety of infectious agents have been postulated to be etiologically involved. These agents have included *Brucella*,[5] *Candida albicans*,[6,7] Epstein-Barr virus,[8,9] *Borrelia burgdorferi*, and human herpesvirus-6[10–12] and share the general properties of being widespread in the human population with somewhat amorphous clinical manifestations. Analysis of most of these reports indicates that the authors have either failed to recognize the ubiquitous nature of the putative pathogens or have failed to study appropriate control populations. In addition to these reports in which the focus has been on a discrete infectious entity, a number of metabolic or environmental factors have also been postulated as playing a role in the pathogenesis of similar clinical syndromes.[13–17] These factors frequently reflect a particular interest or orientation of the health care provider and have not achieved widespread acceptance as a cause of the illness.

EPIDEMIOLOGY AND CASE DEFINITION

In an effort to define the syndrome better, the Centers for Disease Control and Prevention (CDC) convened an expert panel to develop a case definition for the chronic fatigue syndrome (Table 1).[18] The case definition was subsequently modified to exclude fewer individuals with antecedent psychiatric illnesses and to require stratification of individuals with additional confounding conditions.[19] The case definition includes a constellation of symptoms and signs frequently included in individual

reports of the syndrome. The definition has its greatest utility in epidemiologic studies or in studies of the etiology or therapy of the syndrome. This case definition was applied in a surveillance system initiated by the CDC in 1989 and found to apply to 26 percent of patients referred to the CDC for chronic fatigue.[20] An additional 15 percent of patients met the major but not the minor criteria. The remaining patients were felt to have other chronic medical or psychological problems that could be associated with chronic fatigue. The case definition is much less useful in attempting to make a diagnosis in individual patients or in making disability determinations, since it lacks a severity scale. The epidemiologic definition is useful mainly as a general frame of reference, but it should not be used as a rigid checklist with which to rule the syndrome in or out in an individual patient. The diagnosis remains one of exclusion when other specific causes of chronic fatigue and malaise are eliminated.

Fatigue is a very common complaint in outpatient general medical settings. In a study performed in the general medical clinics of the Brigham and Women's Hospital, 23 percent of patients seen for any reason complained of fatigue. It is estimated that there are roughly 6 million office visits per year in the

TABLE 1. CDC Consensus Definition for the Chronic Fatigue Syndrome[a]

Major criteria
1. New onset of persistent or relapsing, debilitating fatigue or easy fatigability in a person who has no previous history of similar symptoms, that does not resolve with bedrest, and that is severe enough to reduce or impair average daily activity below 50 percent of the patient's premorbid activity level for a period of at least 6 months
2. Other clinical conditions that may produce similar symptoms must be excluded by thorough evaluation based on history, physical examination, and appropriate laboratory findings

Minor criteria
  Symptom criteria
  1. Mild fever (oral temperature between 37.5 and 38.6°C, if measured by the patient) or chills
  2. Sore throat
  3. Painful lymph nodes in the anterior or posterior cervical or axillary distribution
  4. Unexplained generalized muscle weakness
  5. Muscle discomfort or myalgia
  6. Prolonged generalized fatigue after levels of exercise that would have been easily tolerated in the patient's premorbid state
  7. Generalized headaches
  8. Migratory arthralgia without joint swelling or redness
  9. Neuropsychologic complaints including
     a. Photophobia
     b. Transient visual scotomata
     c. Foregetfulness
     d. Excessive irritability
     e. Confusion
     f. Difficulty thinking
     g. Inability to concentrate
     h. Depression
  10. Sleep disturbance (hypersomnia or insomnia)
  11. Description of the initial symptom complex as initially developing over a period of a few hours to a few days
  Physical criteria
  1. Low grade fever (oral temperature between 37.6 and 38.6°C or rectal temperature between 37.8 and 38.8°C)
  2. Nonexudatuve pharyngitis
  3. Palpable or tender anterior or posterior cervical or axillary lymph nodes. (Note: lymph nodes greater than 2 cm in diameter suggest other causes.)

[a] In order to make the diagnosis of chronic fatigue syndrome, both of the major criteria must be present. In addition, patients must exhibit at least 6 of the 11 symptom criteria and at least 2 of the 3 physical criteria; or 8 or more of the symptom criteria.

(Modified from Holmes et al.,[18] with permission.)

United States for chronic fatigue syndrome.[21] Chronic fatigue syndrome has been reported throughout the world, although the incidence and prevalence vary from study to study and from country to country.[22–31] These differences are more likely due to cultural differences and/or to differences in case definitions and case finding methodologies rather than to differences in distribution of one or more putative etiologic agents. In most reports of chronic fatigue syndrome, patients are primarily between the ages of 20 and 45 and are more frequently women than men.[8,9] Cases may appear sporadically without any clear epidemiologic association,[8,9] or they may appear in temporally and geographically defined clusters.[28,32] It is not clear that there are any specific clinical, epidemiologic, or demographic features that distinguish sporadic and ''epidemic'' clusters of chronic fatigue syndrome.

PRESENTATION AND CLINICAL MANIFESTATIONS

About half of the patients with chronic fatigue syndrome note a discrete flulike illness as the initiating event in the process. Whether or not an initiating event can be identified, most patients note the onset of malaise and fatigue in which the most distinctive features are its waxing and waning nature and the association with mild cognitive deficits.[8,9] The medical history is the most important aspect of the initial evaluation of individuals presenting with chronic fatigue. Details related to travel, occupational and animal exposure, and HIV-1 risk should be especially carefully ascertained. In most cases, the past medical history will be unremarkable, although a greater proportion of individuals with chronic fatigue syndrome will have a past history suggestive of atopy than might be expected in the general population.[21] Some individuals will have a past history suggestive of histrionic behavior and/or of multiple undiagnosed ''viral'' illnesses. Although such a history has been viewed by some practitioners as being exclusionary, the frequency of such findings in both the general population and in individuals with chronic fatigue syndrome should not lead one to discount the diagnosis. In addition, evidence of preexisting or concurrent affective disorders should be sought. If disorders of sleep patterns or of bowel habits suggestive of depression are noted, psychiatric consultation and use of antidepressant medications may be indicated (see below).

The physical examination is most useful if it is abnormal; in this situation, an abnormal physical finding should steer the thought process toward an alternative diagnosis. Although fever, pharyngitis, and lymphadenopathy are often cited as being extremely prominent features of the syndrome by patients, one of the hallmarks of the syndrome is the absence or minimal degree of such signs on physical examination. In fact, if a temperature of more than 100.4°C, or a bona fide localized or generalized adenopathy is encountered, it is much more likely that another process is responsible for the observed signs. In that case, the differential diagnosis of chronic fatigue syndrome should be expanded to include entities associated with fever of unknown origin. Patients being evaluated for chronic fatigue should also be examined for evidence of HIV-1 infection, such as oral thrush or hairy leukoplakia, and for the presence of rheumatologic or thyroid disorders. In the vast majority of cases, the physical examination will be normal.

LABORATORY FINDINGS

There are no specific laboratory tests that establish or support the diagnosis of chronic fatigue syndrome, and the laboratory should be used sparingly in the evaluation of individuals presenting with fatigue. Laboratory studies should be used primarily to investigate specific diagnostic possibilities raised by the history and physical examination. In most situations, patients with fatigue will have been seen by several health care providers before they are referred to infectious disease specialists for con-

TABLE 2. Core Laboratory Evaluation of Patients with Chronic Fatigue

Complete blood cell count with differential
Erythrocyte sedimentation rate
Serum hepatic aminotransferses
PPD
ELISA for HIV-1 (if suggested by history or physical examination)
Thyroid function studies
Serologic evaluation for primary EBV or CMV infection (if atypical lymphocytes are noted or if hepatic transaminases are elevated)
Serologic studies for hepatitis A, B, or C infection (if hepatic transaminases are elevated)

sultation (Table 2). In these situations, routine laboratory studies will have been performed one or more times in the past, and it will not be necessary to repeat the laboratory studies. In most cases it is prudent to obtain a complete blood count with a differential and an erythrocyte sedimentation rate. If an atypical lymphocytosis is detected, serologic studies for primary cytomegalovirus (CMV) and Epstein-Barr virus (EBV) infection should be performed (see Chs. 117 and 118). Liver and thyroid function should be evaluated in most cases. If elevations in hepatic transaminases are detected, serologic studies for hepatitis A, B, and C should be considered. If there is a history of possible sexual or parenteral exposure to HIV-1, an ELISA for HIV-1 should be performed. In most patients, a purified protein derivative (PPD) should be placed. If there are no unusual clinical or epidemiologic features in an individual case, and if the laboratory studies mentioned above are normal, it is usually not necessary to perform additional laboratory studies. In particular, EBV, CMV, *Borrelia burgdorferi,* and unfocused serologic studies for other infectious agents are seldom indicated outside the context of research studies. In addition, skin testing for hypersensitivity to common environmental agents and extensive studies of cellular and humoral immunologic function are rarely warranted. There is no justification for the routine use of broad panels of laboratory studies in the evaluation of most patients with chronic fatigue.

ETIOLOGY AND PATHOGENESIS

The etiology(ies) and pathogenesis of chronic fatigue syndrome remain unclear. As noted above, multiple infectious agents have been put forward from time to time as potential etiologic agents for chronic fatigue syndrome (Table 3). Each of these agents has passed in and out of favor over the past decade with differing periods and degrees of support. In most cases, an initial association between an infectious agent or a pathophysiologic hypothesis and chronic fatigue syndrome is made on the basis of an uncontrolled or a poorly controlled study, and, over the next 1–2 years, the agent or pathogenic theory receives much publicity in the lay press. As additional controlled data are obtained and/or as therapeutic trials fail to support the initial hypothesis, one theory may be supplanted by another in the achievement of popularity in the lay press. At present there are insufficient data to affix a specific etiology to all, or even most, cases of chronic fatigue syndrome.

The symptoms of chronic fatigue syndrome are similar to those experienced during recovery from viral infections such as infectious mononucleosis or influenza or in the setting of therapy with cytokines such as interferon or interleukin-2. Therefore, it has been speculated that some or all of the symptoms are reflective of an overproduction of one or more cytokines that can be triggered by a specific infectious agent. An alternative hypothesis is that any of a number of infectious agents might establish a regulatory imbalance of cytokines and that the symptoms of chronic fatigue syndrome reflect an inability of the host to reestablish the appropriate balance of cytokines. These theories have been further supported by an array of reports of immune deficiency observed in association with chronic fatigue syndrome.[33] These abnormalities, which include defects in cyto-

TABLE 3. Proposed Etiologies for Chronic Fatigue Syndrome

Etiology	References
Neuropsychiatric	
Neurasthenia	3, 34, 35
Cardiac	
DaCosta Syndrome	4
Endocrinological	
Hypoglycemia	13
Neuroendocrine axis disturbance	35
Rheumatologic	
Fibromyalgia/fibrositis	36
Environmental	
Total allergy syndrome	14–16
Mercury based dental fillings	17
Infectious Agents	
Brucella	5
Epstein-Barr virus	25, 26
Human herpesvirus-6	10, 12, 37
Candida albicans	6, 7
Borrelia burgdorferi	38
HTLV-II	39, 40
Human spumavirus	41
Enteroviruses	42, 43

kine elaboration after stimulation with mitogens and antigens, defects in natural killer cell activity, and imbalances in lymphocyte surface phenotypic markers,[11,33,44] have led some to propose that chronic fatigue syndrome be renamed the *chronic fatigue and immunodeficiency syndrome* (CFIDS). In virtually all of these reports, there is considerable overlap between the findings in patients with chronic fatigue syndrome and those in matched control donors; and it is not clear that the magnitude of any of the immunologic abnormalities correlates either with the clinical severity or the clinical course of the disease. Thus, as in the case of serologic surveys for multiple infectious agents, sophisticated surface phenotypic or functional immunologic assays are rarely warranted outside the setting of research trials.

Recently, increasing interest has focused on the concept that, in some patients, the symptomatology of chronic fatigue syndrome is a reflection of abnormalities in the neuroendocrine axis.[45] In a series of well-controlled studies, patients with chronic fatigue syndrome were demonstrated to have reduced basal evening levels of glucocorticoids, and decreased 24-hour urinary cortisol excretion. Patients with chronic fatigue syndrome also exhibited increased sensitivity to exogenous ACTH. The significance of these findings in terms of pathogenesis is, as yet, uncertain, but the similarity of many of the symptoms of chronic fatigue syndrome to those of adrenal insufficiency render the findings highly provocative. In addition to the abnormalities in the neuroendocrine axis, chronic fatigue syndrome patients exhibit abnormalities in monoamine metabolism with a decrease in basal plasma levels of 3-methoxy-4-hydroxyphenylglycol and an increase in the basal plasma level of 5-hydroxyindoleacetic acid.[46] As in the case of the neuroendocrine abnormalities cited above, the significance of these findings is not yet certain, but they do support the concept that identifiable metabolic abnormalities are present in some patients with chronic fatigue syndrome.

MANAGEMENT

Support

Once other diagnostic entities have been excluded, management is, at present, largely supportive. The major aspect of this support rests with reassuring the patient about three issues: (1) other serious medical problems have been excluded; (2) even though the etiology of the pathogenesis has not yet been delineated, the fatigue and the malaise experienced by the patient are real; and (3) in most cases the illness follows a waxing and waning course, but gradually subsides. Much of the difficulty with the syndrome from the point of view of patients rests on the lack of diagnostic historical features and physical or laboratory findings. This, along with the absence of a defined medical or surgical therapeutic approach, leaves patients with the perception that the illness is purely psychological. Because it is not infrequent that patients with chronic fatigue syndrome have a history suggestive of concurrent or preexisting affective disorder, psychiatric consultation is often helpful. Patients with chronic fatigue syndrome are often highly resistant to psychiatric referral; referral can be facilitated if it is presented as an attempt to enlist additional help in forming a diagnostic and therapeutic team for a physiologic illness rather than as a statement that chronic fatigue syndrome is primarily a psychiatric illness.

Activity

Patients should be encouraged to continue to function at activity levels that are tolerable within the limits of their fatigue. In that symptomatology waxes and wanes, there will be periods during which activity is more easily maintained than others. Individuals should be encouraged to be physically and mentally active when the disease permits, but to decrease activity when symptoms flare. There is little objective evidence that forced rest or that gentle exercise exacerbates or ameliorates the illness. Because the illness runs a variable course, patients should be cautioned about ascribing cause and effect relationships between events, diet, or activities and disease manifestations. Prior to the onset of the illness, many patients will have been in high-pressure employment or family situations. In most cases, such situations are incompatible with recommendations to modulate activity based on symptoms. Thus, assistance should be provided to patients to arrange modifications of employment that allow increased flexibility. In some situations this can be arranged without a change in employers. In others, a more profound change in a work situation is required. Disability should be used only as a last resort. Loss of employment is itself often extremely psychologically debilitating to individuals with high premorbid career aspirations. Disability insurers find chronic fatigue syndrome an extremely challenging syndrome in that there are no specific diagnostic tests or reliable severity scales with which to classify the syndrome. As noted previously, the CDC case definition should not be used to make disability determinations. In most cases, a narrative report, coupled with a psychiatric evaluation, is much more useful than a plethora of normal laboratory findings.

Pharmacologic Therapy

Many therapeutic approaches have been recommended. These range from drugs suggested by putative etiologic agents such as acyclovir,[47] nystatin,[48] or intravenous immunoglobulin[49,50,51] to the more imaginative treatment programs suggested by "clinical ecologists"[14–16,52] and by dentists who advocate replacement of dental fillings containing mercury amalgams.[17] Support for the use of any of these approaches on the basis of well-controlled, blinded, clinical trials is difficult to obtain. In the case of acyclovir and nystatin, well-controlled trials have clearly demonstrated a lack of efficacy.[47,48] Although one trial suggested benefits from intravenous immunoglobulin,[51] two additional trials[49,50] have failed to show benefit, and the use of intravenous immunoglobulin is accompanied by significant morbidity and expense. Thus its use is not recommended. Evaluation of therapeutic interventions is complicated by the subjective nature of the symptoms, the waxing and waning course of the illness, and, often, the commercial implications of successful therapy for the provider. Thus, patients should be cautioned about testimonials given by former patients on behalf of specific therapies or providers.

Many patients, particularly those in whom myalgias and arthralgias are prominent features of the clinical syndrome, benefit from nonsteroidal anti-inflammatory agents. The agent chosen and the dose used should be individualized for each patient. Antidepressants are beneficial to some patients. No single drug in this class is clearly superior to others, and it is often necessary to try several in sequence before the best drug for a given patient is identified. Patients to receive antidepressant medication should be carefully selected, and management is often facilitated by the involvement of a psychiatrist who is facile with both chronic fatigue syndrome and affective disorders. Patients with chronic fatigue syndrome often experience adverse subjective symptoms from psychoactive agents at unexpectedly low doses, and these reactions should be anticipated if such agents are used. As in the case of the initial psychiatric referral, many patients are resistant to the suggestion that psychoactive drugs might be beneficial. Their use may be accepted if patients understand that medications are being used to treat the symptoms of a physiologic process rather than as drugs to treat a primarily mental illness.

SUMMARY

Over the next several years, the understanding of chronic fatigue syndrome will likely continue to sharpen as diagnostic criteria are refined and as additional hypothesis-driven research is undertaken. In the meantime, it seems most appropriate to view the syndrome as a clinical entity with a collection of possible infectious and noninfectious etiologies. It is unlikely that a single infectious agent will be identified that will account for all, or even most, cases. Most patients can be managed by an internist or family practitioner without the need for ongoing intervention by an infectious disease specialist. Reassurance that the symptoms are real and that the illness is not reflective of an undiagnosed underlying problem is much more important than an extensive array of laboratory studies. The use of expensive pharmacologic or immunologic therapy should be discouraged. With supportive treatment, many patients recover without sequelae.

REFERENCES

1. Straus SE. History of the chronic fatigue syndrome. Rev Infect Dis. 1991;13: S2–7.
2. Manningham R. The Symptoms, Nature, Causes and Cure of the Febricula or Little Fever: Commonly Called the Nervous or Hysteric Fever; the Fever on the Spirits; Vapours, Hypo, or Spleen. 2nd ed. London: J. Robinson; 1750: 52–3.
3. Beard G. Neurasthenia, or nervous exhaustion. Boston Med Surgical J. 1869; 3(new series):217–20.
4. DaCosta JM. On irritable heart: A clinical study of a form of functional cardiac disorder and its consequence. Am J Med Sci. 1871;121:17–52.
5. Evans AC. Brucellosis in the United States. Am J Public Health. 1947;37: 139–51.
6. Truss CO. The role of Candida albicans in human illness. J Orthomol Psychiatry. 1981;10:228–38.
7. Crook WG. The Yeast Connection: A Medical Breakthrough. 3rd ed. Jackson, TN: Professional Books, 1983.
8. Jones JF, Ray CG, Minnich LL, et al. Evidence for reactive Epstein-Barr virus infection in patients with persistent, unexplained illnesses: Elevated anti-early antigen antibodies. Ann Intern Med. 1985;102:7–16.
9. Straus SE, Tosato G, Armstrong G, et al. Persisting illness and fatigue in adults with evidence of Epstein-Barr infection. Ann Intern Med. 1985;102: 7–16.
10. Daugherty SA, Henry BE, Peterson DL, et al. Chronic fatigue syndrome in northern Nevada. Rev Infect Dis. 1991;13(Suppl 1):S39–44.
11. Landay AL, Jessop C, Lennette ET, et al. Chronic fatigue syndrome: Clinical condition associated with immune activation. Lancet. 1991;338:707–12.
12. Buchwald D, Cheney PR, Peterson DL, et al. A chronic illness characterized by fatigue, neurologic and immunologic disorders, and active herpesvirus type 6 infection. Ann Intern Med. 1992;116:103–13.
13. Yager J, Young RT. Non-hypoglycemia is an epidemic condition. N Engl J Med. 1974;291:907–8.
14. Stewart DE, Raskin J. Psychiatric assessment of patients with "20th century disease" ("total allergy syndrome"). Can Med Assoc J. 1985;133:1001–6.
15. Bell IR, King DS. Psychological and physiological research relevant to clinical ecology. Overview of current literature. Clin Ecol. 1962;1:15–25.
16. Brodsky CM. "Allergic to everything"—a medical subculture. Psychosomatics. 1983;24:731–42.
17. Ziff S. Silver Dental Fillings: The Toxic Time Bomb. New York: Amora Press; 1984.
18. Holmes GP, Kaplan JE, Gantz NM, et al. Chronic fatigue syndrome: A working case definition. Ann Intern Med. 1988;108:387–9.
19. Schluederberg A, Straus SE, Peterson P, et al. Chronic fatigue syndrome research: Definition and medical outcome assessment. Ann Intern Med. 1992; 117:325–31.
20. Klonoff DC. Chronic fatigue syndrome. Clin Infect Dis. 1992;15:812–23.
21. Nelson C, McLemore T. The National Ambulatory Medical Care Survey: United States, 1975–81 and 1985 Trends. DHHS publication No. (PHS) 88-1754. Vital and Health Statistics, Series 13, No. 93. Hyattsville, MD: National Center for Health Statistics; 1988.
22. Behan PO, Behan WMH, Bell EJ. The postviral fatigue syndrome—an analysis of the findings in 50 cases. J Infect. 1985;10:211–22.
23. Ho-Yen DO, McNamara I. The epidemiology of post viral fatigue syndrome. Scott Med J. 1988;33:368–9.
24. Lloyd AR, Hickie I, Boughton CR, et al. Prevalence of chronic fatigue syndrome in an Australian population. Med J Aust. 1990;153:522–8.
25. Murdoch JC. Myalgic encephalomyelitis (ME) syndrome—an analysis of the clinical findings in 200 cases. NZ Fam Physician. 1987;14:51–4.
26. Ho-Yen DO, McNamara I. General practitioners' experience of the chronic fatigue syndrome. Br J Gen Pract. 1991;41:324–6.
27. Tobi M, Morag A, Ravid Z, et al. Prolonged atypical illness associated with serological evidence of persistent Epstein-Barr virus infection. Lancet. 1982; 1:61–4.
28. Holmes GP, Kaplan JE, Stewart JA, et al. A cluster of patients with a chronic mononucleosis-like syndrome: Is Epstein-Barr virus the cause? JAMA. 1987; 257:2297–302.
29. Sharpe MC, Archard LC, Banatvala JE, et al. A report—Chronic fatigue syndrome: Guidelines for research. J R Soc Med. 1991;84:118–21.
30. van Greure CH, Bouic PJ. Aberrant in vitro HLA-DR expression in patients with chronic fatigue. S Afr Med J. 1990;78:219–20.
31. Lloyd AR, Wakefield D, Boughton C, et al. What is myalgic encephalomyelitis? (Letter). Lancet. 1988;1:1286–7.
32. Bell KM, Cookfair D, Bell DS, Reese P, Cooper L. Risk factors associated with chronic fatigue syndrome in a cluster of pediatric cases. Rev Infect Dis. 1991;13:S32–8.
33. Jones JF. Serologic and immunologic responses in chronic fatigue syndrome with emphasis on the Epstein-Barr virus. Rev Infect Dis. 1991;13(Suppl 1): S26–31.
34. Acheson ED. The clinical syndrome variously called benign myalgic encephalomyelitis, Iceland disease and epidemic neuromyasthenia. Am J Med. 1959; 26:569–95.
35. Henderson DA, Shelokov A. Epidemic neuromyasthenia—clinical syndrome? N Engl J Med. 1959;260:757–64, 814–8.
36. Yunus MB. Diagnosis, etiology, and management of fibromyalgia syndrome: An update. Comprehens Ther 1988;14:8–20.
37. Gold D, Bowden R, Sixbey J, et al. Chronic fatigue: A prospective clinical and virologic study. JAMA. 1990;264:48–53.
38. Krupp LB, Mendelson WB, Friedman R. An overview of chronic fatigue syndrome. J Clin Psychiatry. 1991;52:403–10.
39. DeFreitas E, Hilliard B, Cheney PR, et al. Retroviral sequences related to human T-lymphotropic virus type II in patients with chronic fatigue immune dysfunction syndrome. Proc Natl Acad Sci USA. 1991;88:2922–6.
40. Palca J. Does a retrovirus explain fatigue syndrome puzzle? Science. 1990; 249:1240–1.
41. Martin WJ. Chronic fatigue syndrome (Letter). Science 1992;255:663.
42. Gow JW, Behan WM, Clements GB, et al. Enteroviral RNA sequences detected by polymerase chain reaction in muscle of patients with postviral fatigue syndrome. Br Med J. 1991;302:692–6.
43. Cunningham L, Bowles NE, Lane RJM, et al. Persistence of enteroviral RNA in chronic fatigue syndrome is associated with the abnormal production of equal amounts of positive and negative strands of enteroviral RNA. J Gen Virol. 1990;71:399–402.
44. Buchwald D, Komaroff AL. Review of laboratory findings for patients with chronic fatigue syndrome. Rev Infect Dis. 1991;13:S12–8.
45. Demitrack MA, Dale JK, Straus SE, et al. Evidence for impaired activation of the hypothalamic-pituitary-adrenal axis in patients with chronic fatigue syndrome. J Clin Endocrinol Metab. 1991;73:1224–34.
46. Demitrack MA, Gold PW, Dale JK, et al. Plasma and cerebrospinal fluid monoamine metabolism in patients with chronic fatigue syndrome: Preliminary findings. Biol Psychiatry. 1992;32:1065–77.
47. Straus SE, Dale JK, Tobi M, et al. Acyclovir treatment of the chronic fatigue syndrome: Lack of efficacy in a placebo-controlled trial. N Engl J Med. 1988; 319:1692–8.
48. Dismukes WE, Wade JS, Lee JY, et al. A randomized, double-blind trial of nystatin therapy for the candidiasis hypersensitivity syndrome. N Engl J Med. 1990;323:1717–23.
49. Peterson PK, Shepard J, Macres M, et al. A controlled trial of intravenous immunoglobulin G in chronic fatigue syndrome. Am J Med. 1990;89:554–60.
50. Lloyd A, Hickie I, Wakefield D, et al. A double-blind, placebo-controlled trial of intravenous immunoglobulin therapy in patients with chronic fatigue syndrome. Am J Med. 1990;89:561–8.

51. Lloyd AR, Hickie C, Wakefield D. Immunologic and psychologic therapy for patients with chronic fatigue syndrome: A double-blind, placebo-controlled trial. Am J Med. 1993;94:197–203.
52. American Academy of Allergy: Provocative and neutralization testing. J Allergy Clin Immunol. 1981;67:336–8.

108. CAT SCRATCH DISEASE

GERALD W. FISCHER

Cat scratch disease (CSD) is a syndrome that is typified by regional lymphadenopathy after a cat scratch or bite distal to the involved lymph node. In addition, many patients have atypical presentations other than regional adenopathy. In 1889, Parinaud[1] described cases of oculoglandular fever associated with conjunctivitis, enlargement of regional lymph nodes, and low-grade fever that persisted for weeks. He believed that the disease was contracted from animals and may have described the first cases of CSD. Although tularemia had been associated with Parinaud's oculoglandular syndrome, it became clear that there were other causes as well and that CSD was a common cause of this syndrome.[2] In the early 1930s, Dr. Robert Debré in Paris began to recognize an illness with regional lymphadenopathy that occurred after patients were scratched by cats.[3] Shortly thereafter, Dr. Frank Hanger and Dr. Harry Rose, using aspirated pus from a patient with suppurative CSD adenitis, prepared a skin test antigen that gave positive intradermal reactions in patients with CSD. The first reports on CSD were published in the 1950s,[3,4] and by the early 1980s CSD had become a well-described entity, with over 700 articles published by investigators around the world.[5]

EPIDEMIOLOGY

Cat scratch disease occurs worldwide, and in temperate climates it is seasonal, with most cases occurring between August and January. While most of the reported patients are less than 21 years old, this may reflect a reporting bias from pediatricians. A review of cat owners in Connecticut demonstrated that 43 percent of CSD patients were more than 20 years of age, and 52 percent were females.[6] About 90 percent of patients have a history of exposure to cats, and a cat scratch or bite will have occurred in 75 percent of these individuals. Family outbreaks have been observed in households with cats.[7] Generally, the cases occur within a few weeks of each other, and the animal implicated is usually a kitten. This may suggest that the infectious agent is transmitted from cat to human for only a limited period of time. The mode of transmission is presumably direct contact, since the lymphadenopathy generally follows a scratch, bite, or lick from a young cat. Rarely, a dog, monkey, thorn, or other agent will be implicated in a CSD case. Cats show no clinical evidence of illness.

PATHOLOGY

The lymphatic system is primarily involved, and early in the course of infection lymph nodes show lymphoid hyperplasia. Later, scattered granulomas appear, and some may contain central areas of necrosis with rare multinucleated giant cells. As the process progresses, stellate areas of necrosis coalesce to form one or more abscesses. If the lymph node capsule ruptures, pus extends into the contiguous tissue and may be surrounded eventually by fibrosis. Since the histopathologic appearance of CSD may resemble that of other infections such as tularemia, lymphogranuloma venereum, and fungal and mycobacterial infections, the histopathology cannot be considered diagnostic for CSD. Warthin-Starry silver stain can be used to demonstrate the bacteria recently associated with CSD, but these bacteria may only be found early in the course of infection.

ETIOLOGY

The causative agent of CSD has been controversial. However, substantial evidence points to *Rochalimaea henselae* as a major cause of cat scratch disease. Although it has been proposed that the genus *Rochalimaea* be transferred to the genus *Bartonella* (see Ch. 170), the name *Rochalimaea* will be retained here. Using IFA, antibody to *R. henselae* has been found in 84 percent of 60 Connecticut patients with suspected CSD compared with 3.6 percent of healthy controls.[6] In that study, cats from case households had higher prevalence of antibodies to *Rochalimaea* (81 percent) than cats from other households (46 percent). Of 41 patients with suspected CSD, 88 percent had an IFA antibody titer of at least 1:64.[7] In 24 patients from Hawaii with CSD, 23 (96 percent) had IFA titers to *R. henselae* of at least 1:64 whereas none of 18 controls had titers exceeding 1:16.[7a] ELISA antibodies are under development and appear to support the results of IFA.[8,9] The organism has been found in lymph nodes of patients with cat scratch disease by culture,[10] PCR amplification of DNA,[10a] and immunocytochemical labeling.[10b] *Rochalimaea henselae* has been cultured from the blood of young cats that have been implicated in transmitting either cat scratch disease[7a,11] or bacillary angiomatosis.[11b] Bacteremia appears to be chronic in young cats and not associated with obvious illness.[11b] DNA of *R. henselae* has been detected by PCR in five of five lots of CSD skin test antigen in one study[12] and in two of two lots in another study.[13] Appearance of the organism on Warthin-Starry stain is consistent with *Rochalimaea* spp. although the stain is not specific.

Patients with CSD may have other manifestations that also occur with *R. henselae* infection, including hepatic[14] and bone[15] infections. Syndromes due to *Rochalimaea* spp. other than CSD, such as cutaneous bacillary angiomatosis, bacillary peliosis, and septicemia, are described in Chapter 170.

Isolation of *Afipea felis* from CSD lesions prompted initial interest in this organism as the major cause of the syndrome.[16,17] A patient with presumed CSD meningoencephalitis was said to have seroconverted to *A. felis* and not to *R. henselae*.[18] The current evidence suggests that *A. felis* causes few, if any, cases of CSD. However, because CSD is a syndrome, it is possible that more than one agent could produce the clinical findings.

CLINICAL MANIFESTATIONS

Chronic regional lymphadenopathy is the most common clinical feature of CSD and usually develops about 2 weeks after the scratch or contact (Table 1). In spite of having impressive lym-

TABLE 1. Clinical Features of CSD in 908 Patients

Signs and Symptoms	Percentage	Average Duration	Range
Adenopathy	>90	3 M	0.5–12 M
Adenopathy alone	52	3 M	0.5–12 M
Inoculation site	59–93[a]	7 D	7–240 D
Fever (>38.3°C)	32–60[a]	6 D	1–60 D
Malaise, fatigue	29	13 D	1–210 D
Headache	13	4 D	1–7 D
Anorexia, weight loss, emesis	14	5 D	3–30 D
Splenomegaly	12	11 D	7–300 D
Sore throat	9	2 D	1–5 D
Rash	5	9 D	5–14 D
Parotid swelling	2	—	7–28 D
Conjunctivitis	4.5	—	1–11 D

Abbreviations: M: months; D: days.
[a] Includes data from Carithers.[22]

(Data from Moriarty and Margileth.[23])

phadenopathy, the patient usually appears well. An inoculation site (a scratch, a primary lesion, or both) may be detected in over two-thirds of patients when actively sought. About 3–10 days will elapse from the time of the scratch or cat contact until primary skin papule or pustule forms. Most primary lesions persist for about 1–3 weeks. Low-grade fever lasting for several days occurs in about 30 percent of patients. Malaise or fatigue are noted in about 25 percent and headache and sore throat in about 10 percent of patients.

Whether or not there is a local cutaneous lesion, lymphadenitis becomes the major manifestation of CSD. The enlarged, tender lymph nodes are most commonly found in the head or neck area. The axillary nodes are frequently involved; less commonly, the epitrochlear, inguinal, femoral, and, rarely, supraclavicular nodes may be enlarged (Fig. 1). Single-node involvement occurs in almost half of the patients, involvement of multiple nodes in the same site occurs in about 20 percent. About one-third of patients have lymphadenopathy involving several sites. Node enlargement usually persists for 2–4 months but has been known to last for up to 2 years. Suppuration of the involved node occurs in about 10 percent of patients. Transient exanthemata (maculopapular, petechial, or erythema multiforme or nodosum) have been observed in CSD patients, usually lasting for less than 2 weeks.

Atypical manifestations of CSD may also be seen (Table 2). The oculoglandular syndrome of Parinaud presents as an ocular granuloma or conjunctivitis with preauricular lymphadenopathy. Most patients are only mildly ill and recover without any residua. Encephalitis or encephalopathy and, rarely, radiculitis or neuroretinitis are more serious forms of CSD.[19–21] Children with central nervous system involvement with CSD usually experience sudden onset of neurologic symptoms, often accompanied by fever; this usually occurs within 1–6 weeks of the onset of lymphadenopathy. Recovery may be rapid, although severe

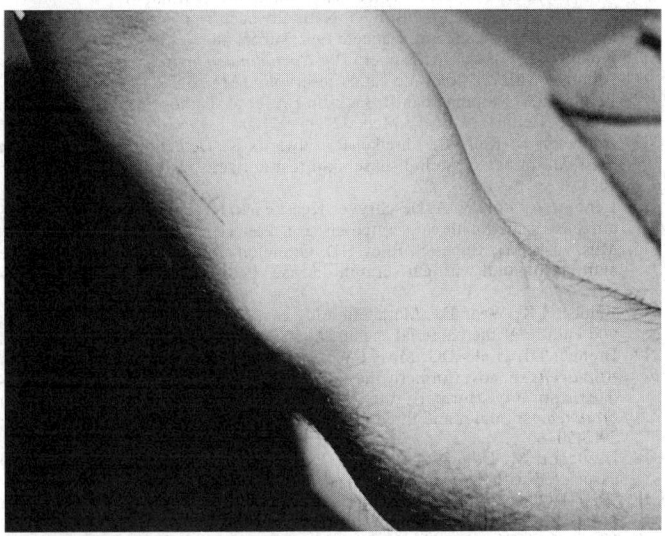

FIG. 1. Epitrochlear lymphadenitis due to CSD.

TABLE 2. Atypical Manifestations of CSD Seen in 1250 Patients

	Percent	Duration[a]
Unusual manifestations	11.6	—
Oculoglandular disease	6	3–28 weeks
Encephalopathy	2	7–240 days
Severe, chronic, systemic disease	2	3–21 months
Arthralgias/arthritis	<1	4–84 days
Erythema nodosum	<1	3–42 days

[a] Based on 423 patients from 1984 to 1986.

(Adapted from Moriarty and Margileth,[23] with permission.)

manifestations with coma or seizures may last for several weeks, with gradual complete recovery generally occurring in 1–6 months. The spinal fluid is usually normal, but there may be minimal pleocytosis or elevation of protein. Electroencephalograms show diffuse slowing or focal abnormalities in most patients.

Three previously healthy children, aged 3, 8, and 10 years, were described as having hepatic granuloma due to CSD.[14] Illness presented as fever of at least 39°C for more than 3 weeks. Ultrasound or computed tomography showed multiple hepatic nodules, which on biopsy were fibrotic areas containing multiple discrete granulomata. Bacilli were seen in the liver of two patients and in an axillary lymph node of the third, who had typical CSD in that location. No liver function abnormalities or hepatomegaly was detected. All three patients recovered without sequelae.

A bone lesion consistent with bacterial osteomyelitis may occur in children.[15] Biopsy may reveal granulomas, and silver stains may be helpful to identify the small bacilli. An elevated sedimentation rate and a positive bone scan make osteitis due to CSD difficult to differentiate clinically from pyogenic osteomyelitis. While history of cat exposure and scratches may suggest a diagnosis of CSD, it is imperative to consider the possibility of other causes of osteomyelitis.

DIAGNOSIS

The diagnosis of CSD is suggested by regional lymphadenopathy that develops slowly over 2–3 weeks in a patient with cat contact and/or scratches. The presence of a primary inoculation papule or pustule at the scratch site strengthens the diagnosis. Other causes of lymphadenopathy must be considered and ruled out.

It is likely, however, that CSD has other presentations, and many individuals may be asymptomatic or have very mild clinical illness.[6] Historically the diagnosis of a typical CSD case required fulfillment of three of four criteria, whereas all four were necessary in an atypical case, including (1) a history of animal (usually dog or cat) contact, with the presence of a scratch or a primary dermal or eye lesion; (2) aspiration of sterile pus from the node (a presumptive diagnostic test) or culture and laboratory data that exclude other etiologic possibilities; (3) a positive CSD skin test; and (4) a node biopsy revealing histopathology consistent with CSD. However, now that the usual etiologic agent of CSD appears to be R. henselae, diagnosis more plausibly will depend upon serology or by culture of the agent from lymph node aspirate. Details of culture techniques are given in Chapter 170.

Tenderness of the node favors CSD or a bacterial adenopathy rather than a neoplasm. Acute lymphadenitis due to bacteria generally develops over 3–4 days. Sonography may be helpful to detect early suppuration of the bubo and to direct needle aspiration when indicated. Early in the disease, a total white blood cell count may show mild leukocytosis and an increased number of polymorphonuclear cells, with eosinophilia in 10–20 percent of patients. The sedimentation rate is usually elevated during the first few weeks.

The cat scratch antigen skin test is positive in 90 percent of patients who are clinically suspected of having CSD and who have had cat contact and/or scratches. However, the skin test only reflects previous exposure to the agent. A negative skin test often occurs if the patient has been ill for less than 3–4 weeks. About 5 percent of patients with typical CSD will have a negative CSD skin test. Since the reaction may persist for years, a positive test may not reflect concurrent disease. Positive reactions have been noted in veterinarians (12–29 percent), healthy persons (4–5 percent), and family contacts of CSD patients. Two negative skin tests at 4-week intervals suggest a disease other than CSD if the patient is not anergic.

The differential diagnosis of CSD includes many known causes of lymphadenopathy. In children and adolescents, lymphogranuloma venereum, syphilis, typical or atypical tuberculosis, other forms of bacterial adenitis, sporotrichosis, tularemia, brucellosis, histoplasmosis, sarcoidosis, toxoplasmosis, infectious mononucleosis, and benign or malignant tumors should be considered. If the patient has an ocular lesion and preauricular adenopathy, which would suggest the oculoglandular syndrome of Parinaud, CSD is the most common cause.[24,25]

SKIN TEST

The skin test used today is essentially unchanged from that described by Hanger and Rose. The antigen is made from pus aspirated from the patient's lymph node and is not commercially available. The purulent material is tested for sterility, diluted in saline, heated to 56°C for 72 hours, and then recultured to ensure sterility. A positive test is considered to be at least 5 mm of induration at 48–72 hours. Equivocal reactions can be biopsied to look for subcutaneous granulomas formation. Since there is no current method of assessing biologic activity, skin test antigen potency is difficult to standardize. Clinicians interested in CSD have assessed their preparation by skin testing patients with several antigen lots. Despite several decades of apparent safety, contemporary use of this antigen is of some concern. Potential transmission of infectious agents not killed by mild heating includes human immunodeficiency virus (HIV), hepatitis B, non-A, non-B hepatitis, and Kreutzfeldt-Jakob disease. Potential antigen donors should be generally well and tested serologically for HIV and hepatitis B. This antigen should be used only with all the procedures appropriate for an experimental biologic fluid, including approval by the local institutional review board. As methods for detection of *R. henselae* infection become more generally available, the CSD skin test is likely to be abandoned in order to avoid the potential hazard of occult viruses and the potential unreliability of an unstandardized test.

TREATMENT

Specific antimicrobial therapies for CSD have not been proven to be efficacious, despite the fact that *R. henselae* is sensitive in vitro to many common antibiotics. Controlled trials will be necessary to determine if antibiotics hasten resolution of lymphadenitis or clinical illness. The adenopathy is benign and will subside spontaneously within several months. Careful follow-up examination is important to reassess the size of the bubo and to reassure the patient that the node(s) are slowly receding. If suppuration occurs, aspiration should be considered to relieve the pain and hasten recovery. Needle aspiration is generally preferred to incision and drainage. After washing the skin with an iodophor skin cleanser, aspiration may be accomplished by inserting an 18- or 19-gauge needle tangentially through normal skin at the base of the node. Rarely, reaspiration may be necessary. Characteristically, CSD lymphadenitis is not responsive to antimicrobials, and they are not recommended at this time. However, in more severely ill patients, antibiotic therapy based on the antimicrobial susceptibility of *R. henselae* may be appropriate (see Ch. 170).

Application of moist soaks to the primary skin or eye lesion may effect drainage and shorten the duration of the adenopathy. Excisional biopsy of the ocular granuloma is rarely necessary. Excisional biopsy of the node may be necessary in selected patients, particularly adults, because of persistent pain or for diagnostic purposes.

PROGNOSIS

Complications and sequelae in typical cases are uncommon. One episode appears to confer lifelong immunity. Rarely, a recurrence of sinus track drainage from the nodes originally involved may occur. If the adenopathy is massive (>5 cm), chronic adenopathy may persist for 1–2 years.

REFERENCES

1. Parinaud H. Conjonctivite infectieuse transmise par les animaux. Ann Ocul. 1889;101:252–3.
2. Cassady JV, Culbertson CS. Cat-scratch disease and Parinaud's oculoglandular syndrome. Arch Ophthalmol. 1953;50:68–74.
3. Debré R, Lamy M, Jammet M, et al. La maladie des griffes de chat. Bull Mem Soc Med Hop (Paris). 1950;66:76–9.
4. Daniels WB, MacMurray FG. Cat scratch disease, report of one hundred sixty cases. JAMA. 1954;154:1247–51.
5. Wear DJ, Margileth AM, Hadfield TL, et al. Cat scratch disease: A bacterial infection. Science. 1983;221:1403–5.
6. Zangwill KM, Hamilton DH, Perkins BA, et al. Cat scratch disease in Connecticut: Epidemiology, risk factors, and evaluating of a new diagnostic test. N Engl J Med. 1993;329:8–12.
7. Regnery RL, Olson JG, Perkins BA, Bibb W. Serological response to *Rochalimaea henselae* antigen in suspected cat-scratch disease. Lancet. 1992;339:1443–5.
7a. Demers DM, Vincent JM, Bass JW, et al. Serologic evidence of *Rochalimaea henselae* (Rh) infection and cat scratch disease (CSD) in humans scratched by Rh bacteremic kittens. Pediatric Res. 1994;35(Abstract 1050):177A.
8. Barka NR, Hadfield T, Patnaik M, et al. EIA for detection of *Rochalimaea henselae*-reactive IgG, IgM, and IgA antibodies in patients with suspected cat scratch disease. J Infect Dis. 1993;167:1503–4.
9. Edwards KM, Goral S, Kelly CS, et al. Serologic studies in patients with cat scratch disease. In: Program and Abstracts of the 33rd Interscience Conference on Antimicrobial Agents and Chemotherapy, 1993. American Society for Microbiology, Washington, D.C., p. 454.
10. Dolan MJ, Wong MT, Regnery RL, et al. Syndrome of *Rochalimaea henselae* suggesting cat scratch disease. Ann Intern Med 1993;118:331–6.
10a. Anderson B, Sims K, Regnery T, et al. Detection of *Rochalimaea henselae* DNA in specimens from patients with cat-scratch disease by PCR. J Clin Microbiol. 1994;32:942–8.
10b. Min K-W, Reed JA, Welch DF, et al. Morphologically variable bacilli of cat scratch disease are identified by immunocytochemical labeling with antibodies to *Rochalimaea henselae*. Am J Clin Pathol. 1994;101:607–10.
11. Regnery RL, Martin M, Olson JG. Naturally occurring *Rochalimaea henselae* infection in domestic cat. Lancet. 1992;340:557–8.
11b. Koehler JE, Glaser CA, Tappero JW. *Rochalimaea henselae* infection. A new zoonosis with the domestic cat as reservoir. JAMA. 1994;271:531–5.
12. Perkins BA, Swaminathan B, Jackson LA, et al. Pathogenesis of cat scratch disease [Letter]. N Engl J Med. 327:1599–1600.
13. Anderson B, Kelly C, Threlkel R, Edwards K. Detection of *Rochalimaea henselae* in cat scratch disease skin test antigens. J Infect Dis. 1993;168:1034–6.
14. Lenoir AA, Storch GA, Deschryver-Kecskemeti K, et al. Granulomatous hepatitis associated with cat scratch disease. Lancet. 1988;1:1132–6.
15. Muszynski MJ, Eppes S, Riley HD. Granulomatous osteolytic lesion of the skull associated with cat scratch disease. Pediatr Infect Dis. 1987;6:199–201.
16. English CK, Wear DJ, Margileth AM, et al. Cat-scratch disease. Isolation and culture of the bacterial agent. JAMA. 1988;259:1347–52.
17. Brenner DJ, Hollis DG, Moss CW, et al. Proposal of *Afipia* gen. nov., with *Afipia felis* sp. nov. (formerly the cat scratch disease bacillus), *Afipia clevelandensis* sp. nov. (formerly the Cleveland Clinic Foundation strain), *Afipia broomeae* sp. nov., and three unnamed genospecies. J Clin Microbiol. 1991;29:2450–60.
18. Drancourt M, Donnet A, Pelletier J, Raoult D. Acute meningoencephalitis associated with seroconversion to *Afipia felis*. Lancet. 1992;340:558.
19. Tsao CY. Generalized tonic-clonic status epilepticus in a child with cat-scratch disease and encephalopathy. Clin Electroencephalogram. 1992;23:65–7.
20. Ulrich GG, Waecker NJ, Meister SJ, et al. Cat scratch disease associated with neuroretinitis in a 6 year old girl. Ophthalmology. 1992;99:346–9.
21. Revol A, Vighetto A, Jouvet A, et al. Encephalitis in cat scratch disease with persistent dementia. J Neurol Neurosurg Psychiatry. 1992;55:133–5.
22. Carithers HA. Cat-scratch disease: An overview base on a study of 1,200 patients. Am J Dis Child. 1985;139:1124–33.
23. Moriarty RA, Margileth AM. Cat scratch disease. Infect Dis Clin North Am. 1987;1:575–90.
24. Margileth AM. Cat scratch disease as a cause of the oculoglandular syndrome of Parinaud. J Pediatr. 1957;20:1000–5.
25. Carithers HA. Oculoglandular disease of Parinaud. Am J Dis Child. 1978;132:1195–1200.

Page numbers followed by f indicate figures; those followed by t indicate tables.

A

Abdomen
anatomy, 705–707, 706f, 707f
intra-abdominal infections. *See* Intra-abdominal infections
Abdominal abscess. *See* Intra-abdominal abscess
Abdominal aorta
graft infections, 789
mycotic aneurysms, 770
Abdominal infections. *See* Intra-abdominal infections
Abdominal pain
and/or diarrhea with eosinophilia, syndrome of, 1005–1008
differential diagnosis, 1006–1008
etiology, 1006t
food-borne disease, 1013–1014, 1015
peritonitis, 714
splenic abscess, 727
vaginal disorders, 1082
and vulvovaginitis, 1082
and Whipple's disease, 1031
Abdominal surgery
perforation: and intraperitoneal abscess, 721
prophylaxis recommendations, 2751t
Abortion
prophylaxis recommendations, 2751t
septic, 1093
anaerobic, 2163t
Campylobacter, 1952
Abscesses
brain, 887–900. *See also* Brain abscess
breast, 2163t
Brodie's, 1049, 1772, 1773f
dental
anaerobic, 2163t
Streptococcus intermedius, 1862
and fever, 541
hepatic, 724–727. *See also* Hepatic abscess
injection site, 926
intra-abdominal. *See* Intra-abdominal abscess
intraperitoneal, 721–722
lung, 642–646. *See also* Lung abscess
melioidosis, 2006
pancreatic, 723–724
pelvic. *See* Pelvic abscess
perinephric, 662, 682f, 682–683
periodontal, 596, 598, 2163t, 2164
peritonsillar. *See* Peritonsillar abscess
pilonidal anaerobic, 2163t, 2165
psoas, 933
renal, 682
soft tissue, 922–927
in the course of bacteremia, 927
factitial (self-induced), 926
injection site, 926
splenic, 727. *See also* Splenic abscess
Streptococcus intermedius, 1862
subphrenic, 541, 1863
tuboovarian. *See* Tuboovarian abscess

vaginal cuff, 1094
visceral, 724–727
Absidia, 2311t
dysentery, 994
pneumonia, 619t
Acanthamoeba, 2394t, 2408–2414
brain abscess, 890
in AIDS, 890
clinical manifestations, 2394t, 2411
contact lens infections, 1114, 2410, 2411, 2413, 2414
encephalomyelitis, 877t
epidemiology, 2410
keratitis, 184, 1114, 2411, 2412f, 2413, 2413f
prevention, 2414
treatment, 1118, 2414
laboratory diagnosis, 2413
meningitis, 835
chronic, 865t
pathogenesis and pathology, 2411
phase microscopy, 179
transmission, 2394t
treatment, 461t, 2413–2414
Acanthamoeba astronyx, 2409
Acanthamoeba castellani, 2409
Acanthamoeba culbertsoni, 2409
Acanthamoeba glebae, 2409f
Acanthamoeba hatchetii, 2409
Acanthamoeba palestinensis, 2409
Acanthamoeba polyphaga, 2409, 2412f
Acanthamoeba rhysodes, 2409
Acarina, 2564
Acedapsone: for leprosy, 398
dosage, 397t
Acetaminophen
for fever, 533, 547
hepatotoxicity, 1148
Acetylcholinesterase deficiency: and paroxysmal nocturnal hemoglobinuria, 71
N-Acetylneuraminic acid (NANA): and *Escherichia coli*, 946
Acetyltransferase, 282
Achlorhydria: and *Salmonella*, 2019
Acholeplasma laidlawii: and HIV/AIDS, 1703
Achromobacter, 2110–2111
β-lactamase, 216t
Achromobacter xylosoxidans, 2111
Acidaminococcus fermentans, 2204
Acid-fast bacilli, 2214, 2244. *See also* Mycobacterial infections
isolation, 2576–2577
Acid hydrolases, 79t
Acid proteases, 79t
Acinetobacter, 2009–2013
bacteremia, 2011
β-lactamase, 268
characteristics, 2010t
clinical manifestations, 2010–2011
endocarditis, 756
epidemiology, 2010
genitourinary infection, 2011
genospecies, 2009, 2010t

history, 2009–2010
intracranial infection, 2011
keratitis, 1113
microbiology, 2009–2010
nomenclature, 2010t
pathogenesis, 2010
resistance, 2012
respiratory tract infection, 2011
soft tissue infection, 2011
treatment, 2011–2012
aminoglycosides, 285t
antimicrobials of choice, 202t
penicillins, 237t
quinolones, 367t
rifampin, 318t
Acinetobacter anitratus: and granulocytopenia, 2676
Acinetobacter calcoaceticus, 1010t, 2009
Acinetobacter calcoaceticus-baumannii complex, 2009
Acinetobacter lwoffi, 2009, 2010t
Acne vulgaris
Pseudomonas aeruginosa, 1997
treatment
clindamycin, 343
topical antibacterials, 383
Acquired immunodeficiency syndrome (AIDS), 1164–1305. *See also* Human immunodeficiency virus
adenovirus and, 1386
amebiasis and, 2397, 2399
anal squamous cancer, 1246
antibody testing, 1194–1195
Aspergillus and, 2306, 2309
Babesia and, 2500
bacillary angiomatosis, 557–558, 920, 939, 1229, 1742–1743, 1743f
treatment, 1746
B-cell lymphomas: EBV and, 1370
brain abscess, 887, 888t, 890, 896–897
Candida, 890
Listeria, 890
Toxoplasma gondii, 887, 1237, 1239, 2458
candidiasis, 2290–2291
diarrhea, 970, 970t
esophagitis, 1182, 1229
in children, 1186, 1186t
incidence, 1182t, 1183
fluconazole for, 408–409, 2301
prophylaxis, 1286t
thrush, 1227
treatment, 403, 2301
case definition
1983 (CDC), 1218
1985 (CDC), 1174–1175, 1218
1987 (CDC), 1174–1175, 1218t, 1219
1993 (CDC), 1174–1175, 1175t, 1218t, 1219
WHO, 1218, 1218t
CDC surveillance case definition (1987), 1218t

CDC surveillance case definition (1993), 1175t, 1218t, 1219
CD4+ measures, 1175, 1175t, 1182, 1218t, 1219, 1219t, 1221, 1222f, 1222–1223, 1223t, 1281. *See also* Human immunodeficiency virus, and CD4+
cervical cancer and, 1227, 1246, 1390
in children, 1184–1187, 1186–1187
LIP/PLH complex, 1184, 1186t, 1186–1187
clinical drug trials, 163
clinical manifestations, 1170–1171, 1217–1253. *See also* Human immunodeficiency virus, clinical findings
CMV and, 557, 1221, 1351
adrenalitis, 1360
diarrhea, 970, 970t, 1230
encephalopathy, 1359–1360
enterocolitis, 1230
esophagitis, 963, 964
gastrointestinal, 1229–1230, 1359
incidence, 1182t
lymphadenitis, 941–942
meningitis, 872, 1239–1240
prophylaxis, 1286t
retinitis, 1240, 1359, 1359f
treatment, 1360
CNS infection, 829
Coccidioides immitis, 557, 2370
meningitis, 872
pneumonia, 1236
treatment, 1283t, 1289
cohort studies, 162
and complement, 66
conjunctivitis, 1106
cotton-wool spots, 1240
counseling, 1194–1195
Cryptococcus neoformans, 2332, 2334, 2335
CNS, 2334, 2335
respiratory, 2334, 2335
treatment, 2337
fluconazole, 408–409, 2337
Cryptosporidium, 2500–2501, 2503
clinical features, 2504–2505
gastric, 1230, 2503, 2503f, 2504
immune response and, 2505
incidence, 1182t, 2501
pathogenesis and pathology, 2503f, 2503–2504, 2504f
prevention, 2508
pulmonary, 1236, 2503–2504, 2504f
treatment, 2507–2508
cutaneous manifestations, 557. *See also specific infections*
diagnosis, 138, 156
diarrhea, 970, 970t
in drug abusers, 2705
drug reactions and, 558
EBV and, 1210
B-cell lymphomas, 1370
treatment, 1288

Acquired immunodeficiency syndrome (AIDS) *(Continued)*
  Encephalitozoon, 2514, 2516, 2518–2519
  encephalomyelitis, 879
  endocarditis: heart pathology, 746
  enterococcal meningitis, 1829
  epidemiology (outside U.S.), 1164–1174. *See also* global perspectives on *below*
  epidemiology (U.S.), 158–159, 1174–1191
    in adults, 1176–1184
    AIDS indicator diseases, 1182t, 1182–1183
    in children, 1184, 1186f, 1186t, 1186–1187
    demography, 1180, 1180t
      in children, 1186, 1186t
    exposure categories, 1178–1180, 1179f
    geographic distribution, 1180–1181, 1181f
    mortality, 1184, 1185f
    total reported cases, 1179f
    transmission modes, 1187–1191
  esophagitis, 964
  fever, 547
  global perspectives on, 1174
    Asia, 1166–1167, 1167f
    industrialized countries, 1165
    Latin America and the Caribbean, 1167, 1168f
    North Africa and the Middle East, 1167–1168
    size of problem, 1164–1168, 1165f
    sub-Saharan Africa, 1165t, 1165–1166, 1166t
  granulomatous hepatitis, 1161
  Haemophilus influenzae, 53–54
    pneumonia, 621, 629, 1235, 1235t
    prophylaxis, 1286t
  in health care workers, 2633–2634, 2634t. *See also* Human immunodeficiency virus, in health care setting
  herpes zoster and, 557
  herpetic proctitis, 1060, 1228, 1231, 1339
  histoplasmosis, 557, 872, 1182t, 1235–1236, 1281, 2341, 2346–2348. *See also* *Histoplasma capsulatum*
    treatment, 1283t, 1289, 2350–2351
  HSV and, 557
  human herpesvirus-6 and, 1212, 1334
  immunology, 1203–1217
  impact of epidemic, 1171–1172
  incidence prevalence (U.S.): in adults, 1175–1176
  indicator diseases, 1174t, 1175, 1182–1183, 1223f
  influenza vaccines and, 1561, 1562, 1562t
  interferon-γ use in, 130
  Isospora belli, 2510–2511
    diarrhea, 970, 970t
    enterocolitis, 1230
    incidence, 1182t
  Kaposi's sarcoma, 557, 1240–1244
    clinical appearance, 1241, 1241t
    clinical course, 1242–1243
    diagnosis of cutaneous, 1242
    epidemiology, 1240–1241
    evaluation, 1242–1243

    gastrointestinal, 1241–1242
    oral, 1242
    pathophysiology, 1241, 1241t, 1602
    prognostic factors, 1241–1242, 1242, 1243t
    pulmonary, 1242
    staging, 1242
    therapy, 1243t, 1243–1244
      local, 1243–1244
      systemic, 1244
  keratitis, 1114
  and *Legionella pneumophila*, 2089, 2090
  and leishmaniasis: visceral (kala azar), 2431, 2432
  Listeria and, 1881
    brain abscess, 890
  lymphadenitis, 941–942
  management of opportunistic infections, 1280–1294. *See also* Human immunodeficiency virus, therapy
    candidiasis, 1283t, 1288
    CMV, 1283t, 1287–1288
    coccidioidomycosis, 1283t, 1289
    cryptococcosis, 1283t, 1288–1289
    cryptosporidiosis, 1289
    EBV, 1288
    enteric pathogens, 1289
    general principles, 1282, 1283t
    histoplasmosis, 1283t, 1289
    HSV, 1283t, 1287
    isosporiasis, 1289
    Kaposi's sarcoma, 1290
    lymphoma, 1290
    Microsporidia, 1289
    mycobacteria, 1283t, 1289
    PML, 1288
    Pneumocystis carinii, 1282–1286, 1283t
    Rochalimaea, 1283t, 1290
    Toxoplasma gondii, 1283t, 1286–1287
    Treponema pallidum, 1289–1290
    VZV, 1283t, 1287
  measles and, 1522
    vaccine use, 1524
  meningitis: chronic, 872
  microsporidia, 2516, 2517t, 2518–2519, 2519t
  molluscum contagiosum and, 1228, 1330
  mortality rates, 1184, 1185f
  mucormycosis and, 2313, 2316
  mucositis, 603
  myalgia, 934
  mycobacterial (atypical) infections in, 557, 2268, 2269. *See also* specific mycobacteria
  Mycobacterium avium-intracellulare, 389, 557, 1221, 1234–1235, 1281, 2250–2264
    brain abscess, 890
    diagnosis, 2253
    differential diagnosis, 2253
    epidemiology, 2251–2252
    gastric, 1230
    immunity and, 2252
    incidence, 1182t, 1183, 1234–1235, 2251
    lymphadenitis, 941
    manifestations, 2255f, 2255t, 2255–2256, 2256f
    pneumonia, 621
    probability of developing, 1223f

    prophylaxis, 1286t, 1289, 2258
    treatment, 131, 1283t, 1289, 2257–2258
  Mycobacterium kansasii and, 557, 1234
  Mycobacterium tuberculosis, 159, 542, 1171, 1171f, 1171t, 1177, 1221, 1231–1232, 1234. *See also Mycobacterium tuberculosis*
    in Africa, 1171, 1171f, 1171t
    chemoprophylaxis, 1286t, 2229, 2230–2231
    cutaneous manifestations, 557
    epidemiology, 2215, 2216, 2217, 2218
    extrapulmonary, 2231, 2232f
    gastrointestinal, 2238
    genitourinary, 2238
    miliary, 2233–2234
    multidrug-resistance, 389, 2213
    probability of developing, 1223f, 2217
    scrofula, 2239
    treatment, 2228–2229
  Mycoplasma incognitus and, 1212, 1703, 1707
  myocarditis, 800–801
  neoplasia, 1240–1246, 1245t
    anal squamous, 1246
    cervical, 1246
    early reports, 1240–1241
    Hodgkin's disease, 1246
    KS, 1240–1244. *See also* Kaposi's sarcoma *above*
    non-Hodgkin's lymphoma, 1244–1245
  neurologic complications
    aseptic meningitis, 1236–1240
    peripheral neuropathy, 1236
  neurosyphilis, 835
  Nocardia, 2275, 2277
  non-Hodgkin's lymphoma, 1244–1245
    CNS, 1244
    peripheral, 1244–1245
    therapy, 1245
  opportunistic infections, 137–138. *See also* management of opportunistic infections *above*
    management, 1280–1294
    spectrum. *See* specific infections throughout
  otitis media and, 581
  outside U.S., 1191–1192. *See also* global perspectives on *above*
  paracoccidioidomycosis and, 2387
  parvovirus B19 and, 1439, 1440, 1443
  PCR assays, 27
  pericarditis, 805
  peripheral neuropathy, 1236
  Pneumocystis carinii, 127, 621, 629, 1182, 1182t, 1233, 1233t, 1281, 1591, 2475–2483, 2669
    in children, 1186t, 1186–1187
    choroiditis, 1240
    clinical manifestations, 2478
    course, 2480
    extrapulmonary, 2478, 2479f
    incidence, 1182t, 1183, 1221, 1222f, 1282, 2476
    pathology and pathogenesis, 2476–2478
    prognosis, 2480
    prophylaxis, 1285, 1286t, 2482–2483

    treatment, 1282–1286, 1283t, 2480–2482
  pneumonia
    acute, 629
    bacterial, 1183, 1231, 1233t, 1235, 1235t
    chronic, 648
    community-acquired, 629
    Pneumocystis carinii. *See Pneumocystis carinii above*
  prevention and control strategies, 166, 1192–1194, 2639–2647
  progressive multifocal leukoen-cephalopathy and, 1238, 1239, 1400, 1402, 1404
    incidence, 1182t, 1400
    treatment, 1288, 1404
  Pseudomonas aeruginosa, 1981, 1985, 1987, 1991, 1996
  pulmonary disease, 1231–1236, 1232t
    radiography, 1232, 1233t
  pyomyositis, 929–930
  rashes, 557–558. *See also specific infections*
  reported cases
    U.S., 1175–1176
    worldwide, 1164–1165
  retinitis, 1240
  Rhodococcus and, 1876–1877
  and *Salmonella*, 2019, 2020, 2024
    bacteremia, 2027–2028
    brain abscess, 890
    incidence, 1182t
    therapy, 2027–2028, 2642
  seborrheic dermatitis, 2384
  sexual transmission. *See* Human immunodeficiency virus, epidemiology
  Shigella and, 970, 970t, 2642
  stomatitis, 603
  surveillance (U.S.), 160, 1174t, 1174–1175, 1175t
  tertiary prevention, 168
  Toxoplasma gondii and, 126, 557, 1182, 1237–1238, 1238–1239, 2455, 2457–2461, 2462, 2464–2465
    brain abscess, 887, 1237, 1239, 2458
    chorioretinitis, 1240, 2460
    clinical manifestations, 2459–2461, 2460f
    CNS, 1238, 1239, 2459–2460, 2466–2467, 2467t
    encephalitis, 1238, 2455, 2460, 2460f
    incidence, 1182t
    myocarditis, 2459
    myositis, 2459
    pneumonia, 1236, 2460
    probability of developing, 1223f
    prophylaxis, 1286t, 1286–1287
    reactivation, 2458
    serology, 1238–1239, 2464–2465, 2469–2470
    treatment, 131, 473, 1283t, 1286–1287, 2466f, 2466–2467, 2467t
  transmission. *See* Human immunodeficiency virus, transmission
  treatment, 412t, 1267–1280. *See also* Human immunodeficiency virus, therapy *and specific infections*
    didanosine, 419–421, 420t
    ditiocarb, 456

experimental agents, 437t
foscarnet, 422–424
ganciclovir, 425
GM-CSF and, 451
immunoglobulin, 454
IMREG-1, 456
interferon-γ, 453
interferons, 429, 452–453
interleukin-2, 453
LF 1695, 456
ribavirin, 429, 431
stavudine, 420t, 432
zalcitabine, 420t, 434–435
zidovudine, 420t, 435–437
vaccine recommendations, 2785, 2785t
vaccine research, 1294–1306. *See also* Human immunodeficiency virus, vaccine research
virology. *See* Human immunodeficiency virus
wasting syndrome, 934, 1175, 1182, 1182t, 1226
in children, 1186, 1186t
WHO case definition, 1218t
Acradinium-ester–labeled nucleic acid probe: for gonococcal infections, 182
Acremonium: nail infections, 2383
Acremonium chrysogenum, 247
Acrocyanosis, 551t
Acrodermatitis chronica atrophicans, 2143, 2147
Acrotheca aquaspera, 2324
Actin, 79
Actinobacillus, 2106–2107
classification and site of infection, 2107t
identification, 186
Actinobacillus actinomycetemcomitans, 2106–2107, 2280
biochemical reactions, 2107t
clinical manifestations, 2047
description, 2046
endocarditis, 756
periodontitis, 594
therapy, 601
prevention and treatment, 2047
Actinobacillus equi: animal bites, 2766
Actinobacillus equuli, 2106
Actinobacillus hominis, 2106, 2107
Actinobacillus lignieresii, 2106
animal bites, 2766
Actinobacillus suis, 2106
Actinobacillus ureae, 2106
Actinomadura madurae: actinomycetoma, 2327, 2328f, 2329f, 2330f
Actinomadura pelletieri, 2327, 2330
Actinomyces, 2158t, 2206, 2280–2288
abdominal, 999t, 1002, 2283f, 2283–2284
brain abscess, 890
canaliculitis, 1131
treatment, 1134
clinical manifestations, 2281–2282
CNS disease, 2284–2285
diagnosis, 2285f, 2285–2286
disseminated, 2285
encephalitis, 876
epidemiology, 2280–2281
female genital infections, 2165
hepatic abscess, 724
incidence, 2162
and intra-abdominal abscess, 729
lacrimal sac infection, 1131

mediastinitis, 815t
musculoskeletal, 2285
as normal flora, 2159t
oral-cervicofacial, 2281f, 2281–2282
oral colonization, 593, 594t
pathogenesis, 2161, 2281
pathology, 2281
pelvic disease, 2284
and PID, 1096
pneumonia
chronic, 647t
radiology, 650t
soft tissue, 926
sulfur granules, 2285–2286
thoracic disease, 2282f, 2282–2283
treatment, 2286
metronidazole, 329
tetracyclines, 307, 308t
Actinomyces bovis, 2280
Actinomyces israelii, 2280
epidural abscess, 905
erythromycin for, 335
intra-abdominal, 729
Actinomyces meyeri, 2280
Actinomyces naeslundii, 2280
Actinomyces odontolyticus, 2280
Actinomyces pyogenes, 1873, 2280
Actinomyces viscosus, 2280
oral colonization, 593, 594t
Actinomycetomas, 2284–2285, 2327
Actinomycosis, 2280–2288. *See also Actinomyces*
Actinomycotic granuloma, 2284–2285
Acumentin, 80
Acute phase response, 30t, 33–34, 530, 534–535
class 1 proteins, 117
class 2 proteins, 117
cytokines and, 117
fever and, 34, 530, 534–535
increased phagocyte number and function, 34
inflammation, 34
metabolic changes, 34
soluble defensive molecules, 34
Acute respiratory disease (ARD): pharyngitis, 567
Acute retroviral syndrome (HIV), 1224t, 1224–1225
ACV. *See* Acyclovir
Acycloguanosine. *See* Acyclovir
Acyclovir, 412t, 413–417, 1335
adverse reactions, 415, 1342
and bone marrow transplantation: prophylactic, 2721t
clinical studies, 415–417
dosage, 414–415, 518t–519t
drug interactions, 415, 520t
ganciclovir, 425
for EBV, 1372
for granulocytopenics, 2681
for herpes B virus, 1381
for HSV, 415–416, 1283t, 1287, 1342
mechanism of action, 413
for neutropenics, 2688t, 2690
pharmacokinetics, 414–415
pharmacology, 518t–519t
resistance, 193, 413–414, 423–424, 432–433, 1342
spectrum of activity, 412t, 413, 414t, 1335
structure, 414f
for transplant recipients: prophylactic, 2714
for VZV, 416–417, 1283t, 1287, 1349

Addison's disease: and tuberculosis, 2233, 2240
Adenine arabinoside. *See* Vidarabine
Adenitis
cervical, 604
mesenteric, 1004–1005
Yersinia pseudotuberculosis and *Y. enterocolitica*, 1004–1005, 2077
Adeno-associated viruses, 1386
Adenoidectomy: for otitis media, 583
Adenopathy. *See also* Lymphadenopathy
and acute retroviral syndrome (HIV), 1224t
mediastinal tuberculous, 2239
Adenosine deaminase (ADA) deficiency, 134t, 150, 151t
Adenoviridae, 1382–1387. *See also* Adenovirus
classification, 1315t
shape and size, 1316f
Adenovirus, 1382–1387
arthritis, 1036t
and bone marrow transplantation, 2720
bronchiolitis, 612t, 613
bronchitis, acute, 606, 606t
capsomeres, 1382–1383
cellular immunity and, 129
classification, 1383, 1384t
clinical syndromes, 1384t, 1384–1386
CNS infection, 1386
common cold, 562, 562t
conjunctivitis, 1105–1106
croup, 574, 574t
cultures, 173
cutaneous manifestations, 550t
description, 1382–1383, 1383f
diagnosis, 1386
enteric: diagnosis, 181
epidemiology, 1383–1384
fibers, 1383, 1383f
hemorrhagic cystitis, 1385
hepatitis, 1137
in transplant recipients, 2728
hexons, 1383, 1383f
infantile diarrhea, 966, 1385
intussusception, 1385–1386
keratoconjunctivitis, 1105, 1115, 1385
epidemic, 1385
treatment, 1118
laryngitis, 573t
lymphadenitis, 940t
oncogenic potential, 1383, 1384t
pathogenesis, 1383, 1384f
pentons, 1383, 1383f
pharyngoconjunctival fever, 566, 1385, 1789
pneumonia
atypical, 630, 1704
differential diagnosis, 1698
prevention, 1386
products and host target, 125t
respiratory infection, 1384t, 1384–1385
and Reye syndrome, 1558
serotypes, 1384t
diseases caused by, 1384t
sinusitis, 585, 585t
structure, 1382–1383, 1383f
type 1, 1383, 1384, 1384t
type 2, 1383, 1384, 1384t
type 3, 1384, 1384t, 1386
type 4, 1384, 1384t
vaccine, 2773–2774
indications for adults, 2784t
type 5, 1383, 1384, 1384t

type 6, 1383, 1384t
type 7, 1384, 1384t, 1385, 1386
vaccine, 2773–2774
indications for adults, 2784t
type 8, 1384
type 9, 1384
type 11, 1384, 1384t
type 12, 1386
type 21, 1384, 1384t, 1386
urinary tract infections, 668
Adenylate cyclase toxin (*Bordetella pertussis*), 3t, 4, 6, 23
Adenyltransferases, 282, 283
Adherence, microbial, 11–19, 1753. *See also specific organisms*
adhesin identification, 11–12, 12t
adhesin-receptor interaction, 13f, 13t, 13–14, 14f
Entamoeba histolytica, 15–16, 16f
HIV gp120/160, 14–15
receptor identification, 12t, 12–13
tissue tropism and, 31
toxins, 4
Adherence assay, 11–12, 12t
Adhesins, 11
classes, 12t
experimental identification, 11–12, 12t
interactions with receptors, 13f, 13t, 13–14, 14f
receptor identification, 12t, 12–13
Adrenal glands
histoplasmosis, 2346–2347
tuberculosis, 2240
Adrenalitis: cytomegalovirus, 1360
Adrenal steroids: for antibiotic-associated colitis, 983
Adrenocorticotropic hormone: and acute phase response, 35
Adriamycin: for Kaposi's sarcoma, 1244
Adult respiratory distress syndrome (ARDS)
neutropenia and, 88
and sepsis syndrome, 693, 696
Streptococcus intermedius and, 1863
Adult T-cell leukemia/lymphoma, 1581–1582
clinical illness, 1581f, 1581–1582, 1582f
diagnosis, 1582
HTLV and, 1579, 1581, 1582
incidence, 1581
infectious complications, 1582
skin lesions, 1581, 1581f
treatment, 1582
Adult T-cell leukemia virus, 1579. *See also* Human T cell lymphotropic viruses
Aedes
and arboviruses, 1456, 1457
and California encephalitis, 1568, 1569
and dengue, 1465, 1466t, 1468
and equine encephalitis, 1456
reservoirs, 2794
and Rift Valley fever, 1568
and yellow fever, 1465, 1466t, 1467
Aerobacter. See Enterobacter
Aerobic bacteria: classification, 1752
Aerobic gram-negative bacilli: meningitis, 834–835
antimicrobial therapy, 850t, 852–853
Aeromonas, 2107–2108
classification and site of infection, 2107t
diarrhea: infantile, 967

Aeromonas (Continued)
  enterotoxin, 5
  toxin, 950
  treatment
    aminoglycosides, 285t
    quinolones, 367t
Aeromonas caviae, 2108
Aeromonas hydrophila, 2108
  β-lactamase, 216t
  carbapenems for, 264t
  cellulitis, 915
  myonecrosis, 933
  symmetric peripheral gangrene, 553
  wound infections: in trauma patients, 2758
Aeromonas shigelloides. See *Plesiomonas shigelloides*
Aeromonas sobria, 2108
Aeromonas veronii, 2108
Aerosol transmission: viral diseases, 1319
Afipia: taxonomy, 1742f
Afipia felis, 557, 938–939, 1745
  and cat scratch disease, 938–939, 1310
African Burkitt's lymphoma: EBV and, 1364, 1369–1370
African histoplasmosis, 2348
African swine fever, 2144
African tick typhus. See *Rickettsia conorii*
African trypanosomiasis, 2450–2455.
    See also *Trypanosoma brucei*
  immunodeficiency and, 138
  keratitis, 1114
Agammaglobulinemia, 49
  enteroviral meningoencephalitis and, 1629
  Staphylococcus aureus and, 1762
  Streptococcus pneumoniae and, 1816, 1817t
  X-linked, 49, 51
  Giardia lamblia, 2489
Agar diffusion assays, 197, 197f
Age. See also Children; Elderly
  and drug pharmacokinetics, 201
  and host defense mechanisms, 35
  renal function and, 201
  and vulvovaginitis, 1081–1082
Agglutination, 185, 191
  for bacteria, 192t
  heterophile, 192t
  for *Toxoplasma gondii*, 2463–2464
Aging: cellular immunity and, 133
Agranulocytosis
  congenital (Kostmann syndrome), 154
  infantile genetic, 89
Agrobacterium, 2111
  classification and site of infection, 2107t
Agrobacterium radiobacter, 2111
Agrobacterium tumefaciens, 2111
  pathogenicity, 23
AIDS. See Acquired immunodeficiency syndrome
AIDS dementia complex, 1589, 1601–1602
  CMV and, 1360
AIDS-related complex, 1218
  lymphadenitis, 942
Air-borne transmission, 166
Ajellomyces dermatitidis, 2354
Alanine aminotransferase (ALT): hepatitis, 1139, 1140f

Albendazole, 460t, 479–480
  adverse reactions, 479–480
  for cysticercosis, 2549
  dosage, 461t, 462t, 466t, 467t
    pediatric, 461t, 462t, 466t, 467t
  for echinococcosis, 2551
  for microsporidia, 2521
  spectrum of activity, 479
Alcaligenes, 2111–2112
  classification and site of infection, 2107t
Alcaligenes faecalis, 2112
Alcaligenes odorans, 2112
Alcaligenes piechaudii, 2112
Alcaligenes xylosoxidans
  and cystic fibrosis, 659
  subsp. *denitrificans*, 2111
  subsp. *xylosoxidans*, 2111
Alcoholic liver disease, 1148–1149
Alcohol use and abuse
  avoidance: in liver disease, 1149
  and cephalosporin adverse effects, 254–255
  cirrhosis: and peritonitis, 709
  and defective chemotaxis, 90
  hepatitis: aminotransferases, 1140f
  and pneumonia, 621
  and *Streptococcus agalactiae* bacteremia, 1839, 1839t
  and *Streptococcus pneumoniae*, 1817, 1817t, 1818t
Aldesleukin, 453
Aleppo evil, 2434–2435
Alexin, 58
Alkaline phosphatase deficiency: and paroxysmal nocturnal hemoglobinuria, 71
Allergic reactions. See also Drug-induced disorders
  penicillins, 239, 239t
  tetracyclines, 309
Allodermanyssus sanguinensis: and rickettsialpox, 1727
Allopurinol, 477
  for *Leishmania*, 2430, 2433
  for *Trypanosoma cruzi*, 2448
Allopurinol ribonucleoside, 477
Allylamines, 401
Alopecia areata, 2380
Alpha-adrenergic blockers: for septic shock, 701
Alpha₁-antichymotrypsin: and acute phase response, 117
Alpha₁-antitrypsin, 34
  and acute phase response, 117
Alpha₁-glycoprotein: and acute phase response, 117
Alpha₂-macroglobulin, 34
α-Melanocyte-stimulating factor: and fever reduction, 532
α-toxin: *Staphylococcus aureus*, 1759
Alphaviruses, 1455–1459. See also *individual viruses*
  arthritis, 1036, 1036t
  clinical manifestations, 1458
  complement fixation test, 1455
  description, 1455–1456
  diagnosis, 1458
  encephalitis
    clinical manifestations, 1458
    epidemiology, 1456
  epidemiology, 1456–1457
  fever, rash, and polyarteritis syndromes
    clinical manifestations, 1458
    epidemiology, 1456–1457

genome, 1455
hemagglutination-inhibition test, 1455
history, 1455
pathogenesis, 1457
structure, 1455
treatment and prevention, 1458–1459
Alternaria, 2391
Alternaria alternata: sinusitis, 586t
Alveolar cyst disease, 2550–2551
Amanita muscaria, 1015t
Amanita pantherina, 1015t
Amanita phalloides, 1015, 1015t
Amanita verna, 1015, 1015t
Amanita virosa, 1015, 1015t
Amantadine, 412t, 417–419
  adverse reactions, 418–419
  clinical studies, 419
  dosage, 418, 518t–519t
    in renal failure, 418t
  drug interactions, 418–419, 520t
  for influenza, 1560
    prophylaxis, 1563
  mechanism of action, 417, 1319
  pharmacology, 418, 518t–519t
  resistance, 417–418
  spectrum of activity, 417
  structure, 417f
  for viral pharyngitis, 571
Amapari virus, 1572
Ambisome, 404–405
Amblyomma americanum
  and ehrlichiosis, 1747t, 1748, 1749, 2565
  and *Francisella tularensis*, 2061
Amblyomma cajennense: and *Rickettsia rickettsii*, 1721
Amblyomma hebraeum, 1725
Amdinocillin
  dosage, 506t–507t
    in renal disease, 238t, 507t
  pharmacology, 506t–507t
Amebiasis, 2394t, 2395–2408. See also *Entamoeba histolytica*
  diagnosis, 2395t
Amebic infections. See also *specific amebae*
  antiparasitic agents, 458, 459t, 461t, 467–468
  dysentery, 989
  Entamoeba histolytica, 2394t, 2395–2408. See also *Entamoeba histolytica*
  free-living, 2408–2414. See also *specific species*
  lung abscess, 643
  meningitis, 835
    antimicrobial therapy, 849t, 850t, 854
    clinical presentation, 844
    diagnosis, 849
  phase microscopy, 179
Amebomas, 2400, 2402
American trypanosomiasis, 2442–2450.
    See also *Trypanosoma cruzi*
Amifloxacin: structure, 365f
Amikacin, 280
  antimicrobial activity, 285t, 286
  clinical trials, 228
  combination therapy, 287t
    for mycobacteria, 396t
    synergism, 207
    trimethoprim, 359
  for cystic fibrosis infections, 660

dosage, 297t, 510t–511t
    in children and neonates, 299t, 510t, 851t
    in hepatic failure, 390t
    for meningitis, 850t, 851t
    in renal dysfunction, 298t, 511t
  for mycetoma, 2330
  for *Mycobacterium avium-intracellulare*, 2258
  for *Mycobacterium tuberculosis*, 394–395
  neuromuscular blockade, 295
  for nontuberculous mycobacteria, 396
  ototoxicity, 294
  pharmacology, 510t–511t
  for Pseudomonads, 2004t
  resistance, 200, 220, 284, 284t
  for sepsis syndrome, 699, 699t
  source and chemistry, 280t
  structure, 281f
  susceptibility testing, 194, 194t
Amino acids: and acute phase response, 535
Aminocyclitol, 280
Aminoglycosides, 205–206, 279–306.
    See also *specific drugs*
  absorption, 209
  administration, 289–290
  adverse reactions, 289–290, 290t, 290–295
  animal models of efficacy, 287–288
  chemistry, 280, 280t
  clinical indications, 295t, 295–296
    prophylaxis, 296
    specific therapy, 295t, 296
  cochlear toxicity, 294
  combination therapy
    animal models, 288, 289t
    resistance prevention, 288
    synergism, 207
  distribution, 290
  dosage, 296–300, 510t–511t
    in cystic fibrosis, 299
    in gonorrhea, 299
    in infective endocarditis, 299
    multiple daily, 296–298
      loading, 296–297, 297t
      maintenance, 297t, 297–298
      and renal dysfunction, 297–298, 298t
    for neonates and children, 299, 299t, 510t
    once-daily, 298–299, 299t
    in renal dysfunction, 511t
  drug interactions, 520t
  empiric therapy, 295t, 295–296
  energy-dependent phase, 282, 283
  enzymatic inactivation, 218, 218t, 282
  excretion, 290
  future use, 300
  for intra-abdominal peritonitis/abscess, 288–289
  mechanism of action, 282, 283
  for *Mycobacterium leprae*, 2249
  nephrotoxicity, 290t, 291f, 291–294, 292t, 293t
    clinical, 292–293
    experimental, 291–292
    pathway, 291f
    risk factors, 293t
    serum levels and, 293–294
  neuromuscular blockade, 295
  for nontuberculous (atypical) mycobacteria, 396
  ototoxicity, 294–295

for peritonitis, 710, 717
and pH, 206
pharmacokinetics, 290
pharmacologic preparations, 300, 300t
pharmacology, 227–228, 289–290,
   510t–511t
   animal models, 228
   clinical trial data, 228
   in vitro models, 228
for pneumonia, 632t
   nosocomial, 2603
for *Pseudomonas aeruginosa*, 228,
   279, 285t, 295t, 296
for pyelonephritis, 676
resistance, 214, 215t, 218, 218t, 219,
   227–228, 283–284
   altered aminoglycoside uptake, 283
   altered ribosome-binding sites, 283
   combination therapy to prevent,
      288
   enterococci, 283–284
   enzymatic modification, 283
   epidemiology, 284, 284t
   inner membrane permeability and,
      219
   phosphorylation, acetylation, and
      adenylation, 218, 218t
   viridans streptococci, 1851
sources, 280, 280t
structure, 280, 281f, 282t
synergy, 287, 287t
vestibular toxicity, 294–295
in vitro activity, 283–286, 285t
Aminopenicillins, 236, 243–244. *See
   also specific formulations*
dosage, 238t, 241t
   in neonates, 242t
   in renal disease, 238t
pharmacokinetics, 238t
structure, 243f
Aminopeptidase N, 13
Aminophylline: quinolone interaction
   with, 370
Aminoquinolines, 469–472
Aminosalicylic acid: drug interactions,
   520t
Aminotransferases
   anoxic liver damage, 1149
   hepatitis, 1139, 1140f
Amithiozone. *See* Thiacetazone
Amnionitis
   anaerobic gram-negative bacilli,
      2199
   Haemophilus influenzae, 2043
Amocarzine, 482
   for onchocerciasis, 2536
Amorolfine
   for dermatophytosis, 2382
   topical, 401
Amoxicillin, 244
   for actinomycosis, 2286
   adverse reactions, 244, 272–273,
      275–276
   with aminoglycosides, 289t
   antibiotic-associated colitis (AAC),
      979
   for bacilli and anaerobes, 237t
   for *Bacteroides fragilis*, 2200t, 2201
   for *Borrelia burgdorferi*, 2151
   for *Chlamydia trachomatis*, 1688
   for cystic fibrosis infections, 660
   dosage, 241t, 506t–507t
      in children, 506t
      in neonates, 242t, 506t
      in renal disease, 238t, 507t

drug interactions, 370
for endocarditis prophylaxis, 797t
for Enterobacteriaceae and
   Pseudomonas, 237t
for *Helicobacter pylori*, 1961
for leptospirosis, 2140
MICs against cocci, 237t
for otitis media, 582, 583
pharmacokinetics, 238t
pharmacology, 238
prophylactic use, 240
for *Pseudomonas pseudomallei*, 2006
for pyelonephritis, 676
for *Salmonella*, 2028
for sinusitis, 589t
structure, 243f
for *Treponema pallidum*, 2129t
for urinary tract infections, 676
   in pregnancy, 679
Amoxicillin-clavulanate, 269
   activity, 268t
   for *Bacteroides fragilis*, 2200t, 2201
   dosage, 506t–507t
   for *Nocardia*, 2277
   pharmacology, 506t–507t
   for pneumonia, 632t
   for sinusitis, 589t
   susceptibility testing, 194t
   for urinary tract infections in preg-
      nancy, 679
Amphotericin B, 404
   absorption, 209
   for amebic infections, 2413
   antiparasitic use, 459t, 466, 477–478
   for *Aspergillus*, 2309
   for *Blastomyces dermatitidis*, 406,
      2362, 2363
   and bone marrow transplantation: pro-
      phylactic, 2719
   for candidiasis, 2299, 2300–2301
   for *Coccidioides immitis*, 406, 1283t,
      1289, 2371
   colloidal dispersion, 404
   combination therapy: synergism, 207
   for *Cryptococcus neoformans*, 406,
      1283t, 1288, 2336–2337
   deoxycholate, 404
      toxicity, 405
   dosage, 461t, 463t, 518t–519t
      pediatric, 461t, 463t
   drug interactions, 520t
      foscarnet, 422
   for endocarditis, 764
   for endophthalmitis, 1126
   for esophagitis, 964t
   fever from, 545
   for granulocytopenics, 2680
   for *Histoplasma capsulatum*, 406,
      1283t, 1289, 2350
   for *Leishmania*, 2430, 2433, 2438
   lipid complex, 404
   for meningitis, 854, 869
   for mucormycosis, 2316–2317
   for mycetoma, 2330
   for neutropenics, 2688t
   for *Paracoccidioides brasiliensis*,
      2388
   for peritonitis, 717
      in peritoneal dialysis, 720t, 721
   pharmacology, 518t–519t
   for *Prototheca*, 2391
   for sporotrichosis, 2323
   structure, 402f
   for suppurative thrombophlebitis, 768
   susceptibility testing, 193

topical, 401t
transfusion pulmonary reactions and,
   95
for transplant recipients: prophylactic,
   2715
Ampicillin, 243–244
   adverse reactions, 239t, 272–273,
      275–276
   antibiotic-associated colitis (AAC),
      979
   antimicrobial spectrum, 241t
   for bacilli and anaerobes, 237t
   for bacterial vaginosis, 1079
   combination therapy
      aminoglycosides, 287t, 289t
      antagonism, 208
      erythromycin, 337
   dosage, 241t, 506t–507t
      in children, 506t, 851t
      for meningitis, 849t, 850t, 851t
      in neonates, 242t, 506t
      in renal disease, 238t, 506t
   for endocarditis
      culture-negative, 764
      Enterobacteriaceae, 763
      Haemophilus influenzae, 763
      prophylactic, 797t
      streptococcal, 760
   for Enterobacteriaceae and
      Pseudomonas, 237t
   for enterococcal infections, 1831,
      1831t
   for epiglottitis, 592
   for leptospirosis, 2140
   for *Listeria*, 1884
   MICs against cocci, 237t
   for *Mobiluncus*, 2052
   for *Nocardia*, 2277
   for peritonitis, 716
      in peritoneal dialysis, 720t
   pharmacokinetics, 238t
   pharmacology, 506t–507t
   prophylactic, 240
      for endocarditis, 797t
      for meningitis, 857
   for pyelonephritis, 676
   resistance, 200
      Haemophilus influenzae, 2042–2043
      Salmonella, 2027
   for sinusitis, 589t
   for *Streptococcus agalactiae*, 1841,
      1841t
   susceptibility testing, 194t
   trade names, 237t
   for *Vibrio cholerae*, 1939
Ampicillin-sulbactam
   antimicrobial activity, 285t
   for *Bacteroides fragilis*, 2200t, 2201
   dosage, 506t–507t
   for endocarditis: staphylococcal, 763
   pharmacology, 506t–507t
   for pyelonephritis, 676
   susceptibility testing, 194t
Amputation surgery: prophylaxis recommendations, 2751t
Amyloid A protein, 34
Amyloidosis
   and fever, 546
   leprosy and, 2248
Anaerobic bacteria, 2156–2209
   animal bites, 2766, 2766t
   antimicrobial associated pseudomem-
      branous colitis, 2163t, 2166
   arthritis, 1034, 1034t, 1035
   bacteremia, 2163t, 2165

Bacteroides, 2195–2204
β-lactamase producing, 2169t, 2171
Bifidobacterium, 2207
cellulitis
   clostridial, 923
   differential diagnosis, 924t
   nonclostridial, 923
classification, 1752
clinical conditions as clues to infection, 2167
Clostridium
   botulinum, 2178–2182
   difficile, 2189–2192
   gas gangrene, 2182–2195
   perfringens, 2182–2189
   tetani, 2173–2178
clues to infection, 2166t, 2166–2167
   as clue to other conditions, 2167
CNS infections, 2162, 2163t, 2164
cocci, 2204–2206
   clinical manifestations, 2205
   isolation, 2204–2205
   taxonomy and microbiology, 2204
   treatment, 2205–2206
conjunctivitis, 1104–1105
defined, 2156–2157
diagnosis, 2167–2169
   alternatives to conventional
      methods, 2168–2169
   direct examination of samples,
      2167–2168
endocarditis, 756
   treatment, 763–764, 764
enteric flora, 947
epidemiology, 2161
Eubacterium, 2207
exogenous infections, 2161
facultative, 1752. *See also specific
   bacteria*
female genital tract infections, 2163t,
   2165
gram-negative cocci, 2199
Fusobacterium, 2195–2204
gram-negative bacilli, 2195–2204
gram-negative cocci: as normal flora,
   2159t
gram-positive bacilli, 2206–2208
gram-positive cocci, 2204–2206
   as normal flora, 2159t
growth or biochemical characteristics,
   189
head and neck infections, 2163t, 2164
historical review, 2157
infections produced by, 2162t,
   2162–2166, 2163t. *See also
   specific anaerobes and infections*
intra-abdominal infections, 2163t,
   2165
intra-abdominal specimen collection
   and processing, 178
intra-amniotic infection syndrome,
   1090
intraperitoneal abscess, 721
Lactobacillus, 2207–2208
Loesche classification, 2156–2157
lung abscess, 642, 2163t
mediastinitis, 815t
Mobiluncus, 2208
necrotizing pneumonia, 642–643,
   643f
as normal flora, 2157–2160, 2159t
osteomyelitis, 2163t, 2166
overview, 2156–2173
pathogenesis, 2161, 2161t

Anaerobic bacteria *(Continued)*
 pathology, 2161–2162
 pathophysiology, 2161–2162
 and peritonitis, 712–713
 pharyngitis (Vincent's angina), 569
 pleuropulmonary infections, 2163t,
  2164–2165
 predisposing conditions, 2161, 2161t
 prevention, 2171, 2171t
 Prevotella, 2195–2204
 primary inoculation, 2168
 Propionibacterium, 2207
 prosthetic joint infections, 1052, 1052t
 resistance, 2171
 role in normal physiology of host,
  2160
 role in pathophysiologic states, 2160
 Rothia dentocariosa, 2208
 soft tissue infections, 2163t,
  2165–2166
 specimen collection and transport,
  2167, 2168f
 streptococcal myonecrosis, 924t, 933
 strict vs. moderate, 2156–2157
 superoxide dismutase, 2157
 susceptibility testing, 2169–2171,
  2170t
 synergistic nonclostridial myonecrosis, 924t, 933
 taxonomy, 2157, 2158t, 2159t
 treatment, 2169–2171, 2170t. *See also*
   specific anaerobes
  antimicrobials of choice, 203t,
   2170t
  carbapenems, 264t
  chloramphenicol, 312t
  clindamycin, 343
  fusidic acid, 278
  metronidazole, 329t, 330t, 332
  penicillins, 241t
  quinolones, 368t
  rifampin, 324
Anaerobiospirillum, 2158t
 bacteremia, 2165
Anaerorhabdus, 2158t
Anaerovibrio, 2158t
Analgesics: for urinary tract infections,
  675
Anal intercourse
 gonorrhea, 1910, 1913, 1914, 1916,
  1920, 1920t
 and HIV transmission, 1169, 1189,
  1193
 lesions, 1056, 1059, 1060
Anal squamous cancer
 and HIV/AIDS, 1246
Anaphylatoxin inactivator (carboxypeptidase B), 58t, 63t
Anaphylaxis
 penicillins, 239, 239t
 tetracyclines, 309
Anatomic barriers, 31–32
 eye, 32
 genitourinary tract, 32
 intestinal tract, 32
 mucous membranes, 31–32
 respiratory tract, 32
 skin, 31–32
 virulence factors for overcoming, 7–8
Ancef. *See* Cefazolin
Ancylostoma braziliense, 2555
Ancylostoma caninum, 2555
Ancylostoma duodenale, 2525t,
  2529–2530
 clinical syndrome, 2530

 diagnosis, 2530
 epidemiology, 2529–2530
 life cycle, 2529
 penetration, 7
 pulmonary infiltrates with eosinophilia,
  631
 treatment, 463t, 2530
  mebendazole, 478–479
  pyrantel pamoate, 480
Anemia
 aplastic: chloramphenicol and,
  313–314
 hemolytic
  Babesia, 2499
  CMV, 1358
  EBV, 1368
  herpesviruses, 1334t
  from nitrofurantoin, 378
  from sulfonamides, 356
  and HIV, 1226
 iron deficiency: hookworm and, 2530
 and leishmaniasis: visceral (kala azar),
  2432
 megaloblastic: intestinal tapeworms,
  2546
 Plasmodium, 2420
 from zidovudine, 436
Aneurysms
 mycotic, 769–773. *See also* Mycotic
  aneurysms
 Treponema pallidum, 2125
Angiokeratomas: differential diagnosis,
  1395
Angioneurotic edema: epiglottitis vs., 591
Angiostrongylus cantonensis, 2555–2556
 meningitis, 835, 2555
  chronic, 865t
  clinical presentation, 844
  diagnosis, 849
 treatment, 461t
Angiostrongylus costaricensis, 2553t,
  2556
 diagnosis, 1006t, 1007
 treatment, 461t
Anichkov's myocytes, 1801
Animal bites, 165, 604, 2766–2768
 anaerobic, 2163t
 antimicrobial susceptibility, 2766t
 bacterial etiology, 2765t
 to head and neck, 603, 604
 management, 2767, 2767t
 Pasteurella, 2069
 rabies, 1527–1528, 1529–1531, 1530f,
  1531f, 1532f
Anisakis, 2553t, 2554–2555
 clinical syndrome, 2554–2555
 diagnosis, 1006t, 2555
 treatment, 461t, 2555
Ankle: infectious arthritis, 1033, 1033t
Ankylosing spondylitis: and Reiter syndrome, 1071
Anogenital warts, 1392f, 1392–1393. *See
  also* Human papillomavirus
 diagnosis, 1395
 treatment, 1394–1395
Anopheles: and *Plasmodium*, 2417
Anopheles albimanus, 2417
Anopheles freeboni, 2417
Anopheles funestus, 2417
Anopheles gambiae, 2417
Anoplura, 2558–2560
Anorectal disease and lesions
 gonorrhea, 1910, 1913, 1914, 1916,
  1919, 1920
 HSV, 1337, 1339

 Pseudomonas aeruginosa, 1995
 STDs, 1060
Anorexia
 hepatitis, 1138
 and peritonitis, 714
Anoscopy: for human papillomavirus
  diagnosis, 1395
Ansamycin. *See* Rifabutin
Anspor. *See* Cephradine
Anthrax, 1885–1889. *See also Bacillus
  anthracis*
Anthrax toxin, 3t, 4, 6, 1887
Anthrax vaccine, 1889, 2774
 adverse reactions, 2774
 indications for adults, 2784t
Antiadhesin antibodies, 13, 16, 2771
Antibacterials, 233–400. *See also specific
   drug categories and individual
   drugs*
 aminoglycosides, 279–306
  pharmacologic tables, 510t–511t
 antimycobacterials, 389–400
  pharmacologic tables, 516t–517t
 azalides: pharmacologic tables,
  512t–513t
 aztreonam, 266–268
 β-lactam allergy, 272–278
 β-lactamase inhibitors, 268–270
 carbapenems, 264–266
 cephalosporins, 247–264
  pharmacologic tables, 508–509t
 chloramphenicol, 310–314
  pharmacologic tables, 512t–513t
 clindamycin, 341–343
 drug interactions, 520t–527t. *See also
   individual drugs*
 fusidic acid, 278–279
  pharmacologic tables, 514t–515t
 generic-trade names, 493t–499t
 for immunocompromised host
  empirical, 2688t, 2688–2689, 2690t
  duration, 2690–2691
  prophylactic, 2692–2693
 lincomycin, 341–343
 lincosamides: pharmacologic tables,
  512t–513t
 macrolides, 334–340
  pharmacologic tables, 512t–513t
 methenamine, 379–380
 metronidazole, 329–334
  pharmacologic tables, 512t–513t
 monobactams, 266
 nitrofurantoin, 376–379
 penicillins, 233–246
  pharmacologic tables, 506t–507t
 pharmacologic tables, 506t–517t
  aminoglycosides, 510t–511t
  antimycobacterials, 516t–517t
  azalides, 512t–513t
  cephalosporins, 508t–509t
  chloramphenicol, 512t–513t
  fusidic acid, 514t–515t
  lincosamides, 512t–513t
  macrolides, 512t–513t
  metronidazole, 512t–513t
  other β-lactams, 510t–511t
  penicillins, 506t–507t
  polymyxins, 514t–515t
  quinolones, 516t–517t
  sulfonamides, 514t–515t
  teicoplanin, 514t–515t
  tetracyclines, 512t–513t
  trimethoprim, 514t–515t
  urinary tract agents, 516t–517t
  vancomycin, 514t–515t

  polymyxins: pharmacologic tables,
   514t–515t
  quinolones, 364–376
   pharmacologic tables, 516t–517t
  rifamycins, 317–329
  sulfonamides, 354–357
   pharmacologic tables, 514t–515t
  teicoplanin, 351
   pharmacologic tables, 514t–515t
  tetracyclines, 306–310
   pharmacologic tables, 512t–513t
  topical, 381–389
  trade-generic names, 499t–505t
  trimethoprim, 357–360
   pharmacologic tables, 514t–515t
  urinary tract agents, 376–381,
   516t–517t, 675
   pharmacologic tables, 516t–517t
  vancomycin, 346–350
   pharmacologic tables, 514t–515t
Antibiotic-associated colitis. *See* Colitis,
  antibiotic-associated
Antibiotic efflux: promotion of, 219
Antibiotic prophylaxis, 167
Antibiotics. *See* Antibacterials; Anti-
  infective therapy
Antibodies. *See also* Immunoglobulin(s)
 adhesin, 13, 16
 affinity maturation, 42
 agglutination, 42
 antiadhesion, 42
 antibody-dependent cellular cytotoxicity, 41
 antiendotoxin, 41
 antigen-binding diversity, generation
  of, 43f, 43–45, 44f
 antimicrobial function, 41–42
 autoantibodies, 42
 B-cell activity regulation, 49
 B-cell ontogeny and differentiation,
  48–49
 B-cell receptor complex, 45–47, 46f
 B1 cells, 49
 cellular mechanisms in production,
  42–49
 CNS infections and, 829
 complement activation, 41
 cryoglobulinemia, 42
 deficiencies, 49–54. *See also specific
   deficiencies*
  ataxia-telangiectasia, 52–53
  bone marrow transplantation and, 53
  combined T-cell and, 52–53
  common clinical features, 49–50
  common variable immunodeficiency, 51
  diagnosis, 50
  HIV-related, 53–54
  malignancies and, 53
  primary: immunoglobulin for, 454
  protein wasting states and, 53
  pure, 51–52
  secondary, 53–54
  severe combined immunodeficiency,
   52
  sickle cell anemia and, 53
  splenectomy and, 53
  transient hypogammaglobulinemia
   of infancy, 51
  Wiskott-Aldrich syndrome, 52
  X-linked agammaglobulinemia, 51
 detection tests, 191, 192t, 193t
  bacterial serologic, 192t
  fungal serologic, 193t
  nonspecific, 192t

distribution and catabolism, 40
and HIV, 1213
    impaired responses, 1209–1210
    neutralized response, 1213
and HIV vaccine research,
    1294–1296, 1295f
hypergammaglobulinemia, 42
immune complexes, 42
immunopathology caused by, 42
inhibition of adherence, 12
intestinal, 948
isotypic switching, 42
memory cells, 42
natural, 31
neutralization
    of microbial toxins, 41
    viruses, 41–42
phagocytosis, 41
primary response, 42
rheumatoid factor, 42
secondary response, 42
and *Streptococcus pneumoniae*,
    1814–1816
    deficiencies, 1816, 1817t
surface molecules of B cell, 45, 45t
T-cell–dependent B-cell activation, 47
T-cell–independent B-cell activation,
    47–48
and urinary tract infections, 666–667
virulence factors and, 8
Antibody coating of bacteria (ACB): in
    urine, 672
Antibody-dependent cellular cytotoxici-
    ty, 41
and HIV, 1213
    vaccine research, 1294
IgE-directed, 39
T helper cells and, 116
Antibody testing. *See also specific tests*
    HIV, 1254–1261. *See also* Human
        immunodeficiency virus, anti-
        body testing
Antibody titers: and FUO, 539
Anticoagulation
    drug interactions: sulfonamides, 356
    for endocarditis: prosthetic valve, 787
    for sepsis syndrome, 701
Anti-complement immunofluorescence
    (ACIF): for CMV, 1352
Antidiarrheal agents: for antibiotic-
    associated colitis, 983
Antiendotoxin antibodies, 41
Antifungals, 401–410. *See also individual
    drugs*
    allylamines, 401
    amphotericin B, 404
    azoles, 401
    benzoic acid, 401
    drug interactions, 520t–527t. *See also
        individual drugs*
    fluconazole, 408–409
    flucytosine, 406
    generic-trade names, 493t–499t
    griseofulvin, 404
    imidazoles, 406–409
    for immunocompromised host
        empirical, 2688t, 2689–2690
        prophylactic, 2693
    itraconazole, 404, 408
    ketoconazole, 404, 407
    morpholine derivatives, 401
    oral
        for deep mycoses, 404–405
        for superficial mycoses, 404
        for thrush, 403

pharmacologic tables, 518t–519t
polyenes, 403
salicylic acid, 401
terbinafine, 404
topical, 401t, 401–403
    for cutaneous use, 401–403
    for vaginal use, 403, 403t
trade-generic names, 499t–505t
Whitfield's ointment, 401
Antigen-binding diversity, 43f, 43–45,
    44f
    quaternary association, 45
    somatic mutation, 45
    VDJ recombination, 44–45
Antigen detection. *See also speciifc
    methods*
    and choice of anti-infective therapy,
        200
    genital lesions, 1060
    HIV, 1261, 1261t
    pneumonia, 625–626
Antigenicity, 165
Antigenic variation: pathogenicity and,
    20
Antigen-presenting cells (APC)
    HIV and, 1208
    and MHC class II, 104
    superantigens and, 110–111
Antigen receptor complex: T cell, 105
Antigen(s)
    immune complexes, 42
    and normal flora, 31
Antihistamines: for otitis media, 582
Anti-infective therapy, 199–530. *See
    also specific categories of
    drugs and individual drugs*
    aminoglycosides, 279–306
        pharmacologic tables, 510t–511t
    antifungal agents, 401–410
        pharmacologic tables, 518t–519t
    antimycobacterials, 389–400
        pharmacologic tables, 516t–517t
    antiparasitic agents, 458–492
    antiviral agents, 411–452
        pharmacologic tables, 518t–519t
    azalides: pharmacologic tables,
        512t–513t
    aztreonam, 266–268
    for bacterial vaginosis, 1079t,
        1079–1080
    β-lactam allergy, 272–278
    β-lactamase inhibitors, 268–270
    for bone marrow transplantation,
        2719
    for brain abscess, 893–895
    for bronchiolitis, 616
    for bronchitis
        acute, 607–608
        chronic, 611
    carbapenems, 264–266
    cephalosporins, 247–264
        pharmacologic tables, 508t–509t
    chloramphenicol, 310–314
        pharmacologic tables, 512t–513t
    clindamycin, 341–343
    combination therapy, 206–209
        adverse effects, 209
        antagonism, 208–209
        cost, 209
        decreased toxicity, 207
        disadvantages of inappropriate,
            208
        in impaired hosts, 208
        indications, 206
        initial therapy, 207

polymicrobial infections, 206–207
prevention of resistance, 206
for sepsis syndrome, 698, 699t
synergism, 208
in vitro results, 206, 207f
for cystic fibrosis, 659–660
determination of activity
    anaerobic bacteria, 195
    assays, 196–197
    bactericidal tests, 195–196
    β-lactamase test, 198
    bioassay, 197, 197f
    broth test, 195–196
    combination studies, 196, 196f
    dilution tests, 195
    disk diffusion, 195
    disk elution, 195
    E-test, 195
    high-pressure liquid chromatogra-
        phy, 197–198
    immunoassay, 197
    methods, 195
    selection of antimicrobials,
        193–195, 194t
    serum bactericidal test, 196
    susceptibility tests, 191–193
drug interactions, 520t–527t
for endocarditis, 760–764
    prophylaxis, 793–799
    prosthetic valve, 786t, 786–787
for esophagitis, 964t
fusidic acid, 278–279
    pharmacologic tables, 514t–515t
generic-trade names, 493t–499t
for granulocytopenics, 2680–2681
for immunocompromised host,
    2686–2691
immunomodulators, 450–458
    cimetidine, 455
    colony-stimulating factors,
        450–452
    glucocorticoids, 455
    immunoglobulins, 453–455
    inflammatory cytokine blockers,
        455
    interferons, 452–453
    interleukins, 453
    pentoxifylline, 455
    thymosin, 455–456
for infectious arthritis, 1037–1038
lincomycin, 341–343
lincosamides: pharmacologic tables,
    512t–513t
for lung abscess, 645–646
macrolides, 334–340
    pharmacologic tables, 512t–513t
for meningitis
    acute, 849–854
    chronic, 868
methenamine, 379–380
metronidazole, 329–334
    pharmacologic tables, 512t–513t
monobactams, 266
for neutrophil defects, 94
nitrofurantoin, 376–379
nosocomial pneumonia from use of,
    2601
for pelvic inflammatory disease, 1096,
    1096t
penicillins, 233–246
    pharmacologic tables, 506t–507t
perioperative prophylactic: for
    surgical wound prevention,
    2747–2748, 2749–2752
for peritonitis, 715–718

pharmacologic tables, 492–530. *See
    also* pharmacology *below*
    aminoglycosides, 510t–511t
    antifungal agents, 518t–519t
    antimycobacterials, 516t–517t
    antiviral agents, 518t–519t
    azalides, 512t–513t
    cephalosporins, 508t–509t
    chloramphenicol, 512t–513t
    drug interactions, 520t–527t
    fusidic acid, 514t–515t
    lincosamides, 512t–513t
    macrolides, 512t–513t
    metronidazole, 512t–513t
    other β-lactams, 510t–511t
    penicillins, 506t–507t
    polymyxins, 514t–515t
    quinolones, 516t–517t
    sulfonamides, 514t–515t
    teicoplanin, 514t–515t
    tetracyclines, 512t–513t
    trimethoprim, 514t–515t
    urinary tract agents, 516t–517t
    vancomycin, 514t–515t
pharmacology, 225–232. *See also*
    pharmacologic tables *above*
    aminoglycosides, 227–228
    antiretrovirals, 231–232
    β-lactams, 226–227
    drug exposure and response,
        225–232
    fluoroquinolones, 228–231
    optimal modes of administration,
        226
for pleural empyema, 640–641
for pneumonia
    acute, 631–632, 632t
    chronic, 653–656
    necrotizing, 645–646
polymyxins: pharmacologic tables,
    514t–515t
principles, 199–210
    choice of proper agent, 199–206
        age and, 201
        determination of susceptibility,
            200–201, 202t–203t
        genetic or metabolic abnormali-
            ties, 203
        identification of infective organ-
            ism, 200
        pregnancy, 204
        previous adverse reactions,
            201
        renal and hepatic function, 204t,
            204–205
        site of infection, 205–206
    choice of route of administration,
        209
    combination therapy, 206–209. *See
        also* combination therapy
        above
    monitoring patient response,
        209–210
for prostatitis, 681
for prosthetic joint infections,
    1054–1055
quinolones, 364–376
    pharmacologic tables, 516t–517t
resistance mechanisms, 212–225
    alteration of bacterial membranes,
        219
    alteration of cell wall precursor tar-
        gets, 220
    alteration of ribosomal target sites,
        220

Anti-infective therapy *(Continued)*
  alteration of target enzymes, 220
    β-lactams, 220
    quinolones, 221
    sulfonamides, 221
    trimethoprim, 221
  aminoglycoside enzymes, 218, 218t
  β-lactamases, 214–218. *See also*
    β-lactamases
  bypass of antibiotic inhibition, 221
  chloramphenicol acetyltransferase,
    218–219
  controlling, 221f, 221–222
  DNA integration elements, 214
  enzymatic inhibition, 214–218,
    215t
  erythromycin esterase, 219
  inner membrane permeability, 219
  major means, 215t
  molecular genetics, 212–214
  outer membrane permeability, 219
  plasmids, 212–213, 213f
  promotion of antibiotic efflux, 219
  transposable genetic elements,
    213–214, 214f
  rifamycins, 317–329
  for sepsis syndrome, 697–699, 699t
  for subdural empyema, 901–902, 902t
  sulfonamides, 354–357
    pharmacologic tables, 514t–515t
  for suppurative thrombophlebitis,
    766–767
  synergism: for sepsis syndrome, 698,
    699t
  teicoplanin, 351
    pharmacologic tables, 514t–515t
  tetracyclines, 306–310
    pharmacologic tables, 512t–513t
  topical antibacterials, 381–389
  topical antifungals, 401–403
  trade-generic names, 499t–505t
  for transplant recipients, 2714t,
    2714–2715
    bone marrow, 2721, 2721t
  for travelers to carry, 2796
  trimethoprim, 357–360
    pharmacologic tables, 514t–515t
  for urethritis, 1069–1070
  urinary tract agents, 376–381,
    516t–517t, 675–678
    pharmacologic tables, 516t–517t
  vancomycin, 346–350
    pharmacologic tables, 514t–515t
  for vulvovaginal candidiasis, 1076t,
    1076–1077
Anti-inflammatory agents: for bacterial
  meningitis, 854–856
Antilymphocyte serums: for transplantation, 2711
Antimalarial drugs, 2422–2425
  chemoprophylaxis, 2424t, 2424–2425
  chloroquine-resistant
    P. falciparum, 2424
    P. vivax, 2424–2425
    P. falciparum (chloroquine-suscep-
      tible), 2424, 2424t
    P. ovale, P. vivax and *P. malariae*,
      2424, 2424t
  mechanism of action, 2422
  in pregnancy, 2425–2426
  resistance, 2415, 2422–2424, 2423f,
    2424t
  in treatment, 2425–2426
  unique targets for, 2422
Antimony: for leishmaniasis, 130

Antimycobacterials, 389–400. *See also*
  individual drugs
  drug interactions, 520t–527t. *See also*
    individual drugs
  generic-trade names, 493t–499t
  for *Mycobacterium leprae*, 397–398,
    2248–2249
    acedapsone, 398
    adverse reactions, 399
    aminoglycosides, 2248
    clofazimine, 398
    dapsone, 397, 2248
    ethionamide, 398, 2248–2249
    newer agents, 2249
    prothionamide, 398, 2248–2249
    rifabutin, 398
    rifampin, 2248
    rifapentine, 398
    sulfoxone, 398–399
    thiacetazone, 398
  for *Mycobacterium tuberculosis*,
    389–395, 2226–2227
    amikacin, 394–395
    amithiozone, 395
    β-lactams, 395
    capreomycin, 394
    in childhood, 2229
    choice of regimen, 2227–2228
    course and observation, 2228
    cycloserine, 394
    ethambutol, 393, 2226, 2227
    ethionamide, 394
    first-line, 389–393, 2226
    in HIV/AIDS, 2228–2229
    and immunosuppresive therapy,
      2229
    isoniazid, 390–391, 2226, 2227
    kanamycin, 394, 395
    in liver disease, 2229
    nine-month regimen, 2227
    noncompliance, 2227
    para-aminosalicylic acid, 394
    in pregnancy, 2229
    pyrazinamide, 392–393, 2226
    quinolones, 395
    retreatment, 2228
    rifabutin, 392
    rifampin, 391–392, 2226, 2227
    second-line, 394–396, 2226–2227
    six-month regimen, 2227
    streptomycin, 393, 2226, 2227
    in uremia and end-stage renal
      disease, 2229
    vincomycin, 394, 395
  for nontuberculous (atypical)
    mycobacteria, 395–397, 396t
    aminoglycosides, 396
    clofazimine, 396
    isoniazid, 395
    macrolides, 396
    rifabutin, 395–396
    rifampin, 395–396
    sulfonamides, 396
    tetracyclines, 396
  pharmacologic tables, 516t–517t
  trade-generic names, 499t–505t
Antinuclear antibody
  and fever, 544
  test: for arthritis, 1037
Antiparasitic agents, 458–492. *See also*
  specific agents
  albendazole, 479–480
  allopurinol, 477
  allopurinol ribonucleoside, 477
  for amebae, 458, 467–468

  aminoquinolines, 469–472
  amocarzine, 482
  amphotericin B, 477–478
  for Apicomplexa, 469–476
  artemisinin, 472
  atovaquone, 475
  azithromycin, 475
  for *Balantidium coli*, 458, 467–468
  benznidazole, 477
  bithionol, 483
  for cestodes (tapeworms), 482–483
  chloroquine, 469–471
  cinchona alkaloids, 471
  clindamycin, 475
  dapsone, 474
  dehydroemetine, 468
  diethylcarbamazine, 481
  dihydrofolate reductase inhibitors, 474
  diloxanide furoate, 468
  doxycycline, 472
  eflornithine, 476
  emetine, 468
  Fansidar, 473–474
  Fansimef, 474
  flubendazole, 480
  furazolidone, 469
  halofantrine, 472–473
  hydroxynaphthoquinones, 475
  for intestinal flagellates, 458, 467–468
  for intestinal nematodes (round-
    worms), 478–481
  iodoquinol, 468
  ivermectin, 481–482
  ketoconazole, 477–478
  for luminal protozoa, 458, 467–468
  macrolide antibiotics, 475
  mebendazole, 478–479
  mefloquine, 471–472
  meglumine antimoniate, 477
  melarsoprol, 476
  metrifonate, 482–483
  metronidazole, 458, 467–468
  niclosamide, 483
  nifurtimox, 476–477
  niridazole, 483
  nitroimidazoles, 458, 468
  oxamniquine, 483
  paromomycin, 468
  pentamidine, 477
  pentavalent antimony, 477
  piperazine, 480–481
  for *Plasmodium*, 469–476
  for platyhelminths, 482–483
  praziquantel, 482
  primaquine, 470–471
  proguanil, 474–475
  pyrantel pamoate, 480
  pyrazolopyrimidines, 477
  pyrimethamine, 473–474
    combination therapy, 473–474
  pyrvinium pamoate, 480
  quinacrine, 469
  quinidine, 471
  quinine, 471
  4-quinoline-carbinolamines, 471–472
  roxithromycin, 475
  spiramycin, 475
  stibogluconate sodium, 477
  sulfonamides, 473–475
  suramin, 476–478
  for systemic nematodes, 481
  tetracycline, 472
  thiabendazole, 480
  for trematodes (flukes), 482–483
  trimethoprim-sulfamethoxazole, 474

  trimetrexate, 475
  for trypanosomatidae, 476–478
  for vaginal flagellates, 458, 467–468
Antipyretics, 533
Antiretrovirals. *See also specific drugs*
  pharmacology
    clinical trial data, 231–232, 232f
    in vitro and animal models, 231
Antiserum: for sepsis syndrome,
  701–702
Antistreptolysin O (ASO), 1786
  and arthritis, 1037
  and rheumatic fever, 1037
Anti-T-cell monoclonal antibodies:
  immunodeficiency from,
  136
Antithymocyte globulins
  immunodeficiency from, 136
  for transplantation, 2711
Antitoxins, 2771
Antiviral agents, 411–452. *See also*
  individual drugs
  acyclovir, 413–417
  administration, 411–413
  amantadine, 417–419
  combination therapy, 413
  didanosine, 419–421
  dosage, 412t
  drug interactions, 520t–527t. *See also*
    individual drugs
  famciclovir, 421–422
  foscarnet, 422–424
  ganciclovir, 424–426
  general principles, 411, 413
  generic-trade names, 493t–499t
  idoxuridine, 426
  for immunocompromised host: pro-
    phylactic, 2693
  interferons, 426–430
  investigative, 437, 437t
  mechanism of action, 411, 413
  penciclovir, 421–422
  pharmacologic tables, 518t–519t
  resistance, 411
  ribavirin, 430–431
  rimantadine, 417–419
  sorivudine, 431–432
  stavudine, 432
  topical administration, 413
  trade-generic names, 499t–505t
  valaciclovir, 413–417
  vidarabine, 433–434
  zalcitabine, 434–435
  zidovudine, 435–437
Aorta
  Salmonella infections, 2022
  Treponema pallidum, 2125
  tuberculosis, 2240
Aortic regurgitation: and endocarditis,
  765
Aortic valve
  bicuspid: and infective endocarditis,
    741
  infections, 741. *See also* Endocarditis,
    infective
Apalcillin: pharmacology, 506t–507t
Aphthous stomatitis, 602–603
Aphtovirus, 1637
Apicomplexa, 2393t. *See also specific*
  parasites
  antiparasitic agents, 459t, 469–476
Aplastic crisis, transient: parvovirus
  B19, 1441, 1442t, 1442–1443
  differential diagnosis, 1443
Apodemus: and hantaviruses, 1569

Apophysomyces, 2311t
mucormycosis, 2312
Appendicitis
actinomycosis and, 2283
anaerobic, 2163t, 2165
differential diagnosis, 728–729
and intra-abdominal abscess, 727–728
and intraperitoneal abscess, 721
Streptococcus intermedius, 1863
treatment, 727
Aprinocid: for *Toxoplasma gondii*, 2469
ARA-A. *See* Vidarabine
*Arachnia propionica. See Propionibac-
terium propionicus*
Arachnida, 2558
ARAM, 109
Arboviruses, 2558t. *See also specific
viruses*
differential diagnosis: enteroviral
meningitis, 1622
group A. *See* Alphaviruses
group B. *See* Flaviviruses
meningitis, 832
Arcanobacterium haemolyticum, 1872t,
1873–1874
pharyngitis, 567, 569, 1789, 1872t
treatment, 571
Archae, 1752
Archaebacteria, 1752
Arcobacter, 1948
Arcobacter butzleri, 1948
clinical manifestations, 1952
Arcobacter skirrowi, 1948
Arenaviridae, 1572–1579. *See also
Arenaviruses and specific
viruses*
classification, 1315t
shape and size, 1316f
Arenaviruses, 1572–1579. *See also individual viruses*
arthritis, 1036t
characteristics, 1572, 1573t
clinical manifestations, 1575–1576
diagnosis, 1576–1577
epidemiology and epizootology, 1572,
1574
intrauterine infection, 1576
pathogenesis, 1574–1575
humans, 1575
nonhuman primates, 1575
rodents, 1574–1575
prevention and treatment, 1577
Argas cooleyi: and Sixgun City virus,
1448
Argasidae, 2565
Argentine hemorrhagic fever
characteristics, 1573t
clinical manifestations, 1576
epidemiology, 1574
intrauterine infection, 1576
pathogenesis, 1575
prevention and treatment, 1577
ribavirin, 431
Arginine vasopressin: and fever reduction, 532
Argyll Robertson pupil, 2124, 2125
Arizona
mycotic aneurysms, 772
taxonomy, 2014
Arizona hinshawii
mycotic aneurysms, 772
snake bites, 2767
Armadillos: paracoccidioidomycosis in,
2386
Artemether: for *Plasmodium*, 2425

Artemisinin (qinghaosu), 459t, 472
for *Plasmodium*, 2425
for *Toxoplasma gondii*, 2469
Arterial catheters: bacteremia from,
2595–2596, 2596t
Arterial infections: *Salmonella*, 2022
Arteriovenous fistulas, dialysis-access:
infections, 790
Arteriovenous malformations, pulmonary: and brain abscess,
889
Arthralgia
parvovirus B19, 1439, 1440, 1442
differential diagnosis, 1443
rubella, 1461
and Whipple's disease, 1031
Arthritis
actinomycosis, 2285
acute bacterial, 1034–1035
clinical features, 1035, 1035f,
1035t
etiology, 1034t, 1035t
blastomycosis, 2359–2360
Borrelia burgdorferi, 1035, 2147
diagnosis, 1037
Brucella, 1035
Candida albicans, 1036, 2297
chlamydial, 1686
chronic monoarticular, 1035t,
1035–1036, 1036f
Haemophilus influenzae, 1034, 1034t,
1035, 2042
herpesviruses, 1334t
and HIV, 1228
infectious, 1032–1039
anaerobic gram-negative bacilli,
2200
antimicrobial therapy, 1037
aminoglycosides, 295t
approach to, 1037–1038
clinical features, 1032–1033, 1033f,
1033t
course, 1038
differential diagnosis, 1037
gram-negative anaerobes, 2200
laboratory findings, 1033
pathogenesis and predisposing factors, 1032, 1032t
pathology, 1034
radiology and imaging, 1033–1034
syndromes, 1034–1037
Neisseria gonorrhoeae, 1032, 1033,
1033f, 1034, 1035, 1918
diagnosis, 1037
and HIV, 1228
parasitic, 1037
parvovirus B19, 1439, 1440, 1442
postinfectious, 1032
reactive. *See* Reiter syndrome
rubella, 1461
Salmonella, 2023–2024
reactive, 2024
septic
in the elderly, 2741
Serratia, 1972
Streptococcus agalactiae, 1839
Streptococcus pneumoniae, 1821
Staphylococcus aureus, 1773–1774
streptococcal, group C and G, 1854
Streptococcus agalactiae, 1840
tuberculous, 2237
viral, 1036–1037
etiology, 1036t
Arthroderma, 2375
Arthropathy: from quinolones, 374

Arthroplasty: prophylaxis recommendations, 2751t
Arthropods, 2558
diseases borne by, 2558t, 2791t–2792t.
See also specific diseases
reservoirs, 2792t, 2794
Arthus reaction: β-lactams, 272
ART test, 2127, 2127t
Arylsulfatase, 79t
Asbestosis pneumonia, 648
Ascaris lumbricoides, 2525t, 2528–2529
clinical syndromes, 2529
diagnosis, 1006, 1006t, 2529
epidemiology, 2529
life cycle, 2528f, 2528–2529
pneumonia, 619t, 631
treatment, 461t, 2529
albendazole, 479
mebendazole, 478–479
piperazine, 480
pyrantel pamoate, 480
Aschoff's nodule, 1801
Ascites
culture-negative neutrocytic, 708
peritonitis, 708
Aspartate aminotransferase (AST):
hepatitis, 1139, 1140f
Aspergilloma, 2307, 2307f
Aspergillus, 2306–2311
appearance in tissue, 2289t
and bone marrow transplantation, 2719
brain abscess, 2308
in the immunocompromised, 890
and CGD, 155
chemoprophylaxis, 2309
and chronic granulomatous disease,
92
clinical manifestations, 2307–2309
CNS, 2308
cutaneous, 2308, 2308f
diagnosis, 2309, 2309f
ear, 2307
encephalitis, 876
endocarditis, 757, 2308
diagnosis, 751
treatment, 764
endophthalmitis, 1123, 2307
in drug abusers, 2704–2705
treatment, 1126
epidemiology, 2306
epidural abscess, 905
eye, 2307
and granulocytopenia, 2676–2677
granulomatous hepatitis, 1161
in HIV/AIDS, 2309
host defense, 2306
hyphae, 2307, 2307f
and immunodeficiency, 150t
Job syndrome and, 156
keratitis, 1113
lacrimal sac infection, 1131
lung, 2307–2308, 2308f
mycotic aneurysms, 772
myocarditis, 800
orbital cellulitis, 1132, 1133
otitis, 580, 2307
paranasal sinus, 1134
pathology, 2306–2307, 2307f
pericarditis, 805
pneumonia, 619t, 631, 2307–2308
chronic, 647t
and granulocytopenia, 2678
in HIV/AIDS, 1236
nosocomial in the immunocompromised, 631

radiology, 650t, 655f
in transplant recipients, 2727t
serology, 193t
sinusitis, 586t, 2307
in the immunocompromised, 1132
symmetric peripheral gangrene, 553
in transplant recipients, 2712, 2723,
2728
treatment, 2309
amphotericin B, 406
wound infections: in trauma patients,
2758
Aspergillus amstelodami, 2306
Aspergillus avenaceus, 2306
Aspergillus caesiellus, 2306
Aspergillus candidus, 2306
Aspergillus carneus, 2306
Aspergillus clavatus, 2306
Aspergillus flavus, 2306
in cancer patients, 2668
diagnosis, 2309f
hypertrophic spinal pachymeningitis,
906
and leukemia, 2672
serology, 193t
Aspergillus fumigatus, 2306. *See also
Aspergillus*
in cancer patients, 2668
and cystic fibrosis, 659, 660
serology, 193t
sputum, 176f, 2309
Aspergillus nidulans, 2327, 2330
Aspergillus niger, 193t
Aspergillus oryzae, 2306
Aspergillus restrictus, 2306
Aspergillus sydowi, 2306
Aspergillus terreus, 2306
Aspergillus ustus, 2306
Aspergillus versicolor, 2306
Aspiration: and lung abscess, 642
Aspiration pneumonia, 630, 648
radiology, 650t
Aspirin
for fever, 533, 547
hepatotoxicity, 1148
Assam fever, 2431–2434
Asterixis: hepatic encephalopathy, 1139
Asthma
Chlamydia pneumoniae and, 1698
rhinovirus and, 1659
Astrocytes: HIV and, 1204
Astroviruses, 1672–1674
clinical manifestations, 1673
diagnosis and treatment, 1673
epidemiology, 1673, 1673t
pathogenesis, 1673
virology, 1672, 1673f
winter vomiting disease, 969
Ataxia-telangiectasia, 50, 52–53, 134t,
151t
diagnosis, 153
immunoglobulin for, 454
Atevirdine/detavirdine, 437t
Atherosclerosis: *Chlamydia pneumoniae*
and, 1699–1700
Athlete's foot, 2378
Atovaquone, 459t, 475
for *Pneumocystis carinii*, 475, 1283t,
1284, 1286, 2481
structure, 475f
for *Toxoplasma gondii*: in HIV/AIDS,
2467, 2467t
Atrial myxomas: and fever, 544
Atrioventricular block: *Borrelia
burgdorferi*, 2148

Attributable risk, 160
Auchmeromyia, 2562
Augmentin. *See* Amoxicillin-clavulanate
Auramine-rhodamine stain, 184t
Autoantibodies, 42
Autoclave, 2579
Autoclave tape, 2579
Autoimmune diseases. *See also specific diseases*
    antibody deficiencies and, 49
    and fever, 544t, 544–545
    hepatitis, 1157t, 1157–1158
Avipoxvirus, 1325
Axillary lymphadenitis, acute, 936
Azalides: pharmacologic tables, 512t–513t
Azathioprine
    immunodeficiency from, 136
    and infection susceptibility, 2668–2669, 2711
Azidothymidine. *See* Zidovudine
Azithromycin, 334, 338–340
    adverse reactions, 340
    antimicrobial activity, 339
    antiparasitic use, 475
    for *Chlamydia trachomatis*, 1688
    for *Cryptosporidium*, 2507
    dosage, 512t–513t
    drug interactions, 340, 520t
    for *Haemophilus ducreyi* (chancroid), 2048
    for *Legionella pneumophila*, 2093, 2093t
    mechanism of action, 339
    for *Mycobacterium avium-intracellulare*, 2258
    for *Mycoplasma pneumoniae*, 1710, 1710t
    for *Neisseria gonorrhoeae*, 1921, 1921t
    for nontuberculous mycobacteria, 396
    pharmacology, 339–340, 512t–513t
    resistance, 339
    structure, 339f
    for *Toxoplasma gondii*: in HIV/AIDS, 2467, 2467t
    for urethritis, 1070
    uses, 340
Azlocillin, 245
    for bacilli and anaerobes, 237t
    clinical trials, 230–231
    combination therapy
        aminoglycosides, 289t
        synergism, 207
    dosage, 241t, 506t–507t
        in neonates, 242t, 507t
        in renal disease, 238t, 507t
    for Enterobacteriaceae and *Pseudomonas*, 237t
    MICs against cocci, 237t
    pharmacokinetics, 238t
    pharmacology, 506t–507t
    structure, 244f
    susceptibility testing, 194t
Azoles, 401
Azotemia: from amphotericin B, 405
AZT. *See* Zidovudine
Aztreonam, 266–268
    adverse reactions, 267
    with aminoglycosides, 287t
    antimicrobial activity, 285t
    clinical use, 267–268
    dosage, 510t–511t
        in children and neonates, 510t
        for meningitis, 850t
        in renal insufficiency, 511t

drug interactions, 520t
    for meningitis, 850t, 853
    for peritonitis, 716–717
    pharmacokinetics, 267, 510t–511t
    pharmacology, 510t–511t
    for Pseudomonads, 2004t
    for *Pseudomonas aeruginosa*, 267, 1994
        endocarditis, 1984
        meningitis, 1989
    for pyelonephritis, 676
    for *Salmonella*, 2026
    for sepsis syndrome, 699, 699t
    structure, 266f
    susceptibility testing, 194, 194t
    in vitro activity, 267, 267t
Azurophil granules, 79, 79t, 86, 87–88

B

Babesia, 2394t, 2497–2500
    animal reservoirs, 2791, 2792t
    clinical manifestations, 2394t, 2498–2499
    and complement, 66
    description, 2497–2498
    diagnosis, 2394t, 2499, 2499f
    differential diagnosis: ehrlichiosis, 1750
    enteric symptoms, 1000t
    epidemiology, 2498
    and fever, 543
    pathogenesis, 2499
    prevention, 2499–2500
    transmission, 2394t, 2627
    treatment, 2499–2500
Babesia bigemina, 2497
Babesia bovis, 2497, 2498
Babesia canis, 2497
Babesia divergens, 2497, 2498, 2499
Babesia equi, 2497
Babesia felis, 2497
Babesia major, 2497
Babesia microti, 2497
    clinical manifestations, 2498–2499
    description, 2498
    diagnosis, 2499f
    enteric symptoms, 1003
    epidemiology, 2498
    fever, 543
    transfusion-related, 2627
    transmission, 2791
    treatment, 461t, 2499–2500
Babesia rodhaini, 2498
Bacampicllin: pharmacology, 506t–507t
Bacillary angiomatosis, 1741, 1742–1744. *See also Rochalimaea henselae* and *Rochalimaea quintana*
    cutaneous, 1742–1743, 1743f
    diagnosis, 1229
    and HIV/AIDS, 557–558, 920, 939, 1229, 1743, 1743f
        treatment, 1283t, 1290
    lymphadenitis, 939
    rash, 557
    rDNA sequencing, 28
Bacillary dysentery, 987–988, 2033–2039. *See also Shigella*
Bacillary epithelioid angiomatosis. *See* Bacillary angiomatosis
Bacillary peliosis, 1741, 1743
Bacilli. *See also* Gram-negative bacilli; Gram-positive bacilli
    classification, 1752

Bacillus, 1890–1894
    bacteremia and septicemia, 1892–1893
    endocarditis, 1892
    ocular infections, 1891, 1892f
    pneumonia, 1892
    quinolones for, 368t
    soft tissue and musculoskeletal infections, 1893
Bacillus abortus. *See Brucella abortus*
Bacillus abortus var. *lipolyticus*. *See Corynebacterium bovis*
Bacillus alvei, 1890t
    pneumonia, 1892
Bacillus anthracis, 1885–1889
    animal reservoirs, 2792t
    chancriform lesions, 913, 913f
    clinical manifestations, 913, 1887–1888
    control and prevention, 1888–1889
    cutaneous, 913, 913f, 1887, 1888
    diagnosis, 1888
    edema factor, 3t, 6, 22t
    epidemiology, 1886
    gastrointestinal, 999t, 1002, 1888, 1889
    history, 1885–1886
    immunization, 1889
    lethal factor, 3t, 6, 22t
    lymphadenitis, 940t
    meningitis, 1888
    microbiology, 1886, 1887f
    pathogenesis, 913, 1887
    pathology, 1888
    and pneumonia, 622t
    protective antigen, 3t, 6, 22t
    respiratory, 1887–1888
    serology, 1888
    skin lesions, 913, 913f
    toxin, 3t, 4, 6, 1887
    transmission, 164
    treatment, 913, 1889
        erythromycin, 338
        sulfonamides, 355t
    vaccines, 1889, 2774
    virulence determinants, 22t
Bacillus anthracoides, 1890t
    meningitis, 1893
Bacillus cereus, 1890, 1890t
    cereolysin, 1890
    clinical manifestations, 1890–1891
    cutaneous: in the immunocompromised, 920
    diarrhea: diagnosis, 180
    diarrheal toxin, 1890
    emetic toxin, 1890
    endophthalmitis, 1121, 1125
        in drug abusers, 2705
    enterotoxin, 950, 1013, 1890
    epidemiology, 1890
    food-borne, 1012t, 1013, 1016, 1020, 1891
        foods implicated, 1017t
        laboratory diagnosis, 1018, 1018t, 1891
    keratitis, 1113
    loop fluid-inducing/skin test/necrotic toxin, 1890
    meningitis, 1893
    neurotoxin, 949t, 949–950
    ocular infections, 1891, 1892f
    phosphatidylcholine hydrolase, 1890
    pneumonia, 1892
    soft tissue and musculoskeletal infections, 1893
    specimen collection, 180

Bacillus circulans, 1890t
    meningitis, 1893
Bacillus laterosporus, 1890t
Bacillus licheniformis, 1890
    food poisoning, 1891
Bacillus megaterium, 1890, 1890t
    meningitis, 1893
Bacillus perfringens. *See Clostridium botulinum*
Bacillus polymyxa, 385, 1890
Bacillus pseudodiphtheriticum. *See Corynebacterium pseudodiphthericum*
Bacillus pumilus, 1890t
Bacillus sphaericus, 1890t
    meningitis, 1893
    pneumonia, 1892
Bacillus stearothermophilus: and heat sterilization, 2579, 2580, 2580f
Bacillus subtilis, 1890, 1890t
    food poisoning, 1891
    and heat sterilization, 2579, 2580f
    meningitis, 1893
    ocular infections, 1891
    pathogenicity, 23
    respiratory infections, 1893
    var. *niger*: and heat sterilization, 2579
Bacitracin, 382, 383–384
    for antibiotic-associated colitis, 983, 984
    drug interactions, 520t
    spectrum of activity, 383–384
BACTEC system
    for mycobacteria, 2214
    for *Mycobacterium avium-intracellulare*, 2253
    nonradiometric, 177
    for tuberculosis, 189–190, 192
Bacteremia. *See also* Septicemia
    Acinetobacter, 2011
    Aeromonas, 2108
    aminoglycosides for, 295t
    anaerobic, 2163t, 2165
        cocci, 2205
        gram-negative bacilli, 2199
    Bacillus, 1892–1893
    and bone marrow transplantation, 2719
    burn wounds, 2763
    Campylobacter, 1951–1952
    and cell-mediated immune defects, 2681
    Clostridium, 2184
    complement and, 72
    defined, 690, 690t
    in the elderly, 2739–2740
    and endocarditis, 743
    enterococcal, 1828
    Erysipelothrix, 1895
    Escherichia coli, 1971–1972
    Flavobacterium, 2113
    Francisella tularensis, 2063
    Haemophilus influenzae, 2042
    intravascular devices, source, 2587–2599
        arterial lines, 2595–2596, 2596t
        central venous catheters, 2592
            long-term, 2594t, 2594–2595
        contamination
            of infusate, 2587
            at insertion site, 2588t, 2588–2589, 2589t
            at junction, 2587

device-specific issues, 2591–2596
diagnosis, 2590f, 2590t, 2590–2591
microbiology, 2589t, 2589–2590
pathogenesis, 2587–2589, 2588f
peripheral IV cannulization, 2591t,
   2591–2592
prevention, 2596
pulmonary artery catheters, 2595
total parenteral nutrition,
   2592–2594, 2593t
transducer domes, 2595–2596
transducers, 2595
in traumatized patient, 2758
Listeria, 1881
meningitis, 838
Neisseria meningitidis, 1900
Pasteurella, 2069
peritonitis, 708
Pseudomonas aeruginosa,
   1987–1988
   treatment, 1987–1988
Salmonella, 2022
and HIV/AIDS, 2027–2028
therapy, 2027
Salmonella choleraesuis, 2022
Serratia, 1972
and skin infections, 921–922
   Haemophilus influenzae, 921–922
   Neisseria gonorrhoeae, 921
   Neisseria meningitidis, 921
   Pseudomonas aeruginosa, 921
   Salmonella typhi, 921
   Staphylococcus aureus, 921
specimen collection and processing,
   177–178
in spinal cord injured patients, 2736
Staphylococcus epidermidis
   in the immunocompromised, 1781
   nosocomial, 1778–1779
streptococcal
   group C and G, 1855–1856
   viridans, 1849
Streptococcus agalactiae
   adult, 1839
   neonatal, 1838
Streptococcus intermedius group,
   1862–1863
Streptococcus pyogenes, 1796–1797
in transplant recipients, 2726–2727
in trauma patients, 2757t
Bacteria
classification, 1752–1753
growth or biochemical characteristics
   anaerobic, 189
   facultative anaerobic, 185, 189
   gram-negative bacilli, 188f, 189
   gram-negative cocci, 188f, 189
   gram-positive bacilli, 186, 189
   gram-positive cocci, 186
   overview, 1752–1754
Bacterial diseases, 1752–2288. *See also*
      specific genera and species
Achromobacter, 2110–2111
Acinetobacter, 2009–2013
Actinobacillus, 2106–2107
Actinomyces, 2280–2288
Aeromonas, 2107–2108
Agrobacterium, 2111
Alcaligenes, 2111–2112
   xylosoxidans subsp. *xylosoxidans*,
      2111
anaerobes, 2156–2209. *See also*
      Anaerobic bacteria
   cocci, 2204–2206
   general concepts, 2156–2173

gram-negative bacilli, 2195–2204
gram-positive bacilli, 2206–2208
animal bites, 2765t, 2766–2767
arthritis, 1034–1035
Bacillus, 1890–1894
   anthracis, 1885–1889
Bacteroides, 2195–2204
Bartonella bacilliformis, 2209–2210
Bifidobacterium, 2207
in blood. *See* Bacteremia
and bone marrow transplantation,
   2718–2719
Bordetella, 2078–2084
Borrelia
   burgdorferi (Lyme disease),
      2143–2155
   relapsing fever, 2141–2143
Brucella, 2053–2060
burn wounds, 2762–2763
   treatment, 2763–2764, 2764t
Calymmatobacterium granulomatosis,
   2210–2213
Campylobacter, 1948–1956
Capnocytophaga, 2103–2106
Cardiobacterium, 2108–2109
CDC group DF-3, 2109–2110
CDC group EF-4, 2110
CDC group IVc-2, 2112
and cell-mediated immune defects,
   2681
Chromobacterium, 2109
Citrobacter, 1974
Clostridium
   botulinum, 2178–2182
   difficile, 2189–2192
   gas gangrene, 2182–2195
   perfringens, 2182–2189
   tetani, 2173–2178
conjunctivitis, 1104t, 1104–1105
Corynebacterium, 1872–1876
   diphtheriae, 1865–1872
cutaneous manifestations, 550t
cytokine and T cell protection, 121t
Edwardsiella, 1974
Eikenella, 2112
endophthalmitis, 1121t, 1121–1122
Enterobacter, 1973
Enterobacteriaceae, 1964–1980. *See
   also* Enterobacteriaceae
enterococcal, 1826–1831
Erwinia, 1975
Erysipelothrix rhusiopathiae,
   1894–1896
Escherichia coli, 1969–1972
Eubacterium, 2207
and fever, 541–542
Flavimonas (CDC group Ve-2),
   2112–2113
Flavobacterium, 2113
Francisella tularensis, 2060–2068
Fusobacterium, 2195–2204
Gardnerella vaginalis, 2050–2051
gram-negative bacilli, 1934–2117.
      See also Gram-negative
      bacilli
   anaerobic, 2195–2204
gram-negative cocci, 1896–1934. *See
      also* Gram-negative cocci
gram-positive bacilli, 1865–1896. *See
      also* Gram-positive bacilli *and
      individual organisms*
gram-positive cocci, 1754–1865. *See
      also* Gram-positive cocci *and
      individual organisms*
and granulocytopenia, 2676

Haemophilus, 2045–2050
   influenzae, 2039–2045
Hafnia, 1973
Helicobacter pylori, 1956–1964
keratitis, 1111t, 1112–1113
Klebsiella, 1972–1973
Lactobacillus, 2207–2208
Legionella, 2097–2103
   pneumophila, 2087–2097
Leptospira, 2137–2141
and leukemia/lymphoma, 2676, 2676t,
   2681
Listeria monocytogenes, 1880–1885
meningitis. *See* Bacterial meningitis
Mobiluncus, 2051–2052, 2208
Moraxella, 1926–1928
mycobacterial, 2213–2273
   avium-intracellulare, 2250–2264
   haemophilum, 2269
   kansasii, 2266–2268
   leprae, 2243–2250
   malmoense, 2269
   marinum, 2268
   rapidly growing, 2269–2270
   scrofulaceum, 2268
   simiae, 2268
   szulgai, 2268–2269
   tuberculosis, 2213–2243
   ulcerans, 2269
   xenopi, 2269
myocarditis, 800, 800t
Neisseria, 1928–1930, 1929t
   gonorrhoeae, 1909–1926
   meningitidis, 1896–1909
Nocardia, 2273–2280
Ochrobactrum, 2113–2114
Oligella, 2113
orchitis, 1101
overview, 1752–1754
Pasteurella, 2068–2070
pathogenicity, 1753
pericarditis, 805t, 805–806
Plesiomonas shigelloides, 2110
Prevotella, 2195–2204
Propionibacterium, 2207
prostatitis
   acute, 1099, 1099t
   chronic, 1099, 1099t
Proteus, 1974
Protomonas, 2114
Pseudomonas, 2003–2009
   aeruginosa, 1980–2003
   cepacia, 2007–2008
   mallei, 2006–2007
   pseudomallei, 2004–2006
pulmonary disease: HIV/AIDS and,
   1234–1235, 1235t
Rhodococcus, 1876–1877
Rothia dentocariosa, 2208
Salmonella, 2013–2033
serologic tests, 192t
Serratia marcescens, 1973
Shigella, 2033–2039
Sphingobacterium, 2114
Spirillum minus, 2155–2156
spirochetes, 2117–2156. *See also*
      Spirochetes
staphylococcal
   S. aureus, 1754–1777
   S. epidermidis and other coagulase-
      negative organisms, 1777–1784
Streptobacillus moniliformis,
   2084–2086
streptococcal
   classification, 1784–1785

enterococci, 1826–1831
glomerulonephritis, 1805–1808
group C, 1852–1856
group G, 1853–1856
intermedius group, 1754–1865
Leuconostoc, 1832
rheumatic fever, 1799–1805
S. agalactiae (group B), 1835–1845
S. bovis, 1832
S. pneumoniae, 1785t, 1811–1826
S. pyogenes, 1786–1799
viridans, 1845–1851
transfusion-related, 2627–2628
in transplant recipients, 2712t
Treponema carateum (pinta), 2133,
   2135–2136
Treponema pallidum
   subsp. *endemicum* (bejel; endemic
      syphilis), 2133, 2136–2137
   subsp. *pallidum* (syphilis),
      2117–2133
   subsp. *pertenue* (yaws), 2133–2135
in urine. *See* Bacteriuria
vaginosis. *See* Bacterial vaginosis
Vibrio, 1934–1948
   cholerae, 1934–1945
   parahaemolyticus, 1945–1946
Weeksella, 2114
Yersinia, 2070–2078
   enterocolitica, 2076–2078
   pestis, 2070–2076
   pesudotuberculosis, 2076–2078
zoonoses, 2791t
Bacterial membranes: alterations of,
   219
Bacterial meningitis, 833t, 834t,
   834–835
adjunctive therapy, 854–856
antimicrobial therapy, 849t, 850t,
   850–853
bacteremia, 838
blood-brain barrier alterations, 839
cerebral blood flow alterations,
   841–842
clinical presentation, 843, 843t
CSF examination, 845t, 846, 846t
diagnosis, 845t, 846, 846t
increased intracranial pressure, 841
management
   anti-inflammatory agents, 854–856
   initial, 848f, 849
   reduction of intracranial pressure,
      856
   surgical intervention, 856
meningeal invasion, 838–839
pathogenesis and pathophysiology,
   837f, 837–842, 838t
prevention, 857–858
radiography, 846, 847f
subarachnoid space inflammation,
   840t, 840–841
Bacterial overgrowth syndromes,
   972–973
and tropical sprue, 1026, 1027f
Bacterial vaginosis, 1078f, 1078–1080,
   2050–2051. *See also*
      Gardnerella vaginalis
complications, 1080
epidemiology, 1078–1079
features, 1075t
pathophysiology, 1079
and posthysterectomy infections, 1094
treatment, 1079t, 1079–1080
Bactericidal permeability increasing
   (BPI) protein, 87

Bactericidal tests, 195–196
Bacteriocins, 7, 30
Bacterium actinomycetem comitans. See Actinobacillus actinomycem-comitans
Bacterium lipolyticus. See Corynebacterium bovis
Bacterium tularense. See Francisella tularensis
Bacteriuria. *See also* Urinary tract infections
   in adults, 668
   asymptomatic, 662
   in children, 668
   defined, 662
   in the elderly, 668, 2737
   in pregnancy, 678–680
   presumptive diagnosis, 669–670
   prevention, 2611–2612
   screening tests, 176
   significant, 662
   suprapubic aspiration, 175
   treatment: methenamine, 380, 2612
Bacteroides, 2158t, 2195–2201. *See also individual species*
   and actinomycosis, 2280
   animal bites, 2767
   antimicrobial susceptibility, 2170t
   bacteremia, 2165, 2199
   brain abscess, 2197
   clenched-fist injuries, 2768
   clinically significant, 2159t
   complement and, 2197
   as enteric flora, 947
   enzymes, 2197
   epidermal cysts, 920
   head and neck infections, 2164
   hepatic abscess, 724
   human bites, 2768
   immunity, 2197
   intra-abdominal infections, 2198–2199
   lung abscess, 644
      treatment, 645
   mediastinitis, 815t
   necrotizing fasciitis, 923
   oral cavity infections, 2198
   oral colonization, 593, 594t
   pleuropulmonary infection, 2164
   pneumonia, 619t
   resistance, 2197
   sinusitis, 585t, 2198
   suppurative thrombophlebitis, 769
   synergistic necrotizing cellulitis, 926
   treatment, 2170t
      fusidic acid, 278
      quinolones, 368t
   vaginal flora, 1074
   and vaginosis, 1079
   virulence, 2196, 2197, 2197t
Bacteroides bile esculin (BBE agar), 2168
Bacteroides bivius: postpartum endometritis, 1091
Bacteroides caccae, 2195t
Bacteroides distasonis, 2195t
   intra-abdominal infections, 2199
   metronidazole for, 329
Bacteroides forsythus, 2195t, 2196
Bacteroides fragilis, 2162, 2195t, 2195–2201
   after gynecologic surgery, 1093–1094
   antimicrobial susceptibility, 2170t
   bacteremia, 2165, 2199
   β-lactamase, 215, 216t

brain abscess, 889
cellular immunity and, 128
characteristics, 2196t
cholangitis, 732
cholecystitis, 730
   treatment, 731
clinically significant types, 2195t
decubitus ulcer infections, 919
endocarditis, 756, 2199
   treatment, 763–764
enterotoxin, 950
identification, 189
incidence, 2162
intra-abdominal infections, 2165, 2198–2199
intraperitoneal abscess, 721
lipopolysaccharide, 2162
lung abscess, 644, 645
meningitis, 2197
mycotic aneurysms, 772
as normal flora, 2159t, 2196
and normal physiology, 2160
osteomyelitis, 2200
pathogenesis, 2196
pelvic abscess, 1095
peritonitis, 710–711, 711–712
   treatment, 716
resistance, 220, 255, 2197
septic arthritis, 2200
skin infections, 2199
snake bites, 2767
soft tissue infections, 2166, 2199
subdural empyema, 900
succinic acid, 2197
superoxide dismutase, 2197
surgical wound infections, 2745, 2746, 2747t
taxonomy, 2195, 2195t
treatment, 285t, 2170t, 2200t, 2200–2201
   antimicrobials of choice, 201t
   azithromycin, 335t
   β-lactamase inhibitors, 268t
   carbapenems, 264t
   cephalosporins, 255t, 257, 258, 259
   clarithromycin, 335t
   clindamycin, 341t, 341–342, 343
   erythromycin, 335t
   fusidic acid, 278
   metronidazole, 329, 329t, 332
   mezlocillin, 245
   penicillins, 237t
   quinolones, 368t
   rifampin, 324
   tetracyclines, 308t
   trimethoprim, 357
virulence, 2196, 2197, 2197t
Bacteroides gingivalis. See Porphyromonas
Bacteroides gracilis, 2195t
   antimicrobial susceptibility, 2170t
   incidence, 2162
   treatment, 2170t, 2200
Bacteroides heparinolyticus, 2767
Bacteroides intermedius. See Prevotella intermedia
Bacteroides melaninogenicus
   metronidazole for, 329t
   pathology, 2161
Bacteroides oralis: endocarditis, 756
Bacteroides ovatus, 2195t
   virulence, 2196
Bacteroides thetaiotaomicron, 2195t
   incidence, 2162

intra-abdominal infections, 2165, 2199
   resistance, 2197
Bacteroides uniformis, 2195t
Bacteroides urealyticus, 2112, 2195t
   oral cavity infections, 2198
   pleuropulmonary infections, 2198
Bacteroides vulgatus, 2195t
   intra-abdominal infections, 2199
Bactisubtil: and *Bacillus* bacteremia, 1893
Baghdad boil, 2434–2435
Bairnsdale ulcers, 2269
Balanitis
   Candida albicans, 2293
   circinate: Reiter syndrome, 1072
   etiology, 1059
   and HIV transmission, 1188
Balantidium coli, 2394, 2511
   dysentery, 987, 989
   diagnosis, 990
   transmission, 2394t
   treatment, 458, 461t, 467–468
   metronidazole, 332
Bamle disease, 1625–1626
Bancroftian filariasis, 2533–2535
Bannwarth syndrome, 2143, 2148
Banzi: transmission, clinical syndromes, and geographic distribution, 1466t
Bare lymphocyte syndrome, 134t
Barium enema
   and endocarditis, 743t, 794t
   for enteric infection diagnosis, 955
Barmah Forest virus: arthritis, 1036
Bartholin cyst abscess: anaerobic gram-negative bacilli, 2199
Bartholinitis, 1085
   Chlamydia trachomatis, 1069
Bartholin's gland, 1085
Bartonella: and *Salmonella*, 2019
Bartonella bacilliformis, 1742, 2209–2210
   clinical manifestations, 2209–2210
   cutaneous manifestations, 550t, 558
   description, 2209
   enteric symptoms, 999t, 1002
   epidemiology, 2209
   Oroya fever, 2209–2210
   pathogenesis, 2209
   prevention and treatment, 2210
   verruga peruana, 2209, 2210
Bartonella elizabethae, 1741, 1745
Bartonella henselae, 1741–1747
   and bacillary angiomatosis, 1741, 1742–1743, 1743f
   and bacillary peliosis, 1741, 1743
   blood cultures, 178
   cat scratch disease, 1310–1311, 1744. *See also* Cat scratch disease
   fever, 542, 543
   and HIV/AIDS, 543, 920, 1229
   lymphadenitis, 938–939, 940t
   classification, 1741, 1742f
   clinical manifestations, 1743f, 1743–1744, 1744f
   conjunctivitis, 1105
   cutaneous manifestations, 550t, 557–558, 920, 1742–1743, 1743f
   diagnosis
      microbiologic, 1744–1745, 1745f
      noncultural, 1745–1746
   differential diagnosis, 1742
   epidemiology, 1741–1742

and HIV/AIDS, 1743, 1743f
   cat scratch disease, 543, 920, 1229
   differential diagnosis, 1742
   treatment, 1746
   in HIV/AIDS, 1283t, 1290
Bartonella quintana, 1741–1747
   classification, 1741, 1742f
   clinical manifestations, 1720t, 1743f, 1743–1744, 1744f
   cutaneous manifestations, 550t, 557–558, 920, 1742–1743, 1743f
   diagnosis
      microbiologic, 1744–1745, 1745f
      noncultural, 1745–1746
   differential diagnosis, 1742
   epidemiology, 1741–1742
   treatment, 1746
   in HIV/AIDS, 1283t, 1290
Bartonella vinsonii, 1741
Bartonellosis, 2209–2210. *See also Bartonella bacilliformis*
Basal cell carcinoma: differential diagnosis, 2437
Basidiobolus, 2311t, 2317–2319
Basidiobolus haptosporus, 2317
Basilar skull fracture meningitis: antibiotic prophylaxis, 857–858
Battey bacillus. *See Mycobacterium avium-intracellulare*
Bayliascaris procyonis, 2556
   treatment, 461t
Bazin's disease, 2240
B7/BB1, 108–109
B-cell lymphomas
   EBV and, 1370
   HIV and, 1601–1602
B cells
   abnormalities: and HIV, 1209–1210
   allelic exclusion, 48
   antibody production, 36. *See also* Antibodies
   antigen presentation, 36
   B1, 49
   B7 marker, 45t
   cytokines and, 117, 119–120
   deficiencies, 133, 151t, 153. *See also specific deficiencies*
   developmental stages, 46f
   immature stage, 48
   isotypic exclusion, 48
   mature, 48
   and MHC II, 104
   pre-, 48
   receptor complex, 45–47
   surface molecules, 45, 45t
   T cells and, 119–120
   tolerance, 48, 49
   VDJ joining, 48
BCG-osis: granulomatous hepatitis, 1161
   mycobacteriosis, 2231
BCG vaccine, 167, 2231, 2774
   adverse reactions, 2774
   ant tuberculin test, 2219
   and granulomatous hepatitis, 1161
   indications for adults, 2784t
   for leprosy, 2247
   for travelers, 2799
Beau's lines, 2567
Bebaru virus, 1457
Beef tapeworm, 2525t, 2547. *See also Taenia saginata*

Behçet's disease
  genital lesions, 1057
  meningitis, 871
  pharyngitis, 569
Bejel (endemic syphilis), 2133,
  2136–2137
Bell's palsy
  Borrelia burgdorferi and, 2148
  HSV and, 1341
Benzathine penicillin, 240
Benznidazole, 459t, 475, 477
  dosage, 467t
  for *Trypanosoma cruzi*, 2447–2448
Benzodiazepines: for *Clostridium tetani*,
  2176, 2177
Benzoic acid, 401
Benzoxazinorifamycins, 324
Benzoyl peroxide, 382, 384t
Benzylpenicillin G. *See* Penicillin G
Benzylpenicillin skin test, 275, 276
β-lactamases
  anaerobic bacteria, 215
  Bush classification, 215t
  and cephalosporins, 250–251
  contribution to β-lactam antibiotic
    resistance, 218
  determined by chromosomal genes,
    217–218
  distribution in clinical isolates, 217
  enzymatic inhibition, 214–218
  extended-spectrum (ESBL), 251
  gram-negative bacteria, 215, 215t
  gram-positive bacteria, 215
  inhibition by β-lactam inhibitors, 268t
  inhibitors, 268–270. *See also specific*
    formulations
  properties of plasmid-determined, 216t
  Pseudomonas aeruginosa, 215, 216t,
    218, 268
  and resistance, 214–218
    to cephalosporins, 250–251
  Staphylococcus aureus, 1759
  tests, 198
β-lactams. *See also* Cephalosporins;
    Penicillin(s) *and specific*
    drugs
  allergy, 272–278
    amoxicillin, 275–276
    ampicillin, 275–276
    classification of reactions, 272–273
    desensitization, 276, 276t
    diagnosing, 275
    Gell and Combs classification, 272,
      273t
    idiopathic reactions, 272–273
    Levine classification, 273
    penicillins, 275–276
    risk factors, 274–275
    type II (cytotoxic antibodies), 272
    type III (immune complexes), 272
    type I (immediate hypersensitivity),
      272
    type IV (cell-mediated hypersensi-
      tivity), 272
  alteration of target enzymes, 220
  cross-reactivity among, 276–277
  immunochemistry, 273–274
  for *Mycobacterium tuberculosis*,
    395
  for peritonitis, 716–717
  pharmacology, 226–227
    animal models, 226–227
    clinical trial data, 227, 227f
    in vitro models, 226
  resistance, 194, 220

β-lysin: virulence factors and, 8
β-toxin: *Staphylococcus aureus*, 1759
Bicampicillin: for sinusitis, 589t
Bifidobacterium, 2158t, 2206, 2207
  as normal flora, 2159t, 2206
Bifidobacterium adolescentis,
  1875–1876, 2207
Bifidobacterium dentium, 2207
  incidence, 2163
Bifonazole: for dermatophytosis, 2382
Bile secretions: peritonitis, 712
Bilharzial dysentery, 989
Biliary carcinoma: fever in, 544
Biliary tract infections
  anaerobic, 2163t, 2165
  Clostridium, 2185
  and fever, 541
  and intraperitoneal abscess, 721
Bilophila, 2158t
Bilophila wadsworthia, 2201
  incidence, 2162
  intra-abdominal infections, 2165
  treatment, 2170t
Bioassays, antimicrobial, 197, 197f
Biocef. *See* Cephalexin
Biologic gradient, 164
Bioluminescence: for bacteriuria, 176
Bipolaris, 2391
  brain abscess, 890
  mycotic aneurysms, 772
  phaeohyphomycosis of paranasal
    sinus, 1132
Bipolaris hawaiiensis: sinusitis, 586t
Bipolaris spicifera: sinusitis, 586t
Birds
  microorganisms harbored by, 2792t
  migration patterns, 2794
Bismuth subsalicylate (Pepto-Bismol):
    for diarrhea, 972, 2802
Bites
  animal, 165, 604, 2766–2768
    antimicrobial susceptibility, 2766t
    bacterial etiology, 2765t
    management, 2767, 2767t
    to neck and face, 603, 604
    Pasteurella, 2069
    rabies, 1527–1528, 1529–1531,
      1530f, 1531f, 1532f
  dog and cat: bacterial isolates, 2765t
  human, 2768
    anaerobic, 2163t
    Eikenella, 2112
    management, 2768
    to neck and face, 603, 604
  venomous snakes, 2767–2768
Bithionol, 460t, 483
  dosage, 463t
    pediatric, 463t
  for liver flukes, 2542
BK virus, 1400–1406
  clinical manifestations, 1401–1402,
    1402t
  description, 1400
  epidemiology, 1400
  and neoplasia, 1402
  pathogenesis, 1401
  in pregnancy, 1401–1402, 1402t
  prevention and treatment, 1404
  in transplant recipients, 2723
    bone marrow, 1402, 1402t, 2720
    renal, 1402, 1402t, 2724
"Black Death," 2073
Black dots
  chromomycosis, 2325f, 2326
  ringworm, 2380

Black eschars: mucormycosis, 2316
Blackflies
  and *Mansonella*, 2536
  and onchocerciasis, 2535
Black piedra, 2385
Black vomit (yellow fever), 1471
Bladder infections. *See* Urinary tract
    infections
Bladder worm, 2544, 2545t
Blastocystis hominis, 2394t, 2511–2512
  diarrhea in AIDS, 970, 970t
  transmission, 2394t
  treatment, 461t
    iodoquinol, 468
    metronidazole, 458
Blastomyces dermatitidis, 2353–2365
  acute infection, 2357, 2357f
  appearance in tissue, 2289t
  bone and joint infections, 2356t,
    2359–2360, 2360f
  brain abscess, 890
  cellular immunity, 2355–2356
  in children, 2360–2361
  chronic or recurrent infection,
    2357–2360
  clinical manifestations, 2356t,
    2356–2362, 2357f, 2394t
  CNS infection, 2356t, 2360, 2360f
  conjunctivitis, 1105
  cutaneous manifestations, 550t, 552,
    2355, 2356t, 2358–2359,
    2359f, 2360f
  description, 2354, 2354f
  diagnosis, 2361–2362
    cellular immunity testing, 2362
    cultures, 2361–2362
    direct examination, 2361
    histopathology, 2361, 2362f
    serologic, 2362
  differential diagnosis, 2322, 2326,
    2345
  epidemiology, 2354f, 2354–2355
  genitourinary tract infection, 2356t,
    2360
  growth, 190
  history, 2354
  and HIV/AIDS, 2361
    meningitis, 872, 2360
    pulmonary, 1236
  humoral immunity, 2356
  immunity, 2355–2356
  in the immunocompromised, 2361
  keratitis, 1113
  meningitis: and HIV, 872, 2360
  pathogenesis and pathology, 2355
  polymorphonuclear leukocytes, 2355
  in pregnancy, 2361
  pulmonary, 2355, 2356t, 2357, 2358f,
    2359f
    chronic, 647t, 2356t, 2357, 2358f
    in HIV/AIDS, 1236
    radiology, 654f, 2357f, 2358f
  serology, 193t
  skin, 2356t, 2358–2359, 2359f,
    2360f
  sputum, 175f
  subcutaneous nodules, 2356t, 2359
  treatment, 2362–2363
    amphotericin B, 406, 2362, 2363
    itraconazole, 408, 2363
    ketoconazole, 406, 407, 2363
  WI-1 protein, 2356
Blastomycosis
  keloidal, 2392
  North American, 1123

South American, 2386–2389. *See*
    also Paracoccidioides
    brasiliensis
Blastoschizomyces capitatus, 2392
Bleach: for HIV disinfection, 2583
Bleomycin: fever from, 545
Blepharitis
  anterior, 1130
  and chronic granulomatous disease,
    92
  herpes simplex virus, 1338, 1339
  laboratory findings, 1133
  posterior (Meibomian gland dysfunc-
    tion), 1130
  staphylococcal, 1130
Blepharoconjunctivitis
  Moraxella lacunata, 1104–1105,
    1928
  Pseudomonas aeruginosa, 1991
  staphylococcal, 1130
Blindness
  from ethambutol, 393
  river, 1113, 2525t, 2535–2536
Blood: specimen collection and process-
    ing, 170t–171t, 177–178
Blood-brain barrier
  antibiotic therapy and: brain abscess,
    893
  viral meningitis and, 836
Blood cultures
  endocarditis, 751, 752t
    culture-negative, 758–759
    prosthetic valve, 784t, 785
  and FUO, 539
  pneumonia, 625–626
Blood flukes (schistosomiasis),
    2538–2541. *See also*
    Schistosoma
Blood infections. *See* Bacteremia
Blood transfusions. *See* Transfusion-
    related infections
Blue bloaters, 609
Blue-green algae, 2512
Body substance isolation, 2576t, 2577t,
    2578
Boerhaave syndrome, 814
Bolivian hemorrhagic fever
  characteristics, 1573t
  clinical manifestations, 1576
  epidemiology, 1574
  intrauterine infection, 1576
  pathogenesis, 1575
  prevention and treatment, 1577
Bone infections, 1032–1056. *See also*
    Joint infections; Musculo-
    skeletal infections *and specific*
    infections
  actinomycosis, 2285
  African histoplasmosis, 2348
  anaerobic gram-negative bacilli, 2200
  Blastomyces dermatitidis, 2356t,
    2359–2360, 2360f
  Coccidioides immitis, 2367–2368,
    2369f
    treatment, 2372
  in drug abusers, 2698
  gram-negative anaerobes, 2200
  mycetoma, 2329, 2329f
  osteomyelitis, 1039–1052
  prostheses, 1051–1055
    bacteriology, 1052, 1052t
    clinical presentation, 1052–1053,
      1053t
    diagnosis, 1053f, 1053–1054
    pathogenesis, 1052–1053

Bone infections (Continued)
prevention, 1054–1055
therapy, 1054
suppressive antibiotic,
1054–1055
Pseudomonas aeruginosa,
1992–1994
treatment, 1992–1994
quinolones for, 372
sporotrichosis, 2322
Bone lesions: Aspergillus, 2308
Bone marrow
AIDS and, 1206
biopsy: and FUO, 541
progenitors, 122
toxicity
chloramphenicol, 313
interferons, 428
Bone marrow aspiration
for Leishmania: visceral (kala azar),
2432
for Trypanosoma brucei, 2453
Bone marrow cultures: for Salmonella,
2021
Bone marrow transplantation
and antibody deficiencies, 53
aspergillosis and, 2306
bacterial infections and, 2718–2719
for chronic granulomatous disease, 93,
95
CMV infections, 2674, 2720, 2720t
ganciclovir for, 426
enteroviral meningoencephalitis and,
1629
fungal infections and, 2719–2720,
2720t
G-CSF for, 450
GM-CSF for, 451
graft-vs.-host disease, 2674, 2717,
2718, 2720–2721
hepatitis C virus and, 2674
HSV infections, 1340
for immunoglobulin deficiencies, 51
immunoglobulins and, 454
infections and, 2673–2674, 2674f,
2710, 2717–2722
prophylaxis, 2721, 2721t
risk factors, 2717–2718, 2718f
temporal patterns, 2717–2718,
2718f
interstitial pneumonia and, 2720–2721
Pneumocystis carinii and, 2721
polyomaviruses and, 1402, 1402t
respiratory syncytial virus and,
1510–1511
Staphylococcus epidermidis bacteremia and, 1781
Streptococcus pneumoniae and, 2669
Toxoplasma gondii and, 2460, 2721
viridans streptococcal infections, 1849
VZV infection, 1348, 2674, 2720
Bordetella, 2078–2082
clinical manifestations, 2080–2081
complications, 2081
description, 2078–2080
diagnosis, 2081
epidemiology, 2080
multilocus enzyme electrophoresis,
27
prevention, 2081–2082
treatment, 2082
vaccine
acellular, 2082
duration, 2080
whole cell, 2082

Bordetella avium, 2078–2079
Bordetella bronchiseptica, 4, 5,
2078–2079
clones, 21t
description, 2079
Bordetella parapertussis, 4, 5,
2078–2082
clones, 21t
description, 2079
Bordetella pertussis, 2078–2082
adenylate cyclase toxin, 5, 23, 2079,
2080
adherence, 2
bronchitis, acute, 606, 607
chemoprophylaxis, 167
clinical manifestations, 2080–2081
clones, 21
complications, 2081
cough, 2081
dermonecrotic toxin, 23, 2079, 2080
description, 2078–2080
diagnosis, 2081
epidemiology, 2080
filamentous hemagglutinin, 23, 24,
2079
fimbrial protein (FIM), 23, 24
fluorescein-labeled antibody (FA),
2081
immunofluorescence, 185
lipopolysaccharide, 2079–2080
nasopharyngeal cultures, 169, 172
O antigen, 2079
pertactin, 23
pertussis toxin, 3, 3t, 4, 6, 23, 2079,
2080
phase variation, 2080
toxins, 3, 3t, 4, 6, 23, 23f, 23t, 2079
tracheal cytotoxin, 5, 2079, 2080
treatment, 2082
chloramphenicol, 312t
erythromycin, 335, 335t, 338t
vaccine, 2080, 2082
virulence factors, 2, 5
virulence regulation, 23, 23f, 23t
Boric acid: for vulvovaginal candidiasis,
1077
Bornholm disease, 1625–1626
Borrelia, 2141–2155. See also individual
species
cutaneous manifestations, 550t
Borrelia burgdorferi, 2143–2155
animal model, 2146
animal reservoirs, 2145, 2790, 2792t,
2794
antibody titers, 2149, 2149f
Babesia and, 2499
Bannwarth syndrome, 2143, 2148
Bell's palsy, 2148
blood cultures, 170t
cardiac manifestations, 2148
and chronic fatigue syndrome, 1306,
1307
clinical manifestations, 2146–2148
clones, 21
congenital infection, 2148
conjunctivitis, 1105
cutaneous manifestations, 550t, 556,
2146f, 2146–2147. See also
erythema chronicum migrans
below
description, 2143–2145
differential diagnosis, 2151
ehrlichiosis, 1750
enteroviral meningitis, 1622
Streptobacillus moniliformis, 2085

early signs and symptoms, 2147t
electron micrograph, 2144f
ELISA, 2149, 2149f
encephalomyelitis, 877
enteric symptoms, 999t
epidemiology, 159, 2145
erythema chronicum migrans, 556,
2143, 2146f, 2146–2147,
2566, 2566f
and fever, 542
keratitis, 1115
laboratory diagnosis, 2148–2151,
2149f, 2150f, 2151t
meningitis, 835
antimicrobial therapy, 850t, 854
chronic, 870
clinical presentation, 844
CSF exam, 847–849
diagnosis, 847f, 847–849
musculoskeletal manifestations,
2147
arthritis, 1035
diagnosis, 1037
myocarditis, 800, 802
myositis, 934
neurologic manifestations, 2148
outer-surface proteins, 2143, 2144
pathogenesis, 2145–2146
prevention, 2152
rash, 556
sensu stricto, 2145
staging, 2146
tick vector, 2145, 2565
transfusion-related, 2627
treatment, 2151–2152
azithromycin, 340
tetracyclines, 307
Western blot, 2149, 2150f
Borrelia garinii, 2145
Borrelia hermsii, 2141
and fever, 542
Borrelia pakeri: and fever, 542
Borrelia recurrentis, 2141
clinical manifestations, 2142, 2142t
description, 2141
diagnosis, 2142, 2142f
enteric fever-like symptoms, 1002
epidemiology, 2141
and fever, 542
pathophysiology, 2141–2142
transmission, 2141
treatment and prevention, 2142–2143
Borrelia turicatae: and fever, 542
Borrelia vincentii: noma (gangrenous
stomatitis), 602
Boston exanthem, 1624
Botryomyces caespitosus, 2324
Botryomycosis, 2285
differential diagnosis, 2329
in the immunocompromised, 920
Botulinum toxin, 2, 3t, 5, 949t, 949–950,
1014, 2179
neuritis, 878
Botulism, 2178–2182. See also
Clostridium botulinum
Boutin de Crete (d'Alep; de Biskra),
2434–2435
Boutonneuse fever, 1720t, 1725. See also
Rickettsia conorii
differential diagnosis: rickettsialpox,
1727
signs and symptoms, 1723t
Bovine leukemia virus, 1579, 1591
Bovine papular (pustular) stomatitis,
1329

Bovine transfer factor: for
Cryptosporidium, 2507
Bovine viral diarrhea virus, 1455
Bowel carcinoma: anaerobes and, 2165
Bowel flora, normal, 32
Bowel strangulation: and peritonitis, 712
Bowenoid papulosis, 1388t, 1393, 1393f.
See also Human papillo-
mavirus
Bowen's disease, 1388t, 1393. See also
Human papillomavirus
Brain. See also Central nervous system
anatomy, 822f, 822–831, 823f
relationship to spinal cord, 822f,
822–824, 823f
Brain abscess, 887–900
anaerobic, 2162, 2163t, 2164
antibiotic therapy, 893–895
approach to patient, 896
AIDS, 896–897
Aspergillus, 890, 2308
Bacillus, 1893
Bacteroides, 2197
Brucella, 890
Candida: in AIDS, 890
clinical manifestations, 890
Clostridium perfringens, 890, 2185
corticosteroids for, 897
CT, 826, 891–893, 892f, 893f
dark-walled fungi, 2391
diagnosis, 891–893
differential diagnosis, 891
in drug abusers, 2704
Entamoeba histolytica, 890, 2401
epidemiology, 887
Fusobacterium, 2197
general management, 896–897
in HIV/AIDS
approach to patient, 896
Candida, 890
Listeria monocytogenes, 890
Toxoplasma gondii, 887, 1237,
1239, 2458
laboratory findings, 891–893
Listeria monocytogenes, 890
in AIDS, 890
in the immunocompromised, 890
lung abscess and, 643
microbiologic etiology, 888t, 889t,
889–891
mycoplasma, 1717
Nocardia asteroides, 890
in the immunocompromised, 890
in transplant recipients, 2729
pathogenesis, 888, 888t
pathology, 889
predisposing conditions, 888t
Prevotella, 890, 2197
prognosis, 897, 897t
Pseudomonas aeruginosa, 1988–1989
in the immunocompromised, 890
treatment, 1989
radiology (CT and MRI), 891–893,
892f, 893f, 894f, 896t
specimen collection, 179
staging, 896t
Streptococcus intermedius, 1863
surgical therapy, 895–896
Toxoplasma gondii: in HIV/AIDS,
887, 1237, 1239, 2458
Brain biopsy: for meningitis, 867
Brain edema
bacterial meningitis and, 841
and CNS infections, 830
therapy, 830t

Brainerd diarrhea, 1015
Brain herniation: and CNS infections, 829f, 830
Brain lymphoma: and HIV/AIDS, 1182t
Brain tumors
  differential diagnosis: brain abscess, 891
  infections and, 2673
Branched-chain cDNA hybridization: hepatitis C virus, 1481
Branhamella
  β-lactamase, 216t
  mediastinitis, 815t
Branhamella catarrhalis. See Moraxella catarrhalis
Brazilian hemorrhagic fever, 1573t
Brazilian purpuric fever, 2040, 2044, 2046
Breakbone fever. *See* Dengue
Breast abscess, anaerobic, 2163t
Breast-feeding
  and HBV transmission, 1424
  and HIV transmission, 1168, 1189
Breast implants: *Staphylococcus epidermidis* infections, 1782
Breast milk: antimicrobials and, 204
Brill-Zinsser disease, 1719, 1720t, 1735, 1736–1737. *See also Rickettsia prowazekii*
  enteric symptoms, 999t, 1003
Brodie's abscess, 1049
  Staphylococcus aureus, 1772, 1773f
Bromoderma, 2356
Bronchial aspirate microscopy, 184
Bronchial cleft cysts, 604
  lymphadenopathy vs., 941
Bronchial infections, 606–662. *See also specific infections*
Bronchial washings, 170t, 173–174
  microscopic examination of pathogens, 172t
Bronchiectasis, anaerobic, 2163t
Bronchiolitis, 612–619
  Acinetobacter, 2011
  asthmatic, 612
  capillary (obstructive), 612
  clinical manifestations, 615
  complications, 616
  diagnosis, 615–616
  epidemiology, 613
  etiology, 612t, 612–613, 613f
  laboratory findings, 615
  obliterans, 616–617
    organizing pneumonia (BOOP): radiology, 650t, 651f
  parainfluenza, 1490, 1490t
  pathophysiology, 613–615, 614f
  respiratory syncytial virus, 1504t, 1507–1508
  therapy, 616
Bronchitis
  acute, 606–608
    catarrhal. *See* Bronchiolitis
    clinical presentation, 607, 607f
    diagnosis, 607
    etiology, 606, 606t
    exacerbations, 608–612
    pathogenesis, 606–607
    treatment, 607–608
  Chlamydia pneumoniae, 1698
  chronic, 608–612
    and acute exacerbations, 610–611
    antimicrobial therapy, 611
    clinical presentation, 609–610
    etiology and pathology, 608–609

    management, 611
    radiology, 610
    rhinovirus and, 1659
    sputum analysis, 610
  influenza virus, 1557, 1557t
  recurrent asthmatic, 608
Bronchoalveolar carcinoma pneumonia: radiology, 650t, 652f
Bronchoalveolar lavage (BAL)
  for *Pneumocystis carinii*, 2477, 2479
  for pneumonia, 624–625
    chronic, 652
    in HIV/AIDS, 1232
    nosocomial, 2602
Bronchodilators: for bronchiolitis, 616
Bronchopleural fistula: *Mycobacterium tuberculosis*, 2235
Bronchopneumonia
  interstitial. *See* Bronchiolitis
  spastic. *See* Bronchiolitis
Bronchopulmonary aspergillosis, 2307
Bronchoscopy
  and endocarditis, 743t, 794t
  fiberoptic: for pneumonia, 624–626
  and FUO, 541
  for Kaposi's sarcoma, 1241–1242
  nosocomial infection control, 2584
  for pneumonia, 656–657
  specimen collection and processing, 170t, 173–174
  therapeutic: for pneumonia, 656–657
Broth test, 195–196
Brovavir. *See* Sorivudine
Broviac catheter infections, 788, 2594
Brown recluse house spider: necrotizing skin lesions, 918
Brucella, 2053–2060
  animal reservoirs, 2792t
  arthritis, 1035, 2056
  blood cultures, 177
  brain abscess, 890
  cardiac manifestations, 2056
  cellular immunity and, 124
  and chronic fatigue syndrome, 1306
  clinical manifestations, 2055
  complications, 2055–2056
  cutaneous manifestations, 2056
  description, 2053
  diagnosis, 2056–2057
  differential diagnosis
    for *Chlamydia psittaci*, 1695
    scrub typhus, 1740
  endocarditis, 756
  enteric fever, 999t, 1002
  epidemiology, 2053–2054, 2054f
  gastrointestinal manifestations, 2055–2056
  genitourinary manifestations, 2056
  hematologic manifestations, 2056
  history, 2053
  host immunity, 2055
  immunodeficiency and, 138
  immunofluorescence, 185
  lymphadenitis, 940t
  meningitis, 870, 2056
  musculoskeletal specimen collection, 180
  mycotic aneurysms, 772
  neurologic manifestations, 2056
  pathogenesis, 2054–2055
  and pneumonia, 622t
  prevention, 2054f, 2057
  pulmonary manifestations, 2056
  serum agglutination test (SAT), 2057
  skeletal manifestations, 1035, 2056

  taxonomy, 2053
  treatment, 2057
    antimicrobials of choice, 202t
    chloramphenicol, 312t
    rifampin, 322–323
    tetracyclines, 307
    trimethoprim-sulfamethoxazole, 360
  vaccine, 2057
Brucella abortus, 2053
  epidemiology, 2053–2054
  granulomatous hepatitis, 1161
  pathogenesis, 2054, 2055
  serology, 192t
  vaccine self-innoculation, 2055
Brucella canis, 2053, 2054, 2055
Brucella melitensis, 2053, 2054
  GI complications, 2055–2056
  pathogenesis, 2054, 2055
Brucella neotomae, 2053
Brucella ovis, 2053, 2055
Brucella suis, 2053, 2054, 2056
Brudzinski's sign: bacterial meningitis, 843, 843t
Brugia malayi, 2533–2535, 2536
  clinical features, 2534
  diagnosis, 2534
  epidemiology, 2534
  life cycle, 2533–2534
  lymphadenitis, 940t
  lymphangitis, 943
  pathology, 2534
  treatment, 462t
    diethylcarbamazine, 481
    and tropical pulmonary eosinophilia, 2536
Brugian filariasis, 2533–2535
Brugia timori, 2533–2535
  diethylcarbamazine for, 481
  epidemiology, 2534
Buboes
  Haemophilus ducreyi (chancroid), 939, 2047
  inguinal
    differential diagnosis, 1684
    LGV, 1684
    of nonvenereal origin, 939
    of venereal origin, 939
  plague, 2072–2073, 2073f
Bubonic plague, 2070, 2072t, 2072–2073, 2073f, 2074f, 2074f. *See also Yersinia pestis*
  inguinal adenopathy, 939
Buccal mucosa. *See also* Oral cavity
  viridans streptococci in, 1846
Buccal space infections, 598. *See also* Oral disease
Budd-Chiari syndrome: hepatic involvement, 1149
Bulbar paralytic poliomyelitis, 1616
Bullae
  defined, 551, 552
  genital, 1057, 1057t. *See also* Genital lesions
  Pseudomonas aeruginosa, 921
  and systemic infections, 550t, 551t
Bullous impetigo, 911
  lesions, 555
Bullous pemphigoid: pharyngitis, 569
Bunyaviridae, 1567–1572. *See also individual viruses*
  characteristics, 1568, 1568t
  classification, 1315t
  clinical manifestations, 1569–1570
  diagnosis, 1570–1571
  epidemiology, 1568–1569

  prevention and treatment, 1571
  shape and size, 1316f
  transmission to humans, 1569
Bunyavirus, 1567–1572
  characteristics, 1568t
Burkitt's lymphoma
  EBV and, 1364, 1369–1370
  and HIV/AIDS, 1182t
Burns
  antibody deficiency and, 53
  wound infections, 2761–2765
    Acinetobacter, 2011
    diagnosis, 2763–2764, 2764t
    enterococcal, 1829
    organisms in biopsies, 2762t
    pathophysiology, 2761–2762
    prevention, 2762–2763
    Pseudomonas aeruginosa, 1996
    pulmonary complications, 2764
    treatment, 2763–2764, 2764t
      aminoglycosides, 295t
      topical antibacterials, 383
Bursitis
  septic, 1033
  Staphylococcus aureus, 1774
Buruli ulcers, 2269
Buschke-Loewenstein tumors, 1393
Bussuquara: transmission, clinical syndromes, and geographic distribution, 1466t
Butnostomum phlebotomum, 2555
Butoconazole
  dosage, 403t
  structure, 402f
  for vulvovaginal candidiasis, 1076t
Butyrivibrio, 2158t
BV-ARA-U. *See* Sorivudine
BvgAS regulon, 23
BvgS protein, 24
BW882C87, 437t

C

Cabassou virus, 1457
Cadmium poisoning, 1014
Calabar swellings, 2535
Calcineurin, 110
Calciphylaxis, 918
Calcium: and neutrophils, 85, 86
Calcofluor stain, 184t
Caliciviridae, 1666–1672. *See also* Norwalk-like agents
  classification, 1315t, 1667
  Norwalk virus, 1666–1672
  shape and size, 1316f
  virology, 1667f, 1667–1668, 1668f, 1668t
  winter vomiting disease, 968
Caliciviruses. *See* Caliciviridae
California encephalitis viruses, 1567
  characteristics, 1568t
  clinical manifestations, 1569–1570
  diagnosis, 1570
  encephalomyelitis, 876
  epidemiology, 1568
  meningitis, 832
  serology, 191
  transmission to humans, 1569
Calliphora, 2563
Calmette-Guérin bacillus (BCG), 189, 2231, 2774
  and granulomatous hepatitis, 1161
  for leprosy, 2247
  for travelers, 2799
  and tuberculin test, 2219

Calnexin: and MHC class I, 102
Calomys: and South American hemorrhagic fevers, 1573t, 1574
Calymmatobacterium granulomatosis,
  2210–2213
  clinical manifestations, 2211f,
    2211–2212, 2212f
  description, 2211
  diagnosis, 2212, 2212f
  differential diagnosis, 1395, 1684,
    2122
  epidemiology, 1056, 2211
  geographic distribution, 2211
  treatment, 2212
Campylobacter, 1948–1956, 2158t. See
    also individual species
  animal reservoirs, 2792t
  antibody deficiencies and, 49
  bacteriology, 1953
  characteristics, 1948–1949
    differential, 1949t
  clinical manifestations, 1951–1952
  diagnosis, 1953
  differential diagnosis
    amebiasis, 2402
    Cryptosporidium, 2504
  direct microscopy, 1953, 1953f
  epidemiology, 160, 1949–1950
  immunity and, 1951
  and immunodeficiency, 150t
  pathogenesis, 1950–1951
  pathology, 1950–1951
  surveillance, 160
  taxonomy, 1948–1956
  therapy, 1953–1954
  in travelers, 2800–2801
Campylobacter cinaedi. See
    Helicobacter cinaedi
Campylobacter coli
  characteristics, 1949t
  clinical manifestations, 1952
  epidemiology, 1949–1950
  growth, 1949t
  therapy, 1954
Campylobacter concisus, 1948
Campylobacter cryaerophila, 1948
Campylobacter fennelliae. See
    Helicobacter fennelliae
Campylobacter fetus
  bacteriology, 1953
  endocarditis, 755
  enteric fever, 999t, 1001–1002
  metronidazole for, 329
  prognosis, 1954
  virulence factors, 952
Campylobacter fetus subsp. *fetus*
  characteristics, 1949t
  clinical manifestations, 1952, 1952t
  epidemiology, 1949–1950
  growth, 1949t
  immunity, 1951
  pathogenesis, 1951
Campylobacter fetus subsp. *venerealis*:
    clinical manifestations, 1952,
    1952t
Campylobacter hyointestinalis
  characteristics, 1949t
  clinical manifestations, 1952
  epidemiology, 1949–1950
  growth, 1949t
Campylobacter jejuni, 1948–1956
  characteristics, 1948–1949
    differential, 1949t, 1957t
  clinical manifestations, 1951–1952,
    1952t

culture, 1948, 1949f
  cytotoxicity, 951
  dysentery, 987, 988–989
  in the elderly, 2740
  epidemiology, 1949–1950
  food-borne, 1012t, 1013, 1016, 1020
    laboratory diagnosis, 1018t,
      1018–1019
    therapy, 1019
  growth, 1949t
  Guillain-Barré syndrome and, 162,
    878, 1014, 1952, 1954
  hosts, 946
  immunity, 1951
  pathogenesis, 1950–1951
  pathology, 1950–1951
  prognosis, 1954
  quinolone resistance, 373
  and Reiter syndrome, 1071
  specimen collection, 180
  toxin, 950
  treatment, 1953–1954
    antimicrobials of choice, 202t
    azithromycin, 335t
    carbapenems, 264t
    clarithromycin, 335t
    erythromycin, 335, 335t, 337–338,
      338t
    quinolones, 367t
    tetracyclines, 308t
  virulence factors, 952
  waterborne, 1015–1016, 1016t
Campylobacter laridis
  characteristics, 1949t
  growth, 1949t
Campylobacter nitrofigilis, 1948
Campylobacter pylori. See Helicobacter
    pylori
Campylobacter sputorum subsp.
    bubulus, 1953
Campylobacter sputorum subsp. *sputo-*
    rum, 1953
Campylobacter upsaliensis, 1949t
  clinical manifestations, 1952
  epidemiology, 1949–1950
  growth, 1949t
Canadian vole agent, 1741
Canaliculitis, 1131
  laboratory findings, 1133
  lacrimal: actinomycosis, 2282
  treatment, 1134
Cancer. *See also* Neoplasia *and specific*
    tumors
  infections in patients with. *See*
    Neoplasia, infections in
    patients with
Candida, 2289–2306. *See also individual*
    species
  clinical manifestations, 2291–2299
    cutaneous, 2293–2296
    deep organ involvement, 2296–2299
    disseminated, 2298–2299
    treatment, 2299–2301
Candida albicans, 2290
  abdominal: treatment, 2300
  adherence, 2291
  agglutination tests, 185
  appearance in tissue, 2289t
  arthritis, 1036, 2297
  balanitis: diagnosis, 1059
  and bone marrow transplantation, 2719
  brain abscess: in AIDS, 890
  canaliculitis: treatment, 1134
  in cancer patients, 2668
  candidemia, 2298–2299, 2299f

cardiac, 2296
  catheter-associated, 2291, 2593, 2595
  cell-mediated immunity and, 2290,
    2295
  and chronic fatigue syndrome, 1306
  clinical manifestations, 2291–2299
  CNS, 2296
    treatment, 2300
  costochondritis, 2297
  cutaneous, 550t, 556–557, 2293–2296
    balanitis, 2293
    chronic mucocutaneous (CMC),
      2295f, 2295–2296
    in disseminated candidiasis, 2294,
      2294f
    erosio interdigitalis blastomycetica,
      2293, 2294f
    folliculitis, 2293, 2294f
    generalized, 2293, 2293f
    intertrigo, 2294
    paronychia and onychomycosis,
      2294, 2294f, 2295f
    differential diagnosis, 2380
    perianal, 2294–2295, 2295f
    in transplantation, 2726
  cytokine and T cell protection, 121t,
    128
  deep organ involvement, 2296–2299
  description, 2290
  diarrhea
    in AIDS, 970, 970t
    chronic, 993–994
  disseminated, 2298–2299
    in leukemics, 2679
    and skin infections, 556, 922
      in leukemics, 2679
    in transplant recipients, 2715, 2727
    treatment, 2300
    urinary tract infections and,
      2612–2613
  ecology, 2290
  in the elderly, 2740
  encephalitis, 876
  endocarditis, 744, 757, 758,
    2296–2297
    diagnosis, 751
    drug abusers, 756
    prosthetic valve, 786
    treatment, 764, 786, 2300
  endophthalmitis, 1122
    in drug abusers, 2704–2705
    treatment, 1125–1126
  enteritides, 993–994
  epidemiology, 2290
  esophagitis, 962, 963f, 2292f,
    2292–2293
    and adult T-cell leukemia/lymphoma,
      1582
    and granulocytopenia, 2678
    and HIV/AIDS, 1181–1182, 1229
      in children, 1186, 1186t
      incidence, 1182t, 1183
    in transplant recipients, 2728
  fever, 543
  folliculitis, 912
  fungemia, 922
  gallbladder, 2298
    treatment, 2300
  and granulocytopenia, 2676–2677
  granuloma, 2295, 2295f
  growth, 190
  hepatic, 2298
    abscess, 724
    granulomatous hepatitis, 1161
    and leukemia, 2679

and HIV/AIDS, 2290–2291
    diarrhea, 970, 970t
    esophagitis, 1181–1182, 1229
      in children, 1186, 1186t
      incidence, 1182t, 1183
    oral, 1226–1227
    prophylaxis, 1286t
    pulmonary, 1235
      incidence, 1182t
    treatment, 1283t, 1288, 2301
    vaginal, 1227
  humoral immunity and, 2291
  and immunodeficiency, 150t
  Job syndrome and, 156
  keratitis, 1113
  lacrimal sac infection, 1131
  and leukemia, 2672–2673
    hairy cell, 2673
  in liver transplantation, 2723
  macrophage inhibition factor and,
    2295
  mediastinitis, 815t
  meningitis, 870
    treatment, 868
  mucocutaneous, 2292–2296
    chronic, 135, 556, 962, 2295f,
      2295–2296
    treatment, 2301
  mucous membrane infections,
    2291–2299
  mycotic aneurysms, 772
  myositis, 2298
  in neutropenics, 2672t
  ocular, 2298, 2298f
    treatment, 2301
  ophthalmitis, 922
  oral, 2292, 2292f
    HIV/AIDS and, 1226–1227
    and leukemia, 2678
    and risk for *P. carinii*, 1222
    specimen collection, 172
    thrush, 2292, 2292f
    treatment, 2301
  osteomyelitis, 2297, 2297f
  otitis externa, 580
  pathogenesis, 2290–2291
  pathology, 2290–2291
  pericarditis, 805
  peritonitis, 712, 2298
    treatment, 717, 721, 2300
  pneumonia, 619t
    nosocomial in the immunocompro-
      mised, 631
  prophylaxis, 2299–2301
  pseudomembranous. *See* oral *above*
  pulmonary: and HIV/AIDS, 1235
    incidence, 1182t
  rash, 556–557
  in renal transplantation, 2723
  respiratory tract, 2296
  serology, 193t
  sexually transmitted, 1055–1056
  spinal cord injury and, 2733
  splenic, 2298
    abscess, 727
  suppurative thrombophlebitis, 768
  thrush. *See* oral *above*
  total parenteral nutrition and, 2593
  in transplant recipients, 2712, 2723
    prophylaxis, 2715
  treatment, 2299–2301
    abdominal, 2300
    CNS, 2300
    disseminated, 2300
    endocarditis, 2300

fluconazole, 408–409, 1283t, 1288
flucytosine, 406
gallbladder, 2300
in HIV/AIDS, 1283t, 1288
ketoconazole, 1283t, 1288
in men, 1077
mucocutaneous, 2301
ocular, 2301
peritonitis, 2300
thrush, 403, 1288, 2301
urinary tract infections,
2300–2301
vulvovaginitis, 404
urethritis: diagnosis, 1065
urinary specimens, 175f
urinary tract infections, 2297
treatment, 2300–2301
complications, 2612–2613
vaginitis, 1075, 2293, 2293f
vascular infection, 2298
vulvovaginitis, 1075–1077, 2293
clinical features, 1076
diagnosis, 1076
features, 1075t
and HIV, 1227
treatment, 1076t, 1076–1077
male partners, 1077
oral therapy, 1076
recurrent infection, 1077
topical, 1076–1077
Candida glabrata, 2290
appearance in tissue, 2289t
and granulocytopenia, 2676
growth, 190
vaginitis, 1075
Candida guilliermondii, 2290
Candida krusei, 2290
and bone marrow transplantation,
2719
and granulocytopenia, 2676
growth, 190
prophylaxis, 2300
Candida lustaniae, 2290
Candida parapsilosis, 2290
endocarditis, 757
growth, 190
infusion-related sepsis, 2587
Candida pseudotropicalis, 2290
Candida rugosa, 2290
Candida stellatoidea, 2290
Candida tropicalis, 2290, 2299
and bone marrow transplantation,
2719
in cancer patients, 2668
endocarditis, 757
growth, 190
in leukemics, 2679
in neutropenics, 2672t
vaginitis, 1075
Candidemia, 2298–2299, 2299f
Canine parvovirus (CPV), 1440
Canine space infections, 598
Capillaria philippinensis, 2553t,
2556–2557
diagnosis, 1006t, 1007, 2557
treatment, 461t, 2557
albendazole, 479
mebendazole, 479
Capillaries, CNS
anatomy, 826
injury, 826–827
Capnocytophaga, 2103–2106, 2167
and actinomycosis, 2280
characteristics, 2104
clinical manifestations, 2104–2105

group DF-2. *See Capnocytophaga
canimorsus*
periodontitis, 594
taxonomy, 2103–2104
treatment, 2104–2105
metronidazole, 329, 329t
Capnocytophaga canimorsus, 2103, 2104,
2105
animal bites, 2766
cutaneous manifestations, 550t
rash, 556
susceptibility, 2766t
Capnocytophaga cynodegmi, 2103, 2105
animal bites, 2766
Capnocytophaga gingivalis, 2103,
2104–2105
Capnocytophaga ochracea, 2103,
2104–2105
Capnocytophaga sputigena, 2103,
2104–2105
Capreomycin
dosage, 516t–517t
in hepatic or renal failure, 390t, 517t
drug interactions, 520t
for *Mycobacterium tuberculosis*, 394
pharmacology, 516t–517t
Caprine arthritis-encephalitis virus
(CAEV), 1591
Capripoxvirus, 1325
Capsids, viral, 1315, 1315t
helical, 1315, 1317f
icosahedral, 1315, 1317f
Capsule, bacterial, 1754
Captopril: tetanus toxin and, 5
Carbamazepine: drug interactions, 310
Carbapenems, 264–266. *See also*
Imipenem; Meropenem
comparative activity, 264t
cross-reactivity, 277
for neutropenics, 2688t
postantibiotic effect (PAE), 265
resistance, 219
structure, 274f
Carbenicillin, 205–206, 233, 244
adverse reactions, 239t
antibiotic-associated colitis (AAC), 979
β-lactamase, 216t
combination therapy
aminoglycosides, 287t, 289t
synergism, 207
dosage, 241t, 506t–507t
in children, 506t
in neonates, 242t, 506t
in renal disease, 204, 238t, 507t
for endocarditis, 764, 1984
pharmacology, 238, 506t–507t
for Pseudomonads, 2004t
for *Pseudomonas aeruginosa*
endocarditis, 1984
meningitis, 1989
structure, 244f
Carbenicillin indanyl sodium: pharmacology, 506t–507t
CARB (1–4) β-lactamase, 216t
Carbohydrate malabsorption, 953
Carboxy penicillins, 236, 244–245
dosage, 238t, 241t
pharmacokinetics, 238t
structure, 244f
Carboxypeptidase B, 58t, 63t
Carbuncles: *Staphylococcus aureus*,
1763, 1764f
Carcinogenesis
ganciclovir, 425
metronidazole, 331, 467–468

Cardiac catheterization: endocarditis, 752
Cardiac disorders and infections. *See
also specific disorders*
Borrelia burgdorferi and, 2148
Candida albicans, 2296
influenza virus, 1558
Mycoplasma pneumoniae and, 1707
Cardiac myocytes: HIV and, 1204–1205
Cardiobacterium hominis, 2108–2109
biochemical reactions, 2107t
classification and site of infection,
2107t
endocarditis, 756
identification, 186
Cardiomyopathy: *Trypanosoma cruzi*,
2446
Cardiothoracic surgery
endocarditis: prophylaxis, 796, 797t
mediastinitis and, 814t, 814–815
microbiology, 815t
prophylaxis, 817
prophylaxis recommendations, 2751t
Cardiovascular embolism: and endocarditis, 746
Cardiovascular graft infections, 789–790
clinical features, 789
diagnosis, 789
microbiology, 789, 789t
morbidity and mortality, 790
pathogenesis, 789
prevention, 790
treatment, 790
rifampin, 323
Cardiovascular infections, 741–821. *See
also specific infections*
dialysis-access arteriovenous fistulas,
790
endarteritis, 769–773
endocarditis, 740–765. *See also*
Endocarditis, infective
prophylaxis, 793–799
prosthetic valve, 783–788
graft. *See also* Cardiovascular graft
infections
intravascular, 741–783
mediastinitis, 814–821
"mycotic aneurysms," 769–773
myocarditis, 800–804
pacemakers, 790–791
pericarditis, 805–808
right atrial indwelling catheters, 788
suppurative thrombophlebitis,
765–769
vascular grafts, 789–791
Cardiovascular reactions
to peritonitis, 713
rabies, 1533, 1534t
syphilis, 2125–2126
Cardioviruses, 1637
Carey Coombs murmur: rheumatic fever,
1802
Carindacillin, 245. *See also* Indanyl carbenicillin
Carotid artery
erosion, 600
mycotic aneurysms, 770
Carrión's disease, 2209. *See also
Bartonella bacilliformis*
Cartilage-hair hypoplasia, 134t
Carumonam: pharmacology, 510t–511t
Case-control studies, 162
Case fatality rate, 164
Case series, 162
Castaneda principle: endocarditis diag-
nosis, 751

Castellani's paint: for dermatophytosis,
2382
Catalase
and hydrogen peroxide, 84
Staphylococcus aureus, 1759
Cataract surgery
Aspergillus and, 2307
and endophthalmitis, 1121
Staphylococcus epidermidis infections,
1782
Cat bites
Capnocytophaga, 2105
Pasteurella, 2069
Cathepsin, 79t
Catheter-related infections, 2587–2599.
See also specific catheters
arterial, 2595–2596, 2596t
Bacillus, 1892–1893
in cancer patients, 2670f, 2670–2671
central venous, 2592
long-term, 2594t, 2594–2595
diagnosis, 2590f, 2590t, 2590–2591
and HIV/AIDS, 1235
infection prophylaxis: topical antibacterials, 382
in leukemia/lymphoma, 2679, 2680
microbiology, 2589t, 2589–2590
pathogenesis, 2587–2589
contamination at insertion site,
2588t, 2588–2589
contamination at junction, 2587
contamination of infusate, 2587
peripheral IV cannulization, 2591t,
2591–2592
Proteus mirabilis, 1974
pulmonary artery, 2595
right atrial indwelling, 788
risk factors, 2588t, 2588–2589
hospital-related, 2589t
Serratia, 1972
Staphylococcus epidermidis,
1779–1780
suppurative thrombophlebitis,
765–769
total parenteral nutrition, 2592–2594
in traumatized patient, 2758
urinary tract
after catheter removal, 2608
Candida, 2297
chronic renal inflammation and,
2610
complications
long-term catheterization, 2610
short-term catheterization, 2610
treatment, 2612–2613
duration of catheterization,
2608–2610, 2609t
in the elderly, 2738
entry, 2607–2608
epidemiology, 2607
long-term catheterization,
2609–2610
obstructions and, 2610
Oligella, 2113
pathogenesis, 2607–2608
prevention, 2610–2612
avoidance of catheterization,
2610–2611
of bacteriuria, 2611–2612
Pseudomonas aeruginosa,
1994–1995
risk factors, 2608
short-term catheterization,
2608–2609
urinary stones and, 2610

Cat hookworm, 2555
Cat(s). *See also* Cat bites; Cat scratch disease
  microorganisms harbored by, 2792t
Cat scratch disease, 1310–1311, 1744
  clinical manifestations, 1310f, 1310t, 1310–1311
    atypical, 1311t
  diagnosis, 1311–1312
  differential diagnosis, 1311–1312
  epidemiology, 1310
  etiology, 1310
  and fever, 542
  lymphadenitis, 938–939
  oculoglandular syndrome, 938
  pathology, 1310
  skin test, 1312
  treatment, 1312
Cat tapeworm, 2547
Cattle: microorganisms harbored by, 2792t
Cavernous sinus infections, 1131–1133
Cavernous sinus thrombosis
  differential diagnosis: orbital cellulitis, 1133
  MRI and CT, 1134
  septic, 600–601, 910, 910t
  treatment, 1135
CAZ β-lactamase, 217
CDC base agar, 2168
CD2 cells, 108
  NK cells and, 122
CD3 cells, 109, 110
CD4 cells, 47, 105–107, 108, 109. *See also* T cells
  cryptococcosis and, 2332, 2333
  Cryptosporidium, 2506
  and cytokines, 116
  cytotoxicity, 121
  deficiency, 134t
  and HIV/AIDS
    binding, 12, 12t, 13, 14–15, 15f, 1204, 1586, 1586f, 1587f, 1588f, 1597f
    depletion, 1205–1208, 1206t, 1586, 1586f, 1588f, 1599
    apoptosis and, 1207
    superantigens and, 1207, 1207f
    functional impairment, 1208
    measures, 1175, 1175t, 1182, 1221, 1222–1223, 1223f, 1223t, 1281
  idiopathic lymphocytopenia, 1182
  Leishmania and, 2430
  memory, 111, 132
  and *Mycobacterium avium-intracellulare*, 2252
  and *Mycobacterium tuberculosis*, 2218
  and *Pneumocystis carinii*, 127, 2477
  protection from infection, 121t, 126, 127, 128
  recombinant soluble: for HIV, 1268–1269
  T cell suppression, 120
CD5 cells, 45t, 49
CD8 cells, 105–107, 108, 109, 111. *See also* T cells
  and cytokines, 116
  cytotoxic, 121–122
  deficiency, 134t
  histoplasmosis and, 2341
  HIV and, 1204, 1208–1209
  intraepithelial lymphocytes (IEL), 112

protection from infection, 121t, 126, 127, 129
  T cell suppression, 120
CD19 cells, 45, 45t
CD21 cells, 45, 45t, 63t
  and B cells, 120
CD22 cells, 45, 45t
CD23 cells, 108
  and B cells, 120
CD25 cells, 47
CD26 cells, 108
CD27 cells, 108
CD28 cells, 47, 108–109
CD31 cells. *See* Platelet/endothelial cell adhesion molecule-1 (PECAM-1)
CD40 cells, 45t, 47, 48, 109, 119, 120
CD44 cells, 108, 111
  and cytokines, 115
CD45 cells, 45t, 109–110, 111
  and cytokines, 115
CD48 cells, 108
CD54 cells, 108
CD58 cells. *See* LFA-3
CD69 cells, 110
CD72 cells, 45t, 47
CD73 cells, 108
CD14 cells: and septic shock, 117
CD18 cells: deficiency: and leukocyte adhesion deficiency, 154
CD57 cells: NK cells and, 122
CDC group DF-3, 2109–2110
  classification and site of infection, 2107t
CDC group EF-4, 2110
  classification and site of infection, 2107t
CDC group IVc-2, 2112
  classification and site of infection, 2107t
CDC group M4. *See Oligella urethralis*
CDC group NO-1, 2114
CDC group Vd. *See Ochrobactrum anthropi*
CDC group Ve-2, 2107t, 2112–2113
CDC group WO-1, 2114
CD3γ deficiency, 134t
CD3ε deficiency, 134t
CD4-PE40, 437t
CD45RA, 111
CD45RO, 109, 111
Ceclor. *See* Cefaclor
Cedecea davisae, 1975t
Cedecea lapagei, 1975t
Cedecea neteri, 1975t
Cefaclor, 257
  chemistry, 249
  dosage, 250t, 508t–509t
    in children and neonates, 508t
    in renal insufficiency, 253t, 509t
  pharmacology, 251, 252t, 508t–509t
  for sinusitis, 589t
  structure, 248f
  in vitro activity, 255t, 257
Cefadroxil, 256
  for bacterial vaginosis, 1079t
  dosage, 250t, 508t–509t
    in children and neonates, 508t–509t
    in renal insufficiency, 253t, 509t
  pharmacology, 251, 508t–509t
  in vitro activity, 255t
Cefadyl. *See* Cephapirin
Cefamandole, 256
  antibiotic-associated colitis (AAC), 979

clinical trials, 227
  dosage, 250t, 508t–509t
    in children, 508t
    in renal insufficiency, 253t, 509t
  pharmacology, 252t, 508t–509t
  resistance, 251
  structure, 248f
  in vitro activity, 255t, 256
  warfarin interaction, 2750
Cefazolin, 256
  antibiotic-associated colitis (AAC), 979
  dosage, 250t, 508t–509t
    in renal insufficiency, 253t, 509t
  for endocarditis
    prophylaxis, 788, 797t
    staphylococcal, 760
    streptococcal, 760
  for peritonitis: in peritoneal dialysis, 720t
  pharmacology, 252t
  prophylactic
    for endocarditis, 797t
    for mediastinitis, 817
    perioperative use, 2749
    in trauma patients, 2759
  structure, 248f
  susceptibility, 2748f
  in vitro activity, 255t, 256
Cefdinir, 259
Cefepime, 259
  chemistry, 249
  pharmacology, 252t
  structure, 248f
  in vitro activity, 255t
Cefixime, 259
  antibiotic-associated colitis (AAC), 979
  chemistry, 249
  dosage, 250t, 508t–509t
    in children, 508t
    in renal insufficiency, 253t, 509t
  for *Neisseria gonorrhoeae*, 1921, 1921t, 1922
  pharmacology, 251, 252t, 508t–509t
  for sinusitis, 589t
  structure, 248f
  in vitro activity, 255t, 260
Cefmenoxime, 259
  chemistry, 248
  clinical trials, 230
  hematologic reactions, 254
  pharmacology, 227, 227f, 252t
Cefmetazole, 257
  dosage, 250t
  hematologic reactions, 254
  pharmacology, 252t
  structure, 248f
  in vitro activity, 255t, 257, 258
Cefobid. *See* Cefoperazone
Cefonicid, 256
  dosage, 250t, 508t–509t
    in renal insufficiency, 253t, 509t
  pharmacology, 508t–509t
Cefoperazone, 259
  adverse reactions, 254
  chemistry, 249
  clinical trials, 227
  dosage, 250t, 508t–509t
    in renal insufficiency, 509t
  pharmacology, 252, 252t, 508t–509t
  for Pseudomonads, 2004t
  resistance, 251
Ceforanide, 256
Cefotaxime, 258–259

antibiotic-associated colitis (AAC), 979
  chemistry, 248
  combination therapy: aminoglycosides, 287t
  dosage, 250t, 508t–509t
    in children and neonates, 508t–509t, 851t
    in renal insufficiency, 253t, 509t
  for epiglottitis, 592
  for *Haemophilus influenzae*, 2043
  for meningitis, 850t, 851, 851t, 852
    dosage, 850t
  for *Neisseria meningitidis*, 1903t, 1904, 1904t
  ototoxicity, 294
  pharmacology, 252t, 508t–509t
  for Pseudomonads, 2004t
  structure, 248f
  susceptibility testing, 194, 194t
  in vitro activity, 255t, 260
Cefotetan, 257
  for *Bacteroides fragilis*, 2200t, 2201
  chemistry, 247
  dosage, 250t, 508t–509t
    in children, 508t
    in renal insufficiency, 253t, 509t
  hematologic reactions, 254
  pharmacology, 252t, 508t–509t
  in vitro activity, 255t, 258
Cefoxitin, 257
  antibiotic-associated colitis (AAC), 979
  for *Bacteroides fragilis*, 2200t, 2201
  chemistry, 247
  combination therapy
    aminoglycosides, 287t
    for mycobacteria, 396t
  dosage, 250t, 508t–509t
    in children, 508t
    in renal insufficiency, 253t, 509t
  for *Mobiluncus*, 2052
  for mycobacteria, 395
  for necrotizing pneumonia, 645–646
  for *Neisseria gonorrhoeae*, 1921, 1922t
  for odontogenic infections, 602t
  pharmacology, 252t, 508t–509t
  for PID, 1096t
  structure, 248f
  in vitro activity, 255t, 257, 258–259
Cefpiramide, 259
  dosage, 250t
  pharmacology, 252, 252t
Cefpirome, 259
  chemistry, 249
  dosage, 250t
  pharmacology, 252t
  structure, 248f
  in vitro activity, 255t
Cefpodoxime, 259
  antibiotic-associated colitis (AAC), 979
  dosage, 250t, 508t–509t
    in children, 508t
    in renal insufficiency, 253t, 509t
  pharmacology, 251–252, 252t, 508t–509t
  structure, 248f
  in vitro activity, 255t
Cefprozil, 257
  dosage, 250t, 508t–509t
    in children, 508t
    in renal insufficiency, 253t, 509t
  pharmacology, 252t, 508t–509t
  in vitro activity, 255t, 257

Cefrozil: structure, 248f
Cefsulodin: for Pseudomonads, 2004t
Ceftazidime, 259
    with aminoglycosides, 289t
    antimicrobial activity, 285t
    for *Bacteroides fragilis*, 2200t, 2201
    chemistry, 249
    dosage, 250t
        for meningitis, 849t, 850t
        in renal insufficiency, 253t
    for endocarditis: *Pseudomonas aerug-
        inosa*, 763
    for meningitis, 849t, 850t, 853
    for *Neisseria meningitidis*, 1904,
        1904t
    nephrotoxicity, 254
    for peritonitis: in peritoneal dialysis,
        720t
    pharmacology, 252t
    for Pseudomonads, 2004t
    for *Pseudomonas aeruginosa*
        bacteremia, 1988
        eye infections, 1992
        malignant otitis externa, 1990
        pneumonia, 1984
    for *Pseudomonas pseudomallei*, 2006
    for sepsis syndrome, 699, 699t
    structure, 248f
    susceptibility testing, 194, 194t
    in vitro activity, 255t, 260
Ceftibuten, 259
    dosage, 250t
    pharmacology, 252, 252t
    structure, 248f
    in vitro activity, 255t
Ceftin. *See* Cefuroxime axetil
Ceftizox. *See* Ceftizoxime
Ceftizoxime, 258–259
    for *Bacteroides fragilis*, 2200t, 2201
    chemistry, 248
    dosage, 250t, 508t–509t
        in children, 508t
        in renal insufficiency, 253t, 509t
    for odontogenic infections, 602t
    pharmacology, 252t, 508t–509t
    for Pseudomonads, 2004t
    structure, 248f
    susceptibility testing, 194, 194t
    in vitro activity, 255t, 260
Ceftriaxone, 259
    adverse reactions, 254
    antimicrobial activity, 285t
    chemistry, 248
    clinical trials, 227
    dosage, 508t–509t
        in children and neonates, 508t, 851t
        for meningitis, 850t, 851t
        in renal insufficiency, 509t
    for epiglottitis, 592
    for *Haemophilus influenzae*, 2043
    for infections arthritis, 1037
    for meningitis, 850t, 851, 851t, 853,
        857
    prophylaxis, 320
    for *Neisseria gonorrhoeae*, 195, 1914,
        1921, 1921t, 1922
    for *Neisseria meningitidis*, 1903t,
        1904, 1904t
    prophylaxis, 1905
    pharmacology, 252, 252t, 508t–509t
    resistance: *Streptococcus pneumoniae*,
        1821–1822
    for *Salmonella*, 2026
    structure, 248f
    susceptibility testing, 194, 194t

for *Treponema pallidum*, 2129t
for viridans streptococci, 1851
in vitro activity, 255t, 260
Cefuroxime, 256–257
    chemistry, 247, 249
    dosage, 250t, 508t–509t
        in children, 508t
        in renal insufficiency, 253t, 509t
    for endocarditis: prophylaxis, 788
    for meningitis, 851
    for *Neisseria meningitidis*, 1904, 1904t
    pharmacology, 252t, 508t–509t
    for sinusitis, 589t
    structure, 248f
    in vitro activity, 255t, 256–257, 257
Cefuroxime axetil, 257
    activity, 258
    dosage: in renal insufficiency, 253t
    pharmacology, 251, 252t
Cefzil. *See* Cefprozil
Celiac artery mycotic aneurysms, 771
Cell-mediated immunity, 102–149. *See
        also* CD *and* T cells
    anaerobes and, 2162
    Babesia and, 2499
    Bacteroides and, 2197
    Blastomyces dermatitidis and,
        2355–2356, 2362
    bone marrow transplantation and,
        2718
    and *Brucella*, 2055
    Candida albicans and, 2290, 2295
    CNS infections and, 829
    Coccidioides immitis and, 2367
    cryptococcosis and, 2332–2333
    Cryptosporidium and, 2505–2506
    cytokines, 112–122, 130–131. *See
        also* Cytokines
    defects, 132–139. *See also* T cells,
        deficiencies
        bacteremia, 2681
        infections and, 2681–2682
            microbiology, 2681
            therapy, 2682
        meningitis, 2682
        pulmonary infections, 2681–2682
        skin and soft tissue infections, 2682
    and endocarditis, 745–746
    Entamoeba histolytica and, 2399
    and Epstein-Barr virus, 129,
        1366–1367
    and *Francisella tularensis*, 2063
    Giardia lamblia and, 2488–2489
    hepatitis C virus and, 1477
    and herpes simplex virus and, 1337
    histoplasmosis and, 2340, 2341–2342
    and HIV, 1213–1214. *See also* Human
        immunodeficiency virus
        (HIV), and CD4+
    and infections in patients with neopla-
        sia, 2666t, 2668–2669
    and *Legionella pneumophila*,
        2090–2091
    Leishmania and, 2428, 2429–2430
    in leukemia/lymphoma: infections
        and, 2681–2682
    lymphokines, 112–118. *See also*
        Lymphokines
    major histocompatibility complex,
        102–105. *See also* Major his-
        tocompatibility complex
    and measles virus, 1521
    mononuclear phagocytes, 122–124
    and *Mycobacterium tuberculosis*,
        2218–2219

NK cells, 122. *See also* NK cells
Nocardia and, 2275
paracoccidioidomycosis and, 2387
Pneumocystis carinii and, 2477
and pneumonia, 620–621
in pregnancy, 35
respiratory syncytial virus and,
    1506–1507
and *Salmonella*, 2019
against specific infections, 124–130
Staphylococcus aureus and, 1762
T cells, 105–112, 119–120, 121t. *See
    also* T cells
Cellulitis, 914–916
    Acinetobacter, 2011
    clinical features, 914–915
    clostridial anaerobic, 923
        clinical features, 923
        crepitant, 2185
        differential diagnosis, 923, 924t, 932
        treatment, 923
    dissecting of scalp, 915
    in drug abusers, 2697
    in the elderly, 2739
    etiology, 915–916
    gangrenous, 917–919, 918t
        clinical features, 917–918
        differential diagnosis, 918–919
        pathology and pathogenesis, 917
        in predisposed host, 917–918
        progressive bacterial synergistic
            gangrene, 917, 917f, 918t
        Pseudomonas aeruginosa, 920
        streptococcal, 917–918, 918t
        treatment, 918–919
    group A streptococcal, 555
    Haemophilus influenzae, 921–922,
        2042
    in the immunocompromised, 915
    nonclostridial anaerobic, 923
        differential diagnosis, 924t, 933
    orbital, 1131–1133
        and dacryocystopyocele, 1131
        differential diagnosis, 1133
        etiology, 1131–1133
        laboratory findings, 1133–1134
        treatment, 1134–1135
    pelvic, 1094
    perianal
        group A streptococcal, 555
        and leukemia, 2678
    postseptal. *See* orbital *above*
    preseptal, 1131
    Pseudomonas, 918t
    spinal cord injury and, 2733
    Staphylococcus aureus, 914, 1765
    Streptococcus agalactiae, 1840
    Streptococcus pyogenes, 1794, 1794f
    synergistic necrotizing, 922, 926
        clinical features, 926
        differential diagnosis, 918t, 924t
        treatment, 926
    treatment, presumptive, 916
    vaginal cuff, 1094
        Trichomonas vaginalis, 2494
    Vibrio vulnificus, 1946
Cell wall precursor targets: alteration in
    resistance, 220
Centipeda, 2158t
Central European encephalitis, 1467
    clinical manifestations, 1472
    epidemiology, 1469
    prevention and treatment, 1473
    transmission, clinical syndromes, and
        geographic distribution, 1466t

Central nervous system (CNS)
    anatomy, 822f, 822–831, 823f
        vascular, 824–826
    brain-spinal cord relationship, 822f,
        822–824, 823f
    drug toxicity. *See* Neurotoxicity
    dysfunction: and infections in patients
        with neoplasia, 2670
    fever and, 546
    specimen collection and processing,
        171t, 178t, 178–179
    vascular anatomy, 824–826
        arteries, 824–826, 825f
        capillaries, 826
        spinal cord, 826
        veins, 825f, 825–826
Central nervous system infections,
    822–909. *See also specific
    infections*
    actinomycosis, 2284–2285
    adenovirus, 1386
    anaerobic cocci, 2205
    anaerobic gram-negative bacilli, 2197
    Aspergillus, 2308
    Blastomyces dermatitidis, 2356t,
        2360, 2360f
    brain abscess, 887–900
    brain herniation and, 829f, 830
    Campylobacter, 1952
    Candida albicans, 2296
        treatment, 2300
    Clostridium, 2185
    cranial nerves and, 823, 823f
    Cryptococcus neoformans, 2333, 2334
    CSF and, 827f, 827–828
    in drug abusers, 2703–2704
    edema and, 830
        therapy, 830t
    encephalitis, 874–878
    epidural abscess, 904–907
    Histoplasma capsulatum, 2347
    influenza virus, 1558
    intracranial circulation and, 824–827
    meningitis. *See also* Meningitis
        acute, 832–865
        chronic, 865–874
    mucormycosis, 2315–2316
    Mycobacterium tuberculosis,
        2234–2235
    Mycoplasma pneumoniae, 1707
    myelitis, 874–878
    neuritis, 874, 878–879
    Nocardia, 2276
    Plasmodium, 2421–2422
    Pseudomonas aeruginosa, 1988–1989
        treatment, 1989
    response, 829–830
    routes, 828
    Salmonella, 2023
    schistosomiasis, 2541
    slow infections, 881–887
        Creutzfeldt-Jakob disease, 881–883
        fatal familial insomnia, 881,
            883–884
        Gerstmann-Straussler-Scheinker
            syndrome, 881, 883
        handling infectious material,
            884–885
        kuru, 881
        treatment, 883
    Streptococcus intermedius group, 1863
    subdural empyema, 900–903
    suppurative intracranial phlebitis,
        907–909
    therapy: for edema, 830t

Central nervous system infections
(*Continued*)
in transplant recipients, 2728t, 2728–2729
in traumatized patient, 2757–2758
vaccinia virus, 1326
vascular supply and, 826–827, 827f
Central venous catheters
bacteremia from, 2592
exchange over guideline, 2592
long-term: bacteremia from, 2594t, 2594–2595
suppurative thrombophlebitis, 766, 767
Cephalexin, 256
antibiotic-associated colitis (AAC), 979
for bacterial vaginosis, 1079t
chemistry, 249
for cystic fibrosis infections, 660
dosage, 250t, 508t–509t
in children and neonates, 508t
in renal insufficiency, 253t, 509t
pharmacology, 252t, 508t–509t
structure, 248f
for urinary tract infections: in pregnancy, 679
in vitro activity, 255t
Cephaloridine, 247
dosage: in renal dysfunction, 204
nephrotoxicity, 254
structure, 248f
Cephalosporinase, 251
β-lactamase, 216t
Cephalosporins, 247–264. *See also specific formulations*
adverse reactions, 253t, 253–254
disulfiran-like, 254–255
GI toxicity, 254
hematologic, 254
hypersensitivity, 253–254
nephrotoxicity, 254
neutropenia, 89
antimicrobial activity: aminoglycosides compared with, 285t
chemistry, 247f, 247–249, 248f
classification, 249, 250t
cross-reactivity, 276–277
with penicillins, 253–254
dosage, 250t, 252t, 508t–509t
in children, 250t, 508t
in neonates, 508t
oral, 250t
parenteral, 250t
in renal insufficiency, 253t, 509t
drug interactions, 521t
for enterococcal infections, 1829
first-generation, 255t, 255–256. *See also specific formulations*
clinical use, 256
oral antibacterial activity, 255t
parenteral antibacterial activity, 255t
pharmacology, 508t–509t
indications, 194
mechanism of action, 249–250
for *Moraxella catarrhalis*, 1928
for *Neisseria meningitidis*, 1903t, 1904, 1904t
perioperative prophylactic use, 2750
for peritonitis, 716
pharmacology, 251–253, 252t, 508t–509t
resistance, 250–251
second-generation, 256–258. *See also specific formulations*

clinical use, 257–258
pharmacology, 508t–509t
for pneumonia, 632t
skin test, 277
for *Streptococcus pyogenes*, 1790–1791
structure, 247f, 248f, 274f
and sugar level testing, 203
third-generation, 258–260. *See also specific formulations*
clinical use, 260
for meningitis, 850t, 851t, 852
for neutropenics, 2688t
perioperative prophylactic use, 280
for peritonitis, 710, 717
pharmacology, 508t–509t
for pneumonia, 632t
nosocomial, 2603
for sepsis syndrome, 699, 699t
Cephalosporium acremonium, 247
Cephalothin, 247, 255–256
with aminoglycosides, 287, 287t
antibiotic-associated colitis (AAC), 979
chemistry, 247
dosage, 250t, 508t–509t
in children and neonates, 508t
in renal dysfunction, 204, 509t
for endocarditis
staphylococcal, 760
streptococcal, 759, 762
pharmacology, 252, 252t, 253, 508t–509t
resistance, 251
structure, 248f
susceptibility testing, 194t
Cephapirin, 256
dosage, 250t, 508t–509t
in children and neonates, 508t
in renal insufficiency, 253t, 509t
pharmacology, 252, 508t–509t
structure, 248f
Cephradine, 256
dosage, 250t, 508t–509t
in children and neonates, 508t
in renal insufficiency, 253t, 509t
pharmacology, 251, 252t, 508t–509t
structure, 248f
in vitro activity, 255t
CEP-1 β-lactamase, 216t
Cercariae, 2557
Cercopithecine herpesvirus 1, 1379–1382.
See also Herpes B virus
Cerebellar ataxia: VZV, 1347
Cerebral angiography: for bacterial meningitis, 842
Cerebral blood flow: bacterial meningitis and, 841–842
Cerebral edema
bacterial meningitis and, 841
and CNS infections, 830
therapy, 830t
Cerebral embolism: and endocarditis, 746, 749
Cerebral infarction: brain abscess vs., 891
Cerebral malaria
pathogenesis, 2419
treatment: steroids, 2426
Cerebral mass lesions: *Histoplasma capsulatum*, 2347
Cerebral ventricles: anatomy, 826, 827f
Cerebritis
Listeria monocytogenes, 1882t, 1883, 1883t, 1884f

in transplant recipients, 2728
Cerebrospinal fluid (CSF)
and CNS infections, 827f, 827–828
cryptococcosis, 2334–2335
examination
bacterial meningitis, 846
encephalitis, 876
and FUO, 539
viral meningitis, 845–846
meningitis
antimicrobial therapy, 853–854
chronic, 867t, 869
examination, 845–846
mumps virus, 1497, 1497t, 1499
shunt infections, 843
antimicrobial therapy, 853
Staphylococcus epidermidis, 1780
treatment, 1780
rifampin, 323, 1780
specimen collection and processing, 171t, 178t, 178–179
Trypanosoma brucei, 2451, 2452, 2453
Cerebrovascular system. *See also* Central nervous system
anatomy
arteries, 824, 825f
capillaries, 826
veins, 825–826, 826f
and CNS infections, 826, 827f
Ceruloplasmin
and acute phase response, 535
and FUO, 539
and inflammation, 34
Cervical adenitis, 603, 604, 937
Mycobacterium avium-intracellulare, 938, 2255
Mycobacterium scrofulaceum, 938, 2255
Cervical carcinoma, 1388t, 1389. *See also* Human papillomavirus
HIV/AIDS and, 1183, 1227, 1246, 1390
Cervical CMV, 1354, 1354t
Cervical discharge, normal, 1084
Cervical dysplasia: and HIV/AIDS, 1175, 1183, 1227, 1246
Cervical ectropion (erosion/eversion), 1084
Cervicitis, 1084–1085
chlamydial, 1085, 1686–1687, 1687f
HIV and, 1687
etiology, 1084f, 1084–1085
gonococcal, 1084f, 1084–1085, 1915, 1916, 1916f
diagnosis, 1919–1920
herpetic, 1085
hypertrophic, 1084
infectious, 1081
treatment, 1085
quinolones, 371
Cervicofacial infections: actinomycosis, 2281
Cervix
examination, 1083
inflammation, 1083
strawberry: *Trichomonas vaginalis*, 2494
Cesarean delivery
postpartum endometritis, 1091
Streptococcus agalactiae, 1840
prophylaxis recommendations, 2751t
Cestodes, 2525t, 2544–2553, 2545t
anatomy, 2544
antiparasitic agents, 460t, 482–483

biology, 2544–2546
coracidium larva, 2544
diagnosis, 1006t, 2547–2548
embryonated, 2544
immunology, 2546
intestinal
Diphyllobothrium latum (fish tapeworm), 2546–2547
Dipylidium caninum (dog/cat tapeworm), 2547
Hymenolepis diminuta (rat tapeworm), 2547
Hymenolepis nana (dwarf tapeworm), 2547
Taenia saginata (beef tapeworm), 2547
Taenia solium (pork tapeworm), 2547
invasive, 2548–2551
Echinococcus (hydatid and alveolar cyst disease), 2550–2551
Taenia solium, 2548–2550
life cycle, 2544–2546, 2545f, 2546f
oncosphere, 2544
pathogenesis, 2546
plerocercoid cyst (sparganum), 2544, 2545
prevention, 2551–2552
procercoid larva, 2544
proglottids, 2544
rostellum, 2544
treatment, 2548. *See also individual species*
Chagas disease, 2442–2450. *See also Trypanosoma cruzi*
Chagoma, 2443
Chalazion, 1130
treatment, 1134
Chancre
Treponema pallidum, 552, 1057, 1058f, 2121f, 2121–2122
Trypanosoma brucei, 2451
Chancriform lesions, 913
differential diagnosis, 2122, 2211
Chancroid, 2047–2048. *See also Haemophilus ducreyi*
Changuinola virus, 1448
Chaperone proteins, 24
Charcot's joints, 2125
Chédiak-Higashi syndrome, 90–91, 150, 151t
diagnosis, 154
neutrophil dysfunction, 90–91, 153, 154
prophylaxis and, 94
Staphylococcus aureus and, 1762
Cheeks, slapped (erythema infectiosum), 1442
Chemicals: food-borne disease, 1014–1016
poisoning, 1012
Chemical sterilization, 2581
Chemiluminescent probes, 184
for mycobacteria, 190
Chemokine α family: characteristics, sources, and effects, 114t
Chemokine β family: characteristics, sources, and effects, 114t
Chemokinesis, 82, 86
Chemoprophylaxis, 167
Chemosterilizers, 2581
Chemotaxis, 86
defects, 90–95
abnormal phagocytosis, 91
abnormal respiratory burst, 92–93
extrinsic, 90

granule abnormalities, 93–94
　in intracellular killing, 91–92
　intrinsic, 90–91
Chemotherapy patients. *See also*
　　　Neoplasia *and specific drugs*
　　　and tumors
　esophagitis in, 963–964
　infections in, 2666–2675. *See also*
　　　Neoplasia, infections in
　　　patients with
Cheyletiella, 2564
C$_H$ genes, 44–45
Chickenpox, 1345–1351. *See also*
　　　Varicella-zoster virus
　clinical manifestations, 1347–1348
　differential diagnosis, 1349
　　rickettsialpox, 1727
　epidemiology, 1346
　in the immunocompromised, 1348
　pathogenesis, 1347
　therapy, 1349
Chiggers, 2564
　and scrub typhus, 1740
Chikungunya, 1455
　arthritis, 1036, 1036t
　clinical manifestations, 1458
　diagnosis, 1458
　differential diagnosis, 1472
　epidemiology, 1456–1457
　myocarditis, 800
　pathogenesis, 1457
Children. *See also* Neonatal disease;
　　　Neonates
　bacteriuria in, 668, 672–673, 673f
　diarrheal diseases in: mortality rates,
　　　945
　drug dosages for. *See* Pediatric drug
　　　dosages
　fever of unknown origin (FUO), 537t
　HIV/AIDS in, 1184–1187, 1186t,
　　　1186–1187
　　demographic characteristics, 1186t
　　testing indications, 1194
　nitrofurantoin use, 379
　subdural empyema in, 902, 902t
　urinary tract infections in, 668
　vaccine indications for, 2783, 2786t,
　　　2787–2788. *See also*
　　　Vaccines
Child sexual abuse, 1056, 1081–1082
　gonorrhea and, 1919
Chills
　in endocarditis, 747, 748t
　and sepsis, 691
Chilopoda, 2558
Chimpanzee coryza virus (CCA), 1502.
　　　See also Respiratory syncytial
　　　virus
Chinese hamster ovary (CHO) cells:
　　　adhesin and, 16
Chinese liver fluke, 2541–2542
"Chinese restaurant" syndrome, 1014,
　　　1015, 1019
Chlamydia
　elementary body (EB), 1677
　genome, 1678
　life cycle, 1677–1678
　overview, 1676–1679
　reticulate body, 1677–1678
　species, 1677t. *See also individual*
　　　species
Chlamydial diseases, 1676–1701. *See*
　　　also individual species
　characteristics, 1677t, 1697t
　endocarditis. *See Chlamydia psittaci*

and fever, 543
LGV. *See Chlamydia trachomatis*;
　　　Lymphogranuloma venereum
　overview, 1676–1679
　pneumonia. *See individual species*
　trachoma. *See Chlamydia trachomatis*
　treatment: quinolones, 367t
　TWAR strain. *See Chlamydia pneu-*
　　　moniae
　venereal. *See Chlamydia trachomatis*
Chlamydia pneumoniae, 1696–1701
　asthma and, 1698
　and atherosclerosis, 1699–1700
　bronchitis, 1698
　　acute, 606
　characteristics, 1677t, 1697t
　clinical disease, 1698–1699
　complement fixation, 1699
　differential diagnosis, 2345
　elementary body, 1696, 1697f
　epidemiology, 1696–1698
　and erythema nodosum, 1700
　fever, 543
　incidence, 1697, 1697t, 1698f
　laboratory diagnosis, 1699, 1699t
　major outer membrane protein
　　　(MOMP), 1696
　microbiology, 1696, 1697f, 1697t
　microimmunofluorescence test, 1699,
　　　1699t
　myocarditis, 800
　overview, 1676–1678
　periodicity, 1697
　pharyngitis, 567t, 569
　pneumonia, 619t, 1698–1699, 1704
　　atypical, 629–630
　　differential diagnosis, 1698
　　incidence, 1698–1699
　　serology, 625–626
　　sputum analysis, 623
　　treatment, 632
　polymerase chain reaction, 1699
　prevalence, 1696–1697, 1697f
　reticulate body, 1678
　serology, 192t
　sinusitis, 585, 1698
　transmission, 1697–1698
　treatment, 1699
　　quinolones, 367t, 371
Chlamydia psittaci, 1676, 1678,
　　　1693–1696
　animal reservoirs, 2792t
　characteristics, 1677t, 1697t
　clinical features, 1694–1695
　cutaneous manifestations, 550t
　diagnosis, 1695
　differential diagnosis, 1695
　endocarditis, 751, 758
　　treatment, 764
　enteric symptoms, 999t, 1003
　epidemiology, 1693–1694
　fever, 543, 1694
　hepatitis, 1694
　Horder's spots, 1694
　laboratory findings, 1695
　macrophages and, 124
　myocarditis, 800
　pathology, 1695
　pneumonia, 619t, 622t, 1694
　　atypical, 630
　prevention, 1695
　serology, 192t
　treatment, 1695
Chlamydia trachomatis, 1677f, 1678f,
　　　1679–1693

antigen detection, 1682t, 1682–1683,
　　　1683f
antigenic and chemical composition,
　　　1680–1681
bartholinitis, 1069, 1085
biovars, 1677, 1677t, 1680–1681. *See*
　　　also Lymphogranuloma
　　　venereum *and* trachoma *below*
cervicitis, 1085, 1686–1687, 1687f
characteristics, 1677t, 1697t
clinical manifestations, 1683–1689
conjunctivitis, 1106, 1114, 1685
　diagnosis, 1107–1108
　differential diagnosis, 1685
　neonatal, 1679, 1688–1689
　　treatment, 1689
cultures, 1682
cytokine protection, 121t
cytologic diagnosis, 1682
diarrhea: in AIDS, 970, 970t
direct fluorescent antibody (DFA) test,
　　　1682
and ectopic pregnancy, 1687
EIA diagnosis, 185
elementary body, 1679
endocervicitis, 1095
endometritis, 1687
epididymitis, 1069, 1101, 1685
genital infection in women,
　　　1686–1687
and HIV transmission, 1188
host range, 1678
immunity, 1681
immunofluorescence, 185
inclusion conjunctivitis, 1106, 1114
　adult, 1685
　diagnosis, 183, 1108
　neonatal, 1688–1689
　　treatment, 1688
and infertility, 1687
keratitis, 1114
laboratory diagnosis, 1681–1683
life cycle, 1677, 1679–1680, 1680f
lymphogranuloma venereum (LGV),
　　　1680, 1684–1685. *See also*
　　　Lymphogranuloma venereum
　isolation in cell culture, 1682
　pathogenesis, 1681
　serology, 1683
　treatment, 1684–1685
microimmunofluorescence test, 1682
nasopharyngeal specimens, 172
Neisseria gonorrhoeae coinfection,
　　　1915
neonatal infections
　inclusion conjunctivitis, 1688–1689
　pneumonia, 1689
　prevention and treatment, 1689
nucleic acid hybridization, 1682–1683
ocular trachoma, 1683–1684
　treatment, 1684
　WHO grading scheme, 1683t
oculogenital disease in adults,
　　　1685–1688
　treatment, 1688
otitis media, 581
overview, 1676–1678
pathogenesis, 1681
perinatal infections, 1688–1689
　inclusion conjunctivitis, 1688–1689
　pneumonia, 1688–1689, 1689f
　prevention and treatment, 1689
peritonitis, 709
PID, 183, 1095, 1687
　treatment, 1688

pneumonia, 619t, 1688
　atypical, 630
　infant, 1689, 1689f
　　prevention and treatment, 1689
postpartum endometritis, 1091
and pregnancy complications,
　　　1687–1688
prevention, 1689–1690
　perinatal infections, 1689
　screening indications for women,
　　　1690t
proctitis, 1686
　and HIV/AIDS, 1231
　treatment, 1688
proctocolitis, 1686
prostatitis, 1685
and Reiter syndrome, 1071
reticulate body, 1677, 1679–1680
salpingitis, 1069, 1687
serology, 192t, 1683
serovar A photomicrograph, 1677f
sexually reactive arthritis, 1686
specimen collection and processing,
　　　171t, 182–183
strains, 1677t
susceptibility, 1678
trachoma, 1106, 1114, 1679, 1680,
　　　1683–1684
　clinical manifestations,
　　　1683–1684
　cytologic diagnosis, 1682
　immunity, 1681
　laboratory diagnosis, 1681–1682
　pathogenesis, 1681
　treatment, 1684
　vaccine research, 1681
　WHO grading system, 1683t
treatment
　azithromycin, 335t, 340
　clarithromycin, 335t, 339, 340
　erythromycin, 335t, 338, 338t
　oculogenital disease in adults,
　　　1688
　perinatal infections, 1689
　quinolones, 367t, 371
　sulfonamides, 355t
　trimethoprim, 357
urethritis, 1067–1068
　asymptomatic, 1065, 1068–1069
　clinical manifestations,
　　　1066–1067
　diagnosis, 1065–1066
　female, 1069, 1686–1687
　male, 1685
　postgonococcal, 1068
　treatment, 1069–1070, 1688
　　sulfonamides, 357
urogenital infections, 1685
Chlamydospores, 2326
Chlorambucil: immunodeficiency from,
　　　136
Chloramphenicol, 310–314, 384t
　adverse reactions, 313–314
　　in diabetics, 203
　　in G6PD deficiency, 203
　　gray baby syndrome, 314
　　hematologic, 313–314
　　optic neuritis, 314
　in anemics, 203
　antibiotic-associated colitis (AAC)
　　　from, 979
　for *Bacteroides fragilis*, 2200t, 2201
　for brain abscess, 895
　combination therapy
　　antagonism, 208–209

Chloramphenicol (*Continued*)
dosage, 512t–513t, 850t
for meningitis, 850t, 851t
in neonates and children, 201, 512t, 851t
in renal dysfunction, 204–205, 513t
drug interactions, 314, 521t
vancomycin, 349
for endocarditis, anaerobic, 764
for enteric fever, 1003
for epiglottitis, 592
for *Francisella tularensis*, 2066
for *Haemophilus influenzae*, 2043, 2044
indications, 314, 314t
mechanism of action, 311
for peritonitis, 715
pharmacologic tables, 512t–513t
pharmacology, 312f, 312–313, 512t–513t
for Pseudomonads, 2004t
for *Pseudomonas pseudomallei*, 2006
in renal and hepatic insufficiency, 313
resistance, 215t, 218–219, 311–312, 851
coagulase-negative staphylococci, 1778
Salmonella, 2026
for *Rickettsia rickettsii*, 1724
for *Salmonella*, 2026, 2026t
for scrub typhus, 1741
structure, 310–311, 311f
and sugar level testing, 203
susceptibility testing, 194t
in vitro activity, 311–312, 312t
for *Yersinia pestis*, 2075
Chloramphenicol acetyltransferase, 218–219
Chlorhexidine, 382
Chlorine dioxide sterilization, 2581
Chloroquanide. *See* Proguanil
Chloroquine
adverse reactions, 470
for amebiasis, 2404t
antiparasitic use, 459t, 469–471
dosage, 464t
pediatric, 464t
prophylactic, 464t, 465t
drug interactions, 521t
for *Histoplasma capsulatum*, 2351
for *Plasmodium*, 2422, 2425
resistance, 2422–2425, 2423f, 2424t
for travelers, 2801
side effects, 2424
structure, 470f
Chlorpropamide: interactions with sulfonamides, 356
Chlortetracycline, 306, 384t
dosage, 512t–513t
and pH, 206
pharmacology, 309f, 310, 512t–513t
structure, 307f
Cholangiocarcinoma: liver flukes and, 2541
Cholangiopancreatography, endoscopic retrograde (ERCP): and pancreatitis, 723
Cholangitis, 732–733
antimicrobial therapy, 733
ascending: and fever, 541
bacteriology, 732
complications, 732
differential diagnosis, 732–733
laboratory findings, 732

liver transplantation and, 2725
pathogenesis, 732
radiography, 732
Salmonella, 2022
sclerosing: and HIV/AIDS, 1230
Streptococcus intermedius, 1863
surgery, 733
symptoms and signs, 732
Cholecystectomy: prophylaxis recommendations, 2751t
Cholecystitis, 729–732
acalculous
and HIV/AIDS, 1230
in trauma patients, 2758
acute, 729–732
antimicrobial therapy, 731
bacteriology, 730–731
complications, 731
differential diagnosis, 731
emphysematous, 731
laboratory findings, 730
pathogenesis, 729, 730f
pathology, 729–730, 730t
radiography, 731
surgery, 731–732
symptoms and signs, 729
and fever, 541
Cholecystography, 731
Cholecystostomy, 732
Choledochojejunostomy: and infections in transplant recipients, 2710
Cholelithiasis, 730
spinal cord injury and, 2735–2736
Cholera, 1934–1945. *See also Vibrio cholerae*
Cholera toxin, 3t, 5, 949t, 950, 1934–1935, 1936
attachment and entry, 4
structure, 1936f
Cholera vaccine, 2774
adverse reactions, 2775
indications for adults, 2784t
research, 1941
for travelers, 2797, 2797t
Cholestatic liver disease, 1149
Cholesteatoma: anaerobic, 2163t
Cholestyramine: for antibiotic-associated colitis, 983–984
Chorea: and rheumatic fever, 1803, 1804
Chorioamnionitis. *See* Intra-amniotic infection syndrome
Chorioretinitis
CMV, 1359, 1359f
Mycobacterium tuberculosis, 2240
Toxoplasma gondii, 2455, 2459
in immunocompetent, 2461, 2461f
pathology, 2458–2459
serology, 2465
Treponema pallidum, 2125
tuberculous, 2240, 2240f
Choroiditis
Borrelia burgdorferi, 2148
Histoplasma capsulatum, 2348
Chromobacterium typhiflavium, 2107t, 2112–2113
Chromobacterium violaceum, 2109
Chromoblastomycosis. *See* Chromomycosis
Chrombodies, 2326
Chromomycosis, 2324–2327
clinical manifestations, 2324–2326, 2325f
diagnosis, 2326
differential diagnosis, 2322, 2437
epidemiology, 2324

etiology and mycology, 2324
pathology, 2326
treatment, 2326
flucytosine, 406
Chronic care facilities: diarrhea in, 970
Chronic fatigue and immunodeficiency syndrome (CFIDS), 1308
Chronic fatigue syndrome, 1306–1310
case definition, 1306t, 1306–1307
clinical manifestations, 1307
differential diagnosis: *Borrelia burgdorferi*, 2151
epidemiology and case definition, 1306–1307
etiology and pathogenesis, 1307–1308, 1308t
history, 1306
laboratory findings, 1306t, 1307
management, 1308–1309
pharmacologic, 1308–1309
Chronic granulomatous disease. *See* Granulomatous disease, chronic
Chronic obstructive pulmonary disease (COPD)
histoplasmosis and, 2345
influenza virus and, 1557, 1557t
and pneumonia, 621
and *Streptococcus pneumoniae*, 1817, 1817t
Chronic pulmonary disease: and nosocomial pneumonia, 2601
Chrysomyia, 2562
Chrysops: and loiasis, 2535
CH$_{50}$ test, 156
Churg-Strauss syndrome
pneumonia, 647t
pulmonary infiltrates with eosinophilia, 631
Ciclopirox: topical, 401t
Ciguatera poisoning, 1012t, 1015, 1015t, 1017
fish implicated, 1017t
laboratory diagnosis, 1018t
management, 1019–1020
Ciguatoxin, 1015
Cilastatin, 265
Ciliary dysentery, 989
Ciliary neurotropic factor (CNTF), 530
Ciliophora, 2393t
Cimetidine, 455
drug interactions, 310
quinolones, 370
for hepatitis, 1150
Cinchona alkaloids, 471
Cineangiography: for endocarditis, 752
Cinnoline, 365f
Cinoxacin, 364
dosage, 370t, 516t–517t
pharmacology, 516t–517t
susceptibility testing, 194t
Ciprofloxacin
adverse reactions, 203
antibiotic-associated colitis (AAC), 979
antimicrobial activity, 285t, 364, 367t, 369t, 371, 373
and bone marrow transplantation: prophylactic, 2721t
for *Campylobacter*, 1953
clinical trials, 230
combination with rifampin
for endocarditis, 321
for osteomyelitis, 322
for cystic fibrosis infections, 660

dosage, 370t, 516t–517t
for meningitis, 850t
drug interactions, 370
for *Haemophilus ducreyi*, 2048
for *Legionella pneumophila*, 2093, 2093t
for meningitis prophylaxis, 320, 857
for *Mycobacterium avium-intracellulare*, 2257, 2258
for *Mycobacterium tuberculosis*, 395
for *Mycoplasma pneumoniae*, 1710, 1710t
for *Neisseria gonorrhoeae*, 1921, 1921t, 1922
for *Neisseria meningitidis* prophylaxis, 1905
for peritonitis, 717
pharmacokinetics, 369t
pharmacology, 516t–517t
in vitro models, 229
for Pseudomonads, 2004t
for *Pseudomonas aeruginosa*, 1990, 1992, 1994, 1995
endocarditis, 1984
for *Salmonella*, 2028
structure, 365f
for travelers' diarrhea, 972
Circadian temperature rhythm, 530
exaggerated, 548
Circumcision: and HIV transmission, 1170
Cirrhosis
alcoholic: and peritonitis, 709
chronic hepatitis and, 1155
defective chemotaxis in, 90
pruritus: rifampin for, 325
Citrobacter, 1974
β-lactamase, 215, 218, 268
diarrhea: infantile, 967
endocarditis, 755
infusion-related sepsis, 2587
toxin, 950
treatment
aminoglycosides, 285t
β-lactamase inhibitors, 268t
nitrofurantoin, 377
quinolones, 367t
and urinary tract infections, 2613
Citrobacter amalonaticus, 1974, 1975t
Citrobacter diversus, 1974, 1975t
brain abscess, 890
meningitis, 1974
treatment
carbapenems, 264t
penicillins, 237t
rifampin, 318t
Citrobacter freundii, 1974, 1975t
mycotic aneurysms, 772
resistance, 221, 251
toxin, 5, 6, 950
treatment
carbapenems, 264t
cephalosporins, 255t, 257
penicillins, 237t
rifampin, 318t
trimethoprim, 357
Cladophialophora ajelloi, 2324
Cladosporium, 2391
Cladosporium carrionii
chromomycosis, 2324–2326
treatment, 2326
Cladosporium trichoides, 2391
brain abscess, 890
Claforan. *See* Cefotaxime

Clam digger's itch, 2557
Clarithromycin, 334, 338–340
    adverse reactions, 340
    antimicrobial activity, 339
    combination therapy: for mycobacteria, 396t
    dosage, 512t–513t
    drug interactions, 340
    for *Legionella pneumophila*, 2093, 2093t
    mechanism of action, 339
    for *Mycobacterium avium-intracellulare*, 2257, 2257t, 2258
    for *Mycobacterium leprae*, 399, 2249
    for *Mycoplasma pneumoniae*, 1710, 1710t
    for nontuberculous mycobacteria, 396
    pharmacology, 339–340, 512t–513t
    resistance, 339
    structure, 339f
    for *Toxoplasma gondii*: in HIV/AIDS, 2467, 2467t
    uses, 340
Clavulanate, 268–269
    adverse reactions, 269
    with amoxicillin. *See* Amoxicillin-clavulanate
    pharmacology, 268–269
    structure, 268f
    with ticarcillin. *See* Ticarcillin-clavulanate
Clavulinic acid: for tuberculosis, 395
Cleaning: defined, 2579
Clenched-fist injuries (CFIs), 2768
    Eikenella, 2112
    treatment, 2201
Cleocin. *See* Clindamycin
Clethrionomys glareolus: and hantaviruses, 1569
Clinafloxacin, 365f
Clindamycin, 334, 341–343, 384t
    adverse reactions, 342–343, 1284
    antibiotic-associated colitis (AAC), 979, 993
    antimicrobial activity, 341t, 341–342
    antiparasitic use, 459t, 475
        dosage, 461t, 464t
            pediatric, 461t, 464t
    for *Babesia*, 2500
    for bacterial vaginosis, 1079, 1079t
    for *Bacteroides fragilis*, 2200t, 2201
    for brain abscess, 893
    for clostridial infections, 2192
    dosage, 512t–513t
        in renal dysfunction, 204–205, 513t
    drug interactions, 343, 521t
    for endocarditis
        anaerobic, 764
        prophylaxis, 797t
        staphylococcal, 762
    for *Gardnerella vaginalis*, 2051
    for intra-abdominal infections, 289
    for necrotizing pneumonia, 645
    for *Neisseria gonorrhoeae*, 1922, 1922t
    for odontogenic infections, 602t
    for peritonitis, 715–716, 717
        in peritoneal dialysis, 720t
    and pH, 206
    pharmacology, 342, 512t–513t
    for PID, 1096t
    for *Pneumocystis carinii*, 343, 1284, 2481
    resistance, 341–342
        coagulase-negative staphylococci, 1778

structure, 341f
    for suppurative thrombophlebitis, 769
    for *Toxoplasma gondii*, 1283t, 1287
        in HIV/AIDS, 2467, 2467t
    uses, 343
Clinical trials, 163
Clitocybe, 1015t
Clofazimine
    adverse reactions, 398
    combination therapy: for mycobacteria, 396t
    dosage, 398, 516t–517t
        for leprosy, 397t
    drug interactions, 521t
    for *Mycobacterium avium-intracellulare*, 2257, 2258
    for *Mycobacterium leprae*, 397t, 398, 2248
    pharmacology, 516t–517t
    structure, 398f
Clonorchis sinensis, 2525t, 2538t, 2541
    clinical syndromes, 2541
    diagnosis, 1006t, 1007, 2541
    treatment, 463t, 2541
        albendazole, 479
        artemisinin, 472
        praziquantel, 482
Clostridial anaerobic cellulitis, 923
    clinical features, 923
    differential diagnosis, 923, 924t
    pathogenesis and pathology, 922–923
    treatment, 923
Clostridial myonecrosis (gas gangrene), 931–933, 2163t, 2166, 2166t, 2186–2189
    antitoxin for, 2188
    clinical features, 931, 932f, 2187f, 2187–2188
    diagnosis, 2188
    differential diagnosis, 918t, 924t, 932, 2188
    epidemiology, 2186–2187
    etiology, 932, 2186
    history, 2186
    laboratory findings, 932
    pathogenesis and pathology, 931
    perfringolysin O (α toxin), 2186
    phospholipase C (α-toxin) and, 2186
    prognosis, 2189
    spontaneous nontraumatic (*C. septicum*), 931
    treatment, 932–933, 2188–2189, 2189f
    uterine, 2185, 2186
Clostridium, 2158t. *See also individual species*
    α-toxin, 2183
    antimicrobial susceptibility, 2170t
    bacteremia, 2184
    β-lactamase, 215
    biliary tract infections, 2185
    brain abscess, 890, 2185
    cholecystitis, 730
    clinically significant, 2159t
    CNS infections, 2185
    differential features, 2183t
    as enteric flora, 947
    enteric infections, 2189–2192, 2190t
    female genital tract infections, 2185
    histotoxic syndromes, 2183t
    and IgA, 8
    intra-abdominal infections, 2184–2185
    microbiology, 2182–2184
    myonecrosis (gas gangrene). *See* Clostridial myonecrosis

Nagler reaction, 2183
    as normal flora, 2159t
    pleuropulmonary infections, 2185
    snake bites, 2767
    soft tissue infections, 2185–2186
    spore formation, 2183
    treatment, 2170t
        antimicrobials of choice, 201t
        chloramphenicol, 312t
        metronidazole, 329t
        quinolones, 368t
Clostridium baratii, 2179
Clostridium bifermentans: gas gangrene, 2186
Clostridium botulinum, 2178–2182
    antitoxin, 2181
    characteristics, 2179
    clinical manifestations, 2180, 2180t
    C2 toxin, 5
    diagnosis, 2180–2181
    differential diagnosis, 2180, 2183t
        poliovirus, 1617
    epidemiology, 2161, 2179
    fish products and, 2179
    food-borne, 1012, 1014, 1016, 2179, 2180
        foods implicated, 1017t
        laboratory diagnosis, 1018t, 1019
    hepatitis, 1147, 1148
    history, 2179
    infant, 5, 2180
    neuritis, 878
    pathogenesis, 2179–2180
    prevention, 2181
    toxin, 2, 3t, 5, 949t, 950, 1014, 2179, 2180
        neuritis, 878
        treatment, 2181
    types A, B, E, F, 2179, 2180
        symptoms, 2180t
    types C and D, 2179
    type G, 2179
    virulence determinants, 22t
    wound, 2179, 2180
        in drug abusers, 2704
        treatment, 2181
Clostridium butyricum, 2179
    necrotizing enterocolitis of newborn, 991
Clostridium difficile
    antibiotic-associated colitis (AAC), 978–987, 2166. *See also* pseudomembranous colitis *below*
    characteristics, 2190t
    clinical diagnosis, 981–982, 2166
    clinical manifestations, 980, 2166
    epidemiology, 946, 979–980, 2161
    laboratory diagnosis, 980–981, 2166
    and leukemia, 2679
    pathogenesis, 979–980, 2161
    pathology, 978f, 978–979, 2161, 2166
    prevention, 985
    treatment, 982–984, 2166
        adrenal steroids, 983
        antibiotics, 982–983
        antidiarrheal agents, 983
        bacitracin, 983
        cholestyramine, 983–984
        colestipol, 983–984
        metronidazole, 983, 2166
        relapses or recurrence, 984
        surgical, 984
        vancomycin, 982–983, 2166

diarrhea
    and AAC, 980, 2166. *See also* antibiotic-associated colitis *above*
    in AIDS, 970, 970t
        diagnosis, 180
        in hospitals, 970
        in institutionalized elderly, 970
    differential diagnosis, 2183t
    Cryptosporidium, 2504
    in the elderly, 2740
    isolation, 2577
    pseudomembranous colitis, 992–993
        clindamycin and lincomycin and, 342
        dysentery, 992f, 992–993
        vancomycin for, 346, 350
    specimen collection, 180
    stool culture, 955
    toxins, 6, 950
        and AAC, 979–980
    treatment
        carbapenems, 264t
        fusidic acid, 278
        quinolones, 368t
        rifampin, 324
Clostridium fallax: gas gangrene, 2186
Clostridium histolyticum, 2183
    differential features, 2183t
    gas gangrene, 2186
Clostridium novyi, 2183
    differential features, 2183t
    gas gangrene, 932, 2186
Clostridium paraperfringens: neutropenic enterocolitis, 2191
Clostridium perfringens, 2183–2184
    α-toxin, 2162, 2183, 2183t, 2184t
    antimicrobial susceptibility, 2170t
    bacteremia, 2184
    β-toxin, 2183t, 2184t
    biliary tract infections, 2185
    cellulitis, 923
        clinical features, 923
        differential diagnosis, 923, 924t
        pathogenesis and pathology, 923
        therapy, 923
    cholangitis, 732
    and colon cancer, 2184
    cytotoxin (toxin B): and AAC, 979–980, 981
    decubitus ulcer infections, 919
    differential features, 2183t
    enteric infection, 2189–2192, 2190t
    enteritis necroticans, 2183t, 2189–2191, 2190t
        clinical features, 2190–2191
        epidemiology, 2190
    enterotoxin, 1013, 2183t, 2184t, 2186t, 2191
        and food poisoning, 2191
        toxin A. *See also* toxin A *below*
            cytotoxicity, 951
        toxin B: and AAC, 979–980, 981
    epidemiology, 2161
    episiotomy, 1093
    food-borne, 1012t, 1013, 1017, 1020, 2183t, 2189, 2190t, 2191–2192
        clinical features, 2192
        diagnosis, 2192
        epidemiology, 2191–2192
        foods implicated, 1017t
        laboratory diagnosis, 1018t, 1018–1019

Clostridium perfringens (Continued)
gas gangrene, 931–933, 2186–2189.
See also Clostridial myonecrosis
uterine, 2185
and HIV/AIDS, 2184
myocarditis, 800
Nagler reaction, 2183
neutropenic enterocolitis, 2189, 2190t,
2191
peritonitis, 711
oxygen therapy, 718
treatment, 716
pleuropulmonary infection, 2185
resistance, 220
septic abortion, 1093
serologic types (A–E), 2184, 2184t
soft tissue infections, 2185–2186
toxins, 3t, 950, 2161–2162, 2183t,
2183–2184, 2184t, 2186,
2186t. *See also* enterotoxin
above
treatment, 2170t
azithromycin, 335t
carbapenems, 264t
chloramphenicol, 312t
clarithromycin, 335t
clindamycin, 343
erythromycin, 335t
metronidazole, 329t, 332
penicillins, 237t
quinolones, 368t
tetracyclines, 308t
trimethoprim, 357
tubo-ovarian and pelvic abscesses,
2185
type A, 2183t, 2191. *See also* food-
borne *above*
type C, 2183t, 2190. *See also* enteritis
necroticans *above*
cytotoxicity, 951
and underlying disease, 2167
Clostridium ramosum, 2183
incidence, 2163
soft tissue infections, 2185
Clostridium septicum, 2183
bacteremia, 2184
cellulitis, 923
differential features, 2183t
gas gangrene, 931–932, 2186, 2187
incidence, 2163
myonecrosis, 923
neutropenic enterocolitis, 2190t, 2191
and underlying disease, 2167
Clostridium sordellii
antitoxin, 978
bacteremia, 2184
differential features, 2183t
episiotomy, 1093
female genital tract infections, 2185
gas gangrene, 2186
neutropenic enterocolitis, 2191
Clostridium sphenoides: neutropenic
enterocolitis, 2191
Clostridium sporogenes: neutropenic
enterocolitis, 2191
Clostridium tertium, 2183
bacteremia, 2184
neutropenic enterocolitis, 2190t, 2191
and underlying disease, 2167
Clostridium tetani, 2173–2178
cephalic, 2174, 2175, 2175f
characteristics, 2174, 2174f
clinical manifestations, 2174–2176,
2175f, 2176f

diagnosis, 2176
differential diagnosis, 2176, 2183t
rabies, 1535
in drug abusers, 2704
epidemiology, 2161, 2173–2174,
2174f
generalized, 2174–2175
history, 2173
localized, 2174, 2175
management protocol for generalized
tetanus, 2177–2178
neonatal, 2173, 2174, 2175–2176,
2176f
neuritis, 878
opisthotonos, 2175, 2175f
pathogenesis, 2174
prophylaxis, 2177
risus sardonicus, 2175, 2175f
tetanus-diphtheria vaccine, 2177
for travelers, 2797t, 2798
tetanus immunoglobulin, 167, 454,
2176, 2783
tetanus toxin (tetanospasmin), 2, 4, 5,
22t, 2174
neuritis, 878
tetanus toxoid vaccine, 50, 2177,
2775t, 2780t, 2781, 2782t
treatment, 2176–2177
trismus ("lockjaw"), 2175
virulence determinants, 22t
*Clostridium welchii. See Clostridium
perfringens*
Clotrimazole, 401, 401t, 403
for candidiasis, 2299, 2301
dosage, 403t
for esophagitis, 964t
structure, 402f
for transplant recipients: prophylactic,
2715
for *Trichomonas vaginalis*, 2495
for vulvovaginal candidiasis, 1076t
Clotting factors: virulence factors and, 8
Cloxacillin, 94, 243
for cellulitis, 916
dosage, 241t, 506t–507t
in neonates, 242t, 506t
in renal disease and dialysis, 238t,
507t
for furuncles, 912
MICs against cocci, 237t
pharmacokinetics, 238t
pharmacology, 506t–507t
structure, 242f
Clue cells, 1083
Clutton's joints: *Treponema pallidum*,
2126
CMI. *See* Cell-mediated immunity
CMI test: and FUO, 540–541
CMV. *See* Cytomegalovirus
Coagglutination tests, 185
CSF, 179
Coagulase: *Staphylococcus aureus*,
1759
Coagulopathy: in sepsis syndrome, 695f,
695–696
Cocci. *See also* Gram-negative cocci;
Gram-positive cocci
classification, 1752
Coccidioides immitis, 2289, 2365–2375
appearance in tissue, 2289t
arthritis, 1035
arthroconidia (hyphae), 2365–2366
brain abscess, 890
chronic pulmonary, 2367, 2368f
clinical manifestations, 2367–2370

cutaneous, 550t, 552, 557, 2369,
2369f
description, 2365–2366, 2366f
diagnosis, 2370–2371
mycologic, 2370
serologic, 2370–2371
skin testing, 2371
differential diagnosis
Bartonella, 1742
histoplasmosis, 2345
disseminated: ketoconazole for, 407
ecology, 2366
endophthalmitis
in AIDS, 1123
treatment, 1126
epidemiology, 2366
extrapulmonary: and HIV/AIDS,
1182t
granulomatous hepatitis, 1161
growth, 190
and HIV/AIDS, 557, 2390
extrapulmonary, 1182t
meningitis, 872
pneumonia, 1236
treatment, 1283t, 1289
in the immunocompromised,
2369–2370
immunologic characteristics,
2366–2367
immunoprophylaxis and immunotherapy, 2373
lymphadenitis, 940t
meningitis, 869, 2368–2369
and HIV, 872
in the immunocompromised, 872
treatment, 868
musculoskeletal, 2367–2368, 2369f
specimen collection, 180
mycotic aneurysms, 772
obstetric and gynecologic, 2369
pathology, 2366
pediatric, 2369
pericarditis, 805
peritonitis, 709
pneumonia, 619t, 622t
chronic, 647t
in HIV/AIDS, 1236
radiology, 650t, 654f
primary infection, 2367, 2367f
serology, 193t, 2370–2371
skin testing, 2370–2371
sputum, 175f, 2370
treatment, 2371–2373
amphotericin B, 406, 1283t, 1289,
2371
bone and joint infection, 2372
chemotherapy, 2371
CNS infection, 2372–2373
fluconazole, 2371, 2372
in HIV/AIDS, 1283t, 1289
itraconazole, 1283t, 1289
ketoconazole, 1283t, 1289, 2371,
2372
disseminated, 407
pulmonary cavity, 2371–2372
Coccidioidin, 2370
Cochlear toxicity: aminoglycosides, 294
Coenurosis, 2544, 2545t, 2551
Coenurus cerebralis: meningitis, 870
Cogan syndrome: ocular involvement,
1115
Cohort studies, 162–163
Cokeromyces, 2311t
Cold, common, 561–566
attack rates, 562

clinical characteristics, 563–564, 1487t
coronavirus, 562, 562t, 1487t,
1487–1488
diagnosis, 564
etiology, 562, 562t
laryngitis and, 573t
pathogenesis, 563
pharyngitis with, 568
rhinoviruses, 562, 562t, 563, 564,
1487t, 1658f, 1658–1659
seasonal incidence, 562
and sinusitis, 586
transmission, 562–563
treatment, 564–565
future, 565
Cold agglutinins, 192t
and *Mycoplasma pneumoniae*, 1708,
1709
Colestipol: for antibiotic-associated colitis, 983–984
Colicin V plasmid: *Escherichia coli*,
1969, 1971
Colistimethate
drug interactions, 521t
pharmacology, 514t–515t
Colistin: anaerobic gram-negative bacilli
resistance, 2196t
Colitis
antibiotic-associated, 978–987,
992–993
clinical diagnosis, 981–982
clinical manifestations, 980
laboratory diagnosis, 980–981
and leukemia, 2679
microbiology, epidemiology, and
pathogenesis, 979–980
pathology, 978f, 978–979
from perioperative prophylactic
use, 2750
prevention, 985
treatment, 982–985
adrenal steroids, 983
antibiotics, 982–983
antidiarrheal agents, 983
bacitracin, 983
cholestyramine, 983–984
colestipol, 983–984
evaluation of new therapies, 984
metronidazole, 983
relapse or recurrence, 984
surgical, 984
Balantidium coli, 2511
Campylobacter, 1950, 1951
Entamoeba histolytica, 2400, 2400t
granulomatous: and fever, 545–546
hemorrhagic: *Escherichia coli*, 1014
ischemic: antibiotic-associated vs.,
981–982
Trichuris trichiura, 2527
ulcerative
antibiotic-associated vs., 981
and fever, 546
postdysenteric, 994
Collagenase, 79t
Collagen-vascular diseases. *See also*
specific diseases
and fever, 537t, 544, 545
myocarditis, 804t
Colon: normal flora, 2159t, 2160
Colon cancer
fever, 544
Streptococcus bovis and, 1832
Colonic lesions: amebiasis, 2398, 2398f
Colonic mucins: *Entamoeba histolytica*
and, 15–16, 16f

Colonoscopy
  for antibiotic-associated colitis, 981
  and endocarditis, 743t, 794t
  nosocomial infection control, 2584
Colon surgery: prophylaxis recommen-
    dations, 2751t
Colony-stimulating factors, 79. *See also
    specific factors*
  for neutropenia, 89
  for sepsis syndrome, 701, 702–703
  therapeutic, 450–452
Colorado tick fever virus, 1446–1447
  classification and virology, 1446
  cutaneous manifestations, 550t
  diagnosis, 1447
  differential diagnosis: ehrlichiosis,
    1750
  meningitis, 832
  serology, 191
Colpitis macularis: *Trichomonas
    vaginalis*, 2494
Colposcopy: for human papillomavirus
    diagnosis, 1395
Coltivirus, 1447
Coma
  Plasmodium, 2421
  rabies, 1533
  trauma patient, 2757
Comamonas acidovorans, 2003
  classification, 2004t
  infections caused by, 2004t
  keratitis, 1113
Comamonas terrigena, 2004t
Comamonas testosteroni, 2004t
  infections caused by, 2004t
Combination therapy, 206–209. *See also
    specific drugs*
Combined immunodeficiency, 133, 135
Commensal host-parasite relationships,
    30, 31
Common cold. *See* Cold, common
Common variable immunodeficiency,
    49, 51, 133, 151t
  diagnosis, 153
Common warts, 1388t, 1389, 1390,
    1392. *See also* Human papillo-
    mavirus
Community-based disease prevention,
    166
Community-based surveillance, 161–162
Community intervention trials, 163
Complement, 32
  activation, 59–64
  alternative pathway, 58, 58t
    activation, 60–62
    deficiencies, 68t, 68–69
  anaphylatoxin inactivator
      (carboxypeptidase B), 58t,
      63t
  and bacterial meningitis, 838,
      839–840
  and *Bacteroides*, 2197
  C1
    activation, 59, 62
    deficiency, 67, 68t, 152t, 156
    esterase inhibitor (C1-INH), 62,
        63t
  C1-INH, 58t
    deficiency, 68t, 70–71
  C1q, 58t, 65
    activation, 59
    deficiency, 152t
  C1qR, 63t, 64
  C1r, 58t, 64
    deficiency, 152t

C1s, 58t, 64
  activation, 59, 60
  deficiency, 152t
C2, 58t, 59, 62, 64, 102
  deficiency, 67, 68, 68t, 71, 152t,
      156
  treatment, 73
C3, 58t, 59, 64, 65, 83
  activation, 60–61, 61f
  and acute phase response, 117
  deficiency, 68t, 69, 71, 90, 152t
    and defective opsonization, 91
    treatment, 73
  regulation of convertases, 62, 63
  and renal disorders, 73
C3a, 63t, 64, 65
C3b, 60–61, 63, 64, 65, 83
  deficiency: and *Streptococcus
      pneumoniae*, 1816
C3b receptor (CR1), 62, 63t, 64
C3bBb, 61–62
C4, 58t, 59, 63, 64, 102
  activation, 59–60
  deficiency, 67, 68, 68t, 72, 152t,
      156
C4a, 65
C4aR, 63t
C4 BP, 58t
C4b, 61
C4b2a, 60
C4bp, 62, 63t
C5, 58t, 59, 64
  activation, 62
  deficiency, 67, 68t, 69, 70, 72, 90,
      152t
C5a, 64, 82, 88
  and renal disorders, 73
C5aR, 63t
C5b, 62
C5b8, 62
C6, 58t, 62, 63, 64
  deficiency, 67, 68t, 69, 70, 72, 152t
    and renal disorders, 73
C7, 58t, 62, 63, 64
  deficiency, 68t, 69, 70, 72, 152t
C8, 58t, 62, 63, 64
  deficiency, 67, 68t, 69, 70, 72, 152t
    and renal disorders, 73
C9, 58t, 62, 63, 64
  deficiency, 68t, 69, 152t
C4B: deficiency, 152t
C5(b9): and renal disorders, 73
CD59, 63, 63t
  deficiency, 68t
  and paroxysmal nocturnal hemo-
      globinuria, 71
classical pathway, 58, 58t
  activation, 59–60
    by antibodies, 41, 59
  deficiencies, 67–68, 68t
CNS infections and, 829
CR3, 63t, 64, 65, 83
  deficiency, 68t
CR1 (CD35), 62, 63t, 64
CR2 (CD21), 63t, 64
CR4 (CD11c/CD18), 63t, 64
D, 58t
DAF
  deficiency, 68t
  and paroxysmal nocturnal hemo-
      globinuria, 71
deficiencies, 66–71, 68t, 156. *See also
    individual CD above*
  alternative pathway, 68t, 68–69
  classical pathway, 67–68, 68t

  and defective opsonization, 91
  hereditary angioedema–C1
      inhibitor, 70–71
  late, 69
  meningococcal infection and, 67,
      67f, 69t, 69–70
  meningococcemia and, 1902
  paroxysmal nocturnal hemoglobin-
      uria, 71
discriminating between host and
    microbial cell surfaces, 63–64
in disease states, 71–73
evaluation and treatment of disorders,
    73–74
factor B, 58t, 59, 63, 64
factor H, 58t, 62, 63, 63t, 64
  deficiency, 68t
factor I, 58t, 62, 63t, 64
  deficiency, 68t
functions mediated by, 64–65
HRF, 63t
  deficiency, 68t
and infectious diseases, 72
membrane attack complex, 58, 58t
  assembly, 62
  regulation, 63
microbial interactions with, 65–66
protein families, 58, 58t, 64. *See also
    specific proteins*
receptors, 64
and renal disorders, 72–73
and rheumatologic disorders, 72
SP-40/40 (clusterin), 58t, 63t
synthesis, catabolism, and distribution,
    59
virulence factors and, 8
vitronectin, 58t, 63, 63t
Complementarity-determining regions
    (CDR), 105–110. *See also
    entries commencing with the
    term* CD
Complement cascade, 32, 60f
  virulence factors and, 8
Complement fixation
  for alphaviruses, 1455
  for bacteria, 192t
  for CMV, 1352
  for *Coccidioides immitis*, 2370, 2371
  for fungi, 193t
  for *Histoplasma capsulatum*, 2349
  for influenza virus, 1554–1555
  for *Mycoplasma pneumoniae*, 1708,
      1709
  for paracoccidioidomycosis, 2388
  for Reye syndrome, 1559–1560
  for *Toxoplasma gondii*, 2463–2464
  for *Trypanosoma cruzi*, 2446, 2447
Complement receptor 1 (CR1), 62, 63t,
    64
Complement receptor 2 (CR2). *See*
    CD21 cells
Computed tomography (CT)
  bacterial meningitis, 841–842, 846,
      847f
  brain abscess, 891–893, 892f, 893f
    therapeutic stereotactic surgery,
        895–896
  Creutzfeldt-Jakob disease, 882
  endocarditis: prosthetic valve, 785
  epidural abscess, 904, 904f
  and FUO, 540
  hepatic abscess, 725–726, 726f
  infectious arthritis, 1034
  intracranial masses in HIV/AIDS,
      1237–1238, 1238f

  intraperitoneal abscess, 721–722
  mediastinitis, 816
  meningitis, 868
  mycotic aneurysms, 771–772
  neck and head infections, 601
  orbital cellulitis, 1134
  osteomyelitis, 1045
  pancreatic abscess, 723–724
  perinephric and intrarenal abscesses,
      682, 682f
  pleural empyema, 639
  sinusitis, 587
  splenic abscess, 727
  subdural empyema, 901, 901f, 903
  trauma patients, 2758
  urinary tract infections, 682
Concentration-time curve, 225
Condoms
  and gonorrhea prevention, 1923
  and HIV transmission prevention,
      1169, 1192–1193
Condylomata acuminata, 1388t, 1389,
    1392f, 1392–1393, 1393f. *See
    also* Human papillomavirus
  Buschke-Loewenstein tumors, 1393
  condylomatous carcinoma, 1393
  course, 1057
  diagnosis, 1059, 1392, 1392f, 1393f,
      1395
  differential diagnosis, 1395
  erythroplasia of Queyrat, 1393
  giant, 1393
  spiked, 1392
  treatment, 412t, 1394–1395
    interferons, 429, 452, 1394
Condylomata lata, 552
  in children, 1056
  diagnosis, 1059
  differential diagnosis, 1395
Condylomatous carcinoma, 1393
Congenital infections. *See* Neonatal
    disease
Conidiobolus, 2317
Conjunctival papillomas, 1388t. *See also*
    Human papillomavirus
Conjunctival petechiae
  endocarditis, 747, 747f
  Neisseria meningitidis, 1900
Conjunctivitis, 1103–1110
  acute hemorrhagic (AHC), 1629–1631
    clinical manifestations, 1630, 1630f
    differential diagnosis, 1631
    enteroviruses type 70, 1629–1631
    epidemiology, 1629–1630
    laboratory diagnosis, 1631
    seroepidemiology, 1630
    transmission, 1630
  adenoviral, 1385
  Bacillus, 1891
  bacterial, 1104t, 1104–1105
  Borrelia burgdorferi, 2148
  chlamydial, 1106, 1114, 1685
    adult, 1685
    diagnosis, 183–184, 1107–1108
    differential diagnosis, 1685
    neonatal, 1679, 1688–1689
    treatment, 1688
  clinical manifestations, 1103–1104
  differential diagnosis, 1107
  etiology, 1104t
  fungal, 1104t, 1105, 1105t
  and FUO, 539
  glaucoma vs., 1106t
  gonococcal, 1104–1105, 1916, 1916f
    diagnosis, 183–184

Conjunctivitis (Continued)
Haemophilus aegyptius, 2043–2044
Haemophilus influenzae, 2043–2044
herpes simplex virus, 1106, 1338
neonatal, 1107
recurrence, 1339
treatment, 1108
laboratory findings, 1107–1108
Listeria, 1883
Moraxella lacunata, 1927t
noninfectious, 1107
ophthalmia neonatorum, 1106–1107
prophylaxis, 1108
parasitic, 1104t, 1106
Reiter syndrome, 1071
Salmonella typhi, 998, 1000t
treatment, 1108
uveitis vs., 1106t
viral, 1104t, 1105f, 1105–1106
Contact isolation, 2576, 2577t
Contact lenses
Acanthamoeba infection, 1114, 2410,
2411, 2413, 2414
and conjunctivitis, 1107
Pseudomonas aeruginosa infections,
1991
Copper pennies, 2326
Copper poisoning, 1014
Coprinus atramentarius, 1015, 1015t
Coprococcus, 2158t
Cordylobia, 2562
Cornea
biopsy, 1116
scrapings, 1116
Corneal abscess: Bacillus, 1891
Corneal clouding: and keratitis, 1112,
1112f
Corneal edema: and keratitis, 1111
Corneal infections: Acanthamoeba, 184,
2410
Corneal inflammation. See Keratitis
Corneal transplantation: from rabies,
1537
Corneal ulcers
anaerobic, 2163t
diagnosis, 184
Pseudomonas aeruginosa, 1991
ring, 1114
Coronary artery embolism: and endocarditis, 749
Coronaviridae, 1486–1489. See also
Coronavirus
classification, 1315t
shape and size, 1316f
Coronavirus, 1486–1489
bronchitis, acute, 606, 606t
clinical manifestations, 1487t,
1487–1488
common cold, 562, 562t, 1487t,
1487–1488
description, 1486–1487, 1487f
epidemiology, 1488
laryngitis, 573t
pharyngitis, 567t
prevention, 1488
receptor, 1317t
strain 229E, 1486, 1487f, 1488
strain OC38, 1486
strain OC43, 1486–1487, 1488
Coronaviruslike particles (CVLPs),
1487, 1488
Cortical vein thrombosis, 907
Corticosteroids
for bacterial meningitis, 855
for Bordetella pertussis, 2082

for brain abscess, 897
for chronic bronchitis, 611
for EBV, 1372
for endophthalmitis, 1126
for fever, 533
and HBV infection course, 1417, 1427
for hepatitis, 1150
immunodeficiency from, 136,
2668–2669, 2756
and infection susceptibility,
2668–2669
for keratitis, 1118
and meningococcal therapy, 1904
for Mycobacterium tuberculosis, 2228
for Nocardia, 2277
for Pneumocystis carinii, 455,
1284–1285, 2477, 2482
for pneumonia, 655–656, 657
for septicemia, 700
and septic shock, 131
for Toxoplasma gondii, 1287
in HIV/AIDS, 2467
for transplantation, 2711
vancomycin interaction, 349
Corynebacterium, 1872–1876
and bone marrow transplantation,
2719
endocarditis: rifampin for, 322
lymphadenitis, granulomatous, 938
mediastinitis, 815t
oral colonization, 593, 594t
treatment
aminoglycosides, 287t
fusidic acid, 278
urinary tract infections, 667
Corynebacterium aquaticum, 1874–1875
Corynebacterium bovis, 1874
Corynebacterium diphtheriae, 1865–1872
anterior nasal, 1868
clinical manifestations, 1868–1870
conjunctivitis, 1105
cultures, 173
cutaneous, 916, 1870
clinical features, 916
differential diagnosis, 916
therapy, 916
description, 1865–1866
diagnosis, 1870
differential diagnosis
epiglottitis, 591
poliovirus, 1617
DNA probes, 27
endocarditis, 756
vancomycin for, 350
epidemiology, 1866f, 1866–1867
faucial, 1868, 1869f
gravis, 1865, 1866
history, 1865
identification, 186
immunization: 1864,1865
intermedius, 1865, 1866–1867
keratitis, 1112
laryngeal, 1869–1870
lymphadenitis, 940t
lysogenic phase, 1865
membranous ulcers, 916
clinical features, 916
differential diagnosis, 916
treatment, 916
mitis, 1865, 1866
myocarditis, 800
nasopharyngeal cultures, 169
neuritis, 878
pathogenesis, 1867f, 1867–1868,
1868f

pharyngitis, 567t, 569, 1789
prevention, 1871
primary cutaneous, 916
respiratory tract, 1868–1870
superinfection of eczematized skin
lesions, 916
toxin, 2, 3t, 4–5
tracheobronchial, 1869–1870
treatment, 1870–1871
erythromycin, 335, 335t, 338t
penicillins, 237t
quinolones, 368t
sulfonamides, 355t
trimethoprim, 357
virulence determinants, 22t
wound, 916
Corynebacterium equi. See Rhodococcus
equi
Corynebacterium group D2, 1872t,
1875–1876
Corynebacterium group E, 1875–1876
Corynebacterium group G2, 1876
Corynebacterium group JK. See
Corynebacterium jeikeium
Corynebacterium haemolyticum. See
Arcanobacterium hemolyticum
Corynebacterium hofmannii. See
Corynebacterium pseudo-
diphtheriticum
Corynebacterium jeikeium, 1872t, 1876
cutaneous manifestations, 1872t
and AIDS, 557
and granulocytopenia, 2676, 2678,
2679
Corynebacterium kutscheri, 1875
Corynebacterium matruchotii: keratitis,
1113
Corynebacterium minutissimum, 1875
erythrasma, 919, 1872t
Corynebacterium ovis. See Corynebac-
terium pseudotuberculosis
Corynebacterium pseudodiphtheriticum,
1872t, 1874
endocarditis, 756, 1872t
Corynebacterium pseudotuberculosis,
1872t, 1873
granulomatous lymphadenitis, 938,
1872t
Corynebacterium pyogenes. See
Actinomyces pyogenes
Corynebacterium striatum, 1875
Corynebacterium ulcerans, 1872t, 1873
pharyngitis, 567, 569, 1872t
Corynebacterium vaginale. See
Gardnerella vaginalis
Corynebacterium xerosis, 1874–1875
Coryneforms. See Diphtheroids
Cost assessment, 166
Costochondritis: Candida albicans, 2297
Cotrimoxazole. See Trimethoprim-
sulfamethoxazole
Cotton-wool spots: and HIV/AIDS, 1240
Cough
as barrier, 32
Bordetella pertussis, 2081
bronchitis
acute, 607
chronic, 609
and common cold, 564
and tuberculosis transmission,
2216–2217
whooping. See Bordetella pertussis
Counterimmunoelectrophoresis (CIE)
endocarditis, 750
Neisseria meningitidis, 1903

pneumonia, 625–626
Streptococcus agalactiae, 1840
Cowpox, 1325–1328. See also Vaccinia
virus
Coxiella burnetii, 1727–1735
animal reservoirs, 2792t
Biotzere strain, 1728
chronic Q fever, 1731
clinical manifestations, 1729–1733
Corazon strain, 1728
description, 1728, 1728f
differential diagnosis, 1695
Dod strain, 1728
endocarditis, 751, 757–758, 1731,
1732f
treatment, 764
enteric symptoms, 999t
epidemiology, 1719, 1720, 1720t,
1728–1729
fever, 543
granulomatous hepatitis, 1161, 1731
in the immunocompromised, 1732
Kawasaki disease and, 1733
neurologic manifestations, 1731–1732
phase variation, 1728
pneumonia, 619t, 622t, 1729–1730,
1730f, 1731f
radiology, 1730f
serology, 625–626
prevention, 1733
self-limited febrile illness, 1729
strains, 1728
taxonomy, 1748
tick vector, 1728, 2565
treatment
quinolones, 373
rifampin, 322, 323
vaccine research, 1733
vertebral osteomyelitis, 1732–1733
Coxsackieviruses, 1620–1636. See also
Enteroviruses
characteristics, 1620–1621
classification, 1606t, 1607
clinical spectrum of infection, 1621t
conjunctivitis, 1105
cutaneous manifestations, 550t, 551,
552, 553
diarrhea, infantile, 966
encephalitis, 874, 1621t, 1623
epidemic pleurodynia, 1621t,
1625–1626
clinical manifestations, 1626
diagnosis, 1626
epidemiology, 1625
history, 1625
management and prognosis, 1626
pathogenesis, 1625–1626
serotypes, 1621t, 1625
epidemiology, 1609, 1609t
exanthems, 1621t, 1623–1624
herpetiform, 1624
petechial, 1624
roseoliform, 1624
group A
bronchitis, acute, 606, 606t
classification, 1607
clinical spectrum of infection, 1621t
differential diagnosis: VZV, 1349
epidemic pleurodynia, 1625
myocarditis, 800
and Reye syndrome, 1558
group B
classification, 1607
clinical spectrum of infection,
1621t

epidemic pleurodynia, 1625–1626
epidemiology, 1609, 1609t
hepatitis, 1632
laboratory diagnosis, 1611
meningitis, 832
myocarditis, 800, 801
myopericarditis, 1626–1627
pancreatitis, 1632
pericarditis, 804
pleurodynia, 934
receptors, 1607
respiratory disease, 1625
and Reye syndrome, 1558
and Guillain-Barré syndrome, 1623
hepatitis, 1137
herpangina, 1621t, 1625
clinical manifestations, 1625
differential diagnosis, 1625
laboratory diagnosis, 1625
serotypes, 1621t, 1625
laryngitis, 573t
lymphadenopathy, 1632
meningitis, 832, 1621t, 1621–1623
clinical manifestations, 1622
differential diagnosis, 1622
laboratory diagnosis, 1622
management and prognosis,
1622–1623
meningoencephalitis in agammaglobulinemic and immuno-
compromised, 1629
clinical manifestations, 1629
myelitis, 874
myocarditis, 800, 803
myopericarditis, 1621t, 1626–1627
clinical manifestations, 1627
diagnosis and differential diagnosis,
1627
epidemiology, 1626–1627
management, 1627
pathogenesis, 1627
serotypes, 1621t, 1626
myositis, 1632
in newborn, 1627–1629
clinical manifestations, 1628
diagnosis and differential diagnosis,
1628
epidemiology, 1627–1628
management, 1628
pathophysiology, 1628–1629
paralysis, 1621t, 1623
parotitis, 1500
pericarditis, 804
pharyngitis, 567t
respiratory disease, acute, 1621t,
1624–1625
serotype A4
hemolytic-uremic syndrome,
1632
myopericarditis, 1626–1627
serotype A9
herpetiform exanthems, 1624
serotype A10
acute lymphonodular pharyngitis,
1625
serotype A16
herpetiform exanthems (hand-foot-
and-mouth) syndrome, 1624,
1631–1632
myopericarditis, 1626–1627
serotype A21
acute hemorrhagic conjunctivitis,
1630
respiratory disease, 1624–1625
transmission, 1610

serotype A24
acute hemorrhagic conjunctivitis
(AHC), 1629–1631
serotype B2: hemolytic-uremic
syndrome, 1632
serotype B4: hemolytic-uremic syndrome, 1632
Cox's organism. *See Coxiella burnetii*
Crab louse. *See Phthirus pubis*
Crack addicts. *See* Drug abusers
CR3 adhesin, 16
Cranial fossae: anatomy, 822, 823f
Cranial nerve(s)
anatomy, 823f
and CNS infections, 823, 823f
Craniotomy: prophylaxis recommendations, 2752t
C-reactive protein, 34
and acute phase response, 117,
534–535, 539
brain abscess, 891
test, 191t
Creatinine: clearance formula, 297
and aminoglycoside dosage, 297, 298t
Creatinine kinase: in myocarditis, 802
Creeping eruption, 2555
Crepitant myositis, 933
Crepitant wounds. *See also* Soft tissue
infections
differential diagnosis, 924t
Creutzfeldt-Jakob disease, 881–883,
1674
clinical manifestations, 881–882
diagnosis, 882
keratitis, 1116
nosocomial infection prevention, 2584
specimen handling, 884
Crimean-Congo hemorrhagic fever virus,
1567
characteristics, 1568t
clinical manifestations, 1570
differential diagnosis, 1472
epidemiology, 1568–1569
prevention and treatment, 1571
ribavirin for, 431
serology, 191
transmission to humans, 1569
Crohn's disease
differential diagnosis, 981
and fever, 545–546
Cross-sectional surveys, 163
Crotamiton, 466t
Croup, 573–579, 1489–1496. *See also*
Laryngotracheobronchitis,
acute
Moraxella catarrhalis, 1927
spasmodic, 574, 577
Crustacea, 2558
Crusts: genital, 1057t, 1059. *See also*
Genital lesions
Cryoglobulinemia, 42
essential mixed: hepatitis B virus and,
1420
hepatitis C virus and, 1480
mixed (type II), 42
hepatitis and, 1139
Cryosurgery: for chromomycosis, 2326
Cryotherapy
for anogenital warts, 1394, 1395
for cutaneous warts, 1393
Cryptococcus neoformans, 2289,
2331–2340
and adult T-cell leukemia/lymphoma,
1582
appearance in tissue, 2289t

brain abscess, 890
in AIDS, 890
in the immunocompromised, 890
bronchoscopy, 174
and cell-mediated immune defects,
2681, 2682
cellular host defense mechanisms,
2332–2333
clinical manifestations, 2334
CNS infection, 2334
CNS localization, 2333
cutaneous, 2334, 2334f
manifestations, 550t
description, 2331
diagnosis, 2334–2336
blood and CSF findings, 2334–2335
histopathology, 2335
serologic, 2335–2336
smear and culture, 2335, 2335f
differential diagnosis, 2336, 2336f
Bartonella, 1742
disseminated: in transplantation, 2727
ecology, 2331–2332
EIA diagnosis, 185
encephalitis, 874–875, 876
endophthalmitis
in AIDS, 1123
treatment, 1126
epidemiology, 2331–2332
epidural abscess, 905
growth, 190
in HIV/AIDS, 1182, 2332, 2333, 2335
extrapulmonary, 1182t
meningitis, 872, 1239, 2334, 2338
respiratory, 629, 1235, 2334, 2335
treatment, 1283t, 1288–1289, 2337
fluconazole, 409, 2337
humoral host defense, 2333
hydrocephalus, 2336
identification, 2331
and immunodeficiency, 150t
Job syndrome and, 156
latex agglutination test, 185
and leukemia, hairy cell, 2673
lymphadenitis, 940t
meningitis, 869, 2332, 2334, 2338
and cell-mediated immune defects,
2681, 2682
and HIV, 872, 1239, 2334, 2338
in the immunocompromised, 872
in transplant recipients, 2723
treatment, 2337–2338
fluconazole, 409, 868
microscopy, 184
musculoskeletal specimen collection,
180
myelitis, 874–875
myocarditis, 800
neurologic disease: HIV/AIDS and,
1239
pathophysiology, 2332f, 2332–2333
perfect states, 2331
pericarditis, 805
pneumonia, 619t
and AIDS, 629, 1235, 2334, 2335
chronic, 647t, 648
radiology, 650t, 654f
treatment, 2337
polysaccharide, 2333
predisposing factors to infection, 2332
prognosis, 2338
respiratory tract infection, 2334
in HIV/AIDS, 629, 1235, 2334,
2335
treatment, 2337

serology, 193t
serotypes, 2331
sinusitis, 586t
sputum, 175f
in transplant recipients, 2712,
2728–2729
treatment, 2336–2338
amphotericin B, 406, 1283t, 1288,
2336–2337
fluconazole, 1283t, 1288
flucytosine, 407, 1283t, 1288, 2337
in HIV/AIDS, 1283t, 1288–1289,
2337
itraconazole, 408, 2337
in non-AIDS patients, 2336–2337
var. *gattii*, 2331
Cryptosporidium, 2394t, 2500–2510
animal reservoirs, 2792t
and cell-mediated immune defects,
2681
clinical features, 2394t, 2504–2505
cytokine protection, 121t
description, 2501
diagnosis, 2395t, 2506f, 2506–2507,
2507f
diarrhea, 2503, 2504
in AIDS, 970, 970t
chronic, 972, 994
in day care centers, 971
diagnosis, 181
differential diagnosis: amebiasis, 2402
dysentery, 994
enterocolitis: and HIV/AIDS, 1230
epidemiology, 2501–2503
and HIV/AIDS, 2500–2501, 2502
clinical features, 2504–2505
diarrhea, 970, 970t
gastric, 1230, 2503, 2503f, 2504
immune response and, 2505
incidence, 1182t, 2501
pathogenesis and pathology, 2503f,
2503–2504
prevention, 2508
pulmonary, 1236, 2503–2504, 2504f
treatment, 2507–2508, 2642
immune response and, 2505–2506
immunofluorescence, 185
life cycle, 2501, 2501f
oocysts, 2501, 2501f
pathogenesis and pathology, 2503f,
2503–2504, 2504f
prevention, 2508
sporozoites, 2501, 2501f
transmission, 2394t, 2791
waterborne, 2794
treatment, 462t, 469, 2507–2508
azithromycin, 475
paromomycin, 468
Cryptosporidium baileyi, 2501
Cryptosporidium meleagridis, 2501
Cryptosporidium muris, 2501
Cryptosporidium parvum, 2501
treatment: aminoglycosides, 295t
CSF-VDRL test, 181, 2128
Ctenocephalides felis: and murine typhus,
1737
CTLA-4, 109
C2 toxin (*C. botulinum*), 3t, 5
CTX-1 β-lactamase, 217
Culex
and arboviruses, 1456, 1457
and flaviviruses, 1466t
and Japanese encephalitis, 1466t, 1468
and St. Louis encephalitis, 1466t,
1467, 1469

Culiseata: California encephalitis, 1568
Culiseata melanura: and arboviruses, 1456, 1457
Cultures. *See* Specimen collection and processing
Cunninghamella
  mucormycosis, 2312, 2313
  pneumonia, 619t
Cunninghamella bertholletiae: sinusitis, 586t
Curvularia, 2391
  brain abscess, 890
  keratitis, 1113
  phaeohyphomycosis of paranasal sinus, 1132
Curvularia lunata, 2327
  sinusitis, 586t
Cutaneous larva migrans, 2555
  pulmonary infiltrates with eosinophilia, 631
  treatment, 462t
Cutaneous neoplasia: Kaposi's sarcoma, 1242
Cutaneous nodules: helminthic, 2553t
Cutaneous reactions. *See* Rashes; Skin lesions and infections
Cutaneous warts, 1388t, 1389, 1390, 1391f, 1392. *See also* Human papillomavirus
  treatment, 1393–1394
Cyanobacterium-like bodies, 2512. *See also Cyclospora*
  dysentery, 994
Cyclacillin
  pharmacology, 506–507t
  for sinusitis, 589t
Cyclic nucleotides: and neutrophil degranulation, 85
Cyclophosphamide: immunodeficiency from, 136
Cycloserine
  adverse reactions, 394
  combination therapy: for mycobacteria, 396t
  dosage, 394, 516t–517t
    in hepatic or renal failure, 390t, 517t
  drug interactions, 521t
  for *Mycobacterium avium-intracellulare*, 2257
  for *Mycobacterium tuberculosis*, 394
  pharmacology, 516t–517t
Cyclospora, 2512
  dysentery, 994
  stool examination, 181
  treatment, 466t
Cyclosporine, 136
  and infection susceptibility, 2668–2669, 2711
Cylindrocarpon: mycetoma, 2327
Cysticercosis, 2544, 2545t, 2547, 2548–2550
  meningitis, 870, 2549
  myalgia, 935
  neural, 2548, 2549
    albendazole for, 479
  treatment, 2549
Cysticercus cellulosae
  dacryocystitis, 1131
  endophthalmitis, 1124
  myositis, 932
  treatment, 466t
Cystic fibrosis, 657–662
  aminoglycoside use, 299
  clinical manifestations, 658
  heart-lung transplantation for, 1987

hypergammaglobulinemia, 42
  microbiology, 659
  pathogenesis, 658–659
  and pneumonia, 621
  Pseudomonas aeruginosa and, 658–659, 1985–1987
    treatment, 1986–1987
  transmembrane regulator (CFTR), 658
  treatment, 659–660
Cystic hygromas, 604
  lymphadenopathy vs., 941
Cystidine monophospho-*N*-acetyl neuraminic acid (CMP-NANA), 66
Cystitis. *See also* Urinary tract infections
  adenoviral hemorrhagic, 1385
  Candida, 2297
  defined, 662
  in the elderly, 2738
  Escherichia coli, 1970–1971
  treatment
    nitrofurantoin, 377–378
    quinolones, 370
Cystoscopy: and endocarditis, 743t
Cystourethrography: voiding, 683–684
Cysts
  bronchial cleft, 604
    lymphadenopathy vs., 941
  Entamoeba histolytica, 2396, 2396f
  epidermal infected, 920–921
  Giardia lamblia, 2487, 2488f
  hydatid disease, 2544, 2550–2551
  pharyngeal cleft, 604
  Pneumocystis carinii, 2475, 2476f
  thyroglossal duct, 604
Cytochrome $_{b558}$, 79, 84, 85
Cytokine-induced platelet-activating factor synthesis: and sepsis syndrome, 696
Cytokines, 30t, 33f, 33–34, 112–122, 114t–115t, 130–131. *See also specific cytokines*
  and acute phase response, 117
  amplifying and attenuating immune responses, 112–113
  and antimicrobial activity of immunity, 120–122, 121t
  and B cell activation, 119–120
  biochemical properties, 113
  cascade, 33f, 33–34
  and cytotoxic T cells, 121
  definitions, 112
  and ELAM-1, 696
  endogenous pyrogenic: and hypothalamus, 532f, 532–533
  endothelial cells and, 82
  exogenous: in treatment of infectious diseases, 130–131
  and fever, 117
  and hematopoiesis, 118
  and HIV, 1210
    regulation of expression, 1210–1211
  immunologic response pathways regulated by, 117–118
  Leishmania and, 2430
  and macrophage activation, 124
  and MHC, 104
  for neutrophil defects, 94
  physicochemical characteristics, 114t–115t
  and pneumonia, 620
  priming neutrophils, 86
  production
    by B cells, 117

    by mononuclear phagocytes, 115–116
    by NK cells, 117
    by T cells, 116
    prophylactic: for immunocompromised host, 2693t, 2693–2694
  pyrogenic, 531
    measurement of circulating, 533–534
  receptors, 45t, 113, 116
  and sepsis, 693–695, 694t
  and septic shock, 117–118
  structure, 113
  and T-cell proliferation and maturation, 118–119
  therapeutic use, 94, 131
    for immunodeficiency, 138
  as vaccine adjuvants, 131
Cytolytic vaginosis, 1080–1081
Cytomegalic inclusion disease virus. *See* Cytomegalovirus
Cytomegalovirus (CMV), 1351–1364
  acalculous cholecystitis: and HIV/AIDS, 1229–1230
  adrenalitis, 1360
  anti-complement immunofluorescence (ACIF), 1352
  and bone marrow transplantation, 2674, 2720, 2720t
    ganciclovir for, 426
  and cell-mediated immune defects, 2681
  cellular immunodeficiency and, 132, 133
  cervical infection, 1354t, 1354–1355
  in children, 1356
  and chronic fatigue syndrome, 1307
  classification, 1330t
  clinical manifestations, 1356–1360
    in children, 1356
    in the immunocompromised, 1358–1360
      mononucleosis, 1357–1358
      neonatal infections, 1356–1357
  clinical syndromes, 1334t
  complement fixation (CF) test, 1352
  congenital, 1354t, 1354–1355
    inclusion disease (CID), 1356
  CSF specimens, 179
  cultivation, 1352
  cutaneous manifestations, 550t, 551
  cytokine and T cell protection, 121t
  description, 1352–1353
  diagnosis, 1333, 1352
  diarrhea: in AIDS, 970, 970t, 1230
  differential diagnosis
    Cryptosporidium, 2504
    Toxoplasma gondii, 2459
  disseminated: in transplantation, 2727
  ELISA, 1352
  endophthalmitis, 1124
    treatment, 1126
  enteritis: in transplant recipients, 2728
  enterocolitis: and HIV/AIDS, 1230
  epidemiology, 1332, 1353–1356
  epididymitis, 1360
  esophagitis, 963
    and HIV/AIDS, 963, 964
  gastritis
    and HIV/AIDS, 1229–1230
    in transplant recipients, 2727–2728, 2729
  and granulocytopenia, 2677
  granulomatous hepatitis, 1161
  growth, 190–191, 191f

  in health care workers, 2661, 2662
  hemolytic anemia, 1358
  hepatitis, 1137, 1146–1147, 1357
    in the immunocompromised, 1147, 1358–1359
    liver transplantation and, 2725–2726
    in transplant recipients, 2728, 2729
  and HIV/AIDS, 557, 1221, 1351. *See also* immunocompromised host *below*
    acalculous cholecystitis, 1229–1230
    diarrhea, 970, 970t, 1230
    encephalopathy, 1359–1360
    enterocolitis, 1230
    epidemiology, 1356
    esophagitis, 963, 964
    gastrointestinal, 1229–1230
    incidence, 1182t
    lymphadenitis, 941
    management, 2642
    meningitis, 872, 1239–1240
    probability of developing, 1223f
    prophylaxis, 1286t
    retinitis, 1124, 1239–1240, 1240, 1287–1288, 1359, 1359f
      incidence, 1182t
      treatment, 1360
    treatment, 1283t, 1287
    viral proteins, 1593
  in homosexuals, 1353–1354
  in the immunocompromised host, 1332t, 1355–1356, 2561, 2662. *See also* HIV/AIDS *above*
    cancer patients, 1356
    clinical manifestations, 1358–1360
    encephalopathy, 1359–1360
    endocrinopathies and glandular involvement, 1360
    gastrointestinal, 1359
    hepatitis, 1358–1359
    HIV/AIDS, 1356. *See also* HIV/AIDS *above*
    meningoencephalitis, 1359–1360
    myelopathy, 1359–1360
    pneumonia, 1358
    retinitis, 1359, 1359f
    transplant recipients, 1355–1356
    treatment, 1360
  immunodeficiency and, 138
  immunoglobulin prophylaxis, 1361
  immunosuppressive therapy and, 135
  incidence and prevalence, 1353
  interferon-γ, 129
  and Kaposi's sarcoma, 1352
  laboratory diagnosis, 1352
  latency, 1332t
  lymphadenitis, 940t
    and AIDS, 941
  meningitis, 833
    and HIV, 872, 1239–1240
  mononucleosis, 1357, 1372
  myelopathy, 1360
  myocarditis, 801
  neonatal
    clinical manifestations, 1356–1357
    epidemiology, 1354t, 1354–1355
  NK cells and, 122, 128
  nosocomial, 2660–2662
    from blood products, 95, 1333, 1353, 2626–2627, 2660–2661
    management of exposed personnel, 2662

prevention, 2661–2662
risks, 2660–2661
transmission mechanisms, 2661
oncogenicity, 1352
oophoritis, 1360
pancreatitis, 1360
papillary stenosis: and HIV/AIDS, 1230
perinatal, 1354t, 1354–1355
pharyngitis, 567t
pneumonia, 1357
and AIDS, 629, 1358
and bone marrow transplantation, 2720–2721
bronchoalveolar lavage, 624
and granulocytopenia, 2678
and heart-lung transplantation, 2725
in the immunocompromised, 1358
in transplant recipients, 2710, 2723, 2727
treatment, 412t, 1360
ganciclovir, 425, 1360
in pregnancy, 1354t, 1354–1355
prevention, 1334t, 1334–1335, 1361
active immunization, 1361
passive immunization, 1361
primary infections, 1332t
product and host target, 125t
receptor, 1317t
recurrence, 1332t
and renal transplantation, 1358, 2710t, 2711, 2711t
prophylaxis, 1361
resistance, 193, 1287
retinitis, 1359, 1359f
and HIV/ AIDS, 1124, 1287–1288, 1359, 1359f
and HIV/AIDS
incidence, 1182t
treatment, 412t, 1283t, 1287–1288, 1360
foscarnet, 423–424, 1273, 1360
seroepidemiology, 1333t
serology, 1352–1353
sexually transmitted, 1332, 1353–1354
spreading/shedding mechanisms, 1320f
structure, 1330t
systemic spread, 1320f
throat cultures, 173
thrombocytopenia, 173
from transfusions, 95, 1333, 1353, 2626–2627, 2660–2661
transmission, 1333t
by blood, 95, 1333, 1353, 2626–2627, 2660–2661
perinatal, 1354t, 1354–1355
sexual, 1332, 1353–1354
transplantation, 1354–1356, 2660, 2729
in transplant recipients, 1354–1356, 1358, 2660, 2709, 2710, 2710t, 2712, 2713, 2713t, 2722, 2723, 2729
allograft rejection and, 1355–1356
culture monitoring, 2714
diagnosis and control, 2713
immunosuppressive drugs and, 1355, 2711
prophylaxis, 1361, 2714–2715
treatment, 1334t, 1334–1335, 1360–1361
acyclovir, 417

experimental agents, 437t
foscarnet, 423–424, 1273, 1283t, 1287–1288, 1360–1361
ganciclovir, 424–426, 1283t, 1287–1288, 1360
in HIV/AIDS, 1283t, 1287–1288
immunoglobulin, 454
resistance, 1287
universal precautions, 2662
vaccine research, 1361
Cytometric indirect immunofluorescence: for HIV, 1261
Cytotoxic antibodies
β-lactams, 272
penicillins, 239, 239t
Cytotoxins
enteric, 949t, 949–951
Enterobacteriaceae, 1966
Cytovene. *See* Ganciclovir

D
DaCosta's syndrome, 1306, 1308t
Dacryoadenitis, 1131
chronic, 1131
Dacryocystitis, 1131
acute, 1131
and orbital cellulitis, 1132
Bacillus, 1891
chronic, 1131
treatment, 1134
Dacryocystopyocele, 1131
Dactylaria gallopava: brain abscess, 890
Dakar bat virus: transmission, clinical syndromes, and geographic distribution, 1466t
Dandruff, 2384
Dapsone
adverse reactions, 398, 474, 1284, 2481
antiparasitic use, 474
combination therapy: with pyrimethamine, 474
dosage, 398, 514t–515t
drug interactions, 521t
for leprosy, 397, 474, 2248, 2249
dosage, 397t
prophylaxis, 2247
resistance, 2248
for mycetoma, 2330
pharmacology, 514t–515t
for *Pneumocystis carinii*, 1284, 2481
prophylaxis, 397, 1286, 1286t, 2482
dosage, 465t
structure, 397f
for *Toxoplasma gondii*, 2469
in HIV/AIDS, 2467, 2467t
Darkfield microscopy, 184
CSF, 179
Treponema pallidum, 181, 1060, 2126–2127, 2127f
Darmbrand, 991–992
Day care centers: diarrhea in, 970–971
ddC. *See* Zalcitabine
ddI. *See* Didanosine
DDS. *See* Dapsone
Deafness
CMV infection and, 1357
and fever, 546
Decay accelerator factor (DAF), 62, 63t
Decongestants: for otitis media, 582
Decontamination
for cancer patients, 2692, 2692t, 2693
defined, 2579

for HIV material, 2643
for transplant recipients, 2715
Decubitus ulcers
anaerobic, 2163t, 2165
Bacteroides fragilis, 2199
Deep fascial space infections
clinical presentation, 598–600
pathways, 598f
Deep venous thrombosis/throm-bophlebitis
and lung abscess, 644
spinal cord injury and, 2734
Deerfly fever, 2060
Deer tick
and babesiosis, 2498, 2500
and *Borrelia burgdorferi*, 2145, 2565
Defense mechanisms, host. *See* Host defense mechanisms
Defensins, 79t, 87
Dehydroemetine, 459t, 468
adverse reactions, 468
for amebiasis, 2404t
dosage, 461t
pediatric, 461t
for hepatic abscess, 726
Deinocerites: and equine encephalitis, 1456
Dejerine-Sotta's disease, 2245
Delaviridine: for HIV, 1273
Delayed-type hypersensitivity (DTH)
and cell-mediated immunity, 102
test, 138, 150, 152
Delhi boil, 2434–2435
Delta hepatitis. *See* Hepatitis D virus
Demeclocycline
dosage, 512t–513t
pharmacokinetics, 309t
pharmacology, 512t–513t
structure, 307f
Demodex: and AIDS, 557
Demodex brevis, 2564
blepharitis, 1130
Demodex folliculorum, 2564
blepharitis, 1130
Dendrid. *See* Idoxuridine
Dendritic cells, 108–109
HIV and, 1204, 1210–1211
Dengue, 1466, 1466t, 1468, 1469–1470, 1470f, 1471, 1472, 1473
antiadhesin antibodies, 13
clinical manifestations, 1471
complement and, 72
cutaneous manifestations, 550t, 552
diagnosis, 1472
differential diagnosis: scrub typhus, 1741
enteric symptoms, 999t
epidemiology, 1468
hemorrhagic fever, 1466, 1469–1470, 1470f, 1471, 1473
clinical manifestations, 1471
epidemiology, 1468
pathogenesis, 1469, 1470f
prevention and therapy, 1473
history, 1466
lymphadenitis, 940t
myocarditis, 800
prevention and therapy, 1473
serology, 191
shock syndrome (DSS), 1469–1470, 1470f, 1471, 1473
transmission, clinical syndromes, and geographic distribution, 1466t

Densovirus, 1440
Dental abscesses
anaerobic, 2163t
Streptococcus intermedius, 1862
Dental caries
pathogenesis, 594–595
Streptococcus intermedius, 1862
Streptococcus mutans, 593, 1846, 1847
therapy, 601–602
Dental infections
anaerobic, 2163t
anaerobic cocci, 2205
Dental procedures: and endocarditis, 743t, 794t
prophylaxis, 797t
Dental sepsis: and brain abscess, 888, 888t
Dentoalveolar infections, 596
Deoxyguanosine: structure, 414f
2-Deoxystreptamine: structure, 281f
Dependovirus, 1440
Dermacentor
and ehrlichiosis, 1747t, 2565
and flaviviruses, 1466t
Dermacentor andersoni
and Colorado tick fever, 1446
and *Coxiella burnetii* (Q fever), 1728, 2565
and *Francisella tularensis*, 2061
and *Rickettsia rickettsii*, 1721, 1722, 2565
Dermacentor variabilis, 2565, 2565f
and ehrlichiosis, 1747t, 1748, 2565
and *Francisella tularensis*, 2061
and *Rickettsia rickettsii*, 2565
Dermanyssus gallinae, 2564
Dermatitis
schistosomiasis, 2539, 2540
seborrheic: *Pityrosporum*, 2384
Dermatobia, 2562
Dermatoblepharitis, 1130
bacterial, 1130
infectious, 1130
Dermatology. *See* Skin
Dermatophagoides farinae, 2565
Dermatophagoides pteronyssinus, 2565
Dermatophytosis, 2375–2386
anthropophilic, 2375t, 2376–2377
clinical features, 2377
deep infections, 2380–2381, 2381f
epidemiology, 2375–2377
geophilic, 2375t, 2376
"id" reactions, 2380
laboratory diagnosis, 2381
onychomycosis, 2380
pathogenesis, 2377
tinea capitis, 2379–2380, 2380f
tinea corporis, 2378, 2378f
tinea cruris, 2378
tinea faciei, 2379, 2379f
tinea imbricata, 2378–2379, 2379f
tinea manus, 2379
tinea pedis, 2377–2378
treatment, 2381–2382
zoophilic, 2375t, 2375–2376
Dermonecrotic toxin: *Bordetella pertussis*, 23
Descriptive studies: in epidemiology, 161
Desciclovir: for EBV, 1372
Desulfomonas, 2158t
Desulfovibrio, 2158t
Devil's grippe, 1625–1626

Dexamethasone
  for cerebral edema, 830t
  and complement, 59
  for cysticercosis, 2549
  for *Haemophilus influenzae*, 131
  for meningitis, 854, 855–856
  topical, 384t
  for typhoid fever, 455
DF-3, 2107t, 2109–2110
DHPG. *See* Ganciclovir
Diabetes mellitus
  antimicrobial therapy issues in, 203
  foot infections, 919–920
    anaerobic, 2163t
    limb-threatening, 919
    non-limb-threatening, 919
  mucormycosis and, 2313
  and pneumonia, 621
    chronic, 648
  Staphylococcus aureus infections,
      1762
  and *Streptococcus agalactiae*, 1839,
      1839t, 1840
  and surgical wound infections, 2746
Diabetic ketoacidosis: peritonitis vs., 714
Diacylglycerol (DAG), 110
  and PKC activation, 86
  release, 45
Dialysis. *See also* Hemodialysis;
      Peritoneal dialysis
  arteriovenous fistulas infections, 790
  hepatitis and, 2620–2621
    prevention and control, 2620–2621
Dialysis-adjusted drug dosage
  aminoglycosides, 297–298, 298t, 511t
  antifungal agents, 519t
  antimycobacterials, 517t
  antiviral agents, 519t
  azalides, 513t
  aztreonam, 511t
  carumonam, 511t
  cephalosporins, 509t
  chloramphenicol, 513t
  fusidic acid, 515t
  imipenem, 511t
  lincosamides, 513t
  loracarbef, 511t
  macrolides, 513t
  metronidazole, 513t
  penicillins, 238t, 507t
  polymyxins, 515t
  quinolones, 517t
  sulfonamides, 515t
  teicoplanin, 515t
  trimethoprim, 515t
  urinary tract agents, 517t
  vancomycin, 515t
Diaminodiphenylsulfone: hemolysis
      from: in G6PD deficiency, 203
Diaminophenyl sulfone. *See* Dapsone
Diarrhea
  with abdominal pain and eosinophilia,
      syndrome of, 1005–1008
    differential diagnosis, 1006–1008
    etiology, 1006t
  adenoviral infant, 1385
  Aeromonas, 2107–2108
  amebiasis, 987, 989, 2400, 2401, 2402
  bacterial overgrowth syndromes,
      972–973
  Balantidium coli, 2511
  Brainerd, 1015
  Campylobacter, 151, 1951
  in children: mortality rates, 945
  in chronic care facilities, 970

from clindamycin and lincomycin,
    342
Cryptosporidium, 2503, 2504
in day care centers, 970–971
diagnosis and management of infec-
    tious, 953–955, 954f
dysentery. *See* Dysentery
in the elderly, 2740
enterohemorrhagic *E. coli*, 988
environmental factors, 945–946
epidemic: in newborn nurseries,
    965–966
epidemiology, 945–946
food-borne disease, 1013–1014, 1015
Giardia lamblia, 971, 972, 2488,
    2489, 2489t
  in AIDS, 970, 970t
in HIV/AIDS, 948, 970, 970t, 1230,
    1230t
  acute retroviral syndrome, 1224t
in hospitals, 970
Legionella pneumophila, 2090–2091
and leukemia, 2679
mortality rates from, 945
noninflammatory, 965–973
  acute
    in adults, 969–970
      differential diagnosis, 972
    chronic, 972
    differential diagnosis, 972
Norwalk virus, 1669, 1670
nosocomial, 970–971
Plesiomonas shigelloides, 2110
popular names for, 945, 971
Pseudomonas aeruginosa, 1995
Salmonella, 2019, 2020, 2021
specimen collection and processing,
    171t, 180–181
travelers', 971t, 971–972, 972t
treatment: quinolones, 371
trichinosis, 2532
Vibrio cholerae, 180, 1936–1938
  non-01, 1947
Vibrio mimicus, 1947
Vibrio parahaemolyticus, 1945
watery, 953t
  diagnosis, 953t
  etiology, 953t
  weanling, 966–968
and Whipple's disease, 1031
Diazepam: for *Clostridium tetani*, 2176,
    2177
Dibekacin, 280
  for nontuberculous mycobacteria, 396
  source and chemistry, 280t
Dick test, 1789
Diclazuril sodium: for *Cryptosporidium*,
    2507
Dicloxacillin, 243
  for cellulitis, 916
  for cystic fibrosis infections, 660
  dosage, 241t, 506t–507t
    in children, 506t
    in neonates, 506t
    in renal disease and dialysis, 238t
  for furuncles, 912
  MICs against cocci, 237t
  pharmacokinetics, 238t
  pharmacology, 506t–507t
  structure, 242f
  trade names, 237t
Didanosine, 419–421, 1267, 1271, 1602
  adverse reactions, 421, 421t, 1271,
    1271t
  clinical studies, 421

dosage and pharmacology, 420–421,
    518t–519t, 1271t
drug interactions, 421, 421t, 522t
  for HIV, 1271, 1271t, 1272f
    for ZDV failure, 1275
  mechanism of action, 420
  resistance, 420, 1272f
  spectrum of activity, 419–420
  structure, 420f
Dideoxynucleoside analogs. *See also*
      specific drugs
  current recommendations, 1276,
    1276t
  dosages, 1271t
  for HIV, 1269–1272, 1270f
  in pregnancy, 1275–1276
  toxicities, 1271t
  zidovudine (ZDV), 1269–1271, 1271t,
    1272f
Dientamoeba fragilis, 2394t
  clinical manifestations, 2394t
  diagnosis, 1006t
  transmission, 2394t
  treatment, 462t, 468
Dieterle stain, 184t
Diethylcarbamazine, 460t, 481
  adverse reactions, 481
  dosage, 462t, 467t
    pediatric, 462t, 467t
  for filariasis, 2534
  for keratitis, 1118
  spectrum of activity, 481
  structure, 481f
Diflucan. *See* Fluconazole
DiGeorge syndrome, 129, 134t, 135, 150,
    151t
  diagnosis, 153
Digestive tract, selective decontamina-
    tion (SDD): for pneumonia
    prevention, 2604
Digoxin: erythromycin interaction with,
    337
Dihydrofolate reductase inhibitors,
    473–474
Diiodohydroxyquin. *See* Iodoquinol
Diloxanide furoate, 459t, 468
  for amebiasis, 2404, 2404t
  dosage, 461t
    pediatric, 461t
Dilution tests, 195
Dimethylsulfoxide (DSMO), 426
Diminazene: for *Babesia*, 2500
Diphtheria, 1865–1872. *See also*
    Corynebacterium diphtheriae
Diphtheria antitoxin, 1870–1871
Diphtheria-tetanus-pertussis (DTP)
    vaccine, 2082, 2771, 2775,
    2775t, 2781
  adverse reactions, 2773t, 2778, 2779
  contraindications, 2779, 2787t
  indications
    for adults, 2784t
    for children and infants, 2775t,
      2780t
    for HIV infected, 2785t
  reportable events, 2786t
Diphtheria toxin, 2, 3t, 4–5, 1867
  attachment and entry, 4
  mechanism of action, 4–5,
    1867–1868
  neuritis, 878
Diphtheria vaccine, 167, 1866, 1867,
    1871, 2775, 2775t
  adverse reactions, 2775
  booster doses, 2775

DTP. *See* Diphtheria-tetanus-pertussis
    vaccine
  morbidity reduction, 2772t
Diphtheroids, 1872–1876. *See also indi-
      vidual bacteria*
  clinical manifestations, 1872t
  endocarditis
    prosthetic valve, 783–784
    treatment, 786–787
  meningitis, 835
  microbiology, 1872–1873
Diphyllobothrium dalliae, 2547
Diphyllobothrium dendricitum, 2547
Diphyllobothrium klebanovskii, 2547
Diphyllobothrium latum, 2525t, 2545t,
    2546–2547
  diagnosis, 2546, 2548
  treatment, 466t, 2546, 2548
    niclosamide, 483, 2548
    praziquantel, 482, 2548
    vitamin B$_{12}$ deficiency and, 947
Diphyllobothrium pacificum: treatment:
      praziquantel, 482
Diphyllobothrium ursi, 2547
Diplobacillus, 1926
*Diplococcus. See Streptococcus pneumo-
      niae*
Diplococcus mucosus. See Acinetobacter
Diplopoda, 2558
Dipstick test
  for bacteriuria, 176
  for HIV, 1260
Dipylidium caninum, 2547
  diagnosis, 2548
  treatment, 466t
    niclosamide, 483
Direct fluorescence antibody (DFA) test
  for *Chlamydia trachomatis*, 182, 1682
  for respiratory viruses, 172
Direct immunofluorescence, 185
Direct transmission, 165
Dirofilaria, 2553t, 2556
Dirofilaria immitis: pulmonary infil-
      trates with eosinophilia, 631,
      2556
Dirofilaria repens, 2556
Dirofilaria subdermata, 2556
Dirofilaria tenuis, 2556
Dirofilaria ursi, 2556
Disease: defining in epidemiology,
    159–160, 163
Disease prevention and control, 166–168
  assessment of risk, feasibility, cost,
      and effectiveness, 166
  individual, institutional, and commu-
      nity based strategies, 166
  primary, 167
  secondary, 167
  tertiary, 167–168
Disease-specific isolation, 2576t, 2577t,
    2578
Disease surveillance, 161–162
Disinfection
  defined, 2579
  high-level, 2581, 2581t
  intermediate-level, 2581, 2581t
  low-level, 2581, 2581t
  and nosocomial infection prevention,
    2579, 2581t, 2581–2583,
    2582t
Disk elution, 195
Disseminated intravascular coagulation
    (DIC)
  rashes, 553
  and sepsis syndrome, 695f, 695–696

Disulfiran-like reactions: to cephalo-
    sporins, 254–255
Dithromycin, 340
Diuretics: for sepsis syndrome, 701
Diversity-generating (D_H) segment
    genes, 44
Diverticulitis
    actinomycosis and, 2283
    and intra-abdominal abscess, 728–729
    and intraperitoneal abscess, 721
    perforated, 729
DNA amplification
    for *Plasmodium*, 2425
    for *Pneumocystis carinii*, 2479
DNA fingerprinting
    aspergillosis, 2306
    Mycobacterium tuberculosis, 2215,
        2217
DNA integration elements: in resistance,
    214
DNA probes, 25–26
    for amebiasis, 2400, 2401
    for *Chlamydia*, 182–183
    and choice of anti-infective therapy,
        200
    for *Histoplasma capsulatum*, 2348
    for HIV, 1262
    hybridization, 184–185
    for *Leishmania*, 2429
    for mycobacteria, 2214
    for *Mycobacterium avium-intracellu-
        lare*, 2214
    for myocarditis, 803
    for pneumonia, 626
    for urethritis, 1065–1066
DNA viruses, 1325–1446. *See also indi-
        vidual viruses*
    Adenoviridae, 1382–1387
    classification, 1314–1315, 1315t
    Hepadnaviridae (HBV and HDV),
        1406–1439
    Herpesviridae, 1330–1382
        CMV, 1351–1364
        EBV (infectious mononucleosis),
            1364–1377
        herpes B virus, 1379–1382
        HHV-6 and 7, 1377–1379
        HSV, 1336–1345
        overview, 1330–1336
        VZV, 1345–1351
    Papovaviridae, 1387–1406
        papillomaviruses, 1387–1400
        polyomaviruses, 1400–1406
    Parvoviridae, 1439–1446
    Poxviridae, 1325–1330
        molluscum contagiosum, 1329–1330
        monkeypox, 1329
        parapoxvirus, 1329
        vaccinia, 1325–1328
        variola (smallpox), 1328–1329
    shapes and sizes, 1316f
    structure, 1314–1315, 1316f
Dobutamine: for sepsis syndrome, 700,
    700t
Doderlein cytolysis, 1080–1081
Döderlein's bacilli, 32
Dog bites
    anaerobic, 2163t
    Capnocytophaga, 2105. *See also
        Capnocytophaga canimorsus*
    Pasteurella, 2069
    rabies, 1527–1528, 1530, 1531, 1538t,
        1539
    vaccination, 2793–2794
Dog hookworm, 2555

Dog(s): microorganisms harbored by,
    2792t
Dog tapeworm, 2547. *See also
        Dipylidium caninum*
Dog tick. *See Dermacentor variabilis*
Domoic acid poisoning, 1012, 1015
Donovan bodies, 2211, 2212, 2212f
Donovanosis, 2210–2213. *See also
        Calymmatobacterium granu-
        lomatosis*
Dopamine: for sepsis syndrome, 700,
    700t
Dot-blot immunobinding assay: for HIV,
    1260
Down syndrome: *Staphylococcus aureus*
    and, 1762
Doxycycline
    adverse reactions, 310
    antiparasitic use, 459t, 472
        prophylaxis dosage, 465t
        pediatric, 465t
    for bartonellosis, 2212
    for *Borrelia burgdorferi*, 2151
    for *Brucella*, 2057
    for cervicitis, 1085
    for *Chlamydia psittaci*, 1695
    for *Chlamydia trachomatis*, 1684,
        1688
    combination therapy: for mycobacteria,
        396t
    dosage, 307t, 512t–513t
    drug interactions, 310
    for endocarditis, 764
        Coxiella burnetii, 1731
    for *Legionella pneumophila*, 2093,
        2093t
    for leptospirosis, 2140
    for LGV, 1684
    MICs
        for aerobic and facultative anaerobic
            infections, 308t
        for anaerobic infections, 308t
    for *Mycoplasma pneumoniae*, 1710,
        1710t
    for *Neisseria gonorrhoeae*, 1921,
        1921t, 1922t
    for nontuberculous mycobacteria, 396
    pharmacokinetics, 309t
    pharmacology, 308–309, 512t–513t
    for PID, 1096t
    for *Plasmodium*
        prophylaxis, 2424t
        for travelers, 2801
    for Reiter syndrome, 1071–1072
    for *Rickettsia rickettsii*, 1724
    structure, 307f
    tissue distribution, 309
    for *Toxoplasma gondii*, 2469
    for *Treponema pallidum*, 2129t
    for urethritis, 1070
Dracontiasis, 2533
Dracunculus medinensis, 2533
    clinical features, 2533
    epidemiology, 2533
    life cycle, 2533
    prevention, 2533
    and pyomyositis, 929
    treatment, 466t, 2533
        metronidazole, 332, 458
Drangedal disease, 1625–1626
Drechslera, 2391
Droplet spread, 165
Drug abusers
    Bacillus infections in, 1890
        bacteremia, 1892

endocarditis, 1892
    ocular, 1891–1892
bone and joint infections in, 2698
cell-mediated immunity in,
    2696–2697
CNS infections in, 2703–2704
Eikenella in, 2112
endocarditis in, 741, 756–757,
    2698–2700
    clinical manifestations, 749
    gram-negative bacilli, 754
    Pseudomonas aeruginosa,
        1983–1984
    S. aureus, 754
hepatitis in, 2702–2703
    HAV, 1643
    HBV, 1421
    HCV, 1482, 2702
    HDV, 2618
    vaccine, 2623
HIV/AIDS in, 1165, 1166–1167,
    1168f, 1176, 1177f, 1179f,
    1189, 1224, 2696, 2697, 2705.
    See also Human immuno-
    deficiency virus, epidemi-
    ology
    prevention, 1193
host defenses, 2696–2697
infections in, 2696–2709. *See also
    specific infections*
melioidosis in, 2005–2006
noncardiac vascular infections in,
    2700–2701, 2701f
ocular infections in, 2704–2705
osteomyelitis in, 1041, 1049
    Pseudomonas aeruginosa
        symphysis pubis, 1993
pulmonary infections in, 2701–2702,
    2702f
skin and soft tissue infections in,
    2697–2698
splenic abscess in, 2703
STDs in, 2705
streptococcal cellulitis in, 1794
Drug-induced disorders
    acyclovir, 415
    albendazole, 479–480
    amantadine, 418–419
    β-lactam allergy, 272–278
    cephalosporins, 253t, 253–254
    chloramphenicol, 313–314
    chloroquine, 470
    clindamycin, 342–343
    clofazimine, 398
    conjunctivitis, 1107
    cycloserine, 394
    dapsone, 398, 474
    dehydroemetine, 468
    didanosine, 421, 421t
    dideoxynucleoside analogs,
        1269–1270, 1271, 1271t,
        1272–1273
    diethylcarbamazine, 481
    erythromycin, 337
    ethambutol, 393
    ethionamide, 394
    Fansidar, 473–474
    foscarnet, 421t, 422–423
    furazolidone, 469
    fusidic acid, 279
    ganciclovir, 421t, 423–424
    genital lesions, 1056
    granulomatous hepatitis, 1162
    hepatitis, 1147–1148, 1148t
    imipenem, 265

immunodeficiency, 135–137
    interferons: antiviral use, 428
    isoniazid, 390, 390t
    mefloquine, 472
    melarsoprol, 476
    methenamine, 380
    metronidazole, 331t, 331–332,
        467–468
    myocarditis, 804t
    neutropenia, 89
    nifurtimox, 476–477
    nitrofurantoin, 378–379
    para-aminosalicylic, 394
    penicillin, 239f, 239t, 239–240
    pentamidine, 478
    primaquine, 470–471
    quinacrine, 469
    quinine, 471
    quinolones, 373–374
    ribavirin, 430–431
    rifabutin, 392
    rifampin, 319–320, 392
    rimantadine, 418–419
    stavudine, 421t, 432
    streptomycin, 393
    sulfonamides, 356–357
    suramin, 476
    teicoplanin, 351
    tetracyclines, 309–310
    thiabendazole, 480
    trimethoprim, 359
    trimethoprim-sulfamethoxazole, 359,
        474
    vancomycin, 348–349
    vidarabine, 433
    zalcitabine, 434
    zidovudine, 421t, 436
Drug interactions, 520t–527t. *See also
        individual drugs*
    rifampin, 319–320, 320t
    tetracyclines, 310
Drug-resistant dihydrofolate reductase
    (DHFR), 221
Drug(s)
    adverse reactions to. *See Drug-
        induced disorders*
    generic-trade names, 493t–499t
    trade-generic names, 499t–505t
Drug therapy. *See Anti-infective therapy
        and specific drugs*
d4T. *See* Stavudine
DTH skin test, 138, 150, 152,
    2349–2350
DTP vaccine, 2082, 2771, 2775, 2775t,
    2778, 2781. *See also individ-
    ual components*
    adverse reactions, 2773t, 2775
    contraindications, 2779, 2787t
    indications
        for adults, 2784t
        for children and infants, 2775t,
            2780t, 2783
        for HIV infected, 2785t
    reportable events, 2786t
Dubin-Johnson syndrome: hepatic
    involvement, 1149
Duck embryo vaccine (DEV), 1534,
    1536
Dumdum fever, 2431–2434
Duncan syndrome, 151t, 153
Duodenal aspiration
    Giardia lamblia, 2490
    microsporidia, 2520
Duodenal biopsy: *Giardia lamblia*, 2490
Duodenal string test: *Salmonella*, 2021

Duodenal ulceration: *Helicobacter pylori*, 1959t, 1959–1960
Duricef. *See* Cefadroxil
Duvenhaga virus, 1528t, 1529
Dwarfism, short-limbed, 134t
Dwarf tapeworm, 2545t, 2547. *See also Hymenolepis nana*
Dysentery, 953t
  acute, 987–990
  amebic, 989
  approach to diagnosis, 990
  bacillary, 988, 2033–2039. *See also Shigella*
  bilharzial, 989
  Campylobacter jejuni, 989
  ciliar, 989
  diagnosis, 953t, 987f, 987–990
  differential diagnosis, 988t
  E. coli
    enterohemorrhagic, 988
    enteroinvasive, 988, 988t, 2033
  epidemiology, 987
  etiology, 953t
  food-borne disease, 1014
  gonococcal proctitis, 990
  parasitic, 989
  salmonellosis, 989
  spirillar, 990
  Trichuris trichiura, 2527
  typhoid fever, 989
  vibriosis, 989
  yersiniosis, 989–990
Dysgonic fermentor-2 (DF-2). *See Capnocytophaga canimorsus*
Dysgonic fermentor-3 (DF-3), 2107t, 2109–2110
Dyspepsia, nonulcer (NUD): *Helicobacter pylori* and, 1959
Dysphagia: in esophagitis, 962
Dysuria: urethritis, 1064, 1067

E

Ear
  microscopic examination of pathogens, 172t
  swimmer's, 580
Ear infections. *See also* Otitis
  Aspergillus, 2307
  Pseudomonas aeruginosa, 1989–1991
    treatment, 1990–1991
Eastern equine encephalitis virus, 1455–1459
  clinical manifestations, 1458
  diagnosis, 1458
  encephalomyelitis, 876
  epidemiology, 1456
  pathogenesis, 1457
  prevention and treatment, 1458–1459
  serology, 191
Eaton agent, 1704. *See also Mycoplasma pneumoniae*
Ebola virus, 1543–1546
  clinical manifestations, 1544–1545
  diagnosis, 1545
  epidemiology, 1544
  pathogenesis and pathology, 1545
  prevention and treatment, 1545
  Reston subtype, 1544
  Sudan subtype, 1544
  transmission, 1544
  waste management, 2582
  Zaire subtype, 1544
EBV. *See* Epstein-Barr virus
Ecchymoses, 553

Echinococcus, 2525t, 2545t, 2550–2551
  diagnosis, 1006t, 2550
  epidural abscess, 905
  hydatid and alveolar cyst disease, 2550–2551
  treatment, 2551
    praziquantel, 482
Echinococcus granulosus, 2545t, 2550–2551, 2553
  pneumonia
    chronic, 647t, 648
    radiology, 650t
  treatment, 466t, 2551
    albendazole, 479
    mebendazole, 479
Echinococcus multilocularis, 2545t, 2550–2551
  treatment, 466t, 2551
    albendazole, 479
    mebendazole, 479
Echinococcus vogeli: albendazole for, 479
Echocardiography
  endocarditis, 751–752, 752t
  mycotic aneurysms, 772
  myocarditis, 802
  pericarditis, 807
Echoviruses. *See also* Enteroviruses
  arthritis, 1036t
  characteristics, 1620–1621
  classification, 1606t, 1607
  clinical spectrum of infection, 1621t
  cutaneous manifestations, 550t, 551
  diarrhea: infantile, 966
  encephalitis, 874, 1621t, 1623
  epidemic pleurodynia, 1625
  epidemiology, 1609, 1609t
  exanthems, 1621t, 1623–1624
    petechial, 1624
    roseoliform, 1624
    rubelliform and morbilliform, 1623–1624
  laboratory diagnosis, 1611
  lymphadenopathy, 1632
  meningitis, 832, 1621t, 1621–1623
    clinical manifestations, 1622
    differential diagnosis, 1622
    laboratory diagnosis, 1622
    management and prognosis, 1622–1623
  meningoencephalitis in agammaglobulinemic and immunocompromised, 1629
    clinical manifestations, 1629
  myelitis, 874
  myopericarditis, 1626–1627
  myositis, 1632
  in newborn, 1627–1629
    clinical manifestations, 1628
    diagnosis and differential diagnosis, 1628
    epidemiology, 1627–1628
    management, 1628
    pathophysiology, 1628–1629
  paralysis, 1621t, 1623
  respiratory disease, acute, 1621t, 1625
  and Reye syndrome, 1558
  type 11
    herpetiform exanthems, 1624
    respiratory disease, 1625
  type 9: exanthems, 1624
  type 22: hemolytic-uremic syndrome, 1632
  type 1: receptor, 1317t
  winter vomiting disease, 968

ECM, 2143
Econazole, 401t, 403
  structure, 402f
  for vulvovaginal candidiasis, 1076t
Ecthyma, 913
  clinical features, 913
  and sepsis, 692
  Streptococcus pyogenes, 1792–1793, 1793f. *See also* Pyodermas
Ecthyma gangrenosum, 551t, 921
  and leukemia, 2678
  Pseudomonas aeruginosa, 554, 692, 914, 921, 1987, 1996
    treatment, 1996
  and sepsis, 692
  and systemic infections, 551t
Ecthyma infectiosum, 550t, 552, 1439t, 1439–1446. *See also* Parvovirus B19
  manifestations, 1442
Ectoparasites, 2558–2567
  chiggers, 2564
  diseases borne by, 2558t
  eradication, control, prevention, 2558
  lice (pediculosis), 2558–2560
  mites, 2564–2565
  myiasis, 2562–2564
  overview, 2558
  scabies, 2560–2562
  ticks, 2565–2567. *See also* Tick-borne diseases
Ectothrix infections, 2379
Ectropion, 1084
Eczema
  acute vesicular, 2381
  herpeticum, 552
  tinea manus vs., 2379
  vaccinatum, 1327
Edema factor: *Bacillus anthracis*, 3t, 6, 22t
Education: and infection control, 2572–2573
Edwardsiella, 1974
Edwardsiella hoshinae, 1974
Edwardsiella ictaluri, 1974
Edwardsiella tarda, 1974, 1975t
EF-4, 2107t, 2110
Effectiveness assessment, 166
Eflornithine, 459t, 475, 476
  dosage, 467t
    for *Pneumocystis carinii*, 2481
    for *Trypanosoma brucei*, 2454, 2454t
Egg yolk-neomycin (EYN) agar, 2168
Ehrlichia: taxonomy, 1742f, 1747t, 1748
Ehrlichia canis, 1747t, 1748, 1749
Ehrlichia chaffeensis, 1747t, 1747–1752
  canine model, 1749
  clinical manifestations, 1749t, 1749–1750
  course, 1750
  description, 1748, 1748f
  diagnosis, 1750
  differential diagnosis, 1750, 1750t
    murine typhus, 1739
  epidemiology, 1748–1749
  pathogenesis and pathology, 1749
  tick vector, 2565
  treatment and prevention, 1750–1751
Ehrlichia equi, 1747t, 1748, 1751
Ehrlichia ewingii, 1747t, 1748
Ehrlichia phagocytophila, 1747t, 1748, 1751
Ehrlichia platys, 1747t
Ehrlichia rusticii, 1747t, 1748, 1749

Ehrlichia sennetsu, 1747t, 1748, 1749, 1751
  fever, 543
Ehrlichiosis, human granulocytic, 1751
Eikenella corrodens, 2112, 2280
  biochemical reactions, 2107t
  bites, 604, 2766, 2766t
  brain abscess, 890
  classification and site of infection, 2107t
  clenched-fist injuries, 2768
  endocarditis, 756
  human bites, 2768
  identification, 186
  mediastinitis, 815t
  soft tissue infections, 2166
  susceptibility, 2766t
  treatment, 2201
ELAM. *See* Endothelial leukocyte adhesion molecule
Elastase, 79t
ELB agent, 1737. *See also Rickettsia typhi*
Elbow: infectious arthritis, 1033, 1033t
Elderly
  adverse drug reactions in, 203
  bacteremia in, 2739–2740
  bacteriuria in, 2740
  cellular immunity in, 133
  diarrhea (infectious) in, 2740
  endocarditis in, 2740
  FUO in, 2741
  infections in, 2737–2742
  meningitis in, 2740–2741
  pharmacologic concerns with, 2741
  pneumonia in, 2738
    community-acquired, 628–629
  pressure sores in, 2739
  renal function in, 201
  septic arthritis in, 2741
  skin infections in, 2739
  Streptococcus pneumoniae in, 1817, 1817t
  tuberculosis in, 2738–2739
  urinary tract infections in, 668, 2737–2738
Electrocardiogram (ECG): pericarditis, 807
Electroencephalography (EEG): brain abscess, 891
Electrolyte disorders: from penicillins, 239t, 240
Electrolyte therapy
  for diarrhea, 2802
  for peritonitis, 718
Electrophoresis: multilocus enzyme, 27
Electrosurgery: for anogenital warts, 1394
Elephantiasis nostras, 942
El Tor biotype (*Vibrio cholerae*), 1934
EMB. *See* Ethambutol
Embolism
  cardiovascular: and endocarditis, 746
  cerebral: and endocarditis, 746, 749
  endocarditis: prosthetic valve, 784t, 784–785
  pulmonary
    in drug abusers, 2700
    and endocarditis, 746, 749
    pneumonia, 647t
    poliovirus, 1616
  splenic artery: and endocarditis, 749
Embryologic cysts, infected: neck and head, 603
Emetine, 468

EMJH medium, 178
Emmonsia: pneumonia, 647t
Emmonsia parva var. *crescens*, 2391
Empyema
    actinomycosis, 2282–2283
    anaerobic, 2163t
        gram-negative bacilli, 2198
    Aspergillus, 2307
    Mycobacterium tuberculosis, 2235
    Nocardia, 2275
    pleural, 638–641. *See also* Pleural
        empyema
    Salmonella, 2023
    subdural, 900–903. *See also* Subdural
        empyema
    in traumatized patient, 2757
Enanthem, 553
Encephalitis, 874–878
    adenovirus, 1386
    amebic, 2409–2410, 2411,
        2412–2413
        treatment, 2413–2414
    arboviral, 1455–1459. *See also*
        Arboviruses *and specific*
        viruses
    clinical findings, 875–876
    coxsackieviruses, 874, 1621t, 1623
    differential diagnosis, 1340
        poliovirus, 1617
    EBV mononucleosis, 1368–1369
    enteroviral, 1621t, 1623
        differential diagnosis, 1623
    etiology, 876–877, 877t
    herpesviruses, 1334t
    HSV, 1340
        CNS response, 828
        treatment, 412t, 416, 1342
    Japanese, 1466, 1466t, 1468, 1471
    laboratory findings, 876
    Listeria monocytogenes, 1882t,
        1882–1883, 1883t
    measles virus, 1521
    mumps virus, 1497, 1497t, 1498
    pathogenesis, 874–875
    pathology, 874–875
    poliovirus, 874, 1616
    St. Louis, 1466t, 1467, 1468–1469,
        1471–1472
    tick-borne, 1466t, 1467, 1469,
        1472
    toxoplasmosis: in HIV/AIDS, 1238,
        1239, 2457
    treatment, 877–878
    vaccinia virus, 1326
    varicella-zoster virus, 1347
    viral
        animal reservoirs, 2792t
        differential diagnosis, 1623
    von Economo's, 1466
Encephalitozoon, 2514–2522
    diagnosis, 2520–2521
    and HIV/AIDS, 2514, 2516,
        2518–2519
    keratitis: in AIDS, 1114
    in non-HIV infected, 2517
    prevention, 2522
    treatment, 2521–2522
Encephalitozoon cuniculi, 2514, 2515,
        2517t
    diagnosis, 2520
    in HIV infected, 2519t
    treatment, 465t
Encephalitozoon hellem, 2514, 2515,
        2516
    diagnosis, 2520–2521

in HIV/AIDS, 2517t, 2518, 2519,
    2519t
treatment, 465t
Encephalomyelitis. *See also* Encepha-
        litis; Myelitis
    Borrelia burgdorferi, 2148
    etiology, 876–877, 877t
    nonviral, 877t
    postvaccinial: rabies vs., 1535
    treatment, 877–878
    viral, 876–877, 877t
Encephalomyocarditis virus, 1637
    receptor, 1317t
Encephalopathy
    Bordetella pertussis, 2081
    CMV: in the immunocompromised,
        1359–1360
    hepatic, 1139
    HIV, 828, 1175, 1237
        in children, 1186, 1186t
        CMV and, 1359–1360
        incidence, 1182t
    from melarsoprol, 476
    rubella, 1462
Endarteritis, infective, 769–773
    clinical manifestations, 771
    epidemiology, 769–770
    etiology, 772
    laboratory findings, 771–772
    pathogenesis, 770
    pathology, 770–771
    therapy, 772–773
    Treponema pallidum, 2120, 2120f,
        2125
Endocarditis, bacterial. *See also*
        Endocarditis, infective
    use of term, 740
Endocarditis, infective, 740–765
    Actinobacillus, 2106
    acute, 740
    anaerobic bacteria, 756, 2199
        bacilli: treatment, 763–764
        gram-negative, 2199
    Aspergillus, 2308
        treatment, 2309
    Bacillus, 1892
    and brain abscess, 888, 888t
    Brucella, 2056
    Candida albicans, 2296–2297
        treatment, 2300
    Cardiobacterium, 2108
    chlamydial, 758
        treatment, 764
    Chlamydia psittaci, 758, 1694
    clinical manifestations, 748t, 748–749
        in drug addicts, 749
    Corynebacterium: treatment, 322
    Corynebacterium jeikeium, 1876
    Corynebacterium pseudodiph-
            theriticum, 756, 1872t, 1874
    Coxiella burnetii, 757–758, 1731,
            1732f
    culture-negative, 758
        treatment, 764
    defined, 740
    diagnostic criteria, 752t
    differential diagnosis: rheumatic fever,
            1803
    in drug abusers, 741, 756–757,
            2698–2700, 2704
        Bacillus, 1892
        clinical manifestations, 749
        gram-negative bacilli, 754
        Pseudomonas aeruginosa,
            1983–1984, 2699

    Staphylococcus aureus, 754,
            2698–2700
    in the elderly, 2740
    Enterobacteriaceae: treatment, 763
    enterococcal, 1828
        treatment, 761–762
        vancomycin, 347, 349
    epidemiology, 740–742
    Erysipelothrix, 1895
    etiology, 752t, 753–758
        culture-negative, 758
        in drug addicts, 756–757
    experimental, 795–796
    and fever, 541
    Flavobacterium, 2113
    fungal, 757
        treatment, 764
    gram-negative anaerobes, 2199
    gram-negative bacilli, 755–756
    gram-positive bacilli, 756
    Haemophilus: spp. other than *influen-*
            zae, 2046–2047
        treatment, 2047
    Histoplasma capsulatum, 2347
        treatment, 2351
    hypergammaglobulinemia, 42
    immunologic factors in, 745–746
    incidence: after various procedures,
            794t, 794–795
    laboratory findings, 749–752
        special diagnostic tests, 751–752
    Listeria monocytogenes, 756
    and lung abscess, 644
    meningitis and, 831
    meningococcal: treatment, 764
    myalgia, 934
    mycotic aneurysms and, 770
    Neisseria gonorrhoeae, 1919
        treatment, 764
    nonbacterial thrombotic, 742–745,
            744t
    pathogenesis, 742f, 742–746
    pathology, 746–747
        CNS, 747
        eye, 747, 747f, 748f
        heart, 746
        kidney, 746
        lung, 747
        mycotic aneurysms, 746–747
        skin, 747, 748f
        spleen, 747
    pathophysiology, 742–746
    polymicrobial, 758
    prophylaxis, 793–799
        in cardiac surgery, 796
        in children, 797
        common errors in, 797
        current recommendations, 797t,
            798
        drug dosage timing and strength,
            796–797
        evidence of efficacy, 795–796
        malpractice and, 797–798
        prosthetic heart valves, 796
    prosthetic valve, 783–788
        Actinobacillus, 2106
        blood cultures, 785
        clinical manifestations, 784t,
            784–785
        coagulase-negative staphylococci,
            1779
        diagnosis, 784–785
            special studies, 785
        enterococcal, 1828
        epidemiology, 741, 783–784

    incidence, 783
    laboratory findings, 785
    management, 785–788
        antibiotics, 785–787, 786t
        anticoagulation, 787
        surgical, 787, 787t
    microbiology, 783t, 783–784
    mortality, 786
    pathogenesis
        early, 784
        late, 784
    pathology, 784, 784f
    prophylaxis, 787–788, 796
    Pseudomonas aeruginosa,
        1983–1984
    Staphylococcus epidermidis, 1779
    treatment: rifampin, 321
    viridans streptococci, 1848
Pseudomonas aeruginosa, 1983–1984
    treatment, 763, 1984
Q fever, 757–758
    treatment, 764
rashes, 554–555
rheumatic fever, 1802
risk estimation, 794t, 794–795
Salmonella, 2022
skin lesions, 922
Spirillum minus, 757
and splenic abscess, 727
staphylococcal, 752t, 754–755,
        1767–1770
    coagulase-negative, 1779
    S. aureus, 1767–1770
    treatment, 762–763
Staphylococcus aureus, 1767–1770
    clinical manifestations, 1767–1768,
            1768f
    diagnosis, 1769
    echocardiography, 1769
    epidemiology, 1767
    laboratory findings, 1768
    management, 1769–1770
    septicemia vs., 1768–1769, 1769t
    septicemia with, 1768, 1769t
    septicemia without, 1768, 1769t
    treatment, 1769–1770
        vancomycin, 347, 349
Staphylococcus epidermidis, 754–755,
        1779
    prosthetic valve, 783–784
    treatment, 321–322, 763, 786
streptococcal, 744t, 744–745, 752t,
        753–754, 753–755
    group C and G, 1855
    treatment
        penicillin-resistant, 761–762
        penicillin-sensitive, 760
    viridans, 1847–1849
        treatment, 1848, 1848t
Streptococcus agalactiae, 1840
    treatment, 1841t
Streptococcus intermedius group, 1863
Streptococcus pneumoniae, 754, 1821
    treatment, 764
subacute, 740
    defective chemotaxis in, 90
transient bacteremia and, 743, 744t
treatment, 759–765
    aminoglycosides, 295t, 299
    antimicrobial, 760–764
        anaerobic bacilli endocarditis,
            763–764
        chlamydial endocarditis, 764
        culture-negative endocarditis,
            764

Endocarditis, infective (Continued)
Enterobacteriaceae or Pseudomonas endocarditis, 763
enterococcal endocarditis, 761–762
fungal endocarditis, 764
gonococcal endocarditis, 764
meningococcal endocarditis, 764
penicillin-resistant streptococcal endocarditis, 761–762
penicillin-sensitive streptococcal endocarditis, 760
pneumococcal endocarditis, 764
Q fever endocarditis, 764
staphylococcal endocarditis, 762–763
fusidic acid, 279
quinolones, 372–373
rifampin, 321–322
surgical, 765
teicoplanin, 351
tests for monitoring, 759
vancomycin, 347, 349, 350
viral, 758
Endocarditis, nonbacterial thrombotic (NBTE), 742–743
and infective endocarditis, 742–743, 743–745
Endocervicitis
chlamydial, 1686
gonococcal, 1095, 1915
diagnosis, 1919
Endocervix
examination, 1083, 1084
normal flora, 2159, 2159t
Endocrinopathies: CMV, 1360
Endocytosis, reverse, 86
Endogenous infection, 164
Endogenous pyrogens, 530–531. See also specific pyrogens
and hypothalamus, 532f, 532–533
Endometritis
anaerobic gram-negative bacilli, 2199
Chlamydia trachomatis, 1687
Haemophilus influenzae, 2043
Neisseria gonorrhoeae, 1917
PID and, 1095, 1917. See also Pelvic inflammatory disease
postabortal, 1093
postpartum
diagnosis, 1091
etiology, 1091
Streptococcus agalactiae, 1840
treatment, 1091
Endomyocardial biopsy: for myocarditis, 803
Endomyometritis: postpartum, 1091
Endoparametritis: postpartum, 1091
Endophthalmitis, 1120–1129
Aspergillus, 2307
Bacillus, 1891, 1892f
bacterial, 1121t, 1121–1122
Candida, 2298, 2298f
cataract surgery and, 1121
in drug abusers, 2704–2705
etiology, 1121t
fungal, 1121t, 1122–1123
laboratory findings, 1125
noninfectious, 1124–1125
parasitic, 1121t, 1124
Pseudomonas aeruginosa, 1991
treatment, 1992
Staphylococcus epidermidis, 1782
treatment, 1125–1126
viral, 1121t, 1123–1124

CMV, 1124
HSV, 1123
rubella, 1124
rubeola, 1124
VZV, 1124
Endoplasmic reticulum (ER): and MHC class I, 102, 103
Endoscopy
for esophagitis, 962, 963t
and FUO, 541
infection prevention in, 2584–2585
for Kaposi's sarcoma, 1241–1242
Endothelial cells, 34
and cytokines, 82
and inflammatory response, 550
Endothelial leukocyte adhesion molecule (ELAM-1)
cytokines and, 696
sepsis and, 696
Endothelial relaxing factor. See Nitric oxide
Endothelin: and septic shock, 118
Endothrix infections, 2379
Endotoxic shock, 6
Endotoxins, 2
Enterobacteriaceae, 1968
and fever, 530
priming neutrophils, 86
Enoxacin
antimicrobial activity, 367t, 369t
dosage, 370t, 516t–517t
in renal dysfunction, 369, 370t, 517t
drug interactions, 370
multiple-dose regimen, 229f
for peritonitis, 717
pharmacokinetics, 369t
pharmacology, 516t–517t
in vitro models, 229
structure, 365f
Entamoeba histolytica, 2394t, 2395–2408
adherence, 2398, 2399
antigen, 2398
brain abscess, 890, 2401
cathepsin B proteinase, 2398
clinical manifestations, 2394t, 2400t, 2400–2401
colitis, 2400, 2400t
colonic lesions, 2398, 2398f
and complement, 66
cysteine proteinase, 2398, 2399
cysts, 2396, 2396f
description, 2395–2396, 2396f
diagnosis, 955, 2401–2403
extraintestinal amebiasis, 2402–2403
intestinal amebiasis, 2401–2402
diarrhea, 987, 989, 2400, 2401, 2402
in AIDS, 970, 970t
diagnosis, 990
differential diagnosis: Cryptosporidium, 2504
endoscopy indications, 2402, 2402t
enteric symptoms, 1000t, 1002
epidemiology, 2396–2397
extraintestinal disease, 2400t, 2401
diagnosis, 2402–2403, 2403f
galactose adhesin, 15–16, 16f
hepatic abscess, 724, 2398, 2399, 2401, 2402–2403
treatment, 726
chloroquine, 470
hepatic necrosis, 2398
history, 2395
host immunity, 2399

intestinal disease, 2400t, 2400–2401
diagnosis, 2401–2402
invasiveness, 16, 952
life cycle, 2396–2397
mature cyst, 2396, 2396f
pathology and pathogenesis, 2397–2398, 2398f
pleural, 639
pneumonia: chronic, 647t
prevention, 2404
pulmonary infiltrates with eosinophilia, 631
receptors, 12
rectocolitis, 2400, 2400t
risk factors, 2397, 2397t
skin gangrene, 917
specimen collection, 180
abscesses, 178
toxic megacolon, 2400
transmission, 2394t
treatment, 461t, 2403–2404
aminoglycosides, 286, 295t
antimicrobial agents, 2403t
diloxanide, 468
iodoquinol, 468
metronidazole, 458
paromomycin, 468
regimens, 2404t
trophozoites, 2396, 2396f, 2397, 2399
waterborne, 1015, 1016t
Entamoeba polecki, 462t
metronidazole for, 458, 462t
Enteric fever, 953t, 998–1004
clinical features, 998–1001, 999t–1000t
differential diagnosis, 1001–1004
epidemiology, 999t–1000t, 1001
etiology, 953t, 999t–1000t
frequency of symptoms, 1000t
laboratory findings, 999t–1000t, 1000–1001
pathogenesis, 998
Salmonella, 2020–2022
diagnosis, 2021–2022
Salmonella paratyphi, 2021–2022
Salmonella typhi, 2021–2022
systemic infections mimicking, 1002–1004
treatment, 1003–1004
quinolones, 371
Enteric immunity, 948
Enteric infections. See also Gastrointestinal infections
and arthritis, 1033
Clostridium, 2189–2192, 2190t
control, 955–956
diagnosis, 953–955, 954f
epidemiology, 945–946
host factors, 946–948
gastric acidity, 946–947
genotypes, 946
human milk and serum, 948
intestinal immunity, 948
intestinal motility, 947
normal flora, 947–948
personal hygiene, 946
inflammatory (invasive), 952–953, 953t
management, 954f, 955–956
microbial factors, 948–952, 949t
attachment, 951
invasiveness, 951–952
toxins, 948–951, 949t
virulence factors, 952
mortality rates, 945

noninflammatory (enterotoxin), 952–953, 953t
occurrence, 945
penetrating, 953, 953t
prevention, 955–956
principles and syndromes, 945–962
types, 952–953, 953t
Enteric isolation, 2577, 2577t
Enteric microflora: normal, 947–948
loss of, 947–948
Enteritides, inflammatory, 987–998
acute dysentery, 987–990
chronic, 993–994
candidiasis, 993–994
E. coli, 993
gastrointestinal tuberculosis, 993
histoplasmosis, 994
parasites, 994
phycomycosis, 994
South American blastomycosis, 994
syphilis, 994
darmbrand, 991–992
enteritis necroticans, 991–992
necrotizing enterocolitis in the newborn, 990–991
pig-bel, 991–992
pseudomembranous enterocolitis, 992f, 992–993
Enteritis. See also Gastroenteritis; Gastrointestinal infections
Campylobacter, 1951
Enteritis necroticans, 991–992, 2189–2191, 2190t
clinical and pathologic features, 2190–2191
diagnosis, 2191
epidemiology, 2190
treatment, 2191
Enterobacter, 1973
after gynecologic surgery, 1093–1094
β-lactamase, 215, 218, 268
and bone marrow transplantation, 2719
catheter infections, 2595
cholecystitis, 730
endocarditis, 755
as enteric flora, 947–948
in the immunocompromised: treatment, 2666
infusion-related sepsis, 2587
mycotic aneurysms, 772
necrotizing fasciitis, 923
nosocomial, 1964
peritonitis, 711
pneumonia, 619t, 621
nosocomial, 2600
in the immunocompromised, 631
radiology, 650t
prostatitis, 680
resistance, 1972
sepsis: in trauma patients, 2759
suppurative thrombophlebitis, 768
surgical wound infections, 2744t
toxin, 950
treatment
aminoglycosides, 285t
antimicrobials of choice, 202t
β-lactamase inhibitors, 268t
carbenicillin, 244
chloramphenicol, 312t
in the immunocompromised, 2666
penicillins, 237t
rifampin, 323–324
tetracyclines, 308t
urinary tract infections, 667

Enterobacter aerogenes, 1973, 1975t
  cephalosporins for, 255t
  resistance: aminoglycosides, 283–284,
      284t, 286
  treatment
      aminoglycosides, 295t
      quinolones, 367t
      rifampin, 318t
  and tropical sprue, 1025
Enterobacter agglomerans, 1972, 1973,
      1975, 1975t
  rifampin for, 318t
Enterobacter amnigenus, 1975t
Enterobacter asburiae, 1975t
Enterobacter cloacae, 1972, 1973, 1975t
  and burn wounds, 2762, 2762t
  cephalosporins for, 255t
  and granulocytopenia, 2676
  resistance, 251
      aminoglycosides, 284t
  treatment
      aztreonam, 267
      carbapenems, 264t
      rifampin, 318t
  and tropical sprue, 1025
Enterobacter gergoviae, 1973, 1975t
Enterobacter hafnia. See *Hafnia*
Enterobacter hormaechi, 1975t
Enterobacteriaceae, 1964–1980. *See also*
      specific genera and species
  and actinomycosis, 2280
  adhesins, 1966
  antibacterial susceptibility testing,
      194t
  antigenic structure, 1965
  β-lactamase, 216t
  brain abscess, 889
      in the immunocompromised, 890
  capsules, 1968–1969
  Citrobacter, 1974
  colonization factor antigen, 1966
  and cystic fibrosis, 659
  cytotoxins, 1966
  Edwardsiella, 1974
  endocarditis, 755
      treatment, 763
  endotoxins, 1968
  Enterobacter, 1973
  enterotoxins, 1967–1968
  epidemiology, 1964–1965
  Erwinia, 1975
  Escherichia coli, 1969–1972. *See also*
      Escherichia coli
  fimbriae, 1966
  folliculitis, 912
  and granulocytopenia, 2676
  Hafnia, 1973
  H antigen, 1964
  iron acquisition, 1968
  K antigen, 1964
  Klebsiella, 1972–1973
  Klebsielleae, 1972–1973
  and lipopolysaccharide binding protein,
      1968
  lipopolysaccharide (LPS), 1964,
      1968
  lung abscess, 644
  mediastinitis, 815t
  miscellaneous, 1975t
  necrotizing fasciitis, 923
  nosocomial infections, 1964
  O antigen, 1964
  pancreatic abscess, 723
  P fimbriae, 1966
  plasmids, 1969

pneumonia, 619t
  chronic, 647
  nosocomial, 2600, 2601
      in the immunocompromised, 631
  prostatitis, 1099
  Proteae, 1973–1974
  Proteus, 1974
  in renal transplantation, 2723
  resistance, 1969
      plasmid-independent, 1969
      plasmids and, 1969
      R-plasmids, 1969
  Serratia marcescens, 1973
  splenic abscess, 727
  structure, 1965
  suppurative thrombophlebitis, 768
  taxonomy, 1964t
  toxins, 1967–1968
  in trauma patients, 2757
      prevention, 2759
  treatment
      aminoglycosides, 285t
          combination therapy, 287t, 288,
              289t
      cephalosporins, 256–257
      trimethoprim, 358, 359
  urogenital colonization, 666
  vaginal infection, 1080
  and *Vibrio cholerae*, 1935
  virulence, 1965–1969
      factors, 1965–1969
  wound infections: in trauma patients,
      2758
Enterobacter sakazakii, 1973, 1975t
Enterobacter taylorae, 1972, 1975t
Enterobius vermicularis, 2525t, 2528
  clinical syndromes, 2528
  diagnosis, 2528
  epidemiology, 2528
  life cycle, 2528
  treatment, 462t, 2528
      albendazole, 479
      mebendazole, 479
      piperazine, 480
      pyrantel pamoate, 480
  vaginal infection, 1080
Enterococcal infections, 1826–1831. *See*
      also individual species
  antimicrobial susceptibility, 1829t,
      1829–1830
      testing, 194t
  bacteremia, 1828
      in the elderly, 2739
  β-lactamase, 215
  biliary tract, 2165
  classification, 1827, 1827t
  clinical manifestations, 1828–1829
  decubitus ulcer, 919
  endocarditis, 752t, 753–754, 1828
      in addicts, 757
      treatment, 761–762
  epidemiology, 1827–1828
  group B: postpartum endometritis,
      1091
  growth, 185
  intra-abdominal and pelvic infections,
      1828
  mediastinitis, 815t
  meningitis, 1829
  microbiology, 1826–1827, 1827t
  neonatal sepsis, 1829
  osteomyelitis, 1042
  pathogenesis, 1827
  peritonitis, 708
  prostatitis, 1099

resistance, 194, 220, 1829t,
      1829–1830
      aminoglycosides, 283–284
  respiratory tract infections, 1829
  surgical wound infections, 2744t
  in trauma patients, 2757
      sepsis, 2759
  treatment, 1830–1831, 1831t
      aminoglycosides, 287, 287t
      antimicrobials of choice, 202t
      chloramphenicol, 312t
      combination therapy, 287t, 288,
          1830, 1831
      erythromycin, 335t
      tetracyclines, 308t
  urinary tract infections, 1828
      nosocomial, 2608–2609, 2609t
      in trauma patients, 2758
  virulence, 1827
  wound and tissue infections,
      1828–1829
Enterococcus: in renal transplantation,
      2723
Enterococcus avium, 1827
  endocarditis, 1828
Enterococcus casseliflavus, 1827
  endocarditis, 1828
  resistance, 220
Enterococcus cecorum, 1827
Enterococcus columbae, 1827
Enterococcus dispar, 1827
Enterococcus durans, 1827
  endocarditis, 753, 1828
  growth, 186
Enterococcus faecalis, 1827
  antimicrobial susceptibility, 1829t
  and burn wounds, 2762t
  endocarditis, 744, 744t, 753, 1828
      in the elderly, 2740
      treatment, 760
          vancomycin, 347, 349
  and granulocytopenia, 2678
  growth, 186
  orbital cellulitis, 1132
  resistance, 220, 222
  treatment
      aminoglycosides, 295t
          combination therapy, 289t
      carbapenems, 264t
      mezlocillin, 245
      nitrofurantoin, 377
      penicillins, 237t
      quinolones, 368t
      rifampin, 318t
      sulfonamides, 355t
      teicoplanin, 351
      trimethoprim, 357
Enterococcus faecium, 1827
  antimicrobial susceptibility, 1829t
  endocarditis, 753, 1828
      treatment, 761
  growth, 186
  resistance, 220, 222, 2750
  treatment
      aminoglycosides, 289t
      quinolones, 368t
Enterococcus flavescens, 1827
Enterococcus gallinarum, 1827
  endocarditis, 1828
  resistance, 220
Enterococcus hirae, 1827
Enterococcus raffinosus, 1827
  endocarditis, 1828
      treatment, 761
Enterococcus saccharolyticus, 1827

Enterococcus seriolicida, 1827
Enterococcus sulfureus, 1827
Enterocolitis
  HIV/AIDS and, 1230t, 1230–1231
  necrotizing
      in neutropenic, 729
      in the newborn, 990–991
      Pseudomonas aeruginosa, 1995
  neutropenic
      Clostridium, 2190t, 2191
      and intra-abdominal abscess, 729
  pseudomembranous, 992t, 992–993
      Pseudomonas aeruginosa, 1995
      Yersinia enterocolitica, 2077
Enterocytozoon, 2514
Enterocytozoon bieneusi, 2514, 2515,
      2516, 2517t
  diagnosis, 2520
  in HIV infected, 2517t, 2518, 2519t
  in non-HIV infected, 2517t, 2518
  treatment, 2521
Enterotoxins, 948–951, 949t. *See also*
      individual toxins of specific
      bacteria
  Bacillus cereus, 1013
  C. perfringens, 1013
  cholera, 3t, 4, 5, 949t, 950,
      1934–1935, 1936, 1936f
  Enterobacteriaceae, 1967–1968
  Escherichia coli, 946, 948–950, 949t,
      1967–1968
  and fever, 530
  heat-labile, 3t, 5
  mechanism of action, 5
  noninflammatory enteric infection,
      953t
  Salmonella, 2018
  staphylococcal, 6, 555, 1012t,
      1012–1013, 1795
  S. aureus, 530, 1760
  T cells and, 110
  Yersinia enterocolitica, 1013–1014
Enteroviruses, 1620–1636. *See also*
      specific viruses
  antibody response, 1608
      deficiencies, 49
  classification, 1606t, 1606–1607
  clinical spectrum of infections, 1621t,
      1621–1632
  coxsackieviruses, 1606t, 1607,
      1620–1636. *See also*
          Coxsackieviruses
  croup, 574, 574t
  cultures, 173
  dual infections, 1608
  echoviruses, 1606t, 1607, 1620–1636.
      See also Echoviruses
  encephalitis, 1621t, 1623
  encephalomyelitis, 876
  endemic and epidemic behavior, 1609,
      1609t
  epidemiology, 1609–1610
      molecular, 1609–1610
  genomes, 1607
  host cell susceptibility, 1607
  immunity and immune response,
      1608–1609
  and immunodeficiency, 150t
  incidence of infection, 1610
  incubation period, 1610
  laboratory diagnosis, 1610–1611
  meningitis, 832, 1621t, 1621–1623
      antimicrobial therapy, 850t
      clinical presentation, 842
      CSF examination, 844–845

Enteroviruses *(Continued)*
  molecular biology, 1607
  mutation, 1608
  newer, 1606t, 1607, 1621t, 1631–1632
    clinical spectrum of infection, 1621t, 1621–1625
    meningitis, 1621t, 1621–1623
  pathogenesis, 1608
  penetration, 1607
  polioviruses, 1606t, 1606–1607, 1613–1620. *See also* Polioviruses
  prevention and treatment, 1611
  receptors, 1607
  replication, 1607
  transmission, 1610
  type 70
    acute hemorrhagic conjunctivitis (AHC), 1629–1631
      clinical manifestations, 1630, 1630f
      complications, 1630–1631
      differential diagnosis, 1631
      epidemiology, 1629–1630
      laboratory diagnosis, 1631
      seroepidemiology, 1630
      transmission, 1630
    infections, 1621t
    laboratory diagnosis, 1611
    transmission, 1610
  type 71
    characteristics, 1631
    clinical manifestations, 1631–1632
    differential diagnosis, 1632
    epidemiology, 1631
    infections, 1621t, 1631–1632
    laboratory diagnosis, 1632
  type 72. *See* Hepatitis A virus
  type 68: infections, 1621t
  type 69: infections, 1621t
  types 68–71
    clinical spectrum of infection, 1621t
    geographic distribution, 1621t
    virions, 1607
Entomophthoramycosis, 2311, 2317–2319
  clinical manifestations, 2317–2318, 2318f
  diagnosis, 2318
  differential diagnosis, 2318
  epidemiology, 2317
  etiology, 2311t, 2317
  pathogenesis, 2317
  therapy and prevention, 2318–2319
Environmental Protection Agency
  on infectious waste disposal, 2582, 2583t
  on microbicidal chemicals, 2581–2582
Enzymatic inhibition: in resistance, 214–218, 215t
Enzyme immunoassay (EIA), 185, 197
  for *Bartonella*, 1745–1746
  for caliciviruses, 1670–1671
  for *Chlamydia*, 182–183, 185
  for gonococcal infections, 182
  for HIV, 1219, 1253, 1254f, 1254t, 1254–1257, 1255t, 1256f
    correlation with Western blot, 1256t
    current methodology, 1254t, 1255, 1256f
    false-negative, 1256, 1256t
    false-positive, 1256t, 1256–1257
    first generation, 1254–1257
    Murex SUDS, 1260–1261

    saliva-based (Orasure), 1261
    second generation, 1257
    third generation, 1257
    type 2, 1257
  for HSV, 183, 185
  for respiratory viruses, 172
Enzyme-linked immunoassay (ELISA)
  anthrax, 1888
  arenaviruses, 1576–1577
  Blastomyces dermatitidis, 2362
  Borrelia burgdorferi, 1249, 2149, 2149f
  and choice of anti-infective therapy, 200
  of circulating pyrogenic cytokines, 533–534
  CMV, 1352
  Cryptosporidium, 2502, 2507
  echinococcosis, 2550
  endocarditis, 750
  Entamoeba histolytica, 2399, 2402
  Francisella tularensis, 2066
  Giardia lamblia, 2490
  hantaviruses, 1570
  hepatitis C virus, 1156, 1480–1481
  HIV, 1213, 1219, 1225, 2647
  influenza virus, 1554–1555
  leishmaniasis
    cutaneous, 2437
    visceral (kala azar), 2433
  leptospirosis, 2140
  measles, 1523
  microsporidia, 2521
  mumps virus, 1499
  mycetoma, 2329
  paracoccidioidomycosis, 2388
  parvovirus B19, 1443
  Plasmodium, 2425
  pneumonia, 623, 625
  rotavirus, 1450
  rubella, 1462
  Toxoplasma gondii, 2462, 2463, 2464, 2465
  Trypanosoma brucei, 2453
  Trypanosoma cruzi, 2446, 2447
  urethritis, 1065–1066
  visceral larva migrans, 2554
Enzymes
  alteration of target, 220
  aminoglycoside, 218, 218t, 283
  β-lactams, 220
  quinolones, 221
  sulfonamides, 221
  trimethoprim, 221
Eosinophil chemotactic factor of ana-phylaxis (ECF-A), 96
Eosinophilia, 96
  with abdominal pain and diarrhea, syndrome of, 1005–1008
    differential diagnosis, 1006–1008
    etiology, 1006t
  from cephalosporins, 254
  helminthic, 2553
    meningitis, 2555–2556
  myalgias with, 934
  pulmonary infiltrates with, 630–631
    pneumonia, 647t
  trichinosis, 2532
  tropical pulmonary, 631, 2536
    treatment, 462t
  visceral larva migrans, 2554
Eosinophilic folliculitis: and HIV, 1229
Eosinophilic gastroenteritis, 2553t
  diagnosis, 1006t

Eosinophilic meningitis (*Angiostrongy-lus cantonensis*), 2553t, 2555–2556
Eosinophil major basic protein (MBP), 96
Eosinophil peroxidase, 96
Eosinophils, 95–96
Epidemic (louse-borne) typhus. *See Rickettsia prowazekii*
Epidemic pleurodynia: coxsackieviruses, 1621t, 1625–1626
  clinical manifestations, 1626
  diagnosis, 1626
  epidemiology, 1625
  management and prognosis, 1626
  pathogenesis, 1625–1626
  serotypes, 1621t, 1625
Epidemiologist, hospital, 2573, 2574f. *See also* Epidemiology team
Epidemiology of infectious diseases, 158–168
  biology and statistics, 160f, 160–161
  case-controlled studies, 162
  case series, 162
  clinical trials, 163
  cohort studies, 162–163
  community intervention trials, 163
  cross-sectional surveys, 163
  definitions, 159–160
  determining appropriate methods, 161
  disease prevention and control, 166–168
    assessment of risk, feasibility, cost, and effectiveness, 166
    individual, institutional, and community based strategies, 166
    primary, 167
    secondary, 167
    tertiary, 167–168
  disease surveillance, 161–162, 2572
  experimental studies, 163
  goals of analysis, 158–159
  host-agent relationship, 163–165, 165t
  observational studies, 161–163
  outbreak investigations, 163
  routes of transmission, 165–166
  types of studies, 161, 161t
Epidemiology team
  educational role, 2572–2573
  and hospital employee health, 161–162, 2572
  hospital epidemiologist, 2573, 2574f
  infection control committee, 2573, 2575
  monitoring antimicrobial utilization, 2573
  organization, 2573, 2574f
  outbreak investigation, 2572
  surveillance, 161–162, 2572
Epidermal cysts: infected, 920–921
Epidermodysplasia verruciformis, 1388t, 1389, 1392. *See also* Human papillomavirus
  treatment, 1395
Epidermoid cysts: differential diagnosis, 1395
Epidermolytic toxins: *Staphylococcus aureus*, 1759–1760
Epidermophyton floccosum, 2375, 2375t, 2376, 2377, 2378
Epididymitis, 1100–1101
  blastomycosis, 2360
  Chlamydia trachomatis, 1069, 1685
  cytomegalovirus, 1360

  and HIV, 1101–1102
  Neisseria gonorrhoeae, 1069, 1685, 1916
    treatment, 1922
  nonspecific bacterial, 1100–1101
  sexually transmitted, 1101
  Ureaplasma, 1715t
Epididymo-orchitis, 1101
  mumps virus, 1497t, 1498
Epidural abscess, 904–907
  anaerobic, 2163t
  anatomy, 822f
  bacteriology, 902t, 904
  differential diagnosis: brain abscess, 891
  etiology and antibiotic therapy, 902t
  intracranial, 904
    clinical features, 904
    diagnosis, 904, 904f
    therapy, 904
  spinal, 904–906
    bacteriology, 904–905
    clinical features, 905
    diagnosis, 905, 905f
    etiology and pathogenesis, 905
    pathology, 905
    therapy, 905–906
  therapy, 902t, 904
Epiglottitis, 590–593
  and croup, 576
  differential diagnosis, 591
  Haemophilus influenzae, 2041–2042
  immunity and, 592
  therapy, 592
Epinephrine: for sepsis syndrome, 700
Epiphora: dacryocystitis and, 1131
Episiotomy, 1092, 1092f
  myonecrosis, 1093
Epithelial hyperplasia of the oral cavity (Heck's disease), 1388t, 1393
Epithelioid angiomatosis. *See* Bacillary angiomatosis
Epitrochlear lymphadenitis: acute suppu-rative, 937
Epizootic diarrhea of infant mice (EDIM), 967
Epstein-Barr nuclear antigen (EBNA), 1365, 1369
Epstein-Barr virus (EBV), 1364–1377
  adherence, 12
  antiadhesin antibodies, 13
  antibodies
    EBV-specific, 1371, 1371t
    heterophile, 1370, 1370t
  arthritis, 1036t
  and B-cell lymphomas, 1370
  biologic properties, 1364–1365
  B-lymphocyte CR2 receptor, 12
  and bone marrow transplantation, 2720
  and Burkitt's lymphoma, 1364, 1369–1370
  cardiac complications, 1369
  cell-mediated immunity and, 129, 1366–1367
  and chronic fatigue syndrome, 1306, 1307
  chronic infection, 1369
  classification, 1330t
  clinical manifestations, 1334t, 1367–1370
  and complement, 66
  cutaneous manifestations, 550t, 553
  dacryocystitis, 1131
  description, 1364–1365

detection, 1371
differential diagnosis, 1372
  CMV mononucleosis, 1357
  scrub typhus, 1741
encephalitis, 876
epidemiology, 1365–1366
fever, 543
granulomatous hepatitis, 1163
hematologic complications, 1368
hematologic findings, 1370, 1370t
hepatic complications, 1369
hepatitis, 1137, 1147
  in transplant recipients, 2730
heterophile antibodies, 1370, 1370t
histopathology, 1366
history, 1364
and HIV/AIDS, 1210
  B-cell lymphomas, 1370
  treatment, 1288
  viral proteins, 1593
HLA-A11 and, 129
humoral responses, 1366–1367
hypergammaglobulinemia, 42
immunization, 1373
in the immunocompromised host,
  1332t
immunodeficiency and, 137
immunosuppressive therapy and, 135
incidence of infection, 1365
infectious mononucleosis, 1367–1370
  complications, 1368–1369
  course, 1369
  manifestations, 1367t
  symptoms and signs, 1367t,
    1367–1368, 1368t
  in transplant recipients, 2730
keratitis, 1115–1116
laboratory diagnosis, 1370–1372
latency, 1332, 1332t
lymphadenitis, 940t
lymphocytosis, 1370, 1370t
lymphomas and, 136
meningitis, 833, 842
mortality, 1369
and nasopharyngeal carcinoma, 1332,
  1332t, 1333, 1369–1370
neurologic complications, 1368t,
  1368–1369
nosocomial, 2663
  management of exposed personnel,
    2663
  prevention, 2663
  risks, 2663
  transmission mechanisms, 2663
pathogenesis, 1333, 1366–1367
pharyngitis, 567t, 568
physical properties, 1364
prevention, 1334t, 1334–1335, 1373
primary infections, 1332t
product and host target, 125t
public health impact, 1366
pulmonary complications, 1369
receptors, 1317t, 1365
recurrence, 1332t
and Reye syndrome, 1558
seroepidemiology, 1333t
serology, 191
serum antibody prevalence, 1365
shedding, 1365t, 1365–1366
spectrum of illness, 1367
splenic rupture, 1368
structure, 1330t
throat cultures, 173
transfusion-related, 2627
transmission, 1333t, 1365–1366

in transplant recipients, 2709, 2712,
  2723, 2730
  diagnosis and control, 2713
treatment, 1334t, 1334–1335,
  1372–1373
  acyclovir, 413, 417
  foscarnet, 422–424
  in HIV/AIDS, 1288
tropism, 1331
tumorogenic, 1332
Equine infectious anemia virus, 1591
Erosio interdigitalis blastomycetica:
  Candida albicans, 2293,
    2294f
Erwinia, 1975
Erysipelas, 914
  clinical features, 914, 914f
  differential diagnosis, 914
  eyelid, 1130
  gangrenous, 552
  group C streptococcal, 1793
  Streptococcus pyogenes, 555, 1793f,
    1793–1794
  treatment, 914
Erysipeloid, 915, 1894–1896
  of Rosenbach, 1895
Erysipelothrix rhusiopathiae, 915,
  1894–1896
  animal reservoirs, 2792t
  clinical manifestations, 1895, 1895f
  differential diagnosis, 1894
  endocarditis, 756
  epidemiology, 1894–1895
  pathogenesis, 1895
  treatment and prevention, 1895–1896
Erythema, diffuse, 552
  genital, 1057t, 1059. *See also* Genital
    lesions
Erythema: Kawasaki syndrome, 2567
Erythema chronicum migrans, 2143,
  2146f, 2146–2147, 2147t,
  2566, 2566f
  differential diagnosis: erysipelas, 914
Erythema gangrenosum, 552
Erythema induratum, 2240
Erythema infectiosum (fifth disease),
  552, 1386, 1439, 1442
  arthritis, 1036t
  differential diagnosis, 1443
Erythema marginatum, 552
  rheumatic fever, 1803
Erythema migrans, 556
Erythema multiforme, 551, 551t, 552t
  differential diagnosis, 552t
  herpesviruses, 1334t
  HSV and, 1341
  and infectious diseases, 551–552
  Mycoplasma pneumoniae and, 1706
  pathogenesis, 1333
  and systemic infections, 551t
Erythema nodosum, 551t, 552t
  Chlamydia pneumoniae and, 1700
  Coccidioides immitis, 2367
  differential diagnosis, 552t
    meningococcal, 554
  granulomatous hepatitis, 1162
  and *Mycobacterium tuberculosis*,
    2220, 2222
  Mycoplasma pneumoniae and, 1706
  Yersinia enterocolitica, 2077
Erythema nodosum leprosum, 399, 2247
Erythematous urticarial eruptions: from
    vaccinia, 1327
Erythrasma, 919
  clinical features, 919

Corynebacterium minutissimum, 919,
  1872t, 1875
  of groin, 2378
Erythrocyte sedimentation rate (ESR)
  endocarditis, 749–750
  infectious arthritis, 1033
Erythromycin, 334–338
  adverse reactions, 337
  antibiotic-associated colitis (AAC)
    from, 979
  antimicrobial activity, 334–336, 335t
  for *Bordetella pertussis*, 2082
  for *Borrelia burgdorferi*, 2151
  for *Borrelia* relapsing fever, 2143
  for *Campylobacter*, 1953
  clinical pharmacology, 336t, 336–337
  combination therapy
    antagonism, 208–209
  for *Coxiella burnetii* pneumonia,
    1730
  dosage, 512t–513t
    in renal dysfunction, 204–205, 513t
  drug interactions, 337
  for erysipelas, 914
  esterase, 219
  for *Francisella tularensis*, 2066
  for furuncles, 912
  for *Haemophilus ducreyi*, 338t, 2048
  for impetigo, 911
  for *Legionella pneumophila*, 2093,
    2093t
  for *Legionella* spp., 2102
  major uses, 337–338, 338t
  for *Mobiluncus*, 2052
  for *Mycoplasma pneumoniae*, 1710,
    1710t, 1711
  and pH, 206
  pharmacology, 512t–513t
  for pneumonia, 632t
  resistance, 219, 221–222, 334–336
    coagulase-negative staphylococci,
      1778
    Francisella tularensis, 2066
    Streptococcus pneumoniae, 1821
  for *Streptococcus pyogenes*, 1790,
    1793
  structure, 334f
  susceptibility testing, 194t
  topical, 384t
  for urethritis, 1070
Erythromycin estolate: pharmacology,
  512t–513t
Erythromycin ethyl succinate: pharmacology, 512t–513t
Erythromycin gluceptate: pharmacology,
  512t–513t
Erythromycin lactobionate: pharmacology,
  512t–513t
Erythromycin stearate: pharmacology,
  512t–513t
Erythroplasia of Queyrat, 1393
Erythropoietin, 113
  recombinant, 452
  therapeutic use, 452
Eschar: rickettsial, 553
Escherichia coli, 1969–1972
  adherence, 2, 31
  adhesin, 11f
  adhesins, 13
  after gynecologic surgery, 1093–1094
  α-hemolysins, 1966
  bacteremia, 1971–1972
  β-hemolysins, 1966
  β-lactamase, 215, 216t
  biliary tract, 2165

and bone marrow transplantation,
  2719
and burn wounds, 2762t
in cancer patients, 2668
chemotaxis, 23
cholangitis, 732
cholecystitis, 730
clones, 21
colicin V plasmid, 1969, 1971
colonization factor antigen (K88;K99),
  951
cytotoxins, 950–951, 1966
differential diagnosis, 1970
  amebiasis, 2402
diffusely adherent (DAEC): pathogenic
  mechanisms and serogroups,
    949t, 951
Dr hemaglutinin, 664, 665t
in drug abusers, 2697, 2698
dysentery, 987–988, 2033
in the elderly, 2740
endocarditis, 755
  treatment, 763
enteric infections, 993, 1969–1970
enteroadherent (EAEC), 1969, 1970
enteroaggregative (EAggEC): pathogenic mechanisms and
  serogroups, 949t, 951
enterohemorrhagic (EHEC), 1969,
  1970. *See also* O157:H7
  below
  cytotoxin, 950
  diagnosis, 955
  diarrhea, 988
  hemolytic-uremic syndrome and,
    6
  pathogenic mechanisms and
    serogroups, 949t
  serotypes, 966t, 989
enteroinvasive (EIEC), 1969, 1970
  dysentery, 987–988, 2033
  pathogenic mechanisms and
    serogroups, 949t, 951
  serotypes, 988, 988t
  toxin, 950
enteropathogenic (EPEC), 24, 946,
  1969, 1970
  chronic diarrhea, 993
  cytotoxins, 1967
  necrotizing enterocolitis of newborn,
    990–991
  in newborn nurseries, 965–966,
    966t
  pathogenic mechanisms and
    serogroups, 949t
enterotoxigenic (ETEC), 22t,
  1969–1970
  attachment, 951
  diagnosis, 955
  diarrhea in adults, 969
  food-borne, 1012t, 1013, 1016
  infantile diarrhea, 966
  pathogenic mechanisms and
    serogroups, 949t, 951
  serotypes, 966t
  toxins, 1967. *See also* enterotoxins
  below
  travelers' diarrhea, 971t, 971–972,
    972t
  waterborne, 1015, 1016t
  weanling diarrhea, 967
enterotoxins, 949t, 950, 1967
  epidemiology, 946
  heat-labile, 1967–1968
  heat-stable, 1967

Escherichia coli (Continued)
  epidural abscess, 904
  extraintestinal, 7
  F adhesin, 664, 665t
  fimbriae, 951
  food-borne, 1012, 1012t, 1013
    foods implicated, 1017t
    laboratory diagnosis, 1018t,
      1018–1019
  G fimbriae, 664, 665t
  and granulocytopenia, 2676
  guanylin, 5
  hemolysin, 4, 22t
  hepatic abscess, 724
  interaction with host tissue, 1967f
  interleukin-1 and, 1968
  intra-amniotic infection syndrome,
    1090
  K88 adherence antigen receptor, 946
  K1 antigen, 24, 966, 966t, 1965,
    1968–1969, 1971
  and leukemia, 2672
    chronic lymphocytic, 2673
  mediastinitis, 815t
  meningitis, 834
    bacteremia, 838
    blood-brain barrier alteration, 839
    CSF examination, 846
    meningeal invasion, 838–839
    neonatal, 1971
  M fimbriae, 664, 665t
  multilocus enzyme electrophoresis, 27
  mycotic aneurysms, 772
  N-acetylneuraminic acid (NANA)
    and, 946
  necrotizing fasciitis, 923
  in neutropenics, 2672t
  as normal enteric flora, 949t
  and normal physiology, 2160
  O157:H7 strain, 27, 1970
    cytotoxin, 950
    dysentery, 2033
    food-borne, 1012t, 1014, 1020
      laboratory diagnosis, 1018t,
        1018–1019
    infantile diarrhea, 966
    specimen collection, 180
    waterborne, 1015, 1016t
  orchitis, 1101
  osteomyelitis, 1041
  pancreatic abscess, 723
  Pap fimbriae, 24
  pap genes, 17
  pap operon, 17, 17f
  pathogenicity, 22t, 22–23
    mechanisms, 949t, 949–950
  penetration, 2, 7
  peritonitis, 708, 711, 713, 715
    in peritoneal dialysis, 719
    treatment, 716
  P fimbriae, 11f, 16–18, 17f, 664–665,
    665t, 1966, 1971
  phase variation, 1966
  pneumonia, 619t
    necrotizing, 644
    nosocomial, 2600
      in the immunocompromised, 631
    sputum analysis, 623f
  postpartum endometritis, 1091
  prophylaxis, 1970
  prostatitis, 680
  in renal transplantation, 2723
  resistance, 200, 2750
    aminoglycosides, 283, 284t
    aminopenicillins, 243

  nitrofurantoin, 377
  quinolones, 366
  trimethoprim, 358
  respiratory tract infections, 1971
  serogroups, 949t, 966, 966t
  serotypes, 966, 966t
  S fimbriae, 664, 665t, 666
  and *Shigella*, 2033
  specimen collection, 180
  STb (STbEC), 948, 949t
  stool culture, 955
  suppurative thrombophlebitis, 768
  surgical wound infections, 2744t,
    2745, 2747t
  symmetric peripheral gangrene, 553
  toxins, 3t, 5
    heat-labile, 3, 3t, 4, 5, 22t
    heat-stable, 3t, 5, 22t
    shiga-like, 3t, 6, 22t
  in trauma patients, 2757
  in travelers, 2801
  treatment
    aminoglycosides, 285t
    aminopenicillins, 243
    antimicrobials of choice, 202t
    aztreonam, 267t
    β-lactamase inhibitors, 268t
    carbapenems, 264t
    cephalosporins, 255, 255t, 257
    chloramphenicol, 312t
    neomycin, 384
    nitrofurantoin, 377–378
    penicillins, 237t
    quinolones, 367t, 371
    rifampin, 318t
    sulfonamides, 355t, 357
    tetracyclines, 307, 308t
    trimethoprim, 357
  and tropical sprue, 1025
  type 1 fimbriae, 664–665, 665t, 666,
    1966
  urinary tract infections, 1970–1971
    in the elderly, 2737
    nosocomial, 2608–2609, 2609t
  uropathogenic, 24, 665–667, 667–668
    adhesins, 665, 665t
  vascular graft infections, 789, 790t
  verotoxigenic, 1014, 1018, 1018t
  virulence factors, 2, 22t, 22–23, 1968
  virulence regulation, 23t, 24
Escherichia fergusonii, 1975t
Escherichia hermannii, 1975t
Escherichia vulneris, 1975t
E-selectin, 81, 82, 123
  and septic shock, 118
Esophageal disease: HIV/AIDS and,
  1229
Esophageal perforation: and mediastinitis, 814, 814t
Esophageal ulceration: tetracyclines, 310
Esophagitis, 962–964
  anti-infective agents for, 964t
  approach to, 964
  candidal, 962, 963f, 2292f, 2292–2293
    and HIV/AIDS, 1229
  in chemotherapy patients, 963–964
  cytomegalovirus, 963
    and HIV/AIDS, 1229
  endoscopy for, 962, 963t
  etiology, 962t, 962–963
  herpes simplex virus, 963, 1340
    and HIV/AIDS, 1229, 1340
  herpesviruses, 1334t
  in HIV/AIDS, 964
    candidal, 1229

  CMV, 1229
  HSV, 1229, 1340
  symptoms, 962
  in transplant patients, 964
Esophagus: tuberculosis, 2238
Estrogen: and host resistance, 35
E-test, 195
Ethambutol
  adverse reactions, 393
  for atypical mycobacterial infections,
    2267, 2268, 2269
  combination therapy: for mycobacteria,
    396t
  dosage, 393, 516t–517t
    in hepatic or renal failure, 390t,
      517t
  for *Mycobacterium avium-intracellu-
    lare*, 2257, 2258
  for *Mycobacterium tuberculosis*, 393,
    1289, 2226, 2227, 2228, 2229
  pharmacology, 516t–517t
  structure, 393f
Ethanol: tetracycline interactions with,
  310
Ethionamide
  adverse reactions, 394
  combination therapy: for mycobacteria,
    396t
  dosage, 394, 516t–517t
    in hepatic or renal failure, 390t,
      517t
  drug interactions, 522t
  for *Mycobacterium avium-intracellu-
    lare*, 2257
  for *Mycobacterium leprae*, 398
  for *Mycobacterium tuberculosis*, 394
  pharmacology, 516t–517t
Ethylene oxide sterilization, 2580–2581
  side effects, 2581
Eubacteria, 1752. *See also* Bacteria
Eubacterium, 2158t, 2206, 2207
  mediastinitis, 815t
  as normal flora, 2159t
  treatment: tetracyclines, 308t
Eubacterium lentum, 2207
  and normal physiology, 2160
  peritonitis, 711, 715
  treatment: chloramphenicol, 312t
Eubacterium nodatum
  female genital infections, 2165
  incidence, 2162
  and underlying disease, 2167
Eucalyptus camaldulensis, 2331
Eucalyptus tereticornis, 2331
Eugonic fermenter (EF-4), 2107t, 2110
Eukaryotic cells: protozoan penetration,
  24–25
Eumycetoma, 2327
European bat virus, 1528t, 1529
European blastomycosis. *See Cryptococcus neoformans*
Ewingella americana, 1975t
Exanthems
  chickenpox (VZV), 1347
  coxsackieviruses, 1621t, 1623–1624
    herpetiform, 1624
    petechial, 1624
    roseoliform, 1624
  echoviruses, 1621t, 1623–1624
    petechial, 1624
    roseoliform, 1624
    rubelliform and morbilliform,
      1623–1624
Exanthem subitum, 1377, 1378
  nosocomial, 2663

Exfoliatins: *Staphylococcus aureus*, 1760
Exogenous infection, 164
Exophiala: keratitis, 1113
Exophiala dermatitidis
  brain abscess, 890
  and CGD, 155
Exophiala jeanselmei, 2324
Exophiala (Phaeoanellomyces) werneckii,
  2384–2385
Exophiala spinifera, 2324
Exotoxins, 2
  A, 3t, 4
    Pseudomonas aeruginosa, 3t, 4, 5,
      1982–1983
  pyrogenic, 6
    cutaneous manifestations, 555
  streptococcal pyrogenic (SPE), 1787,
    1788
Experimental studies: in epidemiology,
  161
Exserohilum, 2391
  phaeohyphomycosis of paranasal
    sinus, 1132
Exserohilum meginnisii: sinusitis, 586t
Exserohilum rostratum: sinusitis, 586t
Eye
  barrier to microorganisms, 32
  examination: and FUO, 539
Eye infections, 1103–1136. *See also*
    specific infections
  anaerobic, 2163t
  Aspergillus, 2307
  Bacillus cereus, 1891, 1892f
  Candida albicans, 2298, 2298f
    treatment, 2301
  cavernous sinus, 1131–1133
  conjunctivitis, 1103–1110. *See also*
    Conjunctivitis; Keratocon-
    junctivitis
  chlamydial, 1106, 1685
    neonatal, 1688–1689
    treatment, 1688
  in drug abusers, 2704–2705
  endophthalmitis, 1120–1129. *See also*
    Endophthalmitis
  Histoplasma capsulatum: treatment,
    2351
  HIV/AIDS and, 1239–1240
  keratitis, 1110–1120. *See also*
    Keratitis; Keratoconjunctivitis
  laboratory features, 1133–1134
  lacrimal apparatus, 1130–1131
  microsporidia, 2513
  Moraxella catarrhalis, 1927
  orbital, 1131–1133
  periocular, 1129–1136
  Pseudomonas aeruginosa, 1991–1992
    treatment, 1991–1992
  specimen collection and processing,
    171t, 183–184
  Staphylococcus epidermidis, 1782
  Toxoplasma gondii, 2461, 2461f
    serology, 2465
    treatment, 2467–2468
  treatment, 1134–1135
    aminoglycosides, 295t
Eyelid infections, 1129–1130
Eye surgery: endophthalmitis after, 1121

F

Fab fragments, 37
Fabry's disease, 546
Facial infections. *See* Orofacial infec-
  tions

F-actin, 79
Factitious illness: and fever, 548
Factor B, 58t, 59, 63, 73
Factor D, 73
Factor H, 58t, 62, 63, 63t, 64
  deficiency, 152t
Factor I, 58t, 62, 63t
  deficiency, 152t
Factor VII: and sepsis syndrome, 695
Factor X: and sepsis syndrome, 695
Factor XII: and sepsis syndrome,
  695–696
Facultative anaerobic bacteria: growth or
  biochemical characteristics,
  185f, 186, 189
Faget sign (yellow fever), 1471
Fallopian tube occlusion: prophylaxis
  recommendations, 2751t
Famciclovir, 421–422
Familial Mediterranean fever
  differential diagnosis
    erysipelas, 914
    peritonitis, 714
  fever of, 546
    pattern, 538
Famvir. See Famciclovir
Fansidar, 355, 459t, 473–474. See also
  Pyrimethamine-sulfadoxine
Fansimef, 474
Fasciitis: necrotizing, 923–926
Fasciola hepatica, 2525t, 2538t, 2541
  clinical syndromes, 2542
  diagnosis, 1006t, 1007, 2542
  granulomatous hepatitis, 1161
  resistance: praziquantel, 482
  treatment, 463t, 2542
    bithionol, 483
Fasciolopsis buski, 2525t, 2538t,
  2542–2543
  clinical syndromes, 2542
  diagnosis, 1006t, 1007–1008,
    2542–2543
  treatment, 463t, 2543
    praziquantel, 482
Fastidious anaerobe agar (FAA), 2168
Fat, dietary: and tropical sprue, 1026
Fatal familial insomnia, 881, 883–884
Favus, 2375, 2376, 2380
Fc receptors
  IgA, 39, 40t, 41
  IgE, 39, 40t, 40–41
  IgG, 39, 40, 40t
    and phagocytosis, 41
    immunoglobulin, 40–41
Feasibility assessment, 166
Febrile response, 532
Fecal-oral transmission
  amebiasis, 2404
  Campylobacter, 1950
  Giardia lamblia, 2487, 2491
  hepatitis A virus, 1643, 1645
  hepatitis E virus, 1664
  rotavirus, 1449
  Salmonella, 2015, 2016
  viral diseases, 1319
Feline panleukopenia virus (FPV), 1440
Female genitalia: examination,
  1082–1084
Female genital tract infections. See also
  Sexually transmitted diseases
  and specific infections
  anaerobic, 2163t, 2165
    gram-negative bacilli, 2199
    specimen collection, 2168t
    treatment, 2201

lesions. See Genital lesions
Streptococcus agalactiae, 1840
tuberculosis, 2238
Female pelvic infections, 1090–1096
  after gynecologic surgery, 1093–1095
    cuff abscess, 1094
    cuff cellulitis, 1094
    osteomyelitis pubis, 1095
    pathogens, 1093t, 1093–1094
    pelvic abscess, 1094–1095
    pelvic cellulitis, 1094
    risk factors, 1094
    septic pelvic thrombophlebitis,
      1095
  anaerobic cocci, 2205
  episiotomy, 1092f, 1092–1093
  intra-amniotic infection syndrome,
    1090
  intrapartum, 1090–1093
  PID, 1095–1096. See also Pelvic
    inflammatory disease
  postabortal, 1093
  postpartum, 1091
  puerperal ovarian vein throm-
    bophlebitis, 1091–1093
Fenticonazole: for vulvovaginal candidiasis, 1076t
Fetal infections. See Neonatal disease;
  Pregnancy
Fetus
  antimicrobials and, 204
  cellular immunity in, 132–133
Fever, 530–561
  acute phase response, 34, 530,
    534–535. See also Acute
    phase response
  and acute retroviral syndrome (HIV),
    1224t
  African swine, 2144
  antipyretics, 533
  Brazilian purpuric, 2040, 2044, 2046
  central, 546
  Chlamydia psittaci, 1694
  continuous, 538
  cytokines and, 117
  ehrlichiosis, 1749, 1749t
  in endocarditis, 747, 748t
    prosthetic valve, 784, 784t
  enteric, 998–1004
  febrile response, 532
  food-borne diseases, 1013–1014
  Fort Bragg, 2138
  and granulomatous hepatitis, 545,
    1162
  Haverhill, 2085
  hyperthermia vs., 531. See also
    Hyperthermia
  hypothalamic, 531
  influenza virus, 1556
  intermittent, 532, 538
  Malta, 2053
  Marseilles, 1725
  Mediterranean spotted, 373, 1725
  meningitis, 842t, 843t
  Meuse, 1741
  Oroya, 1002, 1742, 2209–2210
  pathogenesis, 530–536
    endogenous pyrogenic cytokines
      and hypothalamus, 532f,
      532–533
    endogenous pyrogens, 530–531
    pyrogens, 530
    scheme, 532f
  Pel-Ebstein pattern, 544
  pharyngoconjunctival, 566, 1385

and pneumonia, 621–622
Pontiac, 2087, 2091, 2099
pyrogenic cytokines: measurement of
  circulating, 533–534
Q, 1719, 1720, 1720t, 1727–1735. See
  also Coxiella burnetii
and rash, 549–561
  approach to patient, 549–550
  in bacillary angiomatosis, 557
  Borrelia burgdorferi and, 556
  in candidiasis, 556–557
  Capnocytophaga canimorsus and,
    556
  characteristics of lesion, 551
  differential diagnosis, 551–553
  diffuse erythema, 552
  enanthem, 553
  erythema multiforme, 552t
  erythema nodosum, 552t
  in HIV/AIDS, 557–558
  host defense properties of skin,
    550–551
  in immunocompromised hosts,
    557–558
  macular, 551–552
  maculopapular, 551–552
  Neisseria gonorrhoeae and, 554
  Neisseria meningitidis and,
    553–554
  nodular, 552
  papular, 551–552
  pathogenesis, 551
  petechial purpuric lesions, 553
  Pseudomonas aeruginosa and, 554
  in rickettsial infections, 556
  in septicemia, 553
  Staphylococcus aureus and, 555
  in streptococcal infections, 555–556
  in subacute bacterial endocarditis,
    554–555
  systemic infections, 550t, 551t
  in toxic shock syndrome, 555
  vesiculobullous eruptions, 552–553
rat-bite, 2084–2086, 2155–2156
relapsing (Borrelia), 2141–2143
remittent, 532, 538
Rickettsia prowazekii (louse-borne
  typhus), 1736
San Joaquin Valley, 2365
scrub typhus, 1740
and sepsis, 691
in spinal cord injured patients, 2736
spotted rickettsial, 1719, 1720t,
  1721–1727. See also
  Rickettsia rickettsii
and STDs, 1057
therapeutic use, 533
and transplant recipient infections,
  2714
treatment, 533
typhoid. See Salmonella typhi
of unknown origin (FUO), 536–549
  abscesses and, 541
  acute rheumatic fever and, 542
  in adults, 537t
  amyloidosis and, 546
  atrial myxomas and, 544
  autoimmune disease and, 544t,
    544–545
  babesiosis and, 543
  bacterial infections and, 541–542
  biliary system infections and, 541
  causes, 541–543
  in children, 537t
  chlamydial infections and, 543

  classic, 536, 537t
  CNS disorders and, 546
  collagen-vascular disease and, 537t
  deafness and, 546
  defined, 536
  in elderly, 2741
  exaggerated circadian temperature
    rhythm, 548
  Fabry's disease and, 546
  factitious illness and, 548
  familial Mediterranean fever and,
    546
  fungal diseases and, 543
  and granulocytopenia, 2675
  granulomatous diseases and,
    545–546
    hepatitis, 545
  HIV-associated, 536, 537t
  hypersensitivity and, 544–545
  hypertriglyceridemia and, 546
  infections and, 537t, 541–543
  infective endocarditis and, 541
  inflammatory bowel disease and,
    545–546
  inherited disorders and, 546
  invasive procedures, 540
  Kawasaki syndrome and, 542
  laboratory tests, 539–540
  leptospirosis and, 542
  and leukemia/lymphoma, 2675
  leukemias and, 544
  liver tumors and, 544
  lymphomas and, 544
  malaria and, 543
  management, 548
  medical history, 538
  miscellaneous causes, 548
  neoplasia and, 537t, 543–545, 544t
  neutropenic, 536, 537t
  noninvasive procedures, 540
  nosocomial, 536, 537t
  osteomyelitis and, 541
  parasitic disease and, 543
  physical examination, 538–539
  prolonged, 538t
  rat-bite fever and, 542
  relapsing fever and, 542
  renal cell carcinoma and, 544
  rickettsial infections and, 542
  sarcoidosis and, 545
  skin testing, 540–541
  spinal cord injury and, 2736
  spirochetal infections and, 542
  temperature pattern, 538
  temporal arteritis and, 546
  toxoplasmosis and, 543
  in transplant recipients, 2715
  trypanosomiasis and, 543
  tuberculosis and, 542
  urinary tract infections and, 541–542
  urticaria and, 546
  viral infections and, 543
  Whipple's disease and, 542
Fever therapy, 533
FIAC, 437t
FIAU, 437t
Fiberoptic bronchoscopy
  and lung abscess, 645
  for pneumonia, 624–626
    chronic, 652
Fibrin deposition: and endocarditis, 742,
  745
Fibrinogen
  and acute phase response, 117
  and FUO, 539

Fibrinolysis: and sepsis syndrome, 696
Fibroblast: and inflammatory response, 550
Fibromyalgia: differential diagnosis, 2151
Fibronectin: and host defense, 32, 33, 34
Fifth disease (erythema infectiosum), 552, 1386, 1439, 1442. *See also* Parvovirus B19
Filamentous hemagglutinin: *Bordetella*, 23, 24, 2079
Filariasis, 2525t, 2533–2535. *See also specific species*
   treatment, 462t, 2534
Filobasidiella neoformans
   var. *bacillispora*, 2331
   var. *neoformans*, 2331
Filoviridae, 1543–1546. *See also individual viruses*
   characterization, 1544
   classification, 1315t
   Ebola virus, 1543–1546
   Marburg virus, 1543–1546
Filoviruses: serology, 191
Fimbriae, 12t, 16–18
Fimbrial protein (FIM): *Bordetella pertussis*, 23, 24
First disease. *See* Measles virus
Fish-borne disease, 2792t
   anisakiasis, 2554–2555
   eosinophilic meningitis, 2555
   Erysipelothrix, 1895
   tapeworms, 2546–2547
Fish poisoning, 1014, 1015t. *See also Clostridium botulinum*
Fish tapeworm, 2546–2547. *See also Diphyllobothrium latum*
Fitz-Hugh Curtis syndrome
   Neisseria gonorrhoeae and, 1917
   and peritonitis, 709
Five-day fever, 1741
Fixed drug eruptions
   genital lesions, 1056, 1081
   tetracyclines, 309
FK506: immunodeficiency from, 136
Flagellae: fimbriae vs., 16
Flat warts, 1388t, 1390, 1392. *See also* Human papillomavirus
Flavimonas oryzihabitans (CDC group Ve-2), 2112–2113
   classification and site of infection, 2107t
Flaviviridae, 1465–1486. *See also individual viruses*
   flaviviruses, 1465–1474
   hepatitis C virus, 1474–1486
   shape and size, 1316f
Flaviviruses, 1455, 1465–1474, 1466t. *See also individual viruses*
   clinical manifestations, 1470–1471
   dengue, 1466, 1466t, 1468, 1469–1470, 1470f, 1471, 1472, 1473
   dengue hemorrhagic fever, 1469–1470, 1470f, 1471, 1473
   diagnosis, 1472
   epidemiology, 1467–1469
   history, 1465–1467
   Japanese encephalitis, 1466, 1466t, 1468, 1471
   pathogenesis, 1469–1470
   prevention and therapy, 1472–1473
   St. Louis encephalitis, 1466t, 1467, 1468–1469, 1471–1472

tick-borne encephalitis, 1466t, 1467, 1469, 1472
   yellow fever, 1465, 1466t, 1467–1468, 1469, 1470–1471, 1472
Flavobacterium, 2113
   catheter infections, 2595
   CDC groups IIk-2 and IIk-3. *See Sphingobacterium*
   classification and site of infection, 2107t
Flavobacterium II-b: animal bites, 2766
Flavobacterium indologenes, 2113
Flavobacterium meningosepticum, 2113
   meningitis: vancomycin for, 350
   rifampin for, 324
Flavobacterium multivorum. See Sphingobacterium multivorum
Flavobacterium odoratum, 2113
Flea-borne diseases
   bubonic plague, 2071
   murine typhus, 1737
Fleckfieber. *See* Typhus, epidemic
Fleroxacin
   antimicrobial activity, 367t, 369t, 372
   dosage, 516t–517t
   pharmacokinetics, 369t
   pharmacology, 516t–517t
   structure, 365f
Flexal virus, 1572
Flora, microbial
   alterations in: and infections in patients with neoplasia, 2671f, 2671–2672, 2672t
   anaerobes as, 2157–2160, 2159t
      and normal physiology, 2160
   normal indigenous
      as defense mechanism, 30t, 30–31
      enteric, 947
      oral cavity, 2159, 2159t
Floxacillin: drug interactions, 370
Flubendazole, 480
Flucloxacillin: structure, 242f
Fluconazole, 408–409
   for *Blastomyces dermatitidis*, 2363
   and bone marrow transplantation: prophylactic, 2719, 2721t
   for *Candida albicans*, 408–409, 1283t, 1288, 2299, 2300, 2301
      thrush, 403
   for candidal vulvovaginitis, 404
   for *Coccidioides immitis*, 2371
   for *Cryptococcus neoformans*, 1283t, 1288, 2337
   drug interactions, 522t
   for esophagitis, 964t
   for granulocytopenics, 2680, 2681
   for meningitis, 868
   for neutropenics, 2688t, 2690
   pharmacology, 518t–519t
   structure, 402f
Flucytosine, 406
   combination therapy: synergism, 208
   for *Cryptococcus neoformans*, 406, 1283t, 1288, 2336–2337
   for endophthalmitis, 1125
   for peritonitis, 720
   pharmacology, 518t–519t
Fluid therapy
   for enteric infections, 955
   for food poisoning, 1019
   for peritonitis, 718
   for sepsis syndrome, 699–700
   for *Shigella*, 2036–2037
   for *Vibrio cholerae*, 1937, 1937t, 1938t, 1938–1939

Flukes. *See also individual species*
   blood (schistosomiasis), 2538–2541
   intestinal, 2538t, 2542–2543. *See also* Intestinal flukes
   liver, 2538t, 2541–2542. *See also* Liver flukes
   lung, 2538t, 2543. *See also* Lung flukes
Flumadine. *See* Rimantadine
Fluorescein isothiocyanate (FITC), 185
Fluorescence activated flow cytometry (FACS), 50, 152–153
   for leukocyte adhesion deficiency, 154
Fluorescent calcophor stain: for fungi, 190
Fluorescent treponemal antibody test. *See* FTA-abs test
Fluoride: cariostatic effects, 601
5-Fluorocytosine
   for candidiasis, 2300, 2301
   for chromomycosis, 2326
   dosage: in renal dysfunction, 204
   for endocarditis, 764
   for granulocytopenics, 2680
   structure, 401t
   susceptibility testing, 193
Fluoroquinolones
   drug interactions, 522t
   for enterococcal infections, 1830
   for keratitis, 1117
   pharmacology, 228–231. *See also* Quinolones
   for urethritis, 1070
5'-Fluorouracil
   for anogenital warts, 1394
   drug interactions: sorivudine, 432
Fly-borne diseases, 2558t. *See also specific diseases*
   Francisella tularensis, 2061
Flying: advice while traveling, 2800
Fly larvae (myiasis), 2562–2564
FMLP, 79t, 80
Foam cells (Virchow's cells), 2246
Folinic acid (folate)
   for *Toxoplasma gondii*, 2467, 2467t, 2468
      in HIV/AIDS, 2467, 2467t
   and trimetrexate, 475
   for tropical sprue, 1029
Follicular dendritic cells, 48
Folliculitis, 912
   bacterial: and HIV, 1229
   Candida albicans, 2293, 2294f
   eosinophilic
      and HIV, 1229
      pustular, 912
   and HIV, 1229
   mupirocin for, 386
   Pityrosporum, 2384
   Pseudomonas aeruginosa, 1996
   Staphylococcus aureus, 1763, 1763f
Fonsecaea compacta, 2324
Fonsecaea pedrosoi
   chromomycosis, 2324–2326
   treatment, 2326
Food-borne disease, 1012–1025. *See also* Gastrointestinal infections
   anisakiasis, 2554
   attack rates, 1018t
   caliciviruses, 1669
   Campylobacter, 1949–1950
   from chemicals, 1014–1015
      abdominal cramps and diarrhea (with 6–24 hours), 1015

chronic diarrhea (within 1–3 weeks), 1015
   mushrooms, 1015, 1015t
   nausea/vomiting and abdominal cramps (within 1 hour), 1014
   paresthesias (within 1 hour), 1014–1015
   paresthesias (within 1–6 hours), 1015
   clinical features, 1012–1016
   Clostridium botulinum, 1012, 1014, 1016, 2179, 2180
   Clostridium perfringens, 1012t, 1013, 1017, 1020, 2183t, 2189, 2190t, 2191–2192
   epidemiology, 1012, 1016–1018
      food-specific attack rates, 1017t–1018t, 1017–1018
      geographic location, 1017
      seasonality, 1017
      sources and associations, 1016–1017
   etiology, 1012t, 1017t
   fish and shellfish poisoning, 1015t
   by geography, 1017, 1017t
   Giardia lamblia, 2487
   hepatitis A virus, 1644–1645
   intestinal tapeworms, 2546
   laboratory diagnosis, 1018t, 1018–1019
   Listeria, 1881–1882
   from microorganisms, 1012t, 1012–1014
      abdominal cramps and diarrhea (within 8–16 hours), 1013
      abdominal cramps and watery diarrhea (within 16–72 hours), 1013
      bloody diarrhea without fever (within 72–120 hours), 1014
      fever, abdominal cramps, and diarrhea (within 16–48 hours), 1013–1014
      fever and abdominal cramps (within 16–48 hours), 1013–1014
      nausea/vomiting, diarrhea, and paralysis (within 18–36 hours), 1014
      nausea/vomiting (within 1–6 hours), 1012–1013
   mushroom poisoning, 1015, 1015t
   outbreak investigations, 163
   pathogenesis, 1012t, 1012–1016
   prevention, 1020
   Salmonella enteritidis, 1016, 1020
   Salmonella typhi, 2015
   seasonality, 1017, 1017t
   Shigella, 2035
   staphylococcal, 1012t, 1012–1013, 1774
   streptococcal pharyngitis, 1787
   therapy, 1019–1020, 1020t
   Toxoplasma gondii, 2457
   travel and, 2800
   trichinosis, 2531–2532
   Vibrio cholerae, 1012t, 1013, 1017, 1941–1942
   Vibrio parahaemolyticus, 1012t, 1013, 1016, 1017, 1945, 1946
   waterborne, 1015–1016, 1016t. *See also* Waterborne disease
   Yersinia enterocolitica, 2076, 2077
Food poisoning. *See also* Food-borne disease; Gastrointestinal infections

Bacillus cereus, 1890, 1891
Bacillus licheniformis, 1891
Bacillus subtilis, 1891
Clostridium botulinum, 1012, 1014, 1016
Clostridium perfringens, 1012t, 1013, 1017, 1020, 2190t, 2191–2192
Staphylococcus aureus, 1774
Foot
    diabetic infections, 919–920
    "green," 1997
    Pseudomonas aeruginosa osteochondritis, 1993
    tropical immersion syndrome, 1997
Foot and mouth disease viruses, 1637
Foramen of Luschka: anatomy, 827f, 828
Foramen of Magendie: anatomy, 827f, 828
Foramen of Monro: anatomy, 827f, 828
Foreign body
    aspiration: and mediastinitis, 814t
    vaginitis, 1080
Formaldehyde
    from methenamine, 379, 380
    sterilization, 2580, 2581
Formyl-methionyl-leucyl-phenylalanine (FMLP) receptor, 79
Fortaz. *See* Ceftazidime
Fort Bragg fever, 2138
Foscarnet, 412t, 422–424
    adverse reactions, 421t, 422–423
    and bone marrow transplantation, 2720
    clinical studies, 423–424
    for CMV, 1360–1361
        in HIV/AIDS, 1283t, 1287–1288
        retinitis, 423–424, 1273, 1287, 1360–1361
    dosage
        in renal insufficiency, 423t
    dosage and pharmacology, 422, 518t–519t
    drug interactions, 421t, 422, 522t
    for endophthalmitis, 1126
    for esophagitis, 964t
    for granulocytopenics, 2681
    for HIV, 1273
    for HSV, 422–424, 1287
    nephrotoxicity, 2720
    resistance, 422
    spectrum of activity, 422, 1335
    structure, 423f
Foscavir. *See* Foscarnet
Fournier's gangrene, 925, 1795, 2166
Fowl: microorganisms harbored by, 2792t
Fowlpox, 1325
Fractional bactericidal concentration (FBC), 196
Fractional inhibitory concentration (FIC), 196
Fraction reduction: prophylaxis recommendations, 2751t
Francisella philomiragia, 2061, 2065
    characteristics, 2061t
Francisella tularensis, 2060–2068
    animal reservoirs, 2792t
    biogroup *novicida*, 2060, 2061, 2062, 2065
        characteristics, 2061t
    biogroup *palaeartica* (Type B), 2060–2061, 2062, 2066
        characteristics, 2061t
    biogroup *tularensis* (Type A), 2060–2061, 2062
        characteristics, 2061t

clinical manifestations, 2063–2065, 2064f, 2065f
complications and outcome, 2065–2066
conjunctivitis, 1105
cutaneous manifestations, 550t
cytokine protection, 121t
description, 2060–2061, 2061t
diagnosis, 2066
differential diagnosis
    Chlamydia psittaci, 1695
    Colorado tick fever, 1447
    ehrlichiosis, 1750
enteric-like fever, 1002
epidemiology, 2061–2062, 2062f
glandular, 2063
granulomatous hepatitis, 1161
history, 2060
holartica. *See* biogroup *paleartica* (Type B) *above*
immunofluorescence, 185
lymphadenitis, 936, 940t
neartica. *See* biogroup *tularensis* (Type A) *above*
oculoglandular syndrome, 938, 940t, 2063–2064
pathogenesis, 2062–2063
pharyngeal, 2064
and pneumonia, 622t
pneumonic, 2065, 2065f
prevention, 2066–2067
serology, 192t
subsp. *holartica japonica*, 2061
subsp. *mediaasiatica*, 2061
treatment, 2066
    aminoglycosides, 285t, 286, 295t
    antimicrobials of choice, 202t
typhoidal, 2064–2065
ulceroglandular syndrome, 939, 940t, 1310, 2063, 2064f
vaccine research, 2067
Friedlander's pneumonia, 622. *See also* *Klebsiella pneumoniae*
FTA-abs test, 181, 1061, 2127t, 2128
    for neurosyphilis, 846–847
    for yaws, 2135
FTC, 437t
Fumagillin: for microsporidia, 2522
Fungal infections, 2288–2393. *See also* *specific genera and species*
    appearance in tissue, 2289t
    Aspergillus, 2306–2311
    Blastomyces dermatitidis, 2353–2365
    Blastoschizomyces capitatus, 2392
    and bone marrow transplantation, 2719–2720, 2720t
    brain abscess, 890
    burn wounds: treatment, 2764t
    Candida, 2289–2306
    and cell-mediated immune defects, 2681
    chromomycosis, 2324–2327
    Coccidioides immitis, 2365–2375
    conjunctivitis, 1104t, 1105, 1106t
    Cryptococcus neoformans, 2331–2340
    cutaneous, 550t, 2375–2386. *See also* *specific species*
    cytokine and T cell protection, 121t
    dark-walled, 2391
    dermatophytosis, 2375–2386
    Emmonsia parva var. *crescens*, 2391
    endocarditis, 757
        diagnosis, 751
        treatment, 764

endophthalmitis, 1121t, 1122–1123
    treatment, 1125
entomophthoramycosis, 2317–2319
epidemiology, 2289
and fever, 543
Fusarium, 2392
Gomori methenamine silver stain, 2289
and granulocytopenia, 2676–2677
granulomatous hepatitis, 1161
growth or biochemical characteristics, 190
Histoplasma capsulatum, 2340–2353
HIV/AIDS and. *See also* *specific species*
    pulmonary disease, 1235–1236
keratitis, 1111t, 1113
and leukemia/lymphoma, 2676–2677, 2681
Loboa loboi, 2392
Malassezia furfur, 2392
microscopy, 184
mucormycosis, 2311–2317
mycetoma, 2327–2330
mycology, 2288–2289
myocarditis, 800, 800t
osteomyelitis, 1050
otitis, 580
overview, 2288–2289
Paracoccidioides brasiliensis, 2386–2389
Penicillium marneffii, 2390–2391
pericarditis, 805, 805t
prostatitis, 1099
Pseudallescheria boydii, 2389–2390
Rhinosporidium seeberi, 2391–2392
Scedosporium prolificans, 2390
serologic tests, 193t
sexual spores, 2289
Sporothrix schenckii, 2321–2324
sporulation, 2289
sputum cultures, 173
superficial, 2375–2386
susceptibility testing, 192–193
in transplant recipients, 2712t
Trichosporon beigelii, 2392
Fungal meningitis: specimen collection, 179
Fungemia
    cultures, 178
    skin infections, 922
Funisitis, necrotizing: *Treponema pallidum*, 2126
Furazolidone, 459t, 469
    adverse reactions, 469, 2490
    dosage, 463t
        pediatric, 463t
    drug interactions, 522t
    for *Giardia lamblia*, 2490, 2490t
    hemolysis from: in G6PD deficiency, 203
Furin: gp160 and, 14
Furosemide: for sepsis, 701
Furuncles, 912, 1763
    clinical features, 912
    recurrence, 1763
    Staphylococcus aureus, 1763
    treatment, 912–913
        rifampin, 322
Fusarium, 2392
    and bone marrow transplantation, 2719
    cutaneous manifestations, 550t
    and granulocytopenia, 2676
    mycetoma, 2327, 2330
    nail infections, 2383

Fusarium solani: keratitis, 1113
Fusidic acid, 278–279, 387
    activity, 278
    adverse reactions, 279
    for antibiotic-associated colitis (AAC), 983
    clinical use, 278–279
    dosage, 279t, 514t–515t
        in children, 514t
        in renal dysfunction, 205, 515t
    mechanism of action, 278
    pharmacology, 278–279, 514t–515t
    structure, 278
    topical, 384t
Fusidium coccineum, 278, 387
Fusobacterium, 2158t
    and actinomycosis, 2280
    animal bites, 2767
    antimicrobial susceptibility, 2170t
    bacteremia, 2199
    β-lactamase, 215
    brain abscess, 2197
    characteristics, 2196t
    cholecystitis, 730
    clenched-fist injuries, 2768
    clinically significant, 2159t, 2195t
    endocarditis, 2199
    hepatic abscess, 724
    human bites, 2768
    mediastinitis, 815t
    as normal flora, 2159t, 2196
    oral colonization, 593, 594t
    osteomyelitis, 2200
    peritonitis, 711, 715
        treatment, 716
    pleuropulmonary infections, 2164, 2198
    pneumonia, 619t
    septic arthritis, 2200
    sinusitis, 585t, 2198
    soft tissue infections, 2166
    taxonomy, 2195t, 2195–2196
    treatment, 2170t, 2200
        chloramphenicol, 312t
        metronidazole, 329t
        quinolones, 368t
        tetracyclines, 308t
    virulence, 2197, 2197t
Fusobacterium necrophorum, 2195t, 2196
    endocarditis, 756, 2199
    incidence, 2163
    Lemierre's disease (postanginal septicemia), 569, 2198
    odontogenic infections, 2164, 2198
    oral and respiratory infections, 2198
    suppurative jugular thrombophlebitis, 600
    Vincent's angina, 643
Fusobacterium nucleatum, 2195t, 2196
    endocarditis, 756
    human bites, 2768
    incidence, 2162
    lung abscess, 644
    noma (gangrenous stomatitis), 602
    odontogenic infections, 2198
    penicillins for, 237t
    pleuropulmonary infections, 2198
fyn kinases, 109, 110

G

G-actin, 79, 80
Gadolinium diethylenetriamine pentaacetic acid (Gd-DTPA) MRI: for brain abscess, 893

Galactose adhesin: *Entamoeba histo-lytica*, 15–16, 16f
Galactosyl ceramide: and gp120, 15
Galactosyl cerebroside: and gp120, 15
Gal-gal receptors, 16–17
Gallbladder infections
 actinomycosis, 2284
 Candida albicans, 2298
  treatment, 2300
 Cryptosporidium, 2504
 and fever, 541
Gallium imaging
 endocarditis, 750
 and FUO, 540
 hepatic abscess, 725
 intraperitoneal abscess, 721, 722f, 723f
 osteomyelitis, 1044–1045
Gallstones
 cholangitis, 732
 cholecystitis, 731
Gammagard, 453–454
Gammaglobulin, 167, 2782. *See also* Immunoglobulin(s), thera-peutic
Gammaimmune N, 453–454
Gammar-IV, 453–454
γ-toxin: *Staphylococcus aureus*, 1759
Ganciclovir, 412t, 424–426, 1335
 adverse reactions, 421t, 423–424
 and bone marrow transplantation, 2720, 2721t
 clinical studies, 423–424
 for CMV, 424–426, 1283t, 1287–1288, 1360
 dosage, 518t–519t
  in renal insufficiency, 425t
 drug interactions, 421t, 425, 522t–523t
  immunoglobulin, 454
  zidovudine, 436
 for endophthalmitis, 1126
 for esophagitis, 964t
 mechanism of action, 424
 neutropenia from: G-CSF for, 451
 pharmacokinetics, 425
 pharmacology, 518t–519t
 resistance, 193, 423–424
 spectrum of activity, 414t, 424, 1335
 structure, 414f
 for transplant recipients, 2714
Gangrene
 bacterial synergistic, 2165
 Fournier's, 925, 1795, 2166
 gas (clostridial myonecrosis), 931–933, 2163t, 2166. *See also* Gas gangrene
 gram-negative anaerobic cutaneous. *See* Cellulitis, synergistic necrotizing
 group A streptococcal, 555
 infected vascular, 933
 infectious, 917–919, 918t
  differential diagnosis, 918–919
  in predisposed host, 918
  treatment, 918–919
 progressive bacterial synergistic, 917, 917f, 918t
 pulmonary, 643
 streptococcal, 917, 918t
  scrotal, 925
 Streptococcus pyogenes, 1794–1795
 symmetric peripheral, 551t, 553
 and systemic infections, 551t

Gangrenous cellulitis, 917–919, 918t
 clinical features, 917–918
 differential diagnosis, 918t, 918–919
 pathology and pathogenesis, 917
 in predisposed host, 918
 progressive bacterial synergistic, 917
 Pseudomonas aeruginosa, 921
 streptococcal, 917
 treatment, 918–919
Gangrenous stomatitis, 602
Gardnerella vaginalis, 2050–2051
 bacteremia, 2051
 balanitis, 1059
 clinical manifestations, 2050–2051
 cultures, 1077
 cytolytic toxin, 2050
 description, 2050
 diagnosis and identification, 2051
 differential diagnosis, 2051
 epidemiology, 2050
 history, 2050
 pathogenesis, 2050
 peritonitis, 711
 postpartum endometritis, 1091
 prevention, 2051
 resistance, 2050, 2051
 specimen collection and processing, 171t, 183
 treatment
  metronidazole, 329
  susceptibility, 2051
 urinary tract infections, 2050–2051
 vaginal flora, 1074, 1093
 vaginosis, 1077–1078, 2050
Gas gangrene (clostridial myonecrosis), 931–933, 2163t, 2166, 2186–2189
 antitoxin for, 2188
 clinical features, 931, 932f, 2187f, 2187–2188
 diagnosis, 2188
 differential diagnosis, 918t, 924t, 932, 2188
 epidemiology, 2186–2187
 etiology, 932, 2186
 history, 2186
 laboratory findings, 932
 pathogenesis and pathology, 931, 2186
 perfringolysin O (α toxin), 2186
 phospholipase C (α-toxin) and, 2186
 spontaneous nontraumatic (*C. septicum*), 931
 treatment, 932–933, 2188–2189, 2189f
 uterine, 2185, 2187
Gas sterilization, 2580–2581
Gasterophilus, 2562
Gastric acidity
 and antimicrobials, 201
 and enteric infections, 946–947
 and nosocomial pneumonia, 2601–2602
Gastric lymphoma: *Helicobacter pylori*, 1959t, 1960
Gastric ulceration: *Helicobacter pylori*, 1959t, 1960
Gastritis: CMV
 and HIV/AIDS, 1229–1230, 1359
 in the immunocompromised, 1359
Gastroenteritis. *See also* Enteritis; Gastrointestinal infections
 Plasmodium, 2420
 quinolones for, 371
 and Reiter syndrome, 1071

Salmonella
 clinical manifestations, 2020
 pathophysiology, 2019
 therapy, 2027, 2027t
Salmonella enteritidis, 2021
Salmonella typhimurium, 2019, 2020
 use of term, 945
Gastrointestinal drainage: for peritonitis, 718
Gastrointestinal endoscopy: and endo-carditis, 743t, 794t
Gastrointestinal hemorrhage: poliovirus, 1616
Gastrointestinal infections, 945–1032. *See also specific infections*
 abdominal pain and/or diarrhea with eosinophilia, syndrome of, 1005–1008
 antibody deficiencies and, 49
 Bacillus anthracis, 999t, 1002, 1888
 Brucella, 2055–2056
 CMV
  and HIV/AIDS, 1229–1230, 1359
  in the immunocompromised, 1359
 colitis. *See also* Colitis
  antibiotic-associated, 978–987
 control, 955–956
 diagnostic approach, 953–955, 954f
 diarrhea. *See also* Diarrhea
  noninflammatory, 965–973
 Entamoeba histolytica, 2400t, 2400–2401
 enteric fever, 998–1004
 enteritides: inflammatory, 987–998. *See also* Enteritides, inflam-matory
 epidemiological and environmental factors, 946
 esophagitis, 962–964. *See also* Esophagitis
 food-borne, 1012–1025
 gastric acidity and, 946–947
 histoplasmosis, 2347
 HIV/AIDS and, 1229–1230
 host factors, 946t, 946–948
 intestinal immunity and, 948
 intestinal motility and, 947
 major syndromes of deranged physi-ology, 952f, 952–953, 953t
 mesenteric adenitis, 1004–1005
 microbial factors, 948–952, 949t
  attachment, 951
  invasiveness, 951–952
  other virulence factors, 952
  toxins, 948–951, 949t
 mucormycosis, 2315
 Mycobacterium avium-intracellulare: and HIV/AIDS, 2256
 Mycobacterium tuberculosis, 2238
 nausea/vomiting, 965–973. *See also* Nausea/vomiting
 normal enteric microflora and, 947–948
 occurrence and scope, 945
 personal hygiene and, 946
 prevention, 955–956
 principles and syndromes, 945–962
 Pseudomonas aeruginosa, 1995
  treatment, 1995
 in transplant recipients, 2727–2728
 treatment, 955–956
  quinolones, 371–372
  trimethoprim, 360
 tropical sprue, 1025–1030
 Whipple's disease, 1030–1032

Gastrointestinal neoplasia
 Helicobacter pylori and, 1959t, 1960
 Kaposi's sarcoma, 1241–1242
Gastrointestinal reactions: to peritonitis, 713
Gastrointestinal toxicity
 cephalosporins, 254
 nitrofurantoin, 378
 penicillins, 239t, 240
 quinolones, 374
 tetracyclines, 310
 vidarabine, 433
Gastrospirillum hominis, 1962
Gaucher's disease: and osteomyelitis, 1049
Gel diffusion test: for endocarditis, 750
Gelsolin, 80
Gemella, 2158t
Gemella haemolysans: endocarditis, 754
Gemella morbillorum, 1846t, 1847t, 2204
 biochemical characteristics, 1847t
Genes
 bacterial, 1753
 libraries, 25–26
 virulence: identification and charac-terization, 25–26
Genetics
 and autoimmune hepatitis, 1157
 clonal nature of pathogens, 21
 disorders
  antimicrobial therapy issues in, 203
  fever and, 546
 and HIV, 1170
 poliovirus, 1617
Genital anatomy
 female, 1092f
  examination, 1082–1083
 male, 1098, 1098f
Genitalia: normal flora, 2159, 2159t
Genital lesions, 1055–1063. *See also* Genitourinary tract infections
 age and, 1055–1056
 antigen and genome detection, 1060
 bartonellosis, 2211f, 2211–2212, 2212f
 condylomata acuminata, 1388t, 1389, 1392f, 1392–1393, 1393f
 crusts, 1057t, 1059
 cultures, 1061
 differential diagnosis, 1395, 2211
 diffuse erythema, 1057t, 1059
 direct microscopic examination, 1060
 fever and, 1057
 from foscarnet, 423
 Haemophilus ducreyi (chancroid), 940, 2047–2048
 herpes simplex virus, 1338f, 1338–1339
  and HIV transmission, 1188
 lymphadenitis, 940t
 number of lesions, 1057
 recurrence, 1056, 1337, 1339–1340
 treatment, 412t
  acyclovir, 415–416, 1342
  interferons, 429
 herpesviruses, 1334t
 history taking, 1055–1057
 and HIV transmission, 1168, 1188–1189
 incubation period, 1056
 laboratory examinations, 1060–1061
 morphology, 1057t, 1057–1059
 pain, 1056
 papules, 1057t, 1058–1059

pruritus, 1056
pubic hair, 1059
serology, 1060–1061
sexual history and, 1056
travel and, 1056
ulcers, 1057t, 1057–1058, 1058f
vaginal discharge and, 1057
verrucous, 1059
vesicles and bullae, 1057, 1057t
Genitourinary tract
barrier to microorganisms, 32
female, 1092f
examination, 1082–1083
male, 1098
host defenses, 1098
Genitourinary tract infections. *See also*
Sexually transmitted diseases;
Urinary tract infections
actinomycosis, 2284
anaerobic gram-negative bacilli, 2199
treatment, 2201
Blastomyces dermatitidis, 2356t, 2360
Brucella, 2056
chlamydial, 1685. *See also Chlamydia
trachomatis*
Entamoeba histolytica, 2401
HIV/AIDS and, 1188, 1227–1228
Mycoplasmas, 1713t, 1713–1717
Neisseria gonorrhoeae, 1915–1916
female, 1915–1916
male, 1915, 1915f
Salmonella, 2023
specimen collection and processing,
171t, 181–183
Streptococcus agalactiae, 1840
tuberculosis, 2237t, 2237–2238
in AIDS, 2238
female, 2238
male, 2238
venereal. *See* Sexually transmitted
diseases
Genome detection: genital lesions, 1060
Gen-Probe system, 184–185
Gentamicin, 280
antimicrobial activity, 285t, 286, 296
for cellulitis, 916
clinical trials, 228
combination therapy, 287t
antagonism, 208
synergism, 207
for cystic fibrosis infections, 660
dosage, 297t, 510t–511t
in children and neonates, 299t,
510t, 851t
in cystic fibrosis, 299
once daily, 299t
in renal dysfunction, 298, 298t,
511t
for endocarditis
culture-negative, 764
Enterobacteriaceae, 763
prosthetic valve, 786, 786t, 787
staphylococcal, 760, 762
streptococcal, 759, 760
for enterococcal infections, 1831,
1831t
for *Francisella tularensis*, 2066
for *Gardnerella vaginalis*, 2051
for intra-abdominal infections,
288–289
for keratitis, 1117
for meningitis, 850t, 851t, 853
for necrotizing pneumonia, 646
for *Neisseria gonorrhoeae*, 1922,
1922t

nephrotoxicity, 293
neuromuscular blockade, 295
ototoxicity, 294
for peritonitis: in peritoneal dialysis,
720t
pharmacology, 510t–511t
for PID, 1096t
for Pseudomonads, 2004t
for *Pseudomonas aeruginosa*,
1991–1992
resistance, 220, 284, 284t
coagulase-negative staphylococci,
1778
enterococci, 1831
for sepsis syndrome, 699, 699t
prophylaxis, 702
source and chemistry, 280t
structure, 281f
for suppurative thrombophlebitis, 768
susceptibility testing, 194, 194t
topical, 384t
in vitro trials, 228
Gentian violet: for candidiasis
thrush, 2301
vulvovaginal, 1076
German measles, 1459–1465. *See also*
Rubella virus
Gerstmann-Straussler-Scheinker syndrome, 881, 883, 1674
clinical manifestations, 883
diagnosis, 883
specimen handling, 884
Getah virus, 1457
Giant cell arteritis: and fever, 546
Giant roundworm. *See Ascaris lumbricoides*
Giardia lamblia, 2394t, 2487–2493
animal reservoirs, 2792t
antibody deficiencies and, 49
axonemes, 2487
clinical manifestations, 2394t, 2489,
2489t
cyst, 2487, 2488f
description, 2487, 2488f
diagnosis, 955, 2489–2490
diarrhea, 2488, 2489, 2489t
in AIDS, 970, 970t
chronic, 972
in day care centers, 971
differential diagnosis: *Entamoeba histolytica*, 2402
dysentery, 987, 994
EIA diagnosis, 185
epidemiology, 2487–2488
food-borne, 1012
immune response, 2488–2489
and immunodeficiency, 150t
life cycle, 2487
pathogenesis, 2488–2489
prevention, 2490–2491
specimen collection, 180
transmission, 2394t
traveler precautions, 2491
treatment, 463t, 2490, 2490t
albendazole, 479
furazolidone, 469
metronidazole, 330t, 458
quinacrine, 469
trophozoite, 2487, 2488f
venereal transmission, 2487, 2491
waterborne, 1015, 1016t, 2487, 2794
Giemsa stain, 184t
Gilbert syndrome: hepatic involvement,
1149
Gingival crevice

bacterial colonization, 593, 594t
viridans streptococci on, 1846
Gingivitis
acute necrotizing ulcerative (Vincent's
disease)
anaerobic gram-negative bacilli
and, 2198
clinical presentation, 596, 598
specimen collection, 172
anaerobic gram-negative bacilli, 2196,
2198
clinical presentation, 596, 598
defective chemotaxis in, 90
HIV/AIDS and, 1227
and lung abscess, 642
microbiology, 594
neutrophil defect and, 153
Gingivostomatitis
herpesviruses, 1334t
and leukemia, 2678
Glanders, 2006–2007. *See also
Pseudomonas mallei*
Glaucoma
acute angle closure: conjunctivitis vs.,
1106t
surgery: endophthalmitis after, 1121
Glaucomys volans: and *Rickettsia
prowazekii*, 1735
Glomerulonephritis
and endocarditis, 746, 749
hepatitis and, 1139
membranoproliferative: and endocarditis, 746
membranous: hepatitis B virus and,
1420
streptococcal, 1786, 1805–1808
clinical features, 1807
diagnosis, 1807–1808
differential diagnosis, 1807
epidemiology, 1806t, 1806–1807
etiology, 1806
history, 1805–1806
laboratory findings, 1807
pathology, 1806
prevention, 1808
prognosis, 1808
therapy, 1808
Glossina: and African trypanosomiasis,
2450, 2452
Gloves: and isolation, 2577t
Glucagon: for septic shock, 701
Glucocorticoids
rifampin and, 320
for *Salmonella*, 2026
therapeutic, 455
Glucose-6-phosphate dehydrogenase
(G6PD) deficiency
drug-induced hemolysis and, 203
chloramphenicol, 314
dapsone, 397
melarsoprol, 476
nitrofurantoin, 378
primaquine, 471
quinine, 471
and hepatitis, 1139
neutrophil dysfunction, 93
β-Glucuronidase, 79t
Glutathione peroxidase, 84
Glycolytic pathway: and neutrophil
degranulation, 85
Glycoproteins, 34
viral adherence, 13
Gnathostoma spinigerum, 2553t
cutaneous larva migrans, 2555
eosinophilic meningitis, 2556

treatment, 463t
Goats: microorganisms harbored by,
2792t
Gomori's methenamine silver stain, 184t
Gonococcal infections, 1909–1926. *See
also Neisseria gonorrhoeae*
Gonococcemia, 1917–1919. *See also
Neisseria gonorrhoeae*
skin lesions, 921
Gonorrhea, 1909–1926. *See also
Neisseria gonorrhoeae*
Gonyaulax catenella, 1014
Gonyaulax tamarensis, 1014
*Gordona bronchialis. See Rhodococcus
bronchialis*
Gowns: and isolation, 2577t
gp39 (CD40 ligand), 47
gp41, 14
HIV, 1204t, 1594t, 1595, 1597, 1599,
1600f
gp91*phox*, 84, 85
and chronic granulomatous disease,
92, 92t
gp120: HIV, 14–15, 15f, 1204, 1204t,
1207, 1208, 1594t,
1594–1595, 1596, 1599
and vaccine research, 1294, 1295f,
1296, 1297t, 1298–1299,
1300t
gp 130, 532
biologic properties, 535t
gp160: HIV, 14–15, 15f
and vaccine research, 1297, 1297t,
1299, 1300, 1300t
G proteins: pertussis toxin and, 6
Gradient of infection, 164
Graft-vs.-host disease
bone marrow transplantation and,
2674, 2717, 2718, 2720–2721
immunodeficiency and, 150
Gram-negative anaerobes. *See also individual species*
bacilli, 2195–2204
treatment, 2200–2201
antibiotic, 2200t, 2200–2201
hyperbaric oxygen, 2200
rifampin, 323–324
surgical, 2200
Gram-negative bacilli, 1934–2117. *See
also individual species*
Achromobacter, 2110–2111
Acinetobacter, 2009–2013
Actinobacillus, 2106–2107
Aeromonas, 2107–2108
Agrobacterium, 2111
Alcaligenes, 2111–2112
xylosoxidans subsp. *xylosoxidans*,
2111
anaerobic, 2195–2204
Bordetella, 2078–2084
Brucella, 2053–2060
Campylobacter, 1948–1956
Capnocytophaga, 2103–2106
Cardiobacterium, 2108–2109
CDC group DF-3, 2109–2110
CDC group EF-4, 2110
CDC group IVc-2, 2112
Chromobacterium, 2109
Eikenella, 2112
endocarditis, 755–756
Enterobacteriaceae, 1964–1980
Citrobacter, 1974
Edwardsiella, 1974
Enterobacter, 1973
Erwinia, 1975

Gram-negative bacilli (Continued)
   Escherichia coli, 1969–1972
   Hafnia, 1973
   Klebsiella, 1972–1973
   Klebsielleae, 1972–1973
   miscellaneous, 1975t
   Proteae, 1973–1974
   Proteus, 1974
   Serratia marcescens, 1973
   Flavimonas (CDC group Ve-2), 2112–2113
   Flavobacterium, 2113
   Francisella tularensis, 2060–2068
   Gardnerella vaginalis, 2050–2051
   glucose fermenters, 2106–2110
   glucose nonfermenters, 2110–2115
   growth or biochemical characteristics, 186, 188f
   Haemophilus, 2045–2050
     influenzae, 2039–2045
   Helicobacter pylori, 1956–1964
   Legionella, 2097–2103
     pneumophila, 2087–2097
   Mobiluncus, 2051–2052
   new CDC groups, 2114–2115
   Ochrobactrum, 2113–2114
   Oligella, 2113
   Pasteurella, 2068–2070
   Plesiomonas shigelloides, 2110
   Protomonas, 2114
   Pseudomonas, 2003–2009
     aeruginosa, 1980–2003
     cepacia, 2007–2008
     mallei, 2006–2007
     pseudomallei, 2004–2006
   Salmonella, 2013–2033
   Shigella, 2033–2039
   Sphingobacterium, 2114
   Streptobacillus moniliformis, 2084–2086
   treatment
     antimicrobials of choice, 202t
     penicillins, 241t
   Vibrio, 1934–1948
     cholerae, 1934–1945
     parahaemolyticus, 1945–1946
   Weeksella, 2114
   Yersinia, 2070–2078
     enterocolitica, 2076–2078
     pestis, 2070–2076
     pesudotuberculosis, 2076–2078
Gram-negative bacteria. See also individual species
   bacilli, 1934–2117. See also Gram-negative bacilli
   β-lactamases, 215, 215t, 250–251
   characteristics, 1753
   chloramphenicol for, 312t
   cocci, 1896–1934. See also Gram-negative cocci
   and complement, 66
   identification scheme, 188f
   resistance
     aminoglycosides, 284, 284t
     to cephalosporins, 250–251
   susceptibility testing, 200
   treatment
     aminoglycosides, 285t
     quinolones, 367t
     tetracyclines, 308t
Gram-negative cell walls, 1753, 1753f
Gram-negative cocci, 1896–1934. See also individual species
   growth or biochemical characteristics, 186, 188f

Moraxella, 1926–1928
Neisseria, 1928–1930, 1929t
   gonorrhoeae, 1909–1926
   meningitidis, 1896–1909
   treatment
     antimicrobials of choice, 202t
     penicillins, 241t
Gram-positive bacilli, 1865–1896. See also individual species
   Bacillus, 1890–1894
     anthracis, 1885–1889
   Corynebacterium, 1872–1876
     diphtheriae, 1865–1872
   endocarditis, 756
   Erysipelothrix rhusiopathiae, 1894–1896
   growth or biochemical characteristics, 186, 189
   Listeria monocytogenes, 1880–1885
   penicillins for, 241t
   Rhodococcus, 1876–1877
Gram-positive bacteria. See also individual species
   bacilli, 1865–1896. See also Gram-positive bacilli
   β-lactamases, 215, 251
   characteristics, 1752–1753
   chloramphenicol for, 312t
   cocci, 1754–1865. See also Gram-positive cocci
   identification scheme, 187f
   resistance: to β-lactams, 220
   treatment
     aminoglycosides, 285t
     quinolones, 368t
     tetracyclines, 308t
Gram-positive cell walls, 1753, 1753f
Gram-positive cocci, 1754–1865. See also individual species
   enterococci, 1826–1831
   growth or biochemical characteristics, 186
   Leuconostoc, 1832
   staphylococci
     S. aureus, 1754–1777
     S. epidermidis and other coagulase-organisms, 1777–1784
   streptococci
     classification, 1784–1785
     glomerulonephritis, 1805–1808
     group A. See Streptococcus pyogenes
     group C, 1852–1856
     group G, 1853–1856
     intermedius group, 1861–1865
     rheumatic fever, 1799–1805
     S. agalactiae (group B), 1835–1845
     S. bovis, 1832
     S. pneumoniae, 1811–1826
     S. pyogenes, 1786–1799
     viridans, 1845–1851
   treatment
     antimicrobials of choice, 202t
     penicillins, 241t
Gram stain, 184, 184t
   of anaerobes, 2168
   and choice of anti-infective therapy, 200
   in classification of bacteria, 1752–1753
Granulocyte colony-stimulating factor (G-CSF), 79, 113
   actions, 30t, 34
   characteristics, sources, and effects, 115, 115t, 116, 123

and hematopoiesis, 118
receptor, 113
recombinant, 450–451
   and bone marrow transplantation, 2719
   for burn wounds, 2763
   for immunocompromised host, 2693t, 2693–2694
   for neutropenia, 89
   for sepsis, 701
   therapeutic use, 450–451. See also recombinant above
     adverse reactions, 451
     dosage, 451
Granulocyte-macrophage colony-stimulating factor (GM-CSF), 79, 82, 113
   actions, 30t, 34
   characteristics, sources, and effects, 115, 115t, 123
   and eosinophils, 95
   and hematopoiesis, 118
   HIV and, 1212
   and IgE Fc receptors, 40
   NK cells and, 122
   receptor, 113
   recombinant, 451–452
     for bone marrow transplantation, 2717, 2719, 2721t
     for immunocompromised host, 2693t, 2693–2694
     for neutropenia, 89, 450–451
     for sepsis, 701
   and sepsis, 694t
   therapeutic use, 451–452. See also recombinant above
     adverse reactions, 451–452
     dosage, 451
Granulocytes: transfusions, 94–95
   for neutrophil defects, 94–95
   for sepsis syndrome, 701, 702–703
   prophylactic, 702
Granulocytic phagocytes, 78–101
   chemotactic defects, 90–95
   eosinophils, 95–96
   leukocyte adhesion deficiency syndromes, 89–90
   neutropenia, 88–89
   neutrophils, 79–88. See also Neutrophils
Granulocytopenia
   bacterial infections and, 2676, 2676t
   empiric therapy of infections, 2687–2688
   fungal infections and, 2676–2677
   and infections in patients with neoplasia, 2666t, 2666–2668, 2667f, 2667t, 2668f, 2675–2681
     characteristics, 2677t, 2677–2679
     therapy, 2679–2681
   oropharyngeal infections and, 2678
   parasitic infections and, 2677
   protozoal infections and, 2677
   pulmonary infections and, 2678–2679
   septicemia, 2677–2678
   skin and soft tissue infections and, 2679
   viral infections and, 2677
   from zidovudine, 436
Granulocytosis, 80
Granuloma inguinale, 2210–2213. See also Calymmatobacterium granulomatosis

Granuloma of the pudenda, ulcerating. See Calymmatobacterium granulomatosis
Granuloma pudendi tropicum. See Calymmatobacterium granulomatosis
Granuloma pyogenicum, 1130
Granulomas
   actinomycotic, 2284–2285
   Francisella tularensis, 2063
   schistosomiasis, 2540, 2541
Granulomatosis
   infantiseptica: Listeria monocytogenes, 1161, 1882, 1882t, 1883, 1883t, 1884t
   talc: in drug abusers, 2701
Granulomatous angiitis: meningoencephalitis, 871
Granulomatous corynebacterial lymphadenitis, 938
Granulomatous disease, chronic (CGD), 92–93, 151t, 155
   Aspergillus and, 2308
   of childhood: rifampin for, 323
Granulomatous disease, chronic (GCD)
   antibiotic prophylaxis in, 93
   autosomal recessive, 151t
   carriers, 93
   diagnosis, 93, 155
   interferon-γ for, 453
   management, 93
   and Salmonella, 2019
   Staphylococcus aureus and, 1762
   transfusion-related complications, 95
   X-linked, 151t
Granulomatous diseases. See also specific diseases
   and fever, 545–546
Granulomatous hepatitis, 1159–1164
   diagnosis, 1163
   diseases characterized by, 1160–1162
   fever and, 545, 1162
   infectious diseases and, 1160–1162, 1161t
   noninfectious diseases and, 1162, 1162t
   pathophysiology, 1160, 1160f
   syphilitic, 1161–1162, 2123, 2126
   treatment, 1163
   tuberculosis, 2238
Granulomatous lymphangitis: chronic, 943
Granulomatous prostatitis, 1100
Granuloma venereum. See Calymmatobacterium granulomatosis
Gray baby syndrome: from chloramphenicol, 314
Great Pox. See Treponema pallidum
Green foot: Pseudomonas aeruginosa, 1997
Green nail syndrome: Pseudomonas aeruginosa, 1997
Grille, 2379
Griseofulvin, 404
   drug interactions, 522t
   for onychomycosis, 404
   pharmacology, 518t–519t
   for ringworm, 404
   side effects, 2382
   structure, 402f
Groin
   lesions. See Genital lesions
   vascular graft infections, 789, 789t

Guanarito virus, 1572
　characteristics, 1573t
　epidemiology, 1574
　prevention and treatment, 1577
Guanosine: structure, 430f
Guillain-Barré syndrome
　and *Campylobacter*, 162, 879, 1014,
　　　1952, 1954
　and CMV, 1357
　coxsackieviruses and, 1623
　differential diagnosis
　　botulism, 2181
　　poliovirus, 1617
　and HIV/AIDS, 1236
　influenza virus and, 1558
　Miller Fisher variant, 2181
　neuritis, 878, 879
Guinea worm, 2533. *See also Dracun-*
　　　culus medinensis
Gummatous syphilis, 2125–2126
　hepatic, 1161, 2125–2126
Gut-associated lymphoid tissue (GALT),
　　　948
Gymnodinium breve, 1015
Gynecologic infections. *See also* Female
　　　genital tract infections; Geni-
　　　tourinary tract infections
　anaerobic, 2163t
Gynecologic surgery
　and endocarditis, 743t
　female pelvic infections after,
　　　1093–1095
　　cuff abscess, 1094
　　cuff cellulitis, 1094
　　osteomyelitis pubis, 1095
　　pathogens, 1093t, 1093–1094
　　pelvic abscess, 1094–1095
　　pelvic cellulitis, 1094
　　risk factors, 1094
　　septic pelvic thrombophlebitis,
　　　1095
　prophylaxis recommendations, 2751t
Gyromitra, 1015, 1015t

H

Haber-Weiss reaction, 87
HACEK organisms, 2106, 2107,
　　　2108–2109, 2112. *See also*
　　　individual species
　biochemical reactions, 2107t
　and fever, 541
Haemagogus
　and arboviruses, 1457
　and yellow fever, 1467
Haemaphysalis: and flaviviruses, 1466t
Haemophilus, 2039–2050
　influenzae, 2039–2045
　spp. other than *influenzae*,
　　　2045–2050
　　clinical manifestations, 2046–2047
　　description, 2046, 2046t
　　endocarditis, 2046–2047
　　　treatment, 2047
　　epidemiology and pathogenesis,
　　　2046
　　prevention and treatment, 2047
Haemophilus aegyptius, 2046
　conjunctivitis, 2043–2044
　endocarditis, 755
Haemophilus aphrophilus, 2046
　biochemical reactions, 2107t
　clinical manifestations, 2046
　description, 2046
　differential characteristics, 2046t

endocarditis, 755, 2046–2047
epidemiology and pathogenesis,
　　　2046
Haemophilus b vaccine, 2775–2776
Haemophilus ducreyi, 2046
　buboes, 939, 2047
　clinical manifestations, 2047–2048
　cultures, 1061
　description, 2046
　diagnosis, 1060, 2048
　differential diagnosis, 1395, 2046t,
　　　2048, 2122, 2211
　in drug abusers, 2705
　epidemiology, 1056
　identification, 186
　lymphadenitis, 940t
　lymphadenopathy, 1684, 2047–2048
　prevention, 2048
　resistance, 2048
　treatment, 2048
　　erythromycin, 338t, 2048
　　rifampin, 323
　ulcers, 1057, 2047
Haemophilus felis: animal bites, 2766
Haemophilus haemolyticus, 2046
　description, 2046
　differential characteristics, 2046t
Haemophilus influenzae, 2039–2045
　antibody deficiencies and, 49
　arthritis, 1034, 1034t, 2042
　bacteremia, 2042
　　in the elderly, 2739
　　and skin infections, 921–922
　β-lactamase, 198, 216t
　biogroup *aegyptius*, 2046. *See also*
　　　Haemophilus aegyptius
　brain abscess, 889
　carriage, 2039t, 2039–2040
　and C3 deficiency, 69
　and cell-mediated immune defects,
　　　2681
　cellulitis, 921–922, 2042
　chemoprophylaxis, 167
　and chronic bronchitis, 610
　clones, 21, 21t
　colonization, 2039
　and complement, 66
　　activation, 41
　　deficiency, 2041
　conjunctivitis, 1104–1105, 2043–2044
　　neonatal, 1107
　CSF specimens, 179
　and cystic fibrosis, 658, 659
　dacryocystitis, 1131
　description, 2039
　dexamethasone for, 131
　endocarditis, 755
　　treatment, 763
　epidemiology, 2039t, 2039–2040
　epiglottitis, 591, 592, 2040,
　　　2041–2042
　　isolation, 2576
　E-test, 195
　fimbriae, 838
　growth, 186
　and HIV/AIDS, 53–54
　　pneumonia, 621, 629, 1235, 1235t
　　prophylaxis, 1286t
　identification, 186
　and IgA, 8, 20
　immunity and, 2040–2041
　and immunodeficiency, 150t
　Job syndrome and, 156
　LPS, 839–840, 840
　maternal sepsis, 2043

meningitis, 833t, 833–834, 834t,
　　　2040, 2041
　antimicrobial therapy, 850t, 851,
　　　853, 854, 855–856
　bacteremia, 838
　blood-brain barrier alteration, 839
　chemoprophylaxis, 856–857
　clinical presentation, 843
　CSF examination, 845–846, 846t
　immunoprophylaxis, 858, 858t
　rifampin, 320–321, 324
　subarachnoid space inflammation,
　　　840–841
　mucosal colonization, 837–838
　and multiple myeloma, 2669, 2673
　nasopharyngeal cultures, 169
　natural antibodies, 31
　neonatal sepsis, 2043
　nontypeable diseases, 2043–2044
　　diagnosis and treatment, 2044
　orbital cellulitis, 1132
　　treatment, 1134
　osteomyelitis, 1041
　otitis media, 581, 581t, 582, 2043
　pathogenesis, 2039t, 2039–2040
　pericarditis, 805
　and phagocytes, 88
　pleural empyema, 637
　pneumonia, 619t, 2042, 2043
　　community-acquired, 629
　　in the elderly, 2738
　　and HIV/AIDS, 621, 629, 1235,
　　　1235t
　　and influenza virus, 1556t, 1557,
　　　1557t
　　nontypeable, 2043
　　radiology, 626
　　serology, 625
　　spinal cord injury and, 2733
　　sputum analysis, 623, 623f
　　in trauma patients, 2757
　　treatment, 632
　　type b, 2042
　polymorphonuclear leukocytes and,
　　　2041
　polyribosyl-ribitol capsular polysac-
　　　charide (PRP), 2040, 2041
　polysaccharide, 165
　polysaccharide vaccine: epiglottitis
　　　prevention, 592
　resistance, 194–195, 201, 220, 851,
　　　2042–2043
　sickle cell anemia and, 53
　sinusitis, 585, 585t, 2043
　skin lesions, 921–922
　splenectomy and, 2669
　subdural empyema, 900
　surveillance, 162
　tracheitis, 578
　treatment, 2042–2043
　　aminoglycosides, 285t, 286
　　aminopenicillins, 243
　　amoxicillin-clavulanate, 269
　　antimicrobials of choice, 202t
　　azithromycin, 335t, 339, 340
　　β-lactamase inhibitors, 268t
　　carbapenems, 264t
　　cephalosporins, 255t, 257, 258, 259
　　chloramphenicol, 312, 312t
　　clarithromycin, 335t, 340
　　erythromycin, 335t, 338
　　mezlocillin, 245
　　neomycin, 384
　　penicillins, 237t
　　piperacillin, 245

quinolones, 367t, 370
rifampin, 318t, 320–321
sulfonamides, 355t
tetracyclines, 307, 308t
trimethoprim, 357
type B strain, 165, 2039t, 2039–2040
　diagnosis and treatment,
　　　2042–2043
　diseases, 2040, 2041–2042
　immunity, 2040–2041
　vaccine, 2044, 2044t, 2775–2776
　　adverse reactions, 2776
　　HbOC, 858, 858t, 2044t, 2775,
　　　2776
　　indications for adults, 2784t
　　for meningitis, 858, 858t
　　morbidity reduction, 2772t
　　PRP-D, 2044t, 2775
　　PRP-OMPC, 858, 858t, 2044t,
　　　2775
　　PRP-T, 2044t, 2775
　　splenectomy and, 53
　　type B toxoid conjugate: antibody
　　　response, 50
　V factor, 2039
　virulence, 20
　Wiskott-Aldrich syndrome and, 52
　X factor, 2039
Haemophilus parainfluenzae, 2046
　clinical manifestations, 2046–2047
　description, 2046
　differential characteristics, 2046t
　endocarditis, 755, 2046–2047
　epidemiology and pathogenesis, 2046
　human bites, 2768
　identification, 186
　treatment: aminopenicillins, 243
Haemophilus paraphrophilus, 2046
　clinical manifestations, 2046, 2047
　description, 2046
　differential characteristics, 2046t
　endocarditis, 755
　epidemiology and pathogenesis, 2046
　identification, 186
Haemophilus pertussis. See Bordetella
　　　pertussis
Haemophilus segnis, 2046
Haemophilus test medium (HTM), 2047
Haemophilus vaginalis. See Gardnerella
　　　vaginalis
Hafnia, 1973
Hafnia alvei, 1975t
Hageman factor. *See* Factor XII
Hairy cell leukemia
　cellular immunodeficiency and, 137
　infections and, 2673
　infection susceptibility and, 137
Halofantrine, 459t, 472–473
　dosage, 473
　for *Plasmodium*, 2425
Haloprogin: topical, 401t
Halothane
　and fever, 547
　hepatotoxicity, 1148
Hand-foot-and-mouth disease, 1623,
　　　1624, 1631–1632
　differential diagnosis, 1624
Hand surgery: prophylaxis recommenda-
　　　tions, 2752t
Handwashing: and isolation, 2577t
Hansen's disease, 2243–2250. *See also*
　　　Mycobacterium leprae
Hantaan virus, 1567
　animal reservoirs, 2793
　characteristics, 1568t

Hantaan virus *(Continued)*
clinical manifestations, 1570
serology, 191
treatment: ribavirin, 431
Hantaviruses, 1567
animal reservoirs, 2793, 2794
characteristics, 1568t
clinical manifestations, 1570
epidemiology, 1569
pneumonia, 622t
transmission to humans, 1569
Hantavirus pulmonary syndrome (HPS)
characteristics, 1568t
clinical manifestations, 1570
epidemiology, 1569
prevention and treatment, 1571
Haptoglobin, 34
and acute phase response, 117
and FUO, 539
Hartmanella. See Acanthamoeba
Harvest mite, 2564
HAV. *See* Hepatitis A virus
Haverhill fever, 2085
Hawaii virus, 1667, 1668
characteristics, 1668t
diagnosis, 1670–1671
pathogenesis, 1669, 1669f
winter vomiting disease, 968
HBV. *See* Hepatitis B virus
HCV. *See* Hepatitis C virus
HCV Sapporo agent: characteristics,
1668t
HCV UK 1–4 agent: characteristics,
1668t
Headache
Coxiella burnetii, 1731–1732
ehrlichiosis, 1749t
Head infections, 604. *See also* Orofacial
infections
actinomycosis, 2281
anaerobic, 2163t, 2164
specimen collection, 2168t
mediastinitis and, 814
bacteriology, 815t
postsurgical wounds, 604
Head irradiation, 604
Head surgery: prophylaxis recommendations, 2751t
Head trauma
and brain abscess, 888, 888t
sepsis, 2759
Health care workers
CMV in, 2661, 2662
EBV in, 2663
hepatitis in, 2621–2623, 2622f
HAV, 2618
HBV, 1423, 2617, 2618
prevention, 1431–1432, 2784
HCV, 2618
HDV, 2618
HIV/AIDS in, 2633–2634,
2633–2639, 2634t
case reports, 2634
ethical, legal, and policy issues in
management, 2649–2650
management of adverse exposures,
2643–2647, 2644t–2645t
postexposure antiretroviral chemoprophylaxis, 2646
prospective/longitudinal studies of
incidence, 2636t, 2636–2637,
2637t
right to refuse care, 2648
risk factors, 2637, 2637t
serologic surveillance, 2647

seropositivity, 2634–2638
studies in prevalence, 2634–2636,
2635t
HSV in, 2656–2657
Mycobacterium tuberculosis in,
2217–2218
protection in handling traumatized
patient, 2759–2760
VZV in, 2660
Hearing loss: CMV infection and, 1357
Heart
cardiovascular infections. *See*
Cardiovascular infections
congenital disease
and brain abscess, 888t, 889
and infective endocarditis, 741
degenerative lesions: and endocarditis,
741
endocarditis. *See also* Endocarditis,
infective
pathologic changes, 746
myocarditis. *See* Myocarditis
Heart block: *Borrelia burgdorferi*, 2148
Heart failure
and endocarditis, 755
surgical therapy, 765
Neisseria meningitidis and, 1901
and pneumonia, 621
Heart-lung transplantation
aspergillosis and, 2306
CMV in, 2710t
for cystic fibrosis, 660
infections and, 2722, 2724t, 2725
Heart murmurs: in endocarditis, 747–748,
748t
Heart transplantation
bacteremia and, 2727
CMV in, 2710t
HSV infections, 1340
infections and, 2722, 2722f, 2724,
2724t
for *Trypanosoma cruzi*, 2446
Heart valve replacement: for endocarditis,
765
prosthetic valve infections, 787, 787t
Heat exhaustion: travel and, 2800
Heat-shock protein, 102
Heat sterilization, 2579–2580, 2580f
Heavy chains
antigen-binding diversity, 43–44, 44f
immunoglobulin, 37, 43–44, 44f
Heavy metal poisoning
diarrhea, 972
food-borne, 1012t
laboratory diagnosis, 1018t, 1019
management, 1020
Heck, focal epithelial neoplasia of,
1388t, 1393. *See also* Human
papillomavirus
Heine-Medin disease. *See* Poliovirus
*Helicobacter. See also individual
species*
microbiology, 1956–1957
Helicobacter acinonyx, 1956
Helicobacter cinaedi, 1948, 1956
characteristics, 1949t
clinical manifestations, 1952
growth, 1949t
stool culture, 955
therapy, 1954
Helicobacter felis: biochemical characteristics, 1957t
Helicobacter fennelliae, 1948, 1956
characteristics, 1949t
clinical manifestations, 1952

growth, 1949t
stool culture, 955
Helicobacter heilmanii, 1962
Helicobacter mustelae, 1956
biochemical characteristics, 1957t
Helicobacter nemestrinae, 1956
Helicobacter pylori, 1956–1964
acute infection, 1959
adherence, 2
biochemical characteristics, 1957t
chronic infection, 1959
clinical features, 1959t, 1959–1960
cytotoxicity, 951
diagnosis, 1960, 1961t
duodenal ulceration, 1959t, 1959–1960
epidemiology, 1957
gastric acidity and, 947
gastric carcinoma, 1959t, 1960
gastric lymphoma, 1959t, 1960
gastric ulceration, 1959t, 1960
microbiology, 1956–1957
natural history of infection, 1959f
pathology and pathogenesis,
1957–1959
seroprevalence, 1958f
toxin, 6
treatment, 1960–1961
azithromycin, 335t
clarithromycin, 335t
erythromycin, 335t
metronidazole, 329
quinolones, 371
and tropical sprue, 1026
upper GI lesions, 1959, 1959t
virulence factors, 2
Heligmosomoides polygyris: cellular
immunity and, 127
Helminths, 2525–2557. *See also
individual species*
Angiostrongylus costaricensis, 2556
Anisakis, 2554–2555
antiparasitic agents, 460t
approach to patient, 2526
biology, 2525
Capillaria philippinensis, 2556–2557
cellular immunity and, 127
cestodes (tapeworms), 2525t,
2544–2553, 2545t. *See also*
Cestodes
intestinal, 2546–2548
Diphyllobothrium latum (fish
tapeworm), 2546–2547
Dipylidium caninum (dog/cat
tapeworm), 2547
Hymenolepis diminuta (rat tapeworm), 2547
Hymenolepis nana (dwarf tapeworm), 2547
Taenia saginata (beef tapeworm),
2547
Taenia solium (pork tapeworm),
2547
invasive, 2548–2551
Echinococcus (hydatid and
alveolar cyst disease),
2550–2551
Taenia solium, 2548–2550
classification, 2525t
cutaneous larva migrans (creeping
eruption), 2555
Dirofilaria, 2556
eosinophilia and, 96, 2553
eosinophilic meningitis
(*Angiostrongylus cantonensis*), 2555–2556

epidemiology, 2526
flukes. See trematodes *below*
host-parasite relationship, 2526
IgE and, 39
meningitis
antimicrobial therapy, 850t, 854
clinical presentation, 844
diagnosis, 849
nematodes, 2525t. *See also*
Nematodes
intestinal (roundworms),
2526–2531, 2527t
Ascaris lumbricoides,
2528–2529
Enterobius vermicularis, 2528
hookworm (*Ancylostoma duodenale*; *Necator americanus*),
2529–2530
Strongyloides stercoralis,
2530–2531
Trichuris trichiura, 2526–2528
tissue, 2531–2537
Brugia malayi, 2533–2535, 2536
Brugia timori, 2533–2535
Dracunculus medinensis, 2533
Loa loa, 2535
Mansonella, 2536
Onchocerca volvulus, 2535–2536
Trichinella spiralis, 2531–2533
tropical pulmonary eosinophilia,
2536
Wuchereria bancrofti,
2533–2535, 2536
ocular larva migrans (*Toxocara canis*),
2554
overview, 2525–2526
Phocanema, 2554–2555
trematodes (flukes), 2525t, 2538t,
2538–2544. *See also*
Trematodes
blood (schistosomiasis), 2538–2541
intestinal, 2538t, 2542–2543
Fasciolopsis buski, 2538t,
2542–2543
Heterophyes heterophyes, 2538t,
2543
liver, 2538t, 2541–2542
Clonorchis sinensis, 2538t, 2541
Fasciola hepatica, 2538t,
2541–2542
Opisthorchis, 2538t, 2541
lung (*Paragonimus westermani*),
2538t, 2543
Nanophetus salmincola, 2557
swimmer's itch, 2557
visceral larva migrans (*Toxocara
canis*; *T. cati*), 2553–2554
Hemagglutination-inhibition (HAI)
for alphaviruses, 1455
for bacteria, 192t
for influenza virus, 1554–1555
Hemagglutinin: fusion activity, 131
Hemagluttination assays, 12
Hematologic abnormalities
Brucella and, 2056
drug-induced
cephalosporins, 254
chloramphenicol, 313–314
nitrofurantoin, 378
endocarditis, 749
HIV and, 1209, 1225–1226
Hematopoiesis
constitutive, 118
cyclic, 154
cytokines and, 118

Hematopoietic cytokine receptor super-
    family, 113
Hematopoietic growth factor: for the
    immunocompromised,
    2693–2694
Hemodialysis
    aminoglycoside dosage in, 297, 298t
    and hepatitis infections, 2620
        HBV, 2617, 2620
        HCV, 2620
    for HIV patients, 2584
    and osteomyelitis, 1049
    Staphylococcus epidermidis shunt
        infections, 1782
Hemodynamic monitoring: catheter
    infections, 2595–2596, 2596t
Hemoglobins
    penicillin binding, 206
    tetracycline binding, 206
Hemoglobinuria, paroxysmal nocturnal,
    71
Hemolysins, 7
Hemolytic anemia
    Babesia, 2499
    CMV, 1358
    EBV, 1368
    herpesviruses, 1334t
    from nitrofurantoin, 378
    from sulfonamides, 356
Hemolytic phospholipase: attachment
    and entry, 4
Hemolytic-uremic syndrome
    Aeromonas, 2108
    coxsackieviruses, 1632
    echoviruses, 1632
    enterohemorrhagic *E. coli* and, 6
    epidemiology, 159
    Escherichia coli food poisoning and,
        1014
    Shigella dysenteriae and, 6
Hemophiliacs: HIV in, 1169, 1189, 1224,
    2625–2636
Hemoptysis: and cystic fibrosis, 658
Hemorrhage
    gastrointestinal: poliovirus, 1616
    retinal: and endophthalmitis, 1121
    "splinter," 748, 922
Hemorrhagic fevers, viral
    arenaviruses, 1572–1579
        characteristics, 1573t
        South American, 1572, 1573t,
            1574, 1576, 1577
    cutaneous manifestations, 550t, 553
    filoviruses, 1543–1546
        Ebola, 1543–1546
        Marburg, 1543–1546
Hemorrhagic fever with renal syndrome
    (HFRS)
    characteristics, 1568t
    clinical manifestations, 1570
    epidemiology, 1569
    etiology, 1568t, 1569
    prevention, 1571
    treatment, 1571
        ribavirin, 431
Hemorrhagic telangiectasia, hereditary:
    and brain abscess, 889
Hemothorax: and pleural empyema,
    637
Hendersonula, 2380, 2381, 2382–2383
Hendersonula toruloidea, 2382–2383,
    2383f
    clinical features, 2383, 2383f
Henoch-Schönlein purpura: differential
    diagnosis, 1522

Hepadnaviridae, 1406–1439. *See also*
        Hepatitis B virus *and*
        Hepatitis D virus
    arthritis, 1036t
    classification, 1315t
    shape and size, 1316f
Heparin
    and catheter infections, 2595
    vancomycin interaction with, 349
Hepatic abscess, 724–727
    anaerobic, 2163t
    bacteriology, 724–725
    and chronic granulomatous disease,
        92
    clinical manifestations, 725, 725f,
        726f
    diagnosis, 725f, 725–726, 726f
    Entamoeba histolytica, 2398, 2399,
        2401, 2402–2403
    etiology, 724
    and fever, 541
    liver transplantation and, 2725
    neutrophil defect and, 153
    pathogenesis, 725
    prognosis, 726
    specimen collection and processing,
        178
    Streptococcus intermedius, 1863
    treatment, 726–727
Hepatic encephalopathy, 1139
Hepatic failure: antituberculous drug
        dosage in, 390t
Hepatic function: age and, 201
Hepatic infections
    actinomycosis, 2283
    Candida albicans, 2298
Hepatic insufficiency: chloramphenicol
        use in, 313
Hepatic necrosis, amebic, 2398
Hepatic tuberculosis, 2238
Hepatitis, 1136–1164
    active chronic. *See* autoimmune *below*
    acute viral, 1136–1164. *See also*
            individual viruses
        aminotransferases, 1139, 1140f
        anorexia, 1138
        bilirubin, 1140
        cholestasis, 1140–1141
        clinical manifestations, 1137–1141
        course, 1138f
        in dialysis units, 2620–2621
            prevention and control,
                2620–2621
        differential diagnosis, 1141–1149
            alcoholic liver disease,
                1148–1149
            anoxic liver injury, 1148
            cholestatic liver disease, 1149
            chronic vs., 1146
            EBV, 1372
        in drug abusers, 2702–2703
        eosinophilic degeneration, 1140,
            1141f
        etiology, 1137, 1141–1149
        fulminant, 1137, 1139, 1150
            HAV, 1647
            HEV, 1664–1665
        glomerulonephritis, 1139
        HAV, 1141, 1142f, 1636–1656
        HBV, 1141–1144, 1143f, 1406–1439
        HCV, 1136–1137, 1144–1145,
            1145f, 1474–1486
        HDV, 1144, 1144f
        HEV, 1136–1137, 1145–1146,
            1663–1666

    incubation period, 1137
    jaundice, 1138
    laboratory findings, 1139–1140,
        1140f
    and leukemia, 2679
    liver biopsy, 1140, 1140f
    lobular disarray, 1140, 1140f
    malaise, 1138
    management, 1149–1150
        alcohol avoidance, 1149
        fulminant cases, 1150
        hospitalization, 1149
        rest, 1149
    mixed cryoglobulinemia, 1139
    monitoring, 1150
    nausea/vomiting, 1138
    nosocomial, 2616–2624
        dialysis units, 2620–2621
        employee health, 2621–2623,
            2622f
        epidemiology, 2617
        HAV, 2617–2618
        HBV, 2618, 2619t, 2619–2620,
            2623–2624
        HCV, 2618
        HDV, 2618
        HEV, 2618–2619
        perinatal and reproductive trans-
            mission, 2621
        person-to-person transmission,
            2619t, 2619–2620
        from transfusions, 2624–2625
        vaccine prophylaxis, 2623–2624
    nosocomial prevention, 2584
    pathologic findings, 1140f,
        1140–1141, 1141f
    perinatal and reproductive trans-
        mission, 2621
    physical findings, 1139
    prevention, 1150–1151
    pruritus, 1138
    serologic tests, 1142f, 1146
    serum sickness-like syndrome, 1138
    symptoms, 1137–1139
    in transplant recipients, 2728
    traveler's prevention, 2799
    treatment, 1150
        fulminant, 1150
alcoholic: aminotransferases, 1140f
autoimmune, 1157–1158
    classification, 1157t
    type 1, 1157, 1157t
    type 2 (ALKM-1), 1157t,
        1157–1158
Borrelia relapsing fever, 2141
Chlamydia psittaci, 1694
cholestatic: from HAV, 1646–1647
chronic viral, 1153–1159. *See also*
        individual viruses
    aminotransferases, 1140f
    consequences, 1146t
    differential diagnosis, 1154
        acute vs., 1146
    extrahepatic manifestations, 1146t
    HBV, 1153t, 1154–1155
    HCV, 1153t, 1156–1157
    HDV, 1153t, 1155–1156
    persistent and active (use of terms),
        1154
CMV, 1137, 1146–1147, 1357
    in the immunocompromised, 1147,
        1358–1359
    liver transplantation and, 2725–2726
comparison of viral agents, 1474,
    1474t

Coxiella burnetii, 1731
coxsackieviruses, 1632
    neonatal, 1628
delta. *See* Hepatitis D
drug-induced, 1147–1148, 1148t. *See
        also* Hepatotoxicity
    erythromycin, 337
    rifampin, 319
EBV, 1137, 1147
enterically transmitted NANB. *See*
        Hepatitis E virus
enteric symptoms, 999t, 1003
epidemic non-A, non-B. *See* Hepatitis
        E virus
granulomatous, 1159–1164
    diagnosis, 1163
    diseases characterized by,
        1160–1162
    and fever, 545, 1162
    infectious diseases and, 1160–1162,
        1161t
    noninfectious diseases and, 1162,
        1162t
    pathophysiology, 1160, 1160f
    syphilitic, 1161–1162, 2123,
        2125–2126
    treatment, 1163
    tuberculosis, 2238
gummatous, 1161, 2125–2126
herpes simplex: in transplant recipi-
        ents, 2728, 2729
herpesviruses, 1334t
infectious. *See* Hepatitis A virus
leptospirosis, 1147
lupoid. *See* autoimmune *above*
non-A, non-B (NANB). *See also*
        Hepatitis C virus; Hepatitis E
        virus
    comparisons, 1474t
    history, 1474
nonviral infectious, 1147
posttransfusion. *See* Hepatitis C virus
Q fever, 1147
serum. *See* Hepatitis B virus
Treponema pallidum, 1147, 1161,
    2123
tuberculosis, 2238
yellow fever, 1137, 1147
Hepatitis A antigen (HAAg), 1641
Hepatitis A immunoglobulin, 454, 1151,
    1649–1650. *See also* Hepatitis
        A virus, immunization
    dosage, 1650
    for health care workers, 2621–2622
    recommendations, 1649t, 1650
Hepatitis A vaccine, 1650–1651, 2776,
    2799. *See also* Hepatitis A
        virus, immunization
Hepatitis A virus, 1136, 1141, 1142f,
    1636–1656
    age and, 1643
    age-specific prevalence, 1641–1642,
        1642f
    antigenic composition, 1639, 1640f
    biology in cell culture, 1640–1641
    and cholestasis, 1646–1647
    classification, 1637
    clinical features, 1141, 1142f, 1646,
        1647f
    complications, 1646–1647
    in drug abusers, 2702
    electron micrograph, 1637f
    epidemic patterns, 1643
    epidemiology, 1141, 1641–1643
    extrahepatic manifestations, 1647

Hepatitis A virus (Continued)
  fecal-oral transmission, 1643, 1645
  food-borne, 1012, 1644–1645
  fulminant, 1647
  gender and, 1643
  genome and proteins, 1638–1639,
    1639f
  history, 1636–1637
  in homosexuals, 1141, 1643
  host range, 1641
  immunity, 1648
  immunization, 1649–1651
    active, 1650–1651
    dose, 1649–1650
    passive, 1649
    recommendations, 1649, 1649t
  incidence (U.S. 1952–1991), 1641f
  incubation period, 1645, 1645f, 1646f
  infectivity duration, 1643–1644
  laboratory diagnosis, 1647–1648
  and leukemia, 2679
  nosocomial, 2617–2618
    prevention, 2584
  pathogenesis, 1645–1646
  physicochemical properties,
    1637–1641, 1638t
  prevention, 1648–1651
  relapses, 1647
  resistance to physical and chemical
    agents, 1638
  risk factors, 1643, 1643f
  seasonal patterns, 1643
  serology, 191, 1141, 1142f, 1647f
  Shanghai epidemic (1988), 1642,
    1642t
  strains, 1639, 1640f
  structure, 1637f, 1637–1638, 1638t
  surveillance, 1641
  therapy and general management,
    1651
  transmission, 1643–1645
    food-borne and waterborne, 1012,
      1016, 1016t, 1644–1645
    person-to-person, 1644
    from transfusions, 2624–2625
  viral replication, 1645
  viremia, 1644
  waterborne, 1016, 1016t, 1644–1645
Hepatitis B core antigen (HBcAg), 1154,
    1408, 1411f, 1414, 1415,
    1418
  antibody to, 1143, 1414, 1414f, 1415,
    1415f, 1416, 1416f
    tests, 1426, 1426t
  immunization, 1418
Hepatitis B e antigen (HBeAg), 1143,
    1154, 1407, 1409–1410,
    1411f, 1416, 1416f, 1418,
    1424
  antibody to, 1143, 1154, 1414f, 1416f,
    1417
  health care worker carriers, 2619t
  tests, 1426, 1426t, 1427
Hepatitis B immunoglobulin (HBIG),
    454, 1151, 1428, 2770, 2782
  for neonates, 2621
  postexposure, 1430–1431
    for health care workers, 2622
    neonates, 1431
  preexposure, 1428
Hepatitis B surface antigen (HBsAg),
    159, 1137, 1142, 1143f, 1407,
    1408f, 1409, 1410, 1411f,
    1413–1415, 1416, 1416f,
    1418

antibody to, 1143, 1414, 1414f, 1415f,
    1416f
  tests, 1426, 1426t
chronic carrier state, 1143, 1154,
    1415–1417, 1416f, 1422
  chronic HBV vs., 1155
  and extrahepatic disease, 1420
  health care workers, 2619t, 2620
clinical contamination, 2617
and HDV coinfection, 1419
immunization, 1418, 2776
pregnancy screening, 2621
prevalence, 1421
self-limited primary infection,
    1142–1144, 1414f
tests, 1426, 1426t, 1427
Hepatitis B vaccine, 159, 167, 1137,
    1428–1429, 2776–2777
  adverse reactions, 2773t, 2777
  antibody response, 50
  contraindications, 2787t
  indications, 2776
    for adults, 2783, 2784t
    for children and infants, 2775t,
      2776, 2780t, 2783
    for health care workers, 2784
    for HIV infected, 2785t
    for neonates, 2621
    for occupational exposures, 2784
    in pregnancy, 2777
    for travelers, 2799
  licensed formulations, 1429t
  morbidity reduction, 2772t
  for nosocomial prevention,
    2623–2624
  plasma-derived, 1428–1429
  recommendations for risk groups,
    1429t
Hepatitis B virus, 1136–1137,
    1141–1144, 1143f, 1406–1439
  acute, 1418–1419. See also primary
    infection below
    clinical manifestations, 1424–1425
    management, 1427
    self-limited HBsAg primary infec-
      tion, 1413–1415, 1414f
    self-limited without HBsAg, 1415,
      1415f
  adherence, 12
  arthritis, 1032, 1036, 1036t
  carrier state, 1137, 1412–1413
  chronic, 1141, 1143, 1153, 1153t,
    1154–1155, 1412–1413,
    1418–1419. See also persis-
    tent infection below
    active (CAH), 1418, 1425
    clinical manifestations, 1425
    epidemiology, 1137
    exogenous factors altering,
      1417–1418
    in food handlers, 1432
    HBsAg-negative, 1417
    HBsAg-positive, 1415–1417, 1416f
    HCV and, 1154
    HDV and, 1154
    in health care workers, 1432
    management, 1155, 1427–1428
    persistent (CPH), 1418, 1425–1426
    treatment: thymosin, 455
  clinical manifestations, 1141, 1143f,
    1424–1425
    acute, 1424–1425
    persistent, 1425
  cohort studies, 162
  course of infection, 1413–1418

cryoglobulinemia, 42
cutaneous manifestations, 550t, 551
Dane particle, 1415, 1416f, 1424
  tests, 1426
diagnosis, 1426–1427
in drug abusers, 2702–2703
epidemiology, 1141–1142,
    1421–1424
  persistent, 1421–1422
  primary, 1421, 1421t
extrahepatic disease, 1420–1421
fulminant, 1137, 1139, 1424–1425
genome structure, 1407, 1408f
glomerulonephritis, 1139
HDV coinfection, 1419, 1420f
and hepatocellular carcinoma,
    1419–1420
history, 1407
HIV coinfection, 1155
host range, 1413
immune complexes, 42
immunizations, 1428–1431. See also
    Hepatitis B immunoglobulin;
    Hepatitis B vaccine
  postexposure, 1430–1431
    of newborns, 1431
  preexposure
    with HBV vaccine, 1428–1430,
      1429t
    passive, 1428
infection control, 42
interferon-γ and, 131
and leukemia, 2679
management, 1427–1428. See also
    treatment below
  acute, 1427
  chronic, 1427–1428
    food handlers, 1432
    health care workers, 1432
  neonatal, 1423, 1424, 1425
    prevention, 2621
  nosocomial, 2618, 2619t, 2619–2620
    prevention, 1431–1432, 2584
    vaccine prophylaxis, 2623–2624
  pathogenesis of diseases associated
    with, 1418–1421
  persistent infection. See chronic above
  polyarteritis nodosa, 1139
  P (pol/polymerase) gene, 1407
  prevention, 1428–1432
    blood product contamination, 1432
    environmental measures,
      1431–1432
    in hospitals, 1431–1432
    immunization, 1428–1431
  primary infection. See acute above
  protective immunity against, 1418
  relapsing, 1425
  replication steps, 1412f
  serology, 191, 1142f, 1142–1143,
    1143f
    markers, 1426t
  S (surface/envelope) gene, 1407
  structure
    viral genome, 1407, 1408f
    virion, 1407, 1409f, 1409–1410,
      1410f
  tissue tropism, 1413
  transmission, 1422–1424. See also
    nosocomial above
    from occupational blood exposure,
      2644t
    from transfusions, 2625
  in transplant recipients, 2709
    diagnosis and control, 2713

treatment, 412t. See also management
    above
  experimental agents, 437t
  interferons, 428, 452
  zidovudine, 435
viral forms
  in blood, 1410–1411, 1411f
  in cells and liver, 1411–1413, 1412f
virion structure, 1407, 1409f,
    1409–1410
virology, 1407–1413
X gene, 1407, 1593
X protein: and HIV infection, 1212
Hepatitis C antigen, 1144, 1146, 1154
  antibody, 1144–1145, 1146, 1154
Hepatitis C virus, 1136–1137, 1145,
    1145f, 1474–1486
  acute, 1478
    clinical manifestations, 1479
  antibody, 1145, 1146
  bone marrow transplantation and,
    2674
  chronic, 1137, 1153, 1153t,
    1156–1157, 1478–1479, 1479f
    clinical manifestations, 1480
    treatment, 1483
    vertical transmission, 1156
  clinical manifestations, 1479–1480
  cryoglobulinemia, 42
  and cryoglobulinemia, 1480
  diagnosis, 1480–1481
  in drug abusers, 1482, 2702, 2703
  epidemiology, 162, 163, 1481–1483
  extrahepatic manifestations, 1480
  fulminant, 1479–1480
  genetic variation among strains, 1475,
    1476f
  glomerulonephritis, 1139
  and HBV chronicity, 1154
  and hepatocellular carcinoma, 1479
    clinical manifestations, 1480
  history, 1474
  immune complexes, 42
  influenza vaccines and, 1561
  and leukemia, 2679
  natural history of infection,
    1477–1478, 1478f
  nonparenteral transmission, 1482f,
    1482–1483
  nosocomial, 2618
    in dialysis units, 2620
    prevention, 2584
      in health care workers, 2622
  occupational blood exposure manage-
    ment, 2644t–2645t
  parenterally transmitted, 1482
  pathogenesis, 1476–1479
  persistence and immunity,
    1476–1477
  persistent. See chronic above
  prevalence and incidence, 1481–1482
  prevention, 1483
  primary. See acute above
  replication, 1476
  RNA detection, 1481
  serology, 191, 1142f, 1480–1481
    chronic, 1156
  structure and genome organization,
    1474–1475, 1475f
  from transfusions, 1482, 2625
  in transplant recipients, 2709, 2723,
    2728
  treatment, 412t
    interferons, 429, 452
Hepatitis delta antigen (HDAg), 1419

Hepatitis D virus, 1136–1137, 1143–1144, 1144f
  chronic, 1137, 1153, 1153t, 1155–1156
  coinfection with HBV, 1419, 1420f
  course and serology, 1144f
  diagnosis, 1144
  in drug abusers, 2702–2703
  epidemiology, 1144
  fulminant, 1137
  and HBV. *See also* Hepatitis B virus
    chronicity, 1154
    coinfection and superinfection, 1144
  and leukemia, 2679
  nosocomial, 2618
    prevention, 2584
  serology, 191, 1146
  from transfusions, 2625
  in transplant recipients, 2728
  treatment: interferons, 428
Hepatitis E virus, 1136–1137, 1145–1146, 1663–1666
  antibody, 1145
  clinical manifestations, 1664–1665, 1665f
  diagnosis, 1666
  in drug abusers, 2702
  epidemiology, 1145, 1664, 1665f
  fecal-oral transmission, 1664
  genome, 1663, 1664f
  geographic distribution, 1664, 1665f
  history, 1663
  immunity, 1664
  nosocomial, 2618–2619
    prevention, 2584
  pathogenesis, 1664
  serology, 191
  treatment and prevention, 1666
  vaccine research, 1666
  virology, 1663f, 1663–1664, 1664f
Hepatobiliary disorders: HIV/AIDS and, 1229–1230
Hepatocellular carcinoma
  hepatitis B virus and, 1153t, 1419–1420
  hepatitis C virus and, 1479
    clinical manifestations, 1480
Hepatoma: fever, 544
Hepatomegaly: schistosomiasis, 2540
Hepatotoxicity, 1147–1148, 1148t. *See also specific drugs*
  isoniazid, 203, 390, 390t
  ketoconazole, 407
  nitrofurantoin, 378
  penicillins, 239t, 240
  rifampin, 319, 391
  tetracyclines, 310
Herbicola-Lathyri bacteria, 1973, 1975
Herd immunity, 167
Hereditary angioedema–C1 inhibitor deficiency, 70–71
Hereditary angioneurotic edema, 70
Hereditary factors: host defense, 31
Hernia surgery: prophylaxis recommendations, 2751t
Heroin addicts. *See also* Drug abusers
  osteomyelitis in, 1049
Herpangina: coxsackieviruses, 1621t, 1625
  clinical manifestations, 1625
  differential diagnosis, 1625
  laboratory diagnosis, 1625
  serotypes, 1621t, 1625

Herpes B virus, 1379–1382
  classification, 1330t, 1380
  clinical manifestations, 1334t, 1380–1381, 1381f
  diagnosis, 1333, 1381
  epidemiology, 1380
  history, 1379–1380
  prevention and treatment, 1334t, 1334–1335, 1381
  primary infections, 1332t
  structure, 1330t
  transmission and seroepidemiology, 1333t, 1380
Herpes simplex virus (HSV), 1336–1345
  asymptomatic, 1057
  and bone marrow transplantation, 2720
  and cancer, 1341
  cell-mediated immunity and, 1337
    deficiency, 132–133
    therapy, 2682
  cervicitis, 1085
  clinical manifestations, 1337–1341
  complications, 1340–1341
    in compromised host, 1340–1341, 1341f
    encephalitis, 1340
    neonatal infections, 1340
  conjunctivitis, 1106, 1338
    neonatal, 1107
    treatment, 1108
  CSF specimens, 179
  cutaneous manifestations, 550t, 552. *See also* genital *and* orofacial *below*
    in transplantation, 2726
  cytokine and T cell protection, 121t, 128, 129
  dermatoblepharitis, 1130
  description, 1336
  diagnosis, 1333, 1341–1342
  differential diagnosis: VZV, 1349
  EIA diagnosis, 185
  encephalitis, 875, 1340
    CNS response, 828
    treatment, 412t, 1342
      acyclovir, 415–416
  endophthalmitis, 1123
    treatment, 1126
  epidemiology, 1056, 1332, 1336–1337
  and erythema multiforme, 1341
  esophagitis, 963
    and HIV/AIDS, 964, 1229
    in transplant recipients, 2728
  genital, 1338f, 1338–1339. *See also* type 2 *below*
    differential diagnosis, 1395, 2122
    and HIV transmission, 1188
    lymphadenitis, 940t
    and neonatal transmission, 2657, 2657t
    nongenital lesions, 1060
    number of lesions, 1057
    recurrence, 1056, 1337, 1339–1340
    treatment, 412t
      acyclovir, 415–416
      interferons, 429
  and granulocytopenia, 2677, 2679
  growth, 191, 191f
  hepatitis
    in the immunocompromised, 1147
    in transplant recipients, 2728, 2729
    and HIV/AIDS, 1340
      esophagitis, 964, 1229
      genital, 1188

  incidence, 1182t
  mucocutaneous, 1228
  orofacial, 1228
  perirectal, 1281, 1340
  proctitis, 1060, 1228, 1231, 1339
  prophylaxis, 1286t
  treatment, 1283t, 1287, 2642
  viral proteins, 1593
  and idiopathic neurologic syndromes, 1341
  in the immunocompromised, 1340–1341, 1341f
    complications, 1340–1341, 1341f
    hepatitis, 1147
    treatment, 412t
      acyclovir, 415–416
  immunosuppressive therapy and, 135
  keratitis, 1115
    differential diagnosis, 2411
    disciform, 1115
    recurrence, 1337, 1339
    treatment, 1118
      interferons, 429
  keratoconjunctivitis: treatment, 412t, 1126
  keratouveitis, 1115
  labialis, 1337. *See also* orofacial *above and* type 1 *below*
    recurrence, 1339
    treatment: acyclovir, 416
  latency, 1332, 1337
  lymphadenopathy, 1684
    inguinal, 939
  meningitis, 833, 842
    CSF examination, 845
    therapy, 849–850
  monoclonal antibodies in diagnosis, 1341
  mucocutaneous
    diagnosis, 1341, 1341f, 1342
    treatment, 412t
      acyclovir, 416
  neonatal, 1337, 1340, 2657
    prevention, 1343, 2657, 2657t
    treatment, 412t, 2657
  neuritis, 878
  NK cells and, 122, 128
  nosocomial, 1337, 2656–2657
    management of personnel exposed, 2657
    prevention, 2657, 2657t
    risks, 2656
    transmission mechanisms, 2656–2657
  orofacial, 1337. *See also* labialis *above and* type 1 *below*
    and HIV/AIDS, 1228
    and leukemia, 2678
    recurrence, 1339
    treatment, 1342
  pathogenesis, 1337
  perirectal: and HIV/AIDS, 1281, 1340
  pharyngitis, 568, 1338
  prevention, 1342–1343
    acyclovir, 1342–1343
  primary infections, 1337–1339
  proctitis: and HIV/AIDS, 1060, 1228, 1231, 1339
  product and host target, 125t
  reactivation: and leukemia, 2672
  receptor, 1317t
  recurrent infections, 1337, 1339–1340
  relationship to other diseases, 1341

  resistance, 193
    acyclovir, 413–414, 423–424, 432–433
  and Reye syndrome, 1558
  serology, 1342
  seroprevalence, 1333t
  specimen collection and processing, 171t, 183
  spreading mechanisms, 1321
  throat cultures, 173
  tonsillitis, 1337
  transmission, 1333t, 1336–1337
  in transplant recipients, 2709, 2713t, 2729
    culture monitoring, 2714
    diagnosis and control, 2713
    prophylaxis, 2714
  treatment, 412t, 1334t
    acyclovir, 413, 415–416, 1283t, 1287, 1342–1343
    cimetidine, 455
    experimental agents, 437t
    foscarnet, 422–424, 1287
    ganciclovir, 424–426
    in HIV/AIDS, 1283t, 1287
    trifluridine, 432–433
    vidarabine, 433–434, 1342
  tropism, 1331
  type 1. *See also* labialis *and* orofacial *above*
    characteristics, 1336, 1336t
    classification, 1330t
    clinical syndromes, 1334t
    diagnosis, 1341–1342
    in the immunocompromised host, 1332t
    latency, 1332t
    prevention and treatment, 1334t, 1334–1335
    primary infections, 1332t, 1337–1339, 1338f
    recurrence, 1332t, 1337, 1339–1340
    seroepidemiology, 1333t
    structure, 1330t
    transmission, 1333t, 1337
  type 2. *See also* genital *above*
    characteristics, 1336, 1336t
    classification, 1330t
    clinical syndromes, 1334t
    diagnosis, 1341–1342
    in the immunocompromised host, 1332t
    latency, 1332t
    prevention and treatment, 1334t, 1334–1335
    primary infections, 1332t, 1338f, 1338–1339
    recurrence, 1332t, 1337, 1339–1340
    sexual transmission, 1337
    structure, 1330t
    transmission and seroepidemiology, 1333t
  vaccine research, 1342
  vulvar, 1057, 1058f
  vulvovaginitis, 1080
  whitlow, 1339, 1339f
Herpesviridae, 1330–1382
  arthritis, 1036t
  classification, 1315t, 1330, 1330t
  clinical syndromes, 1334, 1334t
  CMV, 1351–1364. *See also* Cytomegalovirus
  diagnosis, 1333–1334

Herpesviridae (Continued)
  EBV (infectious mononucleosis),
      1364–1377. See also
      Epstein-Barr virus
  epidemiology, 1332–1333
  genomes, 1330t
  glycoproteins, 1330
  herpes B virus, 1379–1382
  HHV-6 and 7, 1377–1379. See also
      Human herpesvirus-6
  HSV, 1336–1345. See also Herpes
      simplex virus
  and immunodeficiency, 150t
  latency, 1332, 1332t
  meningitis, 833
    clinical presentation, 842
  nosocomial infections, 2656t,
      2656–2666. See also specific
      viruses
  nucleocapsids, 1330
  pathogenesis, 1333
  prevention and treatment, 1334t,
      1334–1335
  products and host target, 125t
  replication, 1319, 1331
  seroepidemiology, 1333t
  shape and size, 1316f
  spreading/shedding mechanisms,
      1320f, 1321
  structure, 1330t, 1330–1331
  transformation, 1332, 1332t
  transfusion-related, 2626–2627
  transmission, 1332–1333, 1333t
  in transplant recipients, 2729–2730
  treatment
      foscarnet, 422–424
      interferons, 429
      penciclovir, 421–422
  tropism, 1331–1332
  virion, 1330
  VZV, 1345–1351. See also Varicella-
      zoster virus
Herpesvirus, human-6. See Human her-
      pesvirus-6
Herpesviruses. See Herpesviridae and
      specific viruses
Herpes zoster, 1333, 1345–1351. See
      also Varicella-zoster virus
  clinical manifestations, 1348–1349
  epidemiology, 1346–1347
  therapy clinical manifestations,
      1349–1350
Herpetic whitlow, 1339, 1339f
Herpetiform aphthous ulcers, 603
Herpetiform exanthems: coxsackieviruses,
      1624
Herplex. See Idoxuridine
Hetacillin: pharmacology, 506–507t
Heterophile agglutination, 192t
Heterophyes heterophyes, 2538t, 2543
  diagnosis, 1007
  treatment, 463t, 2543
      praziquantel, 482
HEV. See Hepatitis E virus
Hexachlorophene, 382
Hexapoda, 2558
Hickman catheter infections, 788,
      2594, 2670, 2670f, 2671f,
      2679
Hidradenitis suppurativa, 920
High-pressure liquid chromatography
      (HPLC), 197–198
  for mycobacteria, 190
Hip: infectious arthritis, 1033, 1033t
Hippocratic facies: and peritonitis, 714

Hip replacements: Staphylococcus
      aureus infections, 1773,
      1781–1782
Histamine
  and bronchiolitis, 615
  eosinophils and, 96
Histamine fish poisoning, 1012t, 1015t
  fish implicated, 1017t
Histamine-sensitizing factor. See
      Pertussis toxin
Histocompatible antigens: and infections,
      31
Histoplasma capsulatum, 2340–2353
  African, 2348
  antigen detection, 2349
  appearance in tissue, 2289t
  arthritis, 1036
  brain abscess, 890
  cutaneous, 550t, 552, 557, 2347,
      2347f
      treatment, 2351
  cytokine protection, 121t, 124
  diagnosis, 2348–2350
      antigen detection, 2349
      serologic, 2349
      skin testing, 2349–2350
      staining, 2349, 2349f
  differential diagnosis, 2345, 2437
      Bartonella, 1742
      cryptococcosis, 2336
  ecology, 2340–2341
  endocarditis: treatment, 2351
  endophthalmitis, 1123
  enteric symptoms, 1000t
  enteritides, 994
  epidemiology, 2340–2341
  extrapulmonary: and HIV/AIDS,
      1182t
  fever, 543
  granulomatous hepatitis, 1161
  growth, 190
  histo spots, 2348
  and HIV/AIDS, 557, 1281, 2340,
      2341, 2346–2348
      extrapulmonary, 1182t
      meningitis, 872, 2347–2348
      pneumonia, 1235–1236
      progressive disseminated,
          2346–2348
          treatment, 2350–2351
      treatment, 1283t, 1289, 2350–2351
  host defense mechanism, 2341–2342
  lymphadenitis, 936, 940t, 2345
  mediastinal granulomatosis and fibro-
      sis, 2345
      treatment, 2351
  meningitis, 869–870
      diagnosis, 869–870
      and HIV/AIDS, 872, 2347–2348
      in the immunocompromised, 872
      treatment, 868, 2351
  morphogenesis, 2341, 2342f
  mycology, 2341
  ocular, 2348
      treatment, 2351
  pathogenesis, 2341–2342, 2343f,
      2344f
  pericarditis, 805
      treatment, 2351
  pneumonia, 619t, 622t
      chronic, 647t, 648
      in HIV/AIDS, 1235–1236
      radiology, 650t, 653f
      treatment, 2350
  polymerase chain reaction, 2341

presumed ocular syndrome, 1123
  prevention, 2351–2352
  progressive disseminated, 2346–2348
      acute, 2347f, 2347–2348
      chronic, 2346
      and HIV/AIDS, 2346–2348
          treatment, 2350–2351
      subacute, 2346–2347
      treatment, 2350–2351
  pulmonary, 2341
      acute primary, 2342–2345, 2345t
      chronic, 2345–2346
      treatment, 2350
  restriction fragment length polymor-
      phism (RFLP), 2341
  sclerosing mediastinitis, 817–818
  serology, 193t, 2349
  in transplant recipients, 2712
  treatment, 2350–2351
      amphotericin B, 406, 1283t, 1289,
          2350
      in HIV/AIDS, 1283t, 1289,
          2350–2351
      itraconazole, 408, 1283t, 1289,
          2350
      ketoconazole, 407, 2350
  vaccine research, 2352
  var. duboisii, 2348
Histoplasmin skin test, 2349–2350
Histoplasmoma, 2345
  treatment, 2351
Histoplasmosis, 2340–2353. See also
      Histoplasma capsulatum
Histo spots, 2348
His-Werner fever, 1741
HIV. See Human immunodeficiency
      virus
HIVID. See Zalcitabine
HLA. See Human leukocyte antigens
HMS-1, 216t, 268
Hodgkin's disease
  cellular immunodeficiency and, 137,
      2668
  cryptococcosis and, 2332
  defective chemotaxis in, 90
  fever, 538, 544
  granulomatous hepatitis, 1162
  Histoplasma capsulatum and, 2347
  pulmonary infiltrates with eosinophilia,
      631
  total lymphoid irradiation for: immun-
      odeficiency from, 136–137
  Toxoplasma gondii and, 2460
  treatment, 1290
Hog cholera virus, 1455
Homeless: Mycobacterium tuberculosis
      among, 2218
Homosexuals
  amebiasis in, 2397, 2404
  anogenital warts in, 1392, 1393
  anorectal lesions, 1060
  Campylobacter in, 1950
  CMV in, 1353–1354
  cohort studies, 162
  diarrhea: in AIDS, 970, 970t
  Giardia lamblia in, 2487, 2491
  hepatitis A virus in, 1141, 1643
  hepatitis B virus in, 1421, 1423
      chronic carriage, 1422
      vaccine, 1429, 2623
  HIV/AIDS in, 1165, 1167, 1168f,
      1176, 1176f, 1178, 1179f,
      1182t, 1220–1221, 1591. See
      also Human immunodeficien-
      cy virus, epidemiology

acute retroviral syndrome, 1224
  health care workers, 2633, 2634t
  Kaposi's sarcoma, 1240–1245. See
      also Kaposi's sarcoma
  predictors of progression to disease,
      1223t
  prevention, 1193
  proctitis, 1231
  HSV in, 1337, 1339
  HTLV in, 1581
  Neisseria gonorrhoeae in, 1913, 1914,
      1916, 1920
  Neisseria meningitidis in, 1902
  proctitis in, 1231, 1686
  stool examination, 955
Hookworm, 2529–2530. See also
      Ancylostoma duodenale;
      Necator americanus
Hordeolum
  external (sty), 1130
  internal, 1130
  S. aureus, 1130
Horder's spots: Chlamydia psittaci, 1694
Hormodendrum compactum, 2324
Hormodendrum pedrosoi, 2324
Hormones
  and host defense mechanisms, 35
  and normal flora, 31
Horses: microorganisms harbored by,
      2792t
Hospital employee health. See also
      Health care workers
  and infection control, 2573
Host-agent relationship: epidemiology,
      163–165, 165t
Host defense mechanisms, 30–158
  acute phase response, 30t, 33–34
      increased phagocyte number and
          function, 34
      inflammation, 34
      metabolic changes, 34
      soluble defensive molecules, 34
  age and, 35
  antibodies, 31, 36–57. See also Anti-
      bodies
      antimicrobial function, 41–42
      cellular mechanisms in production,
          42–49
      deficiency states, 49–54
      immunoglobulins, 36–41. See also
          Immunoglobulin(s)
      immunopathology caused by, 42
  cell-mediated immunity, 102–149. See
      also Cell-mediated immunity;
      T cells
      cytokines, 112–122, 130–131
      defects, 132–139
      hematopoiesis, 118
      lymphokines, 112–118
      major histocompatibility complex,
          102–105
      mononuclear phagocytes, 122–124
      NK cells, 122
      against specific infections,
          124–130
      T cells, 105–112, 119–120, 121t
  complement, 32, 58–78
      activation, 59–64
      deficiencies, 66–71
      in disease states, 71–73
      evaluation and treatment of disor-
          ders, 73–74
      functions mediated by, 64–65
      microbial interactions with, 65–66
      protein families, 64

receptors, 64
  synthesis, catabolism, and distribu-
    tion, 59
cytokines, 30t, 33f, 33–34
deficiency evaluation, 149–158. *See*
    also Immunodeficiency *and*
    specific deficiencies
fibronectin, 32
general (nonspecific), 30–35, 31t
granulocytic phagocytes, 78–101. *See*
    also Granulocytic phagocytes;
    Phagocytosis *and specific*
    cells
hereditary factors, 31
hormones and, 35
immunoglobulins, 36–41. *See also*
    Immunoglobulin(s)
  deficiency states, 49–54
impairment and exaggeration of non-
    specific immunity, 34–35
natural antibodies, 31
natural barriers, 31–32
  eye, 32
  genitourinary tract, 32
  intestinal tract, 32
  mucous membranes, 31–32
  respiratory tract, 32
  skin, 31–32
normal indigenous microbial flora,
    30t, 30–31
phagocytosis, 32–33
skin, 550–551
steady-state components of immunity,
    32–33
stress and, 35
tissue tropisms, 31
Host factors influencing exposure,
    infection, and disease, 165,
    165t
Host-parasite relationships, 30
  commensal, 30, 31
  parasitic, 30
  symbiotic, 30
HPMPC, 437t
HSV. *See* Herpes simplex virus
HTLV. *See* Human T cell lymphotropic
    viruses
Human bites
  anaerobic, 2163t
  Eikenella, 2112
  to head and neck, 603, 604
  management, 2768
Human B-lymphotropic virus (HBLV).
    See Human herpesvirus-6
Human caliciviruses, 1667–1671. *See*
    also Caliciviruses
Human foamy virus, 1580t
Human herpesvirus-6, 1377–1379
  in adults, 1378–1379
  and chronic fatigue syndrome, 1306
  classification, 1330t, 1378
  clinical manifestations, 1334t,
    1378–1379
  cutaneous manifestations, 550t, 551
  diagnosis and treatment, 1379
  epidemiology, 1332, 1378
  exanthem subitum (roseola infantum),
    1378
  and HIV/AIDS, 1212, 1334, 1601
    viral proteins, 1593
  immunodeficiency and, 137
  meningitis, 833
  nosocomial, 2663
  prevention and treatment, 1334t,
    1334–1335

primary infections, 1332t
serology, 191
structure, 1330t, 1378, 1378f
transmission and seroepidemiology,
    1333t
Human herpesvirus-7, 1334, 1379
  classification, 1330t
  clinical syndromes, 1334t
  epidemiology, 1332
  meningitis, 833
  nosocomial, 2663
  prevention and treatment, 1334t,
    1334–1335
  structure, 1330t
Human immunodeficiency virus (HIV),
    1164–1305, 1584–1606. *See*
    also Acquired immuno-
    deficiency syndrome
Acholeplasma laidlawii and, 1703
acute retroviral syndrome, 1224t,
    1224–1225
adherence, 12, 13
advanced disease. *See* Acquired
    immunodeficiency syndrome
Agrobacterium and, 2111
AIDS dementia, 1601
AIDS-indicator diseases, 1174t, 1175,
    1182–1183, 1223f
anal squamous cancer, 1246
antiadhesin antibodies, 13
antibody-dependent cellular cytotoxi-
    city and, 1213
antibody testing, 1194–1195,
    1254–1261
  application, 1263, 1263t
  dot-blot immunobinding assay,
    1260
  EIA, 1254f, 1254t, 1254–1257,
    1255t, 1256f, 1256t
  guidelines, 1195
  in health care setting, 2647–2648,
    2648t
  IFA, 1258–1259, 1259t
  indications, 1194–1195
  latex agglutination, 1260
  radioimmunoprecipitation assay,
    1259–1260
  Western blot, 1257–1259, 1258f,
    1259t
antigen detection, 1261, 1261t
anti-p24, 1225
arthritis, 1036t, 1037
Aspergillus, 2309
asymptomatic phase, 1600
bacillary angiomatosis, 557–558,
    920, 939, 1229, 1742–1743,
    1743f
  treatment, 1746
and B-cell lymphomas, 1601–1602
in black Americans, 1180, 1180t
bladder dysfunction, 1101–1102
from blood products, 1169, 1189,
    1190–1191, 2625–2626. *See*
    also in health care setting *and*
    transmission *below*
management of needles and sharp
    objects, 2642–2643
occupational exposure manage-
    ment, 2644t–2645t
prevention, 1193, 2641t,
    2641–2642
botryomycosis, 557
Campylobacter and, 1950
case definition, 1174t, 1175, 1175t
  1993 (CDC), 1175t

and CD4+
  binding, 12, 12t, 13, 14–15, 15f,
    1204, 1586, 1586f, 1587f,
    1588f, 1598f
  depletion, 1205–1208, 1206t,
    1586–1587, 1588f, 1599, 1600
    apoptosis and, 1207
    superantigens and, 1207, 1207f
  functional impairment, 1208
  measures, 1175, 1175t, 1182, 1218t,
    1219, 1219t, 1221, 1222f,
    1222–1223, 1223t, 1281
and CD8, 1204, 1208–1209
  suppression by, 1213–1214
cellular activation, 1204–1205
cervical cancer and, 1227, 1246, 1390
cervical dysplasia and, 1175, 1227
characteristics, 1591–1597
in children, 1169, 1184–1187, 1186t,
    1186–1187. *See also* epidemi-
    ology *above and* transmission
    below
classification, 1219, 1219t
chlamydial cervicitis and, 1687
and chronic fatigue syndrome, 1307
classification of diseases, 1218–1219
  CDC, 1219
  pediatric, 1219
  Walter Reed, 1219, 1219t
clinical expression, 1170–1171, 1171f,
    1172t
clinical findings, 1224–1240. *See also*
    Acquired immunodeficiency
    syndrome *and specific*
    infections
  acute retroviral syndrome, 1224t,
    1224–1225
  constitutional disease, 1226
  cutaneous manifestations, 1228–1229
  gastrointestinal manifestations,
    1229–1231
  genital tract disorders, 1227–1228
  immune thrombocytopenia and
    hematologic manifestations,
    1225–1226
  Kaposi's sarcoma, 1240–1244
  malignancies, 1240–1245
  musculoskeletal complications,
    1228
  neurologic complications, 1236t,
    1236–1240
  non-Hodgkin's lymphoma,
    1244–1245
  ocular disease, 1240
  oral disease, 1226–1227
  peripheral neuropathy, 1236
  persistent generalized lym-
    phadenopathy, 1225
  pulmonary disease, 1231–1236,
    1232t
  renal disease, 1231
clinical manifestations of infection,
    1217–1253. *See also* clinical
    findings *above*
CNS infection, 1601–1602
  injury mechanisms, 1589f,
    1589–1590
cofactors, 1601
control problems, 1590
corneal, 1116
counseling, 1194–1195
  guidelines, 1195
  in health care setting, 2647, 2648,
    2648t
  health care workers, 2647, 2648t

CSF specimens, 179
cultures, 1261–1262
cutaneous manifestations, 550t, 557,
    1228–1229
  bacillary angiomatosis, 1229
  viral infections, 1228
cytometric indirect immunofluores-
    cence, 1261
cytotoxic T-cell response, 1213–1214
decontamination, 2643
detection of infection, 1253–1263
  antigen detection, 1261, 1261t
  application of antibody screening,
    1262, 1263t
  DNA and RNA detection, 1262
  dot-blot immunobinding assay,
    1260
  enzyme immunoassays, 1254f,
    1254t, 1254–1257, 1256f
  HIV-1 antibody assays, 1254–1261
  indirect immunofluorescence assay,
    1259, 1259t
  latex agglutination, 1260
  other antibody tests, 1260–1261
  radioimmunoprecipitation assay,
    1259–1260
  serology, 1253f, 1253–1254
  surrogate markers, 1262–1263
  viral culture, 1261–1262
  Western blot, 1257–1259, 1258f,
    1259t
DF-3 coccobacillus and, 2109–2110
diagnosis of infection, 1219–1220,
    1220f
dideoxynucleoside analogs,
    1269–1272, 1270f. *See also*
    therapy *below and specific*
    drugs
  current recommendations, 1276,
    1276t
  dosages, 1271t
  in pregnancy, 1275–1276
  toxicities, 1271t
differential diagnosis: enteroviral
    meningitis, 1622
dipstick test, 1260
disinfection guidelines, 2583–2584
dissemination, 1586, 1586f
DNA probes, 1262
dot-blot immunobinding assay, 1260
in drug abusers, 1165, 1166–1167,
    1168f, 1176, 1177f, 1179f,
    1189, 1224, 2696, 2697, 2705
dynamics of spread, 1168–1171
  biologic variables, 1169f, 1170
  demography, 1169
  economic and political factors,
    1170
  factors influencing, 1169, 1169t
  sexual behavior, 1169, 1169f
  transmission modes, 1168–1169,
    1187–1191
EBV proteins and, 1593
EIA diagnosis, 1220, 1254f, 1254t,
    1254–1257, 1256f
ELISA diagnosis, 1213, 1220, 1225,
    2647
ELISPOT test, 1261
encephalopathy, 1175, 1237
  in children, 1186, 1186t
  incidence, 1183t
env gene, 1587, 1592, 1594, 1594t,
    1597
enzyme immunoassays, 1254f, 1254t,
    1254–1257, 1255t, 1256f

52 INDEX

Human immunodeficiency virus (HIV)
(Continued)
correlation with Western blot, 1256t
currently licensed tests, 1254t
false-negative, 1256t
false-positive, 1256t
first generation, 1254–1257
for HIV-2, 1257
Murex SUDS, 1261
for p24 antigen, 1261
saliva-based (Orasure), 1261
second generation, 1257
third generation, 1257
epidemiology (outside U.S.),
1164–1174. *See also* global
perspective on infection *above*
epidemiology (U.S.), 1174–1191,
1580t. *See also* global perspectives *above*
in adults, 1176–1184
AIDS indicator diseases, 1182t,
1182–1183
clinical manifestations of infection,
1182–1184
demographic characteristics, 1180,
1180t
in children, 1186, 1186t
exposure categories, 1178–1180,
1179f
geographic distribution,
1180–1181, 1181f
in health care setting, 2632–2656.
See health care setting *below*
mortality, 1184, 1185f
serologic monitoring, 1176f,
1176–1178, 1177f
spectrum and progression of infection, 1181–1182
tuberculosis and, 1183–1184
and epididymitis, 1101–1102
and fever, 536, 537t
former names, 1580t
gag gene, 1587, 1592, 1594, 1594t,
1597
gastrointestinal manifestations,
1229–1231
enterocolitis, 1230t, 1230–1231
esophageal disease, 1229
stomach, small bowel, and hepatobiliary disorders, 1229–1230
genes and gene products, 1594t,
1594–1596. *See also*
individual genes
accessory, 1594t, 1595–1596
structural, 1594t, 1594–1595
genetic variation, 1596–1597
genital tract disorders, 1227–1228
genomes: plasticity and complexity
of, 1587, 1589
genomic organization, 1592, 1593f
global perspectives on infection,
1164–1174
Asia, 1166–1167, 1167f,
1191–1192
in eastern Europe, 1191–1192
industrialized countries, 1165
Latin America and the Caribbean,
1167, 1168f, 1191
North Africa and the Middle East,
1167–1168
size of problem, 1164–1168, 1165f
sub-Saharan Africa, 1165f,
1165–1166, 1166t
gp41, 1204t, 1594t, 1595, 1598, 1599,
1600f

gp120, 14–15, 15f, 1204, 1204t, 1207,
1208, 1594t, 1594–1595,
1596, 1599
and vaccine research, 1294, 1295f,
1296, 1297t, 1299, 1300t
gp160, 14–15, 15f
and vaccine research, 1297, 1297t,
1299, 1300, 1300t
HBV coinfection, 1155
in health care setting, 2632–2656
antibody testing, 2647–2648, 2648t
body fluids implicated in transmission, 2633
decontamination and sterilization,
2643
duty to warn, 2648
impact on training and recruitment
of personnel, 2649
legal and ethical issues, 2647–2649
management of employees sustaining adverse exposures,
2643–2647, 2644t–2645t
management of needles and sharp
objects, 2642–2643
management of opportunistic infections, 2642
mucous membrane exposures, 2633
occupational/nosocomial transmission, 2632–2633, 2633t
partner notification, 2648
patient confidentiality, 2648
patient testing, 2647–2648, 2648t
percutaneous exposures,
2632–2633
prevention, 2639–2647, 2640t,
2641t
provider-to-patient transmission,
2638t, 2638–2639
risk factors, 2637t, 2637–2638
serologic surveillance, 2647
support services and waste disposal,
2643, 2643t
testing indications, 1195,
2647–2648, 2648t
transmission routes, 2632–2633
universal precautions, 2639–2641,
2640t, 2641t
in health care workers, 1190,
2633–2639. *See also* epidemiology *above and* transmission
below
antibody seropositivity, 2634–2638
case reports, 2634
counseling, 2647, 2648t
ethical, legal, and policy issues in
management, 2649–2650
management of adverse exposures,
2643–2647, 2645t–2646t
postexposure antiretroviral chemoprophylaxis, 2646
prevention, 1194
prospective/longitudinal studies of
incidence, 2636t, 2636–2637,
2637t
right to refuse care, 2648
serologic surveillance, 2647
studies of prevalence, 2634, 2635t,
2636
testing indications, 1195
hematologic manifestations,
1225–1226
in hemophiliacs, 1169, 1189, 1224,
2625–2636. *See also* epidemiology *above and* transmission
below

in heterosexuals. *See* epidemiology
above and transmission *below*
in Hispanic Americans, 1180, 1180t
history, 1218, 1584, 1591
Hodgkin's disease and, 1245–1246
in homosexuals, 1165, 1167, 1168f,
1174, 1176, 1177f, 1178,
1179f, 1182t, 1220–1221
acute retroviral syndrome, 1224
predictors of progression to disease,
1223t
hospital waste disposal, 2582,
2583–2584
HSV proteins and, 1593
HTLV and
coinfection, 1583
protein enhancement, 1593, 1601
human herpesvirus-6 and, 1212, 1334,
1601
viral proteins, 1593
human papillomavirus and, 1390
hypergammaglobulinemia, 42
idiopathic CD4+ T lymphocytopenia,
1182
IFA diagnosis, 1220
immune depletion, 1586–1587, 1588f.
See also CD4+ *above*
immune response to, 1212t,
1212–1214
antibody-dependent cellular cytotoxicity, 1213
cell-mediated, 1213–1214
cytotoxic T-cell response,
1213–1214
humoral, 1213
neutralizing antibody response,
1213
noncytolytic suppression by CD8+
T cells, 1214
immune thrombocytopenia,
1225–1226
immunology, 1203–1217
immunopathogenic mechanisms of
infection, 1205–1212
B cell abnormalities, 1209–1210
CD8+ T-cell abnormalities,
1208–1209
CD4+ T-cell depletion, 1205f,
1205–1208, 1206t, 1207f
cofactors in pathogenesis,
1211–1212
cytokine production, 1210
cytokine regulation of HIV
expression, 1211–1212
dendritic cells, 1210–1211
functional impairment of CD4+ T
cells, 1208
impaired antibody responses,
1209–1210
lymphoid tissue and pathogenesis,
1212
lymphomas and, 1210
monocyte/macrophage abnormalities, 1209
NK cells, 1210
T-cell abnormalities, 1205–1209
impact of epidemic, 1171–1172
incidence and prevalence (U.S.): in
adults, 1175–1176
indirect immunofluorescence assay,
1259, 1259t
Western blot and, 1259t
and infective endocarditis, 741
isolation, 2577
Japanese encephalitis and, 1470

Kaposi's sarcoma, 1240–1244, 1602.
See also Acquired immunodeficiency syndrome, Kaposi's
sarcoma
therapy, 1243t, 1243–1244
latex agglutination, 1260
and leishmaniasis, 2428
visceral (kala azar), 2431, 2432
life cycle, 1267, 1268f, 1597–1599,
1598f, 1599f, 1600f
long terminal repeat (LTR), 1203,
1593f, 1593–1595, 1597
lymphadenitis, 941–942
lymphoid organs and, 1586, 1587f
macrophage tropism, 1589–1590
malignancies, 1240–1246
management of opportunistic infections, 1280–1294. *See also*
therapy *below and specific*
infections
candidiasis, 1283t, 1288
CMV, 1283t, 1287–1288
coccidioidomycosis, 1283t, 1289
cryptococcosis, 1283t, 1288–1289
cryptosporidiosis, 1289
EBV, 1288
enteric pathogens, 1289
general principles, 1282, 1283t
in health care setting, 2642
histoplasmosis, 1283t, 1289
HSV, 1283t, 1287
isosporiasis, 1289
Kaposi's sarcoma, 1290
lymphoma, 1290
Microsporidia, 1289
mycobacteria, 1283t, 1289
PML, 1288
Pneumocystis carinii, 1282–1286,
1283t
prospective monitoring, 1281
Rochalimaea, 1283t, 1290
Toxoplasma gondii, 1283t,
1286–1287
Treponema pallidum, 1289–1290
VZV, 1283t, 1287
meningitis, 833
chronic, 872
clinical presentation, 842
CSF examination, 845
mortality rates, 1184, 1185f
myalgia, 934
and *Mycobacterium tuberculosis*, 159,
542, 1171, 1171f, 1171t, 1177,
1183–1184, 1221, 1231–1232,
1234
in Africa, 1171, 1171f, 1171t
in Asia, 1171t
coinfection, 1175
multidrug resistance, 389, 1183
myocarditis, 800–801
natural history of infection, 1220f,
1220–1224, 1221f, 1223f,
1585f
predictors of progression to AIDS,
1223t, 1224
and natural killer (NK) cells, 1210,
1214
nef gene, 1591, 1594t, 1595, 1596
neonatal, 1168–1169, 1186t,
1186–1187. *See also* children
and epidemiology *above and*
transmission *below*
antiretroviral therapy and,
1275–1276
prevention, 1194

surveys, 163
transmission, 1189–1190
neoplasia, 1240–1246, 1245t. *See also*
    Kaposi's sarcoma
neurologic complications, 1236t,
    1236–1240
    CMV, 1239–1240
    Cryptococcus neoformans, 1239
    encephalopathy, 1237
    intracranial mass lesions, 1237t,
        1237–1239, 1238f
    progressive multifocal leukoen-
        cephalopathy, 1239
    toxoplasmosis, 1238–1239
neurologic disease, 1601–1602. *See
    also* neurologic complications
    above
neuropathies, 878–879
neutropenia: G-CSF for, 451
non-Hodgkin's lymphoma, 1240,
    1244–1245
    CNS, 1244
    peripheral, 1244–1245
    therapy, 1245
nosocomial, 1169, 2632–2656. *See
    also* health care setting *above
    and* transmission *below*
    prevention, 2583–2584, 2639–2647
number of reported cases
    U.S., 1175–1176
    worldwide, 1164–1165
ocular disease, 1240
opportunistic infections, 1600–1601
    management, 1280–1294. *See also*
        management of opportunistic
        infections *above*
    spectrum, 1281–1282. *See also*
        specific infections
        throughout
oral disease
    candidiasis, 1226–1227
    gingivitis, 1227
    hairy leukoplakia, 1227
    periodontitis, 1227
    ulcers, 1227
    and orchitis, 1101–1102
outside U.S., 1191–1192. *See also*
    global perspective on infection
    above
p24 antigen detection, 1261, 1261t
particle agglutination test, 1260
pathogenesis of infection, 1586, 1587f
pathogen-host relationships,
    1599–1600
pediatric
    classification, 1219, 1219t
    staging, 1219, 1219t
Penicillium marneffii and, 2390
perinatal, 1186t, 1186–1187
peripheral neuropathy, 1236
persistence, 1586, 1586f
    paradox of, 1586–1587
persistent generalized lymphadenopa-
    thy, 1225
pharyngitis, 567t, 568
pityrosporum folliculitis and, 2384
Pneumocystis carinii, 127, 621, 629,
    1182, 1182t, 1233t,
    2475–2483
pneumonia, 621
    bacterial, 1183, 1231, 1233t, 1235,
        1235t
    chronic, 648
    *Pneumocystis carinii. See
        Pneumocystis carinii* above

pol gene, 1587, 1592, 1594, 1594t,
    1597
polio vaccine use, 1616
polymerase chain reaction (PCR),
    1262
    in pregnancy, 1169, 1189–1190. *See
        also* neonatal *above*
    antiretroviral therapy and,
        1275–1276
    prevention, 1194
prevention of transmission, 166,
    1192–1194
    in health care setting, 2639–2647
primary infection, 1182
progression to disease, 1170–1171,
    1182, 1600–1601. *See also*
    Acquired immunodeficiency
    syndrome
    median time, 1205f, 1220f, 1221
    and prostatitis, 1101–1102
in prostitutes. *See* epidemiology *above
    and* transmission *below*
Pseudallescheria boydii and, 2390
pulmonary disease, 1231–1236, 1232t.
    See also pneumonia *above*
    algorithm for evaluating, 1233f
    fungi, 1235–1236
    mycobacteria, 1233–1235
    pyogenic bacteria, 1235, 1235t
    radiography, 1232, 1233t
pyomyositis, 929–930
radioimmunoprecipitation assay,
    1259–1260
receptor, 12, 1317t
renal disease, 1231
replication stages, 1267, 1268f
retinitis, 1240
reverse transcriptase enzyme, 1204,
    1204t, 1594, 1594t
    inhibition, 1269–1271
    non-nucleoside inhibitors,
        1272–1273
rev gene, 1591, 1594t, 1595, 1596
RNA detection, 1262
R region, 1592, 1593f
St. Louis encephalitis virus and, 1470
and *Salmonella typhi*, 2024
serology, 191, 1220, 1220f, 1253f,
    1253–1254
    algorithm, 1256f
sexual transmission, 1187–1189. *See
    also* epidemiology *above*
    anal intercourse and, 1169
    behavior and, 1169
    genital ulcers and, 1168, 1188
    infectiousness of source partner,
        1187–1188
    prevention, 1192–1193
    STDs and, 1168–1170, 1188
    susceptibility of recipient partner,
        1188–1189
    worldwide, 1168–1170
shedding in semen, 1102
and splenic abscess, 727
sporotrichosis and, 2322
staging
    clinical, 1219, 1219t
    pediatric, 1219, 1219t
    Walter Reed system, 1219, 1219t
Staphylococcus aureus and, 557
sterilization, 2643
    guidelines, 2583–2584
and *Streptococcus pneumoniae*, 1221,
    1235, 1235t, 1816, 1817t
    vaccination, 1823

and strongyloidiasis, 2530
structure, 1591, 1592f
surrogate markers, 1262–1263
surveillance (U.S.), 1174t, 1174–1175,
    1217–1219, 1218t
tat gene, 1587, 1591, 1594t, 1595
taxonomy, 1585f
testing, 1194–1195, 1253–1263. *See
    also* detection of infection
    above and specific tests
    of hospital patients, 2647–2648,
        2648t
    therapy, 1267–1280, 1602–1603
    delaviridine, 1273
    didanosine (ddI), 1271, 1271t,
        1272f, 1602
        for ZDV failure, 1275
    dideoxynucleoside analogs,
        1269–1272, 1270f. *See also
        specific drugs*
    dosages, 1271t
    toxicities, 1271t
    foscarnet, 1273
    gene, 1602–1603
    inhibition by immunoglobulins,
        1269
    inhibition of reverse transcription,
        1269–1271
    interference with attachment,
        1268–1269
    interferon-α, 1273
    need to individualize, 1276–1277
    nevirapine, 1272–1273
    non-nucleoside reverse transcrip-
        tase inhibitors, 1272–1273
    opportunistic infections. *See* man-
        agement of opportunistic
        infections *above*
    protease inhibitors, 1273
    stavudine (d4T), 1271t, 1272
    survival prolongation questions,
        1273
    timing initial antiretroviral,
        1274–1275
    zalcitabine (ddC), 1271t,
        1271–1272, 1272t, 1602
        for ZDV failure, 1275
    zidovudine (ZDV), 1269–1271,
        1271t, 1272f, 1590, 1602. *See
        also* Zidovudine
    current recommendations, 1276,
        1276t
    ddI and ddC for failure of, 1275
    initiating, 1275
    in pregnancy, 1275–1276
    resistance, 1590
    and survival, 1273–1274
from transfusions. *See* blood product
    above
transmission, 1168–1169, 1187–1191
    blood product, 1189, 1190–1191,
        2625–2626
    prevention, 1193
    breast-feeding, 1169, 1190, 1191
    chancroid and, 2047, 2048
    drug injection, 1189
        prevention, 1193
    in health care settings, 1190–1191,
        2632–2656
    prevention, 1194
    occupational/nosocomial,
        2632–2633, 2633t
    other modes, 1191
    perinatal, 1168, 1190
    prevention, 1194

saliva and, 1188, 1191
semen, 1102
sexual, 1187–1189. *See also* sexual
    transmission *above*
    prevention, 1192–1193
Trichomonas vaginalis and, 1188,
    2493
in transplant recipients, 2713t
    diagnosis and control, 2713, 2714
in trauma patients, 2757, 2759
Treponema pallidum and, 557, 1227,
    2119
    coinfection, 2119, 2131
Trypanosoma cruzi and, 2446
tuberculin testing and, 2220
type 2, 1164, 1192, 1203
    in Africa, 1166, 1192
    and CMV, 1171
    enzyme immunoassays, 1257
    epidemiology, 1580t
    former names, 1580t
    genes and gene products, 1594t
    genomic organization, 1593f
    history, 1591
    in India, 1167
    LTR, 1594
    and vaccine research, 1299
    vpx gene, 1203, 1594t, 1595, 1596
universal precautions, 1194,
    2639–2641, 2640t
U3 region, 1592, 1593f
U5 region, 1592, 1593f
urologic manifestations, 1101–1102
vaccine research, 1294–1306
    adjuvants, 1298
    animal models, 1298–1300
        chimpanzees, 1298–1299
        rhesus macaque monkeys,
            1299–1300
    antibody-dependent cellular cyto-
        toxicity and, 1294
    candidate vaccines, 1296–1298,
        1297t
    cellular immunity and, 1295
    deleterious immune responses and,
        1295–1296
    envelope proteins, 1296, 1297t
        human trials, 1300t,
            1300–1301
    human trials, 1300t, 1300–1302
        internal or core antigens, 1300t,
            1301
        perinatal studies, 1301
        recombinant gp120 vaccines,
            1300t, 1300–1301
        recombinant gp160 vaccines,
            1300, 1300t
        studies in seropositives
            (immunotherapy), 1302
        vaccinia virus vector, 1300t,
            1301
    immune response and, 1294–1296
    internal or core antigens: human tri-
        als, 1300t, 1301
    internal or core proteins,
        1296–1297, 1297t
    live attenuated virus vaccines,
        1298
    live vectors, 1297, 1297t
        human trials, 1300t, 1301
    neutralizing antibodies and, 1294,
        1295f
    whole virus vaccines, 1296
        human trials, 1300t
variation and cell tropism, 1205

Human immunodeficiency virus (HIV)
(*Continued*)
varicella-zoster virus and, 1228, 1348
reactivation, 1182, 1228
retinitis, 1240
treatment, 1283t, 1287
vif gene, 1591, 1594t, 1595, 1596,
1597
virion infectivity factor (*vif*), 1203,
1204t
virology, 1203–1205, 1584–1606
cellular targets of infection,
1204–1205
genomic organization, 1203–1204
life cycle, 1204, 1204t
variation and potential cell tropism,
1205
virus particle, 1591–1592.1592f
in vitro antibody production (IVAP)
assays, 1261
vpr gene, 1591, 1594t, 1595, 1596,
1597, 2103
vpu gene, 1203, 1204t, 1591, 1594t,
1595, 1596, 1597
vpx gene, 1203, 1594t, 1595, 1596
Walter Reed staging system, 1219,
1219t
waste disposal, 2643, 2643t
wasting syndrome, 934, 1175, 1182,
1182t, 1226
in children, 1186, 1186t
Western blot, 1213, 1220, 1225,
1257–1259, 1258f, 1259t
enzyme immunoassays correlation
with, 1256t
false-positive, 1259t
and indirect immunofluorescence
assay, 1259t
in women, 1166, 1166t, 1167,
1168–1169, 1174, 1175, 1177,
1178, 1179f, 1180, 1180t,
1183, 1188. *See also* epidemiology, pregnancy *and* sexual
transmission *above*
genital tract disorders, 1227–1228
testing indications, 1194
Human leukocyte antigens (HLA),
102–105
A, 102
B, 102
B27
and infection predisposition, 31
and postinfectious arthritis, 1032
and Reiter syndrome, 1071
C, 102
D, 102
DP, 102
DQ, 102
DR, 102
E, 102
F, 102
G, 102
Plasmodium and, 2421
Human papillomaviruses (HPV),
1387–1400
anogenital warts (condylomata acuminata), 1388t, 1389, 1392f,
1392–1393, 1393f
treatment, 1394–1395
carriage, 1057
and cervical dysplasia, 1227, 1389
cervicitis, 1085
clinical manifestations, 1390,
1392–1393
conjunctivitis, 1106

cutaneous warts, 1388t, 1389, 1390,
1391f, 1392
treatment, 1393–1394
diagnosis, 1395–1396
epidemiology, 1388–1389
epidermodysplasia verruciformis,
1388t, 1389, 1392
treatment, 1395
and neoplasia, 1389–1390
pathogenesis, 1390, 1391f
prevention, 1396
recurrent respiratory papillomatosis,
1388t, 1389, 1393
treatment, 1395
transmission, 1389
treatment, 412t, 1393–1396
experimental agents, 437t
interferons, 429
types and disease association, 1388,
1388t
virology, 1388
vulvovaginitis, 1080
Human parainfluenza virus (HPIV),
1489–1496. *See also*
Parainfluenza virus
Human parvovirus B19. *See* Parvovirus
B19
Human rabies immunoglobulin (HRIG),
1537, 1537t, 1539, 1540
Human rhinovirus 14: receptor, 1317t
Human T cell leukemia virus. *See* Human
T cell lymphotropic viruses
Human T cell lymphotropic viruses, type
III. *See* Human immunodeficiency virus
Human T cell lymphotropic viruses
(HTLV-I/II), 1579–1584
adult T-cell leukemia/lymphoma,
1581–1582
clinical illness, 1581f, 1581–1582,
1582f
diagnosis, 1582
incidence, 1581
infectious complications, 1582
treatment, 1582
arthritis, 1036t, 1037
classification, 1579, 1580t
CSF specimens, 179
discovery, 1579, 1591
encephalomyelitis, 877
epidemiology, 1580–1581
geographic distribution, 1580
history, 1579, 1591
and HIV/AIDS, 1211
interactions, 1582
viral proteins, 1593
influenza vaccines and, 1561
rex gene, 1579
serology, 191
tax gene, 1579, 1593
transfusion-related, 1581, 2626
transmission, 1580–1581
blood products, 1581, 2626
mother to child, 1580
sexual, 1580–1581
treatment: zidovudine, 435–437
type I
adult T-cell leukemia/lymphoma,
1581–1582
epidemiology, 1580t, 1580–1581
neurologic complications, 1582
type II
epidemiology, 1580t, 1580–1581
myelopathy, 1582
neoplasia and, 1582

Human tetanus immunoglobulin (HTIG).
See Tetanus immunoglobulin
Humoral immunity. *See also* Antibodies;
B cells; Immunoglobulin(s)
anaerobes and, 2162
Blastomyces dermatitidis and, 2356
bone marrow transplantation and,
2718
Candida albicans and, 2291
cryptococcosis and, 2333
deficiencies, 49–54. *See also*
Antibodies, deficiencies
and endocarditis, 745–746
and enteroviruses, 1608–1609
and Epstein-Barr virus, 1366–1367
and *Francisella tularensis*, 2063
Giardia lamblia and, 2488
and HIV, 1209–1210
and infections in patients with neoplasia, 2666t, 2669
and Lyme disease, 2145
and *Pneumocystis carinii*, 2476
and respiratory syncytial virus,
1505–1506
and rotavirus, 1450
Staphylococcus aureus and, 1762
virulence factors for avoiding or disrupting, 8
Hutchinson's teeth: *Treponema pallidum*,
2126
Hyalomma: and Crimean-Congo hemorrhagic fever, 1568, 1568t,
1569
Hyaluronidase: *Staphylococcus aureus*,
1759
Hybridization, subtractive, 26
Hybrid resistance, 122
Hydatid cyst disease, 2544, 2550–2551.
*See also Echinococcus granu-
losus*
Hydradenitis suppurativa:
Staphylococcus aureus,
1763–1764
Hydradenoma papilliferum: differential
diagnosis, 1395
Hydration. *See also* Fluid therapy
for urinary tract infections, 674
Hydrocephalus
communicating, 828
Cryptococcus neoformans, 2336, 2338
obstructive, 828
Hydrochloroquine: drug interactions,
523t
Hydrogen peroxide
bactericidal properties, 87, 96
formation, 84
Hydroxyeicosatetraenoic acids (HETE),
82
Hydroxyl radical, 87, 88
bactericidal activity, 87
Hydroxynaphthoquinones
antiparasitic use, 475
for *Toxoplasma gondii*, 2469
Hydroxystilbamidine: for *Blastomyces
dermatitidis*, 2363
Hygiene: and enteric infections, 946
Hymenolepis diminuta, 2547
praziquantel for, 482
Hymenolepis nana, 2545t, 2547
treatment, 466t, 2547, 2548
niclosamide, 483, 2548
praziquantel, 482, 2548
Hyperbaric oxygen
for anaerobic gram-negative bacilli,
2200

for gas gangrene, 2188–2189
for osteomyelitis, 1048–1049
Hypergammaglobulinemia, 42
and acute phase response, 534
and endocarditis, 750
Hyperimmunoglobulinemia E with
impaired chemotaxis. *See* Job
syndrome
Hyperimmunoglobulinemia M:
immunoglobulin for, 454
Hyperpyrexia, 533
Hypersensitivity
adverse reactions, 253–254
cell-mediated: from β-lactams, 272
delayed-type (DTH): and cell-mediated
immunity, 102
drug-induced, 203, 356
isoniazid, 390
nitrofurantoin, 378
rifampin, 391
and fever, 544–545
immediate-type
from β-lactams, 272
IgE and, 39
Hypersensitivity pneumonitis, 647t
pulmonary infiltrates with eosinophilia,
631
Hypertension: and urinary tract infections, 673
Hypertensive airways disease, 608. *See
also* Bronchitis, chronic
Hyperthermia
fever vs., 531. *See also* Fever
malignant, 531
therapeutic, 533
Hypertriglyceridemia: and fever, 546
Hypertrophic spinal pachymeningitis,
906
Hyperventilation
for cerebral edema, 830t
and sepsis, 692
Hypochlorous acid, 87
Hypogammaglobulinemia
acquired. *See* Common variable
immunodeficiency
transient, of infancy, 51
ureaplasma/mycoplasma, 1716–1717
Hypopyon, 1112, 1112f
Hypotension: and sepsis, 693
Hypothalamic fever, 531
Hypothalamus
and core temperature, 531
endogenous pyrogenic cytokines and,
532f, 532–533
thermoregulatory center, 531
Hypoxemia: croup and, 575, 576
Hysterectomy
infections after, 1093–1094
cuff cellulitis, 1094
pelvic cellulitis, 1094
for postabortal infections, 1093
prophylaxis recommendations, 2751t
and vaginal examination, 1082

I

Ibotenic acid: in mushrooms, 1015,
1015t
Ibuprofen
for fever, 547
for septic shock, 701
ICAM-1, 82, 123
rhinovirus, 12t, 13, 14, 14f, 1656,
1660
and T cells, 111, 121

ICAM-2, 82, 123
and T cells, 121
ICAM-3
and T cells, 107, 108, 121
Ichthyosis: and HIV, 1229
Idoxuridine, 426
structure, 423f
Id reactions, 2381
IDU. *See* Idoxuridine
Ileal bypass surgery: and anaerobes, 2160
Ilheus: transmission, clinical syndromes, and geographic distribution, 1466t
Iliac lymphadenitis, suppurative, 937–938
Imidazoles, 406–409
for *Paracoccidioides brasiliensis*, 2388–2389
Imipenem
for *Acinetobacter*, 2012
activity, 264t, 264–265
adverse reaction, 265
antibiotic-associated colitis (AAC), 979
antimicrobial activity, 285t
for *Bacteroides fragilis*, 2200t, 2201
chemistry, 264
clinical use, 265–266
combination therapy
aminoglycosides, 287t
for mycobacteria, 396t
with rifampin, 323–324
for cystic fibrosis infections, 660
dosage, 510t–511t
in children, 510t
for meningitis, 850t
in renal dysfunction, 204, 511t
drug interactions, 523t
mechanism of action, 265
for meningitis, 850t, 853
for mycobacteria, 395
for necrotizing pneumonia, 646
for *Nocardia*, 2277
for odontogenic infections, 602t
for peritonitis, 716, 717
pharmacology, 265, 510t–511t
for Pseudomonads, 2004t
for *Pseudomonas aeruginosa*, 264t, 265, 1984
endocarditis, 1984
meningitis, 1989
for pyelonephritis, 676
resistance, 219
for sepsis syndrome, 699, 699t
structure, 264f
susceptibility testing, 194, 194t
Immersion foot syndrome, tropical, 1997
Immotile cilia syndrome. *See* Kartagener syndrome
Immune complexes
antibody-antigen, 42
β-lactam allergy, 272
circulating: and endocarditis, 746, 750
Immune globulin. *See* Immunoglobulin(s), therapeutic
Immune status: and brain abscess, 890
Immune thrombocytopenia: HIV/AIDS and, 1225–1226
Immunity. *See also* Host defense mechanisms
steady-state components, 32–33
Immunization, 167, 2770–2790. *See also* Vaccines
active, 167

adjuvants, 2770, 2771
administration route, 2771
adverse responses, 2772, 2773, 2773t
age and, 2771
antibodies and, 41
antibody characteristics, 2771
assessing need for, 2785
childhood, 167
constituents, 2770
contraindications and precautions, 2787t
currently available, 2773t, 2773–2783
definitions, 2770
determinants of immunogenicity, 2770–2771
dose, 2770
general principles, 2772t, 2772–2773
immune response
measurement, 2772
mobilization, 2771–2772
temporal course, 2772
immunologic basis, 2770
information sources on, 2788
MHC polymorphism and, 2770
parent and patient education, 2785
passive, 167
record keeping, 2785
responses: reporting, 2786, 2786t
simultaneous administration and intervals between, 2785–2786
standards for pediatric, 2786t, 2787–2788
for travel, 167, 2783, 2784t, 2796–2799, 2797t
Immunoassays, 184–185
antimicrobial, 191, 197
enzyme, 185
Immunocompromised host
Aeromonas in, 2108
amebic encephalitis in, 2409, 2410, 2411
Aspergillus in, 2308
Babesia in, 2497
Bacillus in, 1893
Blastomyces dermatitidis in, 2361
brain abscess etiology in, 890
cancer patients, 2666–2675. *See also* Neoplasia
Capnocytophaga in, 2104
cellulitis in, 915
CMV in
cancer victims, 1356
clinical manifestations, 1358–1360
encephalopathy, 1359–1360
endocrinopathies and glandular involvement, 1360
gastrointestinal, 1359
meningoencephalitis, 1359–1360
myelopathy, 1359–1360
pneumonia, 1358
retinitis, 1359, 1359f
transplant recipients, 1355–1356, 1358
Coccidioides immitis in, 2369–2370
Coxiella burnetii (Q fever) in, 1732
cryptococcosis in, 2332
Cryptosporidium in, 2505
deep dermatophyte infections in, 2380–2381
empirical therapy for infections, 2686–2691
antibiotic foundations for initial therapy, 2688t, 2688–2689, 2690t
antifungal, 2689–2690

candidates, 2687
clinically defined infections, 2691
duration, 2690–2691
guidelines, 2687–2691
preantibiotic evaluation, 2688
rationale and evolving concepts, 2686–2687, 2687t
enteroviral meningoencephalitis in, 1629
fever and rash in, 557–558
herpes simplex virus in, 1340–1341, 1341f
treatment, 412t, 416
histoplasmosis in, 2342
HIV/AIDS. *See* Acquired immunodeficiency syndrome; Human immunodeficiency virus
infections in, 2666–2696. *See also* specific infections
cancer patients, 2666–2675
empirical therapy, 2686–2691. *See also* empirical therapy for infections *above*
leukemia/lymphoma patients, 2675–2686
prevention, 2691–2694
Isospora belli in, 2510
Legionella pneumophila in, 2092
Legionella spp. infections in, 2101
leukemia/lymphoma patients, 2675–2686
Listeria in, 1881
measles in, 1522
meningitis in: chronic, 872
microsporidiosis in, 2516
mucormycosis in, 2313
mucositis in, 603
Mycoplasma pneumoniae in, 1707
myocarditis in, 800–801
opportunistic pathogens and, 1754
paracoccidioidomycosis in, 2387
parainfluenza virus in, 1492
parvovirus B19 in, 1441, 1443
pleural empyema in, 637
Pneumocystis carinii in, 2477, 2478
pneumonia in: nosocomial, 631
poliovirus in, 1616–1617
polyomaviruses in, 1402, 1402t
prevention of infection, 2691t, 2691–2694
antibiotics, 2692–2693
antifungals, 2693
antivirals, 2693
efficacy of regimens, 2692t
future goals, 2694
hematopoietic growth factors and, 2693t, 2693–2694
Pneumocystis carinii, 2693
Protomonas in, 2114
Pseudallescheria boydii in, 2390
Pseudomonas aeruginosa in, 1981, 1987, 1995
respiratory syncytial virus in, 1510–1511
Rhodococcus in, 1876
Salmonella in, 2019, 2020, 2023
treatment, 2027
skin infections in: post-traumatic opportunistic, 920
sporotrichosis in, 2322
Staphylococcus epidermidis bacteremia in, 1781
stomatitis in, 603
Streptococcus pneumoniae in, 1815
vaccination, 1823

Toxoplasma gondii in, 2455
clinical manifestations, 2459–2461
diagnosis, 2464–2465
prevention, 2469–2470
treatment, 2466f, 2466–2467, 2467t
transplant recipients. *See* Transplant recipients
Trypanosoma cruzi in, 2446
vaccines for, 2784, 2784t, 2785t
viral infections in, 411
viridans streptococcal infections in, 1847, 1849
VZV in, 1332t, 1347, 1348, 2658, 2660
prevention, 1350
treatment, 412t, 416
Immunodeficiency
cell-mediated, 132–139. *See also* Cell-mediated immunity, defects
clinical evaluation for suspected, 138–139, 149–158
common variable, 51
Giardia lamblia, 2489
and pneumonia, 621
congenital, 151t–152t
cytokine therapy, 138
directed tests, 152t
drug-induced, 135–137
evaluation, 149–158
HIV/AIDS. *See* Acquired immunodeficiency syndrome; Human immunodeficiency virus
humoral, 49–54. *See also* Immunoglobulin(s), deficiencies
index of suspicion, 149, 150t, 151t–152t
infectious processes and, 137–138
initial evaluation, 149–150, 152t
malnutrition and, 137
neoplasia and, 137. *See also* Chemotherapy patients
primary, 133–135, 134t
radiation-induced, 135–137
screening evaluations, 152t
severe combined, 52
T cell, 150, 152–153. *See also* T cells, deficiencies
Immunodiffusion tests, 191
for fungi, 193t
Immunofluorescence
for anaerobes, 2168
for bacteria, 192t
direct, 185, 191
for *Giardia lamblia*, 2490
for HIV, 1220
cytometric indirect, 1261
indirect
for *Babesia*, 2499
for *Toxoplasma gondii*, 2463
for *Trypanosoma cruzi*, 2446, 2447
for microsporidia, 2521
for *Pneumocystis carinii*, 2479
Immunogenicity, 165
Immunoglobulin A, 39
agglutination, 42
antiadhesion effects, 42
and bacterial meningitis, 838
deficiency, 151t
diagnosis, 50, 150
and enteric infections, 948
selective, 52, 948
distribution, 40
Fc receptors, 39, 40t, 41
functional properties, 37t

Immunoglobulin A *(Continued)*
Haemophilus influenzae and, 8, 20
and immunization, 2772
and intestinal immunity, 948
secretory component, 39
structure, 38f
testing for, 153
tests for *Toxoplasma gondii*, 2464, 2465
and urinary tract infections, 666
viral neutralization, 41
virulence factors and, 8
Immunoglobulin D, 39
function, 45t
functional properties, 37t
Immunoglobulin E, 39
antibody-dependent cellular cytotoxicity, 39
β-lactam reactions, 272, 274
and bronchiolitis, 615
Fc receptors, 39, 40t, 40–41
functional properties, 37t
HIV/AIDS and, 54
and immediate-type hypersensitivity, 39
tests for *Toxoplasma gondii*, 2464, 2465
Immunoglobulin G, 39
agglutination, 42
and complement activation, 41, 59
deficiencies, 39
diagnosis, 50
subclass (IgG₁ and IgG₂), 52
treatment, 50–51
distribution, 40
Fc receptors, 40, 40t
and phagocytosis, 41
functional properties, 37t
and HIV: IFA, 1259, 1259t
and immunization, 2772
rheumatoid factor, 42
and *Staphylococcus aureus*, 1761
structure, 38f
subclasses, 39
testing for, 153
tests for *Toxoplasma gondii*, 2464, 2465
and urinary tract infections, 666
viral neutralization, 41
Immunoglobulin M, 38–39
agglutination, 42
and complement activation, 41, 59
deficiencies: diagnosis, 50
function, 45t
functional properties, 37t
and HIV: IFA, 1259, 1259t
and immunization, 2772
rheumatoid factor, 42
testing for, 153
tests for *Toxoplasma gondii*, 2464, 2465
and urinary tract infections, 666
viral neutralization, 41
X-linked hyper-IgM syndrome, 51–52
Immunoglobulin(s). *See also* Antibodies
agglutination, 42
allotypes, 37
α: function, 45t
β: function, 45t
classes, 37t, 37–39. *See also individual immunoglobulins*
deficiencies, 49–54. *See also individual immunogloglobulins*
ataxia-telangiectasia, 52–53
bone marrow transplantation and, 53

combined T-cell and, 52–53
and defective opsonization, 91
diagnosis, 50
HIV-related, 53–54
malignancies and, 53
protein wasting states and, 53
secondary, 53–54
severe combined immunodeficiency, 52
sickle cell anemia and, 53
splenectomy and, 53
Wiskott-Aldrich syndrome, 52
distribution and catabolism, 40
and endocarditis, 746
Fab fragments, 37
FC receptors, 40t, 40–41
functional properties, 37t
heavy chains, 37
constant region, 37
for HIV inhibition, 1269
intravenous (IVIG), 50. *See also therapeutic below*
bone marrow transplantation and, 53
for IgA deficiency, 52
for IgG deficiency, 50
isotypes, 36. *See also specific isotypes*
switching: cytokines and T cells in, 119–120
light chains, 37
structure and chemistry, 36–37
therapeutic, 453–455, 2782–2783
currently available, 2773t
defined, 2770
for HAV, 1649t, 1649–1650
for HBV, 1428
for HIV, 2782
for immunocompromised host, 2693t, 2693–2694
for Kawasaki syndrome, 2568–2569, 2782
postexposure, 2785
for travelers, 2799
for viral meningitis, 854
viral neutralization, 41
Immunomodulators, 450–458
cimetidine, 455
colony-stimulating factors, 450–452
FDA approved, 450t
glucocorticoids, 455
immunoglobulins, 453–455
inflammatory cytokine blockers, 455
interferons, 452–453
interleukins, 453
pentoxifylline, 455
thymosin, 455–456
Immunophilins, 110
Immunosuppression. *See also Chemotherapy patients; Transplant recipients and individual drugs*
infection susceptibility and, 135–137
rifampin and, 319
transplant recipient infections, 2710–2711
CMV, 1355
and *Trypanosoma cruzi*, 2446
ureaplasma/mycoplasma and, 1716–1717
Immunotherapy: for anogenital warts, 1394
Impetigo, 909–911, 1763
bullous, 911
clinical features, 911
lesions, 555

Staphylococcus aureus, 1765
treatment, 911
clinical features, 910
contagiosa, 1791
differential diagnosis, 911
VZV, 1349
etiology, 911
group A streptococcal, 555, 1763
pathology and pathogenesis, 909–910
Staphylococcus aureus, 1763, 1764f
treatment
fusidic acid, 387
mupirocin, 386
presumptive, 911
topical antibacterials, 382
Incidence, 160
Incineration: of infectious waste, 2583
Indanyl carbenicillin, 245
dosage, 241t
in renal disease, 238t
pharmacokinetics, 238t
Indian tick typhus, 1725
Indirect immunofluorescence
for *Babesia*, 2499
for HIV, 1259, 1259t
Western blot and, 1259t
for *Toxoplasma gondii*, 2463
for *Trypanosoma cruzi*, 2446, 2447
Indirect transmission, 165–166
Indium-111 studies
brain abscess, 892
endocarditis, 750
and FUO, 540
hepatic abscess, 725
intraperitoneal abscess, 721, 722f
myocarditis, 803
osteomyelitis, 1044–1045
Indomethacin
for fever, 547
for septic shock, 701
Infantile genetic agranulocytosis, 89
Infantile paralysis. *See* Poliovirus
Infection
chain of, 164
defined, 19, 163, 690, 690t
in epidemiology, 159–160
endogenous, 164
exogenous, 164
gradient of, 164
Infection control, 2572–2575
antimicrobial utilization, 2573
education, 2572–2573
future challenges, 2575
hospital employee health, 2573
hospital epidemiology program, 2573–2575, 2574f
JCAHO, 2575
new product evaluation, 2573
outbreak investigation, 2572, 2572t
policy development, 2573
quality assessment, 2573
surveillance, 2572
in trauma patients, 2760
Infection control committee, 2573, 2575
Infectious disease: defined, 19–20
Infectious mononucleosis
CMV, 1357, 1372
differential diagnosis, 1372
EBV, 1367–1370. *See also* Epstein-Barr virus
enteric symptoms, 999t, 1003
herpesviruses, 1334t
Infectiousness, 164
Infectious waste disposal, 2582–2583
HIV material, 2643, 2643t

Infectivity, 164
Inferior petrosal sinus thrombosis, 907, 908t
Infertility: chlamydial infections and, 1687
Inflammation: neutrophils and, 80–83, 81f, 82f
Inflammatory bowel disease
diagnosis, 1006t
differential diagnosis: amebiasis, 2401
and fever, 545–546
perforation: and intraperitoneal abscess, 721
Inflammatory cytokine blockers: therapeutic, 455
Inflammatory responses: monocytes and, 123–124
Influenza virus, 1546–1567
antigenic drift, 1549
antigenic shift, 1549–1550
antigenic variation, 1549–1550
arthritis, 1036t
and bone marrow transplantation, 2720
bronchiolitis, 612t, 613, 613f
bronchitis, acute, 606, 606t
cardiac complications, 1558
classification, 1546
clinical features, 1555–1556
CNS complications, 1558
common cold, 562, 562t
complement-fixing (CF) test, 1554–1555
complications, 1556–1559
conjunctivitis, 1106
cytokine and T cell protection, 121t, 129–130
diagnosis, 1559–1560
epidemiologic, 1560
rapid, 1560
differential diagnosis, 1695
EIA diagnosis, 185
electron micrograph, 1547f
ELISA, 1554–1555
envelope, 1548–1549
epidemics, 1550f, 1550–1551, 1551t
proposed mechanism, 1552, 1552f
epidemiology, 1549–1553
and diagnosis, 1560
hemagglutination-inhibiting (HAI) test, 1554–1555
hemagglutinin, 1318f, 1548
binding site, 13
history, 1546
and HIV/AIDS: prophylaxis, 1286t
immunodeficiency and, 137
immunology, 1554–1555
interferon response, 1554
laryngitis, 573t
morphologic characteristics, 1547f, 1547–1548, 1548t
mortality rates, 1552–1553, 1553f, 1554f
M protein, 1548–1549
myalgia, 934
myositis, 1558
neuraminidase, 1548
nonpulmonary complications, 1558
nucleocapsid (ribonucleoprotein), 1549
pandemic, 1551–1552, 1552f
parotitis, 1500
pathologic characteristics, 1554, 1555f
pathophysiology, 1553–1555

peplomers, 1548
pharyngitis with, 567t, 568
pneumonia
  differential diagnosis, 1698
  nosocomial, 2600
    prevention, 2605
  prevention, 1560–1563. See also vaccines below
    chemoprophylaxis (amantadine or rimantadine), 1563
    nosocomial, 1563
  pulmonary complications, 1556t, 1556–1558, 1557t, 1704
    croup, 1557
    exacerbation of chronic pulmonary disease, 1557
    frequency, 1557–1558
    in the immunocompromised, 1557
    primary influenza pneumonia, 1556t, 1556–1557
    secondary bacterial pneumonia, 1556t, 1557, 1557t
    treatment, 1560
  receptors, 12, 13, 31, 1317t
  and Reye syndrome, 1558–1559, 1559t
  serology, 1559–1560
  sinusitis, 585, 585t
  and Streptococcus pneumoniae, 1817, 1817t
  therapeutic cytokines for, 131
  and toxic shock syndrome, 1558
  transmission, 1553
  treatment, 1560
    amantadine and rimantadine, 417, 419, 1560
    antivirals, 1560
    pulmonary complications, 1560
    ribavirin, 430, 431, 1560
    thymosin, 455
  type A, 1546
    antigenic subtypes, 1549, 1549t
    croup, 574, 574t, 576
    epidemics, 1550, 1551t
    genes and protein products, 1547, 1548t
    myocarditis, 800
    in other species, 1553
    pneumonia, 619t
      atypical, 630
    prophylaxis: amantadine, 419
    treatment, 412t
      amantadine and rimantadine, 417, 419
      ribavirin, 430, 431
    in U.S. (1957–1988), 1551t
  type B, 1546
    croup, 574, 574t
    myocarditis, 800
    pneumonia, 619t
      atypical, 630
    treatment: ribavirin, 431
  type C, 1546
  vaccines, 167, 1560–1563, 2777
    adverse reactions, 1561, 2777
    composition, 1561, 1561t
    for cystic fibrosis, 660
    and HIV/AIDS, 1561, 1562, 1562t
    live, 1562–1563
    recommendations, 1561–1562, 2776
      for adults, 2784t
      for HIV infected, 2785t
      for travelers, 2797t, 2799
  virion, 1547, 1547f

virus isolation, 1559
virus shedding, 1553f, 1553–1554
Inguinal adenopathy. See Lymphadenopathy, inguinal
Inguinal buboes, 940t
  of nonvenereal origin, 939
  of venereal origin, 939
INH. See Isoniazid
Injection site abscesses, 926
Inositol triphosphate (IP₃)
  and PKC activation, 86
  release, 45
  and T cell activation, 110
Insects. See also Arthropods
  travel and, 2800
Insertion elements: and pathogenicity, 22
Insertion sequences: and resistance, 213
Insomnia, fatal familial, 883–884
Institution-based disease prevention, 166
Integrin-modulating factor (IMF-1), 82
Integrins, 12t, 81, 81f, 82
  eosinophils and, 96
  regulation, 82
Integrons, 214
Intensive care units (ICUs): as reservoirs of microorganisms, 2756
Intercellular adhesion molecule. See ICAM
Interferon-α, 34
  actions, 30t
  adverse reactions, 428, 1273
  antiviral action, 426–430
  2b: and common cold, 565
  and B cells, 120
  biologic properties, 535t
  characteristics, sources, and effects, 114t, 115
  clinical studies, 428
  and fever, 530, 532f
  formulations available, 452
  as HIV marker, 1223
  mechanism of action, 426–427
  and MHC II, 104
  and muscle proteolysis, 935
  pharmacokinetics, 427–428
  recombinant, 452–453, 530. See also therapeutic use below
  synergism in combination therapy, 426–427
  and T-cell proliferation, 119
  therapeutic use, 452–453
    for anogenital warts, 1394–1395
    for EBV, 1372
    for hepatitis, 412t, 428, 429, 1150
      HBV, 1427
      HCV, 1156–1157, 1483
    for herpesviruses, 429
    for HIV, 429, 1273
    for Kaposi's sarcoma, 1244, 1273
    for papillomaviruses, 429
    for respiratory syncytial virus, 1512
    for respiratory viruses, 429–430
Interferon-β, 113
  adverse reactions, 428
  characteristics, sources, and effects, 114t, 115
  clinical studies, 428
  and fever, 530, 532f
  mechanism of action, 426–427
  and MHC II, 104
  pharmacokinetics, 427–428
  recombinant. See therapeutic use below
  therapeutic use
    antiviral action, 426–430

for hepatitis C virus, 1483
  synergism in combination therapy, 426–427
Interferon-γ, 34, 82, 83, 113
  actions, 30t
  antiparasitic use, 459t
  and B cells, 120
  biologic properties, 535
  characteristics, sources, and effects, 114t, 116, 117, 124
  and Chlamydia trachomatis, 1681
  and CMV, 129
  and cytotoxic T cells, 121
  deficiency, 132, 133
  and Francisella tularensis, 2063
  injurious effects, 131
  Leishmania and, 2430, 2431
  and macrophages, 124
  and MHC II, 104
  recombinant, 453. See also therapeutic use below
  and sepsis, 693, 694t
  therapeutic use, 130, 131, 453
    for hepatitis, 428–429
    in HIV/AIDS, 130–131
    for the immunocompromised, 2693t, 2694
      prophylactic, 2693t, 2693–2694
    in immunodeficiency, 138
    for Leishmania, 2430, 2433, 2438
    for neutrophil defects, 94
    protection from infection, 121t, 125, 126, 127, 128, 129
    for Toxoplasma gondii, 2469
    for Trypanosoma cruzi, 2448
  and Toxoplasma gondii, 2458
  and viral meningitis, 836
Interferon(s). See also individual interferons
  for anogenital warts, 1394
  antiviral use, 426–430
    adverse reactions, 428
    classification, 426, 427t
    clinical studies, 428
    drug interactions, 428
    for hepatitis, 428–429
    for herpesviruses, 429
    for HIV, 429
    mechanism of action, 426–427
    pharmacokinetics, 427–428
    for respiratory viruses, 429–430
  and fever, 530, 532f
  and HBV infection course, 1417
  and influenza virus, 1554
  therapeutic, 452–453
Interleukin-1, 34, 79, 530
  actions, 30t
  and acute phase response, 117
  α, 82, 530
    and hypothalamus, 532
    sources, 11r
  and bacterial meningitis, 839–840, 840
  β, 82, 530
    and hypothalamus, 532
  biologic properties, 535t
  characteristics, sources, and effects, 114t, 115, 116, 117, 123
  and complement, 59
  and Escherichia coli, 1968
  and fever, 117, 530, 531, 534
  and hypothalamus, 532f, 532–533
  injurious effects, 131
  and meningococcal infections, 1904
  and muscle proteolysis, 935

and Mycobacterium avium-intracellulare, 2252
  and pneumonia, 620
  and pulmonary endothelial injury, 696
  receptor antagonist (IL-1ra)
    characteristics, sources, and effects, 114t, 115, 123
    inflammatory effects, 131–132
  recombinant, 530
  and sepsis, 693, 694t, 696
  and septic shock, 118
  therapeutic use, 453
  and thymocytes, 107
  and tissue injury, 88
Interleukin-2, 113
  actions, 30t
  aging and, 133
  and B cells, 120
  characteristics, sources, and effects, 114t, 116
  deficiency, 134t, 151t
  HIV and, 1208
  and HSV, 107
  NK cells and, 122
  and pulmonary vascular leak syndrome, 696
  receptor, 113
  and sepsis, 694t
  and T-cell proliferation, 118
  therapeutic use, 130, 131, 453
    in HIV/AIDS, 131
    in immunodeficiency, 138
  and thymocytes, 107
  and Toxoplasma gondii, 2458
Interleukin-3, 79
  actions, 30t
  characteristics, sources, and effects, 114t, 116
  and eosinophils, 95
  and hematopoiesis, 118
  HIV and, 1211
  and IgE Fc receptors, 40
  and intestinal parasites, 128
  receptor, 113
  therapeutic use, 452
Interleukin-4, 113
  actions, 30t
  and B cells, 120
  characteristics, sources, and effects, 114t, 116
  and cytotoxic T cells, 121
  HIV and, 1211
  and IgE Fc receptors, 40
  and intestinal parasites, 128
  and MHC II, 104
  protection from infection, 121t, 125
  receptor, 113
  and sepsis, 694t
  and T-cell proliferation, 118, 119
  and thymocytes, 107
Interleukin-5, 113
  and B cells, 120
  characteristics, sources, and effects, 114t, 116
  and eosinophils, 95
  and helminthic infections, 96
  and IgE Fc receptors, 40
  receptor, 113
  and sepsis, 694t
Interleukin-6, 34, 82, 113
  actions, 30t
  and acute phase response, 117, 534
  and B cells, 120
  characteristics, sources, and effects, 114t, 115, 117, 123

Interleukin-6 *(Continued)*
  and complement, 59
  and fever, 530, 534
  and hematopoiesis, 118
  HIV and, 1210, 1211
  and hypothalamus, 532
  and meningococcal infections,
      1904
  and muscle proteolysis, 935
  and *Mycobacterium avium-intra-
      cellulare*, 2252
  receptor, 113
  and sepsis, 695
  and septic shock, 118
  and T-cell proliferation, 118
  and *Toxoplasma gondii*, 2458
  and viral meningitis, 836
Interleukin-7, 113
  characteristics, sources, and effects,
      114t
  and cytotoxic T cells, 121
  receptor, 113
  and T-cell proliferation, 118
  and thymocytes, 107
Interleukin-8, 82
  actions, 30t
  and B cells, 120
  characteristics, sources, and effects,
      114t, 115
  and pneumonia, 620
  and sepsis, 694t, 694–695
Interleukin-9
  characteristics, sources, and effects,
      114t, 116
  and hematopoiesis, 118
  receptor, 113
  and T-cell proliferation, 118
Interleukin-10, 113
  actions, 30t
  and B cells, 120
  characteristics, sources, and effects,
      114t, 115, 116, 117, 123
  and cytotoxic T cells, 121
  and hematopoiesis, 118
  protection from infection, 125, 129
  for sepsis, 132
  and *Toxoplasma gondii*, 2458
Interleukin-11, 113, 530
  and acute phase response, 534
  and B cells, 120
  characteristics, sources, and effects,
      114t
  and hypothalamus, 532
Interleukin-12, 34
  actions, 30t
  characteristics, sources, and effects,
      114t, 115, 117
  and cytotoxic T cells, 121
  protection from infection, 121t, 125,
      126
  and T-cell proliferation, 119
Interleukin-13: characteristics, sources,
      and effects, 114t, 116,
      117
Interleukin(s), 112. *See also individual
      interleukins*
  HIV and, 1211
  therapeutic use, 453
Interphalangeal joint: infectious arthritis,
      1033, 1033t
Intertrigo
  Candida albicans, 2294
  infectious, 1081
  spinal cord injury and, 2733
Intestinal carcinoma: fever, 544

Intestinal cestodes (tapeworms),
      2546–2548. *See also individ-
      ual species*
Intestinal flagellates: antiparasitic agents,
      458, 467–468
Intestinal flora, normal, 2159, 2159t
Intestinal flukes, 2538t, 2542–2543
  Fasciolopsis buski, 2538t, 2542–2543
  Heterophyes heterophyes, 2538t, 2543
Intestinal immune system, 112
  and gastrointestinal infections, 948
  and tropical sprue, 1026
Intestinal motility: and gastrointestinal
      infections, 947
Intestinal perforation: and peritonitis,
      710
Intestinal roundworms, 2526–2531,
      2527t. *See also* Roundworms,
      intestinal
Intestinal tract
  barrier to microorganisms, 32
  infections. *See* Gastrointestinal infec-
      tions
Intra-abdominal abscess
  actinomycosis and, 729
  aminoglycosides for, 288–289
  anaerobic gram-negative bacilli, 2196
      treatment, 2201
  appendicitis and, 727–728
  diverticulitis and, 728–729
  and fever, 541
  hepatic, 724–727
  liver transplantation and, 2725
  necrotizing enterocolitis in neu-
      tropenics and, 729
  pancreatic, 723–724
  regional enteritis and, 729
  sources, 727–729
  splenic, 727
Intra-abdominal infections, 705–740. *See
      also specific infections*
  actinomycosis, 2283f, 2283–2284
  anaerobic, 2163t, 2165
      cocci, 2205
      gram-negative bacilli, 2198–2199
      specimen collection, 2168t
      treatment, 2201
  cholangitis, 732–733
  cholecystitis, acute, 729–732
  Clostridium, 2184–2185
  enterococcal, 1828
  gram-negative anaerobes, 2198–2199
  intraperitoneal abscesses, 721–722
  liver transplantation and, 2725–2726
  Salmonella, 2022
  specimen collection and processing,
      171t, 178
  in spinal cord injured patients,
      2735–2736
  Streptococcus intermedius group, 1863
  in transplant recipients, 2727–2728
  treatment
      aminoglycosides, 288–289
      quinolones, 371–372
  visceral abscess, 724–727
      hepatic, 724–727
      pancreatic, 723–724
      splenic, 727
Intra-amniotic infection syndrome (IAIS),
      1090
Intracranial hypertension: bacterial
      meningitis and, 841
  reduction, 856
Intracranial infections: *Acinetobacter*,
      2011

Intracranial mass lesions: HIV/AIDS
      and, 1237t, 1237–1239, 1238f
Intracranial pressure, increased. *See*
      Intracranial hypertension
Intracranial thrombophlebitis, suppura-
      tive, 907–909
  antibiotic therapy, 902t
  bacteriology, 902t
  clinical features, 907
  diagnosis, 907, 908f
  pathology, 907
  treatment, 907–908
Intraepithelial lymphocytes (IEL), 112
Intraepithelial neoplasia, 1388t. *See also*
      Human papillomavirus
Intraperitoneal abscesses, 721–722
  bacteriology, 721
  clinical manifestations, 721
  diagnosis, 722, 722f, 723f
  etiology, 721
  pathogenesis, 722
  prognosis, 722
  treatment, 722
Intrarenal abscess, 662
  diagnosis and therapy, 682, 682f
Intrarenal reflux, 672–673
Intraurethral catheters, 2611
Intrauterine devices
  actinomycosis and, 2281, 2284
  and peritonitis, 709
  and PID, 1095
Intravascular devices. *See also* Catheter-
      related infections
  bacteremia from, 2587–2599
      arterial lines, 2595–2596, 2596t
      central venous catheters, 2592
          long-term, 2594t, 2594–2595
      contamination
          of infusate, 2587
          at insertion site, 2588t,
              2588–2589, 2589t
          at junction, 2587
      device-specific issues, 2591–2596
      diagnosis, 2590f, 2590t, 2590–2591
      microbiology, 2589t, 2589–2590
      pathogenesis, 2587–2588, 2588f
      peripheral IV cannulization, 2591t,
          2591–2592
      prevention, 2596
      pulmonary artery catheters, 2595
      total parenteral nutrition,
          2592–2594, 2593t
      transducer domes, 2595–2596
      transducers, 2595
Intravascular infections, cardiac, 741–783.
      See also Cardiovascular infec-
      tions
  endocarditis, infective, 740–765. *See
      also* Endocarditis, infective
  mycotic aneurysms, 770–774
  suppurative thrombophlebitis,
      765–769
Intravenous drug abusers. *See* Drug
      abusers
Intravenous drug administration, 209
Intraventricular drug administration, 209
Intussusception, adenoviral, 1385–1386
Invasin gene, 7
Invasive organisms, 7
inv operon, 7
Iodochlorhydroxyquin, 468, 971
Iodophors, 382
Iodoquinol, 459t, 468
  dosage, 461t, 462t
      pediatric, 461t, 462t

Ionophores, 86
Iota toxin, 3t
Iridocyclitis
  Bacillus, 1891
  VZV and, 1348
Iritis: *Borrelia burgdorferi*, 2148
Iron: and microorganisms, 31–32
Isepamicin, 280
  source and chemistry, 280t
ISI 2105, 437t
Islet-activating protein. *See* Pertussis
      toxin
Isohemagglutinin tests, 153
Isolation, 2575–2579
  body substance, 2576t, 2577t, 2578
  category-specific, 2576t, 2576–2578,
      2577t
  comparison of methods, 2576t
  contact, 2576, 2577t
  disease-specific, 2576t, 2577t, 2578
  drainage/secretion precautions, 2577,
      2577t
  enteric precautions, 2577, 2577t
  essential elements, 2577t
  respiratory, 2576, 2577t
  strict, 2576, 2577t
  tuberculosis (acid-fast bacilli),
      2576–2577, 2577t
  universal precautions, 2576t, 2577t,
      2578
Isoniazid
  adverse reactions, 203, 390, 390t
  antimicrobial activity, 389
  dosage, 391, 516t–517t
      for children, 516t
      in hepatic and renal failure, 390,
          390t, 517t
  drug interactions, 390, 523t
  hepatotoxicity, 390, 390t, 1148,
      2229–2230
      in prophylaxis, 2229–2230
  for *Mycobacterium avium-intracellu-
      lare*, 2257, 2257t
  for *Mycobacterium tuberculosis*, 391,
      1289, 2226, 2227, 2227t,
      2228, 2229, 2230, 2231, 2232,
      2233, 2234, 2239
      for the elderly, 2739
      miliary, 2233
      prophylaxis, 1283t, 1289, 2229
      resistance, 2214, 2226
      tuberculous meningitis, 2234
  for nontuberculous (atypical)
      mycobacteria, 395, 2267,
      2268, 2269
  pharmacology, 390, 516t–517t
  resistance, 389
  structure, 389f
  and sugar level testing, 203
Isoproterenol: for sepsis syndrome, 700,
      700t
Isospora belli, 2394t, 2510–2511
  clinical manifestations, 2394t
  diagnosis, 1006t, 1007–1008
  diarrhea
      in AIDS, 970, 970t
      chronic, 972, 994
  differential diagnosis
      amebiasis, 2402
      Cryptosporidium, 2504
  enterocolitis: and HIV/AIDS, 1230
  and HIV/AIDS, 2510–2511
      diarrhea, 970, 970t
      enterocolitis, 1230
      incidence, 1182t

transmission, 2394t
treatment, 463t, 469, 473
   in HIV/AIDS, 1289
   trimethoprim-sulfamethoxazole,
      360, 474, 1289
Isoxazolyl penicillins, 243
   dosage, 241t
      in neonates, 242t
      in renal disease and dialysis, 238t
   pharmacokinetics, 238t
   structure, 242f
   trade names, 236t
ITPA index: *Treponema pallidum*, 2128
Itraconazole, 404, 408
   for *Blastomyces dermatitidis*, 408,
      2362–2363
   for candidiasis: vulvovaginitis, 404
   for chromomycosis, 2326
   for *Coccidioides immitis*, 1283t, 1289
   for *Cryptococcus neoformans*, 408,
      2337
   for dermatophytosis, 2382
   dosage, 518t–519t
      in renal dysfunction, 205
   drug interactions, 523t
   for esophagitis, 964t
   for *Histoplasma capsulatum*, 408,
      1283t, 1289, 2350
   for *Leishmania*, 2431
   for microsporidia, 2522
   for paracoccidioidomycosis,
      2388–2389
   pharmacology, 518t–519t
   for pityriasis versicolor, 2383
   structure, 402f
   for vulvovaginal candidiasis, 1076,
      1076t
IUDR. *See* Idoxuridine
Iveegam, 454
Ivermectin, 460t, 481–482
   dosage, 462t, 466t
      pediatric, 462t, 466t
   for filariasis, 2534
   for onchocerciasis, 481, 1126, 2536
   spectrum of activity, 481
Ixodes
   and encephalitis, 1466t, 1467, 1469
   and flaviviruses, 1466t, 1467, 1469
   reservoirs, 2794
Ixodes dammini (scapularis), 2565, 2566f
   and babesiosis, 2498, 2500
   and *Borrelia burgdorferi*, 2145, 2565,
      2566
   and ehrlichiosis, 1748
Ixodes pacificus: and *Borrelia burg-*
   dorferi, 2145, 2565
Ixodes ricinus: and Colorado tick fever,
   1446
Ixodidae, 2565

J

Jail fever. *See* Typhus, epidemic
Jamestown Canyon virus, 1567
   characteristics, 1568t
   clinical manifestations, 1570
   epidemiology, 1568
   meningitis, 832
Janeway lesions, 554, 747, 748f,
   748–749, 922, 1768f
J5 antisera: for immunocompromised
   host, 2693t, 2693–2694
Japanese encephalitis, 1466t,
   1466–1467, 1468, 1471
   clinical manifestations, 1471

epidemiology, 1468
history, 1466–1467
and HIV/AIDS, 1470
pathogenesis, 1470
serology, 191
transmission, clinical syndromes, and
   geographic distribution, 1466t
vaccine, 167, 2777
   adverse reactions, 2777
   indications for adults, 2784t
   for travelers, 2777, 2797t,
      2798–2799
Japan small round-structured viruses
   (SRSV)
   characteristics, 1668, 1668t
   diagnosis, 1670–1671
Jarisch-Herxheimer reaction
   Borrelia relapsing fever, 2143
   rat-bite fever treatment, 2086
   syphilis treatment, 2130–2131
Jaundice
   hepatitis, 1138
   leptospirosis, 2137, 2139
Jaw osteomyelitis, 601
JC virus, 1288, 1400–1406. *See also*
   Leukoencephalopathy, progressive multifocal
   in bone marrow transplant recipients,
      1402, 1402t
   clinical manifestations, 1401–1402,
      1402t
   description, 1400
   diagnosis, 1402–1404
   epidemiology, 1400
   and neoplasia, 1402
   pathogenesis, 1401
   in pregnancy, 1401–1402, 1402t
   prevention and treatment, 1404
   in renal transplant recipients, 1402,
      1402t, 2723
   tropism, 1322
J5 lipopolysaccharidase, 41
Job syndrome, 91, 150, 151t
   diagnosis, 150
   features, 155–156
   Staphylococcus aureus and, 1762
Jock itch, 2378
Joint fluid aspiration: prosthetic joint
   infections, 1053
Joint infections, 1032–1056. *See also*
   Bone infections *and specific*
   infections
   anaerobic
      gram-negative bacilli, 2200
      specimen collection, 2168t
   arthritis, 1032–1039
   Blastomyces dermatitidis, 2356t,
      2359–2360, 2360f
   Borrelia burgdorferi, 2147
   Coccidioides immitis, 2367–2368,
      2369f
      treatment, 2372
   in drug abusers, 2698
   prostheses, 1051–1055
      bacteriology, 1052, 1052t
      clinical presentation, 1052–1053,
         1053t
      diagnosis, 1053f, 1053–1054
      pathogenesis, 1052–1053
      prevention, 1054–1055
      therapy, 1054
         suppressive antibiotic,
            1054–1055
   Pseudomonas aeruginosa, 1992–1994
      treatment, 1992–1994

quinolones for, 372
rheumatic fever, 1803
sporotrichosis, 2322
Joint pain: and prosthetic infections,
   1053
Jugular thrombophlebitis, suppurative,
   600
Jungle yellow fever, 1467
Junin virus, 1572
   characteristics, 1573t
   epidemiology, 1574
   pathogenesis, 1575
   prevention and treatment, 1577
   serology, 191

K

Kala azar, 2428t, 2431–2434. *See also*
   Leishmania donovani
   clinical manifestations, 2432
   diagnosis, 2432–2433
   differential diagnosis, 2433
   epidemiology, 2431
   immunology and pathology,
      2431–2432
   prevention, 2433–2434
   treatment, 2433
Kanamycin, 280
   antimicrobial activity, 285t
   combination therapy, 287t
   dosage, 510t–511t
      in children and neonates, 510t
      in hepatic or renal failure, 390t,
         511t
   for *Mycobacterium tuberculosis*,
      395
   neuromuscular blockade, 295
   ototoxicity, 294
   pharmacology, 510t–511t
   resistance
      anaerobic gram-negative bacilli,
         2196t
      enterococci, 1830
   source and chemistry, 280t
   structure, 281f
Kanamycin-vancomycin laked blood
   agar (KVLB), 2168
K antigen
   Escherichia coli, 24, 966, 966t, 1965,
      1968–1969
   Klebsiella, 1972
Kaposi's sarcoma
   CMV and, 1352
   differential diagnosis, 2210
   HIV/AIDS and, 1240–1244,
      1590–1591, 1602
      clinical appearance, 1241, 1241t
      diagnosis of cutaneous, 1242
      epidemiology, 1170, 1240–1244
      gastrointestinal, 1229–1230,
         1241–1242
      incidence, 1182t, 1183
      management, 1242–1244
      oral, 1242
      pathophysiology, 1241, 1602
      probability of developing, 1223f
      prognostic variables, 1241–1242,
         1243t
      pulmonary, 1242
      spindle cells, 1602
      staging and clinical course,
         1242–1243
      therapy, 1243t, 1243–1244, 1290
         local, 1243–1244
         systemic, 1244

treatment
   in HIV/AIDS, 1243t, 1243–1244,
      1290
   interferon-α, 1244, 1273, 1290
Kartagener syndrome
   chemotactic defect, 91
   and pneumonia, 621
Katayama fever, 2539, 2540
   enteric symptoms, 1000t, 1003
Kawasaki syndrome, 2567–2569
   cardiac involvement, 2568
   clinical features, 2567t, 2567–2568,
      2568t
   Coxiella burnetii and, 1733
   diagnosis, 2567, 2567t
   differential diagnosis, 1765
   epidemiology, 2567
   erythema, 552
   etiology and pathogenesis, 2568
   and fever, 542
   laboratory findings, 2568
   lymphadenopathy, 941
   pathology, 2568
   pharyngitis, 569
   strawberry tongue, 553
   treatment, 2568–2569
      immunoglobulin, 454
Kefurox. *See* Cefuroxime
Kefzol. *See* Cefazolin
Kelftab. *See* Cephalexin
Kell-related antigen K_x: and GCD, 95
Keloidal blastomycosis, 2392
Kemerova virus, 1448
Kenya tick typhus, 1725
Keratinocyte: and inflammatory
   response, 550
Keratitis, 1110–1120
   Acanthamoeba, 1114, 2408, 2411,
      2412f, 2413, 2413f
      prevention, 2414
      treatment, 1118, 2414
   adenoviral, 1385
   bacterial, 1111t, 1112–1113
   Borrelia burgdorferi, 2148
   Chlamydia trachomatis, 1114
   clinical manifestations, 1111–1112,
      1112f
   etiology, 1111, 1111t
   fungal, 1111t, 1113
   herpes simplex virus, 1115
      disciform, 1115
      recurrence, 1337, 1339
      treatment, 1118
         interferons, 429
   laboratory investigations, 1116
   other causes, 1114–1115
   parasitic, 1111t, 1114
   Pseudomonas aeruginosa, 1112, 1113,
      1991
   treatment, 1116–1118
   Treponema pallidum, 2126
   varicella-zoster virus, 1115, 1348
      treatment, 1118
         interferons, 429
   viral, 1111t, 1115–1116
Keratoacanthoma, giant, 2356
Keratoconjunctivitis. *See also* Conjunctivitis; Keratitis
   adenovirus, 1105, 1115, 1385
   epidemic: differential diagnosis,
      1631
   herpes simplex virus
      recurrence, 1339
      treatment, 412t
   herpesviruses, 1334t

Keratoconjunctivitis *(Continued)*
  phlyctenular: and *Mycobacterium tuberculosis*, 2220, 2222
  sicca (Sjögren's syndrome), 1107
Keratoderma
  blenorrhagicum: Reiter syndrome, 1071
  palmar plantar, 2379
Keratoplasty, 1116
Kerion, 2380
Kernig's sign: bacterial meningitis, 843, 843t
Ketoconazole, 404, 407
  antiparasitic use, 459t, 477–478
  for *Blastomyces dermatitidis*, 407, 2362–2363
  for *Candida albicans*, 2299, 2300, 2301
    in HIV/AIDS, 1283t, 1288, 2301
    vulvovaginitis, 404
  for chromomycosis, 2326
  for *Coccidioides immitis*, 407, 1283t, 1289, 2371
  for dermatophytosis, 2382
  dosage, 518t–519t
    in renal dysfunction, 205, 519t
  drug interactions, 523t
  for esophagitis, 964t
  for granulocytopenics, 2680
  for *Histoplasma capsulatum*, 407, 2350–2351
  for *Leishmania*, 2431, 2435
  for neutropenics, 2688t, 2690
  for paracoccidioidomycosis, 2388
  pharmacology, 518t–519t
  for pityriasis versicolor, 2383
  structure, 402f
  susceptibility testing, 193
  for thrush, 403
  topical, 401t
  for vulvovaginal candidiasis, 1076, 1076t
Keyhole limpet hemocyanin, 153
Kidney. *See entries commencing with the terms* Nephr- *and* Renal
Kikuchi's disease, 941
Kingella, 1930
  characteristics, 2010t
  endocarditis, 756
Kingella dentrificans, 1930
  identification, 1927t
Kingella indologenes, 1930
  identification, 1927t
  laboratory identification, 1927t
Kingella kingae, 1930
  biochemical reactions, 2107t
  endocarditis, 756
  identification, 1927t
Kinyoun stain, 184t
  for mycobacteria, 2214
Kissing bugs: and American trypanosomiasis, 2442
Klebsiella, 1972–1973
  after gynecologic surgery, 1093–1094
  β-lactamase, 215
  biliary tract, 2165
  and bone marrow transplantation, 2719
  cholecystitis, 730
  diarrhea: infantile, 967
  in drug abusers, 2697, 2698
  endocarditis, 755
    treatment, 763
  enterotoxin, 5
  mediastinitis, 815t

meningitis, 834
mycotic aneurysms, 772
necrotizing enterocolitis of newborn, 991
necrotizing fasciitis, 923
prostatitis, 680
  in renal transplantation, 2723
resistance, 1972, 2750
suppurative thrombophlebitis, 768
symmetric peripheral gangrene, 553
toxin, 950
treatment
  fluoroquinolones, 228–229
  penicillins, 237t
  quinolones, 367t
and tropical sprue, 1026
urinary tract infections, 667
  in the elderly, 2737
  nosocomial, 2608–2609, 2609t
Klebsiella ornithinolytica, 1975t
Klebsiella oxytoca, 1975t
  β-lactamase, 215
  carbapenems for, 264t
Klebsiella ozaenae, 1972–1973, 1975t
Klebsiella planticola, 1975t
Klebsiella pneumoniae, 1972–1973
  aminoglycoside resistance, 218, 284t
  β-lactamase, 216t, 217
  in cancer patients, 2668
  and granulocytopenia, 2676
  human bites, 2768
  and leukemia, 2672
  lung abscess, 642, 644
  in neutropenics, 2672t
  orchitis, 1101
  peritonitis, 708, 711
    in peritoneal dialysis, 719
  pneumonia, 619t, 622
    community-acquired, 629
    necrotizing, 644
    nosocomial, 2600
      in the immunocompromised, 631
    radiology, 626
  sinusitis, 585
  treatment
    aminoglycosides, 285t, 288, 295t
      combination therapy, 289t
    antimicrobials of choice, 202t
    aztreonam, 267t
    β-lactamase inhibitors, 268t
    carbapenems, 264t
    cephalosporins, 255, 255t, 257
    chloramphenicol, 312t
    rifampin, 318t
    tetracyclines, 308t
    trimethoprim, 357
Klebsiella rhinoscleromatis, 1972, 1975t
  rifampin for, 324
Klebsielleae, 1972–1973. *See also specific species*
Klefex. *See* Cephalexin
Kluyvera ascorbata, 1975t
Kluyvera cryocrescens, 1975t
Knee
  infectious arthritis, 1032, 1033t
    in the elderly, 2741
  replacements: *Staphylococcus aureus* infections, 1773, 1781–1782
Koch's postulate: applied to gene virulence, 26–27
Koch's tuberculin, 2219
Koplik spots, 1519, 1521, 1522–1523
Korean hemorrhagic fever, 2793
Kostmann syndrome, 154
Kotonkan virus, 1529

Krause, gland of, 1130
Kunjin: transmission, clinical syndromes, and geographic distribution, 1466t
Kuru, 881, 1674
  specimen handling, 884
Kyasanur Forest disease: transmission, clinical syndromes, and geographic distribution, 1466t
Kyzylagach virus, 1457

L

Labetalol: for *Clostridium tetani*, 2176, 2177
Laboratory studies, 169–198
  agglutination, 185
  detection of antibodies, 191, 192t, 193t
  determination of antimicrobial activity, 193–198
    anaerobic bacteria, 195
    assays, 196–197
    bactericidal tests, 195–196
    β-lactamase test, 198
    bioassay, 197, 197f
    broth test, 195–196
    combination studies, 196, 196f
    dilution tests, 195
    disk diffusion, 195
    disk elution, 195
    E-test, 195
    high-pressure liquid chromatography, 197–198
    immunoassay, 197
    methods, 195
    selection of antimicrobials, 193–195, 194t
    serum bactericidal test, 196
    susceptibility tests, 191–193
  diarrhea: specimen collection and processing, 171t, 180–181
  direct immunofluorescence, 185
  DNA probe hybridization, 184–185
  enzyme immunoassays, 185
  genital infections: specimen collection and processing, 171t, 181–183
  growth or biochemical characteristics, 185–189
    bacteria, 185–189
      aerobic, 186
      anaerobic, 189
      facultative anaerobic, 185f, 186, 189
      gram-negative bacilli, 186, 188f
      gram-negative cocci, 186, 188f
      gram-positive bacilli, 186.189
      gram-positive cocci, 186, 187
    fungi, 190
    mycobacteria, 189–190
    viruses, 190–191, 191f
  identification of organisms, 183–191
    immunoassays, 184–185
    microscopy, 184
      stained, 184, 184t
      unstained, 184
  musculoskeletal infections: specimen collection and processing, 171t, 179–180
  ocular infections: specimen collection and processing, 171t, 183–184
  respiratory tract: specimen collection and processing, 169–175, 170t, 172t

septicemia: specimen collection and processing, 170t, 177–178
specimen collection and processing, 169, 170t–171t
  guidelines, 169–183
urinary tract: specimen collection and processing, 170t, 175–177
Lacrimal apparatus infections, 1130–1131
Lacrimal drainage: evaluation, 1133
La Crosse virus, 1567
  characteristics, 1568t
  clinical manifestations, 1569–1570
  encephalomyelitis, 876
  epidemiology, 1568
  meningitis, 832
β-Lactamases. *See* β-lactamases
Lactate dehydrogenase virus: receptor, 1317t
D-Lactic acidosis: and anaerobes, 2160
Lactic dehydrogenase (LDH): hepatitis, 1139–1140, 1140f
Lactobacillus, 2158t, 2207–2208
  endocarditis, 756
  as enteric flora, 947
  mediastinitis, 815t
  as normal flora, 2159t
  and normal physiology, 2160
  oral colonization, 593, 594t
  vaginal flora, 1074, 1093
Lactobacillus acidophilus, 2208
  for bacterial vaginosis, 1080
  vaginal flora, 1074
  for vulvovaginal candidiasis, 1077
Lactoferrin, 79t, 87, 88
Lactose intolerance
  diagnosis, 953
  and tropical sprue, 1027
Laennec's cirrhosis: and fever, 547
Lagophthalmous leprosy, 2248
Lagos bat virus, 1528t, 1529
Lambert-Eaton myasthenic syndrome (LEMS), 2180
Laminectomy: prophylaxis recommendations, 2751t
Laminin, 79t
Lamivudine, 437t
Landry-Guillain-Barré syndrome, 829. *See also* Guillain-Barré syndrome
Langerhans cells
  HIV and, 1205
  and inflammatory response, 550
Laparoscopy: and FUO, 541
Laparotomy
  and FUO, 541
  for postabortal infections, 1093
  prophylaxis recommendations, 2751t
Larva migrans
  cutaneous (creeping eruption), 2555
  ocular, 2554
  visceral, 2553–2554
Laryngeal edema, allergic: epiglottitis vs., 591
Laryngeal infections
  Corynebacterium diphtheriae, 1869
  diphtheria, 1869–1870
Laryngitis
  acute, 572–573
    diagnosis, 573
    etiology, 573t
    treatment, 573
  Moraxella catarrhalis, 1927
  Mycobacterium tuberculosis, 2240

Laryngotracheobronchitis, acute (croup), 573–579, 1489–1496. *See also* Parainfluenza virus
  clinical manifestations, 575–576
  complications, 577
  diagnosis, 576–577, 577f
  differential diagnosis, 591
  epidemiology, 575
  etiology, 574t, 574–575
  incidence, 574
  influenza virus and, 1557
  laboratory findings, 576
  pathophysiology, 575
  physiologic correlations, 575, 576f
  respiratory syncytial virus, 574, 574t, 1504t
  treatment, 577–578
Laser therapy: for anogenital warts, 1394
Lassa virus
  characteristics, 1572, 1573t
  clinical manifestations, 1576
  diagnosis, 1576–1577
  electron micrograph, 1573f
  epidemiology, 1574, 2800
  intrauterine, 1576
  lymphadenitis, 940t
  pathogenesis, 1575
  prevention, 1577
  serology, 191
  treatment, 1577
    ribavirin, 430, 431
  waste management, 2582
Lateral pharyngeal space infection, 600
Lateral sinus thrombosis, 908, 908t
Latex agglutination test, 185
  for *Coccidioides immitis*, 2371
  for cryptococcosis, 2336
  CSF, 179
  for fungi, 193t
  for HIV, 1260
  for *Neisseria meningitidis*, 1903
  for pneumonia, 625
  for *Streptococcus agalactiae*, 1840
Latino virus, 1572
lck kinases, 109
LCM virus. *See* Lymphocytic choriomeningitis virus
LCR-1 β-lactamase, 216t
Lebombo virus, 1448
Leclercia adencarboxylata, 1975t
Lectinophagocytosis, 83
Lectins, 12t
  inhibition, 16
Legionella. See also individual species
  buffered charcoal yeast extract agar (BCYE), 2092, 2093, 2102
  clones, 21
  direct fluorescent antibody (DFA) stains, 2102
  genes, 26
  inhibiting phagocytosis, 7
  multilocus enzyme electrophoresis, 27
  penetration, 7
  pneumophila, 2087–2097. *See also Legionella pneumophila*
  replication mechanisms, 25
  spp. other than *pneumophila*, 2097–2103. *See also individual species*
    clinical manifestations, 2099f–2101f, 2101–2102
    description, 2098
    diagnosis, 2102

epidemiology, 2098–2099, 2101
  treatment, 2102
  toxin, 6–7
Legionella anisa, 2097t, 2098t
  epidemiology, 2098
Legionella birminghamensis, 2097t, 2098t
  epidemiology, 2098
Legionella bozemanii, 2097t, 2098t
  clinical manifestations, 2101, 2101f
  epidemiology, 2099
  nosocomial pneumonia, 2101, 2101f
Legionellaceae, 2087–2103
Legionella cincinnatiensis, 2097t, 2098t
Legionella dumoffii, 2097t, 2098t
  clinical manifestations, 2101
  epidemiology, 2098, 2099
Legionella feelei, 2097t, 2098, 2098t
Legionella gormanii, 2097t, 2098t
Legionella hackeliae, 2097t, 2098t
  epidemiology, 2098
Legionella jordanis, 2097t, 2098t
Legionella lansingensis, 2097t, 2098t
Legionella longbeachae, 2097t, 2098t
  epidemiology, 2098, 2099
Legionella maceachernii, 2097t, 2098, 2098t
  diagnosis, 2102
Legionella micdadei, 2097t, 2098, 2098t
  clinical manifestations, 2099f–2100f, 2101
  diagnosis, 2102
  epidemiology, 2098–2099
  and phagocytes, 88
  pneumonia, 619t
    nosocomial, 2099f–2100f, 2101
    radiology, 627
  in transplant recipients, 2712
  treatment
    erythromycin, 337
    rifampin, 322
Legionella oakridgensis, 2097t, 2098t
Legionella pneumophila, 2087–2097
  aerosolization, 2088–2089
  antibody detection, 2092t, 2093
  aspiration, 2088, 2089
  bronchoscopy, 174
  buffered charcoal yeast extract agar (BCYE), 2092, 2093
  catalase, 2087
  and cell-mediated immune defects, 2681
  clinical features, 2091–2092
    chest radiography, 2092
    extrapulmonary disease, 2092
    Legionnaire's disease, 2091–2092
    Pontiac fever, 2091
  clones, 21, 21t
  and complement, 66
  cooling towers and, 2088, 2094
  cultures, 2092t, 2092–2093
  cytokine protection, 121t, 127
  description, 2087f, 2087–2088
  direct fluorescence antibody stain, 2092t, 2093
  DNA probe, 2092t, 2093
  ecology, 2088
  enteric symptoms, 999t, 1003
  epidemiology, 2088–2089
  evaporative condensers and, 2088, 2094
  extracellular products, 2088
  fimbriae (pili), 2087
  history, 2087

and HIV/AIDS, 2089, 2090
  immunization research, 2094
  immunofluorescence, 185
  incidence, 2089
  38-kD metalloprotease, 2088
  laboratory diagnosis, 2092t, 2092–2093
  lipopolysaccharide, 2087
  lung tissue exam, 174–175
  macrophages and, 124
  morphology, 2087–2088
  myocarditis, 800
  outer membrane protein, 2087
  pathogenesis, 2089–2091, 2090f, 2091f
  pathology, 2089
  penetration, 7
  pericarditis, 805
  and phagocytes, 88
  pleural fluid, 174
  pneumonia, 619t, 622, 622t, 2090–2092
    atypical, 630, 1704
    community-acquired, 628
    differential diagnosis, 1698
    necrotizing, 644
    nosocomial, 2089, 2094, 2600
    radiology, 627
    serology, 625–626
    slowly resolving, 629
    sputum analysis, 623
    treatment, 631, 632
  polar flagella, 2087
  polymorphonuclear leukocytes and, 2090
  prevention, 2094
  prognosis, 2094
  replication mechanisms, 25
  reservoir disinfection, 2094
  serogroups, 2087
  serology, 192t
  sinusitis, 585
  sources of infection, 2088
  sputum, 173
  transmission, 164, 2088–2089
  in transplant recipients, 2712
  treatment, 2093t, 2093–2094
    aminoglycosides, 286
    antimicrobials of choice, 202t
    azithromycin, 335t
    clarithromycin, 335t, 339
    erythromycin, 335t, 337, 338t
    quinolones, 372
    rifampin, 322
  urinary antigen, 2092t, 2093
  virulence, 2090–2091
Legionella sainthelensi, 2097t, 2098t
Legionella tusconensis, 2097t, 2098t
Legionella wadsworthii, 2097t, 2098t
  epidemiology, 2098
Legionnaire's disease, 2091–2092. *See also Legionella pneumophila*
Leishmania, 2394t, 2428–2442
  amastigotes, 2429, 2429f
  cellular immunity and, 125
  classification, 2428, 2428t
  clinical manifestations, 2394t
  and complement, 66
  description, 2428–2429, 2429f
  diagnosis, 2395t
  differential diagnosis, 2326
  diffuse cutaneous, 2428t, 2434
    interferon-γ and antimony for, 130
  DNA probes, 2429
  geographical distribution, 2394t

gp63 protein, 2429
  immunodeficiency and, 138
  immunology, 2429–2430
  interferon-γ and, 130, 2430
  kala azar. *See* visceral *below*
  keratitis, 1114
  lipophosphoglycan (LPG), 2429
  mucosal, 2428t
    clinical manifestations, 2437
  new world cutaneous, 2428t, 2435–2438, 2436f, 2437f
    clinical manifestations, 2436–2437
    diagnosis, 2437
    differential diagnosis, 2437–2438
    epidemiology, 2435
    pathogenesis and immunology, 2435–2436
    treatment and prophylaxis, 2438
  old world cutaneous, 2428t, 2434–2435
    clinical manifestations, 2434–2435
    diagnosis, 2435
    epidemiology, 2434
    pathogenesis and immunology, 2434
    treatment and prophylaxis, 2435
  promastigote, 2429, 2429f
  recidivans, 2434
    treatment, 2435
  treatment, 475, 477–478, 2430–2431, 2435
    amphotericin B, 477–478
    ketoconazole, 477–478
    meglumine antimoniate, 477
    pentavalent antimony, 477
    pyrazolopyrimidines, 477
    rifampin, 323
    stibogluconate sodium, 477
  visceral (kala azar), 2428t, 2431–2434
    clinical manifestations, 2432
    diagnosis, 2432–2433
    differential diagnosis, 2433
    epidemiology, 2431
    immunology and pathology, 2431–2432
    post-kala-azar dermal leishmaniasis, 2432
    prevention, 2433–2434
    treatment, 2433
Leishmania aethiopica, 2428t
  cutaneous, 2434–2435
Leishmania amazonensis, 2428t, 2431–2434
  rifampin for, 323
Leishmania archibaldi, 2428t
Leishmania braziliensis, 2428t
  cutaneous disease, 2435–2438
  treatment, 463t
Leishmania chagasi, 2428t
  cutaneous disease, 2435–2438
  and HIV/AIDS, 1281
  visceral, 2431–2434
Leishmania donovani, 2428t, 2429, 2430
  amastigote, 2429f
  blepharoconjunctivitis, 1106
  cutaneous, 2434–2435
  cytokine and T cell protection, 121t
  lymphadenitis, 940t
  macrophages and, 124
  promastigote, 2429f
  treatment, 463t
  visceral, 2431–2434
Leishmania donovani sensu lato, 2431
Leishmania gamhani, 2428t
Leishmania guyanensis, 2428t

Leishmania infantum, 2428t
  cutaneous, 2434–2435
  visceral, 2431–2434
Leishmania major, 2428t, 2429, 2431
  cellular immunity and, 126
  cutaneous, 2434–2435
  cytokine and T cell protection, 121t
Leishmania mexicana, 2428t, 2429, 2431
  cutaneous disease, 2435–2438
  treatment, 463t
Leishmania panamensis, 2428t
  cutaneous disease, 2435–2438
Leishmania pifanoi, 2428t
Leishmania tropica, 2428, 2428t
  cutaneous, 2434–2435
  treatment, 463t
  visceral, 2431–2434
Leishmania venezuelensis, 2428t
Leishmanin skin test, 2435, 2437
Lemierre's disease, 569, 2169
  Fusobacterium and, 2198
Leminorella grimontii, 1975t
Leminorella richardii, 1975t
Lentiviruses, 1584–1606. *See also*
    Human immunodeficiency
      virus
  arthritis, 1036t
  genomes: plasticity and complexity
      of, 1587, 1589
  history, 1584, 1586
  natural history of infections, 1585f,
      1586
  overview, 1584–1590
  taxonomy, 1585f
Leporipoxvirus, 1325
Lepromin intradermal skin test, 2246
Leprosy, 2243–2250. *See also*
    Mycobacterium leprae
Leptomyxid, 2408–2414
Leptosphaeria senegaliensis, 2327
Leptospira, 2137–2141
  anicteric, 2138f, 2138–2139
  animal reservoirs, 2792t
  clinical manifestations, 2138–2139
  CSF specimens, 179
  cutaneous manifestations, 550t
  description, 2137
  differential diagnosis
    enteroviral meningitis, 1622
    scrub typhus, 1741
  enteric symptoms, 999t, 1002
  epidemiology, 2137
  and fever, 542
  hepatitis, 1147
  icteric (Weil syndrome), 2138f, 2139
  laboratory diagnosis, 2139–2140
  lymphadenitis, 940t
  pathogenesis, 2137–2138
  pathology, 2137–2138
  and pneumonia, 622t
  serology, 192t
  stages, 2138, 2138f
  symptoms, 2139t
  treatment and prevention, 2140
Leptospira icterohaemorrhagiae:
    meningitis, 870–871
Leptotrichia, 2158t
  bacteremia, 2165
Leptotrichia buccalis, 2167
Leptotrombidium deliense: and scrub
    typhus, 1740
Lepus: and *Francisella tularensis*, 2061
Lethal factor (anthrax), 6
Leucomax, 451
Leuconostoc, 1832

Leucovorin. *See also* Folinic acid
  for *Toxoplasma gondii*, 1283t
Leukemia
  acute
    altered cell-mediated immunity:
        infections and, 2681–2682
    granulocytopenia: infections and,
        2675–2681
    infections and, 2672–2673,
        2675–2686
      bacterial, 2676, 2676t, 2681
      characteristics, 2677t,
          2677–2679
      fungal, 2676–2677, 2681
      meningitis, 2682
      oropharyngeal, 2678
      parasitic, 2677, 2681
      protozoal, 2677, 2681
      pulmonary, 2678–2679,
          2681–2682
      septicemia, 2677–2678, 2681
      skin and soft tissue, 2679
      therapy, 2679–2681, 2682
      viral, 2677, 2681
    lymphoblastic, 2675
    lymphocytic, 2668
    nonlymphocytic, 2667, 2667f,
        2675
  adult T-cell, 1581–1582. *See also*
      Adult T-cell leukemia/lym-
      phoma
  Aspergillus and, 2308
  childhood: chloramphenicol and,
      313–314
  chronic lymphocytic
    antibody deficiency and, 53
    immunoglobulin for, 454
    infections and, 2673
    and *Streptococcus pneumoniae*,
        1816, 1817t
  and fever, 544
  hairy: infections and, 2673
  pulmonary infiltrates with eosinophilia,
      631
Leukemia inhibitory factor (LIF), 530
  and hypothalamus, 532
  receptor, 113
Leukine, 451
Leukocidin: *Staphylococcus aureus*,
    1759
Leukocyte adhesion deficiency (LAD),
    47, 89–90, 95, 151t, 153
  diagnosis, 150, 154–155
  eosinophils and, 96
  type 1, 154
  type 2, 154–155
Leukocytes
  granulocytes. *See* Granulocytic
      phagocytes
  transfusions, 95
    complications, 95
Leukocytosis: and acute phase response,
    534
Leukoencephalitis, hemorrhagic, 891
Leukoencephalopathy, progressive multi-
    focal, 1400–1406
  clinical manifestations, 1401
  diagnosis, 1402–1403, 1403f
  epidemiology, 1401
  and HIV/AIDS, 1238, 1239, 1400,
      1402
    incidence, 1182t, 1400
    treatment, 1288, 1404
  pathogenesis, 1322, 1401
  prevention and treatment, 1403

Leukopenia
  and acute retroviral syndrome (HIV),
      1224t
  herpesviruses, 1334t
Leukorrhea, 1081
Leukotriene B4 (LTB4), 82
Leukotriene C, 96
  and bronchiolitis, 615
Leukotriene D, 96
Leukotriene E, 96
Levamisole, 91
  for candidiasis, 2301
LFA-1 adhesin, 16, 47, 82, 108, 123
  deficiency, 47
  T cells and, 107, 111
    cytotoxic, 121
LFA-3 adhesin
  and cytokines, 115
  and paroxysmal nocturnal hemoglo-
      binuria, 71
  T cells and, 108, 111
    cytotoxic, 121
Lice
  diseases borne by. *See* Louse-borne
      diseases
  human, 2558–2560. *See also specific
      lice*
  treatment, 463t
Ligands: adhesins and, 11
Ligase chain reaction (LCR), 27
Light chains
  antigen-binding diversity, 43f, 43–44
  immunoglobulin, 37, 43f, 43–44
Limulus lysate assay
  bacterial meningitis, 846
  for gonococcal endotoxin, 1065
Lincocin. *See* Lincomycin
Lincomycin, 334, 341–343
  antibiotic-associated colitis (AAC),
      979
  antimicrobial activity, 341
  dosage, 512t–513t
    in renal dysfunction, 204–205, 513t
  and pH, 206
  pharmacology, 512t–513t
  resistance, 341–342
Lincosamides. *See also* Clindamycin;
    Lincomycin
  pharmacologic tables, 512t–513t
  resistance, 215t, 220
Lindane, 463t, 466t
  for lice, 2560
  for scabies, 2562
Lipids: priming neutrophils, 86
Lipid solubility: of antimicrobials, 205
Lipomelanotic reticuloendotheliosis,
    937
Liponyssoides sanguineus, 2564
Lipopolysaccharidase-binding protein
    (LPS-BP), 34, 117
  and septic shock, 117
Lipopolysaccharide (LPS)
  and bacterial meningitis, 839–840
  binding protein, 1968
  Enterobacteriaceae, 1964, 1968
  and fever, 117, 530
  in gram-negative bacteria, 1753
  and sepsis, 692f
  vaccine: for pneumonia prevention,
      2604
Lipoteichoic acid
  gram-positive bacteria, 1753
  viridans streptococci, 1847
Lipovnik virus, 1448
Listeria

and leukemia, hairy cell, 2673
in transplant recipients, 2712
Listeria monocytogenes, 1880–1885
  brain abscess, 890
    in AIDS, 890
    in the immunocompromised, 890
  cellular immunity and, 125, 126,
      127
    deficiencies, 132, 133, 2681
    therapy, 2682
  cerebritis, 1882t, 1883, 1883t, 1884f
  clinical manifestations, 1882–1883,
      1883t
  CNS infection, 829
  cutaneous manifestations, 550t, 553
  differential diagnosis: *Bartonella*,
      1742
  encephalitis, 1882t, 1882–1883,
      1883t
  endocarditis, 756
  epidemiology, 1881–1882
  focal infections, 1882t, 1883t,
      1883–1884
  food-borne, 1016
  granulomatosis infantiseptica, 1161,
      1882, 1882t, 1883t, 1884t
  granulomatous hepatitis, 1161
  identification, 189
  keratitis, 1112
  lymphadenitis, 940t
  meningitis, 834, 835, 1882t,
      1882–1883, 1883t
    antimicrobial therapy, 850t, 852
    clinical presentation, 843
    CSF examination, 845, 846
    in the elderly, 2740, 2741
  microbiology, 1880–1881, 1881f
  miliary granulomatosis (granulomato-
      sis infantiseptica), 1161
  mycotic aneurysms, 772
  myocarditis, 800
  NK cells and, 122
  oculoglandular syndrome, 938
  pathogenesis, 1882
  penetration, 7
  phospholipase C, 25
  in pregnancy, 1882, 1882t, 1883t
  replication mechanisms, 25
  resistance, 220
  sepsis, 1882, 1882t, 1883t
  toxin, 7
  in transplant recipients, 2728
  treatment, 1884–1885
    aminoglycoside combination
        therapy, 287t
    aminopenicillins, 243
    carbapenems, 264t
    erythromycin, 335, 335t
    penicillins, 237t
    quinolones, 368t
    rifampin, 318t
    sulfonamides, 355t
    trimethoprim, 357
  virulence factors, 2
Listeriolysin O, 25, 1882
Listerolysin, 7
Lithium carbonate: and neutrophils, 80
Liver. *See also entries commencing with
    the term* Hepatic
  infections. *See* Hepatic infections
  primary tuberculosis of, 2238
Liver biopsy
  cholestasis, 1140–1141
  and endocarditis, 743t, 794t
  and FUO, 541

hepatitis
acute viral, 1140, 1140f, 1146
granulomatous, 1160, 1160f, 1163
meningitis, 867
Liver disease
alcoholic, 1148–1149
anoxic injury, 1148
cholestatic, 1149
Mycobacterium tuberculosis treatment, 2229
Liver failure: and *Streptococcus agalactiae* bacteremia, 1839, 1839t
Liver flukes, 2525t, 2538t, 2541–2542
Clonorchis sinensis, 2538t, 2541
Fasciola hepatica, 2538t, 2541–2542
Opisthorchis, 2538t, 2541–2542
Liver transplantation
aspergillosis and, 2306
bacteremia and, 2727
CMV in, 2710t
for fulminant hepatitis, 1150
for hepatic failure, 1150
for hepatitis C, 1150
infections and, 2722, 2724t, 2725–2726
Liver tumors: and fever, 544
LJ 10627
postantibiotic effect (PAE), 266
Lmp2 gene, 103
Lmp7 gene, 103
L-N test, 177
Loa loa, 2535
clinical features, 2535
diagnosis, 2535
epidemiology, 2535
life cycle, 2535
lymphadenitis, 940t
prevention, 2535
treatment, 462t, 2535
diethylcarbamazine, 481
ivermectin, 481
mebendazole, 479
Lobectomy: for pneumonia, 657
Loboa loboi, 2392
differential diagnosis, 2322, 2326, 2437
Lobo's disease, 2392
Lochgoilhead fever, 2099
Lomefloxacin
antimicrobial activity, 367t, 369t
dosage, 370t, 516t–517t
in renal dysfunction, 369, 370t, 517t
pharmacokinetics, 369t
pharmacology, 516t–517t
animal models, 228, 230f
structure, 365f
Lomotil, 971
Lone Star tick. *See Dermacentor americanum*
Loperamide, 2802
Lorabid. *See* Loracarbef
Loracarbef, 257
chemistry, 249
dosage, 250t, 510t–511t
in children, 510t
in renal insufficiency, 253t, 511t
pharmacology, 252t, 510t–511t
for sinusitis, 589t
structure, 248f
in vitro activity, 255t, 257, 258
Lorazepam: for *Clostridium tetani*, 2176, 2177

Louping ill: transmission, clinical syndromes, and geographic distribution, 1466t
Louse-borne diseases, 2558t. *See also specific diseases*
Borrelia relapsing fever, 2141
relapsing fever, 2141–2143
rickettsial. *See Rickettsia prowazekii*
Lower extremity: graft infections, 789
LS-2616. *See* Linomide
L-selectin, 81, 111, 123
Lucilia, 2562
Lucio's reaction, 2247
treatment, 2247
Ludwig's angina
anaerobic gram-negative bacilli, 2198
clinical presentation, 599f, 599–600
and mediastinitis, 814
Lues, 2118
Lumbar puncture: meningitis, 866
Lung abscess, 642–646
amebic, 643
anaerobic, 642, 2163t
gram-negative bacilli, 2198
necrotizing pneumonia, 642–643, 643f
and brain abscess, 888, 888t
and chronic granulomatous disease, 92
clinical manifestations, 642–643
complications, 643
diagnosis, 645
differential diagnosis, 645
in drug abusers, 2701
microbiologic characteristics, 644t, 644–645
Nocardia, 2275
nonanaerobic, 643
pathogenesis, 642
pathology, 642
predisposing causes, 642
prognosis, 646
secondary, 643, 643f
therapy, 645–646
Lung biopsy
for *Pneumocystis carinii*, 2479
for pneumonia, 625
acute, 625
chronic, 652
in HIV/AIDS, 1232
Lung cancer treatment: infections and, 2667
Lung collapse therapy: for *Mycobacterium tuberculosis*, 2235–2236
Lung flukes. *See also Paragonimus westermani*, 2525t, 2538t, 2543
Lung infections. *See* Lung abscess; Pulmonary infections
Lung(s). *See also* entries commencing with the term Pulmonary
abscess. *See* Lung abscess
microscopic examination of pathogens, 172t
specimen collection and processing, 170t, 174–175
Lung transplantation: infections and, 2710, 2724t, 2725
Lutzomyia: and *Leishmania*, 2429
LXA-1 β-lactamase, 216t
Lyme (borreliosis) disease, 2143–2155. *See also Borrelia burgdorferi*
Lymphadenitis, 936–942, 940t
acute, 936
axillary, 937

due to pyogenic bacteria, 937
nonpyogenic, 938–939
suppurative epitrochlear, 937
cat scratch disease, 938–939, 1310t, 1311
cervical, 603, 604, 937
Mycobacterium avium-intracellulare and, 938, 2255
Mycobacterium scrofulaceum, 938, 2255, 2268
suppurative streptococcal, 1789
Toxoplasma gondii, 2459
chronic, 936–937
clinical features, 936–940, 940t
dermatopathic, 936–937
differential diagnosis, 940–942
etiology, 940t, 940–942
generalized
AIDS and, 941–942
systemic infections and, 939–940
granulomatous
corynebacterial, 938
histoplasmosis, 2345
Histoplasma capsulatum, 936, 940t, 2345
inguinal buboes
differential diagnosis, 2211
of nonvenereal origin, 939
of venereal origin, 939
mesenteric tuberculous, 2239
oculoglandular (Parinaud) syndrome, 938
pathogenesis and pathology, 936–937
presumptive treatment, 942
scrofula (tuberculous cervical), 938, 2239
subpectoral, 937
suppurative epitrochlear, 937
suppurative iliac, 937–938
Lymphadenopathy
Borrelia burgdorferi, 2147, 2147t
in cat scratch disease, 1310t, 1310–1311
chancroid (*Haemophilus ducreyi*), 1684, 2047–2048
coxsackievirus, 1632
EBV mononucleosis, 1367, 1368t
echoviruses, 1632
Francisella tularensis, 2063
HSV, 1684
immunoblastic syndrome, 941
inguinal, 1684
differential diagnosis, 1684
urethritis, 1064
LGV, 1684
mediastinal tuberculous, 2239
persistent generalized
differential diagnosis, 1225
HIV/AIDS and, 1225
and non-Hodgkin's lymphoma, 1225
scrub typhus, 1740
sinus histiocytosis with massive, 941
syphilis, 1684
Toxoplasma gondii, 940t, 2459
Trypanosoma brucei, 2451, 2452, 2453
Lymphadenopathy-associated virus (LAV). *See* Human immunodeficiency virus
Lymphangiography: and FUO, 540
Lymphangitis, 942, 943
acute, 942–943
chronic granulomatous, 943
clinical features, 942–943

differential diagnosis, 943
etiology, 943, 943t
group A streptococcal, 555
pathology and pathogenesis, 942
presumptive therapy, 943
Streptococcus pyogenes, 1797
Lymph nodes
biopsy: for meningitis, 867
examination: and FUO, 539
Lymphocyte-function-associated adhesin. *See* LFA adhesin
Lymphocytes
B. *See* B cells
T. *See* T cells
Lymphocytic choriomeningitis virus
animal reservoirs, 2792t
arthritis, 1032, 1036, 1036t
characteristics, 1572, 1573t
clinical manifestations, 1575–1576
CSF specimens, 179
cutaneous manifestations, 550t
diagnosis, 1576, 1577
differential diagnosis: enteroviral meningitis, 1622
encephalomyelitis, 876
epidemiology, 1572, 1574
intrauterine infection, 1576
meningitis, 832–833
clinical presentation, 842
pathogenesis, 1575
prevention and treatment, 1577
serology, 191
Lymphocytosis-promoting factor. *See* Pertussis toxin
Lymphogranuloma venereum (LGV), 1684–1685
buboes, 939, 940t, 1684
clinical manifestations, 1684
conjunctivitis, 1106
differential diagnosis, 1684, 2122
epidemiology, 1056
fever, 543
isolation in cell culture, 1682
oculoglandular syndrome, 939, 940t
pathogenesis, 1681
serology, 1683
treatment, 1684–1685
erythromycin, 338t
trimethoprim-sulfamethoxazole, 360
Lymphoid irradiation: immunodeficiency from, 136–137
Lymphoid tissue: and HIV pathogenesis, 1212
Lymphokine production deficit, 134t
Lymphokines, 112–118. *See also* Cytokines
definitions, 112
Lymphoma
acute
altered cell-mediated immunity: infections and, 2681–2682
granulocytopenia: infections and, 2675–2681
infections and, 2675–2686
bacterial, 2676, 2676t
characteristics, 2677t, 2677–2679
fungal, 2676–2677
meningitis, 2682
oropharyngeal, 2678
parasitic, 2677
protozoal, 2677
pulmonary, 2678–2679
septicemia, 2677–2678

Lymphoma (*Continued*)
skin and soft tissue, 2679, 2682
therapy, 2679–2681, 2682
viral, 2677
adult T-cell, 1581–1582. *See also*
Adult T-cell leukemia/lym-
phoma
antibody deficiency and, 53
biliary obstruction: infections and,
2669
EBV and, 136
and fever, 544
granulomatous hepatitis, 1162
and HIV/AIDS, 1210
CNS, 1238
gastric, 1230
incidence, 1182t
treatment: infections and, 2667
Lymphomatoid granulomatosis pneumonia, 647t
Lymphosarcoma: antibody deficiency
and, 53
Lymphotoxin
α, 102
characteristics, sources, and effects,
114t
β, 102
characteristics, sources, and effects,
115t
recombinant, 530
and cytotoxic T cells, 121
and T-cell proliferation, 119
Lysins, 2771
Lysozyme, 79t, 87
Lyssavirus, 1528
type 1, 1528t
type 2, 1528t

M

Macaca: herpes B virus in, 1380
MacCallum's patch, 1801
Machupo virus, 1572, 1575
characteristics, 1573t
diagnosis, 1576–1577
epidemiology, 1574
pathogenesis, 1575
serology, 191
MacMARCKS, 110
Mac-1 receptor, 82
deficiency, 89–90
Macrolides, 334–340. *See also specific
formulations*
antiparasitic use, 459t, 475
drug interactions, 523t
for nontuberculous (atypical)
mycobacteria, 396
pharmacologic tables, 512t–513t
resistance, 215t, 220
for *Toxoplasma gondii*, 2469
Macronodular lesions: and systemic
infections, 551t
Macropapular eruptions: *Neisseria
meningitidis*, 1900, 1901f
Macrophage activating factor: and
*Mycobacterium avium-intra-
cellulare*, 2252
Macrophage colony-stimulating factor
(M-CSF), 79, 113
characteristics, sources, and effects,
115, 115t, 123
and hematopoiesis, 118
HIV and, 1211
recombinant, 452
therapeutic use, 452

Macrophage inhibition factor: *Candida
albicans*, 2295
Macrophages, 102
abnormalities: and HIV, 1209
activation, 123, 124
cytokines and, 124
cytokines released by, 115
monocytes vs., 122
and *Pneumocystis carinii*, 127
tissue, 122–124
Macular lesions, 551–552
Pseudomonas aeruginosa, 921
systemic infections manifesting, 550t
Macules: defined, 551
Maculopapular lesions, 551–552
Pseudomonas aeruginosa, 921
systemic infections manifesting, 550t
Madarosis, 1130
Madura foot, 2327–2330. *See also*
Mycetoma
Madurella grisea, 2327, 2330
Madurella mycetomatis, 2327, 2330
Maedi virus, 1584, 1585f, 1586, 1591.
See also Visna-maedi virus
Mafenide, 355
for burn wounds, 2762–2763
topical, 384t
Maggots, 2558, 2562–2564
Magnetic resonance imaging (MRI)
bacterial meningitis, 846
brain abscess, 892–893, 894f
cavernous sinus thrombosis, 1134
Creutzfeldt-Jakob disease, 882
epidural abscess, 904, 905, 905f
and FUO, 540
Gd-DTPA: brain abscess, 893
hepatic abscess, 725
infectious arthritis, 1034
intracranial masses in HIV/AIDS,
1237–1238, 1238f
intraperitoneal abscess, 722
mycotic aneurysms, 771–772
myocarditis, 803
orbital cellulitis, 1134
osteomyelitis, 1045
septic intracranial thrombophlebitis,
908, 908f
splenic abscess, 727
subdural empyema, 901, 901f, 903
Majocchi's granuloma, 2381
differential diagnosis, 2322, 2356
Major histocompatibility complex
(MHC), 102–105. *See also*
Human leukocyte antigens
anchor residues, 103
class I, 102–104, 103f
class II, 104
and normal flora, 31
and T-cell–dependent B-cell activation, 47
deficiency, 134t
distribution and regulation of expression, 104–105
genes and molecules, 102
and peptides, 107
structure and assembly, 102–104
and T cells, 107
Malabsorption
differential diagnosis: amebiasis,
2402
Giardia lamblia, 2489, 2489t
postinfectious tropical. *see* tropical
sprue *below*
and tropical sprue, 1026–1028,
1027f

Malaria, 2415–2427. *See also
Plasmodium*
Malassezia furfur, 2383–2384, 2392
folliculitis, 912
fungemia cultures, 178
infusion-related sepsis, 2587
suppurative thrombophlebitis, 768
Malathion, 463t
for lice, 2560
Malayan filariasis, 2533–2535
Male genitalia. *See also* Penis; Testes
anatomy, 1098, 1098f
lesions. *See* Genital lesions
tuberculosis, 2238
Malignancies. *See* Neoplasia *and specific
tumors*
Malignant hyperthermia, 531
Malnutrition
and immunodeficiency, 137
protein-energy
hookworm and, 2530
and immunodeficiency, 137
Maloprim, 474
Malta fever, 2053
Mammary artery, internal (IMA) grafts:
and mediastinitis, 815
Mandibular osteomyelitis, 601
Mandol. *See* Cefamandole
Mannan-binding protein (MBP), 59
deficiency, 91
Mannitol: for cerebral edema, 830t
Mannose-binding protein, 34
α-Mannosidase, 79t
Mansonella, 2536
Mansonella ozzardi, 2536
treatment, 462t
diethylcarbamazine, 481
Mansonella perstans, 2536
treatment, 462t
mebendazole, 479
Mansonella streptocerca, 2536
Mansonia: and equine encephalitis, 1456
Marburg virus, 1543–1546
clinical manifestations, 1544–1545
diagnosis, 1545
epidemiology, 1544
pathogenesis and pathology, 1545
prevention and treatment, 1545
transmission, 1544
waste management, 2582
Marie-Charcot-Tooth disease, 2245
Marin County virus, 1667
Market men's disease, 2060
Marseilles fever, 1725
Masks: and isolation, 2577t
Mast cells: and inflammatory response,
550
Masticator space infections: clinical
presentation, 598, 599f
Mastigophora, 2393t
Mastitis: *Staphylococcus aureus*, 1764
Mastoid air cell system: anatomy, 583f
Mastoiditis, 583–584
and brain abscess, 887, 888t
clinical manifestations, 584
management, 584
pathogenesis, 583–584
Pseudomonas aeruginosa, 1991
treatment, 1991
Mastomys: and Lassa fever, 1573t, 1574
Maxillary sinusitis, 601
Maxillofacial trauma, 603, 604
Mayaro virus, 1455
diagnosis, 1458
epidemiology, 1457

MC virus, 1667
Measles virus, 1519–1526
in adults, 1522
arthritis, 1036t
atypical, 1522
cutaneous manifestations,
550t
chemical and antigenic composition,
1519
clinical manifestations, 1521f,
1521–1522
complications, 1521
conjunctivitis, 1106
cutaneous manifestations, 550t,
551
description, 1519
diagnosis, 1522–1523
diseases associated with, 1520
encephalitis/myelitis, 874
endophthalmitis, 1124
epidemiology, 1519–1520
growth in tissue culture, 1519
hepatitis, 1137
and HIV/AIDS, 1522
vaccine use, 1524
host range, 1519
immunity, 1520–1521
in the immunocompromised, 1522
and immunodeficiency, 137
cell-mediated, 2681
isolation, 2576
keratitis, 1115
Koplik spots, 1519, 1521,
1522–1523
lymphadenitis, 940t
modified form, 1521–1522
morphology, 1519
and multiple sclerosis, 1520
myocarditis, 800
pathogenesis, 1520–1521
in pregnancy, 1522
prevention, 1523–1524
and Reye syndrome, 1558
serology, 191
and SLE, 1520
spreading/shedding mechanisms,
1320f
spread of infection, 1520
subacute sclerosing panencephalitis,
1124, 1520
systemic spread, 1320f
T cell protection, 121t
and tuberculosis, 1522
vaccine, 1523–1524, 2777–2778
adverse reactions, 2773t, 2778
contraindications, 2787t
indications, 2777–2778, 2783
for adults, 2784t
morbidity reduction, 2772t
reportable events, 2786t
for travelers, 2797t, 2798
Mebendazole, 460t, 478–479
adverse reactions, 479
for ascariasis, 2529
dosage, 461t, 462t, 466t, 467t
pediatric, 461t, 462t, 466t, 467t
drug interactions, 523t
for echinococcosis, 2551
for enterobiasis, 2528
for hookworm, 2530
spectrum of activity, 478–479
structure, 478f
for *Trichuris trichiura*, 2527–2528
Meckel's diverticulitis, 727
Mediastinal anatomy, 813f, 813–814

Mediastinitis, 814–821
  actinomycosis, 2283
  acute, 814–817
    antibiotic prophylaxis, 817
    bacteriology, 815t, 815–816
    clinical manifestations, 815–816
    complications, 817–818
    diagnosis, 815–816
    epidemiology and pathogenesis, 814
    etiology, 813–814, 814t
    secondary to cardiothoracic surgery, 814–815
    secondary to head and neck infections, 814
    treatment, 817
  anatomic considerations, 813–814, 814f
  granulomatous (fibrosing). See sclerosing below
  and heart transplantation, 2724
  sclerosing, 813, 817–818
    complications, 817t
    tuberculosis, 2239
Medical Waste Tracking Act, 2582
Medications. See Anti-infective therapy and specific drugs
Mediterranean spotted fever, 1725
  quinolones for, 373
Medlar bodies, 2326
Mefloquine, 459t, 471–472
  adverse reactions, 472
  for Plasmodium, 2424, 2424t, 2425
    for travelers, 2801
  prophylaxis dosage, 465t, 2424t
    pediatric, 465t
  pyrimethamine and sulfadoxine with (Fansimef), 474
  structure, 472f
Mefoxin. See Cefoxitin
Megacolon
  toxic: Entamoeba histolytica, 2400, 2402
  Trypanosoma cruzi, 2446, 2448
Megaesophagus: Trypanosoma cruzi, 2446
Megakaryocytes: HIV and, 1204
Megamonas, 2158t
Megasphaera, 2158t
Megasphaera elsdenii, 2204
Meglumine antimoniate (Glucantime), 459t, 477
  dosage, 463t
    pediatric, 463t
  for Leishmania, 2430, 2433, 2438
Meibomian gland dysfunction (posterior blepharitis), 1130
Melarsoprol, 459t, 476
  adverse reactions, 476, 2454
  dosage, 467t
  for Trypanosoma brucei, 2454
Meleney's ulcer, 918
Melioidosis, 2004–2006. See also Pseudomonas pseudomallei
Membrane attack complex, 58, 58t, 65
  assembly, 62
  meningococcal infections and, 70
  regulation, 63
Membrane cofactor protein (MCP), 62, 63t
Membrane permeability
  inner, 219
  outer, 219
Meningeal biopsy: meningitis, 867
Meningeal carcinomatosis, 871

Meningismus: bacterial meningitis, 843, 843t
Meningitis, 832–874
  Acinetobacter, 2011
  acute, 832–865. See also individual infectious agents
    adjunctive therapy, 854–856
      for bacteria, 854–856
      for viruses, 854
    aerobic gram-negative bacilli, 834–835
      antimicrobial therapy, 850t, 852–853
    amebic, 835
      antimicrobial therapy, 849t, 850t, 854
      clinical presentation, 844
      diagnosis, 849
    Angiostrongylus cantonensis, 835
      clinical presentation, 844
      diagnosis, 849
    antimicrobial therapy, 849–854
      for bacteria, 850–853
      dosages, 848t, 850t
      empiric, 848t
      for neonates and children, 849t
      for protozoa and helminths, 854
      specific, 848t
      for spirochetes, 853–854
      for viruses, 849–850
    arboviruses, 832
    bacterial, 833t, 834t, 834–835. See also individual bacteria
      adjunctive therapy, 854–856
      anti-inflammatory agents for, 854–856
      antimicrobial therapy, 850t, 850–853
      bacteremia, 838
      blood-brain barrier alterations, 839
      cerebral blood flow alterations, 841–842
      clinical presentation, 843, 843t
      CSF examination, 846, 846t
      diagnosis, 846, 846t
      increased intracranial pressure, 841
      meningeal invasion, 838–839
      mucosal colonization and systemic invasion, 837–838, 838t
      pathogenesis and pathophysiology, 837f, 837–842, 838t
      prevention, 857–858
      radiography, 846, 847f
      reduction of intracranial pressure for, 856
      subarachnoid space inflammation, 840t, 840–841
      surgical intervention, 856
      survival within subarachnoid space, 839–840
    basilar skull fracture: antibiotic prophylaxis, 857–858
    Borrelia burgdorferi, 835
      antimicrobial therapy, 850t, 854
      clinical presentation, 844
      diagnosis, 847f, 847–849
    chronic and, 831
    clinical presentation, 842–844
    coxsackieviruses, 1621t, 1621–1623
      clinical manifestations, 1622
      differential diagnosis, 1622

    laboratory diagnosis, 1622
    management and prognosis, 1622–1623
  CSF examination, 845–847
  CSF shunt infections
    antimicrobial therapy, 853
    clinical presentation, 843
  diagnosis, 844–849
  differential diagnosis, 832t
  echoviruses, 832, 1621t, 1621–1623
    clinical manifestations, 1622
    differential diagnosis, 1622
    laboratory diagnosis, 1622
    management and prognosis, 1622–1623
  encephalitis and, 832
  enteroviruses, 832, 1621t, 1621–1623
    clinical presentation, 842
  epidemiology, 832–835
  etiology, 832–835. See also individual infectious agents
  Haemophilus influenzae, 834
    antimicrobial therapy, 850t, 851
    chemoprophylaxis, 856–857
    immunoprophylaxis, 858, 858t
  helminthic, 835
    antimicrobial therapy, 850t, 854
    clinical presentation, 844
    diagnosis, 849
  herpesviruses, 833
    clinical presentation, 842
  HIV, 833
    clinical presentation, 842
  Listeria monocytogenes, 835
    antimicrobial therapy, 850t, 852
  lymphocytic choriomeningitis virus, 832–833
    clinical presentation, 842
  management
    adjunctive therapy, 854–856
    antimicrobial therapy, 849–854
    dosages for neonates and children, 849t
    empiric therapy, 848t
    initial, 848f, 849
    recommended antimicrobial dosages, 848t, 850t
    specific therapy, 848t
  mumps virus, 832
    clinical presentation, 842, 842t
  Neisseria meningitidis, 834, 1896, 1900
    antimicrobial therapy, 850t, 851–852
    chemoprophylaxis, 857
    immunoprophylaxis, 858
  pathogenesis, 836–842
  pathophysiology, 836–842
  prevention, 857–858
    bacterial, 857–858
    viral, 856
  protozoal, 835
    antimicrobial therapy, 850t, 854
    clinical presentation, 844
    diagnosis, 849
  spirochetal, 835
    antimicrobial therapy, 850t, 853–854
    clinical presentation, 844
    diagnosis, 846–847
  staphylococcal, 835
    antimicrobial therapy, 850t, 853

  Streptococcus agalactiae, 834
    antimicrobial therapy, 850t, 852
    prevention, 857
  Streptococcus pneumoniae, 834
    antimicrobial therapy, 850t, 852
    chemoprophylaxis, 857
    immunoprophylaxis, 858
  Treponema pallidum, 835
    antimicrobial therapy, 850t, 853–854
    clinical presentation, 843–844
    diagnosis, 846–847
  viral, 832. See also individual viruses
    adjunctive therapy, 854
    antimicrobial therapy, 849–850
    clinical presentation, 842
    CSF examination, 845
    diagnosis, 845
    pathogenesis and pathophysiology, 836
    prevention, 856
  aseptic, 832
  and fever, 547
  and HIV/AIDS, 1236–1237
  Bacillus, 1893
  Bacillus anthracis, 1888
  Bacteroides fragilis, 2197
  Borrelia burgdorferi, 2148
    acute, 835. See also acute, Borrelia burgdorferi above
    chronic, 870
  and brain abscess, 888
  Brucella, 870, 2056
  Candida, 2296
    chronic, 870
  and cell-mediated immune defects, 2681, 2682
    therapy, 2682
  chronic, 865–874
    acute and, 831
    benign lymphocytic, 871
    Borrelia burgdorferi, 870
    Brucella, 870
    Candida, 870
    coccidioidal, 869
    cryptococcal, 869
      in HIV/AIDS, 1239
    CSF characteristics, 866–867, 867t
    cysticercosis, 870
    differential diagnosis, 865f, 869–872
    Histoplasma, 869–870
    history, 865
    in HIV/AIDS, 872, 1236–1239
    in the immunocompromised, 872
    infectious agents, 865t, 869–871
    laboratory evaluation, 866t, 867–868
    neoplastic, 871
    noninfectious causes, 865t, 871–872
    physical examination, 865f, 865–866
    radiography, 868
    sarcoid, 871
    Sporothrix schenckii, 870
    therapeutic trials, 868
    Treponema pallidum, 870
    tuberculous, 868–869
  Citrobacter diversus, 1974
  CMV, 833, 1358
    and HIV, 872, 1239–1240
  Coccidioides immitis, 2368–2369
    treatment, 2372

Meningitis *(Continued)*
  cryptococcal, 2332, 2336
    and cell-mediated immune defects, 2681, 2682
      therapy, 2682
    chronic, 869
    treatment: fluconazole, 409
  CSF specimens, 178, 178t
  in drug abusers, 2704
  in the elderly, 2740–2741
  enterococcal, 1829
  eosinophilic *(Angiostrongylus cantonensis)*, 2555–2556
  epidemiology, 159
  Epstein-Barr virus, 833, 842
  Escherichia coli: neonatal, 1971
  Flavobacterium, 2113
  Haemophilus influenzae, 2041
    acute, 834. *See also* acute, *Haemophilus influenzae* above
  herpesviruses, 1334t
  Histoplasma capsulatum, 2347
    treatment, 2351
  in HIV/AIDS
    acute, 833, 842
    chronic, 872, 1236–1239
  leptospirosis, 2139
  and leukemia/lymphoma, 2682
  Listeria monocytogenes, 834, 835, 1881, 1882t, 1882–1883, 1883t
    acute, 835
    antimicrobial therapy, 850t, 852
    clinical presentation, 843
    CSF examination, 845, 846
  Mollaret's: HSV and, 1341
  mumps virus, 1497, 1497t, 1498
  Mycobacterium tuberculosis, 2234–2235
    clinical features, 2234, 2234f
    pathology, 2234
    treatment, 2234
  mycoplasmal neonatal, 1717
  poliovirus, 1615
  Pseudomonas aeruginosa, 1988–1989
    treatment, 1989
  rifampin prophylaxis, 320–321
  Salmonella, 2023
  sporotrichosis, 2322
    treatment, 2323
  streptococcal
    group C and G, 1855
    viridans, 1849–1850
  Streptococcus agalactiae
    acute, 834
    adult, 1840
    neonatal, 1838, 1839
    treatment, 1841t
  Streptococcus pneumoniae, 833t, 834t, 835, 1818
    acute, 834
    antimicrobial therapy, 850t, 852
    bacteremia, 838
    blood-brain barrier alteration, 839
    chemoprophylaxis, 857
    clinical presentation, 843
    CSF examination, 845–846, 846t
    immunology, 1814
    immunoprophylaxis, 858
    intracranial hypertension, 841
    treatment, 1822
  in transplant recipients, 2728
  treatment. *See also under specific infectious agents*
    aminoglycosides, 295t

  quinolones, 373
  rifampin, 324
  tuberculous, 2234–2235
    clinical features, 2234, 2234f
    pathology, 2234
    spinal, 2235
    treatment, 2234–2235
      glucocorticoids, 455
  varicella-zoster virus, 833, 1348
  viral (aseptic), 832
  Yersinia pestis, 2072t, 2074, 2075
Meningococcal vaccine, 167, 1896, 1903t, 1905–1906, 2778
  adverse reactions, 2778
  booster doses, 2778
  indications for adults, 2784t
  for travelers, 2778, 2797t, 2798
Meningococcemia, 1900. *See also Neisseria meningitidis*
  chronic, 1901–1902
  complement deficiency and, 1902
  cutaneous manifestations, 555, 921
  differential diagnosis: gonorrhea, 1919
  specimen collection and processing, 177
  with and without meningitis, 1900
Meningococcus. *See Neisseria meningitidis*
Meningoencephalitis
  adenovirus, 1386
  amoebic, 2409–2410, 2411
    treatment, 461t
  Campylobacter, 1952
  CMV, 1358
    in the immunocompromised, 1359
  cryptococcal, 2332, 2336
  enteroviral: in agammaglobulinemic and immunocompromised, 1629
  mumps virus, 1497, 1497t, 1498
  Naegleria, 835, 2408, 2410, 2412
  Neisseria meningitidis, 1900
  use of term, 874
Meningoencephalomyelitis: use of term, 874
Meningopolyneuritis, tick-borne, 2148
Menstruation: toxic shock syndrome and, 162
Meropenem, 266
  activity, 264t
  antibacterial activity, 266
  antimicrobial activity, 285t
  chemistry, 266
  mechanism of action, 266
  for meningitis, 853
  pharmacology, 266
  postantibiotic effect (PAE), 266
  for *Pseudomonas aeruginosa* meningitis, 1989
  resistance, 266
  structure, 266f
  toxicity, 266
Mesenteric adenitis, 1004–1005
  clinical features, 1004t, 1004–1005
  differential diagnosis, 1005
  epidemiology, 1005
  etiology, 1004
  laboratory findings, 1004–1005
  pathogenesis, 1004
  therapy, 1005
Mesenteric lymphadenitis, 727–728
Metabolic disorders
  antimicrobial therapy issues in, 203
  from foscarnet, 422–423
  peritonitis and, 714

Metacarpal joint: infectious arthritis, 1033, 1033t
Metagonimus yokogawai
  diagnosis, 1007
  treatment, 463t
    praziquantel, 482
Metallo protease toxins, 3t
Metazoa
  cellular immunity and, 124, 127–128
  cytokine and T cell protection, 121t, 127–128
Methacycline
  dosage, 512t–513t
  pharmacokinetics, 309t
  pharmacology, 512t–513t
  structure, 307f
Methacycline: pharmacology, 309f
Methadone: zidovudine interaction with, 436
Methenamine, 379–380
  adverse reactions, 380
  antimicrobial activity, 379
  for bacteriuria, 380, 2612
  clinical uses, 380
  dosage, 516t–517t
  drug interactions, 523t
  and pH, 206
  pharmacology, 379–380, 516t–517t
  structure, 379, 379f
Methicillin, 233, 242–243
  adverse reactions, 239t
  dosage, 241t, 506t–507t
    in children, 506t
    in neonates, 242t, 506t
    in renal disease and dialysis, 238t, 507t
  MICs against cocci, 237t
  pharmacokinetics, 238t
  pharmacology, 237–238, 506t–507t
  resistance, 194
    Staphylococcus aureus, 240, 251, 1756, 1757, 1758
    Staphylococcus epidermidis, 1778
    Staphylococcus haemolyticus, 1778
  structure, 242f
  trade names, 236t
  vancomycin interaction with, 349
Methotrexate: immunodeficiency from, 136
Methylbenzethomium chloride: for *Leishmania*, 2435
Methylobacterium extorquens. See Protomonas extorquens
Methylobacterium mesophilicum, 2114. *See also Protomonas extorquens*
Metrifonate, 460t, 482–483
  for schistosomiasis, 2541
Metronidazole, 329–334
  adverse reactions, 331, 331t, 467–468
  for amebiasis, 2404, 2404t
  for anaerobic infections, 332
  for antibiotic-associated colitis, 983, 984
  antibiotic-associated colitis (AAC) from, 979
  antiparasitic use, 458, 459t, 460t, 467–468
  for bacterial vaginosis, 1079t, 1079t
  for *Bacteroides fragilis*, 2200t, 2201
  for brain abscess, 893
    anaerobic gram-negative, 2201
  clinical uses, 332–333
  for *Clostridium tetani*, 2177

  dosage, 330t, 330–331, 512t–513t
    antiparasitic use, 461t, 462t, 463t, 467t
      pediatric, 461t, 462t, 463t, 467t
    in renal dysfunction, 205, 513t
  for dracunculiasis, 2533
  drug interactions, 331–332, 523t
  effect on normal fecal flora, 332
  for *Gardnerella vaginalis*, 2051
  for *Giardia lamblia*, 2490, 2490t
  for *Helicobacter pylori*, 1961
  for hepatic abscess, 726
  for intra-abdominal infections, 289
  mechanism of action, 330
  for necrotizing pneumonia, 645
  for parasites, 332
  for periodontitis, 601
  for peritonitis, 716
  pharmacologic tables, 512t–513t
  pharmacology, 330
  prophylactic use, 333
  resistance, 329–330, 458
    Helicobacter pylori, 1961
  for sepsis syndrome, 699, 699t
  spectrum of activity, 329t, 329–330
  for suppurative odontogenic infections, 602
  for suppurative thrombophlebitis, 769
  teratogenicity, 204, 2490
  topical, 384t
  for *Trichomonas vaginalis*, 329, 330t, 331, 458, 467t, 2495–2496
    in pregnancy, 2495
    resistance, 2495–2496
  trimethoprim combination therapy, 359
  for vulvovaginal candidiasis, 1076t
Meuse fever, 1741
Mezlocillin, 245
  antimicrobial activity, 241t, 285t
  for bacilli and anaerobes, 237t
  combination therapy
    synergism, 207
  dosage, 241t, 506t–507t
    in children, 506t
    in neonates, 242t, 506t
    in renal disease, 238t, 507t
  for Enterobacteriaceae and *Pseudomonas*, 237t
  MICs against cocci, 237t
  pharmacokinetics, 238t
  pharmacology, 506t–507t
  structure, 244t
  susceptibility testing, 194t
MHA-TP test, 181, 1061, 2127t, 2128
  for yaws, 2135
Mice
  and arenaviruses, 1572, 1573t, 1574
  and hantaviruses, 1569
  and Lassa fever, 1573t
  and lymphocytic choriomeningitis, 1572, 1573t
  and rickettsialpox, 1727
  transgenic, 1322
Miconazole, 401, 403
  for candidiasis, 2299
  dosage, 403t, 518t–519t
    in renal dysfunction, 205, 519t
  drug interactions, 524t
  pharmacology, 518t–519t
  for *Pseudallescheria boydii*, 2390
  structure, 402f
  topical, 401t

Microbial flora. *See* Flora, microbial
Microbiology laboratory. *See* Laboratory
    studies
Micrococcus, 1755, 1811
    keratitis, 1112
Micrococcus melitensis. See Brucella
    melitensis
Microhemagglutination tests: for
    syphilis, 181
Microscopy, 184
    stained, 184, 184t
    unstained, 184
Microsporidia, 2513–2524. *See also*
    specific parasites
    classification, 2514
    clinical manifestations, 2517t
    conjunctivitis: in AIDS, 1106
    description, 2513, 2513f, 2514f
    diagnosis, 2519–2521, 2520f
        cytologic, 2519–2520
        electron microscopy, 2521
        histologic, 2520–2521
        immunologic, 2521
        molecular, 2521
        stool examination, 2519–2520
        tissue culture, 2521
    diarrhea: in AIDS, 970, 970t
    differential diagnosis: *Cryptosporidi-
        um*, 2504
    enterocolitis: and HIV/AIDS, 1230
    epidemiology, 2515–2517
    and HIV/AIDS, 2516, 2517t,
        2518–2519, 2519t
        conjunctivitis, 1106
        diarrhea, 970, 970t
        enterocolitis, 1230
        keratitis, 1114
    merogony, 2513
    in non-HIV infected, 2517t,
        2517–2518
    pathology, 2514–2515, 2515f
    phases I–III, 2513
    prevention, 2522
    sporogony, 2513
    treatment, 465t, 2521–2522
Microsporidium
    stool examination, 180, 181
Microsporidium africanum, 2517, 2517t
Microsporidium ceylonensis, 2517,
    2517t
Microsporum, 2375, 2375t
Microsporum audouinii, 2375, 2375t
Microsporum canis, 2375, 2375t
Microsporum ferrugineum, 2375t, 2376
Microsporum nanum, 2375, 2375t
Microsporum persicolor, 2375t, 2376
Microsporum rivalieri, 2375t, 2376
Microtus pennsylvanicus: and han-
        taviruses, 1569
Middleburg virus, 1457
Midges: and *Mansonella*, 2536
Migration inhibitory factor (MIF): and
        *Mycobacterium avium-intra-
        cellulare*, 2252
Miliary granulomatosis: *Listeria mono-
        cytogenes*, 1161
Miliary tuberculosis, miliary, 2332t,
        2332–2334. *See also*
        Mycobacterium tuberculosis
Milk, human: and protection from
        enteric infections, 948
Milker's nodule, 1325, 1329
Minimal bactericidal concentration
        (MBC), 195, 200, 225, 226f
Minimal fungicidal concentration

(MFC), 225
Minimal inhibitory concentration (MIC),
    200, 225, 226f
Minimal lethal concentration (MLC),
    195, 200
Minimum lethal dose: toxins, 7
Mink encephalopathy, transmissible,
    1674
Minocycline
    adverse reactions, 310
    combination therapy: for mycobacteria,
        396t
    dosage, 512t–513t
    for leprosy, 399
    for *Mycobacterium leprae*, 2249
    for *Nocardia*, 2277
    for nontuberculous mycobacteria, 396
    pharmacokinetics, 309t
    pharmacology, 308–309, 512t–513t
    structure, 307f
MIR-1 β-lactamase, 216t, 217
Mite-borne diseases, 2558t, 2564. *See
        also specific diseases*
Mites, 2564–2565
    animal, 2564
    follicle, 2564
    food, 2564
    grain, 2564
    harvest, 2564
    house dust, 2565
    "itch." *See Sarcoptes scabiei*
    and rickettsialpox, 1727
    and scrub typhus, 1740
    treatment and prevention, 2565
Mitral annulus, calcified: and infective
        endocarditis, 741
Mitral valve
    infections, 741. *See also* Endocarditis,
        infective
    prolapse: and endocarditis, 742,
        794–795
    stenosis: and rheumatic fever, 1801
Mitsuokella, 2158t
MMR vaccine, 1500, 1523. *See also
        individual viruses*
    adverse reactions, 2773t
    contraindications, 2787t
    indications
        for adults, 2784t
        for children and infants, 2775t,
            2783
        for HIV infected, 2784
    reportable events, 2786t
Mobiluncus, 1079, 2051–2052, 2158t,
        2206, 2208
    clinical manifestations, 2052
    description, 2051
    diagnosis and identification, 2052
    epidemiology, 2051
    female genital infections, 2199
    pathogenesis, 2052
    therapy and susceptibility, 2052
Mobiluncus curtisii, 2051–2052
Mobiluncus mulieris, 2051–2052
Moellerella wisconsinis, 1975t
Mokola virus, 1528t, 1529
Molds, 2288–2289, 2289t. *See also*
        Fungal infections
Molecular cloning: of virulence genes,
        25–26
Molecular genetics: antibiotic resistance,
        212–214
Molecular research: microbial patho-
        genicity, 19–29
    attributes of pathogens, 20–21

clonal nature of pathogens, 21, 21t
    intracellular parasites, 24–25
    plasmids, phages and insertion ele-
        ments, 22, 22t
    regulation, 22–24, 23f, 23t
    understanding virulence, 27–28
    virulence genes, 25–27
Moll, gland of: infection, 1130
Mollaret's meningitis: HSV and, 1341
Molluscum contagiosum, 1329–1330
    blepharitis, 1130
    in children, 1056
    conjunctivitis, 1106
    diagnosis, 1059, 1061f
    and HIV/AIDS, 1228, 1330
Mollusks: poisoning, 1014–1015, 1015t
Moniliasis. *See Candida albicans*, vulvo-
        vaginitis
Moniliformis moniliformis: treatment, 466t
    pyrantel pamoate, 480
Monkeypox, 1329
Monkeys: arenaviruses in, 1573t, 1575
Monobactams, 266. *See also* Aztreonam
    antimicrobial activity, 285t
    cross-reactivity, 277
    for neutropenics, 2688t
    structure, 274f
Monocid. *See* Cefonocid
Monoclonal antibodies
    for bacterial meningitis, 856
    for immunocompromised host, 2693t,
        2693–2694
    inhibition of adherence, 12, 13, 16
Monocytes, 122–124
    abnormalities: and HIV, 1209
    cytokines released by, 115
    macrophages vs., 122
    recruitment, 123
    regulation of immune and inflamma-
        tory responses, 123–124
Monokines, 112
    regulation of immune and inflamma-
        tory response, 123–124
Mononuclear phagocytes, 33, 34, 102,
        112, 122–124
    produced by cytokines, 115–116
    recruitment and activation, 123
    regulation of immune and inflamma-
        tory responses, 123–124
Mononucleosis
    aminotransferases, 1140f
    CMV, 1357, 1372
    differential diagnosis, 1372
    EBV, 1364–1377. *See also* Epstein-
        Barr virus
        differential diagnosis, 1372
    herpesviruses, 1334t
Monosodium glutamate: reactions, 1012,
        1017t
Montgomery County agent: winter vom-
        iting disease, 968
Montpellier sign, 2434
Moraxella, 1926–1928, 1927t. *See also
        individual species*
    characteristics, 2010t
Moraxella atlantae, 1928
    identification, 1927t
Moraxella catarrhalis, 1926–1928
    β-lactamase producing, 1928
    blepharitis, 1130
    and chronic bronchitis, 610
    conjunctivitis: neonatal, 1107
    and cystic fibrosis, 659
    endocarditis, 755
    growth characteristics, 1929t
    identification, 186, 1927t

keratitis, 1113
    otitis media, 581, 581t, 582
    pneumonia
        community-acquired, 628
        and HIV/AIDS, 1235, 1235t
    sinusitis, 585t
    treatment
        amoxicillin-clavulanate, 269
        azithromycin, 335t, 339
        β-lactamase inhibitors, 268t
        cephalosporins, 255, 255t, 257
        clarithromycin, 335t
        erythromycin, 335t, 338
        quinolones, 367t, 372
Moraxella lacunata, 1928
    conjunctivitis, 1104–1105, 1928
    identification, 1927t
Moraxella morganii: cephalosporins for,
        255t
Moraxella nonliquefaciens, 1928
    identification, 1927t
Moraxella osloensis, 1928
    arthritis, 1034
    identification, 1927t
Moraxella phenylpyruvica, 1928
    identification, 1927t
Moraxella urethralis. See Oligella
        urethralis
Morbidity and Mortality Weekly Report
        (MMWR), 2788
Morbilliform exanthems
    echoviruses, 1623–1624
    enteroviral, 1623–1624
Morbillivirus. *See* Measles virus
Mo-1 receptor, 82
    deficiency, 89–90
Morganella, 1974
    resistance, 251
    treatment
        aminoglycosides, 285t
        carbenicillin, 244
        penicillins, 237t
Morganella morganii, 1974
    keratitis, 1113
    treatment
        carbapenems, 264t
        quinolones, 367t
        rifampin, 318t
    urinary tract infections, 2609t, 2610
Morison's pouch, 706, 706f
Morpholine derivatives, 401
Mortierella, 2311t
Mosquito-borne diseases, 2558t. *See also
        specific diseases*
    arboviruses, 1456, 1457
    California encephalitis, 1568, 1568t
    encephalitis: transmission, clinical
        syndromes, and geographic
        distribution, 1466t
    equine encephalitis, 1456
    filariasis, 2533–2534
    flaviviruses, 1465–1473, 1466t
    Plasmodium, 2417
    reservoirs, 2794
Mountain fever. *See* Colorado tick fever
Mouse acquired immunodeficiency
        syndrome, 1207
Mouse mammary tumor virus (MMTV):
        superantigens and, 1207
Mouth
    microscopic examination of
        pathogens, 172t
    normal flora, 2159t, 2159–2160
    surgery prophylaxis recommenda-
        tions, 2751t

Moxalactam, 259
chemistry, 249
dosage, 508t–509t
in children and neonates, 508t
in renal dysfunction, 204, 509t
hematologic reactions, 254
pharmacology, 508t–509t
for Pseudomonads, 2004t
structure, 248f
Moxam. *See* Moxalactam
M proteins, 6, 110, 1754
Streptococcus pyogenes, 1786f,
1786–1787, 1792, 1793, 1800
and glomerulonephritis, 1806
and rheumatic fever, 1800–1801
T cells and, 110
Mucicarmine stain, 184t
Mucocutaneous infections. *See also*
Mucous membranes; Skin
lesions and infections
Candida albicans, 2292–2296
HSV, 1341, 1341f, 1342
Mucocutaneous lymph node syndrome.
See Kawasaki syndrome
Mucor, 2311t
dysentery, 994
pneumonia, 619t
sinusitis, 586t
specimen collection, 176f
Mucormycosis, 2311–2317
appearance in tissue, 2289t
classification of agents, 2311t, 2312
clinical manifestations, 2313–2316
CNS, 2315–2316
craniofacial, 1133
cutaneous, 2315
diagnosis, 2316, 2316f
differential diagnosis, 2316
in drug abusers, 2704
endophthalmitis, 1123, 2313
epidemiology, 2312
gangrenous cellulitis, 918
gastrointestinal, 2315
and granulocytopenia, 2676, 2679
and HIV/AIDS, 2313, 2316
hyphae, 2316
necrotizing cutaneous, 406, 918t
orbital cellulitis, 1133, 2313, 2314f
treatment, 1134
pathogenesis, 2312–2313
pneumonia: nosocomial in the
immunocompromised, 631
prevention, 2316–2317
pulmonary, 2313, 2315
rhinocerebral, 2313, 2314f, 2315f
treatment, 2316–2317
amphotericin B, 406
Mucositis: in the immunocompromised,
603
Mucous membranes. *See also*
Mucocutaneous infections;
Skin lesions and infections
*and specific mucous mem-
branes*
barrier to microorganisms, 31–32
lesions: genital, 1055–1063. *See also*
Genital lesions
Paracoccidioides brasiliensis, 2387,
2387f
Muerto Canyon virus, 1567
characteristics, 1568t
epidemiology, 1569
prevention and treatment, 1571
transmission to humans, 1569
Multilocus enzyme electrophoresis, 27

Multiple myeloma
antibody deficiency and, 53, 2669
Haemophilus influenzae and, 2669,
2673
and infection susceptibility, 2669,
2673
and *Streptococcus pneumoniae*, 1816,
1817t, 2669, 2673
Multiple sclerosis
coronaviruses and, 1488
measles virus and, 1488
Multivariate regression analysis, 160
Mumps vaccine, 167, 1500, 2778
adverse reactions, 2773t, 2778
contraindications, 2787t
indications for adults, 2784t
morbidity reduction, 2772t
Mumps virus, 1496–1501
arthritis, 1036t
clinical manifestations, 1497t,
1497–1498
complications, 1498–1499
conjunctivitis, 1106
dacryocystitis, 1131
diagnosis, 1499
differential diagnosis, 1499–1500
enteroviral meningitis, 1622
encephalitis/myelitis, 874
epidemiology, 1496
history, 1496
immunology, 1499
isolation, 2576
meningitis, 832
clinical presentation, 842, 842t
CSF examination, 845
immunoprophylaxis, 856
myocarditis, 800
orchitis, 1101
parotitis, 603
pathogenesis, 1496–1497
pathology, 1497
prevention, 1500
serology, 191
spreading/shedding mechanisms,
1320f
systemic spread, 1320f
therapy, 1500
virology, 1496
Mupirocin
clinical uses, 386
for impetigo, 911
mechanism of action, 385
pharmacokinetics, 386
resistance, 385–386
spectrum of activity, 385t, 385–386
for *Staphylococcus aureus*, 1758
for *Streptococcus pyogenes*, 1793
structure, 385f
topical, 384t
Murein sacculus, 234
Murine typhus. *See* Typhus, murine
Mus. See also Mice
and lymphocytic choriomeningitis,
1572, 1573t
and rickettsialpox, 1727
Muscimol: in mushrooms, 1015, 1015t
Muscle
degeneration: soft tissue infections,
933
proteolysis, 933
Musculoskeletal biopsies, 179
Musculoskeletal infections. *See also*
Bone infections; Joint infections
actinomycosis, 2285

Bacillus, 1893
Borrelia burgdorferi, 2147–2148
Brucella, 2056
Coccidioides immitis, 2367–2368,
2369f
Mycobacterium tuberculosis,
2236–2237
Mycoplasma pneumoniae, 1707
specimen collection and processing,
171t, 179–180
Mushroom poisoning, 1012t, 1015,
1015t
laboratory diagnosis, 1018t
management, 1020
Mutagenicity
ganciclovir, 425
metronidazole, 331
Myalgias
and acute retroviral syndrome (HIV),
1224t
cysticercosis, 935
with eosinophilia, 934
epidemic, 1625–1626
HIV, 934
infective endocarditis, 934
influenza, 934
soft tissue infections, 934
toxoplasmosis, 934
trichinosis, 934
Myasthenia gravis: differential diagnosis,
2180
Mycetoma, 2327–2330
clinical manifestations, 2327–2329,
2328f
diagnosis, 2329, 2329f
differential diagnosis, 2326,
2329–2330
epidemiology, 2327
etiology, 2327
pathogenesis and pathology, 2327
treatment and prognosis, 2330
Mycobacterial infections. *See also*
specific mycobacteria
atypical. *See* nontuberculous *below*
brain abscess: in the immunocompromised, 890
cellular immunity and, 125, 126, 127
and complement, 66
diarrhea: in AIDS, 970, 970t
growth or biochemical characteristics,
189–190
HIV/AIDS and. *See also specific
mycobacteria*
extrapulmonary: incidence, 1182t
nontuberculous, 557, 1233–1234,
1234–1235
pulmonary disease, 1233–1235
leprosy, 2243–2250. *See also*
Mycobacterium leprae
malmoense, 2269
nontuberculous, 2264–2273. *See also*
specific mycobacteria
characteristics, 2264–2266
classification and nomenclature,
2264, 2265t
clinical syndromes, 2266t
diagnosis, 2265–2266
epidemiology, 2264–2265, 2265t
and HIV, 557, 1233–1234,
1234–1235. *See also specific
species*
microbiology, 2264
osteomyelitis, 1050
pathology, 2265
pneumonia, 619t

reservoirs, 2265t
skin tests, 2264
rapidly growing, 2269–2270
sputum cultures, 173
treatment. *See also* Antimycobacterials *and specific drugs and
mycobacteria*
leprosy, 397–398
nontuberculous (atypical),
395–397, 396t
quinolones, 368t
rifampin, 320
trimethoprim, 360
tuberculosis, 389–395
tuberculosis, 2213–2243. *See also*
Mycobacterium tuberculosis
Mycobacterium abscessus, 2270
characteristics, 2265t
treatment, 396t
Mycobacterium africanum, 2213
Mycobacterium asiaticum, 2269
Mycobacterium avium-intracellulare,
2250–2264
brain abscess: in AIDS, 890
CD4 cells and, 2252
cellular immunity and, 125
cervical lymphadenitis, 938, 2255
classification, 2252
clinical manifestations, 2253–2256,
2266f
in HIV/AIDS, 2255f, 2255t,
2255–2256, 2256f
non-AIDS patients, 2253–2255,
2254f
signs and symptoms, 2253t
and cystic fibrosis, 659
cytokine protection, 121t
diagnosis, 2252–2253
differential diagnosis, 2253, 2255
Bartonella, 1742
Cryptosporidium, 2504
DNA probes, 2214
epidemiology, 2251–2252
gastrointestinal: and HIV/AIDS, 2256,
2256f
glycopeptidolipids, 2252
hairy cell leukemia and, 137
and HIV/AIDS, 389, 557, 1221,
1234–1235, 1281, 2250
brain abscess, 890
clinical manifestations, 2254–2256,
2255f, 2255t, 2256f
diagnosis, 2253
differential diagnosis, 2253
epidemiology, 2251–2252
gastric, 1230
immunity and, 2252
incidence, 1182t, 1183, 1234–1235,
2251
lymphadenitis, 941
pneumonia, 621
probability of developing, 1223f
prophylaxis, 1286t, 1289, 2258
treatment, 131, 1283t, 1289,
2257–2258
host immunity, 2252
identification, 189, 190
intestinal, 999t
keratitis, 1113
and leukemia, hairy cell, 2673
lymphadenitis, 940t
and HIV/AIDS, 941
microbiology, 2252
osteoarticular, 1050
pathogenesis, 2252

pneumonia
    chronic, 647t
    and HIV/AIDS, 621
    radiology, 650t, 654f
    prophylaxis, 2258
        and HIV/AIDS, 1286t, 1289, 2258
        rifabutin, 1286t, 1289
    signs and symptoms
        AIDS, 2254t
        non-AIDS, 2253t
    treatment, 395–396, 396t, 396–397,
            2256–2258
        aminoglycosides, 285t, 295t
        azithromycin, 340
        clarithromycin, 339, 340
        in HIV/AIDS, 131, 1283t, 1289,
            2257–2258
        interferon-γ, 453
        in non-AIDS patients, 2257, 2257t
        quinolones, 368t
        rifabutin, 324, 395–396
Mycobacterium bovis, 2213, 2214
    characteristics, 2265t
    and HIV/AIDS, 1234
    identification, 189
    INH resistance, 2214
    reservoirs, 2265t
    transmission, 2216
Mycobacterium chelonae, 2270. See also
        Mycobacterium fortuitum
    characteristics, 2265t
    clinical syndromes, 2266t
    and HIV/AIDS, 1234
    keratitis, 1113
    reservoirs, 2265t
    skin infections: in transplantation,
        2726
    treatment, 395–396, 396t, 2270
        quinolones, 368t, 373
        rifampin, 318t
*Mycobacterium chelonei. See
        Mycobacterium chelonae*
Mycobacterium flavescens, 2269
    characteristics, 2265t
    reservoirs, 2265t
Mycobacterium fortuitum, 2270. See also
        Mycobacterium chelonae
    arthritis, 1035
    characteristics, 2265t
    clinical syndromes, 2266t
    keratitis, 1113
    osteoarticular, 1050
    reservoirs, 2265t
    treatment, 395–396, 2270
        quinolones, 368t
        rifampin, 318t
Mycobacterium fortuitum-chelonae,
        2270. See also *Mycobacterium
        chelonae*; *Mycobacterium for-
        tuitum*
    identification, 189
    musculoskeletal specimen collection,
        180
Mycobacterium gastri, 2269
    characteristics, 2265t
    reservoirs, 2265t
Mycobacterium genavense: identifica-
        tion, 189
Mycobacterium gordonae, 2269
    characteristics, 2265t
    DNA probes, 2214
    and HIV/AIDS, 1234
    keratitis, 1113
    osteoarticular, 1050
    reservoirs, 2265t

Mycobacterium haemophilum, 2269
    cutaneous manifestations, 550t
    and HIV/AIDS, 1234
    identification, 189
    treatment, 395
Mycobacterium kansasii, 2266–2268
    arthritis, 1035
    characteristics, 2265t, 2266
    clinical syndromes, 2266t, 2267
    differential diagnosis, 2322
    DNA probes, 2214
    epidemiology, 2264, 2265t, 2266
    and HIV/AIDS, 557, 1234
    identification, 189
    pathology, 2265
    pulmonary infection, 2266t,
        2266–2267, 2267f
        chronic, 647t
    treatment, 395–396, 396, 396t,
        2267–2268
        erythromycin, 335
        quinolones, 368t
Mycobacterium leprae, 2243–2250
    amyloidosis, 2248
    armadillos and, 2244
    borderline, 2245, 2246, 2246f
        lepromatous (BL), 2245
        tuberculoid (BT), 2245
    cellular immunity and, 126, 127
    clinical manifestations, 2245f,
        2245–2246, 2246f
    cytokine and T cell protection, 121t
    defective chemotaxis in, 90
    deformity, 2247
    differential diagnosis, 2247
    diffuse lepromatosis, 2245
    epidemiology, 2244–2245
    eye, 2248
    Fernandez reaction, 2246
    foam cells (Virchow's cells), 2246
    granulomatous hepatitis, 1161
    histology, 2245–2246
    identification, 189
    immunologic spectrum, 2246
    lepra type-1 reactions (downgrading
        and reversal reactions), 2247
        therapy, 2247
    lepra type-2 reactions (erythema
        nodosum leprosum), 2247
        therapy, 2247
    lepromatous, 2245, 2245f, 2246
        histology, 2246
        immunology, 2246
        multidrug therapy, 2248, 2249
        ocular involvement, 2248
        testicular involvement, 2248
    lepromin intradermal skin test, 2246
    Lucio's reaction, 2247
    microbiology, 2244
    Mitsuda reaction, 2246
    morphologic index, 2244
    nerve abscesses, 2247
    neuritis, 878, 2245
    phenolic glycolipid (PGL), 2244,
        2245
    plantar ulceration, 2245, 2247
    prophylaxis, 2247
    testes, 2248
    transmission, 2244
    treatment, 2248–2249
        acedapsone, 398
        adverse reactions, 399
        aminoglycosides, 2249
        antimicrobial, 2248–2249
        clarithromycin, 339

clofazimine, 398, 2248, 2249
    dapsone, 397, 474, 2248, 2249
    ethionamide, 398, 2248–2249
    immunotherapy, 2248
    interferon-γ, 453, 2248
    interleukin-2, 453, 2248
    newer agents, 2249
    prothionamide, 398, 2248–2249
    of reactions, 2247
    regimens, 2249
    response, 2249
    rifabutin, 398
    rifampin, 320, 397t, 2248, 2249
    rifapentine, 324, 398
    sulfoxone, 398–399
    thiacetazone, 398
    tuberculoid, 2245, 2246
    treatment, 2249
Mycobacterium lepraemurium: cellular
        immunity and, 125
Mycobacterium malmoense, 2269
    characteristics, 2265t
    identification, 189
Mycobacterium marinum, 2268
    arthritis, 1035
    characteristics, 2265t
    differential diagnosis, 2322, 2326,
        2356
    granulomatous lymphangitis, 943
    and leukemia, hairy cell, 2673
    musculoskeletal specimen collection,
        180
    osteoarticular, 1049–1050
    reservoirs, 2265t
    treatment, 395–396, 396t
        tetracyclines, 307
Mycobacterium microti, 2213
Mycobacterium paratuberculosis, 2269
Mycobacterium phlei, 2269
Mycobacterium scrofulaceum, 2268
    cervical lymphadenitis, 938, 2255,
        2268
    characteristics, 2265t
    clinical syndromes, 2266t
    identification, 189
    reservoirs, 2265t
    treatment, 396, 396t
        erythromycin, 335
Mycobacterium simiae, 2268
    characteristics, 2265t
    reservoirs, 2265t
Mycobacterium smegmatis, 2270
    characteristics, 2265t
    reservoirs, 2265t
Mycobacterium szulgai, 2268–2269
    characteristics, 2265t
    reservoirs, 2265t
    treatment, 395
Mycobacterium szulgai: identification,
        189
Mycobacterium terrae, 2269
    characteristics, 2265t
    reservoirs, 2265t
Mycobacterium thermoresistibile, 2269
Mycobacterium triviale
    characteristics, 2265t
    reservoirs, 2265t
Mycobacterium tuberculosis, 2213–2243,
        2265t
    in adolescence, 2221–2222
    age influence on infection, 2221–2222
    antimicrobial susceptibility testing,
        191–192, 2214–2215
    arthritis, 1032, 1035, 1035t
        diagnosis, 1037

BACTEC radiometry, 189–190, 2214
brain abscess: in AIDS, 890
bronchogenic carcinoma and,
        2225–2226
bronchogenic spread, 2219, 2223,
        2225
bronchoscopy, 173
caseous, 2219, 2223, 2225
cell-mediated immunity and, 125,
        127, 2218–2219
    defects, 2681, 2682
cervical lymphadenitis (scrofula),
        2255
    and HIV, 938
chemoprophylaxis, 2229t, 2229–2231
    of contacts, 2230
    drug regimens, 2229
    and HIV/AIDS, 1283t, 1289,
        2230–2231
    INH hepatotoxicity risk,
        2229–2230
    isoniazid, 1283t, 1289
    in nursing homes, 2231
    of positive tuberculin reactions,
        2230
    of quiescent, previously untreated
        pulmonary tuberculosis, 2230
    of tuberculin converter, 2230
in childhood, 2221
chronic pulmonary
    apical localization, 2221
    endogenous vs. exogenous reinfec-
        tion, 2221
    epidemiology, 2221
CNS, 829, 2234–2235
conjunctivitis, 1105
in correctional facilities, 2218
CT, 2225
cultures, 2214
cutaneous, 2239–2240
    and AIDS, 557
    classification, 2240t
    differential diagnosis, 2322, 2326,
        2437
cytokine and T cell protection, 121t
differential diagnosis
    cryptococcosis, 2336
    histoplasmosis, 2345
    lung abscess, 645
    from other mycobacteria, 2214
    paracoccidioidomycosis, 2388
disseminated: and splenic abscess,
        727
DNA probes, 27, 2214
in drug abusers, 2701–2702, 2704
in the elderly, 2738–2739
encephalitis/myelitis, 874
endobronchial, 2223–2224
enteric symptoms, 999t, 1003
enteritides, 993
epidemiology, 2215–2218
    recent morbidity and mortality
        trends, 2215f, 2215–2216,
        2216f, 2216t
epididymitis, 1100–1101
erythema nodosum and, 2220
extrapulmonary, 2231–2240
    bronchopleural fistula, 2235
    CNS, 2234–2235
    cutaneous, 2239–2240
    empyema, 2235
    gastrointestinal, 2238
    genitourinary, 2237t, 2237–2238
    and HIV/AIDS, 2231, 2232f
    laryngitis, 2240

Mycobacterium tuberculosis (Continued)
late complications of collapse therapy, 2235–2236
lymphadenitis (scrofula), 2239,
2255
miliary, 2232–2234, 2332t. *See also*
miliary *below*
otitis, 2240
pericarditis, 2236
peritonitis, 2238–2239
pleurisy, 2235
renal, 2237–2238
skeletal, 2236–2237
exudative, 2219
female genital, 2238
and fever, 542
fiberoptic bronchoscopy, 2225
fibrosing mediastinitis, 2239
gastrointestinal, 993, 2238
differential diagnosis, 994
and HIV/AIDS, 2238
genitourinary, 2237t, 2237–2238
female genital, 2238
and HIV/AIDS, 2238
male genital, 2238
Gohn focus, 2220
granulomatous hepatitis, 1161
hepatic, 2233
history, 2213
and HIV/AIDS, 159, 542, 1171,
1171f, 1171t, 1177, 1221,
1231–1232, 1234, 1281–1282,
2213, 2222
in Africa, 1171, 1171f, 1171t
in Asia, 1171t
brain abscess, 890
chemoprophylaxis, 1286t, 2229,
2230–2231
coinfection, 2216
cutaneous manifestations, 557
diagnosis, 2225
epidemiology, 2215
extrapulmonary tuberculosis, 2231,
2232f
gastrointestinal, 2238
genitourinary, 2238
meningitis, 872
miliary tuberculosis, 2233–2234
multidrug-resistance, 389, 1184,
2213
pneumonia, 621
probability of developing, 1223f,
2217
pulmonary, 2224, 2224t
treatment, 1283t, 1289, 2228–2229,
2642
in homeless shelters, 2218
in hospitals, 2217–2218
hypertrophic spinal pachymeningitis,
906
identification, 189–190
immunodeficiency and, 138
cell-mediated, 2681, 2682
immunologic features, 2218–2219
influence of chemotherapy on spread
of infection, 2217
institutional spread, 2217–2218
intestinal, 999t
isolation, 2576–2577
keratitis, 1113, 1115
Kinyoun stain, 2214
Koch phenomenon, 2221
laryngitis, 2223, 2240
late hematogenous, 2222
lower lobe, 2223–2224

lower lung field, 2223
lymphadenitis (scrofula), 936, 940t,
2239
mesenteric, 2239
peripheral nodes, 2239
lysis centrifugation, 2214
male genital, 2238
measles and, 1522
mediastinal lymphadenopathy, 2239
meningitis, 868–869, 2234–2235
clinical features, 2234, 2234f
in the elderly, 2740
and HIV, 872
in the immunocompromised, 872
pathology, 2234
spinal, 2235
treatment, 2234
glucocorticoids, 455
microbiology, 2213–2215
in midadulthood, 2222
miliary, 2232–2234, 2332t
acute, 2232–2233
chorioretinitis, 2240
cryptic, 2233
endophthalmitis, 1121
and hematologic abnormalities,
2233
and HIV/AIDS, 2233–2234
late generalized, 2233
nonreactive, 2233
pleurisy and, 2235
treatment, 2235
primary hepatic, 2233
modes of spread, 2216–2217
morbidity and mortality trends
(recent), 2215f, 2215–2216,
2216f
age distribution, 2216f
incidence of active tuberculosis in
certain groups, 2216t
WHO 1990 worldwide case rates,
2216t
MRI, 2225
multidrug-resistance (MDR-TB), 389,
2218. *See also* resistance
below
and HIV/AIDS, 389, 1184, 2213
outbreaks, 2218
neuritis, 878
Nocardia and, 2275
nonreactive, 2219
nosocomial, 2217–2218
controlling, 2218
in old age, 2222
otitis, 2240
pancreatic abscess, 723
pathogenesis, 2220–2222
evolution of primary infection,
2220–2221
pericarditis, 805, 806, 806f
treatment, 807–808
peritonitis, 708–709, 710, 2238–2239
and phagocytes, 88
phlyctenular keratoconjunctivitis and,
2220
pleural, 640
pleurisy, 2235
pneumonia, 619t
and AIDS, 629
bronchoalveolar lavage, 625
chronic, 647t
HIV and, 621
sputum analysis, 623
polymerase chain reaction, 2215
primary (childhood) infection, 2221

progressive lower lobe, 2223
progressive primary, 2220, 2222
proliferative (productive), 2219
prostatitis, 1100
pulmonary, 2222–2226
in adolescence and adults,
2223–2226
in AIDS, 2224, 2224t
and cancer, 2225–2226
in childhood, 2222–2223
chronic, 2221
classification, 2226
diagnosis, 2225
at autopsy, 2225
epidemiology, 2221
fiberoptic bronchoscopy, 2225
laboratory findings, 2224–2225
lower lobe and endobronchial,
2223–2224
physical examination, 2224
and pleurisy, 2235
postprimary, 2223
primary after childhood, 2223
roentenography, 2224–2225
silicotuberculosis, 2225
symptoms, 2224
treatment, 2226–2231. *See also*
treatment *below*
tuberculomas, 2224
Ranke complex, 2220
reinfection, 2221
endogenous vs. exogenous, 2221
renal, 2237–2238
resistance, 164, 192
multidrug, 389, 2218
and HIV/AIDS, 389, 1183, 2213
primary, 2226
secondary, 2226
restriction fragment length polymorphism, 2215
risk of infection, 2217
risk of progression from infection to
active disease, 2217
roentgenographic findings,
2224–2225
screening programs, 167
silicotuberculosis, 2225
Simon focus, 2220
skeletal, 1050, 2236–2237
peripheral osteoarticular, 2237
Pott's disease, 2236–2237
sputum, 2214, 2225
susceptibility testing, 191–192,
2214–2215
transmission, 2216–2217
in transplant recipients, 2712
treatment, 389–395, 2226–2231
amikacin, 394–395
aminoglycosides, 286, 295t, 300
amithiozone, 395
β-lactams, 395
capreomycin, 394
chemoprophylaxis, 2229t,
2229–2231
in childhood, 2229
corticosteroids, 2228
course and observation, 2228
cycloserine, 394
ethambutol, 393, 1289, 2226, 2227,
2228, 2229
ethionamide, 394
first-line antimycobacterials,
389–393, 2226
four-drug regimen, 2227, 2227t,
2230

glucocorticoids, 455
in HIV/AIDS, 1283t, 1289,
2228–2229
in the immunocompromised,
2687
and immunosuppresive therapy,
2229
isoniazid, 391, 1289, 2226, 2227,
2228, 2229, 2230, 2231, 2232,
2233, 2234, 2237, 2239
kanamycin, 395
in liver disease, 2229
nine-month regimen, 2227
noncompliance, 2227
para-aminosalicylic acid, 394
in pregnancy, 2229
pulmonary disease, 2226–2231
pyrazinamide, 392–393, 1289,
2226, 2227, 2227t, 2228,
2230, 2232, 2233, 2234
quinolones, 368t, 372, 395
retreatment, 2228
rifabutin, 324, 392
rifampin, 391–392, 2226, 2227
rifapentine, 324
second-line antimycobacterials,
394–396, 2226–2227
selecting a regimen, 2227–2228
six-month regimen, 2227
streptomycin, 393, 2226, 2227,
2227t, 2228, 2229, 2230
three-drug regimen, 2227, 2232
in uremia and end-stage renal
disease, 2229
viomycin, 395
tuberculin test, 2219–2220
booster effect, 2219
dosage, 2219
false-positive and false-negative
reactions, 2219–2220
and HIV, 2220
interpretation, 2219–2220
reversion of reactivity to negative,
2220
technical aspects, 2219
tuberculomas
intracranial, 2224
pulmonary, 2224
vaccination, 167, 2231
vaginal infection, 1080
Weigart focus, 2221
in young adulthood, 2221–2222
Zehl-Nielsen stain, 2214
Mycobacterium ulcerans, 2213, 2269
characteristics, 2265t
clinical syndromes, 2266t
and HIV/AIDS, 1234
identification, 189
reservoirs, 2265t
treatment, 396t
Mycobacterium xenopi, 2269
characteristics, 2265t
and HIV/AIDS, 1234
identification, 189
reservoirs, 2265t
treatment, 395
Mycobutin. *See* Rifabutin
Mycology, 2288–2289. *See also* Fungal
infections
Mycoplasma buccale: taxonomy,
1702f
Mycoplasma diseases, 1701–1718. *See
also individual species*
antibody deficiencies and, 49
characteristics, 1701t

description of organism, 1701f, 1701t,
   1701–1702
  characteristics, 1701t
encephalitis, 875
genital, 1703, 1713–1718. *See also
  individual species*
  isolation and identification,
   1713–1714
  properties, 1713t
hemagglutinin response, 42
overview, 1701–1704
pathogenesis, 1703
photomicrograph, 1701f
quinolones for, 367t, 372
specimen collection and processing,
  171t, 183
taxonomy and distribution, 1702f,
  1702–1703
in transplant recipients, 2712t
T-strain. *See Ureaplasma urealyticum*
Mycoplasma faucium: taxonomy, 1702f
Mycoplasma fermentans
HIV and, 1212, 1703, 1707
identification, 1713
incognitus strain, 1703
isolation and identification, 1713
properties, 1713t
taxonomy, 1702f
Mycoplasma genitalium, 1703
identification, 1713
isolation and identification, 1713
properties, 1713t
taxonomy, 1702f
urethritis, 1067, 1714–1716
Mycoplasma hominis, 1703
clinical manifestations, 1714–1717,
  1715t
colonization, 1714
epidemiology, 1714
in heart transplantation, 2724
hypogammaglobulinemia, 1716–1717
identification, 1713, 1714
immunosuppression, 1716–1717
isolation and identification, 1713
neonatal meningitis and brain abscess,
  1717
pelvic inflammatory disease, 1716
postabortal and postpartum fever,
  1715t, 1716
properties, 1713t
pyelonephritis, 1715t, 1716
resistance
  transposon, 214
serotyping, 1714
taxonomy, 1702f
in transplant recipients, 2726
treatment, 1717
  quinolones, 367t
vaginosis, 1079, 1714, 1715t, 1717
Mycoplasma incognitus, 1703
HIV and, 1212, 1703, 1707
taxonomy, 1702f
Mycoplasma lipophilum: taxonomy,
  1702f
Mycoplasma orale: taxonomy, 1702f
Mycoplasma penetrans: properties,
  1713t
Mycoplasma pneumoniae, 1702,
  1704–1713
bronchitis, acute, 606, 607
cardiac complications, 1707
and chronic bronchitis, 610
clinical manifestations, 1705f,
  1705–1707
CNS infection, 830

cold agglutinins, 1708, 1709
complement fixation, 1708, 1709
croup, 574, 574t
cultures, 173
cutaneous manifestations, 550t, 1706
description, 1704–1705
diagnosis, 1708–1710, 1709f, 1709t
differential diagnosis, 2345
enteric symptoms, 999t, 1003
epidemiology, 1705
extrapulmonary involvement, 1706
and Guillain-Barré syndrome, 878
history, 1704
immunology, 1707–1708
musculoskeletal complications, 1707
myocarditis, 800
neurologic complications, 1707
otitis media, 581
pathology and pathophysiology, 1708
pericarditis, 805
pharyngitis, 567t, 569, 1789
pneumonia
  atypical, 630
  community-acquired, 629
  differential diagnosis, 1698
  radiology, 627
  serology, 625–626
  treatment, 631
prevention, 1711
properties, 1713t
Raynaud's phenomenon, 1706, 1708
respiratory infection, 1705f,
  1705–1706. *See also* pneumonia *above*
risk factors, 1707
serology, 192t
sickle cell disease and, 1707, 1707f
taxonomy, 1702f
transmission, 1705
treatment, 1710t, 1710–1711
  azithromycin, 335t, 340
  clarithromycin, 335t, 339, 340
  erythromycin, 335t, 337, 338t
  pneumonia, 631
  quinolones, 372
vaccine research, 1711
Mycoplasma primatum
properties, 1713t
taxonomy, 1702f
Mycoplasma salivarium
properties, 1713t
taxonomy, 1702f
Mycoplasma spermatophilum: properties,
  1713t
Mycoses. *See* Fungal infections
Mycostatin: for burn wounds, 2764,
  2764t
Mycotic aneurysms, 769–773
classification, 769t
clinical manifestations, 771
differential diagnosis: brain abscess,
  891
in drug abusers, 2700, 2701, 2701f
endocarditis and, 746–747, 749
epidemiology, 769–770
etiology, 772
laboratory findings, 771–772
pathogenesis, 770
pathology, 770–771
therapy, 772–773
Myelitis, 874–878
clinical findings, 875–876
etiology, 876–877, 877t
herpesviruses, 1334t
laboratory findings, 876

pathogenesis, 874–875
pathology, 874–875
transverse
  differential diagnosis, 1617
  etiology, 877
  treatment, 877–878
  varicella-zoster virus, 874, 1347, 1348
Myelodysplasia: HIV and, 1209
Myeloma. *See* Multiple myeloma
Myelopathy
cytomegalovirus, 1360
HTLV, 1582
Myeloperoxidase-dependent reactions,
  87
Myeloperoxidase-independent reactions,
  87
Myeloperoxidase (MPO), 79t, 87
deficiency, 93–94, 151t, 154
Myelosuppression: from ganciclovir,
  425
Myiasis, 2558, 2562–2564
clinical manifestations, 2563, 2563f
epidemiology, 2563
ophthalmomyiasis, 2563
treatment, 2563–2564
Myocarditis, 800–804
Chagas disease, 2443–2444
Chlamydia psittaci, 1694
clinical manifestations, 802
CMV, 1358
Corynebacterium diphtheriae, 1869
Dallas criteria, 803
diagnosis, 803, 804t
infectious etiology, 800t, 800–801
influenza virus, 1558
Kawasaki syndrome, 2568
pathology and pathogenesis, 801f,
  801–802, 802f
poliovirus, 1616
rheumatic fever, 1802
Toxoplasma gondii: and HIV/AIDS,
  2459
treatment, 804
Myonecrosis
Aeromonas hydrophila, 933
anaerobic streptococcal, 933
  differential diagnosis, 924t
clostridial (gas gangrene), 931–933,
  2163t, 2166, 2166t,
  2186–2189. *See also*
  Clostridial myonecrosis
  differential diagnosis, 918t, 924t
episiotomy, 1093
synergistic nonclostridial anaerobic.
  See Cellulitis, synergistic
  necrotizing
Myopathy: from zidovudine, 436
Myopericarditis
coxsackieviruses, 1621t, 1626–1627
  clinical manifestations, 1627
  differential diagnosis, 1627
  epidemiology, 1626–1627
  management, 1627
  neonatal, 1628
  pathogenesis, 1627
herpesviruses, 1334t
viral: differential diagnosis, 1627
Myosin, 80
Myositis
Aeromonas hydrophila myonecrosis,
  933
anaerobic streptococcal myonecrosis,
  933
Borrelia burgdorferi, 2147
Candida albicans, 2298

clostridial, 2186
coxsackieviruses, 1632
Cysticercus cellulosae, 933
echoviruses, 1632
enteroviral, 1632
infected vascular gangrene, 933
influenza virus and, 1558
necrotizing cutaneous. *See* Cellulitis,
  synergistic necrotizing
nonclostridial (crepitant), 933
parasitic, 934–935
soft tissue infections, 929–936
Streptococcus pyogenes, 930–931,
  1795, 1795f
synergistic nonclostridial anaerobic
  myonecrosis, 933
Toxoplasma gondii: and HIV/AIDS,
  2459
Myringitis, bullous: *Mycoplasma pneumoniae* and, 1706
Myringotomy: for otitis media, 583
Myristoylated, alanine-rich C-kinase
  substrate (MARCKS), 110
Myrmesia. *See* Plantar warts
Myxoma virus, 1325

N

N-acetylglucosamine (NAG), 234
cephalosporins and, 249
N-acetylmuramic acid (NAM), 234
cephalosporins and, 249
NADPH oxidase, 84
*Naegleria aerobia. See Naegleria
  fowleri*
Naegleria fowleri, 2394t, 2408–2414
clinical manifestations, 2394t, 2411
description, 2408–2409, 2409f
encephalitis, 876
epidemiology, 2410
laboratory diagnosis, 2412
meningitis, 835, 2408, 2410
  antimicrobial therapy, 850t
pathogenesis and pathology,
  2410–2411
phase microscopy, 179
transmission, 2394t
treatment, 461t, 2413
  artemisinin, 472
trophozoites, 2408, 2409f, 2410f
*Naegleria invadens. See Naegleria
  fowleri*
Nafcillin, 243
adverse reactions, 239t
aminoglycoside combination therapy,
  287t, 289t
for cellulitis, 916
dosage, 241t, 506–507t
  in children, 506t, 851t
  for meningitis, 850t, 851t
  in neonates, 242t, 506t
  in renal disease and dialysis, 238t
for endocarditis
  prosthetic valve, 786t
  staphylococcal, 762
for gangrenous cellulitis, 918
indications, 194
MICs against cocci, 237t
pharmacokinetics, 238t
pharmacology, 506–507t
staphylococcal resistance, 194
structure, 242f
for suppurative thrombophlebitis, 768
for toxic shock syndrome, 1767
trade names, 236t

Naftifine
   structure, 402f
   topical, 401t
Nail infections. *See* Onychomycosis
Nairovirus, 1567
   characteristics, 1568t
Nalidixic acid, 364
   adverse reactions, 374
   antimicrobial activity, 367t, 369t
   in breast milk, 204
   dosage, 370t, 516t–517t
   drug interactions, 524t
   pharmacology, 516t–517t
   resistance, 219, 221
   for *Salmonella*, 2026
   for *Shigella*, 2037, 2037t
   structure, 365f
   and sugar level testing, 203
Naloxone: for sepsis syndrome, 701
Nannizzia, 2375
Nanophyetus salmincola, 2553t, 2557
   diagnosis, 2557
   treatment, 463t, 2557
      praziquantel, 482
Naphthyridine: structure, 365f
Nasal collapse: leprosy, 2247
Nasolacrimal duct obstruction: management, 1134
Nasopharyngeal carcinoma: Epstein-Barr
      virus and, 1332, 1332t,
      1369–1370
Nasopharynx
   microscopic examination of
      pathogens, 172t
   specimen collection and processing,
      169, 170t, 172, 172t
Nasotracheal suctioning: and endocar-
      ditis, 743t
Natamycin: for keratitis, 1117
National Childhood Vaccine Injury Act,
      2785, 2786
Natural killer (NK) cells, 34, 102
   and HIV, 1210, 1214
Nausea/vomiting
   food-borne disease, 1012–1013,
      1014
   gastrointestinal infections and,
      965–973
   hepatitis, 1138
   and peritonitis, 714
   winter vomiting disease, 968–969
Ndumu virus, 1457
Nebraska calf diarrhea virus (NCDV),
      967, 1451
Necator americanus, 2529–2530
   clinical syndrome, 2530
   diagnosis, 2530
   epidemiology, 2529–2530
   life cycle, 2529
   penetration, 7
   treatment, 463t, 2530
      mebendazole, 478–479
      pyrantel pamoate, 480
Neck
   irradiation, 604
   postsurgical wounds, 604
Neck infections, 604
   actinomycosis, 2281
   anaerobic, 2163t, 2164
      specimen collection, 2168t
   mediastinitis and, 814
      bacteriology, 815t
Neck surgery: prophylaxis recommenda-
      tions, 2751t
Neck trauma: and mediastinitis, 814t

Necrotizing cellulitis, synergistic, 918t,
      924t, 926
Necrotizing enterocolitis, 991–992
   in neutropenics: and intra-abdominal
      abscess, 729
   in the newborn, 990–991
   Pseudomonas aeruginosa, 1995
Necrotizing fasciitis, 922, 923–926. *See
      also* Streptococcal gangrene
   anaerobic, 2165–2166
   Bacillus, 1893
   clinical features, 925
   in drug abusers, 2698
   Staphylococcus aureus, 1765
   Streptococcus pyogenes, 1794–1795
   treatment, 925–926
   type I, 923
   type II (hemolytic streptococcal gan-
      grene), 923
Necrotizing myositis: group A strepto-
      coccal, 930–931
Negishi: transmission, clinical syn-
      dromes, and geographic
      distribution, 1466t
Negri bodies: rabies, 1535
Neisseria, 1928–1930, 1929t. *See also
      individual species*
   biochemical and growth characteris-
      tics, 1929t
   characteristics, 2010t
   endocarditis, 755
   and immunodeficiency, 150t
Neisseria canis, 1930
   animal bites, 2766
*Neisseria catarrhalis. See Moraxella
      catarrhalis*
Neisseria cinerea, 1928, 1929
   growth characteristics, 1929t
Neisseria elongata, 1928, 1929
   endocarditis, 755
   growth characteristics, 1929t
   identification, 1927t
Neisseria flava: endocarditis, 755
Neisseria flavescens, 1929, 1930
   endocarditis, 755
   growth characteristics, 1929t
Neisseria gonorrhoeae, 1909–1926
   aminoglycosides for, 299
   anorectal, 1910, 1913, 1914, 1916,
      1919
      diagnosis, 1920
   antigenic variations, 24
   arthritis, 1032, 1033, 1033f, 1034,
      1035, 1918
      diagnosis, 1037
      and HIV, 1228
   bacteremia: and skin infections, 921
   bartholinitis, 1085, 1915
   β-lactamase, 198, 216t
   cervicitis, 1084f, 1084–1085, 1915,
      1916, 1916f
      diagnosis, 1919–1920, 1920t
   chromosomal mutations and transfor-
      mation, 1912
   clinical manifestations, 1915–1919
   and complement, 66
   conjunctivitis, 1104–1105, 1916,
      1916f
      diagnosis, 183–184
      neonatal, 1107
   culture, 1919–1920
   cutaneous manifestations, 550t,
      553–554, 921
   dermatitis-arthritis syndrome, 921
   description, 1909–1910

   diagnosis, 1919–1920
      Limulus lysate assay, 1064–1065
   disseminated, 1917–1919
      arthritis, 1034, 1035, 1918
      cutaneous manifestations, 555,
         1060, 1918, 1918f
      treatment, 1922
   in drug abusers, 2705
   EIA diagnosis, 185
   endocarditis, 755
      treatment, 764
   endocervicitis, 1095, 1915
   endotoxin: *Limulus* lysate assay,
      1064–1065
   epidemiology, 1913–1914
   epididymitis, 1069, 1101, 1915
      treatment, 1922
   E-test, 195
   genetics, 1912
   gonococcemia: specimen collection
      and processing, 177
   gram-stained smears, 1920, 1920t
   growth characteristics, 185, 1910,
      1929t
   and HIV transmission, 1188
   identification, 186
   and IgA, 8, 20
   incidence, 1913, 1913f, 1913t
   joint infections, 1032
   keratitis, 1112, 1113
   microbiology, 1909–1912
   neonatal, 1919
   opacity proteins (protein II),
      1910–1911, 1911f
   ophthalmia neonatorum, 1913
   outer membrane, 1910–1912
   pathology, 1912–1913, 1913f
   pediatric, 1919
      treatment, 1922–1923
   pelvic inflammatory disease, 183,
      1095, 1917, 1917f
      treatment, 1921–1922, 1922t
   penicillinase-producing (PPNG),
      1914, 1914f
   peptidoglycan, 1912
   perihepatitis, 1917
   peritonitis, 709, 710
   and phagocytes, 88
   pharyngitis, 569, 1789, 1916
      cultures, 173, 181, 570
   pili, 24, 1910, 1911f
   plasmids, 1912
   porin (protein I), 1910, 1911f
   in pregnancy, 1917
   prevention and control, 1923
   proctitis, 990
      and HIV/AIDS, 1231
   prostatitis, 680
   racial incidence, 1913
   rashes, 554
   reduction-modifiable protein (Rmp;
      protein III), 1911, 1911f
   resistance, 195, 220, 251, 1914, 1914f
      aminoglycosides, 283
      tetracycline-resistant (TRNG),
         1914, 1914f
      transposon, 214
   specimen collection and processing,
      171t, 181
   strain typing, 1912
   surface structures, 1910–1912, 1911f
   tetM, 1912
   transmission, 1913–1914
   treatment, 1921–1923
      aminoglycosides, 285t, 286

      aminopenicillins, 243
      antimicrobials of choice, 202t
      β-lactamase inhibitors, 268t
      carbapenems, 264t
      cephalosporins, 255t, 257, 258, 259
      in children, 1922–1923
      chloramphenicol, 312t
      for disseminated infection, 1922
      for epididymitis, 1922
      erythromycin, 335, 335t
      fusidic acid, 278
      penicillin, 237t, 240, 241t
      for PID, 1921–1922
      piperacillin, 245
      quinolones, 367t, 371
      rifampin, 318t
      of sexual partners, 1923
      spectinomycin, 299
      sulfonamides, 355t
      tetracyclines, 308t
      trimethoprim, 357
      trimethoprim-sulfamethoxazole,
         360
      for uncomplicated disease in adults,
         1921, 1921t
   urethritis, 1915, 1915f
      asymptomatic, 1065, 1068–1069
      clinical manifestations, 1066–1067
      complications, 1069
      diagnosis, 1067, 1919–1920,
         1920t
      exudate, 1064–1065, 1065f
      incubation period, 1915, 1915f
      postgonococcal, 1068
      treatment, 1069–1070
      in women, 1069, 1915–1916
   vaccine research, 1923
   virulence regulation, 24
Neisseria lactamica, 1928, 1929
   growth characteristics, 1929t
   identification, 186
Neisseria meningitidis, 1896–1909
   antigenic structure, 1897–1898
   arthritis, 1034
   bacteremia: and skin infections, 921
   biochemical characteristics,
      1896–1899
   capsular polysaccharide, 1897,
      1897t
   carrier state, 1898–1899
      treatment, 1905
   and C3 deficiency, 69
   chemoprophylaxis, 167
   clinical manifestations, 1900f,
      1900–1902, 1901f, 1902f
   clones, 21
   and complement, 65, 66
      deficiency, 67, 67f, 69t, 69–70,
         156, 1902
   conjunctivitis, 1104–1105
   CSF specimens, 179
   cutaneous manifestations, 550t, 553,
      554, 921
   disseminated intravascular coagula-
      tion, 1904–1905
   epidemiology, 159, 1899–1900
   fimbriae, 837–838
   growth characteristics, 1929t
   identification, 186
   IgA and, 31
   immunologic response to antigens,
      1898
   keratitis, 1112
   laboratory diagnosis of infection,
      1902–1903

lipooligosaccharide, 1904
meningitis, 833t, 834, 834t
  antimicrobial therapy, 850t,
    851–852
  bacteremia, 838
  chemoprophylaxis, 857
  CSF examination, 845–846, 846,
    846t
  immunoprophylaxis, 858
  meningococcemia, 1900. *See also*
    Meningococcemia
  chronic, 1901–1902
  morphology, 1896–1897
  mucosal colonization, 837–838
  nasopharyngeal cultures, 169
  noncapsular cell wall antigens,
    1897–1898
  pericarditis, 805
  and phagocytes, 88
  polysaccharide, 165
  rashes, 553–554
  resistance, 220
  respiratory infections, 1902
  seasonality, 159
  sickle cell anemia and, 53
  splenectomy and, 2669
  surveillance, 162
  symmetric peripheral gangrene, 553,
    554
  systemic. *See also* Meningococcemia
    invasion, 838
  treatment, 1903–1906
    antibiotic, 1903t, 1903–1904,
      1904t
    antimicrobials of choice, 202t
    carbapenems, 264t
    cephalosporins, 257, 258, 259,
      1903t, 1904, 1904t
    chemoprophylaxis of carrier,
      1905
    chloramphenicol, 312t
    erythromycin, 335, 335t
    fusidic acid, 278
    immunoprophylaxis, 1905. *See also*
      vaccines *below*
    penicillin, 237t, 240, 241t, 1903,
      1903t
    piperacillin, 245
    quinolones, 367t
    rifampin, 318t, 1903t, 1905
    sulfonamides, 355t, 357, 1903,
      1905
    supportive care, 1904–1905
    tetracyclines, 308t
    trimethoprim, 357
  urethritis, 1902
  vaccines, 167, 858, 1896, 1903t,
    1905–1906, 2778
Neisseria mucosa, 1929
  endocarditis, 755
  growth characteristics, 1929t
Neisseria perflava, 1930
  endocarditis, 755
Neisseria pharyngis: endocarditis, 755
Neisseria polysaccharea, 1929
  growth characteristics, 1929t
Neisseria sicca, 1929
  endocarditis, 755
  growth characteristics, 1929t
Neisseria subflava, 1929
  growth characteristics, 1929t
Neisseria weaveri, 1928
  animal bites, 2766
  growth characteristics, 1929t
  identification, 1927t

laboratory identification, 1927t
Nematodes. *See also individual species*
  cellular immunity and, 128
  diagnosis, 1006t, 1006–1007
  IgE and, 39
  intestinal (roundworms), 2526–2531,
    2527t. *See also individual
    species*
    antiparasitic agents, 460t, 478–481
    Ascaris lumbricoides, 2528–2529
    Enterobius vermicularis, 2528
    hookworm (*Ancylostoma duode-
      nale*; *Necator americanus*),
      2529–2530
    Strongyloides stercoralis,
      2530–2531
    Trichuris trichiura, 2526–2528
  systemic: antiparasitic agents, 460t,
    481
  tissue, 2531–2537
    Brugia malayi, 2533–2535, 2536
    Brugia timori, 2533–2535
    Dracunculus medinensis, 2533
    Loa loa, 2535
    Mansonella, 2536
    Onchocerca volvulus, 2535–2536
    Trichinella spiralis, 2531–2533
    tropical pulmonary eosinophilia,
      2536
    Wuchereria bancrofti, 2533–2535,
      2536
Neomycin, 280, 382, 384, 384t
  adverse reactions, 289, 292,
    384–385
  dosage, 510t–511t
    in children and neonates,
      510t–511t
    in renal insufficiency, 511t
  for hepatitis, 1150
  mechanism of action, 384
  neuromuscular blockade, 295
  ototoxicity, 294
  pharmacology, 510t–511t
  source and chemistry, 280t
  spectrum of activity, 384
  structure, 281f
  topical, 384t
Neonatal disease. *See also* Children
  adenovirus, 1386
  American trypanosomiasis, 2442
  bacteriuria, 668
  Borrelia burgdorferi, 2148
  chickenpox (VZV), 1347–1348
  CMV, 1354t, 1354–1355
    clinical manifestations, 1356–1357
  conjunctivitis, 1106–1107
  coxsackievirus, 1627–1629
  echovirus, 1627–1629
  epidemic diarrhea in nurseries,
    965–966
  Escherichia coli meningitis, 1971
  HBV, 1423, 1424, 1425
    postexposure HBIG, 1431
  hepatitis, 2621
  herpes simplex virus, 1337, 1340
    prevention, 1343, 2657, 2657t
    treatment, 412t
  HIV transmission, 1168–1169
  HTLV transmission, 1580
  Listeria, 1881
  Moraxella catarrhalis, 1927
  necrotizing enterocolitis, 990–991
  Neisseria gonorrhoeae, 1919
  parvovirus B19, 1441, 1443
  rubella, 1460, 1461–1462, 1462t

Salmonella, 2016, 2020
sepsis
  enterococcal, 1829
    group C and G streptococcal, 1855
  Staphylococcus epidermidis, 1782
  Streptococcus agalactiae, 1835
    early-onset, 1837, 1838–1839
    incidence, 1837
    late-onset, 1839
    transmission, 1837
  Streptococcus pneumoniae bac-
    teremia, 1813
subdural empyema, 902, 902t
Toxoplasma gondii, 2455
  clinical manifestations, 2461–2462
  prevention, 2470
  serology, 2465, 2470
  treatment, 2468
Treponema pallidum, 2119, 2126,
  2126t
Trichomonas vaginalis, 2494
viral, 1319
Neonatal drug dosages. *See* Pediatric
  drug dosages
Neonates. *See also* Children
  cellular immunity in, 132–133
Neoplasia. *See also specific neoplasms*
  and antibody deficiencies, 53
  aspergillosis and, 2306
  Corynebacterium jeikeium and, 1876
  EBV and, 1332, 1332t, 1369–1370
  enteric symptoms, 1000t
  eosinophilia with abdominal pain
    and/or diarrhea, 1006t, 1008
  and fever of unknown origin (FUO),
    537t, 543–545, 544t
  HIV/AIDS and, 1240–1246, 1245t.
    See also Acquired immunode-
    ficiency syndrome *and
    specific tumors*
  human papillomavirus and, 1388t,
    1389–1390
  and immunodeficiency, 137
  infections in patients with, 2666–2675.
    See also specific neoplasms
    acute leukemia, 2672–2673,
      2675–2686
    acute lymphoma, 2675–2686
    alterations in microbial flora and,
      2671f, 2671–2672, 2672t
    bone marrow transplantation,
      2673–2674, 2674f,
      2717–2722
    brain tumors, 2673
    cellular immune dysfunction and,
      2668–2669
    chronic lymphocytic leukemia,
      2673
    CMV, 1356
    CNS dysfunction and, 2670
    empirical therapy, 2686–2691
    granulocytopenia and, 2666–2668,
      2667f, 2667t, 2668f,
      2675–2686
    hairy leukemia, 2673
    humoral immune dysfunction and,
      2669
    medical procedures and,
      2670–2671
    myeloma, 2673
    obstructive phenomena and, 2670
    phagocytic defense defects and,
      2666–2668
    predisposing factors, 2666, 2666t
    prophylaxis, 2691–2694

splenectomy and, 2669–2670
    vascular catheters and, 2670f,
      2670–2671, 2671f
  Kaposi's sarcoma. *See* Kaposi's
    sarcoma
  leukemia. *See* Leukemia
  lymphoma. *See* Lymphoma
  and meningitis, 871
  and nonbacterial thrombotic endo-
    carditis (NBTE), 742
  pleural fluid, 640
  pneumonia and, 647t
  polyomavirus and, 1402, 1402t
  and *Streptococcus agalactiae* bac-
    teremia, 1839, 1839t
Neotestudina rosatii, 2327
Nephritis
  chronic interstitial, 662–663, 663f
  microsporidia, 2513
  shunt, 42
  tuberculous interstitial, 2238
Nephropathy
  and HIV/AIDS, 1231
  reflux, 672
Nephrotic syndrome: antibody deficiency
  and, 53
Nephrotoxicity
  aminoglycosides, 280, 291–294
    clinical, 292–293, 293t
    experimental, 291f, 291–292, 292t
    serum levels and, 293–294
  amphotericin B deoxycholate, 405
  cephalosporins, 254
  drug-induced, 203
  foscarnet, 422
  penicillins, 240
  tetracyclines, 310
  vancomycin, 349
Nerve growth factor (NGF), 113
Netilmicin, 280
  antimicrobial activity, 285t, 286
  combination therapy, 287t
  dosage, 297t, 510t–511t
    in children and neonates, 299t, 510t
    in renal dysfunction, 298t, 511t
  multiple-dose regimen, 229f
  neuromuscular blockade, 295
  ototoxicity, 294
  pharmacology, 510t–511t
  for sepsis syndrome, 699, 699t
  source and chemistry, 280t
  structure, 281f
  susceptibility testing, 194t
  in vitro models, 228
Neupogen, 450–451
Neuralgia, post-herpetic, 1348
Neuritis, 874, 878–879
  clinical findings, 878–879
  laboratory findings, 879
  pathogenesis and pathology, 878
  treatment, 879
Neurocysticercosis, 2548, 2549
  albendazole for, 479
Neurodegenerative diseases, transmissible (TNDs), 881–887,
  1674
  Creutzfeldt-Jakob disease, 881–883,
    1674
  fatal familial insomnia, 881, 883–884,
    1674
  Gerstmann-Straussler-Scheinker
    syndrome, 881, 883, 1674
  handling infectious material, 884–885
  kuru, 881, 1674
  treatment, 884

Neurologic disease. *See also specific disorders*
 Borrelia burgdorferi, 2148
 Brucella, 2056
 Corynebacterium diphtheriae, 1869
 Coxiella burnetii, 1731–1732
 endocarditis and, 749
 HIV/AIDS and, 1236t, 1236–1240
  CMV, 1239–1240
  Cryptococcus neoformans,
   1239
  progressive multifocal leukoencephalopathy, 1239
  toxoplasmosis, 1238–1239
 HTLV, 1582
 Mycoplasma pneumoniae, 1707
 rabies, 1533, 1534t
 syphilis. *See* Neurosyphilis
Neuromuscular blockade: aminoglycosides, 295
Neuroretinitis, diffuse unilateral,1124
Neurosurgery prophylaxis recommendations, 2752t
Neurosyphilis. *See also Treponema pallidum,*835,843-844
 chronology, 2124f
 classification, 2124t
 clinical manifestations, 2124t, 2124–2125
 diagnosis, 2123–2124
 differential diagnosis, 2125
 gummatous, 835
 HIV coinfection, 843–844
 meningitis, 835
 meningovascular, 2124–2125
 parenchymatous, 2124
 tests, 2128
 treatment, 2129t, 2130
Neurotoxicity
 foscarnet, 423
 ganciclovir, 425
 interferons, 428
 isoniazid, 390
 metronidazole, 331
 penicillins, 239t, 240
 quinolones, 374
 tetracyclines, 310
 vancomycin, 349
 vidarabine, 433
Neurotoxins, enteric, 949t, 949–951
Neutropenia, 88–89, 89t, 153, 154
 acquired, 89
 candidiasis, 2672t
 clostridial infections, 2191
 congenital chronic: G-CSF for, 451
 cyclic, 89, 151t, 154
  fever, 538, 547
  G-CSF for, 451
 diagnosis, 154
 enterocolitis
  Clostridium, 2190t, 2191
  necrotizing, 729
 Escherichia coli, 2672t
 and fever of unknown origin (FUO), 536, 537t
 hereditary, 89
 Pseudomonas aeruginosa infections and, 1985, 1995
 staphylococcal infections, 2672t
  S. epidermidis bacteremia, 1781
 streptococcal infections, 2672t
  S. pneumoniae, 1817, 1817t
 treatment
  G-CSF, 450–451

of infections, 2687t, 2687–2694, 2688t
 quinolones, 373
Neutrophils, 79–88
 and acute phase response, 534
 azurophil, 79, 79t
 defects in function, 88–89, 89t, 153–156
  burns and, 2762
  diagnosis, 153–156
 degranulation, 85–86
 delivery to inflammatory site, 80–83, 81f, 82f
 development, 79
 emigration, 82
 kinetics, 80
 microbial defenses against, 88
 microbicidal mechanisms, 87–88
 morphologic and structural characteristics, 79f, 79t, 79–80, 80f
 neutropenia, 88–89, 89t, 153, 154. *See also* Neutropenia
 oxidative burst, 84–85, 85f
 peroxidase-positive granules, 79, 79t
 phagocytosis, 83f, 83–84
 postphagocytic events, 84–86
 priming of responses, 86–87
 signal transduction, 86
 therapy for defects, 94–95
 and tissue injury, 88
Neutrophil specific granule deficiency, 151t, 155
Nevirapine, 437t
 for HIV, 1272–1273
Niacin poisoning, 1014
Niclosamide, 460t, 483, 2548
 dosage, 463t, 466t
  pediatric, 463t, 466t
 structure, 483f
 for tapeworms, 2547, 2548
Nifurtimox, 475, 476–477
 adverse reactions, 476–477, 2447
 dosage, 467t
 for *Trypanosoma cruzi,* 2447, 2448
Nikkomycin Z: for *Histoplasma capsulatum,* 2351
Nikolsky sign, 555, 1765
Niridazole, 483
Nitric oxide
 and sepsis, 694
 and septic shock, 118
Nitroblue tetrazolium (NBT) slide test: for chronic granulomatous disease, 93
Nitrofurantoin, 376–379
 adverse reactions, 378–379
  GI and skin, 378
  hematologic, 378
  hepatic reactions, 378
  peripheral neuropathy, 378–379
  pulmonary, 378
 antimicrobial activity, 376–377
 clinical uses, 377–378
 for cystitis, 377–378
 dosage, 516t–517t
 drug interactions, 524t
 for enterococcal infections, 1830
 hemolysis from: in G6PD deficiency, 203
 pediatric use, 379
 and pH, 206
 pharmacology, 377, 516t–517t
 in pregnancy, 379
 prophylactic use, 378
 for pyelonephritis, 378

resistance, 377
 structure, 376–377, 377f
 and sugar level testing, 203
 susceptibility testing, 194t
Nitrogen, liquid: for chromomycosis, 2326
Nitroimidazoles
 for amebiasis, 2404, 2404t
 antiparasitic use, 458, 467–468
Nitzchia pungens, 1015
NK cells, 122
 cytokines produced by, 117
 deficiency, 132, 134t
  from immunosuppressive therapy, 136
 protection from infection, 121t, 126, 127, 128
NK-stimulating factor. *See* Interleukin-12
N-nucleotides, 106
Nocardia, 2273–2280
 cellular immunity and, 124
  defects, 2681
   therapy, 2682
 and CGD, 155
 classification, 2273
 clinical manifestations, 2275–2276, 2276f
 cutaneous manifestations, 552
 diagnosis, 2275–2276
 differential diagnosis, 2322
 encephalitis, 876
 endophthalmitis, 1122
 and HIV/AIDS, 2275, 2277
 identification, 2273f, 2273–2274, 2274f
 and immunodeficiency, 150t
 keratitis, 1113
 lung abscess, 642, 643
 meningitis, 835
  in the immunocompromised, 872
 microbiology, 2273–2274
 pathogenesis, 2274–2275
 pathology, 2275, 2275f
 pneumonia, 2275–2276, 2276f
  chronic, 647t
   radiology, 650t
  in transplant recipients, 2727t
 prognosis, 2277–2278
 susceptibility testing, 2277
 treatment, 2276–2277
  quinolones, 368t
Nocardia asteroides, 2273, 2273f, 2275, 2276, 2276f, 2277
 actinomycetoma, 2327
 brain abscess, 890
  in the immunocompromised, 890
  in transplant recipients, 2729
 epidural abscess, 905
 in transplant recipients, 2729
 treatment
  erythromycin, 335
  sulfonamides, 355t, 357
  trimethoprim, 357
Nocardia brasiliensis, 2273, 2274, 2276
 actinomycetoma, 2327, 2330
 cellular immunity and, 128
 granulomatous lymphangitis, 943
Nocardia farcinica, 2273, 2274, 2277
Nocardia nova, 2273
Nocardia otitidiscaviarum (caviae), 2273, 2274, 2276
 actinomycetoma, 2327
Nocardia transvalensis, 2273, 2274, 2277

Nocardiopsis dassonvillei, 2274
Nodular lesions, 552
Nodules: defined, 551
Noma, 602, 2165
Noma neonatorum: *Pseudomonas aeruginosa,* 1997
Non-Hodgkin's lymphoma: HIV/AIDS and, 1240, 1244–1245
 CNS, 1244
 peripheral, 1244–1245
 probability of developing, 1223f
 therapy, 1245, 1290
Nonoxynol-9: and gonorrhea prevention, 1923
Nonsteroidal anti-inflammatory drugs (NSAIDs)
 drug interactions: quinolones, 370
 for Reiter syndrome, 1072
Norepinephrine: for sepsis syndrome, 700, 700t
Norfloxacin
 adverse reactions, 203, 374
 antimicrobial activity, 367t, 369t, 370–371, 371, 373
 and bone marrow transplantation: prophylactic, 2721t
 dosage, 370t, 516t–517t
  in renal dysfunction, 369, 370t, 517t
 for peritonitis, 717
 pharmacokinetics, 369t
 pharmacology, 516t–517t
 structure, 365f
 susceptibility testing, 194t
North American blastomycosis, 1123
North Asian tick-borne rickettsiosis, 1719, 1720t. *See also Rickettsia sibirica*
Norwalk-like agents
 characteristics, 1667–1668, 1668t
 diagnosis, 181, 1671
 epidemiology, 1669
 immune responses, 1669–1670
 pathogenesis, 1669, 1669f
 treatment and prevention, 1671
 waterborne, 1016, 1016t
 winter vomiting disease, 968–969
Norwalk virus, 1666–1672
 characteristics, 1667–1668, 1668t
 clinical manifestations, 1670, 1670f
 diagnosis, 1670–1671
 diarrhea, 1669, 1670
 in the elderly, 2740
 epidemiology, 1669
 food-borne, 1012t, 1013
  foods implicated, 1017t
 genome, 1668, 1668f
 history, 1667
 immune responses, 1669–1670
 pathogenesis, 1669
 treatment and prevention, 1671
 virology, 1667–1668, 1668f
 waterborne, 1016
 winter vomiting disease, 968–969
Norwegian (crusted) scabies, 1059, 2561–2562
Nose
 Aspergillus, 2307
 surgery prophylaxis recommendations, 2751t
 tuberculosis, 2240
Nosema, 2514
 and HIV/AIDS, 2516–2517
 keratitis, 1114
 in non-HIV infected, 2517–2518

Nosema conori, 2514, 2515, 2517, 2517t
  neuritis, 878
Nosema corneum, 2514, 2517t
  treatment, 465t
Nosema ocularum, 2514, 2517t
Nosocomial infections, 2572–2666
  Acinetobacter pneumonia, 2011
  AIDS in health care workers,
      2633–2634, 2634t. *See also*
      HIV in health care setting
      below
  arenaviruses, 1577
  bacteremia due to intravascular
      devices, 2587–2599
    arterial lines, 2595–2596, 2596t
    central venous catheters, 2592
      long-term, 2594t, 2594–2595
    contamination
      of infusate, 2587
      at insertion site, 2588t,
        2588–2589, 2589t
      at junction, 2587
    device-specific issues, 2591–2596
    diagnosis, 2590f, 2590t, 2590–2591
    microbiology, 2589t, 2589–2590
    pathogenesis, 2587–2589, 2588f
    peripheral IV cannulization, 2591t,
        2591–2592
    prevention, 2596
    pulmonary artery catheters, 2595
    total parenteral nutrition,
        2592–2594, 2593t
    transducer domes, 2595–2596
    transducers, 2595
  Citrobacter, 1974
  control of, 2572–2575. *See also*
      Infection control
  cytomegalovirus, 2660–2662
    management of exposed personnel,
        2662
    prevention, 2661–2662
    risks, 2660–2661
    transmission mechanisms, 2661
  diarrhea, 970–971
  disinfection, 2579, 2581t, 2581–2583,
      2582t
  Enterobacter, 1964, 1972
  Enterobacteriaceae, 1964
  enterococcal, 1827–1829
    bacteremia and endocarditis, 1828
    intra-abdomninal and pelvic, 1828
    urinary tract, 1828
    wound and tissue, 1828–1829
  Epstein-Barr virus, 2663
    management of exposed personnel,
        2663
    prevention, 2663
    risks, 2663
    transmission mechanisms, 2663
  fever of unknown origin (FUO), 536,
      537t
  in health care workers. *See also* HIV
      in health care workers *below*
    CMV, 2662
    EBV, 2663
    HIV, 2633–2639
    HSV, 2656–2657
    VZV, 2660
  hepatitis, viral, 2616–2624
    dialysis units, 2620–2621
      prevention and control,
        2620–2621
    employee health, 2621–2623, 2622f
    epidemiology, 2617
    HAV, 2617–2618

HBV, 1431, 2618, 2619t,
    2619–2620
  prevention, 1431–1432
  vaccine prophylaxis, 2623–2624
HCV, 2618
HDV, 2618
HEV, 2618–2619
perinatal and reproductive trans-
    mission, 2621
person-to-person transmission,
    2619t, 2619–2620
vaccine prophylaxis, 2623–2624
herpes simplex virus, 2656–2657
  management of personnel exposed,
      2657
  prevention, 2657, 2657t
  risks, 2656
  transmission mechanisms,
      2656–2657
herpesviruses, 2656t, 2656–2666. *See
    also specific viruses*
  transfusion-related, 2626–2627
HIV in health care setting, 2632–2656
  antibody testing, 2647–2648, 2648t
  body fluids implicated, 2633
  counseling, 2647, 2648, 2648t
  decontamination and sterilization,
      2643
  duty to warn, 2648
  impact on training and recruitment
      of personnel, 2649
  legal and ethical issues, 2647–2649
  management of employees sustain-
      ing adverse exposures,
      2643–2647
  management of needles and sharp
      objects, 2642–2643
  management of opportunistic in-
      fections, 2642
  mucous membrane exposure, 2633
  occupational transmission,
      2632–2633
  partner notification, 2648
  percutaneous exposure, 2632–2633,
      2633t
  prevention, 2639–2647, 2640t,
      2641t
  provider-to-patient transmission,
      2638t, 2638–2639
  serologic surveillance, 2647
  support services and waste dis-
      posal, 2643, 2643t
  transmission routes, 2632–2633
  universal precautions, 2639–2641,
      2640t, 2641t
HIV in health care workers,
    2633–2639
  case reports, 2634
  counseling, 2647, 2648t
  ethical, legal, and policy issues in
      management, 2649–2650
  postexposure antiretroviral chemo-
      prophylaxis, 2646
  prospective/longitudinal studies of
      incidence, 2636t, 2636–2637,
      2637t
  right to refuse care, 2648
  risk factors, 2637, 2637t
  serologic surveillance, 2647
  seropositivity, 2634–2638
  studies in prevalence, 2634–2636,
      2635t
human herpesviruses 6 and 7, 2663
infectious waste disposal, 2582–2583
influenza, 1563

isolation, 2575–2579. *See also*
    Isolation
  Klebsiella, 1972
  Listeria, 1881
  Mycobacterium tuberculosis,
      2217–2218
    controlling, 2218
  Ochrobactrum, 2114
  parainfluenza virus, 1492
  parvovirus B19, 1441
  in plasma exchange, 2628
  prevention
    Creutzfeldt-Jakob disease, 2584
    current concerns, 2583–2584
    disinfection, 2579, 2581t,
        2581–2583, 2582t
    endoscopes, 2584–2585
    hepatitis viruses, 2584
    HIV, 2583–2584
    infectious waste disposal,
        2582–2583
    intravascular devices, 2596
    respiratory, 2604–2605
    sterilization, 2575–2581, 2582t
  Proteus mirabilis, 1974
  Pseudomonas aeruginosa bacteremia,
      1987–1988
  respiratory, 2599–2607
    diagnosis, 2602–2603
    etiologies, 2600, 2600t
    incidence and mortality,
        2599–2600, 2600t
    pathogenesis, 2601–2602
    predisposing factors, 2601, 2601t
    prevention, 2604–2605
    treatment, 2603–2604
  respiratory syncytial virus, 1509,
      1510–1511
  Serratia, 1972
  sterilization, 2579–2581
  Streptococcus pneumoniae, 1817,
      1817t
  transfusion-related, 2624t, 2624–2628
    Babesia microti, 2627
    bacteria, 2627–2628
    Borrelia burgdorferi, 2627
    CMV, 2626–2627
    EBV, 2627
    herpesviruses, 2626–2627
    HIV, 2625–2626
    HTLV, 2626
    parvovirus B19, 2627
    prevention, 2628
    protozoa, 2627
    Pseudomonas, 2627, 2628
    retroviruses, 2625–2626
    rickettsial infections, 2627
    spirochetes, 2627
    Toxoplasma gondii, 2627
    Treponema pallidum, 2627
    Trypanosoma cruzi, 2627
    viral hepatitis, 2624–2625
    viruses, 2624–2627
    Yersinia enterocolitica, 2628
  urinary tract, 2607–2616
    after catheter removal, 2608
    complications
      long-term catheterization, 2610
      prevention, 2612
      short-term catheterization, 2610
      treatment, 2612–2613
    duration of catheterization,
        2608–2610, 2609t
    entry, 2607–2608
    epidemiology, 2607

long-term catheterization,
    2609–2610
noncatheter, 2612
pathogenesis, 2607–2608
prevention, 2610–2612
  avoidance of catheterization,
      2610–2611
  of bacteriuria, 2611–2612
  patient-patient transmission,
      2612
  Pseudomonas aeruginosa,
      1994–1995
  risk factors, 2608
varicella-zoster virus, 2658–2660
  investigating epidemics, 2658,
      2660
  management of exposed personnel,
      2660
  prevention, 2658, 2659f
  risks, 2658
  transmission mechanisms, 2658
Novobiocin
  and pH, 206
NPS-1 β-lactamase, 216t
Nucleic acid hybridization tests,
    184–185
  pneumonia, 623
Nucleic acids, viral, 1314–1315, 1315t
Nucleocapsid, viral, 1315, 1315t
5'-Nucleotidase, 79t
Nurseries: epidemic diarrhea in,
    965–966, 966t
Nursing homes. *See also* Nosocomial
    infections
  diarrhea in, 970–971
Nuttaliellidae, 2565
Nystatin
  for candidiasis, 2299, 2301
  dosage, 403t, 518t–519t
  for esophagitis, 964t
  pharmacology, 518t–519t
  for sepsis syndrome, 702
  structure, 402f
  for thrush, 403
  topical, 401t, 403
  for transplant recipients, 2715
  for vulvovaginal candidiasis, 1076,
      1076t

O

O antigen, 1753
  and complement, 65
Obesity: and surgical wound infections,
    2746
Obliterative endarteritis: *Treponema
    pallidum*, 2120, 2120f,
    2125
Obodhiang virus, 1529
Observational studies: in epidemiology,
    161
Obstetrics. *See* Pregnancy
Occupational exposures
  anthrax, 1886
  Erysipelothrix, 1895
  health care. *See* Health care workers
  leptospirosis, 2137
  and pneumonia, 648
  vaccines for, 2783–2784, 2784t
Ochrobacterium: classification and site
    of infection, 2107t
Ochrobacterium anthropi, 2111,
    2113–2114
Ockelbo disease: arthritis, 1036, 1036t
Ocologlandular syndrome, 940t

Octreotide acetate: for *Cryptosporidium*, 2507
Ocular infections. *See* Eye infections
Ocular larva migrans (*Toxocara canis*), 2554
Ocular surgery: *Staphylococcus epidermidis* infections, 1782
Ocular telangiectasia, 52
Ocular trachoma. *See* Trachoma
Oculoglandular syndrome, 938, 1310
  cat scratch disease and, 1310, 1311, 1311t
  conjunctivitis, 1106
  Francisella tularensis, 938, 940t, 2063–2064
  Listeria monocytogenes, 938
Odds ratios, 160, 160f
Odontogenic infections, 593–602
  anaerobic, 2163t, 2164
    gram-negative bacilli, 2198
  anatomic considerations, 595–596, 596f, 597f, 598f
  clinical presentations, 596–600
    buccal, canine, and parotid spaces, 598
    deep fascial space infections, 598–600
    dentoalveolar, 596
    gingivitis and periodontal infections, 596, 598
    lateral pharyngeal space, 600
    Ludwig's angina, 599, 599f
    masticator spaces, 598, 599f
    pericoronitis, 598
    periodontal abscess, 598
    periodontitis, 598
    retropharyngeal, danger, and pretracheal spaces, 600
    submandibular and sublingual spaces, 598–600, 599f
  complications, 600–601
    maxillary sinusitis, 601
    osteomyelitis of the jaws, 601
    septic cavernous sinus thrombosis, 600–601
    suppurative jugular thrombophlebitis, 600
  diagnosis, 601
  gram-negative anaerobes, 2198
  imaging, 601
  microbiology, 593–594, 594t, 595f
  pathogenesis, 594–595
  periodontitis, 598. *See also* Periodontitis
    treatment, 601–602
  specimen collection and processing, 601
  therapy, 601–602
Odynophagia: in esophagitis, 962
Oesophagostomum: albendazole for, 479
Ofloxacin
  adverse reactions, 203, 374
  antimicrobial activity, 285t, 367t, 369t, 370–371, 371, 373, 374
  for *Chlamydia trachomatis*, 1688
  dosage, 370t, 516t–517t
    in renal dysfunction, 369, 370t, 517t
  for *Mycobacterium leprae*, 399, 2249
  for *Mycobacterium tuberculosis*, 395
  for *Mycoplasma pneumoniae*, 1710, 1710t
  for *Neisseria gonorrhoeae*, 1922, 1922t
  for *Neisseria meningitidis*, 1905

pharmacokinetics, 369t
pharmacology, 516t–517t
  for *Pseudomonas aeruginosa*: otitis externa, 1990
  structure, 365f
  for urethritis, 1070
Ohara's disease, 2060
OHIO-1 β-lactamase, 216t
OKT3: immunodeficiency from, 136
Oligella, 2113
  classification and site of infection, 2107t
Oligella ureolytica, 2113
Oligella urethralis, 1928, 2113
  laboratory identification, 1927t
Oligosaccharides, 1753
Oliguria: and sepsis, 693
Omenn syndrome, 134t, 135, 138
Omeprazole: for *Helicobacter pylori*, 1961
Omsk hemorrhagic fever: transmission, clinical syndromes, and geographic distribution, 1466t
Onchocerca volvulus, 1113, 2525t, 2535–2536
  clinical features, 2535–2536
  diagnosis, 2536
  epidemiology, 2535
  keratitis, 1113, 2535–2536
    treatment, 1118
  life cycle, 2535
  lymphadenitis, 940t
  pathology, 2535
  prevention, 2536
  treatment, 462t, 2536
    amocarzine, 482
    diethylcarbamazine, 481, 1126
    ivermectin, 481, 1126
    suramin, 476
Oncostatin M, 530
  and hypothalamus, 532
Oncoviruses, type C, 1579–1584. *See also* Human T cell lymphotropic viruses
Onychomycosis, 2383
  Candida albicans, 2294, 2294f
  clinical features, 2383, 2383f
  dermatophytosis, 2380
  distal and subungual (DLSO), 2380
  griseofulvin for, 404
  and HIV, 1229
  superficial white (SWO), 2380
O'nyong-nyong fever, 1455
  arthritis, 1036, 1036t
  clinical manifestations, 1457
  differential diagnosis, 1472
  epidemiology, 1457
Oophoritis
  cytomegalovirus, 1360
  mumps virus, 1497t, 1498
Operative wounds: infection prophylaxis: topical antibacterials, 382
Ophthalmia, sympathetic, 1124
Ophthalmia neonatorum, 1106–1107
  chemoprophylaxis, 167
  diagnosis, 1107
  gonococcal, 1913, 1919
  Moraxella catarrhalis, 1927
  prophylaxis, 1108
  Pseudomonas aeruginosa, 1991
Ophthalmic artery: anatomy, 824
Ophthalmic surgery prophylaxis, 2751t
Ophthalmitis: *Bacillus*, 1891
Ophthalmomyiasis, 2563

Opisthorchis, 2538t, 2541
  diagnosis, 1006t
Opisthorchis felineus, 2541
Opisthorchis viverrini, 2541
  treatment, 463t
    praziquantel, 482
Opportunism, 20–21
Opportunistic infections. *See also* Immunocompromised host
  characteristics, 1754
  in HIV/AIDS. *See* Acquired immunodeficiency syndrome
  immunosuppressive therapy and, 135
Opsonin-independent phagocytosis, 33
Opsonins, 78, 2771
Optic neuritis: from chloramphenicol, 314
Oral cavity
  Capnocytophaga colonization, 2103–2104
  epithelial hyperplasia of the (Heck's disease), 1388t, 1393
  normal flora, 2159t, 2159–2160
  specimen collection and processing, 169, 170t, 172
Oral-cervicofacial disease: actinomycosis, 2281f, 2281–2282
Oral contraceptives: leukorrhea, 1081
Oral disease
  actinomycosis, 2281
  anaerobic, 2163t
    gram-negative, 2197–2198
  aphthous stomatitis, 602–603
  Candida albicans, 2292, 2292f
    treatment, 2301
  HIV/AIDS and, 1226–1227
    candidiasis, 1226–1227
    gingivitis, 1227
    hairy leukoplakia, 1227
    periodontitis, 1227
    ulcers, 1227
  Kaposi's sarcoma, 1242
  sexually transmitted, 1059–1060
  Streptococcus intermedius group, 1862
  ulcers
    HIV/AIDS and, 1227
    neutrophil defect and, 153
Oral drug administration, 209
Oral flora, indigenous, 593, 594t
Oral hairy leukoplakia: HIV/AIDS and, 1182, 1227
Oral sex. *See* Orogenital sex
Orbital apex syndrome, 1132
Orbital cellulitis
  and dacryocystopyocele, 1131
  differential diagnosis, 1133
  etiology, 1131–1133
  laboratory findings, 1133
  Pseudomonas aeruginosa, 1991
  treatment, 1134–1135
Orbital infections, 1131–1133
Orbivirus, 1447–1448
Orchitis, 1101
  bacterial, 1101
  and HIV, 1101–1102
  viral, 1101
Orf, 1329
Oriental liver fluke, 2541
Oriental sore, 2434–2435
Ornidazole, 468
Ornithodoros: and *Borrelia* relapsing fever, 2141, 2143
Ornithonyssus bacoti, 2564
Ornithosis. *See Chlamydia pneumoniae*

Orofacial infections
  anaerobic, 2163t
  nonodontogenic, 602–603
    aphthous stomatitis, 602–603
    chronic bacterial parotitis, 603
    in the immunocompromised, 603
    mucositis, 603
    noma (gangrenous stomatitis), 602
    salivary gland, 603
    suppurative parotitis, 603
    viral parotitis, 603
  odontogenic, 593–602. *See also* Odontogenic infections
Orogenital sex
  and HIV transmission, 1189
  Neisseria gonorrhoeae, 1916
  Neisseria meningitidis and, 1902
Oropharyngeal histoplasmosis, 2346
Oropharyngeal infections. *See also* Pharyngitis
  and leukemia/lymphoma, 2678
Oropouche, 2794
Oroya fever, 1002, 1742, 2209–2210
Orthomyxoviridae
  arthritis, 1036t
  classification, 1315t
  influenza virus, 1546–1567. *See also* Influenza virus
  shape and size, 1316f
Orthopaedic surgery prophylaxis, 2751t
Orthopoxviruses, 1325
Orthoreoviruses, 1447
Osler nodes, 554, 747, 748, 922
Osteoarthritis: and infectious arthritis, 1032
Osteoarticular diseases. *See also* Bone infections; Joint infections
  sporotrichosis, 2322
    treatment, 2323
  tuberculosis, 2237
Osteochondritis: *Pseudomonas aeruginosa*, 1992
  treatment, 1993
Osteogenesis imperfecta tarda: Job syndrome and, 156
Osteomyelitis, 1039–1052
  actinomycosis, 2282
  anaerobic, 2163t, 2166
    cocci, 2205
    gram-negative bacilli, 2200
  Bacillus, 1893
  Borrelia burgdorferi, 2147
  Brodie's abscess, 1049
  Candida albicans, 2297, 2297f
  in children, 1041
  chronic, 1042–1043
    Pseudomonas aeruginosa, 1993
  and chronic granulomatous disease, 92
  Cierney-Mader classification, 1039, 1039t, 1039–1040, 1040f
  classification, 1039, 1039t, 1040
  contiguous focus
    with generalized vascular insufficiency, 1042, 1044f
    treatment, 1045–1047, 1047f, 1048f
    without generalized vascular insufficiency, 1041–1043, 1043f
  diagnosis, 1043–1045
    CT, 1045
    long bone, 1044
    MRI, 1045
    radiography, 1044

radionuclide, 1045
Staphylococcus aureus, 1772, 1773
vertebral, 1045, 1046f
diffuse, 1039, 1040f
enterococcal, 1829
and fever, 541
fungal, 1050
Gaucher's disease and, 1049
hematogenous, 1040–1041, 1041f,
1042f
treatment, 1045
in hemodialysis patients, 1049
in heroin addicts, 1049
of the jaw, 601
localized, 1039–1040, 1040f
medullary, 1039, 1040f
neonatal, 1041
nontuberculous mycobacterial infections and, 1050
overview, 1039–1040
Pseudomonas aeruginosa, 1992–1994
chronic contiguous, 1993–1994
symphysis pubis, 1993
treatment, 1992–1993
pubis, 1095
Bacteroides fragilis, 2200
in sickle cell disease, 1049
skeletal tuberculosis and, 1049–1050
and soft tissue infections, 926
in spinal cord injured patients, 2732t,
2735
Staphylococcus aureus, 1771–1773
Staphylococcus epidermidis, 1049,
1781
streptococcal group C and G, 1854
Streptococcus agalactiae, 1839, 1840
Streptococcus pneumoniae, 1821
superficial, 1039, 1040f
treatment, 1045–1049
acute hematogenous, 1045
aminoglycosides, 295t
bone concentrations, 1048, 1049t
contiguous focus, 1045–1047,
1047f, 1048f
hyperbaric oxygen, 1048–1049
rifampin, 322
trimethoprim-sulfamethoxazole,
360
vertebral, 1045
tuberculous, 2237
vertebral, 1041
Coxiella burnetii, 1732–1733
diagnosis, 1045, 1046f
Pseudomonas aeruginosa,
1992–1993
Staphylococcus aureus, 1772
treatment, 1045
Otitis
aminoglycosides for, 295t
anaerobic gram-negative, 2198
antibody deficiencies and, 49
Mycobacterium tuberculosis, 2240
Treponema pallidum, 2125
treatment, 2130
Otitis externa, 579–580, 582
acute diffuse (swimmer's ear), 580
chronic, 580
clinical manifestations and management, 580
fungal, 580
malignant, 580
Pseudomonas aeruginosa, 1989,
1990
treatment, 1990
pathogenesis, 580

Otitis media, 580–583
acute, 582
anaerobic, 2163t, 2164
gram-negative bacilli, 2198
and brain abscess, 887, 888t
chronic, 582–583
diagnosis and clinical course, 582
epidemiology, 580–581
Haemophilus influenzae, 2043
immunology, 581–582
microbiology, 581
Moraxella catarrhalis, 1927
pathogenesis, 581
Pseudomonas aeruginosa, 1991
respiratory syncytial virus, 1508
rhinovirus, 1659
Streptococcus pneumoniae, 1818
treatment, 582–583
amoxicillin-clavulanate, 269
tuberculous, 2240
Otomycosis: *Aspergillus*, 2307
Ototoxicity: aminoglycosides, 294–295
Outbreak investigations, 163
and infection control, 2572, 2572t
Outcome variables: epidemiology, 159
Ovarian vein: puerperal thrombophlebitis
(POVT), 1091–1092
Overlap syndrome: pneumonia, 647t
Oxacillin, 243
adverse reactions, 239t
for bacilli and anaerobes, 237t
dosage, 241t, 506t–507t
in children, 506t
for meningitis, 850t
in neonates, 242t, 506t
in renal disease and dialysis, 238t,
507t
for endocarditis: staphylococcal, 762
for Enterobacteriaceae and
Pseudomonas, 237t
indications, 194
MICs against cocci, 237t
pharmacokinetics, 238t
pharmacology, 506–507t
staphylococcal resistance, 194
structure, 242f
for toxic shock syndrome, 1767
trade names, 236t
Oxacillinase β-lactamase, 216t
Oxacillin-hydrolyzing enzymes OXA,
268
Oxamniquine, 460t, 483
dosage, 466t
pediatric, 466t
for schistosomiasis, 2541
OXA(1–9) β-lactamase, 216t
Oxantel, 480
Oxidative burst: neutrophil, 84–85, 85f
Oxolinic acid, 364
pharmacology, 516t–517t
structure, 365f
Oxygen, singlet: and neutrophils, 87
Oxygen metabolites: and neutrophils, 87
Oxygen radicals: and cerebral edema,
841
Oxygen therapy
for bronchiolitis, 616
hyperbaric
for gas gangrene, 932
for osteomyelitis, 1048–1049
for peritonitis, 718
Oxymino-β-lactamase, 216t
Oxytetracycline, 307
dosage, 512t–513t
pharmacokinetics, 309t

pharmacology, 512t–513t
structure, 307f
Ozaenia, 1972

P

Pacemakers
infections, 790–791
Staphylococcus epidermidis,
1782
surgery prophylaxis, 2751t
Pachymeningitis: hypertrophic spinal,
906
Paecilomyces
and CGD, 155
keratitis, 1113
Panaeolus, 1015t
Pancreas transplantation: infections and,
2722, 2723, 2726
Pancreatic abscess, 723–724
bacteriology, 723
clinical manifestations, 723
diagnosis, 723–724
etiology, 723
pathogenesis, 723
prognosis, 724
treatment, 724
Pancreatic duct infections: and fever, 541
Pancreatic tuberculosis, 2238
Pancreatitis
CMV, 1360
coxsackievirus, 1632
Cryptosporidium, 2505
from didanosine, 421, 1271
and intraperitoneal abscess, 721
mumps virus, 1497t, 1498
and pancreatic abscess, 723–724
pleural fluid, 640
Pancytopenia: HIV and, 1209
Panencephalitis, subacute sclerosing:
measles and, 1124, 1520
Panniculitis: *Borrelia burgdorferi*, 2147
Panophthalmitis
Bacillus, 1891
Borrelia burgdorferi, 2148
Pantoea agglomerans, 1975t
PapC protein, 24
PapD protein, 24
Pap fimbriae, 24
Papillary stenosis: and HIV/AIDS, 1230
Papillomaviruses, 1387–1400. *See also*
Human papillomavirus
pap operon, 17, 17f
Papovaviridae, 1387–1406. *See also*
individual viruses
classification, 1315t
papillomaviruses, 1387–1400
polyomaviruses, 1400–1406
shape and size, 1316f
Pap smear
for human papillomavirus diagnosis,
1395
for *Pneumocystis carinii*, 2479
Papular acrodermatitis, infantile: hepatitis
B virus and, 1420
Papular lesions, 551–552
systemic infections manifesting, 550t
Papules
defined, 551
genital, 1057t, 1059. *See also* Genital
lesions
Papulonecrotic tuberculids, 2240
Para-aminobenzoic acid: structure,
354f
Para-aminosalicylic acid

adverse reactions, 394
dosage, 394, 516t–517t
in hepatic or renal failure, 390t,
517t
drug interactions, 524t
for *Mycobacterium tuberculosis*, 394
pharmacology, 516t–517t
Paracoccidioides brasiliensis,
2386–2389
appearance in tissue, 2289t
clinical manifestations, 2386–2387
description, 2386, 2386f
differential diagnosis, 2388
dysentery, 994
ecology, 2386
enteritides, 994
epidemiology, 2386
laboratory diagnosis, 2388
cultures, 2388
histologic, 2388
serologic, 2388
skin tests, 2388
lung lesions, 2387, 2387f
lymphadenitis, 940t
mucosal lesions, 2387, 2387f
pneumonia
chronic, 647t, 648
radiology, 650t
skin lesions, 2387
treatment, 2388–2389
amphotericin B, 2388
imidazole compounds, 2388–2389
ketoconazole, 407
sulfonamides, 2388
Paracoccidioidin skin test, 2386
Paragonimus kellicoti: praziquantel for,
482
Paragonimus westermani, 2525t, 2538t,
2543
brain abscess, 890
clinical syndromes, 2543
pleural, 639
pneumonia, 619t
radiology, 650t
treatment, 463t, 2543
bithionol, 483
praziquantel, 482
Parainfluenza virus, 1489–1496
antigenic variation, 1490
and bone marrow transplantation,
2720
bronchiolitis, 612t, 612–613, 613f
bronchitis, acute, 606, 606t
cellular immunity and, 130
characterization, 1489–1490, 1490f
classification, 1489, 1489t
clinical manifestations, 1491–1492
common cold, 562, 562t
croup, 574, 574t
description, 1489t, 1489–1490
diagnosis, 1492–1493
epidemiology, 1490t, 1490–1491
history, 1489
immune response, 1491
in the immunocompromised, 1492
laryngitis, 573t
nosocomial, 1492
pathogenesis, 1491
pharyngitis, 567
pneumonia, 619t
atypical, 630
primary infection, 1492
reinfection, 1492
and Reye syndrome, 1558
sinusitis, 585, 585t

Parainfluenza virus (Continued)
  treatment, 1493
  type 1, 1489, 1490, 1490t
    clinical manifestations, 1491
    croup, 1490, 1490t
    epidemiology, 1490, 1490t
    pathogenesis, 1491
  type 2, 1489, 1490, 1490t
    clinical manifestations, 1491
    epidemiology, 1490–1485
    pathogenesis, 1491
  type 3, 1489, 1490, 1490t
    carrier state, 1491
    clinical manifestations, 1492
    epidemiology, 1490t, 1491
    nosocomial, 1492
    parotitis, 1500
    pathogenesis, 1491
    reinfection, 1492
    vaccine research, 1493
  type 4: epidemiology, 1491
  type 4A, 1489, 1490, 1490t
  type 4B, 1489, 1490, 1490t
  vaccine development, 1493
Paralysis
  coxsackievirus, 1621t, 1623
  echovirus, 1621t, 1623
  infantile. See Poliovirus
  rabies, 1533
  tick, 2566
Paralytic ileus: poliovirus, 1616
Paramyxoviridae, 1489–1526. See also
    individual viruses
  classification, 1315t, 1489, 1489t
  measles virus, 1519–1526
  mumps virus, 1496–1501
  parainfluenza virus, 1489–1496
  respiratory syncytial virus, 1501–1519
  shape and size, 1316f
Paramyxoviruses, 1486, 1489t. See also
    Mumps virus; Parainfluenza
    virus
  arthritis, 1036t
Paranasal sinus
  Aspergillus, 2307
  infections: and subdural empyema,
    900
  microscopic examination of
    pathogens, 172t
  phaeohyphomycosis of, 1132
Paranasal sinusitis: and orbital cellulitis,
    1132
Parana virus, 1572
Parapoxvirus, 1325, 1329
Paraquat: pharyngitis, 569
Parasites. See also Helminths; Protozoa
  arthritis, 1037
  and complement, 66
  conjunctivitis, 1104t, 1106
  diarrhea: and HIV/AIDS, 1230
  dysentery, 989
  endophthalmitis, 1121t, 1124
  enteric symptoms, 1000t
  enteritides, 994
  and fever, 543
  food-borne, 1012
  hypergammaglobulinemia, 42
  keratitis, 1111t, 1114
  and leukemia/lymphoma, 2677, 2681
  metronidazole for, 332
  myocarditis, 800, 800t
  myositis, 934–935
  penetration, 7
  pericarditis, 805, 805t
  zoonoses, 2792t

Parasitic host-parasite relationships, 30
Paravaccinia (milker's nodule), 1325,
    1329
Parenteral drug administration, 209
Parenteral nutrition, total: bacteremia
    from, 2592–2594, 2593t
Paresis, 2124
Paresthesias: food-borne diseases,
    1014–1015
Parietal peritoneum, 707–708
Parinaud's oculoglandular syndrome,
    938, 1310
  cat scratch disease and, 1310, 1311,
    1311t
  conjunctivitis, 1106
  Francisella tularensis, 938, 940t,
    2063–2064
  Listeria monocytogenes, 938
Paromomycin, 280, 289
  adverse reactions, 468
  for amebiasis, 2404, 2404t
  antimicrobial activity, 285t, 286
  antiparasitic use, 459t, 468
    dosage, 461t, 462t, 463t
      pediatric, 461t, 462t, 463t
  for Cryptosporidium, 2507
  for Giardia lamblia, 2490, 2490t
  for Leishmania, 2435
  source and chemistry, 280t
  structure, 281f
Paronychia
  Candida albicans, 2294, 2294f, 2295f
  Pseudomonas aeruginosa, 1997
Parotid space infections, 598
Parotitis
  anaerobic gram-negative bacilli,
    2198
  chronic bacterial, 603
  differential diagnosis of viral, 1500
  gram-negative anaerobes, 2198
  mumps virus, 603, 1497, 1497t, 1500
  suppurative, 603
Paroxysmal nocturnal hemoglobinuria,
    71
Pars planitis, idiopathic, 1124
Particle agglutination test: for HIV, 1260
Parvoviridae, 1439–1446. See also
    Parvovirus B19
  classification, 1315t
  shape and size, 1316f
Parvovirus B19, 1386
  aplastic crisis, 1439t, 1442t,
    1442–1443
  arthropathy, 1036t, 1439t, 1442
  clinical manifestations, 1439t,
    1442–1443
  diagnosis, 1443–1444
  differential diagnosis, 1443
  ecthyma infectiosum, 550t, 552,
    1439t, 1442
  epidemiology, 1441–1442
  fetal infection, 1441, 1443
  and HIV/AIDS, 1439, 1440, 1443
  in the immunocompromised, 1441,
    1443
  isolation, 2576
  pathogenesis, 1440–1441
  prevention, 1444
  serology, 191
  transfusion-related, 1432, 2627
  transmission, 1441–1442
  treatment, 1444
  virology, 1440
Pasteurella, 2068t, 2068–2070
  clinical manifestations, 2069–2070

description, 2068–2069
  epidemiology, 2069
  pathogenesis, 2069
  prevention and therapy, 2070
Pasteurella aerogenes, 2069
Pasteurella canis, 2069
  animal bites, 2766
Pasteurella dagmatis, 2069
  animal bites, 2766
Pasteurellae, 2068–2070
Pasteurella haemolytica, 2069
Pasteurella multocida
  animal reservoirs, 2792t
  arthritis, 1035
  bites, 604, 2766, 2767
    treatment, 2766t, 2767t
  clinical manifestations, 2069
  differential diagnosis: Bartonella,
    1742
  epidemiology, 2069
  pathogenesis, 2069
  pneumonia, 622t
  prevention and therapy, 2070
  soft tissue infections, 2166
  subsp. multocida, 2069
  subsp. septica, 2069
Pasteurella pneumotropica, 2069
Pasteurella sensu stricto, 2068t,
    2068–2070. See also specific
    species
Pasteurella septica: animal bites,
    2766
Pasteurella stomatis, 2069
  animal bites, 2766
Pasteurella ureae, 2069
Pasteurization, 2579
Pastia's lines, 1788
Pathogenicity, 164. See also Pathogens
  insertion elements and, 22
  molecular research, 19–29
  phages and, 22, 22t
  plasmids and, 22, 22t
  regulation, 22–24, 23f, 23t
  viral, 1319
Pathogens. See also Pathogenicity
  attributes, 20–21
  clonal nature, 21, 21t
  defined, 20
  as intracellular parasites, 24–25
Peau d'orange: erysipelas, 914
Pediatric drug dosages, 506t–519t. See
    also specific drugs
  adjustments, 201
  aminoglycosides, 299, 299t, 510t
  antifungal agents, 518t
  antimycobacterials, 516t
  antiviral agents, 518t
  azalides, 512t
  aztreonam, 510t
  carumonam, 510t
  cephalosporins, 250t, 508t, 509t
  chloramphenicol, 512t
  fusidic acid, 514t
  imipenem, 510t
  lincosamides, 512t
  loracarbef, 510t
  macrolides, 512t
  metronidazole, 512t
  penicillins, 242t, 506t
  polymyxins, 514t
  quinolones, 516t
  sulfonamides, 514t
  teicoplanin, 514t
  trimethoprim, 514t
  urinary tract agents, 516t

vancomycin, 514t
Pediculosis, 2558–2560. See also indi-
    vidual species
  body, 2559–2560
  clinical manifestations, 2559–2560
  epidemiology, 2559
  head, 2559f, 2559–2560
  pubic, 2559, 2560
  treatment, 2560
Pediculus humanus
  Borrelia relapsing fever, 2141
  capitis, 2558, 2559, 2559f, 2560
    treatment, 463t
  corporis, 2558, 2559, 2560
    and epidemic typhus, 1735
    treatment, 463t
Pefloxacin
  adverse reactions, 203, 374
  antimicrobial activity, 367t, 369t, 373
  dosage, 370t, 516t–517t
  for Mycobacterium leprae, 2249
  pharmacokinetics, 369
  pharmacology, 516t–517t
  structure, 365f
Pelvic abscess
  anaerobic, 2163t
  female, 1094–1095
  Streptococcus intermedius, 1863
Pelvic cellulitis, 1094
Pelvic infections
  actinomycosis, 2281, 2284
  enterococcal, 1828
Pelvic inflammatory disease,
    1095–1096
  anaerobic, 2163t, 2199
  chlamydial, 183, 1687
  diagnosis, 1096
  gonococcal, 183, 1095, 1917, 1917f
    treatment, 1921–1922, 1922t
  HIV and, 1227
  mycoplasma, 1715t, 1716
    treatment, 1717
  prognosis, 1096
  risk factors, 1095
  sexually transmitted, 183, 1095, 1917,
    1917f
  specimen collection and processing,
    171t, 183
  treatment, 1096, 1096t, 1688,
    1921–1922, 1922t
Pelvic node obstruction, 1081
Pelvic thrombophlebitis, septic, 767,
    1095
  and nosocomial pneumonia, 2601
  treatment, 767
Penciclovir, 421–422
  spectrum of activity, 414t
  structure, 414f
Penicillinase-resistant penicillins,
    242–243. See also specific for-
    mulations
  clinical use, 241t
  dosage, 238t, 241t
  pharmacokinetics, 238t
  structure, 242f
  trade names, 236t
Penicillin-binding proteins, 220, 234,
    247, 250, 1757
  cephalosporins, 249
  and β-lactam resistance, 220, 234, 236
Penicillin G, 205–206, 236, 240–242
  adverse reactions, 239t
  for anthrax, 1889
  antibiotic-associated colitis (AAC),
    979

antimicrobial spectrum, 240, 241t
for bacilli and anaerobes, 237t
benzathine: pharmacology, 506–507t
for *Borrelia burgdorferi*, 2151
for brain abscess, 895
for cellulitis, 916
for clostridial infections, 2188, 2191, 2192
for diphtheria, 1871
dosage, 241t, 506t–507t
  in children, 506t, 851t
  for meningitis, 850t, 851t
  in neonates, 242t, 506t, 851t
  in renal disease and dialysis, 204, 238t, 507t
for endemic syphilis, 2136
for endocarditis
  enterococcal, 762
  prophylaxis, 795
  prosthetic valve, 786, 786t
for enteritis necroticans, 2191
for Enterobacteriaceae and *Pseudomonas*, 237t
for enterococcal infections, 1830, 1831t
for gangrenous cellulitis, 918
for gas gangrene, 932, 2188
for infections arthritis, 1037
for leptospirosis, 2140
for lymphangitis, 943
for mediastinitis, 816
for meningitis, 850t, 851t, 851–852, 854
MICs against cocci, 237t
for necrotizing pneumonia, 646
for *Neisseria meningitidis*, 1903t, 1904
for odontogenic infections, 602t
for peritonitis, 710, 716
pH and, 201
pharmacokinetics, 238t
pharmacology, 238, 506–507t
for pinta, 2136
procaine: pharmacology, 506–507t
prophylactic use, 240
for rheumatic fever, 1805
for streptococcal infections
  glomerulonephritis, 1807
  group C and G, 1856
  for *S. agalactiae*, 1841, 1841t
  for *S. intermedius*, 1863
  for *S. pneumoniae*, 1822
  for *S. pyogenes*, 1790
  viridans, 1850–1851
    endocarditis, 1848, 1848t
    meningitis, 1850
structure, 242f
for suppurative thrombophlebitis, 769
susceptibility testing, 194t
trade names, 236t
for *Treponema pallidum*, 2129, 2129t
Penicillin N, 247
Penicillin(s), 233–246. *See also specific formulations*
for actinomycosis, 2286
adverse reactions, 239f, 239t, 239–240, 272–278, 275–276
aminoglycosides compared with, 285t
aminopenicillins, 243–244
  dosage, 238t, 241t
  pharmacokinetics, 238t
  structure, 243f
for bacilli and anaerobes, 237t

for *Capnocytophaga*, 2105
carboxy, 244–245
  dosage, 238t, 241t
  pharmacokinetics, 238t
  structure, 244f
chemistry, 233
classification, 236t, 236–237, 237t
clinical use, 240, 241t
combination therapy
  aminoglycosides, 287t, 289t
  antagonism, 208–209
  synergism, 207
dosage, 241t, 506t–507t
  in elderly, 201
  in neonates, 242t, 507t
  in renal disease and dialysis, 204, 238t, 239, 507t
drug interactions, 524t
  cephalosporins, 253–254
Eagle effect, 1796
for endocarditis
  culture-negative, 764
  Enterobacteriaceae, 763
  prophylaxis, 795
  Pseudomonas aeruginosa, 763
  streptococcal, 759, 761–762
for Enterobacteriaceae, 237t
for *Erysipelothrix*, 1895
for *Gardnerella vaginalis*, 2051
haptenization, 273
for impetigo, 911
indanyl carbenicillin, 245
isoxazolyl, 243
for *Listeria*, 1884
mechanism of action, 233–234
  bacterial wall cells, 234
  penicillin-binding proteins, 234
MIC against cocci, 237t
for *Mobiluncus*, 2052
natural, 240–242. *See also specific formulations*
  clinical use, 241t
  dosage, 238t, 241t
  pharmacokinetics, 238t
  properties, 240–242
  structure, 242f
neutropenia from, 89
outer membrane permeability, 219, 236
for *Pasteurella*, 2069
penicillinase-resistant, 242–243
  clinical use, 241t
  dosage, 238t, 241t
  pharmacokinetics, 238t
  structure, 242f
  trade names, 236t
for peritonitis, 716
pharmacokinetics, 238t
pharmacology, 237–239, 238t, 506t–507t
for pneumonia, 632t
prophylactic use, 240
for *Pseudomonas aeruginosa*, 237t
for rat-bite fever, 2086
resistance, 200, 220, 234–236, 235f, 241t
  anaerobic gram-negative bacilli, 2200
  Neisseria gonorrhoeae, 1914, 1914f
  Streptococcus pneumoniae, 1821
  viridans streptococci, 1850
for streptococcal pharyngitis, 570–571
structure, 233, 233f, 274f

and sugar level testing, 203
for suppurative odontogenic infections, 602
ureidopenicillins, 245
  dosage, 238t, 241t
  pharmacokinetics, 238t
  structure, 244f
Penicillin V, 236, 242
absorption, 209
for diphtheria, 1871
dosage, 241t, 506t–507t
  in children, 506t
  in renal disease and dialysis, 238t, 507t
for erysipelas, 914
for impetigo, 911
MICs against cocci, 237t
pH and, 201
pharmacokinetics, 238t
pharmacology, 238, 506–507t
for streptococcal pharyngitis, 570
for *Streptococcus pyogenes*, 1790
structure, 242f
trade names, 236t
for Whipple's disease, 1031
Penicillium chrysogenum, 233
Penicillium marneffii, 2390–2391
  and HIV/AIDS, 1236
Penicillium melini: sinusitis, 586t
Penicilloyl-polylysine (PPL) skin test, 275
Penis
  Francisella tularensis ulcer, 2063, 2064f
  lesions. *See* Genital lesions
  pearly papules, 1059
  prostheses: *Staphylococcus epidermidis*, 323
Pentamidine, 459t, 475, 477
  adverse reactions, 478, 1284, 2481
  dosage, 463t, 467t
    pediatric, 463t, 467t
  drug interactions, 524t
  for *Leishmania*, 2430, 2435, 2438
  for neutropenics, 2688t
  for *Pneumocystis carinii*, 478, 1283t, 1284, 2480–2481
    prophylaxis, 1285–1286, 1286t, 2482
  spectrum of activity, 478
  structure, 478f
  for *Trypanosoma brucei*, 2454
Pentatrichomonas hominis, 2493
Pentavalent antimony, 477
  adverse reactions, 477
  for *Leishmania*, 2430, 2438
  side effects, 2430
Pentazocine abuse, 1983
Pentoxifylline, 455
  for bacterial meningitis, 856
Peptic ulcer perforation
  and intraperitoneal abscess, 721
  and peritonitis, 710, 714
Peptides: and MHC class II, 104
Peptide transporter genes (*TAP*1 and *TAP* 2), 103, 103f
Peptidoglycan, 234, 1753
  cephalosporins and, 249
  Gram staining, 1753
  Staphylococcus aureus, 1758f, 1758–1759, 1761
  Streptococcus pneumoniae, 1811
Peptococcus, 2158t. *See also* *Peptostreptococcus*
  as enteric flora, 947

human bites, 2768
mediastinitis, 815t
peritonitis, 711, 715
  treatment, 716
pneumonia, 619t
treatment
  chloramphenicol, 312t
  tetracyclines, 308t
Peptococcus niger, 2204
Peptostreptococcus, 2158t, 2204–2206. *See also Peptococcus*
antimicrobial susceptibility, 2170t
bacteremia, 2165
bites, 604
clinically significant, 2159t
clinical manifestations, 2205
as enteric flora, 947
epidermal cysts, 920
female genital infections, 2165
mediastinitis, 815t
necrotizing fasciitis, 923
oral colonization, 593, 594t
parotitis, 2198
peritonitis, 711, 715
pleuropulmonary infection, 2164
pneumonia, 619t
sinusitis, 585t, 2198
treatment, 2170t, 2205–2206
  chloramphenicol, 312t
  penicillin MICs, 237t
  tetracyclines, 308t
Peptostreptococcus anaerobius, 2204
Peptostreptococcus asaccharolyticus, 2204
Peptostreptococcus hydrogenalis, 2204
Peptostreptococcus intermedius, 2204
Peptostreptococcus magnus, 2204, 2205
Peptostreptococcus micros, 2204
  intra-abdominal infections, 2165
Peptostreptococcus prevotii, 2204, 2205
Peptostreptococcus productus, 2204
Peptostreptococcus saccharolyticus, 2204
Peptostreptococcus tetradius, 2204
Percutaneous drainage
  hepatic abscess, 726
  intraperitoneal abscess, 722
  pancreatic abscess, 724
  for perinephric and intrarenal abscesses, 682
Perfloxacin
  for leprosy, 399
  for *Pseudomonas aeruginosa* meningitis, 1989
Perforin: and cytotoxic T cells, 121
Perhydroxy radical, 84
Perianal infections. *See also* Anorectal disease and lesions
  actinomycosis, 2283
  Candida albicans, 2294–2295, 2295f
Periapical infections
  actinomycosis, 2281, 2282
  anaerobic abscess, 2163t, 2198
  anaerobic granuloma, 2163t
Periarteritis nodosa: diagnosis, 1006t
Pericardial effusion: and pericarditis, 806
Pericardiectomy: for tuberculous pericarditis, 2236
Pericardiocentesis: for tuberculous pericarditis, 2236
Pericarditis, 805–808
  clinical manifestations, 806–807
  diagnosis, 805t, 807, 807t
  Histoplasma capsulatum, 2343

Pericarditis (Continued)
  treatment, 2351
  infectious etiology, 805, 805t
  influenza virus, 1558
  Mycobacterium tuberculosis, 2236
    treatment, 2236
      glucocorticoids, 455
  Neisseria meningitidis, 1901
  noninfectious causes, 807t
  pathology, pathogenesis, and
      pathophysiology, 805–806,
      806f
  Staphylococcus aureus, 1770
  streptococci group C, 1856
  Streptococcus pneumoniae, 1821
  treatment, 807–808
Perichondritis of auricle: Pseudomonas
    aeruginosa, 1991
Pericoronitis, 598
Perifolliculitis capitis, 915
Periglomerular fibrosis, 663
Perihepatitis
  Neisseria gonorrhoeae and, 1917
  and peritonitis, 709
Perineal irritation: vulvovaginitis, 1082
Perineal phlegmon, 925
Perinephric abscess, 662, 681–682
  diagnosis and therapy, 682, 682f
Periocular infections, 1129–1136. See
    also Eye infections
Periodontal abscess, 596, 598
  anaerobic, 2163t, 2164
Periodontal disease
  anaerobic
    specimen collection, 2168t
  Capnocytophaga, 2104
  clinical presentation, 596, 598
  and leukemia, 2678
  and lung abscess, 642
  neutrophil defect and, 153
  pathogenesis, 594–595
  Streptococcus intermedius, 1862
Periodontal surgery: and endocarditis,
    743t, 794t
  prophylaxis, 797
Periodontitis
  Actinobacillus, 2106
  clinical presentation, 598
  HIV/AIDS and, 1227
  juvenile
    defective chemotaxis in, 90
    microbiology, 594
    therapy, 601
  microbiology, 594
  therapy, 601–602
Periorbital edema, 309
Peripheral IV cannulization: bacteremia
    from, 2591t, 2591–2592
Peripheral neuropathy
  from didanosine, 421
  HIV/AIDS and, 1236
  from nitrofurantoin, 378–379
Peripheral vascular surgery prophylaxis,
    2751t
Perirectal infections
  actinomycosis, 2283
  anaerobic abscess, 2163t
Peritoneal cavity
  anatomy, 706f, 706–708, 707f
  permeability, 707
  serous membrane, 707
Peritoneal dialysis
  aminoglycoside dosage in, 298, 298t
  penicillin dosage in, 238t, 238–239
  and peritonitis, 710, 719–720

chronic ambulatory (CAPD),
    719–720, 1780
  Staphylococcus epidermidis
    catheter-associated, 1780
Peritoneal inflammation. See Peritonitis
Peritoneal reflections, 706, 706f
Peritonitis, 707–721
  Candida albicans, 2298
    treatment, 2300
  enterococcal, 1828
  Mycobacterium tuberculosis,
      2238–2239
  Pasteurella, 2069
  during peritoneal dialysis, 719–720
    acute dialysis, 720–721
    antibiotic therapy, 720, 720t
    chronic dialysis, 719–721
  primary, 708–710
    bacteriology, 708–709
    clinical manifestations, 709
    diagnosis, 709–710
    etiology, 708
    pathogenesis, 709
    prognosis, 710
    treatment, 710
  secondary, 710–719
    cardiovascular response, 713
    clinical manifestations, 714
    diagnosis, 714
    GI response, 713
    local response, 714
    metabolic response, 714
    microbiology, 710–712
    pathogenesis, 712–713
    pathophysiology, 713–714
    physical findings, 714
    prevention, 719
    prognosis, 714–715
    renal response, 714
    respiratory response, 713
    symptoms, 714
    treatment, 715–719
      aminoglycosides, 717
      antimicrobial, 715–718
      antimicrobial trials, 717t,
          717–718
      blood and plasma transfusion,
          718
      cephalosporins, 716
      chloramphenicol, 715
      clindamycin, 715–716
      GI drainage, 718
      hyperbaric oxygen, 718
      metronidazole, 716
      operative support, 718
      penicillins, 716
      quinolones, 717
      respiratory support, 718
      tetracyclines, 716
      water and electrolytes, 718
    staphylococcal: vancomycin for,
        350
  Streptococcus intermedius, 1863
  Streptococcus pneumoniae, 1821
  treatment
    aminoglycosides, 288–289
    primary, 710
    quinolones, 371–372
    secondary, 715–719. See also
        secondary, treatment above
Peritonsillar abscess (quinsy), 569
  anaerobic, 2163t, 2164
    gram-negative bacilli, 2198
  treatment, 571
Peritonsillitis, 569

treatment, 571
Permethrin, 463t
  dosage, 466t
  for scabies, 2562
Peromyscus maniculatus: and han-
    taviruses, 1569
Person-to-person transmission, 164
Pertactin: Bordetella pertussis, 23
Pertussis toxin, 3, 3t, 4, 6, 23, 2079,
    2080
  attachment and entry, 4
Pertussis vaccine, 2778–2779
  adverse reactions, 2779
  contraindications, 2778–2779
  DTP, 2082, 2771, 2775, 2775t. See
      also DTP vaccine
Petechiae
  conjunctival: endocarditis, 747, 747f
  endocarditis, 555, 922
    prosthetic valve, 784t, 785
  endocarditis and, 747, 748
  enteroviral exanthems, 1624
  purpuric lesions, 553
  scarlet fever, 553
  systemic infections manifesting, 550t
Petriellidium boydii. See Pseudalle-
    scheria boydii
P fimbriae
  Enterobacteriaceae, 1966
  Escherichia coli, 11f, 12t, 16–18,
      664–665, 665t, 1966, 1971
pH
  and antimicrobials, 32, 201, 205–206
  urinary: and urinary tract infections,
      674
Phaeohyphomycosis
  differential diagnosis, 2326
  of paranasal sinus, 1132
Phages: and pathogenicity, 22, 22t
Phagocyte oxidase, 84–85
Phagocytes
  deficiencies, 151t
    and infections in patients with neo-
        plasia, 2666–2668
  mononuclear, 122–124
  and pneumonia, 620
  virulence factors directed at, 8
Phagocytosis, 32–33
  cytokines and, 33–34
  frustrated, 86
  neutrophil, 83f, 83–84
  opsonin-independent, 33
Pharygoconjunctival fever, 566, 1375
Pharyngeal cleft cysts, 604
Pharyngeal gonorrhea, 1909, 1910,
    1916
Pharyngeal tularemia, 2064
Pharyngitis, 566–572
  acute lymphonodular: coxsackievirus,
      1625
  and acute retroviral syndrome (HIV),
      1224t
  anaerobic (Vincent's angina), 569,
      1789
    treatment, 571
  arcanobacterial, 569, 1789, 1872t,
      1874
    treatment, 571
  chlamydial, 569
  clinical presentation, 568–569
  with common cold, 568
  Corynebacterium diphtheriae, 569,
      1789, 1868
  Corynebacterium ulcerans, 567, 569,
      1872t

cultures, 173
  diagnosis, 569–570
  differential diagnosis, 1789
  EBV mononucleosis, 568, 1367,
      1368t, 1789
  epidemiology, 567
  etiology, 566–567, 567t, 1789
  gonococcal, 569, 1789, 1916
    cultures, 173, 182, 570
  herpangina, 568
  herpes simplex virus, 568, 1338
  herpetic, 568
  HIV, 568
  with influenza, 568
  mycoplasmal, 569
  Neisseria meningitidis, 1789, 1902
  noninfectious, 569
  pathogenesis, 567–568
  peritonsillitis/peritonsillar abscess
      (quinsy), 569, 2163t, 2164,
      2171
    treatment, 571
  pharyngoconjunctival fever, 566
  prevention, 571
  streptococcal, 566
    group C and G, 1787, 1853–1854
      complications, 1854
      presentation, 568–569
    Streptococcus pyogenes, 1787–1791
      clinical manifestations,
          1788–1789
      epidemiology, 1787–1788,
          1788f, 1806, 1806t
      therapy, 1790–1791
    treatment, 570–571
  treatment, 570–571
  viral: treatment, 571
  yersinial, 569
    treatment, 571
    Y. enterocolitica, 2077
    Y. pestis, 2074
Phase microscopy, 184
Phenothiazines: neutropenia from,
    89
Phenotypic variation: virulence factors
    and, 8
Phenoxymethyl penicillin. See Penicillin
    V
Phenylethylalcohol (PEA) agar, 2168
Phenytoin
  hepatotoxicity, 1148
  isoniazid interaction with, 390
Pheochromocytoma: and fever, 547
Phialophora, 2391
  keratitis, 1113
Phialophora jeanselmei, 2327
Phialophora pedrosoi, 2324
Phialophora verrucosa, 2324
Phlebitis. See also Thrombophlebitis
  suppurative intracranial, 907–909
Phlebotomus
  and bartonellosis, 2209
  and Leishmania, 2429
  and orbiviruses, 1448
Phlebovirus, 1567
  characteristics, 1568t
Phlyctenular keratoconjunctivitis: and
    Mycobacterium tuberculosis,
    2220, 2222
Phocanema, 2554–2555
Phormia, 2562
Phosphatidylinositol 4,5-biphosphate
    (PIP$_2$), 110
Phospholipase C, 110
  and neutrophils, 86

Phosphonoacetic acid (PAA): for EBV, 1372
Phosphotransferase, 282
Photosensitivity: tetracyclines, 309
Phrenicocolic ligament, 706, 706f
Phthiriasis palpebrarum, 1130
Phthirus pubis, 1059, 2558, 2559, 2559f
  blepharitis, 1130
  clinical manifestations, 2560
  epidemiology, 2559
  treatment, 463t, 2560
Phycomycosis, 2311. *See also* Mucormycosis
  enteritides, 994
Pia mater: anatomy, 821
Pichinde virus, 1572
Picornaviridae. *See also individual viruses*
  arthritis, 1036t
  characteristics, 1606–1607
  classification, 1315t, 1606, 1606t
  coxsackieviruses, 1620–1636
  echoviruses, 1620–1636
  enteroviruses, 1620–1636
  hepatitis A virus, 1636–1656
  hepatitis E virus, 1663–1666
  poliovirus, 1613–1620
  rhinovirus, 1656–1663
  shape and size, 1316f
Piedra
  black, 2385
  white, 2385
Piedraia hortae, 2385
Pig-bel, 991–992
Pig coronavirus TGEV: receptor, 12, 13
Pili, 1754. *See also* Fimbriae
  Neisseria gonorrhoeae, 24, 1910, 1911f
Pilonidal abscess: anaerobic, 2163t, 2165
Pink phantom. *See Protomonas extorquens*
Pink puffers, 609
Pinta, 2133, 2135–2136
Pintids, 2135
Pinworms. *See Enterobius vermicularis*
Piperacillin, 245
  adverse reactions, 239t
  antimicrobial activity, 241t, 285t
  for bacilli and anaerobes, 237t
  for *Bacteroides fragilis*, 2200t, 2201
  combination therapy
    aminoglycosides, 287t
    synergism, 207
  dosage, 241t, 506–507t
    in children and neonates, 506t
    in neonates, 242t
    in renal disease, 238t, 507t
  for Enterobacteriaceae and *Pseudomonas*, 237t
  MICs against cocci, 237t
  for odontogenic infections, 602t
  for peritonitis, 720t
  pharmacokinetics, 238t
  pharmacology, 506–507t
  structure, 244f
Piperacillin-tazobactam, 270
  antimicrobial activity, 285t
  for *Bacteroides fragilis*, 2200t, 2201
  dosage, 506–507t
  pharmacology, 506–507t
Piperazine, 460t, 480–481
  for ascariasis, 2529
  drug interactions, 524t
Piritrexin: for *Toxoplasma gondii*, 2469

Pittsburgh pneumonia agent. *See Legionella micdadei*
Pityriasis versicolor, 2383–2384
  clinical features, 2384
  etiology, 2383–2384
  pathogenesis, 2384
  treatment, 2384
Pityrosporum, 2383–2384
  folliculitis, 2384
  seborrheic dermatitis, 2384
Pityrosporum orbiculare, 2383–2384
Pityrosporum ovale, 2383–2384
Pixuna virus, 1457
Plague, 2070–2076. *See also Yersinia pestis*
  bubonic, 2072–2073, 2073f, 2074f
  pneumonic, 2074
  septicemic, 2073–2074, 2074f
Plague vaccine, 2779
  indications for adults, 2784t
  for travelers, 2797t, 2799
Plane warts, 1388t, 1390, 1392
Plantar warts, 1388t, 1389, 1390, 1392. *See also* Human papillomavirus
Plaque
  cutaneous: defined, 551
  dental, 594–595
Plasma transfusions
  nosocomial infections, 2628
  for peritonitis, 718
Plasmids
  and pathogenicity, 22, 22t
  and resistance, 212–213, 213f
Plasminogen activator inhibitor-1: and septic shock, 118
Plasmodium, 2394t, 2415–2427
  anemia: pathogenesis, 2420
  anopheline vector, 2417
  antimalarial drugs, 2422–2425
    chemoprophylaxis, 2424t, 2424–2425
    mechanism of action, 2422
    resistance, 2415, 2422–2425, 2423f, 2424t
    unique targets for, 2422
  blood cultures, 170t
  cerebral malaria: pathogenesis, 2419
  chemoprophylaxis
    chloroquine-resistant
      P. falciparum, 2424
      P. vivax, 2424–2425
    P. falciparum (chloroquine-susceptible), 2424, 2424t
    P. ovale, P. vivax and *P. malariae*, 2424, 2424t
  "chilling stage," 2421
  chloroquine-resistant, 2422–2425, 2423f, 2424t
    prophylaxis, 465t
  clinical manifestations, 2394t, 2421–2422
    differences between nonimmune and semi-immune individuals, 2422
  CNS dysfunction, 2421–2422
  coma, 2421
  cytokine and T cell protection, 121t, 127
  description, 2415
  diagnosis, 2395t, 2425
  differential diagnosis, 1472
    Babesia, 2499
    based on peripheral blood smear, 2415t

enteric symptoms, 1000t, 1002, 1003
  epidemiology, 2415–2418
  falciparum. See Plasmodium falciparum
  fever, 543
    pattern, 538
  gametes, 2416
  gametocytes, 2416
  gastroenteritis, 2420
  geographic distribution, 2394t
  and granulocytopenia, 2677
  hemolysis, 2421
  history, 2415
  HLA antigen and, 2421
  "hot stage," 2421
  hypnozoites, 2416–2417, 2417
  laboratory findings, 2421
  life cycle, 2415–2416, 2416f
    adaptive features, 2416–2417
    ligands and receptors, 2418t
    molecular insights to, 2418, 2418t
  malariae, 2421. *See also Plasmodium malariae*
    treatment. *See* treatment *below*
  merozoites, 2416
  ookinetes, 2416
  ovale, 2415, 2415t, 2421, 2421. *See also Plasmodium ovale*
    treatment. *See* treatment *below*
  pathogenesis, 2418–2421
    anemia, 2420
    cerebral malaria, 2419
    complications, 2419–2420, 2420t
    gastroenteritis, 2420
    host factors, 2421
    hyperparasitemia, 2418–2419
    hypoglycemia and, 2418
    lipid peroxidation and, 2418–2419
    peripheral sequestration, 2418, 2420f
    pulmonary edema, 2420
    renal failure, 2419–2420
    sickle cell hemoglobin and, 2418, 2420f
  prophylaxis, 464t–465t
    chloroquine, 464t, 469–471
      dosage, 464t
    doxycycline: dosage, 464t
    mefloquine, 465t, 471–472
    for travelers, 2801
  pulmonary edema: pathogenesis, 2420
  renal failure, 2422
    pathogenesis, 2419–2420
  resistance, 2415, 2422–2425, 2423f, 2424t
    prophylaxis and, 2424
  rosetting, 2418
  and *Salmonella*, 2019
  seizures, 2421
  sickle cell hemoglobin and, 2417–2418
    protective effects, 2418, 2420f
  sporozoites, 2415, 2416f
  "sweating stage," 2421
  tissue schizonts, 2416
  transfusion (or shared needles) transmission, 2417, 2627
    treatment, 2425
  transmission, 2394t, 2415, 2417
  treatment, 464t, 469–472, 2425
    aminoquinolines, 464t, 469–472
    antibodies against TNF-α, 2426
    artemisinin, 472, 2425
    atovaquone, 475

    chloroquine, 464t, 469–471, 2424t, 2425
      dosage, 464t, 2424t
    dihydrofolate reductase inhibitors, 473
    dosage, 2424t
    doxycycline, 472, 2424t, 2425
      dosage, 464t, 2424t
    Fansidar, 473–474, 2424, 2425
      dosage, 2424t
    Fansimef, 474
    halofantrine, 472–473
    hydroxychloroquine sulfate: dosage, 464t
    mefloquine, 464t, 471–472, 2425
    pediatric dosage, 2424t
    in pregnancy, 2425
    primaquine, 470–471
    Proguanil, 474
    pyrimethamine, 474
      combination formulas, 473–474, 2424, 2424t
    quinidine, 464t, 471, 2425
    quinine, 471, 2426
    steroids for cerebral malaria, 2426
    sulfonamides, 473
    tetracycline, 472
    trimethoprim, 360
    vaccine research, 2426
  tumor necrosis factor and, 2421
    treatment against, 2426
  vivax, 2415, 2415t, 2418, 2421. *See also Plasmodium vivax*
    treatment. *See* treatment *above*
  zygotes, 2416
Plasmodium falciparum
  chemoprophylaxis
    chloroquine-resistant, 2424
    chloroquine-susceptible, 2424, 2424t
  cutaneous manifestations, 550t
  cytoadherence, 2415, 2417f, 2418, 2419f
  description, 2415t
  differential diagnosis, 2415t
  effect on RBC, 2415, 2417f
  pathogenesis, 2417f, 2418–2421, 2419f
    cytoadherence, 2417f, 2418, 2419f
  pathology, 2420–2421
  peripheral sequestration, 2418, 2420f
  sickle cell hemoglobin and, 2418, 2420f
  treatment, 469–471, 472–473, 473, 474–475
    chloroquine-resistant, 2425
    chloroquine-susceptible, 2425
    sulfonamides, 357
    trimethoprim-sulfamethoxazole, 360
Plasmodium malariae
  chemoprophylaxis, 2424, 2424t
  description, 2415t
  pathogenesis, 2421
  treatment, 469–471, 2425
Plasmodium ovale
  chemoprophylaxis, 2424, 2424t
  description, 2415t
  differential diagnosis: based on peripheral blood smear, 2415t
  pathogenesis, 2421
  prevention, 2424, 2424t
  treatment, 469–471, 2424t, 2425
    eradication of persistent hypnozoites, 2425

Plasmodium vivax, 2415, 2415t, 2418, 2421
  chemoprophylaxis, 2424, 2424t
    chloroquine-resistant, 2424–2425
  description, 2415t
  differential diagnosis: based on peripheral blood smear, 2415t
  pathogenesis, 2421
  prevention, 2424, 2424t
  treatment, 469–471, 474, 2424t, 2424–2425
    chloroquine-resistant, 2425
    eradication of persistent hypnozoites, 2425
Platelet-activating factor (PAF), 96
  actions, 30t
  and sepsis, 696
Platelet deposition: and endocarditis, 742, 745
Platelet/endothelial cell adhesion molecule-1 (PECAM-1), 81, 81f, 82
Platyhelminths. *See also* Cestodes; Trematodes
  antiparasitic agents, 482–483
PLC-231, 110
Pleistophora, 2514, 2517t
  diagnosis, 2520–2521
  in HIV infected, 2519, 2519t
  in non-HIV infected, 2517t, 2518
Plesiomonas shigelloides, 2110
  classification and site of infection, 2107t
  enterotoxin, 5
Pleural decortication: for empyema, 640
Pleural drainage: for empyema, 640
Pleural effusion, 638–641
  clinical presentation, 638f, 638–640, 639f
  etiology, 637–638
  examination, 625
  Legionella pneumophila, 2092
  pathogens, 638–639
  and pneumonia, 625
  prognosis, 641
  treatment, 640–641
  tuberculosis and, 2235
    treatment, 2235
Pleural empyema, 638–641
  clinical presentation, 638f, 638–640, 639f
  etiology, 637–638
  exudate, fibropurulent, and organizing phases, 638
  pathogens, 638
  prognosis, 641
  Staphylococcus aureus, 1770–1771
  treatment, 640–641
Pleural fluid
  microscopic examination of pathogens, 172t
  specimen collection and processing, 170t, 174
Pleurisy
  epidemic benign, 1625–1626
  tuberculous, 2235
    treatment, 2235
Pleurodynia, epidemic, 1625–1626
  clinical manifestations, 1626
  diagnosis, 1626
  epidemiology, 1625
  etiology, 1625
  history, 1625
  management, 1626
  pathogenesis, 1625–1626

Pleurodynia syndromes, 934
Pleuropulmonary amebiasis, 2401
Pleuropulmonary infections, 606–662. *See also* Pulmonary infections
  anaerobes
    cocci, 2205
    gram-negative, 2198
  Clostridium perfringens, 2185
  effusions and empyema. *See* Pleural effusion; Pleural empyema
PMEA, 437t
Pneumococcal vaccine, 167, 2779–2780
  antibody response, 50
  for HIV infected, 2785
  indications, 2779–2780, 2783
    for adults, 2784t
    for travelers, 2799
Pneumococcus, 1811–1826. *See also* *Streptococcus pneumoniae*
Pneumoconiosis: chronic, 647t, 648
Pneumocystis carinii, 2394t, 2475–2487
  adherence, 2476
  and adult T-cell leukemia/lymphoma, 1582
  antibody deficiencies and, 49
  BAL, 1233
  and bone marrow transplantation, 2721
  bronchoalveolar lavage (BAL) for, 2477, 2479
  bronchoscopy, 174
  in cancer patients, 2669
  and CD4 cells, 127, 2477
  cellular immunity and, 127
    defects, 2681
    therapy, 2682
  chest radiography, 2478, 2478f
  clinical manifestations, 2394t, 2478, 2478f, 2479f
  course and pathogenesis, 2480
  cyst, 2475, 2476f
  description, 2475, 2476f
  diagnosis, 2395t, 2478–2480
  in drug abusers, 2701
  endophthalmitis, 1123
  epidemiology, 2475–2476
  extrapulmonary, 2478, 2479f
  hairy cell leukemia and, 137
  and heart-lung transplantation, 2725
  HIV/AIDS and, 127, 621, 629, 1182, 1182t, 1233, 1233t, 1281, 1591, 2475–2483, 2669
    in children, 1186t, 1186–1187
  choroiditis, 1240
  clinical manifestations, 2478
  course and pathogenesis, 2480
  extrapulmonary, 2478, 2479f
  incidence, 1182t, 1183, 1221, 1222f, 1282, 2476
  pathology and pathogenesis, 2476–2478
  probability of developing, 1223f, 1282
  prognosis, 2480
  prophylaxis, 1284–1286, 1286t, 2482–2483
  toxoplasmosis vs., 2460
  treatment, 1282–1286, 1283t, 2480–2482
  immunodeficiency and, 133, 138, 150t. *See also* cellular immunity *above*
  and leukemia, hairy cell, 2673
  lung tissue exam, 174

major surface glycoprotein (MSG), 2475
  Papanicolaou stain, 2479
  pathology and pathogenesis, 2476–2478, 2477f
  pneumonia, 619t, 1704
    bronchoalveolar lavage, 624
    differential diagnosis, 2336
    in HIV/AIDS. *See* HIV/AIDS *above*
    nosocomial
      in the immunocompromised, 631
    sputum analysis, 623
  pneumothorax and, 2480
  polymerase chain reaction, 2476, 2479
  precyst, 2475
  prophylaxis, 466t, 1221, 1273–1274, 1284–1286, 1286t, 2482–2483
    dapsone, 397, 1286, 1286t, 2482
    in HIV/AIDS, 1284–1286, 1286t, 2482–2483
    for immunocompromised host, 2693
    pentamidine, 1285–1286, 1286t, 2482
    pyrimethamine, 1286, 1286t
    trimethoprim-sulfamethoxazole, 1285, 1286t, 2482
  pulmonary infiltrates with eosinophilia, 631
  taxonomy, 2475
  transmission, 2394t
  in transplant recipients, 2709, 2722
  treatment, 466t, 473, 1282–1286, 1283t, 2480–2482
    atovaquone, 475, 1283t, 1284, 1286, 2481
    clindamycin, 343, 1284, 2481
    corticosteroids, 455, 1284–1285, 2482
    dapsone, 1284, 2481
    eflornithine, 2481
    in HIV/AIDS, 1282–1286, 1283t, 2480–2482
    pentamidine, 478, 1283t, 1284, 2480–2481
    primaquine, 1284, 2481
    trimethoprim, 357, 360, 1283t, 1284
    trimethoprim-sulfamethoxazole, 360, 474, 1282, 1283t, 2480, 2481
    trimetrexate, 475, 1283t, 1284, 2481
  trophozoite, 2475, 2476f
  Wiskott-Aldrich syndrome and, 52
  X-linked hyper-IgM syndrome and, 51
Pneumonectomy: for pneumonia, 657
Pneumonia. *See also* Pneumonitis
  Acinetobacter, 2011
  actinomycosis, 2282f, 2282–2283
  acute, 619–638
    antigen detection, 625–626
    aspiration, 630
    atypical, 629–630
    BAL, 624–625
    blood cultures, 625–626
    clinical evaluation, 621–622
    community-acquired, 627–629
      in the elderly, 628–629
      HIV/AIDS and, 629

severe, 629–630
  slowly resolving, 629
  environmental factors, 622t
  etiology, 619t. *See also specific agents*
  fiberoptic bronchoscopy, 624–626
  history taking, 621
  host defenses, 619–621, 620t
  lung biopsy, 625
  nosocomial
    in the immunocompromised, 631
  nosocomial in the immunocompromised, 621
  pathogenesis, 619–621
  physical examination, 621–622
  pleural effusion examination, 625
  pulmonary infiltrates with eosinophilia, 630–631
  radiologic examination, 626f–627f, 626–627, 627f
  radionuclide studies, 628
  serology, 625–626
  sputum examination, 622f, 622–624, 623f
  syndromes, 627–629
  therapy, 631–632, 632t
  transtracheal aspiration, 624
adenovirus, 1386
anaerobic necrotizing, 642–643, 643f
Aspergillus, 2307–2308, 2308f
aspiration, 631
  anaerobic, 2163t
    gram-negative bacilli, 2198
  nosocomial, 2601
  poliovirus, 1616
  Pseudomonas aeruginosa, 1985
  radiology, 626
  spinal cord injury and, 2732
  Streptococcus intermedius, 1863
atypical. *See also specific causative agents*
  differential diagnosis, 1698
  Eaton agent and, 1704
  etiology, 619t, 630, 1704
  Mycoplasma pneumoniae, 1704–1713
Bacillus, 1892
bacterial
  and HIV/AIDS, 1183, 1231, 1233t, 1235, 1235t
  and influenza virus, 1556t, 1557, 1557t
Blastomyces dermatitidis, 2355, 2356t, 2357, 2358f, 2359f
  chronic, 647t, 2356t, 2357, 2358f
  in HIV/AIDS, 1236
  and bone marrow transplantation, 2720–2721
  in cancer patients, 2668
Candida, 2296
  and cell-mediated immune defects, 2681–2682
Chlamydia pneumoniae, 1696, 1697t, 1698f, 1698–1699
  diagnosis, 1699, 1699t
  incidence, 1699
  treatment, 1699
Chlamydia psittaci, 619t, 622t, 630, 1694
Chlamydia trachomatis, 1688
  infant, 1689, 1689f
chronic, 647–658
  age and, 647–648
  clinical features, 648–649
  diagnosis, 649–655

drug use and, 648
epidemiology, 647–648
etiology, 647, 647t. *See also specific agents*
invasive procedures, 652
laboratory studies, 649
occupation and, 648
race and, 647–648
radiologic patterns, 649, 650t, 651f–656f, 656f
serology, 652
sex and, 647–648
signs, 649
skin tests, 651
symptoms, 648–649
therapy, 653–656
  antimicrobials, 653–656
  bronchoscopy, 656–657
  corticosteroids, 655–656
  supportive measures, 656
  surgery, 656–657
travel and, 648
and chronic granulomatous disease, 92
community-acquired
  acute, 627–629
  in the elderly, 628–629
  HIV/AIDS and, 629
  severe, 629
  slowly resolving, 629
Coxiella burnetii, 1729–1730, 1730f, 1731f
  treatment, 1729
Cryptococcus neoformans
  differential diagnosis, 2334
  and HIV/AIDS, 1239, 2334, 2335
cytomegalovirus. *See also*
  Pneumonitis, CMV
  treatment, 412t
  ganciclovir, 425
differential diagnosis: peritonitis, 714
in drug abusers, 2701–2702
Escherichia coli, 1971
Francisella tularensis, 2065, 2065f
Haemophilus influenzae, 619t, 2042, 2043
  and influenza virus, 1556t, 1557, 1557t
Histoplasma capsulatum, 619t, 622t
  chronic, 647t, 648
  in HIV/AIDS, 1235–1236
  radiology, 650t, 653f
  treatment, 2350
and HIV/AIDS
  bacterial, 1183, 1231, 1233t, 1235, 1235t
  Blastomyces dermatitidis, 1236
  in children, 1184, 1186t, 1186–1187
  community-acquired, 629
  cryptococcal, 1240, 2334, 2335
  Histoplasma capsulatum, 1235–1236
  Pneumocystis carinii. See
    Pneumocystis carinii
  Toxoplasma gondii, 1236, 2460
influenza virus, 1556t, 1556–1557
  and secondary bacterial, 1556t, 1557, 1557t
Klebsiella, 1972
Legionella pneumophila, 2091–2092
lymphoid interstitial: in children with HIV/AIDS, 1184, 1186t, 1186–1187
measles virus, 1521
melioidosis, 2005

Moraxella catarrhalis, 1927
necrotizing: anaerobic gram-negative bacilli, 2198
Neisseria meningitidis, 1911
Nocardia, 2275–2276, 2276f
nosocomial, 2599–2607
  Acinetobacter, 2011
  diagnosis, 2602–2603
  in the elderly, 2738
  Enterobacteriaceae, 631, 2600, 2601
  Escherichia coli, 631, 1971, 2600
  etiology, 2600, 2600t
  in the immunocompromised, 631
  incidence and mortality, 2599–2600, 2600t
  Klebsiella, 1972
  Legionella pneumophila, 2089, 2094, 2600
  pathogenesis, 2601–2602
  predisposing factors, 2601, 2601t
  prevention, 2604–2605
  Serratia marcescens, 631, 2600
  in trauma patients, 2757
  treatment, 2603–2604
parainfluenza virus, 1490, 1490t
plague, 2074
Pneumocystis carinii. See
  Pneumocystis carinii
Pseudomonas aeruginosa, 1984–1985
respiratory syncytial virus, 1504t, 1507–1508
  nosocomial, 1509
Salmonella, 2023
in spinal cord injured patients, 2732t, 2733
Staphylococcus aureus, 1770, 1771f
  hematogenous, 1770, 1771f
  and influenza virus, 1556t, 1557, 1557t
  inhalation, 1770
Streptococcus agalactiae
  adult, 1840
  neonatal, 1838
Streptococcus pneumoniae, 1814, 1818–1821
  complications, 1821
  diagnosis, 1819, 1820f, 1821
  immunology, 1814
  and influenza virus, 1556t, 1557, 1557t
  physical findings, 1819
  predisposing factors, 1818t
  radiographic findings, 1819
  symptoms, 1818–1819
Streptococcus pyogenes, 1797
Toxoplasma gondii: and HIV/AIDS, 1236, 2460
in transplant recipients, 2727
  etiology, 2727t
in traumatized patient, 2757, 2757t
treatment
  aminoglycosides, 295t
  ticarcillin-clavulanate, 269
viridans streptococci, 1850
Pneumonic plague, 2072t, 2074
Pneumonitis. *See also* Pneumonia
  CMV, 135. *See also* Pneumonia, cytomegalovirus
    and AIDS, 629, 1358
    bronchoalveolar lavage, 624
    in the immunocompromised, 1358
    treatment, 412t
  herpesviruses, 1334t
  and sepsis, 693

varicella-zoster virus, 1347
  treatment, 1349–1350
Pneumothorax
  Aspergillus and, 2308
  and cystic fibrosis, 658
Pneumovirus, 1502. *See also* Respiratoy syncytial virus
P-nucleotides, 106
Podofilox: for anogenital warts, 1394
Podophyllin: for anogenital warts, 1394
Polioencephalitis, 875, 1616
Polio vaccine, 1613–1614, 1618–1619, 2771, 2780
  adverse reactions, 2773t, 2780
  contraindications, 2787t
  disease associated with, 1614
  IPV, 1614, 1618–1619, 2780
  morbidity reduction, 2772t
  OPV, 1614, 1618–1619, 2780
  recommendations
    for adults, 2784t
    for HIV infected, 2784
    for infants and children, 2780t, 2783
  reportable events, 2786t
  for travelers, 2797t, 2797–2798
Poliovirus, 1613–1620. *See also*
    Enteroviruses
  abortive poliomyelitis, 1615
  adherence, 12
  aspiration pneumonia, 1616
  bulbar paralytic poliomyelitis, 1616
  classification, 1606t, 1606–1607, 1613
  clinical features, 1614–1616, 1615f
  CNS response, 828
  complications, 1616
  differential diagnosis, 1617
    rabies, 1535
  epidemiology, 1614
    in other countries, 1619
  GI hemorrhage, 1616
  history, 1613
  host range and virulence, 1613–1614
  incubation period, 1614–1615
  laboratory diagnosis, 1617
  management, 1618
  myocarditis, 1616
  nonparalytic poliomyelitis, 1615
  OPV-associated poliomyelitis, 1614
  in other countries, 1619
  paralytic ileus, 1616
  pathogenesis, 1614
  pathology, 1614
  polioencephalitis, 875, 1616
  postpoliomyelitis syndrome, 1617–1618
  prevention, 1618–1619
  prognosis, 1617
  pulmonary edema, 1616
  pulmonary embolism, 1616
  receptor, 12, 13, 1317t
  respiratory failure, 1616
  and Reye syndrome, 1558
  risk factors, 1616–1617
    age, sex, and pregnancy, 1616
    genetic factors, 1617
    immunodeficiency, 1616–1617
    injections or trauma, 1617
    strenuous exercise, 1617
    tonsillectomy, 1617
  spinal paralytic poliomyelitis, 1615–1616
  spreading/shedding mechanisms, 1320f, 1321

systemic spread, 1320f
transmission, 1610
type 1, 1613
Polyacrylamide gel electrophoresis with silver stain (PAGE-SS): for rotavirus, 1451
Polyarteritis nodosa
  hepatitis B virus and, 1139, 1420
  pneumonia, 647t
Polyarthralgia: *Mycoplasma pneumoniae*, 1707
Polyarthritis
  rheumatic fever, 1802
  Yersinia enterocolitica, 2077
Polyenes, 403
Polygam, 454
Polymerase chain reaction (PCR), 27, 28, 185, 1314
  bacterial meningitis, 846
  Bartonella, 1746
  Borrelia burgdorferi, 2150, 2151
  and FUO, 541
  hepatitis C virus, 1481
  Histoplasma capsulatum, 2341
  HIV, 185, 1262
  Mycobacterium tuberculosis, 2215
  myocarditis, 803
  Neisseria gonorrhoeae, 1919
  Neisseria meningitidis, 1903
  Pneumocystis carinii, 2476, 2479
  pneumonia, 626
  Toxoplasma gondii, 2463, 2465
  Trypanosoma cruzi, 2447
Polymethylmethacrylate cement: and joint infections, 1052–1053
Polymorphonuclear leukocytes (PML), 34, 200. *See also*
    Polymorphonuclear neutrophils
  Blastomyces dermatitidis, 2355
  and enteric infections, 952–953, 953t
  Staphylococcus aureus and, 1755, 1762
Polymorphonuclear neutrophils (PMN).
    See also Polymorphonuclear leukocytes
  cervicitis, 1084
  urethritis, 1064–1065
  vaginal infections, 1083
Polymorphous lesions: and systemic infections, 551t
Polymyositis: and HIV, 1228
Polymyxin B, 385
  dosage, 514t–515t
  drug interactions, 524t
  mechanism of action, 385
  pharmacology, 514t–515t
  spectrum of activity, 385
  topical, 384t
Polymyxin(s), 382
  absorption, 209
  pharmacologic tables, 514t–515t
  for Pseudomonads, 2004t
  resistance, 215t
  trimethoprim combination therapy, 359
Polyneuropathy
  acute inflammatory (AIPN). *See*
    Guillain-Barré syndrome
  chronic inflammatory demyelinating (CIDP): and HIV/AIDS, 1236
Polyomaviruses, 1400–1406. *See also*
    individual viruses
Polysaccharide vaccines, 2771. *See also*
    Meningococcal vaccine;
    Pneumococcal vaccine

Pompholyx, 2381
Pontiac fever, 2087, 2091, 2099. *See also Legionella pneumophila*
Popliteal graft infections, 789, 789t
Populations: epidemiological definition, 159–160
Porins, 251
Pork tapeworm, 2525t. *See also Taenia solium*
Porphyria: differential diagnosis, 714
Porphyromonas, 2158t
  animal bites, 2767
  characteristics, 2196t
  clinically significant, 2159t, 2195t
  female genital infections, 2165
  identification, 189
  incidence, 2162
  mediastinitis, 815t
  as normal flora, 2196
  odontogenic infections, 2198
  oral cavity infections, 2198
  oral colonization, 593, 594t
  osteomyelitis, 2200
  periodontitis, 594
  pleuropulmonary infection, 2164
  soft tissue infections, 2166
  taxonomy, 2195, 2195t
Porphyromonas asaccharolytica, 2195t
  oral cavity and respiratory infections, 2198
  peritonitis, 713
Porphyromonas bivia: peritonitis, 711
Porphyromonas endodontalis, 2195t
Porphyromonas gingivalis, 2195t, 2196
  collagenase, 2197
  odontogenic infections, 2198
  pathology, 2162
  virulence, 2197, 2197t
Porphyromonas ruminicola: peritonitis, 711
Postabortal fever: *Mycoplasma*, 1715t, 1716
Postabortal infections: pelvic, 1093
Postantibiotic effect (PAE)
  carbapenems, 265
  LJ 10627, 266
  meropenem, 266
Post-herpetic neuralgia, 1348
Postinfectious tropical malabsorption. *See Tropical sprue*
Postpartal fever: *Mycoplasma*, 1715t, 1716
Postpartal infections: pelvic, 1091
Postpoliomyelitis syndrome, 1617–1618
Postural drainage
  for chronic bronchitis, 611
  for lung abscess, 646
Potassium hydroxide (KOH): for oral thrush, 172
Pott puffy tumor, 587
Pott's disease, 2236–2237
  abscess and sinus formation, 2236–2237
  paraplegia, 2237
  treatment, 2237
Powassan virus, 1467
  epidemiology, 1469
  transmission, clinical syndromes, and geographic distribution, 1466t
Poxviridae, 1325–1330
  classification, 1315t, 1325
  molluscum contagiosum, 1329–1330
  monkeypox, 1329
  parapoxvirus, 1329
  shape and size, 1316f

vaccinia, 1325–1328
variola (smallpox), 1328–1329
Poxviruses
  arthritis, 1036t
  cellular immunity and, 129
  classification, 1315t, 1325
  products and host target, 125t
PPD test. *See* Purified protein derivative (PPD) test
p22*phox*, 84, 85
  and chronic granulomatous disease, 92, 92t
p47*phox*, 85
  and chronic granulomatous disease, 92, 92t
  deficiency, 92
p67*phox*, 85
  and chronic granulomatous disease, 92, 92t
  mutations, 92
PPL skin test, 275
Pranobex: for cutaneous warts, 1393
Praziquantel, 460t, 482, 2548
  adverse reactions, 482
  for cysticercosis, 2549
  dosage, 463t, 466t
    pediatric, 463t, 466t
  for heterophyiasis, 2543
  for intestinal flukes, 2543
  for intestinal tapeworms, 2547
  for liver flukes, 2542
  for lung flukes, 2543
  for schistosomiasis, 2542
  spectrum of activity, 482
  structure, 482f
  for tapeworms, 2548
Prednisone: for transplantation, 2711
Pregnancy
  anaerobic infections, 2163t
  antimicrobial use in, 204
    antimalarials, 2426
    for *Chlamydia*, 1688
    for *Giardia lamblia*, 2490
    for *Mycobacterium tuberculosis*, 2229
    nitrofurantoin, 379
    for *Plasmodium*, 2426
    for syphilis, 338, 2129–2130
    for *Toxoplasma gondii*, 2468
    trimethoprim, 360
    for urinary tract infections, 679–680
  arenaviruses in, 1576
  BKV virus in, 1401–1402
  Blastomyces dermatitidis in, 2361
  cellular immunity in, 35
  chlamydial infections and, 1688
    ectopic, 1687
  CMV in, 1354
  and endocarditis, 743t
  gonorrhea in, 1917
  hepatitis in
    HBV screening, 2621
    HEV, 1664–1665
  HIV transmission, 1169
    antiretroviral therapy and, 1275–1276
  HSV in, 1340, 1343, 2657, 2657t
  influenza vaccines and, 1562
  JC virus in, 1401–1402
  Listeria monocytogenes in, 1881, 1882, 1882t, 1883t
  measles in, 1522
  mumps virus in, 1499
  polyomavirus in, 1401–1402, 1402t

Streptococcus agalactiae in, 1836–1837
  diagnosis, 1841
  prevention, 1842t, 1842–1843
Toxoplasma gondii in, 2455, 2457, 2461, 2468
  serology, 2465–2466
Treponema pallidum in, 2126, 2129–2130
  treatment, 338, 2129–2130
  urinary tract infections in, 678–680
    epidemiology, 678–680
  vaccines in, 2784, 2784t
    for travelers, 2799
Preisz-Nocard bacillus. *See Corynebacterium pseudotuberculosis*
Prekallikrein: and sepsis syndrome, 695–696
Premature infants
  bacteriuria in pregnancy and, 679
  immunoglobulin for, 454
Prereduced anaerobically sterilized (PRAS) biochemicals, 2168–2169
Pressure sores
  in the elderly, 2739
  spinal cord injury and, 2733–2734
Pretracheal space infection, 600
Prevalence, 160
Prevention of disease, 166–168
  assessment of risk, feasibility, cost, and effectiveness, 166
  individual, institutional, and community-based, 166
  primary, 167
  secondary, 167
  tertiary, 167–168
Prevotella, 2158t
  animal bites, 2766
  brain abscess, 890, 2197
  characteristics, 2196t
  clinically significant, 2159t, 2195t
  female genital infections, 2165, 2199
  identification, 189
  incidence, 2162
  lung abscess, 644
  mediastinitis, 815t
  as normal flora, 2196
  odontogenic infections, 2198
  oral cavity infections, 2198
  oral colonization, 593, 594, 594t
  phospholipase A, 2197
  pleuropulmonary infection, 2164
  sinusitis, 2198
  skin infections, 2199
  soft tissue infections, 2166, 2199
  taxonomy, 2195, 2195t
  treatment, 2201
    metronidazole, 329t
  vaginal flora, 1074
  and vaginosis, 1079
Prevotella bivia, 2195t
Prevotella buccae, 2195t, 2196
  oral cavity and respiratory infections, 2198
Prevotella denticola, 2195t
Prevotella disiens, 2195t
  female genital infections, 2199
  oral cavity and respiratory infections, 2198
Prevotella intermedia, 2195t
  gingivitis, 594
  periodontitis, 594
  pleuropulmonary infections, 2198

Prevotella melaninogenica, 2195t, 2196
  endocarditis, 756, 2199
  intra-abdominal infections, 2199
  noma (gangrenous stomatitis), 602
  odontogenic infections, 2198
  osteomyelitis, 2200
  parotitis, 2198
  pathogenesis, 2196
  periodontitis, 594
  peritonitis, 711, 713
  pleuropulmonary infections, 2198
  skin and soft tissue infections, 2199
  treatment
    chloramphenicol, 312t
    penicillins, 237t, 240, 241t
  virulence, 2196, 2197t
Prevotella oralis, 2195t, 2196
  oral cavity and respiratory infections, 2198
Prevotella oris, 2195t
  oral cavity and respiratory infections, 2198
Primaquine, 459t, 470–471
  clindamycin combination therapy, 343
  dosage, 464t
    pediatric, 464t
    for *Pneumocystis carinii*, 465t
  drug interactions, 524t
    quinacrine, 469
  for *Plasmodium*
    prophylaxis, 2424t
    for travelers, 2801
  for *Pneumocystis carinii*, 1284, 2481
  structure, 470f
Primary prevention of disease, 167
Prion protein (PrP), 1674–1675
  PrP^C, 1675
  PrP^{Sc}, 1675
Prions, 1674–1676
  infection control, 2584
  molecular biology and properties, 1674–1675
Prisons: *Mycobacterium tuberculosis* in, 2218
Probenecid
  drug interactions
    ganciclovir, 425
    quinolones, 370
    zidovudine, 436
  for *Treponema pallidum*, 2129t
Procaine, 240
  sulfonamide interactions with, 356–357
  for *Treponema pallidum*, 2129t
Procrit, 452
Proctitis
  chlamydial, 1686
  gonococcal, 990
  herpetic: and HIV/AIDS, 1060, 1228, 1231, 1339
  in HIV/AIDS, 1231
    herpetic, 1060, 1228, 1230, 1339
  in homosexuals, 1231, 1686
  treatment, 1688
Proctocolitis: *Chlamydia trachomatis*, 1686
Profilin, 80
Profloxacin: for *Mycobacterium avium-intracellulare*, 2258
Progressive bacterial synergistic gangrene, 917, 917f, 918t
Progressive multifocal leukoencephalopathy: HIV/AIDS and, 1239

Proguanil, 474–475
　for travelers, 2801
Prokaryotes, 1752
Propamidine isethionate: for
　　microsporidia, 2522
Properdin
　deficiency, 68–69, 73, 152t, 156
　　treatment, 73
　pathway, 58
Propionibacterium, 2159, 2206, 2207
　as normal flora, 2158–2159, 2159t,
　　2206
　and normal physiology, 2160
　taxonomy, 2158t
　treatment
　　chloramphenicol, 312t
　　tetracyclines, 308t
Propionibacterium acnes, 2159, 2206,
　　2207
　brain abscess, 890
　endocarditis, 756
　endophthalmitis, 1122
　　treatment, 1125
　incidence, 2162
　as normal flora, 2158–2159, 2206
　treatment
　　metronidazole, 329, 332
　　topical antibacterials, 383
　　trimethoprim, 357
Propionibacterium avidum, 2159
Propionibacterium granulosum, 2159
Propionibacterium propionicus, 2280
　canaliculitis, 1131, 1133
　　treatment, 1134
　incidence, 2162
　pneumonia, 647t
Prosector's wart, 2216
Prospect Hill virus, 1569
Prostaglandin E$_2$ (PGE$_2$): and fever, 532,
　　532f, 533
Prostaglandins: and fever, 34
Prostatectomy: and endocarditis, 794t
Prostatic abscess, 1100
Prostatic antibacterial factor, 1098
Prostatic resection, transurethral: and
　　endocarditis, 743t
Prostatitis, 1098–1100
　bacterial
　　acute, 1099, 1099t
　　chronic, 680–681, 1099, 1099t
　　prostatic antibacterial factor and,
　　　1098
　blastomycosis, 2360
　Chlamydia trachomatis, 1685
　classification, 1098–1099, 1099t
　granulomatous, 1100
　and HIV, 1101–1102
　infectious, 680–681
　　acute, 680
　　chronic bacterial, 680–681, 1099,
　　　1099t
　　management, 681
　　nonbacterial, 681
　nonbacterial, 1099t, 1099–1100
　quinolones for, 371
Prostatodynia, 681, 1099t, 1099–1100
Prostatosis, 681
Prosthetic bone and joint infections,
　　1051–1055
　bacteriology, 1052, 1052t
　clinical presentation, 1052–1053,
　　1053t
　diagnosis, 1053f, 1053–1054
　pathogenesis, 1052–1053
　prevention, 1054–1055

Staphylococcus epidermidis,
　　1781–1782
　therapy, 1054
　　suppressive antibiotic, 1054–1055
Prosthetic valve endocarditis, 783–788
　blood cultures, 785
　clinical manifestations, 784t,
　　784–785
　diagnosis, 784–785
　　special studies, 785
　epidemiology, 783–784
　incidence, 783
　laboratory findings, 785
　management, 785–788
　　antibiotics, 785–787, 786t
　　anticoagulation, 787
　　surgical, 787, 787t
　microbiology, 783t, 783–784
　mortality, 786
　pathogenesis
　　early, 784
　　late, 784
　pathology, 784, 784f
　prophylaxis, 787–788, 797
*Protaminobacter rubra. See Protomonas
　　extorquens*
Proteae, 1973–1974
Protease inhibitors, 34
　for HIV, 1273
Protective antigen (anthrax), 6
Proteae. *See also specific species*
Protein
　of bacterial membrane, 1753, 1754
　penicillin-binding, 234
Protein binding: of antimicrobials, 205
Protein-energy malnutrition
　hookworm and, 2530
　immunodeficiency and, 137
Protein kinase C (PKC): diacylglycerol
　　and, 45
Protein-losing enteropathy: antibody
　　deficiency and, 53
Proteinuria, 669
　endocarditis, 750
Protein wasting states: and antibody
　　deficiencies, 53
Proteobacteria, 1742f
Proteosome, 102, 103, 107
Proteus, 1974
　after gynecologic surgery,
　　1093–1094
　β-lactamase, 216t, 217, 268
　decubitus ulcer infections, 919
　in drug abusers, 2697
　endocarditis, 755
　as enteric flora, 947
　and granulocytopenia, 2676
　mediastinitis, 815t
　mycotic aneurysms, 772
　necrotizing fasciitis, 923
　peritonitis, 711
　　in peritoneal dialysis, 719
　snake bites, 2767
　suppurative thrombophlebitis, 768
　symmetric peripheral gangrene, 553
　treatment
　　antimicrobials of choice, 202t
　　carbenicillin, 244
　　cephalosporins, 257
　　chloramphenicol, 312t
　　neomycin, 384
　　nitrofurantoin, 377–378
　urinary tract infections, 667
　　nosocomial, 2609t
　vascular graft infections, 789t

Proteus mirabilis, 1974
　β-lactamase, 216t, 217
　blepharitis, 1130
　catheter-related infections, 1974
　endocarditis: treatment, 763
　and IgA, 8
　osteomyelitis, 1049
　prostatitis, 680
　resistance, 1974
　　aminoglycosides, 284t
　surgical wound infections, 2744t
　treatment
　　aminoglycosides, 285t
　　antimicrobials of choice, 202t
　　β-lactamase inhibitors, 268t
　　carbapenems, 264t
　　cephalosporins, 255, 255t, 257
　　chloramphenicol, 312t
　　penicillins, 237t
　　polymyxin B, 385
　　quinolones, 367t
　　rifampin, 318t
　　sulfonamides, 355t
　　trimethoprim, 357
　urinary tract infections, 1974
　　nosocomial, 2608–2609, 2609t,
　　　2610
*Proteus morganii. See Morganella
　　morganii*
Proteus myxofaciens, 1974
Proteus rettgeri. See Providencia rettgeri
Proteus vulgaris, 1974
　aminoglycoside resistance, 284t
　treatment
　　β-lactamase inhibitors, 268t
　　carbapenems, 264t
　　cephalosporins, 255t
　　penicillins, 237t
　　quinolones, 367t
　　rifampin, 318t
Prothionamide: for *Mycobacterium
　　leprae*, 398, 2248–2249
Protomonas extorquens, 2114
　classification and site of infection,
　　2107t
Prototheca, 2391
Protozoa, 2393–2524
　Acanthamoeba, 2408–2414
　amebae, free-living, 2408–2414
　Babesia, 2497–2500
　Balantidium coli, 2511
　Blastocystis hominis, 2511–2512
　cellular immunity and, 124
　　defects, 2681
　classification, 2393, 2393t
　clinical syndromes, 2394t
　and complement, 66
　Cryptosporidium, 2500–2510
　Cyclospora, 2512
　cytokine and T cell protection, 121t
　diagnosis, 1006t
　　tests, 2395t
　diarrhea: diagnosis, 180
　Entamoeba histolytica, 2395–2408
　enteric symptoms, 1000t, 1003
　geographic distribution, 2394t
　Giardia lamblia, 2487–2493
　immunodeficiency and, 138
　Isospora belli, 2510–2511
　Leishmania, 2428–2442
　Leptomyxid, 2408–2414
　and leukemia/lymphoma, 2677, 2681
　luminal: antiparasitic agents, 458,
　　467–468
　macrophages and, 124

　malaria, 2415–2427. *See also
　　Plasmodium*
　meningitis, 835
　　antimicrobial therapy, 850t, 854
　　clinical presentation, 844
　　diagnosis, 849
　microscopy, 184
　microsporidia, 2513–2524
　Naegleria fowleri, 2408–2414
　overview, 2393–2395
　penetration mechanisms, 24–25
　Plasmodium, 2415–2427
　Pneumocystis carinii, 2475–2487
　Sarcocystis, 2511
　Toxoplasma gondii, 2455–2475
　transfusion-related infections, 2627
　transmission, 2394t
　in transplant recipients, 2712t, 2722,
　　2723f
　Trichomonas vaginalis, 2493–2497
　Trypanosoma, 2442–2455
　　brucei (African trypanosomiasis;
　　　sleeping sickness),
　　　2450–2455
　　cruzi (American trypanosomiasis;
　　　Chagas disease), 2442–2450
Providencia, 1974
　endocarditis, 755
　resistance, 251
　suppurative thrombophlebitis, 768
　treatment
　　aminoglycosides, 285t
　　antimicrobials of choice, 202t
　　penicillins, 237t
Providencia alcalifaciens, 1974, 1975t
Providencia rettgeri, 1974, 1975t
　treatment
　　cephalosporins, 255t
　　quinolones, 367t
　　rifampin, 318t
Providencia rustigianii, 1975t
Providencia stuartii, 1974
　rifampin for, 318t
　treatment: cephalosporins, 255t
　urinary tract infections, 2609, 2609t,
　　2610
pRTP1 plasmid vector, 26
Pruritus
　genital lesions, 1056
　hepatitis, 1138
　rifampin for, 325
P-selectin, 123
PSE (1–4) β-lactamase, 268, 268t
Pseudallescheria boydii, 2289,
　　2389–2390
　arthritis, 1036
　brain abscess, 890
　clinical manifestations, 2390
　diagnosis, 2390, 2390f
　endophthalmitis, 1123
　and granulocytopenia, 2676
　hypertrophic spinal pachymeningitis,
　　906
　in the immunosuppressed, 2390
　keratitis, 1113, 1991
　mycetoma, 2327
　sinusitis, 586t
　treatment, 2390
Pseudobuboes
　bartonellosis, 2211
　differential diagnosis, 1684
Pseudocowpox (milker's nodule), 1325,
　　1329
Pseudoerysipelas, 915
Pseudolithiasis, 254

Pseudomembranous colitis
Clostridium difficile-related, 992f, 992–993
clindamycin/lincomycin and, 342, 993
treatment: vancomycin, 347, 350, 993
and leukemia, 2679
Pseudomonads: taxonomy, 2003. *See also Pseudomonas*
Pseudomonas, 2004t, 2013. *See also individual species*
antibacterial susceptibility, 2004t
testing, 194t
classification, 2004t
infections caused by, 2004t
prostatitis, 1099
taxonomy, 2013
transfusion-related, 2627, 2628
Pseudomonas aeruginosa, 1980–2003
acne vulgaris, 1997
adhesins, 1981
alkaline protease, 1982
arthritis, 1034
bacteremia, 692, 1987–1988
and skin infections, 921
treatment, 1987–1988
β-lactamase, 215, 216t, 218, 268
blepharitis, 1130, 1991
bone and joint infections, 1992–1994. *See also* osteomyelitis *below*
treatment, 1992–1994
and bone marrow transplantation, 2719
brain abscess, 1988–1989
in the immunocompromised, 890
treatment, 1989
bullae, 921
and burn wounds, 1996, 2672t
in cancer patients, 2668
cellular immunity and, 128
cellulitis, 919t
classification, 2004t
clinical manifestations, 1983–1997
CNS infections, 1988–1989. *See also specific disorders*
treatment, 1989
colonization, 1980, 1981
conjunctivitis, 1104–1105
contact lenses infections, 1991
cutaneous manifestations, 552, 1987. *See also* ecthyma gangrenosum *below*
in cystic fibrosis, 658, 659, 1985–1987
prophylaxis, 1986
treatment, 1986–1987
cytotoxin, 1982
decubitus ulcer infections, 919
dialysis-access AVFs, 790
diarrhea, 1995
treatment, 1995
in drug abusers, 2697, 2698
endocarditis, 756–757, 1983, 2699, 2700
ear infections, 1989–1991. *See also* otitis externa *and* otitis media *below*
treatment, 1990–1991
ecthyma gangrenosum, 554, 921, 1987, 1996
treatment, 1996
elastase, 1982
endocarditis, 755, 1983–1984

in drug abusers, 756–757, 1983, 2699, 2700
treatment, 763, 1984
endophthalmitis, 1125, 1991, 1992
treatment, 1992
endoscope contamination, 2585
endotoxin, 1982–1983
epidemiology, 1980–1981
epididymitis, 1100
epidural abscess, 904
exoenzyme S, 1983
exotoxin A, 3t, 4, 5, 1982–1983
eye infections, 1991–1992. *See also specific disorders*
treatment, 1991–1992
fibronectin and, 32
Fisher-Devlin-Gnabasik immunotyping, 1981
folliculitis, 912
gangrenous cellulitis, 918, 921
gastrointestinal infections, 1995
treatment, 1995
glycocalyx (mucoid exopolysaccharide), 1981–1982
and granulocytopenia, 2676, 2678
green foot, 1997
green nail syndrome, 1997
growth, 185–186, 1980
hemolysins, 1982
and HIV/AIDS, 1981, 1985, 1987, 1991, 1996
hospital-acquired, 1980
in the immunocompromised: treatment, 2666
international antigenic typing system (LATS), 1981
invasion, 8
Job syndrome and, 156
keratitis, 1112–1113, 1991
and leukemia, 2672
lipopolysaccharides, 1982, 1983
macular or maculopapular lesions, 921
mastoiditis, 1991
treatment, 1991
mediastinitis, 815t
meningitis, 834, 1988–1989
treatment, 1989
microbiology, 1980
mycotic aneurysms, 772
necrotizing enterocolitis of newborn, 991
noma neonatorum, 1997
opportunism, 20
orchitis, 1101
osteochondritis, 1993
treatment, 1993
osteomyelitis, 1041, 1992–1994
chronic contiguous, 1993–1994
treatment, 1993–1994
treatment, 1993–1994
otitis externa, 580, 1989
malignant, 1989–1990
treatment, 1990
otitis media, 1991
suppurative, 1991
paronychia, 1997
pathogenesis, 1981–1983
perichondritis of auricle, 1991
peritonitis, 710, 711
in peritoneal dialysis, 719
treatment, 716
and phagocytes, 88
phospholipase c, 1982
pili, 1981

pneumonia, 619t
chronic, 647
in drug abusers, 2701
and HIV/AIDS, 1235, 1235t
necrotizing, 644
nosocomial, 2600, 2601
in the immunocompromised, 631
prevention, 2604
serology, 625
proteases, 1982
pyocyanin, 1982
pyoderma, 1996
radionecrosis, 604
rashes, 554, 1996
in renal transplantation, 2723
resistance, 219, 221, 251
aminoglycosides, 283–284, 284t
and cystic fibrosis, 1986
meropenem, 266
neomycin, 384
quinolones, 366
respiratory infections, 1984–1985
treatment, 1985
rhamnolipid, 1982
sepsis: in trauma patients, 2759
septicemia: antiserum, 701
sinusitis, 585, 1991
treatment, 1991
skin infections, 921, 1996–1997. *See also specific disorders*
treatment, 1996–1997
snake bites, 2767
soft tissue infections, 1996–1997
treatment, 1996–1997
sternoarticular pyarthrosis, 1993
subcutaneous nodules, 554
suppurative thrombophlebitis, 768
surgical wound infections, 2744t
symphysis pubis infections, 1993
toe web infection, 1997
in transplant recipients, 2712, 2723
in trauma patients, 2757
treatment, 1983–1997
aminoglycosides, 228, 279, 285t, 295t, 296, 1988, 1991–1992, 1994–1995
combination therapy, 287t, 288, 289t, 295–296, 1992, 1993
antimicrobials of choice, 202t
azlocillin, 245
aztreonam, 267, 1984, 1989, 1994
β-lactamase inhibitors, 268t
carbenicillin, 245, 1984, 1989
ceftazidime, 1984, 1988, 1990, 1992
cephalosporins, 247, 259
chloramphenicol, 312t
ciprofloxacin, 1990, 1992, 1994, 1995
combination therapy, 207, 287t, 288, 289t, 295–296, 1988
aminoglycosides, 287t, 288, 289t, 295–296, 1992, 1993
fluoroquinolones, 228–231
gentamicin, 1991–1992
imipenem, 264t, 264–265, 1984
in the immunocompromised, 2666
meropenem, 264t, 266
penicillins, 237t, 1993–1994
piperacillin, 245
polymyxin B, 385
postantibiotic effect (PAE) of carbapenems, 265
quinolones, 367t, 372
rifampin, 318t, 323, 1988

sulfonamides, 355t
ticarcillin, 244–245
tobramycin, 1984, 1994
trimethoprim, 358
urinary tract infections, 667, 1994–1995
in the elderly, 2737
nosocomial, 2609t, 2610
prevention, 2613
treatment, 1994–1995
vesicles, 921
wound infections, 1996
burn, 1996, 2672t
surgical, 2744t
Pseudomonas alcaligenes
antimicrobial susceptibility, 2004t
classification, 2004t
infections caused by, 2004t
Pseudomonas cepacia, 2007–2008
antimicrobial susceptibility, 2004t
and chronic granulomatous disease, 92
clinical manifestations, 2008
and cystic fibrosis, 659
description, 2007–2008
epidemiology, 2008
and granulocytopenia, 2676
and immunodeficiency, 150t
infections caused by, 2004t
pathophysiology, 2008
pneumonia: necrotizing, 644
treatment, 2008
aminoglycosides, 285t
imipenem, 264t, 265
quinolones, 367t
trimethoprim-sulfamethoxazole, 360
Pseudomonas delafieldii, 2004t
Pseudomonas diminuta, 2004t
Pseudomonas fluorescens, 385
classification, 2004t
infections caused by, 2004t
transfusion-related, 2627, 2628
Pseudomonas gladioli: infections caused by, 2004t
Pseudomonas mallei, 2003, 2006–2007
antimicrobial susceptibility, 2004t
classification, 2004t
clinical manifestations, 2007
description, 2006–2007
diagnosis, 2007
epidemiology and prevalence, 2007
lymphadenitis, 940t
prognosis, 2007
treatment, 2007
Pseudomonas maltophilia. See Xanthomonas maltophilia
Pseudomonas mendocina, 2004t
Pseudomonas mesophilica. See Protomonas extorquens
Pseudomonas orzihabitans, 2107t, 2112–2113
Pseudomonas paucimobilis, 2004t
Pseudomonas pickettii, 2004t
Pseudomonas pseudoalcaligenes, 2004t
Pseudomonas pseudomallei, 2003, 2004–2006
acute localized suppurative infection, 2005
acute pulmonary infection, 2005
acute septicemic infections, 2005–2006
chronic suppurative infection, 2006
clinical manifestations, 2005–2006
description, 2004

diagnosis, 2006
enteric symptoms, 1002
epidemiology and prevalence, 2004–2005
lymphadenitis, 940t
pneumonia, 622t, 2006
  chronic, 647t
prognosis, 2006
resistance, 2006
septicemia, 999t
treatment, 2006
  chloramphenicol, 312t
  tetracyclines, 307, 308t
  trimethoprim-sulfamethoxazole, 360
Pseudomonas putida
  antimicrobial susceptibility, 2004t
  infections caused by, 2004t
Pseudomonas shigelloides. See Plesiomonas shigelloides
Pseudomonas stutzeri
  antimicrobial susceptibility, 2004t
  classification, 2004t
  infections caused by, 2004t
  keratitis, 1113
Pseudomonas vesicularis, 2004t
Pseudomonic acid. *See* Mupirocin
Pseudoparalysis: differential diagnosis, 1617
Psilocybe, 1015t
Psittacosis, 1693–1696. *See also Chlamydia psittaci*
Psoas abscess, 933
Psorophora: and equine encephalitis, 1456
Pubic hair infestations, 1059, 2558, 2559, 2559f
Puerperal fever, 1091
Puerperal infections: streptococcal group C and G, 1855
Puerperal ovarian vein thrombophlebitis (POVT), 1091–1092
Puerperal sepsis: *Streptococcus pyogenes*, 1797
Pulmonary abscess. *See* Lung abscess
Pulmonary artery catheters: bacteremia from, 2595
Pulmonary edema
  in drug abusers, 2701
  Plasmodium, 2420
  poliovirus, 1616
Pulmonary embolism
  in drug abusers, 2700
  and endocarditis, 746, 749
  pneumonia, 647t
  poliovirus, 1616
Pulmonary eosinophilia, tropical, 631, 2536
  treatment, 462t
Pulmonary gangrene, 643
Pulmonary infections. *See also* Respiratory tract infections
  abscess. *See* Lung abscess
  actinomycosis, 2281–2282, 2282f
  anaerobic: specimen collection, 2168t
  Aspergillus, 2307–2308, 2308f
  Blastomyces dermatitidis, 2355, 2356t, 2357, 2358f, 2359f
  burns and, 2764
  Coccidioides immitis, 2367, 2368f
    treatment, 2371–2372
  in drug abusers, 2701–2702, 2702f
  Histoplasma capsulatum
    acute primary, 2342–2345, 2345t
    chronic, 2345–2346

treatment, 2350
HIV/AIDS and, 1231–1236, 1232t
  fungi, 1235–1236
  mycobacteria, 1233–1235
  Pneumocystis carinii, 1233
  pyogenic bacteria, 1235, 1235t
  Toxoplasma gondii, 1236, 2460
and leukemia/lymphoma, 2678–2679, 2681–2682
mucormycosis, 2313, 2315
mycobacterial, 2266t, 2266–2267, 2267f. *See also specific mycobacteria*
Paracoccidioides brasiliensis, 2387, 2387f
schistosomiasis, 2540
sporotrichosis, 2322
  treatment, 2323
Staphylococcus aureus, 1770–1771
in transplant recipients, 2727, 2727t
Pulmonary infiltrates with eosinophilia, 630–631
  pneumonia, 647t
Pulmonary infiltration, diffuse: radiographs, 652–653
Pulmonary manifestations
  Brucella, 2056
  influenza virus, 1556t, 1556–1558, 1557t
    treatment, 1560
  rabies, 1533, 1534t
  in sepsis, 693
Pulmonary neoplasia: Kaposi's sarcoma, 1242
Pulmonary nodules: helminthic, 2553t
Pulmonary reactions: nitrofurantoin, 378
Pulmonary surfactant protein A, 59
Pulmonary surfactant protein D, 59
Pulmonary vascular endothelial injury: in sepsis syndrome, 696
Pulmonic stenosis: cutaneous manifestations, 550t
Purified protein derivative (PPD) test, 2219–2220
  booster effect, 2219
  dosage, 2219
  for the elderly, 2738–2739
  false-positive and false-negative reactions, 2219–2220
  and FUO, 540
  and HIV, 2220
  interpretation, 2219–2220
  meningitis, 867, 869
  for other mycobacteria, 2264
  and pneumonia, 651
  reversion of reactivity to negative, 2220
  in transplant recipients, 2712, 2713
Purine nucleoside phosphorylase (PNP) deficiency, 134t, 150, 151t
Purpura
  bubonic plague, 2073
  systemic infections manifesting, 550t, 551t
Purpura fulminans, 553. *See also* Gangrene, symmetric peripheral
Pustules
  defined, 551
  vesicles vs., 552
Puumula virus
  characteristics, 1568t
  clinical manifestations, 1570
  epidemiology, 1569
Pyelonephritis

acute, 662, 663f
  antimicrobial therapy, 675–676
  defined, 662
chronic, 662–663, 663f
  defined, 662–663
  radiology, 683, 683f
mycoplasma, 1715t, 1716
treatment
  aminoglycosides, 295t
  nitrofurantoin contraindicated, 378
  quinolones, 371
Pyodermas
  anaerobic, 2165
  gangrenosum, 918t
    differential diagnosis, 2356
  group A streptococcal. *See also Streptococcus pyogenes* below, 555, 1791- 1793
  group C and G streptococcal, 1792
  primary, 909–919. *See also sepcific infections*
    bullous impetigo, 911
    carbuncles, 912
    cellulitis, 914–916
    chancriform lesions, 913
    ecthyma, 913
    erysipelas, 914
    folliculitis, 912
    furuncles, 912
    impetigo, 911
    membranous ulcers, 916
    soft tissue, 926–927
    staphylococcal scalded skin syndrome, 911
    staphylococcal scarlet fever, 911
    toxic shock syndrome, 911–912
  Pseudomonas aeruginosa, 1996
    sporotrichosis vs. bacterial, 2322
  Staphylococcus aureus, 912, 1765
  Streptococcus pyogenes
    clinical manifestations, 1792–1793, 1793f
    complications, 1793
    epidemiology, 1791–1792, 1792f, 1806, 1806t
    therapy and prevention, 1793
  treatment
    fusidic acid, 387
    topical antibacterials, 382–383
Pyogenic dermatitis: and chronic granulomatous disease, 92
Pyogranulomas: *Blastomyces dermatitidis*, 2361
Pyomyositis, 929–930
  clinical features, 930
  differential diagnosis, 930
  etiology, 929t, 930
  HIV and, 929–930
  invasive stage, 930
  pathogenesis and pathology, 929–930
  Staphylococcus aureus, 1774
  streptococci group C, 1856
  suppurative stage, 930
  treatment, 930
  tropical, 929
Pyorrhea: anaerobic gram-negative bacilli and, 2198
Pyrantel pamoate, 460t, 480
  dosage, 461t, 480
    pediatric, 461t, 462t
  drug interactions, 525t
  for enterobiasis, 2528
  for hookworm, 2530

Pyrazinamide
  adverse reactions, 392–393
  dosage, 392f, 516t–517t
    in hepatic failure, 390t
    in renal dysfunction, 205, 517t
  mechanism of action, 392f
  for *Mycobacterium tuberculosis*, 389, 390t, 392–393, 1289, 2226, 2227, 2227t, 2230, 2232, 2233, 2234, 2239
    miliary, 2233
    tuberculous meningitis, 2234
  pharmacology, 516t–517t
  structure, 392f
Pyrazolopyrimidines, 477
Pyrenochaeta romeroi, 2327
Pyridopyrimidine: structure, 365f
Pyrimethamine, 459t, 473
  combination therapy, 474
    with dapsone, 474
      dosage, 464t, 466t
    with sulfadoxine, 473. *See also* Pyrimethamine-sulfadoxine
    with sulfadoxine and mefloquine, 474
  dosage, 466t
  for *Pneumocystis carinii* prophylaxis, 1286t, 1287
  structure, 473f
  for *Toxoplasma gondii*, 1283t, 1287, 2467, 2468
    in HIV/AIDS, 2467, 2467t
  for transplant recipients: prophylactic, 2715
Pyrimethamine-sulfadoxine (Fansidar), 355, 459t, 473–474
  adverse reactions, 473–474
  drug interactions, 525t
  for *Plasmodium*, 2425
    prophylaxis, 2424, 2424t
  for *Toxoplasma gondii*, 2469
    ocular, 2467–2468
Pyrimethamine-sulfadoxine-mefloquine (Fansimef), 474
Pyrogenic cytokines, 531
  and hypothalamus, 532f, 532–533
  measurement of circulating, 533–534
Pyrogenic exotoxins, 6
  cutaneous manifestations, 555
  and Kawasaki syndrome, 2568
Pyrogens, 530. *See also specific pyrogens*
  endogenous, 530–531
  and fever, 117
  exogenous, 530
Pyrvinium pamoate, 480
Pyuria, 669, 671
PZA. *See* Pyrazinamide

Q

Q fever, 1719, 1720, 1720t, 1727–1735. *See also Coxiella burnetii*
Qinghaosu, 459t, 472
  for *Plasmodium*, 2425
  for *Toxoplasma gondii*, 2469
Qβ replicase-based probe amplification, 27
Queensland tick typhus, 1719, 1720t. *See also Rickettsia australis*
  differential diagnosis, 1727
Quellung reaction, 185
  Neisseria meningitidis, 1896
  Streptococcus pneumoniae, 1811

Quinacrine, 459t, 469
  adverse reactions, 469
  dosage, 463t
    pediatric, 463t
  drug interactions, 469, 525t
  for *Giardia lamblia*, 2490, 2490t
Quinidine
  antiparasitic use, 459t, 471
  dosage, 464t
    pediatric, 464t
Quinidine gluconate: for *Plasmodium* prophylaxis, 2424t
Quinine
  adverse reactions, 471
  antiparasitic use, 459t, 471
    dosage, 464t
      pediatric, 464t
  clindamycin combination therapy, 343
  drug interactions, 525t
  structure, 471f
Quinine dihydrochloride: for *Plasmodium* prophylaxis, 2424t
Quinolones, 364–376, 471–472. *See also specific formulations*
  absorption, 368–369, 369t
  adverse reactions, 373–374
  alteration of target enzymes, 221
  antimicrobial activity, 366–368, 367t, 369t
    aminoglycosides compared with, 285t
    against anaerobic bacteria, 368t
    against gram-positive bacteria, 368t
  for bone and joint infections, 372
  clinical uses, 370–373
  for *Coxiella burnetii* pneumonia, 1729
  dosage, 370t, 516t–517t
    in renal and hepatic insufficiency, 369–370, 370t, 517t
  drug interactions, 370
  elimination, 369
  for GI and abdominal infections, 371–372
  mechanism of action, 364–366
  for *Mycobacterium tuberculosis*, 395
  for *Mycoplasma pneumoniae*, 1710
  for peritonitis, 717
  pharmacokinetics, 369t
  pharmacology, 228–231, 368–369, 369t, 516t–517t
    animal models, 228, 230f
    clinical trials, 229–230, 231f
    in vitro models, 229, 230f
  for prostatitis, 371
  for *Pseudomonas aeruginosa* endocarditis, 763
  resistance, 215t, 221, 229, 366, 373
  for respiratory tract infections, 372
  for *Salmonella*, 2026, 2027, 2028
  for sexually transmitted diseases, 371
  for skin and soft tissue infections, 372–373
  structure, 364, 365f
  tissue distribution, 369, 369t
  for transplant recipients, 2714
  for urinary tract infections, 370–371
Quinsy, 569
  anaerobic, 2163t, 2164
    gram-negative bacilli, 2198

treatment, 571
Quintan, 1741

R
Rabbit fever, 2060
Rabbit(s): microorganisms harbored by, 2792t
Rabies
  in raccoons, 1530, 1530f, 1531f, 1540–1541, 2394
Rabies antiserum, 1537, 1539
Rabies hysteria, 1535
Rabies immunoglobulin (RIG), 454, 1537, 1537t, 1539, 1540, 2770, 2782–2783
Rabies-related viruses, 1529
Rabies vaccine, 1536t, 1536–1537, 1539–1540, 2780–2781
  adverse reactions, 1536, 2780–2781
  antibody response, 1529
  duck embryo vaccine (DEV), 1534, 1536, 1540
  human diploid cell (HDCV), 1536, 1539, 1540, 1540t, 2780, 2798
  IMOVAX RABIES I.D., 1540
  nerve tissue (NTV), 1536, 1540
  recommendations for adults, 2784t
  RVA, 1536t, 1539–1540, 1540t, 2780
  suckling mouse brain (SMBV), 1534, 1536, 1540
  for travelers, 2797t, 2798
Rabies virus, 1527–1543
  animal reservoirs, 2792t
  antiserum of of equine origin (ARS), 1537, 1539
  canine, 1527–1528, 1530, 1531, 1539
  classification, 1528t, 1528–1529
  clinical manifestations, 1532–1535, 1533f
  CNS response, 828
  coma, 1533
  complications, 1533–1534, 1534t
  CSF specimens, 179
  diagnosis, 1534–1535
  differential diagnosis, 1535
  environmental stability, 1529
  epidemiology, 1529–1532
    animal rabies, 1529–1531, 1530f, 1531f
    human rabies, 1531–1532, 1532f
  ERIG serum, 1537, 1539
  human immunoglobulin (HRIG), 454, 1537, 1537t, 1539, 1540, 2770, 2782
  immunity, 1529
  immunoglobulin, 1537
  incubation period, 1532
  local wound treatment, 1539
  morphology and antigenic structure, 1529
  myocarditis, 800
  Negri bodies, 1535
  neurologic period, acute, 1532–1533
  paralytic, 1533, 1535
    differential diagnosis, 1535
  passive antibody administration, 1539
  pathogenesis, 1529
  postexposure prophylaxis, 1537t, 1537–1540
    rationale for, 1537–1539, 1538f, 1539f
  preexposure prophylaxis, 1540, 1540t
  prevention, 1535–1541
    in animals, 1540–1541

prodrome, 1532
  rapid fluorescent focus inhibition test (RFFIT), 1534
  receptor, 1317t, 1320–1321
  recovery, 1534
  spreading/shedding mechanisms, 1320, 1320f
  systemic spread, 1320f
  T cells and, 110
  treatment, 1535
    rifampin, 324
  vaccine. *See* Rabies vaccine
  virology, 1528–1529
  viruses related to, 1529
rac1 protein, 85
rac2 protein, 85
Radial nerve: leprosy damage, 2247
Radiation therapy
  immunodeficiency from, 135–137
  and infection susceptibility, 2666, 2667, 2668
  for Kaposi's sarcoma, 1244
  pneumonia from, 647t
  upper respiratory tract, 603
Radiculitis, 875
Radioactive labeling: of microbes, 12
Radioallergosorbent test (RAST): for β-lactam reactions, 275
Radioimmunoassay (RIA)
  for caliciviruses, 1670–1671
  of circulating pyrogenic cytokines, 533–534
  for parvovirus B19, 1443
Radioimmunoprecipitation assay
  for *Bartonella*, 1745
  for HIV, 1259–1260
Radiology
  and FUO, 540
  pleural empyema, 638f, 638–639, 639f
  pneumonia, 626f–627f, 626–627
    chronic, 649, 650t, 651f–656f
    Streptococcus pneumoniae, 626, 626f, 1819
  urinary tract infections, 682–684
Radionuclide studies
  and FUO, 540
  infectious arthritis, 1034
  neck and head infections, 601
  osteomyelitis, 1044–1045
  pneumonia, 628
  prosthetic joint infections, 1053–1054
RAG-1 gene, 43
RAG-2 gene, 43
RAG-1 protein, 105
RAG-2 protein, 105
Rahnella aquatis, 1975t
Ramichloridium obovoideum: brain abscess, 890
Ramoplanin: for enterococcal endocarditis, 761
Ramsay Hunt syndrome: VZV and, 1348
Ranitidine
  for *Helicobacter pylori*, 1961
  quinolone interactions with, 370
RANTES, 123
*Rap*1A protein, 85
Rapid fluorescent focus inhibition test (RFFIT), 1534
Rashes. *See also* Skin lesions and infections *and specific lesions*
  and acute retroviral syndrome (HIV), 1224t
  approach to patient, 549–550
  Babesia, 2499

bacillary angiomatosis, 557
bacterial endocarditis, 554–555
bacterial meningitis, 843
Borrelia burgdorferi, 556
Borrelia relapsing fever, 2142
Candida albicans, 556–557
Capnocytophaga canimorsus, 556
CMV, 1358
Coccidioides immitis, 2369, 2369f
Coxiella burnetii (Q fever), 1728
diffuse erythema, 552
drug-induced
  β-lactam, 272–273, 275, 276
  nitrofurantoin, 378
  quinolones, 374
  rifampin, 319
  tetracyclines, 309
  trimethoprim, 359
  vancomycin, 348–349
enanthem, 553
erythema multiforme, 552t
erythema nodosum, 552t
Francisella tularensis, 2065
history taking, 549
HIV/AIDS, 557–558
  in the immunocompromised hosts, 557–558
Kawasaki syndrome, 2567
Lyme disease, 2143, 2146, 2146t, 2147
macular lesions, 551–552
measles virus, 1519, 1521, 1521f
murine typhus, 1738
Neisseria gonorrhoeae, 554
Neisseria meningitidis, 553–554, 1900, 1901f
  from nitrofurantoin, 378
nodular lesions, 551–552
papular lesions, 551–552
parvovirus B19 and, 1439, 1440, 1442
petechial purpuric lesions, 553
physical examination, 550
Pseudomonas aeruginosa, 554, 1996
rickettsial infections, 556, 1720t, 1721. *See also* Rickettsial infections *and individual species*
  Rickettsia rickettsii, 1720t, 1721, 1723, 1723f, 1723t, 1724f
rose spots, 2021
scarlet fever, 1788–1789
schistosomiasis, 2539
septicemia, 553
sexually transmitted diseases, 1060. *See also* Genital lesions
staphylococcal scalded skin syndrome, 555
Staphylococcus aureus, 555
Streptobacillus moniliformis, 2085
streptococcal infections, 555–556
systemic infections manifesting, 550t, 551t
toxic shock syndrome, 555
Trypanosoma brucei, 2452
vesiculobullous eruptions, 552–553
yellow fever, 1470
Rasmussen's aneurysm, 2224
Rat-bite fever
  animal reservoirs, 2792t
  enteric symptoms, 999t
  fever of, 542
  Spirillum minus, 2155–2156. *See also Spirillum minus*
  Streptobacillus moniliformis, 2084–2086. *See also Streptobacillus moniliformis*

Rat-borne diseases. *See also* Rat-bite fever; *Rattus*
  bubonic plague, 2071
  hantaviruses, 1569
Rat lung worm. *See Angiostrongylus cantonensis*
Rattus
  and bubonic plague, 2071
  and murine typhus, 1737
Rattus norvegicus: and hantaviruses, 1569
Raynaud's phenomenon: *Mycoplasma pneumoniae* and, 1706, 1708
rDNA sequencing, 28. *See also* DNA
Receptors
  adhesins and, 11–12
  classes, 12t
  experimental identification, 12t, 12–13
  interactions with adhesins, 13f, 13t, 13–14, 14f
  tissue tropism and, 31
Recombinant clones, 25–26
Recombinant immunoblot assay (RIBA): for hepatitis C virus, 1480
Rectal biopsy
  for *Campylobacter*, 1950, 1951
  for enteric infection diagnosis, 955
Rectal mucosal cells: HIV and, 1204
Red bug, 2564
Reduviid bugs: and American trypanosomiasis, 2442
Reflux nephropathy, 672
Regional enteritis: and intra-abdominal abscess, 729
Regulon, 23
Rehydration. *See* Fluid therapy
Reiter syndrome, 1070–1072, 1686
  Campylobacter and, 1954
  Chlamydia trachomatis and, 1071, 1686
  clinical features, 1071
  Cryptosporidium, 2505
  diagnosis, 1037
  differential diagnosis, 1919
  and HIV, 1228
  HLA-B27 antigen and, 1071
  laboratory findings, 1071
  poststreptococcal, 1803
  Salmonella and, 2024
  Shigella and, 2037
  therapy, 1071–1072
  Yersinia enterocolitica, 2077
Relapsing fever, 2141–2143. *See also Borrelia*
  differential diagnosis: ehrlichiosis, 1750
  fever of, 542
Relative risk, 160, 160f
Renal abscesses, 682
Renal cell carcinoma: and fever, 544
Renal disease
  candidal, 2299
  HIV/AIDS and, 1231
  Mycobacterium tuberculosis, 2237–2238. *See also* Renal tuberculosis
  treatment in end-stage, 2229
Renal dysfunction
  complement and, 72–73
  drug dosage in, 204t, 204–205, 506t–519t. *See also specific drugs*
    aminoglycosides, 297–298, 298t, 511t

antifungal agents, 519t
antimycobacterials, 390t
antiviral agents, 519t
azalides, 513t
aztreonam, 511t
carumonam, 511t
cephalosporins, 253t, 509t
chloramphenicol, 313, 513t
imipenem, 511t
loracarbef, 511t
macrolides, 513t
metronidazole, 513t
penicillins, 238t, 507t
polymyxins, 515t
quinolones, 517t
rifampin, 319, 390t, 517t
sulfonamides, 356, 515t
teicoplanin, 351, 515t
tetracyclines, 310
trimethoprim, 515t
urinary tract agents, 517t
vancomycin, 515t
  in endocarditis, 746
  peritonitis and, 714
Renal epithelial cells: HIV and, 1204
Renal failure
  leptospirosis, 2137
  Plasmodium, 2419–2420, 2422
  and *Streptococcus agalactiae* bacteremia, 1839, 1839t
  Vibrio cholerae and, 1939
Renal function
  age and, 201
  antimicrobial use and, 204–205
Renal infarctions: and endocarditis, 749
Renal papillary necrosis, 663f, 663–664
  defined, 662
  radiology, 683, 684f
Renal transplantation
  aspergillosis and, 2306
  CMV infection, 1358, 2710t, 2711, 2711t
    prophylaxis, 1361
  HSV infections, 1340, 1341f
  infections and, 2710, 2722, 2723–2724, 2724t
  mycotic aneurysms and, 770–771
  polyomaviruses and, 1402, 1402t
  Pseudomonas aeruginosa urinary tract infections and, 1994
Renal tuberculosis, 2237t, 2237–2238
Reoviridae, 1446–1455. *See also individual viruses*
  classification, 1315t
  Colorado tick fever, 1446–1447
  orbivirus, 1447–1458
  reovirus, 1447–1458
  replication, 1318
  rotavirus, 1448–1455
  shape and size, 1316f
Reovirus, 1447–1448
  M cells, 1319
  spread, 1321
  type 3: receptor, 1317t
Reproductive organ diseases, 1055–1103. *See also* Female genital tract infections; Sexually transmitted diseases *and specific infections*
  bartholinitis, 1085
  cervicitis, 1084–1085
  epididymitis, 1100–1101
  female pelvic infections, 1090–1096
  genital skin and mucous membrane lesions, 1055–1063

orchitis, 1101
prostatitis, 1098–1100
skenitis, 1085
urethritis, 1063–1074
vulvovaginitis, 1075–1081
Resistance mechanisms, 212–225. *See also subentry* resistance *for individual organisms and drugs*
  alteration of cell wall precursor targets, 220
  alteration of ribosomal target sites, 220
  alteration of target enzymes, 220
    β-lactams, 220
    quinolones, 221
    sulfonamides, 221
    trimethoprim, 221
  alterations of bacterial membranes, 219
  aminoglycosides, 218, 218t, 283–284
  azithromycin, 339
  β-lactamases, 214–218. *See also* β-lactamases
  bypass of antibiotic inhibition, 221
  cephalosporins, 250–251
  chloramphenicol, 215t, 218–219, 311–312
  chloramphenicol acetyltransferase, 218–219
  clindamycin, 341–342
  combination therapy to prevent, 206
  controlling, 221f, 221–222
  DNA integration elements, 214
  enzymatic inhibition, 214–218, 215t
  erythromycin, 334–336
  erythromycin esterase, 219
  inner membrane permeability, 219
  isoniazid, 389
  major means, 215t
  molecular genetics, 212–214
  outer membrane permeability, 219
  penicillins, 234–236, 235f, 241t
  plasmids, 212–213, 213f
  promotion of antibiotic efflux, 219–220
  quinolones, 373
  rifampin, 215t
  sulfonamides, 355–356
  susceptibility testing, 200–201
  tetracyclines, 214, 215t, 219, 220, 307–308
  transposable genetic elements, 213–214, 214f
  vancomycin, 346
Respiratory burst
  abnormal, 92–93
  enzyme, 84
Respiratory equipment: as source of infection, 2601
Respiratory failure
  poliovirus, 1616
  respiratory syncytial virus, 1511
Respiratory infections. *See* Respiratory tract infections
Respiratory isolation, 2576, 2577t
Respiratory papillomatosis, 1388t, 1389. *See also* Human papillomavirus
  treatment, 1395
Respiratory support: for peritonitis, 718
Respiratory syncytial virus, 1501–1519
  antigenic variation, 1503
  and bone marrow transplantation, 2720

bronchiolitis, 612t, 612–613, 613f
  clinical manifestations, 615
  and immune response, 615
  therapy, 616
bronchitis, acute, 606, 606t
characteristics, 1502, 1502f
classification, 1502
clinical manifestations, 1507–1509
  in older children and adults, 1508t, 1508–1509, 1509f
  uncommon, 1509
  in young children, 1507f, 1507–1508
common cold, 562, 562t
complications, 1509–1511
  acute, 1511
  in children with underlying diseases, 1509–1510, 1510t
  in the immunocompromised, 1510–1511
  long-term, 1511
croup, 574, 574t, 1504f
description, 1502–1504
epidemiology, 1504t, 1504–1505, 1505f
HEp-2 cells, 1502–1503, 1503f
history, 1502
immunity, 1505–1507
immunization, 1512–1513
immunodeficiency and, 137
infection in animals, 1503–1504
laboratory propagation, 1502–1503, 1503f
laryngitis, 573t
long-term, 1511
nosocomial, 1509
otitis media, 1508
pathogenesis, 1505–1507
pneumonia, 619t
  atypical, 630, 1704
  differential diagnosis, 1698
  in the elderly, 2738
  nosocomial, 2600
  prevention, 2605
prevalence and incidence, 1504–1505
repeat infections, 1505
prevention, 1512–1513, 2605
seasonality, 1504
treatment, 412t, 1511–1512
  ribavirin, 429–430, 431
vaccine research, 1512–1513
Respiratory tract
  barrier to microorganisms, 32
  specimen collection and processing, 169–175, 170t, 172t
Respiratory tract infections. *See also* Pulmonary infections
  Acinetobacter, 2011
  adenoviruses, 1384–1385
  Bacillus anthracis, 1887–1888
  Candida albicans, 2296
  Chlamydia pneumoniae, 1698
  Corynebacterium diphtheriae, 1868–1870
  Cryptococcus neoformans, 2334
  Cryptosporidium, 2505
  enterococcal, 1829
  Escherichia coli, 1971
  isolation, 2576
  measles virus, 1521
  Moraxella catarrhalis, 1927
  Mycoplasma pneumoniae, 1705f, 1705–1706
  Neisseria meningitidis, 1902

Respiratory tract infections *(Continued)*
  nosocomial, 2599–2607
    diagnosis, 2602–2603
    etiologies, 2600, 2600t
    incidence and mortality,
      2599–2600, 2600t
    pathogenesis, 2601–2602
    predisposing factors, 2601, 2601t
    prevention, 2604–2605
    treatment, 2603–2604
  Pasteurella, 2069
  pleuropulmonary and bronchial,
      606–662. *See also specific
      infections*
    bronchiolitis, 612–619
    bronchitis
      acute, 606–608
      acute exacerbations, 608–612
      chronic, 608–612
    cystic fibrosis, 657–662
    empyema, 638
    lung abscess, 642–646
    pleural effusion, 638–641
    pneumonia
      acute, 619–638
      chronic, 647–657
    Pseudomonas aeruginosa,
      1984–1985
    treatment, 1985
  streptococcal: group C and G, 1855
  treatment
    quinolones, 372
    trimethoprim, 359
  upper, 561–606. *See also specific
      infections*
    acute laryngitis, 572–573
    acute laryngotracheobronchitis
      (croup), 573–579
    anaerobic
      cocci, 2205
      gram-negative bacilli,
        2197–2198
    bites (human and animal), 603
    cervical adenitis, 603
    common cold, 561–566
    embryologic cysts, infected, 603
    epiglottitis, 590–593
    irradiation and postsurgical
      wounds, 603
    mastoiditis, 583–584
    maxillofacial trauma, 603
    orofacial infections
      nonodontogenic, 602–603
      odontogenic, 593–602
    otitis externa, 579–580, 582
    otitis media, 580–583
    pharyngitis, 566–572
    sinusitis, 585–590
    suppurative thyroiditis, 603
  viral. *See also specific viruses*
    interferons for, 429–430
Restriction fragment length polymor-
    phism: *Mycobacterium
    tuberculosis*, 2215
Reticular dysgenesis, 134t, 150, 151t
Reticuloendothelial system (RES): viral
    diseases and, 1321
Reticuloendotheliosis: lipomelanotic,
    937
Retinal hemorrhage: and endophthalmi-
    tis, 1121
Retinitis
  cytomegalovirus, 1239, 1359, 1359f
    and HIV/ AIDS, 1124, 1287–1288
    and HIV/AIDS: incidence, 1182t

  treatment, 412t, 423–424, 1283t,
      1287–1288, 1360
    foscarnet, 423–424, 1273, 1360
  herpesviruses, 1334t
  VZV, 1240
Retinochoroiditis: *Toxoplasma gondii*,
    1124
Retrobulbar neuritis: from ethambutol,
    393
Retroperitoneal space, 706
Retropharyngeal space infections
  clinical presentation, 600
  and mediastinitis, 814
Retrovir. *See* Zidovudine
Retroviridae, 1579–1606. *See also
    individual viruses*
  classification, 1315t
  HIV, 1590–1606. *See also* Human
      immunodeficiency virus
  HTLV, 1579–1584. *See also* Human
      T cell lymphotropic viruses
  lentiviruses, 1584–1606
  shape and size, 1316f
  transfusion-related, 2625–2626
  type C oncoviruses, 1579–1584
Reverse endocytosis, 86
Reverse transcriptase, 1318
  inhibition: for HIV, 1269–1271
Reverse transcriptase inhibitors, non-
    nucleoside: for HIV,
    1272–1273
Reye syndrome, 1558–1559
  clinical features, 1558–1559, 1559t
  dengue and, 1473
  encephalitis, 875
  epidemiology, 1558
  influenza virus and, 1558–1559
  pathology, 1559
  pathophysiology, 1559
  VZV and, 1348
Rhabdomyolysis: acute, 935
Rhabdoviridae, 1526–1543. *See also
    individual viruses*
  classification, 1315t
  rabies virus, 1527–1543
  shape and size, 1316f
  vesicular stomatitis virus,
    1526–1527
Rhesus rotavirus (RRV) vaccine, 1452
Rheumatic fever, 1799–1805
  anti-inflammatory therapy, 1805t
  antistreptolysin O and, 1801
  clinical manifestations, 1802f,
    1802–1803
  diagnosis, 1803–1804, 1804t
  epidemiology, 1801–1802
  etiology, 1800–1801
  fever of, 542
  heart-reactive antibodies, 1800
  history, 1799–1800
  Jones criteria, 1804, 1804t
  in other countries, 1801–1802
  pathogenesis, 1800–1801
  pathology, 1801
  prevention, 1790–1791, 1804–1805
  reactivation, 1804
  tonsillitis and, 1801
  treatment and prognosis, 1790, 1804,
    1805t
  vaccine research, 1805
Rheumatic heart disease: and infective
    endocarditis, 741
Rheumatoid arthritis
  chloroquine for, 470
  defective chemotaxis in, 90

  differential diagnosis: rheumatic fever,
    1803
  and fever, 545
  and infectious arthritis, 1032
  ocular manifestations, 539
  pleural fluid, 640
Rheumatoid factor, 42
  arthritis, 1037
  and endocarditis, 745, 750
Rheumatoid syndrome: and C3
    deficiency, 69
Rheumatologic disorders
  and complement, 72
  and HIV, 1228
Rh immunoglobulin, 2783
Rhinitis
  chronic atrophic (ozaenia), 1972
  Treponema pallidum, 2126
Rhinocerebral infection: mucormycosis,
    2313, 2314f, 2315f
Rhinocladiella aquaspersa, 2324
Rhinocladiella compacta, 2324
Rhinocladiella pedrosoi, 2324
Rhinoscleroma. *See Klebsiella rhinoscle-
    romatis*
Rhinosporidium seeberi, 2289,
    2391–2392
  conjunctivitis, 1105
  differential diagnosis, 2366
Rhinoviruses, 1656–1663
  adherence, 12
  and asthma precipitation, 1659
  binding site, 13
  bronchiolitis, 612t, 612–613
  bronchitis
    acute, 606, 606t
    exacerbations of chronic, 1659
  characteristics, 1656t, 1656–1657
    antigenic, 1657
    biologic, 1656–1657
  classification, 1656
  clinical manifestations, 1658f,
    1658–1659
  common cold, 562, 562t, 563, 564,
    1487t, 1658f, 1658–1659
    characteristics, 1487t
  complications, 1659
  croup, 574, 574t
  diagnosis, 1659
  epidemiology, 1657
  ICAM-1, 12t, 13, 14, 14f, 1656, 1660
  immunity, 1658
  infection and illness rates, 1657
  laryngitis, 573t
  morphology and structure, 1656
  otitis media, 1659
  pathogenesis, 1657–1658
  pharyngitis, 567t
  prevalence, 1657
  receptor, 12, 13, 1656
  seasonality, 1657
  serology, 1659
  sinusitis, 585, 585t, 1659
  transmission, 1657
  treatment and prevention,
      1659–1661
    combined antiviral antimediator,
      1660
    environmental measures,
      1660–1661
    vaccine research, 1659–1660
    viral isolation, 1659, 1660f
Rhipicephalus
  and ehrlichiosis, 1747t, 1748, 1749
  and *Rickettsia rickettsii*, 1721

Rhizomucor: mucormycosis, 2311–2317,
    2312f. *See also* Mucormycosis
Rhizopus, 2311t
  and bone marrow transplantation,
    2719
  dysentery, 994
  gangrenous cellulitis, 918
  mucormycosis, 2311–2317, 2312f. *See
    also* Mucormycosis
  pneumonia, 619t
  sinusitis, 586t
Rhizopus oryzae, 2311t, 2312
Rhodnius polixus, 2443f
Rhodococcus, 1872t, 1876–1877
Rhodococcus aurantiacus, 1877
Rhodococcus bronchialis, 1877
Rhodococcus equi, 1872t, 1876–1877
  brain abscess: in AIDS, 890
  pneumonia
    and AIDS, 629, 655f, 1235, 1235t,
      1872t
    chronic, 647t
    radiology, 655f
  rifampin for, 323
Rhodococcus erythropolis, 1877
Rhodococcus luteus, 1877
Rhodococcus rhodochrous, 1877
Rhodococcus rubrepertinctus, 1877
*rho*GDI protein, 85
Ribavirin, 412t, 430–431
  adverse reactions, 430–431
  for arenaviruses, 1577
  for bronchiolitis, 616
  for Bunyaviridae infections, 1571
  clinical studies, 431
  dosage and pharmacology, 518t–519t
  drug interactions, 526t
  for influenza, 1560
  mechanism of action, 430
  pharmacokinetics, 430
  for respiratory syncytial virus, 1510,
    1511
  spectrum of activity, 430
  structure, 430f
Ribosomal resistance, 220
Ribosomal target sites: alteration of, 220
Rickettsia africae, 1725
Rickettsia akari, 1725, 1727
  cutaneous manifestations, 550t, 1727
  diagnosis, 1727
  differential diagnosis, 1727
  epidemiology, 1719, 1720t, 1727
  lymphadenitis, 940t
Rickettsia australis, 1725
  clinical features, 1720t
  cutaneous manifestations, 553
  epidemiology, 1720t
Rickettsia belli, 1721
Rickettsia burnetii. See Coxiella burnetii
Rickettsia conorii, 1725
  clinical features, 1720t, 1723t
  epidemiology, 1720t
  lymphadenitis, 940t
Rickettsia diaporica, 1728. *See also
    Coxiella burnetii*
Rickettsia japonica, 1725
Rickettsial infections, 1719–1752. *See
    also individual species*
  cellular immunity and, 124
  clinical manifestations, 1719, 1720t
  cutaneous manifestations and rashes,
      550t, 553, 556, 1720t, 1721.
      See also specific species
  description of pathogen, 1719, 1720f
  developments in the field, 1719–1720

diagnosis, 1719
enteric symptoms, 999t
epidemiology, 1719, 1720t
and fever, 542
myocarditis, 800, 802
overview, 1719–1720
pathology, 1719
replication mechanisms, 25
rifampin for, 323
serology, 192t
taxonomy, 1742f, 1748
transfusion-related, 2627
Weil-Felix reaction, 1719, 1724, 1736,
1737, 1740
Rickettsialpox, 1719, 1720t, 1727. *See
also Rickettsia akari*
Rickettsia montana, 1721
*Rickettsia orientalis. See Rickettsia
tsutsugamushi*
Rickettsia parkeri, 1721
Rickettsia prowazekii, 1735–1737
Brill-Zinsser disease, 1719, 1720,
1720t, 1735, 1736–1737
diagnosis, 1737
clinical manifestations, 1736
cutaneous manifestations, 550t
description, 1735
diagnosis, 1736
epidemiology, 1719, 1720, 1720t,
1735
pathogenesis, 1735–1736
pathology, 1735–1736
prevention, 1736
recrudescent. *See* Brill-Zinsser disease
above
treatment, 1736
vaccine, 1736
for travelers, 2797t, 2798
*Rickettsia quintana. See Bartonella quin-
tana*
Rickettsia rhipicephali, 1721
Rickettsia rickettsii, 1721–1727
animal reservoirs, 2792t
clinical features, 1720t, 1723f, 1723t,
1723–1724, 1724f
cutaneous manifestations, 550t, 552,
556, 1721, 1723f, 1723t,
1723–1724, 1724f
description, 1721
diagnosis, 1724
differential diagnosis
Colorado tick fever, 1447
ehrlichiosis, 1750, 1750t
measles virus, 1522
murine typhus, 1739
Streptobacillus moniliformis, 2085
encephalitis/myelitis, 874–875
epidemiology, 1719, 1720t,
1721–1722, 1722f
lipopolysaccharide, 1721
myocarditis, 800
enteric symptoms, 1003
pathogenesis, 1722–1723
prevention, 1725
tick vector, 2565
treatment, 1724–1725
Rickettsia sibirica, 1725
clinical features, 1720t
epidemiology, 1720t
Rickettsia tsutsugamushi
clinical manifestations, 1740
cutaneous manifestations, 550t
description, 1740
diagnosis, 1740
differential diagnosis, 1740–1741

epidemiology, 1719, 1720t, 1740
lymphadenitis, 940t, 1740
myocarditis, 800, 1740
pathogenesis and pathology, 1740
prevention, 1741
treatment, 1741
Rickettsia typhi, 1719, 1720t,
1737–1739
animal reservoirs, 2792t
clinical manifestations, 1738
cutaneous manifestations, 550t
description, 1737
diagnosis, 1738–1739
encephalitis/myelitis, 874–875
epidemiology, 1719, 1720t, 1737
fever, 543
laboratory findings, 1738
pathology and pathogenesis,
1737–1738
treatment and prevention, 1739
Rifabutin, 318, 324
adverse reactions, 392
dosage, 516t–517t
for *Mycobacterium avium-intracellulare*, 2257
for *Mycobacterium leprae*, 398
for *Mycobacterium tuberculosis*, 324,
392
for nontuberculous (atypical)
mycobacteria, 395–396
pharmacology, 516t–517t
zidovudine interaction with, 436
Rifampicin. *See* Rifampin
Rifampin
adverse reactions, 319–320,
391–392
for anaerobic infections, 324
antibiotic-associated colitis (AAC)
from, 979
antimicrobial activity, 318t, 318–319,
391
for *Brucella*, 322–323, 2057
for chancroid, 323
for chronic granulomatous disease of
childhood, 323
clinical trials, 231
combination therapy
aminoglycosides, 289t
for mycobacteria, 396t
trimethoprim, 359
for *Coxiella burnetii* pneumonia,
1730
for CSF shunt infections, 323
for cutaneous leishmaniasis, 323
dosage, 392, 516t–517t
for children and neonates, 851t
in hepatic or renal failure, 390t,
517t
for meningitis, 850t, 851t
drug interactions, 203, 319–320, 320t,
392, 392t, 525t
isoniazid, 390
zidovudine, 436
for endocarditis, 321–322
prosthetic valve, 786, 786t
staphylococcal, 762
for furuncles, 913
for gram-negative anaerobes, 323
for *Legionella pneumophila*, 322,
2093, 2093t
for meningitis, 324
prophylaxis, 320–321, 857
for mycobacterial infections, 320,
2267, 2268, 2269
leprosy, 320, 397t, 2248

nontuberculous (atypical), 320,
395–396
tuberculosis, 318, 320, 391–392,
2213, 2226–2228, 2232,
2239
miliary, 2233
for *Neisseria meningitidis*, 1903t
for osteomyelitis, 322
pharmacology, 317–318, 391,
516t–517t
for pruritus, 325
for *Pseudomonas aeruginosa*, 318t,
323, 1988
for rabies, 324
resistance, 215t, 319, 321, 397
Neisseria meningitidis, 1905
for *Rhodococcus*, 323
for Rickettsia, 323
for septic arthritis, 322
for staphylococcal infections, 322
methicillin-resistant, 322
for streptococcal carriage, 322, 1758
structure, 317, 317f, 391f
for urethritis, 323
for urinary tract infections, 323
for vascular graft infections, 323
Rifamycins, 317–329. *See also*
Rifampin
mechanism of action, 317
Rifapentine, 324
for *Mycobacterium leprae*, 398
Rifaximin, 324–325
Rift Valley fever virus, 1567
characteristics, 1568t
clinical manifestations, 1570
differential diagnosis, 1472
epidemiology, 1568–1569
prevention, 1571
serology, 191
transmission to humans, 1569
Right atrial indwelling catheter infections,
788
clinical manifestations, 788
microbiology, 788
pathogenesis, 788
therapy, 788
Rimantadine, 412t, 417–419
adverse reactions, 418–419
clinical studies, 419
drug interactions, 418–419
for influenza, 1560
prophylaxis, 1563
mechanism of action, 1319
pharmacokinetics, 418
resistance, 417–418
spectrum of activity, 417
structure, 417f
Ringworm, 2289, 2375, 2378, 2378f
black-dot, 2380
differential diagnosis, 2378
scalp, 2379–2380, 2380f
treatment, 403–404
Rio Bravo: transmission, clinical syndromes, and geographic
distribution, 1466t
Risk assessment, 166
Ritter's disease, 1765
cutaneous manifestations, 555
River blindness, 1114, 2525t,
2535–2536. *See also
Onchocerca volvulus*
RMP. *See* Rifampin
RMSF. *See* Rocky Mountain spotted
fever
RNA glycosidase toxins, 3t

RNA viruses, 1446–1674. *See also
individual viruses*
Arenaviridae, 1572–1579
Astroviridae, 1672–1674
Bunyaviridae, 1567–1572
Calciviridae, 1666–1672
Norwalk virus, 1666–1672
classification, 1314–1315, 1315t
Coronaviridae, 1486–1489
Filoviridae, 1543–1546
Marburg and Ebola hemorrhagic
fevers, 1543–1546
Flaviviridae, 1465–1486
flaviviruses, 1465–1474
hepatitis C virus, 1474–1486
Orthomyxoviridae, 1546–1567
influenza virus, 1546–1567
Paramyxoviridae, 1489–1526
measles virus, 1519–1526
mumps virus, 1496–1501
parainfluenza virus, 1489–1496
respiratory syncytial virus,
1501–1519
Picornaviridae, 1606–1666
coxsackieviruses, 1620–1636
echoviruses, 1620–1636
enteroviruses, 1620–1636
hepatitis A virus, 1636–1656
hepatitis E virus, 1663–1666
overview, 1606–1613
poliovirus, 1613–1620
rhinovirus, 1656–1663
Reoviridae, 1446–1455
Colorado tick fever, 1446–1447
orbivirus, 1447–1458
rotavirus, 1448–1455
replication, 1318
Retroviridae, 1579–1606
HIV, 1590–1606
HTLV, 1579–1584
lentiviruses, 1584–1590
type C oncoviruses, 1579–1584
Rhabdoviridae, 1526–1543
rabies virus, 1527–1543
vesicular stomatitis virus,
1526–1527
shapes and sizes, 1316f
structure, 1314–1315, 1316f
Togaviridae, 1455–1465
alphaviruses, 1455–1459
rubella virus (German measles),
1459–1465
Ro 24-7429, 437t
Ro 31-8959, 437t
Rocephin. *See* Ceftriaxone
*Rochalimaea henselae. See Bartonella
henselae*
*Rochalimaea quintana. See Bartonella
quintana*
Rocha-Lima inclusions, 2210
Rocio fever: transmission, clinical
syndromes, and geographic
distribution, 1466t
Rocky Mountain spotted fever, 1719,
1720t, 1721–1725. *See also
Rickettsia rickettsii*
Rodent-borne diseases, 2792t. *See also
specific rodents*
arenaviruses, 1572, 1573t, 1574–1575
Francisella tularensis, 2061
Rokitansky-Aschoff sinuses, 729–730
Romaña's sign, 2445, 2445f
Romberg sign: *Treponema pallidum*, 2125
Root canal infection: anaerobic, 2163t,
2164

Rosai-Dorfman disease
  HHV-6 and, 1378
  lymphadenopathy, 941
Roseola infantum. *See* Exanthem
    subitum
Roseoliform exanthems: enteroviral,
    1624
Rose spots, 921, 998, 1000, 1000t
  Salmonella, 2021
  and systemic infections, 551t, 552
Ross River virus, 1455
  arthritis, 1036, 1036t
  clinical manifestations, 1457
  differential diagnosis, 1472
  epidemiology, 1457
Rotavirus, 1447, 1448–1455
  clinical manifestations, 1450
  description, 1448f, 1448–1449
  diagnosis, 181, 1450–1451
  diarrhea
    infantile, 966, 971
    noninflammatory in adults, 969
    in travelers, 2801–2802
    weanling, 966–968
  electron micrograph, 1448f
  epidemiology, 1449–1450
  immune response, 1450–1451
  pathogenesis, 1449
  prevention, 1451–1452
  SA-11: receptor, 1317t
  treatment, 1451
  vaccines, 1451–1452
  waterborne, 1016, 1016t
Rothia dentocariosa, 2208
  endocarditis, 756
Roth spots
  of endocarditis, 747, 748f, 749
  and endophthalmitis, 1121
Roundworms, intestinal, 2526–2531,
    2527t. *See also individual
    species*
  Ascaris lumbricoides, 2528–2529
  Enterobius vermicularis, 2528
  hookworm (*Ancylostoma duodenale;
    Necator americanus*),
    2529–2530
  Strongyloides stercoralis,
    2530–2531
  Trichuris trichiura, 2526–2528
Roundworms, tissue
  Dracunculus medinensis, 2533
  filariasis, 2533–2535
  Mansonella, 2536
  onchocerciasis, 2535–2536
  Trichinella spiralis, 2531–2533
  tropical pulmonary eosinophilia,
    2536
Roxithromycin, 340, 475
R-plasmids: Enterobacteriaceae, 1969
RPR test, 2127, 2127t
  lepromin test and, 2246
RTX (repeat in toxin), 7
Rubella vaccine, 167, 1463, 2781
  adverse reactions, 2773t, 2781
  for children, 2783
  complications, 1462
  contraindications, 2787t
  effects on fetus, 1462, 2783
  efficacy, 1462
  morbidity reduction, 2772t
  recommendations for adults, 2784t
  reportable events, 2786t
Rubella virus, 1455, 1459–1465
  arthritis, 1032, 1036, 1036t
  clinical manifestations, 1461

congenital, 1460
  clinical manifestations, 1461–1462,
    1462t
  conjunctivitis, 1106
  cutaneous manifestations, 550t, 551
  diagnosis, 1462
  differential diagnosis: EBV, 1372
  endophthalmitis, 1124
  epidemiology, 1460–1461
  hepatitis, 1137
  lymphadenitis, 940t
  maintenance of immunity, 1460–1461
  pathogenesis, 1461
  postnatal, 1461
    complications, 1461
  reinfection, 1460
  and Reye syndrome, 1558
  serology, 191
  spreading/shedding mechanisms,
    1320f
  systemic spread, 1320f
  treatment, 1462
  vaccine. *See* Rubella vaccine
Rubelliform exanthems
  echoviruses, 1623–1624
  enteroviral, 1623–1624
Rubeola virus, 1519–1526. *See also*
    Measles virus
Rubivirus: arthritis, 1036t
Ruminococcus, 2158t
Rumpel-Leeds test, 1788
Russian spring-summer encephalitis,
    1467
  clinical manifestations, 1472
  epidemiology, 1469
  prevention and treatment, 1473
  transmission, clinical syndromes, and
    geographic distribution, 1466t

S

Sabia virus, 1572
  characteristics, 1573t
Sabin-Feldman dye test: for *Toxoplasma
    gondii*, 2463
Saccharomyces: growth, 190
Saccharomyces boulardii: diarrhea, 984
Saccharomyces cerevisiae: vaginitis,
    1075
Sacroiliac joint: infectious arthritis,
    1033, 1033t
Sacroiliitis
  Brucella, 2056
  Reiter syndrome, 1071
Sagiyama virus, 1457
St. Louis encephalitis virus, 1466t, 1467,
    1468–1469, 1471–1472
  clinical manifestations, 1458,
    1471–1472
  encephalomyelitis, 876
  epidemiology, 1468–1469
  history, 1467
  and HIV/AIDS, 1470
  meningitis, 832
  pathogenesis, 1470
  prevention and treatment, 1473
  serology, 191
  transmission, clinical syndromes, and
    geographic distribution,
    1466t
St. Vitus dance (Sydenham's chorea),
    1801, 1803
Saksenaea, 2311t
  mucormycosis, 2312
Salbutamol: for *Bordetella pertussis*,

2082
Salicylazosulfapyridine, 355
Salicylic acid, 401
  for cutaneous warts, 1393
Salivary gland
  infections, 603
  virus. *See* Cytomegalovirus
Salmonella, 2013–2033
  abdominal infections, 2022
  animal reservoirs, 2792t
  antibody deficiencies and, 49
  arterial infections, 2022
  arthritis, 2023–2024
    reactive, 2024
    septic, 2023–2024
  bacteremia, 2022
    and HIV/AIDS, 2027–2028
    and splenic abscess, 727
    therapy, 2027
  bacterial-mediated endocytosis, 2017
  bacteriophage typing, 2014
  blood cultures, 2021
  bone marrow cultures, 2021
  brain abscess, 890
    in AIDS, 890
  carriage, 2015, 2020
    treatment, 2028
  cellular immunity and, 125, 127
    defects, 2681
  chronic carrier state, 2024
    therapy, 2028
  classification and taxonomy, 2014,
    2014t
  clinical manifestations, 2020–2024
  clones, 21
  CNS infections, 2023
  diarrhea
    in hospitals, 970
    infantile, 966
  differential diagnosis: *Cryptospori-
    dium*, 2504
  dysentery, 989
    diagnosis, 990
  in the elderly, 2740
  empyema, 2023
  endocarditis, 755, 2022
  endoscope contamination, 2585
  enteric fever, 2020–2022
    diagnosis, 2021–2022
  enterocolitis, 989
    and HIV/AIDS, 1230
  enterotoxins, 5, 2018
  epidemiology, 159, 2015–2017
  food-borne, 1012t, 1013, 1016, 1020,
    2015, 2016
    foods implicated, 1017t
    laboratory diagnosis, 1018t, 1019
  gastric acidity and, 947
  gastroenteritis
    clinical manifestations, 2020
    pathophysiology, 2019
    therapy, 2027, 2027t
  H antigen, 2014
  history, 2013–2014
  and HIV/AIDS, 2019, 2020, 2024
    bacteremia, 2027–2028
    brain abscess, 890
    incidence, 1182t
    therapy, 2027–2028, 2642
  inhibiting phagocytosis, 7
  intestinal motility and, 947
  inv operon, 7
  and leukemia, hairy cell, 2673
  localized infections, 2022–2023
  M cells, 2017

meningitis, 834
  microbiology, 2014–2015
  multilocus enzyme electrophoresis, 27
  mycotic aneurysms, 772
  myocarditis, 800
  necrotizing enterocolitis of newborn,
    991
  nontyphoidal
    therapy, 2027
    waterborne, 1015–1016, 1016t
  O antigen, 2014
  osteomyelitis, 1049, 2023
  pathogenesis, 2017t, 2017–2020
    bacterial factors, 2018–2019
    GI host-pathogen interactions, 2017
    host factors, 2019, 2019t
    immunity, 2019–2020
    infectious dose, 2017
    survival within phagocytes,
      2017–2018
  penetration, 2, 7
  Peyer's patches, 2017, 2021
  pneumonia, 2023
  polymorphonuclear leukocytes and,
    2018
  and Reiter syndrome, 1071
  replication mechanisms, 25
  resistance, 2026–2027
    trimethoprim, 358
  rose spots, 2021
  serotypes, 2014
  and sickle cell disease, 2019, 2023
  soft tissue infections, 2022–2023
  spacious phagosomes, 2018
  stool examination, 180
    cultures, 2015
  surveillance, 160
  toxin, 950
  in travelers, 2802
  treatment, 2026–2028
    aminoglycosides, 285t
    antimicrobials of choice, 202t
    cephalosporins, 255t
    chronic carrier state, 2028
    and HIV/AIDS, 2027–2028
    penicillins, 237t
    quinolones, 367t, 371
    sulfonamides, 355t
    trimethoprim, 357, 360
  urogenital infections, 2023
  vaginal infection, 1080
  vascular infection, 2022
  Vi antigen, 2014, 2018
  virulence factors, 2, 8
  Widal test, 2022
Salmonella arizonae: epidemiology,
    2016
Salmonella chester: epidemiology, 2016
Salmonella choleraesuis
  bacteremia, 2022
  endocarditis, 755
  enteric fever, 998, 999t
  mycotic aneurysms, 772
  osteomyelitis, 2023
  pathogenesis, 2018
  taxonomy, 2014
Salmonella dublin
  bacteremia, 2022
  epidemiology, 2016, 2016t
  pathogenesis, 2018
  soft tissue infections, 2023
Salmonella enteritidis
  endocarditis, 755
  epidemiology, 2016, 2016t
  food-borne, 1016, 2016

gastroenteritis, 2021
hosts, 946
mycotic aneurysms, 772
pathogenesis, 2018
risk of infection, 160
Salmonella hadar, 2016, 2016t
Salmonella heidelberg, 2016t
Salmonella javiana, 162, 2016
Salmonella montevideo, 2016t
Salmonella muenchen, 2016
Salmonella newport
epidemiology, 2016t
pathogenesis, 2017
Salmonella oranienburg, 162
Salmonella paratyphi, 2014
chloramphenicol for, 312t
enteric fever, 998, 999t, 2021–2022
epidemiology, 2015
osteomyelitis, 2023
symptoms, 998
Salmonella poona, 2016, 2016t
Salmonella pullorum, 2017
Salmonella thompson, 2016t
Salmonella typhi, 164
bacteremia: and skin infections, 921
carriage, 2015, 2020
chronic carrier state, 2024
conjunctivitis, 998, 1000t
cutaneous manifestations, 550t, 921
differential diagnosis
amebiasis, 2402
for *Chlamydia psittaci*, 1695
scrub typhus, 1740
typhus, 2013
dysentery, 990
endocarditis, 2022
enteric fever, 998–1004, 2021–2022
clinical features, 998–1001,
999t–1000t
differential diagnosis, 1001–1004
epidemiology, 1001
pathogenesis, 998
therapy, 1003–1004
epidemiology, 2015–2016
and HIV, 2024
hosts, 946
immunity, 2021
immunodeficiency and, 138
lymphadenitis, 940t
pathogenesis, 2017, 2018
and phagocytes, 88
resistance, 2015
rose spots, 921, 998, 1000t
symptoms, 998
taxonomy, 2014
travel and, 2015
treatment, 2026, 2026t
chloramphenicol, 312t
glucocorticoids, 455
quinolones, 370
urogenital infections, 2023
vaccines, 955, 2024–2026
adverse reactions, 2025
for travelers, 2024–2026, 2797t,
2798
Ty21a, 2025
Vi polysaccharide, 2025
Vi antigen, 952, 1965, 2014, 2018
Salmonella typhimurium
and complement, 65
cytokine protection, 121t
endocarditis, 755
epidemiology, 948, 2016, 2016t
flagellae, 18
gastroenteritis, 2019, 2020

lipopolysaccharide, 2018
osteomyelitis, 2023
pathogenesis, 2018, 2019
and phagocytes, 88
replication mechanisms, 25
resistance, 219
virulence regulation, 23t, 24
Salmon River tick fever virus, 1447
Salpingitis
Chlamydia trachomatis, 1069, 1687
Haemophilus influenzae, 2043
Neisseria gonorrhoeae, 1917
PID and, 1095, 1917. *See also* Pelvic
inflammatory disease
Sandfly-borne disease
bartonellosis, 2209
Leishmania, 2429
Sandoglobulin, 454
Sanitizer: defined, 2579
San Joaquin Valley fever, 2365
Saperconazole: for chromomycosis,
2326
Sarcocystis, 2394t, 2511
clinical manifestations, 2394t
transmission, 2394t
Sarcodina, 2393t
Sarcoidosis
defective chemotaxis in, 90
differential diagnosis, 2437
and fever, 545
granulomatous hepatitis, 1162
meningitis, 871
pneumonia
chronic, 647t
radiology, 652f
pulmonary infiltrates with eosinophilia,
631
Sarcomas: infections and, 2667
Sarcophaga, 2563
Sarcoptes scabiei, 2560–2562
and AIDS, 557
clinical manifestations, 2561f,
2561–2562
epidemiology, 2561
prevention, 2562
treatment, 466t, 2562
var. *canis*, 2562, 2564
var. *hominis*, 2560–2562
Sarocomastigophora, 2393t
Saxitoxin, 1014
Scabies, 2560–2562. *See also Sarcoptes
scabiei*
animal, 2562
clinical manifestations, 2561f,
2561–2562
epidemiology, 2561
human, 2561
Norwegian (crusted), 1059,
2561–2562
treatment and prevention, 2562
Scarlet fever
septic, 1789
strawberry tongue, 553, 1788–1789
Streptococcus pyogenes, 555,
1788–1789
toxic, 1789
toxins, 6, 1788
*Scedosporium (Monosporium) prolifi-
cans*, 2389, 2390
Schistosoma, 2525t, 2538t, 2538–2541
acute infection, 2540
chronic infection, 2540–2541
clinical syndromes, 2540–2541
cytokine protection, 121t
diagnosis, 1006t, 1007, 2541

dysentery, 989
epidemiology, 2538–2539
life cycle, 2538, 2539f
pathogenesis, 2539–2540
pneumonia, 647t
pulmonary infiltrates with eosinophilia,
631
and *Salmonella*, 2019
treatment, 466t, 2541
artemisinin, 472
niridazole, 483
praziquantel, 482
Schistosoma haematobium, 2525t, 2538t,
2538–2541
clinical syndrome, 2540
diagnosis, 1006t, 1007, 2541
epidemiology, 2538–2539
IgE and, 39, 41
pathogenesis, 2539
treatment, 466t, 2541
metrifonate, 482
Schistosoma intercalatum
clinical syndromes, 2540
epidemiology, 2538
pathogenesis, 2539
Schistosoma japonicum, 2525t, 2538t,
2538–2541
brain abscess, 890
clinical syndromes, 2540, 2541
diagnosis, 1006t, 1007
dysentery, 989
epidemiology, 2538
pathogenesis, 2539
treatment, 466t
praziquantel, 482
Schistosoma mansoni, 2525t, 2538t,
2538–2541
cellular immunity and, 127
clinical syndromes, 2540, 2541
diagnosis, 1006t, 1007
dysentery, 989
epidemiology, 2538
granulomatous hepatitis, 1161
pathogenesis, 2539
penetration, 7
treatment, 466t, 2541
oxamniquine, 483
praziquantel, 482
Schistosoma mekongi, 2538t,
2538–2541
clinical syndromes, 2540
epidemiology, 2538
treatment, 466t, 2541
Schistosomiasis, 2538–2541. *See also
individual species*
travel and, 2800–2801
Schizophyllum commune: sinusitis,
586t
Schultz-Charlton reaction, 1788
Scleral abscess: *Pseudomonas
aeruginosa*, 1991
Sclerosing mediastinitis, 817–818
complications, 817t
Sclerosis
multiple. *See* Multiple sclerosis
progressive systemic: pneumonia,
647t
Sclerotia, 2326
Scombroid fish poisoning, 1012t, 1015t
fish implicated, 1017t
Scopulariopsis: and granulocytopenia,
2677
Scopulariopsis brevicaulis, 2383
Scrapie, 1321, 1674
scr kinases, 109

Scrofula, 2239
and HIV/AIDS, 2239
lymphadenitis, 936, 938, 940t, 2239,
2255
Scrotum: idiopathic gangrene of, 925
Scrub typhus, 1719, 1720t, 1740–1741.
*See also Rickettsia tsutsuga-
mushi*
differential diagnosis, 1472
rickettsialpox, 1727
enteric symptoms, 999t
Scytalidium, 2380, 2382–2383
Scytalidium dimidiatum, 2382–2383
Scytalidium hyalinum, 2382–2383
Seal finger, 915, 1895, 1895f
Sealpox, 1329
Sebaceous cysts: anaerobic, 2165
Sebaceous gland carcinoma: of the eye-
lid, 1130
Seborrheic dermatitis
clinical features, 2384
and HIV, 1229
Pityrosporum, 2384
treatment, 2384
Sebum, 31
Secondary attack rate, 164
Secondary prevention of disease, 167
Second disease. *See* Scarlet fever
Seizures
Bordetella pertussis, 2081
from foscarnet, 423
Plasmodium, 2421
rabies, 1533
Selectins, 81, 81f, 123
Selenomonas, 2158t
bacteremia, 2165
tetracyclines for, 308t
Self-sustaining sequence replication
(3SR), 27
Semen: and HIV transmission, 1102
Semliki Forest virus, 1457
receptor, 1317t
Sendai virus: receptor, 1317t
Sensitivity: in epidemiology, 159
Seoul virus
characteristics, 1568t
clinical manifestations, 1570
epidemiology, 1569
transmission to humans, 1569
Sepik: transmission, clinical syndromes,
and geographic distribution,
1466t
Sepsis. *See also* Sepsis syndrome;
Septicemia
defined, 690, 690t
Haemophilus influenzae, 2043
Listeria monocytogenes, 1882, 1882t,
1883t
severe: defined, 690t, 690–691
in traumatized patient, 2759
Sepsis syndrome, 690–705
ARDS, 696
clinical approach, 696–697, 697t
clinical manifestations, 691t, 692f,
692–693, 693t
coagulopathy in, 695f, 695–696
cytokine-induced platelet-activating
factor synthesis, 696
defined, 690, 690t
epidemiology, 691
host defenses, augmentation of,
702–703
pathophysiology, 693t, 693–695,
694t
prophylaxis, 702

Sepsis syndrome *(Continued)*
  pulmonary vascular endothelial injury, 696
  therapy
    adjunctive, 700–701
    anticoagulation, 701
    antimicrobial, 697–699, 699t
    antiserum, 701–702
    colony-stimulating factors, 701, 702–703
    corticosteroids, 700
    diuretics, 701
    granulocyte transfusion, 701, 702–703
    naloxone, 701
    sympathomimetic amines, 700, 700t
    volume replacement, 699–700
Septata intestinalis, 2514, 2515, 2516
  diagnosis, 2520–2521
  in HIV infected, 2519, 2519t
  treatment, 465t, 2521
Septic arthritis: rifampin for, 322
Septicemia. *See also* Bacteremia; Fungemia; Viremia
  Bacillus, 1892–1893
  defined, 690t, 691
  and leukemia/lymphoma, 2677–2678, 2681
  postanginal (Lemierre's disease), 569
  rashes, 553
  specimen collection and processing, 170t, 177–178
  Staphylococcus aureus
    clinical manifestations, 1767–1768, 1768f
    diagnosis, 1769
    echocardiography, 1769
    endocarditis vs., 1768–1769, 1769t
    epidemiology, 1767
    laboratory findings, 1768
    management, 1769–1770
  Yersinia enterocolitica, 2077
Septicemic plague, 2072t, 2073–2074, 2074f
Septic intracranial thrombophlebitis: bacteriology, 902t
Septic pelvic thrombophlebitis, 1095
Septic shock
  corticosteroids and, 131
  cytokines and, 117–118
  defined, 690t, 691
  refractory: defined, 690t, 691
Séreny test, 2033
Seroincidence surveys, 162
Serology, 191–193, 192t, 193t
  endocarditis, 751
  genital lesions, 1060–1061
  hepatitis
    acute viral, 1142f, 1146
    chronic, 1156
    HAV, 1141, 1142f
    HBV, 191, 1142f, 1142–1143, 1143f, 1426t
    HCV, 191, 1142f, 1156, 1480–1481
    HIV, 1189, 1220, 1220f, 1225, 1253f, 1254–1261
      algorithm for management, 1256f
  infectious arthritis, 1037
  meningitis, 866t
  pneumonia, 625–626, 626
    chronic, 652
  syphilis, 181, 192t, 2127t, 2127–2129
  Toxoplasma gondii, 2463, 2464–2466
  viral, 191

Seroprevalence survey, 163
Serratia, 1973
  β-lactamase, 268
  catheter infections, 2595
  and immunodeficiency, 150t
  infusion-related sepsis, 2587
  and nosocomial urinary tract infections, 2613
  peritonitis, 711
  pneumonia, 619t, 1973
  resistance, 251, 1972
  suppurative thrombophlebitis, 768
  treatment
    cephalosporins, 255t
    penicillins, 237t
Serratia ficaria, 1975t
Serratia fonticola, 1975t
Serratia grimesii, 1975t
Serratia liquefaciens, 1973, 1975t
Serratia marcescens, 1973, 1975t
  and chronic granulomatous disease, 92, 155
  endocarditis, 755
  and granulocytopenia, 2676
  keratitis, 1113
  meningitis, 834
  pneumonia: nosocomial in the immunocompromised, 631
  resistance, 219, 1973
    aminoglycosides, 284t
  treatment
    aminoglycosides, 285t, 295t, 296
    antimicrobials of choice, 202t
    carbapenems, 264t
    chloramphenicol, 312t
    neomycin, 384
    polymyxin B, 385
    quinolones, 367t
    rifampin, 318t, 323–324
    sulfonamides, 355t
    trimethoprim, 357
Serratia odorifera, 1973, 1975t
Serratia plymuthica, 1975t
Serratia proteamaculans, 1975t
Serratia rubidaea, 1973, 1975t
Serum alkaline phosphatase test: hepatic abscess, 725
Serum amyloid A: and acute phase response, 117, 535
Serum antimicrobial dilution titer, 209–210
Serum bactericidal test, 196
Serum bactericidal titer, 209–210
Serum concentrations: of antimicrobials, 205, 209
Serum resistance: virulence factors and, 8
Serum sickness
  differential diagnosis, 1803
  penicillins, 239
Serum sickness-like syndrome: hepatitis, 1138
70-kD stress (heat shock) protein, 34
Severe combined immunodeficiency, 52, 106, 134t, 135, 150, 151
  diagnosis, 138–139
  and *Pneumocystis carinii*, 2477
  treatment
    bone marrow transplants, 51
    immunoglobulin, 454
Sexually transmitted diseases, 1055–1103. *See also individual diseases and agents*
  anorectal lesions, 1060
  and arthritis, 1032

bartholinitis, 1085
bartonellosis, 2211
cervicitis, 1084–1085
Chlamydia trachomatis, 1684–1685
CMV, 1353–1354
condylomata acuminata, 1388t, 1389
in drug abusers, 2705
epidemiology, 160, 163
epididymitis, 1100–1101
extragenital dermatologic manifestations, 1059–1060
female pelvic infections, 1090–1096
generalized rashes, 1060
genital skin and mucous membrane lesions, 1055–1063
  diffuse erythematous, 1059
  history, 1055–1057
  morphology, 1057t, 1057–1059
  pain, 1056
  papules, 1059
  pruritus, 1056
  pubic hair, 1059
  travel and, 1057
  ulcers, 1057–1058, 1058f
  verrucous, 1059
  vesicles and bullae, 1057
hepatitis B virus, 1421, 1423
and HIV transmission, 1168–1170, 1188–1189. *See also* Human immunodeficiency virus, sexual transmission
HSV, 183
HTLV, 1580–1581
inguinal buboes, 939
lymphogranuloma venereum, 1684–1685
mycoplasmal colonization, 1714
Neisseria gonorrhoeae, 1913–1914
oral lesions, 1059–1060
orchitis, 1101
pelvic inflammatory disease, 183, 1095, 1917, 1917f
  treatment, 1921–1922, 1922t
prostatitis, 1098–1100
screening programs, 167
skenitis, 1085
surveillance, 160
treatment
  aminoglycosides, 295t
  quinolones, 371
  trimethoprim, 360
Treponema pallidum, 2119
Trichomonas vaginalis, 2493–2494
urethritis, 1063–1074
vulvovaginitis, 1075–1081
Shanghai fever, 921, 1995
Shank fever, 1741
Sheep: microorganisms harbored by, 2792t
Sheep pox, 1325
Shellfish: microorganisms harbored by, 2792t
Shellfish poisoning, 1014, 1015t
  amnesic (ASP), 1014, 1015t
  hepatitis, 1642
  laboratory diagnosis, 1018t
  neurotoxic (NSP), 1014, 1015t, 1017t
  paralytic (PSP), 1012t, 1014, 1015t, 1017t
Shiga bacillus, 2034. *See also Shigella dysenteriae*
Shiga-like toxins, 3t, 6, 22t, 950, 1014
Shiga-like Vero cell cytotoxin, 950, 1014
Shiga toxin, 3t, 6, 2034, 2037

Shigella, 2033–2039
  anatomic location of infection, 2034
  antibody deficiencies and, 49
  apoptosis, 25
  β-lactamase, 215
  clinical course, 2036–2037, 2037t
  communicability, 2033–2034
  control, 2037–2038
    environmental, 2037
    immunologic, 2037–2038
  cyclic patterns of disease, 2034–2035
  diagnosis, 2035
  diarrhea
    in AIDS, 970, 970t
    infantile, 966
  differential diagnosis
    amebiasis, 2402
    Cryptosporidium, 2504
    dysentery, 987–988
    diagnosis, 990
  E. coli and, 2033, 2034f
  in the elderly, 2740
  epidemiology, 2034–2035
  food-borne, 1012t, 1013, 1016, 1020
    foods implicated, 1017t
  group and type identification, 2033
  and HIV/AIDS, 970, 970t, 2642
  hosts, 946
  incidence by geography and host, 2035
  invasiveness, 951–952, 2034
  isolation, 2033
  laboratory findings, 2036, 2036f
  microbiology, 2033
  modes of spread and reservoirs in nature, 2035
  outbreak investigations, 163
  pathogenesis, 2033–2034
  physical examination, 2036
  and Reiter syndrome, 1071
  replication mechanisms, 25
  resistance: trimethoprim, 358
  stool examination, 180
  surveillance, 160
  toxigenicity, 2034
  in travelers, 2802
  treatment, 2036–2037, 2037t
    antimicrobials of choice, 202t
    cephalosporins, 255t
    chloramphenicol, 312t
    penicillins, 237t
    quinolones, 367t, 371
    sulfonamides, 355t
    tetracyclines, 308t
    trimethoprim, 357, 360
  *vir*R locus, 24
  virulence regulation, 23t, 24
  waterborne, 1015–1016, 1016t
Shigella dysenteriae
  cyclic pattern of disease, 2034
  cytotoxin, 950
  enterotoxin, 950
  and hemolytic-uremic syndrome, 6
  toxin, 3t, 6, 22t, 2034
  virulence determinants, 22t, 22–23
Shigella flexneri
  cyclic pattern of disease, 2034
  enterotoxin, 950
  gastric acidity and, 947
  invasiveness, 951–952
  MXi/Spa protein, 24
  toxin, 2034
Shigella sonnei
  clones, 21, 21t
  cyclic pattern of disease, 2034

enterotoxin, 950
invasiveness, 952
toxin, 2034
Shinbone fever, 1741
Shingles, 1345, 1346–1347, 1348, 1349.
See also Varicella-zoster virus
Shock
"cold," 693
Neisseria meningitidis and, 1901,
1904
septic. *See also* Septic shock
defined, 690t, 691
"warm," 693
"Shock lung," 693. *See also* Adult respiratory distress syndrome
Short bowel syndrome: and anaerobes,
2160
Shoulder: infectious arthritis, 1033,
1033t
SHV-1 β-lactamase, 217, 251, 268,
268t
SHV-2 β-lactamase, 217, 268t
SHV-3 β-lactamase, 216t, 268t
SHV-4 β-lactamase, 217, 268t
SHV-5 β-lactamase, 216t, 217, 268t
Sialadenitis, 603
Siberian tick typhus, 1727
Sickle cell disease
and antibody deficiencies, 53
Bacillus infections and, 1890
differential diagnosis
peritonitis, 714
rheumatic fever, 1803
and hepatitis, 1139
crisis and, 1149
Mycoplasma pneumoniae and, 1707,
1707f
osteomyelitis and, 1049
and *Salmonella*, 2019, 2023
and *Streptococcus pneumoniae*: vaccination, 1822–1823
Sickle cell hemoglobin: and
Plasmodium, 2417–2418
protective effects, 2418, 2420f
Siderophores, 1753
Sigmodon: and South American hemorrhagic fevers, 1573t, 1574
Sigmoidoscopy: and endocarditis, 743t,
794t
Silicosis pneumonia
chronic, 648
radiology, 650t
Silicotuberculosis, 2225, 2231
Silver nitrate: for burn wounds, 2762,
2764t
Silver sulfadiazine, 355, 384t
for burn wounds, 2763, 2764, 2764t
Simian immunodeficiency virus (SIV),
1591
genomic organization, 1593f
and HIV vaccine research, 1301
taxonomy, 1585f
Simian T-cell leukemia virus, 1579,
1591
Simulium: and onchocerciasis, 2535
Sindbis virus, 1455
arthritis, 1036, 1036t
differential diagnosis, 1472
epidemiology, 1456, 1457
pathogenesis, 1457
receptor, 1317t
Sinus histiocytosis with massive
lymphadenopathy: HHV-6
and, 1378
Sinusitis, 585–590

actinomycosis, 2282
anaerobic, 2163t, 2164
gram-negative bacilli, 2198
antibody deficiencies and, 49
Aspergillus, 2307
Chlamydia pneumoniae, 1698
clinical presentation, 586–587,
587f
dark-walled fungi, 2391
diagnosis, 587–588, 588f
epidemiology, 585–586
etiology, 585, 585t, 586t
frontoethmoidal
and brain abscess, 888, 888t
and subdural empyema, 900
Haemophilus influenzae, 2043
maxillary, 601
Moraxella catarrhalis, 1927
paranasal: and orbital cellulitis,1132
pathogenesis, 586
prevention, 589
Pseudomonas aeruginosa, 1991
treatment, 1991
rhinovirus, 1659
sphenoidal
and brain abscess, 888, 888t
and subdural empyema, 900
Streptococcus pneumoniae, 1818
in traumatized patient, 2757
treatment, 588–589
antimicrobial, 588–589
sinus lavage, 589
surgical, 589
Sinus lavage, 589t
Sinus of Valsalva: mycotic aneurysms,
770
Sinus radiography, 587, 588f
Sipoma, 2379
Sisomicin, 280
combination therapy, 287t
source and chemistry, 280t
structure, 281f
Sixgun City virus, 1448
Sixth disease. *See* Exanthem subitum
Sjögren's syndrome
antibody deficiencies and, 49
keratoconjunctivitis, 1107
Skeletal infections. *See* Bone infections;
Joint infections;
Musculoskeletal infections
Skene's gland, 1085
Skenitis, 1085
Skin. *See also* Rashes; Skin lesions and
infections
acidity, 31
barrier to microorganisms, 31–32
host defense properties, 550–551
inflammation, 31
normal flora, 2159, 2159t
vaccinia complications, 1326–1327
Skin biopsy: meningitis, 867
Skin lesions and infections, 909–944.
See also Rashes; Soft tissue
infections *and specific*
infections
adult T-cell leukemia/lymphoma,
1581, 1581f
African histoplasmosis, 2348
amebic, 2411
anaerobic
cocci, 2205
gram-negative bacilli, 2199
treatment, 2201
Aspergillus, 2308, 2308f
bacillary angiomatosis in AIDS, 920

Bacillus anthracis, 913, 913f,
1887–1888
bacteremias and, 921–922
Haemophilus influenzae, 921–922
Neisseria gonorrhoeae, 921
Neisseria meningitidis, 921
Pseudomonas aeruginosa, 921
Salmonella typhi, 921
Staphylococcus aureus, 921
bartonellosis, 2211
Blastomyces dermatitidis, 550t, 552,
2355, 2356t, 2358–2359,
2359f, 2360f
Brucella, 2056
bubonic plague, 2072–2073, 2073f
bullous impetigo, 911
candidiasis (systemic) and, 922,
2293f, 2293–2294, 2294f
carbuncles, 912
cellulitis, 914–916
chancriform lesions, 913
chickenpox (VZV), 1347
chromomycosis, 2324, 2325f, 2326
Coccidioides immitis, 2369, 2369f
cryptococcosis, 2334, 2334f
differential diagnosis, 2336
diabetic foot, 919–920
diffuse erythema, 552
diphtheria, 916, 1870
in drug abusers, 2697–2698
ecthyma, 913
in the elderly, 2739
enanthem, 553
epidermal cysts, 920–921
erysipelas, 914
Erysipelothrix, 1895
erythema multiforme, 552t
erythema nodosum, 552t
erythrasma, 916–919
folliculitis, 912
Francisella tularensis, 2063
fungemias and, 922
furuncles, 912
gangrenous cellulitis, 917–919,
918t
genital, 1055–1063. *See also* Genital
lesions
gram-negative anaerobes, 2199
and granulocytopenia, 2678
herpesviruses, 1334t
hidradenitis suppurativa, 920
Histoplasma capsulatum, 2347, 2347f
treatment, 2351
HIV/AIDS and, 1228–1229
impetigo, 911
infectious gangrene, 917–919, 918t
infective endocarditis and, 922
leishmaniasis, 2434, 2435, 2436f,
2436–2437
and leukemia/lymphoma, 2679, 2682
Lyme disease, 2143, 2145–2146,
2146t, 2147
macular, 551–552
maculopapular, 551–552
melioidosis, 2005
membranous ulcers, 916
mucormycosis, 2315
mycetoma, 2327, 2328f
Mycobacterium tuberculosis,
2239–2240, 2240t
classification, 2240
Mycoplasma pneumoniae, 1706
nodular, 552
onchocerciasis, 2535–2536
papular, 551–552

Paracoccidioides brasiliensis, 2387
petechial purpuric, 553
pinta, 2135–2136, 2136f
post-traumatic opportunistic in the
immunocompromised, 920
Prototheca, 2391
Pseudomonas aeruginosa, 1996–1997
treatment, 1996–1997
pyodermas, primary, 909–919
Reiter syndrome, 1070–1072
schistosomiasis, 2539
secondary bacterial, 919–921
self-induced, 921
in sepsis, 692–693
in spinal cord injured patients, 2732t,
2734–2735
sporotrichosis, 2321f, 2321–2322,
2323f
staphylococcal scalded skin syndrome, 555, 911, 912f
staphylococcal scarlet fever, 911
Staphylococcus aureus, 1763–1767
localized, 1763f, 1763–1765,
1764f
with diffuse rash, 1765
management of localized, 1765
Streptobacillus moniliformis, 2085
streptococcal group C and G, 1854
Streptococcus agalactiae, 1840
Streptococcus pyogenes, 550t,
555–556
superficial, 909–922
ulcers, 919–920
systemic bacterial and mycotic
infections and, 921–922
toxic shock syndrome, 911–912
in transplant recipients, 2726, 2726t
treatment
aminoglycosides, 295t
quinolones, 372–373
verruga peruana, 2210
vesiculobullous eruptions, 552–553
yaws, 2134, 2134f, 2135f
Skin rashes. *See* Rashes *and specific*
rashes
Skin tests
for fever of unknown origin (FUO),
540–541
for pneumonia, 651
PPL, 275
purified protein derivative (PPD),
2219–2220. *See also* Purified
protein derivative (PPD) test
SLE. *See* Systemic lupus erythematosus
Sleeping sickness, 2450–2455. *See also*
Trypanosoma brucei
Slim disease. *See* Wasting syndrome
Slow-reacting substance of anaphylaxis,
96
SLT. *See* Shiga-like toxins
Small bowel. *See also* Gastrointestinal
infections
biopsy: for enteric infection diagnosis,
955
HIV/AIDS disorders, 1229–1230
transplantation: infections and, 2726
tuberculosis, 2238
Smallpox. *See* Variola virus
Smallpox vaccine, 2781
for travelers, 2797
Smoking
and chronic bronchitis, 608–609, 611
and surgical wound infections, 2746
Snail-borne disease: schistosomiasis,
2538t, 2538–2539

Snakes
    travel and, 2800
    venomous bites, 2767–2768
Snow Mountain virus, 1667, 1668
    characteristics, 1668, 1668t
    diagnosis, 1670–1671
    epidemiology, 1669
    food-borne, 1013
    waterborne, 1016
    winter vomiting disease, 968
Snowshoe hare virus: meningitis, 832
Sodium dichloroisocyanurate (NaDCC):
        for HIV disinfection,
        2583–2584
Sodoku, 2155
Soft tissue infections, 909–944. *See also*
        Skin lesions and infections
        and specific infections
    abscesses in the course of bacteremia,
        927
    Acinetobacter, 2011
    actinomycosis, 926, 2281
    Aeromonas, 2108
    anaerobic, 2163t, 2165–2166
        cocci, 2205
        gram-negative bacilli, 2199
        nonclostridial cellulitis, 923
        specimen collection, 2168t
        synergistic nonclostridial
            myonecrosis, 933
        treatment, 2201
    Bacillus, 1893
    Clostridium, 2185–2186
        anaerobic cellulitis, 923
        gas gangrene (clostridial myone-
            crosis), 931–933
    crepitant wounds: differential diagnosis,
        924t
    cysticercosis, 935
    in drug abusers, 2697–2698
    factitial (self-induced) abscesses, 926
    Fournier's gangrene, 925
    gram-negative anaerobes, 2199
    injection site abscesses, 926
    and leukemia/lymphoma, 2679, 2682
    lymphadenitis, 936–942. *See also*
        Lymphadenitis
    lymphangitis, 942, 943. *See also*
        Lymphangitis
    muscle degeneration, 933
    muscle proteolysis, 933
    myalgias, 934
        with eosinophilia, 934–935
        HIV, 934
        infective endocarditis, 934
        influenza, 934
        toxoplasmosis, 934
    myositis, 929–936
        Aeromonas hydrophila myonecrosis,
            933
        anaerobic streptococcal myonecrosis,
            933
        Cysticercus cellulosae, 933
        group A streptococcal, 930–931
        infected vascular gangrene, 933
        nonclostridial (crepitant), 933
        parasitic, 934–935
        synergistic nonclostridial anaerobic
            myonecrosis, 933
    necrotizing fasciitis, 923–926
    nonclostridial anaerobic cellulitis, 923
    osteomyelitis and, 926
    Pasteurella, 2069
    pleurodynia syndromes, 934
    Pseudomonas aeruginosa, 1996–1997

    treatment, 1996–1997
    psoas abscess, 933
    pyodermas
        primary, 926–927
        spreading, 1765
    pyomyositis, 929–930
    quinolones for, 372–373
    rhabdomyolysis, 933
    Salmonella, 2022–2023
    in spinal cord injured patients, 2732t,
        2734–2735
    Staphylococcus aureus, 1765
    streptococcal group C and G, 1854
    Streptococcus agalactiae, 1840
    subcutaneous tissue infections and
        abscesses, 922–927
    synergistic necrotizing cellulitis, 926
    trichinosis, 934
Somatostatin: and fever reduction, 532
Sore throat: and common cold, 564
Sorivudine, 431–432
    for EBV, 1372
    structure, 423f
    for VZV, 431–432
South African tick bite fever, 1725
South American blastomycosis,
        2386–2389. *See also*
        Paracoccidioides brasiliensis
South American hemorrhagic fevers,
        1572, 1573t, 1574, 1576, 1577
    characteristics, 1572, 1573t
    clinical manifestations, 1576
    diagnosis, 1576–1577
    epidemiology, 1574
South American trypanosomiasis. *See*
        Trypanosoma cruzi
Southampton virus, 1668
Southern hybridization, 27
Sparfloxacin
    antimicrobial activity, 367t, 369t
    for leprosy, 399
    structure, 365f
    for tuberculosis, 395
Sparganosis, 2544, 2545, 2545t, 2551
Specificity: in epidemiology, 159
Specimen collection and processing,
        169, 170t–171t
    CNS infections, 171t, 178t, 178–179
    diarrhea, 171t, 180–181
    genital infections, 171t, 181–183
    guidelines, 169–183
    intra-abdominal infections, 171t, 178
    musculoskeletal infections, 171t,
        179–180
    ocular infections, 171t, 183–184
    respiratory tract, 169–175, 170t, 172t
    septicemia, 170t–171t, 177–178
    urinary tract, 170t, 175–177
Spectinomycin
    antimicrobial activity, 285t, 286
    dosage, 510t–511t
    drug interactions, 525t
    for gonorrhea, 299
    pharmacology, 510t–511t
    source and chemistry, 280t
    structure, 281f
Spelunkers: histoplasmosis in,
        2341
Spermicides: and gonorrhea prevention,
        1923
Sphingobacterium, 2114
    classification and site of infection,
        2107t
Sphingobacterium multivorum, 2114
Sphingobacterium spiritivorum, 2114

Spinal cord. *See also* Central nervous
        system
    abscess: in drug abusers, 2704
    injuries, infections and, 2732–2737
        bacteremia, 2736
        evaluation, 2732t, 2732–2733
        fever, 2736
        intra-abdominal, 2735–2736
        osteomyelitis, 2735
        pneumonia, 2733
        predisposing factors, 2732
        skin and soft tissue infections,
            2734–2735
        urinary tract infections, 2733–2734
    relationship to brain, 822f, 822–824,
        823f
    vascular anatomy, 827
Spinal meninges: anatomy, 824, 824f
Spinal pachymeningitis, hypertrophic,
        906
Spinal paralytic poliomyelitis,
        1615–1616
Spinal subdural empyema, 902t, 902–903
    treatment, 902t
Spiramycin, 459t, 475
    dosage, 466t
        pediatric, 466t
Spirillar dysentery, 990
Spirillum minus, 2155–2156
    bacteriology, 2155
    clinical manifestations, 2156
    cutaneous manifestations, 550t
    diagnosis, 2156
    dysentery, 990
    endocarditis, 757
    enteric symptoms, 999t, 1002
    epidemiology, pathogenesis, and
        pathology, 2155–2156
    fever, 542
    lymphadenitis, 940t
    lymphangitis, 943
    therapy, 2156
Spirochetes, 2117–2156. *See also specif-
        ic spirochetes*
    antimicrobial therapy, 850t, 853–854
    Borrelia
        burgdorferi (Lyme disease),
            2143–2155
        relapsing fever, 2141–2143
    classification, 1752
    clinical presentation, 844
    diagnosis, 846–850
    and fever, 542
    Leptospira, 2137–2141
    Spirillum minus, 2155–2156
    transfusion-related, 2627
    Treponema carateum (pinta), 2133,
        2135–2136
    Treponema pallidum
        subsp. *endemicum* (bejel; endemic
            syphilis), 2133, 2136–2137
        subsp. *pallidum* (syphilis),
            2117–2133
        subsp. *pertenue* (yaws), 2133–2135
Spirometra mansonoides, 2545, 2545t,
        2551
Spleen
    abscess. *See* Splenic abscess
    Babesia and, 2498, 2499
    Candida albicans infection, 2298
    infarction: and endocarditis, 747
    rupture: EBV mononucleosis, 1368
    trauma, 2758–2759
Splendore-Hoeppli phenomenon, 2286,
        2327

Splenectomy
    and antibody deficiencies, 53
    Babesia and, 2498, 2499
    and infections in patients with neopla-
        sia, 2669–2670
    and *Streptococcus pneumoniae*
        infections, 1816
    in trauma patients, 2758–2759
Splenic abscess, 727
    bacteriology, 727
    clinical manifestations, 727
    diagnosis, 727, 728f
    in drug abusers, 2703
    etiology, 727
    pathogenesis, 727
    Salmonella, 2022
    treatment, 727
Splenic artery embolism: and endocar-
        ditis, 749
Splenomegaly
    endocarditis, 749
    in *Leishmania*, 2430, 2431
"Splinter" hemorrhages, 922
    endocarditis, 748
Spondweni: transmission, clinical
        syndromes, and geographic
        distribution, 1466t
Spondylitis
    Brucella, 2056
    tuberculous (Pott's disease),
        2236–2237
        treatment, 2237
Sporanox. *See* Itraconazole
Sporothrix cyanescens, 2321
Sporothrix schenckii, 2289, 2321–2324
    appearance in tissue, 2289t
    arthritis, 1035, 1035f, 1036f
        diagnosis, 1037
    clinical manifestations, 2321–2322
    conjunctivitis, 1105
    cutaneous manifestations, 552, 2321f,
        2321–2322
        and AIDS, 557
    description, 2321
    diagnosis, 2323, 2323f
    differential diagnosis, 2326, 2437
    endophthalmitis, 1123
    epidemiology, 2321
    extracutaneous, 2322, 2322f
        multifocal, 2322
    granulomatous lymphangitis, 943
    keratitis, 1113
    meningitis, 870
    musculoskeletal specimen collection,
        180
    oculoglandular syndrome, 938
    pneumonia
        chronic, 647t
        radiology, 650t
        serology, 193t
        sinusitis, 586t
        treatment, 2323
            amphotericin B, 406
Sporotrichosis, 2321–2324. *See also*
        Sporothrix schenckii
Spotted fevers: rickettsial, 1719, 1720t,
        1721–1727. *See also*
        Rickettsia rickettsii
Sprue
    temperate, 1028
    tropical, 1025–1030
Spumaviruses, 1580t
Sputum examination
    Aspergillus fumigatus, 176f, 2309
    Blastomyces dermatitidis, 2361

chronic bronchitis, 610
Coccidioides immitis, 175f, 2370
Klebsiella, 1972
microscopic, 172t, 184
Pneumocystis carinii, 2479
pneumonia
  acute, 622f, 622–624, 623f
  chronic, 651
  nosocomial, 2602
  Streptococcus pneumoniae,
    1819–1820, 1820f
specimen collection and processing,
  169, 170t, 173, 174f,
  175f–176f
Squamous cell carcinoma
differential diagnosis
  blastomycosis, 2356, 2359
  genital ulcers, 2211
  lung radiographs, 656f
  wart conversion to, 1383, 1389
src kinase, 118
SSKI: for sporotrichosis, 2323
Staphylococcal enterotoxins, 6, 1012t,
  1012–1013, 1795
cutaneous manifestations, 555
S. aureus, 530, 1760
Staphylococcal exfoliative toxin, 6,
  2224t
Staphylococcal infections, 1754–1784.
  See also individual species
and actinomycosis, 2280
antibacterial susceptibility testing,
  194t
blepharitis, 1130
  treatment, 1134
coagulase-negative, 1777–1784. *See
  also Staphylococcus epidermidis*
  quinolones for, 368t
  surgical wound infections, 2744t
coagulase-positive. *See
  Staphylococcus aureus*
endocarditis, 752t, 754–755
  treatment, 762–763
enterotoxins, 6, 555, 1012t,
  1012–1013, 1795
food-borne, 1012t, 1012–1013
  laboratory diagnosis, 1018, 1018t
keratitis, 1112, 1113
mediastinitis, 815t
meningitis, 835
  antimicrobial therapy, 850t, 853
orchitis, 1101
peritonitis, 708, 710
  vancomycin for, 350
prosthetic joints, 1052, 1052t
rifampin for, 318t, 322
S. aureus, 1754–1777. *See also
  Staphylococcus aureus*
S. epidermidis and other coagulase-
  organisms, 1777–1784. *See
  also Staphylococcus epidermidis*
vulvovaginitis, 1080
Staphylococcal protein A, 8
Staphylococcal scalded skin syndrome,
  911, 1765
  clinical features, 911, 912f
  and conjunctivitis, 1107
  differential diagnosis, 1765
  epidemiology, 1765
  lesions, 555
  treatment, 911
Staphylococcal scarlet fever, 555, 911
Staphylococcal toxins

enterotoxins, 6, 555, 1012t, 1012–1013,
  1795
  S. aureus, 530, 1760
  T cells and, 110
Staphylococci. *See also* Staphylococcal
  infections *and specific species*
β-lactamase, 215
growth, 186
resistance, 194
Staphylococcus aureus, 1754–1777
adhesion, 1760–1761
α-toxin, 1759
antibiotic susceptibility, 1755–1757.
  See also resistance *below*
  history, 1755–1756
  to other antibiotics, 1757
  to penicillin, 1755
  testing, 200–201
arthritis, 1032, 1033, 1034, 1034t
bacteremia
  in the elderly, 2739
  and skin infections, 921
β-lactamases, 1759
β-toxin, 1759
bites, 604
  animal, 2766
    susceptibility, 2766t
    treatment, 2767t
  human, 2768
blepharitis, 1130
  treatment, 1134
blood cultures, 177
and bone marrow transplantation,
  2719
botryomycosis, 557
brain abscess, 889
bullous impetigo, 555, 911
and burn wounds, 2762, 2762t
  treatment, 2764t
in cancer patients, 2668
carriers, 1757–1758
catalase, 1759
catheter-associated
  in cancer patients, 2670
  in trauma patients, 2758
and cell-mediated immunity, 1762
  defects, 2682
cellulitis, 914, 1765
cell wall: and infectivity, 1758f,
  1758–1759
and CGD, 155
chemotaxis defects and, 1762
and chronic granulomatous disease,
  92
clinical manifestations, 1755t,
  1762–1774
  overview, 1762–1763
clumping factor, 1759
coagulase, 1759
and complement activation, 41
conjunctivitis, 1104–1105
  neonatal, 1107
control measures, 1758
cutaneous manifestations, 550t, 557,
  1763–1767
  in drug abusers, 2697, 2698
  localized, 1763–1765
    with diffuse skin rash,
      1765–1767
    management, 1765
  in transplantation, 2726
and cystic fibrosis, 658–659
dacryoadenitis, 1131
dacryocystitis, 1131
  treatment, 1134

δ-toxin, 1759
dermatoblepharitis, 1130
in diabetics, 1762
dialysis-access AVFs, 790
in drug abusers, 2697, 2698
  cutaneous manifestations, 2697,
    2698
  endocarditis, 746, 756–757,
    2698–2699, 2700
  endophthalmitis, 2705
  mycotic aneurysms, 2701
endocarditis, 743, 744–745, 746, 754,
  1767–1770
  clinical manifestations, 1767–1768,
    1768f
  diagnosis, 1769
  in drug abusers, 746, 756–757,
    2698–2699, 2700
  echocardiography, 1769
  epidemiology, 1767
  heart pathology, 747
  laboratory findings, 750, 1768
  management, 1769–1770
  prosthetic valve, 784
  septicemia vs., 1768–1769, 1769t
  treatment, 762–763, 786
    rifampin, 321–322
endophthalmitis, 1121
  in drug abusers, 2705
  treatment, 1125
enterotoxins, 530, 1760
enzymes, 1759
epidemiology, 1757–1758
epidermal cysts, 920–921
epidermolytic toxins (ET),
  1759–1760
epidural abscess, 904, 905
exfoliatins, 1760
fibronectin and, 32
folliculitis, 912, 1763, 1763f
food-borne, 1012, 1774
  foods implicated, 1017t
furuncles/carbuncles, 914, 1763, 1764f
γ-toxin, 1759
and granulocytopenia, 2678
growth, 186
in heart transplantation, 2724
hepatic abscess, 724–725
and HIV, 557, 1235, 1235t
hordeolum, 1131
host determinants of infection,
  1760–1762
humoral immunity and, 1762
hyaluronidase, 1759
hydradenitis suppurativa, 1763–1764
identification, 1755, 1756t
in the immunocompromised: treatment, 2666
and immunodeficiency, 150t
impetigo, 909–910, 1763, 1764f
  treatment
    mupirocin, 386
    topical antibacterials, 382
injection site abscess, 926
intracellular killing, 1762
invasion, 1761
Job syndrome and, 156
keratitis, 1112, 1114
leukocidin, 1759
lung abscess, 643, 646
  treatment, 646
lymphadenitis, 940t
mastitis, 1764
mediastinitis, 815t

meningitis, 835
  antimicrobial therapy, 850t, 853
  in drug abusers, 2704
methicillin-resistant, 220, 240, 251,
  1758. *See also* resistance
    below
  and surgical wound infections,
    2748
  treatment
    in the immunocompromised,
      2666
    mupirocin, 385
    rifampin, 322
    vancomycin, 347, 349
MIC:MBC ratio, 1757
microbiology, 1755
  and infectivity, 1758–1760
morphology, 1755, 1756f
mycotic aneurysms, 770, 772
  in drug abusers, 2701
myocarditis, 800, 802
nasal carriage
  elimination, 1758
  rifampin for, 322
  topical antibacterials for, 383
necrotizing fasciitis, 923
necrotizing pneumonia, 643, 643f,
  646
in neutropenics, 2672t
neutrophil defect and, 153
nosocomial
  catheter-associated, 2670, 2758
  pneumonia, 2600
  prevention, 1758, 1758t
nuclease, 1759
opsonization, 1761
  defects, 1762
orbital cellulitis, 1132
organ infection, 1770–1774
osteomyelitis, 926, 1041, 1771–1773
  treatment, 1047–1048, 1048t
    rifampin, 322
otitis media, 581, 581t
pathogenicity, 20
peptidoglycan, 1758f, 1758–1759,
  1761
pericarditis, 1770
peritonitis, 719
phage susceptibility, 1757
and phagocytes, 88
pleural empyema, 637, 1770–1771
pneumonia, 619t, 621
  chronic, 647
  community-acquired, 628
  in the elderly, 2738
  and granulocytopenia, 2678
  hematogenous, 1770, 1771f
  and influenza virus, 1556t, 1557,
    1557t
  inhalation, 1770
  necrotizing, 644
  nosocomial, 2600
    in the immunocompromised, 631
  radiology, 626, 627f
  spinal cord injury and, 2733
  sputum analysis, 623f
  in trauma patients, 2757
  treatment, 632
polymorphonuclear leukocytes and,
  1762
polysaccharide layer, 1759
predisposing factors to infection, 1762
prevention: nosocomial, 1758, 1758t
primary pyodermas, 926–927
prosthetic joints, 1052, 1052t

Staphylococcus aureus (Continued)
protein A, 1759, 1761
pulmonary infections, 1770–1771
pyomyositis, 929–930, 1774
radionecrosis, 604
rashes, 555
resistance, 1756–1757, 2750. *See also
    methicillin-resistant above*
  to aminoglycosides, 283
  β-lactamase-mediated, 1756
  borderline oxacillin (borsa), 1757
  to clindamycin, 1757
  to erythromycin, 1757
  to fluoroquinolones, 1757
  intrinsic, 1756–1757
  to lincomycin, 1757
  to methicillin, 220, 240, 251
  to other antibiotics, 1757
  to quinolones, 366, 373
  to rifampin, 1757
  tolerance to killing action of
      β-lactam antibiotics, 1757
  transfer, 1757
right atrial catheters, indwelling, 788
scalded skin syndrome (SSSS), 555,
    1765
sepsis: in trauma patients, 2759
septic arthritis, 1773–1774
septic bursitis, 1774
septicemia, 1767–1770
  clinical manifestations, 1767–1768,
      1768f
  diagnosis, 1769
  echocardiography, 1769
  endocarditis vs., 1768–1769, 1769t
  epidemiology, 1767
  laboratory findings, 1768
  management, 1769–1770
septic vasculitis, 1770
sinusitis, 585
  in trauma patients, 2757
spinal subdural empyema, 902
splenic abscess, 727
spreading pyodermas, 1765
superantigens, 1760, 2568
suppurative intracranial phlebitis,
    907
suppurative lymphadenitis, 937–938
suppurative thrombophlebitis, 768
surgical wound infections, 2744,
    2744t, 2746, 2747, 2747t
symmetric peripheral gangrene, 553
teichoic acid, 1759, 1761
tolerance, 1757
toxic shock syndrome, 555, 1765–1767
  clinical manifestations, 1766,
      1766t, 1767f
  diagnosis, 1766t
  management and prevention, 1767
  menstrual, 1765–1766
  nonmenstrual, 1766
  pathogenic factors, 1766–1767
  toxin (TSST), 1759–1760
toxins, 6, 950, 1759–1760
  cytotoxicity, 951
  enterotoxins, 530, 1760
  and Kawasaki syndrome, 2568
tracheitis, 578
in trauma patients, 2757
treatment, 285t
  aminoglycosides, 286, 295t
    combination therapy, 287t, 289t
  antimicrobials of choice, 202t
  β-lactamase inhibitors, 268t
  cephalosporins, 255t, 257

chloramphenicol, 312t
clindamycin and lincomycin, 341,
    341t
erythromycin, 335t
fusidic acid, 278, 387
imipenem, 264t, 265
in the immunocompromised, 2666
neomycin, 384
penicillin MICs, 237t
quinolones, 368t, 372
rifampin, 318t, 322
sulfonamides, 355t
teicoplanin, 351
tetracyclines, 308t
trimethoprim, 358
vancomycin, 347, 349
urinary tract infections: in the elderly,
    2737
vaginal flora, 1074, 1080
vaginitis, 1080
vascular graft infections, 789t,
    789–790
virulence determinants, 22t
virulence regulation, 23t
wound infections, 1764–1765
  in trauma patients, 2758
Staphylococcus auricularis, 1778t
Staphylococcus capitis, 1777, 1778t
Staphylococcus caprae, 1778t
Staphylococcus cohnii, 1777, 1778t
Staphylococcus epidermidis, 1777–1784
  antibiotic susceptibility, 1778
  bacteremia
    in the elderly, 2739
    in the immunocompromised, 1781
    nosocomial, 1778–1779
  blepharoconjunctivitis, 1130
  and burn wounds, 2762, 2762t
  in cancer patients, 2668, 2670
  catheter-associated, 1779–1780
    in cancer patients, 2670
    peritoneal dialysis, 1780
    right atrial, 788
  clinical manifestations, 1777t,
      1778–1782
  colonization, 1778
  CSF shunt infections, 1780
  ecology, 1777
  endocarditis, 754–755, 1779
    prosthetic valve, 783–784
    renal pathology, 746
    treatment, 763, 786
    rifampin, 321
  endophthalmitis, 1125
  epidemiology, 1778
  epidural abscess, 904
  exopolysaccharide, 1778
  food-borne, 1013
  genetics and, 1777–1778
  and granulocytopenia, 2676, 2678
  growth, 186
  in heart transplantation, 2724
  identification, 1755, 1756t, 1777
  in the immunocompromised
    bacteremia, 1781
    treatment, 2666
  keratitis, 1112
  mediastinitis, 815t
  meningitis, 835
    antimicrobial therapy, 850t
    in neutropenics, 2672t
    nosocomial nature, 1778
  ocular infections, 1782
  osteomyelitis, 1049, 1781
  pediatric infections, 1782

peritonitis, 719
  peritoneal dialysis catheter-associ-
      ated, 1780
prosthetic joint infections, 1781–1782
resistance, 1777–1778
  erythromycin, 219
right atrial catheters, indwelling, 788
spinal subdural empyema, 902
suppurative intracranial phlebitis, 907
suppurative thrombophlebitis, 768
surgical wound infections, 2744,
    2746
in transplantation, 2726
treatment
  aminoglycosides, 295t
    combination therapy, 287t, 289t
  azithromycin, 335t
  β-lactamase inhibitors, 268t
  clarithromycin, 335t
  erythromycin, 335t
  fusidic acid, 278
  in the immunocompromised, 2666
  penicillin MICs, 237t
  rifampin, 318t, 321
  teicoplanin, 351
  trimethoprim, 357
  vancomycin, 347, 349
urinary tract infections, 1780t,
    1780–1781
  nosocomial, 2608–2609, 2609t
vascular graft infections, 789t,
    789–790, 1782
virulence factors, 1777–1778
Staphylococcus haemolyticus, 1777,
    1778t
  resistance, 1778
Staphylococcus hominis, 1778t
Staphylococcus intermedius
  animal bites, 2766, 2766t
  susceptibility, 2766t
Staphylococcus lugdunensis, 1777, 1778t
Staphylococcus pasteurii, 1778t
Staphylococcus saccharolyticus, 1777,
    1778t
Staphylococcus saprophyticus, 1755,
    1777, 1778t
  growth, 186
  identification, 1756t
  nitrofurantoin for, 377–378
  proteins, 1778
  urinary tract infections, 1778, 1780t,
      1780–1781
Staphylococcus schleiferi, 1778t
Staphylococcus simulans, 1777, 1778t
Staphylococcus warneri, 1777, 1778t
Staphylococcus xylosus, 1778t
Statistics: in epidemiology, 160
Stavudine, 432
  adverse reactions, 421t, 432, 1272
  drug interactions, 421t, 432
  for HIV, 1271t, 1272
  mechanism of action, 432
  resistance, 432
  spectrum of activity, 432
  structure, 420f
Steel factor: characteristics, sources, and
    effects, 115t
Stem cell factor (SCF), 113
  actions, 30t
Sterilization
  autoclave, 2579
  chemical, 2581
  defined, 2579
  flash, 2580
  gas, 2580–2581

heat, 2579–2580, 2580f
  for HIV material, 2643
  and nosocomial infection prevention,
      2579–2581, 2582t
Sternoarticular pyarthrosis: *Pseudomo-
    nas aeruginosa*, 1993
Sternoclavicular joint: infectious arthri-
    tis, 1033, 1033t
Stevens-Johnson syndrome
  from β-lactams, 272–273, 275
  defined, 551
  Mycoplasma pneumoniae and, 1706
Stibogluconate sodium, 477
Stibogluconate sodium (Pentostam), 459t
  for *Leishmania*, 2430, 2433, 2438
Still's disease
  fever and, 538, 538t, 539, 545
  keratopathy, 539
STM. *See* Streptomycin
Stomach. *See also* entries commencing
    with the term Gastric
  HIV/AIDS and disorders of,
      1229–1230
  normal flora, 2159t, 2160
  perforation: and peritonitis, 710
  tuberculosis, 2238
Stomatitis
  aphthous, 602–603
  and chronic granulomatous disease, 92
  gangrenous, 602
  in the immunocompromised, 603
Stonefish venom: cellulitis, 915
Stool examination, 180–181
  Balantidium coli, 2511
  Blastocystis hominis, 2511–2512
  blue-green algae, 2512
  Campylobacter, 1953, 1953f
  Cryptosporidium, 2506
  cultures, 955
  dysentery, 990
  Entamoeba histolytica, 2400,
      2401–2402
  enteric infections, 953–955
  food poisoning, 1018t
  and FUO, 539
  Giardia lamblia, 2487, 2489–2490
  hookworm, 2530
  intestinal flukes, 2542–2543
  intestinal tapeworms, 2547
  Isospora belli, 2511
  microsporidia, 2519–2520
  pH, 955
  Salmonella, 2015
  Vibrio cholerae, 1937, 1937t, 1938,
      1939
Stoxil. *See* Idoxuridine
Strand displacement amplification
    (SDA), 27
Stratum corneum, 550
Strawberry cervix: *Trichomonas
    vaginalis*, 2494
Strawberry tongue, 553, 1788
Streptidine, 281f
Streptobacillus moniliformis, 2084–2086
  arthritis, 1034
  bacteriology, 2085
  brain abscess, 890
  clinical manifestations, 2085
  cutaneous manifestations, 550t
  diagnosis, 2085–2086
  endocarditis, 756
  enteric symptoms, 999t, 1002
  epidemiology, 2085
  lymphadenitis, 940t
  therapy and prevention, 2086

Streptococcal infections, 1835–1845
  and actinomycosis, 2280
  agalactiae, 1835–1845. *See also*
      Streptococcus agalactiae
  alpha-hemolytic, 186, 1785, 1811
    in cancer patients, 2668
  anaerobic
    myonecrosis, 933
      differential diagnosis, 924t
    treatment
      antimicrobials of choice, 203t
      tetracyclines, 308t
  antibacterial susceptibility testing,
      194t
  antigen detection kits, 173
  anti-streptolysin O (ASO), 1786
  beta-hemolytic, 186, 1785,
      1852–1856. *See also* group C
      and group G *below*
    microbiology, 1852–1853
  bites, 604
  classification, 1784–1785
  clones, 21
  and complement, 65
  dacryoadenitis, 1131
  dacryocystitis, 1131
  endocarditis, 744t, 744–745, 752t,
      753–754
    treatment
      penicillin-resistant, 761–762
      penicillin-sensitive, 760
  enterococci, 1826–1831. *See also*
      Enterococcal infections
  fever and rash, 555–556
  gangrene, 917, 918t, 922, 923,
      1794–1795. *See also*
      Necrotizing fasciitis
    differential diagnosis, 918t
    scrotal, 925
  glomerulonephritis, 1805–1808
    clinical features, 1807
    diagnosis, 1807–1808
    epidemiology, 1806t, 1806–1807
    etiology, 1806
    history, 1805–1806
    laboratory findings, 1807
    pathology, 1806
    prevention, 1808
    prognosis, 1808
    therapy, 1808
  group A, 1785t, 1786–1799. *See also*
      Streptococcus pyogenes
  group B, 1785, 1835–1845. *See also*
      Streptococcus agalactiae
  group C, 1785t, 1852–1856. *See also*
      individual species
    arthritis, 1854
    bacteremia, 1855–1856
    classification, 1785t
    clinical manifestations, 1853–1856
    endocarditis, 1855
    epidemiology, 1853
    meningitis, 1855
    microbiology, 1852–1853, 1853t
    neonatal sepsis, 1855
    osteomyelitis, 1854
    pharyngitis, 1853–1854
      complications, 1854
    puerperal infections, 1855
    respiratory tract infections, 1855
    skin and soft tissue infections,
        1854
    therapy, 1856
  group D, 186, 1785t. *See also*
      Enterococcal infections

  classification, 1785t
  endocarditis, 752t, 753
  group G, 1853–1856. *See also*
      individual species
    arthritis, 1854
    bacteremia, 1855–1856
    classification, 1785t
    clinical manifestations, 1853–1856
    endocarditis, 1855
      in drug abusers, 2698
    epidemiology, 1853
    meningitis, 1855
    microbiology, 1853
    neonatal sepsis, 1855
    osteomyelitis, 1854
    pharyngitis, 1853–1854
      complications, 1854
    puerperal infections, 1855
    respiratory tract infections, 1855
    skin and soft tissue infections,
        1854
    therapy, 1856
  growth, 186
  intermedius group, 1785, 1861–1865.
      See also Streptococcus
      intermedius group
  and Kawasaki syndrome, 2568
  keratitis, 1112
  Lancefield classification, 1785, 1786,
      1827, 1835, 1852, 1853, 1861
  Leuconostoc, 1832
  mediastinitis, 815t
  microaerophilic, 2204–2206
    clinical manifestations, 2205
    treatment, 2205–2206
  M protein, 6, 110, 1754
    in neutropenics, 2672t
  nonhemolytic, 186, 1785
  nutritionally variant (deficient),
      1851–1852
  oral colonization, 593, 594t
  orchitis, 1101
  pharyngitis, 172–173
  pneumococcal, 1811–1826. *See also*
      Streptococcus pneumoniae
  prosthetic joints, 1052, 1052t
  pyogenes, 1786–1799. *See also*
      Streptococcus pyogenes
  rheumatic fever, 1799–1805
    clinical manifestations, 1802f,
        1802–1803
    diagnosis, 1803–1804, 1804t
    epidemiology, 1801–1802
    etiology, 1800–1801
    history, 1799–1800
    pathogenesis, 1800–1801
    pathology, 1801
    prevention, 1804–1805
    treatment and prognosis, 1804,
        1805t
  toxic strep syndrome, 555
  toxins, 6
  treatment. *See specific species*
  vascular graft, 789t
  viridans, 186, 1846–1851
    bacteremia, 1849
    and bone marrow transplantation,
        2719
    classification, 1785, 1785t, 1846,
        1846t
    clenched-fist injuries, 2768
    clinical manifestations, 1847–1850
    dental caries, 1847
    endocarditis, 752t, 753–754,
        1847–1849

    in addicts, 756
      prosthetic valve, 783–784
      treatment, 349–350, 1848,
          1848t
    epidemiology, 1846–1847
    fibronectin, 1847
    and granulocytopenia, 2678
    human bites, 2768
    identification, 1846, 1846t
    lipoteichoic acid (LTA), 1847
    meningitis, 1849–1850
    microbiology, 1846, 1846t
    pancreatic abscess, 723
    pathogenicity, 1847
    pneumonia, 1850
    prosthetic joints, 1052, 1052t
    resistance, 1851
    tolerance, 1851
    treatment, 1850–1851
      aminoglycosides, 295t
      chloramphenicol, 312t
      clindamycin, 341t, 341–342
      combination therapy, 287t,
          289t
      erythromycin, 335t
      penicillin, 237t, 241t
      rifampin, 318t
Streptococcal pyrogenic exotoxin (SPE),
    1787, 1788
  T cells and, 110
  and toxic shock syndrome, 1795
Streptococcal scarlet fever toxins, 6
Streptococcal toxic shock syndrome,
    923, 1793, 1795–1796. *See*
    also Toxic shock syndrome,
    Streptococcus pyogenes
Streptococcus adjacens, 1785t,
    1851–1852
  endocarditis, 754, 1851
  specimen collection and processing,
      177
  treatment, 1852
Streptococcus agalactiae, 1835–1845
  adult infections, 1839t, 1839–1841
  antigenic determinants, 1836, 1836t
  arthritis, 1840
  bacteremia
    adult, 1839
    in the elderly, 2739
    neonatal, 1838–1839
    treatment, 1841, 1841t
  CAMP test, 1835
  classification, 1785t, 1835
  clinical manifestations, 1838–1841
    in adults, 1839t, 1839–1841
    uncommon manifestations,
        1840–1841
  colonization, 1836t, 1836–1837
  description, 1835–1836
  diagnosis, 1841
  endocarditis, 754, 1840
    in drug abusers, 2698–2699
  epidemiology, 1836–1837
  erysipelas, 914
  female genital tract, 1840
  history, 1835
  identification, 1835
  incidence and serotype distribution,
      1837
  intra-amniotic infection syndrome,
      1090
  meningitis, 833t, 834, 834t
    antimicrobial therapy, 850t,
        852
    bacteremia, 838

    chemoprophylaxis, 857
    CSF examination, 846, 846t
    prevention, 857
  morphology, 1835
  neonatal infection, 1835, 1837
    early-onset, 1837, 1838–1839
    incidence, 1837
    late-onset, 1839
    prevention, 1842
    transmission, 1837
    treatment, 1841, 1841t
  osteomyelitis, 1041, 1840
    treatment, 1841
  pathogenesis, 1837–1838
  pneumonia, 1840
  postpartal
    bacteremia, 1839–1840
    endometritis, 1091, 1092
    incidence, 1837
  in pregnancy, 1836–1837. *See also*
      neonatal infection *above*
    diagnosis, 1841
    prevention, 1842
  prevention, 1842t, 1842–1843
  serology, 1835–1836, 1836t
  serotype I, 1836, 1836t, 1837
  serotype II, 1836, 1836t, 1837
  serotype III, 1836, 1836t, 1837, 1838
    and late-onset neonatal infection,
        1839
  sialic acid, 1838
  skin and soft tissue infections,
      1840
  Todd-Hewitt broth, 1835
  toxins, 530
  transmission, 1836–1837
    neonatal, 1837
  treatment, 1841t, 1841–1842
    aminopenicillins, 243
    antimicrobials of choice, 202t
    azithromycin, 335t
    cephalosporins, 255t
    chloramphenicol, 312t
    clarithromycin, 335t, 339
    erythromycin, 335t
    imipenem, 264, 264t
    nitrofurantoin, 377
    penicillin, 237t, 240, 241t
    quinolones, 368t
    rifampin, 318t
    tetracyclines, 308t
  vaccine research, 1843
Streptococcus anginosus, 1785t, 1846t,
    1847t, 1861–1865, 2204. *See*
    also Streptococcal infections,
    viridans
  brain abscess, 890
  differentiation, 1862f
  endocarditis, 754
  subdural empyema, 900
Streptococcus bovis, 1785t, 1832,
    1846
  biotypes, 1832
  and colon cancer, 1832
  endocarditis, 744t, 753, 1832
    treatment, 759–760
  treatment, 759–760, 1832
    antimicrobials of choice, 202t
    quinolones, 368t
Streptococcus constellatus, 1785t, 1846t,
    1847t, 1861–1865, 2204. *See*
    also Streptococcal infections,
    viridans
  and ARDS, 1863
  brain abscess, 890

Streptococcus constellatus (Continued)
  differentiation, 1862f
  growth, 186
Streptococcus crista, 1785t, 1846, 1846t,
    1847t. *See also* Streptococcal
    infections, viridans
  biochemical characteristics, 1847t
Streptococcus defectivus, 1785t,
    1851–1852
  endocarditis, 745, 753–754, 754, 1851
  specimen collection and processing,
    177
  treatment, 1852
Streptococcus dysgalactiae, 1852–1856,
    1853t. *See also* Streptococcal
    infections, group C
Streptococcus equi, 1852–1856, 1853t.
    See also Streptococcal infec-
    tions, group C
Streptococcus equisimilis, 1852–1856,
    1853t. *See also* Streptococcal
    infections, group C
  arthritis, 1854
Streptococcus gordonii, 1785t, 1846t,
    1847, 1847t. *See also* Strepto-
    coccal infections, viridans
  biochemical characteristics, 1847t
  tolerance, 1851
Streptococcus intermedius group, 1785t,
    1861–1865, 2204
  abdominal infections, 1863
  and ARDS, 1863
  bacteremia, 1862–1863
  bacteriology, 1861, 1861t
  brain abscess, 890
  clinical manifestations, 1862–1863
  CNS infections, 1863
  endocarditis, 1862–1863
  growth, 186
  normal habitat, 1861–1862
  oral infections, 1862
  pathogenicity, 1862
  taxonomy, 1861, 1862f
  therapy, 1863
  thoracic infections, 1863
Streptococcus milleri, 1846t, 1847t. *See
    also* Streptococcal infections,
    viridans
  in drug abusers, 2697
  endocarditis, 1847
  hypertrophic spinal pachymeningitis,
    906
  subdural empyema, 900
Streptococcus milleri group. *See
    Streptococcus intermedius*
    group
Streptococcus mitior, 1846t, 1847t. *See
    also* Streptococcal infections,
    viridans
  endocarditis, 753–754
  treatment, 759
Streptococcus mitis, 1785t, 1846, 1846t.
    See also Streptococcal infec-
    tions, viridans
  biochemical characteristics, 1847t
  endocarditis, 744, 744t, 753–755, 1847
  and granulocytopenia, 2676
  meningitis, 1849
  oral colonization, 593, 594t, 1846
  periodontitis, 594
*Streptococcus morbillorum. See Gemella
    morbillorum*
Streptococcus mutans, 1785t, 1846,
    1846t, 1847t. *See also* Strepto-
    coccal infections, viridans

adherence, 31
biochemical characteristics, 1847t
and dental caries, 593
endocarditis, 744, 744t, 745, 753–754
oral colonization, 593, 594t
Streptococcus oralis, 1785t, 1846, 1846t,
    1847t. *See also* Streptococcal
    infections, viridans
  biochemical characteristics, 1847t
Streptococcus parasanguis, 1785t, 1846t,
    1847t. *See also* Streptococcal
    infections, viridans
  biochemical characteristics, 1847t
Streptococcus parvulus, 2204
Streptococcus pneumoniae, 1785t,
    1811–1826
  acute phase reactants, 1811
  agammaglobulinemia and, 1816,
    1817t
  agglutination tests, 185
  alcoholism and, 1817, 1817t
  antibiotic susceptibility, 1821–1822
  antibody deficiencies and, 49, 1816,
    1817t
  antibody to pneumococcal capsule,
    1814–1816, 1815f, 1816f
  arthritis, 1034, 1034t
  autolysin, 1814
  bacteremia, 1813
    in the elderly, 2739
  brain abscess, 889
  and C3 deficiency, 69
  and cell-mediated immune defects,
    2681
    therapy, 2682
  cellulitis, 915
  cell wall polysaccharides (CWPS),
    1815
  and chronic bronchitis, 610
  clinical manifestations, 1817–1821
  colonization, 1813, 1816
  complement and, 72
    activation, 1814
    deficiencies, 67, 1816, 1817t
  conjunctivitis, 1104–1105
    neonatal, 1107
  C-reactive proteins, 1811
  Danish numbering system, 1812
  in the elderly, 1817, 1817t
  endocarditis, 754, 1821
    treatment, 764
  enteric symptoms, 999t
  epidemiology, 1812–1813, 1813f
  epidural abscess, 904–905
  E-test, 195
  and granulocytopenia, 2676, 2678
  growth, 185, 186
  history, 1811
  and HIV/AIDS, 1221, 1235, 1235t,
    1816, 1817t
    pneumonia, 629, 1183
    prophylaxis, 1286t, 1823
  host defense mechanisms, 1814–1816
  identification, 186
  and IgA, 8
  in the immunocompromised host,
    1815
  and immunodeficiency, 150t
  Job syndrome and, 156
  laryngitis, 573t
  and leukemia, chronic lymphocytic,
    2673
  meningitis, 833t, 834, 834t, 1818
    antimicrobial therapy, 850t, 852
    bacteremia, 838

blood-brain barrier alteration, 839
chemoprophylaxis, 857
clinical presentation, 843
CSF examination, 845–846, 846t
in the elderly, 2740
immunology, 1814
immunoprophylaxis, 858
intracranial hypertension, 841
in trauma patients, 2758
microbiology, 1811–1812, 1812f
multiple myeloma and, 1816, 1817t,
    2669, 2673
myocarditis, 800
neonatal bacteremia, 1813
neuraminidase, 1814
neutropenia and, 1817, 1817t
nosocomial, 1817, 1817t
opsonophagocytosis, 1814
orbital cellulitis, 1132
osteomyelitis, 1821
otitis media, 581, 581t, 582, 583,
    1812, 1818
pathogenic mechanisms, 1813–1814
peptidoglycan, 1811
pericarditis, 804, 1821
peritonitis, 708, 1821
and phagocytes, 88
pleural empyema, 637, 1818
pneumococcal surface protein (PspA),
    1814
pneumonia, 619t, 621, 1818–1821
  antigen detection, 625
  community-acquired, 628
  complications, 1821
  diagnosis, 1819, 1820f, 1821
  in drug abusers, 2701
  in the elderly, 2738
  and empyema, 1821
  and HIV/AIDS, 629, 1183
  immunology, 1814
  and influenza virus, 1556t, 1557,
    1557t
  nosocomial, 2600
  physical findings, 1819
  predisposing factors, 1818t
  radiology, 626, 626f, 627f, 1819
  serology, 625
  slowly resolving, 629
  spinal cord injury and, 2733
  sputum, 622, 622f, 1819–1820,
    1820f
  symptoms, 1818–1819
  treatment, 632–633
polysaccharide, 165
predisposing factors to infection,
    1816–1817, 1817t
prevention, 1822–1823, 1823f, 1823t
Quellung reaction, 1811
replication, 1813
resistance, 195, 220, 251, 1821–1822
septic arthritis, 1821
serotype 3, 1812
sinusitis, 585, 585t, 1818
spleen defenses, 1816
splenectomy and, 2669
subdural empyema, 900
suppurative intracranial phlebitis, 907
symmetric peripheral gangrene, 553
teichoic acid, 1811
in trauma patients, 2757
treatment, 1822
  aminoglycosides, 285t
  aminopenicillins, 243
  azithromycin, 335t, 339
  cephalosporins, 255t, 257–258

chloramphenicol, 312t
clarithromycin, 335t, 339
clindamycin, 341t
erythromycin, 335t, 338t
imipenem, 264, 264t
methicillin, 240
penicillin, 237t, 240, 241t
quinolones, 368t, 372
rifampin, 318t
sulfonamides, 355t
teicoplanin, 351
tetracyclines, 308t
trimethoprim, 357
vancomycin, 347, 349
vaccine, 858, 1815, 1816, 1816f,
    1822–1823, 1823f, 1823t
Streptococcus pyogenes, 1786–1799
  amylase, 1787
  bacteremia, 1796–1797
  carriage: rifampin for, 322
  cellulitis, 914, 1794
  classification, 1785t
  clinical manifestations
    pharyngitis, 1788–1789
    pyoderma, 1792–1793, 1793f
  common cold, 562, 562t
  and complement activation, 41
  cutaneous manifestations, 550t,
    555–556
  dacryocystitis, 1131
  dermatoblepharitis, 1130
  description, 1786–1787
  differential diagnosis: EBV, 1372
  dracryocystitis
    treatment, 1134
  EIA diagnosis, 186
  endocarditis: in drug abusers,
    2698–2699
  epidemiology, 1793
    pharyngitis, 1787–1788, 1788f
    pyoderma, 1791–1792, 1792f
  erysipelas, 555, 914, 1130, 1793f,
    1793–1794
  erythrogenic toxin, 1787, 1788
  esterase, 1787
  extracellular products, 1787
  growth in culture, 1785f
  history, 1786
  human bites, 2768
  hyaluronidase, 1787
  identification, 186
  immune complexes, 42
  immunofluorescence, 184–185
  impetigo, 910
    treatment
      mupirocin, 386
      topical antibacterials, 382–383
  invasive, 1793–1794
    epidemiology, 1793
  lipoteichoic acid (LTA), 1787
  lymphadenitis, 940t
  lymphangitis, 942, 943, 1797
  M proteins, 1786f, 1786–1787, 1792,
    1793, 1800
    and glomerulonephritis, 1806
    and rheumatic fever, 1800–1801
  multilocus enzyme electrophoresis, 27
  myositis, 930–931, 1795, 1795f
  nasopharyngeal cultures, 169
  necrotizing fasciitis, 923, 1794–1795
  necrotizing myositis, 930–931
  nicotinamide adenine dinucleotidase
    (NADase), 1787
  opacity factor (OF), 1787
  orbital cellulitis, 1132

osteomyelitis, 1041
otitis media, 581, 581t
peritonitis, 708
and phagocytes, 88
pharyngitis, 566–567, 567t,
  1787–1791
  clinical manifestations, 568–569,
    1788–1789
  diagnosis, 569–570, 1789–1790
  epidemiology, 1787–1788, 1788f,
    1806, 1806t
  prevention, 571
  scarlet fever, 1788–1789
  suppurative complications, 1789
  treatment, 570–571, 1790–1791
pleural empyema, 637
pneumonia, 1797
  necrotizing, 644
proteinase, 1787
puerperal sepsis, 1797
pyoderma, 1791–1793
  clinical manifestations, 1792–1793,
    1793f
  complications, 1793
  epidemiology, 1791–1792, 1792f,
    1806, 1806t
  immunology, 1792
  therapy and prevention, 1793
rheumatic fever, 1800–1801
scarlet fever, 1788–1789
serology, 192t
somatic constituents, 1786f,
  1786–1787
streptococcal pyrogenic exotoxin
  (SPE), 1787, 1788
streptolysin O, 1787
suppurative lymphadenitis, 937
  axillary, 937
toxic shock syndrome, 27, 1793,
  1795–1796
  case definition, 1796t
  clinical manifestations, 1796
  management, 1796
  pathogenesis, 1795–1796
  therapy, 1796
toxins, 530
  and Kawasaki syndrome, 2568
tracheitis, 578
treatment
  aminoglycoside combination thera-
    py, 287t
  aminopenicillins, 243
  antimicrobials of choice, 202t
  azithromycin, 335t, 339
  cephalosporins, 255t
  chloramphenicol, 312t
  clarithromycin, 335t, 339
  clindamycin, 341, 341t, 341–342
  erythromycin, 335t
  imipenem, 264, 264t
  lincomycin, 341, 341t
  methicillin, 240
  penicillin, 237t, 241t
  quinolones, 368t
  rifampin, 318t, 322
  sulfonamides, 355t
  teicoplanin, 351
  tetracyclines, 308t
  trimethoprim, 357
virulence determinants, 22t
Streptococcus salivarius, 1785t, 1846,
  1846t, 1847t. *See also* Strepto-
    coccal infections, viridans
biochemical characteristics, 1847t
endocarditis, 1847

meningitis, 1849
oral colonization, 593, 594t
Streptococcus sanguis, 1785t, 1846,
  1846t, 1847t. *See also*
    Streptococcal infections, viri-
    dans
biochemical characteristics, 1847t
endocarditis, 744, 744t, 744–745, 745,
  1847
meningitis, 1849
oral colonization, 593, 594t
periodontitis, 594
resistance, 220
tolerance, 1851
Streptococcus sobrinus, 1785t, 1846. *See
  also* Streptococcal infections,
  viridans
Streptococcus suis: endocarditis, 754
Streptococcus vestibularis, 1785t, 1846t,
  1847t. *See also* Streptococcal
  infections, viridans
biochemical characteristics, 1847t
Streptococcus zooepidemicus,
  1852–1856, 1853t. *See also*
  Streptococcal infections,
  group C
arthritis, 1854
Streptolysin O, 1787
Streptomyces, 280, 280t
Streptomyces aureofaciens, 306
Streptomyces avermitilis, 481
Streptomyces capreolus, 394
Streptomyces fradiae, 384
Streptomyces lincolnensis, 341
Streptomyces mediterranei, 391
Streptomyces nodosus, 404
Streptomyces orientalis, 346
Streptomyces rimosus, 306
Streptomyces somaliensis, 2274
  mycetoma, 2327, 2328f, 2329f, 2330
Streptomyces venezuelae, 311
Streptomycin, 280
  adverse reactions, 393
  antimicrobial activity, 282, 285t, 286,
    296
  combination therapy, 287t
    for mycobacteria, 396t
    synergism, 207
  dosage, 297t, 393, 510t–511t,
    516t–517t
    antimycobacterial use, 516t–517t
    in children, 510t, 516t
    in hepatic or renal failure, 390t,
      517t
  for endocarditis
    culture-negative, 764
    prosthetic valve, 786
    streptococcal, 759, 761
  for enterococcal infections, 1831,
    1831t
  for *Francisella tularensis*, 2066
  for mycetoma, 2330
  for *Mycobacterium tuberculosis*, 393,
    2213, 2226, 2227, 2227t,
    2228, 2229, 2230
    resistance, 2226
  neuromuscular blockade, 295
  for nontuberculous mycobacteria, 396
  ototoxicity, 294
  pharmacology, 510t–511t, 516t–517t
  resistance, 200, 283
    enterococci, 1830, 1831
    Mycobacterium tuberculosis, 2226
  source and chemistry, 280t
  structure, 281f, 393

for *Yersinia pestis*, 2075
Stress: and host defense mechanisms, 35
String test: *Giardia lamblia*, 2490
Strongyloides fuelleborni: thiabendazole
  for, 480
Strongyloides stercoralis, 2530–2531
  brain abscess, 890
  and cell-mediated immune defects,
    2681
  clinical syndromes, 2530
  cutaneous larva migrans, 2555
  diagnosis, 955, 1005–1006, 1006t,
    2530
  diarrhea: in AIDS, 970, 970t
  epidemiology, 2530
  life cycle, 2530
  penetration, 7
  peritonitis, 712
  pneumonia, 631
    nosocomial in the immunocompro-
      mised, 631
  treatment, 466t, 2530–2531
    albendazole, 479
    mebendazole, 479
    thiabendazole, 480
  and tropical sprue, 1026
Strychnine poisoning: tetanus vs., 2176
Sty, 1130
Subacute sclerosing panencephalitis:
  measles and, 1124, 1520
Subaortic stenosis, idiopathic hypertrophic (IHSS): and infective
  endocarditis, 741–742
Subarachnoid space
  anatomy, 821–822
  bacterial survival in, 839–840
  induction of inflammation, 840–841
Subclavian artery: mycotic aneurysms,
  770
Subcutaneous abscesses: and chronic
  granulomatous disease, 92
Subcutaneous nodules: *Blastomyces dermatitidis*, 2356t, 2359
Subdural empyema, 900–903
  anaerobic, 2162, 2163t, 2164
  anatomy, 822f
  bacteriology, 900, 902t
  clinical features, 901
  diagnosis, 901, 901f
  differential diagnosis: brain abscess,
    891
  etiology and pathogenesis, 900
  in infants and children, 902, 902t
  pathology, 900
  prognosis, 902
  spinal, 902t, 902–903
  therapy, 901–902, 902t
Sublingual space infections, 598–600
Submandibular space infections,
  598–600
Subpectoral lymphadenitis, 938
Subphrenic abscess
  and fever, 541
  Streptococcus intermedius, 1863
Subtractive hybridization, 26
Succinimonas, 2158t
Succinivibrio, 2158t
Suckling mouse brain vaccine (SMBV),
  1534, 1536
Sucralfate: quinolone interaction with, 370
Suicide plasmid cloning vector, 26
Suipoxvirus, 1325
Sulbactam, 269
  adverse reactions, 269
  clinical use, 269–270

pharmacology, 269
structure, 269f
Sulconazole: topical, 401t
Sulfacarbamide, 354
Sulfacytine: pharmacology, 514t–515t
Sulfadiazine, 354, 356, 357t
  dosage, 514t–515t
  for *Neisseria meningitidis*, 1903t,
    1904
  for *Nocardia*, 2276
  for paracoccidioidomycosis, 2388
  pharmacology, 514t–515t
  for rheumatic fever, 1805
  structure, 354f
  for *Toxoplasma gondii*, 1283t, 1287,
    2467, 2468
    in HIV/AIDS, 2467, 2467t
  with trimethoprim, 359
Sulfadimethoxine, 355
Sulfadimidine, 354
  with trimethoprim, 359
Sulfadoxine, 355, 357t
  dosage, 514t–515t
  pharmacology, 514t–515t
Sulfaguanidine, 355
Sulfamethizole, 354
  dosage, 514t–515t
  pharmacology, 514t–515t
Sulfamethoxazole, 354, 357t
  dosage, 514t–515t
  pharmacology, 514t–515t
  resistance: *Salmonella*, 2027
  structure, 354f
  with trimethoprim. *See* Trimethoprim-
    sulfamethoxazole
Sulfamethoxypridazine, 355
Sulfamylon: for burn wounds, 2762,
  2764, 2764t
Sulfanilamide, 354, 354f
  and sugar level testing, 203
Sulfaphenazole: pharmacology, 514t–515t
Sulfasalazine: pharmacology, 514t–515t
Sulfathalidine, 355
  structure, 354f
Sulfisoxazole, 354, 356, 357t
  clinical use, 357
  dosage, 514t–515t
    in children, 514t
  pharmacology, 514t–515t
  structure, 354f
Sulfonamides, 354–357. *See also
  individual formulations*
  adverse reactions, 356
  alteration of target enzymes, 221
  antimicrobial activity, 355, 355t
  antiparasitic use, 459t, 473–475
  in breast milk, 204
  combination therapy
    synergism, 207
  derivation and nomenclature, 354–355
  distribution, 356, 357t
  drug interactions, 356–357, 525t
  hemolysis from: in G6PD deficiency,
    203
  limited to GI tract, 355
  long-acting, 355
  mechanism of action, 355
  medium-acting, 354
  for *Neisseria meningitidis*, 1903t,
    1904, 1905
  neutropenia from, 89
  for nontuberculous (atypical)
    mycobacteria, 396
  for *Paracoccidioides brasiliensis*,
    2388

Sulfonamides (Continued)
  pharmacologic tables, 514t–515t
  pharmacology, 356
  in renal insufficiency, 356
  resistance, 215t, 221, 355–356
  short-acting, 354
  structure, 354, 354f
  topical, 355
  uses, 357
Sulfoxone: for Mycobacterium leprae, 398–399
Sulfur granules: actinomycosis, 2285–2286
Sunstroke: travel and, 2800
Superantigens, 6
  bacterial, 1754
  Staphylococcus aureus, 1760, 2568
  T cells and, 110
Superior petrosal sinus thrombosis, 908, 908t
Superior sagittal sinus thrombosis, 908, 908t
Superoxide
  anion, 84
  formation, 84
  and neutrophils, 87
Suppurative thrombophlebitis, 765–769
  burn wounds and, 2764
  intracranial, 907–909
    clinical features, 907
    cortical vein, 907
    diagnosis, 907, 908f
    pathology, 907
    treatment, 907–908
    venous sinus, 907, 908t
Suppurative thyroiditis, 603
Supraglottitis, 590–593
Suprapubic aspiration: in urinary tract infections, 670
Suprapubic catheterization, 2611
Suramin, 459t, 476–478
  adverse reactions, 476
  dosage, 467t
  side effects, 2454
  for Trypanosoma brucei, 2454, 2454t
Surgery: prophylaxis recommendations, 2751t–2752t
Surgical wounds
  clean, 2744t
  clean-contaminated, 2744t
  contaminated, 2744t
  postoperative infections, 2742–2756
    aerobic species, 2744t
    airborne contamination, 2745t
    cutaneous bacteria and, 2744, 2745f
    determinants, 2743f, 2743–2748
    direct inoculation, 2745t
    hematologous-lymphatic seeding, 2745t
    host immunity and, 2746
    investigational models of pathophysiology, 2747t
    microenvironment and, 2746–2747, 2747t
    nonwound infections, 2748
    perioperative antibiotics, 2747–2748, 2749–2752
      recommendations, 2750, 2751t–2752t
      regimen selection, 2749
      resistance, 2748, 2748f
      side effects, 2750–2752
      timing and duration, 2749–2750
    prevention and control, 2743–2748
      in practice, 2748t, 2748–2753

species and sources, 2743–2745, 2744t, 2745t
Staphylococcus aureus, 1764–1765
surveillance, 2752–2753
virulence factors, 2746
upper respiratory tract infections, 603
Surveillance, 161–162
  active, 161
  community-based, 161–162
  hospital-wide, 2572
  and infection control, 2572
  passive, 161
  surgical wound infection, 2752–2753
  targeted, 2572
Susceptibility tests, 191–193
  for anaerobic bacteria, 2169–2171, 2170t
  guidelines for selection of agents, 194t
Sweat glands: hydradenitis suppurativa, 1763–1764
Swimmer's ear, 580, 1989
Swimmer's itch, 2557
Swine: microorganisms harbored by, 2792t
Swinepox, 1325
Sydenham's chorea: and rheumatic fever, 1801, 1803
Sylvest's disease, 1625–1626
Sylvilagus: and Francisella tularensis, 2061
Symbiotic host-parasite relationships, 30
Symmetrel. See Amantadine
Sympathomimetic amines: for sepsis syndrome, 700, 700t
Symphysis pubis infections: Pseudomonas aeruginosa, 1993
Synaptobrevin II
  botulinum toxin and, 5
  tetanus toxin and, 5
Synergism, 196
  combination therapy, 207f, 207–208
    aminoglycosides, 287, 287t
    in impaired hosts, 208
Synergistic necrotizing cellulitis, 926
  differential diagnosis, 918t, 924t
Synergistic nonclostridial anaerobic myonecrosis, 933
Synovial fluid examination: infectious arthritis, 1033
Syphilis, 2117–2133. See also Treponema pallidum
  endemic, 2133, 2136–2137
Systemic inflammatory response syndrome (SIRS): defined, 690t, 691
Systemic lupus erythematosus (SLE)
  antibody deficiencies and, 49
  chloroquine for, 470
  and complement deficiency, 72
    C3, 69
  defective chemotaxis in, 90
  differential diagnosis: rheumatic fever, 1803
  influenza vaccines and, 1562
  measles virus and, 1488
  myocarditis, 804t
  pharyngitis, 569
  pleural fluid, 640
  pneumonia, 647t

T
Tabanid flies: and loiasis, 2535
Tabes dorsalis
  differential diagnosis, 714

Treponema pallidum, 2124
Tacaribe virus, 1572
Tache noire: rickettsial, 553, 1725
Taenia, 2525t, 2545t, 2547
  treatment, 2548
  mebendazole, 479
Taenia crassiceps, 2551
Taenia multiceps, 2545t, 2551
Taenia saginata, 2525t, 2545t, 2547
  diagnosis, 2547, 2548
  treatment, 466t, 2547, 2548
    niclosamide, 483
    praziquantel, 482
Taenia serialis, 2551
Taenia solium, 2525t, 2545t
  anatomy, 2546f
  diagnosis, 2547, 2548, 2549
  intestinal, 2547
  invasive, 2548–2550
  meningitis, 870
  treatment, 466t, 2547, 2548, 2549
    praziquantel, 482
Tamiami virus, 1572
Tamm-Horsfall protein (THP), 32, 666
Tampons
  and toxic shock syndrome, 1765, 1767
  and vaginitis, 1080
Tanapox virus, 1325, 1330
Tapeworms, 2525t, 2544–2553, 2545t. See also Cestodes
  beef. See Taenia saginata
  diagnosis, 2547–2548
  dog. See Dipylidium caninum
  dwarf. See Hymenolepis nana
  fish. See Diphyllobothrium latum
  treatment, 466t, 483, 2548
TAP1 gene, 103, 103f
TAP 2 gene, 103, 103f
Tarbadillo. See Typhus, epidemic
Tatumella ptyseos, 1975t
Taunton virus, 1667, 1668
  characteristics, 1668t
  winter vomiting disease, 968
Tazicef. See Ceftazidime
Tazidime. See Ceftazidime
Tazobactam, 270. See also Piperacillin-tazobactam
  clinical use, 270
  pharmacology, 270
  structure, 270f
T-cell antigen receptors (TCR), 105–106
  allelic exclusion, 106
  α chain, 105, 106
  β chain, 105, 106
  negative selection, 106–107
  positive selection, 106–107
  and T cell activation, 109–110
  and thymocyte selection, 106–107
T cells, 34, 102, 105–112, 119–120, 121t
  abnormalities: and HIV, 1205–1209
    See also CD4+ below
  activation
    by microbial superantigens, 110–111
    phenotypical and functional changes and, 111
    TCR complex and, 109–110
  adhesion receptor–ligand pairs and, 107–108
  aging and, 133
  alternative activation pathway, 108
  antigen receptor complex, 105
  and antimicrobial activity of immunity, 120–122, 121t
  APC ligand pairs and, 108–109

B7/BB1, 108–109
  and B cell activation, 119–120
    dependent, 47
    independent, 47
  B cell antigen presentation, 36
  CD4+, 102, 108, 121–122
    and HIV
      binding, 12, 12t, 13, 14–15, 15f
      depletion, 1205f, 1205–1208, 1206t, 1207f
      functional impairment, 1208
      measures, 1175, 1175t, 1182
  CD8+, 108, 121–122
    abnormalities: and HIV, 1208–1209
    and HIV suppression, 1214
  CD28, 108–109
  count assays, 150, 152
  counterimmunomodulatory functions, 120
  cytokine role in proliferation and maturation of, 118–119
  cytokines produced by, 116
  cytotoxic, 108, 121–122. See also CD8 and HIV, 1213–1214
  deficiencies, 151t. See also Cell-mediated immunity, deficiencies
    antibody deficiencies and, 52–53
    CD4+: and HIV, 1205f, 1205–1208, 1206t, 1207f
    from immunosuppressive therapy, 136
    and viral infections, 128–129
  deficiency, 132–135
  double-negative, 105
  γδ, 34
  generation of T-cell receptor diversity, 105–106
  helper, 108, 116. See also CD4
    and cytokines, 116
    and HIV, 1208
    TH-1, 1208
      and immunization, 2771
      proliferation, 118–119
      protection from infection, 121t
    TH-2, 1208
      and helminthic infections, 96
      and immunization, 2771
      proliferation, 118–119
  helper precursors (THp), 116
  lymphocyte adhesion molecules in trafficking and recirculation, 111–112
  memory, 111, 112, 132
  in mucosal immune system, 112
  and peptides, 107
  postselection maturation, 107
  protection from viruses, 128–129
  scanning surface MHC molecules for foreign peptides, 107
  suppression, 120
  thymocytes
    development, 105f, 105–106
    growth and differentiation factors, 107
    selection via surface αβ-T-cell receptors, 106–107
  triple-negative, 105
  virgin, 111
Technetium-99m studies
  brain abscess, 891–892, 892
  cholecystitis, 731
  and FUO, 540
  hepatic abscess, 725, 725f
  osteomyelitis, 1044–1045
  splenic abscess, 727, 728f

Teeth
  bacterial colonization, 593, 594t
  tetracycline staining, 201, 309–310
Teichoic acid
  gram-positive bacteria, 1753
  Staphylococcus aureus, 1759, 1761
  Streptococcus pneumoniae, 1811
Teichomycin A. *See* Teicoplanin
Teichuronic acid, 1753
Teicoplanin, 350–352
  adverse reactions, 351
  and aminoglycosides
    combination therapy, 287t
    nephrotoxicity, 292
  antibacterial activity, 351–352
  dosage, 514t–515t
    in children and neonates, 514t
    in renal dysfunction, 351
  for enterococcal infections, 1831
    endocarditis, 761
    resistance, 1830
  for meningitis, 853
  pharmacokinetics, 351
  pharmacologic tables, 514t–515t
  resistance, 220
    enterococci, 1830
  uses, 351–352
Temafloxacin
  adverse reactions, 374
  structure, 365f
TEM-1 β-lactamase, 217, 218, 251, 268,
    268t
TEM-2 β-lactamase, 216t, 251, 268, 268t
TEM-3 β-lactamase, 217, 268t
TEM-10 β-lactamase, 217
TEM-12 β-lactamase, 217
Temocillin
  dosage, 506t–507t
    in renal disease, 238t, 507t
  pharmacology, 506–507t
Temperate sprue, 1028
Temperature
  core: hypothalamic control, 531
  exaggerated circadian rhythm, 548
  and microbial pathogenicity, 23t, 24
  oral, 531
  pattern of fever of unknown origin
    (FUO), 538
  rectal, 531
Temporal arteritis: and fever, 546
Tenosynovitis, infectious, 1033
Terbinafine, 404
  for dermatophytosis, 2382
  structure, 402f
  topical, 401t
Terconazole, 403
  dosage, 403t
  structure, 402f
Tertiary prevention of disease, 167–168
Testes
  anatomy and physiology, 1098, 1098f
  carcinoma: infections and, 2667
  leprosy, 2248
  orchitis, 1101
  tuberculosis, 2238
Tetanolysin, 2174
Tetanospasmin, 5, 2174. *See also*
    Tetanus toxin
Tetanus, 2173–2178. *See also*
    Clostridium tetani
Tetanus-diphtheria vaccine, 2177. *See
    also* Tetanus toxoid, vaccine
  DTP, 2082, 2771, 2775, 2775t. *See
    also* DTP vaccine
  for travelers, 2797t, 2798

Tetanus immunoglobulin, 167, 454,
    2176, 2770, 2783
Tetanus toxin, 2, 4, 5, 22t, 2174
  neuritis, 878
Tetanus toxoid
  antibody response, 50
  vaccine, 2177, 2192, 2775t, 2780t,
    2781, 2782t
    DTP, 2082, 2771, 2775, 2775t,
    2778–2779. *See also* DTP
    vaccine
    morbidity reduction, 2772t
    recommendations for adults,
    2784t
    reportable events, 2786t
tetM resistance gene, 220
Tetracyclines, 206, 306–310
  adverse reactions, 201, 309–310
    in pregnancy, 204
  for amebiasis, 2404t
  antibiotic-associated colitis (AAC)
    from, 979
  antiparasitic use, 459t, 472
    dosage, 461t, 462t, 464t
      pediatric, 461t, 464t
  for bartonellosis, 2212
  Borrelia relapsing fever, 2142
  for *Chlamydia psittaci*, 1695
  for *Coxiella burnetii*: pneumonia,
    1729
  for cystic fibrosis infections, 660
  dosage, 307t, 512t–513t
    antiparasitic use, 461t, 462t, 464t
      pediatric, 461t, 464t
    for malaria, 464t
    pediatric, 512t
      antiparasitic use, 461t, 464t
    in renal dysfunction, 204–205,
    513t
  drug interactions, 310, 526t
  for *Francisella tularensis*, 2066
  for *Helicobacter pylori*, 1961
  for *Legionella pneumophila*, 2093,
    2093t
  for leptospirosis, 2140
  major indications, 310, 311t
  mechanism of action, 307
  minimum inhibitory concentration
    for aerobic and facultative anaero-
    bic infections, 308t
    for anaerobic infections, 308t
  for *Mycoplasma pneumoniae*, 1710,
    1710t, 1711
  nomenclature and brand names,
    306–307
  for nontuberculous (atypical)
    mycobacteria, 396
  for periodontitis, 601
  for peritonitis, 716
  pharmacokinetics, 309t
  pharmacologic tables, 512t–513t
  pharmacology, 308–309
  for PID, 1096t
  for *Pseudomonas pseudomallei*, 2006
  for rat-bite fever, 2086
  in renal dysfunction, 309
    dosage, 204–205, 513t
  resistance, 214, 215t, 219, 220,
    307–308
    coagulase-negative staphylococci,
    1778
    Neisseria gonorrhoeae, 1914,
    1914f
    Salmonella, 2027
    Streptococcus agalactiae, 1841

Streptococcus pneumoniae, 1821
    transposon, 214
  for *Rickettsia prowazekii* (louse-borne
    typhus), 1736
  for *Rickettsia rickettsii*, 1724
  for scrub typhus, 1741
  structure, 306–307, 307f
  and sugar level testing, 204
  susceptibility testing, 194t
  tissue distribution, 309
  topical, 384t
  for *Toxoplasma gondii*, 2469
  for urethritis, 1069–1070
  for *Vibrio cholerae*, 1939, 1943
  in vitro activity, 307–308, 308t
  for *Yersinia pestis*, 2075
Texas cattle fever, 2497
TFT. *See* Trifluridine
TGF. *See* Tumor growth factor-β
Thalidomide: for erythema nodosum
    leprosum, 399, 2247
Thayer-Martin medium (MTM), 182
Theophylline
  adverse reactions: influenza vaccine
    and, 1561
  drug interactions
    erythromycin, 337
    isoniazid, 390
    quinolones, 370
Thermoregulatory center: of hypo-
    thalamus, 531
Thiabendazole, 460t, 480
  adverse reactions, 480
  dosage, 461t, 462t, 466t
    pediatric, 461t, 462t, 466t
  for dracunculiasis, 2533
  drug interactions, 526t
  spectrum of activity, 480
  for strongyloidiasis, 2530
Thiacetazone
  dosage: in hepatic or renal failure,
    390t
  for *Mycobacterium leprae*, 399
  for *Mycobacterium tuberculosis*, 389,
    395
Thiamphenical, 311
Third disease. *See* Rubella virus
Thoracic aorta: mycotic aneurysms, 770
Thoracic infections
  actinomycosis, 2282f, 2282–2283
  Streptococcus intermedius group,
    1863
Thoracoscopy
  for pleural empyema, 640
  pneumonia, 625
3TC (lamivudine), 437t
Throat
  infections. *See specific infections*
  microscopic examination of
    pathogens, 172t
  specimen collection and processing,
    169, 170t, 172–173
  streptococcal cultures, 1789–1790
Thrombocytopenia
  and acute retroviral syndrome (HIV),
    1224t
  CMV, 1358
  EBV, 1368, 1370
  herpesviruses, 1334t
  immune: HIV/AIDS and,
    1225–1226
  rubella, 1461
Thrombocytopenic purpura
  immune: immunoglobulin for, 454
  thrombotic: and HIV, 1226

Thrombocytosis: from cephalosporins,
    254
Thrombophlebitis
  from cephalosporins, 253
  puerperal ovarian vein (POVT),
    1091–1092
Thrombophlebitis, suppurative, 765–769
  intracranial, 907–909
    bacteriology, 902t
    clinical features, 907
    cortical vein, 907
    diagnosis, 908, 908f
    pathology, 907
    treatment, 908
    venous sinus, 908, 908t
  jugular, 600
  and lung abscess, 644–645
  pelvic, 1095
Thrush. *See Candida albicans,* oral
Thymocytes. *See also* T cells
  development, 105f, 105–106
  growth and differentiation factors,
    107
  selection via surface αβ-T-cell recep-
    tors, 106–107
Thymomas
  antibody deficiency and, 53
  immunodeficiency and, 137
Thymosin, 455–456
Thyroglossal duct cysts, 604
Thyroiditis
  and fever, 545
  suppurative, 603, 604
Ticarcillin, 244–245
  adverse reactions, 239t, 244–245
  antibiotic-associated colitis (AAC),
    979
  antimicrobial spectrum, 241t, 285t
  for bacilli and anaerobes, 237t
  combination therapy
    aminoglycosides, 289t
    synergism, 208
  dosage, 241t, 506t–507t
    in children, 506t
    in neonates, 242t, 506t
    in renal disease, 204, 238t, 507t
  for Enterobacteriaceae and
    Pseudomonas, 237t
  MICs against cocci, 237t
  for peritonitis, 716
  pharmacokinetics, 238t
  pharmacology, 506–507t
    animal models, 226
  for *Pseudomonas aeruginosa* endo-
    carditis, 1984
  structure, 244f
  teratogenicity, 204
Ticarcillin-clavulanate, 269
  antimicrobial activity, 285t
  for *Bacteroides fragilis*, 2200t, 2201
  dosage, 506t–507t
  for odontogenic infections, 602t
  for peritonitis, 716
  pharmacology, 506–507t
  for pyelonephritis, 676
  for sepsis syndrome, 699, 699t
Tick bites, 2565–2566
  granuloma, 2565
  uncomplicated, 2565–2566
Tick-borne diseases, 2558t, 2565. *See
    also specific diseases*
  Babesia, 2498, 2500
  Borrelia burgdorferi, 2143, 2145,
    2565, 2566, 2566f
    prevention, 2152

Tick-borne diseases (*Continued*)
  Borrelia relapsing fever, 2141, 2143
  Colorado tick fever, 1446–1447
  Crimean-Congo hemorrhagic fever, 1568, 1568t
  ehrlichiosis, 1747t, 1748–1749, 2565
  encephalitis, 1466t, 1467, 1469, 1472
    clinical manifestations, 1472
    epidemiology, 1469
    history, 1467
    prevention and treatment, 1473
    transmission, clinical syndromes, and geographic distribution, 1466t
    vaccine: for travelers, 2799
  meningopolyneuritis, 2148
  rickettsial, 1720t, 1721, 1725, 2565. *See also* Rickettsial infections *and individual species*
  Rickettsia rickettsii, 1721
Tick paralysis, 2566
  differential diagnosis: botulism, 2181
Tick(s), 2565–2567
  clinical manifestations, 2565–2566
  epidemiology, 2565
  eradication and prevention, 2566
Tinea barbae, 2379
Tinea capitis, 2376, 2379–2380, 2380f
Tinea circinata, 2377
Tinea corporis, 2376, 2378, 2378f
Tinea cruris, 2376, 2378
Tinea faciei, 2379, 2379f
Tinea imbricata, 2377, 2378–2379, 2379f
Tinea incognito, 2377, 2379
Tinea infection: and HIV, 1229
Tinea manus, 2379
Tinea nigra, 2384–2385
Tinea pedis, 2376, 2377–2378
  differential diagnosis, 2378
Tinea versicolor, 2383–2384
Tinidazole, 468
  dosage, 461t, 467t
    pediatric, 461t, 463t, 467t
  for *Giardia lamblia*, 2490, 2490t
Tin poisoning, 1014
Tioconazole
  for dermatophytosis, 2382
  dosage, 403t
  for vulvovaginal candidiasis, 1076t
Tissierella, 2158t
Tissue concentrations: of antimicrobials, 205
Tissue injury: neutrophils and, 88
Tissue nematodes, 2531–2537. *See also* Nematodes, tissue
Tissue tropisms: host defense, 31
TLE-1 β-lactamase, 216t
TLE-2 β-lactamase, 216t
TNF-α. *See* Tumor necrosis factor-α
TNF-β. *See* Lymphotoxin
TOB-1 β-lactamase, 216t
Tobramycin, 280
  adverse reactions, 293, 294
  antimicrobial activity, 285t, 286, 296
  clinical trials, 227, 228
  combination therapy, 287t
    for mycobacteria, 396t
    synergism, 207
  for cystic fibrosis infections, 660
  dosage, 297t, 510t–511t

  in children and neonates, 299t, 510t, 851t
    for meningitis, 850t, 851t
    once daily, 299t
    in renal dysfunction, 298t, 511t
  neuromuscular blockade, 295
  ototoxicity, 294
  pharmacology, 510t–511t
  for *Pseudomonas aeruginosa*, 1984, 1994, 2004t
    endocarditis, 763
  resistance, 200, 220, 284, 284t
  for sepsis syndrome, 699, 699t
  source and chemistry, 280t
  structure, 281f
  susceptibility testing, 194
Toe web infection: *Pseudomonas aeruginosa*, 1997
Togaviridae, 1455–1465. *See also* *individual viruses*
  alphaviruses, 1455–1459
  arthritis, 1036t
  classification, 1315t
  rubella virus (German measles), 1459–1465
  shape and size, 1316f
  structure, 1455
Tolbutamide: sulfonamide interactions with, 356
Tolnaftate, 401
  structure, 402f
  topical, 401t
Toluidine blue stain, 184t
Tongue
  bacterial colonization, 593, 594t
  histoplasmosis, 2346, 2346f
  strawberry, 553, 1788
  viridans streptococci on, 1846
Tonsillectomy
  and endocarditis, 743t, 794t
  poliovirus and, 1617
  prophylaxis recommendations, 2751t
Tonsillitis, 643
  herpes simplex virus and, 1338
  and rheumatic fever, 1801
Topical antibacterials, 381–389. *See also* *specific drugs*
  for acne vulgaris, 383
  advantages, 382t
  agents in clinical use, 384t
  bacitracin, 383–384
  for burn wound infections, 383
  fusidic acid, 387
  general uses, 381–382
  mupirocin, 385–387
  neomycin, 384
  polymyxin B, 385
  prophylactic use, 382
    catheter-related infections, 382
    clean wounds, 382
    operative wounds, 382
  for pyodermas, 382–383
  for *S. aureus* nasal carriage, 383
  for skin disinfection, 381–382
Topical antifungals, 401–403
Topical sulfonamides, 355
Topoisomerases, 365
TORCH syndrome: differential diagnosis, 2462
Torula histolytica. *See Cryptococcus neoformans*
Torulopsis. *See Cryptococcus neoformans*
Torulopsis glabrata. *See Candida glabrata*
Tosufloxacin, 365f

Total hemolytic complement (CH$_{50}$) test, 156
Total parenteral nutrition: bacteremia from, 2592–2594, 2593t
Total protective environment: for cancer patients, 2692, 2692t
Toxic epidermal necrolysis (TEN), 911. *See also* Staphylococcal scalded skin syndrome
  differential diagnosis, 1765
Toxic erythema: and systemic infections, 551t
Toxic shock-like syndrome: influenza virus, 1558
Toxic shock syndrome
  differential diagnosis: measles virus, 1522
  rash, 555
  staphylococcal, 1765–1767
    clinical manifestations, 1766, 1766t, 1767f
    diagnosis, 1766t
    epidemiology, 162
    management and prevention, 1767
    menstrual, 1765–1766
    nonmenstrual, 1766
    pathogenic factors, 1766–1767
    skin infections, 911–912
    vaginal carriage, 1757
  strawberry tongue, 553
  Streptococcus pyogenes, 27, 555, 1793, 1795–1796
    case definition, 1796t
    clinical manifestations, 1796
    management, 1796
    pathogenesis, 1795–1796
    therapy, 1796
  vaginitis and, 1080
Toxic shock syndrome toxin (TSST), 6, 1759–1760, 1766
  and fever, 530
  and Kawasaki syndrome, 2568
  T cells and, 110
Toxins, 2–7, 22t. *See also specific toxins*
  anthrax, 3t, 4, 6, 1887
  antibody neutralization, 41
  attachment and entry, 4
    and gastrointestinal infections, 951
  bacterial, 1753
  bacteriocins, 7
  Bordetella pertussis, 3, 3t, 4, 6, 23, 23f, 23t, 2079
  characteristics, 3t
  classification, 2–3
  Clostridium botulinum, 2, 3t, 5, 878, 949t, 950, 1014, 2179, 2180
  Clostridium difficile, 6, 950, 979–980
  cytotoxins, 949t, 949–951
  diphtheria, 2, 3t, 4–5
  endotoxin, 2. *See also* Endotoxins
  enteric, 948–951, 949t
  Enterobacteriaceae, 1967–1968
  Escherichia coli, 3t, 5
    cytotoxins, 950, 1951
    enterotoxins, 948–950, 949t, 1967
      heat-labile, 1967–1968
      heat-stable, 1967
    heat-labile, 3, 3t, 4, 5, 22t
    heat-stable, 3t, 5, 22t
    shiga-like, 3t, 6, 22t
  exotoxin, 2. *See also* Exotoxins
    pyrogenic, 6. *See also* Pyrogenic exotoxins

  gastrointestinal infections, 949t, 949–951
  Helicobacter pylori, 6
  hemolysins, 7
  Legionella, 6–7
  Listeria monocytogenes, 7
  mechanism of action, 4–7
  neurotoxins, 949t, 949–951
  potency measurement, 7
  role in clinical disease, 4–7
  RTX (repeat in toxin), 7
  shiga, 6
  shiga-like, 6
  Shigella, 3t, 6, 22t, 2034
  staphylococcal, 6
  Staphylococcus aureus, 6, 530, 950, 1759–1760, 2568
  streptococcal, 6, 530
  structure, 2–3
  synthesis and release, 3–4
  tetanus, 2, 4, 5, 22t, 878, 2174
  Vibrio cholerae, 3t, 4, 5, 949t, 950, 1934–1935, 1936, 1936f
  zonula occludens (ZOT), 5
Toxocara, 2553t, 2553–2554. *See also* Visceral larva migrans
  endophthalmitis, 1124
  treatment, 1126
Toxocara canis
  clinical manifestations, 2554
  diagnosis, 1006t, 1006–1007, 2554
  differential diagnosis, 2554
  granulomatous hepatitis, 1161
  human infection, 2554
  life cycle in dog, 2553–2554
  ocular larva migrans, 2554
  visceral larva migrans, 2553t, 2553–2554
Toxocara cati
  diagnosis, 1006t, 1006–1007
  granulomatous hepatitis, 1161
  visceral larva migrans, 2553–2554
Toxoid: defined, 2770
Toxoplasma gondii, 2394t, 2455–2475
  acute disease
    clinical manifestations, 2459–2461
    treatment, 2466–2467
  agglutination test, 2463–2464
  animal reservoirs, 2792t
  and bone marrow transplantation, 2721
  bradyzoite, 2457
  brain abscess
    in HIV/AIDS, 887, 1237, 1239, 2458
    in the immunodeficient, 890, 896–897
  and cell-mediated immune defects, 2681
  cellular immunity and, 125
    deficiencies, 132, 133
  clinical manifestations, 2394t, 2459–2462
    acute, 2459–2461
    in the immunocompetent, 2459
    in the immunodeficient, 2459–2461. *See also* HIV/AIDS *below*
  CNS infection, 829
  congenital disease
    clinical manifestations, 2461–2462
    prevention, 2470

serology, 2465, 2470
treatment, 2468
cytokine and T cell protection, 121t,
126–127
description, 2456f, 2456–2457
diagnosis, 2395t, 2462–2466
agglutination test, 2463–2464
antigen demonstration, 2463
antigen-specific lymphocyte transformation, 2463
complement fixation test,
2463–2464
double-sandwich IgM ELISA,
2464
histologic, 2462
IFA, 2463
IgA ELISA, 2464
IgE ELISA, 2464
IgG avidity test, 2464
IgG ELISA, 2464
IgM-IFA, 2464
IgM immunosorbent assay, 2464
indirect hemagglutination, 2463
isolation, 2462
lymphocyte typing, 2463
polymerase chain reaction, 2463
Sabin-Feldman dye test, 2463
serology, 2463
differential diagnosis, 2460
EBV, 1372
scrub typhus, 1741
diffuse, 2458
endophthalmitis: treatment, 1126
epidemiology, 2457
and fever, 543
hairy cell leukemia and, 137
in heart transplantation, 2724
and HIV/AIDS, 1182, 1237–1238,
1238–1239, 2455, 2457–2461,
2462, 2464–2465
brain abscess, 887, 1237, 1239,
2458
chorioretinitis, 2459, 2460
clinical manifestations, 2459–2461,
2460f
CNS, 1238, 1239, 2459–2460,
2466–2467, 2467t
encephalitis, 1237, 1239, 2457,
2460, 2460f
incidence, 1182t
myocarditis, 2459
myositis, 2459
pneumonia, 1236, 2460
probability of developing, 1223f,
2458
prophylaxis, 1286t, 1286–1287
reactivation, 2458
retinitis, 1240, 2460
serology, 1238–1239, 2464–2465,
2469–2470
treatment, 131, 473, 1283t,
1286–1287, 2466f,
2466–2467, 2467t. See also
treatment below
immunity, 2457–2458
immunodeficiency and, 138
in the immunodeficient. See also
HIV/AIDS above
brain abscess, 890, 896–897
clinical manifestations, 2459–2461
meningitis, 872
nosocomial pneumonia, 631
serologic screening, 2469–2470
treatment, 2466f, 2466–2467, 2467t
invasion, 25

life cycle, 2456f, 2456–2457
lymphadenopathy, 940t, 2459
macrophages and, 124
myalgia, 934
myocarditis, 800, 802, 802f
neonatal infection, 133
NK cells and, 122
ocular disease
in the immunocompetent, 2461,
2461f
pathology, 2458–2459
serology, 2465
treatment, 2467–2468
oocyst, 2456
pathogenesis, 2457–2458
pathology, 2458–2459
pneumonia, 619t
and HIV/AIDS, 1236
in pregnancy
serology, 2465–2466
treatment, 2468
prevention, 2469–2470
prophylaxis, 1286–1287
pulmonary, 2458
retinochoroiditis, 1124
serology, 2463, 2464–2466
congenital disease, 2465
in the immunocompetent, 2464
in the immunodeficient, 2464–2465
ocular disease, 2465
in pregnancy, 2465–2466
and prevention, 2469–2470
sporozoites, 2455
tachyzoite, 2456, 2456f
tissue cyst, 2457
transfusion-related, 2627
transmission, 2394t, 2457
in transplant recipients, 2709, 2712,
2713t, 2729
diagnosis and control, 2713
treatment, 466t, 469, 1283t,
1286–1287, 2466–2469
aprinocid, 2469
atovaquone, 475, 2467, 2467t, 2469
azithromycin, 340, 475, 2467,
2467t, 2469
clarithromycin, 340, 2467, 2467t
clindamycin, 343, 475, 1283t,
1287, 2467, 2467t, 2468
combination therapy, 2467t, 2468,
2469
congenital disease, 2468
corticosteroids, 1286, 2467
dapsone, 2467, 2467t, 2469
doxycycline, 2467
folinic acid (folate), 2467, 2467t,
2468
hydroxynaphthoquinones, 2469
in the immunocompetent, 2466
in the immunodeficient, 2466f,
2466–2467, 2467t. See also
HIV/AIDS above
immunotherapy, 2469
interferon-γ, 2469
investigational, 2469
leucovorin, 1283t
macrolides-azalides, 2469
ocular disease, 2467–2468
Piritrexin, 2469
in pregnancy, 2468
pyrimethamine, 1283t, 1287
pyrimethamine/sulfadoxine
(Fansidar), 2467, 2467t, 2468,
2469
qinghaosu, 2469

roxithromycin, 475, 2469
specific drugs, 2468–2469
spiramycin, 475
sulfadiazine, 1283t, 1287
sulfonamides, 357, 473
tetracyclines, 2469
trimethoprim, 2469
trimethoprim-sulfamethoxazole,
360, 2469
trimetrexate, 475, 2469
ToxR protein, 24
TPHA test, 2127t, 2128
TPI test, 2127t, 2128
Trabulstella guamrnis (sp?), 1975t
Tracheal aspirates, 169, 170t
Tracheal cytotoxin, 6, 2079, 2080
Tracheitis, bacterial, 578
Tracheobronchial infections: diphtheria,
1869–1870
Tracheobronchitis
Acinetobacter, 2011
Mycoplasma pneumoniae, 1706
respiratory syncytial virus, 1504t,
1507–1508
Trachoma, 1106, 1114, 1679,
1683–1684. See also
Chlamydia trachomatis
clinical manifestations, 1683–1684
cytologic diagnosis, 1682
immunity, 1681
laboratory diagnosis, 1681–1682
pathogenesis, 1681
treatment, 1684
vaccine research, 1681
WHO grading system, 1683t
Transesophageal echocardiography
(TEE)
bacteremia from: and endocarditis,
794t
endocarditis, 751–752
prosthetic valve, 785
and FUO, 540
Transferrin, 34
virulence factors and, 8
Transforming growth factor-β (TGF-β),
30t, 34, 113
and fever, 117
HIV and, 1211
and *Mycobacterium avium-intracellulare*, 2252
receptor, 113
Transfusion-related infections, 2624t,
2624–2628
American trypanosomiasis, 2442,
2444, 2445, 2627
treatment, 2448
Babesia, 2500, 2627
bacterial, 2627–2628
Borrelia burgdorferi, 2627
CMV, 95, 1333, 1353, 2626–2627,
2660–2661
EBV, 2627
hepatitis, viral, 2624–2625
HAV, 2624–2625
HBV, 1423, 2625
prevention, 1432
HCV, 1482, 2625
HDV, 2625
herpesviruses, 2626–2627
HIV, 1169, 1189, 2625–2626
prevention, 1193
testing indications, 1194
HTLV, 1580, 1581, 2626
parvovirus B19, 1441, 2627
prevention, 2628

protozoal, 2627
Pseudomonas, 2627, 2628
retroviruses, 2625–2626
rickettsial, 2627
spirochetal, 2627
Toxoplasma gondii, 2627
in transplant recipients, 2726–2727
Treponema pallidum, 2627
Trypanosoma cruzi, 2627
viral, 2624–2627
Yersinia enterocolitica, 2628
Transfusions
granulocytes, 94–95
for peritonitis, 718
Transgenic mice, 1322
Transmissible neurodegenerative
diseases (TNDs), 881–887
Creutzfeldt-Jakob disease, 881–883
fatal familial insomnia, 881, 883–884
Gerstmann-Straussler-Scheinker
syndrome, 881, 883
handling infectious material, 884–885
kuru, 881
treatment, 884
Transmission
air-borne, 166
direct, 165
fecal-oral. See Fecal-oral transmission
food-borne, 1012–1025. See also
Food-borne disease;
Waterborne disease
indirect, 165–166
sexual, 1055–1103
transplacental, 165
vector-borne, 165–166
vehicle-borne, 165
vertical. See Neonatal disease;
Pregnancy
Transplacental transmission, 165. See
also Neonatal disease
Transplant recipients. See also specific
organs
abdominal infections in, 2727–2728
aspergillosis and, 2306
Aspergillus in, 2728
bacteremia in, 2726–2727
Blastomyces dermatitidis in, 2361
blood-borne infections in, 2726–2727
nonbacterial, 2727
chest infections in, 2727
CMV in, 1355–1356, 1358, 2729
CNS infections in, 2728t, 2728–2729
Coccidioides immitis in, 2369–2370
Cryptococcus neoformans in,
2728–2729
EBV in, 2730
esophagitis in, 964
GI infections in, 2727–2728
graft-vs.-host reaction, 1355, 2710
hepatitis in, 2728
HBV, 2617
herpesviruses in, 2729–2730
HIV in, 2713t
diagnosis and control, 2713, 2714
host-vs.-graft reaction, 1355, 2710
HSV in, 2729
immunodeficiency in, 135–136
and infections, 2710–2711
infections in, 2709–2717. See also
specific infections
bone marrow recipients, 2717–2722
contributing factors, 2709t
culture monitoring, 2714
diagnosis and control, 2713t,
2713–2714

Transplant recipients (Continued)
etiologies, 2711–2713, 2712t, 2713t
fever and, 2714
heart-lung recipients, 2724t, 2725
heart recipients, 2724, 2724t
host factors, 2709
immunosuppression and, 2710–2711
kidney recipients, 2723–2724, 2724t
liver recipients, 2724t, 2725–2726
lung recipients, 2724t, 2725
pancreas recipients, 2726
prophylaxis, 2714t, 2714–2715
small bowel recipients, 2726
solid organ recipients, 2722–2732
time of occurrence, 2722–2723, 2723f
type of transplantation, 2709–2710, 2710t
Leishmania in, 2428
Listeria monocytogenes in, 2728
Nocardia asteroides in, 2729
pulmonary infections in, 2727, 2727t
skin and wound infections in, 2726, 2726t
Toxoplasma gondii in, 2460, 2729
VZV in, 2729–2730
Transposons, 22, 25–26
conjugative, 214
and resistance, 213, 213f, 283
Transtracheal aspiration, 170t
for pneumonia, 624
acute, 624
nosocomial, 2602
Traumatized patient
catheter-acquired bacteremia in, 2758
CNS infections in, 2757–2758
empyema in, 2757
infections in, 2756–2761. See also *specific infections*
etiologies, 2756–2759
health care worker protection, 2759–2760
increased risk, 2756
prevention, 2759
signs and symptoms, 2756
pneumonia in, 2757, 2757t
sepsis in, 2759
sinusitis in, 2757
urinary tract infections in, 2758
wound infections in, 2758–2759
Travelers
advice on return, 2802
advice while traveling, 2798–2802
acclimatization, 2800
flying, 2800
food and beverages, 2800
insects, 2800
schistosomiasis, 2800–2801
sleeping sickness, 2801
snakes, 2800
sunstroke and heat exhaustion, 2800
water, 2800
CDC information guide, 2768, 2796
diarrhea, 971t, 971–972, 972t, 2801–2802
enteroxigenic *E. coli*, 971t, 972t
etiology, 971t
drugs to carry, 2796
FUO, 538
hepatitis in
HEV, 1664, 2619
prevention, 2799

malaria prophylaxis, 2800–2801
medical kit, 2796
pneumonia, 648–649
preparation, 2795–2796
pretravel advice, 2795–2796
protection, 2795–2803
Salmonella in, 2015
vaccine indications, 167, 2783, 2784t, 2796–2799, 2797t
BCG, 2799
cholera, 2797, 2797t
influenza, 2797t, 2799
Japanese B encephalitis, 2797t, 2798–2799
measles, 2797t, 2798
meningococcal meningitis, 2797t, 2798
plague, 2797t, 2799
pneumococcal, 2799
poliomyelitis, 2797t, 2797–2798
during pregnancy, 2799
rabies, 2797t, 2798
smallpox, 2797
tetanus-diphtheria, 2797t, 2798
tick-borne encephalitis, 2799
typhoid, 2024–2026, 2797t, 2798
typhus, 2797t, 2799
yellow fever, 2797, 2797t
Trematodes (flukes). See also *specific flukes*
antiparasitic agents, 460t, 463t, 482–483
blood (schistosomiasis), 2538–2541
diagnosis, 1006t, 1007
intestinal, 2538t, 2542–2543
Fasciolopsis buski, 2538t, 2542–2543
Heterophyes heterophyes, 2538t, 2543
liver, 2538t, 2541–2542
Clonorchis sinensis, 2538t, 2541
Fasciola hepatica, 2538t, 2541–2542
Opisthorchis, 2538t, 2541–2542
lung (*Paragonimus westermani*), 2538t, 2543
Nanophetus salmincola, 2557
swimmer's itch, 2557
Trench fever, 1720t, 1741, 1742. See also *Rochalimaea quintana*
Trench mouth (Vincent's disease), 567, 569, 643, 1789
clinical presentation, 596, 598
specimen collection, 172
Treponema carateum (pinta), 2133, 2135–2136
characteristics, 2133t
clinical manifestations, 2135, 2136f
diagnosis, 2135–2136
epidemiology and pathogenesis, 2135
geographic distribution, 2134f
history, 2135
prevention and treatment, 2136
Treponema hyodysenteriae, 990
Treponemal tests, 181, 2127t, 2128
Treponema pallidum, 2117–2133
Argyll Robertson pupil, 2124, 2125
ART test, 2127, 2127t
atypical presentation, 2126
biopsy specimen, 2127
blood cultures, 170t
cardiovascular, 2125
cellular immunodeficiency and, 132
chancre, 552, 1057, 1058f, 2121f, 2121–2122

differential diagnosis, 2122
multiple, 2121
Charcot's joints, 2125
classification, 2118
clinical manifestations, 2121–2126
Clutton's joints, 2126
congenital
clinical manifestations, 2126, 2126t
endophthalmitis, 1121, 2126
keratitis, 1114, 2126
treatment, 2129
CSF-VDRL test, 181, 2128
darkfield examination, 2126–2127, 2127f
differentiation from nonvenereal treponematoses, 2133t
disseminated. See secondary *below*
in drug abusers, 2705
enteritides, 994
epidemiology, 1056, 2119, 2119f
fibronectin and, 20
follicular syphilids, 2123
FTA-abs test, 2127t, 2128
gummatous, 2125–2126
gun barrel sight, 2125
hepatic gummas, 1161, 2125–2126
hepatitis, 1147, 1161, 2123
history, 2118–2119
and HIV/AIDS, 557, 1227, 2131
coinfection, 2119, 2131
neurosyphilis, 843–844
proctitis, 1231
treatment, 2130
Hutchinson's teeth, 2126
hypertrophic spinal pachymeningitis, 906
immunity, 2131
isolation, 2129
ITPA index, 2128
keratitis, 1114
laboratory diagnosis, 2126–2129
latent, 2120
clinical manifestations, 2123
congenital, 2126
diagnosis, 2123
early, 2123
late, 2123
late (tertiary), 2120. See also *cardiovascular; gummatous; neurosyphilis*
clinical manifestations, 2123–2126
treatment, 2129t, 2130
lymphadenitis, 940t
lymphadenopathy, 1684
meningitis, 835
antimicrobial therapy, 850t, 853–854
chronic, 870
clinical presentation, 843–844
diagnosis, 847–848
meningovascular, 835, 844
MHA-TP test, 2127t, 2128
natural course of untreated, 2120–2121
neurosyphilis, 835, 843–844
chronology, 2124f
classification, 2124t
clinical manifestations, 2124t, 2124–2125
diagnosis, 847–848
differential diagnosis, 2125
gummatous, 835
HIV coinfection, 843–844
meningovascular, 2124–2125
parenchymatous, 835

tests, 2128
treatment, 2129t, 2130
nontreponemal reaginic tests, 2127, 2127t
obliterative endarteritis, 2120, 2120f, 2125
ocular manifestations, 2125
Oslo study, 2121
otitis, 2125
treatment, 2130
papulosquamous syphilids, 2123
paresis, 2124
pathogenesis, 2119–2120
pathology, 2120, 2120f
pharyngitis, 567t
in pregnancy. See also *congenital above*
treatment, 2129–2130
primary, 2120
clinical manifestations, 2121f, 2121–2122
treatment, 2129, 2129t
proctitis: and HIV/AIDS, 1231
pustular syphilids, 2122
receptors, 31
rhinitis, 2126
Rosahn study, 2121
RPR test, 2127, 2127t
lepromin test and, 2246
"saber shin," 2126
secondary, 2120
clinical manifestations, 2122, 2122f, 2122t, 2123f
cutaneous manifestations, 550t, 552, 2122f, 2122–2123
differential diagnosis, 2211
Streptobacillus moniliformis, 2085
granulomatous hepatitis, 1161, 2123
hypergammaglobulinemia, 42
iridocyclitis, 1121–1122
keratitis, 1114
treatment, 2129t
serologic tests, 181, 192t, 1061, 2127t, 2127–2128
false-positive, 2128t, 2128–2129
specimen collection and processing, 171t, 181
tabes dorsalis, 2124
tertiary
differential diagnosis, 2326
granulomatous hepatitis, 1161
TPHA test, 2127t, 2128
TPI test, 2127t, 2128
transfusion-related, 2627
treatment, 2129t, 2129–2131
erythromycin, 335
in pregnancy, 338
and HIV/AIDS, 1289–1290
Jarisch-Herxheimer reaction, 2131
late syphilis, 2130
metronidazole, 329
neurosyphilis, 2130
otitis, 2130
persistent infection, 2130
repeat, 2130
treponemal tests, 181, 2127t, 2128
Tuskegee study, 2121
VDRL test, 2127, 2127t
lepromin test and, 2246
Treponema pallidum subsp. *endemicum* (bejel; endemic syphilis), 2133, 2136–2137
characteristics, 2133t

clinical manifestations, 2136
diagnosis, 2136
epidemiology and pathogenesis, 2136
geographic distribution, 2134f
history, 2136
prevention and treatment, 2136–2137
Treponema pallidum subsp. *pallidum* (syphilis), 2117–2133. *See also Treponema pallidum*
Treponema pallidum subsp. *pertenue* (yaws), 2133–2135
characteristics, 2133f
clinical manifestations, 2134f, 2134–2135, 2135f
diagnosis, 2135
differential diagnosis, 2326, 2437
epidemiology and pathogenesis, 2133–2134
geographic distribution, 2134f
history, 2133
prevention and management, 2135
Triazoles, 407
Tribec virus, 1448
Trichinella spiralis, 2531–2533, 2553
clinical features, 2532, 2532t
diagnosis, 1006t, 1006–1007, 2532–2533
enteric symptoms, 1000t, 1003
epidemiology, 2532
food-borne, 1012
life cycle, 2532
myalgia, 934
dysentery, 934
orbital cellulitis, 1133
pathology, 2532
prevention, 2533
T cell protection, 121t
treatment, 466t, 2533
mebendazole, 479
thiabendazole, 480
Trichloroacetic acid: for anogenital warts, 1394
Trichobilharzia, 2557
Trichomonas tenax, 2493
Trichomonas vaginalis, 2394t, 2493–2497
balanitis, 1059
clinical features, 2394t, 2494, 2494f
description, 2493
diagnosis, 2395t, 2494–2495, 2495t
dysuria, 1069
epidemiology, 2493–2494
and HIV transmission, 1188
hydrogenosomes, 2493
male asymptomatic, 2494
Neisseria gonorrhoeae coinfection, 1915
neonatal, 2494
specimen collection and processing, 171t, 183
strains, 2493
strawberry cervix, 2494
transmission, 2394t
treatment, 467t, 2495–2496
clotrimazole, 2495
metronidazole, 329, 330t, 332, 458, 467t, 2495–2496
resistance, 2495–2496
in pregnancy, 2495
urethritis, 1068
diagnosis, 1065
vaginitis emphysematosa, 2494
vulvovaginitis, 1077
differential diagnosis, 1077

features, 1075t
wet mounts, 1083, 1083f
Trichophyton, 2375t, 2375–2376
laboratory diagnosis, 2381
Trichophyton concentricum, 2375, 2375t, 2376, 2377, 2378–2379
Trichophyton erinacei, 2375t, 2376
Trichophyton gourvilii, 2375t, 2376
Trichophyton interdigitale, 2376
Trichophyton megnini, 2375, 2375t
Trichophyton mentagrophytes, 2375, 2375t, 2377–2378, 2380, 2381
Trichophyton quinckeanum, 2375, 2375t, 2377
Trichophyton rubrum, 2375, 2375t, 2377–2378, 2379f
skin infections: in the immunocompromised, 920
spinal cord injury and, 2733
Trichophyton schoenleinii, 2375, 2376, 2379
Trichophyton simii, 2375t, 2376
Trichophyton soudanense, 2375, 2375t, 2380
Trichophyton tonsurans, 2375t, 2376, 2377, 2380
Trichophyton verrucosum, 2375, 2375t, 2377, 2379
Trichophyton violaceum, 2375t, 2376
Trichophyton yaoundei, 2375t, 2376
Trichosporon
and bone marrow transplantation, 2719
and granulocytopenia, 2676
Trichosporon beigelii, 2385, 2392
Trichostrongylus: treatment, 467t
pyrantel pamoate, 480
thiabendazole, 480
Trichrome stain, 184t
Trichuris trichiura, 2525t, 2526–2528
clinical syndromes, 2527
diagnosis, 2527
epidemiology, 2527
life cycle, 2527, 2527f
treatment, 467t, 2527–2528
mebendazole, 478–479
Tricuspid valve endocarditis: *Pseudomonas aeruginosa*, 1983–1984
Trifluorothymidine. *See Trifluridine*
Trifluridine, 412t
structure, 423f
Trigeminal neuralgia: HSV and, 1341
Trimethoprim, 357–360
adverse reactions, 359, 474, 1284
alteration of target enzymes, 221
antimicrobial activity, 357–358, 358t
combination therapy, 359
synergism, 207–208
dosage, 514t–515t
drug interactions, 359, 526t
for GI tract infections, 360
for malaria, 360
mechanism of action, 357, 357f
for mycobacterial infections, 360
for nontuberculous mycobacteria, 396
pharmacology, 359, 514t–515t
for *Pneumocystis carinii*, 360, 1283t, 1284, 2480, 2481
dosage, 465t, 1283t
prophylaxis dosage, 465t, 1286t
prophylactic
for neutropenics, 360
for *Pneumocystis carinii*, 465t, 1286t

resistance, 200, 215t, 221, 358
for respiratory tract infections, 359
for sexually transmitted diseases, 360
structure, 357, 357f
susceptibility testing, 194t
for *Toxoplasma gondii*, 2469
for urinary tract infections, 359
uses, 359–360
Trimethoprim-sulfadiazine, 359
Trimethoprim-sulfamethoxazole
adverse reactions, 1282, 2480
antibiotic-associated colitis (AAC) from, 979
antimicrobial activity, 285t, 357–358, 358t
antiparasitic use, 459t, 474
and bone marrow transplantation: prophylactic, 2721, 2721t
for brain abscess, 893, 895
for *Brucella*, 2057
for chronic granulomatous disease, 93
for cystic fibrosis infections, 660
dosage, 462t, 514t–515t
in children, 514t, 851t
for meningitis, 850t, 851t
pediatric, 462t
drug interactions, 526t–527t
amantadine: 417
for endocarditis, 764
for enterococcal infections, 1829
for *Isospora belli*, 360, 474, 1289, 2511
for *Legionella pneumophila*, 2093, 2093t
for lower urinary tract infections, 676–677
for meningitis, 850t, 851t, 852
for mycetoma, 2330
for necrotizing pneumonia, 646
for neutropenics, 2688t, 2691, 2692t, 2693
for neutrophil defects, 94
for *Nocardia*, 2277
for nontuberculous mycobacteria, 396
for peritonitis, 720t
pharmacology, 514t–515t
for *Pneumocystis carinii*, 360, 474, 1282, 1283t, 2480
prophylaxis, 1285, 1286t, 2482
for Pseudomonads, 2004t
for *Pseudomonas pseudomallei*, 2006
for pyelonephritis, 676
resistance: *Streptococcus pneumoniae*, 1821
for sepsis syndrome: prophylaxis, 702
for *Shigella*, 2037, 2037t
for sinusitis, 589t
susceptibility testing, 194t
for *Toxoplasma gondii*, 2469
in HIV/AIDS, 2467, 2467t
prophylaxis, 1287
for transplant recipients: prophylactic, 2714
for travelers' diarrhea, 972
for urinary tract infections, 359
in the elderly, 2737
for Whipple's disease, 1031
Trimetrexate, 475
dosage, 465t
for *Pneumocystis carinii*, 475, 1283t, 1284, 2481
for *Toxoplasma gondii*, 2469
Trioleandomycin, 340
Tripelennamine abuse, 1983

Trombiculid mites: and scrub typhus, 1740
Tropheryma whippelii, 1030
and fever, 542
Tropical immersion foot syndrome, 1997
Tropical pulmonary eosinophilia, 2536
treatment, 462t
Tropical spastic paresis, 1579
Tropical sprue, 1025–1030
clinical manifestations, 1026–1028
diagnosis, 1028–1029
epidemiology, 1025
etiology, 1025–1026
intestinal abnormalities, 1028
morphology, 1028
pathogenesis, 1027f
treatment, 1029
Tropism, viral, 1322. *See also specific viruses*
Trypanosoma, 2394t, 2442–2455
African trypanosomiasis (sleeping sickness), 2450–2455. *See also Trypanosomoa brucei*
Chagas disease (American trypanosomiasis), 2442–2450. *See also Trypanosomoa cruzi*
diagnosis, 2395t
and fever, 543
replication mechanisms, 25
salivaria, 2442
stercoraria, 2442
transmission, 2394t
treatment, 476–478
melarsoprol, 476
Trypanosoma brucei, 2450–2455
chancre, 2451
clinical course, 2452–2453
clinical manifestations, 2394t
description, 2450–2451
diagnosis, 2395t, 2453, 2453f
East African. *See Trypanosoma brucei rhodesiense*
epidemiology, 2451–2452
lymphadenitis, 940t
pathogenesis and pathology, 2451
prevention, 2454–2455
stage I and II, 2451, 2452
transmission, 2450–2451
treatment, 476–478, 2453t, 2453–2454
variant antigen types (VATs), 2451
West African. *See Trypanosoma brucei gambiense*
Trypanosoma brucei brucei, 2442, 2450
Trypanosoma brucei gambiense, 475–476, 2442, 2452–2454
clinical course, 2452–2453
comparison with *rhodesiense*, 2452t
diagnosis, 2395t, 2453
distribution, 2443f
epidemiology, 2452
fever, 543
myocarditis, 800
neuritis, 878
treatment, 475–476, 2453t, 2453–2454
eflornithine, 476
pentamidine, 478
suramin, 476
Trypanosoma brucei rhodesiense, 475, 2442, 2452–2454
clinical course, 2453
comparison with *gambiense*, 2452t
diagnosis, 2395t, 2453, 2453f
distribution, 2443f

Trypanosoma brucei rhodesiense
　　(Continued)
　epidemiology, 2452
　fever, 543
　myocarditis, 800
　neuritis, 878
　treatment, 475, 2453t, 2453–2454
Trypanosoma cruzi, 475, 2442–2450
　autoantibodies, 42
　clinical course, 2445f, 2445–2446
　and complement, 66
　cytokine and T cell protection, 121t
　diagnosis, 2446–2447
　distribution, 2443f
　epidemiology, 2444–2445
　heart transplantation and, 2446
　and HUV/AIDS, 2446
　immunodeficiency and, 138
　immunosuppression and, 2446
　life cycle and transmission,
　　2442–2443, 2443f
　lymphadenitis, 940t
　megadisease, 2444, 2445
　myocarditis, 800, 802, 2443, 2444f
　neuritis, 878
　pathology, 2443–2444, 2444f
　prevention, 2448
　Romaña's sign, 2445, 2445f
　transfusion-related, 2442, 2444, 2445,
　　2627
　travel and, 2800
　treatment, 476–478, 2447–2448
　　benznidazole, 477
　　nifurtimox, 476–477
　　pyrazolopyrimidines, 477
　trypomastigote, 2443, 2443f
　vector, 2443f
Trypanosomatidae: antiparasitic agents,
　459t, 476–478
Tryparsamide
　dosage, 467t
　for *Trypanosoma brucei*, 2454, 2454t
Tsetse flies: and African trypanosomia-
　sis, 2450, 2452
T-strain mycoplasma. *See Ureaplasma*
　urealyticum
Tsukamurella aurantiacus. See
　Rhodococcus aurantiacus
Tubercle bacillus, 2213, 2214. *See also*
　Mycobacterium tuberculosis
Tuberculids, 2240
Tuberculin test, 2219–2220. *See also*
　Purified protein derivative
　test
Tuberculomas
　intracranial, 2224, 2235
　pulmonary, 2224
Tuberculosis, 2213–2243. *See also*
　Mycobacterium tuberculosis
Tuberculosis (acid-fast bacilli) isolation,
　2576–2577
Tuberculous cervical lymphadenitis, 938
Tuboovarian abscess
　anaerobic gram-negative bacilli,
　　2199
　Clostridium perfringens, 2185
　Haemophilus influenzae, 2043
　management, 1096
　Neisseria gonorrhoeae, 1917
　and PID, 1095, 1917
Tularemia, 2060–2068. *See also*
　Francisella tularensis
Tumor necrosis factor-α, 30t, 34, 82,
　102, 113
　and acute phase response, 117, 535

and bacterial meningitis, 839
and B cells, 120
biologic properties, 535t
characteristics, sources, and effects,
　114t, 115, 116, 117, 123, 124
and complement, 59
and fever, 117, 530–531, 532, 532f,
　533, 534
and *Francisella tularensis*, 2063
in HIV/AIDS, 130–131, 1210, 1211
and hypothalamus, 532, 533
injurious effects, 131
and meningococcal infections, 1904
and *Mycobacterium avium-intracellu-*
　lare, 2252
Plasmodium, 2421
　treatment against, 2426
and pneumonia, 620
protection from infection, 121t, 125,
　127
and pulmonary endothelial injury, 696
recombinant, 530
and sepsis, 693t, 693–695, 694t, 696,
　702
and septic shock, 117
T cell activation and, 110
therapeutic use, 130
and thymocytes, 107
and tissue injury, 88
Tumors. *See Neoplasia and specific*
　tumors
Tunga penetrans, 2563
Turista. *See* Travelers' diarrhea
Tylosis, 2379
Tympanocentesis, 169
Tympanomastoidectomy: for *Pseudomo-*
　nas aeruginosa otitis media,
　1991
Tympanostomy tubes: for otitis media,
　583
Typhlitis. *See* Enterocolitis, neutropenic
Typhobacillosis of Landouzy, 2233
Typhoidal tularemia, 2064–2065
Typhoid fever. *See Salmonella typhi*
"Typhoid state," 2021
Typhoid vaccine, 167, 955, 2781–2782
　for adults, 2784t
　adverse reactions, 2782
　for travelers, 2797t, 2798
Typhus
　classic. *See* epidemic *below*
　epidemic (louse-borne), 1719, 1720,
　　1720t, 1735–1737. *See also*
　　Rickettsia prowazekii
　　enteric symptoms, 999t, 1003
　recrudescent. *See* Brill-Zinsser
　　disease
　exanthematicus. *See* epidemic *above*
　Indian tick, 1725
　Kenya tick, 1725
　murine (endemic), 1719, 1720t,
　　1737–1739. *See also*
　　Rickettsia typhi
　scrub, 1719, 1720t, 1740–1741. *See*
　　also Rickettsia tsutsugamushi
Typhus vaccine: for travelers, 2797t, 2799

U

Ulceroglandular syndrome, 939, 940t
　Francisella tularensis, 939, 940t,
　　1310, 2063, 2064f
Ulcers. *See also specific ulcers*
　genital, 1057, 1057t, 1058f. *See also*
　　Genital lesions

membranous, 916
　superficial skin, 919–920
Ulnar nerve: leprosy damage, 2247
Ultracef. *See* Cefadroxil
Ultrasonography
　cholecystitis, 731
　and FUO, 540
　hepatic abscess, 725–726
　intraperitoneal abscess, 721–722
　neck and head infections, 601
　orbital cellulitis, 1134
　pancreatic abscess, 723–724
　pleural empyema, 639
　splenic abscess, 727
　urinary tract infections, 683–684
Umbilical vein catheter infections,
　2592
Umbilications: genital, 1059
Una virus, 1457
Uncinaria stenocephala, 2555
Undecylenate: topical, 401t
Uniocular cyst disease, 2550–2551
Universal precautions, 2576t, 2577t,
　2578
　for CMV, 2662
　for HIV, 1194, 2639–2641, 2640t
　isolation and, 2577t
Upper respiratory tract infections,
　561–606. *See also* Respiratory
　　tract infections, upper
Urea: for dermatophytosis, 2382
Ureaplasma urealyticum, 1703,
　1713–1718
　antibody deficiencies and, 49
　bartholinitis, 1085
　clinical manifestations, 1714–1717,
　　1715t
　diagnosis, 183
　epidemiology, 1714
　hypogammaglobulinemia,
　　1716–1717
　identification, 1713
　immunosuppression, 1716–1717
　isolation and identification, 1713
　nongonococcal urethritis, 1714–1716,
　　1715t
　　antibiotic studies, 1715
　　antibody studies, 1714–1715
　　inoculation studies, 1715–1716
　　isolation studies, 1714
　pelvic inflammatory disease, 1716
　postpartum endometritis, 1091
　properties, 1713t
　resistance
　　transposon, 214
　serotyping, 1714
　taxonomy, 1702f
　treatment, 1069–1070, 1717
　　erythromycin, 335
　urethritis, 1067
　　asymptomatic, 1068
　　diagnosis, 1066
　　nongonococcal, 1714–1716, 1715t.
　　　See also nongonococcal
　　　urethritis *above*
　　treatment, 1069–1070
Ureidopenicillins, 236, 245. *See also*
　　specific formulations
　dosage, 238t, 241t
　pharmacokinetics, 238t
　structure, 244f
Uremia
　and endocarditis, 749
　Mycobacterium tuberculosis treat-
　　ment, 2229

Urethra
　antimicrobial protection, 32
　asymptomatic infection, 1068–1069
　catheterization: and endocarditis, 743t
　colonization, 175
　dilatation: and endocarditis, 743t
　examination, 1064
　noninfectious irritation, 1066
　normal flora, 2159t, 2160
　specimen examination, 1064–1066,
　　1065f
　swabs, 1064
　warts, 1392
Urethral syndrome, 671
　Chlamydia trachomatis, 1686–1687
　　treatment, 1688
　Neisseria gonorrhoeae, 1069
Urethritis, 1063–1074
　Acinetobacter, 2011
　asymptomatic infection, 1068–1069
　candidal, 2297
　Chlamydia trachomatis, 1067–1068,
　　1685
　　asymptomatic, 1065, 1068–1069
　　postgonococcal, 1068
　　sulfonamides for, 357
　　in women, 1686–1687
　complications, 1069
　differential diagnosis, 1685
　infectious, 1066–1068
　Neisseria gonorrhoeae, 1066–1068,
　　1905–1916, 1915f
　　diagnosis, 1919, 1920t
　Neisseria meningitidis, 1902
　nongonococcal
　　Chlamydia trachomatis,
　　　1067–1068, 1685. *See also*
　　　Chlamydia trachomatis above
　　differential diagnosis, 1685, 1915,
　　　1915f
　　erythromycin for, 338t
　　etiology, 1067–1068, 1685
　　mycoplasma/ureaplasma,
　　　1714–1716
　　　antibiotic studies, 1715
　　　antibody studies, 1714–1715
　　　inoculation studies, 1715–1716
　　　isolation studies, 1714
　　and Reiter syndrome, 1071
　　Trichomonas vaginalis, 2494
　　uncommon causes, 1068
　noninfectious, 1066
　postgonococcal, 1068
　reexposure, 1071
　Reiter syndrome, 1070–1072
　　clinical features, 1071
　　laboratory findings, 1071
　　therapy, 1071–1072
　syndrome in women, 1069
　treatment, 1069–1070
　　quinolones, 370–371
　　rifampin, 323
　　of sexual partners of men, 1069
　Trichomonas vaginalis, 2494
Urethroprostatitis: *Ureaplasma*, 1715t
Urinary bladder perforation: and peri-
　tonitis, 710
Urinary cultures, 670–671
Urinary diversions, 2611
Urinary pH: and urinary tract infections,
　674
Urinary tract: specimens
　collection and processing, 170t,
　　175–177
　microscopy, 184

Urinary tract agents, 376–381, 675–678. *See also* Urinary tract infections, antimicrobial therapy
  pharmacologic tables, 516t–517t. *See also specific drugs*
Urinary tract calculi, 2610
  Ureaplasma, 1715t
  and urinary tract infections, 667
Urinary tract infections, 662–690. *See also* Genitourinary infections
  Acinetobacter, 2011
  alterations in renal function, 669
  antimicrobial therapy, 376–381, 516t–517t, 675. *See also specific drugs*
    for acute pyelonephritis, 675–676
    for asymptomatic bacteriuria, 677
    classification, 676–679
    for frequency, urgency, and dysuria syndrome, 677
    for lower tract infections, 676–677
    methenamine, 379–380
    nitrofurantoin, 376–379
    pharmacologic tables, 516t–517t
    for reinfection, 678
    for relapsing infections, 677–678
    response to, 675
    serum, tissue, and urine concentrations, 516t, 675
  Brucella, 2056
  Candida albicans, 2297
    treatment, 2300–2301
  catheter-associated, 2607–2613. *See also* nosocomial *below*
    Candida, 2297
    in the elderly, 2738
    infections, 668
  in children, 672–673, 673f
  chronic, 662
  clinical manifestations, 669
  definitions, 662
  diagnosis, 669–672
    by culture, 670–671
    localization of site, 671–672
    with low number of organisms, 671, 671f
    presumptive, 669–670, 670t
  in the elderly, 668, 2737–2738
  enterococcal, 1828
  epidemiology, 668–669
    in adults, 668
    in children, 668
    in the elderly, 668
    in patients with other conditions, 668–669
    in pregnancy, 678–679
  Escherichia coli, 1970–1971
  and fever, 541–542
  intrarenal abscess, 682
    diagnosis and therapy, 682, 682f
  management, 673–678, 685f
    analgesics, 675
    antimicrobial therapy, 675
    hydration, 674
    nonspecific therapy, 674–675
    in pregnancy, 679–680
    prostatitis, 681
    surgical, 684
    urinary pH, 674
  microsporidia, 2520
  natural history, 673
    in adults, 673
    in children, 672–673, 673f
    hypertension and, 673

  nosocomial, 2607–2616
    after catheter removal, 2608
    chronic renal inflammation and, 2610
    complications
      long-term catheterization, 2610
      short-term catheterization, 2610
      treatment, 2612–2613
    duration of catheterization, 2608–2610, 2609t
    in the elderly, 2737–2738
    enterococcal, 1828
    entry, 2607–2608
    epidemiology, 2607
    long-term catheterization, 2609–2610
    noncatheter, 2612
    obstructions and, 2610
    pathogenesis, 2607–2608
    prevention, 2610–2612
      avoidance of catheterization, 2610–2611
      of bacteriuria, 2611–2612
      patient-patient transmission, 2612
    risk factors, 2608
    short-term catheterization, 2608–2609
    urinary stones and, 2610
  papillary necrosis, 663f, 663–664
  pathogenesis, 664–667
    ascending route, 664
    hematogenous route, 664
    host-parasite interactions, 665t, 665–667
    lymphatic route, 664
  pathology, 662–664
  perinephric abscess, 682
    diagnosis and therapy, 682, 682f
  in pregnancy, 678–680
    epidemiology, 678–679
    management, 679–680
  prostatitis, 680–681
    acute, 680
    chronic bacterial, 680–681
    management, 681
    nonbacterial, 681
  Proteus mirabilis, 1974
  Pseudomonas aeruginosa, 667, 1994–1995
    treatment, 1994–1995
  pyelonephritis
    acute, 662, 663f
    chronic (chronic interstitial nephritis), 662–663, 663f
  radiologic evaluation, 682–684, 683f, 684f
  reinfection, 675
    treatment, 678
  relapse, 675
    treatment, 677–678
  Salmonella, 2023
  in spinal cord injured patients, 2732t, 2733–2734
  Staphylococcus epidermidis, 1780t, 1780–1781
  Streptococcus agalactiae, 1840
  superinfection, 675
  symptoms, 669
  in traumatized patient, 2758
  treatment
    quinolones, 370–371
    rifampin, 323
    trimethoprim, 359

Urinary tract obstruction: and urinary tract infections, 667
Urine
  antibody coating of bacteria (ACB), 672
  antimicrobial concentrations, 675
  antimicrobial protection, 32
  cultures: and FUO, 539
  sterility, 670
Urogenital tract. *See* Genitourinary tract
Urologic surgery
  and endocarditis, 743t
  prophylaxis recommendations, 2751t
Urticaria
  and fever, 546
  giant: differential diagnosis, 914
  tetracyclines, 309
Usher proteins, 24
Usutu: transmission, clinical syndromes, and geographic distribution, 1466t
Uterine gas gangrene: *Clostridium perfringens*, 2185
Uterine perforation: and peritonitis, 710
Uveitis
  conjunctivitis vs., 1106t
  idiopathic, 1124
  leprosy, 2248
  Listeria, 1883
  Treponema pallidum, 2125
Uveomeningoencephalitis, 871

V

Vaccine Adverse Events Relating System (VAERS), 2786
Vaccines, 167, 2770–2790. *See also* Immunization *and specific vaccines*
  adenovirus, types 4 and 7, 2773–2774
  adverse responses, 2772, 2773, 2773t
  anthrax, 1889, 2774
  BCG, 2774
  cholera, 2774
  currently available, 2773t, 2773–2782
  cytokines and, 131
  defined, 2770
  development, 2772–2773
  diphtheria, 167, 1866, 1867, 1871, 2775, 2775t
  DTP, 2082, 2771, 2775, 2775t, 2778–2779, 2781
  for enteric infection prevention, 955
  fimbriae and, 18
  Haemophilus b, 2044, 2044t, 2775–2776
  HAV, 1650–1651, 2776, 2799
  HBV, 159, 167, 1137, 1428–1429, 2776–2777
  HIV/AIDS and, 53–54, 2784–2785, 2785t
  indications, 2783–2788
    in adults, 2783, 2784t
    in children, 2783
    in the immunocompromised, 2784, 2784t, 2785t
    for occupational exposures, 2783–2784, 2784t
    postexposure, 2785
    in pregnancy, 2784, 2784t
    routine, 2783
    for travelers, 2783, 2784t, 2796–2799, 2797t

  influenza virus, 167, 1560–1563, 2777
  Japanese encephalitis, 167, 2777
  live vs. killed, 2771
  measles, 1523–1524, 2777–2778
  meningococcal polysaccharide, 2778
  mumps, 167, 1500, 2778
  pertussis, 2778–2779
  plague, 2779
  pneumococcal polysaccharide, 2779–2780
  polio, 1613–1614, 1618–1619, 2771, 2780
  rabies, 1536t, 1536–1537, 1539–1540, 2780–2781
  rubella, 167, 1463, 2781
  smallpox, 2781
  tetanus toxoid, 2177, 2192, 2775t, 2780t, 2781, 2782t
  typhoid, 2781–2782
  VZV, 167, 1350, 2782
  yellow fever, 167, 1472–1473, 2782
Vaccinia immunoglobulin, 2783
Vaccinia necrosum, 1326–1327
Vaccinia virus, 1325–1328
  accidental infection, 1327
  arthritis, 1036t
  conjunctivitis, 1106
  cutaneous manifestations, 550t
  cytokine and T cell protection, 121t, 129
  eczema vaccinatum, 1327
  erythematous urticarial eruptions, 1327
  generalized, 1327
  and HIV vaccine research, 1297, 1297t, 1299, 1300t, 1301
  product and host target, 125t
  receptor, 1317t
  therapeutic cytokines for, 131
  vaccines and vaccination techniques, 1325–1326
    CNS complications, 1326
    dermal complications, 1326–1327
    Elstree strain, 1326
    EM63 strain, 1326
    immunity from, 1326
    New York Board of Health strain, 1326
    passive immunity, 1326
  vaccinia necrosum, 1326–1327
Vagina
  antimicrobial protection, 32
  examination, 1082–1083
  normal flora, 1074–1075, 2159f, 2159t, 2160
Vaginal complaints
  approach to, 1082–1084
  history, 1081
Vaginal cuff
  abscess, 1094
    anaerobic, 2163t
  cellulitis, 1094
Vaginal discharge examination, 1083f, 1083–1084
Vaginal flagellates: antiparasitic agents, 458, 467–468
Vaginal speculum, 1082
Vaginitis
  candidal, 2293, 2293f
  chlamydial, 1686
  desquamative (purulent), 1081
  emphysematosa, 1081
    Trichomonas vaginalis, 2494

Vaginitis (*Continued*)
foreign body, 1080
Trichomonas vaginalis, 2494
Vaginosis, bacterial, 1078f, 1078–1080
complications, 1080
epidemiology, 1078–1079
features, 1075t
pathophysiology, 1079
treatment, 1079t, 1079–1080
Valaciclovir, 413–417
Valtrex. *See* Valaciclovir
Vancomycin, 346–350
absorption, 209
adverse reactions, 348–349, 2750
and aminoglycosides
combination therapy, 287t, 289t, 296
nephrotoxicity, 292
for antibiotic-associated colitis (AAC), 982–983, 984, 993
antibiotic-associated colitis (AAC) from, 979
antimicrobial activity, 347
for brain abscess, 895
for cellulitis, 916
dosage, 514t–515t
in children and neonates, 514t, 851t
for meningitis, 849t, 850t, 851t
in renal dysfunction, 204, 515t
drug interactions, 349, 527t
for endocarditis
enterococcal, 761–762
prophylaxis, 788, 797t
prosthetic valve, 786t, 786–787
staphylococcal, 762, 1779
streptococcal, 761–762
viridans streptococci, 1849
for enterococcal infections, 1830
for meningitis, 849t, 850t, 851t, 852, 853
neutropenia from, 89
for neutropenics, 2688t
perioperative prophylactic use, 2749
for peritonitis, 720t
pharmacology, 347, 348f, 514t–515t
protein binding, 347
resistance, 200, 215t, 220, 2750
anaerobic gram-negative bacilli, 2196t
enterococci, 1830
Leuconostoc, 1832
Streptococcus pneumoniae, 1822
for sepsis syndrome, 702
structure, 346
susceptibility testing, 194t
uses and doses, 349–350
Vantin. *See* Cefpodoxime proxetil
Varicella. *See* Chickenpox; Varicella-zoster virus
Varicella-zoster immune plasma (ZIP), 1350
Varicella-zoster immunoglobulin (VZIG), 454, 1350
for nosocomial prevention, 2658, 2660
for transplant recipients, 2729–2730
Varicella-zoster virus (VZV), 1345–1351
arthritis, 1036t
and bone marrow transplantation, 1348, 2674, 2720
classification, 1330t, 1346
clinical manifestations
chickenpox, 1347–1348
in the immunocompromised, 1348
herpes zoster, 1348–1349

clinical syndromes, 1334t
conjunctivitis, 1106
CSF specimens, 179
cutaneous manifestations, 550t, 552
dermatoblepharitis, 1130
diagnosis, 1333, 1349
differential diagnosis, 1349
measles virus, 1522
peritonitis, 714
encephalitis/myelitis, 874, 1347, 1348
endophthalmitis, 1124
treatment, 1126
epidemiology, 1332, 1346–1347
chickenpox, 1346
herpes zoster, 1346–1347
and granulocytopenia, 2677, 2679
hepatitis, 1137
in the immunocompromised, 1147
in transplant recipients, 2728
history, 1345–1346
and HIV/AIDS, 1228, 1348
reactivation, 1182, 1228
retinitis, 1240
treatment, 1283t, 1287, 2642
immunization, 167, 2782
in the immunocompromised, 1332t, 1347, 1348, 2658, 2660
hepatitis, 1147
prevention, 1350
treatment, 416
immunoglobulin, 2783
immunosuppressive therapy and, 135
iridocyclitis, 1348
keratitis, 1116, 1348
treatment, 1118
interferons, 429
latency, 1332t
meningitis, 833, 1348
neuritis, 878
nosocomial, 2658–2660
investigating epidemics, 2658, 2660
management of exposed personnel, 2660
prevention, 2658, 2659f
risks, 2658
transmission mechanisms, 2658
pathogenesis, 1333, 1347
pneumonitis, 1347
treatment, 1349–1350
post-herpetic neuralgia, 1348
prevention, 1334t, 1334–1335, 1350
primary infections, 1332t
and Ramsay Hunt syndrome, 1348
recurrence, 1332t, 1333, 1346–1347, 1348–1349
and cell-mediated immune defects, 2681
and HIV/AIDS, 1182, 1228
replication, 1346
resistance, 193
and Reye syndrome, 1348, 1558
spreading/shedding mechanisms, 1320f, 1321
structure, 1330t
systemic spread, 1320f
transmission and seroepidemiology, 1333t
in transplant recipients, 2729–2730
diagnosis and control, 2713
skin infections, 2726
treatment, 412t, 1334t, 1334–1335, 1349–1350
acyclovir, 416–417, 1283t, 1287, 1349

experimental agents, 437t
foscarnet, 422–424
ganciclovir, 424–426
in HIV/AIDS, 1283t, 1287
sorivudine, 432
vidarabine, 433, 1349
tropism, 1331
vaccine, 167, 1350, 2782
zoster ophthalmicus, 1347, 1348
Variola virus, 1325, 1328–1329
arthritis, 1036t
clinical illness, 1328–1329
eradication, 159
laboratory diagnosis of smallpox, 1328
Vascular adhesion protein-1 (VAP-1), 112
Vascular catheters: and infections in patients with neoplasia, 2670f, 2670–2671, 2671f
Vascular cell adhesion molecule-1 (VCAM-1), 96
Vascular gangrene, 933
Vascular infections
Candida albicans, 2298
cardiac, 741–821. *See also* Cardiovascular infections
graft, 789–790
in drug abusers, 2700–2701, 2701f
graft
Staphylococcus aureus, 1782
Staphylococcus epidermidis, 1782
Salmonella, 2022
Vascular surgery: prophylaxis recommendations, 2751t
Vascular system
cardiac infections. *See* Cardiovascular infections
cerebral. *See* Cerebrovascular system
Vasculitis
and fever, 544
pneumonia: chronic, 647t
Staphylococcus aureus, 1770
VCAM, 123
VCAM-1, 111
and septic shock, 118
VDJ gene, 44, 44f
antigen-binding diversity and, 45
VDRL test, 181, 1061, 2127, 2127t
lepromin test and, 2246
neurosyphilis, 846–847
for yaws, 2135
Vector-borne transmission, 165–166
Vecuronium: for *Clostridium tetani*, 2176
Veillonella, 2158t, 2204–2206
chloramphenicol for, 312t
mediastinitis, 815t
and normal physiology, 2160
oral colonization, 593, 594t
and tropical sprue, 1025
Veillonella alcalescens, 2204
Veillonella atypica, 2204
Veillonella dispar, 2204
Veillonella parvula, 2204
Velosef. *See* Cephradine
Venereal disease research laboratory test. *See* VDRL test
Venezuelan equine encephalitis virus, 1455–1459
clinical manifestations, 1458
diagnosis, 1458
encephalomyelitis, 876
epidemiology, 1456
pathogenesis, 1457

prevention and treatment, 1458–1459
serology, 191
Venezuelan hemorrhagic fever
characteristics, 1573t
clinical manifestations, 1576
epidemiology, 1574
Venoglobulin-I, 454
Venoglobulin-S, 454
Venotomy: for suppurative thrombophlebitis, 768
Venous sinus thrombosis, 907, 908t
Vero toxins. *See* Shiga-like toxins
Verotoxins: *Escherichia coli*, 1014
Verruca vulgaris: treatment, 1395
interferons, 429
Verrucous carcinoma: wart conversion to, 1383, 1389
Verrucous lesions: genital, 1059
Verruga peruana, 1742, 2209, 2210
Vertebral osteomyelitis, 1041
diagnosis, 1045, 1046f
treatment, 1045
Vertical transmission. *See* Neonatal disease; Pregnancy
Very late antigens (VLA), 111
Vesicles
defined, 551
genital, 1057, 1057t. *See also* Genital lesions
Pseudomonas aeruginosa, 921
pustules vs., 552
systemic infections manifesting, 550t
Vesicobullous eruptions, 552–553
Vesicopustular lesions, 552–553
Vesicoureteral reflux: and urinary tract infections, 667, 672, 673f, 674
Vesicular stomatitis virus, 1526–1527
adhesin, 11f
diagnosis, 1527
epidemiology, 1526
Indiana
clinical manifestations, 1527
epidemiology, 1526
New Jersey
clinical manifestations, 1527
epidemiology, 1526
receptor, 1317t
types, 1526, 1526t
virology, 1526
Vesicular stomatitis with exanthem, 1624
Vesiculobullous eruptions, 552–553
Vesiculoviruses, 1526–1527, 1528
Vestibular adenitis, 1081
Vestibular toxicity: aminoglycosides, 294–295
Viannia, 2429. *See also* Leishmania
Viannia braziliensis, 2429, 2435–2438
Viannia guyenensis, 2436
Viannia panamensis, 2428t, 2435–2438
Viannia peruviana, 2435
VI antigen: *Salmonella typhi*, 952, 1965, 2014, 2018
Vibrio alginolyticus, 1945, 1946
cellulitis, 915
clinical manifestations, 1946
differential diagnosis, 1946
prevention, 1947
treatment, 1947
Vibrio cholerae, 1934–1945
adherence, 2, 31
antigenic structure, 1935
β-lactamase, 216t
BVg protein, 23
carriers, 1942

"classic" biotype, 1934, 1936
classification, 1935, 1935t
clinical manifestations, 1936–1938
cytotoxicity, 951
description, 1935–1936
diagnosis, 1939
diarrhea, 180, 1936–1938
    diagnosis, 180
dysentery, 989
El Tor biotype, 1934, 1936, 1941
Enterobacteriaceae and, 1935
enterotoxin, 3t, 4, 5, 949t, 950,
        1934–1935, 1936, 1936f
    "B" subunits, 1936
epidemiology, 1941–1942
F (flagellar) antigens, 1935, 1935t
fluid replacement, 1937, 1938–1939
    IV solutions, 1937, 1937t, 1938
    oral, 1938, 1938t
fluid volume depletion, 1938t
food-borne, 1012t, 1013, 1017,
        1941–1942
    foods implicated, 1017t
genetics, 1935–1936
Hikojima, 1935, 1935t
host defenses, 1939–1941
Inaba, 1935, 1935t, 1936, 1938, 1941
local immune defenses, 1940–1941
manner of spread, 1941–1942
morphologic characteristics, 1935,
        1935f
nonimmune defenses, 1939–1940
non-O1, 1947
    clinical manifestations, 1947
    diarrhea in adults, 969
    epidemiology, 1947
    food-borne, 1012t, 1013, 1016,
            1017, 1017t
    laboratory findings, 1947
    prevention, 1947
    toxin, 5
O antigens, 1935, 1935t, 1940
O 139 Bengal, 1935, 1936, 1938,
        1942
Ogawa, 1935, 1935t, 1936, 1938, 1941
O1 strain
    food-borne, 1012t, 1013, 1016,
            1017, 1017t
    waterborne, 1015, 1016t
pathophysiology, 1938
prevention, 1942
serotypes, 1935, 1935t
"sicca," 1937
specimen collection, 180
stool
    composition, 1937, 1937t
    culture, 955, 1937, 1937t, 1939,
            1939t
    examination, 1938
    "rice water," 1938
strain variations, 1936
survival of organism, 1936
systemic immune defenses, 1940
toxin, 3t, 5, 949t, 950. See also entero-
        toxin above
toxin coregulated pili (TCP), 951
ToxR protein, 24
treatment, 1938–1939, 1942–1943,
        1943f
    chloramphenicol, 312t
    tetracyclines, 307
    trimethoprim, 357
vaccine, 2774
    adverse reactions, 2774
    indications for adults, 2784t

research, 1941
    for travelers, 2797, 2797t
    virulence factors, 2, 22
    virulence regulation, 23t, 24
Vibrio damsella, 1945, 1946
Vibrio extorquens. See Protomonas
        extorquens
Vibrio fetus. See Campylobacter fetus
Vibrio fluvialis, 1945, 1946
Vibrio hollisae, 1945, 1946
Vibrio mimicus, 1947
    clinical manifestations, 1947
    laboratory findings, 1947
Vibrio parahaemolyticus, 1945–1946
    classification, 1935
    clinical manifestations, 1945
    cytotoxin, 951
    diarrhea: in AIDS, 970, 970t
    differential diagnosis, 1945–1946
    dysentery, 987, 989
    epidemiology, 1945
    food-borne, 1012t, 1013, 1016, 1017,
            1945, 1946
        foods implicated, 1017t
        laboratory diagnosis, 1018t, 1019
    laboratory findings, 1945
    prevention, 1946
    stool culture, 955
    treatment, 1946
Vibrio shigelloides. See Plesiomonas
        shigelloides
Vibrio vulnificus, 1945, 1946
    cellulitis, 915, 1946
    clinical manifestations, 1946
    cutaneous manifestations, 550t, 553
    differential diagnosis, 1946
    food-borne, 1016, 1019
    prevention, 1947
    septicemia, 989
    treatment, 1947
        tetracyclines, 307
    wound infections: in trauma patients,
            2758
Vidarabine, 433–434
    adverse reactions, 433, 1342
    clinical studies, 433–434
    drug interactions, 433, 527t
    for HBV, 1427–1428
    for HSV, 1342
    mechanism of action, 433
    pharmacokinetics, 433
    spectrum of activity, 412t, 433
    structure, 423f
    for VZV, 433, 1349
Videx. See Didanosine
Villus tip cells: destruction of, 952
Vinblastine: for Kaposi's sarcoma, 1244
Vincent's angina, 567, 569, 643, 1789
    clinical presentation, 596, 598
    specimen collection, 172
Vincristine: for Kaposi's sarcoma, 1244
Viomycin
    dosage, 516t–517t
        in hepatic or renal failure, 390t, 517t
    for Mycobacterium tuberculosis, 395
    pharmacology, 516t–517t
VIRA-A. See Vidarabine
Viral diseases, 1314–1674. See also indi-
        vidual viruses
    Adenoviridae, 1382–1387
    aerosol transmission, 1319
    alphaviruses, 1455–1459
    arthritis, 1036–1037
        etiology, 1036t
    Astroviridae, 1672–1674

and bone marrow transplantation,
        2720
Bunyaviridae, 1567–1572
Calciviridae, 1666–1672
and cell-mediated immune defects,
        2681
Colorado tick fever, 1446–1447
conjunctivitis, 1104t, 1105f,
        1105–1106
Coronaviridae, 1486–1489
coxsackieviruses, 1620–1636
CSF specimens, 179
cutaneous manifestations, 550t
    HIV/AIDS and, 1228–1229
cytokine and T cell protection, 121t,
        128–130
cytomegalovirus, 1351–1364
DNA viruses, 1325–1446. See also
        DNA viruses
droplet transmission, 1319
encephalitis, 874–878
    animal reservoirs, 2792t
    CSF specimens, 179
    differential diagnosis: brain
            abscess, 891
encephalomyelitis, 876–877, 877t
endophthalmitis, 1121t, 1123–1124
enteroviruses, 1620–1636
Epstein-Barr virus, 1364–1377
fecal-oral transmission, 1319
    and fever, 543
Filoviridae, 1543–1546
Flaviviridae, 1465–1486
flaviviruses, 1465–1474
food-borne, 1012
German measles. See Rubella virus
Hepadnaviridae, 1406–1439
hepatitis A virus, 1636–1656
hepatitis B and D viruses, 1406–1439
hepatitis C virus, 1474–1486
hepatitis E virus, 1663–1666
herpes B virus, 1379–1382
herpes simplex virus, 1336–1345
Herpesviridae, 1330–1382
human herpesviruses 6 and 7,
        1377–1379
human immunodeficiency virus,
        1590–1606
human T cell lymphotropic viruses
        (HTLV-I/II), 1579–1584
immunodeficiency and, 137
influenza virus, 1546–1567
of joints, 1032
keratitis, 1111t, 1115–1116
lentiviruses, 1584–1590
and leukemia/lymphoma, 2677, 2681
Marburg and Ebola hemorrhagic
        fevers, 1543–1546
measles virus, 1519–1526
meningitis, 832
    acute, 832–834
    adjunctive therapy, 854
    clinical presentation, 842
    CSF examination, 845
    diagnosis, 845
    immunoprophylaxis, 856
    pathogenesis and pathophysiology,
            836
    prevention, 856
molluscum contagiosum, 1329–1330
monkeypox, 1329
mumps virus, 1496–1501
myocarditis, 800, 800t
Norwalk virus, 1666–1672
oncoviruses, 1579–1584

orbivirus, 1447–1458
orchitis, 1101
Orthomyxoviridae, 1546–1567
overview, 1314–1325
papillomaviruses, 1387–1400
Papovaviridae, 1387–1406
parainfluenza virus, 1489–1496
Paramyxoviridae, 1489–1526
parapoxvirus, 1329
Parvoviridae, 1439–1446
    and peptides, 107
pericarditis, 804–805, 805t
poliovirus, 1613–1620
polyomaviruses, 1400–1406
Poxviridae, 1325–1330
Reoviridae, 1446–1458
reovirus, 1446–1458
Retroviridae, 1579–1606
Rhabdoviridae, 1526–1543
rhinovirus, 1656–1663
RNA viruses, 1446–1674. See also
        RNA viruses
rotavirus, 1448–1455
rubella virus, 1459–1465
spreading mechanisms, 1320f,
        1320–1321
Togaviridae, 1455–1465
transfusion-related, 2624–2627
    CMV, 2626–2627
    EBV, 2627
    hepatitis, 2624–2625
    herpesviruses, 2626–2627
    HIV, 2625–2626
    HTLV, 2626
    parvovirus B19, 2627
    retroviruses, 2625–2626
in transplant recipients, 2712t
tropism, 1321–1322
vaccinia (cowpox), 1325–1328
varicella-zoster virus, 1345–1351
variola (smallpox), 1328–1329
vertical transmission, 1319
vesicular stomatitis virus, 1526–1527
zoonoses, 2791t
Viral hemorrhagic fever, 1543–1546
    characteristics, 1544
    clinical manifestations, 1544–1545
    diagnosis, 1545
    epidemiology, 1544
    etiology, 1543, 1544. See also Ebola
            virus; Marburg virus
    pathogenesis and pathology, 1545
    prevention and treatment, 1545
    transmission, 1544
Virazole. See Ribavirin
Virchow's cells, 2246
Viremia, 1321
    and meningitis, 836
    primary, 1321
    secondary, 1321
Viridans streptococcal infections, 186,
        1846–1851. See also Strepto-
        coccal infections, viridans
Virion-attachment protein (VAP), 1316
Virions, 1314
Virology, 1314. See also Viral diseases
Viroptic. See Trifluridine
Virulence, 164, 1319
    clinical correlations and applications,
            27–28
    defined, 19, 20
    determinants, 1322
    genes and
        identification and characterization,
                25–26

Virulence (Continued)
  molecular form of Koch's postulate, 26–27
Virulence factors, 2–29
  adherence, 11–19. See also Adherence, microbial
  for avoiding or disrupting humoral defenses, 8
  defined, 20
  gastrointestinal infections, 948–951, 949t
  molecular perspective of pathogenicity, 19–29. See also Molecular research, microbial pathogenicity
  nontoxin directed at phagocytic cells, 8
  for overcoming anatomic barriers, 7–8
  toxins, 2–7. See also Toxins
Viruses
  attachment, 1316–1317
  capsid symmetry, 1315, 1315t, 1317f
  classification, 1314–1316, 1315t
  disease caused by. See Viral diseases
  entry pathway into cells, 1317, 1318f
  genetic information, 1314
  growth or biochemical characteristics, 190–191, 191f
  interactions
    with cells, 1316–1319, 1317t, 1318f
    with environment, 1322–1323, 1323f
    with host, 1319–1322, 1320f
  nucleic acids, 1314–1315, 1315t
  receptors, 1316, 1317t, 1318f
  replication, 1317–1319
  structure, 1314–1316, 1316f, 1317f
Visceral abscess
  hepatic, 724–727
  pancreatic, 723–724
  splenic, 727
Visceral larva migrans, 2253–2254, 2553t. See also Toxocara
  clinical manifestations, 2554
  diagnosis, 1006t, 1006–1007, 2554
  differential diagnosis, 2554
  enteric symptoms, 1000t, 1003
  human infection, 2554
  life cycle in dog, 2553–2554
  prevention, 2554
  pulmonary infiltrates with eosinophilia, 631
  treatment, 467t, 2554
    albendazole, 479
    thiabendazole, 480
Visna-maedi virus, 1584, 1585f, 1586, 1591
  natural history of infection, 1585f
  taxonomy, 1585f
Vitamin B₁₂-binding protein, 79t
Vitamin C: and common cold prophylaxis, 564–565
Vitamin deficiency: immunodeficiency and, 137
Vitronectin, 58t, 63t
VLA-4, 111, 123
VLA-5, 111
VLA-6, 111
Vogt-Koyanagi-Harada syndrome: meningitis, 871
Voles
  and Francisella tularensis, 2061
  and hantaviruses, 1569
Volhynia fever, 1741
Volume replacement. See also Fluid therapy

for food poisoning, 1019
  for sepsis syndrome, 699–700
Vomiting. See Nausea/vomiting
von Economo's encephalitis, 1466
v-sag protein, 106
Vulvar lesions. See Genital lesions
Vulvar vestibulitis, 1081
Vulvar warts, 1392, 1392f
Vulvitis: focal, 1081
Vulvovaginal abscess: anaerobic, 2163t
Vulvovaginitis, 1075–1081
  abdominal pain and, 1082
  age and, 1081–1082
  approach to, 1082–1084
  bacterial vaginosis, 1078f, 1078–1080
    complications, 1080
    epidemiology, 1078–1079
    pathophysiology, 1079
    treatment, 1079t, 1079–1080
  candidiasis, 1075–1077
    clinical features, 1076
    diagnosis, 1076
    treatment, 1076t, 1076–1077
      male partners, 1077
      oral therapy, 1076
      recurrent infection, 1077
      topical, 1076–1077
  examination of female genitalia, 1082–1084
  foreign body vaginitis, 1080
  herpes simplex virus, 1080
  history taking, 1081
  human papillomavirus, 1080
  laboratory examination, 1083f, 1083–1084
  mode of onset, 1082
  noninfectious, 1081
  odor, 1082
  perineal irritation, 1082
  related considerations and conditions, 1081
  sexual history, 1082
  staphylococcal, 1080
  trichomoniasis, 1077
  typical features, 1075t
VZV. See Varicella-zoster virus

W

Waldenstrom's macroglobulinemia, 53
Warfarin
  adverse reactions: influenza vaccine and, 1561
  drug interactions
    erythromycin, 337
    metronidazole, 332
    rifampin, 320
    sulfonamides, 356
Warthin-Starry-staining bacilli, 1744
Warts
  cutaneous, 1388t, 1389, 1390, 1391f, 1392. See also Human papillomavirus
    treatment, 1393–1394
  prosector's, 2216
Wasting syndrome (HIV/AIDS), 934, 1175, 1182, 1182t, 1226
  in children, 1186, 1186t
Waterborne disease
  amebiasis, 2404
  caliciviruses, 1669
  Cryptosporidium, 2502–2503, 2794
  food poisoning, 1015–1016, 1016t
  Giardia lamblia, 1016, 1016t, 2487
  hepatitis A virus, 1644–1645

hepatitis E virus, 1664
  outbreak investigations, 163
  schistosomiasis, 2538
  Shigella, 2035
  streptococcal pharyngitis, 1787
  travel and, 2800–2801
  Vibrio cholerae, 1941–1942
Water-rat trappers' disease, 2060
Weanling diarrhea, 966–968
Weeksella, 2114
  classification and site of infection, 2107t
Weeksella virosa, 2114
Weeksella zoohelcum, 2114
Wegener's granulomatosis
  pneumonia
    chronic, 647t
    radiology, 650t
  trimethoprim-sulfamethoxazole for, 360
Weight loss: and Whipple's disease, 1031
Weil-Felix reaction: rickettsial infections, 1719, 1724, 1736, 1737, 1740
Weil's disease, 2138
Wesselsbron: transmission, clinical syndromes, and geographic distribution, 1466t
Western blot
  for Borrelia burgdorferi, 2149, 2150f
  for echinococcosis, 2550
  for HIV, 1213, 1220, 1225, 1257–1259, 1258f, 1259t. See also Human immunodeficiency virus, Western blot
    correlation with EIA, 1256t
    false-negative, 1259
    false-positive, 1259t
    indeterminate, 1258–1259
    and indirect immunofluorescence assay, 1259t
    nonreactive, 1258
    radioimmunoprecipitation assay and, 1259–1260
    reactive, 1258
  for mycetoma, 2329
Western equine encephalitis virus, 1455–1459
  clinical manifestations, 1458
  diagnosis, 1458
  encephalomyelitis, 876
  epidemiology, 1456
  pathogenesis, 1457
  prevention and treatment, 1458–1459
  serology, 191
West Nile virus
  lymphadenitis, 940t
  transmission, clinical syndromes, and geographic distribution, 1466t
Whale finger, 1895
Whataroa virus, 1457
Wheezing: differential diagnosis, 616
"Whiff" test, 1078, 1083
Whipple bacillus, 1030, 1030f
Whipple's disease, 1030–1032
  clinical and laboratory findings, 1030–1031
  diagnosis, 955, 1031
  endophthalmitis, 1122
  and fever, 542
  pathogenesis, 1030
  pathology, 1030, 1030f
  rDNA sequencing, 28, 1030
  treatment, 1031–1032

trimethoprim-sulfamethoxazole, 360
Whipworm. See Trichuris trichiura
White piedra, 2385
Whitfield's ointment, 401
Whitlow: herpetic, 1339, 1339f
Whitmore's bacillus. See Pseudomonas pseudomallei
Whooping cough, 2078–2082. See also Bordetella pertussis
  adenovirus and, 1385
Widal's reaction: in typhoid fever, 1000–1001
Widal test: for Salmonella, 2022
Wild hare disease, 2060
Wilson's diseases: hepatic involvement, 1149
Winterbottom sign, 2452, 2453
Winter vomiting disease, 968–969
Wiskott-Aldrich syndrome, 50, 52, 134t, 135, 138, 151t
  bone marrow transplants for, 51
  immunoglobulin for, 454
  Staphylococcus aureus and, 1762
Wohlfahrtia, 2563
Wolfring, gland of, 1130
Wolinella, 2158t
Wollan agent: winter vomiting disease, 968
Wood tick: and Rickettsia rickettsii, 2565
Wor Ditchling agent: winter vomiting disease, 968
Worm infections. See Helminths
  pinworms. See Enterobius vermicularis
  roundworms. See Roundworms, intestinal
  tapeworms. See Cestodes
  whipworm. See Trichuris trichiura
Wound infections
  anaerobic, 2163t
  animal and human bites, 2765–2769
    management, 2767, 2767t, 2768
  burns, 2761–2765. See also Burns, wound infections
  clostridial myonecrosis (gas gangrene), 2186–2187. See also Clostridial myonecrosis
  Clostridium botulinum, 2179, 2180, 2181
  enterococcal, 1828–1829
  Pseudomonas aeruginosa, 1996
  specimen collection and processing, 179–180
  Staphylococcus aureus, 1764–1765
  surgical postoperative, 2742–2756. See also Surgical wounds
  topical antibacterial prophylaxis, 382
  in transplant recipients, 2726
  in traumatized patient, 2758–2759
Wrist: infectious arthritis, 1033, 1033t
Wuchereria bancrofti, 2525t, 2533–2535, 2536
  arthritis, 1037
  blood cultures, 170t
  clinical features, 2534
  diagnosis, 2534
  epidemiology, 2534
  life cycle, 2533–2534
  lymphadenitis, 940t
  lymphangitis, 943
  pathology, 2534
  treatment, 462t
    diethylcarbamazine, 481
    ivermectin, 481

Wuchereria bancrofti (*Continued*)
and tropical pulmonary eosinophilia, 2536

X

Xanthomonas maltophilia, 2004t
classification, 2004
and cystic fibrosis, 659
and granulocytopenia, 2676
imipenem for, 264t, 265
treatment
aminoglycosides, 285t
quinolones, 367t
Xenodiagnosis: for *Trypanosoma cruzi*, 2446
Xenopsylla cheopis: and murine typhus, 1737
Xerosis: and HIV, 1229
X-linked agammaglobulinemia, 49, 50, 51, 135, 151t
bone marrow transplants for, 51
diagnosis, 153
immunoglobulin for, 454
X-linked hyper-IgM syndrome, 49, 51–52, 119, 151t
diagnosis, 153
X-linked immunodeficiency syndrome, 129, 134t, 135, 138
immunoglobulin for, 454
X-linked lymphoproliferative syndrome, 151t
Xylohypha trichoides. See Cladosporium trichoides

Y

YadA adhesin, 25
Yato-byo, 2060
Yaws, 2133–2135
Yeasts, 2288–2289, 2289t. *See also* Fungal infections
Yellow fever, 1465, 1466t, 1467–1468, 1469, 1470–1471, 1472
black vomit, 1471
clinical manifestations, 1470–1471
cutaneous manifestations, 550t
diagnosis, 1472
differential diagnosis, 1472
epidemiology, 1467–1468
Faget sign, 1471
hepatitis, 1137, 1147
history, 1465
jungle, 1467
pathogenesis, 1469
prevention and therapy, 1472–1473
serology, 191
transmission, clinical syndromes, and geographic distribution, 1466t
vaccine, 167, 1472–1473, 2782
boosters, 2782
recommendations for adults, 2784t
for travelers, 2797, 2797t
Yersinia, 2070–2078. *See also individual species*

animal reservoirs, 2792t
cellular immunity and, 124
conjunctivitis, 1105
penetration, 2, 7, 25
and Reiter syndrome, 1071
virulence
determinants, 22t
factor, 2
regulation, 23t
YopH protein, 25
Yersinia enterocolitica, 2070, 2076–2078
ail locus, 8
clinical manifestations, 2077
description, 2076
diagnosis, 2077
diarrhea, 180
differential diagnosis: amebiasis, 2402
dysentery, 990
enteric fever, 999t, 1001–1002
epidemiology, 2076–2077
food-borne, 1012t, 1013–1014, 1016, 1020
laboratory diagnosis, 1018t, 1019
hepatic abscess, 724
history, 2076
invasin gene, 7–8
lymphadenitis, 936
mesenteric adenitis, 1004–1005
clinical features, 1004t, 1004–1005
epidemiology, 1005
laboratory findings, 1004–1005
pathogenesis, 2077
pharyngitis, 567t, 569, 1789
treatment, 571
prevention, 2078
stool culture, 955
toxin, 5
transfusion-related, 2628
treatment, 2077–2078
quinolones, 367t
V antigen, 2076
W antigen, 2076
waterborne, 1016, 1016t
Yad A, 8
Ysc protein, 24
Yersinia frederiksenii, 2078
Yersinia intermedia, 2078
Yersinia kristensenii, 2078
Yersinia pestis, 2070–2076
animal reservoirs, 2792t
bubonic plague, 2072t, 2072–2073, 2073f, 2074f
clinical manifestations, 2072–2075
description, 2071
diagnosis, 2075
DNA probes, 27
epidemiology, 2071f, 2071–2072, 2072f
immunofluorescence, 184–185
laboratory findings, 2075
lymphadenitis, 940t
meningitis, 2072t, 2074, 2075

pathogenesis, 2072
pneumonic plague, 2072t, 2074
prevention, 2076
reservoir and vector control, 2076
septicemic plague, 999t, 2072t, 2073–2074, 2074f
treatment, 2075
aminoglycosides, 285t, 286
antimicrobials of choice, 202t
vaccines, 2076
V antigen, 2071
W antigen, 2071
Yersinia philomiragia. See Francisella philomiragia
Yersinia pseudotuberculosis, 2070, 2076–2078
clinical manifestations, 2077
description, 2076
diagnosis, 2077
enteric fever, 999t, 1001–1002
epidemiology, 2076–2077, 2077
lymphadenitis, 936
mesenteric adenitis, 1004–1005, 2077
clinical features, 1004t, 1004–1005
epidemiology, 1005
laboratory findings, 1004–1005
treatment, 2078
Yokonella regensburgei, 1975t
YopH protein, 25
Young syndrome: and pneumonia, 621

Z

Zalcitabine, 434–435, 1267, 1271–1272, 1602
adverse reactions, 434, 1271t, 1272
clinical studies, 434
dosage and pharmacology, 434, 518t–519t, 1271, 1271t
drug interactions, 421t, 434, 527t
for HIV, 1271t, 1271–1272, 1272f
for ZDV failure, 1275
resistance, 1271
structure, 420f
ZAP-70, 109
ZDV. *See* Zidovudine
Zeiss, gland of: infection, 1130
Zenacef. *See* Cefuroxime
Zeta-associated protein (ZAP-70), 109
Zhiel-Neelsen stain, 184t
Zidovudine, 412t, 435–437, 1267, 1269–1271, 1602
adverse reactions, 421t, 436, 1271t
animal models, 231
clinical studies and trials, 231, 436–437
for *Cryptosporidium*, 2507
dosage and pharmacology, 435–436, 518t–519t, 1271t
drug interactions, 421t, 436, 527t
ganciclovir, 425
for HIV

combination vs. monotherapy, 1274–1275
current recommendations, 1276, 1276t
ddI and ddC for failure of, 1275
postexposure prophylaxis, 2646
in pregnancy, 1275–1276
resistance, 1590. *See also* resistance *below*
and survival, 1273–1274
mechanism of action, 435
neutropenia from: G-CSF for, 451
and non-Hodgkin's lymphoma: avoidance, 1245
resistance, 435, 1271, 1272f, 1590
structure, 420f
zalcitabine combined with, 435
Ziehl-Nielsen stain
for mycobacteria, 2214
for Nocardia, 2274
Zika: transmission, clinical syndromes, and geographic distribution, 1466t
Zinc
deficiency: immunodeficiency and, 137
and inflammation, 34
poisoning, 1014
Zonula occludens toxin (ZOT), 5
Zoonoses, 2790–2795
animal, avian, and aquatic hosts, 2794
animal reservoirs (North America), 2792t
arthropod reservoirs and vectors, 2792t, 2794
bacterial, 2791t
in continental U.S., 2791, 2792–2793
diagnostic approaches, 2794–2795
distribution in nature, 2793–2794
geoclimactic conditions and, 2793–2794
global experience with, 2793
human influence on ecosystem and biosystem, 2794
importance in infectious disease practice, 2790–2793
migration patterns of animals and birds, 2794
parasitic, 2792t
viral, 2791t
Zoster ophthalmicus, 1347, 1348. *See also* Varicella-zoster virus
acyclovir for, 416–417
Zoster sine herpete, 833
Zovirax. *See* Acyclovir
Zygodontomys: and South American hemorrhagic fevers, 1573t, 1574
Zygomycetes: wound infections in trauma patients, 2758
Zygomycosis, 2311. *See also* Mucormycosis